Pancreatic
Amylase
Calcium (total and ionized)
Triglycerides
Lipase
Glucose

Parathyroid
Albumin
Alkaline phosphatase
Magnesium
Creatinine
PTH (whole molecule, amino terminal)
Protein, total
Calcium (total and ionized)
Phosphorus
Urinary calcium

Prenatal Screening
CBC
BUN
Uric Acid

ABO and Rh typing
Urinalysis
Toxoplasmosis Ab
CMV Ab
Hepatitis B surface Ag
HIV antibody
Cervical Pap smear
Cervical culture/amplification for GC,
   Chlamydia, group B Streptococci
Glucose
Creatinine
Free T4
Erythrocyte Antibody screen
Urine culture
Rubella titer
VDRL
Herpes simplex I & II Ab

Renal
Basic Metabolic Panel
Magnesium
Albumin
24-hr urine protein

Creatinine clearance
Phosphorus
Protein, total
24-hr creatinine
CBC

Thyroid Screening
Thyroxine (free T4)
TSH (third or fourth generation)

Toxicology Screening (Urine)
Amphetamines
Benzodiazepines
Marijuana metabolites
Methaqualone
Phencyclidine
Barbiturates
Cocaine metabolites
Methadone
Opiate metabolites
Propoxyphene

AMA DESIGNATED DISEASE/ORGAN PANELS*

80048 Basic Metabolic Panel
Calcium
Carbon Dioxide
Chloride
Creatinine
Glucose
Potassium
Sodium
Urea Nitrogen (BUN)

80076 Hepatic Function Panel
Albumin
Alkaline Phosphatase
Alanine Amino Transferase (ALT)
Aspartate Amino Transferase (AST)
Direct Bilirubin
Total Bilirubin
Total Protein

80069 Renal Function Panel
Albumin
Calcium

Carbon Dioxide
Chloride
Creatinine
Glucose
Phosphorus
Potassium
Sodium
Urea Nitrogen (BUN)

80053 Comprehensive Metabolic Panel
Albumin
Alkaline Phosphatase
Alanine Amino Transferase (ALT)
Asparate Amino Transferase (AST)
Calcium
Carbon Dioxide
Chloride
Creatinine
Glucose
Potassium
Sodium

Total Bilirubin
Total Protein
Urea Nitrogen (BUN)

80074 Acute Hepatitis Panel
Hepatitis A Antibody, IgM
Hepatitis B Core Antibody, IgM
Hepatitis B Surface Antigen
Hepatitis C Antibody

80051 Electrolyte Panel
Carbon Dioxide
Chloride
Potassium
Sodium

80061 Lipid Panel
Triglycerides
HDL-cholesterol, Direct
Total cholesterol
LDL-cholesterol, Calculated

*CPT 2006, Current Procedural Terminology,
Standard Edition, American Medical Association,
Chicago, IL

References
*Department of Practice Parameters: Principles of
Practice Parameters. Chicago, American Medical
Association, 1995, pp 1-18.
Glenn GC, Altshuler CH, Gambino R, et al: Practice
Parameter on Laboratory Panel Testing for Screening
and Case Finding in Asymptomatic Adults. Arch
Pathol Lab Med 1996; 120:929-941.
Henry JB, Howantiz PJ: Organ panels and the
relationship of the laboratory to the physician. *In*
AMA Council on Scientific Affairs: Laboratory Tests in
Medical Practice. Chicago, 1980.

Henry's
Clinical Diagnosis
AND Management BY
Laboratory Methods

TWENTY-FIRST EDITION

21st Edition
Associate Editors

Naif Z. Abraham Jr MD PhD
Staff Pathologist, Director of Chemistry,
Hematology, Immunology, and Microbiology
Department of Pathology
Veterans Affairs Medical Center;
Assistant Professor, Upstate Medical University
Syracuse, NY, USA

Martin H. Bluth MD PhD
Director of Research
Assistant Professor
Departments of Surgery and Pathology
SUNY Downstate Medical Center
Brooklyn, NY, USA

Robert E. Hutchison MD
Professor of Pathology, Director of Clinical
Pathology and Director of Hematopathology
Department of Pathology
Upstate Medical University
Syracuse, NY, USA

Mark S. Lifshitz MD
Director, Clinical Laboratories
NYU Medical Center
Clinical Professor, Department of Pathology
New York University School of Medicine
New York, NY, USA

H. Davis Massey MD PhD
Assistant Professor of Pathology
Virginia Commonwealth University
Richmond, VA, USA

Jonathan L. Miller MD PhD
Professor and Vice Chairman
Department of Pathology
The University of Chicago
Chicago, IL, USA

Gregory A. Threatte MD
Professor of Pathology
Director of Core Laboratories and Outreach
Upstate Medical University
Syracuse, NY, USA

Elizabeth Unger MD PhD
Team Leader
Human Papillomavirus Laboratory
National Center for Infectious Diseases
Atlanta, GA, USA

Gail L. Woods MD
Professor of Pathology
Department of Pathology
University of Arkansas for Medical Sciences
Little Rock, AR, USA

Commissioning Editor: Michael Houston
Development Editor: Russell Gabbedy
Project Manager: Kathryn Mason
Editorial Assistants: Sven Pinczewski and Katie Sotiris
Designer: Stewart Larking
Illustration Manager: Bruce Hogarth
Illustrators: Anne Erickson and Oxford Illustrators
Marketing Managers (UK/USA): Leontine Treur and Kathy Neely

Henry's
Clinical Diagnosis
AND Management BY
Laboratory Methods

TWENTY-FIRST EDITION

Richard A. McPherson MD

Harry P. Dalton Professor and Chairman
Division of Clinical Pathology
Virginia Commonwealth University;
Director
Clinical Pathology
Medical College of Virginia Hospitals
Richmond, Virginia, USA

Matthew R. Pincus MD PhD

Professor
Department of Pathology
State University of New York Health Sciences
Center at Brooklyn;
Chairman
Department of Pathology and Laboratory Medicine
New York Harbor Veterans Affairs Health Care System
Brooklyn and New York, New York, USA

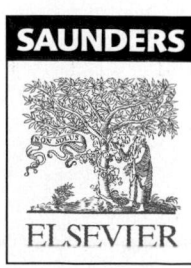

SAUNDERS

ELSEVIER

SAUNDERS
ELSEVIER

An imprint of Elsevier Inc.

© 2007 21st Edition

© 2001, 1996, 1991, 1984, 1979, 1974, 1969, 1962 by W.B. Saunders Company

© 1953, 1948, 1943, 1939, 1935, 1931, 1927, 1923, 1918, 1914, 1912, 1908 by W.B. Saunders Company

Copyright renewed 1990 by Israel Davidsohn and Benjamin B. Wells

Copyright renewed 1975 by Mrs. Anne Ophelia Todd Dowden

Copyright renewed 1970, 1967, 1963 by Mrs. Arthur Hawley Sanford

Copyright renewed 1958, 1955 by Arthur Hawley Sanford

Copyright renewed 1951, 1946, 1942, 1940, 1936 by Edith B. Todd

ISBN-13: 978-1-4160-0287-1
ISBN-10: 1-4160-0287-1

British Library Cataloguing in Publication Data
A catalogue record for this book is available from the British Library

Library of Congress Cataloging in Publication Data
A catalog record for this book is available from the Library of Congress

Notice

Medical knowledge is constantly changing. Standard safety precautions must be followed, but as new research and clinical experience broaden our knowledge, changes in treatment and drug therapy may become necessary or appropriate. Readers are advised to check the most current product information provided by the manufacturer of each drug to be administered to verify the recommended dose, the method and duration of administration, and contraindications. It is the responsibility of the practitioner, relying on experience and knowledge of the patient, to determine dosages and the best treatment for each individual patient. Neither the Publisher nor the author assume any liability for any injury and/or damage to persons or property arising from this publication.

The Publisher

Printed in China
Last digit is the print number: 9 8 7 6 5 4 3 2 1

Contents

I The Clinical Laboratory

Edited by Mark S. Lifshitz MD,
Matthew R. Pincus MD PhD, Gregory A. Threatte MD

II Clinical Chemistry

Edited by Matthew R. Pincus MD PhD,
Mark S. Lifshitz MD

VIII Molecular Pathology

Edited by Elizabeth Unger MD PhD,
Matthew R. Pincus MD PhD

IX Clinical Pathology of Cancer

Edited by Richard A. McPherson MD,
Matthew R. Pincus MD PhD, Martin H. Bluth MD PhD

APPENDICES

Edited by Naif Z. Abraham Jr MD PhD

Dedication

To
our wives,
Stephanie Sammartino McPherson
and Naomi Pincus

and children,
Jennifer and Marianne McPherson

for their love and support in the undertaking of this work, for which we are deeply grateful.

Dr John Bernard Henry: A Tribute

Henry's Clinical Diagnosis and Management by Laboratory Methods is a highly acclaimed text in the field of clinical pathology and has served as a major resource for practitioners in all fields of medicine. It has chronicled the dramatic and revolutionary changes in diagnostic medicine for almost a century. It was first written under the title *A Manual of Clinical Diagnosis* in 1908 by the legendary James C. Todd MD, who edited the first six editions, and was joined on the sixth edition by Dr Arthur H. Sanford MD. Dr Sanford continued with four more editions of this book on his own and was joined on the 11th edition by Dr George G. Stillwell and on the 12th edition by Dr Benjamin B. Wells. The 13th edition was edited by Dr Wells and Dr Israel Davidsohn, a pioneer in the field of clinical and diagnostic immunology, and was renamed Clinical Diagnosis by Laboratory Methods. This change in title reflected the major shift in medical diagnostic testing from disparate laboratories, many using indigenous methodologies, to the central diagnostic laboratories using standardized testing with appropriate method verification.

In 1969, Dr John Bernard Henry joined Dr Davidsohn in the editorship of the 14th edition of this textbook. This was a most fortunate development. Dr Henry, as Professor of Pathology at the State University of New York Upstate Medical Center in Syracuse and Director of the Clinical Pathology service at this medical center, was a pioneer in the organization of the clinical pathology laboratories and an innovator in introducing state-of-the-art methods into the centralized diagnostic laboratory. Dr Henry has been and continues to be an outstanding teacher who has been central to the training of multiple generations of leaders in the field of laboratory medicine. His major focus has always been on the patient, and he established the principle that the ultimate verification of the validity of the result of any test is whether it leads to appropriate and effective therapeutic intervention. This principle requires close interactions between the clinical pathologist and the clinician. Thus, as an editor of this textbook, in addition to promoting discussions of the exciting new developments in testing methodologies that span a vast panorama from spectrophotometry to microscopic diagnosis to molecular biological approaches such as polymerase chain reaction, Dr Henry also emphasized the clinical aspects of the diseases that are diagnosed by them. This synthesis and the broad coverage of the vast area encompassing the field of clinical pathology ensured that this book succeeded in serving as the standard reference text for both laboratorians and clinicians.

Both Drs Davidsohn and Henry edited the 15th edition of this book, published in 1974. Dr Davidsohn died in 1979 at the age of 84, and Dr Henry became the editor for the 16th-20th editions. In the 16th edition, reflecting his emphasis on patient care and the emerging importance of using laboratory tests to follow the progression of disease and the efficacy of therapy, Dr Henry gave this book its current title, Clinical Diagnosis and Management by Laboratory Methods. Under his guidance, this textbook has continued to maintain and expand its tradition of informing the reader of the most recent developments in laboratory testing for the diagnosis and treatment of diseases and of describing how testing is used both to screen for the presence of disease and to monitor progress in the management of disease.

It is a great honor for both of us that we have inherited the mantle of so prolific and distinguished a medical scholar as Dr John Bernard Henry. Both of us have benefited immensely from our close association with him over the past several decades. It is with great humility and respect that we assume editorship of this flagship textbook that has been molded by him and by all of the other outstanding leaders in the field of diagnostic medicine. We feel most fortunate to be able to continue to interact with Dr Henry. We are and will always be deeply indebted to him for his massive contributions to the fields of clinical pathology and diagnostic medicine, his outstanding example as a physician and teacher, and his profound contributions as editor of this textbook that have ensured that this book has taken its place among the most significant textbook contributions in modern medicine.

In tribute to him and his leadership over the last seven editions of this book, it will henceforth be permanently titled *Henry's Clinical Diagnosis and Management by Laboratory Methods.*

Richard A. McPherson MD
Matthew R. Pincus MD PhD

List of Contributors

Naif Z. Abraham Jr MD PhD
Staff Pathologist, Director of Chemistry,
Hematology, Immunology, and Microbiology, Department
of Pathology, Veterans Affairs Medical Center
Assistant Professor, Upstate Medical University
Syracuse, NY, USA

Yoshihiro Ashihara PhD
Vice President, Board Member
Research & Development Division
Fujirebio Inc.
Tokyo, Japan

Katalin Banki MD
Assistant Professor of Pathology
Director of Special Hematology
Department of Pathology
SUNY Upstate Medical University
Syracuse, NY, USA

Wendy V. Beadling MS MT(ASCP)SBB
Assistant Supervisor, Blood Bank
Clinical Pathology
SUNY Upstate Medical University
Syracuse, NY, USA

Jennifer Beane BA BE
PhD Candidate
Bioinformatics Program
Boston University
Boston, MA, USA

Sylva Bem MD
Clinical Assistant Professor
Department of Pathology
Division of Hematopathology
SUNY Upstate Medical University
Syracuse, NY, USA

Jonathan Ben-Ezra MD
Professor of Pathology
Department of Pathology
Virginia Commonwealth University School of
Medicine
Richmond, VA, USA

Gary E. Blank PhD
Associate Professor of Clinical Chemistry
Department of Pathology
University of Pittsburgh
Pittsburgh, PA, USA

Martin H. Bluth MD PhD
Director of Research
Assistant Professor
Departments of Surgery and Pathology
SUNY Downstate Medical Center
Brooklyn, NY, USA

Jay L. Bock MD PhD
Professor and Acting Chair
Department of Pathology
State University of New York at Stony Brook
Stony Brook, NY, USA

Michael J. Borowitz MD PhD
Professor of Pathology
Department of Pathology
Johns Hopkins University/Medical Center
Baltimore, MD, USA

Paul W. Brandt-Rauf MD PhD DPH
Chairman
Department of Environmental Health Sciences
Mailman School of Public Health
Columbia College of Physicians and Surgeons
New York, NY, USA

David J. Bylund MD
Staff Pathologist
Department of Pathology
Scripps Clinic - Torrey Pines
La Jolla, CA, USA

Robert P. Carty PhD
Associate Professor
Department of Biochemistry
SUNY Health Science Center at Brooklyn
Brooklyn, NY, USA

Laura Cooling MD MS
Clinical Assistant Professor
Associate Director, Transfusion Medicine
Department of Pathology
University of Michigan Hospitals
Ann Arbor, MI, USA

xii

Michael Costello PhD
Technical Director
Advocate Shared Services Laboratory
Advocate Lutheran General Hospital
Park Ridge, IL, USA

Ann C. Croft MT(ASCP)
Supervisor
Bacteriology Laboratory
ARUP Laboratories
Salt Lake City, UT, USA

Judy A. Daly PhD
Clinical Professor
Department of Pathology
University of Utah School of Medicine
Salt Lake City, UT, USA

Robertson D. Davenport MD
Associate Professor of Pathology
Medical Director, Blood Bank and Transfusion Service
Ann Arbor, MI, USA

Robert P. De Cresce MD MBA MPH
Chairman, Department of Pathology
Director, Rush Medical Laboratories
Rush University Medical Center
Chicago, IL, USA

Julio C. Delgado MD
Assistant Professor of Pathology
University of Utah;
Associate Director, Laboratory of Immunology
ARUP Laboratories
Salt Lake City, UT, USA

Charles DeLisi PhD
Professor, Senior Associate Provost
Curriculum & Teaching
Boston University
Boston, MA, USA

D. Robert Dufour MD
Chief, Pathology and Laboratory Medicine Service
Veteran Affairs Medical Center
Washington, DC, USA

M. Tarek Elghetany MD
Professor and Vice-Chairman
Department of Pathology
University of Texas Medical Branch
Galveston, TX, USA

Amal F. Farag MD
Assistant Professor of Medicine
Department of Endocrinology
New York Harbour Healthcare System
Brooklyn, NY, USA

Andrea Ferreira-Gonzalez PhD
Professor and Director
Molecular Diagnostics Laboratory
Department of Pathology
Medical College of Virginia
Virginia Commonwealth University
Richmond, VA, USA

Daniel Fink MD
Associate Clinical Professor of Pathology
Department of Pathology
Columbia University Medical Center
New York, NY, USA

Louis M. Fink MD
Director, Core Laboratory Services
Nevada Cancer Institute
Las Vegas, NV, USA

Thomas R. Fritsche PhD MD ABMM
Director of Laboratories
JMI Laboratories
North Liberty, IA, USA

Carleton T. Garrett MD PhD
Division Chief
Pathology
Virginia Commonwealth University
Richmond, VA, USA

Susan S. Graham MS MT(ASCP)SH
Associate Professor and Chair
Department of Clinical Laboratory Science
SUNY Upstate Medical University
Syracuse, NY, USA

Wayne W. Grody MD PhD
Professor, Division of Molecular Pathology and Medical Genetics
Director, Diagnostic Molecular Pathology Laboratory
Departments of Pathology & Laboratory Medicine, Pediatrics, and Human Genetics
UCLA School of Medicine
Los Angeles, CA, USA

Helena A. Guber MD
Assistant Professor of Medicine
Department of Endocrinology
New York Harbour Healthcare System
Brooklyn, NY, USA

Geraldine S. Hall PhD
Professor of Pathology
Division of Pathology and Laboratory Medicine
Cleveland Clinic Foundation
Cleveland, OH, USA

Rosemarie E. Hardin MD
Resident
Department of Surgery
SUNY Downstate Medical Center
Brooklyn, NY, USA

John Bernard Henry MD
Distinguished Service Professor of Pathology
SUNY Upstate Medical University
Syracuse, NY, USA

Timothy Hilbert MD PhD JD
Assistant Professor of Pathology
New York University School of Medicine
New York, NY, USA

Charles E. Hill MD PhD
Assistant Professor
Department of Pathology and Laboratory Medicine
Emory University School of Medicine
Atlanta, GA, USA

Henry A. Homburger MD
Professor of Laboratory Medicine
Mayo Clinic College of Medicine
Consultant
Mayo Clinic
Rochester, MN, USA

Charlene A. Hubbell BS MT(ASCP)SBB
Adjunct Associate Professor, Clinical Laboratory Science
College of Health Professions
Supervisor, Histocompatibility, Immunogenetics and
Progenitor Cell Bank
State University of New York, Upstate Medical University
Syracuse, NY, USA

Robert E. Hutchison MD
Professor of Pathology, Director of Hematopathology and
Director of Clinical Pathology
SUNY Health Science Center
Syracuse, NY, USA

Peter C. Iwen MS PhD M(ASCP) SM(AAM)
Associate Professor
Pathology and Microbiology
University of Nebraska Medical Center
Omaha, NE, USA

Mark L. Jaros MBA MT(ASCP)
Administrative Director
Department of Pathology/Rush Medical Laboratories
Rush University Medical Center
Associate Professor, College of Allied Health
Rush University
Chicago, IL, USA

Jeffrey Jhang MD
Assistant Professor of Clinical Pathology
Department of Pathology
Columbia University Medical Center
New York, NY, USA

Rohan John MD
Resident
Department of Pathology
Rush University Medical Center
Chicago, IL, USA

Aran Kadar MD
PGY4/4th Year Resident
The Pulmonary Center
Boston University Medical Center
Boston, MA, USA

Yasushi Kasahara PhD
Visiting Professor
Department of Clinical Pathology
School of Medicine
Showa University
Tokyo, Japan

Mukhtar I. Khan MD
Assistant Professor of Medicine
Department of Endocrinology, Diabetes, and Metabolism
SUNY Upstate Medical University
Syracuse, NY, USA

Carl R. Kjeldsberg MD
Professor of Pathology
University of Utah School of Medicine
CEO and Chair, Board of Directors
ARUP Laboratories
Salt Lake City, UT, USA

Michael J. Klein MD
Professor of Pathology
Head, Section of Surgical Pathology;
Senior Scientist, Center for Metabolic Bone Disease
The University of Alabama School of Medicine
Birmingham, AL, USA

Katrin M. Klemm MD
Assistant Professor
Department of Pathology
University of Alabama
Birmingham, AL, USA

Joseph A. Knight BS MS MD
Professor of Pathology
Department of Pathology
University of Utah School of Medicine
Salt Lake City, UT, USA

Anthony S. Kurec MS DLM(ASCP)
Administrator, University Pathologists Laboratories, LLP
Clinical Associate Professor
SUNY Upstate Medical University
Syracuse, NY, USA

Richard S. Larson MD PhD
Senior Associate Dean for Research,
Associate Professor of Pathology
Department of Pathology
University of New Mexico HSC
Albuquerque, NM, USA

P. Rocco LaSala MD
Fellow, Medical Microbiology
Department of Pathology
University of Texas Medical Branch
Galveston, TX, USA

Peng Lee MD PhD
Assistant Professor
Department of Pathology
New York University Medical Center
Staff Pathologist
New York Harbor VA Medical Center
Brooklyn and New York, NY, USA

H. Peter Lehmann MD
Professor, Department of Pathology
Louisiana State University Medical Center
New Orleans, LA, USA

Mark S. Lifshitz MD
Director, Clinical Laboratories
NYU Medical Center
Clinical Professor, Department of Pathology
New York University School of Medicine
New York, NY, USA

James S. Lo MT(ASCP) PhD DABCC
Director, Pulmonary Function Blood Gas Laboratory and
Assistant Laboratory
Director, Department of Pathology Vassar Brothers Medical
Center
Affiliate Professor of Medical Technology, Department of
Medical Laboratory Sciences
Marist College
Poughkeepsie, NY, USA

Irina Lutinger MPH DLM(ASCP)
Senior Administrative Director
Clinical Laboratories
Tisch Hospital, Labs
NYU Medical Center
New York, NY, USA

Richard A. Marlar PhD
Professor of Pathology
Associate Director, Coagulation and Special Coagulation
Laboratories
Veteran Affairs Medical Center;
Oklahoma City, OK, USA

H. Davis Massey MD PhD
Assistant Professor of Pathology
Virginia Commonwealth University
Richmond, VA, USA

Sharad Mathur MD
Assistant Professor
Department of Pathology and Laboratory Medicine
University of Kansas Medical Center;
Chief, Pathology and Laboratory Medicine Service
V A Medical Center
Kansas City, MO, USA

Rex M. McCallum MD
Clinical Professor of Medicine, Division of Rheumatology
Associate Medical Director of the Private Diagnostic Clinic
Senior Clinical Advisor, Duke Department of Medicine
Duke University School of Medicine
Durham, NC, USA

Richard A. McPherson MD
Harry P. Dalton Professor and Chairman
Division of Clinical Pathology
Virginia Commonwealth University;
Director
Clinical Pathology
Medical College of Virginia Hospitals
Richmond, VA, USA

W. Greg Miller PhD
Professor of Pathology
Department of Pathology
Virginia Commonwealth University
Richmond, VA, USA

Herb Miller PhD MT (ASCP)
CLS (NCA)
Chairman and Director
Department of Clinical Laboratory Sciences
College of Health Sciences
Rush University
Chicago, IL, USA

Jonathan L. Miller MD PhD
Professor and Vice Chairman
Department of Pathology
The University of Chicago
Chicago, IL, USA

Paul D. Mintz MD
Professor, Departments of Pathology and Internal
Medicine
Director, Division of Clinical Pathology/Clinical
Laboratories
University of Virginia Health System
Charlottesville, VA, USA

Robert M. Nakamura MD
Senior Consultant and Chairman Emeritus
Department of Pathology
Scripps Clinic
La Jolla, CA, USA

Walter W. Noll MD
Professor of Pathology
Department of Pathology
Dartmouth-Hitchcock Medical Center
Lebanon, NH, USA

Frederick S. Nolte PhD
Professor, Pathology and Laboratory Medicine
Emory University School of Medicine
Atlanta, GA, USA

Man S. Oh MD
Professor of Medicine
Department of Medicine
State University of New York
Brooklyn, NY, USA

Michael A. Pfaller MD
Professor and Director, Molecular Epidemiology and
Fungus Testing Laboratory
Departments of Pathology and Epidemiology
University of Iowa College of Medicine and College of
Public Heath
Iowa City, IA, USA

Matthew R. Pincus MD PhD
Professor, Department of Pathology
State University of New York Health Sciences Center at
Brooklyn;
Chairman, Department of Pathology and Laboratory
Medicine
New York Harbor Veterans Affairs Health Care System
Brooklyn and New York, NY, USA

Alvaro A. Pineda MD
Emeritus Professor of Laboratory Medicine
Mayo Clinic College of Medicine
Rochester, MN, USA

Steven W. Pipe MD
Associate Professor
Department of Pediatrics
University of Michigan
Ann Arbor, MI, USA

Margaret A. Piper PhD MPH
Senior Consultant
Technology Evaluation Center
Blue Cross Blue Shield Association
Atlanta, GA, USA

Herbert F. Polesky MD
Former Professor of Laboratory Medicine and Pathology
University of Minnesota School of Medicine
Minneapolis, MN, USA

A. Koneti Rao MBBS
Professor of Medicine, Thrombosis Research and
Pharmacology
Assistant Dean, MD PhD Program
Division of Hematology and Thromboembolic Diseases
Temple University School of Medicine
Philadelphia, PA, USA

Roger S. Riley MD PhD
Director of Coagulation and Professor of Pathology
Department of Pathology
Virginia Commonwealth University
Richmond, VA, USA

Rhonda K. Roby MPH
Senior Forensic Specialist
Applied Biosystems
Foster City, CA, USA

Lazaro Rosales MD
Associate Professor of Pathology
Director of Hemapheresis and Deputy Director of
Transfusion Medicine
Department of Pathology
Upstate Medical University
Syracuse, NY, USA

Susan D. Roseff MD
Medical Director, Transfusion Medicine
Virginia Commonwealth University Medical Center
Associate Professor
Department of Pathology
Virginia Commonwealth University School of Medicine
Richmond, VA, USA

Martin J. Salwen MD
Distinguished Service Professor
Department of Pathology
State University of New York
Brooklyn, NY, USA

Kimberly W. Sanford MD MT(ASCP)
Chief Resident
Department of Pathology
Virginia Commonwealth University School of Medicine
Richmond, VA, USA

Katherine I. Schexneider MD
Medical Director, Blood Bank
Naval Medical Center Portsmouth
Portsmouth, VA, USA

Alvin H. Schmaier MD
Professor of Internal Medicine and Pathology
Director, Coagulation Laboratory
Department of Internal Medicine and Pathology
University of Michigan
Ann Arbor, MI, USA

Rangaraj Selvarangan BVSc PhD
Assistant Professor of Pediatrics
University of Missouri School of Medicine;
Director of Clinical Microbiology and Virology
Laboratories
Children's Mercy Hospital
Kansas City, MO, USA

James W. Sharp MBA MD
Director of Laboratories
Department of Pathology
Vassar Brothers Medical Center
Medical Director, Medical Technology Program
Department of Medical Laboratory Sciences
Marist College
Poughkeepsie, NY, USA

Michael B. Smith MD
Assistant Professor and Director
Division of Clinical Microbiology
Department of Pathology
University of Texas Medical Branch
Galveston, TX, USA

Avrum Spira MD
Assistant Professor
MED Pulmonary Center
Boston University
Boston, MA, USA

Constance K. Stein PhD
Associate Professor
Department of Pathology
Upstate Medical University
Syracuse, NY, USA

Martin Steinau PhD
Division of Viral and Rickettsial Diseases
National Center for Infectious Diseases
Atlanta, GA, USA

Robert L. Sunheimer MS MT (ASCP) SC SLS
Associate Professor
Department of Clinical Laboratory Science
SUNY Upstate Medical University
Syracuse, NY, USA

Scott Tenner MD MPH FACP FACG
Division of Gastroenterology, Maimonides Medical Center
Assistant Professor of Medicine, Mount Sinai School of Medicine
Director, Medical Education and Research
BrooklynGI.com
Brooklyn, NY, USA

Courtney D. Thornburg MD
Lecturer, Department of Pediatrics and Communicable Diseases
University of Michigan
Ann Arbor, MI, USA

Gregory A. Threatte MD
Professor and Chairman
Department of Pathology
SUNY Upstate Medical University
Syracuse, NY, USA

Philip M. Tierno Jr PhD
Director, Clinical Microbiology and Immunology
Associate Professor, Departments of Microbiology and Pathology
New York University Medical Center
New York, NY, USA

Elizabeth Unger MD PhD
Team Leader
Human Papillomavirus Laboratory
National Center for Infectious Diseases
Atlanta, GA, USA

Neerja Vajpayee MD
Clinical Assistant Professor
Department of Pathology
Division of Hematopathology
SUNY Upstate Medical University
Syracuse, NY, USA

David S. Viswanatha MD FRCPC
Senior Associate Consultant
Division of Hematopathology Mayo Clinic;
Associate Professor
Mayo Clinic College of Medicine
Rochester, MN, USA

Carlos Alberto von Mühlen MD PhD
Full Professor of Rheumatology and Internal Medicine
Pontifical Catholic University School of Medicine
Porto Alegre, RS, Brazil

David H. Walker MD
Professor and Chairman
Department of Pathology
University of Texas Medical Branch
Galveston, TX, USA

Robert A. Webster PhD
Assistant Professor
Departments of Pathology, Biochemistry, and Clinical Laboratory Science
Associate Director, Rush Medical Laboratories
Director, Core Laboratory
Rush University Medical Center
Chicago, IL, USA

Ruth S. Weinstock MD PhD
Professor of Medicine and Chief, Endocrinology, Diabetes and Metabolism
Department of Medicine
SUNY Upstate Medical University
Syracuse, NY, USA

David S. Wilkinson MD PhD
Professor and Chair
Department of Pathology
Virginia Commonwealth University
Richmond, VA, USA

Jeffrey L. Winters MD
Assistant Professor of Laboratory Medicine
Department of Transfusion Medicine
Mayo Clinic College of Medicine
Rochester, MN, USA

Brent L. Wood MD PhD
Associate Professor of Laboratory Medicine
Department of Laboratory Medicine
University of Washington
Seattle, WA, USA

Gail L. Woods MD
Director, Clinical Laboratories
Professor of Pathology
Department of Pathology
University of Arkansas for Medical Sciences
Little Rock, AR, USA

Margaret Yungbluth MD
Staff Pathologist
Department of Pathology
St Francis Hospital
Evanston, IL, USA

Edmond J. Yunis MD
Professor of Pathology
Harvard Medical School
Boston, MA, USA

Michael E. Zenilman MD
Clarence and Mary Dennis Professor and Chairman
Department of Surgery
SUNY Downstate Medical Center
Brooklyn, NY, USA

Shourong Zhao MD MS
Fellow of Hematopathology
Department of Pathology
Virginia Commonwealth University Health System
Richmond, VA, USA

Preface

The role of clinical pathology and laboratory medicine continues to grow as the single largest component of objective scientific data within the medical record of patients. The ever-increasing ease with which conventional laboratory analyses can be provided and the broadening diversity of measurements with esoteric assays contribute to clinical management from prenatal days to newborn screening through childhood, adulthood, and into geriatric ages. This life-long trail of medical observations and laboratory test results is now being organized into a continuous and contemporaneous electronic medical record. The challenge for future medicine lies in how best to use all of this information to provide counseling to patients about behavior modifications and disease risk amelioration based on a wide range of medical data with an expanding core of genetic testing, in addition to traditional measures of organ function and metabolism revealed through chemical, hematological, microbiological, and other laboratory disciplines.

The expansion in knowledge of the human genome and its conversion into proteomic phenotypes of the human body present a range of opportunities for exploring health and disease as never before practiced. The methods of examination both for nucleic acids and protein expression of genes will surely transform the way that laboratories provide clinical diagnostic services for decades to come. Numerous applications to clinical testing have already come to fruition in microbiology, coagulation, tissue typing, genetic diseases, cancer and hematologic malignancies. The environment provided by clinical laboratories that demands rigor in analysis, quality control, professional competencies, and cost-effective operations will also foster the application of this new knowledge and these new methods into accepted standard of practice. We should expect that the most successful future practitioners of laboratory medicine will be those well versed in and prepared to pursue advances in informatics, basic analytic methods, communications with clinical colleagues, and participation in national and international efforts to standardize and implement complex changes in our profession. It is at multiple levels of society that the laboratory can serve from individual patient testing through public health initiatives for disease prevention, and extending to industry and government policies for health care and its reform to support best practices and promote health and well being in a climate of limited financial resources.

The 21st edition of this book comes at nearly the century mark since its inception with its first publication in 1908. It has remained throughout that time as the authoritative source of information for residents, students, and other trainees in the discipline of clinical pathology and laboratory medicine and for physicians and laboratorians in that practice. The 21st edition incorporates new discoveries and applications in all chapters to fulfill its mission of being a comprehensive textbook that is up-to-date and readable. Most notable in the format of this edition is the use of color throughout the book with inclusion of many more images and graphical figures than before. One of our goals has been to present laboratory findings in a rendition as close as possible to actual practice as encountered in the real-life conditions of working at the bench. This approach has allowed each author the opportunity to incorporate figures that illustrate diagnostic principles and interpretations.

Part I, The Clinical Laboratory, deals with the organization, purposes, and practices of analysis, interpretation, and management within the clinical laboratory. Overall, we have reorganized this section, for the sake of clarity, by considering, in order, pre-analytical, analytical and post-analytical aspects of laboratory testing. Specifically, issues of administrative organization and operations are discussed in Chs 1 and 2. The approach to proper specimen collection, transport, and handling and other pre-analytical variables are described in Ch. 3. Principles of analysis, instrumentation, and automation are covered in Chs 4 and 5. Extension of laboratory services beyond that of a central laboratory in a hospital to the arena of outpatients along with the regulations covering those near-patient

services and the growth of new technologies to support them is the subject of Ch. 6. The post-analysis processes of reporting, medical decision-making, and interpretation of results are crucial to the utility of laboratory testing (Ch. 7). Selection and interpretation of laboratory information and results to achieve the most cost-effective and efficient medical problem solving with clinical laboratory testing is explored in Ch. 8. Statistical analysis (Ch. 9) is immensely important to all phases of monitoring laboratory processes and decision making with some of its most explicit applications in the area of quality control (Ch. 10). The multitude of laboratory results and their reporting can only be managed by sophisticated information systems that are an essential part of any clinical laboratory (Ch. 11) and that are becoming more important as the tools by which integration of clinical information at multiple levels can be made available to the physician client. The choice of instrumentation, clinical laboratory automation, and computer systems in a laboratory largely determine its productivity (increased volume and variety of complex measurements/examinations) and selection of the most expeditious laboratory service responsive to providers' and patients' needs in terms of access, cost, and quality. The financial impact and solutions to challenges for pathologists and all laboratorians from managed care with capitated reimbursements and/or discounted service contracts are paramount to the survival of both the laboratories themselves and to the institutions they serve (Ch. 12). A relatively new challenge facing laboratories is preparedness and appropriate responses to threats of bioterrorism on local, regional, and national levels (Ch. 13). These themes run through all 76 current, new, updated and/or augmented, strengthened chapters that embrace each topic in a compelling manner from patient specimen collection and processing to the reporting of results.

Part II, Clinical Chemistry, is now organized systematically to present laboratory examinations according to the diseases of organ systems. It begins with the evaluation of renal function, water, electrolytes, metabolic intermediates and molecules of nitrogen exchange, and acid-base balance, that are so important in monitoring patients for critical care as well as in the management of patients with kidney and pulmonary disorders (Ch. 14). This subject leads into the increasingly important laboratory evaluation of bone metabolism and bone loss (Ch. 15). Ever stronger emphasis is now placed on carbohydrates in the laboratory diagnosis and management of diabetes mellitus and other disorders (Ch. 16). Ch. 17 is a new presentation on studies of lipids and their abnormalities that are so important in cardiovascular disease risk assessment, while Ch. 18 deals with the immediate evaluation of heart disease and cardiac injury. The role of specific proteins of the blood and electrophoretic interpretations are emphasized in Ch. 19, while clinical enzymology is covered in Ch. 20. Assessment of liver function is presented in Ch. 21 and that of gastrointestinal and pancreatic disorders in Ch. 22. Toxicological analysis and therapeutic drug monitoring are discussed in Ch. 23 with the complementary methods of evaluating endocrine function in Ch. 24. Ch. 25, on reproductive and pregnancy testing, and Ch. 26, on vitamins and trace metals, complete Part II.

Part III, Urine and Other Body Fluids, covers basic examination of urine (Ch. 27). A special area of consideration is analysis of body fluids such as cerebrospinal fluid, synovial fluid, and serous fluid (Ch. 28).

Part IV, Hematology, updates the examination of blood and bone marrow (Ch. 29), hematopoiesis (Ch. 30), and erythrocytic (Ch. 31) and leukocytic (Ch. 32) disorders. The rapidly growing area of flow cytometric analysis in hematology is emphasized (Ch. 33). Immunohematology (Ch. 34) and transfusion medicine (Ch. 35) address pre-transfusion testing and problem-solving of untoward or unexpected reactions as well as therapy with blood products (components and derivatives). Chs 36 and 37 cover therapeutic applications of apheresis including collection, processing, and dispensing progenitor/stem cells from bone marrow, peripheral blood, and cord blood coupled with tissue banking.

In recognition of recent major advances in our understanding of thromboembolic phenomena that have resulted in effective new treatment protocols, we have added a new section, Part V, Hemostasis and Thrombosis. This section provides expanded coverage to the growing body of knowledge in the areas of coagulation and fibrinolysis (Ch. 38) and to that of platelet function with emphasis on von Willebrand disease (Ch. 39). Over the past decade, major advances in coagulation have led to effective treatment of many different disease conditions, including myocardial infarction and stroke, with a generation of very effective new anti-coagulants. Use of these new agents requires careful monitoring of many features of the coagulation system. Accordingly, this section discusses not only the fundamentals of hemostasis but also discusses the new agents used to treat thrombotic disease, their mechanisms of action, and methods for monitoring their effects. Assessment of risk for thrombosis is discussed in Ch. 40, and the role for the laboratory to play in guiding antithrombotic therapy is detailed in Ch. 41.

Part VI, Immunology and Immunopathology, is updated and expanded in all chapters in its description of the functions of the immune system and immunologic disorders (Ch. 42) along with a comprehensive account of the different types of immunoassays that are in practice throughout the world (Ch. 43). Detailed explanations and laboratory evaluations are provided for the cellular immune system (Ch. 44), humoral immunity (Ch. 45), complement and mediators of inflammation (Ch. 46), and the major histocompatibility complex (Ch. 47) and its role in transplantation and specific diseases (Ch. 48). Immunodeficiency disorders require special diagnostic approaches that are outlined in Ch. 49. Autoimmunity is highlighted in presentations of systemic rheumatic diseases (Chap 50), vasculitis (Ch. 51), and organ-specific diseases (Ch. 52). This section is rounded out with a discussion of allergic diseases that involves a fine correlation between laboratory testing and diagnosis (Ch. 53).

Part VII, Medical Microbiology, deals with infectious agents from viral infections (Ch. 54) through chlamydia, rickettsia, and mycoplasma (Ch. 55) and extending to classical medical bacteriology (Ch. 56) testing for antimicrobial susceptibility (Ch. 57), and spirochetal infections (Ch. 58). The discussion of mycobacteria (Ch. 59) underscores tuberculosis with emerging drug resistance and widespread infection among immuno-suppressed patients. Mycotic diseases (Ch. 60) and medical parasitology (Ch. 61) are also essential considerations in international medicine. The classical techniques of culturing microbiological organisms with identification and antimicrobial susceptibility testing through functional bioassays is rapidly changing with the evolution of new molecular diagnostic methods that will both enhance and replace the conventional methods (Ch. 62). Because of its significance in achieving maximum patient and physician benefit from the laboratory, specimen collection and handling for diagnosis of infectious diseases (Ch. 63) are of special importance. New illustrations and photographs of organisms and methods are particularly prominent in this section. Finally, a new chapter on microbiologic aspects of bioterrorism (Ch. 64) ends the section.

Part VIII, Molecular Pathology, is newly organized for in depth presentations on basic principles of nucleic acid chemistry and their analysis (Chs 65 and 66) with emphasis on the very important methods of nucleic acid amplification (Ch. 67) and hybridization technologies (Ch. 68). Included are the applications and methods of cytogenetics (Ch. 69) with modern techniques for karyotyping. These chapters embrace basic principles and techniques and the procedures for establishing a molecular diagnostics laboratory (Ch. 70). They also include special applications to hematopoietic neoplasms (Ch. 71), molecular diagnosis of genetic diseases, and molecular diagnostic techniques used for forensic identity as well as comprehensive parentage testing through DNA fingerprinting (Ch. 73).

Part IX, Clinical Pathology of Cancer, is a new section that highlights the significant role played by the laboratory in diagnosis and monitoring of malignancies and their treatments. It is vital that all pathologists become aware of the revolution that has taken place in molecular and cell biology and that has resulted in the sequencing of the entire human genome. These discoveries now allow identification of not only the presence of disease but of disease susceptibility, especially cancer. They have likewise given rise to new techniques, including gene microarrays and proteomics that allow rapid evaluation of gene and protein expression. The proteomic approach has developed to the point where patterns of component proteins in serum have been found to characterize specific cancerous states and also the presence of other diseases. Both conventional tumor markers measured in serum (Ch. 74) and newly discovered oncoprotein markers are discussed with applications of the emerging area of proteomics

(Ch. 75). Finally, the prospects for early detection, prognosis, and planning of treatment regimens for cancer by detailed knowledge of alterations in the human genome are clearly on the horizon. We have therefore included these new genome-based approaches as applied to the detection and monitoring of cancer at early stages in the last chapter of this section on molecular diagnosis of neoplasia (Ch. 76). We feel that this information is critical because, in the near future, the clinical laboratory will be called upon to analyze specimens for genomic evaluation in diagnosis of diseases, susceptibility to disease, and even evaluation of the most effective treatment of diseases, as is now being performed for optimal treatment of viral diseases such as hepatitis and AIDS. Therefore, it is incumbent on pathologists to understand the basis for molecular diagnostics and how the human genome was sequenced.

After achieving a sound understanding of analytic principles and interpretation of laboratory examinations and pitfalls in their interpretation due to interferences, physiologic state, or drug interactions, it is also necessary to have strategies for offering tests to provide the appropriate level of care to screen for disease, confirm diagnosis, establish prognosis, and monitor the effects of treatment. For several decades, it has been a popular practice for physicians to order panels of multiple individual tests to screen for abnormalities of many different organs that might not otherwise be suspected. This practice was standardized several years ago by joint action of the American Medical Association and the United States Department of Health and Human Services with the establishment of a group of multi-test panels such as the basic metabolic panel and the comprehensive metabolic panel (inside front cover). Two predominant forces have driven the design of these panels. One is the technologic ease with which multi-channel chemistry analyzers can generate many results quickly and relatively inexpensively. The other force is a restriction on the amount of reimbursement provided for testing and the definition of medical necessity to guide the utilization of test ordering based on initial clinical diagnosis instead of screening widely in the absence of symptoms. The balance between technological capabilities and limitations in reimbursement is due for a reshuffling in the next several years as technological capabilities soar beyond those of today and open the floodgates to inexpensive testing of analytes in numbers that are orders of magnitude greater. The arenas where this change is most likely to occur include genetic testing of many types. In particular, the use of tandem mass spectrometry is making the simultaneous detection of multiple genetic diseases feasible in newborn screening. The state of Virginia has increased the number of screening tests from nine to twenty-eight effective March 2006 for infants under 6 months of age. Previously, screening for individual metabolic diseases was driven largely by the financial impact of detecting and treating cases to prevent the disease and thereby saving state revenues for life-long institutionalization. Today's technologies have drastically changed that equation so that cost is much less of a factor and humanitarian purposes are much more important in deciding what should be tested.

This model of mega-analyte testing is now also being explored in gene expression arrays and can also be anticipated in protein studies (proteomics) as well. Are we equipped professionally to interpret the results of hundreds to tens of thousands of individual results on a single patient? Probably not without advances in statistical analysis and decision making to distinguish between true positive and random false positive results from so many interrogations of the human body. Also needed will be efficient and clear means of communicating these complex results and their interpretations to physicians and their patients.

These are wonderful challenges for the clinical laboratory to have. They reflect the vitality of participating in medicine of the future and the integral role that laboratory medicine will always play in health care. We have attempted to point out areas in laboratory medicine where further investigative work is needed and to stimulate the reader to perform research in these areas (e.g., protein arrays containing multiple antibodies to different signal transducing proteins in serum for detection of cancer). We hope that one effect of this textbook will be to stimulate investigative studies that will advance diagnostic efficacy. We enthusiastically welcome any comments, reactions, or suggestions regarding this book to make the next edition even better.

It is a privilege and an honor to serve as editors for this the 21st edition.

Richard A. McPherson MD
Matthew R. Pincus MD PhD
April 2006

Acknowledgements

We gratefully acknowledge the outstanding contributions made by our expert colleagues and collaborators who served as associate editors: Mark S. Lifshitz MD, Naif Z. Abraham MD PhD, Gregory Threatte MD, Robert E. Hutchison MD, Jonathan L. Miller MD PhD, H. Davis Massey MD PhD, Gail L. Woods MD, Elizabeth Unger MD PhD, and Martin H. Bluth MD PhD. Each of them has made an extensive contribution to the quality of this book both through development of textual matter and through the exercise of practiced review of the chapters under their guidance. They have our deepest appreciation for their efforts in this edition.

We are also grateful to Frederick R. Davey MD for his earlier efforts in past editions as an associate editor. It is with sadness that we note the passing of our good friend and colleague, Chester J. Herman MD PhD, also a former associate editor. He will be remembered for his intellectual curiosity and for his leadership in promoting molecular diagnostic testing.

We acknowledge gratitude to Helene M.A. Paxton MS, Susanna Cunningham-Rundles MD PhD, Maurice R.G. O'Gorman PhD, Eric Wagner PhD, Haixiang Jiang PhD, Michael M. Frank MD, Armead H. Johnson PhD, Carolyn Katovich Hurley PhD, Robert J. Hartzman MD, and Judith A. Wade BSc for the opportunity to revise their prior chapters from the 20th edition for this, the 21st one. We also acknowledge our gratitude to Katherine I. Schexneider MD, for her contributions to this book. She has further enhanced this edition with a companion book, *Review Manual to Henry's Clinical Diagnosis and Management by Laboratory Methods*, also published by Elsevier.

All of our students, residents, and colleagues have over decades contributed enormously to the development of our knowledge in human disease and in the use of laboratories for diagnosis and patient management. To them we are grateful for all their questions and the stimuli they have provided. We are especially grateful for the mentorship and encouragement provided in our careers by Alfred Zettner MD, Cecil Hougie MD, Abraham Braude MD, James A. Rose MD, Robert P. Carty PhD, Donald West King MD, George Teebor MD, Phillip Prose MD, Fred Davey MD and Gerald Gordon MD. We will remember them always and the standards for excellence they set.

The myriad changes in format for this edition would not have been possible without the outstanding professional efforts of our editors at Elsevier: Natasha Andjelkovic, Joanne Husovski, and Russell Gabbedy. Kathryn Mason, Michael Houston, and Stewart Larking were also integral to realizing the development and implementation of this project. We are eternally grateful to them and to all the staff of Elsevier. They have made this endeavor a joy. We also acknowledge very special thanks to Anne Erickson, who has done many of the illustrations with a fine eye to beauty in presentation and ease of comprehension.

We are grateful to all the authors for accepting the challenge to participate in the education of future and present laboratorians by distilling the essential information from each of their fields of expertise and creating readable and authoritative text for our audience.

Most of all, we are perpetually grateful to John Bernard Henry, MD, for his leadership and magnificent contributions to the last seven editions of this book. We also wish to express our heart-felt gratitude for the encouragement and guidance he has provided to us personally and professionally in our careers.

At the completion of the task of writing and editing this 21st edition, we remain humbly grateful to all the individuals who have played a role in making it possible. To those we have named and to those not recognized, we thank you.

Richard A. McPherson MD
Matthew R. Pincus MD PhD

PART I

The Clinical Laboratory

Edited by

Mark S. Lifshitz MD, Matthew R. Pincus MD PhD,
Gregory A. Threatte MD

CHAPTER 1

General Concepts and Administrative Issues

Anthony S. Kurec MS DLM(ASCP), Mark S. Lifshitz MD

KEY POINTS

• Effective laboratory management requires leaders to provide direction and managers to get things done. Strategic planning, marketing, human resource management and quality management are all key elements of a laboratory organization.

• Most laboratory errors occur in the pre-analytic and post-analytic stage. Six Sigma is a tool that can be used to reduce laboratory errors.

• Laboratory services are provided in many different ways and can be thought of as a continuum from point-of-care tests producing immediate answers, to highly sophisticated reference laboratory tests that may take days or weeks to complete.

• Clinical laboratories are highly regulated; many laboratory practices are the direct result of federal or state/local legislation. At the federal level, laboratory activities are regulated through the Clinical Laboratory Improvement Amendments of 1988.

• Biological, chemical, ergonomic and fire hazards cannot be completely eliminated from the laboratory, but they can be contained to avoid harm to staff. Safety strategies include engineering controls (e.g., safety features built into the overall design of a product), personal protective equipment and work practice controls (like hand washing).

The laboratory plays a central role in healthcare. How critical is the laboratory? By one estimate, 70% of all medical decisions are based on laboratory results (Silverstein, 2003), though laboratory costs account for only 3.5% of total healthcare dollars (IOM, 2000). The laboratory is a $30–35 billion industry that offers high clinical value at relatively low cost.

The purpose of the laboratory is to provide physicians and other healthcare professionals with information to: (1) detect disease or predisposition to disease; (2) confirm or reject a diagnosis; (3) establish prognosis; (4) guide patient management; and (5) monitor efficacy of therapy (Kurec, 2000). The laboratory also plays a leading role in education and research, information technology design and implementation, and quality improvement. To successfully achieve its goal, a laboratory must use (1) medical, scientific, and technical expertise; (2) resources such as personnel, laboratory and data processing equipment, supplies, and facilities; and (3) organization, management, and communication skills. The goal of this chapter is to provide a fundamental understanding of general concepts and administrative issues that are the basis of sound laboratory practices. A more detailed discussion of these topics is available elsewhere (Nigon, 2000; Snyder, 1998).

Leadership and Management

An organization is only as good as its people, and people are guided by leaders and managers. The terms leadership and management are often used interchangeably but represent different qualities (Table 1–1).

Leadership provides the direction of where one (or an organization) is going, whereas *management* provides the 'road' to get there. The old adage of, 'If you don't know where you are going, any road will get you there,' illustrates why leadership must set clear goals and strategic objectives. Effective management uses certain skills to work with and through other people to get things done. It requires an optimal mix of dedicated people and task-oriented leaders to achieve these goals. These skills fall under four primary management functions: (1) planning and prompt decision-making, (2) organizing, (3) leading, and (4) controlling.

Leadership is a pattern of behaviors used to engage others to complete tasks in a timely and productive manner. Leadership styles include: directing, coaching, supporting, and delegating (CareerTrack, 1988). A supportive leader provides physical and personal resources so that an individual can accomplish their duties. A directive leader presents rules, orders, or other defined instructions to the individual. The former approach offers flexibility and encourages creative problem solving whereas the latter approach offers concise and detailed instructions on how to complete a task. Other styles are also defined by these qualities: delegating provides low support and direction whereas coaching provides high support and direction. A leader may adopt any one of the behavior styles periodically to suit a situation, but in general, one style usually dominates.

Management uses the human, financial, physical, and information resources available to an organization in the most efficient and effective manner (Griffin, 1987). Some basic managerial responsibilities are listed in Table 1–2. Managers can be stratified as first-line managers (supervisors, team leaders, chief technologists), middle managers (operations manager, division head), and top managers (director, CEO, CFO). Each managerial level dictates the daily activities and skill sets required for that position. Top-level managers concentrate on strategizing and planning for the next 1–5 years, while the first-line manager is more concerned about completing the day's work. A top-level manager may or may not possess technical skills that a first-line manager uses every day. Middle managers are engaged in a variety of technical and nontechnical activities.

Strategic Planning

To survive and even thrive in a competitive environment, a laboratory must constantly re-evaluate its goals and services and adapt to market forces (e.g., fewer qualified laboratory personnel, reduced budgets, stricter regulatory mandates, lower reimbursements, and new sophisticated technologies). This requires a leader to make strategic decisions. For example, a standalone laboratory may consider two totally different strategies; it may grow by repositioning itself as a 'hub' providing reference work to smaller local labs or it may downsize to a 'stat'-only facility. The former strategy seeks to enhance net revenue whereas the latter one tries to lower costs. The process by which these decisions are made is called strategic planning and can be defined as: (1) deciding on the objectives of the organization and changing or modifying existing objectives; (2) allocating resources used to attain objectives; and (3) establishing policies that govern the acquisition, use and disposition of these resources (Lifshitz, 1996). Strategic planning is usually based on long-term projections and a global view that can impact all levels of a laboratory's operations. It is different

Table 1–1 Leader versus Manager Traits

Leader	Manager
Administrator	Implementer
Organizer and developer	Maintains control
Risk-taker	Thinks short term
Inspiration	Asks how and when
Thinks long term	Watches bottom line
Asks what and why	Accepts status quo
Challenges status quo	Is good soldier
Does the right thing	Does things right

Adapted from Ali, 2001.

Table 1–2 Basic Management Responsibilities

Operations management

Quality assurance

Policies and procedures

Strategic planning

Benchmarking

Productivity assessment

Legislation/regulations/HIPPA compliance

Medicolegal concerns

Continuing education

Staff meetings

Human resource management

Job descriptions

Recruitment and staffing

Orientation

Competency assessment

Personnel records

Performance evaluation/appraisals

Discipline and dismissal

Financial management

Departmental budgets

Billing

CPT coding

ICD-9 coding

Compliance regulations

Test cost analysis

Fee schedule maintenance

Marketing management

Customer service

Outreach marketing

Advertising

Website development

Client education

Table 1–3 SWOT Analysis for a New Hospital Outreach Program

Strengths

1. Use current technology/instrumentation
2. Have excess technical capacity
3. Increased test volume will decrease cost per test
4. Strong leadership support
5. Financial resources available

Opportunities

1. Opening of a new physician healthcare facility
2. Department of Health mandates lead testing on all children under 2 years old
3. Have access to hospital marketing department
4. Hospital X is bankrupt; laboratory will close

Weaknesses

1. Staffing shortage
2. Morale issues
3. Inadequate courier system
4. Need to hire additional pathologist
5. Limited experience in providing multi-hospital/client LIS services
6. Turnaround times are marginal

Threats

1. Competition from other local hospital labs
2. Competition from national reference labs
3. Reimbursement decreasing
4. Three local hospitals have consolidated their services including laboratory
5. Several new patient service centers (phlebotomy stations) already opened

are opportunities and threats. This process is a particularly useful tool when developing a marketing strategy (Table 1–3) and should be used to help develop a marketing program (Table 1–4).

Quality Systems Management

A key management goal is to ensure that quality laboratory services are provided; this, in turn, depends on modern equipment, well-trained staff, well-designed physical environment, and a good management team. In recent years, quality issues and medical error rates have become the focus of increasing attention. A 1999 study by the Institute of Medicine (IOM) concluded that 44 000 to as many as 98 000 Americans die each year because of medical errors (Silverstein, 2003; Kohn, 1999). Among those errors, 50% were failure to use appropriate tests, and of those, 32% were due to failure to act on test findings, and 55% were due to avoidable delays in rendering a diagnosis. The frequency of laboratory errors ranges from 0.05–0.61%, though the distribution of errors among the testing stages is similar, with most (32–75%) occurring in the pre-analytical stage and far fewer (13–32%) in the analytical stage (Bonini, 2002). Pre-analytic errors include hemolyzed, clotted or insufficient samples, incorrectly identified or unlabeled samples, wrong collection tube drawn and improper specimen storage; analytic errors include calibration error and instrument malfunction; post-analytic errors include reports sent to wrong physician, long turn-around time and missing reports. Thus, it is clear there are opportunities to improve the quality of laboratory services.

Total Quality Management (TQM) and *Continuous Quality Improvement* (CQI) are useful approaches to quality leadership and management (Juran, 1988; Deming, 1986). TQM is a systems approach that focuses on teams, processes, statistics, and delivery of services/products that meet or exceed customer expectations (Brue, 2002). CQI is an element of TQM that strives to continually improve practices and not just meet established quality standards. Table 1–5 compares traditional quality thinking with TQM. TQM thinking strives to continually look for ways to reduce errors ('defect prevention') by empowering employees to assist in solving problems and getting them to understand their integral role within a greater system ('universal responsibility').

Another quality tool – *Six Sigma* – is popular in the business world and has been adapted to the laboratory (Brue, 2002). This is a hands-on process with the single mantra of 'improvement': improved performance, improved quality, improved bottom line, improved customer satisfaction, and improved employee satisfaction. In the Six Sigma process, the number of defects per million opportunities (DPMO) is measured. A defect is

from tactical planning, which is the detailed, often day-to-day operations needed to meet the strategic goals that have been set. For example, a global strategy to develop an outreach business may prompt other questions like: 'Should we perform more reference work in-house? Do we need additional instrumentation and/or laboratory automation? Are our information technology tools adequate? Is staffing adequate to satisfy service expectations?' So, there is a risk associated with determining a strategy. A wrong decision may burden a laboratory with unnecessary costs, systems or equipment, making it that much harder to change course in response to future market forces or new organizational strategies.

A variety of techniques can be used to facilitate the strategic planning process; these include Histograms/Graphs/Scattergrams, Brainstorming, Fishbone Diagrams, Storyboarding, Pareto Analysis, and Delphi Analysis (Kurec, 2004a). Another way to evaluate the risks associated with new strategies is the *Strengths, Weaknesses, Opportunities,* and *Threats* (SWOT) analysis. Generally, environmental factors internal to the laboratory are classified as strengths and weaknesses and external environmental factors

Table 1–4 Example of Issues to Consider when Establishing a Marketing Program

Assessment	Remember the four Ps of marketing: • Product • Price • Place • Promotion What are the customer needs? Who is the competition? Do you have the right testing menu, equipment, and facilities? Do you have enough personnel? Do you have adequate financial resources? Do you know what it costs to do a laboratory test (test–cost analysis)?
Define your customer segments	Physicians, nurses, dentists, other healthcare providers Other hospital labs, physician office labs (POLs) Insurance companies Identify unique socioeconomic and/or ethnic groups Look for population shifts and location (urban, rural, suburban) Colleges, universities, and other schools Nursing homes, home health agencies, and clinics Veterinarians and other animal healthcare facilities Researchers, pharmaceutical companies, clinical trials
Process	Develop a sales/marketing plan and team Set goals Ensure infrastructure (courier service, LIS capabilities, customer service personnel, etc.) is adequate Develop additional test menu items Educate laboratory personnel in customer service Support and maintain existing client services Advertise/public relations

How to market?	Review test menu for comprehensive services (niche testing, esoteric testing, other unique services that could be provided to an eclectic group)
	Place advertisements
	Develop brochures, specimen collection manuals, and other customer-related material
	Develop website
	Attend/participate in community health forums
	Identify specific target customers:
	    Other hospital labs, independent labs, reference labs
	    College/school infirmaries, health clinics, county laboratory facilities, industrial/occupational facilities (pre-employment, drug screening)
	    Nursing homes, extended care facilities
	    Drug/alcohol rehabilitation centers, correctional facilities
	    Physician offices (POLs), groups, and specialties (pediatrics, dermatology, family medicine, etc.)

Table 1–5 Quality Management: Traditional versus TQM Thinking

Traditional thinking	TQM thinking
Acceptable quality	Error-free quality
Department focused	Organization focused
Quality is expensive	Quality lowers costs
Defects caused by workers	Defects caused by system
Management controls worker	Worker empowered
Status quo	CQI
Manage by intuition	Manage by fact
Intangible quality	Quality defined
We–They relationship	Us relationship
End process focus	System process
Reactive systems	Proactive systems

anything that does not meet customer requirements; for example, a laboratory result error, delay in reporting or a quality control problem. So, if a laboratory analyzes 1000 reports and finds 10 that are reported late, it has a 1% defect rate; this is equivalent to 10 000 DPMO. Six Sigma refers

Table 1–6 Six Sigma Steps

Six Sigma step	Example
Define project goal or other deliverable that is critical to quality	Emergency department results in less than 30 minutes from order
Measure baseline performance and related variables	Baseline performance: 50% of time results are within 30 minutes, 70% within 1 hour, 80% within 2 hours, etc. Variables: staffing on each shift, order to laboratory receipt time, receipt to result time, etc.
Analyze data using statistics and graphs to identify and quantify root cause	Order to receipt is highly variable because samples are not placed in sample transport system immediately and samples delivered to laboratory are not clearly flagged as emergency
Improve performance by developing and implementing a solution	Samples from emergency department are uniquely colored to make them easier to spot among routine samples
Control the factors related to the improvement, verify impact, validate benefits, and monitor over time	New performance: results available 90% of time within 30 minutes

to the goal of reducing defects to near zero. The sigma or standard deviation expresses how much variability exists in products or services. By reducing variability one also reduces defects. Thus, one sigma represents 691 463 defects per million opportunities (DPMO) or a yield (i.e., percentage of products without defects) of only 30.854% whereas the goal of Six Sigma is to reach 3.4 DPMO, or 99.9997% yield (Brue, 2002). Most organizations operate at or near four sigma (6210 DPMO). To put this in perspective, per CLIA'88 guidelines, most proficiency testing (PT) requires an 80% accuracy rate. This translates to 200 000 defects per million tests or 2.4 sigma. The reported PT accuracy rate for CLIA participating laboratories was 97% or 3.4 sigma (Garber, 2004). Six Sigma practices can be applied to patient care and safety (Berte, 2004). Examples, based on College of American Pathologists (CAP) Q-Probes and Q-Tracks programs, show the relationship of applying Six Sigma to some common performance quality indicators. In these studies, the median variance (50th percentile) for test order accuracy was 2.3% or 23 000 DPMO; patient wristband error was 3.13% or 31 000 DPMO; blood culture contamination was 2.83% or 28 300 DPMO; and pathology discrepancy rate was 5.1% or 51 000 DPMO (Berte, 2004). By lowering defects, quality of care is improved and cost savings are realized by eliminating waste (e.g., supplies and materials for reruns), unnecessary steps, and/or staff time (Sunyog, 2004). By some estimates, the cost of doing business is reduced by 25–40% in moving from three sigma to six sigma performance. An example of the Six Sigma process is provided in Table 1–6.

Human Resource Management (HR)

Recruiting, hiring, training and retaining qualified personnel have become a major challenge for today's manager. Over the last 20–30 years, almost 70% of accredited Medical Technology programs have closed, resulting in a 22% reduction in the number of graduating students. In 2002, average vacancy rate for staff medical technologists was about 7% (Ward-Cook, 2003). Some common reasons why there are difficulties in recruiting and/or retaining staff are low wages, perceived dangerous work environment, staffing shortages, lack of public and professional recognition, and stress. This has made recruitment a much tougher undertaking and has necessitated implementation of more creative recruitment incentives as well as competitive salaries, comprehensive benefits, and a non-hostile work environment. Today's job market draws from around the world; thus a greater understanding of cultural, ethnic, and gender-related traits is necessary to achieve a well-rounded pool of job applicants (Kurec, 2004b).

Labor accounts for 50–70% of a laboratory's costs, so a new or replacement staff position, or *full-time equivalent* (FTE), must be justified. It is appropriate to review the authority level, experience, education, and job responsibilities of a position and compare them to any related changes in technology, required skills, or other environmental factors. This is to ensure that the position is still necessary and the duties are essential and current. Another question to consider is whether an unfilled position would negatively impact on the department or the hospital. For example, an unfilled phlebotomist position may delay morning blood collection and result availability.

Once the justification review is complete, a criterion-based job description should be developed (Kurec, 1998). The criterion-based job description should focus on roles and not specific tasks, as the latter may require changes rather frequently depending on operations. A criterion-based job description not only includes title, grade, and qualifications, but clear identification of responsibilities, accountability, and internal and external organizational relationships. This provides a clear guide of what the expectations are for both the employee and employer.

Laboratory Design and Service Models

Laboratory services are provided in many different ways and can be thought of as a continuum from point-of-care tests producing immediate answers, to highly sophisticated reference laboratory tests that may take days or weeks to complete. Radical changes in healthcare have forced laboratories to re-evaluate what services to offer and how to deliver them. This has led to a variety of laboratory testing service models (Table 1–7). In some instances, financial pressures have led hospitals to form external relationships, like networks, where laboratory resources are centralized. Similarly, laboratories have changed their internal design in an effort to consolidate sections and/or services. Laboratory testing has also been pushed out to point-of-care (POCT) to shorten turnaround time for critical results and enhance patient convenience. These types of changes have fostered organizational changes within the laboratory environment and its external relationships with other hospital departments, other healthcare providers, and the community it services.

The *functional design of a laboratory* and its relationship to other testing sites within a facility has evolved over time. The traditional hospital laboratory was designed with discrete hematology, chemistry, microbiology and blood bank sections. However, in recent years the boundaries between these areas have been obscured. In an effort to lower costs and respond more rapidly to clinical needs, there has been realignment of intralaboratory services along the lines of highly automated, rapid response 'core' facilities, semiautomated or manual test processing, and peripheral stat laboratories and/or point of care testing sites. In the past, testing locations were defined by discipline (i.e., hepatitis testing was always done in serology); now, laboratories are defining test location based on technology (hepatitis tests

run on an automated platform along with other immunoassays in chemistry). These trends have been made possible by technologic advances in pre-analytic sample handling (e.g., bar coding, automated centrifuges, de-capper), analyzers (e.g., consolidating multiple analytic modalities into a single, integrated platform), and post-analysis (e.g., reporting laboratory results via networked computer systems, the internet, autofaxing). These advances have produced three distinct approaches to core laboratory testing: single platform (single analyzer), workcell (two or more linked instruments), and total laboratory automation (workcell with pre- and post-analytic processing). These configurations will be further discussed in Chapters 2 and 5.

Regionalization is a consolidation process on a grander scale. In this 'hub and spoke' model, a single core laboratory serves as the hub with one or more other laboratories serving as the spokes. It requires significant up-front resources to initiate a regionalized laboratory, considerable space requirements, commitment from senior personnel, and long-term, continuing education for the staff in dealing with this change. This type of format requires a highly cooperative environment among all parties involved and can take years to fully implement. In this model, two or more hospital laboratories form an interlaboratory alliance and come to agreement on the location of laboratories, retention of staff, instrumentation used, and information management system. Often, a large, core laboratory facility is centrally located to accommodate the routine and the more esoteric tests. Stat or rapid-response laboratories are located at individual hospitals to handle urgent test requests. This model works particularly well where a large, comprehensive laboratory already exists among a number of smaller community-based hospitals. A variation of this model is one that focuses on specialization and laboratory expertise. For example, one hospital laboratory may have well-established microbiology/virology/mycology laboratories with experienced staff that are capable of handling routine and highly specific testing. Sending all but the most basic microbiology tests to the 'core microbiology laboratory' could take advantage of existing laboratory skills and equipment. Similar opportunities may exist for other laboratory sections such as cytogenetics, molecular diagnostics, cytology, or histocompatibility. The advantages of such a consolidation are standardization of procedures, equipment, quality-control programs, and reporting formats (Zeiger, 1997). Reducing equipment redundancy, maximizing specimen throughput, and utilizing staff more effectively can achieve significant cost savings. One laboratory consolidation of services allowed for a 25% reduction in labor (Szumski, 1999); bulk purchase of common supplies reduces costs; and multiple purchasing agreements can be consolidated. The challenges in implementing and succeeding with this model include specimen transportation, resistance to change, personnel issues, morale issues, 'lost identity' of the laboratory, and union problems, and thus require careful consideration in the planning process.

Physical design considerations are important regardless of the type of laboratory. Location of specimen processing area, patient registration and data entry, specimen testing workflow, short- and long-term storage, and laboratory information system (LIS) connectivity requirements must be considered. Spatial requirements in relationship to other hospital services (proximity to emergency department, intensive care units, and surgical operating suite) should be viewed as a multidisciplinary process. Robotics, pneumatic tubes, computers, including intranet and internet accesses, and facsimile machines are the new tools used in modern laboratories and must be accounted for in the design plans. Electrical power, temperature/humidity controls, water and drainage sources, and air circulation/ventilation issues must be considered for placement and adequate quantity. Regulatory compliance codes must be carefully reviewed and implemented appropriately to ensure safety, ergonomic, and comfort needs (Table 1–8). To ensure one meets local, state, and federal codes, a qualified and experienced architect who has experience in designing clinical laboratories should be consulted when considering laboratory relocation or renovation designs. This also minimizes costly change orders and maximizes functionality and workflow.

Regulation, Accreditation, and Legislation

Clinical laboratories are among the most highly regulated healthcare entities; many laboratory practices are the direct result of federal or state/local legislation (Table 1–9). Understanding these laws is necessary to avoid legal or administrative repercussions that may limit a laboratory's operations or shut it down completely. To operate (and receive reimbursement for services), laboratories must be licensed and may also need to be accredited. Licensure is mandatory; it is a federal and/or state requirement to operate a laboratory. Accreditation is voluntary, though it may satisfy licensure requirements in some states.

Table 1–7 Laboratory Design and Service Model Examples

Traditional 'closed' laboratory	The traditional hospital laboratory has discrete sections in hematology, chemistry, microbiology, and blood bank, generally separated into rooms or sections
'Open' laboratory	The discrete services are placed in one large room with portable walls that can be adjusted as needed based on volume
Core laboratory	A common type of consolidation has been hematology and chemistry laboratories ('chematology') (Bush, 1998). Advantages include handling stat requests, improving off-shift workflow, and avoiding chronic staffing problems
Regional laboratory	Specific low-volume or expensive laboratory services currently provided by more then one regional hospital laboratory, that are consolidated into one hospital laboratory. For example, consolidation of all virology or PCR testing into one hospital laboratory
Reference laboratory	Traditional full service laboratory that handles all types of testing, especially esoteric tests
Point-of-care	Laboratory testing that is brought to the patient's bedside. Test menu is generally limited to a few basic chemistry and hematology tests (e.g., glucose, pregnancy, activated clotting time, blood gases)
Stat laboratory	Rapid response laboratory that is often located in or near an emergency department or surgical suite. Provides critical laboratory tests such as hematocrits and blood gases
Limited service	Laboratory provides limited menu of routine (like CBC, chemistry panel, prothrombin time) and/or specialty services (like fertility testing) on a stat or non-stat basis. Includes downsized hospital labs that retain stats and some routine tests but send most work to an off-site core laboratory

Table 1–8 Laboratory Physical Design Considerations (Painter, 1993; Mortland, 1997)

1. In developing a needs assessment, identify space for offices, personal facilities, storage, conference/library area, and students
2. Routinely review all floor plans and elevations for appropriate usage and ensure space and function are related. Handicap accessibility may be required
3. Develop and use a project scheduler
4. Fume hoods and biological safety cabinets must be located away from high traffic areas and doorways
5. Modular furniture allows for flexibility in moving or reconfiguration of the laboratory according to current and anticipated needs
6. Conventional laboratory fixtures may be considered in building depreciation, whereas modular furniture is not
7. Base cabinets (under laboratory counters) provide 20–30% more storage space than suspended cabinets
8. Noise control in open labs may be obtained by installing a drop ceiling. Installation of utilities above a drop ceiling adds to flexibility in their placement
9. In general, space requirements are 150–200 net square feet (excludes hallways, walls, custodial closets, etc.) per FTE, or 27–40 net square feet per hospital bed
10. Rooms over 100 square feet must have two exits; corridors used for patients must be 8 feet wide, while those not used for patients must be 3 feet 8 inches wide
11. An eyewash unit must be within 100 feet of work areas
12. Suggested standard dimensions in planning and designing a laboratory:

Laboratory counter width	2 feet 6 inches
Laboratory counter to wall clearance	4 feet
Laboratory counter to counter clearance	7 feet
Desk height	30 inches
Keyboard drawer height	25–27 inches
Human body standing	4 square feet
Human body sitting	6 square feet
Desk space	3 square feet

At the federal level, laboratory activities are regulated through the Clinical Laboratory Improvement Amendments of 1988 (CLIA'88, Federal Register, 55, 1990; http://www.cms.hhs.gov/clia/). Prior to CLIA'88, there were no consistent federal regulatory standards for most laboratories, only sporadic state initiatives that carried various levels of authority. CLIA'88 was enacted in response to reports of inaccurate PAP smear results and overall concerns about laboratory quality standards. CLIA '88 provides minimum standards that are enforced by the federal government or by designees (Table 1–10) that have standards 'deemed' equivalent to or stricter than CLIA. To test human samples, a clinical laboratory must be CLIA certified indicating that it meets personnel, operational, safety, and quality standards set by the government. One aspect of CLIA is that it applies various standards based on test complexity (Table 1–11). Detailed, current guidelines may be found at the website: http://www.phppo.cdc.gov/clia/regs/toc.aspx.

There are a variety of government agencies and nongovernment organizations that directly or indirectly impact on laboratory operations. Tables 1–12 and 1–13 provide some common examples but are by no means all inclusive. The responsibilities assumed by these agencies represent federal, state, and professional guidelines and/or mandates that are designed to protect the public from shoddy laboratory testing practices or unnecessary exposure to biological, chemical, or radioactive elements. They also ensure the availability of quality blood products, access to laboratory testing as needed, and provide a safe work environment for employees. Professional associations provide guidelines that are often accepted as standard care of practice by governmental agencies. For example, Table 1–14 provides suggested time limits for record and specimen retention based on CAP guidelines.

Safety

The clinical laboratory can potentially expose staff to a variety of hazards through contact with patients, specimens, equipment and routine daily tasks. These include biological, chemical, ergonomic and fire hazards. Though potential hazards cannot be completely eliminated, they can be contained to avoid harm to staff. Laboratories are obligated to identify hazards, implement safety strategies to contain the hazards, and continually

Table 1–9 Various Laboratory Regulations and their Significance

1983 **Prospective Payment System (PPS)** for Medicare patients established payment based on diagnosis related groups (DRGs). Hospitals are paid a fixed amount per DRG, regardless of actual cost, thereby creating an incentive to discharge patients as soon as medically possible. For inpatients, labs become cost centers instead of revenue centers (Social Security Amendments P.L. 98-21)

1984 **Deficit Reduction Act** (P.L. 93-369) – established outpatient laboratory fee schedule to control costs; froze Part B fee schedule

1988 **Clinical Laboratory Improvement Act of 1988 (CLIA 88)**; amended 1990; 1992; established that all laboratories must be certified by the federal government with mandated quality assurance, personnel and proficiency testing standards based on test complexity. Up until this time, the federal government only regulated the few labs conducting interstate commerce or independent or hospital labs that wanted Medicare reimbursement. CLIA applies to all sites where testing is done, including doctor offices and clinics

1989 **Physician Self-referral Ban** (Stark I; PL 101-239) – prevents physicians from referring Medicare patients to self-owned laboratories
Ergonomic Safety and Health Program Management Guidelines – establishes OSHA guidelines for employee safety

1990 **Three-Day Rule** initiated by CMS. Payment for any laboratory testing done 3 calendar days before admission as an inpatient is not reimbursed since it is considered to be part of the hospital stay. (Omnibus Reconciliation Act); directs HHS to develop an outpatient DRG system
Occupational Exposure to Hazardous Chemicals in Laboratories – establishes OSHA guidelines to limit unnecessary exposure to hazardous chemicals

1992 **Occupational Exposure to Blood Borne Pathogens** – establishes OSHA guidelines to limit unnecessary exposure to biologic hazards

1996 **Health Insurance Portability and Accountability Act (HIPPA)** – directs how healthcare information is managed. This law protects patients from the inappropriate dispersion (oral, written, or electronic) of personal information and is the basis for many of the privacy standards currently in place

1997 **OIG Compliance Guidelines** for Clinical Laboratories help laboratories develop programs that promote high ethical and lawful conduct, especially regarding billing practices and fraud and abuse

2001 **CMS National Coverage Determinations** (NCDs) replaced most local medical review policies (LMRPs) used to determine whether certain laboratory tests are medically necessary and therefore reimbursable. Prior to this, each Medicare intermediary had its own medical necessity guidelines

2003 **Hazardous Material Regulations** dealing with shipment of blood and other potentially biohazardous products (DOT)

Table 1–10 CLIA 'Deemed Status'

States
  New York
  Washington
Organizations
  College of American Pathologists
  Joint Commission on Accreditation of Health Care Organizations
  American Association of Blood Banks
  American Society for Histocompatibility and Immunogenetics
  Commission on Office Laboratory Accreditation
  American Osteopathic Association

audit existing practices to determine whether new ones are needed. Frequent safety reviews, disaster drills, and general employee awareness help maintain a safe work environment.

Good safety practices benefit the laboratory as well as employees. Injuries affect staff morale and threaten the emotional and physical health of the party involved. Injuries are also expensive in terms of lost workdays and wages, damaged equipment, and medical treatment. An injured person may be absent for an indefinite period of time and often cannot work at peak efficiency upon return. While inexperience may be a cause for some accidents, others may be a result of ignoring known risks, haste, carelessness, fatigue, or mental preoccupation (failure to focus attention or concentrate on what is at hand).

Table 1–11 CLIA Categories Included and Excluded (Sliva, 2003)

Test categories (based on analyst/operator and complexity to run test)
  Waived (e.g., blood glucose, urine pregnancy)
  Moderate complexity
  High complexity
Not categorized (because they do not produce a result)
  Quality control materials
  Calibrators
  Collection kits (for HIV, drugs of abuse, etc.)
Not currently regulated (by CLIA)
  Non-invasive testing (e.g. bilirubin)
  Breath tests (e.g., alcohol, *H. pylori*)
  Drugs of abuse testing in the workplace
  Continuous monitoring/infusion devices (e.g., glucose/insulin)

Several strategies exist to contain hazards (Table 1–15). *Engineering controls* are safety features built into the overall design of a product; for example, an electrical circuit breaker or a protective sheath on a phlebotomy needle. *Personal protective equipment (PPE)* and barriers like gloves and face shields physically separate the user from a hazard. *Work practice controls* include general procedures and preventive measures that reduce or eliminate exposure to hazards, such as segregating biological waste and hand washing. The most effective safety programs use all three strategies.

Biological Hazards

Biological hazards expose an unprotected individual to bacteria, viruses, parasites, or some other biological entity that results in infection. Exposure occurs from ingestion, inoculation, tactile contamination, or inhalation of infectious material from patients or their body fluids/tissues, supplies or materials that they have come in contact with, contaminated needles, or aerosol dispersion. There is also the potential for inadvertent exposure to the public through direct or indirect contact with infectious bodily fluids or tissues, contaminated laboratory equipment, improperly processed blood products, and inappropriately disposed waste products.

The spread of hepatitis B virus (HBV), human immunodeficiency virus (HIV), and tuberculosis (TB) has focused the responsibility on each healthcare organization to protect its employees, patients, and the general public from infection. In 1987, concern about HIV prompted the Centers for Disease Control (CDC) to update its 1983 'Guidelines for Isolation Precautions in Hospitals' (Garner, 1983) with the release of its 'Universal Precautions,' which recommends that blood and body fluid precautions be consistently used for all patients regardless of their blood-borne infection status (CDC Recommendations and Reports, 1989). Such guidelines are meant to minimize occupational exposures. The Occupational Safety and Health Administration (OSHA) defines occupational exposures as 'reasonably anticipated skin, eye, mucous membrane, or percutaneous contact with blood or other potentially infectious materials that may result from the performance of an employee's duties' (Federal Register, 29CFR, 1910.1030, 1992). Blood and most other body fluids including semen, vaginal secretions, pericardial fluid, peritoneal fluid, synovial fluid, pleural fluid, amniotic fluid, saliva, tears, cerebrospinal fluid, urine, and breast milk of all patients may be considered potentially infectious for HIV, HBV, HCV, and other blood-borne pathogens. In addition, any unfixed tissue samples, whole organs, or blood slides may also be considered potentially infectious. Prior to these requirements, laboratory-associated infections occurred from mouth pipetting, consumption of food in laboratory, spills or splashes on unprotected skin, membranes, or open cuts, and needlesticks. Aerosol contamination was related to inoculating loops (flaming a loop), spills on laboratory counters, expelling a spray from needles, and centrifugation of infected fluids (Sewell, 1995).

While many laboratories require wearing of gloves when performing phlebotomies, OSHA strongly recommends that gloves should be used routinely as a barrier protection especially when the healthcare worker has cuts or other open wounds on their skin; when the worker anticipates hand contamination; when performing skin punctures; or during phlebotomy training (OSHA Correspondence, 1991). All other phlebotomy access procedures may require use of gloves as determined by local policy. Employees must wash their hands after removal of gloves, after any contact with blood or body fluids, or between patients. Gloves should not be washed and reused since microorganisms that adhere to gloves are difficult to remove (Doebbeling, 1988). Masks, protective eyewear, or face shields must be worn to prevent exposure from splashes to the mouth, eyes, or nose. All protective equipment that has the potential for coming into

Table 1–12 Various Laboratory-Related Governmental Agencies

CMS	Centers for Medicare and Medicaid Services (formerly known as HCFA) oversees the largest healthcare program in the US processing over 1 billion claims per year. Medicare (see Chapter 12) provides coverage to approximately 40 million Americans over the age of 65, some people with disabilities, and patients with end-stage renal disease (ERSD) with a budget of $309 billion (2004). Medicaid provides coverage to approximately 50 million individuals with low income through a state–federal partnership that costs $277 billion (2004). CMS sets quality standards and reimbursement rates that apply to the laboratory and are often used by other third-party payers (www.cms.hhs.gov/)
DOT	Department of Transportation has the responsibility of regulating biohazardous materials that include blood and other human products. Laboratory specimens sent to reference laboratories must be packaged per guidelines set by this agency (www.dot.gov/)
EPA	Environmental Protection Agency sets and enforces standards for disposal of hazardous laboratory materials, such as formalin, xylene, and other potential carcinogens (www.epa.gov)
EEOC	Equal Employment Opportunity Commission oversees and enforces Title VIII dealing with fair employment practices related to the Civil Rights Act of 1964 and the Equal Employment Opportunity Act of 1972. Hiring laboratory staff falls under the same rules as most businesses (www.eeoc.gov/)
FDA	Food and Drug Administration is part of HHS and regulates the manufacture of biologics (like blood donor testing and component preparation) and medical devices (like laboratory analyzers) and test kits through its Office of In-Vitro Diagnostic Device Evaluation and Safety. FDA inspects blood donor and/or component manufacturing facilities irrespective of other regulatory agencies and/or accrediting organizations (www.fda.gov/)
HHS	US Department of Health and Human Services oversees CMS, OIG and FDA
NARA	National Archives and Records Administration provides a number of databases including access to the Federal Register where laboratory regulations are published (www.gpoaccess.gov/fr/index.html)
NRC	Nuclear Regulatory Commission develops and enforces federal guidelines that ensure the proper use and operation of non-military nuclear facilities. Laboratory tests that use radioactive materials (like radioimmunoassays) must adhere to guidelines set by this agency (www.nrc.gov/)
NIDA	National Institute on Drug Abuse strictly regulates standards for performing and maintaining appropriate quality control for drugs of abuse testing (www.nida.nih.gov/)
NIOSH	National Institute of Occupational Safety and Health is in the Department of Health and Human Services and provides research, information, education, and training in the field of occupational safety and health. NIOSH makes recommendations regarding safety hazards but has no authority to enforce them (www.cdc.gov/niosh/homepage.html)
NIH	National Institute of Health is an agency of the Department of Health & Human Services (HHS) and is a world leader in medical research. It publishes a variety of clinical practice guidelines some of which are applicable to the laboratory such as those for diabetes and lipid testing (www.nih.gov)
NIST	National Institute of Standards and Technology is a branch of the Commerce Department and has contributed to the development of many healthcare products. In addition, they have developed standards for calibration, weights and measures, and SI units (www.nist.gov)
OIG	Office of the Inspector General is part of HHS and is responsible for auditing, inspecting and identifying fraud and abuse in CMS programs like laboratory testing. OIG's focus is usually noncompliance with reimbursement regulations like medical necessity
OSHA	Occupational Safety and Health Administration is in the Department of Labor and develops and enforces workplace standards to protect employees' safety and health. Recommendations from OSHA include guidelines addressing blood-borne pathogens, chemical safety, phlebotomies, latex gloves, ergonomics, and any other potentially hazardous situation that may be found in the workplace (www.osha.gov/)
State DOH	State Departments of Health vary in the extent to which they regulate laboratories. Some states, like New York, license all labs and have mandatory proficiency testing and laboratory inspection programs; others have neither. New York and Washington have CLIA 'deemed' status

Table 1–13 Various Laboratory-Related, Nongovernmental Organizations

AABB	Formerly known as American Association of Blood Banks, AABB is a peer professional group that offers a blood bank accreditation program that can substitute for (but coordinate with) a CAP inspection. It has CLIA-deemed status (www.aabb.org)
ASCP	American Society of Clinical Pathology is a professional organization and is the largest organization for laboratory professionals offering certification for various specialties (www.ascp.org)
CAP	College of American Pathologists offers the largest proficiency survey program in the US and has a peer-surveyed laboratory accreditation program that has CLIA-deemed status. CAP accreditation is recognized by JCAHO as meeting its laboratory standards (www.cap.org)
CLSI	Clinical and Laboratory Standards Institute (formerly NCCLS) is a peer professional group that develops standardized criteria regarding laboratory practices; accrediting and licensing entities often adopt these as standards, e.g., procedure manual format (www.clsi.org)
COLA	COLA (originally the Commission on Office Laboratory Accreditation) is a nonprofit organization sponsored by the American Academy of Family Physicians, the American College of Physicians, the American Medical Association, the American Osteopathic Association, and the College of American Pathologists. It has CLIA-deemed status and its accreditation is recognized by JCAHO. It originally organized to provide assistance to Physician Office Labs (POLs), but has recently expanded its product line to other services (www.cola.org)
JCAHO	Joint Commission on Accreditation of Healthcare Organizations is an independent, not-for-profit entity that accredits nearly 16 000 healthcare organizations and programs in the US based on a comprehensive set of quality standards. It has CLIA-deemed status and may substitute for federal Medicare and Medicaid surveys; it also fulfills licensure requirements in some states and general requirements of many insurers. JCAHO usually surveys the laboratory as part of an overall healthcare facility survey (www.jcaho.org/)

Table 1–14 Suggested Guidelines for Record and Specimen Retention*

Record/specimen type	Retention
Records	
Requisitions	2 years
Quality control	2 years
Instrument maintenance	2 years
Blood bank donor/recipient records	Indefinitely
Blood bank employee signatures/initials	10 years
Blood bank quality control	5 years
Reports	
Clinical pathology laboratory reports	2 years
Autopsy forensic reports	Indefinitely
Surgical pathology (and bone marrow) reports	10 years
Cytogenetics reports	20 years
Specimens	
Serum/other body fluids	48 hours
Blood smears – routine	7 days
Pathology/bone marrow slides	10 years
Pathology Blocks	10 years
Microbiology smears	7 days
Blood bank donor/recipient specimens	7 days post-transfusion
Cytogenetics slides	3 years
Cytogenetics diagnostic images	20 years

* College of American Pathologists (CAP), Northfield, IL (March 2001) and/or CLIA'88 guidelines (Federal Register 55, 1990; 57, 1992); check with other organizations (like AABB) or local regulatory agencies for current requirements that may differ from those above.

Table 1–15 Laboratory Hazard Prevention Strategies

Work practice controls	Handwashing after each patient contact Cleaning surfaces with disinfectants Avoiding unnecessary use of needles and sharps and not recapping Red bag waste disposal Immunization for hepatitis Job rotation to minimize repetitive tasks Orientation, training and continuing education No eating, drinking, or smoking in laboratory Warning signage
Engineering controls	Puncture-resistant containers for disposal and transport of needles and sharps Safety needles that automatically retract after removal Biohazard bags Splash guards Volatile liquid carriers Centrifuge safety buckets Biological safety cabinets and fume hoods Mechanical pipetting devices Computer wrist/arm pads Sensor-controlled sinks or foot/knee/elbow-controlled faucets
Personal protective equipment (PPE) and barriers	Non-latex gloves Gowns and laboratory coats Masks including particulate respirators Face shields Protective eyewear (goggles, safety glasses) Eyewash station Chemical-resistant gloves; sub-zero (freezer) gloves; thermal gloves

contact with infectious material, including laboratory coats, must be removed before leaving the laboratory area and never taken home or outside the laboratory (such as during lunch or personal breaks). Laboratory coats must be cleaned on site or handled professionally. Eating, drinking, smoking, applying cosmetics, or touching contact lenses are prohibited in working laboratory areas. It is helpful for all employees to know what areas (offices, conference rooms, lounges) and equipment (telephones, keyboards, copy machines, etc.) are designated as laboratory work areas as they can be potentially contaminated.

Table 1–16 outlines some common materials that may be used for decontamination. A 10% solution (volume/volume with tap water, made daily) of common household bleach makes a very effective and economical disinfectant, inactivating hepatitis B virus (HBV) in 10 minutes and HIV in 2 minutes (CLSI M29-A3, 2005). Prewashing removes concentrated amounts of proteins, which is required before effective decontamination is achieved. Furthermore, all laboratory surfaces must be made of nonporous material that allows for easy cleaning and decontamination.

About 600 000–800 000 needlestick and other percutaneous injuries are estimated to occur each year (Bachman, 2003). OSHA has revised blood-borne pathogen standards to reflect the need for healthcare (laboratory) workers to evaluate and use medical safety devices that provide a barrier between the user and a contaminated needle. The Needlestick Safety and Prevention Act of 2000 (Pub. L. 106–430, 2000) revises the Bloodborne Pathogens Standard (Federal Register 29CFR 1910.1030, 1992) requiring employers to identify, evaluate, and implement safer medical sharps devices. It prohibits the removal of needles from a blood tube holder after a venipuncture and requires maintaining a sharps injury log. Table 1–17 provides the healthcare worker with information regarding needlestick injury.

Chemical Hazards

OSHA has determined that there are over 32 million workers exposed to 575 000 potentially hazardous chemicals in the work place (OSHA, 1994; Federal Register 29CFR 1910.1200, 1983). It is estimated that 40 000–50 000 manufacturing workers and 38 000 non-manufacturing workers experience chemically related illnesses a year. Another 14 000 non-manufacturing workers are injured and 102 fatalities occur. The chemical-related chronic disease rate is about 17 000, with over 25 000 cancer cases and almost 13 000 cancer deaths per year. To minimize the

Table 1–16 Common Decontamination Agents

Heat (250°C for 15 minutes)
Ethylene oxide (450–500 mg/L @ 55–60°C)
2% Glutaraldehyde
10% Hydrogen peroxide
10% Formalin
5.25% Hypochlorite (10% bleach)
Formaldehyde
Detergents
Phenols
Ultraviolet radiation
Ionizing radiation
Photo-oxidation

Table 1–17 Risk of Infection: What Healthcare Personnel Need to Know

Risk of infection depends on	The pathogen involved
	Type of exposure
	Amount of blood involved
	Amount of virus in the exposed blood
If exposed to blood, immediately	Wash with soap and water
	Flush splashes to nose, mouth or skin with water
	Irrigate eyes with clean water, saline, or sterile irrigants
What is the risk after an exposure If	vaccinated against hepatitis B (HBV): no risk; unvaccinated have a risk factor of 6–30%
	Exposure to hepatitis C (HCV) blood: risk is 1.8%
	HIV needlestick/cut exposure: 0.3%
	HIV exposure to eyes, nose, or mouth: 0.1%
	HIV exposure to nonintact skin: 0.1%; intact skin: no risk
Treatment	HBV: all healthcare workers should receive vaccination
	HCV: no vaccine available and no treatment to prevent infection
	HIV: no vaccine available. Antiretroviral drugs available if appropriate. Post-exposure treatment (if appropriate) should begin within 24 hours and no later than 7 days

Adapted from *Exposure to blood*. CDC, July 2003.

incidence of chemically related occupational illnesses and injuries in the workplace, OSHA published its 'Hazard Communication Standard' (Federal Register 29CFR 1910.1200; 1983) and 'Chemical Hygiene Plan' (Federal Register 29CFR 1910.1450; 1993), requiring the manufacturers of chemicals to evaluate the hazards of the chemicals they produce and to develop hazard communication programs for employees and other users that are exposed to hazardous chemicals (Table 1–18). These OSHA standards are based on the premise that employees have the *right-to-know* what chemical hazards they are potentially exposed to and what protective

Table 1–18 Chemical Hazard Communications Plan

1. Written hazard communication program
2. Maintain inventory of all chemicals with chemical and common name if appropriate
3. Manufacturer must assess and supply information about chemical or physical hazards (flammability, explosive, aerosol, flashpoint, etc.)
4. Employers must maintain Material Safety Data Sheets (MSDS) in English
5. MSDS must list all ingredients of a substance greater than 1%, except for known carcinogens if greater than 0.1%
6. Employers must make MSDS available to employees upon request
7. Employers must ensure labels are not defaced or removed and post appropriate warnings
8. Employers must provide information and training ('right-to-know')
9. OSHA permissible exposure limit, threshold limit, or other exposure limit value
10. Designate responsible person(s) for the program

measures the employer needs to take to minimize hazardous exposure. Many states have also developed individual guidelines and regulations mandating that employers develop and implement safety and toxic chemical information programs for their workers that are reviewed with all employees each year (e.g., the Right-to-Know Law in New York State [Chap. 551, Art. 48, 12 NYCRR Part 820]).

Ergonomic Hazards

OSHA presented guidelines (Federal Register 54, 29CFR 1910, 1989) to address ergonomic hazards in the workplace and assist employers in developing a program to prevent work-related problems. Cumulative trauma disorders are a collective group of injuries involving the musculo-skeletal and/or nervous systems in response to long-term repetitive twisting, bending, lifting, or assuming static postures (Riggle, 1991). These injuries may evolve from environmental factors such as constant or excessive repetitive actions, mechanical pressure, vibrations, or compressive forces on the arms, hands, wrists, neck, or back. Human error may also be a causative factor when individuals push themselves too hard beyond their limits or when productivity limits are set too high.

Among laboratory personnel, cumulative trauma disorders are usually related to repetitive pipetting, keyboard use, or resting their wrist/arms on sharp edges, such as a laboratory counter. These actions can cause carpal tunnel syndrome (compression and entrapment of nerve from wrist to hand), tendonitis (inflammation of tendon), or tenosynovitis (inflammation or injury to synovial sheath) (Gile, 1994). Awareness and prevention are key to managing these disorders. Work practice and engineering controls and various hand, arm, leg, back, and neck exercises may reduce these problems (Prinz-Lubbert, 1996). The cost of implementing programs to help employees understand and avoid ergonomic hazards can be financially justified. Back injuries are the second most common cause for employee absenteeism after the common cold and can cost employers up to $16 000 per episode (Prinz-Lubbert, 1996).

References

Ali M, Brookson S, Bruce A, et al: Managing for Excellence. London, DK Publishing, 2001, pp 86–149.

Bachman A: Evaluation of safer needles. Adv for Admin Lab 2003; 12(10):22–24.

Berte LM: Patient safety: getting there from here – quality management is the best patient safety program. Clin Leadersh Manag Rev 2004; 18(6):311–315.

Bonini P, Plebani M, Ceriotti F, et al: Errors in laboratory medicine. Clin Chem 2002; 48:691–698.
A review of the literature on laboratory errors, including an analysis of the type and/or volume of pre-analytical, analytical and post-analytical errors as well as transfusion errors.

Brue G: Six Sigma for Managers. New York, McGraw-Hill, 2002, pp 1–50.

CareerTrack Seminars: The One-Minute Manager. Boulder, Blanchard Training & Development, 1988, pp 11–13.

Centers for Disease Control: Recommendations and reports: Guidelines for prevention of transmission of human immunodeficiency virus and hepatitis B

virus to health care and public-safety workers. MMWR 1989; 38(No. S-6).

CLSI: Protection of Laboratory Workers From Occupationally Acquired Infections; Approved Guideline, 3rd ed. CLSI document M29-A3. Clinical and Laboratory Standards Institute, 2005.

Deming EW: Out of Crisis. Cambridge, MA, MIT, Center for Advanced Engineering Study, 1986.

Doebbeling BN, Pfaller MA, Houston AK, Wenzel RP: Removal of nosocomial pathogens from the contaminated glove. Ann Intern Med 1988; 109:394.

Federal Register, 29CFR 1910.1200: Hazard Communication Standard, 1983.

Federal Register 54, 29CFR 1910: Ergonomic Safety and Health Program Management Guidelines, 1989.

Federal Register 55, 42CFR 493: Clinical Laboratory Improvement Act, 1990.

Federal Register 56, 29CFR 1910.1030: Occupational Exposure to Blood Borne Pathogens, 1992.

Federal Register 57, 42CFR 493: Clinical Laboratory Improvement Act, 1992.

Federal Register 55, 29CFR 1910.1450: Occupational Exposure to Hazardous Chemicals in Laboratories, 1993.

Garber C: Six Sigma, its role in the clinical laboratory. Clin Lab News April 2004; 10–14.

Garner JS, Simmons BP: Guidelines for isolation precautions in hospitals. Infect Control 1983; 4:245.

Gile TJ: Ergonomics for the laboratory. CLMR 1994; 8(1):5–18.

Griffin RW: Management, 2nd ed. Boston, Houghton Mifflin Co., 1987, pp 5–69.

Institute of Medicine (IOM): Medicare Laboratory Payment Policy. National Academy of Sciences, 2000, pp 1–57.

Juran J: Juran on Planning for Quality. New York City, The Free Press, 1988.

Kohn LT, Corrigan JM, Donaldson MS (eds): To Err is Human. Building a Safer Health System. Committee on Quality of Health Care in America. Institute of Medicine. Washington DC, National Academy Press, 1999.

Kurec AS: Staffing and scheduling of laboratory personnel. *In* Snyder JR, Wilkinson DS (eds):

Management in Laboratory Medicine, 3rd ed. Philadelphia, Lippincott, 1998, pp 221–243.

Kurec AS: The role and function of the clinical laboratory. *In* Kurec AS, Schofield S, Watters MC (eds): The CLMA Guide to Managing a Clinical Laboratory, 3rd ed. Wayne, PA, CLMA, 2000, pp 1–20.

Kurec AS: Don't waste my time. A guide to common sense meetings. Clin Leadersh Manag Rev 2004a; 18:273–281.

Kurec AS: Employee selection. *In* Garza LS (ed): Clinical Laboratory Management. Washington, DC, ASM Press, 2004b, pp 277–290.

Lifshitz MS, De Cresce RP: Strategic planning for automation. *In* Kost GJ (ed): Clinical Automation, Robotics, and Optimization. New York, John Wiley & Sons, Inc., 1996, pp 471–496.
An overview of the laboratory strategic planning process with special emphasis on how to assess the environment, define objectives and audit operations and technology.

Mortland KK: Facility redesign for your future laboratory requirements. Clin Lab Manage Rev 1997; 11(3):145–152.

New York State Public Health Law, Chapter 551, Article 28 of the New York State Labor Laws, Part 820 Title 12 of the New York Codes, Rules and Regulations, Right-to-Know Law; 1987.

Nigon DL: Clinical Laboratory Management. New York. McGraw-Hill Companies, 2000.
Covers fundamental principles of laboratory management and provides many practical examples and case studies that help illustrate concepts.

Occupational Safety and Health Administration Regulations CPL 2.244B, Glove Wearing, 1991.

Occupational Safety and Health Administration Regulations: Hazard Communication. 1994; 59:6126–6184.

Painter P: Laboratory Design Workshop, Clinical Laboratory Management Association Annual Meeting, 1993.

Prinz-Lubbert P, Giddens J: Working smarter with ergonomics. Adv Admin Lab 1996; 5:18–24.

Riggle M: Cumulative trauma in the workplace. Phys Ther Forum 1991; (April):11–12.

Sewell DL: Laboratory-associated infections and biosafety. Clin Microb Rev 1995; 8(3):389–405.

Silverstein MD: An Approach to Medical Errors and Patient Safety in Laboratory Sciences, A White Paper. Quality Institute Conference, Atlanta, April 13–15, 2003; pp 1–23.

Sliva C: Update 2003: FDA and CLIA. IND Roundtable 510(k) Workshop April 22, 2003.

Snyder J, Wilkinson DS: Management in Laboratory Medicine, 3rd ed. Philadelphia, Lippincott, 1998.
Comprehensive reference dealing with all aspects of laboratory management, including leadership, human resource management, marketing, safety, etc.

Sunyog M: Lean management and Six-Sigma yield big gains in hospital's immediate response laboratory. Clinical Leadership and Management Review 2004; 18:255–258.

Szumski R: Laboratory restructuring: the Calgary experience. Presentation: MDS Diagnostic Sector, 1999; 1–24.

Ward-Cook K, Chapman S: 2002 Wage and vacancy survey of Medical Laboratories. Lab Med 2003; 34(10):702–707.

Zeiger B, Jenkins E: Motoring for success at Henry Ford Health System: Implications for regionalization of lab services. CLMA Vantage Point 1997; 1:1–3.

I

CHAPTER 2

Optimizing Laboratory Workflow and Performance

Mark S. Lifshitz MD, Robert P. De Cresce MD MBA, Irina Lutinger MPH DLM(ASCP)

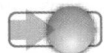

KEY POINTS

- An effective testing process requires integration of pre-analytic, analytic, and post-analytic steps.

- An understanding of workflow is a fundamental prerequisite to any performance optimization strategy.

- A variety of techniques should be used to collect workflow data. These include: sample and test mapping, tube analysis, workstation analysis, staff interviews, and task (process) mapping.

- Though technology is a critical component of every laboratory, it is only a tool to reach a goal. Technology alone does not improve performance and workflow; its success or failure depends on how it is implemented and whether it was truly needed.

- Consolidation, standardization and integration are key strategies that can optimize workflow. Managing test utilization may also change overall operational needs and workflow patterns.

The clinical laboratory is a complex operation that must smoothly integrate all three phases of the testing process: pre-analysis, analysis, and post-analysis. Pre-analysis refers to all the activities that take place prior to testing, such as test ordering and sample collection. The analysis stage includes the laboratory activities that actually produce a result such as running a sample on an automated analyzer. Post-analysis includes patient reporting and result interpretation. Collectively, all of the interrelated laboratory steps in the testing process describe its workflow; this, in turn, occurs within the overall design of a laboratory operation as described in its policies and procedures.

The steps in the testing process can be generally categorized according to testing phase, role (responsibility), or laboratory technology (Fig. 2–1). Note that the testing process and the grouping of steps vary somewhat from one facility to another. Depending on the laboratory service model and technology used, some steps may fall into one category or another. For example, centrifugation may be performed in a physician office (pre-analysis) or in the laboratory as part of a total automation workcell (analysis). Depending on the technology selected, a laboratory may automate some or many of the steps identified in Figure 2–1. Information technology is the essential 'glue' that binds together these steps. A more detailed discussion of each testing phase is covered in Chapters 3–8. This chapter will explore the interrelationship of laboratory workflow, technology and performance.

Understanding Workflow

To fully understand a laboratory's workflow, one must audit all phases of the testing process. Only then can one determine how to optimize performance and to what degree technologic or nontechnologic solutions are needed. Table 2–1 provides some of the issues to consider.

Data are of paramount importance in any workflow analysis. While laboratory data are rather easy to produce because they are readily available from automated analyzers and information systems, they may not be complete, valid, or in the format required. Since laboratory data play a central role in laboratory decision-making (e.g. determining which analyzer to acquire), they have to be accurate; otherwise, one may make wrong downstream decisions that can negatively impact on operations.

One must understand how data are collected by each of these systems and whether they are valid. For instance, do the test statistics pulled from an analyzer provide information on how many patient reportable tests are done or do they count how many total tests are done (with quality control, repeats, etc.)? Are panel constituents counted individually, is only the panel counted, or are both counted? Are the 'collect' times on turnaround time reports that measure 'collect to result' accurate? Or are samples indicated as 'collected' on a patient floor before they are actually collected, thereby making the turnaround time appear longer than actual? Ultimately, there is no substitute for carefully reviewing data to determine whether they make sense. Sometimes, this requires manually verifying data collected electronically or directly observing a work area. For example, it may be necessary to observe when samples arrive in the laboratory to determine how long a delay exists before staff assign a receipt time in the computer. By doing so, one can then determine the accuracy of the sample receipt time.

Data Collection Techniques

There are many types of data that can be used to assess workflow. While some of the fundamental data analysis techniques are described below, they may have to be supplemented with additional data collection to analyze unique characteristics of a laboratory's operation. It is always useful (some would say imperative) to check that the data collected reflect actual laboratory experience rather than anomalies created by unusual workflow patterns or laboratory information system (LIS) programs or definitions.

Sample and Test Mapping

One fundamental data collection technique is to analyze the distribution of samples and tests over time (Fig. 2–2). Depending on what is mapped, the time interval can be a day (e.g., hour increments for frequently ordered tests like those in general chemistry) or a week (e.g., daily increments for tests batched several times a week). The goal is to identify overall workload patterns in order to assess whether resources are appropriately matched to needs and whether turnaround time or other performance indicators can be improved. It is important that the workload measured reflects actual experience. For example, if phlebotomists remotely mark specimen's 'received' or the laboratory actually orders the tests in the LIS, the measured workload distribution may not accurately reflect the underlying processes. As part of the exercise it is also important to map routine samples versus stat ones and map locations that may have special needs like the emergency department. In addition to sample mapping, one should map key tests and the number or 'density' of tests per sample. This is of special interest in the chemistry section. Outpatient samples typically have a greater test density than inpatient ones so an equal number of inpatient and outpatient samples may be associated with different inpatient and outpatient workload. In automated chemistry, sample mapping more closely reflects staffing needs since much of the labor is associated with handling and processing tubes rather than actually performing the assays. In contrast, test mapping more closely reflects instrument needs, i.e., the test throughput it needs to complete its workload in a timely manner. By mapping samples and tests and relating them to turnaround time and staffing, a laboratory can identify production bottlenecks and alter workflow to achieve a better outcome. Very frequently laboratories discover that delays are less the result of instrument issues, per se, but rather workflow patterns which are not matched to instrument capabilities.

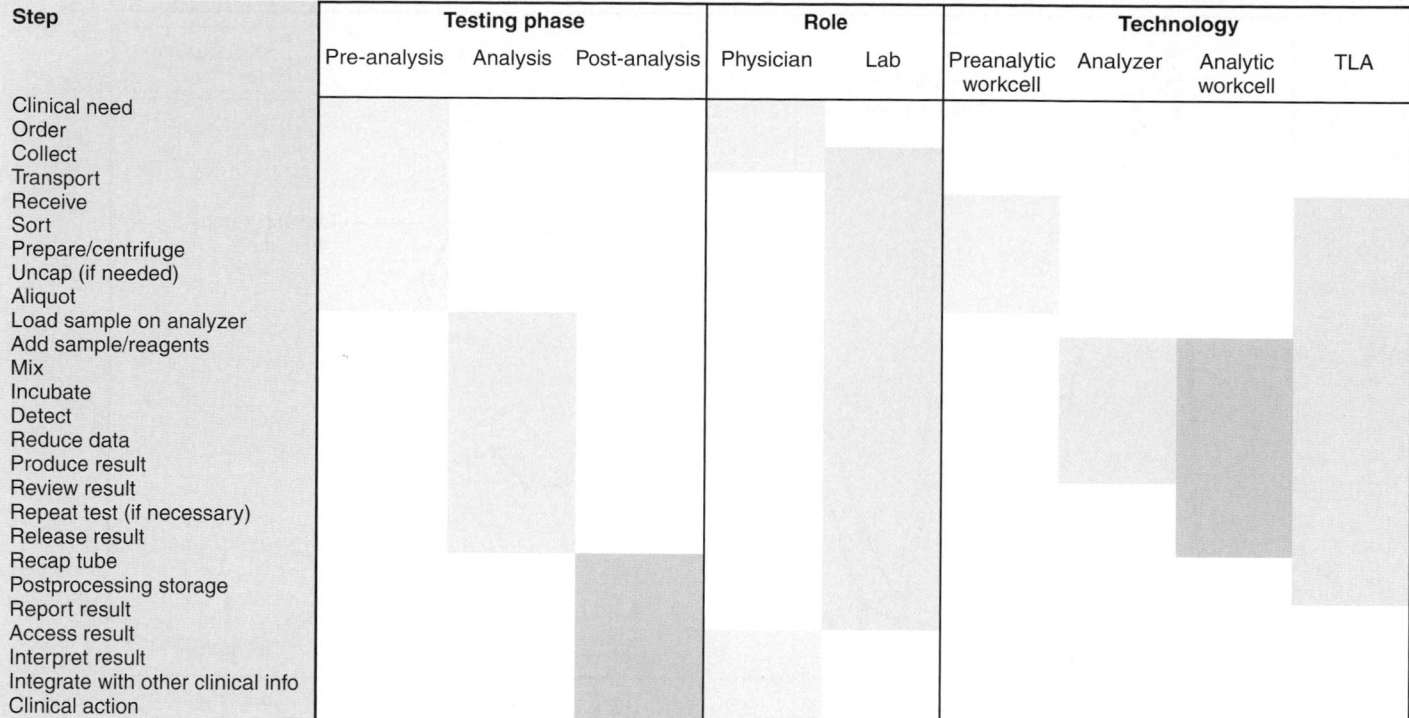

Figure 2–1 Laboratory testing process. Note that the steps can be categorized according to testing phase, role (responsibility), or laboratory technology as indicated by the shading. TLA = total laboratory automation.

Table 2–1 Issues to Consider When Auditing Operations	
Test ordering	Where are orders placed – in the laboratory, patient unit, or office? Are inpatient orders handled differently than outpatient ones? Is there a paper or electronic requisition?
Sample collection	Who collects the samples – laboratory or physician? When are they collected – all hours or just a.m.? Are samples bar coded at the site of collection or in the laboratory? How are the labels generated? Is there a positive patient ID system? Does the label contain all the information needed to process the sample?
Transportation	How are samples delivered – by messenger, automatic carrier transport or combination? Do all laboratories participate? Are all patient care areas served? How are stats handled? What impact do stats have? Is there a separate system for emergency department and intensive-care units?
Sample receipt	Is there a central receiving area? How are samples distributed to each laboratory? Does physical layout promote efficient sample flow? How are stat samples distinguished from routine ones? How are problem samples handled? Are samples sorted by workstation or department?
Sample processing	Are samples centrifuged centrally or in distributed locations? Are stats handled differently? Are samples aliquoted? If so, where? Is a separate sample drawn for each workstation?
Testing	How many workstations are used? How does capacity relate to need? How are samples stored and retrieved? How long are samples kept? When and why are samples repeated? Are repeat criteria appropriate?
Reporting	How are results reported? Electronically? Remote printer? How are stat and critical values reported and are criteria appropriate? How many calls for reports does the laboratory receive and why? How are point-of-care tests reported?

Tube Analysis

Part of the laboratory's daily work is related to processing collection tubes or containers. 'Tube labor' includes sorting and centrifuging; aliquoting; racking, unracking, loading and unloading samples on analyzers; retrieving tubes for add-on tests; manual dilutions or reruns (depending on instrument); and storing tubes. While the time to perform a tube task may seem insignificant, it has to be repeated many times per day and this can add up to a substantial amount of time. For example, at an average of 10 seconds per tube, it will take a laboratory 3.3 hours to sort 1200 tubes per day. While automation can often reduce this labor, redesigning the workflow may be a less expensive and more efficient alternative. To the extent a laboratory reduces the number of tubes and/or the number of tasks associated with each tube, it can reduce tube labor and positively impact workflow and staffing needs. Reducing tube labor is one of the main goals of consolidating chemistry and immunodiagnostic tests into a single analyzer or workcell. While sample mapping provides information about how many containers are received in a specified interval, a tube analysis helps to further analyze how many additional 'tube-related' tasks have to be done. These include the number of containers other than tubes (e.g. fingerstick collections that may require special processing or aliquoting) and the number of reruns (i.e., repeats) that are due to instrument flags and/or laboratory policies (Table 2–2).

Workstation Analysis

A typical laboratory is divided into stations in order to allocate work and schedule staff. Some workstations consist of a variety of tasks or tests that are grouped together for purposes of organizing work for one or more staff. For example, all manual or semiautomated chemistry tests may be grouped into a workstation, even though testing might actually be performed at different sites or equipment around the laboratory. More typically, a workstation is one physical location, e.g., a fully automated analyzer or group of analyzers such as hematology cell counters or a chemistry workcell. Regardless of how a laboratory is organized, it is important to understand where, when and how the work is performed. This is the goal of a workstation analysis.

Instrument Audit. A key component of any workstation is equipment. By performing an instrument audit (Table 2–3), one can better understand how each analyzer is used, its associated costs, and what potential opportunities might exist to improve performance. The operating characteristics of each instrument should be detailed as part of this process. Examples include the maximum number of samples that can be processed per hour, the number of samples that can be loaded at a single time, and the number of reagent containers and assays that can be stored on-board. Instrument throughput (tests/hour) should also be studied by conducting timing studies and reviewing various statistical reports that can be extracted from the instrument and LIS. Most chemistry analyzers are test-

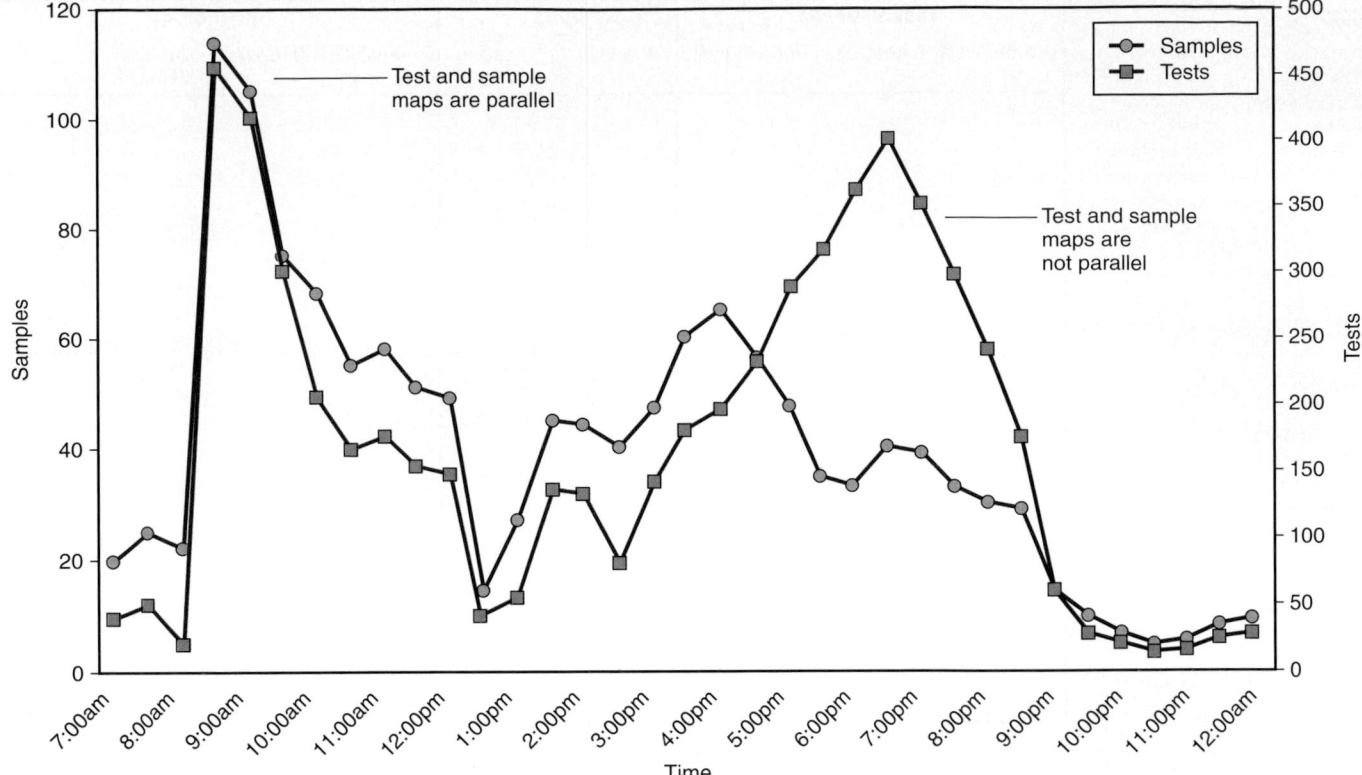

Figure 2–2 Sample and test mapping. Note that the morning volume peak is due to inpatients and the density is roughly 4 tests per sample. The evening peak is largely due to outpatients and density is far greater, about 10 tests per sample. Test density fluctuates during the day; thus both sample and test mapping are necessary to accurately evaluate workload.

Table 2–2 Chemistry Tube Analysis

	Analyzer A	Analyzer B
Total tubes run	500	500
Mechanical error	13	15
Dilution	7	20
Clot/low volume	20	30
Total instrument-related reruns	40 (32% of total reruns)	65 (65% of total reruns)
Delta check	62	21
Panic value	23	14
Total lab criteria-related reruns	85 (68% of total reruns)	35 (35% of total reruns)
Total reruns	125	100
% Reruns	25%	20%

Chemistry 'reruns' are caused by different factors and can be a source of nonproductive technologist time and/or turnaround time delays. Most of Analyzer A reruns are related to overly tight limits for delta checks and panic values that flag too many test results for technologist review and rerun. Most of Analyzer B reruns are related to instrument flags due to a narrow linear range for many methods and a large sample volume requirement per test. A nontechnologic solution (i.e. altering laboratory rerun/review criteria to reduce the number of tubes flagged for rerun) benefits Analyzer A; however, only a technologic solution (i.e., a new analyzer) can lower the number of reruns in Analyzer B.

Table 2–3 Instrument Audit

Instrument model
Vendor
Date acquired
Method of acquisition
  Purchased
  Leased
  Reagent rental
Service cost per year
Supplies cost per year
  Reagents
  Controls, calibrators
  Consumables
Total test volume per year
  Patient samples
  Controls and calibrators
Test menu
Hours of operation
  Days
  Shifts
Number of staff trained
Operating mode
  Batch versus continuous
  Primary system versus backup

based systems, that is, they perform a specific number of tests per hour irrespective of how many tests are ordered on each sample. On the other hand, some of these systems are affected by test mix (for example, the relative proportion of electrolytes, general chemistries and immunoassays) and this is the major reason that actual throughput experienced in the laboratory may be lower than what is claimed by the vendor. The latter may assume an ideal test mix that cannot be achieved in a given laboratory. It is important to understand how test mix affects an analyzer's throughput and whether there is a way to redistribute work so as to enhance throughput. An instrument that was well suited for the laboratory's test mix and volume when initially acquired may no longer provide adequate throughput given a change in test mix. Last, labor considerations should not be ignored – must the instrument be attended at all times or does it have walkaway capability? This information can be very useful in identifying processing bottlenecks and assist in redesigning workflow.

Tests Assayed. A careful review of the laboratory's test offering should be done during a workstation analysis. Are the tests performed appropriate for the facility given the volume and frequency of test analysis? Just because a laboratory can perform a test does not mean that it should. For example, if a test is performed only once a week but requires considerable equipment, training, or labor input, it may make more sense to send it to a reference laboratory where it is performed more frequently. Sometimes the best way to improve turnaround time and lower the cost of a test is not to perform it in the first place. Unfortunately, this option can be easily overlooked if one only focuses on how to improve the way existing tests are performed instead of analyzing how to provide clinicians with more timely laboratory information.

Processing Mode and Load Balancing. These can affect both the cost and timeliness of testing. Samples can be processed in batches or run continuously as they arrive in the laboratory. When grouped into batches, samples are run at specific intervals (e.g., once a shift, once a day, every other day) or whenever the batch grows to a certain size (e.g., every 20 samples). Batch processing is often less expensive than continuous processing because the setup costs (quality control, labor, etc.) are spread over many specimens (see Table 12–2); however, batch processing produces less timely results. Sometimes batch processing is a limitation of the instrument that is used. A batch analyzer cannot be interrupted during operation; thus, a newly arrived sample cannot be processed immediately if the instrument is already in use. Most currently available general chemistry and immunoassay analyzers are random access analyzers that continuously process samples. These analyzers can randomly access sample and reagents and can accommodate an emergency sample at any time. The characteristics of these analyzers are discussed more fully in Chapter 5. Continuous processing is facilitated by load balancing, a technique of spreading testing over a longer period of time to better match instrumentation throughput. For example, outpatient work, which does not require a rapid turnaround time, can be sequenced into the workflow during off hours. This improves testing efficiency, reduces the labor content of individual tests, and reduces throughput requirements (and capital cost) of instruments. The feasibility of load balancing can only be evaluated if accurate test mapping and tube analysis are performed.

Interviews

Data collection is not complete without interviewing staff. This exercise provides an opportunity for staff to participate in analyzing workflow and improving performance. It also identifies issues that would not be readily apparent from data collection alone. For example, many hospitals require electronic order entry on patient care units. While this may eliminate paper requisitions, laboratory staff members may still be placing orders for 'add-on' tests that are called into the laboratory (or added electronically), processing special requests, and troubleshooting incorrect orders, unacceptable samples, or misaligned bar code labels applied by nonlaboratory staff during sample collection. This residual work is likely to be transparent

since it probably will not appear on reports, logs or computer printouts. Thus, 'computer generated orders' may still be associated with considerable manual laboratory labor that may only be identified through interviews.

Interviews are particularly valuable in understanding what occurs outside the laboratory. Test ordering patterns or habits can significantly impact on a laboratory's ability to meet clinician needs. Visits to patient care units and discussions with nursing unit staff can identify pre-processing improvements that cost little to implement but save considerable money downstream.

Early patient discharge can be a challenging task for hospitals trying to shorten length of stay. A full understanding of the discharge process requires interviewing all related staff. One issue that sometimes emerges is the sample collection time for patients awaiting discharge pending a laboratory result. In order to avoid delays in providing results for discharge patients, some facilities develop elaborate 'stat' systems to collect, identify, and process these samples as well as report results during the busiest time of the day – the early morning. Sometimes, dedicated (stat instrument) or new technology (point-of-care device) is used for this purpose. However, one can ensure that results are available in the chart during early morning clinical rounds, by simply collecting laboratory samples from patients on the evening prior to discharge. Thus, not all solutions require technology. A careful mix of workflow restructuring and appropriate technology is usually the correct approach and the most cost-effective solution.

Task Mapping

No workflow study is complete without mapping the tasks or processes involved in performing a test (Middleton, 1996). A rigorous review will detail every specimen handling step, each decision point, and redundant activities. Task mapping can be applied to any segment of a laboratory's workflow be it technical or clerical. A full understanding of the tasks involved usually requires thorough staff interviews as discussed above. Task mapping should be an ongoing activity and also undertaken whenever one contemplates adding a workstation, test, new technology or any significant change to laboratory process. When implementing change, it is important to avoid unnecessary or additional steps that are inadvertently added in the name of 'efficiency'; task mapping helps identify these steps. Mapping also helps compare processes before and after change (Figs 2–3 and 2–4).

Workflow Analysis

Workflow analysis assimilates all of the previously discussed data and transforms them into valuable information. This step can be done manually or, as will be described below, using commercially available software for

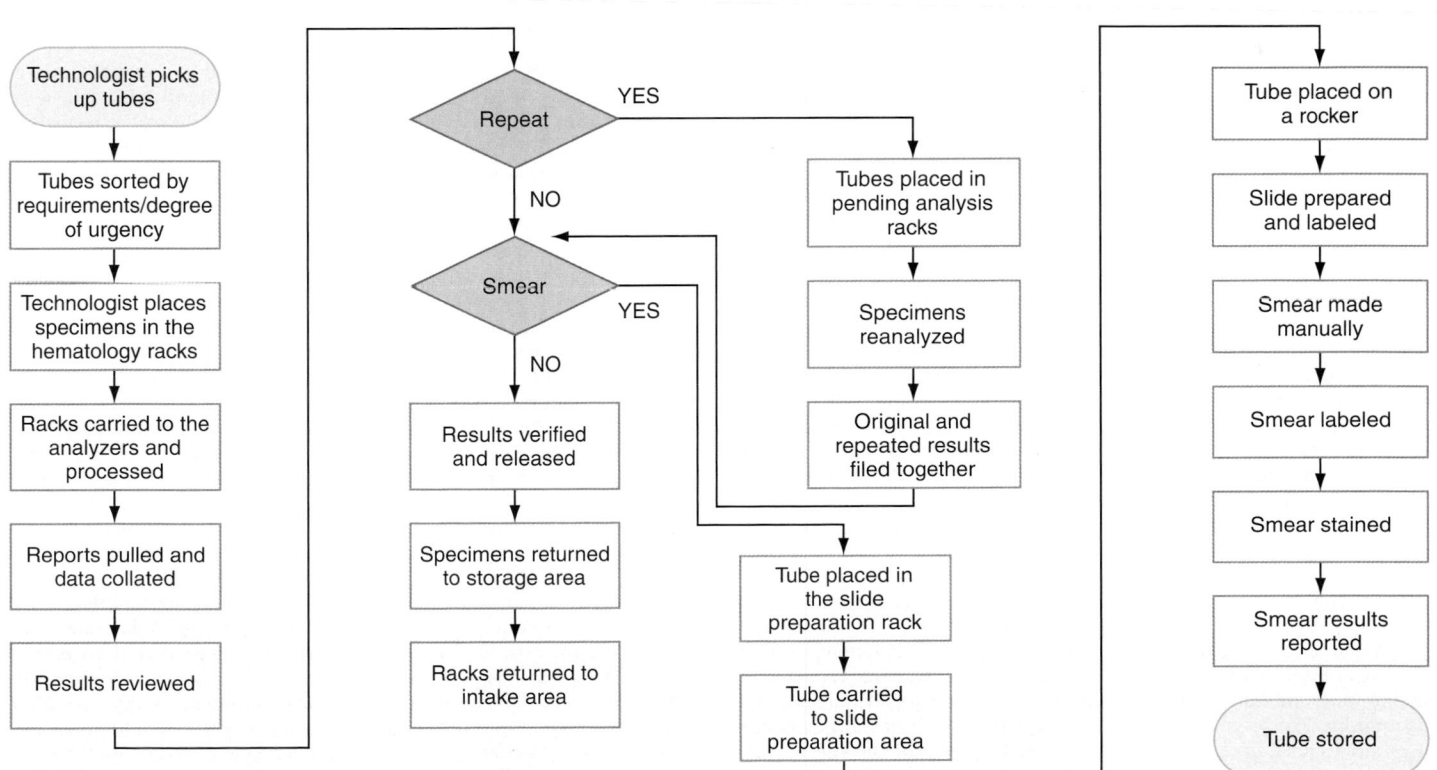

Figure 2–3 Task mapping: original workflow for hematology cell counting

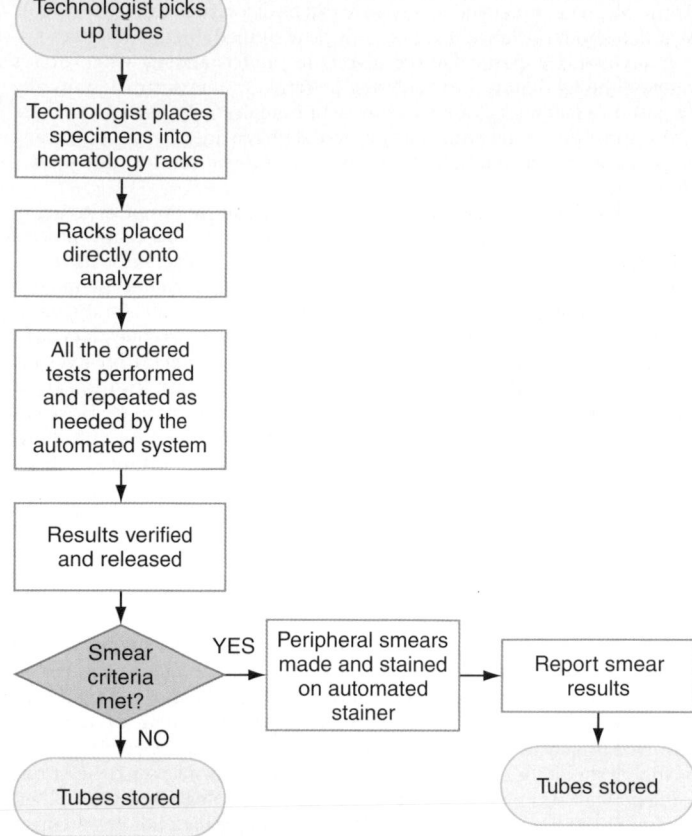

Figure 2–4 Task mapping: improved workflow for hematology cell counting subsequent to workcell implementation. Note the reduction in steps as compared to Figure 2–3.

Table 2–4 Interrelated Variables Simulated by Workflow Software Models

Equipment configuration

Facility design

Labor by shift and day

Throughput

Routine maintenance

Downtime

Sample volume (distribution and peak demand)

Sample container type

Review policy and rerun rates

Batch size

Workflow Modeling

While the above analyses are critical to understanding current and proposed workflow designs, they usually provide a somewhat static picture, i.e. each describes a single data element and often how it changes over time. However, in practice, workflow consists of many interrelated variables and it is difficult to understand (or to evaluate in the laboratory) how a change in one variable affects another one. Further, though workflow studies can be very beneficial, they also consume resources that may not be available in every laboratory. To address this need, technology vendors have developed workflow simulations. By using sophisticated workflow modeling software, one can analyze these complex interrelationships to better predict the outcome of a given workflow design (Table 2–4). Workflow modeling can help identify bottlenecks, and the impact of staffing changes or different equipment configurations on cost and turnaround time. It can also be used to better understand how a given analyzer responds to changes in test volume and test mix. For example, one can simulate the impact of increasing routine test volume on an instrument's turnaround time for stat samples (Mohammad, 2004). As with all workflow analyses, however, software modeling must be based on accurate data collection techniques.

Since most simulation programs are proprietary products, they may not allow modeling of all available instruments. While this is a drawback, workflow simulation is still a powerful tool and inferences can be drawn about more efficient processing and testing regardless of the model instrument involved. More importantly, these programs readily highlight the deficiencies in a laboratory's current operations and can point to specific areas where the greatest improvements are achievable.

Understanding Technology

No discussion of workflow is complete without examining the role of technology (De Cresce, 1988). Laboratory technology refers largely to three functional areas: testing equipment (i.e., analyzers), pre-analytic processors, and information technology (IT). While the former two areas are specific to the laboratory, information technology is not, and its design and role is often determined by factors outside the laboratory. For example, the manner in which a laboratory information system is used for data retrieval and reporting (i.e., whether or not physicians directly access the LIS to view results) depends on whether there is a hospital information system to serve this purpose (see Ch. 11). In the latter case, laboratory data are accessed and reported through a secondary system. Also, the laboratory system may be part of a broader approach or single IT vendor solution within the healthcare center and not a standalone product to be selected by the laboratory. Under these circumstances, the technology selected, while optimal for the general institution, may not be optimal for the laboratory. Changes in hospital-wide systems are rarely made to accommodate efficiencies in ancillary services like the laboratory. These systems are primarily geared towards easy access to clinical information by caregivers and accurate billing by the hospital finance department.

The Role of Technology: Principles and Pitfalls

Technology has radically changed the clinical laboratory over the last 20 years and continues to be the driving force behind many new developments. Periodically, a *breakthrough* technology is introduced that revolutionizes laboratory medicine (Table 2–5). Examples include the random access chemistry analyzer, automated immunodiagnostics system, chemistry and immunodiagnostics integrated workcell and molecular diagnostics. Each change profoundly altered how a laboratory functions and the type of information it provides clinicians. While breakthrough technologies offer a large potential benefit, they also cost more. Over time,

part of the analysis. A comprehensive workstation analysis should identify bottlenecks and highlight areas where improvements are necessary.

How is this done? The easiest way, and one that does not require computer support, is to follow the path of a specimen or group of specimens through the entire process. This should begin at or near the bedside to see how physicians are ordering tests and proceed from that point to specimen acquisition and delivery to the laboratory. A flow sheet should be created which follows the sample from initial order to arrival in the laboratory. A separate task force is usually assigned to the prelaboratory phase since there are usually multiple departments and staff involved; the laboratory often has little or no direct control over this critical portion of workflow, especially when nonlaboratory staff collect samples.

Specimen transit through the laboratory should then be documented, noting areas where batch processing occurs. For example, one should identify minimum and maximum centrifugation time for applicable specimens (like those that have to be aliquoted). If specimens require 10 minutes for loading and spinning, this should not be assumed to be the average time since a sample queue may form during peak periods. Using the sample arrival mapping done in data collection, an average time can be assigned by time of day. If this is being done manually, it is best to select a number of key times and average them, if possible. Similarly, one should note whether there is a delay in loading specimens on the analyzer. There are many other examples of physical bottlenecks that need to be identified and quantified. While it is not always possible to completely eliminate bottlenecks, it is possible to mitigate their impact through new technology, alternative processing modes (e.g., random access versus batch processing) and workflow redesign.

Nonphysical bottlenecks should also be identified and quantified. A classic example is the mode of result verification. Batching results for a technologist to review and accept is every bit as much a bottleneck as is waiting for a centrifuge to process a sample. In contrast, LIS autoverification (where results are automatically released based on preset criteria) can reduce test turnaround time without requiring a major reorganization of the laboratory. However, the degree to which autoverification enhances workflow depends on the manner in which it is implemented and the algorithms defined to qualify a result for this feature. This, in turn, may depend on the LIS used. These issues are discussed further in Chapter 11.

Table 2–5 Breakthrough Technology

Changes fundamental workflow

Consolidates workstations

Saves labor

Improves service

Sets new performance standard

Premium pricing

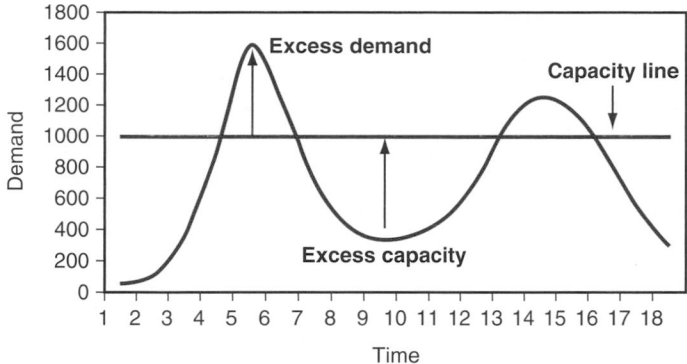

Figure 2–5 Test demand versus instrument capacity. Note that demand exceeds capacity during peak periods thereby creating backlogs. In many facilities, short backlogs are acceptable. If not clinically acceptable, the laboratory should explore ways to more evenly match capacity and demand; for example, by altering blood collection schedules. New technology should be the last approach that is considered.

a breakthrough technology is adopted by multiple vendors, competition develops, prices fall and its use becomes widespread among laboratories, in other words, it becomes a *current* or *derivative technology*. Early adopters of breakthrough technology often pay more and receive less benefit than those who wait until it becomes a current technology. By thoroughly understanding the role of technology one can determine how to best use it in the clinical laboratory. The following issues should be considered when evaluating technology.

Is technology needed? While technology is an integral part of a modern laboratory, it is not the solution to every problem. Often a nontechnologic solution provides a faster, better and less expensive workflow approach than a technologic one. Knowing when to introduce a nontechnologic solution instead of a technologic one can be the difference between a targeted cost-effective solution and an expensive one that does not fully address the initial problem, provides unnecessary functionality, or provides necessary functionality but at an unnecessary cost. For example, a laboratory may experience a sharp morning spike in samples thereby creating workflow backlogs (Fig. 2–5). Instead of purchasing more equipment to provide additional capacity during peak periods, the laboratory should look for ways to distribute work more evenly during the shift. The key is to avoid delivering large sample batches to the laboratory. One approach might be to rearrange phlebotomy draw schedules so that blood draws begin earlier and are spread out over a longer period (Sunyog, 2004). Another approach is to have phlebotomists send samples to the laboratory after every few patients instead of waiting to collect a large batch from an entire floor. Thus one should analyze and re-engineer processes to the greatest possible degree before embarking on a technology solution; this approach may yield an inexpensive solution that is quicker and easier to implement. Sometimes, nontechnologic solutions, while preferable, are out of the direct control of the laboratory staff and consequently do not receive the attention deserved. Thus, a technology solution is selected because it can be implemented without the support of other departments.

Technology is a means to an end, not an end. Technology alone does not improve performance and workflow; it is only a tool to reach a goal. Ultimately, new technology succeeds or fails based on how it's implemented. This, in turn, depends on people and the ability to clearly analyze how technology and workflow can be optimally integrated in their setting. What works for one location may not work for another. Sometimes this means changing longstanding practices or staff schedules. For example, if four chemistry analyzers are consolidated into two, staff needs to be reallocated to take into account fewer workstations and/or peak testing needs. Similarly, batching certain tests on a new high throughput analyzer does not take full advantage of its continuous processing capabilities and in some instances may yield a lower throughput than the analyzer it replaces.

Last, manually transcribing physician orders from paper requisitions into a hospital or laboratory information system provides far less functionality and error reduction capability than direct electronic order entry by physicians. Because technology has to be 'customized' for each site, laboratories implement the same technology in different ways and experience different outcomes. Never assume that improvements and results at another facility will automatically occur in one's own facility. The most successful implementations undertake a total workflow reassessment to evaluate how best to integrate technology. By critically evaluating existing practices, one can avoid perpetuating inefficient processes even with new equipment.

Overbuying – the cardinal sin. More than anything else, overbuying increases costs that burden an operation over the life of the technology. While it is tempting to overbuy 'just in case' capacity needs grow (such as new outreach work), these needs may not materialize or may occur slowly over time and allow for an incremental and more cost-effective approach. A new instrument in the laboratory rarely, if ever, directly translates into new testing volume. The market demand for testing is generally independent of the laboratory's capacity to test, though greater capacity may allow the laboratory to more aggressively market services. There are different types of overbuying. For example, one may buy three analyzers instead of two or an analyzer that performs 1000 tests per hour instead of a device that runs 500 tests per hour. Alternatively, a total laboratory automation solution may be implemented instead of one based on several smaller workcells or stand-alone analyzers. In all instances, overbuying increases costs. All of the above examples increase depreciation costs, require more service and maintenance, and can lead to ineffective labor utilization and suboptimal workflow. Buying more analyzers than necessary can also increase reagent costs in that each instrument has to be calibrated, controlled, and cross-correlated with other devices running the same test. Reagent waste (due to outdating) may also increase if low volume tests are set up on all of the analyzers.

Overbuying should not be confused with excess capacity that is sometimes unavoidable when implementing necessary backup systems. Ultimately, it is the laboratory service model that determines whether backup is needed. For some tests (e.g., cardiac markers) the laboratory may need a backup system, while for others (e.g., tumor markers) it may not. Also, a stat laboratory's backup needs will differ from those of a reference laboratory. A well-designed workflow can balance a laboratory's need for some backup without unnecessary overbuying. For a laboratory that needs a 1000 test/hour capacity, this may mean selecting two 500 test per hour analyzers instead of two running 1000 tests per hour. Alternatively, it may mean selecting one 1000 test per/hour analyzer and using a laboratory nearby (that is interfaced to the first laboratory's information system) for backup. Last, it may mean selecting two 1000 test per/hour analyzers but only running one at a time. This last solution is rarely successful since it duplicates expensive technology and increases maintenance costs. A simple analogy to the family car is often instructive – people rarely buy two automobiles to do what one can do most of the time. Instead, they rely on alternative sources such as renting, public transportation, or taxis to fill occasional needs. Ultimately, the goal is to 'right-buy', that is, to avoid over- or underbuying technology.

Do you understand what you are buying? There is a difference between 'buying' technology and being 'sold' technology by vendors. The former approach requires an analysis by the laboratory to identify what it needs and a thorough understanding of the technology under consideration, whereas the latter relies more heavily on the vendor to provide a solution to the laboratory. The risk of being 'sold' a technology is that it might not be the optimal solution. Most instruments work and do what they are advertised to do. Unfortunately, 'what they do' may not be what one needs.

The type of technology is also important. Current technology is generally easier to understand and a less risky strategy than breakthrough technology though it might also provide less reward. Breakthrough technology is, by definition, a new technology and it may be difficult to fully understand whether it is appropriate in a given laboratory setting, how best to implement, or how significant a financial impact it makes.

Other issues to consider relate to technology itself and whether it currently offers all the features required by a laboratory. A vendor may promote certain enhancements or capabilities scheduled for the future, especially when marketing analyzers. These may include tests in development, instrument or computer hardware improvements, new versions of software, or automatic upgrades to a next generation system. While these future enhancements may seem attractive, they may not materialize, so they should not be a primary reason for choosing technology. A better approach is to delay purchasing the system until it can offer the laboratory the capabilities it needs. Another potential mistake is overestimating a technology's lifetime or usefulness, since it will underestimate its true cost. In the end, the question each laboratorian should ask is not 'does technology work?' but rather 'docs this technology work for me?'

Optimizing Performance

Optimizing performance refers to the process by which workflow (including laboratory design) and technology are integrated to yield an operation that best meets the clinical needs and financial goals of the organization: high quality at low cost. In practice, there are times that workflow changes improve service levels *and* reduce cost. For example, consolidating chemistry systems may lower capital and operating costs and also improve turnaround time. Other times, there is a tradeoff between cost and quality. For example, a phlebotomy staff reduction, while lowering costs, may lengthen the time necessary to complete morning blood collection. This, in turn, may delay when test results become available but may not be significant if results are not needed until later in the day. On the other hand, if a patient's discharge is contingent on reviewing the result in the morning, a testing delay could increase length of stay. Ultimately, these decisions need to be analyzed within the framework of the overall institution, taking into account the downstream impact of these actions and their effect on other departments.

Optimizing performance is an ongoing process that requires one to constantly assess and reassess workflow and needs. This requires periodic data collection and analysis. Table 2–6 provides examples of workflow

Table 2–6 Workflow Metric Examples

Metric	Comments
Turnaround time (TAT) studies	
Collection to receipt	Is collection time correct? How long does it take for samples to reach laboratory? Is tube transport system functioning properly? Are messenger pickups reliable?
Receipt to result	How long does testing take once the laboratory receives a sample? Is it held in a central receiving area before it is brought to the technologist?
Order (or collection) to result	This is what the physician perceives as total turnaround time. Is it accurate? How long does it take for a released laboratory result to appear in the hospital information system? Are there networking issues external to the laboratory that delay the appearance of results?
Stat and routine TAT by hour	Is stat TAT longer in a.m. when routine samples from morning collection arrive? What is the difference in TAT for routine and stats? Are some tests affected more than others?
Monthly volume statistics	
'Billable' tests	How many orderable tests are performed? What is the trend? Has total volume or a specific test's volume changed enough to warrant a re-evaluation of workflow or testing capacity? Should any tests be sent to a reference laboratory instead of performed in-house?
'Exploded' tests	Exploding chemistry panels into individual components provides a more accurate assessment of general testing 'load' on analyzers and reagent usage than orderable tests alone. Has volume changed? Is it related to a specific location or new service?
By location	Has testing volume changed in specific nursing units or outpatient settings? Has the volume of inpatient and outpatient testing changed?
Reference laboratory tests	Are certain tests increasing in volume and, if so, why and at what cost? Are total monthly costs changing? (Tests with the highest cost/year are not always the highest volume ones.) Should certain tests be screened for appropriateness? Does it make sense to perform any of these tests in-house ('buy versus make' decision)?
Sample and test mapping	
Tubes per hour	Tube handling in chemistry has a direct impact on staff, and includes centrifugation, aliquoting and storage
Tests per hour by department or workstation	This is needed to compare 'testing demand' versus 'instrument capacity' and can help determine optimal instrument configuration

metrics that are useful to monitor. Ultimately, the degree to which any of these reports is useful depends on the accuracy of the data. While there are many different approaches to optimizing performance, some of the more common ones are discussed here and in Table 2–7.

Consolidation, integration and standardization are three key interrelated strategies that have assumed increasing importance in recent years as laboratories have become affiliated with one another through large healthcare networks. These concepts are also relevant to a single facility.

Consolidation. Testing can be consolidated from multiple sites or workstations in a single facility or selected tests from many facilities can be centralized in one or more locations. Consolidation creates larger sample batches or runs; this improves testing efficiency since fixed quality control and calibration costs are distributed over more samples. This, in turn, lowers per unit costs. Consolidation may yield larger reference laboratory test volume. A 'make versus buy' analysis can determine whether it is economically feasible to in-source tests previously sent to a reference laboratory (Kisner, 2003). Consolidation may also improve turnaround time by making it cost-effective to perform tests more frequently or to use a more automated technology. Some tests may not be appropriate to consolidate. For example, blood gases and other point-of-care tests may have to be performed in multiple sites in a hospital in order to provide the necessary turnaround time demanded by clinicians. Similarly, there may be little benefit to performing routine hospital CBCs in a central off-site location instead of the main hospital rapid response laboratory. In contrast, it may be beneficial to consolidate across facilities those tests that are less time-sensitive (e.g., tumor markers) or that require special skills and/or dedicated equipment at each site (e.g., microbiology services). To successfully consolidate tests from multiple facilities, a central site must control new costs (by minimizing additional staff or equipment to perform the tests) and provide better or comparable quality and service to what had been provided (Carter, 2004). It must also foster a collaborative approach to ensure that all of the sending facility's needs are met, including common physician concerns such as longer turnaround time and limited ability to access information or interact with a remote laboratory. A successful consolidation should be transparent to the clinician.

Standardization. Standardized policies, methods and equipment benefit laboratories in several ways. Direct benefits, like lower costs, can be realized when the laboratory aggressively negotiates with one vendor to supply all chemistry or hematology equipment and reagents. Indirect benefits are due to the simplified operations that result from standardization that make it easier to cross-train staff or implement policies and procedures. Standardization is a gradual process that can take several years to complete. Rapid transition is usually not possible due to vendor contract lock-ins; a buy-out of an existing contract is usually too expensive and can partially or completely offset any intended saving from a new contract. Sometimes, the unique needs of a location may preclude it from standardizing with other laboratories, or a single vendor may not offer a product line that is suitable for each facility. In these instances it is still possible to significantly lower costs and/or improve performance albeit using a more varied or limited approach.

Integration. Integration is the process by which services at one location are coordinated, shared and/or connected to those at another to provide a seamless operation. Though integration is often a by-product of consolidation and standardization, the latter two strategies are not a prerequisite to successful integration. For example, consider a laboratory information system that links several facilities. While a single seamless operation can be created with a single vendor's system, it is also possible to network systems from different vendors, albeit with greater difficulty and possibly less functionality. Other integration examples include cross-training staff among different laboratory sections or facilities and interfacing point-of-care laboratory data to the main laboratory system.

Managing utilization. Thus far, strategies to optimize performance have focused on ways to do work better and at lower cost. While this is important, it does not address the most basic question – is the work, i.e., test, necessary? After all, the least expensive test is the test that is not done. Lowering test volume may also change overall operational needs and workflow patterns. Keep in mind that inpatient laboratory work is generally not reimbursed (see Ch. 12) so each laboratory test is an added cost to the hospital. Thus, lowering inpatient utilization has a direct impact on costs. In contrast, outpatient testing is generally reimbursed by a third-party payer or the patient. Despite this, the amount reimbursed may not be sufficient to cover the cost of the test. This is especially true for expensive new reference laboratory tests where the laboratory may only receive $0.20–0.30 for each dollar spent. So, selectively controlling outpatient utilization can also be a financial benefit. Appropriate utilization of tests does not only mean lowering utilization. In some instances, tests that should be ordered may

Table 2–7 Strategies to Optimize Performance

Strategy	Example
Consolidate	*One facility*: run stat and routine samples together on the same analyzer; run routine and specialty tests on the same platform; collapse number of analyzers and workstations and use workcell, if applicable. Consolidation can reduce 'tube labor' *Multiple facilities*: centralize selected low volume, high cost tests/services at a single location, e.g., molecular diagnostics (HIV viral load), blood donor collection
Standardize	*Equipment*: all equipment purchased from one vendor yields larger volume discounts, lower costs for reagents and analyzers, especially in chemistry and immunodiagnostics *Method*: uniform reference range for all laboratories promotes seamless testing environment for in- and outpatients with data comparability and trending results across laboratories; also provides system backup without excess redundancy *Policies*: simplifies procedure manuals and compliance documents in that these can be shared *Staff*: standardized operations make it easier to share staff among facilities *LIS*: database management is simplified
Integrate	*Computer*: network LIS system with other data systems to promote seamless flow, e.g., sending point of care results into the LIS *Courier*: use single service to deliver samples among multiple sites
Strategic sourcing	Long-term strategy: competitively bid equipment, supplies, reference laboratory services, etc., taking into account payment terms, delivery charges, value added services and product cost
Rapid repricing	Short-term strategy: renegotiate pricing with existing vendors
'Make versus buy'	Review all send-out tests and low volume in-house tests to identify which tests to 'buy' (i.e., send out or outsource) and which ones to 'make' (i.e., do in-house) based on cost and turnaround time. Also, review services like couriers
Review laboratory policies and tasks	Critically review laboratory policies and procedures to determine their relevance and appropriateness: Can delta check limits be narrowed or eliminated to reduce the number of test repeats and verifications without compromising quality? Are critical call values clinically appropriate or do they generate unnecessary calls to physicians? Can non-urgent expensive tests be batched twice weekly instead of every day? Do clinicians need certain tests daily that are only available several times a week? Are quality control and maintenance procedures excessive?
Make maximum use of simple and/or existing IT solutions	Rule-based autoverification process eliminates need for technologist to manually release each result (Crolla, 2003); sample racking storage system eliminates most of the time spent looking for samples
Cross-train staff	Train technologists to perform automated chemistry and hematology tests instead of chemistry or hematology alone
Adjust skill mix	Adjust skill level (and compensation) of staff to match task performed: use laboratory helpers instead of technologists to centrifuge samples or load samples on analyzers
Adjust staff scheduling	Use part-time phlebotomists to supplement peak blood collection periods instead of full-time ones that are underutilized once morning collection is finished
Change laboratory layout	Design open laboratory that allows all automated testing to run in the same location and promotes cross-training of staff
Manage utilization	Require pathologist or director approval to order select costly reference laboratory tests and/or restrict usage of various tests to specialists

not be ordered, and this could potentially impact on patient care and lengthen stay.

There are different strategies a laboratory may use to manage utilization depending on the type of test (Lewandrowski, 2003). Over the years, laboratories have realized large cost savings through productivity improvements. As a result, it is far easier and less costly to run a $0.10 test than to determine whether each one is appropriate. While this is true for many high volume tests (like CBCs and basic metabolic panels) it is not true for many new, complex and costly reference laboratory tests such as cancer diagnostics and viral genotyping. Thus, a different strategy is needed to manage utilization of costly reference laboratory tests than to manage CBCs. For example, reference laboratory utilization can be managed by reviewing each order (for certain tests) and its cost with the clinician based on guidelines developed with the clinical services. This cost avoidance strategy not only ensures that clinical indications are met; it also educates physicians about the cost, and challenges each one to evaluate the cost–benefit of using it. In contrast, high volume tests like a CBC require a broader strategy that restricts or guides ordering frequency electronically through various clinical pathways or guideline-based decision support systems (van Wijk, 2002). For example, a comprehensive or basic metabolic panel might be limited to one order per admission if the patient is stable. There is little to be saved by eliminating one low-cost laboratory test from a panel of five other tests. The most significant cost saving is realized when a phlebotomy is altogether eliminated. This usually requires rethinking the frequency of laboratory orders across all clinical services and changing practice patterns to reduce the number of times a patient's blood is collected. Test repetition is a common component of overall test utilization and is costly (van Walraven, 2003).

A laboratory-based diagnostic algorithm can assist with medical decision-making and reduce test utilization. With this approach, a physician requests the laboratory to perform a diagnostic work-up (for example, thyroid function evaluation), instead of ordering specific tests. Thus, the laboratory determines the appropriate tests to run and in what order (Yang, 1996).

References

Carter E, Stubbs JR, Bennett B: A model for consolidation of clinical microbiology laboratory services within a multihospital health-care system. Clin Leadersh Manag Rev 2004; 18:211–215.

Crolla LJ, Westgard JO: Evaluation of rule-based autoverification protocols. Clin Leadersh Manag Rev 2003; 17:268–272.

De Cresce RP, Lifshitz MS: Integrating automation into the clinical laboratory. *In* Lifshitz MS, De Cresce RP (eds): Perspectives on Clinical Laboratory Automation. New York, WB Saunders Company, 1988, pp 759–774.
General overview of how to analyze workflow and evaluate technology, including many practical considerations.

Kisner HJ: Make versus buy: a financial perspective. Clin Leadersh Manag Rev 2003; 17:328–330.

Lewandrowski K: Managing utilization of new diagnostic tests. Clin Leadersh Manag Rev 2003; 17:318–324.

Middleton S, Mountain P: Process control and on-line optimization. *In* Kost GJ: Handbook of Clinical Automation, Robotics and Optimization. New York, John Wiley & Sons, 1996, pp 515–540.
Provides an overview of task and process mapping using flow diagrams. Also discusses how to integrate automation, information systems and staff to optimize performance.

Mohammad AA, Elefano EC, Leigh D, et al: Use of computer simulation to study impact of increasing routine test volume on turnaround times of STAT samples on ci8200 integrated chemistry and immunoassay analyzer (abstract). Clin Chem 2004; 50:1952–1955.

Sunyog M: Lean management and six-sigma yield big gains in hospital's immediate response laboratory. Clin Leadersh Manag Rev 2004; 18:255–258.

Van Walraven C, Raymond M: Population-based study of repeat laboratory testing. Clin Chem 2003; 49:1997–2005.

van Wijk MAM, van der Lei J, Mosseveld M, et al: Compliance of general practitioners with a guideline-based decision support system for ordering blood tests Clin Chem 2002; 48:55–60.

Yang JM, Laposata M, Lewandrowski KB: Algorithmic diagnosis. *In* Kost GJ: Handbook of Clinical Automation, Robotics and Optimization. New York, John Wiley & Sons, 1996, pp 911–928.

CHAPTER 3

Pre-Analysis

Herb Miller PhD MT(ASCP) CLS(NCA), Mark S. Lifshitz MD

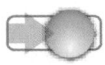

KEY POINTS
- Errors and variables in the pre-analysis stage can affect test results.

- Patient variables include physical activity, diet, age, sex, circadian variations, posture, stress, obesity, smoking and medication.

- Strict adherence to proper technique and site selection can minimize collection variables such as hemolysis, hemoconcentration, clots and other causes for sample rejection or erroneous results.

- Blood collection containers are color-coded based on additive or preservative and each is only suitable for specific tests. Failure to use the proper tubes or filling tubes in the wrong sequence can produce erroneous results.

- Blood collection staff must be adequately trained in safety and confidentiality issues.

- Blood, urine and other body fluid constituents can change during transport and storage. The extent of these changes varies by analyte.

Pre-analysis refers to all the steps that must take place before a sample can be analyzed. Over the years, technologic advances and quality assurance procedures have significantly reduced the number of analytic-based errors. This has exposed the pre-analysis stage as a major source of residual 'error' and/or variables that can affect tests results. Pre-analytic factors include patient-related variables (diet, age, sex, etc.), specimen collection techniques, specimen preservatives and anticoagulants, specimen transport, processing and storage. Potential sources of error, or failures in this process, include sample misidentification, improper timing, improper fasting, improper anticoagulant/blood ratio, improper mixing, incorrect order of draw, and hemolysed or lipemic specimens. Table 3–1 lists 10 of the most common errors associated with specimen collection.

There is a downstream impact of pre-analytic issues on laboratory resources, hospital costs and overall quality. By some estimates, specimen collection errors cost the average 400-bed hospital about $200 000/year in re-collection costs. Proper collection technique is also essential to minimize injury to the phlebotomist and patient. A single post-needlestick treatment can cost $500–3000 and poor technique can result in patient injury such as nerve and arterial damage, subcutaneous hemorrhage, infection, and even death. CDC estimates 385 000 needlestick injuries per year (CDC, 2004). Many go unreported. This chapter discusses the pre-analytic process with special emphasis on the clinical impact of variables and sources of failure.

Pre-Collection Variables

In preparing a patient for phlebotomy, care should be taken to minimize factors related to activities that might influence laboratory determinations. These include diurnal variation, exercise, fasting, diet, ethanol consumption, tobacco smoking, drug ingestion, and posture.

Diurnal variation may be encountered when testing for hormones, iron, acid phosphatase, and urinary excretion of most electrolytes such as sodium, potassium and phosphate (Dufour, 2003). Table 3–2 presents several tests affected by diurnal variations, posture and stress.

Exercise. Physical activity has transient and long-term effects on laboratory determinations. Transient changes may include an initial decrease followed by an increase in free fatty acids. Alanine may increase as much as 180% and lactate as much as 300%. Exercise may elevate creatine phosphokinase (CK), aspartate aminotransferase (AST), and lactate dehydrogenase (LD), and activate coagulation, fibrinolysis, and platelets (Garza, 1989). These changes are related to increased metabolic activities for energy purposes and usually return to pre-exercise levels soon after exercise cessation. Long-term effects of exercise may increase CK, aldolase, AST, and LD values. Chronic aerobic exercise is associated with lower plasma concentration of muscle enzymes such as CK, AST, ALT and LDH. Decreased levels of serum gonadotropin and sex steroid concentrations are seen in long- distance athletes while prolactin levels are elevated (Dufour, 2003).

Diet. An individual's diet can greatly affect laboratory test results. The effect is transient and easily controlled. Glucose and triglycerides, absorbed from food, increase after eating (Dufour, 2003). After 48 hours of fasting, serum bilirubin concentrations may increase. Fasting 72 hours decreases plasma glucose levels in healthy women to 45 mg/dL (2.5 mmol/L), while men show an increase in plasma triglycerides, glycerol, and free fatty acids, with no significant change in plasma cholesterol. When determining blood constituents such as glucose, triglycerides, cholesterol, and electrolytes, collection should be in the basal state (Garza, 1989). Eating a meal, depending on fat content, may elevate plasma potassium, triglycerides, alkaline phosphatase and indoleacetic acid (5-HIAA). Stool occult blood tests, which detect heme, are affected by the intake of meat, fish, iron and horseradish, a source of peroxidase causing a false-positive occult blood reaction (Dufour, 2003). Physiologic changes may include hyperchylomicronemia, thus increasing turbidity of the serum or plasma and potentially interfering with instrument readings.

Certain foods or *diet regimens* may affect serum or urine constituents. Longtime vegetarian diets are reported to cause decreased concentrations of low-density lipoproteins (LDL), very-low-density lipoproteins (VLDL),

Table 3–1 Ten Common Errors in Specimen Collection

1. Misidentification of patient
2. Mislabeling of specimen
3. Short draws/wrong anticoagulant to blood ratio
4. Mixing problems/clots
5. Wrong tubes/wrong anticoagulant
6. Hemolysis/lipemia
7. Hemoconcentration
8. Exposure to light/extreme temperatures
9. Improperly timed specimens/delayed delivery to laboratory
10. Processing errors: incomplete centrifugation, incorrect log-in, improper storage

Table 3–2 Tests Affected by Diurnal Variation, Posture and Stress

Cortisol	Peaks 4–6 a.m.; lowest 8 p.m. to 12 a.m.; 50% lower at 8 p.m. than at 8 a.m.; increased with stress
Adrenocorticotropic hormone (ACTH)	Lower at night; increased with stress
Plasma renin activity	Lower at night; higher standing than supine
Aldosterone	Lower at night
Insulin	Lower at night
Growth Hormone	Higher in afternoon and evening
Acid Phosphatase	Higher in afternoon and evening
Thyroxine (T_4)	Increases with exercise
Prolactin	Higher with stress; higher levels at 4 and 8 a.m. and 8 and 10 p.m.
Iron	Peaks early to late morning; decreases up to 30% during the day
Calcium	4% decrease supine

total lipids, phospholipids, cholesterol and triglycerides. Vitamin B_{12} deficiency can also occur, unless supplements are taken (Young, 2001). A high meat or other protein-rich diet may increase serum urea, ammonia, and urate levels. High protein, low carbohydrate diets, such as the Atkins diet, greatly increase ketones in the urine and increases the serum BUN. Food with a high unsaturated to saturated fatty acids ratio may show decreased serum cholesterol, while a diet rich in purines will show an increased urate value. Foods such as bananas, pineapples, tomatoes, and avocados are rich in serotonin. When ingested, elevated urine excretion of 5-hydroxyindoleacetic acid may be observed. Beverages rich in caffeine elevate plasma free fatty acids and cause catecholamine release from the adrenal medulla and brain tissue. Ethanol ingestion increases plasma lactate, urate, and triglyceride concentrations. Elevated high-density lipoprotein (HDL) cholesterol, γ-glutamyl transferase (GGT), urate, and mean corpuscular volume (MCV) have been associated with chronic alcohol abuse.

Serum concentrations of cholesterol, triglycerides, and apoB lipoproteins are correlated with *obesity*. Serum lactate dehydrogenase activity, cortisol production, and glucose increase in obesity. Plasma insulin concentration is also increased, but glucose tolerance is impaired. In obese men, testosterone concentration is reduced (Young, 2001).

Tobacco smoking. Tobacco smokers have high blood carboxyhemoglobin levels, plasma catecholamines, and serum cortisol. Changes in these hormones often result in decreased numbers of eosinophils, while neutrophils, monocytes, and plasma fatty free acids increase. Chronic effects of smoking lead to increased hemoglobin concentration, erythrocyte counts (RBCs), MCV, and increased leukocyte counts (WBC). Increased plasma levels of lactate, insulin, epinephrine, growth hormone and urinary secretion of 5-hydroxyindoleacetic acid are also seen. Vitamin B_{12} levels may be substantially decreased and have been reported to be inversely proportional to serum thiocyanate levels. Smoking also affects the body's immune response. Immunoglobulins IgA, IgG and IgM are lower in smokers and IgE levels are higher. Decreased sperm counts and motility and increased abnormal morphology have been reported in male smokers when compared to non-smokers. (Young, 2001).

Stress. Mental and physical stress induce the production of ACTH, cortisol, and catecholamines. Total cholesterol has been reported to increase with mild stress, and high-density-lipoprotein cholesterol to decrease as much as 15% (Dufour, 2003). Hyperventilation affects acid-base balance, and elevates leukocyte counts, serum lactate, or free fatty acids.

Posture of the patient during phlebotomy can have an effect on various laboratory results. An upright position increases hydrostatic pressure, causing a reduction of plasma volume and increased concentration of proteins. Albumin and calcium levels may become elevated as one changes position from supine to upright. Elements that are affected by postural changes are albumin, total protein, enzymes, calcium, bilirubin, cholesterol, triglycerides, and drugs bound to proteins. Incorrect application of the tourniquet and fist exercise can result in erroneous test results. Using a tourniquet to collect blood to determine lactate concentration may result in falsely increased values. Prolonged tourniquet application may also increase serum enzymes, proteins, and protein-bound substances, including cholesterol, calcium, and triglycerides, due to hemoconcentration. After bed rest in the hospital a patient's hemoglobin can decrease from the original admitting value enough to falsely lead a physician to suspect internal hemorrhage or hemolysis (Dufour, 2003). Patients should be advised to avoid changes in their diet, the consumption of alcohol and strenuous exercise 24 hours before having their blood drawn for laboratory testing.

Age of the patient has an effect on serum constituents. Young defines four age groups: newborn, childhood to puberty, adult, and elderly adult (Young, 2001). In the newborn much of the hemoglobin is hemoglobin F, not hemoglobin A, as seen in the adult. Bilirubin concentration rises after birth and peaks at about 5 days. In cases of hemolytic disease of the newborn (HDN), bilirubin levels continue to rise. This often causes difficulty in distinguishing between physiologic jaundice and HDN. Infants have a lower glucose level than in adults because of their low glycogen reserve. With skeletal growth and muscle development, the serum alkaline phosphatase and creatinine levels, respectively, also increase. The high uric acid level seen in a newborn decreases for the first 10 years of life then increases, especially in boys, until the age of 16 (Young, 2001). Most serum constituents remain constant during adult life until the onset of menopause in women and middle age in men. An increase of about 2 mg/L (0.02 mmol/L) per year in total cholesterol and triglycerides until midlife has been reported. The increase in cholesterol seen in postmenopausal women has been attributed to the decrease in estrogen levels. Uric acid levels peak in men in their 20s but do not peak in women until middle age. The elderly secrete less triiodothyronine, parathyroid hormone, aldosterone, and cortisol. After age 50, men experience a decrease in secretion rate and concentration of testosterone and women have an increase in pituitary gonadotropins, especially FSH (Young, 2001).

Sex After puberty, men generally have a higher alkaline phosphatase, aminotransferase, creatine kinase and aldolase level than women; this is due to the larger muscle mass of men. Women have lower levels of magnesium, calcium, albumin, hemoglobin, serum iron and ferritin. Menstrual blood loss contributes to the lower iron values (Young, 2001).

Specimen collection

The Test Order

Laboratory tests are usually ordered electronically (e.g., computer) or in writing (e.g., paper requisition). This information is conveyed through written or computer order entry. Online computer input is the most error-free means of requesting laboratory tests. The clinician initiates the request for a laboratory measurement or examination by completing a written order for desired laboratory measurements or examinations in the patient's medical record or chart. Verbal requests are made in emergency situations and should be documented on a standard form; after the blood is drawn, an official laboratory request or computerized order should be placed (Garza, 2002). Physician direct order entry and result acquisition through user-friendly networked computers are realistic approaches to providing prompt and accurate patient care. Patient demographics include the patient's name, sex, age, date of birth (DOB), date of admission, date on which measurement or examination was ordered, hospital number, room number, physician, and physician's pharmacy code number. Computerized laboratory information systems (LIMS) common in today's laboratories are used to generate requisitions and specimen labels. Some systems also generate requisitions with the number of tubes and type of tubes required for collection.

Most laboratories facilitate test ordering by providing a written or computerized medical information system which lists available tests, type of specimen required, collection method, color of blood collection tube used, amount of blood/body fluid required, turnaround time, reference intervals, test codes, costs, diagnostic information, etc. All specimens must be clearly labeled. Preprinted bar code labels applied after proper patient identification and after the specimen is collected, avoid transcription, pre-analytic, errors. Frequently the laboratory receives requests for 'add-ons.' These are additional tests requested to be performed on a specimen that has previously been collected. Problems are encountered when the specimen is not the proper type for the add-on requested test. This is usually due to the presence or absence of a particular anticoagulant or additive. All add-on requests must be documented.

Medicolegal concerns include proper identification of the patient, proper labeling of the specimen, patient consent issues, patient privacy issues, and chain of custody. Laboratories should have clearly written policies for the above issues. In addition, there should be policies on what to do when a patient refuses to have blood drawn, what to do if the patient was unable to be drawn, what to do if a patient is unavailable, and how to deal with a combative patient. The Health Insurance Portability and Accountability Act (HIPAA), addresses the security and privacy of health data and protects the confidentiality of all patient record information including all laboratory data. Employees must be trained to comply with HIPAA.

Time of Collection

Sometimes, samples have to be collected at a specific time. Failure to follow the time schedule can lead to erroneous results and misinterpretation of a patient's condition. The most common tests in this category are the ASAP and stat collections. ASAP means 'as soon as possible' and stat is an American medical term meaning 'immediately' (from the Latin *statim*). The exact definitions of these terms vary from one laboratory to another. Stat specimens are collected and analyzed immediately. They have the highest priority and are usually ordered from the emergency department and critical care units (Strasinger, 2003). Timed specimens are ordered for a variety of reasons, usually to monitor changes in a patient's condition, to determine the level of a medication, or to measure how well a substance is metabolized. For example, a physician may want to monitor a cardiac marker to determine if it is rising or decreasing. In therapeutic drug monitoring, trough and peak levels of a drug may be ordered. Trough specimens reflect the lowest level in the blood and are generally drawn 30 minutes before the drug is administered. The peak specimen is drawn shortly after the medication is given; the actual collection time varies by medication. Drug manufacturers provide the length of time that must pass between the trough and the peak collection times. Measuring how well the body metabolizes glucose involves a 2-hour postprandial specimen and/or a glucose tolerance test. Two-hour postprandial specimens are drawn 2 hours after the patient eats a meal. Results are compared with those of the fasting level. In a glucose tolerance test, multiple samples are drawn over time, one sample before and several after the administration of a standardized glucose solution. This test is used to diagnose diabetes mellitus by determining how well the body metabolizes glucose over a given time period.

Collection-Associated Variables

On occasion when there is a problem finding a vein for phlebotomy, or when the vein is transfixed, the specimen may be hemolysed. *Hemolysis* can also be caused by using a needle that is too small, pulling a syringe plunger back too fast, expelling the blood vigorously into a tube, shaking or mixing the tubes vigorously, or performing blood collection before the alcohol has dried at the collection site. Hemolysis is present when the serum or plasma layer is pink. Hemolysis can falsely increase blood constituents such as potassium, magnesium, iron, lactate dehydrogenase, phosphorus, ammonium, and total protein (Garza, 2002). Table 3–3 shows changes in serum concentration (or activities) of selected constituents due to lysis of erythrocytes.

In order to avoid problems with hemoconcentration and hemodilution, the patient should be seated in a supine position for 15 to 20 minutes before the blood is drawn. (Young, 2001). Extended application of the tourniquet can cause hemoconcentration which increases the concentration of analytes and cellular components. When using blood collection tubes that contain various anticoagulants/additives, it is important to follow the proper order of draw and to thoroughly mix an anticoagulated tube of blood after it has been filled. Failure to mix a tube containing an anticoagulant will result in *failure to anticoagulate* the entire blood specimen and small clots may be formed. Erroneous cell counts can result. If a clot is present it may also occlude, or otherwise interfere with an automated analyzer. It is very important that the proper anticoagulant be used appropriate for the test ordered. Using the wrong anticoagulant will greatly affect the test results.

Table 3–3 Changes in Serum Concentration (or Activities) of Selected Constituents due to Lysis of Erythrocytes (RBC)

Constituent	Ratio of concentration (or activity) in RBC to concentration (or activity) in serum	Change of concentration (or activity) in serum after lysis of 1% RBC, assuming a hematocrit of 0.50 (%)
Lactate dehydrogenase	160 : 1	+ 272.0
Aspartate aminotransferase (AST)	40 : 1	+ 220.0
Potassium	23 : 1	+ 24.4
Alanine aminotransferase (ALT)	6.7 : 1	+ 55.0
Glucose	0.82 : 1	− 5.0
Inorganic phosphate	0.78 : 1	+ 9.1
Sodium	0.11 : 1	− 1.0
Calcium	0.10 : 1	+ 2.9

Modified from Caraway WT, Kammeyer CW: Chemical interference by drug and other substances with clinical laboratory test procedures. Clin Chem Acta 1972; 41:395; and Laessig RH, Hassermer DJ, Paskay TA, et al: The effects of 0.1 and 1.0 percent erythrocytes and hemolysis on serum chemistry values. Am J Clin Pathol 1976; 66:639–644, with permission.

Table 3–4 Reasons for Specimen Rejection

Hemolysis/lipemia

Clots present in an anticoagulated specimen

Nonfasting specimen when test requires fasting

Improper blood collection tube

Short draws, wrong volume

Improper transport conditions (ice for blood gases)

Discrepancies between requisition and specimen label

Unlabeled or mislabeled specimen

Contaminated specimen/leaking container

Each collection tube containing an anticoagulant has a specific manufacture's color code. *Icteric* or *lactescent serum* provides additional challenges in laboratory analysis. When serum bilirubin approaches 430 mmol/L (25 mg/L), interference may be observed in assays for albumin (4-hydroxyazobenzene-2-carboxylic acid [HABA] procedure), cholesterol (using ferric chloride reagents), and total protein (biuret procedure). Artifactually induced values in some laboratory determinations result when triglyceride levels are elevated (turbidity) based on absorbance of light of various lipid particles. Latescence occurs when serum triglyceride levels exceed 4.6 mmol/L (400 mg/dL). Inhibition of assays for amylase, urate, urea, CK, bilirubin, and total protein may be observed. To correct for artifactal absorbance readings, 'blanking' procedures (the blank contains serum, but lacks a crucial element to complete the assay), or dual-wavelength methods may be used. A blanking process may not be effective in some cases of turbidity and ultracentrifugation may be necessary.

Specimen Rejection

All specimens must be collected, labeled, transported and processed according to established procedures that include sample volume, special handling needs and container type. Failure to follow specific procedures can result in specimen rejection. Inappropriate specimen type, wrong preservative, hemolysis, lipemia, clots, etc., are reasons for rejection. Specimen rejection is not only costly and time-consuming, but may cause harm to the patient. It is therefore essential to thoroughly train staff in all aspects of specimen collection, transportation and processing. Table 3–4 lists various reasons for specimen rejection.

Blood Collection Overview

Venipuncture is accomplished using a needle/adapter assembly attached to an evacuated glass/plastic test tube with a rubber/plastic stopper. Blood may also be collected in a syringe and transferred to the appropriate specimen container (evacuated tube system). A syringe may be helpful when procuring a specimen from the hand, ankle, or small children. In addition, patients with small or poor veins may experience collapse of veins with use of an evacuated tube system. However, the latter system is recommended to limit exposure to accidental needlesticks to the phlebotomist.

Stoppers are color coded to distinguish whether the tube contains a specific anticoagulant or additive, or is a special tube made chemically clean (e.g., for lead or iron determinations), or a plain tube with no additives. Table 3–5 lists the most frequently used anticoagulants/additives based on color-coded tube stoppers. Tubes come in various sizes, such as 2, 5, 7, or 10 mL. The use of anticoagulants allows for analysis of whole blood specimens or plasma constituents obtained by centrifugation and separation of the plasma. Plasma contains fibrinogen, which is missing from serum. Many laboratories have converted from glass to plastic collection tubes to minimize exposure to biohazardous material (e.g., blood) and broken glass; lower biohazard waste disposal costs; and comply with Occupational Safety and Health Administration (OSHA) guidelines mandating substitution. This change from glass to plastic has required a modification in the order of draw. Historically, tubes with additives, including gel tubes, were drawn after the citrate tube (blue top) to avoid interference with coagulation measurements. The order of draw was: blood-culture tubes, plain nonadditive red top tubes, coagulation (citrate) tubes, and sequentially additive tubes with gel, EDTA, and oxalate/fluoride. Now that plastic blood-collection tubes are used, the order of draw has been revised (Table 3–6). Plastic serum tubes, with or without a clot activator or gel separator, are now drawn *after* the citrate tube and before the other additive tubes, though a provision within NCCLS guidelines (H3-A5) affords the option to draw glass non-additive serum tubes before citrate ones (Ernst, 2004).

Anticoagulants and Additives

Ethylenediamine tetra-acetic acid (EDTA) is the anticoagulant of choice for hematology cell counts and cell morphology. It is available in lavender top tubes as a liquid or spray-dried in the di- or tripotassium salt form (K_2EDTA in plastic, spray-dried, and K_3EDTA in liquid form in glass tubes). K_3EDTA is a liquid and will dilute the sample ~ 1–2%. K_2EDTA is spray-dried on the walls of the tube and will not dilute the sample. Pink top tubes also contain EDTA. The EDTA is spray-dried K_2EDTA. Pink tubes are used in immunohematology for ABO grouping, Rh typing and antibody screening. These tubes have a special crossmatch label for information required by the AABB and approved by the FDA for blood bank collections. White top tubes also contain EDTA and gel. They are mostly used for molecular diagnostic testing. For coagulation testing, a light blue top tube containing 0.105 M or

Table 3–6 Order of Draw: Evacuated Tube and Syringe

1. Blood-culture tubes (yellow)
2. Sodium-citrate tube (blue stopper)
3. Serum tubes with or without clot activator or gel separator
4. Heparin tubes with or without gel (green stopper)
5. EDTA tubes (lavender stopper)
6. Glycolytic inhibitor tubes (gray stopper)

0.129 M (3.2% and 3.8%) sodium citrate is commonly used because it preserves the labile coagulation factors. Black top tubes also contain buffered sodium citrate and are generally used for Westergren sedimentation rates. They differ from the light blue top tubes in that the ratio of blood to anticoagulant is 4 : 1 in the black top tubes and 9 : 1 in the light blue top tubes.

Heparin, mucoitin polysulfuric acid, is an effective anticoagulant in small quantities without significant effect on many determinations. Heparin was originally isolated from liver cells by scientists looking for an anticoagulant that could work safely in humans. Heparin is available as lithium heparin (LiHep) and sodium heparin (NaHep) in green top tubes. Heparin accelerates the action of antithrombin III, neutralizing thrombin and preventing the formation of fibrin. Heparin has an advantage over EDTA as an anticoagulant, as it does not affect levels of ions such as calcium. However, heparin can interfere with some immunoassays. Heparin should not be used for coagulation or hematology testing. Heparinized plasma is preferred for potassium measurements to avoid an elevation due to the release of potassium from platelets as the blood clots (Garza, 2002). Lithium heparin may be used for most chemistry tests except for lithium and folate levels; for lithium, a royal blue sodium heparin, Na_2EDTA, can be used instead. Sodium heparin cannot be used for assays measuring sodium levels but it is recommended for trace elements, leads and toxicology. Sodium heparin is the injectable form used for anticoagulant therapy.

Gray top tubes are generally used for glucose measurements since they contain a preservative or antiglycolytic agent, such as sodium fluoride and lithium iodoacetate. Sodium fluoride prevents glycolysis for 3 days and iodoacetate does the same for about 24 hours (Strasinger, 2003). In bacterial septicemia, fluoride inhibition of glycolysis is neither adequate nor effective in preserving glucose concentration.

Red top tubes have no additive so blood collected in these tubes clots. Red top tubes are used for most chemistry, blood bank and immunology

Table 3–5 Tube Color and Anticoagulant/Additive

Stopper color	Anticoagulant/additive	Specimen type/use	Mechanism of action
Red (glass)	None	Serum/chemistry and serology	N/A
Red (plastic/Hemogard)	Clot activator	Serum/chemistry and serology	Silica clot activator
Lavender (glass)	K_3EDTA in liquid form	Plasma/hematology	Chelates (binds) calcium
Lavender (plastic)	K_2EDTA/spray-dried	Plasma/hematology	Chelates (binds) calcium
Pink	Spray-dried K_2EDTA	Plasma/blood bank	Chelates (binds) calcium
White	EDTA and gel	Plasma/molecular diagnostics	Chelates (binds) calcium
Light blue	Sodium citrate	Plasma/coagulation	Chelates (binds) calcium
Light blue	Thrombin and soybean trypsin inhibitor	Plasma/coagulation	Good for fibrin degradation products
Black	Sodium citrate	Plasma/sed rates – hematology	Chelates (binds) calcium
Light green/black	Lithium heparin and gel	Plasma/chemistry	Inhibits thrombin formation
Green	Sodium heparin, lithium heparin	Plasma/chemistry	Inhibits thrombin formation
Royal blue	Sodium heparin, Na_2EDTA	Plasma/chemistry/toxicology	Heparin inhibits thrombin formation Na_2EDTA binds calcium
Gray	Sodium fluoride and lithium iodoacetate	Plasma/glucose testing	Inhibits glycolysis
Yellow	Sterile containing sodium polyanetholesulfonate (SPS)	Serum/microbiology culture	Aids in bacterial recovery by inhibiting complement, phagocytes and certain antibiotics
Yellow	Acid citrate dextrose (ACD)	Serum/blood bank, HLA phenotyping and paternity testing	RBC preservative
Tan (glass)	Sodium heparin	Plasma/lead testing	Inhibits thrombin formation
Tan (plastic)	K_2EDTA	Plasma/lead testing	Chelates (binds) calcium
Yellow/gray and orange	Thrombin	Serum/chemistry	Clot activator
Red/gray and gold	Clot activator separation gel	Serum/chemistry	Silica clot activator

assays. Integrated serum separator tubes are available for isolating serum from whole blood. During centrifugation, blood is forced into a thixotropic gel material located at the base of the tube. The gel undergoes a temporary change in viscosity during centrifugation and lodges between the packed cells and the top serum layer (Strasinger, 2003). Pediatric-sized tubes are also available. Advantages of serum separator tubes are (1) ease of use, (2) shorter processing time through clot activation, (3) higher serum yield, (4) minimal liberation of potentially hazardous aerosols, (5) only one centrifugation step, (6) use of the same tube as that into which the patient specimen was drawn, and (7) ease of a single label. A unique advantage is that centrifuged specimens can be transported without disturbing the separation. Some silica gel serum separation tubes may give rise to minute particles that can cause flow problems during analysis. Filtering the serum solves the problem.

A few specialized tubes exist. Red/gray and gold top tubes contain a clot activator and separation gel. These tubes are referred to as SSTs, or serum separator tubes, and are mostly used for chemistry tests.

Therapeutic drug monitoring specimens should not be collected in tubes that contain gel separators as some gels absorb certain drugs causing a falsely lowered result. Significant decreases of phenytoin, phenobarbital, lidocaine, quinidine and carbamazepine have been reported when stored in Vacutainer SST tubes, while no changes were noted in theophylline and salicylate levels. Storage in standard red top Vacutainer collection tubes without barrier gels did not affect measured levels of the above therapeutic drugs (Dasgupta, 1994). Studies indicate that this absorption is time dependent and therefore speed in processing minimizes absorption. The acrylic based gels do not exhibit the absorption problems associated with silicone and polyester gels (Garza, 2002). Studies of the Vacutainer SST II tubes indicate that most drugs are stable for 24 hours with the new gel. SST II tubes have been reported to be effective in collecting blood for therapeutic drug monitoring (Bush, 2001).

Tubes containing gels are not used in Blood Bank or for immunologic testing as the gel may interfere with the immunologic reactions (Strasinger, 2003). Clotting time for tubes using gel separators is approximately 30 minutes, while tubes that have clot activators, such as thrombin, will clot in 5 minutes. Plain red-stoppered tubes with no additives take about 60 minutes to clot completely (Strasinger, 2003).

Anticoagulants may affect the transport of water between cell and plasma, thereby altering cell size and constituent plasma concentration. Oxalate anticoagulants may shrink red cells, thus, blood anticoagulated with oxalate cannot be used to measure hematocrit. Combined ammonium/potassium oxalate does not have the same effect. EDTA, citrate and oxalate chelate calcium, thereby lowering calcium levels. Fluoride, used for glucose determinations, prevents glycolysis by forming an ionic complex with Mg^{++}, thereby inhibiting the Mg^{++} dependent enzyme, enolase. (Young, 2001). Table 3–7 lists anticoagulants/additives and their effect on various blood tests.

Blood Collection Devices

The most common blood collection system uses a vacuum to pull blood into a container; it consists of: a color-coded evacuated collection tube, a double-headed needle and an adapter/holder. Small tubes are available for pediatric and geriatric collections. The blood collection holder accommodates various sizes (gauge) of blood collection needles. Needles vary from large (16 gauge) to small (23 gauge) in size. There are several types of holders designed to eject the needle after use. Recent Occupational Safety and Health Administration (OSHA) policies require that the adapters be discarded with the used needle (OSHA: Needlestick Safety Prevention Act, 2002). Pediatric inserts are available for adapters and accommodate the smaller diameter pediatric blood collection tubes. Also available are a variety of safety needles that cover the needle after use, or retract the needle before it is discarded.

Winged infusion sets (butterfly needles) can be used when blood has to be collected from a very small vein. Butterfly needles come in 21, 23 and 25 gauge. These needles have plastic wings attached to the end of the needle that aid in the insertion of the needle into the small vein. Tubing is attached to the back end of the needle that terminates with an adapter for attachment to a syringe or evacuated collection holder. Every effort must be made to protect the phlebotomist from being stuck with a used needle when using a butterfly infusion set.

Blood collected in a syringe can be transferred to an evacuated tube. Special syringe safety shield devices are available to avoid unnecessary contact with the blood sample. If blood requires anticoagulation, speed becomes an important factor and the blood must be transferred before clot formation begins. Once the blood has been transferred, the anticoagulated the tube must be thoroughly mixed to avoid small clot formation.

Table 3–7 Anticoagulant/Additive Effect on Various Blood Tests

Additive	Test	Effect
EDTA	Alkaline phosphatase	Inhibits
	Creatine kinase	Inhibits
	Leucine aminopeptidase	Inhibits
	Calcium and iron	Decrease
	PT and PTT	Increase
	Sodium and potassium	Increase
	Platelet aggregation	Prevents
Oxalate	Acid phosphatase	Inhibits
	Alkaline phosphatase	Inhibits
	Amylase	Inhibits
	LDH	Inhibits
	Calcium	Decrease
	Sodium and potassium	Increase
	Cell morphology	Distorts
Citrate	ALT, AST	Inhibits
	Alkaline phosphatase	Inhibits
	Acid phosphatase	Stimulates
	Amylase	Decrease
	Calcium	Decrease
	Sodium and potassium	Increase
	Labile coagulation factors	Preserves
Heparin	Triiodothronine	Increase
	Thyroxine	Increase
	PT and PTT	Increase
	Wright's stain	Causes blue background
	Lithium (LiHep tubes only)	Increase
	Sodium (NaHep tubes only)	Increase
Fluorides	Acid phosphatase	Decrease
	Alkaline phosphatase	Decrease
	Amylase	Decrease
	Creatine kinase	Decrease
	ALT and AST	Decrease
	Cell morphology	Distorts

Several additional pieces of phlebotomy equipment are necessary. A tourniquet, usually a flat latex strip or piece of tubing, is used to occlude the vein before blood collection and is discarded after each phlebotomy. OSHA guidelines state that gloves be worn when performing phlebotomy and changed between patients. Gloves are available in various sizes and made of various materials to avoid latex sensitivity experienced by some individuals. Other supplies include gauze pads, alcohol or iodine wipes for disinfection of the puncture site, and a Band-Aid® to prevent bleeding after the completion of the phlebotomy.

Blood Storage and Preservation

During storage, the concentration of a blood constituent in the specimen may change as a result of various processes, including adsorption to glass or plastic tubes, protein denaturation, evaporation of volatile compounds, water movement into the cells resulting in hemoconcentration of the serum and plasma, and continuing metabolic activities of leukocytes and erythrocytes. These changes occur, though to varying degree, at ambient temperature and during refrigeration or freezing. Storage requirements vary widely by analyte.

Stability studies have shown that clinically significant analyte changes occur if serum or plasma remains in prolonged contact with blood cells. After separation from blood cells, analytes have the same stability in plasma and serum when stored under the same conditions. Glucose concentration in unseparated serum and plasma decreases rapidly in the first 24 hours and more slowly thereafter. This decrease is more pronounced in plasma. Lactate levels increase with a greater rise seen in plasma than in serum. Chloride and TCO_2 show a steady decrease over 56 hours with the degree of change more pronounced in plasma. K^+ is reported to be stable for up to 24 hours, after which a rapid increase takes place. The degree of change is slightly more pronounced in plasma. Unseparated serum and plasma yield clinically significant increases of total bilirubin, sodium, urea, nitrogen, albumin, calcium, magnesium and total protein. These changes are attributed to movement of water into cells after 24 hours, resulting in hemoconcentration (Boyanton, 2002). Other studies found potassium, phosphorus, and glucose to be the analytes that were least stable in serum not removed from the clot within 30 minutes. Albumin, bicarbonate, chloride, C-peptide, HDL-cholesterol, iron, LDL-cholesterol, and total protein were found to be unstable after 6 hours when the serum was not separated from the clot (Zhang, 1998).

When serum and plasma are not removed from the cells, lipids (like cholesterol) and some enzymes increase over time with the change more pronounced in plasma than serum. LD activity continuously increases over 56 hours. AST, ALK and CK were found to be stable over 56 hours. GGT activity in plasma, with and without prolonged contact with cells, was found to be 27% lower than in serum at 0.5 hours; however, plasma GGT activity steadily increases with prolonged exposure to cells. Creatinine increases by 110% in plasma and 60% in serum after 24 hours (Boyanton, 2002).

Serum and plasma may yield significantly different results for an analyte. For example, when serum and EDTA plasma results for parathyroid hormone (PTH) are compared from specimens frozen within 30 minutes of collection, EDTA plasma results are significantly higher (> 19%) than those obtained from serum (Omar, 2001). The effect of freeze–thaw cycles on constituent stability is an important consideration. In plasma or serum specimens, the ice crystals formed cause shear effects that are disruptive to molecular structure(s), particularly to large protein molecules. Slow freezing allows larger crystals to form, causing more serious degradative effects. Thus, quick-freezing is recommended for optimal stability.

Importance of Policies and Procedures

It is essential to establish institution-specific phlebotomy policies and procedures that include: personnel standards with qualifications, dress code and evaluation procedures; safety protocols including immunization recommendations, universal precautions, needlestick and sharps information, personal protective equipment; test order procedures; patient identification, confidentiality and preparation, and documentation of problems encountered during blood collection; needlestick site selection and areas to be avoided (mastectomy side, edematous area, burned/scarred areas, etc.); anticoagulants required and tube color; order of draw; special requirements for patient isolation units; and specimen transport. The laboratory should have available all CDC, CAP, NCCLS, OSHA, and JCAHO guidelines as well as other government regulations pertaining to laboratory testing. All employees must be trained about safety procedures and a written blood-borne pathogen exposure control plan must be available. See Chapter 1 for a more complete discussion of safety. The Occupational Safety and Health Administration (OSHA: Bloodborne Pathogens Standard) concluded that the best practice for prevention of needlestick injuries following phlebotomy is the use of a sharp with engineered sharps injury protection (SESIP) attached to the blood tube holder and the immediate disposal of the entire unit after each patient's blood is drawn (OSHA, 2001). Information on exposure prevention can be found on the Exposure Prevention Information Network (EPINet), a database coordinated by the International Healthcare Worker Safety Center at the University of Virginia (http://www.healthsystem.virginia. edu/internet/epinet/). OSHA further mandates that employers make available, closable, puncture-resistant, leak-proof sharps containers that are labeled and color-coded. The containers must have an opening that is large enough to accommodate disposal of the entire blood collection assembly (i.e. blood tube, holder and needle). These containers must be easily accessible to employees in the immediate area of use and if employees travel from one location to another (one patient room to another) the employees must be provided with a sharps container that is conveniently placed at each location/facility. Employers must maintain a sharps injury log to record percutaneous injuries from contaminated sharps while at the same time protecting the confidentiality of the injured employee.

Blood Collection Techniques

Table 3–8 summarizes the technique for obtaining blood from a vein (CLSI H3-A5, 2003).

Arterial Puncture

Arterial punctures are technically more difficult to perform than venous punctures. Increased pressure in the arteries makes it more difficult to stop bleeding, with the undesired development of a hematoma. In order of preference, the radial, brachial, and femoral arteries can be selected. Unacceptable sites are those that are irritated, edematous, near a wound,

Table 3–8 Venous Puncture Technique

1. Verify that computer-printed labels match requisitions. Check patient identification band against labels and requisition forms. Ask the patient for their full name
2. If a fasting specimen is required, confirm that the fasting order has been followed
3. Position the patient properly. Assemble equipment and supplies
4. Ask the patient to make a fist. Select a suitable vein for puncture. Cleanse the venipuncture site. Allow the area to dry. Apply a tourniquet several inches above the puncture site
5. Anchor the vein firmly
6. Enter the skin with the needle at approximately a 15-degree angle to the arm, with the bevel of the needle up:
   a. Follow the geography of the vein with the needle
   b. Insert the needle smoothly and fairly rapidly to minimize patient discomfort
   c. If using a syringe, pull back on the barrel with a slow, even tension as blood flows into the syringe. Do not pull back too quickly to avoid hemolysis or collapsing the vein
   d. If using an evacuated system, as soon as the needle is in the vein, ease the tube forward in the holder as far as it will go, firmly securing the needle holder in place. When the tube has filled, remove it by grasping the end of the tube and pull gently to withdraw
7. Release the tourniquet when blood begins to flow. Never withdraw the needle without removing the tourniquet
8. Withdraw the needle, and then apply pressure to the site. Apply adhesive bandage strip over a cotton ball or gauze to adequately stop bleeding and to avoid a hematoma
9. Mix and invert tubes with anticoagulant; do not shake the tube. Check condition of the patient. Dispose of contaminated material in designated containers (sharps container) using Universal Precautions
10. Initial the labels and record the time specimens were drawn
11. Deliver tubes of blood for testing to appropriate laboratory section or central receiving and processing area

Table 3–9 Modified Allen Test

1. Have the patient make a fist and occlude both the ulnar (opposite the thumb side) and radial arteries (closest to the thumb) by compressing with two fingers over each artery
2. Have the patient open their fist and observe if the patient's palm has become bleached of blood
3. Release the pressure on the ulnar artery (farthest from the thumb) only and note if blood return is present. The palm should become perfused with blood. Adequate perfusion is a positive test indicating that arterial blood may be drawn from the radial artery. Blood should not be taken if the test is negative. Serious consequences may result if this procedure is not followed and may result in the loss of the hand or its function

or in an area of an arteriovenous (AV) shunt or fistula (McCall, 1993). Arterial spasm is a reflex constriction that restricts blood flow with possible severe consequences on circulation and tissue perfusion. Radial artery puncture can be painful and associated with symptoms such as aching, throbbing, tenderness, sharp sensation, and cramping. At times, it is either impractical or impossible to obtain arterial blood from a patient for blood gas analysis. Under these circumstances, another source of blood can be obtained, recognizing that arterial blood provides a more accurate result. Although venous blood is more readily obtained, it usually reflects the acid–base status of an extremity, not the body as a whole.

Before blood is collected from the radial artery in the wrist, one should do a modified Allen test (Table 3–9) to determine whether the ulnar artery can provide collateral circulation to the hand after the radial artery puncture.

The radial and brachial arteries are the preferred vessels for arterial puncture. The femoral artery is relatively large and easy to puncture, but one must be especially careful in older individuals, since the femoral artery can bleed more than the radial or brachial. Because the bleeding site is hidden by bedcovers, it may not be noticed until bleeding is massive.

Table 3–10 Arterial Puncture Procedure

1. Prepare the arterial blood gas (ABG) syringe according to established procedures. The needle (18–20 gauge for brachial artery) should pierce the skin at an angle of approximately 45–60 degrees (90 degrees for femoral artery) in a slow and deliberate manner. Some degree of dorsiflexion of the wrist is necessary with the radial artery, for which a 23–25 gauge needle is used. The pulsations of blood into the syringe confirm that it will fill by arterial pressure alone. If the plunger is pulled back and air is aspirated, immediately withdraw the syringe

2. After the blood specimen is collected gently rotate the syringe, mixing blood and heparin. Place in ice water (or other coolant that will maintain a temperature of 1–5°C) to minimize leukocyte consumption of oxygen. After the arterial puncture, compression with a sterile gauze pad on the puncture site should be applied for a minimum of 2 minutes and preferably for 5 minutes (timed). Apply an adhesive bandage

The radial artery is more difficult to puncture but complications occur less frequently. The major complications of arterial puncture include thrombosis, hemorrhage, and possible infection. When performed correctly, no significant complications are reported except for possible hematomas.

Arterial Puncture Technique

The artery to be punctured is identified by its pulsations and cleansed with 70% aqueous isopropanol solution followed by iodine. A non-anesthetized arterial puncture provides an accurate measurement of resting pH and P_{CO_2} in spite of the theoretical error possible from patient hyperventilation caused by the pain of the arterial puncture. The use of butterfly infusion sets is not recommended. Using 19-gauge versus 25-gauge needles does not vary the P_{CO_2} or P_{O_2} more than 1 mmHg. The amount of anticoagulant should be 0.05 mL liquid heparin (1000 IU/mL) for each milliliter of blood. Using too much heparin is probably the most common pre-analytic error in blood gas measurement (Garza, 2002). Table 3–10 lists the procedure for arterial puncture (CLSI H11-A4, 2004).

Skin Puncture

Skin puncture is the method of choice in pediatric patients, especially infants. The large amount of blood required from repeated venipunctures may cause iatrogenic anemia, especially in premature infants. Venipuncture of deep veins in pediatric patients may also rarely cause (1) cardiac arrest, (2) hemorrhage, (3) thrombosis, (4) venous constriction followed by gangrene of an extremity, (5) damage to organs or tissues accidentally punctured, and (6) infection. Accessible veins in sick infants must be reserved exclusively for parenteral therapy. Skin puncture is useful in adults with (1) extreme obesity, (2) severe burns, and (3) thrombotic tendencies. Skin puncture is often preferred in geriatric patients because skin is thinner and less elastic; thus a hematoma is more likely to occur from a venipuncture.

In newborns, skin puncture is frequently used to collect a sample for bilirubin testing. Screening tests for inherited metabolic disorders and bleeding time tests are also performed on blood collected from skin puncture. Standardization of the bleeding time procedure that controls for blood pressure and depth of stick is essential in order to obtain useful information. Heel punctures are most frequently used for metabolic disease screening. In the older pediatric population, ear lobe blood is available, but in neonates and infants, it is impractical to sample the ear lobe, therefore the heel is more often used. A deep heel prick is made at the distal edge of the calcaneal protuberance following a 5- to 10-minute exposure period to prewarmed water. The best method for blood gas collection in the newborn still remains the indwelling umbilical artery catheter. Table 3–11 lists the steps for a skin puncture (CLSI H4-A5, 2004).

Central Venous Access Devices

Central venous access devices (CVADs) provide ready access to the patient's circulation, eliminating multiple phlebotomies, and are especially useful in critical care and surgical situations. Indwelling catheters are surgically inserted in the cephalic vein, or internal jugular, subclavian, or femoral veins and can be used to draw blood, administer drugs or blood products, and provide total parenteral nutrition. Continuous, real-time, intra-arterial monitoring of blood gases and acid–base status has been accomplished with fiberoptic channels containing fluorescent and absorbent chemical analytes (Smith, 1992).

Table 3–11 Skin Puncture Technique

1. Select an appropriate puncture site. For infants, this is most usually the lateral or medial plantar heel surface. In older infants, the palmar surface of the last digit of the second, third, or fourth finger may be used. Other sites for skin puncture are the plantar surface of the big toe, the lateral side of a finger adjacent to the nail, and the ear lobe. The site of puncture must not be edematous or a previous puncture site

2. Warm the puncture site with a warm, moist towel no hotter than 42°C; this increases the blood flow through arterioles and capillaries and results in arterial-enriched blood

3. Cleanse the puncture site with 70% aqueous isopropanol solution. Allow the area to dry. Do not touch the swabbed area with any nonsterile object

4. Make the puncture with a sterile lancet, or other skin-puncturing device, using a single deliberate motion nearly perpendicular to the skin surface. For a heel puncture, hold the heel with the forefinger at the arch and the thumb proximal to the puncture site at the ankle. If using a lancet the blade should be no longer than 2.4 mm to avoid injury to the calcaneus (heel bone)

5. Discard the first drop of blood by wiping it away with a sterile pad. Regulate further blood flow by gentle thumb pressure. Do not milk the site, as this may cause hemolysis and introduce excess tissue fluid

6. Collect the specimen in a suitable container by capillary action. Closed systems are available for collection of nonanticoagulated blood and with additives for whole blood analysis. Open-ended, narrow-bore disposable glass micropipets are most often used up to volumes of 200 μL. Both heparinized and nonheparinized micropipets are available. Use the appropriate anticoagulant for the test ordered. Mix the specimen as necessary

7. Apply pressure and dispose of the puncture device

8. Label the specimen container with date, time of collection, and patient demographics

9. Indicate in the report that test results are from skin puncture

Table 3–12 Order of Draw from Catheter Lines

1. Draw 3–5 mL in a syringe and discard
2. Blood for blood culture
3. Blood for anticoagulated tubes (lavender, green light blue, etc.)
4. Blood for clot tubes (red, SST, etc.)

CVA Collection Technique

Blood specimens drawn from catheters may be contaminated with whatever was administered or infused via the catheter. The solution (usually heparin) used to maintain patency of the vein must also be cleared before blood for analysis is collected. Sufficient blood (minimum of 2–5 mL) must be withdrawn to clear the line so laboratory data are reliable. Specialized training is therefore necessary before using a catheter line for collecting blood specimens. To obtain a blood specimen from the indwelling catheter 5 mL of intravenous fluid is first drawn and discarded. In a separate syringe the amount of blood required for the requested laboratory procedure(s) is then drawn. Strict aseptic technique must be followed to avoid site and/or catheter contamination. Coagulation measurements such as prothrombin time (PT), activated partial thromboplastin time (APTT), and thrombin time (TT), are extremely sensitive to heparin interference, so that even larger volumes of presample blood must be withdrawn before the laboratory results are acceptable for these tests. The appropriate volume to be discarded should be established by each laboratory.

The laboratory is sometimes asked to perform blood culture studies on blood drawn from indwelling catheters. Because the indwelling catheters are in place for a few days, this procedure is not recommended because organisms that grow on the walls of the catheter can contaminate the blood specimen. Lines, such as central venous pressure lines (CVP lines) are specifically inserted and used for immediate blood product infusion and are less likely to become contaminated. Determination of catheter contamination requires special handling and careful analysis of multiple samples from the catheter and peripheral blood. Table 3–12 lists the order of draw from catheter lines.

Urine and other Body Fluids Collection

Urine

Collection and preservation of urine for analytical testing must follow a carefully prescribed procedure to ensure valid results. Laboratory testing of urine generally falls under three categories: chemical, bacteriologic, and microscopic examination. There are also several kinds of collection for urine specimens: random, clean catch, timed, 24-hour and catheterized. Random specimens may be collected at any time, but a first-morning-voided aliquot is optimal for constituent concentration as it is usually the most concentrated and has a lower pH due to decreased respiration during sleep. Random urine specimens should be collected in a chemically clean receptacle, either glass or plastic. A clean-catch, midstream specimen is most desirable for bacteriologic examinations. Proper collection of a clean-catch specimen requires that the patient first clean their external genitalia with an antiseptic wipe, they next begin urination, stop midstream, discard this first portion of urine, then collect the remaining urine in a sterile container. The vessel is tightly sealed, labeled with the patient's name and date of collection, and submitted for analysis. A Urine Transfer Straw Kit for midstream specimens (BD Vacutainer Systems) can be used to remove an aliquot from the sterile collection container and transported to the laboratory. The system consists of an adapter that attaches to a yellow evacuated sterile tube. The vacuum draws the urine into the sterile tube. The adapter assembly must be treated like a needle assembly system and be discarded into a biohazard container. A similar product is available for cultures; it uses a sterile, gray top tube containing 6.7 mg/L of boric acid and 3.335 mg/L of sodium formate, and the adapter device described above (BD Vacutainer Systems).

Timed specimens are obtained at designated intervals, starting from 'time zero.' Collection time is noted on each subsequent container. Urine specimens for a 24-hour total volume collection are most difficult to obtain and require patient cooperation. Incomplete collection is the most frequent problem. In some instances, too much sample is collected. In-hospital collection is usually supervised by nurses and is generally more reliable than outpatient collections. Pediatric collections require special attention to avoid stool contamination. One can avoid problems in collecting 24-hour specimens by giving patients complete written and verbal instructions with a warning that the test can be invalidated by incorrect collection technique. The preferred container is unbreakable, 4-L (approximately), plastic, and chemically clean with the correct preservative already added. One should remind the patient to *discard* the first morning specimen, record time, and collect every subsequent voiding for the next 24 hours. An easy approach is to instruct the patient to start with an empty bladder and to end with an empty bladder. Overcollection occurs if the first morning specimen is included in this routine. The total volume collected is measured and recorded on the request form, the entire 24-hour specimen is thoroughly mixed and a 40-mL aliquot is submitted for analysis.

It is difficult to determine whether a collection is complete. If results appear clinically invalid, this is cause for suspicion. Since creatinine excretion is based on muscle mass, and since a patient's muscle mass is relatively constant, creatinine excretion is also reasonably constant. Therefore, one can measure creatinine on several 24-hour collections to assess the completeness of the specimen and keep this as part of the patient's record. One- and 2-hour timed collection specimens may suffice in some instances depending on the analyte being measured. Urobilinogen is subject to diurnal variation with the highest levels reached in the afternoon. Commonly, urine is collected from 2–4 p.m. when a quantification of urobilinogen is requested.

Special Urine Collection Techniques

Catheterization of the urethra and bladder may cause infection, but is necessary in some patients (e.g., for urine collection when patients are unable to void or control micturition). Suprapubic aspiration is performed with a syringe and needle above the symphysis pubis through the abdominal wall into a full bladder. This method is used to obtain otherwise problematic anaerobic cultures. Ureteral catheters can also be inserted via a cystoscope into the ureter. Bladder urine is collected first, followed by a bladder washing. Ureteral urine specimens are useful in differentiating bladder from kidney infection, or for differential ureteral analysis, and may be obtained separately from each kidney pelvis (labeled left and right). First morning urine is optimal for cytologic examination.

Urine Storage and Preservation

Preservation of a urine specimen is essential in order to maintain its integrity. Unpreserved urine specimens are subject both to microbiologic

Table 3–13 Changes in Urine with Delayed Testing

Result	Reason
Change in color	Breakdown or alteration of chromogen or other urine constituent (e.g. hemoglobin, melanin, homogentisic acid, porphyrins)
Changes in odor	Bacterial growth, decomposition
Increased turbidity	Increased bacteria, crystal formation, precipitation of amorphous material
Falsely low pH	Glucose converted to acids and alcohols by bacteria producing ammonia. CO_2 lost
Falsely elevated pH	Breakdown of urea by bacteria forming ammonia
False negative glucose	Utilization by bacteria (glycolysis)
False negative ketone	Volatilization of acetone. Breakdown of acetoacetate by bacteria
False negative bilirubin	Destroyed by light. Oxidation to biliverdin
False negative urobilinogen	Destroyed by light
False positive nitrite	Nitrite produced by bacteria after specimen is voided
False negative nitrite	Nitrite converts to nitrogen and evaporates
Increased bacteriuria	Bacteria multiply in specimen before analysis
Disintegration of cells/casts	Unstable environment, especially in alkaline urine, hypotonic urine or both

decomposition and to inherent chemical changes. Table 3–13 lists common changes that occur as urine decomposes. To prevent growth of microbes, the specimen should be refrigerated promptly after collection and, when necessary, contain the indicated chemical preservative. For some determinations, addition of a chemical preservative can affect assay outcome; thus, refrigeration may be more appropriate. When a preservative is added to the empty collection bottle a warning label is placed on the bottle. Warnings are necessary (e.g., acid burns to patient's genitals are not an unknown occurrence with the use of concentrated acids as preservatives). Light-sensitive compounds are protected in amber plastic bottles. Precipitation of calcium and phosphates occurs unless the urine is acidified adequately before analysis.

It is particularly important to use *freshly* voided and concentrated urine to identify casts, and red and white blood cells, as these undergo decomposition upon storage at room temperature or with decreased concentration (< 1.015 specific gravity). They disappear rapidly in hypotonic and alkaline urine. Bilirubin and urobilinogen decrease, especially after exposure to light. Glucose and ketones may be consumed, while bacterial contamination and loss of CO_2 increases the pH. Turbidity precipitates, and color changes. Ideally specimens should be delivered to the laboratory and analyzed within 1 hour of collection.

Urine may be frozen in aliquots to be assayed at a later date for chemical analysis only. When repeat testing is expected, the specimen should be stored in multiple aliquots to circumvent specimen degradation as a result of repeated freeze–thawing of a single specimen. Preservatives may also be added, depending on the substance to be tested. Sodium fluoride can be added to 24-hour urines for glucose determinations to inhibit bacterial growth and cell glycolysis, but not growth of yeast. About 0.5 g of sodium fluoride is added to a 3- to 4-L container. Sodium fluoride may inhibit reagent (enzyme embedded) glucose strip tests. Tablets containing formaldehyde, mercury, and benzoate (95-mg tablet/20 mL urine) have also been used; however these preservatives elevate specific gravity (0.002/one tablet/20 mL). Boric acid in a concentration of 1 g/dL preserves urine elements such as estriol and estrogen for up to 7 days. Boric acid maintains the pH at about 6.0 and preserves protein and formed elements well without interfering with routine testing except for pH. Boric acid is bacteriostatic, not bactericidal, and it does not inhibit the growth of yeasts. Boric acid has been reported to interfere with drug and hormone analysis (Strasinger, 2001). For catecholamines, vanillylmandelic acid (VMA), or 5-hydroxyindoleacetic acid (5-HIAA) collections, 10 mL of 6N HCl is added to a 3- to 4-L container. The HCL establishes a pH of approximately < 3.0 that is good for chemical testing. However, the low pH destroys formed elements and enhances uric acid precipitation. The concentrated acid also adds a risk of potential chemical burns; the patient should be warned about this potential danger and the container should be labeled accordingly. Table 3–14 lists preservatives commonly used for 24-hour urine specimens. The National Committee for Clinical Laboratory Standards for urinalysis and collection, transportation, and preservation of urine specimens approved guidelines

Table 3-14 24-Hour Urine Collection Preservatives

Preservative	Tests
None (refrigerate)	Amino acids, amylase, chloride, copper, creatinine, delta ALA, glucose, heavy metals (arsenic, lead, mercury), histamine, immunoelectrophoresis, lysozyme, methylmalonic acid, microalbumin, mucopolysaccharides, porphobilinogen, porphyrins, potassium, protein, protein electrophoresis, sodium, urea, uric acid, xylose tolerance
10 g boric acid	Aldosterone, cortisol
10 mL 6N HCL	Calcium, catecholamines, citrate, cystine, 5-HIAA, homovanilic acid, hydroxyproline, magnesium, metanephrines, oxalate, phosphorus, VMA
0.5 g sodium fluoride	Glucose
Equal amounts of 50% alcohol, Saccomanno's fixative, SurePath or Preserve CT	Cytologic examination

provide useful information on various preservatives recommended for 24-hour urine collections (NCCLS, 2001).

Other Body Fluids

Cerebrospinal Fluid

Lumbar punctures (LPs) are performed to collect cerebrospinal fluid (CSF) for laboratory evaluation to establish a diagnosis of infection (bacterial, fungal, mycobacterial, or amebic meningitis), malignancy, subarachnoid hemorrhage, multiple sclerosis, or demyelinating disorders. The most common site for lumbar puncture is between the 3rd and 4th lumbar vertebrae, or between the 4th and the 5th lumbar vertebrae. A serious complication of an LP is cerebellar tonsillar herniation in patients with elevated intracranial pressure, and it should be avoided unless CSF findings are expected to improve treatment or outcome. Patients with spinal cord tumors with paresis may progress to paralysis following LP. Patients with sepsis in the lumbar region (skin infection, cellulitis, or epidural abscess) should not have an LP performed, to avoid introduction of infection. Other complications of lumbar puncture include asphyxiation in infants due to hyperextending the head forward, thus occluding the trachea, paresthesia, headache, and rarely, hematomas. CSF is also collected by cisternal puncture. A needle is inserted into the cisternal subarachnoidea, or small space, that serves as a reservoir for CSF between the atlas and the occipital bone in the back of the head, or by lateral cervical puncture (Kjeldsberg, 1993). Specimens can also be collected from ventricular cannulas (shunts) when present.

Before CSF is collected, the pressure should be between 90–180 mmHg; this is measured by allowing fluid to rise in a sterile, graduated manometer. Holding one's breath, abdominal compression, congestive heart failure, inflammation of the meninges, obstruction of intracranial venous sinuses, mass lesions, or cerebral edema may cause the pressure to be elevated (> 180 mmHg). When pressure is normal, 20 mL of specimen may be removed. On closing, the pressure should be between 10–30 mmHg. A marked decrease in pressure following this procedure suggests cerebellar herniation or spinal cord compression; thus, no additional CSF should be collected. Patients with partial or complete spinal block may have low pressure (< 80 mmHg), falling to zero after removal of only 1 mL. Again, no additional fluid should be removed. Not more than 2 mL can be removed when the pressure is greater than 200 mmHg. Three aliquots are generally collected in separate, sterile tubes labeled appropriately with name, date, and sequential tube collection number, and distributed. Hospital policies differ as to which tube is distributed to which laboratory for analysis. It is generally recommended that Tube #1 goes to chemistry for glucose and protein analysis, or to immunology/serology; Tube #2 goes to microbiology for culture and Gram stain; Tube #3 goes to hematology for cell counts. Tube #3 is the least likely to be contaminated by a bloody tap at collection.

Synovial Fluid

Synovial fluid found in the joint cavities is an ultrafiltrate of plasma that is passed through fenestrations of the subsynovial capillary endothelium into the synovial cavity. Once in the cavity, it is combined with hyaluronic acid, a glycosaminoglycan secreted by the synovial lining cells. Synovial fluid differs from the other serous fluids in that it contains hyaluronic acid (mucin) and may contain crystals. Synovial fluid is collected by arthrocentesis, an aspiration of the joint using a syringe, moistened with an anticoagulant, usually 25 units of sodium heparin per mL of synovial fluid. Oxalate, powdered EDTA and lithium heparin should not be used as they can produce crystalline structures similar to monosodium urate (MSU) crystals. Once removed, the synovial fluid is usually transferred to three tubes – one sterile, one containing EDTA or heparin and one red top tube – and 5–10 mL of fluid is added to each. The sterile tube is sent to microbiology, the anticoagulated tube is sent to hematology and the red top tube, after centrifugation, is used for chemical analysis. Some hospitals transfer synovial fluid to DIFCO ESP aerobic and anaerobic bottle for microbiologic examination.

Pleural Fluid, Pericardial Fluid, and Peritoneal Fluid

Pleural fluid is an ultrafiltrate of the blood plasma. It is formed continuously in the pleural cavity. This cavity, normally containing from 1–10 mL of fluid, is formed by the parietal pleura, lining the chest wall, and the visceral pleura, covering the lung. Each lung is enveloped by this double-membrane of contiguous mesothelial layers. Pleural fluid acts as a natural lubricant for the contraction and expansion of the lungs during respiration. It is reabsorbed by the lymphatics and the venules in the pleura (Miller, 1999).

Thoracentesis is a surgical procedure to drain fluid (effusions) from the thoracic cavity and is helpful in diagnosing inflammation or neoplastic disease in the lung or pleura. Pericardiocentesis and peritoneocentesis refer to the collection of fluid from the pericardium (effusion) and the peritoneal cavities (ascites), respectively. These cavities normally contain less than 50 mL of fluid.

The patient, sitting in an upright position, with arms and head extended on an overbed table, is prepared with a local anesthetic after appropriate cleansing of the site. A 50-mL syringe is fitted with a stopcock and rubber tubing to assist in the aseptic collection process. Specimens are obtained for chemical, microbiologic, and cytologic examination and transferred to collection tubes with appropriate additive(s). For most chemical evaluations, no additive is used and the specimen is allowed to clot. Bacteriologic and cytologic specimens may be collected in EDTA or sterile sodium heparin (without preservatives). Special studies for *Mycobacterium*, anaerobic bacteria, or viruses may require special handling procedures. Special handling procedures must be reviewed prior to collection.

Specimen Transport

Transport of blood, urine, body fluids and tissue specimens from the collection site to the laboratory is an important component of processing. For blood samples, it comprises approximately one-third of the total turnaround time (TAT) (Howanitz, 1992). Excessive agitation of blood specimens must be avoided to minimize hemolysis. Specimens should be protected from direct exposure to light, which causes breakdown of certain analytes (e.g., bilirubin). For analysis of unstable constituents such as ammonia, plasma renin activity, and acid phosphatase, specimens must be kept at 4°C immediately after collection and transported on ice. Routine urine is collected in a sterile, disposable, 200-mL plastic container. Pediatric urine collectors are flexible, polyethylene bags, which may be sealed for transportation. All laboratory specimens must be transported in a safe and convenient manner to prevent biohazard exposure or contamination of the specimen. Broken or leaking specimens are a biohazard to those who may come in contact with them and require collection of a new specimen; this can delay treatment of the patient and add to the cost.

The stability of the constituents must be determined prior to transporting specimens. The laboratory usually provides this information along with instructions for specimen preparation and shipping. Polystyrene or other high-impact plastic-type containers are commonly used. Specimens requiring refrigeration must be maintained between 2–10°C and can be appropriately carried in an insulated container. Large-volume urine specimens should be collected in a leak-proof, 3- to 4-L container. Stool specimens are transported in a cardboard container and placed in a polyethylene bag. To mail a specimen in the frozen state, solid carbon dioxide (dry ice) may be packed in a polystyrene container with the specimen, which can be kept frozen at temperatures as low as -70°C.

The OSHA blood-borne pathogen standard (OSHA: 1910.1030) requires specimens of blood or other potentially infectious materials (OPIM) to be placed in a container that prevents leakage during collection, handling, processing, storage, transport, and/or shipping. This container must be labeled or color-coded according to specific standards (OSHA: 1910.1030(g)(1)(i)). Furthermore, according to the standard, if contamination of the outside of the primary container occurs, or if the specimen could puncture the primary container, the primary container must be placed in a secondary container that is puncture-resistant in addition to having the above characteristics (OSHA: 1910.1030(d) (2) (xiii)).

Labeling is required on all containers used to store, transport, ship, or dispose of blood or other potentially infectious materials, except as noted in the OSHA standard. For example, if individual containers of blood or OPIM are placed in a larger container during storage, transport, shipment or disposal, and that larger container is either labeled with the OSHA 'BIOHAZARD' label or color-coded, the individual containers are exempt from the labeling requirement. OSHA accepts the Department of Transportation's (DOT's) 'INFECTIOUS SUBSTANCE' label in lieu of the 'BIOHAZARD' label on packages where the DOT requires its label on shipped containers, but requires the 'BIOHAZARD' label where OSHA regulates a material but DOT does not. If the DOT-required label is the only label used on the outside of the transport container, the OSHA-mandated label must be applied to any internal containers containing blood or OPIM. The accepted 'BIOHAZARD' label is fluorescent orange.

For local, on-site transport, pneumatic tube systems provide a rapid, efficient, and cost-effective way of transporting laboratory specimens to a specific location. For laboratory use, blood specimens are placed in a carrier with liners to prevent leakage and padding to ensure that specimen containers remain intact. The advantages of a pneumatic tube system are improved turnaround time (TAT), reliability, minimal training, low maintenance, availability 24 h/day, 7 days/week, and improved staff utilization. Studies have shown that most routine chemical and hematologic evaluations are not substantially affected by rapid transport, including blood gases, red cell packs, and lactate dehydrogenase values (Hardin, 1990; Keshgegian, 1992).

Specimen Processing

Processing of specimens includes three distinct phases: precentrifugation, centrifugation, and postcentrifugation. Continuing appraisal of all specimen handling activities is an important pre-analytical component of total quality control. Appropriate guidelines must be established and adhered to by laboratory personnel in each phase of specimen handling to ensure the generation of reliable and medically meaningful measurement and examination results.

Precentrifugation Phase

Ideally, all measurements should be performed within 45 minutes to 1 hour after collection. Whenever this is not practical, the specimen should be processed to a point at which it can be properly stored in order to preclude alterations of constituents to be measured. With the exception of blood gases and ammonia determinations, plasma or serum is preferred for most determinations. In clinical chemistry, serum and plasma are interchangeable except for a few measurements. Serum is required for protein electrophoresis and immunofixation assays, just as plasma is necessary for fibrinogen and other coagulation measurements. Serum is most commonly the specimen of choice, owing to its simplicity in collection and handling. Additionally, interference from anticoagulants is obviated. Plasma may be used in medical emergencies since samples do not have to clot prior to centrifugation. Usually, a greater volume of plasma than serum is obtained from a given volume of whole blood owing to the clot formation process.

Blood should be stoppered in the original container until ready for separation. For plasma preparation, centrifuge blood within 1 hour after collection, for 10 minutes at a relative centrifugal force (RCF) of $850-1000 \times$ gravity (g), keeping the container stoppered to prevent evaporation of plasma or serum water. Adequate time for clotting must be allowed to prevent latent fibrin formation, which may cause undesirable clogging of automated chemistry analyzers. Loosening the clot by 'trimming' or 'ringing' the tube may cause some hemolysis and should be avoided. When glass tubes are used, they should be centrifuged in an aerosol-contained vessel. Serum or plasma must be stored at $4-6\,°C$ if analysis is to be delayed more than 4 hours. One recent study suggests that this may not be necessary (Melanson, 2004). Many laboratories store samples for 7 days in case a test is added.

Centrifugation Phase

A centrifuge uses centrifugal force to separate phases of suspensions by different densities. It is most frequently used in processing blood to derive plasma or serum fractions. Urine and other body fluids may be centrifuged to concentrate particulate matter as sediment to be examined and to minimize interference in other determinations from the same material. Conditions for centrifugation should specify both the time and the centrifugal force. In selecting a centrifuge, one should look for the highest possible centrifugal force and not the rotational speed. The relative centrifugal force (RCF) in gravity units (g), i.e., multiples of the gravitational force, may be calculated by the use of the following formula:

$$RCF = 1.118 \times 10^{-5} \times r \times (rpm)^2$$

1.118×10^{-5} is a constant; r is the radius, expressed in centimeters, between the axis of rotation and the center of the centrifuge tube; and rpm is the speed in revolutions per minute.

The RCF can also be obtained from a nomogram that gives the RCF without the need to calculate it from the above formula.

Several principles must be observed to avoid damage to the centrifuge, or the specimen, and danger to personnel. Tubes, carriers, or shields of equal weight, shape, and size should be placed in opposing positions in the centrifuge head to achieve appropriate balance. Tubes must be balanced across the center of rotation and each bucket must be balanced with respect to its pivotal axis (Seamonds, 2001). Specimens must be placed with regard for a geometrically symmetrical arrangement, using water-filled tubes to attain balance.

Equipment

A wide variety of centrifuges and accessories are available to meet specific needs in the clinical laboratory. These include tabletop, general laboratory centrifuges; horizontal head, fixed-angle, or angle-head; high-speed centrifuges; portable floor models, undercounter models; microcentrifuges; refrigerated and unrefrigerated types; and ultracentrifuge models. Ultracentrifuges are high speed and capable of reaching a centrifugal force of 165 000 times gravity. These centrifuges require refrigeration chambers to compensate for the considerable heat produced. Ultracentrifuges are used to clear serum of chylomicrons, which is necessary to avoid interference with clinical testing (Bermes, 2001). An example of a centrifuge designed for fast speed and quick turnaround time is the StatSpin Express 3 (StatSpin, 2005), a microprocessor-controlled, high-speed bench-top centrifuge designed to rapidly separate blood in evacuated tubes. This centrifuge accelerates rapidly and brakes very fast, decreasing specimen processing time. The centrifuge operates at a fixed speed of 8500 rpm, produces a RCF of $4440 \times (g)$ and can be operated with a 120- or 180-second spin cycle.

Centrifuge capacities vary with model type and centrifuge head. Specimen volume (per tube), number of tubes to be centrifuged, speed required for adequate separation, and durability of equipment should be considered. For every laboratory procedure requiring centrifuge operation, a written specification identifying centrifuge type, temperature, the g forces required, and the length of centrifugation time is required. Calibration of the centrifuge must be part of the quality assurance process. Speed settings must be calibrated using revolutions per minute, and RCFs must be calculated using the above formula or a nomogram. Any significant changes will indicate deterioration effects, such as wearing of brushes or bearing problems. Timers must also be checked for accuracy.

References

BD Vacutainer Systems, Franklin Lakes, NJ 07417. Online. Available: http://www.bd.com.

Bermes EW, Young DS: General laboratory techniques, procedures, and safety. *In* Burtis CA, Ashwood ER (eds): Tietz Fundamentals of Clinical Chemistry, 5th ed. Philadelphia, WB Saunders, 2001, pp 2–29.

Boyanton L, Blick K: Stability studies of twenty-four analytes in human plasma and serum. Clin Chem 2002; 48(12):2242–2247.

This article studies plasma and serum analyte stability over 56 hours in samples removed from cells and allowed to remain on cells. No significant changes were found in the serum and plasma specimens removed from the cells within 30 minutes of collection. The article provides an excellent historical bibliography of the major studies performed on this topic.

Bush V, Blennerhasset J, Wells A, Dasgupta A: Stability of therapeutic drugs in serum collected in vacutainer serum separator tubes containing a new gel (SST II). Ther Drug Monit 2001; 23(3):259–262.

Caraway WT, Kammeyer CW: Chemical interference by drug and other substances with clinical laboratory test procedures. Clin Chem Acta 1972; 41:395.

Centers for Disease Control and Prevention: Workbook for Designing, Implementing, and Evaluation a Sharps Injury Prevention Program, Introduction. Division of Healthcare Quality Promotion – (DHOP Home) Privacy Policy – Accessibility. Published date: June 4, 2004; Reviewed date: July 28, 2004. Online. Available: http://www.cdc.sharpssafety/wk_overview.html.

I

This excellent Internet publication available for free download includes an overview of sharps risks and prevention, organizational steps for development of prevention programs, recommendations for selection of sharps injury prevention devices and education and training materials. The appendices contain useful worksheets for all aspects of sharps injury and prevention documentation.

Clinical and Laboratory Standards Institute (CLSI, formerly NCCLS). Procedures for the Collection of Diagnostic Blood Specimens by Venipuncture: Approved Standard, 5th ed. Document H3-A5. Wayne, PA, NCCLS, 2003.

Clinical and Laboratory Standards Institute (CLSI, formerly NCCLS). Procedures for the Collection of Arterial Blood Specimens; Approved Standard, 4th ed. Document H11-A4. Wayne, PA, NCCLS, 2004.

Clinical and Laboratory Standards Institute (CLSI, formerly NCCLS). Procedures and Devices for the Collection of Diagnostic Capillary Blood Specimens; Approved Standard, 5th ed. Document H4-A5. Wayne, PA, NCCLS, 2004.

Dasgupta A, Dean R, Saldana S, et al: Absorption of therapeutic drugs by barrier gels in serum separator blood collection tubes. Volume and time dependent reduction in total and free drug concentrations. Am J Clin Path 1994; 101(4):456–461.

Dufour DR: Sources and control of preanalytical variation. *In* Kaplan LA, Pesce AJ, Kazmierczak SC (eds): Clinical Chemistry: Theory, Analysis, Correlation, 4th ed. St. Louis, Mosby, 2003, pp 64–82.

Ernst DJ, Calam R: NCCLA simplifies the order of draw: A brief history. MLO 2004; 36:26–27.

Garza D, Becan-McBride K: Phlebotomy Handbook, 2nd ed. Norwalk, CT, Appleton & Lange, 1989, pp 79–82.

Garza D, Becan-McBride K: Phlebotomy Handbook: Blood Collection Essentials, 6th ed. Upper Saddle River, Prentice Hall, 2002, pp 163, 205, 263, 341.

This handbook presents a complete discussion of all aspects related to phlebotomy. Included are safety procedures, equipment, step-by-step procedures, management and legal issues. It contains an excellent, basic discussion of the circulatory system with colored diagrams.

Hardin G, Quick G, Ladd DJ: Emergency transport of AS-1 cell units by pneumatic tube system. J Trauma 1990; 30:346–348.

Howanitz PJ, Steindel SJ, Cembrowski GS, et al: Emergency department stat test turnaround times. A College of American Pathologists' Q-Probes study for potassium and hemoglobin. Arch Pathol Lab Med 1992; 116:122–128.

Kjeldsberg CR, Knight AK: Cerebral Spinal Fluid in Body Fluids, 3rd ed, Chicago, American Society of Clinical Pathology, 1993, p 65.

Keshgegian AA, Bull GE: Evaluation of a soft-handling computerized pneumatic tube specimen delivery system. Am J Clin Pathol 1992; 97:535–540.

Laessig RH, Hassermer DJ, Paskay TA, et al: The effects of 0.1 and 1.0 percent erythrocytes and hemolysis on serum chemistry values. Am J Clin Pathol 1976; 66:639–644.

McCall RE, Tankersley CM: Phlebotomy Essentials. Philadelphia, JB Lippincott Company, 1993, pp 202–206.

Melanson SF, Hsieh B, Flood J et al: Evaluation of add-on testing in the clinical chemistry laboratory of a large academic medical center. Arch Pathol Lab Med 2004; 128:885–889.

Miller HJ: Pleural effusions. *In* Davis B, Bishop M, Mass D (eds): Principles of Laboratory Utilization and Consultation. Philadelphia, WB Saunders, 1999.

National Committee for Clinical Laboratory Standards. Urinalysis and Collection, Transportation, and Preservation of Urine Specimens: Approved Guideline, 2nd ed. GP 16-A2. Villanova, PA, NCCLS, 2001.

National Committee for Clinical Laboratory Standards (NCCLS): Online. Available: http://www.nccls.org and http://www.nccls.org/Template.cfm?section=About_NCCLS

Occupational Safety and Health Administration (OSHA): Occupational Safety Bloodborne Pathogens Standard 29 CFR 1910.1030. 2001. Online. Available: http://www.osha.gov/SLTC/bloodbornepathogens/index.html.

Occupational Safety and Health Administration (OSHA): Occupational Safety Bloodborne Needlestick Safety Prevention Act, OSHA: Revised Standards 2002.

Omar H, Chamberlin A, Walker V, Wood PJ: Immulite 2000 parathyroid hormone assay: Stability of parathyroid hormone in EDTA blood kept at room temperature for 48 hours. Ann Clin Biochem 2001; 38(Pt 5):561–563.

Seamonds B, Elizabeth AB: Basic laboratory principles and techniques. *In* Burtis, CA, Ashwood, ER (eds): Tietz Fundamentals of Clinical Chemistry, 5th ed. Philadelphia, WB Saunders, 2001, pp 3–44.

Smith BE, King PH, Schlain L: Clinical evaluation-continuous real-time intra-arterial blood gas monitor during anesthesia and surgery by fibro-optic sensor. Int J Clin Monitor Comput 1992; 9:45–52.

StatSpin Operator's Manual: StatSpin Express Centrifuge Model Number M500-22. 85 Morse Street, Norwood, Massachusetts 02062, USA (800), StatSpin, Inc., http://www.statspin.com, 2005.

Strasinger SK, DiLorenzo MS: Urinalysis and Body Fluids, 4th ed. Philadelphia, FA Davis, 2001, pp 23–32.

Strasinger SK, DiLorenzo MS: The Phlebotomy Workbook, 2nd ed. Philadelphia, FA Davis, 2003, pp 115, 164, 95, 96.

This text contains a comprehensive presentation of all aspects of phlebotomy. It is an excellent teaching guide and discusses state of the art equipment and techniques. The book is divided into three parts: general phlebotomy, safety and healthcare information; techniques for blood collection; and medical terminology, anatomy and physiology. Contained within the various chapters are excellent summary tables and quick reference charts. It also provides an extensive description of the various blood collection tubes and anticoagulants/additives they contain and information on pre-analytic factors affecting laboratory results.

Young MB, Bermes EW: Specimen collection and other preanalytical variables. *In* Burtis CA, Ashwood ER (eds): Tietz Fundamentals of Clinical Chemistry, 5th ed. Philadelphia, WB Saunders, 2001, pp 30–54.

This chapter contains many of the most important pre-analysis factors that affect laboratory results. Dr Young has also written a series of reference books that contain peer-reviewed information regarding test interactions; they are published by AACC Press, Washington DC and include: Young DS, Friedman RG: Effects of Disease on Clinical Laboratory Tests, 4th ed, 2001; Young DS: Effects of Drugs on Clinical Laboratory Tests, 5th ed, 2000; and Young DS: Effects of Preanalytical Variables on Clinical Laboratory Tests, 2nd ed, 1997.

Zhang DJ, Elswick RK, Miller WG, Bailey JL: Effect of serum–clot contact time on clinical chemistry laboratory results. Clin Chem 1998; 44: 1325–1333.

CHAPTER 4

Analysis: Principles of Instrumentation

Robert L. Sunheimer MS MT(ASCP)SC SLS, Gregory Threatte MD, Mark S. Lifshitz MD, Matthew R. Pincus MD PhD

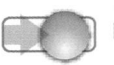

KEY POINTS

• Many analytical determinations made in clinical laboratories are based upon measurements of radiant energy that is absorbed or transmitted. The devices used to measure absorbed or transmitted light energy are photometers and spectrophotometers.

• The basic components of spectrophotometers include: radiant energy source, wavelength selector, cuvet holder, photodetector, signal processors and readout devices.

• A reflectometer is used to measure analytes by measuring the quantity of light reflected by a liquid sample that has been dispensed onto a grainy or fibrous solid support.

• Nephelometers are used to detect light that is scattered at various angles, whereas turbidimetry measures a reduction in light transmission due to particle formation.

• A flow cytometer measures light patterns produced as particles pass single-file through a laser light source. The flow cytometer is used to count and sort cells. It is also a key component of hematology analyzers and the technology used to differentiate white blood cells.

• Electrochemical principles are used to measure numerous analytes in biological fluids. Specific electrochemical techniques include; potentiometry, amperometry, coulometry, conductivity and anodic stripping voltammetry.

• Analytes measured by electrochemical techniques include electrolytes, blood gases, pH, metabolites, e.g., glucose and urea nitrogen, ionized calcium, lead and chloride in sweat.

• Chromatography is a separation technique based on the different interactions of specimen compounds with a mobile phase and a stationary phase, as the compound travels through a support medium.

• Mass spectrometers have become increasingly important clinical instruments, especially in emerging fields such as proteomics. Mass spectrometry (MS) is based on fragmentation and ionization of molecules. The relative abundance of each of the ions yields a characteristic mass spectrum of the parent molecule. The basic components of a mass spectrometer include: ion source, a mass analyzer and an ion detector.

A fundamental understanding of the principles of instrumentation used in clinical laboratories is essential. These instruments must provide the clinician with the best possible data to be of value to the patient. Without a thorough understanding of the necessary principles associated with an analyzer the operators will be ill equipped to perform maintenance procedures, calibrations, and troubleshoot problems that may arise.

The goal of this chapter is to provide the reader with a brief and broad description of the essential principles of analytical instruments in the clinical laboratory. For a more comprehensive review of this topic, the reader is referred to references on clinical instrumentation at the end of this chapter.

Principles of Instrumentation

Spectrophotometry

Absorption spectroscopy has provided scientists with a means to perform both qualitative and quantitative methods for measuring analytes in body fluids. Bouguer initially developed the principles of absorption spectroscopy in the early 1700s. Two other scientists, Lambert and Beer, continued to develop the fundamental principles of absorption spectroscopy, commonly known as Beer's law. Before reviewing the laws of spectroscopy, it is prudent to gain an understanding of light and the effects of its interactions with matter.

Many spectrophotometric methods use EMR, which can take several forms, the most recognizable being light and radiant heat. Other manifestations of EMR include gamma rays and X-rays as well as microwaves, radiofrequency radiation and ultraviolet radiation. The energies involved with the specific regions of the electromagnetic spectrum (EMS) and their corresponding wavelengths change dramatically from radio waves to gamma radiation.

Some properties of EMR can be described by means of a classical sinusoidal wave model. Parameters associated with this waveform include wavelength, frequency, velocity and amplitude as shown in Figure 4–1A. Electromagnetic radiation requires no supporting medium for its transmission and passes readily through a vacuum.

The sine wave model does not provide the total picture when discussing the absorption and emission of radiant energy. Electromagnetic radiation also exists as a stream of discrete particles, or packets (also bundles) of

A

Electric field

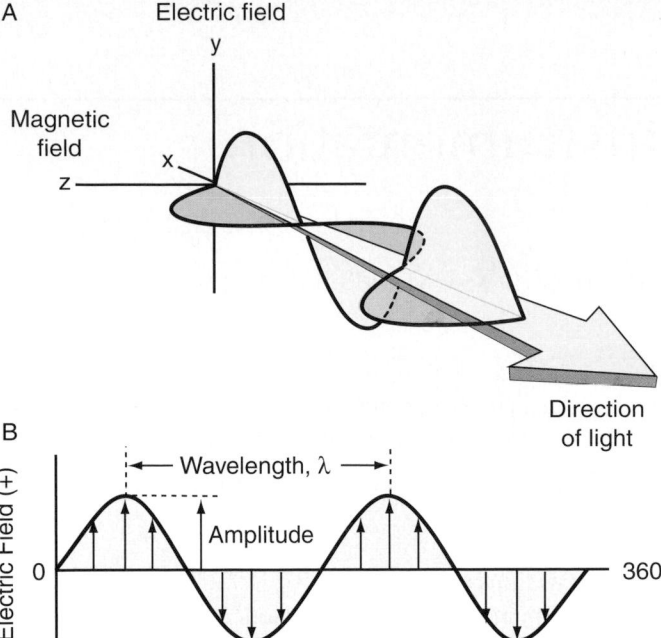

Magnetic field

Direction of light

B

$(-)$ Electric Field $(+)$

Wavelength, λ

Amplitude

0

360

Time or Distance

Figure 4–1 Diagram of a beam of monochromatic, plane-polarized light. A, Magnetic (*y*-axis) and electric (*x*-axis) field vectors at right angle to one another. B, Two-dimensional view of the electric vector.

energy called photons. The energy of the photons is proportional to the frequency of the radiation. This dual nature of EMR is considered complementary and applies to the behavior of streams of electrons, protons and other elementary particles.

The wave model allows us to represent EMR as both an electric and magnetic field that can undergo in-phase, sinusoidal oscillation at right angles both to each other and to the direction of propagation. The electric and magnetic field for a monochromatic beam of plane-polarized light (with oscillation of either the electric or magnetic fields within a single plane)* in a specific direction of propagation is shown in Figure 4–1*B* (Skoog, 1998).

The electric vector or component of the waveform is shown in two-dimensional format. Remember that a vector has both magnitude and direction. The electric field vector at a certain point in time and space is proportional to its own magnitude.

Time or distance of wave propagation is plotted on the abscissa. Most of the instrument principles widely used in the laboratory involve the electric component of radiation and will represent the focus of discussion throughout this chapter. An exception will be nuclear magnetic resonance (NMR). In this technique, the magnetic component produces the desired effect.

Several wave parameters will be described. *Amplitude* of the sine wave is shown as the length of the electronic vector at maximum peak height. A *period, p,* is defined as the time in seconds required for the passage of successive maxima or minima through a fixed point in space. The number of oscillations of the waveform in a second is called *frequency, ν.* The unit of frequency is hertz (Hz), which corresponds to one cycle per second. Frequency is also equal to $1/p$. A *wavelength, λ* is the linear distance between any two equivalent points on a successive wave. A widely used unit for wavelength in the visible spectrum is the nanometer, nm (10^{-9} m). Electromagnetic radiation in the X-ray or gamma region may be expressed in terms of angstrom units, Å (10^{-10} m). Finally, due to its much longer wavelength, EMR in the infrared region may have units corresponding to the micrometer, μm (10^{-6} m).

Example 4–1. 1 nm = 10^{-9} m = 10^{-7} cm; other units sometimes used include:

1 μm = 10^{-6} m = 10^{-4} cm

1 Å = 10^{-10} m = 10^{-8} cm.

Velocity of propagation

Velocity of propagation, v_i in meters per second is determined by multiplying frequency by wavelength. Thus:

$$v_i = \nu \lambda_i \quad (4–1)$$

The frequency of light is determined by the source and does not change, whereas the velocity depends upon the composition of the medium through which it passes. Therefore, Equation 4–1 implies that the wavelength of radiation is also dependent upon the medium.

The velocity of light traveling through a vacuum is independent of wavelength and is at its maximum. This velocity is represented by the symbol *c*, and is equivalent to 2.99792×10^8 m/s. Equation 4–1 can then re written as:

$$c = \nu \lambda = 3.00 \times 10^8 \text{ m/s} = 3.00 \times 10^8 \text{ m s}^{-1} = 3.00 \times 10^{10} \text{ cm/s} \quad (4–2)$$

Example 4–2. What is the wavelength in nm for EMR having a frequency of 1.58×10^{15} Hz?

Solution

$$\lambda = c/\nu$$

$$\lambda \text{ (nm)} = \frac{3.00 \times 10^8 \text{ m/s}}{1.58 \times 10^{15} \text{ Hz}}$$

$$\lambda \text{ (nm)} = 190$$

In any medium containing matter, the propagation of radiation is slowed by the interaction between the EMR field of the radiation and the electrons bound in the atoms of that matter. Since the radiant frequency does not vary and is fixed by the source, the wavelength must decrease as radiation passes from air to a slower medium.

Energy of EMR

One should note the following safety concern: optical devices that emit high frequency EMR generate very high energies and can damage the eyes. Examples include deuterium and xenon lamps.

Wavelength and frequency are related to the energy of a photon, *E*, by Planck's* constant *h*, 6.626×10^{-34} J s, and c, the velocity of light in a vacuum (3.00×10^8 ms^{-1}):

$$E = h\nu = hc/\lambda \quad (4–3)$$

where:

E is the energy of a photon in Joules or eV

h is Planck's constant (6.626×10^{-34} J s)

ν is frequency in Hz (cycles/s).

Quite often the energies of photons are stated in terms of an electron volt (eV). An eV is defined as the energy acquired by an electron that has been accelerated through a potential of 1 volt. The conversion factors between Joules and eV is as follows:

1 J = 6.24×10^{18} eV

1 eV = 1.602×10^{-19} J

To illustrate the difference in energies of photons in the EMS, compare the energy of photons in the ultraviolet (UV) region versus the visible region of the EMS.

Example 4–3. What is the energy in Joules and eV of EMR equivalent to (a) 190 nm? (b) 520 nm?

Solution

(a)

$$E = hc/\nu$$

$$E = \frac{(6.626 \times 10^{-34} \text{ J s}) (3.0 \times 10^8 \text{ m/s})}{190 \text{ nm} (10^{-9} \text{ m/nm})}$$

$$E = 1.046 \times 10^{-18} \text{ J}$$

Or to convert to eV use the conversion of 1 J = 6.24×10^{18} eV.

Therefore the number of eVs is 6.53.

(b)

$$E = hc/\nu$$

$$E = \frac{(6.626 \times 10^{-34} \text{ J s}) (3.0 \times 10^8 \text{ m/s})}{520 \text{ nm} (10^{-9} \text{ m/nm})}$$

$$E = 3.82 \times 10^{-19} \text{ J or 2.38 eV}$$

The relationship of frequency, wavelength and photon energy throughout the EMS can be seen in Figure 4–2. This graphic illustrates for example that very high-energy gamma photons have extremely short wavelengths and very high frequencies (Rubinson, 2000). The converse is true for television and radio wave parameters.

Scattering of Radiation

Transmission of radiation in matter can be viewed as a momentary retention of the radiant energy by atoms, ions, or molecules followed by

---

* Unpolarized radiation has waves in many planes.

* Also expressed in units 6.626×10^{-27} erg s

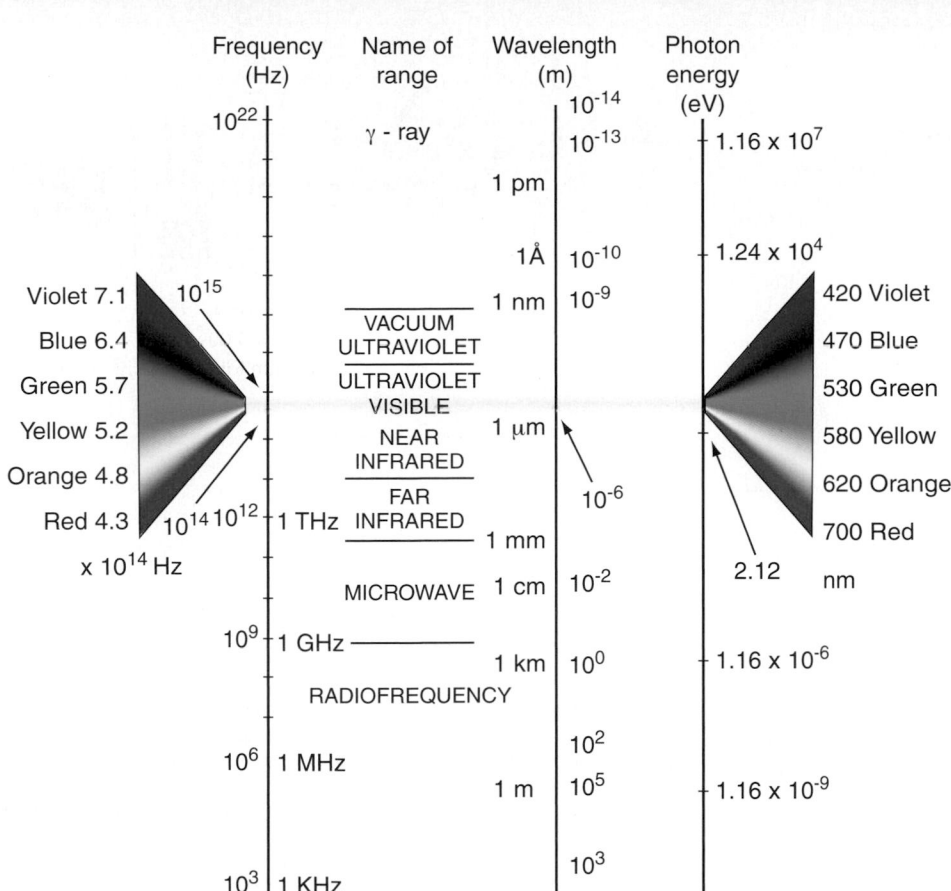

re-emission of the radiation in all direction as the particles return to their original state. Destructive interference removes most but not all of the re-emitted radiation involving atomic or molecular particles that are small relative to the wavelength of the radiation. The exception is the radiation that travels in the original direction of the beam; the path of the beam appears to be unaltered because of the interaction. It has been shown that a very small fraction of the radiation is transmitted at all angles from the original path and that the intensity of this scattered radiation increases with particle size.

Rayleigh Scattering

Scattering by molecules or aggregates of molecules with dimensions significantly smaller than the wavelength of the radiation is referred to as *Rayleigh scattering*. The intensity is proportional to the inverse fourth-power of the wavelength, the square of the polarizability of the particles and the dimensions of the scattering particles. In Rayleigh scattering the wavelengths of the absorbed and emitted photons are the same. An example of Rayleigh scattering is the blue color of the sky, which results from the increased scattering of the shorter wavelength of the visible spectrum.

Tyndall Effect

The Tyndall effect occurs with particles of colloidal dimensions and can be seen with the naked eye. Measurements of scattered radiation are used to determine the size and shape of polymer molecules and colloidal particles.

Raman Scattering

Raman scatter involves absorption of photons producing vibrational excitation. Emission or scatter at longer wavelengths occurs. Raman scatter always varies from the excitation energy by a constant energy difference.

Beer–Lambert Law

If monochromatic EMR (P_o) is directed toward a cuvet containing an absorbing species, the amount of light (P) transmitted (T) is equal to:

$$T = P/P_o \qquad (4\text{–}4)$$

and percent transmittance is equal to $100T$.

Lambert proved that for monochromatic radiation that passes through an absorber of constant concentration, there is a logarithmic decrease in the radiant power as the path length increases arithmetically. The absorbance (A) of a solution was determined to be equivalent to:

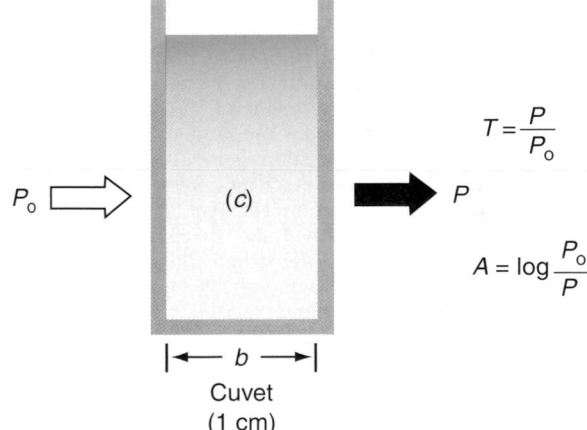

$$T = \frac{P}{P_o}$$

$$A = \log \frac{P_o}{P}$$

Cuvet
(1 cm)

Figure 4–3 Attenuation of monochromatic light by an absorbing solution.

$$A = \log P_o/P \qquad (4\text{–}5)$$

The relationship between transmittance, T or percent transmittance ($P/P_o \times 100$) and absorbance is shown in Figure 4–3. Absorbance and percent transmittance are inversely related as given by:

$$A = 2 - \log \%T \qquad (4\text{–}6)$$

Example 4–4. What is the absorbance of a solution whose transmittance is 10%?

Solution

$$A = 2 - \log \%T$$
$$A = 2 - \log 10\%T = 2 - 1 = 1$$

Beer's followed with studies on the relationship between radiant power and concentration. His approach was to keep the path length and wavelength constant while determining the relationship of radiant power, P and concentrations of the absorbing species. Based on previous work by Lambert, Beer discovered that for monochromatic radiation, absorbance is directly proportional to the path length, b, through the medium and the

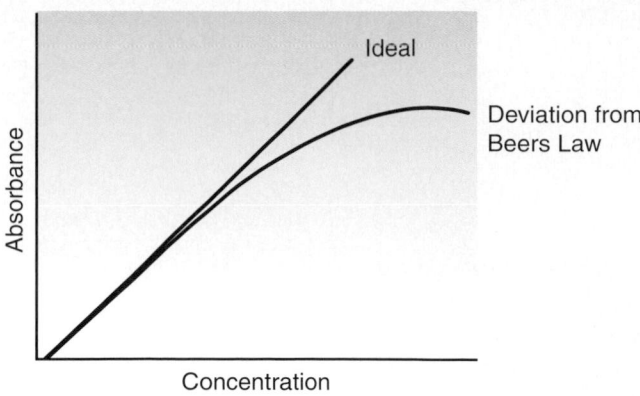

Figure 4–4 A plot of absorbance versus concentration illustrating deviation from Beer's law.

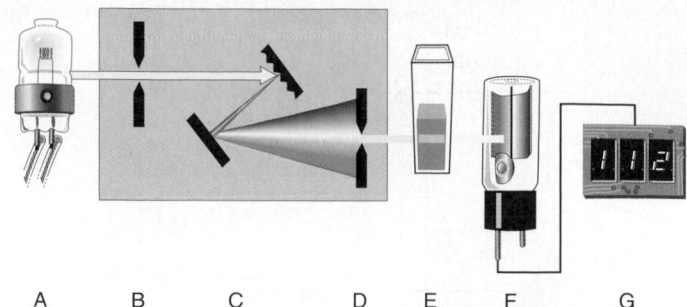

Figure 4–5 Components of a single-beam spectrophotometer. A, exciter lamp; B, entrance slit; C, monochromator; D, exit slit; E, cuvet; F, photodetector; G, LED display.

concentration, c, of the absorbing species. The work culminated in the Beer–Lambert law or simply Beer's law.

The principles established are represented by the following:

$$A = -\log T = \log P_o/P = abc \qquad (4\text{–}7)$$

where a is absorptivity in $L\,g^{-1}\,cm^{-1}$, b is path length of 1 cm, and c is concentration in units of g/L.

When the concentration in Equation 4–7 is expressed in moles per liter and the path length is in centimeters, the term applied is *molar absorptivity* and given the symbol ε, epsilon, and is equivalent to the extinction coefficient ('a') times gram molecular weight of the absorbing species.

$$A = \varepsilon bc \qquad (4\text{–}8)$$

where units for ε are $L\,mol^{-1}\,cm^{-1}$.

The graph of absorbance versus concentration shows the intercept at zero and a linear plot with a slope equivalent to 'ab'. Absorption spectroscopy is used best for solutions whose absorbance values are less than 2.0. Absorbance values greater than 2.0 may yield erroneous results due to other interactions of light with matter, e.g., variations in the refractive index of a solution. This may cause a deviation from Beer's law resulting in a bending of the linear plot as shown in Figure 4–4.

Deviations from Beer's law may be caused by changes in instrument functions or chemical reactions. Instrument deviation is commonly a result of the finite band pass of the filter or monochromator. Beer's law assumes monochromatic radiation, but truly monochromatic radiation is best achieved using only unique line emission sources. If absorptivity is constant over the instrument band pass, then Beer's law is followed within close limits.

Deviations from Beer's law become apparent at higher concentration, i.e., higher absorbance. In Figure 4–4, the curved line bends toward the concentration axis as opacity is approached. This lack of adherence to Beer's law in a negative direction is undesirable because of the somewhat large increase in the relative concentration error.

Deviation from Beer's law can occur with shifts or changes in chemical or physical equilibrium involving the absorbing species. Changes in solution pH, ionic strength and temperature can result in such deviations.

Components of a Spectrophotometer

A typical photometer or spectrophotometer contains six basic components in either a single or double beam configuration. The six components include: (1) a stable source of radiant energy; (2) a filter that isolates a specific region of the electromagnetic spectrum; (3) a sample holder; (4) a radiation detector; (5) a signal processor and (6) a readout device. Each component of a typical photometer is shown in Figure 4–5.

The following steps outline the function of each component in any absorption-type photometer as it detects light and provides information to the operator.

1. The light source provides the energy that the sample will modify or attenuate by absorption. The light is polychromatic, i.e., all visible wavelengths present.
2. A wavelength selector or filter isolates a portion of the spectrum emitted by the source and focuses it on the sample.
3. The sample in a suitable container, e.g., cuvet, absorbs a fraction of the incident light and transmits the remainder.
4. The light that passes through the cuvet and sample strikes the cathode of a photodetector and generates an electrical signal.
5. The electrical signal is processed electronically, e.g., amplified, digitized.
6. The processed signal is electronically coupled to the display unit, e.g., LED, X–Y strip chart recorder, meter.

Radiant Energy Sources

Radiant energy sources or lamps provide polychromatic light and must generate sufficient radiant energy or power to measure the analyte of interest. A regulated power supply is required to provide a stable and constant source of voltage for the lamp. Radiant energy sources are of two types: *continuum* and *line*. A continuum source emits radiation that changes in intensity very slowly as a function of wavelength. Line sources emit a limited number of discrete lines or bands of radiation, each of which spans a limited range of wavelengths.

Continuum sources find wide applications in the laboratory. Examples of continuum sources include tungsten, deuterium and xenon. For testing in the visible region of the EMS tungsten or tungsten–halogen lamps are widely used. The filament in the tungsten–halogen lamp is maintained at a higher temperature than in the normal tungsten lamp. This takes advantage of the Wien and Sefan relationship to provide a source with a maximum wavelength near the center of the visible spectrum (whiter) and with a greater energy output (brighter). Introducing a halogen gas into the lamp envelope counteracts the problem of increased atom vaporization from the high-temperature filament.

The deuterium lamp is routinely used to provide ultraviolet (UV) radiation in analytical spectrometers. The voltage applied is typically about 100 volts, which gives the electrons enough energy to excite the deuterium atoms in a low-pressure gas to emit photons across the full UV range.

The strong atomic interaction in a high-pressure xenon discharge lamp produces a continuous source of radiation, which covers both the UV and visible range. The discharge light is normally pulsed for short periods with a frequency that determines the average intensity of the light from the source and also its lifetime.

In atomic emission line sources, the electrons move between atomic energy levels. If the atom is free of any interaction with other atoms, the amount of energy liberated can be very precise, and all of the photons share a very clearly defined wavelength. This is the characteristic sharp 'line' emission from an electronic discharge in a low-pressure gas. Line sources that emit a few discrete lines find wide use in atomic absorption, molecular and fluorescent spectroscopy. Mercury and sodium vapor lamps provide sharp lines in the ultraviolet and visible regions and are used in several spectrophotometers. For atomic absorption spectroscopy applications, the hollow cathode lamp provides atomic emission from free metal atoms by using the heat of a gaseous discharge (e.g., in neon) to vaporize metal atoms into the discharge. Typically, each lamp is specific to a particular metal. However, some lamps use two, three or more metals, although the emission from each of these is reduced.

A laser source is very useful in analytic instrumentation because of its high intensity, narrow bandwidth, and the coherent nature of its outputs. Several specific uses include high-resolution spectroscopy, in kinetic studies of processes with lifetimes in the range of 10^{-9} to 10^{-12} s, in the detection and determination of extremely small concentrations of species in the atmosphere, and in the induction of isotopically selective reactions.

Wavelength Selectors

A critical component of all spectrometers is the device used to select the appropriate wavelength. There are several types of wavelength selectors including filters, prisms, grating monochromators and recently holographic gratings. The quality of these selectors is described by their nominal wavelength, spectral bandwidths and bandpass. *Nominal wavelength* represents the wavelength in nanometers at peak transmittance. Spectral

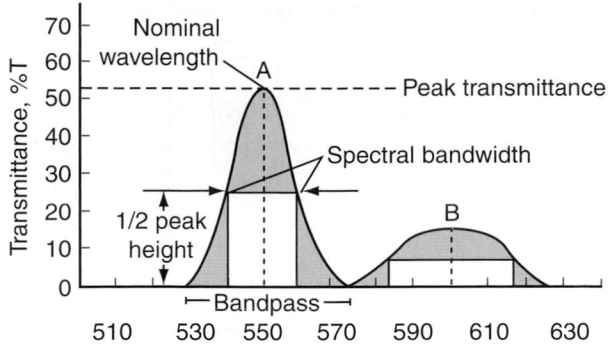

Figure 4–6 Comparison of spectral characteristics of two types of filters: A, interference filter and B, absorption filter. The spectral bandwidth of filter A is much less than filter B and therefore allows fewer wavelengths of light through.

bandwidth is the range of wavelengths above one-half peak transmittance. It is sometimes called the half power point or full width at half peak maximum (FWHM). The total range of wavelengths transmitted is the *bandpass*. Figure 4–6, summarizes these characteristics of wavelength selectors. This figure also summarizes the difference in wavelength selectivity between interference (left) and absorbance filters (right) as we now discuss.

Filters

An important component of the spectrophotometer is the wavelength filter. Its purpose is to deliver monochromatic light, or at least as narrow a range of wavelengths of light as possible, to the sample or to the photodetector. Remember, the purpose of absorption spectroscopy is to detect how much light is absorbed by the sample. This is measured as the absorbance and is directly proportional to the concentration of the sample (see Beer's law above). The percent transmittance is the ratio of the amount of light transmitted through the sample to the amount of light transmitted in the absence of the sample (e.g., buffer or solvent without the sample). Theoretically, it should be possible to determine this ratio without any filter at all. However, under these circumstances, most of the light that enters the sample in the cuvet will not be absorbed so that, to determine absorbance, it would be necessary to measure a small difference between two large numbers, i.e., the amount of light transmitted in the absence (control) and presence of the sample. Therefore, to obviate this condition, it becomes necessary to filter out as much 'extraneous' light as possible to enable accurate measurements of absorbance.

There are two approaches to filtering light waves. The first is to limit the wavelengths of light that enter the sample with appropriate filters, so-called pre-sample filters. The second is to allow multi-wavelength light to pass through the sample and then to break up this light into its component wavelengths using a high-resolution prism, and focus each of these component wavelengths on specific detectors, essentially one for each of the component wavelengths. If a sample absorbs light at one wavelength, then the ratio of the light transmittance of this wavelength of the sample to that for the control can be used to compute the percent transmittance and absorbance. This arrangement is termed post-sample filtering.

Pre-Sample Filters (Bender, 1987). There are fundamentally two types of these filters: absorption and interference filters. Absorption filters simply absorb regions of the electromagnetic spectrum and only allow a limited domain of this spectrum to pass through to the sample cuvet. The simplest sort of absorption filters consist of different forms of glass. One form of glass only allows transmission of wavelengths of light of over 400 nm while a second form allows transmission only of light of wavelengths under 600 nm. If both glasses are arranged serially, they allow for transmission of light of wavelengths of only between 400–600 nm, with a peak at 500 nm. As a refinement of this approach, the older spectrophotometers utilize colored glass or transparent plastic materials. These colors are arranged in a circle or wheel so that light of a relatively narrow range of wavelengths is transmitted when each colored sector is in the light path. For example, if light in the green portion of the visible spectrum is desired, the wheel is turned so that the green filter is placed in the light path. The spectral bandwidth of these absorption filters ranges from about 30–50 nm (Fig. 4–6).

This bandwidth is rather large but is quite adequate for determining the concentration of compounds in solution; absorbance filters are less adequate for scanning the absorption spectra of individual compounds

and macromolecules or for accurately determining low concentrations of molecules. To achieve the latter goals, it becomes necessary to use interference filters.

In the simplest interference filter, light on the path to the sample cuvet enters a magnesium fluoride chamber that is coated with micro-mirrors on the interior. As shown in Figure 4–7A, light enters evenly spaced ports or slits on the left. Only light that enters each slit can continue; the rest is absorbed by the chamber. Light entering a slit, at an angle to the horizontal, travels across the chamber and is reflected back to the opposite wall. In Figure 4–7A, if the path length ab equals bc, and the path length equals the desired wavelength of the light, it can be shown from the theory of optics that the light whose wavelength equals that of the path length or integral multiples of this path length will undergo constructive interference (i.e., the waves will add to one another exactly) with incoming light at slits above it. For example, in Figure 4–7A, light of wavelength L = ab, reflected from b to c, will be exactly in phase with light of wavelength L or integral multiples of L, entering the slit at c; all other wavelengths will destructively interfere with light entering slit c. The light is then reflected again at c to d and back again to e where, again, it will add to (constructively interfere with) only light waves of the same wavelength or integral multiples of it. Eventually, only light at the desired wavelength will be transmitted through the opposite wall at slits f and h.

It is important to note that, since integral multiples of the wavelengths of incident light will constructively interfere with the transmitted light in the chamber, more than one wavelength of light can be transmitted from the chamber. The actual quantitative relationship between the wavelengths (L) transmitted by the chamber, the angle of incidence, q, of the light entering a slit, the refractive index, R, of MgF_2 (1.38) and the distance, d, across the chamber, is:

$$ML = 2dR\sin(q) \tag{4–9A}$$

M is any integer. Note that this equation predicts that for any given distance, d, many wavelengths, of integral multiples to the fundamental wavelength where M = 1, can be transmitted. In practice, many of these other wavelengths can be excluded by using such techniques as placing the appropriate glass filters in series with the interference chamber.

The above arrangement successfully transmits (close to) monochromatic light at a particular wavelength. However, it does not allow for scanning of wavelengths to obtain the absorption spectra of different samples. To accomplish this, another, similar arrangement is used. In this case, however, advantage is taken of another principle from the theory of optics, the principle of light diffraction. As shown in Figure 4–7B, when monochromatic light is allowed to enter two slits on one surface of a chamber, very much like the one shown in Figure 4–7A except that there is no material (MgF_2) in the chamber, the two light waves interfere with one another such that if a screen is placed on the opposite surface of the chamber, there will be discrete regions of light and dark bands (Bender, 1987). The light bands are from light waves that have added constructively to one another and are transmitted while the dark bands are from destructive interference of the light waves and no light waves are transmitted. The position of the bands and distance between the bands depends on the wavelength of the light that enters the two apertures and on the angle of incidence of both beams. Since, for a given angle of incidence, the position of the light bands for transmitted monochromatic light depends exclusively on the wavelength of the light, if exit apertures are placed on the opposite surface only where the light bands occur for light of a desired wavelength, only light of that wavelength will be emitted from the chamber. This effect can be enhanced by placing multiple entry apertures next to one another in a sawtooth or grating pattern such that adjacent apertures are at a fixed distance, d, from one another as shown in Figure 4–7B.

Now, polychromatic light is composed of multiple different monochromatic wavelengths of light. When polychromatic light is allowed to pass through the two apertures, as in Figure 4–7B, each of the wavelengths will constructively and destructively interfere with itself as described above. Two different wavelengths of light will interfere only destructively with one another unless they are integral multiples of one another as discussed in the case of the MgF_2 chamber above. This allows us to 'trap' the light of the desired wavelength by placing the exit apertures where the light bands are known to occur on the opposite surface for that monochromatic wavelength. A limiting factor for selecting truly monochromatic light is the size of the aperture that can allow some 'stray' light from adjacent light bands for very close wavelengths to exit.

As with the MgF_2 interference chamber described above, another source of contaminating light can occur from light of wavelengths that are integral multiples of the desired wavelength. The relationship that

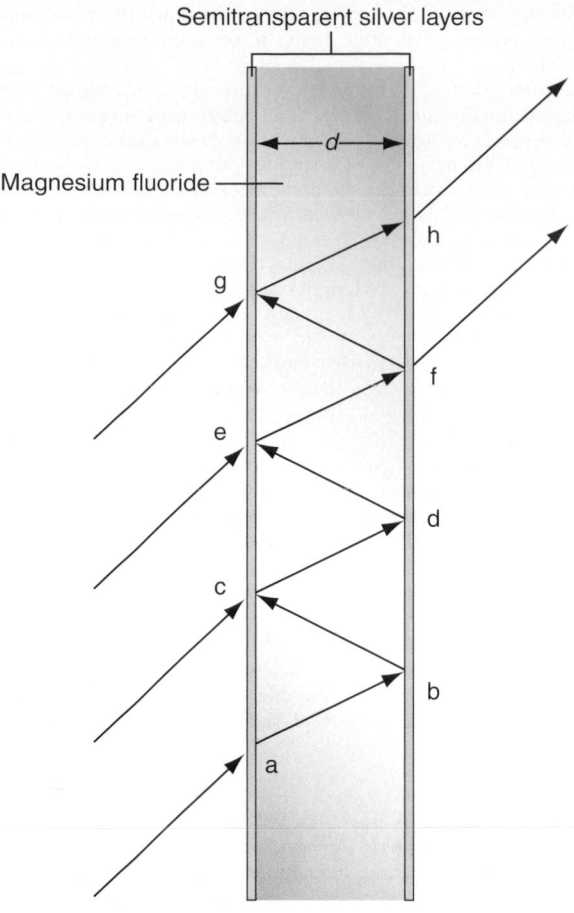

Semitransparent silver layers

Magnesium fluoride

A

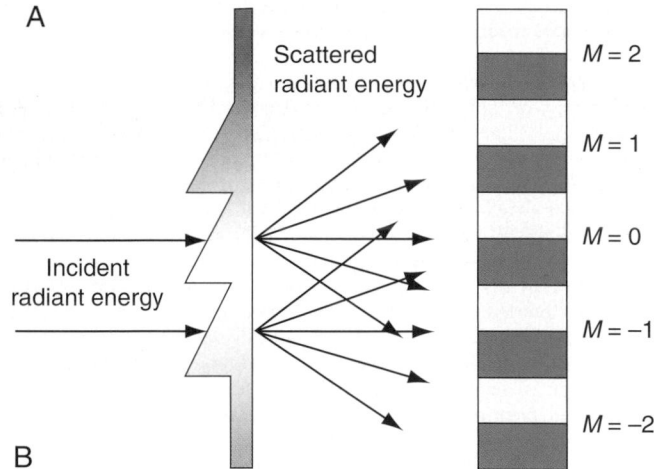

Scattered
radiant energy

Incident
radiant energy

$M = 2$

$M = 1$

$M = 0$

$M = -1$

$M = -2$

B

Figure 4–7 *A*, An interference MgF_2 filter. Light enters the filter at regularly spaced apertures at the same angle of incidence at each aperture. Going from the bottom of the figure, the light entering at a travels to b where there is a mirror reflecting it to c. Path lengths ab = bc. If these are, in turn, equal to the desired wavelength (or integral multiples of it), light of the desired wavelength arriving at c will be exactly in phase with light from the light source of that wavelength and will result in constructive interference. It will be out of phase with all other wavelengths and will therefore destructively interact with them. This summation process takes place multiple times until only light of the desired wavelength escapes through exit apertures such as at f and h (after Bender, 1987). *B*, A diffraction filter. When light enters multiple apertures, as in part *A*, each of which is equidistant from its two neighbors, light of each of the wavelengths interferes both constructively and destructively with itself giving rise to light (yellow) and dark (blue) bands or fringes that can be observed on a screen. The position and spacing of these bands depend only on the wavelength and the angle of incidence. As shown in this figure, if apertures are placed only at the points where light (yellow) fringes occur in the figure, only light of a specific wavelength will pass through this exit aperture.

describes the wavelength as a function of the distance is similar to that for the MgF_2 chamber, i.e.,

$$ML = d\sin(q) \tag{4–9B}$$

Here, however, d is the distance between two adjacent entry slits on the near surface (towards the light source), *not* the distance across the chamber as with the MgF_2 chamber. Note that for a given distance, d, and angle of incidence, q, there are multiple solutions to this equation. For example, if the desired wavelength is 800 nm, $d\sin(q) = 800$. But this is for $M = 1$, $L = 800$ nm. Another solution is $M = 2$, $L = 400$ nm, and another $M = 3$, $L = 266.67$ nm, etc. As discussed for the MgF_2 chamber, these other wavelengths can be filtered out by the use of appropriate glass or other filters.

Note that the system shown in Figure 4–7B allows for continuous scanning of the absorption spectrum for any analyte. Wavelengths can be continuously changed, most often using electronic devices, by changing the position of the aperture on the exit side of the chamber or by changing the angle of incidence of the entering light by altering the angle of the near surface of the chamber. Filters that have this capacity are called monochromators. Both interference systems in Figure 4–7 have spectral bandwidths of approximately 1.5% of the wavelength at peak transmittance, much lower than the absorption filters as illustrated in Figure 4–6.

Post-Sample Filters. A different approach to obtaining monochromatic light and an accurate determination of absorbance is simply to allow the light to pass through the sample unfiltered. The light is then passed through a prism where it is broken into its constituent wavelengths. The action of a prism depends on the refraction of radiation by the prism material. The dispersive power depends on the variation of the refractive index with wavelength. A ray of radiation that enters a prism at an angle of incidence is bent toward the normal (vertical to the prism face), and at the prism–air interface it is bent away from the vertical. As we describe in the section on photomultipliers below, each wavelength is focused onto a photodiode array such that each photodiode responds to only a specific set of wavelengths. The amount of transmitted light in the presence of the sample is compared with that in the absence of the sample. Photodiode arrays are examples of devices that convert photon energy into electrical currents in a system where photons excite the outer electrons in metal to move in the so-called conduction band generating a current.

Sample Containers (Cuvets)

Sample containers, i.e., cells or cuvets, are used to hold samples and must be made of material that is transparent to radiation in the spectral region of interest. In the ultraviolet region (below 350 nm) cuvets are made from fused silica or quartz. Silicate glasses can be used in the region between 350–2000 nm. Plastic containers have also found application in the visible region. Generally, the path length of cuvets is 1 cm, although much smaller path lengths are used in automated systems. However, to increase sensitivity, some cuvets are designed to have path lengths of 10 cm, increasing the absorbance for a given solution by a factor of 10 (Beer's law; Equation 4–7).

Many double beam spectrophotometers are designed with two cuvet holders; one for the sample and the other for the solvent. If two cuvets are used, they should be optically matched for more accurate results. Matched pairs are obtainable from a manufacturer, but their optical performance should be verified prior to use by running identical samples in each cell. One cell should then be reserved for the sample solution and the other for solvent. Cells should be scrupulously cleaned before and after each use.

Photodetectors

It is necessary to determine how much light passes through the sample in the cuvet. To accomplish this task, advantage is taken of the photoelectric effect that forms the basis of the quantum theory. Photons of specific wavelength excite the outer shell electrons of metals at their resonance frequencies to high energy states in which they move through the so-called 'conduction band,' in which electrons move through the outer shells of the metal, thereby causing a current. This current, the magnitude of which is directly related to the intensity of the incident light, can then be detected and digitized.

Photomultiplier Tubes (PMT). Perhaps the most common type of photon detector is the photomultiplier. Photomultiplier tubes are commonly used when radiant power is very low, which is characteristic of very low analyte concentrations. The operating principle is similar to the phototube with one significant difference, which is that a PMT has multiple dynodes that result in 10^6–10^7 electrons passing through the anode. The response of the PMT begins when incoming photons strike a photocathode. Electrons are ejected from the surface of the photocathode. A

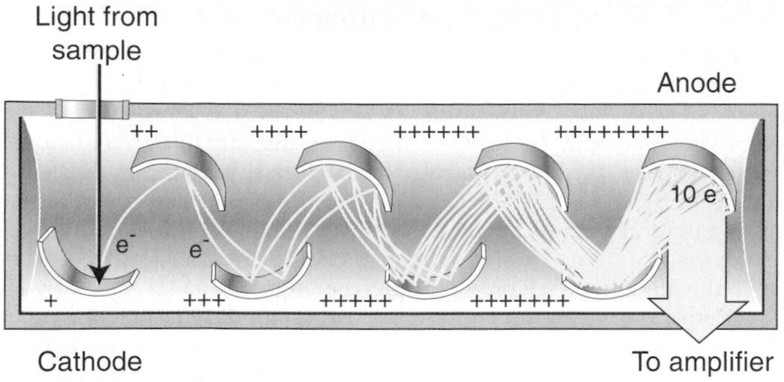

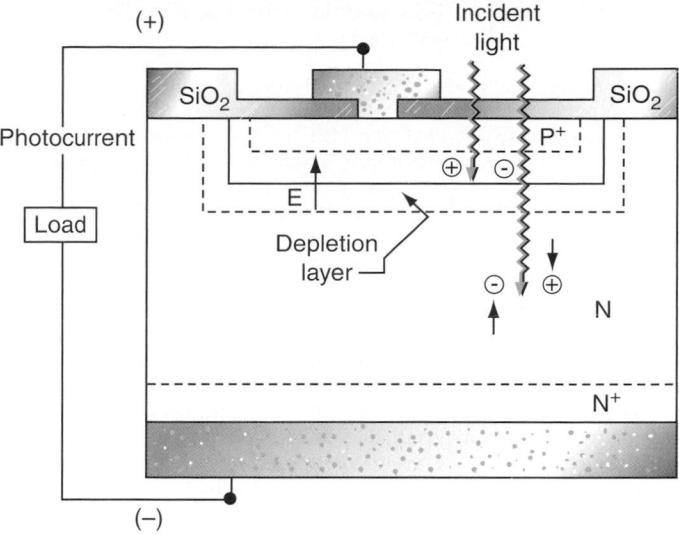

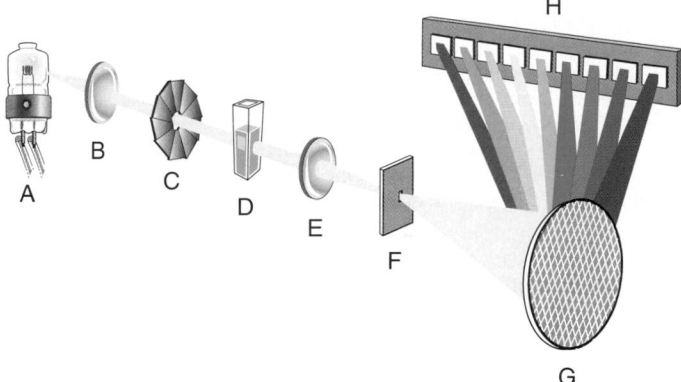

Figure 4–8 Schematic of a photomultiplier tube. In this diagram a tenfold amplification of the initial signal is produced at the anode. (Redrawn from Simonson MG: *In* Kaplan LA, Pesce AJ [eds]: Nonisotopic Alternatives to Radioimmunoassay. New York, Marcel Dekker, 1981.)

Figure 4–9 Schematic of a semiconductor photodiode used as a detector in many spectrometers.

Figure 4–10 Photodiode array. A, lamp; B, lens; C, shutter; D, cell; E, lens; F, slit; G, grating; H, photodiode array

PMT has several additional electrodes called dynodes, each having a potential that is approximately 90 V higher than the previous one. Upon striking a dynode, each photoelectron causes emission of several additional electrons; these, in turn, are accelerated toward a second dynode, which is 90 V more positive than the previous dynode, which further amplifies the incident signal. This process, shown in Figure 4–8, continues within the PMT until all the electrons are collected at the anode where the resulting current is passed to an electronic amplifier.

Photomultiplier tubes are highly sensitive to ultraviolet and visible radiation. They also have very fast response time. These tubes are limited to measuring low-power radiation because intense light causes irreversible damage to the photoelectric surface.

Photovoltaic or Barrier Layer Cell.
A variant method of detecting photon-induced current is the photovoltaic cell. This is a basic phototransducer that is used for detecting and measuring radiation in the visible region. This cell typically has a maximum sensitivity at about 550 nm and the response falls off to about 10% of the maximum at 350 and 750 nm. It consists of a flat copper or iron electrode upon which is deposited a layer of semiconductor material, such as selenium. The outer surface of the semiconductor is coated with a thin transparent metallic film of gold or silver, which serves as the second or collector electrode. When radiation of sufficient energy reaches the semiconductor, covalent bonds are broken, with the result that conduction electrons and holes are formed. The electrons migrate toward the metallic film and the holes toward the base upon which the semiconductor is deposited. The liberated electrons are free to migrate through the external circuit to interact with these holes. The result is an electrical current of a magnitude that is proportional to the number of photons that strike the semiconductor surface and a photocurrent that is directly proportional to the intensity of the radiation that strikes the cells.

These types of photodetectors are rugged, low cost and require no external source of electrical energy. Low sensitivity and fatigue are two distinct disadvantages of these cells. For routine analyses at optimum wavelengths, these photocells provide reliable analytical data.

Vacuum Phototubes.
A vacuum phototube has a semicylindrical cathode and a wire anode sealed inside an evacuated transparent envelope. The concave surface of the electrode supports a layer of photoemissive material that tends to emit electrons when it is irradiated. When a potential is applied across the electrode, the emitted electrons flow to the wire anode generating a photocurrent that is generally about one-tenth as great as the photocurrent associated with photovoltaic cells for a given radiant intensity. The number of electrons ejected from a photoemissive surface is directly proportional to the radiant power of the beam that strikes the surface. All of the electrons are collected at the anode. Several types of photoemissive surfaces are used in commercial phototubes. These include; (1) highly sensitive bi-alkali materials made up of potassium, cesium and antimony, (2) red sensitive material using multialkalis for example Na/K/Cs/Sb, (3) ultraviolet sensitive with UV transparent windows; and (4) flat response type substances using Ga/As compositions.

Silicon Diode Transducers.
Silicon diode transducers are more sensitive than vacuum phototubes but less sensitive than the PMTs described above. Photodiodes have spectral ranges from about 190–1100 nm. These devices contain positively (p) and negatively (n) charged semiconductive materials adjoining one another embedded on a silicon chip. A power supply is attached to this arrangement so that its positive pole connects to the *n*-type and its negative pole to the *p*-type material. This arrangement results in a depletion layer that reduces the conductance of the junction to nearly zero. If radiation is allowed to

impinge on the chip, holes and electrons formed in the depletion layer are swept through the device to produce a current that is proportional to radiant power (Skoog, 1998). This process is shown in Figure 4–9.

Multichannel Photon Transducers.
In the discussion of post-sample filters, it was noted that unfiltered light emerging from the sample could be broken up into its constituent wavelengths using prisms; these different wavelengths are then directed to electronic detectors such that the intensity of light of each of the constituent wavelengths can be quantitated. Here, we describe some of these multiwavelength photodetectors.

A multichannel transducer consists of an array of small photoelectric-sensitive elements arranged either linearly or in a two-dimensional pattern on a single semiconductor chip. The chip, which is usually silicon and typically has dimensions of a few millimeters on a side, also contains electronic circuitry that makes it possible to determine the electrical output signal from each of the photosensitive elements either sequentially or simultaneously. The alignment of a multichannel transducer is generally in the focal plane of a spectrometer so that various elements of the dispersed spectrum can be converted and measured simultaneously. There are several types of multichannel transducers currently used, and they include (1) photodiode arrays (PDAs), (2) charge-injection devises (CIDs) and (3) charge-coupled devices (CCDs).

Photodiode Arrays. By using the modern fabrication techniques of microelectronics, it is now possible to produce a linear (one-dimensional) array of several hundred photodiodes set side-by-side on a single integrated circuit (IC), or 'chip,' Figure 4–10. Each diode is capable of recording the intensity at one point along the line, and together they provide a linear profile of the light variation along the array.

A multiplex method is used to sort all of the signals received from the PDA. It records each signal individually, and then feeds the signals sequentially to a single amplifier. The output of the PDA is a histogram profile, along the array, of the charge leaked by each photodiode. This mirrors the variation of light intensity across the array. Thus, the PDA detection occurs in three main stages:

1. initialization
2. accumulation of charge at each pixel-integration time
3. read-out signals.

In comparison to the PMT, the PDA has a lower dynamic range and higher noise. It is most useful as a simultaneous multichannel detector (Skoog, 1998).

Charge-transfer devices. Recent developments in solid-state detection techniques have now produced very effective two-dimensional array detectors that operate on a charge-transfer process, as an alternative to photodiodes. The term 'charge-transfer device' (CTD) is a generic term that describes a detection system in which a photon, striking the IC semi-conductor material, releases electrons from their bound state into a mobile state. The released charge, consisting of negative electrons and positive holes then drifts to, and accumulates at, surface electrodes. An array of these surface electrodes divides the detector into separate, light-sensitive, 'pixels.' The charge that accumulated at each electrode is proportional to the integrated light intensity falling on that particular pixel.

There are two distinct classes of CTDs and they are charge-injection devices (CIDs) and charge-couple devices (CCDs). In a CCD, all of the charge packets are moved 'in-step' along the array row from one pixel to the next as in a 'bucket chain.' At the end of the row, the charge packets are fed sequentially into an *on-chip* low noise amplifier, which then converts the charge into a voltage signal. The overall signal profile across the two-dimensional array is recorded one row at a time, thus giving a series of voltage signals corresponding to all of the pixels in the detection area.

In a CID, the charge accumulated in each pixel can be measured independently and nondestructively by using a network of 'sensing' electrodes, which can monitor the presence of the accumulated charge. This is an important factor that differentiates CID systems from CCD and PDA systems in which the whole of the detection area is 'read' destructively in a single process.

Signal processors and readout

The processing of an electrical signal received from a transducer is accomplished by a device that amplifies, rectifies AC to DC (or the reverse), alters the phase of the signal and filters it to remove unwanted components. In addition, the signal processor may need to perform mathematical operations on the signal such as differential calculations, integration, or conversion to a logarithm. Several readout devices have been used and include digital meters, d'Arsonval meters, recorders, light emitting diodes (LEDs), cathode-ray tubes (CRTs) and liquid crystal displays (LCDs).

Quality Assurance in Spectrophotometry

There are several photometric parameters that must be monitored periodically by the users. Monitoring these parameters is mandated by most regulatory agencies and accrediting organizations. The parameters routinely monitored include:

- wavelength or photometric accuracy
- absorbance check
- linearity
- stray light.

Accuracy is the closeness of a measurement to its true value. Wavelength accuracy implies that a photometer is measuring at the wavelength that it is set to. Photometric accuracy can be assessed quite easily using special glass-type optical filters. Two examples of commonly used filters include didymium and holmium oxide. Didymium glass has a broad absorption peak around 600 nm and holmium oxide has multiple absorption peaks with a sharp peak occurring at 360 nm.

An absorbance check is performed using glass filters or solutions that have known absorbance values for a specific wavelength. The operator simply measures the absorbance of each solution at a specified wavelength and compares the results with the stated values. Each user should establish a tolerance for the measurements based upon accepted criteria.

Linearity is defined as the ability of a photometric system to yield a linear relationship between the radiant power incident upon its detector and the concentration, i.e., Beer's law. The linearity of a spectrometer can be determined using optical filters or solutions that have known absorbance values for a given wavelength. Linearity measurements should be evaluated for both slope and intercept.

Stray light is described as any light that impinges upon the detector that does not originate from the polychromatic light source. Stray light can have a significant impact on any measurement made. Stray light effect can be evaluated by using special cutoff filters.

Types of photometric instruments

There are several instrument designs and configurations used for absorption photometry. Each has unique terminology associated with its design. The terminology is not universal among users but is presented here as a guide. A *spectroscope* is an optical instrument used for visual identification of atomic emission lines. It has a monochromator, usually a prism or diffraction grating, in which the exit slit, is replaced by an eyepiece that can be moved along the focal plane. The wavelength of an emission line can then be determined from the angle between the incident and dispersed beam when the line is centered on the eyepiece.

A *colorimeter* uses the human eye as the detector. The user compares the observed color of the unknown sample to a standard or a series of colored standards of known concentrations. *Photometers* consist of a light source, a filter and a photoelectric transducer as well as a signal processor and readout. Some manufacturers used the term colorimeter or photoelectric colorimeters for photometers. These photometers used filters for isolation of specific wavelengths and not gratings or prisms.

A *spectrometer* is an instrument that provides information about the intensity of radiation as a function of wavelength or frequency. Spectrophotometers are spectrometers equipped with one or more exit slits and photoelectron transducers that permit the determination of the ratio of the power of two beams as a function of wavelength as in absorption spectroscopy. Most spectrophotometers use a grating monochromator to break up the light into a spectrum as discussed above in the section on pre-sample filters.

Single-beam spectrophotometers are the simplest types of absorption spectrometer. These instruments are designed to make one measurement at a time at one specified wavelength. In using a single-beam instrument, the absorption maximum of the analyte must be known in advance. The wavelength is then set to this value. The reference material (solvent blank) is positioned into the radiation path, and the instrument is adjusted to read 0%T when a shutter is placed so as to block all radiation from the detector, and to read 100%T when the shutter is removed. After these adjustments have been made, the sample is placed in the path, the absorbance is measured and the concentration is determined using Beer's law or by the use of either a calibration curve for the material or proper algebraic methods.

A double-beam spectrophotometer splits or chops the monochromatic beam of radiation into two components. One beam passes through the sample and the other through a reference solution or blank. In this design, the radiant power in the reference beam varies with the source energy, monochromator transmission, reference material transmission, and detector response, making the difference between the sample and reference beam largely a function of the sample. The output of the reference beam can be kept constant, and the absorbance of the sample can be recorded directly as the electrical output of the sample beam.

There are two fundamental instrument designs for double-beam spectrophotometers, (1) double-beam in space and (2) double-beam in time. A double-beam in space design uses two photodetectors, one for the sample beam and the other for the reference beam. The two signals generated are directed to a differential amplifier, which then passes on the difference between the signals to the readout device. A schematic of the double-beam in space system is shown in Figure 4–11.

A double-beam in time instrument uses one photodetector and alternately passes the monochromatic radiation through the sample cuvet and then to the reference cuvet using a *chopper*. A chopper is the term used for a device such as rotating sector mirror that breaks up or rotates the

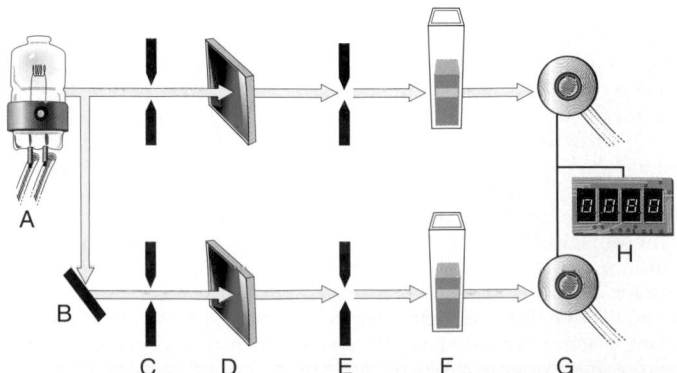

Figure 4–11 Double-beam in space design of spectrophotometer. A, exciter lamp; B, mirror; C, entrance slits; D, monochromators; E, exit slits; F, cuvets; G, photodetectors; H, light-emitting diode (LED).

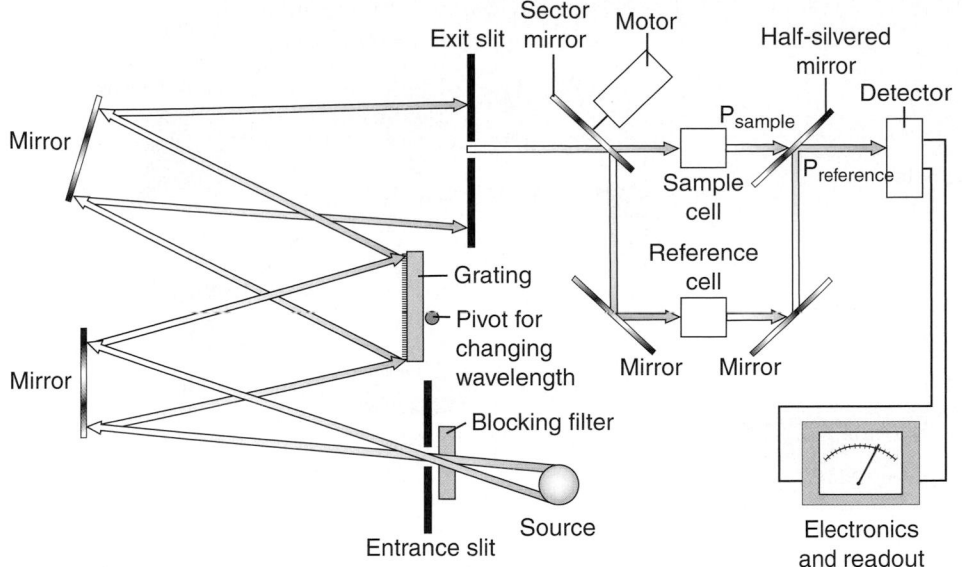

Figure 4–12 Double-beam in time design of spectrophotometer.

radiation beams. Each beam, consisting of a pulse of radiation separated in time by a dark interval, is then directed onto an appropriate detector. A schematic of the double-beam in time system is shown in Figure 4–12.

A scanning double-beam system includes a double beam spectrophotometer and a recorder that can provide an X–Y plot of absorbance versus wavelength for given test sample. This type of configuration is ideal for determining the wavelength spectrum of an analyte in solution. The spectrophotometer has an automatically driven wavelength cam that can rotate at a predetermined speed. The recorder can be calibrated to the wavelength of the monochromator to facilitate the identification of each peak maxima.

Reflectometry

Measurement of analytes in biological fluids using reflectometry has been used for decades. Two clinical applications include urine dipstick analysis and dry slide chemical analysis. The instruments used for these applications include a reflectometer. A reflectometer is a filter photometer that measures the quantity of light reflected by a liquid sample that has been dispensed onto a grainy or fibrous solid support.

There are two types of reflectance, (1) specular and (2) diffuse. Specular reflectance occurs on a polished surface where the angle of incidence of the radiant energy is equal to the angle of reflection. Polished surfaces, for example a mirror, are used to direct and manage radiant energy but are not used to determine concentration. Diffuse reflectance occurs on nonpolished surfaces i.e., grainy or fibrous surface as noted above. The reflected radiant energy tends to go in many directions. Diffuse reflection occurs within the layers and depends on the properties and characteristics of the layers themselves. A colored substance absorbs the wavelength of its color and reflects all other wavelength at many different angles. Therefore the amount of a substance present can be measured as an indirect function of the reflected light.

A typical reflectometer used in a clinical laboratory detects only a constant fraction of the diffuse reflected light. Thus the reflectance of a sample is represented by:

$$R_{(\text{diffuse reflectance})} = \frac{R'_{(\text{fraction of diffuse reflectance of sample})}}{R'_{(\text{fraction of diffuse reflectance of a standard})}} \qquad (4\text{–}10A)$$

The amount of light reflected by a solution dispensed onto a white granular or grainy surface is inversely related to the concentration of the samples as give by:

$$R_{\text{density}} = -\log\left(\frac{R_{\text{sample}} - R_{\text{black}}}{R_{\text{standard}}}\right) \times R_{\text{white}} \qquad (4\text{–}10B)$$

where:
R_{density} is the corrected reflectance density of the sample
R_{sample} is the measured reflectance of the sample
R_{black} is the reflectance of a black reference
R_{white} is the reflectance of a white reference
R_{standard} is the reflectance of a standard solution.
The ideal reflectance value of a pure white standard of ceramic material

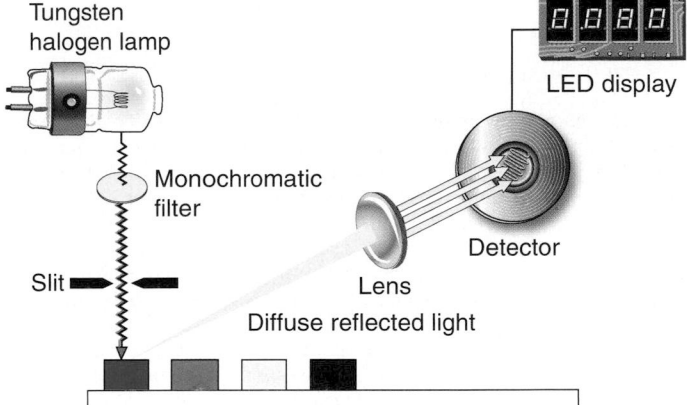

Figure 4–13 Components in a typical reflectometer used to measure analytes on urine dipstick. The different colored blocks represent different tests performed in urinalysis; the blue represents the quantitation of analyte using reflectance, i.e., the reflectance of light focused on the sample and reflected at an angle (yellow beam), where it is detected.

is *one*, i.e., all light is reflected and conversely the ideal reflectance value of pure black material is *zero* i.e. all light is absorbed.

The relationship of percent reflectance and concentration of an analyte is nonlinear. Several algorithms have been developed for linearizing this relationship. The specific algorithm used depends upon the reflection characteristics of the composition material of the pad or film, the nature of the ilumination and the geometry of the instrument.

Reflectometers

The components of a reflectometer are very similar to those of a photometer as shown in Figure 4–13. A tungsten-quartz halide lamp serves as a source of polychromatic radiation. A monochromator e.g. stationary filter or filter wheel for multiple analytes is used to isolate the wavelength of interest. Next, the monochromatic light passes through a slit and is directed onto the surface of urine dipstick pad or dry slide depending upon the instrumentation being used. Solid-state photodiodes are typically used to detect the reflected radiant energy. Special optical devices, for example fiber optics or ellipsoidal mirrors, may be used to direct radiant energy onto the detector. A computer or microprocessor is used to convert nonlinear reflectance signals into direct readout concentration units.

Molecular Luminescence Spectroscopy (Fluorometry)

Principle. Luminescence is based on an energy exchange process that occurs when certain compounds absorb electromagnetic radiation, become excited and return to an energy level lower than or equal to their original level. Because some energy is lost before emission from the excited state by

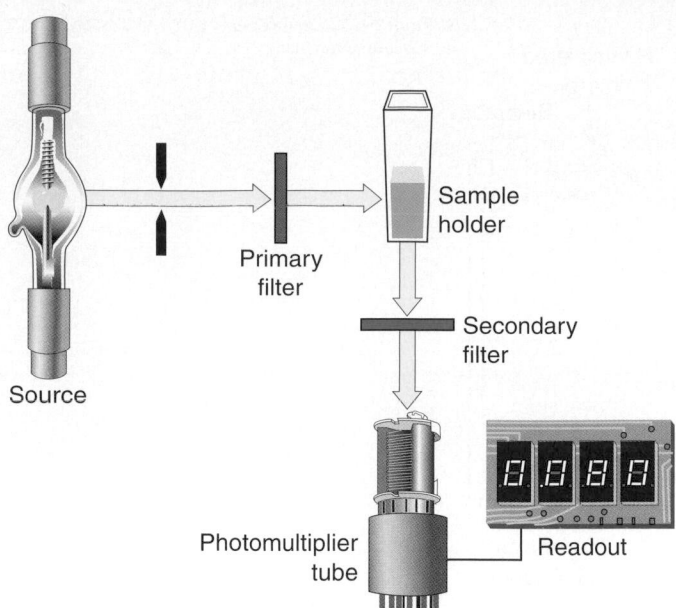

Figure 4–14 Components of a fluorometer. (From Bishop ML, Duben-Engelkirk JL, Fody EP: Clinical Chemistry: Principles, Procedures, Correlations. Philadelphia, JB Lippincott Company, 1992, with permission.)

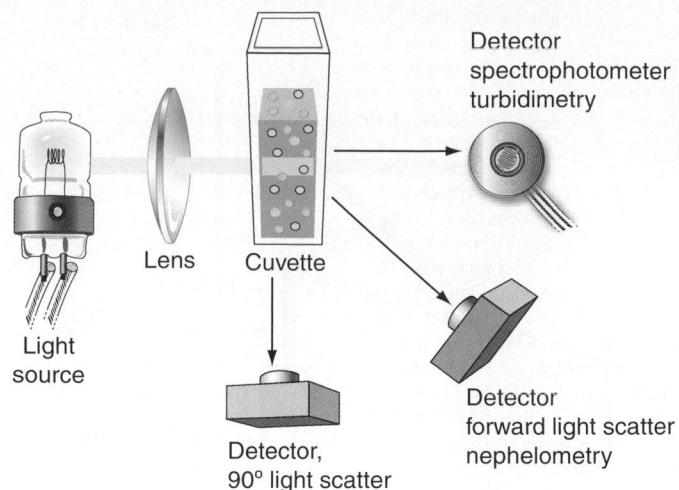

Figure 4–15 Optical arrangements of nephelometry and turbidimetry. Note that nephelometry detects (right-angle or forward) scattered light and turbidimetry measures a reduction of light transmitted in the forward direction. (Modified from Bishop ML, Duben-Engelkirk JL, Fody EP: Clinical Chemistry: Principles, Procedures, Correlations. Philadelphia, JB Lippincott Company, 1992, with permission.)

collision with the solvent or other molecules, the wavelength of the emitted light is longer than that of the exciting light. Most uncharged molecules contain even numbers of electrons in the ground state. The electrons fill molecular orbits in pairs with their spins in opposite directions. No electron energies can be detected by application of a magnetic field to such spin patterns, and this electronic state is called the singlet state. Similarly, if an electron becomes excited by electromagnetic radiation and its spin remains paired with the ground state, it creates a singlet excited state. The lifetime of the excited state is the average length of time the molecule remains excited before emission of light. For a singlet excited state, the lifetime of the excited state is on the order of 10^{-9} to 10^{-6} s. The light emission from a singlet excited state is called *fluorescence.* When the spins of the electrons in the excited state are unpaired, the electron energy levels will be split if a magnetic field is applied, and this electronic state is called a triplet state. Triplet state lifetimes range from 10^{-4} to 10 s (Willard, 1988). Light emission from an excited triplet state is called *phosphorescence.*

Luminescence is widely used because of its high sensitivity – the signal-to-noise ratio is very high, that is, the signal can be compared to nearly zero background noise. High specificity is a function of using two spectra, the excitation and emission spectra, and the possibility of measuring the lifetime of the fluorescent state. Two compounds that are excited at the same wavelength but emit at different wavelengths are readily differentiated with this technique.

Components of Fluorometers and Spectrophotofluorometers. Instruments designed for fluorescence measurement have the following basic components: a light source, an excitation (primary) monochromator, a cuvet, an emission (secondary) monochromator, and a photodetector (Fig. 4–14). The exciter lamp is a high-intensity light source such as a mercury vapor lamp or a xenon arc lamp. Simple instruments use mercury vapor lamps that do not require any special power supply. Mercury vapor lamps produce discrete and intense resonance lines that are not ideal for compounds with absorption bands at wavelengths not coinciding with these emission bands. For such compounds, xenon arc lamps producing an intense continuous spectrum between 300–1300 nm are appropriate. These lamps are used in nearly all commercial spectrophotofluorometers. In fluorescence measurements, the emitted light is detected at a right angle to the incident light to eliminate potential interference by the excitation signal. Phototubes or photomultiplier tubes (PMT) are required for fluorescence measurements because the signals are generally of low intensity. Newer fluorometers on the market today use diode-array and CTDs, which allow the rapid recording of both excitation and emission spectra and are particularly useful in chromatography and electrophoresis.

Time-resolved fluorescence assays minimize problems inherent in other fluorescent assays such as overlapping excitation or emission spectra of compounds present in the sample with the fluorophore. The label most commonly used is a chelate of europium (Eu^{3+}). Energy is absorbed by the organic ligand, leading to an excited state as the electrons migrate from the ground state singlet to the excited singlet state. The excitation may lead to any vibrational multiplet of the excited state S_1. The molecule rapidly returns to the lowest energy levels in S_1 by a nonradiative process. The energy is transferred to the metal ion, which becomes excited and subsequently emits characteristic radiation. The radiative transition of excited Eu^{3+} after an energy transfer from triplet state, results in an emission wavelength of 613 nm. The fluorescence lifetime of Eu^{3+} chelate is 10–1000 µs compared to nanoseconds for the most commonly used fluorophore. Therefore, Eu^{3+} with its longer emission lifetime makes it more attractive to use over a fluorophore like fluorescein with a lifetime of 4.5 ns. Time-resolved fluorescence instruments are similar to a typical fluorometer except the time-resolved fluorometers use a time-gated measure on only a portion of the total emission spectra.

Chemiluminescence applications have increased dramatically owing to the increased sensitivity over fluorescence. The primary application has been in the area of immunoassays where several chemiluminescence compounds have been used as antigen labels. Chemiluminescence differs from fluorescence and phosphorescence, in that the emission of light is created from a chemical or electrochemical reaction and not from absorption of electromagnetic energy. The chemical reaction yields an electronically excited compound that emits light as it returns to its ground state or that transfers its energy to another compound, which then produces emission. Chemiluminescence involves the oxidation of an organic compound, e.g., dioxetane, luminol, or acridinium ester, by an oxidant (hydrogen peroxide, hypochlorite, or oxygen). These oxidation reactions may occur in the presence of catalysts, such as enzymes (alkaline phosphatase, horseradish peroxidase, or microperoxidase), metal ions (Cu^{2+} or Fe^{3+} phthalocyanine complex), and hemin. The excited products formed in the oxidation reaction produce chemiluminescence on return to the singlet state. A luminometer is used to detect chemiluminescence; it contains a PMT that provides a very strong electrical output signal. A typical signal from a chemiluminescent compound rises rapidly with time and reaches a maximum when reagent and analyte are completely mixed. An exponential decay of the signal follows until baseline is reached.

Nephelometry and Turbidimetry

Nephelometry and turbidimetry are used to measure the concentration of large particles (such as antigen–antibody complexes, prealbumin and other serum proteins) that because of their size cannot be measured by absorption spectroscopy. Nephelometry detects light that is scattered at various angles; scattered light yields a small signal that must be amplified. In contrast, turbidimetry measures a reduction in light transmission due to particle formation; thus, it detects a small decrease in a large signal (Fig. 4–15).

Principle. Nephelometry and turbidimetry are based on the scattering of radiation by particles in suspension. When a collimated light beam strikes a particle in suspension, portions of the light are absorbed, reflected, scattered, and transmitted. Nephelometry is the measurement of the light scattered by a particulate solution. Three types of light scatters occur based on the relative size of the light wavelength (Gauldie, 1981). If the wavelength

(λ) of light is much larger than the diameter (d) of the particle ($d < 0.1\lambda$), the light scatter is symmetric around the particle. Minimum light scatter occurs at 90 degrees to the incident beam and was described by Rayleigh (Rayleigh, 1885). If the wavelength of light is much smaller than the particle diameter ($d > 0.1\lambda$), then the light scatters forward owing to the destructive out-of-phase backscatter, as described by the Mie theory. If the wavelength of light is approximately the same as the particle size, more light scatters in the forward direction than in other directions, as defined by the Rayleigh–Debye theory. A common application of nephelometry is the measurement of antigen–antibody reactions. Because most antigen–antibody complexes have a diameter of 250–1500 nm and the wavelengths used are 320–650 nm, light is scattered forward ((Rayleigh–Debye type).

Nephelometer. A typical nephelometer consists of a light source, a collimator, a monochromator, a sample cuvet, stray light trap, and a photodetector. Light scattered by particles is measured at an angle, typically 15–90 degrees to the beam incident on the cuvet (Fig. 4–15). Light scattering depends on the light wavelength and the particle size. For macromolecules with size close to or larger than the light wavelength, measurement of the forward light scatter increases the sensitivity of nephelometry. Light sources include a mercury-arc lamp, a tungsten-filament lamp, a light-emitting diode, and a laser.

Lasers produce stable, nearly ideal monochromatic light of narrow bandwidth and emit radiant energy that is coherent, parallel, and polarized. A laser beam can be maintained as a very slim cylinder only a few micrometers in cross-section. A typical helium–neon laser lamp consists of a helium-pumping electrode (cathode) and a hollow glass laser core surrounded by a laser plasma tube (anode). Both the plasma tube and the core are filled with free helium and neon gases. The electrical discharge between the cathode and the anode is confined to the hollow glass core to keep it concentrated for maximum energy transfer. Two mirrors are positioned at the ends of the laser tube. One of them is fully reflective and the other partially transparent. When the electrode is charged, the helium atoms are excited to a higher energy state and then transfer this energy to the neon atoms by collision. In turn, the excited neon atoms emit photons. Photons bounce back and forth between the two end mirrors, stimulating other atoms to emit further photons, resulting in an amplification process. The amplified light eventually emerges as a laser beam through the partially transparent mirror. With the high-intensity monochromatic beam, a substantial increase in sensitivity has been seen with lasers over conventional light sources. Disadvantages of laser sources include cost, safety and cooling requirements, and limited availability of wavelengths.

Turbidimetry. The measurement of the reduction in light transmission caused by particle formation is termed turbidimetry. Light transmitted in the forward direction is detected. The amount of light absorbed by a suspension of particles depends on the specimen concentration and on the particle size. Solutions requiring quantitation by turbidimetry are measured using visible photometers or visible spectrophotometers. Higher sensitivity has been achieved using photodetectors that can detect small changes in photon signals. Sensitivity comparable to nephelometry can be attained using low wavelengths and high-quality spectrophotometers. Many clinical applications exist for turbidimetry. Various microbiology analyzers measure turbidity of samples to detect bacterial growth in broth cultures. Turbidimetry is routinely used to measure the antibiotic sensitivities from such cultures. In coagulation analyzers, turbidimetric measurements detect clot formation in the sample cuvets. Turbidimetric assays have long been available in clinical chemistry to quantify protein concentration in biological fluids, such as urine and cerebrospinal fluid (CSF).

Refractometry

Refractometry is based on light refraction. When light passes from one medium into another, the light beam changes its direction at the boundary surface if its speed in the second medium is different from that in the first. The angle created by the bending of the light is called the *critical angle*. The ability of a substance to bend light is called *refractivity*. The refractivity of a liquid depends on the wavelength of the incident light, the temperature, the nature of the liquid medium, and the concentration of the solute dissolved in the medium. If the first three factors are held constant, the refractivity of a solution is an indirect measurement of total solute concentration. Refractometry can be used to measure protein concentration, specific gravity of urine and column effluent of high-performance liquid chromatography analysis.

Osmometry

Osmometry is the measurement of the osmolality of an aqueous solution such as serum, plasma, or urine. As osmotically active particles e.g. glucose, urea nitrogen and sodium are added to a solution causing its osmolality to increase, four other properties of the solution are also affected. These properties are osmotic pressure, boiling point, freezing point, and vapor pressure. They are called colligative properties of the solution because they can be related to each other and to the osmolality. As the osmolality of a solution increases, (1) the osmotic pressure increases, (2) the boiling point is elevated, (3) the freezing point is depressed, and (4) the vapor pressure is depressed. Osmometry is based on measuring changes in the colligative properties of solutions that occur owing to variations in particle concentration. Freezing-point depression osmometry is the most commonly used method for measuring the changes in colligative properties of a solution. It is based on the principle that addition of solute molecules lowers the temperature at which a solution freezes.

Principle of Freezing Point Osmometry. The freezing point is the temperature at which water and ice are in equilibrium and is related to solute concentration. It is described by the following equation:

$$\rho T_f = K_f\, m \tag{4–11}$$

where:
ρT_f = the change in freezing point temperature
K_f = the freezing point constant of the solvent
m = the molality.

A 1.0 mOsm solution has a freezing point depression of 0.00186°C when compared to pure solvent (usually water). Thus, the osmolality of blood (about 285 mOsm/kg), has a freezing point of −0.53°C.

Freezing Point Osmometer. A freezing-point osmometer consists of a sample chamber containing a stirrer and a thermistor (temperature-sensing device) connected to a readout device. The sample is rapidly supercooled to several degrees below its freezing point in a refrigeration chamber containing, for example, ethylene glycol. The sample is then agitated with the stirrer to initiate freezing. As ice crystals form, heat is released from the solution; this raises the temperature of the sample. The rate at which this heat of fusion is released from the ice being rapidly formed reaches equilibrium with the rate of heat removed by the colder temperature of the sample chamber. This equilibrium temperature, known as the freezing point of the solution, stays constant for several minutes once it is reached. This freezing point is detected by the thermistor, and the osmolality of the sample is converted to units of milliosmoles per kilogram of water.

Flow Cytometry

A flow cytometer measures multiple properties of cells suspended in a moving fluid medium. As each particle passes single-file through a laser light source, it produces a characteristic light pattern that is measured by multiple detectors for scattered light (forward and 90 degrees) and fluorescent light (if the cell is stained with a fluorochrome). Flow cytometry is used to count and sort cells, as well as viral particles, DNA fragments, bacteria and latex beads. It is a core component of hematology cell counters and the technology used to differentiate white blood cells.

In flow cytometry, the term *particle* describes any object flowing through the instrument. An *event* is anything that is interpreted by the instrument to be a single particle. An *event* may be determined correctly or incorrectly by a flow cytometer. Methods have been developed to compensate for measurement of unwanted *events*. An example is the correction for measuring the simultaneous passing of two particles. To be analyzed, particles must be in suspension as single cells. If not, they can be made suitable for flow cytometry by the use of mechanical disruption or enzymatic digestion. Size restrictions also apply; cells or particles must be from 1–30 μ in diameter. Specialized flow cytometers are designed to handle smaller particles such as DNA fragments or bacteria.

Instrument Components. The system shown in Figure 4–16 has all of the design features of a flow cytometer with cell sorting capabilities. The cell suspension aliquots are introduced into the flow chamber using air pressure. As the cells pass through the flow chamber, a low-pressure sheath fluid surrounds them. This outer fluid stream creates a laminar flow forcing the specimen to the center, and results in a single-file alignment of the individual cells. This process is called *hydrodynamic focusing*. A laser beam passes through each cell as it flows through the chamber. Forward light scatter is proportional to cell size, and 90-degree or right-angle scatter is related to cell granularity and nuclear irregularity. If the cells are labeled with appropriate fluorochromes, fluorescent signals proportional to the amount of bound label can be measured. Green fluorescence usually means that the dye fluorescein was used as a marker; red fluorescence usually means that a dye such as phycoerythrin was used as the contrasting marker. These dyes are usually attached to antibodies to specifically target selective antigens on cells or particles.

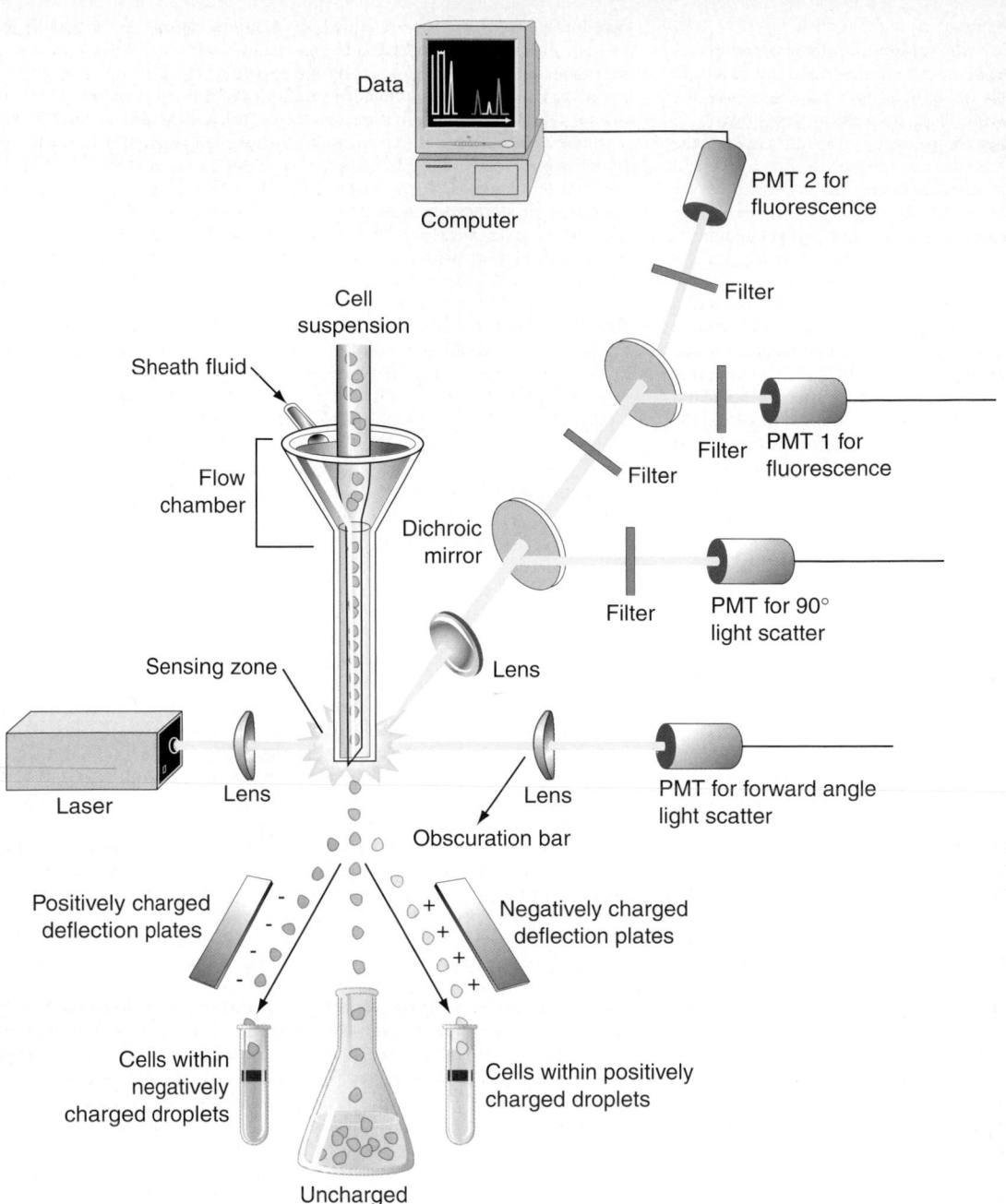

Figure 4–16 Components of a flow cytometer and a cell sorter. (Redrawn from Ward KM, Lehmann CA, Leiken AM: Clinical Laboratory Instrumentation and Automation; Principles, Applications, and Selection. Philadelphia, WB Saunders Company, 1994, with permission.)

Forward light scatter is directed to the forward scatter photodetector. At right angles to the laser beam are mirrors that divide the right-angle light scatter among the remaining photodetectors, e.g., a right-angle scatter detector and two fluorescence detectors. Across the forward lens is an obscuration bar that blocks the laser beam after it passes through the stream. Only light from the laser that has been refracted or scattered as it strikes a particle in the stream is diverted enough from its original direction to avoid the obscuration bar and strike the forward-positioned lens and the photodiode behind it. Granulocytes, monocytes, and lymphocytes are separated based on size and granularity patterns, determined by simultaneously analyzing forward and right-angle light scatter. For example, granulocytes with irregular nuclei scatter more light to the side than do lymphocytes with their spherical nuclei. Cell subpopulations can be identified by using electronic gating and analyzing fluorescence patterns (based on labels used for specific cells).

FACS, an acronym for *'fluorescence-activated cell sorter,'* describes a flow cytometer's ability to physically sort cells in a liquid suspension. To do so, the instrument design has to be modified to electrically charge cells of interest. This is done by first vibrating the sheath stream to break it into drops. The stream of drops flows past two charge (high-voltage) plates where cells of interest are electrically charged with a voltage pulse. Then the flow stream enters an electrical field where charged cells are deflected

into suitable collection containers. Unwanted cells are not charged and not deflected upon passing through the field.

Electrochemistry

Electrochemistry involves the measurement of the current or voltage generated by the activity of specific ions. Analytical techniques include potentiometry, coulometry, voltammetry, and amperometry.

Potentiometry

The measurement of potential (voltage) between two electrodes in a solution forms the basis for a variety of procedures for measuring analyte concentration. Electrical potentials are produced at the interface between a metal and ions of that metal in a solution. Such potentials also exist when a membrane semipermeable to that ion separates different concentrations of an ion. To measure the electrode potential, a constant-voltage source is needed as the reference potential. The electrode with a constant voltage is called the *reference electrode*, whereas the measuring electrode is termed the *indicator electrode*. Concentration of ions in a solution can be calculated from the measured potential difference between the two electrodes. The measured cell potential is related to the molar concentration by the Nernst equation:

$$E = E^o - RT/nF \ln a_{red}/a_{ox} = E^o - 2.302\ RT/nF \log a_{red}/a_{ox} \quad (4-12)$$

where:

  E = the cell potential measured
  E^o = the standard reduction potential
  n = the number of electrons involved in the reaction
  a_{red} = activity of the reduced species
  a_{ox} = activity of the oxidized species
  F = faraday (96 485 C/mol)
  T = absolute temperature
  R = molar gas constant.

Substituting molar concentration for activity and common logarithm for natural log:

$$E = E^o - (0.0592/n)\ \log C_{red}/C_{ox} \tag{4–13}$$

where:

  C_{red} = concentration of reduced species
  C_{ox} = concentration of oxidized species.

The Nernst equation is useful for predicting the electrochemical cell potential given the concentrations of oxidized and reduced species for a given electrode system.

Reference Electrodes. In many electroanalytical applications, e.g. measuring pH; it is desirable that the half-cell potential of one electrode be known, constant, and completely insensitive to the composition of the solution under study. An electrode that fits this description is called a reference electrode.

An ideal reference electrode should be: (1) reversible and obey the Nernst equation; (2) exhibit a potential that is constant with time; (3) return to its original potential after being subjected to small currents; and (4) exhibit little hysteresis, i.e., lag with temperature cycling. The standard hydrogen electron (SHE) exhibits many of these qualities but is not practical to use in clinical laboratory instrumentation. Thus, the calomel and silver/silver chloride reference electrodes are widely used for clinical measurements.

The calomel electrode (saturated calomel electrode, SCE) consists of mercury in contact with a solution that is saturated with mercury (I) chloride (calomel) and that also contains a known concentration of potassium chloride. The silver/silver chloride electrode consists of a silver electrode immersed in a solution of potassium chloride that has been saturated with silver chloride. Silver/silver chloride electrodes have the advantage in that they can be used at temperatures greater than 60°C, whereas calomel electrodes cannot. On the other hand, mercury (II) ions react with fewer sample components than do silver ions (which can react with proteins for example); such reactions can lead to plugging of the junction between the electrode and analyte solution.

Ion-Selective Electrode. An ion-selective electrode (ISE) is an electrochemical transducer capable of responding to one specific ion. An ISE is very sensitive and selective for the ion it measures. It consists of a membrane or other barrier separating a reference solution and a reference electrode from the solution to be analyzed. The complexity of ion-selective electrode design depends on the membrane/barrier composition that determines its ionic selectivity. Many types of ISEs are available including glass electrode, liquid membrane electrode, precipitate-impregnated membrane electrode, solid-state electrode, gas electrode, and enzyme electrodes.

pH Electrode. Glass electrodes were the first and are still the most common electrodes for measuring hydrogen ion activity (pH or negative log of the hydrogen ion concentration). A pH electrode consists of a small bulb made of layers of hydrated and nonhydrated glass, which contains a chloride ion buffer solution. The buffer has a known hydrogen ion concentration. An internal electrode, usually silver/silver chloride, serves as an internal reference electrode. A saturated calomel electrode is used as an external reference electrode. One theory suggests that the sodium ions in the hydrated glass layer drift out. Sodium ions have a large ionic radius. Specimens containing hydrogen ions, which have a smaller ionic radius, replace the sodium ions. The result is a net increase in the external membrane potential. This potential propagates through the thin, dry membrane to the inner hydrated surface of the glass. Chloride ions in the inner buffer solution respond by migrating to the internal glass layer. Potentials generated at the pH electrode are referenced to the external reference electrode (saturated calomel), and the difference or change is displayed as pH units.

P_{CO_2} Electrode. The P_{CO_2} electrode is a pH electrode contained within a plastic jacket. This plastic jacket is filled with a sodium bicarbonate buffer and has a gas-permeable membrane (Teflon or silicone) across its opening. When whole blood containing dissolved CO_2 contacts the Teflon membrane, CO_2 from the blood passes through and mixes with the buffer. A chemical reaction, shown here, occurs that results in a decrease in pH.

The hydrogen ion activity is measured by a potentiometric pH indicator system.

$$CO_2 + H_2O \rightleftharpoons HCO_3^- + H^+ \tag{4–14}$$

Coulometry

Coulometry measures the quantity of electricity (in coulombs) needed to convert an analyte to a different oxidation state. By definition a coulomb is the quantity of electricity or charge that is transported in 1 second by a constant current of 1 ampere. For a constant current of I amperes for t second, the number of coulombs Q is given by the expression:

$$Q = It \tag{4–15}$$

A Faraday is the charge in coulombs associated with one mole of electrons. The charge of the electron is 1.6018×10^{-19} C, thus 1 Faraday is equal to 96 485 C/mol.

Coulometry is used to measure chloride ion in serum, plasma, CSF and sweat samples. In measuring chloride with coulometry, a constant current is applied across the two silver electrodes, which liberate silver ions into the specimen at a constant rate. Chloride ions in the sample combine with the released silver ions to produce insoluble silver chloride. A pair of indicator and reference electrodes senses the excess silver ions and stops the titration. The number of silver ions released by ionization, which is exactly equal to that of chloride ions in the sample, can be calculated from Faraday's law:

$$Q = It = znF \tag{4–16}$$

where:

  z = the number of electrons involved in the reaction
  n = the number of moles of analyte in the sample
  F = Faraday's constant (96 485 C/mol of electrons)

Amperometry

Amperometry is the measurement of the current flow produced by an oxidation–reduction reaction. Several immobilized enzyme electrodes use this principle as well as P_{O_2} electrodes (discussed below) and chloride titrators. The measurement of chloride in samples involves the use of two electrochemical methods; coulometry (discussed above) and amperometry. In the chloride titrator, a pair of silver electrodes serves as the indicator electrodes. When all of the chloride has been consumed, the silver appears in excess, causing an increase in current. This is referred to as amperometric end point detection.

P_{O_2} Gas-Sensing Electrode. The most widely used oxygen-sensing electrode (to determine partial pressure of oxygen in blood) uses an amperometric or current-sensing electrolytic cell as the indicator system.

The P_{O_2} electrode uses a gas-permeable membrane, usually polypropylene, which allows dissolved oxygen to pass through. This membrane also prevents other blood constituents (that may interfere with the electrode) from passing through. Once the oxygen permeates the membrane it reacts with the polarized platinum cathode and is reduced according to the following reaction:

$$O_2 + 4H^+ + 4e' \rightleftharpoons 2H_2O \tag{4–17}$$

This, in turn, produces a change in the current through the cell, and the change is directly proportional to the partial pressure of oxygen present in the specimen.

Voltammetry

Voltammetry is a method in which a potential is applied to an electrochemical cell and the resulting current is measured. The most important advantages of voltammetry are sensitivity and the capability for multi-element measurements. Analytes can be detected in the parts-per-billion range. With careful selection of testing conditions and methods, several analytes can be measured simultaneously in a single voltammetric study. Voltammetry consumes minimal analyte, unlike coulometry that converts all of the analyte to another state. *Anodic stripping voltammetry* is an electrochemical technique used to measure heavy metals such as lead. It allows sample to be preconcentrated at the electrode and this enables the method to detect very low analyte levels.

Conductance

The principles of conductance have several applications associated with clinical laboratory procedures. Examples include monitoring water purity, measuring analytes in blood such as urea nitrogen, as components of detectors used in high-performance liquid chromatography (HPLC), gas chromatography (GC), cell counters and capillary electrophoresis.

Electrolytic conductivity is a measure of the ability of a solution to carry an electric current. Solutions of electrolytes conduct an electric current by the migration of ions under the influence of a potential gradient. The ions

INITIAL CONDITIONS:

Figure 4–17 Isoelectric focusing (see text). (Redrawn from Schoeff LE, Williams RH: Principles of Laboratory Instruments. St Louis, Mosby, 1993, with permission.)

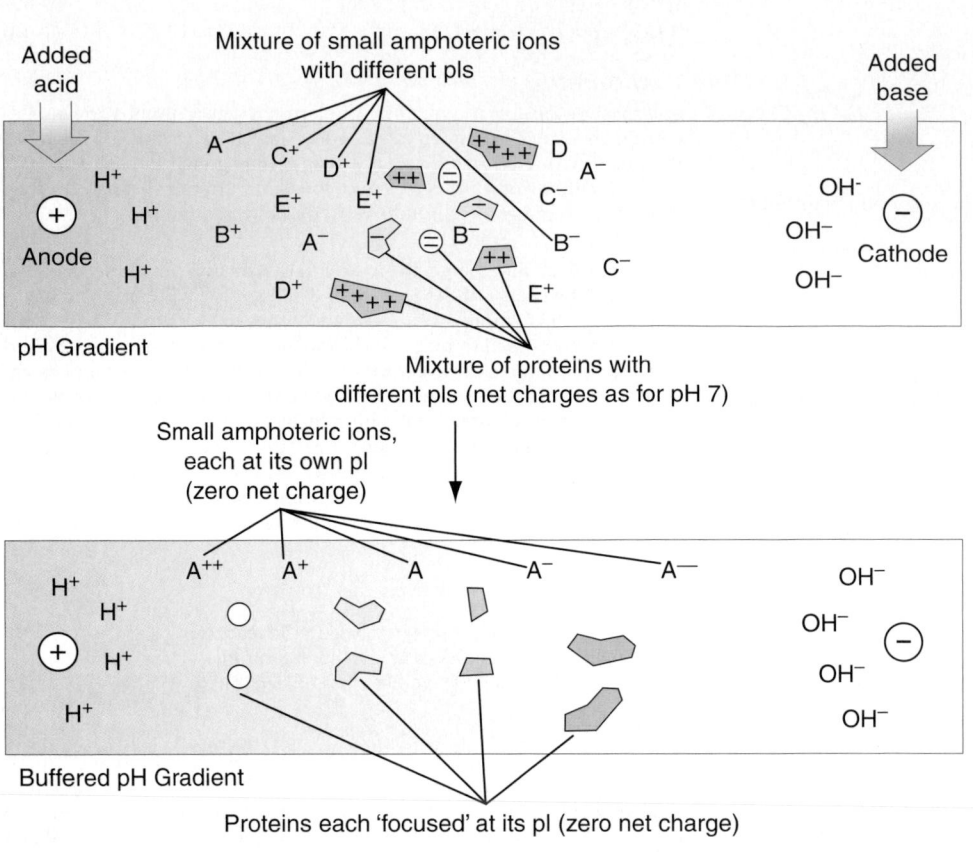

CHAPTER: 4 Analysis: Principles of Instrumentation

move at a rate dependent on their charge and size, the microscopic viscosity of the medium and magnitude of the potential gradient. Thus, for an applied potential, E, maintained constant but at a value that exceeds the deposition potential of the electrolyte, the current, I, that flows between the electrodes immersed in the electrolyte varies inversely with the resistance of the electrolytic solution, R. The reciprocal of resistance, $1/R$, is called the conductance, G, and is expressed in reciprocal ohms, or mhos.

Impedance

Electrical impedance measurement is based on the change in electrical resistance across an aperture when a particle in conductive liquid passes through this aperture. Electrical impedance is used primarily in the hematology laboratory to enumerate leukocytes, erythrocytes, and platelets. In a typical electrical impedance instrument by Coulter, aspirated blood is divided into two separate volumes for measurements. One volume is mixed with diluent and delivered to the cell bath, where erythrocyte and platelet counts are performed. As the blood passes through the aperture, the electric current between the electrodes changes each time a cell passes through. This produces a voltage pulse, the size of which is proportional to the cell size. The number of pulses is directly related to the cell count. Particles measuring between 2–20 fL are counted as platelets, whereas those measuring greater than 36 fL are counted as erythrocytes. The other blood volume is mixed with diluent and a cytochemical-lytic reagent that lyses only the red blood cells. A leukocyte count is performed as the remaining cells pass through an aperture. Particles greater than 35 fL are recorded as leukocytes.

Electrophoresis and Densitometry

Electrophoresis is the separation of charged compounds based on their electrical charge. When a voltage is applied to a salt solution (usually sodium chloride), an electrical current is produced by the flow of ions, cations toward the cathode, and anions toward the anode. Conductivity of a solution increases with its total ionic concentration. The greater the net charges of a dissolved compound, the faster it moves through the solution toward the oppositely charged electrode. The net charge of a compound, in turn, depends on the solution pH. Electrophoresis separations often require high voltages (50–200 V DC); therefore, the power supply should supply a constant DC voltage at these levels. The buffer solution must have

a carefully controlled ionic strength. A dilute buffer causes heat to be generated in the cell, while a high ionic strength does not allow good separation of the fractions. Common support media for electrophoresis in clinical work include cellulose acetate, agarose, and polyacrylamide gels. Total volume of specimen applied depends on the sensitivity of the detection method. For clinical work, 1 µL of serum may be applied. Once the electrophoresis is completed, the support medium is treated with a dye to identify the separated fractions. The most common dyes used for the visualization step include Amido Black, Ponceau S, Fat Red 7B, and Sudan Black B. To obtain a quantitative profile of the separated fractions, densitometry is performed on the stained support medium.

A *densitometer* measures the absorbance of the stain on a support medium. The basic components of a densitometer include a light source, monochromator, and movable carriage to scan the medium over the entire area, an optical system, and a photodetector. Signals detected by the photodetector are related to the absorbance of the sample stain on the support, which is proportional to the specimen concentration. The support medium is moved through the light beam at a fixed rate so that a graph may be constructed that represents multiple density readings taken at different points. Most densitometers have a built-in integrator to find the area under the curve so that all sample fractions can be quantified.

Isoelectric Focusing

Proteins are polymers of amino acids that can be anions or cations depending on the pH environment. At a specific pH, a protein will have a net charge of zero when the positive charge and the negative charge of its amino acids cancel each other out. At this pH value, known as the protein's isoelectric point (pI), the protein is isoelectric. Isoelectric focusing (IEF) techniques are performed similarly to other electrophoresis methods except that the separating molecules migrate through a pH gradient. This pH gradient is created by adding acid to the anodic area of the electrolyte cell and adding base to the cathode area (Fig. 4–17). A solution of ampholytes (mixtures of small amphoteric ions with different pIs) is placed between the two electrodes. These ampholytes have high buffering capacity at their respective isoelectric points. The ampholytes close to the anode carry a net positive charge, and those close to the cathode carry a net negative charge. When an electrical voltage is applied, each ampholyte will rapidly migrate

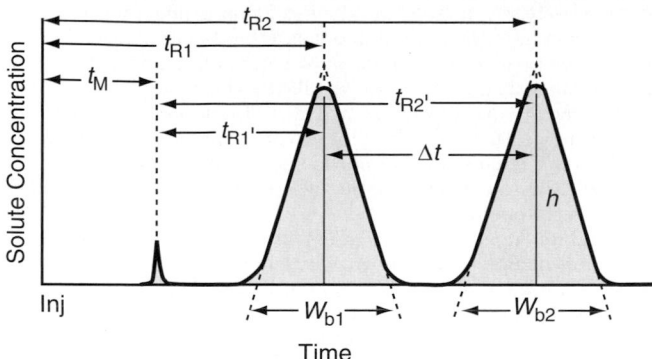

Figure 4–18 Chromatogram for the separation of two compounds. Note the uncorrected retention time (t_{R1} and t_{R2}) is from injection (Inj) to peak; the corrected time ($t_{R1'}$ and $t_{R2'}$) takes into account the retention time of a nonretained compound (t_M). (Redrawn from Ravindranath B: Principles and Practice of Chromatography. New York, John Wiley & Sons, 1989, with permission.)

to the area where the pH is equal to its isoelectric point. With their high buffering capacity, the ampholytes create stable pH zones for the more slowly migrating proteins. The advantage of isoelectric focusing techniques lies in their ability to resolve mixtures of proteins. Using narrow-range ampholytes, macromolecules differing in isoelectric point by only 0.02 pH units can be identified. Isoelectric focusing has been useful in measuring serum acid phosphatase isoenzymes. Its application has also been extended to detect oligoclonal immunoglobulin bands in CSF and isoenzymes of creatine kinase and alkaline phosphatase in serum.

Chromatography

Chromatography is a separation method based on the different interactions of the specimen compounds with the mobile phase and with the stationary phase, as the compounds travel through a support medium. The compounds interacting more strongly with the stationary phase are retained longer in the medium than those that favor the mobile phase. Chromatographic techniques may be classified according to their mobile phase: gas chromatography and liquid chromatography. Figure 4–18 shows a typical chromatogram representing the concentration of each detectable compound eluting from the column as a function of time. Retention time (t_R) is the time it takes a compound to elute. This value is characteristic of a compound and is related to the strength of its interaction with the stationary phase and the mobile phase. The retention time therefore can be used to determine a compound's identity. In this example, two compounds are separated and their retention times are represented by (t_{R1}) and (t_{R2}). These are uncorrected retention times and are measured from the injection time, $t = 0$. A column's ability to separate two compounds depends on several factors that include: (1) the difference in retention of the compounds or capacity factor, k', and (2) selectivity factor, α and (3) number of theoretical plates.

The value of k' can be calculated by the following equation:

$$k' = (t_{R1} - t_m)/t_m \text{ or } t_{R1'}/t_m \tag{4–18}$$

where:

t_m is the retention time of a nonretained compound
$t_{R1'}$ is the corrected retention time.

Another measurement derived from the calculated capacity factor is the selectivity factor (α) or relative retention of two solutes. A ratio of both capacity factors is used to calculate the selectivity factor. To measure the width of each peak, draw tangents along the sides of the peak to the baseline. W_b represents the distance between the two intersected lines. Another useful concept is theoretical plates. This describes the process by which the sample is transported down the column. In each 'plate,' the sample equilibrates between the stationary and mobile phase. The analyte moves down the column as the equilibrated mobile phase transfers sample from one plate to another. To calculate the number of theoretical plates (N), use the following equation:

$$N = 16(t_R/W_b)^2 \tag{4–19}$$

A plate number has no units, and the larger the value of N for a column, the greater its separation efficiency. The combined effects of solvent efficiency and column efficiency are expressed in the resolution (R_s) of the column:

$$R_s = (t_{R2} - t_{R1})/0.5(W_{b1} + W_{b2}) \tag{4–20}$$

The concentration of unknown compound can be derived by integration of peak areas or using the method of internal standardization.

Gas Chromatography

Gas chromatography (GC) is useful for compounds that are naturally volatile or can be easily converted into a volatile form. GC has been a widely used method for decades owing to its high resolution, low detection limits, accuracy, and short analytical time. Applications include various organic molecules including many drugs (see Ch. 23). Retention of a compound in GC is determined by its vapor pressure and volatility, which, in turn, depends on its interaction with the stationary phase. Two types of stationary phases commonly used in GC are solid absorbent (gas–solid chromatography [GSC]) and liquids coated on solid supports (gas–liquid chromatography [GLC]). In GSC, the same material (usually alumina, silica, or activated carbon) acts as both the stationary phase and the support phase. Although this was the first type of stationary phase developed, it is not as widely used as other types, primarily because of the strong retention of polar and low volatile solutes by the column (Ravindranath, 1989). GLC uses liquid phases such as polymers, hydrocarbons, fluorocarbons, liquid crystals, and molten organic salts to coat the solid support material. Calcine diatomaceous earth graded into appropriate size ranges is often used as a stationary phase because it is a stable inorganic substance. The use of fused silica capillary columns in which the stationary phase is chemically bonded onto the inner surface of the column has become very popular with chromatographers. The advantage of this type of column is that the stationary phase does not leave the solid support and bleed into the detector, and a uniform monomolecular layer of the stationary phase is obtained through the bonding procedure.

Components of a typical GC system are illustrated in Figure 4–19. Its basic design consists of five components: a gas cylinder as a mobile phase source, a sample injector, a column, a detector, and a computer for data acquisition. These systems may be automated to provide the user with a more precise and efficient separation. Carrier gases (mobile phase), which must be chemically inert, include helium, hydrogen and nitrogen. Other substances used as mobile phases include steam and supercritical fluids. Examples of these are carbon dioxide, nitrous oxide, and ammonia. The carrier gas should be of high purity, and the flow must be tightly controlled to ensure optimum column efficiency and reproducibility of test results. Samples are introduced into the GC using a hypodermic

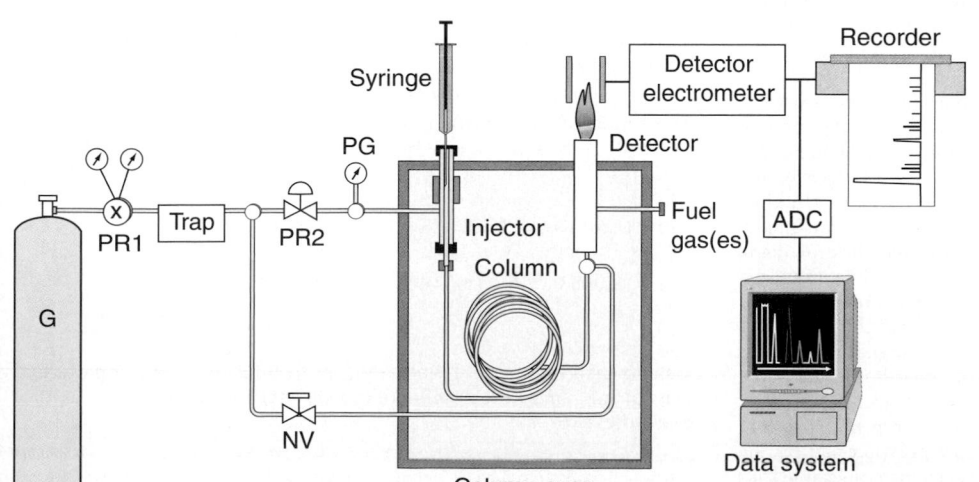

Figure 4–19 Components of a gas chromatographic system. G, gas cylinder; PR1 and PR2, regulators; PG, pressure gauge; NV, valve for adjusting the gas flow rate. (Redrawn from Ravindranath B: Principles and Practice of Chromatography. New York, John Wiley & Sons, 1989, with permission.)

syringe or an automated sampler. A needle pierces an elastic septum contained within the injector port. Each injection port is heated to very high temperatures. Samples are vaporized and swept onto the column. If the molecule of interest is not volatile enough for direct injection, it is necessary to derivatize it into a more volatile form. Most derivatization reactions belong to one of three groups: silylation, alkylation, and acylation. Silylation is the most common technique that replaces active hydrogens on the compounds with alkylsilyl groups. This substitution results in a more volatile form that is also less polar and more thermally stable.

Retention of compounds in a GC column can also be adjusted by changing the column temperature. The column temperature affects the volatility of the compounds and thus the degree of their interaction with the stationary phase. By proper selection of the starting temperature and temperature gradient during the procedure, good resolution of both weakly and strongly retained compounds may be achieved. The GC column, enclosed in a temperature-controlled oven, can be a packed column or capillary column. Packed columns are usually 1–5 m long and 2–4 mm in diameter, and are filled with a stationary phase. Capillary columns range from 5–100 m in length, 0.1–0.8 mm in diameter, and have a stationary phase located on their interior surface (Bartle, 1993). Capillary columns generally have higher efficiency and better detection limits. However, packed columns have a larger specimen or sample capacity, making them more useful in purification work. Examples of detectors used in GC include a flame ionization detector, a thermal conductivity detector, a nitrogen-phosphorus detector, an electron capture detector, a flame photometric detector, and a mass spectrometric detector. Flame ionization detectors (FID) are widely used and are capable of detecting almost all organic compounds and many inorganic compounds. This type of detector measures the ions produced by the compounds when burned in a hydrogen–air flame. An electrode producing an electric current collects the ions. The analog signal from the detector is then converted into a result (Tipler, 1993).

Liquid Chromatography

GC as a separation technique has some restrictions that make liquid chromatography a suitable alternative. Many organic compounds are too unstable or are insufficiently volatile to be assayed by GC without prior chemical derivatization. Liquid chromatography techniques use lower temperatures for separation, thereby achieving better separation of thermolabile compounds. These two factors allow liquid chromatography to separate compounds that cannot be separated by GC. Finally, it is easier to recover a sample in liquid chromatography than in gas chromatography. The mobile phase can be removed, and the sample can be processed further or reanalyzed under different conditions.

There are many forms of liquid chromatography available, and the selection of an appropriate form depends on a variety of factors. These factors include analysis time, type of compound, and detection limits. Paper, thin-layer, ion-exchange, and exclusion liquid chromatography often result in poor efficiency and a very long analysis time owing to low mobile phase flow rates. High-performance liquid chromatography (HPLC) emerged in the late 1960s as a viable form of liquid chromatography that provided advantages over other forms of liquid chromatography and gas chromatography. HPLC uses small, rigid supports and special mechanical pumps producing high pressure to pass the mobile phase through the column. HPLC columns can be used many times without regeneration. The resolution achieved with HPLC columns is superior to that of other forms of liquid chromatography, analysis times are usually much shorter, and reproducibility is greatly improved. All of these attributes of HPLC render it a better method of separation over other forms of liquid chromatography.

There are five commonly used separation techniques in liquid chromatography. They include adsorption, partition, ion-exchange, affinity, and size exclusion. Each is characterized by a unique combination of stationary phase and mobile phase. In *adsorption (liquid–solid) chromatography*, the compounds are adsorbed to a solid support such as silica or alumina. Although this was the first type of column liquid chromatography developed, it is not widely used owing to the strong retention of many compounds by the supports, making them difficult to elute from the column. *Partition (liquid–liquid) chromatography* separates compounds based on their partition between a liquid mobile phase and a liquid stationary phase coated on a solid support. Partition chromatography includes normal-phase liquid chromatography, which uses a polar liquid stationary phase, and reverse-phase liquid chromatography, which uses a nonpolar stationary phase. *Ion-exchange chromatography* uses column packings that have charge-bearing functional groups attached to a polymer matrix. The mechanism in this type of chromatography is the exchange of sample ions and mobile-phase ions with the charged group of the stationary phase. *Affinity chromatography* uses immobilized biochemical ligands as the stationary phase to separate a few solutes from other unretained solutes. This type of separation uses the so-called lock-and-key binding that is widely present in biological systems. *Size-exclusion chromatography* separates molecules according to the difference in their size. The support material has a certain range of pore sizes. As solutes travel through, the small molecules can enter the pores, whereas the larger ones cannot and will elute first from the column.

Liquid chromatography is similar in many aspects to GC, and therefore, the instrumentation is similar. A typical liquid chromatography system consists of a liquid mobile phase, a sample injector (manual or automatic), a mechanical pump, a column, a detector, and a data recorder (Fig. 4–20). The liquid mobile phase is pumped from a solvent reservoir through the column. A mechanical pump must provide precise and accurate flow, often working at high pressures (typically up to 6000 PSI). The pump must have low internal volume and be constructed of material that does not react with the solvent. Sample injection is achieved using a syringe and depositing the sample into a loop. The injection may be performed manually or automatically using a microprocessor control autosampler. Most analytical separations are performed using packed column. There are many types of packing material available. Selection of the appropriate packing material is largely dependent on the type of compound(s) to be separated. In liquid chromatography, the physical properties of the sample and mobile phase are often very similar. Two basic types of detectors have been developed. One is based on the differential measurement of a physical property common to both the sample and mobile phase; examples include refractive index, conductivity, and electrochemical detectors. The other is based on the measurement of a physical property that is specific to the sample, either with or without the mobile phase; examples include absorbance and fluorescent detectors.

A widely used clinical application of HPLC is the separation and quantitation of hemoglobin, in particular HbA_{1c}. The systems available for this type of analysis are automated and complete the analysis in less than 5 minutes.

Mass Spectrometry

Mass spectrometry (MS) is based on fragmentation and ionization of molecules using a suitable source of energy. The resulting fragment masses and their relative abundance yield a characteristic mass spectrum of the parent molecule. Before a compound can be detected and quantified by mass spectrometry it must be isolated by another method, either GC or HPLC. Mass spectrometry typically involves the following major steps: (1) conversion of the parent molecule into a stream of ions (usually singly charged positive ions); (2) separating the ions by mass-to-charge ratio (m/z), where m is the mass of the ion in atomic mass units and z is its charge; and (3) counting the number of ions of each type or measuring current produced when the ions strike a transducer. Because most of the ions formed are singly charged, the m/z is usually simply the mass of the ion. MS is also described in Chapter 23 (see especially Figs 23–5 and 23–6).

Atomic weights (amu and Da)

Atomic and molecular weight are generally expressed in terms of atomic mass units (amu) or daltons (Da). The amu or Da is based upon a relative scale in which the reference is the carbon isotope $^{12}_{6}C$, which is assigned a mass of exactly 12 amu. Therefore the amu or Da is defined as $1/12$ of the mass of one neutral $^{12}_{6}C$ atom. From this definition we derive the following equality:

$$1 \text{ amu} = 1 \text{ Da} = 1.66054 \times 10^{-27} \text{ kg/atom } ^{12}C$$

Also 1 mole of $^{12}_{6}C$ weighs 12.0000 g.

Example 4–5. What are the masses in Da for $^{12}C^{1}H_4$ and $^{13}C^{1}H_4$?

Solution

$^{12}C^{1}H_4$

$m = 12.000 \times 1 + 1.007825 \times 4 = 16.031$ Da

$^{13}C^{1}H_4$

$m = 13.00335 \times 1 + 1.007825 \times 4 = 17.035$ Da

Mass-to-charge ratio

Mass-to-charge ratio (m/z) is obtained by dividing the atomic or molecular mass of anion m by the number of charges z that the ion bears.

Example 4–6

$^{12}C^{1}H_4^{+}$

$m/z = 16.035/1 = 16.035$

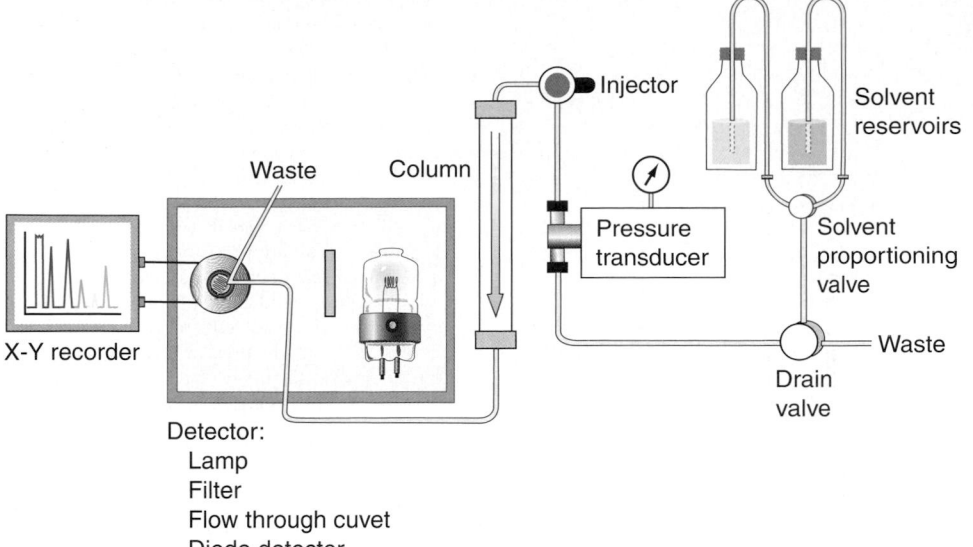

Figure 4–20 Components of a high-performance liquid chromatograph.

$^{13}C^1H_4^{2+}$

$m/z = 17.035/2 = 8.518$

Many ions produced in mass spectrometers are singly charged; thus the term mass-to-charge ratio is often shortened to the more convenient term mass. Strictly speaking, this abbreviation is incorrect, but it is widely used in mass spectrometry literature. This term also represents the x-axis for MS spectrums of molecules plotted against their relative abundance (y-axis).

Basic Components

All spectrometers have three basic components: an ion source, a mass analyzer, and an ion detector. The inlet unit admits samples to the mass spectrometer. When the instrument is part of a GC/MS arrangement, the inlet unit must be heated to maintain the volatile compounds in the vapor state upon coming into the ion source unit. It must also strip away most of the carrier gas to adapt to the high-vacuum condition required for mass spectrometry operation.

Ion source unit. The ion source unit is maintained at high temperature and vacuum to provide adequate conditions for ionizing the vaporized sample molecules. Several types of energy sources are available to ionize the sample molecules in mass spectrometry. One commonly used source is a beam of electrons produced by a heated filament. The process of bombarding the sample with electrons is called *electron-impact ionization*. Other processes of ionization include *chemical ionization*, in which the sample molecules are ionized by a reagent gas that has been ionized by an electron beam, and *fast atom bombardment*, in which a solid sample is ionized by a beam of atoms such as argon.

Most laboratorians are familiar with the use of mass spectrometers for drug and other low molecular weight compound analysis. Two examples are confirmation of positive drug screens and amino acid analysis. These techniques required the coupling of a gas chromatograph and a mass spectrometer (GCMS). This conventional approach had several limiting factors associated with it. These limitations include the need to separate analyte from specimen matrix and the need to make stable volatile derivatives, amenable to ionization by electron impact (EI) or chemical ionization (CI). Although these conventional techniques produced highly specific and sensitive analyses they were also technically demanding and lacked the ruggedness required for the clinical laboratory. However, the increased focus on protein analysis, molecular diagnostics and genetic related testing has ushered in a new wave of mass spectrometers possessing the capabilities of evaluating complex compounds such as proteins.

The *matrix-assisted laser desorption ionization (MALDI)* source consists of a solid mixture of analyte and matrix (including organic chromophore) on a sample plate, along with a laser light and ion optics (Fig. 4–21A). (This technique is further described in Ch. 76.) When the chromophore absorbs the laser light, it vaporizes and lifts the analyte ions from the surface into a gas phase directly above the target plate and into the analyzer. The MALDI technique is considered an offline ionization technique because the sample is purified, deposited, and dried on the sample plate before analysis (Skoog, 1998). *Surface-enhanced laser desorption ionization (SELDI)* is a technique that measures proteins from complex biological specimens such as serum, plasma, intestinal fluids, urine, cell lysates and cellular secretion products (see also Ch. 76). Proteins are captured by adsorption, partition, electrostatic interaction, or affinity chromatography on a solid-phase protein chip surface. A laser ionizes samples that have been co-crystallized with a matrix on a target surface. The protein chip chromatographic surfaces in SELDI are uniquely designed to retain proteins from complex mixtures according to their specific properties. After the addition of a matrix solution, proteins can be ionized with a nitrogen laser and their molecular masses measured by TOF MS (Fig. 4–21B) (see also Fig. 23–5). The protein chip arrays are the heart of the SELDI-TOF MS technology and distinguish it from other MS-based systems. Each array is composed of different chromatographic surfaces that, unlike HPLC or GC, are designed to retain, not elute, proteins of interest. The protein chip arrays have an aluminum base with several spots composed of a chemical (anionic, cationic, hydrophobic, hydrophilic, or metal ion) or biochemical (immobilized antibody, receptor, DNA, enzymes, etc.) active surface. Each surface is designed to retain proteins according to a general or specific physicochemical property of the proteins. Chemically active surfaces retain whole classes of proteins, and surfaces to which a biochemical agent, such as an antibody or other types of affinity reagent, is coupled are designed to interact specifically with a single target protein (Skoog, 1998).

Mass spectrometer analyzer unit. The output of the ion source is a stream of positive or negative gaseous ions that are then accelerated into the mass analyzer that sorts the parent molecular ions and their fragment ions according to their mass-to-charge ratio. This is accomplished in several different ways. *Time-of-flight (TOF)* analyzer consists of a metal flight tube and the m/z ratios of the ions are determined by accurately and precisely measuring the time it takes the ions to travel from the MALDI or SELDI sources to the detector. Given that all ions of different m/z receive the same kinetic energy, low m/z ions will reach the detector sooner than high m/z ions. In *the quadrupole mass spectrometer* (Fig. 4–22A) (and Fig. 23–5), direct electrical current and radiofrequency voltages of selected magnitudes are applied to two pairs of metallic rods. Only ions of specific mass-to-charge ratio can pass undeflected to the end of the rods, where they are detected. All other ions have unstable trajectories along the path and are deflected toward the rods, never reaching the detector. An advantage to this design is that this system can perform tandem mass-spectrometry scan modes in the same analyzer. The *ion-trap mass spectrometer* (Fig. 4–22B) functions as a mass analyzer and an ion source unit. Three electrodes, in a ring shape and two end caps, produce ions in the cavity until selectively ejected to the ion detector as the scanning radiofrequency voltage on the ring electrode varies. A major advantage of the ion-trap analyzer is its ability to get full mass spectra at very low sample concentrations (Karasek, 1988). In the *magnetic sector mass spectrometer*, a very high voltage accelerates the ions out of the ion source unit onto a magnetic field. The exiting path curvature of an ion depends on its mass-to-charge ratio, the magnetic field strength, and the applied voltage. The magnetic field or the voltage can be varied to allow selective ions to exit the magnetic field.

Ion detector. The ion detector in mass spectrometers are usually an electron multiplier or an ion–photon conversion detector. In an *electron multiplier*, the ions strike the detector's first dynode, which triggers the

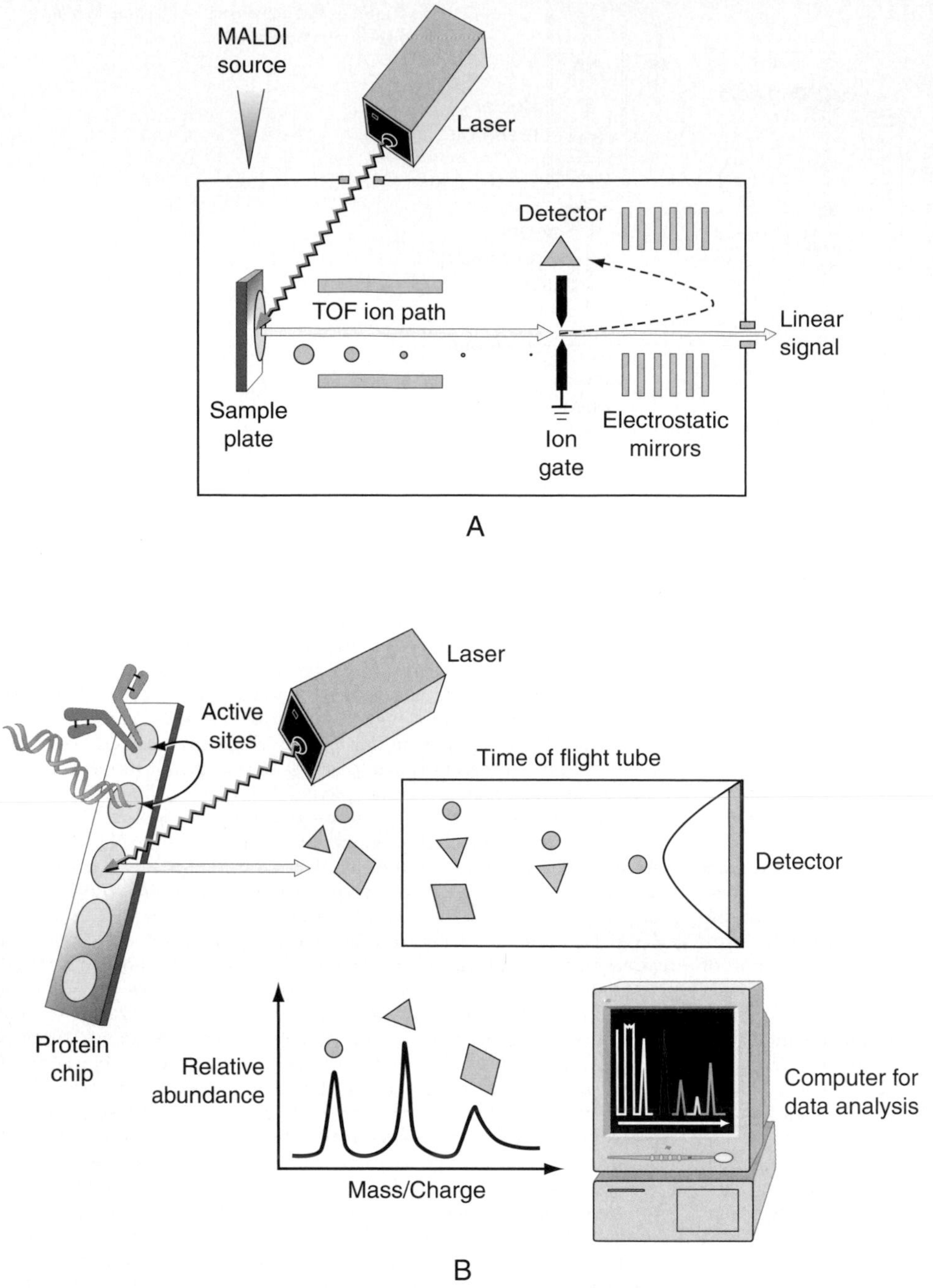

Figure 4–21 Diagrams of two systems widely used for proteomic research. *A*, MALDI time of flight mass spectrometer, and *B*, SELDI time of flight mass spectrometer.

release of secondary electrons. A cascade of electrons occurs similarly to that in a photomultiplier tube, resulting in an amplification of about a millionfold. In an *ion–photon conversion detector*, the ions strike a phosphor that emits a photon for each corresponding ion. A conventional photomultiplier tube then amplifies the signal in the usual fashion. The computerized data unit controls the multiple operating parameters of the instrument components, and stores and analyzes a vast amount of acquired data. The built-in libraries of reference mass spectra for known compounds can be searched by computer and compared with the sample spectrum for identification. As emphasized in Chapter 23, each compound or macromolecule has a unique mass spectrum, a 'fingerprint' of the molecule. A typical mass spectrum is shown in Figure 23–6.

Scintillation Counter

Scintillations are flashes of light that occur when gamma rays or charged particles interact with matter. Chemicals used to convert their energy into light energy are called scintillators. If gamma rays or ionizing particles are absorbed in a scintillator, some energy absorbed by the scintillator is emitted as a pulse of visible light or near-UV radiation. A photomultiplier tube detects light either directly or through an internally reflecting optic fiber. A scintillation counter is an instrument that detects scintillations using a photomultiplier tube and counts the electrical impulses produced

by the scintillations. An application for scintillation counting is radioimmunoassay (RIA). Two types of scintillation methods exist: crystal scintillation and liquid scintillation.

Crystal scintillation generally is used to detect gamma radiation. When a gamma ray penetrates the sodium iodide (NaI) crystal, which contains 1% thallium, it excites the electrons of iodide atoms and raises them to higher energy states. When the electrons return to ground state, energy is emitted as UV radiation. The UV radiation is promptly absorbed by the thallium atoms and emitted as photons in the visible or near-UV range. The photons pass through the crystal and are detected by a photomultiplier tube. A pulse-height analyzer sorts out the pulse signals from the photomultiplier tube according to their pulse height and allows only those within a restricted range to reach the rate meter for counting.

Liquid scintillation is primarily used to count radionuclides that emit beta particles. A sample is suspended in a solution or 'cocktail' consisting of a solvent such as toluene, a primary scintillator such as 2,5-diphenyloxazole (PPO), and a secondary scintillator such as 2,2'-*p*-phenylenebis (5-phenyloxazole) (POPOP). Beta particles from the radioactive sample ionize the primary scintillator of the solvent. A secondary scintillator absorbs the photons emitted by the primary scintillator and re-emits them at a longer wavelength. The secondary scintillator facilitates more effective energy transmission from the beta particles, especially when a large amount of quenching is present. Quenching is a process that results in a

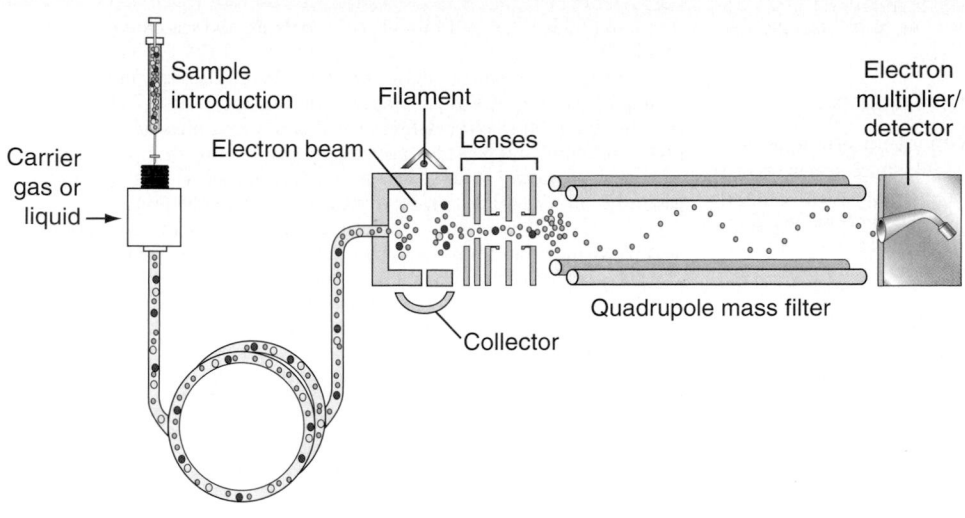

A

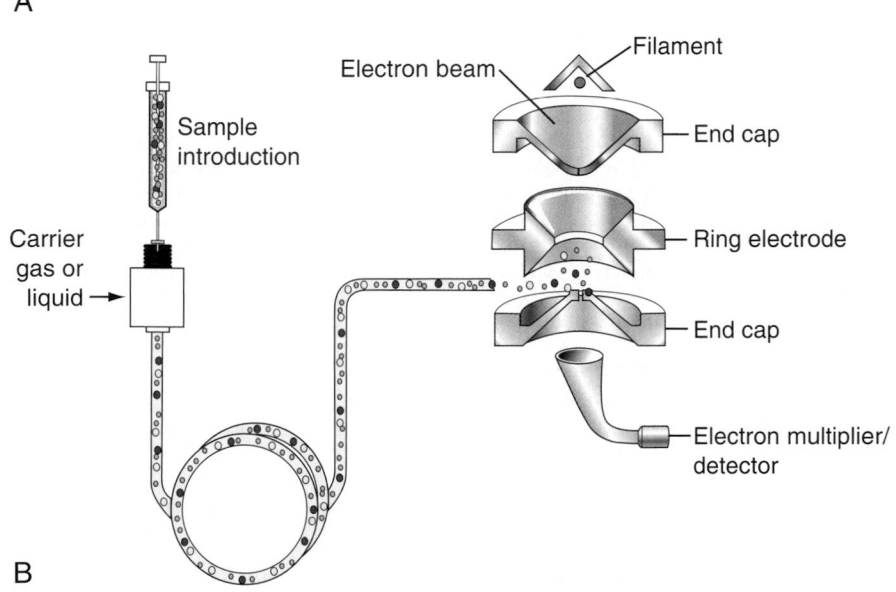

B

Figure 4–22 Mass spectrometer: *A,* quadrupole type; *B,* ion-trap type. (Redrawn from Schoeff LE, Williams RH: Principles of Laboratory Instruments. St Louis, Mosby, 1993, with permission.)

reduction of the photon output from the sample. This phenomenon may be due to chemical quenching, in which impurities in the sample compete with the scintillators for energy transfer, or color quenching, in which colored substances such as hemoglobin absorbs the light photons produced by scintillation. The light photons produced in the sample are detected and amplified by the photomultiplier tubes in the same manner as for the crystal scintillation counter.

Capillary Electrophoresis

Capillary electrophoresis (CE) represents another alternative in separation techniques. A typical capillary electrophoresis system, as shown in Figure 4–23, consists of a fused silica capillary, two electrolyte buffer reservoirs, a high-voltage power supply, and a detector linked to a data acquisition unit. The sample is introduced into the capillary inlet. When a high voltage is applied across the capillary ends, the sample molecules are separated by electro-osmotic flow, a bulk flow resulting from excess positive ions at the inner capillary surface moving toward the cathode. The positive ions in the specimen emerge early at the capillary outlet because the electro-osmotic flow and the ion movement are in the same direction. Negative ions in the specimen also move toward the capillary outlet but at a slower rate. As the sample ions migrate toward the capillary outlet, different types of detectors, including optical, conductivity, electrochemical, mass spectroscopy, or radioactivity detectors, are used to detect them. Advantages of CE over conventional electrophoresis and HPLC are its short analytical time, resolving power, and microsample volumes (Love, 1994). Using nanoliter quantities of specimen, complex mixtures of molecules can be separated with a theoretical plate number approaching one million. Separations may be completed in less than 10 minutes by applying very high voltage. The application of high voltage is made possible by the capillary's high surface-to-volume ratio that allows for efficient heat transfer through the capillary wall. Applications of capillary

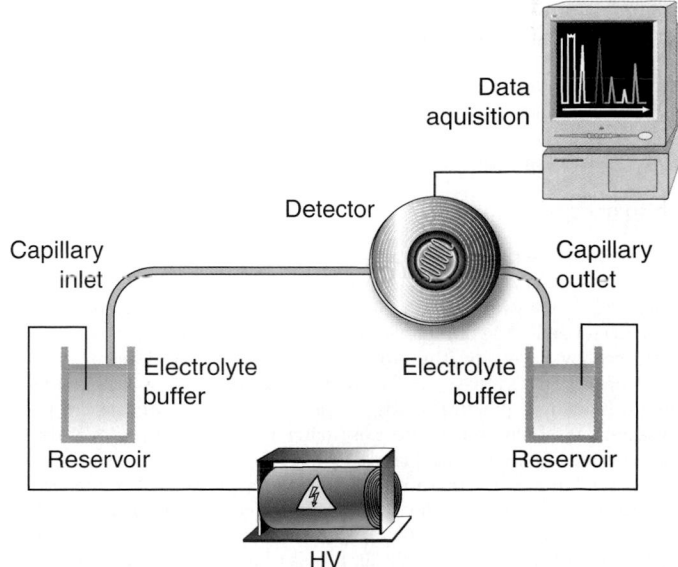

Figure 4–23 Capillary electrophoresis system. HV, high-voltage source. (Redrawn from Ward KM, Lehmann CA, Leiken AM: Clinical Laboratory Instrumentation and Automation; Principles, Applications, and Selection. Philadelphia, WB Saunders Company, 1994, with permission.)

electrophoresis include separation of serum proteins and hemoglobin variants.

Nuclear Magnetic Resonance Spectroscopy

Nuclear magnetic resonance spectroscopy (NMR) is a technique for determining the structure of organic compounds. Unlike mass spectroscopy (MS), NMR is non-destructive, though it does require a larger sample volume than MS. While NMR is widely used as a diagnostic imaging technique, it has only been adapted for a limited number of clinical laboratory analyses, the most popular being lipoprotein particle measurements (see Ch. 17).

Nuclear magnetic resonance is a phenomenon that occurs when the nuclei of certain atoms are immersed in a static magnetic field and exposed to a second oscillating magnetic field, i.e., the magnetic component of electromagnetic radiation (EMR). Some nuclei experience this phenomenon and others do not, depending upon whether they possess a property called spin. The spin of a proton causes an NMR signal. The nucleus of a hydrogen atom does spin and because hydrogen atoms occur very frequently, they are useful in determining structure.

When EMR is used to bombard molecules, the hydrogen atoms present will absorb photons of different energies depending upon the location of the hydrogen atom. For example in compounds containing hydrogen and chloride, the proton near two chloride atoms produces a different NMR than the proton located near a single chloride and single hydrogen. The energy absorbed by the spinning nuclei can be plotted versus the frequency of the applied EMR to obtain an NMR spectrum of the molecule.

In lipoprotein subclass measurements, the NMR signal originates in the protons of the terminal methyl groups of the lipid carried in the particles (primarily the cholesterol ester and triglyceride of the particle core, and the phospholipids of the particle shell). The signals from these different lipids combine to produce one signal with a characteristic frequency and shape related to particle size, i.e., the diameter of the phospholipids shell, excluding the influence of the apolipoprotein attached to the particle.

Basic components of an NMR spectrometer are the magnet that is used to separate the nuclear spin energy state and a transmitter, that supplies the radio frequencies (rf) or irradiating energy. A sample probe contains coils for coupling the sample with the rf field (s) and a computer is used to evaluate the data.

General Analytical Methods and Issues

Perhaps the most fundamental aspect of the analytical process is the preparation of high quality reagents that will be used in the analytical procedure. In this process the quality of water, purity of the chemical, the selection of correct glassware or plastic ware, the correct preparation of reagents are all important for the proper operation of laboratory equipment and the performance of testing procedures. In this section several topics will be presented that relate to analytical process and will ultimately impact on the results of a test performed on a patient's specimen.

Chemicals

The chemicals used to prepare reagents for chemical testing exist in varying degrees of purity. Proper selection of chemicals is important so that the desired results may be attained. Chemicals acquired for reagent preparation are characterized by a grading system. The grading of any chemical is greatly influenced by its purity. The type and quantity of impurities are usually stated on the label affixed to the chemical container. Less pure grades of chemicals include practical grade, technical grade and commercial grade. These grades of chemicals are unsuitable for use in most quantitative assays performed in a clinical laboratory.

Most qualitative and quantitative procedures performed in the clinical laboratory require the use of chemicals that meet the specifications of the American Chemical Society (ACS). These chemicals are classified as either analytical grade or reagent grade. Examples of other designations of chemicals that meet high standards of purity include spectrograde, nanograde, and HPLC grade. These are often referred to as ultrapure chemicals.

Pharmaceutical chemicals are produced to meet the specifications defined in *The United States Pharmacopoeia* (USP), *The National Formulary* and *The Food Chemical Index*. The specifications define impurity tolerances that are not injurious to health.

The International Union for Pure and Applied Chemistry (IUPAC) has developed standards and purity levels for certain chemicals. These include atomic weight standard (grade A); ultimate standard (grade B); primary standard (grade C), working standard (grade D) and secondary substances (grade E).

A very good source of highly purified chemicals, especially reference materials, is the National Institute of Standard and Testing (NIST) (Gaithersburg, MD). NIST define their chemical and physical properties for each compound and provides a certificate documenting their measurements. NIST also provides Standard Reference Material (SRMs) in solid, liquid or gaseous form. The solids may be crystalline, powder or lyophilized.

There are two professional organizations that can provide laboratory staff with guidelines for proper chemical selection and reagent preparation. They are the College of American Pathologists (CAP, Northfield, IL 60093) and Clinical and Laboratory Standard Institute (CLSI), formerly the National Committee for Clinical Laboratory Standard (NCCLS) (Wayne, PA 19087-1898).

Water

Water has numerous uses in the clinical laboratory. Water is used to prepare reagents, as diluent for controls and calibrators, to flush and clean internal components of analyzers, to serve as a heating bath for cuvets and to wash and rinse laboratory glassware. For most of these uses the source of the water must be of the highest purity, whereas the water required for rinsing glassware may be of a lesser purity.

Types of Water Purity

CLSI and CAP have defined three grades of water purity. They are type I, II and III. The criteria for each type are outlined in CLSI guidelines (NCCLS, 1997). When selecting a water purification system the purchaser must pay strict attention to these criteria so that all of the appropriate filters and components necessary to produce type I water are included. Also, special attention must be given to the 'feed-water' which is usually the laboratory tap water. The feed-water may contain unique contaminants, or may have a high mineral content (hardness), which will often require the inclusion of additional components in the water processing system.

Purification

Many laboratories produce or purify their own water. There are several means available to produce reagent-grade water. Most water filtration systems use a prefilter to begin the process. This prefilter has feed-water running through it to trap any particulates before sending it on to the next component. At this point in the water filtration process water may be distilled or passed through a reverse osmosis filter. Distillation is the process by which a liquid is vaporized and condensed and is used to purify or concentrate a substance or separate a volatile substance from a less volatile substance. Water that has been distilled does not meet the specific resistivity requirements of CAP type I water. Reverse osmosis (RO) is a process where water is forced through a semipermeable membrane that acts as a molecular filter. The RO filter removes 95–99% of organic compounds, bacteria, and other particulate matter and about 95% of all ionized and dissolve minerals, but not as many gaseous impurities. Reverse osmosis alone does not produce type I water but like distillation if additional filters such as ion-exchange and carbon particulate filters are added to the system, type I water may be produced.

Ion-exchange filters remove ions to produce mineral-free deionized water. Deionization is accomplished by passing water through insoluble resin polymers that contain either anion- or cation-exchange resins. These exchange resins replace H^+ and OH^- ions for impurities present in ionized form in the water. Another type of material used is a mixed bed resin that contains both anion and cation-exchange materials. Deionizers are capable of producing water that has specific resistance exceeding 1–10 Mohm•cm ($M\Omega$ cm).

Carbon filters containing activated charcoal may be added to the water purification system to help remove several types of organic compounds that may still be in the water. When these filters are used CLSI/CAP considers the end-product to contain minimal organic material.

A particulate filter may be added at the end of the system. This filter with a mean pore size down to about 0.22 μm will serve to trap any remaining particulates as large as or larger than the pore size.

Monitoring Water Purity

Because water is such an integral part of laboratory analysis, its purity must be monitored on a consistent basis. The frequency of water testing is dependent upon many factors including the composition of the feed-water, availability of staff to perform the water testing, and the amount of water the laboratory uses during a given period of time. At the very least, resistivity and bacterial content of the water should be monitored on a regular basis. In addition, pH, silica content and organic contaminants may be determined. Depending upon the laboratory's resources some or all of these parameters should be checked on a periodic basis.

Most water filtration systems will have an in-line resistivity meter available. Resistivity measurements are used to assess the ionic content of purified water. The higher the ion concentration in water the lower the resistivity value will be. CLSI/CAP requires that type I water have a resistivity of greater than 10 MΩ•cm.

Monitoring bacterial contamination can be accomplished quite easily. The water should be allowed to run for at least 1 minute to flush the system. Next an aliquot of water is taken depending upon the procedure used and plated on an appropriate media. After an appropriate incubation time determine the number of colony-forming units on the agar plate. The most commonly found organisms in water after the purification process is complete are gram-negative rods.

Once Your System has been installed

Most water purification systems are designed for easy access to end-product type I water. Therefore it is advisable to use only type I water for most applications in the laboratory. Type II or III water could be used for rinsing glassware and cleaning exterior surfaces. If a procedure, for example heavy metal testing or HPLC, requires the use of specially prepared water then type I water should not be used. Ultra pure water can be purchased from NERL Diagnostics Corporation (East Providence, RI 02914).

Measurement of Mass

Mass is the quantity of matter contained within an object. The weight of a body is the gravitational acceleration exerted on it and unlike mass, varies with altitude. The weight is equal to mass times gravity. In the laboratory we are measuring the mass of an object.

Types of Balances

There are several different types of balances available depending upon what needs to be weighed. For example, to weigh a fecal fat specimen an appropriate balance to use would be a top loading precision balance capable of accurately weighing kilogram amounts. Preparation of standards for toxicology assays requires microgram quantities, thus a single-pan microbalance would be appropriate.

Unequal-Arm Substitution Balances

Unequal-arm substitution balances are typically single-pan types and commonly used in laboratories, though almost all of these balances are being replaced by electronic-type balances. This single-pan, mechanical, unequal-arm balance operates on the principle of removing weights rather than adding them. A fixed mass counterweight is used to balance the combined mass of the pan and the removable weights across two arms of unequal weight. When a sample is placed on the weighing pan, the internal weights in 1-g or 10-g increments are moved one at a time by the operator turning a set of knobs. This is continued until the system returns to equilibrium, at which time the sum of the weights removed is equal to the weight of the object.

Magnetic Force Restoration Balance

Another widely used balance is the single-pan balance that relies on magnetic force restoration. The restoring force is the force required to put the balance back into equilibrium. The unknown mass is placed on the pan and this system goes out of equilibrium. The operator who adjusts the internal weights restores partial equilibrium. The null detector optics circuit senses when equilibrium is near and provides a signal to the sensor motor to generate a restoring current until, equilibrium is reached. At this time the unknown mass is equal to the mass of the weights removed plus the value of the restoring current.

Top-Loading Balances

Single-pan top-loading balances operate on the same principle as single-pan analytical balances (i.e., weighing by substitution). Damping is accomplished by magnetic rather than an air-release mechanism. These balances are especially suitable for rapidly weighing larger masses (up to 10 000 g) that do not require as much analytical precision, such as large-volume reagent preparation.

Electronic Balances

There are several electronic balance designs. One design uses a strain gauge load cell. This is a small thin device, which changes electrical resistance when it is stretched or compressed. Typically, several strain gauges are used in a Wheatstone bridge arrangement and they are glued onto the load cell in a protected location. A load cell is usually in the shape of a beam or plate. When the beam or plate is displaced it bends a tiny amount, and this tiny bending is detected by the strain gauges. The amount of bending might be only a thousandth of an inch, but that is enough for a strain gauge to measure.

Another electronic balance design operates on the principle of electro-magnetic force (EMF) compensation. A coil, placed between the poles of a cylindrical electromagnet, is mechanically connected to a weighing pan. Mass placed on the pan produces a force that displaces the coil within the magnetic field. A regulator generates a compensation current just sufficient to return the coil to its original position. The more mass placed on the pan, the larger the deflecting force, and the stronger the current required to correct the deflection of the coil. The measuring principle is based on a strict linear relationship between compensation current and force produced by the load placed on the pan.

There are several additional features that may be available on some models of electronic balances. For example, some electronic balances include an electronic vibration damper. Any excess vibration can be detected when variation of the pointer or oscillation of the number in the last decimal place of the digital display is observed. Another feature available in some models is built-in taring. This allows the weight of the weighing container to be 'zeroed.' Also electronic balances can be interfaced with computers to provide calculations such as weight averaging and statistical analysis of multiple weighing. The fundamental design of electronic balances allow for faster weighing which is advantageous when doing multiple readings, e.g., pipet calibrations.

Calibration

Laboratory balances require calibration at regular intervals. The NIST states that there is no fixed calibration interval for scientific applications. Calibration intervals should coincide with the requirements of the laboratory's licensing and accrediting organizations.

The mass standard and test weight accuracy classes for weights used in calibrating balances have been updated and replace the older requirements specified by NBS class S and class S1 weights. The new mass standards and test weight accuracy classes appropriate for laboratory balances include American Society for Testing and Materials (ASTM) class 1 and 2. Refer to ASTM E617-97 for specific information regarding range, readability and best uncertainly applicable to these classes.

NIST class 1 weights (extra-fine accuracy) are available up to 250 mg and may be used for high-precision, e.g., single-pan and electronic, balances that are precise to four decimal places. The range of weight for class 2 balances may be in excess of 1000 g.

Handling Weights Used for Testing Accuracy

Meticulous care must be used when handling class 1 or 2 weights. The operator must avoid direct contact with the weights by using clean gloves or special lifting tools, e.g., forceps. Hand contact with the weights can cause corrosion. The weights should not be dragged across any surface, including the stainless steel weighing pan. Usually the weights are sent in a covered box and should always be stored in that box.

Environmental Concerns for Best Weighing Accuracy

There are several aspects of the environment that may impact on the performance of a laboratory balance. They include temperature, air drafts, floor vibrations, table instability and static electricity. Minimizing the effects of the environment on your weighing procedures can often be done quite easily. For example if there are air drafts in the room, a shroud or enclosure can be placed around the balance. A marble table can be used to reduce table vibrations or instability.

Balance Specifications

There are several important specifications that an operator should be knowledgeable about concerning balances. They include:
* capacity – which represents the maximum load one can weigh
* accuracy – is dependent on the smallest mass one will be weighing
* linearity – the ability of a balance to provide accurate output over its full range
* resolution (readability) – the smallest increment of weight that may be discernible.

Laboratory accrediting agencies require verification of accuracy of balances at various time intervals. There are several sources available to guide the laboratory through this requirement.

Types of Glassware

The most common type of glassware encountered in volume measurements is borosilicate glass. This glass is characterized by a high degree of thermal resistance, has low alkali content, and is free from the magnesium–lime–zinc group of elements, heavy metals, arsenic, and antimony. Commercial brands are known as Pyrex® (Corning; Corning, NY) and Kimax® (Kimble; Vineland, NJ). The caustic conditions in storing concentrated alkaline solutions in borosilicate glass will etch or dissolve the glass and destroy the calibration. Borosilicate glassware with heavy walls, such as bottles, jars, and even larger beakers, should not be heated with a direct flame or hotplate. Glass should not be heated above its strain point (Pyrex® is 515°C) because rapid cooling strains and cracks glass easily when heated again. In the case of volumetric glassware, heating can destroy the calibration.

Corex® (Corning, NY)* brand glassware is a special alumina-silicate glass strengthened chemically rather than thermally. Corex is six times stronger than borosilicate glass (e.g., Corex® pipets have a typical strength of 30 000 psi, compared with 2000–5000 psi for borosilicate pipets) and will outlast conventional glassware by 10-fold. Corex® also resists clouding and scratching better.

Low actinic glassware is a glass of high thermal resistance with an amber or red color added as an integral part of the glass. The density of the red color is adjusted to permit adequate visibility of the contents, yet give maximum protection to light-sensitive materials, such as bilirubin standards. Low actinic glass is commonly used in containers used to store control material and reagents.

Types of Plasticware

Several types of plasticware are used in clinical laboratories. For example pipet tips, beakers, flask, cylinder and cuvets. Polypropylene, polyethylene, Teflon, polycarbonate and polystyrene are all examples of types of plastics used for laboratory plasticware.

Plastic pipet tips are made primarily of polypropylene. This type of plastic may be flexible or rigid, is chemically resistant and can be autoclaved. These pipet tips are translucent and come in a variety of sizes. Polypropylene is also used in several tube designs including specimen tubes, and test tubes. Specially formulated polypropylene is used for cryogenic procedures and can withstand temperatures down to −190°C.

Polyethylene is widely used in plasticware too, including test tubes, bottles, graduated tubes, stoppers, disposable transfer pipets, volumetric pipets and test tube racks. Polyethylene may bind or absorb proteins, dyes, stains and picric acid.

Polycarbonate is used in tubes for centrifugation, graduated cylinders and flasks. The usable temperature range is broad, −100 to +160°C. It is a very strong plastic but is not suitable for use with strong acids, bases and oxidizing agents. Polycarbonate may be autoclaved but with limitations (refer to furnished instructions).

Polystyrene is a rigid, clear type of plastic that should not be autoclaved. It is used in an assortment of tubes, including capped graduated tubes and test tubes. Polystyrene tubes will crack and splinter when crushed. This type of plastic is not resistant to most hydrocarbons, ketones, and alcohols.

Teflon is widely used for manufacturing stirring bars, tubing, cryogenic vials, and bottle cap liners. Teflon is almost chemically inert and is suitable for use at temperatures ranging from −270 to +255°C. This type of plastic is resistant to a wide range of chemical classes including acids, bases, alcohol and hydrocarbons.

Volumetric Laboratoryware

Pipets

There are many kinds of pipets available for use in a clinical laboratory, each intended to serve a specific function. They are used for reconstitution of controls and calibrators, preparing serum or plasma dilutions and aliquoting specimens. Thus, a high degree of accuracy and precision is required. Manual pipets fall into two general categories: transfer (volumetric) and measuring. Three subclassifications include, to contain (TC), to deliver (TD) and to deliver/blow-out (TD/blow-out).

Class A Designation

Class A glassware including pipets is manufactured and calibrated to deliver the most accurate volume of liquid. Class A specifications are defined by NIST. The College of American Pathologists (CAP) specifies that volumetric pipets must be of certified accuracy (Class A) or the volumes of the pipets must be verified by calibration techniques, e.g., gravimetric or photometric. The letter 'A' appears on all pipets that conform to the standards of Class A glassware. Volumetric glassware designated as Class A has been manufactured to Class A tolerances as established by the American Society for Testing and Materials (ASTM) E694 (West Conshohocken, Pennsylvania) for volumetric apparatus. Other standards include ASTME 542 for calibration of volumetric apparatus, ASTME 288 for volumetric flasks.

Types of Pipets

Pipets designed to contain (TC) are often referred to as rinse-out pipets because they must be refilled or rinsed out with the appropriate solvent after the initial liquid has been drained from the pipet. TC pipets contain an exact amount of liquid that must be completely transferred for accurate measurement. Examples of TC pipets are Sahli hemoglobin and Long-Levy pipets. These pipets do not meet Class A certification criteria.

To deliver or TD pipets are designed to drain by gravity. TD pipets must be held vertically and the tip placed against the side of the container and must not touch the liquid in it. The stated volume is obtained when draining stops. This type of pipet should not be blown out. Examples of TD pipets include Mohr, serological and volumetric transfer pipets. These pipets are designed to meet the requirements of Class A type pipets.

Volumetric TD pipets have an open-ended bulb, which holds the bulk of the liquid. On one side of the pipet is a long glass tube with a line indicating the extent to which the pipet is to be filled. The other end is tapered for smooth delivery of liquid. These pipets should be allowed to drain freely and not be shaken, or hit against the container. Any disruption of the free-flowing liquid may result in an inaccurate delivery of the liquid.

Some TD pipets are designed so that most of the contents are allowed to drain freely, after which the remaining fluid in the tip is blown out. These pipets are not rinsed out. Examples of pipets designed to be blow-out type pipets include Ostwald-Folin and serological pipets. TD/blow-out pipets are identified by the presence of one or two frosted bands near the mouthpiece of the pipet. It is vital to remember that one should never pipet or blow out solutions by mouth. It is always necessary to use an appropriate pipetting aid, e.g., bulb.

Serologic glass or plastic pipets are long tubes with uniform diameters. They have volume graduations extending to the delivery tip of the pipet. The last volume of liquid blown out is included in the delivery volume. The design of the Mohr TD pipet is different from that of the serological pipet. Mohr pipets are not graduated to the tip. The accuracy of the Mohr pipets is valid only when the pipet is filled. If smaller volumes are dispensed, the accuracy decreases proportionally.

Micropipets

The two most widely used types of micropipets are the air displacement and positive displacement. These pipets are capable of delivering liquid volumes from 1–1000 μL. Some micropipets are designed to deliver a fixed volume while others can deliver variable amounts of sample.

Air-displacement pipets are piston-operated devices. A disposable, one-time use polypropylene tip is attached to the pipet barrel. The pipet tip is placed into the liquid to be aspirated and drawn into and dispensed from this tip.

Positive-displacement pipets use a capillary tip that may be siliconized glass, glass or plastic. This type of pipet is useful if a reagent reacts to plastics. Positive-displacement pipets use a Teflon-tipped plunger that fits tightly inside the capillary. These capillary tips are reusable and carry-over is negligible if the pipet is properly maintained. Some procedures require a washing or flushing step in between samples.

Pipet Calibration

Monitoring the performance of pipetting devices is not only mandatory in most states that issue licenses to laboratories that perform diagnostic testing but it is also very wise. Micropipets should be verified for accuracy and precision before they are put into use and monitored during the course of the year. The frequency of verification depends in part on the amount of use and requirements by the licensing and/or accrediting agency. Proper maintenance of air-displacement pipets is very important. This type of pipet has a fixed stroke length that must be maintained. These pipets also have seals to prevent air from leaking into the pipet when the piston is moved. These seals require periodic greasing to maintain their integrity.

Positive-displacement micropipets need to have their spring checked and the Teflon tip replaced periodically. A slide wire is used to quickly check the plunger setting. This check does not replace the scheduled precision and accuracy checks.

---

* Corning Glass no longer manufactures Corex® glassware.

There are several procedures used by laboratories to verify precision and accuracy of micropipets. Most of these procedures are time-consuming especially the procedures that require the weighing of water. No matter, this verification procedure must be done to assure proper performance of the laboratory micropipets.

CLSI has provided an acceptable procedure for determining pipet accuracy and precision (I8-P, NCCLS, 1984). This gravimetric procedure is labor intensive but does provide a low-cost means of complying with the regulations set forth by the various accrediting agencies.

More expensive procedures for calibrating micropipets include:
- commercial photometric pipet calibration products
- calibration services providers
- Pipet Tracker™ (Labtronics Inc., Canada).

One of the major concerns when considering the cost attributed to pipet calibration procedures is technologist time. The technologist time required for the photometric procedures is often 50–60% less than the inexpensive manual weighing techniques.

Volumetric Flasks

Volumetric flasks represent a special type of glassware in the laboratory. These flasks are often used to prepare standards for quantitative procedures. Therefore the accuracy must be optimal. Volumetric flasks used for the preparation of standards and other solutions requiring optimal accuracy must meet Class A specifications as defined by NIST. These specifications are imprinted on the flasks. Volumetric flasks are used to contain (TC) an exact volume when the flask is filled to the *mark*. A Teflon or ground-glass stopper should be used to seal the flask. Volumetric flasks should not be used for reagent storage.

Calibration of Volumetric Glassware

According to the strictest of standards, every piece of volumetric glassware in the clinical laboratory should be coded and a record kept of its calibration. Any piece of glassware that does not meet Class A tolerance should be rejected. To prepare a piece of glassware for calibration, thoroughly wash and dry it using appropriate cleaning procedures. CLSI can provide the laboratory with an appropriate procedure to calibrate volumetric flasks.

Thermometry

Thermometers and other types of temperature sensing devices are used in the laboratory to monitor the temperatures in refrigerators, freezers, water baths, heating blocks, and incubators. Special applications of thermometry include osmometry, refrigerated centrifuges, refrigerated reagent compartments of automated analyzers, warming compartments of automated analyzers and circulating waters baths for cuvet compartments in automated analyzers. All of these temperature-monitoring applications have the same requirements, and they are, accurate measurements and a constant temperature.

Appropriate quality control procedures must be carried out and documented routinely for all of these temperature-monitoring devices. Any temperature sensitive device that fails to perform within established tolerances must be replaced. Because many assays performed in the laboratory are enzymatic in nature even the slightest deviation from the optimal temperature required to perform the assay may result in an erroneous result.

Types of Thermometers

The two types of liquid-in-glass thermometers most widely used are total immersion and partial immersion. A total immersion thermometer requires that the bulb and entire column of liquid be immersed into the medium measured. These thermometers are used to monitor freezers and refrigerators. Partial immersion thermometers must have the bulb and stem immersed to the immersion line or defined depth on the thermometer. This type of thermometer is often used for water baths and heating blocks.

Special applications of temperature-sensing devices

Thermistors are used in several types of instruments found in the laboratory including freezing point depression osmometers. A thermistor is a transducer that converts changes in temperature (heat) to resistance. It consists of a small bead constructed of a fused mixture of metal oxides, attached to two leads and encapsulated in glass. The metal oxide mixture has a large negative temperature coefficient of resistance. Thus a small decrease in temperature causes a relatively large increase in the resistance of the thermistor.

A thermocouple is a sensor that consists of two dissimilar metals, joined together at one end. When the junction of the two metals is heated or cooled a voltage is produced that can be correlated back to the temperature. Thermocouples come in several designs including beaded wire, probes and surface probes. An important feature of most thermocouples used in laboratory analyzers is their fast response times. The response time of a thermocouple is defined as the time required by a sensor to reach 63.2% of a step change in temperature under a specified set of conditions. Five time constants are required for the sensor to approach 100% of the step change value.

Laboratory applications for thermocouple use include gas and liquid chromatography, surface temperature measurements in heating compartments in automated analyzers, thermo-cuvets, and circulating water baths in chemistry analyzers

Mercury-free laboratories

There are initiatives nationwide to make laboratories mercury-free. For example in June 1998 a landmark agreement was put together between the American Hospital Association (AHA) and the US Environmental Protection Agency (EPA) (JCAHO, 2002). A memo of understanding was signed between the two organizations in an effort to decrease and eventually eliminate hospital pollution practices over a 5- to 10-year period. One of the goals is to eliminate mercury waste.

Mercury is contained in numerous chemical reagents used by the laboratory and of course in mercury thermometers. The cost associated with proper disposal of mercury and the impact of mercury in the environment make replacing mercury thermometers a sound idea. Several alternatives exist for replacement thermometers that provide the necessary accuracy for laboratories procedures. They include:
- thermometers containing an organic red-spirit and pressurized with nitrogen gas
- thermometers containing blue biodegradable liquid (isoamyl benzoate and dye)
- a red liquid thermometer filled with kerosene
- bimetal digital thermometers
- digital thermometers with stainless steel stems.

Thermometer Calibration

Monitoring the temperature accuracy of thermometers is necessary to ensure the reliability of procedures requiring temperature regulation. Thermometers may be purchased with a certificate to indicate traceability to standards provided by NIST. Also, many commercially available thermometers meet or exceed NIST and American National Standards Institute (NY, NY)/Scientific Apparatus Makers Association (UK) (ANSI/SAMA) tolerance for accuracy.

Noncertified thermometers can be calibrated by using a NIST SRM® 934 thermometer or a NIST SRM® 1968 gallium melting point cell. The SRM® 934 clinical laboratory thermometer is calibrated per specifications by International Temperature Scale 1990 (ITS-90) at 0, 25, 30, and 37°C. A gallium melting point cell consists of about 25 g of very pure (99.99999%) gallium metal that has a single fixed melting point at 29.7646°C (as defined by ITS-90). The gallium is sealed in an inert plastic crucible and surrounded in a stainless steel envelop (Strouse, 1997).

Temperature monitoring devices should be verified for accuracy at 6- or 12-month intervals. Guidelines and procedures for proper monitoring and tolerances are available (NCCLS approved standard I2-A2, 1990).

Water Baths

For general clinical laboratory use, constant temperature water baths must offer variable temperature control from +5°C above ambient temperature to 100°C, with accurate control to ± 0.2°C. Water baths can be circulating or noncirculating. The circulating water baths provide the best temperature control. Another important consideration in the selection of a constant temperature bath is that the model be large enough to accommodate the desired working volume.

Maintenance

Maintenance of a constant temperature water bath is improved by filling it with type II (or type I) water. This prevents the accumulation of mineral deposits from regular tap water, which can affect the temperature-sensing elements and generally lead to poor heat transfer. However, if an accumulation of these minerals does occur, a weak hydrochloric acid solution will dissolve the deposits. Frequent cleaning and fresh water will prevent overgrowth of bacteria and algae. Also a 1 : 1000 dilution of thimerosal (Merthiolate) can be added to help prevent bacterial growth. Overheating and subsequent damage can occur if the bath goes dry. At higher temperatures the bath should be covered, both to maintain proper temperature control and to prevent rapid evaporation to dryness.

Quality Control

A thermometer calibrated against another certified by NIST must be a component of any water bath. The temperature should be noted and recorded for each assay. This function by the operator ensures that indeed the temperature of the bath is the same as the reading of the thermometer.

Heating Blocks, Dry-Bath Incubators and Ovens

Heating blocks and dry-bath incubators are commonly used for incubating liquids at higher temperatures. Most incubators are constructed of an aluminum alloy that is capable of distributing the heat in a uniform manner. Their heating efficiency is less than a circulating water bath but will maintain a constant temperature within $\pm 0.5°C$. A certified thermometer or NIST calibrated thermometer must be present in the heating block to monitor the temperature.

Heating ovens are used in chromatography procedures, to dry chemicals, and assist in extraction, and are used to dry membrane or gels in electrophoresis. Several different designs are available depending upon the desired temperature and purpose. Oven designs include programmable, vacuum or standard laboratory type. Temperature control is usually within $\pm 1°C$. The oven must have a certified thermometer or NIST calibrated thermometer available to monitor the interior temperature.

Mixing

Mixing is an operation intended to form a homogeneous mass or create a uniform heterogeneous system. Mixing is used to bring solids into solution; to bring phases into intimate contact, for instance, in extraction procedures; to wash suspended solids; to homogenize liquid phases; and to perform many other operations. A serious consequence of inadequate mixing can be failure to completely resuspend protein that settles out under long-term frozen storage of serum controls, resulting in invalid data. In some instances, excessive mixing may cause denaturation of protein or hemolysis. A phase separation occurs when serum (or plasma) specimens stand for a period of time and must be thoroughly mixed before analysis. The concentration of even small molecules in such a system will be heterogeneous as proteins settle and become more concentrated, thus effective water concentration decreases in this layer. This produces a water concentration gradient throughout the system and, consequently, a concentration gradient of all components.

Single-Tube Mixers

A vortex mixer is capable of a variable speed oscillation that results in a swirling motion to liquid contents of a test tube or other container. The angle of contact and degree of pressure can be regulated for optimal mixing action. A very effective mixing action is created by a multiple touch sequence (i.e., touching and withdrawing the tube from the neoprene oscillating cup of the mixer). The operator must be careful not to fill the container too full or to mix the liquid contents too fast, since spillage can occur.

Multiple-Tube Mixers

Various mixers are available that handle a number of tubes and tube sizes, and with different types of mixing motions. A Thermolyne Maxi-Mix (Sybron Corporation, Dubuque, IA) can conveniently be used for vortex mixing one tube or several tubes at one time. Changing the pressure of the container against the replaceable foam rubber top varies mixing action. Circular motion on a tilted disk provides continuous inversion of contents in tubes, which are clip-mounted at the circumference of the rotating disk. Rotational speed can be varied to provide gentle or more vigorous mixing. Control sera are conveniently reconstituted on this type of mixer. Tube shakers that operate by tilting back and forth at variable speeds provide thorough mixing of whole blood samples.

Aqueous Solution

The concentration of a solution may be expressed as molarity (M), normality (N), and less frequently (m) molality. Accurate preparation of reagents requires fundamental knowledge of solution chemistry, basic mathematics and techniques.

Molarity

Molarity (M) is equal to the number of moles of solute per liter of solution (solvent). A mole of a substance is the number of grams equal to the atomic or molecular weight of the substance. The atomic or molecular

weight of a substance is the actual mass of the chemical particle (atom or molecule) relative to the mass of the carbon atom. One mole of any substance will contain approximately 6.02×10^{23} particles (Avogadro's number). Thus a one molar solution contains 1 mole of solute per liter of solution.

Example 4–7. How many grams of NaCl are required to prepare 1 liter of a 0.5 M solution? The gram molecular weight (GMW) of NaCl is 58.5?
Solution

$$GMW \times M = g/L$$
$$58.5 \times 0.5 = 29.25\ g/L$$

Therefore weigh out 29.25 g of NaCl and transfer it to a 1-L volumetric flask. Add water to the 1-L mark on the flask.

Millimoles

When small concentrations are used, they are frequently expressed in millimoles per liter (1000 mmol = 1 mol). For example, to prepare 10 mL of a 10 mmol (0.01 moles) NaOH solution, 4 mg NaOH are diluted to 10 mL.

Normality

Normality (N) is equal to the number of gram equivalents of solute per liter of solution and is dependent on type of reaction involved, e.g. acid–base, oxidation. One-gram equivalent weight of an element or compound equals the gram molecular weight divided by number of replaceable hydrogens or hydroxyls (also valence):

Gram equivalent weight = GMW/Number of replaceable hydrogens, hydroxyls or valence
1 N = Number of gram equivalents of solute/L of solution

Example 4–8. What is the gram equivalent weight of $Ca(OH)_2$ (GMW = 74)?
Solution

Gram equivalent weight = 74/2 = 37
1 mole = 2 equivalents

Example 4–9. What is the gram equivalent weight of H_2SO_4 (GMW = 98)?
Solution

Gram equivalent weight = 98/2 = 49
1 mole = 2 equivalents

Example 4–10. How many milliliters of concentrated H_2SO_4 (specific gravity, 1.84, percent purity, 96.2%) are required to prepare 1 liter of a 1 normal solution?
Solution

Step 1: compute GEW H_2SO_4 = 98/2 = 49.
Step 2: compute the number of grams of H_2SO_4 in 1 liter = 98 g/L.
Step 3: compute number of grams of H_2SO_4 per milliliter of solution = SG $\times$ % assay = $1.84 \times 96.2 = 1.77$.
Step 4: compute numbers of milliliters of concentrated H_2SO_4 required preparing 1 liter of a 1 normal solution:

$$\frac{1.77\ g}{1\ mL} = \frac{49\ g}{X\ mL}$$

$$X = 27.6\ mL$$

Molal

In the laboratory, we sometimes measure the physical properties of solutions; for example, when we measure the osmolality of serum or urine. The molality of the solution is determined instead of the molarity. A molal solution is one mole of solute in one kilogram of solvent. Molal solutions are based on weight, not volume. Since the density of water at room temperature is approximately 1 gram per milliliter, 1000 grams of water occupies about 1 liter. Therefore, a 1 molal aqueous solution is approximately the same as a 1 molar solution.

Example 4–11. How many grams of NaOH are needed to make a 2.00 molal solution?
Solution

Step 1: determine the GMW of NaOH = 40g.
Step 2: compute the number of grams of NaOH required to prepare the solution by using the following formula:

$$Molality = \frac{Grams\ of\ solute/GMW\ of\ solute}{1.0\ kg\ of\ solvent}$$

$$2\ Molal = \frac{X\ g\ of\ NaOH/40.00\ g}{1.0\ kg\ of\ solvent}$$

$$X = 80\ g\ of\ NaOH$$

Dilutions

Dilution procedures are not performed as frequently as in the past owing to the improvements in computers and instruments where the system performs the dilution automatically. But, there are occasions when a dilution has to be prepared and a brief review follows.

A laboratory procedure may involve the addition of one substance to another to reduce the concentration of one of the substances. This mixture is called a dilution. Laboratory staff often confused the terminology associated with dilutions and ratios. The term ratio is the more general and refers to an amount of one thing relative to an amount of something else with no other implications. Dilution, as the term is used in laboratories, is more specific. It refers to a number of parts of a substance in the total number of parts of mixture containing the substance. The implication is how the mixture was made or how it is to be made. The following are examples of ratios followed by dilutions:

Ratios

1. The serum to saline ratio is 1 : 9.
2. The saline to serum ratio is 9 : 1.
3. The serum to total volume ratio is 1 : 10.

Note that a colon is used as the ratio symbol.

Dilutions

1. Make a 1 to 10 dilution of serum in saline.
2. Make a 1 in 10 dilution of serum in saline.
3. Make a 1/10 dilution of serum with saline.

Example 4–12. Prepare a 1 ml to 10 ml dilution of a serum sample.

Solution. Pipet 1.0 ml of serum and add 9.0 ml of saline for a total volume of 10 ml.

A clinical application may involve the dilution of a patient serum sample because the bilirubin result exceeds the upper limit of linearity. The technologist decides to make a 1 to 2 dilution of the sample and assay the diluted sample. To prepare the dilution the technologist pipets 100 μL of patient serum and adds 100 μL of water for a total volume of 200 μL. The sample is assayed for bilirubin and the analyzer prints out a value 12 mg/dL. Before reporting the patient's bilirubin result the technologist must multiply the analyzer value times 2 (the dilution factor) and then report the value of 24 mg/dL.

Acids, Alkalis, and pH

An acid molecule yields hydrogen ions (protons) in aqueous solutions; an alkali accepts these. At room temperature in pure water:

$$[H^+] = [OH^-] = 1 \times 10^{-7} \text{ molar}$$

In all aqueous solutions, both acid and alkaline:

$$K_w = [H^+] \times [OH^-] = 10^{-14}$$

In an acid solution, $[H^+]$ is greater than 10^{10-7} mol. In an alkaline solution, $[H^+]$ is less than 10^{10-7} mol. pH is the exponent that must be applied to 10 in order to give the value of $1/H^+$. That is:

$$pH = \log_{10} 1/H^+$$

When pH is	H^+ is	and OH^- is
1	10^{-1}	10^{-13}
2	10^{-2}	10^{-12}
4	10^{-4}	10^{-10}
6	10^{-6}	10^{-8}
10	10^{-10}	10^{-4}
13	10^{-13}	10^{-1}

A change of one pH unit indicates a 10-fold change in H^+ concentration.

Buffer Solution

The theory of buffers and their preparation can be found in Appendix 1. For most commonly used buffers, the amounts of salts of the acids and bases have been predetermined and may be found in reference books, e.g., Bates, 1973, which contains a very good discussion of the theoretical aspects of buffers and extensive information of how to prepare several buffer solutions.

References

ASTM: E288-03 Standard Specification for Laboratory Glass Volumetric Flasks. ASTM International. Online. Available: http://www.astm.org.

ASTM: E542-01 Standard Practice for Calibration of Laboratory Volumetric Apparatus. ASTM International. Online. Available: http://www.astm.org.

ASTM: E694-99 Standard Specification for Laboratory Glass Volumetric Apparatus. ASTM International. Online. Available: http://www.astm.org.

For referenced ASTM standards, visit the ASTM website, or contact ASTM Customer Service at service@astm.org. For Annual Book of ASTM Standards volume information, refer to the standard's Document Summary page on the ASTM website.

Bartle KD: Introduction to the theory of chromatographic separations with reference to gas chromatography. *In* Baugh PJ (ed): Gas Chromatography; A Practical Approach, 1st ed. New York, Oxford University Press, 1993, pp 9–10.

Bates RG: Determination of pH – Theory and Practice, 2nd ed. New York, John Wiley and Sons, 1973.

Bender GT: Principles of Chemical Instrumentation. Philadelphia, WB Saunders Company, 1987.

Clinical and Laboratory Standard Institute (CLSI), formerly the National Committee for Clinical Laboratory Standard (NCCLS) (Wayne, PA 19087-1898).

Provides comprehensive guidelines and procedures for basic laboratory methods.

Gauldie J: Principles and clinical applications of nephelometry. *In* Kaplan LA, Pesce AJ (eds): Nonisotopic Alternatives to Radioimmunoassays. New York, Marcel Dekker Inc, 1981, pp 289–291.

Joint Commission on Accreditation of Health Care Organizations (JCAHO): Eliminating Mercury in Hospitals. Environmental Best Practices for Health Care Facilities. US Environmental Protection Agency, November 2002.

Karasek FW, Clement RE: Basic Gas Chromatography–Mass Spectrometry: Principles and Techniques. Amsterdam, Elsevier, 1988.

Love JE, Ward KM: Electrophoretic instrumentation systems. *In* Ward KM, Lehmann CA, Leiken AM (eds): Clinical Laboratory Instrumentation and Automation: Principles, Applications, and Selection. Philadelphia, WB Saunders Company, 1994, pp 173–174.

NCCLS: Determining Performance of Volumetric Equipment, NCCLS Proposed Standard I8-P, Villanova, PA, NCCLS, 1984.

NCCLS: Temperature Calibration of Water Baths, Instruments, and Temperature Sensors, 2nd ed. NCCLS Approved Standard I2-A2, Villanova, PA, NCCLS, 1990.

NCCLS: Preparation and Testing of Reagent Water in the Clinical Laboratory, 3rd ed. NCCLS Approved Guideline C3-A3, Villanova, PA, NCCLS, 1997.

Ravindranath B: Principles and Practice of Chromatography. Chichester, England, Ellis Horwood, 1989, pp 89–127.

Rayleigh, Lord B: On waves propagated along the plane surface of an elastic solid. Proc London Math Soc 1885; xviv:4–11.

Rubinson KA, Rubinson JF. Contemporary Instrumental Analysis. NJ, Prentice Hall, 2000.

Schoeff LE, Williams RH: Principles of Laboratory Instruments. St Louis, Mosby, 1993.

Skoog DA, Holler FJ, Nieman TA: Principles of Instrumental Analysis, 5th ed. Philadelphia, Harcourt Brace & Company, 1998.

Provides a comprehensive explanation of instrument principles for nearly all clinical laboratory equipment.

Strouse GF, Furukawa GT, Mangum BW, et al: NIST Standard Reference Materials for Use as Thermometric Fixed Points. Gaithersburg, MD, NIST, 1997.

Tipler A: Gas chromatography instrumentation, operation, and experimental considerations. *In* Baugh PJ (ed): Gas Chromatography; A Practical Approach, 1st ed. New York, Oxford University Press, 1993, pp 63–67.

Willard HH, Merritt LL, Dean JA, et al: Instrumental Methods of Analysis. Belmont, CA, Wadsworth, Inc, 1988.

CHAPTER 5

Analysis: Clinical Laboratory Automation

Robert L. Sunheimer MS MT(ASCP)SC SLS, Gregory Threatte MD

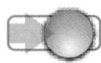

KEY POINTS
• Laboratory testing has undergone revolutionary changes over the past decade so that all routine chemistry and hematology testing is completely automated.

• This includes specimen processing; all tubes are initially bar coded; they can be directly placed on autoanalyzers which not only read which tests to perform but can directly sample from tubes and enter all results in the laboratory computer system, which is linked directly to the hospital information system.

• The three stages of laboratory testing are pre-analytical, analytical and post-analytical. Several examples of how these stages have been automated are presented in this chapter.

• Instrument manufacturers are attempting to design systems that will offset the staff shortages, provide a safer working environment for technologists and provide the test menus and throughputs being demanded by the clinicians.

Introduction

Automation in the clinical laboratories has been available since the mid-1950s with the introduction of the Technicon Auto Analyzer® for laboratory use. The primary driver of automation has been the need to create automated systems capable of reducing or eliminating the many manual tasks required to perform analytical procedures. Continued development has led to, at first, the consolidation of most high-volume chemistry measurements onto single platforms and more recently to the consolidation of chemistry and immunoassay systems onto single platforms. By eliminating manual steps, the opportunity to reduce error is enhanced since the potential for error due to fatigue or erroneous sample identification is reduced.

In parallel with these automation steps in chemistry, the 1960s witnessed remarkable growth in hematology laboratories with the introduction of automated electronic cell counting instruments that drastically changed measurements previously performed with pipets, hemocytometers, and microscopes. After initially improving accuracy and precision with red cell measurements, subsequent development and adaptations including flow cytometric technology have now allowed both the automation of most white blood cell differentials as well as a more flow cytometric based classification of hematopoietic neoplasms.

The 1970s saw the introduction and implementation of laboratory information systems, automating the process of information flow in the clinical laboratory and eliminating the expected 5% transcription error rate seen when laboratory results were manually transcribed into various medical record formats. The 1990s saw the introduction of intralaboratory transportation systems, including specimen carriers and a conveyor taking samples between instruments, and including processing stations such as centrifugation, decapping/capping and storage, leading to the concept of total laboratory automation.

At the time of the last publication of this book, the American laboratory automation industry included three independent laboratory automation companies (LAB-InterLink, Inc., Labotix Automation Inc., and AutoMed, Inc.). Since then, AutoMed now provides support primarily to its parent company, MDS, Inc., which controls more than 30% of the Canadian laboratory market. LAB-Interlink, first bought Labotix, and then later declared bankruptcy, leaving many customers with expensive systems that could no longer be supported. As a result, hospital administrators have become increasingly cautious, making new systems more difficult to justify.

The system vendors that remain in the American market are largely aligned with major in vitro diagnostic instrument manufacturers or provide modular products automating only a portion of an automation solution. In spite of this lack of independent vendors, the need for reduced turnaround time, reduced error rate and decreased dependency on manual labor makes the need for automation as strong as ever.

Overall, the scope and magnitude of the drivers of automation have taken a direction similar to all other technologies. A list of factors that serve to drive automation is shown in Table 5–1. In this chapter several of these drivers will be discussed in the context of how automation in the clinical laboratory has changed over time to become what it is today. Several analytical systems will be selected as examples of how manufacturers responded to the demands of the laboratory. The cause and impact of change on the three stages of laboratory testing will be presented, beginning with pre-analytical, then analytical and finally post-analytical stages. The demands of the laboratory are paced in part by the needs of clinicians and patients, and this has provided the majority of drivers that push the changes seen in laboratory automation today.

Automated Analysis

The measurement of samples using automated instrumentation has undergone an evolutionary process since the Technicon Auto Analyzer®. It

Table 5–1 Factors that Serve to Drive Laboratory Automation
Turnaround times (TAT) demands
Specimen integrity
Staff shortages
Economic factors
Less maintenance
Less calibration
Less downtime
Faster start-up times
24/7 uptime
Throughput
Computer and software technology
Primary tube sampling
Increasing the number of different analytes on one system
Increasing the number of different methods on one system
Reducing laboratory errors
Number of specimens
Types of fluids
Safety
Environmental concerns, i.e., biohazard risks

Table 5–2 Examples of Sample Processing Tasks
ID/labeling
Sorting
Centrifuging
Decapping
Aliquoting
Recapping/storage/retrieval

began with a single channel analyzer using continuous flow analysis and measured one analyte on a batch of samples, i.e., one sample, one test. These samples were measured in a sequential fashion, i.e., one sample after another. The specimen throughput rates were approximately 40–60 per hour. Technicon continued to develop upon their systems, which evolved into multiple channel instruments, e.g., SMAC II® that produced specimen throughput rates as high as 150 per hour with test throughput of approximately 3750 test per hour depending upon the test configuration. One major disadvantage to this type of instrument configuration was that all testing was performed in a parallel fashion. This resulted in the measurement of every analyte configured on the system for every sample. This inflexibility in testing led to the development of analyzers that provided 'discrete' testing, i.e., measured only the tests requested on a sample.

The next generation of automated analyzers included centrifugal analyzers and modular analyzer configurations. Centrifugal analyzers were discrete, batch-type systems. A significant limitation at the time was the throughput rates. Because the analyzers were configured to measure one analyte at a time, the only way to improve upon throughput was to purchase multiple systems so that several tests could be run simultaneously depending upon how many systems the laboratory purchased.

The solution to the drawbacks associated with centrifugal analysis was to design a modular system that could be configured to measure multiple analytes on multiple samples and the process be controlled by a computer rather than humans. This is the essence of *random access testing*. Modular instruments allow the user to add-on additional units, e.g., ISE and/or immunoassay modules.

The ultimate result of combining modular design with random access testing was to increase specimen throughput rates to hundreds per hour and test throughput rates to thousands per hour.

Pre-Analytical Stage

The three stages of laboratory testing are pre-analytical, analytical and post-analytical. Improving efficiency and productivity during the pre-analytical stage of laboratory testing was not the main focus of laboratory staff at the outset. Likewise the post-analytical stage received very little attention. This lack of attention to improvements for these two stages are due in part to the lack of technologies that would later be developed and serve to change the scope of each of these stages. Also many of the drivers of automation that now exist were not a priority in the early days of clinical laboratories.

The pre-analytical stage is concerned primarily with sample or specimen processing. For decades specimens drawn within a facility were brought to the laboratory usually by the blood drawers or 'runners.' If the specimens were obtained from outside the laboratory facility a courier service was often used. Courier service is a batch process that requires scheduling from a given pick-up point. These individuals represented the first link between patient and laboratory, and were also a source of problems that would result in some remarkable changes and innovations to the process of laboratory

testing as a whole. One example of an early solution to replacing humans as specimen carriers was the introduction of pneumatic tubes.

Pneumatic tube delivery systems were installed to provide point-to-point delivery of specimens to the laboratory and offered several advantages over human transport. The tubes are sent very quickly to the laboratory encased in a carrier lined with a foam-type material to reduce breakage. Pneumatic tube systems are designed to prevent hemolysis by avoiding significant elevations of g forces during acceleration and deceleration.

Electric track vehicles can transport a larger number of specimens than pneumatic tubes. The electric tracks require a station for loading and unloading specimens and this may pose a problem in facilities with limited space. Like couriers, electric tracks allow for batching of specimens.

Later robots or mobile robots of many designs were used by laboratories to transport specimens from within and outside of the facility. Samples are usually batched for pick-up and delays in time of pick-up notification occurred.

Conveyors or track systems are used in some laboratory facilities, especially if the laboratory receives a very large number of samples. Conveyor or track systems are designed to transport specimens in a horizontal fashion and upward or vertically to another floor.

Once the specimens arrive at the laboratory processing workstation several tasks need to be done. These tasks are listed in Table 5–2. Several novel approaches were used and culminated into what is termed 'pre-analytical modules.' These modules are available from several instrument manufacturers. There were many earlier attempts to process specimens with minimal human involvement prior to the development of pre-analytical modules. Many of these devices are still used.

Labeling specimens by hand requires a substantial amount of time and proved to be a large source of laboratory error. Labeling went beyond the specimen tube and included pour-off tubes, sample cups, dilution cups and send-out containers. The use of printed bar code labels facilitated this process tremendously. Later as computers became more sophisticated and communication between computers improved, the bar code label system improved processing time and reduced pre-analytical errors.

Manual sorting or separating of samples was needed because of the diverse type of testing most laboratories engaged in. Specimen tubes of all shapes and sizes would be received in the processing area of a clinical laboratory and the technologist would have to sort tubes by stopper color, size, tests ordered, instrument design requirements and tube destinations.

In the earlier days of clinical laboratories each red top tube was double spun so that clot removal was optimal. This step required manual decapping of the specimen tubes. The invention of the serum separator tube eliminated the need for this double spin technique, and decapping at this stage was not necessary. A specimen would have to be decapped to process aliquots, poured off into sample cups or to be introduced into the analyzer. The decapping of tubes posed health hazards to the technologist via aerosol dispersal from the tubes, and direct contact with the blood.

Centrifugation of blood collection tubes required the technologist to manually load tube carriers and place them into the centrifuge. The tubes would then be removed from the centrifuge and re-sorted, aliquots would be processed and the samples distributed to their destinations or target area. This whole process was fraught with potential safety hazards, opportunities for mistakes and large increases in sample processing time.

Many specimens required aliquots to be poured off, also known as splitting of the samples. The aliquots were used by instrument operators, sent to other laboratories sections, sent out to reference laboratories and used for dilutions. Like other manual processing steps, aliquoting blood specimens was a potential source of hazards for the laboratory staff, errors and increased processing time.

When the samples were no longer needed for testing they were stored in a refrigerator or freezer. All of the samples were stored in an organized fashion in the event that they were needed again for retesting. Manual storage and retrieval of samples created big problems for some laboratories. Samples were often lost, not stored properly, and hard to locate.

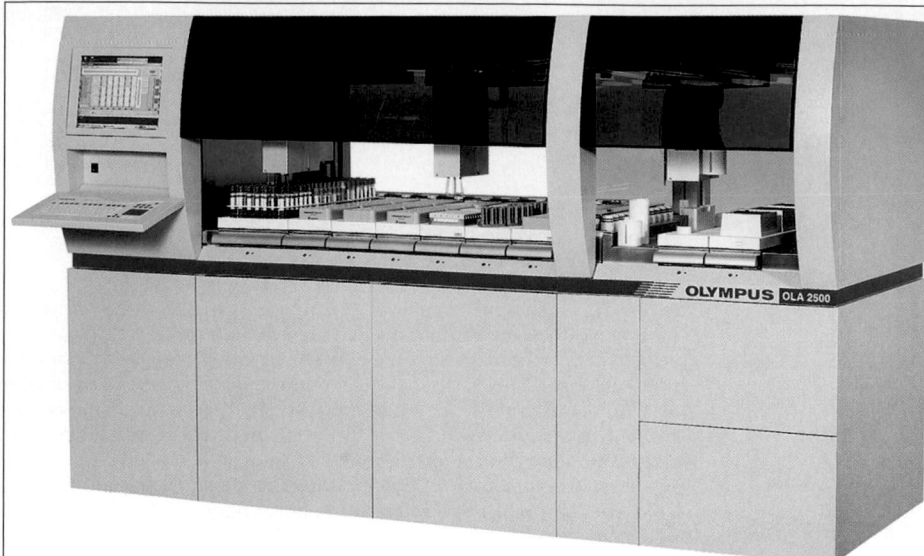

Figure 5–1 Olympus® OLA 2500™ Lab Automation System. This system consists of a decapper, sorter, archiver and aliquotter with throughput of 650 tubes per hour. (From Olympus with permission.)

Automated Approaches to Specimen Processing

Two goals for automating specimen processing are (1) to minimize non-value-added steps in the laboratory process, e.g., sorting tubes, and (2) to increase available time for value-added steps in the tasks that technologists perform that help make a difference in the quality of the test result and ultimately, the diagnosis.

Advantages for automating laboratory testing include:
- increasing the quality of the pre-analytical steps
- reducing error rates
- reducing operator exposure to potentially hazardous biological material
- eliminating repetitive stress injuries.

There are several front-end sample processing systems available to improve upon all of the shortcomings associated with manual sample processing. The system designs may be integrated specimen processing or modular. Some modular systems are designed to exist as stand-alone front-end processors.

Integrated specimen processing systems allow the user to perform some or the entire specimen handling tasks. These systems process only certain types of samples and specimen containers. This inflexibility with specimen containers resulted in many laboratories, especially hospital laboratories, to purchase modular specimen processing systems. Each module has its own on-board computer that is linked to a master controller computer systems. Also modular systems can accommodate several different specimen types, e.g., whole blood, serum and plasma, with their respective specimen containers.

Whatever the configuration, each automated pre-analytical system attempts to provide the user with some or all of the tasks necessary to prepare samples for testing. These tasks include:
- pre-sorting
- centrifugation
- volume checks
- clot detection
- decapping
- secondary tube labeling
- aliquoting
- destination sorting into analyzer racks.

The stand-alone system automates one portion of front-end processing. Stand-alone systems automate the sample sorting, sample uncapping, and aliquot functions of the front-end samples processing. A centrifuge is not included in this design. If serum or plasma is required the sample must be carried to the centrifuge by the technologist. Examples of stand-alone automated units are the Roche Diagnostic PSD1 decapper/sorter and Roche Diagnostic VSII aliquoter/sorter (Roche Diagnostics, Indianapolis, IN). These units are featured as *task targeted automation*, a concept that is characterized by state-of-the-art automation of pre- and post-analytical steps. Samples are processed by these units and then hand carried to their respective workstation or targets. The PSD1 and VSII are designed to increase the quality of pre-analytical steps, reduce operator exposure to hazardous biological material and eliminate repetitive stress injuries.

Archiving and retrieval of specimens in an automated fashion is also available in stand-alone designs. Automated sample archiving systems use bar-coded specimens that are scanned and placed in numbered positions in numbered racks. Retrieval of specimens is initiated by entering the patient's sample accession number or a medical record number into the archival system's database. The rack number and position in the rack are determined and displayed for the user. Some systems include a refrigerator for sample storage and automatic disposal of samples at predetermined times.

Olympus (Olympus American Inc., Diagnostic System Group, Melville, NY) has designed a fully automated pre- and post-analytical sample handling system that can serve as a stand-alone unit or modular unit to be utilized in configurations that fit the laboratory's volume and workflow patterns. The OLA 2500™ Lab Automation System (Fig. 5–1) has several unique features that include:
- A camera station that recognizes tube types and tube sizes, and can be used for sample material recognition as well as sample volume calculations.
- The aliquoting unit uses disposable tips to eliminate any carryover. It also can generate up to six daughter tubes from each mother tube.
- Archiving can be performed either in parallel to sorting or as a batch.

Modular systems are designed to automate the entire process. The automated modular system decaps specimens, prepares aliquots, sorts (mother and daughter samples) and transports specimens via a track system. A sample sensor or transducer senses liquid levels, separator gels and detects short samples. The Roche **MODULAR** PRE-ANALYTICS (Fig. 5–2) combines many of the pre-analytical steps, which are coordinated using an *intelligent process management* component.

Analytical Stage

The analytical stage of testing has evolved to a very sophisticated level due to the progress in technology, improvements in computer technology, and as a result of many of the drivers of automation listed earlier. The tasks in the analytical stage of laboratory testing are listed in Table 5–3.

Sample Introduction

Automatic sampling may be accomplished using several different physical mechanisms. Peristaltic pumps and positive-liquid displacements pipets are two examples. Peristaltic pumps are an example of older technology but are still used in some instrument designs, e.g., electrolyte measurements. Positive-liquid displacement pipets are usually a single pipet that transfers samples from cups or tubes to the next analytical process. Most positive displacement pipets function in one of two ways. Either they dispense aspirated samples into the reaction container or they flush out samples together with diluent.

The movement of the sample from the sample cup or tube to its destination via the sample probe is accomplished in several different ways. Some analyzers use a robotic-like arm that pivots back and forth, picking up a sample and depositing it into a reaction vessel or onto the surface of a porous pad. Other systems may use a worm gear device that pulls the sample probe from one point to another.

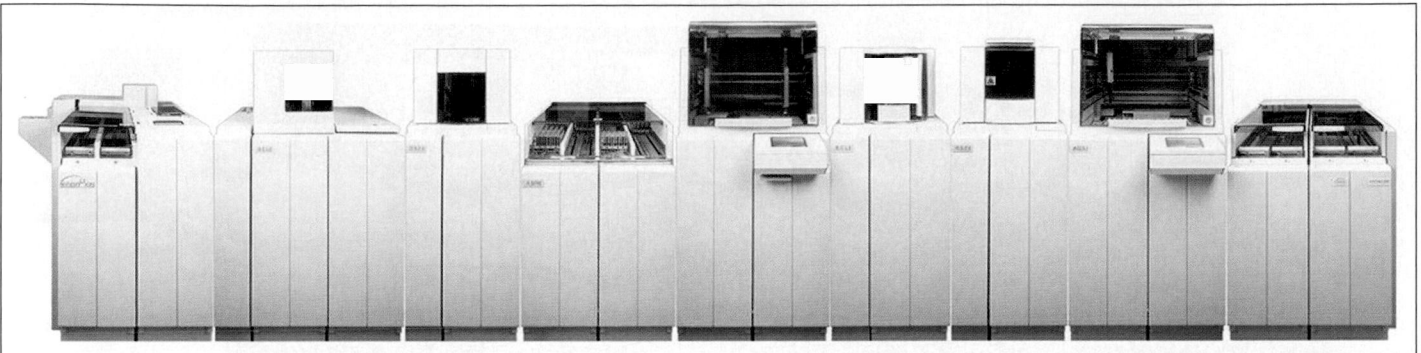

Figure 5–2 Roche **MODULAR** PRE-ANALYTICS with 'intelligent process management,' and modules that provide bar code labels, centrifuge, destopper, aliquotter, restopper and sorter. (From Roche Diagnostics with permission.)

Table 5–3 Tasks Included in the Analytical Stage of Laboratory Testing

Sample introduction and transport to cuvet or dilution cup

Addition of reagent

Mixing of sample and reagent

Incubation

Detection

Calculations

Readout and result reporting

In most analyzers samples are pipetted using a thin, stainless steel probe. The probe may be required to pierce a rubber stopper or pass directly into a test tube or cup. A given quantity of sample is aspirated into the probe and the probe is moved toward an appropriate container for dispensing. A potential source of problems with this type of sample probe is the formation of a clot in a sample that subsequently attaches to the probe. These clots may plug the probe making continued use impossible. Also, the clot may occupy sample volume and thus cause an error in the measurement. Because of the sticky nature of serum or plasma, the clot may adhere to the sample probe and as the sample probe swings towards its next destination, the whole clot and sample vessel may move along with it. This could result in an instrument malfunction and/or sample probe misalignment. Several sample probe designs have a clot detector capability and reject a sample that is clotted. Another feature associated with sampling is the ability of the sample probe to detect the presence of a liquid. These liquid level sensors detect the presence of a short sample and will not allow the analyzer to continue processing this sample. The pipet and liquid level sensor travel a specified distance into the sample container to determine if liquid is present or not.

Another problem associated with reusable pipet probes is carry-over. Carry-over is contamination of one sample by the previous sample. This contamination may cause serious variation in results for subsequent tests. Several instrument modifications have been used to reduce carry-over. One method used is to aspirate a wash solution in between each pipetting. Another technique used is to back flush the probe using a wash solution. The wash solution flows through the probe in a direction opposite to that of the aspiration, into a waste container. This technique also tends to minimize the risk of pulling a small clot further into the system.

Many samplers use disposable plastic pipet tips to transfer samples. This has the distinct advantage of eliminating carry-over associated with contamination within the sample probe and from sample to sample. A downside to the use of disposable tips is the increased cost associated with performing the assays.

Reagents

Reagents used in automated analyzers require attention to several concerns that include:
- handling, preparation and storage
- proportioning
- dispensing.

Most laboratories use bulk reagents that are ready for use with little or no preparation. If the reagent is lyophilized, most analyzers will automatically dispense the proper diluent to dissolve the dried reagents. Chemistry analyzers that use unit test reagents (i.e., where there is sufficient reagent present for the performance of a single test) may require some reagent preparation. For dry slide analysis where a thin film is impregnated with the appropriate reagent, preparation consists of wetting the reagent with water, buffer, or sample. Another type of unit test reagent is a container or test tube consisting of premeasured liquid or powdered material to which water, buffer, or sample is added.

Reagents that come either wet or dry are maintained within the reagent compartments and a complete inventory is established on real-time basis within the computer. Most of the methodologies used in the laboratory require only a single reagent, while several require two or more. As a reagent becomes depleted, the computer signals the operator that the reagent container is empty and a new one should be added. The amount of inventory for reagents that needs to be available within the analyzer depends upon the volume of testing done for any given analyte. On-board reagent storage compartments are refrigerated to maintain reagent stability.

Reagent identification and inventory processes are accomplished by use of bar-coded labels. The bar code label may also contain additional information such as expiration dates, lot numbers, and number of tests the contents of the container may provide. Some analyzers may couple a liquid level sensor onto the reagent probe, which will alert the operator as to whether a sufficient quantity of reagent exists to complete the tests.

For immunoassay tests the bar-coded reagent label stores critical information about calibrators. Examples of stored information include but are not limited to the concentration of calibrants, expected detector responses, calibration curve algorithms and tolerances for acceptability of calibration. This information is often referred to as *master lot* or *master calibration*.

An important classification category for all automated analyzers is based upon reagents. Automated analyzers are categorized as *open* or *closed* reagent systems. This distinction is often a key determinant as to whether a laboratory will select an analyzer or not. An *open* reagent system is described as a system in which reagents other than the instrument manufacturer's reagents can be used. Also, in an *open* reagent system the operator may change the parameters necessary to run the particular test. *Open* reagent systems provide the users with more flexibility and adapt easily to new methods and analytes. A *closed* reagent system is described as a system where the operator can only use the manufacturer's reagents. Usually reagents for *closed* reagent systems are more expensive, but *closed* reagent systems may save on expenses because reconstitution or preparation of the reagents for use does not require technologist time. Also the possibility of increased imprecision associated with the reconstitution of reagents in an *open* reagent system is negated with a *closed* reagent system. One problem with a closed system is that it may not be possible to introduce desired new tests that are not performed on the closed system.

The correct proportion of reagent(s) and sample must be constant to achieve precise and accurate results. For unit test applications the reagents are already apportioned in the appropriate amounts, thus only the sample needs to be added. Methods requiring the addition of bulk reagents pose an additional means of increasing imprecision. When bulk reagents are used, proportioning is accomplished by volumetric addition.

The delivery of bulk reagents requires automated volumetric dispensing devices. For random-access analyzers, syringes or volumetric overflow devices are used. These devices volumetrically proportion reagent and sample into a test tube or other type of container.

Another mechanism used for proportioning reagents and sample is the continuous-flow technique. The sample and reagents are proportioned by their relative flow rates. Devices using continuous flow include peristaltic pumps. Many instrument designs use electronic valves to control the time reagents can flow. The flow rate is controlled by the air pressure applied to

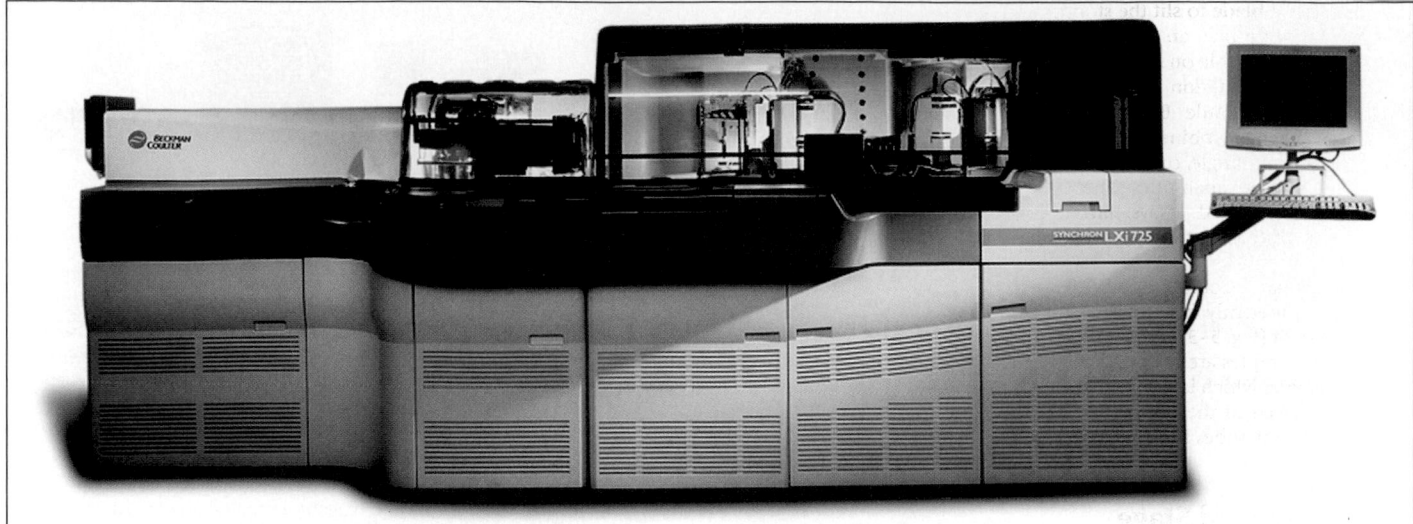

Figure 5–3 Beckman Coulter™ SYNCHRON LX®i725 clinical system has a large test menu (146 assays) and will accept user-defined chemistry. (From Beckman Coulter Brea CA with permission.)

the reagent container and the flow resistance in the tubing connected to the reaction vessel.

Liquid reagents are aspirated, delivered and dispensed into mixing chambers or reaction vessels by pumps or positive-displace syringes. These pumps are connected to the reagent containers using plastic tubing. On command from the computer each pump draws a given amount of reagent or diluent out of the container and transports it via the tubing to its destination where it is dispensed.

Syringe devices are widely used in automated systems for both reagent and sample delivery. Most are positive-displacement devices, and the volume of reagent delivered is computer controlled. If the reagent syringe is to be used for more than one reagent, adequate flushing in between is essential to reduce carry-over of reagent.

Mixing

There are many examples of unique mixing devices and techniques used in automated systems. They include the following:
- magnetic stirring
- rotating paddles
- forceful dispensing
- the use of ultrasonic energy
- vigorous lateral displacement.

Dry slide analyzers do not require mixing of sample and reagents. The sample is allowed to flow through the layers containing reagents.

Incubation

Warming components or solutions in automated analyzers is accomplished by heating air, water or metal. The warming process must be constant and accurate. Electronic thermocouples and thermistors are used to monitor and maintain required temperatures in analyzers. Circulating water baths are used in several instruments as the warming mechanism. Thus these analyzers require a water purification and delivery system, which is usually external to the analyzer and is an additional cost to consider. In some analyzers the cuvets or reaction vessels are allowed to incubate within a chamber containing circulating air. Heated metal blocks are a widely used device for incubating cuvets, test tubes or plastic pouches containing solutions. The timing for each incubation period is monitored by the instrument's computer system and represents an extremely complex process given the throughput for these systems.

Two novel approaches for incubating reaction mixtures have been developed and released on current automated chemistry analyzers. Bayer Diagnostics (Tarrytown, NY) uses an elongated cuvet path length and a fluorocarbon oil incubation bath to maximize result accuracy by enhancing absorbance values, while using microvolume technology for samples and reagents. This design feature is found in their model ADVIA® chemistry systems.

Beckman Coulter uses a Peltier thermal electric module in the shape of a ring to maintain a constant temperature for analysis. Peltier modules are small solid-state devices that function as heat pumps. The Peltier thermal ring consisting of 125 quartz glass cuvets is made of copper. Each cuvet is surrounded on three sides by copper. Temperature is maintained by the use of heating and sensing elements in physical contact with a copper core filled with Freon 134A, and is controlled by the *reaction heat controller board* assembly, mounted in the wheel's handle. Calibration information is stored on two electrically erasable programmable read-only memory ICs (EEPROMs) on the *reaction heater controller* board and the *heater/sensor board*.

Detection

Absorption spectroscopy has been the principal means of measurement in automated analyzer design to measure a wide variety of compounds. Reflectance photometry has been adapted to dry slide analysis and has been used in chemistry laboratories for decades. Fluorescent compounds, e.g., fluorescein, as signal generators have been used for measurement of drugs, hormones and vitamins in several immunoassay analyzers. In the past decade chemiluminescence compounds such as acridinium have replaced fluorescent compounds because of improvements in sensitivity. Electrochemiluminescence methods have also been incorporated into automated systems. Automated electrolyte measurements have been accomplished using ion selective electrodes. All of these means of detection have been discussed elsewhere in this edition. In this section the focus will be on new approaches to measuring compounds with automated analyzers.

Novel approaches to measurement designs include not only addition of new measurement principles but also inclusion of two or more unique detectors in one analytical system. Most of the integrated chemistry analyzers being marketed today incorporate several measuring platforms. Each platform requires a distinct detector. The Roche COBAS Integra 800 incorporates a photometer, ISE, FPIA optics and turbidimetric optics.

The Beckman Coulter™ SYNCHRON LX®i725 Clinical System includes a luminometer, photometer, electrochemical detectors and near infrared detector (Fig. 5–3). Infrared detection is used for the near infrared particle immunoassay (NIPIA) method to measure high-sensitivity C-reactive protein (hs-CRP). A 940 nm light-emitting diode produces light that is directed into a cuvet to measure hs-CRP.

Other Unique Features Located in New Automated Instrument Designs

The majority of chemistry analyzers use a high intensity polychromatic light source, usually quartz/halogen lamp. Some analyzers use a xenon light source; this lamp lasts longer (5-year life span) because its operating voltage is maintained at a lower level than in other lamps. The xenon lamp provides a very intense polychromatic light useful for many and varied analyses.

All fully automated general chemistry analyzers are capable of sampling directly from the collection tube. Direct tube sampling along with bar code reading has eliminated the need to transfer samples into another container, reduced errors, and minimized technologist exposure to potentially biohazardous material. Tubes are typically decapped before sampling; however, some chemistry systems like the Beckman Coulter™ SYNCHRON LX®i725 Clinical System offer cap-piercing technology. The analyzer uses a blade to slit the stopper and the sample probe pierces the stopper to withdraw an aliquot of sample. Note that cap-piercing technology is available on all high throughput hematology analyzers.

Laboratory automation can consolidate multiple workstations into a single unit. The Dade Behring Dimension® Xpand Plus™ integrated chemistry system combines comprehensive chemistry and stat immunoassay testing on a single, compact system with the smallest footprint for an instrument of its capabilities. The Dimension® Xpand Plus™ features a large menu of varied assays, fast time for first results, stat interrupt capabilities, throughput of approximately 400 tests per hour and reagent flexibility.

The Beckman Coulter™ SYNCHRON LX®i725 Clinical System is constructed differently from the Dimension® Xpand Plus™. The SYNCHRON LX®i725 system (Fig. 5–3) is designed as a self-contained integrated modular system. The samples are placed in a load area and are shuttled to the *closed tube aliquot unit*, which is similar to a small track design. An aliquot of each sample is placed in the immunoassay analytical unit for processing; the rack and primary tubes are then released for general chemistry testing.

Post-Analytical Stage

The electrical signal generated by the detector, representing analyte concentration, is directed into the analyzer's microprocessor or computer. The instrument computer represents a means to accomplish several tasks, which include signal processing, data handling and process control.

Signal processing involves the conversion of an analog signal derived from the detector to a digital signal, which is usable by all communication devices. The processing of data by computers has allowed automation of nonisotopic immunoassays, reflectance photometry and other nonlinear assays because computer algorithms can transform nonlinear standard input signals into linear calibration plots.

Data processing by computers includes data acquisition, calculations, monitoring and displaying data. In addition to transforming data into linear calibration plots, computers can perform statistics on patient and control values. Computers can perform corrections on data, subtract blank responses and determine first-order linear regression for slope and intercept. Computers can monitor patient results against reference values. They can also test control data against established QC protocols. Computer monitors can display all types of information including patient results, QC data, maintenance and instrumentation operation checks.

The computer has a profound impact on the entire process of automated laboratory instruments. Within the analyzer the computer commands and times the electromechanical operations so that they can be done in a uniform manner, in repeatable fashion and in the correct sequence. These operations include activating pipetting devices, moving cuvets from one point to another, moving sample tubes and dispensing reagents, to name a few.

A computer provides a means of communication between the analyzer and operator. Instrument computers can display information usable by the operator, such as warnings that something may not be working properly or that a specific reaction has exceeded method-defined parameters.

Chemistry analyzer computers can display graphical information such as Levy–Jennings QC charts and calibration curves. They can also 'flag' data that do not meet some predefined criteria. The operator can reprogram the computer to meet a specific need, such as adding a new test or changing an operating parameter.

A computer has the ability to be linked to other computers, which has drastically improved automation efforts. Instrument computers can be linked via interfaces, e.g., RS232, to laboratory information systems (LIS) to provide a means of transmitting information either in a unidirectional or bidirectional format. Instrument computers are now being equipped with the means to link to the internet via a TCP/IP (transmission control protocol/internet protocol). Instrument manufactures have designed analyzer computers that will link up from the laboratory's to the company's own manufacturing site. This link-up is in real time and serves to monitor the instrument's performance at all times. If a problem with the analyzer does develop, the manufacturer can see real-time data to help the laboratory resolve the problem in the shortest time possible.

There are several other features available in newer instrument designs that are worth noting. On-board troubleshooting is available on many systems through the analyzer's computers. In the event a problem occurs technologists may access the systems help protocols, which guide them through a step-by-step procedure in an effort to resolve the problem. Some of these on-board troubleshooting programs are quite sophisticated and include video and graphics. Another on-board feature available in some systems is a training program. This is an effective feature that serves to augment staff training of new users to the system.

Automated System Designs Available for Laboratories

Total Laboratory Automation (TLA)

The idea of totally automating a clinical laboratory has its roots in Japan and was first tried in the early 1980s. The early designs used one-arm robots, conveyor belts and modifications to existing chemistry analyzers to perform as many of pre-analytical and analytical tasks as possible with no human intervention. Each laboratory workstation was coupled to the conveyor belts so that samples could be moved from one workstation to another. Continued research and modifications to these earlier systems led to the development of commercial TLA systems designed for hospital-based laboratories.

A TLA approach can be described as the combination of several instruments, consolidated instruments, workcells, integrated workcells or integrated modular workcells that are coupled to a specimen management and transportation system as well as a process control software component to automate a large percentage of laboratory work.

An example of a TLA is the Roche Diagnostics system that includes a modular pre-analytics (MPA) and platform C (i.e. the chemistry analyzer). The Roche TLA consists of an integrated tract device that connects all of the laboratory workstations, including front-end processing, instrumentation and archiving, together to create a continuous, inclusive network that serves to automate nearly every step involved in the testing of each sample. TLA can incorporate testing specimens for chemistry, hematology, coagulation and immunochemistry.

The advantage of TLA includes a decrease in labeling errors, reduced turnaround times and reduction in full-time equivalents (FTEs). Laboratories using a high degree of automation thus have the ability to bring new assays into the laboratory by using some of the staff no longer needed for automated testing.

The major drawbacks of TLA are the needs for substantial financial investment and increased floor space (Wilson, 2003). Initial investment monies may reach millions of dollars and floor space requirements may exceed 4000 square feet. Another factor that requires attention by the planners because of the complex nature of TLA is the need for highly technical personnel to operate and troubleshoot the system. Other challenges to TLA include infrastructure remodeling, personnel team building and software interfacing. In addition, several of these systems do not allow for interruption of the workflow to analyze emergency (*stat*) samples (Battisto, 2004).

Modular Integrated Systems

In the USA only about 7% of laboratories are considered to be able to benefit from TLA. A hospital with fewer than 600 beds may not be suitable for TLA. Therefore, modular automation provides a more attractive approach for hospital laboratories and physician group laboratories because the systems are smaller, require less initial capital investment and require less planning than TLA (Sarkozi, 2003). Modular systems can be configured to include several different platforms, e.g., hematology and immunochemistry. Also, the combination of modules can include multiple identical models of analyzers, pre- and post-analytical modules. These modules are linked into a single testing platform that interconnects by use of a track or other 'connector'-type device. Individual modules can be added to the entire system to reflect changes in either workload or testing patterns.

Configuration(s) of Automated Modules

Workstation Consolidation

Workstations represent a unique environment within a laboratory facility dedicated to one type of testing, e.g., hematology and immunoassays. All of the stages of specimen testing are carried out for a particular discipline at its respective workstation. One approach taken to improve workflow has been to consolidate workstation data management. This design allows a technologist to monitor a variety of analyzers (typically from the same vendor) from a single workstation.

Workcells

A workcell is described as a combination of a specimen manager with instruments or consolidated instruments of chemistry and immunoassay reagents that provide a broad spectrum of analytical tests. Modular workcells

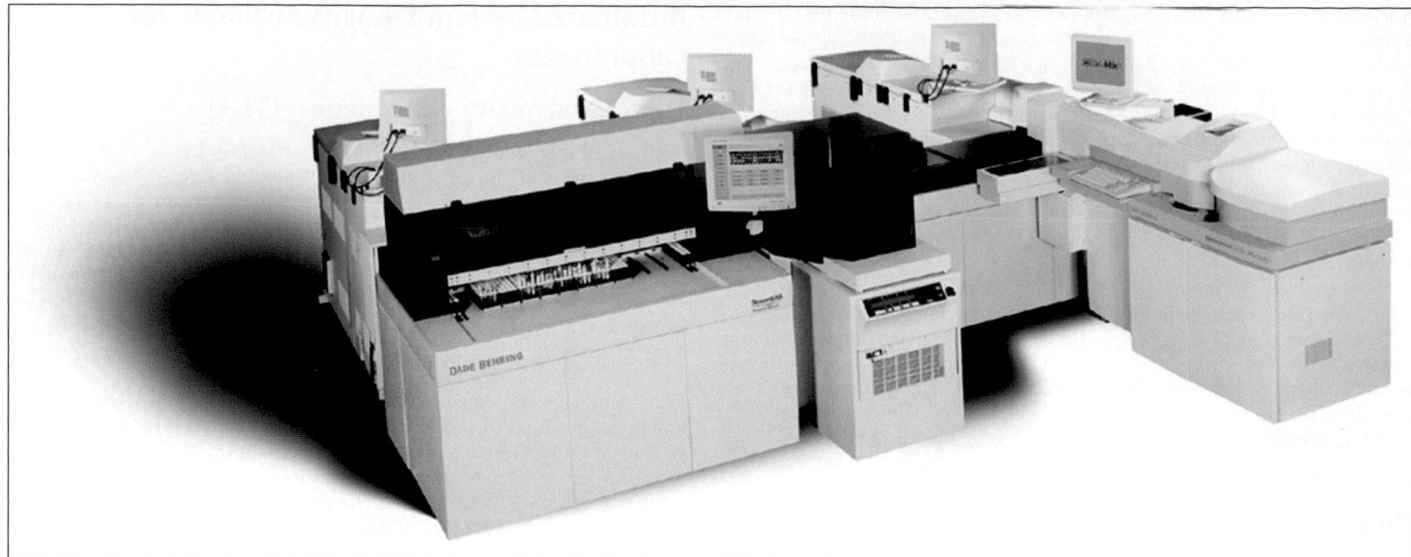

Figure 5–4 Dade Behring StreamLab® Analytical Workcell links multiple dimensions system via a single operator interface and features automated pre- and post-analytical function. (From Dade Behring Inc. Newark Del with permission.)

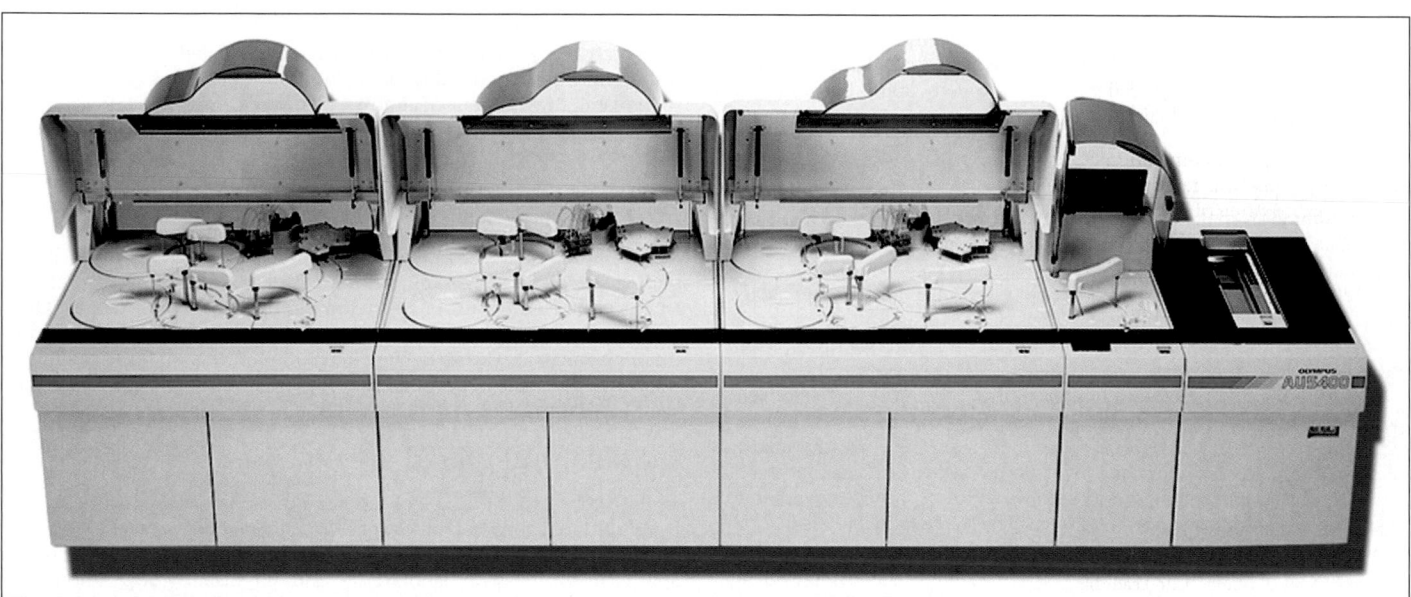

Figure 5–5 Olympus AU5400™ fully automated integrated system is available as a two or three photometric unit version including one single or double cell ISE unit. Throughput of 300–800 samples per hour depending upon configuration. (From Olympus, with permission.)

are workcells where the instruments used are configured to interface directly with the specimen manager. The Dade Behring StreamLAB® (Fig. 5–4) is an example of this type of workcell. The StreamLAB® integrates pre-analytical and multiple analytical components, e.g., Dimension® systems via a single operator interface. Dade Behring offers an optional centrifugation module.

Fully Integrated Systems

The trend in automation design is to integrate several modules into one continuous system that will allow the user to assay photometric chemistry, immunoassay chemistries, both homogeneous and heterogeneous and electrochemistries. The tests menu for fully integrated systems exceeds 100 tests and includes immunoassays, routine chemistries and ion-selective electrodes. All modular integrated systems use random access technology that allows for the analysis of different chemistry assay types.

The Olympus AU5400™ Integrated Chemistry-Immunoassay analyzer (Fig. 5–5) is an example of this trend toward combining instrument platforms. This system is a true random access analyzer with test throughput rates exceeding 3000 photometric test/hour. For ISE measurements the throughput rate is approximately 600 samples/hour. A distinct advantage with these modular systems is the ability to be able to link two or more modules, thereby increasing throughput.

The Bayer modular automated ADVIA® 1650 Chemistry System has a full track system integrated with other testing modules via the ADVIA®

WorkCell or ADVIA® LabCell automated sample transportation system. The processing system automatically sends general chemistry specimens to the ADVIA® 1650 chemistry analyzer and immunoassay specimens to the ADVIA® Centaur.

Another approach to modular integrated automation is exemplified by the Roche **MODULAR** ANALYTICS shown in Figure 5–6. **MODULAR** ANALYTICS incorporates most of the tests other integrated systems offer but can increase the test menu by linking one more module, e.g., Roche Diagnostic E170. The E170 module offers 25 heterogeneous immunoassays. Therefore if the laboratory integrated all available modules including the control unit and core load unit, the **MODULAR** ANALYTIC can provide a very large test menu and very high specimen and test throughput rates.

Other Enhancements to Integrated Automated Systems

Instrument Connectors

Olympus developed a unit called the AU-Connector that enables clinical chemistry and immunoassay analysis to be consolidated into one single workstation without compromising function or performance of the connected systems. The AU-Connector uses *intelligent sample management* and tube presorting capabilities to keep all the analyzers working at full

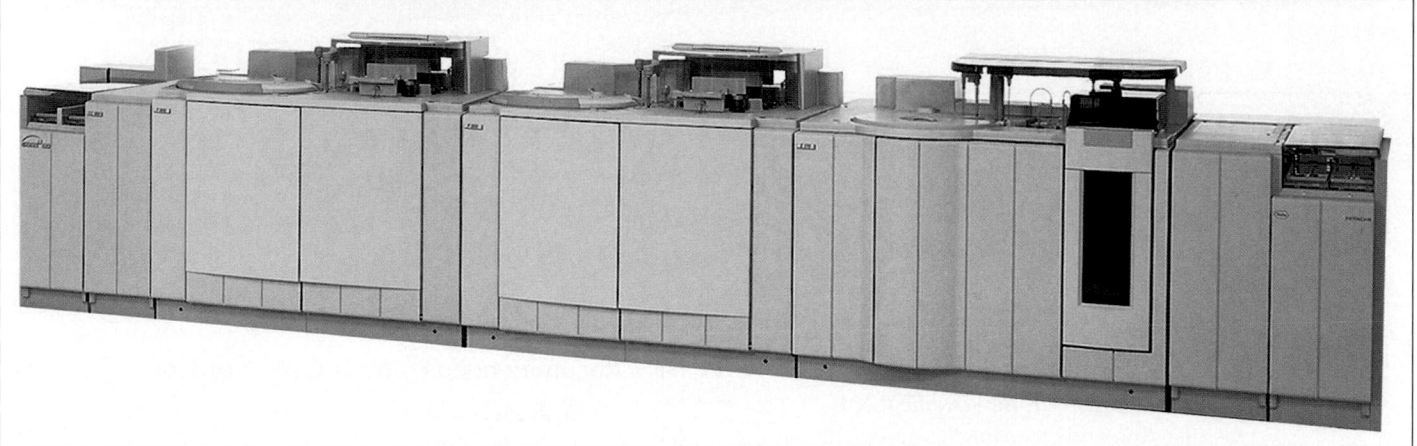

Figure 5–6 Roche **MODULAR** ANALYTICS provides five different analyzer modules, 197 applications producing throughputs rates ranging from 170–10 000 tests/hour. (From Roche Diagnostics with permission.)

potential. The AU-Connector does not use a track device, which can create additional throughput bottlenecks and increase turnaround times.

Middleware

Middleware allows laboratories to connect their existing LIS and instrumentation to facilitate automatic information processing and performs tasks not currently done with laboratories' existing hardware and software. Middleware packages provide several features and functionality including:

- automatic verification of test results through rules-based decision processing
- automation and customization of work and information based on a laboratory's specific needs
- automatic tracking of data and location of samples requiring storage
- automatic sample interference testing and detection
- provision for real-time reflexive testing
- automatic comparison of current results with previous results on a patient's test (delta checking).

On the Horizon

The drivers of automation listed above are continually changing and evolving and this will lead to new approaches to the delivery of healthcare.

The test menus will grow even larger, and new technologies will be needed to measure these analytes. These new technologies will need to be incorporated into existing systems. Another demand that systems manufactures will need to address is to be able to link different instruments or modules to their systems. A standardized interface will be required to accomplish this and LIS will need to adjust their processors as well. Increased emphasis on employee safety and support by legislative efforts will cause instrument manufactures to continue to develop their products to reduce exposure to technologist. As the field of proteomics evolves, so will the methods and instruments required for measurement. Proteomic systems are currently coming to the marketplace and in time this type of testing will find a place in the clinical laboratories. Automated systems manufacturers, for example Roche Diagnostic, are currently marketing automated sample processing systems for PCR analysis. The automated sample processing is accomplished using the MagNA Pure LC (MP, Roche Applied Science, Indianapolis, Ind) instrument. The assay is completed using the Roche COBAS analyzer. This analyzer can function as a stand-alone and linked to Roche Preanalytics.

References

Battisto DG: Hospital clinical laboratories are in a constant state of change. Clin Leadersh Manag Rev 2004; 18(2):86–99.
Provides valuable information that is current for laboratories contemplating changes in their facilities.

Kaplan L, Pesce A, Kazmierczak S: Clinical Chemistry: Theory, Analysis and Correlation, 4th ed. St Louis, Mosby, 2003.
Provides substantial amount of detailed information for all aspects of pre-analytical, analytical and post-analytical stages of laboratory testing.

Sarkozi L, Simson E, Ramanathan L: The effects of total laboratory automation on the management of

a clinical chemistry laboratory. Retrospective analysis of 36 years. Clinica Chimica Acta 2003; 329(1–2): 89–94.

Wilson LS: New benchmarks and design criteria for laboratory consolidations. Clin Leadersh Manag Rev 2003; 17(2):90–98.
Shows the results of a consolidation project serving a multihospital system.

CHAPTER 6

Point-of-Care and Physician Office Laboratories

Gregory A. Threatte MD

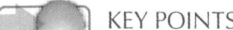

KEY POINTS

• Point-of-care testing refers to the scope of laboratory tests that are performed where patient care is delivered. This includes physician office testing as well as various hospital locations outside the laboratory, such as the emergency department, operating room, and intensive-care unit.

• When performed in a physician office, simple tests (like urine dipstick and whole blood glucose meters) are exempt from most regulations involving personnel, proficiency testing, and rigorous quality assurance requirements. These are referred to as 'waived' tests under the Clinical Laboratories Improvement Act (CLIA). In hospitals, these tests fall under the laboratory certificate of the parent hospital or healthcare facility and are generally subject to stricter requirements.

• Special personnel requirements are necessary (including those for laboratory director) if a physician office laboratory performs moderate-complexity testing.

• Key components of a hospital point-of-care testing program include method validation, training nonlaboratory staff, and clear policies and procedures to establish who is responsible for each part of the program. Laboratory oversight is mandatory.

Point-of-care (POC) testing (also known as near-patient testing, alternative-site testing, patient-focused testing) is used in a variety of settings such as the emergency department, operating suites, clinics, health maintenance organizations (HMOs), physician offices, and nursing homes (Kurec, 1993). POC brings laboratory testing to the site of the patient rather than obtaining a specimen and sending it to the laboratory. Real-time measurements of a patient's status may be obtained in a short period of time allowing the healthcare provider to address acute patient needs (Zaloga, 1991; Woo, 1993). The 'biologic half-life' of laboratory data for chronically ill patients generally shows minimal changes, whereas the clinical conditions of acutely ill patients are more variable (Geyer, 1992). POC is recognized by the Joint Commission on Accreditation of Healthcare Organizations, and the Clinical Laboratories Improvement Act of 1988 (CLIA'88; Federal Register 55, 42CFR, 1990; 57, 42CFR, 1992; 68, 42CFR, 2003).

In previous editions of this book, this chapter has been devoted to physician office laboratories (POLs). As shown in Figure 6–1A, the number of POLs in August of 2004 has grown to 103 378 from the 95 000 laboratories indicated in a similar figure in the 20th edition. However, Figure 6–1B, also obtained from the CMS CLIA database at http://www.cms.hhs.gov/clia, shows that at present, 80% of registered laboratories are now of the waived or provider performed microscopy procedures (PPMP) certificate type. Large POLs are likely registered in either the Compliance or Accreditation classifications similar to hospitals and commercial laboratories and are subject to the same standards, regulations, protocols and procedures (see Ch. 1). This chapter will focus on the regulations and procedures recommended for small POLs and point-of-care testing sites where more waived and PPMP testing is expected to occur.

In an analysis of the marketplace for clinical diagnostic equipment, Breindel has reported that the chemistry laboratory instrument market is expected to decline at a 2.7% adjusted annual growth rate (AAGR) due to cost containment and consolidation in central laboratories. Meanwhile,

POC testing equipment is expected to experience an 8.1% AAGR through 2007 (Breindel, 2003). Advances in medical technology, such as prepackaged reagent systems, microprocessor-controlled reactions and calibrations, and miniaturization of components, are leading to a modern generation of laboratory instruments that require less technical skill on the part of the operator. Between 1992 and 2003, the FDA granted waived status to 994 test systems (CMS, 2003) and there are currently more than 40 assays that can be done in this category, ranging in scope from glucose to bladder tumor antigen cancer detection. New systems such as these will work their way into both POC and POLs, blurring their technological differences. However, differences in regulatory requirements will remain and must be observed.

Laboratory Regulation

Clinical Laboratories Improvement Act

Under the CLIA, a laboratory is 'A facility for the … examination of materials derived from the human body for the purpose of providing information for the diagnosis, prevention, or treatment of any disease or impairment of, or the assessment of the health of, human beings. These examinations also include procedures to determine, measure, or otherwise describe the presence or absence of various substances or organisms in the body' (Federal Register 57, 42CFR, 1992). This includes healthcare providers using equipment as basic as urine dipsticks or bedside glucose monitors. Currently, in-vivo and externally attached patient-dedicated monitoring devices, e.g., pulse oximetry, S_vO_2 pulmonary artery catheters, and apnographs, are not subject to CLIA. Should it be determined at a later date that they are subject to the CLIA, proper notice and opportunity for public comment will be provided.

Under this definition, 'laboratories' are prohibited from soliciting or accepting human specimens for analysis unless a certificate issued by the Secretary of the Department of Health and Human Services (HHS) is held for each procedure that is to be performed. All laboratories are required to be registered with the federal government and pay biennial license fees to have a valid CLIA identification number before performing any laboratory analysis used in patient care. With the evolving technology, the primary difference between the POL and POC testing will be that in the POL, this certification will held by the POL, while POC testing will be performed under the laboratory certificate of the parent hospital or healthcare facility.

Certification and Licensing Requirements

CLIA certification relies on laboratory standards that vary according to the complexity of the measurements performed. Simple tests that the Centers for Disease Control and Prevention (CDC) have determined to have low patient risk even if performed incorrectly are waived from most regulations. These types of procedures will include those that have been approved by the Food and Drug Administration (FDA) for home use, or are so simple and accurate as to render the likelihood of erroneous results negligible. All laboratories must be certified under one of the five types of CLIA certificates listed in Table 6–1.

A three-tiered approach was initially implemented classifying all laboratory tests, based on the complexity of testing. The three categories

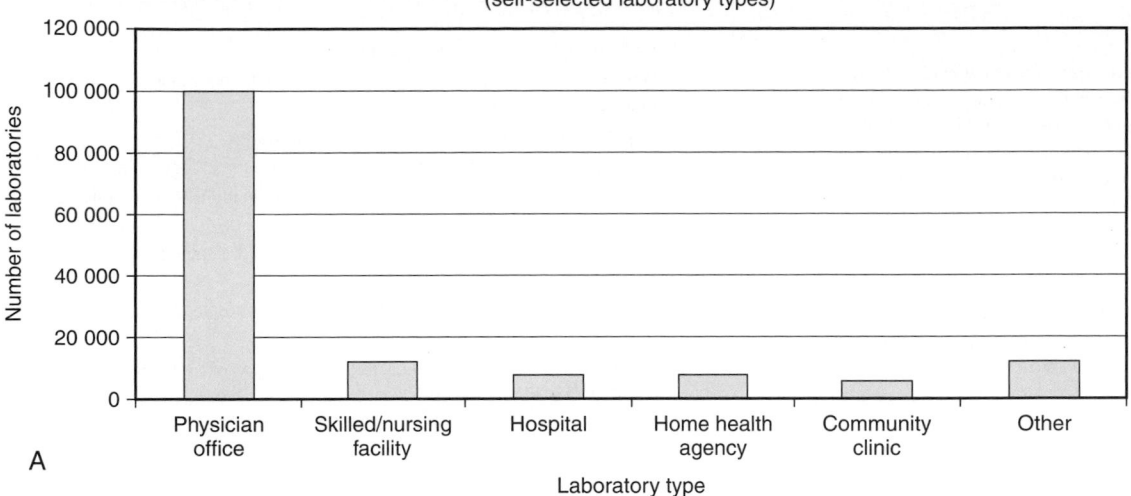

Total CLIA laboratories registered
(self-selected laboratory types)

A

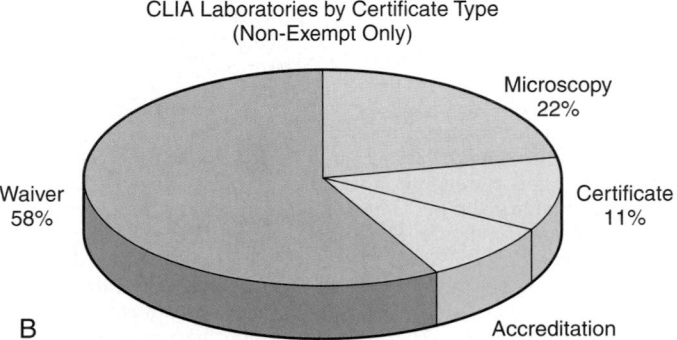

CLIA Laboratories by Certificate Type
(Non-Exempt Only)

Microscopy
22%

Certificate
11%

Waiver
58%

Accreditation
9%

B

Figure 6–1 *A*, The number of POLs in August of 2004 relative to hospital, skilled nursing facilities, and independent laboratories (from the CMS CLIA Database, August, 2004 at http://www.cms.hhs.gov/clia/statregi.pdf). *B*, Relative proportion of registered laboratories by certification type (from the CMS CLIA Database, August, 2004 at http://www.cms.hhs.gov/clia/statcer.pdf).

Table 6–1 Types of CLIA Certificates

Certificate of Waiver

Certificate issued to a laboratory to perform only waived tests

Certificate for Provider-Performed Microscopy Procedures (PPMP)

Certificate issued to a laboratory in which a physician, midlevel practitioner or dentist performs no tests other than the microscopy procedures. This certificate permits the laboratory to also perform waived tests

Certificate of Registration

Certificate issued to a laboratory that enables the entity to conduct moderate or high complexity laboratory testing or both until the entity is determined by survey to be in compliance with the CLIA regulations

Certificate of Compliance

Certificate issued to a laboratory after an inspection that finds the laboratory to be in compliance with all applicable CLIA requirements

Certificate of Accreditation

Certificate issued to a laboratory on the basis of the laboratory's accreditation by an accreditation organization approved by HCFA

Obtained at http://www.cms.hhs.gov/clia/downloads/types_of_clia_certificates.pdf

---

are certificate of waiver or 'waived' tests, moderate complexity tests, and high complexity testing. Laboratories performing only waived tests would be exempt from personnel proficiency testing, and the more rigorous quality assurance requirements that are required with more complex testing. HHS retains the right to conduct spot checks to make sure that these laboratories are performing only waived tests. The original exempt tests included urinalysis dipstick or tablet reagent analysis of pH, specific gravity, glucose, protein, bilirubin, hemoglobin, ketone, leukocytes, nitrite, and urobilinogen. Also exempt were whole blood glucose using devices approved by the FDA specifically for home use, spun microhematocrits, hemoglobin by copper sulfate method or by self-contained single-analyte instruments with direct measurement and

readout (e.g., HemoCue), fecal occult blood, urine pregnancy tests by visual color comparison, visual color ovulation tests for human luteinizing hormone, and the erythrocyte sedimentation rate. Laboratories performing only waived tests must register and pay a biennial fee.

It is important to understand that the original list of waived tests specified by Congress included only the short list of generic tests listed above. In addition, provision was made so that manufacturers could add specific methods to the waived list through a certification process maintained by both the Centers for Disease Control (CDC) and the FDA. The incentive to manufacturers allowing them to appeal to a larger market has led to a rapid influx of devices and methods that are now classified as waived. The list of approved waived tests is updated regularly and can be found at http://www.cms.hhs.gov/clia/downloads/cr4136.waivetbl.pdf. An alphabetical list of waived tests can be found at http://www.accessdata.fda.gov/scripts/cdrh/cfdocs/cfClia/analyteswaived.cfm. Office laboratories appear to be shifting from moderately complex testing to waived testing, most likely because of this rapidly broadening menu (Roussel, 1996; Binns, 1998; LaBeau, 1998), and the same measurements are appropriate for the POC arena.

A fourth category, provider-performed microscopy procedures (PPMP), was created in 1993 and expanded in 1995. This category includes the following procedures: all urine sediment examinations; direct wet mount preparations for the presence or absence of bacteria, fungi, parasites, and human cellular elements; all potassium hydroxide (KOH) preparations; pinworm examinations; fern tests; postcoital direct, qualitative examinations of vaginal or cervical mucous; nasal smears for granulocytes; fecal leukocyte examinations; and qualitative semen analysis (limited to the presence or absence of sperm and detection of motility).

Only certain professionals are permitted to perform the procedures under this PPMP category if exemption from the moderate complexity designation is to be retained. This includes licensed physicians, dentists, and midlevel practitioners such as nurse practitioners, nurse midwifes, and physician assistants under the supervision of a physician, or in an independent practice, only if authorized by the State in which the practice is located. With PPMP, the specimen must be examined, during the patient visit, on a specimen obtained from either the provider's own patient, or from a patient of a group medical practice of which the provider is a member or an employee.

Table 6–2 Personnel Requirements in a Laboratory Performing Moderately Complex Testing

Director	Responsible for the overall management and direction of the laboratory but does not have to be on-site at all times. Broad range of experience and education is acceptable. For example, a physician with 1 year of experience directing/supervising a non-waived laboratory or 20 Continuing Medical Education credits in laboratory practice would qualify, as would a person with a bachelor's degree and 2 years' laboratory training/experience plus 2 years' supervisory experience in non-waived testing. The director could, depending on education and experience, qualify for all other positions
Testing personnel	Responsible for specimen processing, test performance and reporting test results. Minimum requirement is a high school diploma or equivalent and training for the testing performed
Technical consultant	Responsible for the technical and scientific oversight of the testing. Minimum requirement is a bachelor's degree with 2 years' laboratory training or experience in non-waived testing
Clinical consultant	Provides clinical consultation. Minimum requirement is a doctoral degree with board certification

From CDC Moderate Complexity Testing Overview at http://www.phppo.cdc.gov/clia/moderate.aspx.

Table 6–3 Point of Care Checklist

1. Equipment, if needed, must be evaluated
2. Persons performing the test must be trained, competency assessed, and this must be documented
3. A written procedure must be available and followed
4. Calibrations and quality control samples must be run at regular intervals
5. All patient results must be documented and the relationship to quality control measures must be clear
6. Appropriate action must be taken and documented on all out-of-range QC results
7. Appropriate action must be documented on all abnormal patient results

By congressional law, CLIA'88, a regulated test is any measurement used in the diagnosis, treatment and management of a patient.

The primary instrument for performing the test under the PPMP certificate is the microscope, limited to bright-field or phase-contrast microscopy. The specimen has to be labile or a delay in performing the test could compromise the accuracy of the test result. In general, control materials are not available to monitor the entire testing process and limited specimen handling or processing is required.

In moderately complex testing, a laboratory performs only waived tests and one or more tests designated as moderately complex by the FDA. To determine at which complexity level a particular method has been categorized, refer to the CDC, Division of Laboratory Systems website at http://www.phppo.cdc.gov/dls/clia/testcat.asp. Manufacturers of moderately complex tests must submit their testing system to the FDA for classification. Therefore, this list will be continuously updated along with the waived test list.

Laboratories must submit an application to HHS or its designee on a form prescribed by HHS detailing the number, type, and methodologies employed for each measurement or examination, as well as the qualifications of the persons directing, supervising, and performing these procedures. Each laboratory location must complete a separate application except for mobile sites, and not-for-profit and governmental agencies. Certificates may be valid for up to 2 years, and any changes in the information required in the application must be submitted to HHS or its designee within 30 days of any change in ownership, name, location, or director. Changes in method complexity require notification within 6 months of the change. This application may be through an approved accrediting body or state agency if the accrediting standards of the agency are equal to or more stringent than those of HHS and if the agency is authorized to inspect the laboratory as frequently as required and submit to HHS required records and information.

Laboratory Directorship

Laboratories that perform under a Certificate of Waiver or with a certificate for provider-performed microscopy procedures (PPMP) can perform waived testing without the overhead of having personnel who meet established qualifications in training, experience, job performance, and competency. However, if any moderate complexity tests or measurements are performed, CLIA requires that the laboratory be directed by a laboratory director, and/or a laboratory consultant with at least the director's credentials listed in Table 6–2. This director is to be responsible for determining the qualification of individuals performing and reporting test results, as well as ensuring compliance with all applicable regulations. The director is also responsible for the analytical performance of all assays, and must monitor the ongoing proficiency, accuracy, and precision. If more than one individual in the practice qualifies as a laboratory director, the laboratory is required to designate one as being responsible. It must be demonstrated that the laboratory director is providing effective direction over the operation of the laboratory, and if they do not provide on-site direction, they must provide

consultation by phone or delegate to qualified personnel specific responsibility as required by regulation. Online courses are available that allow physicians to qualify as a director of a moderately complex laboratory by obtaining the 20 hours of continuing education credit and can be found at the CMS website at http://www.cms.hhs.gov/clia.

For point-of-care testing, a separate certification is usually not necessary when it is performed under the supervision of the laboratory director responsible for laboratory services in a healthcare facility. Point-of-care testing that occurs within a healthcare facility, in sites that are located in contiguous buildings on the same campus, and under common direction can be performed under the certificate of the parent organization. When assays and procedures are performed in a situation such as this, the terms 'waived' and 'complexity' no longer have meaning. The test menu is no longer restricted to just waived testing; however, more frequent inspections and higher scrutiny are received in return. Since the parent organization typically has a certificate that allows testing at all levels of complexity, it is the responsibility of the laboratory director to insure that the test methodology used in the point-of-care site is appropriate for the skills and training of those performing the test. What inspectors do not tolerate could be called 'rogue testing.' This occurs when a clinic or service sets up a test without the knowledge and supervision of the laboratory director. With the new tracer methodology used by accrediting agencies such as JCAHO, if an inspector finds a lab result and traces it back to a laboratory that is not adequately supervised by the laboratory director, a citation may be issued to the discredit of the healthcare facility.

Recommended Point-of-Care Protocol

Table 6–3 shows the recommended steps that should be taken when point-of-care tests are set up. In the first step, the equipment must be obtained and evaluated. Professional laboratorians usually have a good sense of what is available on the market. Point-of-care instrumentation tends to be hand-held, durable units with easy analysis, simple quality control (QC), varied reporting methods, low throughput, and higher unit cost. The easy analysis and simple QC make these methods more likely to be classifiable as waived, allowing less-well-trained operators. At regular intervals, cross-correlation between POC methods and central laboratory methods should be obtained to ensure that differences between POC devices and central laboratory results are minimized and not mistaken for changes in patient status.

In the second step, persons performing the test must be trained and competency assessed, and this must be documented. Training documentation should include both the date of initial training as well as any additional inservices and competency assessments. This documentation can include the performance of controls and/or proficiency samples as a measure of competency assessment.

Next, a written procedure must be available and followed. These procedures should adhere to the manufacturer's recommended steps, be simple, easy to follow, and functional rather than a collection of articles, package inserts, and instrument protocols that are too disorganized for the inexperienced operator. The procedure manual should include specimen requirements, procedures for specimen collection, identification and processing, assay methodology, reference intervals, quality control, and reporting methods. Since this is standard practice in laboratories, it should be fairly easy to have a procedure designed by the central laboratory staff.

Calibrations and quality control samples must be run at regular intervals. This is often the most difficult task to implement with nonlaboratory staffs that have not been indoctrinated in the importance of controls and calibrations. For this reason, many instruments designed for the point-of-care arena have features that block the reporting of results when appropriate calibrations and controls have not been performed. Some instruments can even lockout staff who have not been properly trained and issued a code recognizable to the machine.

All patient results must be documented and the relationship to quality control measures must be clear. Inspectors are not pleased when they find evidence of test results being used 7 days a week and controls being run Monday through Friday by only a small fraction of the users. In addition, if laboratory analyzers are in use, records of preventive maintenance and any corrective maintenance must be kept. Finally, if the POC is being operated under the certificate of a central laboratory, it is a requirement that these point-of-care tests be enrolled in a proficiency testing program, such as that provided by the College of American Pathologists (CAP), in which results of proficiency samples are sent periodically to the proficiency testing service. These results are compared with those of a peer group to ascertain the accuracy of the specific tests.

Appropriate action must be taken and documented on all out of range QC results. Often it is best to have POC staff call the central laboratory when controls fail because it creates the opportunity to review procedural steps and have a better-trained POC staff. Quality has costs, but the lack of quality can cost even more.

Appropriate action must be documented on all abnormal patient results. In this day of wireless networks, it is better to have POC results transmitted to the computer and included with laboratory results generated centrally for comparison. If this is not available, results should at least be written in the chart rather than being acted upon without proper documentation.

Experience has shown that a point-of-care site operates far more efficiently when a person of sufficient authority is designated as being responsible for the site. With a responsible person in charge, there will be quicker reporting of suspected equipment malfunctions, controls will be more reliably performed, and it is less likely that untrained individuals will attempt to perform testing.

Compliance

In addition to CLIA, there are additional regulatory procedures that all laboratories must adhere to, particularly in the outpatient setting. First, all testing for which Medicare is billed must be medically necessary. Screening tests and other measures of wellness are generally not covered. Medical necessity determination is implemented by Medicare, Medicaid, and other insurance carriers through the use of Current Procedural Terminology (CPT) codes used in conjunction with the International Classification of Disease (ICD) codes. When the ICD-9 code does not warrant the CPT-4 code, payment is rejected. Even worse, if it is determined that a laboratory deliberately added codes to obtain a higher payment than it deserves or payment for work that it has not done, it can be charged with fraud, which is a felony and subjected to fines. Errors are assumed to be deliberate unless there is a compliance program in place that actively seeks to uncover billing errors.

Another potential pitfall is Stark regulations. The Stark laws are named after their original sponsor Representative Fortney Pete Stark (D-CA), and were intended to prevent unnecessary self-referrals intended to boost revenue. Under Stark, physicians are prohibited from referring Medicare patients to laboratories in which the physician (or close family member) has a financial interest. Since this prohibition would be detrimental to most POLs, it is important to understand the 'safe harbors' that allow legitimate self-referral.

References

Binns HJ, LeBailly S, Gardner HG: The physicians' office laboratory: 1988 and 1996 survey of Illinois pediatricians. Arch Pediatr Adolesc Med 1998; 152:585–592.
Survey results contrasting physician office laboratories before and after the implementation of CLIA'88. Shows the changes that offices made as a result of the increased regulation.
Breindel B: B-168 The U.S. Clinical Diagnostic Equipment Market. Norwalk, CT, Business Communications Company, Inc., 2003.
Article detailing trends and projections in the US clinical diagnostic equipment market. Includes the consideration of cost control pressures and the likely responses from equipment manufacturers.
CMS: Questions and Answers for CMS-2226-F (January 24, 2003 Regulation – Medicare, Medicaid, and CLIA Programs; Laboratory Requirements

Relating to Quality Systems and Certain Personnel Qualifications; Final Rule). Online. Available: http://www.cms.hhs.gov/clia/default.asp and http://www.cms.hhs.gov/clia/cms2226fqa.pdf.
Federal Register, 55, 42CFR 493; Clinical Laboratory Improvement Act, 1990.
Federal Register, 57, 42CFR 493; Clinical Laboratory Improvement Act, 1992.
Federal Register, 68, 42CFR 493; Clinical Laboratory Improvement Act, 2003.
Most recent changes to CLIA'88 regulatory framework.
Geyer SJ: Joining the technological evolution of healthcare. Med Lab Observ 1992; 24:2–7.
Kurec AS: Implementing point-of-care. Clin Lab Sci 1993; 6:225–227.
LaBeau KM, Simon M, Steindel SJ: Clinical laboratory test menu changes in the Pacific Northwest: 1994 to 1996. Clin Chem 1998; 44:833–838.

Roussel PL: Impact of CLIA on physician office laboratories in rural Washington state. J Fam Pract 1996; 43:249–254.
Study showing the impact of CLIA'88 on rural office laboratory practice in the State of Washington. Shows that laboratories that performed only waived testing increased from 1% to 34%; laboratories performing tests of moderate complexity declined from 76% to 53%.
Woo J, McCabe JB, Chauncey D, et al: The evaluation of a portable clinical analyzer in the emergency department. Am J Clin Pathol 1993; 100:599–605.
Zaloga GP: Monitoring versus testing technologies: Present and future. Med Lab Observ 1991; 23:20–31.

I

CHAPTER 7

Post-analysis: Medical Decision-Making

Rohan John MD, Mark S. Lifshitz MD, Jeffrey Jhang MD, Daniel Fink MD,

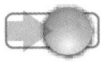

KEY POINTS

• Reference intervals distinguish normal from abnormal patient populations. False-positive and false-negative results occur when there is overlap between these populations.

• The ability of a test to discriminate disease from no disease (accuracy) is described by the sensitivity and specificity of the test. Sensitivity is the probability of a positive result in a person with the disease (true positive rate). Specificity is the probability of a negative result in a person without disease (true negative rate).

• Screening tests require high sensitivity so that no case is missed. Confirmatory tests require high specificity to be certain of the diagnosis.

• Altering a test cutoff has a reciprocal effect on sensitivity and specificity. A cutoff can be lowered to include all cases (100% sensitivity) but this reduces the specificity (i.e., increases false positives).

• Receiver operating characteristic (ROC) curves plot true positive rate versus false positive rate and graphically present the range of sensitivities and specificities at all test cutoffs. If two tests are compared, the more accurate test is closer to the upper left-hand corner of the ROC curve.

• The likelihood ratio of a test relates the true-positive rate to the false-positive rate. It is the likelihood of a test result in disease to the same result in the absence of disease.

• Predictive value describes the probability of disease or no disease for a positive or negative result, respectively. The predictive value of a positive test increases with disease prevalence.

• Evidence-based medicine is a process by which medical decisions can be made using as many objective tools as possible; it integrates the most current and best medical evidence with clinical expertise and patient preferences.

Laboratory tests are ordered to detect, diagnose, or monitor disease, or predisposition to disease. Asymptomatic individuals are screened for unsuspected disease and symptomatic patients are tested to confirm or identify disease. After the laboratory produces a result, it must be interpreted so that a medical decision can be made. Results are interpreted as normal or abnormal and these, in turn, influence the decision to do nothing if the patient is considered healthy or to follow up with additional tests or treatment if disease is suspected or confirmed. The following chapter (Ch. 8) discusses how to interpret particular laboratory abnormalities and their significance in various diseases. However, a general and more basic question facing clinicians is whether an 'abnormal' result truly reflects disease, and whether a 'normal' result necessarily indicates a disease-free state. Many clinicians use experience to intuitively decide how to interpret a test result and whether or not to act on it. To some extent this decision is guided by the degree of clinical suspicion of the disease. However, one must also consider a variety of other factors, including some less well understood, to accurately interpret results and

make sound decisions. These include pre-analytical variables (Ch. 3), analytical error, biological variability, and the inherent ability of a test to discriminate between patients with and without disease. The purpose of this chapter is to discuss the diagnostic usefulness of laboratory tests in medical decision-making, in general, and the importance of using objective means to interpret results and make decisions.

Reference Intervals

To interpret a test, one must first compare the result to a reference ('normal') interval. While the procedure for establishing reference intervals is discussed elsewhere (Ch. 9), it is important to understand how reference intervals affect clinical test interpretation. A reference interval is usually defined as the range of values that represents the central 95% tendency of measurements from a population of nondiseased or 'normal' individuals.

Note that a reference interval is the laboratory's attempt to separate 'normal' and 'abnormal' patient populations to help a clinician interpret results and make a decision. For purposes of the following discussion, the terms *normal*, *negative*, *healthy* and *nondiseased* are used synonymously as are *abnormal*, *positive*, and *diseased*. In some instances, only one end of the reference interval merits consideration so that a single cutoff is used to separate normal and abnormal patients. For example, a PSA level of 4 ng/mL might be used to distinguish patients that require no further follow-up ('normal') from those that require a biopsy ('abnormal'). Or, a cardiac troponin I (cTnI) of 0.1 ng/mL might be used to distinguish patients with noncardiac chest pain that can be released from the emergency department ('nondiseased') from those that have myocardial damage ('diseased') and must be admitted. Note that the terms 'disease' and 'no disease' in this discussion do *not* relate to just any disease, but only to the disease that is supposed to be identified by a particular test; for example, prostate cancer in the case of PSA or myocardial damage in the case of troponin.

In other instances, a reference interval has two cutoffs – one at the lower end and one at the upper end. This reference interval distinguishes three patient populations: abnormal patients with low values, normal patients, and abnormal patients with high values. Most reference intervals fall into this category. For example, TSH is used to distinguish hypothyroid (high TSH value) and hyperthyroid patients (low TSH value) from those that are euthyroid.

Random Variability. What accounts for the spread of a reference interval or the fact that consecutive values from the same patient are often different? For the most part, it is due to random variability from analytical and biological factors. Analytical variability is a function of assay imprecision or reproducibility. If the same sample is run many times, some variation is expected; this variability is expressed as a coefficient of variation (CV) (discussed further in Ch. 9). Biological variability occurs between individuals as well as within the same individual. *Inter-individual* variation occurs because each individual usually has a unique 'set value' that is normal for him/her. For example, creatine kinase (CK) level is related to muscle mass. Thus, an entire population of subjects will express a range of CK values according to each individual's muscle mass. In practice, we do not know what each individual's 'set point' is, but we can

Table 7–1 Inter-individual and Intra-individual Biological Variability for Common Analytes

Analyte	Inter-individual CV (%)	Intra-individual CV (%)	Index of individuality	Method CV (%)
Alanine aminotransferase	50.2	23.7	0.47	3.2
Albumin	8.9	2.8	0.31	3.4
Alkaline phosphatase	33.4	4.4	0.13	6.5
Apolipoprotein A	17.8	7.0	0.39	4.8
Apolipoprotein B	27.6	9.5	0.34	2.7
Aspartate aminotransferase	29.1	15.1	0.52	3.4
β-Carotene	67.4	24.2	0.36	7.4
Bicarbonate	13.3	11.0	0.83	2.4
Bilirubin, total	43.9	24.6	0.56	3.0
C peptide	65.7	28.4	0.43	7.2
Calcium, ionized	3.6	2.4	0.67	1.4
Calcium, total	4.7	3.3	0.70	2.2
Chloride	3.1	1.9	0.61	1.0
Cholesterol, total	22.3	8.2	0.37	2.3
Creatinine	18.7	6.8	0.36	1.0
Creatinine, urine	61.3	43.0	0.70	2.2
Fibrinogen, plasma	25.6	16.2	0.63	3.9
Folate	64.3	22.6	0.35	3.6
Gamma-glutamyl transferase	59.8	16.2	0.27	1.7
Glucose, plasma	12.5	8.3	0.66	1.7
Glycohemoglobin, blood	9.6	1.5	0.16	3.1
HDL-cholesterol	28.3	12.4	0.44	2.5
Homocysteine	36.6	18.0	0.49	6.0
Iron	41.6	29.0	0.70	3.2
Iron binding capacity, total	15.5	6.9	0.45	3.3
Insulin, plasma	55.9	25.2	0.45	13.0
Lactate dehydrogenase	21.6	7.9	0.37	6.0
Phosphorus	15.8	9.2	0.58	2.0
Potassium	7.7	5.4	0.70	0.5
Protein, total	6.2	3.5	0.56	0.9
Selenium	13.2	5.1	0.39	4.8
Sodium	1.6	1.3	0.81	0.7
Triglycerides	56.8	28.8	0.51	4.7
Urea nitrogen	32.1	18.0	0.56	3.7
Uric acid	27.1	9.0	0.33	0.7
Varicella antibody	43.2	13.7	0.32	6.7
Vitamin A	30.7	9.5	0.31	2.5
Vitamin B$_{12}$	41.6	13.4	0.32	6.2
Vitamin E	35.1	11.3	0.32	2.9

From: Lacher, 2005.

Table 7–2 Clinically Significant Difference Between Two Consecutive Patient Results

Analyte	Change
Total T$_4$	2.2 µg/dL
Free T$_4$	0.5 ng/dL
Total T$_3$	35 ng/dL
Free T$_3$	0.1 ng/dL
TSH	0.75 mIU/L
Thyroglobulin	1.5 ng/mL

From: Baloch, 2003.

much lower than the biological variability and hence much less of a factor in affecting the overall random variability of measurements.

Random variation is also evident in repeated measurements on the same patient, where greater variability is seen between consecutive samples than from a single sample that is repeated. While the within-sample variation is determined by analytical variability, the between-sample variation includes analytical and biologic variability. Thus the CV$_{between}$ is always greater than the CV$_{within}$. It is important to understand this concept when asking a laboratory to repeat (duplicate) a sample measurement (i.e., within sample variability) or when trying to determine whether two consecutive sample measurements are different from one another (i.e., between sample variability). The between sample CV is shown for some commonly measured analytes in Table 7.1 where it is referred to as the intra-individual CV. Note that this degree of random variability is far greater for some analytes (e.g., ALT) than others (e.g., sodium). Keep in mind that changes in some analytes are clinically more significant than changes in others. For example, a change in serum potassium in a hospitalized patient may justify immediate treatment. On the other hand, even a moderate increase in serum cholesterol may not necessitate any therapeutic change until repeat testing at the next scheduled visit. For some analytes, guidelines have been published as to what constitutes a clinically significant difference between two consecutive patient sample results. As an example, Table 7–2 provides this information for various thyroid function tests (Baloch, 2003).

In general, how does one decide if two consecutive measurements on the same patient are statistically different? For this, the difference between the two measurements must be greater than the expected random variability or variance of each measurement. For each measurement, random variability yields results that are within 4 variances or 2 standard deviations (SD) of the mean, 95% of the time (SD = the square root of the variance). For two measurements this is equal to 2.83 SD and is calculated by adding the maximum variance (variance = SD^2) of both measurements and then deriving the SD. (The combined maximum *variance* from two measurements (95% of the time) is $(2\,SD)^2 + (2\,SD)^2$ or 4 variances + 4 variances = 8 variances; the corresponding number of SDs is the square root of 8 or 2.83 SD.) Note that this is valid only when the repeat testing is performed under the same laboratory conditions (and it only considers the random error due to analytical variability, not biological variability).

Classifying Patients in the Truth Table. Ideally, a distribution of test results from normal ('nondiseased') patients would be completely distinct from those of abnormal ('diseased') patients. In such a situation (Fig. 7–1) any reference cutoff point between the two distributions will discriminate perfectly between the two patient populations. Thus a test result would reflect with certainty whether disease is present or absent. Unfortunately, even near perfect tests are exceedingly rare. In general, tests do not yield distinct populations of results from patients with and without disease. Instead, tests yield a continuum of results and some overlap of values between patients with and without disease (Fig. 7–2). In this area of overlap (at both the low and high cutoffs), the test cannot discriminate disease from no disease. This is the inherent limitation of nearly all laboratory tests.

Based on test results from these overlapping populations, patients can be classified into four groups (Fig. 7–2 and Table 7–3). Patients correctly classified as abnormal are called true positives (TP) and those correctly classified as normal are called true negatives (TN). Note that these true results are non-overlapping areas of the two patient populations. Patients incorrectly classified as normal are false negatives (FN) and those incorrectly classified as abnormal are false positives (FP). False results occur because the two populations overlap, i.e., because a test cannot completely discriminate all abnormal patients from normal ones. As seen in Figure 7–3, where for ease of illustration a single cutoff is used to discriminate disease from normal populations, varying the cutoff changes

determine what the range of values should be for a population and use this as a guide to interpret a given patient's result. *Intra-individual* variation is due to biological changes that cause analyte levels to fluctuate over time. For example, serum estrogen levels vary from day to day depending on the menstrual cycle; serum cortisol shows diurnal variation, being highest in the morning and decreasing later in the day; and vitamin D shows seasonal variation with lower values in winter. Most other analytes show some level of physiologic variation, including that related to changes such as exercise or food intake. Table 7–1 provides estimates of inter-individual and intra-individual biological variation for common analytes. As expected, the intra-individual variation is generally less than the inter-individual variation. The index of individuality is the ratio of the *intra*-individual CV to *inter*-individual CV. A low index (< 0.6) means that results from a given individual fluctuate within a narrow range of the reference interval. In such instances, serial changes in an individual's analyte may be more useful in detecting disease than comparing each of the measurements with the reference interval (Lacher, 2005). Table 7–1 also shows that the method CV or degree of analytical variability is usually

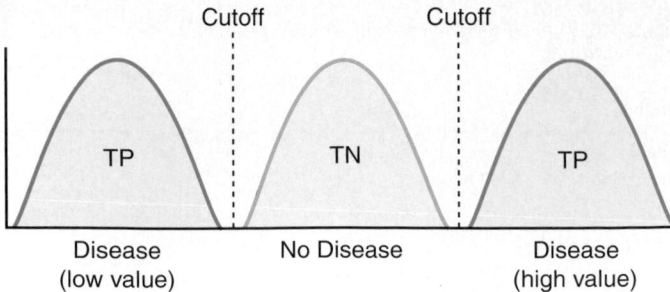

Figure 7–1 Distribution of test results from non-overlapping populations of patients with and without disease (see Table 7–3).

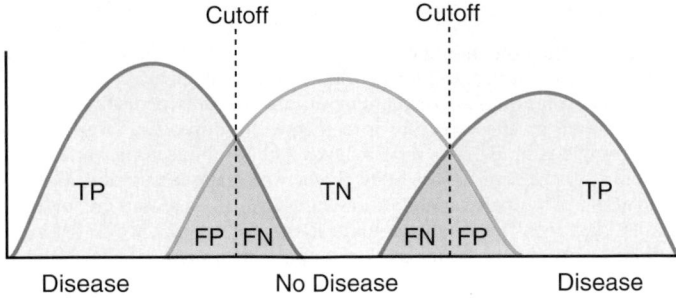

Figure 7–2 Distribution of test results from overlapping populations of patients with and without disease (see Table 7–3).

Table 7–3 Truth Table: Classifying Patients

Result	Disease	No disease	Total
Positive	True positive (TP)	False positive (FP)	TP + FP
Negative	False negative (FN)	True negative (TN)	FN + TN
Total	TP + FN	FP + TN	TP + FP + FN + TN

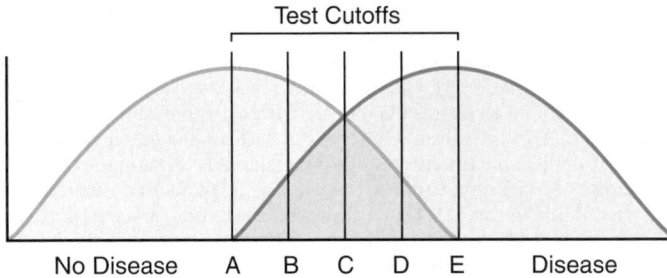

Figure 7–3 Effect of varying the test cutoff on overlapping populations of patients with and without disease.

the number of true and false results in a given population. When a reference interval has two cutoffs as in the TSH example, overlapping populations at both the low and high cutoffs produce false results. Changing the proportion of false results will, in turn, affect the discriminatory power or diagnostic accuracy of the test.

Diagnostic Accuracy

Accuracy is the ability of a test to discriminate between two states, i.e., disease and no disease, and is described by two key parameters: sensitivity and specificity (Galen, 1975).

Sensitivity is the ability of a test to detect disease and is expressed as the proportion of persons with disease in whom the test is positive (Table 7–4). Thus a test that is 90% sensitive will give positive results in 90% of diseased patients (TP) and negative results in 10% of diseased patients (FN).

Specificity is the ability to detect absence of disease and is expressed as the proportion of persons without disease in whom the test is negative (Table 7–4). Thus a test that is 90% specific will give negative results in 90% of patients without disease (TN) and positive results in 10% of patients without disease (FP).

A test with a higher sensitivity identifies a greater proportion of persons with disease, and a test with a higher specificity excludes a greater proportion of persons without disease. Sensitivity is also the true-positive

Table 7–4 Sensitivity, Specificity, Predictive Value and Efficiency

Definition	Example
Sensitivity (%) = [TP/(TP + FN)] × 100	Cardiac marker gives positive results in 196 of 200 acute MI patients. TP = 196; FN = 4 Sensitivity (%) = 196/(196 + 4) = 98%
Specificity (%) = [TN/(TN + FP)] × 100	Cardiac marker gives negative results in 180 of 200 healthy patients. TN = 180; FP = 20 Specificity (%) = 180/(180 + 20) = 90%
Predictive value (PV)	In a population of 1000 hospital patients, 50 have an acute MI (prevalence = 50/1000). This means 950 patients do not have acute MI. Based on above sensitivity and specificity: TP = 50 AMI patients × 0.98 sensitivity = 49 FN = 50 − 49 = 1 TN = 950 non-AMI × 0.90 specificity = 855 FP = 950 − 855 = 95
Predictive value of a positive test (%) = [TP/(TP + FP)] × 100	PV positive cardiac marker = 49/(49 + 95) = 34%
Predictive value of a negative test (%) = [TN/(TN + FN)] × 100	PV negative cardiac marker = 855/(855+1) ≈ 100%
Efficiency (%)= [(TP + TN)/(TP + TN + FP + FN)] × 100	(49 + 855)/(49 + 1 + 855 + 95) = 90%

TP = true positive; TN = true negative; FP = false positive; FN = false negative.

rate and the inverse, 1 − sensitivity, is the false-negative (FN) rate. If the sensitivity is 95%, 5 out of 100 individuals with the disease will test negative. Specificity is the true-negative rate, and the inverse, 1 − specificity, is the false-positive (FP) rate. If the specificity is 95%, 5 out of 100 individuals without disease will test positive.

Sensitivity and Specificity in Diagnostic Testing

Effect of Altering the Test cutoff. Sensitivity and specificity measure the extent to which a test correctly identifies persons with and without disease. While tests are described with a given sensitivity and specificity, these measures vary depending on the analyte level (cutoff) selected to distinguish positive from negative results. This is important to remember because we often assume sensitivity and specificity are fixed characteristics of a test, but they are not. Figure 7–3 illustrates why altering a cutoff changes a test's sensitivity and specificity as it relates to overlapping normal and abnormal patient populations. Note that when the cutoff is lowered (i.e., the cutoff line is moved to the left), more diseased patients are classified as abnormal. Thus, changing the cutoff from C to B increases sensitivity. If the cutoff is moved to A, then all diseased persons will have a positive test, and the sensitivity will be 100%. While it sounds as if it might be very useful to have a test that is 100% sensitive, the increased sensitivity comes at a price: decreased specificity. Thus the number of nondiseased persons with a positive test (false positives) increases from point C to B and to A. On the other hand, if the cutoff is raised (i.e., the cutoff line is moved to the right), more nondiseased patients are classified as normal. Thus, changing the cutoff from C to D increases specificity. If the cutoff is moved to E, then all nondiseased persons will have a negative test, and the specificity will be 100%. The increased specificity also comes with a price: decreased sensitivity and more false-negative results. Thus, when a cutoff is altered there is an inverse relationship between sensitivity and specificity and a trade-off between the number of false-positive and false-negative results. Of course, this is only true because there is an overlap in the distributions of results from persons with and without disease. If there were no overlap, there would be no false results.

The Need for High Sensitivity versus High Specificity. False-positive and false-negative results can lead to misdiagnosis and a financial or clinical cost. For example, a false-positive result may cause the inappropriate admission of a patient. Similarly, a false-negative result may lead to a patient's release from the emergency department despite a life-threatening disorder. Manufacturers are constantly trying to develop new tests that can better discriminate between normal and abnormal populations and therefore yield higher sensitivity and specificity. For example, cTnI is more sensitive than CK-MB at distinguishing normal patients from those with myocardial damage. Troponin is also far more specific than CK-MB since it is only present in cardiac muscle, unlike CK-MB that can give a false-positive result due to skeletal muscle damage. However, for a given test it is rarely possible to eliminate false results entirely because there is always some overlap of the biologic process between diseased and nondiseased persons. Thus, for a given test it is not usually possible to enhance sensitivity or specificity without decreasing the specificity or sensitivity, respectively. In most situations the cost of either a false-positive or a false-negative result supersedes the other, and the cutoff that delineates normal from abnormal can be shifted to reduce the more significant of the two costs. When sensitivity should be high as when PSA is used to screen for prostate cancer, the cutoff might be lowered to include all potential cases. However, some balance is necessary because many persons without cancer (including some with prostatitis and nodular hyperplasia) will also have a positive result. The current cutoff of 4.0 ng/mL includes a majority of persons with prostate cancer (true-positive PSA), but also many without (false-positive PSA). Hence one will have to perform a number of unnecessary prostate biopsies (false-positive cost) to confirm the few with prostate cancer. In general a high sensitivity is required when it is extremely important not to miss any disease.

On the other hand, high specificity is required when one must be sure of the diagnosis, even if the disease may not be treatable. Clinical suspicion may be high or low but is superseded by the seriousness of the disease and the need to be absolutely certain of the diagnosis. A highly specific test excludes persons without disease (eliminates false positives). By simply increasing the cutoff one could exclude persons without the disease (increase specificity), although this would also exclude some with the disease (Fig. 7–3). Highly specific tests are often used in combination with highly sensitive ones so that the decreased sensitivity that occurs as a consequence of improving specificity does not lead to missed cases (false negatives). Thus, a high specificity is applied after including all those who might potentially have disease (as well as some who do not have disease). For example, to detect HIV infection, an ELISA for broadly reacting antibodies against HIV antigens is an appropriate initial test. However, some non-HIV individuals with cross-reactive antibodies might test positive (false positives). So a highly specific test, like the Western blot, can then be used to confirm HIV infection and to exclude those non-HIV individuals who initially tested positive, i.e., false positive. In many instances, such a confirmatory test, besides being highly specific, is also highly sensitive. However, because such tests are more cumbersome or expensive, they are not used as screening tests. Drug screening is another example wherein highly sensitive tests are used to screen for drugs and highly specific ones (like GC/MS) are used to confirm positive results.

Declining Accuracy. The diagnostic accuracy of a test tends to diminish as the test becomes more widely used in a population. Initial validation studies are often performed on a small group of individuals in whom disease is clearly absent or present. Those who lack the disease are often selected from a population of subjects in overall good health. In practice, however, patients exhibit a spectrum of illness, including early or mild disease that overlaps with nondiseased individuals including those with other diseases, some of which might cause an abnormal test result. Thus, the proportion of false test results is often higher in clinical practice than is claimed by the manufacturer from more limited studies in healthy individuals.

Probability of Disease

When evaluating the diagnostic capability of a test, both the sensitivity and specificity are important. For example, a test may be 100% sensitive and yet be useless in its ability to discriminate patients with disease from those without disease, i.e., it may always be positive. Such a test would have a specificity of 0%. While this example is an exaggeration, it does demonstrate that a positive (or negative) result does not always indicate the presence or absence of disease in a patient. Therefore a clinician needs to know more about the test, i.e., when a test is positive, what is the likelihood that the patient has disease; and when a test is negative, what is the likelihood that the patient does not have disease. This is commonly called the predictive value of a test. For example, how likely is it that an elevated PSA implies the patient has cancer, or, how likely is it that an undetectable cTnI excludes myocardial damage? Whatever the test result, there is always at least some degree of uncertainty of the true state of the patient. This diagnostic uncertainty is objectively expressed as a quantitative probability of disease (Sox, 1986), a measure of the likelihood that the patient does or does not have disease. To determine this information, one must consider predictive value theory also known as Bayes theorem.

Bayes theorem applies population data from the test directly to an individual subject, and calculates the probability of disease given the test result. Information from the test result is incorporated into the pre-test probability of disease to produce a post-test probability of disease.

Table 7–5 Post-Test Probability (Predictive Value) from Bayes Theorem

Post-test probability (predictive value or PV) depends on diagnostic accuracy and disease prevalence

Post test probability of disease (PV of a positive test) = (Prevalence × Sensitivity)/[(Prevalence × Sensitivity) + (1 − Specificity) (1 − Prevalence)]	A test for rheumatoid factor (RF) is positive in 95 of 100 patients with rheumatoid arthritis (RA) (sensitivity of 95%), but is also positive in 10 of 100 non-RA patients (specificity of 90%). The RA pre-test probability (prevalence) is 5% in a rheumatology practice.
	Post-test probability of disease = (0.05 × 0.95)/[(0.05 × 0.95) + (1 − 0.9)(1 − 0.05)] = 0.0475/(0.0475 + 0.095) = 0.33 or 33%
Post-test probability of no disease (PV of a negative test) = [(1 − Prevalence)(Specificity)]/[(1 − Prevalence)(Specificity) + (1 − Sensitivity)(Prevalence)]	For the same test conditions.
	Post-test probability of no disease = [(1 − 0.05) × 0.9]/[(1 − 0.05) × 0.9 + (1 − 0.95) × 0.05] = 0.855/(0.855 + 0.0025) = 0.997 or 99.7%

Pre-test probability or *a priori* probability is the prevalence of disease in the patient's clinical setting. For example, the prevalence of myocardial damage among subjects with chest pain is higher in the Cardiac Care Unit (CCU) than it is in the emergency department.

Post-test probability or *a posteriori* probability is the probability of disease in the post-test situation and is commonly referred to as the predictive value of the test.

Thus Bayes theorem describes the relationship between the post-test and pre-test probability of disease or no disease using the sensitivity and specificity of the test. The probability (post-test) of disease or no disease is calculated as shown in Table 7–4.

The predictive value of a positive test (sometimes, although incorrectly, referred to as positive predictive value) may be understood as the probability that a positive test indicates disease. It is the proportion of persons with a positive test who truly have the disease (Table 7–4). *The predictive value of a negative test* (sometimes, although incorrectly, referred to as negative predictive value) is the probability that a negative test indicates absence of disease. It is the proportion of persons with a negative test who are truly without disease (Table 7–4).

Understand that while the sensitivity and specificity describe a test (e.g., *what percent of diseased patients have abnormal results?*), the predictive value describes the state of the patient (e.g., *how likely is it that a given patient's positive result indicates disease?*). The predictive value depends on sensitivity, specificity, and prevalence of the disease being tested. Tables 7–5 and 7–6 illustrate how disease prevalence, test accuracy, and predictive value of a test are interrelated (Bayes theorem).

Predictive Value and Prevalence. The predictive value of a positive test is highly dependent on the prevalence of the disease being tested. The higher the prevalence, or pre-test probability, the higher will be the post-test probability, or predictive value of a positive test. Consider a test with a sensitivity of 90% and a specificity of 90% for a disease with a prevalence of 0.1%. Based on the formula, the predictive value of a positive result (PV+) would be 0.9%. If the prevalence increases to 5.0%, the PV+ increases to 32%. Thus the predictive value of a positive test increases as the prevalence increases. This effect of prevalence on predictive value is shown in Table 7–6. Predictive value theory quantitates a concept that is intuitively obvious – a positive result is more likely to truly reflect disease if it comes from a population of patients with a high prevalence of disease.

The impact of prevalence on predictive value theory has a practical application in that it enables one to derive a higher predictive value from a test result performed in a high prevalence setting as compared to a low prevalence setting. For example, consider serum CK-MB measurement for a patient in the emergency department. The predictive value of an abnormal CK-MB might be only 10%. On the other hand, if cardiac damage is strongly suspected, the patient might be transferred to the CCU, where on repeat testing, an elevated serum CK-MB will have a much higher predictive value. In the restricted setting of a CCU, the prevalence of acute MI is higher. We can also examine this situation from a pre-test probability point of view. For the patient to be in the CCU (instead of still in the emergency department), the clinical suspicion of myocardial damage must be significantly higher. Since pre-test probability determines post-test probability, the stronger pre-test suspicion translates into a stronger prediction of disease.

Table 7–6 Predictive Value of a Positive Test: The Effect of Prevalence and Accuracy

Prevalence (%)	Predictive value of a positive test (%)	
	Sensitivity 90% Specificity 90%	Sensitivity 99% Specificity 99%
0.01	0.09	0.9
0.1	0.9	9
5	32.1	83.9
50	90.0	99

For a disease with a low prevalence, even a test with high sensitivity and specificity will yield a low predictive value because the majority of positive test results will be false positives. For example, consider a disease with a prevalence of 1 in 10 000 and a test that is 99% sensitive and 99% specific. The PV+ will be only about 1% since 99 of every 100 who test positive have false-positive results. One can see that the accuracy of tests for rare conditions must be very high in order to reliably predict disease. Thus, besides requiring a near perfect sensitivity, tests that are used to screen for rare diseases have more utility in selected populations that offer a higher pre-test probability.

On the other hand, the predictive value of a negative test decreases as the prevalence of disease increases. However, the effect is small, especially when the sensitivity and specificity are high. Prevalence influences the predictive value of a negative test to a noticeable extent only when the starting prevalence is high.

Predictive Value and Accuracy. Keep in mind that improved accuracy (i.e., sensitivity and specificity) enhances the predictive value of a test. The formula for predictive value (Table 7–5) from Bayes theorem shows that sensitivity and specificity influence the predictive value. Further, Table 7–6 shows that the predictive value of a positive test increases with increasing prevalence and improved accuracy. Specificity has the biggest impact on the predictive value of a positive test, whereas sensitivity is what determines the predictive value of a negative test. This is also appreciated from Table 7–4 where it can be seen that the number of false positives directly influences the predictive value of a positive test whereas the numbers of false negatives have the same effect on a negative test.

When a test cutoff changes, the accuracy (i.e., proportion of false results) and predictive value also change. Consider D-dimer testing to exclude deep vein thrombosis in patients presenting to the emergency department. In the reference population a value greater than 400 U/ml is considered abnormal and indicative of thrombosis. For a patient in the emergency department with symptoms suggestive of thrombosis, an even lower D-dimer value will predict thrombosis to the same extent as the > 400 U/ml value does in the general population. (Recall that post-test probability is dependent on pre-test probability.) Consider that a cutoff of 400 U/ml is not 100% sensitive and excludes some patients with thrombosis, thereby yielding false negatives. As one cannot risk neglecting a possible case of thrombosis, a lower value of 200 U/ml could be selected to decrease the proportion of false negatives, and greatly improve the predictive value of a negative test. A negative test could then be used to exclude thrombosis and obviate the need for additional costly diagnostic studies like an ultrasound of the leg.

Receiver Operator Characteristic (ROC) Curves

Based on the above discussion, it is clear that sensitivity and specificity are inversely related and are altered by the cutoff of a test. Thus the obvious question confronting a laboratorian is 'what cutoff should be used and is one preferable to another?' Receiver operator characteristic (ROC) curves help answer this question.

ROC analysis is based on signal detection theory, developed in the context of electronic or radar signal detection to discriminate signal from noise. Radar *operators* used certain *characteristics* to decipher the significance of images *received* on the radar screen. *Curves* were then generated to represent the accuracy of the generated signal.

An ROC plot is a complete measure of the accuracy of a test, the ability of a test to discriminate between the two alternative outcomes, disease and no disease (Zweig, 1993). An extension of sensitivity and specificity, the curve is a graphic representation of the varying sensitivities and specificities that are possible by varying a test's cutoff. A single sensitivity and specificity provide only a single view (based on a particular cutoff) of a test's ability to discriminate between the absence and presence of disease. By simply altering the cutoff, it is possible to determine many different combinations of sensitivity and specificity for a given test. In some

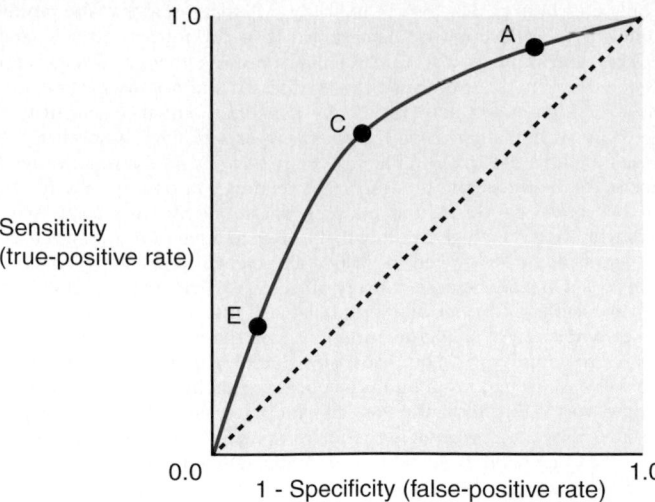

Figure 7–4 ROC curve: effect of varying the cutoff value for separating disease from no disease (also see Fig. 7–3).

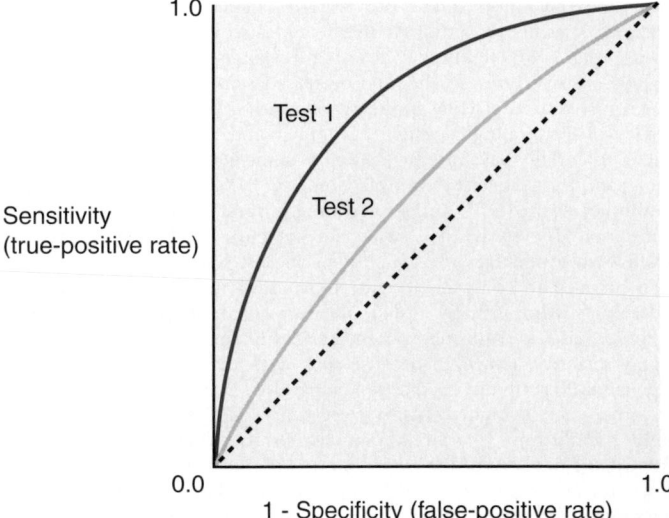

Figure 7–5 ROC curves for two tests. Note Test 1 is always superior to Test 2 since it has higher sensitivity than Test 2 (i.e., it is always above and to the left of Test 2).

instances, a higher sensitivity might be preferred and one would want to know the specificity at the new cutoff. On the other hand, the cutoff might be increased to reduce the number of false positives, and one would want to know the new sensitivity. The advantage of the ROC curve is that it depicts the entire spectrum of sensitivity–specificity pairs using all possible cutoffs. Note that each sensitivity value is paired with a single specificity value.

The ROC curve is generated by plotting the sensitivity (*y*-axis) versus 1 − specificity (*x*-axis), or the true-positive rate versus the false-positive rate, respectively (Fig. 7–4). Each point on the ROC curve represents the sensitivity and specificity for a possible diagnostic cutoff. The curve clearly shows the unavoidable trade-off between sensitivity and specificity as the cutoff is varied. When sensitivity increases, specificity decreases. In Figure 7–4, point A has the highest sensitivity but the lowest specificity, while point E has the highest specificity but the lowest sensitivity. These correspond to changes in the cutoffs observed in Figure 7–3. Point E on the ROC curve corresponds to the highest cutoff in Figure 7–3 while point A corresponds to the lowest cutoff. The central cutoff point (C) provides the best combination of sensitivity and specificity on the ROC curve.

A test that perfectly discriminates between disease and no disease will follow the upper left-hand corner. At this point, the true-positive rate (or sensitivity) is 100%, and the false-positive rate is 0 (or 100% specificity). A test with no discrimination is the diagonal (45°) line. ROC curves from most tests fall between these two lines. The higher the Y point, the fewer false negatives; and the farther the X point, the more false positives. ROC curves provide an easy comparison of the performance of two or more tests. Thus a curve closer to the upper left-hand corner is associated with a more accurate test. In Figure 7–5, Test 1 provides greater diagnostic accuracy than Test 2 since Test 1 has a higher sensitivity than Test 2 at each

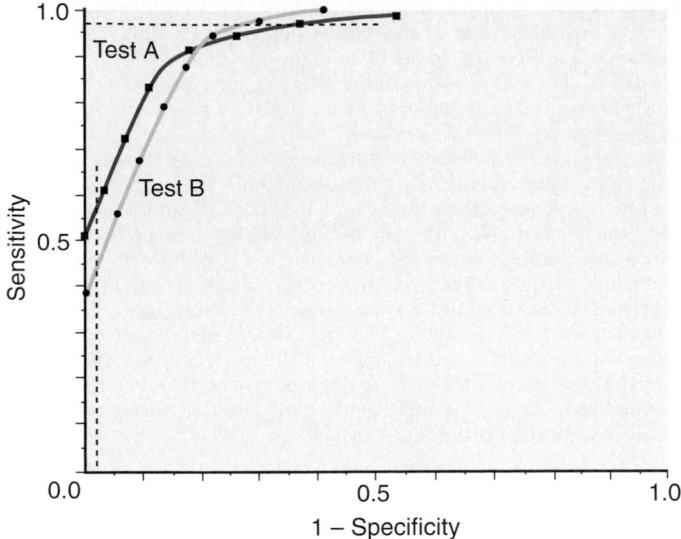

Figure 7–6 ROC curves for two tests. Note that the curves cross. See text for interpretation.

Table 7–7 Likelihood Ratio (LR)

Definition

Probability of test result in persons with disease/probability of same result in persons with no disease

Example

LR of positive test = Sensitivity/ (1 – Specificity)	From Table 7–5, using the test for RF that is positive in 95 of 100 RA patients (sensitivity of 95%) but also positive in 10 of 100 non-RA patients (specificity of 90%)
	LR of a positive test – (95/100)/(10/100) = 9.5
LR of negative test = (1 – Sensitivity)/Specificity	The same test for RF is negative in 90 of 100 non-RA patients but also negative in 5 of 100 RA patients
	LR of a negative test = (5/100)/(90/100) = 0.06

point on the curve. Visually, two tests are easily contrasted by their relative positions.

On a single curve, the point closest to the upper left-hand corner represents the cutoff with the most diagnostic accuracy. A cutoff is selected depending on whether a higher sensitivity or a higher specificity is more desirable. In practice, the cutoff with maximum sensitivity and specificity is generally selected as the decision limit. As with other measures of diagnostic accuracy, prevalence of disease does not affect the curve.

Sometimes the curves of two tests cross (Fig. 7–6) indicating that one test is superior at high sensitivities and the other is superior at high specificities. The best test would then depend on the clinical need. Screening tests need very high sensitivity. In the example (Fig. 7–6), Test B is the best screening test. At a sensitivity of 97%, Test B has a lower false-positive rate than Test A (28% versus 40%). Confirmatory (definitive diagnoses) tests need high specificity. Test A is the best confirmatory test. At a false-positive rate of 2% (specificity of 98%), Test A has a higher sensitivity than Test B (59% versus 47%).

The area under the ROC curve is a single number that describes the overall accuracy of a test. It is a quantitative description of how close the curve is to the upper left-hand corner, and represents the accuracy of a test over the entire range of sensitivity and specificity, not just at a given cutoff or a portion of the plot. An area of 1.0 represents a perfect test, while an area of 0.5 (the curve being the 45° diagonal) represents a test with no ability to discriminate. The mathematical value of the area is obtained from computer programs that use statistical methods to compare two tests.

The ROC curve should be visually studied to determine the point that provides the sensitivity and specificity that is most useful for clinical decisions. When curves cross (Fig. 7–6), one must consider that the curves have different accuracies in different portions of the plot.

The area under the curve has direct predictive implications. A value of 0.9 means that 90% of the time, two randomly selected subjects (one healthy and one diseased) will be correctly classified by the test. This value is not the same as the sensitivity or the predictive value of the test. With respect to test accuracy, an area of > 0.9 is considered excellent, an area < 0.7 is considered poor, and a value in between is considered fair to good.

Efficiency of a Test

Test efficiency is the ability of a test to correctly identify the true outcome, in other words, true positives and true negatives. It is expressed as the percentage of true results (Table 7–4), or the proportion of true positives and true negatives among all results. While sensitivity and specificity refer to the ability of a test to distinguish between presence and absence of disease, efficiency measures the ability to detect all true results. Thus true positives and true negatives are treated equally just as the false positives and false negatives are weighted equally. In practice, one of the false results (FP or FN) is often more clinically significant than the other and efficiency does not take this into account. Thus a test introduced to identify all patients with a certain disease can have a very high efficiency but it may not meet clinical needs because the false-negative rate is too high.

Sometimes it is preferable to select the cutoff with the highest efficiency and this can be visualized by graphing efficiency versus cutoff. Note that a cutoff can be selected to reduce either false positives or false negatives, depending on which goal is more important.

Like predictive value, test efficiency is influenced by disease prevalence so one must cautiously interpret efficiency when prevalence is very low or very high. At extremes of prevalence (much greater or much less than 50%), but particularly when the prevalence is very low, the cutoff can be altered to yield no false results in any one category. Thus, a test with a reportedly high efficiency may have poor sensitivity or specificity.

Likelihood Ratios

When interpreting results, a clinician considers not only whether a test result is normal or abnormal, but also how high or low the value is in relation to the reference limit. For example, an ALT of 60 U/L (with an upper limit of 55 U/L) is generally treated differently than an ALT of 2000 U/L since the former is far less indicative of liver disease than the latter. The likelihood ratio quantitates what a clinician may know intuitively – the further a result is from the reference limit, the more likely it is to indicate disease.

The likelihood ratio (LR) is the ratio of two probabilities: the probability of a test result when disease is present (true positive) divided by the probability of the same test result when disease is absent (false positive). In other words, the calculation gives the odds or likelihood of a test result occurring in a diseased patient as opposed to a healthy one. The higher the likelihood ratio of a positive test, the more useful is the information from a positive test. For example, consider the measurement of serum lipase to detect acute pancreatitis. The lipase value might be elevated (higher than the cutoff of 200 U/L) in 90 of 100 individuals with acute pancreatitis, but also similarly elevated in 10 of 100 individuals with other causes of abdominal pain. The likelihood ratio is 9, which means that an abnormal lipase is 9 times more likely in individuals with pancreatitis than those without, or, 9 times as many patients with pancreatitis than with other abdominal diseases will have an elevated lipase. The likelihood ratio refers to the likelihood of the test result, given the disease. This is not the same as the likelihood of pancreatitis being 9 times greater, given an abnormal lipase. The latter would be the predictive value of a positive lipase.

LR can be derived from sensitivity and specificity (Table 7–7). Like these other measures of test accuracy, the LR is an assessment of the test status or performance, and not disease status in the patient being tested. The LR is also not influenced by disease prevalence. The LR can be calculated for multiple test result levels. Thus, a result's degree of abnormality can be taken into account and medical decisions can be made at a point where there are fewer false negative and positive results.

The LR can also be derived from the ROC curve. The slope of the ROC curve – sensitivity/(1 – specificity) – at any cutoff value yields the LR of a positive test at that value. From Table 7–7, the LR is the true-positive rate (sensitivity) divided by the false-positive rate (1 – specificity). Over a broader range of the curve, the LR is the change in sensitivity divided by the change in specificity. As is the situation with the area under the curve, the use of the derived LR without appreciation of the actual curve can be misleading. A high LR may not necessarily imply a useful test because a test could have a high LR yet have a very low sensitivity.

Another and more practical way to understand LR is from the standpoint of pre- and post-test probability. The LR and pre-test probability (prevalence) can be used to calculate post-test probability (predictive value). This is illustrated in the examples in Table 7–8. For a positive test, any LR > 1 will increase the post-test probability. The larger the LR, the greater is the difference between pre-test and post-test probability.

Table 7–8 Likelihood Ratio (LR) and Probability of Disease

The LR and pre-test probability (prevalence) can be used to calculate post-test probability (predictive value). This is best understood by expressing probability in terms of odds

Definitions

Odds = Probability/ (1 – Probability)	Step 1. Pre-test probability is converted to pre-test odds in order to calculate post-test odds of disease or no disease (see examples)
Post-test odds = Pre-test odds × LR	Step 2. Post-test odds is calculated. Note as LR of a positive or negative result increases, so do the odds that the result will predict disease or no disease, respectively
Probability = Odds/ (1 + Odds)	Step 3. Odds are converted back into probability in order to calculate the post-test probability (predictive value) of a positive or negative test

Example 1

From Table 7–5, the rheumatoid arthritis pre-test probability (prevalence) is 5% in a rheumatology practice. From Table 7–7, the LR of a *positive* rheumatoid factor test is 9.5. Note that the probability of disease increases from 5% (pre-test) to 33% (post-test) because of the positive test result

Pre-test odds of disease = Pre-test probability/(1 – Pre-test probability)	Pre-test odds = 0.05/0.95 = 0.053 to 1
Post-test odds of disease = Pre-test odds of disease × LR of a positive test	Post-test odds = 0.053 × 9.5 = 0.5 to 1
Post-test probability = Odds/(1 + Odds)	Post-test probability = 0.5/1.50 = 0.33 or 33%

Example 2

From Table 7–7, the LR of a *negative* rheumatoid factor test is 0.06. While the probability of disease increases from 5% (pre-test) to 33% (post-test) because of the positive test result (Example 1), the probability of disease decreases from 5% (pre-test) to 0.3% (post-test) because of the negative test result

Pre-test odds of disease = Pre-test probability/(1 – Pre-test probability)	Pre-test odds = 0.05/0.95 = 0.053 to 1
Post-test odds of disease = Pre-test odds of disease × LR of a negative test	Post-test odds = 0.053 × 0.06 = 0.003 to 1
Post-test probability = Odds/ (1 + Odds)	Post-test probability = 0.003/1.003 = 0.003 or 0.3%

Regardless of prevalence, a high LR increases the probability that a positive test result predicts disease. The converse applies for a negative test result, for which any LR < 1 will decrease the post-test probability. The smaller the LR, the greater is the difference between pre-test and post-test probability. Thus, tests likely to be useful in clinical practice are those for which a positive result has a high LR and a negative result has a low LR.

Diagnostic Accuracy and Clinical Need

In order to help clinicians predict disease, the clinical laboratory must provide a diagnostically accurate test. A test that poorly discriminates between presence and absence of disease is unlikely to offer predictive power. The laboratory can alter test sensitivity or specificity to meet clinical goals. In general, screening tests require a very high sensitivity to avoid excluding someone with disease. This is true when evaluating babies for neonatal hypothyroidism or when assessing adults with chest pain in the emergency department for myocardial infarction. In either situation, the suspicion of disease may not be high, but the seriousness of the disease in question and the availability of therapeutic intervention dictate that no case be missed. This approach may yield many costly, albeit unavoidable, false-positive results. A test with a high sensitivity is also used to exclude disease, because it has a high predictive value for a negative test.

Confirmatory tests, like those for HIV, require high specificity. This is particularly true when there is little clinical evidence to support the disease or when there is a need to be certain of the diagnosis because the disease is serious and a false-positive result carries a high cost.

The diagnostic accuracy of the test together with prevalence provides a probability of disease (predictive value of a positive test). Improved diagnostic accuracy improves predictive power. Additionally, the predictive value of a positive test is enhanced when the prevalence (or pre-test probability) is high. An elevated PSA in an elderly male with an enlarged prostate confers a higher probability of cancer than does an elevated PSA in the general male population. As a corollary, for a rare disease, most positive results will be false positives.

The pre-test probability of disease (prevalence) affects post-test probability but also influences test interpretation. Thus, a positive test has a greater effect when the pre-test probability is low, and a negative test has greater effect when the pre-test probability is high. If a clinical diagnosis is strongly suspected, a positive test adds little to the clinical evaluation. Additionally, if the pre-test probability is very high, even a negative test may have little effect on patient management, unless the sensitivity of the test is 100%. The most benefit obtained from a test is when there is moderate uncertainty of disease, i.e., when the pre-test probability is intermediate. Similar benefit is obtained when the pre-test probability is close to a medical decision point so that the test will considerably influence the course of action.

Evidence-Based Medicine

Historically, medical decisions have relied heavily on clinical experience, expert opinions and other subjective or uncontrolled sources of information. This has also been true in laboratory medicine where there is often an inadequate foundation of evidence to support existing practices (Price, 2000, 2003). For example, there may not be a clear understanding of why a test is ordered, i.e., what clinical question is it trying to answer? Alternatively, there may not be any information on whether or when a test impacts on patient outcome such as morbidity, mortality, cost-benefit, patient satisfaction, risk and discomfort (Bruns, 2001). For example, does point-of-care testing improve patient diagnosis and discharge in the emergency department? (Kendall, 1998; Price, 2003; Bruns, 2001; Westgard, 2004; Trenti, 2003). Studies of clinical effectiveness in the clinical laboratory are hard to find because they are expensive and difficult to design (McQueen, 2001; Price, 2003). In addition, laboratory consultation is often based on the tradition of clinical and laboratory experience and less on a systematic approach to determining the current best evidence (Price, 2003; Guyatt, 1992).

In contrast to traditional approaches, evidence-based medicine (EBM) is a process by which medical decisions can be made using as many objective tools as possible. This, in turn, can help reduce the uncertainty of medical decision-making. EBM is a systematic practice that integrates the most current and best evidence with clinical expertise and patient preferences when making medical decisions (Sackett, 2000). EBM places emphasis on critically analyzing information from the literature and developing knowledge for medical practice (Sackett, 1983; Elstein, 2004, 1980; Sackett, 1991; Ludmerer, 2004). EBM encourages the cultivation of continuous learning and sharing of medical knowledge at all levels of training from medical student to attending physicians (Ludmerer, 2004). Since its introduction, EBM has grown to become a key tool for all healthcare providers.

There are five steps to practicing evidence-based medicine (Price, 2000, 2003; Sackett, 2000): (1) Ask a clinical question based on a patient encounter; (2) acquire information by searching resources; (3) analyze and critically evaluate the information and reach a conclusion that answers the clinical question; (4) apply the information to individual patients; (5) audit the effectiveness and monitor the literature.

A clinical encounter of a patient with a healthcare provider generally results in a clinical question that necessitates one or more laboratory tests – whether for screening, diagnosis, prognosis, or monitoring of treatment (McQueen, 2001). The question that is developed should be specific to a decision that must be made for that patient. The question compares an intervention such as ordering a diagnostic test, with the accepted practice. The clinical question can be described in four parts and summarized with the acronym PICO (Elstein, 2004; Sackett, 2000): *Problem (P)*: What is the problem of interest for the specific patient? *Intervention (I)*: What intervention is being considered? *Comparison (C)*: What are the alternatives that the intervention can be compared to? *Outcome (O)*: Is there a quantifiable clinical outcome that can be measured?

For example, a 55-year-old man, who recently returned from a trip to Europe, complains of swelling of the right leg, which upon examination, is warm, red, and swollen. The clinical question can be summarized as follows: *Problem*: Is D-dimer a good 'rule-out' test for deep vein thrombosis in a middle-aged man with a risk factor for thrombosis (like lengthy travel)? *Intervention*: D-dimer test. *Comparison*: Venous ultrasound or venography as the reference method. *Outcome*: Predictive value of D-dimer in 'ruling out' deep vein thrombosis.

A second example might be: A 58-year-old man with atrial fibrillation arrives in the emergency department with gastrointestinal bleeding due to a warfarin overdose. *Problem*: Is vitamin K effective in correcting coagulopathy caused by a warfarin overdose? *Intervention*: Vitamin K administration. *Comparison*: Fresh frozen plasma may be the alternative treatment. *Outcome*: Correction of bleeding and prothrombin time.

The strategy for answering these questions must be determined prior to searching the resources in order to prevent the introduction of selection bias. Information sources include textbooks, journals, electronic textbooks, and summary journals. Textbooks may provide an introduction to the pathophysiology of the disease, but they do not contain the current best evidence. Journal articles provide more up-to-date information than textbooks, but are also outdated by the time the articles have been written, accepted, and published. Randomized clinical controlled trials (RCTs) that are double-blinded are the most valuable of the journal articles because they are the least biased. However, RCTs are very dependent on the methods employed in the blinding and treatment of subjects (Lijmer, 1999).

Secondary articles and meta-analysis (a statistical technique to integrate results from multiple studies) summarize the best current evidence and provide practice guidelines. The Centre for Evidence-Based Medicine (http://www.cebm.net), Cochrane Collaboration/Cochrane Library (http://www.cochrane.org), Up-to-Date (http://www.uptodate.com/), and Best Clinical Evidence (Godlee, 2004) are sources that present summarized information. The Evidence-Based Medicine (ebm.bmjjournals.com) series of journals are also an excellent resource for up-to-date summaries. Although convenient, a summary article should be evaluated with caution since an 'expert' may introduce bias regarding which studies are assessed and the value applied to particular articles. Medical decision-making tools help to critically analyze each step in the process and have been summarized (Guyatt, 2002).

References

Baloch Z, Carayon P, Conte-Devolx B, et al: Guidelines Committee, National Academy of Clinical Biochemistry. Laboratory medicine practice guidelines. Laboratory support for the diagnosis and monitoring of thyroid disease. Thyroid 2003; 13(1):3–126.

Bruns DE: Laboratory related outcomes in healthcare. Clin Chem 2001; 47(8):1547–1552.

Elstein AS, Frazier HS, Neuhauser D, et al: Clinical Decision Analysis, 1st ed. Philadelphia, WB Saunders Company, Harcourt Brace Jovanovich, Inc., 1980.

Elstein AS: On the origins and development of evidence-based medicine and medical decision-making. Inflamm Res 2004; 53(Suppl 2):S184–S189.

Galen RS, Gambino SR: Beyond Normality: The Predictive Value and Efficiency of Medical Diagnoses. New York: John Wiley & Sons, Inc., 1975.

This book serves as an introduction to understanding the interpretation of a diagnostic test. The basics of diagnostic test accuracy and predictive value of tests are well outlined.

Godlee FE: Clinical Evidence Concise, 11th ed. Richmond, VA, BMJ Publishing Group, 2004.

Guyatt G, Cairns J: Evidence-based medicine: A new approach to teaching the practice of medicine. JAMA 1992; 268(17):2420–2425.

Guyatt G, Rennie D: User's Guide to the Medical Literature: A Manual for Evidence-Based Clinical Practice, 4th ed. Chicago, IL, American Medical Association, 2002.

Kendall JB, Reeves B, Clancy M: Point of care testing: Randomized controlled trial of clinical outcome. BMJ 1998; 316:1053–1057.

Lacher DA, Hughes JP, Carroll MD: Estimate of biological variation of laboratory analytes based on the Third National Health and Nutrition Examination survey. Clin Chem 2005; 51(2):450–452.

Lijmer JG, Mol BW, Heisterkamp S, et al: Empirical evidence of design-related bias in studies of diagnostic tests. JAMA 1999; 282(11):1061–1066.

Ludmerer KM: Learner centered medical education. NEJM 2004; 351(12):1163–1164.

McQueen MJ: Overview of evidence-based medicine: Challenges for evidence-based laboratory medicine. Clin Chem 2001; 47(8):1536–1546.

General overview of the practice of EBM as it relates to the laboratory, including examples and useful resources.

Price CP: Evidence-based laboratory medicine: Supporting decision-making. Clin Chem 2000; 46(8):1041–1050.

Price CP: Application of the principles of evidence-based medicine to laboratory medicine. Clin Chim Acta 2003; 333:147–154.

Sackett DL: Interpretation of diagnostic data: How to do it with pictures. Can Med Assoc J 1983; 129:429–432.

Sackett DL, Haynes RB, Guyatt GH, et al: Clinical Epidemiology: A Basic Science for Clinical Medicine. Boston/Toronto/London, Little and Brown, 1991.

Sackett DL, Straus SE, Richardson WS, et al: Evidence-Based Medicine: How to Practice and Teach EBM. 2nd ed. London, Churchill Livingstone, 2000.

Comprehensive, easy-to-read primer on all facets of EBM that includes many examples.

Sox HC Jr: Probability theory in the use of diagnostic tests. An introduction to critical study of the literature. Ann Intern Med 1986; 104:60–66.

The article provides an understanding of the expression of diagnostic uncertainty as the probability of disease. Issues in diagnostic accuracy and the influence of pre-test probability on post-test interpretation are also discussed.

Trenti T: Evidence-based laboratory medicine as a tool for continuous laboratory improvement. Clin Chim Acta 2003; 333:155–167.

Westgard JO, Darcy T: The truth about quality: medical usefulness and analytic reliability of laboratory tests. Clin Chim Acta 2004; 346(1):3–11.

Zweig MH, Campbell G: Receiver-operating characteristic (ROC) plots: A fundamental evaluation tool in clinical medicine. Clin Chem 1993; 39:561–577.

An in-depth article on the concept, use and application of ROC curves in clinical testing. A comparison with other measures of test accuracy is part of the discussion.

CHAPTER 8

Interpreting Laboratory Results

Matthew R. Pincus MD PhD, Naif Z. Abraham Jr. MD PhD

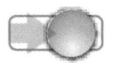 KEY POINTS

- Accurate differential diagnoses can be made from a systematic study of the laboratory profiles of patients in a large majority of cases.

- There are basically four types of anemia: iron deficiency, anemia of chronic disease, hemolytic anemia and macrocytic/nutritionally deficient anemia. These can be readily distinguished from one another both by the hematological profile and simple laboratory testing.

- By examining the urinary sodium, potassium and osmolarity, the causes of hypo- and hypernatremia can be readily determined.

- Liver function tests can distinguish among six different diseases of the liver: hepatitis, cirrhosis, biliary disease, space-occupying lesions of the liver, passive congestion and fulminant hepatic failure.

- Renal failure can be readily diagnosed by observing elevated BUN and creatinine; it is possible to pinpoint the site of renal failure, i.e., glomerular or tubular, from the ratio of serum to urine osmolality.

- Blood gas determinations allow determination of the causes of metabolic vs. respiratory acidosis or alkalosis; there is a critical relationship between the partial pressure of oxygen and carbon dioxide such that, in respiratory diseases, high levels of carbon dioxide block oxygenation of venous blood, leading to respiratory crisis.

- Elevation of tropinin in serum is diagnostic of myocardial infarction (or, less commonly, of unstable angina).

- Elevations of several serum analytes, like C-reactive protein, indicate inflammatory disease. Elevations of serum amylase and lipase point to acute pancreatitis.

- Two types of endocrine disease are discussed: thyroid and adrenal. Serum levels of T_4 (or better, free T_4) and thyroid-stimulating hormone (TSH) can be used to diagnose primary or secondary hypo- or hyperthyroidism; serum levels of cortisol and adrenocorticotropic hormone (ACTH) can be used to diagnose primary or secondary hypo- or hyperadrenalism.

Interpreting and Correlating Abnormal Laboratory Values

General Considerations

The major purpose of performing analyte determinations in the clinical laboratory is to aid in the diagnosis and management of patients with disease and individuals in health assessment. In this regard, the clinical pathologist is often called upon as a consultant to explain abnormal laboratory values, especially those that do not seem to correlate with one another, and to recommend or even to order laboratory tests that may lead to the correct diagnosis in the work-up of patients for particular medical problems. In addition, evaluation of laboratory test results on individual patients by the clinical pathologist can not only reveal the (infrequent) occurrence of laboratory errors, but can help in the selection of appropriate, cost-effective tests from a wide variety of increasingly complex test choices (Witte, 1997; Dighe, 2001; Bonini, 2002).

For evaluation of test results, the laboratory computer is an invaluable aid. Virtually all such systems perform daily checks for patient values that lie significantly outside of their established reference intervals or that have undergone large changes over a 24-hour period. These are often reported as 'failed delta checks.' Thus patients with significantly abnormal laboratory findings can be identified.

This chapter presents an approach to interpretation of laboratory values that will enable laboratorians to aid in the establishment of clinical diagnoses and to assist in clinical management. This discussion is by no means comprehensive and cannot possibly cover every conceivable illness afflicting patients. Rather, this presentation is concerned with general approaches to interpreting abnormal values and discussion of the most common causes of such findings so that the reader has a framework for interpreting abnormal values.

The reader may prefer to complete the Clinical Chemistry (Part II) and Hematology (Part IV) sections of this book before reading this section, which gives an overview of both of these vital diagnostic areas. Alternatively, the reader may decide to read this chapter to obtain the overview first prior to reading the several chapters in Chemistry and Hematology, Parts II and IV, respectively.

Fundamental Principles in Interpretation of Values

Before embarking on a discussion of specific conditions giving rise to abnormal values, certain precepts should always be followed, encapsulated as follows:

1. Never rely on a single (out-of-reference range) value to make a diagnosis. It is vital to establish a *trend* in values. A single sodium value of, for example, 130 mEq/L does not necessarily indicate hyponatremia. This single abnormal value may be spurious and may reflect such factors as improper phlebotomy technique, laboratory variability, etc. Rather, a series of low sodium values in successive serum samples from a given patient does indicate this condition. Thus it is vital to follow trends in particular values.
2. Osler's Rule. Especially if the patient is under the age of 60 years, try to attribute all abnormal laboratory findings to a single cause. Only if there is no possible way to correlate all abnormal findings should the possibility of multiple diagnoses be entertained.

Abnormalities in the Hematology Profile

Often, in laboratory reports, the first section contains the hematology profile, including the CBC or complete blood count. Comprehensive discussions of clinical hematopathology are given in Part IV. Here, we discuss very basic patterns of abnormalities to provide an overall reference frame for interpreting values and for the ordering of further examinations. Though this part of the book is concerned with clinical chemistry or chemical pathology, we discuss the hematology profile because the interpretation of hematopathologic results often depends on the results of quantitative determinations performed in clinical chemistry.

Anemias

Anemia, a common hematological disorder, is defined pathophysiologically as a decrease in the oxygen-carrying capacity of the blood. All oxygen-carrying capacity of the blood is due to the binding of oxygen to hemoglobin contained uniquely in red blood cells. Since anemia can cause tissue hypoxia, it often produces such symptoms as fainting, fatigue, pallor, and difficulty in breathing.

Practically, the best indicator for this condition is a low red blood cell count or number of red blood cells per volume of whole blood. While the reference range for the red cell count varies with age, sex and population, it encompasses values from around $4-6 \times 10^6$ red blood cells per cubic millimeter (cu mm) or microliter. This range may change somewhat depending on population. Red blood cell counts below the lower limit of the reference range suggest the presence of anemia. In addition, red blood cells occupy a well-defined range in terms of the percent of the volume which they occupy of whole blood or the hematocrit. Generally, normal adult hematocrit values range from about 36–45% (normal values for females are generally slightly lower than those for males). In addition, the concentration of hemoglobin in whole blood is about 12–15 g/dL or approximately 33–36 g/dL in red blood cells, i.e., the mean corpuscular hemoglobin concentration. Normal values are also dependent upon patient age and altitude of residence. Normally, the hematocrit is about three times the value of the hemoglobin concentration, which in turn, is about three times the value of the red blood cell count.

If anemia has been diagnosed, it is then mandatory to determine the cause of the anemia. An excellent history and physical examination is required for appropriate test selection, diagnosis, and the best possible patient care and treatment. In addition, a review of the peripheral blood film with respect to red and white cell morphology is often helpful.

To narrow further the differential diagnosis and facilitate appropriate test selection, a number of classification schemes for anemia have been developed, with no single ideal scheme available. A particularly useful approach utilizes the common red cell indices of mean corpuscular volume (MCV), in conjunction with the red cell distribution width (RDW) and the reticulocyte count (percent reticulocytosis) or reticulocyte production index (RPI). Taken together, these indices help to form a working hypothesis for the underlying cause of the anemia.

Electronic determination of MCV directly from red cell distribution data allows for classification on the basis of red blood cell size as macrocytic (MCV generally > 100 μm³ [100 fL]), microcytic (MCV generally < 80 μm³ [80 fL]), or normocytic (MCV generally between 80–100 μm³ [fL]). The RDW (percent) is a parameter that helps to further classify an anemia and reflects the variation of red blood cell size (anisocytosis). RDW generally varies between about 12–17, and is dependent upon the patient's age,

Table 8–1 Common Types of Anemias and Their Diagnostic Work-ups*

Anemia	Cause	Common analyte abnormality
1. Hypoproliferative, microcytic	Iron deficiency	Low ferritin Increased IBC Decreased serum iron Reduced Fe/TIBC ratio Generally increased RDW
2. Hypoproliferative, microcytic	Anemia of chronic disease	Generally high ferritin Normal IBC Decreased serum iron Normal Fe/TIBC ratio Generally normal RDW
3. Hyperproliferative, normocytic	Hemolytic anemia	Schistocytosis Increased reticulocytes Low haptoglobin Elevated carboxyhemoglobin Elevated LD Elevated indirect bilirubin Generally increased RDW
4. Hypoproliferative, normocytic	Aplastic anemia	Leukopenia Thrombocytopenia Hypocellular bone marrow Generally normal RDW
5. Hypoproliferative, normocytic	Renal failure	Elevated BUN and creatinine Low erythropoietin Burr cells may be present Generally normal RDW
6. Hypoproliferative, macrocytic		
A. Megaloblastic	B_{12} and/or folate deficiency	Low B_{12} and/or folate Hyperlobulated polymorphonuclear leukocytes Macro-ovalocytes Increased RDW
B. Nonmegaloblastic	Hypothyroidism	Elevated TSH Normal RDW

* In this table, low is equivalent to depressed, and high is equivalent to elevated. Ferritin, haptoglobin, LD, bilirubin, BUN, creatinine, erythropoietin, TSH and T_4 are all expressed as concentrations. All of these analytes are measured in serum.

IBC = iron-binding capacity; TIBC = total IBC; RDW = red cell distribution width; Fe = iron; LD = lactate dehydrogenase; BUN = blood urea nitrogen; TSH = thyroid-stimulating hormone.

sex, and ethnic subgroup. It can be helpful in differentiating causes of microcytosis, since moderate to severe iron deficiency anemia is associated with an increased RDW, while thalassemia and anemia of chronic disease (ACD) are associated with a normal RDW.

Peripheral blood reticulocytosis is a measure of bone marrow response in the face of anemia. A similar measure, the RPI, corrects the reticulocyte count with respect to: (1) the proportion of reticulocytes present in a patient without anemia, and (2) the premature release of reticulocytes into the peripheral circulation. Bone marrow response to anemia may be appropriate (hyperproliferative) with an RPI > 3 generally indicating marrow red cell hyperproliferation; however, the anemia may be due to defective red blood cell production or marrow failure (hypoproliferative) which is generally indicated by an RPI < 2. Thus, although these red cell indices are not pathognomonic of a particular type of anemia, the combination of MCV, RDW, and RPI examined together will often significantly narrow the differential diagnosis and facilitate further test selection. Table 8–1 illustrates common examples of anemia and their diagnostic work-up using these red cell indices as well as other helpful analytic abnormalities.

Microcytic Anemia

Common microcytic anemias include iron deficiency anemia (IDA) and the thalassemias. Some hemoglobinopathies and the anemia of chronic disease (ACD) may also be microcytic. In our discussion, we will focus on *iron deficiency anemia* and the *anemia of chronic disease*, a common differential diagnosis for patients with microcytic anemia. Both anemias appear to be disorders involving iron metabolism.

In IDA, there is a primary deficiency of iron available to the red cell (usually due to blood loss, but other causes include dietary deficiency, malabsorption, and pregnancy); chronic blood loss should always lead to further investigation since it is commonly associated with malignancy. ACD, however, appears to be due to defective iron utilization/metabolism and is associated with chronic nonhematologic disorders such as chronic infections, connective tissue disorders, malignancy, and renal, thyroid, and pituitary disorders.

To distinguish between IDA and ACD, a number of different laboratory measurements are very useful in addition to the RDW. The diagnosis is typically made using additional serum or whole blood laboratory tests. However, because IDA is always accompanied by loss of iron that is stored bound to the protein ferritin in bone marrow macrophages, the diagnosis can always in principle be made with a bone marrow biopsy with an iron stain that shows the absence of marrow iron. This procedure is, of course, invasive and should only be performed as a last resort.

Serum Ferritin Levels. Normally, there is an equilibrium between intracellular and extracellular ferritin. The lower the stored iron becomes, the lower is the intracellular ferritin and, consequently, the lower the extracellular ferritin becomes. The level of extracellular ferritin can be directly measured by determining the serum ferritin level, which is readily and accurately performed on serum aliquots, using ELISA (enzyme-linked immunosorbent assay) techniques, described in Chapter 43. Overall, therefore, serum ferritin levels give an excellent measure of available iron stores, noninvasively. Because, in ACD, iron stores are abundant, serum ferritin levels are characteristically normal to elevated. In contrast, in IDA, in which iron stores become depleted, serum ferritin levels are characteristically decreased. Thus, serum ferritin level is one assay that can be used in differentiating IDA from ACD.

One caveat in using serum ferritin values to provide this distinction is the fact that ferritin also happens to be an acute phase reactant. Acute phase reactants are proteins (discussed in Ch. 19) that rise in response to an acute process, usually an acute inflammatory condition. So, if a patient has an acute infection, the serum ferritin level may be spuriously elevated. The net effect may be a ferritin in the reference interval. Usually, in IDA, accompanied by an acute process, this level is in the low reference range.

Use of Serum Iron and Iron-Binding Capacity. In addition to ferritin levels, serum iron and serum iron-binding capacity (IBC) can be measured. On average, serum iron is, of course, reduced in iron deficiency anemia and normal or sometimes low in the anemia of chronic disease. The iron-binding capacity is a direct measure of the protein transferrin, which transports iron as Fe^{2+} from the gut to iron storage sites in bone marrow. In iron deficiency anemia, the serum iron is reduced, and the iron-binding capacity increases.

However, both serum iron and transferrin are subject to wide fluctuations because of such factors as diet and do not always reliably reflect iron stores. Also, transferrin is a beta-protein, i.e., it migrates in the beta-region in serum protein electrophoresis, and is an acute phase reactant. Thus its serum levels can change (usually decrease, as a so-called 'negative acute phase reactant') in inflammatory conditions. There is considerable overlap between serum levels of iron and iron-binding capacity in iron deficiency anemia and the anemia of chronic disease. A somewhat more reliable discriminating measure of iron deficiency anemia is the *ratio* of serum iron to the total iron-binding capacity (TIBC). This ratio is around 1 : 3 for normal individuals while in iron-deficiency anemia, it is significantly reduced to values of around 1 : 5 or lower. Again, there is considerable overlap even in this ratio for patients with iron deficiency anemia and the anemia of chronic disease, so the values should always be interpreted with care.

Use of Red Blood Cell Distribution Width. Finally, use of automated procedures for determination of cell counts and indices enable us to obtain average erythrocyte sizes and size distributions. In iron deficiency anemia, there is a marked dispersion in cell volumes (sizes) so that the *red cell distribution width* (RDW) increases, whereas it generally remains within normal limits in the anemia of chronic disease. Normal RDWs occur in the range of 12–17%. Unfortunately, the standard deviations for normals, and for patients with iron deficiency anemia or the anemia of chronic disease can overlap significantly, tending to limit the validity of using the RDW exclusively for distinguishing between these conditions.

The major laboratory findings that distinguish IDA from ACD are summarized as entries 1 and 2 in Table 8–1. Note that most of the major tests used to distinguish these two conditions are performed in the clinical chemistry laboratory. This emphasizes the strong interdependence of both of these services in obtaining definitive diagnoses through laboratory measurements.

Normocytic Anemia

Common causes of normocytic anemia include acute hemorrhage, hemolytic anemia, marrow hypoplasia, renal disease, and ACD. It may seem paradoxical that acute hemorrhage presents as normocytic anemia since it involves major blood loss that is associated with loss of iron stores. However, iron depletion requires time to develop; acutely, major blood loss presents as normocytic anemia.

Hyperproliferative Normocytic Anemias

Hyperproliferative normocytic anemias, associated with an *increased* reticulocyte count, include both *hemolytic anemia* and *the anemia associated with acute blood loss*, while *hypoproliferative anemias*, associated with a *decreased* reticulocyte count, include such causes as bone marrow aplasia/hypoplasia, renal disease, and ACD. As mentioned above, a history and physical as well as examination of the patient's peripheral blood film are helpful in establishing a differential diagnosis. In this section we will focus on the most common causes of normocytic anemia: hemolytic anemia, aplastic anemia, and the anemia associated with renal disease.

Hemolytic Anemia. Hemolysis is defined as the destruction of the red cell membrane causing hemoglobin release. This may occur slowly as a normal physiological process or may be accelerated in pathological states. Many different underlying causes exist for the decrease in survival/increase in destruction of red blood cells. These include membrane defects (e.g., hereditary spherocytosis), enzyme defects (e.g., glucose-6-phosphate dehydrogenase [G6PD] deficiency), hemoglobinopathies (e.g., sickle cell disease or beta-thalassemia), immune destruction (e.g., autoimmune hemolytic anemia or hemolytic transfusion reaction), and nonimmune destruction. The latter includes destruction due to infectious agents, toxic agents/drugs, physical agents, hypersplenism, and those classified as *microangiopathic hemolytic anemias* – a group of anemias due to mechanical destruction of red blood cells caused by such factors as fibrin deposition within blood vessels, prosthetic heart valves, etc.

Specific laboratory measurements that readily confirm the diagnosis of hemolytic anemia are based on the natural events that occur subsequent to hemolysis. After erythrocyte membrane breakdown, hemoglobin is extruded. This hemoglobin becomes bound to the alpha-2 fraction protein, haptoglobin. The hemoglobin–haptoglobin complex becomes catabolized by macrophages that engulf these complexes by receptor-mediated endocytosis. Thus an excellent laboratory test for hemolytic anemia is a *low* haptoglobin value. Extremely sensitive and rapid ELISA assays for haptoglobin are available for this purpose.

When hemoglobin is extruded, large amounts of it become oxidized to methemoglobin. The heme portion dissociates and then becomes oxidized ultimately to bilirubin. The first step in this process is the oxidative opening of the porphyrin ring of heme with the attendant liberation of carbon monoxide (CO). CO may be measured easily by gas chromatographic techniques or even more conveniently by co-oximetry, based on spectrophotometry (Ch. 4), as carboxyhemoglobin. Elevated CO levels in normochromic, normocytic anemias are an excellent indicator of hemolytic anemia.

Since there is an increased production of bilirubin, which is unconjugated (Ch. 21), there will be at least a transient elevation of serum indirect bilirubin. This elevation, in the presence of normal liver function, will be modest, usually in the range of about 2–2.5 mg/dL. (The upper limit of normal is around 1.2 mg/dL.)

As mentioned above, the reticulocyte count will be elevated (increase in polychromasia on the blood film), with erythroid hyperplasia present in the bone marrow, indicative of increased red cell production. The peripheral blood film may show evidence of the particular type of red cell damage associated with the particular type of hemolytic anemia (e.g. sickle cells in sickle cell disease or schistocytes/helmet cells in microangiopathic hemolytic anemia). There is also a noticeable difference in red cell size (anisocytosis) and shape (poikilocytosis) due to the presence of damaged and/or young cells. Because of the often-marked changes in size and/or shape, the RDW is usually elevated. A number of nucleated red blood cells may also be identified.

Plasma and urine may contain free hemoglobin or its degradation products. Free hemoglobin may be present acutely in the plasma (hemoglobinemia) or urine (hemoglobinuria), while hemosiderin may be present in the urine (hemosiderinuria) in more chronic episodes of hemolysis. LD (lactate dehydrogenase), an enzyme within the red cell, is often increased and is a relatively sensitive, although nonspecific finding. Also, because it is the chief intracellular ion, potassium ion becomes elevated in serum. Finally, a direct antiglobulin test (DAT)/direct Coombs' test can be used to detect immunoglobulin attached to the red cell surface. A positive test suggests an autoantibody or alloantibody may be responsible for the anemia. The final diagnosis will ultimately depend upon the results of specific tests for specific etiologies (e.g., a positive DAT for immune mechanism, or a positive G6PD screening test for G6PD deficiency); the selection of these tests will be dependent upon the clinical evaluation as well as the preliminary laboratory data.

Laboratory findings that are diagnostic of hemolytic anemia are summarized in entry 3 of Table 8–1. Note that virtually all of the quantitative diagnostic testing for hemolytic anemia, i.e., serum and urine hemoglobin, haptoglobin, carboxyhemoglobin, indirect bilirubin, and LD are performed in the clinical chemistry laboratory, again emphasizing the strong interdependence of the clinical chemistry and hematology laboratories.

Microangiopathic Hemolytic Anemia (MHA). As previously mentioned, red cell fragments (schistocytes) may be present on peripheral blood films due to mechanical (prosthetic heart valve) or thermal (severe burns) destruction. Mechanical rupture of red cells within the microvasculature may also occur by physical damage to red cells in the microvasculature of bone marrow. This may be due to space-occupying lesions, such as metastatic tumors or leukemia or lymphoma, to myelofibrosis or to the intravascular deposition of fibrin strands upon endothelial cell surfaces. Since red blood cells are damaged and destroyed, this process leads to so-called microangiopathic (i.e., lesions in the microvasculature) hemolytic anemia.

Besides the space-occupying lesions, other causes of this type of anemia include disease states in which fibrin is deposited on endothelial surfaces, also resulting in the shearing and fragmentation of newly synthesized red blood cells as in disseminated intravascular coagulopathy (DIC). In addition, other disease states may give rise to microangiopathic hemolytic anemia in which there may be an immunologic component, i.e., antibodies to determinants on endothelial cells or on other structures in the microvasculature, resulting in immune complex deposits with or without fibrin deposits. These states include thrombotic thrombocytopenic purpura (TTP), and the hemolytic anemic/uremic syndrome (HUS). Since these two conditions involve the microvasculature in general, other tissues are frequently affected. Thus, in both HUS and TTP, damage to the renal microvasculature occurs resulting in renal failure and is associated with elevated BUN and creatinine as described in Abnormalities in Clinical Chemistry below. In TTP, there is also involvement of the cerebral circulation giving rise to behavioral changes and other neurological sequelae. In addition, platelets are also affected giving rise to thrombocytopenia.

MHA may also occur with other immune-mediated disorders, e.g., connective tissue disorders such as disseminated lupus erythematosus where, again, endothelial damage from the attachment of immune complexes and complement produces fibrin deposition on endothelial surfaces.

Importantly, since microangiopathic hemolytic anemia results from traumatic destruction of newly formed red blood cells in the microvasculature where both red and white blood cell precursors are being formed, often both red and white blood cell precursors are released into the circulation. Thus, all of the findings of hemolytic anemia are present, in addition to which a significant number of precursor cells are seen in the peripheral blood such as nucleated red blood cells, myelocytes and metamyelocytes, a pattern termed the leukoerythroblastic picture.

As discussed below, in DIC and occasionally in TTP, laboratory findings include thrombocytopenia, increased prothrombin time, activated partial thromboplastin time, thrombin time, fibrin degradation products and D-dimer levels, but low fibrinogen levels. BUN and creatinine are also elevated.

Hypoproliferative Normocytic Anemias

Bone Marrow Hypoplasia/Aplastic Anemia. This is a *hypoproliferative* anemia, with MCV and RDW usually within normal limits, and which typically affects all peripheral blood elements (red cells, white cells, and platelets – see below). Immature white cells and red cells are not usually present on peripheral blood films. Bone marrow biopsy is commonly performed to obtain the diagnosis and typically shows severely hypoplastic/ aplastic marrow with severe depletion of all hematopoietic marrow precursors. Aplastic anemia may be primary/inherited or secondary/ acquired, with the latter due to chemical toxin, infection, radiation, or immune dysfunction. Serum iron may be elevated, due to lack of erythropoiesis. The typical hematological findings in this condition are summarized in entry 4 of Table 8–1. Importantly, none of the quantitative serum diagnostic tests for hemolytic anemia, such as haptoglobin, carboxyhemoglobin, and indirect bilirubin elevation, are positive in this condition.

Myelodysplastic Syndrome. Another less common condition but nonetheless an important cause of hypoproliferative normocytic anemia is the myelodysplastic syndrome (MDS). This syndrome, which often presents as a normocytic anemia, although it can also on occasion present as a mildly macrocytic or as microcytic anemia, is refractory to treatment, e.g., transfusions of packed red blood cells. It may present simply as a refractory anemia, in its early stages and is thought to progress then to refractory anemia with ringed sideroblasts and eventually to so-called 'preleukemic' stages, in particular, refractory anemia with an excess of

blasts (generally in the myeloid or lymphoid lines) and an excess of blasts in transformation. The condition may also present initially as a refractory cytopenia that involves all three (erythroid, granulocytic, megakaryocytic) hematopoietic cell lines. As might be surmised from this latter observation, MDS appears to be a clonal stem cell disorder that is characterized by ineffective hematopoiesis. Further discussion of this fascinating disease can be found in Chapter 32.

Anemia of Renal Failure. Another normocytic, hypoproliferative anemia is the anemia of chronic renal failure. Loss of the kidneys' excretory function produces an increase in BUN and creatinine, as discussed below, as well as a build-up of metabolic byproducts. The resulting uremia appears to be responsible for changes in red cell shape, with burr cells (echinocytes) and ellipsoidal cells commonly present on peripheral blood films. Identification of burr cells on peripheral blood films during the course of illness may signal the development of renal dysfunction. In addition to a decreased excretory function, there is a decrease in the kidneys' ability to produce erythropoietin, resulting in impaired erythropoiesis, such that the marrow's response to hypoxia becomes inadequate. Distinguishing this condition from aplastic anemia (entry 4 in Table 8–1), white cell and platelet counts usually remain within normal limits. The typical findings in this condition are summarized in entry 5 of Table 8–1. Again, as in bone marrow hypoplasia/aplastic anemia (entry 4, Table 8–1), none of the quantitative serum diagnostic tests for hemolytic anemia, such as haptoglobin, carboxyhemoglobin, and indirect bilirubin elevation, are positive in this condition.

Macrocytic Anemia

Macrocytic anemia can be diagnosed from the hemogram from a low red blood cell count and a high mean corpuscular volume (MCV), often exceeding 100 fl. By far the most common cause of macrocytic anemia is nutritional deficiency, i.e., vitamin B_{12} and/or folate deficiency. Lack of either factor is thought to disrupt DNA synthesis but not RNA synthesis, such that the nucleus and cytoplasm of the cell no longer mature in synchrony. Morphologically, the cell cytoplasm matures, while the nucleus remains immature, and the cell appears megaloblastic. This lack of synchrony produces hypersegmented neutrophils (five-lobed nuclei in more than 5% of the neutrophils or any neutrophil with six or more lobes) and large, oval-shaped red cells termed macroovalocytes, both of which are present on blood films of patients with megaloblastic anemia. In addition, the RDW is typically increased, and the reticulocyte count is decreased.

If macrocytic anemia is diagnosed, the first serum analytes whose concentrations should be determined are B_{12} and folate for which rapid and accurate ELISA assays are performed. If these analytes are both found to be within the reference range, assays for thyroid function should be performed since hypothyroidism is a cause of macrocytosis. As discussed below in the endocrine function testing section, elevated thyroid-stimulating hormone (TSH) with low or normal thyroxine (T_4) serum levels confirm the diagnosis of primary hypothyroidism. Since certain therapeutic drugs, particularly azathymidine (AZT) used in the treatment of the acquired immune deficiency syndrome (AIDS), are known also to induce macrocytic anemia, it is important to ascertain whether a patient is being treated with such drugs.

In this era of the automated complete blood count (CBC), it is possible also that red cell precursor forms, such as nucleated red blood cells, may be counted as mature erythrocytes. Therefore, in a patient with a 'macrocytic' anemia with normal B_{12}, folate and thyroid hormone levels, it is important to check the reticulocyte and nucleated red blood cell count to determine if these are significantly elevated. If so, the possibility of a hemolytic anemia should be considered. Thus the diagnostic work-up for hemolytic anemia described in the preceding section should be instituted.

Other possible causes of macrocytic anemia include post-hemorrhagic states (differentiated by an elevation of the reticulocyte count and polychromasia); alcoholism (associated with folate deficiency), liver disease and myelodysplasia. Note again that the definitive tests for determining the cause of macrocytic anemia, i.e., B_{12}, folate, and thyroid function tests, are often performed in the clinical chemistry section.

The major clinical laboratory findings for macrocytic anemia are summarized as entries 6A and B in Table 8–1. Note that macrocytic anemias are divided into megaloblastic (entry 6A), typical of B_{12} and folate deficiency, and non-megaloblastic (entry 6B), typical of hypothyroidism. Whether or not the macrocytic anemia is megaloblastic can be determined only by bone marrow biopsy. This procedure is not necessary in most cases since the cause of the macrocytosis can be determined by the assays described above.

Table 8–1 summarizes some of the pertinent findings and specific determinations used to distinguish and diagnose common anemias previously discussed. Note that this table is a guide as to what specific tests should be ordered and, by implication, what tests need not be ordered. For example, a microcytic anemia should be worked up with orders for ferritin levels, TIBC, and Fe/TIBC ratios, but generally there is no need to order B_{12} and folate levels. Conversely, there is no need to order ferritin, TIBC, etc., for a macrocytic anemia, for which B_{12} and folate levels should be ordered.

Quantitative White Blood Cell Abnormalities

The white blood cell count (WBC) encompasses several types of commonly circulating nucleated cells: granulocytes (principally mature neutrophils, basophils, and eosinophils), lymphocytes, and monocytes. It should be noted that absolute concentrations (and not percentages) of these cells are significant in interpreting the WBC. An increase above the normal physiological level in the WBC, termed leukocytosis, may primarily involve any of these white cells, depending upon which cell type is chiefly elevated (i.e., neutrophilia, basophilia, eosinophilia, monocytosis, and lymphocytosis). Likewise, a decrease in the WBC, termed leukopenia, may also center on a single cell series (i.e., neutropenia, monocytopenia, and lymphocytopenia). Absolute decreases in the eosinophils and basophils are difficult to identify because of the low numbers present normally. Certain differential diagnoses are commonly associated with certain WBC changes (e.g., infection and/or inflammation with neutrophilia; allergic reactions and parasitic infections with eosinophilia). In addition, elevations may be due to a benign process (e.g., infection) or a malignant process (e.g., leukemia). Occasionally, plasma cells may be found in the peripheral blood. Here, we note several quantitative patterns and their associations that correlate with abnormal chemical findings.

Again, clinical history and physical findings are important in diagnosis and management of the patient. In addition, the complete blood count (CBC) and white cell differential are important laboratory findings used, in conjunction with the clinical impression, to formulate the differential diagnosis. In adults, the reference range for the white count is approximately 4000–7000 white cells/mm³; approximately two-thirds of the white cells are neutrophils and slightly less than one-third are lymphocytes.

Infection: the Most Common Cause of Elevated White Blood Cell Count (WBC)

An elevated WBC between about 10 000–20 000/µL commonly points to an infectious/reactive process. In general, *neutrophilia* is associated with infection (bacterial, fungal, viral), inflammatory states (trauma, surgery), certain drugs (e.g., corticosteroids) as well as myeloproliferative conditions. Exceptions to the neutrophilia seen in bacterial infections are tuberculosis, brucellosis, pertussis, where the predominant cells are lymphocytes, and infections, mainly in newborns, with *Listeria monocytogenes*, for which a monocytic response is predominant.

Eosinophilia is commonly associated with allergic reactions, parasitic infections, and hematologic malignancies (Brigden, 1997; Rothenberg, 1998; Brito-Babapulle, 2003). *Basophilia* is also commonly associated with hematologic malignancies (e.g., chronic myelogenous leukemia or CML), but may be seen in some inflammatory states and allergic reactions. *Lymphocytosis* is commonly associated with acute viral infections, such as infectious mononucleosis (EBV infection), chronic infections, such as tuberculosis, brucellosis, and pertussis, as well as hematologic disease and immune stimulation. *Monocytosis* is commonly associated with hematologic disease, such as chronic myelomonocytic leukemia, as well as with some infectious processes, such as tuberculosis, rickettsia and listeria.

Elevated WBC Due to Leukemoid Reaction

In patients who do not have leukemia, very high white blood cell counts (generally greater than 50×10^9/L) may produce a peripheral blood film appearance similar to leukemia. This is termed a *leukemoid reaction*. The more common type of leukemoid reaction is granulocytic although lymphocytic reactions may also occur. The granulocytic type usually reveals reactive neutrophils present in the peripheral blood film, with a left shift in the neutrophil series (i.e., immature forms such as bands, metamyelocytes and myelocytes). Changes in the cells' cytoplasmic appearance, such as toxic granulation and Dohle body production (Ch. 32), are also commonly present. Causes of the granulocytic type of reaction include bacterial infection (e.g., diphtheria), malignancy (Hodgkin's disease), and reactive conditions such as rebound granulocytosis.

Although these changes are helpful, C-reactive protein (CRP), an acute phase plasma protein, rapidly rises and falls with the onset and resolution of inflammation. CRP appears to be an earlier and more sensitive indicator of acute inflammation and infection (Seebach, 1997) and can now be quickly measured using present-day analyzers.

Leukemoid reaction must be distinguished from chronic myelogenous leukemia (CML) and other myeloproliferative conditions. Importantly, *the*

enzyme, neutrophil alkaline phosphatase, will be normal or elevated in a granulocytic leukemoid reaction but is decreased in CML.

Elevated WBC Due to Chronic Myelogenous Leukemia (CML)

At present, definitive *diagnosis of CML* rests upon the demonstration of the Philadelphia chromosome (i.e., the *BCR/c-abl* translocation between chromosome #9 and #22) by either cytogenetics or molecular techniques (e.g., see Silver, 2003; George, 2003; Sattler, 2003). Detection of molecular or cytogenetic abnormalities is also of diagnostic (and can be of prognostic) significance in other hematologic diseases including acute myeloid leukemia, acute lymphoblastic leukemia, T cell leukemia/lymphoma and myelodysplasia (Glassman, 1997). Molecular techniques are now also currently utilized to detect very early stages of disease, as well as to detect minimal residual disease, that is, disease that may only be apparent at the molecular level. For example, quantitative polymerase chain reaction can be used to monitor *BCR/c-abl* translocation levels in CML patients being treated with the kinase inhibitor Gleevec (Hughes, 2003).

Elevated WBC Due to Chronic Lymphocytic Leukemia (CLL)

When the lymphocytes appear normal, but are significantly increased in number in an older individual, the possibility of *chronic lymphocytic leukemia (CLL)* must be considered. Again, molecular techniques, such as flow cytometric, immunophenotypic and cytogenetic/fluorescence in situ hybridization analysis (Oscier, 2004; Shanafelt, 2004) can help establish the diagnosis. In CLL, the neoplastic B lymphocytes will be found to express an unusual (but characteristic) human leukocyte differentiation antigen designated CD5, which is typical for this disease. Other CD antigens can also be detected by flow cytometry and have become useful in resolving other hematologic diagnostic problems.

Leukocytosis Due to Acute Leukemias

Both acute myeloid and lymphoid leukemias present often as markedly elevated white cell counts. In lymphoblastic leukemia, numerous lymphoblasts are seen on the peripheral smear. The myeloid leukemias can present in a myriad of forms including myeloblastic, promyelocytic, monoblastic/monocytic, myelomonocytic, erythroblastic and megakaryoblastic. Again, flow cytometric, immunophenotypic and karyotypic/molecular analysis can help establish the diagnosis, as well as define prognosis (Winton, 2004). These are discussed fully in Chapter 32. Here, we point out that blast forms of any kind on a peripheral blood smear raise the strong diagnostic possibility of an acute leukemia.

Low White Cell Counts

Aplastic Anemia. Low WBC, if accompanied by marrow hypoplasia and two out of three of the following findings – anemia (with corrected reticulocyte count < 1%), neutropenia (neutrophil count < 500/µL), and thrombocytopenia (platelet count < 20 000/µL) – may be part of generalized pancytopenia secondary to marrow failure (Guinan, 1997; Marsh, 2003). Also known as aplastic anemia, this condition may be primary/inherited or acquired/secondary. Known causes of the acquired type include drugs/toxins, infections (including hepatitis), radiation, and immune dysfunction (Gordon-Smith, 2002). Cytogenetic study may be utilized to rule out myelodysplasia; if unsuccessful, molecular techniques such as fluorescent in situ hybridization (FISH) may be necessary for chromosome analysis (Guinan, 1997). The primary/inherited types may not always be present at birth (i.e., congenital) and diagnosis of this type of marrow failure relies heavily on clinical assessment in conjunction with appropriate laboratory evaluation (Alter, 1999, 2002).

Gram Negative Sepsis as a Cause of Leukopenia. Leukopenia may also be seen in other conditions including Gram-negative sepsis. Interestingly, Gram-negative sepsis with a low WBC is often accompanied by a cholestatic pattern in the liver (i.e., a mild rise in bilirubin and alkaline phosphatase).

Coagulation Disorders

This vast and complex topic is discussed in Part V. For our review, we focus on four hematologic parameters that may be important in correlation with test results in chemistry determinations: the platelet count, the bleeding time, the activated partial thromboplastin time (APTT), reflecting the function of the intrinsic coagulation system, and the prothrombin time (PT), reflecting the function of the extrinsic coagulation system. Diminished values of the platelet count and/or abnormalities in platelet aggregation can lead to abnormal bleeding times. Elevated PTs and/or APTTs are not generally associated with abnormal bleeding times except mainly in factor VIII deficiency with concomitant deficiency of von Willebrand factor. This latter factor is needed for platelet aggregation.

Historically, the bleeding time (BT) was utilized as a screening test for platelet function. It should be noted that the BT, at present, is not felt to correlate accurately with or to predict bleeding (DeCaterina, 1994; Gerwirtz, 1996) and is now uncommonly used to screen for platelet function abnormalities (Kottke-Marchant, 2002).

Remember that the anticoagulant *heparin*, which accelerates the inactivation of thrombin and other coagulation factors (such as factor Xa), *preferentially blocks the intrinsic system, leading to prolonged APTTs* but not significant elevations in PTs. On the other hand, the vitamin K antagonist, *coumadin*, preferentially *blocks factor VII* in the extrinsic system leading to *prolonged PTs but not APTTs.*

If the PT or the APTT becomes elevated, in the absence of treatment with heparin or coumadin, and the platelet count is normal, it is important to perform mixing studies of the patient's plasma with normal plasma to determine if the coagulation time normalizes, i.e., whether there is a factor deficiency. A not infrequent cause of factor deficiency is liver failure, discussed subsequently and in Chapter 21. Thus liver function measurements should also be checked in these instances. If mixing studies do not completely correct the prolonged coagulation times, the presence of coagulation inhibitors, such as circulating lupus anticoagulant or antifactor antibodies should be suspected.

If the platelet count diminishes and the APTT and PT both rise, the diagnosis of disseminated intravascular coagulation (DIC) should be entertained. This diagnosis is confirmed by the finding of elevated fibrin split products (FSP) and, more specifically, the D-dimer, discussed in Chapter 39, the D–D fragment of fibrin that results from the proteolytic action of plasmin upon the fibrin clot that forms during intravascular coagulation. D-dimer is detected in an assay utilizing a very specific monoclonal antibody to this crosslinked fibrin degradation product. DIC is an extremely dangerous condition and must be diagnosed rapidly.

In this condition, there is an abnormal activation of *both* coagulation cascades and a consumption of platelets. This activation may be caused by Gram-negative sepsis (activation of the cascades may be from bacterial endotoxins), cancer, chronic inflammatory states such as in collagen vascular diseases, leukemia (especially acute promyelocytic leukemia), complications of pregnancy, blood transfusion complications, liver failure, and physical trauma such as burns, drowning, and CNS injuries, etc. DIC causes the formation of microemboli that can result in widespread tissue infarction or ischemia with attendant abnormal chemical values, e.g., elevated liver function enzymes, elevated BUN and creatinine, suggestive of renal failure, even elevation of cardiac enzymes such as creatine phosphokinase and its cardiac-specific MB fraction, indicative of myocardial damage. Thus low platelet counts, elevated APTT and PT, together with chemical abnormalities suggestive of multisystem dysfunction, strongly suggest DIC. Anticoagulant therapy must be instituted rapidly to block further embolization and tissue destruction.

Abnormalities in Clinical Chemistry: Chemical Pathology

Electrolyte Abnormalities

Figure 8–1 summarizes the basic mechanisms by which the kidneys control electrolyte and water balance. Functionally, keep in mind that the *purpose of the kidneys is to conserve fluids or, tantamount to this, to concentrate the urine.* The mechanism by which this conservation of fluids is effected is by the building up of high sodium chloride gradients in the interstitial space between the descending and ascending limbs of the loop of Henle using the countercurrent multiplier mechanism. In this mechanism, sodium chloride is extruded into the interstitial space such that NaCl concentrations become greater towards the tip of the loop of Henle. The ascending limb of the loop of Henle is impermeable to water as are the distal convoluted tubules and collecting ducts. However, under the effect of antidiuretic hormone (ADH), the collecting ducts are made permeable to water, allowing it to flow into the interstitial space and to penetrate the vasa recta. The entire driving force for this process is the high concentrations of NaCl in the interstitium. Any interference with the countercurrent multiplier will block reabsorption of water because the ion gradients are eliminated.

As also shown in Figure 8–1, sodium ion, 70% of which is reabsorbed in the proximal convoluted tubule, can be further reabsorbed in the distal convoluted tubules and collecting ducts under the effect of aldosterone from the zona glomerulosa of the adrenal cortex. This hormone promotes

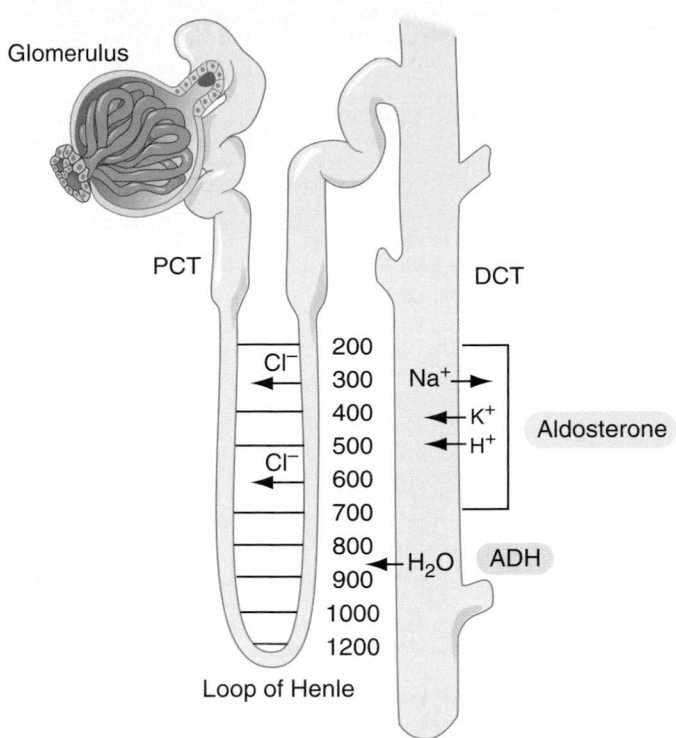

Figure 8–1 A schematic representation of a nephron showing the fundamental mechanism of water and salt conservation by the kidneys. Filtration occurs at the glomerulus (upper left, showing capillaries in red), and the filtrate passes through the proximal convoluted tubule (PCT), where about 70% of the total filtered sodium is reabsorbed. In the loop of Henle, the countercurrent multiplier mechanism is operative. Chloride ion (Cl−) is extruded from the ascending limb into the interstitial space (shown in the upper middle part of the figure). Sodium ion passively follows. The cells of the ascending limb of the loop of Henle are impermeable to water, and the cells of the descending limb are impermeable to chloride ions. The result of this system is that high concentrations of NaCl are built up at the tip of the loop of Henle. The numbers beside the loop of Henle are osmolalities at different levels along the loop that, in humans, reach a maximum of 1200 mOsm as shown in the figure. At the top of the loop, the filtrate becomes isotonic (where the 300 mOsm mark occurs) and then hypotonic due to the continuous extrusion of chloride ions. The hypertonic interstitium allows water to diffuse in from the collecting ducts (CD) provided that antidiuretic hormone (ADH, labeled and highlighted in color in the figure) is secreted. More sodium ion can be conserved in the distal convoluted tubule (DCT) provided aldosterone (labeled and highlighted in color) is secreted, resulting in the one-to-one exchange of Na+ for K+ and H+.

the 1 : 1 exchange of sodium for potassium or hydrogen ion. Sodium levels in serum depend almost completely on the interplay between aldosterone and ADH. With these simple considerations in mind, the most common causes of hyponatremia and hypernatremia are now summarized with an explanation of how to identify them.

Hyponatremia
The four most common causes of hyponatremia are given in Table 8–2, together with a fifth, rare, cause, Bartter's syndrome. A sixth, metabolic cause, diabetes mellitus, is also presented in this table. In all forms of hyponatremia, the chloride ion concentration is also generally low since chloride is the chief counterion for sodium.

Basic Principle
All confirmed serum sodium abnormalities must be followed up with urinalysis on the patient who should be fluid restricted. This urinalysis should include the urine sodium and urine osmolality. For conditions 1 and 2 in Table 8–2, the serum sodium tends to correct over a 24-hour period when the patient is fluid restricted.

Overhydration. In this condition, the most common cause of which is the consumption of large amounts of water or hypotonic fluids due to such causes as psychogenic polydipsia, serum sodium is reduced below 135 mEq/L. Since the consumed water is excreted by the kidneys, the urine is also dilute in this ion. In fact, *the osmolality of urine will be low, i.e., < 300 mOsm*. Often accompanying hyponatremia in overhydration are *low values of the hematocrit and low values of BUN*, discussed subsequently. This triad of findings strongly suggests overhydration as the cause. Urinalysis in the fluid-restricted patient will reveal urinary sodiums of < 25 mEq/L and low osmolalities. The potassium may also be low although it often

Table 8–2 Common Causes of Hyponatremia and Electrolyte Patterns in Serum and Urine with Normal Renal Function*

Cause	Serum Na	Urine Na (UNa)	Urine osmolality	Serum K	24-Hour UNa
1. Overhydration	Low	Low	Low	Normal or low	Low
2. Diuretics	Low	Low	Low	Low	High
3. SIADH†	Low	High	High	Normal or low	High
4. Adrenal failure	Low	Mildly elevated	Normal	High	High
5. Bartter's syndrome	Low	Low	Low	Low	High
6. Diabetic hyperosmolarity‡	Low	Normal	Normal	High	Normal

* All Na and K values are concentrations except for 24-hour UNa, which is the total number of milliequivalents of Na excreted in 24 hours in the urine.

† Secretion of inappropriate levels of antidiuretic hormone.

‡ In this condition, serum glucose is markedly elevated.

Table 8–3 Common Causes of Hypernatremia and Electrolyte Patterns in Serum and Urine with Normal Renal Function*

Cause	Serum Na	Urine Na (UNa)	Urine osmolality	Serum K	24-Hour UNa
1. Dehydration	High	High	High	Normal	Varies
2. Diabetes insipidus	High	Low	Low	Normal	Low
3. Cushing's disease or syndrome	High	Low	Normal	Low	Low

* All Na and K values are concentrations except for 24-hour UNa, which is the total number of milliequivalents of Na excreted in 24 hours in the urine.

remains within the reference range. Since mainly water is excreted in urine in this condition, the total 24-hour sodium excretion will be low (cause no. 1 in Table 8–2).

Use and/or Abuse of Diuretics. Loop diuretics block the chloride pump in the loop of Henle, thereby blocking the formation of the ion gradients via the countercurrent multiplier, necessary for water conservation. Thus water is lost. Also, because sodium is no longer retained because it follows chloride in the loop, it also is depleted from serum. The 24-hour sodium excretion is high, unlike in overhydration (entry 2 in Table 8–2). The pattern resembles overhydration (dilute serum and urine) except that loop diuretics cause severe potassium depletion unless the diuretic is combined with a potassium-sparing diuretic like triamterene. Combined hyponatremia and hypokalemia with a high urinary sodium and potassium 24-hour excretion point to diuretic use. Of course, a history will generally also reveal use of diuretics.

Syndrome of Inappropriate ADH (SIADH) Secretion (entry 3, Table 8–2). In this condition, secondary to head trauma, seizures, other CNS diseases, and neoplastic conditions especially lung, breast and ovarian cancers, that secrete ADH-like hormones, the serum sodium is depressed due to the excess retention of water in the collecting ducts. This results in depletion of water in the renal tubules, thereby concentrating the urine. Therefore, while the serum is dilute in sodium (hypotonic), the urine is concentrated to levels > 40 mEq/L, and the urine osmolality exceeds 300 mOsm while the serum osmolality < 280 mOsm. This pattern clearly is diagnostic of SIADH.

Aldosterone Deficit (entry 4, Table 8–2). This condition is secondary to Addison's disease and AIDS-related hypoadrenalism. Without aldosterone, the Na^+–K^+ and Na^+–H^+ exchange in the distal convoluted tubules and collecting ducts does not occur. Therefore, serum sodium concentration is reduced while serum potassium concentration increases, and there is a mild metabolic acidosis. Urinary sodium increases but not to the high levels seen in SIADH, and the osmolality of urine is also not so elevated as in SIADH.

Bartter's Syndrome (entry 5, Table 8–2). This condition resembles diuretic use except that the hyponatremia is not corrected with fluid restriction. The cause of this rare condition is unknown, but sodium chloride gradients cannot form in the loop of Henle. This results in retention of chloride ion that is not available for the countercurrent mechanism. Thus the ion gradients that normally form in the loop of Henle cannot exist. In this condition, there is a persistent hyponatremia, hypokalemia and a high 24-hour sodium and potassium excretion.

Diabetic Hyperosmolar State. In patients with *diabetes mellitus*, if they are in a hyperosmolar state, i.e., where the serum glucose is markedly elevated, say around 700 mg/dL, the hyperosmolality of serum causes efflux of cellular water, with a consequent *osmotic dilution of serum sodium.* Roughly, for *each 100 mg/dL increase in serum glucose, there is a 1.6 mEq/L decrease in the serum Na^+ concentration.* Since transport of glucose into cells is accompanied by concurrent transport of potassium into cells, low insulin levels also cause high serum potassium. So, the net effect of *diabetic hyperosmolar states is a low serum sodium and a high serum potassium.* This resembles *hypo*aldosteronism (cause 4 in Table 8–1), but the presence of abnormally high glucose levels signals the possibility of diabetes mellitus as the cause.

Pseudohyponatremia

This condition is usually caused by the presence of excess lipids in serum. No sodium ions are dissolved in lipids, which can take up a considerable volume of serum. If the absolute amount of sodium in a given volume of serum is determined, as is performed when using such methods of sodium determination as *flame photometry*, this value is divided by the sample volume to get the concentration. But part of this volume is lipid that has no sodium. So a falsely low value of sodium can be obtained. This artifact is eliminated by the use of ion-selective electrodes that directly determine the concentration of sodium and do not depend upon knowledge of the volume of serum.

Hypernatremia

Table 8–3 summarizes the three basic causes of hypernatremia. Note that each cause is the counterpart of a cause for hyponatremia. These causes are summarized as follows.

Dehydration. This can be caused by excess renal loss with high positive free water clearance (i.e., loss of water in excess of NaCl), excess sweating and low water intake. The serum sodium is elevated, as is the hematocrit (possibly masking a true anemia), *and* the urine sodium is also high due to increased renal excretion of NaCl.

Diabetes insipidus (DI). DI may be central (neurogenic) (i.e., due to decreased vasopressin secretion) or nephrogenic (i.e., due to decreased renal response). Functionally, this condition is the reverse of SIADH, i.e., water retention in the tubules is not adequate. While this condition is not completely understood, and may be multifactorial, current research suggests that either mutation and/or changes in protein expression of 'water channel molecules' (renal aquaporins) and/or the vasopressin V2 renal collecting tubule cell receptor may play a role in both pathological water loss, such as in nephrogenic DI, and pathological water retention, such as in SIADH (Schrier, 2003; Brown, 2003; Nguyen, 2003; Nielsen, 2002). The pattern is elevated serum sodium but dilute urinary sodium due to the functionally inadequate levels of ADH.

Hyperaldosteronism. This condition may result from adrenal hyperplasia, Cushing's syndrome and Cushing's disease. The levels of circulating aldosterone are inappropriately high, causing excessive reabsorption of Na and excretion of K^+ and H^+ ions. The patient will be hypernatremic and hypokalemic and exhibit a mild metabolic alkalosis.

Hypokalemia

Many of the causes of hypokalemia overlap with those of hyponatremia including overhydration; use of loop diuretics; SIADH; and Bartter's syndrome, as discussed above. In addition to these causes overlapping with those of hyponatremia, there are the following states that lead uniquely to hypokalemia.

1. Infusion of insulin to diabetics. This results in rather large influxes of potassium into cells, lowering it in serum.
2. Alkalosis. Red blood cells are themselves excellent buffers. They are capable of exchanging potassium for hydrogen ions. Thus, in acidosis, H^+ ions enter red cells in exchange for K^+ ions. *Conversely, in alkalosis, H^+ ions leave red cells (to neutralize excess base) while K^+ ions enter the red cells.*
3. Vomiting. The major loss is both H^+ and K^+ from the stomach.

Hyperkalemia

Among the major causes are those that also cause hypernatremia, e.g., dehydration and diabetes insipidus, and, additionally, the following:

acidosis and diabetes mellitus (as discussed above); and hemolysis. Any kind of cell damage, such as rhabdomyolysis, and especially hemolysis of erythrocytes, can cause hyperkalemia. In hemolysis, all of the intracellular K^+ is extruded into plasma. Another analyte that is concentrated in red cells that rises with K^+ in hemolysis is lactate dehydrogenase (LD). Concomitant elevations of potassium and LD in serum should be taken as indications of hemolysis either artifactually after a blood sample has been taken from the patient or, less commonly, hemolysis from an underlying hemolytic condition.

Renal Disease (Schnerman, 1998)

There are four analytes that aid in the diagnosis of this condition: BUN, creatinine, calcium and phosphate. It is amazing that neither BUN nor creatinine has any inherent relationship to kidney function, but both fortuitously are superb indicators of renal condition.

BUN

BUN is blood urea nitrogen. The formula for urea is $H_2N–CO–NH_2$. There are two moles of nitrogen per mole of urea. This is the end product of NH_3 metabolism in the liver as discussed in Chapter 21. Urea is excreted by the renal tubules at a rate that is roughly proportional to the glomerular filtration rate (GFR). Note, therefore, that the *retained* urea, i.e., plasma or serum urea or BUN, is approximately *inversely* proportional to the GFR, i.e.

$$BUN \propto 1/GFR \qquad (8\text{--}1)$$

Creatinine

Creatinine is secreted but is also reabsorbed to an approximately equal extent so that the *net* effect is that the amount filtered is the amount excreted. The total amount of creatinine filtered then is its urinary concentration, $U_{cr} \times$ the volume of urine, V, over a given time. The total plasma that delivered this quantity of creatinine to the glomerulus is the total amount of creatinine filtered divided by the plasma concentration, P_{cr}. This quantity is also the creatinine clearance, C_{cr}. So the glomerular filtration rate is:

$$GFR = C_{cr} = U_{cr} \times V/P_{cr} \qquad (8\text{--}2)$$

Suppose the BUN is abnormally high (reference range = 10–20 mg/ml). There are two possible reasons for this. The first is *prerenal* where renal plasma flow is reduced, from such lesions as renal artery stenosis, renal vein thrombosis and the like. This causes a reduction in the GFR. From Equation 8–1, the BUN will then rise. However, the serum creatinine levels (P_{cr} in Equation 8–2), reference range 0.5–1.0 mg/dL, will generally remain within normal limits or may be mildly elevated because, from Equation 8–2, low GFR will result in lower urine flow (V in Equation 8–2). P_{cr} and U_{cr} will remain generally within normal limits. Thus there will be a disproportionate rise in BUN over creatinine. The normal BUN/creatinine ratio is 10–20 : 1, and in prerenal disease it rises to well above 20 : 1.

The second cause of elevated BUN is true *renal* disease. Here again there will be a rise in BUN due to low GFRs. Now, however, creatinine filtration will be compromised so that its serum level will rise correspondingly. Thus, in true renal disease, *both* BUN and creatinine rise together, maintaining the BUN/creatinine at 10–20 : 1 (Newman, 1999). This pattern also occurs in so-called *postrenal* disease, i.e., obstructive uropathy due to renal or ureteral stones (nephro- or urolithiasis), prostatic enlargement from benign prostatic hypertrophy or prostatic carcinoma, urinary tract infection, bladder stasis, urothelial carcinomas, etc.

Pinpointing the Lesion. Suppose a patient is found to have a BUN of, say, 60 mg/dL and a creatinine of 3.5 mg/dL. True renal failure can therefore be diagnosed. Now consider the kidney to be two compartments, one a filtration compartment (glomerulus) and the other a concentration compartment (renal tubules). If renal failure is present, where is the lesion – in the filtration or concentration compartment?

As discussed previously, the function of the kidneys is to *conserve* fluids or to concentrate the urine. Therefore, if a patient is on a fluid-restricted diet, the osmolality of urine (Uosm) should be significantly higher than the osmolality of plasma (Posm). In fact, Uosm/Posm is > 1.2 for normal individuals. If a 24-hour urine specimen collection from the above patient on a fluid-restricted diet is measured for Uosm, we can determine where the lesion has occurred. If Uosm/Posm < 1.2, then the urine is not being concentrated so that there *must* be a tubular lesion. On the other hand, if there is a normal ratio, then, by exclusion, the lesion must be glomerular. Causes of glomerular lesions are many: glomerulonephritis, pyelonephritis, diabetes, and infarction number among these; tubular lesions also have many causes including pyelonephritis, diabetes, papillary necrosis, acute tubular necrosis (ATN), infarction, shock, ischemia, etc. It

is remarkable that from a blood specimen of only 100 µL and several urine aliquots, not only can we determine the presence of renal failure, but we can localize the lesion and all of this virtually noninvasively.

Calcium and Phosphate

The kidneys play an important role in the regulation of calcium levels. In renal failure, calcium levels tend to fall while phosphate levels correspondingly tend to rise. The topic of calcium and phosphorus metabolism is discussed in detail in the context of evaluating endocrine function (Ch. 24). Here, we discuss these two analytes for diagnostic purposes.

Remember that calcium is the most abundant cation in the body, most of it stored in bone as a calcium hydroxyphosphate in hydroxyapatite. Calcium complexes with phosphate in several different forms, depending on the ionization state of phosphate, i.e.,

$$H_3PO_4 \rightleftharpoons H_2PO_4^- + H^+ \qquad (8\text{--}3)$$
$$H_2PO_4^- \rightleftharpoons HPO_4^{2-} + H^+ \qquad (8\text{--}4)$$
$$HPO_4^{2-} \rightleftharpoons PO_4^{3-} + H^+ \qquad (8\text{--}5)$$

The most insoluble calcium phosphate forms are those with the most basic phosphates (i.e., those in Equation 8–5). Thus alkaline conditions promote calcium deposition in bone while acidic conditions promote leaching of calcium from bone. Therefore, alkalosis promotes hypocalcemia while acidosis promotes hypercalcemia.

Note also that there is an equilibrium between soluble calcium phosphate and insoluble calcium phosphate in bone. We represent this equilibrium as:

$$Ca + P \rightleftharpoons (CaP) \text{ insoluble} \qquad (8\text{--}6)$$

where the left side is all soluble calcium phosphate salts and the right side is the insoluble salt forms. The equilibrium constant, K_{sp}, for this equilibrium is:

$$K_{sp} = (Ca) \times (P)/(CaP) \text{ insoluble} \qquad (8\text{--}7)$$

Since (CaP) insoluble is constant in concentration, the product of soluble Ca × soluble P is a constant, called the solubility constant. Thus there is an *inverse* relationship between Ca and P. Hypocalcemic states are almost always accompanied by hyperphosphatemic states and vice versa.

Of the soluble calcium, in the numerator of Equation 8–7, there are two forms, calcium bound to albumin and globulin in chelate form and so-called ionized or nonchelated calcium. Biologically active calcium is in the ionized form. Therefore, serum levels of ionized calcium are considered to be the best measure of hypo-, normo- or hypercalcemia.

The kidneys are vital in calcium metabolism and regulate calcium levels in two ways: parathyroid hormone stimulates the renal tubules to *excrete* phosphate. By Equation 8–7, the serum calcium level must then rise. Also, the kidneys are vital to the formation of active vitamin D in the synthesis of 1,25-dihydroxycholecalciferol, necessary for the absorption of calcium in the gut.

In renal disease, where there is tubular failure, phosphate excretion is inhibited due to the nonresponsiveness of the tubules to parathyroid hormone. Therefore, phosphate levels rise while calcium levels fall. In addition, active vitamin D production is reduced, lowering absorbed calcium. *Hypocalcemia and hyperphosphatemia*, in the face of elevated BUN and creatinine, indicative of renal disease, strongly suggest *tubular failure*.

Other Causes of Hypocalcemia. Besides alkalosis and renal failure, hypocalcemia may be caused by hypoparathyroidism, also leading to hyperphosphatemia. Rarely, such as in medullary thyroid carcinomas and other APUD (amine precursor uptake and decarboxylase activity) cell tumors, the elaboration of calcitonin, a well-known calcium-lowering hormone, may lead to decreased serum calcium levels. These causes may be encapsulated in the acronym, CHAR (Calcitonin, Hypoparathyroidism, Alkalosis, Renal failure).

Causes of Hypercalcemia. Besides acidosis, the possible causes of this condition may be summarized by Bakerman's 'CHIMPS' mnemonic (Bakerman, 1994), or Cancer, Hyperthyroidism, Iatrogenic causes, Multiple myeloma, hyperParathyroidism, and Sarcoidosis.

Blood Gas Abnormalities

We have discussed the effects of acidosis and alkalosis on serum calcium levels. The actual diagnosis of acidosis or alkalosis, however, depends on measurement of the pH of arterial blood. The topic of arterial blood gases is discussed in Chapter 14. Here we focus on how to interpret abnormal results and to correlate them with other laboratory findings.

Blood gas determinations refer to the quantitative measurement of the pH of arterial blood, the P_{CO_2}, the bicarbonate, the P_{O_2}, oxygen saturation and base excess. Three of these quantities are interdependent on one another,

Table 8–4 Patterns of pH, P_{CO_2} and Bicarbonate in Different Conditions

	Condition	pH	Bicarbonate	P_{CO_2}	Typical causes
1.	Metabolic acidosis	< 7.40	Low	Low	Diabetic ketoacidosis; lactic acidosis
2.	Metabolic alkalosis	> 7.40	High	High	Vomiting
3.	Respiratory acidosis	< 7.40	High	High	COPD; paralysis of respiratory muscles
4.	Respiratory alkalosis	> 7.40	Low	Low	Anxiety; acute pain

COPD = chronic obstructive pulmonic disease.

i.e., the P_{CO_2}, the bicarbonate and the pH, by the Henderson–Hasselbalch equation, i.e.,

$$pH = 6.1 + \log[(HCO_3^-)/(H_2CO_3)] \qquad (8–8)$$

Since the H_2CO_3 concentration in blood is directly proportional to the P_{CO_2}, i.e., at room temperature, $H_2CO_3 = 0.03 \times P_{CO_2}$, Equation 8–8 can be written as:

$$pH = 6.1 + \log[(HCO_3^-)/(0.03 \times P_{CO_2})] \qquad (8–9)$$

Note that if bicarbonate, in the numerator of Equation 8–9, becomes consumed as in metabolic acidosis, the respiratory rate will increase, thereby decreasing the P_{CO_2}, causing the denominator of this equation to fall, resulting in compensation. If the P_{CO_2} increases as in respiratory acidosis, the kidneys retain bicarbonate so that *both* numerator and denominator increase so as to maintain the ratio relatively constant.

In interpreting blood gas results, the first number to note is the pH. Regardless of the values of the bicarbonate and P_{CO_2}, if the pH is less than 7.4, the patient is acidotic; if greater than 7.4, the patient is alkalotic; if equal to 7.4, the patient is neither. Once the diagnosis of acidosis or alkalosis is made, then the bicarbonate or the P_{CO_2} can be used to decide whether it is of metabolic or respiratory origin.

Table 8–4 summarizes the four basic abnormal states: metabolic and respiratory acidosis and metabolic and respiratory alkalosis. In metabolic acidosis, the primary problem is production of acid as in diabetic ketoacidosis, lactic acidosis (e.g., from Gram-negative sepsis) and renal failure. This acid is buffered by bicarbonate, which is therefore consumed. To compensate for the bicarbonate loss, the breathing rate increases to lower the P_{CO_2}. So a low pH combined with a low bicarbonate and a low P_{CO_2} point to metabolic acidosis as shown in condition 1 of this table. As shown in condition 2 of the table, the opposite condition, metabolic alkalosis, results in reversal of the levels shown in condition 1. The most common cause of metabolic alkalosis is vomiting with a loss of HCl from the stomach and an attendant rise in bicarbonate.

When CO_2 is abnormally retained by the lungs as in chronic obstructive pulmonic disease (COPD), the denominator of Equation 8–9 increases, causing the pH of blood to fall. To compensate, the kidneys retain bicarbonate, thus increasing the numerator of this equation. If the blood pH is below 7.4 and the CO_2 and bicarbonate are both *increased* (condition 3 in Table 8–4), the acidosis is of respiratory origin. Note the mirror image condition (opposite levels) for respiratory alkalosis in condition 4 of this table. Besides COPD, the major causes of respiratory acidosis include diseases, like myasthenia gravis, in which there is partial paralysis of the accessory muscles of breathing; pneumonia; and central nervous system diseases affecting the brainstem in areas involved in respiratory control. Respiratory alkalosis is due mainly to hyperventilation, often of psychogenic origin. Here, the P_{CO_2} is reduced because of the rapidity of breathing.

The pH of blood can affect the levels of electrolytes in serum. In acidosis, besides bicarbonate buffering, red cells also buffer the excess H^+ ions by exchanging these for intracellular K^+ ions, the net effect being a mild hyperkalemia. An attendant hypokalemia occurs in alkalosis. Remember also that acidosis can cause a mild hypercalcemia; alkalosis can cause a mild hypocalcemia and especially affect the ionized calcium moiety.

Anion Gap

All sodium ions must be neutralized by counterions, most of which in blood are constituted by chloride and bicarbonate ions, and, to a lesser degree, by phosphate, sulfate and protein carboxylate groups. Normal serum sodium is about 140 mEq/L, chloride is usually around 100 mEq/L and bicarbonate around 24 mEq/L. The anion gap is then defined as $Na^+ -$ ($Cl^- + HCO_3^-$), which, for normal individuals is around 16. This 16 mEq/L

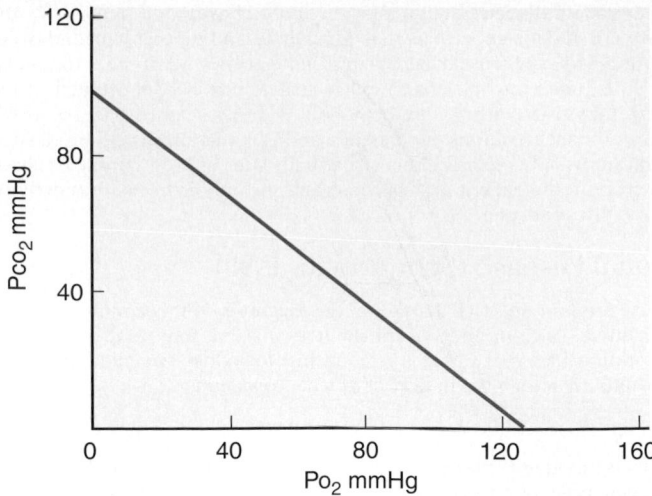

Figure 8–2 The effect of increased P_{CO_2} on the P_{O_2} in the alveolus and in arterial blood. This figure demonstrates that as the P_{CO_2} increases, there is a greater than a one-to-one decrease of P_{O_2}.

really comprises the other counterions that neutralize sodium but are not measured in serum.

If an individual has a metabolic acidosis, in which the rise in H^+ ion concentration is accompanied by a corresponding rise in Cl^- ions, the acid will be buffered by bicarbonate (converted to H_2CO_3). The bicarbonate value will therefore decrease, but there will be a 1 : 1 increase in chloride ion. Thus there will be no change in the anion gap. If the metabolic acidosis is due to the presence of an acid whose counterion is not Cl^-, such as acetoacetic acid (in diabetic acidosis) or lactic acid as in sepsis or hypoperfusion, then bicarbonate is reduced, as above, but there is no corresponding increase in Cl^-. Therefore, there is an increase in the anion gap which can reach values of 25–30 mEq/L. The presence of a widened anion gap signifies the presence of a metabolic acidosis due to a non-chloride-containing acid.

Low Anion Gaps. *Consistently* low anion gaps, typically in the range of 1–3 mEq/L, signify the presence of high levels of basic protein, often a myeloma protein. Basic protein contains ammonium ions, the counterions for which are chloride. Now the 'invisible' ion is ammonium while there is a measurable increase in chloride ion. This tends to decrease the anion gap. Persistently low anion gaps are a serious sign of possible malignancy, i.e., myeloma.

Oxygenation

Blood gases also give an excellent measurement of tissue perfusion through measurement of the P_{O_2} and the oxygen saturation of hemoglobin. Normal P_{O_2} values should be 90–100 mmHg while O_2 saturation should be 100%. Low values of either or both of these numbers flag underlying pathology. The major causes of low values for these measurements are myocardial infarction, pulmonary embolus, severe pulmonary interstitial disease (e.g., interstitial pneumonia) and tissue anoxic states secondary to hypoperfusion as in septicemia and severe congestive heart failure. In pulmonary embolus, there is blockage of the pulmonary circulation by the embolus, despite adequate ventilation, giving rise to ventilation/perfusion inequalities.

Hypercarbia as a Cause of Hypoxia. Another major cause of hypoxic states in arterial blood is CO_2 retentive states as in severe COPD. This occurs because, as CO_2 builds up in alveoli, it reduces the volume of O_2 in the air space. At P_{CO_2} values of over 50 mmHg, the effect on alveolar P_{O_2}, represented as $P_{A O_2}$, becomes important, as illustrated in Figure 8–2. Oxygen, unlike CO_2, is not soluble in water or membranes, so that there is a difference of about 10–15 mmHg pressure between alveolar and arterial O_2 (represented as $P_{a O_2}$), called the A–a gradient. Thus the $P_{a O_2}$ is even lower than the decreased $P_{A O_2}$. It is important to remember that the total oxygen breathed in, called the $P_{I O_2}$, is *partitioned*, therefore, between the alveolar sac and the arterial blood. This relationship may be written as,

$$P_{I O_2} = P_{A O_2} + P_{a O_2} \qquad (8–10)$$

For each mole of O_2 consumed, approximately 0.8 mole of CO_2 is produced. The ratio of CO_2 produced to O_2 consumed is called the respiratory quotient or the RQ. The $P_{a O_2}$ may be written as $P_{a CO_2}/RQ$. Overall, Equation 8–10 can be rewritten as:

$$P_{A O_2} = P_{I O_2} - P_{a CO_2}/RQ \qquad (8–11)$$

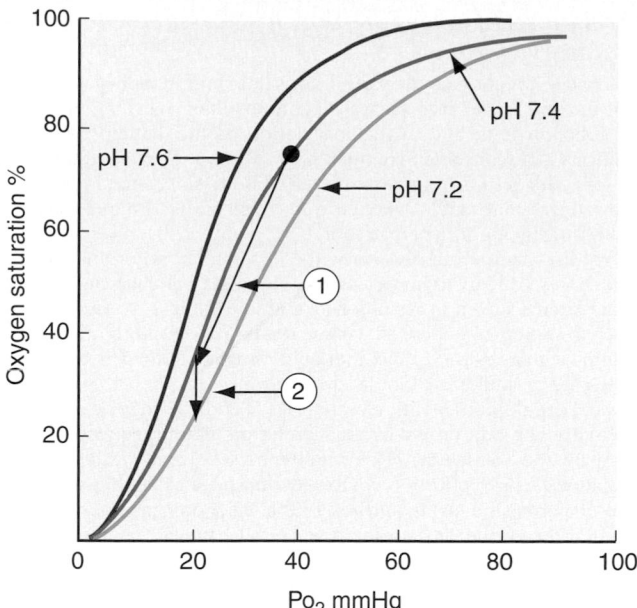

Figure 8–3 The effects of decreasing Po_2 in the allosteric zone of the oxygen–hemoglobin dissociation curve. On the pH 7.4 (middle) curve, if the Po_2 drops from 80 to 60 mmHg, there is little effect on the oxygen saturation. However, a drop from 40 to 20 mmHg results in a large drop in oxygen saturation from about 80% to 30% (arrow 1 in the figure). With this low oxygen saturation, there is a marked tissue lactic acidosis from anaerobic metabolism. The increased acidosis results in a drop in blood pH to 7.2, shifting the oxygen–hemoglobin dissociation to the right (pH 7.2 curve). Now, for a Po_2 of 20 mmHg, the oxygen saturation drops even further (arrow 2 in the figure) to about 20%, setting a vicious cycle in motion.

For an RQ of 0.8:
$$P_AO_2 = P_IO_2 - 1.25 \times P_aCO_2 \qquad (8\text{–}12)$$

This equation states that for each increment in the P_aCO_2, there will be a more than one-to-one decrease in the P_AO_2. This will result in severe oxygen deficits.

Figure 8–3 is the oxygen–hemoglobin dissociation curve. Note that the curve is sigmoidal due to the allosteric nature of the binding of oxygen to hemoglobin. For Po_2 values between 70–100 mmHg, the saturation of hemoglobin is close to 100%. But at Po_2 values < 70 mmHg, there is a steep drop in the saturation fraction so that small drops in Po_2 lead to large decreases in percent saturation. Compounding this effect is the disproportionate decrease in Po_2 whenever Pco_2 increases as described previously.

While these detrimental events transpire, tissue perfusion severely diminishes because of the diminished oxygen saturation of arterial blood. The result is tissue acidosis (mainly from lactic acid as a result of anaerobic metabolism). Acidosis shifts the oxygen–hemoglobin dissociation to the right as in Figure 8–3, causing even lower saturation for a given Po_2, causing further diminished tissue perfusion and more tissue acidosis. This vicious cycle can be corrected by placing the patient on a respirator to cause increased expiration of CO_2.

The pattern of arterial blood gas determinations for this type of patient will be low arterial blood pH, low Po_2, low oxygen saturation, high Pco_2, and low bicarbonate. This pattern is not typical of the four basic patterns given in Table 8–4 because, on top of a fundamental respiratory acidosis (high Pco_2), there is a superimposed tissue metabolic lactic acidosis, causing low bicarbonate. These findings, together with the low Po_2, indicate the immediate need for ventilation of the patient on a respirator.

Unlike the two conditions, myocardial infarction and pulmonary embolus, the treatment of the acute hypercarbic state is *not* to administer oxygen *unless* the patient is being adequately ventilated. Hypercarbia induces a CO_2 – induced inhibition of the respiratory centers in the pons and the medulla oblongata in the brainstem. In fact, the only impetus to breathe is the hypercarbia-induced hypoxia, causing chemoreceptors in the aortic arch to send signals to the respiratory center in the brain to continue breathing. *Administration of oxygen to patients with this condition without ventilation can cause cessation of respiration and the acute demise of the patient.*

Glucose Abnormalities

The normal reference interval for fasting serum glucose is generally between 70–110 mg/dL. As described in Chapter 16, the two basic abnormalities that occur with serum glucose levels are hyperglycemia,

almost always associated with diabetes mellitus, and hypoglycemia due to iatrogenic (overdose with insulin in the diabetic patient) or to other underlying causes (such as reactive hypoglycemia due to 'hypersensitivity' to insulin, insulinoma, etc.). To establish hyperglycemia, it is vital to determine whether the patient has (1) a fasting serum glucose level greater than or equal to 126 mg/dL, or (2) a serum glucose level greater than or equal to 200 mg/dL and classic symptoms of diabetes, or (3) a 2-hour postload plasma glucose concentration greater than or equal to 200 mg/dL during an oral glucose tolerance test (Sacks, 1999). Any one of the above findings is diagnostic, if it can be confirmed by repeat testing on a subsequent day (Sacks, 1999).

In the glucose tolerance test, described in Chapter 16, after giving the patient, who has not eaten for 12 hours overnight, a well-defined amount of glucose orally, the blood and urine glucose levels are followed. Normally, serum glucose levels rise and then fall within about a 2-hour period. If the glucose levels remain elevated, however, the diagnosis of diabetes mellitus may again be made. Also, if glucose is detected in the urine at any point, evidence for this condition is also obtained, although absence of urinary glucose does not in any way rule out diabetes mellitus.

High levels of serum glucose also result in the glycosylation of hemoglobin. Glycosylated hemoglobin levels change slowly over time and therefore constitute a stable and reliable indicator of serum glucose levels over the past 2–3 months. Glycosylated hemoglobin levels that are greater than 7% are considered to be indicative of diabetes mellitus, and efficacy of treatment is gauged by whether this serum level is reduced to less than 7. Of all of the methods for diagnosing and especially for monitoring treatment of diabetes mellitus, measurement of glycosylated hemoglobin levels is perhaps the most accurate and should be measured in conjunction with blood glucose determinations (Blincko, 2001; Krishnamurti, 2001; Kilpatrick, 2004).

Other Abnormal Laboratory Findings in Diabetes Mellitus

As discussed in the electrolyte section above, under the influence of insulin, whenever glucose is transported into the cell, it is accompanied by potassium. In diabetes, in the absence of insulin, blood glucose is elevated as is potassium. Due to increased metabolism of fats, there is a build-up of acetoacetic acid, leading to a metabolic acidosis. In diabetes where the blood glucose becomes exceptionally elevated, i.e., > 300 mg/dL, serum osmolality becomes dangerously high and can cause nonketotic, hyperosmolar coma. In this condition, red (and white) cell water flows from the cells into the vascular volume, tending to dilute analytes such as sodium. Thus the nonketotic, hyperosmolar coma patient may have a hyperosmolar serum, hyperglycemia, hyperkalemia and hyponatremia. In ketotic states, the patient will have, additionally, a metabolic acidosis and a large anion gap.

In *hypoglycemia*, serum glucose levels of < 60 mg/dL on a series of random fasting serum specimens strongly indicate this condition. Glucose tolerance tests show that after an initial sharp rise of serum glucose levels, there is an abnormally rapid drop to levels substantially below 60 mg/dL. If hypoglycemia is suspected, it is advisable to give the patient a 5-hour glucose tolerance test because the hypoglycemic 'dip' often is not seen until after 3 hours. Glucose tolerance tests on patients with suspected hypoglycemia should be performed with great caution because the procedure can induce severe reactive hypoglycemia causing loss of consciousness and even shock.

Liver Function Tests

Liver function is discussed in depth in Chapter 21. In that chapter, a detailed breakdown is given of different patterns in abnormal liver function tests. The reader will find it virtually impossible to memorize these patterns without a basic understanding of the underlying principles. We can reduce the most common liver test abnormalities to a set of six conditions summarized in Table 8–5. The principles for these patterns are explained as follows.

1. All *acute injuries and/or necrotic lesions* in the liver primarily cause a marked rise in the levels of the aminotransferases, aspartate aminotransferase (AST) and alanine aminotransferase (ALT). Cell injury and necrosis also cause the rise of other enzymes such as lactate dehydrogenase (LD). These include acute hepatitis (e.g., infectious and chemically induced), infarction, and trauma. The biliary tract is always affected so that direct bilirubin rises from interference with bile flow. Because of biliary tract injury, the enzyme alkaline phosphatase rises along with gamma-glutamyl transferase (GGT) and 5'-nucleotidase (5'-N). Hepatocyte injury causes loss of conjugation of transported bilirubin, so that indirect (unconjugated) bilirubin also rises.

Table 8–5 Six Fundamental Patterns of Liver Function Tests

Condition	AST	ALT	LD	ALP	TP	Albumin	Bilirubin	Ammonia
1. Hepatitis	H	H	H	H	N	N	H	N
2. Cirrhosis	N	N	N	N–sl H	L	L	H	H
3. Biliary obstruction	N	N	N	H	N	N	H	N
4. Space-occupying lesion	N or H	N or H	H	H	N	N	N–H	N
5. Passive congestion	Sl H	sl H	sl H	N–sl H	N	N	N–sl H	N
6. Fulminant failure	Very H	H	H	H	L	L	H	H

H = high; N = normal; L = low; sl = slightly; AST = aspartate aminotransferase; ALT = alanine aminotransferase; LD = lactate dehydrogenase; ALP = alkaline phosphatase; TP = total protein.

Because, generally, in hepatitis, much less than 80% of the liver is destroyed, total regeneration will occur and enough tissue is present to enable adequate levels of protein synthesis and ammonia fixation as urea. Therefore, the total protein and albumin and ammonia levels remain normal. These typical results are summarized in condition 1 of Table 8–5.

2. *Cirrhosis of the liver* is characterized by two cardinal features: fibrosis, preventing regeneration of liver tissue wherever this has occurred and nodules of regenerating liver tissue, which are the only source of any kind of hepatocytic function. Thus, in cirrhosis, almost the *reverse* pattern occurs from the one seen in condition 1 in Table 8–5 for hepatitis. Because, in panhepatic cirrhosis, there is destruction of > 80% of liver tissue, with no regeneration of damaged liver tissue, the AST/ALT aminotransferases and LD levels (all from the regenerating nodules) tend to be normal or low or occasionally mildly elevated. However, the total protein and albumin are both abnormally low. The ammonia levels are elevated. Because there is insufficient viable liver tissue remaining, and because fibrosis destroys the cholangioles, both indirect and direct bilirubin tend to be elevated. These findings are summarized in condition 2 of Table 8–5.

3. *Acute biliary obstruction* caused by stones in the biliary tree or by neoplasms that block bile excretion, results in elevations in direct bilirubin and biliary tract alkaline phosphatase, along with the enzymes, GGT and 5'-N (see above). All other liver function test results are normal. For simple biliary obstruction, therefore, the pattern is as shown in condition 3 of Table 8–5.

4. *Space-occupying lesions* of the liver are characterized, for reasons that are not well understood, by isolated elevations of the enzymes, alkaline phosphatase and LD. This pattern is shown in condition 4 of Table 8–5. The most common cause of this condition is metastatic carcinoma to the liver.

5. *Passive congestion* of the liver is characterized by a mild elevation of aminotransferases (AST/ALT) and LD and, in more severe cases, elevations of total bilirubin and alkaline phosphatase. This pattern is also seen in infectious mononucleosis, where the rise in bilirubin may be marked. The general passive congestion pattern is shown in condition 5 of Table 8–5.

6. *Acute fulminant hepatic failure* from a variety of causes which include Reye's syndrome and hepatitis C (Gill, 2001; Schiodt, 2003), is discussed in Chapter 21. This condition is *total liver failure*. The overall pattern (Sunheimer, 1994) is shown in condition 6 of Table 8–5. It appears as a *combination* of hepatitis and cirrhosis. Here AST and ALT reach exceptionally high values, often in excess of 10 000 IU/L. At the same time, total protein and albumin are markedly reduced, and the ammonia levels are abnormally elevated, causing hepatic encephalopathy. LD, alkaline phosphatase and bilirubin are also elevated. Besides the marked rise in AST and ALT, combined with hyperammonemia, there is a characteristic disproportional rise of AST over ALT, further confirming the diagnosis. It is vital to recognize this pattern because the underlying condition is a medical emergency which must be treated promptly.

Correlations of Liver Function Test Results with Other Laboratory Findings

In severe liver failure, secondary to cirrhosis or to fulminant hepatic failure, it is not uncommon to find electrolyte abnormalities and abnormalities in renal function tests, and in the coagulation profile. Patients with either conditions 2 or 6 in Table 8–5, often have ascites, with marked third space fluid loss. This results in increased levels of both ADH and aldosterone to retain intravascular water. Depending on which levels 'win out,' the patient may become hypo- or hypernatremic.

Severe liver failure can also cause the hepatorenal syndrome, i.e., renal dysfunction secondary to hepatic failure. This disease is characterized by the typical patterns shown in conditions 2 and 6 in Table 8–5. As discussed in the renal section above, renal failure results in elevations in BUN and creatinine with a 10–20 : 1 ratio, indicative of renal failure. The Uosm/Posm ratio is < 1.2 : 1, indicating tubular dysfunction.

Severe coagulopathies with elevated APTTs and PTs may be seen due to the absence of production of coagulation factors. Not infrequently, DIC will accompany the liver failure. This condition must be distinguished from low coagulation factor production combined with hepatosplenomegaly due to portal hypertension as in cirrhosis. The splenomegaly may result in sequestration of platelets, so that the overall pattern may resemble DIC but not be true DIC. To clinch the diagnosis of DIC, there should be elevations of both D-dimer and fibrin split products (FSP) levels. Also, in severe liver failure, abnormal red cell forms, called target cells, may be seen in the peripheral blood smear.

Patients with cirrhosis and acute fulminant hepatic failure tend to be immunocompromised. Many of these patients have defective T cell function but produce an excess of (ineffective) immunoglobulin. Thus these patients tend to have low serum albumin levels from diminished albumin synthesis but elevated serum immunoglobulins.

Cardiac Function Tests

Diagnosis of Myocardial Infarction (MI) and Acute Coronary Syndrome

These are discussed at length in Chapter 18. Because acute MI (AMI) requires rapid and accurate diagnosis, especially now that new treatment options with thrombolytic agents are available, the clinical laboratory has been called upon to provide serum diagnostic tests that can make this diagnosis at an early stage. Until recently, laboratory diagnosis was based on serial determinations of the MB fraction of creatine phosphokinase (CK-MB); confirmation of the diagnosis was provided by the so-called 'flipped ratio' of the isozymes of lactate dehydrogenase (LD) 24–36 hours after the initial acute event and/or by observation of the characteristic time courses for elevations of the three enzymes, CK, aspartate aminotransferase (AST) and LD.

These approaches have been replaced mainly by two other analytes, myoglobin (MY) and especially troponin (Tn), that provide more rapid and specific diagnostic capabilities. MY is an oxygen-binding/transport protein found in both cardiac and skeletal muscle. Its relatively small size and function allow for early release from irreversibly damaged cells. However, current methods of measurement cannot distinguish MY's tissue of origin. Therefore, its use is confined to screening patients for possible AMI; positive results suggest further work-up for AMI.

Troponin is a regulatory protein complex in muscle tissue; it comprises three subunits designated troponin I (TnI), troponin T (TnT), and troponin C (TnC). Different genes encode TnI in skeletal and cardiac muscle, giving rise to isoforms that differ significantly in sequence. In addition, cardiac TnI contains an additional 31 amino acid residues on its N-terminal. Rapid and accurate immunoassays for TnT and cardiac TnI have been developed (Moss, 1999, Apple, 1999). In AMI, cardiac TnI becomes elevated 4–8 hours after onset of chest pain, reaches a peak at about 12–16 hours and remains elevated for 5–9 days. Values at or above 1.5 ng/dL are considered to be suggestive of AMI.

Because troponin levels rise relatively rapidly and remain elevated for prolonged times, troponin determinations have replaced the so-called 'flipped ratio' of the two isozymes of LDH, LD1 and LD2 (LD2 : LD1 ratio rises to > 0.75 and often exceeds 1.0) which occurs only about 36 hours after the onset of symptoms.

TnT does not have tissue-specific sequence differences. Nonetheless, it has proved to be effective in the diagnosis of AMI. One problem with use of TnT is that it may be elevated in patients with renal disease (Diris, 2004) although this does not affect use of TnT in predicting the prognosis of patients with acute coronary syndromes (Aviles, 2002). Overall, both troponin determinations have sensitivities and specificities that exceed

90%, and elevated serum troponin levels 12 hours after the onset of chest pain have 100% sensitivity in diagnosing MI.

It should be noted that CK-MB remains useful in diagnosing AMI. This is an isozyme of creatine phosphokinase (CK), which has three isozymes composed of two chains (called the M and B chains) which are MM, MB and BB. The MB fraction is predominantly found in cardiac muscle (Roberts, 1997). To diagnose AMI from CK-MB serum levels, it is important to show both a rise in the *concentration* of CK-MB and in the *ratio* of CK-MB to total CK (also called the cardiac index) (Thompson, 1988; Woo, 1992). Because there is a small amount of CK-MB in skeletal muscle, diseases of skeletal muscle that cause the level of CK-MM to rise to high values will also cause the levels of CK-MB to rise to high *absolute* concentrations in serum, that can cause false-positive values for CK-MB. In addition, to increase both the sensitivity and specificity of CK-MB in the diagnosis of acute AMI, it has been found necessary to perform *serial* determinations of MB fraction (at 3- to 4-hour intervals over a 12- to 16-hour period) that show a progressive rise that reaches a peak, followed by a fall to low levels. This pattern is virtually 100% diagnostic of myocardial infarction (Lott, 1984; Wu, 1999). Importantly, CK-MB generally rises 4–6 hours, and sometimes only 2 hours, after the onset of chest pain, and peaks within 12 hours. Therefore, MY and CK-MB have been recommended (Wu, 1999; Alpert, 2000; Fromm, 2001; Lewandrowski, 2002) for use as early markers of AMI since both markers are released soon after AMI, with MY, and sometimes CK-MB, increasing as early as 1–2 hours after onset of AMI.

However, elevated TnT and, especially TnI, levels are more specific for cardiac injury than are elevated CK-MB levels. Like CK-MB, they rise within 4–6 hours, and sometimes within 2 hours, after the onset of chest pain. Furthermore, single elevated troponin levels are diagnostic of acute MI and unstable angina and do not require follow-up levels or computation of cardiac indices to confirm these diagnoses, making troponin more effective diagnostically and more cost-effective than CK-MB. As an added bonus, troponin, unlike CK-MB, also serves as a marker for unstable angina. Thus many medical centers use troponin as the preferred marker for MI.

Current protocols for the laboratory diagnosis of AMI vary. In some medical centers TnI or TnT is used exclusively while in other centers, both troponin and CK-MB are used together. Based on earlier recommendations from a conference on standards in laboratory practice (Wu, 1999) concerning laboratory diagnosis of AMI, for patients who present with chest pain and nondiagnostic ECG changes, many centers use both an early marker of myocardial damage, e.g., CK-MB or myoglobin, together with a definitive marker, i.e., troponin (high specificity and sensitivity), for cardiac damage. For patients with diagnostic clinical findings of AMI before treatment is begun, troponin and/or CK-MB may be ordered to document infarction, to monitor the extent of the disease, to detect possible reinfarction and to monitor therapeutic efficacy. In addition, troponin and/or CK-MB can be used to detect perioperative AMI during surgical procedures.

Diagnosis of Congestive Heart Failure

Until recently, this condition was diagnosed strictly on the basis of symptomatology and/or as a result of procedures such as echocardiography. However, a new biomarker has been discovered, B-type natriuretic peptide (BNP), that has been approved as a definitive test for this condition and appears to be an excellent marker for early heart failure; this test may also be both diagnostically and prognostically significant in patients presenting with acute dyspnea and chest pain. The differential diagnosis in these patients includes dyspnea caused by chronic heart failure (signs and symptoms of which are typically nonspecific) versus other causes of acute dyspnea (e.g., pneumonia, carcinoma, effusion, asthma). Normal levels (i.e., a high negative predictive value for this test) appear useful in excluding a cardiac etiology in these patients. Levels of BNP may also be an independent predictor of arrhythmia, stroke, and death (Clerico, 2004; Ishii, 2003; Mueller, 2004; Prahash, 2004; Wang, 2004; Winter, 2004).

Pancreatic Function Tests

Elevations in serum pancreatic amylase and lipase are definitive markers for pancreatic disease. The most common cause for such increases in the serum levels of these enzymes is pancreatitis. In acute pancreatitis, both enzymes are elevated. Since amylase can also be produced by the salivary glands, amylase is slightly less specific than lipase as a marker for pancreatitis. Elevations in the latter enzyme are definitive for pancreatic disease.

Markers for Inflammatory Conditions

As discussed previously in the hematology section, increases in the white blood cell count, especially with a predominance of neutrophils, indicate acute infection. In most acute inflammatory conditions, as noted previously, acute phase reactant proteins are also found to be increased. These proteins occur in the alpha (including alpha-1-antitrypsin, alpha-2-macroglobulin) and beta (including ferritin and C-reactive protein) regions of the serum protein electrophoretogram as discussed in Chapter 19 on serum protein electrophoresis. In this regard, quantitative determinations for serum C-reactive protein (CRP) are very helpful in recognizing acute inflammatory states.

Recently, specific antibodies to CRP have allowed for highly sensitive measurement of CRP (termed high-sensitivity CRP or hs-CRP) at lower concentrations than were previously measurable (Roberts, 2000). Currently, elevated levels of hs-CRP appear to serve as an early marker of inflammation and may have utility in assessing cardiovascular risk for stroke and MI (Abrams, 2003; Ridker, 2003; Libby, 2004).

Fibrinogen, also an acute phase reactant, may additionally increase. Often, the platelet count tends to rise, and platelets themselves have been considered as 'acute phase reactants.' In addition, in both acute and chronic inflammatory conditions, erythrocytes exhibit increased mobilities. Thus there is an increase in the erythrocyte sedimentation rate (ESR).

Finally, one common cause of acute inflammation is gout, i.e., hyperuricemia, or elevations of uric acid in serum. Uric acid crystals cause a severe, acute arthritic condition (gout). Serum levels of uric acid > 7.5 mg/dL are indicative of this condition. Less constant findings are the presence of uric acid crystals in the urinary sediment (Ch. 27) or in joint fluid (Ch. 28).

Endocrine Function Testing

We noted that abnormal functioning of the thyroid and adrenal cortex can give rise to important abnormal laboratory findings. Hypothyroidism, for example, can give rise to macrocytic anemia, while hypoadrenalism gives rise to electrolyte abnormalities, i.e., hyponatremia and hyperkalemia and an acidosis; hyperadrenalism produces the opposite effect, i.e., hypernatremia, hypokalemia and an alkalosis. It is therefore important to confirm that these endocrine glands are malfunctioning. The important topic of endocrine function testing is discussed in Chapter 24. Here we present simple principles for the laboratory diagnosis and identification of the site of origin of thyroid and adrenal dysfunction.

Thyroid Function

Thyroid function tests are the most commonly ordered tests for endocrine function. It is important to note that in a hospital population (as opposed to an ambulatory population) thyroid screening tests may be diagnostically misleading. This is due to endocrine stress responses (as well as medications) that may affect hormone levels (Van den Berghe, 2003). The thyroid gland synthesizes thyroid hormone, tetraiodothyronine, or T_4, with four iodines, which requires iodine uptake by the gland. This activity is strongly stimulated by the peptide hormone, thyroid-stimulating hormone (TSH), from the pituitary. In the periphery, T_4 is converted to T_3 (three iodines). Of prime importance, *high T_4 causes inhibition of TSH secretion, while low T_4 causes elevation of TSH.* In *primary hyperthyroidism* (*primary thyroid gland disease*), *excess T_4* is secreted by the *thyroid gland*, which is the source of the problem. As a result, TSH is decreased and T_4 is elevated. If, however, there is a primary lesion in the pituitary gland, e.g., hyperplasia or adenoma, then TSH is oversecreted. Because TSH is elevated, T_4 secretion is elevated. This is *secondary hyperthyroidism* (*secondary to pituitary disease*).

Conversely, if *pituitary TSH is reduced* (*pituitary problem*), *T_4 becomes low*. This is *secondary hypothyroidism*. On the other hand, if T_4 secretion by the thyroid is low causing *primary hypothyroidism, TSH increases*. Importantly, often, in subclinical hypothyroidism, T_4 can be within the reference range, but TSH is elevated. In ambulatory patients, elevated TSH in the presence of low levels of T_4 is diagnostic of primary hypothyroidism.

Adrenal Function

As discussed in depth in Chapter 24, the adrenal gland is divided anatomically into two endocrine glands: the adrenal cortex and the adrenal medulla. Adrenal cortical hormones are steroid hormones of three basic types: mineralocorticoids, like aldosterone, that regulate sodium and potassium ions in the distal convoluted tubule as discussed above; the glucocorticoids, like cortisol, that are gluconeogenic, and the sex hormones, i.e., the estrogens and androgens. The adrenal medulla is a neuroendocrine gland that secretes epinephrine and norepinephrine that act on the sympathetic nervous system. By far the most commonly ordered serum analyte used to measure adrenal cortical function is *cortisol*. Cortisol secretion by the adrenal cortex is stimulated by the pituitary hormone, adrenocorticotropic hormone, ACTH. ACTH secretion is stimulated by the hypothalamic hormone, corticotropin-releasing factor (CRH). Its serum levels are under diurnal control such that serum ACTH levels peak at about

200 pg/mL in the morning hours (about 7:00 a.m.) while they decline to their lowest values of around 100 pg/mL at midnight. Cortisol secretion follows ACTH secretion such that its serum levels are highest at 8:00–9:00 a.m. Cortisol inhibits ACTH secretion by the pituitary gland both by directly blocking pituitary ACTH secretion and by inhibiting CRH secretion by the hypothalamus.

Therefore, if the adrenal cortex hypersecretes cortisol secondary to such conditions as adrenal hyperplasia, adenoma or carcinoma, serum cortisol levels increase and block ACTH secretion. This condition is called *primary hyperadrenalism*. Serum cortisol levels are elevated, but ACTH levels decrease.

On the other hand, as with thyroid hormone secretion, if ACTH levels are elevated by an ACTH pituitary tumor (Cushing's disease) or as ectopic ACTH secretion, e.g., by a nonpituitary tumor (Cushing's syndrome), cortisol levels will also rise giving rise to *secondary hyperadrenalism*. Both cortisol and ACTH are elevated in this condition. In cases of Cushing's disease or syndrome, the diurnal variation of serum ACTH is absent.

In addition to measurements of serum cortisol, it is often desirable to measure urinary free cortisol in cases of hypercortisolemia. Normally, almost all cortisol is bound to serum protein, mainly transcortin, while, in hypercortisol states, cortisol exceeds the capacity of transcortin to bind to it and is consequently filtered by the kidneys. The reference range for morning serum cortisol is ~ 10–25 µg/dL, and for urinary free cortisol, ~ 24–108 µg/24 h for healthy males.

In cases of *hypercortisolism*, especially where ACTH levels may remain in the reference range or have 'borderline' high or low values, it is often desirable to perform the *dexamethasone suppression test*. Dexamethasone is a potent glucocorticoid that strongly suppresses normal pituitary ACTH secretion. This can be accomplished with low-dose dexamethasone. If low dose dexamethasone results in diminished serum cortisol levels and low values for urinary free cortisol, pituitary function is most likely normal while the adrenals are hypersecreting cortisol, i.e., *primary hyperadrenalism*. This test may further be used to distinguish the possible source of primary hyperadrenalism, i.e., hyperplasia vs. adenoma or carcinoma. High-dose dexamethasone will generally lower serum cortisol levels in adrenal hyperplasia, while it will have no effect in adrenal adenoma or carcinoma.

Conversely, in *pituitary failure*, serum ACTH levels decrease as do serum cortisol levels since ACTH stimulation of the adrenal gland decreases. This condition is referred to as *secondary hypoadrenalism*. If the *adrenal gland function is compromised* (*primary adrenal insufficiency*) serum cortisol levels decrease, resulting in less inhibition of pituitary secretion of ACTH and, consequently, in elevated serum levels of ACTH. This condition is referred to as *primary hypoadrenalism* or *Addison's disease*.

Examples of Clinical Cases with Clinicopathological Correlations

Given the above overview of many salient features of the causes of the more common abnormal laboratory findings, the laboratory results from a number of different patients are now presented to illustrate how analyte levels change in different disease states and how these analyte concentrations are used to diagnose these conditions.

Case A. A 64-year-old white male, was found unconscious in his home after suffering a cerebrovascular accident (CVA) and brought to the emergency medicine department. His hematocrit was 44%, but red blood cell count was 4.3 million/µL (lower limit of normal, 4.6 million/µL) with an MCV of 104 fL; a series of serum sodium values ranged from 164–175 mEq/L; admission BUN was 33 mg/dL; creatinine was 1.5 mg/dL. The total serum osmolality was 357 mOsm (upper limit of normal, 290 mOsm) while the urine osmolality was 1008 mOsm (upper limit of normal, 1000 mOsm), and the random urine sodium was 228 mEq/L.

A liver panel showed a marginally elevated AST at 41 IU/L (upper limit of normal, 39 IU/L), elevated but continually decreasing LD (admission value of 426 IU/L; upper limit of normal, 200 IU/L), GGT of 72 U/L (upper limit of normal, 43 IU/L), total protein of 7.8 g/dL (normal) but a low albumin of 2.8 g/dL (normal 3.5–5.0 g/dL). Lipase was mildly elevated at 127 IU/L (upper limit of normal, 60 IU/L). Occult blood was found in his stool which was found positive for *Clostridium difficile*. Urine was nitrite positive (indicative of bacteriuria) and was markedly positive for hemoglobin, red cells and white cells.

After infusion of half-normal saline, the hematocrit was reduced to 34% but then rose to 38% with a persistently elevated MCV. The sodium and the BUN were reduced to within the reference range.

Evaluation. The basic diagnosis of this patient's condition is hypernatremia. This patient was dehydrated as shown by the markedly elevated serum sodium (average value of 169 mEq/L), high normal hematocrit, and elevated BUN. Note that the diagnosis of dehydration was confirmed by the finding of a high serum *and* urinary (228 mEq/L) sodium and a high urinary osmolality of 1008 mOsm (Table 8–3).

The red blood cell count was low, which seems to contradict the high normal hematocrit. This apparent discrepancy may be explained by the macrocytosis, causing each erythrocyte to occupy a greater than normal volume. Yet the total number of cells was reduced. The low red cell count indicates a true anemia. The macrocytosis was caused by a nutritional (vitamin B_{12}) deficiency. All of these findings may be attributed to malnutrition and insufficient fluid consumption, a not-uncommon finding in the elderly, especially in this stroke victim.

Note that the BUN and creatinine were mildly elevated in a pattern with a ratio > 20 : 1 suggesting a prerenal (low perfusion) etiology. The renal tubules were evidently functioning well, as evidenced by the high urine-to-serum osmolality ratio (1008/357 = 2.8, which is greater than 1.2 : 1). Hypoperfusion may have also caused the mild abnormalities found in some of the liver function tests and the elevated pancreatic lipase.

Note also that the total protein was normal even though the albumin, the most abundant serum protein, was low. Because of possibly two infectious diseases identified in urine and stool examinations, the patient may have produced elevated levels of immunoglobulins.

Accompanying the CVA was a peptic ulcer, so-called Cushing's ulcer, known to be associated with this condition; hence the occult blood in this patient's stool. *C. difficile* is known to infect patients with chronic debilitating disease. The urinary tract infection was responsible for the high red cell count and hemoglobin in this patient's urine.

The next case illustrates a more complex electrolyte disorder.

Case B. A 31-year-old white male patient with known Type 1 diabetes mellitus, end-stage renal disease secondary to diabetic nephropathy, and a history of alcoholism, was admitted with acute abdominal pain in the mid-epigastrium, with a serum glucose of 736 mg/dL; it rose as high as 933 mg/dL; serum sodium of 134 mEq/L, which decreased to as low as 124 mEq/L; potassium of 7.1 mEq/L, BUN of 64 mg/dL and a creatinine of 18 mg/dL. These values were confirmed and found to follow a consistent trend. Serum osmolality was 316 mOsm. Blood gas values on admission were pH of 7.58, Po_2 of 121 mmHg, O_2 saturation of 99%, Pco_2 of 20 mmHg, and bicarbonate of 20 mEq/L. The anion gap rose in one day from 13 (high end of normal) to 20. Serum lipase was elevated at 469 IU/L (upper limit of normal is 60 IU/L). There was no urine output, and the patient was subjected to peritoneal dialysis.

Evaluation. This diabetic patient was evidently in a hyperosmolar state due to abnormally elevated glucose levels. The low serum sodium and high serum potassium might appear to be due to low circulating aldosterone or renal tubular failure. However, there was no urine output so no filtration could occur. The end-stage renal disease is reflected in the BUN and especially in the creatinine value (18 mg/dL). The BUN/creatinine ratio of about 4 confirms the diagnosis of true renal failure.

As noted in the discussion on glucose, in diabetes mellitus with high serum glucose levels, there is an efflux of cell water that causes dilution of serum analytes such as sodium. Whenever glucose is transported into cells under the influence of insulin, it is accompanied by potassium. Low insulin levels can therefore result in hyperkalemia. This mechanism was operative in this patient. Though the anion gap increased after admission, it was normal on admission. Thus this patient was in a nonketotic, hyperosmolar state but subsequently became ketotic.

The admission blood gas picture suggests a respiratory alkalosis since the arterial blood pH was 7.57 (alkalosis) but the Pco_2 was low at 20 mmHg and the bicarbonate was low at 20 mEq/L (condition 4 in Table 8–4). This is an unusual finding in a patient with diabetes mellitus in whom a finding of metabolic acidosis is more frequently encountered.

An explanation for this finding may be found in the serum lipase, which was markedly elevated, denoting pancreatitis, a common finding in patients with a history of alcoholism. The sharp epigastric pain caused increased respiration (respiratory rate on admission was 25/min) precipitating a *lowering* of the Pco_2, which was partially compensated by a lowering of the bicarbonate.

Treatment of this patient with dialysis, hydration and insulin corrected the abnormal laboratory findings, and the patient was discharged on chronic dialysis.

The next case presents multiple disorders, including electrolyte disorders, all related to liver failure.

Case C. A 38-year-old white female, with a past medical history of multiple abdominal surgical procedures over a 7-year period, sporadic alcohol abuse, pancreatitis, and a 30 pack-year history of smoking, was brought to the emergency department in shock and acute abdominal distress. Significant laboratory values included: white blood cell count of $12.1 \times 10^3/\mu L$, red cell count of $3.07 \times 10^6/\mu L$, hematocrit of 34.6%, and red cell indices that showed macrocytosis and hypochromia (low mean corpuscular hemoglobin concentration). Vitamin B_{12} and folate levels were normal. The peripheral blood smear showed a leukoerythroblastic pattern. Serum glucose was low at 38 mg/dL; total protein was 4.3 g/dL, albumin 1.5 g/dL. Lactate levels were elevated. The alkaline phosphatase was elevated at 241 IU/L (upper limit of normal, 129 IU/L), and the bilirubin was mildly elevated at 1.6 mg/dL (upper limit of normal, 1.2 mg/dL). Serum ammonia was found to be elevated at 146 micromolar (upper limit of normal, 30 micromolar). Screens for hepatitis A, B, and C were all negative. Multiple blood, urine and throat cultures were negative. Exploratory laparotomy revealed abdominal adhesions and cholestasis. Postoperatively, the patient became encephalopathic; her liver function deteriorated as evidenced by dramatic elevations of AST and ALT from normal levels to 1660 and 545 IU/L, respectively; of LD to 2190 IU/L; bilirubin to 14.5 mg/dL; and ammonia to 177 micromolar. A liver–spleen scan performed on the fifth hospital day showed no dye uptake in the liver, consistent with functional liver failure. The serum sodium, normal on admission, increased within 5 days to 166 mEq/L together with chloride levels that rose to 123 mEq/L, a pattern that persisted throughout the hospital course despite aggressive intravenous infusion of half-normal saline. Serum potassium was consistently < 3.5 mEq/L. The BUN and creatinine both rose to abnormally high levels with a ratio of < 20 : 1, suggesting renal failure. Plasma aldosterone was elevated at 13.2 ng/dL (upper limit of normal = 8.5 ng/dL). The platelet count dropped rapidly while the APTT and PT rose to values at least twice those of the corresponding normal controls, while her level of fibrin split products (FSP) became abnormally elevated. Her condition worsened, and the patient expired on the eighth hospital day.

Evaluation. Although a complex patient presentation, the fundamental problem with this patient lay in the dramatically abnormal liver function test profile. Note how there was an acute elevation in the aminotransferases (transaminases) with the AST/ALT ratios significantly greater than 1. There were concurrent rapid elevations in the bilirubin and the LD. At the same time, the total protein and albumin were abnormally low. The ammonia levels rose rapidly (despite high doses of lactulose). The pattern is that of fulminant hepatic failure shown in condition 6 in Table 8–5. This condition is a medical emergency and is associated with fatal encephalopathy and severe disseminated coagulopathy (DIC) as evidenced by the low platelet counts, elevated PT and APTT and FSP levels. This condition can cause multiple system infarcts, resulting in multiple organ failure.

The patient's peripheral blood picture showed a macrocytosis but, concurrently, a leukoerythroblastic picture. This pattern suggests that the macrocytosis was caused by an increased number of erythrocyte precursor forms. This condition was most likely caused by disseminated intravascular coagulopathy (DIC) that causes microangiopathic hemolytic anemia with a leukoerythroblastic picture. It is also possible that, with the persistently elevated white cell count and the elevated lactate levels, Gram-negative sepsis affecting bone marrow may have also contributed to the leukoerythroblastic picture. Though cultures were consistently negative, the patient was being treated with broad-spectrum antibiotics, the effects of which may have blocked growth of the organism(s) in culture. As noted previously, patients with liver failure from either cirrhosis or acute fulminant hepatic failure are generally immunocompromised.

In both panhepatic cirrhosis and fulminant hepatic failure there is severe third-space fluid loss associated with ascites that invariably develops. We noted previously that, to retain vascular volume, both aldosterone and ADH rise. It appears that aldosterone became elevated to markedly high values, causing abnormal sodium retention and potassium loss in this patient.

Almost always accompanying both cirrhosis and acute fulminant hepatic failure is renal failure, generally manifested by the hepatorenal syndrome. In fulminant hepatic failure, an additional possible cause is acute tubular necrosis.

References

Abrams J: C-reactive protein, inflammation, and coronary risk: An update. Cardiol Clin 2003; 21:327–331.

Alpert JS, Thygesen K, Antman E, Bassand JP, et al: Myocardial infarction redefined – A consensus document of the Joint European Society of Cardiology/American College of Cardiology Committee for the Redefinition of Myocardial Infarction. J Am Coll Cardiol 2000; 36:959–969.

Alter BP: Bone marrow failure syndromes. Clin Lab Med 1999; 19:113–133.

Alter BP: Bone marrow failure syndromes in children. Pediatr Clin N Am 2002; 49:973–988.

Apple FS, Henderson AR: Cardiac function. *In* Burtis CA, Ashwood ER (eds): Tietz Textbook of Clinical Chemistry, 3rd ed. Philadelphia, PA, WB Saunders, 1999, pp 1178–1203.

Aviles RJ, Askari AT, Lindahl B, et al: Troponin T levels in patients with acute coronary syndromes, with or without renal dysfunction. N Engl J Med 2002; 346:2047–2052.

Bakerman S, Strausbauch P: ABC's of Interpretive Laboratory Data, 2nd ed. Myrtle Beach, SC, Interpretive Laboratory Data, 1994.
This is an excellent review of not only the use of laboratory testing but also of the underlying methodology.

Blincko S, Edwards R: Current issues in glycated haemoglobin measurement. Clin Lab 2001; 47:377–385.

Bonini P, Plebani M, Ceriotti F, Rubboli F: Errors in laboratory medicine. Clin Chem 2002; 48:691–698.
This is an important review of laboratory errors and how to recognize them.

Brigden M, Graydon C: Eosinophilia detected by automated blood cell counting in ambulatory North American outpatients: Incidence and clinical significance. Arch Pathol Lab Med 1997; 121:963–967.

Brito-Babapulle F: The eosinophilias, including the idiopathic hypereosinophilic syndrome. Br J Haematol 2003; 121:203–223.

Brown D: The ins and outs of aquaporin-2 trafficking. Am J Physiol Renal Physiol 2003; 284:F893–F901.

Clerico A, Emdin M: Diagnostic accuracy and prognostic relevance of the measurement of cardiac natriuretic peptides: A review. Clin Chem 2004; 50:33–50.
This is an up-to-date review of the use of BNP in the diagnosis of congestive heart failure. It is especially relevant in view of the wide attention this analyte has been receiving.

DeCaterina R, Lanza M, Manca G, Strata GB, et al: Bleeding time and bleeding: An analysis of the relationship of the bleeding time test with parameters of surgical bleeding. Blood 1994; 84:3363–3370.

Dighe AS, Soderberg BL, Laposata M: Narrative interpretations for the clinical laboratory evaluations: An overview. Am J Clin Pathol 2001; 116(Suppl 1):S123–S128.

Diris JH, Hackeng CM, Kooman JP, et al: Impaired renal clearance explains elevated troponin T fragments in hemodialysis patients. Circulation 2004; 109:23–25.

Fromm Jr RE, Roberts R: Sensitivity and specificity of new serum markers for mild cardionecrosis. Curr Probl Cardiol 2001; 26:246–284.

George TI, Arber DA: Pathology of the myeloproliferative diseases. Hematol Oncol Clin North Am 2003; 17:1101–1127.

Gerwirtz AS, Miller ML, Keys TF: The clinical usefulness of the preoperative bleeding time. Arch Pathol Lab Med 1996; 120:353–356.

Gill RQ, Sterling RK: Acute liver failure. J Clin Gastroenterol 2001; 33:191–198.

Glassman AB: Cytogenetics: An evolving role in the diagnosis and treatment of cancer. Clin Lab Med 1997; 17:21–37.

Gordon-Smith EC, Marsh JC, Gibson FM: Views on the pathophysiology of aplastic anemia. Int J Hematol 2002; 76(Suppl 2):163–166.

Guinan EC: Clinical aspects of aplastic anemia. Hematol Oncol Clin North Am 1997; 11:1025–1044.

Hughes T, Branford S: Molecular monitoring of chronic myeloid leukemia. Semin Hematol 2003; 40(Suppl 2):62–68.

Ishii J, Cui W, Kitagawa F, et al: Prognostic value of combination of cardiac troponin T and B-type natriuretic peptide after initiation of treatment in patients with chronic heart failure. Clin Chem 2003; 49:2020–2026.

Kilpatrick ES: HbA1c measurement. J Clin Pathol 2004; 57:344–345.

Kottke-Marchant K, Corcoran G: The laboratory diagnosis of platelet disorders: An algorithmic approach. Arch Pathol Lab Med 2002; 126:133–146.

Krishnamurti U, Steffes MW: Glycohemoglobin: A primary predictor of the development or reversal of complications of diabetes mellitus. Clin Chem 2001; 47:1157–1165.

Lewandrowski K, Chen A, Januzzi J: Cardiac markers for myocardial infarction. Am J Clin Pathol 2002; 118(Suppl 1):S93–S99.
This is an excellent review of the different biomarkers for myocardial infarction and their usefulness in diagnosing this condition.

Libby P, Ridker PM: Inflammation and atherosclerosis: Role of C-reactive protein in risk assessment. Am J Med 2004; 116(Suppl 6A):9S–16S.

Lott JA: Serum enzyme determinations in the diagnosis of acute myocardial infarction: An update. Hum Pathol 1984; 15:706–716.

Marsh JC, Ball SE, Darbyshire P, et al: Guidelines for the diagnosis and management of acquired aplastic anemia. Br J Haematol 2003; 123:782–801.

Moss DW, Henderson AR: Clinical enzymology. *In* Burtis CA, Ashwood ER (eds): Tietz Textbook of Clinical Chemistry, 3rd ed. Philadelphia, WB Saunders, 1999, pp 617–721.

Mueller C, Scholer A, Laule-Kilian K, et al: Use of B-type natriuretic peptide in the evaluation and management of acute dyspnea. N Engl J Med 2004; 350:647–654.

Newman DJ, Price CP: Renal function and nitrogen metabolites. *In* Burtis CA, Ashwood ER (eds): Tietz Textbook of Clinical Chemistry, 3rd ed, Philadelphia, WB Saunders, 1999, pp 1204–1270.
This is an excellent discussion of the laboratory evaluation of renal function using BUN and creatinine and how the kidneys regulate nitrogen-containing metabolites.

Nielsen S, Froklar J, Marples D, et al: Aquaporins in the kidney: From molecules to medicine. Physiol Rev 2002; 82:205–244.

Nguyen MK, Nielsen S, Kurtz I: Molecular pathogenesis of nephrogenic diabetes insipidus. Clin Exp Nephrol 2003; 7:9–17.

Oscier D, Fegan C, Hillmen P, et al: Guidelines on the diagnosis and management of chronic lymphocytic leukemia. Br J Haematol 2004; 125: 294–317.

Prahash A, Lynch T: B-type natriuretic peptide: A diagnostic, prognostic, and therapeutic tool in heart failure. Am J Crit Care 2004; 13:46–53.

Ridker PM: High-sensitivity C-reactive protein and cardiovascular risk: Rationale for screening and primary prevention. Am J Cardiol 2003; 92(Suppl):17K–22K.

Roberts R: Rapid MB CK subform assay and the early diagnosis of myocardial infarction. Clin Lab Med 1997; 17:669–683.

Roberts WL, Sedrick R, Moulton L, et al: Evaluation of four automated high-sensitivity C-reactive protein methods: Implications for clinical and epidemiological applications. Clin Chem 2000; 46:461–468.

Rothenberg ME: Eosinophilia. N Engl J Med 1998; 338:1592–1600.

Sacks DB: Carbohydrates. *In* Burtis CA, Ashwood ER (eds): Tietz Textbook of Clinical Chemistry, 3rd ed, Philadelphia, WB Saunders, 1999, pp 750–808.

Sattler M, Griffin JD: Molecular mechanisms of transformation by the BCR-ABL oncogene. Semin Hematol 2003; 40(Suppl 2):4–10.

Schiodt FV, Lee WM: Fulminant liver disease. Clin Liver Dis 2003; 7: 331–349.

Schnermann JB, Sayegh SI: Kidney Physiology. New York, Lippincott-Raven, 1998.

Schrier RW, Cadnapaphornchai MA: Renal aquaporin water channels: From molecules to human disease. Prog Biophys Mol Biol 2003; 81:117–131.

Seebach JD, Morant R, Ruegg R, et al: The diagnostic value of the neutrophil left shift in predicting inflammation and infectious disease. Am J Clin Pathol 1997; 107:582–591.

Shanafelt TD, Call TG: Current approach to diagnosis and management of chronic lymphocytic leukemia. Mayo Clin Proc 2004; 79: 388–398.

Silver RT: Chronic myeloid leukemia. Hematol Oncol Clin North Am 2003; 17:1159–1173.

Sunheimer R, Capaldo G, Kashanian F, et al: Serum analyte pattern characteristic of fulminant hepatic failure. Ann Clin Lab Sci 1994; 24:101–109.

This paper summarizes serum liver function analyte patterns that have been found to occur in this uncommon but fatal disease. It corelates analyte patterns with tissue pathological findings.

Thompson WG, Mahr RG, Yohannan W, Pincus MR: Use of creatine kinase MB isoenzyme for diagnosing myocardial infarction when total creatine kinase activity is high. Clin Chem 1988; 34:2208–2210.

Van den Berghe G: Endocrine evaluation of patients with critical illness. Endocrinol Metab Clin N Am 2003; 32:385–410.

Wang TJ, Larson MG, Levy D, et al: Plasma natriuretic peptide levels and the risk of cardiovascular events and death. N Engl J Med 2004; 350:655–663.

Winter WE, Elin RJ: The role and assessment of ventricular peptides in heart failure. Clin Lab Med 2004; 24:235–274.

Winton EF, Langston AA: Update in acute leukemia 2003: A risk adapted approach to acute myeloblastic leukemia in adults. Semin Oncol 2004; 31(Suppl 4):80–86.

Witte DL, VanNess SA, Angstadt DS, et al: Errors, mistakes, blunders, outliers, or unacceptable results: How many? Clin Chem 1997; 43:1352–1356.

Woo J, Zaman S, Patel L: The diagnostic value of specific CK-MB assay in acute myocardial infarction. *In* Miyai K, Kanno T, Ishikawa E (eds): Progress in Clinical Biochemistry, London, Elsevier, 1992, pp 243–246.

Wu AH, Apple FS, Gibler WB, et al: National Academy of Clinical Biochemistry standards of laboratory practice: Recommendations for the use of cardiac markers in coronary artery diseases. Clin Chem 1999; 45:1104–1121.

CHAPTER 9

Laboratory Statistics

Richard A. McPherson MD

KEY POINTS

• For statistical analyses, nominal variables can take on only a limited number of values (or categories) whereas continuous variables are used to report quantitative data.

• Independent variables are considered input (cause) and dependent variables are considered output (effect).

• Distributions of continuous data are described by a measure of central tendency (e.g., mean or median) and dispersion (standard deviation). Gaussian distributions derive from a mathematical formula and hence are parametric. A common application of descriptive statistics is to establish reference ranges.

• Statistical tests such as comparisons of different groups of data points are either parametric (i.e., assume Gaussian distributions; example is Student t-test) or nonparametric (i.e., make no assumption of distributions; example is test based on rank-order).

• Confidence intervals are preferable over point estimates to express level of certainty in the calculation of any statistical parameter.

• Nominal data are conveniently analyzed with proportions using the chi-square test.

• The effect of multiple factors in a model system can be assessed through analysis of variance (ANOVA).

• Regression analysis between two continuous variables is usually done by least squares fit to a straight line. Applications of regression analysis are common in comparing different analytic methods for validation in clinical laboratories.

allocation of data points into a range of percentiles (e.g., interquartile range). These approaches are everyday phenomena in clinical laboratories for the monitoring of all quantitative assays. Reference ranges are initially set up with these techniques. Methods of quality control for precision and proficiency testing for accuracy also are based on these principles. For data that are not continuous but take on only two or a few discrete values (e.g., positive or negative), the analysis might consist of counting up the number in each category and looking at the proportion of all values by category.

Comparison of data typically asks the question whether one group is different from another group. These comparisons are usually done by t-test or by analysis of variance depending on whether two or more groups of continuous data are compared. If the data are discrete, comparison is done by chi-square analysis. When data can take on a range of different values, it is convenient to do a correlation between two different data sets with a straight line fit. The newcomer to statistical analysis frequently poses the question: Which statistical test is best? The question of which test to use depends largely on whether the data are continuous or discrete, and whether continuous data follow particular distributions. However, statistics is based on convention so that the investigator should try very diligently to understand the importance of differences between tests and whether possible findings and conclusions are likely to reflect accurately the nature and significance of the question being asked. In contrast to the investigator who is interested in finding the right test for data already collected, the statistician is more interested in helping the investigator plan the experiment and collection of data so that statistical tests are most valid. This chapter relies heavily on common clinical laboratory examples for which specific statistical tests are applied to demonstrate some useful choices.

Introduction

The quantification of information in meaningful summaries and comparisons is the domain of statistical analysis. The first task in analysis is to provide a description of the magnitude of the observations and how close to one another the different measurements are. Descriptive statistics provides a consistent framework for calculating or estimating the central tendency of continuous data in the familiar forms of mean, median, and mode. The variation in data is generally described by the mathematical calculation of variances and standard deviations or by the simple

Definitions

Variables: The things that we measure, count, or otherwise delineate are termed *variables* because the values they can assume vary. Variables are usually considered to fall in one of the following scales:

• *Nominal scale* where a variable can take on only a limited number of values, usually called categories (or characters). Examples of nominal variables are gender (male or female), risk factors (smoker or nonsmoker), etc.

- *Ordinal scale* where the variable takes on specific values that have some inherent order such as magnitude but without equivalent distances between categories (e.g., trace amount, 1+, 2+, etc. of protein in urine).
- *Interval scale* where a variable takes on values in a quantitative range with defined differences between points. It is conventional to treat most numerical laboratory measurements as *continuous variables* even though they may be reported as *discrete* values (e.g., glucose values of 123 or 124 mg/dL, but not 123.857... mg/dL).

Coefficient of variation (CV): The standard deviation (SD) of a set of data points divided by the mean result expressed either as a percentage or as a decimal fraction.

Confidence interval (CI): The interval that is computed to include a parameter such as the mean with a stated probability (e.g., commonly 90%, 95%, or 99%).

Degrees of freedom (df): A parameter related to the sample size (n). Df indicates the number of quantities free to vary and is usually $n - 1$ for applications such as the *t*-test. For the chi-square test, it is the number of rows minus one times the number of columns minus one. Df is employed in calculating the *p*-value for a statistical test.

Gaussian normal distribution: A spread of data in which elements are distributed symmetrically around the mean with most values close to the center. It is explicitly described by a mathematical equation and so is a parametric distribution. Random scatter or random selection of a population often results in a Gaussian normal distribution. This type of distribution is often a criterion for completely valid application of many parametric tests.

Linear regression: The mathematical process for calculating the best straight line to fit the relationship observed between two variables measured on the same items. *Simple* or *least squares linear regression* yields the best fit for x and y data sets by minimizing the sum of the squared y-axis (vertical distance) differences between each data point (x,y) and the line. This approach assumes the x-axis data to be nearly perfect or without error. Uneven distribution of data points across the entire range may significantly alter the reliability of linear regression. *Deming linear regression* does not assume the x-axis data to be free of error, but instead uses the weighted sum of squared y-axis and x-axis differences between the data points and the line. The *correlation coefficient (r)* describes how well the line fits the data (r ranges from -1 to 1).

Mean: Sum of all results divided by the number of results. Also related are the *median*, which is the middle value that divides the distribution of data points into upper and lower halves (also called the 50th percentile); and the *mode*, which is the most common value. The mean, median, and mode are all measures of central tendency.

Parametric statistics: Statistical measures that are calculated based on the assumption that the data points follow a Gaussian distribution and include parameters such as mean, variance, standard deviation.

Nonparametric statistics are based on rank or order of data.

Null hypothesis (H_0): The proposal that there is no difference in a comparison. The alternative hypothesis is that there is a difference. When the critical value of a statistic is exceeded, rejection of the null hypothesis occurs thereby favoring the acceptability of the alternative hypothesis.

Significance level (p or α): The probability that a difference between groups occurred by chance alone, by convention set at less than 0.05.

Statistical power ($1 - β$): The probability that a difference between groups will be detected by the study, generally set at least to 80%.

Standard deviation (SD): The square root of the sum of the squared differences of each data point from the mean divided by $n - 1$ for samples (divided by n for populations). The SD is a predictable measure of dispersion from the mean in a Gaussian normal distribution.

Standard deviation index (SDI): The difference between the value of a data point and the mean value divided by the group's SD. The *z-transformation* is the expression of a result from the mean in SD units. The Z-value is the probability of a result being z SDs from the mean value. The SDI is commonly used in reporting performance in proficiency testing for an individual laboratory compared to peers.

Student t-test: Statistical test for comparing means between two sample groups. The test can be either paired (e.g., two separate measurements on the same individuals before and after some intervention) or unpaired. Values of t and df yield a level of statistical significance (*p*-value).

Type I error (alpha error, α): Incorrectly rejecting the null hypothesis and stating that two groups are statistically different when they really are not.

Type II error (beta error, β): Incorrectly failing to reject the null hypothesis and stating that two groups are not statistically different when they really are.

Variables

Statistical questions are often posed in terms of input versus output, cause and effect, or correlation between two or more variables. The input or cause is considered an *independent variable* because it is already determined and so is not influenced by other factors. Examples of independent variables are age, gender, temperature, time, etc. In contrast, *dependent variables* are those things that might change in response to the independent variable. Examples of dependent variables are blood glucose concentration, enzyme activities, presence or absence of malignancy, etc. Of course we can change our thinking and switch which is the independent and which is the dependent variable if the experimental question changes. For graphical display, the independent variable is plotted along the horizontal (x) axis or abscissa, while dependent variables are plotted along the vertical (y) axis or ordinate. With a single independent variable (e.g., time) on the x-axis, more than one dependent variable can be plotted on the y-axis to demonstrate different relationships simultaneously. The relationship observed between an independent variable and dependent variables is used to predict future outcomes of the dependent ones based on what values the independent variable assumes.

Preparing to Analyze Data

Most statistical calculations today are done automatically by computer with software programs that present multiple sophisticated options for analysis and even graphical displays of the data. To prepare data for these automated analyses, it is always necessary to enter them into readable format for the program. This process can entail either automated transfer from one electronic data set to the statistical program or manual entry from printed sheets of data. Manual entry is obviously fraught with opportunity for typographical errors, but even automated transfer of data can have erroneous entries, especially when translating older data sets that have been stored on media that might have been corrupted (e.g., magnetic tapes re-examined decades later). Even converting data strings to columns and rows of data points can leave some values in the wrong places. Consequently it is good practice always to examine the data set for accuracy before performing the statistical analysis. This examination could be done by proof reading every entry or by double entry of each value and automatic comparison for discrepancies, although both of these approaches could be impractical when the data sets contain hundreds, thousands, or more values. At the very least, visual examination of the plotted values gives a quick idea if some serious data entry errors occurred. For example, an incorrectly entered value of 50.0 for potassium (instead of 5.0) can be immediately identified by scanning all values on a graphical plot. The person preparing to perform statistical analyses, should do this visual test to identify and correct the most obvious errors and to search for any systematic errors that might also have arisen in data transfer and entry.

Descriptive Statistics

When multiple data points are collected, it is useful to provide a summary of those results that makes it easier to understand than simply listing all values. The methods used to summarize data are termed *descriptive statistics* because they describe what the magnitude of results is and how the data points differ from one another. In the case of categorical variables, this description can be a simple count of discrete values (e.g., how many men and how many women had blood drawn in a clinic?). For continuous variables, it is conventional to use some measure of *central tendency* about which the data points cluster, and a measure of how far apart they are *dispersed* from one another (e.g., what are the ages of the patients who had blood drawn?).

Central Tendency

The most widely recognized measure of central tendency is probably the *mean* or average value that is calculated by adding up the values of all the individual data points and dividing that sum by the total number of data points, expressed mathematically as:

$$\text{mean} = \bar{x} = (x_1 + x_2 + \dots x_n) \div n = \frac{1}{n}\sum_{i=1}^{n} x_i \qquad (9\text{--}1)$$

Because this technique derives the mean value from a defined formula, it is termed a *parametric method*. An alternative measure of central tendency is

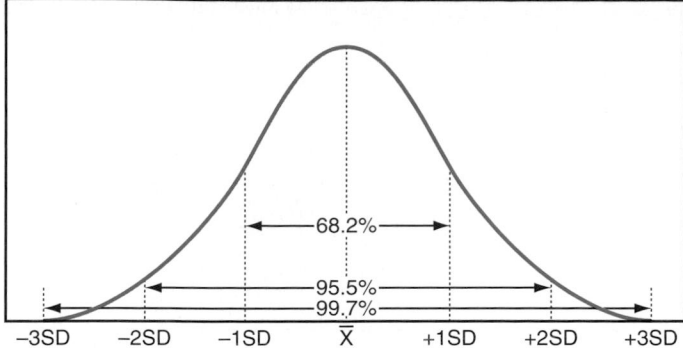

Figure 9–1 Idealized Gaussian (normal) distribution showing areas under the curve corresponding to mean ± 1, 2, and 3 standard deviations.

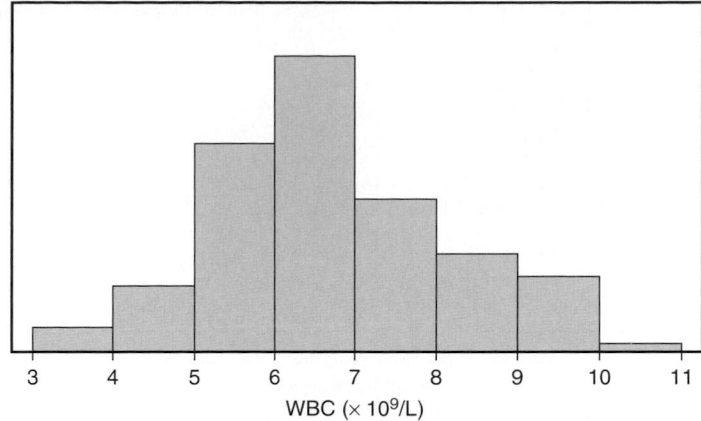

Figure 9–2 Distribution of white blood cells in the blood of 85 healthy individuals.

the *median*, which divides all the data points exactly in half with one half being larger and one half lower. The median is also called the 50th percentile. It is not calculated from a formula because it is taken from a straight count of the data points, so it is termed a *nonparametric method*. The third commonly used measure of central tendency is the *mode*, which is the most common value, i.e., the value of the variable that has the greatest number of data points. The mode is not a very useful measure for describing or comparing data sets, but it does have a role in understanding when a data set consists of two or more different populations that result in more than one mode. If there are two separate populations, then it is called a bimodal population, etc. In general, parametric methods allow a great deal of further calculations for application of many different statistical tests that are based on specific formulas. The advantage of nonparametric methods is that they do not assume or require that the data points follow any particular distribution for them to be applicable. Parametric methods can be applied to data sets that deviate from preferred distributions, but those calculations and conclusions may not be fully warranted if the deviations are extreme.

Gaussian (Normal) Distribution

The Gaussian (also called normal) distribution is a symmetric, bell-shaped curve centered about the mean value (Figure 9–1). It is described by the mathematical formula:

$$P(x) = \frac{1}{\sigma\sqrt{2\pi}} e^{-\left(\frac{(x-\bar{x})^2}{2\sigma^2}\right)} \qquad (9\text{–}2)$$

where σ is the standard deviation of the ideal Gaussian population (Dawson-Saunders, 1994). It corresponds to the distance from the mean to the *x* value at which the curve has an inflection point.

The area under this curve within ± 1 σ from the mean is approximately 68.2% of the total area, meaning that 68.2% of data points from a Gaussian distribution should fall within ± 1 σ of the mean. Similarly 95.5% of the data points will be within ± 2 σ of the mean, and 99.7% will be within ± 3 σ of the mean.

Dispersion

A common parametric measure (based on the Gaussian distribution) of the dispersion of data points about the mean value of a population under examination is the standard deviation, mathematically calculated as:

$$\text{standard deviation} = SD = \sqrt{\frac{\sum_i (x_i - \bar{x})^2}{n-1}} \qquad (9\text{–}3)$$

The quantity under the square root sign is termed *variance*. Use of the standard deviation assumes that the data follow a bell-shaped curve that can be described mathematically by the formula for a normal or Gaussian distribution. To the extent that the data are normally distributed, then the standard deviation is a good estimate of the dispersion.

Two additional terms derive from the standard deviation. One is the *coefficient of variation (CV)*, which is calculated as the SD divided by the mean. The CV is often expressed as a percentage, although it can also be expressed as a decimal fraction less than 1. For a situation where the mean = 25 and the SD = 5, the CV = 20%, or 0.20. The other term is the *standard deviation index (SDI)*, which is the distance that an individual data point is away from the mean value divided by the SD. The main use for the SDI is in such applications as proficiency testing where performance of any one laboratory is standardized according to the dispersion of data in the performance by all laboratories.

A common clinical laboratory application of the normal distribution is to calculate the central 95% of values obtained from a healthy population when trying to establish the reference range for an analyte. This range is of course easily calculated as mean ± 2 SD for a truly Gaussian normal population. An example of this application is calculation of the central 95% of values of white blood cell count in a group of 85 healthy medical students (Fig. 9–2). The bar graph plot is roughly bell shaped and symmetrical although there is a slight asymmetry that can probably be ignored. The mean value is 6.60×10^9 cells/L with a SD of 1.457×10^9 cells/L, and the calculated central 95% range is 3.69–9.52×10^9 cells/L. This is a small group of individuals compared to what might be used for actual reference range calculations, but it does show a few persons with WBCs higher than this range and some lower, so this estimate of central 95% appears appropriate.

Another way of thinking about these calculations is that the persons tested represent only a sample of all persons to whom we are interested in generalizing these findings (Daniel, 1999). The mean value actually observed would probably be somewhat different if another group of 85 healthy people were tested. Based on the values observed and their spread, a confidence interval can be placed around the mean such that we can be certain by a desired percent that the true mean of WBCs from all healthy persons falls in that range. The confidence limit is calculated as:

$$\text{confidence interval} = \bar{x} \pm z\frac{SD}{\sqrt{n}} \qquad (9\text{–}4)$$

where the critical factor *z* derives from transformation of the problem to a standard normal distribution. The quantity $\frac{SD}{\sqrt{n}}$ is termed the *standard error of the mean*. In this example, let the confidence interval be 95%, for which $z = 1.96$. The 95% confidence interval around the mean value is

$6.60 \pm 1.96 \times \frac{1.457}{\sqrt{85}}$ or 6.295–6.914×10^9 cells/L. Note that this range is

the 95% confidence interval on the mean value alone, whereas the calculations above yielded the central 95% of all the data points. Confidence intervals are used to give an idea of how broad the estimate of something is. It can be made more certain by using 99% confidence intervals (i.e., 99% confident that the true mean falls in the interval), in which case $z = 2.575$ for the calculation and the 99% confidence interval is

broader at $6.60 \pm 2.575 \times \frac{1.457}{\sqrt{85}}$ or 6.193–7.007×10^9 cells/L.

Nonparametric Measures

The median value of WBC for this group of healthy persons is 6.4×10^9 cells/L, which is also roughly the same as the mean value. For a perfectly Gaussian normal distribution, values of the mean, median and mode are exactly the same. Delineation of the range from the 2.5-percentile to the 97.5-percentile also gives an estimate of the central 95% range (for the example of WBC, it is 3.94–9.89×10^9 cells/L, which is really the exact range for this specific population). This is a nonparametric estimate of the range because it does not use a calculation, but only divides up the data points according to their order. Many applications of median use the central 50% of data points from the 25th percentile to the 75th percentile (also called interquartile range) to describe central tendency by nonparametric method.

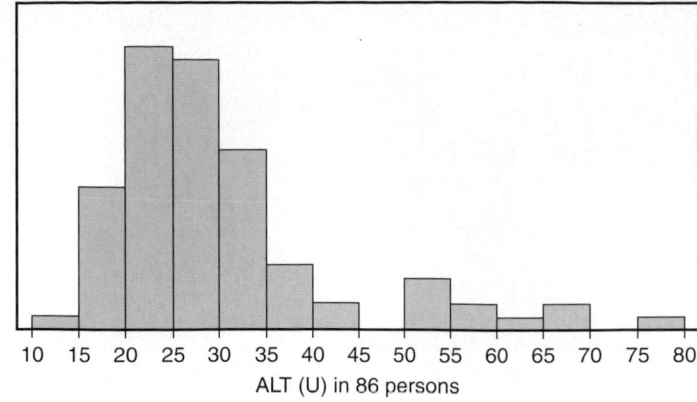

Figure 9–3 Distribution of alanine aminotransferase in the serum of 86 healthy individuals.

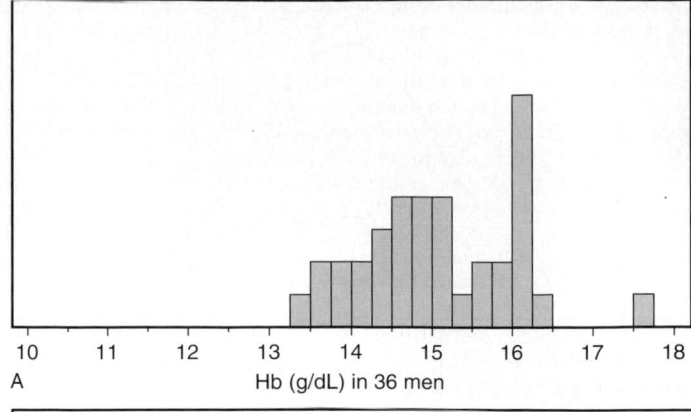

A Hb (g/dL) in 36 men

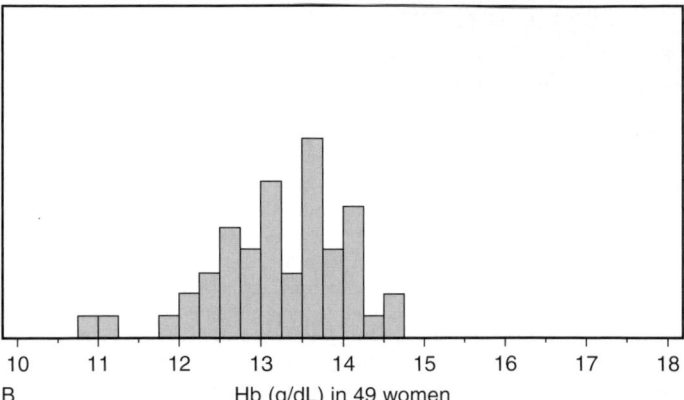

B Hb (g/dL) in 49 women

Figure 9–4 Distribution of hemoglobin in the blood of A. healthy men and B. healthy women.

Sometimes the parametric method of mean ± 2 SD produces an erroneous estimate of the central 95% range. An example of this situation arises with the distribution of alanine aminotransferase (ALT) activities in the serum of apparently healthy individuals (Fig. 9–3). In this population, the mean value is 30.1 U, the SD is 12.69 U, and the calculated reference range (mean ± 2 SD) is 4.73–55.48 U. This range is not appropriate because the actual lowest value observed in the group was much higher (12 U). This estimate of the lower end of the range (4.73 U) is far too low. Similarly the estimate of the upper end (55.48 U) is too low and excludes about 10% of the data points instead of only 2.5%. Another clue that the parametric method may not work here is that the median value is 27.0 U, which is somewhat different from the mean. The reason for this discrepancy is apparent upon looking at the distribution, which is *skewed* to the right with many values tailing off at the upper end. In this case, a much more useful estimate of the central 95% can be obtained simply from the 2.5-percentile to the 97.5-percentile range. It is 15.2–68.0 U. The form of this distribution for ALT is sometimes termed *log-normal*, because it can be converted to a normal distribution by using the values of log ALT instead. The *geometric mean* is calculated from the data after log transformation.

Comparative Statistics

One of the questions frequently asked by statistical means is whether one group is different from another group in some characteristic. The question boils down to a comparison of the central tendency of one group versus that of the other and the scatter that each group exhibits about the central values. If the scatter of data is extreme, then calculated differences between mean values of two groups might not be important, but rather the result of adding in the extreme values. Another way to think about these comparisons is that of signal-to-noise ratio. If there is little noise (scatter of data), then the difference in the signal from each group is more believable.

Student *t*-Test

The most common method for comparison of a continuous variable between groups is probably the Student *t*-test (Dawson-Saunders, 1994). The pseudonym Student was used by William Gosset, a statistician working for the Guinness brewery, who wanted to keep his work for optimizing productivity unrecognized by competing companies. The *t*-test is based on a parametric calculation of the *t* statistic as:

$$t = \frac{\bar{x}_1 - \bar{x}_2}{SD_{12}\sqrt{\frac{1}{n_1} + \frac{1}{n_2}}} \qquad (9-5)$$

where $\bar{x}_1$ is the mean value in group 1,
n_1 is the number of values in group 1
$\bar{x}_2$ is the mean value in group 2,
n_2 is the number of values in group 2, and
SD_{12} is the standard deviation of groups 1 and 2 combined.

Fortunately the calculation of *t* statistics is conveniently performed by computers in modern times, so the analyst now has the responsibility of vouching for the accuracy of data input and the correct choice of statistical tests and their validity for the situation.

There are some specific assumptions about the data sets that are also necessary for applicability. For example, it is necessary to have sufficient numbers of data points in each group to make a valid comparison with approximately equal numbers in each. The spread of the data points should be equivalent (usually assessed by whether the variances of the groups are equivalent). The selection of data points should be independent of one another; for example, it would be inappropriate to include the same patient twice in one group. The issue of independence is usually handled experimentally by a random selection of subjects or patients. Randomization of treatments is an exacting process for important research such as clinical trials. For laboratory use, it is more likely that data come from patients that present themselves to the hospital or clinic for testing rather than being a random sample of all people in a city or from a country. The more random the selection process, the more likely that results can be generalized to a much larger target population for which inference is desired.

The statistical question for consideration is reduced to two mutually exclusive hypotheses that include all the possible situations. The null hypothesis (H_0) states that there is no difference between groups. The alternative hypothesis (H_{alt}) is that the difference between mean values is significant. If the *t* statistic has a sufficiently high value, we can reject the null hypothesis and consequently must accept the alternative hypothesis that there is a significant difference. If the *t* value is on the low side, we cannot reject the null hypothesis, but neither can we accept it. This decision is somewhat like that of the verdict from a trial in which the possible outcomes are 'guilty' and 'not guilty.' The innocence of the defendant is never established, and similarly the null hypothesis is never proven. We could end up thinking that the null hypothesis is correct (particularly since the alternative hypothesis now seems unlikely), but the test we performed did not strictly lead to that conclusion.

Consider the distribution of hemoglobin values in the whole blood of 36 healthy males and 49 healthy females (Fig. 9–4A and B). Visual inspection of the bar graphs for hemoglobin (Hb) shows that the females generally have lower values (mean 13.2 g/dL, SD 0.80 g/dL) than the males (mean 15.1 g/dL, SD 0.96 g/dL). Only a portion of the males and females overlap one another in hemoglobin values. In this example, the value of $t = 9.898$. One other factor must be taken into account, the degrees of freedom, which is obtained from the total number of data points minus 2 or $df = n_1 + n_2 - 2 = 36 + 49 - 2 = 83$.

Significance

The value of the *t* statistic is assessed for significance according to the degrees of freedom. One way to approach the assessment is look up the value of *t* for which the degrees of freedom yield a probability (*p*) value that is to be applied for significance using a table of values. More often the software does this calculation automatically. Generally p-values of 0.05 or less are required to claim statistical significance. A p-value of 0.05 (also called alpha) means that the difference observed between the two groups could have occurred one time in 20 with the particular spread of data actually observed. The value of alpha is also thought of as the risk that we are willing to take to conclude falsely that there is a significant difference when in fact none exists (type I error). The use of alpha = 0.05 is merely an arbitrary convention, but it is ingrained in the minds of reviewers and protocols for evaluating studies. Of course, if the p-value is much smaller, such as 0.01 or 0.001, then the statistical significance of a difference between group means is that much more credible.

Even though an observed difference between groups might have an extraordinarily impressive p-value ($p = 0.001$ means that the result should happen by chance only 1 in 1000 times), it is incumbent upon the investigator to conclude whether the observation is *clinically significant*. The statistical significance of any difference can always be amplified, no matter how insignificant it is for decision-making, simply by increasing the number of data points (see the formula for calculating t, Equation 9–5).

A potential problem arises when a large number of comparisons are done in studies where no clear hypothesis is stated, but instead the data are mined for whatever might fall out upon examination. In that case the minimal level of significance should be adjusted to reflect the large number of tests that could conceivably discover 'significant results' by chance alone. After all, if a p-value of 0.05 is used, then by doing 20 different comparisons, one ought to find on average some comparison with a statistically significant difference regularly. The Bonferroni correction is done to lower the risk of such false discovery. It consists of dividing the usually accepted p-value by the number of comparisons. Thus for 5 different comparisons, the correction is p-value = 0.05/5 = 0.01 as the acceptable threshold value for significance.

For this particular example comparing hemoglobin values between males and females, the p-value is less than 0.0001, so we can reject the null hypothesis and conclude that there is a significant difference between groups. Most statisticians would not report this level, but would be satisfied with saying the p-value was less than 0.001. Another condition to denote is whether this test is two-sided or one-sided, meaning that the question being asked is whether one group is simply different from the other (two-sided) as opposed to the question whether one group is only higher than the other group (one-sided). Most journals require the use of two-sided t-tests because they are more demanding.

Sample Size

Suppose the two groups being compared showed a difference that was not quite statistically significant with a p-value of 0.06. One way to achieve statistical significance is to increase the number of subjects studied. This will be the case if the difference remains the same, because the t-value will be increased by greater n. A pilot study can be done in a clinical trial to establish roughly what the difference between groups is and what the scatter of the data is. These pieces of information are then used in a formula to calculate the *sample size* necessary to bring the results to statistical significance. Calculation of sample size also takes into account another factor called beta, which is the risk you have of missing a true effect by chance (type II error). The *power of the study* is 1 – beta. When beta is set to 0.20, the power of the study is 0.80, which says that the number of subjects calculated for use will yield a statistically significant result 80% of the time with the specified difference between groups and scatter of data.

The t-test used for this example was *unpaired* because the comparison was between different individuals. If the experimental design included a comparison of values on the same individuals before and after a treatment, then it is appropriate to use a *paired* t-test. A paired test is potentially a more powerful mathematical tool because it looks only at the change between the values within each person and is not influenced by variation in background values between individuals.

Nonparametric Tests

If the assumption about normality of the data is not valid, other nonparametric tests can be used to compare distributions between groups. The *Wilcoxon signed-ranks test* is such a technique. By that method, all values of both groups are given a numerical rank according to their magnitude. In the case of ties for the same value, both are assigned the intermediate rank (e.g., if 4th and 5th places are tied, then both are given the rank 4.5). All ranks are summed in each group and divided by the number of data points in each group. The difference between the rank scores is then given a probability. This technique is easily done by

Table 9–1 Observed Values of Contamination in Blood Cultures

Result	Baseline period	Post-training
Number of cultures contaminated	53	32
Number of cultures not contaminated	978	891

Table 9–2 Expected Values of Contamination in Blood Cultures

Result	Baseline period	Post-training
Number of cultures contaminated	44.8	40.2
Number of cultures not contaminated	986.2	882.8

computer software and may be quite useful when assumptions required for a parametric method are not met by a data set.

Analyzing Discrete Data: Testing Proportions

The analysis of discrete data takes on a different form from that of continuous variables that can be expressed as distributions. With discrete data, answers are typically dichotomous: either something is present or absent, patient gender is male or female, the patient lived or died. Consider the fictitious example of an intervention to lower contamination rates in blood culture collection. (This is a universal problem in all laboratories, but these data are only hypothetical.) Before the intervention, baseline information over a 2-month period showed that 53 cultures were considered contaminated and 978 were not. After training and implementation of the new collection process, a second 2-month period showed 32 contaminated cultures and 891 that were not. These nominal data are conveniently expressed in a 2×2 display termed a contingency table of observed values (Table 9–1). These data consist of simple counts in one category or another. The question to be asked is whether the proportion of contaminated cultures was significantly different in the two time periods.

Chi-Square Test

The statistical test to be used is the chi-square test. It is calculated as:

$$\chi^2 = \sum \frac{(\text{Observed} - \text{Expected})^2}{\text{Expected}} \quad (9\text{–}6)$$

where the observed values are as listed above and the expected values are calculated from the overall assortment of counts (Dawson-Saunders, 1994). In this example, the expected number of contaminated cultures in the baseline period is the total number of cultures done in that period ($53 + 978 = 1031$) times the proportion of contaminated cultures in both time periods together (proportion calculated as $[53 + 32]/[53 + 978 + 32 + 891] = 0.0435$), or $1031 \times 0.0435 = 44.8$. Calculation of the other expected values follows similarly, resulting in a contingency table of expected values (Table 9–2). Then calculation of the χ^2 value is done by summing the squares of the differences (this converts all differences to positive values) between expected and observed values and dividing by the expected value in each cell of the table. In this example:

$$\chi^2 = \frac{(53 - 44.8)^2}{44.8} + \frac{(978 - 986.2)^2}{986.2} + \frac{(32 - 40.2)^2}{40.2} + \frac{(891 - 882.8)^2}{882.8}$$

$$= 3.3 \quad (9\text{–}6A)$$

With one degree of freedom ([number of rows – 1][number of columns – 1]), the p-value is 0.07, which does not meet the universal threshold of at least 0.05 for statistical significance. It is fair to say that a trend toward less contamination was observed after the intervention, but that it was not quite statistically significant. It is important to keep in mind that for χ^2 testing to be valid, each cell must have a minimum value of 5 observations.

Trend Evaluation and Correlative Statistics

The relationship between an independent variable and a dependent variable is demonstrated by plotting them on a scattergram or a plot with the independent (input) variable on the x-axis and the dependent (output) variable on the y-axis. If there is no relationship between the two variables, the data scatter randomly over the graph. If there is a relationship, it can be described mathematically by finding a line that is the best fit through all the data points. This line can be calculated by the least squares approach in which the vertical distances from each point to the calculated line are minimized for the entire population of values. This statistical method is referred to as *linear regression* (National Committee for Clinical Laboratory Standards, 2003).

Linear Regression

The general form for the equation of a straight line is:

$$y = a + bx \qquad (9\text{–}7)$$

in which the slope 'b' indicates how the value of y changes when x changes. When b = 1, the relationship of change between x and y is one to one. The intercept 'a' indicates how the relationship between x and y is offset or biased by a constant factor. The calculation is easily done by any of several different statistical programs that also provide information about the goodness of fit of the line. This approach is commonly used when comparing an existing method (A) with a new method (B) for the same analyte (Fig. 9–5A). This example shows a strong correlation between method A and method B because the data points fall very close to the line, which is described by the equation: *Method B = 0.62 + 0.99 × Method A*. The slope of 0.99 is almost perfect, and the intercept of 0.62 is quite small on the scale of possible values. In fact the 95% confidence limits on b are −0.47 to 1.72, which includes the value 0, indicating that the intercept is not significantly different from 0.

The vertical (y axis) distances from each data point to the best fit line are termed the *residuals*. The most valid line fits are associated with relatively constant values of the residuals over the entire range of values. If the residuals grow larger at one end of the graph, then the line fit is less certain in that portion of the range. The *standard error of regression* (also called *standard error of the estimate*) denoted $S_{y.x}$ is used to estimate the variation that could be expected from doing the regression again with another sample of data points. The $S_{y.x}$ is calculated as the square root of the sum of

residuals squared, divided by n − 2. It is important that data points from patient specimens be spread over the entire analytic range to yield the most valid comparison of methods unbiased by over- or under-representation of data in any region (National Committee for Clinical Laboratory Standards, 2002).

In laboratory practice, regression or correlation analysis is frequently used to compare the performance of a new method with an old method. In this situation, the old method could have worse precision than the new one, and so it would not be appropriate to base a judgment just on how the new method compares with the old one as a 'gold standard.' A common approach to this issue is Deming regression analysis, named for W Edwards Deming (1900–1993), a mathematician influential in principles of quality improvement. In Deming regression, the best line is obtained by minimizing the sum of squares of both x and y distances from the data points to the line (Cornbleet, 1979). In addition, Deming regression applies a weighting factor (λ) that incorporates the relative variances of both the z and y data. The result is more heavily weighted in favor of the data set with better precision.

The relationship between method A and method B is further described by the *correlation coefficient (r)*, which can range in value from −1 to +1. A value of 0 indicates no relationship, and a value of 1 indicates perfect relationship (−1 is also a perfect but inverse relationship). Other values between −1 and +1 indicate intermediate relationships. The square of the correlation coefficient is termed the *coefficient of determination* (r^2), which describes the amount of variation observed in the dependent variable that is due to the relationship between the two variables. In this example, r = 0.9976 and r^2 = 0.9952, both of which are very high values showing an extremely strong relationship between method A and method B that accounts for 99.52% of the variation. The p-value on this correlation is less than 0.0001.

In contrast with the very good correlation between method A and method B, the performance of method C versus method A (Fig. 9–5B) is not nearly as good. By simple visual examination, the data points are scattered further from the line, and the line is shifted upwards. The value of r = 0.8757, somewhat less than between method A and method B, but still a strong correlation with p-value less than 0.0001. The value of r^2 = 0.7668, so 76.68% of the variation can be accounted for by the relationship between method C and method A. The equation for this line is *Method C = 10.2 + 0.84 × Method A*, so the change in values using method C compared to method A is slightly lower (slope of 0.84). There is also a significant upward bias by method C (intercept of 10.2 with 95% confidence limits of 2.8 to 17.6).

Method Comparisons

These two examples show somewhat different relationships, although both are statistically significant. It is up to the person assessing the performance to determine which is sufficient for the application. The comparison of method A with method B is extraordinarily strong both by visual review and by statistical analysis, and so it can comfortably be said that those methods are equivalent for purposes of replacing one with the other in clinical practice. On the other hand, the comparison of method A with method C is messier because of the larger amount of data scatter. The smaller slope suggests that the two methods do not react equivalently with the analyte, and furthermore there is a positive bias by method C. With expectations for excellent precision and accuracy on modern instrumentation, method C would probably be rejected if method B were a viable alternative. And yet the level of correlation observed between method A and method C might be very welcome to researchers trying to ask a different question relating to cause and effect between biological processes that have inherently high levels of variation.

A special example of regression analysis termed *logistic regression* is employed when the outcome is a dichotomous or binary variable for continuous independent (predictor) variables.

Analysis of Variance

When the mean values of more than two different groups are to be compared, the process is termed *analysis of variance (ANOVA)* (Dawson-Saunders, 1994). This analysis can be thought of as extending the t-test beyond two independent samples to three or more. The null hypothesis in this situation is that the mean values of all groups are the same. The alternative hypothesis is that not all the means are equal (some could be the same, but others different). The test statistic is the F-ratio of the mean squares among all groups (MS_A) to the error mean square (MS_E):

$$F\text{-}ratio = \frac{MS_A}{MS_E} \qquad (9\text{–}8)$$

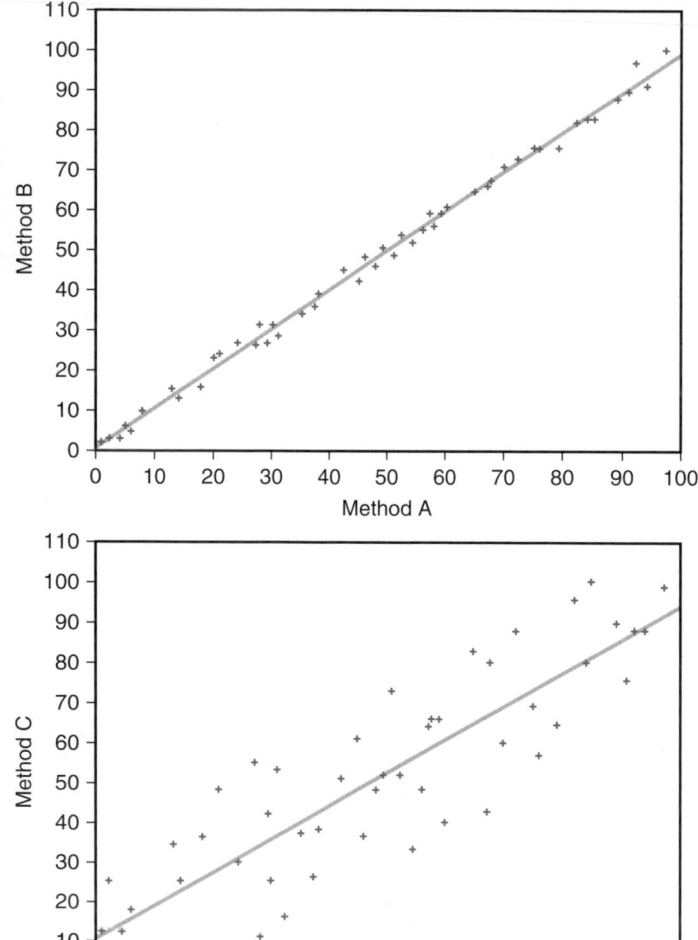

Figure 9–5 A: Regression analysis between method A and method B; strong correlation. B: Regression analysis between method A and method C; weaker correlation.

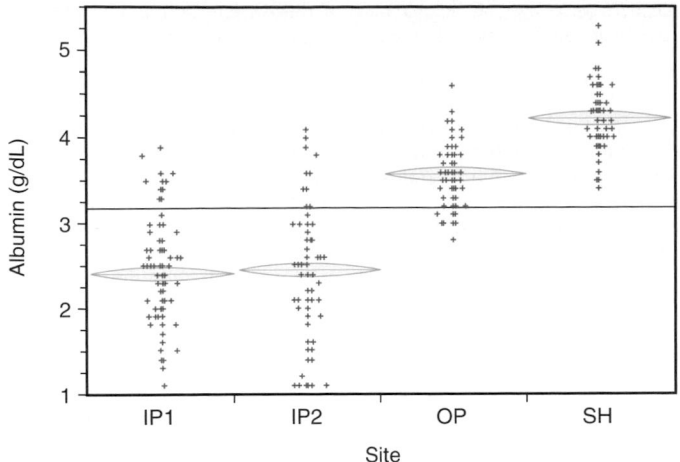

Figure 9–6 Analysis of variance. Serum albumin at different patient sites (IP1, IP2, inpatient wards 1 and 2; OP, outpatient; SH, student health).

It compares the variance of the group means versus the mean of all the data (numerator) and the variance of individual data points within each group (denominator). If the group means differ from one another (signal) more than the variation within groups (noise), then the F-ratio will exceed a critical value for significance.

An example of ANOVA is the comparison of serum albumin values from patients at two inpatient sites, an outpatient clinic, and a student health clinic (Fig. 9–6). One hundred consecutive specimens from each site were recorded. The horizontal line shows the grand mean of all 400 values of 3.17 g/dL. Within each group, the diamonds indicate group means (midline) and 95% confidence intervals on those means (upper and lower vertices). The F-ratio = 279 for which the p-value < 0.0001, so the null hypothesis can be rejected with the conclusion that at least some of the means are different. This approach is more conservative and realistic than comparing each group with every other group using a series of different t-tests (with four groups, there could be six comparisons). The problem with too many comparisons is the possibility of 'accidentally finding significance' that is not true. To extend ANOVA, comparisons of group means by such procedures as Tukey's honestly significant difference (HSD) can be done. In this example, Tukey's HSD indicates that IP1 and IP2 are not different from one another, but that OP and SH are both different from all other groups. At this stage, the investigator is free to elaborate on potential reasons for these observed differences without putting further statistical significance on the individual differences.

Some conditions should be met for parametric ANOVA to be completely valid mathematically:
- The data were collected using random sampling where all observations are independent of one another.
- The data in each group are normally distributed.
- Each group has an equal number of data points.
- Each group has equal variances.

If this set of ideal criteria is not met, other methods are available for comparisons. The Mann–Whitney test can be used to compare medians. The Wilcoxon and Kruskal–Wallis test for rank sums are nonparametric alternatives. This example of serum albumin shows greater variances for the inpatient groups than for the outpatients, so nonparametric analysis could be more appropriate. (The Wilcoxon test also showed significant differences among the groups of this example.) This case dealt with one variable, and so it was one-way ANOVA. To deal with two variables, the procedure can be extended to two-way ANOVA.

Analysis of Covariance

Sometimes the way a comparison is set up by selection of subjects into different groups can lead to a confounding effect from another variable besides the variable of primary interest. In that case, it is revealing to perform *analysis of covariance (ANCOVA)* to account for potential influence from the covariable.

As an example of ANCOVA, consider the comparison of serum calcium measurements in 61 male and 41 female healthy adults to establish whether different reference ranges of calcium would be necessary for males and females. Simple one-way ANOVA similar to that in Figure 9–6 yielded a statistically significant (p = 0.0045) difference between the group means of calcium (males 9.3 mg/dL, females 9.1 mg/dL). (This ANOVA with only two groups is equivalent to an unpaired t-test.) This finding and

previous studies were consistent, so it probably is appropriate to have gender-specific reference ranges for serum calcium, but does that make sense from a physiologic view? It is also well recognized that serum albumin influences total calcium levels by binding some of the calcium. A linear regression for these subjects confirmed that relationship. The effects of gender and the covariable albumin on calcium are sorted out by ANCOVA. In this example, the effect on calcium from gender was completely accounted for by the effect of albumin on calcium and the different distribution of albumin in males versus females. ANCOVA can be enlightening to discover and eliminate by statistical analysis those covariables that might not be known and planned for in the design of an experiment. Further discussion of ANCOVA can be found in more advanced texts on statistics (Matthews, 1988).

Method Validation and Process Control

Statistical analysis is integral to the validation of new laboratory methods and to the monitoring of analytic and workflow processes in clinical laboratories (Lott, 1998).

Reference Ranges

The examples depicted in Figures 9–2, 9–3, and 9–4 demonstrate some of the issues encountered when establishing reference ranges through application of descriptive statistics. The basic aim is to establish a range of values within which the majority of healthy people will fall, while excluding individuals with disease. The simplest approach is to use the central 95% of data points from the healthy individuals by calculating mean ± 2 SD whenever the distribution is normal or bell-shaped as for WBC in Figure 9–2. This parametric approach fails to provide a complete reference range when the data are skewed as for ALT in Figure 9–3. In this case, the central 95% can be determined nonparametrically by using the range 2.5-percentile to 97.5-percentile, which excludes 2.5% at both upper and lower ends. The distribution of ALT actually appears to have two subpopulations in these healthy people. Consequently basing reference ranges solely on observed ranges in apparently healthy persons might not be the best approach. In fact, some new recommendations for ALT set the upper range much lower than wide-based population studies would suggest. The new guidelines try to eliminate persons who might have mild, asymptomatic liver changes such as steatosis (Prati, 2002). This approach is similar to the strategy used for setting desirable or healthy levels of cholesterol and lipid fractions (National Cholesterol Education Program, 2002) and for glucose (Report of the Expert Committee on the Diagnosis and Classification of Diabetes Mellitus, 2003). In the future, recommendations from other consensus groups or professional organizations will probably be even more active in setting desirable ranges for other analytes in place of population-based reference ranges.

Finally, healthy subgroups of people should be recognized by separate reference ranges whenever major differences occur according to factors such as age or gender (Fig. 9–4).

Accuracy

The performance of a new method can be assessed for accuracy (e.g., the ability to correctly detect and quantify an analyte) by assaying patient specimens or interlaboratory survey materials with known values. The example of a strong correlation between methods in Figure 9–5A indicates that the analyte reacts in a nearly one-to-one manner by each method (slope ~ 1) with essentially no bias (intercept ~ 0). In contrast, the correlation depicted in Figure 9–5B has a slope different from 1, indicating that the analyte reacts differently with the two methods. One explanation for this type of discrepancy occurs when tumor markers are measured by two immunoassays that employ different antibodies that potentially recognize different epitopes. A bias such as that shown by method C versus method A in Figure 9–5B also suggests a basic methodologic difference that impacts on accuracy, albeit in a predictable way that could be compensated for with calibration adjustment.

The accuracy of any assay depends heavily on the calibrators, how they are originally constituted, how they remain stable over time, and how they compare with calibrators from other vendors (see Ch. 10). The best situation is to have an assay calibrated against internationally distributed standards such as from the World Health Organization or other professional group. Using calibrators with such traceability and standardized units of measurement, it is feasible to use values from different assays interchangeably for the same patient or to compare outcomes in different groups of patients being monitored with different methods.

After implementation of a method, periodic proficiency survey testing of unknown specimens is usually reported in terms of SDIs away from the mean of all laboratories. For example, if the mean of creatinine measurements is 11 mg/dL for all participants with SD of 2 mg/dL, then a laboratory reporting a value of 8 mg/dL would have SDI = $(8 - 11)/2 = -1.5$.

Precision

The reproducibility of an assay is conveniently expressed with the coefficient of variation (CV) that allows the observed SD to be normalized by the magnitude of the signal being measured. It should be kept in mind that assays typically have different CVs for different ranges of analyte values. Therefore it is good practice to establish CVs for an assay at high, low, and mid-range values.

Analytical Sensitivity

The lowest value that an assay can reliably detect is termed *the analytical sensitivity*. A common approach to making this judgment is to measure a zero standard multiple times (e.g., 10 times) and calculate the SD of the signal detected, which is noise. Then set the lowest reliable detection threshold at three or four times that SD. This approach is often individualized within laboratories. This characteristic is also termed the detection limit. Another use of the term analytical sensitivity refers to the change in response of an assay for a given change in the amount or concentration of the analyte (Giacomo, 1984). In this respect, a highly sensitive assay has the characteristic of readily detecting small changes in analyte at concentrations in the mid-range of measurement.

Analytical Specificity

The major interferents in laboratory measurements are hemolysis, icterus, and lipemia due either to interference with optical absorbances (or light scattering) or to actual chemical interactions (e.g., peroxidase activity of hemoglobin in many immunoassays that use horseradish peroxidase as indicator). Beyond these endogenous interferents, drugs can also interact with various chemical or immunologic assays. The magnitude of these interactions (or lack of) is typically documented by addition of known, large amounts of the substances to serum samples that are tested for recovery of the analyte in the serum.

Acceptability of a Method

The final decision of whether to accept a method as valid depends on a combination of factors. Do the statistical tests show a new method to perform analytically as it should with good accuracy and precision? Does the new method provide useful medical information that is not otherwise available? Is the method feasible to do (easy to perform, low cost, rapid)? Does the maximum error fall within medically acceptable limits? The final decision is a professional judgment based on all of these items.

References

Cornbleet PJ, Gochman N: Incorrect least-squares regression coefficients in method-comparison analysis. Clin Chem 1979; 25:432–438.

Daniel WW: Biostatistics: A Foundation for Analysis in the Health Sciences, 7th ed. New York, John Wiley & Sons, 1999.

This book is a more rigorous text on the use of statistical analysis in medicine and life sciences.

Dawson-Saunders B, Trapp RG: Basic & Clinical Biostatistics, 2nd ed. Norwalk, Appleton & Lange, 1994.

This very readable book provides excellent descriptions of statistical procedures applied to multiple examples in the life sciences and medicine.

Giacomo P: International Vocabulary of Basic and General Terms in Metrology. Geneva, International Organization for Standardization, 1984, pp 4–40.

Lott JA: Process control and method evaluation. *In* Snyder JR, Wilkinson DS (eds): Management in Laboratory Medicine, 3rd ed. Philadelphia, Lippincott, 1998, pp 293–325.

This book is a comprehensive source for all aspects of management in the clinical laboratory.

Matthews DE, Farewell VT: Using and Understanding Medical Statistics, 2nd edition. Basel, Switzerland, Karger, 1988.

National Cholesterol Education Program: Detection, Evaluation, and Treatment of High Blood Cholesterol in Adults (Adult Treatment Panel III), Final Report. National Heart, Lung, and Blood Institute, National Institutes of Health, Bethesda, NIH, 2002.

National Committee for Clinical Laboratory Standards: Method Comparison and Bias Estimation Using Patient Samples; Approved Guideline. Document EP9-A2 [ISBN 1-56238-472-4] Wayne, PA, NCCLS, 2002.

National Committee for Clinical Laboratory Standards: Evaluation of the Linearity of Quantitative Measurement Procedures: A Statistical Approach; Approved Guideline. Document EP6-A [ISBN 1-56238-498-8] Wayne, PA, NCCLS, 2003.

This and all the NCCLS guidelines have been developed through a consensus process involving international representatives from industry, government, and user laboratories to yield recommendations that can be applied worldwide. As of January 1, 2005, NCCLS has been renamed Clinical and Laboratory Standards Institute (CLSI).

Prati D, Taioli E, Zanella A, et al: Updated definitions of healthy ranges for serum alanine aminotransferase levels. Ann Inn Med 2002; 137:1–10.

Report of the Expert Committee on the Diagnosis and Classification of Diabetes Mellitus. Diabetes Care 2003; 26(Suppl 1):S5–S20.

Quality Control

W. Greg Miller PhD

KEY POINTS

• Quality control specimens are assayed on a regular schedule to verify that a laboratory procedure is performing correctly.

• Interpretation of quality control results is based on criteria that are sensitive to bias, imprecision, and trend in bias.

• In the event of an incorrect quality control result, corrective action is taken to fix the method problem, and all patient results from the time of the previous acceptable QC result are repeated.

• Because of commutability limitations, QC specimens should not be used to verify that two methods produce the same results for patient samples.

• Proficiency testing provides external evaluation that a laboratory is using a method correctly and in conformance with the manufacturer's specifications.

Introduction

The purpose of a clinical laboratory test is to evaluate the pathophysiologic condition of an individual patient to assist with diagnosis and/or to monitor therapy. To have value for clinical decision-making, an individual laboratory test result must have total error small enough to reflect the biological condition being evaluated. The total error of a result is influenced by the following:
• biological/physiological variability within an individual
• pre-analytical variability in sample collection, transportation, processing, and storage
• analytical variability in test performance
• interfering substances such as drugs or metabolic components.

This chapter addresses quality control of the analytical measurement process to ensure analytical variability meets accuracy and precision requirements that have been established for a measurement procedure and are considered appropriate for patient care. Quality control (also called statistical process control) is a process to statistically sample a measurement procedure to verify it is performing according to pre-established specifications.

Analytical Variability and Calibration

Figure 10–1 illustrates the meaning of accuracy and imprecision for a measurement. In this figure, the horizontal axis represents the numeric value for an individual result, and the vertical axis represents the number of replicate measurements made on the same sample. The red line shows the dispersion of individual results for repeated assays of the same specimen, which is the imprecision (or random bias) of the measurement. The imprecision frequently follows a Gaussian (normal) distribution and is described by the standard deviation (SD). Note that results near the average value (mean) occur more frequently than results further away from the mean. The difference between the average value and the true value for an analyte in the sample is the systematic bias (or accuracy) of the method. Accuracy is established by calibration and can be affected by interferences due to nonspecificity of the method for the analyte.

Figure 10–2 illustrates that method calibration can reduce the systematic bias to zero (within tolerance limits). Note that calibration has no effect on imprecision. All methods have an inherent imprecision. Individual patient results from a correctly calibrated method will have variability consistent with the inherent imprecision of the method. The primary purpose of quality control is to statistically sample the measurement process to verify the method continues to perform within the specifications consistent with acceptable systematic bias and imprecision.

Overview of Statistical Process Control

Statistical process control samples the measurement procedure by assaying QC materials for which the correct result is known in advance. If the result for a QC material is within acceptable limits of the known value, the measurement procedure has been verified to be performing as expected, and results for patient samples can be reported with good probability that they are correct. If QC results are not within acceptable limits, patient results are not reported and corrective action is necessary. Good laboratory practice requires verification that a method is performing correctly at the time patient results are measured.

Figure 10–3 summarizes statistical process control and emphasizes its role as a component of an integrated quality management system. The key elements of statistical process control are sampling the measurement system using QC specimens for which the expected result is known. If the

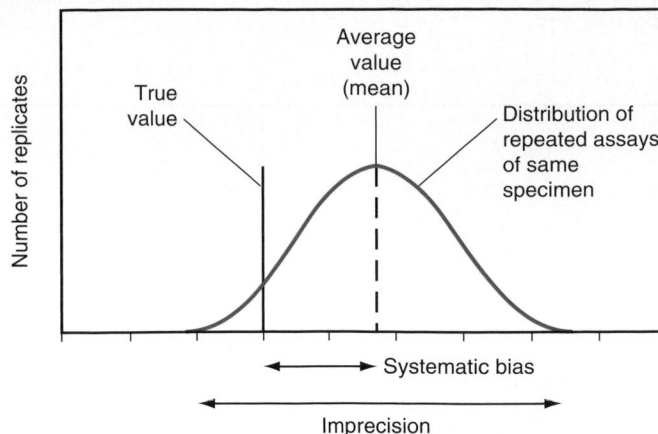

Figure 10–1 Illustration of imprecision and systematic bias (accuracy).

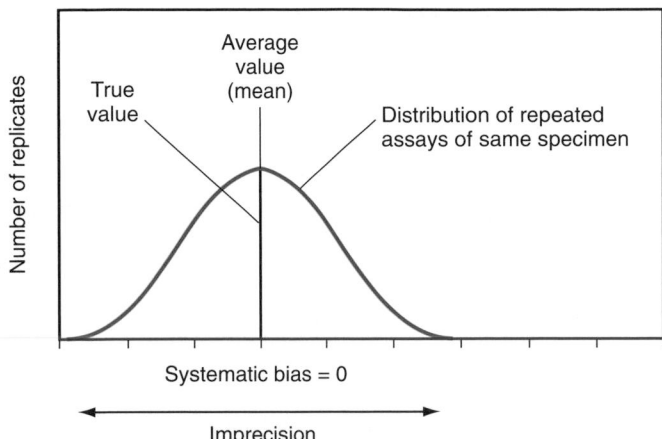

Figure 10–2 Calibration to correct systematic bias.

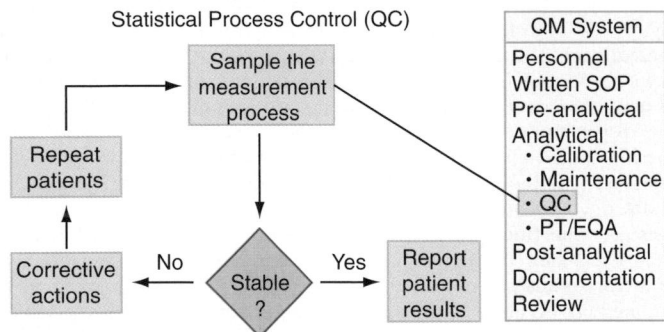

Figure 10–3 Overview of statistical process control (QC) and its integration into a quality management (QM) system. (Reprinted with permission from Miller WG: Quality control. *In* Clarke WA, Dufour DR: (eds): Contemporary practice in clinical chemistry, Washington DC, AACC Press, 2006.)

QC results indicate a stable measurement process, then the patient results have a high probability of being correct. If the QC results fail evaluation criteria, then the patient results may not be reliable for clinical use. In the latter case, corrective action must be taken to fix the analytical process, and repeat assay of the patient samples performed.

Statistical process control is part of the analytical component of the overall quality management system. The quality management system integrates good laboratory practices to assure correct results for patient care. Well-trained and competent personnel are critical for all aspects of laboratory medicine including quality control. Written standard operating procedures (SOP) are required for all aspects of laboratory operation including pre-analytical, analytical, and post-analytical components. For statistical process control, the SOP should include all aspects of the program including the selection of QC materials, how frequently to sample the measurement process, how to determine statistical parameters to describe method performance, criteria for acceptability of QC results, corrective action when problems are identified, and the documentation and review processes. The SOP should include who is authorized to establish acceptable process control limits and interpretive rules for release

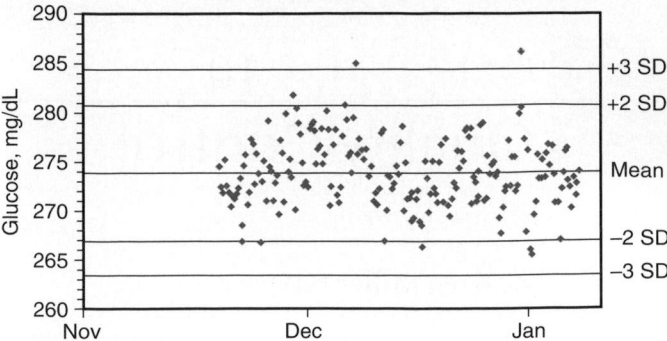

Figure 10–4 Levey–Jennings (Shewhart) plot of QC results (*N* = 199) for a single lot of QC material used for a 49-day period.

of results, who should review performance parameters including statistical quality control results, and who can authorize exceptions to or modify an established quality control policy or procedure.

Figure 10–4 shows a Levey–Jennings (Levey, 1950), also called Shewhart (Shewhart, 1931), plot, which is the most common presentation for evaluating QC results. This format shows each QC result sequentially over time and allows a quick visual assessment of method performance. The mean value represents the target value for the result, and the SD lines represent the expected imprecision for the method. Assuming a Gaussian (normal) distribution of imprecision, the results are distributed as expected with results scattered uniformly around the mean, and with results observed more frequently closer to the mean than near the extremes of the distribution. However, a few results are greater than 2 SD and two results slightly exceed 3 SD. For a large number of repeated assays, the number of results expected within the SD intervals is as follows:

- ± 1 SD = 68.3% of observations
- ± 2 SD = 95.4% of observations
- ± 3 SD = 99.7% of observations.

Interpretation of an individual QC result is based on its probability to be part of the expected distribution of results for the method when the method is performing correctly. A later section has more details regarding interpretive rules for evaluation of QC results.

Implementing Statistical Process Control

Selection of QC Materials

Generally, two different concentrations are necessary for adequate process control. For quantitative methods, QC materials should be selected to provide analyte concentrations which monitor the analytical measurement range of the method. It is important to confirm that method performance is stable near the limits of the assay. Most quantitative assays have a linear response over the analytical measurement range, and one can be confident the performance over the range is acceptable if the results near the assay limits are acceptable. In the case of nonlinear method response, it may be necessary to use additional controls at intermediate concentrations. Critical concentrations for clinical decisions, e.g. therapeutic drugs, TSH, PSA, may also warrant QC monitoring. In the case of analytes which have poor precision at low/normal concentrations, such as troponin I or bilirubin, the concentration must be chosen to provide adequate standard deviation (SD) for practical evaluation. For procedures with extraction or pretreatment, at least one control must be capable of detecting defects in the extraction or pretreatment step.

This chapter is primarily focused on QC procedures for quantitative methods. However, the principles can be adapted to most qualitative procedures, with allowances for the lack of numeric results. For tests based on qualitative interpretation of quantitative measurements, e.g. drugs of abuse, it is desirable to monitor near the threshold concentrations to ensure appropriate discrimination between negative and positive responses. Similarly for other qualitative tests, e.g. human chorionic gonadotropin, a negative and positive control are necessary, and it is good practice to use a positive control that is relatively near the threshold to adequately control for discrimination between negative and positive. For qualitative procedures with graded responses, e.g. dipstick urinalysis, a negative, and at least one positive that has a value in the intermediate graded response region are required. For qualitative tests based on other properties, e.g. electrophoretic procedures, stain adequacy, immunofluorescence, organism identification, it is necessary to ensure the QC procedure will appropriately discriminate normal from pathologic conditions.

The QC materials selected must be manufactured to provide a stable product which can be used for an extended time period, preferably 1 or more years for stable analytes. Use of a single lot for an extended period allows reliable interpretive criteria to be established which will permit efficient identification of an assay problem, avoid false alerts due to poorly defined expected ranges for the QC results, and minimize limitations in interpreting values following reagent and calibrator lot changes.

There are limitations inherent in currently available QC materials. One limitation is that the QC material is frequently noncommutable with native clinical samples. A commutable QC material (or other reference material such as a method calibrator or PT material) is one that reacts in a measurement system to give a result that would be comparable to that expected for a native patient sample with the same amount of analyte. QC materials are typically noncommutable with native patient samples because the serum or other biological fluid matrix is usually altered from that of a native patient sample (Miller, 2003). The matrix alteration is due to the processing of the biological fluid during product manufacturing, the use of partially purified human and nonhuman analyte additives to achieve the desired concentrations, and various stabilization processes which alter proteins, cells and other components. The impact of the matrix alteration on the recovery of an analyte in an assay system is not predictable, is typically different for different lots of QC material, is different for different analytical methods, and can be different for different lots of reagent within the same analytical method.

A second limitation of QC materials is deterioration of the analyte during storage. Analyte stability during unopened refrigerated or frozen storage is generally excellent, but slow deterioration eventually limits the shelf life of a product and can introduce a gradual drift into monitoring data. Analyte stability after reconstitution or vial opening and exposure to air can be an important source of variability in QC results, and can vary substantially among analytes in the same vial. User variables to be controlled are the time spent at room temperature and the time spent uncapped with the potential for evaporation. An expiration time after opening should be established for each QC material and may be different for different analytes in the same control product. For QC materials reconstituted by adding a diluent, the vial-to-vial variability can be minimized by standardizing the pipetting procedure; e.g., use the same pipet or filling device (preferably an automated device) and have the same person prepare the controls whenever practical.

Another limitation is that analyte concentrations in multiconstituent control materials may not be at levels optimal for all assays. This limitation is caused by solubility considerations and potential interactions between different constituents, particularly at higher concentrations. It may be necessary to use supplementary QC materials to adequately monitor the analytical measurement range.

Frequency to Assay QC Materials

The frequency to assay QC specimens is a function of several parameters:
- the analytical stability of the method
- how much error can be tolerated without impact on patient care
- the number of patient samples measured in a period of time
- the need to verify and document the reliability of clinical results at the time they are reported.

The stability of the measurement system is the fundamental determinant of how frequently a QC specimen needs to be assayed. The more stable the system, the less frequently a statistical process control evaluation needs to be performed. Minimum laboratory practice, consistent with the USA CLIA regulations section 493.1256 (Department of Health and Human Services, 2003), is to assay controls at least once per 24 hours, or more frequently if specified by the method manufacturer, or if the laboratory determines that more frequent QC assays are necessary for the performance characteristics of a method. Some types of tests have more stringent requirements. For example, USA CLIA section 493.1267 requires that blood gas measurements assay at least one control every 8 hours that includes both high and low levels in the course of 24 hours; in addition a control must be run with each patient sample unless the instrument automatically calibrates at least every 30 minutes. Methods that have automated internal (self-contained) control procedures may use less frequent assay of external QC materials.

The need to verify the clinical acceptability of results may support more frequent process control sampling than based strictly on method stability characteristics, or on regulatory minimum requirements. More frequent QC sampling is appropriate to avoid the situation of discovering a methodological problem after the physician has acted on the laboratory

Table 10–1 Common Sources of Measurement Variability

Source	Time interval for fluctuation	Likely statistical distribution
Pipet volume	Short	Gaussian
Instrument temperature control	Short or long	Gaussian or other
Electronic noise in the measuring system	Short	Gaussian
Calibration cycles	Short to long	Gaussian or shift (periodic step)
Reagent deterioration in storage	Long	Drift
Reagent deterioration after opening	Intermediate	Cyclic, periodic drift/step
Calibrator deterioration in storage	Long	Drift
Calibrator deterioration after opening	Intermediate	Cyclic, periodic drift/step
Control material deterioration in storage	Long	Drift
Control material deterioration after opening	Intermediate	Cyclic, periodic drift/step
Environmental temperature and humidity	Variable	Variable
Reagent lot changes	Intermediate to long	Shift (random step)
Calibrator lot changes	Intermediate to long	Shift (random step)
Instrument maintenance	Variable	Gaussian, cyclic or shift (periodic step)
Deterioration of instrument components	Variable	Variable

results. For example, QC sampling performed on a 24-hour cycle might be performed at 9 a.m. If the QC results indicate a method problem, the erroneous condition could have started at any time during the previous 24 hours. If the problem had occurred at 3 p.m. the previous day, out of control results would have been reported for 18 hours, and the medical implication of those erroneous results must be considered. The cost of a medical error, or simply the cost of repeating the questionable patient samples, could be more expensive than a more frequent QC sampling schedule that would have detected the error condition in a more timely manner.

Establishing QC Target Value and SD that Represent a Stable Measurement Operating Condition

QC target values and acceptable performance limits are established to optimize the probability of detecting a measurement defect which is large enough to impact clinical care, while minimizing the frequency of 'false alerts' due to statistical limitations of the criteria used to evaluate the QC results. The measurement system must be correctly calibrated and operating within acceptable performance specifications, before the statistical parameters to be used to establish QC interpretive rules can be determined. Some sources of measurement variability are listed in Table 10–1. Measurement variability includes sources with short time interval frequencies, many of which can be described by Gaussian error distributions, and intermittent and longer time interval sources which can cause cyclic fluctuations over several days or weeks, gradual drift over weeks or months, and more abrupt shifts in results. Acceptance criteria for QC results must adequately account for all sources of variability in results that are expected to occur when the measurement system is performing to specifications.

A QC material must have a reliable target value for an analyte. This requires adequate statistical sampling of both the QC material and the typical sources of measurement variability during a period of time when the method is calibrated correctly and is exhibiting the expected imprecision associated with a stable measurement condition. The experimental design objective is to include all sources of variability in the measurement process to ensure a representative mean value. This objective is rarely met, because of longer-term variability components and the practical inability to account for all influences at the time of target value assignment. The generally accepted minimum protocol for target value assignment is to use the mean value from assaying a QC material a minimum of 20 times, on 20 different days (CLSI, 2006). Note that it is preferable to use a single bottle of QC material for the expected duration of its open vial use to account for analyte stability effects, rather than use a fresh bottle on each day of testing. If a 20-day protocol is not practical, provisional target values can be established with fewer data but should be updated when additional replicate results are available. When applicable, more than one method calibration should be represented in the 20-day sample to adequately include the variability associated with the calibration process.

Some QC materials are provided by the method manufacturer with pre-assigned target values and ranges that can be used to confirm the method meets the manufacturer's specifications. Such assigned values can be used initially by the laboratory. It is recommended that both the target value and SD be re-evaluated and adjusted by the laboratory after adequate replicate results have been obtained, because the QC interpretive rules used in a single laboratory should reflect performance for the method in that laboratory. The acceptability limits suggested by a manufacturer may reflect sources of variability, such as between instrument, between reagent lots and between calibrator lots, that may be greater than the variability expected for a method used in an individual laboratory. QC materials with assigned target values are available from third party manufacturers (i.e., manufacturers not affiliated with the method manufacturer). Caution should be used with third party QC materials that have preassigned values, because the target values and SD may have been assigned using protocols that do not adequately reflect method performance, and noncommutability may limit applicability of those values for some methods.

Once a target value has been assigned to a QC material, a standard deviation (SD) must be assigned that represents the typical imprecision of the method when it is performing according to its design specifications. An SD is the conventional way to express the method variability, even though there are non-Gaussian components of variability in the QC results, because the statistical packages in instrument and laboratory computer systems are designed for QC data analysis based on mean and SD parameters. An SD based on the data from the 20-day target value assignment, or a 30-day monthly summary, has a large uncertainty (typically 30% for $N = 20$; CLSI, 2006) and is very unlikely to include all sources of variability expected over a longer time interval.

When previous experience with a method exists, it is recommended to determine the SD for stable measurement performance from the cumulative SD over a 6- to 12-month period to ensure all expected sources of variation are represented. Figure 10–5 illustrates the fluctuation in SD when calculated for monthly intervals compared to the relatively stable value observed for the cumulative SD after a period of 6 months. Note that the cumulative SD is not the average of the monthly values. Different sources of long-term variability, which occur at different times during the use of a method, may not be represented in a monthly SD. However, the cumulative SD includes contributions from all sources of variability as they occur and as they are reflected in the individual QC results. Consequently, the cumulative SD will typically be larger than the monthly values, and better represents the actual variability of the method. If the imprecision expected during normal stable operation is underestimated, then the acceptable range for QC results will be too small and the false alert rate will be unacceptably high. If the imprecision for the stable condition is overestimated, then the acceptable range will be too large and a significant measurement error might go undetected.

It is important to include all valid QC results in the calculation of SD. A valid QC result is one that was, or would have been, used to verify acceptable assay performance and reporting of patient results. Only QC results that were, or would have been, responsible for not releasing patient results should be deleted (with documentation) from summary calculations. If selective editing of QC results occurs, the method SD will be inappropriately small, which will produce inappropriately small evaluation limits and an increase in false QC alerts with concomitant reduction in the effectiveness of statistical process control.

When a method has been established in a laboratory, and a new lot of QC material is being introduced, the target value for the new lot is used with the cumulative SD from the previous lot to establish acceptable ranges for the new lot of QC material. This practice is appropriate because in most cases the measurement imprecision is a property of the method and equipment used and is unlikely to change with a different lot of QC material. If the target values for the old and new lots are substantially different, there may be a different imprecision observed, and an adjustment to the SD may be necessary as additional experience with the new lot is accumulated.

If a new method is introduced for which there is no historical performance information, then the SD for stable performance must be

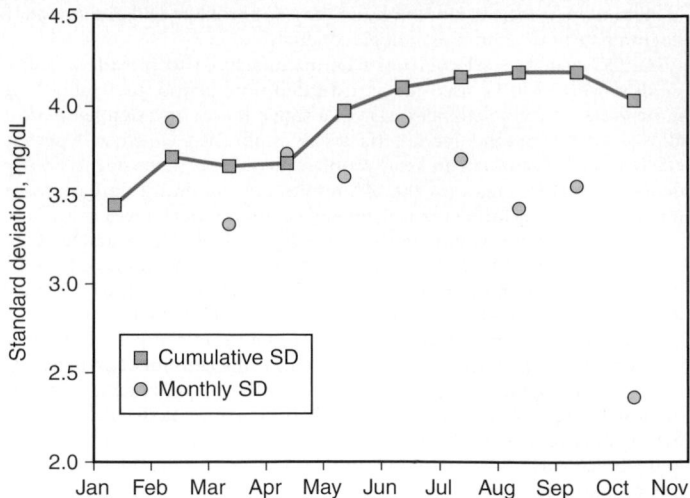

Figure 10–5 Cumulative SD vs. single monthly values calculated from the data in Figure 10–7.

Table 10–2 Abbreviation Nomenclature to Express QC Rules Based on Gaussian (Normal) Distribution of Imprecision

Rule	Meaning	Detects
1_{2S}	One observation exceeds 2 SD from the target value	Imprecision or systematic bias
1_{3S}	One observation exceeds 3 SD from the target value	Imprecision or systematic bias
2_{2S}	Two sequential observations, or observations for two QC specimens in the same run, exceed 2 SD from the target value in the same direction	Systematic bias
$2_{2.5S}$	Two sequential observations, or observations for two QC specimens in the same run, exceed 2.5 SD from the target value in the same direction	Systematic bias
R_{4S}	Range between two observations in the same run exceeds 4 SD	Imprecision
10_m	Ten sequential observations are on the same side of the target value (mean)	Systematic bias, trend
8_{1S}	Eight sequential observations for the same material exceed 1 SD in the same direction from the target value	Systematic bias, trend

established using data available from the method validation and target value assignment of the QC materials. Additional information on expected method performance can be obtained from the method manufacturer, and from the method's performance in interlaboratory QC and/or proficiency testing programs. In this case, the initial SD and evaluation criteria will need to be monitored closely and adjustments made as additional experience allows the inherent measurement imprecision from all sources to be reflected in the cumulative SD.

Establishing Rules to Evaluate QC Results

The choice of criteria for interpretation of QC results are based on the probability of detecting a significant analytical error condition with an acceptably small false-alert rate. The desired process control performance characteristics must be established for each analyte before the appropriate QC evaluation rules can be selected.

The conventional way to express QC interpretive rules is with an abbreviation nomenclature popularized among clinical laboratories by Westgard (Westgard, 1981) and summarized in Table 10–2. Note that fractional standard deviation intervals are permissible as in the $2_{2.5S}$ example. Other techniques such as cumulative sum or exponentially weighted moving averages are also used to monitor for bias trends over longer time periods (Ryan, 1989).

Power function graphs were developed (Westgard, 1979) to express the probability that a QC interpretive rule will detect an analytical error. Westgard's statistical model assumed Gaussian (normal) error distributions

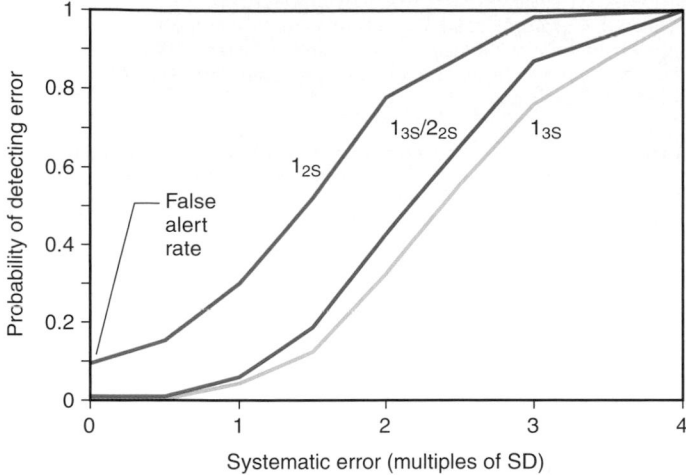

Figure 10–6 Power function graph for ability of different QC interpretive rules to detect systematic error using two controls in a run. The systematic error is expressed in number of SD from the target value. (After Westgard 1979, with permission.)

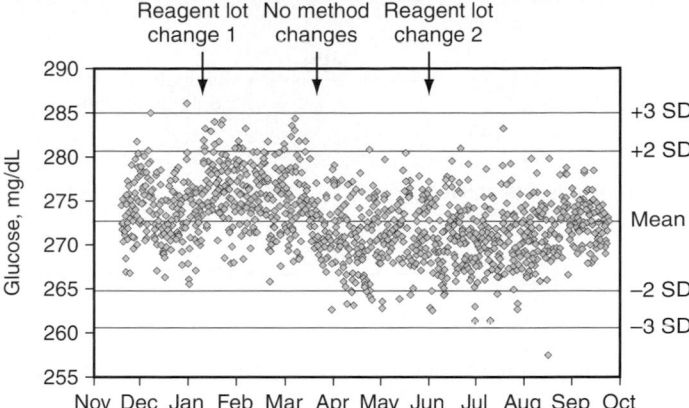

Figure 10–7 Levey–Jennings (Shewhart) plot of QC results ($N = 1232$) for a single lot of QC material used for a 10-month period. (Reprinted with permission from Miller WG: Quality Control. *In* Clarke WA, Dufour DR (eds): Contemporary practice in clinical chemistry. Washington DC, AACC Press, 2006.)

Table 10–3 Empirical Multi-rule for the QC Data in Figure 10–7

Multi-rule components	Type of variability detected
1_{3S}	Imprecision or bias
$2_{2.5S}$	Bias
R_{4S}	Imprecision
$8_{1.5S}$	Bias trend

and, despite the fact that non-Gaussian error distributions exist in measurement systems, has provided useful guidelines for selecting rules to interpret QC results. Other literature reports have addressed rules selection criteria using other statistical models and assumptions regarding distribution of errors (Parvin, 1997a,b; Westgard, 1992; Linnet, 1989).

Figure 10–6 shows a power function graph which plots the probability of detecting a measurement error (y-axis), which is the probability that a particular interpretive rule will be violated, vs. a systematic bias of known magnitude in a result (x-axis). When evaluating interpretive rules, it is common practice to express the magnitude of an error in multiples of the standard deviation for the method (i.e., standard deviation intervals, SDI). For example, the 1_{2S} rule is violated if a single QC result is > 2 SD from the target value. From Figure 10–6, for the 1_{2S} rule, a result with a systematic bias of 1 SD (x-axis) has a 0.35 probability (y-axis) to exceed a total of 2 SD from the target value (1 SD from the bias, plus 1 SD from the imprecision in the results). Thus, a 1_{2S} interpretive rule has a 35% probability of detecting a systematic error which is 1 SD in magnitude. The three lines in Figure 10–6 represent the probabilities of the different interpretive rules to detect systematic biases of various magnitudes. Similar graphs can be determined for other interpretive rules for both systematic bias and imprecision error conditions.

Note in Figure 10–6 that none of these interpretive rules has a 100% probability of detecting a systematic bias until the error becomes relatively large. The 1_{2S} rule has a good probability of detecting errors (e.g., almost 90% probability of detecting a 2.5-SD bias) but a high false-alert rate indicated by the y-intercept (note the pointer showing that, due to imprecision, there is a 10% probability of indicating an error condition for zero bias). Because of this high false-alert rate, it is not recommended to use a 1_{2S} rule. The 1_{3S} rule has a low false-alert rate, but a lower probability of detecting an error (e.g., a 55% probability of detecting a 2.5-SD bias). It is recommended to improve the efficiency of QC interpretive rules by combining two or more rules and applying them simultaneously as a multi-rule criterion. For example, the $1_{3S}/2_{2S}$ multi-rule identifies an error condition if either one control exceeds ± 3 SD from the target value, or if two controls exceed ± 2 SD in the same direction from the target value. In Figure 10–6, the $1_{3S}/2_{2S}$ multi-rule has a low false-alert rate similar to the 1_{3S} rule, but an improved probability of detecting an error (e.g. a 65% probability of detecting a 2.5-SD bias and a 90% probability of detecting a 3.2-SD bias). In this multi-rule example, the 1_{3S} component is sensitive to imprecision or large systematic bias, while the 2_{2S} component is sensitive to systematic bias.

A challenge for selecting interpretive rules for QC results is that the different types of variability listed in Table 10–1 occur in most contemporary automated assay systems and introduce longer-term cyclic and step fluctuations in performance. These types of variability are not adequately described by Gaussian models for rules selection. Because almost all QC software used in instrument and laboratory computer systems is based on SDI interpretation, it is necessary to estimate an SD that approximates the long-term variability from both Gaussian and non-Gaussian influences. Thus data collected over a significant time period are necessary to determine an SD that represents typical variability when the method is stable and performing correctly.

Figure 10–7 shows results for a single lot of QC material used for a 10-month period for an automated glucose method. The glucose method stability and performance over the 10 months was considered acceptable for clinical use. The data for the first 49 days is the same as in Figure 10–5 and represents the initial experience with this lot of QC material. Examination of these data shows several fluctuations that cannot be described by a Gaussian statistical model. The first reagent lot change caused a step shift to higher values. The second reagent lot change had no effect on the QC results. Between March and April there was a transition to lower values which did not correspond to any maintenance or calibration events. Throughout the 10-month period, there were intervals of several weeks' duration when the imprecision was either better or worse than other time periods (also see Fig. 10–5). If the acceptance criteria had been based on the SD for the initial period, the subsequent longer-term fluctuations would have caused a large number of false alerts and a large amount of effort and expense troubleshooting what was actually the inherent variability in the method's technology when it was stable and performing as expected.

An empirical approach is frequently used to establish interpretive rules that will adequately encompass the observed variability in a method, and allow the laboratory director to base criteria on the clinical requirements for test performance. Table 10–3 gives an example of an empirically developed multi-rule based on the data in Figure 10–7. This multi-rule was selected based on a decision that the observed long-term method performance was acceptable for clinical requirements, and the combined acceptance criteria should identify potential method issues with a false-alert rate < 1%. This multi-rule had 0.6% false alerts when applied to the data in Figure 10–7 using the mean from the Nov–Jan period as the target value and the cumulative SD for the 10-month period to represent overall imprecision. If a 2_{2S} rule had been used instead of a $2_{2.5S}$ rule (across runs in this example), the false-alert rate would have increased from 0.6% to 1.8%. An $8_{1.5S}$ rule was used to provide detection of bias trends because it had zero false alerts compared to 0.5% for an 8_{1S} rule, and the SD was small enough that a bias trend of this magnitude would not adversely affect clinical interpretation of patient results. A rule that evaluates sequential results on one side of the mean can have a high false-alert rate when a method's actual error distributions are not Gaussian. For example, a 10_m rule for the data in Figure 10–7 would have increased the false-alert rate by 10.6%. Many contemporary analyzers are very stable and may produce QC results on one side of the mean for extended periods of time; however, the magnitude of the difference from the target value is small and may not imply a problem with the method nor with clinical interpretation of the patient results.

In practice it is frequently necessary to use empirical judgment to set QC rules that fit the actual data seen over a long enough time period to adequately accommodate the variability observed when the method is working correctly. Caution should be used when selecting QC interpretive rules based only on Gaussian models of imprecision because the rules may not correctly accommodate all the types of variability observed for

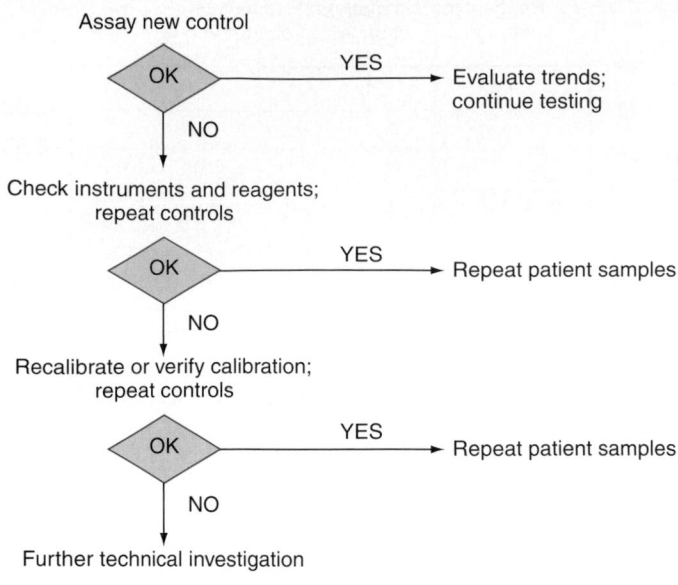

Figure 10–8 Generalized troubleshooting sequence following a QC alert. (Reprinted with permission from Miller WG: Quality Control. *In* Clarke WA, Dufour DR: (eds): Contemporary practice in clinical chemistry. Washington DC, AACC Press, 2006.)

Table 10–4 Example of Empirical Criteria for Patient Test Result Agreement between Repeated Assays; and for Agreement for a Single Patient Sample Measured on Multiple Instruments (for Selected Chemistry Analytes)

Analyte	Acceptance criteria (difference between results)
Albumin	0.4 g/dL
ALP	10 U/L or 10%*
ALT	10 U/L or 10%*
Amylase	15 U/L or 10%
AST	10 U/L or 10%*
Bilirubin, total	0.3 mg/dL or 10%*
Calcium, total	0.5 mg/dL
Chloride	4 mmol/L
Cholesterol	5%
CK	10 U/L or 10%
CO_2	4 mmol/L
Creatinine	0.2 mg/dL or 10%*
GGT	10 U/L or 10%
Glucose	6 mg/dL or 5%*
Iron	10 µg/dL or 10%
Lactate	0.32 mmol/L
LD	10 U/L or 10%
Magnesium	0.3 mg/dL
Phosphorus	0.4 mg/dL
Potassium	0.3 mmol/L
Protein, total	0.4 g/dL
Sodium	4 mmol/L
Triglycerides	10%
Urea nitrogen (BUN)	3 mg/dL or 10%*
Uric acid	0.4 mg/dL

* Whichever is greater.

many analytical systems. Whatever statistical approach is used, the balance between false alerts and the probability of detecting an error is improved when multiple rules are used in combination. When establishing rules to interpret QC results, it is important to remember that statistical process control can only verify that a measurement system is producing results that conform to the expected variability when the system is properly calibrated and in a stable operating condition. QC rules are intended to detect changes in calibration and changes in imprecision that are significant enough to require correction before patient results are reported.

It may be determined in the process of reviewing statistical parameters for QC data that a method's variability is too large to meet medical requirements. If the method is performing in a stable condition, the observed variability is an inherent limitation of the current technology. In this case, the only solutions are to improve the method performance or to use a different method. If the method performance cannot be improved and a better method is not available, the laboratory must accept the method limitations and communicate them to patient care providers. It is important in this circumstance not to make the QC limits or interpretive rules artificially stringent. This incorrect approach will not improve method performance, but will increase the QC false-alert rate, and decrease the efficiency and practicality of the statistical QC process.

Corrective Action when a QC Result Indicates a Measurement Problem

A QC alert occurs when a QC result fails an evaluation rule which indicates that an analytical problem may exist. A QC alert means there is a high probability the assay is producing results which are unreliable for patient care. When this condition occurs, it is necessary to take corrective action to investigate the cause for the QC alert. Figure 10–8 presents a generalized troubleshooting sequence. Repeating the QC measurement is not recommended because, with properly designed control rules, it is more likely that a measurement system problem exists, than the QC result was a statistical outlier. However, QC materials can deteriorate after opening because of improper handling and storage or due to labile analytes. Thus, repeating the measurement on a new specimen of the QC material may establish that the alert was caused by a deteriorated QC material rather than a method problem. In this situation, if the QC alert is resolved, testing of patient samples can resume. One caution is to consider a developing trend. If the repeat result is very near the acceptability limits, it means the method's results are close to unacceptability, and may indicate an impending problem that should be investigated as soon as possible. It is very important to include a trend-detecting QC rule, such as the $8_{1.5S}$ (in the Table 10–3 example), an exponentially weighted moving average, or a cumulative sum, in the multi-rule sequence.

When repeat testing of a new QC specimen does not resolve the alert situation, the instrument and reagents should be inspected for component deterioration, mechanical problems, etc. When the problem is identified and corrected, controls should be assayed to verify the correction, and any affected patient samples repeated. In many cases it will be necessary to recalibrate (or verify calibration), confirm correct method performance by assaying controls, then repeat patient samples.

In some cases, there may not be adequate patient specimen volume (quantity not sufficient; QNS) for repeat testing. In these situations, no results can be reported unless it is documented that the impact of the method defect on the original results was small enough to have minimal effect on clinical interpretation. A protocol to evaluate the clinical impact of the methodological problem is to repeat those specimens which have adequate volume. The repeated specimens must represent the concentration range of the QNS specimens, must represent the time span since the previous acceptable QC results, and should include a significant number of the total specimens originally assayed while the method was in the unstable condition. If the repeat results for this sample group are within established criteria for repeat testing of patient specimens, the original results for the QNS specimens can be reported. Otherwise, the original results for the QNS specimens are considered erroneous and no results can be reported. The laboratory director must establish acceptable criteria to determine if two sets of results agree adequately to permit reporting of original results for those specimens with inadequate volume to repeat the testing. As an example, Table 10–4 lists empirical criteria used in the author's laboratory for this purpose. The criteria for acceptability of repeated tests are based on method characteristics, population served and clinical requirements of the medical services.

Verifying QC Evaluation Parameters Following a Reagent Lot Change

Changing method reagent lots can have an unexpected impact on QC results. Careful reagent lot cross-over evaluation of QC target values is

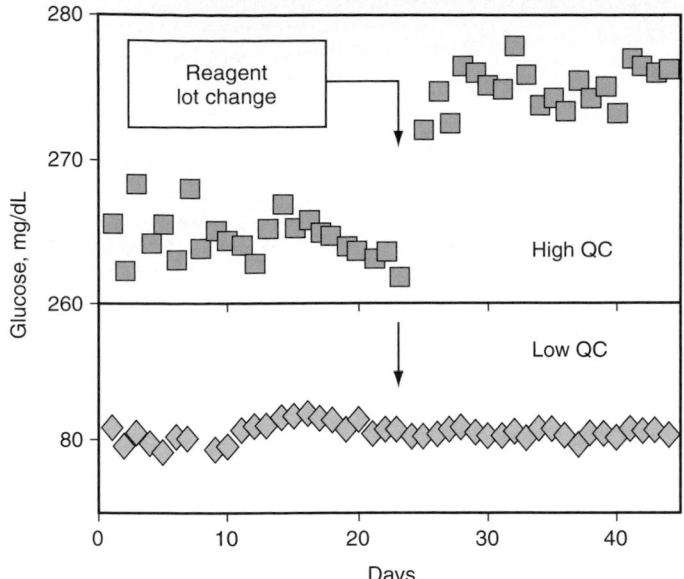

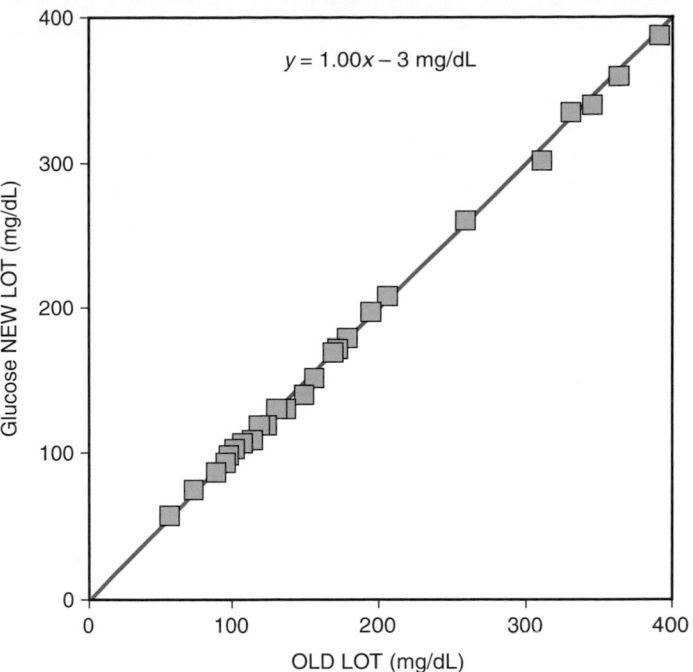

Figure 10–9 Levey–Jennings (Shewhart) graph showing impact of a reagent lot change on matrix interaction with QC materials. (Reprinted with permission from Miller WG: Quality Control. *In* Clarke WA, Dufour DR: (eds): Contemporary practice in clinical chemistry. Washington DC, AACC Press, 2006.)

Figure 10–10 Deming regression analysis of results from a patient sample comparison between old and new lots of reagent.

Table 10–5 Example of Empirical Acceptance Criteria for Deming Regression Parameters for Agreement between Results for Approximately 10 Patients' Samples

Analyte	Slope (difference from 1.0)	*y*-Intercept (±)
Albumin	5%	0.3 g/dL
ALP	6%	20 U/L
ALT	6%	10 U/L
Amylase	6%	20 U/L
AST	6%	10 U/L
Bilirubin, total	7%	0.2 mg/dL
Calcium, total	10%	1 mg/dL
Chloride	10%	15 mmol/L
Cholesterol	3%	10 mg/dL
CK	6%	25 U/L
CO_2	10%	3 mmol/L
Creatinine	5%	0.15 mg/dL
GGT*	6%	10 U/L
Glucose	5%	5 mg/dL
Iron	5%	7 µg/dL
Lactate	5%	0.3 mg/dL
LD	6%	25 U/L
Magnesium	10%	0.2 mg/dL
Phosphorus	5%	0.4 mg/dL
Potassium	6%	0.3 mmol/L
Protein, total	5%	0.3 g/dL
Sodium	10%	15 mmol/L
Triglycerides	10%	25 mg/dL
Urea nitrogen (BUN)	5%	2 mg/dL
Uric acid	5%	0.3 mg/dL

necessary. Because the matrix interaction between a QC material and a reagent can change with a different reagent lot, the QC results may not be a reliable indicator of a method's performance for patient specimens following a reagent lot change. In the example in Figure 10–9, the QC values for the high-level control shifted following the change to a new lot of reagents, but there was no change in results for the low-level control.

It is well documented that QC materials, and proficiency testing materials which are prepared similarly, have unpredictable matrix interactions with different methods and potentially with different reagent lots within the same method (Miller, 2003). For this reason, it is not possible to determine if the QC change in Figure 10–9 was caused by a calibration error with the new lot of reagent or by a difference in matrix interaction between the QC material and the new vs. old reagent lots. Note that it is also possible for the agreement in QC results for the other concentration QC material to have been an artifact caused by a different matrix interaction that masked a possible calibration error ('false negative'). Consequently, it is recommended to use native patient samples to verify the consistency of results between an old and new lot of reagents.

Figure 10–10 shows results for native patient samples assayed using both the old and new lots of reagent, represented in Figure 10–9, both of which have been calibrated according to the method manufacturer's instructions. The patient results span the analytical measurement range and have nearly identical values as indicated by the slope of 1 and small intercept of –3 mg/dL from the Deming regression analysis (Cornbleet, 1979; Linnet, 1993). Regression analysis is commonly used to compare results between two different reagent lots for the same method, between two instruments using the same method, or between two different methods. These data verify that the new reagent lot calibration agrees with the previous lot, and that current patient results can be directly compared with previous results. These data also confirm that the shift in QC target value seen in Figure 10–9 was due to a difference in matrix interaction with the new reagent lot.

There are no well-established guidelines for the number of patient samples to use in this type of comparison when reagent lots are changed. The Clinical and Laboratory Standards Institute (formerly known as NCCLS) guideline EP9 recommends a minimum of 40 patient samples for comparison of performance between two methods (CLSI, 2002a). This number is intended for validation of a new method, and is not practical for verification of reagent lot changes. The laboratory should use enough patient samples to represent the analytical measurement range for the assay, and establish acceptance criteria consistent with the number of samples used and the clinical requirements for the method. Table 10–5 lists empirical acceptance criteria used in the author's laboratory for agreement between results for 10 patients' samples measured using both old and new lots of reagent. Ideally the slope should be 1 with a zero intercept. However, the criteria need to reflect the relatively large confidence intervals associated with a small number of observations.

Figure 10–11 illustrates the recommended procedure to verify method performance when changing reagent lots, and to confirm or adjust the target value for a QC material when a different matrix interaction is observed with a new reagent lot. The first step is to verify that the calibration of the new reagent lot produces results for native patient samples that are consistent with the previous lot. If a problem is identified, the calibration of the new reagent lot must be investigated and corrected. Once the results for patients are acceptable, the second step evaluates results for the QC material to determine if the target value is correct for use with the new lot of reagent(s). If the target value has changed, it must be adjusted to reflect the correct value to be used with the new lot of reagents. In making this adjustment, the laboratory is compensating for the altered

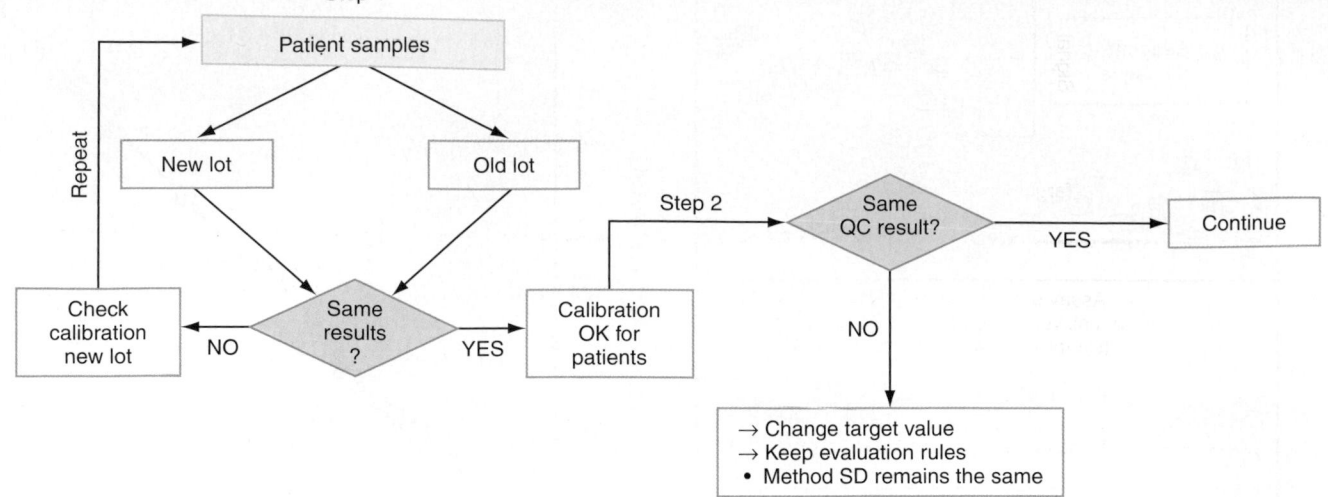

Figure 10–11 Strategy for assessment of potential matrix impact on QC materials following a reagent lot change.

matrix interaction of the QC material with a different lot of reagent(s). The native patient sample results, not the QC results, are the basis to verify the method calibration is consistent with that of the previous reagent lot.

The SD used to evaluate QC results will not typically change when a new lot of reagent(s) is put into service. The SD represents the expected variability when the method is stable and performing according to specifications. In most cases, the variability of a method will be the same with any lot of reagent(s); however, there may be occasional exceptions requiring adjustment of the SD. The QC material has not changed; however, the matrix bias between the QC material and the new reagent(s) may be different from that of the previous lot of reagent(s). Thus, when necessary, adjustment of the QC target value keeps the expected variability centered around the new QC target value so the QC interpretive rules will remain valid.

Verifying Method Performance Following Use of a New Lot of Method Calibrator

Figure 10–12 shows an example where a new lot of method calibrator caused a 20% increase in the values of the QC results. When a new lot of calibrator is used, with no change in reagents, there is no change in matrix interaction between the QC material and the reagents. In this case, the QC results provide a reliable indication of calibration status with the new lot of calibrator. If the QC results indicate a bias following use of a new lot of calibrator, the problem needs to be corrected to ensure consistent results for patient samples.

Some methods are packaged as kits which include reagents, calibrators and QC materials. In this case, the QC results could fail to identify a calibration shift, and it is required to assay native patient samples with the old and new kits to verify consistency of patient results. When possible, it is recommended to avoid changing lots of QC material at the same time as changing lots of reagents or calibrators.

Calibration Issues in Quality Control

Calibration of the analytical measurement system is a key component in achieving quality results. The principal reason to perform statistical process control is to verify that the calibration and the variability of the analytical system remain within limits expected for stable method performance. Specific techniques for calibration are unique to individual methods and will not be covered here. However, some general principles for implementing calibration procedures, and for verifying calibration uniformity among multiple methods can contribute to stability and clinical reliability of laboratory results.

Calibration of methods is most often performed by the laboratory using calibrator materials provided by the method or instrument manufacturer. In some cases, e.g., point of care devices, methods are calibrated during the manufacturing process and the laboratory performs a verification of that calibration. In either situation, traceability of result accuracy to the highest order reference system is provided by the method manufacturer. The method manufacturer's calibrator material and assigned target values are designed to produce accurate results with native patient samples assayed

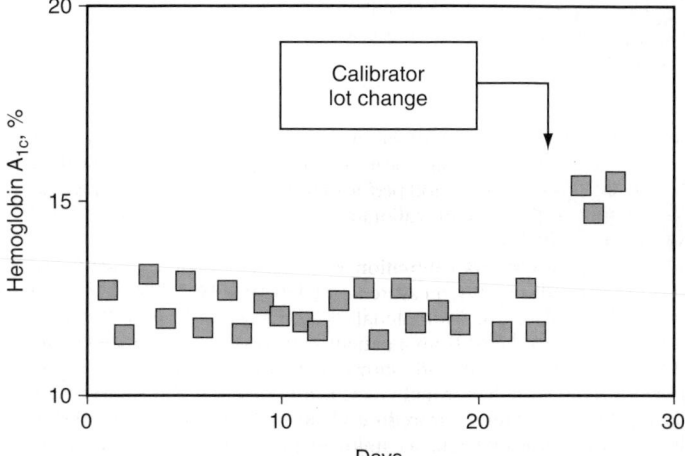

Figure 10–12 Levey–Jennings (Shewhart) graph showing impact of a calibrator lot change on QC results.

using that particular manufacturer's method. One manufacturer's product calibrator is not intended to be commutable with other methods, and laboratories should not use calibrator materials intended for one method with any other method. Use of a calibrator with a method for which it was not specifically intended can produce miscalibration and erroneous patient results.

In some cases, national and international reference materials may be used for calibration of routine methods. In most cases, these reference materials are intended for use with higher-order reference measurement procedures and may not be suitable to use directly with routine field methods. Laboratories should not use national or international reference materials to directly calibrate a routine method (or to verify the calibration of a routine method) unless commutability with native patient samples has been verified for that specific routine method. If the reference material is noncommutable, the routine method could actually be miscalibrated and produce erroneous patient results (Koch, 1988; Naito, 1993; Thienpont, 2003; Miller, 2003).

Optimal long-term stability of patient results is achieved if recalibration is only performed when the relationship between analytical measurement system response and specimen concentration has changed. Performing a method recalibration when the analytical system response has not changed introduces imprecision into the overall long-term method performance. This imprecision occurs because the new calibration will produce a slightly different relationship between analytical system response and specimen concentration. The size of the change will be governed by the inherent error budget of the assay system. The USA CLIA regulations section 493.1255 require calibration or calibration verification at least every 6 months, or more frequently if recommended by the method manufacturer (Department of Health and Human Services, 2003). Recalibration should be performed when necessitated by drift in method stability, which can be

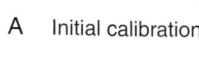

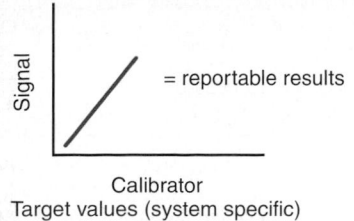

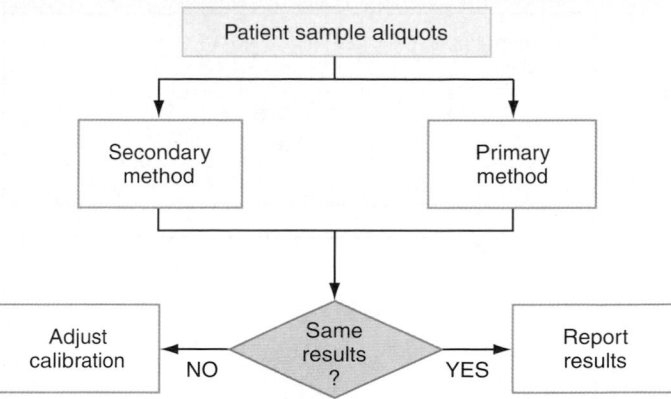

Figure 10–14 Process to evaluate agreement between methods, and to adjust calibration, if necessary, to achieve equivalent results from different methods.

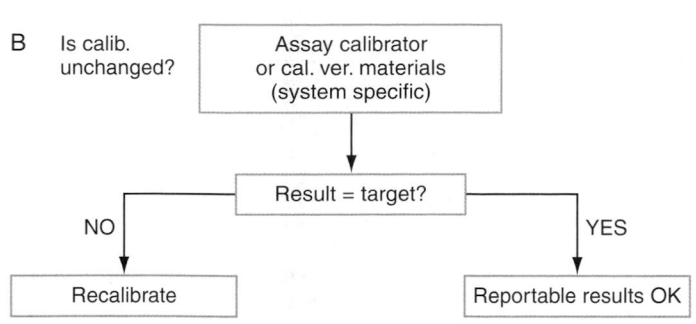

Figure 10–13 *A*, Calibration, and *B*, Calibration verification using recovery of method calibrators or other system-specific materials certified for calibration verification.

detected by QC results or other monitoring parameters, by changes in reagent lots, or following significant instrument maintenance. When there has been no change in method performance parameters, it is recommended to verify that the current calibration is valid rather than perform a recalibration.

Figure 10–13*A* shows calibration of a method which establishes the relationship between the measurement signal and the quantitative value of analyte in the calibrator materials. This relationship is used to convert the measurement signal from a patient sample into a reportable value for the analyte. Figure 10–13*B* shows that verification of the method calibration can be performed to confirm that the calibration has not changed. One common procedure to verify calibration is to assay the method calibrator materials as 'unknowns.' Recovery of the target values indicates the measurement system calibration has not changed, and there is no reason to perform a recalibration because the same relationship between measurement signal and the quantitative value of analyte in the calibrators would be re-established. The laboratory must establish criteria for agreement with the calibrator target value. Conservative criteria for agreement, such as ±1 or ±1.5 SD from the target value, should be considered to avoid misinterpretation of the calibration status.

Another approach to verify calibration is to assay materials, provided by some routine method manufacturers, which are specifically intended for this purpose. It is important to recognize that such method manufacturer provided materials typically have matrix characteristics and target values which limit their use to only the specific methods claimed in the package insert, and cannot be used with any other manufacturer's methods. These calibration verification materials may have target values assigned which are specific for stated reagent lots, or may have values certified by the manufacturer to be suitable for all reagent lots. As discussed previously, national or international reference materials can only be used to verify calibration if they have been demonstrated to be commutable with native clinical specimens for the routine field method of interest. The reference material certificate of analysis should be reviewed for commutability documentation.

Third party QC materials are usually not suitable to verify calibration. These materials are typically not validated for commutability among different routine methods, and do not have target values that are traceable to reference systems.

Another approach to verify calibration is to perform a method comparison using native patient samples measured with another method known to be correctly calibrated.

Using Patient Data in Quality Control Procedures

Results from patient samples are used in four principal ways to support the QC processes in the laboratory:

- to delta check with a previous result for a patient
- to verify consistency of patient results when changing lots of reagent or calibrator for a method
- to verify consistency of patient results when an analyte is measured using more than one instrument or method in a healthcare system
- in a statistical process control scheme which uses the mean (or median) of patient results to monitor method performance

The second bullet has been described in the previous sections on changing reagent or calibrator lots. Because of the noncommutability of most QC materials, it is highly recommended to reanalyze specific patient samples to determine if they give the same results as those prior to the change in reagent lots.

Delta Check With a Previous Result for a Patient

Some types of laboratory errors can be identified by comparing a patient's current test result to a previous result for the same analyte. This comparison is called a 'delta check.' Specimen mix-ups and specimens altered by dilution with i.v. fluid are examples of errors that can be detected using delta checks. The previous result must be a specified time in the past such that the result is not likely to have changed physiologically during the interval. This limitation restricts the analytes which can be effectively monitored with a delta check. The difference between results must be sufficiently large to avoid excessive numbers of false alerts; however, as the difference threshold becomes larger, the number of potential problems missed also increases. Kazmierczak (2003) has reviewed delta check and other patient data based quality control procedures.

Verify Consistency Between More than One Instrument or Method

Another common use of patient results in a QC process is to verify consistency of patient results when an analyte is measured using more than one instrument or method within the same health delivery system. Good laboratory medicine requires that multiple instruments or methods for the same analyte be calibrated to give the same results for patient samples whenever possible. It may be necessary to modify the calibration settings of one measurement system to match another system's results. This strategy allows a common reference range to be used, provides continuity in results between encounters in different locations, and avoids clinical confusion regarding interpretation of laboratory results. The USA CLIA regulations section 493.1281 require that the relationship between test results performed using different methods or performed at multiple sites be evaluated twice a year (Department of Health and Human Services, 2003).

As illustrated in Figure 10–14, native patient sample aliquots are measured using two or more methods (or instruments) to confirm agreement or to adjust the calibration of different methods to achieve agreement in results for patient samples. Such an analysis design is frequently called a round robin. One method/instrument is chosen to represent the primary method to which others will be adjusted to achieve equivalent results. The primary method should be chosen based on quality and reliability of results with consideration of: its calibration traceability to national or international standards; its performance stability; its specificity for the analyte; and its susceptibility to interfering substances. An alternative approach to evaluate agreement between a larger number of methods/instruments in a round robin group is to use the mean of all the methods.

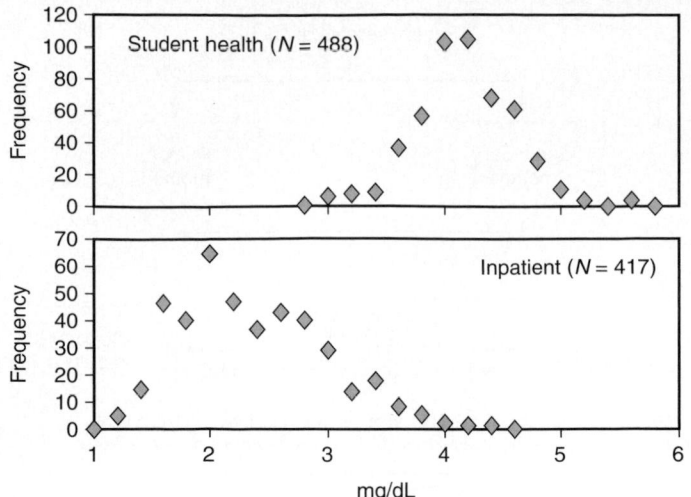

Figure 10–15 Histograms for distribution of sequential patient results for albumin from a student health outpatient clinic and a hospital general medicine inpatient unit.

Each method is evaluated for agreement with the mean, and calibration adjustments made to any methods/instruments as necessary to produce equivalent results among the group.

As mentioned previously for evaluating consistency following reagent lot changes, there are no well-established guidelines for the number of samples to use for verifying consistency of patient sample results. The laboratory will need to establish the frequency of evaluation and number of samples based on the stability of the methods, the frequency of reagent and calibrator lot changes, and the clinical requirements of the health delivery system. Common practices include splitting one or more individual patient samples, or a small pool from several samples, on a weekly basis for high-volume methods, a monthly or quarterly basis for lower-volume or very stable methods, or the regulatory minimum of every 6 months. A larger number of samples is recommended if the monitoring is performed less frequently. When establishing interpretation criteria, the laboratory needs to consider the limited statistical power for the number of results available, and to utilize trend monitoring techniques. For example, if one patient sample is tested weekly, the evaluation criteria for agreement will need to allow for the expected imprecision of the methods used, and rely more on the persistence of a trend to identify a method that may be performing differently from others in the group. Table 10–4 provides, as an example, empirical criteria used in the author's laboratory for evaluation of agreement based on a single patient sample assayed weekly among multiple instruments. A result outside the criteria is not acted on unless the situation persists for 2 or more weeks or the difference is large.

Results for QC materials should not be used for the purpose of verifying consistency of patient sample results assayed using different instruments or methods. This limitation is due to the common occurrence of noncommutability of QC materials between different methods. Even when more than one instrument/method from the same manufacturer is used, QC results should be used cautiously because there can be differences in the measured value for QC materials between different reagent lots, or due to differences in measurement details between different instrument models. It is recommended to use patient samples to verify agreement between multiple instruments.

Using Patient Data for Statistical Process Control

An additional use of patient results in a statistical QC process is to use the mean (or median) of patient results to monitor method performance. For a sufficiently large number of results, the mean (or median) value is frequently stable enough to be used as an indicator of method consistency over time. This approach can be used on a periodic basis by extracting data for a time period, e.g., 3–12 months, calculating the mean and SD for the distribution of results, and comparing one time period to another to determine if any changes have occurred. This type of periodic evaluation can identify changes in calibration stability or in overall imprecision for a method. The mean and SD can also be compared for consistency between multiple methods for the same analyte.

Selection of patient populations to sample must be made with consideration of the physiological homogeneity of results. Important considerations include parameters likely to influence the reference range: disease status, pediatric vs. adult, gender, and ethnic differences. Figure 10–15 shows an example of the potential impact of a nonhomogeneous sample of

Table 10–6 Proficiency Testing Participant Evaluation Report

Shipment date: 10/13/2003
Evaluation date: 11/21/2003

Test Units Method	Specimen	Reported result	Mean	SD	N labs	SDI	Limits of acceptability Lower	Upper
Calcium	1	9.6	9.92	0.23	587	−1.4	8.9	11.0
mg/dL	2	8.8	8.86	0.26	592	−0.2	7.8	9.9
Arsenazo	3	7.5	7.65	0.23	587	−0.7	6.6	8.7
dye	4	8.2	8.43	0.23	590	−1.0	7.4	9.5
Vitros 950	5	10.8	18.87	0.25	589	−0.3	9.8	11.9
Iron	1	190	192.5	7.0	397	−0.4	154	232
μg/dL	2	65	65.0	3.4	394	0.0	51	78
Pyridyl	3	74	69.2	3.2	395	+1.5	55	83
azo dye	4	**124**	**107.9**	**4.6**	395	**+3.5**	**86**	**130**
Vitros 950	5	277	260.9	8.8	396	+1.8	208	314

patients for distribution of albumin results for hospital general medicine inpatients compared to a student health outpatient clinic. The histograms are very different because the two patient groups differ in severity of disease, and in recumbent vs. supine position for blood collection, which influences vascular water volume and concentration of albumin.

Automated approaches have been described to determine the mean (or median) for groups of sequential patient results for use as a continuous process control parameter. These methods are called 'average of normals (AON)' or 'moving average' techniques and are suitable for use in higher-volume assays in chemistry and hematology (Westgard, 1996; Smith, 1996; Cembrowski, 1984; Ye, 2000; Kazmierczak, 2003). In general, these approaches evaluate sequential patient results over time intervals such as several hours to 1 or more days. The patients are typically grouped by age, gender and ethnicity to obtain homogeneous subgroups, and the results may be trimmed to remove extreme values so the remaining results are more reflective of patients without disease conditions that influence a particular analyte. The mean, or other statistical parameter, for a group of results is tracked to monitor method performance. Statistical procedures such as cumulative sum or exponentially weighted moving average are used to monitor trends in method calibration status (Ryan, 1989). These approaches can be very useful to supplement traditional QC sampling techniques to monitor a method's stability, and to monitor calibration uniformity between multiple methods in a laboratory system. Patient result based process control algorithms are useful for high-volume settings, but have not been widely adopted, because of lack of consensus guidelines for their use, and lack of computer support from instrument manufacturers and laboratory information system vendors.

Proficiency Testing

The process of external evaluation of method performance is referred to as proficiency testing (PT) or external quality assessment (EQA). PT allows a laboratory to verify that its results are consistent with those of other laboratories using the same or similar methods for an analyte, and thus to confirm it is using a method correctly. PT providers circulate a set of specimens among a group of laboratories. Each laboratory includes the PT specimens along with patient samples in the usual assay process. The results for the PT specimens are reported to the PT provider for evaluation.

Table 10–6 is an example of a typical evaluation report sent to a participating laboratory. Each reported result is compared to the mean result from all laboratories using the same method (called a peer group). The report also includes the SD for the peer group distribution of results, the number of laboratories in the peer group, and the standard deviation interval (SDI) which expresses the reported result as the number of SD it is from the mean value. The limits of acceptability are established by regulation in many countries, or are established by the PT provider for tests without regulatory criteria. The evaluation criteria are either a number of standard deviations from the mean value, a fixed percent from the mean value, or a fixed concentration from the mean value. In Table 10–6, the calcium acceptability criteria are ± 1 mg/dL from the mean value, and the iron criteria are ± 20% from the mean value.

Peer group evaluation allows a laboratory to verify that it is using a method according to the manufacturer's specifications and producing patient results that are consistent with those of other laboratories using the same method. In Table 10–6, the calcium results are in close agreement with the peer group mean (SDI ranges from − 0.2 to − 1.4). However, the iron results show more variability with one result + 3.5 SDI. Although that iron result is within the acceptability criteria, it is recommended to investigate the method because that SDI indicates a high probability of a method problem which may need to be corrected (see Interpretation of PT Results, below).

Many QC material manufacturers also provide a data analysis service which peer groups methods and calculates group statistics for performance evaluation. As with PT evaluation, this type of interlaboratory QC data analysis allows a laboratory to verify that it is producing patient results that are consistent with those of other laboratories using the same method.

Proficiency testing is an important component of a quality management program. In many countries, there are regulations requiring PT and specifying the evaluation criteria for acceptable performance. PT evaluation criteria are designed to evaluate the total error of a single measurement. The acceptability limits for PT include bias and imprecision components expected within a laboratory plus other error components that are unique to PT specimens such as: between laboratory variation in calibration; filling imprecision of the PT material vials; stability variability in the PT material both in storage/shipping and after reconstitution or opening in the laboratory; and variable matrix interaction with different lots of reagents within a peer group. Consequently, the acceptability limits for PT specimens are frequently larger than what might be expected for clinically acceptable total error with native patient samples.

PT is not offered for some analytes either because the test is new to the clinical laboratory or the analyte stability makes it difficult to include in a PT material. In these situations, the laboratory should use an alternative approach to periodically verify acceptable performance of the method. The Clinical and Laboratory Standards Institute has a guideline document which provides several approaches to verify method performance when formal PT is not available (CLSI, 2002b).

Noncommutability of PT Materials and Peer Group Grading

Peer group evaluation is used for PT because of limitations caused by noncommutability of the materials typically used as PT specimens. As discussed under the heading 'Selection of QC Materials' and 'Verifying QC Evaluation Parameters Following a Reagent Lot Change', the manufacturing process for QC and PT materials frequently introduces changes to the serum or other fluid matrix constituents such that the measurement response is different from that of a native patient sample (Miller, 2003). Matrix interference is unique to each combination of method and processed PT (or QC, or reference) materials, and can be quantitatively different for different method/material combinations for the same analyte. Several investigations have reported > 60% incidence of noncommutable materials for many different analytes (Ross, 1998; Miller, 1993, 2003, 2005).

Figure 10–16 illustrates the effect of noncommutable materials on interpretation of PT results. In this example, pooled native patient sera and PT specimens were assayed by the duPont Dimension analyzer and by the Abell–Kendall reference method for cholesterol (Naito, 1993). The Abell–Kendall method is known to be unaffected by matrix-induced changes in PT specimens (Ellerbe, 1990). The patient samples showed excellent agreement between the two methods (average bias = 0.2%). However, the PT materials had a large negative bias (− 9.5%) with this method. This apparent bias for the PT specimens was due to noncommutability of the PT specimens between the duPont method and the reference method. If the routine method accuracy vs. the reference method was erroneously evaluated, and the calibration was erroneously adjusted based on PT results, the results for native patient samples would then be incorrect. The PT results were still valuable to judge the performance of laboratories using the duPont method, because the matrix interference was uniform within this peer group. Thus, if an individual laboratory's results agreed with those of the peer group, the individual laboratory could conclude the method was performing as expected. However, the accuracy of the duPont method for patient samples could not be evaluated from the PT results. A separate evaluation splitting native patient samples between the field method and reference method would be necessary to evaluate accuracy for patient samples.

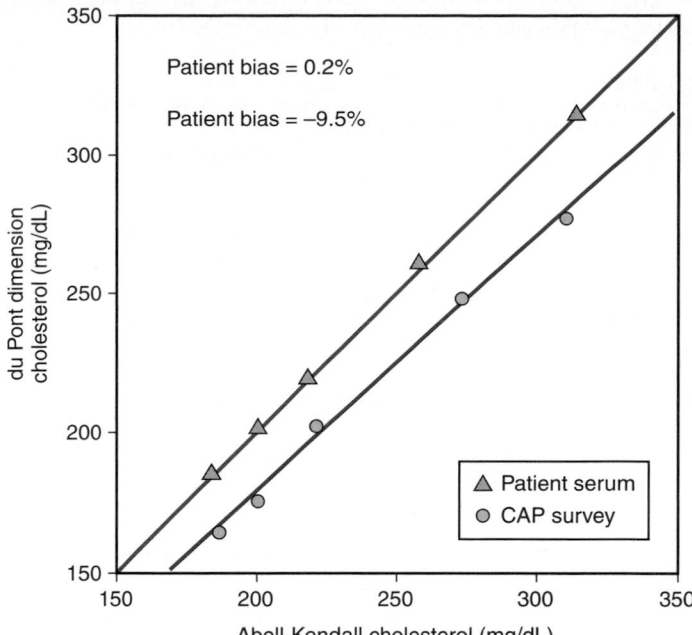

Figure 10–16 Example of noncommutability between PT materials and native patient samples for a specific method. (After Naito 1993, with permission.)

Reporting PT Results when One Method is Adjusted to Agree with Another Method

It is good laboratory practice (and consistent with USA CLIA regulations section 493.1281; Department of Health and Human Services, 2003) to adjust the calibration of different methods for the same analyte, used within a health delivery system, so the results for patient samples are the same irrespective of which method was used. In this situation, it is important to report PT results correctly so they can be properly evaluated against the peer group target value. The peer group target value reflects the method calibration established by the method manufacturer. For an individual laboratory's PT result to be evaluated against the peer group mean, that individual result must be reported to the PT provider with any user-applied calibration adjustment removed so the reported result is consistent with the manufacturer's nonadjusted calibration. The most convenient way to remove a calibration adjustment is to first assay the PT specimens with the method calibration adjustment in the measurement system as would be the usual assay process for patient samples. After the assay, adjust the PT results 'in reverse' by mathematically removing the calibration adjustments. One should not recalibrate the instrument with a new set of calibrators for the purpose of assaying PT specimens, because this practice would violate regulations requiring the PT material to be assayed in the same manner as patient samples.

For example, a laboratory has performed a native patient sample comparison between glucose Method A used in the main laboratory and Method B used in a satellite laboratory. Method B gives consistently 10% higher results. Method B is then adjusted to agree with Method A by putting the adjustment factor 0.9 in the Method B instrument to automatically multiply each measured result by 0.9 to lower the reported result by 10%. When reporting PT results from Method B, it is necessary to remove the 0.9 factor to allow the reported result to be compared to the peer group mean of measured results from all laboratories using Method B. Removing the 0.9 factor is accomplished by multiplying the reported PT result from Method B by the factor 1.1 to increase its numeric value by 10% to the nonadjusted value which was actually measured by the instrument according to the manufacturer's defined calibration procedure. This process allows the PT result measured by Method B to be appropriately evaluated by comparison to its peer group. It permits the PT specimen to be assayed in the same manner as the patient samples, and the numeric result reported to the PT provider to reflect the actual measured result using the manufacturer's recommended calibration settings.

Interpretation of PT Results

An individual laboratory's PT results can confirm that the method's results are in agreement with other laboratories using the same method or measurement principle. This condition verifies that the laboratory is using

Table 10–7 Examples of Causes for PT Failures

Condition	Examples
Technical problem with a method	Calibration problem
	Inadequate maintenance causing increased imprecision
	Deterioration of reagents
	Deterioration of other components
	Inadequate environmental control in the laboratory
Incorrect procedure	Incorrect dilution process
	Incorrect calculation of result
	Specimen allowed to evaporate
Incorrect handling of the PT specimen	Incorrect reconstitution
	Incorrect mixing
	Incorrect storage conditions
Incorrect reporting of PT result	Failure to convert measurement units to those required for the PT report
	Failure to identify correct method used
	Transcription error on report form
Problem with the PT material	Analyte not stable in PT material
	Interfering substance in PT material
	Specimen mishandled during shipping to laboratory

After Hoeltge, 1987.

the method correctly and in conformance with the manufacturer's specifications.

If an unacceptable PT result is identified, it is necessary to investigate the method for possible causes and take any corrective action necessary. Even when a PT result is within the acceptability criteria, it is good laboratory practice to investigate PT results that are greater than approximately 2.5 SDI from the peer group mean. When the SDI is 2.5, there is only a 0.6% probability of the result being within the expected distribution for the peer group; consequently, there is a good probability of a method problem which may need to be corrected. In addition, PT result(s) that have been near the failure limit for more than one PT event, even if the result(s) have passed the PT acceptance criteria, should initiate a review for systematic problems with the method. These practices support identification of potential problems before they progress to more serious situations.

Common causes for PT failure are listed in Table 10–7. Incorrect handling and reporting are potentially unique to PT events and may not reflect the same process used in the laboratory for patient results. Nonetheless, these situations reflect attention to detail which is a necessary attribute for quality laboratory testing. Occasionally the PT material may have a defect which causes it to perform inappropriately for all or a subgroup of methods. In this case, the PT provider will identify the situation and not grade participants for that specimen.

Investigation of an unacceptable PT result, and any corrective action taken, must be documented and reviewed by the appropriate supervisory individual (usually the laboratory director). PT results are always received several weeks after the date of testing. Consequently, a review of quality control, reagent logs, calibration and maintenance records for the date of the test and the preceding several weeks or months is necessary. If review of these records suggests a stable operating condition, and review of the PT material handling and documentation does not identify a cause for the erroneous PT result, it may be concluded the PT failure was a random event. The investigative steps, data reviewed, and conclusions from the review must be documented in a written report of the unacceptable PT result.

PT providers also include a summary report which includes the mean and SD for all the peer groups represented by the participant's results; similar reports are available from interlaboratory QC programs. Summary reports are very useful but must be interpreted with knowledge of the limitations of noncommutable specimens. The peer group mean and SD are useful to evaluate the uniformity of results between laboratories in the same peer group, to confirm an individual laboratory is using the method correctly as designed by the manufacturer, and to evaluate the consistency of an individual laboratory's method performance relative to the peer group over extended periods of time from one PT event to the next (trend monitoring). The summary information also allows evaluation of the imprecision of various method groups, and the number of users of each method group identifies methods which are in common use.

The frequent occurrence of noncommutability of PT materials makes it incorrect to use PT summary reports to compare an individual laboratory's result to the peer group mean for another method group, to compare method peer group mean values to each other, or to compare an individual method peer group value to a value assigned by a reference measurement procedure. The noncommutability limitation also prevents evaluation of the accuracy (trueness) of a method peer group for native patient samples, and makes it invalid to use PT (or QC) results to infer the agreement for patient results between different methods for the same analyte.

Accuracy-Based PT Programs

In special cases, PT providers have used commutable specimens in PT programs. Commutable specimens have typically been prepared by pooling native clinical samples with minimal processing or additives to avoid any alteration of the sample matrix. To achieve specimens with abnormal levels of analytes, donors can be identified with known pathologic conditions, or blood and serum units from a general donor population can be prescreened for selected analytes. When commutable PT specimens can be prepared, then the results from all laboratories reflect results that would be expected if native patient samples were sent to each of the different laboratories. Thus, agreement between laboratories (called harmonization) and between different methods can be correctly evaluated. The agreement between an individual laboratory result and the reference measurement result (accuracy), and the agreement between a method group mean value and the reference measurement result (called trueness) can be evaluated when a reference measurement procedure is available for an analyte.

For example, the College of American Pathologists Glycohemoglobin Survey has for many years used pooled freshly collected whole blood from both normal and diabetic donors. The target values for the pooled blood are assigned by reference measurement procedures for hemoglobin A_{1c}. In this survey, the accuracy of individual laboratory results, and the trueness of method group mean values, can be evaluated because the PT materials are commutable with native patient specimens. The method group trueness can be used by the respective method manufacturers to monitor the effectiveness of their calibration processes.

PT programs have included a commutable specimen on an occasional basis to evaluate individual laboratories and method groups for agreement with reference measurement procedures and for harmonization of results between laboratories and method groups (Miller, 2003, 2005; Palmer-Toy, 2005; Steele 2005). It has been challenging to prepare commutable materials for use in large PT programs. The Clinical and Laboratory Standards Institute has consensus protocols to validate commutability (CLSI, 2001, 2005), and other approaches for validation have been published (Baadenhuijsen, 2002; Franzini, 1993; Rej, 1993; Bretaudiere, 1981).

References

Baadenhuijsen H, Steigstra H, Cobbaert C, et al: Commutability assessment of potential reference materials using a multicenter split-patient-sample between-field-methods (twin-study) design: study within the framework of the Dutch project 'Calibration 2000,' Clin Chem 2002; 48:1520–1525.

Bretaudiere J-P, Dumont G, Rej R, Bailly M: Suitability of control materials. General principles and methods of investigation. Clin Chem 1981; 27:798–805.

Cembrowski GS, Chandler EP, Westgard JO: Assessment of 'average of normals' quality control procedures and guidelines for implementation. Am J Clin Pathol 1984; 81:492–499.

CLSI: Preparation and Validation of Commutable Frozen Human Serum Pools as Secondary Reference Materials for Cholesterol Measurement Procedures; Approved Guideline C37-A. Wayne, PA, Clinical and Laboratory Standards Institute, 1999.

CLSI: Method Comparison and Bias Estimation Using Patient Samples; Approved Guideline EP9-A2. Wayne, PA, Clinical and Laboratory Standards Institute, 2002a.

CLSI: Assessment of Laboratory Tests When Proficiency Testing is Not Available; Approved Guideline GP29-A. Wayne, PA, Clinical and Laboratory Standards Institute, 2002b.

CLSI: Evaluation of Matrix Effects; Approved Guideline, 2nd ed. EP14-A2. Wayne, PA, Clinical and Laboratory Standards Institute, 2005.

CLSI: Statistical Quality Control for Quantitative Measurements: Principles and Definitions; Approved Guideline C24-A3. Wayne, PA, Clinical and Laboratory Standards Institute, 2006.
Consensus document describing the principles and implementation guidelines for a statistical quality control system.

Cornbleet PJ, Gochman N: Incorrect least-squares regression coefficients in method comparison analysis. Clin Chem 1979; 25:432–438.

Department of Health and Human Services, 42 CFR Part 493, Medicare, Medicaid, and CLIA Programs;

Laboratory Requirements Relating to Quality Systems and Certain Personnel Qualifications; Final Rule. USA Federal Register 68(16):3639–3714, 24 January 2003.

Clinical Laboratory Improvement Amendments of 1988; final rule containing the regulatory requirements for quality practices in laboratories in the USA.

Ellerbe P, Myers GL, Cooper GR, et al: Comparison of results for cholesterol in human serum obtained by the reference method and by the definitive method of the National Reference System for Cholesterol. Clin Chem 1990; 36:370–375.

Franzini C: Commutability of reference materials in clinical chemistry. J Int Fed Clin Chem 1993; 5:169–173.

Hoeltge GA, Duckworth JK: Review of proficiency testing performance of laboratories accredited by the College of American Pathologists. Arch Pathol Lab Med 1987; 111:1011–1014.

Kazmierczak SC: Laboratory quality control: using patient data to assess analytical performance. Clin Chem Lab Med 2003; 41:617–627.

Review of the strengths and limitations of specimen based QC, and the usefulness of several patient data based QC practices.

Koch DD, Hassemer DJ, Wiebe DA, Laessig RH: Testing cholesterol accuracy: performance of several common laboratory instruments. JAMA 1988; 260:2552–2557.

Levey S, Jennings ER: The use of control charts in the clinical laboratory. Am J Clin Pathol 1950; 20:1059–1066.

Linnet K: Choosing quality-control systems to detect maximum clinically allowable errors. Clin Chem 1989; 35:284–288.

Linnet K: Evaluation of regression procedures for methods comparison studies. Clin Chem 1993; 39:424–432.

Miller WG, Kaufman H, McLendon WW: College of American Pathologists Conference XXIII: matrix effects and accuracy assessment in clinical chemistry. Arch Pathol Lab Med 1993; 117(4):343–436.

Miller WG: Specimen materials, target values and commutability for external quality assessment (proficiency testing) schemes. Clin Chim Acta 2003; 327:25–37.

Review of commutability issues for QC and PT materials, the impact of noncommutability on use and interpretation of results, and examples of results using commutable materials for QC and PT applications.

Miller WG, Myers GL, Ashwood ER, et al: Creatinine measurement: state of the art in accuracy and inter-laboratory harmonization. Arch Pathol Lab Med 2005; 129:297–304.

Report of the value added when a commutable PT material was used, and the impact of noncommutable materials on interpretation of PT results.

Naito HK, Kwak YS, Hartfiel JL, et al: Matrix effects on proficiency testing materials: impact on accuracy of cholesterol measurement in laboratories in the nation's largest hospital system. Arch Pathol Lab Med 1993; 117:345–351.

Palmer-Toy DE, Wang E, Winter WE, et al: Comparison of pooled fresh frozen serum to proficiency testing material in College of American Pathologists surveys: cortisol and immunoglobulin E. Arch Pathol Lab Med 2005; 129(3):305–309.

Parvin CA: Quality-control (QC) performance measures and the QC planning process. Clin Chem 1997a; 43:602–607.

Parvin CA, Gronowski AM: Effect of analytical run length on quality-control (QC) performance and the QC planning process. Clin Chem 1997b; 43:2149–2154.

Rej R: Accurate enzyme activity measurements. Two decades of development in the commutability of enzyme quality control materials. Arch Pathol Lab Med 1993; 117:352–364.

Ross JW, Miller WG, Myers GL, Praestgaard J: The accuracy of laboratory measurements in clinical chemistry. A study of 11 routine chemistry analytes in the College of American Pathologists Chemistry Survey with fresh frozen serum, definitive methods, and reference methods. Arch Pathol Lab Med 1998; 122:587–608.

Ryan TP: Statistical Methods for Quality Control. New York, Wiley, 1989.

Shewhart WA: Economic control of quality of manufactured product. New York, Van Nostrand, 1931.

Smith FA, Kroft SH: Exponentially adjusted moving mean procedure for quality control. An optimized patient sample control procedure. Am J Clin Pathol 1996; 105:44–51.

Steele BW, Wang E, Klee GG, et al: Analytical bias of thyroid function tests: Analysis of a College of American Pathologists fresh frozen serum pool by 3900 clinical laboratories. Arch Pathol Lab Med 2005; 129(3):310–317.

Thienpont LM, Stockl D, Friedecky B, et al: Trueness verification in European external quality assessment schemes: time to care about the quality of the samples. Scand J Clin Lab Invest 2003; 63:195–201.

Westgard JO, Groth T: Power functions for statistical control rules. Clin Chem 1979; 25:863–869.

Westgard JO: Charts of operational process specifications ('OP-Specs charts') for assessing the precision, accuracy, and quality control needed to satisfy proficiency testing criteria. Clin Chem 1992; 38:1226–1233.

Westgard JO, Barry PL, Hunt MR: A multi-rule Shewhart chart for quality control in clinical chemistry. Clin Chem 1981; 27:493–501.

Initial paper describing the commonly used 'Westgard Rules' approach to interpreting QC results.

Westgard JO, Smith FA, Mountain PJ, Boss S: Design and assessment of average of normals (AON) patient data algorithms to maximize run lengths for automatic process control. Clin Chem 1996; 42:1683–1688.

Ye JJ, Ingels SC, Parvin CA: Performance evaluation and planning for patient-based quality control procedures. Am J Clin Pathol 2000; 113(2):240–248.

I

CHAPTER 11

Clinical Laboratory Informatics

Mark S. Lifshitz MD, Gary E. Blank PhD, Katherine Schexneider MD

KEY POINTS

- The laboratory information system (LIS) is typically part of a hospital or healthcare system network of clinical, registration, patient management, and financial systems that exchange information with one another.

- A comprehensive electronic patient record must address various global issues including how to establish positive patient identification, maintain patient confidentiality and synchronize data among disparate systems.

- The LIS supports workflow and information flow in all steps of the laboratory testing process, including patient registration, test ordering, sample collection, testing and reporting.

- Informatics plays a key role in assisting physicians to manage laboratory orders (e.g., clinical pathways and decision support systems) and results (e.g., clinical alerts, interpretive reports, and reflex tests). Together, these approaches maximize the usefulness of the laboratory to clinicians.

- Communication protocols have been developed to standardize data exchanges among various applications. Health Level Seven (HL7) is the most prevalent communication standard in healthcare. Logical Observation Identifier Names and Codes (LOINC) is a nomenclature standard that provides a set of universal names and codes for identifying laboratory test results. It can be used to identify a test in an HL7 message.

Clinical laboratory informatics has been defined as 'that aspect of the practice of pathology which focuses on the management (generation, collection, organization, validation, processing, storage, integration, interpretation, communication, and presentation) of information and systems in support of patient care decision-making, education, and research (Balis, 1993). It constitutes an ever-expanding portion of the practice of clinical pathology. Informatics permeates every aspect of the clinical laboratory operation and all steps in the pre-analytic, analytic and post-analytic stages.

The clinical laboratory has always been one of the most data-intensive areas of a hospital and, thus, one of the first departments to computerize information handling and test generation. For years, laboratories have used information systems (LIS) to communicate with laboratory analyzers and systems external to the laboratory like hospital information systems (HIS) or billing systems. In some instances, the LIS was the only clinical system used by physicians to order and view results. Radical changes have occurred in recent years. The LIS is no longer a standalone system or one that communicates with one or two external systems. The LIS is now part of a hospital or enterprise (healthcare system) network of clinical, registration, patient management, and billing systems. The laboratory exchanges information with these systems and must rely on them to send

it accurate patient information (like test orders); in return, the LIS provides clinicians with laboratory results. The ability to meet clinical needs depends as much on how well the LIS is integrated with other information systems as it does on how quickly the laboratory can produce a result. This, in turn, depends on two key elements: hardware, i.e., the communication backbone and how robustly it transmits data; and software, i.e., the LIS and external applications, specifically how the database files are built and how accurately they exchange information. Table 11–1 summarizes the key functions of many of the external systems that exchange data with the LIS and Figure 11–1 provides an overview of facilities and locations that interact with the LIS.

Clinical informatics includes all aspects of information technology, including hardware, software and communications. A comprehensive review of every facet of informatics is beyond the scope of this discussion. The purpose of this chapter is to review how informatics applies to the clinical laboratory with special emphasis on information flow and key developments and trends.

Information Flow

In the ideal world, all patient information would be held in electronic format and flow seamlessly from one system to another. While informatics is heading in the direction of a comprehensive (national) electronic medical record, many issues need to be addressed in order to reach that goal. First and foremost is a convention for identifying a patient to insure that all information is correctly associated with a patient. This is a fundamental patient safety issue. Other issues concern patient confidentiality (and patient permission to access medical records) and synchronization of information among different systems within a healthcare enterprise (Aller, 2001).

What follows is a brief overview of the information flow: the various steps that process and exchange information and key issues that pertain to each. Note that information flow and workflow are closely related – one impacts on the other. The LIS's main function is to support both of these interconnected activities. Table 11–2 provides an example of how the LIS is used to provide hospital laboratory services. Keep in mind that information flow (Figs 11–2 and 11–3) varies from one facility to another and that approaches and issues discussed in this chapter may not be applicable to all settings.

Patient Registration/Identification (ID)

A permanent and unique patient identification number is the basic organizational element in a patient-centered clinical information system. The registration process assigns the unique identifier, creates a patient record, and defines demographic data that is reused at each patient visit. It also includes information such as physician, patient location, diagnosis and date of service that may vary with each laboratory encounter (for example, every time an outpatient or inpatient has blood collected). The

Table 11.1 Information Systems and Applications Communicating with the Laboratory

System	Function
Hospital information system (HIS)	Clinical system that holds patient information (laboratory, radiology, medications, etc.) for one or more patient admissions. Often used in conjunction with paper history/physical charts though it can be integrated with the electronic medical record
Electronic medical record (EMR)	Popular in outpatient settings. Paperless chart is used to record history, physical and other findings, schedule appointments or follow-up, and manage clinical review of data (like laboratory results)
Enterprise data repository (EDR)	Clinical tool that contains longitudinal patient information collected from all inpatient and outpatient systems. Used to view patient data not to manage patients or order tests
Enterprise data warehouse	This is a research, not a clinical, tool. Provides a view across many different patients (generally anonymized) and permits the recognition of general patterns, and potentially the development of new knowledge about disease
Enterprise patient registration	Enterprise-wide (or hospital-wide) central registration system that assigns a master patient identifier and collects patient demographic information that is automatically sent to various downstream systems like the HIS or LIS. This approach ensures that all patient registration data is standardized among applications, e.g., the patient name is spelled the same and supports access to longitudinal patient information
Outpatient medical necessity	A program that checks for medical necessity of laboratory orders (see Ch. 12) can be a standalone system that is interfaced to an LIS or financial/billing system; or it can be a feature that is built into the order entry application of the LIS or financial/billing system
Financial/billing	The LIS can transmit test charges or tests performed (that are translated into charges by the billing system) in batch or in real time
Reference laboratory	Laboratory orders and results can be interfaced with non-enterprise laboratories
Governmental agencies	Electronic clinical laboratory reporting system (ECLRS) uses HL7/LOINC to automatically transmit communicable disease information from the LIS to the state departments of health or federal agencies. This is an important component of a national surveillance program for bioterrorism (see Ch. 13)
Other communication links	Point-of-care servers, commercial clients (MDs, clinics), other laboratory facilities in a health system network

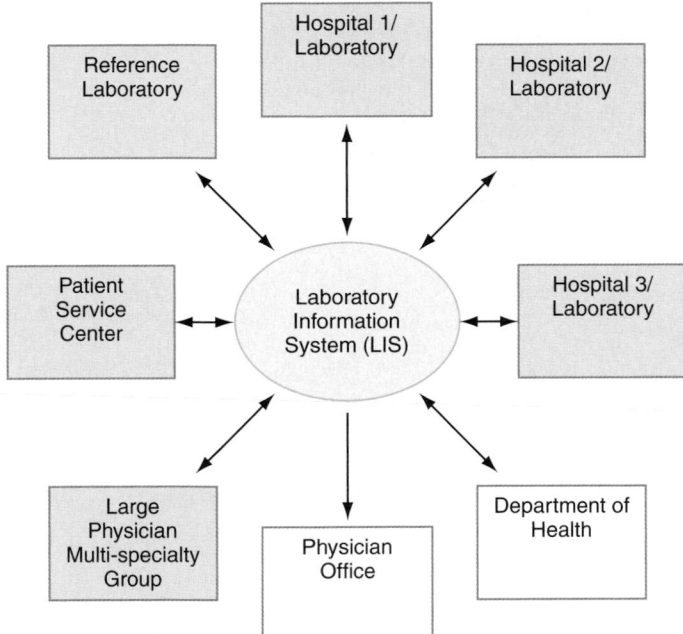

Figure 11–1 Overview: Example of facilities and locations that interact with the LIS bidirectionally (to exchange orders and results – purple shading) or unidirectionally (to receive results only – yellow shading).

LIS assigns a different *requisition* or *order* number to each one of these laboratory encounters.
Patient ID. Patient identification items include *patient name, social security number, age, birth date, sex,* race, address, phone number, *medical record number, master patient index* (see below), and insurance identification and billing information. The italicized items are generally considered key patient identifiers that can be used to positively identify a patient and distinguish one patient from another. This is especially important when deciding whether two patient records belong to the same patient (and should be merged) or are different. Record linkage is of critical importance in a blood bank (where one must search for previous testing and transfusion records), surgical pathology, hematopathology, and cytology. In these settings, it is particularly important to gather date of birth and sex (and, wherever possible, social security number) in addition to patient name. Accurate linkage is often impossible to achieve with only a patient name.

A patient identification number can include a social security number or a unique indexed number generated from and exclusive to the registration system. Every attempt must be made to keep a common reference to a patient's records and to reuse the identification number for recurring visits. Health systems with multiple institutions are gravitating to the introduction of a master (or enterprise master) patient index (EMPI), a number generated for the health system and used throughout all clinical information service modules in all associated facilities. A major benefit of an EMPI is that it can unify all of a patient's records even if each one is identified by a different medical record number. Another major benefit of an EMPI is that it can be used in conjunction with a front-end healthcare system-wide registration system to maintain patient demographics centrally for a variety of information systems, and eliminate the need for each system (laboratory, radiology, physician office) to maintain its own patient demographics. In this way, patient demographics, such as address or insurance, can be updated centrally. Not only does it eliminate repetitive work, it improves accuracy in that a patient's name, for example, appears the same in each system. The EMPI does not preclude each downstream system from using another unique patient identifier since the EMPI can automatically link itself to each of these additional IDs. So, the laboratory can assign the patient its own unique number that is linked to the EMPI. Although there is a need, there is no immediate prospect of a national health identification number that could link a patient's medical records that are currently disseminated across many physicians and facilities.
Positive Patient Identification. A uniquely assigned patient number is of limited use if one cannot positively identify the patient. Thus, a variety of approaches, like bar-coded wristbands have been developed to identify patients in hospital settings. The *Radiofrequency Identification (RFID)* system is a new technology that provides hands-off, zero-error identification. It consists of a patient tag and a computerized scanner or reader. The 'smart' label or tag contains human-readable information, a bar code and an integrated circuit (IC) chip with memory. A small amount of radiofrequency energy ('excitation signal') is released from the scanner, energizing the RFID tag, which then emits a radiofrequency signal ('return signal') transmitting the patient's ID. Though several issues (e.g., data encryption and protocol standardization) are not completely resolved, RFID technology offers several benefits: passive operation and dynamic data storage, features that favor its use in sample collection and tracking, bedside testing, drug management, and infection control.

Test Orders

After patient identification, test requests are entered, indicating when the specimen was (or will be) collected, who collected it, the time of collection, tests to perform, and who ordered the tests. Order comments may include patient status (position, weight, physiological state), sample type (source of a culture – like wound or sputum), notification requirements (like call results), or clinical management attributes (like drug dosage – peak or trough level, times for physiological challenge studies). Laboratory orders should be entered (electronically or on paper) directly by the *physician*. Otherwise, orders must be translated by non-physicians and this may lead to transcription errors.

Table 11.2 Key Steps in Laboratory Information Flow for a Hospital Patient

Step	Description
Register patient	Patient record (e.g., ID#, name, sex, age, location, etc.) must be created in LIS before tests can be ordered. LIS usually automatically receives these data from a hospital registration system (when the patient is admitted)
Order tests	Physician orders tests on a patient to be drawn as part of the laboratory's morning blood collection rounds. The order is entered into the HIS and electronically sent to the LIS
Collect sample	Before morning blood collection, the LIS prints a list of all patients that have to be drawn and the appropriate number of sample bar code labels for each patient order. Each bar code has a patient ID, sample container type (e.g. red top tube) and laboratory workstation (that can be used to sort the tube once it reaches the laboratory). Another and increasingly popular approach is for patient caregivers or nurses to collect the blood sample. Immediately prior to collection, sample bar code labels can be printed (on demand) at the nursing station on an LIS printer
Receive sample	When samples arrive in the laboratory, their status has to be updated in the LIS from 'collected' to 'received'. This can be done by scanning each sample container's bar code ID into the LIS. Once the sample is 'received', the LIS transmits the test order to the analyzer that will perform the test
Run sample	The sample is loaded onto the analyzer and the bar code is read. Having already received the test order from the LIS, the analyzer knows which tests to perform on the patient. No worklist is needed. For manually performed tests, the technologist prints a worklist from the LIS. The worklist contains a list of patients and the tests ordered on each. Next to each test is a space to record the result
Review results	The analyzer produces the results and sends them to the LIS. These results are only viewable to technologists since they have not been released for general viewing. The LIS can be programmed to flag certain results, e.g., critical values, so that a technologist can easily identify what needs to be repeated or further evaluated
Release results	The technologist releases results. (Unflagged results are usually reviewed and released at the same time.) The LIS can also be programmed to automatically review and release normal results or results that fall within a certain range. The latter approach reduces the number of tests that a technologist has to review. Upon release, results are automatically transmitted to the HIS
Report results	Physician can view the results on the HIS screen. Reports are printed when needed from the LIS

CHAPTER 11: Clinical Laboratory Informatics

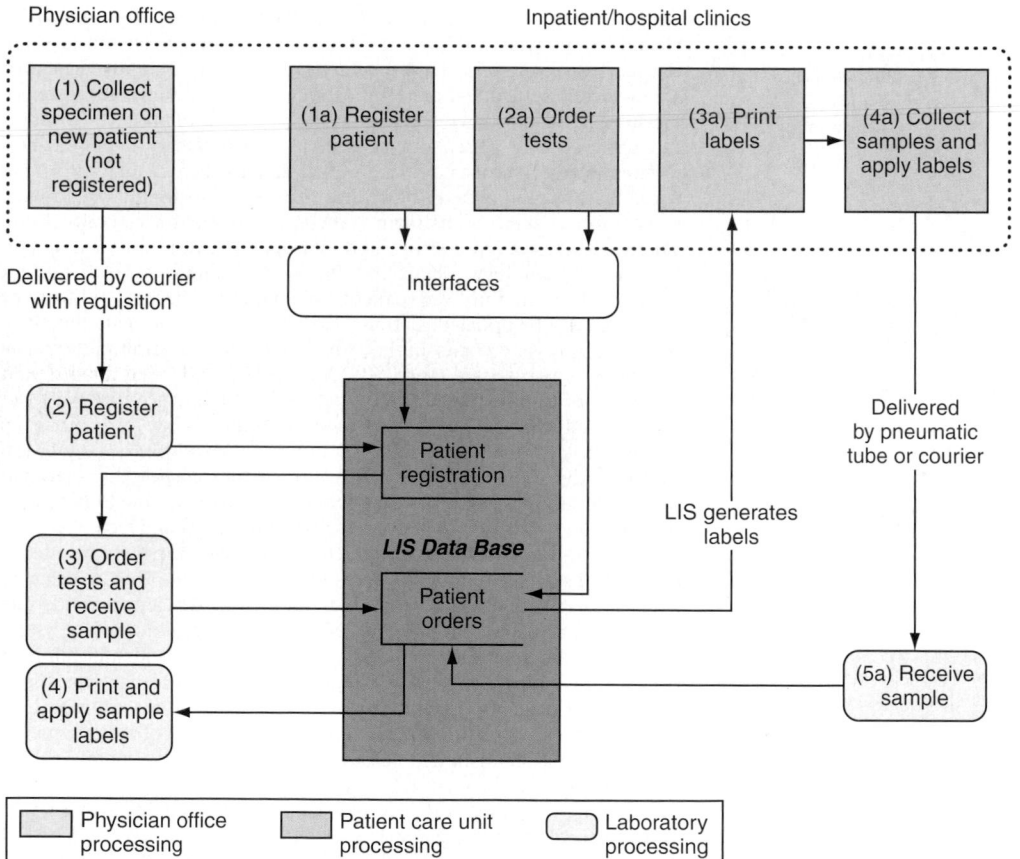

Figure 11–2 LIS role in ADT (registration) and order processing.

Electronic Order Entry. Ideally, the physician at the point of care should enter laboratory orders electronically. This has the greatest impact in reducing order errors (that might otherwise occur using a paper requisition); also, real-time interaction with an information system can be used to promote appropriate test utilization through the use of clinical pathways (clinical order sets or algorithms based on the patient's diagnosis). Computers are very useful and effective for some applications (information retrieval, calculations, data transmission), whereas humans are far more effective for others (judgment, reasoning from incomplete data). Structured, rule-based decision and forecasting (predictive) support systems can improve the quality of care while still supporting human judgment. For example, when a drug is ordered that can potentially impair renal function, the BUN/creatinine level can be displayed. If the values are elevated another drug could be considered. Decision (predictive) support during the order activities can vary from annotations reminding the staff of actions to take in conjunction with the order (e.g., patient should be fasting or order requires pathologist approval) to blocking an unacceptable order because it is ordered too frequently. Orders might also be cross-referenced to other ancillary systems like pharmacy to identify whether the therapeutic drug level request is a peak or trough level based on the last patient dosing. In the outpatient setting, the system might perform medical necessity checking (see Ch. 12) and ask the physician whether or not there are additional diagnosis codes applicable to the patient. These electronic interactions are only effective if physicians who can respond in

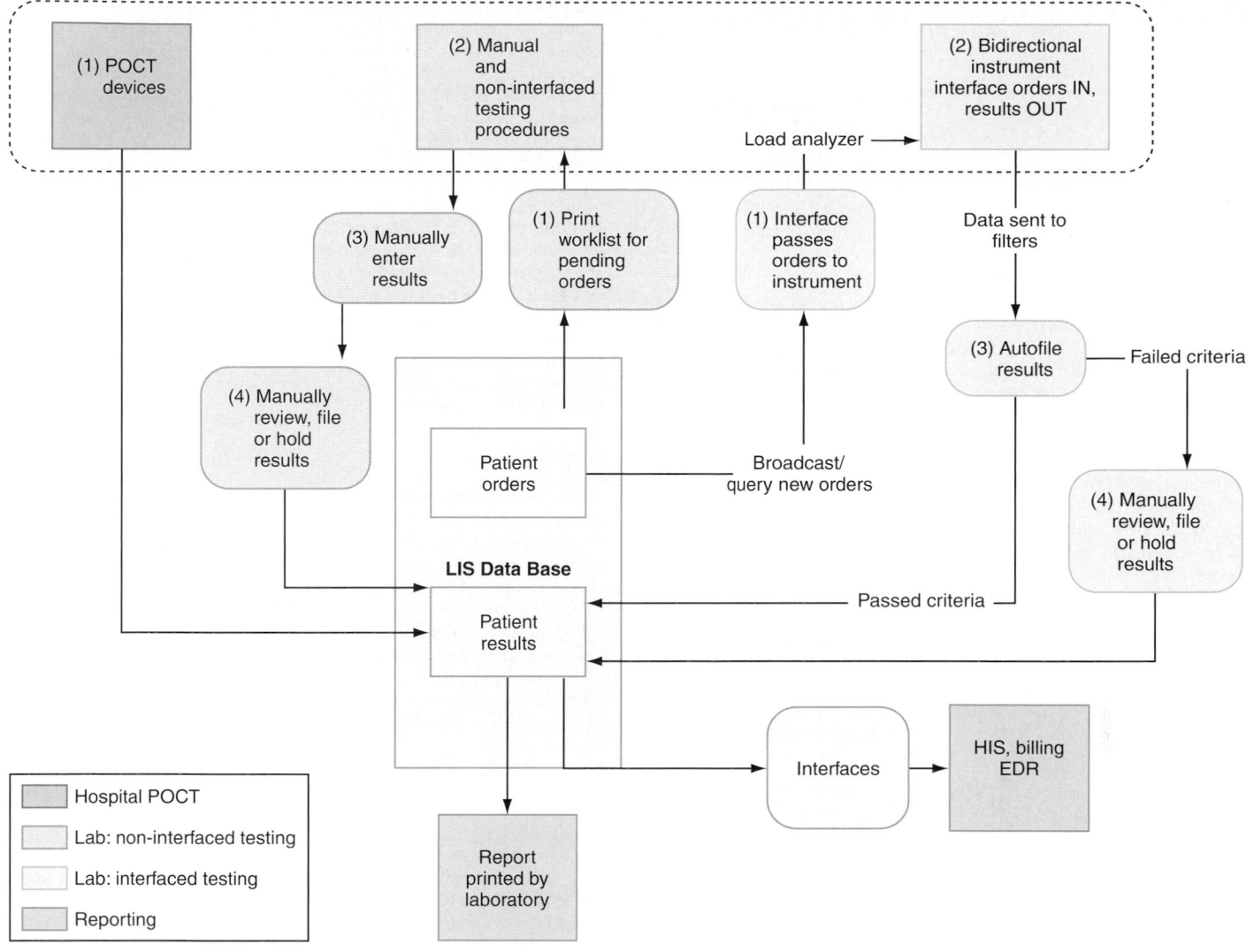

Figure 11–3 LIS role in processing results. Note three approaches to processing results: manual data entry, interfaced (online) instruments and hospital point-of-care testing (POCT). (Workflow steps are numbered for each approach.)

real time place the orders. Inpatient orders are usually placed into a HIS and then transmitted to the laboratory. Outpatient electronic orders are entered into a physician office computer that communicates with the laboratory or entered via a web-based program that sends the order to the laboratory.

Electronic orders can be placed by individually selecting tests from a scroll-down menu of all tests or from menus of common order sets that can be customized by clinical specialty. An electronic service catalog can provide collection requirements and information about test method, diagnostic usefulness and interpretation. The service catalog is rapidly evolving into an online electronic document.

Manual (Paper Requisition) Order Entry. In some hospitals and outreach laboratories, laboratory tests are requested on paper requisitions, which are physically sent to the laboratory for entry. Test requests may be entered as short alphabetic mnemonics (e.g., CBC, CEA, Na) or by numeric codes. Alphabetic codes have a clearer meaning, and may be easier to remember, but numeric codes are faster to enter, less ambiguous, can include a check digit, and are easier to manage in billing systems. Paper requisitions should be preprinted with the physician name and address and populated with tests most frequently ordered. The goal is to minimize the number of tests that have to be handwritten on a form and thus subject to misinterpretation.

Sample Collection and Labeling

Test orders typically fall into two categories: (1) requests for the laboratory to obtain a specimen and (2) requests accompanied by a specimen. In the hospital, test requests received in advance are entered into the HIS and transmitted to the LIS where they are grouped into routine phlebotomy batches. Shortly before the scheduled collection time, labels are printed

that identify the patients to draw and the samples (i.e., container types) to collect. These (typically) bar-coded labels (see below) also include specimen/aliquot volumes and special handling instructions. Collection labels are printed in the order in which the phlebotomist should draw the patients – urgent specimens first, then others in geographic sequence (by floor and bed number). Alternatively, the entire phlebotomist work queue can be stored in a portable device (see below) and labels can be generated at the bedside as a sample is collected from each patient. Collected, uncollected or partially collected orders are indicated as such in the LIS.

When orders are received with a specimen (i.e., when samples are not collected by the laboratory), collection containers may or may not already be labeled with an LIS bar code, depending on whether LIS bar code printing is available on patient care units. Tubes without LIS labels have to be relabeled in the laboratory and this carries a risk that the wrong computer label will be applied to a patient tube.

Portable Collection Devices. Current technology can route collection procedures to the bedside. Using radiofrequency transmission, small handheld devices can be continuously updated with patient orders and even print LIS bar code labels in real time. This has several major benefits: real time audit trail of collection procedure including collection time and collection comments (e.g., difficult draw, no draw, etc.); fewer labeling errors since labels are only printed as needed at the bedside; potential for positive patient confirmation e.g., scanning a patient bar-coded wristband so the handheld device can automatically print labels; and ability to modify orders up to the actual draw time. The latter eliminates the problem of 'add-on tests,' a circumstance wherein no label exists for a sample (test) that is added after the laboratory has already printed and distributed the order labels for the patient.

Sample Labeling. All samples have to be labeled, preferably with a bar code containing the order or requisition number (which is typically the

Table 11.3 Bar Code Symbologies Used In Healthcare

Symbology	Attributes
Code 128	Complete character set of digits, letters (upper and lower case) and ASCII symbols; inherent check digit; can be read bidirectionally
Code 39	All digits and letters (upper case only), some symbols; high security; low density; can be read bidirectionally
Codabar	All digits, limited letters and symbols; low security
Interleaved 2 of 5	Digits only

same for all samples from a given patient encounter or draw). An additional number (called the container or accession number, depending on LIS vendor nomenclature) also prints on the label. It can be assigned to a group of samples (for example, all chemistry containers from the order) or a single sample, depending on how the LIS database is defined. With the former approach, the LIS cannot distinguish between two red top chemistry tubes even though one might be used for a chemistry panel and one for a reference laboratory test. With the latter approach, the LIS can distinguish between both tubes and can determine whether one or both are collected. To minimize labeling errors, the bar code should be attached to the sample at the site of collection, not in the laboratory. The bar code format and label orientation determine compatibility with automated sample handling systems. Robotic systems additionally require that each sample from a patient be uniquely coded. Typical applications in healthcare have used code 39 symbology, but mandates to achieve a national standard are motivating organizations to convert to code 128. Table 11–3 lists attributes of various bar code symbologies found in healthcare environments. Details of the size, placement and orientation of the label on a sample tube are discussed in the National Committee for Clinical Laboratory Standards document AUTO2-A (NCCLS, 2000).

Performing Tests and Releasing Results

High-volume testing is typically performed on analyzers that *bidirectionally communicate* with the LIS. This means that the LIS sends orders to the analyzer and the analyzer sends results back to the LIS. In addition to an accession number, the order may also include collection date/time and patient demographics such as name, birth date and sex. As specimens are logged into the LIS as 'received,' the computer automatically downloads the orders to the instrument. Alternatively, using the host query mode, the instrument reads the sample's bar-coded accession number and asks the LIS what tests to perform on the specimen. Periodically, a 'pending test list' can be checked on the workstation screen to verify that no specimens have been overlooked. Chemistry analyzers typically work in this manner.

Some analyzers *unidirectionally communicate* with the LIS. This means that they do not automatically receive an order from the LIS but they do send results to the LIS. In this instance, a technologist manually enters orders into the analyzer or, in the case of a hematology cell counter, an order is unnecessary since each sample is processed for the same test (e.g., complete blood count). Some instruments (e.g., refractometer) or manual methods are not interfaced at all to the LIS. In these instances, one must prepare a work list that includes controls and standards in addition to specimens. The work list indicates where to position each specimen and/or what tests to perform. Results are manually entered into the LIS.

As results are entered into the laboratory computer, either manually via keyboard or automatically via instrument interface, the computer performs a variety of validity checks. Results that should be numeric are checked; required numbers of decimal places are verified. Reference ranges, specific for the patient's age and sex (and, where available, other factors, including medication and diagnoses), are compared with the result. For laboratories performing veterinary work, species-specific reference ranges are required. Critical (panic) values are flagged by the LIS, identifying those results that have to be communicated (usually called) immediately to the clinician and documented as such in the LIS. Results are also compared with a given patient's previous results to determine whether a significant change has occurred (so-called 'delta check'). A delta check flag may be the first indication of a patient sample mix-up, or may reflect a change in physiological status. Coded comments are checked to be sure the code is listed in the proper dictionary. Some results are processed through laboratory-defined calculations. For example, LDL-cholesterol is automatically calculated from the total cholesterol, triglycerides and HDL-cholesterol values. Algorithms can be used to generate interpretive comments; for example, the LIS can produce a different comment depending on which tests are positive in a hepatitis B panel. Certain results may cause a test to be automatically ordered on the same sample (e.g., a positive RPR test might generate a confirmatory FTA-ABS) to expedite diagnostic work-ups, improve patient care, and reduce unnecessary testing (e.g., having the computer order direct bilirubin only if the total bilirubin is elevated).

Autovalidation protocols can be used to automatically release (or 'post') results received from the analyzer without technologist review. For example, the LIS can be programmed to release all tests falling within the reference range. This way, the physician can view results as soon as the analyzer completes them. Quality control values are checked against defined limits for each test method, lot number, and level of control, and complex multirule algorithms can readily be applied (see Ch. 10). One of the most important advantages of an LIS is that it closes the loop between the test order and the result entry: an order without a corresponding result appears on the incomplete test list, compelling the technologist to seek out and resolve the discrepancy.

Reporting

Advances in communications technology have provided many innovative methods for communicating laboratory results to the clinician beyond the traditional printed report, including: inquiry/display terminals, voice output, beeper activation, fax, e-mail, web-based applications, and wireless links to hand-held workstations. Printed reports can be formatted many different ways to present only the most recent results, the results for a single specimen, or cumulative results that include all results from patient admission or other date interval. Laboratory results can be electronically reported to a variety of clinical systems, including the HIS, enterprise data repository (EDR) or electronic medical record (see Table 11–1 and Fig. 11–5). These systems generally allow the user to customize the way the results are displayed. Data warehouses provide a view across many different patients and permit the recognition of general patterns, and potentially the development of new knowledge about disease (Elevitch, 1999). The laboratory report also serves an important medicolegal role and must meet all regulations applicable to medical records.

Interpretive reports are an essential component of laboratory practice and can be used to help transform laboratory data into clinically useful information. The LIS may be used to transmit pathologist-generated comments; may automatically produce interpretations on reports based on a predefined algorithm; or may serve as a complex expert system, suggesting interpretive comments to the pathologist. Full potential of these systems in medical quality assurance will be realized only when clinical action is taken, and then is recorded, in information systems, allowing the computer to verify that a pathognomonic laboratory result actually resulted in appropriate therapeutic intervention. Recent advances in Web browser technology greatly facilitate the display of laboratory values on physician office or personal computers, improving efficiency.

Another important benefit of an LIS is that it can be used, alone or in conjunction with other systems (like an HIS), to provide clinical alerts. In its most basic form, a clinical alert is a laboratory value that is flagged as high or low on the report. However, a single set of clinical alerts does not take into account a patient's underlying condition, i.e., what is 'normal' may differ widely from one patient to another. Thus, an elevated creatinine level in an end-stage renal disease patient may qualify as a 'call value' even though it may be 'normal' for that patient. To address this issue, some systems allow one to customize clinical alerts by physician or specialty to more accurately identify patients who may have results that are potentially serious given their condition. Sophisticated algorithms have also been designed to recognize critical pathological changes over time in patients who normally have abnormal laboratory results (Fritsche, 2002).

World Wide Web (www) Access to Patient Results. Intranets, or confidential private 'Webs,' are versatile and powerful tools for disseminating laboratory data, based on dynamic Web content. With its intrinsic multimedia capability, Web technology can format data in many ways by using hypertext markup language (HTML). HTML can generate new content automatically in response to user commands, and thus is capable of automating report generation and facilitating custom data searches (Yearworth, 1998; Lowe, 1996). Dynamic content means customized clinical reports can be 'created on the fly' and represents a value-added standard of care that the laboratory may offer to its clients. The ultimate challenge with intranet technology is how to securely and completely integrate it with outside networks servicing physicians and other facilities.

Table 11.4 Relational Database Structure

Patient Registration Data

Patient ID #	First name	Last name	Age	Sex
P1234	John	Smith	33	M
P3456	Mary	White	58	F

Test Order Data

Order #	Patient ID #	Date	Physician	Test
O34782	P1234	04/12/2005	Jones	Hemoglobin
O34783	P3456	04/12/2005	White	Hematocrit

Test Result Data

Order #	Test	
O34782	Hemoglobin	15
O34783	Hematocrit	33

Reference Range Data

Test	Adult Male	Adult Female	Child	Units
Hemoglobin	14–18	12–16	11–16	g/dL
Hematocrit	42–52	37–47	31–43	%

Though each table has unique data it also contains at least one data item that relates it to another table. (Matching data fields are shaded in same color.) Thus data from all four tables can be extracted to produce a single patient report that contains patient name and ID, order #, physician, test, result and reference range.

The LIS

What is it?

At its core, the LIS is a collection of data that is structured using one of several different database architectures. One common approach is the relational database, a collection of data items organized as a set of tables from which data can be accessed or reassembled in many different ways without having to reorganize the database tables. The standard user and application program interface to a relational database is the *structured query language (SQL)*. SQL statements are used both for interactive queries for information from a relational database and for gathering data for reports. In addition to being relatively easy to create and access, a relational database has the important advantage of being easy to expand. After the original database is created, a new data category can be added without having to modify all existing applications.

A relational database is a set of tables (conceptually similar to a spreadsheet) containing data organized in predefined categories. Each table (which is sometimes called a *relation*) contains one or more data categories in columns. Each row contains a unique instance of data for the categories defined by the columns (Table 11-4). For example, the Patient Registration table may have separate columns for Patient ID #, Patient first name, Patient last name, Date of birth, etc. Each row in the table describes a separate patient. The Test Order table may have a column for Patient ID #, Date of order, Physician name, and the Test # for every item ordered. A third table may have a list of tests with separate columns for the Test #, Test name and Sample type. Note that each of these tables contains at least one key data element that relates it to another table. For example, Patient ID # links the Patient Registration table with the Test Order table and test Order # links the Test Order table with the Test Result table. Using this approach, data from multiple tables can be extracted and displayed as a single view. For example, the Order Entry Screen can present patient demographics, along with order information and the Patient ID.

When creating a relational database, one can define the range of possible values in a data column and apply restrictions to the data values. For example, one might limit the number of tests that can be ordered per patient visit, require five characters in a zip code field or allow only two digits and one decimal place to be entered in the result field for calcium. By creating these limitations one can ensure that the data entered is valid.

A typical LIS database contains many different interrelated tables that have to be populated by the laboratorian. For example, there are tables for test names and reference ranges as well as one for client information. The functionality of an LIS and its impact on workflow is directly related to the

Table 11.5 LIS Functions

Pre-analysis	Patient registration (if not received from external system)
	Test ordering
	Customized requisitions (e.g., outreach clients)
	Phlebotomy draw lists
	Bar-coded collection labels and aliquot labels
	Specimen tracking/racking system
Analysis	Instrument worklist (via interface and automatic download)
	Manual worklist
	Manual results entry
	Automated results entry via interface
	Result validation and manual or automatic release
	Quality control
Post-analysis	Requisition-based patient reports (final, partial)
	Cumulative patient reports
	Corrected report
	Results inquiry
	Electronic reporting to external interfaced systems, e.g., HIS, billing
Management	Pending (incomplete) list
	Turnaround time reports
	Workload statistics
	Ad hoc report writer
	HIS and instrument integrity monitoring tools

manner in which these files are created. Thus, it is extremely important to understand how these tables relate to each other in order to optimize workflow.

Special Functions of the LIS

A typical clinical laboratory LIS consists of a variety of modules: general laboratory (e.g., specimen collection and processing, chemistry, hematology, serology); microbiology; and blood bank. In practice, some laboratories use separate blood bank information systems. An LIS serves many functions, some of which are listed in Table 11–5. In addition to supporting the information flow steps outlined above, the LIS provides specialized functions for management and certain laboratory sections.

Microbiology

The microbiology section of the laboratory requires unique data management. A microbiologist must have an efficient method of entering organism names and antimicrobial sensitivities and must be able to transmit complex information through instrument interfaces. A single specimen can result in multiple organism isolates, each of which can have one or more sets of biochemical characterizations (for internal use) and susceptibility results (for external reporting). Susceptibility reporting is often formatted to influence clinical practice; for example, expensive and toxic antimicrobials may be omitted from the report if the organism is susceptible to inexpensive and safe agents, or at least the inexpensive, efficacious drugs can be listed first. Epidemiology reports, antimicrobial susceptibility patterns, and other specialized summaries are also needed. The LIS can be used to automatically and electronically transmit communicable disease reports to public health agencies (White, 1999) (see Communication Standards below).

Infection Control. By correlating patient demographics including hospital location with microbiology results, the laboratory can help detect nosocomial infections (Wright, 2004). Automated surveillance has been used to detect outbreaks (Stern, 1999) and provide disease reporting to the health department (Backer, 2001; Effler, 1999) and is expected to play a pivotal role detecting episodes of bioterrorism (Lazarus, 2001). Real-time notification can provide patient unit and infection control staff with reports of patients requiring isolation as well as the organisms identified and their antimicrobial susceptibility patterns. A surveillance program deployed across multiple institutions' LIS systems, promotes consistent standards of healthcare for patients receiving inter-institutional services, mitigates exposure upon entry into sister facilities, and can cut the time and need for survey work-ups.

Blood Bank

The blood bank LIS qualifies as a healthcare device requiring Food and Drug Administration (FDA) approval for deployment, and particular attention must be devoted to any changes regarding the blood bank regarding software, system validation, and FDA regulatory requirements. This includes interfaces with chemistry and serology instruments that process donor-screening tests (hepatitis, human immunodeficiency virus [HIV], and other assays for infectious disease). The blood bank must track not just patient specimens, but also blood components and the matching of these two. Blood component and derivative unit inventories must be maintained, with careful attention to expiration dates and special characteristics of each unit (e.g., special antigen typing). Special units for particular patients, including autologous, directed and phenotyped units, have imposed complex new record-keeping and crosschecking requirements. Before blood can be issued, a unit tag must be attached to the unit, confirming the identity of the patient for whom this blood is intended. On issue, records must be kept of reinspection of unit, who picked up the unit, and so on. Patient histories must be maintained for prolonged periods, particularly on problem patients, to avoid infusing incompatible blood into a patient who has unexpected antibodies that have fallen below the level of detection. Additional requirements apply to the donor center, including maintaining a donor database and permanent deferral lists, processing and testing of donor units, and conducting inventories, among others. As in the microbiology laboratory, the clinical pathology staff in the blood bank manage a complex data system, and must be familiar with how the LIS supports their operations.

Point-of-Care Testing

Point of care testing (POCT) data can be transmitted to an LIS via a manually initiated upload. Point to point interfaces between the LIS and workstations are prohibitively expensive and complicated to maintain. A more cost-effective alternative utilizes a single interface to a data server interjected between the disparate POCT workstations of different vendors. Devices can communicate with the server via a wired or wireless network connection. All data exchanged with the LIS is mediated through the server, and interface costs are reduced, since fewer interfaces are required for multiple POCT connections. This common data path allows a single user access to data from multiple devices and simplifies laboratory oversight and quality control review. A variety of vendors offer information solutions that accept data from different types of POCT devices or even a user that manually enters results for POCT tests like urine dipstick. The goal is to centralize all POCT results.

Management Tools

The laboratory and other computer databases throughout the hospital are powerful tools for medical quality assurance, as they provide the pathologist or manager with detailed and accurate accounts of laboratory activities. The LIS can draw from its database to provide time-stamped audit trails of what has happened to every specimen at each processing step. It can track clinician or internal laboratory problems and generate data on turnaround time (by test, shift, technologist and ordering location), laboratory workload distribution (including test and sample mapping) and a variety of other activities. Data extracted from the LIS can be used to analyze workflow and optimize performance (see Ch. 2). Workload recording, productivity assessment, and management index reports (e.g., the Laboratory Management Index Program, College of American Pathologists, Northfield, IL) are valuable management tools. These reports can be used for tracking internal, longitudinal trends and for benchmarking: comparing laboratory fiscal performance with that of comparable laboratories (see Ch. 12). Occasionally, the laboratory staff will need to design ad hoc reports; for example, 'Give me all the patients with sodium of greater than 150, between the ages of 62 and 75, who were on the oncology ward.' This ad hoc query capacity should address all fields in the database files and format its output for downloading into a personal computer. The LIS security functions ensure that each staff member has access to only those functions appropriate for his or her job duties, training, and level of licensure. In addition, they provide an extensive audit trail suitable for documenting legal inquiries, including each individual involved with specimen log-in, processing, resulting, reporting, inquiry, and client service. Quality assurance software programs have been developed to assess the appropriateness of laboratory use and its cost-effectiveness based on patient condition (severity), outcome and detailed electronic medical record data (Connelly, 1997).

Billing

In many institutions, the LIS produces billing transactions for every test performed. These may be issued at the time of test order, specimen collection or receipt, or result completion. To ensure regulatory compliance, billing systems must be able to accurately capture tests that are added or deleted from the initial order. Billing interfaces operate in batch mode (sending a daily batch of all transactions) or dynamically, as the charge qualifies. The latter approach minimizes delays in processing. Laboratory billing regulations are very complex (see Ch. 12). In some instances, improved billing accuracy and compliance may justify the LIS purchase.

LIS Selection, Implementation and Management

New vendor LIS installations usually occur as part of a hospital or health-system migration to a single company's platform or because of significant or anticipated changes in service volume or complexity that cannot be met by the current vendor's system. LIS upgrades from existing vendors are usually related to new software versions or technology and can be just as challenging to successfully implement as a completely new LIS.

Selection. Selecting an LIS can be a daunting process. One approach is to begin with a gap analysis, a study of the differences between the capabilities of an existing system and a proposed one. In a gap analysis, LIS software features are divided into existing, new, and future needs and these, in turn, can be weighted as meeting or failing to meet the organization's compliance and performance requirements. The assessment requires a multidisciplinary approach involving laboratory, information technology, and end-user departments. While the gap analysis can identify acceptable vendor solutions, the decision to implement a solution hinges on local budgetary, staffing, and concurrent project considerations. The gap analysis is typically followed by site visits, which provide further insight into the project timeline and expected resources needed for deployment. Site visits are the most valuable tool in the selection process when the sites mirror one's own configuration or projected business plan. Site visits should explore key areas like system performance, staff overhead, system flexibility, system stability, and vendor responsiveness.

Implementation. Laboratory staff managing the LIS implementation must have a firsthand knowledge of policies, procedures and workflow and understand how to define the LIS database to achieve optimal performance. The most challenging part of any implementation is determining how to structure the LIS and its many interrelated data elements. Sometimes this requires experimenting with different approaches (and a mini-database of tests, clients, etc.) to fully appreciate the implications of one design versus another.

Next, data are collected such as test names, reference ranges, physicians and other clients, etc. Generally, collecting the data and deciding how to build the database usually takes longer than actually entering the data. After the database has been built and the new workflow has been developed, staff is trained. To minimize the need for support staff, a 'train the trainer' approach works effectively. In this instance supervisors or lead technologists are trained, and they instruct their staff. The LIS is a critical component of the hospital information complex and deserves a dedicated support staff knowledgeable about the laboratory's operation to deploy and maintain the service.

Validation. The laboratory quality management program requires all new and modified processes to be thoroughly tested and documented. Thus, all changes to the LIS must be validated regardless of whether they are major (e.g., new or upgraded LIS, new interface to the HIS) or minor (new instrument interfaced to the LIS, new coded test) modifications. Changes must be migrated from development ('test area') to production ('live area') through a change control procedure. Given the LIS's central role in the laboratory and the many process improvement projects occurring in laboratories, validation testing has become an ongoing and sometimes very laborious task. Automating the software validation process allows the LIS support staff to keep pace with new revisions and releases. Software designed to expedite the testing of these revisions exercises the application software and documents the outcome. The audits address local change control and licensing agency documentation requirements. However, there is no substitute for actively reviewing the documentation to determine whether performance criteria have been met. For example, when a new interface is established to transmit laboratory results to the HIS, one should view actual printed HIS reports to validate that the information is accurate, understandable and appears in the proper section of the report.

Management. The laboratory must prepare, execute and routinely update and test a plan to recover from a disaster. Figure 11–4 compares several *disaster recovery strategies* with respect to cost and system availability. Every organization must determine to what degree, if any, it can tolerate recovery time ('downtime') and design a strategy to meet needs. For example, a hospital laboratory may require a more 'fail safe' system than an outpatient or specialized reference laboratory that does not operate 24 hours a days. A *disaster recovery plan* is needed to document the procedures and activities associated with a potential loss of LIS service. This plan must be updated periodically and tested to ensure that laboratory operations can proceed if the LIS fails.

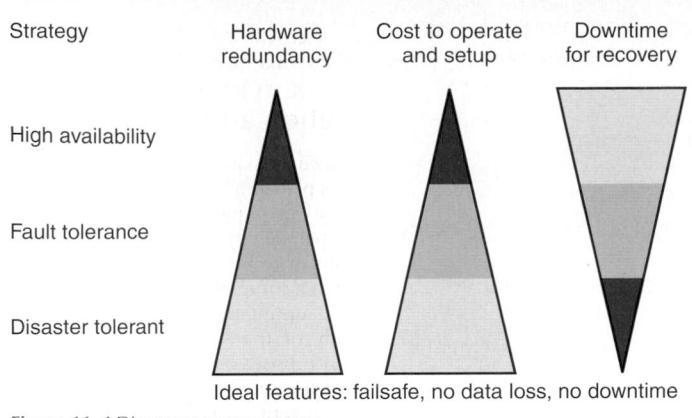

Figure 11–4 Disaster recovery strategy.

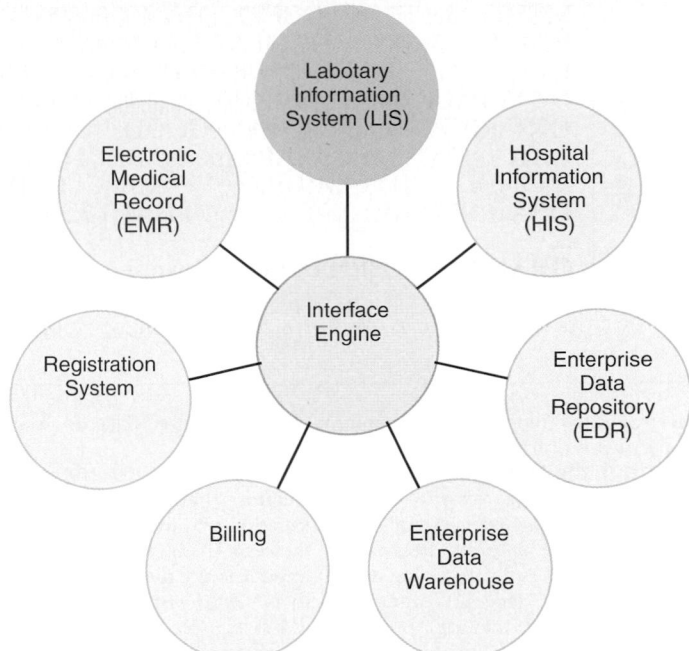

Figure 11–5 The LIS exchanges information with other systems via an interface engine (see text). Note that the LIS receives patient demographics and admission/discharge/transfer information (from the registration system) and electronic test orders for inpatients (from HIS) and outpatients (from EMR). It also sends patient results to a variety of systems.

HIPAA mandates strict patient confidentiality and this, in turn, requires management to ensure the integrity and safety of the LIS data. To achieve these goals, one must *control access and maintain patient confidentiality*. This is accomplished in several ways, including defining password protection that restricts a user to only job-related LIS functions; logging all inquires to patient data; limiting the number of users authorized to modify the database; and maintaining security systems to guard against phone line or network access by hackers. An erroneous database alteration can significantly affect laboratory operations (e.g., incorrect collection tube) or the clinical interpretation of test results (e.g., incorrect reference range). Thus, there must be a procedure to review all database modifications before and after they are moved to the production area. Also, periodically, one should review laboratory reports to detect any unanticipated changes.

Communication Standards and their Applications

LIS systems must exchange data with many other information systems. Each system stores its information in a unique way that supports its special function (e.g., billing, registration, HIS, etc.). Historically, each time data had to be exchanged between two disparate systems, a separate custom interface had to be developed by each system's vendor. This 'point-to-point' (e.g., LIS–HIS) interface was time-consuming, complex, and expensive to maintain. To address this issue, communication protocols have been developed to standardize the exchange of information. The intent is to standardize data exchanges rather than applications. These standards have two important benefits: (1) they simplify and shorten interface development and (2) they reduce the number of interfaces, by eliminating 'point-to-point' data exchange and replacing it with an interface engine (Fig. 11–5). The interface engine is a data 'traffic cop'; it is a powerful computer system that serves as a clearinghouse to exchange or 'route' data among various information systems. It can also manipulate data to make sure that they are in the correct format for each system. Consider the following example. Without communication standards and an interface engine, a hospital might have to develop several interfaces to transmit laboratory results: LIS–HIS, LIS–Billing, and LIS–Enterprise Data Repository. Each interface would have to be separately developed and maintained and each new information system would require another interface. With an interface engine, there is only one laboratory interface: LIS–Interface Engine. If a new information system is added, it, too, can receive laboratory results from the interface engine without any need on the part of the laboratory to develop a new interface.

There are different communication standards to address the various steps in data transmission. For instance, in order for a technologist to view data on the LIS that has been uploaded by an analyzer, the data must travel sequentially through a variety of devices that control this activity: analyzer, network terminal server device, network switch (or hub), LIS, network, and PC. Transmitting data through all these steps would be very complicated and laborious to develop without standard data communication protocols.

Users, vendors and consultants voluntarily adopt standard communication protocols. Some of the more popular protocols include HL7 (Health Level 7), used to interface laboratory data at the application level (e.g., HIS–LIS), ASTM (American Society for Testing and Materials) frequently used to interface laboratory data between analyzers and laboratory information systems, and TCP/IP (a combination of Transmission Control Protocol and Internet Protocol) used to connect information systems to network devices, other information systems, interface engines, analyzers,

Table 11.6 Data Record Formats Typically Used in LIS Data Transmission

Record type (flat file formats)	Typical application	Attributes
Fixed length, column oriented	Import into word processor or spreadsheet	One record per transaction, fixed content and order
Variable length, comma delimited	Import into word processor or spreadsheet	One record per transaction, shorter than column oriented, fixed content and order
Record-centric	Instrument (ASTM) or HIS (HL-7) interface	Multiple records needed for a transaction, unsuitable for ad hoc report utilities. Fixed order within a record
Field-centric	Instrument or HIS interface (XML)	Maximum flexibility in transaction content and order, unsuitable for ad hoc report utilities

PCs and printers. For purposes of data exchange, records can be formatted in a variety of styles. These are illustrated in Table 11–6.

Health Level Seven (HL7)

The healthcare industry has created several standards to facilitate the exchange of information among inpatient and outpatient computer applications such as patient registration (i.e., ADT – hospital admissions, discharges and transfers), clinical information systems (e.g., HIS), billing, clinical laboratory and radiology. The most prevalent such standard is Health Level Seven (HL7) (http://www.hl7.org); it is also the name of the organization that developed and continues to modify this standard. The Open System Interconnection (OSI) model of the International Organization for Standardization (ISO) is a networking standard that defines how data are moved from one application to another application on a different computer. OSI separates data networking into seven steps or levels, each pertaining to either software or hardware. The last step or highest layer is Level Seven and it addresses three software issues: defining the data to be exchanged, timing the exchanges, and communicating errors between applications. HL7 defines the standards for Level 7 data exchange in healthcare. HL7 is commonly used to interface a laboratory information system with a hospital information system or a reference laboratory. It is also used in conjunction with LOINC (see below) to

Transaction

```
MSH|^~\&|LIS|HC1|OCF|OCF|20040906000031||ORU^R01|13|P|2.2|
PID|||123456789^^^HC1||PATIENT^NEW^||19561016|M|^^|||||||000001269264249^^^HC1|195529345|
PV1|||IP|4G^G0422-06||||51900^PHYSICIAN^FIRST^^^^^^MPACCOMM|15160^DOCTOR^SECOND^^
^^^^MPACCOMM|||||||IP|||||||||||||||||200409040000||
ORC|RE||P286688||||||||51900^GOOD^DO^^^^^^MPACCOMM||||^|
OBR|1||12579528|GASAP^Arterial Blood Gas(ICU) ^GASAP|||200409052355|||||||200409052356|^^
|51900^DOCTOR^ORDER^^^^^^MPACCOMM||||X14004||||PI|F||^^^^R|^~^~^|^12579528|||||
OBX|1|NM|PHAP^pH-Arterial^PHAP|1|7.39||7.35—7.45||||F|||200409052359|NICUL^NEW ICU LAB ||
···
OBX|6|NM|FIO2P^Fraction of Inspired O2^FIO2P|1|100|%|||||F|||200409052357|NICUL^NEW ICU LAB ||
```

Figure 11–6 HL7 result transaction for arterial blood gas order. Note the message is divided into segments: Message Header (MSH); Patient Identification (PID); Patient Visit (PV1); Common Order (ORC); Order (OBR); and Result (OBX). The blood gas has six results; each is included in a separate OBX, though only the first and sixth results are presented here.

electronically report various communicable disease data to state departments of health and federal agencies.

Defining the Data to Exchange. HL7 compiles data into *messages* that are constructed according to specific standards. There are two types of messages. A *display message* contains information that the sender formats to only display or print. Because the message is not subdivided into discrete data fields, the receiving system cannot capture the information or manipulate the data. In contrast, a *record-oriented message* consists of discrete elements that can be captured by the receiving system and manipulated into its own reports. Each message is subdivided into *segments* and each segment is further divided into *fields*. Every transaction or event is defined by its own unique message format. For example, there are separate messages for Laboratory Order, Laboratory Result, Result Query, and ADT. Figure 11–6 demonstrates how an HL7 laboratory result message is divided into segments and data fields.

Timing the Data Exchange and Error Tracking. Trigger events determine when a message is sent. A message may be sent by itself or it may be batched with other messages and sent at one time. For example, a laboratory result message may be sent to the clinical information system as soon as it becomes available. On the other hand, laboratory test billing messages may be batched before they are sent to the financial system once a day. HL7 can also define whether a message is a response to a query or an unsolicited update. For example, every time a test is ordered on the clinical system, a laboratory order message (unsolicited update) can be sent to the laboratory system. HL7 also defines how error messages are communicated. When information is exchanged between two systems, the receiving system must validate that it has all required information and return a message to the first system indicating that the transmission was successful or that an error occurred and data are missing.

LOINC

LOINC is an acronym for Logical Observation Identifier Names and Codes. Strictly speaking, it is not a communication standard, but rather a nomenclature standard (McDonald, 2003). LOINC is growing in popularity, particularly where there is a need to exchange data at a national level, and has been adopted by large reference laboratories, hospitals and various governmental agencies. It provides a set of universal names and codes for identifying laboratory and clinical test results. The purpose is to facilitate the exchange and pooling of results, such as blood hemoglobin or serum potassium for clinical care, outcomes management, and research. For example, state health departments can more readily compile information regarding transmissible diseases if each laboratory reports the information electronically using the same LOINC code, instead of many different test names or codes to describe each test.

There are over 25 000 laboratory-related LOINC codes (http://www.regenstrief.org/loinc). Each LOINC record includes fields for specifying a variety of characteristics (Tables 11–7 and 11–8). In order to assist local facilities to map their local test codes to the LOINC ones, a mapping program called Regenstrief LOINC Mapping Assistant (RELMA™) is available at no cost (http://www.regenstrief.org/loinc). Though LOINC codes were initially developed for single test observations (like a serum potassium result), they can also be used to order the test. The LOINC database also contains several common standardized *panels* like arterial blood gas, hemogram and differential count. Some instrument vendors have started to supply LOINC codes as part of the result that is sent to the LIS. This decreases mapping work that would otherwise have to be done by the laboratory.

LOINC and HL7 complement each other. The LOINC database is meant to provide the test code for the observation identifier field (OBX-3) in HL7 laboratory result messages (Fig. 11–7) and DICOM messages (see below).

Table 11.7 Parts of a LOINC name

Part	Example
Component (analyte)	Potassium, hemoglobin, hepatitis C antigen
Property measured	Mass concentration, enzyme activity
Timing	Point in time, period of time (e.g., 24 hours)
System (specimen, organ)	Urine, serum, whole blood
Scale	Quantitative, ordinal (1+, 2+), qualitative (cloudy), nominal (*E. coli*)
Method (if required)	Radioimmunoassay (RIA) (only used to differentiate methods that give clinically significant different results)

Table 11.8 LOINC Examples

Code	Component	Property	Timing	Specimen	Scale
2951-2	Sodium	SCNC	PT	SER/PLAS	QN
3665-7	Gentamicin^Trough	MCNC	PT	SER	QN

LOINC name	Meaning of name
SODIUM:SCNC:PT:SER/PLAS:QN	Sodium: substance concentration: random point in time: serum/plasma: quantitative
GENTAMICIN^TROUGH: MCNC:PT:SER:QN	Gentamicin trough level: mass concentration: random point in time: serum: quantitative

Note: a colon separates each part of the LOINC name and a ^ separates subparts.

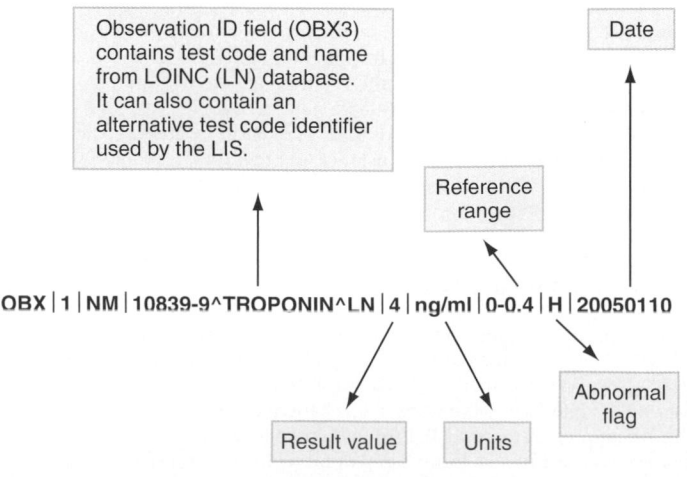

Figure 11–7 How LOINC is used in an HL7 result message.

Note that the HL7 result message contains separate fields for reporting various result data. In addition to the OBX-3 field that identifies the test, there are separate fields for the result value, units of measure, flags, etc.

Other Standards

The *Clinical Context Object Workgroup (CCOW)* standard (http://www.ccow-info.com/), based on context management architecture (CMA), allows information in separate healthcare applications to be synchronized so that each application automatically and seamlessly refers to the same patient, test or event. Thus one can view an inpatient's current laboratory data in the HIS and then toggle to the electronic data repository to view last year's outpatient laboratory data on the same patient (without having to select the patient again). This standard can be used in conjunction with a single sign-on procedure that simultaneously logs in a user to multiple applications. This enhances security and convenience due to a single username and password. Overall, CCOW is a secure means of deploying interoperability between old and new technologies and multiple vendors.

Digital Image Communications in Medicine (DICOM) (http://www.hl7.org/standards/dicom.htm) is the emerging world standard for exchanging medical images and related information across vendor platforms. The Visible Light Supplement 15 is an extension of DICOM designed for pathology and laboratory medicine that specifies a diagnostic encoding structure for gross and microscopic images and associated data. An additional pathology-related module, Structured Reporting Supplement, will incorporate laboratory medicine and pathology-specific concepts such as accession numbers, reference ranges and systematized nomenclature of medicine (SNOMED) (http://www.snomed.at/) International codes into the DICOM repertoire. It is designed to complement the visible light standard, which encodes information such as capture device specifications, magnification, gross and microscopic descriptions, and diagnostic information. These two supplements are intended to function together to provide a completely interoperable data format for seamless information interchange across disparate laboratory information systems.

A convergence of informatics standards is providing a path to true interoperability of the comprehensive patient electronic medical record. For example, HL7, DICOM and LOINC are interrelated standards for healthcare data. Similarly, for searchable data, extensible markup language (XML) holds great promise for becoming the standard by which textual information is encoded into a searchable format (Dolin, 1998; Sokolowski, 1999). (XML describes the data that HTML displays.) With the creation of a unified electronic medical record, one may achieve worldwide interchange capability for all categories of medical information. The potential glue to facilitate this interchange, SNOMED-RT, a product of the College of American Pathologists, is intended as a multilingual comprehensive lexicon of medical terminology. Since the SNOMED vocabulary is being translated into many languages, it may eventually be used with the above standards to convert complete medical records from one language to another.

References

Aller RD: Connectivity from source to action. Clin Chemistry 2001; 47(8):1521–1525.

Backer HD, Bissel SR, Vugia DJ: Disease reporting from an automated laboratory-based reporting system to a state health department via local county health departments. Public Health Rep 2001; 116:257–265.

Balis UJ: Informatics training in U.S. pathology residency programs. Results of a survey. Am J Clin Pathol 1993; 100(Suppl 1):S44–S47.

Connelly DP: Outcomes and informatics. Arch Pathol Lab Med 1997; 121: 1176–1182.

Dolin RH, Rishel W, Biron PV, et al: SGML and XML as interchange formats for HL7 messages. Proc AMIA Symp 1998; :720–724.

Effler P, Ching-Lee M, Bogard A, et al: Statewide system of electronic notifiable disease reporting from clinical laboratories: comparing automated reporting with conventional methods. JAMA 1999; 282:1845–1850.

Elevitch FR: Prospecting for gold in the data mine. Clin Lab Med 1999; 19:373–384.

Fritsche L, Schlaefer A, Klemens B, et al: Recognition of critical situations from time series of laboratory results by case-based reasoning. J Am Med Inform Assoc 2002; 9:520–528.

Lazarus R, Kleinman KP, Dasevsky I, et al: Using automated medical records for rapid identification of illness syndromes (syndromic surveillance): the example of lower respiratory infection. BMC Public Health 2001; 1:9.

Lowe HJ, Antipov I, Walker WK, et al: WebReport: A World Wide Web based clinical multimedia reporting system. Proc AMIA Annu Fall Symp 1996; 314–318.

McDonald CJ, Huff SM, Suico JG, et al: LOINC, a universal standard for identifying laboratory observations: a 5-year update. Clinical Chemistry 2003; 49:624–633.
An excellent and well-written overview of LOINC including its purpose and structure; also includes useful examples that explain LOINC coding.

NCCLS: Laboratory Automation: Bar Codes for Specimen Container Identification; Approved Standard. Document AUTO2-A [ISBN 1-56238-414-7, ISSN 0273-3099] Wayne, PA, NCCLS, 2000.

Sokolowski R, Dudeck J: XML and its impact on content and structure in electronic health care documents [in process citation]. Proc AMIA Symp 1999: 147–151.

Stern, L, Lightfoot D: Automated outbreak detection: a quantitative retrospective analysis. Epidemiol Infect 1999; 122:103–110.

White MD: Evaluation of vocabularies for electronic laboratory reporting to public health agencies. J Am Med Inform Assoc 1999; 6:185–194.

Wright MO, Perencevich EN, Novak C, et al: Preliminary assessment of an automated surveillance system for infection control. Infect Control Hosp Epidemiol 2004; 25:325–332.

Yearworth M, Battle S: Workflow management for multimedia information in clinical laboratories. Comput Meth Progr Biomed 1998; 55:1–9.

CHAPTER 12

Financial Management

Mark L. Jaros MBA MT(ASCP), Mark S. Lifshitz MD, Robert P. De Cresce MD MBA MPH

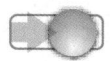

KEY POINTS

• Costs can be described in different ways depending on whether they directly relate to laboratory operations (direct/indirect), change proportionally with test volume (variable/fixed), relate to staffing (salary/nonsalary), or are related to useful life of supplies or equipment (operating/capital). Cost per reportable result is a key indicator.

• Reimbursement for laboratory services comes mostly from third party payers such as Medicare (government) and managed care companies (nongovernment/private insurance) and payments are almost always less than charges.

• Inpatient laboratory testing charges are usually not reimbursed; they are considered to be part of a per diem rate (i.e., general hospital daily room reimbursement rate) or diagnosis-related group (DRG) rate (i.e., set rate for the entire hospital stay, regardless of actual length of stay). Thus, inpatient laboratory testing is considered a 'cost center.' In contrast, outpatient laboratory charges are reimbursed separately; thus testing is considered a 'revenue center.'

• For reimbursement purposes, CPT codes describe tests and ICD-9 codes describe the clinical diagnosis. Medical necessity requirements may limit reimbursement to those tests associated with specific predefined diagnoses.

• Budgeting is the process of planning, forecasting, controlling and monitoring the financial resources of an organization.

• A variety of financial tools are used to evaluate a capital project such as purchasing a chemistry analyzer. These measure how long it takes to recoup an investment (payback), how much it generates in today's dollars (net present value) and its rate of return (internal rate of return).

• Laboratory equipment can be acquired in different ways, including purchase and lease. Each has pros and cons.

Every organization, no matter the products or services it provides, must be concerned with the management, oversight and accounting of its monetary resources. To sustain a viable entity, an organization cannot only recoup the cost of operations, but must have a positive net income in order to reinvest in itself to remain competitive. The laboratory is no exception. To be successful in the financial management of the laboratory, the director/manager must be able to identify and categorize costs,

understand the relationship between revenue and reimbursement, become familiar with the budget process and use financial ratios and information to make sound decisions. Credibility with administrators and colleagues, demands the director/manager be comfortable and confident when explaining financial issues or justifying the need for additional resources.

Industry Overview

Most industries in the United States are subject to traditional free-market competition. However, this principle does not apply to healthcare because few of the many people who use healthcare pay directly for it. Most people are beneficiaries of some form of health insurance. This, in combination with the increasing number of uninsured or underinsured, has led to a system that provides services even when no one pays adequately for them. Most medical claims are paid by a 'third party' such as the government (Medicare, Medicaid) or a private insurance company. Thus, someone other than the patient usually pays a physician (Snyder, 1998).

The healthcare industry is one of the largest industries in the United States and continues to be a growing sector of the gross domestic product (GDP), having increased from 5.1% ($27 billion) in 1960 to 14.9% ($1.5 trillion) in 2002 (CMS, 2004). Hospitals continue to be a driving force behind escalating healthcare costs. Most US hospitals are tax exempt, not-for-profit entities. Though not-for-profit implies a profit is not made, it actually means profits are not distributed to owners or shareholders; instead, profits are reinvested in the organization. Historically, not-for-profit status led hospital administrators to be less profit conscious than counterparts in other businesses. However, today's hospitals are having a difficult time just covering operating costs, given dwindling reimbursement and increasing supply and labor costs. With scarce money left for capital reinvestment in equipment, buildings, facilities and technology, hospitals are aggressively seeking ways to produce a profit to invest for the future.

Defining and Identifying Costs

A cost (expense) is the supply, labor and overhead money spent on a product or service. It is important to understand costs in order to accurately price tests and other services, to determine when and how to offer new tests and to determine whether to acquire new outreach client business or a managed care contract. Costs can be classified in different ways (see Table 12–1).

Direct costs are expenses that can easily be traced directly to an end product. In the laboratory setting, the end product is a billable test.

Table 12–1 Cost Classification

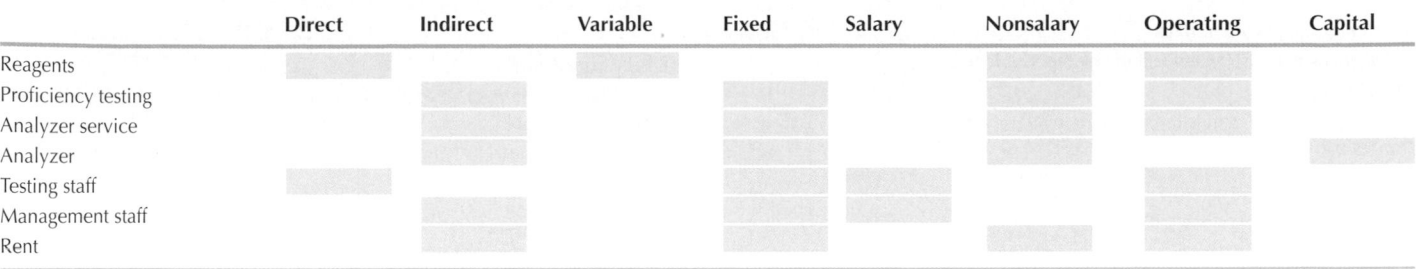

	Direct	Indirect	Variable	Fixed	Salary	Nonsalary	Operating	Capital
Reagents	▪		▪			▪	▪	
Proficiency testing		▪		▪		▪	▪	
Analyzer service		▪		▪		▪	▪	
Analyzer		▪		▪		▪		▪
Testing staff	▪				▪		▪	
Management staff		▪		▪	▪			
Rent		▪		▪		▪	▪	

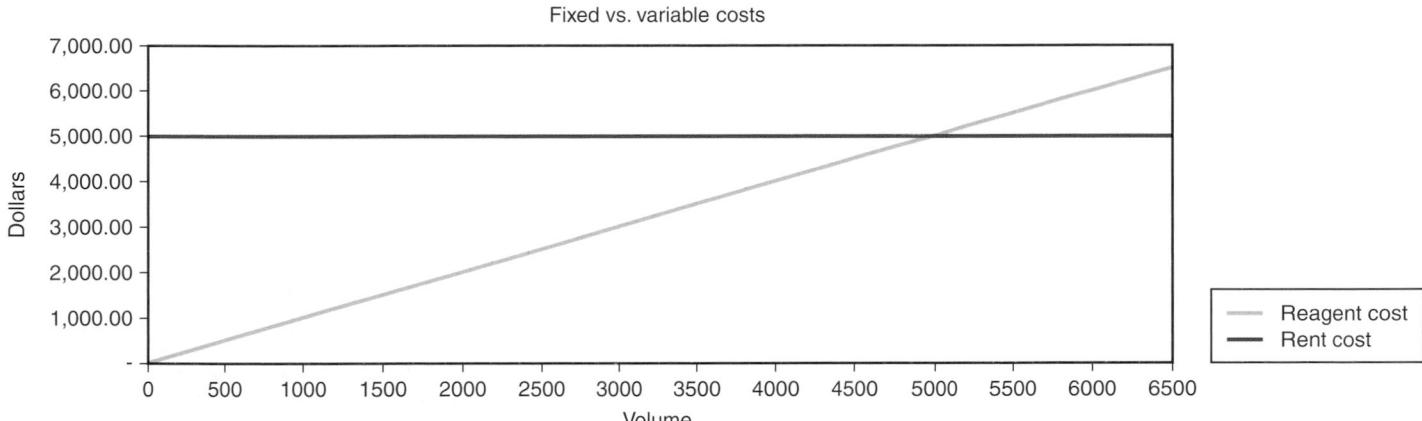

Figure 12–1 Fixed vs. variable costs. Fixed costs like rent remain constant. Variable costs like reagents are directly proportional to test volume.

Examples are reagents, consumables and hands-on technologist time. In contrast, *indirect costs* are not directly related to a billable test, but are necessary for its production. Indirect costs are often referred to as overheads. Examples are proficiency testing and utility expenses.

Variable costs change proportionately with the volume of tests. As test volume grows, so do reagent costs. If the reagent cost per test is $1.00, when 1000 tests are performed the reagent cost is $1000; when 20 000 tests are performed the reagent cost is $20 000. *Fixed costs* do not change with the volume of tests performed. If a laboratory pays $5000 per month to rent its space, this expense remains the same if the laboratory produces 1000 or 20 000 tests a month (Fig. 12–1). Because fixed costs do not vary with activity, the goal is to produce as much as possible from fixed costs in order to achieve economies of scale. The more produced, the lower the *fixed cost per activity*. In the preceding scenario, if the laboratory produced 1000 tests the fixed cost per test is $5; with 20 000 tests the fixed cost per test falls to $0.25. Note that even some fixed costs have a variable component. For example, if an instrument's capacity is 20 000 tests per month and the volume increases beyond that, another instrument will have to be purchased, increasing the fixed costs per test. Fixed costs that change with increments of volume are called *step costs*.

Salary costs need to be looked at differently from *nonsalary costs* because salary costs have fringe benefits associated with them. Salary expenses are approximately 50–70% of the laboratory budget. Salary expenses are generally fixed and therefore it is important to strive for economies of scale. The hourly pay or salaried wage of an employee is not the entire cost of employment. Fringe benefits such as Social Security, health insurance, tuition reimbursement, pension plans and life insurance can represent an additional 16–28% expense above the base salary (Travers, 1997). Furthermore, the total cost of employment is not just the salary and fringe benefits. There are associated costs with the recruitment, interview and selection process. Once an employee is hired, orientation, training and ongoing growth and development costs are incurred.

Operating costs are the expenses incurred to produce a product or service. Many items have only a one-time use, and once used the item has no further value. Examples of one-time operating costs are reagents, electricity, disposable pipets and the salary expense in the production of a test. Other items, such as analytical equipment, computers and the physical plant, have a useful life greater than one production cycle. These items are capital items. To qualify as a *capital* item, the item must meet three criteria: time, price and purpose. To meet the time criterion, the item must have a useful life of more than 1 year. The institution must designate a minimum dollar amount, usually $1000–5000, that once exceeded,

qualifies an item as capital. Last, the purpose of acquiring capital items is usually to replace old damaged equipment with safer and more efficient models, and to add new equipment to support new products or services. With time, capital equipment loses its value. The annual loss of a capital item's value is called *depreciation* and is an annual expense, a capital cost that is deducted from a business's revenue. Depreciation is not a cash expense, i.e., you do not 'pay it' each year but it is a real expense since it recognizes the 'wearing out' of an asset that was acquired with cash and will eventually have to be replaced. If an analyzer has not yet been fully depreciated, it still has 'book value'. Note that operating and capital costs are budgeted separately (see below).

The cost of producing a test can be derived in different ways. *Microcosting* determines the total direct labor and supply costs of producing a test, and is the starting point to determine the fully-loaded cost and ultimately the price for a test. Most testing in the clinical laboratory is performed in batches or continuous 'runs' of many samples during one or more shifts. A run can be a group of tests that are performed once or many times during a shift or entire 24-hour period. A run includes all quality control and calibration costs needed to produce patient results. When microcosting a test, it is important to consider how a test is performed since labor and supply costs vary according to workflow and laboratory policy for quality control and repeats. The *cost per reportable* result (CPRR) distributes the total direct costs of a run over the patient 'reportable' results for that run. Testing efficiency is defined as the total reportable patient results/total test results. Thus, the more repeats and controls performed, the lower the efficiency and the higher the CPRR. As testing efficiency increases, the CPRR decreases. The *incremental cost* is the cost of producing one additional test that, typically, does not require additional salary or capital. For example, the incremental cost of running a chemistry test is usually the cost of dispensing reagent for one additional test, assuming there are no sample collection costs. Other associated costs, like technologist time, equipment, quality control, etc. are fixed costs that are incurred irrespective of the additional test. The incremental cost is usually the lowest possible cost incurred to produce a result. It is best used to assess how much it costs to produce small increments in test volume. As volume grows, a laboratory may need additional staff and equipment and these costs would have to be included in the incremental costing analysis. Incremental costing is especially useful when trying to determine whether additional outreach work is profitable or not. The *fully loaded cost* for a test is the total direct and indirect costs. The allocation of indirect costs is usually done using a formula. The goal of allocating indirect costs is to apply the costs based on the strongest correlation between the indirect cost and to what it is being

Table 12–2 Test Cost Analysis*

Test: Prostate-Specific Antigen

A. Microcosting: Instrument run of one reportable test

Direct labor

Determine the total 'hands-on' time in minutes required to perform an instrument 'run' of one patient test. Assume labor cost is $20 per hour

	Minutes	Expense
Prepare specimen	5	
Prepare reagents	10	
Prepare instrument	10	
Computer and/or worksheet set-up	5	
Documentation of results/QC/maintenance	10	
Clean-up	10	
Total direct labor	50	$16.67

Direct supplies

List all consumables needed to perform the test. Note 4 tests (1 sample and 3 controls) are needed to produce 1 patient reportable result. Calibration costs should be added if they are required with each run

	Unit cost	Units	Expense
Reagent ($700 kit/100 tests)	$7	4	$28.00
Disposable pipets ($10/100 pipets)	$0.10	4	$0.40
Disposable reagent cups ($10/200 cups)	$0.05	4	$0.20
Low, medium and high control material (0.05mL/test @ $20/mL)	$1	3	$3.00
Total direct supplies			$31.60
Total direct costs			$48.27
Cost per reportable (Total direct cost/ Reportable results)	$48.27/1		$48.27
Testing efficiency (Reportable patient results/Tests)	1 result/4 tests		25%

B. Microcosting: Instrument run of 15 reportable tests

Direct labor

For a group of tests run on automated analyzers, use direct labor expense from microcosting. For manual batch testing, direct labor costs may apply to each batch; additional labor time studies may be necessary to derive accurate data

	Minutes	Expense
Total direct labor per batch (same as microcosting in this example)	50	$16.67

Direct supplies

Note: 18 tests (15 samples and 3 controls) are needed to produce 15 reportable results. Fixed costs (controls) are spread over more than 1 sample, in contrast to first example

	Unit cost	Units	Expense
Reagent ($700 kit/100 tests)	$7	18	$126.00
Disposable pipets ($10/100 pipets)	$0.10	18	$1.80
Disposable reagent cups ($10/200 cups)	$0.05	18	$0.90
Low, medium and high control material (0.05mL/test @ $20/mL)	$1	3	$3.00
Total direct supplies			$131.70
Total direct costs			$148.37
Cost per reportable (Total direct cost/ Reportable results)	$148.37/15		$9.89
Testing efficiency (Reportable patient results/Tests)	15 results/21 tests		71%

C. Incremental cost: Cost for one more test

	Units	Expense
Reagent ($700 kit/100 tests)	1	$7
Disposable pipets ($10/100 pipets)	1	$0.10
Disposable reagent cups ($10/200 cups)	1	$0.05
Total		$7.15

Table 12–2 Test Cost Analysis* (cont'd)

	Unit cost	Units	Expense
D. Fully loaded cost			
Direct cost (cost per reportable result for typical size run) from Example B above			$9.89
Indirect cost (estimated by typical hospital as 2.5 direct costs)			$24.73
Fully loaded cost			$34.62
E. Contribution margin			
Example of charging a 20% mark-up for laboratory tests			
Fully loaded cost plus 20% mark-up (test charge at list price)	$34.62 × 1.2		$41.54
Fully loaded cost from Example D above			($34.62)
Contribution margin			$6.92

* This analysis is for illustration purposes only.

applied. For example, utilities could be based on departmental square footage, while human resources costs could be based on number of employees in the department. *Make vs. buy* decisions should be considered when the fully loaded cost of the test is more than the price offered by a commercial or reference laboratory. If it costs more to produce a test than to buy it from another supplier, the test should be considered for outsourcing. When analyzing make vs. buy decisions, cost is only one factor to consider. Turnaround-time, methodology and reliability of the potential alternative supplier should also be considered. The price charged for a test needs to be marked up (increased) from the fully loaded cost in order to realize a profit. The *contribution margin* is the balance remaining after the fully loaded costs are deducted from the price charged for a test. Table 12–2 demonstrates various ways to determine the cost of a test and how to establish its charge.

The *total cost of ownership* (TCO) for a laboratory is the life cycle cost of its capital assets. It focuses attention on the sum of all costs of owning and maintaining all assets for a specific service or product, as opposed to the initial capital or operating costs. In the laboratory, TCO includes acquisition, setup (construction, training), support (ordering supplies, dealing with back orders), ongoing maintenance (scheduled and unscheduled downtime), service, and operating expenses (reagents, controls, repeat testing, inventory control, proficiency testing, testing personnel, supervisory personnel) of a specific workbench and its associated testing instrumentation. TCO is useful in determining make vs. buy decisions, but determining an accurate TCO can be very difficult.

Revenue

Revenue is the total price of services rendered or products sold. It is the money a business is entitled to receive for the services and products it produces. In healthcare, revenue should not be confused with reimbursement or cash collected. *Gross patient revenue* is the total charges at a facility's full-established rates (list price) for the provision of inpatient and outpatient care before deductions from revenue are applied. *Net patient revenue* is the gross inpatient and outpatient revenue minus all related deductions. *Deductions* from revenue include contractual adjustments, provision for bad debts, charity care, and other adjustments and allowances that reduce gross patient revenue. *Contractual adjustments* are the difference between billings at full-established rates and amounts received or receivable from third-party payers under formal contract agreements. For example, if the list price of a test is $10 but the contracted payment from the insurance company is $6, the adjustment is $4 (Harmening, 2003). If all deductions and contractual allowances are correct, net patient revenue should equal cash collected, or $6 in the above example.

In healthcare, it is important to distinguish between inpatient and outpatient care because they are reimbursed differently. Inpatient laboratory testing charges are usually not reimbursed separately; they are considered to be part of a per diem rate (i.e., general hospital daily room reimbursement rate) or diagnosis-related group (DRG) rate (i.e., set rate for the entire hospital stay, regardless of actual length of stay). Thus, inpatient laboratory testing is considered a 'cost center.' The hospital is paid the same rate regardless of how many tests are provided. In contrast, outpatient laboratory testing is a revenue center since each test is separately reimbursed, usually by a third party (Table 12–3). Thus there is a financial

Table 12–3 Reimbursement Comparison for PSA* by Payer Type

	List price	Reimbursement terms	Amount paid	Contractual allowance
Inpatient				
Managed care (HMO)	$41.54	No separate reimbursement for laboratory tests since they are included in the contracted per diem rate	0	N/A
Medicare	$41.54	No separate reimbursement for laboratory tests since they are included in the DRG rate	0	N/A
Outpatient				
Indemnity insurance	$41.54	Usual and customary charge (UCC) is $38; insurance pays 80% of UCC	$30.40	$11.14
Managed care (PPO)	$41.54	Contract pays 110% of Medicare fee schedule ($25.70 for PSA)	$28.27	$13.27
Managed care (HMO)	$41.54	No separate reimbursement for laboratory tests because of capitation arrangement: laboratory receives per member per month payment irrespective of usage	N/A	N/A
Medicare	$41.54	Medicare fee schedule	$25.70	$15.84

* Reimbursement amounts are for illustrative purposes only and may not accurately reflect current Medicare reimbursement.

disincentive to perform inpatient tests and an incentive to perform outpatient ones.

Payers and Reimbursement

Hospitals in early America served a different purpose from those of today. A visiting physician usually provided healthcare at home, and care was administered by family members, midwives and servants. Early hospitals were founded to shelter older adults, the dying, orphans, those with mental illness and vagrants, and to protect the citizens of a community from contagious diseases and the dangerously insane. Many of today's county, municipal or religious order hospitals were originally a combination of these almshouses and isolation hospitals (Sultz, 2004).

The transformation of hospitals from charitable institutions to complex technical organizations came about due to the passage of the Hill-Burton Hospital Construction Act of 1946 and the growth of private hospital insurance. The Hill-Burton Act provided federal money to the states to plan and construct new facilities. The first private health insurance policy was formed by a group of teachers and Baylor Hospital in Dallas, Texas to provide coverage for certain hospital expenses. This arrangement created the model for the development of what was to become Blue Cross Insurance. The development of health insurance to provide reimbursement for routine medical care carried gigantic implications. The original concept of any insurance was to guard against the low risk of a rare occurrence such as premature death or accident. Today's health insurance provides for coverage of routine, predictable services as well as the unforeseen illnesses and injuries (Sultz, 2004).

Private Insurance

Private health insurance falls into two main categories, indemnity and managed care. Indemnity plans, also known as fee-for-service, are traditional insurance plans that give patients absolute freedom to choose their physicians and medical facilities. The insurance companies require the patients to fulfill a yearly deductible, usually between $300 and $500 per

person per year. After the deductible is fulfilled, the insurance company pays a certain coinsurance rate of the usual and customary charge (UCC). The UCC is set by the payer and can be less than the actual billed charge, in which case the patient may be responsible for the balance. Generally, the coinsurance is 70%/30% or 80%/20%, where the insurance company pays the higher percentage and the insured the lower. Indemnity plans were the mainstay of the health insurance world prior to the 1980s. Today, managed care is the norm. Some employers still offer indemnity plans despite their high premium payments in order to allow their employees the freedom to choose medical services.

As an alternative to indemnity health insurance, managed care was introduced in 1973 with the passage of the Health Maintenance Organization Act. This Act encouraged and funded the development of health maintenance organizations (HMOs) as a strategy to contain the rising cost of healthcare. HMOs utilized managed care features that coupled healthcare reimbursement with delivery of service and allowed the payers significant economic control over how, where and what services were delivered. Common features in managed care are: specific physicians and hospitals are selected to care for members, referrals are usually necessary from a case manager for specialty or inpatients services, and providers share in the financial risk through capitation agreements and per diem rates (Sultz, 2004).

Capitation agreements pay the service provider (e.g., physician) a fixed dollar amount per member per month (PMPM). From this amount the provider agrees to cover all care for plan members. For example, if a laboratory signs a capitation agreement to accept $1.50 PMPM for the outpatient testing needs of 2000 HMO members, the laboratory receives $3000 per month; $36 000 per year. If it costs the laboratory more than $36 000/year to provide the services, it realizes a financial loss; if it costs less than $36 000 it realizes a profit. In a capitation testing agreement, a laboratory assumes the risk of spending more than it is paid. One key to managing this risk is gaining access to test utilization of plan members and accurately assessing laboratory costs.

Per diem or per day rates are negotiated with hospitals to provide all the necessary care and services for managed members requiring inpatient care. The reimbursement for any laboratory testing during the inpatient stay is included in the per diem amount. As with capitation, if it costs more to provide the inpatient services than the per diem rate, the hospital is at financial risk.

Sometimes, a service is separately negotiated, i.e., it is not included as part of the capitation or per diem rate. This is called a 'carve out.' Esoteric and expensive tests (chromosome analysis, certain molecular testing) should be targeted as carve outs from capitation outpatient laboratory testing agreements. A negotiated fee-for-service price for these tests is more appropriate. By excluding these tests from capitation, one can avoid huge financial losses due to unexpectedly high utilization of these costly services.

Government Payers

Medicare is federal health insurance for individuals age 65 and older, individuals who are permanently disabled and those with end-stage renal disease who have met the specified waiting period. Medicare was established in 1965 by Title XVIII of the Social Security Act. It is administered by the Centers for Medicare and Medicaid Services (CMS), a division of the US Department of Health and Human Services (HHS). Coverage is provided under Parts A, B and C and claims are processed by CMS approved contractors. These contractors are usually private health insurers that serve as fiscal intermediaries (generally processing Part A claims) and carriers (generally processing Part B claims). In order for a laboratory to qualify for Medicare/Medicaid reimbursement, the laboratory must maintain CLIA (Clinical Laboratory Improvements Amendments of 1988) certification (Washington G-2, 2004).

Medicare Part A covers inpatient hospitalization, hospice care, skilled nursing care and home healthcare. Coverage is automatic for those who are eligible. Prior to the Tax Equity and Fiscal Responsibility Act of 1982 (TEFRA), inpatient hospitalization was reimbursed on a retrospective cost based system. This system paid hospitals for all costs incurred during an inpatient stay. After TEFRA, the system switched to a prospective payment system (PPS) which reimbursed hospitals based on preset payments for services provided to patients with similar diagnoses. With this diagnosis-related group (DRG) payment system, hospitals are reimbursed the same amount for the same DRG no matter how many discreet units of services are provided. Thus, hospitals can earn a profit or realize a loss on each inpatient stay, depending on whether their costs are lower or higher than the DRG payment. The aim of TEFRA, with its fixed DRG reimbursements, was to force hospitals to contain costs by reducing the length of stay (LOS) and eliminate unnecessary and/or overutilized services (Washington G-2, 2004).

Medicare Part B covers outpatient laboratory tests, physician professional services, and other medical services and devices. Coverage is not automatic. Eligible beneficiaries must enroll for Part B coverage and pay premiums. Beneficiaries must pay an annual deductible and a 20% copayment for all Part B services, except for clinical laboratory testing which is covered in full, provided certain conditions are met (see below).

The Part B fee schedule plays an important role in reimbursement since it is a baseline that nongovernment payers use to establish their own rates. For example, a private insurance company may set its fee schedule at 110% of the Part B fee schedule.

Medicare Part C is an alternative to the traditional Part B fee-for-service program. It is designed to reduce patient 'out of pocket' costs by providing services through health maintenance organizations and other service models. Medicare Part C is known as Medicare+Choice and is not available in all States (Washington G-2, 2004).

Medicaid is a Federal program that offers healthcare coverage for select low-income families. It was authorized in 1965 as a Federal/State sponsored program designed to pay medical costs for certain families with low income or inadequate resources. Eligibility includes people who are aged, blind, or disabled, and those in families with dependent children. Although Medicaid is a Federal program, it is under the jurisdiction of each individual state. This means each state determines who is eligible, the range of health services offered and how they are reimbursed. It is a common misconception that Medicaid covers healthcare costs for all low-income persons. Medicaid does not provide paid medical assistance to every single poor person. To receive medical assistance, a person must meet eligibility requirements.

Reimbursement Coding Systems

In order to be paid, a medical claim must describe the patient's medical condition (or diagnosis) and list the services (or tests) provided. This information is conveyed via a standardized coding system, recognized by all government and private payers: *Healthcare Finance Administration Common Procedural Coding System* (*HCPCS*) codes describe the test or service and the *International Classification of Disease, 9th Revision with Clinical Modifications* (ICD-9-CM) codes describe the patient's condition or diagnosis. These standards allow data to be accurately communicated among physicians, patients and third-party payers.

HCPCS was developed in 1983 and consists of two levels of codes. Level I is the *Current Procedural Terminology* (*CPT*) coding system and is used to identify nearly all clinical laboratory tests and most medical services. CPT codes are assigned by the American Medical Association (AMA) and are reviewed and updated annually to keep current with changes in technology and medical practice. Each CPT code has five digits and a description of the test or service (CPT, 2003). For example, the CPT code for a prostate-specific antigen (PSA) test is 84153.

Level II consists of HCPCS/National Codes assigned by the government. CPT does not contain all the codes needed to report services or to describe special circumstances that may apply to Medicare. HCFA (Healthcare Financing Administration, predecessor of CMS) developed this second level of codes to fill the gap. HCPCS Level II codes begin with a single letter (A through V) followed by four digits. These codes are updated annually by CMS. An example of Level II coding is prostate-specific antigen for cancer screening, G0103 (CMS, 2004). Note that CMS treats this test differently than the PSA CPT code above, even though the tests are identical to the laboratory. This allows CMS to assign different criteria for reimbursement, based on why a test is ordered.

The ICD-9 (International Classification of Disease, 9th Revision) was originally developed by the World Health Organization (WHO) as a classification system for reporting mortality and morbidity statistics by physicians throughout the world. The ICD-9-CM is a US clinically modified revision of the WHO's ICD-9. This modification is maintained and updated by the National Center for Health Statistics. These modifications assist healthcare providers to index patient records, retrieve case data for clinical studies and submit claims for healthcare services (Physician ICD-9-CM, 2001).

Why Accurate Coding is Important

Correct coding is important for three reasons. First, one should be paid for services rendered. Insufficient or incorrect coding yields lower reimbursement than is rightfully due. Second, one must not receive more reimbursement than is rightfully due. Coding for services not provided or assigning a code that recoups more reimbursement (this practice is known

as 'up-coding') is illegal and constitutes fraud. Third, one must comply with *Medical Necessity* regulations established by CMS for Medicare patients. These policies define under what conditions a test is considered 'medically necessary' and thus reimbursable. Certain tests are only considered 'medically necessary' if they are associated with specific diagnoses. Thus, reimbursement depends on whether the diagnosis or medical condition code (ICD-9 code) supports the test code (HCPCS code). For example, 'malignant neoplasm of the prostate,' supports the medical necessity of doing a PSA test, so Medicare would pay for the test; in contrast, 'congestive heart failure' is not considered a medically necessary reason for a PSA test, so the test would not be reimbursed. Note that a physician (or other provider) can order any test on a patient, even if it is not 'medically necessary'; it just will not be reimbursed.

Most laboratory fee schedules are set by the local Medicare contractor (fiscal intermediary or carrier). Historically, each contractor established separate guidelines for determining which tests were subject to medically necessary diagnosis codes. These *local medical review policies* (LMRP) differed from one carrier to another, making it very difficult to submit and process claims. In some instances, a diagnosis code valid for a test from one carrier would not be considered medically necessary by another carrier. In an effort to standardize all carrier reimbursement guidelines for specific outpatient laboratory tests, 23 tests have been assigned *national coverage decisions* (NCD); these medical necessity guidelines apply to all carriers in the country. See Table 12–4 for the list of NCD tests (CMS, 2004).

Coding at any level should be as specific as possible. The National Correct Coding Initiative (NCCI) outlines correct coding practices based on the codes defined in the AMA's CPT Manual. Most analytes or tests have a specific CPT like that of PSA. However, sometimes a new test does not have its own code. When that happens, the test must be identified by the method used to perform the analysis (like 82486-Chromatography or 83519-Immunoassay, RIA). A method code is usually reimbursed at a lower rate than a CPT code specific to a test.

Tests that are performed together, i.e., as a panel, must be coded correctly. There are nine AMA approved panels (see Table 12–5). When these panels are performed, they must be coded with a unique panel code and not by each individual test's CPT code. Reimbursement is much lower

Table 12–4 National Coverage Determinations for Laboratory Testing (CMS, 2004)

General testing category	CPT codes included
Alpha-fetoprotein	82105
Blood counts	85004, 85007, 85008, 85013, 85014, 85018, 85025, 85027, 85032, 85045, 85049
Blood glucose testing	82947, 82948, 82962
Carcinoembryonic antigen	82378
Collagen crosslinks, any method	82523
Digoxin therapeutic drug assay	80162
Fecal occult blood test (FOBT)	82270
Gamma glutamyl transferase	82977
Glycated hemoglobin/glycated protein	82985, 83036
Hepatitis panel/acute hepatitis panel	80074
Human chorionic gonadotropin (HCG)	84702
Human immunodeficiency virus (HIV) testing (diagnosis)	86689, 86701, 86702, 86703, 87390, 87391, 87534, 87535, 87637, 87538
Human immunodeficiency virus (HIV) testing (prognosis including monitoring)	87536, 87539
Lipids	80061, 82465, 83715, 83716, 83718, 83721, 84478
Partial thromboplastin time	85730
Prostate-specific antigen	84153
Prothrombin time	85610
Serum iron studies	82728, 83540, 83550, 84466
Thyroid testing	84436, 84439, 84443, 84479
Tumor antigen by immunoassay CA 125	86304
Tumor antigen by immunoassay CA 15-3/CA 27.29	86300
Tumor antigen by immunoassay CA 19-9	86301
Urine culture, bacterial	87086, 87088, 87184, 87186

Table 12–5 AMA Organ or Disease Oriented Panels (CPT, 2003)

CPT	Panel	Required components	
80048	Basic metabolic panel	Calcium	(82310)
		Carbon dioxide	(82374)
		Chloride	(82435)
		Creatinine	(82565)
		Glucose	(82947)
		Potassium	(84132)
		Sodium	(84295)
		Urea nitrogen (BUN)	(84520)
80050	General health panel	Comprehensive metabolic panel	(80053)
		Blood count, complete (CBC)	(85025) or (85027) and (85004)
		OR	
		Blood Count, complete (CBC)	(85027) and (85007) or (85009)
		Thyroid-stimulating hormone	(84443)
80051	Electrolyte panel	Carbon dioxide	(82374)
		Chloride	(82435)
		Potassium	(84132)
		Sodium	(84295)
80053	Comprehensive metabolic panel	Albumin	(82040)
		Bilirubin, total	(82247)
		Calcium	(82310)
		Carbon dioxide	(82374)
		Chloride	(82435)
		Creatinine	(82565)
		Glucose	(82947)
		Phosphatase, alkaline	(84075)
		Potassium	(84132)
		Protein, total	(84155)
		Sodium	(84295)
		Transferase, alanine amino	(84460)
		Transferase, aspartate amino	(84450)
		Urea nitrogen (BUN)	(84520)
80055	Obstetric panel	Blood count, complete (CBC)	(85025) or (85027) and (85004)
		OR	
		Blood count, complete (CBC)	(85027) and (85007) or (85009)
		Hepatitis B surface antigen	(87340)
		Antibody, rubella	(86762)
		Syphilis test, qualitative	(86592)
		Antibody screen, RBC	(86850)
		Blood typing, ABO	(86900)
		Blood typing, Rh	(86901)
80061	Lipid panel	Cholesterol, total	(85465)
		HDL cholesterol	(83718)
		Triglycerides	(84478)
80069	Renal function panel	Albumin	(82040)
		Calcium	(82310)
		Carbon dioxide	(82374)
		Chloride	(82435)
		Creatinine	(82565)
		Glucose	(82947)
		Phosphorus, inorganic	(84100)
		Potassium	(84132)
		Sodium	(84295)
		Urea nitrogen (BUN)	(84520)
80074	Acute hepatitis panel	Hepatitis A antibody, IgM	(86709)
		Hepatitis B core antibody, IgM	(86705)
		Hepatitis B surface antigen	(87340)
		Hepatitis C antibody	(86803)

Table 12–5 AMA Organ or Disease Oriented Panels (CPT, 2003) *(cont'd)*

CPT	Panel	Required components	
80076	Hepatic function panel	Albumin	(82040)
		Bilirubin, total	(82247)
		Bilirubin, direct	(82248)
		Phosphatase, alkaline	(84075)
		Protein, total	(84155)
		Transferase, alanine amino	(84460)
		Transferase, aspartate amino	(84450)

for a panel than it is for the sum total reimbursement of each test. Coding for each individual test component as opposed to the one panel code is considered 'unbundling,' which is a fraudulent billing practice (CMS, 2004).

Professional pathology physician services (like test interpretation, slide review, etc.) are not included in the laboratory fee schedule. They are paid by the Medicare physician fee schedule, which uses a resource-based relative value scale (RBRVS) to determine the payment based on a service's relative value unit (RVU). These amounts are adjusted to reflect local economic factors. Unlike the laboratory fee schedule, these professional services are subject to the annual deductible and the 20% copayment (Washington G-2, 2004).

Medicare Reimbursement

Medicare is the largest insurance program in the country. In many hospitals it accounts for 25–40% of all revenue. Outpatient services are reimbursed differently from inpatient ones.

Medicare Inpatients. Diagnosis-related groups (DRGs) are a patient classification system used to reimburse inpatient (Part A) hospital costs for Medicare patients. While the costs associated with inpatient clinical laboratory tests are included in the DRG, it does not cover physician services (Part B). After a Medicare patient has been discharged from the hospital, the patient's medical record is reviewed by health information management coders and assigned appropriate ICD-9-CM and HCPCS codes for one or more diagnoses and procedures for the inpatient stay. These codes along with the patient's demographic information are grouped by decision trees (this process is computerized) into a specific DRG. There are currently more than 500 DRGs. CMS assigns a weight to each DRG based on the severity of the diagnoses, types of procedures performed, number of laboratory tests, volume and type of drugs administered and the presence of complications or comorbidity conditions. CMS assigns each hospital a specific rate that is calculated based on type of facility (community hospital vs. teaching hospital), setting (urban vs. rural) and location (West Coast vs. Midwest). The CMS assigned rate for the DRG is multiplied by the hospital's assigned rate to determine reimbursement for the hospital stay. This amount is payment-in-full for the inpatient hospitalization. If it costs the hospital more than the reimbursed amount to treat the patient, the hospital must absorb the cost. The patient cannot be billed for any nonreimbursed Part A services (Washington G-2, 2004).

Medicare Outpatients. For many years after the enactment of DRGs, each outpatient service continued to be reimbursed individually (Harmening, 2003). However, the reimbursement system changed when CMS started to implement an outpatient prospective payment system (OPPS) with the introduction of the Ambulatory Payment Classification (APC) system in 2000. Under this system, virtually all hospital-based outpatient services (like ED and clinic visits, oncology treatment, surgery, etc.) provided to Medicare patients are reimbursed on a prospective basis based on a preset rate, similar to DRGs. Clinical laboratory tests are *not* included in the APC, and are still reimbursed individually based on CMS fee schedule with some exceptions (Varnadoe, 1996).

Under certain conditions, Medicare does not pay for laboratory tests (Table 12–6). If a laboratory expects Medicare to deny payment because a test does not meet medical necessity requirements, it must inform the patient before the service is provided. An *advanced beneficiary notice (ABN)* is used to document that the beneficiary was told the test might not be covered by Medicare, the reason(s) for the possible denial, and the decision by the patient to pay for the test if Medicare does not reimburse or to refuse the test entirely. The use of ABNs became mandatory January 1, 2003 (Washington G-2, 2004).

An important consideration for hospitals that have laboratories which perform outpatient testing on Medicare patients is the *72 hour rule*. This rule states that a hospital cannot bill an outpatient (Part B) claim for laboratory tests performed within 72 hours of an inpatient admission. The outpatient testing that is performed 72 hours prior to the admission must

Table 12–6 National Coverage Determinations for Laboratory Testing (CMS, 2004)

Category	Medicare coverage	ABN necessary?
LMRP or NCD tests	Provider paid according to outpatient fee schedule, if medical necessity met	No, unless test is not 'medically necessary'
FDA cleared or 'homebrew' tests not included above	Provider paid according to outpatient fee schedule, if medical necessity met	No, unless test is not 'medically necessary'
Investigational use only or research tests (i.e., not FDA cleared)	Not covered, no payment	Yes
Health and wellness screening	Not covered, with few exceptions: PAP smears covered every 2 years for all women and every year for those with high cancer risk or abnormal smear. PSA covered every year for men older than 50	Yes, unless it is one of the allowable exceptions

Table 12–7 Pro Forma Laboratory Budget

Category	Current year	Assumptions	Change	Projection for new year
Revenue	$3 000 000	4% growth	$120 000	$3 120 000
Total tests	370 000	4% growth	14 800	384 800
Revenue/test	$8.11			$8.11
Expenses				
Salaries	$950 000	3% cost of living increase	$28 500	$978 500
Laboratory supplies	$421 000	4% growth (no price increase)	$16 840	$437 840
Reference lab fees	$250 000	4% growth 1% price increase (on projected $260 000)	$10 000 $2600	$262 600
Phlebotomy supplies	$35 500	4% growth	$1420	$36 920
Maintenance contracts	$40 000	No change		$ 40 000
Total expense	$1 696 500		$59 360	$1 755 860
Cost per test	$4.59			$4.56

be included with the inpatient claim and is reimbursed according to the assigned DRG for that stay. Hospital laboratories must identify outpatient Medicare services that are affected by this rule and make sure they are not billed separately. A nonhospital independent laboratory is not subject to the 72 hour rule (CMS, 2004). Thus preadmission tests performed 2 days before hospitalization are not reimbursed if performed in the admitting hospital's laboratory but are reimbursed if done in an independent laboratory.

Financial Performance and Monitoring

Budgeting

Budgeting is the process of planning, forecasting, controlling and monitoring the financial resources of an organization. The *operational budget provides a target of* day-to-day revenues and expenditures that are to be achieved in the forthcoming year.

Different budget planning strategies are used based on the type and seasonality of the business; however, all use a method to forecast and project what will occur in the next budget cycle. Projections are made for the expected increases and decreases in revenues and expenses based on historical information and adjustments for inflation, loss of business, new business, new product lines, etc. The laboratory typically uses a *pro forma* budget. It provides in a pro forma or 'predetermined set form' the expected annual revenue and expense based on various projections and assumptions, including test volume. It uses actual costs, ratios and percent calculations to extrapolate from historical data what the new budget will be. Table 12–7 is an example of a pro forma budget.

In contrast to the pro forma budget, which uses baseline data from one year to develop data for the next, a *zero-based budget* has no baseline. A zero-based budget requires management to annually evaluate all services and products to determine which should be funded or eliminated. Each department manager must justify its budget as if all of its activities are new. It assumes no existing program is entitled to automatic budget approval, but must prove its financial merit when compared to the organization's other programs. Programs are ranked and funded by merit priority to the level of the organization's available funds. Laboratories use a zero-based approach to propose a new service (e.g., blood donor program, outpatient blood collection center, etc.) or laboratory section (e.g., mycology) or test (PCR assay) (Travers, 1997).

The capital budget is used to fund large capital projects like acquiring an instrument or information system, or remodeling the laboratory. These projects may cost thousands or millions of dollars and require several years to plan or implement. The laboratory's proposed projects must compete with those of other hospital departments for limited capital dollars. Each project is evaluated (see below) and ranked based on a variety of financial and clinical factors. The operational budget must be linked to the capital budget, for it is the revenues generated by operations that are used to fund the needed capital items and projects. Operational budgets must generate surplus revenue to fund capital projects; a business must reinvest in itself to remain competitive.

Variance Analysis

The operational budget should be reviewed periodically, usually monthly, to determine how closely the projected budget matches actual revenues and expenses. A *variance* is the difference between the projected budget and the actual revenue and expenses (Budget − Actual = Variance). Both positive variances (less than expected revenue or expenses) and negative variances (more than expected revenue or expenses) need to be analyzed. By analyzing a variance, one can identify whether it can be controlled or not. Once the cause is determined, one can take necessary action to improve performance and more accurately prepare future budgets.

If revenues (and expected test volume) are within budget but laboratory supplies show a negative variance, one must investigate the reason for the discrepancy. For example, technologists may be repeating tests too frequently, running too many controls, or scheduling work inefficiently, in many small batches. This is an example of a variance that can be controlled by the laboratory if it changes its practices. Actions to consider are increasing the frequency of instrument maintenance to reduce problems that require repeats and controls, staff education to reinforce policies of when repeats and controls are needed, and rescheduling work into more efficient batch sizes.

An example of an uncontrollable variance is if a hospital decides to eliminate the cardiac chest pain service. In this scenario, there would be a positive reagent expense variance (i.e., less money spent on reagents than expected) related to doing fewer cardiac marker tests. There is nothing a laboratory manager can do to correct this variance. However, this does not absolve the manager from ignoring it. One must verify the amount of the variance and determine if it is appropriate for the amount of lost business. When forecasting for the next budget cycle, one should decrease projected revenues and expenses attributed to the loss of the cardiac services.

Financial Reporting and Statements

Managerial accounting is used to prepare and monitor budgets. Revenue and expenses are organized into logical groupings known as cost centers that represent a laboratory section (like microbiology, core lab, blood bank) or function (phlebotomy). Each cost center is subdivided into a variety of expense and revenue categories. Salary and nonsalary expense categories are grouped separately. Periodic review, at least monthly, of the cost center's accounts is needed to monitor the variances and put corrective action in place to keep the organization on its expected financial plan. Table 12–8 is an example of a laboratory cost center's accounts.

Financial accounting is a system used to report business information to external entities such as the Internal Revenue Service (IRS) or its stockholders. Generally accepted accounting principles (GAAP) are used to standardize this information. Balance sheet, income statement and statement of cash flows are the financial statements most commonly used to assess an organization's financial position. Banks and investors rely heavily on these statements to determine whether to lend a business money or purchase shares of stock.

Table 12–8 Cost Center: Microbiology

		Current month			Year to date		
		Revenue					
Account number	**Account name**	**Actual**	**Budget**	**Variance**	**Actual**	**Budget**	**Variance**
20100	Inpatient revenue	$1 414 245	$1 403 172	$11 073	$289 2427	$2 764 597	$127 830
20 200	Outpatient revenue	$906 343	$894 405	$11 938	$1,699 418	$1,748 169	$(48 751)
TOTAL REVENUE		$2 320 588	$2 297 577	$23 011	$4 591 845	$4 512 766	$79 079
		Expenses					
40100	Salary, management	$22 045	$21 811	$234	$43 310	$43 622	$(312)
40200	Salary, technical	$85 161	$105 410	$(20 249)	$170 437	$210 820	$(40 383)
40201	Overtime	$3385	$3907	$(522)	$6713	$7814	$(1101)
Total salary expense		$110 591	$131 128	$(20 537)	$220 460	$262 256	$(41 796)
41580	Laboratory supplies	$109 961	$96 114	$13 847	$193 102	$188 461	$4 641
41590	Medical surgical supplies	$1682	$1715	$(33)	$3964	$3362	$602
41890	Service contracts	$75	$355	$(280)	$150	$710	$(560)
42010	Minor equipment	$1112	$1083	$29	$2568	$2166	$402
45300	Sendout test expense	$14 973	$13 750	$1223	$28 812	$27 500	$1312
46300	Accreditation expense	$–	$100	$(100)	$–	$200	$(200)
Total nonsalary expense		$127 803	$113 117	$14 686	$228 596	$222 399	$6197
TOTAL EXPENSE		$238 394	$244 245	$(5851)	$449 056	$484 655	$(35 599)

The *balance sheet* is the statement of an organization's financial position at a specific point in time. This statement is usually generated at the end of an organization's fiscal year or at the end of the calendar year. It records the organization's assets (what it owns), its liabilities (what it owes) and its equity or net worth (what is left after subtracting what it owes from what it owns). From this statement is derived the fundamental accounting equation: Assets = Liabilities + Equity (Net worth). This statement is used to assess an organization's level of indebtedness to what it owns.

The *income statement*, also known as the statement of profit and loss, summarizes the organization's revenues and expenses over an accounting period, usually quarterly or annually. The income statement records all of a laboratory's gross patient revenue, less allowances for a given period, and deducts the expenses for that same period to arrive at net income before taxes (NIBT). Taxes are only paid if the organization is for-profit. Net income is realized when net revenues exceed expenses. A net loss is realized when expenses exceed net revenues. Note that revenue does not necessarily equate to cash generated. Many times a test is performed and recorded as income though the payment (cash) may not be received for several months. The income statement records the organization's ability to make a profit; it does not reflect its cash position.

The *statement of cash flows* shows the amount of cash generated by an organization over a period of time, usually a calendar or fiscal year. Cash outflows (cash paid out) are subtracted from cash inflows (cash received) to calculate the net change in cash for the period. Excess cash in a given period can be reinvested in the organization, used to make additional debt payments or placed in easily liquidated securities for emergency use. If the net cash position for a period is negative, the organization must meet its cash obligations by using cash reserves from previous periods. If this trend is not reversed, the organization will eventually run out of cash.

Benchmarking and Productivity Measures

Benchmarking and productivity measures go hand in hand. It does no good to collect productivity data if they are not compared with a standard or evaluated for trends over time. Benchmarking is the measurement of an organization's products or services against specific standards for comparison and improvement (Wallace, 1998). Benchmarking can be internal or external.

Internal benchmarking trends an organization's productivity over time. Productivity is the relationship between input (labor and supplies) and output (product or service) (Travers, 1997). It is usually expressed as a ratio of the product or service to the various inputs used for the production of the product or service. See Table 12–9 for common productivity ratios used in the laboratory. The purpose of trending internal productivity is to determine if internal standards are being met, exceeded or not met. If adjustments to workflow or personnel are made, the next period's benchmarking data can

Table 12–9 Common Productivity Measures for Clinical Laboratories

Productivity measure	Target*	Quarter 1	Quarter 2
Billable tests/paid FTE	>3680	3798	3500
Billable tests/worked FTE	>4000	4128	4080
Worked FTE/paid FTE	>92%	95.2%	90%
Labor cost/billable test	<$5.00	$4.68	$5.01
Supply cost/billable test	<$1.00	$0.99	$1.01
Overtime/worked straight time	<3%	2.7%	3.5%

FTE = full time equivalent or 2080 paid hours in a year; paid FTE = all salaries paid (benefit time plus worked time).

* Target is for illustration purposes only. It should not be considered a laboratory standard.

be used to determine if the adjustments were the probable cause for improvements or for decreased productivity.

External benchmarking compares a laboratory's productivity to that of other laboratories. Its purpose is to identify top performers in a particular field. Top performers can be contacted to find out what processes or resources have been used to achieve high productivity. This information may guide a laboratory to make similar changes that could result in higher productivity. Professional organizations such as the College of American Pathologists (CAP) or the University Healthcare Consortium (UHC) offer external laboratory specific benchmarking programs. Caution should always be used when interpreting external benchmarking information. Although clinical laboratories are similar, no two are exactly alike and, despite best efforts, sometimes data are collected and reported differently. A laboratory may never be able to achieve as high productivity as its peers due to factors beyond the laboratory's control. Labor availability, the disease and acuity mix of the patients, access to technology and automation will each have an effect on how productive a laboratory is, and how much more productive it can become.

Evaluating a Capital Project

A hospital has limited capital; it cannot fund all projects so it must prioritize them based on a variety of factors including clinical need and financial impact. Whether or not money is borrowed to finance these projects, it may be necessary for the project or investment to pay for itself and even generate excess cash to fund other projects. The following section discusses different ways to evaluate a capital project in order to answer the question: 'Is it a good investment'? Table 12–10 compares these methods.

Table 12–10 Financial Evaluation of a New Automated Analyzer

Given

Investment (cost of analyzer)		$200 000
Discount rate (rate of inflation or interest rate of borrowed money)		10.00%
Useful life of analyzer	5 years	
Annual depreciation expense	$200 000/5 years	$40 000
Annual revenue	100 000 tests at $5.00/test	$500 000
Annual labor expense	100 000 tests at $2.50/test	$250 000
Annual supply expense	100 000 tests at $2.00/test	$200 000
Annual net revenue (Annual revenue – Annual expense)	$500 000 – ($250 000 + $200 000)	$50 000
Net revenue per test (Test revenue – Test expense)	$5.00 – ($2.50 + $2.00)	$0.50

Calculations

PAYBACK PERIOD = Investment/ Annual net revenue	$200 000/$50 000	4 years
BREAKEVEN		
Per year = Depreciation/Net revenue per test	$40 000/$0.50	80 000 tests
Life of analyzer = Investment/(Net revenue per test)	$200 000/$0.50	400 000 tests
RETURN ON INVESTMENT (ROI) = Annual net revenue/ Investment	$50 000/$200 000	25% per year

NET PRESENT VALUE (NPV) = Present value of the sum of future net revenue (cash flows) minus investment. Note: Present value interest factor (PVIF) for each year based on 10% discount rate is multiplied by net revenue to determine present value. PVIF is available from any financial data resource. NPV can also be calculated with financial calculator

Today's investment	($200 000)	
Year 1 Net revenue × PVIF	$50 000 × 0.9091 = $45 455	
Year 2 Net revenue × PVIF	$50 000 × 0.8264 = $41 320	
Year 3 Net revenue × PVIF	$50 000 × 0.7513 = $37 565	
Year 4 Net revenue × PVIF	$50 000 × 0.6830 = $34 150	
Year 5 Net revenue × PVIF	$50 000 × 0.6209 = $31 045	
Present value of sum of future net revenue	$189 535	
NPV		$(10 465)

INTERNAL RATE OF RETURN (IRR) = Discounted interest rate at which NPV = 0. Note: financial calculator is used to determine IRR by entering cash flow and discount rate

Today's investment	($200 000)	
Year 1 Net revenue × PVIF	$50 000 × 0.9265 = $46 326	
Year 2 Net revenue × PVIF	$50 000 × 0.8585 = $42 923	
Year 3 Net revenue × PVIF	$50 000 × 0.7954 = $39 769	
Year 4 Net revenue × PVIF	$50 000 × 0.7369 = $36 847	
Year 5 Net revenue × PVIF	$50 000 × 0.6828 = $34 140	
Present value of sum of future net revenue	$200 000	
NPV	$0	
IRR		8%

Payback Period

The payback period is commonly used to evaluate a capital project. The payback is the length of time required for an investment's net revenue to cover the cost of the initial investment (Brigham, 1998).

Because laboratory equipment or technology can become obsolete in a very short period of time, it is important to recover the investment cost as soon as possible. Once the initial investment is recovered, net revenue (Revenue – Expense) from this investment represents a profit to the organization. The sooner a capital project's payback period is reached, the sooner an organization can realize a profit from the investment.

Breakeven Point

The breakeven point of a capital project is reached when the volume of sales is such that total revenue equals total costs (fixed and variable) and therefore profit is zero. Before the breakeven point is reached the project is operating at a loss; after it is reached the project is realizing a profit (Brigham, 1998). As with the payback period, the sooner the breakeven point is reached the better it is for the organization.

Return on Investment (ROI)*

The rate of return for a capital project is the ratio of net income it generates to the total investment of the project (Travers, 1997). ROI is a standard for evaluating how wisely management uses its capital dollars, whether from its own cash reserves or from borrowing activities. The higher the rate of return the better the capital dollars are used. ROI is the formal means of expressing the phrase 'better bang for your buck.'

Net Present Value (NPV)*

Money loses its value over time; $10 000 today is more valuable than $10 000 3 years from now. This concept is known as the time value of money. The payback period and return on investment calculations do not consider the time value of money. They assume that the value of future cash flows remains constant. To address this shortcoming, the net present value calculation is used to determine if a project's cash flows (i.e., cash it generates in the future) are sufficient to repay the original investment, taking into account that money loses value over time. Thus, cash received in the future has to be *discounted* (i.e., the value has to be reduced) in order to determine how much it is worth in today's dollars. The discount rate is usually the inflation rate (if no money was borrowed to finance the project) or the interest rate on a loan used to fund the project. *Net present value (NPV)* is defined as the present value of future cash flows, which have been discounted at the interest rate used to fund the capital project (Brigham, 1998).

When the NPV is a positive number, the project will generate enough cash to pay for the original investment. When the NPV is a negative number, the project cost is not recouped and/or the future cash flows are not sufficient to cover the interest costs for borrowing the money.

Internal Rate of Return*

The internal rate of return also discounts cash flow into today's value. It determines the actual rate of return the investment earns. The *internal rate of return (IRR)* is the discount rate at which the present value of a capital project's expected cash inflows equals the present value of its costs, or in other words when the NPV equals zero.

Identifying a project's IRR is necessary to ensure that its rate is higher than the cost of the capital borrowed for the project. The higher the IRR, the faster the project pays for itself. Hospitals and corporations use the IRR as one way to rank projects.

Interpretation of Financial Calculations

While the preceding calculations are important tools, an organization should not make its capital decisions based strictly on the outcome of the equations. As with all budgeting activities, there is an element of the unknown in the assumptions. Predicting future cash flows for replacement instrumentation is usually more reliable than predicting it for new product lines or technology. Assigning an expected life to a piece of capital equipment is also an educated estimate. Having a good sense of how reliable the predictions are will determine how much credence should be given to the calculations.

If only the payback period, breakeven analysis and ROI were considered when evaluating the example in Table 12–10, the project would look acceptable. However, when the NPV and IRR are also considered, it does not look as good. The NPV is unfavorable and the IRR is much less than

---

* Note: Financial calculators and financial software packages are programmed to calculate ROI, NPV and IRR. The NPV and IRR are very tedious calculations requiring multiple steps and the use of discount tables. It is not recommended to do these calculations manually.

Table 12–11 Capital Acquisition Options

	Advantages	Disadvantages
Purchase	Ownership	Risk of obsolescence; opportunity cost
Operating (true) lease	Hedging obsolescence; flexibility in financing; cancelable	Nonownership; interest/financing cost
Financial lease	Ownership; flexibility in financing	Noncancelable; interest/financing cost
Rental	Hedging obsolescence; flexibility in length of use	High cost; nonownership

the ROI because the cost of capital is high (10%). Does this mean the project should not go forward? Not necessarily. Depending on other issues, it may be determined that this new chemistry analyzer is absolutely essential to support the mission of the organization.

There are other inherent drawbacks to these calculations. As mentioned earlier, some of the calculations take into account the time value of money and others do not. The time value of money is a very important consideration when the cost of capital is high (as with the example in Table 12–10) or during periods of high inflation. The rate of return calculations yield a percentage but the actual dollars it represents is not immediately apparent. A capital project that yields an ROI of 15% might initially look better than one that yields 10%. However, the size of the projects may differ considerably. For example, in the former, an initial investment of $10 000 could produce $1500 in net revenue, while in the latter project, an initial investment of $200 000 produces $20 000 in net revenue. None of these financial calculations should be considered in isolation but used in aggregate to assist in the analysis of capital projects.

Capital Acquisition Methods

When evaluating a capital project, the method for acquiring the equipment is also an important consideration. Table 12–11 summarizes the advantages and disadvantages of acquisition methods: purchase, leasing and renting. Just as there is not a single best financial calculation when evaluating a project, there is not a single best acquisition method. The method selected depends on the individual needs, characteristics and financial philosophy of the organization.

The concept of purchasing the needed equipment is easy to understand, but is it the wisest use of an organization's money? If the capital (money) needed to fund the project is currently invested in a security that is earning a higher interest rate than the rate needed to borrow money, it makes financial sense to borrow the needed capital. Conversely if capital earns a lower interest rate than the borrowing rate, it makes sense to use the organization's capital.

Once the equipment is purchased, it is an asset of the organization and is depreciated by a method appropriate for such a piece of equipment. The depreciation expense is noted in the income statement, but will probably not be included in the monthly operational budget documents. (It will depend on each organization as to whether depreciation is listed on the monthly budget reports.) The operational expense for the equipment will be the supplies, maintenance and labor to support it.

There are many different variations and contract terms that could be associated with a leasing agreement. Being certain to 'read the fine print' never rings truer than when considering an equipment leasing arrangement. Nonetheless, no matter how complicated the terms of a leasing contract are, there are only two types of leases.

An *operating lease* (also known as a 'true' lease) allows an organization (lessee) full use of the equipment for a predetermined time. The time period is usually 1–3 years, but always less than the useful life of the equipment. A termination clause could be included in the agreement. Equipment maintenance is included in an operating lease. The lessee has no right to ownership during or after the lease period. No equity is established during the term. The owner (lessor) retains full ownership of the equipment and the full responsibilities for it. The leasing agreement may or may not contain an option to allow the lessee to purchase the equipment at the end of the term. This is only an option; however, and

should not be misinterpreted as established equity over the course of the agreement. If there is a purchase option it is usually for the equipment's fair market value at the end of the lease period. If the original lessee decides not to purchase the equipment at the end of the lease term, the lessor could re-lease it to the original lessee, or to another organization as the equipment still has useful life (Brigham, 1998)

The other lease type is a financial lease. With a *financial* lease (also known as a capital lease or lease-purchase), the lessee eventually gains ownership of the equipment. The lease period corresponds to the economic life of the equipment. Through the lease payments, the lessor recovers the cost of the equipment plus an interest factor to ensure a return on their investment. A financial lease is not cancelable and equipment maintenance is not included (Brigham, 1998).

Renting equipment is not the same as leasing it. The major differentiators are: renting does not carry an option for later purchase, there is no predetermined specified length of time for renting, it can be terminated at any time, and maintenance and repair are the responsibility of the owner, not the renter (Travers, 1997). A reagent rental agreement is a misnomer; it is not a rental but a lease. These agreements require the lessee to purchase reagents that are specific for a particular piece of equipment. The price of the reagents is marked up by a certain amount to cover the 'rent' of the equipment. The mark-up is a lease payment to cover the cost of the capital. Whether or not the equipment will be owned at the end of the reagent rental agreement will determine if the agreement was a financial lease. Recent federal legislation requires vendors to clearly state the proportion of annual payments that are allocated to the capital portion of the lease. This simplifies the analysis of competing lease agreements.

Creating Financial Value/Conclusions

Financial oversight of any organization is not easy. For a clinical laboratory this oversight is especially difficult because in order to remain competitive it must offer state-of-the-art technologies that are often complex, expensive and quick to become obsolete. This combined with the strict coding criteria for submitting claims that yield a predetermined fixed reimbursement rate leaves little opportunity for the laboratory to cover costs, let alone make a profit.

The equation for net profit is defined as revenue minus expenses. Therefore the only way to increase net profit is to either increase net revenue or to decrease expenses. In a managed care environment, increasing patient volume (and gross revenue) does little to increase net profit because variable expenses increase proportionally with the larger volume. For an increase in gross revenue to have a positive impact on net profit, the newly generated revenue must have a closer relationship to what is billed and to what is collected. The best way to achieve this is by providing testing to clients that is paid based on a fee schedule instead of a DRG, APC, per diem or capitation. Many laboratories attempt to do this by offering commercial or reference outreach programs. The target markets for outreach business are physician offices, clinics and other laboratories or hospitals. If a laboratory has excess capacity for testing and can perform this additional testing without adding fixed costs, the increase in this revenue should increase the net profit. This of course also assumes the prices charged for the tests cover the expenses for this outreach testing. Once the increase in volume requires the addition of fixed costs (more labor, equipment, space, etc.), careful evaluation of this new volume needs to be performed to ensure the increase can cover the new costs.

Expense reduction seems to be more the norm when trying to increase net profit in a managed care environment. Eliminating as much of the fixed cost as possible is the most effective way to accomplish this. While it is very important to negotiate favorable pricing for supplies, reagents and other variable cost items, reducing their unit cost several cents or even several dollars will not have as great an impact as eliminating unneeded or underutilized fixed costs. Achieving economies of scale through maximum use and efficiency of an organization's fixed costs is critical in realizing substantial cost reductions.

Effective financial management requires careful planning, analysis and critical thinking when decisions need to be made of how best to acquire capital equipment, assign pricing and reduce costs. Keeping abreast of the various payer requirements ensures the laboratory is reimbursed appropriately for the services rendered. When applied with common sense, these tools and knowledge base will promote the financial success of a clinical laboratory operation.

References

Brigham EF, Houston JF: Fundamentals of Financial Management, 8th ed. Philadelphia, PA, The Dryden Press, Harcourt Brace College Publishers, 1998.

An introduction to finance textbook written for the undergraduate business student.

Center for Medicare and Medicaid Services (CMS): Medicare's National Level II Codes HCPCS, 17th ed. Dover, DE, American Medical Association, 2004.

Center for Medicare and Medicaid Services. Online. Available: http://www.cms.hhs.gov/statistics/nhe/, March 24, 2004.

CPT: Current Procedural Terminology, Standard Edition. Chicago, IL, American Medical Association, 2003.

Harmening DM: Laboratory Management Principles and Processes. Upper Saddle River, NJ, Prentice-Hall, Inc., 2003.

A textbook designed to balance theory and practical applications of laboratory management.

Physician ICD-9-CM. Salt Lake City, UT, Medicode, 2001.

Snyder JS, Wilkinson DS: Management in Laboratory Medicine, 3rd ed. Philadelphia, Lippincott, 1998.

A textbook developed to prepare medical technology students and pathology residents for the basic through intermediate levels of management.

Sultz HA, Young KM: Health Care USA Understanding Its Organization and Delivery, 4th ed. Boston, Jones and Bartlett, 2004.

A text describing the changing roles of the components of the healthcare system in addition to the technical, economic, political and social forces responsible for these changes.

Travers EM: Clinical Laboratory Management. Baltimore, Williams & Wilkins, 1997.

A comprehensive basic textbook for training healthcare professionals for clinical laboratory management roles.

Varnadoe LA: Medical Laboratory Management and Supervision. Philadelphia, PA, FA Davis Company, 1996.

A text directed toward laboratory professionals that have expertise in the clinical operations of the laboratory but who have no previous knowledge of the administrative and management aspects.

Wallace MA, Klosinski DD: Clinical Laboratory Science Education & Management. Philadelphia, PA, WB Saunders Company, 1998.

A textbook presenting the basic tenets of education and management for practical application in the field of laboratory medicine.

Washington G-2 Reports: 2004 MEDICARE Reimbursement Manual for Laboratory and Pathology Services, 2004.

CHAPTER 13

Biological, Chemical and Nuclear Terrorism: Role of the Laboratory

Philip M. Tierno Jr PhD, Mark S. Lifshitz MD

KEY POINTS

• Level A laboratories, also known as sentinel laboratories, may be the first to identify an unusual organism or cluster of isolates that may signal a bioterrorism event.

• The responsibility of a Level A laboratory is to 'rule out' suspected biological agents rather than perform complete identification or highly complex analyses.

• Suspect samples must be handled safely and legally (using chain of custody).

• Specific protocols (and presumptive identification criteria) must be applied for each biological agent.

• Category A (highest priority) biological agents are easily disseminated, can cause high mortality and can cause public panic. They include: bacterial (anthrax, plague, tularemia), viral (smallpox, viral hemorrhagic fever) and toxin-mediated (botulism) agents.

• Level A laboratories play mostly a supportive role in the management of hospitalized patients who are victims of a chemical terror attack.

Bioterrorism

Introduction

On September 11, 2001, following the unimaginable terrorist attacks on New York City and Washington DC the Centers for Disease Control (CDC) recommended that healthcare professionals increase surveillance for any unusual disease occurrences, or clusters of disease, asserting that these may be sentinel indicators of bioterrorist (BT) attack. As predicted, anthrax cases were reported in several states, thereby justifying the CDC's suspicions that a bioterrorist was at large. Over the years, it has become clear that germ warfare is equally attractive to terrorist cells, organizations, and even disgruntled individuals as it is to countries. It delivers the greatest impact for the smallest amount of money, and it is relatively easy to carry out. It also comes with a big bonus – it has a dramatic psychological effect on the population. Compared to nuclear weapons or conventional armaments, biological weapons are relatively cheap and easy to make. For anyone with a rudimentary understanding of microbiology and the requisite materials, making biological agents of death in quantity is little more technically demanding than brewing beer. The microorganisms involved are often readily obtainable in nature, like the anthrax bacillus that abounds in soil throughout most of the world, or can be easily acquired from other sources such as a country's pharmaceutical and agricultural industries, or academic institutions. Toxic ricin, for example, which strikes at the central nervous system, can be extracted from the same castor beans that are the source of castor oil.

The United States Department of Defense and the Center for Disease Control has published a list of the most likely biological weapons (NATO, 1996). They fall into three categories. The first includes deadly bacteria such as anthrax and plague. The second comprises viruses, such as those that cause smallpox, encephalitis, and hemorrhagic fevers like Ebola, Lassa and Rift Valley fever. The last group is made up of toxins that attack the central nervous system, such as botulinum, fungal toxins, and ricin.

An effective national strategy to detect, prevent, and limit bioterrorism should consider the following:

• A coordinated plan is needed to network all federal, state and municipal antibioterrorism programs. All first responders must be adequately educated and equipped to deal with any biowarfare or bioterrorism event.

• Military and law enforcement personnel and medical and health practitioners, especially first responders, should be vaccinated whenever possible so that they can more effectively carry out their respective missions.

• Research and development of new wave (sub-particle) vaccines, blocking agents and antibiotics are needed to prevent and treat disease caused by biological weapons.

• Vaccination programs for the general public should be instituted to protect against the likeliest biological weapons.

• The public should be kept informed about germ warfare and should be instructed to report unusual neighborhood activities to local authorities. 'Bioterrorism watches' could be introduced on the model of 'neighborhood crime watches.'

• All physicians and healthcare providers should be familiar with the symptoms and treatment of the diseases caused by the likeliest biological warfare agents. All hospitals and medical facilities should develop emergency preparedness plans and establish disaster policies to deal with any bioterror event or other disaster. Included with such plans is the development of a clinical laboratory preparedness and response plan.

• A nationwide epidemiological surveillance program should link all medical facilities with the CDC or another assigned federal, state, or local agency in order to identify clusters of cases (sentinel events). Small clusters may signal a terrorist practicing before a larger-scale act is carried out.

The keynote to all this is vigilance. Any complacency or overconfidence will surely prove fatal, sooner or later. The bottom line is that we must remain on alert for animal and human epidemics and keep searching for better ways to respond to them, whether they are of natural or unnatural origin (Tierno, 2004).

This chapter explains how a Level A laboratory responds to a bioterror event as part of a health facility's larger emergency preparedness plan. This chapter excludes some common potential bioterror agents such as *Salmonella*, *Shigella*, *E. coli* 0157, *Campylobacter*, *Vibrio*, etc. since they are well known and routinely cultured by Level A laboratories (see Part 7, Medical Microbiology). Instead it focuses on several more likely bioterror agents with which a Level A laboratory may be less familiar.

Role of a Level A Laboratory

The Laboratory Response Network (LRN) is a new laboratory testing and referral system formed as an outgrowth of the CDC's Health Alert Network

Table 13–1 Biological Safety Level (BSL) Practices

BSL-1 practices: for work with agents of minimal hazard

Restrict or limit access when working

Prohibit eating, drinking and smoking

Prohibit mouth pipetting

Needles and sharps precautions

BSL-2 practices: for agents of moderate hazard

BSL-1 practices plus:
  Use BSC-Class II
    Type A1: 30% air exhausted to room
    Type A2: 30% air exhausted to outside
    Type B1: 70% air exhausted to outside
    Type B2: 100% air exhausted to outside
  Use leakproof containers

BSL-3 practices: for agents of serious or potential lethal hazard

BSL-2 practices plus:
  Use BSC-Class II 100% air exhausted to outside through double HEPA filtration or HEPA plus incineration. Cabinet is gas tight and sealed, operation performed through rubber gloves
  Use PPE (personal protection equipment)

Table 13–2 Category A Agents

Highest priority of agents that pose a national security risk

Characteristics	Agents
Easily disseminated and/or transmitted from person to person	Anthrax (*Bacillus anthracis*)
	Botulism (*Clostridium botulinum*)
Can result in high mortality rates with a major public health impact	Plague (*Yersinia pestis*)
	Smallpox (variola major)
Might cause public panic	Tularemia (*Francisella tularensis*)
	Viral hemorrhagic fevers – filoviruses (i.e., Ebola, Marburg) and arenaviruses (i.e., Lassa, Machupo)

Table 13–3 Category B Agents

Characteristics	Agents
Moderately easy to disseminate	Brucellosis (*Brucella* species)
Moderate morbidity and low mortality	Epsilon toxin of *Clostridium perfringens*
May require enhanced (CDC) diagnostic capacity	Food safety threats (i.e., *Salmonella* sp., *Escherichia coli* 0157:H7, *Shigella*)
	Glanders (*Burkholderia malleri*)
	Meliodosis (*Burkholderia pseudomallei*)
	Psittacosis (*Chlamydia psittaci*)
	Q Fever (*Coxiella burnetii*)
	Ricin toxin from (*Ricinus communis*) (castor beans)
	Staphylococcal enterotoxin B
	Typhus fever (*Rickettsia prowazekii*)
	Viral encephalitis (alphaviruses: Venezuelan equine encephalitis, eastern and western equine encephalitis)
	Water safety threats (i.e., *Vibrio cholerae*, *Cryptosporidium parvum*)

(HAN). Its purpose is to prepare for and provide a coordinated, rapid response to bioterrorism and other public health emergencies. The LRN consists of four types of laboratories, designated Levels A, B, C and D.

Safety Issues

Level A laboratories must always operate in compliance with accepted biological safety level 2 (BSL-2) requirements, including regulations, policies and procedures for handling blood-borne pathogens (Table 13–1). When handling any potential pathogen, all Level A laboratories should utilize BSL-3 practices for all culture manipulations that might produce aerosols. Level B laboratories operate in compliance with all the BSL-2 requirements and *always* practice BSL-3 safety procedures. Level C laboratories operate in compliance with all BSL-3 safety requirements and are certified as BSL-3 facilities. Their staff is specially trained to handle highly pathogenic and potentially lethal agents.

It is of paramount importance to practice good laboratory safety. For example, staff that process viral cell cultures are at risk of contracting unsuspected bioterror agents, such as smallpox or hemorrhagic fever viruses (BSL-4 agents). To minimize exposure, staff must practice universal precautions and use biological safety cabinets (BSCs) to set up cultures (Gilchrist, 2000; NCCLS, 2001; CDC, 2001).

Laboratory Designations

Level A facilities are also known as sentinel laboratories, in that they may identify an unusual organism that may be highly suspect and therefore may be first to signal a bioterrorism event has occurred. Alternatively, the Level A laboratory might report a cluster of isolates of the same organism for a number of patients that may be unusual and thus signal an event. Most clinical laboratories fall into this category. The cardinal responsibility of a Level A laboratory is to 'rule out' suspected agents of bioterror rather than perform complete identification or highly complex analyses. Once a Level A laboratory reports a finding to a state or municipal public laboratory, it may be instructed to forward the microbe to a Level B or C laboratory so that it can be 'confirmed' using advanced methods. For example, if an agent is suspected of being *Bacillus anthracis* but cannot be ruled out by the Level A laboratory, it must be shipped out to a Level B or C facility.

Level D laboratories are even more advanced and may help develop and evaluate new tests for future use in Level B and C laboratories. They can usually type confirmed bioterror agents or may perform more sophisticated molecular testing on strains. Level D laboratories also archive organisms for future studies or reference (Gilchrist, 2000; CDC, 2001; NCCLS, 2001).

Once a Level A laboratory decides it cannot 'rule out' an agent, it is common policy for the laboratory to notify the infection control officer or hospital epidemiologist, who, in turn, notifies the local health department. The laboratory should be prepared to follow instructions for shipping the suspect agent according to the Infectious Substance Guidelines provided by the Department of Transportation or International Air Transport Association. It is not the responsibility of the Level A laboratory to declare that a bioterrorist event has taken place. Such responsibility rests with the state and or federal authorities.

Because environmental specimens usually become evidence in a legal case, these specimens require full chain of custody management that is the domain of Level B and C laboratories. Such environmental samples may also pose a hazard for patients in a hospital setting; therefore in no case should Level A laboratories accept or process environmental specimens. It is the FBI's responsibility to manage the investigation of environmental samples that are submitted to Level B and C laboratories.

Law Enforcement Issues

The Level A laboratory may play a role in a criminal investigation. If a specimen is suspected or known to possess a biological threat, it is important to preserve the original specimen, plates, cultures, etc. If the laboratory is contacted by the FBI or other law enforcement agencies, the Level A laboratory must notify state health authorities as well as the hospital infection control officer or epidemiologist. Any information relevant to analysis of potential evidence *cannot* be released to the public and should *only* be conveyed to the appropriate law enforcement officials and health authorities.

Chain of custody is a legal document that describes how evidence is handled from the time it is acquired and through all subsequent examinations and storage. The laboratory should have a written chain of custody policy and appoint one person to serve as an 'evidence custodian,' i.e. one who controls storage of evidence and documents access to it on a chain of custody form that is securely stored under lock and key. The Laboratory Response Network (LRN) suggests completing a 'receipt of property' form each time the laboratory receives evidence. This form should contain a unique identifier, the quality and quantity of each item, a description of each item and as much information as possible regarding the submitter, etc. (Gilchrist, 2000; CDC/NIH, 2001; NCCLS, 2001).

Biological Agents/Diseases

The Center for Disease Control and Prevention (CDC) and other governmental agencies list biological agents/diseases in three categories (A, B, and C) according to priority of risk and ease of ability to disseminate to the population. Some representative examples in each category are listed in Tables 13–2, 13–3, and 13–4 (Gilchrist 2000; USAMRIID, 2001;

Table 13–4 Category C Agents

Characteristics	Agents
Availability	Hantavirus
Ease of production and dissemination	Nipah virus
Potential for high morbidity and mortality	Other emerging pathogens that could be engineered for mass dissemination
Potential major health impact	

Tierno, 2002). Table 13-5 summarizes diagnosis and treatment issues related to the bioterror agents discussed below. The role of the Level A laboratory is described in Tables 13–6 through 13–14 for each agent discussed below.

Anthrax (Table 13–6)
History and Background
Bacillus anthracis, the etiologic agent of anthrax, is a rod-shaped Gram-positive bacterium that produces a spore. Ordinarily these bacteria grow in a vegetative form but when conditions are not ideal for growth they sporulate. Thus, they can survive even under adverse conditions. The vegetative forms are relatively easy to kill with simple germicides, such as alcohol or peroxide, or even heat, but spores are very resistant to both

Table 13–6 *Bacillus anthracis:* Level A Laboratory Role

Presumptively identify based on criteria below and then submit culture to a Level B or C laboratory for final identification

Direct smears	Samples such as blood, CSF, skin (eschar) show encapsulated Gram-positive rods single or in chains. Generally, spores not seen
Culture smears	Large Gram-positive bacilli (1–1.5 by 3–5 μm) which may be Gram-variable after 72 hours; spores can be found in culture especially under non-CO_2 atmosphere but are nonswollen and are terminal or subterminal
Colonies on sheep blood agar plates	Rapidly growing 2–5 mm (overnight at 35°C), nonhemolytic, nonpigmented, dry 'ground-glass' surface colonies with irregular edges with comma-shaped projections (Medusa head). There is a sticky (tenacious) consistency of the colony when teased with a loop
Other criteria	Nonmotile, catalase positive, urease negative, nitrate positive, encapsulated bacillus which can be lysed by gamma phage (gamma phage typing is usually performed by Level B or C laboratory)

Table 13–5 Bioterrorism Agents: Diagnosis and Treatment

Agent	Diagnosis	Tests and specimens	Treatment
Anthrax	Clinical evaluation and laboratory findings	*Culture:* blood, CSF, wounds (definitive) *Nasal culture:* determines extent of spore spread in population *Immunohistochemical (IHC):* tissue *PCR:* can confirm diagnosis if culture is negative *Serology:* ELISA, IFA	Antibiotics including penicillin, quinolones, tetracycline. Treat inhalation anthrax for 60 days. Can combine antibiotics (30 days) and vaccine (3 doses at 0, 14 and 28 days). Full vaccination regimen is 6 doses at 0, 2, 4 weeks and 6, 12, 18 months followed by yearly boosters
Plague	Clinical evaluation and laboratory findings	*Culture:* sputum, blood, lymph *Direct FA:* respiratory secretions *Serology:* F1–V antigen (fusion protein) assay	Antibiotics including tetracycline; quinolones, streptomycin, gentamicin, and chloramphenicol for 10–14 days. Prophylaxis: medication for 7 days. Formalin-killed vaccine given 0, 1 and 4–7 months. Boosters every 1–2 years
Brucella	Difficult with many rule-outs; laboratory required	*Culture:* nasal, sputum, respiratory specimens (can also use PCR); blood culture is definitive test *Serology:* IFA, ELISA and microagglutination (gold standard) to detect antibodies	Combination antibiotics (6 weeks): doxycycline and rifampin or quinolone and rifampin. Prophylaxis requires 3 weeks. Numerous vaccines (both killed or live attenuated) available with no proven success
Tularemia	Difficult with many rule-outs; laboratory required Key symptom: pneumonia with nonproductive cough	General laboratory tests not helpful *Culture:* bacterium does not grow on ordinary media, needs cysteine blood or chocolate agar *Capsular AG detection or PCR:* whole unclotted blood *Direct FA and PCR:* nasal, induced respiratory specimens *IHC:* tissue sometimes helpful *Serology:* ELISA AB	Treatment: antibiotics like gentamicin, streptomycin, ciprofloxacin Prophylaxis: doxycycline Vaccine: live attenuated available
Botulism	Clinical evaluation; routine laboratory tests are no value; toxin assay may be useful if toxin present in serum	*PCR and toxin assay:* use nasal induced respiratory secretions and blood	Supportive treatment. Antitoxin can be administered up to 24 hours after exposure: two types, trivalent and pentavalent. Also available is a pentavalent toxoid vaccine
Smallpox	Clinical findings (exanthems)	*Cell or chick embryo culture:* skin lesions ideal; nasal swabs, respiratory secretions, serum specimens can also be cultured *Electron microscopy:* identifies virus *PCR:* Use same specimens as above *Agar gel precipitation:* skin lesions *Serology:* tests are available	Vaccinia immune globulin (VIG) must be used in conjunction with vaccinia vaccine if exposure occurs beyond a 3-day time frame. Within 3 days only vaccinia vaccine need be given by scarification. Cidofovir offers promise
VEE	Difficult with many rule-outs; laboratory required	*PCR or culture in cells/suckling mice:* nasal, induced respiratory secretions and serum *Serology:* ELISA, IFA and hemagglutination inhibition; detect AB	Some drugs show promise. At present no specific therapy. Treatment geared towards relieving symptoms. Some vaccines show promise (i.e., TC-84)
VHF	Clinical evaluation; key finding is vascular involvement, i.e., petechiae, bleeding, postural hypotension, edema, etc.	*General:* leukopenia, thrombocytopenia; elevated AST *Serology:* ELISA, IFA and PCR; detect different VHFs	Management of hypotension and fluid loss. Aggressive supportive care needed. Ribavirin and immune globulin therapy show some promise. Several vaccines under development

chemicals and heat. *B. anthracis* spores survive for decades. This is a key point since spores cause infection. In nature, anthrax is usually associated with grazing animals such as sheep, goats, cattle and wildlife that acquire spores as they feed on vegetation or meat from infected animals. *B. anthracis* is present in soil throughout the world; in the US it is found mostly along old cattle trails in Texas, Louisiana, Mississippi, Arkansas, New Mexico, Oklahoma and some Midwestern states. However, anthrax is rare in the US because it is controlled in animal populations by vaccination programs. Spores occur when the pH of a richly organic soil is higher than 6.0 and rainfall gives way to drought conditions. When herbivorous animals contract the infection they can transmit the infection to humans by direct contact with animal products such as hair, wool, hides, bones, etc. Certain occupations are at increased risk for contracting anthrax, such as animal handlers, agricultural workers and veterinarians. About 90% of all human anthrax cases reportedly occur in millworkers handling imported goat hair. Humans can be infected three ways: (1) via the skin (cutaneous) through scratches or abrasions, (2) by inhalation of spores, or (3) by eating contaminated insufficiently cooked meat or meat products. The word anthracis comes from the Greek word meaning 'coal' and was so named because the microbe can cause a black scab (eschar) to form on the skin of cutaneous anthrax victims. For the same reason, it is sometimes called the 'black carbuncle' (Tierno, 2002).

Anthrax is the single greatest biowarfare threat because it is easy to cultivate spores, although production of a weaponized spore is not so simple. The media sometimes refer to 'weapons grade' anthrax versus 'non-weapons grade.' Criteria for weapons grade are: small spore size, usually 1–3 microns; lack of clumping (usually accomplished by adding a polymer that prevents the natural tendency of spores to clump); amount of spores present; and an effective delivery system. By this description, the anthrax unleashed on the US in the fall of 2001 was near weapons grade because it fulfilled two of the four criteria. The spores were small and dispersed well in the air, but particles were present in limited quantities and delivered via the mail. If enough product had been made and if it had been effectively delivered, it would have been considered weapons grade.

In nature, spores in soil tend to clump together making it very difficult for a person to contract inhalation anthrax naturally. In order for a terrorist to weaponize anthrax spores he must first prevent clumping of particles and then he must deliver the weapon in sufficient quantity. Clearly both of these tasks are very difficult. Even a crop-duster would have to be retrofitted quite extensively in order to deliver spores effectively. To be an effective weapon the anthrax spores must remain airborne in a concentration that is high enough to be inhaled deep into the lungs. Based on the available data, it appears that number varies from about 8000–40 000 spores. A few studies suggest that inhalation of small numbers of spores, around 500 over an 8-hour period, did not make goat mill workers develop disease. Although there are three types of infections that *B. anthracis* can cause (skin, inhalation, gastrointestinal) a bioterrorist would be most interested in causing inhalation anthrax because of the high mortality rate associated with it. In nature, however, approximately 95% of human cases of anthrax are cutaneous infections (Lew, 2000; Tierno, 2002).

Anthrax spores can survive inside macrophages, eventually vegetating and growing to such numbers that they cause the cells to burst and release bacilli into the bloodstream. These bacteria produce four virulence factors, three are toxins that cause systemic symptoms: protective antigen toxin, the lethal factor and the edema factor. Last, it produces a capsule that protects it from destruction by the body's leukocytes. Once systemic symptoms occur, antibiotics are useless, since they have no effect on the circulating toxins (Tierno, 2002).

Clinical Features

Inhalation Anthrax. This form is a biphasic disease. The *initial* phase is characterized by mild flu-like symptoms (e.g. malaise, fatigue, low-grade fever) followed by a period of apparent wellness for about a day. This is immediately followed by the *acute* phase, which eventually leads to more serious symptoms (e.g. acute respiratory distress). The incubation period can vary from 1–5 days, depending on the number of spores inhaled, but can be as long as 60 days. Shock and death usually occur 24–36 hours after the onset of respiratory distress. The fatality rate of inhalation anthrax approaches 90% even with antibiotic therapy. However, this figure will probably change for the better owing to the availability of newer antibiotics and superior intensive care treatment facilities. Inhalation anthrax is not spread via person-to-person transmission.

Cutaneous Anthrax. This skin form of anthrax occurs after spores are introduced beneath the skin by inoculation or contamination of a pre-existing lesion or break in the skin. The incubation period is 2–7 days (rarely after 1 day) but more often occurs between 2–5 days. The lesion begins as small, painless, pimples on exposed skin and progresses to vesicles and eventually an ulceration that develops a black scab (eschar) at the center (within 2–6 days). Untreated cutaneous anthrax can have a fatality rate of up to 20%, but fatalities are rare (1%) with proper antibiotic treatment. While anthrax is not transmitted from person to person, secondary lesions can develop from direct exposure to vesicle secretions.

Gastrointestinal Anthrax. This form of anthrax occurs by ingesting contaminated meat, in particular raw or undercooked, from infected animals. As of this writing, there has never been a case of gastrointestinal (GI) anthrax reported in the US. The incubation period is 2–7 days. There are two types of GI anthrax characterized by different symptoms: intestinal (e.g. nausea, vomiting, diarrhea) and oropharyngeal (e.g. neck swelling, difficulty swallowing). Shock and toxemia can characterize both forms of the disease, especially in the terminal stages. The fatality rate is 25–60%. Inhalation, cutaneous and GI anthrax can be complicated by meningitis, which occurs in about 5% of the cases (Lew, 2000).

Practical Considerations

- Hand washing is the single most important protective measure. Spores are effectively removed with soap and water.
- Any article suspected of being contaminated with spores should be sanitized with a 1 : 10 dilution of household bleach. Let bleach remain in contact for at least 30 minutes before rinsing. If heavy spore contamination is suspected use concentrated bleach to decontaminate the article.
- N95 respirator masks are protective against spore aerosols.
- Any cut, scratch, or abrasion should be covered with a dressing that has been coated with 1% tincture of iodine. If the cut or abrasion is not too extensive, apply tincture of iodine to its surface. Iodine is an outstanding antiseptic and can be sporicidal. No contusion is too small to warrant attention.
- Homes that have central air conditioning fitted with HEPA (high-efficiency particulate air) will remove more than 99.97% of particles 0.3 microns or larger. Since anthrax spores tend to clump they will be efficiently trapped by HEPA filters. Alternatively an air purifier outfitted with a HEPA filter will serve to keep a 'safe-room' free of spores.

Plague (Table 13–7)

History and Background

'Black Death' or the 'plague' that befell Europe in the 14th century killed more than 25 million people or about 25% of the population. This period is called the 'second' pandemic. The first of three pandemics started in AD541 and continued through to the eighth century with an estimated 40 million deaths. The third and last pandemic began in China in the 1860s and spread to Africa, Europe, and the Americas. The plague is a zoonotic disease that primarily infects rodents and is caused by the bacterium *Yersinia pestis*, transmitted by a rat flea (*Xenopsylla cheopis*, the oriental flea, or *Pulex irritans*, the human flea). In the past, human epidemics originated by contact with fleas of infected rodents. The great plagues spread from

---

Table 13–7 *Yersinia pestis*: Level A Laboratory Role

Presumptively identify based on criteria below and then submit culture to a Level B or C laboratory for final identification

Direct smears	More likely to see bipolar staining ('safety pin') from clinical specimens (blood, sputum, aspirates, etc.) than from cultures. Bipolarity is better seen using Wayson or Wright–Giemsa stains. Beware that bipolar staining is not always observed and is not unique to *Y. pestis*
Culture smears	Plump Gram-negative rods (1–2 by 0.5 μm) single or in short chains
Colonies on sheep blood agar plates	Grow at 35°C (faster at room temperature) as gray-white, nonhemolytic, translucent, pinpoint colonies at 24 h, but by 48 h colonies are 1–2 mm in diameter, becoming yellowish with age. Growth occurs with or without CO_2. Colonies can appear as 'fried egg' or with 'hammered copper' shiny surface. On MacConkey, grow as pinpoint nonlactose fermenting colonies after 24 h; slightly larger at 48 h
Other criteria	The bacterium is nonmotile at both 35–37°C and room temperature (*Y. pestis* is the only *Yersinia* that is nonmotile at room temperature). It is oxidase and urease negative; catalase positive; growth in broth is flocculent and described as 'stalactite' and clumps at side and bottom of tube

rats to man in crowded unsanitary urban areas. Man is only accidental to the usual cycle: rodent–flea–rodent. In the US, most naturally occurring human cases of plague (about 12/year) are concentrated in the southwest and pacific states (Perry, 1997; Tierno, 2002).

In a biowarfare scenario, the plague bacillus could be delivered by contaminated fleas as vectors causing the bubonic plague or, more likely spread by an aerosol that would cause pneumonic plague. In nature, a rat flea regurgitates the bacterium upon biting its host. Cats are also susceptible and can transmit the pneumonic plague to humans. Unlike anthrax, which cannot be transmitted person-to-person, pneumonic plague can be transmitted via large aerosol droplets from a coughing patient.

Yersinia pestis can be killed by polymorphonuclear cells, but they can survive in monocytes, where they produce a capsule to resist phagocytosis. These bacteria can then rapidly reach the lymph system, bloodstream and disseminate to all organs, causing hemorrhage and necrosis.

Fewer than 100 organisms are necessary to cause human infection. Studies have shown that the bacteria can remain alive for up to 1 year in soil and up to 270 days in live tissue. The bacterium is killed after heat exposure (15 minutes at 72°C/160°F) and within several hours of exposure to sunlight (Tierno, 2002).

Clinical Features

There are three clinical forms: bubonic, characterized by swelling of the lymph nodes (buboes); pneumonic, in which the lungs are extensively involved; and septicemic, in which the bloodstream is infected with *Yersinia pestis*. The mortality rate of untreated pneumonic plague is 100% and that of untreated bubonic plague is about 50%.

Bubonic plague. The incubation period of 2–10 days is characterized by malaise, high fever and tender lymph nodes (buboes) that enlarge and eventually necrose. Septicemia may occur and bacteria can also spread to the central nervous system, lungs (this produces the pneumonic disease which can then be spread person to person), and the rest of the body, eventually causing death.

Pneumonic Plague. The 1- to 3-day incubation period is shorter than that of bubonic plague. Symptoms are high fever, cough, chest pain and bloody sputum; pneumonia can lead to respiratory and circulatory collapse (Perry, 1997).

Practical Considerations

- Pneumonic plague patients transmit infection by large particle droplets (greater than 5 microns) generated by coughing, talking or sneezing. A simple surgical-type mask can protect workers or family members. 'Droplet Precautions' should be maintained for 3 complete days of antibiotic therapy, after which a person is no longer contagious.
- Since 'droplets' only occur within 3–5 feet from a patient, central air conditioning systems do not need to be fitted with HEPA filters, i.e., do not need to provide bacteria and particle free air.
- If an outbreak occurs, it is important to control fleas, rats and other animals like cats. Insecticides and repellants are widely available.
- Hand washing is an essential prevention strategy.
- Since *Y. pestis* does not have a spore form, surfaces can be decontaminated with a simple germicide like 10% bleach solution. Skin can be decontaminated using any germicidal soap product. Alcohol-based hand sanitizers like Purell can also be effective.
- Clothing should be washed with a germicidal detergent and hot water (155°F) even though exposure is unlikely to occur from re-aerosolization of bacteria from contaminated clothing.
- Stand clear (further than 3–5 feet) of individuals taking a coughing fit or producing sputum with or without blood.

Brucellosis (Table 13–8)
History and Background

Brucellosis is a systemic zoonotic disease caused by: *Brucella melitensis, B. suis, B. abortus* and *B. canis*. These bacteria ordinarily cause disease in domestic animals, such as goats, sheep and camels (*B. melitensis*); cattle (*B. abortus*); and pigs (*B. suis*). The primary pathogen of dogs, *B. canis* rarely causes disease in humans. Natural infection in humans occurs when bacteria are inhaled as aerosols, ingested in raw unpasteurized infected milk or meat, or introduced into abrasions in skin or through contact with conjunctival surfaces. Human disease is called undulant fever, Malta fever, Bang's disease, Gibraltar fever, and Mediterranean fever and occurs worldwide. In developed countries, human infection is associated with the meat packing and dairy industries. Several studies report that human brucellosis is underdiagnosed and under-reported. By some estimates, 25–30 cases go unrecognized for every reported case. As a biological warfare agent, brucellae would likely be delivered via the aerosol route. Brucellae are intracellular bacteria; they are able to survive phagocytosis

Table 13–8 *Brucella* species: Level A Laboratory Role

Presumptively identify based on criteria below and then submit culture to a Level B or C laboratory for final identification and/or confirmation, although most Level A laboratories are able to completely identify *Brucella*

Direct smears	Blood and/or bone marrow most often submitted. *Brucella* appear as faintly staining, small Gram-negative coccobacilli (0.5–0.7 by 0.6–1.5 μm) mostly seen as single cells appearing like 'fine sand'
Culture smears	Similar to above
Colonies on sheep blood (SBA) and chocolate (CA) agars	Usually not visible or are pinpoint at 24 hr; at 48 h colonies are tiny, nonpigmented, smooth with an entire edge, and are nonhemolytic on SBA. Growth of some strains is enhanced by CO_2 tension. Some strains grow on MacConkey; Thayer-Martin can be used as a selective medium. Blood cultures are held for 21 days for suspect cases
Other criteria	These coccobacilli are catalase, urease, and oxidase positive (*B. canis* is variable). They are nonmotile and do not require X and V factors. Brucellosis is one of the most commonly reported laboratory-acquired infections. Automated systems are not useful nor are they recommended for identification. <u>Remember that sniffing culture plates of *Brucella* can result in infection</u>

and thus can be carried from lymph tissue to blood and deposited in numerous organs. Inside the phagocytes the bacteria grow and eventually their host cells are killed and a new crop of bacteria are released. The 'undulant' fever pattern observed with this disease corresponds to the release of bacteria into the blood, thereby causing fever. As these bacteria are eliminated, the fever subsides only to recur when another crop of bacteria are released. Relapses are common. *Brucella* species have two morphologically different colony types: 'smooth' and 'rough.' The smooth form is more pathogenic because of the presence of a capsule which protects the bacterium from phagocytosis and destruction. *B. melitensis* and *B. suis* are more virulent than the other two species and have better intracellular survival. On the other hand, *B. abortus* and *B. canis* have an insidious onset but cause milder disease and fewer complications (Shapiro, 1998, 1999; Tierno, 2002).

Clinical Features

The incubation period can be 1–8 weeks but is usually 3–4 weeks. Onset is insidious with malaise, fever, chills, sweats, headache, fatigue, myalgias, and arthralgias. Fever usually rises in the afternoon; it falls during the night and is accompanied by drenching sweat. Swollen lymph, spleen and liver may also be present. The 'undulant fever' can occur over weeks, months or even years. Yet, there are many days when a patient has no fever and feels relatively well, only to experience another cycle of waxing and waning fever. Patients are often diagnosed with a fever of unknown origin. Cough occurs in about 20% of cases but the X-ray appears normal. Mortality rate is about 6% for *B. melitensis* but 1% for the other species. Most deaths are associated with endocarditis or meningitis. Gastrointestinal symptoms occur in up to 70% of adult cases though less frequently in children.

Practical Considerations

- Although *Brucellae* species have a long incubation period and slow onset, the characteristic *'undulant fever'* syndrome helps make a diagnosis so that treatment can start.
- *Brucella* has such a low fatality rate (especially with proper antibiotic therapy) that it is not a very effective biological weapon.
- Brucellosis cannot be transmitted person to person so that patient isolation is not required. However, contact precautions are indicated if there is a draining lesion.
- *Brucella* species have no spore form so they are readily killed with any common germicide. Pasteurization (at 155°F) kills bacteria in contaminated food.
- Brucellosis is contracted through eye contact (i.e. rubbing or touching your eyes) so hand washing with germicidal soap or alcohol-based hand sanitizers is an important protective strategy.

Tularemia (Table 13–9)
History and Background

The causative agent of tularemia (also known as 'rabbit fever') is *Francisella tularensis*. These bacteria are Gram-negative bacilli that are nonmotile and

Table 13–9 *Francisella tularensis*: Level A Laboratory Role

Presumptively identify based on criteria below and then submit culture to a Level B or C laboratory for final identification

Direct smears	Gram stain of blood, biopsy material, scrapings, or aspirates may be difficult to interpret because bacteria are tiny, pleomorphic, poorly staining Gram-negative coccobacilli seen mostly as single cells
Culture smear	Very tiny (0.2–0.5 by 0.7–1.0 μm) poorly staining, pleomorphic, Gram-negative coccobacilli. They are smaller than *Haemophilus influenzae* and *Brucella* spp. Their miniscule size should raise awareness
Colonies on sheep blood (SBA), chocolate (CA) and blood cysteine (BCA) agars	Grow poorly and slowly on SBA as 1–2 mm gray-white, nonhemolytic colonies after 48–72 h. On CA and BCA, colonies are slightly larger 1–3 mm gray-white to bluish-gray with an entire edge and smooth flat surface. Colonies do not subculture well to SBA (viability is usually lost). Subcultures should be made onto CA, BCA or Thayer-Martin agars. CO_2 is not required for growth. No growth occurs on MacConkey or EMB agars
Other criteria	*F. tularensis* is nonmotile, oxidase and urease negative; catalase can be weakly positive or negative. X and V factors are not required. Slow growth in thioglycollate broth with a dense band near top which eventually diffuses downward with time

have no spore form. Humans acquire this zoonotic disease through contact with animals, usually through the inoculation of skin or their mucous membranes with blood or tissue fluids of infected animals or bites from infected ticks, mosquitoes or flies. A less common method of acquiring infection is through inhalation of contaminated dusts or ingestion of contaminated foods or water. A bioterrorist would likely use an aerosol to deliver *Francisella* since it causes *typhoidal (systemic) tularemia*, a disease with > 10% fatality rate.

Since the bacterium is highly contagious, as few as 25 inhaled organisms or as few as 10 administered subcutaneously can cause infection. The smallest break in the skin can serve as a portal of entry. The bacterium is so contagious that numerous cases of tularemia have resulted from laboratory accidents while processing infected clinical or research samples. *Francisella* is distributed worldwide. In the US, the disease has been reported primarily in southern and south-central states.

F. tularensis produces a capsule which allows the organism to avoid immediate destruction by the body's phagocytes. It can survive as an intracellular parasite within cells of the lymph system.

Clinical Features

There are six major syndromes associated with tularemia and they differ by the mode of infection.

1. *Ulceroglandular tularemia* (70–85% of cases) typically presents with a skin ulcer, usually the result of a tick bite, and swollen lymph nodes, fever, chills, headache, sweating and coughing.
2. *Glandular tularemia* (5–12% of cases) is characterized by fever and swollen lymph nodes but no obvious skin lesion.
3. *Typhoidal tularemia* (7–14% cases) presents with acute onset of fever, chills, headache, vomiting and diarrhea. There is usually no skin lesion or swollen lymph nodes but it is associated with primary or secondary pneumonia. This form has the highest mortality rate and is the most likely bioterror form.
4. *Oculoglandular tularemia* (1–2% cases) presents with severe conjunctivitis and swollen lymph nodes, usually the result of self-inoculating the organism into the conjunctivae.
5. *Oropharyngeal tularemia* occurs in patients who have a primary lesion in the oropharynx. Patients present with severe headache and bilateral tonsillitis or severe streptococcal-type sore throat. Persistent swollen lymph nodes in the neck appear after 1–2 weeks.
6. *Pneumonic tularemia* (8–13% cases) is primarily a complication of the other forms, especially typhoidal tularemia. It is also acquired by inhaling infectious aerosols or as a result of blood-borne dissemination. Lymph nodes in the lungs are enlarged. Sometimes, the pneumonia is not evident (Wong, 1999).

In all tularemia syndromes, lymph nodes may remain enlarged for a long time and eventually become necrotic and drain. Fever (usually low grade) is accompanied by malaise, headache, and pain in the regional lymph nodes.

Table 13–10 Botulinum Toxin Exposure: Level A Laboratory Role

Submit specimens immediately to public health laboratory for evaluation and referral, even if criminal activity is not suspected. Level A laboratories should not manipulate specimens, culture, identify or perform toxin assays. Level A laboratory responsibility is limited to advising the medical staff on specimen selection, packing, shipping as well as notifying the recipient laboratory about specimens from a suspected case

	Specimen	Transport
Suspect food samples	25–50 g of food should be submitted in original containers which have been placed in a leakproof sealed system	4°C
Nasal swabs	If aerosolized release is suspected, collect nasal swabs for toxin testing and/or PCR analysis	Room temperature
Stool, enema fluid	Collect 25–50 g of stool into sterile leakproof containers	4°C
Serum	Collect approximately 10 mL for serologic assays	4°C
Other	Collect environmental and/or other samples on swabs	4°C

Note: Level A laboratory responsibility for other suspected toxins such as staphylococcal toxins, mycotoxin, saxitoxin, ricin, etc. should be treated in a similar manner.

Practical Considerations

- Hand washing with germicidal soap or alcohol-based hand sanitizers is the most important protective strategy. Any aerosolized bioterror attack would contaminate the surrounding environment and could lead to secondary exposure through direct contact with skin and mucous membranes. Simple germicides, like bleach, destroy the bacterium on contaminated surfaces.
- Since there are no spore forms, only vegetative ones, bacteria are easy killed by heat (30 min at 145°F). The relatively low fatality rate does not make it a very effective biological weapon. Infected patients rapidly improve on adequate (10–14 days) antibiotic therapy.
- Since tularemia can be transmitted by contact with household pets like cats and dogs, it is important to observe any changing habits or health status of pets. They can be the sentinel event to warn you of an impending disaster, much like the 'canary in the mine.'
- *Francisella* is rarely transmitted by food or water; nevertheless, it is important to be alert to that possibility. Cooking food renders the bacterium harmless as does filtering or heating water.

Botulinum Toxins (Table 13–10)

History and Background

Clostridia are anaerobic, Gram-positive, spore-forming bacilli that elaborate toxins. The most pathogenic species are *Clostridium perfringens* (agent of gas gangrene), *C. tetani* (agent of tetanus) and *C. botulinum* (agent of botulism). The aforementioned diseases are the result of exposure to the protein toxins that the bacteria produce, the most powerful of which is the botulinum toxin. There are seven *C. botulinum* toxins: A, B, C, D, E, F and G. Human illness is caused by four of the seven toxins: types A, B, E and F. The toxins bind to synaptic vesicles of cholinergic nerves, preventing release of acetylcholinesterase at peripheral nerve endings (including neuromuscular junctions). Patients develop acute flaccid descending paralysis. By blocking neurotransmission, the toxins cause palsies and skeletal muscle weakness, common clinical features. *Clostridium botulinum* toxins are among the most toxic substances known to man. A lethal human dose is only one-millionth of a gram (Tierno, 2002; Angulo, 1998).

Several forms of botulism occur in humans. The classic type is *food-borne botulism* which typically occurs in adults and is caused by ingestion of toxin present in contaminated food. *C. botulinum* grows in food and produces its toxin. The usual foods involved are canned alkaline foods that are eaten without cooking, or smoked, and vacuum-packed foods. Under anaerobic conditions, *C. botulinum* spores grow into vegetative forms that produce toxin. *Wound botulism*, the rarest form, occurs when bacteria gain access to a wound site and then produce toxins in vivo. *Infant botulism*, the most common type, occurs when a child consumes food contaminated with *C. botulinum* rather than consuming preformed toxins. Toxin is produced in the infant's gut, de novo, and poisons from within. Some botulism patients do not have an obvious food or wound source; they fall into the 'classification undetermined' group.

As a bioterror weapon, botulism toxin could be purified from large stores of toxin-producing *Clostridium botulinum*. It could then be delivered as an aerosol that causes symptoms like those of food-borne botulism. Another approach might be to sabotage food supplies with toxin, though the latter is not an efficient delivery system (USAMRIID, 2001; Tierno, 2002). We know that botulinum toxins can be weaponized because the Iraqi government admitted to a United Nations inspection team in August 1991 that it had done research on these toxins prior to the Persian Gulf War. It is possible to weaponize any of the seven known botulinum toxins as they would all have the same effect.

Clinical Features

Symptoms usually begin 18–24 hours after ingestion or inhalation of toxin, though it may take several days. Initial symptoms include double vision, lack of coordination of eye muscles, inability to swallow, speech difficulty, generalized weakness and dizziness. These are followed by descending progressive weakness of the extremities and weakness of the respiratory muscles. There is no fever and the patient may be totally alert and oriented. Neurological examination shows flaccid muscle weakness of the tongue, larynx, respiratory muscles and extremities. A patient remains fully conscious until shortly before death from respiratory paralysis or cardiac arrest. Mortality rate is high. Patients who recover do not develop antitoxin in the blood. There is probably a suppression of antibody production caused by the toxins in much the same way that toxic shock syndrome toxin-1 produced by *Staphylococcus aureus* prevents antibody production. In infants, signs of paralysis are called 'floppy baby' syndrome (Tierno, 2002).

Practical Considerations

- Antitoxins and vaccines are available for treatment and prophylaxis.
- Botulinum toxin is *less* toxic and lethal when delivered by inhalation than by a food-borne assault.
- Soap and water can be very effective at removing most toxins from skin, clothing and equipment so that decontamination of a toxin is *not* as critical as decontamination of an infectious microbe. A very mild bleach solution (1 part bleach in 9 parts water) effectively inactivates most protein toxins.
- A protective N95 mask if worn properly is effective against toxin aerosols. However, it is important that a tight fit is achieved since even a small leak could result in significant exposure. Bearded individuals would not be able to achieve a tight fit but would nevertheless reduce their exposure with a mask.
- Because botulinum toxin does not permeate skin, special protective clothing is not as important as it would be for other agents, including chemical attacks.

Smallpox (Table 13–11)
History and Background
Smallpox has the distinct honor of being the greatest single killer in recorded history; it is estimated that this virus has killed about 500 million people.

Table 13–11 Smallpox: Level A Laboratory Role

Smallpox is highest-level emergency; submit specimens immediately to public health laboratory. Virus is highly infectious; avoid manipulation, if necessary use BSL-3 practices. Responsibility of Level A laboratories is limited to advising medical staff on specimen selection, packing and shipping sample, and communicating with reference laboratory. Level A laboratories should not culture, sample or perform assays on specimens suspected of containing the virus. Clinical diagnosis is confirmed by Level D laboratory techniques

	Specimen	Transport	Storage
Biopsy	Aseptically place two to four portions of tissue into sterile, leakproof, freezable container	≤ 6 h/4°C	−20°C to −70°C
Scabs	Aseptically place scrapings/material into sterile, leakproof freezable container	≤ 6 h/4°C	−20°C to −70°C
Vesicular fluid	Collect fluid from separate lesions onto separate sterile swabs. Always include material from base of each vesicle	≤ 6 h/4°C	−20°C to −70°C

The smallpox virus, a.k.a. variola, is a member of the Orthopoxvirus group of viruses. There are two variants of smallpox: variola major, which is associated with a higher mortality rate of 15–40% and variola minor, which causes a milder disease and is associated with a mortality rate of only 1%. Smallpox is the human type of poxvirus. There are other poxviruses that naturally infect animals but they also can cause incidental infection in humans (zoonoses). These viruses share common antigens with smallpox, thus allowing them to be used as vaccines for humans. Thus, vaccinia virus has been the historically chosen animal virus for vaccine production. As the incidence of smallpox waned, there were more complications related to the vaccinations than there were smallpox cases. Some of these complications were severe and included encephalitis and fatal reactions in immunocompromised patients who were vaccinated, sometimes inadvertently. Vaccinia viruses spread easily among unvaccinated immunocompromised patients in close contact. This would still be the case if a massive national vaccination program were to be considered. There would be a large group of immunocompromised patients that simply would not be candidates for the vaccine (Tierno, 2002).

In 1967, the World Health Organization introduced a worldwide campaign to eradicate smallpox. At the time there were 33 countries with endemic smallpox and about 15 million cases per year. By 1979, smallpox was eradicated. Smallpox virus currently exists in only two laboratories, one in the US and the other in Russia. The fate of these remaining stocks is debated. Destroying the stocks will preclude further research in the event of an outbreak. Like plague, smallpox is very contagious from man to man. It is currently assumed that an aerosol infective dose is low and presumably ranges from 10–100 organisms (Tierno, 2002).

How would smallpox be weaponized? There are two ways to spread smallpox: aerosol dispersal and contact. Since smallpox is highly contagious and efficiently spread through air, an aerosol delivery system poses the greatest threat and exposes the most people. However, as learned with anthrax, this is not so easy to do. Smallpox could also be delivered by direct contact. One way could be to self-contaminate a group of volunteers who would then interact with the general population, infecting people over days or weeks as they came in contact with them. If a smallpox outbreak is detected in an area, the CDC and other health authorities would be able to contain the outbreak by immediately vaccinating all individuals surrounding the index case or cases. Post-exposure immunization with smallpox vaccine (vaccinia virus) is effective and is recommended if given within 3 days of exposure. However, even if more than 3 days elapse, vaccination and vaccinia immune globulin may provide protection. It is necessary to establish a ring of immunity around index cases. This is precisely the method used to eradicate smallpox worldwide and should be just cause for some optimism.

Clinical Features
The entry portal for smallpox virus is the mucous membranes of the upper respiratory tract. Smallpox is transmitted by either large or small respiratory droplets, and by contact with skin lesions or secretions. Patients are considered more infectious if they are actively coughing. The incubation period is typically 12 days with a range of 10–12 days. The clinical illness begins with a 2- to 3-day period of vague symptoms such as malaise, fever, headache, chills and backache. The fever can last as long as 5 days or be as short as 1 day. After the fever, an exanthem (eruption of skin or rash) appears which undergoes a papular, pustular and crustular stage. The latter falls off 2–4 weeks after the initial lesion and leaves a pink scar. An important characteristic of smallpox, is that lesions in affected areas appear in the same state. This differs from chickenpox where lesions are not synchronous and occur in crops. Smallpox lesions are distributed centrifugally (more numerous on the face and extremities rather than the trunk) unlike chickenpox. Hence, the smallpox exanthem is very characteristic and a useful diagnostic tool. The fatality rate is 15–40% in unvaccinated patients and < 1% in those vaccinated.

Patients with smallpox are infectious as soon as a rash occurs and remain infectious until scabs fall off approximately 3 weeks later. There is a rare form of smallpox called 'hemorrhagic variola' that is very pathogenic and has a very high mortality rate.

Practical Considerations
- If a major outbreak of smallpox occurs, prepare to stay indoors for a few days or weeks in order to reduce contact with those contaminated; this will contain the epidemic. Households should be stocked with adequate food supplies.
- Generally, respiratory droplets become infectious earlier than skin lesions. In hospitals, both airborne and contact precautions are required to prevent contagion. In contrast to plague precautions, a simple surgical mask is insufficient protection. A special respirator mask, N95 (certified to have at least 95% filter efficiency), is

Table 13–12 VEE or Other Encephalitides: Level A Laboratory Role

Submit samples immediately to public health laboratory for evaluation and referral. Level A laboratory responsibility is limited to advising medical staff on specimen selection, packing and shipping sample, and communicating with reference laboratory

	Specimen	Transport	Storage
Serum	For culture, PCR or serologies (ELISA, HI, FA, etc.)	< 6 h/4°C	−20°C to −70°C
CSF	For culture, PCR or serologies	< 6 h/4°C	−20°C to −70°C
Nasal, respiratory (including induced samples)	For culture and PCR	< 6 h/4°C	−20°C to −70°C
Other	Biopsy, autopsy, stool, etc. for pathology, culture, hematology/chemistry analysis, etc.	< 6 h/4°C	−20°C to −70°C

recommended and must be worn for such protection. Smallpox patients should be quarantined from the time the rash first appears until the scab finally falls off (about 3 weeks).
- If a household member contracts smallpox, all clothing, bed linens or other materials that contacted the patient must be decontaminated with a germicide such as a 1 : 10 bleach solution, steam, or heat.
- Hand washing with germicidal soap is essential after any contact with a smallpox patient or their environment.

Venezuelan Equine Encephalitis (VEE) (Table 13–12)
History and Background
VEE is clinically indistinguishable from other encephalitis viruses such as St Louis encephalitis, eastern and western equine encephalitis, Japanese B-type encephalitis, Russian Far East encephalitis, and even West Nile encephalitis viruses. The first question to consider is why other such agents are not high on the list as potential bioterror weapons? Many can be, but the attack rate, that is, the number of people who would probably get the disease after being exposed to the agent, is much lower than that for VEE. VEE has an attack rate of about 100% (pretty hard to beat). That is precisely the reason the US government weaponized it in the 1950s and 1960s before terminating its offensive biowarfare program. However, it remains a potential weapon and one likely to serve as a surrogate virus to deliver more pathogens. Nevertheless, the Level A laboratory responsibility is similar for all encephalitis viruses such as VEE (USAMRIID, 2001; Tierno, 2002). VEE can be weaponized either as a liquid or dry form for aerosol dispersal. It can be transmitted in three ways: (1) via mosquitoes, though naturally occurring incidence of VEE is low; (2) via aerosol, either liquid or dry form; and (3) via secondary spread from person to person (though this has not yet been conclusively demonstrated).

In nature, VEE is a mosquito-borne viral disease that is neurotrophic causing encephalitis in equine animals and an unremarkable febrile illness in humans. More than 50% of equines that become infected develop encephalitis, while in humans almost 100% of those exposed develop an influenza-like illness. In naturally contracted disease, only 2–4% of patients develop signs of central nervous system involvement and less than 1% die (Tierno, 2002).

In the US, VEE is a rare disease. The disease was first reported in Venezuela in 1936. VEE is prevalent in South and Central America, Trinidad, Mexico, and Panama. In the case of the West Nile encephalitis virus, a sentinel animal (birds) indicated the presence of disease before human infection occurred. In the case of VEE, that would have been horses, but because we vaccinate them there is no sentinel animal system to warn us that a VEE virus attack has occurred. On the other hand, because we have eradicated VEE from the US, any human with the disease would likely signal bioterrorism (Tierno, 2002).

VEE is an arthropod-borne alphavirus that has been incidentally associated with human disease. Eight serologically distinct viruses exist, but only two are important pathogens for humans: variants A/B and C (Tierno, 2002). Most encephalitis viruses are destroyed by heat and are easily killed by ordinary disinfectants.

Clinical Features
The incubation period is 1–5 days, after which there is rapid onset of fever (usually high), headache, dizziness, lethargy, depression, anorexia, chills, myalgia, photophobia, nausea, vomiting, cough, sore throat, and sometimes diarrhea. VEE is indistinguishable from other viruses that cause encephalitis.

Table 13–13 Crimean Congo and Other Hemorrhagic Fevers: Level A Laboratory Role

Submit samples immediately to public health laboratory for evaluation and referral. Some viruses are highly infectious; avoid manipulation, if necessary use BSL-3 practices. Level A laboratory responsibility is limited to advising medical staff on specimen selection, packing and shipping sample, and communicating with reference laboratory

	Specimen	Transport	Storage
Serum	For culture, PCR or serologies (ELISA, HI, FA, etc.)	< 6 h/4°C	−20°C to −70°C
Other	Biopsy, autopsy, etc. for pathology, culture, hematology/chemistry analysis, etc.	< 6 h/4°C	−20°C to −70°C

Table 13–14 Viral Hemorrhagic Fever (VHF) Means of Transmission

VHF agent	Natural means of transmission
Ebola	Contact
Marburg	Contact
Lassa fever	Contact
Argentine (Junin)	Contact and aerosol
Bolivian (Machupo)	Contact and aerosol
Crimean Congo	Ticks and contact
Hantavirus	Contact and aerosol
Rift Valley fever	Mosquito and aerosol
Dengue	Mosquito
Yellow fever	Mosquito

The acute phase of the disease exists from 1–3 days followed by a prolonged period (up to 2 weeks) of lethargy. Full recovery usually occurs after 2 weeks. It is estimated that inoculation with 10–100 viruses can cause infection. In a naturally occurring epidemic, < 5% of patients have a neurologic manifestation, one characterized by convulsions, coma, and paralysis.

Practical Considerations
- VEE has very low lethality and in most victims might manifest as only a flu-like disease. Note: bioterrorists may use any encephalitis virus as a surrogate for a more pathogenic weapon via genetic engineering.
- If an outbreak occurs, the mosquito population must be controlled, similar to the approach used for West Nile virus.
- Hand washing can prevent the otherwise rare person-to-person transmission (via contact spread).
- Simple germicides such as a 10% bleach solution or Lysol, and heat (165°F) easily destroy VEE virus.
- Contaminated clothing can be washed with any detergent.

Crimean Congo and Other Hemorrhagic Fevers (Table 13–13)
History and Background
Crimean Congo hemorrhagic fever (CCHF) is only one of many illnesses referred to as viral hemorrhagic fevers (VHFs). These agents and their natural mode of transmission are listed in Table 13–14. Any one of these hemorrhagic viruses, except dengue (which is only transmissible via mosquito), can be weaponized via an aerosol delivery (USAMRIID, 2001; Tierno, 2002). In general, VHFs are very difficult to weaponize because there is no real carrier state.

CCHF is transmitted by ticks. Several reports describe person-to-person spread of CCHF in hospitals. As few as 1–10 viral particles can cause infection (USAMRIID, 2001). Rift Valley fever (RVF) is transmitted by mosquitoes as well as by aerosols; an inactivated vaccine is available for prevention, and RVF virus is susceptible to the antiviral drug ribavirin. The Ebola and Marburg viruses are transmitted by direct contact with blood, secretions, organs, or semen of infected patients. Argentine, Bolivian and Hantavirus hemorrhagic fevers are also spread by dried rodent excreta (USAMRIID, 2001).

Clinical Features
The general clinical syndrome associated with all of the aforementioned viruses is similar and is called 'viral hemorrhagic fever' or VHF. The most common presenting symptoms are fever, myalgia, low blood pressure,

flushing and ecchymoses anywhere on the body. Typically the onset of CCHF is 3–12 days after tick exposure or inhalation of an aerosol. There can be extensive GI bleeding and extensive ecchymoses. Other symptoms are headache, back pain, nausea, vomiting, delirium, jaundice and hepatomegaly. Mortality for CCHF is 15–30%, but some hemorrhagic fevers, such as Ebola can have a death rate near 90% (Tierno, 2002).

Practical Considerations

- Any individual who may have been exposed to blood, body fluids, secretions, or excretions from a patient with suspected VHF should immediately and thoroughly wash skin surfaces with soap and water; a shower is preferable.
- In hospitals, contact precautions should be instituted to prevent contagion. An N95 mask is recommended and should be worn for protection. Infected patients should be quarantined for the duration of the illness.
- Anyone caring for (or visiting during convalescence) a patient that is stricken with VHF must practice strict 'barrier nursing' techniques (in other words, completely protect oneself from the infected patient by dressing in gown, gloves, mask, eye protection, hat, booties, etc.), because evidence indicates that large droplets or even fomites (inanimate objects) may act as mediators of virus transmission.
- Any contamination of mucous membranes must be immediately diluted with copious quantities of water. If contaminated, eyes can be irrigated with saline or products like Visine.
- Clorox (10% solution) can be used to decontaminate surfaces, equipment, or other articles.
- Deceased individuals should be sealed in leakproof material for prompt burial or cremation.
- Heavily soiled clothing should be discarded, or washed with bleach or a strong germicide-containing detergent.

Chemical Terrorism

History and Background

Chemical weapons were first used in modern warfare during World War I. On April 22, 1915, outside the Belgian village of Ypres, the German army released about 60 tons of chlorine gas from about 6000 pressurized gas cylinders into the winds, which carried clouds of chlorine gas over the Allied forces. A second attack using chlorine gas occurred 2 days later. The end result of both attacks was the grotesque choking death of approximately 10 000 troops. By the end of 1915, a more deadly gas agent, phosgene, was introduced by the Germans; it was 10 times more effective than chlorine. Both gases are considered chemical weapons that affect the lungs; thus they are called 'pulmonary agents.' They damage the membranes that separate air sacs (alveoli) from the capillary blood vessels. Fluid (plasma) leaks into the air sacs, accumulates and prevents air exchange. The victim is usually unable to get enough oxygen and eventually suffocates to death after an agonizing 2- to 24-hour period. Victims initially have shortness of breath with coughing fits, which can be quite severe. The production of large amounts of yellowish (chlorine) to clear (phosgene) frothy sputum occurs prior to death. There is also significant irritation of the eyes, nose, and a burning of the throat (Byrnes, 2003).

By the time the Germans introduced phosgene they were becoming very proficient at producing chemical weapons of various types and were equally proficient at delivering them. Great Britain quickly followed in kind with the use of chemical weapons against the German army. Great skill was needed to deliver gas weapons because if wind direction changed or if the weapon was inappropriately delivered poison gas could fall on one's own troops. This did happen often, especially during the early use of such chemical weapons. By the summer of 1917 the Germans introduced a new type of gas called mustard. Mustard gas is a chemical weapon belonging to a group of agents called 'blistering agents.' As the name implies one of the symptoms is a blistering of the skin and internal organs. The skin, eyes, lungs, the gastrointestinal tract, mucous membranes, bone marrow, and other organs can be severely damaged.

These early weapons forced armies to defend themselves by using gas masks as well as protective suits or outer coverings, both of which hampered efficient fighting on the battlefield. Nevertheless by wars end more than 110 000 tons of chemical weapons were used by both sides and the number of casualties measured over a million including about 100 000 dead.

The Geneva Protocol

Because of the agonizing deaths and horrendous suffering that was inflicted by chemical weapons during World War I, an effort was made to ban their use after the war. The League of Nations met at Geneva and developed a protocol to eliminate chemical weapons during warfare. The 'Protocol for the Prohibition of the Use in War of Asphyxiating, Poisonous, or Other Gases, and of Bacteriological Methods of Warfare' was signed by 38 nations in 1925 (Byrnes, 2003) though it had many loopholes and no provision to punish nations who violate the pact. During World War II, surprisingly, no chemical weapons were used in battle even though the Germans developed new chemical weapons, 'nerve agents,' including tabun, sarin, and soman. Nerve agents are a particularly potent class of chemical weapons and share some interesting properties. The mechanism of action of nerve agents such as sarin is that they disrupt nerve communication with the organs that they stimulate. In other words, the nerve is normal but the transmission of the nerve impulse to the muscle or other organ is faulty, usually causing overactivity. This interferes with basic bodily functions and death can occur in a period as soon as 1–10 minutes after inhalation. If a nerve agent is in liquid form it is characteristically heavier than water. Their vapors are also heavier than air, and they therefore tend to sink toward the ground or the basement of a building. Although nerve agent vapor affects victims in a very short period of time, the range of these effects will vary greatly depending upon the degree of exposure. Exposure to nerve agents will initially affect airways and the portions of the face that come into contact with the agent: the eyes, nose and mouth. The pupils become small (pinpoint), the eyes reddened, and vision becomes blurred. Some patients also experience eye pain, headache, and nausea and vomiting. Rhinorrhea may be an important feature, as is excessive salivation. If a nerve agent is inhaled, airways can become constricted, and they induce coughing fits or shortness of breath. If a sufficient quantity of the agent is inhaled, there can be sudden loss of consciousness followed by convulsions. Within a few minutes a victim stops breathing and becomes flaccid. Even a very small amount of a nerve agent like sarin can produce fasciculations (muscular twitching). Nausea and vomiting may accompany exposure. In case of greater exposure, involuntary defecation and urination may also occur (Byrnes, 2003).

Many new 'nerve agent' chemical weapons were developed from ordinary insecticides and/or pesticides. (People actually use weaker forms of nerve agents every time they tend their garden with insecticides. For example, insecticides like Malathion or sevin, and dozens of others are actually nerve agents. They do the exact same thing to humans that sarin or other more potent nerve agents do, though they require much larger doses and longer contact time to have a similar effect.) In the early 1950s, Great Britain made what was considered a breakthrough discovery of a new nerve agent that was magnitudes greater in its lethal abilities than any other known substance at the time. The agent was called by its code name – VX. This agent was not only more lethal but also more persistent (because it remains a liquid for more than 24 hours) and could enter the body either by inhalation or directly via the skin. Entry through the skin was possible because this agent is nonvolatile and is persistent. The US cooperated with Great Britain on this project, eventually taking over the large-scale production of agent VX. Production and stockpiling of VX continued into the 1960s until an accidental release of VX occurred at the manufacturing facility in Dugway, Utah killing more than 6000 sheep. But probably the most infamous US chemical agent, used primarily during the Vietnam War in the 1960s, was Agent Orange, an herbicide used to defoliate vegetation that offered cover to the enemy. Agent Orange contained varying quantities of dioxin (tetrachlorodibenzo-dioxin), which was later considered to be so dangerous that the EPA, in 1986, prohibited its use anywhere. Animal studies have linked the chemical to non-Hodgkin's lymphomas, sarcomas, and carcinomas as well as a host of other diseases (Byrnes, 2003).

The 1972 Convention on Prohibition of Biological and Chemical Weapons

Throughout recent decades, efforts have been made to limit or ban the use of toxic weapons (both chemical and biological). In 1972, more than 140 countries including the US signed the 'Convention on the Prohibition of the Development, Production, and Stockpiling of Biologic and Toxic Weapons and Their Destruction' which theoretically limited further development or use of biological or chemical weapons (Byrnes, 2003). Unfortunately there are numerous breaches in that accord. To take two relatively recent examples of an ongoing trend, in 1988 Libya built a chemical-weapons plant in the guise of a pharmaceutical factory. Often this occurs with the cooperation of companies that sell so-called dual-use technology to countries like Iraq and Libya. A plant for making pesticides can readily be turned into one for making chemical weapons. Iraq used mustard gas in its long war with Iran, and has used both mustard gas and toxic nerve agents against its own dissident Kurdish population. The 1980s saw the use of chemical warfare agents in Afghanistan, Cambodia, Iran, Iraq, and Laos (Tierno, 2002; Byrnes, 2003).

In March of 1995, a Japanese religious cult, Aum Shinriyko released sarin nerve gas in the Tokyo subway system (Tierno, 2002). Thousands were injured and 11 people were killed. This recent use of chemical weapons on the civilian population underscores the relative availability, and ease of use of such weapons and raises public and governmental awareness.

Weaponization and Delivery of Chemical Agents

Any chemical agent must be weaponized prior to its delivery. In general, the process of weaponization involves numerous steps. First, an agent must be made in sufficient quantity, temporarily stored and stabilized to prevent either evaporation or degradation. Thickeners are added to increase the viscosity of liquid agents and a carrier agent is required to improve dispersion of the chemical. Next the chemical agent must be inserted into an appropriate delivery device such as explosive, pneumatic, or mechanical munitions or dissemination device. Regardless of approach, the goal is to aerosolize the chemical agent to a particulate size of 1–7 microns. This can be accomplished by using either very sophisticated delivery systems such as munitions devices usually only available to governments, or unsophisticated devices like aerosol generators, such as an underarm deodorant or garden sprayers which can be quite an effective dissemination system. The important caveat here is that these unsophisticated devices are readily available to the masses. There are numerous other factors that might affect the weaponization and delivery of a chemical weapon, such as:

- *temperature (air and ground):* generally higher temperatures cause faster evaporation
- *humidity:* high humidity may cause enlargement of particle size, reducing effectiveness
- *precipitation:* heavy rain can dilute and disperse a chemical weapon; snow increases persistence of a chemical weapon
- *wind speed:* can disperse vapors, aerosols and liquids, affecting the target area
- *nature of buildings:* buildings may absorb or adsorb agents; they can also offer protection
- *nature of terrain:* woodlands and hills can create greater turbulence of low-lying clouds of agent.

Categories of Chemical Weapons

There are literally hundreds of chemical agents and poisonous gases that can be used in an attack and potentially new ones under development using newly described genetic engineering methods. Governmental agencies classify chemical weapons in various categories (Table 13–15).

Role of Level A Laboratory: Chemical Terrorism

It goes without saying that timely detection of the relatively quick acting chemical agents that a terrorist might use, such as nerve agents (i.e., sarin and VX), is critical not only to a patient (casualty) but also to the first responder or hazardous material (HAZMAT) unit member responding to an event. The rapid detection of the type of agent as well as its concentration after a terror incident can allow for an effective treatment of the victim including proper antidote selection, as well as allow for an appropriate protective response in order to assure the safety of the public at large. As such, it may be obvious but the most appropriate entity to detect such agents is not the clinical laboratory; instead, it is the bailiwick of the first responder unit or HAZMAT team. These teams use a wide variety of commercially available equipment manufactured for the rapid detection of hazardous chemicals, including the agents of chemical terrorism. Likewise, the military has provided a number of devices that can be used to detect such chemical agents or their vapors. The most portable chemical vapor detector is the chemical agent monitor (CAM). It uses ion mobility spectroscopy to detect nerve, blister, and blood agents. The simplest and most rapid liquid detectors are also products of the military, namely the M8 and M9 papers that can be used to detect mustard or nerve agents. These are mostly rapid screening devices and may show false-positive reactions (Byrnes, 2003). However, colorimetric tubes are the most common detection technology used by HAZMAT teams. Their analytic capabilities are broad and usually include tests for chlorine and phosgene gas (pulmonary agents), cyanide (blood agents), and organophosphates (nerve agents). In addition, HAZMAT teams possess a wide variety of some newer post-9/11 technologies enabling their members to detect virtually ALL necessary chemical agents in a relatively rapid time frame (Byrnes, 2003).

While the role of Level A clinical laboratories may be a secondary one, they can nevertheless still provide some support for detecting chemical agents used in an attack or their degradation products in victims, which can be useful to triage or treat incoming hospital patients. For practical

Table 13–15 Chemical Weapons

Category	Examples	Comments
Nerve agents	Sarin, tabun, soman, VX, malathion, sevin	Interfere with transmission of message from nerve to organ or muscle
Blood agents	Hydrogen cyanide, cyanogen chloride	Usually absorbed after inhalation; in the bloodstream cause lethal damage by acting on the cytochrome oxidase enzyme responsible for cellular respiration. Oxygen starvation occurs because cells are unable to use oxygen. (See Ch. 23)
Blister agents	Nitrogen and sulfur mustards, lewisite	Cause a blistering of skin as well as internal organs and tissues. This destroys the tissue and also causes massive number of mutations by crosslinking DNA and RNA
Heavy metals	Arsenic	Metallic elements form poisonous compounds, disrupting cellular metabolic processes
Pulmonary agents	Chlorine gas, phosgene	Damage the membranes of the lungs causing fluid build up and oxygen deprivation and eventually suffocation
Dioxins	Tetrachlorodibenzo-dioxin	Associated with lymphomas, sarcomas, carcinomas, chloracne, and a host of other diseases. (A major long-term complication is type II diabetes)
Incapacitating or psychotomimetic agents	Quinuclidinylbenzylate, phencyclidine	Cause pseudopsychotic disorders; affect ability to make decisions; cause disorientation, any of which could incapacitate an individual. Death due to respiratory arrest can occur with high doses
Corrosive acids and bases	Sulfuric acid, sodium hydroxide	Cause severe burning and destruction of tissue in exposed areas

purposes we can divide the potential chemical agents that a clinical chemistry laboratory may offer in their analytic repertoire into four major categories: nerve agents, blood agents (cyanide), blister agents (vesicants), and pulmonary agents.

Most modern clinical chemistry laboratories currently have the capacity to provide some specific and useful analytic data to support hospitalized victims of a chemical attack. For example, several automated chemistry analyzers can measure increased cholinesterase activity, which would be a hallmark of patients exposed to nerve agents. This information is used to measure progress and recovery of victims exposed to nerve agents. Gas chromatography–mass spectrometry has been used to detect metabolites of vesicants such as mustard gas or Lewisite (Byrnes, 2003) and is useful to measure the progress of a patient's recovery postexposure. Unfortunately for patients exposed to pulmonary agents such as chlorine or phosgene, the laboratory's role is limited to supportive monitoring such as blood gas analysis (for measuring P_{O_2}). This also applies to patients exposed to a blood agent like cyanide. Gaseous cyanide is lethal in seconds and patients who ingest cyanide need an antidote immediately to prevent anoxia and respiratory arrest. Therefore, the HAZMAT team may be the best means to analyze and identify such agents, and then provide antidotes to poisoned patients in the field, well before they reach a hospital.

In short, Level A laboratories play mostly a supportive role in the management of hospitalized patients who are victims of a chemical terror attack.

Nuclear Terrorism

History and Background of Nuclear Weapons

In 1895, Ernest Roentgen discovered penetrating radiations that produced fluorescence; he named them X-rays. The following year, Henri Becquerel identified that these penetrating radiations (later classified as alpha, beta and gamma rays) are emitted by uranium. In 1905 Albert Einstein formulated his now famous equation $E = mc^2$ which concluded that matter could be converted to energy. These discoveries provided the scientific framework to eventually harness nuclear energy, though this did not occur until World War II. In 1942, Los Alamos, New Mexico, was selected as the central site for a laboratory to research the physics and design of atomic weapons. In approximately 30 months, the 'Manhattan Project' (the name ascribed to the program that resulted in the production of the first atomic weapon) had achieved its goal of producing a nuclear weapon. By 1945 Germany had surrendered, but Japan continued its war effort. On July 26, 1945, the Potsdam Declaration was issued wherein President Harry Truman, Chiang Kai-Shek of China, and Winston Churchill of Great Britain advised the Japanese government to proclaim an unconditional surrender of all Japanese armed forces, cautioning against the alternative. The Japanese government rejected the declaration on July 29th, 1945 (Byrnes, 2003). On the morning of August 6, 1945 a US aircraft named *Enola Gay* dropped *Little Boy*, an enriched uranium bomb, on Hiroshima, Japan (15 kilotons). Several days later *Fat Man* was dropped on Nagasaki. The nuclear age had arrived.

The Potential Threat of Nuclear Terrorism

Since the end of World War II the US has manufactured over 70 000 nuclear weapons, though many have since been retired. Today's weapons are larger (1000 kilotons or 1 megaton) and far more destructive than the 15 kiloton Hiroshima bomb. Although the 'Cold War' with Russia has officially ended and efforts have been made to reduce the number of nuclear weapons, other countries possess or are trying to develop nuclear capabilities. There is concern that such weapons may fall into the hands of terrorists or might be used by rogue nations. While it is possible that terrorists may gain access to nuclear weapons of mass destruction, it is much more likely that they will construct 'dirty bombs' – a combination of conventional explosives and radioactive materials. 'Dirty bombs' are relatively simple to build and detonate. The main purpose of a dirty bomb is not to kill people so much as it is to create widespread panic and psychological fear. The amount of radioactivity a dirty bomb yields depends on the radioactive material used in the device. However, even a small amount of radiation from such a device has the potential to cause a relatively large decontamination cost.

Role of Level A Laboratory: Nuclear Terrorism

The clinical laboratory is not actively involved in detecting radiation contamination. This is more likely done in a hospital emergency department using one or more hand-held radiation survey instruments such as the Ludlum Model 3/Model 44-9 combo Geiger-Mueller detector that is able to detect alpha-, beta-, and gamma-emitting radionuclides. Routine HAZMAT and other first responder teams have such analytical capabilities and are the likely entity to first identify or detect a nuclear event. Clinical chemistry and hematology laboratories merely play a support role for any patients that may require hospitalization.

References

Angulo FJ, St Louis ME: Botulism. *In* Evans AS, Brachman PS (eds): Bacterial Infections of Humans. New York, Plenum, 1998, pp 131–153.

Byrnes ME, King DA, Tierno PM: Nuclear Chemical and Biological Terrorism. Boca Raton, CRC Press, 2003.

This text provides a comprehensive review of the various weapons of mass destruction, along with sound advice and simple actions that can be taken by emergency responders or the general public in order to reduce risks and avoid panic in the event of a terrorist attack.

CDC: NYC DOH response to terrorist attack September 11, 2001. MMWR, 2001; 50:941–948.

CDC/NIH: Biosafety in Microbiological and Biomedical Laboratories, 2nd ed. Wayne, NCCLS, 2001.

Gilchrist MJR, McKinney WP, Miller JM, Weisfeld AS: Cumitech 33, Laboratory Safety, Management and Diagnosis of Biological Agents Associated with Bioterrorism. Washington DC, ASM Press, 2000.

Lew DP: *Bacillus anthracis. In* Mandell GL, Bennett JE, Dolin R (eds): Principles of Infectious Diseases, 5th ed. Philadelphia, Churchill Livingston, 2000, pp 2215–2220.

NATO: Handbook of Medical Aspects of NBC Defensive Operations, Amed P-6(B) Part II Biological. Depts of the Army, Navy and Air Force, 1996.

NCCLS: Protection of Laboratory Workers from Instrument Hazards. Villanova, NCCLS, 2001.

Perry RD, Fetherson JD: *Yersinia pestis* – the etiologic agent of plague. Clin Microl Rev 1997; 10:35–66.

Shapiro RL, Hatheway C, Swerdlow DL: Botulism in the United States: A clinical and epidemiologic review. Ann Intern Med 1998; 129:221–228.

Shapiro DS, Wong JD: Brucella. *In* Murray PR (ed): Manual of Clinical Microbiology, 7th ed. Washington DC, ASM Press, 1999, pp 625–631.

Tierno PM: Protect Yourself Against Bioterrorism. New York, Pocket Books, 2002.

This pocket guide to bioterrorism provides concise information on the 18 most common biologic agents including background, history, and clinical features. It discusses pre-and postexposure management information as well as numerous protective response strategies.

Tierno PM: The Secret Life of Germs, 2nd ed. New York, Simon and Schuster, 2004.

USAMRIID: Medical Management of Biological Casualties Handbook, 4th ed. Fort Detrick, United States Army Medical Research Institute for Infectious Diseases, 2001.

This is the US Army's concise handbook on effective medical countermeasures against the likeliest bacterial, viral and toxic agents to be used as bioterror weapons. It is designed as a quick ready reference and overview rather than a complete resource.

VanPelt C, Verduin CM, Goessens WHF, et al: Identification of *Burkholderia* spp. in the clinical laboratory: comparison of conventional and molecular methods. J Clin Microbiol 1999; 37:2158–2164.

Wong JD, Shapiro DS: Francisella. *In* Murray PR (ed): Manual of Clinical Microbiology, 7th ed. Washington DC, ASM Press, 1999, pp 647–651.

I

PART II
Clinical Chemistry

Edited by

Matthew R. Pincus MD PhD, Mark S. Lifshitz MD

Evaluation of Renal Function, Water, Electrolytes and Acid–Base Balance

Man S. Oh MD

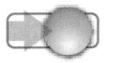

KEY POINTS

- Normal volumes and composition of electrolytes in various body fluid compartments are essential for maintenance of life.

- Maintenance of normal volumes and composition of electrolytes requires participation of various control mechanisms, and the role of the kidney is particularly important.

- The kidney is the most important organ in the maintenance of normal fluid volume and composition, and the initial discussion will be on the normal physiology of the kidney and various tests that are designed to detect abnormal renal function.

- The most important function of the kidney is elimination of the waste products of metabolism, and this function is best represented by the glomerular filtration rate (GFR). Hence, much discussion will be on the methods of measurement of GFR, and various laboratory tests that reflect the level of GFR.

- The two most widely used markers of the adequacy of GFR are plasma concentrations of creatinine and urea nitrogen, and much discussion will involve chemical measurements of these two substances.

- Among the important parameters of normal body fluid composition are the concentrations of protons, sodium, and potassium.

- The section on the disorders of potassium discusses mechanisms, causes and treatment of abnormally high and abnormally low potassium concentrations in the extracellular fluid.

- The section on the disorders of sodium discusses mechanisms, causes and treatment of abnormally high and abnormally low sodium concentrations in the extracellular fluid.

- The section on acid–base disorders discusses mechanisms, causes and treatment of abnormally high (i.e., acidosis) and abnormally low (i.e., alkalosis) proton concentrations in the extracellular fluid.

Introduction

Laboratory tests for evaluation of disorders of renal, water, electrolyte, and acid–base status are the most common procedures performed in clinical chemistry laboratories; collectively, screening tests for these are often grouped together in a basic metabolic panel. Disorders of acid–base balance and electrolytes are seen in a high percentage of hospitalized individuals, and electrolyte disorders are frequent complications of treatment for a variety of common conditions. Renal disease is one of the major sequelae of common disorders such as diabetes and hypertension. Proper interpretation of laboratory tests of renal, electrolyte, and acid–base disorders requires an understanding of the physiology and pathophysiology of these systems. Most central to an understanding of these disorders is knowledge of renal function and how the kidneys regulate extracellular volume.

Volumes and Osmolality of Body Fluid

The body fluid is an aqueous solution containing electrolytes and nonelectrolytes, and consists of intracellular and extracellular compartments.

The intracellular compartment is not a single compartment, but each cell has its own separate environment, communicating with other cells only via interstitial fluid and plasma. Consequently, difference exists among cells in various tissues in their solute content and concentrations. Because cell membranes are permeable to water through the ubiquitous presence of aquaporins (water channels), osmotic equilibrium is maintained so that the osmolality of all cells is the same and in equilibrium with the extracellular osmolality (Agre, 2002; Nielsen, 2002; Goodman, 2002).

Operation of normal metabolic functions of the body requires maintenance of an optimal ionic strength of its environment, primarily the intracellular fluid, where most metabolic activities occur. The homeostatic mechanisms of the body are at work to provide such an environment. Because the extracellular fluid is not the site of major metabolic activity, substantial alteration in its ionic strength may occur without adverse effects on body function. The main function of the extracellular fluid is to serve as a conduit between cells and between organs. The plasma is a route of rapid transit, and the interstitial fluid serves as a slow supply zone. The ability of the extracellular fluid to function efficiently as a conduit requires maintenance of optimal extracellular volume, particularly of vascular volume. An additional important function of the extracellular fluid is regulation of the intracellular volume and its ionic strength. Because of the osmotic equilibrium between the cells and the extracellular fluid, any alteration in extracellular osmolality is followed by an identical change in intracellular osmolality, which is usually accompanied by a reciprocal change in cell volume (Carroll, 1989).

Although cells and organs can be supplied with substrate and relieved of metabolic products with a much slower circulation, normal circulation is required to supply sufficient oxygen for the body's metabolic needs. Normal plasma volume is a prerequisite for maintenance of normal circulation. Because plasma is in equilibrium with the interstitial fluid, the maintenance of normal vascular volume requires normal extracellular volume. A low extracellular volume results in impaired organ perfusion, and an excessive extracellular volume leads to vascular congestion and pulmonary edema.

Volume of Body Fluids

Total body water can be determined by dilution of various substances including deuterium, tritium, and antipyrine. Total body water measured with antipyrine in hospitalized adults without fluid and electrolyte disorders is about 54% of the body weight (Carroll, 1989). The fractional water content is higher in infants and children, and decreases progressively with aging. The water content also depends on the body content of fat; women and obese persons, because of their higher fat content, tend to have less water for a given weight. A useful short cut for the calculation of total body water, using the fact that 54% of body weight in kg is body water, and 1 kg is 2.2 lb, is:

Total body water (L) = Body weight (lb)/4   (14–1)

For an obese subject subtract 10% from the calculated body water, and for a lean person add 10%. For a very obese person, subtract 20%. Women have about 10% less body water than men for the same body weight. Extracellular volume is measured directly, and the intracellular volume is estimated as the difference between total body water and extracellular volume. The measurement of total body water is reliable, but the measurement of extracellular volume is not, because no ideal marker has been found. Markers such as sodium, chloride, and bromide, penetrate the cells to some extent, whereas other markers such as mannitol, inulin, and sucrose, do not penetrate certain parts of the extracellular fluid. Thus, depending on the type of marker used, the extracellular fluid volume could vary from 27–53% of total body water (Carroll, 1989).

Extracellular volume measured with chloride and expressed as percent of total body water varies from 42–53%, greater in older subjects and women. Extracellular volume measured with inulin or sulfate is smaller, about 30–33% of total body water (Carroll, 1989). For discussion in this chapter, a value of 40% of total body water will be considered to represent extracellular volume. Extracellular volume is further divided into three fractions: interstitial (space between cells) volume (28% of total body water), plasma volume (8%), and transcellular water volume (4%) (Table 14–1). Transcellular water includes luminal fluid of the gastrointestinal tract, the fluids of the central nervous system, fluid in the eye as well as the lubricating fluids at serous surface.

Composition of the Body Fluid

Extracellular Composition

The concentrations of electrolytes in plasma are easily measured and their values well known. These concentrations increase by about 7% when

Table 14–1 Volumes of Body Fluid Compartments*

Intracellular volume	24 L (60%)
Extracellular volume	16 L (40%)
Interstitial volume	11.2 L (28%)
Plasma volume	3.2 L (8%)
Transcellular volume	1.6 L (4%)

* A normal man weighing 73 kg (160 lb) with 40 L of total body water is used as a model.

expressed in plasma water, because about 7% of plasma is solids. Thus, plasma sodium is 140 mEq/L but the concentration in plasma water is about 150 mEq/L. The concentrations of electrolytes in interstitial fluid are different from those in the plasma because of difference in protein concentrations between plasma and interstitial fluid. The differences in electrolyte concentrations between plasma and interstitial fluid can be predicted by the Donnan equilibrium (Table 14–2) (Oh, 1995). With normal plasma protein concentrations, the concentrations of diffusible cations are higher in plasma water than in interstitial water by about 4%, while the concentrations of diffusible anions are lower in the plasma than in the interstitial fluid by about 4%. The concentrations of calcium and magnesium in the interstitial fluid are lower than the values predicted by the Donnan equilibrium, because they are substantially protein-bound.

Part of the interstitial space is occupied by a ground substance consisting of glycosaminoglycans – the most abundant glycosaminoglycan is hyaluronan (hyaluronic acid) – and this space excludes distribution of proteins. In the other part, proteins diffuse freely and communicate with lymphatics. The first part is a gel phase, and the second part a free phase. Interspersed within the interstitial space is elastin, which provides the elastic property of the interstitial tissue; this property is necessary for generation of a normal negative pressure of the interstitial space and a positive pressure with the development of edema (Reed, 1992; Aukland, 1993; Burton, 1988).

Intracellular Composition

While sodium, chloride, and bicarbonate are the main solutes in the extracellular fluid, potassium, magnesium, phosphate, and proteins are the dominant solutes in the cell. The intracellular concentrations of sodium and chloride cannot be measured with accuracy, and is estimated by subtracting the amount that is extracellular from the total tissue value. Since concentrations of electrolytes in the extracellular fluid are high, a small error in extracellular water volume measurement will cause a large error in the measurement of intracellular concentration of these ions. The concentration of bicarbonate is calculated from cell pH, and the bicarbonate concentration shown in Table 14–2 is based on the assumption that average cell pH is 7.0.

The electrolyte composition of intracellular fluid is not identical throughout the tissues. For example, the concentration of chloride in muscle is very low, about 3 mEq/L, but it is about 75 mEq/L in erythrocytes. The concentration of potassium in the muscle cell is about 140 mEq/L, but in the platelets only about 118 mEq/L. The concentration of sodium in the muscle and red blood cell is about 13 mEq/L, but in the leukocytes about 34 mEq/L. The main phosphate in the red blood cell is 2,3-DPG, but in the muscle ATP and creatinine phosphate are the main phosphates. Because the muscle represents the bulk of the body cell mass, it is customary to use the electrolyte concentration of the muscle cells as representative of the intracellular electrolyte concentration. Because a substantial part of the anions inside the cell consists of polyvalent ions such as phosphate and protein, the total ionic concentration in the cell in mEq/L is higher than that of the extracellular fluid in order to maintain osmotic equilibrium with the extracellular fluid.

Measurement of Plasma Osmolality

Osmolarity refers to the number of moles of solute in a liter of solution, whereas osmolality refers to the number of moles of solute in a kg of water (solvent). Osmolality is the preferred term, since measurements of both osmolarity and osmolality are based on colligative properties. A colligative property is a physical property that is based on the number of particles dissolved in a given number of water molecules, and examples include freezing point, boiling point, and vapor pressure. The molecular mass of water represents the number of water molecules more accurately than the volume, because water volume changes with temperature, albeit little, but

Table 14–2 Electrolyte Concentrations in Extracellular and Intracellular Fluids

	Plasma		Interstitial fluid		Plasma water		Cell water (muscle)	
	(mEq/L)	(mmol/L)	(mEq/L)	(mmol/L)	(mEq/L)	(mmol/L)	(mEq/L)	(mmol/L)
Na^+	140	140	145.3	145.3	149.8	149.8	13	13
K^+	4.5	4.5	4.7	4.7	4.8	4.8	140	140
Ca^{2+}	5.0	2.5	2.8	2.8	5.3	5.3	1×10^{-7}	0.5×10^{-7}
Mg^{2+}	1.7	0.85	1.0	0.5	1.8	0.9	7.0	3.5
Cl^-	104	104	114.7	114.7	111.4	111.4	3	3
HCO_3^-	24	24	26.5	26.5	25.7	25.7	10	10
SO_4^{2-}	1.0	0.5	1.2	0.6	1.1	0.55	–	–
P	2.1	1.2*	2.3	1.3*	2.2	1.2*	107	57†
Protein	15	1	8	0.5	16	1	40	2.5‡
Organic anions	5	5§	5.6	5.6§	5.3	5.3§	–	–

* The calculation is based on the assumption that the pH of the extracellular fluid is 7.4 and the pK of $H_2PO_4^-$ is 6.8.

† The intracellular molal concentration of phosphate is calculated with the assumption that the pK of organic phosphates is 6.1 and the intracellular pH 7.0.

‡ The calculation is based on the assumption that each mmol of protein has on average 15 mEq, but the nature of cell proteins are not clearly known.

§ The assumption has been that all the organic anions are univalent.

the molecular mass does not. However, the terms, osmolality and osmolarity, are often used interchangeably, because changes in volume of water with temperature are negligible. One should note, however, that 1 kg of water occupies exactly 1 L at 4°C.

One mole of NaCl in solution contains 2 osmoles because NaCl is dissociated to Na^+ and Cl^-. One mole of D-glucose in solution contains 1 osmole since glucose does not dissociate. One mole of Na_3PO_4 in solution contains 4 osmoles, since it will dissociate into 3 Na^+ ions and one PO_4^{3-} ion. To calculate the osmolality of a solution whose solute dissociates into more than one particle, the following equation is used:

$M \times a = Osm/L$

M is molarity; a is the number of particles into which a molecule of the substance dissociates.

When the osmolal concentration of the extracellular fluid increases by accumulation of solutes that are restricted to the extracellular fluid (effective osmols), e.g., glucose, mannitol, and sodium, osmotic equilibrium is re-established as water shifts from the cell to the extracellular fluid (ECF) increasing intracellular osmolality to the same level as the extracellular osmolality (Hill, 1990a; Oh, 1995; Weisberg, 1978). When the extracellular osmolality increases by accumulation of solutes that can enter the cell freely (ineffective osmols), e.g., urea and alcohol, the osmotic equilibrium is achieved by entry of those solutes into the cell. Since most of the solutes normally present in the extracellular fluid are effective osmols, loss of extracellular water (e.g., insensible losses) will increase effective osmolality, and hence cause shift of water from the cells. Reduction in extracellular osmolality either by loss of normal extracellular solutes or by retention of water reduces effective osmolality for the same reasons, and hence causes shift of water into the cells.

Osmolality of serum or plasma can be measured directly with an osmometer as described in Chapter 4 or estimated as the sum of the concentration of all the solutes in the plasma. Because an osmometer does not distinguish between effective and ineffective osmols, effective osmolality can only be estimated. As it happens, urea is the only ineffective osmol that has substantial concentration in the plasma, 5 mOsm/L. In the normal plasma, therefore, total osmolality is nearly equal to effective osmolality. Plasma osmolality is estimated as follows:

Serum osmolality = {Serum Na^+ (mEq/L) $\times$ 2}+ (14–2)
{Glucose (mg/dL)/18}+ {Urea (mg/dL)/2.8}

At normal serum glucose and urea concentrations, osmolality almost equals serum $Na^+ \times 2$, because the opposing errors cancel each other; osmolality of sodium and accompanying anions are overestimated by not considering the osmotic coefficient and assuming that all serum anions are univalent; and on the other hand, osmolality is underestimated by ignoring non-sodium cations and other solutes, and using plasma sodium concentration instead of sodium concentration in plasma water. It should be noted that for the contributions of urea and glucose to serum osmolality, their values in mg/dL are divided by one-tenth of each (2.8 and 18) of their molecular weights (28 and 180), because osmolality is expressed as mOsm/L, not mOsm/dL.

Many of the solutes that may accumulate abnormally in the body are anions of an acid, e.g., salicylate, glycolate, formate, lactate, beta-

hydroxybutyrate. These substances should not be added in estimating plasma osmolality since they are largely balanced by sodium and therefore already included in the value when plasma sodium is multiplied by 2. Nonelectrolyte solutes that accumulate abnormally in the serum, e.g., ethanol, ethylene glycol, methanol, and mannitol, will cause the measured osmolality to exceed the calculated osmolality, producing an osmolal gap (Gennari, 1984; Kruse, 1994). This osmolal gap is a useful clinical clue to the presence of the toxic substances listed above. Accumulation of neutral and cationic amino acids also causes a serum osmolal gap.

Effect of Hyperglycemia on Serum Na^+

The permeability of a membrane for a given solute varies with the cell type. For example, glucose does not accumulate in the muscle. It does not enter the muscle cell freely, and when it enters the cell with the help of insulin, it is quickly metabolized. Thus, glucose is an effective osmol for the muscle cell, e.g., hyperglycemia will cause shift of water from the muscle cell. On the other hand, glucose is an ineffective osmol for the red blood cells, liver, kidney cells, and most brain cells because it enters these cells freely. Glucose is generally categorized as an effective osmol mainly because the muscle cells represent the largest body cell mass as noted previously in this chapter. Accumulation of glucose or mannitol in the extracellular fluid is a well-known cause of hyponatremia because, as discussed in Chapter 8, glucose is osmotically active and induces flow of water from the cells to the extracellular fluid, diluting its electrolytes. The fluid shift affects concentrations of all extracellular electrolytes, but its absolute effect is greatest on serum sodium because of its high concentration. The relationship between change in serum sodium and change in glucose concentration in a normal adult is about 1.5 mEq/L of Na^+ for 100 mg/dL of glucose. This figure is valid, however, only when the volume of distribution of glucose is somewhere between 40–50% of total body water. Volume of distribution of glucose refers to a theoretical volume into which glucose would be evenly distributed when none of the administered glucose is excreted and none metabolized. For example, if 10 g (10 000 mg) of glucose is given to a person, and the serum concentration were to increase by 1000 mg/L (100 mg/dL) (with the assumption that none was metabolized and none excreted), the volume of distribution would be 10 L. Normally, the volume of distribution of glucose is slightly greater than the extracellular volume because some cells such as red blood cells and hepatocytes allow free diffusion of glucose, achieving the same concentration of glucose in that cell as in plasma. As the volume of distribution of glucose in relation to total body water is increased, the effect of glucose on serum sodium decreases progressively. Decreased volume of distribution of glucose has an opposite effect. The change in serum Na caused by hyperglycemia can be estimated with the following formula (Oh, 1995):

ΔNa^+ (mEq/L) = (5.6 − 5.6a)/2 (14–3)

where ΔNa^+ is a reduction in serum Na^+ in mEq/L for each 100 mg/dL increase in glucose, and 'a' the fraction of the volume of glucose distribution over total body water.

In conditions with marked expansion of extracellular volume, e.g., congestive heart failure and other edema forming states, the volume of distribution of glucose represents a much greater fraction of total body water, and hence a fall in serum sodium caused by hyperglycemia would be much less than usual. For example, when the volume of distribution of glucose is 80% of total body water (0.8), the decrease in serum Na^+ for 100 mg/dL rise in glucose would be only 0.56 mEq/L; $(5.6 - 5.6 \times 0.8)/2 = 0.56$. When the glucose volume is 20% of total body water, ΔNa^+ would be 2.2 mEq/L for a 100 mg/dL increase in glucose.

Tonicity

The tonicity of a solution refers to the effect of a particular solution on the volume of cells. A hypertonic solution is one that shrinks the cells, while a hypotonic solution is one that causes swelling of the cells. An isotonic solution is one that does not induce any volume change in the cells. A solution of 0.9% saline (154 mM solution of sodium chloride) is generally isotonic. When the term tonicity is applied to a fluid in vitro, as in the urine, it is used almost interchangeably with total osmolality. Thus, urine with a high concentration of urea is called hypertonic (Pradella, 1988).

Osmolality and Specific Gravity

The specific gravity of a solution is the mass of the solution divided by the solution volume. Whereas osmolality of fluid depends on osmolal concentration of its solute, specific gravity is determined by the weight of the solute relative to the volume it displaces in solution. Plasma protein contributes little to osmolality because of its low molal concentration, but is the major factor determining specific gravity of plasma. Urinary specific gravity and osmolality usually change in parallel, but discrepancy between the two occurs with heavy proteinuria and severe glycosuria (Carroll, 1989).

Regulation of Extracellular Volume

As discussed below, the extracellular volume depends primarily on its sodium concentration, which is closely regulated by two hormones: antidiuretic hormone (ADH) that promotes water retention and aldosterone that promotes sodium retention which in turn causes water to be retained with it, as discussed in Chapter 8. Because the extracellular sodium concentration is maintained within a fairly narrow range through the regulation of ADH release, the extracellular volume depends primarily on its sodium content. In most clinical situations, the extracellular volume correlates well with vascular volume, which in turn correlates positively with the effective vascular volume. Effective vascular volume is an imaginary volume that reflects cardiac output in relation to the tissue's demand for oxygen (Oh, 1995).

Effective vascular volume, rather than the extracellular volume or vascular volume, is the chief determinant of how much extracellular fluid is retained. The location and type of sensors that perceive changes in effective vascular volume is not well known. Most physiologists consider baroreceptors, present in such loci as the atria of the heart and the aortic arch, likely candidates that send neural signals to the central nervous system resulting in increases or decreases of ADH and alter sympathetic tone. However, the preponderance of evidence argues against usefulness of such receptors in chronic states of altered effective vascular volume. For example, in a hypertensive patient with congestive heart failure, both atrial low pressure and arterial high pressure baroreceptors would sense a higher than normal volume. Yet, the neurohumoral responses (e.g., high ADH, high catecholamines, and high renin and angiotensin concentrations) in such states suggest the presence of low effective vascular volume. The kidney of course responds appropriately by reducing urinary excretion of sodium and chloride. These physiological responses to low effective vascular volume sometimes lead to a pathological retention of salt. For example, salt is retained in congestive heart failure despite markedly expanded extracellular volume and vascular volume, because effective vascular volume is decreased.

Theoretically, there are two ways to alter the salt content of the body: to alter the intake of salt or to alter renal salt output. There is no well-developed mechanism that influences salt intake in response to changes in effective vascular volume. Thus, alterations in salt content of the body are achieved primarily through changes in renal salt output. Changes in renal salt output can be achieved through physical and humoral factors. The physical factors for renal salt regulation work through changes in the glomerular filtration rate (GFR) and in peritubular capillary oncotic and hydrostatic pressures. When other factors that influence renal salt output are kept unchanged, the greater the GFR, the greater the amount of sodium filtered and the greater the amount of sodium excreted. In general, however, tubular reabsorption rather than glomerular filtration plays the major role in the regulation of renal excretion of sodium. In advanced renal failure, GFR may be 10% of normal, but patients with renal failure excrete their usual amount of sodium intake like normal people.

Tubular reabsorption of sodium is regulated by humoral factors and physical factors. The latter's influence on sodium reabsorption is limited mainly to the proximal tubule where a great deal of sodium reabsorption occurs passively through the paracellular (between cells) pathway. Increased hydrostatic pressure on the peritubular capillary retards passive fluid reabsorption through the paracellular pathway while it promotes passive back diffusion of fluid into the tubular lumen. Increased oncotic pressure has the opposite effects. For example in congestive heart failure, peritubular hydrostatic pressure is reduced because of the increased renal vascular resistance caused by constriction of both afferent and efferent arterioles. Constriction of afferent arterioles would tend to reduce glomerular capillary hydrostatic pressure. However, the glomerular pressure does not decrease much because the constriction of efferent arterioles is even greater than that of afferent arterioles. The maintenance of the glomerular filtration pressure helps to minimize a fall in GFR in volume depletion states. The result is increase in filtration fraction (the ratio of GFR to renal plasma flow), which increases the concentration of plasma protein in the blood leaving the glomerular capillary through the efferent arterioles to a greater extent than usual. Because the efferent arterioles become peritubular capillaries, the oncotic pressure of the peritubular capillary would be higher than usual. A lower-than-usual hydrostatic pressure and a higher-than-usual oncotic pressure of the peritubular capillary blood in volume depletion states tend to favor reabsorption of salt and water through the paracellular pathway of the proximal tubule, the tubular segment in which passive reabsorption of salt through the paracellular pathway plays a big role in the overall renal tubular salt transport. Normally, the oncotic pressure of the peritubular capillary plasma is about 20% higher than that of the peripheral blood plasma because the filtration fraction is 0.2. In states of volume depletion, the value could be 25 or 30% higher than that of the peripheral plasma.

Humoral factors that influence tubular reabsorption of sodium include angiotensin II, aldosterone, and catecholamines. Angiotensin II directly increases proximal tubular sodium reabsorption through its effect on the sodium–hydrogen exchanger-3 (NHE-3), and also indirectly by increasing aldosterone secretion, which in turn increases sodium reabsorption in the cortical collecting duct. Catecholamines influence sodium reabsorption mainly through their effects on renal blood flow, but may have some direct tubular effect in the proximal nephron.

The role of ADH in the regulation of extracellular volume is modest at most, because of the overwhelming importance of osmolality as the main regulator of ADH secretion. For this reason, *salt content of the body is the main determinant of the extracellular volume.* When sodium is retained, a proportionate amount of water is retained in order to maintain normal serum osmolality. Only when the effective vascular volume depletion is very great, will ADH secretion occur despite hyponatremia. In such settings, extracellular volume could theoretically increase in the absence of sodium retention. However, massive water retention without sodium retention will cause only a modest increase in extracellular volume. For example, if a person with 40 L of total body water gains 10 L of water without a change in sodium content, for example due to inappropriate secretion of ADH or in a person with acute renal failure, serum sodium would decrease from 140 mEq/L to 112 mEq/L ($140 \times 40/50 = 112$), a value that would cause severe morbidity or even death. This would increase the extracellular volume only by 4 L, since the bulk (60%) of retained water would enter the cell. On the other hand, the same fluid volume retained with salt would remain almost exclusively in the extracellular space. In other words, the amount of water that can be retained without salt is limited by severe and fatal hyponatremia. This is the reason why a massive increase in extracellular volume as in severe congestive heart failure is possible only with massive sodium retention. Figure 14–1 shows the nomenclature of the nephron sites.

The ultimate source of energy for reabsorption of sodium at various nephron segments is Na^+–K^+-ATPase located on the basolateral membrane, which transports $3Na^+$ out of the cell in exchange for $2K^+$ into the cell. The resulting reduction in intracellular sodium concentration and the negative cellular electrical potential allow passive diffusion of Na^+ into the cell through the luminal membrane. Four major sites of sodium reabsorption in the nephron utilize four different mechanisms of sodium entry (Fig. 14–2). A number of humoral factors have been proven or suggested as participating in the regulation of renal salt output. Those with well-proven physiological effects are aldosterone, catecholamines, angiotensin II, and perhaps ADH and prostaglandins (Oh, 1995; Biggi, 1995).

Nonrenal Control of Water and Electrolyte Balance

Insensible Loss of Water from the Skin. Water is lost from the skin primarily as a means of eliminating heat. Water loss from the skin without

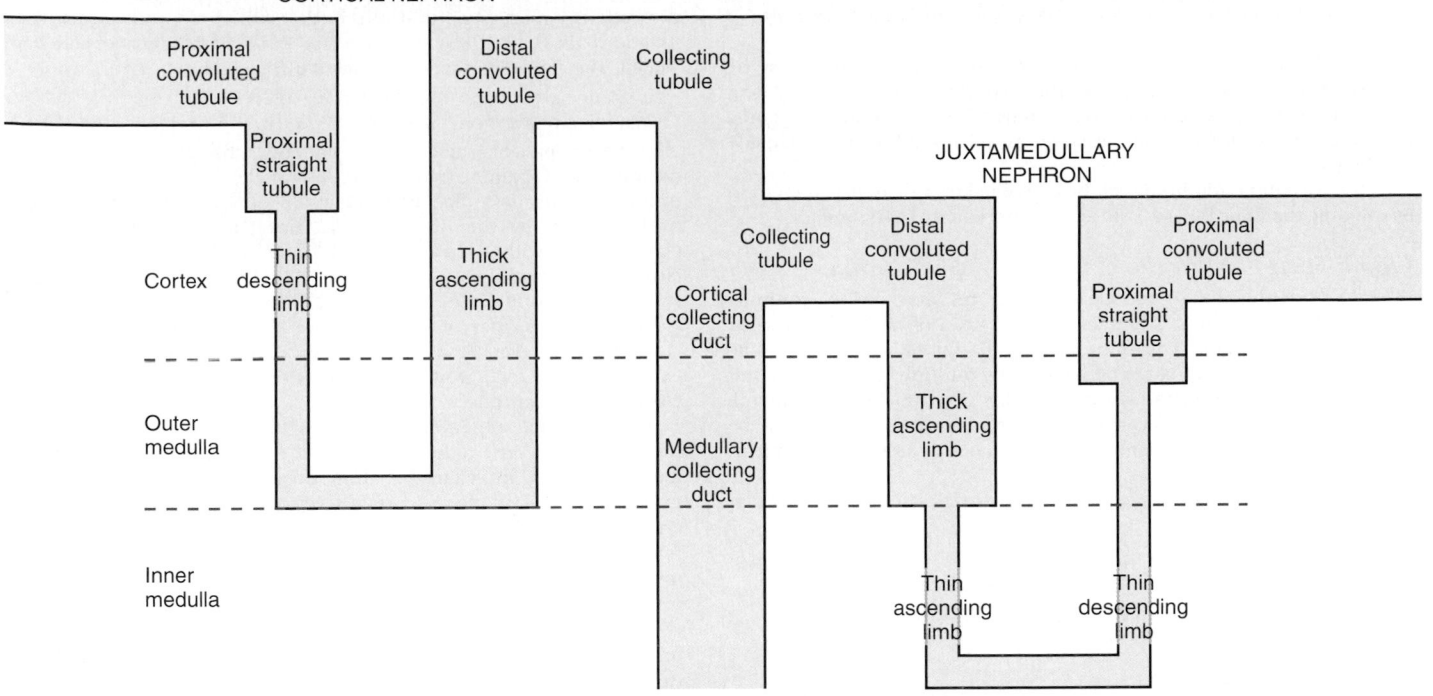

Figure 14–1 Distribution and subdivision of nephrons. There are two major types of nephron: cortical nephrons and juxtamedullary nephrons. The loop of Henle of the cortical nephrons does not enter the inner medulla, and has no thin ascending limb. The juxtamedullary nephron has the thin ascending limb of Henle, which resides in the inner medulla. Both nephrons are further subdivided into eight or nine segments.

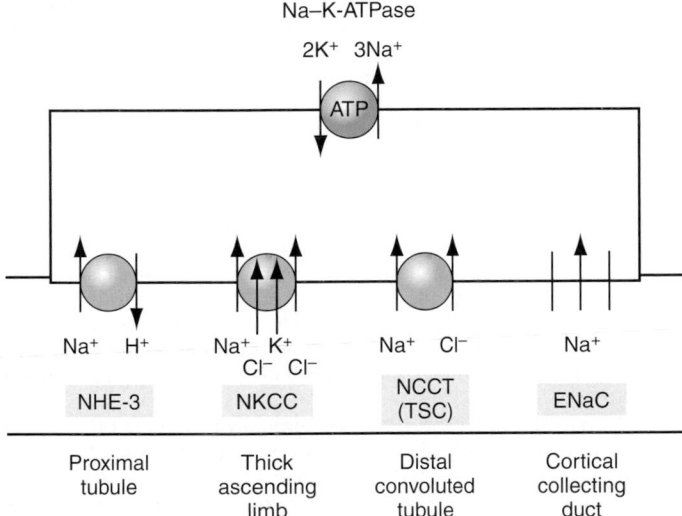

Figure 14–2 Mechanisms of sodium reabsorption at different nephron segments. The main source of energy for sodium reabsorption at all nephron segments is the basolateral Na$^+$–K$^+$-ATPase, which transports 3Na$^+$ out of the cell in exchange for 2K$^+$ into the cell, which creates a low intracellular sodium concentration and negative cellular potential. Both of these conditions allow passive diffusion of Na$^+$ into the cell through the luminal membrane. In the proximal tubule, Na$^+$ entry is accompanied by exit of H$^+$ through the sodium–hydrogen exchanger type 3 (NHE-3). In the thick ascending limb of Henle, a Na$^+$ enters with a K$^+$ and 2Cl$^-$ through the sodium–potassium–chloride cotransporter (NKCC). In the distal convoluted tubule, sodium enters with chloride through the sodium–chloride cotransporter (NCCT), and in the cortical collecting duct, sodium enters through the epithelial sodium channel (ENaC). TSC stands for thiazide-sensitive cotransporter.

sweat is called insensible perspiration. Sweat contains about 50 mEq/L of sodium and 5 mEq/L of potassium. Because the main purpose of water loss from the skin is elimination of heat, water loss from the skin depends mainly on the amount of heat generated in the body:

Water loss from the skin = 30 mL per 100 calories   (14–4)

Loss of Respiratory Water. The water content of inspired air is less than that of the expired air, and hence water is lost during normal ventilation. Because the ventilatory volume is determined by the amount of CO$_2$ production, which is in turn determined by the caloric expenditure,

ventilatory water loss in normal environmental conditions depends also on caloric expenditure:

Respiratory water loss = 13 mL per 100 calories at normal $P\text{CO}_2$ (14–5)

By coincidence, the quantity of water lost during normal respiration is about equal to the metabolic water production. Hence, in calculating water balance, respiratory water loss may be ignored in the measurement of insensible water loss, provided that metabolic water gain is also ignored. Respiratory water loss increases with hyperventilation or fever disproportionately to metabolic water production (Carroll, 1989).

Loss of Water in the Gastrointestinal Tract. The net activity of the gastrointestinal tract to the level of the jejunum is secretion of water and electrolytes. The net activity from jejunum to colon is reabsorption. Most of the fluid entering the small intestine is absorbed in the small intestine, and the remainder by the colon, leaving only about 100 mL of water to be excreted daily in the feces. The contents of the gastrointestinal tract are isotonic with plasma, and any fluid that enters the gastrointestinal tract becomes isotonic. Thus, if water is ingested and vomited, solute is lost from the body.

Measurement of Renal Function

Concept of Clearance

Renal clearance relates the rate of urinary excretion of material to the plasma concentration of that material. It is defined as the volume of plasma that would theoretically have to be 'cleared' of the substance in order to account for the amount of the substance excreted in the urine during a given period (14). In order to calculate clearance, one must know first the amount of the substance excreted in the urine, which is calculated from the urine concentration (U_x) and volume (V), and then know the plasma concentration of the substance (P_x). For example, if a person excreted 1500 mg of creatinine in a day, he would need 150 L of plasma to account for that 1500 mg of creatinine if the plasma concentration were 10 mg/L (1 mg/dL); creatinine clearance (C_{creat}) then, would be 150 L/day. At a plasma concentration of 100 mg/L (10 mg/dL), only 15 L of plasma would be needed to account for the same 1500 mg of creatinine; C_{creat} in this case would be 15 L/day. Customarily, clearance is expressed in mL/min, but any volume and time units can be used. Thus, a clearance of 150 L/day is equal to 6.25 L/hour and 104 mL/min. The formal equation for clearance is:

$$C_x = (U_x V)/P   (14–6)$$

C_x is clearance of a substance x, U_x and P_x are concentrations of the substance in urine and plasma respectively, and V the volume of urine per unit time.

In estimating clearance, concentration and volume units must be consistent. For example, if urine creatinine concentration is 70 mg/dL and volume is 2000 mL/day, urine creatinine must also be expressed in mg/mL, not mg/dL. So the total amount excreted is: 0.7 mg/mL × 2000 mL/day = 1400 mg/day.

A clearance in mL/24 hours can be converted to a clearance in mL/min by dividing the value by 1440, since 24 hours equals 1440 minutes.

Quick Formulas for the Calculation of Clearance

When calculating a 24-hour clearance in mL/min, urine creatinine excretion may be expressed in g/24 hours instead of mg/24 hours while expressing the plasma creatinine as mg/dL instead of mg/mL. The incorrect use of these units can be rectified by multiplying the final result by 1000 (for using g instead of mg) and then by 100 (for using mg/dL instead of mg/mL). A further correction requires dividing the value by 1440 in order to convert a 24-hour clearance value to a value in mL/min as follows (Carroll, 1989):

$$C_x = U_x V \text{ (g/24 hours)}/P_x \text{ (mg/dL)} \times 100\,000 \times 1/1440 \qquad (14\text{--}7)$$

Since $100\,000/1440 = 70$:

$$C_x \text{ (mL/min)} = U_x \text{ (g/day)} \times 70/P_x \text{ (mg/dL)} \qquad (14\text{--}8)$$

Measurement of Glomerular Filtration Rate (GFR)

GFR is generally considered the best overall indicator of the level of kidney function (Smith, 1951). Two different approaches have been utilized for the measurement of GFR. One approach has been to use an endogenous substance, and the other to use an exogenous substance. It is important, whatever molecular marker is used to determine GFR, that it be minimally reabsorbed in and minimally secreted by the renal tubules.

Measurement of GFR with Exogenous Substances

Inulin clearance is widely regarded as the gold standard for measuring glomerular filtration rate (14). Inulin clearance in healthy young adults has mean values of 127 mL/min/1.73 m^2 in men and 118 mL/min/1.73 m^2 in women. GFR declines with age. After age 20–30 years, GFR decreases by approximately 1.0 mL/min/1.73 m^2 per year. The classic method of inulin clearance requires an intravenous infusion and timed urine collections over many hours. Inulin is expensive and not readily available. Consequently, a number of alternative measures for estimating GFR have been introduced (Price, 2000; Gaspari, 1997). The urinary clearance of exogenous radioactive markers such as ^{125}I-iothalamate and ^{99m}Tc-DTPA (diethylene triamine penta-acetic acid) provides good measures of GFR (Biggi, 1995; Brochner-Mortensen, 1969, Christensen, 1986, Fleming, 1991). Plasma clearance of exogenous substances such as iohexol and ^{51}Cr-EDTA has also been used to estimate GFR, and an advantage of this method is that it does not require urine collection (Krutzen, 1984; Russel, 1985; Agarwal, 2003). However, the plasma clearance methods are not as accurate as those that require urine collection. GFR has also been measured with nonradiolabeled iothalamate in blood and urine, and an obvious advantage of this method is avoidance of radioactive materials.

Measurement of GFR with Endogenous Substances

Endogenous substances that are widely used to determine GFR include urea nitrogen, creatinine and cystatin C. The first two are widely used in clinical practice, mainly because of their ready availability.

Creatinine as a Measure of Renal Function

Creatinine is an endogenous substance with a molecular weight of 113 Da. It is produced by the muscle from creatine and creatine phosphate by a nonenzymatic dehydration process. The rate of production is proportionate to the muscle mass (Oh, 1993). An additional source of creatinine is creatine contained in ingested meat. The rate of in vitro conversion of creatine to creatinine in meat is dependent on temperature and acidity; high temperature and low pH increase the conversion. Creatinine is the most widely used marker of GFR for several reasons. First, it is an endogenous substance of a fairly constant rate of production. Second, creatinine is not bound to plasma proteins, and therefore is filtered freely by the glomerulus. It is not reabsorbed by the renal tubules, and only a small amount is secreted by the tubules.

In the use of creatinine clearance the inconvenience of urine collection and uncertainty of its completeness can be avoided by estimating the excretion rate. When renal function is normal and stable, creatinine excretion is almost equal to its production, which depends primarily on muscle mass (Oh, 1993). Muscle mass varies with sex, age, and body weight. The creatinine production rate is estimated by age (A):

Creatinine production (mg/kg/day): $28 - 0.2A$ (men) $\qquad (14\text{--}9A)$
Creatinine production (mg/kg/day): $23.8 - 0.17A$ (women) $\qquad (14\text{--}9B)$

In obese patients and wasted patients, the above formula will overestimate creatinine production. Normally, creatinine excretion in urine is slightly less than its production, because some creatinine is broken down by the intestinal bacteria. The discrepancy increases progressively with decreasing renal function, because the nonrenal clearance of creatinine, which is about 0.04 L/kg/day, remains constant (Oh, 1993). Normally, a 70-kg man would have an extrarenal creatinine clearance of 2.8 L/day or 2 mL/min, less than 2% of the normal renal clearance. However, at a renal clearance of 4 mL/min, 2 mL/min of extrarenal clearance would represent one-third of the total plasma clearance of creatinine.

However, there are several drawbacks to the use of creatinine as a measure of GFR. First, although the rate of production is fairly constant, it has a substantial individual variation, depending mainly on the muscle mass (Oh, 1993). In the presence of severe muscle wasting, production of creatinine could be reduced to less than 25% of the amount predicted from the body weight. Second, creatinine is also derived from dietary meat, and the quantity of meat ingestion can substantially influence the total daily production. Third, creatinine measurement is made most commonly by the alkaline picrate method (see below for more detailed discussion), and a number of chromogens, both endogenous and exogenous, interfere with its measurement by this technique. Finally, creatinine is partially secreted by the proximal tubules via the organic cation pathway, and the tubular secretion is blocked by various drugs including cimetidine, trimethoprim, pyrimethamine, and salicylate (Hilbrands, 1991; Van Acker, 1992). The extent of tubular secretion varies with individuals, and variation is much greater in the presence of renal dysfunction; tubular secretion could be as much as 50% of the amount excreted in the urine in advanced renal failure. In order to obviate the errors due to tubular secretion, creatinine clearance has been obtained with the simultaneous administration of cimetidine, which inhibits tubular secretion of creatinine. However, suppression of creatinine secretion by cimetidine is not complete, and also has wide individual variations.

Creatinine Measurement

The most widely used method of creatinine measurement is based on the Jaffe reaction described more than 100 years ago, which is based on the reaction of creatinine with picrate (Spencer, 1986; Weber, 1991). The alkaline solution enhances the reaction, and hence the term alkaline picrate method. The method of Hare involves the isolation of creatinine by absorption into Lloyd's reagent, and discarding the plasma containing interfering chromogens (Abdul-Karim, 1986). This method is difficult to manipulate and is often messy. The Jaffe reaction has also been adapted for use on autoanalyzers.

Creatinine can also be measured enzymatically by the use of creatinine amidohydrolase or creatinine iminohydrolase (Suzuki, 1984; Fossati, 1994). Creatinine is hydrolyzed by creatinine iminohydrolase to ammonia and N-methylhydantoin. The ammonia then combines with 2-oxoglutarate (alpha-ketoglutarate) and NADH in the presence of glutamate dehydrogenase to produce glutamate and NAD$^+$. The consumption of NADH, measured as decrease in absorbance at 340 nm, then measures the concentration of creatinine. Creatinine can also be measured by converting creatinine to creatine by creatinine amidohydrolase. Creatine is then hydrolysed by imidinohydrolase and sarcosine oxidase to produce hydrogen peroxide. In the presence of horseradish peroxidase, 2,4-dichlorophenolsulfonate is converted to a colorless polymer by hydrogen peroxide, and the concentration of the polymer is then measured at 510 nm.

Several substances such as ketones, glucose, fructose, protein, urea and ascorbic acid also react with picrate, and falsely increase creatinine concentration (Spencer, 1986; Weber, 1991; Kroll, 1983; Molitch, 1980; Watkins, 1967). Interference by glucose with creatinine measurement becomes significant when glucose concentration is very high, as in diabetic ketoacidosis or hyperglycemic coma (Sjoland, 2003). Glucose concentration is extremely high in peritoneal dialysate, and a correction for the level of high glucose is needed when creatinine concentration is measured in the effluent of peritoneal dialysate. The magnitude of glucose interference in creatinine measurement has been shown not only on the glucose concentration but also on the creatinine concentration. The interference by glucose in creatinine measurement does not occur in the enzymatic methods. Bilirubin and hemoglobin also interfere with the alkaline picrate method, resulting in falsely low values (Schoenmakers, 1993). Cephalosporin antibiotics also positively interfere with the alkaline picrate method, resulting in falsely elevated values (Swain, 1977; Kroll, 1983).

Without removing noncreatinine chromogens, the upper limit of normal measured by the Jaffe reaction is 1.6–1.9 mg/dL for adults. The upper limit of normal for serum creatinine measured after removing the chromogens is usually 1.2–1.4 mg/dL. Values for women are 0.1–0.2 mg/dL lower. When serum creatinine is very high, noncreatinine chromogens contribute proportionally less to the total reaction. With normal renal function, noncreatinine chromogens make up 14% (range 4.5–22.3%) of the total, but in advanced renal dysfunction, they contribute only about 5%.

Cimetidine-Enhanced Creatinine Clearance

Tubular secretion of creatinine results in falsely elevated values in creatinine clearance, especially in renal insufficiency, and measurements of creatinine clearance with inhibition of tubular secretion with cimetidine substantially improves the creatinine clearance estimate of GFR in patients with mild to moderate renal impairment (Hilbrands, 1991; Van Acker, 1992). However, tubular secretion of creatinine is not completely blocked by cimetidine, and hence the method still overestimates glomerular filtration rate.

Formulas to Estimate Creatinine Clearance as an Estimate of GFR

With the realization that accurate urine collection is a major limitation in the creatinine clearance as a measure of GFR, attempts have been made to mathematically transform serum creatinine to estimate glomerular filtration rate. In part because of the convenience, these methods are widely used in clinical practice. The two most widely used formulas are the Cockcroft and Gault formula and the MDRD formula (Levey formula).

Cockcroft and Gault Formula (mL/min) (Cockcroft, 1976).

$(140 - \text{Age}) \times (\text{IBW})/(72 \times \text{SCr})$, multiply by 0.85 if female   (14–10)

where IBW is ideal body weight and SCr is serum creatinine concentration. IBW is calculated by the following formula:

Males: IBW = 50 kg + 2.3 kg for each inch over 5 feet   (14–11A)
Females: IBW = 45.5 kg + 2.3 kg for each inch over 5 feet   (14–11B)

The Cockcroft and Gault formula (Cockcroft, 1976) reduces the variability of serum creatinine estimates of GFR caused by difference in creatinine production due to differences in muscle mass based on sex and age. However, because the formula does not take into account differences in creatinine production due to variation in muscle mass caused by disease states, it systematically overestimates glomerular filtration rate in individuals who have relatively low muscle mass in relation to their body weight such as obese, edematous, or chronically debilitated subjects. Moreover, it does not take into account variations caused by extrarenal elimination and tubular secretion.

In the Modification of Diet in Renal Disease (MDRD) study, Levey and co-workers measured GFR by I^{125}-iodothalamate to derive a formula for estimating glomerular filtration rate using six variables: age, race, sex, serum urea nitrogen, serum creatinine, and serum albumin concentration (Levey, 1999). Subsequently, in 2000 the same investigators produced a simplified MDRD formula based on four variables, serum creatinine, age, race, and sex. Few diabetic individuals were included in the original studies and these formulas tested in diabetic patients were found to be inaccurate. Furthermore, the use of logarithms in the formula prevents routine uses in clinical practice.

MDRD Formula (mL/min/1.73 m³)

GFR = $170 \times Cr^{-0.999} \times \text{Age}^{0.176} \times (0.762 \text{ if female}) \times$ (14–12A)
$(1.180 \text{ if black}) \times \text{BUN}^{-0.170} \times \text{Alb}^{0.318}$

The simplified MDRD formula (mL/min/1.73 m³) based on four variables (serum creatinine, age, race and sex) (Levey, 2002):

GFR = $186.3 \times Cr^{-1.154} \times \text{Age}^{-0.203} \times 1.212$ (14–12B)
(for Black) $\times 0.742$ (for women)

Cr = serum creatinine (mg/dL); BUN = blood urea nitrogen (mg/dL); Alb = serum albumin (g/dL). Whereas the Cockcroft and Gault formula includes the body weight, the MDRD formula does not include the body weight, because the result of the latter is expressed in mL/min/1.73 m³ rather than an absolute value as in the former. Following are the formulas used most often for calculating creatinine clearance for children (Schwartz, 1976; Counahan, 1976; Leger, 2002; Pierrat, 2003):

Schwartz Formula.

GFR = $0.55 \times \text{Height (cm)}/\text{Serum creatinine (mg/dL)}$ (14–13A)
GFR = $43 \times \text{Height (cm)}/\text{Serum creatinine (μmol/L)}$ (14–13B)

Modified Counahan Barrett Formula.

GFR = $40 \times \text{Height (cm)}/\text{Serum creatinine (μmol/L)}$ (14–14)

It has been shown repeatedly that GFR estimated from these formulas is not very accurate. However, creatinine clearance values estimated from the formulas are still more accurate than those from direct measurements, mainly because of the inaccurate urine collections and variations in plasma creatinine concentration in the latter. Consequently, K/DOQI (Kidney Disease Outcomes Quality Initiative) guidelines have recommended the use of these formulas instead of direct measurements in calculating creatinine clearance (Levey, 1999).

Urea as Measure of Renal Function

Urea is the main waste product of nitrogen-containing chemicals in the body. It has a molecular weight of 60 Da. However, by custom, the concentration of urea is expressed only in terms of the nitrogen content of urea. For this reason the term serum or urine urea nitrogen is much more widely used. As noted above in the section on osmolality, a molecule of urea contains two nitrogen atoms, and therefore, the molecular weight of urea nitrogen is 28 Da.

Serum urea is widely used as a measure of renal dysfunction, but its value as a measure of GFR is not very good for several reasons. First, urea concentration in the serum depends not only on the renal function but also on the rate of urea production, which depends largely on the protein intake. The rate of protein intake varies widely from individual to individual. Urea is freely filtered at the glomerulus, but is reabsorbed substantially in the proximal tubule and in the inner medullary collecting duct (Oh, 1997). The amount reabsorbed in the proximal tubule varies greatly depending on the status of effective vascular volume. Furthermore, the amount reabsorbed in the inner medullary collecting duct depends on the urine flow rate. Despite these shortcomings, serum urea nitrogen is still widely used as a measure of renal dysfunction. In the presence of normal renal function without volume depletion, urea clearance is about 50% of creatinine clearance, but in the presence of severe volume depletion, its clearance could be as little as 10% of creatinine clearance. As renal failure progresses, urea clearance approaches parity with creatinine clearance.

Measurement of urea

Essentially there are three methods for the measurement of urea. The gold standard, which is used only as a reference method because of its high cost, is isotope dilution mass spectrometry (Kessler, 1999). In the clinical laboratories, urea is measured either by the colorimetric method based on a reaction of urea with diacetyl monoxime or by enzymatic methods (Barbour, 1992; Natelson, 1951; Passey, 1980). In the former, urea reacts directly with diacetyl monoxime under strong acidic conditions to give a yellow condensation product. The reaction is intensified by the presence of ferric ions and thiosemicarbazide. The intense red color formed is measured at 540 nm.

The initial reaction in all enzymatic methods is hydrolysis of urea by urease, which produces ammonia and CO_2. Ammonia and CO_2 produced are measured by various methods to calculate the concentration of urea in the original sample. Measurement of ammonia is most often used. In one of these methods, ammonia produced by urease converts glutamate and ATP to glutamine and ADP. The ADP so produced is consumed in reactions catalyzed sequentially by pyruvate kinase and pyruvate oxidase to generate hydrogen peroxide (Lespinas, 1989). The hydrogen peroxide is then measured as an indirect estimate of urea concentration. In another enzymatic method, as in the one used for creatinine described in the preceding section, ammonia produced from urea hydrolysis reacts with alpha-ketoglutarate and NADH to produce glutamic acid and NAD^+ by glutamate dehydrogenase (Fawcett, 1960). The amount of NADH consumed is measured photometrically to determine the urea concentration. Another urease method involves the indophenol method, in which ammonium produced by urease reacts with hypochlorite to form monochloramine (Higashi, 2000). In the presence of phenol and an excess of hypochlorite, the monochloramine forms a blue-colored compound, indophenol, the concentration of which is determined spectrophotometrically at 630 nm. In yet another enzymatic method, CO_2 produced by urease is measured by thermal conductivity gas chromatography.

Cystatin C

Cystatin C is a 122 amino acid protein with a molecular weight of 13 000 Da, and is an inhibitor of cysteine proteinase. The substance is produced by all nucleated cells, and its production rate is relatively constant from age 4 months to age 70 years, and is proportionate to GFR (Massey, 2004; Laterza, 2002; Ylinen, 1999). The rate of production is not affected by muscle mass, sex, and race. Because of its small size (small for a protein) and a positive net charge, it is freely filtered at the glomerulus at the same concentration as in the plasma. It is completely reabsorbed by the proximal tubule, and in the absence of proximal tubular defect, none is excreted in the urine. Hence appearance of cystatin C signifies proximal tubular damage. There is some evidence that glucocorticoids reduce production of cystatin C (Risch, 2001), and this might result in overestimation of renal function in renal transplantation patients, who are regularly given glucocorticoids. A number of studies made comparison of serum creatinine and serum cystatin C as an indicator of renal function, and general consensus is that cystatin C is better than creatinine. However, cystatin C is not widely used clinically because measurements are difficult and expensive (Massey, 2004). It must be noted that cystatin renal clearance cannot be measured because normally it is completely reabsorbed, and none excreted in the urine. For this reason, serum concentration changes of cystatin are used as indirect estimates of GFR.

Urea Clearance and Urea/Creatinine Ratio in Serum

In the absence of renal dysfunction and severe dehydration, urea clearance is about 50% of creatinine clearance, and hence about 50% of GFR, because about 50% of the filtered urea is reabsorbed. The bulk of urea reabsorption occurs in the proximal tubule, about 40% of the filtered load. Among the distal nephron sites, the inner medullary collecting duct reabsorbs urea extensively along a concentration gradient when urine is being concentrated. Some of the urea reabsorbed from the inner medulla re-enters the tubule at the descending thin limb; this re-entry represents intrarenal recycling of urea. Urea re-entry occurs mainly in the short loop of Henle. Some of the urea reabsorbed from the inner medullary collecting duct is carried away from the medulla by the ascending vasa recta; this amount represents about 10% of the filtered load with normal urine flow, but with marked urine concentration the amount can increase greatly (Lyman, 1986).

A marked reduction in urea clearance occurs when the proximal reabsorption of urea is greatly increased by a reduction in effective vascular volume. Reabsorption of urea in the proximal tubule is passive and depends on a favorable urea concentration gradient. This gradient is created by reabsorption of water in the proximal tubule. Normally, about two-thirds of the filtered water is reabsorbed in the proximal tubule as a result of reabsorption of salt (mainly sodium chloride). Loss of two-thirds of the water in the tubule increases urea concentration in the tubule threefold, creating a favorable gradient for urea diffusion out of the tubule. When the water reabsorption is 90% of the filtered load, the urea concentration would increase to 10 times the plasma concentration. Volume depletion and decreased renal plasma flow without volume depletion, e.g., renal artery stenosis, also reduce the glomerular filtration rate, thereby reducing clearance of both creatinine and urea. Hence, volume depletion decreases creatinine clearance only by reduced filtration, and urea clearance by both reduced filtration and increased reabsorption. Hence, in volume depletion, urea clearance decreases more than does creatinine clearance. Normally the ratio of plasma urea nitrogen to plasma creatinine is about 10 to 1, but in volume depletion the ratio is usually greater than 20 to 1. The prediction of volume status by the urea/creatinine ratio is based on the assumption of constancy of urea and creatinine production, which is often not the case. Glucocorticoids and a high protein diet increase urea production, whereas chronic protein malnutrition decreases it. Creatinine production also varies considerably; marked muscle wasting may reduce its production to less than one-third of a usual value. Nowadays, the main cause of a high BUN/creatinine ratio in the hospital is not dehydration, but adequate protein intake (often by tube feeding) in a patient with severe muscle wasting. Thus, fractional excretion of urea (see below) would be a more reliable index of volume status than plasma urea/creatinine ratio (Carvounis, 2002). Mechanisms by which low effective vascular volume increases the proximal reabsorption of salt and water were explained earlier in the section on the control of extracellular volume.

Glomerular Filtration Rate (GFR), Renal Plasma Flow (RPF), and Filtration Fraction (FF)

As discussed in the preceding section, because inulin is filtered freely at the glomerulus but is neither reabsorbed nor secreted by the tubules, its clearance equals GFR, which is the rate (mL/min) of plasma filtered by the glomerulus from the blood into the tubular system. The clearance of para-aminohippurate (PAH) measures another aspect of renal function. As it happens, whatever PAH that is not filtered at the glomerulus is almost all secreted into the proximal tubule, thereby allowing PAH clearance to be a measure of renal plasma flow, which is the total quantity of plasma perfusing the glomerular capillary. The quantity of plasma filtered as a fraction of the total quantity perfusing the glomerular capillary is the filtration fraction (Smith, 1951). Because inulin clearance represents glomerular filtration rate and PAH clearance the quantity of plasma perfusing the glomerulus:

$$\text{Filtration fraction (FF)} = C_{IN}/C_{PAH} \tag{14–15}$$

where C_{IN} is inulin clearance, and C_{PAH} PAH clearance.

Filtration fraction in man is normally about 0.2. As discussed above in the section on regulation of extracellular volume, when effective vascular volume decreases as in heart failure, renal perfusion diminishes, but GFR decreases to a lesser degree because glomerular capillary pressure is maintained by increased efferent arteriolar tone. The result is an increase in filtration fraction. An increase in glomerular filtration for a given plasma flow, i.e., increased filtration fraction, increases the concentrations of plasma proteins by concentrating the nonfilterable plasma constituents. This increases the oncotic pressure of peritubular capillary blood, thus resulting in increased fluid movement from the tubular interstitium to the capillary. This in turn helps to increase fluid reabsorption from the proximal tubule into the interstitial space. Similarly, increased tone of efferent arterioles in an attempt to maintain a high glomerular capillary pressure tends to reduce the peritubular capillary hydrostatic pressure. This also contributes to increased salt reabsorption by the proximal tubule.

When the effective vascular volume is expanded, the filtration fraction decreases because the increase in renal plasma flow is greater than the increase in GFR. Changes in oncotic pressure and hydrostatic pressure in the peritubular capillary blood and their effects on proximal salt and water reabsorption are the opposite of those encountered in conditions of reduced effective vascular volume (Oh, 1995) described above.

Fractional Excretion (FE)

Fractional excretion is the quantity of a substance excreted in the urine expressed as a fraction of the filtered load of the same substance.

$$F_x = P_x \times \text{GFR} \tag{14–16}$$

where F_x is the amount of a substance x filtered.

$$F_x = P_x \times C_{creat} \text{ (assume that GFR} = C_{creat}) = P_x \times (U_{creat}V/P_{creat}) \tag{14–17}$$

$$E_x = V \times U_x, \tag{14–18}$$

where E_x is the amount excreted in the urine and U_x the urine concentration of substance x.

Hence:

$$\text{FE} = [(V \times U_x)]/[P_x \times (V \times U_{creat}/P_{creat})] \tag{14–19}$$

When V is cancelled on both sides, the equation is simplified as:

$$\text{FE} = (U_x/P_x)/(U_{creat}/P_{creat}) \tag{14–20}$$

or

$$\text{FE} = (U_x/P_x) \times (P_{creat}/U_{creat}) \tag{14–21}$$

Thus, the measurement of fractional excretion can be obtained in a spot urine sample. When the substance excreted in the urine has a clearance less than creatinine clearance, fractional excretion is less than 1. When FE is multiplied by 100, the result is %FE. FE of sodium is often used to distinguish between acute tubular necrosis and prerenal azotemia. A value of FE of sodium of less than 0.01 (less than 1%) suggests prerenal azotemia, while a value greater than 0.01 suggests acute tubular necrosis.

Renal Failure Index (RFI)

Renal failure index is another formula that is used for the differential diagnosis of acute renal failure. It is expressed as $U_{Na+}/(U_{creat}/P_{creat})$. The renal failure index is differentiated from fractional excretion of sodium by the exclusion of plasma Na^+ concentration in the formula. Hence, the value of the renal failure index will be 140 times the value of fractional excretion of Na^+ when the serum Na^+ concentration is 140 mEq/L. When fractional excretion of Na^+ is expressed as a percentage value:

$$\text{FE}_{Na+} \times 1.4 = \text{Renal failure index} \tag{14–22}$$

A word of caution: Both FE of Na^+ and the renal failure index are used only in the differential diagnosis of acute renal failure with oliguria. For example, usual fractional excretion of Na^+ on regular salt intake is less than 0.01, and this does not indicate the presence of prerenal azotemia.

Fractional Reabsorption (FR)

Fractional reabsorption is the quantity of a substance reabsorbed expressed as a fraction of the filtered load. It is estimated from fractional excretion as:

$$\text{FR} = 1 - \text{FE} \tag{14–23}$$

Free Water Clearance and Negative Free Water Clearance

Free water is the volume of water excreted in excess of the amount necessary to keep the urine isotonic to plasma. In other words, it is the volume of water that would have to be removed to make the urine isotonic. Free water clearance, like all other clearances, is expressed as volume per unit time, usually as mL/min. To determine free water clearance, one first determines the total amount of solute in the urine (mOsm), which is measured from urine osmolality and urine volume ($U_{osm} \times V$), and then determine the amount of water required to hold that quantity of solute at the same osmolality as plasma, which is called osmolar clearance. Free water clearance is the difference between osmolar clearance and urine volume (Carroll, 1989).

$$\text{Osmolar clearance } (C_{osm}) = (U_{osm} \times V)/P_{osm} \qquad (14–24)$$

$$\text{Free water clearance } (C_{H_2O}) = V – C_{osm} \qquad (14–25)$$

or

$$C_{H_2O} = V – (U_{osm} \times V/P_{osm}) \qquad (14–26)$$

If the urine is more concentrated than the plasma, then in a sense free water has been removed from isotonic urine, and the term negative free water clearance is used. In other words, it is the amount of water that would have to be added to make the urine isotonic.

$$\text{Negative free water clearance } (Tc_{H_2O}) = C_{osm} – V \qquad (14–27)$$

In the presence of normal renal function, the kidneys usually concentrate the urine, and therefore U_{osm} is greater than P_{osm}, resulting in a negative value for C_{H_2O}. On the other hand, loop diuretics block reabsorption of sodium chloride in the loop of Henle, interfering with both concentration and dilution of urine, and urine is approximately isotonic with little free water or negative free water.

The above discussion concerns the overall mechanisms by which the kidneys control extracellular volume and how measurements of specific chemicals, like BUN and creatinine, in serum and urine are used to measure renal function. The kidneys regulate extracellular volume by regulating the concentrations of ions that are retained in blood. Disorders of renal function result frequently in electrolyte imbalances, while disorders of electrolytes can often be at least partially corrected by normal functioning kidneys. We therefore now discuss causes of electrolyte disturbances.

Disorders of Potassium

Total body K^+ in hospitalized adults is about 43 mEq/kg body weight, and only about 2% of this is found in the extracellular fluid. When the potassium concentrations across the cell membrane are in electrochemical equilibrium, the gradient of K^+ determines and is also predicted by the membrane potential (E_m) according to the Nernst equation (Veech, 1995; Goldman, 1943):

$$E_m \text{ (mV)} = –61 \log (\text{Intracellular } K^+/\text{Extracellular } K^+) \qquad (14–28)$$

The normal ratio of intracellular K^+/extracellular K^+ is about 30, and therefore normal E_m is –90 mV. The membrane potential tends to increase with hypokalemia and to decrease with hyperkalemia. In hypokalemia, both intra- and extracellular K^+ tend to decrease, but the extracellular concentration tends to decrease proportionally more than the intracellular concentration. Hence, the ratio of intracellular K^+/extracellular K^+ tends to increase. In hyperkalemia, the membrane potential tends to decrease because an increase in the extracellular K^+ is proportionally greater than that in the intracellular K^+.

Control of Transcellular Flux of Potassium

Transmembrane electrical gradients cause diffusion of cellular K^+ out of cells and Na^+ into cells. Since the Na^+-K^+ pump, which reverses this process, is stimulated by insulin and catecholamines (through beta-2-adrenergic receptors), alterations in levels of these hormones can affect K^+ transport and its serum levels (Meister, 1993; Feraille, 1999; Sweeney, 1998; Goguen, 1993). Cells can act as buffers. In acidosis, cells can take up H^+ ions in exchange for K^+ ions, and, in alkalosis, cells extrude H^+ ions in exchange for K^+ ions. These effects are summarized in Figure 14–3. The effect of acidosis and alkalosis on transcellular K^+ flux depends not only on the pH but also on the type of anion that accumulates. In general, metabolic acidosis causes greater K^+ efflux than respiratory acidosis. Metabolic acidosis due to inorganic acids, e.g., sulfuric acid and hydrochloric acid, causes greater K^+ efflux than that due to organic acids, e.g., lactic acid and ketoacids, because organic anions accumulate substantially in the cell as well as in the ECF, whereas inorganic anions accumulate mainly in the ECF. Acidosis causes efflux of K^+ from the cell because of a shift of H^+ into the cell in exchange for K^+. A modifying factor appears to be the anion accumulation in the cells. In organic acidosis, much of the H^+ entering the cell is balanced by organic anions, and therefore efflux of K^+ is prevented. In respiratory acidosis, the anion that accumulates in the cell to balance the incoming H^+ is bicarbonate (Perez,

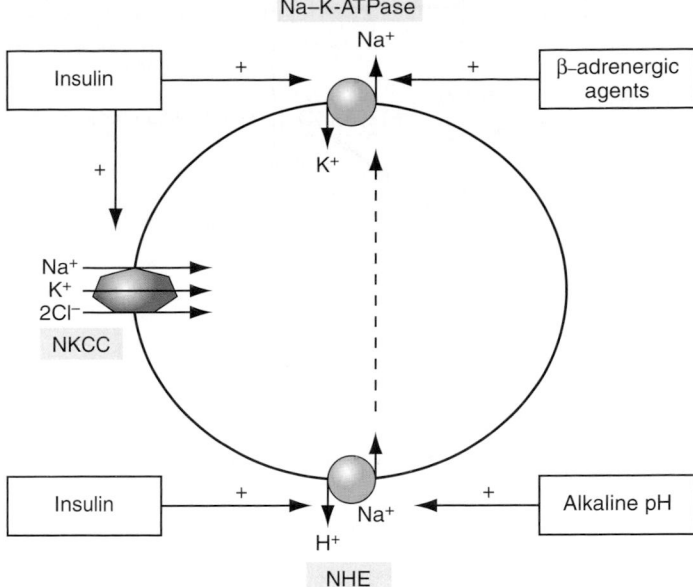

Figure 14–3 Control of transcellular movement of potassium. Potassium enters the cell through Na^+–K^+-ATPase (stimulated by beta-adrenergic agents or insulin) or through NKCC (stimulated by insulin). Stimulation of either transporters increases intracellular movement of potassium. Stimulation of NHE by a high extracellular pH or insulin increases intracellular sodium concentration, which in turn stimulates Na^+–K^+-ATPase. NKCC = Na–K–Cl cotransporter; NHE = Na–H exchanger.

1981). Alkalosis tends to lower serum K^+, because, as noted above, H^+ leaves cells, in exchange for K^+ which enters the cells. As with acidosis, K^+ influx varies with the type of alkalosis. In respiratory alkalosis, with its attendant lower P_{CO_2} and compensatory lower bicarbonate, as discussed below, probably because of a drop in cellular bicarbonate concentration, K^+ influx is not as great as in metabolic alkalosis. When pH is kept normal with proportionately increased concentration of bicarbonate and P_{CO_2}, K^+ tends to move into the cells; accumulation of bicarbonate in the cell must be accompanied by Na^+ and K^+. Similarly, when pH is kept normal with proportionately low bicarbonate and low P_{CO_2}, K^+ tends to move out of the cells.

Control of Renal Excretion of Potassium

About 90% of the daily K^+ intake (60–100 mEq) is excreted in the urine and 10% in the stool. Potassium filtered at the glomerulus is mostly (70–80%) reabsorbed by active and passive mechanisms in the proximal tubule. In the ascending limb of Henle's loop, K^+ is reabsorbed together with Na^+ and Cl^-; the concentration of K^+ at the beginning of the distal convoluted tubule is about 1 mEq/L with fluid volume of about 25 L. Thus, K^+ excreted in the urine is largely what has been secreted into the cortical collecting duct by mechanisms shown in Figure 14–4. Na^+–K^+-ATPase located on the basolateral side of the cortical collecting duct pumps K^+ into the cell while it pumps Na^+ out of the cell. The luminal Na^+ enters the cell through ENaC (epithelial sodium channels), providing a continuous supply of Na^+. This is the most critical step in the reabsorption of Na^+, which is an absolute requirement of secretion of potassium in the cortical collecting duct. Aldosterone is the main regulator of the expression of ENaC on the luminal membrane, and therefore the main determinant of renal excretion of potassium. The negative luminal potential that develops as a result of sodium reabsorption causes reabsorption of chloride through the paracellular channels. Because Na^+ reabsorption is not followed one to one by Cl^- reabsorption, the charge imbalance is corrected by secretion of K^+ through a specialized K^+ channel, the ROMK (renal outer medullary K channel). Aldosterone increases K^+ secretion by increasing passive entry of Na^+ from the lumen to the cell through increased expression of ENaC on the luminal membrane. The resulting increase in cellular concentration of sodium indirectly stimulates Na^+–K^+-ATPase, but aldosterone can also directly stimulate Na^+–K^+-ATPase and ROMK activities. The peritubular K^+ concentration and pH also influence K^+ secretion through their effects on Na^+–K^+-ATPase activity. High serum K^+ concentration and alkaline pH stimulate the enzyme activity, and low serum K^+ and acidic pH inhibit the activity.

When Na^+ is accompanied by anions to which the tubules are less permeable than to chloride, luminal negativity is increased, resulting in

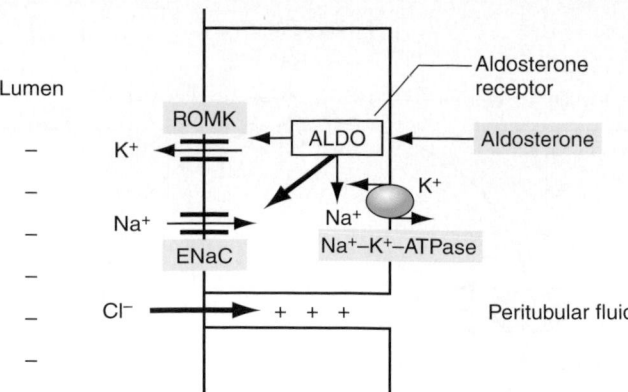

Figure 14–4 Control of potassium secretion at the cortical collecting duct. Sodium enters from the luminal fluid into the cell through ENaC and is transported out of the cell through Na⁺–K⁺-ATPase on the basolateral membrane. These processes create the luminal electrical potential that is more negative than the electrical potential of the peritubular fluid. The electrical charge imbalance created by sodium reabsorption is partly matched by paracellular reabsorption of chloride, and partly by entry of potassium into the lumen through the ROMK, a potassium channel. ENaC = epithelial Na channel; ROMK = renal outer medulla K channel.

enhanced K^+ secretion. Examples of such anions include sulfate, bicarbonate, and anionic antibiotics such as penicillin and carbenecillin. Bicarbonate in the tubular fluid enhances K^+ secretion not only through its effect as a poorly reabsorbable anion but also by enhancing ROMK activity. An increase in renal K^+ excretion in patients who vomit, resulting in excretion of H^+ with increased serum, and ultimately urine, levels of bicarbonate, may be explained by this mechanism. ADH also increases the luminal K^+ channel activity. K^+ secretion is increased by rapid urine flow by maintaining a low luminal K^+ concentration. Renal K^+ wasting during osmotic diuresis could be explained by this mechanism. The more Na^+ presented to the distal nephron, the more can be absorbed and the more K^+ secreted 'in exchange.' The increased Na^+ delivery to the collecting duct also increases renal K^+ excretion by its effect on urine flow (Giebisch, 1998; Halperin, 1998; Giebisch, 2002). A higher urine flow allows greater secretion of potassium into the luminal fluid while reducing back diffusion of potassium into the tubular cells because the luminal concentration would be lower for a given amount of potassium secreted (Oh, 2003).

Plasma Renin Activity (PRA), Plasma Aldosterone Concentration (PA) and Abnormalities in Potassium Metabolism

Because abnormalities in PRA and PA are frequently either responsible for or caused by abnormalities in K^+ metabolism, it is important to understand their relationships (Bock, 1992; Hollenberg, 2000; Laragh, 1995; Hall, 1991). The general principles are:

- Expansion of effective arterial volume caused by primary increase in aldosterone (primary aldosteronism) or by other mineralocorticoids will cause suppression of PRA. When mineralocorticoids other than aldosterone are present in excess, they induce retention of salt and water, and the resulting volume expansion leads to suppression of both PRA and PA
- Increase in PRA will always lead to increase in PA (secondary aldosteronism), unless the rise in PRA is caused by a primary defect in aldosterone secretion. PRA may be high because of:
  – volume depletion secondary to renal or extrarenal salt loss
  – abnormality in renin secretion, e.g., reninoma (hemangiopericytoma of afferent arteriole), malignant hypertension, renal artery stenosis
  – increased renin substrate production, e.g., oral contraceptives.

Elevation in serum K^+ can directly stimulate the adrenal cortex to release aldosterone. When renin is deficient primarily, aldosterone is always low, e.g., hyporeninemic hypoaldosteronism.

Causes and Pathogenesis of Hypokalemia (Table 14–3)

Hypokalemia occurs by one of three main mechanisms: intracellular shift, reduced intake and increased loss. Because the intracellular K^+ concentration greatly exceeds the extracellular concentration, K^+ shift into the cell can cause severe hypokalemia with little change in its intracellular

Table 14–3 Causes of Hypokalemia

Intracellular shift

Alkalosis

Periodic paralysis

Beta-2-agonists

Barium poisoning

Insulin

Nutritional recovery state

Poor intake

Gastrointestinal loss:
   Vomiting
   Diarrhea
   Intestinal drainage
   Laxative abuse

Excessive renal loss

Primary aldosteronism (adrenal adenoma or hyperplasia); PRA is suppressed

Secondary aldosteronism (the increase in aldosterone is secondary to increase in renin)

Malignant hypertension, renal artery stenosis, reninoma

Diuretics

Bartter's syndrome, Gitelman's syndrome

Excess mineralocorticoids other than aldosterone, e.g. Cushing's syndrome, ACTH-producing tumor, licorice

Chronic metabolic acidosis

Delivery of poorly reabsorbed anions to the distal tubule, e.g. bicarbonate, ketone anions, carbenecillin

Miscellaneous causes: Magnesium deficiency, acute leukemia, Liddle's syndrome

concentration (Clemessy, 1995; Matsumura, 2000; Rakhmanina, 1998; Jordan, 1999; Ogawa, 1999; Cannon, 2002; Jurkat-Rott, 2000; Bradberry, 1995; Steen, 1981). Alkalosis, insulin, and beta-2-agonists can cause hypokalemia by stimulating $Na^+–K^+$-ATPase activity (Matsumura, 2000). Intracellular shift of potassium is the cause of hypokalemia in familial hypokalemic periodic paralysis, and defective activity of dihydropyridine-responsive Ca^{2+} channels or voltage-dependent sodium channels has been documented in some patients, but the exact mechanism for hypokalemia is unknown (Jurkat-Rott, 2000; Bradberry, 1995). In barium poisoning, K^+ accumulates in the cell and hypokalemia develops, because of the inhibition of the K^+ channel by barium, resulting in inhibition of K^+ efflux from the cell, in the face of continuous cellular uptake of K^+ through the action of $Na^+–K^+$-ATPase. K^+ accumulates in the cell along with anions as the cell mass increases during nutritional recovery, because K^+ is the main intracellular cation.

Poor intake of K^+ is rarely a cause of hypokalemia by itself, because it is usually accompanied by poor caloric intake, which causes catabolism and release of K^+ from the tissues (Steen, 1981). Vomiting and diarrhea are common causes of hypokalemia (Steen, 1981). Diarrhea causes direct K^+ loss in the stool, but in vomiting hypokalemia is mainly the result of K^+ loss in the urine rather than in the vomitus, since, as discussed above, vomiting causes metabolic alkalosis, and the subsequent renal excretion of bicarbonate leads to renal K^+ wasting.

Renal loss of K^+ is by far the most common cause of hypokalemia. With rare exceptions, hypokalemia due to increased renal wasting of potassium can be attributed to an increased activity of aldosterone or other mineralocorticoids. Increased aldosterone could be a primary disorder as in primary hyperaldosteronism or due to increased renin secretion as in secondary hyperaldosteronism. Even with increased aldosterone, renal K^+ wasting occurs only if it is accompanied by adequate distal delivery of Na^+ (Torpy, 1998; Stowasser, 1995; Abdelhamid, 1995; Vargas-Poussou, 2002; Finer, 2003; Kuncharapty, 1999; Seyberth, 1985; Krozowski, 1999; Heilmann, 1999). In primary aldosteronism, distal delivery of Na^+ is increased because increased NaCl reabsorption in the cortical collecting duct by the action of aldosterone inhibits salt reabsorption in the proximal tubule and Henle's loop. In secondary aldosteronism, hypokalemia occurs only in conditions that are accompanied by increased distal Na^+ delivery. Examples of secondary hyperaldosteronism that result in hypokalemia include renal artery stenosis, diuretic therapy, and malignant hypertension, and congenital defects in renal salt transport such as Bartter's syndrome and Gitelman's syndrome. It must be noted that, in the absence of extrarenal salt loss, renal salt excretion ultimately equals salt intake even in conditions of increased aldosterone or aldosterone deficiency, since prolonged imbalance between the intake and output is impossible; without eventual balance, an individual could not survive volume excess or volume depletion. However, when salt reabsorption is increased at the mineralocorticoid active site (i.e., cortical collecting duct), the amount of salt delivered to this site must be increased when the final salt output eventually equals the intake. When balance is achieved, an increased amount of salt is delivered to the site and an increased amount is reabsorbed, so that the normal amount equaling the intake is excreted; ultimate balance is possible only when the amount entering the body equals the amount leaving the body. This is the mechanism by which salt delivery to the aldosterone site is increased in primary hyperaldosteronism as well as in all cases of secondary hyperaldosteronism that are associated with hypokalemia.

Bartter's syndrome, a rare potassium-losing autosomal recessive condition is caused by defective NaCl reabsorption in the thick ascending limb of Henle (Miyamura, 2003; Finer, 2003; Kunchaparty, 1999; Seyberth, 1985; Schultheis, 1998), whereas in Gitelman's syndrome the defect in NaCl reabsorption is in the distal convoluted tubule (Schultheis, 1998). Defective Na$^+$ reabsorption proximal to the aldosterone effective site in these conditions results in increased delivery of Na$^+$ to the cortical collecting duct and hence in hypokalemia. Heart failure does not lead to hypokalemia despite secondary hyperaldosteronism unless distal delivery of Na$^+$ is increased by diuretic therapy.

Substances that are not aldosterone but have mineralocorticoid activity include corticosterone, deoxycorticosterone (DOC), and synthetic mineralocorticoids such as 9-α-fludrocortisone (Florinef). With licorice intake, mineralocorticoid activity is increased because cortisol, which is normally a potent mineralocorticoid but has a negligible concentration in the cortical collecting duct cells owing to its rapid breakdown by the enzyme 11-beta-hydroxysteroid dehydrogenase, maintains a high intracellular concentration because licorice inhibits the enzyme (Krozowski, 1999; Heilmann, 1999).

Rare causes of renal potassium wasting that are not accompanied by increased mineralocorticoid activity include Liddle's syndrome and chronic metabolic acidosis. Liddle's syndrome is a congenital disorder that is characterized by increased ENaC activity in the collecting duct in the absence of increased aldosterone, resulting in increased sodium reabsorption and enhanced potassium secretion; aldosterone secretion is reduced because salt retention due to the increased ENaC activity leads to physiological suppression of renin secretion (Warnock, 2001).

In chronic metabolic acidosis, hypokalemia develops probably because reduced proximal reabsorption of NaCl allows increased delivery of NaCl to the distal nephron. Direct stimulation of aldosterone secretion by metabolic acidosis is an additional mechanism that contributes to hypokalemia.

Differential Diagnosis of Hypokalemia

The first step in the differential diagnosis is to measure urinary excretion of K$^+$. If urinary K$^+$ excretion is low (< 20 mEq/day or < 0.01 mEq/mg of creatinine), the cause is low intake, extrarenal loss of K$^+$ or intracellular shift. Superacute development of hypokalemia usually suggests intracellular shift as the mechanism. The most common cause of extrarenal loss is diarrhea, which can be suspected by history and a low or negative urine anion gap (urine Na$^+$ + K$^+$ − urine Cl$^-$); the normal urine anion gap is about 40 mmol/24 hours. Intracellular shift is suggested by the history and clinical findings. If urinary excretion is normal or increased (urine K$^+$ > 30 mEq/day or 0.02 mEq/mg of creatinine), the cause is renal loss. Once a renal cause is suspected, the next step should be the measurement of PRA and plasma aldosterone.

High PRA and high aldosterone suggest secondary hyperaldosteronism, which includes diuretic therapy, renal artery stenosis, malignant hypertension, renin-producing tumors, and hereditary defects in renal salt transport (Bartter's syndrome and Gitelman's syndrome). Blood pressure would be normal in subjects with Bartter's syndrome or Gitelman's syndrome, and a normotensive person on diuretic therapy. Blood pressure would be high in all other conditions and in a hypertensive subject on diuretic therapy. Low PRA and high plasma aldosterone suggest primary hyperaldosteronism, which is caused by adrenal adenoma or bilateral hyperplasia. If PRA and plasma aldosterone are low, the likely conditions include Liddle's syndrome, apparent mineralocorticoid excess states (both hereditary and drug-induced), 11-hydroxylase deficiency, and 17-hydroxylase deficiency. Reduction in renal K$^+$ excretion will be achieved with spironolactone in all these conditions except for Liddle's syndrome, which will respond to ENaC blockers such as triamterene and amiloride (Oh, 2003).

Table 14–4 Causes of Hyperkalemia

Pseudohyperkalemia

Thrombocytosis, severe leukocytosis, use of tourniquet with fist exercise, in vitro hemolysis

True hyperkalemia

Due to extracellular shift:
  Acute acidosis (especially inorganic acidosis)
  Catabolic states, periodic paralysis, succinylcholine
  Cationic amino acids
  Exercise while using a beta-blocker
  Digitalis intoxication

Due to excessive ingestion: rare if renal excretion of K$^+$ is normal

Decreased renal excretion:
  Hypoaldosteronism: Addison's disease; selective hypoaldosteronism (hyporeninemic hypoaldosteronism, heparin, congenital adrenal enzyme deficiencies, angiotensin-converting enzyme inhibitors)
  Tubular unresponsiveness to aldosterone (pseudohypoaldosteronism type I and II): congenital, salt-losing nephropathy
  Potassium-sparing diuretics
  Antirejection medications: ciclosporin, tacrolimus
  Severe dehydration

Causes and Pathogenesis of Hyperkalemia

Hyperkalemia may be caused by one of three mechanisms: (a) shift of potassium from the cells to the extracellular fluid (Wasserman, 1997; Perazella, 1999; McIvor, 1985, 1987; Emser 1982), (b) increased potassium intake, and (c) reduced renal potassium excretion (Table 14–4). Hyperkalemic familial periodic paralysis, administration of succinylcholine in paralyzed patients (Delphin, 1987; Cooperman, 1970; Gronert, 1975; Larach, 1987), administration of cationic amino acids such as arginine and lysine, epsilon-aminocaproic acid (this probably becomes a cationic amino acid), rhabdomyolysis or hemolysis, and acute acidosis all cause hyperkalemia by extracellular potassium shift. Rhabdomyolysis and hemolysis cause hyperkalemia only when they are accompanied by renal failure. Although hyperkalemia is not as predictable with organic acidosis as with inorganic acidosis in experimental situations, hyperkalemia is common in diabetic ketoacidosis and phenformin-induced lactic acidosis. The more frequent occurrence of hyperkalemia in clinical organic acidosis may be explained by the longer duration of acidosis and the presence of other factors such as dehydration and renal failure and insulin deficiency in diabetic ketoacidosis (Perez, 1981).

Hyperkalemia can also occur in severe digitalis intoxication by extracellular shift of potassium as digitalis inhibits the Na$^+$–K$^+$-ATPase pump. The kidney's ability to excrete potassium is so great that hyperkalemia rarely occurs solely on the basis of increased intake of potassium. Thus, hyperkalemia is almost always due to impaired renal excretion. There are three major mechanisms of diminished renal potassium excretion: reduced aldosterone or aldosterone responsiveness, renal failure, and reduced distal delivery of sodium. Aldosterone deficiency may be part of a generalized deficiency of adrenal hormones (e.g., Addison's disease) or it may represent a selective process (e.g., hyporeninemic hypoaldosteronism). Hyporeninemic hypoaldosteronism is the most common cause of all aldosterone deficiency states, and by far the commonest cause of chronic hyperkalemia among nondialysis patients (Oh, 1974; Phelps, 1980a). Selective hypoaldosteronism can also occur with heparin therapy, which inhibits steroid production in the zona glomerulosa (Phelps, 1980b). In patients with reduced aldosterone secretion, any agent that limits the supply of renin or angiotensin II may provoke hyperkalemia; for example, ACE (angiotensin-converting enzyme) inhibitors, nonsteroidal anti-inflammatory agents, beta-blockers. The latter may compound the tendency to hyperkalemia by interfering with potassium transport into cells. Renal tubular unresponsiveness to aldosterone (pseudohypoaldosteronism) may be congenital, but it is more often an acquired defect. This defect may involve only potassium secretion (pseudohypoaldosteronism type II) or sodium reabsorption as well as potassium secretion (pseudohypoaldosteronism type I) (Wilson, 2001, 2003; Sebastian, 1981; Brautbar, 1978). Most cases of so-called 'salt-losing nephritis' appear to represent the latter defect. Severe volume depletion may cause hyperkalemia despite secondary hyperaldosteronism because volume depletion causes a marked reduction in delivery of sodium to the cortical collecting duct.

II

Pseudohyperkalemia is defined as an increase in potassium concentration only in the local blood vessel or in vitro, and has no physiological consequences (Stewart, 1979, 1985; Kim, 1990; Zaltzman, 1982; Bellevue, 1975; Iolascon, 1999; Hayward, 1999; Delaunay, 1999; Don, 1990). Prolonged use of a tourniquet with fist exercises can increase the serum potassium level by as much as 1 mEq/L. Thrombocytosis and severe leukocytosis cause pseudohyperkalemia through potassium release from the platelets and white blood cells respectively during blood clotting (Table 14–4).

Differential Diagnosis of Hyperkalemia

The first step in the differential diagnosis of hyperkalemia should be to rule out pseudohyperkalemia. ECG abnormalities of hyperkalemia are absent in pseudohyperkalemia, but the absence of ECG changes does not eliminate true hyperkalemia because ECG changes are rare in chronic hyperkalemia. Pseudohyperkalemia should be suspected in conditions known to cause pseudohyperkalemia, such as thrombocytosis or in vitro hemolysis (pink serum). In pseudohyperkalemia due to thrombocytosis, both serum and plasma K$^+$ should be obtained simultaneously. Once pseudohyperkalemia is ruled out, the next step is to differentiate among the three major causes of hyperkalemia: increased K$^+$ intake, shift of K$^+$ from the cell, and impaired renal excretion. Measurement of a 24-hour urine K$^+$ will distinguish increased intake from the other two causes. Although hyperkalemia due to a shift of K$^+$ from the cell would result in an increased urinary excretion of K$^+$, renal excretion of K$^+$ is often not increased because impaired renal excretion of K$^+$ often contributes to hyperkalemia. A careful dietary history will be sufficient to rule out hyperkalemia due to increased intake, unless the patient is deliberately trying to deceive the physician.

Chronic hyperkalemia is almost always due to impaired renal excretion, and a 24-hour urine K$^+$ measurement is rarely needed to determine impaired renal excretion of K$^+$ as the cause of hyperkalemia. Among the renal causes of hyperkalemia, acute renal failure is the most common cause of acute hyperkalemia, and this will be obvious from serum creatinine and BUN. For differential diagnosis of chronic hyperkalemia of renal causes, the first step is to measure plasma renin activity, plasma aldosterone, and urinary excretion of Na$^+$ and K$^+$. A very low urinary Na$^+$ and a low K$^+$ in the absence of polyuria suggest that the aldosterone effect is normal, but that K$^+$ excretion is impaired because of the reduced availability of Na$^+$ and a marked reduction in collecting duct flow. Markedly increased proximal reabsorption of Na$^+$ due to low effective vascular volume, such as in severe congestive heart failure, can cause hyperkalemia by such a mechanism. If urinary Na$^+$ is adequate (> 20 mEq/L), plasma renin activity and aldosterone should be measured.

Low PRA and low aldosterone suggest hyporeninemic hypoaldosteronism, whereas high PRA and low aldosterone suggest a primary defect in aldosterone secretion such as Addison's disease, heparin therapy, and aldosterone biosynthetic defect. When PRA and aldosterone are both increased, likely culprits are pseudohypoaldosteronism, and very low Na$^+$ delivery to the cortical collecting duct, drugs that impair the ENaC function or the aldosterone action such as potassium-sparing diuretics, e.g., amiloride, triamterene, spironolactone, and certain antibiotics, e.g., trimethoprim, pentamidine (Oh, 2003).

Disorders of Water, Sodium and Antidiuretic Hormone (ADH) Metabolism

Regulation of Thirst and ADH Release

A rise in effective osmolality shrinks the hypothalamic osmoreceptor cells, which then stimulate the thirst center in the cerebral cortex and stimulate antidiuretic hormone (ADH) production in the supraoptic and paraventricular nuclei. Conversely, a decline in effective osmolality causes swelling of the osmoreceptor cells, resulting in inhibition of ADH production. ADH produced in the hypothalamus is carried through long axons and is secreted from the posterior pituitary (McKinley, 1998; Ibata, 1999). Stimulation and inhibition of osmoreceptor cells affect both production by the hypothalamus and secretion by the pituitary of ADH.

Regulation of ADH secretion by a change in effective osmolality is extremely sensitive. A rise in effective osmolality by only 2–3% stimulates ADH secretion sufficiently to result in a maximally concentrated urine, and decline in plasma osmolality of only 2–3% produces maximally dilute urine (< 100 mOsm/L) (Bourque, 1997; Olsson, 1983).

ADH release is also regulated by nonosmotic factors. Low effective vascular volume provokes thirst and ADH release, and high effective vascular volume has the reverse effects (Wells, 1998; Aguilera, 2000; Nielsen, 2002; Schrier, 1979). These effects are mediated through baroreceptors and some humoral factors released in response to reduced blood flow. Alpha catecholamines suppress and beta catecholamines enhance ADH output. Prostaglandins inhibit the effect of ADH on the kidney. Angiotensin II stimulates thirst and ADH release. Lack of glucocorticoid enhances ADH action on the kidney and also increases ADH release. Physical and emotional stress, e.g., major surgery, increase ADH output, possibly in part through emetic stimuli, which are common complications of major surgery and are attributed to the effects of anesthesia and surgical trauma. Many drugs affect ADH release or action, e.g., ethanol inhibits the output of ADH. Lithium and demeclocycline inhibit the effect of ADH on the kidney. Chlorpropamide increases the action of ADH on the kidney. Some drugs may operate through the emetic stimulus, which is one of the most potent physiologic stimuli to ADH release. The urine may become osmotically concentrated in the absence of ADH if effective vascular volume is very low. The combination of reduced GFR and enhanced proximal reabsorption of filtrate reduces urine flow to the collecting duct so greatly that even the limited permeability of the membrane permits withdrawal of sufficient amounts of water to concentrate urine.

There are three classes of ADH receptors: V1 receptors cause rise in vasomotor tone and certain metabolic effects, V2 receptors are associated with antidiuresis and V3 receptors cause stimulation of ACTH secretion in the anterior pituitary (Ma, 1999; Mouri, 1993). The antidiuretic effect of ADH is mediated by its effect on the collecting duct of the kidney to enhance permeability to water and on the outer medullary thick ascending limb of Henle's loop to stimulate salt reabsorption. Vasopressinase, which normally breaks down ADH, may be increased in pregnancy and occasionally causes polyuria (Molitch, 1998). DDAVP, a synthetic analogue of arginine vasopressin, which resists vasopressinase and therefore has a prolonged effect, is useful in polyuria of pregnancy.

Urine Concentration and Dilution

About 180 L of water are filtered daily; 120 L are reabsorbed in the proximal tubule and 35 L in the descending limb of Henle. About 25 L of dilute urine are delivered to the collecting duct at the osmolality of about 60–80 mOsm/L. Because of the conditional expression of aquaporin 2 on the luminal membrane of collecting ducts (the cortical as well as the medullary collecting duct), which depends on the action of antidiuretic hormone (ADH), no water reabsorption occurs in the cortical and outer medullary collecting ducts when ADH is absent. However, a small amount of water (about 5 L during water diuresis) is reabsorbed in the terminal portion of the inner medullary collecting duct even when ADH is totally absent. It seems that aquaporins are present constitutively in this part of the nephron. During the maximal water diuresis, the combined effects of further salt reabsorption in the collecting duct and small additional reabsorption of water in the inner medullary collecting duct allow final excretion of about 20 L of dilute urine at an osmolality of about 40 mOsm/L. It must be noted that the maximal urine output during water diuresis depends greatly on the salt intake, because the maximal urine output can never exceed the amount delivered into the ascending limb of Henle. Even with a mild salt restriction, e.g., 2 g per day, the resulting mild volume depletion increases reabsorption of salt and water in the proximal tubule sufficiently to reduce the volume delivery to the ascending limb of Henle's loop to 12–15 L per day, and the final maximal urine output during water diuresis in a person with salt restriction may be no more than 10–12 L.

In the presence of maximal ADH, urine can be concentrated to as high as 1200 mOsm/L as water is reabsorbed in the cortical and medullary collecting duct, with urine volume as low as 0.5 L a day (Fig. 14–5). In the proximal tubule, water reabsorption passively follows salt reabsorption, whereas in the descending thin limb water reabsorption is unaccompanied by salt reabsorption, but occurs in response to the salt reabsorption which takes place in the ascending limb. The osmolality of urine as it enters the ADH effective site, i.e., the cortical collecting duct, is the same during water diuresis and during antidiuresis, and the value is quite low, about 60 mOsm/L. The urine osmolality is reduced by continuous salt reabsorption without water reabsorption in the ascending thin and thick limbs of Henle and the distal convoluted tubule and connecting tubule. These nephron segments do not express aquaporins, and therefore do not respond to ADH. Urine concentration is achieved by reabsorption of water in the collecting duct through transcellular reabsorption; water first enters the cell through the luminal membrane, and then leaves the cell through the basolateral membranes. Diffusion of water through either membrane requires expression of aquaporins, some of which requires the action of ADH in order to be expressed in the membrane. Aquaporin 3 is

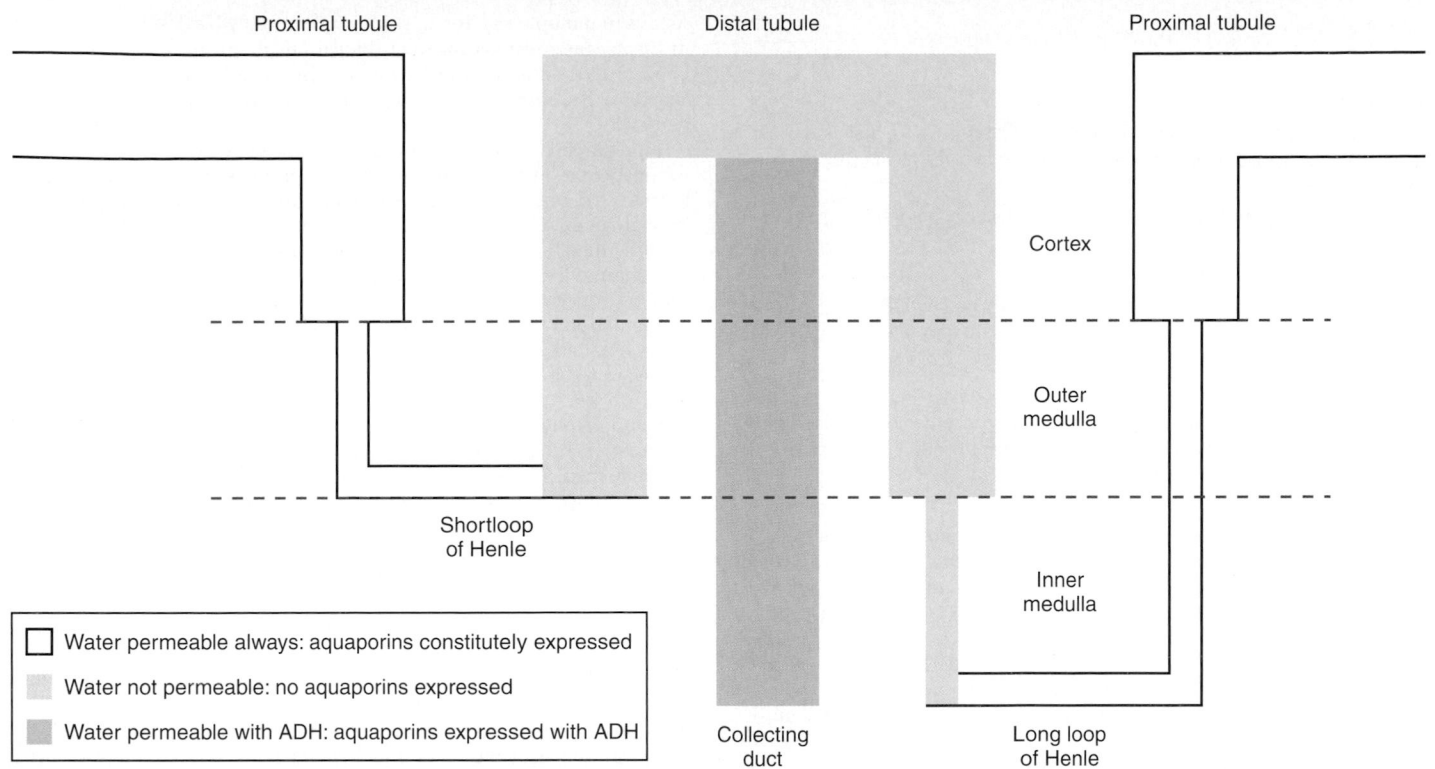

Figure 14–5 Transport of water at various nephron sites. The proximal tubule and the descending thin limb are always water permeable because aquaporins are constitutively expressed at these sites. The ascending thin limb and ascending thick limb of Henle, the distal convoluted tubule, and the connecting tubule have no aquaporins expressed and are always water impermeable. The collecting duct is water permeable with ADH action.

constitutively expressed in the basolateral membrane of the cortical collecting duct and aquaporin 4 is constitutively expressed in the basolateral membrane of the medullary collecting duct. Entry of water in the collecting duct from the lumen into the cell requires the expression of aquaporin 2 on the luminal membrane, and this is an ADH-mediated mechanism.

Increase in urine osmolality from a very low value at the beginning of the cortical collecting duct to an isotonic value at the corticomedullary junction requires only the presence of ADH and the tubular responsiveness to ADH, since the interstitium of the cortex is always isotonic. However, the reabsorption of water in the medullary collecting duct requires not only the ADH action but also the hypertonicity of the medullary interstitium. Maintenance of the medullary hypertonicity is achieved by the counter-current multiplication mechanism. In short, the medullary interstitial fluid becomes progressively hypertonic from the corticomedullary junction toward the tip, achieving a level of about 1200 mOsm/L at the tip. Medullary hypertonicity in the outer medullary area is achieved by the active reabsorption of salt in the thick ascending limb of Henle that is not accompanied by water reabsorption. In the inner medulla, where salt reabsorption in the thin ascending limb of Henle (the inner medulla lacks the thick ascending limb of Henle) is only passive, salt reabsorption without water reabsorption occurs with the help of urea recycling from the inner medullary collecting duct. The mechanism by which urea contributes to the concentration of urine is still hotly debated, and is beyond the scope of this discussion. The fact that the final interstitial osmolality of the medulla is much greater than the initial osmolality of the fluid that enters the medulla is attributed to the countercurrent mechanism, which is made possible by two conditions: (1) the selective reabsorption of salt from the ascending limbs of Henle without water reabsorption and reabsorption of water from the descending limb of Henle unaccompanied by salt reabsorption, and (2) the countercurrent arrangement of the descending and ascending limbs of Henle by looping around of the tubule at the tip of Henle's loop (Hogg, 1986, 1978; Pallone, 2003; de Rouffignac; 1987; Oh, 1997; Sands, 1996; Burg, 1995; Schmidt-Nielsen, 1977; Knepper, 1983; Greger, 1983).

In order for the medullary interstitial fluid to become more concentrated than the plasma despite water diffusion out of the descending limb of Henle, the amount of salt transported out of the ascending limb has to be proportionately greater than the amount of water transported out of the descending limb. As evidence for this, the osmolality of the fluid in the thick ascending limb of Henle at the corticomedullary junction is hypotonic. The physiological purpose of water diffusion out of the descending limb is

to increase the concentration of NaCl in the luminal fluid to a level similar to that of the interstitial fluid so that when the loop of Henle bends at the tip and makes its upward turn, the sodium concentration of the luminal fluid of the ascending limb will be similar to (albeit somewhat lower than) that of the interstitial fluid. Otherwise, sodium reabsorption will stop when the concentration of interstitial sodium is about 1.5 times that of the luminal fluid since about one-half of sodium reabsorption at this site occurs passively through the paracellular pathways, and the energy for the passive reabsorption is the slightly positive luminal potential (about + 10 mV).

Polyuria

Polyuria is arbitrarily defined as urine volume in excess of 2.5 L a day. There are two types of polyuria: osmotic diuresis and water diuresis (Carroll, 1989).

Osmotic Diuresis

Osmotic diuresis is defined as increased urine output due to an excessive rate of solute excretion; the commonly accepted level of solute excretion for osmotic diuresis is a rate in excess of 60 mOsm/h or 1440 mOsm/day in the adult (Carroll, 1989). Urine osmolality is usually greater than that of plasma, but it may be lower than plasma osmolality when it coexists with water diuresis. Solutes commonly responsible for osmotic diuresis include glucose, urea, mannitol, radiopaque media, and NaCl.

Water Diuresis

Water diuresis is characterized by excretion of a large volume of dilute urine. The polyuria is caused by reduced reabsorption of water in the collecting duct. Reasons for reduced water reabsorption in the collecting duct are lack of ADH (Vokes, 1988; Leggett, 1999; Siggaard, 1999; Rutishauser, 1999; Ito, 1997; Halperin, 2001) or unresponsiveness to ADH (nephrogenic diabetes insipidus). Nephrogenic diabetes insipidus (DI) can be either congenital or acquired. Congenital nephrogenic DI is due to either a defective ADH receptor or an aquaporin defect (Weir, 1992; Lam, 2000; Nielsen, 2002; Spruce, 1984; Canada, 2003; Marples, 1995).

The lack of ADH, which could be congenital or acquired (Levine, 1987; Vokes, 1988; Leggett, 1999; Siggaard, 1999; Rutishauser, 1999; Ito, 1997), is either due to primary deficiency (central diabetes insipidus) or physiologic suppression by low serum osmolality (primary polydipsia, dipsogenic diabetes insipidus) (Levine, 1987; Rendell, 1978; Hariprasad, 1980). The deficiency of ADH could be mild, moderate or severe. When

CHAPTER: 14   Evaluation of Renal Function, Water, Electrolytes and Acid–Base Balance

Table 14–5 Causes of Polyuria Due to Water Diuresis

Lack of ADH

Central DI: congenital or acquired (idiopathic cell degeneration, tumors and granulomas, surgery, trauma, infarction, and infection of the pituitary or hypothalamus)

Dipsogenic DI (suppression by excessive water intake): psychogenic, organic brain disease, iatrogenic

Gestational DI: excess vasopressinase.

Failure of the kidney to respond to ADH (nephrogenic DI)

Congenital nephrogenic diabetes insipidus: a defect in ADH receptor, a defect in aquaporin expression

Chronic renal failure

Acquired nephrogenic diabetes insipidus: lithium toxicity, demeclocycline toxicity, methoxyflurane toxicity, amyloidosis, light chain nephropathy, hypercalcemia, hypokalemia, obstructive uropathy.

ADH deficiency is partial, urine osmolality may be fairly close to normal. In a rare instance, ADH is made, but cannot be released in response to a rise in body fluid osmolality because of a defect involving the osmoreceptor cells, e.g., hypothalamic lesions (Leggett, 1999; Siggaard, 1999; Rutishauser, 1999; Ito, 1997). In such instances ADH may be released in response to hypovolemia or to drugs. During pregnancy, ADH deficiency may be caused by excessive production of vasopressinase (gestational DI) (Molitch, 1998). Causes of polyuria including central and nephrogenic DI are listed in Table 14–5.

Primary polydipsia is defined as increased water drinking that is not caused by physiologically stimulated thirst, i.e., in the absence of hyperosmolality or volume depletion (Rendell, 1980; Hariprassad, 1980; Levine, 1987). Primary polydipsia is usually psychogenic in origin, hence the term psychogenic polydipsia (Leadbetter, 1994). In contrast, polydipsia in patients with diabetes insipidus or diabetic patients with severe glycosuria is secondary polydipsia, which is due to thirst stimulation in response to hyperosmolality. In primary polydipsia, increased urine output is due to physiological suppression of ADH secretion, and hence, serum Na^+ is usually at the low range of normal. In contrast, in central or nephrogenic DI serum sodium is in the high normal range. Occasionally, serum sodium is frankly low in severe primary polydipsia, indicating that the capacity of the GI tract to absorb water exceeds the normal capacity of the kidney to excrete water.

Causes and Pathogenesis of Hyponatremia

Hyponatremia, the most common electrolyte disorder, is defined as a reduced plasma sodium concentration to a value less than 135 mEq/L. Generally, clinical concern arises when the concentration is less than 130 mEq/L.

The term pseudohyponatremia, as discussed in Chapter 8, is applied to a spurious reduction in serum sodium concentration due to a systematic error in the measurement. The commonest, yet not widely known, cause of pseudohyponatremia is in vitro hemolysis, a well-known cause of pseudohyperkalemia (Oh, 2003). Since cell lysis does not change osmolality of the plasma, any rise in serum potassium must be met by a reciprocal decrease in serum sodium. However, the reduction in serum Na^+ from hemolysis is somewhat greater than the increase in serum K^+, by a factor of 1.3, because hemoglobin released from the red cells cause additional reduction in serum Na^+ as in hyperproteinemia; this error occurs because hemoglobin is mostly a protein, and it has the same effect as hyperproteinemia in displacing plasma water. This additional error occurs only when samples are diluted before the measurement of serum sodium, just as pseudohyponatremia of hyperlipidemia and hyperproteinemia occurs only when samples are diluted before the measurement. Other causes of pseudohyponatremia include hyperlipidemia, hyperproteinemia, and increased viscosity of the plasma (Weisberg, 1989; Milionis, 2002). The error in measurement in pseudohyponatremia results from the dilution of the sample. Measurements of serum sodium with a flame photometer can result in this type of error because the sample is always diluted. The same error also occurs even with an ion-specific electrode method, if the sample is diluted (indirect method). In pseudohyponatremia, plasma osmolality, which is customarily measured without dilution, is normal. However, a low plasma sodium concentration with a normal plasma osmolality need not indicate the presence of pseudohyponatremia; true hyponatremia may be accompanied by a normal plasma osmolality because of hyperglycemia, azotemia, or the presence of alcohol. In hypergammaglobulinemic states

such as in multiple myeloma, serum sodium may be falsely low because of displacement of serum water by gammaglobulins, but on the other hand the sodium concentration is also truly low because cationic charges of gammaglobulins displace sodium to maintain electrical neutrality.

Hyponatremia induced by acute hyperglycemia is not pseudo-hyponatremia, since sodium concentration in the extracellular fluid is truly low; this occurs as a result of water shift from the cell caused by hyperglycemia. Serum sodium decreases by 1.5 mEq/L for every 100 mg/dL rise in serum glucose, as discussed above (Oh, 2003).

The immediate mechanisms responsible for a reduction in extracellular sodium concentration are: (1) shift of water from the cell caused by accumulation of extracellular solutes, such as glucose, other than sodium salts (Agraharkar, 1997; Akan, 1996; Agarwal, 1994); (2) retention of excess water in the body; (3) loss of sodium (Gowrishankar, 1998; Sonnenblick, 1993); and (4) shift of sodium into the cells. The appropriate physiologic response to hypotonicity is suppression of ADH release, which leads to rapid excretion of excess water and correction of hyponatremia. Persistence of hyponatremia therefore indicates the failure of this compensatory mechanism. In most instances hyponatremia is maintained because the kidney fails to produce water diuresis, but sometimes ingestion of water in excess of the limits of normal renal compensation is responsible. The reasons for inability of the kidney to excrete water include: (1) renal failure, (2) reduced delivery of glomerular filtrate to the distal nephron, and (3) the inappropriate presence of ADH.

The mechanism for impaired water excretion in renal failure is obvious and needs no further explanation. Reduced distal delivery of filtrate results from low glomerular filtration rate and enhanced proximal tubular reabsorption of salt and water, and these states are most commonly caused by volume depletion.

In most cases of hyponatremia the main reason for the fall of serum sodium is abnormal retention of water, which is either ingested as such or administered as hypotonic fluids. However, in certain clinical settings, water retention can occur despite administration of isotonic fluid. The latter phenomenon occurs when urine is excreted containing sodium and potassium at concentrations that exceed the sum of serum concentrations of the two ions; for example, if urine contains sodium at 140 mEq/L and potassium at 100 mEq/L, the combined concentration would be 240 mEq/L, which is clearly hypertonic. Excretion of hypertonic urine in regards to sodium and potassium occurs in the setting of increased urinary sodium excretion in the presence of ADH, such as someone with SIADH (see below) who is given an infusion of normal saline or a person who is given a thiazide diuretic. Excretion of such urine will cause hyponatremia even without net water retention. Loss of potassium has the same effect on serum sodium as loss of sodium. It must be noted that development of hyponatremia with excretion of hypertonic urine occurs only when hypertonicity of urine is caused by increased excretion of sodium or potassium. Hypertonic urine by increased excretion of urea would not produce hyponatremia, for obvious reasons. The physiological requirement for the excretion of hypertonic urine is an increased amount of ADH in the presence of marked sodium diuresis (Halperin, 2001). Clinical examples include: (a) a patient who receives a large amount of isotonic fluid in the immediate postoperative period, (b) a patient with a condition termed secretion of inappropriate antidiuretic hormone (SIADH) who is treated with isotonic fluid, and (c) a patient who receives a thiazide diuretic (Gowrishankar, 1998; Sonnenblick, 1993). The normal dilution of urine requires delivery of adequate amounts of fluid to the diluting segment and the reabsorption of solute without water at that segment. An increased body fluid tonicity causes release of ADH, which allows reabsorption of water in the collecting duct, helping to restore the body fluid tonicity. The response is considered appropriate when ADH is released in response to hypertonicity of the body fluid. However, release of ADH in the presence of hyponatremia is also considered appropriate if the effective vascular volume is reduced. The term, syndrome of inappropriate ADH secretion (SIADH) is therefore reserved for ADH secretion that occurs despite hyponatremia and despite a normal or increased effective vascular volume. Causes of SIADH include tumors, pulmonary diseases such as tuberculosis and pneumonia, central nervous system diseases, drugs, etc (Table 14–6) (Bartter, 1967; Ajaelo, 1998; Fallon, 1998; Gold, 1983; Hensen, 1995; North, 2000; Arlt, 1997; Johnson, 1997; Argani, 1997; Ferlito, 1997; Friedmann, 1993). Hyponatremia in clinical states associated with reduced effective vascular volume such as congestive heart failure and cirrhosis of the liver is caused by a combination of reduced delivery of fluid to the distal nephron and increased secretion of ADH. Salt restriction and diuretics increase severity of hyponatremia. ADH secretion may be present despite hyponatremia in myxedema (Macaron, 1978) and

Table 14–6 Classification of Hyponatremia by Pathogenesis

Due to Na⁺ loss

Thiazide diuretics in the presence of ADH

Saline infusion in the presence of ADH

Due to water retention

Excessive water intake: primary polydipsia

Advanced renal failure

Appropriate ADH secretion: edema-forming states (CHF, nephritic syndrome, ascites). Salt depletion states (GI loss, diuretic therapy, aldosterone deficiency, hypothyroidism)

Inappropriate ADH secretion

Tumors: cancers of the lung, pancreas, duodenum, ureter, bladder, prostate, lymphoma, thymoma, mesothelioma, Ewing's sarcoma

Intrathoracic causes: bacterial and viral pneumonia, tuberculosis, lung abscess, aspergillosis, asthma, positive pressure breathing, pneumothorax, cystic fibrosis

CNS abnormalities: encephalitis, meningitis, brain tumors and abscess, head trauma, subdural hematoma, cerebrovascular accidents, Guillain–Barré syndrome, acute intermittent porphyria, brain atrophy, schizophrenia, hydrocephalus, acute psychosis, multiple sclerosis, cavernous vein thrombosis, lupus cerebritis, Shy–Drager syndrome, Rocky Mountain spotted fever, delirium tremens, seizure disorder

Drugs: arginine vasopressin and its analogs, sulfonylureas, tricyclic antidepressants, clofibrate, carbamazepine, vinca alkaloids, cylophosphamide, selective serotonin reuptake inhibitors, opiates, phenothiazines, haloperidol

Surgical and emotional stress

Emesis

Endocrine causes: glucocorticoid deficiency and myxedema

Table 14–7 Causes of Hypernatremia

Reduced water intake

Defective thirst due to altered mental state or thirst center defect

Inability to drink water

Lack of access to water

Increased water loss (water intake must be impaired)

Gastrointestinal loss: vomiting, osmotic diarrhea

Cutaneous loss: sweating and fever

Respiratory loss: hyperventilation and fever

Renal loss: diabetes insipidus, osmotic diuresis

Increased sodium content of the body (water intake must be impaired)

Increased intake

Hypertonic saline or sodium bicarbonate infusion

Ingestion of sea water

Renal salt retention; usually in response to primary water deficit

---

glucocorticoid deficiency states. It is not clear, however, whether ADH secretion in these conditions is truly inappropriate or appropriate. Finally, mild hyponatremia may be caused by 'resetting of the osmostat' at an osmolality lower than the usual level. In such cases urine dilution occurs normally when the plasma osmolality is brought down below the reset level. Resetting of the osmostat is a form of SIADH, since ADH secretion occurs inappropriately at hyponatremic levels without evidence of reduced effective vascular volume. Patients with chronic debilitating diseases such as pulmonary tuberculosis often manifest this phenomenon (Hill, 1990a). Some authorities believe the existence of a cerebral salt-wasting syndrome, which is defined as renal loss of salt caused by humoral substances released in response to cerebral disorders such as acute subarachnoid hemorrhage. These patients are thought to manifest volume depletion that results in hyponatremia. However, a careful analysis of the existing data does not support the existence of such an entity, and those cases labeled as cerebral salt-wasting syndrome probably represent cases of inappropriate ADH secretion (Oh, 1999).

Causes and Pathogenesis of Hypernatremia

Hypernatremia is defined as an increased sodium concentration in plasma water, and is generally diagnosed at serum sodium levels > 145 mEq/L. Whereas hyponatremia may not be accompanied by hypo-osmolality, hypernatremia is always associated with an increased effective plasma osmolality and hence with a reduced cell volume. However, the extracellular volume in hypernatremia may be normal, decreased or increased.

Hypernatremia is caused by loss of water, gain of sodium, or both (Table 14–7). Loss of water could be due to increased loss or reduced intake, and gain of sodium is due either to increased intake or to reduced renal excretion. Increased loss of water can occur through the kidney (e.g., in diabetes insipidus or osmotic diuresis), the gastrointestinal tract (e.g., gastric suction or osmotic diarrhea), or the skin. Reduced water intake occurs most commonly in comatose patients or in those with a defective thirst mechanism. Less frequent causes of reduced water intake include continuous vomiting, lack of access to water, and mechanical obstruction due to a condition such as esophageal tumor. Gain of sodium in a person with normal perception of thirst, ability to drink water, and availability of water does not result in hypernatremia because a proportional amount of water is retained to maintain normal body fluid osmolality. Whereas the physiological defense against hyponatremia is increased renal water excretion, the physiological defense against hypernatremia is increased water drinking in response to thirst. Because thirst is such an effective and sensitive defense mechanism against hypernatremia, it is virtually impossible to increase serum sodium by more than a few mEq/L if the water-drinking mechanism is intact. Therefore, in a patient with hypernatremia, there will always be reasons for reduced water intake. These reasons include defective thirst mechanism, inability to drink water, and unavailability of water. The excess gain of sodium leading to hypernatremia is usually iatrogenic, e.g., from hypertonic saline infusion, accidental entry into maternal circulation during abortion with hypertonic saline, or administration of hypertonic sodium bicarbonate during cardiopulmonary resuscitation or treatment of lactic acidosis. Reduced renal sodium excretion leading to sodium gain and hypernatremia is usually in response to dehydration caused by primary water deficit. Water depletion due to diabetes insipidus, osmotic diuresis or insufficient water intake leads to secondary sodium retention through volume-mediated activation of sodium-retaining mechanisms in those who continue to ingest or are given sodium. Consequently, in chronic hypernatremia sodium retention plays a more important role than water loss (Carroll, 1989; Oh, 2003).

Whether hypernatremia is due to sodium retention or water loss can be determined by examination of the patient's volume status. For example, if a patient with a serum sodium concentration of 170 mEq/L does not have obvious evidence of dehydration, hypernatremia is not caused entirely by water loss. In order to increase the serum sodium to 170 mEq/L by water deficit alone, one would have to lose more than 20% of total body water.

Acid–Base Disorders

Bicarbonate and CO_2 Buffer System

All body buffers are in equilibrium with protons (H^+) and therefore with pH as shown in the following equation (Ramsay, 1965):

$$pH = pK + \log A^-/HA \tag{14–29}$$

where A^- is a conjugate base of an acid HA.

Because HCO_3^- and CO_2 are the major buffers of the body, pH is typically expressed as a function of their ratio, as discussed in Chapter 8, and shown in the Henderson–Hasselbalch equation:

$$pH = 6.1 + \log HCO_3^-/P_{CO_2} \times 0.03 \tag{14–30}$$

where 6.1 is the pK of the HCO_3^- and CO_2 buffer system, and 0.03 is the solubility coefficient of CO_2.

The equation can be further simplified by combining the two constants, pK and solubility coefficient of CO_2: $pH = 6.1 + \log HCO_3^-/P_{CO_2} \times 0.03 = 6.1 + \log 1/0.03 + \log HCO_3^-/P_{CO_2} = 7.62 + \log HCO_3^-/P_{CO_2}$ (Carroll, 1989). Hence:

$$pH = 7.62 - \log P_{CO_2}/HCO_3^- = 7.62 + \log HCO_3^- - \log P_{CO_2} \tag{14–31}$$

When H^+ is expressed in nM instead of a negative log value (pH), P_{CO_2} can be related to HCO_3^- in an equation:

$$H \text{ (nM)} = 24 \times P_{CO_2} \text{ (mmHg)}/HCO_3^- \text{ (mM)} \tag{14–32}$$

The Henderson–Hasselbalch equation indicates that pH depends on the ratio of HCO_3^-/P_{CO_2}. pH increases when the ratio increases (alkalosis), and pH decreases when the ratio decreases (acidosis). The ratio may be increased by an increase in HCO_3^- (metabolic alkalosis) or by a decrease in P_{CO_2} (respiratory alkalosis). The ratio may be decreased by a decrease in HCO_3^- (metabolic acidosis) or by an increase in P_{CO_2} (respiratory acidosis).

Definition of Acid and Base

Arrhenius's definition.
An acid is a substance that increases the concentration of hydrogen ion (H^+) when dissolved in water and a base is a substance that increases the concentration of hydroxyl ion (OH^-) when dissolved in water.

Bronsted and Lowry's definition.
An acid is a substance that donates a proton in a reaction, while a base is a substance that accepts a proton in a reaction.

Lewis's definition.
An acid is a molecule or ion that accepts a pair of electrons to form a covalent bond, and a base is a molecule that donates a pair of electrons for a covalent bond.

The definition of Bronsted–Lowry is the most widely accepted and most relevant clinically.

Whole Body Acid–Base Balance

Metabolic acidosis occurs either because net acid production is increased or net acid excretion is reduced. Because a typical modern diet results in acid production, the normal function of the kidney is to excrete acid in order to remain in acid–base balance. For these reasons, proper understanding of disorders of acid–base balance requires the knowledge of the sources of acid production as well as the mechanisms by which acids are disposed of.

Net Acid Production

On a typical American diet, the daily production of nonvolatile acid is about 90 mEq/day. The main acids are sulfuric acid (about 40 mEq/day), which originates from metabolism of sulfur-containing amino acids such as methionine and cysteine, and incompletely metabolized organic acids (about 50 mEq/day) (Oh, 1992). The source of sulfuric acid is protein, but the sulfate content varies greatly with the types of protein that are ingested (Lemann, 1959). In general, when sulfur content is expressed as mEq per 100 g of proteins, proteins of animal sources (meat, fish, milk, and egg) contain higher amounts of sulfate for a given amount of protein than proteins of plant origin (cereal, beans, and nuts). The sulfur content is much greater in fruits, vegetables, and potatoes, but these food groups are not important sources of protein in the amounts usually eaten. The total amount of acid/alkali content depends not only on the sulfur content but also on alkali content of food, which is present mainly as salts of organic acids. When both factors are considered, milk has a net alkali value, whereas meat and fish have a net acid value. As a whole, fruits and vegetables contain a large amount of net alkali because they contain large amounts of organic anions. The total amount of organic acids produced normally is much more than 50 mEq/day, but the bulk of organic acids produced in the body is metabolized; only a small amount is lost in the urine as organic anions that escape metabolism (e.g., citrate) or as a metabolic end-product (e.g., urate). On typical American diets, the amount of alkali absorbed from the GI tract is about 30 mEq/day (Lemann, 1959; Oh, 1992). Thus, the net amount of acid produced daily can be estimated as:

Net acid production = (Urine sulfate + Urine organic anions) – (14–33)
Net alkali absorbed from the GI tract

Determination of the net alkali (or acid) content of diet is based on the metabolic fates of the chemicals in the diet after absorption into the body rather than its in vitro states. For example, citric acid in the food is considered neutral, because it would be metabolized to CO_2 and water in the body, whereas K^+ citrate is an alkali because it would be converted to K^+ bicarbonate after metabolism. Similarly, arginine Cl^- is an acid, because metabolism of arginine in the body would result in the formation of HCl (Lemann, 1959). Thus, net alkali value of diet is best determined by the total amount of noncombustible cations (Na^+, K^+, Ca^{2+}, and Mg^{2+}) relative to the total amount of noncombustible anions (Cl^- and P):

Net alkali content = ($Na^+ + K^+ + Ca^{2+} + Mg^{2+}$) – ($Cl^- + 1.8P$) (14–34)

All units are expressed as mEq/day except for P which is expressed as mmol/day multiplied by 1.8, because phosphate valence depends on pH, and at pH 7.4 the average valence of phosphate is 1.8. Only the above six ions are considered in the equation because other noncombustible ions are present in negligible amounts in normal food. Sulfate is not included here because sulfate is formed in the body only after metabolism of sulfur-containing amino acids. The amount of alkali absorbed from the food is not equal to the amount present in the food, because the absorption of divalent noncombustible ions, Ca^{2+}, Mg^{2+}, and P, is incomplete. Hence, traditionally the measurement of the net GI alkali absorption required analysis of the food as well as the stool, which necessitated prolonged

collection of stool (Oh, 1992; Relman, 1961). Thus, the net GI alkali absorption is expressed as:

Net GI alkali absorbed = Net alkali of food – Net alkali of stool (14–35)

The analysis of the food for the measurement of net alkali content is cumbersome and the analysis of the stool is even more cumbersome. Such analyses typically require admitting patients to a special metabolic unit. A new method has been developed to measure net GI alkali absorption. In this method (Oh, 1989), urine electrolytes, instead of diet and stool electrolytes, are measured. The method is based on the principle that noncombustible ions absorbed from the GI tract would eventually be excreted in the urine and therefore that the individual amounts of these electrolytes excreted in the urine would equal those absorbed from the GI tract. Hence,

Net GI alkali absorption = Urine ($Na^+ + K^+ + Ca^{2+} + Mg^{2+}$) – (14–36)
Urine ($Cl^- + 1.8P$)

Twenty-four-hour urine can be collected in outpatient settings, while the subjects are eating their usual diets. The amount of net alkali absorbed on a typical American diet stated earlier, 30 mEq/day, was measured by the analysis of urine electrolytes using the above formula (Oh, 1992).

Net Acid Excretion

The most important function of the kidney in acid–base homeostasis is excretion of acid, which is tantamount to generation of alkali. Acid is excreted in the form of NH_4^+ and titratable acid. Another important function of the kidney is excretion of HCO_3^-. Usually, the main function of renal excretion of HCO_3^- is prevention of metabolic alkalosis, but a small amount of bicarbonate is normally excreted in the urine (about 10 mEq/day). Thus, net acid excretion, which is tantamount to net renal production of alkali, can be determined by subtracting HCO_3^- excretion from acid excretion (Lemann, 1959).

Net acid excretion = Acid excretion – HCO_3^- excretion = (14–37)
NH_4^+ + Titratable acid – HCO_3^-

Normally, about two-thirds of acid excretion occurs in the form of NH_4^+, but in acidosis NH_4^+ excretion may increase as much as 10-fold. Excretion of titratable acid is usually modest because of the limited amount of buffer that produces titratable acid, i.e., phosphate, creatinine, and urate, but may be increased markedly in disease states, e.g., beta-hydroxybutyrate in diabetic ketoacidosis. Maintenance of acid–base balance requires that net acid production equals net acid excretion. Metabolic acidosis develops when net acid production exceeds net acid excretion, and metabolic alkalosis develops when net acid excretion exceeds net acid production.

Metabolic Acidosis

Classification

All metabolic acidoses result from reduction in bicarbonate content of the body, with two minor exceptions: acidosis resulting from dilution of the body fluid by administration of a large amount of saline solution (dilution acidosis) and acidosis that results from shift of H^+ from the cell. Reduction in bicarbonate content may be due to a primary increase in acid production (*extrarenal acidosis*) or due to a primary reduction in net acid excretion (*renal acidosis*) (Table 14–8). In this classification nonrenal loss of bicarbonate or an alkali precursor is considered as part of increased acid production. In extrarenal acidosis, net acid excretion is markedly increased as the kidney compensates to overcome acidosis. On the other hand, net acid excretion may be restored to normal in chronic renal acidosis as acidosis stimulates renal H^+ excretion. Normal net acid excretion in the presence of acidic pH suggests a defect in renal acid excretion, and therefore renal acidosis. If the renal acid excretion capacity is normal, net acid excretion should be supernormal in the presence of acidic pH.

Renal Acidosis

Renal acidosis is further classified into two types: uremic acidosis and renal tubular acidosis (RTA). In uremic acidosis, reduced net acid excretion results from reduced nephron mass, i.e., renal failure, whereas in renal tubular acidosis, reduction in net acid excretion results from a specific tubular dysfunction. Because development of renal acidosis depends on the rate of net acid excretion as well as the rate of net acid production, which varies greatly according to the diet, the level of renal failure at which uremic acidosis develops depends on the dietary intake of acid. On a usual diet, uremic acidosis may develop when GFR falls below 20% of normal (Bommer, 1996; Oh, 1992).

Three types of RTA are recognized: types I, II and IV. Type I RTA, also called classical RTA or distal RTA, is characterized by inability to reduce urine pH below 5.5. Since acidification of urine to a very low urine pH

Table 14–8 Causes of Metabolic Acidosis According to Net Acid Excretion

Renal acidosis: absolute or relative reduction in net acid excretion
Uremic acidosis
Renal tubular acidosis:
Distal renal tubular acidosis (type I)
Proximal renal tubular acidosis (type II)
Aldosterone deficiency or unresponsiveness (type IV)
Extrarenal acidosis: increase in net acid excretion
Gastrointestinal loss of bicarbonate
Ingestion of acids or acid precursors: ammonium chloride, sulfur
Acid precursors or toxins: salicylate, ethylene glycol, methanol, toluene, acetaminophen, paraldehyde
Organic acidosis
L-Lactic acidosis
D-Lactic acidosis
Ketoacidosis.

Table 14–9 Causes of L-Lactic Acidosis

Type A lactic acidosis: due to tissue hypoxia
Circulatory shock
Severe hypoxemia
Heart failure
Severe anemia
Grand mal seizure
Type B lactic acidosis: no tissue hypoxia
Acute alcoholism
Drugs and toxins, e.g., phenformin, antiretroviral drugs
Diabetes mellitus
Leukemia
Deficiency of thiamin or riboflavin
Idiopathic

occurs at the collecting duct, the likely site of defect is the collecting duct, which is a part of the distal nephron, hence the term distal RTA. Because H^+ secretion in the collecting duct is somewhat impaired also in type IV RTA, some authors consider both type I and type IV RTA a form of distal RTA. Still, most authorities use the terms type I RTA and distal RTA synonymously. Type I RTA can develop as a primary disorder or secondary to drug toxicity, tubulointerstitial renal diseases or other renal diseases (Rodriguez Soriano, 2002).

Type II RTA, also called proximal RTA, has defective proximal bicarbonate reabsorption characterized by reduced renal bicarbonate threshold. Urine can be made free of bicarbonate and acidified normally when serum bicarbonate decreases to a low level. Most patients with proximal RTA have evidence of generalized proximal tubular dysfunction, i.e., Fanconi's syndrome, which is manifested by bicarbonaturia, aminoaciduria, glycosuria, phosphaturia, and uricosuria. Of these, renal glycosuria (glycosuria in the presence normal blood glucose) is most useful in diagnosing Fanconi's syndrome. Type II RTA may be a primary disorder or secondary to genetic or acquired renal dysfunction. Hypokalemia is a characteristic finding of both type I and type II RTA, but tends to be more severe in type I than in type II. Type III RTA, a term used to describe a hybrid form of types I and II RTA, is no longer in use.

Type IV RTA is caused by aldosterone deficiency or tubular unresponsiveness to aldosterone, resulting in impaired renal tubular potassium secretion and hence hyperkalemia. Although reduced H^+ secretion in the collecting duct plays a role, the major mechanism of acidosis in type IV RTA is hyperkalemia-induced impairment in ammonia production in the proximal tubule. Type IV RTA is far more common than either type I or type II RTA, and the most common cause of type IV RTA is hyporeninemic hypoaldosteronism.

Organic Acidosis

Among external causes of acidosis, overproduction of endogenous acid, especially that of lactic acid and ketoacids, is the most important mechanism. Only a marked overproduction, well in excess of 1000 mEq/day of lactic acid, leads to acidosis because of the enormous capacity to metabolize organic acids. When organic acids react with bicarbonate, organic anions and CO_2 are formed. Retention of organic anions results in metabolic acidosis with increased anion gap, as defined below. Renal excretion of organic anions results in hyperchloremic acidosis with normal anion gap. The retained organic anions are potential bicarbonate; when they are metabolized, bicarbonate is regenerated. Thus, loss of organic anions in the urine is tantamount to loss of bicarbonate. If an organic anion produced is entirely retained, subsequent metabolism will result in the complete recovery of the lost alkali. Characteristically organic acidosis is rapid in onset and in recovery.

Lactic Acidosis. Lactic acid is produced from pyruvic acid by the action of the enzyme LDH and the cofactor NADH. Metabolism of lactic acid requires its conversion back to pyruvic acid, using the same enzyme and NAD^+ as a cofactor. For this reason, both production and metabolism of lactic acid are reciprocally influenced by the same factors; increased concentration of pyruvic acid and increased ratio of $NADH/NAD^+$ increase lactic acid production and at the same time reduce its metabolism. Consequently, in most cases of lactic acidosis lactic acid production is increased and at the same time its metabolism is reduced. By far the most common cause of lactic acidosis is tissue hypoxia (type A lactic acidosis),

which results from circulatory shock, severe anemia, severe heart failure, acute pulmonary edema, cardiac arrest, carbon monoxide poisoning, seizures, vigorous muscular exercise, etc. (Carroll, 1989; Oh, 2003; Arenas-Pinto, 2003). Lactic acidosis in acute alcoholism and severe liver disease is caused by impaired lactic acid utilization (Luft, 2001). Lactic acidosis that occurs in the absence of tissue hypoxia is called type B lactic acidosis (Table 14–9).

D-Lactic Acidosis. Lactic acidosis, unless specified, refers to the acidosis caused by L-lactic acid, which is the isomer normally produced in the human body because the enzyme LDH, responsible for production of lactic acid, is an L-isomer. The accumulation of D-lactic acid, which is due to production of D-lactic acid by bacteria in the colon, causes D-lactic acidosis, which is characterized by severe acidosis and neurological manifestations. The affected patients behave as if they are intoxicated with alcohol despite normal blood ethanol levels. The mechanism of D-lactic acidosis is the colonic overproduction of D-lactic acid by bacteria. Necessary requirements for overproduction of D-lactic acid in the colon are delivery of a large amount of substrate to the colon, i.e., malabsorption syndrome, and proliferation of D-LDH-forming bacteria in the colon (Uribarri, 1998; Oh, 1979). Treatment of D-lactic acidosis is oral administration of antibiotics.

Ketoacidosis. Ketoacids, acetoacetic acid and betahydroxybutyric acid, are produced in the liver from free fatty acids (FFA), and metabolized by the extrahepatic tissues. Increased production of ketoacids is the main mechanism for ketoacid accumulation, although decreased utilization of ketoacids by the brain with the patient in a coma may accelerate the ketoacid accumulation. Increased production requires a high concentration of FFA and its conversion to ketoacids in the liver. Insulin deficiency is responsible for increased mobilization of FFA from the adipose tissue, and glucagon excess and insulin deficiency stimulate conversion of FFA to ketoacids in the liver. The initial step in ketoacid production from FFA is the entry of FFA into the mitochondria, which requires acylcarnitine transferase. This step is stimulated by glucagon excess. The next step is metabolism of FFA to acetyl CoA, and then finally to ketoacids. Diversion of acetyl CoA to fatty acid resynthesis requires the enzyme acetyl CoA carboxylase, and inhibition of this enzyme by insulin deficiency, glucagon excess and excess of stress-induced hormones further contributes to increased ketoacid synthesis.

The clinical diagnosis of ketoacidosis is usually made with *Acetest*, which detects acetoacetate (AA) but not beta-hydroxybutyrate (BB). Although beta-hydroxybutyrate is the predominant acid in typical ketoacidosis (the usual ratio of BB/AA is about 2.5–3.0), the reaction to Acetest represents a fair estimate of the total concentration of ketoacids as long as the ratio remains within a usual range. When the ratio of BB/AA is greatly increased, Acetest may be negative or only slightly positive despite retention of a large amount of total ketones in the form of BB. Such condition is called beta-hydroxybutyric acidosis, and is commonly seen in alcoholic ketoacidosis (Delaney, 2000; Oh, 1977).

Serum Anion Gap (AG)

Serum anion gap is estimated as: $Na^+ - (Cl^- + HCO_3^-)$ or $(Na^+ + K^+) - (Cl^- + HCO_3^-)$. Since normal serum potassium concentration is quantitatively a minor component of serum electrolytes, the fluctuation in its concentration affects little the overall result, and hence the first of the two equations is more commonly used to estimate the anion gap. The normal value is about 12 mEq/L (8–16 mEq/L). Although the term anion gap implies that there is a gap between cation and anion concentrations, the concentration of total cations in the serum is exactly equal to the concentration of total anions. The anion gap, $Na^+ - (Cl^- + HCO_3^-)$, is

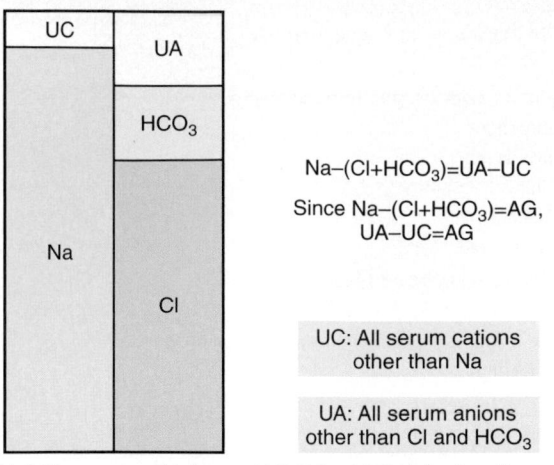

$$Na-(Cl+HCO_3)=UA-UC$$

Since $Na-(Cl+HCO_3)=AG$,
$$UA-UC=AG$$

UC: All serum cations
other than Na

UA: All serum anions
other than Cl and HCO_3

Figure 14–6 The anatomy of anion gap (AG). When UC is defined as all serum cations other than Na, and UA as all serum anions other than Cl or bicarbonate, the serum anion gap can be stated as UA minus UC.

12 mEq/L because the total concentration of unmeasured anions (i.e., all anions other than chloride and bicarbonate) is about 23 mEq/L, and of the total concentration of unmeasured cations (i.e., all cations other than sodium) is about 11 mEq/L.

Let us assume that total serum cations = Na^+ + unmeasured cations (UC), and that total serum anions = Cl^- + HCO_3^- + unmeasured anions (UA). Since total serum cations = total serum anions, Na^+ + UC = (Cl^- + HCO_3^-) + UA. Hence, $Na^+ - (Cl^- + HCO_3^-)$ = UA – UC. Since the anion gap = $Na^+ - (Cl^- + HCO_3^-)$, the anion gap = UA – UC (Fig. 14–6) (Oh, 1977).

It is apparent that a change in the anion gap must involve changes in unmeasured anions or unmeasured cations, or a laboratory error involving the measurement of Na^+, Cl^-, or HCO_3^-. The anion gap can be increased by increased UA or decreased UC or by a laboratory error resulting in a false increase in serum Na^+ or a false decrease in serum Cl^- or HCO_3^-. AG can be decreased by decreased UA or increased UC or by a laboratory error resulting in a false decrease in serum Na^+ or a false increase in serum Cl^- or HCO_3^-. The equation also predicts that a change in UA may not change AG if UC is also changed by the same extent in the same direction.

Decreased AG is most commonly due to reduction in serum albumin concentration, while increased AG is most often due to accumulation of anions of acids, such as sulfate, lactate, or ketone anions. Although bromide is an unmeasured anion, bromide intoxication is accompanied by low serum anion gap because bromide causes a false increase in serum Cl^-. A change in serum Na^+ usually does not cause a change in AG because serum Cl^- usually changes in the same direction. For the same reason, HCO_3^- concentrations cannot be used to predict a change in AG. For example, when serum HCO_3^- concentration increases in metabolic alkalosis, Cl^- concentration almost invariably decreases reciprocally in order to maintain electrical neutrality, so that anion gap is unchanged. When HCO_3^- concentration decreases, Cl^- concentration may remain unchanged or be increased. If bicarbonate is replaced by another anion, Cl^- concentration remains unchanged, hence normochloremic acidosis with increased anion gap. Examples are organic acidosis and uremic acidosis. When bicarbonate concentration decreases without another anion replacing it, electrical neutrality is maintained by a higher Cl^- concentration: hence, hyperchloremic acidosis with normal anion gap. Proper interpretation of serum anion gap requires knowledge of the existence of conditions that influence anion gap even though they may have no direct effect on metabolic acidosis. For example, if a person with hypoalbuminemia develops lactic acidosis, the anion gap could be normal because the low albumin and the lactate accumulation have opposite effects on the anion gap.

Differential Diagnosis

One approach to the differential diagnosis of metabolic acidosis is to calculate the serum anion gap. An increased anion gap suggests organic acidosis, uremic acidosis, and acidosis due to certain toxins (Table 14–10). A normal anion gap suggests renal tubular acidosis and acidosis due to diarrheal loss of bicarbonate. Most cases of uremic acidosis are accompanied by normal anion gap; only in advanced chronic and acute renal failure is anion gap increased. Furthermore, the vast majority of patients with ketoacidosis pass through a phase of hyperchloremic acidosis (normal anion gap) during the recovery phase.

Another approach to the differential diagnosis of metabolic acidosis is to classify the acidosis into renal and extrarenal acidosis. Three major

Table 14–10 Classification of Metabolic Acidosis by Anion Gap

Metabolic acidosis with increased anion gap (normochloremic acidosis)
Ketoacidosis
L-Lactic acidosis
D-Lactic acidosis
Beta-hydroxybutyric acidosis
Uremic acidosis
Ingestion of toxins: salicylate, methanol, ethylene glycol, toluene, acetaminophen

Metabolic acidosis with normal anion gap (hyperchloremic acidosis)
Renal tubular acidosis
Uremic acidosis (early)
Acidosis following respiratory alkalosis
Intestinal loss of bicarbonate
Administration of chloride-containing acid: HCl, NH_4Cl
Ketoacidosis during recovery phase

causes of extrarenal acidosis are organic acidosis, diarrheal loss of bicarbonate, and acidosis due to exogenous toxins. The presence of organic acidosis is usually obvious from clinical findings, e.g., evidence of tissue hypoxia in lactic acidosis, or hyperglycemia and ketonemia in ketoacidosis. Diarrhea as the cause of metabolic acidosis is first suspected from history, but history is often misleading because the severity of diarrhea cannot be easily determined. The measurement of urine anion gap is useful in determining the severity of diarrhea. Urine anion gap, which is measured as: urine (Na^+ + K^+) – urine Cl^-, is reduced or negative when diarrhea is severe. The low urine anion gap in diarrhea is explained by the preferential loss of Na^+ + K^+ in excess of Cl^- because diarrheal fluid contains more Na^+ + K^+ than Cl^-, as some of the cations are balanced by bicarbonate. In other types of metabolic acidosis, urine anion gap is not altered because there is no extrarenal loss of electrolytes that are components of the urine anion gap (Oh, 2002a). History of drug ingestion and acute onset will suggest acidosis due to exogenous toxins.

Once extrarenal acidosis is excluded, renal acidosis is the only alternative diagnosis. Of the two types of renal acidosis, uremic acidosis can be readily diagnosed by the measurement of serum creatinine and BUN. If renal acidosis is confirmed but uremic acidosis is ruled out, the diagnosis must be renal tubular acidosis. Among the three types of RTA, type IV RTA is suspected by the presence of hyperkalemia. Hypokalemia suggests either type I or type II RTA. If spontaneous urine pH is below 5.5, type I RTA is ruled out. If urine pH is higher than 5.5, urine pH should be measured after oral administration of 40 mg of furosemide or 10 mg of torsemide. The latter drug has higher sensitivity and specificity. If the urine pH remains above 5.5, the likely diagnosis is type I RTA. The evidence of Fanconi's syndrome (the best evidence is renal glycosuria) suggests type II RTA.

Compensation of Metabolic Acidosis

Compensation of metabolic acidosis is achieved by hyperventilation that results in decreased P_{CO_2}. The compensation is moderately effective, and the maximal compensation is completed within 12–24 hours. The formula that predicts the expected increase in P_{CO_2} (ΔP_{CO_2}) is as follows:

$$\Delta P_{CO_2} = \Delta HCO_3^- \times 1.2 \pm 2 \quad (\Delta HCO_3^- \text{ is a given} \qquad (14\text{–}38)$$
change in serum HCO_3^- concentration)

Metabolic Alkalosis

Causes and Pathogenesis

At normal serum bicarbonate concentration, bicarbonate filtered at the glomerulus is virtually completely reabsorbed. As serum bicarbonate concentration rises above the normal level, bicarbonate reabsorption is incomplete and bicarbonaturia begins. A slight increase in serum bicarbonate above 24 mEq/L causes marked bicarbonaturia. Hence, when renal tubular bicarbonate handling and GFR are normal, maintenance of a high plasma bicarbonate concentration is extremely difficult unless an enormous amount of bicarbonate is given. Therefore, maintenance of metabolic alkalosis requires two conditions: a mechanism to increase plasma bicarbonate and a mechanism to maintain the increased concentration. Bicarbonate concentration may be increased by administration of alkali, gastric loss of HCl through vomiting or nasogastric suction, or by renal generation of bicarbonate (Table 14–11). Maintenance of high plasma

Table 14–11 Mechanisms and Causes to Increase Extracellular Bicarbonate Concentration

Loss of HCl from the stomach, e.g., gastric suction, vomiting

Administration of bicarbonate or bicarbonate precursors, e.g., sodium lactate, sodium acetate, sodium citrate

Shift of H^+ into the cell, e.g., K^+ depletion

Rapid contraction of extracellular volume without loss of bicarbonate, e.g., contraction alkalosis by the use of loop diuretics

Increased renal excretion of acid, e.g., diuretic therapy, high aldosterone state, potassium depletion, high P_{CO_2}, secondary hypoparathyroidism

Table 14–12 Causes of Respiratory Acidosis

Lung diseases: chronic obstructive lung disease, advanced interstitial lung disease, acute asthma

Thoracic deformity or airway obstruction

Diseases of respiratory muscle and nerve: myasthenia gravis, hypokalemia paralysis, botulism, amyotrophic lateral sclerosis, Guillain–Barré syndrome

Depression of the respiratory center: barbiturate intoxication, stroke hypothyroidism

Table 14–13 Causes of respiratory alkalosis

Diseases of the lung: any intrapulmonary pathology such as pneumonia, pulmonary fibrosis, pulmonary congestion, pulmonary embolism

Hypoxemia

CNS lesions

Gram-negative sepsis

Drugs: salicylate, progesterone

bicarbonate concentration occurs in advanced renal failure or when renal threshold for bicarbonate is increased (Palmer, 1997). The two most common causes for increased renal bicarbonate threshold are volume depletion and K^+ depletion. Metabolic alkalosis corrected by administration of chloride-containing fluid, e.g., NaCl or KCl solution, is called chloride-responsive metabolic alkalosis, e.g., vomiting-induced alkalosis. Patients with chloride-responsive metabolic alkalosis are typically volume depleted (Oh, 2002b). However, in edema-forming conditions, administration of Cl^- may not improve metabolic alkalosis even though the mechanism of high renal bicarbonate threshold is volume depletion. Parathyroid hormone (PTH) normally interferes with bicarbonate reabsorption in the proximal tubule, and therefore renal tubular bicarbonate tends to be increased in hypoparathyroidism.

Compensation

Compensation of metabolic alkalosis is achieved by hypoventilation that results in increased P_{CO_2}. Partly because hypoxemia occurs inevitably with hypoventilation in the absence of oxygen supplement, the compensation is the least effective among the four acid–base disorders. The formula that predicts the expected increase in P_{CO_2} (ΔP_{CO_2}) is as follows:

$$\Delta P_{CO_2} = \Delta HCO_3^- \times 0.7 \pm 5 \quad (\Delta HCO_3^- \text{ is a given change} \qquad (14\text{–}39)$$
in a serum HCO_3^- concentration)

The maximal compensation is completed within 12–24 hours. Observations have shown that no matter how severe the metabolic alkalosis, P_{CO_2} rarely exceeds 60 mmHg unless a complicating independent respiratory disorder that compromises ventilation coexists.

Respiratory Acidosis

Causes and Pathogenesis

The causes are usually quite apparent. They include diseases of the lung (most common), respiratory muscle, respiratory nerve, thoracic cage, and airways, and suppression of the respiratory center by stroke, drugs such as phenobarbital, or severe hypothyroidism (Table 14–12).

Compensation

The normal compensatory response to respiratory acidosis is to increase HCO_3^- concentration in an attempt to minimize the reduction in pH. This occurs in two distinct stages, first by tissue buffering of CO_2, and second by increased renal excretion of acid.

Tissue Buffering

This phase of compensation is extremely fast, and occurs within a second. The chemical reaction is as follows:

$$CO_2 + H_2O \longrightarrow H_2CO_3 \qquad (14\text{–}40)$$
$$H_2CO_3 + KBuff \longrightarrow HBuff + KHCO_3 \qquad (14\text{–}41)$$

KBuff is a non-HCO_3^- buffer, and the reaction proceeds to the right because of the rising P_{CO_2}. Because extracellular fluid has little non-HCO_3^- buffers, most of this buffering occurs in the cell. The increased concentration of cellular HCO_3^- causes an extracellular shift of HCO_3^- in exchange for Cl^-. The relationship between an increase in P_{CO_2} (ΔP_{CO_2}) and the increase in serum levels of HCO_3^- (ΔHCO_3^-) in acute respiratory acidosis is shown in the equation:

$$\Delta HCO_3^- \text{ (mEq/L)} = \Delta P_{CO_2} \text{ (mmHg)} \times 0.07 \pm 1.5 \qquad (14\text{–}42)$$

Renal Compensation

Renal compensation for respiratory acidosis is delayed, but it increases the HCO_3^- concentration to a much higher level. The increased concentration of HCO_3^- is achieved by increased net acid excretion, primarily in the form of NH_4^+. Maximal compensation requires 5 days, but is 90% complete in 3 days. Increased excretion of NH_4^+ is accompanied by Cl^-. As new HCO_3^- is

retained, Cl^- is lost. It follows therefore when respiratory acidosis is corrected, that excretion of HCO_3^- must be accompanied by retention of Cl^-, which is possible only if Cl^- is taken in. Restriction of NaCl intake during the recovery phase of chronic respiratory acidosis results in the maintenance of a high serum HCO_3^-.

The relationship between the increase in P_{CO_2} (ΔP_{CO_2}) and the increase in HCO_3^- (ΔHCO_3^-) in chronic maximally compensated respiratory acidosis is shown in the following equation:

$$\Delta HCO_3^- \text{ (mEq/L)} = \Delta P_{CO_2} \text{ (mmHg)} \times 0.4 \pm 3 \qquad (14\text{–}43)$$

Respiratory Alkalosis

Causes and Pathogenesis

With the exception of respirator-induced alkalosis and voluntary hyperventilation, respiratory alkalosis is always the result of stimulation of the respiratory center. The two most common causes of respiratory alkalosis are hypoxic stimulation of the respiratory center and stimulation through the pulmonary receptors caused by various lung lesions, such as pneumonia, pulmonary congestion, and pulmonary embolism. Certain drugs, e.g., salicylate and progesterone, stimulate the respiratory center directly (Saaresranta, 1999; Bayliss, 1992). Respiratory alkalosis is common in Gram-negative sepsis through an unknown mechanism. Blood pH tends to be extremely high when respiratory alkalosis is caused by psychogenic stimulation of the respiratory center because the condition is usually superacute and therefore there is no time for compensation. Causes of respiratory alkalosis are listed in Table 14–13.

Compensation

Two types of compensation lower plasma HCO_3^- and minimize the increase in blood pH in respiratory alkalosis: tissue buffering and renal compensation.

Tissue Buffering

Compensation by buffering of HCO_3^- is completed within a second with the reactions (Carroll, 1989):

$$HBuff + HCO_3^- \rightarrow H_2CO_3 + Buff \qquad (14\text{–}44)$$
$$H_2CO_3 \rightarrow CO_2 + H_2O \qquad (14\text{–}45)$$

The reactions proceed to the right because CO_2 is lost by hyperventilation. The magnitude of reduction in HCO_3^- content depends on the amount of cellular acid buffers (HBuff) that react with HCO_3^-. As cellular HCO_3^- is consumed in the buffer reaction, extracellular HCO_3^- enters the cell in exchange for cellular Cl^- that enters the extracellular fluid. An additional mechanism of tissue buffering is increased production of lactic acid and other organic acids. Increased lactic acid production is explained in part by the stimulatory effect of alkaline pH on phosphofructokinase, a rate-limiting enzyme for glycolysis. The magnitude of reduction in plasma HCO_3^- concentration by acute compensation is predicted from the following equation:

$$\Delta HCO_3^- \text{ (mEq/L)} = \Delta P_{CO_2} \text{ (mmHg)} \times 0.2 \pm 2.5 \qquad (14\text{–}46)$$

(ΔHCO_3^- (mEq/L) is the expected decrease in plasma HCO_3^- for a given decrease in P_{CO_2} (ΔP_{CO_2}) in mmHg.)

Table 14–14 Formulas for Predicting Normal Acid–Base Compensation

Metabolic acidosis: $\Delta PCO_2 = \Delta HCO_3^- \times 1.2 \pm 2$

Metabolic alkalosis:* $\Delta PCO_2 = \Delta HCO_3^- \times 0.7 \pm 5$

Acute respiratory acidosis: $\Delta HCO_3^- = \Delta PCO_2 \times 0.07 \pm 1.5$

Chronic respiratory acidosis: $\Delta HCO_3^- = \Delta PCO_2 \times 0.4 \pm 3$

Acute respiratory alkalosis: $\Delta HCO_3^- = \Delta PCO_2 \times 0.2 \pm 2.5$

Chronic respiratory alkalosis: $\Delta HCO_3^- = \Delta PCO_2 \times 0.5 \pm 2.5$

ΔHCO_3^- and ΔPCO_2 represent the difference between normal and actual values.

* No matter how high the serum HCO_3^- rises, PCO_2 rarely rises above 60 mmHg in metabolic alkalosis.

Renal Compensation

Renal compensation of respiratory alkalosis is achieved by reduction in net acid excretion (Carroll, 1989; Oh, 2003). This is achieved initially by increased excretion of HCO_3^-, but later by reduced excretion of NH_4^+ and titratable acid. The magnitude of reduction in plasma HCO_3^- concentration due to renal compensation can be predicted from the following equation:

$$\Delta HCO_3^- \text{ (mEq/L)} = \Delta PCO_2 \text{ (mmHg)} \times 0.5 \pm 2.5 \qquad (14\text{–}47)$$

(ΔHCO_3^- [mEq/L] is the expected decrease in plasma HCO_3^- for a given decrease in PCO_2 [ΔPCO_2] in mmHg.)

Among the four types of acid–base disorders, compensation is most effective in respiratory alkalosis; pH after compensation sometimes returns to normal levels. The process is completed within 2–3 days. When complete compensation does occur, one should look for evidence of complicating metabolic acidosis.

Mixed Acid–Base Disorders

The term mixed acid–base disorder refers to a clinical condition in which two or more primary acid–base disorders coexist. They generally present with one obvious disturbance with what appears to be an inappropriate (excessive or inadequate) compensation. The 'inappropriateness' of the compensatory process is the result of a separate primary disorder. The appropriate degrees of compensation for primary acid–base disorders have been determined by analysis of data from a large number of patients, and are expressed in the form of equations in Table 14–14. When the two disorders influence the blood pH in opposite directions, the blood pH will be determined by the dominant disorder. If the disorders cancel out each other's effects, blood pH can be normal. When there is any degree of compensation for acid–base disorders, both PCO_2 and HCO_3^- change in the same direction, i.e., both are high or both are low. If PCO_2 and HCO_3^- have changed in opposite directions, e.g., PCO_2 is high and HCO_3^- is low, or PCO_2 is low and HCO_3^- is high, the presence of a mixed acid–base disorder is certain. Appropriateness of compensation can be determined by consulting Table 14–14. Compensation could be excessive, insufficient, or appropriate. One can also have an approximate idea about the appropriateness of compensation from the degree of pH deviation without consulting the formula for normal compensation.

In general, compensation is most effective in respiratory alkalosis (pH is often normalized), the next best is respiratory acidosis (pH may become normal), and the third best is metabolic acidosis. Compensation is least effective in metabolic alkalosis, probably because hypoxemia, an inevitable consequence of hypoventilation, stimulates ventilation. If a patient has low PCO_2 and low HCO_3^- with normal pH, the likely diagnosis is compensated respiratory alkalosis rather than compensated metabolic acidosis (Carroll, 1989; Oh, 2003).

CHAPTER: 14   Evaluation of Renal Function, Water, Electrolytes and Acid–Base Balance

References

Abdelhamid S, Lewicka S, Vecsei P, et al: A new subset of mineralocorticoid hypertension with excess of 21-deoxyaldosterone and Kelly's-M1 steroid: clinical and morphological findings. J Clin Endocrinol Metab 1995; 80:737–744.

Abdul-Karim RW, Harris JE, Beydoun SN, Cuenca VG: Endogenous creatinine clearance during pregnancy. II. Variations in normal standards based on methodology. Obstet Gynecol 1978; 51:431–432.

Agarwal RA: Am J Kidney Dis 2003; 41:752–759.

Agarwal R, Emmett M: The post-transurethral resection of prostate syndrome: therapeutic proposals. Am J Kidney Dis 1994; 24:108–111.

Agraharkar M, Agraharkar A: Posthysteroscopic hyponatremia: evidence for a multifactorial cause. Am J Kidney Dis 1997; 30:717–719.

Agre P, King LS, Yasui M, et al: Aquaporin water channels—from atomic structure to clinical medicine. J Physiol 2002; 542:3–16.

Aguilera G, Rabadan-Diehl C: Regulation of vasopressin V1b receptors in the anterior pituitary gland of the rat. Exp Physiol 2000; 85:19S–26S.

Akan H, Sargin S, Turkseven F, et al: Comparison of three different irrigation fluids used in transurethral prostatectomy based on plasma volume expansion and metabolic effects. Br J Urol 1996; 78:224–227.

Ajaelo I, Koenig K, Snoey E: Severe hyponatremia and inappropriate antidiuretic hormone secretion following ecstasy use. Acad Emerg Med 1998; 5:839–840.

Arenas-Pinto A, Grant AD, Edwards S, Weller IV: Lactic acidosis in HIV infected patients: a systematic review of published cases. Sex Transm Infect 2003; 79:340–343.

Argani P, Erlandson RA, Rosai J: Thymic neuroblastoma in adults: report of three cases with special emphasis on its association with the syndrome of inappropriate secretion of antidiuretic hormone. Am J Clin Pathol 1997; 108:537–543.

Arlt W, Dahia PL, Callies F, et al: Ectopic ACTH production by a bronchial carcinoid tumour responsive to desmopressin in vivo and in vitro. Clin Endocrinol (Oxf) 1997; 47:623–627.

Aukland K, Reed RK: Interstitial-lymphatic mechanisms in the control of extracellular fluid volume. Physiol Rev 1993; 73:1–78.

Barbour HM, Welch C: Development and evaluation of a kinetic diacetyl monoxime method for urine urea. Ann Clin Biochem 1992; 29:101–104.

Bartter FC, Schwartz WB: The syndrome of inappropriate secretion of antidiuretic hormone. Am J Med 1967; 42:790–799.

Bayliss DA, Millhorn DE: Central neural mechanisms of progesterone action: application to the respiratory system. J Appl Physiol 1992; 73:393–404.

Bellevue R, Dosik H, Spergel G, Gussoff BD: Pseudohyperkalemia and extreme leukocytosis. J Lab Clin Med 1975; 85:660–664.

Biggi A, Viglietti A, Farinelli MC, et al: Estimation of glomerular filtration rate using chromium-51 ethylene diamine tetra-acetic acid and technetium-99m diethylene triamine penta-acetic acid. Eur J Nuc Med 1995; 22:532–536.

Bock HA, Hermle M, Brunner FP, Thiel G: Pressure dependent modulation of renin release in isolated perfused glomeruli. Kidney Int 1992; 41:275–280.

Bommer J, Keller C, Gehlen F, Hergesell O: Acidosis in uremic patients. Clin Nephrol 1996; 46:280–285.

Bourque CW, Oliet SH: Osmoreceptors in the central nervous system. Annu Rev Physiol 1997; 59:601–619.

Bradberry SM, Vale JA: Disturbances of potassium homeostasis in poisoning. J Toxicol Clin Toxicol 1995; 33:295–310.

Brautbar N, Levi J, Rosler A, et al: Familial hyperkalemia, hypertension, and hyporeninemia with normal aldosterone levels. A tubular defect in potassium handling. Arch Intern Med 1978; 138:607–610.

Brochner-Mortensen J, Giese J, Rossing N: Renal inulin clearance versus total plasma clearance of 51Cr-EDTA. Scand J Clin Lab Invest 1969; 23:301–305.

Burg MB. Molecular basis of osmotic regulation. Am J Physiol 1995; 268:F983–F989

Burton RF: The protein content of extracellular fluids and its relevance to the study of ionic regulation: net charge and colloid osmotic pressure. Comp Biochem Physiol A 1988; 90:11–16.

Canada TW, Weavind LM, Augustin KM: Possible liposomal amphotericin B-induced nephrogenic diabetes insipidus. Ann Pharmacother 2003; 37:70–73.

Cannon SC: An expanding view for the molecular basis of familial periodic paralysis. Neuromuscul Disord 2002; 12:533–543.

Carroll HJ, Oh MS: Water, Electrolyte, and Acid–Base Metabolism. Philadelphia, Lippincott Co., 1989.

Carvounis CP, Nisar S, Guro-Razuman S: Significance of the fractional excretion of urea in the differential diagnosis of acute renal failure. Kidney Int 2002; 62:2223–2229.

Christensen AB, Groth S: Determination of 99mTc-DTPA clearance by a single plasma sample method. Clinical Physiol 1986; 6:579–588.

Clemessy JL, Favier C, Borron SW, et al: Hypokalaemia related to acute chloroquine ingestion. Lancet 1995; 346:877–880.

Cockcroft DW, Gault MH: Prediction of creatinine clearance from serum creatinine. Nephron 1976; 16:31–41.

Cooperman LH: Succinylcholine-induced hyperkalemia in neuromuscular disease. JAMA 1970; 213:1867–1871.

Counahan R, Chantler C, Ghazali S, et al: Estimation of glomerular filtration rate from plasma creatinine concentration in children. Arch Dis Child 1976; 51:875–878.

Delaney MF, Zisman A, Kettyle WM: Diabetic ketoacidosis and hyperglycemic hyperosmolar nonketotic syndrome. Endocrinol Metab Clin North Am 2000; 29:683–705.

Delaunay J, Stewart G, Iolascon A: Hereditary dehydrated and overhydrated stomatocytosis: recent advances. Curr Opin Hematol 1999; 6:110–114.

Delphin E, Jackson D, Rothstein P: Use of succinylcholine during elective pediatric anesthesia should be reevaluated. Anesth Analg 1987; 66:1190–1192.

de Rouffignac C, Jamison RL: (eds): Kidney Int 1987; 31:501–672.

Don BR, Sebastian A, Cheitlin M, et al: Pseudohyperkalemia caused by fist clenching during phlebotomy. N Engl J Med 1990; 322:1290–1292.

Emser W: Hypermagnesemic periodic paralysis: treatment with digitalis and lithium carbonate. Arch Neurol 1982; 39:727–730.

Fallon JK, Kicman AT, Hutt AJ, et al: Low-dose MDMA ('ecstasy') induces vasopressin secretion. Lancet 1998; 351:1784.

Fawcett JK, Scott JE: A rapid and precise method for the determination of urea. J Clin Pathol 1960; 13:156–159.

Feraille E, Carranza ML, Gonin S, et al: Insulin-induced stimulation of Na+,K(+)-ATPase activity in kidney proximal tubule cells depends on phosphorylation of the alpha-subunit at Tyr-10. Mol Biol Cell 1999; 10:2847–2859.

Ferlito A, Rinaldo A, Devaney KO: Syndrome of inappropriate antidiuretic hormone secretion associated with head neck cancers: review of the literature. Ann Otol Rhinol Laryngol 1997; 106:878–883.

Finer G, Shalev H, Birk OS, et al: Transient neonatal hyperkalemia in the antenatal (ROMK defective) Bartter syndrome. J Pediatr 2003; 142:318–323.

Fleming JS, Wilkinson J, Oliver RM, et al: Comparison of radionuclide estimation of glomerular filtration rate using technetium 99m diethylenetriaminepentaacetic acid and chromium 51 ethylenediaminetetraacetic acid. Eur J Nuc Med 1991; 18:391–395.

Fossati P, Ponti M, Passoni G, et al: A step forward in enzymatic measurement of creatinine. Clin Chem 1994; 40:130–137.

Friedmann AS, Memoli VA, North WG: Vasopressin and oxytocin production by non-neuroendocrine lung carcinomas: an apparent low incidence of gene expression. Cancer Lett 1993 75:79–85.

Gaspari F, Perico N, Remuzzi G: Measurement of glomerular filtration rate. Kidney Int 1997; 63(Suppl):S151–S154.

Gennari FJ: Current concepts. Serum osmolality. Uses and limitations. N Engl J Med 1984; 310:102–105.

Giebisch G: Renal potassium transport: mechanisms and regulation. Am J Physiol 1998; 274:F817–F833.

Giebisch GH: A trail of research on potassium. Kidney Int 2002; 62:1498–1512.

Goguen JM, Halperin ML: Can insulin administration cause an acute metabolic acidosis in vivo? An experimental study in dogs. Diabetologia 1993; 36:813–816.

Gold PW, Robertson GL, Ballenger JC, et al: Carbamazepine diminishes the sensitivity of the plasma arginine vasopressin response to osmotic stimulation. J Clin Endocrinol Metab 1983; 57:952–957.

Goldman DE: J Gen Phyiol 1943; 27:37–60.

Goodman BE: Transport of small molecules across cell membranes: water channels and urea transporters. Adv Physiol Educ 2002; 26:146–57.

Gowrishankar M, Lin SH, Mallie JP, et al: Acute hyponatremia in the perioperative period: insights into its pathophysiology and recommendations for management. Clin Nephrol 1998; 50:352–360.

Greger R, Schlatter E, Lang F: Evidence for electroneutral sodium chloride cotransport in the cortical thick ascending limb of Henle's loop of rabbit kidney. Pflugers Arch 1983; 396:308–314.

Gronert GA, Theye RA: Pathophysiology of hyperkalemia induced by succinylcholine. Anesthesiol 1975; 43:89–99.

Hall JE: The renin-angiotensin system: renal actions and blood pressure regulation. Compr Ther 1991; 17:8–17.

Halperin ML, Kamel KS: Potassium. Lancet 1998; 352:135–140.

Halperin ML, Bichet DG, Oh MS: Integrative physiology of basal water permeability in the distal nephron: implications for the syndrome of inappropriate secretion of antidiuretic hormone. Clin Nephrol 2001; 56:339–345.

Hariprasad MK, Eisinger RP, Nadler IM, et al: Hyponatremia in psychogenic polydipsia. Arch Intern Med 1980; 140:1639–1642.

Hayward LJ, Sandoval GM, Cannon SC: Defective slow inactivation of sodium channels contributes to familial periodic paralysis. Neurology 1999; 52:1447–1453.

Heilmann P, Heide J, Hundertmark S, Schoneshofer M: Administration of glycyrrhetinic acid: significant correlation between serum levels and the cortisol/cortisone-ratio in serum and urine. Exp Clin Endocrinol Diab 1999; 107:370–378.

Higashi I, Morizono T: Artifactually low serum urea caused by antibodies to bacteria urease. Clin Chem 2000; 46:297–299.

Hilbrands LB, Artz MA, Wetzels JF, Koene RA: Cimetidine improves the reliability of creatinine as a marker of glomerular filtration. Kidney Int 1991; 40:1171–1176.

Hill AR, Uribarri J, Mann J, Berl T: Altered water metabolism in tuberculosis: role of vasopressin. Am J Med 1990a; 88:357–364.

Hill LL: Body composition, normal electrolyte concentrations, and the maintenance of normal volume, tonicity, and acid–base metabolism. Pediatr Clin North Am 1990b; 37:241–256.

Hensen J, Haenelt M, Gross P: Water retention after oral chlorpropamide is associated with an increase in renal papillary arginine vasopressin receptors. Eur J Endocrinol 1995; 132;459–464.

Hogg RJ, Kokko JP: Comparison between the electrical potential profile and the chloride gradients in the thin limbs of Henle's loop in rats. Kidney Int 1978; 14:428.

Hogg RJ, Kokko JP: Urine concentrating and diluting mechanisms in mammalian kidneys. In Brenner, BM, Rector, FC (eds): The Kidney. Philadelphia, WB Saunders Co, 1986, Ch. 8, pp 251–279.

Hollenberg NK: Implications of species difference for clinical investigation: studies on the renin-angiotensin system. Hypertension 2000; 35:150–154.

Ibata Y, Okamura H, Tanaka M, et al: Functional morphology of the suprachiasmatic nucleus. Front Neuroendocrinol 1999; 20:241–268.

Iolascon A, Stewart GW, Ajetunmobi JF, et al: Familial pseudohyperkalemia maps to the same locus as dehydrated hereditary stomatocytosis (hereditary xerocytosis). Blood 1999; 93:3120–3123.

Ito M, Jameson JL, Ito M: Molecular basis of autosomal dominant neurohypophyseal diabetes insipidus. Cellular toxicity caused by the accumulation of mutant vasopressin precursors within the endoplasmic reticulum. J Clin Invest 1997 15(99):1897–1905.

Johnson BE, Chute JP, Rushin J, et al: A prospective study of patients with lung cancer and hyponatremia of malignancy. Am J Respir Crit Care Med 1997; 156:1669–1678.

Jordan P, Brookes JG, Nikolic G, Le Couteur DG: Hydroxychloroquine overdose: toxicokinetics and management. J Toxicol Clin Toxicol 1999; 37:861–864.

Jurkat-Rott K, Mitrovic N, Hang C, et al: Voltage-sensor sodium channel mutations cause hypokalemic periodic paralysis type 2 by enhanced inactivation and reduced current. Proc Natl Acad Sci USA 2000 15(97):9549–9554.

Kessler A, Siekmann L: Measurement of urea in human serum by isotope dilution mass spectrometry: a reference procedure. Clin Chem 1999; 45:1523–1529.

Kim HJ, Chung CH, Moon CO, et al: Determinants of magnitude of pseudohyperkalemia in thrombocytosis. Korean J Intern Med 1990; 5:97–100.

Knepper MA: Urea transport in isolated thick ascending limbs and collecting ducts from rats. Am J Physiol 1983; 245:F634–F639.

Kroll MH, Hagengruber C, Elin RJ: Reaction of picrate with creatinine and cepha antibiotics. Clin Chem 1984; 30:1664–1666.

Krozowski Z, Li KX, Koyama K, et al: The type I and type II 11beta-hydroxysteroid dehydrogenase enzymes. J Steroid Biochem Mol Biol 1999; 69:391–401.

Kruse JA, Cadnapaphornchai P: The serum osmole gap. Crit Care 1994; 9(3):185–197.

Krutzen E, Back SE: Plasma clearance of a new contrast agent, iohexol: a method for the assessment of glomerular filtration rate. J Lab Clin Med 1984; 104:955–961.

Kunchaparty S, Palcso M, Berkman J, et al: Defective processing and expression of thiazide-sensitive Na-Cl cotransporter as a cause of Gitelman's syndrome. Am J Physiol 1999; 277:F643–F649.

Lam GS, Asplin JR, Halperin ML: Does a high concentration of calcium in the urine cause an important renal concentrating defect in human subjects? Clin Sci (Lond) 2000; 98:313–319.

Larach MG, Rosenberg H, Gronert GA, Allen GC: Hyperkalemic cardiac arrest during anesthesia in infants and children with occult myopathies. Clin Pediatr 1997; 36:9–16.

Laragh JH: Renin-angiotensin-aldosterone system for blood pressure and electrolyte homeostasis and its involvement in hypertension, in congestive heart failure and in associated cardiovascular damage (myocardial infarction and stroke). J Hum Hypertens 1995; 9;385–390.

Laterza OF, Price CP, Scott MG: Cystatin C: an improved estimator of glomerular filtration rate? Clin Chem 2002; 48:699–707.

Leadbetter RA, Shutty MS Jr: Differential effects of neuroleptic and clozapine on polydipsia and intermittent hyponatremia. J Clin Psych 1994; 55(Suppl B):110–113.

Leger F, Bouissou F, Coulais Y, et al: Estimation of glomerular filtration rate in children. Pediatr Nephrol 2002; 17:903–907.

Leggett DA, Hill PT, Anderson RJ: 'Stalkitis' in a pregnant 32-year-old woman: a rare cause of diabetes insipidus. Australas Radiol 1999; 43:104–107.

Lemann J Jr, Relman AS: The relation of sulfur metabolism to acid-base balance and electrolyte excretion: the effects of DL-methionine in normal man. J Clin Invest 1959; 38:2215–2223.

Lespinas F, Dupuy G, Revol F, Aubry C: Enzymic urea assay: a new colorimetric method based on hydrogen peroxide measurement. Clin Chem 1989; 35:654–658.

Levey AS, Bosch JP, Lewis JB, et al: A more accurate method to estimate glomerular filtration rate from serum creatinine: a new prediction equation. Modification of Diet in Renal Disease Study Group. Ann Intern Med 1999; 130:461–470.

Levey AS, Greene T, Tusek JW, et al: A simplified equation to predict GFR from serum creatinine (Abstract). J Am Soc Nephrol 2000; 11:A0828.

Levine S, McManus BM, Blackbourne BD, Roberts WC: Fatal water intoxication, schizophrenia, and diuretic therapy for systemic hypertension. Am J Med 1987; 82:153–155.

Litchfield WR, New MI, Coolidge C, et al: Evaluation of the dexamethasone suppression test for the diagnosis of glucocorticoid-remediable aldosteronism. J Clin Endocrinol Metabol 1997; 82:3570–3573.

Luft FC: Lactic acidosis update for critical care clinicians. J Am Soc Nephrol 2001; 12(Suppl 17):S15–S19.

Lyman JL: Blood urea nitrogen and creatinine. Emerg Med Clin North Am 1986; 4:223–233.

Ma XM, Aguilera G: Differential regulation of corticotropin-releasing hormone and vasopressin transcription by glucocorticoids. Endocrinol 1999; 140:5642–5650.

Macaron C, Famuyiwa O: Hyponatremia of hypothyroidism. Appropriate suppression of antidiuretic hormone levels. Arch Intern Med 1978; 138:820–822.

McIvor ME, Cummings CC: Sodium fluoride produces a K+ efflux by increasing intracellular Ca2+ through Na+-Ca2+ exchange. Toxicol Lett 1987; 38:169–176.

McIvor ME, Cummings CC, Mower M, et al: The manipulation of potassium efflux during fluoride intoxication: implications for therapy. Toxicol 1985; 37:233–239.

McKinley MJ, Allen AM, Burns P, et al: Interaction of circulating hormones with the brain: the roles of the subfornical organ and the organum vasculosum of the lamina terminalis. Clin Exp Pharmacol Physiol 1998; 25(Suppl):S61–S67.

Marples D, Christensen S, Christensen EI, et al: Lithium-induced downregulation of aquaporin-2 water channel expression in rat kidney medulla. J Clin Invest 1995; 95:1838–1845.

Massey D: Commentary: clinical diagnostic use of cystatin C. J Clin Lab Anal 2004; 18:55–60.

Matsumura M, Nakashima A, Tofuku Y: Electrolyte disorders following massive insulin overdose in a patient with type 2 diabetes. Intern Med 2000; 39:55–57.

Meister B, Aperia A: Molecular mechanisms involved in catecholamine regulation of sodium transport. Semin Nephrol 1993; 13: 41–49.

Milionis HJ, Liamis GL, Elisaf MS: The hyponatremic patient: a systematic approach to laboratory diagnosis. CMAJ 2002; 166:1056–1062.

Miyamura N, Matsumoto K, Taguchi T, et al: Atypical Bartter syndrome with sensorineural deafness with G47R mutation of the beta-subunit for ClC-Ka and ClC-Kb chloride channels, barttin. J Clin Endocrinol Metab 2003; 88:781–786.

Molitch ME: Pituitary diseases in pregnancy. Semin Perinatol 1998; 22:457–470.

Molitch ME, Rodman E, Hirsch CA, Dubinsky E: Spurious serum creatinine elevations in ketoacidosis. Ann Intern Med 1980; 93:280–281.

Mouri T, Itoi K, Takahashi K, et al: Colocalization of corticotropin-releasing factor and vasopressin in the paraventricular nucleus of the human hypothalamus. Neuroendocrinol 1993; 57:34–39.

Natelson S, Scott ML, Beffa C: A rapid method for the estimation of urea in biologic fluids. Am J Clin Pathol 1951; 21:275–281.

Nielsen S, Frokiaer J, Marples D, et al: Aquaporins in the kidney: from molecules to medicine. Physiol Rev 2002; 82:205–244.

North WG: Gene regulation of vasopressin and vasopressin receptors in cancer. Exp Physiol 2000; 85;27S–40S.

Ogawa T, Kamikubo K: Hypokalemic periodic paralysis associated with hypophosphatemia in a patient with hyperinsulinemia. Am J Med Sci 1999; 318:69–72.

Oh MS: A new method for estimating G-I absorption of alkali. Kidney Int 1989; 36:915–917.

Oh MS: Does serum creatinine rise faster in rhabdomyolysis? Nephron 1993; 63:255–257.

Oh MS: Acid–Base Electrolytes. New York, Ohco, LLC, 2003.
This textbook by a single author contains a great deal of information on all aspects of electrolyte disorders and acid–base balance, including information on the basic physiology of the kidney discussed in depth and the role of the kidney in the body's fluid balance.

Oh MS, Carroll HJ: The anion gap. N Engl J Med 1977; 297:814–817.

Oh MS, Carroll HJ: Whole body acid-base balance. Contrb Nephrol 1992; 100:89–104.
This article has an extensive discussion on all aspects of whole body acid–base balance.

Oh MS, Carroll HJ: In Arieff AI, DeFronzo RA (eds): Fluid, Electrolyte, and Acid–base Disorders, 2nd ed. New York, Churchill Livingstone, 1995.

Oh MS, Carroll HJ: Cerebral salt-wasting syndrome. We need better proof of its existence. Nephron 1999; 82:110–114.

Oh MS, Carroll HJ: Value and determinants of urine anion gap. Nephron 2002a; 90:252–255.

Oh MS, Carroll HJ: Mechanism of chloride deficit in the maintenance of metabolic alkalosis. Nephron 2002b; 91:379–382.

Oh MS, Carroll HJ, Clemmons JE, et al: A mechanism for hyporeninemic hypoaldosteronism in chronic renal disease. Metabolism 1974; 23:1157–1166.

Oh MS, Halperin ML: The mechanism of urine concentration in the inner medulla. Nephron 1997; 75:384–393.

Oh MS, Phelps KR, Traube M, et al: D-lactic acidosis in a man with the short-bowel syndrome. N Engl J Med 1979; 301:249–252.

Olsson K: Central control of vasopressin release and thirst. Acta Paediatr Scand 1983; 305(Suppl):36–39.

Pallone TL, Turner MR, Edwards A, Jamison RL: Countercurrent exchange in the renal medulla. Am J Physiol 2003; 284:R1153–R1175.

Palmer BF, Alpern RJ: Metabolic alkalosis. J Am Soc Nephrol 1997; 8:1462–1469.

Passey RB, Gillum RL, Fuller JB, et al: Evaluation of three methods for the measurement of urea nitrogen in serum as used on six instruments. Am J Clin Pathol 1980; 73:362–368.

Perazella MA, Biswas P: Acute hyperkalemia associated with intravenous epsilon-aminocaproic acid therapy. Am J Kidney Dis 1999; 33:782–785.

Perez GO, Oster JR, Vaamonde CA: Serum potassium concentration in acidemic states. Nephron 1981; 27:233–243.

Phelps KR, Lieberman RL, Oh MS, Carroll HJ: Pathophysiology of the syndrome of hyporeninemic hypoaldosteronism. Metabol 1980b; 29:186–199.

Phelps KR, Oh MS, Carroll HJ: Heparin-induced hyperkalemia: report of a case. Nephron 1980a; 25:254–258.

Pierrat A, Gravier E, Saunders C, et al: Predicting GFR in children and adults: a comparison of the Cockcroft-Gault, Schwartz, and modification of diet in renal disease formulas. Kidney Int 2003; 64:1425–1436.

Pradella M, Dorizzi RM, Rigolin F: Relative density of urine: methods and clinical significance. Crit Rev Clin Lab Sci 1988; 26:195–242.

Price CP, Finney H: Developments in the assessment of glomerular filtration rate. Clin Chim Acta 2000; 297:55–66.

Rakhmanina NY, Kearns GL, Farrar HC 3rd: Hypokalemia in an asthmatic child from abuse of albuterol metered dose inhaler. Pediatr Emerg Care 1998; 14:145–147.

Ramsay AG: Clinical application of the Henderson-Hasselbalch equation. Appl Ther 1965; 7:730–736.

Reed RK, Laurent UB: Turnover of hyaluronan in the microcirculation. Am Rev Respir Dis 1992; 146:S37–S39.

Relman AS, Lennon EJ, Lemann J Jr: Endogenous production of fixed acid and the measurement of the net balance of acid in normal subjects. J Clin Invest 1961; 40:1621–1630.

Rendell M, McGrane D, Cuesta M: Fatal compulsive water drinking. JAMA 1978; 240:2557–2559.

Risch L, Herklotz R, Blumberg A, et al: Effects of glucocorticoid immunosuppression on serum cystatin C concentrations in renal transplant patients. Clin Chem 2001; 47:2055–2059.

Rodriguez Soriano J: Renal tubular acidosis: the clinical entity. J Am Soc Nephrol 2002; 13:2160–2170.

Russel C: J Nucl Med 1985; 25:1243–1247.

Rutishauser J, Kopp P, Gaskill MB, et al: A novel mutation (R97C) in the neurophysin moiety of prepro-vasopressin-neurophysin II associated with autosomal-dominant neurohypophyseal diabetes insipidus. Mol Genet Metab 1999; 67:89–92.

Saaresranta T, Polo-Kantola P, Irjala K, et al: Respiratory insufficiency in postmenopausal women: sustained improvement of gas exchange with short-term medroxyprogesterone acetate. Chest 1999; 115:1581–1587.

Sands JM, Kokko JP: Current concepts of the countercurrent multiplication system. Kidney Int 1996; 57(Suppl):S93–S99.

Schmidt-Nielsen B: Excretion in mammals: role of the renal pelvis in the modification of the urinary concentration and composition. Fed Proc 1977; 36:2493–2503.

Schoenmakers CH, Kuller T, Lindemans J, Blijenberg BG: Automated enzymatic methods for creatinine measurement with special attention to bilirubin interference. Eur J Clin Chem 1993; 31:861–868.

Schrier RW, Berl T, Anderson RJ: Osmotic and nonosmotic control of vasopressin release. Am J Physiol 1979; 236:F321–F332.

Schultheis PJ, Lorenz JN, Meneton P, et al: Phenotype resembling Gitelman's syndrome in mice lacking the apical Na$^+$ Cl$^-$ cotransporter of the distal convoluted tubule. J Biol Chem 1998 273:29150–29515.

Schwartz GJ, Haycock GB, Edelman CM, Spitzer A: A simple measure of glomerular filtration rate in children derived from body length and plasma creatinine. Pediatrics 1976; 58:259–263.

Sebastian A, Rector FC Jr, Schambelan M: Mineralocorticoid-resistant renal hyperkalemia without salt wasting (type II pseudohypoaldosteronism): role of increased renal chloride reabsorption. Kidney Int 1981; 19:716–727.

Seyberth HW, Rascher W, Schweer H, et al: Congenital hypokalemia with hypercalciuria in preterm infants: a hyperprostaglandinuric tubular syndrome different from Bartter syndrome. J Pediatr 1985; 107:694–701.

Siggaard C, Rittig S, Corydon TJ, et al: Clinical and molecular evidence of abnormal processing and trafficking of the vasopressin preprohormone in a large kindred with familial neurohypophyseal diabetes insipidus due to a signal peptide mutation. J Clin Endocrinol Metab 1999; 84:2933–2934.

Sjoland JA, Marcher KS: Creatinine concentration measurement in glucose based peritoneal dialysate. Scand J Clin Lab Invest 2003; 63:203–206.

Smith HW: The Kidney: Structure and Function in Health and Disease. New York: Oxford University Press, 1951, pp 231–238.

Sonnenblick M, Friedlander Y, Rosin AJ: Diuretic-induced severe hyponatremia. Review and analysis of 129 reported patients. Chest 1993; 103:601–660.

Spencer K: Analytical reviews in clinical biochemistry: the estimation of creatinine. Ann Clin Biochem 1986; 23:1–25.

Spruce BA, Baylis PH, Kerr DN, Morley AR: Idiopathic hypergammaglobulinaemia associated with nephrogenic diabetes insipidus and distal renal tubular acidosis. Postgrad Med J 1984; 60:493–494.

Steen B: Hypokalemia—clinical spectrum and etiology. Acta Med Scand 1981; 647(Suppl):61–66.

Stewart GW, Ellory JC: A family with mild hereditary xerocytosis showing high membrane cation permeability at low temperatures. Clin Sci 1985; 69:309–319.

Stewart GW, Corrall RJ, Fyffe JA, et al: Familial pseudohyperkalaemia. A new syndrome. Lancet 1979; 2:175–177.

Stowasser M, Bachmann AW, Jonsson JR, et al: Clinical, biochemical and genetic approaches to the detection of familial hyperaldosteronism type I. J Hypertens 1995; 13:1610–1613.

Suzuki M, Yoshida M: A new enzymatic serum creatinine measurement based on an endogenous creatine-eliminating system. Clin Chim Acta 1984; 143:147–155.

Swain RR, Biggs SL: Positive interference with the Jaffe reaction by cephalosporin antibiotics. Clin Chem 1977; 23:1340–1342.

Sweeney G, Klip A: Regulation of the Na$^+$/K$^+$-ATPase by insulin: why and how? Mol Cell Biochem 1998; 182:121–133.

Torpy DJ, Gordon RD, Lin JP, et al: Familial hyperaldosteronism type II: description of a large kindred and exclusion of the aldosterone synthase (CYP11B2) gene. J Clin Endocrinol Metab 1998; 83:3214–3218.

Uribarri J, Oh MS, Carroll HJ: D-lactic acidosis. A review of clinical presentation, biochemical features, and pathophysiologic mechanisms. Medicine (Baltimore) 1998; 77:73–82.

Van Acker BA, Koomen GC, Koopman MG, et al: Creatinine clearance during cimetidine administration for measurement of glomerular filtration rate. Lancet 1992; 340:1326–1329.

Vargas-Poussou R, Huang C, Hulin P, et al: Functional characterization of a calcium-sensing receptor mutation in severe autosomal dominant hypocalcemia with a Bartter-like syndrome. J Am Soc Nephrol 2002; 13:2259–2266.

Veech RL, Kashiwaya Y, King MT: The resting membrane potential of cells are measures of electrical work, not of ionic currents. Integr Physiol Behav Sci 1995; 30:283–307.

Vokes TJ, Gaskill MB, Robertson GL: Antibodies to vasopressin in patients with diabetes insipidus. Implications for diagnosis and therapy. Ann Intern Med 1988; 108:190–195.

Warnock DG: Liddle's syndrome: genetics and mechanisms of Na$^+$ channel defects. Contrib Nephrol 2001; 136:1–10.

Wasserman K, Stringer WW, Casaburi R, Zhang YY: Mechanism of the exercise hyperkalemia: an alternate hypothesis. J Appl Physiol 1997; 83:631–643.

Watkins PJ: The effect of ketone bodies on the determination of creatinine. Clin Chim Acta 1967; 18:191–196.

Weber JA, van Zanten AP: Interferences in current methods for measurements of creatinine. Clin Chem 1991; 37:695–700.

Weir B: Pituitary tumors and aneurysms: case report and review of the literature. Neurosurg 1992; 30:585–591.

Weisberg HF: Osmotic pressure of the serum proteins. Ann Clin Lab Sci 1978; 8:155–164.

Weisberg LS: Pseudohyponatremia: a reappraisal. Am J Med 1989; 86:315–318.

Wells T: Vesicular osmometers, vasopressin secretion and aquaporin-4: a new mechanism for osmoreception? Mol Cell Endocrinol 1998 15; 136:103–107.

Wilson FH, Disse-Nicodeme S, Choate KA, et al: Human hypertension caused by mutations in WNK kinases. Science 2001; 293:1107–1112.

Wilson FH, Kahle KT, Sabath E, et al: Molecular pathogenesis of inherited hypertension with hyperkalemia: the Na-Cl cotransporter is inhibited by wild-type but not mutant WNK4. Proc Natl Acad Sci USA 2003; 100:680–684.

Ylinen EA, Ala-Houhala M, Harmoinen AP, Knip M: Cystatin C as a marker for glomerular filtration rate in pediatric patients. Pediatr Nephrol 1999; 13:506–509.

Zaltzman M, Bezwoda WR: Hyperkalaemia in prolymphocytic leukaemia – a sometimes spurious result. A case report. S Afr Med J 1982; 6; 61:209–210.

Analytical Techniques

Total calcium measurements include protein-bound calcium and ionized calcium; alternatively, ionized calcium alone can be measured. The total calcium measurement is easier to perform in the laboratory, but this result must be interpreted in clinical context. For example, patients with malignancies often exhibit hypoalbuminemia, a condition that may result in falsely low total calcium levels. When this occurs, the total calcium level (expressed in mg/dL) can be corrected with the following equation:

Total calcium (mg/dL) corrected for hypoalbuminemia = Total calcium (measured) + [(Normal albumin − Patient's albumin) × 0.8]

An albumin of about 4.4 is typically used as the normal value in the above formula. This corrected value is a more accurate assessment of the patient's calcium status. Since albumin is the primary protein that binds calcium, variations in this protein are clinically significant. Only a small percentage of calcium binds to other proteins such as gammaglobulins. Therefore, clinical states such as hypogammaglobulinemia are unlikely to drastically alter the total calcium levels.

Total and Ionized Calcium. Although many total calcium procedures have been reported, only three methods are commonly used: (1) colorimetric analysis with metallochromic indicators; (2) atomic absorption spectrometry (AAS); and (3) indirect potentiometry.

Total calcium is most widely measured by spectrophotometric determination of the colored complex when various metallochromic indicators or dyes bind calcium. Orthocresolphthalein complexone (CPC) and arsenazo III are the most widely used indicators. CPC reacts with calcium to form a red color in alkaline solution, which is measured near 580 nm. Interference by magnesium ions is reduced by the addition of 8-hydroxyquinoline. Arsenazo III reacts with calcium to form a calcium-indicator complex usually measured near 650 nm. The stable reagent exhibits high specificity for calcium at slightly acidic pH.

Atomic absorption spectrophotometry is the reference method for determining calcium in serum. Despite its greater accuracy and precision compared with other methods, very few laboratories continue to use AAS for routine determination of total calcium. This may be because laboratories performing large numbers of sample determinations rely on automated methods that are not widely available for this technique. In addition, the level of equipment maintenance required in this technique is difficult for high-volume laboratories.

In indirect potentiometry, an electrode selective for calcium measures a sample that is also measured against a sodium-selective electrode, and calcium concentrations are proportional to the difference in potential between the electrodes.

Instruments with calcium-selective electrodes provide accurate, precise, and automatic determinations of free (ionized) calcium. Calcium ion-selective electrodes (ISEs) consist of a calcium-selective membrane enclosing an inner reference solution of $CaCl_2$, AgCl and other ions, and a reference electrode.

Reference Interval

The reference interval for total calcium in normal adults ranges between 8.8–10.3 mg/dL (2.20–2.58 mmol/L). Serum is the preferred specimen for total calcium determination, although heparinized plasma is also acceptable. Citrate, oxalate, and ethylenediaminetetraacetic acid (EDTA) interfere with commonly used methods. Other factors that have been reported to interfere with the colorimetric methods include hemolysis, icterus, lipemia, paraproteins, and magnesium.

The reference interval for *ionized (free) calcium* in normal adults is 4.6–5.3 mg/dL (1.16–1.32 mmol/L). Whole blood, heparinized plasma, or serum may be used. Specimens should be collected anaerobically and transported on ice and stored at 4°C to prevent loss of CO_2, glycolysis, and to stabilize pH (since pH changes alter the ionized calcium fraction). Proper collection technique is important to ensure accurate ionized calcium results; a tourniquet left on too long can lower pH at the site of collection and falsely elevate levels.

The reference interval for *urinary calcium* varies with diet. Individuals on an average diet excrete up to 300 mg/day (7.49 mmol/day). Urine specimens should be collected with appropriate acidification to prevent calcium salt precipitation.

Phosphorus

Physiology

Distribution. The total body phosphorus content in normal adults is around 700–800 g. Approximately 80–85% is present in the skeleton; the remaining 15% is in the ECF in the form of inorganic phosphate and intracellularly in the soft tissues as organic phosphates such as phospholipids, nucleic acids, and ATP. The skeleton contains primarily inorganic phosphate, predominantly as hydroxyapatite and calcium phosphate.

In blood, organic phosphate is located primarily in erythrocytes, with the plasma containing mostly inorganic phosphate. Approximately two-thirds of blood phosphorus is organic, while only about 3–4 mg/dL of the total of 12 mg/dL represents the inorganic form. Inorganic phosphate in serum exists as both divalent (HPO_4^{2-}) and monovalent ($H_2PO_4^-$) phosphate anions, both of which represent important buffers. The ratio of $H_2PO_4^-$: HPO_4^{2-} is pH dependent and varies between 1 : 1 in acidosis, 1 : 4 at pH of 7.4, and 1 : 9 in alkalosis. Approximately 10% of the serum phosphorus is bound to proteins; 35% is complexed with sodium, calcium, and magnesium; and the remaining 55% is free. Only inorganic phosphorus is measured in routine clinical settings.

Function. In addition to its role in the skeleton, phosphate has important intracellular and extracellular functions. Phosphate is an important constituent of nucleic acids in that both RNA and DNA represent complex phosphodiesterases. In addition, phosphorus is contained in phospholipids and phosphoproteins. It forms high-energy compounds (ATP) and cofactors (NADP) and is involved in intermediary metabolism and various enzyme systems (adenylate cyclase). Phosphorus is essential for normal muscle contractility, neurologic function, electrolyte transport, and oxygen carrying by hemoglobin (2,3-DPG).

Phosphorus Homeostasis. Most blood phosphate is derived from diet, but some is derived from bone metabolism. Phosphorus is present in virtually all foods. The average dietary intake for adults is about 800–1400 mg, most of which is derived from dairy products, cereals, eggs, and meat. About 60–80% of the ingested phosphate is absorbed in the gut, mainly by passive transport. However, there is also an active energy-dependent process, which is stimulated by $1,25(OH)_2D_3$. Phosphorus is freely filtered in the glomerulus. More than 80% of the filtered phosphorus is reabsorbed in the proximal tubule and a small amount in the distal tubule. Proximal reabsorption occurs by passive transport coupled to sodium (Na–P cotransport). Phosphorus intake and PTH mainly regulate this cotransport. Phosphorus restriction increases reabsorption, and intake decreases it. PTH induces phosphaturia by inhibition of Na–P cotransport. The effect is exerted mainly in the proximal tubule. The hormone binds to specific receptors in the basolateral membrane, resulting in the activation of two pathways – the adenylate cyclase/cyclic AMP/protein kinase A and the phospholipase C/calcium/protein kinase C systems, both of which are involved in the inhibition of Na–P cotransport (Bellorin-Font, 1990).

While PTH lowers serum phosphate, serum levels of phosphate are increased by administration of vitamin D and growth hormone. Vitamin D increases intestinal absorption and renal reabsorption of phosphorus. Growth hormone is a main regulator of skeletal growth. Its presence in the bloodstream reduces renal excretion of phosphates, thereby increasing serum levels.

Analytical Techniques

Most commonly used methods for determination of inorganic phosphate are based on the reaction of phosphate with ammonium molybdate to form phosphomolybdate complex. Direct UV measurement of the colorless unreduced complex by absorption at 340 nm, as originally described by Daly and Ertinghausen in 1972, has been adapted for use on most of the automated analyzers. Alternatively, the phosphomolybdate complex can be reduced by a wide variety of agents (e.g., aminonaphtholsulfonic acid, ascorbic acid, methyl-*p*-aminophenol sulfate, ferrous sulfate) to produce molybdenum blue, which can be measured at 600–700 nm. The formation of phosphomolybdate complex is pH dependent, and the rate of its formation is influenced by protein concentration. Measurements of unreduced complexes have the advantages of being simple, fast, and stable. An enzymatic method has also been described whereby phosphorus undergoes successive enzymatic reactions catalyzed by glycogen phosphorylase, phosphoglucomutase, and glucose-6-phosphate dehydrogenase (G6PD). The NADPH produced can be quantitated fluorometrically or spectrophotometrically. The reaction takes place at neutral pH, thus permitting the measurement of inorganic phosphorus in the presence of unstable organic phosphate.

Serum is preferred because most anticoagulants, except heparin, interfere with results and yield falsely low values. Phosphorus levels are increased by prolonged storage with cells at room temperature. Hemolyzed specimens are unacceptable because erythrocytes contain high levels of organic esters, which are hydrolyzed to inorganic phosphate during storage, and thus yield elevated levels.

Reference Interval

In normal adults, serum phosphorus varies between 2.8–4.5 mg/dL (0.89–1.44 mmol/L). Higher phosphorus levels occur in growing children (4.0–7.0 mg/dL or 1.29–2.26 mmol/L). Serum phosphate is best measured in fasting morning specimens because of a diurnal variation, with higher levels in the afternoon and evening, as well as a reduction in serum phosphate after meals. Levels are influenced by dietary intake, meals, and exercise.

Magnesium

Physiology

Distribution. Magnesium is the fourth most abundant cation in the body after calcium, sodium, and potassium; it is the second most prevalent intracellular cation. The normal body magnesium content in an adult is approximately 1000 mmol or 22.66 g, of which 50–60% is in bone, and the remaining 40–50% is in the soft tissues. One-third of skeletal magnesium is exchangeable and probably serves as a reservoir for maintaining a normal extracellular magnesium concentration.

Only 1% of the total body magnesium (TBMg) is in extracellular fluid. In serum, about 55% of magnesium is ionized or free magnesium (Mg^{2+}), 30% is associated with proteins (primarily albumin), and 15% is complexed with phosphate, citrate, and other anions. The interstitial fluid concentration is approximately 0.5 mmol/L. In CSF, 55% of the magnesium is free or ionized and the remaining 45% is complexed with other compounds (Elin, 1988).

Approximately 99% of the TBMg is in bone matrix or is intracellular. About 60% of this total is within bone matrix and the other 40% is within skeletal muscle, within blood cells, or in the cells of other tissues. Intracellular magnesium concentration is approximately 1–3 mmol/L (2.4–7.3 mg/dL). Within the cell, magnesium is compartmentalized, and most of it is bound to proteins and negatively charged molecules; approximately 80% of cytosolic magnesium is bound to ATP. Significant amounts of magnesium are found in the nucleus, mitochondria, and endoplasmic reticulum. Free magnesium accounts for 0.5–5.0% of the total cellular magnesium, and is the fraction that is probably important as a cofactor supporting enzyme activity.

Function. Magnesium is essential for the function of more than 300 cellular enzymes, including those related to the transfer of phosphate groups, all reactions that require ATP, and every step related to the replication and transcription of DNA and the translation of mRNA. This cation is also required for cellular energy metabolism and has an important role in membrane stabilization, nerve conduction, ion transport, and calcium channel activity. In addition, magnesium plays a critical role in the maintenance of intracellular potassium concentration by regulating potassium movement through the membranes of the myocardial cells. Thus, magnesium deficiency can result in a variety of metabolic abnormalities and clinical consequences including refractory plasma electrolyte abnormalities (especially depressed potassium) and cardiac arrhythmias most often observed after stress such as cardiac surgery (Weisinger, 1998).

Magnesium Homeostasis. Total body magnesium depends mainly on gastrointestinal absorption and renal excretion. The average dietary intake of magnesium fluctuates between 300–350 mg/day, and the intestinal absorption is inversely proportional to the ingested amount. The factors controlling the intestinal absorption of magnesium remain poorly understood.

The kidney is the principal organ involved in magnesium regulation. The renal excretion is about 120–140 mg/24 h for a person on a normal diet. Approximately 70–80% of the plasma magnesium is filtered through the glomerular membrane. Tubular reabsorption of Mg^{2+} is different from that for other ions because the proximal tubule has a limited role and 60–70% of the reabsorption of Mg^{2+} takes place within the thick ascending loop of Henle (Quamme, 1989). Even though the distal tubules reabsorb only 10% of the filtered Mg^{2+}, they are the major sites of magnesium regulation. Many factors, both hormonal and nonhormonal (e.g., parathyroid hormone, calcitonin, glucagon, and vasopressin, and magnesium restriction, acid–base changes, and potassium depletion), influence both the Henle's loop and distal tubule reabsorption. However, the major regulator of reabsorption is the plasma concentration of Mg^{2+} itself. Increased Mg^{2+} concentration inhibits loop transport, whereas decreased concentration stimulates transport regardless of whether or not there is magnesium depletion. The mechanisms appear to be regulated by the Ca^{2+}/Mg^{2+}-sensing receptor, located on the capillary side of the thick-ascending-limb cells, which senses the changes in Mg^{2+} (Quamme, 1997).

Other factors that may also play a role in magnesium regulation include calcium concentration and rate of sodium chloride reabsorption.

In magnesium deficiency, serum levels decrease and this leads to reduced urinary excretion. Later, bone stores of magnesium are affected as the process of equilibration with bone stores takes place over several weeks.

Since serum only contains about 1% of total body magnesium, it may not accurately reflect total stores. In general, a low serum level indicates deficiency and a high level indicates adequate stores. However, the most common result – a normal level – should be interpreted with caution since it does not exclude an underlying deficiency. The most accurate assessment of magnesium status is generally considered to be the loading test wherein magnesium is given intravenously. Magnesium-deficient individuals retain a greater proportion of the load and excrete less in the urine than normal individuals (Papazachariou, 2000). However, the test is uncommonly used because it is difficult to administer.

Analytical Techniques

Total Magnesium. Serum is preferred over plasma for magnesium determination because anticoagulant interferes with most procedures. Serum magnesium is usually measured by photometry. The reference method for total magnesium is atomic absorption spectrophotometry (AAS). Most clinical laboratories use a photometric method on an automated analyzer. These methods use metallochromic indicators or dyes that change color upon selectively binding magnesium from the sample. Some of the chromophores used include calmagite, methylthymol blue, formazan dye, and magon. In the calmagite photometric method, which is the one most commonly used, calmagite forms a colored complex with magnesium in alkaline solution. This complex is stable for over 30 minutes, and its absorbance at 520 nm is directly proportional to the magnesium concentration in the specimen aliquot.

Ionized (Free) Magnesium.

Ionized magnesium can be measured with magnesium ion-selective electrodes (ISEs) that have been incorporated into several commercial clinical analyzers (Huijgen, 1999). These ISEs employ neutral carrier ionophores that are selective for Mg^{2+}. However, in addition to Mg^{2+}, these ISEs also measure Ca^{2+}, thus requiring a chemometric correction to calculate the true free magnesium levels in the sample. Studies have shown significant differences in the measured ionized magnesium on different analyzers that were attributed to the interference from free calcium in the sample as well as to the insufficient specificity and a lack of standardization of the calibrators (Hristova, 1995; Cecco, 1997). Further improvements in the methodology for ISEs for ionized magnesium will improve the performance and increase the availability of Mg^{2+} determination in the clinical laboratory.

As with ionized calcium determinations, ionized magnesium measurements are affected by pH. The rate of change of ionized magnesium measurements is not as significant as that seen in ionized calcium determinations. The changes of magnesium in relation to alterations of pH are similar to those of ionized calcium, although less well characterized. With an increase in pH, ionized magnesium is decreased, and with a decrease in pH, it is increased (Wang, 2002).

Reference Interval

The reference interval for serum *total magnesium* in normal adults ranges between 0.75–0.95 mmol/L (1.7–2.2 mg/dL or 1.5–1.9 mEq/L). There appear to be no significant sex or age differences. Erythrocyte magnesium is about three times that of serum. The magnesium concentration in CSF is 2.0–2.7 mg/dL (1.0–1.4 mmol/L). The reference interval for *ionized magnesium* depends on the analyzer used for its measurement and varies from 0.44–0.60 mmol/L (Hristova, 1995).

Hormones Regulating Mineral Metabolism

The three principal hormones regulating mineral and bone metabolism are parathyroid hormone (PTH), 1,25-dihydroxyvitamin D_3 (1,25$(OH)_2D_3$) and calcitonin. PTH and 1,25$(OH)_2D_3$ are the primary hormones that exert an effect, while calcitonin is less prominent in the cycle that maintains mineral metabolism. In addition, the metabolic effects of calcitonin are less well understood.

Parathyroid Hormone
Physiology

Synthesis. PTH is synthesized and secreted by the chief cells of the parathyroid gland. Intact PTH is a single-chain polypeptide consisting of 84 amino acids with a molecular mass of 9500 Da. It is derived from a

II

larger precursor, pre-pro-PTH, of 115 amino acids, which undergoes two successive cleavages, both at the amino-terminal sequences. This yields, first, an intermediate precursor, pro-PTH, and then the hormone itself. Any pro-PTH that reaches the circulation is immediately converted to PTH and other products.

Secretion. Multiple factors control the release of PTH from the parathyroid glands, but only a small number are known to be physiologically important. PTH secretion is regulated on a time scale of seconds by extracellular ionized calcium and represents a simple negative-feedback loop. Extracellular signals are detected by a calcium-sensing receptor, located on the plasma membrane of the parathyroid cell. Stimulation of this receptor leads to a suppression of the rate of PTH secretion via intracellular signals (inositol triphosphate and diacylglycerol) generated by the active receptor. The receptor is present in parathyroid glands, the calcitonin-secreting cells of the thyroid, brain, and kidney. This G-protein-linked receptor is mutated in the disorders of familial hypocalciuric hypercalcemia, neonatal severe hyperparathyroidism, and autosomal dominant hypocalcemia (Mundy, 1999).

Ionized magnesium has been also shown to influence the secretion of PTH. Hypocalcemic patients with low serum magnesium concentration often require administration of magnesium to increase the serum PTH levels before the serum calcium concentration can be restored to the desired interval. Chronic severe hypomagnesemia such as that seen in alcoholism has been associated with impaired PTH secretion, whereas an acute decrease in the serum magnesium concentration can lead to an increased PTH.

Other levels of PTH control include regulation of PTH gene transcription and parathyroid chief cell mass by vitamin D and extracellular calcium. 1,25-Dihydroxyvitamin D_3 chronically suppresses the synthesis of PTH by interacting with the vitamin D receptors in the parathyroid gland.

Function. The primary physiologic function of PTH is to maintain the concentration of ionized calcium in the ECF, which is achieved by the following mechanisms: (1) stimulation of osteoclastic bone resorption and release of calcium and phosphate from bone; (2) stimulation of calcium reabsorption and inhibition of phosphate reabsorption from the renal tubules; and (3) stimulation of renal production of $1,25\text{-}(OH)_2D_3$, which increases intestinal absorption of calcium and phosphate. The amino-terminal end of the PTH molecule binds to the PTH receptor, which modulates adenylate cyclase and phospholipase C. Activating mutations in this receptor may cause the hypercalcemia and the epiphyseal disorganization seen in Jansen's chondrodysplasia (Bastepe, 2004).

The net effect of PTH actions on bone, kidney, and indirectly on intestine include increased serum total and ionized calcium concentrations and decreased serum phosphate. Its immediate effects on the kidney are to increase renal plasma flow and cause a diuresis. At the level of the distal convoluted tubule, it causes increased reabsorption of calcium and chloride with the exchange of phosphate into the urine. These effects are mediated through its activation of renal adenyl cyclase. As a result, there is an increase in urinary cyclic adenosine monophosphate (cAMP) and in urinary phosphate with a mild secondary hyperchloremic acidosis. In the absence of disease, the increase in serum calcium reduces PTH secretion through a negative-feedback loop, thus maintaining the calcium homeostasis. If this negative-feedback loop is interrupted by an autonomously functioning parathyroid gland sufficiently to increase resting calcium to abnormally high levels, the capacity of the distal tubules to reabsorb calcium is exceeded and hypercalciuria results.

Heterogeneity. PTH metabolism is complex and produces several fragments of varying biological and immunologic reactivity. The intact PTH is the biologically active form and has a half-life in the circulation of less than 4 minutes. The kidney and liver clear intact PTH rapidly. In the liver, intact PTH is cleaved into discrete fragments and smaller peptides that are released into the circulation. The released inactive carboxy-terminal fragments circulate considerably longer than the intact hormone, mainly because they are cleared exclusively by glomerular filtration (Mundy, 1999).

Analytical Techniques

Historically, PTH immunoassays were developed to measure mid-region, N-terminal and C-terminal regions. However, these assays cross-reacted with amino acid sequences present in both mid-region and carboxyl fragments of the intact hormone and measured mostly inactive fragments since they are present in greater concentration than the intact molecule. Since the kidney clears inactive PTH fragments, results from these assays were difficult to interpret, especially in patients with impaired renal function. PTH intact is measured by *noncompetitive immunometric (sandwich)* assays, which, depending on the type of detection system used, are divided into *immunoradiometric* (IRMA), when radiolabeled, and *immunochemiluminometric*, when labeled with a chemiluminescent compound. Most

automated systems use immunochemiluminometric assays. These immunometric assays have several advantages over earlier assays: (1) increased sensitivity and specificity through the use of sequence-specific and affinity-purified antibodies, (2) extended assay concentration range, (3) decreased incubation time, and (4) they do not utilize radioactive compounds

Reference Interval

The reference interval for intact PTH in normal adults is 10–65 pg/mL (ng/L) when a two-site immunometric method is used. Studies have demonstrated that intact PTH is secreted in episodic or pulsatile fashion, with an overall circadian rhythm characterized by a nocturnal rise in intact PTH. Serum is the preferred specimen for measurement of PTH. Prolonged storage of the specimen aliquot causes falsely decreased levels.

Bio-Intact PTH

Physiology

The traditional tests for intact PTH detect and measure both the biologically intact 84-amino-acid PTH molecule (1-84) as well as its minimally active to inactive metabolites. Recall that the intact, biologically active molecule is cleaved within minutes to the many metabolites that have a longer half-life and of which there is a much higher concentration in the circulation at any given time. One of these cleavage products, the 7-84 PTH breakdown fragment, is a weak antagonist to PTH activity and may actually lower patient serum calcium levels. It is therefore important to distinguish between the intact PTH and breakdown products in the setting of patients with chronic renal failure (Brossard, 2000). In uremic patients, the metabolites including the 7-84 breakdown fragment accumulate due to decreased renal clearance, and can therefore give the impression of an elevated PTH (Quarles, 1992).

Recent advances have made available a test for only the biologically active, intact PTH. This third-generation test eliminates interference by the metabolites and is of great clinical utility in patients with impaired renal function. The bio-intact PTH test specifically measures the (1-84) molecule via a two site chemiluminescent assay. This assay yields a higher specificity than the second-generation tests for the biologically active intact PTH, but cost and availability considerations make this a second-line test used primarily in following metabolic bone status in renal insufficiency patients.

The normal ranges for this test show seasonal variation, due in part to lower serum 25(OH)D during the wintertime in the healthy population. Normal values for this test range from 8–50 pg/mL (Nichols Advantage, 2004).

Intraoperative PTH

Historically, parathyroid surgery has consisted of bilateral neck exploration in an attempt to identify enlarged parathyroid glands. In recent years, clinical practice has moved away from this costly and invasive procedure that often requires an overnight hospital stay, to minimally invasive parathyroidectomy with or without the use of a hand-held gamma probe. This procedure consists of preoperative administration of technetium-99m sestamibi 2 hours preoperatively and then performing a parathyroid scan. The parathyroid adenoma, with its increased numbers of cytoplasmic mitochondria, selectively absorbs large amounts of this radioactive substance that then allows for identification of the adenoma(s) with a hand-held gamma probe. This method of identifying the enlarged gland allows for removal of only the hyperfunctional parathyroid gland in cases of parathyroid adenoma. Cases of parathyroid hyperplasia still require bilateral neck exploration. Depending on the size of these enlarged glands, they may or may not be identified on the preoperative parathyroid scan (Goldstein, 2000; Sofferman, 1998; Sokoll, 2000).

Once the hyperfunctioning parathyroid gland is identified via sestamibi scan, and only a single parathyroid gland has been shown to be involved, patients are taken to surgery for minimally invasive parathyroidectomy. This approach has reduced surgical and hospital costs, as well as admission time (Goldstein, 1991).

Prior to surgery, a baseline PTH value is obtained. Following incision, dissection to the radioactive parathyroid gland is then guided by use of a gamma probe. Once identified, the parathyroid gland is removed. Following removal, the surgeon waits about 10–20 minutes and obtains a post-removal PTH value. This post-removal PTH value should decrease to at least 50–75% below the preoperative level or have a 'significant' trend toward normal in patients with markedly elevated preoperative PTH levels. The decrease in PTH levels reassures the surgeon that the adenomatous gland has been removed. If there has been no or minimal decrease in the intraoperative PTH level, the surgeon is obligated to resume neck exploration for additional abnormal glands, and either multiple adenomas or hyperplasia is suggested as the underlying process. Intraoperative PTH testing is recommended for patients undergoing surgery for primary hyperparathyroidism, reoperative hyperparathyroidism and venous/tumor localization presurgery in the angiography suite (Sokoll, 2004).

Analytical Techniques

The intraoperative technique for intact PTH customarily requires blood collected in an EDTA tube (plasma) or a red top tube (serum). The sample is maintained at a cold temperature to minimize breakdown, and is submitted for rapid PTH testing. These immunochemiluminometric assays provide rapid results by modifying certain test parameters on the standard assay. Specifically, increased incubation temperature, continuous shaking of the reaction contents and alterations in sample and reagent volumes are used to expedite antibody–antigen reactions. The end result is a more rapid assay, albeit one that is more costly, less sensitive and more imprecise than the standard assay. These assays correlate well with standard assays and are totally acceptable for measuring large drops in PTH concentration during surgery.

Parathyroid Hormone-Related Peptide
Physiology

Parathyroid hormone-related peptide (PTH-rP) was first discovered in tumors derived from lung, breast, kidney, and other solid tissues. It has since been described as a hormone with paracrine and autocrine functions. PTH-rP is composed of 141 amino acids and shows significant homology with PTH in the first 13 amino acids. It is the product of a large gene on chromosome 12 that is syngeneic to the PTH gene on chromosome 11. This peptide shares the same receptor as PTH. Its actions include binding to and activating the PTH receptor, thus simulating the PTH biological effects on bone, kidney, and intestine. Like PTH, PTH-rP increases bone resorption by stimulating osteoclasts and promotes renal tubular reabsorption of calcium. The net effect is elevated serum calcium concentration. It is now known that PTH-rP is produced by approximately 50% of primary breast cancers and its production may be enhanced by bone-derived factors such as transforming growth factor-β (Yin, 1999). Other malignant tumors also elaborate this peptide. PTH-rP has been implicated as the agent responsible for humoral hypercalcemia in patients with malignancy.

Elevation of PTH-rP has been observed in approximately 50–90% of patients with malignancy-associated hypercalcemia. Increased PTH-rP is seen in squamous cell carcinomas of the lung, esophagus, cervix, and skin as well as other malignancies (e.g., islet cell carcinomas, T-cell and B-cell lymphomas, multiple myeloma). PTH-rP levels are normal in patients with primary hyperparathyroidism, hypoparathyroidism, chronic renal failure, and other conditions with hypercalcemia.

Some benign hyperplasias may also elaborate this peptide, including massive mammary hypertrophy, VIP-secreting tumors, pheochromocytomas, and lactational changes of the breast (Strewler, 1997).

A recent study demonstrated that PTH-rP has therapeutic potential in the treatment of postmenopausal osteoporosis; PTH-rP increased bone mineral density by nearly 5%, a rate that exceeds those of current therapeutic approaches (Horwitz, 2003).

Analytical Technique and Reference Interval

PTH-rP is measured by immunometric assay (usually IRMA) in which antibodies to different sequences of the PTH-rP molecule are used as capture antibodies and radiolabeled signal antibodies. The limit of detection of these assays is between 0.1–1.0 pmol/L (Endres, 1999). The reference interval for PTH-rP is method dependent. In normal individuals, PTH-rP levels range from undetectable to around 2 pmol/L whereas the mean concentration of PTHrP in patients with humoral hypercalcemia of malignancy has been reported to be 22.2 pmol/L.

Calcitonin
Physiology

Synthesis and Metabolism. Calcitonin is synthesized and secreted by the specialized C cells (parafollicular cells) of the thyroid gland and acts on the bones, kidneys, and gastrointestinal tract. Circulating immunoreactive calcitonin is derived from a larger precursor, and the monomeric form is the only biologically active entity. Calcitonin monomer is a 32-amino-acid peptide with a molecular mass of 3500 Da. The ionized calcium concentration is the most important regulator of calcitonin secretion. Increases in ionized calcium lead to an increase in the calcitonin secretion. Other potent calcitonin secretagogues are the gastrointestinal peptide hormones and gastrin in particular (Care, 1971). The latter could explain the presence of a mild postprandial increase in calcitonin concentration.

The calcitonin receptor is structurally similar to the PTH/PTH-rP and secretins receptors; it exists in several isoforms, and its expression seems to be influenced by ambient concentrations of calcitonin itself (Mundy, 1999). Calcitonin is metabolized within minutes of secretion, primarily by the kidney.

Physiologic Role and Clinical Use. Although calcitonin has been viewed as a major calcium-regulating factor because of its calcium-lowering and phosphorus-lowering properties, its precise physiologic role is still unclear. Calcitonin directly inhibits osteoclastic bone resorption by direct binding to osteoclasts. The effect of this binding action is observed within minutes after calcitonin administration. This inhibition is transient and likely has little role in overall calcium homeostasis, although it may be important in the short-term control of calcium loads. Calcitonin also inhibits the action of PTH and vitamin D. While some clinical studies suggest that serum calcium does not appear to be affected in patients with total thyroidectomy, other studies suggest that medullary thyroid carcinoma and excess of calcitonin can give rise to marked hypocalcemia. In the kidney, calcitonin causes increased clearance of calcium and phosphate. The mechanisms of its action on the GI tract have not entirely been elucidated.

In addition to the evaluation of calcitonin in the setting of bony abnormalities, testing for calcitonin is an important adjunct in the evaluation of the patient with nodular thyroid disease, and is often performed in the hopes of identifying the patient with early medullary thyroid carcinoma, which may be seen in the setting of MEN II. Therapeutic success in medullary thyroid carcinoma hinges on its early identification, and slight elevations of calcitonin with subsequent surgical exploration of the thyroid may identify this lesion in its early, nonpalpable stage of development. It is well known that the therapeutic efficacy is poor in cases that are identified as well-developed palpable tumors because many such patients already have metastatic disease (Rieu, 1995; Horvit, 1997).

Therapeutic applications of calcitonin have been explored and include its use in the treatment of osteoporosis and also in the treatment of Paget's disease, the early stages of which are characterized by increased bone resorption.

Analytical Technique and Reference Interval

In the past, serum calcitonin was measured primarily by radioimmunoassay (RIA). However, differences in assay specificity and sensitivity, matrix and nonspecific serum effects, and the heterogeneity of the circulating calcitonin have contributed to contradicting results and discrepancies in the reference values for the hormone. At present, a number of highly sensitive (limit of detection as low as 2 pg/mL), two-site immunometric methods (electroimmunoassays [EIAs] and immunoradiometric assays [IRMAs]) for serum calcitonin are available. These tests are now regarded as the most reliable methods of testing for serum calcitonin.

The reference interval for serum calcitonin in normal adults is less than 25 pg/mL for males, and less than 20 pg/mL for females. Gender, age, growth, pregnancy, lactation, and ingestion of food have been reported to affect the levels of calcitonin.

Vitamin D and Metabolites
Physiology

Synthesis and Metabolism. The steroid hormone $1,25(OH)_2D_3$ is the major biologically active metabolite of the vitamin D sterol family. The vitamin D precursor (cholecalciferol or vitamin D_3) is either ingested in the diet or synthesized in the skin from 7-dehydrocholesterol (provitamin D_3) through exposure to sunlight. The plant-derived form of vitamin D is called vitamin D_2 or ergosterol. Neither form of vitamin D has any significant biological activity; both must be metabolized to hormonally active forms. This activation occurs in two steps, the first of which takes place in the liver and the second of which takes place in the kidney. Cholecalciferol is transported to the liver bound to a specific α_1-globulin. In the liver, vitamin D undergoes hydroxylation to produce 25-hydroxyvitamin D (calcidiol), a metabolite with limited biological activity. Since the liver only loosely regulates this step, circulating levels of 25-hydroxyvitamin D mirror the amounts of vitamin D that are either ingested or synthesized by the skin. The 25-hydroxyvitamin D is then bound by the vitamin D-binding protein and transported to the kidney, where it undergoes further hydroxylation by 1-alpha hydroxylase in the proximal tubular mitochondria to form the more potent metabolite $1,25(OH)_2D_3$ (calcitriol). The renal hydroxylation of 25-hydroxyvitamin D is the major controlling point in vitamin D metabolism, a step that is regulated by serum phosphate, calcium, and circulating PTH concentrations. PTH and phosphate depletion act independently to increase $1,25(OH)_2D_3$

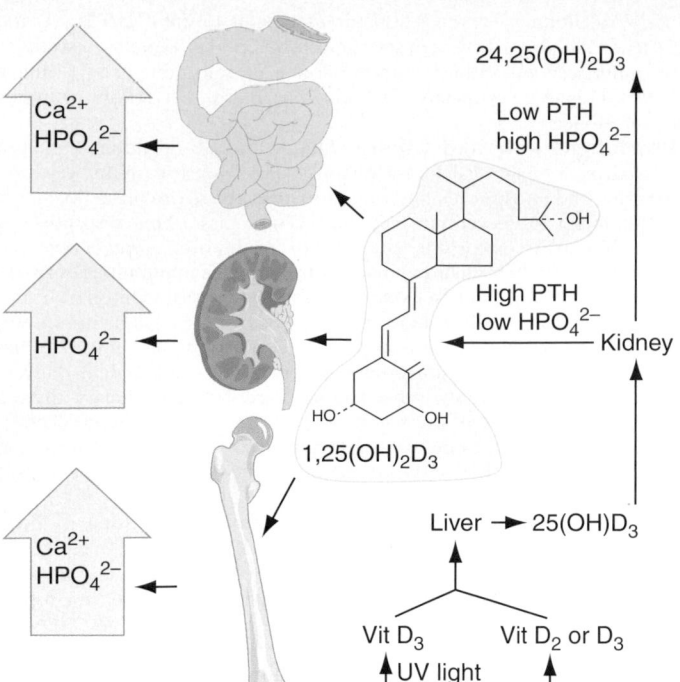

Figure 15–3 Pathways of vitamin D synthesis and their end-organ effects. The large green arrows indicate increases in calcium and phosphate induced by vitamin D (dihydroxycholecalciferol).

production by inducing 1-alpha hydroxylase activity, with PTH being the more potent stimulus. Decreased blood calcium stimulates the parathyroid glands to secrete PTH, which in turn increases production of $1,25(OH)_2D_3$ in the renal proximal tubules. Conversely, a rise in blood calcium suppresses PTH secretion, which lowers the production of $1,25(OH)_2D_3$. The only other known important extrarenal sites of $1,25(OH)_2D_3$ production are in the placenta and in granulomatous tissue. In humans, the half-life of $1,25(OH)_2D_3$ in the circulation is approximately 5 hours. It is excreted as urinary and fecal metabolites (Mundy, 1999). There are several other vitamin D metabolites produced in the kidney, most of which have been shown to be biologically inert. The most notable of these is 24,25-dihydroxyvitamin D_3, produced by the action of 24-alpha hydroxylase in the kidney; it is activated when PTH levels are low or when inorganic phosphate levels are elevated (Fig. 15–3).

Physiologic Role. $1,25(OH)_2D_3$ bound to a vitamin D-binding protein is delivered to the intestine, where the free form is taken up by the cells and transported to a specific nuclear receptor protein. Although the receptor binds several forms of vitamin D, its affinity for 1,25-dihydroxyvitamin D_3 is about 1000 times that of 25-hydroxyvitamin D_3, thus accounting for why the former is so much more biologically active than the latter. As a result of this interaction in the intestine, calcium-binding protein is synthesized. In bone, osteocalcin, osteopontin, and alkaline phosphatase are produced. In the intestine, the net effect of $1,25(OH)_2D_3$ is to transport calcium and phosphate from the lumen of the small intestine into the circulation by stimulating the expression of calcium carrying proteins, thus increasing plasma calcium and phosphate concentrations. It also increases bone resorption and enhances the effects of PTH in the nephron to promote renal tubular calcium reabsorption. $1,25(OH)_2D_3$ is a powerful differentiating agent for committed osteoclast precursors, causing their maturation to form multinucleated cells that are capable of resorbing bone. These pathways enable $1,25(OH)_2D_3$ to provide a supply of calcium and phosphate available at bone surfaces for the formation of normal mineralized bone (Mundy, 1999).

The demonstration that the sites of action of $1,25(OH)_2D_3$ are not limited to its target tissues, namely, the intestine, bone, and kidney, has expanded the therapeutic function of vitamin D. Administration of vitamin D hormone has been shown to be effective in the therapeutic management and prevention of postmenopausal and age-related osteoporosis. There is evidence that besides its calciotropic properties, vitamin D may also be a developmental hormone.

Analytical Techniques

Of the more than 35 metabolites of vitamin D_2 and vitamin D_3, only 25(OH)D and $1,25(OH)_2D$ measurements are clinically important. 25(OH)D is a better marker than vitamin D for evaluation of vitamin D

Table 15–1 Causes of Hypercalcemia

PTH mediated
Primary hyperparathyroidism (most common):
Sporadic
Multiple endocrine neoplasia (types 1 and 2)
Familial hypocalciuric hypercalcemia
Ectopic secretion of PTH by neoplasms (rare)?
Non-PTH mediated
Malignancy associated (most common)
Vitamin D mediated:
Vitamin D intoxication
Increased generation of $1,25(OH)_2D$
Other endocrinopathies:
Thyrotoxicosis
Hypoadrenalism
Immobilization with increased bone turnover
Milk–alkali syndrome
Sarcoidosis
Multiple myeloma

status because of its longer half-life (2–3 weeks vs. 5–8 hours) (Papapoulos, 1982), more limited fluctuation with exposure to sunlight and dietary intake, larger concentration, and ease of measurement. Measurement of $1,25(OH)_2D_3$ is useful in detecting certain states of inadequate or excessive hormone production in the evaluation of hypercalcemia, hypercalciuria, and hypocalcemia, as well as in bone and mineral disorders. Because both vitamin D_2 and vitamin D_3 are metabolized to compounds of similar if not equal biological activity, for clinical purposes, the assays should measure $25(OH)D_2$ and $25(OH)D_3$ or $1,25(OH)_2D_2$ and $1,25(OH)_2D_3$, respectively. At present, most assays for vitamin D metabolites are measured by radioimmunoassay or chemiluminescent immunoassay.

Reference Interval

The reference interval for 25(OH)D in serum is approximately 10–50 ng/mL (25–125 nmol/L) and for $1,25(OH)_2D$ is 15–60 pg/mL (36–144 pmol/L) (Endres, 1999). Levels for 25(OH)D are influenced by sunlight exposure, latitude, skin pigmentation, sunscreen use, and hepatic function. 25(OH)D levels also exhibit seasonal variation. Winter values may be 40–50% lower than summer values because of reduced UV radiation exposure. Concentrations of vitamin D metabolites also vary with age and are increased in pregnancy.

Disorders of Mineral Metabolism

Hypercalcemia

Increased serum calcium is associated with anorexia, nausea, vomiting, constipation, hypotonia, depression, high-voltage T waves on electro-cardiography, and occasionally lethargy and coma. Persistent hypercalcemia or persistently elevated calcium–phosphorus ionic activity product may cause ectopic depositions of calcium in tissues throughout the body. This may take the form of ectopically calcified blood vessel walls associated with necrotic skin lesions in calciphylaxis. It may also lead to calcifications in viable tissues (metastatic calcification), particularly those developing pH gradients with localized relative alkalosis (e.g., pulmonary alveolar walls, renal medullary pyramids, and deep gastric mucosa). The most common causes of hypercalcemia are primary hyperparathyroidism and malignant neoplasms, which account for 80–90% of all patients with hypercalcemia. Less frequent causes include renal failure, diuretics, vitamin A and D intoxication, lithium therapy, milk–alkali syndrome, immobilization, hyperthyroidism and other nonparathyroid endocrinopathies, and familial hypercalciuric hypercalcemia (Table 15–1).

Primary hyperparathyroidism (PHPT) is characterized by excessive secretion of PTH in the absence of an appropriate physiologic stimulus and with no response to the physiologic negative feedback loop of hypercalcemia. This results in a generalized disorder of calcium, phosphate, and bone metabolism. Approximately 100 000 cases of PHPT occur each year in the US, and the incidence increases with age. The disease affects women twice as frequently as it affects men. The majority of the cases are caused by solitary parathyroid adenomas. Other causes include multiple parathyroid adenomas, hyperplasia, and rarely, parathyroid carcinoma. Hypercalcemia in PHPT is characteristically associated with decreased serum phosphate

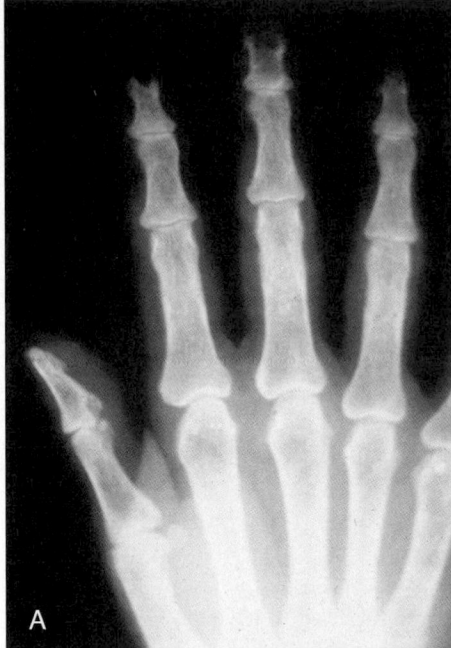

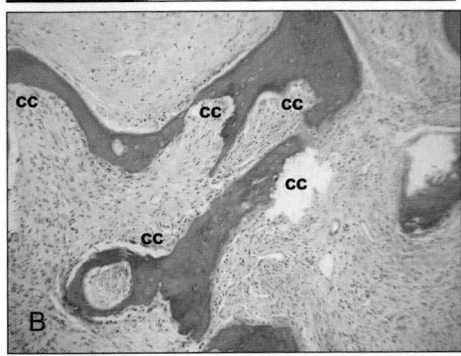

Figure 15–4 Hyperparathyroid bone disease (osteitis fibrosa cystica). *A*, The hand radiograph demonstrates scalloped cortical resorption on the radial (left) side of the phalanges and radiolucency of the terminal phalangeal tufts. *B*, Biopsy of compact bone with advanced hyperparathyroid disease demonstrates conversion of compact to cancellous bone with internal resorption of Haversian systems by osteoclastic cutting cones (CC) and paratrabecular fibrosis (100 ×).

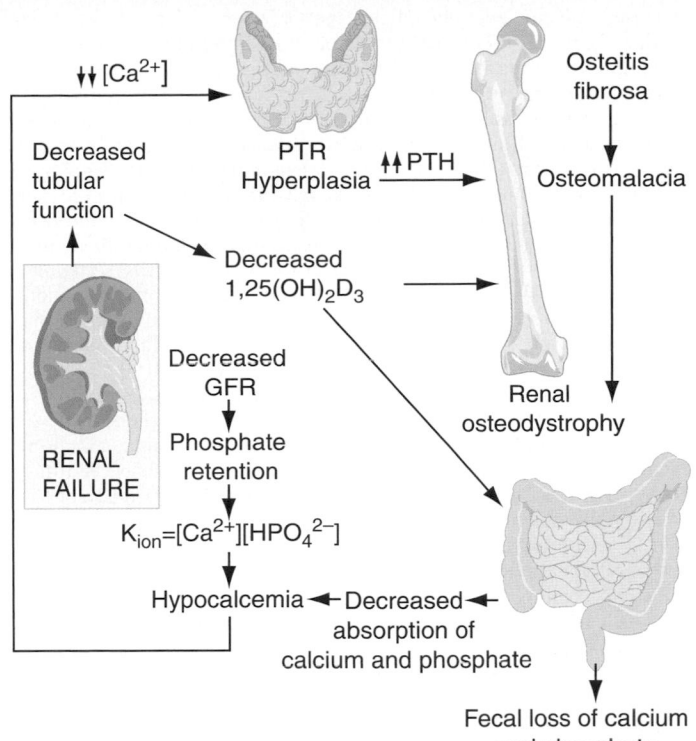

Figure 15–5 Relationships leading to renal osteodystrophy in chronic renal failure.

due to PTH-induced phosphate diuresis and is frequently accompanied by mild acidosis from decreased renal reabsorption of bicarbonate. The hypercalcemia is attributed to (1) the direct action of PTH on bone, causing increased resorption; (2) PTH-activated renal tubular reabsorption; and (3) PTH-stimulated increased renal biosynthesis of $1,25(OH)_2D_3$, which increases intestinal absorption of calcium (Boden, 1990). Half or more of the patients with PHPT are asymptomatic. Symptomatic patients usually present with recurrent nephrolithiasis, chronic constipation, mental depression, neuromuscular dysfunction, recurrent chronic pancreatitis, peptic ulcer, and less frequently with unexplained or premature osteopenia (Deftos, 1993). The unique bone manifestation of PHPT is osteitis fibrosa cystica generalizata. This is characterized by diffuse skeletal radiolucency with focal cystic bone lesions, subperiosteal bone resorption most pronounced in the digits, and osseous deformities on routine X-ray films. Histologically, there is paratrabecular fibrosis and marrow hypervascularity accompanied by increased numbers of osteoclasts causing trabecular scalloping (Howship's lacunae) as a result of accelerated bone resorption (Fig. 15–4A and B). As the disease progresses, there is gradual replacement of the marrow cavity by fibrous tissue. The process is even more pronounced in compact bone, where large aggregates of osteoclasts demonstrate wedge-shaped resorption that enlarges Haversian canals (cutting cones). Fractures that develop through this altered bone tend to heal poorly and result in space-occupying lesions filled with fibrous tissue, multinucleated giant cells, hemorrhage, and hemosiderin; these are sometimes referred to as 'brown tumors' even though they are not neoplastic. Generalized osteitis fibrosa cystica is now very uncommon because serum calcium and phosphate screening usually reveals early parathyroid hyperfunction long before signs or symptoms develop.

PHPT may also be inherited as an autosomal dominant trait and present as a part of *multiple endocrine neoplasia* (MEN). MEN 1 consists of hyperparathyroidism and tumors of the pituitary gland and pancreas. It is often associated with Zollinger–Ellison syndrome, characterized by islet cell tumors with gastrin hypersecretion and peptic ulcer disease. MEN 2A consists of hyperparathyroidism, pheochromocytoma, and medullary carcinoma of the thyroid. Studies have identified the molecular defects in hyperparathyroidism. A gene locus on chromosome 11 has been associated with MEN 1. The same locus appears to be lost in approximately 25% of solitary parathyroid adenomas, implying that the same defect responsible for MEN 1 can also cause the sporadic disease.

Secondary hyperparathyroidism is present when there is resistance to the metabolic actions of PTH, such as in patients with renal failure, vitamin D deficiency (osteomalacia), and pseudohypoparathyroidism. This leads to parathyroid gland hyperplasia and excessive production of PTH. The pathogenesis varies somewhat, depending on the nature and severity of renal disease. However, decreased renal excretion of phosphate as a consequence of impaired glomerular filtration is paramount. In such patients, there is an initial tendency towards hypocalcemia because as phosphate levels rise, calcium levels decrease because their ionic activity product constant makes their serum concentrations inversely related. In addition, in chronic renal failure there is reduced production of $1,25(OH)_2D$ by the kidney. Decreased $1,25(OH)_2D$ causes a reduced response of the skeleton to PTH, and decreased calcium absorption from the intestine, contributing to hypocalcemia. Because of the decreased serum ionic calcium, there is positive feedback to increase parathyroid hormone secretion; this causes parathyroid gland hyperplasia. The initial clinical manifestations include low to normal serum calcium and hyperphosphatemia. Later, in cases with severe secondary hyperparathyroidism, both hypercalcemia and hyperphosphatemia develop. In addition, bone pain, ectopic calcifications, and pruritus may be seen. The complex bone disease occurring in secondary hyperparathyroidism and renal failure is usually termed renal osteodystrophy (Fig. 15–5) and is discussed in greater depth below. Autonomous hyperparathyroidism may sometimes supervene in the setting of chronic parathyroid stimulation. Typical patients are those with chronic renal failure or with some other disease that chronically lowers serum ionized calcium levels and stimulates long-term parathyroid hormone secretion. This chronic parathyroid stimulation results in increased parathyroid mass and diffuse parathyroid hyperplasia. If the increased levels of parathyroid hormone are not diminished by hypercalcemia, whether it occurs in the setting of continued calcium wasting or if the calcium level is corrected (e.g., after renal transplantation), the clinical syndrome is sometimes referred to as *tertiary hyperparathyroidism*. Patients with this syndrome may have parathyroid adenomas, parathyroid hyperplasia, and even parathyroid carcinomas. There is also a tendency for these patients to develop metastatic calcifications because their transiently increased calcium and phosphate levels may exceed the ionic activity product for these ions and cause precipitation of the excess.

Malignant tumors are the most frequent cause of hypercalcemia in the hospital inpatient population. *Malignancy-associated hypercalcemia* can be divided into cases with or without bony metastases. Radiolucent bone lesions indicative of metastatic disease are frequently seen in patients with hematologic malignancies (multiple myeloma, lymphomas, and leukemias), lung carcinoma, renal cell carcinoma, and thyroid carcinoma. Several possible mechanisms have been implicated in the development of malignancy-associated hypercalcemia, including direct tumor lysis, secretion of osteoclast-activating factor by tumor cells, secretion of lymphokines with osteoclast potentiating activity such as interleukin-1 and tumor necrosis factor. Conventional bone X-rays and bone scanning can detect most bony metastases. Hypercalcemia without bony metastases is also known as *humoral hypercalcemia of malignancy* (HHM). Diagnosis in these cases, in general, is more difficult since the primary tumor may be occult. A variety of tumor types have been associated with this syndrome including renal carcinoma, hepatocellular carcinoma, carcinomas of the head and neck, lung carcinomas, and islet cell tumors of the pancreas. The most common cause of HHM is a secretion of PTH-rP by the tumor. The diagnosis is highly suggestive when there is increased urinary cAMP excretion (typically seen in hyperparathyroidism) in the setting of reduced or normal PTH.

Vitamin D intoxication is another cause of hypercalcemia and is usually the result of excessive intake of vitamin supplements over a prolonged period of time. Excess vitamin D causes increased calcium absorption by the intestines, enhanced bone resorption, and hypercalciuria. PTH is suppressed, but the frequent development of renal failure may make it difficult to exclude hyperparathyroidism; 25(OH)D has been implicated as the major metabolite responsible for the syndrome. The diagnosis is supported by careful history-taking, measurements of 25(OH)D, and a prompt response following steroid administration. Clinically, vitamin D intoxication is manifest by weakness, irritability, nausea, vomiting, and diarrhea. Soft tissue calcification is a common feature, since serum phosphorus tends to be elevated. Intoxication may persist for months because of storage of vitamin D in adipose tissue.

Hypercalcemia associated with *granulomatous disorders* is commonly seen in patients with sarcoidosis and less frequently in patients with tuberculosis, silicone-induced granulomas, and fungal diseases such as coccidioidomycosis and candidiasis. Renal failure, soft tissue calcification, nephrolithiasis and severe hypercalcemia are potential manifestations. Different mechanisms in the development of hypercalcemia have been implicated, including enhanced sensitivity to vitamin D, increased concentration of vitamin D metabolites, and unregulated generation of $1,25(OH)_2D$ by macrophages in granulomatous tissue.

Milk–alkali syndrome was first reported in patients with peptic ulcer disease taking large amounts of milk and absorbable alkali (e.g., calcium carbonate). Recently, a rise in the incidence of the syndrome has been reported; this may be due to the widespread use of calcium carbonate preparations in the treatment and prophylaxis of osteoporosis. The syndrome is manifest by hypercalcemia, hypocalciuria, alkalosis, azotemia, and soft tissue calcifications.

Laboratory testing in the differential diagnosis of hypercalcemia includes measurements of serum total and ionized calcium, urine calcium, serum and urine phosphorus, alkaline phosphatase, albumin, intact PTH, PTH-rP, and urine cAMP. Determination of various other analytes can provide valuable information in selected cases (e.g., growth hormone, cortisol, cortisone suppression test, selective venous catheterization with measurement of local PTH concentration, and measurements of vitamin D metabolites). Meaningful interpretation of the relevant laboratory data often requires various special studies in addition to a complete history and physical examination. Renal function tests and studies of acid–base balance may be indicated. Histopathologic examination of bone biopsy specimens from appropriate sites can be of unique value in selected cases.

Hypocalcemia

Chronic hypocalcemia presents with neuromuscular and neurologic manifestations including muscle spasms, carpopedal spasm, peripheral and perioral paresthesias, cardiac arrhythmias, lengthening of the QT interval and low-voltage T waves on the electrocardiogram, and, in severe cases, laryngeal spasm and convulsions. Respiratory arrest may occur. Severe hypocalcemia will eventually result in tetany. There are many causes of hypocalcemia, which can be divided into several major categories: (1) deficiencies in PTH production or secretion, (2) resistance to PTH action, (3) deficiency of vitamin D or vitamin D metabolites, and (4) deficiencies in bone mineralization with normal metabolism of PTH and vitamin D

Table 15–2 Causes of Hypocalcemia

PTH mediated

PTH deficiency:
  Permanent:
    Acquired:
      Postsurgical
    Hereditary:
      Idiopathic hypoparathyroidism
      DiGeorge syndrome (branchial dysgenesis)
      Polyglandular autoimmune syndromes
  Reversible:
    Severe hypomagnesemia
    Longstanding hypercalcemia
PTH resistance:
  Pseudohypoparathyroidism

Vitamin D mediated

Vitamin D deficiency

25(OH)D deficiency

$1,25(OH)_2$ deficiency:
  Reversible inhibition of 1-hydroxylase
  Intrinsic renal defects (chronic renal failure, tubulopathies, Fanconi's syndrome)

Defective response to $1,25(OH)_2D$
  Mutations of vitamin D receptor

(Table 15–2). The most common causes of hypocalcemia are chronic renal failure, hypomagnesemia, hypoparathyroidism, pseudohypoparathyroidism, vitamin D deficiency, and acute pancreatitis. Less frequently, low plasma calcium may be seen in critically ill patients with sepsis, burns, and acute renal failure. Transient hypocalcemia can be observed after administration of a number of drugs, including heparin, glucagon, protamine, as well as after massive transfusions of citrated blood products.

Hypoparathyroidism, hereditary or acquired, is characterized by diminished or absent PTH production by the parathyroid glands, which leads to a fall in plasma calcium and a corresponding hyperphosphatemia. In addition, these patients also have absent or low levels of $1,25(OH)_2D$. In the past, acquired hypoparathyroidism secondary to neck surgeries and thyroidectomies, in particular, was more common than hereditary hypoparathyroidism. With improvement in surgical techniques, however, its incidence has diminished dramatically. Hereditary hypoparathyroidism can occur as an isolated entity with a variable pattern of inheritance (idiopathic hypoparathyroidism), in association with defective development of both the thymus and the parathyroid glands (DiGeorge syndrome or branchial dysgenesis), or as part of a complex hereditary autoimmune syndrome involving failure of the adrenals, ovaries, and the parathyroids, usually referred to as autoimmune polyglandular deficiency. Hereditary hypoparathyroidism is often manifested within the first decade of life. In addition to low or absent PTH and hypocalcemia, certain skin manifestations, such as alopecia and candidiasis frequently occur.

Pseudohypoparathyroidism (PHP), also known as Albright's hereditary osteodystrophy, is a rare genetic disorder in which there is an ineffective PTH action rather than a failure of parathyroid gland hormone production. Clinically, PHP presents with some of the features of hypoparathyroidism such as extraosseous calcifications, extrapyramidal symptoms and signs such as choreoathetotic movements and dystonia, chronic changes in fingernails and hair, lenticular cataracts, and increased intracranial pressure with papilledema. Serum calcium is depressed despite an increased concentration of PTH, suggesting a resistance to PTH. Moreover, whereas infusion of PTH in patients with hypoparathyroidism generally results in a marked increase in both urinary cAMP and phosphaturia, patients with PHP usually respond with subnormal urinary phosphate excretion and cAMP production. This is due to a defect in the stimulatory G protein of adenylate cyclase that is necessary for the action of PTH.

Hypocalcemia associated with hypomagnesemia is associated with both deficient PTH release from the parathyroid glands and impaired responsiveness to the hormone.

Hypocalcemia associated with hypovitaminosis D may occur as a result of inadequate production of vitamin D_3 in the skin, insufficient dietary supplementation, inability of the small intestine to absorb adequate amounts of the vitamin from the diet, and resistance to the effects of vitamin D. The latter may be due to deficient or defective receptors for $1,25(OH)_2D$ or use of drugs that antagonize vitamin D action.

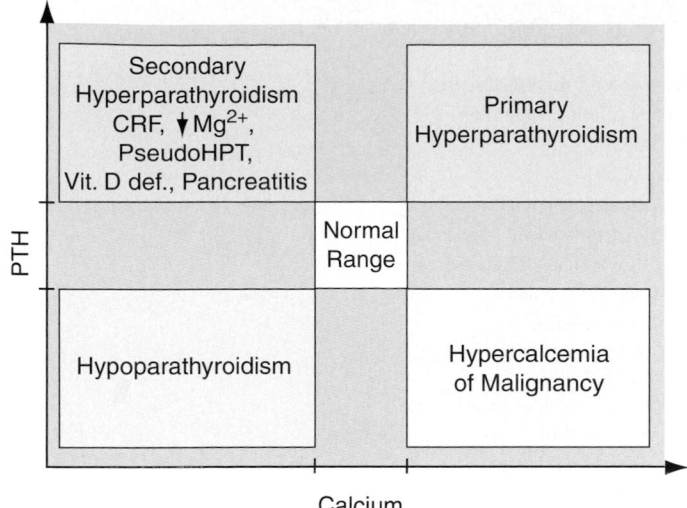

Figure 15–6 Graph correlating alterations in serum calcium levels and parathyroid hormone levels with the diseases most frequently causing these alterations.

Table 15–3 Serum Calcium, Phosphate, and Vitamin D Levels in Various Disorders

Disorder	Calcium	25(OH)D	1,25(OH)D	Phosphate
25(OH)D intoxication	High	High	Low, normal	Normal, high
Primary hyperparathyroidism	High	Normal	Normal, high	Low
Secondary hyperparathyroidism	Low	Low, normal, high	Low, normal, high	Low, normal, high
Tertiary hyperparathyroidism	Normal, high*	Low, normal, high	Low, normal, high	Low, normal, high
Malignancy	High	Normal	Low, normal	Low
Vitamin D deficiency	Low	Low	Low, normal, high	Low
Renal failure	Low	Normal	Low	High
Hyperphosphatemia	Low	Normal	Low	High
Vitamin D rickets type I, II	Low	Normal, high	Low, normal, high	Low
Granulomatous diseases (sarcoid/TB)	High	Low, normal, high	High	Normal, high
Postmenopausal osteoporosis	Normal	Normal	Normal	Normal
Senile osteoporosis	Normal	Normal	Normal	Normal
Osteomalacia	Low, normal	Low, normal	Low	Low, normal, high

* Calcium may be normal in the setting of concurrent $1,25(OH)_2D_3$ deficiency.

Hypovitaminosis D is associated with disturbances in mineral metabolism and secretion of PTH and mineralization defects in the skeleton such as rickets in children and osteomalacia in adults (see below). Decreased levels of vitamin D lead to insufficient intestinal absorption of calcium and hypocalcemia, followed by an increased secretion of PTH (secondary hyperparathyroidism). Increased PTH stimulates calcium release from bone and decreases calcium clearance by the kidney, thus increasing the calcium levels in the circulation. If hypovitaminosis D persists, severe hypocalcemia may occur.

An inherited disorder, characterized by a defective production of $1,25(OH)_2D$ in the kidney, has been described. In this syndrome, known as *pseudovitamin D-deficient rickets* or *vitamin D-dependent rickets type I*, there is a deficiency in the renal 25(OH)D-1α-hydroxylase activity, which results in a low production of $1,25(OH)_2D$ and decreased levels in the circulation, but with a normal response to physiologic doses of calcitriol. In vitamin D-dependent rickets type II, mutations impair the function of the $1,25(OH)_2D$ receptor by altering the binding of the hormone to the receptor, causing elevated levels of circulating $1,25(OH)_2D$. Although administration of high doses of calcitriol produces further increases in the levels of $1,25(OH)_2D$, there is no physiologic response. Another inherited disease associated with impaired vitamin D metabolism is X-linked hypophosphatemic rickets. This condition is characterized by a functional defect in 25(OH)D-1α-hydroxylase, hypophosphatemia, and normal or low serum levels of $1,25(OH)_2D$. Figure 15–6 summarizes the more common etiologies of abnormal calcium levels along with their differential diagnoses.

Tables 15–3 and 15–4 summarize serum calcium, phosphate, vitamin D levels, and other laboratory values in altered metabolic states.

Hyperphosphatemia

Hyperphosphatemia is usually caused by decreased renal excretion in acute and chronic renal failure; increased intake with excessive oral, rectal, or intravenous administration; or an increased extracellular load due to transcellular shift in acidosis. Less common causes include increased tubular reabsorption in hypoparathyroidism; pseudohypoparathyroidism; and increased extracellular load due to cell lysis in rhabdomyolysis, intravascular hemolysis, leukemia, lymphoma, and cytotoxic therapy. In addition, hyperphosphatemia may be seen secondary to overmedication with vitamin D and production of vitamin D by granulomatous diseases such as sarcoidosis and tuberculosis.

No direct symptoms result from hyperphosphatemia. When high levels are maintained for long periods, however, mineralization is enhanced, and calcium phosphate may be deposited in abnormal sites. Ectopic calcification is a frequent complication in patients with chronic renal failure receiving supplements of vitamin D when correction of hyperphosphatemia is inadequate (Weisinger, 1998).

Hypophosphatemia

Hypophosphatemia is observed in 0.25–2.15% of general hospital admissions. Alcohol abuse is the most common cause of severe hypophosphatemia, probably due to poor food intake, vomiting, antacid use, and marked phosphaturia. It is also caused by ingestion of large amounts of nonabsorbable antacids that bind phosphate. Hypophosphatemia is induced by a number of mechanisms, including internal redistribution, increased urinary excretion, decreased intestinal absorption, or a combination of these abnormalities. The most common cause is a shift of phosphorus from extracellular fluid into cells, which can be observed in acute respiratory alkalosis associated with sepsis, salicylate poisoning, alcohol withdrawal, heat stroke, hepatic coma, increased insulin during glucose administration, recovery from diabetic ketoacidosis, and refeeding of malnourished patients. Increased urinary excretion is usually secondary to hyperparathyroidism, renal tubular defects as in Fanconi's syndrome and familial hypophosphatemia, X-linked vitamin D-resistant rickets, aldosteronism, glucocorticoid and mineralocorticoid administration, and

Table 15–4 Laboratory Values in Various Altered States of Calcium Metabolism

	Primary hyperparathyroidism	Humoral hypercalcemia of malignancy	Secondary hyperparathyroidism	Tertiary hyperparathyroidism	Familial hypocalciuric hypercalcemia
Urine calcium	High	High	Normal, high	Normal, high	Low
Serum phosphate	Low	Low	Low, normal, high	Low, normal, high	Low
Urine phosphate	High	High	High	High	High
1,25(OH)D	Normal, high	Low, normal	Low, normal, high	Low, normal, high	Normal, high
PTH intact	High	Low	High	High	High
PTHr protein	Normal	High	Normal	Normal	Normal

Table 15–5 Causes of Abnormal Phosphate Levels

Elevated

Hypoparathyroidism and pseudohypoparathyroidism

Renal failure

Hypervitaminosis D

Cytolysis

Pyloric obstruction

Decreased

Alcohol abuse

Primary hyperparathyroidism

Acute respiratory alkalosis

Myxedema

Exogenous/endogenous steroids

Diuretic therapy

Renal tubular defects

Oncogenic phosphaturia

Diabetic coma

Table 15–6 Causes of Hypomagnesemia

Decreased intake/absorption

Protein calorie malnutrition

Starvation

Alcoholism

Prolonged intravenous therapy

Inadequate parenteral supplementation

Malabsorption (e.g., celiac sprue)

Neonatal gut immaturity

Excessive GI losses:
  Prolonged gastric suction
  Laxatives
  Intestinal or biliary fistula
  Severe diarrhea

Excessive renal losses

Diuretics

Acute tubular necrosis – diuretic phase

Acute renal failure – diuresis

Primary aldosteronism

Hypercalcemia

Renal tubular acidosis

Idiopathic renal wasting

Chronic renal failure with wasting

Miscellaneous

Idiopathic

Acute pancreatitis

Porphyria with SIADH

Multiple transfusions with citrated blood

Endocrine:
  Hyperthyroidism
  Hyperparathyroidism
  Diabetes mellitus with diabetic ketoacidosis
  Hyperaldosteronism

Medications (e.g. cisplatin, ciclosporin, gentamicin, ticarcillin, etc.)

---

diuretic therapy. Hypophosphatemia due to urinary losses is observed in osmotic diuresis, acute volume expansion, and up to 30% of patients with malignant neoplasms such as certain leukemias and lymphomas. In oncogenic hypophosphatemia with osteomalacia, mesenchymal tumors which may be benign or malignant produce hyperphosphaturia by a mechanism in which overproduction of fibroblast growth factor (FGF-23) has been implicated (Nelson, 2003; Folpe, 2004). Increased intestinal loss is seen due to vomiting, diarrhea, and use of phosphate-binding antacids. Decreased intestinal absorption is observed in malabsorption, vitamin D deficiency, and steatorrhea (Table 15–5).

Symptomatic hypophosphatemia is usually observed when plasma phosphorus falls below 0.32 mmol/L. The clinical manifestations include proximal weakness, anorexia, dizziness, myopathy, dysphagia, ileus, respiratory failure due to weakness of the respiratory muscles, impairment of cardiac contractility due to a depletion of ATP in myocardial cells, and metabolic encephalopathy.

Hypermagnesemia

Hypermagnesemia (i.e., plasma Mg^{2+} concentration > 0.9 mmol/L) is rare and usually iatrogenic. Those most at risk are the elderly and patients with bowel disorders or renal insufficiency. Clinical manifestations of hypermagnesemia include hypotension, bradycardia, respiratory depression, depressed mental status, and electrocardiographic (ECG) abnormalities (Weisinger, 1998).

Hypomagnesemia

Magnesium deficiency is found in approximately 11% of hospitalized patients. The usual reason is loss of magnesium from the GI tract or the kidney. Depletion by GI tract occurs during acute and chronic diarrhea, malabsorption, steatorrhea after extensive bowel resection, and in patients with the rare inborn error of metabolism, primary intestinal hypomagnesemia. Excessive Mg^{2+} loss from the kidney is often the basis for magnesium depletion because of sodium reabsorption in the same tubular segments (magnesium transport passively follows that of sodium) or because of a primary defect in renal tubular reabsorption of Mg^{2+}. Factors that can cause Mg^{2+} losses from the urine include thiazide and loop diuretics, increased sodium excretion and volume expansion (parenteral fluid therapy), hypercalcemia and hypercalciuria (hyperthyroidism or malignancy), nephrotoxic drugs (aminoglycoside antibiotics, cisplatin, amphotericin B, ciclosporin). Diabetes mellitus is a common cause of hypomagnesemia, probably secondary to glycosuria and osmotic diuresis. Another important and very common cause for magnesium deficiency is alcohol, which is found in approximately 30% of alcoholic patients admitted to hospital. Sustained and extensive stress including that associated with varied surgical procedures and acute illnesses, may be associated with depressed serum magnesium levels (Table 15–6).

Signs and symptoms of magnesium depletion do not usually appear until extracellular levels have fallen to 0.5 mmol/L or less. Manifestations of significant magnesium depletion are largely due to the associated hypocalcemia and include neuromuscular hyperexcitability characterized by carpopedal spasm, seizures, muscular weakness, depression, psychosis; metabolic abnormalities (carbohydrate intolerance, hyperinsulinism); and cardiac arrhythmias.

Biochemical Markers of Bone Remodeling

The skeleton constantly undergoes a process of remodeling that is essential for bone health. Bone remodeling is a coupled process that begins with resorption of old bone by osteoclasts, followed by the formation of new bone by osteoblasts. Beginning in middle age or earlier, bone loss occurs because resorption exceeds formation, a fact that was identified over 50 years ago by Dr. Alton Fuller, the father of metabolic bone disease. He noted that postmenopausal women had elevated urinary calcium levels and deduced that this reflects a negative calcium balance that can result in osteoporotic fractures. Estrogen deficiency and many other diseases and conditions accentuate bone resorption (Watts, 1999).

Three major diagnostic procedures are available to monitor bone turnover and evaluate metabolic bone disease: bone imaging techniques, bone biopsy, and biochemical markers of bone turnover. While bone density measurement is an important diagnostic tool in osteoporosis, it is difficult for the test to detect increased bone turnover in its early stages or to monitor acute changes. Also, bone densitometry gives a summated measure of mineralized bone matrix; it does not define abnormal distribution of bone loss. Bone biopsy can define the distribution of bone mass and can answer questions about bone mineralization not able to be answered with bone densitometry. However, bone biopsy is invasive and, in the absence of mineralization defects, it provides a relatively static glimpse into long and slowly developing processes; it is not useful in routine clinical management of osteoporosis. In osteoporosis, net bone loss is caused by only a slight imbalance of bone resorption over formation, so conventional markers, such as calcium and PTH, are usually normal. In contrast, bone turnover markers are more sensitive to subtle change and can be used to noninvasively detect and monitor progression of metabolic bone disease. Laboratory assessment of these markers has been the focus of much attention in recent years (Ju, 1997; Souberbielle, 1999).

Bone Resorption Markers

Bone tissue has three components: an organic matrix (called osteoid), bone mineral, and bone cells. Bone resorption markers have included constituents of bone matrix including calcium and collagen degradation products such as hydroxyproline, pyridinium crosslinks, and telopeptides and cellular products such as tartrate-resistant acid phosphatase (TRAP). Urinary calcium is affected by diet and renal function; thus, it is not sensitive or specific for assessment of bone remodeling (Watts, 1999). Tartrate resistant acid phosphatase, a lysosomal enzyme found in osteoclasts, is not considered a useful test. The measurement of the amino acids hydroxyproline and glycosylated (galactosyl and glucosyl-galactosyl) hydroxylysine, is not specific for skeletal collagen, and has been found to correlate poorly with bone resorption, as determined by bone histomorphometry and calcium kinetics. The most useful tests measure pyridinium crosslinks and crosslinked telopeptides.

Pyridinium Crosslinks (Pyridinoline and Deoxypyridinoline)

Collagen fibrils consist of many crosslinked amino acids that effectively stabilize the mature collagen molecule. These include pyridinoline (Pyr), a crosslinked polymer formed from three hydroxylysine residues, and deoxypyridinoline (DPyr) which is formed from two hydroxylysine and one lysine residues. These crosslinks are found in collagen types I, II, and III. While these crosslinks are not unique to bone, they are found in a unique ratio in the bone, a fact that makes these substances ideal candidates as markers for bone breakdown. In the collagen of most other tissues, the ratio of Pyr : DPyr is 10 : 1, while in bone it is 3–3.5 : 1. This difference means that DPyr is more pronounced in bone and metabolic bone disease. DPyr is essentially specific for bone, in that it is only found in relatively significant amounts in bone, and has been shown to correlate well with bone turnover (Robins, 1995). An additional characteristic that makes evaluation of pyridinium-crosslinks ideal is that they are neither metabolized upon their release nor absorbed from the diet. They are excreted in urine in free form (40%) and in peptide-bound form (60%). Since crosslink molecules are only found in mature collagen, their excretion in the urine reflects breakdown of mature collagen and is not an expression of newly synthesized bone collagen (Watts, 1999). Excretion of Pyd and DPyr is increased after menopause and can be utilized to study the effect of hormone replacement therapy on bone turnover (Fledelius, 1994). The clinical applications of measuring these substances include identification of individuals at risk for bone loss, assessment of metabolic bone disease, prediction of bone metastases in cancer patients, and management of antiresorptive therapy. Pyr and Dpyr are measured in urine by HPLC (high pressure liquid chromatography) or immunoassays. Care must be taken to account for the marked diurnal variation that is seen with urinary pyridinolines, with a peak late at night and early in the morning. While a 24-hour urine collection avoids this issue and does not require correction for the creatinine concentration, an early morning fasting sample corrected for creatinine concentration is a more sensitive marker of bone turnover (Bettica, 1992).

Crosslinked Telopeptides

During bone resorption, only 40% of crosslinks are released as free pyridinium crosslinks; the remaining 60% are peptide-attached crosslinks (Risteli, 1993). Type I collagen has two sites with attached crosslinks. These are called telopeptides, and they occur in the amino-terminal and in the carboxy-terminal regions of the collagen molecule. These telopeptides are released into the circulation as collagen is degraded; they are then excreted into the urine. Amino-telopeptides (NTx) and carboxy-telopeptides (CTx) are excreted in the urine and can be measured by immunoassay.

Crosslinked telopeptides have been utilized in estimating relative risks of hip fracture in postmenopausal women, and show promise in predicting such complications of osteoporosis (Chapurlat, 2000; Swaminathan, 2001.).

While baseline levels of crosslinked telopeptides do not necessarily correlate with baseline bone mineral density, their serial measurement has shown the capacity to predict early response to therapy (Fink, 2000). Studies have shown reductions of urinary CTx and NTx in the range of 50–60% in 3–6 months of antiresorptive therapy (Eatell, 2003) and correlation of these reductions with the prediction of long-term bone mass response (Ravn, 2003).

Bone Formation Markers

Bone formation markers include alkaline phosphatase and three by-products of bone matrix synthesis, including osteocalcin and amino- and carboxy-terminal procollagen I extension peptides.

Alkaline Phosphatase (see Ch. 20)

Bone alkaline phosphatase (ALP-B), an osteoblast membrane-bound enzyme, is released into the circulation by phosphatidylinositol glycanase activity and formation of membrane vesicles. Studies have shown that the amount of ALP-B activity in osteoblasts and in bone is proportional to collagen formation; thus, it can provide an index of the rate of bone formation. Human serum contains a variable mixture of ALP isoenzymes from liver, intestine, kidney, and bone. During pregnancy, alkaline phosphatase may be derived from the placenta (Farley, 1994). Certain malignant tumors may also produce a heat-stable ALP isoenzyme. The function of ALP is unknown; however, it has been postulated that ALP probably has a role in the mineralization of newly formed bone. Measurements of total serum ALP are useful to follow disease activity when the amount of bone isoenzyme is exceptionally high such as in Paget's disease or osteosarcoma.

The two major circulating ALP isoenzymes, bone and liver, are difficult to distinguish because they are the products of a single gene and differ only by post-translational glycosylation. Separation of the skeletal ALP can be achieved by heat inactivation, wheat germ agglutinin precipitation, electrophoresis, isoelectric focusing, and two-site immunoradiometric assays. At present, immunoassay is the method of choice because of high specificity and satisfactory precision.

Osteocalcin

Osteocalcin is the major noncollagenous protein of the bone matrix. It is a 49-amino-acid polypeptide that is rich in glutamic acid. Its function is incompletely understood, but may serve as a site of deposition for hydroxyapatite crystals. During bone matrix synthesis, some osteocalcin is released into the circulation and rapidly cleared by the kidney. Osteocalcin can be measured by immunoassay in plasma or serum. However, assays for osteocalcin are not yet standardized, because different antibodies recognize different fragments. Antibodies that recognize both the intact molecule and large amino-terminal mid-molecule fragment appear to provide the best clinical information (Watts, 1999). Recent studies have shown that although vitamin K does not affect the amount of osteocalcin concentration, it does affect the amount of carboxylation. Under-carboxylated osteocalcin has been suggested to be a better predictor of certain outcomes such as fracture (Vergnaud, 1997). Osteocalcin is mainly metabolized in the kidney and to a lesser extent in the liver; the half-life in the circulation is about 5 minutes. Osteocalcin is increased when there is high bone turnover such as occurs in hyperparathyroidism, acromegaly and Paget's disease. It is decreased in hypoparathyroidism, hypothyroidism and in patients on glucocorticoid therapy. Osteocalcin reference intervals are approximately 1.1–11 ng/mL (adult male) and 0.7–6.5 ng/mL (adult female).

Metabolic Bone Disease

Metabolic bone disease may be defined as a general disease of metabolism that affects the entire skeleton. Since the disease is generalized, by definition every bone in the body should reflect these metabolic alterations to some extent. While a very few metabolic disorders (e.g., fluorosis, vitamin A toxicity) may increase bone density, the vast majority of metabolic bone diseases are clinical problems resulting in decreased bone density. The result may be bones with decreased organic matrix with normal mineralization (e.g., osteoporosis), bones with decreased mineral content without a significant decrease in organic matrix (e.g., osteomalacia), and bones with both diminished organic matrix and decreased mineral content (e.g., renal osteodystrophy).

Osteoporosis

Osteoporosis is the most common metabolic disease of bone (Table 15–7). It is a systemic skeletal disorder characterized by decreased organic bone matrix and microarchitectural deterioration of bone tissue, with a subsequent increase in bone fragility and susceptibility to fracture (Ferrari, 1999). While this may be expressed as low bone mineral density as measured by dual-energy X-ray absorptiometry (DEXA), the abnormality in no way reflects abnormal mineralization, since the mineral is normal in both structure and content. Rather, total bone mass is decreased in osteoporosis primarily because of a decrease in bone collagen

Table 15–7 Deficiencies in Organic Bone Matrix

Primary osteoporosis

Idiopathic (children and young adults)

Postmenopausal

Senile

Secondary osteoporosis

Hyperparathyroidism

Hyperadrenocorticism

Hypogonadism

Thyrotoxicosis

Immobilization

Calcium deficiency

Prolonged heparin administration

Miscellaneous (alcoholism, malnutrition, liver disease, rheumatoid arthritis, malabsorption)

Disorders of connective tissue

Osteogenesis imperfecta

Ehlers–Danlos syndrome

Marfan's syndrome

CHAPTER: 15   Biochemical Markers of Bone Metabolism

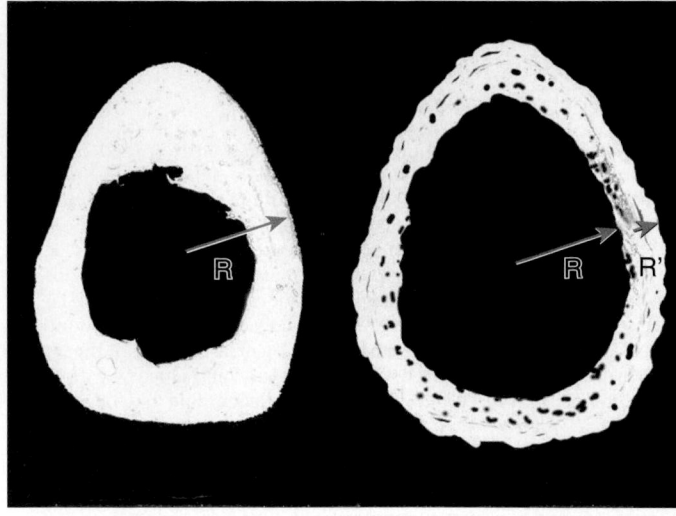

$$\text{Strength} \approx R^3 \qquad \text{Strength} \approx (R+R')^3$$

Figure 15–7 Schematic comparison of femoral cortex in a 30-year-old male (left) and a 75-year-old male (right). Note that the proportionate strength of the bone shaft on the right is greater than that on the left.

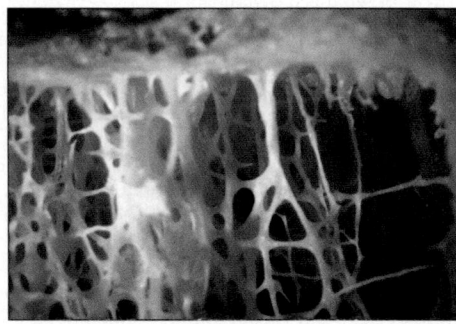

Figure 15–8 Osteoporosis of lumbar vertebra. There is generalized loss of bone. The vertical plates have become more perforated and the number of horizontal cross-braces are decreased markedly in proportion to the vertical plates (compare to Fig. 15–1B).

Bone mass and strength are related to volumetric density, bone size, microarchitecture, and intrinsic tissue quality. These factors are likely to change during bone growth and bone loss, with selective modifications according to the skeletal site. Postmenopausal white and Asian women who are thin or small and have a positive family history are at greatest risk. Other risk factors include cigarette smoking, alcohol abuse, a sedentary lifestyle, and the consumption of too little calcium. Strong evidence indicates that genetic and lifestyle factors are important determinants of peak bone mass.

As bone becomes less dense, it becomes more radiolucent; this appearance may be due to decreased collagen and/or decreased mineral. Collectively, this state is called *osteopenia*, a radiographic term that does not discriminate between the various sorts of metabolic bone disease. This term should not be confused with its use in bone densitometry studies, wherein osteopenia refers to a significant loss of bone density that is about one standard deviation less than is defined as osteoporosis. The radiologic loss of bone mass is due to a loss of compact and cancellous bone, but the most common skeletal problems associated with osteoporosis arise from the loss of cancellous bone. This is as much due to the arrangement of each bone type as it is to actual decreased bone mass.

So long as the bony cortex forms a continuous ring, the strength of the shaft of a long bone is proportional to the distance from the center of the medullary cavity to the outside of the cortex raised to the third power; its stiffness is proportional to this distance raised to the fourth power. Since resorption of compact bone is primarily an endosteal event caused by osteoclasts, this means that as compact bones become more osteoporotic, their shafts become more hollow. The hollowing of the shafts is somewhat compensated for by intramembranous ossification on the cortical surface. Consequently, when the medullary cavity enlarges by endosteal osteoclasis, the diameter of the cortex also enlarges. The enlargement means that the radius from medullary midpoint to outer cortex increases. Since the strength of the intact bone is proportional to this distance raised to the third power, a small increase in appositional bone can biomechanically compensate for a relatively large loss of endosteal bone (Fig. 15–7).

Cancellous (trabecular) bone, on the other hand, is affected earlier by osteoporosis not only because it has less mass but because of its architecture. Cancellous bone is arranged in thin, highly perforated vertically oriented parallel plates braced laterally by even thinner horizontal struts. Only 25% of the cancellous bone compartment is bone by volume; the remaining intertrabecular spaces are filled with fat and marrow (see Fig. 15–1B). Compared with the cortex, the surface to volume ratio in the cancellous bone is very high, giving all bone cells free access to the delicate surfaces of the trabeculae; so cancellous bone is resorbed more rapidly than cortical bone. Furthermore, if osteoclastic resorption progresses at an equal rate in all parts of cancellous bone, the horizontal struts which serve to brace and reinforce the vertical plates are lost earlier because they began with significantly less bone mass than the vertical plates. Resorption of these horizontal braces contributes proportionately more to the morbidity of osteoporosis than the diffuse loss of bone mass. As these struts disappear, the vertical trabeculae form longer and longer vertical line segments that are subject to progressively increased bending forces (Fig. 15–8). Increasing the length of each of these vertical trabecular line segments increases their susceptibility to fatigue

fracture by a factor of the incremental length squared. So if the unprotected length of a vertical plate is doubled, it is four times more likely to fracture. It is not surprising that pain, skeletal deformities and fractures are common sequelae. Osteoporosis may be divided etiologically into primary and secondary types. In primary osteoporosis, there are typical complex associations and patient ages, but the exact etiology of bone loss in not known. The most common type of primary osteoporosis is postmenopausal osteoporosis, which occurs in the setting of hormonal decrease, has its maximal loss of bone mass in the first menopausal decade, and seems to be associated with increased osteoclastic activity. It is manifest mainly as a loss of cancellous bone. So-called 'senile' osteoporosis manifests a decade or more later than the postmenopausal variety and is associated with a decline in osteoblast number proportionate to the demand for their activity; it affects mainly compact bone (Manolagas, 1995). Idiopathic juvenile osteoporosis occurs in the peripubertal period and is associated with increased osteoclastic activity. Unlike the postmenopausal and senile varieties, it is usually self-limited and the skeleton may regain much of its bone mass.

In secondary osteoporosis, there is a known reason for the loss of bone mass that may sometimes be preventable or even reversed. Etiologies include hyperparathyroidism and other endocrinopathies, space-occupying marrow lesions causing increased pressure in the marrow cavity, calcium deficiency, malabsorption, administration of steroids or heparin, and immobilization.

Certain connective tissue disorders such as osteogenesis imperfecta, Marfan syndrome, and Ehlers–Danlos syndrome also result in structural or functional osteoporosis.

Osteomalacia and Rickets

Osteomalacia and rickets are disorders of calcification. Osteomalacia is a failure to mineralize newly formed organic matrix (osteoid) in the mature skeleton. Osteoid formation continues, but the bones gradually become softer as the ratio of osteoid to mineralized bone increases over time.

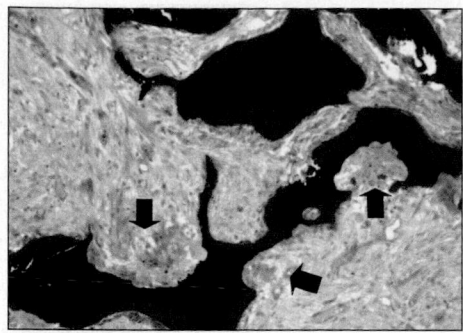

Figure 15–9 Renal osteodystrophy with hyperparathyroidism and osteomalacia. This undecalcified section is stained by the Von Kossa method that stains mineralized bone black and osteoid with Alizarin red. The thick red areas represent seams of newly formed osteoid resulting from renal failure (see Fig. 15–10A). The solid black arrows point to the cutting cones of osteoclasts tunneling into the mineralized substance of the bone trabeculae. Note that these scalloped resorption surfaces occur only in the black areas. The red areas are devoid of osteoclasts and are smooth (250 ×).

Weakness, skeletal pain and deformities, and fractures can occur as the disease progresses. Roentgenographic examination reveals a generalized decrease in skeletal radiodensity. While the skeleton becomes less radiodense, this does not discriminate between absolute loss of mineralization and loss of mineralized organic matrix (osteoporosis).

Rickets, a disease of children, is the designation for osteomalacia that occurs prior to cessation of growth; that is, prior to closure of the epiphyseal plates of long bones. The skeletal deformities in rickets are accentuated as a consequence of compensatory overgrowth of epiphyseal cartilage, wide bands of which remain unmineralized and unresorbed. In severe cases of rickets, decreased growth can be associated with such evident deformities as swelling of the costochondral junctions of the ribs (rachitic rosary), a protuberant sternum, costodiaphragmatic depression (Harrison's sulcus), delayed closure of the anterior fontanelle with frontal bossing, and visibly widened metaphyses of the long bones.

Optimal mineralization requires (1) an adequate supply of calcium and phosphate ions from the extracellular fluid, (2) an appropriate pH (~ 7.6), (3) bone matrix of normal chemical composition and rate of synthesis, and (4) control of inhibitors of mineralization. The major categories of diseases that produce osteomalacia or rickets are vitamin D deficiency states, phosphate depletion, systemic acidosis, and inhibitors of mineralization.

Vitamin D deficiency is particularly important in childhood and may be caused by inadequate dietary intake, intestinal malabsorption, diminished synthesis of active metabolites, increased catabolism, or peripheral resistance to vitamin D action. Dietary deficiency is very uncommon in the US because of the widespread use of fortified milk and bread and vitamin supplements. When vitamin D deficiency occurs in adults, it is usually a consequence of malabsorption. Because vitamin D is a fat-soluble vitamin, its absorption is impaired in celiac disease (nontropical sprue), biliary and pancreatic disease, or steatorrhea from other causes. A systemic resistance to vitamin D can be of major importance in the osteomalacia that accompanies chronic renal disease. On the other hand, hereditary resistance to $1,25(OH)_2D_3$, often called vitamin D-dependent rickets type II, is a rare disorder caused by a variety of defects in the vitamin D receptor.

Renal Osteodystrophy

Renal osteodystrophy refers to the spectrum of bone abnormalities that occur in patients with end-stage renal disease (ESRD): predominantly, osteitis fibrosa cystica, osteomalacia, or a combination of both (see Secondary hyperparathyroidism above – Fig. 15–5). Osteitis fibrosa cystica is characterized by increased bone turnover due to secondary hyperparathyroidism, a consequence of decreased levels of $1,25(OH)_2D_3$ and ionized calcium. (In general, bone dissolution is accelerated and bone formation decreased.) Osteomalacia is characterized by poor mineralization of bone resulting in the accumulation of surface osteoid (unmineralized bone). Osteoclasts cannot penetrate (resorb) these osteoid surfaces since they are only attracted to mineralized surfaces. Thus, osteoclasts dig cutting cones through the few remaining mineralized surfaces into the mineralized cores of old trabeculae. This phenomenon is histologically referred to as 'tunneling resorption' because of the manner in which osteoclasts gain access to mineralized bone (Fig. 15–9).

The defective mineralization process in osteomalacia of ESRD patients can be attributed to low serum calcium levels, the accumulation of aluminum in bone or other as yet unexplained factors. Renal failure patients who are treated orally with aluminum-containing phosphate

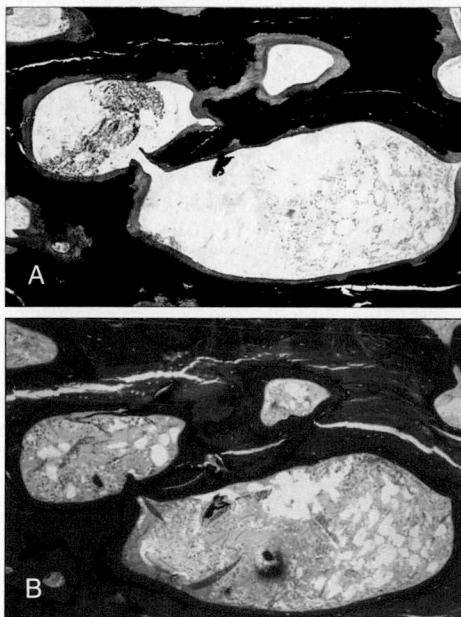

Figure 15–10 Osteomalacia in renal osteodystrophy. A, Von Kossa stain shows previously formed bone in black; newly synthesized, unmineralized osteoid stains magenta. Note that all surfaces are covered with thick magenta osteoid seams (125 ×). B, The same field of the same biopsy stained with solochrome azurine to detect aluminum. Note that the lines corresponding to the demarcation between black and magenta in the Von Kossa section are stained with a dark blue line. This corresponds to aluminum derived from dietary phosphate binders that has been incorporated into the hydroxyapatite matrix of the bone and interferes with further mineralization (125 ×).

binders to control hyperphosphatemia or who undergo hemodialysis using aluminum-containing dialysates can experience osteomalacia because aluminum ion can interfere with normal hydroxyapatite lattice formation. Undecalcified bone biopsies stained for aluminum can distinguish between this and the more usual types of osteomalacia (Fig. 15–10A and B).

Paget's Disease

Paget's disease of bone (osteitis deformans) is a chronic disorder of bone that may be unifocal or multifocal. Although it resembles a metabolic disease because involved bones are structurally and functionally abnormal, it is not a true metabolic disease because uninvolved bones are normal. The cause of Paget's disease is currently unknown; however, it has been suspected to be of viral origin because paramyxovirus-like particles have been identified in the nuclei of osteoclasts from affected bone. A family history of the disorder is sometimes identified. Regardless of its etiology, the disease displays uncoupling of osteoclast and osteoblast function with osteoclastic activity predominating early in the disease and osteoblastic activity predominating late in the disease. The osteoclasts are often large and bizarre, with 50 or more nuclei; there is trabecular scalloping with multiple Howship's lacunae, paratrabecular fibrosis, and marrow hypervascularity. The early histological picture resembles osteitis fibrosa of hyperparathyroidism. As osteoblastic new bone production takes place, the Howship's lacunae are filled in by irregular patches of mature and immature bone; the outlines of the original delimitations of osteoclast resorption are preserved as irregularly disposed reversal cement lines, and the resulting bone comes to resemble a tile mosaic. This results in structurally weak bone that is prone to both deformities and fractures. Patients with extensive bone lesions that have underlying heart disease may develop high output cardiac failure as a complication. Approximately 1% of patients eventually develop bone sarcomas, usually with osteosarcomatous differentiation. Laboratory findings are of some interest. While serum calcium and inorganic phosphorus concentrations are typically normal, they may occasionally become elevated. Serum calcium levels may, in fact, become very elevated if an extensive area of Paget's disease is immobilized. Once osteoblast activity begins, serum alkaline phosphatase increases, and may be used to follow the activity of the bone-synthesizing phase of the disease. Alkaline phosphatase levels rise further if a patient with Paget's disease develops osteosarcoma. Urinary excretion of calcium and phosphorus is normal or increased, whereas excretion of hydroxyproline is usually significantly increased. Paget's disease frequently responds both clinically and pathologically to therapeutic administration of calcitonin.

Bastepe M, Raas-Rothschild A, Silver J, et al: A form of Jansen's metaphyseal chondrodysplasia with limited metabolic and skeletal abnormalities is caused by a novel activating parathyroid hormone (PTH)/PTH-related peptide receptor mutation. J Clin Endocrinol Metab 2004; 89(7):3595–3600.

Bellorin-Font E, Starosta R, Milanes CL, et al: Effect of acidosis on PTH-dependent renal adenylate cyclase in phosphorus deprivation: Role of G proteins. Am J Physiol 1990; 258:F1640–F1649.

Bettica P, Moro L, Robins SP, et al: Bone-resorption markers galactosyl hydroxylysine, pyridinium crosslinks, and hydroxyproline compared. Clin Chem 1992; 38:2313–2318.

Boden SD, Kaplan FS: Calcium homeostasis. Orthop Clin North Am 1990; 21:31.

Brossard JH, et al: Influence of glomerular filtration on non-(1-84) parathyroid hormone (PTH) detected by intact PTH assays. Clin Chem 2000; 46:697–703.

Care AD, Bruce JB, Boelkins LJ, et al: Role of pancreozymin-cholecystokinin and structurally related compounds as calcitonin secretogogues. Endocrinology 1971; 89(1):262–271.

Cecco SA, Hristova EN, Rehak NN, et al: Clinically important intermethod differences for physiologically abnormal ionized magnesium results. Am J Clin Pathol 1997; 108:564–569.

Chapurlat RD, Garnero P, Brart G, et al: Serum type I collagen breakdown product (SerumCTX) predicts hip fracture risk in elderly women: The EPIDOS study. Bone 2000; 27:283–286.

Deftos LJ, Parethemore JG, Stabile BE: Management of primary hyperparathyroidism. Annu Rev Med 1993; 44:19.

Eatell R, et al: Relationship of early changes in bone resorption to the reduction in fracture risk with risedronate. Journal of Bone and Mineral Research 2003; 18(6):1051–1056.

Elin RJ: Magnesium metabolism in health and disease. Dis Mon 1988; 34:161.

Endres DB, Rude RK: Mineral and bone metabolism. In Burtis CA, Ashwood ER (eds): Tietz Textbook of Clinical Chemistry, 3rd ed. Philadelphia, WB Saunders Company, 1999, pp 1395–1457.

Farley JR, Hall SL, Ilacas D, et al: Quantification of skeletal alkaline phosphatase in osteoporotic serum by wheat germ agglutinin precipitation, heat inactivation, and two-site immunoradiometric assay. Clin Chem 1994; 40:1749–1756.

Ferrari S, Rizzoli R, Bonjour JP: Genetic aspects of osteoporosis. Curr Opin Rheumatol 1999; 11:294–300.

Fink et al: Differences in the capacity of several biochemical markers to assess high bone turnover in early menopause and response to alendronate therapy. Osteoporosis International 2000; 11(4):295–303.

Fledelius C, Riis BJ, Overgaard K, Christiansen C: The diagnostic validity of urinary free pyridinolines to identify women at risk of osteoporosis. Calcif Tissue Int 1994; 54(5):381–384.

Folpe AL, Fanburg-Smith JC, Billings SD, et al: Most osteomalacia-associated mesenchymal tumors are a single histopathologic entity: an analysis of 32 cases and a comprehensive review of the literature. Am J Surg Pathol 2004; 28(1):1–30

Goldstein RE, Blevins L, Delbeke D, Martin WH: Efficacy of minimally invasive radioguided parathyroidectomy on efficacy, length of stay, and costs in the management of primary hyperparathyroidism. Ann Surg 1991; 15:716–723.

Goldstein RE, Blevins L, Delbeke D, et al: Effect of minimally invasive radioguided parathyroidectomy on efficacy, length of stay, and costs in the management of primary hyperparathyroidism. Ann Surg 2000; 231(5):732–742.

Horvit PK, Gagel RF: The goitrous patient with an elevated serum calcitonin – what to do? J Clin Endocrinol Metab 1997; 82(2):335–337.

Horwitz MJ, et al: Short-term high dose parathyroid hormone-related protein as a skeletal anabolic agent for the treatment of postmenopausal osteoporosis. J Clin Endocrinol Metab 2003; 88(2):569–575.

Hristova EN, Cecco S, Niemela JE, et al: Analyzer-dependent differences in results for ionized calcium, ionized magnesium, sodium, and pH. Clin Chem 1995; 41:1649–1653.

Huijgen HJ, Sanders R, Cecco SA, et al: Serum ionized magnesium: Comparison of results obtained with three ion-selective analyzers. Clin Chem Lab Med 1999; 37:465–470.

Hsu H. et al: Tumor necrosis factor receptor family member RANK mediates osteoclast differentiation and activation induced by osteoprotegerin ligand. Proc Natl Acad Sci USA 1999; 96:3540–3545.

Ju HSJ, Leung S, Brown B, et al: Comparison of analytical performance and biological variability of three bone resorption assays. Clin Chem 1997; 43:1570–1576.

Kurokawa K, Fukagawa M: Introduction to renal osteodystrophy: Calcium metabolism in health and uremia. Am J Med Sci 1999; 317:355–356.

Lewiecki EM: Management of osteoporosis. Clin and Molec Allergy 2004; 2:9.

Manolagas SC, Jilka RL: Mechanisms of disease: Bone marrow, cytokines, and bone remodeling – emerging insights into the pathophysiology of osteoporosis. N Engl J Med 1995; 332:305.

Mundy GR, Guise TA: Hormonal control of calcium homeostasis. Clin Chem 1999; 45:1347–1352.

Overview of calcium physiology and pathophysiology including roles of PTH, vitamin D, PTH-related peptide, and calcitonin. Also presents physiologic defenses against hypercalcemia and hypocalcemia.

Nelson AE, Bligh RC, Mirams M, et al: Clinical case seminar: Fibroblast growth factor 23: a new clinical marker for oncogenic osteomalacia. J Clin Endocrinol Metab 2003; 88(9):4088–4094.

Nichols Advantage BIO-INTACT PTH assay directional insert, ADS document 7040, 2004.

Papapoulos SE, et al: The effect of renal function on changes in circulating concentrations of 1,25 dihydroxycholecalciferol after an oral dose. Clin Sci 1982; 62(4):427–429.

Papazachariou IM, Martinez-Isla A, Efthimiou E, et al: Magnesium deficiency in patients with chronic pancreatitis identified by an intravenous loading test. Clinica Chimica Acta 2000; 302(1–2):145–154.

Quamme GA: Control of magnesium transport in the thick ascending limb. Am J Physiol 1989; 256:F197–F210.

Quamme GA: Renal magnesium handling: New insights in understanding old problems. Kidney Int 1997; 52:1180–1195.

Quarles LD, et al: Intact parathyroid hormone overestimates the presence and severity of

parathyroid mediated osseous abnormalities in uremia. J Clin Endocrinol Metab 1992; 75:145–150.

Raisz LG: Physiology and pathophysiology of bone remodeling. Clin Chem 1999; 45:1353–1358.

Ravn P, et al: Biochemical markers for prediction of 4-year response in bone mass during bisphosphonate treatment for prevention of postmenopausal osteoporosis. Bone 2003; 33(1):150–158

Rieu M, Lame MC, Richard A, et al: Prevalence of sporadic medullary thyroid carcinoma: the importance of routine measurement of serum calcitonin in the diagnostic evaluation of thyroid nodules. Clin Endocrinol 1995; 42:453–460.

Risteli L, Risteli J: Biochemical markers of bone metabolism. Ann Med 1993; 25:385–393.

Robins SP: Collagen crosslinks in metabolic bone disease. Acta Orthop Scand 1995; 66(Suppl 266):171–175.

Sofferman RA, Standage J, Tang ME: Minimal-access parathyroid surgery using intraoperative parathyroid hormone assay. Laryngoscope 1998; 108:1497–1503.

Sokoll LJ, Drew H, Udelsman R: Intraoperative parathyroid hormone analysis: A study of 200 consecutive cases. Clin Chem 2000; 46: 1662–1668.

Sokoll L, Remaley A, Sena S, et al: National Academy of Clinical Biochemistry Laboratory Medicine Practice Guidelines. Evidence-Based Practice for POCT. Intraoperative PTH. Draft 2 October 15, 2004.

This comprehensive evidence-based review proposes practice guidelines for all intraoperative PTH-related issues including clinical indications, time of draws, method, location of testing and financial impact. Guidelines are organized in clear question and answer format.

Souberbielle JC, Cormier C, Kindermans C: Bone markers in clinical practice. Curr Opin Rheumatol 1999; 11:312–319.

Strewler GJ: Hypercalcemia of malignancy and parathyroid hormone-related protein. In Clark OH, Duh Q-Y (eds), Textbook of Endocrine Surgery. Philadelphia, WB Saunders Company, 1997, pp 426–431.

Swaminathan R: Biochemical markers of bone turnover. Clinica Chimica Acta 2001; 313:95–105.

Vergnaud P, Garnero P, Meunier PJ, et al: Undercarboxylated osteocalcin measured with a specific immunoassay predicts hip fracture in elderly women: The EPIDOS study. J Clin Endocrinol Metab 1997; 82:719–724.

Watts NB: Clinical utility of biochemical markers of bone remodeling. Clin Chem 1999; 45:1359–1368.

This is a thorough overview of bone resorption and formation markers including biological and assay variability issues and clinical uses. The latter are presented in a useful clinical question and answer format like 'is the patient responding to treatment?'

Wang S, McDonnell EH, Sedor FA, Toffaletti JG: pH effects on measurements of ionized calcium and ionized magnesium in blood, Arch Pathol Lab Med 2002; 126(8):947–950.

Weisinger JR, Bellorin-Font E: Magnesium and phosphorus. Lancet 1998; 352:391–396.

Yin JJ, Chirgwin JM, Dallas M, et al: Blockage of TGFβ signaling inhibits PTH-rP secretion by breast cancer cells and the development of bone metastasis. J Clin Invest 1999; 103:197–206.

CHAPTER 16

Carbohydrates

Mukhtar I. Khan MD, Ruth S. Weinstock MD PhD

KEY POINTS

• The diagnosis of diabetes requires a fasting plasma glucose of ≥ 126 mg/dL (7.0 mmol/L) on at least two occasions or a casual plasma glucose level (or 2-h post-glucose load level) of ≥ 200 mg/dL (11.1 mmol/L). Normal fasting plasma glucose is < 100 mg/dL (5.6 mmol/L) and normal glucose levels 2 h post-glucose load are < 140 mg/dL (7.8 mmol/L).

• Oral glucose tolerance tests should be performed to diagnose gestational diabetes.

• Whole blood capillary glucose values obtained with point of care devices are useful for the detection of hyperglycemia and hypoglycemia in individuals with diabetes, and help monitor and direct therapy. They should not be used to diagnose diabetes or hypoglycemic disorders. To establish these diagnoses, confirmation with laboratory measures of plasma glucose are essential because of their greater accuracy.

• HbA$_{1c}$ levels should be performed every 3–6 months in individuals with diabetes to monitor glycemic control using a certified method, traceable to the DCCT reference method. Reliability and accuracy are diminished in the presence of shortened red blood cell survival, lower mean blood cell age or need for transfusions as seen with certain hemoglobinopathies and hemolytic conditions, as well as with uremia.

• Commonly used strips and tablets for ketone testing use sodium nitroprusside, which does not detect beta-hydroxybutyrate. Since beta-hydroxybutyrate levels are high in diabetic ketoacidosis (DKA) and fall with treatment, whereas acetoacetic acid and acetone levels rise with treatment, these strips are not useful to monitor therapy. Calculation of the anion gap is commonly used to monitor recovery from DKA. Enzymatic methods for measuring beta-hydroxybutyrate are also now available.

• Circulating autoantibodies (GAD65, ICA512, IA-2, IAA) may be present before and at the onset of autoimmune type 1 diabetes. These tests should not be used for routine screening of asymptomatic nondiabetic individuals except in a research setting. When performed, assays should be used that have been shown to have the best performance by the Diabetes Antibody Standardization Program.

• Hypoglycemic symptoms with a plasma glucose level of ≤ 50 mg/dL (2.8 mmol/L) in an individual who is not receiving medications for diabetes warrant further evaluation. A careful drug and medical history, and measurements of insulin, C-peptide, proinsulin, insulin autoantibodies, beta-hydroxybutyrate and drug levels (sulfonylureas, repaglinide, nateglinide) during the hypoglycemic episode are recommended to determine the diagnosis.

• Glycogen storage diseases that primarily affect the liver usually manifest with hypoglycemia and hepatomegaly, whereas those affecting muscle commonly cause muscle cramps, weakness, fatigue and exercise intolerance.

Introduction

Carbohydrates are major constituents of physiological systems. They are organic compounds composed of carbon, hydrogen and oxygen $[C_x(H_2O)_y]$, which, along with lipids and proteins, provide energy and contribute to the structure of organisms. Complex carbohydrates are digested into simple sugars, principally glucose, which is used primarily as an energy source or stored as glycogen. The most important dietary hexoses (6 carbon-containing carbohydrates) are D-glucose, D-galactose and D-fructose, but the principal sugar circulating in the bloodstream is glucose. Lactose (glucose and galactose) and sucrose (glucose and fructose) are important disaccharides. Carbohydrates are needed for specific cellular functions (such as ribose in nucleic acids) and can modify proteins and their function by glycosylation. Carbohydrates are measured in whole blood, serum or plasma. In addition, measurements of glucose in urine, cerebrospinal fluid, and other body fluids are important clinically; these are discussed in Part III.

The concentration of glucose in blood is normally controlled within narrow limits by many hormones, the most significant of which, insulin, is produced by the endocrine pancreas. Diabetes mellitus is the most common disease of carbohydrate metabolism. Most individuals with diabetes have either type 1 (beta cell destruction with absolute insulin deficiency) or type 2 (insulin resistance and an insulin secretory defect). Measurements of glycemic control are increasingly important in diabetes, since the development and progression of microvascular and macrovascular complications are associated with glycemia. The material in this chapter will review the aspects of carbohydrate metabolism most critical to the practice of medicine.

Function of the Endocrine Pancreas

The pancreas functions as both an endocrine and exocrine organ in the control of carbohydrate metabolism. As an exocrine gland, it produces and secretes an amylase responsible for the breakdown of ingested complex carbohydrates. Further digestion leads to the production of monosaccharides, which can be absorbed. Once absorbed, the monosaccharides signal the endocrine pancreas, which regulates hormones involved in energy homeostasis. Enteroendocrine cells in the gastrointestinal tract are also stimulated by nutrients to secrete incretins, peptide hormones that affect pancreatic function, gastric emptying and intestinal motility.

The endocrine pancreas secretes four hormones from different cells residing in the islets of Langerhans. Insulin is produced by the beta cells, glucagon by the alpha cells, somatostatin by the delta cells, and pancreatic polypeptide (PP) by the PP or F cells. In insulin-sensitive tissues such as skeletal muscle, fat and liver, insulin stimulates glucose uptake and the formation of glycogen, and inhibits glucose production. Glucagon acts primarily in the liver, where it stimulates glucose production, and, over time, ketogenesis. Somatostatin, on the other hand, inhibits insulin and glucagon secretion, as well as the secretion of a number of other hormones. Nutrient ingestion is the major stimulus for PP secretion. The physiological significance of PP is not clear, but it can reduce appetite and food intake. In the rare reported cases of islet cell tumors producing excess PP, or in PP hyperplasia, some patients have been asymptomatic, whereas other cases are associated with watery diarrhea syndrome (Bellows, 1998; Pasieka, 1999; Tomita, 1980).

The ratio of insulin to glucagon is important in the regulation of carbohydrate metabolism. Anabolism is favored when there is a relative increase in the insulin to glucagon ratio as in the postprandial state, while catabolism is favored with a relative decrease in this ratio as in the fasting state. The ratio of insulin to glucagon is influenced by somatostatin, neural input, intestinal peptides, and the concentration of glucose and other metabolites. The ratio of insulin to glucagon is tightly regulated to keep blood glucose concentrations within the normal range.

In addition to the hormones mentioned above, the pancreatic beta cell secretes a 37-amino-acid protein called islet amyloid polypeptide (IAPP) or amylin. First discovered in 1987, amylin is co-localized and co-secreted with insulin in response to stimulation with nutrients. IAPP can inhibit insulin secretion, slow gastric emptying, and inhibit postprandial glucagon secretion. Oligomeric forms are associated with an increase in beta cell apoptosis. IAPP is first synthesized as a larger precursor peptide, which is processed within the beta cell. High levels of IAPP have been observed in hyperinsulinemic, insulin resistant states, such as impaired glucose tolerance and early type 2 diabetes, and low levels are seen in type 1 diabetes. Amyloid deposits, fibroid material derived from IAPP, are observed in islets in type 2 diabetes. IAPP levels can also be elevated in pancreatic cancer. Amylin assays are not used in clinical practice, but clinical trials of amylin analogues in diabetes are in progress, with the hope that these analogues will improve glycemic control by limiting postprandial glucose excursions (Nyholm, 2001). A synthetic analog of amylin, pramlintide acetate, has recently become available for use by injection prior to major meals in patients with insulin-requiring diabetes.

Insulin

Insulin is a peptide hormone with a mass of ~ 5800 daltons, secreted by the beta cells in the islets of Langerhans in the pancreas. It has a 21-amino-acid A chain and a 30-amino-acid B chain that are linked by two disulfide bonds. Insulin is synthesized initially as a longer single-chain peptide precursor hormone, pre-proinsulin. Proinsulin (~ 9000 daltons), the immediate precursor of insulin, is processed into insulin in the secretory granules of the beta cells by enzymatic removal of the 31-amino-acid peptide segment that connects the A and B chains, known as C-peptide (Figs 16–1 and 16–2). This proteolytic processing is catalyzed by proprotein convertase PC2 and PC1/PC3 which first convert proinsulin into the intermediate metabolites 32,33 split proinsulin and 65,66 split proinsulin, and then, after cleavage by carboxypeptidase H, to des-31,32 split proinsulin and des-64,65 split proinsulin. In adults, small amounts of intact proinsulin and these metabolically active conversion intermediates, especially des-31,32 split proinsulin, are cosecreted with insulin. Healthy infants and preterm neonates, however, have higher proinsulin and 32,33 split proinsulin levels than adults. Proinsulin and its metabolites may crossreact with insulin in some insulin radio-immunoassays. This can be significant, especially since the half-life of proinsulin is at least three times as long as that of insulin. In vivo studies of proinsulin have shown that it has 10–15% of the biological activity of insulin.

Elevated proinsulin levels (intact and partially processed proinsulin) have been found in type 2 diabetes, and are associated with a decreased ability of the beta cells to secrete insulin (Roder, 1998). An increase in proinsulin levels has also been observed in pre-type 1 diabetes, where

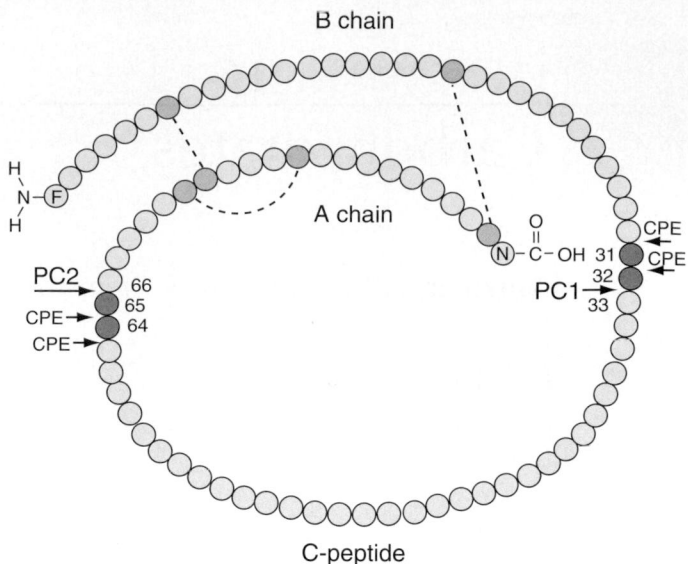

Figure 16–1 Human proinsulin, with cleavage sites for the proprotein convertases PC1 and PC2 and for carboxypeptidase H (CPE). Orange circles represent the two pairs of basic amino acids used for proteolytic processing, and the green circles represent cysteine residues that participate in disulfide bonding. (Diagnosis and classification of diabetes mellitus. Copyright © 2004 American Diabetes Association. From Diabetes Care, Vol. 27, 2004; S5–S10. Reprinted with permission from *The American Diabetes Association*.)

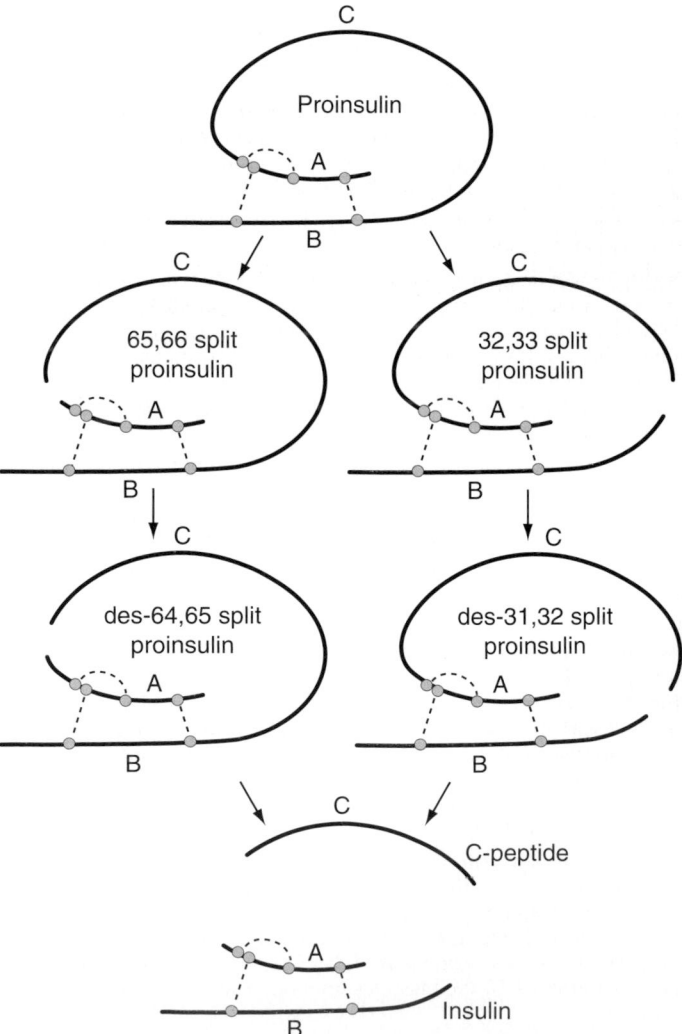

Figure 16–2 Processing of proinsulin to insulin. Green circles represent cysteine residues that participate in disulfide bonding. Copyright by John Wiley and Sons Ltd, reproduced with permission (Temple, 1992).

there is a reduction in beta cell function, and may be the result of beta cell damage from cytokines produced by infiltrating immunocytes (Hostens, 1999). Less common conditions associated with high proinsulin levels include insulinomas. Familial hyperproinsulinemia is a rare condition caused by mutations in the proinsulin gene. In affected Japanese families, this genetic abnormality is associated with impaired glucose tolerance or type 2 diabetes, but in a three-generation Caucasian family with hyperproinsulinemia and mutant proinsulin (Arg65-His), glucose tolerance was normal (Roder, 1996).

C-peptide and insulin are secreted in equimolar amounts into the portal vein, but the ratio in serum is about 5 : 1 to 15 : 1. The molar concentration of C-peptide in blood is higher than that of insulin due primarily to the hepatic clearance of insulin. Approximately 50% of insulin is rapidly removed by its initial passage through the liver, but hepatic extraction of C-peptide is negligible. In cirrhosis, hyperinsulinemia is observed due to decreased hepatic insulin clearance. In healthy individuals, the half-life of both C-peptide and proinsulin is approximately 30 minutes, whereas it is only 4–9 minutes for insulin. In normal individuals, the molar ratio of C-peptide to insulin in the fasting state is 5:1. Whether C-peptide has any significant biological activity is unclear (Wojcikowski, 1990; Ido, 1997).

Disease states occur when insulin concentrations are inappropriate for given blood glucose levels. Insulin deficiency, either absolute or relative, leads to diabetes mellitus. Serum insulin levels should be measured with a concomitant glucose level, since insulin secretion is regulated primarily by glucose. Whereas a high insulin level in the presence of low glucose level suggests inappropriate secretion or administration of insulin, high insulin levels can be observed in insulin-resistant individuals who need to secrete additional insulin to keep blood glucose levels normal.

Unregulated excess insulin secretion causes hypoglycemia. This is seen in insulin-secreting tumors, especially insulinomas, where patients have low serum glucose levels (< 50 mg/dL), and elevated insulin and proinsulin levels with hypoglycemic symptoms (e.g., shakiness, palpitations, diaphoresis, confusion). C-peptide levels are measured in hypoglycemic states to help identify the etiology of the hypoglycemia. *Sera from insulinoma patients have high insulin and C-peptide levels, whereas hypoglycemia from injected or exogenous insulin is characterized by high insulin levels and low C-peptide levels.* Commercially available insulin preparations are free of C-peptide and proinsulin. Since C-peptide is less stable than insulin, serum samples should be separated quickly and frozen.

In people with diabetes mellitus, C-peptide levels at baseline and after glucagon stimulation can be measured by immunoassay to help classify the etiology of the diabetes and provide information concerning beta cell secretory capacity. C-peptide and glucose can be measured after an overnight 8-hour fast and 90 minutes after stimulation by an oral mixed meal, Sustacal (Mead Johnson), as well (DCCT, 1993). These tests are usually not performed in routine clinical practice, but are used in research studies. Low C-peptide levels are characteristic of the absolute insulin deficiency of type 1 diabetes. C-peptide measurement can also be useful in follow-up evaluations after pancreatectomy and post-pancreatic transplantation. Unlike insulin, both C-peptide and proinsulin are primarily degraded in the kidneys and so levels are elevated in renal failure.

Many commercial immunoassays for insulin, C-peptide and proinsulin are now available. The American Diabetes Association Task Force on Standardization of the Insulin Assay reviewed 17 insulin assays, and found significant variability (Robbins, 1996). It was recommended that all assays be standardized to one reference method. Manufacturers were encouraged to publish data concerning the performance of their assays, including accuracy, recovery, precision, specificity, linearity, and LOD/LOQ (lowest measurable concentration statistically different from zero/limits of quantitatation). Laboratory certification was also encouraged. In the US, there is an external quality assessment program for insulin and C-peptide measurements available through the College of American Pathologists (College of American Pathologists, Northfield Headquarters, 325 Waukegan Road, Northfield, Illinois 60093-2750).

Serum insulin measurements may be falsely low in the presence of hemolysis. An insulin-degrading enzyme found in red blood cells as well as in other tissues is responsible for this problem. C-peptide and proinsulin measurements appear to be less affected by hemolysis. Insulin antibodies will also interfere with insulin immunoassays, with both falsely elevated and suppressed levels reported.

Glucagon

Proglucagon is synthesized in the pancreatic alpha cells and the L cells of the distal small bowel. Through differential processing, the glucagon family of gene products is formed. Fasting plasma glucagon concentrations are normally 25–50 pg/mL. Pancreatic glucagon stimulates glucose production.

It is an important regulator of hepatic glycogenolysis, gluconeogenesis and ketogenesis. In type 1 diabetes, over time, progressive glucagon deficiency develops. This deficiency of glucagon results in increased glycemic fluctuations and difficulty recovering from hypoglycemia.

Serum glucagon levels are rarely measured in clinical practice. Glucagonomas are rare islet cell tumors that produce excessive glucagon. Clinically, glucagonomas present with a characteristic necrotizing migratory erythematous rash, stomatitis, glossitis, weight loss, anemia and mild diabetes mellitus. These tumors are usually associated with fasting glucagon levels of over 120 pg/mL, but levels can range from 900–7800 pg/mL. The processing of proglucagon is impaired, and large-molecular-weight forms can be seen. Mild elevations in blood glucagon levels are seen in patients with multifunctional neuroendocrine tumors. Glucagon levels can also be mildly elevated in cirrhosis, diabetes, Cushing's syndrome, pancreatitis, acromegaly and renal insufficiency. In familial hyperglucagonemia, an autosomal dominant disorder, glucagon levels are high in the absence of tumor. Family history is helpful in making this diagnosis.

Incretins

Oral nutrients stimulate the release of incretins from the intestines. The incretin effect, first described over 40 years ago, refers to the greater and earlier insulin response to the oral administration of glucose compared to intravenous glucose. The most important incretins in the regulation of insulin secretion are glucagon-like peptide 1 (GLP-1) and glucose-dependent insulinotropic peptide (GIP), both of which are members of the glucagon superfamily. GIP, originally called gastric inhibitory polypeptide, exerts some beta cell effects in animal models, but does not affect glucagon release or gastric emptying in physiological doses.

In the intestine, GLP-1 is formed from proglucagon, and functions mostly as an incretin to rapidly stimulate insulin secretion in response to a meal. Other effects include the suppression of glucagon and lipase secretion, inhibition of gastric emptying and stimulation of somatostatin secretion. GLP-1 may reduce appetite and have effects on energy intake as well (Flint, 1998). In vitro and animal studies indicate that GLP-1 can inhibit beta cell apoptosis and stimulate beta cell proliferation and neogenesis from precursor duct cells (Drucker, 2003a). Plasma meal-stimulated GLP-1 levels are decreased in type 2 diabetes mellitus (Toft-Nielsen, 2001). GLP-1 (7-37), the most common active form, has a half-life of only 2–3 minutes. It is rapidly cleaved by circulating aminopeptidases to the inactive GLP-1 (9-37). This inactive form represents 80% of the circulating GLP-1. Both forms of GLP-1 are short-lived and cleared by the kidney. Dipeptidyl peptidase-4 (DPP-4) a serine peptidase present on the surface of endothelial cells, inactivates GLP-1 by removing two N-terminal amino acids. Inhibitors of DPP-4 are currently being studied in clinical trials for the treatment of diabetes, as are long-acting GLP-1 analogues. (Drucker, 2003b). A GLP-1 receptor agonist, exenatide, has recently become available for use by injection in patients with type 2 diabetes.

Somatostatin

Somatostatin, a tetradecapeptide with a disulfide bond, was first isolated from the hypothalamus. Somatostatin was originally considered a hypothalamic hormone that inhibited growth hormone secretion, but the discovery of somatostatin in the islets of Langerhans prompted further investigation of its function in the endocrine pancreas. Subsequently, somatostatin was found in the gastrointestinal tract. It inhibits pituitary (growth hormone and thyrotropin), gastrointestinal (gastrin, secretin, vasointestinal peptide) and pancreatic (insulin, glucagon) hormones as well as possesses nonendocrine functions (e.g., inhibition of gastric acid secretion, gastric emptying time and pancreatic enzyme release). The first isolated somatostatin peptide had 14 amino acids and is called somatostatin-14. Subsequently, somatostatin-28 was isolated, which contains an N-terminal extension, and is a more potent inhibitor of other islet hormones.

In the pancreatic islets, somatostatin is produced in the delta cells, which comprise 5–10% of the islet cells. Rare islet cell tumors, somatostatinomas, secrete high levels of somatostatin. Elevated somatostatin levels can also be seen in small cell lung cancer, medullary thyroid cancer and pheochromocytoma. Somatostatin has a very short half-life, and is rarely measured in clinical practice. Two long-acting somatostatin analogues, octreotide and lanreotide, which bind primarily to the somatostatin receptor subtype 2 (SSTR2), are used to treat neuroendocrine tumors as well as other disorders of the pancreas and gastrointestinal tract. Octreotide scintigraphy has also been used for tumor diagnosis, localization and prediction for success of treatment with somatostatin analogues.

II

Specimen Considerations

Measurements of glucose are critical to the diagnosis and management of diseases affecting carbohydrate metabolism. Glucose is measured in whole blood, plasma, serum, cerebrospinal fluid, pleural fluid, and urine for a variety of diagnostic and management purposes (see also Chs 27 and 28). In addition, newer devices can measure glucose from interstitial fluid for continuous monitoring of glucose levels in people with diabetes. How and when specimens are collected and handled as well as the site of collection affect the clinical interpretation of the analytical result.

The standard clinical specimen is venous plasma glucose. Glucose is metabolized at room temperature at a rate of 7 mg/dL/h (0.4 mmol/L/h); at 4°C, the loss is approximately 2 mg/dL/h (Weissman, 1958). The rate of metabolism is higher with bacterial contamination or leukocytosis. A serum specimen is appropriate for glucose analysis if serum is separated from the cells within 30 minutes, but if serum is in contact with cells for longer than 30 min, a preservative such as sodium fluoride that inhibits glycolysis should be added. However, in serum specimens without bacterial contamination or leukocytosis, results remain clinically acceptable even after a delay of up to 90 min before separation of serum and cells. If whole blood is refrigerated, 2 mg of sodium fluoride per milliliter of whole blood prevents glycolysis for up to 48 hours (Chan, 1989). When refrigerated, glucose is stable in serum or plasma for 48 hours. With long-term specimen storage, even at −20°C, glucose values decrease significantly and progressively.

Glucose Measurement Methods

Most measurements of glucose employ enzymatic methods. These enzymatic methods provide specificity and can be packaged to furnish point of care determinations. Three enzyme systems are currently used to measure glucose: glucose dehydrogenase, glucose oxidase and hexokinase. These reactions produce an electrical current that is proportional to the initial glucose concentration or a product that measured spectrophotometrically is proportional to the initial glucose concentration. The assays can be initial rate of change assays, where the velocity of the reaction is dependent on the initial glucose, or end-point assays.

When glucose is measured using a glucose dehydrogenase method, glucose is reduced to produce either a chromophore that is measured spectrophotometrically (Equation 16–1) or by an electrical current (Equation 16–2) (Kost, 1998).

$$\alpha\text{-D-glucose} \rightarrow (\text{mutoarotase}) \rightarrow \beta\text{-D-glucose} \tag{16–1}$$
$$\beta\text{-D-glucose} + NAD \rightarrow (\text{glucose dehydrogenase}) \rightarrow \text{D-gluconolactone} + NADH$$
$$MTT + NADH \rightarrow (\text{diaphorase}) \rightarrow MTTH \text{ (blue color)} + NAD$$
$$\text{Glucose} + \text{Pyrroloquinoline quinone (PQQ)} \rightarrow (\text{glucose dehydrogenase}) \rightarrow \text{Gluconolactone} + PQQH_2 \tag{16–2}$$
$$PQQH_2 + 2[Fe(CN)_6]^{3-} \rightarrow PQQ + 2[Fe(CN)_6]^{4-} + 2H^+$$
$$2[Fe(CN)_6]^{4-} \rightarrow 2[Fe(CN)_6]^{3-} + 2e^-$$

Glucose oxidase, a flavoenzyme, catalyzes the reactions shown below. The peroxidase reaction can be measured spectrophotometrically (Equation 16–3), and can be inhibited by high concentrations of uric acid, ascorbic acid, bilirubin, glutathione, creatinine, L-cysteine, L-dopa, dopamine, methyldopa and citric acid (Zaloga, 1997). In addition, the glucose oxidase reaction can be coupled to ferricyanide/ferricyanide couple to produce an electrical current, as shown below (Equation 16–4). This system is dependent on the partial pressure of O_2 since oxygen will compete in the reaction to form hydrogen peroxide, so that the higher the partial pressure of O_2 the lower the electrically measured glucose (Kurahashi, 1997). Glucose oxidase can also be used in another electrical system, shown below in Equation 16–5.

$$\beta\text{-D-glucose} + O_2 \rightarrow (\text{glucose oxidase}) \rightarrow \tag{16–3}$$
$$\text{D-gluconolactone} + H_2O_2$$
$$\text{gluconolactone} + H_2O \rightarrow \text{gluconic acid}$$
$$H_2O_2 + \text{chromogenic oxygen acceptor (ortho-dianisidine,}$$
$$\text{4-aminophenazone, ortho-tolidine)} \rightarrow (\text{peroxidase}) \rightarrow$$
$$\text{color chromogen} + H_2O$$
$$\beta\text{-D-glucose} + 2[Fe(CN)_6]^{3-} + H_2O \rightarrow (\text{glucose oxidase}) \rightarrow \tag{16–4}$$
$$\text{D-gluconic acid} + 2[Fe(CN)_6]^{4-} + 2H^+$$
$$2[Fe(CN)_6]^{4-} \rightarrow 2[Fe(CN)_6]^{3-} + 2e^-$$
$$\beta\text{-D-glucose} + O_2 \rightarrow (\text{glucose oxidase}) \rightarrow \tag{16–5}$$
$$\text{D-gluconolactone} + H_2O_2$$
$$H_2O_2 \rightarrow 2H^+ + O_2 + 2e^-$$

The hexokinase system assay is the generally accepted reference method for measuring glucose. The reaction is shown below (Equation 16–6). The glucose concentration is proportional to the rate of production of NAD(P)H, which is followed spectrophotometrically. Depending on the source of the glucose-6-phosphate dehydrogenase, the enzyme can require specificity for NADP or from some sources it can use NAD as well. Hemolyzed samples can be problematic since the contents released from the erythrocytes may interfere with the stoichiometric relationship between glucose and NAD(P)H accumulation.

$$\text{Glucose} + MgATP \rightarrow (\text{hexokinase}) \rightarrow \tag{16–6}$$
$$\text{glucose-6-phosphate (G-6-P)} + MgADP$$
$$\text{G-6-P} + NA(P)^+ \rightarrow (\text{glucose-6-phosphate dehydrogenase}) \rightarrow$$
$$\text{6-phosphogluconolactone} + NAD(P)H + H^+$$

Whole blood glucose specimens can be analyzed with point of care devices. These monitoring devices are used in the home, in the physician's office, or at the bedside in the hospital to monitor for hypoglycemia and hyperglycemia. Most of these devices have been calibrated to give results similar to plasma levels and can report either plasma or whole blood readings. Whole blood tends to give approximately 10–15% lower glucose readings than plasma, but the percentage varies based on hematocrit, analysis technique and sample timing (fasting versus post-glucose load). Capillary blood is the source for most of these whole blood glucose measuring devices. Capillary blood glucose is similar to arterial glucose, but can vary markedly from venous samples, depending upon timing relative to food ingestion. For example, a postprandial specimen is higher in the capillary sample than in the venous sample. Capillary glucose tests, using point of care devices, should not be used to diagnose diabetes or hypoglycemic disorders. To establish these diagnoses, confirmation with laboratory measurements of plasma glucose is essential because of their greater accuracy.

Home blood glucose monitoring devices help people with diabetes better self-manage their disease. A wide variety of devices are available for home measurements. Proper training of patients in the use of individual meters is critical in avoiding operator errors, which, in one study, were reported in 12% of users (Schrot, 1999). Errors that may contribute to inaccurate readings in certain devices include the application of an insufficient volume of blood, milking the finger to acquire sufficient blood, the use of outdated test strips, environmental factors (humidity, heat, altitude), the use of a malfunctioning meter, the use of a dirty meter, hypertriglyceridemia, hypotension, and measurements outside of the hematocrit or temperature range. Some blood glucose monitoring devices are influenced by high levels of salicylate, acetaminophen, levodopa, uric acid, bilirubin, lipids or low oxygen levels, and others are altered by touching the reaction area. Most are inaccurate at very high and low glucose values.

Desirable features of home blood glucose monitoring devices, aside from performance characteristics (precision and accuracy) include the following: ease of use, requirement of a small volume of blood, low maintenance, large print readout, rapid testing, appropriate alarms, minimal interfering substances, and memory storage and download capabilities. Some meters now permit alternative site testing (such as forearm, upper arm, thigh), but results from alternative sites may be less accurate when there are rapid changes in glucose levels. Others incorporate electronic logbooks for recording events, insulin doses and carbohydrate intake. This information can be downloaded to a computer to present the data in several displays such as logbook, graphs, charts, and summary statistics.

Interstitial glucose measuring devices have been developed for monitoring glucose levels in people with diabetes. Most of these devices use electrochemical methods to automatically and frequently measure glucose levels in the interstitial fluid of dermis or subcutaneous fat tissue, and require repeated calibration to plasma or whole blood glucose levels. Examinations of these data provide information about glucose patterns over hours to days. This glucose 'trend analyses' can reveal useful findings for modifying treatment, such as unsuspected nocturnal hypoglycemia or postprandial hyperglycemia (Kaufman, 2002).

Interstitial glucose is in slow (5–30 min) equilibrium with capillary blood glucose, and therefore not equal to blood glucose except in stable systems (Zierler, 1999; Cheyne, 2002). Particularly during times when glucose levels are rapidly changing, such as after meal ingestion or recovery from hypoglycemia, interstitial fluid readings will lag behind fingerstick glucose levels. Because the precision and accuracy of the currently available portable continuous glucose monitors are not as high as for the conventional home blood glucose monitoring devices, they may supplement but cannot replace conventional home blood glucose monitoring. Individual glucose readings obtained by fingersticks should be primarily used to direct therapy. Technologies currently under development for noninvasive glucose monitoring include impedance spectroscopy, thermal emission spectroscopy, near infrared spectroscopy, far infrared spectroscopy,

Table 16-1 Diagnosis of Pre-Diabetes and Diabetes Mellitus

	Fasting plasma glucose		2-h Plasma glucose level (after 75-g glucose load)	
	mg/dL	mmol/L	mg/dL	mmol/L
Normal	< 100	< 5.6	< 140	< 7.8
Pre-diabetes				
Impaired fasting glucose	100–125	5.6–6.9		
Impaired glucose tolerance			140–199	7.8–11.0
Diabetes mellitus	≥ 126	≥ 7.0	≥ 200	≥ 11.1

From American Diabetes Association, 2004a.

Table 16–2 Diagnosis of Gestational Diabetes Mellitus

Initial Screening Test for Average-Risk Women

1-h Plasma glucose level (after 50-g glucose load)	Detection of gestational diabetes
> 130 mg/dL (7.2 mmol/L)	90%
> 140 mg/dL (7.8 mmol/L)	80%

Oral Glucose Tolerance Tests (OGTT) for High-Risk Women and Average-Risk Women with Abnormal Screening Test Results

	100-g OGTT Plasma glucose		75-g OGTT Plasma glucose	
	mg/dL	mmol/L	mg/dL	mmol/L
Fasting	≥ 95	≥ 5.3	≥ 95	≥ 5.3
1 hour	≥ 180	≥ 10.0	≥ 180	≥ 10.0
2 hour	≥ 155	≥ 8.6	≥ 155	≥ 8.6
3 hour	≥ 140	≥ 7.8		

Gestational diabetes mellitus diagnosed if ≥ 2 plasma glucose levels are exceeded (American Diabetes Association, 2004b).

ellipsometry, magnetic resonance imaging, and methods using electromagnetic waves.

Diabetes Mellitus

Introduction

Diabetes mellitus is a group of diseases in which blood glucose levels are elevated because of deficient insulin secretion and/or abnormal insulin action. Diabetes is the most common set of disorders of carbohydrate metabolism, affecting approximately 18 million Americans over the age of 20 in 2002. The prevalence of diabetes is increasing, with the prediction of an estimated 33% of males and 39% females born in 2000 in the US being diagnosed with diabetes during their lifetime (Narayan, 2003). This chronic disease is responsible for significant morbidity, mortality and cost. Diabetes is the leading cause of treated end-stage renal disease, the most common cause of nontraumatic amputations, and the foremost cause of new blindness in adults ages 20–74. Nerve damage, known as diabetic neuropathy, occurs in 60–70% of people with diabetes. Most diabetes-related deaths, however, are related to the increased risk of developing atherosclerotic disease. People with diabetes are at least two to four times more likely to have heart disease and cerebrovascular disease than those without diabetes. In 2002 it was estimated that diabetes in the US cost $132 billion, representing $92 billion in direct costs and $40 billion in indirect costs (American Diabetes Association, 2003).

The Expert Committee on the Diagnosis and Classification of Diabetes Mellitus revised the criteria for the diagnosis of diabetes in 1997, with recent modifications by the American Diabetes Association (2004a). A fasting plasma glucose level of ≥ 126 mg/dL (7.0 mmol/L), on at least two occasions, is diagnostic for diabetes (Table 16–1). This test should be performed after an 8-hour fast. Symptoms of hyperglycemia (e.g. polyuria, polydipsia, polyphagia, unexplained weight loss) with a casual plasma glucose level of ≥ 200 mg/dL (11.1 mmol/L) also are sufficient to diagnose diabetes. Pre-diabetes designates conditions in which glucose homeostasis is abnormal, but serum glucose levels are not high enough to be classified as diabetes. This group includes individuals with impaired fasting glucose and impaired glucose tolerance. It is estimated that 41 million Americans have pre-diabetes. They are also at increased risk for cardiovascular and cerebrovascular diseases.

Formal oral glucose tolerance tests are not generally recommended for routine clinical use for the diagnosis of diabetes. If used, the procedure described by the World Health Organization (1985), utilizing a 75-gram glucose load should be followed. For children, 1.75 g glucose/kg up to 75 g is recommended. The exception to these criteria is the diagnosis of gestational diabetes (Table 16–2), the glucose intolerance that develops during approximately 7% of all pregnancies (American Diabetes Association, 2004b). To detect gestational diabetes in high-risk individuals, an oral glucose tolerance test (OGTT) should be performed (the 'one-step' approach). The 'two-step' approach is recommended for women with average risk. This approach uses an initial screening test, followed by an OGTT if the screening test glucose level is elevated.

Prior to performing an OGTT, individuals should ingest at least 150 g/day of carbohydrates for the 3 days preceding the test without limitation in physical activity, and the test should be performed after an overnight 8- to 14-hour fast. The individual should not eat food, drink tea, coffee or alcohol, or smoke cigarettes during the test, and should be seated. Venous glucose samples are preferably collected in gray top tubes containing fluoride and an anticoagulant.

Hemoglobin A_{1c} levels, which are useful for monitoring glycemic control, should not be used to diagnose diabetes. This is because hemoglobin A_{1c} assays are not yet standardized in all laboratories and may not correlate precisely with fasting and 2-hour postprandial glucose levels (American Diabetes Association, 2004a).

Approximately 64 million adults in the US in 2000 had the metabolic syndrome and this number is increasing (Ford, 2004). Of great concern is the increasing prevalence of the metabolic syndrome in US adolescents, affecting over 2 million, with over 30% of overweight adolescents having the metabolic syndrome phenotype (Duncan, 2004). The metabolic syndrome is associated with an increased risk of cardiovascular disease and of developing diabetes. The criteria defining the metabolic syndrome according to the Third Report of the National Cholesterol Education Program Expert Panel on Detection, Evaluation and Treatment of High Blood Cholesterol in Adults are the presence of three or more of the following: (1) impaired fasting glucose, (2) blood pressure ≥ 130/85 mmHg, (3) waist circumference > 102 cm in men and > 88 cm in women, (4) serum triglycerides ≥ 150 mg/dL (1.695 mmol/L), and (5) HDL-cholesterol < 40 mg/dL (1.036 mmol/L) in men and < 50 mg/dL (1.295 mmol/L) in women. Most commonly, these individuals are insulin resistant and have smaller, denser, more atherogenic LDL-cholesterol particles.

The classification of diabetes was revised in 1997, and is shown in Table 16–3 with recent minor modifications (American Diabetes Association, 2004a). The most common forms of diabetes are type 1 and type 2 diabetes (Table 16–4). Type 1 diabetes, characterized by absolute insulin deficiency and beta cell destruction, used to be called juvenile-onset diabetes or insulin-dependent diabetes, but these terms are no longer used. Although this disease is most commonly diagnosed in young people, its onset can occur at any age. Since people with other forms of diabetes also use insulin therapy, the term 'insulin-dependent' is confusing and should not be utilized. Type 2 diabetes, characterized by insulin resistance and an insulin secretory defect, has been referred to as adult-onset or non-insulin-dependent diabetes in the past. These terms are also no longer used. Although the onset of type 2 diabetes is most common in older adults, it can occur at any age, including childhood. Many patients with type 2 diabetes use insulin therapy, so it is no longer referred to as non-insulin-dependent diabetes. Uncommon causes of diabetes include genetic defects of beta cell function and insulin action, pancreatic diseases, endocrinopathies such as Cushing's syndrome, acromegaly and pheochromocytoma, and certain drugs, chemicals and infections (Table 16–3).

Type 1 Diabetes

Type 1 diabetes mellitus represents approximately 10% of all cases of diabetes. There usually is an autoimmune destruction of the insulin-producing beta cells in the islets of the pancreas causing an absolute deficiency in insulin production. The genetic susceptibility to develop type 1 diabetes is related, at least in part, to the inheritance of specific immune response genes associated with HLA-DR/DQ on chromosome 6 as well as other genes and genetic markers. It is then hypothesized that a precipitating event occurs, such as a viral infection, toxin exposure or other environmental influence, which triggers the autoimmune destruction of

II

Table 16–3 Classification of Diabetes Mellitus

I. Type 1 diabetes (beta cell destruction, usually leading to absolute insulin deficiency)
   A. Immune mediated
   B. Idiopathic
II. Type 2 diabetes (may range from predominantly insulin resistance with relative insulin deficiency to a predominantly secretory defect with insulin resistance)
III. Other specific types
   A. Genetic defects of beta cell function
      1. Chromosome 12, HNF-1α (MODY3)
      2. Chromosome 7, glucokinase (MODY2)
      3. Chromosome 20, HNF-4α (MODY1)
      4. Chromosome 13, insulin promoter factor-1 (IPF-1; MODY4)
      5. Chromosome 17, HNF-1β (MODY5)
      6. Chromosome 2, *Neuro*D1 (MODY6)
      7. Mitochondrial DNA
      8. Others
   B. Genetic defects in insulin action
      1. Type A insulin resistance
      2. Leprechaunism
      3. Rabson–Mendenhall syndrome
      4. Lipoatrophic diabetes
      5. Others
   C. Diseases of the exocrine pancreas
      1. Pancreatitis
      2. Trauma/pancreatectomy
      3. Neoplasia
      4. Cystic fibrosis
      5. Hemochromatosis
      6. Fibrocalculous pancreatopathy
      7. Others
   D. Endocrinopathies
      1. Acromegaly
      2. Cushing's syndrome
      3. Glucagonoma
      4. Pheochromocytoma
      5. Hyperthyroidism
      6. Somatostatinoma
      7. Aldosteronoma
      8. Others
   E. Drug or chemical induced
      1. Vacor
      2. Pentamidine
      3. Nicotinic acid
      4. Glucocorticoids
      5. Thyroid hormone
      6. Diazoxide
      7. β-Adrenergic agonists
      8. Thiazides
      9. Dilantin
      10. α-interferon
      11. Others
   F. Infections
      1. Congenital rubella
      2. Cytomegalovirus
      3. Others
   G. Uncommon forms of immune-mediated diabetes
      1. 'Stiff-man' syndrome
      2. Anti-insulin receptor antibodies
      3. Others

Table 16–3 Classification of Diabetes Mellitus (*cont'd*)

   H. Other genetic syndromes sometimes associated with diabetes
      1. Down syndrome
      2. Klinefelter's syndrome
      3. Turner's syndrome
      4. Wolfram's syndrome
      5. Friedreich's ataxia
      6. Huntington's chorea
      7. Laurence–Moon–Biedl syndrome
      8. Myotonic dystrophy
      9. Porphyria
      10. Prader–Willi syndrome
      11. Others
IV. Gestational diabetes mellitus

From: The American Diabetes Association: Diagnosis and classification of diabetes mellitus. Diabetes Care 2004a; 27:S8.

Table 16–4 Characteristics of Type 1 and Type 2 Diabetes Mellitus

	Type 1 diabetes	Type 2 diabetes
Frequency	5–10%	90–95%
Age of onset	Any, but most common in children and young adults	More common with advancing age, but can occur in children and adolescents
Risk factors	Genetic, autoimmune, environmental	Genetic, obesity, sedentary lifestyle, race/ethnicity
Pathogenesis	Destruction of pancreatic beta cells, usually autoimmune	No autoimmunity Insulin resistance and progressive insulin deficiency
C-peptide levels	Very low or undetectable	Detectable
Pre-diabetes	Autoantibodies (GAD65, ICA512, IAA) may be present	Autoantibodies absent (testing not indicated)
Medication therapy	Insulin absolutely necessary; multiple daily injections or insulin pump	Oral agents Insulin commonly needed
Therapy to prevent or delay onset of diabetes	None known Clinical trials in progress	Lifestyle (weight loss and increased physical activity) Oral medications (metformin, acarbose) may be helpful Clinical trials in progress

IA-2β autoantibodies since IA-2β antibodies generally react with IA-2. Although the presence of antibodies may help in the differentiation of type 1 diabetes from other types of diabetes early in the course of the disease, the absence of antibodies does not exclude this diagnosis.

Those individuals at greatest risk of developing type 1 diabetes have high titers of multiple autoantibodies. In family as well as in population studies, the detection of at least two autoantibodies is associated with increased risk of developing type 1 diabetes (Maclaren, 1999, 2003). GAD65 has the highest sensitivity (91%) as a single screening marker for detecting multiple antibody-positive individuals (Krischer, 2003). IAA are more common in young children who develop type 1 diabetes, whereas GAD65 is more common in adults. These antibody assays are being used in type 1 diabetes detection and prevention research. Their use for routine screening of asymptomatic individuals is not recommended at the present time, in part, because effective interventions have yet to be demonstrated (Verge, 1998).

In the past, the autoantibody assays have not been well standardized and the cutoff values for the assays were not firmly established. Quality control programs are important, since almost 50% of blinded samples that are considered 'low positive' are found to be negative on repeat testing of a blinded duplicate aliquot (Eisenbarth, 2003). Fluid phase radioassays for GAD65 and IA-2 in general have better sensitivity and specificity than standard available ELISA assays (Bingley, 2003). For IAA assays, the microradioassays perform best. These assays use a smaller volume of serum and utilize protein A precipitation (Williams, 1997).

The Diabetes Antibody Standardization Program, a collaboration between the Immunology of Diabetes Society and the Centers for Disease

the beta cells. It is only after most of the beta cells are destroyed, that hyperglycemia develops. Antibody markers of beta cell destruction are commonly present before and at the time of the onset of the diabetes. These include antibodies to antigens for which recombinant autoantibody assays are available: antibodies to the 65-kDa isoform of glutamic acid decarboxylase (GAD65), insulin autoantibodies (IAA) and islet cell antigen 512 autoantibodies (ICA512). ICA512 are autoantibodies to parts of the tyrosine phosphatase IA-2 antigen. The tyrosine phosphate IA-2β (phogrin) is a separate but partly homologous antigen to IA-2. The ICA512 (and IA-2) autoantibody assays are used more frequently than assays for

Control and Prevention, has established a Proficiency Testing Service. They have reported their first proficiency evaluation for different assays of GAD65, IA-2 and IAA (Bingley, 2003). Poorest performance (greatest variation) was observed between different IAA assays. In this study, GAD65 and IA-2 antibody values were expressed in common units, WHO units/mL, as suggested by the Immunology of Diabetes Society. Further information about the Diabetes Antibody Standardization Program can be obtained at http://www.idsoc.org.

The 'pre-diabetes' period of gradual and progressive beta cell destruction can last for months, years or decades. During this period, the acute insulin response to intravenous glucose, called the first phase insulin release, becomes depressed or absent. The absence of first phase insulin response is also found in other forms of diabetes. Eventually, in most people with type 1 diabetes, most or all of the beta cells are destroyed, resulting in inadequate or absent insulin secretion. C-peptide levels and endogenous insulin levels are therefore very low or undetectable. People with untreated type 1 diabetes develop diabetic ketoacidosis. Insulin therapy is required for all patients with type 1 diabetes.

Type 2 Diabetes

Type 2 diabetes is the most common type of diabetes, affecting approximately 90% of Americans with diabetes. This disease is familial, but the underlying genetic defects, for most of those affected, have yet to be determined. Risk factors include overweight (BMI* ≥ 25 kg/m^2), sedentary lifestyle, family history of diabetes, advanced age (≥ 45 years), ethnicity (African Americans, Latinos, Native Americans, Asian Americans and Pacific Islanders), polycystic ovary disease, and history of gestational diabetes or delivery pre-diabetes of a baby weighing > 9 lb, hypertension, vascular disease or dyslipidemia (HDL-cholesterol ≤ 35 mg/dL [0.90 mmol/L] and/or triglyceride level ≥ 250 mg/dL [2.82 mmol/L]). This is not an autoimmune disease, so antibody testing is not worthwhile. C-peptide levels are measurable in type 2 diabetes. Of the estimated 18 million Americans with type 2 diabetes, 5 million are undiagnosed. Unlike undiagnosed type 1 diabetes, in which patients are usually symptomatic, the people with new onset of type 2 diabetes can be free of symptoms. It is not unusual to diagnose type 2 diabetes after the onset of complications. Routine screening for high-risk individuals is therefore recommended.

* Body mass index: Weight (kg)/[Height (m)]^2.

The American Diabetes Association (2004c) recommends screening for type 2 diabetes by the individual's healthcare provider if one or more risk factors are present. In general, it is recommended that adults ages 45 and older, especially if they are overweight, be screened for diabetes every 3 years, but screening should be performed earlier and more frequently if the individual is at higher risk. The preferred test is a fasting plasma glucose level. If a random plasma glucose level is ≥ 160 mg/dL (8.9 mmol/L), a fasting plasma glucose should be performed (Table 16–1). It should be remembered that whole blood glucose values, which are measured on some home blood glucose monitoring devices, are 10–15% lower than plasma glucose values. These devices should not be used to diagnose diabetes. If, however, an individual does have a capillary glucose test on one of these machines that reads ≥ 140 mg/dL (7.8 mmol/L), they should be rescreened with a fasting plasma glucose or OGTT using venous samples (Table 16–1).

In recent years type 2 diabetes is being diagnosed in younger individuals, including children. The American Diabetes Association (2004c) recommends screening children and adolescents, beginning at age 10, who are overweight (BMI > 85th percentile or weigh > 120% of ideal) with two of the following three risk factors: family history (type 2 diabetes in first- and second-degree relatives), high-risk race/ethnicity (Native Americans, African Americans, Hispanic Americans, Asians/South Pacific Islanders), signs of insulin resistance (acanthosis nigricans, hypertension, dyslipidemia, polycystic ovary syndrome).

Most people with type 2 diabetes are insulin resistant and have a relative or absolute deficiency in insulin secretion. Most people with type 2 diabetes are also obese. There is inappropriately high hepatic glucose production, and impaired glucose utilization peripherally. Decreased glucose transport can be demonstrated in muscle and adipose tissue. For glucose tolerance to remain normal, the pancreas has to secrete sufficient insulin. If the pancreas is unable to increase insulin secretion, impaired glucose homeostasis or type 2 diabetes results. Hyperglycemia also is toxic to beta cell function and impairs insulin secretion. Over time, there is usually progressive beta cell failure, and the beta cells produce lesser amounts of insulin contributing to increasing insulin deficiency. Although many people with type 2 diabetes can be effectively treated with diet, exercise and oral glycemic control agents, others require insulin therapy.

Hemoglobin A$_{1c}$	Preprandial glucose		Postprandial glucose*	
(%)	mg/dL	mmol/L	mg/dL	mmol/L
ADA† < 7‡	90–130	5.0–7.2	< 180	< 10.0
AACE§ ≤ 6.5	≤ 110	≤ 6.1	≤ 140	< 7.8

Table 16–5 Glycemic Goals

* 1–2 h after beginning meal.
† ADA, American Diabetes Association, 2004d.
‡ < 6% can be considered in individual patients.
§ AACE, American Association of Clinical Endocrinologists, 2002.

Measures of Glycemic Control

It has been established that improved glycemic control is associated with preventing or delaying the progression of microvascular complications in diabetes. The Diabetes Control and Complications Trial (DCCT) demonstrated that lowering glucose levels in patients with type 1 diabetes slows or prevents the development of retinopathy, neuropathy and nephropathy (DCCT Research Group, 1993). A 50–75% decrease in complications was observed in the intensively treated group, in which a hemoglobin A$_{1c}$ (HbA$_{1c}$) of 7.2% was achieved (compared to 9.0% in the conventionally treated group). Reduction in microvascular complications in type 2 diabetes was found in the United Kingdom Prospective Diabetes Study (UKPDS) as well as in a smaller Japanese study (UK Prospective Diabetes Study Group, 1998a,b; Ohkubo, 1995). In the UKPDS, microvascular complications were decreased by 25% in intensively treated patients by lowering the HbA$_{1c}$ from 7.9 % to 7.0%. The standard of care is to measure HbA$_{1c}$ levels every 3–6 months to monitor glycemic control (American Association of Clinical Endocrinologists, 2002; American Diabetes Association, 2004d). Glycemic goals are shown in Table 16–5.

Glycosylated hemoglobin (GHb) is formed nonenzymatically by the two-step reaction shown below. The first reaction is rapid, reversible, dependent on the ambient glucose concentration, and produces a labile aldimine or Schiff base. Over time, the aldimine slowly undergoes Amadori rearrangement and is converted to a stable ketoamine, glycosylated hemoglobin. Most HbA$_{1c}$ assays measure this stable ketoamine, not the labile product which is more prone to be influenced by recent dietary intake.

$$
\begin{array}{ccccc}
\text{HC=O} & & \text{HC=N-}\beta\text{A(Hb)} & & \text{CH}_2\text{-NH}_2\text{BA(Hb)} \\
| & & | & & | \\
\text{HCOH} & & \text{HCOH} & & \text{C=O} \\
| & & | & & | \\
\text{HOCH} & & \text{HOCH} & \text{Amadori} & \text{HOCH} \\
| & \leftarrow & | & \text{rearrangement} & | \\
\text{(Hb)}\beta\text{A-NH}_2 + \text{HCOH} & \rightarrow & \text{HCOH} & \rightarrow & \text{HCOH} \\
| & \text{(rapid)} & | & \text{(slow)} & | \\
\text{HCOH} & & \text{HCOH} & & \text{HCOH} \\
| & & | & & | \\
\text{CH}_2\text{OH} & & \text{CH}_2\text{OH} & & \text{CH}_2\text{OH} \\
& \leftarrow & \text{Aldimine} & & \\
\text{Hb A + Glucose} & \rightarrow & \text{(Schiff base)} & \rightarrow & \text{Glycosylated Hb} \\
& & \text{Labile Pre-A}_{1C} & & \text{(ketoamine)}
\end{array}
$$

$$(16-7)$$

HbA$_{1c}$ is now defined by the International Federation of Clinical Chemistry Working Group on HbA$_{1c}$ as the hemoglobin A that is irreversibly glycosylated at one or both N-terminal valines of the β-chains of the tetrameric hemoglobin molecule, including hemoglobin that may also (but not solely) be glycosylated on lysine residues.

GHb testing provides an index of average blood glucose levels over the past 2–4 months. Although the life span of red blood cells is approximately 120 days, GHb levels represent a 'weighted' average of glucose levels, with youngest erythrocytes contributing to a greater extent than older ones. Approximately 50% of the GHb level is determined by plasma glucose levels over the previous month, and 75% during the previous 2 months (Tahara, 1993). The testing methods have been standardized to the HbA$_{1c}$ assay, which is now the preferred test to use to assess glycemic control. To avoid confusion for the general public, the American Diabetes Association, the American College of Endocrinology, and the National Diabetes Education Program recommend using the term 'A1c' testing when referring to HbA$_{1c}$ equivalent (GHb) or HbA$_{1c}$ results.

The National Glycohemoglobin Standardization Program (NGSP) began in 1996, with the goal of standardizing GHb tests to the high-

Table 16–6 Correlation Between Hemoglobin A$_{1c}$ and Mean Plasma Glucose Levels

Hemoglobin A$_{1c}$ (%)	Approximate mean plasma glucose	
	mg/dL	mmol/L
4	65	3.5
5	100	5.5
6	135	7.5
7	170	9.5
8	205	11.5
9	240	13.5
10	275	15.5
11	310	17.5
12	345	19.5

From Rohlfing CL, Wiedmeyer H-M, Little RR, et al: Defining the relationship between plasma glucose and HbA (lc): analysis of glucose profiles and HbA (lc) in the Diabetes Control and Complications Trial. Copyright © 2002 American Diabetes Association. From Diabetes Care. Vol. 25, 2002; 275–278. Modified with permission from *The American Diabetes Association*.

performance liquid chromatography (HPLC) method reported as HbA$_{1c}$ or HbA$_{1c}$ equivalent as used in the DCCT. There are several types of certified methods available for measuring hemoglobin A$_{1c}$: immunoassay, ion-exchange HPLC, electrophoresis, boronate affinity HPLC, and enzyme methods. Reliable bench-top point of care analyzers, such as one which uses a cassette-based immunoassay method, are also now available (Guerci, 1997). The majority of US laboratories use a certified method and the College of American Pathologists' proficiency testing program, which utilizes whole blood and lyophilized samples (Little, 2001).

To obtain and retain a 'Certificate of Traceability to the DCCT reference method' in the NGSP, the laboratory must annually satisfy precision criteria (CV ≤5%; ≤3% for Level 1 laboratories), bias criteria (95% confidence interval (CI) of differences between test method and Secondary Reference Laboratories (SRL) must fall within ± 1% GHb of the SRL (± 0.75% GHb for Level 1 laboratories) and outlier criteria (greater than mean + 3 SD of absolute differences between pairs). Level 1 laboratories are usually large and involved in research studies. The NGSP website, http://www.missouri.edu/~diabetes/ngsp.html, contains information on certified laboratories, methods, protocols and procedures for obtaining certifications.

GHb assays vary in reliability in the presence of a variety of factors. Interference by carbamylated hemoglobin can occur with uremia, hypertriglyceridemia and hyperbilirubinemia, and salicylates can cause interference by acetylated species. Hemoglobinopathies (HbSS, HbSC, HbCC) associated with high red blood cell turnover and need for transfusions will adversely affect accuracy as will chronic alcohol or opiate use, iron deficiency and lead poisoning (Hoberman, 1982; Tarim, 1999). Vitamins C and E can falsely lower levels by inhibiting glycosylation, but vitamin C can also increase levels for some assays (Davie, 1992; Ceriello, 1991). There may also be sample storage effects. Any condition associated with shortened red blood cell survival, or lower mean red blood cell age, such as hemolysis, recovery from acute blood loss, transfusions or splenectomy, will lower the HbA$_{1c}$ level because of reduced exposure to plasma glucose. Hyperglycemia has been associated with a decrease in erythrocyte survival, suggesting that HbA$_{1c}$ levels in poorly controlled patients may underestimate their mean plasma glucose concentration (Virtue, 2004).

In general, people without diabetes have HbA$_{1c}$ levels between 4–6%. The correlation between HbA$_{1c}$ and average plasma glucose levels for clinical use, based upon data from the DCCT is shown in Table 16–6.

The turnover time of serum proteins, primarily albumin, is much shorter than that of erythrocytes (14–20 days), so their glycosylation reflects glycemic control over narrower periods of time. The nonenzymatic glycation of these serum proteins occurs similarly to that of hemoglobin, with the formation of ketoamine-linked glucose protein. There are several methods for measuring glycosylated proteins or glycosylated albumin, including affinity chromatography and immunoassays. These assays may be useful in patients for whom HbA$_{1c}$ assays are inaccurate, such as those with hemoglobinopathies and hemolytic anemias, but unlike HbA$_{1c}$ levels, their clinical utility has not been firmly established.

Fructosamine assays are the most widely used to assess short-term (3- to 6-week) glycemic control, since the average half-life of the proteins is 2–3 weeks. These assays have the advantage of using serum samples and automated equipment so are simple to perform and low in cost. They are more reliable than other glycosylated protein assays, but can be affected by alterations in serum protein levels that are present during acute illnesses and liver disease. Whether fructosamine values should be corrected for serum protein or albumin concentrations is controversial. The assay should not be performed if the serum albumin level is ≤ 3.0 mg/dL. High uric acid, triglyceride and bilirubin levels and the presence of heparin or hemolysis can also affect the assay.

Ketone Testing

The ketone bodies beta-hydroxybutyric acid, acetoacetic acid and acetone are products of fatty acid degradation. Beta-hydroxybutyric acid and acetoacetic acid are normally present in a 1 : 1 ratio at concentrations of 0.5–1.0 mmol/L each. Ketone testing, using urine or blood, is particularly important for individuals with type 1 diabetes mellitus to detect ketosis. Diabetic ketoacidosis (DKA) is a serious and potentially fatal hyperglycemic condition requiring urgent treatment. It is frequently associated with nausea, vomiting, abdominal pain, electrolyte disturbances and severe dehydration. Type 2 diabetes patients who are poorly controlled, particularly in the presence of extreme stress or severe acute illness, can also develop DKA. Ketone testing may be useful in pregnancy and in determining the etiology of hypoglycemic disorders.

The ratio of beta-hydroxybutyrate acid to acetoacetic acid is greatly increased in DKA due to the altered redox state and elevated levels of NADH in the hepatic mitochondria. The most commonly used strips and tablets use sodium nitroprusside (sodium nitroferricyanide) and turn purple in the presence of elevated levels of acetoacetic acid. Acetone is detected in the presence of glycine. False-negative results can occur with old strips, strips that have had excessive contact with air, and after ingestion of large amounts of vitamin C. False-positive results have been observed with angiotensin-converting enzyme inhibitors and other sulfhydryl medications. Beta-hydroxybutyric acid is not detected by these methods. Since beta-hydroxybutyric acid levels fall and acetoacetic acid and acetone levels rise during the treatment of DKA, these tests are not useful for the monitoring of therapy.

To specifically quantitate beta-hydroxybutyric acid, enzymatic methods are now available for use by hospitals as well as by individuals at home using point-of-care devices. Beta-hydroxybutyric acid can also be measured using electrochemical, chromatographic, electrophoretic and colorimetric methods. For the monitoring of recovery from DKA in the hospital setting, serial measurements of beta-hydroxybutyric acid can be followed, but more commonly, serum electrolytes including bicarbonate with calculation of the anion gap are used.

Hypoglycemia

Hypoglycemia results from an imbalance between glucose utilization and production in such a manner that the rate of glucose utilization exceeds the rate at which glucose is being produced. The symptoms of hypoglycemia can be divided into two categories: neurogenic and neuroglycopenic. Neurogenic symptoms are triggered by the autonomic nervous system. Tremulousness, palpitations and anxiety are catecholamine mediated and diaphoresis, hunger and paresthesias are related to acetylcholine release. The neuroglycopenic symptoms are due to diminished glucose supply to the central nervous system and include dizziness, tingling, difficulty concentrating, blurred vision, confusion, behavioral changes, seizure and coma (Towler, 1993; Schwartz, 1987; Mitrakou, 1991).

Treatment of diabetes mellitus with insulin or agents that increase insulin secretion (insulin secretagogue drugs) such as sulfonylureas is the major cause of hypoglycemia. However, a number of drugs and medical conditions can cause hypoglycemia (Table 16–7). Pancreatic hyper-insulinemic hypoglycemia can be diagnosed by demonstrating that insulin secretion is not suppressed normally when the individual develops hypoglycemia. Measurements of insulin, C-peptide, proinsulin, insulin and insulin receptor autoantibodies, beta-hydroxybutyrate and drugs (i.e., sulfonylurea/meglitinide levels) are recommended to determine the correct diagnosis. Insulin and proinsulin autoantibodies may interfere with the immunoassays for insulin, proinsulin and C-peptide.

'Whipple's triad' initially proposed by Whipple for the diagnosis of hypoglycemic disorders continues to be an important tool in assessing patients with episodes suggestive of low plasma glucose levels. Whipple's triad refers to symptoms consistent with hypoglycemia associated with a documented low plasma glucose level, and relief of symptoms with correction of hypoglycemia (Whipple, 1938). Further evaluation is indicated if a patient presents with symptoms of hypoglycemia and a laboratory plasma glucose level of ≤50 mg/dL (2.8 mmol/L) in the absence of treatment of diabetes mellitus (Service, 1999a). A blood glucose level

Table 16–7 Clinical Classification of Hypoglycemia

Drugs

Insulin

Sulfonylureas

Benzoic acid derivatives (repaglinide)

Nateglinide

Alcohol

Pentamidine

Beta-blockers

Quinine

Salicylates

Sulfonamides

Haloperidol

Propoxyphene

Para-aminobenzoic acid

Critical illnesses

Hepatic failure

Renal failure

Cardiac failure

Sepsis

Malnutrition

Hormonal deficiencies

Glucagon

Epinephrine

Cortisol

Growth hormone

Endogenous hyperinsulinism

Pancreatic beta cell disorders

   Tumor (insulinoma)

   Nontumor (nesidioblastosis or diffuse hyperplasia of the islets)

Autoimmune hypoglycemia

Insulin antibodies

Insulin receptor antibodies

Non-beta cell tumors

Mesenchymal: Fibrosarcoma, mesothelioma, rhabdomyosarcoma, leiomyosarcoma, liposarcoma, lymphosarcoma, hemangiopericytoma

Carcinomas: Hepatomas, adrenocortical tumors, hypernephroma, Wilms' tumor

Neurological and neuroendocrine tumors: Pheochromocytoma, carcinoid tumor, neurofibroma

Hematologic: Leukemias, lymphoma, myeloma

Hypoglycemia of infancy and childhood

Hyperinsulinism

   Transient: Erythroblastosis fetalis, Beckwith–Wiedemann syndrome, uncontrolled diabetes (mother)

   Persistent: Hyperinsulinemic hypoglycemia of infancy

Glycogen storage diseases

Hereditary fructose intolerance

Galactosemia

Defects in gluconeogenesis

Reye's syndrome

Deficiency of glucose transporters

Impaired ketogenesis

Carnitine deficiency

Defects in mitochondrial function

Alimentary hypoglycemia

Post-gastric surgery

Idiopathic (functional) postprandial hypoglycemia

Adapted from:

Cryer PE: Glucose homeostasis and hypoglycemia. *In* Larsen PR, Kronenberg HK, Melmed S, Polonsky KS (eds): Williams Textbook of Endocrinology, 10th ed. Philadelphia, Saunders, 2003, pp 1585–1618.

Lteif AN, Schwenk WF: Hypoglycemia in infants and children. Endocrinol Metab Clin N Amer 1999; 28(3):619–646.

≤ 50 mg/dL (2.8 mmol/L) in infants is considered abnormal and warrants diagnostic assessment (Sperling, 2004; Haymond, 1989).

Hypoglycemic Disorders

Drugs. Medications, particularly insulin and insulin secretagogues such as sulfonylurea drugs, repaglinide and nateglinide, remain the most common causes of hypoglycemia. Elevated insulin with low C-peptide levels are observed when exogenous insulin has been administered. High insulin and C-peptide levels with a positive drug screen for an insulin secretagogue would be expected when these oral agents have been used surreptitiously. It is important that these blood tests be drawn during the hypoglycemic episode. The assays for sulfonylureas and meglitinides should be sent to a laboratory that has the capability to measure very low levels of these drugs, as assays using higher detection limits can lead to an inaccurate diagnosis (Manning, 2003).

Pentamidine used for the treatment of *Pneumocystis carinii* pneumonia causes hypoglycemia by damaging pancreatic beta cells. Hypoglycemia can occur within a few hours to days of administration of pentamidine. The plasma insulin levels are high despite low glucose concentrations, indicating excessive insulin leakage (Bouchard, 1982; Assan, 1995). Sulfonamide-induced hypoglycemia is also associated with increased insulin and C-peptide levels in susceptible individuals (Hekimsoy, 1997). Salicylate-induced hypoglycemia may be due to increased peripheral glucose utilization secondary to uncoupling of oxidative phosphorylation, decreased hepatic glyconeogenesis and increased insulin release (Marks, 1999). Beta-blockers, such as propranolol, can cause hypoglycemia by antagonizing catecholamine-mediated glycogenolysis (Chavez, 1999).

Alcohol consumption can inhibit hepatic gluconeogenesis and increase glycogen phosphorylase activity, depleting hepatic glycogen stores and resulting in hypoglycemia. Alcohol-induced hypoglycemia is usually seen in the setting of a history of alcohol intake of 50–300 g without food intake for the preceding 6 to greater then 36 hours. Alcohol can be detected in the blood or breath. Plasma beta-hydroxybutyrate levels are elevated, and plasma insulin and C-peptide levels are low during the hypoglycemic episode (Arky, 1989; Marks, 1999).

Severe medical illnesses. Widespread hepatic disease as well as severe cardiac failure can result in hypoglycemia. Pathogenic mechanisms can include impaired gluconeogenesis, hepatic congestion with decreased oxygen delivery to hepatocytes, impaired insulin degradation and shunting of portal blood into the systemic circulation (Khoury, 1998). A decrease in glycogen reserves coupled with failure of gluconeogenesis and enhanced glucose utilization may be the cause of hypoglycemia in patients with severe sepsis (Miller, 1980). In addition, patients with very low muscle mass, such as those with spinal muscular atrophy and congenital myopathy, are at risk for hypoglycemia during prolonged fasting (23 hours), presumably related to poor availability of the gluconeogenic substrate alanine. Low plasma insulin and high plasma glucagon levels are observed during the hypoglycemia (Orngreen, 2003).

Hypoglycemia in end-stage renal disease (ESRD) can be related to defective gluconeogenesis as well as impaired hepatic glycogenolysis due to poor nutritional status (Arem, 1989). Alcohol use, use of insulin or sulfonylurea drugs, sepsis, malnutrition, liver disease and cardiac failure can increase the likelihood of hypoglycemic events in a patient with renal failure (Haviv, 2000). Gabapentin has been associated with hypoglycemia in a patient with ESRD on peritoneal dialysis. Plasma insulin and C-peptide levels were elevated during the hypoglycemic episode (Penumalee, 2003).

Hormone deficiencies. Glucose counterregulation, mediated by glucagon, catecholamines, cortisol and growth hormone, is important in preventing hypoglycemia. Glucagon initially stimulates glycogenolysis and later gluconeogenesis to increase plasma glucose levels. Catecholamines increase glycogenolysis, gluconeogenesis, and lipolysis, decrease insulin-mediated glucose uptake and inhibit insulin release. Both growth hormone and cortisol decrease insulin-mediated tissue glucose uptake and increase release of glucose into the circulation. A deficiency in the secretion of these counterregulatory hormones can contribute to low blood glucose levels. Hypoglycemia in adults is rarely attributable to deficiencies of glucagon or catecholamines, but poor glucagon and epinephrine responses to hypoglycemia are common in patients with longstanding diabetes mellitus and are associated with prolonged hypoglycemic episodes. Infants and children with a deficiency of cortisol and growth hormone are prone to develop hypoglycemia, especially during an acute illness. Adults with glucocorticoid or growth hormone deficiency can also develop hypoglycemia usually after a prolonged fast (Smallridge, 1980; Zuker, 1995; Bunch, 2002).

Non-beta cell tumors. Non-islet cell tumor hypoglycemia (NICTH) originates from non-beta cell tumors, mostly of mesenchymal origin. These tumors are associated with increased production of insulin-like growth factor-II (IGF-II). It is believed that elevated levels of IGF-II increase glucose utilization and suppress endogenous glucose production (Chung, 1996; Daughaday, 1989). The diagnosis of NICTH can usually be made by the presence of fasting hypoglycemia, low insulin, proinsulin and C-peptide levels, an elevated IGF-II to IGF-I ratio and low growth hormone and beta-hydroxybutyrate levels. The tumor is usually detected on physical examination and confirmed by radiologic diagnostic studies.

Endogenous Hyperinsulinism. Hypoglycemia from endogenous insulin can be due to: (1) insulin-secreting beta cell tumors (insulinomas), (2) congenital hyperinsulinism (also called nesidioblastosis/islet hypertrophy or noninsulinoma pancreatogenous hypoglycemia syndrome), (3) autoantibodies to insulin in patients who have never been treated with insulin (Hirata, 1994). A supervised 72-hour fast is recommended for the diagnosis of insulinoma with frequent clinical and biochemical monitoring for signs of hypoglycemia. During the hypoglycemic episode blood is drawn for glucose, insulin, proinsulin, C-peptide and beta-hydoxybutyrate levels. Blood or urine screening tests for sulfonylurea/meglitinide drugs are also performed. The diagnostic criteria for an insulinoma are: presence of signs and symptoms of hypoglycemia with plasma glucose level of ≤ 45 mg/dL (2.5 mmol/L), an inappropriately elevated insulin level $\geq 6\,\mu U/mL$ (by radioimmunoassay) or $\geq 3\,\mu U/mL$ (by immunochemiluminometric assay), C-peptide ≥ 0.2 pmol/L, proinsulin ≥ 5 pmol/L, beta-hydroxybutyrate ≤ 2.7 mmol/L, a ≥ 25 mg/dL change in plasma glucose in response to a 1 mg glucagon injection given intravenously and a negative sulfonylurea/meglitinide blood/urine screen (Service, 1995, 1999b).

Autoimmune. Hypoglycemia associated with autoantibodies to insulin in patients who have not received insulin injections is a rare condition called the autoimmune insulin syndrome (AIS). Individuals with autoimmune diseases or recent ingestion of sulfhydryl-containing medications (i.e., methimazole, penicillamine, captopril, imipenem) are at increased risk for AIS. Excessive amounts of insulin secreted after a meal are bound to antibodies and as a result insulin becomes unavailable to target tissues. Hours later the insulin dissociates from the antibodies resulting in hyperinsulinemia and hypoglycemia. Insulin levels are extremely elevated and distinctly higher than in insulinoma. C-peptide levels are incompletely suppressed and a high insulin to C-peptide molar ratio is present. Serum insulin antibodies are elevated (Hirata, 1994; Dozio, 1998; Lidar, 1999; Cavaco, 2001; Vogeser, 2001; Yaturu, 2004).

Antibodies directed against the insulin receptor can cause hypoglycemia or hyperglycemia with extreme insulin resistance. Other autoimmune diseases, such as systemic lupus erythematosus and Hashimoto's thyroiditis, may also be present in these patients. In this condition, insulin receptor antibodies block insulin from attaching to the insulin receptor. In some patients hyperglycemia is seen due to receptor degradation or down-regulation leading to insulin resistance. Hyperglycemia and hypoglycemia can sometimes be seen in the same patient. Plasma glucose, beta-hydroxybutyrate and proinsulin levels are low and insulin levels and the insulin : C-peptide ratio is inappropriately high. The insulin receptor antibodies can be detected by immunoprecipitation assays (Redmon, 1999; Taylor, 1989). Mutations in the insulin receptor gene are another rare cause of hypoglycemia.

Infancy and Childhood. The hypoglycemia of infancy, occurring in the first 72 hours after birth, is usually transient and common in preterm or small for gestational age infants. Infants of women with poorly controlled diabetes mellitus have sustained hyperinsulinism that increases the risk of hypoglycemia during the few days after birth. Other etiologies include pituitary and adrenal disorders. Ketogenic hypoglycemia can be seen in children between 18 months and 5 years of age. Alanine, a gluconeogenic substrate, is found to be low in these patients. Usually an episode of illness or prolonged fasting is associated with the hypoglycemia (Haymond, 1983).

Persistent hyperinsulinemic hypoglycemia of infancy (PHHI) is most commonly due to inability of the pancreatic beta cell to appropriately suppress insulin secretion during hypoglycemia. This condition usually presents during the first year of life, typically during the first few hours to days after birth. Mutations in the beta cell ATP-sensitive K+ channel (K_{ATP} channel) genes SUR1 (the sulfonylurea receptor) and Kir6.2 cause inappropriate insulin release and the most severe forms of PHHI. The noninsulinoma pancreatogenous hypoglycemia syndrome reported in adults is not associated with mutations in either the SUR1 or Kir6.2 genes. These patients usually present with postprandial hypoglycemia. The serum insulin and C-peptide levels are elevated and the drug screens for sulfonylureas and meglitinides are negative (Service, 1999b).

The enzyme glucokinase (GCK) functions as a glucose sensor in the pancreatic beta cell and mediates glucose-stimulated insulin secretion.

Activating mutations of GCK are inherited in an autosomal dominant manner and have been associated with familial hyperinsulinemic hypoglycemia. The hypoglycemia is usually mild (as compared with the autosomal recessive form) and is not limited to infancy. De novo mutations in the GCK gene resulting in hypoglycemia have also been described. In the hyperinsulinism hyperammonia syndrome, hypoglycemia is caused by an activating mutation of the glutamate dehydrogenase gene (GLUD1) located on chromosome 10. It is an autosomal dominant disorder characterized by hypoglycemia and elevated ammonia levels (three to eight times normal). Less severe hypoglycemia is seen in sporadic cases (Sunehag, 2002; Straub, 2001; Cuesta-Munoz, 2004; Stanley, 1998). Hypoglycemia as well as lactic acidosis have been described in a child with a mutation in a subunit of the mitochondrial respiratory chain complex III (Haut, 2003). In addition, mutations in enzymes involved in mitochondrial fatty acid oxidation can cause PHHI (Molven, 2004).

Alimentary. Alimentary (reactive) hypoglycemia occurs several hours after a meal. OGTTs are unreliable in diagnosing this condition. Individuals who have had gastric surgery are at risk. Rapid gastric emptying and the dumping syndrome can trigger an exaggerated insulin response with resultant hypoglycemia. Some individuals without gastrointestinal pathology report spontaneous symptoms suggestive of hypoglycemia 1–4 hours after intake of carbohydrate-rich meals, but have a normal laboratory evaluation. These patients are believed to have idiopathic reactive hypoglycemia. The OGTT is also not useful for the diagnosis of this condition (Lefebvre, 1988). Increased insulin sensitivity has been seen in some patients exhibiting features of postprandial hypoglycemia (Tamburrano, 1989). Contributing factors may also include delayed release of insulin in response to a meal and concomitant alcohol ingestion (Flanagan, 1998).

Inborn Errors of Carbohydrate Metabolism

Normal plasma glucose levels are maintained by absorption of glucose from the diet, synthesis of glucose during gluconeogenesis and the release of glucose from glycogen, the principal storage form of glucose. Glycogen storage diseases or glycogenoses result from defects in glycogen metabolism. These diseases are the consequence of inherited deficiencies of enzymes that control the synthesis or breakdown of glycogen. Abnormal quality or quantity of glycogen is found in these disorders. Liver and muscle are most commonly affected by defects in glycogen metabolism as these tissues have abundant quantities of glycogen. Glycogen storage diseases that primarily affect the liver (hepatic glycogenoses) usually manifest with hypoglycemia and hepatomegaly. Muscle cramps, exercise intolerance, fatigue and weakness are common complaints in glycogen storage diseases affecting muscles (muscle glycogenoses). Glycogen storage diseases types I (glucose-6-phosphatase deficiency), III (debrancher deficiency), IV (brancher deficiency), VI (liver phosphorylase deficiency), IX (phosphorylase kinase deficiency) and type 0 (glycogen synthase deficiency) and glucose transporter-2 (GLUT-2) deficiency mainly affect the liver. Table 16–8 shows the various characteristics of hepatic glycogenoses (Wolfsdorf, 1999; Chen, 2001). Muscle glycogenoses or glycogen storage diseases affecting the muscles (Table 16–9) include type V (muscle phosphorylase deficiency), type VII (muscle phosphofructokinase deficiency), and glycogen storage diseases secondary to defects in phosphoglycerate kinase, phosphoglycerate mutase, lactate dehydrogenase, fructose 1,6-biphosphate aldolase A, pyruvate kinase, muscle phosphorylase kinase, lysosomal acid alpha-glucosidase (type II, Pompe disease) and cardiac-specific phosphorylase kinase (Tsujino, 2000; Chen, 2001; Weinstein, 2002).

Defects in Galactose Metabolism

Galactose is a monosaccharide constituent, together with glucose, of the disaccharide lactose. Milk and milk products are the main sources of galactose. Enzymatic defects of galactokinase, galactose-1-phosphate uridyltransferase and uridine diphosphate galactose-4-epimerase result in the defective metabolism and accumulation of galactose and its metabolites causing galactosemia (Holton, 2001).

Galactosemia with Uridyl Transferase Deficiency. Galactose-1-phosphate uridyl transferase (GALT) deficiency (classic galactosemia) has an autosomal recessive mode of inheritance. The most common mutation of the GALT gene is the Q188R mutation on chromosome 9. GALT deficiency presents early in infancy with symptoms of hypoglycemia, vomiting, diarrhea, irritability, feeding difficulties and failure to thrive. These infants may have jaundice, hepatomegaly and easy bruisability. Initial diagnostic tests may reveal hyperbilirubinemia, elevated liver transaminases, metabolic acidosis, galactosuria, glycosuria, hypoglycemia and abnormal clotting measurements. These patients are at risk of developing cerebral edema. Vitreous hemorrhage and *Escherichia coli* sepsis have also been reported in affected individuals.

Table 16–8 Hepatic Glycogenoses

Type (GSD)	Defect	Clinical features	Laboratory findings	Treatment	Genetics
Ia/von Gierke disease	Glucose-6-phosphatase	Thin extremities, short stature, protuberant abdomen, skin xanthomas, retinal changes, hepatomegaly, hypoglycemic seizures, growth retardation.	Hypoglycemia, lactic acidosis, hyperuricemia, dyslipidemia Diagnosis: Liver biopsy to demonstrate glucose-6-phosphatase activity in both intact and fully disrupted microsomes	High complex carbohydrate feeds during day, total parenteral nutrition, nocturnal nasogastric or gastrostomy tube infusion of glucose at night, uncooked starch Restrict fructose and galactose	Autosomal recessive
Ib	Glucose-6-phosphatase translocase	As for 1a, plus recurrent bacterial infections	As for 1a, plus neutropenia and inflammatory bowel disease	As for 1a, plus granulocyte and granulocyte/macrophage colony-stimulating factors (GM-CSF) for neutropenia	Autosomal recessive
IIIa (also called 'Cori' or 'Forbes' disease	Glycogen debranching enzyme (both in liver and muscle)	Childhood: Hepatomegaly, hypoglycemia, growth retardation Adult: Muscle atrophy, weakness, cardiomyopathy	Childhood: Dyslipidemia, hypoglycemia, ↑ hepatic transaminases, fasting ketosis, normal lactate and uric acid Adult: EMG shows myopathy Diagnosis: Demonstration of abnormal glycogen and abnormal enzyme activity on liver and muscle biopsy	Childhood: Same as 1a, plus high-protein diet. No dietary restriction of fructose and galactose Adult: No effective treatment of myopathy	Autosomal recessive
IIIb	Glycogen debranching enzyme in liver (normal muscle debranching enzyme)	Same as in IIIa, with no muscle symptoms	Same as in IIIa, with no muscle findings	Same as in IIIa	Autosomal recessive
IV (also called Andersen disease, amylopectinosis)	Glycogen branching enzyme	Hepatosplenomegaly, failure to thrive, liver cirrhosis, portal hypertension, ascites, esophageal varices and fatal by 5 years of age. Hypoglycemia rare but may occur in liver cirrhosis Neuromuscular form: Neonate: Hypotonia, muscle atrophy, Childhhood: Myopathy or cardiomyopathy Adulthood: Diffuse central and peripheral nervous system dysfunction (adult polyglucosan body disease)	Tissue deposition of amylopectin-like material Deficiency of branching enzyme in liver Adult polyglucosan body disease: Deficient branching enzyme in leukocytes or nerve biopsy	No specific treatment Maintenance of normoglycemia Liver transplantation in selected cases	Autosomal recessive
VI (also called Hers disease)	Glycogen phosphorylase (in liver)	Hepatomegaly, growth retardation in early childhood, benign course. Hepatomegaly improves with age	Mild hypoglycemia, dyslipidemia, ketosis Normal uric acid and lactic acid Diagnosis: Abnormal enzyme activity in biopsy of affected tissues	High-carbohydrate diet, frequent feedings No specific treatment in most patients	Autosomal recessive
IXa	Phosphorylase kinase (in liver)	Hepatomegaly, protuberant abdomen, growth retardation, delay in motor development	Mild dyslipidemia, mildly elevated liver transaminases, fasting ketosis, mild hypoglycemia Diagnosis: Abnormal enzyme activity in biopsy of affected tissues	High-carbohydrate diet, frequent feeds Course usually benign	X-linked
IXb	Phosphorylase deficiency (in liver and muscle)	Hepatomegaly, growth retardation, muscle hypotonia (in some patients)	Same as in IXa	Same as in IXa	Autosomal recessive
0	Glycogen synthase	Hypoglycemic symptoms in morning. No hepatomegaly Mild growth delay (in few cases)	Fasting hypoglycemia, hyperketonemia Hyperglycemia and elevated lactate level after meals Diagnosis: Mutation analysis of the hepatic glycogen synthase gene	Uncooked starch feeding during night Frequent feedings during day with high protein content	Autosomal recessive

Table 16–8 Hepatic Glycogenoses (*cont'd*)

Type (GSD)	Defect	Clinical features	Laboratory findings	Treatment	Genetics
XI (also called Fanconi–Bickel syndrome)	GLUT 2	Protuberant abdomen due to hepatomegaly and renomegaly, rickets, failure to thrive	Glucosuria, phosphaturia, aminoaciduria, bicarbonate wasting, hypophosphatemia, elevated alkaline phosphatase level Mild fasting hypoglycemia and dyslipidemia Rickets on radiologic studies	No specific therapy Symptomatic replacement of water, electrolytes, vitamin D Restriction of galactose Frequent small meals with corn starch supplement	Autosomal recessive

Adapted from:

Chen YT: Glycogen storage diseases. *In* Scriver CR, Beaudet AL, Sly WS, Valle D, eds: The Metabolic and Molecular Bases of Inherited Disease, 8th ed. New York, McGraw-Hill, 2001. pp 1521–1551.

Wolfsdorf JI, Holm IA, Weinstein DA: Glycogen storage diseases. Phenotypic, genetic, and biochemical characteristics, and therapy. Endocrinol Metab Clin N Amer 1999; 28(4):801–823.

Weinstein DA, Wolfsdorf JI: Glycogen storage diseases: A primer for clinicians. Endocrinologist 2002; 12: 531–538.

Table 16–9 Muscle Glycogenoses

Type	Defect	Clinical features	Laboratory findings	Treatment
V (McArdle disease)	Muscle phosphorylase	Exercise intolerance, muscle cramps Dark red-colored urine after intense exercise Usually presents in 2nd or 3rd decade	Myoglobinuria, ↑ creatinine kinase at rest and increases after exercise, ↑ ammonia and ↑ uric acid with exercise Diagnosis: Enzymatic evaluation of muscle or mutation analysis	↑ Exercise tolerance by aerobic training, or by ingestion of glucose or fructose High-protein diet Vitamin B_6 supplementation
VII (Tarui disease)	Phosphofructokinase	Same as in type V plus: Severe exercise intolerance or myopathy in childhood, compensated hemolytic anemia, more hyperuricemia than type V, acute exercise intolerance post-carbohydrate-rich meals	↑ Creatine kinase and ↑ bilirubin, reticulocytosis, hyperuricemia Diagnosis: Biochemical or histochemical demonstration of enzyme defect	Avoid strenuous exercise for prevention of muscle cramps and myoglobinuria
Phosphoglycerate kinase deficiency	Phosphoglycerate kinase	Same as in type V plus: Hemolytic anemia, CNS dysfunction and/or myopathy	↑ Creatine kinase (not always) Abnormal enzyme assays in muscles	Same as in type VII
Phosphoglycerate mutase deficiency	Phosphoglycerate mutase M subunit	Same as in type V	↑ Serum creatine kinase level	Same as type VII
Lactate dehydrogenase deficiency	Lactic acid dehydrogenase M subunit	Same as in type V plus: Erythematous rash, difficulties in childbirth (uterine stiffness)	↑ Creatine kinase level (not always)	Same as type VII
Fructose-1,6-biphosphate aldolase A deficiency	Fructose-1,6-biphosphate aldolase A	Same as type V plus: Muscle weakness, hemolytic anemia	↑ Creatine kinase (not always)	Same as type VII
Pyruvate kinase deficiency	Pyruvate kinase muscle isozyme	Muscle cramps, fixed muscle weakness	↑ Creatine kinase (not always)	Same as type VII
Muscle phosphorylase kinase deficiency	Muscle phosphorylase kinase (muscle specific)	Same as type V plus: Muscle weakness and atrophy	↑ Creatine kinase (not always)	Same as type VII
II/Pompe disease	Lysosomal acid alpha glucosidase (acid maltase)	*Infant:* muscle weakness, feeding problems, macroglossia, hepatomegaly, cardiomyopathy *Late childhood:* Proximal muscle weakness, swallowing difficulties, respiratory muscle weakness *Adult:* Proximal muscle weakness with pelvic girdle, paraspinal and diaphragm muscle affected seriously	↑ Creatine kinase, ↑ aspartate transaminase, LDH Diagnosis: Decreased or absent acid alpha-glucosidase activity in muscle or cultured skin fibroblasts	*Infant:* No effective treatment *Late childhood and adult:* High-protein diet Ventilatory support

Adapted from:

Chen YT: Glycogen storage diseases. *In* Scriver CR, Beaudet AL, Sly WS, Valle D (eds). The Metabolic and Molecular Bases of Inherited Disease, 8th ed. New York, McGraw-Hill, 2001, pp 1521–1551.

Tsujino S, Nonaka I, DiMauro S: Glycogen storage myopathies. Neurol Clin 2000; 18(1):125–150.

Long-term complications in GALT deficiency include impaired cognition, ovarian failure in females and ataxic neurologic disease. Microbiologic and fluorometric assays are used in the screening of the newborn to detect galactosemia. A fluorescent spot screening test for GALT activity (Beutler test) is available. An abnormal test is followed by a biochemical or molecular confirmation of the diagnosis. The quantitative assays can give false-negative results following blood transfusion. A milder form of galactosemia known as the 'Duarte variant' is also caused by a mutation within the GALT gene and is characterized by decreased red cell enzyme activity, which is generally of no clinical significance. Treatment of GALT deficiency consists of restriction of galactose in the diet (Holton, 2001; Leslie, 2003).

Galactokinase (GALK) deficiency. In GALK deficiency, galactose cannot be converted into galactose-1-phosphate, and this leads to cataract formation. Pseudotumor cerebri is another rare complication observed in this disorder. The diagnosis is made by demonstrating an elevated blood galactose level with normal uridyltransferase activity and absence of galactokinase activity in erythrocytes. A galactose-free diet can reverse cataracts if started in early infancy (Holton, 2001; Bosch, 2002).

Uridine diphosphate galactose-4-epimerase (GALE) deficiency. The benign form is associated with enzyme deficiency limited to erythrocytes and leukocytes. These affected individuals are healthy and no treatment is required. In the severe form, clinical findings are similar to those seen in GALT deficiency with the additional findings of hypotonia and sensorineural deafness. Treatment consists of dietary restriction of galactose (Walter, 1999; Holton, 2001).

Defects in Fructose Metabolism

Essential fructosuria, hereditary fructose intolerance and fructose-1,6-diphosphatase deficiencies are the clinical conditions resulting from defects in fructose metabolism.

Essential Fructosuria. This autosomal recessive disorder results from fructokinase deficiency. Fructokinase catalyzes the conversion of fructose to fructose-1-phosphate. The condition is asymptomatic and is usually diagnosed incidentally by the detection of fructose in urine as a reducing substance. No treatment is necessary.

Hereditary fructose intolerance. A defect of fructose-1,6-biphosphate aldolase B activity in the liver, kidney and intestine results in the failure of conversion of fructose-1-phosphate and fructose-1,6-biphosphate into dihydroxyacetone phosphate, glyceraldehyde-3-phosphate, and glyceraldehydes. Fructose intake leads to accumulation of fructose-1-phosphate and causes symptoms of hypoglycemia and nausea followed by vomiting. Symptoms occur only when fructose-containing foods are ingested. Prolonged exposure to fructose-containing foods can cause frequent hypoglycemic episodes, hepatomegaly, irritability, lethargy, seizures and proximal tubular dysfunction. Hepatic dysfunction can result in prolonged clotting time, elevated transaminases with elevated bilirubin levels and hypoalbuminemia. The diagnosis is supported by clinical suspicion followed by an intravenous fructose tolerance test. Definitive diagnosis can be made by assay of aldolase B activity in a liver biopsy specimen.

Fructose-1,6-biphosphatase deficiency. This autosomal recessive defect in fructose-1,6-biphosphatase results in failure of hepatic glucose generation by gluconeogenic precursors such as lactate, glycerol and alanine. Life-threatening episodes of hypoglycemia, hyperventilation, lactic acidosis, convulsions and coma can be seen in the affected patients. The diagnosis is established by demonstrating enzyme deficiency in a liver or intestinal biopsy specimen. Correction of hypoglycemia and acidosis by intravenous fluids is the treatment of choice during acute attacks. Prolonged fasting can cause symptoms in affected individuals if glycogen stores are depleted. Fructose and sucrose need to be limited in the diet (Steinman, 2001).

Lactic Acidosis

Lactic acid is a product of pyruvic acid metabolism. Approximately 1400 mmol of lactic acid are produced daily in healthy individuals, most of which is derived from glucose via the glycolytic pathway and deamination of alanine (Marko, 2004; Kreisberg, 1980). This enormous amount of lactic acid is eliminated by several mechanisms including buffering by extracellular buffers and removal by the liver and kidneys. Under normal circumstances the rates of lactate entry and exit from the blood are in equilibrium and net lactate accumulation is zero. Excessive accumulation of L-lactic acid is caused by overproduction and/or underutilization of L-lactate (the levorotary form of lactic acid).

Selected causes of lactic acidosis are shown in Table 16–10. Lactic acid production increases during ischemia, seizures, vigorous exercise and some leukemic conditions. High levels of lactic acid produced during strenuous exercise are rapidly cleared both by renal and hepatic mechanisms as well as by aerobic metabolism in muscle (half-life approximately 60 min). A decrease in lactic acid utilization can also lead to accumulation of lactic acid. This is generally seen in diseases of the liver and kidneys. Defects in the removal of lactic acid have been associated

Table 16–10 Selected Causes of L-Lactic Acidosis

Tissue Hypoxia

Septic shock

Cardiogenic shock

Hemorrhagic shock

Acute hypoxemia

Carbon monoxide poisoning

Metabolic/Medical Conditions

Uncontrolled diabetes mellitus

Hepatic insufficiency

Renal insufficiency

Tumors

Leukemia

Lymphoma

Drugs/Toxic Substances

Zidovudine

Metformin

Ethanol

Salicylates

Isoniazid

Cyanide

Methanol

Ethylene glycol

Inborn Errors of Metabolism

Type 1a glycogen storage disease (von Gierke disease)

Fructose-1,6-biphosphatase deficiency

Pyruvate dehydrogenase deficiency

Organic acidurias: Propionic acidemia, methylmalonic acidemia

Mitochondrial diseases:
  KSS (Kearns–Sayre syndrome)
  PEO (progressive external ophthalmoplegia)
  PS (Pearson's syndrome)
  MERRF (myoclonic epilepsy with ragged-red fibers)
  MELAS (mitochondrial encephalopathy, lactic acidosis, and stroke-like episodes)
  MILS (maternally inherited Leigh's syndrome)

with hepatic insufficiency, specific enzymatic defects, and severe acidosis. Metformin, which is widely prescribed for the treatment of type 2 diabetes, rarely causes lactic acidosis. Risk factors for metformin-related lactic acidosis include congestive heart failure, tissue hypoxia, renal insufficiency and sepsis (Salpeter, 2003; Misbin, 2004). Nucleoside reverse transcriptase inhibitors (NRTI) used in the treatment of HIV infection can also induce lactic acidosis (John, 2002; Ogedegbe, 2003).

Lactic acidosis is diagnosed by the presence of high blood lactate levels (> 45 mg/dL or > 5.0 mmol/L), an elevated anion gap and a low blood pH (< 7.35). For accurate measurements of lactate, tourniquet use should be minimal and the patient should not clench their fist at the time of the blood draw. A gray top tube containing fluoride oxalate should be used for sample collection as it blocks further glycolysis.

Treatment of lactic acidosis consists of correction of underlying conditions that initiated the disruption in normal lactate metabolism. Tissue oxygenation, improved fluid status, amplification of cardiac status and treatment of sepsis play important roles in the treatment of lactic acidosis. Dialysis is sometimes necessary for removal of lactate.

D-Lactic acidosis results from excessive accumulation of D-lactic acid (the dextrorotary form of lactic acid). It has been described in patients with jejunoileal bypass or small bowel resection. In these conditions, glucose and other carbohydrates are converted into D-lactic acid in the colon by bacteria. The D-lactic acid is absorbed into the systemic circulation and slowly metabolized. Affected patients present with episodes of metabolic acidosis and encephalopathy. D-Lactate levels can be measured using D-lactate dehydrogenase enzymatic assays (Luft, 2001; Zhang, 2003).

References

American Association of Clinical Endocrinologists: Medical guidelines for the management of diabetes mellitus. Endocr Pract 2002; 8(Suppl 1):40–82.
Describes the diabetes monitoring and management guidelines endorsed by the American College of Endocrinology.

American Diabetes Association: Economic costs of diabetes in the US in 2002. Diabetes Care 2003; 26(3):917–932.

American Diabetes Association: Diagnosis and classification of diabetes mellitus. Diabetes Care 2004a; 27(Suppl 1):S5–S10.

American Diabetes Association: Gestational diabetes mellitus. Diabetes Care 2004b; 27(Suppl 1):S88–S90.

American Diabetes Association: Screening for type 2 diabetes. Diabetes Care 2004c; 27(Suppl 1):S11–S14.

American Diabetes Association: Standards of medical care for patients with diabetes mellitus. Diabetes Care 2004d; 27 (Suppl 1):S15–S35.
Summarizes the criteria for the classification and diagnosis of diabetes, and provides recommendations for assessment of glycemic control, management goals and strategies to prevent complications.

Arem R: Hypoglycemia associated with renal failure. Endocrinol Metab Clin N Amer 1989; 18(1):103–121.

Arky RA: Hypoglycemia associated with liver disease and ethanol. Endocrinol Metab Clin N Amer 1989; 18(1):75–90.

Assan R, Perronne C, Assan D, et al: Pentamidine-induced derangements of glucose homeostasis. Determinant roles of renal failure and drug accumulation. A study of 128 patients. Diabetes Care 1995; 18(1):47–55.

Bellows C, Haque S, Jaffe B: Pancreatic polypeptide islet cell tumor: case report and review of the literature. J Gastrointest Surg 1998; 2(6):526–532.

Bingley PJ, Bonifacio E, Mueller PW, and Participating Laboratories: Diabetes Antibody Standardization Program: First assay proficiency evaluation. Diabetes 2003; 52:1128–1136.
A report of the first proficiency evaluation of the Diabetes Antibody Standardization Program, which includes information concerning the performance of different assays for GAD, IA-2 and insulin autoantibodies.

Bosch AM, Bakker HD, van Gennip AH, et al: Clinical features of galactokinase deficiency: a review of the literature. J Inherit Metab Dis 2002; 25(8):629–634.

Bouchard P, Sai P, Reach G, et al: Diabetes mellitus following pentamidine-induced hypoglycemia in humans. Diabetes 1982; 31(1):40–45.

Bunch TJ, Dunn WF, Basu A, Gosman RI: Hyponatremia and hypoglycemia in acute Sheehan's syndrome. Gynecol Endocrinol 2002; 16(5):419–423.

Cavaco B, Uchigata Y, Porto T, et al: Hypoglycaemia due to insulin autoimmune syndrome: report of two cases with characterisation of HLA alleles and insulin autoantibodies. Eur J Endocrinol 2001; 145(3):311–316.

Ceriello A, Guigliano D, Quatraro A, et al: Vitamin E reduction of protein glycosylation in diabetes. New prospect for prevention of diabetes complications? Diabetes Care 1991; 14:68–72.

Chan AY, Swaminathan R, Cockram CS: Effectiveness of sodium fluoride as a preservation of glucose in blood. Clin Chem 1989; 35:315–317.

Chavez H, Ozolins D, Losek JD: Hypoglycemia and propranolol in pediatric behavioral disorders. Pediatrics 1999; 103(6):1290–1292.

Chen YT: Glycogen storage diseases. In: Scriver CR, Beaudet AL, Sly WS, Valle D (eds). The Metabolic and Molecular Bases of Inherited Disease, 8th ed. New York: McGraw-Hill, 2001, pp 1521–1551.

Cheyne EH, Cavan DA, Kerr D: Performance of a continuous glucose monitoring system during controlled hypoglycaemia in healthy volunteers. Diabetes Technology & Therapeutics 2002; 4(5):607–613.

Chung J, Henry RR: Mechanisms of tumor-induced hypoglycemia with intraabdominal hemangiopericytoma. J Clin Endocrinol Metab 1996; 81(3):919–925.

Cryer PE: Glucose homeostasis and hypoglycemia. In Larsen PR, Kronenberg HM, Melmed S, Polonsky KS (eds): Williams Textbook of Endocrinology, 10th ed. Philadelphia, Saunders, 2003, pp 1585–1618.

Cuesta-Munoz AL, Huopio H, Otonkoski T, et al: Severe persistent hyperinsulinemic hypoglycemia due to a de novo glucokinase mutation. Diabetes 2004; 53(8):2164–2168.

Daughaday WH: Hypoglycemia in patients with non-islet cell tumors. Endocrinol Metab Clin N Amer 1989; 18(1):91–101.

Davie SJ, Gould BJ, Yudkin JS: Effect of vitamin C on glycosylation of proteins. Diabetes 1992; 41:167–173.

Diabetes Control and Complications Trial Research Group: The effect of intensive treatment of diabetes on the development and progression of long-term complications in insulin-dependent diabetes mellitus. N Engl J Med 1993; 329:977–986.

Dozio N, Scavini M, Beretta A, et al: Imaging of the buffering effect of insulin antibodies in the autoimmune hypoglycemic syndrome. J Clin Endocrinol Metab 1998; 83(2):643–648.

Drucker DJ: Glucagon-like peptide 1 and the islet beta-cell: augmentation of cell proliferation and inhibition of apoptosis. Endocrinology 2003a; 144:5145–5148.

Drucker DJ: Enhancing incretin action for the treatment of type 2 diabetes. Diabetes Care 2003b; 26:2929–2940.

Duncan GE, Li SM, Zhou X-H: Prevalence and trends of a metabolic syndrome phenotype among U.S. adolescents, 1999–2000. Diabetes Care 2004; 27:2438–2443.

Eisenbarth GS: Insulin autoimmunity: immunogenetics/immunopathogenesis of type 1A diabetes. Ann NY Acad Sci 2003; 1005:109–118.

Flanagan D, Wood P, Sherwin R, et al: Gin and tonic and reactive hypoglycemia: what is important – the gin, the tonic, or both? J Clin Endocrinol Metab 1998; 83(3):796–800.

Flint A, Raben A, Astrup A, et al: Glucagon-like peptide 1 promotes satiety and suppresses energy intake in humans. J Clin Invest 1998; 101(3):515–520.

Ford ES, Giles WH, Mokdad AH: Increasing prevalence of the metabolic syndrome among U.S. adults. Diabetes Care 2004; 27: 2444–2449.

Guerci B, Durain D, Leblanc H, et al: Multicentre evaluation of the DCA 2000 system for measuring glycated haemoglobin. DCA 2000 Study Group. Diabetes Metab 1997; 23(3):195–201.

Haymond MW: Hypoglycemia in infants and children. Endocrinol Metab Clin N Amer 1989; 18(1):211–252.

Haymond MW, Pagliara AS: Ketotic hypoglycaemia. Clin Endocrinol Metab 1983; 12(2):447–462.

Haut S, Brivet M, Touati G, et al: A deletion in the human QP-C gene causes a complex III deficiency resulting in hypoglycaemia and lactic acidosis. Human Genetics 2003; 113:118–122.

Haviv YS, Sharkia M, Safadi R: Hypoglycemia in patients with renal failure. Renal Failure 2000; 22(2):219–223.

Hekimsoy Z, Biberoglu S, Comlekci A, et al: Trimethoprim/sulfamethoxazole-induced hypoglycemia in a malnourished patient with severe infection. Eur J Endocrinol 1997; 136(3):304–306.

Hirata Y, Uchigata Y: Insulin autoimmune syndrome in Japan. Diabetes Res Clin Pract 1994; 24(Suppl):S153–S157.

Hoberman HD, Chiodo SM: Elevation of the hemoglobin A1 fraction in alcoholism. Alcoholism: Clin Exp Res 1982; 16:260–266.

Holton JB, Walter JH, Tyfield LA: Galactosemia. In Scriver CR, Beaudet AL, Sly WS, Valle D (eds) The Metabolic and Molecular Bases of Inherited Disease, 8th ed. New York: McGraw-Hill, 2001, pp 1553–1587.

Hostens K, Pavlovic D, Zambre Y, et al: Exposure of human islets to cytokines can result in disproportionately elevated proinsulin release. J Clin Invest 1999; 104(1):67–72.

Ido Y, Vindigni A, Chang K, et al: Prevention of vascular and neural dysfunction in diabetic rats by C-peptide. Science 1997; 277(5325):563–566.

John M, Mallal S: Hyperlactaemia syndromes in people with HIV infection. Curr Opin Infect Dis 2002; 15(1):23–29.

Kaufman FR, Austin J, Neinstein A, et al: Nocturnal hypoglycemia detected with the Continuous Glucose Monitoring System in pediatric patients with type 1 diabetes. J Pediatr 2002; 141:625–630.

Khoury H, Daugherty T, Ehsanipoor K: Spontaneous hypoglycemia associated with congestive heart failure attributable to hyperinsulinism. Endocr Pract 1998; 4(2):94–95.

Kost GJ, Vu HT, Lee JH, et al: Multicenter study of oxygen-insensitive handheld glucose point-of-care testing in critical care/hospital/ambulatory patients in the United States and Canada. Crit Care Med 1998; 26(3):581–590.

Kreisberg RA: Lactate homeostasis and lactic acidosis. Ann Intern Med 1980; 92:227–237.

Krischer JP, Cuthbertson DD, Yu L, et al: Screening strategies for the identification of multiple antibody-positive relatives of individuals with type 1 diabetes. J Clin Endocrinol Metab 2003; 88(1):103–108.

Kurahashi K, Maruta H, Usuda Y, et al: Influence of blood sample oxygen tension on blood glucose concentration measured using an enzyme-electrode method. Crit Care Med 1997; 25(2):231–235.

Lefebvre PJ, Andreani D, Marks V, Creutzfeldt W: Statement on postprandial hypoglycemia. Diabetes Care 1988; 11(5):439–440.

Leslie ND: Insights into the pathogenesis of galactosemia. Ann Rev Nutr 2003; 23:59–80.

Lidar M, Rachmani R, Half E, Ravid M: Insulin autoimmune syndrome after therapy with imipenem. Diabetes Care 1999; 22(3):524–525.

Little RR, Rohlfing CL, Wiedmeyer H-M, et al: The National Glycohemoglobin Standardization Program: A five-year progress report. Clin Chem 2001; 47(11):1985–1992.
Summarizes the National Glycohemoglobin Standardization Program, including descriptions of certification criteria and procedures, and progress in standardization nationally and internationally.

Lteif AN, Schwenk WF: Hypoglycemia in infants and children. Endocrinol. Metab Clinics N Amer 1999; 28(3):619–646.

Luft AN, Schwenk WF: Lactic acidosis update for critical care clinicians. J Amer Soc Nephrol 2001; 12(Suppl 17):S15–S19.

Mackin RB: Proinsulin: recent observations and controversies. Cell Molec Life Sci 1998; 54:696–702.

Maclaren N, Lan M, Coutant R, et al: Only multiple autoantibodies to islet cells (ICA), insulin, GAD65, IA-2 and IA-2beta predict immune-mediated (Type 1) diabetes in relatives. J Autoimmunity 1999; 12:279–287.

Maclaren NK, Lan MS, Scatz D, et al: Multiple autoantibodies as predictors of Type 1 diabetes in a general population. Diabetologia 2003; 46(6):873–874.

Manning PJ, Espiner EA, Yoon K, et al: An unusual cause of hyperinsulinaemic hypoglycaemia syndrome. Diabet Med 2003; 20(9):772–776.

Marko P, Gabrielli A, Caruso LJ: Too much lactate or too little liver? J Clin Anesth 2004; 16(5):389–395.

Marks V, Teale JD: Drug-induced hypoglycemia. Endocrinol Metab Clin N Amer 1999; 28(3):555–577.

Miller SI, Wallace RJ Jr, Musher DM, et al: Hypoglycemia as a manifestation of sepsis. Amer J Med 1980; 68(5):649–654.

Misbin RI: The phantom of lactic acidosis due to metformin in patients with diabetes. Diabetes Care 2004; 27(7):1791–1793.

Mitrakou A, Ryan C, Veneman T, et al: Hierarchy of glycemic thresholds for counterregulatory hormone secretion, symptoms, and cerebral dysfunction. Am J Physiol 1991; 260(1 Pt 1):E67–74.

Molven A, Matre GE, Duran M, et al: Familial hyperinsulinemic hypoglycemia caused by a defect in the SCHAD enzyme of mitochondrial fatty acid oxidation. Diabetes 2004; 53:221–227.

Narayan KM, Boyle JP, Thompson TJ, et al: Lifetime risk for diabetes mellitus in the United States. JAMA 2003; 290(14):1884–1890.

Nyholm B, Brock B, Orskov L, et al: Amylin receptor agonists: a novel pharmacological approach in the management of insulin treated diabetes mellitus. Expert Opin Investig Drugs 2001; 10:1641–1652.

Ogedegbe AE, Thomas DL, Diehl AM: Hyperlactataemia syndromes associated with HIV therapy. Lancet Infect Dis 2003; 3(6):329–337.

Ohkubo Y, Kishikawa H, Araki E, et al: Intensive insulin therapy prevents the progression of diabetic microvascular complications in Japanese patients with non-insulin-dependent diabetes mellitus: a randomized prospective 6-year study. Diabetes Res Clin Pract 1995; 28:103–117.

Orngreen MC, Zacho M, Hebert A, et al: Patients with severe muscle wasting are prone to develop hypoglycemia during fasting. Neurology 2003; 61:997–1000.

Pasieka JL, Hershfield N: Pancreatic polypeptide hyperplasia causing watery diarrhea syndrome: a case report. Can J Surg 1999; 42(1):55–58.

Penumalee S, Kissner PZ, Migdal SD: Gabapentin-induced hypoglycemia in a long-term peritoneal dialysis patient. Am J Kidney Dis 2003; 42(6): E3–E5.

Redmon JB, Nuttall FQ: Autoimmune hypoglycemia. Endocrinol Metab Clin N Amer 1999; 28(3):603–618.

Robbins DC, Andersen L, Bowsher R, et al: Report of the American Diabetes Association's Task Force on standardization of the insulin assay. Diabetes 1996; 45:242–256.

Roder ME, Porte D Jr, Schwartz RS, Kahn SE: Disproportionately elevated proinsulin levels reflect the degree of impaired B cell secretory capacity in patients with noninsulin-dependent diabetes mellitus. J Clin Endocrinol Metab 1998; 83(2):604–608.

Roder ME, Vissing H, Nauck MA: Hyperproinsulinemia in a three-generation Caucasian family due to mutant proinsulin (Arg65-His) not associated with impaired glucose tolerance: the contribution of mutant proinsulin to insulin bioactivity. J Clin Endocrinol Metab 1996; 81(4):1634–1640.

Rohlfing CL, Wiedmeyer H-M, Little RR, et al: Defining the relationship between plasma glucose and HbA($_{1c}$): analysis of glucose profiles and HbA($_{1c}$) in the Diabetes Control and Complications Trial. Diabetes Care 2002; 25:275–278.

Salpeter SR, Greyber E, Pasternak GA, Salpeter EE: Risk of fatal and nonfatal lactic acidosis with metformin use in type 2 diabetes mellitus: systematic review and meta-analysis. Arch Intern Med 2003; 163(21):2594–2602.

Schrot RJ, Foulis PR, Morrison AD, Farese RV: A computerized model for home glucose monitoring proficiency testing: efficacy of an innovative testing program. Diabetes Educator 1999; 25(1):48–55.

Schwartz NS, Clutter WE, Shah SD, Cryer PE: Glycemic thresholds for activation of glucose counterregulatory systems are higher than the threshold for symptoms. J Clin Invest 1987; 79(3):777–781.

Service FJ: Hypoglycemic disorders. N Engl J Med 1995; 332(17):1144–1152.
Reviews hypoglycemic disorders, with detailed clinical classification, description of diagnostic testing including a protocol for performing the 72-h fast, and management strategies.

Service FJ: Diagnostic approach to adults with hypoglycemic disorders. Endocrinol Metab Clinics N Amer 1999a; 28(3):519–532.

Service FJ, Natt N, Thompson GB, et al: Noninsulinoma pancreatogenous hypoglycemia: a novel syndrome of hyperinsulinemic hypoglycemia in adults independent of mutations in Kir6.2 and SUR1 genes. J Clin Endocrinol Metab 1999b; 84(5):1582–1589.

Smallridge RC, Corrigan DF, Thomason AM, Blue PW: Hypoglycemia in pregnancy. Occurrence due to adrenocorticotropic hormone and growth hormone deficiency. Arch Intern Med 1980; 140(4):564–565.

Sperling MA, Menon RK: Differential diagnosis and management of neonatal hypoglycemia. Pediatr Clin N Amer 2004; 51(3):703–723.

Stanley CA, Lieu YK, Hsu BY, et al: Hyperinsulinism and hyperammonemia in infants with regulatory mutations of the glutamate dehydrogenase gene. N Engl J Med 1998; 338(19):1352–7.

Steinman B, Gitzelman R, Van den Berghe G: Disorders of fructose metabolism. *In* Scriver CR, Beaudet AL, Sly WS, Valle D (eds): The Metabolic and Molecular Bases of Inherited Disease, 8th ed. New York, McGraw-Hill, 2001, pp 1489–1520.

Straub SG, Cosgrove KE, Ammala C, et al: Hyperinsulinism of infancy: the regulated release of insulin by KATP channel-independent pathways. Diabetes 2001; 50(2):329–339.

Sunehag AL, Haymond MW: Glucose extremes in newborn infants. Clin Perinatol 2002; 29(2):245–260.

Tamburrano G, Leonetti F, Sbraccia P, et al: Increased insulin sensitivity in patients with idiopathic reactive hypoglycemia. J Clin Endocrinol Metab 1989; 69(4):885–890.

Tahara Y, Shima K: The response of GHb to stepwise plasma glucose change over time in diabetic patients. Diabetes Care 1993; 16:1313–1314.

Tarim O, Kucukerdogan A, Gunay U, et al: Effects of iron deficiency anemia on hemoglobin A$_{1c}$ in type 1 diabetes mellitus. Pediatr Int 1999; 41:357–362.

Taylor SI, Barbetti F, Accili D, et al: Syndromes of autoimmunity and hypoglycemia. Autoantibodies directed against insulin and its receptor. Endocrinol Metab Clin N Amer 1989; 18(1):123–143.

Temple R., Clark PM, Hales CN: Measurement of insulin secretion in type 2 diabetes: problems and pitfalls. Diabetic Med 1992; 9:503–512.

Toft-Nielsen MB, Damholt MB, Madsbad S, et al: Determinants of the impaired secretion of glucagon-like peptide-1 in type 2 diabetic patients. J Clin Endocrinol Metab 2001; 86:3717–3723.

Tomita T, Kimmel JR, Friesen SR, et al: Pancreatic polypeptide cell hyperplasia with and without watery diarrhea syndrome. J Surg Oncol 1980; 14(1):11–20.

Towler DA, Havlin CE, Craft S, Cryer P: Mechanism of awareness of hypoglycemia. Perception of neurogenic (predominantly cholinergic) rather than neuroglycopenic symptoms. Diabetes 1993; 42(12):1791–1798.

Tsujino S, Nonaka I, DiMauro S: Glycogen storage myopathies. Neurol Clin 2000; 18(1):125–150.

UK Prospective Diabetes Study Group: Intensive blood-glucose control with sulphonylureas or insulin compared with conventional treatment and risk of complications in patients with type 2 diabetes (UKPDS 33). Lancet 1998a; 352(9131):837–853.

UK Prospective Diabetes Study Group: Effect of intensive blood glucose control with metformin on complications in overweight patients with type 2 diabetes (UKPDS 34). Lancet 1998b; 352(9131):854–865.

Verge CF, Stenger D, Bonifacio E, et al: Combined use of autoantibodies (IA-2 autoantibody, GAD autoantibody, insulin autoantibody, cytoplasmic islet cell antibodies) in type 1 diabetes. Combinatorial Islet Autoantibody Workshop. Diabetes 1998; 47:1857–1866.

Virtue MA, Furne JK, Nuttall FQ, Levitt MD: Relationship between GHb concentration and erythrocyte survival determined from breath carbon monoxide concentration. Diabetes Care 2004; 27:931–935.

Vogeser M, Parhofer KG, Furst H, et al: Autoimmune hypoglycemia presenting as seizure one week after surgery. Clin Chem 2001; 47(4):795–796.

Walter JH, Roberts RE, Besley GT, et al: Generalised uridine diphosphate galactose-4-epimerase deficiency. Arch Dis Child 1999; 80(4):374–376.

Weinstein DA, Wolfsdorf JI: Glycogen storage diseases: A primer for clinicians. Endocrinologist 2002; 12:531–538.
Reviews in detail the major glycogen storage diseases.

Weissman M, Klein B: Evaluation of glucose determinations in untreated serum samples. Clin Chem 1958; 4:420.

Whipple AE: The surgical therapy of hyperinsulinisim. J Int Chir 1938; 3:237–276.

Williams AJ, Bingley PJ, Bonifacio E, et al: A novel micro-assay for insulin autoantibodies. J Autoimmun 1997; 10:473–478.

Wojcikowski C, Blackman J, Ostrega D, et al: Lack of effect of high dose biosynthetic human C-peptide on pancreatic hormone release in normal subjects. Metabolism 1990; 39:827–832.

Wolfsdorf JI, Holm IA, Weinstein DA: Glycogen storage diseases. Phenotypic, genetic, and biochemical characteristics, and therapy. Endocrinol Metab Clin N Amer 1999; 28(4):801–823.

World Health Organization: Diabetes mellitus: Report of a WHO Study Group. (Technical Report Series, No. 727) Geneva, WHO, 1985.

Yaturu S, DePrisco C, Lurie A: Severe autoimmune hypoglycemia with insulin antibodies necessitating plasmapheresis. Endocr Pract 2004; 10(1):49–54.

Zaloga GP: Beware of errors in blood glucose measurement. Crit Care Med 1997; 25(2):212.

Zhang DL, Jiang ZW, Jiang J, et al. D-lactic acidosis secondary to short bowel syndrome. Postgrad Med J 2003; 79(928):110–112.

Zierler, K: Whole body glucose metabolism. Am J Physiol 1999; 276(3 Pt 1):E409–426.

Zuker N, Bissessor M, Korber M, et al: Acute hypoglycaemic coma – a rare, potentially lethal form of early onset Sheehan syndrome. Aust N Z J Obstet Gynaecol 1995; 35(3):318–320.

II

CHAPTER 17

Lipids and Dyslipoproteinemia

Timothy Hilbert MD PhD JD, Mark S. Lifshitz MD

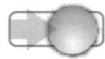

KEY POINTS

• While ultracentrifugation and electrophoretic techniques are of historical significance, most useful lipid and lipoprotein testing methods are now enzymatic, often coupled with detergent precipitation.

• LDL-cholesterol (LDL-C) can be measured directly, but is usually calculated using the Friedewald formula. Calculated values require evaluation of fasting samples.

• LDL-C is currently considered the most important value in assessing cardiac risk, and directing therapy.

• The profile currently recommended for initial screening in adults, age 20 or older, includes total cholesterol (TC), LDL-C, HDL-cholesterol (HDL-C) and Triglycerides. Testing should be repeated at least once every 5 years.

• Other tests including apolipoprotein levels and lipoprotein subclasses may prove valuable in fine-tuning risk assessment, and evaluating response to therapy.

• New guidelines elevate the perceived atherosclerotic risk of diabetes, and support aggressive intervention in diabetics and patients with the recently recognized metabolic syndrome.

Overview

Disorders of lipid metabolism play a major role in atherosclerosis and coronary heart disease (CHD). There is a clear-cut relationship between elevated serum cholesterol and myocardial infarction, and at the tissue level cholesterol deposits occur in areas of endothelial cell damage and are a prominent part of atherosclerotic lesions. While cholesterol may be considered 'bad' because of the above association, it is actually a vital structural component of cell membranes and a precursor of steroid hormones and bile acids. Another lipid, triglyceride, is a major source of energy for cells. Cholesterol and triglycerides are the most important lipids in the study and management of coronary heart disease risk.

Lipids are soluble in nonpolar organic solvents, such as chloroform and ether, but relatively insoluble in polar solvents such as water. Thus, cholesterol and triglycerides travel in plasma not as free-floating molecules, but as part of water-soluble macromolecules called *lipoproteins*. These particles contain cholesterol in two forms: free cholesterol, a polar nonesterified alcohol (about 30%) and cholesterol ester, a hydrophobic form wherein cholesterol is bound to fatty acids (about 70%). The lipoprotein is arranged like a micelle. Hydrophobic lipids, such as cholesterol esters and triglycerides, are located in the core of the particle.

Water-soluble lipids, like free cholesterol and phospholipids are arranged on the surface with polar groups pointing outward. *Apolipoproteins*, the protein moiety of lipoproteins, are also arrayed on the surface (Fig. 17–1).

There are four major lipoprotein classes: chylomicrons (CM), very-low-density lipoprotein (VLDL), low-density lipoprotein (LDL), and high-density lipoprotein (HDL). Several minor lipoproteins have also been identified, including intermediate-density lipoprotein (IDL) and lipoprotein(a) (Lp(a)) (Tables 17–1 and 17–2). Lipoproteins can be differentiated by density, particle size, chemical composition, and electrophoretic mobility. These physical properties are due to differences in protein, triglyceride and cholesterol content and reflect the role of each lipoprotein in lipid metabolism (see below). Each lipoprotein is associated with specific apolipoproteins that play important roles in lipid transport, such as activating or inhibiting the enzymes involved in lipid metabolism, and binding lipoproteins to cell surface receptors. The apolipoprotein composition of the lipoprotein classes is summarized in Table 17–1.

Lipoproteins are commonly differentiated from one another on the basis of their electrophoretic mobility and buoyant density. When plasma lipoproteins are separated by agarose gel electrophoresis CM remains at the origin, HDL migrates fastest in the α-region, followed by VLDL in the 'pre-beta' region and IDL and LDL in the beta region. Ultracentrifugation separates lipoproteins by buoyant density. The density of a lipoprotein particle is determined mostly by its protein and triglyceride content. Lipoproteins with high triglyceride and low protein content (CM and VLDL) are less dense than those with high protein and low triglyceride content (HDL). LDL and IDL are more dense than VLDL but less dense than HDL.

In terms of function, lipoproteins can be separated into two general categories: lower-density predominantly apoB-containing particles (CM, VLDL, IDL and LDL) which distribute cholesterol and triglycerides to the tissues, and the higher-density apoA-containing particle (HDL). HDL is formed in the liver and plays a key role in reverse cholesterol transport, the process by which excess cholesterol is returned from tissues to the liver where it is reused or excreted in bile. This role explains why high serum HDL decreases CHD risk. More than 90% of the protein component of HDL is apoA-I.

In contrast to HDL, lower-density lipoproteins are more heterogeneous. They contain a variety of apolipoproteins, apoB, C, D and E. The predominant apolipoprotein, apoB (B-48 in CM and B-100 in VLDL, IDL and LDL), is one of the ligands which binds to receptors on the surface of macrophages, fat and liver cells. The corresponding receptor is called the LDL receptor even though it can bind particles other than LDL. The LDL receptor has been shown to bind apoB-100, and apoE, but not apoB-48. Unlike HDL which removes excess cholesterol from tissues, this group of

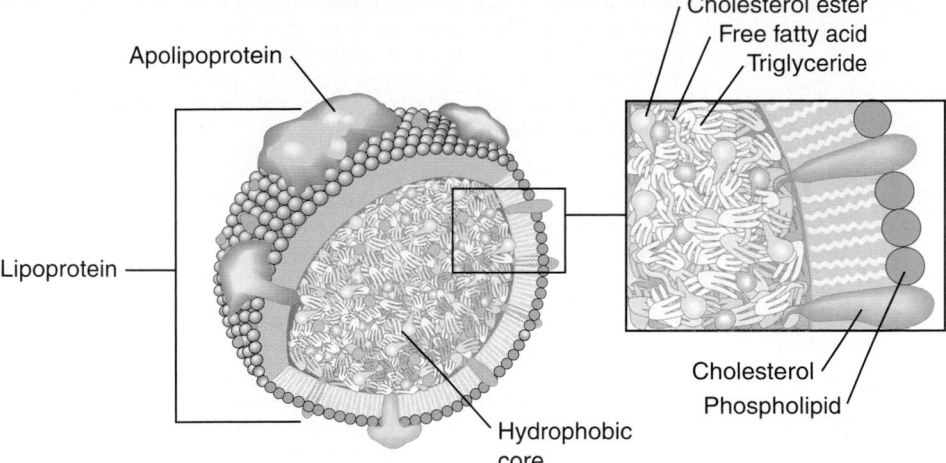

Figure 17–1 Lipoprotein structure.

Apolipoprotein

Lipoprotein

Hydrophobic core

Cholesterol ester
Free fatty acid
Triglyceride

Cholesterol
Phospholipid

Table 17–1 Major Classes of Human Plasma Lipoproteins: Physicochemical Characteristics

Particle	Electrophoretic mobility*	Major apolipoproteins	Diameter (Å)	Density (kg/L)	Sf[†]
Chylomicrons	Origin	ApoB-48, C, E	750–12 000	< 0.95	> 400
VLDL	Pre-β	ApoB-100, C, E	300–700	0.95–1.006	20–400
IDL	β or pre-β	ApoB-100, E		1.006–1.019	12–20
LDL	β	ApoB-100	180–300	1.019–1.063	0–12
HDL$_2$	α	ApoA-I, A-II, C	50–120	1.063–1.125	
HDL$_3$	α	ApoA-II, A-I, C	50–120	1.125–1.210	
Lp(a)	Pre-β	ApoB-100, Apo(a)		1.045–1.080	

* Agarose-gel electrophoresis.
[†] Svedberg flotation rate.

Table 17–2 Chemical Composition of Major Classes of Plasma Lipoproteins

	Protein (%)*	Cholesterol (%)	Cholesterol esters (%)	Triglyceride (%)	Phospholipid (%)
Chylomicrons	1–2	1–3	2–4	80–95	3–6
VLDL	6–10	4–8	16–22	45–65	15–20
IDL			*Intermediate between VLDL and LDL*		
LDL	18–22	6–8	45–50	4–8	18–24
HDL	45–55	3–5	15–20	2–7	26–32

* Percentage of dry weight.
Data from Albers (1974); Fless (1984); Gaubatz (1983); Gotto (1986); Gries (1988).

lipoproteins is mainly involved in delivering lipids to tissues for storage or use in energy production. CM (formed in the intestine from dietary fat) and VLDL (formed in the liver) are triglyceride-rich particles that are metabolized after entering the circulation. Through the action of lipoprotein lipase (LPL), these particles shed triglycerides and cholesterol esters, and are transformed into denser lipoproteins with a higher percentage of cholesterol. LDL is the densest of these particles, and elevated serum LDL-cholesterol (LDL-C) is a primary cardiac risk factor. Treatment of CHD-causing dyslipidemia is generally aimed at lowering LDL.

One way to understand apoB-containing lipoproteins is to view them as a metabolic progression in which CM and VLDL release triglycerides to tissues via interaction with LPL. As a result of this interaction, CM and VLDL become triglyceride depleted, denser and relatively protein and cholesterol rich, giving rise to CM remnants and LDL. These particles are internalized and metabolized by cells, CM by liver cells and LDL by liver cells, as well as cells throughout the body. LDL serves as the major source of cholesterol for tissues. This metabolic progression is presented in Figure 17–2.

A block in any step of the pathway leads to the accumulation of one or more lipoproteins. The number over each step in the pathway represents the functional hyperlipoproteinemia (originally described by Fredrickson,

1967) caused by a block between two intermediates. For example, a block in the progression from CM to CM remnants results in the accumulation of CM – Type 1 or 5 disease – and presents with high triglycerides and normal cholesterol. A block in the conversion of VLDL to IDL and LDL results in Type 4 disease, i.e., VLDL accumulation with elevated triglyceride and frequently elevated cholesterol. Often the cause of Types 1, 5 and 4 diseases is LPL deficiency, and the resulting inability to break down triglycerides. Type 2 disease results from a block in LDL metabolism and may have a genetic basis: a defective apoB protein that does not bind to the LDL receptor or a mutant LDL receptor that does not recognize apoB. Type 2 is further subcategorized based on the triglyceride level. Note that other studies (see below) may be necessary to distinguish Type 2B and Type 3 since both present with elevated cholesterol and triglycerides. This functional classification is presented in Table 17–3.

Note that in reality, the interaction among lipoproteins is far more complex than discussed above and is mediated by a host of apolipoproteins, enzymes and other factors, some of which remain poorly understood. For example, in addition to the LDL receptor, other lipoprotein receptors have been identified, including the VLDL receptor (VLDLR) and apoE receptor-2 (APOER2) that bind apoE, and the scavenger receptor SCARBI. There is

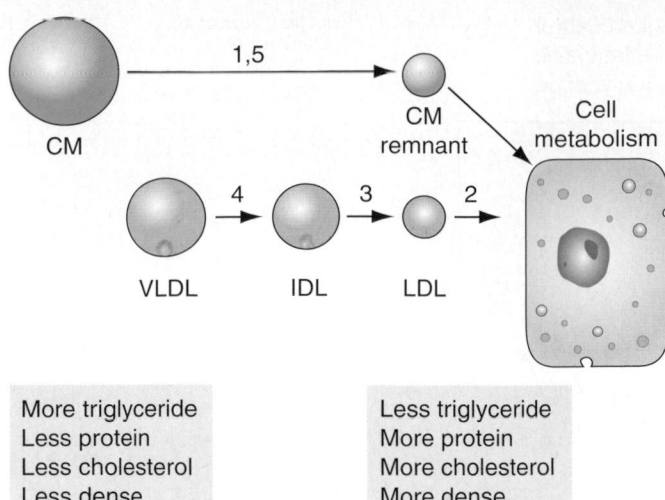

More triglyceride
Less protein
Less cholesterol
Less dense

Less triglyceride
More protein
More cholesterol
More dense

Figure 17–2 Metabolism of lipoprotein particles. The number over each step in the pathway represents the functional hyperlipoproteinemia caused by a block between two intermediates (see Table 17–3).

Table 17–3 Functional Classification: Key Laboratory Findings

Type	Particle	Triglycerides	Cholesterol	Comments
1	CM	Very high	Normal	Low cardiac risk; hereditary
5	CM	Very high	Normal	Low cardiac risk; acquired
4	VLDL	Very high	Low	Lower cardiac risk than types 2 and 3
3	IDL	High	High	High cardiac risk; dietary control; presence of β-VLDL; VLDL-cholesterol/plasma TG ratio > 0.3
2A	LDL	Low	High	High cardiac risk
2B	LDL, VLDL	High	High	High cardiac risk

no ideal system for classifying lipid disorders. They can be categorized in many different ways: primary versus secondary, hereditary versus acquired, as well as by lipoprotein fraction phenotypes. In general, each category is heterogeneous with respect to genetic, clinical and pathologic factors. These are discussed in greater detail at the end of the chapter.

Lipoproteins, Apolipoproteins, and Related Proteins

Classification

Lipoprotein particles are dynamic entities that acquire and shed protein and lipid components as they circulate in the body. As mentioned above, CM and VLDL particles lose triglycerides and become smaller as they are metabolized. Thus, young VLDL and CM particles are larger and less dense than their more mature counterparts. For this reason, it is best not to view each of the lipoprotein classes as a collection of identical particles, but as a heterogeneous group. In fact, distinct lipoprotein subfractions or subclasses have been well described.

Major Lipoproteins
Chylomicrons

Chylomicrons (CM) are large particles produced by the intestine that transport lipids of dietary origin to the tissues of the body. They are very rich in triglycerides, but relatively poor in free cholesterol, phospholipids and protein. The interaction of chylomicrons with lipoprotein lipase at the luminal surface of capillary endothelium results in the depletion of triglycerides and surface elements. The resulting smaller particles, called chylomicron remnants, are removed from circulation by the liver, primarily through the interaction of apoE with receptors including the LDL receptor. Because of the very high lipid/protein ratio, chylomicrons are considerably less dense than water, and float without centrifugation.

When present at high levels chylomicrons result in 'milky' plasma and accumulate as a floating creamy layer when left undisturbed for several hours. The apolipoproteins in chylomicrons include proteins that are present in newly secreted particles (apoB-48, apoA-I, and apoA-IV) and proteins that are acquired from other lipoproteins in circulation (apoC-I, apoC-II, apoC-III, and apoE).

Very-Low-Density Lipoproteins
VLDL particles are produced by the liver and supply the tissues of the body with triglycerides of endogenous, primarily hepatic, origin and cholesterol. As compared to chylomicrons, VLDL particles are smaller and produce turbid plasma when present in excessive amounts. They are rich in triglycerides though to a lesser extent than chylomicrons, and have a higher buoyant density because of their lower lipid/protein ratio. By mass, VLDL particles contain approximately 50% triglyceride, 40% cholesterol and phospholipid, and 10% protein, mostly apoB-100 and apoC, but also apoE. VLDL particles vary widely in size and chemical composition. Larger particles are rich in triglycerides and apoC. Smaller particles have less of these two components. Lipoprotein lipase hydrolyzes VLDL and this produces highly atherogenic, smaller, triglyceride and surface material-depleted particles called VLDL remnants and IDL. These particles can be further metabolized to LDL.

Low-Density Lipoproteins
LDL is produced through the metabolism of VLDL in circulation and constitutes about 50% of the total lipoprotein mass in human plasma. The particles are much smaller than the triglyceride-rich lipoproteins (VLDL and CM), and do not scatter light or alter the clarity of plasma even at greatly increased concentrations. LDL consists of approximately 50% cholesterol, mostly esterified, 25% protein, mostly apoB-100 with traces of apoC, 20% phospholipid, and only traces of triglycerides. While each VLDL and LDL particle is thought to contain only one apoB-100 molecule, the extraordinary size of this protein allows it to be the largest protein component of these particles. The liver takes up most of the LDL in circulation (approximately 75%) with apoB-100 serving as a target for the hepatic receptor. The remaining LDL is delivered to other tissues, or removed from circulation by scavenger cells such as those found in atheromatous plaque. Small LDL particles contain less cholesterol ester, and have a lower cholesterol/apoB ratio. Increased amounts of the small particles have been found in patients with several common forms of dyslipoproteinemia that are associated with CHD.

High-Density Lipoprotein
HDL is a small particle, consisting of mostly protein, cholesterol, and phospholipids, with only traces of triglycerides. Produced by the liver, HDL is involved in reverse cholesterol transport, the process by which excess cholesterol is returned from tissues to the liver. HDL is cleared from circulation through the interaction of apoE with the LDL receptor, although additional receptors have been identified. Discrete HDL particle subpopulations have been identified based on differences in size or charge, including two major ultracentrifugation subclasses, HDL$_2$ and HDL$_3$ (Blanche, 1981; MacKenzie, 1973; Sundaram, 1974). The distinction is significant because HDL$_2$ is thought to be more cardioprotective than HDL$_3$, and people with low levels of HDL$_2$ are thought to be at increased risk for premature CHD. Additionally, HDL has also been subfractionated into particles that contain apoA-I but not apoA-II, and those that contain both apoA-I and apoA-II (Fruchart, 1992; von Eckardstein, 1994). The physiologic function of these particles is not fully understood; however, particles that contain only apoA-I are thought to be most important for the efflux of cholesterol from tissues. A high percentage of HDL$_2$ particles fall into the apoA-I-only category. The laboratory measurement of such particles may eventually prove to be clinically useful.

Minor and Abnormal Lipoproteins
Intermediate-Density Lipoproteins
Formed through the metabolism of VLDL in circulation, IDL can be removed from circulation quickly through interaction with the LDL receptor, or further metabolized to LDL. As expected, the lipid content, size and density of IDL is intermediate between VLDL and LDL, and IDL is sometimes considered a subclass of LDL.

Lipoprotein(a) or Lp(a)
Lp(a) is similar to LDL in terms of density and overall composition, and can be thought of as an LDL particle to which apolipoprotein (a) has been added, linked to apoB-100 via a disulfide bond (Fless, 1984, 1985; Gaubatz, 1983). The electrophoretic mobility of Lp(a) is usually pre-β but can vary between that of LDL (β) and albumin (pre-α). Lp(a) is generally

Table 17–4 Significant Human Apolipoproteins

Apolipoprotein	Major lipoproteins	Mr* (kDa)	Amino acids	Chromosome	Plasma concentration (µmol/L)	Plasma concentration (mg/dL)
A-I	HDL	29	243–245	11	32–46	90–130
A-II	HDL	17.4	154	1	18–29	30–50
A-IV		44.5	396	11		
(a)	Lp(a)	350–700	Variable	6		
B-100	VLDL, IDL, LDL	512.7	4536	2	1.5–1.8	80–100
B-48	CM	240.8	2152	2	< 0.2	< 5
C-I	CM, LDL	6.6	57	19	6.1–10.8	4–7
C-II	CM, LDL	8.9	78 or 79	19	3.4–9.1	3–8
C-III	CM	8.8	79	11	9.1–17.1	8–15
D	HDL	19	169	3		
E	CM, LDL, IDL	34.1	299	19	0.8–1.6	3–6

* Mr, relative molecular mass.

present in much lower concentrations than LDL; however, in normal subjects values can range from < 20–1500 mg/L or more. Increased levels can be familial, showing an autosomal dominant pattern of inheritance, and have been associated with an increased risk of CHD, cerebrovascular disease and stroke. When concentrations in the plasma are increased above 200–300 mg/L, Lp(a) appears electrophoretically as a lipid-staining pre-β band in the plasma fraction containing lipoproteins of density > 1.006 g/mL.

Lp(a) is synthesized in the liver, but the details of its metabolism are not well understood. It binds to the LDL-receptor by virtue of its apoB-100 component, albeit with lower affinity than LDL (Floren, 1981). The removal of apo(a) from Lp(a) increases the affinity of the residual apoB-containing particle for the LDL-receptor (Armstrong, 1985), and it has been suggested that apo(a) may interfere with the uptake of apoB-100-containing particles (Scanu, 1988). At present, neither the function of Lp(a) nor its atherogenic properties are well understood. It has been speculated that Lp(a) or apo(a) might interfere with normal thrombolysis by virtue of its similarity to plasminogen.

LpX Lipoprotein

LpX is an abnormal lipoprotein found in patients with obstructive biliary disease, and in patients with familial lecithin : cholesterol acyltransferase (LCAT) deficiency. Lipids account for more than 90% of its weight (mostly phospholipids, unesterified cholesterol, and very little esterified cholesterol). Proteins, primarily apoC and smaller amounts of albumin, constitute < 10% of LpX by weight.

β-VLDL ('floating β' lipoprotein)

β-VLDL ('floating β' lipoprotein) is an abnormal lipoprotein that accumulates in type 3 hyperlipoproteinemia. It is richer in cholesterol than VLDL and apparently results from the defective catabolism of VLDL. The particle is found in the VLDL density range but migrates electrophoretically with or near LDL.

Important Proteins in Lipoprotein Metabolism

Apolipoproteins

As mentioned previously, apolipoproteins constitute the major protein component of lipoproteins. They are commonly referred to using the nomenclature introduced by Alaupovic (1971). Some significant properties of the apolipoproteins are outlined in Tables 17–4 and 17–5.

Lipolytic Enzymes and Other Proteins

The major enzymatic systems that are known to participate in plasma lipoprotein metabolism are the lecithin : cholesterol acyltransferase (LCAT) and the lipolytic enzymes, lipoprotein lipase (LPL), hepatic triglyceride lipase (HL), and endothelial lipase (EL). Many other proteins are also involved in lipoprotein metabolism. Some significant attributes of these proteins are summarized in Table 17–6.

Lipid Transport and Lipoprotein Metabolism

Triglycerides and cholesterol enter circulation as part of triglyceride-rich lipoprotein particles, chylomicrons (CM) produced in the intestine, and

VLDL produced primarily by the liver. These lipoprotein particles begin to undergo intravascular change almost immediately after entry into the circulation through the action of lipoprotein lipase (LPL). This enzyme hydrolyzes triglycerides and diglycerides, releasing fatty acids and monoglycerides, which are taken up by cells and used as a source of energy. ApoC-II stimulates the hydrolysis of triglycerides. In addition to losing triglycerides by LPL-mediated hydrolysis, CM lose surface lipids and apolipoproteins by transfer of these components to HDL. Overall, chylomicrons lose over 95% of their mass, in the form of triglyceride and the A and C apolipoproteins. The depleted chylomicron remnant particle contains apoB-48 and apoE as its major apolipoproteins. It binds to the surface of hepatocytes and is internalized and degraded by means of a rapid and specific receptor-mediated endocytotic process. ApoE apparently targets the chylomicron remnant to its receptor; however, the process by which this targeting occurs is still not completely understood. It seems to involve several receptor proteins, including the LDL-receptor, LDL-receptor related protein, and SCARB1. The C apolipoproteins inhibit the uptake of chylomicrons, allowing them to remain in the circulation long enough to complete the hydrolysis of triglycerides. In the fasting state, the intestine continues to make apolipoprotein B and secretes 'intestinal VLDL' (small chylomicrons). These particles may constitute up to 10% or 20% of the circulating 'VLDL,' but are probably metabolized as chylomicrons (Byers, 1960; Cenedella, 1974; Green, 1981; Risser, 1978).

VLDL is synthesized in the liver. Like chylomicrons, VLDL is catabolized upon entry into the circulation, in part by lipoprotein lipase, and converted to cholesterol-enriched VLDL remnants. Some of these remnants are removed from circulation by the liver via receptor-mediated endocytosis; others are further catabolized to IDL and LDL (Bachorik, 1988). LDL carries most of the circulating cholesterol and transports cholesterol to hepatic and extrahepatic tissues, where it is taken up by LDL-receptor-mediated endocytosis (Brown, 1981). LDL binds to the LDL-receptor (i.e., via apoB-100) and is subsequently internalized and directed to the lysosome, where apoB-100 is degraded and cholesteryl ester and other lipids are hydrolyzed. LDL-receptors are recycled back to the cell membrane (Fig. 17–3).

The unesterified cholesterol produced via lysosomal hydrolysis becomes available for membrane, hormone and bile acid synthesis. Excess cholesterol is re-esterified by the microsomal enzyme acyl : cholesterol acyl transferase (ACAT) and is stored until it is needed. Cellular cholesterol, when present in sufficient quantity, downregulates the LDL-receptor, reducing the number of cell membrane receptors and consequently the uptake of LDL. About two-thirds of LDL is removed from plasma via hepatic LDL-receptors. While most tissues use cholesterol only for membrane synthesis or store it as cholesteryl ester, the liver can also utilize cholesterol in other ways. The liver excretes cholesterol into the bile both as unesterified cholesterol and after conversion to bile acids, and reuses cholesterol for lipoprotein synthesis, as when it secretes VLDL into the circulation. Steroid-secreting tissues use cholesterol as a precursor of the steroid hormones.

While LDL and chylomicrons deliver lipids to the tissues, HDL is thought to be the vehicle for reverse cholesterol transport, the process by which excess cholesterol is removed from peripheral tissues and transported back to the liver. HDL is secreted from both the liver and the intestine as nascent, disk-shaped particles that contain apolipoproteins,

Table 17–5 Apolipoprotein Functions and Significant Characteristics

Apolipoprotein	Main distribution	Function (if known)	Comments
A-I	HDL	Activates LCAT which esterifies cholesterol in plasma	Synthesized in liver and intestine
A-II	HDL		May inhibit lipoprotein and hepatic lipases and increase plasma triglyceride
A-IV	HDL, CM and free in plasma		May be a cofactor for LCAT
B-100	VLDL and LDL	Carboxy-terminal recognition signal targets LDL to the LDL (apo B, E) receptor	Very large protein, synthesized in liver; found in lipoproteins with lipids of endogenous origin (i.e., not chylomicrons)
B-48	CM	Not recognized by LDL receptor	Synthesized in intestine, encoded by same gene and has same amino terminus as apoB-100. Differential production of the two proteins involves RNA editing
C-I	CM and VLDL		May inhibit hepatic uptake of VLDL and cholesterol ester transfer protein
C-II	CM and VLDL	Activates lipoprotein lipase	Deficiency causes reduced clearance of triglyceride-rich lipoproteins
C-III	VLDL, HDL	Appears to inhibit lipolysis of triglyceride-rich lipoproteins; may regulate clearance rate of remnant particles	
C-IV	CM, HDL		May be involved in lipid absorption
D	HDL	Activates LCAT	
E	CM, VLDL, IDL, remnants and HDL	Recognition factor that targets chylomicron and VLDL remnants to hepatic receptor; also binds to cell surface LDL receptors	E-2, E-3, and E-4 isoforms E-4 is associated with high LDL-C, higher risk of CHD and Alzheimer's disease E-2 associated with type 3 hyperlipoproteinemia
H	HDL, VLDL and CM	Unknown, possibly related to activation of LPL	Antibodies against apoH, or β_2-glycoprotein-I, are a subset of antiphospholipid antibodies, and may be associated with hyperthrombosis and stroke
Apo(a)	Lp(a)		Homologous to plasminogen, may be prothrombotic. Bound to apoB-100 by disulfide linkage

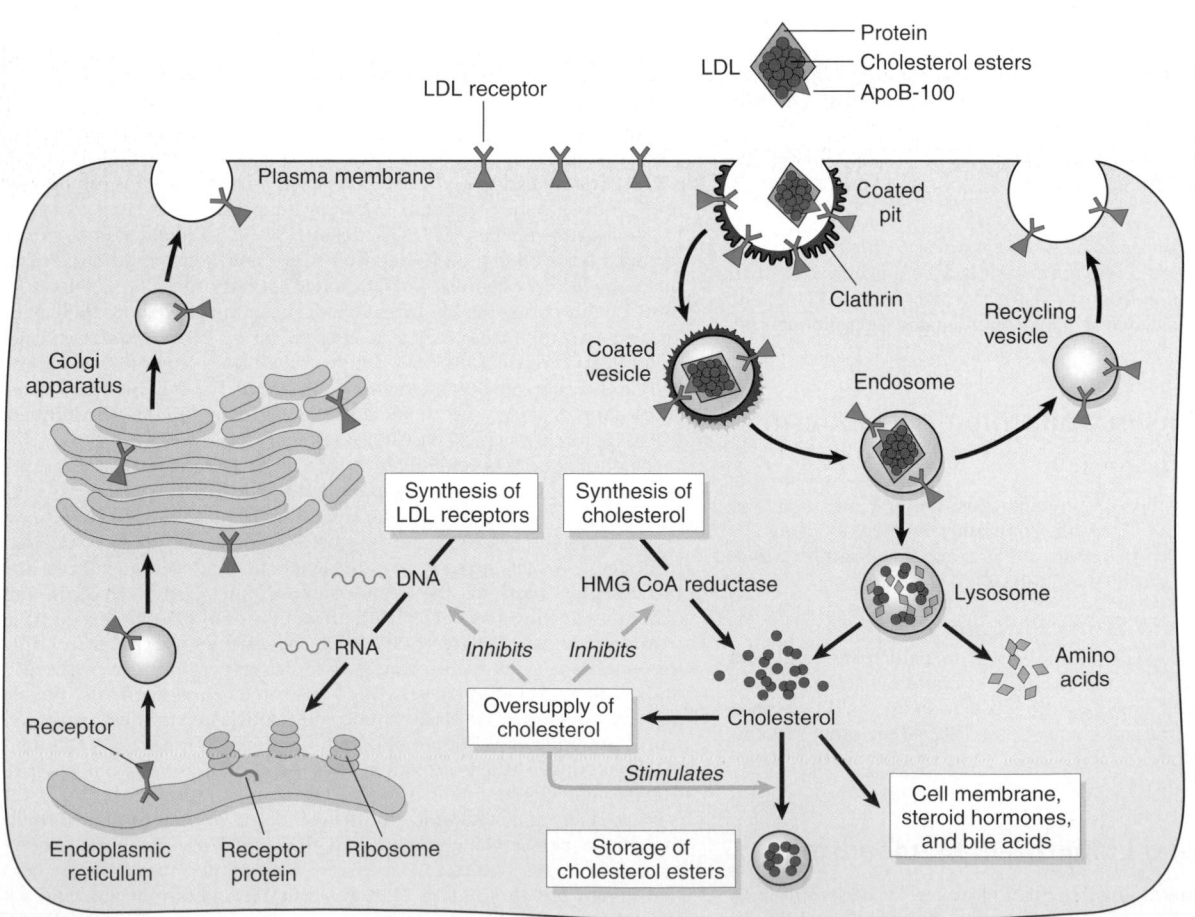

Figure 17–3 The LDL receptor pathway and regulation of cholesterol metabolism.

Table 17–6 Enzymes and Other Proteins Important for Lipoprotein Metabolism

	Gene location	Function	Deficiency	Tissue expression
Lipoprotein lipase (LPL)	8q22	Hydrolysis of TG in lipoproteins (esp. VLDL and CM) releasing free fatty acids and glycerol to tissues. PL and apoC-II are essential cofactors	Large CM and VLDL with very high TG levels	Present on surface of capillary endothelial cells in adipose tissue and skeletal and heart muscles, but not produced by endothelial cells
Hepatic lipase (HL)	15q22-23	Hydrolysis of TG and PL, esp. from HDL$_2$, and may be necessary for HDL metabolism. Also active on lipids in VLDL remnants and IDL. Not very active on newly release VLDL or CM	Increased TC, TG and HDL-C in deficiency	Secreted by hepatocytes, associates with nonparenchymal liver cells
Endothelial lipase (EL)	18q21.1	Hydrolysis of PL and TG in lipoproteins, esp. PL in HDL. Homologous to LPL and EL and pancreatic lipase	Increased levels of HDL$_2$, and large buoyant LDL. Overexpression in mice decreased TC, PL and HDL-C	Expressed in many tissue, including liver. Synthesized by endothelium
Lecithin cholesterol acyltransferase (LCAT)	16q22.1	Catalyzes the esterification of cholesterol, esp. in HDL, by promoting transfer or fatty acids from lecithin to cholesterol. Enables HDL to accumulate cholesterol as CE. Activated by apoA-I	Deficiency results in decreased HDL	Produced in liver and circulates with HDL
Cholesterol ester transfer protein (CETP)	16q21	Transfers CE, PL and TG among lipoproteins, esp. the transfer of CE from HDL to apoB-100-containing lipoproteins in exchange for TG	Deficiency results in large cholesterol-laden HDL	Produced in liver and circulates with HDL
Phospholipid transfer protein (PLTP)	20q12	Transfer of PL to and from HDL. Important for HDL growth and remodeling	Deficiency in mice results in low HDL	Expressed on many cell types
LDL receptor (LDLR)	19p13.2	Binds apoE and apoB-100 and mediates endocytosis of lipoproteins, mostly LDL, but also VLDL, IDL and possibly CM remnants and HDL	Familial hypercholesterolemia results primarily in elevated LDL	Expressed on most cell types, but hepatic receptors clear 70% of LDL
ATP-binding cassette protein A-1 (ABCA1)	9q22-31	Efflux of cholesterol from peripheral cells into HDL. Important for uptake of cholesterol by nascent HDL	Tangier disease, with very low HDL and accumulation of lipids in peripheral cells	Many cell types, prominently in the liver, testis, and adrenal
Scavenger receptor class B, member 1 (SCARB1)	12q24.31	Binds HDL on cell surface, may help in HDL development and clearance of CE from HDL in liver and steroidogenic tissues. May also enable macrophages to bind oxidized LDL	Accumulation of large CE-rich HDL, and accelerated atherosclerosis in mice	Macrophage, adrenal, liver and testis

cholesterol and phospholipid (Havel, 1980; Oppenheimer, 1987; Oram, 1986; Scanu, 1982). The formation of nascent HDL particles is almost exclusively dependent on the synthesis and release of apoA-I. Some HDL also seems to arise de novo in circulation from excess surface material (e.g., free cholesterol, apoA-I, apoA-II, apoC and phospholipid) removed from the triglyceride-rich lipoproteins as they are catabolized. In peripheral tissues, excess cholesterol is exported from cells (including macrophages) partially through the action of the protein ABCA1. This free cholesterol is accumulated by nascent HDL particles and esterified by LCAT. As cholesteryl esters move into the hydrophobic core, the particle becomes spherical and larger, developing eventually into HDL$_3$ and then HDL$_2$. Several plasma enzymes and proteins are involved in this remodeling process, including phospholipid transfer protein (PLTP) and cholesterol ester transfer protein (CETP). CETP catalyses the transfer of cholesterol esters to apoB-100-containing particles in exchange for triglycerides (Tall, 1990). PLTP facilitates the transfer of phospholipids from other lipoproteins to HDL, allowing the particle to grow by acquiring surface phospholipid as it accumulates esterified cholesterol and triglyceride in its core. Once formed, HDL delivers excess lipids, especially cholesterol, to the liver and other tissues (Bachorik, 1987; Glass, 1983; Stein, 1984). This may occur directly when HDL is either taken up by the hepatocytes via

specific receptors or through the action of cell surface receptors and enzymes (HL and EL) that deplete phospholipid and triglyceride without internalizing the HDL particles. Lipids may also return to the liver indirectly or be directed to peripheral tissues via lipoproteins to which they are transferred from HDL by PLTP and CETP.

Although HDL particles may return to the liver soon after formation, the bulk of HDL seems to remain in circulation for several days, continuously exchanging lipids and apolipoproteins with other lipoprotein particles, retrieving additional cholesterol from peripheral tissues, and delivering those lipids to the liver and steroid-producing tissues. This is supported by the fact that apoA-I has a half-life of several days in circulation. Eventually, HDL may be internalized by the liver (probably via the LDL receptor or SCARB1), or small lipid-depleted HDL may be catabolized in the kidney following filtration and cubulin-mediated reuptake in the proximal tubule.

Lipid and Lipoprotein Measurement

Lipoprotein concentrations have been measured and described in several ways. Some of these measurements, including particle mass and mass concentration (the mass of each lipoprotein particle as solute per liter of

Table 17–7 Physiologic Variation of Plasma Lipids, Lipoproteins, and Apolipoproteins

Component	CV$_P$ (%)*	CV$_P$ (%)†
Total cholesterol	5.0	6.4
Triglycerides	17.8	23.7
LDL-cholesterol	7.8	8.2
HDL-cholesterol	7.1	7.5
ApoA-I	7.1	–
ApoB	6.4	–

CV$_P$ = coefficient of physiologic variation.

* Data from patients of a lipid clinic (Kafonek, 1992).

† Data from the National Cholesterol Education Program (NCEP) 1995 Working Group on Lipoprotein Measurement.

solution), are not easily applied for screening or routine clinical purposes. Fortunately, other methods exist to describe the lipoprotein content of blood. Because the cholesterol composition of each lipoprotein class is similar from individual to individual, lipoprotein cholesterol is commonly used to evaluate lipoprotein concentration. For example, it is easier to determine the amount of LDL-C in a specimen than it is to determine the mass of LDL (cholesterol + triglyceride + protein) in solution, yet both measurements provide similar information about the LDL content of plasma. Lipoprotein-cholesterol concentrations correlate well with analytical ultracentrifugation values. Also, because these values have been used in most population studies of cardiovascular risk, they have documented predictive value.

When considering various methods of lipid analysis, several issues should be kept in mind. First, the more complicated the analytical procedures, the greater the variability of the analyses (Bookstein, 1990; Brown, 1990). For example, the measurement of plasma lipoproteins usually requires two steps, separating lipoprotein classes and measuring the class of interest. Both steps contribute to the error in the measurements. Consistent with this, lipoprotein-cholesterol analyses are generally more variable than total cholesterol (TC) analyses because of the additional manipulations required to prepare the lipoprotein-containing fractions. Second, in addition to analytical sources of error, there are significant preanalytical variables that affect measured lipid and lipoprotein levels. In fact, plasma lipoprotein concentrations can change dramatically as a result of normal physiologic variation. In this section, issues of sampling and storage are considered, along with methods for measuring lipids and lipoproteins.

Blood Sampling and Storage

Variation and error can be introduced before or during venipuncture, or when the samples are handled and stored before analysis. Therefore, it is important to standardize conditions under which blood specimens are drawn and prepared for analysis.

Biologic Variation. Physiologic variations in cholesterol, triglyceride, and lipoproteins have been examined in a number of studies (Bookstein, 1990; Brown, 1990; Demacker, 1982; Kafonek, 1992; Warnick, 1979). For cholesterol, the coefficient of physiologic variation within an individual averages about 6.5% but can be higher in certain individuals (Table 17–7). When measured in serial samples from the same person, the cholesterol levels in 95% of the samples will vary by about 13% above or below that person's mean level. As a result, physiologic variation can be several times greater than analytical error, and measurements must be made in several blood samples taken at least a week apart in order to establish the individual's usual lipoprotein concentration.

A variety of biological factors can affect lipid and lipoprotein levels. Cholesterol levels rise with age starting in early adulthood in both sexes. Women have lower levels than men, except in childhood and after the early fifties. Age-related variation is the basis for the National Cholesterol Education Program (NCEP) recommendation that cholesterol screening be repeated every 5 years. Seasonal variation also occurs, such that cholesterol levels are slightly higher in the winter (Robinson, 1992). Also, dietary intake of saturated fat and cholesterol significantly influences plasma lipid levels. The effects of dietary modification take several weeks to become apparent; thus, before ascertaining a person's cholesterol level, it is important that they be on their usual diet for 2 weeks and are neither gaining nor losing weight. Several common

medications significantly alter lipid levels, including oral contraceptives, postmenopausal estrogens, and some antihypertensive drugs. Medical disorders that lead to secondary dyslipoproteinemia, include, thyroid, hepatic, and kidney disease (see Table 17–15, below). In such cases, management of the hyperlipidemia is predominantly a function of treating the underlying disorder. Lifestyle and biological factors that produce short-term deviations from baseline lipid values include fasting, posture, venous occlusion, anticoagulants, recent myocardial infarction, stroke, cardiac catheterization, trauma, acute infection, and pregnancy. It is recommended that lipoprotein measurements be made no sooner than 8 weeks after any form of trauma or acute bacterial or viral infection, and 3–4 months after childbirth.

Fasting. Ideally patients should fast for 12 hours before venipuncture. Chylomicrons are usually present in postprandial plasma and, depending on the type and amount of food ingested, can markedly increase the plasma triglyceride (TG) concentration. The concentrations of LDL- and HDL-cholesterol (LDL-C and HDL-C) also decline transiently after eating, in part as a consequence of CETP-mediated compositional changes that occur during the catabolism of chylomicrons (Cohn, 1988). Chylomicrons are almost completely cleared within 6–9 hours, and their presence after a 12-hour fast is considered to be abnormal. Generally, TC and HDL-C levels can be measured in nonfasting individuals, greatly facilitating screening and monitoring. Fasting has little effect on plasma TC levels, and although nonfasting HDL-C levels can be a few mg/dL lower than fasting levels, this should not lead to misclassification of patients with low HDL levels. When TG and LDL-C are being measured, fasting becomes a requirement. The postprandial appearance of chylomicrons, and compositional changes in LDL lead to the underestimation of LDL-C and can result in the misclassification of truly affected patients. The National Cholesterol Education Program (NCEP) Adult Treatment Panel III (ATP III) (NCEP, 2002) has recommended that patients fast for at least 9 hours before blood specimens are taken for lipid and lipoprotein analysis. This is an accommodation to patients who may be unable or unwilling to fast for 12 hours. The shorter fasting period should produce only minor, and clinically insignificant errors in the estimation of the patient's usual TG, LDL-C and HDL-C levels. A 12-hour fasting period is still considered appropriate when making lipoprotein measurements in clinical and epidemiologic studies.

Posture. When a standing patient reclines, extravascular water transfers to the vascular system and dilutes nondiffusible plasma constituents. Decreases of as much as 10% in the concentrations of TC, LDL-C, HDL-C, apoA-I and apoB (Miller, 1992) have been observed after a 20-minute period of recumbence. The decrease in TG is about 50% greater, suggesting that factors other than simple hemodilution may also operate. These effects are about half as great in a standing subject who sits (Miller, 1992). Postural changes are reversible when the patient resumes the standing position. The position of the patient should therefore be standardized for venipuncture, preferably to the sitting position, which is most commonly used. Current NCEP guidelines recommend that patients be seated for 5 minutes prior to sampling to prevent hemoconcentration. If it is necessary to use the recumbent position, this position should be used each time the patient is sampled to minimize postural change. Prolonged venous occlusion can lead to hemoconcentration and cholesterol increases of 10–15%. Tourniquets should not be applied for more than a minute or two, if possible.

Venous vs. capillary samples. Although it is generally assumed that venous and capillary samples are equivalent, the available information at present is limited and somewhat contradictory. Some investigators have found that cholesterol measurements in the two kinds of samples agreed within about 4% (Koch, 1987) or less (Law, 1997; Lunz, 1987), but others have reported differences of 8–12% (Bachorik, 1990). In general, the measurements in capillary blood samples seem to be a little lower than in venous samples. Additionally, measurements in fingerstick samples tend to be more variable than in venous samples obtained at the same time, probably due to pre-analytical sources of error. Estimates for the biological component of within-subject variations have been made for lipid and lipoprotein in venous and fingerstick samples, and are similar in both kinds of samples for cholesterol, TG, HDL, and LDL (Kafonek, 1996). Although the use of capillary samples may be unavoidable under some conditions, it is well to keep in mind first that the epidemiologic data on which risk levels for lipids and lipoproteins are derived are based on measurements in venous samples, and second, that for various physiologic and methodologic reasons, the measurements in the two kinds of samples may differ.

Plasma vs. serum. Either plasma or serum can be used when only cholesterol, TG and HDL-C are measured, and LDL-C is calculated from these three measurements (see below); however, plasma is preferred when the lipoproteins are measured by ultracentrifugal or electrophoretic methods because the samples can be cooled to 4°C immediately to retard changes that can occur in the lipoproteins at room temperature. When plasma is to be used, blood is cooled in an ice bath as soon as it is drawn, and the cells are removed as soon as possible, generally within 3 hours. The plasma is then stored at 4°C until it is analyzed. Plasma should not remain in contact with the cells overnight. Even in the presence of the anticoagulant, protein aggregation can occur in plasma that is stored in the refrigerator for a few days or frozen for longer periods. This can make it difficult to obtain a homogeneous aliquot for analysis and, furthermore, can interfere with the flow of sample in automated analyzers, resulting in inaccurate or variable results. Protein aggregation occurs less frequently in serum, and serum has been used under certain circumstances, such as when it is necessary to store samples for weeks or months before analysis.

The choice of anticoagulant is also important. Some anticoagulants, such as citrate, exert rather large osmotic effects that result in falsely low plasma lipid and lipoprotein concentrations. Heparin, because of its relatively high molecular weight, has little effect on plasma volume, but can alter the electrophoretic mobilities of the lipoproteins. EDTA is the preferred anticoagulant, even though cholesterol and triglyceride concentrations in EDTA plasma are about 3% lower than in serum (Laboratory Methods Committee of the Lipid Research Clinics Program, 1977). This anticoagulant retards certain kinds of oxidative and enzymatic alterations that occur in the lipoproteins during storage.

Storage Generally, TC, triglycerides, and HDL-C can be satisfactorily analyzed in frozen samples, and LDL-C concentrations can be estimated with the Friedewald equation (Friedewald, 1972). Apolipoproteins can also be measured in frozen samples (see below). Frozen samples are not appropriate for ultracentrifugal analysis, because the triglyceride-rich lipoproteins do not withstand freezing. When serum or plasma must be stored for long periods, it should be maintained at temperatures of −70°C or lower. For short-term storage (up to a month or two), the samples can be kept at −20°C, but they should not be stored in a self-defrosting freezer. The temperature in a self-defrosting freezer actually cycles between about −20°C and −2°C during the defrost cycle and effectively subjects the samples to daily freeze–thaw cycles, which can hasten their deterioration and cause the lipid and lipoprotein measurements to become variable (i.e., less reproducible).

Estimation of Plasma Lipids

Cholesterol and triglycerides are the plasma lipids of most interest in the diagnosis and management of lipoprotein disorders. Phospholipid analyses generally provide little additional information, and are seldom required. Occasionally, they may be requested in cases of obstructive liver disease or disorders associated with abnormally low lipoprotein levels.

Cholesterol

Cholesterol accounts for almost all of the sterol in plasma. It exists as a mixture of unesterified (30–40%) and esterified (60–70%) forms, and the proportion of the two forms is fairly constant within and between normal individuals. TC and lipoprotein-cholesterol concentrations are usually expressed in terms of the sterol nucleus without distinguishing the esterified and unesterified fractions. In general, it is not necessary to distinguish the two forms except in cases in which the contribution of the fatty acid moiety to cholesteryl ester mass must be accounted for, or when the cholesterol/cholesteryl ester mass ratio is of interest.

This discussion considers primarily the enzymatic methods of cholesterol quantification, which have virtually replaced the chemical methods that were used for most clinical and research purposes (Bachorik, 1976; Lipid Research Clinics Program, 1982; Wood, 1980). However, one chemical method, a modification of the Abell–Kendall method (Abell, 1952) continues as the reference method for cholesterol used by the Centers for Disease Control and Prevention (CDC) and a network of secondary reference laboratories (Myers, 1989). In the Abell–Kendall method, cholesteryl esters are hydrolyzed with alcoholic potassium hydroxide (KOH), unesterified cholesterol is extracted with petroleum ether and measured with the Liebermann–Burchard reagent using purified cholesterol standards. This method can be accurate within about 0.5% of true value.

Enzymatic Methods. These measure TC directly in plasma or serum through a series of reactions in which cholesteryl esters are hydrolyzed, the 3-OH group of cholesterol is oxidized and hydrogen peroxide, one of the reaction products, is quantified enzymatically:

$$\text{Cholesteryl ester} + H_2O \xrightarrow[\text{hydrolase}]{\text{Cholesteryl ester}} \text{Cholesterol} + \text{Free fatty acid}$$
(Rx. 17–1)

$$\text{Cholesterol} + O_2 \xrightarrow[\text{oxidase}]{\text{Cholesterol}} \text{Cholest-4-en-3-one} + H_2O_2 \quad \text{(Rx. 17–2)}$$

$$H_2O_2 + \text{Phenol} + \text{4-aminoantipyrine} \xrightarrow{\text{Peroxidase}}$$
$$\text{Quinoneimine dye} + 2H_2O$$
(Rx. 17–3)

The absorbance of the quinoneimine dye produced in Reaction 17–3 is measured at 500 nm.

Enzymatic methods are less subject to interference by nonsterol substances that react in the chemical methods; however, they are not absolutely specific for cholesterol. Cholesterol oxidase (Reaction 17–2) can react with sterols other than cholesterol that are present in plasma, and with plant sterols which are present in appreciable concentrations in the circulation of patients with β-sitosterolemia. These sterols also contribute to the cholesterol values measured via most chemical methods. In addition to sterols, reducing substances such as ascorbic acid and bilirubin can interfere with the enzymatic measurements by consuming H_2O_2 (Naito, 1984; Witte, 1978). Interference by bilirubin is complex and can produce falsely high or low cholesterol values depending on reagent concentrations. Bilirubin itself absorbs light at 500 nm, which would tend to increase measured cholesterol values; however, it is oxidized by H_2O_2, and as a result loses its absorbance at 500 nm. This complicates the application of a serum blank to correct for bilirubin absorbance. Bilirubin may also interfere directly with enzymatic methods by reacting with an intermediate in the peroxidase reaction. On the whole, interference by bilirubin seems to be significant only at concentrations exceeding 5 mg/dL, at which level it has been reported to decrease apparent cholesterol values by 5–15% (Deacon, 1979; Naito, 1984; Pesce, 1977). Sample turbidity as a result of elevated TG concentrations can also interfere with the enzymatic methods (Pesce, 1977). Uric acid and hemoglobin, as well as a large number of other substances, do not significantly affect the cholesterol measurements even at abnormally high plasma concentrations (Deacon, 1979; Pesce, 1977).

In addition to their relative resistance to interference, enzymatic methods have other significant benefits. They consume only microliter quantities of sample and do not require a preliminary extraction step. They are rapid, and if the cholesteryl ester hydrolase step is omitted, they can be used to measure unesterified cholesterol. Finally, enzymatic methods are precise, with coefficients of variation generally in the range of 1–2%. For the most part, they use stabilized pure cholesterol standards or serum calibration standards, for which the stated values are traceable to the CDC reference method for cholesterol (Pesce, 1977). Enzymatic values generally agree with reference values within 1–2% when measured in a laboratory setting with modern equipment. Serum-based calibrators are inherently preferable to pure cholesterol, as they are subject to all analytic reactions undergone by patient samples.

Triglycerides

A wide variety of methods have been used to measure plasma triglycerides (Bachorik, 1977), but the methods most commonly used for clinical or epidemiologic purposes are based on the hydrolysis of triglycerides and the measurement of glycerol that is released in the reaction:

$$\text{Triglyceride} + 3H_2O \xrightarrow{\text{Lipase}} \text{Glycerol} + \text{Fatty acid} \quad \text{(Rx. 17–4)}$$

The reactions are almost universally performed enzymatically (as above); and, as with cholesterol, the enzymatic methods have replaced the earlier chemical methods (Kessler, 1966; Lipid Research Clinics Program, 1982).

One chemical method is still used as the CDC reference method for triglycerides. The CDC-reference method uses a chloroform extraction procedure followed by silicic acid chromatography to isolate the triglycerides. Glycerol is released by saponification (alkaline hydrolysis of triglycerides) and oxidized with sodium periodate:

$$\text{Glycerol} + NaIO_4 \longrightarrow \text{Formaldehyde} + \text{Formic acid} \quad \text{(Rx. 17–5)}$$

The formaldehyde produced is measured by reaction with a sulfuric acid solution of chromotropic acid to produce a pink chromophore. This method is not specific for glycerol. Formaldehyde is also produced indirectly from glycerol-containing phospholipids; however, these and other interfering substances are removed during the extraction (with chloroform) and adsorption (silicic acid chromatography) steps and do not interfere with TG measurements made using the CDC reference method.

Enzymatic methods (Bucolo, 1973). These are now universally used for TG analysis in the clinical laboratory. They are relatively specific, rapid, and easy to use. The analyses are performed directly in plasma or serum, and are not subject to interference by phospholipids or glucose.

Common to most enzymatic methods is the hydrolysis of triglycerides to free fatty acids and glycerol, followed by the phosphorylation of glycerol to glycerophosphate.

$$\text{Triglycerides} \xrightarrow{\text{Lipase}} \text{Glycerol + Fatty acids} \qquad \text{(Rx. 17–6)}$$

$$\text{Glycerol + ATP} \xrightarrow{\text{Glycerokinase}} \text{Glycerophosphate + ADP} \qquad \text{(Rx. 17–7)}$$

However, several methods exist to quantitate the amount of glycerol formed, and therefore the amount of triglyceride in plasma. In one approach, glycerophosphate reacts as follows.

$$\text{Glycerophosphate + NAD} \xrightarrow{\substack{\text{Glycerophosphate} \\ \text{dehydrogenase}}}$$

$$\text{Dihydroxyacetone phosphate + NADH + H+} \qquad \text{(Rx. 17–8)}$$

$$\text{NADH + Tetrazolium dye} \xrightarrow{\text{Diaphorase}} \text{Formazan + NAD}^+ \qquad \text{(Rx. 17–9)}$$

NADH formation can be measured spectrophotometrically at 340 nm. In other methods, Reaction 17–9 has been added so that the absorbance readings can be made in the 500- to 600-nm region of the spectrum, using instruments that are more commonly available in the clinical laboratory.

In a common variation, the glycerophosphate formed in Reaction 17–7 is oxidized by the action of glycerophosphate oxidase:

$$\text{Glycerophosphate + O}_2 \xrightarrow{\substack{\text{Glycerophosphate} \\ \text{oxidase}}} \text{Dihydroxyacetone + H}_2\text{O}_2 \qquad \text{(Rx. 17–10)}$$

The resulting H_2O_2 is measured as described previously for cholesterol methods (Reaction 17–3).

In a third approach, ADP, rather than glycerophosphate formed in Reaction 17–7, is quantitated:

$$\text{ADP + Phosphoenol pyruvate} \xrightarrow{\substack{\text{Pyruvate} \\ \text{kinase}}} \text{ATP + Pyruvate} \qquad \text{(Rx. 17–11)}$$

$$\text{Pyruvate + NADH + H}^+ \xrightarrow{\substack{\text{Lactate} \\ \text{dehydrogenase}}} \text{Lactate + NAD}^+ \qquad \text{(Rx. 17–12)}$$

In this method, the disappearance of NADH is measured at 340 nm.

Enzymatic TG methods generally perform well. The reagents are available commercially as lyophilized preparations that need only be reconstituted before use. Based on recent College of American Pathologists (CAP) surveys, the interlaboratory coefficients of variation (CVs) for TG measurement using a variety of enzymatic methods was of the order of 5–6%. It is prudent before selecting an enzymatic method to evaluate its accuracy and precision over the range of triglyceride concentrations likely to be encountered most frequently (1.299–12.987 mmol/L; 50–500 mg/dL).

Triglyceride Blanks. Enzymatic measurements of triglyceride involve the generation and measurement of glycerol. While phospholipids and glucose do not interfere with enzymatic methods, free glycerol does. Glycerol is normally present in plasma in concentrations below 0.163 mmol/L (1.5 mg/dL), equivalent to a triglyceride concentration of about 14 mg/dL, but can be present in higher concentrations, such as after extremely vigorous exercise, in patients with uncontrolled diabetes, after chance contamination with the glycerol lubricant used on the stoppers of some blood collection tubes, after recent ingestion of glycerol-containing medications, or in a relatively rare disorder, hyperglycerolemia which arises secondary to a mutation in the glycerol kinase gene on chromosome Xp21.3. A blank assay, without the addition of lipase, provides a measure of pre-existing glycerol. Increased readings in the blank indicate the presence of glycerol, and measured TG values can be corrected accordingly. In an alternative procedure, free glycerol is consumed in a preliminary reaction before initiating triglyceride hydrolysis. In this case, the measured value is the equivalent of a blanked triglyceride.

The blanking procedures described above are satisfactory for correcting spurious measurements that arise from many nonglyceride sources, but not for those that result from partial glycerides (diglycerides and mono-glycerides). Partial glycerides are generally present at very low concentrations in fresh plasma or serum, but can form through the slow hydrolysis of triglycerides when samples are stored. It is not clear whether partial glycerides in fresh plasma should be subtracted, but those that form during storage should probably not be subtracted because they arise from triglycerides that were originally present in the sample.

Fortunately, as complex as the blanking problem is, it is usually of little practical importance. Blanks are not determined routinely in many laboratories, and their use continues to be an area of uncertainty. When measured, the magnitude of the blanks encountered in most fresh samples is of the order of 0.056–0.112 mmol/L (5–10 mg/dL), expressed as triglyceride, although they can be higher in samples with high triglyceride concentrations. However, blanks can assume importance in the standardization and quality control of triglyceride measurements, since they can be

of the order of 0.226–0.339 mmol/L (20–30 mg/dL) or more in serum pools used for these purposes, probably owing in part to the partial hydrolysis of triglycerides during the preparation of the pools.

Phospholipids

Most of the phospholipid in human plasma is phosphatidyl choline (70–75%) or sphingomyelin (18–20%). The remaining phospholipids include phosphatidyl serine, phosphatidyl ethanolamine (3–6%) and lysophosphatidyl choline (4–9%). Phospholipid analysis usually provides little additional information in cases of dyslipoproteinemia; however, it may be desirable to measure total phospholipids or even individual phospholipid classes in disorders characterized by altered phospholipid concentration, composition or lipoprotein distribution, including obstructive jaundice, Tangier disease, abeta- or hypobetalipoproteinemia and LCAT deficiency.

Total phospholipids can be most conveniently determined by measuring phospholipid phosphorus. Lipids are extracted from the sample and oxidized completely to convert phospholipid phosphorus to inorganic phosphate, which is then determined colorimetrically. These procedures are reproducible and sensitive and can be adapted to measure total phospholipid phosphorus in 100 µL or less of plasma or serum. Each mole of phosphorus contributes about 4% to the total phospholipid mass; thus phospholipid mass can be determined by multiplying the phospholipid phosphorus concentration (expressed in mg/dL) by 25.

Serum or plasma phospholipids can also be measured enzymatically using commercially available methods. In the method available from WAKO Pure Chemical Industries, Ltd. (Osaka, Japan), lecithin (phosphatidyl choline), sphingomyelin, and lysolecithin are hydrolyzed using phospholipase D, and the choline liberated is oxidized.

$$\text{Phospholipid} \xrightarrow{\text{Phospholipase D}} \text{Choline} \qquad \text{(Rx. 17–13)}$$

$$\text{Choline} \xrightarrow{\substack{\text{Choline} \\ \text{oxidase}}} \text{Betaine + H}_2\text{O}_2 \qquad \text{(Rx. 17–14)}$$

The resulting H_2O_2 produced is measured in a manner similar to that shown in Reaction 17–3.

Analysis of individual phospholipid classes is seldom required for the evaluation of the dyslipoproteinemia and is not discussed in this chapter.

Estimation of Lipoproteins and Lipoprotein Cholesterol

Because lipoproteins share common lipid and apolipoprotein components, the central problem in lipoprotein analysis is the separation of different lipoprotein classes from one another. Many methods have been applied to lipoprotein separation including: ultracentrifugation, adsorption, gel filtration, affinity chromatography, electrophoresis in various media, polyanion and alcohol precipitation, immunochemical procedures, and various combinations of methods. Some of these methods require special skills and equipment, and are not easily adapted for clinical or epidemiologic purposes. This discussion is limited to several procedures that have been used by clinical laboratories.

Ultracentrifugal methods. These take advantage of two properties of the lipoproteins. First, by virtue of their lipid content, lipoproteins have lower densities than the other plasma macromolecules. Second, each class of lipoproteins has a different density. Thus, lipoproteins can be separated from the other plasma proteins, as well as from one another, by ultracentrifugation at the appropriate density. Ultracentrifugation methods are of largely historical and academic interest, and are seldom used clinically.

Electrophoretic Methods. In the past, electrophoresis was widely used in the clinical laboratory to separate and measure lipoproteins. However, because the method has significant limitations (described below), and because it is generally not required for the diagnosis of dyslipoproteinemia, its use in routine clinical practice has diminished in recent years. In general, the cost of the procedure, both in terms of time and money, is rarely justified by the information provided.

The most commonly used support medium for lipoprotein electrophoresis is agarose gel because of its speed, sensitivity, and ability to resolve the lipoprotein classes. Chylomicrons, if present, remain at the origin. Of the remaining major lipoproteins, HDL migrates the fastest, LDL slowest and VLDL at a rate intermediate between HDL and LDL. The electrophoretically separated lipoproteins have been named according to their mobilities: HDL (α-lipoprotein) moves with the α_1-globulins; LDL (β-lipoprotein) migrates with the β-globulins, and VLDL (pre-β lipoprotein) migrates with the α_2-globulins. Different properties of the lipoproteins form the basis for electrophoretic and ultracentrifugal separation, and analogous fractions separated by the two techniques may not be identical.

For example, β-VLDL (found in type 3 hyperlipidemia, see below) is isolated with VLDL by ultracentrifugation but moves electrophoretically with LDL. In the absence of additional information, a sample containing β-VLDL would appear to have an elevated VLDL concentration by ultracentrifugation and an increased LDL concentration by electrophoresis. Another example is that Lp(a) is isolated in the LDL–HDL density range by ultracentrifugation, but it has an electrophoretic mobility similar to that of VLDL. This dichotomy is responsible for naming Lp(a) 'sinking pre-β-lipoprotein.'

Electrophoresis can be performed using unfractionated plasma or in plasma fractions that contain other serum proteins. Lipoprotein electrophoretograms are usually visualized with a lipid-staining dye such as Oil Red O, Fat Red 7B, or Sudan Black B. These lipid stains react primarily with the ester bonds in triglycerides and cholesteryl esters. Lipoproteins rich in free cholesterol and phospholipids (such as LpX) stain very poorly and thus are grossly underestimated by electrophoretic techniques.

Attempts have been made to quantitate the lipoproteins by densitometry. Lipoprotein levels have been expressed in terms of the percentage distribution of lipid-staining material in β-, pre-β-, and α-lipoproteins, or have been converted to lipoprotein-cholesterol concentrations according to calculations that incorporate assumptions about cholesterol content and dye uptake of the lipoproteins. In general, these approaches have not been successful, for reasons that include incomplete resolution of β- and pre-β-lipoproteins, the presence of minor or unusual lipoproteins, and differences in the intensity of staining. Electrophoresis has been used most successfully in conjunction with other methods.

Polyanion Precipitation Methods. Some lipoproteins are precipitated with polyanions such as heparin sulfate, dextran sulfate, phosphotungstate, and others in the presence of divalent cations such as Ca^{2+}, Mg^{2+} and Mn^{2+}. Conditions have been established in which the major classes of lipoproteins can be precipitated in stepwise fashion beginning with the lower-density, lipid-rich lipoproteins (Burstein, 1982). The more dissimilar the lipoproteins are from one another, the better the separation. Thus, it is easier to separate apoB-containing lipoproteins from HDL than it is to separate VLDL from LDL or HDL_2 from HDL_3. Historically, polyanion precipitation was most commonly used to remove apoB-containing lipoproteins prior to the analysis of HDL-C. It required a sample pretreatment and was not fully automated. Most clinical laboratories have replaced precipitation techniques with automated homogeneous assays for HDL-C and LDL-C.

Methods for Determining HDL-C Values

Historically, HDL-C has been measured in the supernatant of samples following the precipitation of apoB-containing lipoproteins by polyanion-divalent cations. Several combinations of polyanion-divalent cations have been used, and not all of them give precisely the same results. HDL-C values determined with heparin sulfate-Mn^{2+} procedures agree closely with those obtained using analytical or preparative ultracentrifugation (Bachorik, 1976; Warnick, 1979). This method was widely used in epidemiologic studies. Dextran sulfate (relative molecular mass 50 000)-Mg^{2+} and sodium phosphotungstate-Mg^{2+} methods gained popularity because they do not interfere with enzymatic cholesterol studies. However, they give results about 5% lower than ultracentrifugation. Heparin-Ca^{2+} appears to give results that are about 10% higher. These differences arise, in part, from the underprecipitation of apoB-containing lipoproteins which leads to the overestimation of HDL-C, or the overprecipitation of HDL which can lead to underestimation of HDL-C. Increased triglycerides interfere with precipitation methods and overestimate HDL-C. Attempts were made to simplify precipitation methods by using dextran sulfate coated magnetic beads to achieve selective separation of HDL from the apoB-containing lipoproteins (Naito, 1995).

Currently, homogeneous assays are the most popular method for measuring HDL-C. Unlike precipitation methods, these fully-automated two-reagent procedures do not require off-line pretreatment and separation (hence the term 'homogeneous') and can be adapted to most chemistry analyzers. Thus, they reduce hands-on time and overall assay costs. Test kits distributed in the US are based on a variety of methods. Usually, the first reagent forms a stable complex with non-HDL lipoproteins, preventing them from participating in the reaction, and the second reagent releases HDL-C that is then measured enzymatically. According to CAP 2005 Surveys, the most common method uses a synthetic polymer together with a polyanion to block non-HDL lipoproteins, followed by a selective detergent to release HDL-C (Genzyme Diagnostics, Cambridge, MA; Beckman Coulter, Inc.). Other methods use polyethylene glycol-modified enzyme (Roche Diagnostics, Indianapolis, IN), or immunoinhibition (Wako Chemicals USA, Inc, Richmond, VA) to block non-HDL lipoproteins. A fourth method (Polymedco Inc., Cortlandt Manor, NY) uses a special reagent to selectively eliminate cholesterol in non-HDL lipoproteins, followed by a second reagent that releases cholesterol from HDL (Denka Seiken Co., Niigata, Japan). These methods are generally not affected by high triglycerides, bilirubin and globulins.

In a comprehensive review (Warnick, 2001), multiple HDL-C homogeneous assays were compared to traditional precipitation and ultracentrifugation procedures. The authors concluded that the new procedures simplify the determination of HDL-C and are accurate, precise and meet NCEP criteria for total error. However, atypical lipoproteins evaluated by homogeneous assay may show discrepant results when compared to the established precipitation method. These differences are seen in patients with hyperlipidemia, or liver or kidney disease where abnormal lipoprotein forms occur. Laboratories that encounter a high proportion of atypical lipoproteins (e.g., lipid clinics or research settings) should thoroughly validate a homogeneous assay for use with their patient population

Methods for LDL-C Measurement

Several methods have been used to measure LDL-C. The first, a reference laboratory procedure, involves ultracentrifugation to separate LDL from other lipoproteins, followed by analysis as described above to measure cholesterol. This method is not extensively discussed here. A much more common second method uses the Friedewald formula to calculate LDL-C. Finally, more recently developed homogeneous methods for measuring LDL-C are now available.

Friedewald Calculation. LDL-C can be determined by using the Friedewald formula, originally described by Friedewald, Levy, and Fredrickson (Friedewald, 1972). Generally, in fasting plasma samples LDL contains the cholesterol that is not present in HDL or VLDL. Thus LDL-C can be determined by the following equation in which concentrations are expressed in mmol/L, and the term [Plasma TG]/2.175 is used to represent VLDL-C.

$$[\text{LDL-cholesterol}] = [\text{Total cholesterol}] - [\text{HDL-cholesterol}]$$
$$- [\text{Plasma TG}]/2.175 \qquad (17\text{--}1)$$

The term [Plasma TG]/5 is used when concentrations are expressed in mg/dL. In this method, the plasma TC, TG, and HDL-C concentrations are determined as described. Because most plasma triglyceride is carried by VLDL, VLDL-C concentration is estimated from the ratio of triglyceride to cholesterol in VLDL:

$$\text{VLDL-C} = \text{Plasma TG}/2.175 \qquad (17\text{--}2)$$

It has been reported that the factor [Plasma TG]/2.825 gives a more nearly accurate estimate of VLDL-C (DeLong, 1986). This is equivalent to Plasma TG/6.5, when concentrations are expressed in mg/dL. However, the factor that gives the best estimate of VLDL-C, and therefore the best estimate of LDL-C, varies among populations and depending upon the triglyceride method used; on balance, the NCEP Working Group on Lipoprotein Measurement preferred the unmodified Friedewald equation (NCEP Working Group on Lipoprotein Measurement, 1995).

The Friedewald formula has significant limitations (Sniderman, 2003). These limitations arise largely from two assumptions upon which the method is based. First, the calculation assumes that essentially all plasma triglycerides are carried in VLDL. Second, the method assumes the triglyceride/cholesterol ratio of VLDL is invariant. Neither assumption is entirely true; as a result, this method is unsuitable for nonfasting samples that contain chylomicrons or samples that contain β-VLDL. As compared to VLDL, the ratio of triglycerides to cholesterol in chylomicrons is much higher. Thus, when CM is present the use of the factor TG/2.175 to account for non-HDL, non-LDL cholesterol can overestimate the amount of cholesterol in VLDL, leading to underestimation of LDL-C. Similarly the ratio of triglyceride to cholesterol in β-VLDL is much lower than in VLDL, and the use of the factor TG/2.175 in the presence of β-VLDL can underestimate VLDL-C and thus overestimate LDL-C. A patient with type 3 hyperlipoproteinemia can be misclassified as having an elevated LDL-C. It is important to distinguish the two conditions because their treatments differ.

Even in chylomicron-free samples the ratio of VLDL-C to triglyceride changes as triglyceride levels increase, and can lead to errors in estimates of VLDL-C. Because VLDL generally only carries about 25% of the TC in plasma, the resulting errors in LDL-C are usually less than 5–10 mg/dl (0.130–0.260) mmol/L). However, the calculation is not suitable for samples with high triglyceride concentrations. Errors in LDL-C become noticeable at triglyceride levels > 2.26 mmol/L (200 mg/dL), and are felt to become unacceptably large at triglyceride levels > 4.52 mmol/L (400 mg/dL). The accuracy of LDL-C calculation also suffers at low LDL-C levels, indicating that calculated LDL-C values may not provide the best assessment of cardiac risk in patients who are already receiving cholesterol-lowering therapy (Sniderman, 2003). Provided that its limitations are appreciated, the Friedewald equation has broad utility, both as a screening tool and for following patients.

Another issue to consider is non-LDL lipoproteins. Generally, LDL contributes most of the cholesterol to the measurement, and IDL and Lp(a) contribute only a few mg/dL each. However, these lipoproteins can contribute significantly to cholesterol measurements in some hyperlipidemia patients. Since Lp(a) levels are not lowered by a number of treatments that effectively lower LDL levels, Lp(a) measurements can, in some circumstances, reveal why a patient does not respond well to LDL-lowering therapy.

Direct LDL-C Measurement. To a large extent the ability to calculate LDL-C has eliminated the need for direct measurements. However, homogeneous direct LDL-C methods are useful when triglycerides are elevated because they are not subject to interference by triglycerides even at relatively high concentrations (= 600 mg/dL) (Bachorik, 2000). Direct assays have been adapted for use on a variety of analyzers and have been extensively reviewed elsewhere (Nauck, 2002; Miller, 2002). While these methods differ significantly, in general they use a combination of two 'reagents.' The first reagent usually selectively removes non-LDL lipoproteins (and/or stabilizes or inhibits LDL from reacting with enzymes) and the second reagent releases cholesterol from LDL so that it can be measured enzymatically.

In one method (Equal Diagnostics, Exton, PA; Genzyme Diagnostics, Cambridge MA), the first reagent uses a detergent polymer mixture to disrupt non-LDL lipoproteins, releasing their cholesterol. The cholesterol is then de-esterified, and acted upon by cholesterol oxidase to generate hydrogen peroxide, which further reacts to form a colorless compound. The second reagent contains a detergent that releases cholesterol from LDL. After de-esterification, the LDL-C proceeds through a similar set of reactions, except that the final step generates a colored compound. The intensity of the color is proportional to the concentration of LDL-C. Another method (Roche Diagnostics, Indianapolis, IN) is based on selective micellar solubilization of LDL by a nonionic detergent, as well as the interaction of a sugar compound with HDL, VLDL and chylomicrons to inhibit the participation in the measurement assay (Sugiuchi, 1998). A third method exploits the fact that reactivity of cholesterol in the different lipoproteins is affected by the hydrophile : lipophile balance (HLB) of solubilizing detergents. In this method non-LDL-C is reacted with cholesterol esterase and cholesterol oxidase at conditions under which LDL-C is inhibited and the resulting peroxide eliminated by catalase. A second reagent then alters the HLB of the detergent, creating conditions under which LDL-C reacts. This reagent also contains azide that inhibits catalase and allows the colorimetric detection of peroxide (see Reaction 17–3) (Polymedco Inc., Cortlandt Manor, NY; Reference Diagnostics, Bedford, MA). In a fourth method, the first reagent contains amphoteric surfactants that protect LDL, and allow the elimination of non-LDL-C and resulting peroxide, as above. The second reagent contains non-ionic surfactants that displace the protecting surfactants and allow measurement of LDL-C (Sigma Diagnostics, St Louis, MO).

While these methods exhibit good precision, they produce discrepancies as compared to the reference ultracentrifugation procedures in a number of circumstances, including presence of abnormal lipoproteins. When the triglyceride level is < 400 mg/dL, homogeneous methods perform no better than the Friedewald calculation for classifying patients into treatment groups (Miller, 2002). However, unlike the calculation, homogeneous assays can provide clinically useful results when triglycerides > 400 mg/dL. Another potential benefit is the convenience of measuring LDL-C in nonfasting individuals though some have recommended against this practice (Miller, 2002). ATP III recommendations do not favor replacing calculated LDL-C with direct LDL-C since the constituents of the calculation have to be measured in any case. Running direct LDL-C would only add to the expense.

Additional Methods in the Study of Dyslipidemia

Measurement of Lipoprotein Subclasses. Subpopulations or subclasses have been identified in VLDL, LDL and HDL by techniques including analytical ultracentrifugation, gradient gel electrophoresis and nuclear magnetic resonance (NMR) spectroscopy (Krauss, 1992, 1987; Otvos, 1992). Some subclass distinctions are of clinical significance, yet the number of subclasses identified varies between methods of separation, and the nomenclature for subclasses is less than uniform. For example, when NMR technology is used to identify lipoprotein subclasses, particle subclass numbers tend to increase with increasing particle size; thus LDL particles of the L2 subclass are larger than L1 particles. When electrophoresis or

ultracentrifugation is used, the opposite is true, and particles tend to decrease in size with higher numbers. Thus, in segmented gradient gel electrophoresis, LDL subclass IV (or LDL_4) particles are smaller than subclass II (LDL_2) particles, and in gradient ultracentrifugation subclass LDL_4 particles are smaller than LDL_3 particles.

Recent interest has focused on the role of subclasses in the development of atherosclerosis, specifically the smallest and least dense LDL particles. This fraction is thought to be more atherogenic than large LDL. Small HDL and large VLDL subclasses have also been associated with an increased incidence of atherosclerosis. The NMR LipoProfile (LipoScience, Raleigh, NC) allows the quantification of lipoprotein particles by subclass based upon their unique NMR-spectral characteristics. This profile provides information about CHD risk by quantifying the subclass distribution of lipoprotein particles (Otvos, 2002). At least partially, the appeal of this technique arises from the idea that the migration of LDL particles into the artery wall is gradient driven, and dependent upon LDL particle number. When large numbers of small LDL particles are present, LDL-C measurements tend to underestimate the number of LDL particles, and thus the atherosclerotic effects of LDL. Triglyceride levels > 100 mg/dL and HDL-C < 60 mg/dL are associated with high levels of small LDL particles; so, when these conditions are present, NMR profiling may be a useful technique for assessing CHD risk. Sensitive electrophoretic methods should provide similar results. These methods are not currently viewed as screening tools. They are more appropriate for refining risk assessment and treatment in patients with previously identified CHD risk, who are under treatment and have LDL-C values at or close to treatment goals. This is consistent with most accepted guidelines, which stress the importance of LDL-C as the primary goal of therapy in most types of dyslipidemia.

Standing Plasma Test. Chylomicrons, if present in appreciable quantities, are detected using the 'standing plasma' test. An aliquot of plasma (2 mL) is placed into a 10×75-mm test tube and allowed to stand in the refrigerator at $4°C$ undisturbed overnight. Chylomicrons accumulate as a floating 'cream' layer and can be detected visually. The presence of chylomicrons in fasting plasma is considered to be abnormal. A plasma sample that remains turbid after standing overnight contains excessive amounts of VLDL; if a floating 'cream' layer also forms, chylomicrons are present as well.

Detection of β-VLDL and Lp(a). As mentioned above, the abnormal lipoprotein β-VLDL ('floating β' lipoprotein), has the density of VLDL, but migrates electrophoretically with LDL in the β-region. It can be detected when the ultracentrifugal fraction of d < 1.006 kg/L is examined electrophoretically. In practice, unfractionated plasma and both ultracentrifugal fractions (< and > 1.006 kg/L) are examined at the same time; each sample thus serves as its own control to establish the relative migration of the lipoprotein bands. In normal plasma, the β (LDL and IDL), pre-β (VLDL), and α (HDL) lipoprotein bands are visible in unfractionated plasma, only the pre-β band is present in the d < 1.006 kg/L fraction, and the β- and α-lipoprotein bands are seen only in the d > 1.006 kg/L fraction. When present, β-VLDL is observed as a band with β-mobility in the d < 1.006 kg/L fraction. Its presence is abnormal, and is usually associated with dysbetalipoproteinemia (type 3 hyperlipoproteinemia), although occasionally it is seen in other disorders. Chylomicrons, which are often seen in type 3 patients, remain at the origin on agarose gel.

Lp(a) has a density similar to LDL, but migrates similarly to VLDL on electrophoresis. Thus it can be detected when the d > 1.006 g/mL protein is examined electrophoretically. When Lp(a) is present in concentrations exceeding 20–30 mg/dL (i.e., when it contributes more than about 10 mg/dL to the LDL-C measurement) an additional band with pre-β mobility is also observed in the d > 1.006 kg/L fraction (hence the name sinking pre-β-lipoprotein). Under these conditions the physician may wish to request a quantitative Lp(a) measurement. Lp(a) can now be measured using immunoturbidimetric methods. When the Lp(a) level is very high, it may be necessary to correct LDL-C for the contribution of Lp(a)-cholesterol. The following relationship has been used to estimate the contribution of Lp(a)-cholesterol to the measured LDL-C value, where the values are given in mg/dL:

$$Lp(a)\text{-cholesterol} = 0.3 \times [Lp(a) \text{ mass}] \qquad (17\text{–}3)$$

$$LDL\text{-}C = TC - [HDL\text{-cholesterol}] - [Plasma\ TG]/5 - (0.3[Lp(a)\ mass]) \qquad (17\text{–}4)$$

VLDL-C/Plasma Triglyceride Ratio. The ratio of VLDL-C to plasma triglycerides may be useful in the evaluation of type 3 hyperlipoproteinemia. This ratio, expressed in mol/mol or (mass/mass), is generally in the range of 0.230–0.575 (0.1–0.25) in samples without β-VLDL, depending on the relative amounts of VLDL, LDL, and HDL present, and on the errors inherent in the VLDL-C and plasma triglyceride measurements. Type 3 subjects have ratios > 0.689 (0.3), usually in the range of 0.689–0.919

Table 17–8 NCEP Guidelines for Acceptable Measurement Error

Analyte	Total error	Bias	CV*
Cholesterol	≤9%	≤3%	≤3%
Triglyceride	≤15%	≤5%	≤5%
HDL-cholesterol	≤13%	≤5%	≤4%[†]
LDL-cholesterol	≤12%	≤4%	≤4%

* Coefficient of variation defined as standard deviation/mean × 100.

[†] Precision criteria applied to HDL-cholesterol levels of 42 mg/dL (1.09 mmol/L) and higher. At lower levels, CV is not used; rather, standard deviation should not exceed 1.7 mg/dL (0.044 mmol/L).

Table 17–9 ATP III Classification for LDL, Total and HDL Cholesterol, and Triglyceride values*

LDL cholesterol	
< 100	Optimal
100–129	Near optimal/above optimal
130–159	Borderline high
160–189	High
≥ 190	Very high
Total cholesterol	
< 200	Desirable
200–239	Borderline high
≥ 240	High
HDL cholesterol	
< 40	Low
≥ 60	High
Triglycerides	
< 150	Normal
150–199	Borderline high
200–499	High
≥ 500	Very high

* NCEP, 2002.

Table 17–10 Major Risk Factors that Modify LDL Goals*

Cigarette smoking

Hypertension (BP ≥ 140/190 or on antihypertensive medication)

Low HDL cholesterol (< 40 mg/dL)

Family history of premature CHD (CHD in a male first-degree relative < 55 years; CHD in a female first-degree relative < 65 years)

Age (men ≥ 45; women ≥ 55)

Diabetes mellitus

Pre-existing CHD

* NCEP, 2002.

(0.3–0.4), although higher ratios can be observed. Again, because of errors in the measurements, the observation of a ratio of 0.689 (0.3) on a single occasion may or may not be significant. Overt type 3 patients manifest both β-VLDL and a VLDL-C/plasma triglyceride ratio of 0.689 (0.3) or greater. Occasionally, a lipid disorder treatment clinic may request the assessment of apoE phenotype to supplement the diagnosis of type 3 hyperlipoproteinemia (see below), since homozygosity for apoE-2 is associated with this disorder. However, not all homozygous patients have type 3 hyperlipoproteinemia, and ultracentrifugation is still required for assessing the presence of β-VLDL.

Apolipoprotein Analysis. Studies have indicated that apoA-I and apoB may be better discriminators of atherosclerotic disease than lipid or lipoprotein determinations. Because apoA-I is present primarily in HDL, while apoB (in fasting samples) is present in VLDL, IDL and LDL, it stands to reason that low apoB and high apoA-I levels, as well as a low apoB to apoA-I ratio should be a good thing. In general, the evidence for this has been more consistent for apoB than for apoA-I, but the reason for this is not clear. A large-scale, placebo-controlled intervention trial, AFCAPS (Gotto, 2000), found that apoB was the best single lipid, lipoprotein, or apolipoprotein measurement to predict both baseline and on-treatment CAD risk, followed by apoA-I. ApoB : A-I ratios may also be useful in assessing risk.

Apolipoproteins are usually measured by immunoassay or immuno-nephelometry. These techniques rely upon the measurement of the turbidity caused by apolipoprotein–antibody complexes (Lopes-Virella, 1980). A potential limitation of this method stems from the inherent turbidity of lipemic samples, or even nonlipemic samples after repeated freezing and thawing. To some extent, automated systems can correct for such turbidity.

The NCEP Guidelines

The Third Report of the National Cholesterol Education Program (NCEP) Expert Panel on Detection, Evaluation, and Treatment of High Blood Cholesterol in Adults (Adult Treatment Panel III, or ATP III) was published in 2002 (NCEP, 2002). It presents the updated NCEP evidence-based guidelines for cholesterol testing and management, and provides detailed information on other topics including the classification of lipids and lipoprotein particles, CHD risk assessment, lifestyle intervention, drug treatment, specific dyslipidemias, and treatment adherence issues. More recently, the NCEP recommendations have been updated in consideration of new clinical trial data (Grundy, 2004).

Reliability of Measurements

NCEP guidelines have shifted the focus from recognizing abnormal and normal cholesterol values to assessing overall cardiovascular risk based on cutoffs for cholesterol, triglycerides, HDL-C, and LDL-C. The adoption of a single set of cutoffs imposes on laboratories the mandate to measure lipids and lipoproteins accurately and precisely. The Laboratory Standardization Panel of NCEP (NCEP, 1995) guidelines are presented in Table 17–8. Note that each test has a single maximum acceptable value for total error that includes assay bias (i.e., a measure of accuracy) and CV (i.e., a measure of imprecision). Total error is calculated as follows:

% total error = % bias + 1.96 (%CV)   (17–5)

For each test, Table 17–8 provides an example of a target bias and CV that, when considered together, would yield the maximum acceptable total error. Note that by using total error, a laboratory can slightly exceed the limit for bias, provided that the CV is sufficiently small to maintain the total error within the guideline (the opposite is also true). For example, cholesterol has a target bias of 3% and a target CV of 3%. A laboratory with a bias of 3.5% and a CV of 2% exceeds the target for bias though it

meets the target for CV. However, the total error of 7.5% (i.e., 3.5% + 1.96 × 2%) is acceptable since it is less than the 9% target.

Testing and Treatment

ATP III introduced several new concepts for the evaluation of hyper-lipidemia. Diabetes mellitus is now considered a risk equivalent, because it confers a high risk of new CHD within 10 years. This means that for the evaluation of elevated cholesterol levels, diabetic patients are treated like patients who already have CHD. Also, ATP III recognized patients with 'metabolic syndrome' (described below) and patients with a high 10-year risk for CHD based upon the Framingham risk projections as candidates for intensive intervention and therapy.

Cholesterol goals. ATP III recommends a complete lipoprotein profile (TC, LDL-C, HDL-C, and triglycerides) as the initial test for evaluating blood cholesterol. Testing should be performed in all adults age 20 or older, and should be repeated at least once every 5 years. If testing is performed in the nonfasting state, then only TC and HDL-C can be used. In such circumstances, if the TC is = 200 mg/dL or the HDL is < 40 mg/dL, then a follow-up profile should be performed. ATP III provides guidelines for acceptable test values and uses LDL-C as the primary target for cholesterol-lowering therapy (Table 17–9). Note that major risk factors (Table 17–10) can modify LDL cholesterol goals (Table 17–11). Therapeutic lifestyle change (TLC) and drug therapy are the two approaches used to reach the LDL-C goal. TLC involves dietary change and increased physical activity, combined with regular follow-up. Regardless of a patient's risk category or LDL goal, TLC represents the first line of therapy, though it may be initially combined with drug therapy when treating high-risk patients. Note that patients in the moderate-risk category are further subdivided (for drug therapy) based on a Framingham Risk Score, which estimates the 10-year risk of cardiac events based on factors in Table 17–10, as well as other factors like TC, and HDL-C (Wilson, 1998). Drug

Table 17–11 Risk-Based LDL-C Goals*

Risk category	LDL goal (mg/dL)	Initiate TLC	Consider drug therapy
CHD and CHD risk equivalents	< 100 *Optional: < 70*	≥ 100	≥ 100 70–100
Moderately high risk (2+) risk factors[†] and a Framingham 10-year risk of 10–20%	< 130 *Optional:*	≥ 130 < 100	≥ 130 100–129
Moderate risk (2+) risk factor[†] and a Framingham 10-year risk < 10%	< 130	≥ 130	≥ 160
Zero to one risk factor[†]	< 160	≥ 160	≥ 190

* NCEP, 2002, and Grundy, 2004.

[†] Note that modifying risk factors are listed in Table 17–10

therapy for hyperlipidemia usually consists of four types of medications: statins, fibric acid derivatives, bile acid resins, and nicotinic acid. Some relevant characteristics of these medications are briefly summarized in Table 17–12.

Metabolic Syndrome. This physiologic syndrome is characterized by a constellation of known and emerging risk factors for CHD. Several organizations including the WHO and NCEP have proposed different definitions for this syndrome; however, risk factors generally include abdominal obesity, atherogenic dyslipidemia (elevated triglycerides, small LDL particles, and low HDL-C), raised blood pressure, insulin resistance (with or without glucose intolerance), and prothrombotic and proinflammatory states. First described as 'syndrome X' in the late 1980s, this condition may be present in 20–25% of adult Americans. In patients with metabolic syndrome, LDL-C is the primary target of therapy; however, patients are usually candidates for more intensive cholesterol-lowering therapy than might be suggested by their LDL-C alone. Other objectives include treatment of the underlying causes (i.e., obesity and physical inactivity), and treatment of associated nonlipid and lipid risk factors (Garber, 2004).

Hypertriglyceridemia. Supported by data from recent meta-analyses, ATP III identifies elevated triglycerides as an independent risk factor for CHD. Factors associated with a high triglyceride level include obesity, physical inactivity, cigarette smoking, excess alcohol intake, high carbohydrate diets (> 60% of energy intake), several diseases (e.g., type 2 diabetes, chronic renal failure, nephritic syndrome), certain drugs (e.g., corticosteroids, estrogens, retinoids, higher doses of β-adrenergic blocking agents) and genetic disorders (familial combined hyperlipidemia, familial hypertriglyceridemia, and familial dysbetalipoproteinemia). In persons with elevated triglycerides, the primary aim of therapy is to achieve the target for LDL-C. In the fasting state most circulating triglyceride is in VLDL remnant lipoproteins, so non-HDL cholesterol (TC – HDL cholesterol) can be used as a secondary target for therapy. Non-HDL cholesterol includes all apoB-containing lipoproteins, but in the fasting state provides a combined assessment of LDL-C and VLDL-C. Treatment plans for hypertriglyceridemia emphasize weight reduction and increased physical activity with borderline high elevations, but include LDL-lowering medications, and triglyceride-lowering drugs (nicotinic acid or fibrate) at higher levels. In rare patients with very high triglyceride levels (> 500 mg/dL) the initial aim of therapy is to prevent acute pancreatitis.

Emerging Risk Factors. ATP III recognizes additional positive risk factors for CHD including: elevations in Lp(a), remnant lipoproteins, small LDL particles, fibrinogen, homocysteine, high-sensitivity C-reactive protein (hs-CRP), impaired fasting plasma glucose (110–125 mg/dL), and pre-existing subclinical atherosclerosis (as evidenced by myocardial ischemia on exercise testing, carotid intimal–medial thickening, and/or coronary artery calcium deposition). The links between some of these factors and CHD are obvious or are discussed elsewhere; however, others require expanded consideration. For example, elevated homocysteine levels have been linked to medications, as well as genetic, disease and lifestyle conditions, and may contribute to CHD at least partially by exerting toxic effects on the endothelium. The links between hs-CRP (a marker of chronic inflammation) and fibrinogen (a marker of prothrombotic states) and CHD at this point remain largely statistical; clear mechanisms have not been established. Elevation of apoB (present in chylomicrons, VLDL, IDL and LDL), decreases in apoA-I (present mostly in HDL), and increases in the apoB/apoA-I ratio have also been associated with increased risk of CHD (Walldius, 2004). While these risk factors are not widely used for screening purposes, they may be useful in defining risk status, and refining treatment in patients already known to be at risk.

Children. Current evidence indicates that atherosclerotic lesions can begin in childhood, and that children with high blood cholesterol levels have a high probability of becoming adults with high blood cholesterol. In an effort to intervene early in the disease course of children with an atherosclerotic predisposition, guidelines for assessing CHD risk in children and adolescents have been promulgated by organizations including NCEP (NCEP Expert Panel on Children and Adolescents) (NCEP, 1992) and American Heart Association (Kavey, 2003). Current recommendations support selectively screening (starting at 2 years of age) children and adolescents with a family history of premature cardiovascular disease, or those with at least one parent with high blood cholesterol. Table 17–13 classifies these children by total and LDL-C levels. These recommendations do not support the universal laboratory screening of children and adolescents

Intervention aimed at reducing risk is recommended when the averaged results of three fasting lipid profiles are above the cutoffs for TC and LDL described above, or with elevated triglycerides (> 150 mg/dL) or decreased HDL-C (< 35 mg/dL). As in adults, intervention focuses on a search for medical causes of lipid abnormalities, TLC and pharmacologic intervention when necessary.

Table 17–12 Hyperlipidemia Drugs

Drug class	Primary effects	Secondary effects	Mechanism	Side effects	Examples
Statins	Lowers LDL-cholesterol (20–60%)	Small decreases in elevated triglyceride Modest increase in HDL-cholesterol	Inhibit HmG-CoA reductase	Rare-GI disturbances, liver problems, rhabdomyolysis	Lovastatin Simvastatin Pravastatin Fluvastatin Atorvastatin
Fibric acid derivatives	Lowers triglycerides (20–50%)	Small increases in HDL (10–15%)	Not clearly defined. May decrease the catabolism of HDL, increase the activity of LPL, and inhibit the hepatic synthesis of VLDL	GI disturbances, increased likelihood of cholesterol gallstones, may increase effects of warfarin, and tendency of statins to cause rhabdomyolysis	Gemfibrozil Fenofibrate
Bile acid resins	Lowers LDL-cholesterol (10–20%)		Bind bile acids in intestine leading to excretion	Mild GI disturbances	Cholestyramine Colestipol Colesevelam
Niacin (nicotinic acid)	Lowers triglycerides (20–50%)	Raises HDL-cholesterol (15–35%) Reduces LDL-cholesterol (10–20% decrease)	May inhibit mobilization of fatty acids in adipocytes via G-protein-coupled receptor, HM74A, leading to decreased VLDL production by liver	GI disturbances, flushing, chills, pruritus, liver problems, gout, elevated blood sugar	Niacin

Table 17–13 Classification of Total and LDL-Cholesterol in Children: Targeted Fasting Screen in Children > 2 Years of Age with Family History of Dyslipidemia or Premature CHD

Category	Total cholesterol (mg/dL)	LDL-cholesterol (mg/dL)
Acceptable	< 170	< 110
Borderline	171–199	111–129
High	≥ 200	≥ 130

After Kavey, 2003.

Lipids, Lipoproteins and Disease

Lipoprotein and lipid levels are used to predict CHD and form the basis of the NCEP guidelines discussed above. However, for many years, the Fredrickson Classification (alluded to in Table 17–3 and in the chapter overview) was used to characterize lipid disorders (Hansen, 1998). The Fredrickson Classification used electrophoresis and a standing plasma test for CM to correlate clinical disease syndromes with laboratory phenotypes (Fredrickson, 1967). Note that each phenotype is not a specific disease but rather a variety of disorders that affect the same lipoproteins and therefore express the same lipid pattern. Thus treatment is usually the same for all disorders falling within the same phenotype. One limitation of this system is that it does not consider low HDL as a risk factor for CHD. In recent years, the Fredrickson Classification has proved less useful given modern analytical techniques and an evolving understanding of the genetics of these disorders. Nevertheless, the nomenclature for a few pathognomonic syndromes (e.g., Type 1, and Type 3 hyperlipidemias) has remained in use. Some pertinent details of the Fredrickson Classification are presented in Table 17–14.

As our understanding of lipids, lipoprotein metabolism, and genetics has evolved, far more complex systems for describing clinical lipid disorders have been conceived. Presently, there is no ideal scheme to categorize these disorders. They can arise from lifestyle or secondary causes as well as mutations in genes encoding apoliporoteins, apolipoprotein receptors, or enzymes of lipoprotein metabolism. Some genes (e.g., *apoA-I, apoC-III,* and *apoA-IV*) are in close proximity and share similar response elements, allowing a single mutation to alter multiple aspects of lipoprotein metabolism. The following disorders of lipoprotein metabolism are categorized based on laboratory findings. Lifestyle factors affecting lipid profiles and causes of secondary hyperlipidemia are listed in Table 17–15 in association with their most common laboratory presentation. As with the genetic dyslipidemias, these factors can produce overlapping and somewhat variable lipoprotein profiles. In Figures 17–4 and 17–5 some of the disorders described below are incorporated into the schemes of forward and reverse cholesterol transport, so that their etiology and pathogenesis may be more readily understood.

Table 17–14 Pertinent Details of the Fredrickson Classification

Type	Refrigerator test	Gel electrophoresis	Clinical presentation
1	Positive; clear plasma	Normal	Eruptive xanthoma; acute, recurrent pancreatitis in early childhood; lipids improve on low-fat diet
2a	Negative; clear plasma	Increased β band	Xanthelasma, tendon xanthoma; premature coronary disease; autosomal dominant familial inheritance; commonly known as familial hypercholesterolemia
2b	Negative; cloudy plasma	Increased β and pre-β band	Isolated xanthelasma may be present; premature coronary disease; autosomal dominant pattern; affected family members must have varied patterns (e.g., isolated hypertriglyceridemia, isolated hypercholesterolemia or combined hyperlipidemia) to meet diagnostic criteria for familial combined hyperlipidemia
3	Occasional cloudy plasma	Increased pre-β band (called 'broad β' band)	Eruptive xanthoma and palmar xanthoma; premature coronary disease; autosomal recessive pattern; a secondary cause of dyslipidemia, such as hypothyroidism, can unmask type 3, and treatment of the secondary condition can return lipids to normal
4	Negative; cloudy plasma	Increased α-2 band	May or may not be associated with premature coronary disease
5	Positive; cloudy plasma	Increased α-2 band	Eruptive xanthoma; may be associated with pancreatitis; may be associated with premature coronary disease

Table 17–15 Lifestyle Factors and Causes of Secondary Dyslipidemia

Lipoprotein profile	Secondary causes	Lifestyle factors
High cholesterol and high LDL-C with or without low HDL-C	Hypothyroidism and nephrotic syndrome Medications such as thiazide diuretics and steroids Chronic obstructive liver disease	Obesity Excess dietary cholesterol and/or saturated fat ApoE-4 may increase susceptibility
High triglycerides with normal total and LDL-C with or without low HDL-C	Medications such as thiazide diuretics, estrogens, corticosteroids, retinoids, ciclosporin, and beta-blockers (without intrinsic sympathomimetic) Insulin resistance/diabetes Chronic renal failure and nephrotic syndrome	Obesity Physical inactivity Cigarette smoking Excess alcohol intake High carbohydrate diets
High cholesterol and high triglycerides with or without low HDL-C	Medications, notably high-dose steroids or ciclosporin Severe hypothyroidism, diabetes/insulin resistance, and nephrotic syndrome	Obesity
Isolated low HDL-C	Medications such as isotretinoin, probucol, and anabolic steroids, beta-blockers and certain progestogens	Physical inactivity Increased body weight High-carbohydrate, low-fat diets
Isolated high HDL-C	Medications such as phenytoin, phenobarbital, rifampicin, griseofulvin, and estrogens	Alcohol intake

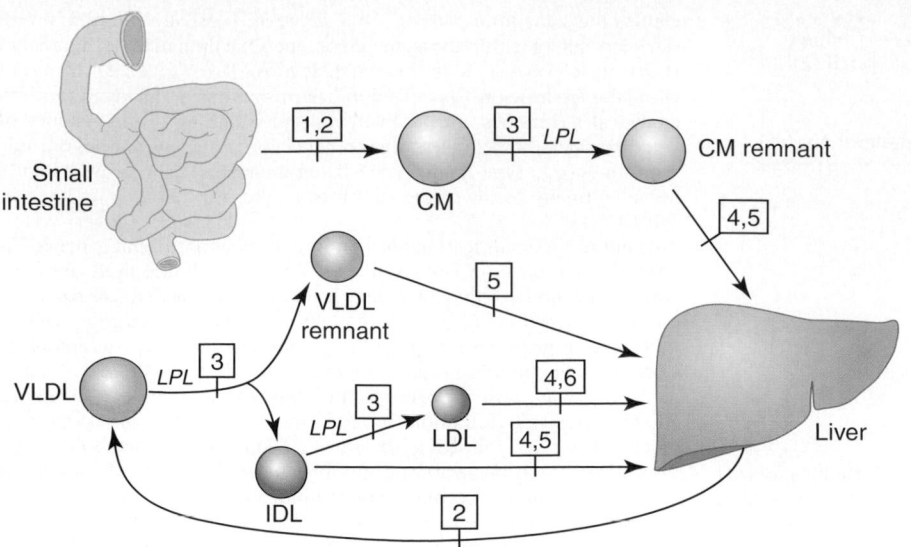

Figure 17-4 Disorders associated with the transport of lipids. LPL = lipoprotein lipase.

1 - Chylomicron retention (Apo B-48 defect)
2 - Hypobetalipoproteinemia / Abetalipoproteinemia
3 - LPL deficiency / Apo C II deficiency
4 - Familial hypercholesterolemia
5 - Dysbetalipoproteinemia (Type III hyperlipoproteinemia, associated with Apo-E-2)
6 - Familial defective Apo B

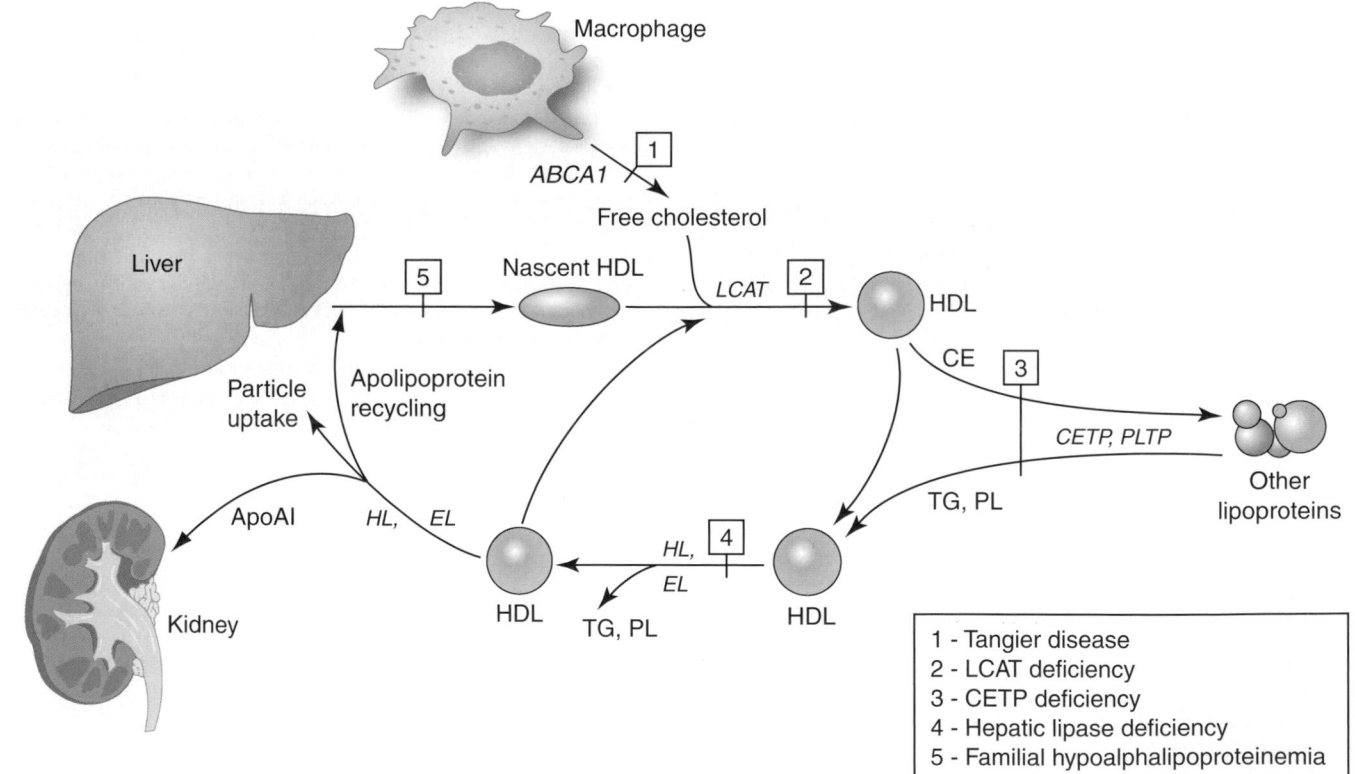

1 - Tangier disease
2 - LCAT deficiency
3 - CETP deficiency
4 - Hepatic lipase deficiency
5 - Familial hypoalphalipoproteinemia

Figure 17–5 Disorders associated with the reverse transport of lipids. ABCA1 = ATP-binding cassette protein A-1; CE = cholesterol ester; CETP = cholesterol ester transfer protein; EL = endothelial lipase; HL = hepatic lipase; LCAT = lecithin : cholesterol acyltransferase; PL = phospholipids; PLTP = phospholipid transfer protein; TG = triglycerides.

High Cholesterol with High LDL-C

These disorders share one feature – hyperbetalipoproteinemia (Fredrickson Type 2A), characterized by elevated LDL-C and normal triglycerides. It is associated with a high cardiac risk that is not surprising given the elevations of LDL, a highly atherogenic particle. This is a commonly encountered laboratory presentation.

Polygenic (Nonfamilial) Hypercholesterolemia is a general term used to describe individuals in whom the cause of hypercholesterolemia is likely multifactorial (Soutar, 1998). While some of the causative factors in this disease are thought to be genetic, before a patient's hypercholesterolemia is labeled 'polygenic', secondary and familial hypercholesterolemia (autosomal dominant) must be ruled out. Approximately 85%

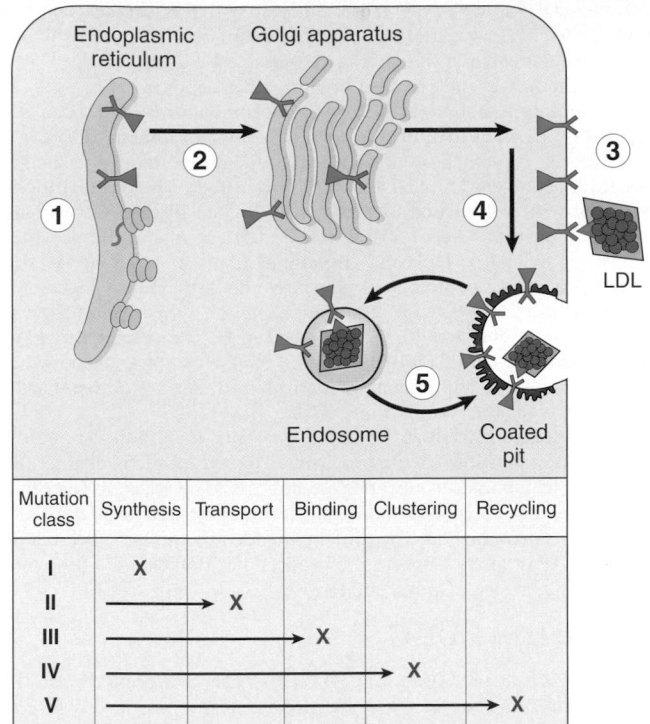

Mutation class	Synthesis	Transport	Binding	Clustering	Recycling
I	X				
II	→	X			
III	→		X		
IV	→			X	
V	→				X

Figure 17–6 Classification of LDL receptor mutations based on abnormal function of the mutant protein. These mutations disrupt the receptor's synthesis in the endoplasmic reticulum, transport to the Golgi complex, binding of apoprotein ligands, clustering in coated pits, and recycling in endosomes. Each class is heterogeneous at the DNA level. (Modified with permission from Hobbs HH, et al: The LDL receptor locus in familial hypercholesterolemia: mutational analysis of a membrane protein. Annu Rev Genet 1990; 24:133–170. copyright 1990 by Annual Reviews.)

of the hypercholesterolemia in the population may fall into this category. Some clinicians use this term to describe patients who develop age-related increases in cholesterol that do not respond to lifestyle modification.

Familial Hypercholesterolemia (FH) is an autosomal dominant disorder caused by one of several mutations in the LDL-receptor gene on chromosome 19. The resulting defective receptors cannot bind or clear LDL from the circulation (Hobbs, 1992). Several hundred mutations have been identified in the *LDL receptor* gene and they affect most aspects of receptor synthesis, transport, and function (Fig. 17–6). This genetic heterogeneity has led to variability in presentation and responsiveness to therapy. Heterozygous FH occurs in 1 in 500 individuals and is associated with premature atherosclerotic disease. Affected heterozygous men usually present in their fourth decade, and women 10–15 years later. Untreated LDL-C levels are typically > 220 mg/dL. Homozygous FH presents in childhood with LDL levels > 400 mg/dL. Vascular deposition of lipid results in premature symptomatic CHD. Additionally, large valvular and supravalvular cholesterol deposits can produce symptomatic aortic stenosis. Other stigmata of the disease include corneal arcus, tendinous xanthomata, and xanthelasma. These stigmata generally develop in early childhood in homozygotes, and by adulthood in heterozygotes. Statins, which inhibit 3-hydroxy-3-methylglutaryl-CoA (HmG-CoA) reductase, may be effective; however, because these drugs may act indirectly by increasing LDL-receptor activity, not all heterozygous patients will normalize their LD-C despite maximum doses of statins. Homozygous patients have two abnormal LDL-receptor genes, making statin drugs ineffective unless combined with apheresis (Ose, 1999).

Familial Defective ApoB is an autosomal dominant disorder of the *apoB* gene on chromosome 2 that interferes with the recognition of apoB-100 by the LDL-receptor (Hansen, 1998). The estimated frequency in the population is 1 in 750. Patients with familial defective apoB have similar physical stigmata to those of FH: tendinous xanthomata, xanthelasma, and premature coronary disease. Untreated LDL-C levels can overlap those seen in FH, but tend to be slightly lower. Statin drugs are effective.

Sitosterolemia is an extremely rare autosomal recessive disorder where phytosterols (plant sterols), are absorbed and accumulate in plasma and peripheral tissues. This disease appears to result from mutations in the *ABCG8* and *ABCG5* genes, both located at chromosome 2p21. Mutations in these genes disrupt the mechanisms by which passively absorbed plant sterols (phytosterols) are pumped back into the intestine and secreted by the liver into the bile. Children present with tendinous xanthomata and normal to high levels of LDL. Premature CHD is present. Cholesterol levels may be normal or elevated. Many common assays do not differentiate between cholesterol and plant sterols, and measurement of plasma phytosterols is necessary to confirm the diagnosis. Treatment consists of restricting dietary phytosterol intake (Patel, 1998).

High Triglycerides with Normal Cholesterol

These disorders are related to elevations of triglyceride-rich particles, namely chylomicrons or VLDL (Fredrickson Types 1 and 4). This commonly encountered laboratory presentation is usually due to hyperprebetalipoproteinemia (VLDL) and may be due to secondary causes such as excess alcohol or high-carbohydrate diet. LDL and LDL-C are typically normal.

Diabetic dyslipidemia consists of atherogenic dyslipidemia (high triglycerides, low HDL and small dense LDL) in persons with type 2 diabetes. Current evidence supports the treatment of LDL-C as the primary target in patients with this disorder. Although cholesterol levels may be within the 'normal' range, treatment is often directed at LDL-C, because diabetes is viewed as a CHD risk equivalent, and thus is associated with a lower than 'normal' target cholesterol value (Table 17–11).

Familial Hypertriglyceridemia occurs along with other lipoprotein abnormalities as part of a number of familial hyperlipidemia syndromes. Isolated hypertriglyceridemia (or Type 4 hyperlipidemia) is a relatively common autosomal dominant disorder, affecting approximately 1 : 300 to 1 : 50 people in the US, depending upon the criteria used for diagnosis. The disorder usually presents in adulthood with fasting triglyceride levels in the 200–500 mg/dL range. The pathophysiology remains elusive, but VLDL triglyceride production is increased in the setting of normal apoB production, resulting in the formation of 'fluffy', triglyceride-rich VLDL particles. Some kindreds have premature CHD; however, it is unclear whether the CHD results from hypertriglyceridemia or from the frequently coexisting exacerbating factors, obesity and insulin resistance (Brunzell, 1983).

Lipoprotein Lipase Deficiency (Hyperlipoproteinemia Type 1 or Hyperchylomicronemia) is a rare, autosomal recessive disorder, which presents in childhood with abdominal pain and pancreatitis. Defective or absent LPL creates an inability to clear chylomicrons, creating the classic 'type 1' chylomicronemia syndrome (Tables 17–3 and 17–14). Fasting triglyceride levels may be > 100 mg/dL, and may rise to > 10 000 mg/dL postprandially. Patients with LPL deficiency do not develop premature CHD, implying that chylomicrons themselves are not atherogenic. Treatment with a low-fat diet to reduce chylomicron input is effective; fat-soluble vitamins should be supplemented and drug therapy can be considered to lower endogenous VLDL production (Brunzell, 1995). Heterozygotes have half-normal LPL activity and occur in the general population at a frequency of 1 in 500. It has been speculated that heterozygous individuals with the defective *LPL* gene constitute a subset of families with familial combined hyperlipidemia (Babirak, 1989).

ApoC-II Deficiency. ApoC-II is an activating cofactor for LPL. Thus, the absence of apoC-II creates a functional LPL deficiency, and presents similarly to LPL deficiency as a rare autosomal recessive form of familial hyperchylomicronemia. The disorder presents in children and young adults as recurrent bouts of abdominal pain and pancreatitis. Several defects in the *apoC-II* gene have been described (Fojo, 1992). Patients can be treated with plasma transfusions during severe hypertriglyceridemia, providing apoC-II, which will activate endogenous LPL.

ApoC-III Excess interferes with the activity of lipoprotein lipase and binds to the carboxy-terminal portion of apolipoprotein B, preventing the binding of lipoproteins to the LDL-receptor. Excess apoC-III, especially within the apoB-containing lipoproteins LDL and VLDL, may be an independent risk factor for CHD. ApoC-III levels can be increased in diabetics, and diabetics with hypertriglyceridemia may have defects in the apoC-III gene (Fredenrich, 1998); however the exact physiologic significance of these mutations has not been elucidated.

High Cholesterol with High Triglycerides

These disorders are related to elevations of LDL and triglycerides (Fredrickson Types 2B and 3). Familial combined hyperlipidemia (2B) is the most common primary hyperlipoproteinemia and presents with a variety of lipoprotein phenotypes within a family. The relatively rare dysbetalipoproteinemia (Type 3) is characterized by an abnormal LDL (IDL) that appears as a broad beta electrophoretic band and distinguishes it from familial combined hyperlipidemia. These disorders are associated with an increased cardiac risk due to the elevated LDL.

Familial Combined Hyperlipidemia (Type 2B) is a relatively common disorder where affected individuals may have simple hypercholesterolemia, simple hypertriglyceridemia, or a mixed defect. Because of the disorder's phenotypic heterogeneity and the lack of a definitive biochemical marker for the disorder, there is considerable overlap and confusion with other forms of hyperlipidemia. The estimated frequency in the population is 1 in 100. Affected families must have more than one pattern of lipid disorder to meet diagnostic criteria for familial combined. The genetic basis is unknown (deGraaf, 1998) and appears to be multifactorial, although inheritance was initially thought to be autosomal codominant. The specific gene or genes explaining the defect have not been fully elucidated.

Dysbetalipoproteinemia (Type 3). ApoE is present on chylomicrons, VLDL, IDL and chylomicron remnants. By binding to the LDL receptor, and probably other receptors, apoE helps to clear these lipoproteins from circulation. There are three common electrophoretic isoforms of apoE, each form attributable to several different genetic mutations. The most common isoform is E-3, followed by E-4 and E-2. ApoE-2 seems to have lower affinity for the LDL receptor, and thus lipoprotein particles accumulate in the blood of patients who are homozygous for E-2. However, while individuals with this genotype are relatively common in the population (1 in 100), the expression of the Type 3 phenotype occurs in only 1 in 10 000 individuals. Thus, the manifestation of the Type 3 hyperlipidemia phenotype is thought to require a second factor in addition to the homozygous E-2 genotype (Mahley, 1995). Secondary factors implicated in the manifestation of disease include obesity, diabetes mellitus, hypothyroidism and medications such as protease inhibitors.

Type 3 hyperlipidemia primarily affects adults, and men more commonly than women. Symptomatic individuals typically have roughly equal elevations of cholesterol and triglycerides and other studies may be needed to distinguish this from familial combined hyperlipidemia. Type 3 has a pathognomonic feature: a broad abnormal band between VLDL and LDL known as 'abnormally migrating beta lipoprotein' or β-VLDL. The cholesterol content in VLDL is also increased, and measurement of the VLDL-C/triglyceride ratio is a useful screen. Normally, the VLDL-C/triglyceride ratio is 0.2; typical Type 3 patients have a ratio > 0.3. Day-to-day variation in lipid levels is more pronounced than usual. Clinical stigmata include palmar xanthoma and tuberoeruptive xanthoma on elbows, knees, and buttocks. Premature atherosclerosis is very prevalent, and unlike familial hypercholesterolemia more often involves abdominal and femoral arteries. The atherosclerosis appears reversible with treatment of the lipid disorder (Kuo, 1988). Patients are responsive to low-fat diets, weight loss, and most classes of lipid-lowering drugs.

Hepatic Lipase Deficiency. Generally resulting from mutations of the *HL* gene, this is a rare familial disorder associated with combined hyperlipidemia, characterized by TC levels of 250–1500 mg/dL and TG levels of 400–8000 mg/dL. Levels of HDL-C are normal or increased. Physical stigmata include palmar and tuberoeruptive xanthoma; the risk of atherosclerosis is thought to be increased. In contrast to Type 3 hyperlipidemia, although β-VLDL is increased, the TC/TG ratio is not increased. The triglyceride content of all lipoproteins is increased three- to fivefold. Families with compound heterozygous mutations have been described (Connelly, 1998).

Isolated Low Total Cholesterol

These uncommon disorders are associated with defective apoB synthesis or metabolism, leading to low or nonexistent levels of apo-B lipoproteins such as CM, VLDL and LDL. Triglycerides and cholesterol are low. Fat-soluble vitamin deficiencies are common. Low-fat diet therapy is required.

Abetalipoproteinemia is a rare, autosomal recessive disorder where apoB is degraded shortly after transcription, resulting in undetectable circulating apoB levels. The premature degradation of apoB is not due to defects in the *apoB* gene or gene product but due to defects in the hepatic microsomal transport protein, which is essential for apoB secretion (Rader, 1993). Neither apoB-48 nor apoB-100 is present in plasma. Patients present in childhood or early adolescence with fat malabsorption, hypolipidemia, retinitis pigmentosa, cerebellar ataxia, and acanthocytosis. Laboratory testing usually shows decreased apoB, triglycerides and TC (typically < 50 mg/dL). Patients develop fat-soluble vitamin deficiencies because of malabsorption of vitamins A, K, and E. Vitamin D does not require chylomicrons for absorption and therefore is typically not deficient. Since both vitamin A and vitamin K have transport systems independent of lipoproteins, clinical deficiency is not as severe as seen with vitamin E, which not only depends upon chylomicrons for absorption but relies upon

VLDL and LDL for delivery to tissues. Children with this disorder respond to a low-fat diet rich in medium-chain fatty acids and supplemented with high-dose fat-soluble vitamins, especially vitamin E. Replacing vitamin E stores improves the retinal and peripheral neuropathic symptoms. Heterozygotes have no symptoms and no evidence of abnormal plasma lipid levels.

Hypobetalipoproteinemia is an autosomal dominant disorder, in some families explained by nonsense or missense mutations in the *apoB* gene leading to very low LDL-C levels (Wu, 1999). The familial form is associated with a decreased risk for cardiovascular disease. Homozygous individuals have TC levels < 50 mg/dL, and present at an early age with fat malabsorption and low plasma cholesterol levels at a young age. They develop progressive neurologic degenerative disease, retinitis pigmentosa, and acanthocytosis, similar to patients with abetalipoproteinemia. Complications from vitamin E deficiency can be prevented by treatment with high-dose vitamin E (100–300 mg/kg/day). Heterozygous individuals have LDL-C levels approximately half that of age- and sex-matched controls, but are otherwise asymptomatic.

Chylomicron Retention Disease presents in childhood with fat malabsorption and low circulating lipids. This syndrome is distinct from abetalipoproteinemia, as only apoB-48 appears to be affected. The genetic abnormality associated with this disorder is associated with the *SARA2* gene on chromosome 5q3. The protein encoded by this gene belongs to a family of GTPases which govern the intracellular trafficking of proteins in protein-coated vesicles (Jones, 2003).

Isolated Low HDL-C

Low HDL levels are associated with CHD, presumably because insufficient HDL is available to participate in reverse cholesterol transport, the process by which cholesterol is eliminated from peripheral tissues.

Familial Hypoalphalipoproteinemia is a common autosomal dominant disorder that occurs in 1 in 400. Affected men have HDL-C levels < 30 mg/dL and women have HDL-C levels < 40 mg/dL. Half of the affected families appear to have hepatic lipase or *apoA-I/C-III/A-IV* gene defects (Breslow, 1995). Mutations in the *ABCA1* gene, the same gene that is mutated in Tangier disease, have also been associated with some cases of hypoalphalipoproteinemia. Premature CHD is typically present.

ApoA-I Deficiency and ApoC-III Deficiency is a rare autosomal recessive condition characterized by a reduction in the formation of HDL. It has been linked to point mutations in the *apoA-I* gene and deletions/gene rearrangements at the *apoA-I/C-III/A-IV* gene locus on the long arm of chromosome 11 (Assman, 1995). HDL-C levels are < 5 mg/dL; both corneal opacification and premature coronary disease are seen.

ApoA-I Variants are rare specific amino acid substitutions in the *apoA-I* gene. They have been shown to increase catabolism of HDL and apoA-I (Breslow, 1995). Homozygous patients generally present with autosomal recessive inheritance of low HDL-C levels (approximately 10 mg/dL), corneal opacifications, xanthomata, and premature coronary disease. Heterozygous individuals may present with low HDL-C. One mutation, *apoA-I-Milano*, shows autosomal dominant inheritance, and is associated with low HDL-C levels but not associated with premature coronary disease (Calabresi, 1997).

Tangier Disease is a rare autosomal recessive disorder characterized by very low cholesterol and elevated triglycerides. In the homozygous state, patients present with low or undetectable HDL in plasma, hepatosplenomegaly, peripheral neuropathy, orange tonsils, and premature coronary disease (Rust, 1999). Recent reports indicate that this disease results from mutations in the *ABCA1* gene. In normal cells, the ABCA1 protein enables cholesterol to exit the cell where it combines with apoA-I to form the HDL. In the absence of ABCA1 activity cholesterol accumulates in cells (Bodzioch, 1999; Rust, 1999). The small amount of HDL that is present in patients with this disorder differs qualitatively from normal HDL. LDL-C is also low; however, the reason for this unique laboratory finding is not fully understood.

Lecithin : Cholesterol Acyltransferase (LCAT) Deficiency occurs in two forms: a classic (or complete) familial LCAT deficiency, and a milder partial deficiency phenotype known as fish-eye disease (Peelman, 1999). Both are very rare, autosomal recessive disorders caused by mutations in the *LCAT* gene. In complete deficiency, HDL-C levels are typically < 10 mg/dL but total cholesterol levels are normal or high. Without LCAT, most cholesterol remains unesterified and HDL synthesis is impeded. Premature CHD has been reported even in cases of partial LCAT deficiency (Kuivenhoven, 1997).

Isolated High HDL-C

Cholesteryl Ester Transfer Protein Gene Defects. HDL is involved in the reverse transport of cholesterol from peripheral tissues to the liver. An important step in this process involves CETP, the plasma protein that facilitates the transfer of cholesteryl esters from HDL to apoB-100-rich proteins (VLDL and LDL) in exchange for triglycerides. CETP deficiency is an autosomal recessive disorder, in which the transfer of cholesterol esters is inhibited. As a result HDL particles are large and laden with cholesterol ester, and apoA-I is increased, as is HDL-C (typically > 100 mg/dL). There is an associated increased risk of CHD (Inazu, 1990). Heterozygotes have moderately increased HDL-C levels. Paradoxically, inhibition of CETP has been proposed as a strategy for therapeutically raising HDL-C levels.

References

Abell LL, Levy BB, Brodie BB, et al: A simplified method for the estimation of total cholesterol in serum and demonstration of its specificity. J Biol Chem 1952; 195:357–366.

Alaupovic P: Apolipoproteins and lipoproteins. Atherosclerosis 1971; 13:141–146.

Albers JJ, Hazzard WR: Immunochemical quantification of human plasma Lp(a) lipoprotein. Lipids 1974; 9:15–26.

Armstrong VW, Walli AK, Seidel D: Isolation, characterization, and uptake in human fibroblasts of an apo(a)-free lipoprotein obtained on reduction of lipoprotein (a)1. J Lipid Res 1985; 26:1314–1323.

Assman G, von Eckardstein A, Brewer HB: Familial high-density lipoprotein deficiency: Tangier's disease. In Scriver CR, Beaudet AL, Sly SW, Valle D (eds): The Metabolic Basis of Inherited Disease, 7th ed. New York, McGraw-Hill, 1995, pp 2053–2072.

Babirak SP, Iverius PH, Fujimoto WY, et al: Detection and characterization of the heterozygote state for lipoprotein lipase deficiency. Arteriosclerosis 1989; 9:326–334.

Bachorik PS: Measurement of low density lipoprotein cholesterol. In Rifai N, Warnick GR, Dominiczak MH (eds): Handbook of Lipoprotein Testing. Washington, DC, AACC Press, 2000.

Bachorik PS, Kwiterovich PO Jr: Apolipoprotein measurements in clinical biochemistry and their utility vis-a-vis conventional assays. Clin Chim Acta 1988; 178:1–34.

Bachorik PS, Wood PDS: Laboratory considerations in the diagnosis and management of hyperlipoproteinemia. In Rifkind BM, Levy RI (eds): Hyperlipidemia: Diagnosis and Therapy. New York, Grune & Stratton, 1977.

Bachorik PS, Rock R, Cloey T, et al: Cholesterol screening: Comparative evaluation of on-site and laboratory-based measurements. Clin Chem 1990; 36:255–260.

Bachorik PS, Virgil DG, Kwiterovich PO: Effect of apolipoprotein E-free high-density lipoproteins on cholesterol metabolism in cultured pig hepatocytes. J Biol Chem 1987; 262:13636–13645.

Bachorik PS, Wood PDS, Albers JJ, et al: Plasma high-density lipoprotein cholesterol concentrations determined after removal of other lipoproteins by heparin/manganese precipitation or by ultracentrifugation. Clin Chem 1976; 22:1828–1834.

Blanche PJ, Gong EL, Forte TM, et al: Characterization of human high-density lipoproteins by gradient gel electrophoresis. Biochim Biophys Acta 1981; 665:408–419.

Bodzioch M, Orso E, Klucken J, et al: The gene encoding ATP-binding cassette transporter 1 is mutated in Tangier disease. Nat Genet 1999; 22:347–351.

Bookstein L, Gidding SS, Donovan M, Smith FA: Day-to-day variability of serum cholesterol, triglyceride and high-density lipoprotein cholesterol levels. Arch Intern Med 1990; 150:1653–1657.

Breslow JL: Familial disorders of high-density lipoprotein metabolism. In Scriver CR, Beaudet AL, et al: (eds): The Metabolic Basis of Inherited Disease, 7th ed. New York, McGraw-Hill, 1995, pp 2031–2052.

Brown MS, Kovanen PT, Goldstein JL: Regulation of plasma cholesterol by lipoprotein receptors. Science 1981; 212:628–635.

Brown SA, Boerwinkle E, Kashanian FK, et al: Variation in concentrations of lipids, lipoprotein lipids, and apolipoproteins A-I and B in plasma from healthy women. Clin Chem 1990; 36:207–210.

Brunzell JD, Albers JJ, Chait AI, et al: Plasma lipoprotein in familial combined hyperlipidaemia and monogenic familial hypertriglyceridaemia. J Lipid Res 1983; 24:147–155.

Brunzell JD: Familial lipoprotein lipase deficiency and other causes of the chylomicronemia syndrome. In Scriver CR, Beaudet AL, Sly WS, Valle D (eds): The Metabolic Basis of Inherited Disease, 7th ed. New York, McGraw-Hill, 1995, pp 1913–1932.

Bucolo G, David H: Quantitative determination of serum triglycerides by the use of enzymes. Clin Chem 1973; 19:476–482.

Burstein M, Legmann P: Lipoprotein precipitation. In Clarkson TB, Kritchevsky D, Pollak OJ (eds): Monographs on Atherosclerosis, Vol II. Basel S, Karger AG, 1982.

Byers SO, Friedman M: Site of origin of plasma triglyceride. Am J Physiol 1960; 198:629–631.

Calabresi L, Franceschini G: High-density lipoprotein and coronary heart disease: Insights from mutations leading to low high-density lipoprotein. Curr Opin Lipidol 1997; 8:219–224.

Cenedella RJ, Crouthamel WG: Intestinal versus hepatic contribution to circulating triglyceride levels. Lipids 1974; 9:35–42.

Cohn JS, McNamara JR, Schaefer EJ: Lipoprotein cholesterol concentrations in plasma of human subjects as measured in the fed and fasted states. Clin Chem 1988; 34:2456–2459.

Connelly PW, Hegele RA: Hepatic lipase deficiency. Crit Rev Clin Lab Sci 1998; 35:547–572.

Deacon AC, Dawson PJG: Enzymic assay of total cholesterol involving chemical or enzymic hydrolysis – a comparison of methods. Clin Chem 1979; 25:976–984.

deGraaf J, Stalenhoef AF: Defects of lipoprotein metabolism in familial combined hyperlipidaemia. Curr Opin Lipidol 1998; 9:189–196.

DeLong DM, DeLong ER, Wood PD, et al: A comparison of methods for the estimation of plasma low- and very low-density lipoprotein cholesterol. The Lipid Research Clinics Prevalence Study. JAMA 1986; 256:2372–2377.

Demacker PNM, Schade RWB, Jansen RTP, et al: Intra-individual variation of serum cholesterol, triglycerides, and high-density lipoprotein cholesterol in normal humans. Artherosclerosis 1982; 45:259–266.

Fless GM, Rolih CQ, Scanu AM: Heterogeneity of human plasma lipoprotein(a). Isolation and characterization of the lipoprotein subspecies and their apoproteins. J Biol Chem 1984; 259:11470–11478.

Fless GM, ZumMallen ME, Scanu AM: Isolation of apolipoprotein(a) from lipoprotein(a). J Lipid Res 1985; 26:1224–1229.

Floren C-H, Albers JJ, Bierman EL: Uptake of Lp(a) lipoprotein by cultured fibroblasts. Biochem Biophys Res Commun 1981; 102:636.

Fojo SS, Brewer HB: Hypertriglyceridaemia due to genetic defects in lipoprotein lipase and apolipoprotein C-II. J Intern Med 1992; 231:669–677.

Fredenrich A: Role of apolipoprotein CIII in triglyceride-rich lipoprotein metabolism. Diabetes Metab 1998; 24:490–495.

Fredrickson DS, Levy RI, Lees RS: Fat transport in lipoproteins – an integrated approach to mechanisms and disorders. N Engl J Med 1967; 276:34–42, 94–103, 148–156, 215–225, 273–281.

Friedewald WT, Levy RI, Fredrickson DS: Estimation of the concentration of low-density lipoprotein cholesterol in plasma without use of the preparative ultracentrifuge. Clin Chem 1972; 18:499–502.

Fruchart JC, Ailhaud G: Apolipoprotein A-containing particles: Physiological role, quantification and clinical significance. Clin Chem 1992; 38:793–797.

Garber AJ: The metabolic syndrome. Med Clin North Am 2004; 88(4):837–846.

Gaubatz JW, Heideman C, Gotto AM Jr, et al: Human plasma lipoprotein(a). Structural properties. J Biol Chem 1983; 258:4582–4589.

Glass C, Pittman RC, Weinstein DB, et al: Dissociation of tissue uptake of cholesterol ester from that of apoprotein A-I of rat plasma high-density lipoprotein: Selective delivery of cholesterol ester to liver, adrenal and gonad. Proc Natl Acad Sci USA 1983; 80:5435–5439.

Gotto AM Jr, Pownall HJ, Havel RJ: Introduction to the plasma lipoproteins. Meth Enzymol 1986; 128:3–41.

Gotto AM, Whitney E, Stein EA, et al: The relation between baseline and on-treatment lipid parameters and first acute major coronary events in the Air Force/Texas Coronary Artery Prevention Study (AFCAPS/TEXCAPS). Circulation 2000; 101:477–484.

Green PHR, Glickman RM: Intestinal lipoprotein metabolism. J Lipid Res 1981; 22:1153–1173.

Gries A, Fievet C, Marcovina S, et al: Interaction of LDL, Lp(a), and reduced Lp(a) with monoclonal antibodies against apoB. J Lipid Res 1988; 29:1–8.

Grundy SM, Cleeman JI, Merz CN, et al: Coordinating Committee of the National Cholesterol Education Program. Implications of recent clinical trials for the National Cholesterol Education Program Adult Treatment Panel III Guidelines. J Am Coll Cardiol 2004; 4:44(3):720–732.

Hansen PS: Familial defective apolipoprotein B-100. Danish Med Bull 1998; 45:370–382.

Havel RJ: Lipoprotein biosynthesis and metabolism. Ann NY Acad Sci 1980; 348:16–29.

Hobbs HH, Brown MS, Goldstein JL: Molecular genetics of the LDL-receptor gene in familial hypercholesterolemia. Hum Mutation 1992; I:445–466.

Inazu A, Brown ML, Hesler CB, et al: Increased high-density lipoprotein levels caused by a common cholesteryl-ester transfer protein gene mutation. N Engl J Med 1990; 323:1234–1238.

Jones B, Jones EL, Bonney SA, et al: Mutations in a Sar1 GTPase of COPII vesicles are associated with lipid absorption disorders. Nat Genet 2003; 34:29–31.

Kafonek SD, Derby CA, Bachorik PS: Biological variability of lipoproteins and apolipoteins in patients referred to a lipid clinic. Clin Chem 1992; 38:864–872.

Kafonek SD, Donovan L, Lovejoy KL, Bachorik PS: Biological variation of lipids and lipoproteins in fingerstick blood. Clin Chem 1996; 42:2002–2007.

Kavey RE, Daniels SR, Lauer RM, et al; American Heart Association: American Heart Association guidelines for primary prevention of atherosclerotic cardiovascular disease beginning in childhood. J Ped 2003; 142(4):368–372.

Kessler G, Lederer H: Fluorometric measurement of triglycerides. In Skeggs LT (ed): Automation in Clinical Chemistry, Technicon Symposia. New York, Mediad, 1966.

Koch TR, Mehta U, Lee H, et al: Bias and precision of cholesterol analysis of physician's office analyzers. Clin Chem 1987; 33:2262–2267.

Krauss RM: Relationship of intermediate and low-density lipoprotein subspecies to risk of coronary heart disease. Am Heart J 1987; 113:578–582.

Krauss RM, Blanche PJ: Detection and quantitation of LDL subfractions. Curr Opin Lipidol 1992; 3:377–383.

Kuivenhoven JA, Pritchard H, Hill J, et al: The molecular pathology of lecithin:cholesterol acyltransferase (LCAT) deficiency syndromes. J Lipid Res 1997; 38:191–205.

Kuo PT, Wilson AC, Kostis JB: Treatment of type III hyperlipoproteinemia with gemfibrozil to retard progression of coronary artery disease. Am Heart J 1988; 116:85–90.

Laboratory Methods Committee of the Lipid Research Clinics Program: Cholesterol and triglyceride concentrations in serum/plasma pairs. Clin Chem 1977; 23:60.

Law WT, Doshi S, McGeehan J, et al: Whole-blood testing for total cholesterol by a self-metering, self-timing disposable device with built in quality control. Clin Chem 1997; 43:384–389.

Lipid Research Clinics Program: Manual of laboratory operations. Lipid and lipoprotein analysis. U.S. Department of Health and Human Services, Publication No. (NIH) 75. Revised September, 1982.

Lopes-Virella MFL, Virella G, Evangs G, et al: Immunocephelometric assay of human apolipoprotein A. J Clin Chem 1980; 26:1205–1208.

Lunz ME, Castleberry BM, James K, et al: The impact of the quality of laboratory staff on the accuracy of laboratory results. J Am Med Assoc 1987; 258:361–363.

MacKenzie SL, Sundaram GS, Sodhi HS: Heterogeneity of human high-density lipoprotein (HDL₂). Clin Chim Acta 1973; 43:223–229.

Mahley RW, Rall SC: Type III hyperlipoproteinaemia (dysbetalipoproteinemia): The role of apolipoprotein E in normal and abnormal lipoprotein metabolism. In Scriver CR, Beaudet AL, Sly WS, Valle D (eds): The Metabolic Basis of Inherited Disease, 7th ed, New York, McGraw-Hill, 1995, pp 1953–1986.

Miller M, Bachorik PS, Cloey TA: Normal variation of plasma lipoproteins: Postural effects on plasma concentrations of lipids, lipoproteins and apolipoproteins. Clin Chem 1992; 38:569–574.

Miller WG, Waymack PP, Anderson FP, et al: Performance of four homogenous direct methods for LDL-cholesterol. Clin Chem 2002; 48(3):489–498.

Myers GL, Cooper GR, Winn CL, et al: The Centers for Disease Control–National Heart, Lung and Blood Institute Lipid Standardization Program. An approach to accurate and precise lipid measurements. Clin Lab Med 1989; 9:105–135.

Naito HK, David JA: Laboratory considerations: Determination of cholesterol, triglyceride, phospholipid, and other lipids in blood and tissues. In Story JA (ed): Lipid Research Methodology. New York, Alan R Liss, 1984.

Naito HK, Kwak YS: The evaluation of a new high-density lipoprotein cholesterol (HDL-C) technology; selective separation of lipoproteins by magnetic separation. Clin Chem 1995; 41:S135.

National Cholesterol Education Program (NCEP): Highlights of the report of the Expert Panel on Blood Cholesterol Levels in Children and Adolescents. Pediatrics 1992; 89:495–501.

National Cholesterol Education Program Working Group on Lipoprotein Measurement: Recommendations on lipoprotein measurement. Publication No. 95-3044, Bethesda, MD, NIH, 1995.

National Cholesterol Education Program Expert Panel: Third Report of the National Cholesterol Education Program (NCEP) expert panel on detection, evaluation, and treatment of high blood cholesterol in adults (Adult Treatment Panel III). Final report. Circulation 2002; 106:3143–3421.
A comprehensive monograph that includes the latest recommendations for screening, evaluating and treating hyperlipidemia.

Nauck M, Warnick GR, Rifai N: Methods for measurement of LDL-cholesterol: a critical assessment of direct measurement by homogenous assays versus calculation. Clin Chem 2002; 48(2):236–254.
A comprehensive review of current LDL-C methods including the advantages and disadvantages of each, performance characteristics and an explanation of the chemistry and technology upon which the assay is based.

Oppenheimer MJ, Oram JF, Bierman EL: Down regulation of high-density lipoprotein receptor activity of cultured fibroblasts by platelet-derived growth factor. Arteriosclerosis 1987; 7:325–332.

Oram JF: Receptor-mediated transport of cholesterol between cultured cells and high-density lipoproteins. Meth Enzymol 1986; 129:645–659.

Ose L: An update on familial hypercholesterolaemia. Ann Med 1999; 31(Suppl 1):13–18.

Otvos J, Jeyarajah E, Bennett DW, Krauss RM: Development of a proton nuclear magnetic resonance spectroscopic method for determining plasma lipoprotein concentrations and subspecies distributions from a single, rapid measurement. Clin Chem 1992; 39:1632–1638.

Otvos JD: Handbook of Lipoprotein Testing, 2nd ed. Washington, DC, AACC Press, 2000, Ch 31 (Measurement of lipoprotein subclass profiles by nuclear magnetic resonance spectroscopy), pp 609–623.

Patel SB, Salen G, Hidaka H, et al: Mapping a gene involved in regulating dietary cholesterol absorption. The sitosterolemia locus is found at chromosome 2p21. J Clin Invest 1998; 102:1041–1044.

Peelman F, Verschelde JL, Vanloo B, et al: Effects of natural mutations in lecithin:cholesterol acyltransferase on the enzyme structure and activity. J Lipid Res 1999; 40:59–69.

Pesce MA, Bodourian SH: Interference with the enzymatic measurement of cholesterol in serum by use of five reagent kits. Clin Chem 1977; 23:757–760.

Rader DJ, Brewer HB: Abetalipoproteinemia. New insights into lipoprotein assembly and vitamin E metabolism from a rare genetic disease. JAMA 1993; 270:865–869.

Risser TR, Reaven GM, Reaven EP: Intestinal contribution to secretion of very low-density lipoproteins into plasma. Am J Physiol 1978; 234:E277–E281.

Robinson D, Bevan EA, Hinohara S, Takahashi T: Seasonal variation in serum cholesterol levels – evidence from the UK and Japan. Atherosclerosis 1992; 95:15–24.

Rust S, Rosier M, Funke H, et al: Tangier disease is caused by mutations in the gene encoding ATP-binding cassette transporter 1. Nat Genet 1999; 22:352–355.

Scanu AM: Lipoprotein(a). A potential bridge between the fields of atherosclerosis and thrombosis. Arch Pathol Lab Med 1988; 112:1045–1047.

Scanu AM, Byrne RE, Mihovilovic M: Functional roles of plasma high-density lipoproteins. CRC Crit Rev Biochem 1982; 13:109–140.

Sniderman AD, Blank D, Zakariana R, et al: Triglycerides and small dense LDL: the twin Achilles heels of the Friedewald formula. Clinical Biochemistry 2003; 36:499–504.

Soutar AK: Update on low-density lipoprotein receptor mutations. Curr Opin Lipidol 1998; 9:141–147.

Stein O, Stein Y, Coetzee GA, Van der Westhuyzen DR: Metabolic fate of low-density lipoprotein and high-density lipoprotein labeled with an ether analogue of cholesteryl ester. Klin Wochenschr 1984; 62:1151–1156.

Sugiuchi H, Irie T, Uji Y, et al: Homogenous assay for measuring low-density lipoprotein cholesterol in serum with triblock co-polymer and α-cyclodextrin sulfate. Clin Chem 1998; 44:522–531.

Sundaram GS, MacKenzie SL, Sodhi HS: Preparative isoelectric focusing of human serum high-density lipoprotein (HPL₃). Biochem Biophys Acta 1974; 337:196–203.

Tall AR: Plasma high-density lipoproteins: Metabolism and relationship to atherogenesis. J Clin Invest 1990; 86:379–384.

von Eckardstein A, Huang Y, Assmann G: Physiological role and clinical relevance of high-density lipoprotein subclasses. Curr Opin Lipidol 1994; 5:404–416.

Walldius G, Jungner I: Apolipoprotein B and apolipoprotein A-I: risk indicators of coronary heart disease and targets for lipid-modifying therapy. J Int Med 2004; 255:188–205.

Warnick GR, Cheung MC, Albers JJ: Comparison of current methods for high-density lipoprotein cholesterol quantitation. Clin Chem 1979; 25:596–604.

Warnick GR, Nauck M, Rifai N: Evolution of methods for measurement of HDL-cholesterol: from ultracentrifugation to homogeneous assays. Clin Chem 2001; 47:1579–1596.
A comprehensive review of all methods used to measure HDL-C with particular emphasis on the new homogeneous assays. It discusses the pros and cons of each assay, accuracy and precision, clinical usefulness as well as the chemistry or technology upon which each is based.

Wilson PW, D'Agostino RB, Levy D, et al: Prediction of coronary heart disease using risk factor categories. Circulation 1998; 97: 1837–1847.

Witte DL, Brown LF, Feld RD: Effects of bilirubin on the detection of hydrogen peroxide by use of peroxidase. Clin Chem 1978; 24:1778–1782.

Wood PD, Bachorik PS, Albers JJ, et al: An investigation of the effects of sample aging on total cholesterol values determined by the automated ferric chloride-sulfuric acid and Liebermann–Burchard procedures. Clin Chem 1980; 26:592–597.

Wu J, Kim J, Li Q, et al: Known mutations of apoB account for only a small minority of hypobetalipoproteinemia. J Lipid Res 1999; 40:955–959.

CHAPTER: **17** Lipids and Dyslipoproteinemia

CHAPTER 18

Evaluation of Cardiac Injury and Function

Jay L. Bock MD PhD

KEY POINTS

• The most important disease affecting the heart is coronary heart disease (CHD), which can lead to an acute blockage of coronary blood flow known as an acute coronary syndrome (ACS). ACS with frank necrosis of any amount of myocardium is known as myocardial infarction (MI).

• The primary tests for diagnosing ACS are electrocardiography (ECG) and laboratory measurement of cardiac markers. Cardiac markers are proteins released into the circulation from damaged heart muscle. The most important cardiac marker today is cardiac troponin (cTn), which derives only from heart muscle.

• Troponin is a complex of three proteins, two of which are suitable as specific cardiac marker tests: cTnI and cTnT. These two proteins have different properties, but their clinical applications are similar. Clinically, MI is now essentially defined as an ACS that causes release of troponin.

• There is a delay of a few hours following MI before cTn is detected in the circulation; it peaks in about 24 h and then declines over several days. Myoglobin is a marker that appears in the circulation faster than cTn, but it is also present in skeletal muscle.

• Patients presenting to an emergency department with symptoms suggesting ACS must be processed rapidly and precisely to provide life-saving interventions as needed, yet avoid wasting resources. Rapid measurements of cTn, and possibly other laboratory markers, play a critical role.

• The clinical laboratory also measures risk factors associated with the development and progression of CHD. Significant laboratory markers of risk include lipids (cholesterol, triglycerides, and specific lipoprotein fractions – see Ch. 17), homocysteine (Hcy), and C-reactive protein (CRP). Hcy is an amino acid that exacerbates thrombosis. CRP is an inflammatory marker that appears to reflect the severity of CHD and may contribute to its pathogenesis.

• CHD and other heart diseases can impair the heart's ability to pump blood, causing the clinical syndrome of heart failure (HF). B-type natriuretic peptide (BNP), a 32-amino-acid peptide secreted by the cardiac ventricles in response to wall-stretch stimuli, is a marker of the presence and severity of HF. BNP testing is particularly useful for aiding the differential diagnosis of patients who present to an emergency department with shortness of breath.

Overview

Heart disease is an affliction intimately tied to high technology. Technology has had a causal role, partly by allowing people to live longer, and partly by enabling a sedentary and overly consumptive lifestyle. During the 20th century heart disease rose from obscurity to become the leading cause of morbidity and mortality in developed nations (see Table 18–1). Diagnosis and treatment of heart disease also depends heavily on advanced technology, including electrophysiologic, imaging, catheterization, surgical, and clinical laboratory modalities. The following major laboratory applications will be the subject of this chapter:

1. Measurement of proteins specific to cardiac myocytes indicate recent damage to cardiac muscle. These tests are used mainly for the diagnosis and management of ischemic events (acute coronary syndromes).
2. Measurement of substances that are damaging to the coronary arteries, or at least have proven association with coronary heart disease (CHD), are used to assess risk and select appropriate preventive measures. The most important laboratory risk factors are lipids, which are discussed in Chapter 17. Of the many other substances that could be discussed, this chapter will focus on two: homocysteine and C-reactive protein.
3. Most recently, measurement of natriuretic peptides released from myocardium have been used in the diagnosis and management of congestive heart failure.

Background

It is ironic that for the heart, an organ that pumps several liters of blood each minute, the most important disease process is *ischemia* – the lack of an adequate blood supply. This is because heart muscle depends on constant nutrition through a system of coronary arteries, which are highly vulnerable to the process of *atherosclerosis*. Atherosclerosis is a chronic process involving damage to endothelium and the build-up of vessel-occluding lesions called *plaque*. In the early stages of atherosclerosis, as coronary blood flow is gradually reduced, there are typically no symptoms or laboratory evidence of cardiac injury. Once the diameter of a coronary artery is reduced to less than 10–20% of its original size, chest pain (angina pectoris) often develops when demand for oxygen increases, particularly during exercise (exertional angina). More rapid reduction in blood flow can occur when plaque stimulates formation of a thrombus in a coronary artery, leading to an *acute coronary syndrome* (ACS). When a thrombus completely cuts off blood flow, the supplied muscle will develop irreversible ischemic damage, and the syndrome is a *myocardial infarction* (MI). When the blockage is not complete, irreversible muscle damage may be avoided, but the patient will experience severe angina, even at rest, and this syndrome is known as *unstable angina* (UA). The broad spectrum of heart disease resulting from impaired coronary blood flow is referred to as *coronary heart disease* (CHD).

MIs can be categorized by whether they are accompanied by characteristic changes on the electrocardiogram (ECG). The more severe MIs, generally involving transmural damage to myocardium, typically cause the rapid appearance of ST-segment elevations and the later appearance of Q waves. These are categorized as ST-elevation MIs (STEMIs). MIs without

Table 18–1 Heart Disease Statistics for the US

- 1 in 5 males and females has some form of cardiovascular diseases (including hypertension)
- 13 200 000 Americans have a history of CHD – of these, 7 800 000 have had an MI and 6 800 000 have had angina pectoris
- 5 000 000 Americans have HF
- 5 000 000 Americans have experienced a stroke
- Cardiovascular disease accounts for 38.5% of all deaths, almost 1 000 000 deaths per year. It claims more lives each year than the next five leading causes of death combined, which are cancer, chronic lower respiratory diseases, accidents, diabetes mellitus, and influenza and pneumonia
- The estimated annual direct and indirect cost of cardiovascular disease is 368 billion dollars
- Although some trends in cardiovascular disease are favorable, other factors, including an alarming increase in the prevalence of obesity and type 2 diabetes, will fuel the epidemic for many years to come

Source: American Heart Association, 2003.

Table 18–2 Clinical (nonlaboratory) risk factors for CHD

- Cigarette smoking (any smoking in the past month)
- Hypertension (blood pressure > 140/90 mmHg or on antihypertensive medication)
- Family history of premature CHD (CHD in male first-degree relative < 55 years, or in female first-degree relative < 65 years)
- Age (men > 45 years; women > 55 years)
- Obesity
- Diabetes mellitus
- Sedentary lifestyle

The definitions given in parentheses are used, along with the HDL-cholesterol level, in a risk estimate formula for targeting a desirable LDL-cholesterol level (National Cholesterol Education Program Expert Panel, 2002) – see Chapter 17.

these changes (non-Q wave MIs or non-ST-elevation MIs [NSTEMIs]) typically involve lesser degrees of muscle damage, possibly only to the subendocardium, but any ACS event carries serious risk for possibly lethal arrhythmias and for future events. Damage to a sizable quantity of cardiac muscle carries the additional risk of compromising the heart's ability to pump blood, leading to the clinical syndrome of *heart failure* (HF), discussed further below.

Cardiac muscle is relatively resistant to ischemia, compared to other cells such as neurons and renal tubular epithelial cells, in which even short duration of ischemia can lead to cell death. In experimental animals, complete blockage of blood flow to an area of the heart does not cause cell death (MI) until at least 20–30 minutes of ischemia; if blood flow had been previously restricted, cell death often is delayed for up to an hour. With complete coronary artery occlusion, there is typically a gradient of ischemia, with oxygen deprivation worst in areas receiving blood flow last (the subendocardial portions of the ventricular wall). Cells near the border between ischemic myocardium and normally perfused myocardium may receive some oxygen supply, and thus may remain viable for several hours. The longer the duration of ischemia, the higher the percentage of cells at risk that will die; 3 hours of ischemia increases cell death to 80% of cells at risk, while 6 hours of ischemia causes death of almost 100% of cells at risk. For this reason, early recognition of persistent ischemia and intervention to restore blood flow are needed to minimize cell death.

The pathobiology of atherosclerosis and ACS remains incompletely understood. Formation of obstructive plaques probably begins with nonobstructive lesions known as *fatty streaks*, which have been observed in the coronary arteries of young individuals dying in combat or accidents (Enos, 1953; Strong, 1999; Berenson, 1992). The lesions are likely triggered by uptake of oxidized low-density lipoprotein (LDL) particles by macrophages, which then invade the coronary endothelium (Ross, 1993; Witztum, 1994; Adams, 2000; Zaman, 2000). Inflammatory cells and mediators play a role in the evolution of the lesion, which eventually becomes a structure containing a lipid core (mainly cholesterol esters) surrounded by numerous macrophages and other inflammatory cells, and covered with a cap of endothelialized connective tissue (Weissberg, 2000; Davies, 2000). Advanced lesions also contain new blood vessels and calcium deposits. Plaques in coronary arteries were formerly regarded as passive, and physiologically irreversible, barriers to blood flow. In recent years their more dynamic role in ACS has been appreciated. A balance of inflammatory mediators, shear forces, and other factors can cause the fibrous cap of the plaque to strengthen or weaken. Erosion of the cap can expose thrombogenic material, leading to deposition of platelets and eventually enlargement of the lesion. More ominous is actual rupture of the plaque, causing thrombosis with sufficient occlusion to result in ACS. A major contributor to this concept of plaque *vulnerability* has been the finding that the cholesterol-lowering statin drugs can diminish the risk of ACS substantially without causing appreciable diminution of the degree of stenosis caused by atherosclerotic lesions (see Ch. 17).

The extent of atherosclerotic disease in the coronary circulation can be identified by coronary angiography and other tests. Blood tests that reflect the actual extent of atherosclerotic disease may be available in the future; for example, measurement of microparticles shed by plaque has been proposed (Heloire, 2003). At present, however, risk of CHD in individuals

is mainly assessed indirectly through the measurement of *risk factors*, each of which appears to play a contributory but not necessarily definitive role (Stampfer, 2004). Several clinical parameters, summarized in Table 18–2, have been established as important risk factors. Additionally, hundreds of laboratory tests have been studied in relation to CHD risk. Of these, several lipid tests, discussed in Chapter 17 have the best-established role in risk assessment. Two newer markers, homocysteine and C-reactive protein, are discussed below.

Next to CHD, and often as a direct consequence of it, the most important heart disease is HF. HF is a clinical syndrome, with prominent symptoms including fatigue, shortness of breath, and edema, resulting from impairment in the heart's pumping ability. It is most commonly caused by damage to the myocardium, as from CHD. Due to the high incidence of CHD and the improving survival of people who suffer from it, HF is a rapidly increasing problem, especially in the elderly. HF can also be caused by mechanical problems, such as valvular disease, which interfere with the pump function of the heart. When the problem relates to filling of the left ventricle during diastole, it is often referred to as diastolic HF.

Diagnosing HF, and monitoring its progression, can be difficult. A defining parameter for systolic HF is the left ventricular ejection fraction (LVEF), which is the fraction of the left ventricle's blood volume that is ejected during systole. It can be measured by echocardiography or radionuclide ventriculography. Symptomatic HF is usually associated with LVEF < 40%, but correlation between LVEF and subjective symptoms is poor. Until recently, no clinical laboratory test had specific utility in disclosing the presence or severity of HF. That situation has changed with the introduction of testing for cardiac natriuretic peptides, discussed below.

Of the myriad other diseases that can affect the heart, brief mention should be made of genetic diseases that, though relatively uncommon, have disproportionate importance because of their potentially life-threatening consequences. The syndrome of hypertrophic cardiomyopathy, described more than a century ago, occurs in 1 in 500 individuals and is the most common cause of sudden death in the young (Taylor, 2004). Over 240 mutations have been tied to this disorder (Gomes, 2004); they affect various proteins of the contractile apparatus, including the troponins, actin, and myosin, and are generally inherited in autosomal dominant fashion. The long-QT syndrome, an abnormality in ventricular repolarization that can cause sudden death, has several distinct variants caused by both autosomal dominant and recessive mutations in ion channels and other proteins (Priori, 2004). Application of molecular diagnostics to these disorders is in its infancy, but evidence already exists that identifying the genotype is not only useful for confirming the diagnosis but may play an important role in guiding specific therapy.

Markers of Myocardial Damage

Historical Development

Biochemical markers of myocardial damage were essentially a serendipitous discovery in the early 1950s, when LaDue and coworkers were investigating the transaminase enzymes then known as GOT (glutamate-oxaloacetate transaminase; now aspartate transaminase, AST) and GPT (glutamate-pyruvate transaminase; now alanine transaminase, ALT) (LaDue, 1954). Surveying a variety of hospital patients, the investigators noted that serum transaminase levels rose sharply after an MI, and thus was born the era of 'cardiac enzymes.' The simple underlying principle, as with other organ markers, is that cell death will cause release of cellular proteins into the circulation. (A more difficult question, still not fully resolved, is the extent to which *reversible* cell damage can cause protein leakage.)

Transaminases have not endured as cardiac markers because of their abundance in liver, skeletal muscle, and other tissues. They were soon superseded for cardiac diagnosis by two other enzymes, lactate dehydrogenase (LD) and creatine kinase (CK) (Hess, 1963; Roe, 1977; Johnston, 1982; Wolf, 1989; Lee, 1986). LD is a zinc-containing enzyme that is part of the glycolytic pathway and found in virtually all cells in the body. CK transfers high energy phosphate between creatine and ADP, mainly in muscle cells, but it is found in all types of muscle and also in brain and other tissues. With both of these enzymes, improved cardiac specificity was achieved through separation of *isoenzymes*. LD is a tetramer of two active subunits, H (for heart) and M (for muscle) with a molecular weight of 134 kDa. Combinations of subunits produce five isoenzymes ranging from LD_1 (HHHH) to LD_5 (MMMM); the intermediate isoenzymes contain differing combinations of H and M subunits (LD_2, HHHM; LD_3, HHMM; LD_4, HMMM). As the subunit names imply, LD_1 is relatively abundant in cardiac muscle, whereas LD_5 is more abundant in skeletal muscle. Patients with MI exhibit a characteristic pattern of 'flipped' LD, where the normal finding $LD_2 > LD_1$ is reversed.

CK is predominantly found as a dimer of catalytic subunits, each with a molecular weight of about 40 kDa; the two subunits are termed M (for muscle) and B (for brain). The three resulting isoenzymes are CK_1 (BB), CK_2 (MB), and CK_3 (MM). CK is found in small amounts throughout the body, but is in high concentrations only in muscle and brain, although CK from brain virtually never crosses the blood–brain barrier to reach plasma. In skeletal muscle, CK-MB comprises 0–1% of the total CK in type 1 fibers and 2–6% of CK in type 2 fibers. During regeneration of skeletal muscle, increased amounts of CK-MB are produced relative to CK-MM, similar to the pattern seen in fetal muscle (Tzvetanova, 1971). In the normal heart, an average of 15–20% of the CK is CK-MB; its distribution is not uniform, with CK-MB percentage greater in the right heart than in the left heart (Marmor, 1980). A single study, however, suggests that CK-MB is not found in normal myocardium, only appearing when the muscle becomes diseased (Ingwall, 1985). CK-BB is the dominant isoenzyme of CK found in brain and in smooth muscle.

In the past, clinical laboratories would commonly analyze both CK and LD isoenzymes to improve overall diagnostic performance, especially since the two enzymes exhibit different kinetics, with changes in LD observable for a much longer time than changes in CK. The isoenzyme analyses were relatively lengthy and tedious, generally involving electrophoretic separation, followed by development of color or fluorescence using suitable substrates, followed by densitometric scanning. Hence these tests could only be performed about once per day, a situation that was acceptable at a time when 'rule out MI' patients were generally admitted to hospital for at least a several-day period of observation.

CK-MB Mass Assay

A major step forward for cardiac diagnosis was the development of *immunometric* assays for proteins using monoclonal antibody technology. This technology allowed introduction of the so-called CK-MB 'mass assay,' where the protein is simply measured as an antigen, without depending on its enzymatic properties (el Allaf, 1986; Mair, 1991). CK-MB mass assay is now widely employed, and can be performed rapidly, usually in well under 1 hour, on a variety of automated platforms. The mass assay also offers better analytical performance, especially in terms of low-end accuracy, than traditional isoenzyme separation. However, the assay still suffers from the fundamental limitation that CK-MB is not specific for myocardium. Interpretation is aided by knowledge of the total CK, which, for reasons of cost, is still measured as enzyme activity. The ratio of (CK-MB mass) to (total CK activity) is often called the 'relative index' (RI) or 'relative percent,' since it is an awkward ratio of different types of measurements in different units. A higher RI is more suggestive of cardiac damage. To be suggestive of MI, a CK-MB mass result should exceed a reference limit for both absolute quantity (typically about 5 ng/mL) and RI (typically about 2%).

Cardiac Troponin

With the advent of immunometric assays it became possible for the first time to look for organ-specific protein markers having no measurable enzymatic activity. This led to the introduction of assays for cardiac troponin (cTn), now the most important laboratory test for cardiac diagnosis.

Troponin (Tn) is a regulatory complex of three proteins that resides at regular intervals in the thin filament of striated muscle. The three

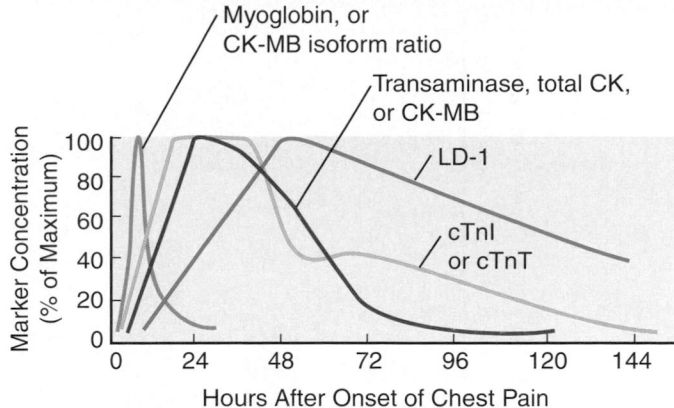

Figure 18–1 Schematic depiction of the kinetics of several cardiac markers following an MI.

individual proteins are: TnT (tropomyosin-binding subunit, 37 kDa), TnI (inhibitory subunit, 24 kDa), and TnC (calcium-binding subunit, 18 kDa). The Ca^{2+} trigger for muscle contraction is transmitted via the Tn complex, which causes a conformational change in another thin-filament component, tropomyosin, then allowing interaction between actin and myosin to proceed. In contrast to most other markers, the forms of Tn found in skeletal and cardiac muscle differ. For TnC, the forms found in type 2 fibers and cardiac muscle are identical, obviating its use as a differential marker. TnI has a cardiospecific form (cTnI) as well as distinct forms in types 1 and 2 skeletal muscle fibers, each coded by a separate gene. Presence of the cardiospecific form in tissue other than cardiac muscle has never been documented (Bodor, 1995). TnT also has distinct forms in myocardium (cTnT), fast-twitch, and slow-twitch skeletal muscle, but here the situation is more complicated, because cTnT has been detected in fetal skeletal muscle and diseased skeletal muscle. However, post-translational modifications cause detectable differences between cTnT produced in myocardium and cTnT produced in diseased skeletal muscle (Apple, 1998, 1999). Hence, an immunochemical test for cTnT with carefully chosen antibodies, such as the current generation (but not earlier generations) of commercial cTnT assay, should also have myocardial specificity approaching 100%. Nevertheless, small increases in circulating cTnT, even with newer assays, have been reported in patients with muscular dystrophy and renal failure who do not have any other evidence for cardiac disease (Muller-Bardorff, 1997; Hammerer-Lercher, 2001a).

Within the cardiac myocytes, cTnT and cTnI are predominantly bound to muscle fibers, as described above, and the bound form is released slowly over the course of 1–2 weeks following myocardial infarction. Thus, although cTnI and cTnT are relatively small proteins that are rapidly cleared, their plasma levels fall slowly after cardiac injury. A small fraction of cTn in the myocardial cell is free within the cytoplasm; this averages 6% for cTnT and slightly lower (2–5%) for cTnI. The free fraction allows early leakage from injured myocardial cells and detection in a time frame similar to that of CK-MB, with cTn reaching a peak at about 24 h following MI. Due to the slow release of the fiber-bound cTn, the rapid decline in circulating cTn right after its peak is typically followed by a plateau and even a small secondary increase. It is important that such an increase *not* be interpreted as evidence of reinfarction. Circulating cTn declines to baseline levels in about 5–10 days, depending on infarct size (Mair, 1997) (Fig. 18–1).

In contrast to other cardiac markers, cTnT and cTnI are nearly absent from normal serum. cTn rarely exceeds 0.1 ng/mL in healthy individuals. However, it is important to note that cTn elevation, though presumably indicating cardiac myocyte damage, need not be caused by *ischemic* damage. Elevations, though generally much smaller than those seen with MI, have been observed with pericarditis, myocarditis, pulmonary embolism, renal failure, sepsis, and other critical illness (Roongsritong, 2004). Small measured elevations in cTn may also be analytical artifacts (see Assay Procedures below).

The high sensitivity and specificity of cTn has led to rethinking of the clinical definition of MI. Previous criteria were those of the World Health Organization, which were mainly intended for epidemiologic purposes (Joint Task Force, 1979). The somewhat vague definition was based on the triad of clinical history, ECG, and changes in 'serum enzymes.' Many patients with ischemic symptoms can have negative or equivocal ECG, negative tests for older markers such as CK-MB, but unequivocal (though often slight) elevation in cTn. Reversible ischemia probably does not cause

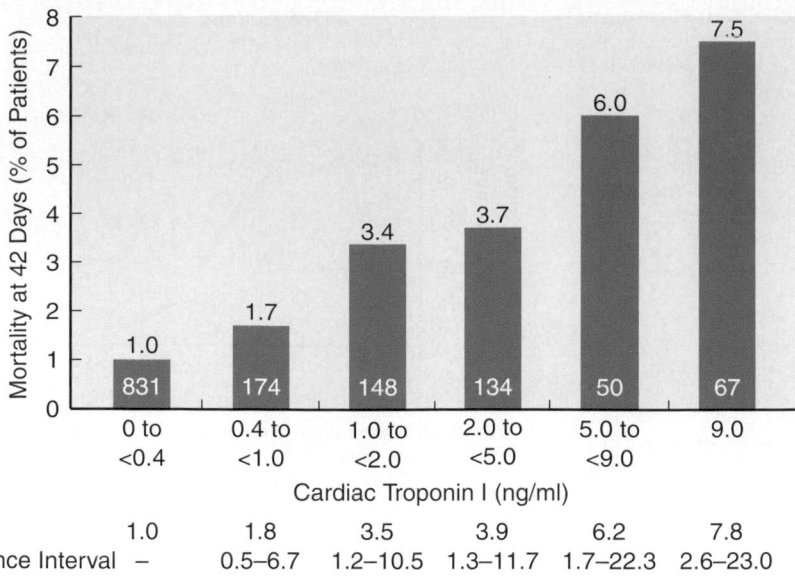

Figure 18–2 Mortality rates of ACS patients as a function of cTnI level. The 1441 patients in the TIMI IIIB study were from 21–76 years of age, had episodes of pain at rest that were presumed to be ischemic in origin and had lasted for at least 5 minutes (but less than 6 hours) within the preceding 24 hours, and had documented evidence of CHD. Patients were excluded from the study if left bundle-branch block was noted on presentation, a documented myocardial infarction had occurred within the previous 21 days, a treatable cause of angina was present, thrombolytic therapy had been administered within the previous 72 hours, or angioplasty had been performed in the previous 6 months. Mortality rates at 42 days are shown for ranges of cTnI measured at enrollment. The numbers at the bottom of each bar are the numbers of patients with cTnI in each range, and the numbers above the bars are percentages. $p < 0.001$ for the increase in the mortality rate (and the risk ratio for mortality) with increasing levels of cTnI at enrollment. (Redrawn from Antman EM, Tanasijeric MJ, Thompson B, et al: Cardiac-Specific troponin I levels to predict the risk of mortality in patients with acute coronary syndromes. N Engl J Med 335:1342–1349, 1996.)

Cardiac Troponin I (ng/ml)	0 to <0.4	0.4 to <1.0	1.0 to <2.0	2.0 to <5.0	5.0 to <9.0	9.0
Risk Ratio	1.0	1.8	3.5	3.9	6.2	7.8
95% Confidence Interval	–	0.5–6.7	1.2–10.5	1.3–11.7	1.7–22.3	2.6–23.0

such elevations, although this has not been established with certainty (Morrow, 2001). These patients, occasionally said to have 'minimum myocardial damage,' 'microinfarctions' or 'infarctlets,' probably have true MIs with a lesser amount of muscle necrosis than could previously be detected. A consensus conference recommended that they should properly have the diagnosis of MI (Joint Committee, 2000).

Apart from nosology, low-positive cTn clearly confers increased risk for complications of CHD (Hamm, 1992, 1997; Polanczyk, 1998; Luscher, 1997; Antman, 1996) (see Fig. 18–2) and may have important implications for therapy. Patients with ischemic symptoms who also have elevations in cTn receive greater benefit from therapies with various antiplatelet and antithrombotic agents (Hamm, 1999; Lindahl, 1997; Morrow, 2000; Newby, 2001).

Myoglobin

Myoglobin is a heme-containing protein that binds oxygen within cardiac and skeletal muscle; there is only a single form common to both muscle types. Lacking cardiac specificity, myoglobin's usefulness derives from its kinetics (see Fig. 18–1). Having a molecular weight of only 18 kDa, it apparently leaks from damaged cells more rapidly than other proteins. Elevated serum levels are apparent within 2–3 h following onset of MI, earlier than with troponin or other markers (Montague, 1995). Myoglobin is cleared mainly by renal filtration; its half-life is approximately 4 hours, but is longer if renal function is impaired. Typically myoglobin peaks about 6 h after MI and returns to baseline after 24 h. In normal individuals, myoglobin levels are related to muscle mass and muscle activity, similar to the pattern for CK. Plasma levels are higher in men than in women. Myoglobin increases with increasing age, reflecting decreased glomerular filtration rate. Day-to-day variation is about 10–15% (Panteghini, 1997). Despite myoglobin's lack of specificity for myocardium, as a test for MI it offers fairly high clinical specificity (> 95%) when patients with renal failure or suspected injury to skeletal muscle are excluded. The sensitivity of myoglobin can be enhanced by considering a result positive if, even though within the reference interval, it represents a large change ('delta myoglobin') from a specimen drawn 1–3 h earlier (Brogan, 1994; Tucker, 1994; Woo, 1995).

Myoglobin testing may occasionally be useful for documenting damage to skeletal muscle, but other markers, such as total CK, are usually more convenient for this purpose. Occasionally testing for myoglobin in serum or urine is useful to determine whether a positive urine dipstick test for 'blood,' based on heme's peroxidase activity, actually reflects myoglobinuria.

Other Markers

Carbonic Anhydrase III (CA III)

CA III is an enzyme present in skeletal but not cardiac muscle, and hence can serve as a sort of 'negative' cardiac marker. It is released from damaged muscle at a fairly fixed ratio to myoglobin. Thus myoglobin is a more specific indicator of myocardial damage when its ratio to CA III is also elevated (Väänänen, 1990; Brogan, 1996; Beuerle, 2000).

Glycogen Phosphorylase (GP)

GP is a widely distributed enzyme that catalyzes the first step in glycogenolysis. A dimer of identical subunits, it has three characterized isoenzymes, named for the tissue in which they are most expressed: GPLL (liver), GPMM (muscle), and GPBB (brain). GPBB is also expressed in myocardium, as well as other tissues, but it is not in skeletal muscle, which only contains GPMM. The potential usefulness of GPBB is that it appears to be released earlier than other markers, and may in fact be released under conditions of reversible ischemia that do not give rise to comparable elevations in other markers (Rabitzsch, 1995; Krause, 1996). However, comparisons with modern cTn assays have been limited and not particularly encouraging (Lang, 2000).

Creatine Kinase Isoforms

High-resolution electrophoresis of serum creatine kinase discloses that the MM and MB isoenzymes are heterogeneous, with MB having two sub-bands, and MM three sub-bands. These species, known as *isoforms*, arise due to the action of carboxypeptidase in serum cleaving the terminal lysine off of the M-subunit (Wevers, 1978; George, 1984). Thus the MB isoenzyme can have 0 or 1 lysine cleaved, whereas the MM isoenzyme can have 0, 1, or 2 lysines cleaved. The cleavage only occurs after the native enzyme is released into the circulation due to tissue damage. In acute MI, the native (tissue) isoforms CK-MB$_2$ and CK-MM$_3$ are released into the blood; it takes several hours before they are converted into CK-MB$_1$ and CK-MM$_1$/MM$_2$ isoforms, respectively. Hence a high ratio of MB$_2$/MB$_1$ or MM$_3$/MM$_1$ suggests that a recent release of enzyme has occurred, as from an MI. This increased ratio is typically observed shortly before the absolute quantity of serum MB exceeds the reference limit. Thus in the first 3–4 hours following symptom onset, improved sensitivity for MI detection is achieved (Puleo, 1994; Bock, 1999). The test can be performed by a commercial, automated, rapid electrophoresis system, but this still represents a dedicated workstation for the clinical laboratory.

Heart Fatty Acid Binding Protein (HFABP)

HFABP is a low-molecular-weight (15 kD) protein that is a relatively early marker of myocardial damage, with kinetics similar to those of myoglobin. It is not cardiac specific and therefore does not seem to offer advantage over myoglobin. However, the ratio of myoglobin to HFABP is much lower in heart than in skeletal muscle and may have diagnostic applicability (Van Nieuwenhoven, 1995; Zanotti, 1999).

Myosin

Myosin comprises the thick filament of the muscle contractile apparatus, and is composed of a pair of heavy chains (200 kD) and one pair each of type I and type II light chains (20–26 kD). Various of these components have been examined as cardiac markers (Uji, 1991; Ravkilde, 1994, 1995; Katus, 1988). It has not been possible to achieve complete cardiac specificity with myosin, and it is not clear that it would offer any important advantages.

Ischemia Modified Albumin (IMA)

IMA is a unique type of cardiac marker, FDA approved in 2003, that is *not a* protein released from damaged myocytes (Bar-Or, 2000, 2001; Bhagavan, 2003; Christenson, 2001). Rather, the test detects a variant form of albumin with a reduced affinity for metal ions near the N-terminus. The variant is measured by a spectrophotometric determination of Co^{2+} binding. It is postulated to arise from interaction of albumin with free radicals at sites of tissue ischemia. The theoretical advantage of this test is that it detects ischemia prior to irreversible cell damage. The change in albumin appears to occur within minutes of ischemia and lasts for about 6 hours. The test is clearly not specific for cardiac ischemia, but appears to have a clinical sensitivity of 80–90% for ACS at the time of presentation, greater than that of an electrocardiogram (Roy, 2004; Sinha, 2004). At the time of this writing, the clinical usefulness of the test has not been well documented.

Assay Procedures

As indicated above, the measurement of cardiac markers has evolved over the years from measurement of total enzyme activity, to electrophoretic or chromatographic isoenzyme separations, to the current era of sophisticated immunoassay technology. At the present time virtually all cardiac marker analysis (excluding IMA) is by immunoassay, and the general difficulties and pitfalls of immunoassay are applicable to all of them. Particular difficulties with cTn, the most important marker and in some ways an especially challenging protein analyte, are worthy of separate discussion.

As a protein complex that degrades as it is released into the circulation, cTn is a highly heterogeneous analyte. Circulating forms that have been identified include a ternary cTnT-I-C complex, binary cTnI-C, free cTnT (but not free cTnI), oxidized forms (cTnI but not cTnT contains cysteine residues that can be oxidized to form an intramolecular disulfide bond), phosphorylated forms, and degraded forms (Wu, 1998; Gao, 1997; Shi, 1999; Morjana, 1998; Katrukha, 1998; Bunk, 2000; Labugger, 2000). Evidently certain epitopes are blocked or modified in some of these forms, because differences of greater than 20-fold have been observed in their reactivity with different commercial assays for cTnI (Wu, 1998; Shi, 1999; Kao, 2001; Datta, 1999; Newman, 1999; Tate, 1999). The problem does not arise in the same way for cTnT because assays are at this time marketed by only one manufacturer.

Another problem is that since the normal level of plasma cTn is very low, even a miniscule degree of assay reactivity caused by interference or technical artifact may be read as a 'positive' result, implying myocardial injury. This may lead to unnecessary invasive procedures such as coronary angiography. Various cTnI assays have in fact been found susceptible to interferences from heterophilic antibodies, fibrin, and other substances (Nosanchuk, 1999; Fitzmaurice, 1998; Roberts, 1997; Dasgupta, 1999, 2001; Parry, 1999; Galambos, 2000). Negative interference due to a frequently occurring serum component has also been reported (Eriksson, 2003)

Reference ranges and decision points have been a matter of some confusion (Jaffe, 2004). As discussed above, when cTn testing was first introduced it was realized that small elevations often did not correlate with any elevation of CK-MB or other conventional (but less sensitive) sign of myocardial necrosis. It was therefore common to set a relatively high, and essentially arbitrary, decision point for cTn as being indicative of MI; lower levels were indeterminate, or taken to mean 'minimal myocardial damage.' The subsequent redefinition of MI altered this thinking, and it was recommended that the upper reference limit for cTn should be the 99th percentile of the healthy population, a level at which assays should ideally achieve a coefficient of variation (CV) within 10% (Joint Committee, 2000). As of 2003–2004, no commercial assay in the US achieved this level of precision (Panteghini, 2004), but a cTnI assay has been recently described that achieved a CV < 10% at 0.027 µg/L, which was below a population upper reference limit (99th percentile) measured at 0.041 µg/L (Venge, 2003). For assays that do not achieve a 10% CV at the 99th percentile, the diagnostic cutoff should be the lowest concentration that produces a 10% CV.

Clinical Protocols

Diagnosis of ACS

Diagnosis of MI has evolved from a somewhat leisurely process spanning several days of a hospital stay to an urgent task carried out largely in the emergency department (ED), sometimes within a specialized chest pain center (Zalenski, 1998). Approximately 8 000 000 emergency department visits in the US each year are for chest pain or other symptoms, including shortness of breath, dizziness, or loss of consciousness, that may suggest ACS (Storrow, 2000). Although diagnosis is often straightforward, the challenge is to achieve a very high level of accuracy. Missed diagnosis of

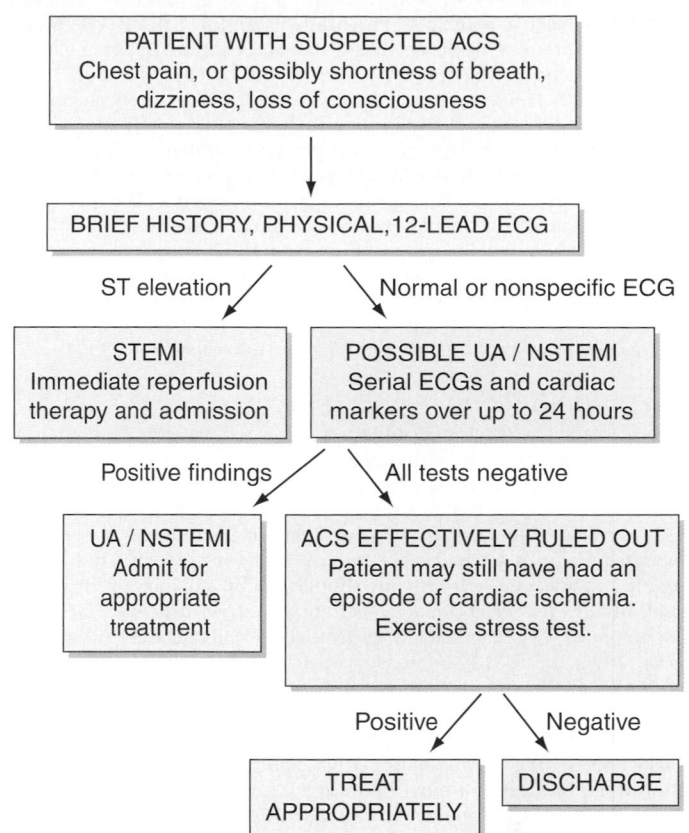

Figure 18–3 Outline of a clinical algorithm for treating patients presenting to an emergency department with symptoms suggesting ACS. The protocol is general, and has to be customized to particular institutions and used with proper clinical judgment. (Adapted from Pearson TA, Mensah GA, Alexander RW, et al: Markers of inflammation and cardiovascular disease application to clinical and public health practice: A statement for healthcare professionals from the centers for Disease Control and Prevention and the American Heart Association. Circulation 107:499–511, 2003.)

ACS, which may occur in about 2% of cases, carries an increased risk of mortality and is the leading cause of malpractice payout for emergency physicians (Pope, 2000; Karcz, 1996). On the other hand, the conservative practice of hospital admission for most patients with suspected ACS spends billions of dollars unnecessarily, because two-thirds of these patients turn out not to have ACS.

Biochemical markers play a secondary role in the initial management of patients with suspected ACS. The earliest decision-making, which should ideally take place within 10 min of the patient's arrival in the ED, is based on history, physical examination, and 12-lead ECG (Braunwald, 2002) (see Fig. 18–3). The ECG may establish the diagnosis of STEMI, at which point the patient is a candidate for immediate thrombolysis and other interventions, as presented in detailed guidelines for this condition (Antman, 2004). Biochemical marker results are not necessary before these interventions, and are in fact likely to be negative at this early time.

If the initial ECG is negative for STEMI, biochemical markers assume increasing importance. Choice of markers and time points for testing vary among institutions, but there is now general agreement that cTn (either I or T) is the preferred marker for definitive diagnosis (Christenson, 2004; Braunwald, 2002) Timing of specimens is based on marker kinetics. Thus, for cTn, which may not rise until several hours after myocyte necrosis, a negative specimen at the time of presentation should be followed with a second specimen at 6–12 h, and possibly, at least when the index of suspicion is high, a third specimen at about 24 h. At centers emphasizing early diagnosis, a specimen in the 1- to 4 h-time frame can also be included, and it is useful to include an early marker, typically myoglobin but possibly CK isoforms, at the 0 and 1- to 4-h time points. The diagnosis of NSTEMI is established by positive biomarker results with appropriate changes over time. Negative biomarker results, but ischemic ECG changes (ST depression or T-wave inversions) or other evidence may establish the diagnosis of UA. These two diagnoses are managed similarly, possibly with invasive artery-opening therapy (Braunwald, 2002).

If after several hours the patient's presenting symptoms have resolved and ECG and biochemical findings have been consistently negative, then an ACS has been effectively ruled out. For increased safety, before discharging such a patient, a provocative test for CHD is commonly performed, such as a simple exercise ECG test, or a more elaborate nuclear imaging or echocardiography stress test (Lindsay, 1998; Farkouh, 1998; Storrow, 2000). These tests must be rapidly and continuously available if the ED is to achieve the desired rapid discharge of low-risk patients. They have the drawbacks of expense and significant numbers of false-positive and false-negative results, depending on the test modality chosen.

Because both clinical care and patient flow through the ED require rapid risk assessment, cardiac marker test results must be available quickly. It is commonly advocated that point-of-care testing be considered when the central laboratory cannot reliably provide results within about 1 h. Both qualitative and quantitative tests for cardiac markers that are suitable for point-of-care testing are now available and have demonstrated effectiveness (Antman, 1997; Brogan, 1998; Muller-Bardorff, 1999)

Other Applications

Cardiac marker tests are performed on most ACS patients even after the diagnosis is established. Although as a universal practice this may be questioned, it has some benefits (Christenson, 2004). It can serve as a noninvasive indicator that reperfusion has occurred, either spontaneously or as a result of therapy. Due to the 'washout phenomenon' a bolus of myocyte proteins is released in the minutes following reperfusion, so blood sampled in the next 60–120 min should exhibit an increase in marker concentration (either absolute or percentage) above a defined threshold. Myoglobin was found to perform better than CK-MB or cTn for this purpose (Ishii, 1994; Zabel, 1993; Tanasijevic, 1997) but, unlike angiography, biomarker measurements cannot distinguish degrees of occluded flow.

Marker concentrations following MI correlate with infarct size, functional impairment, and prognosis (Delanghe, 1992; Glatz, 1994; Hackel, 1984; Mair, 1995; Omura, 1995; Panteghini, 2002; Mutlu, 2004). Clinical application is limited because the correlations are rather weak, especially if only measurements at a single time point are considered, and interpretation is greatly affected by whether reperfusion has occurred. Marker measurements are also useful for detecting the approximately 17% of MI patients who suffer early reinfarction (Marmor, 1981). This is one application where CK-MB appears to be superior to cTn because of its more rapid decline following MI; myoglobin is also useful. cTn may be useful for patient monitoring and prognosis in situations other than ACS, e.g., in heart failure (Missov, 1999; Missov, 1997; Del Carlo, 1999), but protocols are not well established.

Diagnosis of MI following surgical procedures (perioperative MI) was challenging in the pre-troponin era because nonspecific markers are routinely released from damage to skeletal muscle and other noncardiac tissues. cTn is clearly the marker of choice in this situation, but if surgery is being done on the heart itself, the question arises of how much release of cTn is to be expected in the absence of complications. In a study of patients with diverse open heart surgery, 17 patients suffering defined 'cardiac events' post-surgery all had peak cTnI values above 40 ng/mL, some much higher, whereas only 3 of 83 patients without events had cTnI > 40 ng/mL, most much lower (Greenson, 2001). A more recent study found that cTnT > 1.26 ng/mL in a specimen 24 h post-surgery was associated with 6.3-fold higher risk for evolution of new Q-waves (Lehrke, 2004). In a study of patients undergoing coronary artery bypass surgery, 69 subjects who did not develop Q waves had a median peak cTnI post-surgery of 2.1 ng/mL, compared to 17 ng/mL for those who developed Q waves. Cardioversion, whether external or internal, causes minimal to no elevation in cTn (Allan, 1997; Gorenek, 2004; Greaves, 1998; Rao, 1998). Percutaneous interventions can cause minor degrees of elevation which do not indicate adverse prognosis (Shyu, 1998; Attali, 1998; Bertinchant, 1999).

Markers of Coronary Risk

CHD is a chronic disease of aging, and obviously the most desirable approach is to prevent or minimize its development. As summarized in the Background section above, our understanding of the causation of CHD is still incomplete, so definitive preventive measures are not foreseeable at this time. However, many lines of evidence, the most important being large epidemiology studies, have identified several *risk factors* associated with CHD. Most of these risk factors pertain not just to the heart but to the general processes of atherosclerosis and/or thrombosis. Hence they have important implications for stroke and peripheral vascular disease as well.

The major clinical risk factors for CHD (not related to laboratory tests) are summarized in Table 18–2. Of the risk factors that can be determined by the clinical laboratory, the earliest identified, and still one of the most important, is serum cholesterol. It is actually the low-density lipoprotein

(LDL) fraction of cholesterol, which generally contains about 70% of the total circulating cholesterol, that is directly associated with risk; the high-density lipoprotein (HDL) fraction is in fact a *negative* risk factor. The other major lipid class commonly measured in plasma, triglyceride, has been an issue of controversy but is now generally accepted as a significant risk factor. Lipid testing and its relationship to CHD risk assessment are discussed in Chapter 17.

Aside from the lipids, a wide array of plasma constituents have been related to CHD risk. These include various nutrients, hormones, clotting factors, drugs, toxins, oxidants, antioxidants, and markers of inflammation or infection. In this chapter only two markers that appear to be relatively important will be discussed: C-reactive protein and homocysteine.

C-Reactive Protein (CRP)

First isolated in 1930 from the plasma of patients with pneumococcal pneumonia, CRP was so named because it binds to the C-polysaccharide of the pneumococcus. It was later found that the protein appeared in plasma during many infectious or inflammatory conditions, and CRP was the original *acute phase reactant*. Modern molecular studies have determined that CRP is a member of the *pentraxin* family of proteins. It comprises five protomers, each of 206 amino acids, molecular weight 23 kDa, arranged in cyclic symmetry. With the participation of Ca^{2+} ions, it binds various proteins and phospholipids, particularly phosphocholine. It opsonizes particles and also activates complement via the classical pathway, but its actual biological function is unknown (Black, 2004; Szalai, 1999)

In plasma from normal individuals, the median CRP concentration is about 1 mg/L, and the 99th percentile is about 10 mg/L. In individuals with acute illness, cytokines, chiefly interleukin-6, stimulate hepatic production of CRP, and plasma levels increase to 300 mg/L or more. Plasma CRP is increased in a variety of disorders, including most bacterial (but usually not viral) infection. MI is among the acute illnesses associated with elevation of plasma CRP (de Beer, 1982).

In recent years many epidemiologic studies have established that individuals with higher baseline levels of plasma CRP are at increased risk for CHD and stroke. In the relatively early Physicians Health Study, enrolling 22 000 male US physicians to examine cardioprotective effects of aspirin and beta-carotene, plasma CRP averaged 1.51 mg/L in participants who developed MI, 1.38 mg/L in those who developed stroke, and 1.13 mg/L in controls who did not suffer vascular events (Ridker, 1997). In the larger and more recent Reykjavik study, the average baseline CRP was 1.75 mg/L in participants who developed MI, versus 1.25 in those without vascular events (Danesh, 2004). Generally similar findings, as summarized in a 2004 meta-analysis, have been reported from some 20 other epidemiology studies, although the degree of independent risk associated with CRP has varied (Danesh, 2004). A report on the Women's Health Study suggested that CRP was actually more predictive than LDL-cholesterol (Ridker, 2002), whereas the investigators for the Reykjavik study reported that CRP is less predictive than total cholesterol, cigarette smoking, or systolic blood pressure. Differences may relate to the nature of the population studied and means of correction for traditional risk factors.

The elevation of plasma CRP indicated above that confers excess coronary risk is minute compared to the 100- to 1000-fold increases that occur with overt inflammatory or infectious diseases. For this reason, testing of CRP related to cardiac risk has been given the somewhat misleading name 'high-sensitivity CRP' (hsCRP). Actually, even at concentrations around 1 mg/L or less, CRP is a relatively abundant plasma protein, not requiring the most sensitive techniques for accurate measurement. Methods such as nephelometry, which had been established for measuring CRP as an inflammatory marker, have been readily adapted to 'hsCRP' assay, the main differences being in degree of dilution and calibration. Commercial hsCRP assays have adequate precision, and the long-term stability of hsCRP in individual patients appears to be comparable to that of other risk factors, such as blood pressure and cholesterol (Danesh, 2004).

Although diverse evidence points to a role of inflammation in CHD (Paoletti, 2004), a precise mechanism for the relationship of plasma CRP to CHD risk is lacking at this point. A key question still unresolved is whether the elevation in CRP is a cause or a consequence of the disease (or possibly both). The inflammatory response associated with atheromatous lesions may trigger enough cytokine production to be associated with a measurable rise in plasma CRP. CRP may in turn, through its proinflammatory effects, increase plaque vulnerability or have other effects that worsen the severity of CHD. Presence of CRP in human atheromatous lesions has been demonstrated (Reynolds, 1987), and in rats it has been shown that injection of human CRP after ligation of the coronary artery enhances infarct size (Griselli, 1999). Another intriguing possibility is that the risk associated with CRP relates to cytokine production by adipocytes,

Table 18–3 Recommendations of a Joint Committee of the American Heart Association and the Centers for Disease Control and Prevention on CRP Testing to Assess CHD Risk (Pearson, 2003)

- If inflammatory markers are to be used in assessment of CHD risk, hsCRP is the current analyte of choice
- Optimally, hsCRP results should be averaged from two specimens drawn about 2 weeks apart. If a level > 10 mg/L is identified, there should be a search for an obvious cause of infection or inflammation; that result should then be discarded, and another test done 2 weeks later
- Decision intervals are: < 1 mg/L, low risk; 1–3 mg/L, intermediate risk; > 3–mg/L, high risk (approximately corresponding to tertiles in the adult population)
- Patients most likely to benefit from an hsCRP test would be those in whom the risk estimate from established factors is moderate (i.e., approximately 10–20% risk of CHD in the next 10 years), and the physician desires additional information to guide preventive therapy
- The role of hsCRP in secondary prevention (i.e., prevention of disease progression in patients with established CHD) is limited, because it is not likely to alter management (which needs to be aggressive, regardless of additional information provided by CRP or other markers)
- Universal hsCRP screening of the adult population is *not* warranted.

and that CRP is essentially a biochemical marker of the recently recognized metabolic syndrome discussed in Chapter 17 (Ridker, 2004b; Yudkin, 1999).

Given the variations in quantitative risk estimates, the unclear role of CRP in pathogenesis of vascular disease, and the lack of specific treatment for high CRP, the usefulness of the hsCRP test in individual patients has been controversial. A joint committee of the Centers for Disease Control and Prevention and the American Heart Association issued recommendations in 2003, some of which are listed in Table 18–3.

Homocysteine (Hcy)

Hcy (Fig. 18–4) is a sulfur-containing amino acid that is not incorporated into protein but is a metabolic intermediate; it can either be methylated to form methionine, or converted through the transsulfuration pathway to cystathionine and then to cysteine. Hcy can exist in plasma as the species with a free sulfhydryl group, as a disulfide (homocystine), or as a mixed disulfide, linked to a plasma protein via one of its cysteine residues. It is the sum of these, which may be referred to as 'total homocysteine (tHcy),' 'homocyst(e)ine,' or simply 'homocysteine (Hcy)' that is generally measured.

Excessive levels of circulating Hcy generally reflect a diminished level of one of the enzymes involved in its metabolism. The classical syndrome of homocystinuria, first described in 1962 (Carson, 1962; Gerritsen, 1962) is due to a homozygous defect in the enzyme cystathionine-β-synthase (CBS). It results in very high circulating levels of the various forms of Hcy, and of methionine. Clinical manifestations include dislocation of the optic lens, osteoporosis with associated skeletal abnormalities, mental retardation, psychiatric disturbance, and thromboembolic disease, including CHD (Yap, 2003).

The basis of the damaging effects of Hcy is uncertain. At a biochemical level, oxidant stress and inhibition of transmethylation reactions are likely

possibilities. Cellular effects that have been documented in experimental systems include: endothelial injury, alteration of NO metabolism, platelet activation, and smooth muscle proliferation (Thambyrajah, 2000). Some of the toxicity of Hcy may derive from its enzymatic conversion to Hcy thiolactone (Fig. 18–4), which can modify LDL and enhance its uptake by macrophages (McCully, 1993; Vignini, 2004).

Hcy's development as a CHD risk marker in some ways parallels that of cholesterol: the regular occurrence of atherosclerosis in persons with massive elevation, due to an inborn error of metabolism, led to the hypothesis of increased risk in individuals with more moderate elevations. Experimentally induced hyperhomocysteinemia in animals lent support to the hypothesis (McCully, 1993). In humans, mild to moderate elevations in Hcy can have many causes. Genetic causes include a heterozygous defect in CBS, a defect in methionine synthase (rare), or a defect in 5,10-methylenetetrahydrofolate reductase (MTHFR) (generally rare, except for a temperature-sensitive form that is relatively common). Nutritional causes include a deficiency of any of the vitamin cofactors involved in metabolism of Hcy: folate, B_{12}, or pyridoxine (B_6).

Many of the earlier epidemiology studies seemed to confirm a correlation between moderate Hcy levels and CHD. For example, in the Physicians Health Study it was initially reported that having a Hcy level in the upper 5% of the population conferred three- to fourfold higher risk (Stampfer, 1992). However, other studies, including a longer-term follow-up in the Physicians Health Study (Chasan-Taber, 1996), and many of the larger and more recent studies, have shown little or no association between moderate elevations of Hcy and CHD risk. Furthermore, widespread folate supplementation of food has probably tended to diminish average circulating Hcy in the US population, and there are sparse data to support cardioprotective effects of Hcy-lowering therapy. For these reasons there is no general advice for widespread Hcy screening. However, measurement of Hcy may be warranted in individuals who develop CHD despite being at relatively low risk based on traditional risk factors (Homocysteine Studies Collaboration, 2002; Malinow, 1999; Ridker, 2004a).

Hcy has traditionally been measured by chromatographic techniques (Ubbink, 1999; Arndt, 2004; Frick, 2003; Vester, 1991). A method using enzymatic adenosylation followed by immunoassay has been automated on the Abbott IMx analyzer (Shipchandler, 1995), and purely enzymatic methods suitable for automation have also been introduced (Huijgen, 2004; Roberts, 2004; Tan, 2000). Attention must be paid to proper sample collection and storage to prevent an artifactual increase in measured Hcy (Willems, 2004).

Markers of Congestive Heart Failure

Cardiac Natriuretic Peptides

The heretical concept that the heart could be an endocrine organ was enforced by two reports in 1956: that inflating a balloon inside the left atrium of a dog caused an increase in urine flow (Henry, 1956); and that structures resembling secretory granules were visible in electron micrographs of guinea pig atrial cells (Kisch, 1956). In 1981 extracts of rat heart atria (but not ventricles) were found to have a natriuretic effect (de Bold, 1981), and in 1984 a peptide named atrial natriuretic peptide (ANP) was isolated from human heart (Kangawa, 1984) A short time later a similar peptide named brain natriuretic peptide (BNP) was isolated from porcine brain (Sudoh, 1988) It turns out that in humans BNP is produced

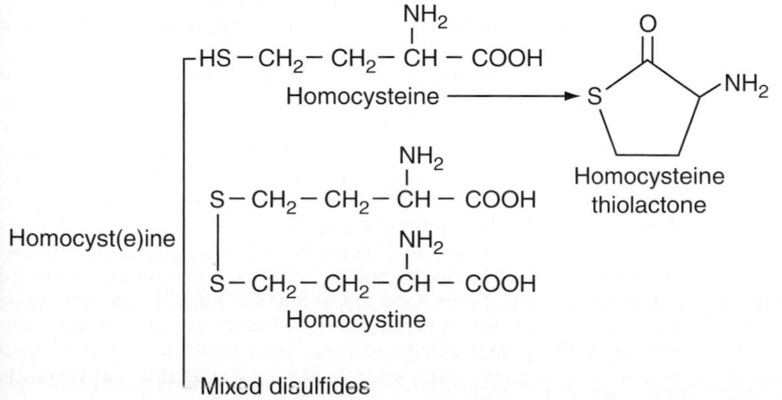

Figure 18–4 Chemical structure of homocysteine and related compounds.

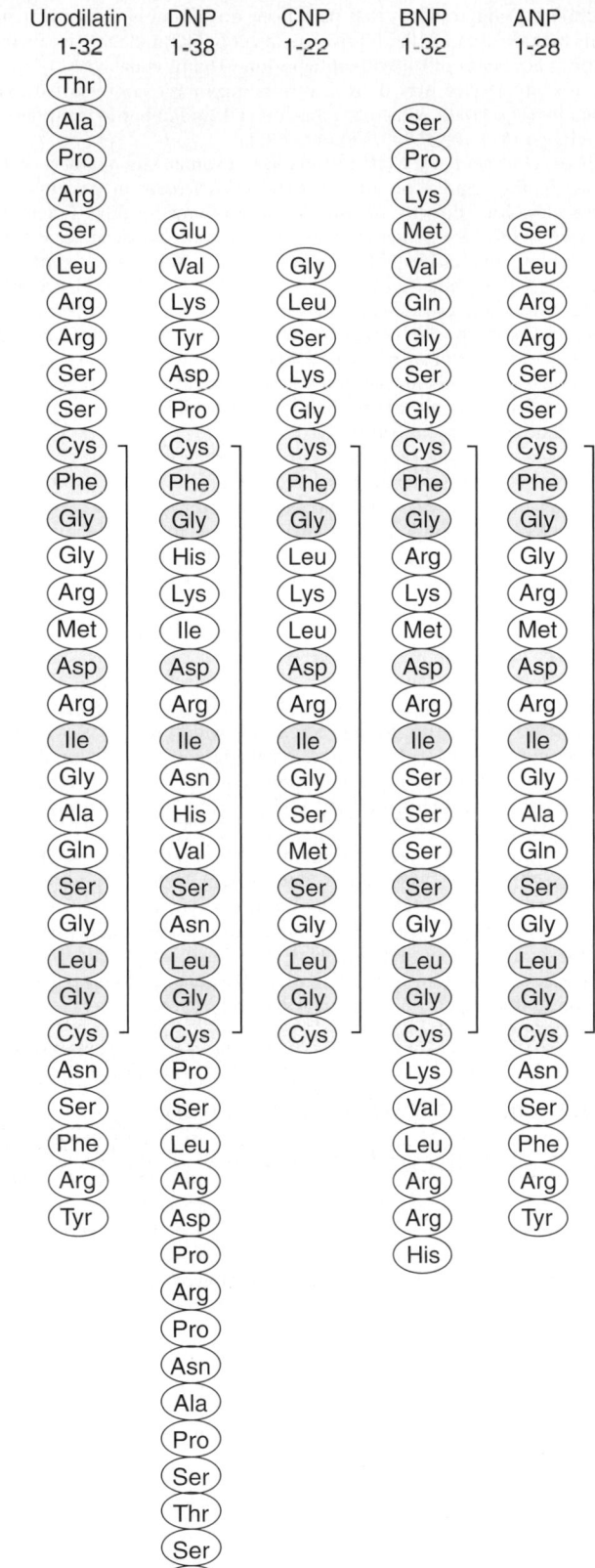

Figure 18–5 Amino acid sequences of the natriuretic peptides. Amino acids preserved through the family are indicated in color.

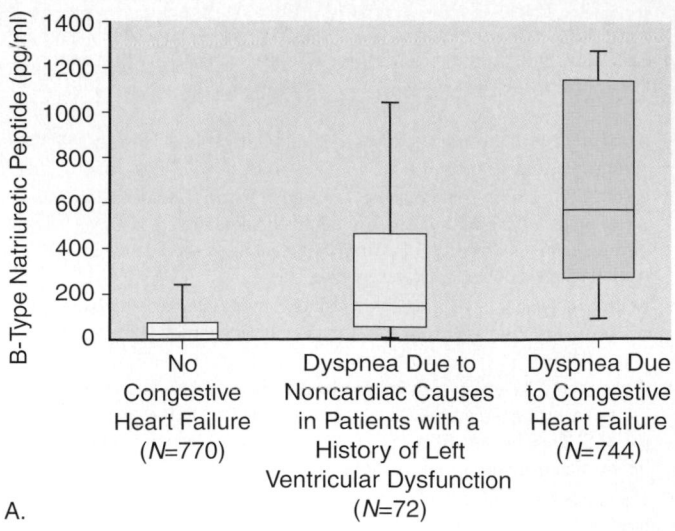

A.

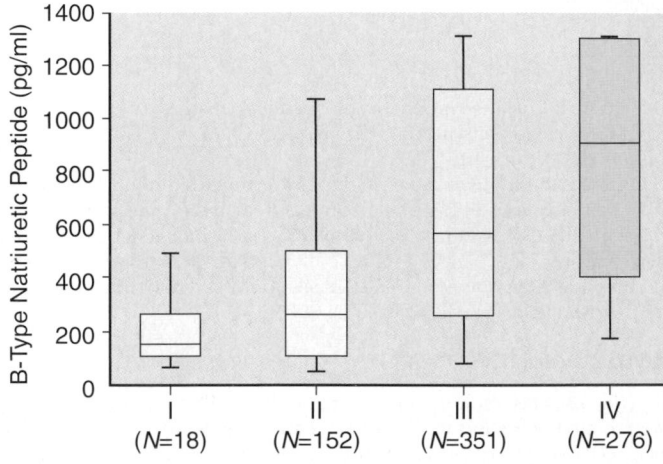

B. New York Heart Association Class

Figure 18–6 Box plots showing median levels of B-type natriuretic peptide in patients presenting to an emergency department with dyspnea, in the Breathing Not Properly study. *A,* Patients in different diagnostic categories. *B,* Patients with HF, classified according to the New York Heart Association criteria. A higher class indicates more severe disease, evidenced by a lesser amount of activity needed to provoke symptoms (American Heart Association, 1994). Boxes show interquartile ranges, and I bars represent highest and lowest values. (Redrawn from Maisel AS, Krishnaswamy P, Nowak RM, et al: Rapid measurement of B-type natriuretic peptide in the emergency diagnosis of heart failure. N Engl J Med 347:161–167, 2002.)

Dendroaspis angusticeps (Schweitz, 1992). DNP immunoreactivity was later reported in human plasma (Schirger, 1999), but this peptide has not been definitively demonstrated in the human (Richards, 2002). Finally, urodilatin is a form of ANP with four additional amino acids at the N-terminus, likely produced in the kidney by alternative splicing of the same gene product (Schulz-Knappe, 1988). Both ANP and BNP have been investigated with regard to testing for HF, and the latter has proved more useful, so further discussion will be confined to the BNP system.

Circulating BNP derives from a 108-amino-acid prohormone, proBNP, which is cleaved within the cardiac myocyte by the endoprotease furin to a 32-amino-acid C-terminal fragment, the active BNP, and an inactive N-terminal fragment, N-BNP or NT-proBNP (Sawada, 1997). Secretion of both fragments is enhanced by ventricular wall stretch and volume overload, as occurs in HF (Tabbibizar, 2002). BNP is removed from the circulation by binding to a clearance receptor and also by action of endopeptidases; its circulating half-life is approximately 22 minutes. The circulating half-life of N-BNP is considerably longer (60–120 min), and its mechanism of clearance is not well understood.

BNP and the other natriuretic peptides exert their effects through two types of G-protein-coupled receptors, resulting in release of the second messenger cyclic guanosine monophosphate (c-GMP). They downregulate the renin–angiotensin–aldosterone system, decrease sympathetic nerve activity in the heart and kidney, increase renal blood flow, and increase sodium excretion via a direct effect on the renal collecting duct (Spevack, 2004; Beltowski, 2002).

mainly in the cardiac ventricle (Mukoyama, 1991), so the hormone is now commonly referred to as B-type natriuretic peptide.

Members of the natriuretic peptide family are illustrated in Figure 18–5. Their notable common feature is a 17-amino-acid ring structure, closed by a cystine bridge, with substantial homology among the family members. C-type natriuretic peptide (CNP), described in 1990, is not produced in the heart but rather in endothelial cells (Sudoh, 1990). D-type natriuretic peptide (DNP) was isolated in 1992 from the green mamba snake,

Plasma levels of BNP are less than 100 pg/mL in most healthy individuals; reference ranges depend on age and gender. The best-established application of BNP measurement is for diagnosing acutely ill patients presenting to emergency service with shortness of breath. Distinguishing HF from lung disease, such as emphysema, in these patients is occasionally difficult, and until now no laboratory test has been specifically applicable. The multinational Breathing Not Properly study enrolled patients presenting to emergency centers with dyspnea, and employed a point-of-care method for measurement of BNP. At a decision point of 100 pg/mL, the BNP test had the following characteristics for diagnosis of HF: sensitivity 90%, specificity 76%, positive predictive value (PPV) 79%, negative predictive value (NPV) 89% (Maisel, 2002). Among patients with a history of ventricular dysfunction, BNP was higher in those whose current symptoms were thought to be caused by HF; it was also higher in patients with more severe failure (Fig. 18–6).

Many other possible applications of BNP testing have been suggested, including monitoring the course and treatment of patients with HF (Cheng, 2001); risk stratification of patients with ACS (de Lemos, 2001; Wiviott, 2004; Jernberg, 2004; Omland, 2002); monitoring disease severity in patients with stable CHD (Weber, 2004); screening for ventricular dysfunction in selected populations (Nielsen, 2003; Bay, 2003); and testing for drug cardiotoxicity (Okumura, 2000). One small study demonstrated fewer adverse events in a patient group treated for HF with use of BNP monitoring than in a control group treated without the use of the test (Troughton, 2000). However, the benefit may have derived from a general impetus for more aggressive management, rather than important discriminatory information provided by the test (Packer, 2003). Mueller et al. randomized 452 patients presenting to an emergency department with dyspnea to a diagnostic strategy with and without use of a bedside BNP measurement. Measurement of BNP appeared to decrease the time to discharge and the total cost of treatment (Mueller, 2004).

A major limitation of BNP is that a wide range of values is observed in patients with and without HF, and all of the determinants of the circulating BNP level have not yet been well established. BNP is increased in conditions of fluid imbalance other than HF, particularly renal insufficiency, which commonly coexists with HF (McCullough, 2004). Also, patients with symptomatic HF, especially when it is chronic and stable, can have 'normal' levels (Tang, 2003). Intra-individual variability is relatively high; in a group of patients with stable, chronic HF, week-to-week variability (CV) for both BNP and N-BNP were 30–40% (Bruins, 2004). At this time it appears that the most appropriate use of the BNP test is as an adjunctive test to rule out HF in the acute setting. In other contexts it should be used judiciously as more information becomes available (Cowie, 2003).

The earliest assay for BNP commercially available in the US was an immunoassay using an instrument most suitable for point-of-care measurement. More recently the test has become available on large, automated immunoassay platforms. Assays of both BNP and N-BNP are available; a clear advantage of one biomarker over the other for any particular application has not been established (Hammerer-Lercher, 2001b).

Besides being a biomarker for HF, BNP has natriuretic, vasodilatory, and other effects that are ameliorative for the syndrome, and is in fact available as the drug nesiritide (Natrecor) for treatment of HF. Due to the short half-life of BNP, measured levels several hours after its administration would reflect endogenous secretion. However, the utility of BNP measurement in the context of its therapeutic administration has not been established at this time.

References

Adams MR, Kinlay S, Blake GJ, et al: Atherogenic lipids and endothelial dysfunction: mechanisms in the genesis of ischemic syndromes. Annu Rev Med 2000; 51:149–167.
Reviews mechanisms involved in the genesis of CHD.

Allan JJ, Feld RD, Russell AA, et al: Cardiac troponin I levels are normal or minimally elevated after transthoracic cardioversion. J Am Coll Cardiol 1997; 30:1052–1056.

American Heart Association: Classification of functional capacity and objective assessment. American Heart Association. Entered 1994. Online. Available: http://www.americanheart.org/presenter.jhtml?identifier=4569 13 October 2004.

American Heart Association: Heart disease and stroke statistics – 2004 update. American Heart Association. Entered 2003. Online. Available: http://www.americanheart.org/downloadable/heart/1079736729696HDSStats2004UpdateREV3-19-04.pdf 13 October 2004.
An extensive compilation of statistics for CHD, HF, other heart diseases, and stroke.

Antman EM, Anbe DT, Armstrong PW, et al: ACC/AHA guidelines for the management of patients with ST-elevation myocardial infarction; A report of the American College of Cardiology/American Heart Association Task Force on Practice Guidelines (Committee to Revise the 1999 Guidelines for the Management of patients with acute myocardial infarction). Entered 4 August 2004. Online. Available: http://www.acc.org/clinical/guidelines/stemi/index.pdf 13 October 2004.
Detailed guidelines for the management of STEMI.

Antman EM, Grudzien C, Mitchell RN, et al: Detection of unsuspected myocardial necrosis by rapid bedside assay for cardiac troponin T. Am Heart J 1997; 133:596–598.

Antman EM, Tanasijevic MJ, Thompson B, et al: Cardiac-specific troponin I levels to predict the risk of mortality in patients with acute coronary syndromes. N Engl J Med 1996; 335:1342–1349.

Apple FS: Tissue specificity of cardiac troponin I, cardiac troponin T and creatine kinase-MB. Clin Chim Acta 1999; 284:151–159.

Apple FS, Ricchiuti V, Voss EM, et al: Expression of cardiac troponin T isoforms in skeletal muscle of renal disease patients will not cause false-positive serum results by the second generation cardiac troponin T assay. Eur Heart J 1998; 19(Suppl N):N30–N33.

Arndt T, Guessregen B, Hohl A, et al: Total plasma homocysteine measured by liquid chromatography-tandem mass spectrometry with use of 96-well plates. Clin Chem 2004; 50:755–757.

Attali P, Aleil B, Petitpas G, et al: Sensitivity and long-term prognostic value of cardiac troponin-I increase shortly after percutaneous transluminal coronary angioplasty. Clin Cardiol 1998; 21:353–356.

Bar-Or D, Curtis G, Rao N, et al: Characterization of the Co(2+) and Ni(2+) binding amino-acid residues of the N-terminus of human albumin. An insight into the mechanism of a new assay for myocardial ischemia. Eur J Biochem 2001; 268:42–47.

Bar-Or D, Lau E, Winkler JV: A novel assay for cobalt-albumin binding and its potential as a marker for myocardial ischemia – a preliminary report. J Emerg Med 2000; 19:311–315.

Bay M, Kirk V, Parner J, et al: NT-proBNP: a new diagnostic screening tool to differentiate between patients with normal and reduced left ventricular systolic function. Heart 2003; 89:150–154.

Beltowski J, Wojcicka G: Regulation of renal tubular sodium transport by cardiac natriuretic peptides: two decades of research. Med Sci Monit 2002; 8:RA39–RA52.

Berenson GS, Wattigney WA, Tracy RE, et al: Atherosclerosis of the aorta and coronary arteries and cardiovascular risk factors in persons aged 6 to 30 years and studied at necropsy (The Bogalusa Heart Study). Am J Cardiol 1992; 70:851–858.

Bertinchant JP, Polge A, Ledermann B, et al: Relation of minor cardiac troponin I elevation to late cardiac events after uncomplicated elective successful percutaneous transluminal coronary angioplasty for angina pectoris. Am J Cardiol 1999; 84:51–57.

Beuerle JR, Azzazy HM, Styba G, et al: Characteristics of myoglobin, carbonic anhydrase III and the myoglobin/carbonic anhydrase III ratio in trauma, exercise, and myocardial infarction patients. Clin Chim Acta 2000; 294:115–128.

Bhagavan NV, Lai EM, Rios PA, et al: Evaluation of human serum albumin cobalt binding assay for the assessment of myocardial ischemia and myocardial infarction. Clin Chem 2003; 49:581–585.

Black S, Kushner I, Samols D: C-reactive protein. J Biol Chem 2004; 279(47):48487–48490.

Bock JL, Brogan GX Jr, McCuskey CF, et al: Evaluation of CK-MB isoform analysis for early diagnosis of myocardial infarction. J Emerg Med 1999; 17:75–79.

Bodor GS, Porterfield D, Voss EM, et al: Cardiac troponin-I is not expressed in fetal and healthy or diseased adult human skeletal muscle tissue. Clin Chem 1995; 41:1710–1715.

Braunwald E, Antman EM, Beasley JW, et al: ACC/AHA guidelines for the management of patients with unstable angina and non-ST-segment elevation myocardial infarction: executive summary and recommendations. A report of the American College of Cardiology/American Heart Association task force on practice guidelines (committee on the management of patients with unstable angina). Entered 2002. Online. Available: http://www.acc.org/clinical/guidelines/unstable/unstable.pdf 8 October 2004.
Extensive guidelines for management of NSTEMI.

Brogan GX Jr, Bock JL: Cardiac marker point-of-care testing in the Emergency Department and Cardiac Care Unit. Clin Chem 1998; 44:1865–1869.

Brogan GX Jr, Friedman S, McCuskey C, et al: Evaluation of a new rapid quantitative immunoassay for serum myoglobin versus CK-MB for ruling out acute myocardial infarction in the emergency department. Ann Emerg Med 1994; 24:665–671.

Brogan GX Jr, Vuori J, Friedman S, et al: Improved specificity of myoglobin plus carbonic anhydrase assay versus that of creatine kinase-MB for early diagnosis of acute myocardial infarction. Ann Emerg Med 1996; 27:22–28.

Bruins S, Fokkema R, Römer JWP, et al: High intraindividual variation of B-type natriuretic peptide (BNP) and amino-terminal proBNP in patients with stable chronic heart failure. Clin Chem 2004; 50:2052–2058.

Bunk DM, Dalluge JJ, Welch MJ: Heterogeneity in human cardiac troponin I standards. Anal Biochem 2000; 284:191–200.

Carson NA, Neill DW: Metabolic abnormalities detected in a survey of mentally backward individuals in Northern Ireland. Arch Dis Child 1962; 37:505–513.

Chasan-Taber L, Selhub J, Rosenberg IH, et al: A prospective study of folate and vitamin B6 and risk of myocardial infarction in US physicians. J Am Coll Nutr 1996; 15:136–143.

Cheng V, Kazanagra R, Garcia A, et al: A rapid bedside test for B-type peptide predicts treatment outcomes in patients admitted for decompensated heart failure: a pilot study. J Am Coll Cardiol 2001; 37:386–391.

Christenson RH, Apple FS, Cannon CP, et al: Biomarkers of acute coronary syndrome and heart failure. Draft guidelines, Version 2. Entered 2004. Online. Available: http://www.nacb.org/lpmg/card_biomarkers_lmpg_draft.stm 13 October 2004. *Draft of a revision of guidelines first published in 1999.*

Christenson RH, Duh SH, Sanhai WR, et al: Characteristics of an albumin cobalt binding test for assessment of acute coronary syndrome patients: a multicenter study. Clin Chem 2001; 47:464–470.

Cowie MR, Jourdain P, Maisel A, et al: Clinical applications of B-type natriuretic peptide (BNP) testing. Eur Heart J 2003; 24:1710–1718.

Danesh J, Wheeler JG, Hirschfield GM, et al: C-reactive protein and other circulating markers of inflammation in the prediction of coronary heart disease. N Engl J Med 2004; 350:1387–1397. *A relatively large study of coronary risk associated with CRP, along with a meta-analysis.*

Dasgupta A, Banerjee SK, Datta P: False positive troponin I in the MEIA assay due to the presence of rheumatoid factors in serum: elimination of this interference by using a polyclonal antisera against rheumatoid factors. Am J Clin Pathol 1999; 112:753–756.

Dasgupta A, Wells A, Biddle DA: Negative interference of bilirubin and hemoglobin in the MEIA troponin I assay but not in the MEIA CK-MB assay. J Clin Lab Anal 2001; 15:76–80.

Datta P, Foster K, Dasgupta A: Comparison of immunoreactivity of five human cardiac troponin I assays toward free and complexed forms of the antigen: implications for assay discordance. Clin Chem 1999; 45:2266–2269.

Davies MJ: The pathophysiology of acute coronary syndromes. Heart 2000; 83:361–366.

de Beer FC, Hind CR, Fox KM, et al: Measurement of serum C-reactive protein concentration in myocardial ischaemia and infarction. Br Heart J 1982; 47:239–243.

de Bold AJ, Borenstein HB, Veress AT, et al: A rapid and potent natriuretic response to intravenous injection of atrial myocardial extract in rats. Life Sci 1981; 28:89–94.

de Lemos JA, Morrow DA, Bentley JH, et al: The prognostic value of B-type natriuretic peptide in patients with acute coronary syndromes. N Engl J Med 2001; 345:1014–1021.

Del Carlo CH, O'Connor CM: Cardiac troponins in congestive heart failure. Am Heart J 1999; 138:646–653.

Delanghe JR, De Buyzere ML, Cluyse LP, et al: Acute myocardial infarction size and myoglobin release into serum. Eur J Clin Chem Clin Biochem 1992; 30:823–830.

el Allaf M., Chapelle JP, el Allaf D, et al: Differentiating muscle damage from myocardial injury by means of the serum creatine kinase (CK) isoenzyme MB mass measurement/total CK activity ratio. Clin Chem 1986; 32:291–295.

Enos WF, Holmes RH, Beyer J: Coronary disease among United States soldiers killed in action in Korea. Preliminary report. JAMA 1953; 152:1090–1093.

Eriksson S, Junikka M, Laitinen P et al: Negative interference in cardiac troponin I immunoassays from a frequently occurring serum and plasma component. Clin Chem 2003; 49:1095–1104.

Farkouh ME, Smars PA, Reeder GS, et al: A clinical trial of a chest-pain observation unit for patients with unstable angina. Chest Pain Evaluation in the Emergency Room (CHEER) Investigators. N Engl J Med 1998; 339:1882–1888.

Fitzmaurice TF, Brown C, Rifai N, et al: False increase of cardiac troponin I with heterophilic antibodies. Clin Chem 1998; 44:2212–2214.

Frick B, Schrocksnadel K, Neurauter G, et al: Rapid measurement of total plasma homocysteine by HPLC. Clin Chim Acta 2003; 331:19–23.

Galambos C, Brink DS, Ritter D, et al: False-positive plasma troponin I with the AxSYM analyzer. Clin Chem 2000; 46:1014–1015.

Gao WD, Atar D, Liu Y, et al: Role of troponin I proteolysis in the pathogenesis of stunned myocardium. Circ Res 1997; 80:393–399.

George S, Ishikawa Y, Perryman MB, et al: Purification and characterization of naturally occurring and in vitro induced multiple forms of MM creatine kinase. J Biol Chem 1984; 259:2667–2674.

Gerritsen T, Vaughn JG, Waisman HA: The identification of homocystine in the urine. Biochem Biophys Res Commun 1962; 9:493–496.

Glatz JF, Kleine AH, Van Nieuwenhoven FA, et al: Fatty-acid-binding protein as a plasma marker for the estimation of myocardial infarct size in humans. Br Heart J 1994; 71:135–140.

Gomes AV, Potter JD: Molecular and cellular aspects of troponin cardiomyopathies. Ann N Y Acad Sci 2004; 1015:214–224.

Gorenek B, Kudaiberdieva G, Goktekin O, et al: Detection of myocardial injury after internal cardioversion for atrial fibrillation. Can J Cardiol 2004; 20:165–168.

Greaves K, Crake T: Cardiac troponin T does not increase after electrical cardioversion for atrial fibrillation or atrial flutter. Heart 1998; 80:226–228.

Greenson N, Macoviak J, Krishnaswamy P, et al: Usefulness of cardiac troponin I in patients undergoing open heart surgery. Am Heart J 2001; 141:447–455.

Griselli M, Herbert J, Hutchinson WL, et al: C-reactive protein and complement are important mediators of tissue damage in acute myocardial infarction. J Exp Med 1999; 190:1733–1740.

Hackel DB, Reimer KA, Ideker RE, et al: Comparison of enzymatic and anatomic estimates of myocardial infarct size in man. Circulation 1984; 70:824–835.

Hamm CW, Goldmann BU, Heeschen C, et al: Emergency room triage of patients with acute chest pain by means of rapid testing for cardiac troponin T or troponin I. N Engl J Med 1997; 337:1648–1653.

Hamm CW, Heeschen C, Goldmann B, et al: Benefit of abciximab in patients with refractory unstable angina in relation to serum troponin T levels. c7E3 Fab Antiplatelet Therapy in Unstable Refractory Angina (CAPTURE) Study Investigators. N Engl J Med 1999; 340:1623–1629.

Hamm CW, Ravkilde J, Gerhardt W, et al: The prognostic value of serum troponin T in unstable angina. N Engl J Med 1992 327:146–150.

Hammerer-Lercher A, Erlacher P, Bittner R, et al: Clinical and experimental results on cardiac troponin expression in Duchenne muscular dystrophy. Clin Chem 2001a; 47:451–458.

Hammerer-Lercher A, Neubauer E, Muller S, et al: Head-to-head comparison of N-terminal pro-brain natriuretic peptide, brain natriuretic peptide and N-terminal pro-atrial natriuretic peptide in diagnosing left ventricular dysfunction. Clin Chim Acta 2001b; 310:193–197.

Heloire F, Weill B, Weber S, et al: Aggregates of endothelial microparticles and platelets circulate in peripheral blood. Variations during stable coronary disease and acute myocardial infarction. Thrombosis Research 2003; 110:173–180.

Henry JP, Pearce JW: The possible role of cardiac atrial stretch receptors in the induction of changes in urine flow. J Physiol 1956; 131:572–585.

Hess JW, MacDonald RP: Serum creatine phosphokinase activity. A new diagnostic aid in myocardial and skeletal muscle disease. J Mich State Med Soc 1963; 62:1095–1099.

Homocysteine Studies Collaboration: Homocysteine and risk of ischemic heart disease and stroke: a meta-analysis. JAMA 2002; 288:2015–2022.

Huijgen HJ, Tegelaers FP, Schoenmakers CH, et al: Multicenter analytical evaluation of an enzymatic method for the measurement of plasma homocysteine and comparison with HPLC and immunochemistry. Clin Chem 2004; 50:937–941.

Ingwall JS, Kramer MF, Fifer MA, et al: The creatine kinase system in normal and diseased human myocardium. N Engl J Med 1985; 313:1050–1054.

Ishii J, Nomura M, Ando T, et al: Early detection of successful coronary reperfusion based on serum myoglobin concentration: Comparison with serum creatine kinase isoenzyme MB activity. Am Heart J 1994; 128:641–648.

Jaffe AS, Katus H: Acute coronary syndrome biomarkers: the need for more adequate reporting. Circulation 2004; 110:104–106.

Jernberg T, James S, Lindahl B, et al: Natriuretic peptides in unstable coronary artery disease. Eur Heart J 2004; 25:1486–1493.

Johnston CC, Bolton EC: Cardiac enzymes. Ann Emerg Med 1982; 11:27–35.

Joint Committee: Myocardial infarction redefined – a consensus document of The Joint European Society of Cardiology/American College of Cardiology Committee for the redefinition of myocardial infarction. J Am Coll Cardiol 2000; 36:959–969. *This document changed the long-established 'WHO criteria' for diagnosis of MI, using any definitive release of cardiac troponin as a basis for diagnosing MI.*

Joint Task Force: Nomenclature and criteria for diagnosis of ischemic heart disease. Report of the Joint International Society and Federation of Cardiology/World Health Organization task force on standardization of clinical nomenclature. Circulation 1979; 59:607–609.

Kangawa K, Matsuo H: Purification and complete amino acid sequence of alpha-human atrial natriuretic polypeptide (alpha-hANP). Biochem Biophys Res Commun 1984; 118:131–139.

Kao JT, Wong IL, Lee JY, et al: Comparison of Abbott AxSYM, Behring Opus Plus, DPC Immulite and Ortho-Clinical Diagnostics Vitros ECi for measurement of cardiac troponin I. Ann Clin Biochem 2001; 38:140–146.

Karcz A, Korn R, Burke MC, et al: Malpractice claims against emergency physicians in Massachusetts: 1975–1993. Am J Emerg Med 1996; 14:341–345.

Katrukha AG, Bereznikova AV, Filatov VL, et al: Degradation of cardiac troponin I: implication for reliable immunodetection. Clin Chem 1998; 44:2433–2440.

Katus HA, Diederich KW, Hoberg E, et al: Circulating cardiac myosin light chains in patients with angina at rest: identification of a high risk subgroup. J Am Coll Cardiol 1988; 11:487–493.

Kisch B: Electron microscopy of the atrium of the heart. I. Guinea pig. Exp Med Surg 1956; 14:99–112.

Krause EG, Rabitzsch G, Noll F, et al: Glycogen phosphorylase isoenzyme BB in diagnosis of myocardial ischaemic injury and infarction. Mol Cell Biochem 1996; 160–161:289–295.

Labugger R, Organ L, Collier C, et al: Extensive troponin I and T modification detected in serum from patients with acute myocardial infarction. Circulation 2000; 102:1221–1226.

LaDue JS, Wróblewski F, Karmen A: Serum glutamic oxaloacetic transaminase activity in human acute transmural myocardial infarction. Science 1954; 120:497–499.

Lang K, Borner A, Figulla HR: Comparison of biochemical markers for the detection of minimal myocardial injury: superior sensitivity of cardiac troponin – T ELISA. J Intern Med 2000; 247:119–123.

Lee TH, Goldman L: Serum enzyme assays in the diagnosis of acute myocardial infarction. Ann Intern Med 1986; 105:221–233.

Lehrke S, Steen H, Sievers HH, et al: Cardiac troponin T for prediction of short- and long-term morbidity and mortality after elective open heart surgery. Clin Chem 2004; 50:1560–1567.

Lindahl B, Venge P, Wallentin L: Troponin T identifies patients with unstable coronary artery disease who benefit from long-term antithrombotic protection. Fragmin in Unstable Coronary Artery Disease (FRISC) Study Group. J Am Coll Cardiol 1997; 29:43–48.

Lindsay J Jr, Bonnet YD, Pinnow EE: Routine stress testing for triage of patients with chest pain: is it worth the candle? Ann Emerg Med 1998; 32:600–603.

Luscher MS, Thygesen K, Ravkilde J, et al: Applicability of cardiac troponin T and I for early risk stratification in unstable coronary artery disease. TRIM Study Group. Thrombin Inhibition in Myocardial ischemia. Circulation 1997; 96:2578–2585.

McCullough P, Joseph K, Mathur VS: Diagnostic and therapeutic utility of B-type natriuretic peptide in patients with renal insufficiency and decompensated heart failure. Rev Cardiovasc Med 2004; 5:16–25.

McCully KS: Chemical pathology of homocysteine. I. Atherogenesis. Ann Clin Lab Sci 1993; 23:477–493.

Mair J: Progress in myocardial damage detection: new biochemical markers for clinicians. Crit Rev Clin Lab Sci 1997; 34:1–66.
Though some new information is missing, gives a relatively complete review of the biochemistry of cardiac markers.

Mair J, Artner-Dworzak E, Dienstl A, et al: Early detection of acute myocardial infarction by measurement of mass concentration of creatine kinase-MB. Am J Cardiol 1991; 68:1545–1550.

Mair J, Wagner I, Morass B, et al: Cardiac troponin I release correlates with myocardial infarction size. Eur J Clin Chem Clin Biochem 1995; 33:869–872.

Maisel AS, Krishnaswamy P, Nowak RM, et al: Rapid measurement of B-type natriuretic peptide in the emergency diagnosis of heart failure. N Engl J Med 2002; 347:161–167.

Malinow MR, Bostom AG, Krauss RM: Homocyst(e)ine, diet, and cardiovascular diseases: a statement for healthcare professionals from the Nutrition Committee, American Heart Association. Circulation 1999; 99:178–182.

Marmor A, Margolis T, Alpan G, et al: Regional distribution of the MB isoenzyme of creatine kinase in the human heart. Arch Pathol Lab Med 1980; 104:425–427.

Marmor A, Sobel BE, Roberts R: Factors presaging early recurrent myocardial infarction ('extension'). Am J Cardiol 1981; 48:603–610.

Missov E, Calzolari C, Pau B: Circulating cardiac troponin I in severe congestive heart failure. Circulation 1997; 96:2953–2958.

Missov E, Mair J: A novel biochemical approach to congestive heart failure: cardiac troponin T. Am Heart J 1999; 138:95–99.

Montague C, Kircher T: Myoglobin in the early evaluation of acute chest pain. Am J Clin Pathol 1995; 104:472–476.

Morjana NA: Degradation of human cardiac troponin I after myocardial infarction. Biotechnol Appl Biochem 1998; 28(Pt 2):105–111.

Morrow DA: Troponins in patients with acute coronary syndromes: biologic, diagnostic, and therapeutic implications. Cardiovasc Toxicol 2001; 1:105–110.

Morrow DA, Antman EM, Tanasijevic M, et al: Cardiac troponin I for stratification of early outcomes and the efficacy of enoxaparin in unstable angina: a TIMI-11B substudy. J Am Coll Cardiol 2000; 36:1812–1817.

Mueller C, Scholer A, Laule-Kilian K, et al: Use of B-type natriuretic peptide in the evaluation and management of acute dyspnea. N Engl J Med 2004; 350:647–654.

Mukoyama M, Nakao K, Hosoda K, et al: Brain natriuretic peptide as a novel cardiac hormone in humans. Evidence for an exquisite dual natriuretic peptide system, atrial natriuretic peptide and brain natriuretic peptide. J Clin Invest 1991; 87:1402–1412.

Muller-Bardorff M, Hallermayer K, Schroder A, et al: Improved troponin T ELISA specific for cardiac troponin T isoform: assay development and analytical and clinical validation. Clin Chem 1997; 43:458–466.

Muller-Bardorff M, Rauscher T, Kampmann M, et al: Quantitative bedside assay for cardiac troponin T: a complementary method to centralized laboratory testing. Clin Chem 1999; 45:1002–1008.

Mutlu B, Yilmaz A, Sonmez K, et al: Prognostic importance of predischarged troponin T levels in acute anterior myocardial infarction. Jpn Heart J 2004; 45:43–52.

National Cholesterol Education Program Expert Panel: Third Report of the National Cholesterol Education Program (NCEP) Expert Panel on Detection, Evaluation, and Treatment of High Blood Cholesterol in Adults (Adult Treatment Panel III) Final Report. Bethesda, MD, National Institutes of Health, 2002. Online. Available: http://www.nhlbi.nih.gov/guidelines/cholesterol/atp3xsum.pdf 13 October 2004.

Newby LK, Ohman EM, Christenson RH, et al: Benefit of glycoprotein IIb/IIIa inhibition in patients with acute coronary syndromes and troponin T-positive status: the PARAGON-B troponin T substudy. Circulation 2001; 103:2891–2896.

Newman DJ, Olabiran Y, Bedzyk WD, et al: Impact of antibody specificity and calibration material on the measure of agreement between methods for cardiac troponin I. Clin Chem 1999; 45:822–828.

Nielsen OW, McDonagh TA, Robb SD, et al: Retrospective analysis of the cost-effectiveness of using plasma brain natriuretic peptide in screening for left ventricular systolic dysfunction in the general population. J Am Coll Cardiol 2003; 41:113–120.

Nosanchuk JS, Combs B, Abbott G: False increases of troponin I attributable to incomplete separation of serum. Clin Chem 1999; 45:714.

Okumura H, Iuchi K, Yoshida T, et al: Brain natriuretic peptide is a predictor of anthracycline-induced cardiotoxicity. Acta Haematol 2000; 104:158–163.

Omland T, Persson A, Ng L, et al: N-terminal pro-B-type natriuretic peptide and long-term mortality in acute coronary syndromes. Circulation 2002; 106:2913–2918.

Omura T, Teragaki M, Takagi M, et al: Myocardial infarct size by serum troponin T and myosin light chain 1 concentration. Jpn Circ J 1995; 59:154–159.

Packer M: Should B-type natriuretic peptide be measured routinely to guide the diagnosis and management of chronic heart failure? Circulation 2003; 108:2950–2953.

Panteghini M, Pagani F: Biological variation of myoglobin in serum. Clin Chem 1997; 43:2435.

Panteghini M, Cuccia C, Bonetti G, et al: Single-point cardiac troponin T at coronary care unit discharge after myocardial infarction correlates with infarct size and ejection fraction. Clin Chem 2002; 48:1432–1436.

Panteghini M, Pagani F, Yeo KT, et al: Evaluation of imprecision for cardiac troponin assays at low-range concentrations. Clin Chem 2004; 50:327–332.

Paoletti R, Gotto AM Jr, Hajjar DP: Inflammation in atherosclerosis and implications for therapy. Circulation 2004; 109:III20–III26.
Discusses the role of inflammation in CHD.

Parry DM, Krahn J, Leroux M, et al: False positive analytical interference of cardiac troponin I assays: an important consideration for method selection. Clin Biochem 1999; 32:667–669.

Pearson TA, Mensah GA, Alexander RW, et al: Markers of inflammation and cardiovascular disease: application to clinical and public health practice: A statement for healthcare professionals from the Centers for Disease Control and Prevention and the American Heart Association. Circulation 2003; 107:499–511.

Polanczyk CA, Lee TH, Cook EF, et al: Cardiac troponin I as a predictor of major cardiac events in emergency department patients with acute chest pain. J Am Coll Cardiol 1998; 32:8–14.

Pope JH, Aufderheide TP, Ruthazer R, et al: Missed diagnoses of acute cardiac ischemia in the emergency department. N Engl J Med 2000; 342:1163–1170.

Priori SG, Napolitano C: Genetics of cardiac arrhythmias and sudden cardiac death. Ann N Y Acad Sci 2004; 1015:96–110.

Puleo PR, Meyer D, Wathen C, et al: Use of a rapid assay of subforms of creatine kinase-MB to diagnose or rule out acute myocardial infarction. N Engl J Med 1994; 331:561–566.

Rabitzsch G, Mair J, Lechleitner P, et al: Immunoenzymometric assay of human glycogen phosphorylase isoenzyme BB in diagnosis of ischemic myocardial injury. Clin Chem 1995; 41:966–978.

Rao AC, Naeem N, John C, et al: Direct current cardioversion does not cause cardiac damage: evidence from cardiac troponin T estimation. Heart 1998; 80:229–230.

Ravkilde J, Botker HE, Sogaard P, et al: Human ventricular myosin light chain isotype 1 as a marker of myocardial injury. Cardiology 1994; 84:135–144.

Ravkilde J, Nissen H, Horder M, et al: Independent prognostic value of serum creatine kinase isoenzyme MB mass, cardiac troponin T and myosin light chain levels in suspected acute myocardial infarction. Analysis of 28 months of follow-up in 196 patients. J Am Coll Cardiol 1995; 25:574–581.

Reynolds GD, Vance RP: C-reactive protein immunohistochemical localization in normal and atherosclerotic human aortas. Arch Pathol Lab Med 1987; 111:265–269.

Richards AM, Lainchbury JG, Nicholls MG, et al: *Dendroaspis* natriuretic peptide: endogenous or dubious? Lancet 2002; 359:5–6.

Ridker PM, Brown NJ, Vaughan DE, et al: Established and emerging plasma biomarkers in the prediction of first atherothrombotic events. Circulation 2004a; 109:IV6–19.
Concise review of many established and proposed risk factors for CHD.

Ridker PM, Cushman M, Stampfer MJ, et al: Inflammation, aspirin, and the risk of cardiovascular disease in apparently healthy men. N Engl J Med 1997; 336:973–979.
One of the earlier major studies to establish CRP as a risk factor for CHD.

Ridker PM, Rifai N, Rose L, et al: Comparison of C-reactive protein and low-density lipoprotein cholesterol levels in the prediction of first cardiovascular events. N Engl J Med 2002; 347:1557–1565.

Ridker PM, Wilson PW, Grundy SM: Should C-reactive protein be added to metabolic syndrome and to assessment of global cardiovascular risk? Circulation 2004b, 109:2818–2825.

Roberts RF, Roberts WL: Performance characteristics of a recombinant enzymatic cycling assay for quantification of total homocysteine in serum or plasma. Clin Chim Acta 2004; 344:95–99.

Roberts WL, Calcote CB, De BK, et al: Prevention of analytical false-positive increases of cardiac troponin I on the Stratus II analyzer. Clin Chem 1997; 43:860–861.

Roe CR: Diagnosis of myocardial infarction by serum isoenzyme analysis. Ann Clin Lab Sci 1977; 7:201–209.

Roongsritong C, Warraich I, Bradley C: Common causes of troponin elevations in the absence of acute myocardial infarction: incidence and clinical significance. Chest 2004; 125:1877–1884.

Ross R: The pathogenesis of atherosclerosis: a perspective for the 1990s. Nature 1993; 362:801–809.
Discussion of the pathogenesis of CHD.

Roy D, Quiles J, Aldama G, et al: Ischemia modified albumin for the assessment of patients presenting to the emergency department with acute chest pain but normal or non-diagnostic 12-lead electrocardiograms and negative cardiac troponin T. Int J Cardiol 2004; 97:297–301.

Sawada Y, Suda M, Yokoyama H, et al: Stretch-induced hypertrophic growth of cardiocytes and processing of brain-type natriuretic peptide are controlled by proprotein-processing endoprotease furin. J Biol Chem 1997; 272:20545–20554.

Schirger JA, Heublein DM, Chen HH, et al: Presence of *Dendroaspis* natriuretic peptide-like immunoreactivity in human plasma and its increase during human heart failure. Mayo Clin Proc 1999; 74:126–130.

Schulz-Knappe P, Forssmann K, Herbst F, et al: Isolation and structural analysis of 'urodilatin,' a new peptide of the cardiodilatin-(ANP)-family, extracted from human urine. Klin Wochenschr 1988; 66:752–759.

Schweitz H, Vigne P, Moinier D, et al: A new member of the natriuretic peptide family is present in the venom of the green mamba (*Dendroaspis angusticeps*). J Biol Chem 1992; 267:13928–13932.

Shi Q, Ling M, Zhang X, et al: Degradation of cardiac troponin I in serum complicates comparisons of cardiac troponin I assays. Clin Chem 1999; 45:1018–1025.

Shipchandler MT, Moore EG: Rapid, fully automated measurement of plasma homocyst(e)ine with the Abbott IMx analyzer. Clin Chem 1995; 41:991–994.

Shyu KG, Kuan PL, Cheng JJ, et al: Cardiac troponin T, creatine kinase, and its isoform release after successful percutaneous transluminal coronary angioplasty with or without stenting. Am Heart J 1998; 135:862–867.

Sinha MK, Roy D, Gaze DC, et al: Role of 'ischemia modified albumin,' a new biochemical marker of myocardial ischaemia, in the early diagnosis of acute coronary syndromes. Emerg Med J 2004; 21:29–34.

Spevack DM, Schwartzbard A: B-type natriuretic peptide measurement in heart failure. Clin Cardiol 2004; 27:489–494.

Stampfer MJ, Malinow MR, Willett WC, et al: A prospective study of plasma homocyst(e)ine and risk of myocardial infarction in US physicians. JAMA 1992; 268:877–881.

Stampfer MJ, Ridker PM, Dzau VJ: Risk factor criteria. Circulation 2004; 109:IV3–IV5.

Storrow AB, Gibler WB: Chest pain centers: diagnosis of acute coronary syndromes. Ann Emerg Med 2000; 35:449–461.

Strong JP, Malcom GT, McMahan CA et al: Prevalence and extent of atherosclerosis in adolescents and young adults: implications for prevention from the Pathobiological Determinants of Atherosclerosis in Youth Study. JAMA 1999; 281:727–735.

Sudoh T, Kangawa K, Minamino N, et al: A new natriuretic peptide in porcine brain. Nature 1988; 332:78–81.

Sudoh T, Minamino N, Kangawa K, et al: C-type natriuretic peptide (CNP): a new member of natriuretic peptide family identified in porcine brain. Biochem Biophys Res Commun 1990; 168:863–870.

Szalai AJ, Agrawal A, Greenhough TJ, et al: C-reactive protein: structural biology and host defense function. Clin Chem Lab Med 1999; 37:265–270.

Tabbibizar R, Maisel A: The impact of B-type natriuretic peptide levels on the diagnoses and management of congestive heart failure. Curr Opin Cardiol 2002; 17:340–345.

Tan Y, Tang L, Sun X, et al: Total-homocysteine enzymatic assay. Clin Chem 2000; 46:1686–1688.

Tanasijevic MJ, Cannon CP, Wybenga DR, et al: Myoglobin, creatine kinase MB, and cardiac troponin-I to assess reperfusion after thrombolysis for acute myocardial infarction: results from TIMI 10A. Am Heart J 1997; 134:622–630.

Tang WH, Girod JP, Lee MJ, et al: Plasma B-type natriuretic peptide levels in ambulatory patients with established chronic symptomatic systolic heart failure. Circulation 2003; 108:2964–2966.

Tate JR, Heathcote D, Rayfield J, et al: The lack of standardization of cardiac troponin I assay systems. Clin Chim Acta 1999; 284:141–149.

Taylor MR, Carniel E, Mestroni L: Familial hypertrophic cardiomyopathy: clinical features, molecular genetics and molecular genetic testing. Expert Rev Mol Diagn 2004; 4:99–113.

Thambyrajah J, Townend JN: Homocysteine and atherothrombosis – mechanisms for injury. Eur Heart J 2000; 21:967–974.

Troughton RW, Frampton CM, Yandle TG, et al: Treatment of heart failure guided by plasma aminoterminal brain natriuretic peptide (N-BNP) concentrations. Lancet 2000; 355:1126–1130.

Tucker JF, Collins RA, Anderson AJ, et al: Value of serial myoglobin levels in the early diagnosis of patients admitted for acute myocardial infarction. Ann Emerg Med 1994; 24:704–708.

Tzvetanova E: Creatine kinase isoenzymes in muscle tissue of patients with neuromuscular diseases and human fetuses. Enzyme 1971; 12:279.

Ubbink JB, Delport R, Riezler R, et al: Comparison of three different plasma homocysteine assays with gas chromatography–mass spectrometry. Clin Chem 1999; 45:670–675.

Uji Y, Sugiuchi H, Okabe H: Measurement of human ventricular myosin light chain-1 by monoclonal solid-phase enzyme immunoassay in patients with acute myocardial infarction. J Clin Lab Anal 1991; 5:242–246.

Väänänen A, Syrjälä H, Rahkila P, et al: Serum carbonic anhydrase III and myoglobin concentrations in acute myocardial infarction. Clin Chem 1990; 36:635–638.

Van Nieuwenhoven FA, Kleine AH, Wodzig WH, et al: Discrimination between myocardial and skeletal muscle injury by assessment of the plasma ratio of myoglobin over fatty acid-binding protein. Circulation 1995; 92:2848–2854.

Venge P, Johnston N, Lagerqvist B, et al: Clinical and analytical performance of the liaison cardiac troponin I assay in unstable coronary artery disease, and the impact of age on the definition of reference limits. A FRISC-II substudy. Clin Chem 2003; 49:880–886.

Vester B, Rasmussen K: High performance liquid chromatography method for rapid and accurate determination of homocysteine in plasma and serum. Eur J Clin Chem Clin Biochem 1991; 29:549–554.

Vignini A, Nanetti L, Bacchetti T, et al: Modification induced by homocysteine and low-density lipoprotein on human aortic endothelial cells: an in vitro study. J Clin Endocrinol Metab 2004; 89:4558–4561.

Weber M, Dill T, Arnold R, et al: N-terminal B-type natriuretic peptide predicts extent of coronary artery disease and ischemia in patients with stable angina pectoris. Am Heart J 2004; 148:612–620.

Weissberg PL: Atherogenesis: current understanding of the causes of atheroma. Heart 2000; 83:247–252.

Wevers RA, Delsing M, Klein Gebbink JA, et al: Post-synthetic changes in creatine kinase isozymes (EC 2.7.3.2). Clin Chim Acta 1978; 86:323–327.

Willems HP, Den HM, Lindemans J, et al: Measurement of total homocysteine concentrations in acidic citrate- and EDTA-containing tubes by different methods. Clin Chem 2004; 50:1881–1883.

Witztum JL: The oxidation hypothesis of atherosclerosis. Lancet 1994; 344:793–795.

Wiviott SD, de Lemos JA, Morrow DA: Pathophysiology, prognostic significance and clinical utility of B-type natriuretic peptide in acute coronary syndromes. Clin Chim Acta 2004; 346:119–128.

Wolf PL: Lactate dehydrogenase isoenzymes in myocardial disease. Clin Lab Med 1989; 9:655–665.

Woo J, Lacbawan FL, Sunheimer R, et al: Is myoglobin useful in the diagnosis of acute myocardial infarction in the emergency department setting? Am J Clin Pathol 1995; 103:725–729.

Wu AH, Feng YJ, Moore R, et al: Characterization of cardiac troponin subunit release into serum after acute myocardial infarction and comparison of assays for troponin T and I. American Association for Clinical Chemistry Subcommittee on cTnI Standardization. Clin Chem 1998; 44:1198–1208.

Yap S: Classical homocystinuria: vascular risk and its prevention. J Inherit Metab Dis 2003; 26:259–265.

Yudkin JS, Stehouwer CD, Emeis JJ, et al: C-reactive protein in healthy subjects: associations with obesity, insulin resistance, and endothelial dysfunction: a potential role for cytokines originating from adipose tissue? Arterioscler Thromb Vasc Biol 1999; 19:972–978.

Zabel M, Hohnloser SH, Koster W, et al: Analysis of creatine kinase, CK-MB, myoglobin, and troponin T time–activity curves for early assessment of coronary artery reperfusion after intravenous thrombolysis. Circulation 1993; 87:1542–1550.

Zalenski RJ, Rydman RJ, Ting S, et al: A national survey of emergency department chest pain centers in the United States. Am J Cardiol 1998; 81:1305–1309.

Zaman AG, Helft G, Worthley SG, et al: The role of plaque rupture and thrombosis in coronary artery disease. Atherosclerosis 2000; 149:251–266.

Zanotti G: Muscle fatty acid-binding protein. Biochim Biophys Acta 1999; 1441:94–105.

CHAPTER 19

Specific Proteins

Richard A. McPherson MD

KEY POINTS

• The primary structure of a protein is its linear sequence of amino acids with different side groups, which determine how the protein folds on itself (secondary and tertiary structures) and how it reacts with other molecules and cells (i.e., its molecular identity).

• Methods to quantitate and fractionate proteins are based on turbidimetry, colorimetry, absorption spectrophotometry, dye binding, column chromatography, electrophoresis, and immunoassays.

• Protein electrophoresis separates proteins according to their electrical charges (usually at pH 8.6).

• The major proteins in plasma that contribute to the electrophoretic pattern are albumin, α_1-antitrypsin, α_2-macroglobulin, haptoglobin, β-lipoprotein, transferrin, complement C3, fibrinogen, and immunoglobulins.

• Several minor components of plasma proteins have clinical utility in diagnosing and monitoring diseases, such as ceruloplasmin, C-reactive protein, prealbumin, and protease inhibitors, and are quantitated by immunoassays.

• Patterns of protein electrophoresis in serum and urine are characteristic of specific diseases primarily involving changes in synthetic rates (liver), loss (renal), or inflammatory states.

• Hereditary deficiency of some plasma proteins leads to significant diseases (e.g., α_1-antitrypsin).

• Proteins in plasma play several roles including maintaining oncotic pressure, transporting small molecules, and promoting or inhibiting inflammatory reactions.

• The major clinical use of serum and urine protein electrophoresis is to screen for monoclonal gammopathies.

Examination of the proteins in plasma can provide information reflecting disease states in many different organ systems. The most frequently performed measurement, that for total protein, is usually performed on serum, which has no fibrinogen and no anticoagulant that may slightly dilute proteins in plasma. Although total protein determination gives the physician some information as to a patient's general status regarding nutrition or severe organ disease (as in protein-losing states), further fractionations yield far more clinically useful information.

Additional quantitation of albumin, for example, is more informative regarding nutritional status, liver synthetic capacity, or protein-losing nephropathy or enteropathy. It also allows the clinician to interpret high or low calcium and magnesium levels, because albumin binds about one-half of each of those ions on a molar basis. The calculated difference between total protein and albumin represents the value of all globulins, a composite of the other fractions that individually may rise several fold in severe disorders.

Protein electrophoresis separates the globulins from albumin and resolves the major proteins of serum into patterns that may be highly specific for some diseases. High-resolution techniques can provide a display of all the components in concentrations down to about 1 g/L (0.1 g/dL in traditional units); however, at that level, quantitation by scanning of stained proteins is not highly reliable and alternative methods should be employed. Such techniques, involving immunologic detection of individual proteins, have the dual advantages of specificity and sensitivity over electrophoresis (Ch. 43).

Yet there is much to be appreciated from visual inspection of an electrophoretogram of proteins, because the human eye is highly efficient at detecting subtle variations in individual proteins as well as alterations in protein patterns. Identification of these patterns is a useful screening method to be followed by more specific confirmatory procedures to identify and quantitate aberrant protein bands. Protein electrophoresis also can be a useful tool for monitoring patients over long periods of time when there are marked alterations in levels of particular proteins such as in myeloma, nephrotic syndrome, cirrhosis, or extensive body burn.

This chapter reviews protein structure, methodologies of measurement and separation, the major plasma proteins (except for coagulation factors, immunoglobulins, and the complement system, which are covered in Chs 38, 45, and 46), and some of the patterns encountered in particular disease states.

Protein Structure

The backbone of all protein molecules is a continuous chain of carbon and nitrogen atoms joined together through *peptide bonds* between adjacent *amino acids*. At one end (the amino-terminus), there is a free amino group, and at the other end (the carboxy-terminus), there is a free carboxyl group. Whereas the peptide backbone is qualitatively invariant between different proteins (its total length is equivalent to the total number of amino acids in a particular protein), proteins have structural identity by virtue of the side groups or residues of the constituent amino acids. The average molecular weight of an amino acid is 120 Da. Serum proteins range in size from roughly 66 kDa to over 700 kDa. These amino acid side chains are conventionally grouped according to chemical nature: *hydrogen* (glycine), *aliphatic* (alanine, valine, leucine, and isoleucine), *hydroxymethylamino* (serine and threonine), *aromatic* (tyrosine, phenyl-alanine, and tryptophan), *imino* (proline and hydroxyproline), *acidic* (aspartate and glutamate), *basic* (arginine, histidine, and lysine), *amides* (asparagine and glutamine), and *sulfur-containing* (cysteine and methionine). These different side chains are charged, polar, or hydrophobic, resulting in the tendency for them to be relatively soluble or insoluble in water, respectively.

The linear sequence of the amino acids in a protein is called its *primary structure*; this sequence of amino acids determines the identity of a protein, what its molecular structure is, what functions it can perform, how it can bind to other molecules, and how it can participate in processes of recognition between molecules and cells. These biological interactions are guided by reactivities between charged groups on one molecule and those on another and similarly by hydrophobic interactions between molecules. Analytic processes such as chromatography, electrophoresis, dye binding, light absorbance, and others also depend on the primary amino acid sequence.

The *secondary structure* refers to specific regular three-dimensional conformations into which portions of the polypeptide chain fold. There are three such structures (Branden, 1991). First is the α-helix, in which the chain forms a regular helix such that the backbone C=O of the *i*th peptide group hydrogen bonds to the N–H of the $(i + 4)$th peptide unit. The second is β-pleated sheets in fully extended structures, in which the chain forms a flat structure such that the side chains of adjacent amino acids point in opposite directions; in this conformation, two or more extended chains can associate so that the maximum number of C=O ● ● ● H–N bonds form between them. β-Pleated sheets can have their individual β-strands in parallel or antiparallel orientations. Finally, a third grouping of structures is the bend conformation, in which the direction of the polypeptide chain reverses itself, thereby allowing long primary structures to bend back on themselves and assume compact conformations.

The core of a protein molecule typically consists of combinations of α-helices and β-strands linked by loops of various lengths and shape. This inner core generally contains hydrophobic amino acids, whereas the loops and other surface portions of the protein molecule are richer in polar and charged amino acids that are hydrophilic. Upon degradation, some proteins (e.g., serum amyloid-associated protein, immunoglobulin light chains, prealbumin) release fragments rich in β-regions. These fragments are capable of coming together spontaneously in vivo to form deposits of β-sheets in fibrils that constitute amyloid. Recent work has shown an association between the genotype of apolipoprotein E (especially the allele *apoE-4*) and the progression of late-onset Alzheimer's disease, in which cerebral plaques of amyloid form within the brain. These genetic findings suggest that Alzheimer's disease may be understood and treated as a disease that has a biochemical basis in β-pleated sheet generation (Roses, 1994; Hayashi, 2004).

Molecular regions with clusters of hydrophobic side groups tend to remain on the interior of a protein that is soluble in water, whereas those regions with clusters of charges or other hydrophilic moieties tend to appear on the protein's surface. Conversely, proteins that are membrane bound usually have a distinct hydrophobic segment that protrudes to anchor the protein molecule in the lipid phase of the membrane. The actual three-dimensional structure or folding pattern of the protein, uniquely determined by its amino acid sequence, is termed its *tertiary structure*. Individual proteins or monomeric subunits may form more stable complexes, such as dimers, trimers, and tetramers, which is termed *quaternary structure*.

The sulfhydryl group on a cysteine residue can form a *disulfide* (covalent) bond with another cysteine within the same protein to hold different segments tightly together. This action helps stabilize the whole structure from disruption by mechanical, thermal, or other forces. These intramolecular disulfide bonds most likely form after spontaneous protein folding along the linear amino acid sequence into thermodynamically most stable conformations. Disulfide bonds can also form between cysteine residues on different molecules, thereby stabilizing multimeric molecular structures (e.g., haptoglobin, von Willebrand's antigen).

The acidic and basic amino acids determine the net charge on a protein and hence its electrophoretic mobility. The charge on carboxyl and amino groups is a function of pH (i.e., whether a hydrogen ion is bound to or dissociated from the group). Combining all the different side groups and their different degrees of dissociation, the pH at which a particular protein has net charge equal to zero is called its *isoelectric point* (pI). Proteins with pI less than 7 are acidic and tend to have carboxyl side groups exposed, whereas those with pI greater than 7 are basic (e.g., histones that, in turn, bind to the external helical structure of DNA that is negatively charged with phosphate groups).

Proteins are synthesized from the amino end to the carboxyl end by ribosomes translating from the information encoded in messenger RNA (mRNA). The initial translation product of some proteins is acted on before secretion by proteolytic enzymes that convert a preform to the mature protein by removal of a signal peptide (generally hydrophobic) that otherwise holds the new protein molecule to the endoplasmic reticulum. Release of a preprotein from the endoplasmic reticulum entails passage through a membrane pore with the participation of various translocation factors (Brodsky, 1998). The correct assembly of a protein may also critically depend on the function of so-called molecular chaperones, which are other proteins that guide the folding of nascent proteins in concert with proteases that remove selective segments to achieve functional conformations (Wickner, 1999). Many genetic diseases are due to harmful mutations in DNA leading to alterations in the amino acid sequence of a protein that may block this complex assembly process or that may render any assembled protein molecules nonfunctional (Kuznetsov, 1998).

Additional modifications to protein structures occur post-translationally (i.e., after joining of the amino acids is complete) (Harding, 1985). *Phosphorylation* consists of the enzymatically regulated attachment of phosphate groups to serine or threonine groups in the peptide backbone, thereby forming phosphoproteins with a more negative charge. *Glycosylation* can occur either spontaneously, in the presence of sugar molecules, or in a directed manner under enzymatic control in which oligosaccharides, frequently terminating with sialic acid (which carries a negative charge), are attached to the protein (Van den Steen, 1998). These species of molecules are termed glycoproteins. Linkages are generally to asparagine residues through *N*-acetylglucosamine or to serine and threonine residues through *N*-acetylgalactosamine. *Proteolysis* results in the cleavage or removal of short segments of the peptide backbone that can open up catalytic sites of a zymogen (e.g., plasminogen to plasmin) or facilitate recognition by a receptor molecule (e.g., proinsulin to insulin). Many of these post-translational steps are unique to eukaryotic cells and do not occur in prokaryotic cells; this point is very important to the biotechnology industry, which uses cloned genes to produce human proteins in bacteria, yeast, or other artificial cell types and so must take additional steps to synthesize accurate molecules (Jenkins, 1996). Post-translational changes in the structure of proteins influence their antigenicity, specific chemical or catalytic activities, abilities to bind to receptors, and electrophoretic mobilities.

Techniques of Protein Separation

Electrophoresis

Modern understanding of the protein composition of serum and plasma derives from the electrophoretic techniques introduced by Tiselius. He separated proteins dissolved in an electrolyte solution by application of an electric current through a U-shaped quartz tube that held the protein solution. At pH 7.6, four serum protein fractions, designated albumin, α, β, and γ, were identified and quantified optically by change in refractive index at the boundaries among these bands. Because separation was achieved in a homogeneous solution without solid support medium, convective forces prevented resolution into distinct zones. Hence, this technique has been termed *moving boundary* or *frontal electrophoresis*. Introduction of filter paper as an anticonvection support medium permitted separation of the protein fractions into discrete bands or zones in a process termed *zonal electrophoresis* . On solid support medium and at pH 8.6, the α fraction further splits into two groups of proteins, $α_1$ and $α_2$. Other support media have been used, such as cellulose acetate membrane, agarose gel, starch gel, and polyacrylamide gel. Cellulose acetate and agarose have predominated in the clinical laboratory because of ease of use, low cost, and commercial availability (Jeppsson, 1979).

Application of samples can be done in wells that are cut into the gel, but this process typically leaves an artifact that can interfere with the scan. A method to get around this problem involves soaking the sample into the gel by means of an overlying template. Each end of the gel is then immersed into separate buffer chambers in which electrodes are mounted. A voltage is applied between the electrodes generating a current that passes through the gel, usually for a period of about 30 minutes, to achieve desired resolution. The ionic strength of the buffer determines the amount of current and the movement of the proteins for a fixed voltage. If ionic strength is low, relatively more current is carried by the charged proteins. If the ionic strength is high, less current is carried by the proteins, which move a shorter distance. If the electrodes are not properly aligned, the current may be denser on one side of the gel than on the other; proteins will migrate further on the side with more current. If the electrophoresis proceeds too long, the proteins may migrate off the gel into the buffer. If there is a break in the electrical circuit and no current passes, the proteins will not move from the point of application. Frequently gels show the 'smile artifact' in which samples at the center of the gel migrate further than those at the edges.

Following electrophoresis, the gel is treated with a mild fixative, such as acetic acid, that precipitates the proteins at the positions to which they have migrated. They are then stained, and the gel is dried and cleared of excess stain. Protein patterns can be inspected visually for qualitative identification of abnormal proteins. Densitometric scanners are used to generate tracings and quantitate the relative percentages of protein in each fraction. Those percentages are then multiplied by the total protein

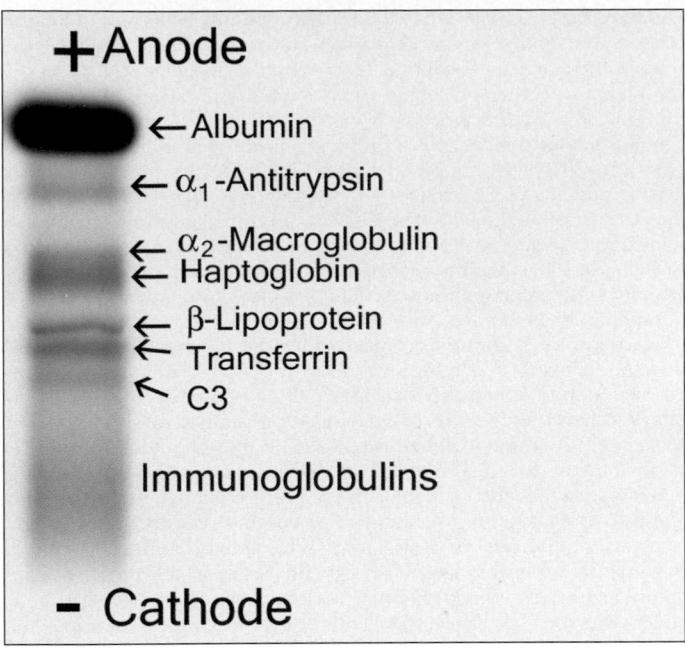

19–1 Positions of major serum proteins in a normal person using electrophoresis in agarose. Individual proteins separate according to their electrical charge between the anode (positive pole) and cathode (negative pole).

(separately measured) in the sample to yield the concentration of protein in each fraction.

When an electrophoretic support medium has a negative charge, the electromotive force to which it is subjected tends to move it toward the anode (positive pole; Fig. 19–1). However, the solid support medium is fixed and so it cannot move. The complementary positively charged ions in the surrounding buffer are free to move under the electromotive force, and they carry with them molecules of the solvent water, which are clustered around their charges. The net result is flow of buffer toward the cathode. This buffer flow is termed *electro-osmosis* or *endosmosis*, which also carries the proteins with it to some extent by mechanical flow, not by charge. The actual distance traveled by a particular protein migrating in an electrical field is determined by the combined magnitudes of the electromotive force (a feature of the protein itself and the pH) and the electro-osmotic force (a function primarily of the support medium). When the electro-osmotic force is greater than the electrophoretic force acting on weakly anionic proteins (e.g., γ-globulins), those proteins move from the application point toward the cathode, even though their charge is slightly negative.

Through critical manipulations of buffer salt composition, endosmotic properties of the medium, and means of sample application, commercially available electrophoretic agarose plates now achieve consistently high-resolution qualities that allow routine separation of all the major serum protein species (Fig. 19–2). Because of variability in chemical formulations of gels, it should not necessarily be expected that each manufacturer's electrophoretic system will yield identical protein separation patterns. Furthermore, optimal separation of isoenzymes generally requires different buffer and gel composition compared with the conditions for best resolution of serum proteins versus lipoproteins versus hemoglobins. A significant variation in conditions for protein electrophoresis is that for optimizing the separation of the γ-region to resolve and detect oligoclonal bands of immunoglobulin in cerebrospinal fluid (CSF). In this case, the endosmosis is set high to maximize the cathodal movement of immunoglobulins from the point of application over a span of the gel that is convenient for visual inspection.

Polyacrylamide is an inert support medium whose porosity is easily adjusted by changing the composition of acrylamide prior to polymerization. Although *polyacrylamide gel electrophoresis* (PAGE) is applicable to standard separation of native proteins, it can also be used for separating proteins according to molecular weight when they are denatured in the presence of sodium dodecyl sulfate (SDS). SDS-PAGE is at present the most widely used protein electrophoretic technique for research in molecular biology. However, its very power for resolving proteins and separating them into multitudinous subunits has virtually excluded it from routine use in the clinical laboratory. Nevertheless, there is promise for clinical application of *two-dimensional electrophoresis* (2-DE), which uses standard separation in one direction followed by SDS-PAGE in the perpendicular direction. 2-DE results in perhaps hundreds of identifiable protein peaks from which it may be possible to obtain important diagnostic information by sophisticated pattern analysis.

Isoelectric focusing affords superior resolution of closely migrating proteins or various forms of a single protein that differ in charge owing to minor modification (e.g., post-translational) (Ch. 4). By this technique, proteins migrate through a gel containing a gradient of pH established with a mixture of ampholytes. As each protein reaches the gel location where the pH is equal to its pI, the net charge on it becomes zero. It no longer has electromotive force acting on it, and it comes to rest. Thus the final pattern is strictly according to pI.

Precipitation

Chemical precipitations of serum proteins have been devised to resolve albumin and the globulins into two or more fractions that can then be measured for protein content. With the addition of sodium sulfate, sodium sulfite, ammonium sulfate, or methanol, the globulins tend to precipitate, leaving albumin in solution. By measuring total protein in the original serum and protein in either the precipitate or the supernatant, values for albumin and globulin can be derived. The ratio of these values

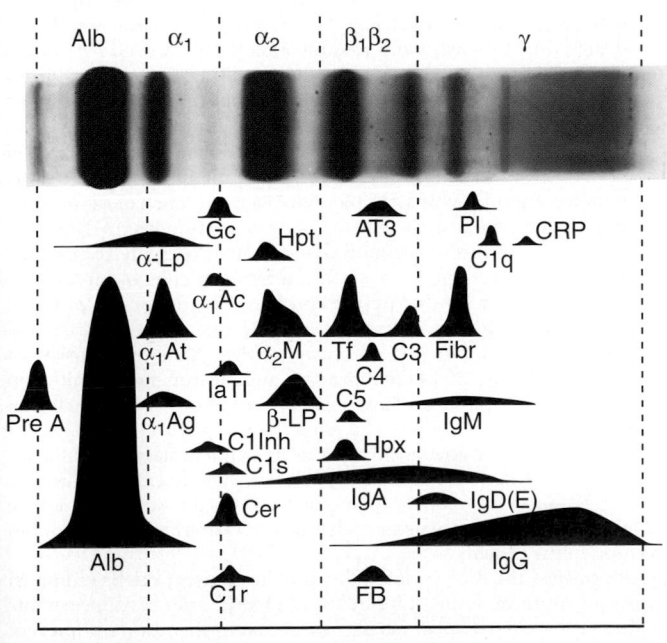

Figure 19–2 Plasma protein electrophoresis pattern in agarose gel is composed of five fractions, each composed of many individual species. Some of the major proteins are shown here in an artist's rendition for clarity. (Adapted from Laurell CB: Electrophoresis, specific protein assays, or both in measurement of plasma proteins? Clin Chem 1973; 19:99, with permission.)
α₁Ac = α₁-antichymotrypsin
α₁Ag = α₁-acid glycoprotein
α₁At = α₁-antitrypsin
α₂-M = α₂-macroglobulin
α-Lp = α-lipoprotein
Alb = albumin
AT3 = antithrombin III
β-Lp = β-lipoprotein
Complement components:
    C1q, C1r, C1s, C3, C4, C5 = as designated
    C1Inh = C1 esterase inhibitor
Cer = cerulosplasmin
CRP = C-reactive protein
Gc = Gc-globulin (vitamin D-binding protein)
FB = factor B
Fibr = fibrinogen
Hpt = haptoglobin
Hpx = hemopexin
Immunoglobulins
    IgA, IgD, IgE, IgG, IgM = as designated
IaTI = Inter-α-trypsin inhibitor
Pl = plasminogen
Pre A = prealbumin
Tf = Transferrin

(A/G ratio) has been used extensively because it accentuates abnormalities in serum protein composition, which in disease generally involve depression of albumin and elevation of one or more globulin fractions. Albumin may be depressed owing to either decreased synthesis (malnutrition, malabsorption, liver failure, diversion to synthesis of other proteins) or increased loss (proteinuria, accumulation of ascites fluid, enteropathy). Globulins may be elevated owing to increased synthesis of many different proteins as part of acute or chronic reactions to disease. The lowering of albumin and elevation of globulins tend to occur simultaneously in disease, thus leading to exaggerated changes in the A/G ratio as the numerator and denominator move in opposite directions. Precipitation methods are not as accurate as zonal electrophoresis, because some α-globulins may fail to precipitate and thus lead to an overestimate of the albumin fraction.

Preparative procedures for the isolation of a single minor protein constituent usually begin with a precipitation step to remove the bulk of other undesired serum proteins. The next step in protein isolation is typically a column that separates on the basis of molecular size (gel filtration) or charge (ion exchange).

Column Separations

Gel filtration media such as Sephadex or agarose beads are rated according to pore sizes, which, in turn, determine what size molecules can pass through the interior of each bead or particle of the column. After application of a sample composed of various-sized proteins in aqueous solvent containing buffer and salt, more of the buffer is applied to drive the sample through the column. Very large molecules tend to flow through interstices of the column without entering the beads and emerge first from the bottom of the column in the void volume. Slightly smaller molecules enter the largest pores before being washed through and so are slightly retarded in passing through the column. Small protein molecules pass into still smaller pores and are retained still longer. Finally, particles the size of dissolved salt penetrate farthest into the interior of gel filtration beads and come out after all the proteins have emerged in an amount of applied buffer called the salt volume. Thus, in gel filtration, the order of protein elution is by molecular weight or size from largest first to smallest last. Because all protein species continuously move through a gel filtration column all at the same time but with different rates, it is necessary to apply the sample in a small and uniform volume in order to optimize separation between peaks. Gel filtration requires that the medium be inert and not interact chemically or by charge with the proteins. It is not a method to be employed for high-resolution separation.

Ion exchange chromatography, on the other hand, takes advantage of the charge on proteins to bind them to beads of a charged support medium such as DEAE or QAE. In *anion exchange chromatography*, proteins are usually applied at a basic pH such as 8.6, at which they are either negatively charged (albumin and α_1-, α_2-, and β-globulins are anions) or have no net charge (γ-globulins). The neutral proteins pass immediately through an anion exchange column, whereas the anionic ones stick to the positively charged column matrix. If a buffer with a higher salt concentration is washed through, anions of the salt displace the anionic proteins and exchange for them by binding to the support medium. The proteins then elute from the column. By using a steadily increasing gradient of salt concentration in the eluting buffer, the proteins can be resolved according to charge. The ones with a small amount of charge will elute first, whereas those with the greatest charge (e.g., albumin) elute only when displaced by higher salt levels.

Alternatively, if pH is lowered while salt concentration is held low, anionic proteins acquire a net neutral or slightly positive charge and pass through the column. A gradient of falling pH can be used to resolve anionic proteins, with the order of elution being roughly β-, α_2-, and α_1-globulins, and albumin. Note that this order of elution is the reverse order of electrophoretic migration at pH 8.6, because in anion exchange chromatography, mobility is retarded according to net negative charge, whereas in electrophoresis the mobility is enhanced by that charge.

Cation exchange chromatography begins at an acid pH with the proteins having positive charge (cations) and adhering to a negatively charged column matrix such as carboxymethylcellulose. They can be displaced by the cations of high salt in an eluting buffer or by increasing the pH, which will reverse the charge on the proteins to negative. By cation exchange, albumin should elute first, followed by α_1-, α_2-, β-, and γ-globulins.

Another separation modality by column is *hydrophobic chromatography*, in which samples are applied at high salt and eluted with low salt. The support medium interacts with proteins according to hydrophobic nature and is a good complementary technique to follow ion exchange chromatography, in which the sample was eluted with high salt.

Affinity chromatography is based on specific binding between a protein of interest and another protein that has been covalently linked to the solid support medium of a column. For example, coagulation factor VIII complexed with von Willebrand factor (vWF) can be selectively removed from the other plasma proteins by passing plasma through a column that contains monoclonal anti-vWF antibody linked to the solid phase matrix. The factor VIII–vWF complex selectively binds to the column as other plasma proteins wash through. The factor VIII is then dissociated from the vWF, thereby allowing it to elute in a purified fraction suitable for transfusion therapy. Such antigen–antibody interactions may be disrupted by high salt concentration, change in pH, or a chemical denaturant, such as urea, in different applications. Other affinity chromatography gels use a binding phenomenon that mimics naturally occurring molecular interactions. Thus, some dyes coupled to agarose are able to bind albumin, thereby removing it selectively from serum. Therapeutic antibodies or their Fab portions are concentrated with affinity columns containing their intended target antigens (e.g., Digibind for digoxin; CroFab for crotalid snake venom). Immunoglobulins can also be absorbed from a sample by staphylococcal protein A coupled to the gel matrix. Many other separation schemes exist that effect a high degree of purification in a single step with affinity chromatography medium coupled to dyes, drugs, nucleotide cofactors, and sugars. A clinical test using affinity chromatography is quantitation of glycosylated hemoglobin using a dihydroxyboronate affinity matrix that selectively binds molecular species of hemoglobin to which glucose has been covalently attached, while allowing the nonglycosylated forms to pass through the column. The glycosylated hemoglobin is then separately eluted and quantitated.

Capillary electrophoresis is a separation method based on flow through a capillary tube that can be tailored to resolution of different molecules based on size, hydrophobicity, or stereospecificity. It is applicable to large molecules such as DNA or proteins as well as to small ones such as hormones or therapeutic drugs. Physically, the method is similar to high-performance liquid chromatography (HPLC), in which solvent is pumped through a column that retains or passes solutes according to chemical interactions. Capillary electrophoresis for serum proteins employs a column with properties similar to agarose, so the separation of proteins is comparable to that from electrophoresis. This analysis can be automated with a detector at the effluent end that detects and quantitates protein bands without the need for staining and separate scanning. Although equipment costs are relatively high for capillary electrophoresis, reagent and labor costs are low and the procedure is fast and very quantitative, leading to the promise of more widespread clinical applications in the future (Chen, 1991; Brinkman, 2004).

Protein Detection and Quantitation

The ultimate reference method for determining concentration of protein is the analysis for *nitrogen content*. Nitrogen is present uniformly along the peptide bonds throughout the length of a protein and more irregularly in the side groups wherever tryptophan, arginine, lysine, histidine, asparagine, or glutamine is present. The Kjeldahl technique consists of an acid digestion to release ammonium ions from nitrogen-containing compounds. The ammonium can then be quantitated by conversion to ammonia gas and titration as a base or by nesslerization, in which double iodides (potassium and mercuric) form a colored complex with ammonia in alkali. Although determination of nitrogen content can be extremely precise, its use for calculation of protein concentration depends on the exact protein composition of a sample, since each protein has a somewhat different nitrogen content according to amino acid composition. However, for a sample of a purified protein, nitrogen content is highly accurate for estimating protein concentration when the nitrogen content on a molar basis is already known for that purified protein. Knowledge of a protein's exact amino acid sequence allows an accurate calculation of what the nitrogen content should be. Because clinical samples consist of unpredictable mixtures of different proteins and measurement of nitrogen content is not a simple procedure, it is not commonly used in clinical laboratories.

Refractive index can be accurate for measuring serum protein concentration as dissolved solute for levels above 2.5 g/dL. Hemolysis, lipemia, icterus, and azotemia produce erroneously high results. Refractive index cannot be used for urine protein measurements because of excess amounts of solutes in relation to the protein.

Specific gravity (and thus, by inference, protein content) can be estimated by pipetting drops of serum or blood into a graded series of copper sulfate solutions. A protein–copper shell forms about the drop to prevent dissolution for a short interval, during which time the drop falls to the bottom, remains stationary, or rises to the top. The protein concentration of a sample is estimated from the specific gravity of the copper sulfate solution in which the drop remains stationary. This technique is simple and has been used widely as a screening test for hemoglobin concentration in whole blood.

Proteins in solution *absorb ultraviolet light* at 280 nm (A_{280}), owing mostly to tryptophan but also owing to tyrosine and phenylalanine (Layne, 1957). For accurate conversion of A_{280} readings to protein concentration, the molar absorptivity must be used, because each protein contains a different amount of these three amino acids. However, the A_{280} of a mixture of proteins is not a perfect measure of protein content, because molar absorptivities vary greatly between different proteins. Because nucleic acids (which absorb strongly at 260 nm and also somewhat at 280 nm) may be present in protein preparations, a better estimate of protein concentration in the presence of nucleic acids is given by the formula:

$$\text{Protein concentration (mg/mL)} = 1.55 \times A_{280} - 0.76 \times A_{260}$$

Direct measurements of absorbance can be used for quantitating proteins in the range of 0.05–1.5 mg/mL.

Turbidimetric methods are often used for a similar concentration range in CSF or urine. Protein forms precipitate on the addition of trichloroacetic acid, sulfosalicylic acid, or other acid reagent. The resulting turbidity can be used for protein quantitation by increment in optical density in comparison with similarly treated standards. However, these techniques are not specific to proteins, because other acid-insoluble substances such as nucleic acids can also precipitate.

A *colorimetric* technique highly specific for proteins and peptides is the *biuret* method by which copper salts in alkaline solution form a purple complex with substances containing two or more peptide bonds. Interferences are minimal, although ammonium ion may acidify the reaction, while hemoglobin and bilirubin absorb in the same region as the biuret complex (540–560 nm). The biuret method is extensively used in clinical laboratories, particularly in automated analyzers in which protein concentration can be measured down to 10 or 15 mg/dL.

Greater sensitivity can be obtained using the *Folin–Ciocalteu reagent* (or phenol reagent, phosphotungstomolybdic acid), which oxidizes phenolic compounds such as tyrosine and, in addition, tryptophan and histidine to give a deep blue color.

Lowry (1951) used the biuret method followed by the phenol reagent, which greatly enhanced color formation, because the phenol reagent can react with biuret complexes involving all the peptide bonds. The *Lowry assay* has been extensively used for consistently accurate determinations of protein concentration.

Further sensitivity for detection down to 1 µg of protein can be obtained using *Coomassie brilliant blue dye*, which is free of interferences from a very wide range of substances.

Comparable sensitivity is also obtained with *ninhydrin*, which develops a violet color by reacting with primary amines. This reagent is widely used for detection of peptides and amino acids after paper chromatogaphy and amino acid analyses from ion exchange columns as well as for detection of drugs on toxicology screens using thin-layer chromatography (Ch. 23).

Quantitation of albumin in the presence of other proteins is possible by virtue of the specific binding of albumin to certain dyes such as bromphenol blue, methyl orange, hydroxybenzeneazobenzoic acid (HABA), bromcresol purple, and bromcresol green (BCG). BCG is extensively used in automatic analyzers for determining serum albumin in parallel with biuret reagent for total protein. Dyes bound to albumin absorb maximally at slightly different wavelengths, thus allowing direct spectrophotometric quantitation of the albumin.

The standard dyes used for staining electrophoresis are Coomassie brilliant blue, Ponceau S, and amido black. For detection of minor components in high-resolution gels, silver staining is very sensitive down to nanogram quantities (Merril, 1981).

In addition, special dyes, such as Oil Red O and Sudan black, stain lipoproteins and periodic acid–Schiff stains glycoproteins separated in special electrophoretic applications.

Because electrophoresis followed by staining does not afford explicit identification of serum proteins, immunologic measurements have been instituted for quantitation of individual proteins (Laurell, 1966). Nephelometry detects the turbidity produced usually within minutes or less by the precipitation of a reagent antibody with its target protein in a serum sample (Maachi, 2004). The major serum proteins are now widely measured by this method on automated immunochemistry analyzers that have supplanted former measurements by radial immunodiffusion. Owing to the specificity of the antibody reagent, nephelometry has great specificity for quantitating individual proteins even in the presence of others. Proteins present in lower concentrations may also be quantitated

Table 19–1 Characteristics of Major Plasma Proteins

Protein	Concentration range (g/L)	Molecular weight	Actions
Prealbumin	0.15–0.36	62 000	Binds thyroxine; transports vitamin A
Albumin	39–51	66 000	Oncotic pressure; amino acid reservoir; carries small molecules
α_1-Antitrypsin	2.0–4.0	54 000	Protease inhibitor
α_2-Macroglobulin	1.5–3.5	725 000	Protease inhibitor
Haptoglobulin	0.4-2.9	100 000 (Type 1–1)	Binds hemoglobin
β-Lipoprotein	2.7–7.4	380 000	Lipid transport
Transferrin	2.0–4.0	80 000	Transports iron
C3	0.6–1.4	185 000	Component of complement system
Fibrinogen	1.0–4.0	340 000	Clot formation
Immunoglobulin A	0.4–3.5	160 000	Surface immunity
Immunoglobulin D	0.1–0.4	180 000	
Immunoglobulin E	50–600 (µg/L)	180 000	Binds to mast cells; hypersensitivity reactions
Immunoglobulin G	7–15	150 000	Humoral immunity
Immunoglobulin M	0.25–2.0	850 000	Humoral immunity primary response

by immunologic methods, such as radioimmunoassay (RIA) or enzyme-linked immunosorbent assay (ELISA).

Specific Plasma Proteins

Major Components

The major serum proteins are those components that are readily resolved and detected on electrophoretic gels stained by conventional clinical laboratory techniques (Table 19–1 and Fig. 19–1).

Prealbumin. Prealbumin is defined electrophoretically as the fraction that migrates in a position faster than albumin toward the anode. Prealbumin has a tetrameric structure with a total molecular weight of 62 000 Da, making it one of the smaller serum proteins. Each monomer can bind a molecule of thyroxine. As such, it is also called thyroxine-binding prealbumin (TBPA) or transthyretin (TTR), although only a small fraction of thyroxine is actually bound to TBPA in normal individuals, because thyroxine-binding globulin has a 100-fold greater affinity for thyroxine (Oppenheimer, 1968). However, there is at least one molecular variant of prealbumin, inherited in a familial pattern, that has a greatly increased affinity for thyroxine resulting in elevated serum thyroxine content, although those individuals have normal free thyroxine concentrations and so are euthyroid (Moses, 1982).

Prealbumin plays a significant role in the metabolism of vitamin A by complexing with the retinol-binding protein (RBP) which, in turn, complexes with vitamin A to transport it through the body (Peterson, 1971). RBP is a small protein of only 182 amino acids, and so it would be rapidly removed from the circulation by filtration through the kidney if it were not held in the plasma by the larger protein prealbumin, which is not cleared into the glomerular filtrate. The complex of retinal, RBP, and transthyretin appears to be assembled in the endoplasmic reticulum of hepatocytes (Gaetani, 2002).

Prealbumin is rich in tryptophan (sometimes called tryptophan-rich prealbumin) and also has considerable β-pleated sheet conformation. A portion of prealbumin is the source of the β-fibrillar amyloid component in type I familial amyloidotic polyneuropathy (Glenner, 1980). This hereditary amyloidosis derives from a mutation in the prealbumin gene that results in a protein (e.g., TTR Met 30 variant) susceptible to proteolytic cleavage creating the β-structured fragments that are the building blocks of amyloid in nerve fibers (Ii, 1991; Saraiva, 1989). More than 80 different mutations in transthyretin are recognized, mostly affecting nerve or heart with amyloid. These pathogenetic variants of prealbumin cannot be distinguished from normal by standard protein electrophoresis. Current diagnosis is based on analysis at the DNA level.

Prealbumin has a relatively short half-life in the circulation (roughly 2 days) compared with other major serum proteins. Its synthetic rate is also exquisitely sensitive to intake of adequate nutrition and to alterations in hepatic function where it is produced. Therefore, prealbumin concentrations in serum fluctuate more rapidly in response to alterations in synthetic rate than do those of other proteins such as albumin. For that reason, quantitation of serum prealbumin has major clinical utility as a marker for nutritional status (Gofferje, 1978). Because of the rapid dynamics of its synthesis and clearance, prealbumin is considered to be a better early indicator of change in nutritional status than other commonly used markers, such as albumin and transferrin, which are more abundant but whose levels respond to other factors as well and at slower time scales.

Because of its compactness, prealbumin crosses more easily into the CSF than do the other serum proteins. Therefore, concentrating CSF prior to electrophoresis allows visualization of a distinct prealbumin band in CSF. CSF normally contains a major peak of albumin plus prealbumin and a small amount of transferrin. Electrophoresis of CSF is usually requested for detection of oligoclonal bands of immunoglobulin, and the presence of a distinct band of prealbumin is used only as a landmark to confirm that the specimen was likely CSF. True prealbumin is generally below the level of detection by serum electrophoresis; instead it is best quantified by immunologic measurements such as nephelometry. A protein band frequently appears in the prealbumin position of patients who have had heparin therapy. In the circulation, heparin activates and releases lipoprotein lipase activity, which attacks triglycerides in lipoprotein fractions, thereby greatly enhancing their electrophoretic migration anodally. Protein stain reveals the apolipoproteins in the prealbumin position but no β-lipoprotein fraction. This is an in vivo effect that does not occur if heparin is added to samples already collected.

Albumin. The single most abundant protein in normal plasma is albumin, usually constituting up to two-thirds of total plasma protein (Peters, 1975). For that reason, depressions in albumin level due to impaired synthesis (e.g., malnutrition, malabsorption, hepatic dysfunction) (Rothschild, 1972) or to losses (e.g., ascites or protein-losing nephropathy or enteropathy) result in serious imbalance of intravascular oncotic pressure. This loss is manifested clinically by the development of peripheral edema (Slater, 1975). However, the congenital absence of albumin (analbuminemia) generally does not lead to such problems, presumably because of lifelong compensatory mechanisms that control hydrostatic pressures (Waldman, 1964). Albumin also serves as a mobile repository of amino acids for incorporation into other proteins. A third function ascribed to albumin is that of a general transport or carrier protein. Many organic and inorganic ligands (e.g., thyroxine, bilirubin, penicillin, cortisol, estrogen, free fatty acids, warfarin [Coumadin], calcium, magnesium, and heme) complex with different regions of the albumin molecule in either covalent (e.g., δ-bilirubin) (Lauff, 1982) or dissociable binding (Koch-Weser, 1976). These binding interactions with very different ligands are possible because of a wide variety of binding sites on the albumin molecule, which consists of 585 amino acids arranged in nine loops held together by the disulfide bonds between cysteine residues (Meloun, 1975). The primary sequence of albumin contains three major regions with three peptide loops each, suggesting that it arose from gene duplication of some ancestral gene in a tandem rearrangement process (Peters, 1977; Sevall, 1986). It is also interesting to note that α-fetoprotein has regions of homology with serum albumin, which may indicate a common ancestral gene origin for these two proteins.

In addition to the genetic abnormality of analbuminemia, there are many hereditary variants of albumin that differ from the most common allotype, albumin A, by single amino acid substitutions. These variants can be either rapid or slow migrating compared with albumin A, leading to two distinct albumin peaks (bisalbuminemia) in the heterozygous state. None of the variant albumins appear to affect health, but one variant does have greatly enhanced affinity for thyroxine, which leads to elevated thyroxine content in the serum of such persons, who nevertheless remain euthyroid (Ruiz, 1982).

Up to 8% of albumin circulating in normal persons becomes glycosylated nonenzymatically, whereas up to 25% becomes glycosylated during hyperglycemia in analogy with glycosylated hemoglobin (Guthrow, 1979). The half-life of circulating albumin is about 17 days, so that measurements of the glycosylated form may be useful in monitoring diabetic control during an interval of a few weeks. Measurement of glycosylated albumin (also called fructosamine) can be very useful for assessing diabetic control in patients with hemolytic anemias (e.g., sickle cell disease, thalassemia, autoimmune hemolysis), whose red cell survival is greatly shortened and in whom measurement of glycosylated hemoglobin is unreliable. Glycosylated albumin measurements may not be reliable for assessing diabetic control in patients with protein-losing nephropathy, in which

albumin clearance is accelerated. Diabetic patients on hemodialysis can be monitored with either glycosylated hemoglobin or glycosylated albumin (Ghacha, 2001).

Analysis of newly synthesized albumin from intracellular sites has revealed the existence of a precursor proalbumin, which has an additional hexapeptide at its amino-terminal end. The primary structure of albumin has 35 cysteine residues, of which 34 form intramolecular disulfide bonds and one remains free. On storage for many days, albumin forms covalently linked dimers through the free cysteines, resulting occasionally in an extra band of albumin on electrophoresis.

Clinical measurements of albumin are very frequent, with determinations of total protein and albumin often included in chemistry panel profiles. The organ- or disease-oriented panels of chemistry tests in current use include the following measurements: comprehensive metabolic panel has albumin and total protein; renal function panel has albumin; hepatic function panel has albumin and total protein.

Elevations of serum albumin concentration are infrequent, although they do occur in dehydration as the plasma water phase shrinks. Following rehydration, the albumin level should fall to within the normal reference range. Elevation of serum albumin may also occur artifactually as the result of prolonged application of a tourniquet for venipuncture. In that instance, the increased hydrodynamic pressure from venous backup forces water and small solutes out of the intravascular space, thereby concentrating cellular elements, micellar forms of lipoproteins, and proteins such as albumin.

Depression of albumin concentrations is frequent in sick individuals, and a review of hospitalized patients reveals a substantial proportion of albumin measurements that are below healthy reference ranges (Fig. 9–6). Although some of these decreases are likely dilutional owing to the administration of intravenous fluids, others are caused by loss of albumin into urine, ascitic fluid, or the gastrointestinal tract in enteropathies or by decreased synthesis in the liver due to either hepatic disease such as cirrhosis or to the secondary effect on synthesis from compromised nutrition or diversion of synthetic capacity to other proteins. This sensitive but nonspecific reduction of albumin in so many different conditions has led to it being termed a 'negative acute phase reactant' (Post, 1991). Measurements of albumin concentrations are vital to the understanding and interpretation of calcium and magnesium levels because these ions are bound to albumin, and so decreases of albumin are directly responsible for depression of their concentrations, too. In some disease states, decreases in albumin are at least partially compensated for by increases in other serum proteins, thereby stabilizing oncotic pressures intravascularly. In particular, cirrhosis shows a major polyclonal increase of immunoglobulins in the γ-fraction (Fig. 19–3A) and nephrotic syndrome shows high levels of α_2-macroglobulin (Fig. 19–3B).

Body fluids that form normally, such as CSF, or pathologically, such as filtrates of plasma (e.g., ascites), contain albumin as the major component, with very little contribution from other plasma proteins. The presence of albumin in the urine is generally considered abnormal even in trace amounts, although some healthy individuals exhibit albuminuria following intense exercise. Progression of diabetic nephropathy can be assessed by the quantitative measurement of albuminuria, as it tends to appear ahead of the other serum proteins in urine during the course of renal glomerular damage. The immunologic measurement of microalbumin in urine is now considered a standard of care for management of diabetes mellitus and the early detection of diabetic complications. The nephrotic syndrome, which is marked by extensive hypoalbuminemia, is often due to diabetic nephropathy or one of several other primary glomerular diseases (Orth, 1998).

α_1-**Antitrypsin.** The major component of the α_1-globulins is the protease inhibitor α_1-antitrypsin (AAT), which has the capacity to combine with and inactivate trypsin (Eriksson, 1965; Berninger, 1985a). The first clue to this function came with the discovery that the serum of some young adults with pulmonary emphysema was deficient in α_1-globulin. Further investigations revealed a similar deficiency of AAT in children with cirrhosis (Sveger, 1976). Usually, there are no appreciable circulating levels of trypsin in blood, but other related proteases, such as elastase, are released from leukocytes responding to irritants or inflammation. AAT is able to neutralize the activity of these proteases, too, and hence is an intrinsic factor in the homeostatic mechanism modulating endogenous proteolysis within the body and preventing inappropriately severe biochemical response to inflammation (Cox, 1986).

The majority of people are homozygous for the normal fully active M allele of AAT, or phenotype MM (Lieberman, 1972). About 10% of white people (and fewer of other races) are heterozygous for M and some other allele of the protease inhibitor or Pi system. More than 2% carry the PiZ allele and exhibit the phenotype MZ. Although these individuals have somewhat

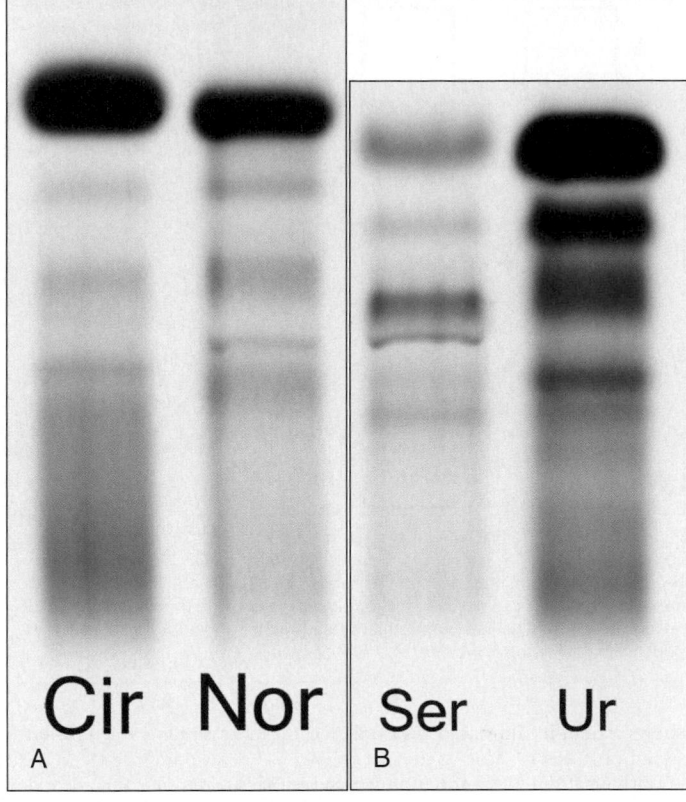

Figure 19–3 *A*, Serum protein electrophoresis in cirrhosis (Cir) shows more rapidly migrating albumin compared to normal serum (Nor) due to the additional negative charge from covalently linked conjugated bilirubin (i.e., δ-bilirubin). The gamma globulins are broadly increased in the polyclonal elevation characteristic of cirrhosis of the liver. *B*, Protein electrophoretic patterns of serum (Ser) and concentrated urine (Ur) in a patient with nephrotic syndrome. Smaller molecular-sized proteins such as albumin are preferentially lost from blood into urine. Larger proteins such as α_2-macroglobulin and β-lipoprotein are retained in the blood and constitute major bands in the serum pattern.

reduced levels of trypsin inhibitory capacity in serum, they are asymptomatic; however, their homozygous ZZ offspring are susceptible to pulmonary or hepatic disease. The ZZ phenotype occurs in about 1 in 4000 individuals. Serum protein electrophoresis may be used to screen for AAT deficiency, but confirmation must be made with ancillary tests such as trypsin inhibitory capacity (TIC) and phenotyping by cross-electrophoresis or isoelectric focusing (Jeppsson, 1982) in order to rule out the presence of some other alleles, such as *PiS* or *PiF*, which migrate differently. These alleles result in a lower TIC but probably are sufficient to prevent the abnormalities seen with the ZZ phenotype, which has a very low TIC corresponding to concentration of antigenic AAT. Screening can also be conducted in suspected cases by nephelometry to quantitate serum levels of AAT. Only the ZZ phenotype yields markedly low levels of AAT. Definitive typing may require analysis of the DNA sequence for the *AAT* gene. At least 75 different alleles exist for *AAT*. About 17 alleles have sufficiently low protein production to lead to pulmonary disease, and only a few are responsible for liver disease (Cox, 1986).

Therapy for pulmonary emphysema secondary to AAT deficiency has been greatly advanced with intravenous replacement of AAT, using concentrates or recombinant protein, to bring circulating levels into ranges sufficient for antielastase protection to the lungs (Snider, 1989). Further replacement has also been successful with AAT inhalation for patients in whom pulmonary disease has not yet become extensive (Hubbard, 1989). Avoidance of cigarette smoking by homozygous individuals is essential, because cigarette smoke is a major source of irritants that trigger leukocytes in the lung to release proteases (Gelb, 1977). The cirrhosis in young children is treated by hepatic transplant, because the liver is the site of AAT synthesis. An interesting aspect of cirrhosis and the ZZ phenotype is the presence of unsialylated mutant type AAT granules in the hepatocytes, implying a defect of secretion in those alleles. Cirrhosis secondary to AAT abnormality has not been improved by replacement therapy. Children with this disorder can develop progressive, severe cholestasis prompting liver transplantation. Following transplant, the recipient takes the AAT phenotype of the donor.

AAT is one of the serum glycoproteins that rise in response to acute inflammation, but such elevations lack clinical specificity. The α_1-fraction never appears completely empty in AAT deficiency, because other proteins (e.g., α-lipoprotein, α_1-acid glycoprotein) migrate there but do not resolve into distinct bands.

α_2-Macroglobulin. AMG is the largest major nonimmunoglobulin protein in plasma, with a molecular weight of 725 000 Da (Roberts, 1985). The serum concentration in normal individuals is comparable to that of the other major protease inhibitor AAT, although women have higher levels than men in response to estrogen (Horne, 1970). The concentration of AMG rises 10-fold or more in the nephrotic syndrome when other lower-molecular-weight proteins are lost (Beetham, 1993). The loss of AMG into urine is prevented by its large size. The net result is that AMG reaches serum levels equal to or greater than those of albumin (~ 2–3 g/dL) in the nephrotic syndrome, which has the effect of maintaining oncotic pressure. There may also be enhanced synthesis of AMG in nephrotic syndrome, which accounts for its absolute increase in concentration. AMG inactivates proteases by complexing with them and forming covalent bonds to them. Its own conformation is thereby altered, which enhances clearance by the reticuloendothelial system. There are at least four molecular forms of AMG that differ in sialic acid, mannose, and galactose content and that can be separated by isoelectric focusing. Other molecular variations probably are the result of proteases linked to AMG prior to removal from the circulation. The spectrum of inhibition by AMG is very wide, including virtually all types of serine, carboxyl, thiol, and metal proteases. AMG complexes with prostate-specific antigen in a form that is not detected by immunoassay for PSA (Ch. 74). Although AMG function is certainly important for maintaining balance in the ebb and flow of proteolysis, no specific deficiency with associated disease has been recognized, and there is no disease state generally attributed to low concentrations of AMG. Mild but distinct elevations of AMG can be observed on serum protein electrophoresis early in the course of diabetic nephropathy.

Haptoglobin. The other major protein migrating in the α_2-region is haptoglobin, which has the function of combining with hemoglobin released by lysis of red cells in order to preserve body iron and protein stores. The circulating half-life of haptoglobin, free of hemoglobin, is roughly 4 days. Hemoglobin–haptoglobin complexes are removed from the circulation within minutes by the reticuloendothelial system, where the hemoglobin is broken down into globin and heme, which further degrades to iron and bilirubin. When the hemoglobin-binding capacity of haptoglobin is exceeded, the free hemoglobin enters the glomerular filtrate as α-chain–β-chain dimers that are subsequently reabsorbed in the proximal renal tubules and converted to hemosiderin.

Haptoglobin has two heavy chains and two light chains linked by disulfide bonds in analogy to the basic structure of immunoglobulins. Some persons have a light chain gene that is duplicated in a head-to-tail arrangement (Type 2). Normal haptoglobin (Type 1–1) gives rise to a single molecular species of molecular weight 100 000. Heterozygous individuals (1–2) have, in addition to Type 1–1 haptoglobin, a series of multimers (e.g., dimers, trimers) by virtue of intermolecular disulfide linkages through the duplicated light chain. Type 2–2 haptoglobin consists of a different series of multimers, because the Type 2 light chain has a different molecular weight from the Type 1 light chain (Konigsberg, 1974).

Haptoglobin can be quantitated in terms of its hemoglobin-binding capacity or by immunologic means, especially nephelometry. Owing to steric hindrance between molecular sites on the multimers, the different phenotypes of haptoglobin yield measurements of antigen- or hemoglobin-binding capacity that may be discrepant with the absolute amount of haptoglobin protein present in a sample. Accordingly, the reference range for haptoglobin is broader for an entire population of different phenotypes than within individual phenotypes. For that reason, interpretation of haptoglobin concentrations is soundest for serial measurements in the same individual. However, very high levels can readily be distinguished from very low ones, which can be important in the first-time evaluation of a patient for hemolysis. Congenital deficiency of haptoglobin appears not to have clinical consequence (Manoharan, 1997).

Serum haptoglobin rises in response to stress, infection, acute inflammation, or tissue necrosis, probably by stimulation of synthesis (see later under Acute Phase Reactants). After a hemolytic episode, haptoglobin concentrations fall as the complexes with hemoglobin are cleared from the circulation. This effect is dramatic following massive hemolysis in situations of hemolytic transfusion reaction, thermal burns, or autoimmune hemolytic anemia. It is also a useful measurement for serially monitoring patients who have a slow but steady rate of red cell breakdown such as by mechanical heart valves, hemoglobinopathies, or exercise-associated trauma. Low haptoglobin concentrations may accompany liver disease when hepatic synthetic capacity is impaired. There are also individuals with congenital deficiency of haptoglobin who apparently use other mechanisms to conserve body iron stores. Serum samples from blood hemolyzed in vitro during phlebotomy or processing show a displaced band of haptoglobin–hemoglobin complex on protein electrophoresis.

It should be noted that myoglobin does not bind to haptoglobin and, therefore, release of large amounts of myoglobin by rhabdomyolysis does not diminish haptoglobin levels in serum. This difference can be useful in the work-up of a positive dipstick test for blood (actually a test for pseudoperoxidase activity of heme in hemoglobin or myoglobin) in urine with no coexisting red cells. In that case, low serum haptoglobin suggests hemoglobinuria (hemolysis), whereas high serum haptoglobin suggests myoglobinuria. Lactate dehydrogenase (LD) isoenzyme 1 in serum is also associated with hemolysis, whereas LD_5 and creatine kinase are released in rhabdomyolysis.

β-Lipoprotein. β-Lipoprotein (low-density lipoprotein [LDL]) migrates with a characteristic sharp leading cathodal edge and feathery trailing region more anodally. Although it is better quantitated by stains for lipid, there is sufficient apoprotein content to be a distinct band on staining for protein. The exact position of the β-lipoprotein band is sensitive to recent ingestion of fatty foods; thus, samples from fasting versus postprandial collections will show the β-lipoprotein in slightly different positions. The other lipoproteins (very-low-density lipoprotein [VLDL], high-density lipoprotein [HDL], and chylomicrons) are relatively small in intensity, and they occur in overlapping electrophoretic positions with other serum proteins so that these fractions are generally not appreciated on protein stain. Administration of heparin activates postheparin lipoprotein lipase, which degrades triglycerides in the circulating lipoprotein fractions. Consequently, heparinized patients transiently demonstrate an anomalous band of β-lipoprotein that can migrate very rapidly and also unevenly across the electrophoretic path, even into the prealbumin region. Elevations of LDL, with greater staining intensity to the β-lipoprotein band, occur in hypercholesterolemia. Lipoproteins are discussed more thoroughly in Chapter 17.

Transferrin. The major β-globulin is transferrin (siderophilin), which transports ferric ions from the iron stores of intracellular or mucosal ferritin to bone marrow, where erythrocyte precursors and lymphocytes have transferrin receptors on their surfaces (Irie, 1987).

Transferrin consists of 687 amino acids with a calculated molecular weight of 79 550 Da (MacGillivray, 1982). Analysis of the amino acid sequence shows that transferrin has two homologous domains that may have arisen by contiguous duplication of an ancestral transferrin gene. Each domain has a binding site with very high affinity for iron. Transcription of mRNA for transferrin synthesis in the liver is regulated by the concentration of iron in the circulation and surrounding the hepatocytes.

In normal serum, transferrin ranges in concentration from 200–400 mg/dL, which is conveniently measured as iron-binding capacity (IBC) (Tsung, 1975). In response to short-term iron deficiency, transferrin levels rise markedly to twice normal levels or higher. Because transferrin is a single molecular species with a tight electrophoretic mobility, an elevated level can have the appearance of a paraprotein (pseudoparaproteinemia) in cases of severe iron deficiency (Zawadzki, 1970). At least some iron deficiency and elevation of transferrin should be expected with pregnancy (Mendenhall, 1970). Administration of iron to deficient patients increases the saturation followed by return of transferrin to normal.

Chronic saturation of transferrin occurs in idiopathic hemochromatosis and transfusional hemosiderosis. Because there is almost no unsaturated IBC in those syndromes, iron cannot be mobilized normally for excretion, resulting in the disorders of deposition that also occur in congenital deficiency of transferrin. Current strategies to screen for hemochromatosis include measurement of serum iron and serum transferrin (usually by nephelometric immunoassay), with the calculation of percent saturation as the best index for identifying previously unrecognized cases. Hemochromatosis is a hereditary disorder that results in cirrhosis, diabetes, cardiomyopathy, arthritis, and other endocrine disorders owing to the toxic effects of excess free iron. Screening for hemochromatosis is desirable because the disease progression can be halted by lowering the body burden of iron by such means as phlebotomy or chelation therapy.

Transferrin may also demonstrate an antibacterial effect by complexing iron and removing it from bacteria that require iron for growth (Reddy, 1970; Weinberg, 1978).

In protein-losing nephropathy of sufficient severity, transferrin is lost from the circulation into the urine, carrying iron with it. This loss may contribute to the development of hypochromic anemia.

Electrophoretic variants of transferrin occur occasionally in serum owing to allotypic variation in the amino acid sequence and hence have a different charge on the molecule. In that case, the heterozygous state

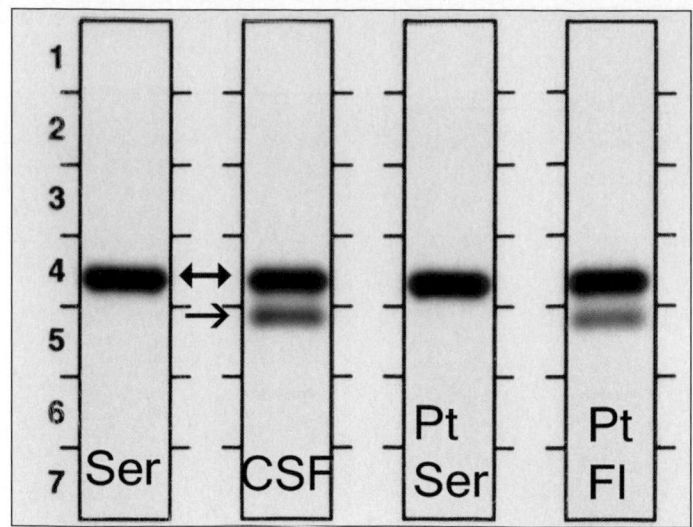

Figure 19–4 Immunofixation with transferrin antibody to test for presence of cerebrospinal fluid. Ser, normal serum showing position of transferrin (Tf; double-headed arrow); CSF, normal position of Tf and asialotransferrin (aTf, single-headed arrow); Pt Ser, patient serum included to rule out electrophoretic variant of Tf; Pt Fl, unknown fluid from patient demonstrating bands of both Tf and aTf that confirm the presence of CSF in that fluid.

shows a doublet in place of a single electrophoretic band for transferrin (Kamboh, 1987).

Transferrin is a glycoprotein in which various sugar molecules are added to newly synthesized protein molecules in the liver. Persons who engage in heavy alcohol consumption demonstrate abnormal carbohydrate-deficient transferrin in their serum (Stibler, 1991). This aberrant transferrin molecule may be due either to failure of glycosyltransferases in hepatocytes or to increased sialidase activity in serum or to a combination of the two (Xin, 1995). Carbohydrate-deficient transferrin can be detected by anion exchange chromatography or isoelectric focusing of isoforms in serum followed by immunoblotting. Other methods include HPLC, capillary zone electrophoresis, mass spectrometry, and turbidimetric immunoassay (Bean, 2001).

A variant of transferrin has been recognized in CSF (Zaret, 1992), aqueous and vitreous humor of the eye (Tripathi, 1990), and perilymph of the ear (Thalmann, 1994). Chemically, it lacks sialic acid in glycosylation compared to the transferrin found in plasma (Hoffman, 1995); it is called asialotransferrin, τ protein, or β_2-transferrin because of slightly different electrophoretic migration (towards the cathode) because it carries less negative charge than plasma transferrin (Blennow, 1995). CSF contains both forms of plasma transferrin and asialotransferrin, whereas plasma contains only one form. Consequently, detection of asialotransferrin in fluid from a fistula or drainage is presumptive evidence for presence of CSF in cases of skull fractures or other head trauma with nasal drainage (Solomon, 1999), or for presence of perilymph in fistula fluid from otologic procedures such as cochlear implants (Delaroche, 1996). Asialotransferrin reacts immunologically as transferrin, and so it can be readily detected by immunoblotting following electrophoresis (Roelandse, 1998). This procedure is easily done by adapting commercially available agarose gel electrophoresis systems already used in many laboratories for direct immunofixation of immunoglobulins (Normansell, 1994); using an antitransferrin antibody demonstrates a single band of transferrin in serum samples, but two bands if the specimen contains CSF (Fig. 19–4). It is necessary to include serum in addition to the test fluid from the patient to rule out allelic variants of transferrin that could cause false positives if not recognized (Sloman, 1993). Presence of CSF in drainage fluid may require surgical repair or antibiotic therapy, so detection of asialotransferrin as a marker for CSF can have substantial clinical impact.

Complement. A separate fraction of β-globulin consists of the C3 component of complement. Although this protein can be resolved easily with a fresh serum sample, in stored specimens and commercial control serum that has been lyophilized, C3 is cleaved to form C3c, which migrates anodally to native C3 as a band nondistinct from other β-globulins. Depression of C3 occurs in autoimmune disorders when the complement system is activated and C3 becomes bound to immune complexes deposited in tissues, thereby removing them from plasma. Thus, C3 (and also C4) concentration is a convenient marker for assessing disease activity in the rheumatic disorders such as lupus erythematosus and rheumatoid arthritis. C4 is not appreciated on serum protein electrophoresis because its concentration is normally only about one-fifth that of C3. Both C3 and C4 are now easily quantitated by nephelometry for monitoring rheumatic disease activity. No particular diagnostic significance is ascribed to higher than normal levels of C3 or C4 except as mild indicators of an acute phase response. The complement system and its inhibitors are discussed further in Chapter 46.

Fibrinogen. Plasma contains 100–400 mg/dL of fibrinogen, which is the most abundant of the coagulation factors and which forms the fibrin clot. With an overall molecular weight of 340 000 Da, fibrinogen is a dimer consisting of three pairs of peptide chains (A-α, B-β, and γ) linked with multiple disulfide bonds near their amino-terminal ends (Doolittle, 1975, 2001). This region of the molecule is termed the E domain or disulfide knot (DSK). The chains extend outward into two other identical domains (D) at their carboxyl ends, where all three chains are intertwined. Thrombin cleaves fibrinopeptides A and B from the amino ends of the A-α and B-β chains, thereby resulting in a fibrin monomer that polymerizes into fibrils that macroscopically form a fibrin clot. Factor XIII then produces covalent bonds between lysine and glutamine residues on adjacent γ-chains of different fibrin molecules, making the fibrin clot essentially a single molecule. A crosslinked clot is refractory to dissolution by chemical denaturants and is mechanically very stable.

Numerous hereditary variants of fibrinogen (dysfibrinogenemias) have been identified, in which a functionally abnormal fibrinogen molecule is synthesized with altered amino acid sequence owing to genetic mutation. Some dysfibrinogenemias exhibit impairment of clotting and a hemorrhagic diathesis, whereas others show increased tendency to thrombosis (Menache, 1973). Congenital afibrinogenemia, in which essentially no fibrinogen is synthesized, results in a hemorrhagic disorder, which paradoxically is not as severe as the hemophilias in terms of joint abnormalities secondary to hemorrhage (hemarthroses).

Fibrinogen levels become elevated with the other acute phase reactants, occasionally to over 1.0 g/L. In such instances, the erythrocyte sedimentation rate (ESR) is also markedly elevated owing to fibrinogen content directly. Fibrinogen levels also rise with pregnancy and use of contraceptive medications. Low levels generally indicate extensive activation of coagulation with consumption of fibrinogen. During this process, plasminogen is also activated into plasmin, which degrades fibrin and fibrinogen into split products that are measured for the assessment of intravascular coagulation. Normally, clots that form are removed by action of plasmin, which, in turn, is inactivated by antiplasmin and the other protease inhibitors.

Fibrinogen is absent from normal serum but should appear in plasma electrophoresis as a distinct band between the β- and γ-globulins (Fig. 19–5). Not infrequently, blood drawn from heparinized patients does not fully clot, so that a fibrinogen band is present on electrophoresis. It can be distinguished by examining the specimen for a fine clot and by repeat electrophoresis of a thoroughly clotted sample. This maneuver is important to distinguish a residual fibrinogen band from a monoclonal spike of immunoglobulin that can migrate in the same electrophoretic position.

Minor Components

The next group of individual proteins are those not usually detected by standard protein electrophoresis owing to low levels in serum. Their quantitation is typically performed by immunologic methods.

Ceruloplasmin. Migrating with the α₂-globulins is a copper-binding protein, ceruloplasmin, whose precise physiologic function is unknown, although it does exhibit oxidase activity in the laboratory (Ch. 21). Synthesized in the liver, it has a molecular weight of 132 000 Da and consists of a single polypeptide chain. Although lower at birth (Al-Rashid, 1971), serum levels are 20–40 mg/dL in normal adults, with twofold elevations found in oral contraceptive therapy and pregnancy (Burrows, 1971), or as an acute phase reactant. Each molecule of ceruloplasmin can bind six atoms of copper, which imparts a blue color to the protein. The combination of this blue with the yellow from other chromogens of plasma imparts a greenish color to plasma with elevated ceruloplasmin concentrations (Schenker, 1971); this green appearance is frequently noted in bags of plasma donated for transfusions. Iron is oxidized from ferrous to ferric ions by ceruloplasmin, which may be a means of releasing iron from ferritin for binding to transferrin (Roeser, 1970).

Wilson's disease (hepatolenticular degeneration) results from disordered copper metabolism, in which hepatic excretion of copper into the bile is impaired leading to toxic deposition of copper in tissues. Normal metabolism of copper includes incorporation by the liver into ceruloplasmin (about six to seven copper atoms per molecule), which is

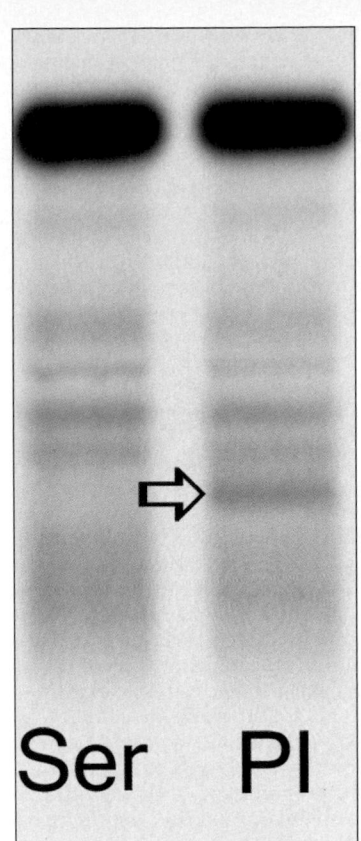

Figure 19–5 Comparison of serum (Ser) and citrated plasma (Pl) from the same individual demonstrates the position of fibrinogen (arrow) in plasma that should not be confused with a monoclonal immunoglobulin.

then secreted into the plasma. In Wilson's disease, this process is impaired and copper that has been absorbed by the body and transported to the liver fails to re-enter the circulation as part of ceruloplasmin. Normal excretion of copper through the bile is diminished, with an overall increase in body copper deposits that are toxic to liver, brain, cornea, kidneys, bones, and parathyroids. Diagnosis is usually made in childhood or adolescence when damage to the liver is first noticed. Other affected persons may present later in life when neurologic changes also occur. Treatment is long-term chelation with penicillamine or, in severe cases, liver transplantation, which may be curative.

Diagnosis of Wilson's disease is based on physical findings (liver disease, neurologic signs, Kayser–Fleischer ring in the cornea), measurement of low serum ceruloplasmin level, and increased copper concentrations in urine and on liver biopsy. The oxidase activity of ceruloplasmin can be used in a colorimetric assay, with p-phenylenediamine as substrate, for quantitation. Additionally, immunochemical methods are used, because the band is too faint to be used reliably on protein electrophoresis. Because no single clinical or laboratory finding is sufficient to make the diagnosis of Wilson's disease, a combination of them is necessary (Ferenci, 2004).

Gc-Globulin. Vitamin D binds to the group-specific component (Gc) globulin (vitamin D-binding protein [DBP]) (Daiger, 1975; Bikle, 1986), which migrates as an α₁-globulin and has a molecular weight of about 51 000 Da. Normal serum concentration is 20–55 mg/dL. It may be decreased in severe liver disease. Gc-globulin has two autosomal codominant alleles expressed as three phenotypes: 1–1, 2–2, and 1–2 (Giblett, 1969). Congenital absence of this protein may be a lethal mutation, owing to impairment of vitamin D transport, because vitamin D has low solubility in aqueous media. Gc-globulin binds vitamin D and its metabolites on a mole-per-mole basis, but in plasma, it probably is not fully saturated. Nephrotic syndrome results in urinary loss of DBP, some of which is complexed with vitamin D. This loss of vitamin D may contribute to subsequent problems of calcium metabolism encountered in nephrotic syndrome (Goldstein, 1981). As a minor component of plasma proteins, Gc-globulin can be quantitated by radioimmunoassay, radioimmunodiffusion, or rocket immunoelectrophoresis (Walsh, 1982; Westwood, 1986). More recent studies with immunonephelometry have shown lower levels of Gc-globulin in trauma patients who develop organ dysfunction and sepsis (Dahl, 2003).

Hemopexin. The β-migrating globulin hemopexin binds heme released by degradation of hemoglobin (Muller-Eberhard, 1970). By this means, this small porphyrin molecule with its iron atom is protected from excretion, thereby contributing to the preservation of body iron stores. Among plasma proteins, hemopexin has the strongest binding affinity for heme, which probably helps to limit the toxicity of free heme (Tolosano, 2002). Normal serum concentration is 50–120 mg/dL so that it must be quantitated by immunologic means. It has a molecular weight of 70 000 Da, of which 20% is carbohydrate and consists of a single polypeptide chain. Although low levels of hemopexin can occur with nonspecific urinary loss or due to decreased synthesis in liver failure, the most profound decreases occur following intravascular hemolysis, when the amount of free hemoglobin exceeds the binding capacity of haptoglobin. The circulating plasma hemoglobin can then degrade to release heme, which is bound molecule per molecule by hemopexin. Heme–hemopexin complexes are cleared from the circulation by hepatocytes, which markedly lowers hemopexin concentration in serum. Excess heme then binds to albumin as methemalbumin. As more hemopexin is made available by new synthesis, heme passes from methemalbumin to hemopexin, which continues to depress the hemopexin level. As such, it can be an additional aid for diagnosing hemolysis at an earlier time, after haptoglobin levels have returned to normal but before full clearance of the heme (Wochner, 1974).

α₁-Acid Glycoprotein. This protein, also known as orosomucoid, has a very high carbohydrate content, which minimizes its visualization by standard protein stains (Alvan, 1986). With a molecular weight of roughly 44 000 Da, it passes into the glomerular filtrate to a large extent, resulting in a half-life of only about 5 days in the circulation. Serum levels are normally 40–105 mg/dL, with elevations during pregnancy (Schmid, 1975). It is an acute phase reactant, but its biological function is not known. As a binder of progesterone, it may be important in the transport or metabolism of that steroid hormone. It also binds some drugs (e.g., lidocaine) and keeps them in an inactive circulating pool. Measurements of this protein have clinical utility in interpreting levels of drugs, such as lidocaine, that may achieve high serum concentrations without expected therapeutic effect owing to being complexed in inactive form to higher than normal amounts of α₁-acid glycoprotein. There are also some genetic polymorphisms of this protein that may be additionally complicated by isomorphic forms from specific tissue sources, although the primary site of its synthesis appears to be the liver.

C-Reactive Protein. This serum constituent was discovered by interacting the serum of patients, who had recovered from pneumococcal infections, with C-polysaccharide of that bacterium. Visible flocculates formed, which allowed extensive study and purification of the C-reactive protein (CRP) from serum in the 1940s. It was found that CRP is present in the serum of patients with disorders other than pneumococcal infections, but that it rises strikingly whenever there is tissue necrosis. Many other substances react with CRP, such as DNA, nucleotides, various lipids, and other polysaccharides (Hokama, 1982). Thus, it appears to serve as a general scavenger molecule. Its molecular weight is between 118 000–144 000 Da, with substantial carbohydrate content. The normal serum concentrations are about 100 ng/mL at birth, 170 ng/mL in children, and 470–1340 ng/mL in adults. Despite these low concentrations, CRP has major significance as a highly sensitive acute phase reactant (Deodhar, 1989). It is generally measured by its capacity to precipitate C-substance or by immunologic methods, including nephelometry, precipitations, RIA, and enzyme immunoassay (Saxstad, 1970; Claus, 1976). By electrophoresis, CRP is a γ-migrating protein that may form a minor but distinct monoclonal-appearing band in patients having a severe inflammatory response. CRP levels are sometimes used as a rapid test for presumptive diagnosis of bacterial infection (high CRP) versus viral infection (low CRP) (Clyne, 1999). CRP is often used by rheumatologists to monitor the progression or remission of autoimmune disease. The gene for CRP has been localized to human chromosome 1 (Whitehead, 1983). Recent epidemiologic studies have shown that a high-sensitivity assay for CRP (hs-CRP) can add to the predictive value of serum lipids for identifying individuals at risk of cardiovascular events, presumably due to the role that inflammation plays in atherogenesis (Ridker, 2000). Persons with high normal CRP concentrations are at greater risk for stroke or myocardial infarction than those with low normal values (discussed in greater detail in Ch. 18).

Protease Inhibitors

In addition to α₁-antitrypsin and α₂-macroglobulin, which have already been considered, other distinct inhibitors of different proteases are present in plasma. They include α₁-antichymotrypsin (AAC) (Berninger, 1985b), inter-α-trypsin inhibitor (IATI) (Daniels, 1975), antithrombin III (AT3), antiplasmin, C1 esterase inhibitor (Prograis, 1985), protein C (Stenflo, 1984), and plasminogen activator inhibitor-1 (PAI-1) (Nilsson, 1984). None of these proteins attains plasma concentrations appreciable on

stained protein electrophoresis. Whereas the other inhibitors show inhibition over a rather wide range of proteases, AAC is highly specific for neutralizing chymotrypsin, which cleaves peptide bonds at the carboxyl side of tyrosine and phenylalanine residues. AAC has a molecular weight of 68 000 Da with about 25% carbohydrate content. Normal serum concentration is 40–60 mg/dL, but AAC can rise rapidly to five times normal as an acute phase reactant that remains elevated throughout a period of inflammation (Kosaka, 1976). AAC complexes with prostate-specific antigen, measured as the bound form of PSA by immunoassay (Ch. 74). It can be lost along with other low-molecular-weight serum proteins in the proteinuria of nephrotic syndrome.

IATI is a glycoprotein of molecular weight 160 000 Da. Its concentration normally is about 50 mg/dL. IATI does not rise appreciably as an acute phase reactant. Its role in disease states is probably similar to that of the major protease inhibitors in preventing autodigestion of tissues by endogenous cellular enzymes (Daniels, 1975).

AT3 is of special clinical interest because of the role it plays in neutralizing thrombin, which normally becomes activated intravascularly from prothrombin during clot formation. This 62 000-Da protein forms a covalently bonded complex with thrombin over a period of several minutes when mixed in solution. On addition of heparin, the complex formation occurs almost instantaneously (Rosenberg, 1975, 1985, 1987). Although AT3 is probably essential for successful therapeutic administration of heparin, only those rare individuals with marked deficiencies seem to have thrombotic disorders (Carvalho, 1976). The action of AT3 extends to other coagulation factors (IX, X, XI, XII, and kallikrein). Serum levels of AT3 may be depressed in severe liver disease or in protein-losing disorders when the similar-sized molecule albumin is lost, and also in disseminated intravascular coagulopathy (DIC). A new experimental protocol for treating DIC involves replacing AT3, by infusion of concentrates, when the patient's AT3 level falls to very low concentrations as part of the consumptive coagulopathy. Presumably, return to normal levels of AT3 has the effect of blocking further thrombosis systemically. AT3 levels are lower in heparin therapy and slightly elevated in oral anticoagulant therapy owing to increased and reduced turnover respectively.

Although AAT, AMG, and AT3 provide the bulk of plasmin-neutralizing activity in serum (Harpel, 1976), there is a distinct antiplasmin that migrates as an α₂-globulin (Lijnen, 1985). This cross-reactivity of serum protease inhibitors for plasmin illustrates the difficulty in sorting out the precise physiologic function of each molecular species, because each one appears capable of substituting for another in different instances. However, antiplasmin binds quantitatively to the majority of plasmin that is generated from plasminogen in human plasma that undergoes clotting. Antiplasmin thus serves as one of the critical checks within the joint coagulation–fibrinolytic system, which maintains hemostasis by balancing clot formation against dissolution. By this mechanism, clot formation and breakdown are generally contained within local regions of the vasculature without extending to the entire circulation. Hereditary deficiency of antiplasmin results in a bleeding disorder owing to relatively unlimited fibrinolysis.

PAI-1 acts to prevent activation of plasminogen, thereby blocking fibrinolysis at an early step. Deficiency of PAI-1 results in less inhibition, leading to greater fibrinolysis and potentially a bleeding disorder. Elevated levels of PAI-1 prevent fibrinolysis, leading to thrombotic disorders and interestingly also to the progression of atherosclerosis. Protein C (with its cofactor protein S) inactivates activated coagulation factors V and VIII. Deficiency of protein C or S (Griffin, 1987) allows prolonged activity in vivo of procoagulant factors leading to thrombotic disorders.

The C1 esterase inhibitor is capable of inhibiting activated complement components C1r and C1s plus some other coagulation and fibrinolytic factors. It rises as an acute phase reactant. Hereditary deficiency of C1 esterase inhibitor allows activation of complement to proceed relatively unabated, a disorder termed hereditary angioedema. The complement system and its inhibitors are described in depth in Chapter 46.

Acute Phase Reactants

The acute phase reactant proteins share the property of showing elevations in concentrations in response to stressful or inflammatory states that occur with infection, injury, surgery, trauma, or other tissue necrosis (Daniels, 1974; Laurell, 1975; Dowton, 1988). They include AAT, α₁-acid glycoprotein, haptoglobin, ceruloplasmin, fibrinogen, serum amyloid A protein, and CRP. Others are factor VIII, ferritin, lipoproteins, complement proteins, and immunoglobulins. It is easy to see how such a response of the plasma proteins would be advantageous to the body: inflammation causes release from leukocytes of proteolytic enzymes in tissue that must be neutralized by enzyme inhibitors to limit their extent of destruction;

scavenger proteins (haptoglobin, CRP) help collect and transport cellular debris and breakdown products to phagocytic cells (reticuloendothelial system) to process them and conserve vital substances (e.g., iron); and healing of wounds requires a large amount of fibrin, which arrives via the circulation as fibrinogen. Thus, the humoral response of the acute phase reactants can be viewed as a phenomenon that is geared to handle extensive insult each time it is triggered even though not all components will be needed on every occasion. The elevation of acute phase reactants is likely a response to the cytokines including interleukin-1, tumor necrosis factor, interferon-γ, and interleukin-6. The total physiologic response includes induction of fever, recruitment of leukocytes, catabolism of muscle, and a shift in protein synthesis patterns with reduction in albumin production.

For clinical use in diagnosis, other parameters may in fact be as sensitive as these and far easier to measure (e.g., fever, leukocytosis, or ESR). However, these proteins provide another dimension of quantitation that can be useful for monitoring the course of a patient by serial determinations (van Oss, 1975). Of course, those patients with congenital deficiencies (Gitlin, 1975), those with other impairment of synthesis due to drugs or organ disease, or newborns who normally have lower levels of many constituents (Gitlin, 1969) may not show the dramatic increases expected. However, a generally useful acute phase reactant for monitoring response is CRP, which is the fastest rising acute phase reactant and one that returns to normal quickly following successful therapies (Fischer, 1976). CRP is frequently applied to the detection and preliminary classification of occult infections, because bacterial infections can stimulate much higher levels of CRP than viral ones. It is also widely used for assessing disease activity in autoimmune disorders, because it is rarely elevated persistently without continued inflammatory response. Elevations of CRP can be up to 1000 times normal levels, which greatly assists in detecting abnormal states compared with the other acute phase reactants that may rise at most only severalfold in such responses, although ferritin levels may occasionally rise to values of over 20 000 ng/mL.

Patterns of Protein Abnormalities

Some of the most frequently encountered patterns of protein abnormalities in electrophoresis are shown as densitometric scans in Figure 19-6. Scanning allows quantitation of each fraction, but visual inspection of the electrophoretic strip provides more detailed information about individual proteins separated in high-resolution systems (Ritzman, 1975). Interpretation of electrophoretic results depends on visual inspection to identify abnormal patterns or aberrant bands and on quantitation by scan to gauge the relative quantities of individual fractions.

Patterns of *hypoproteinemia* due to malnutrition or gross loss of protein show decreases in all fractions, but the most dramatic reduction is often seen in albumin compared with its normally high value as the most abundant serum protein (Fig. 19-7, lane 3). Severe starvation, malabsorption, or the inanition associated with severe chronic disease will show marked reduction in albumin to levels below 20 g/L. The other serum proteins appear even fainter on electrophoresis, including AAT, AMG, haptoglobin, transferrin, and C3. Reduction of staining intensity for the β-lipoprotein parallels a marked decrease in serum cholesterol concentration. The immune system is strongly affected by severe starvation, with decreased synthesis of immunoglobulins resulting in hypogammaglobulinemia and impaired resistance to bacterial and other infections. Protein-losing enteropathy (Fig. 19-6H) shows a variation on the hypoproteinemia pattern in which most fractions are diminished owing to the combination of decreased synthesis and increased loss, although α₂ may be relatively higher owing to a coexisting acute phase response (haptoglobin) or to preferential retention of larger molecules (α_2-macroglobulin).

Specific loss of proteins into the urine such as in *nephrotic syndrome* occurs on a molecular weight basis, with smaller proteins being lost more rapidly than larger ones. Accordingly, albumin appears early in the course of protein-losing nephropathies followed by smaller amounts of AAT, transferrin and, ultimately, immunoglobulins (Fig. 19-8, lanes 1 and 2). The very large molecule AMG is retained, as are the large micelles of β-lipoprotein. The result is complementary patterns of proteins in the serum (decreases in albumin and α_1-, β-, and γ-globulins; increased α_2-macroglobulin and elevated β-lipoprotein) versus those in urine (Fig. 19-3B) (glomerular proteinuria with albumin, α_1-, β-, and γ-fractions present but without α_2-macroglobulin in the urine sample). Tubular proteinuria that is due to impaired renal tubular reabsorption of small proteins shows a pattern of α, β, and γ in the urine with only minimal albumin loss into the urine (Killingsworth, 1982) (Fig. 19-8, lane 4). In

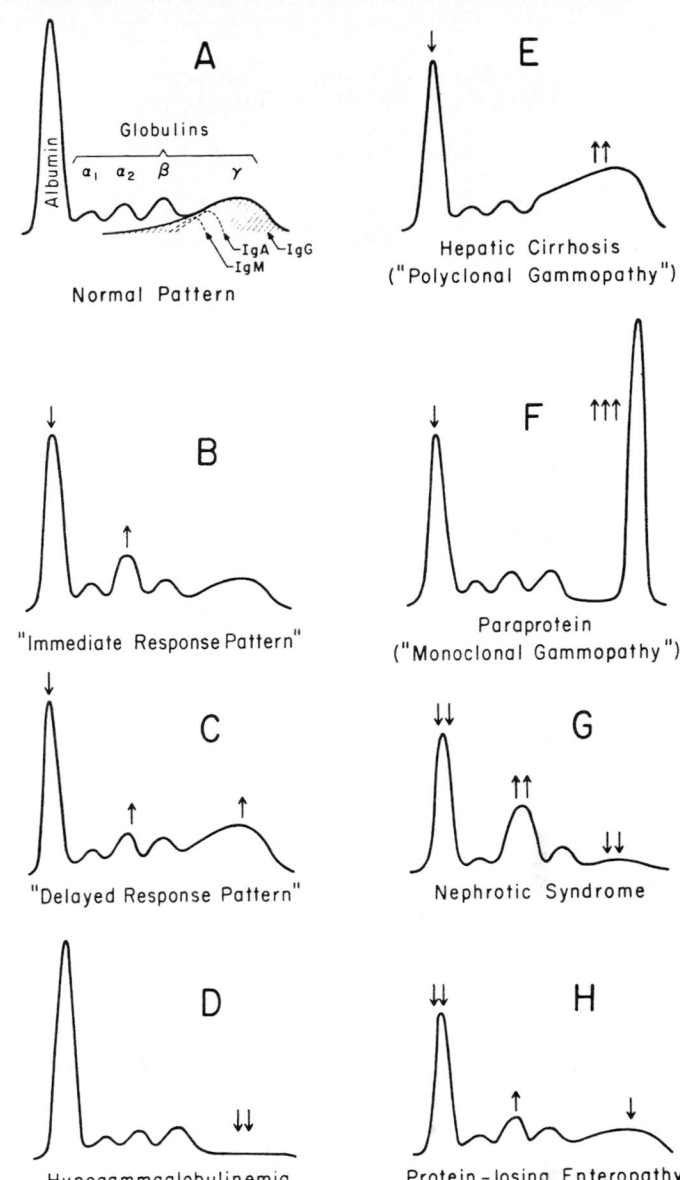

Figure 19–6 Serum protein electrophoresis: clinicopathalogic correlations. (Courtesy of Dr A E Krieg.)

addition to glomerular and tubular patterns of proteinuria (Maachi, 2004), it is important to recognize the important pattern of a monoclonal gammopathy in urine (Fig. 19-8, lane 3, and Fig. 19-9). A similar pattern of a single large band also occurs in hemoglobinuria (Fig. 19-8, lane 5) that must be distinguished from a monoclonal immunoglobulin or free light chains.

Acute phase or *immediate response* patterns have greatest effect on serum protein electrophoresis by increasing the amount of haptoglobin while slightly decreasing the concentration of albumin. Increases in haptoglobin usually indicate some form of response, whether acute or chronic, to stressful stimuli (Fig. 19-7). Other proteins such as AAT can contribute in this response; the minor components such as CRP do not contribute significantly to this protein stain pattern, although immunologic measurement of CRP may show up to 1000-fold elevations. If the haptoglobin has been depleted in a patient as a result of active hemolysis, there can be an independent band of hemoglobin migrating in the β- or α_2-region. Hemolysis of a sample in vitro may show a red-colored band (on the unstained gel) of the haptoglobin–hemoglobin complex that migrates differently from hemoglobin alone. The pattern of delayed response or chronic pattern is an extension of the acute phase response (high haptoglobin, slight reduction in albumin) with greater decrease of albumin and polyclonal increase of immunoglobulins broadening the γ-region.

A striking elevation of transferrin in the β-region sometimes occurs in patients suffering from *iron deficiency anemia*. The increase of transferrin corresponds to increased IBC, and the percent saturation is low (Koerper,

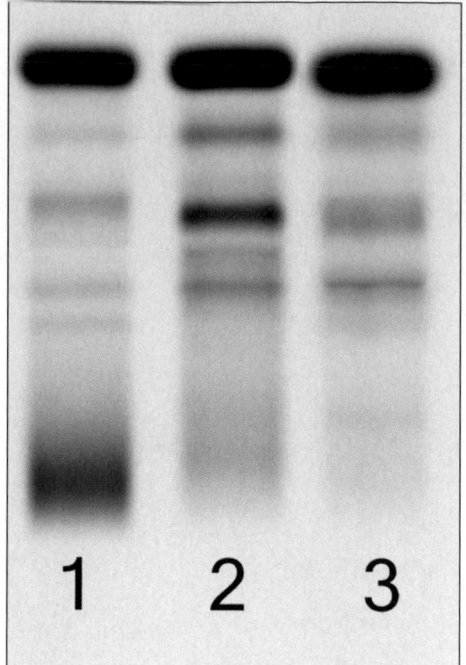

Figure 19–7 Serum protein patterns in: (1) chronic inflammation with decreased albumin and increased γ-globulins; (2) acute inflammation with increased α₂-fraction (haptoglobin) and decreased C3 due to activation and consumption of complement; (3) inanition post-spinal cord injury with hypoproteinemia of several fractions.

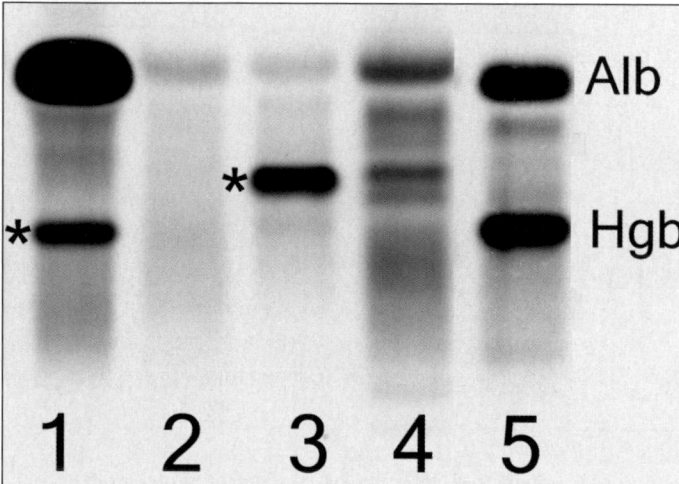

Figure 19–8 Patterns of urine protein electrophoresis in different disorders. (1) Severe glomerular proteinuria with a major band of albumin plus a secondary one of transferrin (*). (2) Trace proteinuria with a faint band of albumin and other diffuse proteins. (3) Immunoglobulin light chains (*). (4) Tubular proteinuria with multiple bands that do not correspond to major serum proteins. (5) Hematuria with a major band of hemoglobin (not to be confused with monoclonal gammopathy) in addition to albumin.

1977). This variation may be confused with a myeloma protein because the transferrin band forms a narrow, clonal-appearing band.

Cirrhosis of the liver creates a protein pattern that is recognizable (Fig. 19–3A). Hepatocellular damage from cirrhosis results in diminished capacity to synthesize albumin. Furthermore, the imbalance of hemodynamic pressures in portal hypertension secondary to cirrhosis leads to the formation of ascitic fluid, which contains almost exclusively albumin. This decreased synthesis, coupled with increased loss, greatly

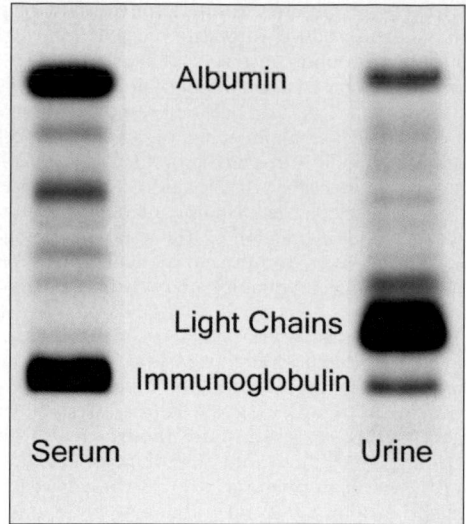

Figure 19–9 Serum and urine protein electrophoretic patterns in a patient with multiple myeloma. Serum demonstrates a predominance of the larger complete immunoglobulin, while the urine has a large amount of the smaller-sized light chains with only a small amount of the whole immunoglobulin.

reduces serum albumin concentrations. The loss of albumin is balanced to some extent by marked polyclonal increase in immunoglobulins with a γ-fraction that may contribute significantly to oncotic pressures. The increase in γ-globulin involves all immunoglobulins; the increase of immunoglobulin A (IgA) in the slow β-region shows a continuum with the γ (also termed β–γ bridging).

In contrast to polyclonal increases, *oligoclonal bands* consist of only a few clones of distinct immunoglobulins that migrate in defined positions. This pattern is seen in serum in cases in which an immunologic disorder is present or in some patients treated with chronic immunosuppression for organ transplantation (Myara, 1991). Oligoclonal bands in the CSF are used to indicate immunologic activity in the central nervous system and occur in infectious diseases or autoimmune or demyelinating disorders (Ch. 45).

Hypogammaglobulinemia is manifested as a nearly to completely absent γ-fraction. It occurs normally in neonates prior to maturation of the immune system. It also occurs in some congenital immunodeficiency states such as Bruton's agammaglobulinemia and other states involving B cell function. Perhaps more commonly, this pattern is seen in adults with lymphoreticular disorders in whom normal plasma cells have been displaced by lymphocytic proliferations and also to some extent after chemotherapy for eradication of malignancies as well as in hypoproteinemic states (Fig. 19–7, lane 3).

The single most important and widespread clinical application of serum protein electrophoresis is for the detection of *monoclonal gammopathies*. This very explicit pattern comes from a paraprotein (immunoglobulin) secreted by a monoclonal proliferation of plasma cells and is generally found without normal amounts of polyclonal γ as normal plasma cells are replaced by the malignant clone (Fig. 19–9). Presence of a paraprotein with normal polyclonal γ suggests a possible plasmacytoma that has not yet spread throughout the bone marrow. The laboratory evaluation of myeloma should include serum and urine protein electrophoreses to detect aberrant clonal bands, immunoelectrophoresis or immunofixation to type the heavy and light chains of the paraprotein, and quantitation of immunoglobulins to provide a baseline for monitoring the patient's response to therapy or disease progression. Other proteins that may sometimes be mistaken for monoclonal bands of immunoglobulin on serum protein electrophoresis include haptoglobin–hemoglobin complexes, C3 and its variants, β-lipoprotein, transferrin, fibrinogen, immune complexes, CRP, and occasionally, α₂-macroglobulin.

Immunoglobulins, disorders of the immune system, and abnormalities of complement are discussed further in Chapters 45, 46, and 49.

References

Al-Rashid RA, Spangler J: Neonatal copper deficiency. N Engl J Med 1971; 285:841–843.

Alvan G: Ethnic differences in reactions to drugs and xenobiotics. Other protein variants with pharmacogenetic consequences: Albumin and orosomucoid. Prog Clin Biol Res 1986; 214:345–355.

Bean P, Harasymiw J, Peterson CM, Javors M: Innovative technologies for the diagnosis of alcohol abuse and monitoring abstinence. Alcoholism Clin Exp Res 2001; 25:309–316.

Comprehensive review of assays for carbohydrate-deficient transferrin and strategies for their use.

Beetham R, Cattell WR: Proteinuria: Pathophysiology, significance and recommendations for measurement in clinical practice. Ann Clin Biochem 1993; 30:425–434.

Berninger RW: Protease inhibitors of human plasma. Alpha 1-antitrypsin. J Med 1985a; 16:23–99.

Berninger RW: Protease inhibitors of human plasma. Alpha 1-antichymotrypsin. J Med 1985b; 16:101–128.

Bikle DD, Halloran BP, Gee E, et al: Free 25-hydroxyvitamin D levels are normal in subjects with liver disease and reduced total 25-hydroxyvitamin D levels. J Clin Invest 1986; 78:748–752.

Blennow K, Fredman P: Detection of cerebrospinal fluid leakage by isoelectric focusing on polyacrylamide gels with silver staining using the PhastSystem. Acta Neurochir (Wien) 1995; 136:135–139.

Branden C, Tooze J: Introduction to Protein Structure. New York, Garland Publishing, Inc, 1991.

Brinkman JW, Bakker SJ, Gansevoort RT, et al: Which method for quantifying urinary albumin excretion gives what outcome? A comparison of immunonephelometry with HPLC. Kidney Int Suppl 2004; 92:569–575.

Brodsky JL: Translocation of proteins across the endoplasmic reticulum membrane. Int Rev Cytol 1998; 178:277–328.

Burrows S, Pekala B: Serum copper and ceruloplasmin in pregnancy. Am J Obstet Gyncecol 1971; 109:907–909.

Carvalho A, Ellman L: Hereditary antithrombin III deficiency. Effect of antithrombin on platelet function. Am J Med 1976; 61:179–183.

Chen FA: Rapid protein analysis by capillary electrophoresis. J Chromatogr 1991; 559:445–543.

Claus DR, Osmand AP, Gewurz H: Radioimmunoassay of human C-reactive protein and levels in normal sera. J Lab Clin Med 1976; 87:120–128.

Clyne B, Olshaker JS: The C-reactive protein. J Emerg Med 1999; 17:1019–1025.

Cox DW: Clinical and molecular studies of alpha 1-antitrypsin deficiency. Prog Clin Biol Res 1986; 214:373–384.

Dahl B, Schiodt FV, Ott P, et al: Plasma concentration of Gc-globulin is associated with organ dysfunction and sepsis after injury. Crit Care Med 2003; 31:152–156.

Daiger SP, Schanfield MS, Cavalli-Sforza LL: Group-specific component (Gc) proteins bind vitamin D and 25-hydroxy-vitamin D. Proc Natl Acad Sci USA 1975; 72:2076–2080.

Daniels JC: Abnormalities of protease inhibitors. In Ritzmann SE, Daniels JC (eds): Serum Protein Abnormalities, Diagnostic and Clinical Aspects. Boston, Little, Brown & Co, 1975.

Daniels JC, Larson DL, Abston S, Ritzmann SE: Serum protein profiles in thermal burns. II. Protease inhibitors, complement factors and C-reactive proteins. J Trauma 1974; 14:153–162.

Delaroche O, Bordure P, Lippert E, Sagniez M: Perilymph detection by beta 2-transferrin immunoblotting assay. Application to the diagnosis of perilymphatic fistulae. Clin Chim Acta 1996; 245:93–104.

Deodhar SD: C-reactive protein. The best laboratory indicator available for monitoring disease activity. Cleveland Clin J Med 1989; 56:126–130.

Doolittle RF: Fibrinogen and fibrin. In Putnam FW (ed): The Plasma Proteins, Vol II, 2nd ed. New York, Academic Press, 1975, p 110.

Doolittle RF, Yang Z, Mochalkin I: Crystal structure studies on fibrinogen and fibrin. Fibrinogen. Ann N Y Acad Sci 2001; 936:31–43.

Dowton SB, Colten HR: Acute phase reactants in inflammation and infection. Semin Hematol 1988; 25:84–90.

Eriksson S: Studies in alpha 1-antitrypsin deficiency. Acta Med Scand 1965; 177(Suppl):1–85.

Ferenci P: Review article: diagnosis and current therapy of Wilson's disease. Aliment Pharmacol Ther 2004;19:157–165.
Up-to-date account of the role of laboratory testing in diagnosing Wilson's disease.

Fischer CL, Gill C, Forrester MG, Nakamura R: Quantitation of 'acute phase proteins'

postoperatively. Value in detection and monitoring of complications. Am J Clin Pathol 1976; 66:840–846.

Gaetani S, Bellovino D, Apreda M, Devirgiliis C: Hepatic synthesis, maturation and complex formation between retinol-binding protein and transthyretin. Clin Chem Lab Med 2002; 40:1211–1220.

Gelb AF, Klein E, Lieberman J: Pulmonary function in nonsmoking subjects with alpha-1-antitrypsin deficiency (MZ phenotype). Am J Med 1977; 62:93–98.

Ghacha R, Sinha AK, Karkar AM: HbA1c and serum fructosamine as markers of the chronic glycemic state in type 2 diabetic hemodialysis patients. Dialysis & Transplantation 2001; 30:214–217.

Giblett ER (ed): Genetic Markers in Human Blood. Oxford, Blackwell Scientific, 1969.

Gitlin D, Biasucci A: Development of gamma G, gamma A, gamma M, C'1 esterase inhibitor, ceruloplasmin, transferrin, hemopexin, haptoglobin, fibrinogen, plasminogen, alpha 1-antitrypsin, orosomucoid, beta-lipoprotein, alpha 2-macroglobulin, and prealbumin in the human conceptus. J Clin Invest 1969; 48:1433–1446.

Gitlin D, Gitlin JD: Genetic alterations in the plasma proteins of man. In Putnam FW (ed): The Plasma Proteins, Vol II, 2nd ed. New York, Academic Press, 1975, p 321.

Glenner GG: Amyloid deposits and amyloidosis. The beta-fibrilloses. N Engl J Med 1980; 302:1283–1292.

Gofferje H: Prealbumin and retinol binding protein, highly sensitive parameters for the nutritional state in respect to protein. Med Lab 1978; 5:38–44.

Goldstein DA, Haldimann B, Sherman D, et al: Vitamin D metabolites and calcium metabolism in patients with nephrotic syndrome and normal renal function. J Clin Endocrinol Metab 1981; 52:116–121.

Griffin JH, Heeb MJ, Schwarz HP: Plasma protein S deficiency and thromboembolic disease. Prog Hematol 1987; 15:39–49.

Guthrow CE, Morris MA, Day JF, et al: Enhanced nonenzymatic glucosylation of human serum albumin in diabetes mellitus. Proc Natl Acad Sci USA 1979; 76:4258–4261.

Harding JJ: Nonenzymatic covalent posttranslational modification of proteins in vivo. Adv Protein Chem 1985; 37:247–334.

Harpel PC, Rosenberg RD: Alpha-2-macroglobulin and antithrombin–heparin cofactor: Modulators of hemostatic and inflammatory reactions. Prog Hemost and Thromb 1976; 3:145–189.

Hayashi H, Kimura N, Yamaguchi H, et al: A seed for Alzheimer amyloid in the brain. J Neurosci 2004; 24:4894–4902.

Hoffmann A, Nimtz M, Getzlaff R, Conradt HS: 'Brain-type' N-glycosylation of asialo-transferrin from human cerebrospinal fluid. FEBS Lett 1995; 359:164–168.

Hokama Y: Methods of assay and role of acute phase C-reactive protein in human diseases. In Nakamura RM, Dito WR, Tucker ES (eds): Immunologic Analysis. Recent Progress in Diagnostic Laboratory Immunology. New York, Masson Publishing, 1982, p 239.

Horne CHW, Weir RJ, Howie PW, Goudie RB: Effect of combined oestrogen–progesterone oral contraceptives on serum levels of alpha-2-macroglobuin, transferrin, albumin, and IgG. Lancet 1970; 1:49–50.

Hubbard RC, Brantly ML, Sellers S, et al: Anti-neutrophil-elastase defenses of the lower respiratory tract in alpha 1-antitrypsin deficiency directly augmented with an aerosol of alpha 1-antitrypsin. Ann Intern Med 1989; 111:206–212.

Ii S, Minnerath S, Ii K, et al: Two-tiered DNA-based diagnosis of transthyretin amyloidosis reveals two novel point mutations. Neurology 1991; 41:893–898.

Irie S, Tavassoli M: Transferrin-mediated cellular iron uptake. J Med Sci 1987; 293:103–111.

Jenkins N, Parekh RB, James DC: Getting the glycosylation right: Implications for the biotechnology industry. Nat Biotechnol 1996; 14:975–981.

Jeppsson J-O, Franzén B: Typing of genetic variants of alpha-1-antitrypsin by electrofocusing. Clin Chem 1982; 28:219–225.

Jeppsson J-O, Laurell CB, Franzén B: Agarose gel electrophoresis. Clin Chem 1979; 25:629–638.

Kamboh MI, Ferrell RE: Human transferrin polymorphism. Hum Hered 1987; 37:65–81.

Killingsworth LM: Clinical applications of protein determinations in biological fluids other than blood. Clin Chem 1982; 28:1093–1102.

Koch-Weser J, Sellers EM: Drug therapy. Binding of drugs to serum albumin. N Engl J Med 1976; 294:311–316.

Koerper MA, Dallman PR: Serum iron concentration and transferrin saturation in the diagnosis of iron deficiency in children: Normal developmental changes. J Pediatr 1977; 91:870–874.

Konigsberg W: Molecular diseases. In Bondy PK, Roenberg LE (eds): Duncan's Diseases of Metabolism, 7th ed. Philadelphia, WB Saunders Company, 1974, p 86.

Kosaka S, Tazawa M: Alpha-1-antichymotrypsin in rheumatoid arthritis. Tohoku J Exp Med 1976; 119:369–375.

Kuznetsov G, Nigam SK: Folding of secretory and membrane proteins. N Engl J Med 1998; 339:1688–1695.

Lauff JJ, Kasper ME, Wu TW, Ambrose RT: Isolation and preliminary characterization of a fraction of bilirubin in serum that is firmly bound to protein. Clin Chem 1982; 28:629–637.
Early account of delta-bilirubin and its relationship to albumin.

Laurell CB: Quantitative estimation of proteins by electrophoresis in agarose gel containing antibodies. Anal Biochem 1966; 15:45–52.

Laurell CB: Electrophoresis, specific protein assays, or both in measurement of plasma proteins? Clin Chem 1973; 19:99–102.

Laurell CB, Jeppsson J-O: Protease inhibitors in plasma. In Putnam FW (ed): The Plasma Proteins, Vol I, 2nd ed. New York, Academic Press, 1975, p 299.

Layne E: Spectrophotometric and turbidimetric methods for measuring proteins. Meth Enzymol 1957; 3:447–445.
Classical paper on protein measurements.

Lieberman J, Gaidulis L, Garoutte B, Mittman C: Identification and characteristics of the common alpha-1-antitrypsin phenotypes. Chest 1972; 62:557–564.

Lijnen HR, Collen D: Protease inhibitors of human plasma. Alpha 2-antiplasmin. J Med 1985; 16:225–284.

Lowry OH, Rosebrough NJ, Farr L, Randall RJ: Protein measurement with Folin phenol reagent. J Biol Chem 1951; 193:265–275.

Maachi M, Felahi S, Regeniter A, et al: Patterns of proteinuria: urinary sodium dodecyl sulfate electrophoresis versus immunonephelometric protein marker measurement followed by interpretation with the knowledge-based system MDI-LabLink. Clin Chem 2004; 50:1834–1837.
This paper presents patterns of proteinuria and new methods for their discrimination.

MacGillivray RTA, Mendez E, Sinha S, et al: The complete amino acid sequence of human serum transferrin. Proc Natl Acad Sci USA 1982; 79:2504–2508.

Manoharan A: Congenital haptoglobin deficiency, letter. Blood 1997; 90:1709.

Meloun B, Moravek L, Kostka V: Complete amino acid sequence of human serum albumin. FEBS Lett 1975; 58:134–137.

Menache D: Abnormal fibrinogens: A review. Thromb Diath Haemorrh 1973; 29:525–535.

Mendenhall HW: Serum protein concentrations in pregnancy. I. Concentrations in maternal serum. Am J Obstet Gynecol 1970; 106:388–399.

Merril CR, Goldman D, Sedman SA, Ebert MH: Ultrasensitive stain for proteins in polyacrylamide gels shows regional variation in cerebrospinal fluid proteins. Science 1981; 211:1437–1438.

Moses AC, Lawlor J, Haddow J, Jackson IMD: Familial euthyroid hyperthyroxinemia resulting from increased thyroxine binding to thyroxine-binding prealbumin. N Engl J Med 1982; 306:966–969.

Muller-Eberhard U: Hemopexin. N Engl J Med 1970; 283:1090–1094.

Myara I, Quenum G, Storogenko M, et al: Monoclonal and oligoclonal gammopathies in heart transplant recipients. Clin Chem 1991; 37:1334–1337.

Nilsson IM, Tengborn LA: A family with thrombosis associated with high level of tissue plasminogen activator. Haemostasis 1984; 14:24.

Normansell DE, Stacy EK, Booker CF, Butler TZ: Detection of beta-2 transferrin in otorrhea and rhinorrhea in a routine clinical laboratory setting. Clin Diagn Lab Immunol 1994; 1:68–70.

Oppenheimer JH: Role of plasma proteins in the binding, distribution and metabolism of the thyroid hormones. N Engl J Med 1968; 278:1153–1162.

Orth SR, Ritz E: The nephrotic syndrome. N Engl J Med 1998; 338:1202–1211.

Peters T: Serum albumin: Recent progress in the understanding of its structure and biosynthesis. Clin Chem 1977; 23:5–12.

Comprehensive review of clinically important structure–function relationships of albumin.

Peters T Jr: Serum albumin. *In* Putnam FW (ed): The Plasma Proteins, Vol II, 2nd ed. New York, Academic Press, 1975, p 133.

Peterson PA: Studies on interaction between pre-albumin, retinol-binding protein and vitamin A. J Biol Chem 1971; 246:44–49.

Post DJ, Carter KC, Papaconstantinou J: The effect of aging on constitutive mRNA levels and lipopolysaccharide inducibility of acute phase genes. Ann NY Acad Sci 1991; 621:66–77.

Prograis LJ, Brickman CM, Frank MM: Protease inhibitors of human plasma. C1-inhibitor (C1-Inh). J Med 1985; 16:303–350.

Reddy S, Adcock KJ, Adeshina H, et al: Immunity, transferrin, and survival in kwashiorkor. Br Med J 1970; 4:268–270.

Ridker PM, Hennekens CH, Buring JE, Rifai N: C-reactive protein and other markers of inflammation in the prediction of cardiovascular disease in women. N Engl J Med 2000; 342:836–843.

Ritzmann SE, Daniels JC (eds): Serum Protein Abnormalities. Diagnostic and Clinical Aspects. Boston, Little, Brown & Co, 1975.

Roberts RC: Protease inhibitors of human plasma. Alpha 2-macroglobulin. J Med 1985; 16:129–224.

Roelandse FW, van der Zwart N, Didden JH, et al: Detection of CSF leakage by isoelectric focusing on polyacrylamide gel, direct immunofixation of transferrins, and silver staining. Clin Chem 1998; 44:351–353.

Roeser HP, Lee GR, Nacht S, Cartwright GE: The role of ceruloplasmin in iron metabolism. J Clin Invest 1970; 49:2408–2417.

Rosenberg RD: Actions and interactions of antithrombin and heparin. N Engl J Med 1975; 292:146–151.

Rosenberg RD, Bauer KA: Thrombosis in inherited deficiencies of antithrombin, protein C, and protein S. Hum Pathol 1987; 18:253–262.

Rosenberg RD, Bauer KA, Marcum JA: Protease inhibitors of human plasma. Antithrombin-III: The heparin–antithrombin system. J Med 1985; 16:351–416.

Roses AD: Apolipoprotein E is a genetic locus that affects the rate of Alzheimer disease expression. Neuropsychopharmacology 1994; 10:55.

Rothschild MA, Oratz M, Schreiber SS: Albumin synthesis. N Engl J Med 1972; 286:748, 816–821.

Ruiz M, Rajatanavin R, Young RA, et al: Familial dysalbuminemic hyperthyroxinemia. A syndrome that can be confused with thyrotoxicosis. N Engl J Med 1982; 306:635-639.

Saraiva M, Alves IL, Costa PP: Simplified method for screening populations at risk for transthyretin met 30 associated familial amyloidotic polyneuropathy. Clin Chem 1989; 35:1033–1035.

Saxstad J, Nilsson L-A, Hanson LA: C-reactive protein in serum from infants as determined with immunodiffusion techniques. Acta Pediatr Scand 1970; 59:676–680.

Schenker JG, Jungreis E, Polishuk WZ: Oral contraceptives and serum copper concentrations. Obstet Gynecol 1971; 37:233–237.

Schmid K: Alpha-1-acid glycoprotein. *In* Putnam FW (ed): The Plasma Proteins, Vol I, 2nd ed. New York, Academic Press, 1975.

Sevall JS: The albumin gene: DNA–protein interaction. Fed Proc 1986; 45:2412–2415.

Slater L, Carter PM, Hobbs JR: Measurement of albumin in the sera of patients. Ann Clin Biochem 1975; 12:33–40.

Sloman AJ, Kelly RH: Transferrin allelic variants may cause false positives in the detection of cerebrospinal fluid fistulae. Clin Chem 1993; 39:1444–1445.

Snider GL: Pulmonary disease in alpha1-antitrypsin deficiency. Ann Intern Med 1989; 111:957–959.

Solomon P, Chen J, D'Costa M, et al: Extracranial drainage of cerebrospinal fluid: A study of beta-transferrins in nasal and lymphatic tissues. Laryngoscope 1999; 109:1313–1315.

Stenflo J: Structure and function of protein C. Semin Thromb Hemost 1984; 10:109–121.

Stibler H: Carbohydrate-deficient transferrin in serum: A new marker of potentially harmful alcohol consumption reviewed. Clin Chem 1991; 37:2029–2037.

Sveger T: Liver disease in alpha 1-antitrypsin deficiency detected by screening of 200,000 infants. N Engl J Med 1976; 294:1316–1321.

Thalmann I, Kohut RI, Ryu J, et al: Protein profile of human perilymph: In search of markers for the diagnosis of perilymph fistula and other inner ear disease. Otolaryngol Head Neck Surg 1994; 111:273–280.

Tolosano E, Altruda F: Hemopexin: structure, function, and regulation. DNA Cell Biol 2002; 21:297–306.

Comprehensive discussion of the chemistry and roles of hemopexin.

Tripathi RC, Millard CB, Tripathi BJ, Noronha A: Tau fraction of transferrin is present in human aqueous humor and is not unique to cerebrospinal fluid. Exp Eye Res 1990; 50:541–547.

Tsung SH, Rosenthal WA, Milewski KA: Immunological measurement of transferrin compared with chemical measurement of total iron-binding capacity. Clin Chem 1975; 21:1063–1066.

Van den Steen P, Rudd PM, Dwek RA, Opdenakker G: Concepts and principles of O-linked glycosylation. Crit Rev Biochem Mol Biol 1998; 33:151–208.

Van Oss CJ, Bronson PM, Border JR: Changes in the serum alpha glycoprotein distribution in trauma patients. J Trauma 1975; 15:451–455.

Waldman TA, Gordon RS, Rosse W: Studies on the metabolism of the serum proteins and lipids in patients with analbuminemia. Am J Med 1964; 37:960–968.

Walsh PG, Haddad JG: 'Rocket' immunoelectrophoresis assay of vitamin D-binding protein (Gc globulin) in human serum. Clin Chem 1982; 28:1781–1783.

Weinberg ED: Iron and infection. Microbiol Rev 1978; 42:45–66.

Westwood SA, Werrett DJ: Group-specific component: A review of the isoelectric focusing methods and auxillary methods available for the separation of its phenotypes. Forensic Sci Int 1986; 32:135–150.

Whitehead AS, Bruns GAP, Markham AF, et al: Isolation of human C-reactive protein complementary DNA and localization of the gene to chromosome 1. Science 1983; 221:69–71.

Wickner S, Maurizi MR, Gottesman S: Posttranslational quality control: Folding, refolding, and degrading proteins. Science 1999; 286:1888–1893.

Wochner RD, Spilberg I, Iio A, et al: Hemopexin metabolism in sickle cell disease, porphyrias and control subjects: Effect of heme injection. N Engl J Med 1974; 290:822–826.

Xin Y, Lasker JM, Lieber CS: Serum carbohydrate-deficient transferrin: Mechanism of increase after chronic alcohol intake. Hepatology 1995; 22:1462–1468.

Zaret DL, Morrison N, Gulbranson R, Keren DF: Immunofixation to quantify beta 2-transferrin in cerebrospinal fluid to detect leakage of cerebrospinal fluid from skull injury. Clin Chem 1992; 38:1908–1912.

Description of assay for a specific marker for CSF in unknown fluid.

Zawadzki Z, Edwards G: Pseudoparaproteinemia due to hypertransferrinemia. Am J Clin Pathol 1970; 54:802–809.

CHAPTER 20
Clinical Enzymology

Naif Z. Abraham Jr MD PhD, Robert P. Carty MD, D. Robert DuFour MD, Matthew R. Pincus MD PhD

KEY POINTS

• Enzymes are protein catalysts utilized by essentially all mammalian cells in specific biochemical reactions in different organs of the body and which may also be physically located in different organelles and structures within a cell.

• Most enzymes have a practical or trivial name as well as a name based upon standardized nomenclature of the International Union of Biochemistry; the latter is based upon the type of reaction catalyzed by the enzyme.

• In addition to certain narrow ranges of pH, temperature, and protein and salt concentration, most enzymes require additional organic molecules and/or inorganic ions for optimal enzyme function.

• An understanding of enzyme kinetics allows for laboratory measurement of plasma enzyme levels as well as determination of possible enzyme inhibition.

• Damaged or dying cells within organs can release enzymes into the circulation; these plasma enzyme levels can be used clinically to develop a differential diagnosis of a patient with respect to specific organ disease and dysfunction.

• Many enzymes have isozymes, i.e., polypeptide chains that differ in sequence but have similar enzymatic activity. Some enzymes are composed of two or more different polypeptide chains, such as the M and B chains of creatine phosphokinase, giving rise to isozymes that differ in chain composition, e.g., the MM, MB and BB forms of CPK. In a number of diseases, specific isozymes become elevated in serum, facilitating diagnosis.

• Examples of the above key point include changes in creatine phosphokinase (CPK)-MB isoform serum levels (a myocardial enzyme) in heart disease, alanine aminotransferase (ALT) serum level changes in liver disease, and changes in serum levels of total creatine phosphokinase with skeletal muscle injury.

General Properties of Enzymes

A catalyst accelerates the rate of a chemical reaction. The acceleration may occur in solution and the process is called homogeneous catalysis. Catalysis on an insoluble surface is termed heterogeneous catalysis. Biological catalysts are called enzymes and for the most part are proteins that exhibit homogeneous catalysis. However, some enzymes are embedded in membrane structures and should be considered insoluble, heterogeneous catalysts.

Enzyme specificity defines the capacity of protein catalysts to recognize and bind only one or a few molecules, the *substrate*(s), excluding all others, a process referred to as *binding specificity*. An enzyme catalyzes a unique chemical process, i.e., a solitary type of covalent bond is broken or formed. This is called *reaction specificity*. Most enzymes exhibit absolute reaction specificity; that is, no minor by-products are formed. Binding specificity permits many biochemical reactions to occur simultaneously within the same biological space. Absolute reaction specificity saves energy because it reduces the pool of unwanted metabolites.

Enzymes are stereoselective because of the asymmetry of their active sites. They recognize only one enantiomeric form (i.e., one of a pair of compounds having a mirror image relationship) of a chiral substrate. Hence, proteases exclusively bind polypeptides made up of L-amino acids (and *not* D-amino acids) and catalyze their hydrolysis. Enzymes exhibit geometric specificity exemplified by the fumarase reaction, in which the Krebs cycle intermediate, fumarate (the *trans* isomer), but not maleate (the *cis* isomer) undergoes hydration.

The concentration of enzyme molecules within a given intracellular or extracellular space depends on its rate of synthesis and degradation. Control of enzyme synthesis occurs at both transcriptional and translational levels. In eukaryotes, cells of different organs express different isoforms of the same enzyme, which alters rates and specificity suitable for selective cellular homeostasis. The presence of substrate, or other inducing molecule, can cause a sudden increase in enzyme levels.

Enzymatic activity is also subject to control through the binding of small molecules that produce conformational changes in the structure of the enzyme. This binding can alter substrate affinity for the enzyme, or change the enzyme's catalytic activity, or both. Generally, enzymes that catalyze rate-determining steps in metabolic pathways are subject to this type of regulation.

Enzymes do not affect the value of the equilibrium constant. In a reversible reaction they accelerate the forward and reverse reactions by the same relative amount. The equilibrium distribution of reactants and products is unchanged whether the equilibrium state has been achieved in the presence or absence of an enzyme.

Almost all known enzymes are proteins or conjugated proteins. A few enzymes are nucleoproteins, which are RNA molecules complexed to proteins.

Enzymes contain a surface region referred to as the *active site* where binding and catalysis occur. It is a cleft or crevice in which are embedded specific groups, suitably oriented, which carry out the roles of binding, and bond-making or bond cleavage. The three-dimensional shape of the active site is a vital determinant in the recognition and specificity process. The *enzyme–substrate complex* is the adduct formed by the physical adsorption of the substrate to the active site. Enzyme–substrate complex formation requires specific alignment of atoms in the active site with

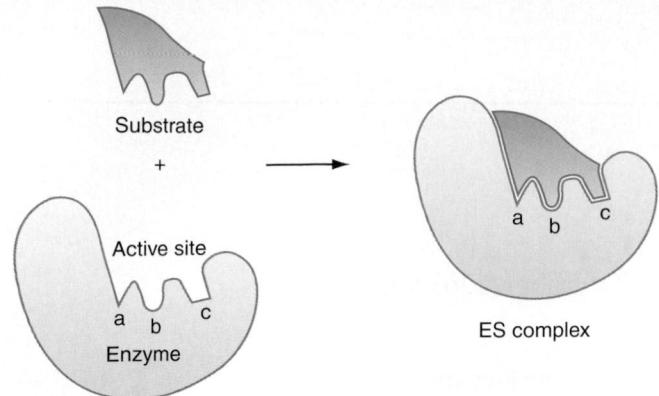

Figure 20–1 The *lock and key* model of substrate binding to the enzyme active site. The enzyme exhibits preformed steric and electronic complementarity to the shape and charge distribution of the substrate. No shape changes or electronic redistributions in either the enzyme or the substrate are necessary for optimal binding. (Redrawn from W.H. Freeman and Company, San Francisco, CA, Lubert Stryer, Stanford University, Biochemistry, 2nd edn., 1981.)

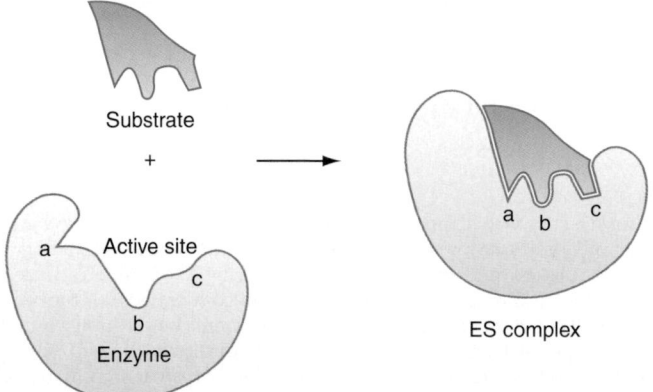

Figure 20–2 The *induced fit* model of substrate binding to the enzyme active site. The induced fit model postulates an initial weak, flexible interaction of the substrate with groups in the enzyme's substrate-binding site. This is sufficient to trigger a conformational rearrangement of the enzyme's surface that exposes additional ligand binding groups that enhance the binding affinity of the substrate for the enzyme. (Redrawn from W.H. Freeman and Company, San Franscisco, CA, Lubert Stryer, Stanford University, Biochemistry, 2nd edn., 1981.)

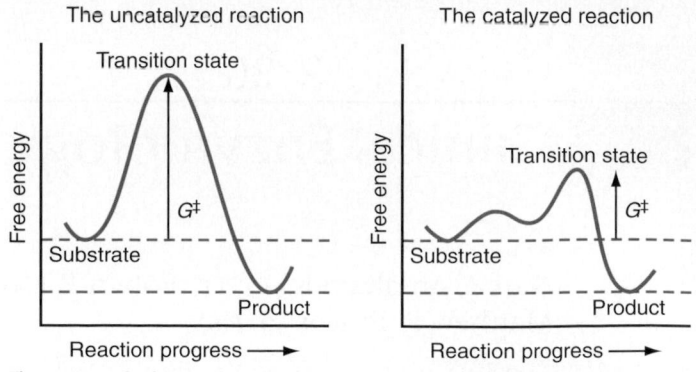

The uncatalyzed reaction   The catalyzed reaction

Figure 20–3 The free energy path of a reactant molecule through its transition state on its way to becoming a product molecule. *A*, The uncatalyzed reaction; *B*, The enzyme-catalyzed reaction. The energy trajectory followed by a molecule undergoing a chemical reaction is the minimum free energy pathway known as the *reaction coordinate*. The transition state, the state of highest free energy, is the point where there is an equal probability that reaction will take place or that the *activated complex* will decompose back to the reactant. The free energy change, $\Delta G^{\ddagger}$, is the energy that the substrate molecule must acquire to reach the activated complex. This energy is less in the catalyzed reaction. The energy diagram on the right (*B*) represents a two-step process characteristic of enzyme-catalyzed reactions in which the covalent change is preceded by a binding step. In a multistep reaction the overall rate is a function of the step with the highest value of $\Delta G^{\ddagger}$.

atoms in the substrate molecule. This complementary arrangement is referred to as the *lock and key* fit of the substrate in the active site and is illustrated in Figure 20–1. Sometimes the shape of the substrate molecule does not exactly match the contour of the active site. Yet the substrate binds tightly because of its capacity to reshape the active site to a conformation that binds the substrate with high affinity. This type of substrate adsorption is described as *induced fit*. It is illustrated in Figure 20–2. Active sites of 'induced fit' enzymes only become complementary *after* the substrate is bound. Some of the favorable binding energy is used in reorganizing the shape of the active site.

The *free energy of activation* is the energy absorbed by reactant molecules before they have a chance to convert to products. The free energy of activation is a barrier to chemical reactivity. When this barrier is large, the rate of a chemical reaction is very slow. The lower the barrier, the faster is the reaction rate. The barrier exists for almost all chemical reactions because, for bonds to be broken, they must be stretched and sometimes bent away from their equilibrium positions. These deformations require energy. Enzymes *lower* the free energy of activation. Most metabolic reactions have very high activation barriers; and in the absence of enzymes, reaction rates are imperceptibly slow. Cells can selectively reduce metabolic reaction rates to near zero by abolishing enzyme activity. This feature of metabolism allows cells to 'turn on' and 'turn off' metabolic pathways during different stages of the cell cycle. Enzymes lower the free energy of activation in various ways. Binding and appropriate orientation of the substrate in the active site increases its proximity to the catalytic groups. Various types of catalysis are used by enzymes. The major types of catalysis are acid–base, electrophilic, nucleophilic, metal ion and electrostatic catalysis. Reductions in the free energy of activation occur through preferential binding of the transition state (or intermediate enzyme–substrate) complex to active site groups. The side chains of different amino acids participate in catalysis. The side chain of histidine is an effective acid–base catalyst, while the side chains of serine, cysteine, lysine, histidine

and aspartic acid participate in covalent catalysis. The side chains of lysine and arginine, as well as metal ions, can act as electrostatic catalysts by stabilizing negative charges that develop during catalysis.

The rate of the reaction is proportional to the concentration of molecules that have attained an energy equal to the free energy of activation, $\Delta G^{\ddagger}$. This energy is higher for the uncatalyzed reaction. The idea that enzymes accelerate chemical reactions by lowering $\Delta G^{\ddagger}$ is illustrated in Figure 20–3, where the free energy needed for a productive reaction is compared between an uncatalyzed and enzyme-catalyzed reaction. Enzymes have developed as extremely efficient catalysts because their active sites have evolved to bind transition states very tightly. It is this tight binding, which stabilizes the transition state and lowers the free energy of activation. Enzymes do not alter the ground state energies of reactants and products of a chemical reaction. The equilibrium state is characterized as a state of lowest energy and the composition of the reactant and product mixture at equilibrium is a reflection of these ground state energies. Enzymes emerge from the catalytic process unaltered, although some undergo transient chemical modification during the reaction.

Nomenclature of Enzymes

The nomenclature of commonly measured enzymes was standardized by the Enzyme Commission (EC) of the International Union of Biochemistry (1979, 1992). Each enzyme has two names, a practical or trivial name and a systematic name. The latter consists of a unique numerical code designation and the nature of the catalytic reaction, as follows: Enzymes are named by citing the name of the substrate molecule, and following that with the suffix, *ase*; sometimes the name also includes a designation of the type of reaction catalyzed.

Examples

1. Ribonucleic acid (RNA) is hydrolyzed by an enzyme called *ribonuclease*.
2. Lactic acid is oxidized to pyruvic acid by an enzyme called *lactic acid dehydrogenase*.

Older trivial names persist in the literature. Examples are trypsin, a protein-hydrolyzing enzyme secreted into the gut, and papain, a plant enzyme that also hydrolyzes proteins. A more systematic classification of enzymes has been implemented in the biochemical literature (International Union of Biochemistry, 1979, 1992). Enzymes have been organized into six major classes by reaction type as shown in Table 20–1.

Many enzymes have *isoenzymes*, i.e., structurally different forms that catalyze the same reaction. Most commonly, different isoenzymes are found in specific organs or tissues; determination of the type of isoenzyme present can then be of use in identifying the tissue damaged and releasing the enzyme. The standard nomenclature of isoenzymes is based on their electrophoretic migration, with the isoenzyme migrating farthest towards the anode designated isoenzyme 1. The most widely recognized isoenzymes are those that are composed of varying combinations of subunits; common examples are creatine kinase (CK), a dimer of M (muscle) and B (brain) subunits, and lactate dehydrogenase (LD), a

Table 20–1 Enzyme Classification

Class		Type of reaction catalyzed
1	Oxidoreductases	Oxidation–reduction reactions
2	Transferases	Transfer of functional groups
3	Hydrolases	Hydrolysis reactions
4	Lyases	Group elimination to form double bonds
5	Isomerases	Isomerizations
6	Ligases	Bond formation coupled with ATP hydrolysis

tetramer of H (heart) and M (muscle) subunits. In other cases, isoenzymes may have the same protein component, but differ based on modifications made by the cell of origin. For example, the bone, renal, and liver isoenzymes of alkaline phosphatase have identical amino acid sequences but differ in carbohydrate composition.

In some cases, isoenzymes may have completely different protein structures. There are distinct cytoplasmic and mitochondrial isoenzymes of both CK and aspartate aminotransferase (AST) with markedly differing structures. Placental and intestinal alkaline phosphatase isoenzymes have a different protein structure than do the 'tissue nonspecific' forms found in liver, bone, and other organs.

Finally, enzymes can be modified by proteases present in serum to produce forms that differ slightly from each other; these are termed *isoforms*. As an example, CK-M subunits are partially metabolized by carboxypeptidase N, removing a lysine residue from the carboxy-terminal end of the molecule and converting the tissue isoform to a differently charged plasma isoform. The relative amount of the tissue and plasma isoforms can be used as a marker of duration of injury to CK-containing cells. The official names and EC numbers of the commonly measured, clinically useful enzymes are given in Table 20–2 (Zollner, 1989).

Enzyme Cofactors

Two-thirds of all enzymes contain cofactors that are a group of heat-stable substances required for catalysis. They are low-molecular-weight organic molecules and inorganic ions. The combination of cofactor plus the protein portion, the *apoenzyme*, forms the complete catalytic entity and is known as the *holoenzyme*. Organic cofactors are bound covalently or noncovalently to the apoenzyme. Covalently bound cofactors are sometimes referred to as *prosthetic groups*. Cofactors are observed in oxidation–reduction, group transfer, and isomerization reactions, and reactions that form covalent bonds. Hydrolytic reactions generally do not require cofactors. Organic cofactors are listed in Table 20–3. Inorganic cofactors that include mainly metal ions are listed in Table 20–4. A *cosubstrate* is an organic cofactor that behaves as a second substrate in an enzyme-catalyzed reaction. Cofactors such as NAD^+ can serve as cosubstrates for many oxidoreductases. A single molecule of

Table 20–3 Organic Cofactors

Coenzyme	Reaction type	Deficiency
Coenzyme A	Acyl transfer	
Thiamine pyrophosphate	Aldehyde transfer	Beriberi
Folic acid coenzymes	One-carbon transfer	Megaloblastic anemia
Cobamide (B_{12}) coenzymes	Alkylation	Pernicious anemia
Nicotinamide coenzymes	Oxidation–reduction	Pellagra
Flavin coenzymes	Oxidation–reduction	
Biotin	Carboxylation	
Lipoic acid	Acyl transfer	
Pyridoxal phosphate	Amino group transfer	
Coenzyme Q	Electron transfer	

Table 20–4 Inorganic Cofactors

Mg^{2+}	Ca^{2+}
Fe^{2+}/Fe^{3+}	Mn^{2+}
Zn^{2+}	Co^{2+}
Cu^+/Cu^{2+}	

NAD^+ may act as a cosubstrate many thousands of times. The product, NADH, must first be oxidized back to NAD^+ before it can participate again as an electron and H atom acceptor. The recycling of the NAD^+–NADH oxidation–reduction couple depends on the ready availability of a chemical system capable of regenerating NAD^+ from NADH. A substrate molecule is usually irreversibly changed in a reaction. In contrast, cosubstrate molecules are recycled.

Factors Affecting Plasma Enzyme Activities

There are a number of mechanisms by which plasma levels of enzymes may be increased. Since enzymes are high-molecular-weight compounds, the most common cause for increased plasma enzymes is death of enzyme-containing cells. As cells die, activation of phospholipases leads to development of holes in the plasma membrane, allowing leakage of cytoplasmic macromolecules such as proteins. Enzymes are also released in the process of normal cell turnover; this is thought to be the source of normal plasma levels of various enzymes. Increased synthesis of enzymes by cells also leads to increased plasma enzyme levels. With increased activity of osteoblasts, plasma levels of bone isoenzyme of alkaline phosphatase increase. This may also be responsible for the increase in muscle-related enzymes seen with increased exercise (Dickerman, 1999).

Table 20–2 Names, Enzyme Numbers, Substrates for Enzymes

Enzyme (IUB group, EC number)	Substrate	Comments
Acetylcholinesterase (hydrolase, EC 3.1.1.7) or AChE	Acetylcholine, acetyl thiocholine; hydrolyzes acetyl-beta-methylcholine	Choline is $HOCH_2CH_2CH_2N(CH_3)_3$, a quarternary amine; many esters with the OH group are substrates
Pseudocholinesterase (hydrolase, EC 3.1.1.8) or PChE	Many aliphatic esters of choline; unlike AChE, does not hydrolyze acetyl-beta-methylcholine but, also unlike AChE, does hydrolyze butyryl-and benzoylcholine	
Acid phosphatase (hydrolase, EC 3.1.3.2)	Cleaves phosphate esters like ALP but at pH of about 5, incl. G6P, phenyl-P, α-glycerophosphate, phenolphthalein-P, thymolphthalein-P, naphthol-P	Cleaves phosphate esters like ALP but at pH of about 5 pH optimum at about 5.0
Alkaline phosphatase (hydrolase, EC 3.1.3.1)	See acid phosphatase	ALP has unusual pH optimum of about 9. Optimum pH varies with substrate and buffer
Angiotensin-converting enzyme (ACE) (hydrolase, EC 3.4.15.1)	Splits C-terminal His–Leu dipeptide of angiotensin I to yield angiotensin 2; also splits hippuryl-His–Leu to hippurate + His–Leu	Considered a nonspecific hydrolase; acts on met- and leu-enkephalin
Lactate dehydrogenase (oxidoreductase, 1.1.1.27)	Pyruvate and other ketoacids + NADH. Also lactate and other α-hydroxy acids + NAD	Moderately specific
5'-Nucleotidase (hydrolase, EC 3.1.3.5)	5'-Ribonucleotides	Wide specificity for 5'-ribonucleotides

IUB = International Union of Biochemistry; EC = Enzyme Commission; ALP = alkaline phosphatase; G6P = glucose-6-phosphate; P = phosphate; NAD = nicotinamide-adenine dinucleotide; NADH = the reduced form of NAD.

Many drugs that stimulate microsomal enzymes, including ethanol and antiepileptic agents, lead to increased plasma γ-glutamyl transferase (GGT). In some cases, release of enzyme from cells occurs without cell death or increased synthesis. As discussed in Chapter 21 on liver function, ethanol causes expression of the mitochondrial isoenzyme of aspartate aminotransferase (AST) on the surface of hepatocytes and increased plasma levels. Ischemia of myocardial cells leads to loss of glycogen phosphorylase BB isoenzyme into plasma. Ingestion of food leads to release of intestinal alkaline phosphatase into lymphatic fluid, and may transiently increase plasma levels of alkaline phosphatase (ALP). A number of liver enzymes (ALP, GGT, leucine aminopeptidase, 5'-nucleotidase [5'-NT]) are bound to the canalicular surface of the hepatocyte. Increased concentrations of bile salts with canalicular obstruction may release fragments of membrane with enzyme attached into the circulation, or may solubilize the membrane-binding domain (Van Hoof, 1997). Finally, increased plasma enzyme levels may be due to decreased clearance of enzymes from the circulation. Some smaller enzymes, such as amylase and lipase, are partially cleared by glomerular filtration; renal failure increases their plasma levels. For many enzymes, autoantibodies against one or more isoenzymes may cause development of enzyme–antibody complexes (often termed *macroenzymes*) that result in enzyme half-lives similar to the 3-week half-life of immunoglobulin G (IgG) (Remaley, 1989). Most commonly, there is no specific clinical feature associated with such macroenzymes; however, it is common to see antibodies against the intestinal isoenzyme of alkaline phosphatase in persons with bacterial infections (Mader, 1994). A similar phenomenon can occur when enzymes are bound to antibodies directed against other antigens, such as LD complexes with antibodies to streptokinase (Podlasek, 1989).

The time course of appearance and disappearance of enzymes with cell injury is dependent on a number of factors. With cell death, defects in cellular membranes enlarge gradually with time; thus, smaller cytoplasmic enzymes will leak from damaged cells sooner than larger ones. For example, with myocardial injury, CK and AST are smaller than LD and appear in plasma sooner. Some enzymes are not cytoplasmic, but are either within mitochondria (isoenzymes of CK and AST) or bound to plasma membranes (such as ALP and GGT); cell death typically does not lead to release of such enzymes. If cell death is due to infarction, caused by interruption of blood flow to a portion of an organ, enzyme released from damaged cells must diffuse away from the nonperfused region before appearing in the circulation. For example, in myocardial infarction, CK peaks later in persons whose coronary arteries are not successfully reperfused by use of thrombolytic agents. The degree of elevation of an enzyme is related to the number of cells injured, the gradient in concentration between the cell and plasma, and the rates of enzyme entry into and clearance from plasma. In myocardial infarction, the amount of CK released is strongly correlated to size of infarction; thus, enzyme levels with one-time injury are related to amount of cell injury occurring. If injury is ongoing, plasma enzyme levels will continue to be elevated for a longer time period. For example, in acute hepatic injury, the time course of enzyme changes can be used to differentiate viral hepatitis, where immunologic damage causes ongoing cell death and prolonged enzyme elevation, from ischemic and toxic injury, where damage is immediate but short-lived and enzyme elevations rapidly return to normal.

Other important determinants of the time course of enzyme changes include the relative gradient in enzyme levels between cells and serum and the rate of clearance of enzyme from plasma. For any given amount of cell damage, the enzyme with the higher gradient between cells and serum will show greater elevation of plasma levels. For example, with hepatocyte injury, AST levels in hepatocytes are higher than those of alanine aminotransferase (ALT), and both are many times higher than levels of LD. Immediately after injury, therefore, AST will show a greater degree of elevation than will ALT, while LD will show the least degree of increase. In cardiac tissue, the gradient of CK between myocardial cells and plasma is several times higher than that for LD, leading to higher peak CK than LD levels. Once enzyme reaches plasma, the rate of clearance also becomes important; for example, the half-life of AST is much shorter than that of ALT, and the half-life of CK is shorter than that of the cardiac isoenzymes of LD. With hepatic injury, therefore, plasma ALT often becomes higher than AST within a short time of injury. Following myocardial infarction, CK returns to normal several days earlier than does LD.

Enzyme Kinetics

The basic objective of clinical enzymology is the determination of the total concentration of specific enzymes in serum and other body fluids. Qualitatively, detecting the presence of enzymes in body fluids is fortunately quite simple because each enzyme has almost total specificity for one or at most a few substrate(s). By adding the substrate, say, to serum, and observing either its disappearance or the appearance of the product, the presence of the enzyme can be ascertained. As is now explained, the rate at which substrate disappears or product appears can be directly used to determine the concentration of enzyme present (Cleland, 1970, 1990; Cornish-Bowden, 1995; Fersht, 1999, Segal, 1993).

Enzymes exhibit saturation, which occurs when the rate becomes unresponsive to further increases in substrate concentration. Ordinary chemical reactions occur with rates proportional to the entire range of reactant concentrations. In an enzyme-catalyzed reaction, at low substrate concentrations, rates are proportional to substrate concentration. At higher concentrations, the rate does not increase in direct proportion. At still higher substrate concentration, the rate becomes constant and unresponsive to any further change in substrate concentration. This led to the proposal that enzyme catalysis is a two-step process, an initial adsorption where the substrate combines with the enzyme to form a noncovalent enzyme–substrate complex, ES, followed by a second step in which the enzyme–substrate complex decomposes into product (P) and free enzyme (E).

$$E + S \underset{k_{-1}}{\overset{k_1}{\rightleftharpoons}} ES \overset{k_2}{\longrightarrow} P + E \tag{20–1}$$

The physical explanation for saturation is that binding reduces the number of active sites available to form the enzyme–substrate complex. When all sites are filled, no further binding can occur until an active site discharges its contents. The step that determines the overall rate is the k_2 step. Adding additional substrate molecules under saturating conditions does not change the rate because all unbound substrate molecules must wait until an active site becomes vacant.

The velocity, v, the rate at which product forms, of an enzyme-catalyzed reaction is defined as:

$$v = \frac{d[P]}{dt} = k_2[ES] \tag{20–2}$$

where t is time.

The differential rate law which gives the rate of change of [ES] with time is the difference between the rate of the k_1 step leading to the formation of the complex and the rates of the steps leading to the disappearance of [ES], the k_{-1} and k_2 steps.

$$\frac{d[ES]}{dt} = k_1[E][S] - k_{-1}[ES] - k_2[ES] \tag{20–3}$$

For a wide variety of enzyme-catalyzed reactions, it has been found that, over long periods of time, after an initial transient phase lasting a few milliseconds, the concentration of the ES complex remains constant provided that $[S] >> [E_T]$ where E_T is the total enzyme concentration. This allows that:

$$\frac{d[ES]}{dt} = 0 = k_1[E][S] - k_{-1}[ES] - k_2[ES] \tag{20–4}$$

The equation of conservation for the enzyme, $E_T = E + ES$, may be used to eliminate [E] from the above equation to give:

$$0 = k_1[E_T][S] - k_1[ES][S] - k_{-1}[ES] - k_2[ES] \tag{20–5}$$

and combining terms and solving for [ES] gives:

$$k_1[E_T][S] = [ES](k_1[S] + k_{-1} + k_2) \tag{20–6}$$

and,

$$[ES] = \frac{k_1[E_T][S]}{k_1[S] + k_{-1} + k_2} \tag{20–7}$$

and dividing top and bottom of the right-hand side by k_1 gives:

$$[ES] = \frac{[E_T][S]}{([S] + \frac{k_{-1} + k_2}{k_1})} \tag{20–8}$$

and finally,

$$[ES] = \frac{[E_T][S]}{[S] + K_M} \tag{20–9}$$

where:

$$K_M = \frac{k_{-1} + k_2}{k_1} \tag{20–10}$$

K_M is known as the *Michaelis constant* and is an experimentally derived quantity. The initial velocity can now be expressed in terms of the measurable variable, [S], and the constant, $[E_T]$. Therefore:

$$v = \frac{d[P]}{dt} = k_2[ES] = \frac{k_2[E_T][S]}{([S] + K_M)} \tag{20–11}$$

When $[E_T] = [ES]$, saturation has occurred, and the rate has reached a maximum. This rate is called the maximal velocity, V_{max}, and:

$$V_{max} = \frac{d[P]}{dt} = k_2[E_T] \tag{20-12}$$

and substituting for $k_2[E_T]$,

$$v_O = \frac{V_{max}[S]}{([S] + K_M)} \tag{20-13}$$

where v_o is the initial velocity. Equation 20–13 is called the *Michaelis–Menten law*, governing most single substrate enzyme-catalyzed reactions. Note in Equation 20–13 that v is written as v_o. This is due to the fact that when rates of enzyme-catalyzed reactions are measured, it is most desirable to measure the *initial velocity* or *rate*, i.e., at the very beginning of the reaction, where the substrate concentration is known. It is also important to measure initial velocities to ensure the absence of product inhibition (at t_o, [P] is zero) and the loss of enzyme due to proteolysis, denaturation or time-dependent adsorption onto glass or plastic surfaces.

In the steady-state development, no assumptions have been made concerning the relative magnitudes of the rate constants. Michaelis and Menten reported the same rate law in 1913 prior to the introduction of the steady-state concept by Briggs and Haldane in 1925. Michaelis and Menten assumed that $k_{-1} \gg k_2$, tantamount to the assertion that the first step achieves equilibrium. Hence, K_M is now assumed to be equal to the equilibrium dissociation constant of the ES complex, K_S, which can be written:

$$K_S = \frac{k_{-1}}{k_1} = \frac{[E][S]}{[ES]} \tag{20-14}$$

The affinity of the substrate for the enzyme is a quantitative measure of the strength of the noncovalent interaction of the substrate and the enzyme in the enzyme–substrate complex. It is defined as the equilibrium constant for the association reaction:

$$E + S \rightleftharpoons ES \tag{20-15}$$

Unfortunately, affinity is most often indexed to the dissociation constant, K_S, for the reaction:

$$ES \rightleftharpoons E + S \tag{20-16}$$

There is a reciprocal relationship between the dissociation constant and the affinity. The higher the value of K_S, the lower is the affinity.

K_M is an experimentally derived constant, whereas K_S is an assumption concerning the meaning of K_M, and:

$$K_M = (k_{-1} + k_2)/k_1 = K_S + k_2/k_1 \tag{20-17}$$

$K_M = K_S$ only when k_2 goes to zero. Hence, K_M is always $\geq K_S$. K_M can never be $< K_S$. K_M only becomes a reasonable measure of the affinity if k_2/k_1 is small. This is not unreasonable because k_1 refers to the substrate-binding step that is generally fast, sometimes occurring at the diffusion controlled limit. However, for some enzymes k_2 is large, and the assumption of equilibrium does not apply. Examples include carbonic anhydrase ($k_2 = 10^6 s^{-1}$, CO_2 is the substrate); catalase ($k_2 = 10^7 s^{-1}$, H_2O_2 is the substrate); and superoxide dismutase ($k_2 = 10^6 s^{-1}$, superoxide anion, $O_2^{\bullet-}$, is the substrate). K_M has the dimensions of concentration. The sum of $k_2 + k_{-1}$ has units of reciprocal time (s^{-1}), and the units of k_1 are reciprocal concentration times reciprocal time ($M^{-1}s^{-1}$). Dividing ($k_{-1} + k_2$) by k_1 leaves 1/reciprocal concentration, or concentration, in the usual case, M.

A plot of initial velocities (v_o) versus substrate concentrations [S] is a rectangular hyperbola and is shown in Figure 20–4.

K_M, defined operationally, is the substrate concentration required to attain half-maximal velocity. This is readily apparent by substituting $v_o = V_{max}/2$ in the Michaelis–Menten rate law:

$$v_O = V_{max}/2 \frac{V_{max}[S]}{([S] + K_M)} \tag{20-18}$$

and,

$$[S] + K_M = 2[S] \tag{20-19}$$

and,

$$K_M = [S] \tag{20-20}$$

At low substrate concentration ([S] $\ll K_M$), the velocity is proportional to [S], and:

$$v_O = \frac{V_{max}[S]}{K_M} \tag{20-21}$$

Since the rate depends on the concentration of substrate only, it is called 'first order in substrate' or a first-order reaction.

At high substrate concentration ([S] $\gg K_M$), the velocity is constant and equal to V_{max}, and:

$$v_O = \frac{V_{max}[S]}{[S]} = V_{max} \tag{20-22}$$

Since the rate is constant (the reaction is at the maximal rate or V_{max}), the reaction is referred to as zero order (it has no concentration dependence). And since $V_{max} = k_2 \times [E]t$, the reaction rate is directly

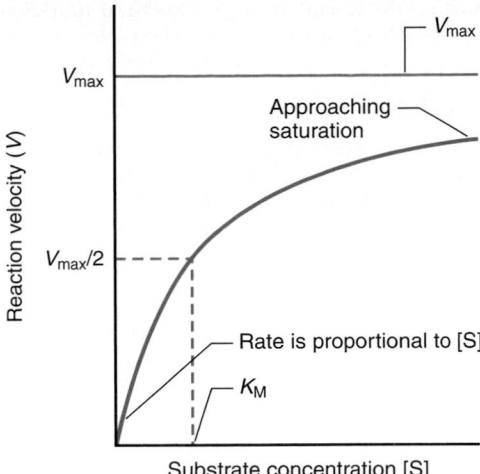

Figure 20–4 The effect of substrate concentration [S] on the velocity (V) of an enzyme-catalyzed reaction. The plot is for an enzyme which obeys Michaelis–Menten kinetics where the maximal velocity is V_{max} and [S] equals K_M where V equals $V_{max}/2$.

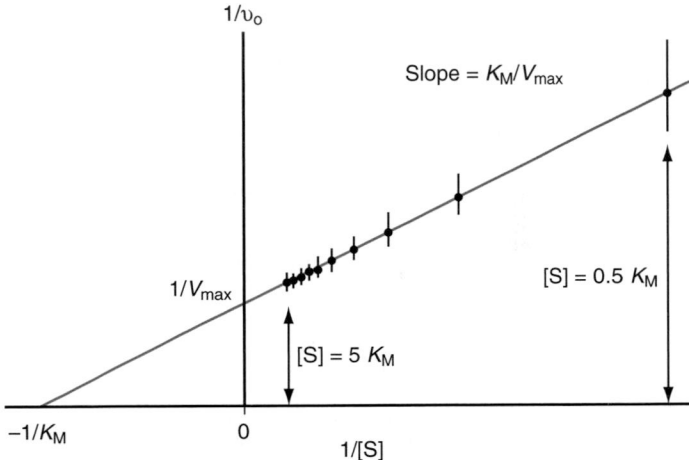

Figure 20–5 The Lineweaver–Burk double reciprocal plot of $1/v_o$ vs. 1/[S]. The substrate concentration range is from 0.5–5 K_M and the vertical lines are weighted error bars. The lowest substrate concentrations give the smallest velocities whose estimates have the greatest uncertainty. These appear on the right side of the plot where 1/[S] is highest. The highest substrate concentrations give the highest velocities whose estimates have the least uncertainty. They appear on the left side of the plot where 1/[S] is lowest. Large errors in $1/v_o$ lead to large errors in K_M and V_{max}.

proportional to the concentration of enzyme, allowing a direct determination of enzyme concentration. Note that this condition can be met simply by adding sufficiently high concentration of substrate so that it is much higher than the known K_M. The initial rate of product formation (or substrate disappearance) will then be directly proportional to the enzyme concentration, which is the objective of clinical enzymology.

All of the above conditions are met by the hyperbolic relationship of the v_o versus [S] curve. Inversion of the Michaelis–Menten equation and separation of terms gives the *Lineweaver–Burk transform*, which provides a linear relationship between the new variables, $1/v_o$ and 1/[S].

$$\frac{1}{v_O} = \left(\frac{K_M}{V_{max}}\right)\frac{1}{[S]} + \frac{1}{V_{max}} \tag{20-23}$$

A plot of $1/v_o$ versus 1/[S] is shown in Figure 20–5. In the v_o versus [S] plot, the rate approaches V_{max} asymptotically. Therefore, V_{max} can only be estimated from such a plot. Since the value of V_{max} is essential for the estimation of K_M, a simple v_o versus [S] plot can only provide rough estimates of the kinetic parameters. The Lineweaver–Burk transform permits a linear extrapolation of the $1/v_o$ versus 1/[S] plot to the ordinate axis where the value of $1/v_o$ at 1/[S] = zero is $1/V_{max}$. Dividing the value of the slope, K_M/V_{max}, by the intercept, $1/V_{max}$, gives a reasonable estimate of K_M. Substrate concentrations must span a range which brackets K_M. Measurements of v_o at low [S] have relatively large errors, yet it is these estimates which are critical in determining accurate values of K_M and V_{max}. Modern computer programs estimate reasonably accurate values for K_M and V_{max} based upon weighted values of the initial velocities. Weights are assigned based on the magnitude of v_o. Nonlinear regression analysis is used to fit the weighted data to a hyperbolic v_o versus [S] curve, and a Lineweaver–Burk plot is used only for visual display of the kinetic data.

Catalytic Efficiency

Catalytic efficiency is assessed in terms of the rate constants of the catalyzed reaction. The catalytic rate constant, k_{cat}, or *turnover number*, is defined as the number of substrate molecules converted to product molecules per molecule of enzyme (or active site) per unit time (seconds) and is expressed as:

$$k_{cat} = V_{max}/E_T \qquad (20\text{--}24)$$

For the simple single-substrate model of Michaelis and Menten, $k_{cat} = k_2$. The meaning of k_{cat}/K_M can be gleaned from a consideration of the catalytic rate when S << K_M. Under these circumstances [E] ≈ [E_T] and:

$$v_O \approx \left(\frac{k_2}{K_M}\right)[E]_T[S] \approx \left(\frac{k_{cat}}{K_M}\right)[E][S] \qquad (20\text{--}25)$$

k_{cat}/K_M has the units of a second-order rate constant (*second order because the rate now depends on the concentration of both enzyme and substrate*) and is a reflection of the frequency of productive encounters of enzyme and substrate molecules in solution. There is an upper boundary to the frequency of encounters that is determined by the temperature and the diffusion coefficients of the substrate and enzyme. This limiting value is 10^8–$10^9\,M^{-1}\,s^{-1}$. If the value of k_{cat}/K_M is at the diffusion controlled limit, every encounter of the enzyme and substrate leads to product formation, and the enzyme has achieved catalytic perfection. Some enzymes have achieved a state of catalytic perfection and these include superoxide dismutase (k_{cat}/K_M = $2.8 \times 10^9\,M^{-1}\,s^{-1}$), acetylcholinesterase (k_{cat}/K_M = $1.5 \times 10^8\,M^{-1}\,s^{-1}$), and catalase ($k_{cat}/K_M$ = $4.0 \times 10^8\,M^{-1}\,s^{-1}$). As part of the evolutionary strategy of reaching perfect catalytic efficiency, enzymes have evolved to bind their substrates rather poorly. For example, a molecule such as NAD$^+$ could potentially bind at its substrate-binding site with a K_S of ≈ 1×10^{-20} M; however, K_M values for NAD$^+$ are of the order of 1×10^{-4} M. The binding constant is close to the intracellular concentration of NAD$^+$, and for many enzymes the in vivo [S] ≈ K_M. Near the K_M, the velocity is sensitive to both increases and decreases in [S]. In addition, the ground state energy of the ES complex is not so low as to constitute a handicap to reaching the transition state of the rate-determining k_2 step. By not binding the substrate very tightly, and preferentially binding the k_2 transition state, enzymes have evolved to minimize the energy required to overcome the activation barriers of the reactions they catalyze.

Another measure of catalytic efficacy of enzymes is the *rate acceleration*. To evaluate this parameter, in addition to k_{cat}, the first-order rate constant for the nonenzymatic conversion of substrate to product, k_{uncat}, must be known. The ratio, k_{cat}/k_{uncat}, gives the rate acceleration, which is often difficult to obtain because the rates of most cellular reactions occur very slowly in the absence of enzymes. For enzymes they are in the range of 10^8–10^{12}, but some are even higher. The rate acceleration for adenosine deaminase, which catalyzes the deamination of adenosine to inosine, is 10^{14}, and the rate acceleration of alkaline phosphatase is 10^{17}. Both adenosine deaminase and alkaline phosphatase have modest k_{cat} values, $10^2\,s^{-1}$. Their unusually large rate accelerations stem from the stability of their substrates at pH 7.0 and 25°C. For example, the half-time for the deamination of adenosine at 20°C and pH 7.0 is approximately 20 000 years, and k_{uncat} is $10^{-12}\,s^{-1}$. The nonenzymatic rate constant for the hydrolysis of phosphate esters under neutral, room temperature conditions is estimated to be $10^{-15}\,s^{-1}$.

Inhibition of Enzymes

The inhibition of enzymes may be reversible or irreversible. In irreversible inhibition a covalent bond is formed between the inhibitor and the enzyme, and enzyme activity cannot be restored by dissociation of the inhibitor. Examples include the inhibition of acetylcholinesterase and pseudo-cholinesterase by chemical warfare agents such as sarin and tabun, which irreversibly phosphorylate the side chain OH group of the active-site serine residue. The first fluorinated anesthetic, fluroxene ($CF_3CH_2OCH=CH_2$), proved to be too toxic for use as a general anesthetic because it irreversibly alkylated a heme ring N atom in the cytochrome P450 monooxygenase responsible for its detoxification. This alkylation led to the complete loss of enzyme.

Reversible inhibition is one of three types; competitive, noncompetitive or uncompetitive:

- *Competitive inhibition* occurs when the inhibitor binds at the same site as the substrate. The molecular basis for the binding of competitive inhibitors at the active site is that the substrate and inhibitor are structurally similar, with the result that the enzyme is 'deceived' into

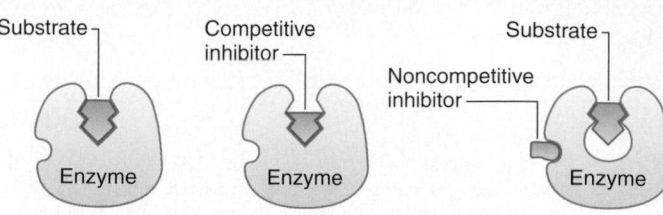

Figure 20–6 The structural difference between a *competitive* and a *noncompetitive* inhibitor. During competitive inhibition the inhibitor occupies the substrate-binding site and prevents the substrate from binding. The noncompetitive inhibitor binds to a site distinct from the active site. Binding of inhibitor to this site alters either K_M or V_{max} or both. Changes in the kinetic parameters occur as a result of conformational changes in the active site brought about by the binding of the noncompetitive inhibitor.

$$E + S \underset{k_{-1}}{\overset{k_1}{\rightleftharpoons}} ES \xrightarrow{k_2} P + E$$
$$+$$
$$I$$
$$K_I \updownarrow$$
$$EI + S \rightleftharpoons EIS$$

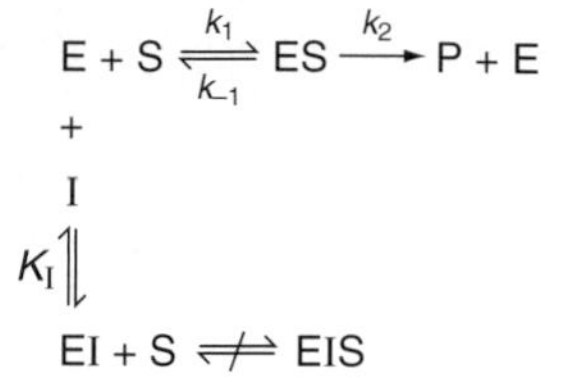

Figure 20–7 The kinetic model for competitive inhibition. The inhibitor, I, binds reversibly to the enzyme and is in rapid equilibrium with it. The binary complex, EI, the enzyme–inhibitor complex, is inactive. The effect of a competitive inhibitor is to reduce the amount of free enzyme available for substrate binding.

recognizing and binding the inhibitor. Examples of competitive inhibition include the inhibition of dihydrofolate reductase by the chemotherapeutic agent, methotrexate, and the inhibition of the Krebs cycle enzyme, succinic dehydrogenase, by malonate.

- *Noncompetitive inhibition* occurs when the inhibitor binds at a site distinct from the substrate-binding site. Both the inhibitor and substrate are capable of binding the enzyme simultaneously. Binding of the inhibitor to this second site may completely abolish enzyme activity or it may only partially reduce it. Hence, noncompetitive inhibition may be either *full* or *partial*. Noncompetitive inhibitors bind to both free E as well as to ES. If the binding of the inhibitor and the substrate are independent of each other, *simple noncompetitive inhibition* exists. If bound substrate alters the affinity of the enzyme for the inhibitor, a condition of *mixed competitive inhibition* exists. These two cases may be distinguished by kinetic analysis. Schematic examples of competitive and noncompetitive inhibition are shown in Figure 20–6. Binding of the noncompetitive inhibitor alters the conformation of the substrate-binding site. The substrate can still bind; however, the binding affinity and/or the catalytic activity is reduced.

- In *uncompetitive inhibition* the inhibitor binds only to the ES complex, and not to free E. No EI complex forms. Binding of the substrate causes a conformational change creating a site for binding of the inhibitor.

The kinetic mechanism for competitive inhibition is shown in Figure 20–7. The inhibitor is assumed to be in rapid equilibrium with free E and the EI complex. Kinetically, the inhibitor reduces the concentration of free E available to combine with S. The equation of conservation of enzyme now reads:

$$[E_T] = [E] + [EI] + [ES] \qquad (20\text{--}26)$$

[EI] is defined in terms of the equilibrium constant, K_I, for the dissociation of the inhibitor from the EI complex, and

$$[EI] = [E][I]/K_I \qquad (20\text{--}27)$$

Since:

$$[E] = K_M[ES]/[S] \qquad (20\text{--}28)$$

$$[EI] = \frac{[E][I]}{K_I} = \frac{K_M[ES][I]}{[S]K_I} \qquad (20\text{--}29)$$

and,

$$[E_T] = [ES]\left[\frac{K_M}{[S]}\left(1 + \frac{[I]}{K_I}\right) + 1\right] \qquad (20\text{--}30)$$

rearranging to solve for [ES] gives:

$$[ES] = \frac{[E]_T[S]}{K_M\left(1 + \frac{[I]}{K_I}\right) + [S]} \qquad (20\text{--}31)$$

and using the expression for the initial velocity, $v_o = k_2[ES]$:

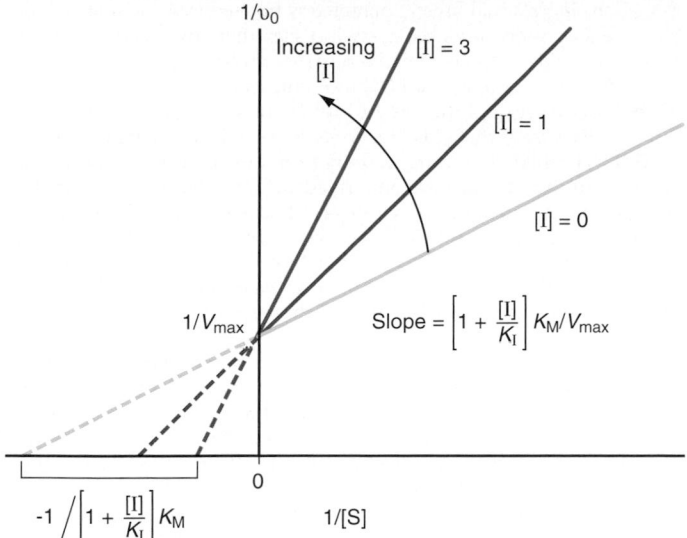

Figure 20–8 The Lineweaver–Burk plot of a Michaelis–Menten enzyme in the presence of a competitive inhibitor. Each line is generated from a plot of $1/v_o$ at different initial $1/[S]$ values in the presence of constant $[I]$. Lines of different slope correspond to different $[I]$ values, including $[I] = 0$. All lines intersect on the $1/v_o$ axis reflecting the fact that at infinite substrate concentration, there is no inhibition.

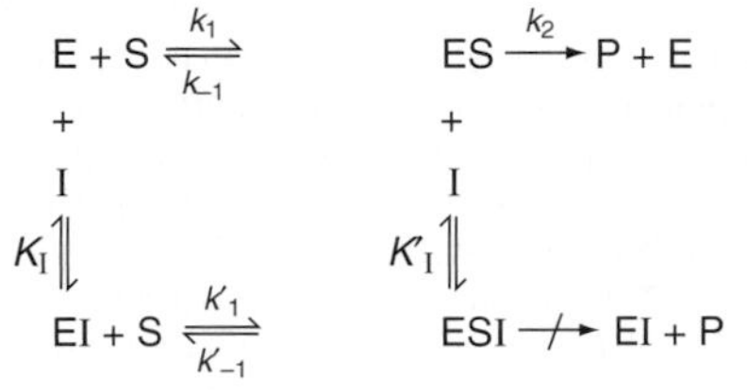

$$E + S \underset{k_{-1}}{\overset{k_1}{\rightleftharpoons}} ES \overset{k_2}{\longrightarrow} P + E$$

$$+ \qquad\qquad +$$

$$I \qquad\qquad I$$

$$K_I \Big\| \qquad\qquad K_I' \Big\|$$

$$EI + S \underset{k_{-1}}{\overset{k_1}{\rightleftharpoons}} ESI \overset{}{\longrightarrow} EI + P$$

Figure 20–9 The kinetic model for noncompetitive inhibition. The inhibitor, I, can bind to either the free enzyme or the enzyme–substrate complex. The inhibitor can form either a binary complex, EI, or a ternary complex, ESI. If bound substrate does not alter the dissociation constant of the inhibitor from the enzyme, *simple* noncompetitive inhibition is the result. If bound substrate alters the binding affinity of the inhibitor, *mixed* noncompetitive inhibition results.

$$v_O = k_2[ES] = \frac{k_2[E]_T[S]}{K_M\left(1 + \dfrac{[I]}{K_I}\right) + [S]} \tag{20–32}$$

Inversion of the above equation gives the Lineweaver–Burk linear transform shown below:

$$\frac{1}{v_O} = \left(1 + \frac{[I]}{K_I}\right)\frac{K_M}{V_{max}}\frac{1}{[S]} = \frac{1}{V_{max}} \tag{20–33}$$

Note that a plot of $1/v_o$ versus $1/[S]$ at different inhibitor concentrations gives linear traces in which the slope, but not the intercept, is altered in the presence of a competitive inhibitor. V_{max} is unchanged, and only K_M is altered. K_M is modified by the coefficient $(1 + [I]/K_I)$. The Lineweaver–Burk plot in the presence of a competitive inhibitor is shown in Figure 20–8. Values for $(1 + [I]/K_I)K_M$ may be obtained by dividing the slopes by the intercept at $1/[S]$ equals zero. K_I may then be estimated from K_M and $[I]$.

The kinetic scheme for *noncompetitive inhibition* is shown in Figure 20–9. If $K_I = K_I'$, the type is referred to as simple noncompetitive inhibition. If $K_I \neq K_I'$, the type is referred to as mixed noncompetitive inhibition. Using the equilibrium assumption and the further assumption that $K_S = K_S'$, the Michaelis–Menten rate law for noncompetitive inhibition is:

$$v_O = \frac{V_{max}[S]}{\left(1 + \dfrac{[I]}{K_I}\right)K_M + \left(1 + \dfrac{[I]}{K_I'}\right)[S]} \tag{20–34}$$

The Lineweaver–Burk equation for simple noncompetitive inhibition is:

$$\frac{1}{v_O} = \left(1 + \frac{[I]}{K_I}\right)\frac{K_M}{V_{max}}\frac{1}{[S]} + \left(1 + \frac{[I]}{K_I}\right)\frac{1}{V_{max}} \tag{20–35}$$

In the presence of inhibitor, both the slope and the intercept increase in value. If the substrate does not modify the affinity of the enzyme for the inhibitor, and vice versa, then for a given inhibitor concentration, the slopes and intercept increment by the same relative amount. When $K_I = K_I'$, the lines on the Lineweaver–Burk plot intersect on the $1/[S]$ axis at a

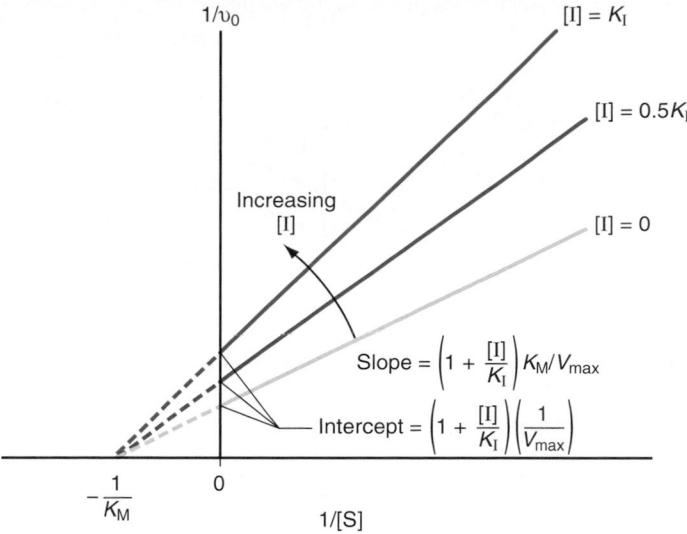

Figure 20–10 The Lineweaver–Burk plot of a Michaelis–Menten enzyme in the presence of a noncompetitive inhibitor. Each line is generated from a plot of $1/v_o$ at different initial $1/[S]$ values in the presence of constant $[I]$. Lines of different slope correspond to different $[I]$ values, including $[I] = 0$. For simple noncompetitive inhibition, all lines intersect on the $1/[S]$ axis at a point which corresponds to $-1/K_M$. For mixed noncompetitive inhibition, all lines would intersect in the second quadrant.

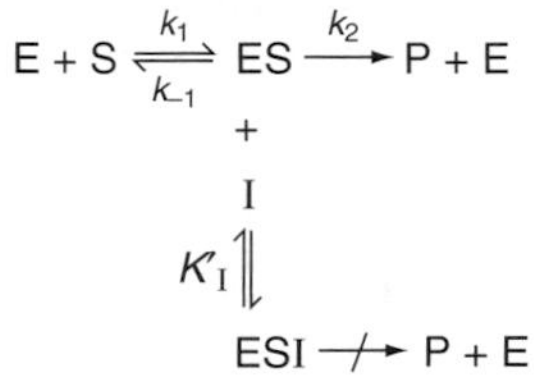

$$E + S \underset{k_{-1}}{\overset{k_1}{\rightleftharpoons}} ES \overset{k_2}{\longrightarrow} P + E$$

$$+$$

$$I$$

$$K_I' \Big\|$$

$$ESI \overset{}{\longrightarrow} P + E$$

Figure 20–11 The kinetic model for uncompetitive inhibition. The inhibitor, I, can bind to the enzyme–substrate complex but not to free enzyme. The inhibitor can only form a ternary complex, ESI; no binary complex, EI, is formed. The inhibitor-binding site only exists after the ES complex is formed. The substrate cannot dissociate from the ESI complex, and the effect of the uncompetitive inhibitor is to block access to or egress from the active site.

point corresponding to $-1/K_M$ as in shown on the double reciprocal plot in Figure 20–10. At any value of $[I]$ including $[I] = 0$, dividing the slope by the intercept gives K_M indicating that, if $K_I = K_I'$ and $K_S = K_S'$; the inhibitor only modifies the k_2 step. If K_I' is not equal to K_I, then *mixed noncompetitive inhibition* results and the lines on the Lineweaver–Burk noncompetitive inhibition plot will intersect in the second ($K_I < K_I'$, K_M decreases) or third ($K_I > K_I'$, K_M increases) quadrant, and not on the abscissa line. V_{max} is lower and the value of $1/[S]$ when $1/v_o$ is zero is:

$$-\left(1 + \frac{[I]}{K_I'}\right)\left(1 + \frac{[I]}{K_I}\right)K_M \tag{20–36}$$

For *uncompetitive inhibition*, the kinetic model takes the form shown in Figure 20–11. K_I' is the dissociation constant of the ESI complex and is equal to $[ES][I]/[ESI]$. The Michaelis–Menten equation for uncompetitive inhibition is:

$$v_O = \frac{V_{max}[S]}{K_M + \left(1 + \dfrac{[I]}{K_I'}\right)[S]} \tag{20–37}$$

At high $[S]$ values where $[S] \gg K_M$, v_o approaches $V_{max}/(1 + [I]/K_I')$. At low $[S]$ values v_o equals $(V_{max}/K_M)[S]$ and the uncompetitive inhibitor is without effect. Inversion and separation of terms gives the Lineweaver–Burk linear transform:

$$\frac{1}{v_O} = \left(\frac{K_M}{V_{max}}\right)\frac{1}{[S]} + \left(1 + \frac{[I]}{K_I'}\right)\left(\frac{1}{V_{max}}\right) \tag{20–38}$$

A plot of $1/v_o$ versus $1/[S]$ gives a distinctive set of parallel lines of equal slope with intercepts on the $1/v_o$ axis equal to $(1 + [I]/K_I')/V_{max}$. The Lineweaver–Burk plot of simple uncompetitive inhibition is represented in Figure 20–12. Replots of $(1 + [I]/K_I')/V_{max}$ versus the intercept values where $1/[S]$ is zero may be used to evaluate K_I'. Alternatively, replots of $-(1 + [I]/K_I')/K_M$ versus the values of $1/[S]$ on the abscissa line where $1/v_o$ is zero will also provide a value for K_I'.

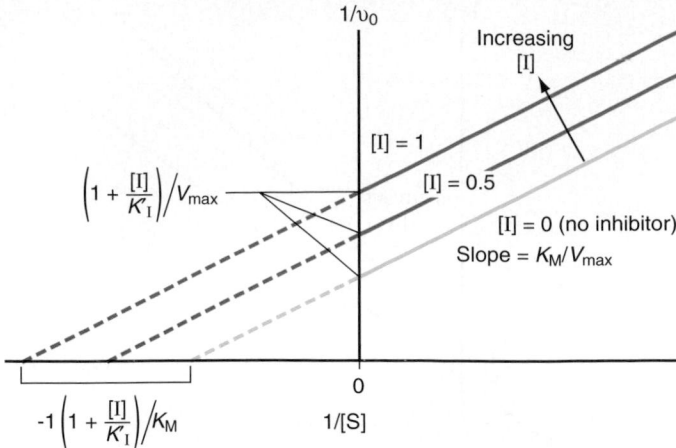

Figure 20–12 The Lineweaver–Burk plot of a Michaelis–Menten enzyme in the presence of an uncompetitive inhibitor. Each line is generated from a plot of $1/v_0$ at different initial $1/[S]$ values in the presence of constant [I]. Lines of identical slope and different values of $1/v_0$ at $1/[S] = 0$ correspond to different [I] values, including [I] = 0. All lines have identical slopes equal to K_M/V_{max}. K_M apparent and V_{max} apparent change by the same relative amount in the presence of an uncompetitive inhibitor.

Table 20–5 Changes in V_{max} and K_M for Various Types of Reversible Inhibitors

Type of inhibition	V_{max} (apparent)	K_M (apparent)
None	V_{max}	K_M
Competitive	V_{max}	$K_M (1 + [I]/K_I)$
Noncompetitive (simple)	$V_{max}/(1 + [I]/K_I)$	K_M
Uncompetitive	$V_{max}/(1 + [I]/K_I')$	$K_M/(1 + [I]/K_I')$

Table 20–5 summarizes the changes in the apparent values of V_{max} and K_M derived from the intercepts and slopes of double-reciprocal Lineweaver–Burk plots for competitive, simple noncompetitive and uncompetitive inhibition.

Assay of Enzymes

The *concentration* of enzyme in a biological fluid such as plasma may be measured either by an assay of enzyme activity or by an immunological technique. Enzyme activity is assayed by estimating the initial velocity under defined conditions and calculating the specific activity, which is a measure of the activity per unit volume of biological fluid (or per unit weight of some blood protein such as hemoglobin). As noted above, the condition that the velocity is directly proportional to the enzyme concentration occurs when $[S] >> K_M$. Thus many enzyme assays are performed under this condition. Sometimes, the condition that $v_o = V_{max}$ is difficult to attain since the value of v_o when [S] is 10 K_M is still only $0.91V_{max}$. Reasons for not carrying out the assay at saturating substrate concentrations include substrate solubility and/or cost of substrate.

In certain deficiency states, the conditions of the in vitro assay may not mirror the in vivo conditions that give rise to the deficiency state. In cases where a genetic defect does not alter normal protein levels of enzyme, and the k_{cat} value is unchanged, by applying the principle that the assay should be carried out at saturating substrate concentration, it is possible that a K_M-type mutation may go undetected because the enzyme, inactive at low substrate levels, exhibits full or nearly full activity at the higher [S] used in the assay. For example, a variant erythrocyte hypoxanthine-guanine-phosphoribosyltransferase (HGPRT) was inactive in assays at low [S], but full activity could be restored by increasing the substrate concentration. The defect was interpreted as a mutation in the substrate-binding site of HGPRT, leading to an increased K_M. To guard against such a false negative, a clinical evaluation should include a determination of the K_M for the mutant enzyme.

In some cases, an enzyme defect may go undetected because the clinical evaluation occurs at an inappropriate time. Administration of the antimalarial, primaquine, to a glucose-6-phosphate dehydrogenase (G6PDH)-deficient individual carrying the common type A– variant (G6PDH A–) causes transient hemolytic anemia. Patients can recover completely from the anemia despite continued drug treatment. The type

A– variant has normal kinetic parameters but reduced thermal stability. The initial episode clears older erythrocytes that have reduced G6PDH activity. The older cells are replaced by new cells that have higher amounts of enzyme. The amount of G6PDH molecules in erythrocytes is a function of erythrocyte age, and the rate of loss of enzyme molecules in type A– variant cells exceeds that in normal cells by a significant margin. The assay for G6PDH activity following recovery from anemia will be substantially higher than that if assays are performed before or during the hemolytic episode, because hemolysis selectively destroys older cells containing lower amounts of enzyme. Recovery results in the replacement of these older cells with new cells with higher levels of G6PDH A– molecules. During and following recovery, the younger set of cells is able to cope with the primaquine treatment because of the presence of higher levels of enzyme activity.

Initial velocity measurements are subject to a variety of errors from other sources. Enzyme inhibitors present in biological fluids may permit underestimation of the amount of enzyme present. Proteases in plasma may attack the enzyme while the velocity estimate is being made. The stability of the enzyme under evaluation must be known and sample storage conditions must be determined. In some cases, plasma must be used for the determination of enzyme activity in blood samples because polyanionic anticoagulants such as citrate, heparin and EDTA inactivate metal-containing enzymes. For example, EDTA inactivates the zinc-containing enzyme, alkaline phosphatase.

The substrate may be subject to attack by other enzymes normally present in biological fluids. Creatine kinase (also known as creatine phosphokinase) activity is often estimated in a coupled assay in which the product of the reverse reaction (CrP + ADP $\rightleftharpoons$ Cr + ATP), ATP, is used to phosphorylate glucose in the hexokinase reaction. The resulting glucose-6-phosphate is oxidized in a third step by G6PDH, which transfers reducing equivalents to NADP+ forming NADPH. Creatine kinase activity is proportional to the increase in absorbance at 340 nm associated with the formation of NADPH. However, if the sample contains adenylate kinase, the creatine kinase substrate, ADP, will also be consumed by this unwanted reaction. This problem cannot be corrected by using saturating concentrations of ADP because the product of the adenylate kinase reaction is also ATP, and the ATP produced in the creatine kinase reaction has to directly determine the amount of glucose-6-phosphate produced to accurately determine the creatine kinase level.

Enzyme damage through proteolysis, and substrate decomposition may be corrected by the use of suitable blanks and preincubation studies. Enzyme levels in plasma or other biological fluids may be estimated under conditions where $[S] << K_M$ by following the first-order disappearance of substrate. In this instance the first-order rate constant is directly proportional to the enzyme concentration in the assay mixture. Since determination of the first-order rate constant requires estimating the remaining substrate concentration at several time points through at least two half-lives, the enzyme must be reasonably stable. Assays may be carried out by following the appearance of product since $-d[S]/dt = d[P]/dt$. If a sensitive method is available for following product formation (as discussed below), this is the preferred method since monitoring substrate disappearance requires measuring small differences between two large values of [S]. Initial velocity estimates eliminate the possibility of product inhibition because $[P_o] = 0$ at t_o, and refer all velocity measurement to the same substrate concentration, $[S_o]$. Often, initial velocities are calculated from estimates of $\Delta P/\Delta t$, where $\Delta P = P_t - P_o$ where P_t is measured at time t_t, and P_o is measured at time t_o. Single point measurements of this type assume linearity of substrate consumption or product appearance up to time t_t. Linearity will depend on the sensitivity of the method, which will determine the magnitude of $-\Delta S$ or ΔP required to give a reproducible and accurate estimate of change. For those enzyme-catalyzed reactions in which the product binds to the enzyme with a higher affinity than the substrate, $\Delta P/\Delta t$ or $-\Delta S/\Delta t$ will be curvilinear, and estimates of the initial velocity are best made from tangents drawn to the substrate or product–time course curves at $t = 0$. These tangents are best determined from continuous traces of substrate disappearance or product formation.

As discussed in more detail below, the use of monoclonal antibodies or polyclonal antibodies raised against an enzyme whose concentration is desired can be employed to determine enzyme concentration in a biological fluid. Correspondence between measurement of enzyme activity and the protein (enzyme) concentration from immunoassays will pertain as long as the enzyme antigen is fully active. Such is not always the case when inherited deficiencies associated with point mutations are involved. In these instances, estimates of enzyme concentration based on immunoassays can exceed those based on measurements of enzyme activity. If the underlying basis of disease is genetic, it is best to estimate enzyme activity from kinetic measurements and compare these to normal values. Some mutations destabilize protein structure, leading to the rapid intracellular proteolysis of the enzyme. In this instance, the results from immunological methods and enzyme activity measurements can concur. The presence of inhibitors in the source biological fluid may lead to underestimation of the amount of enzyme present based on activity but not immunological measurements. Usually, reversible enzyme inhibitors will not interfere with immunological estimates of enzyme concentration.

Another source of error involves sample age. Enzymes whose activity depends on active-site sulfhydryl groups may suffer slow inactivation due to oxidation and/or disulfide exchange reactions. In many instances these processes are irreversible and lead to underestimation of the enzyme concentration by activity measurements. Also, immunoassays are the method of choice when the distribution of isoenzymes in a sample is desired because specific antibodies raised against each individual isoenzyme will identify and quantitate each of the variants present in the sample.

Enzyme Activity

From the discussion above on the kinetics of enzyme-catalyzed reactions, once V_{max} is determined, the concentration of enzyme can be directly computed. That is, since $V_{max} = k_2[F_T]$, then if k_2 is known (as from Lineweaver–Burk plots for the enzyme), $[E_T] = V_{max}/k_2$. However, because often there is more than one isoenzyme of an enzyme present and, in general, each isoenzyme has different values for k_2, V_{max}, which is the total enzyme activity, is reported. It is important to understand that V_{max} contains the k_2 term, and k_2 values depend on the specific substrate being used in the enzyme assay; the substrate used must be specified.

Enzyme activity is reported in terms of enzyme units; two standards are used. Until the 1960s, reporting the rate of reaction of an enzyme was typically based on the method used to measure it. In 1964, a common term, the *International Unit*, IU, was developed to standardize reporting of enzyme activity. The International Commission on Enzymes established by the International Union of Biochemistry defines the International Unit as that amount of enzyme that catalyzes the formation of 1 micromole of product in 1 minute. It applies only under specified conditions of pH, temperature and ionic strength, all factors which influence enzyme activity. With development of the Système International d'Unites (SI) system, and use of moles and seconds as base units, a second definition for the unit of enzyme activity was developed, the katal (kat): 1 kat is defined as the amount of enzyme that catalyzes the conversion of 1 mol of substrate to product in 1 second, under the conditions used in the assay. One IU is equal to 16.7 nkat and 1 katal is equal to 6×10^7 IU.

An important limitation of both terms is that conditions of the assay are often not standardized between laboratories; therefore, although the term 'IU' or 'kat' is used, results are not comparable unless the same assay conditions are used. Thus, reference ranges for normal enzymatic activity can vary from one laboratory to another (Langdon, 1994). For example, at one point, upper limits of normal lipase activity were 300 U/L and 24 U/L at two hospitals in the same geographic area. Similarly, a normal lactate dehydrogenase upper limit at one hospital was reported as 618 U/L, while simultaneously, at a second hospital, it was 172 U/L. In addition, as procedures undergo modification in the same laboratory, normal levels can change two- to threefold over a period of years. Referring physicians can pass along enzyme values different from the values obtained by the receiving physician if estimates were obtained in two different locations. Variability in normal ranges for selected enzymes estimated at different locations may be eliminated by universally setting the upper boundary of normal to 100 and expressing all other values as percentages or ratios. A result that an enzyme level was 10 times normal is useful to a physician. If the result is $10x$ U/L, then the physician must hunt the value of x and calculate the ratio himself. Nowadays, many laboratories provide sample values in U/L and their current normal reference range.

The determination of enzyme activity in biological samples depends on many variables including the assay method used, as well as sample preparation, age and storage conditions. Additional important variables in determining enzyme activity include temperature, pH, concentration of substrate, concentration of cofactors of the assay, use of other enzyme reactions as indicators, and whether the forward or backward reaction is used to measure the enzyme. These variables can lead to significant differences in enzyme activity between methods. For example, LD measured using the forward reaction has approximately one-third the activity of LD measured using the reverse reaction, while lipase measured with colipase present has 5–10 times the activity of lipase measured without its cofactor. As long as the assays are performed with internal consistency in a highly reproducible manner, quantitative results are comparable between one laboratory and another if relative activities are reported.

Measuring Enzyme Activity

In measurement of enzyme activity, either the rate of disappearance of substrate or the rate of appearance of product can be measured. In general, it is easier to measure small increases in product than to measure small decreases in a large amount of substrate. In many instances, however, neither the product nor the substrate of a chemical reaction can be measured conveniently. In such instances, the enzymatic reaction can be 'coupled' to another reaction that uses the product of the enzyme-catalyzed reaction to produce an indicator substance. An example of a typical coupled enzymatic reaction is the Oliver–Rosalki method for measurement of CK activity, illustrated in Equation 20–39, below. The reverse reaction of CK is used, producing adenosine triphosphate (ATP), which is used in a second reaction to produce glucose-6-phosphate (G6P); a third reaction produces the reduced form of nicotinamide-adenine dinucleotide (NAD), NADH, the indicator of the reaction.

> Creatine phosphate + ADP → Creatine + ATP (catalyzed by CK) (20–39)
> Glucose + ATP → G6P + ADP (catalyzed by hexokinase)
> G6P + NAD → 6-Phosphogluconate + NADH (catalyzed by glucose-6-phosphate dehydrogenase)

In coupled reactions, it is critical that the rate-limiting step in the reaction is the amount of ATP generated by the action of CK. One potential problem with CK measurements using this reaction is the presence of other enzymes that can generate ATP. Adenylate kinase, an enzyme found in red blood cells and liver, converts adenosine diphosphate (ADP) to ATP (Equation 20–40); specimens with high adenylate kinase activity will have falsely elevated values for CK activity.

> 2ADP → ATP + AMP (catalyzed by adenylate kinase)   (20–40)

In assays of enzyme activity, some methods use 'end point' measurements, determining the concentration of substrate or product at a specific time after addition of the sample. End point methods are typically used in simple methods, such as bedside glucose testing instruments or with dipstick reactions, such as for glucose or leukocyte esterase in urine. End point methods may give erroneously low results in situations where there is very high enzyme activity. Most enzymatic assays use 'kinetic' methods of measurement (as discussed above), where the rate of change in concentration of substrate or product is determined. (For simplicity's sake, throughout the rest of this section, only measurement systems that detect appearance of product will be described; the same principles, however, would apply to situations where rate of disappearance of substrate was being monitored.) Kinetic methods are more accurate and make it easier to detect changes in reaction conditions and samples requiring dilution. In a kinetic reaction, the rate of reaction can be expressed as $\Delta P/\Delta t$, the change in amount of product per unit time; since the IU and katal represent the amount of enzyme producing a specific amount of product in a given time period, this approach allows direct reporting of enzyme activity in either IU or katal, as desired.

Most enzyme assays use spectrophotometry to measure the amount of product produced; however, a number of other detection methods could be used as appropriate, depending on the product being measured. For example, lipase acts on emulsions of lipid; these are often turbid, so that measuring rate of clearance of turbidity could be used to determine lipase activity. Glucose oxidase, widely used to measure glucose concentration, uses oxygen or an alternative oxygen acceptor. Measuring the change in potential due to alteration in charge on the acceptor can also be used to determine the reaction rate. Urease is widely used to measure urea concentration; urease splits urea to bicarbonate and ammonium ion. The change in conductance of the specimen due to the appearance of the ions in the sample can be used to determine the rate of reaction. (For simplicity's sake in the following discussion, only the term 'absorbance' will be used when discussing measurement of enzyme activity, while recognizing that the same relationship described applies to other measurement methods as well.) Since the concentration of a product can be measured by its absorbance, then $\Delta P/\Delta t \propto \Delta A/\Delta t$. The exact formula for determining enzyme activity from measurement of $\Delta P/\Delta t$ is given in Equation 20–41; in the equation, ε is the molar absorptivity coefficient for the compound and b is the path length of light through the sample (see Ch. 4 for a discussion of absorption spectroscopy). If the molar absorptivity of the product is known, then the equation can be used to directly determine enzyme activity, since all of the other factors are specified as part of the reaction conditions. For example, a common indicator in clinical enzymology is NADH, which has an intense absorption maximum at 340 nm, while NAD^+ does not absorb at that wavelength. The molar absorptivity coefficient for NADH is 6.22×10^3 L mol^{-1} cm^{-1}. If the molar absorptivity of the product is unknown, then it can be determined by plotting $\Delta A/\Delta t$ on the y-axis with the activity of known enzyme calibrators on the x-axis.

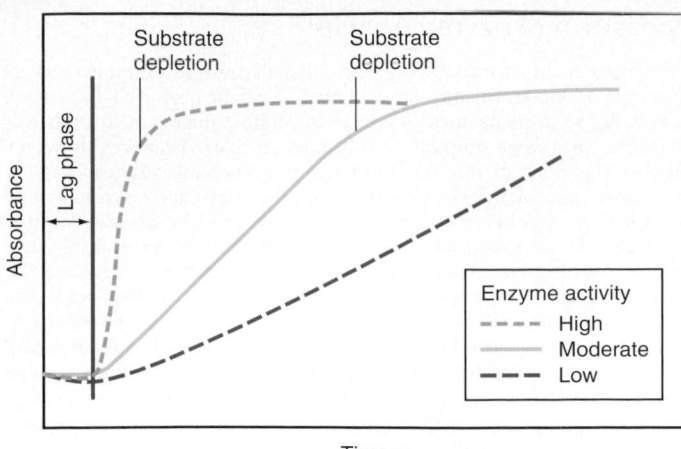

Figure 20–13 Enzyme activity can be calculated from a plot of absorbance versus time when monitoring an enzyme-catalyzed reaction. When reagents and serum are mixed, there may initially be a period of time when mixing and any preliminary chemical reactions occur; this is termed the *lag period*. Following this phase, the reaction will proceed at zero-order kinetics (V_{max}); at this point, the rate of appearance of product (as measured from the slope of the line, $\Delta A/\Delta t$) is directly proportional to the enzyme activity present. As the reaction proceeds and substrate is depleted, the rate of reaction will fall below V_{max} and the plot is no longer linear. At this point, the reaction is no longer zero order with respect to substrate concentration; rate of reaction is now dependent on both amount of substrate (which is declining) and amount of enzyme present, making it difficult to calculate amount of enzyme present. (From Dufour DR: Enzyme kinetics. *In* Dufour DR [ed]: Professional Practice in Clinical Chemistry: A Companion Text. Washington, DC, American Association for Clinical Chemistry, 1999, p 8–1, with permission.)

$$\text{Enzyme activity} = \Delta A/\Delta t \times 1/\varepsilon \times 1/b \times \text{Total volume}/\text{Sample volume} \qquad (20\text{–}41)$$

As discussed above, to measure enzyme activity in a sample, it is necessary to design a measurement system in which the reaction occurs at zero-order kinetics. As discussed earlier, when substrate concentration is $>> K_M$, the reaction is zero order with respect to the substrate and the rate of reaction is at V_{max}. Under these conditions, reaction rate is directly proportional to total amount of enzyme present. With a kinetic enzyme assay system, the rate of reaction is determined by measuring the change in product concentration per unit time, as illustrated in Figure 20–13. The slope of the line ($\Delta A/\Delta t$) is directly related to the activity of enzyme present in the linear portions of the graph. In an enzyme reaction, there is typically a lag phase following mixture of the specimen and reagents, when preliminary reactions and mixing of sample occur. The initial absorbance of the sample is based on the absorbance due to the reagents and the sample, and is considered to be 'zero' in terms of making interpretation of enzyme activity. Once the reaction begins, there will be a period of time when the graph follows a straight line; at this point, the reaction is zero order and enzyme activity can be determined. As the reaction proceeds, substrate is utilized and substrate concentration falls towards K_M; at some point, the reaction will then be first order, and affected both by the amount of substrate (which is not a constant) and by the enzyme activity; at this point, reaction rate no longer reflects only amount of enzyme present. With modern, automated instruments, such graphs need not be created; the instrument simply measures $\Delta A/\Delta t$ at multiple specified time points during a period in which zero-order kinetics typically are present, and verifies that the change in $\Delta A/\Delta t$ is the same throughout the measurement period. If $\Delta A/\Delta t$ decreases during the measurement period, the instrument reports a linearity code, indicating that specimen dilution is required.

Other Factors Affecting Enzyme Activity

Temperature

Enzyme-catalyzed reaction rates are extremely sensitive to temperature changes; to ensure accuracy, the temperature of the reaction mixture must not deviate by more than ±0.1°C from the assigned temperature. In general, every 10°C increase in the temperature leads to an approximate doubling of enzyme activity, although this varies slightly from one enzyme to another. The use of higher temperatures gives faster reaction rates, improving sensitivity, an advantage when the enzyme activities are low. Lower temperatures increase the linear limit of an assay, requiring fewer dilutions. The choice of temperature with most modern instruments is governed by the

capabilities of the instrument. There is a limit to the amount of temperature increase that can be used; most enzymes start to denature and become inactive as the temperature is increased. For example, CK starts to break down at 37°C, and amylase begins to denature at 45°C. Some enzymes remain stable at extremely high temperatures; the Taq polymerase, as discussed in Chapter 67, used in the polymerase chain reaction is stable at 95°C.

pH

Enzymes have a pH optimum for maximal activity; usually, the pH of the reaction conditions is chosen to be that at which the enzyme shows the greatest activity rate. Selection of pH is not always critical; some enzymes have a very broad pH maximum, so that small changes in pH do not appreciably change activity. For example, alkaline phosphatase has maximum activity at pH between 9–10. In some cases, particularly for enzymes with multiple isoenzymes, selection of pH represents a compromise, as different isoenzymes may have maximum activity at differing pH values. In that situation, the pH for the reaction is selected to allow measurement of all isoenzymes.

Salt and Protein Concentration

The ionic strength of solutions affects enzyme activity; if ionic strength is too high, enzyme activity drops. The activity of many enzymes is also affected by protein concentration. When enzyme activity is over the linear limits of the assay, dilution of plasma typically requires use of 'enzyme diluents' containing plasma proteins. Human plasma contains about 70 g protein per liter, but normal urine has almost no protein; use of protein such as albumin increases the activity of urinary amylase and standardizes its measurement. In protein-free solutions, enzymes lose activity rapidly either by denaturation or by adsorption to the walls of the container.

Inhibitors and Interferences

Typically, enzymes are measured in serum samples. Heparinized plasma is generally considered an equivalent sample to serum for most routine analytes, but that may not be the case for enzymes. Heparin may inhibit the activity of some enzymes, notably amylase and aspartate aminotransferase (AST) (using some, but not all, methods). Citrate, used in evacuated collection tubes for coagulation testing and as a preservative in blood products, complexes divalent cations; citrate-containing specimens may cause falsely low results for enzymes such as CK and alkaline phosphatase. Ethylenediaminetetraacetic acid (EDTA) and fluoride inhibit the activity of many enzymes, and should virtually never be used for specimens for enzyme analysis. An exception is in measurement of renin, where EDTA inhibits the action of enzymes that convert prorenin to the active enzyme renin and prevents artifactual increase in renin activity.

Antibody-Based Techniques for Measuring Enzymes

As mentioned briefly earlier, immunoassays can be used to measure the mass of enzyme protein. Most commonly, immunoassays are used to measure one isoenzyme, simplifying its determination. Immunoassays are, in general, less affected by factors that affect enzyme activity, and are often more precise. As with enzyme activity, however, the determination of enzyme mass may vary depending on the reagents used; calibrators often lead to different results for mass activity between different methods. Examples include the MB isoenzyme of CK, the pancreatic isoenzyme of amylase, the prostatic and bone isoenzymes of acid phosphatase, and the bone isoenzyme of alkaline phosphatase. Antibodies can also be used to selectively inhibit or bind particular enzyme subunits. This approach allows the total and isoenzyme measurements to be expressed in the same units. For example, antibodies to CK-M subunits inhibit half of CK-MB isoenzyme and all of CK-MM isoenzyme. Measuring CK activity of a sample after incubation with an anti-M antibody can be used to determine the activity of non-M subunits of CK. Antibodies can also be used as 'capture' antibodies to separate a particular isoenzyme from other forms of the same enzyme, followed by measurement of enzymatic activity. Examples of such capture assays include tests for the bone isoenzyme of alkaline phosphatase and the bone and prostate isoenzymes of acid phosphatase. Some enzymes circulate bound to antiproteases, such as prostate-specific antigen (PSA) (see Ch. 74) and α_1-antichymotrypsin or trypsin and α_1-antitrypsin. Antibodies may differ in their ability to measure free and bound forms. Some enzymes are also bound to α_2-macroglobulin, such as PSA (Otto, 1998) and acid phosphatase (Brehme, 1999); enzyme bound to this antiprotease is usually not enzymatically active and cannot be measured by most immunoassays, since the binding site is hidden from antibody recognition. Finally, in common with other immunoassays, measurement of enzymes by immunoassay can show interferences from substances that bind to reagent antibodies, such as heterophil antibodies (Sosolik, 1997) and rheumatoid factor (Dasgupta, 1999).

Table 20–6 Relative Amounts of Enzymes in Various Organs (Relative to Serum)*

	AST[†]	ALT	LD	CK
Liver	7000	3000	700	
Kidney	4500	1200	500	10
Brain				1700
Spleen	700	150		
Heart	8000	500	600	5000–8000
Skeletal muscle	5000	300	700	20 000–30 000
Smooth muscle				300–600
Red cells	15	7	500	0

* Relative amount is calculated by dividing the activity of enzyme in tissue (in IU/kg of tissue) by the upper reference limit of plasma activity of the enzyme (in IU/L), assuming that 1 L of plasma = 1 kg. Since the data are from multiple publications, the relative amounts between enzymes may be approximate, but the relative amount of a single enzyme in each tissue is accurate.

[†] Total amount in cells; varying amounts represent mitochondrial isoenzyme, which reaches serum in only small amounts.

AST = aspartate transaminase; ALT = alanine aminotransferase; LD = lactate dehydrogenase; CK = creatine kinase.

Specific Enzymes

A number of enzymes are clinically useful in recognition and monitoring of particular disease processes. Many of these are discussed in other chapters of this book. Discussion of enzymes in serum and urine for recognition of renal disease is found in Chapter 14; enzymes of bone metabolism are presented in Chapter 15; enzymes useful in recognition of liver disease are mentioned in Chapter 21; pancreatic enzymes are covered in Chapter 22; enzymes and other proteins that are useful in diagnosing heart disease are discussed in Chapter 18; and enzyme deficiencies that produce hemolytic anemia are summarized in Chapter 31. This chapter covers general aspects of enzymes that are of clinical utility, and specifically discusses markers of muscle injury. A number of enzymes that are covered in other chapters (amylase, glucose-6-phosphate dehydrogenase, lipase, and pyruvate kinase) are not discussed further in this chapter.

The pattern of enzyme changes can often help to indicate the source of injury. In some cases, isoenzymes are relatively specific for a single organ; identification of which isoenzyme is elevated can point to the organ injured. For enzymes with no tissue-specific isoenzymes, the relative amount of different enzymes in plasma provides a clue as to the type of organ injured. For example, LD, AST, and ALT are found in many organs, but the relative amounts in each differ (Table 20–6). If LD is markedly elevated, while AST and ALT are only slightly elevated, this would suggest damage to an organ or tissue (such as red blood cells, white blood cells, or tumors) with a high LD/AST ratio. On the other hand, if AST and ALT are elevated but LD is only slightly elevated, this suggests damage to liver, which has a low LD/AST ratio.

Acid Phosphatase (EC 3.1.3.2)

Biochemistry and Physiology

Acid phosphatases (ACP) belong to the hydrolase class of enzymes (Table 20–1) and occur as several isoenzymes with a common enzymatic function (the hydrolytic breakdown of phosphate monoesters). They all show optimal enzyme activity below a pH of 7.0. They possess some tissue specificity (greatest concentrations occur in prostate, liver, spleen, and bone). The major forms are coded for by different genes, and also possess different molecular weights and structures, as well as differences in sensitivity to tartrate inhibition (Moss, 1995). Lysosomal, prostatic, erythrocyte, macrophage, and osteoclastic ACP are five important types found in humans. Normally, concentrations in serum are low (Moss, 1999; Bull, 2002). The activity of erythrocyte ACP can be distinguished from that of the other ACP isoenzymes in that it is inhibited by 2% formaldehyde solution and 1 mM cupric sulfate solution. This is in contrast to the other isoenzymes, which are not inhibited by these agents. In addition, erythrocyte ACP is not inhibited by 20 mM tartrate solution, which does inhibit the other isoenzymes. Importantly, tartrate-resistant acid phosphatase (TRAP) is present in certain chronic leukemias and some lymphomas, most notably, in hairy cell leukemia, as described in Chapter 32 on leukocytic disorders.

Reference Ranges and Pre-analytical Variation

Reference values depend on age, gender, and hormonal status (in women). Total and tartrate-resistant ACP values are high in children, rising through the first decade to peak at three to four times adult levels in adolescence, paralleling changes in alkaline phosphatase (Chen, 1979). In the late teen years, levels decline to adult values that are constant to approximately 80 years in both genders. Normal men and women up to about age 55 have the same reference ranges for ACP. In women, total and tartrate-resistant acid phosphatase increase after menopause (Schiele, 1988), and increase with use of depo-medroxyprogesterone acetate in premenopausal women (Mukherjea, 1981).

The enzymatic activity of ACP is unstable at normal plasma pH; specimens must be acidified to prevent loss of ACP activity (Theodorsen, 1985). The effect of specimen pH is not as consistently seen with immunoassays for prostatic ACP; some studies have recommended routine use of acidification for all ACP specimens, but it is not clear that this is essential (Panteghini, 1992).

The half-life of prostatic ACP (PACP) is about 1–3 hours (Wadstrom, 1985). The day-to-day variation of acid phosphatase is relatively high; the average variation of the prostatic isoenzyme is 30% (Maatman, 1993), although it may be as high as 100% in patients with prostatic carcinoma (Brenckman, 1981); and the bone isoenzyme variation averages about 35% (Panteghini, 1995).

Measurement

Total acid phosphatase is typically measured by its ability to cleave phosphate groups at an acid pH. Usually the test is utilized for the measurement of prostatic serum ACP in the diagnosis or monitoring of prostatic adenocarcinoma. A variety of substrates and conditions have been used to measure enzymatic activity with increased specificity; these include thymolphthalein monophosphate and alpha-naphthyl phosphate. High bilirubin causes falsely low values for tartrate-resistant acid phosphatase activity, but not for total acid phosphatase (Alvarez, 1999).

Isoenzymes of ACP can be separated by electrophoresis; however, there is usually little interest in isoenzymes other than prostate and bone. Immunoassays (Moss, 1999; Bull, 2002) for both prostatic and bone isoenzymes of acid phosphatase have been developed; the former are widely available.

Causes of Abnormal Results

The main cause of increased ACP is prostate disease; with development of PSA (see Ch. 74), ACP has become less popular for use in prostate cancer. In early prostate cancer, the sensitivity of ACP is inferior to that of PSA (Burnett, 1992), while ACP, like PSA, is elevated in a significant percentage of patients with benign prostatic hyperplasia (Salo, 1990) or prostatic infarction, making ACP of little use for prostate cancer screening (Kaplan, 1985). Almost all patients with prostate cancer and elevated ACP have extracapsular extension or metastases (Salo, 1990; Burnett, 1992), so that an elevated ACP may provide useful information in staging of patients. Occasionally, elevated prostatic ACP may be due to other causes. Urinary tract obstruction/acute urinary retention may cause elevated ACP (Collier, 1986). Extensive prostatic massage, prostatic inflammation, infarction/ ischemia, and prostatic manipulations such as needle biopsy and cystoscopy may also cause a transient increase in serum PACP; testing should be done before any procedures are performed.

After surgical treatment of prostate cancer, ACP falls faster than PSA (Price, 1991), and should become undetectable after complete tumor resection. Since PSA is an androgen-dependent protein, androgen deprivation therapy decreases PSA production, but has no effect on ACP (Price, 1991; Narayan, 1995), suggesting that ACP may be of use in monitoring patients treated in this fashion.

ACP has been used for many years in cases of suspected rape. Fluid collected from the vagina on a cotton swab will give a positive test for ACP if semen is present, provided a stabilizing fluid with an acidic pH is used (Ricci, 1982). Peak values are generally present in the first 12 hours, remaining elevated for up to 4 days.

Alkaline Phosphatase (EC 3.1.3.1)

Biochemistry and Physiology

As with acid phosphatase, alkaline phosphatases (ALP) are a type of hydrolase class of enzyme (Table 20–1). Alkaline phosphatase in the canalicular (biliary) system is discussed in Chapter 21 on liver function. Alkaline phosphatases represent a family of enzymes coded for by different genes. Their physiological role is not yet understood. The most

Table 20–7 Relative Levels of Enzymes, by Gender, Relative to Young Adult Males (1.0)*

Enzyme	Age/gender	8	12	16	22	30	40	50	60
Aspartate aminotransferase	Male	0.75	0.86	0.82	1.00	1.16	1.26	1.21	1.11
	Female	0.73	0.80	0.69	0.89	0.89	1.01	0.77	0.96
Alanine aminotransferase	Male	1.14	1.09	0.89	1.00	1.03	1.11	1.06	0.83
	Female	1.11	0.89	0.83	0.75	0.75	0.75	0.72	0.83
Alkaline phosphatase	Male	3.61	4.76	4.48	1.52	1.00	1.00	0.95	0.95
	Female	3.14	4.10	2.52	0.81	0.86	0.76	1.00	1.38
γ-Glutamyl transferase	Male	0.25	0.29	0.37	0.62	1.00	1.07	1.16	0.99
	Female	0.24	0.28	0.33	0.38	0.52	0.58	0.9	1.09

* Results expressed as upper reference limits as a fraction of the upper reference limits for healthy young males.

Data from Siest G, Henry J, Schiele F, Young DS: Interpretation of Clinical Laboratory Tests: Reference Values and Their Biological Variation. Foster City, CA, Biomedical Publications, 1985.

abundant plasma ALP isoforms are coded for by a single gene on chromosome 1, producing the tissue nonspecific (sometimes called unspecific) isoenzyme found in kidney, liver, and bone; they differ in their carbohydrate side chains. Two other genes on chromosome 2 code for alkaline phosphatase of placental and intestinal origin; another gene on chromosome 2 codes for the so-called germ cell or placental-like isoenzyme, which has some antigenic and physical similarities to placental isoenzyme. In cells, ALP is primarily bound to cell membranes, where it appears to be involved in cleavage of phosphate-containing compounds and may facilitate movement of substances across cell membranes. Hepatocytes produce liver ALP, where it is found attached to the canalicular surface of the cells. Osteoblasts produce bone ALP, which appears to be involved in cleavage of pyrophosphate, an inhibitor of bone mineralization. Intestinal epithelial cells produce intestinal ALP, which is released into the intestine following ingestion of fatty foods.

There appear to be different mechanisms for release of ALP from cells, leading to varying forms of ALP in plasma. With liver injury, ALP synthesis increases, but bile acids dissolve fragments of canalicular cell membrane with attached enzymes (including ALP, GGT, leucine aminopeptidase, and 5'-NT) (Moss, 1997). While in normal serum a single form (of liver or bone origin) of ALP is typically seen, with hepatobiliary disease, both the normal product and the membrane-attachment form (high molecular weight) bound to lipoproteins can be seen (Wolf, 1994). Intestinal isoenzyme of alkaline phosphatase is released in large amounts into duodenal fluid (Deng, 1992), and large amounts enter lymphatic fluid draining the intestinal tract following a meal (Reynoso, 1971). However, much of the isoenzyme apparently becomes bound to red blood cell (RBC) ABO antigens (Bayer, 1980), so that only small amounts reach the plasma except in individuals who possess both the secretor gene and a large amount of H substance (group O or B), where alkaline phosphatase may increase by up to 30 IU/L following a meal (Domar, 1993). ALP is also higher in individuals of group O or B than in A and AB individuals (Agbedana, 1996) because of differences in intestinal ALP levels (Domar, 1993). Curiously, placental ALP is also lower in pregnant women of groups A and AB (Ind, 1994).

The half-life of isoenzymes of ALP differs significantly, so that it is necessary to know the isoenzyme that is elevated to evaluate rate of clearance: intestine, minutes; bone, 1 day; liver, 3 days; and placenta, 7 days. Day-to-day variation in total ALP is 5–10%, although bone isoenzyme shows 20% day-to-day variability.

Reference Ranges and Pre-analytical Variation

Reference ranges for ALP are highly dependent on age and gender (Table 20–7). During childhood, levels gradually rise throughout the first decade, reaching peak values three to four times normal adult levels, higher in boys than in girls. The higher values in children are due to bone isoenzyme. After a peak in the early teens, values gradually decrease to adult levels by the early 20s, and are similar in men and women until age 50. After menopause, bone isoenzyme increases slightly in women, causing a rise in reference limits after age 50. Reference limits are 15% higher in African-American men and 10% higher in African-American women (Manolio, 1992). Pregnancy causes a two- to threefold increase in ALP,

mainly due to placental isoenzyme, but also due to an increase in bone isoenzyme (Valenzuela, 1987).

A number of other factors affect ALP levels as well. High body mass index is associated with a 10% average increase in ALP (Salvaggio, 1991). Oral contraceptives decrease ALP an average of 20% (Dufour, 1998; Schiele, 1998), while fibric acid derivatives decrease total ALP by 25% and liver isoenzyme by 40% (Day, 1993). Antiepileptic agents commonly cause increased total ALP, mainly due to increases in liver isoenzyme; however, in some cases, bone isoenzyme may also be elevated (Nijhawan, 1990). Smoking causes an average 10% increase in total ALP, due to pulmonary production of placental-like ALP (Kallioniemi, 1987). Blood transfusion and cardiopulmonary bypass decrease alkaline phosphatase, often causing low levels (Kyd, 1998); this may be due to chelation of necessary cations by citrate.

Measurement

Although numerous methods exist, alkaline phosphatase activity is usually measured using p-nitrophenyl phosphate as the substrate at alkaline pH. A variety of buffers are used to bind phosphate groups; this increases activity, since inorganic phosphate (as well as some other anions) inhibits ALP. Zinc is a component of the enzyme, and magnesium and other cations activate the enzyme. Chelators present in collection tubes (such as EDTA, citrate, and oxalate) falsely lower ALP activity; in the case of EDTA, activity is often too low to measure. The activity of the enzyme increases slowly on storage, due to loss of inhibitors, but specimens are relatively stable at 4°C for up to 1 week.

A number of methods have been employed to separate ALP isoenzymes. Inhibition by phenylalanine reduces reactivity of intestinal and placental isoenzymes, while levamisole inhibits bone and liver isoenzymes; inhibition assays are poorly reproducible and are seldom used. Heat fractionation has been used for many years to determine the source of an elevated total ALP. The most heat-stable isoenzyme is placental (and germ cell) ALP, while liver isoenzyme is moderately stable and bone isoenzyme is the most heat labile. To achieve reliable results, use of standards of known composition and careful control of both temperature and time are essential. For these reasons, electrophoretic separation has been used for a number of years. Standard cellulose acetate and agarose gel electrophoresis cannot completely resolve bone and liver isoenzymes, making them unsuitable for other than qualitative studies. Since the difference in these isoenzymes is in their carbohydrate side chains, use of neuraminidase (to remove sialic acid) and wheat germ lectin (to bind to other isoenzymes) improves separation of bone and liver forms, allowing their quantitation. High-resolution electrophoresis using poly-acrylamide gel, and isoelectric focusing are capable of resolving multiple bands of alkaline phosphatase. Immunoassays for bone and placental isoenzymes of ALP are available commercially. Bone isoenzyme assays typically show some degree of cross-reactivity with liver isoenzyme, while placental isoenzyme assays have varying cross-reactivity with the germ cell isoenzyme.

Causes of Abnormal Results

The most common causes of increased ALP are liver and bone disease. Hepatic causes of elevated ALP are discussed in more detail in Chapter 21; disorders causing cholestasis more frequently cause elevation of ALP than do hepatocellular disorders. Causes of bone ALP elevation are discussed more fully in Chapter 15. Increased osteoblastic activity in Paget's disease, osteosarcoma, tumors metastatic to bone, and metabolic bone diseases are the most common causes of elevated bone isoenzyme. Occasionally, patients will have elevation of both bone and liver isoenzymes, especially in metastatic carcinoma. Rarely, marked transient elevations of alkaline phosphatase occur, usually in children and often following trivial illness; these may reach several thousand IU/L, and persist for weeks to months before resolving (Steinherz, 1984).

Increases in intestinal alkaline phosphatase may occur in patients with intestinal infarction, inflammation, and ulceration. Increases in placental-like isoenzymes, such as Regan and Nagao, are commonly found in patients with malignancies (ovary, cervical, lung, breast, colon, pancreas) and are due to ectopic production by the neoplasm.

As mentioned before, low ALP may occur transiently after blood transfusions or cardiopulmonary bypass. Prolonged, severely low levels of ALP occur in hypophosphatasia, a rare inherited disorder of bone metabolism (Whyte, 1996). Decreased ALP can also occur in zinc deficiency, since zinc is a necessary cofactor for ALP activity, as well as other conditions.

As discussed in Chapter 74 on tumor markers, placental alkaline phosphatase is a useful tumor marker in serum and cerebrospinal fluid (CSF) for most germ cell tumors.

Angiotensin-Converting Enzyme (EC 3.4.15.1)

Biochemistry and Physiology

Angiotensin I-converting enzyme (ACE), also known as kininase II and peptidyl-dipeptidase A, belongs to the hydrolase class of enzymes (Table 20–1) and is usually involved in the hydrolysis of peptide bonds at a free C-terminus, releasing a dipeptide in the reaction. However, it may also act as an endopeptidase or an aminopeptidase. It is responsible for conversion of angiotensin I to angiotensin II (in the renin–angiotensin–aldosterone system), as well as for inactivation of bradykinin (in the kallikrein–kinin system). Through these systems, ACE modulates peripheral vascular resistance as well as renal and cardiovascular function. Although its catalytic action is somewhat nonspecific in vitro, only angiotensin I, bradykinin, and hemoregulatory peptide Ac-DSKP are definite in vivo substrates (Macours, 2004).

ACE consists of a single polypeptide chain, with two homologous, zinc-binding catalytic sites (ACE is a zinc-metalloprotease). Enzyme activity is lost if zinc is bound to a chelating agent, such as EDTA, or is replaced with a different cation. In cells, ACE is a transmembrane protein, with a large amino-terminal extracellular domain, a very short hydrophobic trans-membrane domain, and a small intracellular carboxy-terminal domain; the cell-bound molecule is referred to as tissue ACE. The two catalytic sites are present in the extracellular domain: One near the amino-terminus and one nearer the carboxy-terminus. Proteolytic cleavage releases the functional enzyme from the cell membrane into the extracellular environment, producing circulating ACE.

The majority of ACE is tissue-bound (> 90%), with much lower levels circulating in plasma. ACE is predominantly found in endothelial cell membranes throughout the body. The lungs and the testes are particularly rich in ACE. Information on the molecular biology and structure of ACE is available (Dzau, 2002; Macours, 2004). There appear to be two distinct forms of ACE: a somatic form (sACE) and a smaller isoform found in testes (tACE). A single gene encodes both forms, by utilizing alternative promoters. sACE is found in many tissues and contains two active sites (as described above), while tACE contains only the C-terminal active site and is exclusively found in testes. Although both active sites of sACE require zinc ion, their biochemical properties are not identical (Dzau 2002, Macours 2004).

Reference Ranges and Pre-analytical Variation

ACE activity is higher in children than in adults; during adolescence, values are higher in boys than in girls (Beneteau-Burnat, 1990), gradually falling to adult levels by 18 years. Men and women have the same values, although not all studies show this pattern. ACE appears to be cleared by the liver; the half-life in plasma is roughly 48 hours. Average day-to-day variation is less than 10%, with no diurnal variation (Thompson, 1986).

A number of other factors affect ACE levels. Smokers have ACE activities about 30% lower than in nonsmokers or former smokers who have stopped smoking for at least 10 years (Ninomiya, 1987). Thyroid hormone stimulates ACE synthesis. Postmenopausal estrogen replacement causes a 20% fall in ACE activity in serum (Proudler, 1995). There are rare families that lack an endogenous inhibitor of ACE activity and, consequently, have markedly elevated serum ACE levels (Luisetti, 1990).

Measurement

ACE is typically measured by its ability to cleave synthetic peptides, releasing hippuric acid or other indicator molecules. A modification of the assay is required in CSF samples because of their much lower ACE activity (Oksanen, 1985).

Causes of Abnormal Results

The most common reason for ordering ACE levels is in diagnosis and monitoring of sarcoidosis. In general, ACE levels are directly related to number of organs affected (Muthuswamy, 1987) and activity of granulomas; mature granulomas tend to produce less ACE than developing ones (Mimori, 1998). In sarcoidosis, there is a general correlation between disease activity and ACE levels (Gupta, 1992); as disease progresses to fibrosis, ACE levels decline. ACE is more likely to be elevated with pulmonary involvement than with purely hilar adenopathy. ACE is also increased in many other granulomatous diseases, although not as frequently as in sarcoidosis. While most individuals with sarcoidosis have elevated ACE, the frequency of elevation in other granulomatous disorders is 10% (Studdy, 1978). For this reason, ACE is not usually considered a diagnostic test, although it may be helpful in patients with primarily ocular involvement, where biopsy cannot be readily performed (Power, 1995).

ACE is frequently elevated in a number of other disorders, including multiple sclerosis (Constantinescu, 1997), Addison's disease (Falezza, 1985), hyperthyroidism (Reiners, 1988), diabetes mellitus (Schernthaner, 1984), alcoholic hepatitis (Borowsky, 1982), peptic ulcer (D'Onofrio, 1984), nephrotic syndrome (Huskic, 1996), and at various stages in patients with bacterial (Kerttula, 1986) and pneumocystis pneumonitis (Singer, 1989). Other pulmonary disorders with a significantly increased ACE are emphysema, asthma, small-cell carcinoma, and squamous cell carcinoma (Ucar, 1997). In chronic renal failure, it is increased only in those on hemodialysis, and rises during the course of a dialysis procedure (Docci, 1988); it is decreased in those with chronic renal failure who are not on dialysis (Le Treut, 1983). In human immunodeficiency virus (HIV) infection, frequency and degree of elevation correlates with stage of disease (Ouellette, 1992). Decreased ACE levels are seen in various malignancies (Romer, 1980; Schweisfurth, 1985), in chronic liver disease (Sakata, 1991), in anorexia nervosa (Matsubayashi, 1988), and in hypothyroidism (Reiners, 1988).

Use of CSF ACE levels for diagnosis and monitoring of neurosarcoidosis has been criticized (Dale, 1999). A number of other diseases cause elevated CSF ACE, among them viral encephalitis, multiple sclerosis, and central nervous system (CNS) syphilis (Schweisfurth, 1987).

Acetylcholinesterase (EC 3.1.1.7) and Cholinesterase (EC 3.1.1.8)

Biochemistry and Physiology

Acetylcholinesterase (true cholinesterase or choline esterase I) and cholinesterase (pseudocholinesterase or choline esterase II) are carboxylic ester hydrolases (class 3, Table 20–1). Acetylcholinesterase (AChE) catalyzes the reaction:

$$\text{Acetylcholine} + H_2O \rightleftharpoons \text{Choline} + \text{Acetate} \tag{20–42}$$

Cholinesterase (PChE) catalyzes the reaction:

$$\text{An acylcholine} + H_2O \rightleftharpoons \text{Choline} + \text{A Carboxylate} \tag{20–43}$$

Acetylcholinesterase and cholinesterase (also called pseudocholinesterase or PChE) are two different enzymes, produced by different tissues, that are able to cleave acetylcholine, one of the body's major neurotransmitters. True cholinesterase has acetylcholine (ACh) as its primary natural substrate, and is also inhibited by it at approximately 10^{-2} mole/liter; it is found in high activity in the CNS, red blood cells (RBCs), lung, and spleen. ACh is a primary neurotransmitter at various sites in the CNS, and AChE rapidly hydrolyses ACh producing rapid termination of neurotransmission. AChE is not normally found in amniotic fluid.

The normal function of the enzyme found in serum, PChE (also called acylcholine acylhydrolase), is not known, but it is important in the cleavage of succinylcholine and mivacurium, muscle relaxants used during surgery. Serum PChE is not inhibited by AChE. PChE production occurs primarily in the liver, although other tissues, such as myocardium and pancreas, can also produce it. While both enzymes hydrolyze acetylcholine, AChE, but not PChE, hydrolyzes acetyl-beta-methylcholine; conversely, PChE, but not AChE, hydrolyzes butyryl- and benzoylcholine.

A number of genetic variants of PChE have reduced affinity (higher K_M) for acetylcholine as well as for competitive inhibitors such as dibucaine and fluoride, when compared to the common U (usual) form; these are termed A (for atypical), F (for fluoride resistant), and S (for silent). The S variant actually represents a number of mutations that may cause absence of enzymatic activity or absence of pseudocholinesterase synthesis. Heterozygous deficiency is found in about 4% of the population, while homozygous deficiency affects 0.3–0.5% of individuals. These variants cause decreased (or, in the case of the S variant, absent) PChE activity when present in homozygous or mixed heterozygous forms (AA, AF, AS, FF, FS, SS). Because of the broad range of normal values, reduced PChE activity is not usually found in common (U) form heterozygotes.

Another way to detect such variants is to measure the percent of enzyme activity remaining after in vitro incubation of serum enzyme with dibucaine or fluoride (termed dibucaine number or DN, and fluoride number, respectively). As mentioned above, the increased K_M of variants produces less effective catalysis than normal; decreased affinity thus exists for dibucaine and fluoride, making these variants more resistant to inhibition than normal. In general, dibucaine inhibits usual (U) plasma cholinesterase activity by approximately 70–90%. Variant cholinesterase activity is more resistant to inhibition, so that heterozygote activity is inhibited by approximately 50–70%, and homozygous variant activity is inhibited by approximately 10–30%. The DN will then reflect percentage inhibition of enzyme activity and will give a rough measure of the enzyme's activity; this in turn will indicate the presence or the absence of a variant form of the enzyme. The DN is calculated using the formula in Equation 20–44. For example, the UU form may show 85% inhibition, or 15% remaining activity, and yield a DN of 85.

Dibucaine (fluoride) number = $100 \times (1 - $ Enzyme activity with inhibitor/Enzyme activity without inhibitor) $\qquad$ (20–44)

Newer molecular biology techniques, such as the use of polymerase chain amplification (as described in Ch. 67) with separation of the reaction products by gel electrophoresis (Cerf, 2002), allow for much more accurate identification of variants, as compared to traditional biochemical analysis.

Reference Ranges and Pre-analytical Variation

PChE values are low in infants and gradually rise to adult levels by 4 months (Karlsen, 1981). Values in men do not change after this point until age 45; in women, they fall by about 10% at menarche and increase by 15% after menopause. A recent study (Abou-Hatab, 2001) found no significant correlation between older patient age and changes in plasma enzyme activities of AChE and PChE; healthy young and older individuals (study age range of 18–85 years) showed similar enzyme activities. Values in men are about 15–20% higher than in women until age 45, when values in women become equal. Oral contraceptives cause a decrease of about 15% in pseudocholinesterase activity (Lepage, 1985). There is about a fourfold range of values in normal individuals. Increased body mass index is associated with an increase in PChE, while low protein intake leads to decreased PChE.

The half-life of PChE has been estimated at between 2–10 days. Average day-to-day variation is about 7% (Moses, 1986), much smaller than that for most other enzymes.

Measurement

Enzyme activity is typically measured using an acylthiocholine ester as a substrate; released thiocholine reacts with Ellman's reagent (dithiobis-nitrobenzoic acid [DTNB]), releasing 5-mercapto-2-nitro benzoic acid, which is measured photometrically. Pseudocholinesterase activity is measured in serum, while acetylcholinesterase activity is measured in a hemolysate of washed RBCs. Acetylcholinesterase may also be determined in amniotic fluid by gel electrophoresis. To measure dibucaine or fluoride numbers, serum is incubated with dibucaine (30 μmol/L) or fluoride (4 mmol/L).

Causes of Abnormal Results

The main reasons for measuring PChE are (1) to monitor exposure to cholinesterase inhibitors, (2) as a liver function test, or (3) for diagnosis of genetic variants. Organophosphate insecticides are irreversible inhibitors of both AChE and PChE, although typically PChE plasma activity falls before AChE activity in RBCs with poisoning (Areekul, 1981). Because of the small individual variation and large interindividual variation in PChE values, it is advisable to obtain baseline values for PChE before individuals are exposed to organophosphates (Trundle, 1988). A decrease of 40% from baseline is needed before symptoms develop, and severe symptoms typically occur with over 80% fall in values; thus, symptoms often occur with PChE values within the reference range. If no baseline values are present, serial determinations are helpful. In one study, 90% of symptomatic organophosphate poisonings were associated with PChE values within the reference range, while postexposure levels showed a rise confirmed toxicity (Coye, 1987). While PChE reflects acute toxicity, AChE (RBCs) better reflects chronic exposure.

In contrast to other hepatocyte enzymes, PChE production by the liver appears to reflect synthetic function rather than hepatocyte injury. Levels of PChE are decreased in acute hepatitis, cirrhosis, and carcinoma metastatic to liver. PChE is decreased in malnutrition, but is normal or increased in nephrotic syndrome. As is the case when monitoring organophosphate exposure, changes in values compared to baseline are more useful than single values, limiting the diagnostic usefulness of PChE as a nutritional or liver injury monitor.

The other common use of PChE measurements is in recognizing the presence of genetic variants. Most commonly, such testing involves family members of individuals having prolonged apnea after use of succinyl-choline or mivacurium (neuromuscular blocking agents/muscle relaxants) during anesthesia. Testing typically involves both total PChE and determination of fluoride and dibucaine numbers to recognize homozygous or compound heterozygous variants that put an individual at risk from exposure to cholinesterase inhibitors. Patients at risk (with variant cholinesterase forms) may more slowly hydrolyze the neuromuscular blocking agent, unexpectedly increasing the duration of respiratory muscle relaxation and prolonging apnea. This is in contrast to the usual rapid

Table 20–8 Relative Percentage of Lactate Dehydrogenase (LD) Isoenzymes in Various Tissues

Tissue	LD$_1$	LD$_2$	LD$_3$	LD$_4$	LD$_5$
Serum	25	35	20	15	5
Heart	45	40	10	5	0
Red cells	40	35	15	10	0
Renal cortex	35	30	25	20	0
Lung	10	15	40	30	5
Skeletal muscle	0	0	10	30	60
Liver	0	5	10	15	70

drug hydrolysis with the usual (U) forms, leading to rapid recovery of the patient.

As mentioned above, measurement of RBC AChE is useful in organophosphate exposure and poisoning. In addition, qualitative analysis of AChE in amniotic fluid may be useful in the diagnosis of neural tube defects, especially in high-risk groups (Muller, 2003). AChE can be identified in amniotic fluid from pregnancies with neural tube defects, as well as some other types of birth defects. AChE is absent in amniotic fluid from normal pregnancies.

Lactate Dehydrogenase (EC 1.1.1.27)

Biochemistry and Physiology

Lactate dehydrogenase (LD) is a class 1 enzyme (oxidoreductase, Table 20–1), acting on a CH–OH group of donors with NAD$^+$ (nicotinamide-adenine dinucleotide, a coenzyme required for the reaction) as acceptor, and catalyzes the transfer of hydrogen:

$$(L)\text{-lactate} + NAD^+ \rightleftharpoons Pyruvate + NADH + H^+ \qquad (20\text{–}45)$$

The enzyme is also capable of oxidizing other (L)-2-hydroxymono-carboxylic acids.

Lactate dehydrogenase (often abbreviated LD) is a zinc-containing enzyme that is part of the glycolytic pathway; it is found in the cytoplasm of all cells and tissues in the body. LD is a tetramer of two active subunits, H (for heart) and M (for muscle) with a molecular weight of 134 kDa. Combinations of subunits produce five isoenzymes ranging from LD$_1$ (HHHH) to LD$_5$ (MMMM); the intermediate isoenzymes contain differing combinations of H and M subunits (LD$_2$, HHHM; LD$_3$, HHMM; LD$_4$, HMMM). There are inherited forms of deficiency of H (Joukyuu, 1989) and M (Kanno, 1980) subunits of LD, associated with low LD levels in plasma and only one isoenzyme on electrophoresis. Another form of LD composed of four C subunits is found in spermatozoa and in semen, but has never been detected in serum, even in individuals with seminoma (Vogelzang, 1982). Rarely, another band detected in electrophoresis and termed 'LD$_6$' can be seen; this probably represents alcohol dehydrogenase, which can also metabolize lactate (Kato, 1984).

The tissue distribution of LD varies primarily in its isoenzyme composition, not in its content of LD (Table 20–6). It is important to note that LD$_1$ and LD$_2$ are expressed at high levels in myocardial tissue and in erythrocytes and at much lower levels in tissues such as liver and muscle; the reverse is true for LD$_4$ and LD$_5$. In myocardial damage, the predominant isoenzymes that become elevated in serum are LD$_1$ and LD$_2$, while in liver or skeletal muscle disease, the LD$_4$ and LD$_5$ isoenzymes become elevated predominantly in serum. In contrast to enzymes such as AST, ALT, and CK, which show marked variation in enzyme activity between tissues, the range in values for LD is only about 1.5-fold between those with the highest amounts (such as liver) and those with lower amounts (such as kidney); most tissues have LD activities that are 500–1000 times greater in tissue than that found in normal serum (see Table 20–6). Thus, a significant elevation of plasma levels occurs with a small amount of tissue damage/breakdown. The tissue distribution of LD isoenzymes is shown in Table 20–8. The specific composition of elevated isoenzyme levels found in plasma will reflect tissue origin. In plasma, the majority of LD comes from breakdown of erythrocytes and platelets, with varying contributions from other organs. LD is apparently eliminated in bile, as injection of radiolabeled LD results in radioactivity in the gallbladder and small intestine (Smith, 1988).

Reference Ranges and Pre-analytical Variation

LD values are highest in newborns and infants; values do not change with age in adults, and there is no gender difference. Persons over age 65 tend to have slightly higher values. Exercise causes, at most, slight increases in total LD; even strenuous exercise causes only a 25% rise in average values (Tanada, 1993). Even trace to slight hemolysis invalidates LD and LD isoenzyme analyses. Contact with the clot increases LD, and physical agitation of specimens, as occurs in most pneumatic tube systems, tends to cause some hemolysis and an increased LD. Hemolysis affects both total LD and the LD_1/LD_2 ratio. Exercise has little effect on LD or its isoenzymes. Extreme exercise can cause LD_1 to become greater than LD_2. Total LD increases transiently after blood transfusion, but returns to baseline within 24 hours (Wiesen, 1998). Delayed separation of red cells from serum does not affect LD values for 1–2 days. Few drugs directly affect LD activity, but granulocyte/macrophage colony-stimulating factor (GM-CSF) appears to increase LD in parallel to the increase in white blood cell (WBC) count (Sarris, 1995).

The half-life of LD isoenzymes varies greatly, from approximately 4–4.5 days for LD_1 to 4–6 hours for LD_5. Day-to-day variation of LD is only 5–10%.

Measurement

LD activity can be measured using either the forward (lactate to pyruvate) or reverse (pyruvate to lactate) direction of the reaction. The vast majority of laboratories use the forward reaction; the reverse reaction, predominantly used in the dry slide method for LD, produces activities that have good correlation with the forward reaction but at measured activities approximately threefold higher, making comparison of results without data conversion difficult.

The reverse (pyruvate-to-lactate) reaction is used in a few laboratories currently, due to faster reaction kinetics, less costly cofactor (NADH) needed, and a smaller specimen volume requirement. Disadvantages of the pyruvate-to-lactate reaction are an early loss of linearity of reaction kinetics, the effect of potent LD inhibitors in some NADH preparations, and the suboptimal concentrations of pyruvate that can be used because of substrate inhibition on the activity of LD. Also, lactate is a more specific substrate for this enzyme; pyruvate is less specific and serves as a substrate for such enzymes as pyruvate dehydrogenase.

Electrophoretic separation of LD isoenzymes is typically used when quantitation of different isoenzymes is required; agarose gel is most commonly used. Quantitation usually uses the forward reaction, allowing detection of fluorescent NADH or a reduced formazan dye in a colorimetric development step. The electrophoretic support and developing agent affect the results, and the reference ranges for the different methods are not the same. Inhibition methods for LD_1 are also available, but only allow quantitation of this isoenzyme; results are often expressed as ratio of LD_1 to total LD. Hydroxybutyrate is preferentially cleaved by LD_1 isoenzyme; until the early 1970s, measurement of 'hydroxybutyrate dehydrogenase' was employed as a diagnostic test for myocardial infarction.

Serum LD is, on average, 30 IU/L higher than plasma LD, owing to release of LD from platelets. With prolonged incubation of plasma containing platelets (separated at $< 1200\,g$ centrifugation), LD can leak from damaged platelets, increasing plasma LD as well (Hollaar, 1979). LD is not stable on storage at 4°C due to cold lability of LD_5. Specimens can be stored for up to 24 hours at room temperature with little change. Three days of storage at room temperature decreases the total LD by about 20%, increases the apparent LD_1 by 20%, and decreases the apparent LD_5 by 18%. If specimens are frozen, LD_5 decreases significantly, and the isoenzyme pattern shifts with an artifactual increase in LD_1 and decrease in LD_5. Serum should not be frozen for assay of LD or for its isoenzymes.

Causes of Abnormal Results

LD is a highly nonspecific test; an abnormal value is not specific for damage to any particular organ. The relative amounts of LD, AST, and ALT (along with CK) may provide clues to the source of LD elevation. If LD is markedly elevated, but AST, ALT, and CK are normal or minimally increased, this suggests damage to cells such as red or white blood cells, kidney, lung, lymph nodes, or tumors. Increases in both CK and LD, with greater increases in AST than ALT, occur with cardiac or skeletal muscle injury. Increases in LD are uncommon in liver disease, usually occurring only transiently with toxic or ischemic liver injury (Cassidy, 1994); in such cases, AST and ALT are typically increased more than LD. In many cases, such as in shock and with metastatic carcinoma, LD is increased due to damage to multiple organs, so that mixed patterns can be seen. Marked elevations of LD (> 5–10 times normal) are seen in megaloblastic anemia, hemolytic anemias, advanced malignancies (particularly lymphoma and leukemia), sepsis or other causes of shock, and cardiopulmonary arrest. LD is often moderately elevated in *Pneumocystis carinii* pneumonia (Smith, 1988), while it is often normal in most other forms of pneumonia (Rotenberg, 1988). While LD is highly sensitive (so that normal values make the diagnosis unlikely) (Quist, 1995), predictive value of LD is not

adequate to establish a diagnosis of *P. carinii* pneumonia in an HIV patient (Grover, 1992). In patients with biliary pancreatitis (inflammation due to gallstones impacted in the bile duct), the LDH : AST ratio is elevated, and appears to indicate the presence of pancreatic necrosis (Isogai, 1998). Note that 10–20% of patients with biliary pancreatitis may present with normal liver function tests (Dholakia, 2004).

In cases where the cause of elevated LD cannot be determined by other means, LD isoenzymes may be useful in determining the source of injury. In normal serum, the LD isoenzymes, in decreasing order of activity, are $2 > 1 > 3 > 4 > 5$. In germ cell tumors (particularly seminoma and dysgerminoma), LD_1 is increased, and can serve as a tumor marker (von Eyben, 2000, 2001).

As noted in Chapter 18 on cardiac function, LD increases in serum over about a 36-hour period during which time the $LD_1 : LD_2$ ratio, which is normally less than 1, increases to values of 1 or above, the so-called 'flipped' ratio. This was employed to confirm the diagnosis of myocardial infarction (MI) but could not be used to make acute diagnoses of MI because of the prolonged time (36 h) required for the flipped ratio to develop. As discussed in Chapter 18, there are better biomarkers, specifically troponin, for the acute diagnosis of MI and in confirmation of the diagnosis (serum troponin levels remain elevated for over 1 week after the acute event). Also, hemolytic anemia, megaloblastic anemia, and renal cortical diseases such as renal infarcts and renal cell carcinoma cause increases in LD_1 and, often, a flipped $LD_1 : LD_2$. In tumors of WBCs (leukemia, lymphoma, multiple myeloma) LD_3 and, often, LD_4 are typically increased, whereas the relative amount of LD_1 and LD_2 is decreased (Copur, 1989; Ricerca, 1988; Pandit, 1990). Pulmonary disease can produce a similar pattern. Increases in LD_5 and, sometimes, LD_4 are typically seen with skeletal muscle injury or with ischemic or toxic hepatic injury. The presence of LD_6 is associated with a poor prognosis (Ketchum, 1984). An isomorphic pattern, in which total LD is increased but isoenzymes are present in normal proportions, and a 'tombstone' pattern, when the relative amount of each isoenzyme is roughly the same, are typically seen in persons with diffuse tissue damage, often accompanied by shock or hypoxemia.

5′-Nucleotidase (EC 3.1.3.5)

Biochemistry and Physiology

5′-Nucleotidase (5′-NT) is a phosphoric monoester hydrolase (class 3 enzyme, Table 20–1), also known as 5′-ribonucleotide phosphohydrolase or NTP, which catalyzes the following reaction:

$$\text{A 5′-ribonucleotide} + H_2O \rightleftharpoons \text{A ribonucleoside} + \text{Phosphate} \tag{20–46}$$

It is a cytoplasmic membrane-bound phosphatase with a wide specificity for 5′-ribonucleotides and a molecular weight of about 70 kDa. It acts only on nucleotides (such as adenosine 5′-triphosphate or ATP and guanosine 5′-triphosphate or GTP), and is believed to function in extracellular adenosine production, nutrient absorption, and cell proliferation. 5′-NT is a metalloprotein, and zinc is believed to be an integral part of the enzyme. It is widely distributed in the body, predominantly attached to cell membranes (similarly to ALP and GGT). Plasma 5′-NT is predominantly derived from the liver. A detailed review of 5′-NT is available (Sunderman, 1990).

Reference Ranges and Pre-analytical Variation

5′-NT is normally present at low activities in children, rises in adolescence, and plateaus until age 40, when levels increase significantly (Moses, 1986); reference values are independent of gender and race. There is a slight increase in 5′-NT during the second and third trimesters of pregnancy (Bacq, 1996). Similarly to ALP and GGT, antiepileptic drugs can increase 5′-NT activity; however, values are usually less than twice the reference limits, and less than 25% of those taking such agents show elevated 5′-NT activity (Fortman, 1985).

Measurement

The measurement of 5′-NT is made difficult because other phosphatases, notably ALP, are capable of cleaving the substrate used to measure the lower activity of 5′-NT present in the sample. Approaches usually utilize large amounts of other, non-nucleoside substrates to 'competitively inhibit' ALP (although they are actually being metabolized by ALP, they prevent ALP from acting on nucleotide phosphates). Although it would be simplest to measure generated phosphate, this cannot be done, since cleavage of other phosphates by ALP would produce incorrect results. Therefore, measurement of the nucleotide released by the action of 5′-NT is required. Most chelating agents such as EDTA inhibit enzyme activity, presumably by making zinc unavailable.

CHAPTER: 20 Clinical Enzymology

As with GGT, 5'-NT is most commonly used to determine if the source of an elevated ALP is from liver or bone. While 5'-NT is more commonly elevated with cholestatic disorders, acute hepatitis causes an increase in 5'-NT synthesis by the liver and slight elevation in 5'-NT in plasma (Fukano, 1990). 5'-NT is increased in ovarian carcinoma (Chatterjee, 1981), and in rheumatoid arthritis, where levels correlate with extent of inflammation as reflected by erythrocyte sedimentation rate (Johnson, 1999). Sapey et al. (2000) prospectively studied ALP, GGT, and 5'-NT in 80 cholestatic patients, correlating intrahepatic (i.e., secondary to intrahepatic parenchymal disease) and extrahepatic (i.e., secondary to biliary tree obstruction) causes with enzyme changes. They found markedly increased levels with extrahepatic causes (compared with intrahepatic disease) and that elevations in GGT and 5'-NT levels were independently linked to cause. The GGT/5'-NT ratio differed significantly between the two groups, with a ratio < 1.9 highly suggestive of (but insensitive to) intrahepatic disease (Sapey, 2000).

Skeletal Muscle Injury – Creatine Kinase/Phosphokinase (CK/CPK)

The basic assay for this enzyme was discussed above under Assay of Enzymes. This enzyme has two major isoenzymes, M and B, each of which has the same activity. CK is composed of three types of dimers: MM (mainly in skeletal muscle), MB (found mainly in cardiac tissue) and BB (found predominantly in brain and intestine). As discussed at length in Chapter 18, because CK-MB is found mainly in myocardial tissue, CK-MB is used as a serodiagnostic test for myocardial infarction (MI). In this section, CK is discussed as a biomarker for skeletal muscle injury.

Skeletal muscle injury can occur from a variety of sources. Direct trauma, as occurs with physical injury (including contact sports), surgery, strenuous exercise, and intramuscular injections are common causes of mild elevations of CK (up to about five to six times reference limits). In these situations, CK typically increases rapidly and then falls quickly, returning to baseline with a half-life of approximately 24 hours. An important clinical disorder associated with acute muscle injury is neuroleptic malignant syndrome, a rare complication of treatment with phenothiazines or other psychotropic agents. Typically, affected individuals present with muscle rigidity, fever, and elevated WBC counts; CK is considered a diagnostic test for this disorder. Prompt recognition and treatment are necessary to prevent death from this syndrome; discontinuation of medications and use of the muscle-stabilizing agent dantrolene are the cornerstones of treatment (Pelonero, 1998).

Chronic damage to muscle causes more persistent elevation of CK, which may be either mild or more extensive. The broad range of normal values and pre-analytical variation seen in total CK values can hamper recognition of mild, ongoing muscle injury. Generally, persistent elevation above the reference limits for an appropriate comparison group despite cessation of any other factors known to affect CK is needed to diagnose muscle injury in asymptomatic individuals. Common causes of chronic muscle injury include medications (particularly HMG-CoA reductase inhibitors and glucocorticoids), congenital myopathies (such as Duchenne's muscular dystrophy), inflammatory disorders (polymyositis and dermatomyositis), hypothyroidism, and alcohol abuse. In chronic myopathies, CK-MB is often increased, reflecting its production by regenerating muscle.

With severe acute damage to muscle, a clinical picture termed rhabdomyolysis may develop. In such situations, CK-MB/total CK may be elevated above normal, in the absence of myocardial infarction (cardiac troponin levels are normal); this is not uncommonly seen in patients with inflammatory muscle disease (Kiely, 2000). In addition to normal cardiac troponin levels with elevated CK levels, two distinct isoforms (representing fast or slow skeletal fiber types) of serum skeletal troponin I may be identified (Simpson, 2002); research is ongoing in this area.

There are no specific criteria for differentiating rhabdomyolysis from lesser degrees of muscle injury; among the more important features are the higher total CK (one suggested diagnostic level is CK > 20 times upper reference limits), the rapid rise and fall of CK, and the appearance of myoglobinuria. Many assays for myoglobin (found in skeletal, smooth, and cardiac muscle) are relatively insensitive, and myoglobin has a short half-life; thus, CK is a more reliable test for establishing the diagnosis. As a form of 'cell lysis syndrome,' rhabdomyolysis is associated with the release of other cell contents, such as potassium, phosphate, and nucleotides that can be converted to uric acid. Qualitative testing for myoglobin in the urine is important since myoglobin is potentially toxic to the kidneys and the patient is at risk for acute renal failure. Myoglobinuria may lead to development of acute tubular necrosis, with appearance of pigmented casts in the urine sediment. If renal failure develops, hyperkalemia, hyperphosphatemia, and hyperuricemia typically also will be present. There is no direct relationship between the degree of elevation of CK and likelihood of development of renal failure (Gabow, 1982; Ward, 1988). Common causes of rhabdomyolysis include drugs (particularly ethanol and cocaine), viral infections, extreme exertion, hyperthermia, trauma including crush injuries, ischemia of the lower extremities, and inflammatory myopathies.

References

General

Brehme CS, Roman S, Shaffer J, et al: Tartrate-resistant acid phosphatase forms complexes with alpha2-macroglobulin in serum. J Bone Miner Res 1999; 14:311–318.

Dasgupta A, Banerjee SK, Datta P: False-positive troponin I in the MEIA due to the presence of rheumatoid factors in serum. Elimination of this interference by using a polyclonal antisera against rheumatoid factors. Am J Clin Pathol 1999; 112:753–756.

Dickerman RD, Pertusi R, Zachariah NY, et al: Anabolic steroid induced hepatotoxicity: Is it overstated? Clin J Sports Med 1999; 9:34–39.

International Union of Biochemistry: Enzyme Nomenclature, 1978: Recommendations of the Nomenclature Committee of the International Union of Biochemistry and the Nomenclature and Classification of Enzymes. San Diego, Academic Press, 1979.

International Union of Biochemistry and Molecular Biology, Nomenclature Committee: Enzyme Nomenclature. Recommendations 1992. San Diego, Academic Press, 1992.

Langdon DE: Enzyme neurosis – a clinician's plan for standardization. Ann Intern Med 1994; 121:234–235.

Mader M, Kolbus N, Meihorst D, et al: Human intestinal alkaline phosphatase-binding IgG in patients with severe bacterial infections. Clin Exp Immunol 1994; 95:98–102.

Moss DW, Henderson AR: Clinical enzymology. *In* Burtis CA, Ashwood ER (eds): Tietz Textbook of Clinical Chemistry, 3rd ed. Philadelphia, WB Saunders, 1999, pp 617–721.

Otto A, Bar J, Birkenmeier G: Prostate-specific antigen forms complexes with human alpha 2-macroglobulin and binds to the alpha 2-macroglobulin receptor/LDL receptor-related protein. J Urol 1998; 159:297–303.

Podlasek SJ, Dufour DR, McPherson RA: Alterations in lactate dehydrogenase isoenzyme pattern after therapy with streptokinase or streptococcal infection. Clin Chem 1989; 35:1763–1766.

Remaley AT, Wilding P: Macroenzymes: Biochemical characterization, clinical significance, and laboratory detection. Clin Chem 1989; 35:2261–2270.

Sosolik RC, Hitchcock CL, Becker WJ: Heterophilic antibodies produce spuriously elevated concentrations of the MB isoenzyme of creatine kinase in a selected patient population. Am J Clin Pathol 1997; 107:506–510.

Van Hoof VO, Deng DT, De Broe ME: How do plasma membranes reach the circulation? Clin Chim Acta 1997; 266:23–31.

Zollner H: Handbook of Enzyme Inhibitors. New York, VCH Publishers, 1989.

Enzyme Kinetics

Cleland WW: Steady state kinetics. *In* Boyer PD (ed): The Enzymes, Vol 2, 3rd ed. San Diego, Academic Press, 1970, pp 1–65.

Cleland WW: Steady state kinetics. *In* Sigman DS, Boyer PD (eds): The Enzymes, Vol 19, 3rd ed. San Diego, Academic Press, 1990, pp 99–158.

Cornish-Bowden A: Fundamentals of Enzyme Kinetics, Revised ed. London, Portland Press, 1995.

Fersht A: Structure and Mechanism in Protein Science. New York, Freeman, 1999, Chapters 3–7.

Segal IH: Enzyme Kinetics, New York, Wiley-Interscience, 1993.

Specific Enzymes

Abou-Hatab K, O'Mahony MS, Patel S, Woodhouse K: Relationship between age and plasma esterases. Age Ageing 2001; 30:41–45.

Agbedana EO, Yeldu MH: Serum total, heat and urea stable alkaline phosphatase activities in relation to ABO blood groups and secretor phenotypes. Afr J Med Med Sci 1996; 25:327–329.

Alvarez L, Peris P, Bedini JL, et al: High bilirubin levels interfere with serum tartrate-resistant acid phosphatase determination: Relevance as a marker of bone resorption in jaundiced patients. Calcif Tissue Int 1999; 64:301–303.

Areekul S, Srichairat S, Kirdudom P: Serum and red cell cholinesterase activity in people exposed to organophosphate insecticides. Southeast Asian J Trop Med Public Health 1981; 12:94–98.

Bacq Y, Zarka O, Brechot JF, et al: Liver function tests in normal pregnancy: A prospective study of 103 pregnant women and 103 matched controls. Hepatology 1996; 23:1030–1034.

Bayer PM, Hotschek H, Knoth E: Intestinal alkaline phosphatase and the ABO blood group system: A new aspect. Clin Chim Acta 1980; 108:81–87.

Beneteau-Burnat B, Baudin B, Morgant G, et al: Serum angiotensin-converting enzyme in healthy and sarcoidotic children: Comparison with the reference interval for adults. Clin Chem 1990; 36:344–346.

Borowsky SA, Lieberman J, Strome S, Sastre A: Elevation of serum angiotensin-converting enzyme level.

Occurrence in alcoholic liver disease. Arch Intern Med 1982; 142:893–895.

Brenckman WD Jr, Lastinger LB, Sedor F: Unpredictable fluctuations in serum acid phosphatase activity in prostatic cancer. JAMA 1981; 245:2501–2504.

Bull H, Murray PG, Thomas D, et al: Acid phosphatases. J Clin Pathol: Mol Pathol 2002; 55:65–72.
Recent review of acid phosphatases, with emphasis on tartrate-resistant acid phosphatase and its function and clinical usefulness in processes involving bone resorption.

Burnett AL, Chan DW, Brendler CB, et al: The value of serum enzymatic acid phosphatase in the staging of localized prostate cancer. J Urol 1992; 148:1832–1834.

Cassidy WM, Reynolds TB: Serum lactic dehydrogenase in the differential diagnosis of acute hepatocellular injury. J Clin Gastroenterol 1994; 19:118–121.

Cerf C, Mesguish M, Gabriel I, et al: Screening patients with prolonged neuromuscular blockade after succinylcholine and mivacurium. Anesth Analg 2002; 94:461–466.

Chatterjee SK, Bhattacharya M, Barlow JJ: Evaluation of 5′-nucleotidase as an enzyme marker in ovarian carcinoma. Cancer 1981; 47:2648–2653.

Chen J, Yam LT, Janckila AJ, et al: Significance of 'high' acid phosphatase activity in the serum of normal children. Clin Chem 1979; 25:719–722.

Collier DS, Pain JA: Acute and chronic retention of urine: Relevance of raised serum prostatic acid phosphatase levels. A prospective study. Urology 1986; 27:34–37.

Constantinescu CS, Goodman DB, Grossman RI, et al: Serum angiotensin-converting enzyme in multiple sclerosis. Arch Neurol 1997; 54:1012–1015.

Copur S, Kus S, Kars A, et al: Lactate dehydrogenase and its isoenzymes in serum from patients with multiple myeloma. Clin Chem 1989; 35:1968–1970.

Coye MJ, Barnett PG, Midtling JE, et al: Clinical confirmation of organophosphate poisoning by serial cholinesterase analyses. Arch Intern Med 1987; 147:438–442.

Dale JC, O'Brien JF: Determination of angiotensin-converting enzyme levels in cerebrospinal fluid is not a useful test for the diagnosis of neurosarcoidosis. Mayo Clin Proc 1999; 74:535.

Day AP, Feher MD, Chopra R, et al: The effect of benzafibrate treatment on serum alkaline phosphatase isoenzyme activities. Metabolism 1993; 42:839–842.

Deng JT, Hoylaerts MF, Van Hoof VO, et al: Differential release of human intestinal alkaline phosphatase in duodenal fluid and serum. Clin Chem 1992; 38:2532–2538.

Dholakia K, Pitchumoni CS, Agarwal N: How often are liver function tests normal in acute biliary pancreatitis? J Clin Gastroenterol 2004; 38:81–83.

Docci D, Delvecchio C, Turci F, et al: Effect of different dialyzer membranes on serum angiotensin-converting enzyme during hemodialysis. Int J Artif Organs 1988; 11:28–32.

Domar U, Karpe F, Hamsten A, et al: Human intestinal alkaline phosphatase; release to the blood is linked to lipid absorption, but removal from the blood is not linked to lipoprotein clearance. Eur J Clin Invest 1993; 23:753–760.

D'Onofrio GM, Levitt S, Ilett KF: Serum angiotensin converting enzyme in Crohn's disease, ulcerative colitis and peptic ulceration. Aust N Z J Med 1984; 14:27–30.

Dufour DR: Effects of oral contraceptives on routine laboratory tests. Clin Chem 1998; 44:A137.

Dzau VJ, Bernstein K, Celermajer D, et al: Pathophysiologic and therapeutic importance of tissue ACE: A consensus report. Cardiovasc Drugs Ther 2002; 16:149–160.
Report from a recent consensus conference examining the actions of angiotensin-converting enzyme in the pathology of cardiovascular disease and the use of tissue ACE inhibitors as antihypertensive agents in these patients.

Falezza G, Lechi Santonastaso C, Parisi T, et al: High serum levels of angiotensin-converting enzyme in untreated Addison's disease. J Clin Endocrinol Metab 1985; 61:496–498.

Fortman CS, Witte DL: Serum 5′-nucleotidase in patients receiving anti-epileptic drugs. Am J Clin Pathol 1985; 84:197–201.

Fukano M, Amano S, Hazama F, et al: 5′-Nucleotidase activities in sera and liver tissues of viral hepatitis patients. Gastroenterol Jpn 1990; 25:199–205.

Gabow PA, Kaehny WD, Kelleher SP: The spectrum of rhabdomyolysis. Medicine (Baltimore) 1982; 61:141–152.

Grover SA, Coupal L, Suissa S, et al: The clinical utility of serum lactate dehydrogenase in diagnosing *Pneumocystis carinii* pneumonia among hospitalized AIDS patients. Clin Invest Med 1992; 15:309–317.

Gupta SK, Chakraborty M, Mitra K: Serum angiotensin converting enzyme in respiratory diseases. Indian J Chest Dis Allied Sci 1992; 34:19–24.

Hollaar L, Van der Laarse A: Interference of the measurement of lactate dehydrogenase (LDH) activity in human serum and plasma by LDH from blood cells. Clin Chim Acta 1979; 99:135–142 1979.

Huskic J, Kulenovic H, Culo F: Serum angiotensin-converting enzyme activity in patients with endemic nephropathy. Nephron 1996; 74:120–124.

Ind TE, Iles RK, Carter PG, et al: Serum placental-type alkaline phosphatase activity in women with squamous and glandular malignancies of the reproductive tract. J Clin Pathol 1994; 47:1035–1037.

Isogai M, Yamaguchi A, Hori A, Kaneoka Y: LDH to AST ratio in biliary pancreatitis – a possible indicator of pancreatic necrosis: Preliminary results. Am J Gastroenterol 1998; 93:363–367.

Johnson SM, Patel S, Bruckner FE, et al: 5′-Nucleotidase as a marker of both general and local inflammation in rheumatoid arthritis patients. Rheumatology 1999; 38:391–396.

Joukyuu R, Mizuno S, Amakawa T, et al: Hereditary complete deficiency of lactate dehydrogenase H-subunit. Clin Chem 1989; 35:687–690.

Kanno T, Sudo K, Takeuchi I, et al: Hereditary deficiency of lactate dehydrogenase M-subunit. Clin Chim Acta 1980; 108:267–276.

Kaplan LA, Chen IW, Sperling M, et al: Clinical utility of serum prostatic acid phosphatase measurements for detection (screening), diagnosis, and therapeutic monitoring of prostatic carcinoma; assessment of monoclonal and polyclonal enzymes and radioimmunoassays. Am J Clin Pathol 1985; 84:334–339.

Karlsen RL, Sterri S, Lyngaas S, et al: Reference values for erythrocyte acetylcholinesterase and plasma cholinesterase activities in children, implications for organophosphate intoxication. Scand J Clin Lab Invest 1981; 41:301–302.

Kato S, Ishii H, Kano S, et al: Evidence that 'lactate dehydrogenase isoenzyme 6' is in fact alcohol dehydrogenase. Clin Chem 1984; 30:1585–1586.

Kerttula Y, Weber TH: Serum angiotensin converting enzyme in pneumonias. J Clin Pathol 1986; 39:1250–1253.

Ketchum CH, Robinson CA, Hall LM, et al: Clinical significance and partial biochemical characterization of lactate dehydrogenase isoenzyme 6. Clin Chem 1984; 30:46–49.

Kiely PD, Bruckner FE, Nisbet JA, Daghir A: Serum skeletal troponin I in inflammatory muscle disease: Relation to creatine kinase, CKMB and cardiac troponin I. Ann Rheum Dis 2000; 59:750–751.

Kyd PA, Vooght KD, Kerkhoff F, et al: Clinical usefulness of bone alkaline phosphatase in osteoporosis. Ann Clin Biochem 1998; 35:717–725.

Lepage L, Schiele F, Gueguen R, et al: Total cholinesterase in plasma: Biological variations and reference limits. Clin Chem 1985; 31:546–550.

Le Treut A, Chevet D, Guenet L, et al: Serum angiotensin-converting enzyme levels in patients with chronic renal failure. Pathol Biol (Paris) 1983; 31:182–185.

Luisetti M, Martinetti M, Cuccia M, et al: Familial elevation of serum angiotensin converting enzyme activity. Eur Respir J 1990; 3:441–446.

Maatman TJ: Comparative analysis of fluctuation of serum tumor markers in advanced cancer of prostate. Urology 1993; 42:672–676.

Macours N, Poels J, Hens K, et al: Structure, evolutionary conservation, and functions of angiotensin- and endothelin-converting enzymes. Int Rev Cytol 2004; 239:47–97.
Recent overview of both angiotensin-converting enzyme and endothelin-converting enzyme examining the structure and biological role of these molecules.

Manolio TA, Burke GL, Savage PJ, et al: Sex- and race-related differences in liver-associated serum chemistry tests in young adults in the CARDIA study. Clin Chem 1992; 38:1853–1859.

Matsubayashi S, Tamai H, Kobayashi N, et al: Angiotensin-converting enzyme and anorexia nervosa. Horm Metab Res 1988; 20:761–764.

Mimori Y: Sarcoidosis: Correlation of HRCT findings with results of pulmonary function tests and serum angiotensin-converting enzyme assay. Kurume Med J 1998; 45:247–256.

Moses GC, Tuckerman JF, Henderson AR: Biological variance of cholinesterase and 5′-nucleotidase in serum of healthy persons. Clin Chem 1986; 32:175–177.

Moss DW: Physicochemical and pathophysiological factors in the release of membrane-bound alkaline phosphatase from cells. Clin Chim Acta 1997; 257:133–140.

Moss DW, Raymond FD, Wile DB: Clinical and biological aspects of acid phosphatase. Crit Rev Clin Lab Sci 1995; 32:431–467.

Mukherjea M, Mukherjee P, Biswas R, et al: Effect of medroxyprogesterone acetate contraception on human serum enzymes. Int J Fertil 1981; 26:35–39.

Muller F: Prenatal biochemical screening for neural tube defects. Childs Nerv Syst 2003; 19:433–435.

Muthuswamy PP, Lopez-Majano V, Ranginwala M, et al: Serum angiotensin-converting enzyme (SACE) activity as an indicator of total body granuloma load and prognosis in sarcoidosis. Sarcoidosis 1987; 4:142–148.

Narayan P, Tewari A, Jacob G, et al: Differential suppression of serum prostatic acid phosphatase and prostate-specific antigen by 5-alpha-reductase inhibitor. Br J Urol 1995; 75:642–646.

Nijhawan R, Wierzbicki AS, Tozer R, et al: Antiepileptic drugs, hepatic enzyme induction and raised serum alkaline phosphatase isoenzymes. Int J Clin Pharmacol Res 1990; 10:319–323.

Ninomiya Y, Kioi S, Arakawa M: Serum angiotensin converting enzyme activity in ex-smokers. Clin Chim Acta 1987; 164:223–226.

Oksanen V, Fyhrquist F, Somer H, et al: Angiotensin converting enzyme in cerebrospinal fluid: A new assay. Neurology 1985; 35:1220–1223.

Ouellette DR, Kelly JW, Anders GT: Serum angiotensin-converting enzyme level is elevated in patients with human immunodeficiency virus infection. Arch Intern Med 1992; 152:321–324.

Pandit MK, Joshi BH, Patel PS, et al: Efficacy of serum lactate dehydrogenase and its isozymes in monitoring the therapy in patients with acute leukemia. Indian J Pathol Microbiol 1990; 33:41–47.

Panteghini M, Pagani F: Biological variation in bone-derived biochemical markers in serum. Scand J Clin Lab Invest 1995; 55:609–616.

Panteghini M, Pagani F, Bonora R: Pre-analytical and biological variability of prostatic acid phosphatase and prostate-specific antigen in serum from patients with prostatic pathology. Eur J Clin Chem Clin Biochem 1992; 30:135–139.

Pelonero AL, Levenson JL, Panduranji AK: Neuroleptic malignant syndrome: A review. Psychiatr Serv 1998; 49:1163–1172.

Power WJ, Neves RA, Rodriguez A, et al: The value of combined serum angiotensin-converting enzyme and gallium scan in diagnosing ocular sarcoidosis. Ophthalmology 1995; 102:2007–2011.

Price A, Attwood SE, Grant JB, et al: Measurement of prostate-specific antigen and prostatic acid phosphatase concentrations in serum before and 1–42 days after transurethral resection of the prostate and orchidectomy. Clin Chem 1991; 37:859–863.

Proudler AJ, Ahmed AI, Crook D, et al: Hormone replacement therapy and serum angiotensin-converting-enzyme activity in postmenopausal women. Lancet 1995; 346:89–90.

Quist J, Hill AR: Serum lactate dehydrogenase (LDH) in *Pneumocystis carinii* pneumonia, tuberculosis, and bacterial pneumonia. Chest 1995; 108:415–418.

Reiners C, Gramer-Kurz E, Pickert E, et al: Changes of serum angiotensin-I-converting enzyme in patients with thyroid disorders. Clin Physiol Biochem 1988; 6:44–49.

Reynoso G, Elias EG, Mittelman A: The contribution of the intestinal mucosa to the total serum alkaline phosphatase activity. Am J Clin Pathol 1971; 56:707–712.

Ricci LR, Hoffman SA: Prostatic acid phosphatase and sperm in the post-coital vagina. Ann Emerg Med 1982; 11:530–534.

Ricerca BM, Storti S, Campisi S, et al: Serum lactate dehydrogenase isoenzyme pattern in non-Hodgkin's lymphomas. Int J Biol Markers 1988; 3:237–242.

Romer FK, Emmertsen K: Serum angiotensin-converting enzyme in malignant lymphomas, leukaemia and multiple myeloma. Br J Cancer 1980; 42:314–318.

Rotenberg Z, Weinberger I, Davidson E, et al: Significance of isolated increases in total lactate dehydrogenase and its isoenzymes in serum of patients with bacterial pneumonia. Clin Chem 1988; 34:1503–1505.

Sakata T, Takenaga N, Endoh T, et al: Diagnostic significance of serum angiotensin-converting enzyme activity in biochemical tests with special reference of chronic liver diseases. Jpn J Med 1991; 30:402–407.

Salo JO, Rannikko S, Haapiainen R: Serum acid phosphatase in patients with localised prostatic cancer, benign prostatic hyperplasia or normal prostates. Br J Urol 1990; 66:188–192.

Salvaggio A, Periti M, Miano L, et al: Body mass index and liver enzyme activity in serum. Clin Chem 1991; 37:720–723.

Sapey T, Mendler M-H, Guyader D: Respective value of alkaline phosphatase, gamma-glutamyl transpeptidase and 5′ nucleotidase serum activity in the diagnosis of cholestasis: a prospective study of 80 patients. J Clin Gastroenterol 2000; 30:259–263.

Sarris AH, Majlis A, Dimopoulos MA, et al: Rising serum lactate dehydrogenase often caused by granulocyte- or granulocyte-macrophage colony stimulating factor and not tumor progression in patients with lymphoma or myeloma. Leuk Lymphoma 1995; 17:473–477.

Schernthaner G, Schwarzer C, Kuzmits R, et al: Increased angiotensin-converting enzyme activities in diabetes mellitus: Analysis of diabetes type, state of metabolic control and occurrence of diabetic vascular disease. J Clin Pathol 1984; 37:307–312.

Schiele F, Artur Y, Floc'h AY, et al: Total, tartrate-resistant, and tartrate-inhibited acid phosphatases in serum: Biological variations and reference limits. Clin Chem 1988; 34:685–690.

Schiele F, Vincent-Viry M, Fournier B, et al: Biological effects of eleven combined oral contraceptives on serum triglycerides, gamma-glutamyl-transferase, alkaline phosphatase, bilirubin and other biochemical variables. Clin Chem Lab Med 1998; 36:871–878.

Schweisfurth H, Schioberg-Schiegnitz S, Kuhn W, et al: Angiotensin I converting enzyme in cerebrospinal fluid of patients with neurological diseases. Klin Wochenschr 1987; 65:955–958.

Schweisfurth H, Schmidt M, Brugger E, et al: Alterations of serum carboxypeptidases N and angiotensin-I-converting enzyme in malignant diseases. Clin Biochem 1985; 18:242–246.

Simpson JA, Labugger R, Hesketh GG, et al: Differential detection of skeletal troponin I isoforms in serum of a patient with rhabdomyolysis: markers of muscle injury? Clin Chem 2002; 48:1112–1114.

Singer F, Talavera W, Zumoff B: Elevated levels of angiotensin-converting enzyme in *Pneumocystis carinii* pneumonia. Chest 1989; 95:803–806.

Smith RL, Ripps CS, Lewis ML: Elevated lactate dehydrogenase values in patients with *Pneumocystis carinii* pneumonia. Chest 1988; 93:987–992.

Steinherz PG, Steinherz LJ, Nisselbaum JS, et al: Transient, marked, unexplained elevation of serum alkaline phosphatase. JAMA 1984; 252:3289–3292.

Studdy P, Bird R, James DG: Serum angiotensin-converting enzyme (SACE) in sarcoidosis and other granulomatous disorders. Lancet 1978; 2:1331–1334.

Sunderman FW Jr: The clinical biochemistry of 5′-nucleotidase. Ann Clin Lab Sci 1990; 20:123–139.

Tanada S, Higuchi T, Nakamura T, et al: Evaluation of exercise intensity indicated by serum lactate dehydrogenase activity in healthy adults. Acta Biol Hung 1993; 44:153–160.

Theodorsen L: Collection and storage of samples for the determination of prostatic acid phosphatase in serum. Scand J Clin Lab Invest Suppl 1985; 179:57–65.

Thompson PJ, Kemp MW, McAllister WA, et al: Angiotensin-converting enzyme. Investigation of diurnal variation, the effect of a large dose of prednisolone, and prednisolone pharmacokinetics in patients with sarcoidosis. Am Rev Respir Dis 1986; 134:1075–1077.

Trundle D, Marcial G: Detection of cholinesterase inhibition. The significance of cholinesterase measurements. Ann Clin Lab Sci 1988; 18:345–352.

Ucar G, Yildirim Z, Ataol E, et al: Serum angiotensin converting enzyme activity in pulmonary diseases: Correlation with lung function parameters. Life Sci 1997; 61:1075–1082.

Valenzuela GJ, Munson LA, Tarbaux NM, et al: Time-dependent changes in bone, placental, intestinal, and hepatic alkaline phosphatase activities in serum during human pregnancy. Clin Chem 1987; 33:1801–1806.

Vogelzang NJ, Lange PH, Goldberg E: Absence of sperm-specific lactate dehydrogenase-x in patients with testis cancer. Oncodev Biol Med 1982; 3:269–272.

von Eyben FE: A systematic review of lactate dehydrogenase isoenzyme 1 and germ cell tumors. Clin Biochem 2001; 34:441–454.
Review of lactate dehydrogenase isoenzyme 1 as a possible serum marker in patients with germ cell tumors.

von Eyben FE, Liu FJ, Amato RJ, Fritsche HA: Lactate dehydrogenase isoenzyme 1 is the most important LD isoenzyme in patients with testicular germ cell tumor. Acta Oncol 2000; 39:509–517.

Wadstrom J, Wenk M, Huber P: Serum half life of prostatic acid phosphatase. Urol Res 1985; 13:131–132.

Ward MM: Factors predictive of acute renal failure in rhabdomyolysis. Arch Intern Med 1988; 148:1553–1557.

Whyte MP, Walkenhorst DA, Fedde KN, et al: Hypophosphatasia: Levels of bone alkaline phosphatase immunoreactivity in serum reflect disease severity. J Clin Endocrinol Metab 1996; 81:2142–2148.

Wiesen AR, Byrd JC, Hospenthal DR, et al: Transient abnormalities in serum bilirubin and lactate dehydrogenase levels following red blood cell transfusions in adults. Am J Med 1998; 104:144–147.

Wolf PL: Clinical significance of serum high-molecular-mass alkaline phosphatase, alkaline phosphatase–lipoprotein-X complex, and intestinal variant alkaline phosphatase. J Clin Lab Anal 1994; 8:172–176.

CHAPTER 21

Evaluation of Liver Function

Matthew R. Pincus MD PhD, Philip Tierno PhD, D. Robert Dufour MD

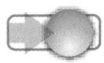

KEY POINTS

• The liver is composed of three systems: the hepatocyte, concerned with metabolic reactions and macromolecular, especially protein, synthesis and degradation; the biliary system, involved with the metabolism of bilirubin and bile salts; and the reticuloendothelial system, concerned with the immune system and the production of heme and globin metabolites (e.g., bilirubin).

• The function of each of these systems can be measured conveniently and virtually noninvasively by determining the serum levels of specific analytes, in the so-called liver function test profile.

• One of the most common causes of acute liver injury is viral hepatitis, mainly hepatitis A, B and C, all of which induce acute elevations of serum alanine and aspartate aminotransferases (AST and ALT, respectively).

• Diagnosis of viral hepatitis can be made by screening for viral antigens, especially in hepatitis B, and for IgM and IgG directed against specific viral antigens. Confirmation of the diagnosis of a particular form of viral hepatitis is carried out using suitable molecular diagnostic techniques such as real-time PCR (RT-PCR) using primers encoding specific viral gene sequences.

• The diagnosis of specific liver diseases including hepatitis, cirrhosis, acute biliary obstruction, space-occupying lesions, autoimmune diseases and fulminant hepatic failure, can be made from specific patterns of serum liver function tests and from the presence of specific antibodies in serum.

Normal Liver Function

The liver is the largest and most complex organ of the gastrointestinal tract. Overall, it comprises three systems: first, the *biochemical hepatocytic system*, which is responsible for the vast majority of all metabolic activities in the body, including protein synthesis, aerobic and anaerobic metabolism of glucose and other sugars, glycogen synthesis and breakdown, amino acid and nucleic acid metabolism, amino acid and dicarboxylic acid inter-conversions via transaminases (aminotransferases), lipoprotein synthesis and metabolism, xenobiotic metabolism, e.g., drug metabolism, usually involving the cytochrome P450 oxidation system, storage of iron and vitamins such as A, D, and B_{12}, and synthesis of hormones such as angiotensinogen, insulin-like growth factor I and triiodothyronine. It is also the site of clearance of many other hormones such as insulin, parathyroid hormone (PTH), estrogens and cortisol. Uniquely, the liver is the site for metabolism of ammonia to urea.

It should also be noted that all of the albumin in the body is synthesized in the liver as are all of the coagulation factor proteins with the exception of von Willebrand factor synthesized in endothelial cells and megakaryocytes.

Patients with liver disease may have signs or symptoms related to disturbance of any of the above functions.

The second major hepatic system is the *hepatobiliary system* concerned with the metabolism of bilirubin, a process that involves transport of bilirubin into the hepatocyte, its conjugation to glucuronic acid and its secretion into bile canaliculi, and the enterohepatic system. Lastly, there is the *reticuloendothelial system*, i.e., *Kupffer cells*. These are a form of macrophage involved (a) with the immune system, including being a major site of defense against intestinal bacteria and the primary location for removal of antigen–antibody complexes from the circulation, and (b) with the breakdown of hemoglobin from dead erythrocytes, giving rise to bilirubin, which, together with bilirubin from the spleen, enters the hepatocyte.

Because, in liver disease, clinical symptoms often lag behind the progression of disease, it is important to detect the presence and even the onset of these conditions. Fortunately, evaluation of liver function can often be achieved by determination of serum analytes in a test profile known as 'liver function tests,' many of whose components are not unique to liver but, when evaluated together, allow for accurate diagnosis. An outline of liver function tests and their interpretation has been presented in Chapter 8.

This chapter reviews the most common laboratory tests for evaluation of liver function and injury, methods used for their measurement, testing for causes of liver injury, and patterns of laboratory abnormalities seen in specific liver diseases.

Metabolic Functions

Bilirubin

Normal Bilirubin Metabolism

Bilirubin is the major metabolite of heme, the iron-binding tetrapyrole ring, found in hemoglobin, myoglobin, and cytochromes. Approximately 250–350 mg of bilirubin is produced daily in healthy adults, about 85% derived from turnover of senescent red blood cells (Chowdhury, 1988; Berk, 1994a; Berlin, 1981). In macrophages mainly in the spleen, methemoglobin from red cells is split to give free globin chains and heme. The porphyrin ring of heme is oxidized by microsomal heme oxygenase, producing the straight-chain compound biliverdin, releasing iron. In this ring-opening reaction, one mole of CO (carbon monoxide) is released, which is transported ultimately as carboxyhemoglobin, whose serum levels can be useful in the diagnosis of hemolytic anemia, as discussed in Chapter 8. Biliverdin is then reduced to bilirubin (Fig. 21–1) by the NADPH-dependent enzyme, biliverdin reductase. Bilirubin is then transported mainly in the portal system, bound mainly to albumin, to the liver where it enters the hepatocyte on its membrane surface in contact with the sinusoids, as shown in Figure 21–2.

As free bilirubin enters hepatocytes, additional bilirubin dissociates from albumin. This process is highly efficient; clearance of unconjugated

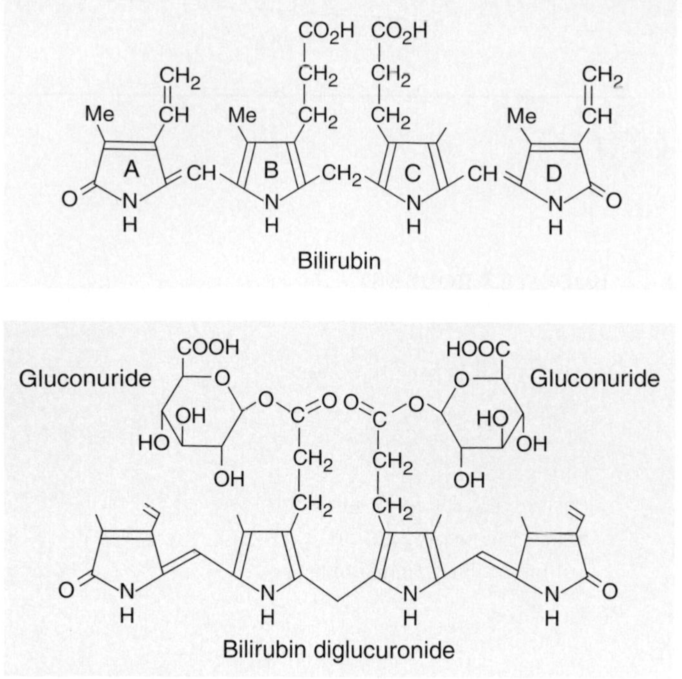

Figure 21–1 Structures of critical molecules in the metabolism of bilirubin to its diglucuronide. Bilirubin is transported into the hepatocyte, where it is converted into the diglucuronide form and secreted into canaliculi (Crawford, 1988b).

small fraction of free bilirubin. Light can cause photoisomerization of bilirubin, from a *trans*-form to a more compact *cis*-form, making it much more water soluble allowing it to be excreted in urine (Onishi, 1986); this forms the basis for phototherapy in treatment of neonatal (unconjugated) hyperbilirubinemia. The pathway for clearance of bilirubin by the liver is illustrated in Figure 21–2. Note that unconjugated bilirubin enters the hepatocyte at the membrane surface adjacent to the sinusoids, opposite the face which is in contact with bile canaliculi.

There are two mechanisms by which bilirubin enters hepatocytes: one is by passive diffusion and the other by receptor-mediated endocytosis. As summarized in Figure 21–2, once in the hepatocyte, bilirubin is 'handed-off' from one protein complex to another in a chain. First, it complexes with the so-called Y and Z proteins and then binds sequentially to a protein complex called ligandin. From this complex, it is transported to the smooth endoplasmic reticulum (SER). In the SER, bilirubin becomes the substrate of the enzyme, glucuronyl transferase, which catalyzes the esterification of the propionic acid side chains of bilirubin with glucuronic acid (present as uridine diphosphoglucuronic acid) to form mainly the diglucuronide conjugate, shown in Figure 21–1 (Chowdhury, 1988). Some monoglucuronide and a small amount of triglucuronide also form. The ratio of monoconjugated to diconjugated pigment in bile is 1:4, whereas the ratio is nearly 1:1 in plasma, suggesting that monoconjugates reflux into plasma more readily.

As schematized in Figure 21–2, the conjugated bilirubin is then transported to the canalicular face of the hepatocyte at which it is directly secreted, by an energy-dependent mechanism, into the canaliculi; only conjugated bilirubin can be directly excreted into the canaliculi while unconjugated bilirubin cannot traverse this membrane.

Once bilirubin is excreted into the canaliculi and ultimately into the intestinal tract, it is further metabolized by intestinal bacteria which effect its deconjugation and oxidation or reduction with the formation of compounds collectively called urobilinogen and urobilin, which can then be reabsorbed from the gut. The majority of urobilinogen absorbed is re-excreted by the liver. A minor fraction may be excreted in the urine. Larger quantities are found in the urine in conditions leading to hyperbilirubinemia or in conditions in which the liver cannot readily secrete urobilinogen absorbed from the gut. Ultimately, intestinal urobilinogen is converted to stool pigments such as stercobilin; their absence leads to clay-colored stools, often an early sign of impaired bilirubin metabolism.

bilirubin at normal values is about 5 mg/kg/day or, for a 75-kg individual, about 400 mg/day (Berk, 1994b). The half-life of unconjugated bilirubin is short; 60% of labeled bilirubin appears within hepatocytes within 5 minutes of injection (Bloomer, 1973). Clearance rate increases with an increasing concentration of unconjugated bilirubin up to at least 4 mg/dL (Berk, 1994b).

In its most common isomeric (*trans-*) form, bilirubin is highly insoluble in water, and most of it is transported bound to albumin, with only a

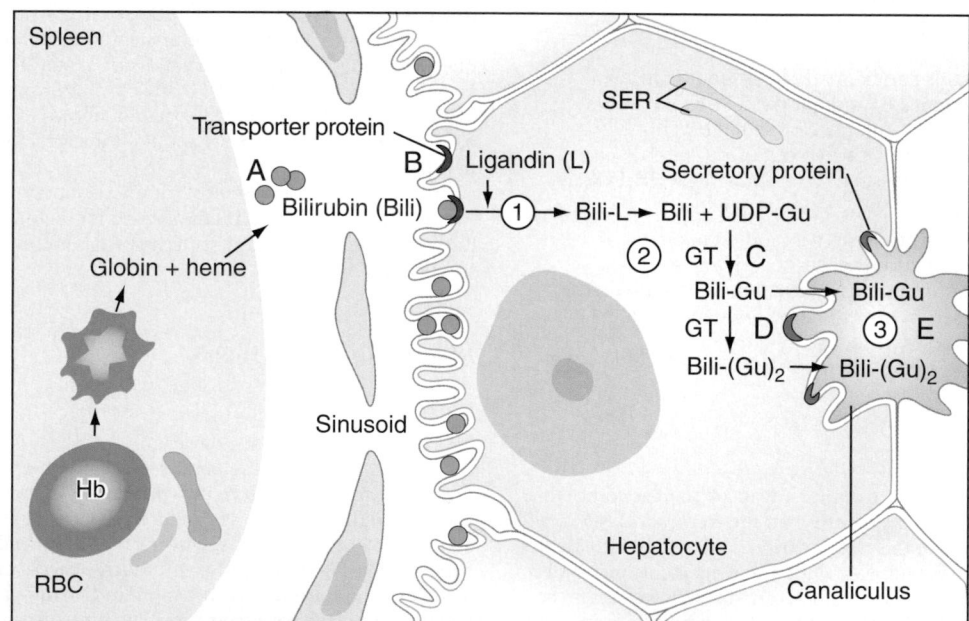

Figure 21–2 Schematic summary of the pathway of bilirubin (labeled as Bili and also shown in brown circles) transport and metabolism. Bilirubin (Bili) is produced from metabolism of heme, primarily in the spleen, and is transported to the liver bound to albumin. It enters the hepatocyte by binding to a transporter protein (red crescents) and crosses the cell membrane (circled 1 in the figure) thus entering the cell. It binds to Y and Z proteins (not shown) and then to ligandin for transport to the smooth endoplasmic reticulum (SER). In the SER, bilirubin is conjugated to glucuronic acid by UDP-glucuronyl transferase 1 (circled 2 in the figure), producing mono- and diglucuronides of bilirubin – Bili-Gu and Bili-(Gu)$_2$. Conjugated bilirubin is then secreted into the canaliculi (circled 3 in the figure) by the ATP-binding cassette transporter protein MRP2/cMOAT/ABCC2, shown as blue crescents in the figure. In overproduction disease (**A**), such as in hemolytic anemia, unconjugated bilirubin is produced at rates that exceed the ability of the liver to clear it, leading to a usually transient increase in unconjugated bilirubin in serum. In both Gilbert's and the Crigler–Najjar syndromes, mutations in the gene encoding UDP glucuronyl transferase (UDPGT1A1), shown at C in the figure, result in build-up of unconjugated bilirubin in hepatocytes and ultimately in serum. In Gilbert's syndrome, there may also be a defect in the bilirubin transporter protein shown at B in the figure. Mutations in the MRP2/cMOAT/ABCC2 gene result in defective secretory proteins resulting in the build-up of conjugated bilirubin in hepatocytes and, ultimately, in serum, resulting in the Dubin–Johnson syndrome (**D**), an autosomal recessive disease. Conjugated hyperbilirubinemia is also found in the Rotor syndrome, possibly virus-induced. In adults, blockade of any of the major bile ducts, especially the common bile duct, by stones or space-occupying lesions such as tumors (**E**) are the most common causes of conjugated hyperbilirubinemia.

When conjugated bilirubin is present in serum, it can become covalently bound to albumin, producing biliprotein or delta-bilirubin (Lauff, 1982; McDonagh, 1984). While conjugated bilirubin has a half-life of less than 24 hours, delta-bilirubin has a half-life similar to that for albumin at 17 days (Fevery, 1986), causing prolonged jaundice during recovery from hepatocellular injury (Van Hootegem, 1985) or biliary obstruction (Kozaki, 1998). Conjugated bilirubin, being water soluble, can be filtered by the glomerulus and appear in urine, where it may be detected with dipstick examination; urobilinogen measurement adds little to standard tests of liver function or injury, however (Binder, 1989). Urinary bilirubin is elevated in most patients with increased serum conjugated bilirubin (Binder, 1989).

Derangements of Bilirubin Metabolism. As shown in Figure 21–2, in each step in the processing of bilirubin, there is a possible lesion leading to elevated serum levels of unconjugated or conjugated bilirubin. Each of these is discussed in turn.

Causes of Elevated Serum Levels of Unconjugated Bilirubin

Hemolysis. As discussed in Chapter 8, in hemolytic anemias, unconjugated bilirubin rises due to abnormally high levels of hemoglobin released from erythrocytes. If the rate of bilirubin formation exceeds the rate of the liver clearance, i.e., a state of *overproduction of bilirubin*, there will be a rise in the bilirubin level in serum. Virtually all of this bilirubin will be unconjugated bilirubin. This is particularly likely to occur in neonates, whose glucuronyl transferase activity is low. Thus, one manner of confirming a diagnosis of hemolytic anemia is the finding, in adults, of elevated indirect bilirubin levels in serum. Usually, these levels are not dramatically elevated and are generally in the 1.5–3.0 mg/dL range.

Gilbert's Syndrome and the Crigler–Najjar Syndrome are Caused by Gene Mutations and Deletions. In Gilbert's syndrome, characterized by a mild unconjugated hyperbilirubinemia, the most common genetic lesion appears to be the insertion of two bases into the promoter region of the UGT1A1 gene resulting in lower transcriptional rates (Maruo, 2004; Kraemer, 2002) and an overall lower enzymatic activity (reduced to about 30% of normal). In the more serious Crigler–Najjar syndrome, frequently characterized by high serum levels of unconjugated bilirubin, multiple mutations are found to occur in this gene including shifts in the reading frames, stop codons and critical amino acid substitutions, all of which give rise to a spectrum of dysfunctional proteins from mildly dysfunctional to completely nonfunctional proteins (Kraemer 2002).

In *Gilbert's syndrome*, which occurs in a significant fraction (3–5%) of the population, the genetic defect may be necessary but not sufficient since, in an earlier study (Persico, 1999), a significant percentage of males with this defect were found to have hyperbilirubinemia while no females with this enzyme deficit were found to have elevated serum bilirubin levels (Bosma, 1995). In some patients with Gilbert's syndrome, the rate of organic anion uptake has been found to correlate negatively with serum bilirubin (Persico, 1999), suggesting that an additional defect may be present to cause hyperbilirubinemia that may be related to a transport deficit in the sinusoidal membrane of the hepatocyte. In this condition, total bilirubin, virtually all of which is unconjugated, is typically elevated to 2–3 mg/dL; levels can increase further with fasting but seldom exceed 5 mg/dL. Since passive diffusion of bilirubin into hepatocytes occurs, this condition is rarely serious and may result in mild elevations of bilirubin such as those seen in hemolytic anemia as described above.

Gilbert's syndrome has perhaps been overdiagnosed, since it is most frequently diagnosed in young adults ranging in age from 20–30 years. However, normal bilirubin ranges are age-dependent and actually reach their highest levels in adolescents and young adults (Rosenthal, 1984) as discussed further below.

In the more serious or type I forms of the *Crigler–Najjar syndrome*, e.g., homozygously nonfunctioning proteins, the unconjugated hyperbilirubinemia becomes marked, almost always exceeding 5 mg/dL causing jaundice, and sometimes exceeding 20 mg/dL. Affected infants develop severe unconjugated hyperbilirubinemia, which typically leads to kernicterus, deposition of bilirubin in the brain, particularly affecting the basal ganglia, mainly the lenticular nucleus, causing severe motor dysfunction and retardation. In the less severe type II form, enzyme activity is approximately 10% of normal, and survival to adulthood is possible (Berk, 1994c). The danger of kernicterus is a certainty at levels exceeding 20 mg/dL. It is vital to treat these infants with phototherapy, as discussed above, to cause excretion of the unconjugated bilirubin.

Causes of Elevated Serum Levels of Conjugated Bilirubin

Excretion Deficits: Dubin–Johnson Syndrome. In another inborn error of metabolism, called the Dubin–Johnson syndrome, there is a blockade of the excretion of bilirubin into the canaliculi, owing to defects in the ATP-binding cassette (ABC) canalicular multispecific organic anion transporter, MRP2/cMOAT/ABCC2 (Paulusma, 1997; Tsujii, 1999; Gottesman, 2001). This protein is a member of a family of approximately 100 different transporter proteins that share homology within the ATP-binding cassette (ABC) region and contain transmembrane domains involved in recognition of substrates, which are transported across, into, and out of cell membranes and include proteins involved in multiple drug resistance (MDR) to chemotherapeutic agents in cancer treatment. Some protein members utilize ABCs to regulate ion channels. Several genetic diseases result from transporter mutations including the Dubin–Johnson syndrome, cystic fibrosis, age-related macular degeneration, Tangier disease, and progressive familial intrahepatic cholestasis (Gottesman, 2001).

Dubin–Johnson syndrome is associated with increased plasma conjugated bilirubin, typically with mild jaundice (total bilirubin 2–5 mg/dL), and intense dark pigmentation of the liver due to accumulation of lipofuscin pigment. Thus conjugated bilirubin accumulates within the hepatocyte and eventually back-diffuses into the circulation where it is detected in serum. This inborn error can sometimes be confused with the Rotor syndrome, possibly of viral origin, where there is also a block in the excretion of conjugated bilirubin but without liver pigmentation (Berk, 1994d). In these cases, liver biopsy often will reveal cytosolic inclusion bodies within hepatocytes.

Biliary Obstruction. In adults, cholelithiasis is the most common cause of hyperbilirubinemia. This condition results from the presence of bile stones (that are composed either of bilirubin or cholesterol) most commonly in the common bile duct (choledocholithiasis). Most frequently, patients presenting with this condition are parous white females in early middle age (giving rise to the semi-mnemonic, 'fair, fecund, fortyish female'). Biliary obstruction due to cholelithiasis results in the elevation of total bilirubin, with > 90% being direct bilirubin. In over 90% of such patients, there is a concomitant rise in alkaline phosphatase. The levels of this enzyme are variable but are frequently above 300 IU/L.

Inflammatory conditions of the biliary tract, such as ascending cholangitis, also give rise to elevated serum levels of direct bilirubin and alkaline phosphatase, as discussed later in this chapter. The rise in direct bilirubin often exceeds 5 mg/dL. In Gram-negative sepsis, there can be what appears to be a mild inflammation of the biliary tract, resulting in mild elevations of direct bilirubin to levels of 2–3 mg/dL. There is a concomitant elevation of alkaline phosphatase to levels of 200–300 IU/L.

In hepatitis, in which there is toxic destruction of hepatocytes due to viral, chemical or traumatic causes, focal necrosis and/or cellular injury result both in blocking conjugation of bilirubin and in excretion of conjugated bilirubin. Thus there is an elevation of *both* direct and indirect bilirubin. Serum levels of bilirubin are variable, depending on the severity of infection and the extent of disease. In viral hepatitis, such as hepatitis B, as discussed subsequently, serum bilirubin levels often reach levels of 5–10 mg/dL or greater.

Aside from liver disease, elevations of conjugated bilirubin may occur with a few other disorders. Septicemia, total parenteral nutrition, and certain drugs such as androgens commonly cause increased conjugated bilirubin, but the mechanism is not understood (Zimmerman, 1979). Fasting causes increases in unconjugated bilirubin in normal individuals, but to a lesser degree than seen in Gilbert's syndrome.

Laboratory Tests for Bilirubin

Bilirubin is typically measured using diazotized sulfanilic acid which forms a conjugated azo compound with the porphyrin rings of bilirubin resulting in reaction products that absorb strongly at 540 nm. Because unconjugated bilirubin reacts slowly, accelerants such as caffeine or methanol are used to measure total bilirubin. Deletion of these accelerants allows determination of direct-reacting, or direct, bilirubin.

Until the early 1980s, it was accepted that direct bilirubin was equal to conjugated bilirubin. The introduction of dry slide technology, using differential spectrophotometry to measure conjugated and unconjugated bilirubin separately, led to the observation that the sum of these two entities did not equal total bilirubin and to the characterization of delta-bilirubin. Approximately 70–80% of conjugated bilirubin and delta-bilirubin, and a small percentage of unconjugated bilirubin, are measured in the direct bilirubin assay (Lo, 1983; Doumas, 1991). While there are good data supporting measurement of conjugated bilirubin instead of estimating it from direct bilirubin (Arvan, 1985; Doumas, 1987), the direct bilirubin assay is still widely used. The accuracy of direct bilirubin assays is dependent on sample handling and reagent composition. Prolonged exposure to light causes photoisomerization, increasing direct-reacting bilirubin (Ihara, 1997). Use of wetting agents or incorrect pH buffers increase the amount of unconjugated bilirubin measured as direct bilirubin (Doumas, 1991). Typically, direct bilirubin should be 0–0.1 mg/dL in normal individuals, with rare values of 0.2 mg/dL in the absence of liver or biliary tract disease.

Reference values for total bilirubin are both age and gender dependent. Bilirubin levels typically reach peak values around age 14–18, falling to stable adult levels by age 25 (Rosenthal, 1983; Notter, 1985; Zucker, 2004). Values are higher in males than in females at all ages (Rosenthal, 1983; Notter, 1985; Carmel, 1985; Dufour, 1998a; Zucker, 2004). Strenuous exercise causes significant increase in bilirubin values compared to those seen in sedentary individuals or those with chronic exercise (Dufour, 1998b). African Americans have bilirubin levels significantly lower than those of other ethnic groups.

Other Metabolic Tests

Ammonia Is Metabolized Exclusively in the Liver. Ammonia is derived mainly from amino acid and nucleic acid metabolism. Some ammonia is also produced from metabolic reactions such as the action of the enzyme glutaminase on glutamine, resulting in the production of glutamic acid and ammonia. As it happens, ammonia can be metabolized only in the liver because the liver uniquely contains the critical enzymes for the Krebs–Henseleit or urea cycle, in which ammonia, a toxic substance, is ultimately converted into urea, a nontoxic compound that is readily excreted. In this cycle, ammonia, with the enzyme carbamoyl phosphate synthetase, is condensed with CO_2 and ATP to form carbamoyl phosphate that then, in the rate-determining step, carboxamidates the delta-amino group of ornithine to form citrulline using the enzyme, ornithine carbamoyltransferase (OCT), an enzyme that is unique to the liver. Congenital deficiency of this or other urea cycle enzymes leads to increased levels of ammonia in serum and in cerebrospinal fluid (Batshaw, 1994).

A unique feature of liver tissue is its ability to regenerate. To abolish liver tissue function, over 80% of the liver must first be destroyed. If most of the liver is destroyed as a result of such conditions as cirrhosis (Stahl, 1963), or, less commonly, acute fulminant hepatic failure, including Reye's syndrome (Heubi, 1984; Sunheimer, 1994), the urea cycle enzymes are no longer present, resulting in the toxic build-up of ammonia and some of the amino acid intermediates in the urea cycle, like arginine, that has known neurotoxic effects. The result is the increase of ammonia and these amino acid intermediates in the circulation and in the central nervous system, giving rise to hepatic encephalopathy. In addition, in most cirrhotics, intrahepatic portal-systemic shunting occurs, thereby causing ammonia to bypass the liver and resulting in elevated serum ammonia concentrations. Elevated serum levels of ammonia therefore often indicate some form of liver failure, although other conditions can also induce increases in serum ammonia levels.

In patients with cirrhosis or fulminant hepatic failure, there is some dispute as to whether ammonia itself is the cause of the observed metabolic encephalopathy; possibly other toxins that accumulate as a result of absent hepatic detoxification are the cause. One of the arguments often used is that there is no clear correlation between the severity of the encephalopathy and the serum ammonia concentrations (Lewis, 2003). Countering this argument is the finding that, although venous ammonia levels do not correlate with the degree of encephalopathy (Stahl, 1963), *arterial* levels of ammonia do generally correlate with degree of encephalopathy. Furthermore, in patients with cirrhosis or fulminant hepatic failure, lowering the serum ammonia invariably diminishes the severity of the encephalopathy (Pincus, 1991). An important mechanism by which ammonia can cause toxicity to the central nervous system is its ability to lower the concentration of gamma-aminobutyric acid (GABA), a critically important neurotransmitter in the central nervous system, by reacting with glutamic acid to form glutamine via reversal of the glutaminase-catalyzed reaction (Butterworth, 1987). This depletes glutamic acid in the CNS. However, GABA is formed directly from the decarboxylation of glutamic acid so that GABA levels consequently decrease, with potentially serious effects on neurotransmission. Since ammonia causes the accumulation of glutamine in the central nervous system, there is the suggestion that, at least in valproic acid-induced hyperammonemia, cerebrospinal fluid levels of glutamine can be used in the diagnosis and management of hepatic encephalopathy.

Most commonly, elevated serum ammonia concentrations in hepatic encephalopathy are reduced with the agent, lactulose, which is metabolized by specific gut bacteria to lactic acid. The acid so produced in the intestinal lumen traps ammonia as ammonium ion which can no longer diffuse across the intestinal membrane and is thus excreted. Ammonia-producing bacteria in the intestine are removed by treatment with antibiotics such as neomycin.

Assays for Ammonia. Ammonia is typically measured by enzymatic assays using glutamate dehydrogenase, which catalyzes the reaction of alpha-ketoglutarate and ammonia to form glutamate, with oxidation of NADPH to NADP as the indicator (decrease in absorbance at 340 nm). Ammonia is also measured in a dry slide method using alkaline pH buffers to convert all ammonium ions to ammonia gas, with bromphenol blue as the indicator (Huizenga, 1994). Because ammonia is a product of cellular metabolism, methods used in specimen collection and trans-portation are critical in preventing artifactually increased levels. Arterial blood is the preferred specimen for measurement of ammonia. Although venous blood is not recommended, if used, tourniquets should be used minimally, and fist clenching and relaxing avoided during collection. Specimens should be kept in ice water until separation of cells from plasma (Howanitz, 1984; da Fonseca-Wollheim, 1990).

Lipids

Cholesterol and Other Lipids (Ch. 17). Since the liver is vital in lipoprotein synthesis and interconversions, hepatic disorders often cause derangements in lipoprotein metabolism. Though none of these abnormalities is used to diagnose liver pathology, it is important to recognize that they may result from liver disease. In *severe liver injury* including *cirrhosis*, these abnormalities include a decrease in the HDL, particularly the HDL_3 (but often not the HDL_2), fraction and in other altered lipoprotein distributions due, in part, to deficiencies of lecithin : cholesterol acyltransferase (LCAT) (the enzyme that esterifies cholesterol), and lipoprotein lipases, resulting in hypertriglyceridemia (triglyceride levels ranging from 250–500 mg/dL). In addition, the decreased synthesis of LCAT and lipoprotein lipases causes increases, in blood and in the HDL fraction, of unesterified cholesterol, and also in increased levels of phospholipids, including lecithins, in blood and in the VLDL fraction, and increased serum triglycerides. Overall, the resulting lipoprotein pattern is that of the so-called abnormally migrating beta-lipoprotein, typical of Type III hyperlipoproteinemia (Ch. 17). However, in cirrhotics with poor nutrition, despite the critical enzyme deficiencies, low levels of cholesterol (< 100 mg/dL) may be found.

In contrast, in *alcohol-induced liver injury*, alcohol induces increased expression of apoA-I protein. Thus, HDL, especially HDL_3, may be elevated if alcohol ingestion continues.

Since, in cirrhosis, apoA-I protein decreases, serum levels of this protein have been used to diagnose this disease using the so-called PGA index (Teare, 1993), a combination of apoA-I protein with gamma-glutamyl transferase activity, discussed below, which increases, and the prothrombin time, which also increases (the so-called PGA index). This index differs for alcoholic hepatitis, enabling the distinction to be made between these two conditions without the necessity of liver biopsy.

In *cholestasis*, regurgitation of biliary contents into the bloodstream results in the build-up of lipoprotein X (LpX), discussed in Chapter 17, and elevations of biliary lipids. Since LpX carries high levels of unesterified cholesterol, cholesterol levels in serum can become markedly elevated (Turchin, 2005).

Bile Salts. Bile salts, which are products of cholesterol metabolism, facilitate absorption of fat from the intestine. They are stored in the gallbladder and released to the intestine after meals through gallbladder contraction mediated by cholecystokinin. They are not usually used in the diagnosis of abnormal liver function but are important in that they constitute a substantial amount of bile in bilirubin excretion and can therefore be of use in diagnosing cholestasis. Also, in severe biliary obstruction, the build-up of bile salts in serum causes symptomatic illness in the form of intractable itching, although this has been disputed (Jones, 1999). The primary bile salts, cholate and chenodeoxycholate, are produced in the liver; they are excreted into the biliary and enterohepatic systems, and, in the intestinal tract, they are metabolized by bacteria, producing secondary bile salts, i.e., lithocholate, deoxycholate, and ursodeoxycholate (Carey, 1988) by bacterial 7-alpha-dehydroxylation in the intestinal lumen. Ursodeoxycholate, an end-product of bile salt metabolism in man, is produced by isomerization of secondary bile salts and has been found to be therapeutic in cholestatic diseases (Rost, 2004). These bile salts are conjugated, in the microsomal system discussed above, to glycine and taurine and are also sulfated and glucuronidated. Conjugation of bile salts to taurine and sulfates increases with the severity of cholestasis in conditions causing obstruction to bile outflow. Recirculation of bile salts to the liver occurs by reabsorption from the terminal ileum where deoxycholate is almost completely reabsorbed, and chenodeoxycholate is about 75% reabsorbed. In cirrhosis, there is a disproportionate decrease in cholic acid and a reduced ratio of primary to secondary bile salts. With cholestasis, secondary bile salts are not formed; thus, the ratio of primary to secondary bile salts is markedly increased.

Renal clearance of bile salts is negligible in normal patients, but in cholestasis, renal excretion of bile salts, mainly in the form of sulfates and glucuronides, is enhanced. Fasting bile salts, when normal, can exclude the presence of parenchymal liver disease in patients with Gilbert's syndrome (Vierling, 1982), discussed above. It should also be recognized that defective production of bile salts, which help solubilize the contents of bile, in the liver may predispose to the formation of bilirubinate or cholesterol stones and post-hepatic biliary obstruction.

Analysis of bile salts must be on serum taken from patients who are in the fasting state or on serum taken at a specified time after meals, since food ingestion causes a significant increase in bile acid levels. Bile salts can be measured by many techniques, but chromatographic methods, particularly high-performance liquid chromatography, HPLC, discussed in Chapter 23, are most widely used and allow separation of different bile salts.

Drug Metabolism

Many xenobiotics, such as drugs, are metabolized in the liver mainly in the microsomes of hepatocytes. There are complex series of reactions, many of which are dependent on cytochrome P450, that is involved in the oxidation of these compounds. Whether or not specific exogenous compounds are converted to metabolites depends on the isoforms of cytochrome P450, such as CYP1A and CYP2B (cytochrome P450 1A and 2B, respectively). Often, the conversion of xenobiotics into metabolites using this system involves two phases: phase I reactions involve oxidations/hydroxylations and phase II reactions conjugate the metabolite (or parent compound) to polar compounds such as glucuronic acid, glycine, taurine, and sulfate. In more severe liver disease, which involves microsomal damage, this ability to metabolize xenobiotics is compromised. Thus the ability of hepatocytes to metabolize drugs can be used to measure liver damage. This is generally accomplished by administering a known dose of radiolabeled (usually ^{13}C-labeled) drug and measuring the $^{13}CO_2$ exhaled over time in a patient's breath. Two categories of breath tests have been developed based on the rate-limiting step in metabolism. The first group, which includes drugs like aminopyrine, caffeine and diazepam, all are metabolized at rates that are independent of hepatic blood flow to the liver and depend only on the enzymatic activity of different cytochromes P450 (e.g., CYP1A). The second group is composed of drugs like methacetin, phenacetin and erythromycin whose rates of metabolism depend on the rate of blood flow, i.e., their rates of metabolism are fast compared with their rates of delivery to the liver. These types of dynamic tests appear not to be so useful in initial diagnosis of hepatic disease; rather, they are more useful in estimating the extent of liver damage in known liver disease (Nista, 2004). Some interferences that complicate the interpretations of the results of these tests include dependence of the demethylation of aminopyrine (the methyl group is oxidized to CO_2) on vitamin B_{12}; in cases of vitamin B_{12} deficiency, less than normal amounts of $^{13}CO_2$ will be exhaled because of low B_{12} levels, not necessarily liver damage. Rates of caffeine metabolism generally decrease with increasing age but are increased by smoking, findings that can complicate the interpretation of test results.

Synthetic Functions

Protein Synthesis

The liver is the site of synthesis for most plasma proteins. (The major exceptions are immunoglobulins and von Willebrand's factor.) Greater than 90% of all protein and 100% of albumin synthesis occur in the liver. Thus extensive destruction of liver tissue will result in low serum levels of total protein and albumin. In cirrhosis, besides hepatocyte destruction, another cause of diminished protein production is portal hypertension, which decreases delivery of amino acids to the liver. Two vital measurements of liver function, therefore, are total protein and albumin levels in serum. However, it should always be kept in mind that there are other major causes of low serum total protein and albumin; these are renal disease, malnutrition, protein-losing enteropathies, and, less commonly, chronic inflammatory diseases. These alternative causes must always be considered when evaluating liver function status.

In liver diseases in which there is widespread injury or necrosis, such as in fulminant hepatic failure and cirrhosis, plasma levels of liver-synthesized proteins fall such that proteins with longer half-lives tend to decrease more slowly. Albumin has a half-life of about 20 days, so that decreases in its serum levels occur more slowly than those of proteins with shorter half-lives. Among the liver-produced proteins with short half-lives are factor VII (4–6 hours), transthyretin (1–2 days), and transferrin (6 days).

Determination of serum protein levels is based usually on the biuret method. This method reflects the ability of the peptide backbone C=O groups of proteins to form color complexes with copper that absorb strongly at 540 nm. Some methods utilize a dye-binding method in which the proteins form a complex with the dye Coomassie blue. Albumin forms a unique color complex with the dyes bromcresol green and bromcresol purple such that they absorb maximally at slightly different wavelengths, thus allowing direct spectrophotometric quantitation (Ihara, 1991). The reference range for total serum protein levels is generally in the 6–7.8 g/dL range. At least 60% of this should be albumin, the normal range for which is about 3.5–5 g/dL.

Serum protein electrophoresis and quantitative immunoglobulins may reveal characteristic changes in liver disease as discussed in Chapter 19.

Typically, in cirrhosis, albumin is significantly decreased, as are the alpha-1, alpha-2 and beta (principally transferrin) bands. However, there is often a polyclonal increase in immunoglobulins, producing the characteristic beta–gamma 'bridging' pattern as discussed in Chapter 19. In autoimmune hepatitis, albumin is typically decreased, accompanied by a marked polyclonal increase in IgG. Primary biliary cirrhosis is accompanied by a polyclonal increase in IgM.

Albumin

Albumin is the major protein produced by the liver; liver synthesis is increased by low plasma oncotic pressure, and is decreased by cytokines, particularly interleukin-6. While normal albumin synthesis is about 120 mg/kg/day, the rate of synthesis can approximately double with low oncotic pressure. A decrease in albumin is one of the major prognostic features in patients with cirrhosis. Albumin measurements are discussed above and more fully in Chapter 19. It is also a transport protein for many substances, both endogenous (e.g., bilirubin and thyroid hormone) and exogenous (e.g., drugs). Low serum albumin levels due to liver disease are almost always caused by massive destruction of liver tissue and are seen primarily in cirrhosis, most often secondary to alcoholism. The diminution in albumin is paralleled by a fall in total serum protein. Because albumin is the osmotically active intravascular colloid, hypoalbuminemia often results in edema. In cirrhosis, where increased resistance to blood flow in the sinusoids causes portal hypertension, the combined effect of elevated hydrostatic pressure in the portal system and the low colloid osmotic pressure results in ascites, a frequent finding in cirrhosis.

Other Serum Proteins

While most of the proteins discussed in Chapter 19 are produced by the liver, two bear special importance in detecting congenital liver disorders.

Alpha-1-Antitrypsin (AAT). Alpha-1-antitrypsin, the most abundant $alpha_1$-globulin, is the most important protease inhibitor in plasma. While its name indicates that it inhibits trypsin, it also is an inhibitor of other serine proteases, such as elastin. AAT is coded for by the *Pi* gene on chromosome 14; there are several genetic variants due to point mutations, leading to single amino acid substitutions (Chappell, 2004). The most common variant, M, is associated with normal serum AAT levels. The mutations present in the S and Z variants prevent normal protein glycation, leading to accumulation of AAT within hepatocytes and reduced plasma AAT levels (Propst, 1994). In the United States, the overwhelming genotype is Pi^{MM}, where Pi is protease inhibitor. The other genotypes, Pi^{ZZ}, Pi^{SS}, Pi^{SZ}, Pi^{MZ}, and Pi^{MS}, all contain measurable activity of antiprotease, except a rare null genotype Pi$^-$. If the antiprotease activity of the MM phenotype is used as the reference, then the activity in phenotype ZZ is 15%, SS is 60%, MZ is 57.5%, and MS 80%. Adults with Pi^{ZZ} are the most prone to develop emphysema relatively early in life as a result of uninhibited trypsin activity on alveolar wall elastin. Patients with Pi^{ZZ} tend to accumulate the Z protein in periportal hepatocytes where it forms discrete cytoplasmic bodies and may also develop neonatal hepatitis. Curiously, although infants may die of the hepatic injury, it resolves in most infants and progresses to cirrhosis in only about 3% (Sveger, 1988). In adults, there is an increased likelihood of liver injury in patients heterozygous or homozygous for the Z variant of AAT that may be due to accumulation of AAT in the endoplasmic reticulum that induces autophagy and apoptosis of hepatocytes (Teckman, 2004). AAT phenotyping can be performed using isoelectric focusing (Propst, 1994). Since AAT is an acute phase reactant, its serum levels can be normal in MZ heterozygotes.

Ceruloplasmin. The major copper-containing protein in serum, ceruloplasmin, is also the enzyme present in highest circulating concentration. Ceruloplasmin is a ferroxidase, essential for converting iron to the ferric state to allow binding to transferrin. Low levels of ceruloplasmin are found in Wilson's disease, a rare congenital disorder (1 in 30 000 individuals) associated with one of many mutations in the gene on chromosome 13 coding for a cellular adenosine triphosphatase (ATPase), ATP7B, a new member of the cation-transporting p-type ATPase family (Bull, 1993). This protein is principally expressed in the liver and promotes copper secretion into plasma, coupled with ceruloplasmin synthesis, and into the biliary tract. More than 200 mutations of this Wilson's disease gene have been detected resulting in impairment of ATP7B function and intracellular copper accumulation (Langner, 2004). Excess intracellular copper becomes deposited in lysozomes in hepatocytes and induces free-radical reactions including lipid peroxidation and membrane instability. Resultant liver damage can lead to chronic active hepatitis, cirrhosis or, uncommonly, fulminant hepatic failure. In addition, steatosis and inflammation can also result in this condition. Copper becomes deposited in the central nervous system, especially in the lenticular nucleus of the basal ganglia, causing neuropsychiatric disease; it can also be deposited at the edge of the iris, forming the observed Keyser–Fleischer rings.

The diagnosis of Wilson's disease is made on the basis of typical clinical and laboratory findings, including low serum ceruloplasmin, which can be measured either by immunoassay or enzymatic assay, increased urinary copper excretion, and increased hepatic copper content. While ceruloplasmin is characteristically low in Wilson's disease, factors increasing ceruloplasmin synthesis (e.g., cytokines, pregnancy, estrogens) may cause normal ceruloplasmin levels in up to 15% of patients overall, and as many as 35% with hepatic manifestations of Wilson's disease (Dufour, 1997), particularly acute Wilsonian hepatitis (Berman, 1991). Genetic testing is the most reliable means to establish the diagnosis, but is difficult, since over 200 mutations have been shown to cause disease.

Clotting Factors

As mentioned earlier, except for the von Willebrand factor, which is made by endothelial cells and megakaryocytes, coagulation proteins are synthesized in the liver. In addition, inhibitors of coagulation are synthesized in the liver, such as antithrombin III, alpha-2-macroglobulin, alpha-1-antitrypsin, C1 esterase inhibitor, and protein C. In addition, fibrin degradation products are catabolized in the liver. Low levels of antithrombin III in patients with cirrhosis and hepatitis may be caused by decreased synthesis, increased consumption, or an alteration in the transcapillary flux ratio (Kelly, 1987). The most common coagulopathy seen in liver failure, i.e., cirrhosis and acute fulminant hepatic failure, is disseminated intravascular coagulopathy (DIC) as discussed in Chapter 8 and throughout Part V of this book. This condition is characterized by an increased consumption of clotting factors and platelets, causing thrombocytopenia and elevations of both the prothrombin (PT) and partial thromboplastin (PTT) times. The mechanism has been postulated to be decreased synthesis of clotting inhibitory factors, decreased clearance of activated clotting factors, or release of tissue thromboplastin from hepatocytes (Kelly, 1986). Fibrin split products, detected in DIC, have been found in up to 80% of patients with liver disease without evidence of fibrinolysis (Van de Water, 1986). It is important that the diagnosis of DIC be made certain by determination of elevated blood D-dimer levels as described in Part V on hemostasis and thrombosis. In some cases of liver failure, platelet counts are decreased because of sequestration in an enlarged spleen due to hepatosplenomegaly. This condition combined with elevated levels of the PT and PTT caused by low levels of synthesis of coagulation factors can masquerade as DIC. In these cases, D-dimer levels are not elevated, excluding this diagnosis.

Perhaps the most frequently ordered laboratory test for detecting liver-associated coagulation abnormalities is the prothrombin time (PT) and its associated measurement, the international sensitivity ratio, as described in Part V. The PT measures the efficacy of the extrinsic clotting system in which factor VII is activated by tissue factor as discussed in Part V; since factor VII is uniquely synthesized in the liver, its measurement can be used to evaluate liver function status. Often, the PT is computed as the INR, the international standardized ratio, that attempts to standardize all PT measurements relative to a 'gold standard' PT measuring method, using the international sensitivity index (ISI), as described in Part V.

Some Caveats in Using the PT and INR to Evaluate Liver Function. Since PT and PTT measure the status of the coagulation cascades (extrinsic and intrinsic, respectively), any coagulation disorders will give rise to abnormal PTs and/or PTTs independent of liver function. In addition, in patients with cholestasis, i.e., disease of the biliary tract, with no hepatocytic dysfunction, e.g., cirrhosis or fulminant hepatic failure, absorption of the fat-soluble vitamin K from the gut may be impaired because of low levels of bile salts that allow membrane transport of this vitamin. Since factors II, VII, IX and X depend on vitamin K for biosynthesis via carboxylation, coagulation abnormalities often result. Therefore, in patients with cholestasis, normal serum levels of inactive precursor forms of these four coagulation factors can be detected as discussed further below. Correction of the prothrombin time by the administration of vitamin K is usually possible when factor V is normal in patients with cholestatic liver disease.

Also, use of the INR in evaluating liver function can give misleading results. As discussed in Part V, the INR is based on PT values for patients treated with coumadin (which blocks mainly the extrinsic system). Thus its appropriateness for evaluating non-coumadin-induced coagulopathies has been questioned, especially in view of the finding that PT increases much less with lower international sensitivity index (ISI) in patients with liver disease than in patients being treated with coumadin (Kovacs, 1994; Ts'ao, 1994; Johnston, 1996; Robert, 1996).

Prothrombin Times Are Used to Compute the MELD Score. The PT is an integral part of the MELD (model for end-stage liver disease) score in evaluating priority for liver transplantation in liver disease (Trotter, 2004). This score is a computed number based on the values of bilirubin, creatinine and INR. While this score appears to predict accurately the 3-month mortality

for cirrhotic patients awaiting liver transplantation (Farnsworth, 2004), it must be used with caution both because reference ranges of these analytes differ among different laboratories making standardization difficult and because of the caveats in using INR values as described above.

Des-Gamma-Carboxy Prothrombin (DCP)

The vitamin K-dependent coagulation factors (II, VII, IX, X) are synthesized in the liver and require a vitamin K-mediated post-translational modification (gamma-carboxylation of a number of terminal glutamic acid residues to gamma-carboxyglutamic acid) to occur prior to secretion into the blood, which is necessary for functional activity of these factors in the coagulation cascade. The unmodified precursor of prothrombin, DCP, has been found to be elevated in the sera of patients with hepatocellular carcinoma. DCP is measured using two monoclonal antibodies, 19B7 and MU-3. Increases of DCP in patients with hepatocellular carcinoma predict decreased survival times (Nagaoka, 2003). However, assays for DCP do not have the same general use as alpha-fetoprotein, discussed below, for diagnosing and following this disease.

Tests of Liver Injury

Plasma Enzyme Levels

As metabolically complex cells, hepatocytes contain high levels of a number of enzymes. With liver injury, these enzymes may leak into plasma and can be useful for diagnosis and monitoring of liver injury. While enzymes are discussed further in Chapter 20, an understanding of the cellular location of enzymes and patterns of enzyme change is critical in understanding the findings in various types of liver disease.

Cellular Locations of Enzymes

Within the hepatocyte, the commonly measured enzymes are found in specific locations; the type of liver injury will determine the pattern of enzyme changes. Figure 21–3 illustrates the locations of the most important hepatocytic enzymes. Cytoplasmic enzymes include lactate dehydrogenase (LD), aspartate aminotransferase (AST), and alanine aminotransferase (ALT). Mitochondrial enzymes, such as the mitochondrial isoenzyme of AST, are released with mitochondrial damage. Canalicular enzymes, such as alkaline phosphatase and gamma-glutamyl transferase (GGT), are increased by obstructive processes.

Mechanisms of Enzyme Release

Enzymes are released from hepatocytes as a result of injury to the cell membrane that directly causes extrusion of the cytosolic contents. In addition, agents like ethanol cause release of mitochondrial AST from hepatocytes and its expression on cell surfaces (Zhou, 1998a). Accumulation of bile salts with canalicular obstruction causes release of membrane fragments with attached canalicular enzymes (Schlaeger, 1982; Moss, 1997). Increased synthesis of GGT, and to a lesser extent alkaline phosphatase, can occur with medications that induce microsomal enzyme synthesis, notably ethanol, phenytoin, and carbamazepine (Aldenhovel, 1988).

Aminotransferases (Transaminases). There are two diagnostically very useful enzymes in this category, aspartate aminotransferase (AST), also known as serum glutamate oxaloacetate transaminase (SGOT) and alanine aminotransferase (ALT), formerly called serum glutamate pyruvate transaminase (SGPT). These enzymes catalyze reversibly the transfer of an amino group of either aspartate (AST) or alanine (ALT) to alpha-ketoglutarate to yield glutamate plus the corresponding ketoacid of the starting amino acid, i.e., oxaloacetate or pyruvate, respectively. Both enzymes require pyridoxal phosphate (vitamin B_6) as a cofactor. Using ALT as an example, alanine reacts with pyridoxal phosphate to yield pyruvate plus pyridoxine. Pyridoxine then reacts with alpha-ketoglutarate to yield glutamate plus regenerated pyridoxal phosphate.

At the core of these reactions is the cofactor, pyridoxal phosphate, vitamin B_6. In many of the serum assays for ALT and AST, it is assumed that the patient's serum provides a sufficient complement of pyridoxal phosphate, a circumstance that does not always apply. In a most poignant case illustrating this point, a patient, a known alcoholic, was admitted to a hospital with a presumptive diagnosis of alcoholic hepatitis, a condition described at length below. His admission clinical chemistry profile showed normal to low serum levels of ALT and AST. This finding is unusual in alcoholic hepatitis, since, as we discuss below, both enzymes become significantly elevated such that AST levels are higher than those for ALT. During the course of the next 24 hours, he was treated for his condition, with apparent clinical improvement. However, a repeat liver function profile showed marked elevations of both enzymes to levels greater than 200 IU/L. This presented a diagnostic dilemma,

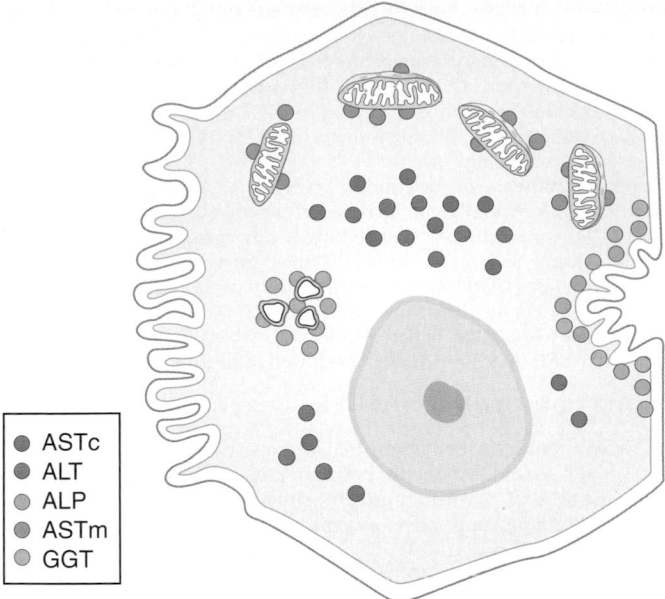

- ● ASTc
- ● ALT
- ● ALP
- ● ASTm
- ● GGT

Figure 21–3 Location of hepatocellular enzymes. The major diagnostic hepatocellular enzymes are located at various sites in the hepatocyte, giving rise to different patterns of enzyme release with different causes of injury. Alanine aminotransferase (ALT) and the cytoplasmic isoenzyme of aspartate aminotransferase (ASTc) are found primarily in the cytosol. With membrane injury as in viral or chemically-induced hepatitis, these enzymes are released and enter the sinusoids, raising plasma AST and ALT levels. Mitochondrial aspartate aminotransferase (ASTm) is released primarily with mitochondrial injury, as caused by ethanol as in alcoholic hepatitis. Alkaline phosphatase (ALP) and gamma-glutamyltransferase (GGT) are found primarily on the canalicular surface of the hepatocyte. Bile acids accumulate in cholestasis and dissolve membrane fragments, releasing bound enzymes into plasma. GGT is also found in the microsomes, represented as rings in the figure; microsomal enzyme-inducing drugs, like phenobarbital and dilantin, can also increase GGT synthesis and raise plasma GGT activity.

which was resolved when it was realized that, as part of the protocol for treatment of alcoholic hepatitis, the patient had received vitamin supplements including vitamins B_6 and B_{12}. Since the serum assays for both ALT and AST required vitamin B_6 supplied by the patient's serum and the patient, an alcoholic, was vitamin B_6-deficient (common in alcoholics), the assays for both enzymes showed normal-to-low levels due to the absence of vitamin B_6. Upon therapeutic intervention, when vitamins were administered, sufficient serum levels of vitamin B_6 were present to allow for full enzyme activities. This clinical history illustrates the central role of pyridoxal phosphate in enzyme catalysis by AST and ALT and the importance of understanding the chemical basis for enzyme assays.

AST and ALT have respective blood half-lives of 17 and 47 hours and have upper reference range limits of around 40 IU/L. (See Ch. 20 for the definition of international units or IU.) AST is both intra- and extra-mitochondrial, while ALT is completely extramitochondrial. Mitochondrial AST isoenzyme has a half-life of 87 hours (Panteghini, 1990). AST is ubiquitously distributed in the body tissues, including the heart and muscle, whereas ALT is found primarily in the liver, although significant amounts are also present in kidney.

Total cytoplasmic AST is present in highest activity in hepatocytes, with cell AST level approximately 7000 times that in plasma. ALT is also present in highest activity in hepatocytes, with cell ALT level approximately 3000 times that in plasma. With pyridoxine deficiency, hepatic synthesis of ALT is impaired; a similar phenomenon occurs in hepatic fibrosis and cirrhosis. The enzyme changes seen in hepatic injury can be readily explained by differing hepatic activity levels and half-lives of enzymes. With most forms of acute hepatocellular injury, such as hepatitis, AST will be higher than ALT initially, due to the higher activity of AST in hepatocytes. Within 24–48 hours, particularly if ongoing damage occurs, ALT will become higher than AST, based on its longer half-life.

An exception to these observations occurs in acute alcohol-induced hepatocyte injury as in alcoholic hepatitis. Studies suggest that alcohol induces mitochondrial damage, resulting in the release of mitochondrial AST, which, besides being the predominant form of AST in hepatocytes, has a significantly longer half-life than do extramitochondrial AST and ALT. This frequently results in the disproportionate elevation of AST over ALT giving an ALT/AST quotient, also called the DeRitis ratio, of 3–4 : 1 in alcohol-induced liver disease. There is some disagreement as to whether cessation of alcohol

consumption reduces this ratio. In one early study, serum mitochondrial AST was measured in cirrhotic and noncirrhotic patients who abuse alcohol (Nalpas, 1986). Patients with chronic alcohol abuse, regardless of the extent of their underlying liver disease, had more consistent mitochondrial AST elevations than other patients; values dropped more than 50% with abstinence for more than 1 week. On the other hand, in more recent studies, involving over 300 patients, it was found that high AST/ALT ratios suggest advanced alcoholic liver disease (Nyblom, 2004). It should also be noted that many alcoholics are vitamin B_6-deficient, causing lower rates of synthesis of ALT and suppression of existing ALT activity.

In chronic hepatocyte injury, mainly in cirrhosis, ALT is more commonly elevated than AST; however, as fibrosis progresses, ALT activities typically decline, and the ratio of AST to ALT gradually increases, so that by the time cirrhosis is present, AST is often higher than ALT (Williams, 1988; Sheth, 1998). However, in end-stage cirrhosis, the levels of both enzymes are generally not elevated and may be low due to massive tissue destruction. In acute fulminant hepatic failure, as discussed below and in Chapter 8, the serum levels of both aminotransferases are markedly increased and are such that AST : ALT ratio is often significantly greater than 1 (Sunheimer, 1994).

Overall, ALT activity is more specific for detecting liver disease in nonalcoholic, asymptomatic patients. Mild elevations are often seen in hepatitis C infections. AST is used for monitoring therapy with potentially hepatotoxic drugs; a result more than three times the upper border of normal should signal stopping of therapy. Chronic elevation of aminotransferase activities in asymptomatic patients may have several causes, including alcohol or medication use, chronic viral hepatitis, or nonalcoholic fatty liver disease. Weight reduction may lower ALT in overweight patients whose ALT is elevated (Palmer, 1990). Ursodeoxycholic acid lowers ALT as well as GGT (see below) when these are found to be elevated in blood donors (Bellentani, 1989).

Assays for AST and ALT. There are several variants of assays for these enzymes. In one, alanine for ALT or aspartate for AST is added to force the reaction to the right yielding glutamate. Production of the latter is then coupled to the enzyme, glutamate dehydrogenase, in the so-called indicator reaction, yielding alpha-ketoglutarate. In this reaction, NAD is converted to NADH that can be measured as an increase in absorbance at 340 nm. These reactions must be evaluated over short time periods because one of the substrates for these enzymes, alpha-ketoglutarate, is regenerated by the indicator reaction. Another variant for AST involves coupling the oxaloacetate (OAA) that forms from aspartate in the reaction, to malate dehydrogenase, which converts OAA to malate, and in which NADH is converted to NAD that is measured by a decrease in absorbance at 340 nm. For ALT, conversion of alanine to pyruvate allows for coupling to the pyruvate dehydrogenase complex in which pyruvate is converted to acetyl coenzyme A and in which NAD is converted to NADH that can be directly measured by an increase in absorbance at 340 nm. As noted above, it is vital that pyridoxal phosphate be present in sufficient quantity to allow these reactions to proceed.

Lactate Dehydrogenase. As described in Chapter 20, this cytosolic glycolytic enzyme catalyzes the reversible oxidation of lactate to pyruvate. Five major LD isozymes exist, consisting of tetramers of two forms, H and M, the former having high affinity for lactate, the latter for pyruvate. Progressing from HHHH to MMMM, the five possible isozymes are labeled LD_1–LD_5. LD_1 and LD_2 predominate in cardiac muscle, kidney, and erythrocytes. LD_4 and LD_5 are the major isoenzymes in liver and skeletal muscle. The upper reference range limit for total LD activity in serum is around 150 IU/L (see Ch. 20 for the definition of international units or IU). Serum LD levels become elevated in hepatitis; often, these increases are transient and return to normal by the time of clinical presentation (Dufour, 1988c; Fuchs, 1998; Singer, 1995) because LD isozymes originating in liver (LD_4 and LD_5) have a relatively low activity in hepatocytes relative to plasma (about 500 times) and a half-life of approximately 4–6 hours.

More important is the large increase of total LD to levels of 500 IU/L or more, combined with a significant increase in alkaline phosphatase (ALP), discussed below and in Chapter 20, to levels > 250 IU/L, in the absence of other dramatic abnormalities in liver function enzyme levels, especially AST and ALT. These selective increases often accompany space-occupying lesions of the liver, such as metastatic carcinoma, primary hepatocellular carcinoma, or, rarely, benign lesions, such as hemangiomata. The source of the LD, most often the LD_5 isozyme, is not clear since it can originate either from hepatocytes, from the tumor, or from both. The rise in ALP is due to blockage of local canaliculi and ductules by the masses in the liver as discussed below. Assays for LD are described in Chapter 20.

Enzymes Primarily Reflecting Canalicular Injury

As shown in Figure 21–3, these enzymes are located predominantly on the canalicular membrane of the hepatocyte and include alkaline phosphatase, gamma-glutamyl transferase and 5′-nucleotidase. In contrast to cytoplasmic enzyme activities, canalicular enzyme activities within hepatocytes are typically quite low; focal hepatocyte injury seldom causes significant increases in canalicular enzyme levels.

Alkaline Phosphatase (ALP). Alkaline phosphatase is present in a number of tissues, including liver, bone, kidney, intestine, and placenta, each of which contains distinct isozymes which can be separated from one another by electrophoresis. Total ALP in serum is mainly present in the unbound form and, to a lesser extent, complexed with lipoproteins or rarely with immunoglobulins.

ALP in the liver, which has a half-life of about 3 days, is a hepatocytic enzyme that is found on the canalicular surface and is therefore a marker for biliary dysfunction. The bone isozyme is particularly heat-labile, allowing it to be distinguished from the other major forms. In addition, small intestinal and placental ALP are antigenically distinct from liver, bone, and kidney ALP. The bulk of ALP in the serum of normal patients is made up of liver and bone ALP.

In obstruction of the biliary tract from stones in the ducts or ductules, or infectious processes resulting in ascending cholangitis, or from space-occupying lesions, biliary tract ALP rises rapidly to values sometimes in excess of 10 times the upper limit of normal. The reasons for this increase are probably a combination of increased synthesis and decreased excretion of ALP. In obstructive cholestasis, ALP most commonly rises to twice the upper limit of normal or greater, roughly paralleling the rate of rise in serum bilirubin. If obstruction is partial, ALP usually increases as much as with complete obstruction, often out of proportion to the increase in conjugated bilirubin (dissociated jaundice). Passive congestion of the liver can occasionally result in moderate ALP elevations, more so than abnormal bilirubin levels. ALP is also moderately elevated in most instances of jaundice resulting from hepatic injury. When the resulting cholestasis is relieved, serum ALP levels fall to normal more slowly than bilirubin.

A high-molecular-weight ALP appears in serum in cholestasis. This ALP is attached to fragments of canalicular membrane. Bile salts solubilize the enzymes from the sinusoidal and canalicular membranes. In serum, the membrane-bound enzymes aggregate with lipids and lipoproteins. This may explain the relationship that has been observed, for instance, with lipoprotein X (LpX) (see Ch. 17). Another form of high-molecular-weight ALP, which migrates differently on electrophoresis from the isozyme just described, has been found in malignant disease involving the liver (Viot, 1983).

Intestinal ALP is increased in a variety of disorders of the intestinal tract and in cirrhosis. Serum intestinal ALP is detected in over 80% of cirrhotic patients as compared with 10% of normal controls. The measurement of this enzyme activity was suggested as one method of discriminating intrahepatic from extrahepatic jaundice, because intestinal ALP may be absent in extrahepatic obstruction, but it lacks adequate sensitivity and specificity (Collins, 1987). Assays for ALP are described in Chapter 20.

Gamma-Glutamyl Transferase (GGT). This enzyme regulates the transport of amino acids across cell membranes by catalyzing the transfer of a glutamyl group from glutathione to a free amino acid. Its major use is to discriminate the source of elevated ALP, i.e., if ALP is elevated and GGT is correspondingly elevated, then the source of the elevated ALP is most likely biliary tract. The highest values, often greater than 10 times the upper limit of normal, may be found in chronic cholestasis due to primary biliary cirrhosis or sclerosing cholangitis. It is also elevated in about 60–70% of those who chronically abuse alcohol, with a rough correlation between amount of alcohol intake and GGT activity (Whitehead, 1978). Levels often decline slowly with abstention from alcohol, and remain elevated for at least 1 month after abstinence begins (Belfrage, 1977; Moussavian, 1985). GGT has a half-life of 10 days, but, in recovery from alcohol abuse, the half-life may be as long as 28 days. It tends to be higher in obstructive disorders and with space-occupying lesions in the liver than with hepatocyte injury (Kim, 1977).

The gene for human GGT has been cloned and the nucleotide sequence identified (Rajpert-De Meyts, 1988). GGT can be detected in three major forms in serum (Wenham, 1985), but such determinations are not readily available. A high-molecular-weight form is present in normal serum as well as in biliary obstruction and more frequently in malignant infiltration of the liver. An intermediate-molecular-weight form consists of two fractions, the major one detected in liver diseases and the other one found in biliary obstruction. Determination of these fractions lacks both sufficient sensitivity and specificity to be worthwhile (Collins, 1987). The third form is a low-molecular-weight compound of uncertain importance.

Serum levels of GGT differ from those of ALP during pregnancy, in which GGT remains normal even during cholestasis in pregnancy. GGT is often increased in alcoholics even without liver disease; in some obese people; and in the presence of high concentrations of therapeutic drugs, like acetaminophen and phenytoin and carbamazepine (increased up to five times the reference limits), even in the absence of any apparent liver injury. Possibly, increases in GGT occur to restore glutathione used in the metabolism of these drugs, which may account for the elevated GGT activities assayed. Glutathione is conjugated to these drugs via the glutathione S-transferase system, and the complex is then excreted.

Most assays for GGT utilize the substrate, gamma-glutamyl-*p*-nitroanilide. In the reaction catalyzed by GGT, *p*-nitroaniline is liberated and is chromogenic, enabling this colored product to be measured spectrophotometrically.

Other Enzymes. 5'-Nucleotidase activity is increased in cholestatic disorders with virtually no increase in activity in patients with bone disease. Measurement of 5'-nucleotidase can corroborate the elevation of ALP from a hepatic source. Other enzymes, such as leucine aminopeptidase (LAP) can also be used for the same purpose but virtually never are. Isocitrate dehydrogenase and OCT – unique to the liver – activities are elevated in hepatocellular injury, and parallel ALT and AST. Again, like LAP, they are virtually never used in routine laboratory assays.

Alpha-Fetoprotein (AFP)

AFP is synthesized by embryonic hepatocytes and fetal yolk sac cells and peaks in the second trimester of pregnancy, reaching levels that constitute up to one-third of fetal serum protein. The function of AFP is not known. It may be immunosuppressive, preventing fetal destruction by circulating maternal antibodies.

As discussed in Chapter 25, AFP becomes elevated to abnormal levels in fetal neural tube deficits. The reasons for this correlation are unclear. It is important to note that normal AFP levels vary considerably with gestational age. Therefore, the decision that the serum level of this protein is abnormally high will depend upon the reference interval for the gestational age of the patient.

Shortly after birth, AFP levels fall, reaching the adult normal range at around 1 year of age. After acute hepatic injury, a rise in AFP (typically 100–200 ng/dL) from regenerating hepatocytes usually occurs. Often, however, these typical elevations after acute hepatic insults do not occur after surgical resection of the liver. Regeneration is therefore not a sufficient impetus for elevated AFP levels to occur.

As discussed in Chapter 74, AFP has been found to be an important marker for hepatocellular carcinoma (HCC). Elevated levels occur in over 90% of patients with this disease. As noted above, elevated levels can also occur after acute liver disease and also fibrosis, making this marker somewhat nonspecific. However, at levels > 400 ng/dL, there is a high probability of HCC, but at these levels of AFP, the tumor is widespread so that its use as an early detector of HCC is limited. Serum levels of AFP in HCC are also dependent on the extent and degree of differentiation of the tumor and the age of the patient.

Autoimmune Markers

Antimitochondrial Antibody Is a Marker for Primary Biliary Cirrhosis (PBC). Occasionally, autoimmune disease may be the primary cause of liver injury. The most common autoimmune liver disease is primary biliary cirrhosis (PBC), which occurs primarily in women, usually in the fifth decade, often accompanied by other autoimmune diseases (especially Sjögren's syndrome). This condition, which is discussed at length in Chapter 52, causes fibrosis of the bile canaliculi in the portal triads. Bile eventually seeps into hepatocytes, causing necrosis. Granulation tissue replaces hepatocytes so that the fibrosis eventually spreads into the liver parenchyma, giving rise to the pattern of fibrosis and regenerating nodules. A similar course occurs in secondary biliary cirrhosis as a result of other underlying conditions such as choledocholithiasis, carcinoma of the head of the pancreas, and occasionally, hepatitis and sepsis.

A vital difference between primary and secondary biliary cirrhosis is that the former uniquely appears to be part of a generalized autoimmune condition. Over 90% of patients with primary biliary cirrhosis are found by immunofluorescence to have serum antibodies that react with liver, kidney, stomach and thyroid tissue. These circulating antibodies, which can be detected in serum using an enzyme-linked immunosorbent assay (ELISA), are directed against mitochondrial antigens (antimitochondrial antigen or AMA) from the inner mitochondrial membrane, called M2, which has been found to be dihydrolipoamide acetyltransferase, a component of the pyruvate dehydrogenase multienzyme complex (Krams, 1989; Coppel, 1988; Kaplan, 1984). Antimitochondrial antibodies have been found in a variety of disease states, but there are two anti-M2 antibodies in primary biliary cirrhosis that uniquely react either with a protein of molecular mass 48 kilodaltons (kD) or 62 kD (Manns, 1987; Fussey, 1988). In other disorders, AMA against M1 antigen has been found in syphilis, anti-M5 in collagen vascular diseases, anti-M6 in iproniazid-induced hepatitis, and anti-M7 in cardiomyopathies (Berg, 1986). AMA with anti-M2 specificity are 100% specific for primary biliary cirrhosis.

ANCA is a Marker for Primary Sclerosing Cholangitis. Primary sclerosing cholangitis (PSC) is an autoimmune disease associated with destruction of extrahepatic as well as intrahepatic bile ducts. Approximately two-thirds of patients with PSC have circulating perinuclear antineutrophil cytoplasmic antibodies (p-ANCAs) with specificities against antigens such as bactericidal/permeability-increasing protein, cathepsin G, and/or lactoferrin (Mulder, 1993; Roozendaal, 1998). Up to 75% also have other autoantibodies such as antinuclear antibodies (ANAs) or anti-smooth muscle antibodies (ASMAs) (Chapman, 1986). Unlike primary biliary cirrhosis, PSC occurs primarily in young to middle-aged men, often associated with inflammatory bowel disease, particularly ulcerative colitis.

Serum Markers for Autoimmune Hepatitis. Autoimmune hepatitis is responsible for as much as 3–5% of chronic hepatitis, and occasionally may present as acute hepatitis. There are several variants of autoimmune hepatitis, associated with various markers (Czaja, 1995a,b). In the US, the most common variant, type 1, is associated with antinuclear antibodies (ANAs) most commonly, and also with antibodies to actin (often detected as ASMAs). Titers of AMAs and/or ASMAs greater than 1 : 80 support the diagnosis in patients with hepatitis (Johnson, 1993). Type 2 autoimmune hepatitis typically affects children, and is much more common in Europe than in the US, where it is rarely encountered. ANAs and ASMAs are often negative in type 2, while antibodies to liver–kidney microsomal antigens (anti-LKM$_1$) are positive in the majority of cases. Lower level titers of ANAs or ASMAs are commonly seen in other forms of liver disease, particularly hepatitis C, in which they may be found in up to 40% of cases (Czaja, 1995a,b).

Markers of Hepatitis Virus Infection

Numerous viruses cause liver damage. Some, like the hepatitis A, B and C viruses and the arboviruses, are hepatotoxic, but others, like EBV, CMV, VZV, HSV, HH6, HIV, adenovirus, and echovirus, induce transient to moderately aggressive hepatitis. Even newly identified hepatitis G causes only a self-limited form of hepatitis. In actuality, viruses are the cause of 80–90% of acute and chronic hepatitis. While a variety of such viruses can affect the liver, most viral-induced liver pathology is caused by five viruses that are known to cause hepatocyte injury, and are termed 'hepatitis viruses,' namely, hepatitis A, B, C, D, and E.

Hepatitis A

Hepatitis A virus (HAV) is a member of the picornavirus family of RNA viruses. It is transmitted by the fecal–oral route and typically has an incubation period of 15–50 days with a mean time of about a month, dependent upon the inoculum (Brown, 2003). Epidemics or clusters of HAV infection often occur with conditions of poor sanitation, in day-care centers, with military actions, and from contaminated food. Infection with HAV is almost always self-limiting, although in 5–10% of cases a secondary rise in enzymes occurs. The time course of markers of HAV infection is shown in Figure 21–4. During the incubation period, HAV RNA is present in stool and in plasma, and remains detectable for an average of 18 days after clinical onset of hepatitis (Fujiwara, 1997). The initial immune response to the virus is IgM anti-HAV, which typically develops about 2–3 weeks after infection; increasing AST and ALT develop *after antibody development*. IgM antibodies typically persist for 3–6 months after infection. IgG antibodies develop within 1–2 weeks of IgM antibodies, and typically remain positive for life (Skinhoj, 1977). 'Total' anti-HAV assays detect both IgM and IgG antibodies. The prevalence of total anti-HAV varies, ranging from 5–10% in children below 5 years to 75% in those over age 50 years (Koff, 1995). Following HAV immunization, detectable antibody develops in 2–4 weeks and persists to 5 years in 99% of responders (Totos, 1997). If necessary for epidemiologic purposes, polymerase chain reaction (PCR) assays are available to identify HAV RNA in plasma and stool. There is no need, however, to incorporate the use of PCR for routine diagnostic purposes.

Hepatitis B

Hepatitis B virus (HBV) is a member of the hepadnavirus family, a group of related viruses that cause hepatitis in various animal species. This virus causes infection of the liver with clinical features that are extremely variable, ranging from absent or mild disease to severe liver failure (Horvat, 2003). Hepatitis B is transmitted primarily by body fluids, especially serum; however, it is also spread effectively by sex and can be transmitted from mother to baby. Hepatitis B produces several protein antigens that can be detected in serum: a core antigen (HBcAg), a surface antigen (HBsAg or HBs), and e antigen (HBeAg), related to the core antigen; commercial assays are available for HBsAg and HBeAg. Antibodies to each of these antigens can also be measured, and commercial assays for each are available. The time course of self-limited infection with HBV is illustrated in Figure 21–5. Different groups of tests are recommended for three different clinical situations as follows:

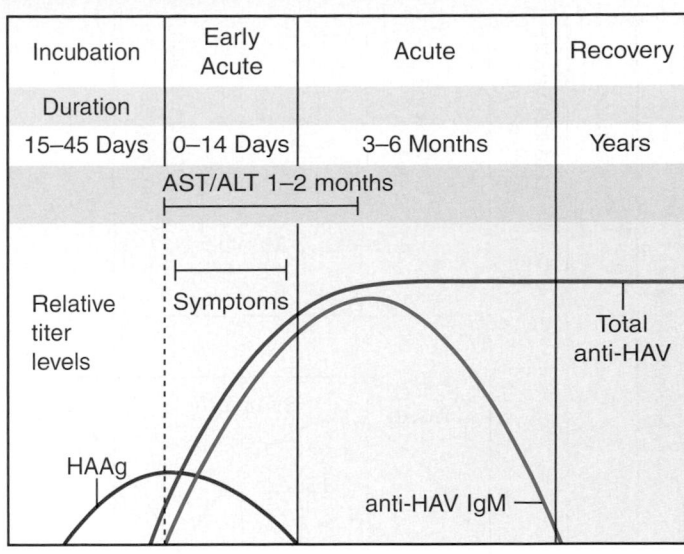

Figure 21–4 Typical time course for appearance of viral antigens and antiviral antibodies in hepatitis A viral (HAV) infection. The appearance of the hepatitis A antigen, HAAg, occurs early on and it is no longer present during the acute phase, during which time jaundice may develop. During the incubation period (which averages 2–3 weeks), HAV RNA is replicating, and viral particles can be detected in stool by immune electron microscopy. Viral RNA is also detectable during this time by real-time PCR. The most effective diagnostic determination of hepatitis A acute infection is the detection of anti-HAV IgM. Also shown in this figure is the rise of the aminotransferases, AST and ALT, which occurs at the beginning of the early acute phase and lasts for several weeks to a month. The patient ceases to be infectious after anti-HAV IgM falls to undetectable levels in 3–6 months post-early phase. Permanent anti-HAV IgG rises over several months and lasts for many years, conferring immunity on the exposed or infected individual. (Adapted from 'Hepatitis A Diagnostic Profile' from Abbott Laboratories Diagnostic Educational Services, North Chicago, IL, 1994, with permission.)

1. *acute HBV hepatitis*: HBsAg, IgM anti-HBc
2. *chronic HBV hepatitis*: HBsAg, IgG anti-HBc, IgG anti-HBs
3. *monitoring chronic HBV infection*: HBs, HBeAg, IgG anti-HBs, IgG anti-HBe, and ultrasensitive quantitative PCR.

The initial serologic marker of acute infection is HBsAg, which typically becomes detectable 2–3 months after infection. After another 4–6 weeks, IgM anti-HBc appears, accompanied by increases in AST and ALT. When symptoms of hepatitis appear, most patients still have detectable HBsAg, although a few patients have neither detectable HBs nor anti-HBs, leaving anti-HBc the only marker of infection ('core window'). IgM anti-HBc typically persists for 4–6 months; however, it may be intermittently present in patients with chronic HBV infection (Czaja, 1988).

In most individuals, HBV hepatitis is self-limited, and the patient recovers; about 1–2% of normal adolescents and adults have persistent viral replication which causes chronic hepatitis. The frequency of chronic HBV infection is 5–10% in immunocompromised patients and 80% in neonates, with the likelihood of chronic infection declining gradually during the first decade of life. With recovery from acute infection, HBsAg and HBCag disappear, and IgG anti-HBs and IgG anti-HBe appear; development of anti-HBs is typically the last marker in recovery, and is thought to indicate clearance of virus. Anti-HBs and anti-HBc are felt to persist for life, although in about 5–10% of cases anti-HBs ultimately disappears (Seeff, 1987). Isolated anti-HBc can also occur during periods of viral clearance in acute and chronic hepatitis, and as a false-positive result. The titer of anti-HBc is important in determining its significance; low titers are typically false-positive results, while high titers almost always (50–80% of cases) indicate immunity to HBV infection as demonstrated by an anamnestic response to hepatitis B vaccine (Aoki, 1993).

The newest assay to assess HBV infections is the ultrasensitive quantitative real-time PCR technology, which is discussed extensively in Part VIII. This quantitative HBV DNA PCR detects a highly conserved region of the surface gene at a level as low as 200 copies of viral genome per mL (0.001 pg/mL) with a range up to 200 000 000 copies/mL. Its primary use is to monitor therapeutic responsiveness in clinically infected patients. Also available is the quantitative digene hybrid capture assay, which employs a signal amplification antibody capture microplate test that utilizes chemiluminescent detection. But this quantitative HBV PCR technique utilizes an RNA probe and has detection limits of 5000 copies/mL

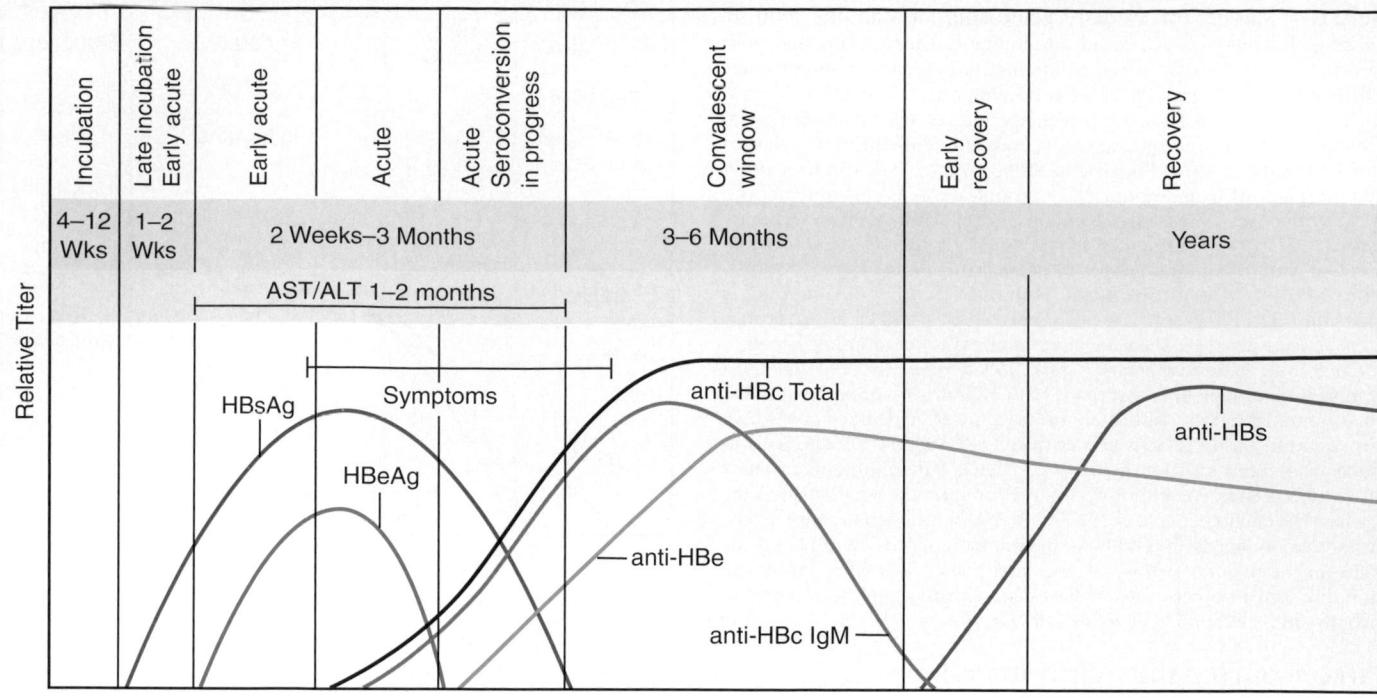

Figure 21–5 Typical time course for appearance of viral antigens and antiviral antibodies in hepatitis B viral (HBV) infection. In the early acute phase, the HBV surface antigen (HBsAg) appears and lasts for several months. Detection of this antigen signifies acute HBV infection. Between the time the titer of HBsAg falls and the titer of anti-HBV IgG, that confers immunity, rises, there is a gap of about 6 months. In this time period, the titers of anti-HBV core antigen (anti-HBc) IgM and IgG rise, indicating acute HBV infection. This is the so-called 'core window.' IgG anti-HBV e antigen (anti-HBe) also rises during this core window period. Permanent immunity is conferred by anti-HBsAg IgG (anti-HBs in the figure). It is difficult to determine the time at which the patient is no longer infectious. Generally, an individual is considered noninfectious when no HBsAg, HBeAg, and no anti-HBcAg IgM can be detected, and the anti-HBsAg IgG has plateaued. Also shown in this figure is the pattern of AST and ALT elevations. These occur in the early acute phase, slightly after HBsAg rises. AST and ALT levels may remain elevated for several weeks to several months, after which time they decline. In HBV chronic active hepatitis, HBsAg is present continuously. AST and ALT generally remain elevated, although they can oscillate throughout the course of the disease. (Adapted from 'Hepatitis B Diagnostic Profile' from Abbott Laboratories, Diagnostic Educational Services, North Chicago, IL, 1994, with permission.)

(0.02 pg/mL) making it less sensitive than the ultraquantitative assay although branched-DNA (b-DNA) assays, discussed in Ch. 67, are also used widely, with detection limits of 2000 copies/mL.

Patients who have clinically recovered from HBV infection and are anti-HBs positive have no detectable HBV DNA using most assays. Using sensitive PCR assays, circulating HBV DNA can be found in a high percentage of anti-HBs-positive patients who have clinically recovered from HBV infection (Yotsuyanagi, 1998; Cabrerizo, 1997), as well as in patients with hepatitis C and isolated anti-HBc (Cacciola, 1999). The significance of finding low levels of HBV DNA is not known, although in patients with concurrent hepatitis C viral infections, it may be associated with more severe liver damage. The e antigen has historically been used to detect presence of circulating viral particles; there is a good correlation between levels of HBeAg and amount of HBV DNA (Hayashi, 1996). In chronic HBV infection, approximately 1–1.5% of patients will spontaneously clear HBeAg each year; some will recover, while others enter a nonreplicative phase in which HBV DNA integrates into the cell genome. This transition phase is often associated with a rise in AST and ALT and, occasionally, jaundice. Rarely, HBeAg may again be detectable in plasma in such patients. Patterns of HBV markers and their interpretation are shown in Table 21–1.

Hepatitis C

Hepatitis C (HCV) is an RNA virus of the flavivirus group. It was the primary etiologic agent of non-A, non-B hepatitis transmitted via blood transfusions and transplantation before 1990. At present, 60% of all new cases occur in injection drug users, but other serum modes of transmission are also seen, such as following accidental needle punctures in healthcare workers, in dialysis patients, and rarely from mother to infant. While sexual transmission is thought to be an inefficient means of transmitting infection it nevertheless accounts for at least 10% of new cases. Monogamous sexual partners of HCV-infected patients rarely become infected, while a history of multiple sexual partners has been recognized as a risk factor. In contrast to HAV and HBV, chronic infection with HCV occurs in about 85% of infected individuals, with an estimated 4 million individuals chronically infected in the US alone (Alter, 1999). About half of HCV chronically-infected individuals with persistent viremia will have elevated ALT levels. Physical symptoms are absent for the first two decades after infection. As the disease progresses, inflammation and liver cell death can lead to fibrosis, and in about 20% of patients, fibrosis will advance to cirrhosis. The risk for hepatocellular carcinoma (HCC) in a patient with chronic HCV is about 1–5% after 20 years. HCC is only seen in patients with cirrhosis (Shuhart, 2003). Laboratory tests for HCV infection and their common uses are summarized in Table 21–2.

HCV has not been grown in culture; HCV genomes can, however, be amplified by recombinant technology. A number of structural and nonstructural antigens have been identified. An immunoassay for the core antigen of HCV has been developed (Aoyagi, 2001) but has been found to be less sensitive than HCV RNA assays (Krajden, 2004). The major diagnostic test for HCV infection has been the second-generation anti-HCV, which detects presence of antibody to one of four different viral

Table 21–1 Interpretations of Patterns of HBV Markers

Interpretation	IgM Anti-HBc	Total Anti-HBc	HBsAg	Anti-HBs	HBeAg	Anti-HBe
Incubation period of HBV infection	–	–	+	–	–	–
Acute HBV infection	+	+	+	–	+	–
Recent, resolving HBV infection	+	+	–	+	–	+
Acute HBV infection in core window	+	+	–	–	–	–
Active chronic HBV infection	–	+	+	–	+	–
Chronic HBV carrier state	–	+	+	–	–	+
Resolved HBV infection	–	+	–	+	–	+
HBV immunity after vaccination	–	–	–	+	–	–

Table 21–2 Interpretation of Patterns of HCV Markers

Interpretation	Anti-HCV	RIBA	HCV RNA
Acute HCV infection	–	–	+
Active HCV infection	+	+	+
Possible HCV clearance	+	+	–
False-positive HCV test	+	–	–
Requires further study	+	Indeterminate*	–

* Indeterminate result; only one band positive, or more than one band and nonspecific reactivity.

antigens an average of 10–12 weeks after infection (Alter, 1992a). A third-generation anti-HCV assay detects antibody at an average of 7–9 weeks after infection (Barrera, 1995). IgM anti-HCV is present in both acute and chronic HCV infection, and is not helpful diagnostically (Brillanti, 1993). Total anti-HCV typically persists for life, although it may disappear with recovery from HCV infection (Seeff, 1994; Beld, 1999).

In high-risk populations, the predictive value of anti-HCV for HCV infection is over 99%, so that further testing is not typically needed to prove viral exposure (Pawlotsky, 1998). In low-risk populations, such as blood donors, the predictive value of positive anti-HCV is only 25%. In low-risk patients, or when needed to confirm HCV exposure, supplemental tests for anti-HCV should be used. The HCV recombinant immunoassay (RIBA-1) test uses recombinant HCV proteins isolated in a dot or strip blot assay; this is analogous to Western blot tests used to confirm positivity in other types of infectious diseases. Using the second-generation RIBA-2 assay, the presence of antibodies to two (of four) or more HCV antigens is considered a positive result, and absence of antibodies is considered negative; antibody to one antigen or antibody to more than one antigen and the nonspecific marker superoxide dismutase are considered indeterminate results. In the third-generation RIBA assay, isolated antibody to the NS5 antigen is virtually never associated with HCV viremia, suggesting that it may indicate a false-positive result (Vernelen, 1994; LaPerche, 1999).

The primary test for confirming persistence of HCV infection is HCV RNA, detected by a variety of amplification techniques. Quantitative assays can typically detect as few as 1000 copies/mL; however, results from different assays are not interchangeable and detection limits vary between methods (Ravaggi, 1997; Lunel, 1999). Qualitative HCV RNA assays generally have lower limits of detection compared to quantitative methods using the same amplification technique, are less expensive, and are more useful for detecting presence or absence of infection.

A World Health Organization (WHO) standard has been developed to improve comparability between methods (Saldanha, 1999) and is based on an international unit or IU/mL of serum or plasma and on recently developed real-time PCR techniques which have a detection range of 5–200 000 000 IU/mL, thereby eliminating the need to do qualitative and quantitative levels. In a recent study (Shiffman, 2003), it has been found, using the international standard, that approximately 90% of serum values for HCV RNA were within 1 log unit irrespective of which virological assay was used. However, some significant differences in results have been found, a few samples giving a maximum of 2 log unit differences (factor of 100). Such discrepant results may have an impact upon the management of patients receiving interferon therapy. These findings suggest that it is important to obtain more than one HCV RNA determination before making treatment decisions (Shiffman, 2003).

With acute infection, HCV RNA is typically present within 2 weeks of infection, but falls with development of antibody; as many as 15% of those with acute HCV infection have negative HCV RNA (Alter, 1992b; Villano, 1999). Viral RNA may be intermittently present for the first year of infection, but then becomes persistently present (Villano, 1999). In later stages of infection, HCV RNA levels generally fluctuate by no more than 0.5–1.0 log around mean values (Nguyen, 1996). HCV has a high rate of mutation, similar to that of other reverse transcriptase viruses such as human immunodeficiency virus (HIV). This produces a number of 'quasispecies' of HCV that may emerge, often associated with fluctuating ALT levels (Yuki, 1997). There are unique species of HCV, termed genotypes. In the US, the most common is genotype 1, divided into subtypes 1a and 1b; these together cause about 65% of HCV infections in Caucasians, but 90–95% of infections in African Americans (Reddy, 1999; McHutchison, 1999). Genotypes 2 and 3 are generally more responsive to treatment (Poynard, 1998; McHutchison, 1998); other strains are responsible for 1–2% of infections. Detection of the unique nucleic acid sequences of each strain by one of several nucleic acid methods (Lau,

1995), discussed at length in Part VIII, is the most reliable means to identify the responsible genotype in an individual.

Hepatitis D

Hepatitis D (delta-agent, HDV) is an RNA virus that can replicate only in the presence of HBsAg; circulating viral particles have viral RNA inside a shell of HBsAg. While HDV is rare in the US, occurring primarily in injecting drug users and hemophiliacs, it is endemic in some parts of the world (London, 1996). In patients with HBV infection, HDV may occur in two forms. If infection with both viruses occurs at about the same time (co-infection), the course of infection is more severe, often follows an atypical course, is a cause of acute fulminant hepatic failure (Sunheimer, 1994) and has a higher fatality rate than HBV infection alone. If HDV infection occurs in the presence of persisting HBV infection (super-infection), there may be a faster progression of disease. The major diagnostic test is presence of anti-HDV; both total and IgM antibody tests are available. Both antibodies may eventually disappear following convalescence. The simultaneous assessment of anti-HBc IgM will help differentiate co-infections (present) from superinfections (absent).

Hepatitis E

Hepatitis E (HEV), an RNA virus with a clinical course similar to that of HAV infection, is common in parts of Asia, Africa, and Mexico, but is rarely seen in the US except in individuals who have traveled to endemic areas (Erker, 1999). Like HAV, it is spread by the fecal–oral route. Person-to-person transmission of HEV appears to be uncommon. When infection occurs in pregnancy, there is an increased fatality rate of about 20%, although in general the fatality rate is between 0.5–4%. HEV infections range from inapparent illness to severe acute hepatitis, sometimes leading to fulminant hepatitis and death. The signs and symptoms cannot be distinguished from those associated with cases of acute hepatitis caused by other hepatotropic viruses (Schlauder, 2003). Antibody tests for HEV are available, but appear to have frequent false-positive results, depending on the antigens used for detecting reactivity (Mast, 1998). There are two serological tests available: anti-HEV IgM which detects recent or current infection, and anti-HEV IgG which detects current or past infection. Because of the current questionable specificity of serological assays, a confirmatory test is required. A PCR amplification of an HEV RNA-specific product using serum, plasma, bile, or feces becomes the definitive indicator of acute infection. However, the PCR test window of detection is from 2–7 weeks after infection.

Hepatitis G

Two other viruses have been suspected, but have not been proven, to cause post-transfusion hepatitis: Hepatitis G virus (HGV, sometimes called G-B) (Laskus, 1997) and transfusion-transmitted virus or TTV (Matsumoto, 1999). While both viruses can be isolated from a high percentage of persons with post-transfusion hepatitis, and viremia is found in at least 1% of blood donors, they do not seem to cause liver disease **in these cases**. To date there are no commercially available serological or PCR assays available to detect these agents. Although acute and chronic HGV can be detected at some research centers with a qualitative PCR assay for HGV RNA, no routine testing is recommended because the clinical significance of HGV remains unknown (Shuhart, 2003). A number of other viruses can cause hepatitis, but typically also affect other organs as well; their tests will not be discussed here.

Diagnosis of Liver Diseases

In Chapter 8, the fundamental patterns of laboratory findings in liver function abnormalities are summarized and are encapsulated in Table 8–5. In this section, the major hepatic disorders are discussed with emphasis on laboratory evaluations that enable diagnoses to be made, often without the need to perform invasive procedures such as liver biopsies.

It is important to remember that in acute hepatitis the principal changes are significant elevations of aminotransferases; in cirrhosis, these tend to remain normal or become slightly elevated while the total protein and albumin are depressed, and ammonia concentrations in serum are elevated. In post-hepatic biliary obstruction, bilirubin and alkaline phosphatase become elevated; and in space-occupying diseases of the liver, alkaline phosphatase and lactate dehydrogenase are elevated. In fulminant hepatic failure, the aminotransferases and ammonia are elevated while total protein and albumin are depressed.

Hepatitis

Hepatitis usually first manifests itself clinically with the symptoms of fatigue and anorexia. Microscopically, cell injury and generally minimal necrosis are caused both by direct virus (or toxic agent)-induced cell damage and by the immune response to the virus. Jaundice may be present. By far the most common cause (> 90% of cases) of hepatitis is viral, with about 50% due to hepatitis B, 25% to hepatitis A, and 20% to hepatitis C. Generally, jaundice is often initially seen as scleral icterus when the patient has total serum bilirubin concentrations above 2 mg/dL. The cause of acute hepatitis is almost always (> 90% of cases) viral, although chemical exposure such as to carbon tetrachloride or chloroform or to drugs such as acetaminophen, especially in children, should be considered. A special category of toxin-induced hepatitis is that induced by alcohol, discussed below.

The cardinal finding in hepatitis is a rise in the aminotransferases to values of more than 200 IU/L and often to 500 or even 1000 IU/L. An exception to this finding is in hepatitis C in which only modest elevations of ALT (but not AST) can occur. The AST/ALT ratio generally favors ALT. The bilirubin is frequently elevated and is composed of both direct and indirect types. Frank jaundice occurs in about 70% of cases of acute hepatitis A (Lednar, 1985), 33% of cases of hepatitis B (McMahon, 1985), and about 20% of acute hepatitis C cases (Hoofnagle, 1997). Elevations of indirect bilirubin are due to the inability of injured hepatocytes to conjugate bilirubin, while the rise of direct bilirubin is due to the blockage of compromised canaliculi secondary to the inflammatory process that occurs in the acute phase. Because of hepatocyte damage, LD levels are mildly elevated to values typically around 300–500 IU/L. Because of inflammation and/or necrosis apoptosis of canalicular and ductular lining cells, the alkaline phosphatase may also be elevated to values of typically 200–350 IU/L. Unless the hepatitis is severe and involves the whole liver, progressing to fulminant hepatic failure, the total protein and albumin are within their normal ranges. The gammaglobulin fractions may be elevated as a result of infection (Lotfy, 2006).

Given the pattern of the above analytes suggestive of hepatitis, screens for specific causes should be made, i.e., a determination of serological markers for hepatitis A, B and C. Screening for antihepatitis A IgM and for HBsAg can be performed within 1 day. If either of these is positive, the diagnosis is established. If negative, further screening for hepatitis B should be undertaken, i.e., determination of serum titers of anti-HBcAg IgM and IgG ('core window'), and anti-HBsAg IgG as described above. If only the latter is positive, it may be difficult to establish whether hepatitis B is the cause of the infection or whether the patient has had past exposure to the virus. Unless the patient has chronic active or persistent hepatitis, in which case HBsAG is continuously present, elevated titers of anti HBsAg IgG occur long after the aminotransferases return to normal levels. Screens for hepatitis C should also be performed. If these are negative, other viral causes should be sought, e.g., cytomegalovirus and Epstein–Barr virus. Especially in the event that a viral hepatitis screen is negative, nonviral causes, such as chemical toxins, should be considered. In addition, less common causes of hepatitis such as Wilson's disease, in which decreased serum ceruloplasmin and increased urinary copper are found, and auto-immune hepatitis, should be considered. Both conditions can present either as acute or chronic diseases; in the chronic forms, both can give rise to chronic active hepatitis and, less commonly, cirrhosis. In the chronic form of autoimmune hepatitis (often accompanied by elevations in ANA titers), polyclonal increases in the gammaglobulins can usually be detected.

Alcoholic Hepatitis. In alcoholic hepatitis, the above-described pattern of abnormal analyte concentrations holds except that AST, much of it mitochondrial AST, often becomes disproportionately elevated over ALT. In addition, there are marked elevations of the enzyme GGT, often out of proportion to elevations in alkaline phosphatase. Unless malnutrition in the alcoholic patient exists, the total protein and albumin are found to be within their reference ranges.

Chronic Hepatitis. In chronic hepatitis, there is ongoing hepatocyte damage, and chronic inflammation in hepatocytes on biopsy. This condition is caused mainly by chronic hepatitis B or C infections, detected by persisting HBsAg or RT-PCR for hepatitis C sequences, respectively, and is a major predisposing factor for cirrhosis and hepatocellular carcinoma, the two leading causes of death from liver disease. Chronic hepatitis may be asymptomatic or mildly symptomatic. There is usually a mild elevation of AST and ALT and, more commonly in hepatitis C, there may be a mild elevation only of ALT.

Chronic Passive Congestion

In chronic passive congestion of the liver, most often secondary to congestive heart failure, back pressure from the right heart is transmitted to the hepatic sinusoids from the inferior vena cava and hepatic veins. Increased pressure causes sinusoidal dilation, which may cause some physical damage to hepatocytes. The result is a mild increase in the aminotransferases and occasionally a mild hyperbilirubinemia. Other analytes that measure liver function are usually within their reference ranges.

Cirrhosis

Cirrhosis of the liver is a condition that results in parenchymal fibrosis and hepatocytic nodular regeneration and can be caused by alcoholism (macronodular or Laennec's cirrhosis), panhepatic hepatitis, chronic active hepatitis, toxins and drugs, and diseases of the biliary tract as in primary and secondary biliary cirrhosis.

In addition, systemic diseases can predispose to cirrhosis. In *hemochromatosis*, for example, excess iron becomes deposited in a variety of tissues including liver and becomes toxic to hepatocytes, predisposing to cirrhosis. This disease is caused by single amino acid substitutions, most commonly tyrosine for cysteine 282, in the protein product of the HFE gene on chromosome 6 (Feder, 1996; Crawford, 1998a). This protein is thought to be involved in the interaction of transferrin with the transferrin receptor (Zhou, 1998b), and amino acid substitutions like C282Y, induce protein malfunction, resulting in abnormal iron deposition in tissues including liver. More recent work suggests that the HFE protein can regulate intracellular iron storage independently of its interaction with transferrin receptor-1 (TfR1) (Carlson, 2005). Testing for this condition involves determination of the serum iron-binding saturation, which is greater than or equal to 45%. This test has high sensitivity but low specificity, diminishing its screening value. Other tests for this condition include determination of iron content of liver biopsy samples and genetic analysis.

As just discussed, in *Wilson's disease*, copper deposits in liver are also toxic and can also lead to a form of chronic active hepatitis and cirrhosis. In *alpha-1-antitrypsin deficiency*, because of continuing proteolysis in hepatocytes, patients have a significantly increased propensity to develop cirrhosis. Chronic hepatitis due to persistent circulating hepatitis B or C virus and autoimmune disease with elevated ANA or ASMA also predispose to cirrhosis.

In general, irrespective of the cause, cirrhosis is a chronic but gradually worsening condition that can occasionally progress to fulminant hepatic failure as discussed below (Sunheimer, 1994). At its inception, it is often focal and may not be evident clinically.

Diagnosing and Following Cirrhosis, Fibrosis and Necroinflammation of the Liver Non-invasively Using Serum Analytes

The definitive diagnosis of fibrosis and/or necrosis and inflammation of the liver is liver biopsy. Because this invasive procedure carries with it a morbidity such as bleeding and pneumathorax and because the liver biopsy itself has the confounding problem of sampling eTrrors, there has been a search to devise means of diagnosis and following these disease processes non-invasively using the levels of serum analytes that measure liver function. The first of these was the "PGA index" (Poynard, 1991), computed from the prothrombin time (PT), and serum levels of gamma-glutamyl transferase and apolipoprotein A1. Ranges of values for each of these analytes are divided into four categories, numbered 0–4, in increasing order of severity. For example, GGT values between 20–49 are scored as 1, values between 50–99 are scored 2, etc. For apo-A1, increasing severity of disease correlates with decreasing concentration of this protein in serum. The prothrombin time increases with severity of disease because the liver is the sole site for synthesis of coagulation factors. These scores are then summed to give the PGA index. Higher PGA scores have been found to correlate with the degree of hepatic fibrosis and with the severity of cirrhosis as judged both by clinical grading and from liver biopsies (Teare, 1993). This index also has a good correlation with the level of pro-collagen type III pro-peptide (PIIIP) in serum, also used to follow active cirrhosis.

More recently, other indices have been developed that appear to be more effective. These include the Fibrotest and the Actitest index (Poynard, 2005) that utilize the measurement of six analyte levels, i.e., apolipoprotein A1, GGT (these two analytes also being in the PGA index), haptoglobin, total bilirubin, alpha-2 macroglobulin and ALT and also include the patient's age and gender. The correlations with liver biopsy results are then performed using an artificial intelligence algorithm. Scores for the Fibrotest component are computed on a scale of 0 to 1.0 corresponding to histopathological staging system, called METAVIR (METAVIR Cooperative Group, 1994), as follows: F0 (no fibrosis): F1 (portal fibrosis); F2, bridging fibrosis with few septae; F3, bridging fibrosis with many septae -F4, frank cirrhosis. Actitest scores are computed likewise on a scale of 0–1.0, using the same parameters except that they are correlated with necroinflammatory activity using a METAVIR grading system (Bedossa, 1996) as follows: A0, no activity; A1, minimal activity; A2, moderate activity; A3, severe activity. These indices are widely used in Europe but thus far not in the United States. There is some disagreement as to the efficacy of these indices in diagnosing and following liver fibrosis and necrosis/inflammatory activity. For example, in one study (Rossi, 2003) on 125 patients with hepatitis C, serum sample were obtained and assayed for the six analytes in the Fibro-and Actitests. Using the cutoffs of < 0.1, to signify minimal fibrosis and > 0.6 to indicate severe fibrosis, of 33 patients with a score of < 0.1, six (18 percent) were found to have significant fibrosis while of 24 patients with scores > 0.6, five (21 percent) were found to have mild fibrosis on biopsy. On the other hand, in another similar study of over 300 patients with Hepatitis C, for whom analyses were performed prior to and after a treatment regimen using anti-viral agents, high values (almost 0.8) for the areas under the receiver-operator curves (see Chapter 7) were found before pre- and post-treatment. The overall sensitivity (Chapter 7) of the method was 90 percent, and the positive predictive value was 88 percent. These values indicate that the index is of value in detecting fibrosis. It has been pointed out that false positive results may occur as the result of treatment for hepatitis C with ribavirin since this drug can induce hemolysis, thereby reducing haptoglobin and increasing unconjugated bilirubin, both of which will change the index in a manner unrelated to increasing liver fibrosis. Other conditions that are unrelated to liver fibrosis that can change the index are Gilbert's Disease, extra-hepatic cholestasis and acute inflammation. With these caveats, Poynard has estimated that 18 percent of discordances between liver biopsy and Fibro- and Actitest results are due to sampling erros on liver biopsy, a known problem with this procedure and that 2 percent were due to the test (Poynard, 2004). Other investigators have concluded from studies that there is a need for standardization of methodologies so that all testing laboratories obtain similar values for individual test results (Rosenthal-Allieri, 2005) and a need for large prospective studies (Afdhal, 2004).

Other indices (reviewed and evaluated in Parkes, 2006) have also been developed and include the FIBROSpect II index based on tissue inhibitors of metalloproteinases, alpha-2 macroglobulin and hyaluranic acid, the latter appearing to give better correlations with liver fibrosis than procollagen type III peptide mentioned above; the international normalized ratio (INR); platelet count; ratio of AST to ALT; AST-platelet ratio index (APRI) and the Forns index that correlates age, platelet count, GGT and cholesterol with extent of liver fibrosis (Forns, 2002). These appear to have similar although somewhat lower sensitivities and/or specificities than the Fibro- and Actitest (Thabut, 2003). It seems clear that these non-invasive tests with proper refinement hold promise of becoming reliable in diagnosing liver fibrosis and necrosis and in following these conditions with respect to treatment efficacy.

Biochemical and Clinical Correlations of Cirrhosis

As cirrhosis progresses to involve most (> 80%) of the liver parenchyma, liver function becomes compromised. Total protein synthesis drops to low levels as does synthesis of albumin. Portal hypertension, together with the drop in colloid osmotic pressure, results in ascites and even anasarca. Compression of the intrahepatic bile ductules and cholangioles results in diminished excretion of bilirubin and bile salts, causing hyper-bilirubinemia and a rise in alkaline phosphatase, GGT and 5'-nucleotidase. The serum concentrations of hepatocyte enzymes, like AST, ALT and LD are either normal or diminished. If injury to viable hepatocytes is ongoing, the levels of these enzymes in serum may become mildly elevated.

In more advanced stages of cirrhosis, serum ammonia levels become significantly elevated and correlate roughly with the degree of encephalopathy. There are four clinically graded levels of hepatic encephalopathy: motor tremors detected as asterixis, in which the hands of the patient when pressed back and then released, move back and forth in a flapping motion; a lethargic, stuporous state; severe obtundation; and frank coma. Lowering ammonia levels reduces the degree of encephalopathy. More recently, earlier signs of encephalopathy have been observed including the sleep disturbance and abnormal results on neuropsychiatric tests.

Since the liver is the site of synthesis of all of the coagulation factors except von Willebrand factor, and there is markedly diminished synthesis of these factors in cirrhosis, coagulation disorders result, as discussed above. Accelerated partial thromboplastin and prothrombin times become prolonged, often accompanied by diminished platelet counts. The latter may be caused by splenic sequestration due to splenomegaly caused by portal hypertension. However, disseminated intravascular coagulopathy may occur in cirrhosis as evidenced by high levels of D-dimer and fibrin split products in serum and may be the cause of the diminished platelet count. Because of derangements in lipid metabolism in the liver, fats enter the circulation and become deposited in erythrocyte membranes, causing these cells to appear as target cells.

Loss of vascular volume from ascites and anasarca can cause low tissue perfusion and lactic acidosis. Volume receptors, sensitive to volume loss, stimulate the secretion of antidiuretic hormone (ADH). The retained water causes serodilution, leading to hyponatremia.

Cirrhosis of the liver is often associated with renal failure as a result of the hepatorenal syndrome. In this condition, which is not well-understood, renal tubular function is compromised. Serum BUN and creatinine rise to markedly elevated levels indicating renal failure. Low tissue perfusion may also cause acute tubular necrosis. In hepatorenal syndrome, restoration of liver function generally reverses the renal failure.

Primary and secondary biliary cirrhosis have been discussed previously in this chapter. The diagnosis of these conditions is made difficult by the changing pattern of serum analyte concentrations used to evaluate liver status. Usually beginning as an obstructive pattern, in which alkaline phosphatase and sometimes bilirubin are elevated the pattern progresses to one which resembles hepatitis due to the toxic effects of bile salts on hepatocytic function. With time, this pattern gives way to a cirrhotic pattern in which the aminotransferases decrease, total protein and albumin decrease, and ammonia rises. In patients with a persistent obstructive pattern indicated by laboratory results, with no evidence of mass lesions or stones causing blockage of bile flow, the presence of anti-M2 antimitochondrial antibody should be ascertained. Increased titers of this antibody are virtually 100% diagnostic of primary biliary cirrhosis. In addition, assays for serum pANCA antibodies should be performed to detect secondary biliary cirrhosis which can also produce a cholestatic pattern.

Survival for patients with primary biliary cirrhosis may be computed using an empirical formula, analogous to the MELD score discussed above, that utilizes the age of the patient, the serum albumin and bilirubin, the prothrombin time (as in the MELD score), and the extent of edema (Dickson, 1989). This formula gives an estimate of the time limit when the patient may undergo liver transplantation.

Posthepatic and Posthepatocytic Biliary Obstruction

Posthepatic biliary obstruction refers to blockage of the intrahepatic, and extrahepatic ducts and/or to the blockage of bilirubin excretion from the hepatocyte into the canaliculi, leading to back-flow of bile into the hepatocyte and ultimately into the circulation. The most common cause of this condition is cholelithiasis. Other causes include primary biliary cirrhosis and primary sclerosing cholangitis as discussed above, inflammation of the biliary tract, as occurs in ascending cholangitis and in Gram-negative sepsis. Drugs, such as the neuroleptics, like chlorpromazine, can cause cholestatic jaundice. Mass lesions such as carcinoma of the head of the pancreas or lymphoma can also cause posthepatic biliary obstruction by blocking the common bile duct at the porta hepatis. These conditions cause elevated bilirubin, most of it direct, ALP and GGT. Often, however, especially in inflammatory conditions in the biliary tract, there is an incomplete obstruction to bile flow, resulting in partial flow of bile. Under these conditions, bilirubin remains normal or is only mildly increased. However, alkaline phosphatase, GGT and 5'-nucleotidase become significantly elevated.

Occasionally, hyperbilirubinemia may be observed in patients who are otherwise normal. The bilirubin is of the indirect type and most often results from hemolysis, most often in hemolytic anemia. Hemolytic anemias may be triggered by hepatic disease. For example, viral hepatitis may precipitate hemolysis in patients with glucose-6-phosphate dehydrogenase deficiency. In Zieve's syndrome, hemolysis occurs in conjunction with alcoholic hepatitis and hyperlipidemia. Wilson's disease is sometimes associated with acute hemolysis. Patients with chronic hepatitis secondary to autoimmune disease may develop severe hemolytic disease, sometimes requiring splenectomy.

Space-Occupying Lesions

In space-occupying lesions of the liver, a high percentage of which are due to metastatic cancer, a smaller percentage to lymphoma, primary hepatocellular carcinoma, and angiosarcoma of the liver, and a small percentage to benign lesions like hemangioma of the liver, the cardinal finding is isolated increases in the two enzymes, LD and alkaline phosphatase. Increases in the latter are caused by encroachments of the mass(es) on canaliculi and cholangioles and even on the main bile ducts. The reasons for increases in LD are not clear. Most commonly, it is the LD_5 fraction that is responsible for the increase. This fraction may be produced by the liver but also may be produced by tumors. Typically, the values for LD are 500–1000 IU/L or more and for alkaline phosphatase, > 500 IU/L. If a malignant tumor spreads widely through the liver, there may be a mild elevation in the aminotransferases, along with hyperbilirubinemia due to bile duct obstruction, and low protein and albumin. The latter findings may not be caused as much by liver dysfunction as by generalized cachexia associated with tumor spread. A number of cancers that originate in the liver can be identified using serodiagnostic tests. For example, as discussed in the alpha-fetoprotein (AFP) section in this chapter, serum levels of AFP are elevated in hepatocellular carcinoma. As discussed in Part IX of this book, angiosarcomas can be diagnosed using specific antibodies to mutated *ras*-p21 protein.

Fulminant Hepatic Failure

In acute fulminant hepatic failure, an uncommon but highly fatal condition, there is massive destruction of liver tissue resulting in complete liver failure. Depending on the nature and extent of the destruction, ultimate liver regeneration frequently does not occur, although if the cell death is limited and if hepatocytes can recover from the acute injury, normal liver function may return. The causes of this condition are largely unknown. Reye's syndrome is an example of this condition in which a child has an acute viral infection with fever and is treated with aspirin. Within 1–2 weeks after the infection and fever have dissipated, the child suddenly becomes encephalopathic secondary to hyperammonemia caused by acute hepatic failure. An adult form of Reye's syndrome has also been described. Other possible causes of fulminant hepatic failure include acute hepatitis B with hepatitis D superinfection, Budd–Chiari syndrome and other hepatic vein thrombotic conditions, vascular hypoperfusion of the liver, ileojejunal bypass for obesity, tylenol intoxication, alcoholism, and cirrhosis. Another significant predisposing condition is the fatty liver of pregnancy (Sunheimer, 1994).

There are two histopathologic forms of fulminant hepatic failure: panhepatic necrosis, in which all hepatocytes have become necrotic, and microvesicular steatosis in which there is sinusoidal enlargement and cholestasis. The latter is most commonly observed in Reye's syndrome and the fatty liver of pregnancy. It is important to note that, since the microvesicular steatosis pattern often shows only minimal changes histologically, liver biopsy is unrevealing. It is necessary to rely on laboratory analysis of liver function for a definitive diagnosis, as described below.

Many of the pathophysiologic sequelae of cirrhosis also occur in fulminant hepatic failure (Sunheimer, 1994). Patients develop ascites and become encephalopathic due to hyperammonemia. Total serum protein and serum albumin are depressed. Virtually all of the patients with fulminant hepatic failure exhibit severe coagulopathies, particularly disseminated intravascular coagulopathy, and virtually all are anemic. All develop renal failure because of the hepatorenal syndrome and acute tubular necrosis.

In addition, many of these patients become hypoglycemic, possibly because of the absence of enzymes involved in glycogenolysis. Lactic acidosis also develops because of poor tissue perfusion. Interestingly, unlike in cirrhosis, in which the patients become hyponatremic, patients with fulminant hepatic failure may become *hyper*natremic and hypokalemic. This observation may be explained by the finding that circulating levels of aldosterone in the serum of some of these patients are quite high (Sunheimer, 1994). Perhaps the failure of the liver to clear aldosterone from the circulation results in the observed high levels of this hormone.

Diagnostic laboratory findings for fulminant hepatic failure are rapid increases in serum levels of the aminotransferases to markedly elevated levels, such that AST, which can reach levels of over 20 000 IU/L, is at least 1.5 times greater in value than ALT. While these enzymes rise in value, the total protein and albumin become markedly depressed. Overall, this pattern resembles hepatitis and end-stage cirrhosis combined except that usually in acute hepatitis, save alcoholic hepatitis, AST and ALT rise in a ratio of about 1 : 1 or in a ratio that favors ALT. Shortly after these patterns occur, serum ammonia increases rapidly, leading to encephalopathy. LD, alkaline phosphatase and bilirubin all increase markedly. All of the changes described previously occur over a period of about 1 week. After another week, the serum AST and ALT return to low, sometimes undetectable, levels. This finding signifies complete destruction of all viable liver tissue (Sunheimer, 1994).

Patients whose AST and ALT undergo the stereotypical changes described should be observed closely for fulminant hepatic failure, especially if there is any indication of encephalopathy. Though supportive therapy can sometimes result in restoration of normal liver function, for most patients in fulminant hepatic failure, the only ultimate cure is liver transplantation.

References

Afdhal NH, Nunes D: Evaluation of liver fibrosis: a concise review. Am J Gastroenterol 2004; 99:1160–1174.

Aldenhovel HG: The influence of long-term anticonvulsant therapy with diphenylhydantoin and carbamazepine on serum gamma-glutamyltransferase, aspartate aminotransferase, alanine aminotransferase and alkaline phosphatase. Eur Arch Psychiatry Neurol Sci 1988; 237:312–316.

Alter HJ: New kit on the block: Evaluation of second-generation assays for detection of antibody to the hepatitis C virus. Hepatology 1992a; 15:350–353.

Alter MJ, Kruszon-Moran D, Nainan OV, et al: The prevalence of hepatitis C virus infection in the United States, 1988 through 1994. N Engl J Med 1999; 341:556–562.

Alter MJ, Margolis HS, Krawczynski K, et al: The natural history of community acquired hepatitis C in the United States. The Sentinel Counties Chronic non-A, non-B Hepatitis Study Team. N Engl J Med 1992b; 327:1899–1905.

Aoki SK, Finegold D, Kuramoto IK, et al: Significance of antibody to hepatitis B core antigen in blood donors as determined by their serologic response to hepatitis B vaccine. Transfusion 1993; 33:362–367.

Aoyagi K, Iida K, Matsunaga Y, et al: Performance of a conventional enzyme immunoassay for hepatitis C virus core antigen in the early phases of hepatitis C infection. Clin Lab 2001; 47:119–127.

Arvan D, Shirey TL: Conjugated bilirubin: A better indicator of impaired hepatobiliary excretion than direct bilirubin. Ann Clin Lab Sci 1985; 15:252–259.

Barrera JM, Francis B, Ercilla G, et al: Improved detection of anti-HCV in post-transfusion hepatitis by a third-generation ELISA. Vox Sang 1995; 68:15–18.

Batshaw ML: Inborn errors of urea synthesis. Ann Neurol 1994; 35:133–141.

Beld M, Penning M, van Putten M, et al: Quantitative antibody responses to structural (core) and nonstructural (NS3, NS4, and NS5) hepatitis C virus proteins among seroconverting injecting drug users: Impact of epitope variation and relationship to detection of HCV RNA in blood. Hepatology 1999; 29:1288–1298.

Belfrage P, Berg B, Hagerstrand I, et al: Alterations of lipid metabolism in healthy volunteers during long-term ethanol intake. Eur J Clin Invest 1977; 7:127–131.

Bellentani S, Tabarroni G, Barchi T, et al: Effect of ursodeoxycholic acid treatment on alanine aminotransferase and gamma-glutamyltranspeptidase serum levels in patients with hypertransaminasemia. Results from a double-blind controlled trial. J Hepatol 1989; 8:7–12.

Berg PA, Klein R, Lindenborn-Fotinos JL: Antimitochondrial antibodies in primary biliary cirrhosis. J Hepatol 1986; 2:123–131.

Berk PD, Noyer C: Structure, formation, and sources of bilirubin and its transport in plasma. Semin Liver Dis 1994a; 14:325–330.

Berk PD, Noyer C: Clinical chemistry and physiology of bilirubin. Semin Liver Dis 1994b; 14:346–351.

Berk PD, Noyer C: The familial unconjugated hyperbilirubinemias. Semin Liver Dis 1994c; 14:356–385.

Berk PD, Noyer C: The familial conjugated hyperbilirubinemias. Semin Liver Dis 1994d; 14:386–394.

Berlin NI, Berk PD: Quantitative aspects of bilirubin metabolism for hematologists. Blood 1981; 57:983–999.

Berman DH, Leventhal RI, Gavaler JS, et al: Clinical differentiation of fulminant Wilsonian hepatitis from other causes of hepatic failure. Gastroenterology 1991; 100:1129–1134.

Binder L, Smith D, Kupka T, et al: Failure of prediction of liver function test abnormalities with the urine urobilinogen and urine bilirubin assays. Arch Pathol Lab Med 1989; 113:73–76.

Bloomer JR, Berk PD, Vergalla J, et al: Influence of albumin on the extravascular distribution of unconjugated bilirubin. Clin Sci Mol Med 1973; 45:517–526.

Bosma PJ, Chowdhury JR, Bakker C, et al: The genetic basis of the reduced expression of bilirubin UDP-glucuronosyltransferase 1 in Gilbert's Syndrome. N Engl J Med 1995; 333:1171–1175.

Brillanti S, Masci C, Miglioli M, Barbara L: Serum IgM antibodies to hepatitis C virus in acute and chronic hepatitis C. Arch Virol Suppl 1993; 8:213–218.

Brown EA, Stapleton JT: Hepatitis A virus. *In* Murray PR (ed): Manual of Clinical Microbiology, 8th ed. Washington, DC, ASM Press, 2003, pp 1452–1463.

Bull PC, Thomas GR, Rommens JM, et al: The Wilson disease gene is a putative copper transporting P-type ATP-ase similar to the Menkes gene. Nat Genet 1993; 5:327–337.

Butterworth RF, Giguere JF, Michaud J, et al: Ammonia: Key factor in the pathogenesis of hepatic encephalopathy. Neurochem Pathol 1987; 6:1–12.

Cabrerizo M, Bartolome J, De Sequera P, et al: Hepatitis B virus DNA in serum and blood cells of hepatitis B surface antigen-negative hemodialysis patients and staff. J Am Soc Nephrol 1997; 8:1443–1447.

Cacciola I, Pollicino T, Squadrito G, et al: Occult hepatitis B virus infection in patients with chronic hepatitis C liver disease. N Engl J Med 1999; 341:22–26.

Carey MC, Cahalane MJ: Enterohepatic circulation. *In* Arias IM, Jakoby WB, Popper H, et al: (eds): The Liver: Biology and Pathobiology, 2nd ed. New York, Raven Press, 1988, pp 573–616.

Carlson H, Zhang AS, Fleming WH, Enns CA: The hereditary hemochromatosis protein, HFE, lowers intracellular iron levels independently of transferrin receptor 1 in TRVb cells. Blood 2005; 105(6):2564–2570. Epub 2004.

Carmel R, Wong ET, Weiner JM, et al: Racial differences in serum total bilirubin levels in health and in disease (pernicious anemia). JAMA 1985; 253:3416–3418.

Chapman RW, Cottone M, Selby WS, et al: Serum autoantibodies, ulcerative colitis and primary sclerosing cholangitis. Gut 1986; 27:86–91.

Chappell S, Guetta-Baranes T, Batowski K, et al: Haplotypes of the alpha-1 antitrypsin gene in healthy controls and Z deficiency patients. Hum Mutat 2004; 24:535–536.

Chowdhury JR, Wolkoff AW, Arias IM: Heme and bile pigment metabolism. *In* Arias IM, Jakoby WB, Popper H, et al: (eds): The Liver: Biology and Pathobiology, 2nd ed. New York, Raven Press, 1988, pp 419–449.

Collins D, Goold MF, Rosalki SB, et al: Plasma intestinal alkaline phosphatase and intermediate molecular mass gamma glutamyltransferase activities in the differential diagnosis of jaundice. J Clin Pathol 1987; 40:1252–1255.

Coppel RL, McNeilage LJ, Surh CD, et al: Primary structure of the human M2 mitochondrial autoantigen of primary biliary cirrhosis: Dihydrolipoamide acetyl transferase. Proc Natl Acad Sci USA 1988; 85:7317–7321.

Crawford DH, Jazwinska EC, Cullen LM, Powell LW: Expression of HLA-linked hemochromatosis in subjects homozygous or heterozygous for the C282Y mutation. Gastroenterology 1988a; 114:1003–1008.

Crawford JM, Hauser SC, Gollan JL: Formation, hepatic metabolism, and transport of bile pigments: A status report. Semin Liver Dis 1988b; 8:105–118.

Czaja AJ: Autoimmune hepatitis: Evolving concepts and treatment strategies. Dig Dis Sci 1995a; 40:435–456.

Czaja AJ, Ming C, Shirai M, Nishioka M: Frequency and significance of antibodies to histones in autoimmune hepatitis. J Hepatol 1995b; 23:32–38.

Czaja AJ, Shiels MT, Taswell HF, et al: Frequency and significance of immunoglobulin M antibody to hepatitis B core antigen in corticosteroid-treated severe chronic active hepatitis B. Mayo Clin Proc 1988; 63:119–125.

da Fonseca-Wollheim F: Preanalytical increase of ammonia in blood specimens from healthy subjects. Clin Chem 1990; 36:1483–1487.

Davies SM, Szabo E, Wagner JE, et al: Idiopathic hyperammonemia: A frequently lethal complication of bone marrow transplantation. Bone Marrow Transplant 1996; 17:1119–1125.

Dickson ER, Grambsch PM, Fleming TR, et al: Prognosis in primary biliary cirrhosis: Model for decision making. Hepatology 1989; 10:1–7.

Doumas BT, Wu TW: The measurement of bilirubin fractions in serum. Crit Rev Clin Lab Sci 1991; 28:415–445.

Doumas BT, Wu TW, Jendrzejczak B: Delta bilirubin: Absorption spectra, molar absorptivity, and reactivity in the diazo reaction. Clin Chem 1987; 33:769–774.

Dufour DR: Gender related differences in liver function and integrity tests. Clin Chem 1998a; 44:A137.

Dufour DR: Effects of habitual exercise on routine laboratory tests. Clin Chem 1998b; 44:A136.

Dufour JF, Kaplan MM: Muddying the water: Wilson's disease challenges will not soon disappear. Gastroenterology 1997; 113:348–350.

Dufour DR, Teot L: Laboratory identification of ischemic hepatitis (shock liver). Clin Chem 1988c; 34:A1287.

Erker JC, Desai SM, Schlauder GG, et al: A hepatitis E virus variant from the United States: Molecular characterization and transmission in cynomolgus macaques. J Gen Virol 1999; 80:681–690.

Farnsworth N, Fagan SP, Berger DH, Awad SS: Child-Turcotte-Pugh versus MELD score as a predictor of outcome after elective and emergent surgery in cirrhotic patients. Am J Surg 2004; 188:580–583.
This is an excellent survey of the efficacy of different predictive methods for patients with cirrhosis.

Feder JN, Gnirke A, Thomas W, et al: A novel MHC class I-like gene is mutated in patients with hereditary haemochromatosis. Nat Genet 1996; 13:399–408.

Fevery J, Blanckaert N: What can we learn from analysis of serum bilirubin? J Hepatol 1986; 2:113–121.

Forns X, Ampurdance S, Llovet JM, et al: Identification of chronic hepatitis C patients without hepatic fibrosis by a simple predictive model. Hepatology 2002; 36:986–992.

Fuchs S, Bogomolski-Yahalom V, Paltiel O, Ackerman Z: Ischemic hepatitis: Clinical and laboratory observations of 34 patients. J Clin Gastroenterol 1998; 26:183–186.

Fujiwara K, Yokosuka O, Ehata T, et al: Frequent detection of hepatitis A viral RNA in serum during the early convalescent phase of acute hepatitis A. Hepatology 1997; 26:1634–1639.

Fussey SP, Guest JR, James OFW, et al: Identification and analysis of the major M2 autoantigens in primary biliary cirrhosis. Proc Natl Acad Sci USA 1988; 85:8654–8658.

Gottesman MM, Ambudkar SV: Overview: ABC transporters and human disease. J Bioenerg Biomembr 2001; 33:453–458.
This is a succinct discussion of the family of transporter proteins that share homology within the ATP-binding cassette (ABC)

region and contain transmembrane domains involved in recognition of substrates, which are transported across, into, and out of cell membranes, including the bilirubin glucuronides that are secreted by an ABC protein in the canaliculi.

Hayashi PH, Beames MP, Kuhns MC, et al: Use of quantitative assays for hepatitis B e antigen and IgM antibody to hepatitis B core antigen to monitor therapy in chronic hepatitis B. Am J Gastroenterol 1996; 91:2323–2328.

Heubi JE, Daugherty CC, Partin JC, et al: Grade 1 Reye's syndrome – outcome and predictors of progression to deeper coma grades. N Engl J Med 1984; 311:1539–1542.

Hoofnagle JH: Hepatitis C: The clinical spectrum of disease. Hepatology 1997; 26(3 Suppl 1):15S–20S.

Horvat RT, Tegtmeier GE: Hepatitis B and D viruses. *In* Murray PR (ed): Manual of Clinical Microbiology, 8th edition. Washington DC, ASM Press, 2003, pp 1480–1494.

Howanitz JH, Howanitz PJ, Skrodzki CA, Iwanski JA: Influences of specimen processing and storage conditions on results for plasma ammonia. Clin Chem 1984; 30:906–908.

Huizenga JR, Tangerman A, Gips CH: Determination of ammonia in biological fluids. Ann Clin Biochem 1994; 31:529–543.

Ihara H, Nakamura H, Aoki Y, et al: Effects of serum-isolated vs. synthetic bilirubin-albumin complexes on dye-binding methods for estimating serum albumin. Clin Chem 1991; 31:1269–1272.

Ihara H, Shino Y, Hashizume N, et al: Effect of light on total and direct bilirubin by an enzymatic bilirubin oxidase method. J Anal Bio Sci 1997; 20:349–354.

Johnson PJ, McFarlane IG, Alvarez F, et al: Meeting report: International Autoimmune Hepatitis Group. Hepatology 1993; 18:998–1005.

Johnston M, Harrison L, Moffatt K, et al: Reliability of the international normalized ratio for monitoring the induction phase of warfarin: Comparison with the prothrombin time ratio. J Lab Clin Med 1996; 128:214–217.

Kaplan MM, Gandolfo JV, Quaroni EG: An enzyme-linked immunosorbent assay (ELISA) for detecting antimitochondrial antibody. Hepatology 1984; 4:727–730.

Kelly DA, Summerfield JA: Hemostasis in liver disease. Semin Liv Dis 1987; 7:182–191.

Kelly DA, Tuddenham EGD: Hemostatic problems in liver disease. Gut 1986; 27:339–349.

Kim NK, Yasmineh WG, Freier EF, et al: Value of alkaline phosphatase, 5'nucleotidase, gamma-glutamyltransferase, and glutamate dehydrogenase activity measurements (single and combined) in serum in diagnosis of metastasis to the liver. Clin Chem 1977; 23:2034–2038.

Koff RS: Seroepidemiology of hepatitis A in the United States. J Infect Dis 1995; 171(Suppl 1):S19–S23.

Kovacs MJ, Wong A, MacKinnon K, et al: Assessment of the validity of the INR system for patients with liver impairment. Thromb Haemost 1994; 71:727–730.

Kozaki N, Shimizu S, Higashijima H, et al: Significance of serum delta-bilirubin in patients with obstructive jaundice. J Surg Res 1998; 79:61–65.

Krams SM, Surh CD, Coppel RL, et al: Immunization of experimental animals with dihydrolipoamide acetyltransferase, as a purified recombinant polypeptide, generates mitochondrial antibodies but not primary biliary cirrhosis. Hepatology 1989; 9:411–416.

Kraemer D, Scheurlen M: Gilbert disease and Type I and II Crigler–Najjar syndrome due to mutations in the same UGT1A1 gene locus. Med Klin (German) 2002; 15:528–532.

Krajden M, Shivji R, Gunadasa K, et al: Evaluation of the core antigen assay as a second-line supplemental test for diagnosis of active hepatitis C virus infection. J Clin Microbiol 2004; 42:4054–4059.

Langner C, Denk H: Wilson disease. Virchows Arch 2004; 445:111–118.

LaPerche S, Courouce AM, Lemaire JM, et al: GB virus type C/hepatitis G virus infection in French blood donors with anti-NS5 isolated reactivities by recombinant immunoblot assay for hepatitis C virus. Transfusion 1999; 39:790–791.

Laskus T, Radkowski M, Wang LF, et al: Lack of evidence for hepatitis G virus replication in the livers of patients coinfected with hepatitis C and G viruses. J Virol 1997; 71:7804–7806.

Lau JY, Mizokami M, Kolberg JA, et al: Application of six hepatitis C virus genotyping systems to sera from chronic hepatitis C patients in the United States. J Infect Dis 1995; 171:281–289.

Lauff JJ, Kasper ME, Wu TW, Ambrose RT: Isolation and preliminary characterization of a fraction of bilirubin that is firmly bound to protein. Clin Chem 1982; 28:629–637.

Lednar WM, Lemon SM, Kirkpatrick JW, et al: Frequency of illness associated with epidemic hepatitis A virus infections in adults. Am J Epidemiol 1985; 122:226–233.

Lewis M, Howdle PD: The Neurology of Liver Failure. QJM 2003; 96:623–633.

Lo DH, Wu TW: Assessment of the fundamental accuracy of the Jendrassik-Grof total and direct bilirubin assays. Clin Chem 1983; 29:31–36.

London WT, Evans AA: The epidemiology of hepatitis viruses B, C, and D. Clin Lab Med 1996; 16:251–271.

Lotfy M, El-Kady IM, Nasif WA, et al: Distinct serum immunoglob pattern in Egyptian patients with chronic HCV infection analyzed by nephelometry. J Immunoassay Immunochem 2006; 27:103–114.

Lunel F, Cresta P, Vitour D, et al: Comparative evaluation of hepatitis C virus RNA quantitation by branched DNA, NASBA, and monitor assays. Hepatology 1999; 29:528–535.

McDonagh AF, Palma LA, Lauff JJ, et al: Origin of mammalian biliprotein and rearrangement of bilirubin glucuronides in vivo in the rat. J Clin Invest 1984; 74:763–770.

McHutchison JG, Gordon SC, Schiff ER, et al: Interferon alfa-2b or in combination with ribavirin as initial treatment for chronic hepatitis C. Hepatitis Interventional Therapy Group. N Engl J Med 1998; 339:1485–1492.

McHutchison JG, Poynard T, Gordon SC, et al: The impact of race on response to anti-viral therapy in patients with chronic hepatitis C. Hepatology 1999; 30:A302.

McMahon BJ, Alward WL, Hall DB, et al: Acute hepatitis B virus infection: Relation of age to the clinical expression of disease and subsequent development of the carrier state. J Infect Dis 1985; 151:599–603.

Manns M, Gerken G, Kyriatsoulis A, et al: Two different subtypes of antimitochondrial antibodies are associated with primary biliary cirrhosis: Identification and characterization by radioimmunoassay and immunoblotting. Hepatology 1987; 7:893–899.

Maruo Y, Addario C, Mori A, et al: Two linked polymorphic mutations [A(TA) 7TAA and T3279G] of UGT1A1 as the principal cause of Gilbert syndrome. Hum Genet 2004; 115:525–526.

Mast EE, Alter MJ, Holland PV, Purcell RH: Evaluation of assays for antibody to hepatitis E virus by a serum panel. Hepatitis E Virus Antibody Serum Panel Evaluation Group. Hepatology 1998; 27:857–861.

Matsumoto A, Yeo AE, Shih JW, et al: Transfusion-associated TT virus infection and its relationship to liver disease. Hepatology 1999; 30:283–288.

Moss DW: Physicochemical and pathophysiological factors in the release of membrane-bound alkaline phosphatase from cells. Clin Chim Acta 1997; 257:133–140.

Moussavian SN, Becker RC, Piepmeyer JL, et al: Serum gamma-glutamyl transpeptidase and chronic alcoholism. Influence of alcohol ingestion and liver disease. Dig Dis Sci 1985; 30:211–214.

Mulder AH, Horst G, Haagsma EB, et al: Prevalence and characterization of neutrophil cytoplasmic antibodies in autoimmune liver diseases. Hepatology 1993; 17:411–417.

Nagaoka S, Yatsuhashi H, Hamada H, et al: The des-gamma-carboxy prothrombin index is a new prognostic indicator for hepatocellular carcinoma. Cancer 2003; 98:2671–2677.

Nalpas B, Vassault A, Charpin S, et al: Serum mitochondrial aspartate aminotransferase as a marker of chronic alcoholism: Diagnostic value and interpretation in a liver unit. Hepatology 1986; 6:608–614.

Nguyen TT, Sedghi-Vaziri A, Wilkes LB, et al: Fluctuations in viral load (HCV RNA) are relatively insignificant in untreated patients with chronic HCV infection. J Viral Hepat 1996; 3:75–78.

Nista EC, Fini L, Armuzzi A, et al: ^{13}C-breath tests in the study of microsomal liver function. Eur Rev Med Pharmacol Sci 2004; 8:33–46.

Notter D: Bilirubin. In Siest G, Schiele F, Henny J, et al: (eds): Interpretation of Clinical Laboratory Tests. Foster City, CA, Biomedical Publications, 1985.

Nyblom H, Berggren U, Balldin J, Olsson R: High AST/ALT ratio may indicate advanced alcoholic liver disease rather than heavy drinking. Alcohol Alcohol 2004; 39:336–339.

Onishi S, Isobe K, Itoh S, et al: Metabolism of bilirubin and its photoisomers in newborn infants during phototherapy. J Biochem (Tokyo) 1986; 100:789–795.

Palmer M, Schaffner F: Effect of weight reduction on hepatic abnormalities in overweight patients. Gastroenterology 1990; 99:1408–1413.

Panteghini M: Aspartate aminotransferase isoenzymes. Clin Biochem 1990; 23:311–319.

Parkes J, Guha IN, Roderick P, et al: Performance of serum marker panels for liver fibrosis in chronic hepatitis C 2006; 44:462–474.

Paulusma CC, Kool M, Bosma PJ, et al: A mutation in the human canalicular multispecific organic anion transporter gene causes the Dubin–Johnson syndrome. Hepatology 1997; 25:1539–1542.

Pawlotsky JM, Lonjon I, Hezode C, et al: What strategy should be used for diagnosis of hepatitis C virus infection in clinical laboratories? Hepatology 1998; 27:1700–1702.

Persico P, Persico E, Bakker C, et al: Hyperbilirubinemia in subjects with Gilbert syndrome (GS) mutations is determined by the rate of hepatic uptake of organic anions. Hepatology 1999; 30:A501.

Pincus JH, Cohan JL, Glaser GH: Neurologic complications of internal disease. In Baker AB, Baker LH (eds): Clinical Neurology, New York, Harper and Row, 1991, pp 10–13.

Poynard T, Aubert A, Bedossa P, et al: A simple biological index for detection of alcoholic liver disease in drinkers. Gastroenterology 1991; 100:1397–1402.

Poynard T, Marcellin P, Lee SS, et al: Randomised trial of interferon alpha2b plus ribavirin for 48 weeks or for 24 weeks versus interferon alpha2b plus placebo for 48 weeks for treatment of chronic infection with hepatitis C virus. International Hepatitis Interventional Therapy Group (IHIT). Lancet 1998; 352:1426–1432.

Poynard T, Munteanu M, Imbert-Bismut F, et al: Prospective analysis of discordant results between biochemical markers and biopsy in patients with chronic hepatitis C. Clin Chem 2004; 50:1344–1355.

Propst T, Propst A, Dietze O, et al: Alpha-1-antitrypsin deficiency and liver disease. Dig Dis 1994; 12:139–149.

Rajpert-De Meyts E, Heisterkamp N, Groffen J: Cloning and nucleotide sequence of human gamma-glutamyl transpeptidase. Proc Natl Acad Sci USA 1988; 85:8840–8844.

Ravaggi A, Biasin MR, Infantolino D, Cariani E: Comparison of competitive and non-competitive reverse transcription-polymerase chain reaction (RT-PCR) for the quantification of hepatitis C virus (HCV) RNA. J Virol Methods 1997; 65:123–129.

Reddy KR, Hoofnagle JH, Tong MJ, et al: Racial differences in response to therapy with interferon in chronic hepatitis C. Consensus Interferon Study Group. Hepatology 1999; 30:787–793.

Robert A, Chazouilleres O: Prothrombin time in liver failure: Time, ratio, activity percentage, or international normalized ratio? Hepatology 1996; 24:1392–1394.

Roozendaal C, Van Milligen de Wit AW, Haagsma EB, et al: Antineutrophil cytoplasmic antibodies in primary sclerosing cholangitis: Defined specificities may be associated with distinct clinical features. Am J Med 1998; 105:393–399.

Rosenthal P, Pincus MR, Fink D: Sex and age-related differences of bilirubin in serum. Clin Chem 1984; 30:1380–1382.

Rosenthal-Allieri MA, Peritore ML, Tran A, et al: Analytical variability of the Fibrotest proteins. Clin Biochem 2005; 38:473–478.

Rossi E, Adams L, Prins A, et al: Validation of the FibroTest biochemical markers score in assessing liver fibrosis in hepatitis C patients Clin Chem 2003; 49:450–454.

Rost D, Rudolph G, Kloeters-Plachky P, Stiehl A: Effect of high-dose ursodeoxycholic acid on its biliary enrichment in primary sclerosing cholangitis. Hepatology 2004; 40:693–698.

Saldanha J, Lelie N, Heath A: Establishment of the first international standard for nucleic acid amplification technology (NAT) assays for HCV RNA. WHO Collaborative Study Group. Vox Sang 1999; 76:149–158.

Schlaeger R, Haux P, Kattermann R: Studies on the mechanism of the increase in serum alkaline phosphatase activity in cholestasis: Significance of the hepatic bile acid concentration for the leakage of alkaline phosphatase from rat liver. Enzyme 1982; 28:3–13.

Schlauder GC, Dawson GJ: Hepatitis E virus. In Murray PR (ed): Manual of Clinical microbiology, 8th edition. Washington DC, ASM Press, 2003, pp 1495–1511.

Seeff LB, Beebe GW, Hoofnagle JH, et al: A serologic follow-up of the 1942 epidemic of post-vaccination hepatitis in the United States Army. N Engl J Med 1987; 316:965–970.

Seeff LB, the NHLBI Study Group: Mortality and morbidity of transfusion-associated non-A, non-B hepatitis and type C hepatitis: An NHLBI multi-center study. Hepatology 1994; 20:A204.

Shepard RL, Kraus SE, Babayan RK, Sirosky MB: The role of ammonia toxicity in the post transurethral prostatectomy syndrome. Br J Urol 1987; 60:349–351.

Sheth SG, Flamm SL, Gordon FD, Chopra S: AST/ALT ratio predicts cirrhosis in patients with chronic hepatitis C virus infection. Am J Gastroenterol 1998; 93:44–48.

Shiffman ML, Ferreira-Gonzalez A, Reddy KR, et al: Comparison of three commercially available assays for HCV RNA using the international unit standard: Implications for management of patients with chronic hepatitis C virus infection in clinical practice. Am J Gastroenterol 2003; 98:1159–66.
This is an important summary of the issues concerning standardized international units for assays for hepatitis C.

Shuhart MC, Gretch DR: Hepatitis C and G viruses. In Murray PR (ed): Manual of Clinical Microbiology, 8th edition. Washington, DC, ASM Press, 2003, pp 1480–1494.

Singer AJ, Carracio TR, Mofenson HC: The temporal profile of increased transaminase levels in patients with acetaminophen-induced liver dysfunction. Ann Emerg Med 1995; 26:49–53.

Skinhoj P, Mikkelsen F, Hollinger FB: Hepatitis A in Greenland: Importance of specific antibody testing in epidemiologic surveillance. Am J Epidemiol 1977; 105:140–147.

Stahl J: Studies of the blood ammonia in liver disease. Its diagnostic, prognostic, and therapeutic significance. Ann Intern Med 1963; 58:1–24.

Sveger T: The natural history of liver disease in alpha-1-antitrypsin deficient children. Acta Paediatr Scand 1988; 77:847–851.

Sunheimer R, Capaldo G, Kashanian F, et al: Serum analyte pattern characteristic of fulminant hepatic failure. Ann Clin Lab Sci 1994; 24:101–109.
This describes the major pathophysiological aspects of fulminant hepatic failure and gives a summary of liver function profiles in different liver disease states.

Teckman JH, An JK, Blomenkamp K, et al: Mitochondrial autophagy and injury in the liver in alpha 1-antitrypsin deficiency. Am J Physiol Gastrointest Liver Physiol 2004; 286:G851–G862.

Teare JP, Sherman D, Greenfield SM, et al: Comparison of serum procollagen III peptide concentrations and PGA index for assessment of hepatic fibrosis. Lancet 1993; 342:895–898.

Thabut D, Simon M, Myers RP, et al: Noninvasive prediction of fibrosis in patients with chronic hepatitis C. Hepatology 2003; 37:1220–1221.

Totos G, Gizaris V, Papaevangelou G: Hepatitis A vaccine: Persistence of antibodies 5 years after the first vaccination. Vaccine 1997; 15:1252–1253.

Ts'ao C, Swedlund J, Neofotistos D: Implications of use of low international sensitivity index thromboplastins in prothrombin time testing. Arch Pathol Lab Med 1994; 118:1183–1187.

Trotter JF, Brimhall B, Arjal R, Phillips C: Specific laboratory methodologies achieve higher model for endstage liver disease (MELD) scores for patients listed for liver transplantation. Liver Transpl 2004; 10:995–1000.

Tsujii H, Konig J, Rost D, et al: Exon–intron organization of the human multidrug-resistance protein 2 (MRP2) gene mutated in Dubin–Johnson syndrome. Gastroenterology 1999; 117:653–660.

Turchin A, Wiebe DA, Seely EW, et al: Severe hypercholesterolemia mediated by lipoprotein X in patients with chronic graft-versus-host disease of the liver. Bone Marrow Transplant 2005; 35:85–89.

Van de Water L, Carr JM, Aronson D, McDonagh J: Analysis of elevated fibrinogen degradation product levels in patients with liver disease. Blood 1986; 67:1468–1473.

Van Hootegem P, Fevery J, Blanckaert N: Serum bilirubins in hepatobiliary disease: Comparison with other liver function tests and changes in the post-obstructive period. Hepatology 1985; 5:112–117.

Vernelen K, Claeys H, Verhaert AH, et al: Significance of NS3 and NS5 antigens in screening for HCV antibody. Lancet 1994; 343:853.

Vierling JM, Berk PD, Hoffman AF, et al: Normal fasting-state levels of serum cholyl-conjugated bile acids in Gilbert's syndrome: An aid to the diagnosis. Hepatology 1982; 2:340–343.

Villano SA, Vlahov D, Nelson KE, et al: Persistence of viremia and the importance of long-term follow-up after acute hepatitis C infection. Hepatology 1999; 29:908–914.

Viot M, Thyss A, Schneider M, et al: Alpha 1 isoenzyme of alkaline phosphatases. Clinical importance and value for the detection of liver metastases. Cancer 1983; 52:140–145.

Vossler DG, Wilensky AJ, Cawthon DF, et al: Serum and CSF glutamine levels in valproate-related hyperammonemic encephalopathy. Epilepsia 2002; 43:54–59.

Wenham PR, Horn DB, Smith AF: Multiple forms of gamma-glutamyl-transferase: A clinical study. Clin Chem 1985; 31:569–573.

Whitehead TP, Clarke CA, Whitfield AG: Biochemical and haematological markers of alcohol intake. Lancet 1978; 1:978–981.

Williams AL, Hoofnagle JH: Ratio of serum aspartate to alanine aminotransferase in chronic hepatitis. Relationship to cirrhosis. Gastroenterology 1988; 95:734–739.

Xu SR, Yao EG, Dong ZR, et al: Plasma ammonia in patients with acute leukemia. Chin Med J 1992; 105:713–716.

Yotsuyanagi H, Yasuda K, Iino S, et al: Persistent viremia after recovery from self-limited acute hepatitis B. Hepatology 1998; 27:1377–1382.

Yuki N, Hayashi N, Moribe T, et al: Relation of disease activity during chronic hepatitis C infection to complexity of hypervariable region 1 quasispecies. Hepatology 1997; 25:439–444.

Zhou SL, Gordon RE, Bradbury M, et al: Ethanol up-regulates fatty acid uptake and plasma membrane expression and export of mitochondrial aspartate aminotransferase in Hep G2 cells. Hepatology 1998a; 27:1064–1074.

Zhou XY, Tomatsu S, Fleming RE, et al: HFE gene knockout produces mouse model of hereditary hemochromatosis. Proc Natl Acad Sci USA 1998b; 95.2492–2497.

Zimmerman HJ: Intrahepatic cholestasis. Arch Intern Med 1979; 139:1038–1045.

Zucker SD, Horn PS, Sherman KE: Serum bilirubin levels in the U.S. population: Gender effect and inverse correlation with colorectal cancer. Hepatology 2004; 40:827–835.

CHAPTER 22

Laboratory Diagnosis of Gastrointestinal and Pancreatic Disorders

Martin H. Bluth MD PhD, Rosemarie E. Hardin MD, Scott Tenner MD, Michael E. Zenilman MD, Gregory A. Threatte MD

KEY POINTS

• *Helicobacter pylori* is recognized as the principal cause of gastrointestinal ulcers and gastritis. Serology tests are used to screen for *H. pylori* and noninvasive breath tests or endoscopic biopsy are used to confirm eradication after treatment.

• Serum amylase is the analyte of choice to diagnose acute pancreatitis. Other markers, including lipase, trypsinogen (and metabolites), AST and ALT, can aid in determining etiology and/or diagnosis. Routine laboratory testing is of little value in identifying patients with chronic pancreatitis. Diagnosis relies on imaging techniques (ERCP).

• Laboratory screening for cystic fibrosis should be limited to sweat chloride testing. Genetic analysis should be used as a confirmatory test in specific cases.

• Chronic diarrhea can often be classified as inflammatory, osmotic or secretory in origin or the result of altered bowel motility. Initial stool tests for blood, microbes, fat and leukocytes help determine subsequent testing algorithms.

• IgA deficiency should be considered in patients suspected of having celiac sprue and incorporated in the interpretation of anti-gliadin, anti-endomysium, anti-reticulin, or anti-transglutaminase antibody results.

• Lactose intolerance increases with age. Screening tests for true disaccharidase deficiencies include oral challenge of suspected disaccharides to reproduce the abdominal symptomatology followed by stool analysis. Definitive diagnosis of disaccharidase deficiencies depends on the demonstration of low specific enzyme activity in the mucosa of small intestinal biopsy material.

• p-ANCA and ASCA can be used to distinguish abdominal pain seen in irritable bowel syndrome from inflammatory bowel disease.

• Carcinoid tumor is the most common type of neuroendocrine tumor of the gastrointestinal tract.

• Intraoperative gastrin measurements are useful in identifying whether the abnormal tissue is completely removed in patients undergoing surgery for gastrinomas.

• Screening with fecal occult blood testing can decrease mortality from colon cancer by 15–35%. A variety of factors can create false-positive or false-negative results.

Over the past two decades the practice of gastroenterology has evolved tremendously. Increased expertise with endoscopic techniques has allowed direct visualization and biopsy of pathological lesions, facilitating confirmation of suspected clinical diagnoses such as gastric and duodenal ulcer disease. Although these endoscopic evaluations are invaluable diagnostic modalities, they are expensive, invasive and require the specialized skill of a gastroenterologist. In recent years, clinical practices have continued to evolve with the advent of new laboratory evaluations for noninvasive diagnosis of gastrointestinal and pancreatic disorders. Examples include fecal immunochemical and DNA testing for detection of colon cancer and various serum antibody testing to aid diagnosis of inflammatory bowel disease. The latter gives one the ability to differentiate Crohn's disease from ulcerative colitis, which was previously impossible using the available routine laboratory testing. Furthermore, new laboratory tests with enhanced sensitivity and specificity are replacing older, previously established tests for diagnosis of diseases. One such example is the replacement of fecal chymotrypsin with fecal elastase levels to detect pancreatic insufficiency. Knowledge of these tests, their sensitivity and specificity profiles as well as awareness of false positives and negatives of these tests is crucial to the interpretation of the results, especially to the clinician responsible for appropriate disease management. New non-invasive serum tests are also being explored for clinical utility as screening methods, such as pepsinogen tests for detection of atrophic gastritis and early gastric carcinoma. In this chapter we will present clinically relevant disorders and discuss the utility of laboratory methods in confirming disease, guiding therapeutic interventions, predicting prognosis and monitoring therapy. In this edition, we have chosen to adapt laboratory evaluations to those that most closely reflect common clinical practice in the era of endoscopy and with the advent of the newer diagnostic tests.

Common Gastroenterological Disorders

Gastric Disorders

Peptic Acid Disease

The practical approach to peptic acid disease requires the integration of data supplied by the clinician, endoscopist, radiologist, clinical pathologist, and surgical pathologist. *Helicobacter pylori* has been recognized as the principal cause of duodenitis and duodenal ulcers, as well as being strongly associated with type B chronic antral gastritis, gastric ulcers, nonulcer dyspepsia, gastric carcinoma, and MALTomas (Veldhuyzen van Zanten, 1994; Wotherspoon, 1998; Peterson, 1991; Thiede, 1997). The use of nonsteroidal anti-inflammatory drugs (NSAIDs) causes or aggravates peptic and gastric inflammation and ulceration. Hypersecretory states are a much rarer cause of acid peptic disease. Data gathered by history and physical examination may initially suggest peptic acid disease. Radiologic and/or endoscopic techniques are employed to confirm the diagnoses. Testing for *H. pylori* and hypersecretory states involves laboratory analysis. (For more information see Ch. 56.)

Since *H. pylori* has been shown to be the most important causative agent for peptic ulcer disease, and is significantly associated with multiple other types of upper gastrointestinal (GI) pathology, there has been tremendous research involving its detection and treatment, and the confirmation of pathogen eradication. Within the last decade there have been numerous Food and Drug Administration (FDA)-approved and commercially available products for the detection of this bacterium. A cogent argument has been made that all patients found to harbor this organism should be treated (Graham, 1997). Although the numbers and types of tests will likely continue to grow, tissue sampling, breath tests, and serology are currently the mainstay in the diagnostic armamentarium.

Testing for *H. pylori* often utilizes the organism's ability to produce urease. Radioactive and nonradioactive breath hydrogen tests are examples of noninvasive means for detecting active *H. pylori* infection. Each is sensitive and specific prior to therapy. The incidental use of proton pump inhibitors, antibiotics, or bismuth-containing antacids may lead to false-negative tests. Treatment of *H. pylori* may not lead to complete eradication of the organism. Hydrogen breath tests may be falsely negative if they are performed too soon after treatment, before the bacterial load is great enough to be detected (Atherton, 1994).

Serum antibodies directed against *H. pylori* can be used to detect exposure to *H. pylori*. Enzyme-linked immunosorbent assay (ELISA) tests are available and reliable (Feldman, 1995a, b; van de Wouw, 1996). Although quantitative levels of these antibodies are not currently routinely utilized in the clinical setting to determine whether there is current or past infection, they have been reported to be highly accurate (Lerang, 1998). At present, serology is generally utilized to screen for *H. pylori* and breath tests are used to confirm eradication after treatment unless endoscopy allows collection of tissue for rapid urease testing or histologic review (Megraud, 1997).

Urease-based chemical tests are routinely used to detect *H. pylori* in biopsy specimens obtained via endoscopy. Fresh biopsy specimens obtained via endoscopy are placed into fluids or gels containing urea. The bacterial urease splits the urea, producing ammonia. The change in pH affects a color indicator, thus providing the basis for the detection. Bacterial load will determine the amount of urease present and can affect the rapidity of response. If the load is too low, the test can be falsely negative (Xia, 1994). The test is inexpensive and easy to perform, but it requires endoscopy with its expense and potential risks.

Office-based serologic quick-test kits are available. The accuracy of these kits has been shown to be dependent on the antibody preparations used. Immunoglobulin G (IgG) preparations perform most consistently. Other test qualities such as reproducibility, cost, and ease of utilization are factors to be considered when reviewing each of the many available brands marketed today (Laheij, 1998). Histologic review of biopsy specimens stained with Warthin–Starry or Giemsa's stain remains one of the most frequently employed techniques to determine active infection. Culture of the organism may be inconsistent and is usually not done in routine clinical settings. Stool studies employing antigen enzyme assays and polymerase chain reaction (PCR) methodologies are also commercially available, but efficacy remains controversial (Makristathis, 1998).

Hypersecretory states are suggested by extensive peptic acid disease, especially in the absence of *H. pylori*, and the use of NSAIDs. Failure to respond to the usual doses of histamine-2 (H_2)-receptor blocking agents and proton pump inhibitors also suggests oversecretion of hydrochloric acid. Although gastric analysis remains the 'gold standard' with regard to the amount of acid secreted, it is invasive and used much less frequently. Care must be taken to avoid the use of antisecretory medications for the appropriate time intervals before such testing. H_2-receptor blockers should be held for 48 hours and proton pump inhibitors should be avoided for 7 days. H_2-receptor blockers are available without prescriptions, so patient education is important and clinicians must remember to review all of the medications their patients utilize.

Gastrin levels, with and without secretin stimulation, can be used to diagnose Zollinger–Ellison syndrome, in many cases sparing the patient gastric analysis. Serum gastrin levels greater than 150 ng/L (normal < 100 ng/L), especially with simultaneous gastric pH values of < 3, are highly suggestive of a gastrinoma. For equivocal results, secretin can be given (2 U/kg) intravenously and serial gastrin levels can be drawn at 2, 5, 10, 15, and 20 minutes. An increase in gastrin of more than 100 ng/L (normal increase < 50 ng/L or 50%) is considered a positive test. Octreotide, a synthetic form of somatostatin, has been used for localization of the tumor(s). Radioactive-labeled octreotide binds to somatostatin receptors and can be subsequently localized by scintigraphy. If such tumors are surgically removed, gastrin levels can be used to assess potential success or future recurrence.

Table 22–1 Differential Diagnosis of Hyperamylasemia and Macroamylasemia

Condition	Serum amylase	Serum lipase	Urinary amylase	$C_{am}:C_{cr}$	Serum macroamylase
Pancreatic hyperamylasemia	High	High	High	High	Absent
Salivary hyperamylasemia	High	Normal	Low or normal	Low or normal	Absent
Macroamylasemia type 1	High	Normal	Low	Very low	High
Macroamylasemia type 2	High	Normal	Low or normal	Low	Moderate
Macroamylasemia type 3	Normal	Normal	Normal	Low or normal	Trace

$C_{am}:C_{cr}$ = amylase clearance : creatinine clearance ratio = (urinary amylase/serum amylase) × (serum creatinine/urinary creatinine).

After Kleinman DS, O'Brien JF: Macroamylase. Mayo Clin Proc 1986, 61:69, with permission.

Pancreatic disorders

Macroamylasemia

Macroamylasemia is the term used to describe a condition of persistently elevated serum amylase activity with no apparent clinical symptoms of a pancreatic disorder. It is attributed to the presence of an amylase–macromolecule complex whose larger size precludes its excretion into urine, prolonging its half-life. Macroamylase is a circulating complex of normal amylase linked to an immunoglobulin in most cases and to a polysaccharide in others. The immunoglobulins involved are IgA and IgG. The composition of macroamylases is heterogeneous. Analysis of the complex after acid dissociation revealed that P-type and S-type isoamylases were present in variable proportions. The molecular weight has been estimated at 150 000 to more than 1 million. Macroamylasemia may also occur in hyperamylasemic patients with undiminished urine amylase and in patients with normal serum and urine amylase activity. Serum lipase may also form a complex with circulating immunoglobulins, resulting in macrolipasemia (Zaman, 1994). Table 22–1 shows the distinguishing features of different types of hyperamylasemia.

Macroamylasemia can occur with a frequency of 1.05% in randomly selected patients, 2.56% among persons with hyperamylasemia, and 0.98% in persons with normal serum amylase (Klonoff, 1980). Macroamylasemia per se is not a disease entity because no clinical symptoms consistently accompany it. It is an acquired and benign condition that may occur in apparently healthy individuals and is found more frequently in men than in women. The age at the time of discovery in most patients is in the fifth through seventh decades. The occurrence of macroamylasemia may be an early sign of disease, either as a marker or as a nonspecific disease-induced dysproteinemia with amylase-binding capability, and it may be regarded as one of the immunoglobulin-complexed enzyme disorders.

Clinically, it is important to differentiate macroamylasemia from other conditions associated with hyperamylasemia. A patient with hyperamylasemia, a very low (< 1%) amylase/creatinine clearance ratio, and normal renal function should be considered for the possibility of having macroamylasemia. Definitive identification of macroamylasemia, however, requires direct demonstration of the existence of macroamylase molecules by ultracentrifugation, chromatography, or other physical techniques. A detection method using chromatography has been in use for many years and a rapid and simple assay based on selective precipitation of macroamylase in a polyethylene glycol solution has also been reported (Levitt, 1982).

Acute Pancreatitis

Since the first description in 1929, serum amylase has remained the universal laboratory diagnostic test in the determination of acute pancreatitis (Elman, 1929). Derived from pancreatic acinar cells, the serum amylase level rises over the first 2–12 hours after the onset of acute pancreatitis, peaks at 48 hours and returns to normal within 3–5 days (Zieve, 1964). In the appropriate clinical setting marked by new-onset sharp, 'boring' epigastric pain radiating to back or flanks associated with nausea and vomiting, the serum amylase helps to confirm the suspected diagnosis of acute pancreatitis with a positive predictive value approaching 100%.

Despite high positive and negative predictive values, there are certain clinical situations where the clinician must entertain a degree of skepticism and be aware of the assay's limitations. The sensitivity is limited in patients with hypertriglyceridemia and alcoholism. The specificity is limited by elevations in amylase from inflammatory intra-abdominal processes, parotid and submandibular salivary gland inflammation. Also, decreased clearance can lead to falsely elevated levels in patients with renal insufficiency and normal persons who harbor proteins or polypeptides that are not associated with disease (Smotkin, 2002). Regardless, the serum amylase is accurate in the appropriate clinical setting. Using a cutoff of greater than three times the upper limit of normal will lead to an increased specificity (Steinberg, 1985).

Although serum lipase is derived from pancreatic acinar cells, it rises slightly earlier than amylase, 4–8 hours after the onset of acute pancreatitis, and peaks earlier, at 24 hours (Steinberg, 1985). The serum lipase also lasts longer in the serum, 8–14 days. For these reasons, serum lipase is more sensitive and specific than the serum amylase. However, the utility of serum lipase in acute pancreatitis has been shown to vary due to discrepancies in measurement method, patient selection, and cutoff point (Tietz, 1993).

There is no additional clinical benefit in the determination of serum lipase in a patient with the clinical symptoms of acute pancreatitis and a serum amylase greater than three times the upper limit of normal. The use of a serum lipase in the diagnosis of acute pancreatitis should be reserved to patients with clinical symptoms consistent with the disease and an amylase that is suspected to be falsely low, such as in alcoholics, patients with hypertriglyceridemia, or presenting late with the disease. Due to the additional cost and lack of benefit in the majority of patients, utilizing serum lipase in conjunction with serum amylase as a routine process in the laboratory evaluation of suspected acute pancreatitis should be considered inappropriate.

It is recognized that amylase and lipase may both arise from sources other than the pancreas (Frank, 1999). Thus, utilizing both assays may optimize accuracy (Corsetti, 1993). Others feel that pancreatic isoamylase determination is the most cost-effective method (Sternby, 1996). Due to a lack of a readily available gold standard measurement for the diagnosis of acute pancreatitis and variability of chemical methods, it is difficult to calculate sensitivity and specificity for these enzymes precisely. Recently, urinary dipstick testing for trypsinogen-2 was shown to have a sensitivity of 94% and a specificity of 95% as compared to serum amylase with a sensitivity of 85% and a specificity of 91% with 300 U/L as the upper limit (Kemppainen, 1997). This may provide a rapid screening test under the correct clinical circumstance. A sensitive assay that detects plasma calcitonin precursors is another method that is currently being investigated for the determination of severity of an acute episode of pancreatitis. Abnormal levels can be detected upon admission, usually within hours after the onset of abdominal pain (Ammori, 2003). Plasma calcitonin precursors have been demonstrated to rise significantly with the onset of severe infection and systemic inflammation, as occurs with acute pancreatitis. Furthermore, this rise occurs in a predictable stepwise fashion allowing this serum assay to potentially serve as a marker for disease severity.

Although a considerable number of other enzymes have been examined for their potential clinical role in the diagnosis and prognosis of acute pancreatitis, none has gained widespread clinical use. Additionally, urinary amylase offers no advantage over serum testing and urinary clearance of amylase is not specific (Lankisch, 1977).

Laboratory testing can help distinguish the etiology in patients with acute pancreatitis. Management decisions to prevent a recurrence of disease depend on the ability to determine the etiology. A meta-analysis showed that an alanine aminotransferase (ALT) and/or aspartate aminotransferase (AST) of more than 150 IU/dL (a threefold elevation) had a positive predictive value of 95% in predicting gallstones as the underlying cause. Despite the high specificity, only half of the patients with gallstone pancreatitis demonstrated a significantly elevated AST/ALT (Tenner, 1994). Due to a combination of low sensitivity and low specificity, it appears that the bilirubin and alkaline phosphatase have a limited role in the diagnosis of gallstone acute pancreatitis. However, in a patient with gallstone pancreatitis, persistent elevations of the serum bilirubin may signal the presence of a persistent common bile duct stone warranting endoscopic retrograde cholangiopancreatography (ERCP) and stone extraction. Because of decreased clearance, the alkaline phosphatase remains elevated for weeks beyond an acute event involving the biliary tree.

Unlike the normal pancreas that becomes inflamed in patients with gallstone pancreatitis, the pancreas in a patient with alcohol-induced acute pancreatitis has been damaged over years of alcohol consumption. The ducts have been altered by the deposition of proteinaceous plugs. The gland itself typically has altered architecture. For this reason, the disease is different. One in four patients with alcohol-induced acute pancreatitis present with a normal amylase (Spechler, 1983). The gland becomes 'burned out.' Although the amylase is affected, the lipase is not as affected.

Table 22–2 Laboratory Tests in Acute Pancreatitis

Laboratory test	Purpose	Usage and limitations
Amylase	Diagnosis	Accurate over three times the upper limit of normal, decreased specificity in renal failure, normally elevated in macroamylasemia, test interference in hypertriglyceridemia, elevated from other sources such as salivary gland and/or intra-abdominal inflammation (not above 3×), can be normal in alcohol-induced acute pancreatitis
Lipase	Diagnosis	Decreased specificity in renal failure, immune complex creates false positives, elevated from salivary gland and intra-abdominal inflammation
Trypsinogen 2	Diagnosis	Limited use, unclear if superior to amylase/lipase
AST/ALT	Etiology	If greater than three times upper limit of normal, gallstones present as etiology in 95% of cases. Low sensitivity
Lipase/amylase ratio	Etiology	Greater than 5 is diagnostic for alcohol acute pancreatitis. Low sensitivity
Carbohydrate deficient transferrin (CDT)	Etiology	Useful in patients who deny alcohol, remains elevated for weeks after binge drinking
Trypsinogen activation peptide (TAP)	Severity	Greater than 30 mmol/L in 6- to 12-hour urine, 100% negative predictive value
Hematocrit	Severity	Greater than 44 on admission, or rising over initial 24 hours associated with pancreatic necrosis
C-reactive protein	Severity	Values over 200 IU/L associated with pancreatic necrosis. Useful after first 36–48 hours

There appears to be four to five times more lipase in the pancreas than amylase (Tietz, 1993). Thus, the lipase/amylase ratio appears to predict alcohol-induced pancreatitis (Tenner, 1992). Using multiples of the upper limit of normal, a ratio of greater than 3 is predictive, while greater than 5 is diagnostic for acute alcohol-induced acute pancreatitis.

In addition to the lipase/amylase ratio, carbohydrate deficient transferrin (CDT) appears useful in the determination of alcoholism. A person who consumes large amounts of alcohol will have a CDT elevation regardless of whether they have been consuming alcohol during the past several days. It is an ideal marker in a patient suspected of being an alcoholic, who denies alcohol use when the alcohol level is normal (Le Moine, 1994).

In the management of acute pancreatitis, difficulty in the early determination of severity complicates the management of a significant proportion of patients. Multiple laboratory tests have been studied in an attempt to define severity early in the course of the disease. Despite intense study, only two tests, trypsinogen activation peptide (TAP) and hematocrit appear to be useful early in the course of the disease.

Inappropriate early activation of trypsin in the acini of the pancreas leads to the release of trypsinogen activation peptide. This protein product is typically not seen at significant levels in the blood or urine. In patients with acute pancreatitis, TAP levels rise. A TAP greater than 30 mmol/L has been shown to be associated with severe disease, with a negative predictive value of 100% (Tenner, 1997). A new ELISA is available from Biotrin (Dublin, Ireland) that can assist in the determination of severity through the use of urine samples.

A hematocrit above 44 or rising over the first 24 hours has been shown to be associated with pancreatic necrosis (Baillargeon, 1998). This is likely related to hemoconcentration from a combination of severe third space losses, fluid sequestration, and poor intravenous hydration. A serum C-reactive protein is useful later (after 36–48 hours after the onset of symptoms) in determining the presence of pancreatic necrosis (Buchler, 1986). Refer to Table 22–2 for a summary of laboratory tests used in the evaluation of acute pancreatitis.

Chronic Pancreatitis

Chronic pancreatitis is marked by progressive destruction of islet cells and acinar tissue, the latter responsible for the maldigestion associated with this disease, due to loss of enzyme secretion responsible for digestion of foodstuffs within the small intestine. Routine laboratory testing is of little value in patients suspected as having chronic pancreatitis. Although the amylase and lipase may be elevated in acute exacerbations, the absence of these enzyme elevations in the serum does not rule out an attack of pain from chronic pancreatitis. Chronic pancreatitis is suspected in the correct clinical setting and presents as mild glucose intolerance to frank diabetes mellitus, chronic abdominal pain, and/or maldigestion/malabsorption. Hyperglycemia may result from disease progression with subsequent pancreatic endocrine dysfunction. As malnutrition progresses, the serum albumin may fall. A serum beta-carotene may be found to be low as malabsorption for lipids develops.

The clinical diagnosis of chronic pancreatitis depends on the finding of structural abnormalities in ductal anatomy found on imaging, typically ERCP. The simplest method of functional testing of the pancreas is assessing the presence of fat in the stool. Unfortunately, maldigestion of fat occurs after 90% of pancreatic lipase secretory capacity is lost. Serum trypsinogen assays are available and may have a diagnostic utility when values are below 20 ng/mL but the levels are only found to be low in patients with advanced disease (typically when steatorrhea is already present) (Jacobsen, 1984). Because of inadequate delivery of fecal elastase to the duodenum, a low level of pancreatic elastase in the stool can be used in the diagnosis of chronic pancreatitis. Although initial studies suggested that the test could not detect chronic pancreatitis in the absence of steatorrhea, more novel tests have shown that the test is accurate in the evaluation of less advanced disease. A novel ELISA for fecal elastase, a pancreas-specific enzyme that is not degraded during intestinal transport and reaches concentration in fecal matter five to six times that found in duodenal juice, has been developed and marketed and appears to be very sensitive for chronic pancreatitis (Loser, 1996). One clinical study found sensitivities of 63%, 100% and 100% for patients with mild, moderate and severe pancreatic insufficiency respectively.

If symptoms suggest this disorder, the anatomy of the gland is reviewed radiographically and insulin and exocrine pancreatic enzymes are replaced as necessary. There is little clinical need to estimate the percentage of exocrine or endocrine function. When pancreatic maldigestion is suspected as the cause for diarrhea, many clinicians will attempt an empiric course of exogenous pancreatic enzymes. If this works, the diagnosis is likely in the appropriate clinical setting.

Cystic Fibrosis

Cystic fibrosis (mucoviscidosis) of the pancreas is an autosomal recessive disease with an incidence of 1 in 1600 Caucasian births and 1 in 17 000 African American births in the United States. Approximately 1 in every 20 Caucasians is a carrier. Cystic fibrosis is characterized by abnormal secretion from the various exocrine glands of the body, including the pancreas, salivary glands, peritracheal, peribronchial, and peribronchiolar glands, lacrimal glands, sweat glands, mucosal glands of the small bowel, and bile ducts. Involvement of the intestinal glands may result in the presence of meconium ileus at birth. Chronic lung disease and malabsorption resulting from pancreatic involvement are the major clinical problems of those who survive beyond infancy.

Because of the multiple alleles at the cystic fibrosis gene (see Ch. 69), laboratory diagnosis still depends largely on the demonstration of increased sodium and chloride in the sweat. Unfortunately, unless the sweat test is correctly performed, it probably is the least reliable test and has a high proportion of false-positive and false-negative results. In children, chloride concentrations of over 60 mmol/L of sweat on at least two occasions are diagnostic. Levels of between 50–60 mmol/L are suggestive in the absence of adrenal insufficiency. Patients in whom cystic fibrosis is suspected on the basis of indeterminate sweat electrolyte results may undergo confirmatory testing by having the sweat electrolytes test repeated following administration of a mineralocorticoid such as fludrocortisone. In these patients, the electrolyte values would remain unchanged, whereas normal controls would show a decrease in sweat electrolytes. Sodium concentrations in sweat tend to be slightly lower than those of chloride in patients with cystic fibrosis, but the reverse is true in normal subjects. Sweat chloride concentrations of more than 60 mmol/L may be found in some patients with malnutrition, hyperhidrotic ectodermal dysplasia, nephrogenic diabetes insipidus, renal insufficiency, glucose-6-phosphatase deficiency, hypothyroidism, mucopolysaccharidosis, and fucosidosis. These disorders are usually easily differentiated from cystic fibrosis by their clinical symptoms. False-negative sweat test results have been seen in patients with cystic fibrosis in the presence of hypoproteinemic edema.

Sweat electrolytes in about half of a group of premenopausal adult women were shown to undergo cyclic fluctuation, reaching a peak chloride concentration most commonly 5–10 days prior to the onset of menses. Peak values were slightly under 65 mmol/L. Men showed random fluctuations up to 70 mEq/L. For this reason, interpretation of sweat electrolyte values in adults must be approached with caution.

Intestinal Disorders

Chronic Diarrhea

Acute diarrhea is self-limited, typically viral, and resolves quickly. Chronic diarrhea is a common complaint of patients presenting to physicians. The differential diagnosis is complex and a variety of laboratory tests can be found to be useful. The definition of chronic diarrhea is greater than three loose stools per day for more than 4 weeks' duration and/or daily stool weight greater than 200 g/day (Thomas, 2003). Using a definition of chronic diarrhea as excessive stool frequency without associated abdominal pain, the prevalence of this disorder in western population is estimated to be approximately 4–5% (Thomas, 2003). Laboratory testing begins with randomly collected stool specimens submitted for blood, fat and microbes (ova and parasites). In addition, detecting the presence of leukocytes in the stool is of importance in determining whether the diarrhea is inflammatory in nature (ulcerative colitis, Crohn's disease, ischemic colitis, invasive microbes). Detection of fecal leukocytes with Wright's stain on microscopy is also of importance. However, a newer method utilizing lactoferrin may be more accurate in the identification of leukocytes and appears to be more sensitive (Guerrant, 1992).

The principal function of the colon is to absorb water from the fecal stream. Approximately 90% of the water that enters the colon is removed during transit. The rectosigmoid colon also stores stool until it is possible to defecate in a socially acceptable fashion. Diarrhea occurs when the amount of water in the colonic lumen (which is the sum of the water reaching it from the small bowel and the water secreted by the colonic mucosa) exceeds the amount of water capable of being absorbed by the colonic mucosa. It can also result from irritation or inflammation of the colon, which interferes with the colon's ability to store feces. An absent or significantly abbreviated colon ensures large volume and loose stools.

The causes of diarrhea are often divided into four major pathogenic groups. These major groups are the inflammatory diarrheas, the osmotic diarrheas, the secretory diarrheas, and the diarrheas that result from altered bowel motility. Specific causes of diarrhea may do so by more than one pathogenic means, and more than one diarrheal etiology can be present in a single patient simultaneously. Although many clinicians use the category 'factitious' as a fifth pathogenic classification for those who self-induce diarrhea, the method or methods employed by the patient involve one of the four aforementioned types.

A brief mention of factitious diarrhea is warranted because it is not uncommon. Analysis of laxatives should be done early in the evaluation. Stool water should be analyzed for osmolality and electrolytes. The osmotic gap is calculated from electrolyte concentrations in stool water by the following formula: $290 - [2 \times (Sodium + Potassium)]$. The sum of the sodium and potassium concentrations is multiplied by a factor of two to account for associated anions. The osmolality of the stool within the distal intestine is estimated to be 290 mOsm/kg (equilibrates with plasma osmolality). If findings suggest secretory diarrhea, osmotic gap less than 50, the patient may have ingested a laxative causing a secretory diarrhea, such as sodium phosphate (Fleet phosphosoda). If stool electrolyte analysis suggests osmotic diarrhea, osmotic gap > 125 mOsm/kg, magnesium laxatives (Maalox) should be suspected.

Similarly, iatrogenic diarrhea is not a separate pathogenic category. Although multiple drugs and other therapies induce diarrhea as an unwanted side effect, the mechanism by which they do so involves inflammation, osmotic load, secretion, altered motility, or some combination thereof. Rectal incontinence is often incorrectly reported as diarrhea. Diarrhea may precipitate incontinence in someone who can control defecation with formed stool. The management of incontinence may be quite different from the management of diarrhea, so it is important to distinguish between the two.

Inflammatory or exudative diarrhea is often bloody, but it does not have to be. The presence of fecal leukocytes on microscopic evaluation may be the only clue to inflammation. In some cases of inflammatory diarrhea, the mucosa of the bowel appears grossly normal, while histologic review of biopsy specimens demonstrates inflammation. A frankly exudative process classic for inflammatory diarrhea is not present in these cases. The overlap of the pathogenic types of diarrhea is thus demonstrated. Semantic arguments aside, it is most reasonable to determine whether blood or fecal leukocytes are present in the stool of a patient with diarrhea. Their presence suggests that inflammation is playing a role in the patient's diarrhea. Crohn's disease, ulcerative colitis, ischemic colitis, invasive infectious organisms, and radiation-induced colitis are common causes of inflammatory diarrhea. The atypical inflammatory bowel diseases such as microscopic colitis or collagenous colitis do not produce exudative diarrhea. Hypersecretion or lessened absorption of water may be the means by which these entities produce diarrhea. Classification via pathogenesis remains controversial.

Osmotic diarrhea occurs when the osmotic load of the fecal stream favors excess water loss. In other words, the osmotic gradient drives water into the colonic lumen creating looser, more voluminous stools. One can calculate a stool osmotic gap by first measuring stool osmolality, sodium, and potassium. A value of greater than 100 mmol/L suggests the presence of a large number of unmeasured osmotic particles causing fluid to be drawn into the colonic lumen. The stool specimen from which these measurements are derived must be very fresh. Fecal bacteria continue to produce osmotic particles as a result of digestion while the specimen awaits processing. These bacterial breakdown products can falsely elevate the fecal osmotic load. The most practical way of determining that the diarrhea is osmotic in the cooperative patient is to fast the patient. A strict fast causes osmotic diarrhea to subside. Uncooperative patients or patients with 'factitious diarrhea' who continue to ingest osmotically active substances will continue to have diarrhea. Such patients may have to be observed during the fast.

Secretory diarrhea result from the active secretion of water into the fecal stream that overwhelms the absorptive process. Multiple toxins, hormones, and medications can cause an active secretion of water and electrolytes in the colonic lumen. Such diarrheas can cause dehydration, electrolyte depletion, and even death. The classic secretory diarrhea is cholera. In developed countries, medications are probably the most common cause of secretory diarrhea. A variety of hormonal causes such as gastrinoma (Zollinger–Ellison syndrome), carcinoid syndrome, medullary thyroid carcinoma, mastocytosis, vasoactive intestinal polypeptide (VIP)-producing tumors (e.g., VIPoma syndrome), and villous adenoma of the rectosigmoid colon have been identified. Analysis of the urine for 5-hydroxyindoleacetic acid for carcinoid syndrome, vanillylmandelic acid for pheochromocytoma and histamine for mastocytosis is rarely helpful. However, if the clinical suspicion exists, the tests should be submitted for analysis. Unlike osmotic diarrheas, the conditions continue to generate diarrhea even when the patient invokes a strict fast. In fact, these patients can dehydrate quickly without continued fluid intake, and such fasting should be under observation when secretory diarrhea is suspected.

Motility disorders can hurry the fecal stream and thwart complete water absorption. Irritable bowel syndrome may involve excessive neural stimulation with resultant decreased stool transit times. Short gut syndromes (e.g., postsurgical) reduce the amount of absorptive colon and can result in diarrhea. Motility disorders are, by far, the most difficult to characterize and quantify. Most current diagnostic methodologies alter the colonic milieu and, presumably, alter motility. Barium studies or the ingestion of radiopaque markers may assist in estimating colonic transit time, but consensus normal values are lacking. Unless there are obvious structural defects, or the diagnosis of irritable syndrome is clear, motility disorders are often suspected by exclusion.

The diagnosis of diarrhea starts with a very thorough history. Whether the diarrhea is bland or bloody, the presence or absence of constitutional symptoms and the duration of the illness are major points in determining the subsequent evaluation. Self-limited, acute diarrhea (less than 2 weeks in duration) without bleeding or constitutional symptoms rarely requires diagnostic testing. Chronic diarrhea, the passage of blood, and constitutional symptoms all suggest the need for making a specific diagnosis. The history is the key to narrowing down the potential diagnosis. The physical examination, although usually less helpful than the history, must still be very comprehensive.

A critical aspect in the evaluation of diarrhea revolves around immuno-competence. In patients with the acquired immunodeficiency syndrome (AIDS), or who have been significantly immunosuppressed, the diagnostic evaluation must consider unusual infections. In any patient with chronic diarrhea it is wise to consider establishing human immunodeficiency virus (HIV) status.

Patients with diarrhea must be queried about their medications, diet, and water supply. Duration of symptoms, stool frequency, urgency, incontinence, daily stool patterns, stool consistency, and stool volume should be estimated. Travel histories, sexual practices, and family histories may be useful. Constitutional symptoms such as fever, weight loss, arthralgias/arthritis, rashes, and the like, may give strong clues as to the diarrheal etiology. If the patient is among others who develop diarrhea simultaneously, a common infectious source should be considered (see Ch. 56). Antibiotic usage, recent surgery, radiation, or chemotherapy, and any change in a patient's usual regimen may shed light on the situation. The clinician should always inquire about potential similar episodes in the past and determine if the diarrhea is recurrent. It helps to know if there are outbreaks of diarrheal illnesses in the community. In patients with similar diarrheal illnesses occurring over the same time period, an infectious cause or common toxin can be suspected. Infectious agents may be sought. Stool culture, enzymes for rotavirus and giardiasis, and ova and parasite examinations should be done in the appropriate clinical setting (see Ch. 61). Table 22–3 shows recommended tests that can be used in the evaluation strategy.

Any diarrheagenic medication that can be stopped should be, especially if it was started or the dosage was increased around the time that the diarrhea began. It should be remembered that the 'active' drug may not be responsible for the diarrhea, but that the carrier substance (e.g., sorbitol) may be. Stools may be alkalinized to test for phenolphthalein if surreptitious laxative use is suspected. It must be remembered that many readily available substances can cause diarrhea, and stool alkalinization, although widely written about, is often of little practical value. It is simple and inexpensive, however, and should be considered under the right clinical conditions.

Stool can be tested for blood, electrolytes, leukocytes, and osmolality. Infectious agents may be sought via enzymatic testing, culture, or direct microscopic evaluation. Fecal fat testing is also relatively simple. The standard method for detecting fat in the stool is using Sudan stain. Sensitivity varies based on the level of observer skill and experience. An alternative method of assessing fecal fat is semiquantitative, the steatocrit. This method correlates well with quantitative fat output as measured using the van de Kamer method (Sugal, 1994). Although 48- to 72-hour quantitative testing of stool for fecal fat remains the gold standard, for practical considerations, this test has been largely abandoned. A fast may be very helpful. Once these data have been collected it is usually possible to classify the diarrhea and begin to find the specific diagnosis, if it has not become evident already. Complicated and expensive diagnostic evaluations for secretory diarrhea should generally not be undertaken unless other more likely causes have been ruled out or unless signs and symptoms are suggestive.

Breath testing is becoming increasingly utilized for the evaluation of chronic diarrhea, abdominal bloating and pain. The most common tests use a probe for carbon-14 or a nonradioactive fermentable sugar. Breath testing assists in the evaluation of a person's difficulty in metabolizing lactose, sucrose and glucose (secondary to bacterial overgrowth). The exact methodology depends on the sugar studied and the sensitivity and specificity desired. The most frequent tests for lactase insufficiency rely on the ingestion of 25 g of lactose.

HIV-Related Diarrhea

The actual causes of diarrhea in the patient with HIV are related to the aforementioned pathophysiologic mechanisms. However, the specific etiologic agents (especially the infectious ones) often differ greatly from those in the immunocompetent patient. Thus, in all patients with chronic diarrhea, it is prudent to consider the possibility of AIDS.

Nosocomial Diarrhea

Clostridium difficile, a Gram-positive, spore-forming anaerobic bacillus, is the most important cause of nosocomial diarrhea in adults with greater than 300 000 cases per year in the US (Malnick, 2000). It is thought to be associated with approximately 25% of all antibiotic-associated cases of diarrhea and 50–75% of cases involving antibiotic-associated colitis (Malnick, 2000). It may present clinically, from a mild watery diarrhea to life-threatening pseudomembranous colitis and toxic megacolon. This can lead to colonic perforation and peritonitis, with a mortality rate as high as 38% (Poutanen, 2004). Patients can present with watery diarrhea, lower abdominal pain/cramping, systemic symptoms such as fever and malaise, or can have occult GI bleeding. The pathogenesis of this disease entity usually involves disruption of the normal colonic flora, typically following a course of antibiotic therapy in hospitalized patients, followed by exposure to a toxigenic strain of *C. difficile*. Broad-spectrum antibiotics such as penicillin, clindamycin and cephalosporins have been particularly implicated; however, any antibiotic can lead to development of *C. difficile* colitis (Malnick, 2000). Clinical suspicion of the disease is confirmed with detection of *C. difficile* toxin A or B virulence factors in stool samples. Both toxin A and B lead to increased vascular permeability and have potential to cause hemorrhage. They induce the production of tumor necrosis factor alpha and inflammatory interleukins that are responsible for the inflammatory response and pseudomembrane formation (Poutanen, 2004).

Direct visualization of the colonic mucosa with the aid of endoscopy is required for diagnosis of pseudomembranous colitis associated with *C. difficile*. However, endoscopy should be avoided in cases of suspected fulminant colitis because of the risk of perforation. Laboratory methods are available for confirmation of *C. difficile* infection. Tissue culture cytotoxicity assays, which take at least 48 hours to complete, for detecting *C. difficile* cytotoxin B in stool specimens are considered the 'gold standard,' with a sensitivity ranging between 94–100% and specificity of

Table 22–3 Laboratory Tests in the Differential Diagnosis of Diarrhea

Test	Method	Use
Initial screening tests		
Fecal leukocytes	Wright's stain or methylene blue	Identify inflammatory diarrhea
Hemoccult test	Peroxidase reaction for hemoglobin	Identify hemorrhagic diarrhea
Fecal osmotic gap	FOG = fecal osmolality – 2 × (fecal Na + K)	Distinguish secretory vs. osmotic diarrhea
Stool alkalinization	Color change after adding NaOH to stool	Phenolphthalein laxative ingestion
Infectious causes		
Stool bacterial culture	Routine culture and sensitivity	Identify *Shigella, Salmonella, Campylobacter*
Stool special culture	Specialized culture and serotyping	Identify *E. coli* 0157:H7, *Yersinia, Vibrio*
Stool *C. difficile* toxin assay	Tissue culture cytotoxicity	Pseudomembranous colitis
HIV serology	ELISA	HIV enteritis
Stool rotavirus screen	Antigen enzyme immunoassay	Rotavirus enteritis
Stool ova and parasites	Wet mount	Enteric parasitic infection
Stool mycobacteria	Acid-fast stain and culture, PCR	*M. tuberculosis*, MAI
Stool protozoans	Iodine or modified acid-fast stain	*Cryptosporidium, Isospora belli*
E. histolytica Ab titers	Serology	*Entameoba histolytica*
Stool *Giardia* antigen	Enzyme immunoassay	*Giardia lamblia*
Endocrine causes		
Urine 5-HIAA	HPLC	Carcinoid syndrome
Blood serotonin	HPLC	Carcinoid syndrome
Serum VIP	RIA	VIPoma
Serum TSH, free T_4	Immunoassay	Hyperthyroidism
Serum gastrin	RIA	Zollinger–Ellison syndrome
Serum calcitonin	RIA	Hypocalcemia-related diarrhea
Serum somatostatin	RIA	Somatostatinoma
Maldigestion		
Lactose tolerance test	See text	Lactase deficiency
Sweat chloride	See text	Pancreatic insufficiency Cystic fibrosis
Stool reducing sugars	Clinitest tablets	Carbohydrate intolerance
Malabsorption		
D-Xylose absorption test	See text	Evaluate surface area of intestinal mucosa
72-Hour fecal fat content	Saponification and titration	Lipid malabsorption
Fecal fat stain	Sudan stain	Lipid malabsorption
Serum carotene	Spectrophotometry	Lipid malabsorption
$^{14}CO_2$ breath test as a test for lipid (fat) malabsorption	See text	Lipid malabsorption
Endomysial antibody	Serology	Celiac disease
Gliadin antibody	Serology	Celiac disease
H_2 breath test	Expired H_2 by gas chromatography	Carbohydrate malabsorption
Bacterial colony count	Small bowel aspirate and quantitative culture	Bacterial overgrowth
Other and miscellaneous		
Serum ionized calcium	Ion-specific electrode	Hypocalcemia-related diarrhea
Serum protein and albumin	Biuret reaction, anionic dyes	IBD, protein-losing enteropathy
Stool alpha-1-antitrypsin	See text	Protein-losing enteropathy
Quantitative immunoglobulins	Nephelometry	Agammaglobulinemia
Colon biopsy	Endoscopic biopsy	Neoplasia, lymphocytic colitis, collagenous colitis
Intestinal biopsy	Endoscopic or open biopsy	Whipple's disease, MAI, abetalipoproteinemia, lymphoma, amyloidosis, eosinophilic gastroenteritis, agammaglobulinemia, intestinal lymphangiectasia, Crohn's disease, tuberculosis, graft-versus-host disease, *Giardia*, other parasitic infections, collagenous colitis, microscopic colitis

PCR = polymerase chain reaction; HPLC = high-performance liquid chromatography; RIA = radioimmunoassay; IBD = inflammatory bowel disease; MAI = *Mycobacterium avium-intracellulare*; HIV = human immunodeficiency virus; ELISA = enzyme-linked immunoabsorbent assay; 5-HIAA = 5-hydroxyindoleacetic acid; Ab= antibody.

approximately 99% (Malnick, 2000). This tissue culture assay can detect as little as 10 pg of toxin in stool specimens (Malnick, 2000). Rapid enzyme immunoassays, which can be completed within several hours, have been developed for the detection of toxin A or B from stool specimens. However, the sensitivity and specificity of these immunoassays are decreased, 65–85% and 95–100% respectively, compared with cytotoxic assays, The ELISA can detect 100–1000 pg of toxin in stool specimens

(Malnick, 2000) In hospitalized patients with greater than six stools per day, ELISA is the optimal diagnostic test (Malnick, 2000). Stool cultures can also be performed but require up to 96 hours for completion. Latex agglutination tests that detect glutamate dehydrogenase, a common clostridial protein, can also be performed but has much lower sensitivity and specificity compared to other available tests, limiting its clinical utility. PCR methods for detection of *C. difficile* toxin A or B are currently being

Table 22–4 Laboratory Tests Available for the Diagnosis of *Clostridium Difficile*-Associated Diarrhea

Test	Advantages	Disadvantages
C. difficile cytotoxin assay	Excellent specificity (99–100%)	Decreased diagnostic sensitivity (80–90%) Test results not available until after 48 h Requires tissue culture facility Detects only toxin B
Immunoassay for detection of toxin A or toxins A and B	Good specificity (95–100%) Test results available within 4 h Technically simple	Reduced sensitivity (65–85%) as compared with cytotoxin assay
Stool culture to isolate *C. difficile* with subsequent cytotoxin assay of isolate	Excellent sensitivity (> 90%) and specificity (> 98%) Enables typing of strain for outbreak investigation	Results not available for at least 72–96 h Labor-intensive Requires tissue culture facility

"*Clostridium difficile*-Associated diarrhea in adults" – Reprinted from *CMAJ* 06-Jul-04; 171(1), Pages 51–58 by permission of the publisher. © 2004 CMA Media Inc.

developed with similar sensitivity and specificity profiles compared to cytotoxic assays (Poutanen, 2004). However, PCR is unable to distinguish between asymptomatic carriage and symptomatic infection. It is currently recommended that these tests be performed on diarrheal stool specimens; in most cases one stool sample is sufficient for diagnosis of *C. difficile* infection (Poutanen, 2004). However, multiple samples may be required for confirmation, and empiric treatment with oral antibiotics may be indicated in patients with clinical evidence of *C. difficile* infection. Refer to Table 22–4 for laboratory tests available for the diagnosis of *C. difficile*-associated diarrhea.

Malabsorption Syndromes

Malabsorption results from either inadequate mucosal absorption of carbohydrates, proteins, fats vitamins or minerals or from the presence of substances in the bowel that cannot be absorbed, for example nonabsorbable sugars such as lactulose and sorbitol. Maldigestion results from an intraluminal defect that leads to the incomplete breakdown of nutrients into their absorbable substrates. This can occur with pancreatic insufficiency and loss of exocrine function. Normal absorption, therefore, cannot occur. These conditions may result in increased osmotic load of the colon, resulting in diarrhea. In addition, patients can have selective malabsorption/maldigestion of specific nutrients resulting in associated clinical sequelae.

Hepatic maldigestion results from interference or obstruction of bile flow. Loss of bile salts interferes with fat emulsification, diminishing the surface area available for lipolytic action. In addition, bile salt activation of lipase activity is lost. Patients are usually jaundiced, pass dark urine, and have other signs of liver disease. Hepatic steatorrhea may coexist with pancreatic steatorrhea, as in patients with a neoplasm obstructing the ampulla of Vater. Malassimilation or the inability to assimilate fats and proteins due to maldigestion also occurs in patients with vasculitis, diabetes mellitus, carcinoid syndrome, hypogammaglobulinemia, and relative vitamin B_6 or B_{12} deficiency.

Enteric malabsorption comprises a variety of conditions that have in common normal digestion but inadequate net assimilation of foodstuffs. This may result from competition by bacteria or altered bacterial flora, as in the blind loop syndrome or diverticulosis of the small bowel, and from obstruction to the flow of lymph, as in lymphoma. It may also result from diseases affecting the small bowel mucosa, such as amyloidosis, inflammation following irradiation (radiation enteritis), diminished mucosal surface area as in gastroileostomy (gastric bypass), or small bowel resection. Depending on the location within the intestinal tract of such pathology, preferential loss of specific substrates may occur. One of the most common clinical scenarios encountered is regional enteritis localized to the distal ileum, the site of vitamin B_{12} and bile acid absorption, which will result in vitamin B_{12} deficiency as well as a decreased pool of circulating bile acids for metabolism. The classic malabsorption syndromes, celiac disease and Whipple's disease, are described below.

Patients with malabsorption syndromes may remain symptomatic. If symptoms arise, the clinical presentation may be specific to the malabsorbed substrate such as with lactase deficiency causing lactose intolerance, or may

be a general consequence of the increased osmotic load to the colon. For example, steatorrhea is a hallmark finding in patients with malabsorption, resulting in fluid, semifluid, or soft and pasty, pale, bulky and foul smelling stools. These stools may be foamy due to the high fat content and may tend to float on water. However, the latter may occur with stools from healthy individuals and is therefore, a nonspecific sign of malabsorption. Normal individuals with a normal fat intake excrete up to 5 g of lipid daily. Steatorrhea may be defined as the presence of more than 5 g of lipid (measured as fatty acids) in feces per 24 hours. Although the source of fecal lipid is largely dietary, gastrointestinal excretions, cellular desquamation, and bacterial metabolism also contribute. Lipids are normally present as soaps and triglycerides. In addition, lipoids are present, including higher alcohols, paraffins, and vegetable carotenoids. Although diet has some effect on it, the pattern of lipids excreted may be very different from the lipids ingested in the diet, and the quantity of fat ingested by a normal individual has a relatively small effect on the total output of fat. According to one study, fecal lipid is equal to a constant (2.93 g) plus 2.1% of the dietary fat intake. On a fat-free diet, the output of fat normally varies from 1–4 g/day.

Another clinical presentation of malabsorption is the development of fat-soluble vitamin (A, D, E, and K) deficiencies. Primary and secondary alterations of the bowel mucosa may also result in deficiencies of water-soluble vitamins. Other evidence of nutritional deficiencies, such as hypoprothrombinemia, glossitis, anemia, edema, ascites, and osteomalacia may be evident in these individuals. These patients are also liable to experience significant weight loss due to diarrhea-induced, large caloric losses leading to cachexia in severe cases.

Classic fat malabsorption is diagnosed by revealing excessive fecal fat. Spot stool specimens can be stained with Sudan stain for detection of fecal fat. The low sensitivity of this test limits its clinical application. However, if positive, it may prompt further evaluation with a 72-hour stool collection (Romano, 1989). A false-negative rate as high as 25% may result with use of the qualitative Sudan III fat staining if steatorrhea is less than 10 g per 24 hours (Romano, 1989). The gold standard however, remains quantifying the amount of fecal fat per 24 hours in a 72-hour stool collection after consumption of a high-fat diet. Normal fat absorption requires normal mucosa, pancreatic enzymes and bile acids. Intraluminal defects as occur with maldigestion or mucosal abnormalities will result in abnormal fat excretion, detectable in the stool specimen. Therefore, the 72-hour fecal stool fat measurement is an accurate diagnostic test for identification of maldigestion/malabsorption with high sensitivity and specificity. The evaluation of stool for fecal fat content remains the definitive test for steatorrhea, an indicator of malabsorption. However, other diagnostic tests include determination of levels of carotenoid, the main precursor of vitamin A in humans, which requires the normal absorption of dietary fat for proper absorption; as well as the breath test and titrimetric methods for detection of malabsorption; and the D-xylose test for differentiation of pancreatic malabsorption from enteric malabsorption. These tests are described in full detail in the latter part of this chapter.

Celiac Sprue

Celiac sprue is a disorder characterized by intestinal malabsorption of nutrients due to sensitivity to the alcohol-soluble portion of gluten known as gliadin. Wheat, rye, barley and, to a lesser extent, oats contain this protein substance and can induce mucosal damage in the gut causing nonspecific villous atrophy of the small intestine mucosa. The prevalence is not clear but estimated to be between 1 : 300 and 1 : 1000 (Catassi, 1994; Not, 1998). Most patients with celiac sprue are asymptomatic. The diagnosis is often made by an astute clinician that notes a patient with thin stature, iron deficiency anemia, weight loss, chronic bloating and/or diarrhea. This disease has variable clinical manifestations and can lead to severe symptoms such as profound malabsorption, steatorrhea, and wasting. There are associations between celiac sprue and type 1 diabetes mellitus, Down syndrome, dermatitis herpetiformis, IgA deficiency, autoimmune thyroid disease, and others (Barr, 1998). Uncontrolled celiac sprue appears to predispose patients to gut carcinomas and lymphomas (Nehra, 1998). There is a genetic predisposition and it is most common in Caucasians of Northern European descent.

Due to the enteropathy associated with the disorder, multiple hematologic and biochemical abnormalities may be found in persons with untreated celiac sprue, including iron deficiency, folate deficiency, and vitamin D deficiency. The peripheral blood film may reveal nonspecific target cells, siderocytes, crenated red cells, Howell–Jolly bodies, and Heinz bodies. Similarly, small bowel absorptive testing will be abnormal, including oral D-xylose testing and fecal fat evaluation.

The gold standard for diagnosis remains biopsy of the small bowel mucosa and identification of classic histologic changes (Trier, 1998). This is done via endoscopy. The lesions may be patchy, and sampling errors can

Table 22–5 Ranges of Sensitivities and Specificities for Commercially Available Serologic Tests for Celiac Sprue

	Adults		Children	
	Sensitivity (%)	Specificity (%)	Sensitivity (%)	Specificity (%)
AGA-IgA	31–100	85–100	90–100	86–100
AGA-IgG	46–95	87–98	91–100	67–100
EMA-IgA	89–100	95–100	100–100	100–100
ARA-IgA	41–92	95–100	29–100	98–100

From Murray JA: Serodiagnosis of celiac disease. Clin Lab Med 1997; 17:452, with permission.

occur. Biopsy is reserved for patients in whom the diagnosis is suspected based on signs or symptoms of the disease, especially in higher-risk populations. Owing to the fact that these patients must utilize a gluten-free diet for the rest of their lives in order to control symptoms and mitigate cancer risk, histologic diagnosis is very important.

In current clinical practice, there are four serologic studies used to assist in the diagnosis of celiac sprue (Table 22–5). These include testing for antibodies to gliadin (AGA-IgA and AGA-IgG), endomysium (EMA-IgA), reticulin (ARA-IgA), and transglutaminase (tTG-IgA), all of which are commercially available. Results of serological testing for celiac disease must be analyzed with caution because this disease is associated with selective IgA deficiency that will give rise to false-negative serum IgA antibody tests (Thomas, 2003). Therefore, IgG serology or total IgA levels should be checked if there is a high clinical suspicion of celiac disease. The sensitivity and specificity of these tests are extremely high when compared to a gold standard of flattened small bowel villi responding to dietary changes (Farrell, 2001). Endomysial antibodies have the best sensitivity and specificity, but they are currently detected via immunofluorescence of sections of monkey esophagus or human umbilical cord and are costly, cumbersome, and subject to interobserver interpretive variability.

Wheat storage protein, gliadin, is available to be used as an antigen in an ELISA. Although serum IgA and IgG AGA levels are frequently elevated in untreated celiac sprue, these tests are of only moderate sensitivity and specificity. The IgG AGA testing is particularly useful in the 2% of patients with celiac disease who appear to be IgA deficient. However, these tests have largely been replaced by EMA. EMA binds to connective tissue surrounding smooth muscle cells. Most laboratories use sections of human umbilical cord. Serum IgA EMA binds to the endomysium to produce a characteristic staining pattern seen on indirect immunofluorescence. The antibody is very sensitive and specific. However, after treatment the titers fall quickly to undetectable levels (Volta, 1995). The epitope against which EMA is directed has been shown to be tissue transglutaminase. Use of IgA anti-tTG assays has been shown to be highly sensitive and specific for the diagnosis of celiac sprue (Dieterich, 1998). An ELISA for IgA anti-tTG is widely available, less costly and easier to perform than the older immunofluorescence assay for IgA EMA. Although IgG endomysium and IgG tTG antibodies may be suitable for serological diagnosis of celiac disease, they cannot be used to monitor the response to dietary modification. Endomysium IgA antibodies disappear following treatment of celiac sprue with a gluten-free diet.

Whipple's Disease

Whipple's disease is a very rare multisystem disease that often presents with arthralgias, diarrhea, and weight loss. It is caused by the Gram-positive rod *Tropheryma whippelii*, an organism yet to be cultured. As this disease can be treated and is no longer uniformly fatal, it is important to make the diagnosis. PCR testing of infected tissue or cerebrospinal fluid (CSF) is the optimal way to confirm the diagnosis and monitor treatment (von Herbay, 1997). Biopsy of the duodenum with periodic acid–Schiff (PAS) staining had been considered pathognomonic for Whipple's disease. It is now recognized that PAS-positive macrophages may be seen in AIDS patients with *Mycobacterium avium* complex. Thus, PCR has gained even more importance in the management of this entity. Long-term antibiotic therapy with central nervous system (CNS) penetration is used to treat patients with Whipple's disease (Singer, 1998; Ramzan, 1997).

Disaccharidase Deficiency

Many of the previously listed conditions causing malabsorption may also be associated with intolerance to disaccharides. Disaccharide absorption is diminished either from primary disaccharidase deficiencies such as

Table 22–6 Markers for Inflammatory Bowel Disease

	Percent frequency	
	p-ANCA	ASCA
Irritable bowel syndrome (normal patients)	<5	<5
Ulcerative colitis	70	15
Crohn's disease	20	65

p-ANCA = perinuclear antineutrophil cytoplasmic antibody; ASCA: anti-*Saccharomyces cerevisiae* antibody.

sucrase–isomaltase deficiency, lactase deficiency, primary alactasia, primary trehalase deficiency, or secondary disaccharidase deficiencies due to celiac disease, tropical sprue, acute viral gastroenteritis, or drugs such as orally administered neomycin, kanamycin, and methotrexate. These secondary disaccharidase deficiencies are usually transient and involve more than one enzyme. Although the incidence of lactose intolerance due to congenital lactase deficiency is low, the prevalence of lactose intolerance in adults is quite high. About 10% of Caucasians, 70–80% of African Americans, and an even greater percentage of Asian people manifest some degree of lactose intolerance even though they were able to digest lactose well as infants. In these disorders, intestinal bacteria ferment unhydrolyzed and unabsorbed carbohydrates, producing gas, lactic acid or other organic acids. Normally, absorption of digested carbohydrates is rapid and fairly complete in the proximal small intestine. Unhydrolyzed disaccharides or monosaccharides unabsorbed because of deficiencies in transport are osmotically active and hence cause secretion of water and electrolytes into the small and large intestines. This can result in protracted diarrhea as well as complaints of bloating and flatulence.

Screening tests for disaccharidase deficiencies include oral challenge of suspected disaccharides to reproduce the abdominal symptomatology, followed by stool analysis. The stools are usually watery, acidic, explosive, and fermentative. Stool pH of less than 5.5 is suggestive, but the measurement of pH is not valid if the patient is taking oral antibiotics. High pH does not exclude the diagnosis. Normal infants between 3–7 days of age commonly have high stool pH. Stools can be analyzed for sugars by chromatography or by one of the semiquantitative nonspecific tests for urinary sugar adapted for stool analysis. The Clinitest tablet (Bayer Diagnostics, Australia) is suitable for this purpose. The presence of 0.25 g/dL reducing substances is considered normal; from 0.25–0.5 g/dL is regarded as suspicious; more than 0.5 g/dL is considered abnormal. In patients with intolerance to sugar, the amount of total reducing substances in the stool usually exceeds 0.25 g/dL feces.

An oral tolerance test using a specific sugar such as lactose or sucrose can be used to establish a specific carbohydrate intolerance. Although the oral tolerance test is fairly specific and sensitive, in some instances, 23–30% false-positive results were noted following administration of lactose – that is, a flat tolerance curve and less than a 20 mg/dL (1.1 mmol/L) increase in blood sugar (Krasilnikoff, 1975). Delayed gastric emptying appears to be the cause of the false-positive result, because duodenal instillation of lactose eliminates the flat tolerance curve.

Definitive diagnosis of disaccharidase deficiencies depends on the demonstration of low specific enzyme activity in the mucosa of small intestinal biopsy material. An assay for disaccharidase has been published (Dahlqvist, 1968).

Inflammatory Bowel Disease

Immunologic mechanisms within the colon are involved in the pathogenesis of inflammatory bowel disease. The underlying antigenic challenge to the immunologic response is not clearly understood. Over the last decade, two antibody tests have become available that assist in the laboratory evaluation of patients with inflammatory bowel disease. Perinuclear-antineutrophil cytoplasmic antibody (p-ANCA) and anti-*Saccharomyces cerevisiae* antibody (ASCA) can be used to distinguish abdominal pain seen in irritable bowel syndrome from inflammatory bowel disease; and subtype inflammatory bowel disease as either ulcerative colitis or Crohn's disease (Sendid, 1998; Shanahan, 1994) (see Table 22–6). These tests have limitations, and interpretation requires careful understanding of the tests. Whereas few normal persons with irritable bowel syndrome will have ANCA, 70% of persons with ulcerative colitis and 20% of persons with Crohn's disease will have significant titers. In patients with inflammatory bowel disease, 65% of patients with Crohn's disease will have ASCA, whereas only 20% of patients with ulcerative colitis will have significant titers. Given the low sensitivity and

Table 22–7 Neuroendocrine Tumors

APUDoma	Hormones	Clinical sequelae
Carcinoid	Serotonin (many others possible)	Abdominal pain, flushing, diarrhea, asthma, edema
Gastrinoma	Gastrin	Ulcers, diarrhea
Insulinoma	Insulin	Hypoglycemia
VIPomas	Vasoactive intestinal polypeptide	Diarrhea, hypokalemia, acidosis, hypochlorhydria
Glucagonoma	Glucagon	Necrolytic migratory erythema, weight loss, diabetes, depression, deep venous thromboses
Somatostatinoma	Somatostatin	Gallstones, diabetes. diarrhea, hypochlorhydria

specificity, the use of these tests should be dependent upon the clinical circumstance. For example, a person with diarrhea and equivocal biopsy findings found to have a positive ANCA is more likely to have inflammatory bowel disease than irritable bowel syndrome. Likewise, if a person with what appears to be ulcerative colitis is found to have a positive ASCA, Crohn's colitis may be present.

Neuroendocrine Tumors

Neuroendocrine tumors of the gastrointestinal tract are relatively rare neoplastic lesions with protean clinical manifestations (Table 22–7). Abdominal pain and diarrhea are two of the commoner clinical symptoms. Due to the fact that they exhibit amine precursor uptake and decarboxylation (APUD) they are also known as APUDomas. The most common of these tumors are the carcinoid tumors, constituting 50% of the total. Gastrinomas comprise 25% of the APUDomas, while 15% are insulinomas and 6% are VIPomas. Glucagonomas are quite rare and make up 2–5% of series. Other even rarer types, such as somatostatinomas, have been identified (Perry, 1996). The chemical measurement of the secretagogues of these tumors generally suggests the diagnosis in the right clinical setting. Localizing the tumors can be quite challenging. Ultrasonography, CT scanning, magnetic resonance imaging (MRI) operative exploration, endoscopy, angiography, and octreotide scanning all have significant technical limitations. With the exception of ultrasonography and MRI, there can be potential morbidity from the testing as well. Although it was initially hoped that octreotide scanning would replace other modes of localization, recent data suggest that it is useful in determining the extent of carcinoids and gastrinomas, while of little use in finding insulinomas or nonfunctional tumors (Kisker, 1997). These tumors are often small, frequently multifocal, and can be located in a variety of organs. They can be malignant or benign. They are similar on histologic examination, so histologic staining is employed to distinguish the types (Perry, 1996). As in all neoplastic lesions, biopsy is essential to confirm the diagnosis. Table 22–7 shows the distinguishing features of the various APUDomas.

Common Tests, Methods and Clinical Applications

Amylase (Total Serum and Urine)

Amylase is a stable enzyme. In serum and urine it is stable for 1 week at room temperature and for at least 6 months under refrigeration in well-sealed containers. It may be kept in the frozen state much longer without appreciable loss of activity. Plasma specimens that have been anticoagulated with citrate or oxalate should be avoided for amylase determination because amylase is a calcium-containing enzyme, and falsely low enzyme activities are obtained from such specimens. Heparinized plasma specimens do not interfere with the amylase assay.

While there are a variety of amylase methods available, regardless of the method chosen, caution must be exercised to avoid contamination of specimens with saliva, because its amylase content is approximately 700 times that of serum. Red cells contain no amylase, so hemolysis generally presents no problem with most of the methods except those coupled-enzyme methods in which the released peroxide is determined by a coupled-peroxidase reaction.

Interpretation

Elevations of serum and urine amylase are observed in a wide variety of disorders. Most of the elevations of serum amylase are due to increased rates of amylase entry into the bloodstream, decreased rates of clearance, or both.

Serum amylase activity rises within 6–48 hours of the onset of acute pancreatitis in about 80% of patients, but is not proportional to the severity of the disease. Values of over 600 Somogyi units/dL, or over four times the upper limit of normal, are highly suggestive of the diagnosis. Activity usually returns to normal in 3–5 days in patients with the milder edematous forms of the disease. Elevated values persisting longer than this suggest continuing necrosis or possible pseudocyst formation.

The urine amylase activity rises promptly, often within several hours of the rise in serum activity, and may remain elevated after the serum activity has returned to the normal range. Values of over 1000 Somogyi units/h are seen almost exclusively in patients with acute pancreatitis. False-negative results are often seen when the urine specimen is taken too soon or too late or in patients with fulminating necrosis in which the production of amylase is decreased or has ceased. In a majority of patients with acute pancreatitis, serum amylase activity is elevated and there is a concomitant increase in urine amylase activity. There may be instances, however, in which the elevated urine amylase is not accompanied by a concomitant increase in serum amylase.

Increased renal clearance of amylase can be used in the diagnosis of acute and relapsing pancreatitis, and the ratio of amylase clearance to creatinine clearance expressed as a percentage has been used diagnostically. This ratio (C_{am}/C_{cr}) can be calculated by the following formula:

Clearance ratio (percent) = (Urine amylase activity/Serum amylase activity) × (Serum creatinine concentration/Urine creatinine concentration) × 100

The normal ratio averages 1–4%, whereas that for patients with pancreatitis usually exceeds 4% and is often in the range of 7–15%. Unfortunately, about one-third of patients with pancreatitis have normal ratios, and elevated ratios may be found in patients with burns, ketoacidosis, renal insufficiency, heart disease, and duodenal perforation, as well as following thoracic surgery. Thus, the ratio adds little to the diagnostic armamentarium.

Approximately 20% of patients with pancreatitis have normal or near-normal amylase activity. In hyperlipemic patients with pancreatitis, normal serum and urine amylase levels are frequently encountered. The spuriously normal levels are believed to be the result of suppression of amylase activity by triglyceride or by a circulating inhibitor in serum.

Lower than normal serum amylase activity may be found in patients with chronic pancreatitis and has also been seen in such diverse and unexpected conditions as congestive heart failure, pregnancy (during the second and third trimesters), gastrointestinal cancer, bone fractures, and pleurisy.

Serum amylase may be elevated in patients with pancreatic carcinoma, but too late to be diagnostically useful. It is also elevated frequently (in over 60% of cases) in patients with diabetic ketoacidosis. Polyacrylamide gel electrophoresis has demonstrated that in this condition, it is usually salivary rather than pancreatic amylase that is elevated. Serum amylase activity may also be elevated in patients with cholecystitis or peptic ulcer, or following gastric resection, renal transplant, viral hepatitis, or ruptured ectopic pregnancy. Very high activity has been reported in patients with carcinoma of the lung. Fewer hyperamylasemic patients may be found to have intestinal obstruction, mesenteric thrombosis, and peritonitis. In some of these patients, pancreatic secretions find their way into the peritoneal cavity and are absorbed into the bloodstream. In others, there may be inflammation involving the pancreas.

Increased ascites fluid amylase levels have been seen in patients with pancreatitis, a leaking pancreatic pseudocyst, pancreatic duct rupture, pancreatic cancer, abdominal tumors that secrete amylase, and perforation of a hollow viscus.

Lipase

The pancreas is the major and primary source of serum lipase. Human pancreatic lipase is a glycoprotein with a molecular weight of 45 000 Da. In contrast to amylase, which is present in both the pancreas and the salivary glands, lipase is not present in the salivary glands. Lipases are defined as enzymes that hydrolyze preferentially glycerol esters of long chain fatty acids at the carbon 1 and 3 ester bonds, producing 2 mol of fatty acid and 1 mol of β-monoglyceride per mole of triglyceride. After isomerization, the third fatty acid can be split off at a slower rate. Lipolysis increases in proportion to the surface area of the lipid droplets, and the absence of bile salts in duodenal fluid with a resultant lack of emulsification renders lipase ineffective.

The presence of colipase and bile salt is required for full catalytic activity and the greatest specificity of the pancreatic lipase. Proteins, bile acids, and phospholipids inhibit serum lipase, colipase reverses this inhibition. Both lipase and colipase are secreted by the pancreas and are, therefore, present in the serum. Colipase is present in the blood of patients with pancreatitis but in variable concentrations and usually below normal and below the amount needed to activate pancreatic lipase fully. To determine accurately and fully the pancreatic lipase activity in patients with pancreatitis it is essential to add colipase to the reagent pack.

Pancreatic lipase must be differentiated from lipoprotein lipase, aliesterase, and arylester hydrolase, which are related but different enzymes. These enzymes' activities may be included in the measurement of lipase activity unless the suitable assay conditions for 'pancreatic' lipase are adapted. Lipase is also present in liver, stomach, intestine, white blood cells, fat cells, and milk.

Calcium is necessary for maximal lipase activity, but at a concentration higher than 5×10^{-3} M, it has an inhibitory effect. It is speculated that the inhibitory effect is due to its interference with the action of bile salts at the water–substrate interface. Like serum albumin, bile salts prevent the denaturation of lipase at the interface. Heavy metals and quinine inhibit lipase activity.

Lipase is filtered by the glomeruli owing to its low molecular weight; it is normally completely reabsorbed by the proximal tubules and is absent from normal urine. In patients with failure of renal tubular reabsorption caused by renal disorders, lipase is found in the urine. Urine lipase activity in the absence of pancreatic disease is inversely related to the creatinine clearance.

Serum lipase is stable up to 1 week at room temperature and may be kept stable longer if it is refrigerated or frozen. The optimal reaction temperature is about 40°C. The optimal pH is 8.8, but other values ranging from 7.0–9.0 have been reported. This difference probably is due to the effect of the difference in types of substrate, buffer, incubation temperature, and concentrations of reagents used. Serum is the specimen of choice for blood lipase assays. Icterus, lipemia, and hemolysis do not interfere with turbidimetric lipase assays.

In acute pancreatitis serum lipase activity tends to become elevated at about the same time as, if not earlier than, the elevation of serum amylase, and it remains elevated for about 7–10 days. Increased lipase activity rarely lasts longer than 14 days, and prolonged increases suggest a poor prognosis or the presence of a cyst.

The combined use of serum lipase and serum amylase is effective in ruling out acute pancreatitis. Although determination of serum lipase has diagnostic advantages over serum amylase for acute pancreatitis, it is not specific for acute pancreatitis. Serum lipase may also be elevated in patients with chronic pancreatitis, obstruction of the pancreatic duct, and nonpancreatic conditions including renal diseases, various abdominal diseases such as acute cholecystitis, intestinal obstruction or infarction, duodenal ulcer, and liver disease, as well as alcoholism, and diabetic ketoacidosis, and in patients who have undergone endoscopic retrograde cholangiopancreatography. Patients with trauma to the abdomen uniformly have increases in both serum amylase and lipase, whereas those with primarily head injury or manipulation of the parotid gland during surgery have a significant increase in serum amylase only. Elevation of serum lipase activity in patients with mumps strongly suggests significant pancreatic as well as salivary gland involvement by the disease.

Serum lipase and amylase tests have been and continue to be widely used in the diagnosis of acute pancreatitis. Both serum amylase and serum lipase are elevated in many patients who have inflammatory or other disorders of organs in the abdominal cavity but no evidence of pancreatitis. It is concluded that the pancreas is exquisitely sensitive to inflammatory or metabolic disturbances in the peritoneum and nearby organs.

Isoamylases

The amylase present in blood and urine of normal individuals is predominantly of pancreatic and salivary origin. Amylase of pancreatic and salivary origin is abbreviated to P-type and S-type amylase (isoenzyme, isoamylase), respectively, whenever such a distinction is needed. These two types of amylase are closely related enzymes, but have organ-specific variations. They have the same amino acid composition and yield similar but not identical peptide maps. Each appears to consist of a single polypeptide chain without subunits. Pancreatic amylase has a molecular weight of 54 000. Higher molecular weights have been reported for salivary amylase. Both amylases contain sulfhydryl groups. Amylases are metalloenzymes containing at least one atom of calcium per molecule; they require this metal for their catalytic activities. The pH for optimal activity ranges from 6.9–7.0. The pH optimum for salivary amylase varies with the anion used as activator, of which chloride is the most important. Optimal chloride concentration is 10 mmol/L, and the activation is

allosteric. Bromide and iodide ions also activate amylase. The isoelectric points (pI) have been reported to be 7.6 and 7.2 for P-type, and 6.4 and 5.8 for S-type isoamylases.

The fractionation of amylase in serum, urine, or other body fluids may be achieved by physical means, such as electrophoresis, chromatography, and isoelectric focusing, and each isoenzyme is then quantitated either by direct densitometry or by amyloclastic or saccharogenic techniques. A simplified, readily adaptable, chromatographic method has been described by Fridhandler (1980). A chemical inhibition assay employing a salivary amylase-specific protein inhibitor is also being used for isoenzyme determinations and is commercially available. The chemical inhibition of isoamylase determination is simple, fast, and suitable for emergency situations. An immunoinhibition method using a monoclonal antibody to inhibit the salivary amylase and subsequently quantitate the remaining pancreatic amylase has been reported (Mifflin, 1985). Because of its simplicity, acceptable analytical precision, and good correlation with the electrophoretic isoamylase method, this method should be further investigated for clinical application.

A great number of reports have supported the finding that in acute pancreatitis, P-type amylase is invariably elevated in both serum and urine. The S-type isoenzyme, however, is decreased to 0–15% of the total activity of serum hyperamylasemia in patients with acute pancreatitis, to 12–25% in those with chronic relapsing pancreatitis, and to near zero in those with carcinoma of the head of the pancreas. The P-type isoenzyme is also elevated in chronic relapsing pancreatitis, hypoparathyroidism, and glomerulonephritis. S-type amylase is increased in the serum of patients with chronic pancreatitis, mumps, pancreatic insufficiency, Sjögren's syndrome, cholelithiasis, common duct narrowing, alcohol ingestion, acute gastroenteritis, acute respiratory insufficiency, chronic renal failure, lung cancer, and with other cancer-associated hyperamylasemias. Isoenzyme studies on serum, urine, and duodenal fluid from patients with cystic fibrosis revealed that two-thirds of the patients had no or little pancreatic amylase.

The relative activity of P-type isoamylase has been reported to be highly useful as a diagnostic index of pancreatic pseudocysts (Warshaw, 1980). The P1 isoamylase (the slowest migrating or least anodic) normally accounts for 80–90% of total amylase activity: P2 and P3 account for 0–4% in both serum and pancreatic juice. The mean ratios of P2/P1 and P3/P1 in fresh pancreatic juice, normal serum, acute pancreatitis serum, chronic pancreatitis serum, and pancreatic cancer serum were always less than 0.25 and less than 0.04, respectively. This ratio was elevated in about 90% of sera from patients with proven pseudocysts but not from others. In several cases, this isoamylase analysis ruled out a pseudocyst correctly, whereas ultrasound or CT scan erroneously indicated the presence of a pseudocyst.

Gastrin

Gastrin is a primary gastrointestinal hormone, produced mainly by the antral G cells, that regulates gastric acid secretion and stimulates growth of the gastric mucosa among other functions. To a lesser extent, gastrin is produced by the G cells of the proximal small intestine and delta cells of the pancreas. Gastrin acts on the parietal cells located in the fundus of the stomach, stimulating the secretion of gastric acid. Gastrin also increases blood flow to the stomach and is responsible for increased gastric and intestinal motility. Other functions include stimulation of gastric pepsinogens and intrinsic factor secretion, release of secretin from the small intestine and secretion of pancreatic enzymes as well as bicarbonate (Henderson, 1994). This hormone is secreted mainly after the detection of digested protein products as well as from antral distention. Maximal stimulation of gastrin secretion occurs within a pH range of 5–7. An acid environment serves as a negative-feedback mechanism for the release of gastrin with 80% reduction in secretion at a pH of 2.5 (Henderson, 1994). This serves to protect the stomach from overacidification from excess stimulation of gastrin. For this reason, individuals on acid suppression therapy for peptic ulcer disease may have elevated gastrin levels.

Three main forms of gastrin exist in human blood and tissues: G34, G17, and G14, known as big gastrin, little gastrin and mini gastrin respectively. All gastrins originate from a single precursor, preprogastrin that is cleaved by the action of trypsin. Preprogastrin yields progastrin, which is subsequently processed to yield glycine-extended gastrin (G34 Gly and G17 Gly) before conversion to the amidated forms G34 and G17 (Wang, 1999). Interestingly, in pathologic cases of increased gastrin production, as with achlorhydric gastritis or gastrinomas, larger molecular forms of gastrin and incompletely processed precursors are present and are beyond the scope of detection by conventional assays. In such cases only little gastrin would be detectable in serum (Goetze, 2003).

Laboratory determination of gastrin levels with available RIA or ELISA assays is indicated for the confirmation of suspected diagnosis of gastrin-secreting tumors, namely, gastrinomas or Zollinger–Ellison syndrome. The antibodies present in these assays are specific for the biologically active C-terminal of the gastrin molecule and they have minimal cross-reactivity with CCK peptides. Prior to determination of gastrin levels, a patient must be fasting for 12 hours because the concentration of G34 doubles and the concentration of G17 quadruples following a meal, altering the results of the assay. Specimens must be frozen immediately because gastrin is unstable in serum. Due to the action of proteolytic enzymes, 50% of the specimen's immunoreactivity may be lost within 48 hours at a temperature of 4°C. It is recommended that specimens should be kept in a freezer at a temperature of −70°C without a self-defrosting cycle, if long-term storage is required. Specimens must be analyzed immediately after thawing, avoiding refreezing and thawing.

Normal reference gastrin levels for fasting individual range up to 100 ng/L. However, it should be noted that fasting serum gastrin levels are increased with increasing age, especially in patients older than 60 years, in part due to unrecognized gastric mucosal atrophy. Approximately 15% of individuals older than 60 years may have gastrin levels between 100–800 ng/L (Henderson, 1994). It should also be noted that reference intervals for infants and children differ from those for adults, so values should be compared to an age-specific reference range for accuracy. Gastrin concentration greater than 1000 ng/L with gastric acid hypersecretion (basal acid secretion > 15 mmol/h) is diagnostic of gastrinomas. In patients with Zollinger–Ellison syndrome (ZE) there is usually a marked elevation, up to 2000 times the normal gastrin level. The secretin stimulation test is a provocative biochemical test that can help confirm the diagnosis of ZE in questionable cases. Infused secretin should cause a drop in gastrin levels, as occurs in normal patients. However, in patients with ZE, there is a dramatic increase in gastrin level, confirming the diagnosis. The mechanism by which secretin stimulates an increase in gastrin levels in these patients is poorly understood; however, it is thought to be due to a direct local effect on the blood flow to the tumor (Ashley, 1999). Limitations include altered results from conditions that may lead to elevated gastrin levels such as gastric ulcer disease, chronic renal failure, hyperparathyroidism, pyloric obstruction, vagotomy, retained gastric antrum, short bowel syndrome, and pernicious anemia. Certain medication can also increase gastrin measurements such as antacids, H₂-blocking agents and proton pump inhibitors, all commonly used in the treatment of patients with peptic ulcer disease. However, these elevations are moderate and certainly not as high as in a patient with a gastrin-secreting tumor.

Assays have traditionally been used to detect elevated gastrin levels associated with diseases such as ZE or gastrinoma. However, the clearly established benefit of rapid intraoperative PTH assays (see Ch. 15) has prompted similar interest in gastrin as an intraoperative guide for therapeutic management, either to confirm adequate removal of gastrin-secreting tissue or to prompt further dissection and possibly more elaborate procedures. Intraoperative testing is of potential use because gastrinomas can be multiple and are often difficult to locate because they can be distributed widely, among for example, stomach, pancreas, and duodenum or periaortic lymph nodes. Gastrin is an appropriate hormone for rapid intraoperative testing because it has a short analyte half-life, approximately 10 minutes, so that changes can be detected shortly after resection of hypersecreting tissue, rapid analysis that can be completed within the time frame of the operative procedure, and a positive clinical utility (Sokoll, 2004). The catabolic breakdown of most peptide hormones follows first-order exponential decay. Therefore, if the entire hormone-secreting tissue is surgically resected, only approximately 12.5% of the baseline concentration would be present in serum after three half-lives (Sokoll, 2004). In one clinical study, patients with ZE or gastrinomas were evaluated with intraoperative gastrin assays, and a drop of gastrin levels to within reference values within 20 minutes of resection was indicative of cure. The sensitivity for intraoperative gastrin assays has been estimated to be 88%. This test may help to identify patients who may benefit from more extensive dissections or operative procedures such as duodenopancreatectomy, a procedure not advocated on all patients because of associated morbidity and mortality (Sokoll, 2004). However, gastrin assays intraoperatively may help to identify patients who would benefit from this surgical intervention, a remarkable advancement in the management of patients with gastrinomas.

Pepsin and Pepsinogen

Pepsinogens are the biologically inactive proenzymes of pepsins that are produced by the chief cells and other cells in the gastric mucosa and are found in two distinct types, pepsinogen I (PGI), also known as pepsinogen A, and pepsinogen II (PGII), also known as pepsinogen C. Pepsinogen secretion is stimulated by the vagus nerve, gastrin, secretin and CCK, and is inhibited by gastric inhibitory peptide (GIP), anticholinergics, histamine H₂-receptor antagonists and vagotomy (Henderson, 1994). PGI is produced in the chief cells and mucous cells of oxyntic glands; PGII is produced in mucous cells in oxyntic and pyloric regions and the duodenum. The ratio of concentration of pepsinogen I to pepsinogen II in serum or plasma of healthy individuals is approximately 4 : 1 (Samloff, 1982). Pepsinogen is converted to the active form, pepsin, by gastric acid that can activate additional pepsinogen autocatalytically. Both groups of pepsinogen are activated at an acid pH below 5 and destroyed by alkaline pH. Both types can be detected in blood. Only type I pepsinogens are present in the urine, and type II is present in semen (Henderson, 1994). Pepsins are responsible for the hydrolysis of proteins to polypeptides. The pepsinogen released from the gastric mucosa is predominantly secreted and constitutes a major component of gastric fluid. Only approximately 1% gets into the peripheral blood. Active pepsin is rapidly inactivated in the bloodstream, whereas pepsinogen is stable in the blood. Pepsinogen is then filtered by the kidneys and is excreted in the urine, where the slightly acidic pH converts the pepsinogen, now called uropepsinogen to uropepsin (Henderson, 1994). Immunoassay is the method used to detect serum pepsinogen. However, the PGI isoform is commonly analyzed in the clinical laboratory since it is the isoform commonly associated with disease.

Serum levels of pepsinogen I are an accurate estimate of parietal cell mass and correlate with acid-secretory capacity of the stomach. Increased pepsinogen levels and associated activity is observed in patients with disease states that lead to increased gastric output or with increased parietal cell mass, namely, gastrinomas, Zollinger–Ellison syndrome, duodenal ulcer disease and acute and chronic gastritis (Henderson, 1994). Decreased levels of pepsinogen are associated with disease states marked by decreased parietal cell mass, namely atrophic gastritis and gastric carcinoma as well as in patients with myxedema, Addison's disease and hypopituitarism (Henderson, 1994). The PGI/PGII ratio decreases linearly with worsening atrophic gastritis. Absence of pepsinogen is noted in patients with achlorhydria. This must be kept in mind when analyzing serum pepsinogen levels, possibly limiting clinical utility of this serum assay. Pepsinogen I levels measured by immunoassay usually range from 20–107 and pepsinogen II levels usually range from 3–19 µg/L.

Pepsinogen assays are being explored for their utility in the noninvasive identification of patients with chronic atrophic gastritis as well as to provide an estimate of the extent of atrophic gastritis, a known precursor of gastric carcinoma. Severe atrophic body gastritis causes a four- to fivefold increase in the risk of gastric carcinoma compared to healthy individuals (Sanduleanu, 2003). This will hopefully identify a sub group of individuals with chronic atrophic gastritis that would benefit from endoscopic evaluations for detection of early-stage gastric tumors. These assays are currently utilized in Japan, an area marked by high prevalence of gastric cancer, as a potential method for widespread screening of high-risk individuals (Miki, 2003). Miki recommended that criteria for diagnosing chronic atrophic gastritis be persons with PGI < 70 µg/liter and PGI/PGII ratio < 3.0. All patients fitting these criteria should then be referred to a gastroenterologist for further endoscopic evaluations. In Japan, the pepsinogen serum screening test has been demonstrated to detect a higher percentage of early cancers compared to conventional methods, and a considerable number of patients have subsequently been candidates for treatments with endoscopic surgery (Mikki, 2003). The most sensitive test for fundic atrophic gastritis is considered to be the PGI/II serum ratio, with 99% sensitivity and 94% specificity (Henderson, 1994). Furthermore, pepsinogen II levels may be a useful marker of prognosis, serving as an independent predictor of tumor biology and survival in patients with gastric carcinoma. The absence of PGII production has been associated with aggressive tumor behavior and shorter overall survival in gastric cancer patients (Fernandez, 2000). Pepsinogen assays may therefore prove to be a useful serum screening method for detection of gastric carcinoma among high-risk individuals.

Trypsinogen

Trypsin is produced in the exocrine pancreas as two proenzymes, known as trypsinogen 1 and trypsinogen 2. The proenzymes are activated in the duodenum by an enterokinase that yields trypsin 1 and trypsin 2 respectively. Trypsin present within the peripheral circulation is inactivated by complexing with either alpha-2-macroglobulin or alpha-1-antitrypsin (AAT). Trypsin, unlike amylase, is solely produced by the pancreatic acinar cells and is therefore a specific indicator of pancreatic damage. Premature activation of the proenzyme to active trypsin within the pancreatic parenchyma is thought to be a key mechanism in the development of acute pancreatitis (Andersen, 2001). Currently, levels of all forms of trypsin are determined by specific immunoassays.

the container and not to overfill the container. Gas, which frequently accumulates, should be released gradually by carefully loosening of the cap. Failure to observe this simple precaution, especially in the case of an overfilled container, can result in an explosive release of contents.

Fecal matter left on the physician's gloved finger at the time of a rectal examination may be transferred to a piece of filter paper for inspection and testing for occult blood. Because of wide variation in bowel habits, intestinal transit time, and bulk of stool, special consideration must be given to methods of timed stool collection. For collection of timed urine specimens, the urinary bladder can be emptied before and at the end of the collection period. The gastrointestinal tract, however, cannot be emptied completely at will. Therefore, the amount of stool collected in a 24-hour period usually correlates very poorly with the amount of food ingested during a similar period of time. For determining the 24-hour fecal excretion of any substance, stool should be collected over a period of at least 3 days, and calculations should be based on the entire specimen divided by the number of days of collection. The accuracy of this method can be enhanced somewhat by having the patient ingest carmine dye (0.3 g) at the beginning and charcoal (1 g) at the end of a collecting period, and collecting the stools from the beginning of the appearance of the dye to the beginning of the appearance of the charcoal. However, *Salmonella cubana* outbreaks in Massachusetts and California were traced to carmine dye. Another method of signaling the collection period involves the use of inert, nonabsorbable stool markers. These are taken in divided uniform doses for several days prior to the beginning of the collection, continuing through the collection period. The concentration of the material found in the stool specimen is then used to determine the quantity of stool containing 1 day's ingestion of the material as an indication of the 24-hour output. For this purpose, chromium sesquioxide (Cr_2O_3) has been used, and its concentration in the feces is determined chemically. The substitution of radioactive chromium or zirconium isotope has made it possible to determine concentration by measuring the radioactivity of the stool, but these methods, as currently used, are too time-consuming for routine determinations.

Fecal specimen sample collection at home is by no means simple and easy unless the patient has been instructed properly. Hoffman (1973) has described a collection method that has the advantages of ease of transportation and storage, absence of requirements for special equipment, and acceptability to patients and laboratory staff.

A pediatric method described by Jelliffe (1973) includes the use of a thick-walled glass tube, which is lubricated by dipping into water and then inserted into the young child's rectum. In about two-thirds of cases, a core of feces can be obtained, which can be poked out with an applicator stick into the container.

Macroscopic Examination of Feces

Inspection of the feces is important because it may lead to a diagnosis of parasitic infestation, obstructive jaundice, diarrhea, malabsorption, rectosigmoidal obstruction, dysentery, ulcerative colitis, or gastrointestinal tract bleeding.

The quantity, form, consistency, and color of the stool should be noted. Normally, 100–200 g of stool is passed per day. When diarrhea is present the stool is watery. Passage of large amounts of mushy, foul-smelling, gray stool that floats on the water is characteristic of steatorrhea. Constipation may be associated with passage of small, firm, spherical masses of stool (scybala). Constipation most often results from the irritable colon syndrome in patients with anxiety or from overuse of laxatives. In such patients, repeated tests for occult blood are called for to detect more serious organic problems such as carcinoma, which may also afflict those patients.

A narrow, ribbon-like stool suggests the possibility of spastic bowel or rectal narrowing or stricture. Clay color suggests diminution or absence of bile or the presence of barium sulfate. Blood, especially blood originating from the lower gut, may cause the stool to be red; beets in the diet may mimic this. Bleeding from the upper gastrointestinal tract is more likely to cause the stool to be black and have a tarry consistency. Bismuth, iron, and charcoal may also cause a black color. Stool that is allowed to stand in the air for a time may darken on the surface. Green stools may result from ingestion of spinach and other green vegetables or calomel, or it may result from the presence of biliverdin, seen in patients taking antibiotics orally. It is not unusual to see seeds and vegetable skins. Parasites are considered in Chapter 61.

Mucus. The presence of recognizable mucus in a stool specimen is abnormal and should be reported. Translucent gelatinous mucus clinging to the surface of the formed stool suggests spastic constipation or mucous colitis. It is seen in stools of emotionally disturbed patients and may result from excessive straining. Bloody mucus clinging to the fecal mass suggests

neoplasm or inflammatory processes of the rectal canal. Mucus associated with pus and blood is found in stools of patients with ulcerative colitis, bacillary dysentery, ulcerating diverticulitis, and intestinal tuberculosis. Patients with villous adenoma of the colon may pass copious quantities of mucus, amounting to 3–4 L in 24 hours. They frequently develop severe dehydration and electrolyte disturbances, especially hypokalemia.

Pus. Patients with chronic ulcerative colitis and chronic bacillary dysentery frequently pass large quantities of pus with the stool, the recognition of which requires microscopic examination. This also occurs in patients with localized abscesses or fistulas communicating with the sigmoid colon, rectum, or anus. Large amounts of pus seldom accompany the stools of patients with amebic colitis and its presence is evidence against this diagnosis. No inflammatory exudate is seen in the watery stools of patients with viral gastroenteritis.

Microscopic Examination of Feces

Fat. The crudest technique is microscopic examination using Sudan III, Sudan IV, or Oil Red O stain. The procedure has been widely employed for screening because of its simplicity. In our experience, results have correlated well with quantitative measurements when aliquots of the same homogenized stool have been analyzed. For this purpose, a small aliquot of stool suspension is placed on a slide and mixed with two drops of 95% ethanol; then two drops of saturated ethanolic solution of Sudan III are added, with further mixing. A coverslip is then applied. Under these conditions fatty acids are present as lightly stained flakes or as needle-like crystals that do not stain and therefore may be missed. Soaps also do not stain but appear as well-defined amorphous flakes or as rounded masses or coarse crystals. Neutral fats, however, appear as large orange or red droplets. When 60 or more stained droplets of neutral fats per high-power field (hpf) are seen, one may be reasonably certain that the patient has steatorrhea. Caution is advisable in interpretation, however, because mineral oil or castor oil may mimic neutral fat. The procedure is then repeated, adding several drops of 36% (v/v) acetic acid to the stool mixture and warming the slide several times over a flame until slight boiling occurs. This converts neutral fats and soaps to fatty acids and melts the fatty acids, causing them to form droplets that stain strongly with Sudan III. The slide is then examined while warm. After this procedure, the presence of up to 100 stained droplets per high-power field is considered normal. Patients with steatorrhea of pancreatic origin are likely to have greater increases in fatty acids and soaps. Some have advocated using Oil Red O because it permits substitution of isopropanol for ethanol.

Meat Fiber. The technique for sampling is identical to that used for Sudan preparations for detection of fecal fat. The stool is mixed thoroughly on a slide with a 10% alcohol solution of eosin, allowed to stain for 3 minutes, and then examined for muscle fibers. The entire area under the coverslip is examined, and only rectangular fibers with clearly evident cross-striation are counted. It appears that examination for meat fibers yields results that correlate well with chemical determination of fat excretion.

Leukocytes. A small fleck of mucus or a drop of liquid stool is placed on a glass microscopic slide with a wooden applicator stick. Two drops of Loffler methylene blue are added and mixed thoroughly and carefully. A coverslip is placed on the mixture, which is allowed to stand for 2–3 minutes for good nuclear staining. Using low-power scanning, rough quantitative counts are made by approximating the average number of leukocytes and erythrocytes. All differential counts should be made under high power, counting 200 cells when possible. Only those cells clearly identified as either mononuclear or polymorphonuclear are included in the differential count. Macrophages and epithelial cells that cannot be clearly identified are ignored. The initial cell counts should be performed at the time of presentation of the specimen.

Fecal Occult Blood Testing

Colon cancer is a leading cause of cancer-related deaths in the US, accounting for approximately 55 000 deaths annually. According to recent cancer statistics, approximately 150 000 new colon cancer cases were diagnosed in 2003. Evidence has demonstrated the clinical usefulness of fecal occult blood testing (FOBT) to detect these cancers at an earlier stage, potentially resulting in decreased mortality. Three randomized, controlled trials have demonstrated that FOBT decreases mortality from colon cancer by 15–35% (Clinical Guideline, 1997). Due to the generally favorable clinical biology of these tumors when detected earlier, with an 80–90% survival rate with local confined disease (Helm, 2003) and the relatively inexpensive, noninvasive nature of FOBT, this may serve as a useful screening technique. Several professional organizations recommend annual of biennial FOBT but universal accepted screening protocols have not been established. The American Cancer Society (ACS) guidelines for colorectal cancer screening, the most widely utilized, recommend annual

FOBT and flexible sigmoidoscopy every 3–5 years beginning at age 50 in asymptomatic, average-risk individuals (Marshall, 1996). The College of American Pathologists Laboratory Testing Strategy Task Force also recommends annual stool blood screening as a standard of practice. The limitations of this testing include the high number of false-positive and false-negative results. The sensitivity of FOBT has been estimated between 30–50%. The true sensitivity of FOBT is difficult to determine because individuals who test negative, do not undergo further colonoscopic evaluation to determine if the FOBT is a true negative. Only approximately 5–10% of positive reactions prove to be caused by an occult malignancy (Simon, 1998). However, following a stepwise approach to colon cancer screening should minimize the clinical effects of limited sensitivity and specificity and offer valuable information nonetheless.

Occult blood can be detected by chemical (guiac), hemoporphyrin or immunological methods. Occult blood may arise anywhere along the intestinal tract and is often the first warning sign of GI malignancy. Other potential sources of occult blood may arise from bleeding esophageal varices, polyps, esophageal or gastric inflammation, hemorrhoids or fissures, IBD, PUD or angiodysplasias of the colon. Laboratory diagnosis of the presence of fecal occult blood generally involves a guiac-smear test (Hemoccult, Searcult, Coloscreen), the most commonly used method at present. Guiac is a naturally occurring phenolic compound that is oxidized to quinone by hydrogen peroxidase, resulting in a detectable color change. These tests detect the pseudoperoxidase activity of heme, either as intact hemoglobin or as free heme (Allison, 1996). These tests are not specific for human hemoglobin, and hemoglobin from red meat, peroxidase from fruits and vegetables and certain medications can lead to false-positive results. The presence of greater than 20 mL/day of blood in the stool results in a positive guiac smear. Stool specimens should be received from three consecutive stools. Two slides should be prepared for each stool sample. Studies have shown that slides should not be rehydrated and should be developed within 7 days of collection. This is a standard protocol for FOBT, recommended by randomized clinical trials. Interestingly, medical institutions are now requiring that stool samples be sent to the laboratory for guiac testing rather than having residents perform the test on the wards, to ensure compliance with this protocol. Most guiac tests performed by residents are completed after a single digital rectal examination. Rehydration increases test sensitivity for detection of colorectal cancer but decreases specificity, resulting in a 10% or greater increase in false-positive results. This prompts further unnecessary invasive and expensive colonoscopic evaluations, making screening impractical. In addition, the test must be performed under appropriate conditions that serve to limit the sensitivity of this test. Factors that can cause inaccuracies in the results include the presence of bleeding gums for example, or ingestion of large amounts of red meat prior to testing. In addition, patients may be using certain medications that will influence the result of FOBT. For example, drugs that can cause GI irritation and subsequent bleeding such as anticoagulants, aspirin, NSAIDs, colchicines or iron supplements may lead to false-positive results. Other drugs that have been implicated include reserpine and oxidizing drugs such as iodine. On the contrary, ingestion of large amounts of vitamin C can lead to a false-negative result. Therefore, patients must be informed of these effects and ideally should avoid such medications or food products prior to FOBT; if not clinically feasible, FOBT should then be interpreted with caution, or avoided altogether as a screening modality in these patients.

A positive result on FOBT should be defined as positivity in one or more slide windows, maximizing the sensitivity of the screening procedure. A positive FOBT then prompts further evaluation for suspected colonic neoplasia. A middle-aged patient determined to have a positive FOBT, without slide rehydration, has an estimated 7–14% probability of having an early stage, Dukes A or B colon cancer (Clinical Guideline, 1997). Further evaluations usually include either sigmoidoscopy with barium enema or full colonoscopy, the latter being the preferred modality. A negative FOBT, however, cannot definitely rule out the presence of colonic neoplasia. If a patient is presenting with signs and symptoms suggestive of colon cancer, further evaluation is warranted, even in the presence of negative FOBT.

Fecal immunochemical testing for human hemoglobin, such as HemeSelect or InSure, has been developed to improve the sensitivity and specificity of guiac testing to detect colonic neoplasia. HemeSelect testing is based on an antigen–antibody reaction involving fixed chicken red blood cells coated with anti-human-hemoglobin antibody (Allison, 1996). Samples demonstrating agglutination are interpreted as positive for occult human blood. InSure is a test which uses monoclonal mouse antihuman hemoglobin antibody with subsequent colorimetric detection and is sensitive enough to detect 50 μg Hb/g feces (Quest Diagnostics). These tests do not react with nonhuman hemoglobin or peroxidase, so food

restrictions are not necessary. Immunochemical InSure tests target the globin portion of hemoglobin, which does not survive passage through the upper GI tract. Therefore, these tests are more specific for lower gastrointestinal, colonic bleeding (Quest Diagnostics).

Fecal DNA testing is a promising technique for detection of occult blood; however, widespread use is not current practice. This test involves collection of a single stool specimen which is then screened for DNA markers originating from cells of cancers present in the gastrointestinal tract that are shed into the stool (Helm, 2003). PCR is used to amplify the fecal DNA to yield an extremely sensitive assay. This is a useful test because neoplastic DNA remains stable in stool, whereas the cells shed from normal epithelium are degraded by enzymes as part of normal cell death (Helm, 2003). APC and p53 are examples of genes serving as DNA markers in stool testing because they control colorectal cell growth and are often affected by colonic neoplasia. Clinical studies have shown that fecal DNA testing has increased specificity, ranging from 93–100% and sensitivity ranging from 71–91% for detection of cancer, considerably more than chemical guiac testing, promising improved laboratory diagnosis of colorectal malignancy. Refer to Figure 22–1 for an algorithm for fecal occult blood testing for early detection of colon cancer.

Fecal Elastase

Elastase 1 is a proteolytic enzyme, produced by the pancreas, with a molecular weight of 28 kD, and represents approximately 6% of pancreatic enzyme secretions. It was initially isolated in 1975 and called protease E (Lankisch, 2004). Pancreatic elastase survives intestinal transit intact and is concentrated in the feces, five- to sixfold the concentration present in pancreatic juice (Lankisch, 2004).

Fecal elastase 1 determination is a novel fecal enzyme test, used for indirect assessment of pancreatic function to aid diagnosis of exocrine pancreatic insufficiency. This test may replace fecal chymotrypsin levels. Interestingly, elastase 1 is increased in acute and relapsing chronic pancreatitis, more so than serum amylase (Henderson, 1994). In addition, elevation of elastase 1 persists longer than serum amylase levels and, therefore, may be more specific for detection of pancreatitis and more accurately follow the clinical course of the disease (Henderson, 1994). Continued investigation will likely define appropriate utility for fecal elastase analysis in particular clinical settings; until then, caution is warranted in interpretation of results.

This ELISA test uses monoclonal antibodies that react with human pancreatic elastase (PE) (Lankisch, 2004). It is therefore, unaffected by pancreatic enzyme replacement therapy, making it a useful diagnostic test. The test is highly sensitive for detection of severe pancreatic insufficiency; however, it lacks high sensitivity for detection of milder forms, a problem common to indirect tests of pancreatic function. Fecal elastase has diagnostic superiority over fecal chymotrypsin levels as well as older test of exocrine pancreatic function, namely, para-aminobenzoic acid (PABA) bentiromide test and pancreolauryl test (Lankisch, 2004).

A single analysis of a 100-mg stool sample is adequate for determination of fecal elastase levels. If borderline values are detected, then a repeat sample may be useful. This test should only be performed on formed stool, important in specimen collection and processing. Based on previous testing, values greater than 200 μg PE-1/g are considered normal, values ranging from 100–200 μg PE-1/g indicate mild to moderate pancreatic insufficiency and values below 100 indicate severe insufficiency (Lankisch, 2004). Using these cutoff estimations, the fecal elastase enzyme test is estimated to be 57–90% specific. Sensitivity of this test is based on severity of pancreatic insufficiency. This test is estimated to be 100% sensitive for detection of severe disease. However, this decreases to between 33–89% for moderate disease and between 0–65% for mild pancreatic insufficiency as per current preliminary studies. Using a cutoff of 200 μg/g stool, the positive predictive value of fecal elastase determination is estimated to be approximately 50% (Luth, 2001).

Fecal elastase determination may be more useful than fecal chymotrypsin levels for diagnosis of pancreatic insufficiency. However, it lacks sensitivity for detecting mild to moderate disease and cannot diagnose chronic pancreatitis with certainty. In addition it is unable to differentiate between pancreatic and nonpancreatic steatorrhea, limiting its clinical utility. Refer to Table 22–8 for summary of the clinical application of fecal elastase-1 estimation for diagnosing chronic pancreatitis and exocrine pancreatic insufficiency.

Lactose Tolerance Test

Following an overnight fast, administer orally 50 g of lactose dissolved in 400 mL of water. Draw fasting blood and blood samples at 30, 60, and 120 minutes after ingestion as for a glucose tolerance test. An optional 5-hour stool specimen can be collected, examining and recording the appearance, consistency, and pH.

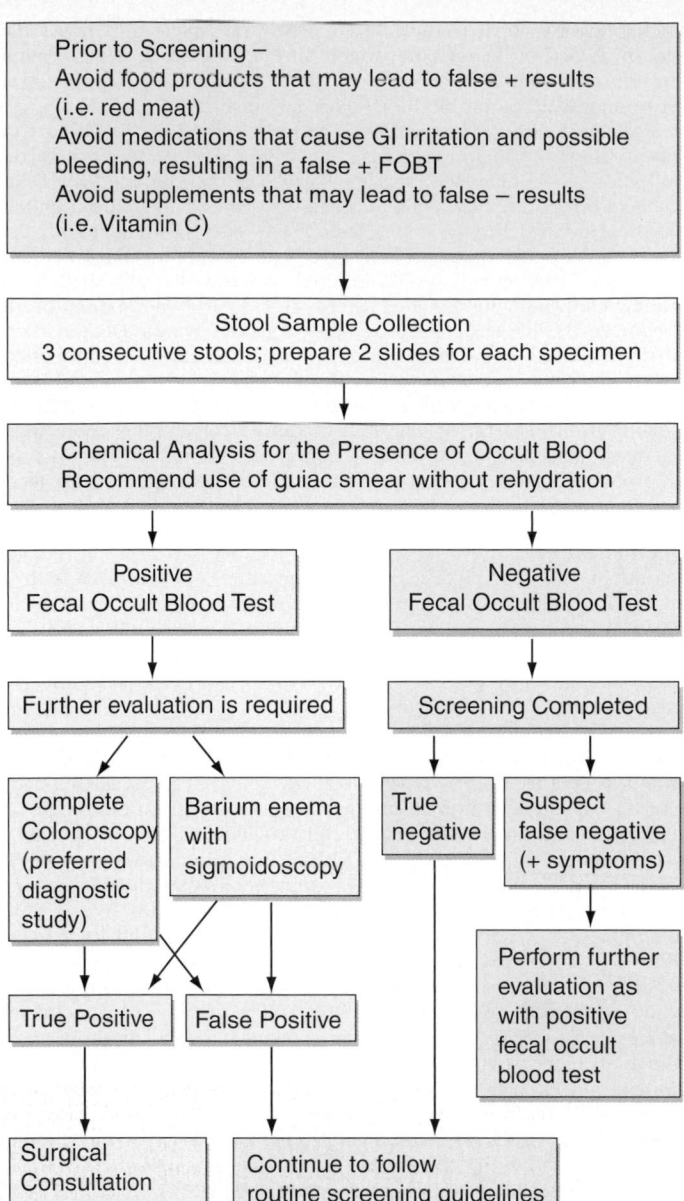

Figure 22–1 Screening for occult colorectal malignancy with fecal occult blood testing (FOBT).

Table 22–8 Value of Fecal Elastase-1 Estimation in Diagnosing Chronic Pancreatitis and Exocrine Pancreatic Insufficiency

Fecal elastase-1 estimation	Morphologic procedures (US, EUS, CT, ERCP)	Interpretation of fecal elastase-1 estimation*
Normal	Normal	Severe exocrine pancreatic insufficiency excluded; mild to moderate impairment possible
Abnormal	Normal	Exocrine pancreatic insufficiency may or may not be present; test not helpful, especially in differentiating steatorrhea/diarrhea
Abnormal	Abnormal	Test confirms chronic pancreatitis but does not indicate whether steatorrhea, and thus pancreatic enzyme substitution-requiring insufficiency, is present
Normal	Abnormal	Two interpretations possible: The patient has chronic pancreatitis on the basis of morphological procedures, but mild to moderate exocrine pancreatic insufficiency was not detected; fecal elastase-1 estimation falsely normal. The abnormal morphologic examination is due to scars following acute pancreatitis; fecal elastase-1 estimation is correctly normal

* Interpretation based on suggestion that diagnosis of chronic pancreatitis should be made on a combination of abnormal results of morphologic examinations and abnormal exocrine pancreatic functions tests.

CT = computed tomography; EUS = endoscopic ultrasound; ERCP = endoscopic retrograde cholangiopancreatography; US = ultrasound.

After Lankisch PG: Now that fecal elastase is available in the United States, should clinicians start using it? Curr Gastroenterol Rep 2004; 6:126–131, with permission.

Patients with lactase deficiency exhibit a peak rise of less than 20 mg/dL in reducing substances expressed as glucose. In all persons with flat tolerance curves, the test should be repeated within 2 days and the less abnormal of the two curves used for interpretation. A control test may be performed, using 25 g glucose and 25 g galactose if the lactose test indicates malabsorption. Some investigators use a 100-g dose, which has been reported by some to yield more definitive results. It may cause symptoms in patients with mild lactase deficiency. In children, the dose of lactose or other sugars is 2 g/kg body weight.

Genetic Markers for Gastrointestinal Disease

The molecular defect underlying cystic fibrosis results in alterations in epithelial cell electrolyte transport. The defect is an autosomal recessive mutation in the CFTR gene located on chromosome 7. The degree of the defect depends on the nature of the mutation. There are several characterized mutations that lead to a milder form of the disease. The classic delta F508 mutation leads to cystic fibrosis when two copies of the gene are inherited. Persons heterozygous for the R117H mutation may develop pancreatic insufficiency. These persons may present as idiopathic chronic pancreatitis (Durie, 2000).

The central enzyme involved in activation of all the digestive proenzymes is trypsin. Trypsin is synthesized and maintained as inactive trypsinogen in secretory granules in the pancreatic acinar cell. Trypsin is stabilized in the pancreatic acini by a serine protease inhibitor, SPINK1. After release into the pancreatic duct, trypsinogen is cleaved by enterokinase on the brush border of the duodenum to active trypsin. Several mutations in trypsin and SPINK1 exist that have recently gained importance in the evaluation of pancreatitis and pancreatic cancer.

Cationic trypsinogen (PRSS1) mutations involving codon 29 and 122 cause autosomal dominant forms of hereditary pancreatitis (Whitcomb, 2000). The number of mutations is limited, and the type of mutation appears to alter the protein, leading to decreased ability to prevent inactivation. Thus a series of events leading to active intra-acinar trypsin occurs.

Mutations in the SPINK1 molecule lead to a similar problem, as the native form leads to stabilization of trypsin. Mutations have been described (N34S) that decrease the ability to promote trypsin degradation. The presence of increased acinar trypsin leads to activation of proenzymes and thus pancreatitis.

Patients with these disorders typically have recurrent acute pancreatitis sometime between infancy and the 4th decade. Chronic pancreatitis and pancreatic cancer develop at a relatively young age. No specific treatment exists for the prevention or treatment of hereditary pancreatitis. Clinical testing is available for the disorders described (Etemad, 2001). There are regulations developed by the Food and Drug Administration for such testing. Ordering genetic testing requires that the physician clearly understand how to interpret the results and anticipate how the results will affect patient management.

Although many other markers are currently being evaluated, none has achieved widespread use at this time. A more extensive discussion of tumor markers is found in Chapter 74.

References

Allison J, Tekawa I, Ransom LJ, et al: A comparison of fecal occult blood tests for colorectal cancer screening. N Engl J Med 2004; 334:155–159.
Evaluation of three commonly used screening tests for fecal occult blood with regard to sensitivity, specificity, and predictive value related to colonoscopy and biopsy findings.

Ammori BJ, Becker KL, Kite P: Calcitonin precursors in the prediction of severity of acute pancreatitis on the day of admission. Br J Surg 2003; 90(2):197–204.

Andersen JM, Hedstrom J, Kemmpainen E, et al: The ratio of trypsin-2-alpha1-antitrypsin to trypsinogen-1 discriminates biliary and alcohol-induced acute pancreatitis. Clin Chem 2001; 47:231–236.

Ashley SW, Evoy D, Daly JM: Stomach. In Schwartz SI, Shires GT, Spencer FC, et al: (eds): Principles of Surgery. New York, McGraw Hill, 1999, pp 1195–1196.

Atherton JC, Spiller RC: The urea breath test for H. pylori . Gut 1994; 35:723–725.

Baillargeon JD, Orav J, Ramagopal V, et al: Hemoconcentration as an early risk factor for necrotizing pancreatitis. Am J Gastroenterol 1998; 83:2130–2136.

Barr GD, Grehan MJ: Coeliac disease. Med J Aust 1998; 169:109–114.

Buchler MW, Malfertheiner P, Schoetensack C, et al: Sensitivity of antiprotease and complement factors and C reactive protein in detecting pancreatic necrosis. Results of a prospective clinical study. Int J Pancreatol 1986; 1:227–235.

Clinical Guideline: Part 1: Suggested technique for fecal occult blood testing and interpretation in colorectal cancer screening. Ann Intern Med 1997; 126(10):808–810.
Guidelines address the technique of screening by using fecal occult blood tests, with emphasis on the interpretation of positive and negative test results and the subsequent work-up of persons with positive results.

Corsetti JP, Cox C, Schulz TJ, Arvan DA: Combined serum amylase and lipase determinations for diagnosis of suspected acute pancreatitis. Clin Chem 1993; 39:2495–2499.

Dahlqvist A: Assay of intestinal disaccharides. Anal Biochem 1968; 22:99–107.

Dieterich W, Laag E, Schopper H, et al: Autoantibodies to tissue transglutaminase as predictors of celiac disease. Gastroenterology 1998; 115:1317–1324.

Durie PR: Pancreatic aspects of cystic fibrosis and other inherited causes of pancreatic dysfunction. Med Clin North Am 2000; 84:609–620.

Elman R, Arneson I, Graham EA. Value of blood amylase estimations in the diagnosis of pancreatic diseases. Arch Surgery 1929; 19:943–948.

Etemad B, Whitcomb DC: Chronic pancreatitis. Diagnosis, classification, and new genetic developments. Gastroenterology 2001; 120:682–707.

Farrell RJ, Kelly CP: Diagnosis of celiac sprue. Am J Gastroenterol 2001; 96:3237–3246.

Feldman RA, Deeks JJ, Evans SJW, et al: Multi-laboratory comparison of eight commercially available Helicobacter pylori serology kits. Eur J Clin Microbiol Infect Dis 1995a; 14:428–433.

Feldman RA, Evans SJW: Accuracy of diagnostic methods used for epidemiological studies of Helicobacter pylori. Aliment Pharmacol Ther 1995b; 9(Suppl 2):21–31.

Fernandez R, Vizoso F, Rodriguez JC: Expression and prognostic significance of pepsinogen C in gastric carcinoma. Ann Surg Oncol 2000; 7(7):508–514.

Frank B, Gottlieb K: Amylase normal, lipase elevated: is it pancreatitis? A case series and review of the literature. Am J Gastroenterol 1999; 94:463–469.

Fridhandler L, Berk JE: Simplified chromatographic method for isoamylase analysis. Clin Chem Acta 1980; 101:135–138.

Goff JS: Two-stage triolein breath test differentiates pancreatic insufficiency from other causes of malabsorption. Gastroenterology 1982; 83:44–46.

Graham DY: Can therapy ever be denied for Helicobacter pylori infection? (editorial). Gastroenterology 1997; 113:S113–S117.

Goetze JP, Rehfeld JF: Impact of assay epitope specificity in gastrinoma diagnosis. Clin Chem 2003; 49(2):333–334.

Guerrant RL, Araujo V, Soares E, et al: Measurement of fecal lactoferrin as a marker of fecal leukocytes. J Clin Microbiol 1992; 30:1238–1242.

Guritzky RP, Rudnitsky G: Bloody neonatal diaper. Ann Emerg Med 1996; 27:662–664.

Helm J, Choi J, Sutphen R, et al: Current and evolving strategies for colorectal cancer screening. Cancer Control 2003; 10(3):193–204.

Henderson AR, Tietz NW, Rinker AD. Gastric, pancreatic and intestinal function. In: Burtis CA, Ashwood ER (eds): Textbook of Clinical Chemistry. Philadelphia, WB Saunders Co., 1994, pp 1576–1644.

Hoffman NE, LaRusso NF, Hoffman AF: An improved method for fecal collection: The field-kit. Lancet 1973; 1:1422.

Jacobsen DG, Currington C, Connery K, Toskes PP: Trypsin like immunoreactivity as a test for pancreatic insufficiency. N Engl J Med 1984; 310:1307–1312.

Jelliffe DB, Jelliffe EFD: Collection of a stool sample. Lancet 1973; 2:618.

Kemppainen EA, Hedstrom JI, Puolakkainen PA, et al: Rapid measurement of urinary trypsinogen-2 as a screening test for acute pancreatitis. N Engl J Med 1997; 336:1788–1793.

Kemppainen E, Hietaranta A, Puolakkainen P, et al: Time course profile of serum trypsinogen-2 and trypsin-2-alpha 1-antitrypsin in patients with acute pancreatitis. Scand J Gastroenterol 2000; 35(11):1216–1220.

Kisker O, Bartsch D, Weinel RJ, et al: The value of somatostatin-receptor scintigraphy in newly diagnosed endocrine gastroenteropancreatic tumors. J Am Coll Surg 1997; 184:487–492.

Klonoff DC: Macroamylasemia and other immunoglobulin-complexes enzyme disorders. West J Med 1980; 133:392–407.

Krasilnikoff PA, Gudman-Hoyer E, Moltke HH: Diagnostic value of disaccharide tolerance tests in children. Acta Paediatr Scand 1975; 64:693–698.

Laheij RJF, Straatman H, Jansen JBMJ, Verbeek ALM: Evaluation of commercially available Helicobacter pylori serology kits: A review. J Clin Microbiol 1998; 36:2803–2809.

Lankisch PG: Now that fecal elastase is available in the United States, should clinicians start using it? Curr Gastroenterol Rep 2004; 6:126–131.

Lankisch PG, Koop H, Otto J, et al: Specificity of increased amylase to creatinine clearance ratio in acute pancreatitis. Digestion 1977; 16:160–164.

LeGrys VA, Burnett RW: Current status of sweat testing in North America. Results of the College of American Pathologists Needs Assessment Survey. Arch Pathol Lab Med 1994; 118:865–867.

Le Moine O, Devaster JM, Deviere et al: Trypsin activity. A new marker of acute alcoholic pancreatitis. Dig Dis Sci 1994; 39:2634–2638.

Lerang F, Huag JB, Moum B, et al: Accuracy of IgG serology and other tests in confirming Helicobacter eradication. Scand J Gastroenterol 1998; 33:710–715.

Levitt MD, Ellis C: A rapid and simple assay to determine if macroamylase is the cause of hyperamylasemia. Gastroenterology 1982; 83:378–382.

Loser C, Mollgaard A, Folsch UR: Fecal elastase 1: a novel highly sensitive and specific tubeless pancreatic function test. Gut 1996; 39:580–586.

Luth S, Teyssen S, Forssmann K, et al: Fecal elastase-1 determination: 'gold standard' of indirect pancreatic function tests? Scand J Gastroenterol 2001; 36(10):1092–1099.

McRury JM, Barry RC: A modified Apt test: a new look at an old test. Pediatr Emerg Care 1994; 10(3):189–191. Erratum in: Pediatr Emerg Care 1994; 10(4):248.

Makristathis A, Pasching E, Schutze K, et al: Detection of Helicobacter pylori in stool specimens by PCR and antigen enzyme immunoassay. J Clin Microbiol 1998; 36:2772–2774.

Malnick S, Zimhony O: Treatment of Clostridium difficile-associated diarrhea. Ann Pharmacother 2000; 36:1767–1775.

Marshall JB: Colorectal cancer screening: present strategies and future prospects. Postgrad Med 1996; 99(3):253–264.

Megraud F: Diagnosis and candidates for treatment of Helicobacter pylori infection: How should Helicobacter pylori be diagnosed? Gastroenterology 1997; 113:S93–S98.

Mifflin TE, Benjamin DC, Bruns DE: Rapid quantitative, specific measurement of pancreatic amylase with the use of a monoclonal antibody. Clin Chem 1985; 31:1283–1288.

Miki K, Morita M, Sasajima M, et al: Usefulness of gastric cancer screening using the serum pepsinogen test method. Am J Gastroenterol 2003; 98(4):735–739.

Murray JA: Serodiagnosis of celiac disease. Clin Lab Med 1997; 17:445–464.

Nehra V: New clinical issues in celiac disease. Gastroenterol Clin North Am 1998; 27:453–465.

Not T, Horvath K, Hill ID, et al: Celiac disease risk in the USA. Scand J Gastroenterol 1998; 494:33–39.

Perry RR, Vinik AI: Endocrine tumors of the gastrointestinal tract. Annu Rev Med 1996; 47:57–68.

Peterson WL: Helicobacter pylori and peptic ulcer disease. N Engl J Med 1991; 324:1043–1048.

Poutanen SM, Simor AE: Clostridium difficile-associated diarrhea in adults. CMAJ 2004; 171(1):51–58.

Radebold K: VIPomas. eMedicine, 2003. Online. Available: http://www.emedicine.com.

Ramzan NN, Loftus E Jr, Burgart LJ, et al: Diagnosis and monitoring of Whipple disease by polymerase chain reaction. Ann Intern Med 1997; 126:520–527.

Romano TJ, Dobbins JW: Evaluation of the patient with suspected malabsorption. Gastroenterol Clin North Am 1989; 18(3):467–483.

Samloff IM: Pepsinogens I and II: Purification from gastric mucosa and radioimmunoassay in serum. Gastroenterology 1982; 82:26–33.

Sanduleanu S, Bruine A, Biemond I, et al: Ratio between serum IL-8 and pepsinogen A/C: a marker for atrophic body gastritis. Eur J Clin Invest 2003; 33(2):147–154.

Sendid B, Quinton JF, Charrier G, et al: Anti-Saccharomyces cerevisiae mannan antibodies in familial Crohn's disease. Am J Gastroenterol 1998; 93:1306–1312.

Shanahan F: Neutrophil autoantibodies in inflammatory bowel disease: are they important. Gastroenterology 1994; 107:586–590.

Simon JB: Fecal occult blood testing: clinical value and limitations. Gastroenterologist 1998; 6(1):66–78.

Singer R: Diagnosis and treatment of Whipple's disease. Drugs 1998; 55:699–704.

Smotkin J, Tenner S: Laboratory diagnostic tests in acute pancreatitis. J Clin Gastroenterol 2002; 34:459–464.

Sokoll LJ, Wians FH, Remaley AT: Rapid intraoperative immunoassay of parathyroid hormone and other hormones: A new paradigm for point-of-care testing. Clin Chem 2004; 50(7):1126–1135.

Spechler SJ, Dalton JW, Robins AH, et al: Prevalence of normal serum amylase levels in patients with acute alcoholic pancreatitis. Dig Dis Sci 1983; 28:865–875.

Steinberg W, Goldstein SS, Davis ND, et al: Diagnostic assays in acute pancreatitis: a study of sensitivity and specificity. Ann Intern Med 1985; 102:576–580.

Sternby B, O'Brien JF, Zinsmeister AR, DiMagno EP: What is the best biochemical test to diagnose acute pancreatitis? A prospective clinical study. Mayo Clin Proc 1996; 71:1138–1144.

Sugal E, Srur G, Vazquez H, et al: Steatocrit: a reliable semiquantitative method for detection of steatorrhea. J Clin Gastroenterol 1994; 19:206–209.

Tenner SM, Steinberg W: The admission serum lipase/amylase ratio. A new index that distinguishes acute episodes of alcoholic from non-alcoholic pancreatitis. Am J Gastroenterol 1992; 87:755–1761.

Tenner S, Dubner H, Steinberg W: Predicting gallstone pancreatitis with laboratory parameters: a meta-analysis. Am J Gastroenterol 1994; 89:1863–1866.

Tenner S, Fernandez-del Castillo C, Warshaw A, et al: Urinary trypsinogen activation peptide (TAP) predicts severity in patients with acute pancreatitis. Int J Pancreatol 1997; 21:105–110.

Thiede C, Morgner A, Alpen B, et al: What role does *Helicobacter pylori* eradication play in gastric MALT and gastric MALT lymphoma? Gastroenterology 1997; 113:S61–S64.

Thomas PD, Forbes A, Green J, et al: Guidelines for the investigation of chronic diarrhea, 2nd ed. Gut 2003; 52(Suppl V):v1–v15.

Provides guidelines to establish an optimal investigative scheme for patients presenting with chronic diarrhea in order to maximize positive diagnosis while minimizing the number and invasiveness of investigations. Also features summary/recommendation tables with sections devoted to noninvasive testing.

Tietz NW, Shuey DF: Lipase in serum: the elusive enzyme: an overview. Clin Chem 1993; 39:746–756.

Trier JS: Diagnosis of celiac sprue. Gastroenterology 1998; 115:211–216.

van de Wouw BAM, de Boer WA, Jansz AR, et al: Comparison of three commercially available enzyme-linked immunosorbent assays and biopsy-dependent diagnosis for detecting *Helicobacter pylori* infection. J Clin Microbiol 1996; 34:94–97.

Veldhuyzen van Zanten SJ, Sherman PM: *Helicobacter pylori* infection as a cause of gastritis, duodenal ulcer, gastric cancer and nonulcer dyspepsia: A systematic overview. CMAJ 1994; 150:177–185.

Vinik A: Vasoactive intestinal peptide tumor (VIPoma). *In* Vinik A (ed): Diffuse Hormonal Systems and Endocrine Tumor Syndromes, Ch 6. Endotext.com, 2004. Online. Available: http://www.endotext.com.

Volta U, Molinaro N, de Franceschi L, et al: IgA anti-endomyseal antibodies on human umbilical cord tissue for celiac disease screening. Save both money and monkeys. Dig Dis Sci 1995; 40:1902–1908.

von Herbay A, Ditton HJ, Schuhmacher F, Maiwald M: Whipple's disease: Staging and monitoring by cytology and polymerase chain reaction analysis of cerebrospinal fluid. Gastroenterology 1997; 113:434–441.

Wang TC, Dockray GJ: Lessons from genetically engineered animal models. I. Physiological studies with gastrin in transgenic mice. Am J Physiol 1999; 277:G6–G11.

Warshaw AL, Lee KH: Aging changes of pancreatic isoamylases and the appearance of 'old amylase' in the serum of patients with pancreatic pseudocysts. Gastroenterology 1980; 79:1246–1251.

Whitcomb DC: Genetic predispositions to acute and chronic pancreatitis. Med Clin North Am 2000; 84:531–547.

Wotherspoon AC: Gastric lymphoma of mucosa-associated lymphoid tissue and *Helicobacter pylori*. Annu Rev Med 1998; 49:289–299.

Xia HX, Keane CT, O'Morain CA: Pre-formed urease activity of *Helicobacter pylori* as determined by a variable cell count technique – clinical implications. J Med Microbiol 1994; 40:435–439.

Zaman Z, Van Orshoven A, Marien G, et al: Simultaneous macroamylasemia and macrolipasemia. Clin Chem 1994; 40:939.

Zieve L: Clinical value of determinations of various pancreatic enzymes in serum. Gastroenterology 1964; 46:62–71.

Toxicology and Therapeutic Drug Monitoring

Matthew R. Pincus MD PhD, Naif Z. Abraham Jr. MD PhD

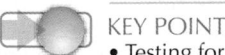
KEY POINTS

• Testing for the presence of drugs in the blood and other body fluids of patients has undergone a vast increase over the past 20 years.

• Testing for the presence of drugs of abuse and/or poisons in patients has become mandatory both in the emergency room and in employment screening.

• Most drugs can be assayed for using homogeneous immunological techniques.

• Gas chromatography–mass spectroscopy (GC-MS), which involves separation of derivatized compounds in the gas phase and detection from their mass-to-charge ratios and fragmentation patterns, is the 'gold standard' for detection and quantitation of drugs in body fluids.

• The mechanisms of action of many therapeutic drugs have been at least partially elucidated. Many of these, such as the anti-inflammatory, anti-asthmatic and immunosuppressive drugs, block specific points in signal transduction pathways.

• Ingestion of poisons cause life-threatening illness; poisons include cyanide, carbon monoxide and a number of metals such as lead, mercury, iron and arsenic. If detected, the effects of these poisons can often be reversed.

Toxicology is the study of substances introduced exogenously into the body. Elsewhere in this textbook, the analytical methods presented are concerned with determining the presence and levels of natural substances involved in normal body function. In this chapter, we discuss the biological effects and methods for detection of exogenous chemical compounds that profoundly influence bodily functions, often in a deleterious way but also for therapeutic benefit.

As it has evolved over the past several years, toxicology has become divided into four areas. The first two areas are the detection of drugs of abuse and the determination of the levels of therapeutic drugs being administered to patients. Also, it has been recognized that certain environmental compounds that are mutagens and carcinogens such as benzpyrene and acetylaminofluorene cause mutations in critical sequences of human DNA, leading to the frank development of cancer. In the ongoing revolution in molecular biology, this field has now expanded into the detection of certain markers such as abnormal DNA sequences or the presence of mutated proteins or of the presence of carcinogens bound to DNA.

Finally, there are a variety of toxins to which individuals become exposed such as carbon monoxide, cyanide, metals, and so forth, and for which detection is vital in order for physicians to be able to reverse the adverse acute physiologic effects. In this chapter, we discuss each of these divisions of toxicology with special reference to the detection of drugs and toxins in body fluids.

Basic Techniques for Detecting Drugs in Serum and Urine

The techniques involved in detecting the presence and/or the level of particular drugs, whether they are drugs of abuse or therapeutic drugs, are of two basic types: immunochemical and chromatographic.

Immunochemical Methods

Much drug testing today is performed using the so-called homogeneous immunoassay. The term homogeneous refers to the fact that these assays are all performed in a single step (i.e., only one antibody is used in the procedure). This technology has revolutionized toxicology because it allows performance of rapid, stat analyses of blood and urine constituents. The technique is shown schematically in Figure 23–1. Here we show examples of two types of assays. In the first, the enzyme-mediated (or multiplied) immunologic technique (EMIT), the drug itself is covalently attached to an enzyme such as alkaline phosphatase (Figure 23–1A-1). When the drug–enzyme complex is incubated with an antibody (usually monoclonal) to the drug, the enzyme activity is markedly decreased as a result of the blocking of the active site of the enzyme by the antibody. When, as in Figure 23–1A-2, exogenous drug (such as in serum) is added to the immune complex, this exogenous drug competes with the drug–enzyme for the antibody. Liberated drug–enzyme results in increased enzymatic activity. Increasing concentrations of drug in serum result in increased observed enzymatic activity. This methodology has been pioneered largely by the Syva Corporation (part of Behring Diagnostics Inc, San Jose, CA) and has been applied both to therapeutic drug monitoring and to detection of drugs of abuse. Fluorescence polarization immunoassay (FPIA) is the second type of homogeneous drug assay, as shown in Figure 23–1B. This is a particularly sensitive and elegant method. Rather than being linked to an enzyme, as in Figure 23–1A, the drug is covalently attached to a fluorescent probe molecule. If a fluorescent molecule is excited with polarized light and is stationary (i.e., it does not 'tumble' in solution), it will emit polarized light as a fluorophore. This emitted light has the same polarization as the exciting light. So, for example, if the exciting light is polarized to the left, the emitted light will also be polarized to the left. If a fluorophore tumbles freely in solution, however, the polarization is lost; that is, the emitted light is now polarized equally to the left and right. However, if the fluorophore is bound to a macromolecule, like an antibody, the polarization is strong because, attached to the nontumbling antibody, it remains relatively stationary. In these assays, the probe-labeled drug is incubated with the antibody. The fluorescence polarization of the probe-labeled drug is, of course, high because the fluorescence probe is relatively immobilized bound to the antibody directed against it (Fig. 23–1B-1). Addition of exogenous drug, as in serum, to the incubated mixture results in displacement of some of the fluorescent probe-labeled drug molecules, as shown in Figure 23–1B-2. These displaced molecules can now tumble freely in solution. The result is a decrease in fluorescence polarization. This decrease is directly related to the concentration of drug in serum.

This assay can detect drug levels in the nanomolar range and is both highly sensitive and specific. Both Abbott Laboratories (Chicago, IL), on the TDX and AXSYM analyzers, and Roche Diagnostic Laboratories (Nutley, NJ), on the COBAS and INTEGRA analyzers, have pioneered this most effective technique in monitoring a wide variety of therapeutic drugs and also drugs of abuse.

Drug Binding to Antibodies

In both of the homogeneous methods discussed previously, there is a nonlinear relationship between the concentration of drug in serum and the response of the system – that is, the color that results from the enzymatic reaction (Fig. 23–1A) or the decrease in fluorescence polarization (Fig. 23–1B). This nonlinearity in response is due to the phenomenon of binding (i.e., the drug must bind to antibody before it is detected). This phenomenon may be expressed by the following equilibrium:

$$D + D^* - Ab \rightleftharpoons D - Ab + D^* \tag{23–1}$$

where D is the drug concentration in serum, D^* is the 'marker' drug (i.e., drug labeled with an enzyme or a fluorescent probe), and Ab is the antibody. The concentration of free D^* is a measure of $D - Ab$, since both are equimolar. The concentration of $D - Ab$ is, in turn, related to D, the more D being present, the more $D - Ab$ is formed. However, because the concentration of Ab is fixed in a given experiment, at sufficiently high concentrations of D, all of the Ab will be saturated, so that at higher concentrations of D, no further $D - Ab$ can form. The relationship between D and $D - Ab$ is given by the Langmuir expression:

$$r = (D - Ab)/(Ab_0) = nkD/(kD + 1) \tag{23–2}$$

where (Ab_0) is the total concentration of antibody, k is the equilibrium constant for formation of the $D - Ab$ complex, n is the number of antibody-binding sites per molecule of antibody, and D is free drug concentration as defined above. Equation 23–2 is very similar to the Michaelis–Menten equation discussed in Chapter 20, except that there is no catalytic step here. This equation shows that the concentration of $D - Ab$ is nonlinear in D except where $kD << 1$. Where $kD >> 1$, saturation is achieved. This equation can be linearized in the form used for a Scatchard plot; that is:

$$r/D = kn - kr \tag{23–3}$$

where r/D is plotted versus r. Given the results for a set of experiments, a least-squares-best-fit line is drawn through the points, and the values of n

and k are determined. Once values for n and k are known, the value of D for any measured value of r can be *directly computed* from Equation 23–3.

Two problems that arise in using Equation 23–3 are that often the antibodies are nonhomogeneous, so that the Scatchard plot is nonlinear, and from possible blockage of free antibody sites by drug molecules in solid-phase immunoassays. The first problem has been solved by Rodbard (1971), wherein the analysis mentioned previously has been applied to multiple-binding equilibria. This analysis is used commonly in microprocessors that analyze the calibration curves in immunoassays. The second problem has been analyzed using a different theoretical approach (Pincus, 1981). Equation 23–3 illustrates the basic principle of how the results of the drug immunoassay on serum are converted into drug concentrations in serum.

Chromatographic Techniques

Chromatographic procedures (see Engelhardt, 2004 for an excellent brief history of liquid chromatography) have been applied mainly to the qualitative detection of drugs of abuse and toxins and less to the determination of the levels of therapeutic drugs. The three major methods are thin-layer chromatography (TLC), high-performance liquid chromatography (HPLC), and gas chromatography–mass spectroscopy (GC-MS). Although GC-MS is considered the 'gold standard' for detection and quantitation of volatile drugs and poisons, newer analytical techniques such as capillary electrophoresis (CE) and liquid chromatography–mass spectroscopy (LC-MS) are being developed. These techniques are all discussed in turn.

Thin-Layer Chromatography

Many compounds can be separated from one another using this method, based on their relative affinities for a polar solid stationary phase (usually a hydrated silicate) and a mobile liquid phase that is nonpolar (such as 10% methanol in chloroform). Depending on these affinities, different compounds adsorb to the hydrated silicate at different positions as the nonpolar solvent migrates up the stationary hydrated silicate. The principle is illustrated in Figure 23–2. For a given solvent system, the ratio of the distance traversed by the compound to the distance traversed by the solvent front is a constant for the compound and can be used to identify the compound in a mixture. This ratio is called the r_f. This technique is central to identifying different drugs of abuse, many of which can be separated from one another using TLC. The method has now been packaged in the form of Toxi-lab (Irvine, CA) kits in which the user is supplied with discrete strips of silicate, extraction solvents, and color-developing solutions.

Toxi-lab Procedures

The best specimen for drug detection, by chromatography, is urine because large quantities of this body fluid can be collected noninvasively. Once a urine specimen is collected, it is subjected to concentration and extraction procedures. In extraction procedures, acidic drugs are separated from basic ones. Almost all drugs of abuse are basic drugs, all of which are amine derivatives. The important 'acid' drugs comprise almost exclusively the barbiturates. In aqueous solution, the basic drugs are charged because of the equilibrium in Equation 23–4A:

$$R - NH_2 + H^+ \rightleftharpoons R - NH_3^+ \tag{23–4A}$$

$$RNH_3^+ OH^- \rightleftharpoons RNH_2 + H_2O \tag{23–4B}$$

in which a primary amine (secondary and tertiary amines exhibit the same equilibrium) is represented by RNH_2. The ammonium ion form (right side of Equation 23–4A) is soluble in water but not in nonpolar organic solvents. However, the amine-free base (left side of Equation 23–4A) is soluble in nonpolar organic solvents. Extraction procedures to isolate the basic drugs are aimed at treating the urine with base so that significant amounts of the basic drugs will be uncharged as the amine-free base (Equation 23–4B). This form can then be extracted into a nonpolar organic phase and then applied to the silicate strip. The reverse process is carried out for acidic drugs (i.e., these are treated with acid and extracted into nonpolar solvents). In practice, a small paper disk is added to the organic extraction mixture, and the solvent is then evaporated so that all basic drugs adsorb onto the paper disk. This disk is then applied to one end of the silicate strip, and the strip is placed in the migrating nonpolar solvent. A separate strip is used for each extraction, the A strip being used for basic drugs, the B strip for acidic drugs. The chief utility of the B strip is in identifying the barbiturates, as discussed subsequently.

Identification of Specific Drugs

After separation of the drugs on the plate, it is necessary to identify them. This objective is achieved by subjecting the drugs to standard color

A. EMIT Scheme

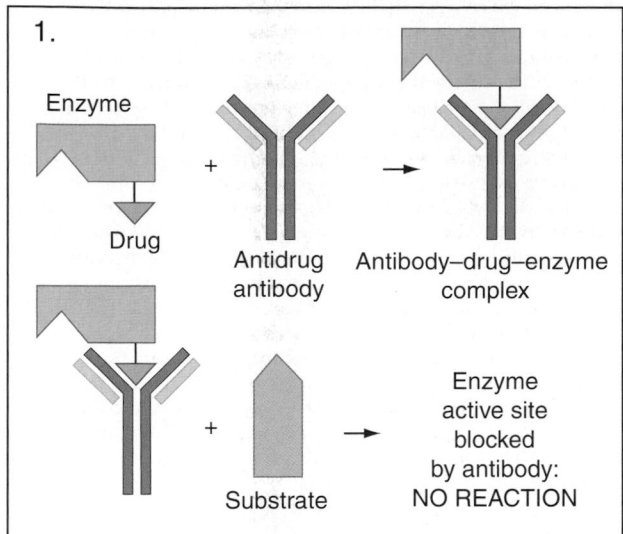

1.

Enzyme

Drug

+

Antidrug antibody

→

Antibody–drug–enzyme complex

+

Substrate

→

Enzyme active site blocked by antibody: NO REACTION

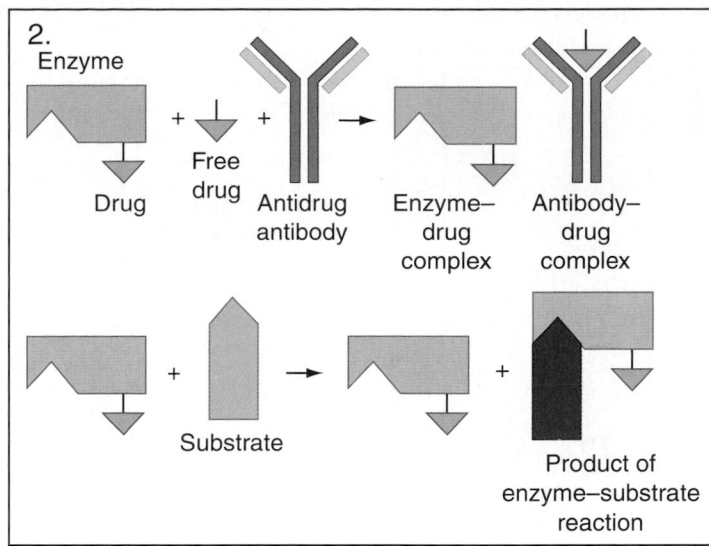

2.

Enzyme

Drug

+

Free drug

+

Antidrug antibody

→

Enzyme–drug complex

Antibody–drug complex

+

Substrate

→

+

Product of enzyme–substrate reaction

B. FPIA Scheme

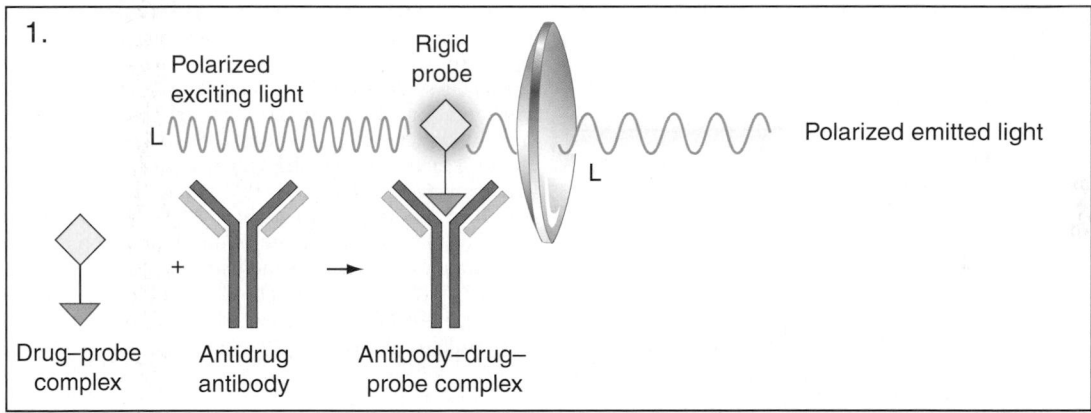

1.

Polarized exciting light

Rigid probe

L

Polarized emitted light

L

Drug–probe complex

+

Antidrug antibody

→

Antibody–drug–probe complex

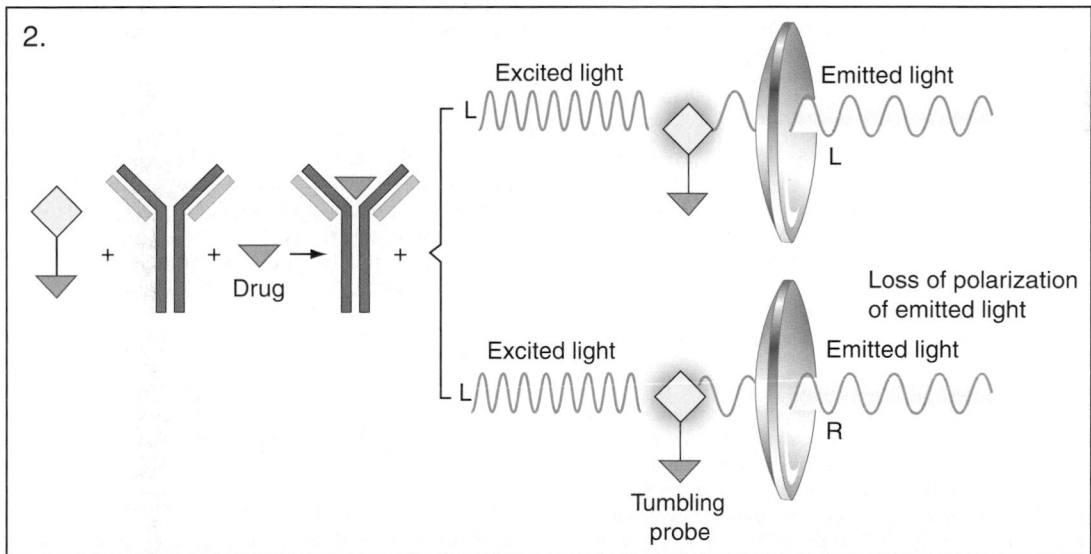

2.

Excited light

Emitted light

L

L

+

+

Drug

→

+

Loss of polarization of emitted light

Excited light

Emitted light

L

R

Tumbling probe

Figure 23–1 Homogeneous methods for detecting qualitatively or quantitatively the levels of drugs in body fluids. *A*, In the enzyme-mediated immunologic technique (EMIT) method, a drug–enzyme complex is used as the marker. When bound to the antidrug antibody, the active site of the enzyme (linked to the drug) is blocked. Therefore, when substrate is added, no reaction will occur, as shown in Part 1. However, if free drug (as in serum) is present, some or most of the enzyme–drug complex is displaced from the antidrug antibody. Now the active sites of the liberated enzyme–drug complexes are free, and the substrate undergoes reactions as indicated in Part 2. *B*, In the fluorescence polarization method (FPIA), the same general approach is used as in *A*, except that, in this method, the drug is attached to a fluorescent label or fluorophore. As shown in the upper scheme, when the drug–label complex is bound to the antidrug antibody, it becomes immobilized ('rigid probe' in the figure). When excited with polarized light (shown as polarized to the left or 'L' in the figure), the fluorophore emits light which is likewise polarized (to the left in the figure). As shown in the lower scheme, when displaced by free drug, as in serum or urine, the drug–probe complex is displaced from the antidrug antibody. It is no longer immobilized and therefore tumbles freely in solution. This results in loss of polarization of the emitted light ('L' and 'R,' for left and right polarization), i.e., in diminished fluorescence polarization.

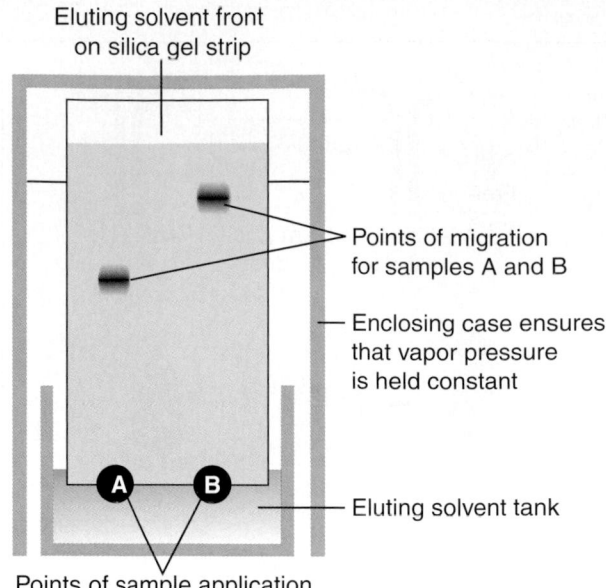

Eluting solvent front
on silica gel strip

Points of migration
for samples A and B

Enclosing case ensures
that vapor pressure
is held constant

Eluting solvent tank

Points of sample application

Figure 23–2 Illustration of the principle of thin-layer chromatography (TLC). Two solutes, A and B, are applied to the polar silicate strip. A is more polar than B and has a higher affinity, therefore, for the polar stationary phase than for the nonpolar mobile phase (usually methanol in chloroform). This relative affinity of A is, moreover, higher than the affinity of B for the polar phase. Therefore, A separates out first on the strip, and B migrates further on the strip.

reactions for each separate compound. In this procedure for basic drugs, the strip is simply dipped successively in three different solvents, which result in characteristic color patterns for each drug. The strip is also subjected to ultraviolet (UV) light, which excites fluorescence in selected compounds. Similar procedures are used for the acidic drugs extracted onto the B strip. As shown in Figure 23–3, which is from the Toxi-lab reference pattern book, each drug can be identified not only by its r_f but also by its color and characteristic color change in different reagents. These patterns are reinforced by the fluorescence characteristics. As an example, notice in Figure 23–3 on the Toxi-lab A worksheet that morphine, the main metabolite of heroin, has a characteristic r_f of 0.14 and a characteristic dark red or purple color in the first solvent that diminishes in intensity and changes color in the second solvent, water. It is nonfluorescent. If one or more of these characteristics differ(s) from this pattern, strong doubt about identification of the spot as morphine would exist. If all criteria are met, the sensitivity and specificity of the method are increased.

Reliability of the Method

Because the identification of each drug depends on use of qualitative color changes and/or the presence of fluorescence, the sensitivity of the method is limited by the ability of the naked eye to detect these changes. Practically, the level of detection is on the order of 1 µg/mL of compound present on the strip. The chief value of the chromatographic method is confirmatory (i.e., confirmation of a positive immunoassay test result). The two methods are often performed together on a single specimen.

The major problems that occur with this method are that extraction procedures are occasionally inefficient, so that insufficient amounts of drug are absorbed onto the disk. Also, the extraction and evaporation procedures are somewhat time-consuming, requiring approximately half an hour for full processing. Furthermore, cocaine has a number of metabolites that are polar (e.g., ecgonine) and that barely migrate from the origin, so that it is sometimes difficult to detect the presence of this drug of abuse because it has been converted completely to the polar metabolites prior to excretion. Some difficulty may also be encountered in distinguishing among various opiates, such as between morphine and other opiates, since the r_f values of these drugs can be close to one another (see Fig. 23–3 Toxi-lab A worksheet). However, experienced personnel can make this distinction in most cases. Also, some nontoxic drugs may give characteristic color changes and r_f values that are similar to those for the drug of abuse. A case in point is certain antihistamines that appear on the A strip to be very similar to amphetamines.

High-Performance Liquid Chromatography

Thin-layer chromatography allows direct qualitative detection of drugs in a panoramic way. HPLC allows quantitative detection of drugs and allows

sharper separation of these same drugs. In HPLC, the stationary phase, which can be *either* polar (silicic acid) or nonpolar (such as the C-18 columns), in reverse-phase chromatography, is composed of uniform, ultrafine particles that vastly increase its adsorptive surface area. This stationary phase is packed into a column. The resistance to flow in this column is high, so that large pressures are required to deliver constant reasonable flow rates. In the Waters HPLC instrument (Waters Corporation, Milford, MA), a constant pressure head is delivered to the column by the use of two pumps that operate so that as one withdraws, the other pushes forward (i.e., the two operate 180 degrees out of phase). The eluate from the column is monitored by a variety of detectors ranging from UV multiwavelength detectors to redox potential electrode detectors. It is the usual practice in performance of quantitative HPLC to use an internal standard – that is, a compound similar in structure to the drug(s) of interest, which is added to the specimen to be analyzed in a known concentration. By knowing how much of this marker compound or internal standard is placed on the column and how much is recovered from the column in the eluate, the percentage recovery from the column can be calculated for this compound and, by extrapolation, for all of the drugs of interest for which concentrations are being quantitated. Thus, losses owing to the column (in addition to losses in extraction procedures) can be corrected for using this technique. Generally, HPLC has been used for the quantitation of specific therapeutic drugs but has found use in detection of cocaine and heroin in urine. The sensitivity of the method is in the nanomolar to micromolar range.

One of the greatest uses of HPLC is in the separation and quantitation of the tricyclic antidepressants and their metabolites. These are among the most commonly prescribed drugs and are also used in excess as drugs of abuse in suicide attempts. It is often necessary to determine the levels not only of the parent tricyclic antidepressant but also of its active and inactive metabolites reviewed subsequently. Figure 23–4 shows a typical separation on a silicate column. Protriptyline, an inactive tricyclic compound, is the internal standard. It is clear that the separation among the metabolites and parent compounds is quite sharp. This separation is completely reproducible. A recent variant of thin-layer chromatography that includes the advantages of HPLC is capillary electrophoresis (CE) (Tagliaro, 1998; Shihabi, 1993). In this method, a capillary tube, lined with silicate, 10–100 µm in internal diameter and 100–1000 mm in length is used as the solid support in an electrophoresis apparatus. Here, the driving force for separation is the voltage (on the order of 25 kV) rather than pressure, as in HPLC. Because of the vast surface area, separations are quite sharp. The system is highly versatile and can be used to separate serum proteins and small molecules. CE possesses a wide analytical spectrum (including biopolymers, pesticides, aromatic compounds, drugs, inorganic ions, etc.) due to high versatility in terms of separation modes. Different analyte selectivity is based on different physicochemical principles of separation without changes in instrumental hardware, a distinct advantage of this technique. Capillary zone electrophoresis, micellar electrokinetic capillary chromatography (MECK), capillary isotachophoresis, capillary isoelectric focusing, capillary electrochromatography, and capillary gel electrophoresis are different separation modes utilized in CE separations. For example, by adding a detergent to the buffer system, as with MECK, micelles will form. A neutral compound (such as a pesticide) will partition into the detergent, forming micelles, and the complex will separate out based on the mobility/charge of the micelle. In addition, new platforms such as chip-based CE and immunoaffinity CE are currently being developed. CE has not yet enjoyed as widespread use as the immunoassay techniques (discussed previously) in clinical toxicology, but is commonly utilized in analytical forensic toxicologic studies as well as in molecular diagnostic studies and may have a significant effect on future clinical laboratory medicine (see Petersen, 2003; Boone, 2003).

Gas Chromatography–Mass Spectroscopy

Testing for drugs of abuse has become one of the most rapidly developing areas in the clinical laboratory in view of the widespread and ever-expanding use of these drugs among large segments of the working population. In view of the increasing requirements for routine drug screening, it has become necessary to have gold standard techniques to confirm the results obtained using screening methods such as EMIT and TLC.

GC-MS has proved to be such a gold standard because of its great sensitivity and its reliability. This methodology, as its name implies, involves two techniques: gas–liquid chromatography and mass spectroscopy. In the former, compounds are directly heated into the gas phase or are derivatized to make them labile to facilitate heating them into the gas phase. They are then passed over a column containing the stationary phase, which often consists of a liquid, usually a hydrocarbon or silicone oil, that coats a solid support in the column and offers a large surface area for adsorption.

TOXI-LAB® A WORKSHEET

A

TOXI-LAB® B WORKSHEET

B

Figure 23–3 A set of typical separations of the major drugs of abuse (and some therapeutic drugs) on Toxi-lab thin-layer chromatography. *Toxi-lab A worksheet:* Typical separation of the basic drugs on the A strip together with characteristic color changes. The third Toxi-lab A strip shows characteristic fluorescence of different drugs. Note that amphetamine and methamphetamine on the lower left are both fluorescent. *Toxi-lab B worksheet:* Left: Typical separation of the more acidic drugs on the B strip with characteristic color changes. The major use of the B strip is to identify the presence of the barbiturates. Right: fluorescence patterns of the drugs on the B strip.

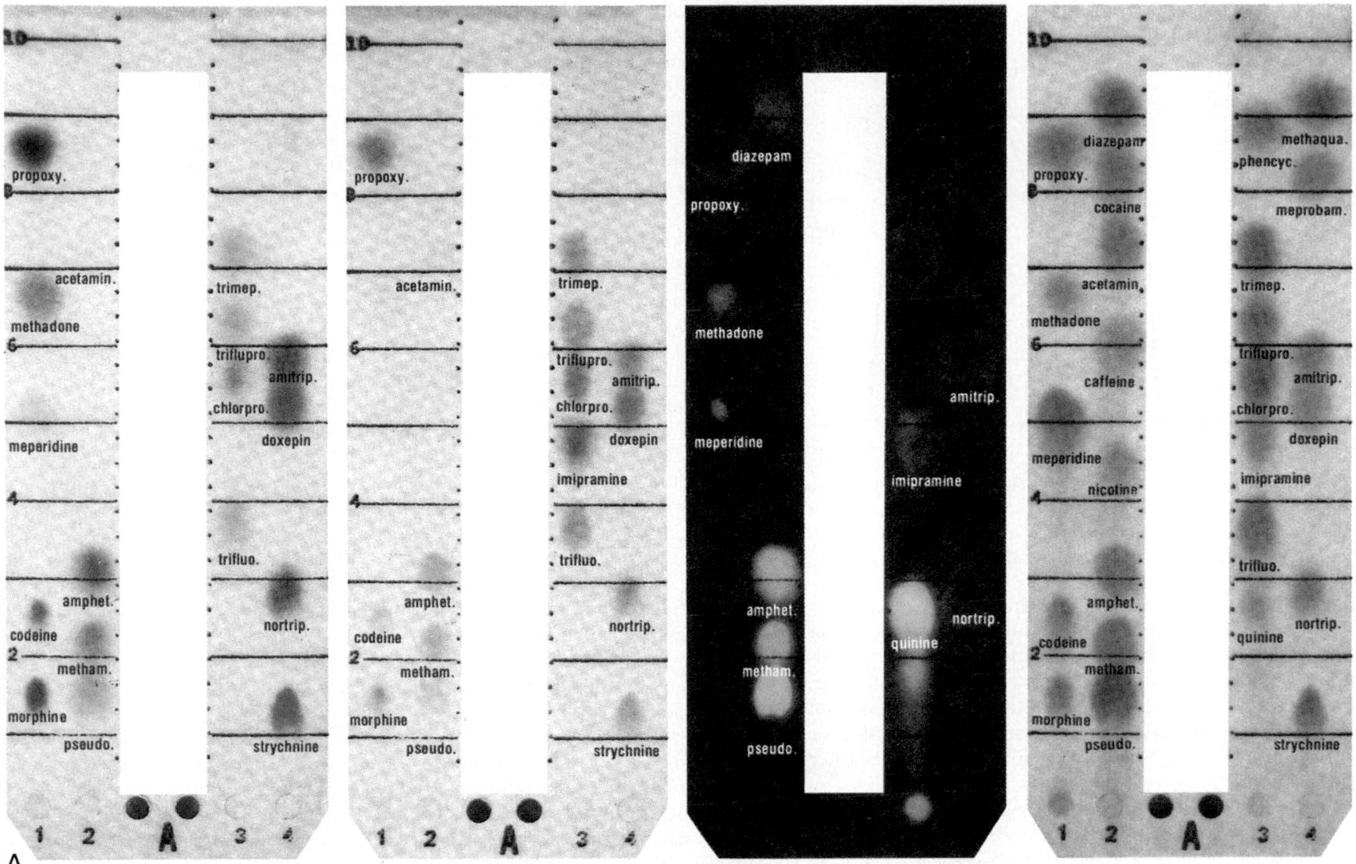

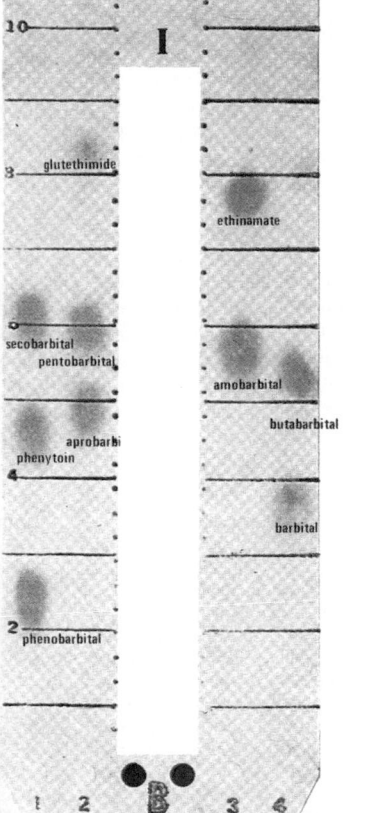

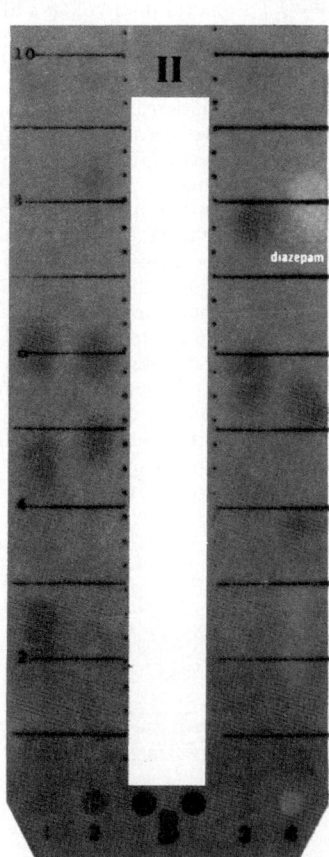

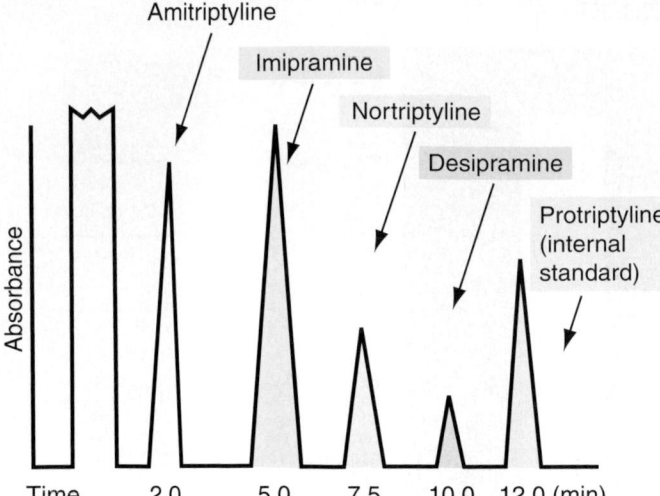

Figure 23–4 Sketch of a typical separation of the major tricyclic antidepressants on high-performance liquid chromatography (HPLC). A complete separation can be effected in 12 minutes. The concentration of each drug is on the order of 100 μg/mL.

Separation is based, much as in TLC, on the ability of each compound to adsorb to the stationary phase, which partially depends on the relative solubilities of the compound in the gas versus the liquid phase. Normally, the compounds eluting from the column could be detected by conventional techniques, as discussed previously, except that once the compounds are in the gas phase, where they are heated, advantage can be taken of another feature of the system – the ability of compounds that are heated to high temperatures to lose or gain electrons.

At high temperatures, the highest energy electrons of a compound (i.e., the ones of lowest ionization potential) can be excited such that the molecule can lose electrons and become charged. This process may be aided by such techniques as electron bombardment in a specially designed chamber that directly creates molecule-ions. Most of these resulting molecule-ions are single cations. Different molecule-ions in general have different sizes and different molecular weights. These molecule-ions decompose into characteristic fragments whose ratios with respect to one another and whose positions of migration relative to one another are also constant. The molecule-ions are then passed through an electric field generated by four rods that are subjected to rapidly alternating currents, the so-called quadrupole detector. Depending on how the field is 'tuned,' certain molecule-ions with specific mass/charge ratios can pass through the field to a detector. Thus, the molecule-ions can be separated on the basis of molecular weight or, more exactly, on their mass/charge ratios. The overall design of GC-MS is shown in Figure 23–5.

The presence of the molecule-ion on the plate is detected by a charge multiplier detector system. The technique of GC-MS has become highly refined. Each molecule-ion created in the gas phase can undergo further changes, such as elimination reactions and rearrangements and further degradation to small fragments that, in turn, ionize and give characteristic decomposition patterns. The patterns of thousands of compounds have now been determined. The position of the parent molecule-ion of the compound and the decomposition fragments give rise to a 'fingerprint'

pattern unique to the compound. These patterns are stored in a computer so that when a pattern for an unknown compound or group of compounds is obtained, the pattern is compared with the stored patterns to identify the compound(s) of interest. The entire methodology has been highly successful in detecting even low levels of cocaine and/or its metabolites in body fluids. A typical cocaine pattern is shown in Figure 23–6. Because single molecule-ion species give rise to significant currents in the detector, it is possible to detect very low levels of drugs, making this technique the ultimate reference method and the best confirmatory testing procedure available at present.

Liquid Chromatography–Mass Spectroscopy (Marquet, 2002; Maurer, 1998; Niessen, 1995, 2003)

As discussed above, GC-MS is the gold standard for the identification of volatile compounds. Nonvolatile compounds, however, can be detected utilizing LC-MS. Unlike GC-MS, however, the coupling of LC with MS requires sophisticated interfaces between the LC and MS components. The interface must volatilize nonvolatile compounds that have been separated on the LC; must remove the liquid solvent from the LC; and must correct flow-rate incompatibility between the LC and MS. Recently, two interface methods, electrospray (ES) and atmospheric pressure chemical ionization (APCI), appear to have become the gold standards for LC-MS. Both interface methods are utilized with atmospheric pressure ionization devices to facilitate removal of the mobile phase. They differ primarily in the range of analytes that can be accommodated and in how the solvent phase is nebulized.

Ionizable analytes of high molecular weight and/or high polarity can be accommodated with ES, while APCI can be used for analytes of less polarity and lower molecular weight. At present, ES appears to have more clinical and forensic applications than APCI in toxicology. LC-MS can be used to confirm positive test results from a screening assay and has been used for confirmation of drugs-of-abuse assays, poisoning detection in acute or chronic intoxication, therapeutic drug identification and quantitation, as well as for pharmacokinetic and drug metabolism studies. Although LC-MS has limitations when compared with GC-MS, it has become a powerful 'mature and validated' (Marquet, 2002) technique in analytical toxicology and a complementary method to GC-MS.

Screening for Drugs of Abuse

In most states of the United States, two levels of testing for drugs of abuse have become recognized: emergency room testing and employment screening/forensic testing. The former involves rapid, stat screening methods: in particular, EMIT (or FPIA) and TLC. The purpose of this type of screening test is to detect the presence of a drug or several drugs of abuse in the patient's urine. Rarely are the more sophisticated chromatographic procedures like HPLC and GC-MS used for this purpose. Forensic testing, on the other hand, requires not only a screen but also an independent confirmatory method, which is almost always chosen to be GC-MS or, less commonly, HPLC. It should be noted that, strictly by law, any confirmatory method is valid, provided it is a completely different method from the primary one. Thus, TLC can confirm EMIT, whereas FPIA cannot confirm it because both EMIT and FPIA are immunochemical methods. Another important legalistic consideration in forensic testing is the so-called chain of custody (Poklis, 2001; DeCresce, 1989). This process is used in the collection of urine from the individual from whom the

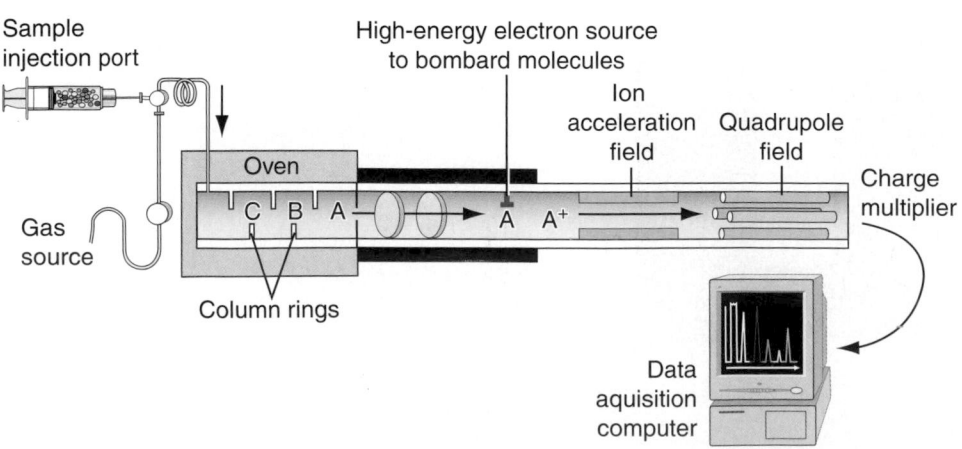

Figure 23–5 A schematic view of the components of gas chromatography–mass spectroscopy (GC-MS) instrumentation. On the left of the figure is the gas chromatographic system where a volatilized compound is moved over a column consisting of rings coated with a liquid by an inert gas. Compounds C, B, and A separate on this column and are maintained in the gas phase by the oven that surrounds the column. The separated compounds then enter the mass spectrometer on the right side of the figure, where they are subjected to bombardment by electrons, resulting in molecule ion species. These ionic species then are accelerated in a field and then passed through an electric quadrupole field. Only those ions with a narrow range of mass/charge ratios (m/e ratios) will pass through the tuned field so that they strike the detector. The electric currents that result are digitalized and stored in a computer that analyzes the data (see Davis, 1989).

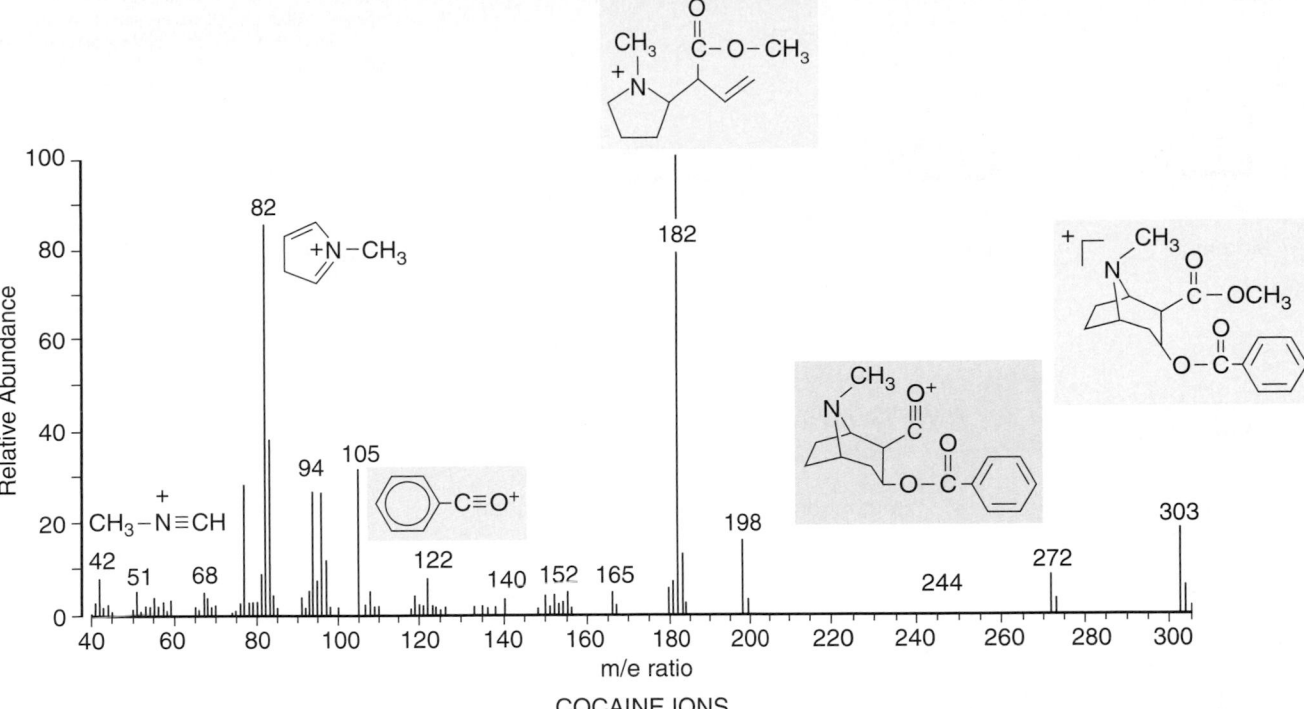

Figure 23–6 Fragmentogram for cocaine using gas chromatography–mass spectroscopy (CG-MS). The specimen is urine. This figure shows the characteristic peaks for cocaine metabolites. (Courtesy of Dr Chip Walls, Onondaga County, NY, Medical Examiners Office.)

specimen is taken. It may begin by observation of specimen collection by one person. Then, that person or another specifically designated individual, usually a police officer (in the case of prisoners or suspects) or some other designated official, accompanies the messenger who brings the specimen from the individual to the laboratory. This individual is a witness to the testing (and must sign a legal document to this effect) of the specific urine sample collected. More than one designated individual may be involved as the witness in this chain.

The Drugs of Abuse (Goldfrank, 2002; Sweetman, 2002)

General Aspects of the Mechanisms of Action

The major drugs of abuse are shown in Figure 23–7. As may be seen in this figure, these drugs, with the exception of the barbiturates, are all basic amino-group-containing compounds that also all contain benzene rings. The steric relationship of the amino group with respect to the aromatic benzene rings is rather similar, especially in cocaine, the opiates, and methadone. As might be expected, these compounds can cross-react with each other's target receptors.

The primary physiologic mechanisms of action of these drugs are not known, but some rudimentary knowledge has been gained over the past several years as to some of the main targets of these drugs. Many of these drugs act directly on dopaminergic neurotransmitter systems, especially the limbic system (sometimes referred to as the smell brain). This system is a more primitive one associated with pleasure seeking. In Figure 23–8, we show possible effects of several of the most important drugs on this system. It appears that the amphetamines, closely related structurally to dopamine and the catecholamines, can both directly act as neurotransmitters at critical synapses *and* can cause release of dopamine from the vesicles at the axonal side of the synapse. Cocaine further appears to stimulate release of dopamine in this system, which may partially be responsible for its producing a pleasant sensation (so-called high) in many individuals (Hurd, 1988). The tricyclic antidepressants also stimulate the dopaminergic pathways except, rather than promoting release of the neurotransmitters, they block reuptake of dopamine into the vesicles on the axonal side of the synapse. It is of great interest that, paradoxically, the tricyclic antidepressants such as imipramine (Tofranil) have been used successfully to treat the effects of cocaine. The major tranquilizers such as haloperidol (Haldol) and chlorpromazine appear to block attachment of dopamine to the dendritic receptors in the synapse,

thereby blocking the stimulatory effects of dopamine. Associated with many dopaminergic neurons are inhibitory neurons that use gamma-aminobutyric acid (GABA) as their neurotransmitters. It appears that many benzodiazepine receptors exist on these neurons, causing the release of GABA at the synapses in this system, reducing the dopaminergic effects of the stimulatory pathways on the limbic system. Thus, some of the tranquilizing effects of diazepam (Valium) and other benzodiazepines can be explained. Widely distributed throughout the central nervous system and periphery are a variety of opioid receptors classified mainly as mu-, delta-, kappa- (the three classic opioid receptor types), and epsilon- (not well characterized, see Tseng, 2001; Snyder, 2003) receptors. The mu-receptors appear to be highly specific for morphine and heroin, both of which produce a general analgesic state. At the moment, there appears to be no direct relationship between these receptors and the dopaminergic pathways. Interestingly, the naturally produced opiate peptide, met-enkephalin, whose amino acid sequence is Tyr–Gly–Gly–Phe–Met, cross-reacts significantly with mu-receptors, although its primary 'target' is epsilon-receptors. It has been shown that Valium may be structurally related to enkephalin, which, in turn, may be structurally related to morphine (Pincus, 1987; Murphy, 1992). It is therefore possible that these compounds have similar effects, at least indirectly, on the dopaminergic pathways.

Cocaine

Cocaine is derived from the coca plant and has enjoyed much popularity as an additive to certain foods. At the beginning of the 20th century, it was used in Coca-Cola, but owing to its addictive effects, this practice was discontinued. Cocaine is a derivative of the alkaloid ecgonine (i.e., the methyl ester of benzoylecgonine), as shown in Figure 23–7. Unfortunately, use of cocaine has now been re-continued in a particularly perverse way in modern times. There has been a virtual epidemic of cocaine abuse and addiction in the US. It is estimated that there are at least 5 million known addicts in the US and a reported 30 million overall users of this drug (Hollander, 2002; DeCresce, 1989). Fatalities from cocaine abuse are now a major cause of death in the US. These fatalities are of two types: direct toxicity of the drug (Johanson, 1989) and crime related to the illicit acquisition of the drug. The normal route of administration of cocaine is nasal (i.e., inhalation, called 'snorting') such that the drug passes through the nasal membranes. The prevalent form of cocaine currently used, called 'crack,' is the free-base form that passes rapidly across the nasal membranes and is highly potent for that reason (i.e., for a given dose, most or all of it enters the bloodstream rapidly). Its half-life is 1–2 hours, and the parent compound and its metabolites are usually cleared from the body within 2 days.

1. OPIATES

Figure 23–7 Chemical structures for the major drugs of abuse. All of the opiates are seen to be basic compounds that are tertiary amines and that contain benzene rings. Notice that, in the barbiturate series, barbituric acid may be considered as a condensation product of urea and malonic acid.

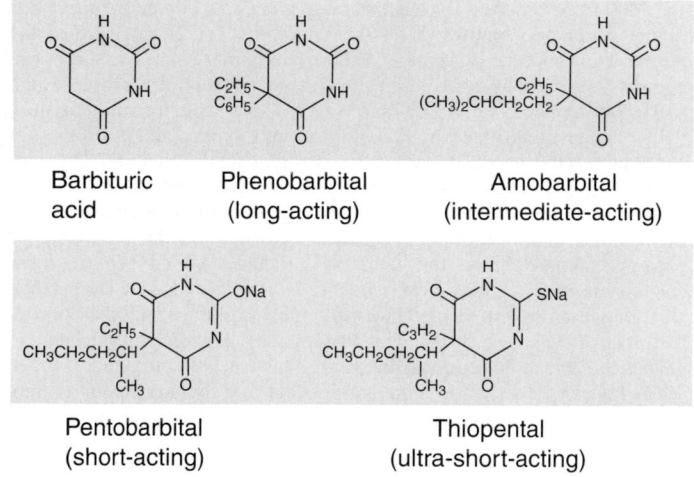

Morphine Codeine Heroin

Naloxone (Narcan) Methadone Propoxyphene (Darvon)

2. TRANQUILIZERS

Diazepam (Valium) Oxazepam

3. BARBITUATES; SEDATIVE - HYPNOTICS

Barbituric acid Phenobarbital (long-acting) Amobarbital (intermediate-acting)

Pentobarbital (short-acting) Thiopental (ultra-short-acting)

Cocaine is used medically to induce local anesthesia during nasopharyngeal surgery. However, in large doses, it induces a euphoric state (the 'high' experienced by the user) and may also induce hallucinatory states. It can also promote violent behavior (Goldfrank, 2002). Many of these results can be explained by cocaine's dopaminergic effects. One study (Azmitia, 1990) suggests that cocaine induces increased calcium ion influxes in dopaminergic neurons. The increased intracellular calcium activates phospholipases that possibly act as second messengers in causing ultimate release of dopamine in synapses. Prolonged action of phospholipases, however, ultimately causes cell death. In the previously mentioned study, in fact, cocaine was found to be neurotoxic. It also has a general cytotoxic effect from formation of an N-oxide free radical produced in the metabolism of this compound in the liver. It appears then that, over time, cocaine induces neuronal loss. In addition, binding of cocaine to cell receptors in the limbic system induces synthesis of cAMP that appears to be critical in activating cell processes involved in dopamine release (Cami, 2003).

Studies (Lange, 1989, 2001; Frishman, 2003) further indicate that prolonged use of cocaine results in cardiotoxicity – that is, cocaine can cause progressive atherosclerosis and causes constriction of the coronary arteries that can, in turn, induce myocardial ischemia and sometimes frank infarction. The pathogenesis of cocaine-induced coronary artery disease is not known. One highly disturbing aspect of cocaine abuse is the fact that it passes readily across the placenta and also into the lactating mammary gland and is readily passed from mothers to nursing infants. Often in the hospital setting, mothers receive the drug from dealers and breastfeed their newborn babies, who are therefore maintained on this drug. Cocaine causes mental retardation, delayed development, and strong drug dependence in newborns. It can also produce malformations in utero. Cocaine has classically not been considered to be an addictive drug, as it does not cause the true physical dependence typical of abusers of barbiturates and opiates. However, the high produced by the drug is extraordinarily reinforcing, so that the drug-seeking behavior of the cocaine and opiate abuser is similar. Recent evidence in experimental animals suggests that cocaine can induce the release of beta endorphins that bind to mu-receptors in the limbic system (Gianoulakis, 2004). This induces a pleasant and positive feeling of reinforcement. Clinically, patients who are overdosed with cocaine may become violent and

Figure 23-7 *(cont'd)* 305

4. DOPAMINERGIC PATHWAY STIMULANTS

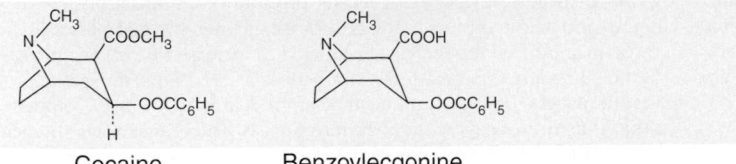

Cocaine

Benzoylecgonine
(less active metabolite)

AMPHETAMINES

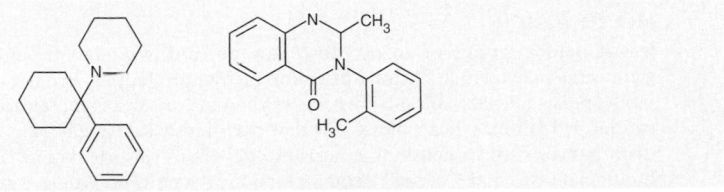

Amphetamine

Methamphetamine

Methylphenidate
(Ritalin - used to treat
hyperactive children)

5. HALLUCINOGENS

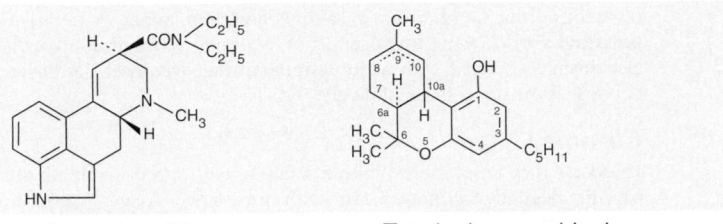

Phencyclidine

Methaqualone

Lysergic acid
diethylamide
(LSD)

Tetrahydrocannabinol

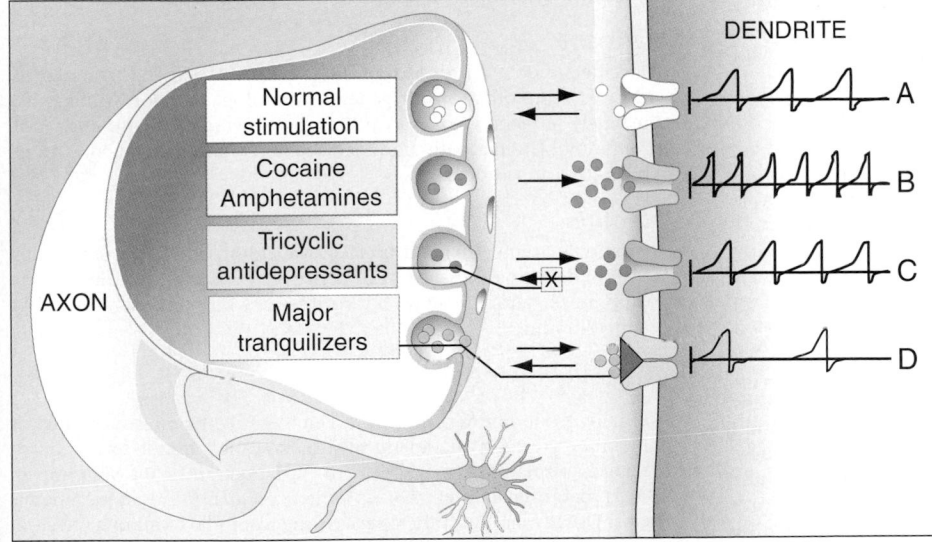

Figure 23-8 Illustration of the possible mechanisms of action of drugs of abuse and some therapeutic drugs on dopaminergic pathways. *A,* Normal neural transmission. A nerve impulse is conducted down the axon to the terminal boutons at the nerve ending. Vesicles, represented by the round gray structure, release their contents of neurotransmitter, here dopamine, represented by small white circles. Dopamine molecules traverse the synaptic cleft and bind to dendritic receptors, initiating action potentials (shown on the right of the figure under 'dendrite') in the dendrites. Notice the arrows showing that dopamine is both released and taken up by the vesicles. *B,* In the presence of cocaine and amphetamines, enhanced release of neurotransmitter (red circles) from vesicles occurs, increasing the rate of firing in the dendrites. Amphetamines can also directly act as neurotransmitters. *C,* Tricyclic antidepressants block (arrow with 'X' in yellow box) the reuptake of the neurotransmitter (purple circles), causing more dopamine to 'recycle' to the dendritic receptors, resulting in increased firing. *D,* Some of the neuroleptics act by blocking (gray wedge) postsynaptic dendritic receptors for dopamine (blue circles), causing decreased firing.

irrational, requiring sedation. Interestingly, many new users of this drug find themselves in a hyperexcitable state with palpitations and use large quantities of Valium to calm themselves. Thus, it is not uncommon to find cocaine and Valium in the urine of cocaine addicts. Occasionally, overdosed patients will become obtunded or comatose. The treatment for these patients is usually supportive. As noted in the previous section, antidepressants, including the tricyclics and fluoxetine (Prozac), have been found to inhibit the actions of cocaine. Thus, treatment with these drugs is often instituted.

Metabolism

The half-life of cocaine, as stated previously, is approximately 1–2 hours. It is metabolized to more polar compounds that have significantly less potency than the parent compound. These metabolites have longer half-lives and, with techniques such as GC-MS, can be detected up to 48 hours after administration of the drug. The immunoassay methods can detect the drug for about 24–36 hours after administration. If a patient has inhaled cocaine free base ('crack'), it is possible to detect the parent compound, cocaine, by TLC up to several hours after administration, owing to the high doses of drug present.

The Opiates (Morphine, Codeine, Heroin)

The structures for these drugs are shown in Figure 23–7 and are quite similar to one another. Morphine is used as a powerful analgesic and acts by binding to mu-receptors in the limbic system (CNS), resulting in an analgesic state. On the molecular level, binding of morphine to these receptors activates a cell signaling cascade via G-protein activation that results in elevated expression of many transcriptionally active proteins such as ERK, *jun* and *fos* and superactivation of adenyl cyclase resulting in high intracellular levels of cAMP (Tso, 2003). Besides being used as a major analgesic, morphine has become important in treating acute congestive heart failure by lowering venous return to the heart (i.e., it is a powerful preload reducer by causing increased splanchnic pooling of blood). Codeine is used as a mild analgesic and as an antitussive. Heroin induces a pleasant, euphoric state and is highly addictive both physically and psychologically. Withdrawal from this drug is exceedingly difficult, with a myriad of symptoms such as hypothermia, palpitations, cold sweats, and nightmares. This is a true physical dependence, the molecular basis for which is not fully understood. It appears that the dependence is strongly linked to the number of surface cell mu-receptors (Tso, 2003).

This class of compounds exhibits certain important paradoxical effects on the parasympathetic nervous system. These drugs exert a pro-cholinergic effect on the eyes and on blood vessels in the periphery (i.e., they cause constriction of pupils and peripheral vasodilation). In contrast, in the gut they lower gastrointestinal (GI) motility (i.e., they exhibit anticholinergic effects in the GI tract). This fact enables rapid diagnosis of heroin or, in general, opiate abuse in a patient brought to the emergency room in an obtunded or a comatose state. These patients typically have severe miosis (pupillary constriction). Although the sign is not useful in acute diagnosis, constipation commonly occurs in these patients.

Administration of heroin occurs via the intravenous route. Addicts are readily recognized by the presence of needle tracks on their arms and hands and by extensive thrombosis of their peripheral veins. The half-life of heroin via the intravenous route is about 3 minutes, and the effects of the drug last approximately 3 hours. The major metabolites are *N*-acetylmorphine and morphine. The half-life of morphine is about 3 hours. Overdoses of heroin are extremely dangerous and can cause severe obtundation, coma, respiratory arrest, and cardiac arrhythmias. One of the most common therapeutic modalities for heroin overdose is treatment intravenously with naloxone (Narcan), a strong competitive antagonist to the action of heroin. The structure of naloxone is shown in Figure 23–7. Heroin addiction, as a chronic problem, is treated pharmacologically with a partial agonist of heroin, methadone.

Methadone

This interesting compound, whose structure is shown in Figure 23–7, is a nonbicyclic drug that binds competitively with morphine to mu-receptors in the brain. However, although it can become addictive, the addictive effects are less than those of equivalent concentrations of heroin, possibly because its binding affinity is lower so that it induces less of an effect than that of heroin. Thus, administration of methadone to heroin addicts allows them to experience the effects of heroin but in a modulated manner. By gradually lowering the methadone dose, physical dependence becomes reduced and it appears that a trough serum methadone level greater than 100 ng/mL is adequate for effective methadone maintenance (Bell, 1988). However, it should be noted that addiction to methadone can also occur. In toxicology laboratories, the most common request received for methadone screens comes from methadone clinics to test whether a patient is administering methadone or has relapsed into taking heroin. As can be seen in Figure 23–3, it is a simple matter to distinguish methadone from the opiates by thin-layer chromatography. Similarly, EMIT or FPIA detect each drug with high specificity.

Amphetamines

These compounds, as can be seen in Figure 23–7, bear a close resemblance to the adrenergic amines such as epinephrine and norepinephrine and may be expected to exert sympathomimetic effects. They also resemble dopamine and may also be expected to have effects on dopaminergic pathways. The amphetamines cause euphoria and increased mental alertness that may be attributed to their effects on these pathways. This group of drugs, however, also exerts pronounced stimulatory effects on alpha- and beta-receptors in the cardiovascular system and in the kidney to cause pronounced adrenergic effects such as increased heart rate, increased blood pressure, palpitations, bronchodilation, anxiety, pallor, and tremulousness. Studies indicate that amphetamines are also competitive inhibitors of the enzyme monoamine oxidase, which inactivates adrenergic neurotransmitters by oxidatively removing their amino groups. Blockage of this enzyme prolongs the effect of epinephrine and norepinephrine with the attendant neurologic and cardiovascular sequelae. One particular amphetamine, 3,4-methylenedioxymethamphetamine (MDMA or 'ecstasy'), a derivative of methamphetamine (see Figure 23–7), has become popular as a recreational drug of abuse because it has euphoric and psychedelic effects but minimal hallucinogenic effects (Gill, 2002).

Clinical Symptoms

The pharmacologic action of amphetamines includes CNS and respiratory stimulation and sympathomimetic activity (e.g., bronchodilation, pressor response, and mydriasis). Loss of weight may also occur as a result of an anorectic effect. Psychic stimulation and excitability, leading to a temporary increase in mental and physical activity, can occur, and nervousness can also be produced.

Acute Toxicity

Initial manifestations of an overdose may be cardiovascular in nature; symptoms may include flushing or pallor, tachypnea, palpitation, tremor, labile pulse rate and blood pressure (hypertension and hypotension), cardiac arrhythmias, heart block, circulatory collapse, and angina. Mental disturbances such as delirium, confusion, delusions, disorientation, and hallucinations may occur. Acute psychotic syndromes may occur characterized by vivid auditory and visual hallucinations, restlessness, homicidal or suicidal tendencies, panic state, paranoid ideation, loosening of associations, combativeness, and changes in affect. A frequent and potential sign of acute intoxication is hyperpyrexia; rhabdomyolysis has also been associated with acute amphetamine overdose. Cardiovascular collapse is the usual cause of death.

Chronic Usage

Tolerance may be produced within a few weeks, and possibly physical or psychic dependence may occur with prolonged usage. Symptoms of chronic abuse include emotional lability, somnolence, loss of appetite, occupational deterioration, mental impairment, and social withdrawal. Trauma and ulcer of the tongue and lip may occur as a result of continuing chewing or teeth-grinding movements. A syndrome with the characteristics of paranoid schizophrenia can occur with prolonged high-dosage use. Aplastic anemia and fatal pancytopenia are rare complications.

Treatment

No specific antidote for amphetamine overdose exists, and treatment of overdose is symptomatic with general physiologic supportive measures immediately implemented. For cardiovascular symptoms, administration of propranolol (Inderal), discussed subsequently under therapeutic drugs, can be used as an antidote.

Detection

Both Toxi-lab (Irvine, CA) and EMIT (Syva, San Jose, CA) procedures are effective in detecting these drugs of abuse. Occasionally, on the Toxi-lab A strip, amphetamines may be confused with antihistamines like diphenhydramine.

Benzodiazepines

Among this group of drugs, shown in Figure 23–7, the most prominent is Valium; they are used therapeutically, as so-called minor tranquilizers. Their mechanisms of action appear to be induction of the secretion of GABA, a neurotransmitter that inhibits conduction in dopaminergic neurons. Usually used as a therapeutic drug to produce calming effects at doses between 2.5–10 mg and to produce muscle-relaxing effects at higher doses, Valium has been used by drug addicts in high dosage to counter the excitatory effects of other drugs of abuse or as a means of inducing tranquil states. Among some drug abusers, benzodiazepines are used to potentiate the effects of heroin (Fraser, 1998). A number of drug abusers have become addicted to Valium when using high doses several times each day. Acutely, benzodiazepine overdose may produce somnolence, confusion, seizures, and coma. Rarely, hypotension, respiratory depression, and cardiac arrest may occur. Chronically, physical and psychological dependence occur. Sudden discontinuance of the drug may lead to anxiety, sweating, irritability, hallucinations, diarrhea, and seizures. Treatment is supportive. Gradual diminution of the benzodiazepine removes physical dependence. The half-life for Valium is 20–70 hours, but the half-life of one of its active metabolites is 50–100 hours.

Phencyclidine (PCP)

This interesting tricyclic compound, shown in Figure 23–7, has numerous effects on a variety of different neural pathways. Used almost exclusively as a drug of abuse, this drug is traded on the streets under the name of angel dust or angel hair. It is peculiar that the use of this drug appears to be periodic. The physiologic effects of PCP appear to be analgesic and anesthetic and, paradoxically, stimulatory. This drug has been found to interact with cholinergic, adrenergic, GABA-secreting, serotoninergic, and opiate neuronal receptors. Thus, a wide variety of bizarre and apparently paradoxical symptoms can be seen in the same patient. This drug has been shown to bind to specific regions of the inner chloride channels of neurons, apparently profoundly affecting chloride transport. It has also been found to bind strongly to a class of neural receptors called sigma-receptors (Schuster, 1994). This receptor also binds strongly to the neuroleptic, antipsychotic drug haloperidol (Haldol), a finding that may implicate the sigma-receptor in some of the clinical findings of severe psychosis in patients suffering from overdose with PCP.

Because of its varied actions, clinically acute manifestations vary from depression to euphoria and can involve catatonia, violence, rage, and auditory and visual hallucinations. Vomiting, hyperventilation, tachycardia, shivering, seizures, coma, and death are also among the common occurrences that result from abuse of this drug. Most fatalities occur from the hypertensive effects of the drug, especially on the large cerebral arteries (Bayorh, 1984). As can be inferred from this spectrum of possible symptoms, diagnosis based on clinical findings is impossible. Only the results of a drug screen can be diagnostic. Treatment of drug abuse with PCP is supportive, with the patient kept in isolation in a darkened, quiet room. Acidification of the urine increases the rate of PCP excretion. As might be expected from the findings regarding the sigma-receptor, treatment with Haldol results in sedation of the violent, hallucinating patient.

Barbiturates: Sedative-Hypnotics

There is an almost bewildering variety of these major sedative drugs. However, all are derivatives of barbituric acid, which may be regarded as the condensation product of urea and malonic acid, as indicated in Figure 23–7. Depending upon the substituents on the $–CH_2$ group of the malonic acid portion, the particular drug may be long acting, as is phenobarbital, with a benzene ring and ethyl group substituents on this carbon; short acting, as is pentobarbital, with neopentyl and ethyl groups at this position; or ultra-short acting, as is the case with thiopental. The long-acting barbiturate phenobarbital is a therapeutic drug used as an anticonvulsant, unlike the short- and ultra-short-acting drugs, and is discussed subsequently under therapeutic drugs. All of the barbiturates are fat soluble and therefore pass easily across the blood–brain barrier. All of them seem to stabilize membranes such that depolarization of the membranes becomes more difficult. For unknown reasons, the short-acting and ultra-short-acting barbiturates seem to inhibit selectively the reticular activating system, involved with arousal; hence their sedative and hypnotic effects. The ultra-short-acting barbiturates rapidly diffuse out of the CNS, accounting for their rapid action. Phenobarbital, however, selectively reduces the excitability of rapidly firing neurons and is therefore a highly effective anticonvulsant. It may be more than coincidental that phenobarbital and the equally effective anticonvulsant phenytoin (Dilantin) bear structural resemblance to one another and may exert similar effects on rapidly firing neurons. The mechanism of action of phenytoin is discussed subsequently.

Clinically, at low doses, the short-acting and ultra-short-acting barbiturates produce sedation, drowsiness, and sleep. They also impair judgment. At higher doses, anesthesia is produced. At very high dose, these drugs can cause stupor, coma, and death. The toxic manifestations of these drugs are depression, Cheyne–Stokes respiration, cyanosis, hypothermia, hypotension, tachycardia, areflexia, and pupillary contraction.

The treatment of drug overdose is supportive and includes the standard treatment for shock. When administered within 30 minutes of drug ingestion, activated charcoal is an effective barbiturate chemoadsorbent.

Diagnosis of drug abuse with short- and ultra-short-acting barbiturates is by immunoassay and TLC screening procedures. HPLC has found some use in this regard but is not a standard method. The barbiturates are weak acids, the N–H protons being somewhat acidic, so that they are acid extracted and placed on the B strip in Toxi-lab (Irvine, CA) procedures.

Their presence is easily detected by Toxi-lab TLC, as shown in Figure 23–3 Worksheet B. Immunoassays for those drugs are also excellent, the one caveat being that high levels of phenobarbital in urine cross-react with the antibodies against the short-acting barbiturates. Thus, it is important that TLC confirms a positive immunoassay result for sedative-hypnotic barbiturates.

Propoxyphene (Darvon)

This analgesic drug has pharmacologic properties very similar to those of the opiates like morphine. This drug can be taken orally so that the sedated, good feelings induced by opiates can be induced without having to have recourse to the intravenous apparatus needed for infusion of heroin. A major cause of drug-related deaths is propoxyphene overdose either alone or in combination with CNS depressants like barbiturates and alcohol. Toxic symptoms are similar to those seen with overdoses of opiates (namely, respiratory depression, cardiac arrhythmias, seizures, pulmonary edema, and coma). Nephrogenic diabetes insipidus may also occur. The treatment for propoxyphene overdose is mainly supportive. Administration of naloxone (Narcan) reverses the toxic effect of the drug.

Methaqualone (Quaalude)

Methaqualone is a 2,3-disubstituted quinazoline (Fig. 23–7) that has sedative-hypnotic properties. This compound also possesses anticonvulsant, antispasmodic, local anesthetic, antitussive, and weak antihistamine actions. Oral administration leads to rapid and complete absorption of the drug, with approximately 80% bound to plasma protein. Peak plasma concentrations are reached in approximately 2–3 hours, and almost all of the drug appears to be metabolized by the hepatic cytochrome P450 microsomal enzyme system, with only a small percentage (< 5%) excreted unchanged in the urine. The serum half-life ranges from 20–60 hours.

The dosages that are used for its hypnotic–sedative actions are 150–300 mg daily. Toxic serum concentrations are generally reached at 10 µg/mL. Tolerance to some of its actions, as well as dependence, occurs, such that abusive dosages can be up to six to seven times greater than those employed therapeutically. Symptoms of overdose can be similar to barbiturate toxicity and produce CNS depression with lethargy, respiratory depression, coma, and death. However, unlike barbiturate overdose, muscle spasms, convulsions, and pyramidal signs (hypertonicity, hyperreflexia, and myoclonus) can result from severe methaqualone intoxication. Treatment for overdose includes supportive therapy as well as delaying absorption of remaining drug with activated charcoal and drug removal by gastric lavage.

Marijuana (Cannabis)

This is one of the oldest and most widely used of the mind-altering drugs. Marijuana is a mixture of cut, dried, and ground portions of the hemp plant *Cannabis sativa*. Hashish refers to a more potent product produced by extraction of the resin from the plant. The principal psychoactive agent in marijuana is considered to be delta-9-tetrahydrocannabinol (THC), a lipid-soluble compound that readily enters the brain and may act by producing cell membrane changes. Delta-9-tetrahydrocannabinol binds to the presynaptic neural cannabinoid receptor, CB1, which releases the inhibitory neurotransmitter, gamma-aminobutyric acid (GABA) in the hippocampus, amygdala and cerebral cortex (Iversen, 2003). Marijuana may be introduced either through the lungs by smoking or through the gastrointestinal tract by oral ingestion in food. Once THC enters the body, it is readily stored in body fat and has a half-life of approximately 1 week. Biotransformation is complex and extensive, and less than 1% of a dose is excreted unchanged. About one-third is excreted in the urine as, primarily, delta-9-carboxy-THC and 11-hydroxy-delta-9-THC. These metabolites may be detected in the urine from 1–4 weeks after the last ingestion, depending on both dosage and frequency of ingestion. Marijuana does not appear, in general, to cause physiologic dependence, but tolerance (see Martin, 2004) and psychological dependence do seem to occur although a proportion of chronic users of this drug can develop physiological dependence on it (Iversen, 2003). Two major physiologic effects of marijuana are reddening of the conjunctivae and increased pulse rate. Muscle weakness and deterioration in motor coordination can also occur. The preponderant changes seen with cannabis intoxication are perceptual and psychic changes. These range from euphoria, relaxation, passiveness, and altered time perception, seen at low doses, to adverse reactions such as paranoia, delusions, and disorientation, which can be seen at high doses in psychologically susceptible individuals. The dosage, the route of administration, the individual's psychological makeup, and the setting are important determinants in each individual's reaction to cannabis intoxication. Thus, high doses in an individual unprepared or unaware of drug consumption may produce a disturbing experience. More commonly, experienced users report mild euphoria, enhancement or alteration of the physical senses, introspection with altered emphasis or importance of ideas, and heightening of subjective experiences. Heavy chronic use may produce bronchopulmonary disorders and, although the relative safety of chronic use is controversial, acute panic reactions, delirium, and psychoses occur rarely (Bryson, 1989). Few users seek treatment, and when this occurs in a distressed patient, medical intervention is generally conservative. However, following an acute episode, psychological evaluation may be necessary in an individual with an underlying psychiatric disturbance. Rarely, marijuana may be ingested by intravenous infusion of a boiled concentrate. Severe multisystem toxicity may be produced by this route of administration. Symptomatology may include acute renal failure, gastroenteritis, hepatitis, anemia, and thrombocytopenia.

Lysergic Acid Diethylamide (LSD, Lysergide)

LSD is a semisynthetic indolalkylamine and a hallucinogen. It is one of the most potent pharmacologic materials known, producing effects at doses as low as 20 µg, and is equally effective by injection or oral administration. LSD is believed to affect multiple sites in the CNS, and may act on a presynaptic serotonin receptor, decreasing the activity of serotonin by inhibiting its release. This process, in turn, may produce a state of CNS hyperarousal. Both the sympathetic and parasympathetic nervous systems are affected. However, the sympathetic effect appears to be greater, and initial symptoms include hypertension, tachycardia, mydriasis, and piloerection.

The usual dosage of LSD is 1–2 µg/kg; LSD produces an experience that begins within an hour of ingestion, usually peaks at 2–3 hours, and generally lasts 8–12 hours, after ingestion. Metabolism occurs in the liver, whereas excretion occurs mainly in the bile.

LSD is the most commonly abused drug in its class and is believed by its users to provide insights and new ways of solving problems. The psychic effects are usually intense, and vary, depending on the user's personality, expectations, and circumstances. LSD acts on all the body senses, but visual effects are most intense. Common perceptual abnormalities include changes in the sense of time, organized visual illusions or hallucinations, blurred or 'undulating' vision, and synesthesias. Mood may become very labile, and dissolution and detachment of ego may occur. LSD toxicity levels are low, and deaths are generally due to trauma secondary to errors in the user's judgment. Panic reactions – a 'bad trip' – are the most common adverse reactions. These may occur in any user and cannot be reliably predicted or prevented. Borderline psychotic and depressed individuals are at risk for the precipitation of suicide or a prolonged psychotic episode by the usage of LSD. Flashbacks, which are poorly understood, also occur days to months after ingestion. This occurs when the user experiences recurrences of a previous hallucinogenic experience in the absence of drug ingestion.

Acute panic reactions may be treated by frequent reassurance and a quiet and calm environment; diazepam may also be effective. However, except for treating specific complications, LSD abuse has no systematic program of treatment.

Therapeutic Drug Monitoring

It has become recognized that it is critical that the serum levels of many of the therapeutic drugs administered to patients be frequently determined, both because of the possible toxic side effects of many of these medications and because, often, lack of patient compliance results in subtherapeutic levels of the drug. Furthermore, it is important for the physician when initiating drug therapy to ascertain when the serum levels of the drug have achieved a stable therapeutic level. It becomes important, therefore, to understand the principles on which drug therapy is based (i.e., pharmacokinetics). Some of the basic principles of pharmacokinetics and then the physiologic effects of specific classes of therapeutic drugs are presented in this section. The ones discussed are those whose specific levels are most commonly followed by clinicians and are most commonly assayed for in clinical laboratories. It should be noted that virtually all therapeutic drugs are assayed from specimens of serum, not urine, most commonly using immunoassay techniques such as FPIA.

Pharmacokinetics (Gerson, 1987a,b)

Figure 23–9 summarizes the two ways in which a therapeutic drug is administered to a patient: discontinuously or continuously. The former method is the most common one. Most patients are treated with medications taken orally at fixed periods. For example, to achieve anti-

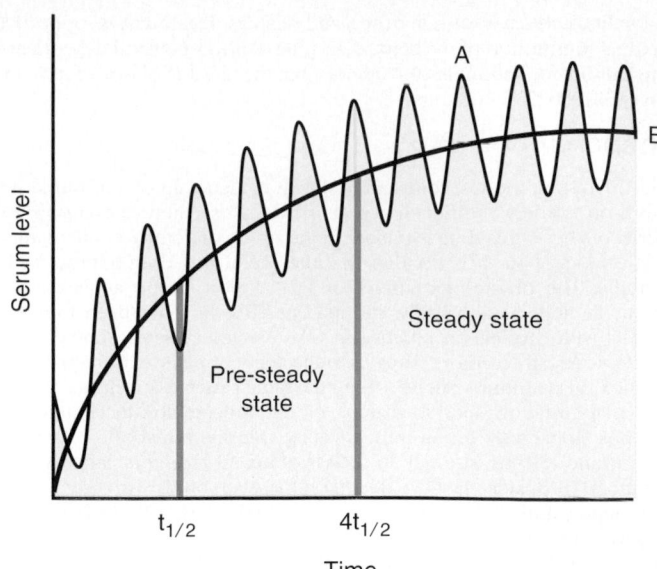

Figure 23–9 Illustration of the time course of drug levels as a function of method of administration. *A*, Discontinuous method. A constant dose is administered at each half-time for the drug. After four halftimes (4t$_{1/2}$), drug levels fluctuate around a constant steady-state level. *B*, Continuous method (intravenous infusion). Convergence to the steady-state limit achieved in *A*.

inflammatory effects, two aspirin tablets of 350 mg each are taken every 4–6 hours. In this case, the aspirin is taken at discrete times between which a certain amount will be excreted before the next dose is given. Sometimes, a patient will be infused with a drug intravenously such as with lidocaine (Xylocaine) in the intensive care unit (ICU) for a cardiac arrhythmia or with heparin to prevent thromboembolic events. In this case, while the drug is metabolized, a constant amount of the drug is being infused. Eventually, with continuous infusion of a drug, a steady-state concentration of the drug is reached once the amount of drug infused in a unit of time equals the amount of drug eliminated in the same unit of time. A steady-state concentration of a drug that is *discontinuously* infused is also reached. However, repeated dosing (equal doses spaced equally apart) produces peak and trough serum concentrations that tend to vary around a steady-state or average concentration.

For both discontinuous and continuous infusions, the ultimate drug level is determined by a battle between the amount infused and the amount excreted. All drugs are eventually excreted. They can be excreted unchanged in urine, or excreted in urine as metabolites of the parent drug. These metabolic conversions occur in the liver. Occasionally, some drugs enter the enterohepatic circulation and are excreted in stool. Regardless of their mode of excretion, many, but not all, drugs have a half-life that is more or less independent of their concentrations. The half-life of a drug is the time taken for half the drug that was initially present in serum to be excreted. The reason that the half-life of a drug is independent of its concentration is that many drugs are excreted according to so-called first-order kinetics. This process may be summarized as follows:

$$D \xrightarrow{k} E \tag{23–5}$$

where D is the drug concentration, and E is the excreted form of the drug. The constant, k, is the rate constant for the disappearance of D. The half-life, called $t_{1/2}$, is related to the rate constant, k, by the following relationship:

$$t_{1/2} = 0.693/k \tag{23–6}$$

As can be seen from this equation, $t_{1/2}$ is a constant and does not depend on drug concentration. Thus, the half-life of the drug determines the time to reach the steady-state or average concentration.

The object of all drug therapy is to achieve a constant serum level of the drug that will be therapeutic. If the half-life for a drug is known, it is possible to compute the divided dose of the drug that should be given and the time interval between doses so that this level will be achieved. As can be seen in Figure 23–9, curve A, at the beginning of drug administration, there are wide fluctuations of the drug level until, after a given period, the fluctuations converge around a constant level. In general, for discontinuous doses, the drug level, at the end of the nth dosing period, can be expressed as the sum of a geometric series:

$$D = (D_0 r \times r^n - D_0 r)/(1 - r) \tag{23–7}$$

where D_o is the desired steady-state level of the drug; r is the fraction of drug remaining after the constant time interval between doses; and n is the number of the dose (e.g., the second dose, third dose, etc.). If the time interval between doses is chosen as the $t_{1/2}$, $r = 1/2$. If the time interval is chosen to be that for $3/4$ of the drug to remain, $r = 3/4$. (This time can be calculated directly from the $t_{1/2}$ as $1/2 t_{1/2}$.) After four timed doses, if, for example, $r = 1/2$, the first term in the numerator of Equation 23–7 is small and, in effect,

$$D = (D_o/2)/(1/2) = D_o \qquad (23–8)$$

After four or more half-lives, when r^n is $(1/2)^4$ or 1/16 (0.06), i.e., small, the steady-state level is approached.

For continuous infusions (Fig. 23–9, curve B), for the simplest case where drug distribution is instantaneous, the rate of drug infusion is constant and the drug is excreted in a first-order manner, then it can be shown that the drug level at any time is given by the following:

$$D = (k_1/k_2)(1 - e^{-k_2 t}) \qquad (23–9)$$

where D is the drug concentration, k_1 is the constant infusion rate, k_2 is the first-order rate constant for excretion of the drug, and t is the time. Because, as shown previously in Equation 23–6, $k_2 = 0.693/t_{1/2}$, after four half-lives when $t = 4t_{1/2}$,

$$D = (k_1/k_2)(1 - e^{-2.772}) \qquad (23–10)$$

where, in effect, D is close to k_1/k_2. Thus, for continuous infusions, assuming no loading dose is given, the ratio of k_1 (the rate of drug infused per unit of time) to k_2 (the rate constant for the first-order disappearance of the drug) is the desired steady-state level of the drug (i.e., where the amount of drug delivered equals the amount of drug eliminated over the same unit of time).

There are two major points from this presentation. First, it is a good rule of thumb to wait for four or more half-lives to achieve the steady-state level of a drug. Second, results of an assay for a drug level in the time period during which this steady state is being achieved should be interpreted with extreme caution, a rule often forgotten in clinical practice. Notice from Figure 23–9 that if assays are performed in the pre-steady-state period (before achievement of four or more half-lives), highly erratic results are obtained owing to the fluctuations in drug concentrations for the discontinuous case, and rising but persistently low values for the continuous case.

The considerations from the preceding paragraphs underlie implementation of effective drug therapy without serious side effects, where it is always necessary to remain within the therapeutic range without causing toxicity to the patient. In addition, a subtherapeutic level must be avoided. Equation 23–8 shows that, in the steady state at the beginning of the dosing period, the dose D_0 is added to the steady state value of D_0, giving a serum level of $2D_0$. This may produce toxicity. Therefore, it may be desirable to lower the periodic dose to less than D_0 but to give these doses at more frequent regular intervals to reach the same steady state value (D_0 in this example). Although it will result in longer times to reach the target steady state value, this procedure results in lower increases in drug levels at the steady state and lower functuations between the peak levels (right after drug administration) and through levels (just before the next dose is administered).

Volume of Distribution

When one is administering drugs, it is of vital importance to know whether the drug is stored in fat or other tissue or whether it is all present in serum. Because a given dose of a drug is known and the concentration of the drug in serum can be determined, one can measure the total volume of body fluid in which the drug is dissolved by the following relation:

$$D = D_o/V_d, \text{ or } V_d = D_o/D \qquad (23–11)$$

where D is the concentration of drug in serum, D_o is the amount of drug administered, and V_d is the volume in which D_o must be dissolved to give the concentration D. This volume, V_d, is referred to as the volume of distribution. If all of the drug is present in serum, V_d is the blood volume that can be determined from conversion tables relating body weight to blood volume. If, however, some of the drug is stored in body tissue, a smaller amount is present in serum, so that the denominator in Equation 23–11 ($V_d = D_o/D$) is reduced and V_d will be larger than the expected blood volume, indicating that some drug is being stored in tissue. If this result occurs, it means that the drug is being released continuously from storage depots (i.e., tissues), which can raise anomalously the level of drug in serum, potentially to toxic levels. Thus, before any drug is administered, the volume of distribution should be known.

Metabolism in the Liver

Many drugs are converted to metabolites, some of which are pharmacologically active and some inactive. Much of this conversion occurs in the extramitochondrial, microsomal system present in hepatocytes. This metabolic system is mainly an oxidative one that utilizes a series of oxidative enzymes that, in turn, utilize a special cytochrome system: cytochrome P450 (Hardman, 2001). This extremely critical cytochrome system has now been strongly implicated as predisposing certain individuals for developing cancer by metabolizing certain environmental compounds such as benzpyrene into frank carcinogens (see below). In addition, genetic polymorphism of the cytochrome P450 enzymes affects an individual's particular response to a drug, including toxicity and an adverse drug reaction (Ingelman-Sundberg, 2004). The excretion of many drugs depends on the integrity of the liver and the cytochrome P450 system. In patients with liver failure due to passive congestion, hepatitis, cirrhosis, and the like, the effective half-life of the drug is increased, making it necessary to *lower* the divided dose of the drug. Conversely, some drugs induce the intracellular synthesis of the microsomal enzymes leading to *diminished* half-life values, so that it may be necessary to *raise* the divided dose.

One example of drug induction of microsomal enzymes is phenobarbital. This drug induces its own metabolism (so that its concentration levels do not obey first-order kinetics). In instances in which the levels of a drug metabolized in the liver are higher than the highest therapeutic value, reductions in the levels may be induced by administering low levels of phenobarbital to induce the microsomal system.

This summary of some of the general principles of drug administration should be helpful in the interpretation of values clinically and permit a better understanding of the subsequent discussion of specific therapeutic drugs, most commonly measured or determined in the laboratory. Tables 23–1 to 23–7 summarize the critical pharmacologic data for the most commonly assayed drugs.

In the following presentation, seven classes of the drugs most commonly assayed for are discussed: cardiotropic, anticonvulsant, antiasthmatic, anti-inflammatory, immunosuppressive, psychotropic and chemotherapeutic. (Antibiotics are discussed in Part VII – Medical Microbiology.) The emphasis in this discussion is on the mechanisms of action of these drugs. Common to most of these drugs is the fact that they interfere with specific steps in signal transduction pathways in cells, which are often remarkably similar to one another. Despite this phenomenon, specific drugs block signal transduction pathway steps that affect only specific cells and seem not to affect signal transduction in other cells.

Cardiotropics (Opie and Gersh, 2001)

These drugs are the ones most commonly used to treat congestive heart failure and cardiac arrhythmias. Despite differences in the structures and properties of the drugs and their specific uses, all of them act on one or another phase of the action potentials in cells that are in the conduction system and in myocytes. Their net effect is to *slow down electrical conduction*. In addition, it is important to remember that the conduction tissue is innervated by both sympathetic and parasympathetic (mainly vagal) nervous systems. The former increases the conduction rate while the latter tends to slow conduction. The actions of each of the cardiotropic drugs are summarized in Figure 23–10. As shown in this figure, there are several major ion currents that control the action potentials of the cells comprising pacemaker tissue of the AV node and the ventricular conduction bands (composed of Purkinje cells): first, rapid sodium influx current, and then a decreased flux (shut off of sodium conductance channels), as outlined in the red area in Figure 23–10; second, a calcium ion influx that prolongs the action potential and then calcium channel shut off, as outlined in the blue area in Figure 23–10; third, potassium ion efflux that promotes repolarization of the cell. As shown in Figure 23–10 there are four classes of drugs that act on one or more of these phases of the action potential resulting in its prolongation. Class I drugs block sodium influx in phase I and include quinidine, procainamide and lidocaine. These agents, especially lidocaine, act by blocking the rapid sodium influx of phase I, decreasing the rate of ventricular diastolic depolarization. Class II drugs include the beta receptor blockers, like propranol, that inhibit the chronotropic effects of adrenergic neuroransmitters like epinephrine and norepinephrine. Class III drugs, like amiodarone, block repolarizing potassium currents, increasing the length of the action potential, as represented by the black curve over the yellow area in Figure 23–10 and increase the refractory period. Class IV drugs, of which verapamil is an important member, slow calcium ion influx, resulting in action potential prolongation. In addition to these classes of drugs, digitalis cardiac glycosides have parasymphathetic-like effects on the cells of the AV node resulting in slowing of conduction. Both digitalis and amiodarone also have marked inotropic effects on the myocardium. Thus both are used in the treatment of congestive heart failure. In damaged myocardium, digitalis blocks sodium-potassium ATPase resulting in transient increases of sodium ion around the sarcolemma resulting in the release of cytosolic calcium ion to the T-system. This allows for increased

CARDIOTROPIC DRUG ACTIONS

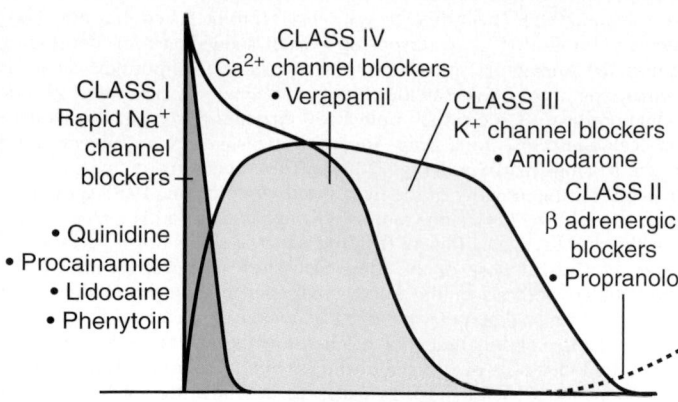

Figure 23–10 Overview of the effects of different anti-arrhythmic agents on the myocardial conduction system. The normal action potential is shown as the black line that first spikes to a high voltage, due mainly to a rapid sodium influx into cells in the conduction system. This component of the action potential, due to sodium ion influx, is shown enclosed in the red area. The actual action potential is prolonged by a succeeding influx of calcium ions shown enclosed under the blue-colored area that overlaps somewhat with the red (sodium influx) area. Termination of the calcium ion influx and efflux of potassium ions results in repolarization shown by the curve bordered by the blue and yellow areas. Class I channel blockers, as listed in the figure, block sodium influx, thereby diminishing the rate of depolarization. Class II blockers, like propranolol, block beta-adrenergic (epinephrine and horepinephrine) stimuli, diminishing the rate of diastolic depolarization. Class III blockers, like amiodorone, block potassium channels, resulting in reduction in potassium efflux, slowing down repolarization. This results in prolongation of the action potential as shown by continuation of the voltage curve over the yellow area in the figure. Class IV blockers, like verapamil, block calcium channels, again prolonging the action potential (blue), although this prolongation is not explicitly shown in the figure. By prolonging the action potential, Class III and IV agents slow down nodal conduction due to prolonged refractoriness of the affected cells. (After Opie LH, Gersh BJ: Drugs for the Heart, 5th ed. Philadelphia, WB Saunders, 2001.)

myocardial contractility. We now discuss the key properties and actions of these cardiotropic durgs.

Digitalis Glycosides

Digoxin. Because they slow conduction in the AV node, the digitalis glycosides are used to treat atrial arrhythmias, in particular atrial flutter and fibrillation. The rationale is to block rapid atrial conduction signals to the ventricles, thereby slowing ventricular response. Their direct positive inotropic effect increases cardiac output in cardiac failure.

Digoxin (Table 23–1) has a rapid onset of action (within 1–2 hours when given orally) and a relatively short half-life (35–40 hours). Most patients will excrete approximately 50–75% of a dose unchanged in the urine. The general range of therapeutic serum levels is from 0.5–2 ng/mL. High concentrations of the drug are found in skeletal and cardiac muscle as well as in liver, brain, and kidneys.

Digitoxin. In contrast, digitoxin has a longer half-life (4–6 days) with a relatively slower onset of action (within 1–4 hours when given orally, with maximal effect in 8 hours); 90–100% of a dose is absorbed, with approximately 95% bound to plasma protein. The general range of therapeutic serum levels is from 9–25 ng/mL. The drug is extensively metabolized in the liver (90%), with digoxin being the active metabolite.

Toxic side effects of the digitalis glycosides include gastric disturbances, nausea, vomiting, and atrial and ventricular arrhythmias. It is crucial that levels of digoxin (or digitoxin) be monitored closely and accurately while the patient is initially being given this drug. As mentioned previously, the therapeutic range for digoxin is from 0.5–2 ng/mL (i.e., the range is narrow). Toxic levels exceed 2 ng/mL, so the difference between therapeutic and toxic doses is small. This difference necessitates careful digoxin assay.

Digoxin toxicity is often treated with Digibind (GlaxoSmithKline, Research Triangle Park, NC), consisting of ovine Fab fragments. This antidote can interfere with determination of digoxin serum levels (Valdes, 1998). Some assays have been reported to determine only the 'free' digoxin level, i.e., that not bound to Digibind Fab, which inactivates digoxin. For other assays that determine total digoxin (i.e., free plus Fab-bound digoxin), it is recommended that an ultrafiltrate of serum be employed to determine the level of free or active digoxin. Alternatively, since Digibind can cause spurious and erroneous results, it has been recommended that, since the half-life of

Table 23–1 Digoxin

Purpose	Treatment of congestive heart failure and atrial fibrillation–flutter
General adult dose	Oral: 0.75–1.5 mg for digitalization, 0.125–0.5 mg/day for maintenance
Usual bioavailability	Approx. 60–85% for tablet or elixir; 90–100% for liquid-filled capsules
Half-life	Approx. 35–40 hours; however, prolonged in patients with decreased renal function
General therapeutic range	0.5–2 ng/mL
General toxic level	> 2 ng/mL, but somewhat variable
Transport	Approx. 20–25% plasma protein bound
Metabolism	Generally, only small amounts are metabolized (liver, lumen of large intestine)
Elimination	Approx. 50–75% unchanged in urine
Steady state	Approx. 7 days in undigitalized patients with normal renal function
Mechanism of action	Causes release of calcium ions in T-system of myocardium; slows AV node conduction
Toxic effects	Gastric disturbances, nausea, vomiting, atrial and ventricular arrhythmias; irregular pulse

Digibind is 15–20 hours, therapeutic levels of digoxin should be determined 2–4 days after the last Digibind dose.

Procainamide (Pronestyl) (Table 23–2) is a class I antiarrhythmic drug that is useful in treating supraventricular or ventricular arrhythmias. One of its major effects is increased refractoriness of the atrium and decreased myocardial excitability. The bioavailability of procainamide is 75–95%. Approximately 15% is bound to plasma protein and approximately 50% is excreted by the kidneys. The half-life is approximately 3.5 hours, with a general range of therapeutic serum level of 4–10 µg/mL. *N*-acetylation to the major active metabolite *N*-acetylprocainamide (NAPA) is the major metabolic pathway of biotransformation. Toxic side effects include a reversible lupus-like syndrome with elevated antinuclear antibody (ANA) titers, urticaria, rash, agranulocytosis, and nephrotic syndrome.

The lupus-like syndrome may be initiated by leukocyte metabolism of procainamide to a chemically reactive metabolite that could then covalently bind to monocyte/macrophage membrane proteins to stimulate production of autoantibodies. In addition, the tertiary amino moiety of the covalently bound procainamide metabolite might mimic a portion of histone protein and result in the production of antihistone antinuclear antibody (Uetrecht, 1988).

Quinidine, also a class I anti-arrhythmic, like procainamide, is used to treat supraventricular and ventricular arrhythmias and tachyarrhythmias. The prevention of ventricular tachycardia or frequent premature ventricular contractions and the maintenance of sinus rhythm after the conversion of atrial flutter or atrial fibrillation are its two major uses (Valdes, 1998).

The bioavailability of quinidine is 90–100%, with approximately 85% of the drug bound to plasma protein. Quinidine is 60–85% metabolized in the liver via hydroxylation reactions, with some metabolites being active. Urinary excretion is approximately 20%. The half-life of quinidine is 5–12 hours, and the general therapeutic range is 2.3–5 µg/mL. Maximal serum levels are reached in 1–3 hours. Toxic side effects of quinidine include cinchonism (vertigo, tinnitus, headache, visual disturbances and disorientation), fever, hepatitis, and blood dyscrasia. Ventricular arrhythmias, AV block, and ventricular fibrillation leading to syncope and sudden death can occur.

Lidocaine (Xylocaine), another class I anti-arrhythmic, can also be used as a local anesthetic. Its major use as an antiarrhythmic is in the acute control and prevention of ventricular arrhythmias after acute myocardial infarction. A loading intravenous dose of 50–100 mg is given over 2–3 minutes to treat ventricular arrhythmias in adults. These dosages may be repeated in 5- to 10-minute intervals of 25–50 mg, up to a maximum of 300 mg in a 1-hour period. Following loading, infusion is then continued at a rate of 1.4–3.5 mg/min for a 70-kg man. In children, 0.5–1 mg/kg can be given every 5 minutes for a maximum of three doses.

Lidocaine is neither highly protein bound nor appreciably stored in body tissues; it has a half-life of approximately 2 hours and a therapeutic serum

Table 23–2 Procainamide

Purpose:	Treatment of supraventricular or ventricular arrhythmias
General adult dose	Oral: 4 g/day, in divided doses, for maintenance therapy
Usual bioavailability	75–95%
Half-life	Approx. 3.5 hours in patients with normal renal function
General therapeutic range	4–10 μg/mL
General toxic level	> 12 μg/mL
Transport	Approx. 15% plasma protein bound
Metabolism	Hepatic: *N*-acetylprocainamide (active), with $t_{1/2}$ approx. 7 hours in patients with normal renal function
Elimination	Approx. 50–60% unchanged in urine
Steady state	Minimum of 12 hours
Mechanism of action	Prolongation of atrial refractory period and decreased myocardial excitability
Toxic effects	Reversible lupus erythematosus-like syndrome, irregular pulse, hypotension, rash, agranulocytosis

range of 1.2–5.5 μg/mL. The time to reach a maximum serum level is generally 5–8 hours. Ninety percent of a dose of lidocaine is metabolized in the liver via *N*-dealkylation. Urinary excretion is 10%. Toxic side effects include convulsions, coma, and respiratory depression (CNS effects), as well as bradycardia and hypotension.

Propranolol, a class II anti-arrhythmic beta-receptor blocking drug that antagonizes the effects of epinephrine on the heart, on the arteries and arterioles of skeletal muscles, and on the bronchus, exerts its effects largely on the AV node and is used to treat sinus tachycardia, atrial tachycardia and ventricular arrhythmias. Overall, blockade of beta-1-receptors increases AV conduction time and reduces heart rate, myocardial contractility and output, and cardiac automaticity. Because it is a vasodilator, it is also used in the treatment of angina pectoris; hypertension; and symptomatic coronary artery disease, particularly after an acute myocardial infarction. Oral dosages vary from 40–320 mg daily, in adults, for antiarrhythmic activity to as high as 480 mg daily in the control of hypertension. Both supine and standing blood pressure are also reduced. Bioavailability of propranolol is approximately 30%. The half-life of propranolol is 3 hours, with a therapeutic serum range of 50–100 ng/mL and with maximum serum levels reached in approximately 6 hours. Approximately 93% is protein bound. Propranolol is metabolized in the liver, with 0.5% excreted in the urine unchanged. Toxic effects include bradycardia, arterial insufficiency (Raynaud's type), hypotension, AV block, nausea, vomiting, pharyngitis, bronchospasm, and thrombotic thrombocytopenic purpura. Marrow suppression occurs rarely.

Amiodarone, chiefly a class III antiarrhythmic drug, markedly prolongs the action potential by blocking potassium channels in cardiac muscle (Fig. 23–10). This prolongs the effective refractory period. Its activity is complex in that it also significantly blocks inactivated sodium channels, thus exhibiting class I action, and also exhibits weak adrenergic and calcium channel-blocking effects. Its indication for use is with life-threatening ventricular arrhythmias. The oral loading dose is 1200–1600 mg/day with a maintenance dose of 200–400 mg/day. Bioavailability is ~ 35–65%. Amiodarone has two components in its half-life: A rapid component of 3–10 days (involving ~ 50% of the drug) and a slow component of 25–110 days. The general therapeutic range is 1–2.5 μg/mL, although this is not well defined, and a toxic level of > 2.5 μg/mL, again not well defined. Approximately 96% is plasma protein bound; the drug undergoes liver metabolism, and shows extensive body distribution due to its hydrophobic (lipid soluble) structure. Excretion is very slow by skin, biliary tract, and lacrimal glands. Toxic effects can be profound and include symptomatic bradycardia, heart block, fatal pulmonary fibrosis, hepatitis, visual field disturbances, photodermatitis, and, importantly, mainly hypothyroidism but sometimes hyperthyroidism.

Verapamil is a class IV antiarrhythmic drug that blocks activated and inactivated calcium channels that are especially prominent in nodal tissue (particularly the AV node). Indications include angina, hypertension, and supraventricular arrhythmias. The oral dose is 120–480 mg/day in three to four divided doses. Bioavailability is ~ 10–20%. The half-life is 2–8 hours but increases to 4.5–12 hours after repeated oral doses. The general therapeutic range is 80–400 ng/mL, although this is not well defined. Approximately 90% is plasma protein bound and the drug undergoes extensive metabolism in the liver, where norverapamil, an active metabolite, is produced. Approximately 75% of the active components are eliminated by the kidney and ~ 25% through the GI tract. Toxic effects include hypotension, ventricular fibrillation, constipation, and peripheral edema.

Anticonvulsants

Anticonvulsants are used in the treatment of seizure disorders, in particular, grand mal, petit mal, and psychomotor seizures and other specialized seizure disorders such as tic douloureux (trigeminal neuralgia). While the mechanism of action of these drugs has not been elucidated, it appears that all of these agents, with the possible exception of phenobarbital, block sodium influx into neurons that have damaged membranes as schematized in Figure 23–11. In addition, several of these agents, especially phenytoin, also block secondary calcium influxes into such cells, which also seems to inhibit the rapid firing of these cells. Another effect of phenobarbital, and possibly also phenytoin, is membrane stabilization through intercalation as also shown in Figure 23–11. Many of the anticonvulsants are effective against grand mal seizures but have no effects or adverse ones on petit mal seizures. *Only ethosuximide (Zarontin) and valproic acid (Depakote) are effective against this condition.* Thus, while the mechanism of action of these drugs appears to be similar, they differ in specificities.

Phenobarbital (Table 23–3), a long-acting barbiturate, is used in the treatment of generalized tonic–clonic seizures and simple partial seizures with motor or somatosensory symptoms, as well as for anxiety and insomnia. It is not used in the treatment of absence seizure (i.e., petit mal), which may be exacerbated by phenobarbital; nor for complex partial seizures, which do not respond well. Phenobarbital is also given for the withdrawal symptoms in infants born to opiate- or barbiturate-addicted mothers. Because phenobarbital enhances the metabolism of bilirubin by enzyme induction, it has been used to treat cases of congenital hyperbilirubinemia (familial nonhemolytic, nonobstructive jaundice). In addition to induction of hepatic microsomal enzymes, barbiturates are believed to stabilize damaged membranes (Fig. 23–11) as well as to raise the threshold for neuronal membrane depolarization. The oral dose of phenobarbital for anxiety in adults is 30–120 mg daily in divided doses; for sleep induction in adults, 100–320 mg daily is generally used. For seizure control, divided doses of 100–200 mg/day in adults or 30–100 mg/day in children are generally used.

Phenobarbital has a long half-life of 4–6 days. Oral doses are almost completely absorbed (90–100% bioavailability), and the optimal serum concentration for seizure control is generally 15–30 μg/mL; 40–60% is metabolized in the liver, whereas 10–40% may be eliminated unchanged in the urine. Approximately 40–60% is plasma protein bound, and the main site of storage is the brain. A steady state is reached in 14–21 days. Toxic side effects include nystagmus, ataxia, stupor, respiratory depression, coma, and hypotension. Barbiturates are contraindicated in patients with acute intermittent porphyria, i.e., partial porphobilinogen deaminase deficiency, since barbiturates enhance the synthesis of delta-aminolevulinic acid synthetase and thus the synthesis of heme pathway intermediates in the liver.

Phenytoin (Dilantin) is used to treat generalized tonic–clonic, simple partial, and complex partial seizures (Table 23–4). It is ineffective in treating myoclonus, absence (petit mal), and atonic seizures. It is usually given intravenously in addition to intravenous diazepam to terminate status epilepticus. Remarkably, phenytoin has no apparent effects on resting neurons or on normally firing neurons. It is thus specific for epileptogenic foci in the CNS (Yaari, 1986). Interestingly, carbamazepine (Tegretol) exerts similar effects, as discussed below. Data on the mechanism of action of this drug strongly suggest that phenytoin blocks sodium and calcium influxes into repeatedly depolarizing neurons in the CNS and also into neurons that are partially depolarized. By reducing sodium and calcium influx into these cells, it reduces their excitability and prolongs their refractory period (Yaari, 1986). In fact, phenytoin appears to bind selectively to fast-firing sodium channels in their refractory states, thereby prolonging their refractory periods (Bazil, 1998). This finding helps explain the ability of phenytoin to block only neurons that are firing rapidly and repetitively.

Although the average daily maintenance dose in adults is 300–400 mg, dosage must be tailored to the patient's response and serum drug concentrations. The usual therapeutic serum concentration is 10–20 μg/mL, with a steady state reached in 5–10 days (for plateau; see Fig. 23–9). The serum half-life is generally 24 hours, but it is dose-dependent. Thus, its

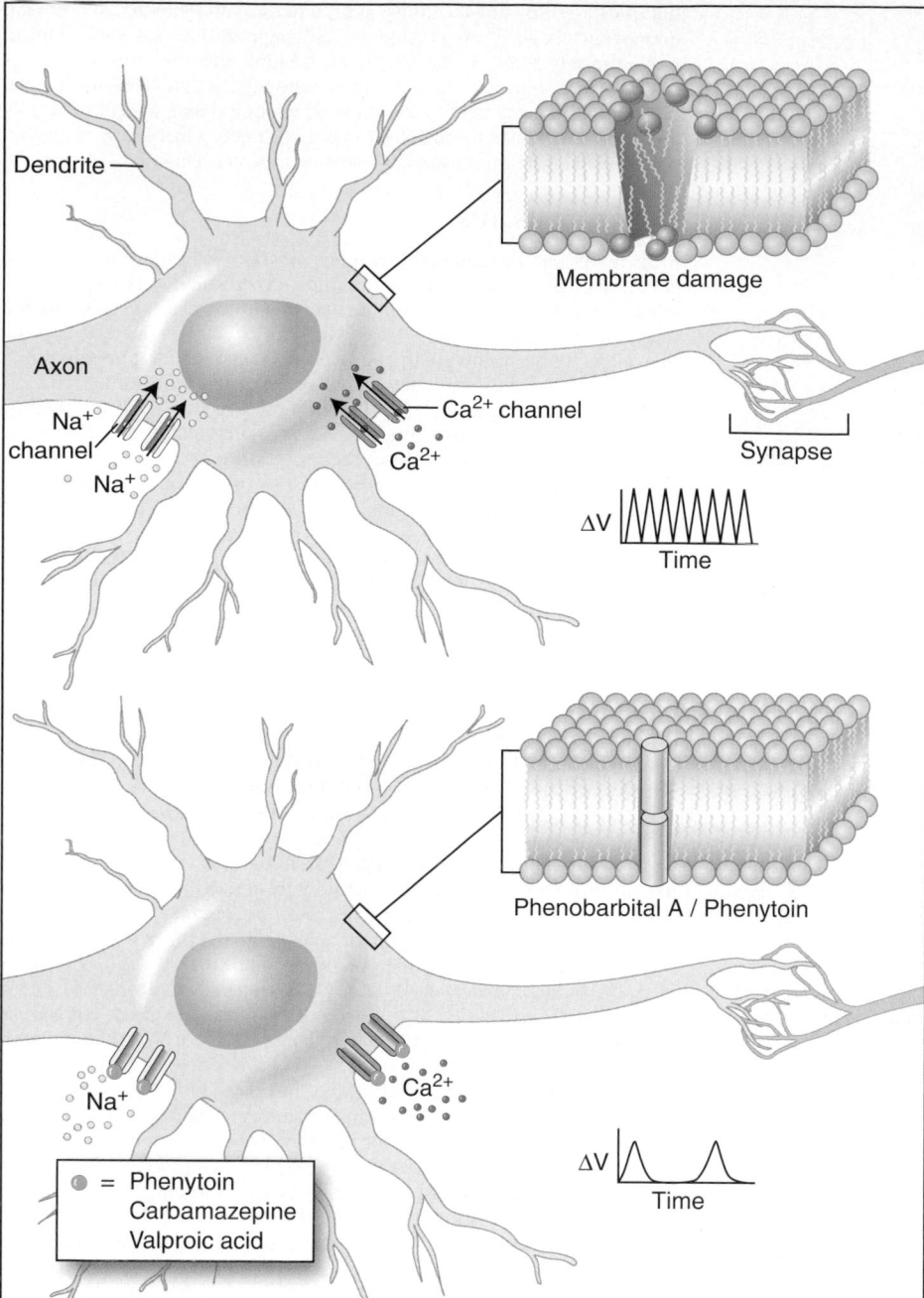

Figure 23-11 Effects of anticonvulsants on neurons. *Upper figure:* Damaged neuronal membranes, as shown in the section on the upper right of the figure, result in sodium (yellow circles) and calcium (red circles) influxes via their respective channels that cause repeated firing shown in the voltage–time curve to the right of the figure. *Lower figure:* Anticonvulsants like phenytoin (Dilantin), carbamazepine (Tegretol) and valproic acid (Depakote), represented by the small blue circles, block sodium and calcium channels, resulting in a substantially diminished rate of firing as shown in the voltage–time curve to the right of the figure. Both phenytoin and phenobarbital, shown as blue cylinders, are also thought to stabilize the damaged neuronal membrane as shown in the membrane section schematized in the upper right drawing.

excretion is not a first-order process. Phenytoin is stored in the brain, metabolized in the liver (95%), and is approximately 90–95% bound to plasma protein. Both aspirin and phenylbutazone can displace phenytoin from serum albumin and can significantly increase the serum concentration of phenytoin. Because phenytoin, like phenobarbital, is a relatively potent enzyme-inducer, certain antibiotics, oral anticoagulants, quinidine, and oral contraceptives may be more rapidly metabolized, thus decreasing their effectiveness.

Because the relationship between serum concentrations and daily dosage is not linear, small increases in dosage can greatly increase therapeutic serum concentrations. Symptoms of toxicity generally occur at serum concentrations greater than 20 μg/mL. Toxic side effects include nystagmus, ataxia, stupor, and coma. Arrhythmias can be produced by rapid intravenous administration.

Fosphenytoin is a water-soluble parenteral formulation of phenytoin that is rapidly converted (half-life of 8–15 minutes) in vivo to phenytoin. The half-life is independent of plasma concentration, and it has identical pharmacodynamic, pharmacokinetic, and clinical properties to phenytoin. This prodrug offers improved flexibility and tolerability for the patient, as compared with intravenous phenytoin, and is indicated for the treatment of partial and generalized seizures in adults where intravenous administration is indicated (Bazil, 1998).

Primidone (Mysoline) is used to treat generalized tonic–clonic, simple partial, and complex partial seizures. Its chemical structure is closely related to the basic structure of the barbiturates, and it is metabolized in the liver into two active metabolites: phenobarbital and phenylethyl-malonamide (PEMA). Thus some of its anticonvulsant effects are due to phenobarbital activity. Unlike phenobarbital, however, primidone may increase the threshold of membrane depolarization within the CNS.

Oral doses range from 250 mg daily to 2 g/day in divided doses. Absorption is rapid and complete (100%), with the usual therapeutic serum concentration being 5–21 μg/mL. A steady state is reached in 4–7 days, and the half-life is approximately 12 hours. Plasma protein binding is relatively low (20%), with most of the drug remaining free in the serum and with little drug being stored in body tissues.

Sedation is a common toxic side effect. Dizziness, ataxia, and skin rashes have also been observed. Primidone, like phenobarbital, is contraindicated in patients with acute intermittent porphyria.

Ethosuximide (Zarontin) is the drug of choice for absence (petit mal) seizures unaccompanied by other types of seizures. It is preferred over valproic acid (see below), at least initially, because hepatotoxicity is a rare but serious side effect of valproic acid. Ethosuximide may depress the motor cortex and may reduce the frequency of neuronal firing, but its molecular site of action is poorly understood.

Table 23–3 Phenobarbital

Purpose	Treatment of generalized tonic–clonic seizures, simple partial seizures, anxiety, insomnia
General adult dose	Oral: 100–200 mg/day for seizure control; 30–120 mg/day for anxiety; 100–320 mg for sleep induction
Usual bioavailability	Approx. 90–100%
Half-life	Approx. 5–6 days in adults; approx. 3–4 days in children
General therapeutic range	15–30 µg/mL for epilepsy control
General toxic level	> 40 µg /mL, although tolerance may develop
Transport	Approx. 40–60% plasma protein bound
Metabolism	Approx. 75% hepatic: p-hydroxyphenobarbital, inactive
Elimination	Approx. 25% unchanged in urine
Steady state	Approx. 14–21 days
Mechanism of action	Stabilizes damaged membranes and raises threshold for neuronal membrane depolarization
Toxic effects	Drowsiness, depression, respiratory depression, coma, sedation, hypotension. Respiratory depression may be caused by rapid intravenous administration

Table 23–4 Phenytoin (Dilantin)

Purpose	Treatment of generalized tonic–clonic seizures, simple partial seizures, complex partial seizures
General adult dose	Oral: 300–400 mg/day maintenance dose
Usual bioavailability	Variable: 30–95%
Half-life	24 plus or minus 12 hours, and dose-dependent
General therapeutic range	10–20 µg/mL
General toxic level	> 20 µg/mL
Transport	Approx. 90–95% plasma protein bound
Metabolism	Hepatic: 5-(p-hydroxyphenyl)5-phenylhydantoin, inactive
Elimination	Approx. 5% unchanged in urine
Steady state	Approx. 7–8 days
Mechanism of action	Appears to block sodium and calcium ion influxes into repeatedly depolarizing CNS neurons
Toxic effects	Nystagmus, ataxia, diplopia, drowsiness, coma; rapid intravenous administration may produce cardiovascular collapse and/or CNS depression

The oral dosage in adults is generally 500–1000 mg daily. Absorption is fairly rapid and complete (100%), with peak serum concentrations occurring in 1–4 hours. A steady state is reached in 8–10 days. The usual therapeutic serum concentration is 40–100 µg/mL, but can be as high as 170–190 µg/mL in children. The serum half-life is generally 60 hours in adults and 30 hours in children. Ethosuximide is essentially free in serum and not protein bound. It is mainly metabolized in the liver (60–90%) to desmethylmethsuximide. Gastrointestinal disturbances are among the most common toxic effects and include nausea, vomiting, and gastric distress. Other effects include drowsiness and ataxia. Rare serious side effects, such as SLE (systemic lupus erythematosus), aplastic anemia, and pancytopenia have been reported.

Carbamazepine (Tegretol) (Table 23–5) is a primary antiepileptic drug and is used in the treatment of generalized tonic–clonic seizures and simple partial and complex partial seizures, as well as in combinations of these seizure types. Absence (petit mal), myoclonic, and atonic seizures may be exacerbated by this drug. This drug is also used to treat tic douloureux (trigeminal neuralgia) and glossopharyngeal neuralgia, and is, in fact, the drug of choice in the treatment of these neuralgias.

Carbamazepine is a tricyclic compound (i.e., iminostilbene) and is chemically related to imipramine, a tricyclic antidepressant. It is believed that a reduction of excitatory synaptic transmission in the spinal trigeminal nucleus is the basis for this drug's antineuralgic action. Its antiepileptic

Table 23–5 Carbamazepine (Tegretol)

Purpose	Treatment of generalized tonic–clonic seizures, simple partial seizures, complex partial seizures; trigeminal neuralgia and glossopharyngeal neuralgia
General adult dose	Oral: 0.8–1.2 g/day maintenance for seizure control; 0.2–1.2 /day for neuralgia
Usual bioavailability	70%
Half-life	Initially approx. 35 hours; approx. 8–20 hours after 3–4 weeks of administration
General therapeutic range	4–12 µg/mL
General toxic level	> 12 µg/mL
Transport	60–70% plasma protein bound
Metabolism	Hepatic: carbamazepine-10,11-epoxide (active); carbamazepine-10,11-transdihydrodiol (inactive)
Elimination	1–2% unchanged in urine
Steady state	3–7 days
Mechanism of action	Decreases sodium and calcium ion influx into repeatedly depolarizing CNS neurons; reduces excitatory synaptic transmission in the spinal trigeminal nucleus
Toxic effects	Drowsiness, ataxia, dizziness, nausea, vomiting, involuntary movements, abnormal reflexes, irregular pulse

action is quite similar to that of phenytoin – that is, it decreases sodium and calcium influx into hyperexcitable neurons (Yaari, 1986; Bazil, 1998).

Oral doses of carbamazepine are completely absorbed, and the usual adult maintenance dose is 0.8–1.2 g/day. Ninety-eight percent is biotransformed in the liver into two active metabolites: a 10,11-epoxide form and a 10,11-dihydroxy form of carbamazepine. The usual therapeutic serum concentration is 4–12 µg/mL, with a steady state reached in 3–4 days. The serum half-life of Tegretol is 8–20 hours (after 3–4 weeks of administration), and 60–70% is plasma protein bound. The more common toxic reactions seen with this drug include drowsiness, ataxia, dizziness, nausea and vomiting, and lightheadedness. Rare hematologic reactions may occur and can be quite serious; they include aplastic anemia, thrombocytopenia, and agranulocytosis.

Valproic acid (Depakene) is commonly used in the treatment of generalized tonic–clonic seizures, absence seizures, myoclonic seizures, and atonic seizures. It is not effective for the treatment of infantile spasms. Although the mechanism of action is not definitely known, valproic acid is thought to enhance the activity of the GABA-mediated inhibitory system. In addition, its action is similar to that of phenytoin and carbamazepine in that it prolongs the refractory state of sodium channels (Hardman, 2001). Absorption of valproic acid is rapid and complete. The average daily maintenance dose of valproic acid in adults is 15–30 mg/kg, when utilized alone, and 30–45 mg/kg in combination with other antiepileptic drugs. The usual therapeutic serum concentration is 50–100 µg/mL, and a steady state is reached in 1–4 days. Most (90–100%) of the drug is metabolized in the liver, while a high percentage (90%) of the drug is plasma protein bound. The serum half-life is 8–15 hours.

Valproic acid has been shown to produce teratogenic effects in experimental animals; these included developmental abnormalities and skeletal defects. Thus, valproic acid should be used with caution in pregnant women. Toxic side effects include sedation, gastric disturbances, hematologic reactions, ataxia, somnolence, and coma. Rare fatal hepatotoxicity has occurred, and severe or fatal pancreatitis has been reported (see Sztajnkrycer, 2002).

Newer Anticonvulsants

Topiramate, lamotrigine (Lamictal), gabapentin (Neurontin), and felbamate are four anticonvulsant agents recently approved for use in this country and are being used for patients whose response to the more established anticonvulsants is less than optimal. Topiramate and lamotrigine are utilized as adjunctive treatment for partial seizures in adults. Topiramate has a half-life of approximately 21 hours, with approximately 15% of the drug protein bound. Lamotrigine has a variable half-life, depending on whether the drug is used as monotherapy or with an inducer.

Approximately 55% of lamotrigine is protein bound. Gabapentin is also utilized as adjunctive treatment for partial seizures and has a half-life of

II

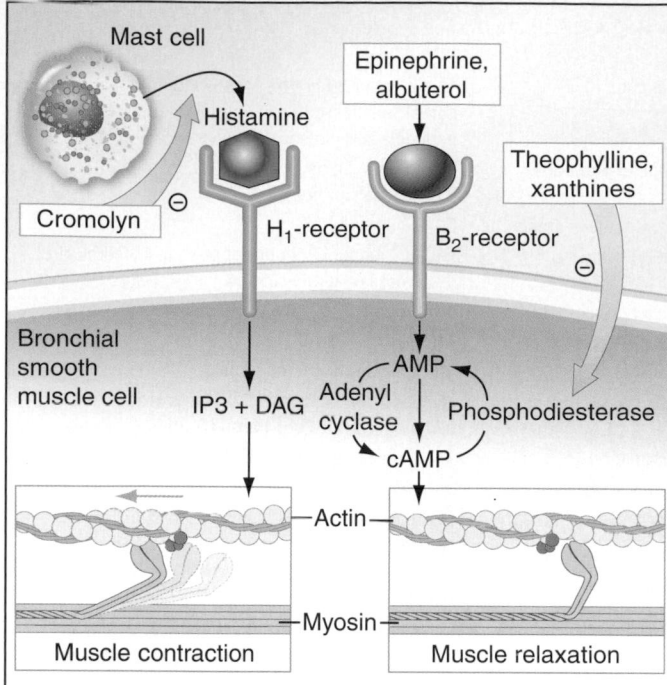

Figure 23–12 Summary of the mechanisms of action of antiasthmatic agents. Three basic mechanisms are shown. Note that all three mechanisms result in promotion of smooth muscle relaxation in the small airways, i.e., fewer actin–myosin cross-bridges, as shown at the bottom of the figure. On the left of the figure, release of histamine from mast cells in response to allergenic stimulation results in histamine–H_1-receptor complexes that promote a signal transduction pathway in which inositol triphosphate (IP3) and diacylglycerol (DAG), both second messengers, are induced and promote smooth muscle contraction. Histamine release is blocked ('–' beside the green arrow) by the drug, cromolyn. In the middle of the figure, epinephrine and albuterol are shown to form complexes with beta-receptors; these complexes induce adenyl cyclase activity such that cyclic AMP (cAMP in the figure) is synthesized; this second messenger *blocks* smooth muscle contraction. On the right of the figure, xanthines, such as theophylline, are shown to block ('–' beside the green arrow) the enzyme, phosphodiesterase, resulting in prolonged lifetimes of cAMP, allowing it to function for prolonged periods in blocking smooth muscle contraction.

5–7 hours with less than 3% protein binding. Therapeutic ranges and toxic concentrations for these drugs have not been determined. Common side effects of topiramate include fatigue, psychomotor slowing, somnolence, and difficulty with concentration and speech. Acute angle glaucoma can also occur (Asconape, 2002). Common side effects of lamotrigine include ataxia, CNS depression, diplopia, dizziness, abnormal thinking, nausea, nervousness, rash, and somnolence. Common side effects of gabapentin include ataxia, dizziness, fatigue, and somnolence. A major toxic effect reported for lamotrigine is Stevens–Johnson syndrome (Warner, 1998; Brodtkorb, 1998). Felbamate has been found to produce a relatively high incidence of aplastic anemia and hepatic failure (Asconape, 2002). Thus, the drug is only utilized in patients failing other treatments where the potential clinical benefits outweigh the potential clinical risks (Bazil, 1998; Brodtkorb, 1998; Asconape, 2002).

Antiasthmatics

Asthma is a form of chronic obstructive pulmonary disease (COPD) that has a variety of causes, some of them allergenic in nature. As indicated in Figure 23–12, at the heart of asthma is bronchoconstriction due to contraction of smooth muscle fibers in bronchioles. This may be induced by allergenic processes in which inflammatory processes result in the release of histamine from mast cells. Histamine, when it binds to H_1 receptors in smooth muscle cells induces second messengers such as inositol triphosphate (IP3) and diacylglycerol (DAG) that ultimately stimulate muscle contraction (Fig. 23–12). Opposing this process is the binding of epinephrine to beta-2-receptors resulting in stimulation of adenylate cyclase that induces synthesis of cyclic AMP (cAMP), a second messenger molecule that blocks muscle contraction. As part of a regulatory process, phosphodiesterase induces hydrolysis of cAMP and thus helps to remove inhibition of smooth muscle contraction.

As indicated in Figure 23–12, there are at least three different therapeutic strategies for blocking bronchiolar smooth muscle contraction. The first is blockade of release of histamine from mast cells by drugs such as cromolyn.

This is not the only inflammatory process that can induce the bronchoconstriction of asthma. Other components of the inflammatory process may also be active in provoking bronchoconstriction. These are summarized in Figure 23–13, which shows that, among the agents promoting bronchoconstriction, the leukotrienes and prostaglandins are quite prominent. To counter these effects, oral anti-inflammatory agents, such as the leukotriene inhibitors zileuton and zafirlukast, have been found to be effective in asthma, since they interrupt the leukotriene/arachidonic acid pathways involved in inflammation and bronchial reactivity. Importantly, steroids have been found to be highly effective in blocking inflammation-induced bronchospasm. As indicated in Figure 23–13, these agents potently inhibit leukotriene, prostaglandin, and platelet-activating factor (not shown in Fig. 23–13) production by both inhibiting phospholipase A_2 and the inducible cyclo-oxygenase 2 isoform. Lipid-soluble steroids, especially in the aerosolized form, avoiding adverse systemic effects, have been found to be among the most effective agents against asthma. These agents include beclomethasone, flunisolide, and triamcinolone. Longer-acting lipid-soluble beta-2 agonists, such as formoterol and salmeterol, are also available and appear to be long acting due to their ability to dissolve into the bronchial smooth muscle membrane.

Second, for severe asthmatic attacks, subcutaneous injection of epinephrine is effective in relieving the bronchoconstriction on an acute basis via the mechanism shown in Figure 23–12. For more chronic treatment, beta-2-receptor-binding drugs including albuterol (Proventil, Ventolin) and terbutaline (Brethine) are effective in reversing this process by the same mechanism. Both of these agents stimulate production of cAMP as shown in the central pathway of Fig. 23–12. Third, as shown in Figure 23–12, blockade of phosphodiesterase by such drugs as theophylline and the xanthines, prevents hydrolysis of cAMP, allowing for continuous inhibition of bronchoconstriction.

Although still a commonly prescribed antiasthmatic drug, theophylline is being replaced with the other antiasthmatics such as steroid and beta-adrenergic bronchial inhalers, used mainly for acute and subacute asthmatic attacks in adults. These latter agents have fewer toxic side effects (Pesce, 1998). However, laboratory assays for therapeutic levels of antiasthmatics have been performed only for theophylline, predominantly because its therapeutic range is narrow, and potential side effects are serious, as now discussed.

Theophylline (Table 23–6) is used as a bronchodilator for the treatment of moderate or severe asthma, both for the prevention of attacks and for the treatment of symptomatic exacerbations. Theophylline also exerts additional actions, including vasodilation, diuresis, positive cardiac inotropic effects, and the stimulation of diaphragmatic contraction. Owing to the latter stimulating effect, theophylline may be of some benefit to some patients with emphysema. Theophylline has also been effective in the treatment of primary apnea of prematurity, in which the absence of respiratory effort lasts more than 20 seconds in newborn infants. The mechanism of action of this latter effect is thought to be due to medullary stimulation by the drug. It has been found that caffeine is more effective for this purpose because it has diminished toxicity (Pesce, 1998). In the treatment of asthma, dosage is calculated on the basis of body weight and depends on the route of administration and the age of the patient. Because the therapeutic index (i.e., the closeness of toxic levels to the therapeutic levels) of theophylline is low, cautious dosage determination is essential. Careful monitoring of patient response and serum theophylline levels is required because theophylline is metabolized at different rates for each patient. Theophylline levels can be estimated at 1 hour after intravenous administration, 1–2 hours after oral administration, or generally 3–8 hours after extended-release administration from appropriately drawn blood samples.

The therapeutic serum level is 10–20 µg/mL, and the mean half-life is approximately 8.7 hours in nonsmoking adults (5.5 hours in smoking adults). However, the half-life may vary widely among individuals, again indicating the need for close supervision of the patient and appropriate monitoring of serum concentrations in each patient. Approximately 60% of the drug is protein bound, and about 90% is metabolized in the liver, with caffeine being one of the inactive metabolites produced. Theophylline crosses the placenta, and may be teratogenic in pregnant females. Other common side effects include tachycardia, arrhythmias, seizures, and gastrointestinal bleeding.

Anti-Inflammatory and Analgesic Drugs

As noted in the preceding section and as shown in Figure 23–13, membrane damage, resulting from immune complexes, trauma, or other stress, induces, among other events, the release of phospholipids. These, in turn, become substrates for phospholipase A_2, which results in the production

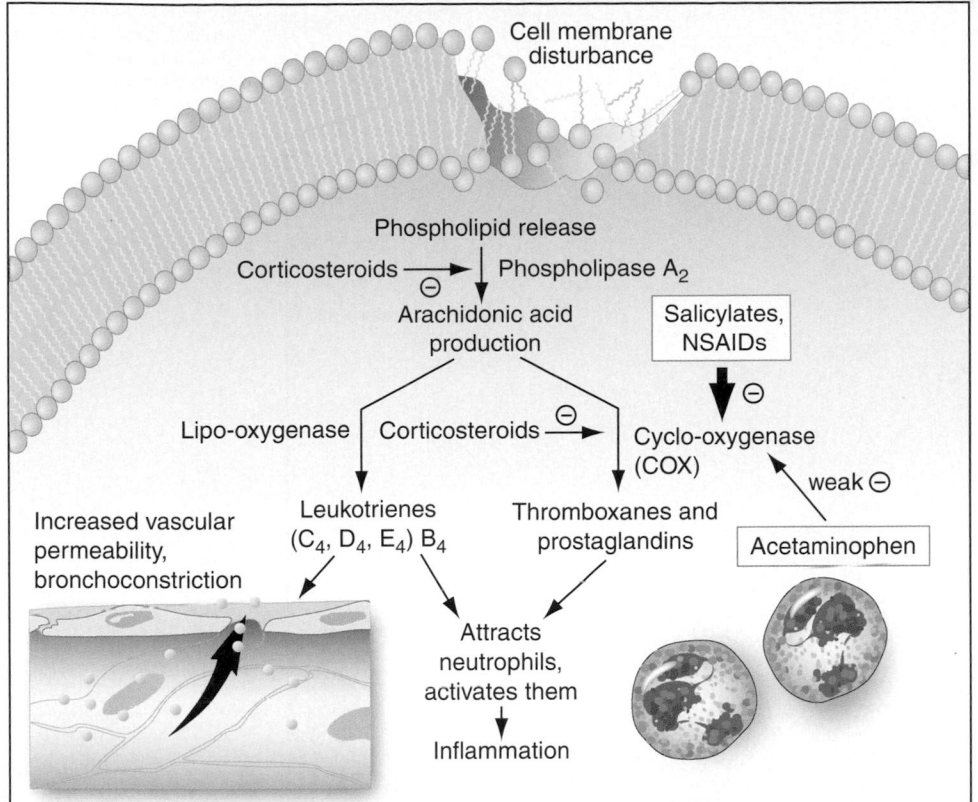

Figure 23–13 Mechanisms of action of anti-inflammatory drugs. The figure shows that the fundamental event in inflammation-induced cell death is membrane damage in cells that results in activation of phospholipase A_2. This enzyme promotes the synthesis of arachidonic acid. This is a substrate for two critical enzymes: lipo-oxygenase, that promotes synthesis of leukotrienes, and cyclo-oxygenase (COX) that promotes synthesis of thromboxanes and prostaglandins. Both classes of compounds promote neutrophil chemotaxis (shown on the lower right of the figure) with resulting phagocytosis of damaged cells and a further destructive inflammatory response. Leukotrienes themselves promote increased vascular permeability, causing increased migration of neutrophils to the damaged cells, and smooth muscle contraction (lower left of figure). In this figure, corticosteroids such as prednisone and cortisone are shown to block (black '–' signs beside arrows) two key enzymes in this signal transduction inflammatory cascade: phospholipase A_2 and cyclo-oxygenase. Corticosteroids also are thought to stabilize damaged membranes. Nonsteroidal anti-inflammatory drugs (NSAIDs) block predominantly cyclo-oxygenase; acetaminophen (Tylenol) blocks mainly COX in the central nervous system and only weakly blocks peripheral COX and is therefore more of an antipyretic than an anti-inflammatory drug.

Table 23–6 Theophylline

Purpose	Treatment and prevention of moderate to severe asthma
General adult dose	Depends on body weight, route of administration, and age and condition of patient
Usual bioavailability	Varies according to form, with about 100% for oral liquids and uncoated tablets
Half-life	Varies: 8–9 hours in nonsmoking adults, 5–6 hours in adults who smoke, and 3–4 hours in children, but may vary widely
General therapeutic range	10–20 µg/mL
General toxic level	> 20 µg/mL
Transport	60% plasma protein bound
Metabolism	Hepatic: caffeine; 1,3-dimethyluric acid; 1-methyluric acid; 3-methylxanthine
Elimination	10% unchanged in urine
Steady state	Five half-lives; 90% of steady state reached in three half-lives
Mechanism of action	Increases intracellular cAMP by inhibiting phosphodiesterase; this causes the smooth muscle of the bronchial airways and pulmonary blood vessels to relax
Toxic effects	Hypotension, syncope, tachycardia, arrhythmias, seizures, gastrointestinal bleeding

of arachidonic acid. This centrally important compound is converted into either leukotriene via lipo-oxygenase or thromboxane and prostaglandin via cyclo-oxygenase (COX). All of these agents provoke chemotaxis of neutrophils, resulting in their activation and, ultimately, in inflammation. In addition, they increase vascular permeability (inducing more influx of neutrophils) and smooth muscle contraction. As noted in the preceding section, and shown in Figure 23–13, corticosteroids are powerful anti-inflammatory agents through the blockade of cyclo-oxygenase.

While steroids are highly effective anti-inflammatory agents, they provoke a number of undesirable side effects including fluid retention, weight gain, osteoporosis, gastrointestinal bleeding and mental changes. Other nonsteroidal drugs, the so-called nonsteroidal anti-inflammatory drugs (NSAIDs) have been found to be effective in blocking inflammation by similar mechanisms as shown in Figure 23–13 without the undesirable side effects of the corticosteroids. Most of these agents block COX specifically and include such drugs as naproxen (Naprosyn), ibuprofen (Advil, Motrin), and piroxicam (Feldene). These agents inhibit two forms of COX, COX-1 and COX-2, the former being involved in maintaining membrane integrity of mucosal cells in the gastrointestinal tract, the latter being involved in the inflammatory process. Since all of the above agents inhibit both forms of COX, they have the undesirable side effect of gastrointestinal tract toxicity and induce GI bleeding. Newer agents, that more selectively inhibit COX-2, have recently become available including celecoxib (Celebrex) and rofecoxib (Vioxx). Because some patients treated with Vioxx have been diagnosed with myocardial infarction, this drug has recently been withdrawn.

Aspirin, a potent cyclo-oxygenase inhibitor, is an effective anti-inflammatory agent and has, in addition, antipyretic and analgesic effects, which also result from cyclo-oxygenase inhibition. The latter two effects are thought to be due to inhibition of COX in the central nervous system (so-called COX-3), mainly in the hypothalamus.

Acetaminophen (Tylenol) inhibits COX-3 but exerts little effect on COX-1 and COX-2. Thus it is non-anti-inflammatory, does not result in gastrointestinal tract bleeding and is an effective analgesic and antipyretic.

Of all of these drugs, therapeutic drug monitoring is performed on only aspirin and Tylenol. We therefore discuss these drugs further.

Acetylsalicylic acid (aspirin) is a nonsteroidal anti-inflammatory compound and is used as an analgesic, an antipyretic and, in larger doses, an anti-inflammatory agent. In lower doses, it exhibits its anticoagulant activity due to its antiplatelet activity through inhibition of COX in platelets, resulting in blockade of platelet plug formation. It can be effective in the treatment of fever, neuralgia, headache, myalgia, and arthralgia, and in the management of some rheumatic diseases.

Oral dosages of aspirin that are generally used for analgesia and antipyresis in adults range from 500 mg as necessary, to a maximum of 4 g/day. Increased dosages (3.5–5.5 g/day) are used for rheumatoid arthritis and osteoarthritis in adults and for juvenile arthritis (up to 3.5 g/day) in children.

The small intestine is the primary site of aspirin absorption, and absorption usually occurs rapidly following oral administration with peak plasma levels established within 1–2 hours. Before entering the system's circulation, aspirin is rapidly hydrolyzed to acetic acid and salicylic acid. Hydrolysis occurs partly by plasma esterase and partly by the liver. Both aspirin and salicylic acid enter the CNS.

Approximately 70–90% of salicylic acid is plasma protein-bound. The serum half-life is dose-dependent and increases with the dose: from approximately 3 hours with 500 mg to approximately 15 hours with 4 g. Salicylic acid is cleared not only by metabolism but also by urinary

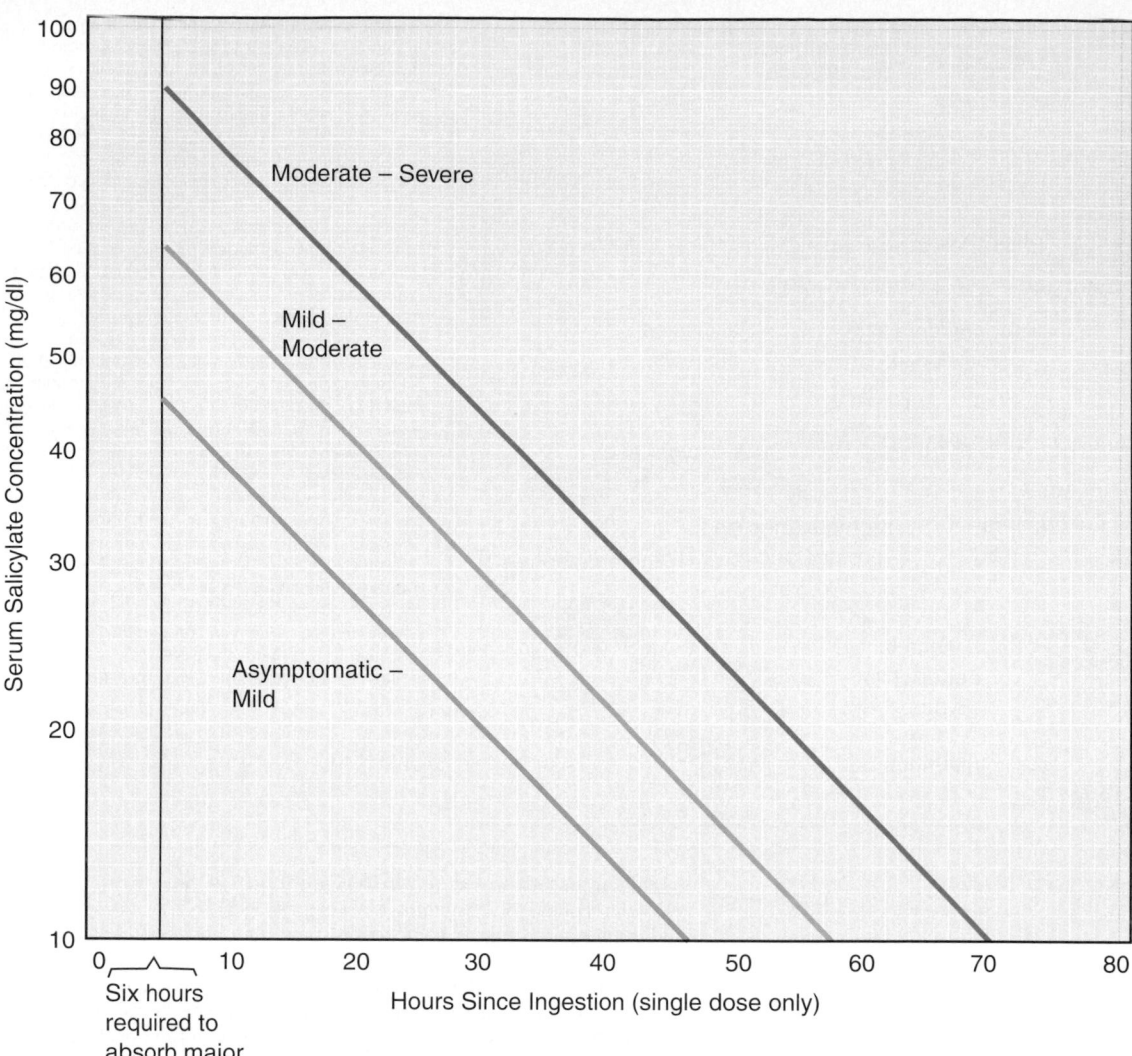

Figure 23–14 Aspirin toxicity levels in children as a function of time. (Howanitz, 1984, modified from Done AK: Pediatrics 1960; 26:800, with permission.)

Serum Salicylate Concentration (mg/dl)

Hours Since Ingestion (single dose only)

Six hours required to absorb major portion of dose

excretion, and as the half-life increases, the rate of urinary excretion decreases. This can produce toxic effects if the dosage interval is not increased appropriately. However, the rate of elimination can vary widely with the patient, necessitating individualization of dosage for large amounts of drug. Tinnitus, muffled hearing, and a sensation of fullness in the ears are the most common signs of chronic aspirin toxicity. In infants, young children, and patients with pre-existing hearing loss, otic symptoms will not occur, and hyperventilation is the most common sign of overdose. As discussed in Chapter 14, overdoses of aspirin can cause metabolic acidosis. Because salicylate itself stimulates central respiratory centers, overdoses cause an increased breathing rate, leading to a respiratory alkalosis. Acute aspirin intoxication is a common cause of fatal drug poisoning in children. Toxic doses produce acid–base disturbances, direct CNS stimulation of respiration, hyperpyrexia and hypoglycemia, gastrointestinal bleeding, and nausea and vomiting. Acute renal failure, CNS dysfunction with stupor and coma, and pulmonary edema may develop. Figure 23–14 summarizes the toxic levels of aspirin in children as a function of time after the toxic dose was taken.

A serious toxic effect of aspirin, mainly in children but also recognized in adults, is hepatotoxicity leading to fulminant hepatic failure, i.e., Reye's syndrome. This occurs when a patient is treated with aspirin for fever during a viral illness. After apparent recovery, the patient becomes seriously ill from hepatic failure with signs and symptoms, including hepatic encephalopathy, described in Chapters 8 and 21. Although once almost always fatal, newer supportive measures have resulted in a significant increase in survival from this life-threatening condition, the basic cause of which is as-yet undetermined.

Acetaminophen (Tylenol) is used as an analgesic and antipyretic to treat fever, headache, and mild to moderate myalgia and arthralgia. Acetaminophen is as effective as aspirin in its analgesic and antipyretic actions and is preferred over aspirin in patients with a bleeding/coagulation disorder or in children requiring only antipyretics or analgesics, because no association between acetaminophen and the incidence of Reye's syndrome

in children has been demonstrated. Furthermore, an accidental overdose in children may be less toxic than with aspirin, since hepatotoxicity is rarely associated with acetaminophen overdose in children under the age of 6.

Oral doses of acetaminophen are rapidly and essentially completely absorbed from the GI tract. Generally, 325–650 mg at 4-hour intervals is prescribed for adults and children over 12, with a maximum of 4 g daily. The plasma half-life is approximately 2 hours, with peak plasma levels of 5–20 µg/mL occurring in 30–60 minutes. The percentage of plasma protein binding is about 20% with therapeutic doses. The major metabolites of acetaminophen produced by the liver are glucuronide and sulfate conjugates, with minor metabolites being deacetylated and hydroxylated derivatives. The latter metabolite is thought to produce hepatotoxicity with overdose.

Toxic doses of acetaminophen occur at acute ingestion levels of 140 mg/kg (White, 1998). Acute manifestations of toxic doses generally occur within 2–3 hours after ingestion and include nausea, vomiting, and abdominal pain. A characteristic sign of toxicity is cyanosis of the skin, mucosa, and fingernails due to methemoglobinemia. However, this is seen more frequently with phenacetin poisoning. CNS stimulation followed by CNS depression may occur in severe poisoning, with vascular collapse, shock, and total seizures occurring. Coma usually precedes death. At very high doses (as with suicide attempts), fulminant hepatic failure may occur, with maximum liver damage not becoming apparent until 2–4 days after drug ingestion (Sunheimer, 1994).

Chronic acetaminophen abuse may produce chronic toxicity and death. Anemia, renal damage, and gastrointestinal disturbances are usually associated with chronic toxicity.

Immunosuppressives (Dancey, 2002; Drosos, 2002; Dunn, 2001; Mueller, 2004; Scott, 2003)

While intact humoral and cell-mediated immunity are essential in preventing infection, there are circumstances when it becomes vital to

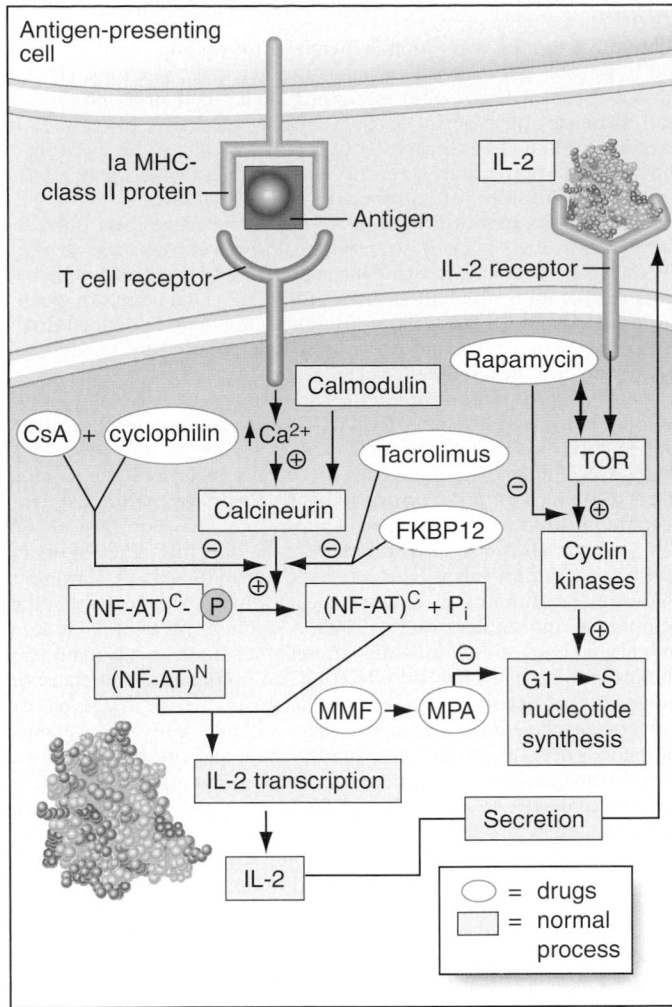

Figure 23–15 Mechanisms and sites of action of immunosuppressive drugs. This figure shows two linked centrally important signal transduction pathways induced by antigen, in this case foreign transplanted cells, for activation of cell-mediated immunity. In the first pathway, antigen is 'presented' to antigen-specific (clonal) T cells by attachment of the antigen to the Ia molecule (MHC-class 2 – or DR in humans – protein). The formation of a ternary complex of antigen (red box), Ia (green receptor on the antigen presenting cell, i.e., macrophage) and the T cell receptor (purple receptor, left upper part of the figure) results in a signal transduction cascade which results in the synthesis of interleukin-2 (IL-2) shown as a space-filling model in the lower left part of the figure. Critical to this pathway is activation, by calcium-activated calmodulin, of the phosphatase, calcineurin, which dephosphorylates cytosolic nuclear factor of activated T cells (NF-AT)^C resulting in its activation; whereupon it translocates to the nucleus and binds to NF-AT from the nucleus (NF-AT)^N, which directly promotes transcription of IL-2. In the second, linked, signal transduction pathway (right side of figure), newly synthesized IL-2 is then secreted by the T cell and acts as an autocrine factor in binding to the extracellular domain of the T cell's IL-2 receptor to form a complex as shown in the upper right part of the figure. This complex induces activation of a second signal transduction cascade in which target of rapamycin (TOR) protein is stimulated and, in turn, activates cyclin kinases that promote activation of cyclins, which in turn promote progression of the cell cycle from G1 to S necessary for blast transformation of clonal T cells that, with macrophages, engulf and destroy the antigen.

All elements of the normal signal transduction pathways are shown as pink boxes. The immunosuppressive drugs and their target proteins, block different parts of these two pathways and are shown as yellow ellipses. Ciclosporin (CsA) and tacrolimus complex, respectively, with cyclophilin and FKBP12 to form inhibitory complexes that block calcineurin in the first pathway. On the other hand, rapamycin blocks TOR, thereby blocking IL-2-induced blast transformation in the second pathway; mycophenolate mofetil (MMF) blocks nucleotide synthesis, thereby blocking G1–S progression in the second pathway. MPA = mycophenolic acid.

suppress functioning of these systems. These include aberrations of the immune system such as in autoimmune disease (e.g., lupus erythematosus, Sjögren's syndrome, etc.) and normal functioning of the immune system as, for example, in tissue transplantation. In the latter circumstance, the most important component of the immune system is cell-mediated immunity. As shown in Figure 23–15, either in host-versus-graft or in graft-versus-host disease, CD4+ T cells become activated when a foreign antigen binds to the (MHC class II) Ia protein on the surface of macrophages (antigen-

presenting cells). Specific T cell clones bind to the antigen using their T cell receptors (CD3), which recognize the antigen–Ia complex. Activation of the T cell receptor results in a signal transduction cascade that ultimately ends in engulfment via receptor-mediated endocytosis of the antigen by the macrophage and destruction in lysosomes. In this cascade, calcium ions are mobilized, resulting in the activation of calcineurin, a phosphatase that forms a complex with calmodulin. Activated calcineurin dephosphorylates cytosolic nuclear factor of activated T cells (NF-AT)^C resulting in its activation, whereupon it translocates to the nucleus and binds to NF-AT from the nucleus (NF-AT)^N. This is a transcriptionally active complex that results in the synthesis of interleukin-2 (IL-2), which becomes secreted as an extracellular mitogen. It binds to the IL-2 receptor of the T cell activating it towards the binding of a protein, called 'target of rapamycin,' or TOR, which serves to activate cyclin kinases that promote progression of the cell cycle from G1 to S and stimulate nucleotide synthesis. This ends in differentiation and proliferation of the T cell and ultimate antigen destruction.

As shown in Figure 23–15, there are specific agents (Isoniemi, 1997; Braun, 1998; Kahan, 1989; Hess, 1988; McEvoy, 2004) that block one or more of these steps and, by so doing, inhibit antigen destruction. The drugs ciclosporin and tacrolimus are cyclic polypeptides that bind to intracellular proteins called immunophilins. Ciclosporin binds to the immunophilin, cyclophilin, while tacrolimus binds to the immunophilin called FKBP12. These complexes then block calcineurin-induced activation of NF-AT, and therefore block IL-2 synthesis, so that antigen destruction cannot occur. On the other hand, another immunosuppressive agent, rapamycin (Sirolimus), has no such effect on T cells but rather binds to the critical TOR protein, disenabling activation of cyclin kinases so that T cell activation cannot proceed. Finally, mycophenolate mofetil (MMF), an antibiotic, is hydrolyzed to free mycophenolic acid in the cell. This agent is a powerful inhibitor of inosine monophosphate dehydrogenase and guanosine monophosphate synthetase, disenabling deoxypurine nucleotide synthesis, which, in turn, disables DNA synthesis. In the same vein, some alkylating agents that are generally used as chemotherapeutic agents, such as cyclophosphamide (Cytoxan), can be used to suppress DNA synthesis in T cells.

It should be noted that the corticosteroids also have immunosuppressive effects on cell-mediated immunity, but are much less specific and, as noted in the previous section, have multiple undesirable side effects. They are, therefore, not the drugs of choice for use in transplantation.

In the following section, we discuss the properties of the more specific immunosuppressive drugs, most of which require monitoring of serum (plasma) levels.

Ciclosporin is a cyclic polypeptide containing 11 amino acids, five of which are methylated. Maximum suppression with ciclosporin occurs during the first 24 hours of antigen stimulation by the allograft. Thus, ciclosporin must be administered in the early phase of the immune response for optimal suppression of T cell function and increased success of transplantation (McEvoy, 2004).

Ciclosporin is indicated to prevent organ rejection in kidney, heart, and liver allogeneic transplants and is the drug of choice for maintenance of kidney, liver, heart, and heart–lung allografts. Ciclosporin (CsA) may also be utilized as a first- or second-line drug in the treatment of acute graft-versus-host disease following bone marrow transplantation, in the active stage of severe rheumatoid arthritis, and for severe, recalcitrant plaque psoriasis. It may also be used in the treatment of other autoimmune diseases and organ transplantation.

Because ciclosporin is variably absorbed from the GI tract, the optimal dose must be carefully determined for each patient individually, and blood levels should be monitored frequently. It has been occasionally found that, while serum levels of the parent drug are low, the metabolites, some of which are active, maintain a therapeutic drug level. Therefore, in patients with apparently low levels of the parent drug, it is necessary to determine the levels of metabolites. Peak blood concentrations occur at approximately 3.5 hours after administration. About 20–40% of a given dose of ciclosporin is absorbed, and it is metabolized on the first pass through the liver. Human cytochrome P450 III A3 of the P450 III gene family appears to be the primary enzyme responsible for ciclosporin metabolism. Since a number of drugs either may induce or may be metabolized by this cytochrome P450 isoenzyme, co-administration of these drugs may be responsible for alterations in ciclosporin levels that can complicate ciclosporin therapy (Kronbach, 1988). Trough whole blood or plasma concentrations, at 24 hours, of 250–800 ng/mL or 50–300 ng/mL, respectively (as determined by immunoassay), are believed to minimize graft rejection and, concurrently, toxic effects.

Adverse effects of ciclosporin may occur on all organ systems of the body. Trough serum levels (determined by radioimmunoassay [RIA]) greater than 500 ng/mL are associated with *ciclosporin-induced nephrotoxicity*, which is the most frequent toxic reaction seen with ciclosporin. Ciclosporin-

CHAPTER: 23 Toxicology and Therapeutic Drug Monitoring

induced nephrotoxicity is accompanied by hyperkalemia and hyperuricemia, hypertension, and gingival hyperplasia.

Other toxic effects include neurologic effects (tremors, seizures, headache, paresthesia, flushing, confusion), dermatologic effects (hirsutism, hypertrichosis, rash), hepatotoxicity, GI effects (diarrhea, nausea, vomiting, anorexia, abdominal discomfort), infectious complications, hematologic effects (leukopenia, anemia, thrombocytopenia), and sensitivity reactions, including anaphylaxis (Philip, 1998). Importantly, there is an increased risk of immunosuppressed states, and the occurrence of lymphoma, especially CNS lymphoma, may also be associated with immunosuppression by ciclosporin. Very recently, it has been found that ciclosporin induces immune system-independent increased invasiveness of adenocarcinoma cells in culture, apparently by activating transforming growth factor-beta (TGF-beta) (Hojo, 1999). This behavior is blocked with monoclonal antibodies to TGF-beta.

Both oral and intravenous preparations of ciclosporin are available. There is variable interpatient and intrapatient absorption of the oral preparation, and absorption can be affected by many factors. It is generally recommended that whole blood be used for drug level monitoring, and that an assay method with high specificity for unchanged drug (vs. metabolites) be used. Thus, the optimal dose must be carefully determined for each patient individually, and blood levels should be monitored frequently, with ciclosporin blood concentrations qualified by biologic fluid (whole blood vs. plasma vs. serum) and assay method (immunoassay vs. HPLC) used. At present, any currently available immunoassay (RIA, FPIA, EMIT) is acceptable for routine monitoring, although it is important that consistent laboratories and methods be used (McEvoy, 2004).

Neoral is a microemulsion formulation of ciclosporin that is miscible in water; it increases the solubility of ciclosporin in the small bowel (Miller, 1998). This preparation has shown superior pharmacokinetics with improved bioavailability and equivalent safety with no apparent increase in toxicity. It appears to offer advantages over oral solutions of CsA, by decreasing intra- and interpatient blood level variability. Intravenous ciclosporin is reserved for patients unable to tolerate oral administration; this route of administration carries a low but definite (0.1%) risk of anaphylaxis, which does not occur following oral administration of the drug.

Tacrolimus (FK-506) is a macrolide lactone antibiotic with a mechanism of action similar to that of ciclosporin, and which is more potent than CsA in its inhibitory effect (McEvoy, 2004). It is currently being utilized in transplant surgery to prevent organ rejection. Similarly to CsA, higher trough concentrations appear to increase the relative risk of toxicity, and therapeutic drug monitoring is recommended. The same monoclonal antibody is used in the two methods available for monitoring. One method is a microparticle enzyme immunoassay and the other method is an enzyme-linked immunosorbent assay (ELISA). Whole blood is the specimen of choice. The toxic potential appears to be similar to the toxic effects of CsA. The most common include nephrotoxicity, neurotoxicity (such as tremor and headache), gastrointestinal effects such as diarrhea and nausea, hypertension, alterations in glucose metabolism (diabetes mellitus), hyperkalemia, and infectious complications. However, unlike CsA, gingival hyperplasia and hirsutism do not occur. Anaphylaxis may occur with intravenous administration, and oral therapy is recommended whenever possible. Tacrolimus appears to be best suited for use in combination with other new immunosuppressive agents.

Rapamycin (Sirolimus) is an antibiotic similar to tacrolimus. Major side effects include GI symptoms (abnormalities in lipid levels) and thrombocytopenia. It does not appear to be nephrotoxic, however.

Mycophenolate mofetil is a derivative of mycophenolate acid, a fungal antibiotic. The use of this drug appears to decrease the rate of renal allograft rejection, but definite differences in patient and allograft survival have not been demonstrated (Isoniemi, 1997). It may be of use in patients who do not tolerate CsA or tacrolimus (FK-506) well. The major side effects include GI symptoms such as diarrhea and nausea, and myelosuppression. Neither nephrotoxicity nor neurotoxicity has been demonstrated.

Leflunamide (LFM), also a deoxy (pyrimidine) nucleotide synthesis inhibitor, is an isoxazole derivative, which inhibits lymphocyte proliferation. It is presently used in the treatment of rheumatoid arthritis, the only condition for which it has been approved for treatment. LFM has not been demonstrated to cause nephrotoxicity or myelosuppression in humans.

Drugs Used in the Treatment of Manic-Depression: Lithium and the Tricyclic Antidepressants

Both lithium and the tricyclic antidepressants are used in the treatment of psychiatric affective disorders.

Lithium

Lithium is a monovalent cation, a member of the group of alkali metals, and is available commercially as the citrate and carbonate salts. Lithium salts are considered to be antimanic agents and are used for the prophylaxis and treatment of bipolar disorder (manic–depressive psychosis). In addition, lithium is considered by some investigators to be the drug of choice for the prevention of chronic cluster headache, and may also be effective in episodic or periodic forms of cluster headache.

Initial oral dosages of lithium for acute mania range from 0.6–1.8 g daily (maximum of 2.4 g) to produce a therapeutic serum level of 0.75–1.5 mEq/L. Once the attack subsides, the dose is reduced rapidly to produce a serum concentration of 0.4–1.0 mEq/L. Oral adult dosages for cluster headaches generally range from 0.6–1.2 g daily in divided doses. In general, serum levels and patient response are used to individualize dosage and must be monitored carefully.

Complete absorption of lithium occurs 6–8 hours after oral administration. Plasma half-life varies from 17–36 hours, and onset of action is slow (5–10 days). Elimination occurs almost entirely by the kidneys, and about 80% of filtered lithium is reabsorbed. Lithium is not protein bound and is distributed in total body water, but shows delayed and varied tissue distribution. Thus, symptoms of acute intoxication may not correlate well with serum levels, since the distribution of the drug into different organs may be slow and/or varied. The exact mechanism of action of lithium is unknown, but lithium, as a monovalent cation, competes with other monovalent and divalent cations (such as sodium, potassium, calcium, and magnesium) at ion channels in cell membranes and at protein-binding sites such as membrane receptors and protein/peptide transport molecules and enzymes that are critical to the synthesis, storage, release, and uptake of central neurotransmitters. Lithium also has a marked inhibitory effect on inositol monophosphatase and on the synthesis of phosphatidylinositides, which are second messengers involved in neurotransmission, and on the synthesis of cAMP, also involved in neurotransmission (Phiel, 2001).

Toxicity may occur acutely, as the result of a single toxic dose, or chronically, from high and/or prolonged dosages or changes in lithium pharmacokinetics. Water loss (resulting from fever, decreased intake, abnormal gastrointestinal conditions such as diarrhea, vomiting, diuretics, or pyelonephritis) is the main contributing factor underlying chronic intoxication. Renal toxicity and hypothyroidism are also known possible side effects of lithium. Thus it is advisable to monitor creatinine and thyroid-stimulating hormone (TSH) periodically in patients who are under continuing treatment with this drug.

Severity of intoxication is not clearly related to serum lithium levels. However, an imprecise prediction of severity of intoxication may be attempted from serum lithium levels obtained 12 hours after the last dose: slight to moderate intoxication with 1.5–2.5 mEq/L, severe intoxication with 2.5–3.5 mEq/L, and potentially lethal intoxication if greater than 3.5 mEq/L. Severity of lithium intoxication also depends on the length of time that the serum concentration remains toxic.

The most common symptoms of mild to moderate intoxication include nausea, malaise, diarrhea, and fine hand tremor. In addition, thirst, polydipsia, and polyuria, as well as drowsiness, muscle weakness, ataxia, and slurred speech may occur. Symptoms of moderate to severe toxicity include hyperactive deep tendon reflexes, choreoathetoid movements, persistent nausea and vomiting, fasciculations, generalized seizures, and clonic movements of whole limbs. These may progress rapidly to generalized seizures, oliguria, circulatory failure, and death with serum levels greater than 3.5 mEq/L.

Tricyclic Antidepressants

The structures of several of these compounds that are related to one another are shown in Figure 23–16. Two other effective tricyclic antidepressant drugs are doxepin (Fig. 23–16) and desyrel (Trazadone), a second-generation tricyclic antidepressant, which does not contain the three fused ring system of the above drugs. The mechanism of action of these tricyclic antidepressants is the blockage of the reuptake of adrenergic and dopaminergic neurotransmitters as discussed above under 'The Drugs of Abuse' (see Fig. 23–8). The action of these excitatory neurotransmitters is thereby prolonged by allowing them to remain at their receptor sites. Besides stimulating dopaminergic pathways, the tricyclics, especially amitriptyline, have anticholinergic effects.

The pharmacologic side effects of the tricyclic antidepressants in fact reflect their anticholinergic activities. These include dry mouth, constipation, blurred vision, hyperthermia, adynamic ileus, urinary retention, and delayed micturition. Other CNS effects include drowsiness, weakness, fatigue, and lethargy, which are most common, as well as

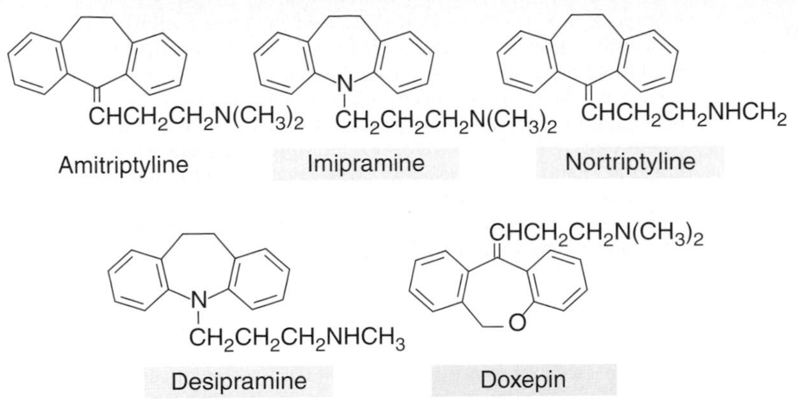

Figure 23-16 Structures of the most commonly used tricyclic antidepressants.

Amitriptyline   Imipramine   Nortriptyline

Desipramine   Doxepin

agitation, restlessness, insomnia, and confusion. Seizures and coma can also occur. Extrapyramidal symptoms may also occur and include a persistent fine tremor, rigidity, dystonia, and opisthotonos.

More recently, other non-tricyclic drugs with strong antidepressant activity have been developed. The most prominent of these is fluoxetine (Prozac). This drug blocks the reuptake of serotonin in central serotonergic pathways and is referred to as a selective serotonin reuptake inhibitor (SSRI). This drug appears not to have some of the side effects, such as the anticholinergic effects, of the tricyclic antidepressants, but has been reported to cause nausea and decreased libido and sexual function. There have also been reports of attempted suicide with some patients being treated with this drug.

It is important to realize that the tricyclic antidepressants are frequently used in suicide attempts by depressed individuals who are being treated for depression with these drugs. The cardinal signs of tricyclic antidepressant overdose are anticholinergic symptoms: dilated pupils and dry skin.

Toxicity. Overdose produces symptoms that are primarily extensions of common adverse reactions with excess CNS stimulation and anticholinergic activity. These include seizures, coma, hypotension, respiratory depression, areflexia, shock, and cardiorespiratory arrest. Agitation, confusion, hypertension, and the parkinsonian syndrome may also occur, as well as hallucinations and delirium. Occasional manifestations include ataxia, renal failure, dysarthria, and vomiting.

Treatment. Symptomatic and supportive care is the general mode of treatment. Gastric lavage, accompanied by instillation of activated charcoal, is usually recommended for removal of the tricyclic from the GI tract. Seizures are generally treated with intravenous diazepam. For overdoses with amitriptyline (Fig. 23-16), use of cholinesterase inhibitors such as neostigmine has proved to be effective in reversing the anticholinergic symptoms.

The Neuroleptics, Antipsychotic Major Tranquilizers

These drugs are used mainly in the treatment of acute schizophrenia and result in suppression of the agitated state. All of the neuroleptics appear to block the action of dopamine and serotonin postsynaptically in the limbic system and motor cortex (see Fig. 23-8). There are specific dopaminergic pathways that connect the substantia nigra of the midbrain to the limbic system and motor cortex, called the mesolimbic-mesocortical pathways. In addition, the substantia nigra connects to the basal ganglia via the nigrostriatal pathway; depletion of dopamine in this pathway results in Parkinson's disease. Thus it may be expected that dopamine antagonists would affect the latter pathway in addition to the mesolimbic-mesocortical pathways. Indeed many of the neuroleptics have, as side effects, dystonias, tardive dyskinesias and frank Parkinsonism, the latter fortunately being much less common. Originally, two classes of neuroleptics, the phenothiazines, typified by chlorpromazine, and the butyrophenones, typified by haloperidol (Haldol), were the drugs of choice. Besides postsynaptic blockade of dopamine, Haldol is known also to bind with high affinity to sigma-receptors in the CNS, and this action may stimulate inhibitory pathways that modulate the activity of the dopaminergic pathways. All compounds in both classes had the undesired extrapyramidal side effects mentioned above.

More recently, newer neuroleptics have been developed that affect the nigrostriatal pathway to a lesser extent but are potent postsynaptic dopamine blockers in the mesolimbic-mesocortical pathways and therefore are effective with fewer of the extrapyramidal side effects of the older drugs. These newer drugs (see also Burns, 2001) include risperdal

(Risperidone) (which does have some documented extrapyramidal side effects), olonzapine (Zyprexa), quetiapine (Seroquel), and aripiprazole (Abilify).

It has been difficult to monitor the levels of any of these drugs in serum because of the large number of metabolites for each drug resulting from extensive metabolism in the liver. Chlorpromazine, for example, has approximately 150 metabolites. The therapeutic efficacy of most of these metabolites is unknown. It is therefore quite difficult to establish ranges for normal serum levels of these drugs. Methods for assay include FPIA and HPLC. It is not clear in FPIA which, if any, metabolites cross-react with the antibody. For chlorpromazine, the estimated therapeutic range is wide, between 50–300 ng/mL. The half-life of the drug is 16–30 hours, and its bioavailability is 25–35%. Normal doses for chlorpromazine are 200–600 mg/day in divided doses. Other drugs in the phenothiazine series include thioridazine and fluphenazine (Prolixin).

Besides the extrapyramidal side effects, mainly the phenothiazines can cause orthostatic hypotension, cholestasis and, rarely, aplastic anemia. Occasionally, contact dermatitis has been reported to occur with phenothiazines. Of great importance is the subset of patients who have been chronically treated with these drugs and develop tardive dyskinesia. In most of these patients, these motor disturbances are irreversible.

Neuroleptics can cause a rare but important adverse reaction termed the neuroleptic malignant syndrome. This can occur in patients who are extremely sensitive to the extrapyramidal effects of these drugs, and may be fatal. Marked muscle rigidity is the first symptom to occur, and may be followed by high fever, altered pulse and blood pressure, and leukocytosis. An excessively rapid inhibition of postsynaptic dopamine receptors is believed to be responsible for this syndrome. Treatment is cessation of the drug.

Chemotherapeutic Agents: Methotrexate and Busulfan

Serum levels of both of these agents are monitored to assess whether therapeutic serum levels are present.

Methotrexate, an antimetabolite consisting of a mixture containing no less than 85% 4-amino-10-methylfolic acid, and related compounds, is a folic acid antagonist (see Table 23–7). It inhibits the enzyme dihydrofolate reductase. This results in the blockade of the synthesis of tetrahydrofolic acid, which is needed for the formation of N-5,10-tetrahydrofolate, an intermediate in the transfer of a methyl group to deoxyuridylate to form thymidylate, needed in DNA synthesis. It has also been suggested that methotrexate may also cause a rise in the intracellular levels of ATP, which blocks ribonucleotide reduction, also resulting in the blocking of DNA synthesis. Methotrexate also appears to inhibit polynucleotide ligase involved in DNA synthesis and repair.

Methotrexate is also an important immunosuppressive agent. Indications are severe, recalcitrant psoriasis and severe, active rheumatoid arthritis; in the latter, it may be used in combination with ciclosporin (Tugwell, 1995). It is also used as an anticancer agent for some neoplastic diseases. Depending on the specific disease entity being treated, dosages given will vary, as will the therapeutic level of the drug. In Table 23–7, the doses and therapeutic drug levels for several different conditions are noted. The serum levels were determined by FPIA.

The kinetics of steady-state levels of this drug are biphasic: a rapid phase with $t_{1/2}$ is 2–3 hours and a slow phase with $t_{1/2}$ is 8–10 hours. Excretion of the drug is also biphasic: 92% is excreted within 24 hours and the remainder over a period of days. Approximately 50% of the drug in blood is bound to serum proteins.

The toxic effects of methotrexate include hematologic effects (i.e., leukopenia and thrombocytopenia), gastrointestinal effects (i.e., ulceration,

Table 23–7 Methotrexate

Condition	Usual dose	Serum level
Psoriasis	i.m. or i.v.: 7.5–50 mg/week Oral: 7.5–30 mg/week	< 10 nM (see Roenigk, 1998)
Refractory rheumatoid arthritis	i.m.: 5–25 mg/week Oral: 7.5–15 mg/week	(See Tugwell, 1987a and b)*
Malignant neoplastic diseases[†]	i.m. or i.v.: 25 mg/m², 1–2 times/week Oral: 2.5–5 mg/day High-dose i.v.: 1.5 g/m² with rescue every 3 weeks (different regimens are available)	Approximately 50 nM

* Baseline monitoring of patient parameters (hemoglobin; white blood cell count; mean corpuscular volume; platelet count; urinalysis; blood urea nitrogen; and serum creatinine, transaminase, and alkaline phosphatase levels) is advocated.

† With high-dose therapy, methotrexate levels are followed, and leucovorin doses are adjusted until serum methotrexate levels are less than 50 nM (see Grem, 1995).

glossitis, stomatitis, nausea, vomiting) hepatic lesions such as cirrhosis; pulmonary lesions such as pulmonary fibrosis; dermatologic effects such as urticaria and vasculitis; and CNS effects from intrathecal methotrexate, including arachnoiditis, leukoencephalopathy, and increased cerebrospinal fluid (CSF) pressure. It is occasionally necessary to administer high doses of methotrexate to individuals with tumors that do not respond to normal doses of this drug. In these cases, the drug leucovorin (citrovorum factor) is given 18–36 hours after the initial methotrexate dose, while monitoring methotrexate levels. Leucovorin is N-5-formyltetrahydrofolate, which is the product of dihydrofolate reductase. Thus, this compound overcomes the blockage caused by methotrexate. The rationale for this regimen is that the rapidly proliferating tumor cells will be killed by the high dose of methotrexate, while many normal cells that are not dividing often can be 'rescued' by leucovorin. Especially in this type of drug regimen, it is essential to monitor the serum levels of methotrexate carefully. In addition, leucovorin should be immediately administered to a patient receiving low-dose methotrexate when methotrexate overdose is suspected (Roenigk, 1998). Serum methotrexate levels should be monitored during this time (Grem, 1995).

Busulfan is an alkylating agent used to treat a variety of leukemias and lymphomas prior to bone marrow transplantation. It is cytotoxic to marrow cells and is used in combination with cyclophosphamide, which is cytotoxic to mature lymphocytes that may be involved in a graft-versus-host reaction (Slattery, 1998). The therapeutic index of the drug is narrow. High plasma levels increase the possibility of development of hepatic veno-occlusive disease (VOD), a potentially fatal complication. Therefore, therapeutic monitoring of busulfan levels, using HPLC or GC-MS, with measurement of the dose interval of this drug, is now routinely performed at bone marrow transplant centers. This decreases the incidence of VOD in patients whose initial serum levels of busulfan are too high and allows increasing doses for patients with too low an initial level of busulfan, thus optimizing therapeutic levels for each patient.

Toxins and Acute Poisoning

In this section, agents that cause chronic or acute injury to the patient are discussed. This injury can be either direct as with the poisons such as cyanide and carbon monoxide or indirect such as with carcinogens that induce mutations in genes that encode proteins that are critical in controlling the cell cycle.

Environmental Carcinogens

Over the past decade or so, attention has been focused on the effects of chemical agents in the environment, carcinogens, which predispose individuals exposed to them to develop tumors in various tissues where these agents accumulate. Many of the individuals who are exposed to these agents work in industries where these agents are produced. Benzpyrene, an aromatic compound produced in cigarettes and also produced in the exhaust of engines, is a known potent carcinogen, and has been implicated in causing lung cancer. Nitrites, used as preservatives in red meats, have been associated with colon cancer. Aflatoxin, produced by the fungus

Aspergillus, has been implicated in causing hepatocellular carcinoma. Aromatic hydrocarbons such as benzene and ionizing radiation have been implicated in causing acute leukemias. Vinyl chloride and the formerly used dye thorotrast have been linked to angiosarcoma. Benzidine dyes, beta-naphthylamine, dimethylbenzanthracene, and other aromatic compounds have been linked to multiple malignancies occurring in humans. Exposure to asbestos has been strongly implicated as a carcinogen in lung cancer and mesothelioma. In animal studies, polychlorinated biphenyls (PCB) and dioxin, the former produced in fires, have been strongly implicated as causing a variety of cancers. A number of carcinogens, like benzpyrene, are inactive in their native forms but are transformed into carcinogens through oxidative reactions catalyzed by cytochrome P450-dependent systems. Thus, to be an active carcinogen, benzpyrene must be converted into benzpyrene diol epoxide. Since only particular isoforms of cytochrome P450 react with particular carcinogens, only those individuals carrying the genes encoding these forms are susceptible (see, e.g., Caraco, 1998). A major effort is now being devoted to identifying those individuals with phenotypes who would be at risk (see Peto, 2001 for overview).

Much interest has now been focused on workers in occupations where carcinogens are present in significant amounts. Steel foundries, shipbuilding and rubber plants, and other industrial plants may produce such carcinogens in significant amounts. In some of these industries, certain cancers occur at rates higher than in the general population (Brandt-Rauf, 1998; Pincus, 2003). Thus, in these exposed populations, it has become desirable to determine the levels of exposure to certain known carcinogens.

Carcinogens are thought to bind to DNA, leading ultimately to mutations in the genetic code, often resulting in synthesis of mutated proteins involved in control of the cell cycle (Brandt-Rauf, 1998; Pincus, 2003). These proteins are called oncogene-encoded proteins or oncoproteins. Mutagenesis, oncogenes and oncoproteins are discussed in Chapter 75.

In populations with histories of exposure to carcinogens, assays have been developed to detect the presence either of these carcinogens or of their DNA adducts. For the detection of most unmodified carcinogens, the method of choice is currently GC-MS. For certain carcinogenic compounds like PCBs, the method of electron capture is used. Halogenated compounds like PCBs are separated on a GC column using an ionized gas as the carrier. Halogenated compounds 'capture' electrons conducted through the carrier gas and are thus detected by the reduced currents.

Often, the presence of carcinogens in blood or urine is hard to detect directly. The carcinogens, however, may be bound to proteins or to DNA intracellularly. These adducts can be detected using Western blotting, which takes advantage of the existence of monoclonal antibodies to carcinogen–DNA adducts (Santella, 1987; Perera, 1988). This technique is sensitive to nanogram quantities of the nucleic acid adduct, which can be conveniently harvested from peripheral lymphocytes. It is also very useful in detecting oncoproteins in the body fluids of patients who have been exposed to carcinogens (De Vivo, 1994) as described in Chapter 75.

Cyanide

The cyanide anion binds avidly to iron in the ferric or trivalent state. Because cyanide forms a relatively stable cyanoferric complex, it is able to inactivate iron-containing enzymes that cycle between the ferrous and ferric states in oxidation–reduction reactions.

Cyanide produces tissue and cellular hypoxia primarily by reversibly binding to cytochrome A_3 and by inhibiting its reoxidation. This inhibits the electron transport system and prevents cellular respiration and ATP (high-energy phosphate) formation. This blockade prevents the utilization of oxygen and aerobic metabolism, producing severe metabolic (lactic) acidosis. Although cyanide binds preferentially to the ferric form of iron, it can also bind to the ferrous iron of hemoglobin, producing cyanohemoglobin, which cannot transport oxygen. Cyanide will also form complexes with other iron-containing enzymes, but its acute poisonous effect is attributable to the inhibition of electron transport and cell death, predominantly in the CNS.

The principal symptoms of cyanide overdose are tachypnea (initially) followed by respiratory depression and cyanosis, hypotension, convulsions, and coma. Death may occur in a matter of minutes because cyanide is a fast-acting toxin. Diagnosis may be difficult, and a high index of suspicion is needed to make the correct diagnosis. Clues include the odor of bitter almonds, the occurrence of an altered mental status and tachypnea in the absence of cyanosis, and an unexplained metabolic acidosis (with an increased anion gap).

Antidotal therapy is based on a two-step strategy. First, to pull the CN⁻ ions away from cytochrome A_3, hemoglobin is converted to methemoglobin

Table 23–8 Influence of Acute Ethanol Ingestion on Ethanol Levels and Behavior

Ounces	Blood concentration	Influence
1–2	10–50 mg/dL (2.2–10.9 mmol/L)	None to mild euphoria
3–4	50–100 mg/dL (10.9–21.7 mmol/L or greater	Mild influence on stereoscopic vision and dark adaptation
	100 mg/dL (21.7 mmol/L)	Legally intoxicated
4–6	100–150 mg/dL (21.7–32.6 mmol/L)	Euphoria; disappearance of inhibition; prolonged reaction time
6–7	150–200 mg/dL (32.6–43.4 mmol/L)	Moderately severe poisoning; reaction time greatly prolonged: loss of inhibition and slight disturbances in equilibrium and coordination
8–9	200–250 mg/dL (43.4–54.3 mmol/L)	Severe degree of poisoning; disturbances of equilibrium and coordination; retardation of the thought processes and clouding of consciousness
10–15	250–400 mg/dL (54.3–86.8 mmol/L)	Deep, possibly fatal coma

(Fe^{3+} state) by using specific oxidants (i.e., amyl nitrite and sodium nitrite). The former is given first because it can be inhaled. Methemoglobin directly competes with ferricytochrome A_3 to form a methemoglobin–CN^- complex. This cyanomethemoglobin complex is relatively nontoxic. In a second step, sodium thiosulfate is given intravenously. This reagent reacts with cyanomethemoglobin to form thiocyanate, which is harmless and is excreted in urine. The first step is necessary simply to remove CN^- from the respiratory chain. Approximately 25–40% of the patient's total hemoglobin is converted to methemoglobin in this step; this methemoglobin is rapidly reconverted to oxyhemoglobin by red cell enzymes. The antidotes that are involved in each step are sold commercially as a cyanide antidote package by Eli Lilly and Company (Indianapolis, IN).

Carbon Monoxide

Carbon Monoxide (CO) intoxication produces tissue hypoxia as a result of decreased oxygen transport. Carbon monoxide disrupts oxygen transport by binding to hemoglobin to form a reversible complex, carboxyhemoglobin. It also produces toxicity by decreasing or inhibiting oxyhemoglobin saturation by shifting the oxyhemoglobin dissociation curve to the right and by binding to other heme-containing proteins such as myoglobin and cytochrome A_3. Binding to cytochrome A_3 inhibits cellular respiration and electron transport, while binding to hemoglobin will decrease the oxygen reserve available to cardiac and skeletal muscle, with cardiac muscle being more severely affected.

Because the brain and heart are most susceptible to carbon monoxide poisoning, carbon monoxide intoxication is commonly manifested through respiratory, neurologic, and cardiac symptoms, with dyspnea being a principal symptom. Others include headache, visual disturbances, tachycardia, syncope, tachypnea, coma, convulsions, and death. Symptomatology correlates somewhat with blood carboxyhemoglobin concentrations. However, diagnosis is difficult, since no pathognomonic symptoms occur except for a cherry red color of the face that is a strong clue to acute CO poisoning. CO poisoning should enter into the differential diagnosis of an acute encephalopathic state in the appropriate circumstances or setting.

A co-oximeter is utilized to make the definitive diagnosis by measuring the concentration of blood carboxyhemoglobin. This instrument is a dedicated spectrophotometer that measures total hemoglobin and the percentage of carboxyhemoglobin, oxyhemoglobin, and methemoglobin by screening at four different wavelengths simultaneously. This accurate and rapid analysis is mandatory to establish the diagnosis and should be performed with minimal delay after CO exposure. Treatment is mainly with 100% oxygen with additional supportive treatment given as necessary.

Alcohols and Glycols

Ethanol (Table 23–8) is probably the most common drug of abuse and is frequently responsible for the presentation of patients with altered mental status to hospitals and emergency rooms. Ethanol is rapidly absorbed from the gastrointestinal tract, has a volume of distribution approximately equal to that of total body water, and diffuses freely in body tissues. It is predominantly metabolized by hepatic alcohol dehydrogenase to acetaldehyde and acetic acid and then, by way of the Krebs cycle, to carbon dioxide and water. The fatal dose is generally 300–400 mL of pure ethanol (600–800 mL of 100 proof whiskey) consumed in less than 1 hour. Peak plasma concentrations are usually reached within 1 hour after ingestion. Table 23–8 summarizes the effects of different levels of ethanol in serum on human function.

Ethanol acts as a sedative-hypnotic and depresses the CNS irregularly in descending order from cortex to medulla. Acute intoxication may be manifested by decreased inhibitions, incoordination, blurred vision, slurred speech, stupor, coma, seizures, and death. Most fatal intoxications occur at blood concentrations greater than 400 mg/dL. Capillary and arterial blood samples most accurately reflect brain ethanol concentrations. Serum ethanol concentrations are usually determined by enzymatic, gas chromatographic, or electrochemical oxidation techniques. In the most accurate assays for ethanol, serum is incubated with alcohol dehydrogenase, which oxidizes ethanol to acetaldehyde, and NAD is converted to NADH. Thus, simple monitoring of the absorbance of the incubated serum at 340 nm gives a direct determination of alcohol present. Acute poisoning is generally treated by supportive therapy, gastric lavage with tap water, or hemodialysis, if indicated (> 500 mg/dL). Symptoms of chronic intoxication, such as acute alcoholic mania, may be treated with diazepam. Phenytoin may be utilized in patients with a history of seizures.

Methanol (wood alcohol) poisoning occurs in patients who ingest methylated spirits or methanol-containing antifreeze. It is rapidly absorbed from the gastrointestinal tract and is metabolized and excreted at approximately 20% of the rate of ethanol. The toxic range is thought to be 60–250 mL, although as little as 15 mL has caused death. Alcohol dehydrogenase metabolizes methanol to formaldehyde and formic acid, which is responsible for ocular toxicity (diminished light sensation or frank blindness), and anion gap metabolic acidosis, which are the principal symptoms of intoxication. Other symptoms include nausea, vomiting, headache, seizures, and coma. GC-MS is used to measure blood methanol levels, with a peak level greater than 50 mg/dL considered toxic. In addition, serum osmolality levels are increased to levels greater than 300 mOsm. Methanol (or ethylene glycol) poisoning should be considered in acutely ill patients with hyperosmolarity, metabolic acidosis, and increased anion gap.

Ethylene glycol (l,2-ethanediol) is used in car radiator antifreeze. It has a half-life of around 3 hours and is metabolized to three major toxic compounds: glycolaldehyde, glycolic acid, and glyoxylic acid. The oxidation of ethylene glycol to glycolaldehyde is catalyzed by liver alcohol dehydrogenase. Both oxalic acid and formic acid are formed in smaller amounts. Oxalic acid itself is a highly toxic compound, which can rapidly precipitate as calcium oxalate crystals in various tissues as well as in urine. The formation of these crystals in urine, although not a constant finding, is an important diagnostic clue to ethylene glycol poisoning. The metabolite that accumulates in the highest concentrations in the blood is glycolic acid, and its concentration in blood and urine appears to correlate directly with symptomatology and mortality. It is the major contributor to the high anion gap seen in metabolic acidosis. The fatal dose of ethylene glycol is around 100 g, and anuria and necrosis are the principal symptoms of acute poisoning. Other symptoms include nausea and vomiting, myoclonus, seizures, convulsions, depressed reflexes, and coma. Definitive diagnosis of ethylene glycol intoxication can be made by measuring serum ethylene glycol and glycolic acid by HPLC.

Treatment of ethylene glycol and methanol toxicity is similar and is based on symptomatology and serum level. The mainstay of treatment is ethanol therapy, since ethanol competes with both methanol and ethylene glycol in metabolism by alcohol dehydrogenase. If this enzyme is saturated by ethanol, methanol and ethylene glycol metabolism is decreased, their toxic products do not build up in the tissues, and the parent compounds may be excreted unchanged in the urine. In addition to ethanol, intravenous alkali (bicarbonate) therapy is generally begun in the acidotic patient, to correct the metabolic acidosis. Dialysis, either hemodialysis or peritoneal dialysis, is also utilized to remove either parent compound and its corresponding toxic metabolic products.

Isopropyl alcohol has a half-life of approximately 3 hours and a volume of distribution similar to that of ethanol. It is readily absorbed through the GI tract, and metabolized at approximately 50% of the rate of ethanol. The metabolism of isopropanol occurs mainly by alcohol dehydrogenase to produce acetone, carbon dioxide, and water. The fatal dose of ingestion is 250 mL. Both isopropyl alcohol and its major metabolite, acetone, are CNS depressants.

CNS depression is the principal symptom of acute isopropanol intoxication. In addition, it produces significant GI irritation, which may be manifested by nausea and vomiting, including hematemesis and melena, abdominal pain, and gastritis. Other symptoms include confusion, coma, hypertension, respiratory failure, and death.

The diagnosis of isopropanol intoxication is difficult to make. Clues to the diagnosis include acetonuria, acetonemia and hyperosmolarity without glycosuria, hyperglycemia, or acidosis. Gas chromatography is generally considered to be the best technique to determine isopropanol blood concentrations. Treatment includes supportive care, activated charcoal with gastric lavage, and hemodialysis in severe poisoning.

Arsenic

Arsenic is used in ant poisons, rodenticides, herbicides and weed killers, insecticides, paints, wood preservatives, ceramics, the production of various metal alloys, livestock feed, as a tanning agent, and in medicines. Inorganic arsenicals, including sodium arsenate and lead or copper arsenite; organic arsenicals, such as carbarsone and tryparsamide; and arsine gas are the major toxicologic forms of arsenic. Arsine gas poisoning generally occurs in the industrial setting, where its production arises from the action of acid or water on arsenic-bearing metals.

Arsenic is readily absorbed through the GI tract and lungs, whereas absorption through the skin occurs more slowly. Twenty-four hours after ingestion, arsenic is distributed to all body tissues. The major route of excretion is through the kidneys. Arsenic can cross the placenta.

The major concern with arsenic ingestion is systemic poisoning, presumably through its reversible interaction with multiple enzyme sulfhydryl groups. This, in turn, leads to the disruption of multiple metabolic systems.

Arsine gas, the most dangerous form of arsenic, may irreversibly attach to sulfhydryl groups of hemoglobin, causing intravascular hemolysis, hemoglobinemia, and consequent acute renal failure, as well as direct nephrotoxicity.

The acute fatal dosage of arsenic trioxide is approximately 120 mg, whereas less than 30 parts per million (ppm) of arsenic gas can produce poisoning. Organic arsenicals release arsenic slowly and have a fatal dose of approximately 0.1–0.5 g/kg.

Acute toxicity is usually manifested within the first hour of ingestion, and generally reflects multiorgan involvement. Gastrointestinal symptomatology is the most common presentation, with burning and dryness of the mouth and throat, difficulty in swallowing, vomiting, and watery or bloody diarrhea containing shreds of intestinal lining or mucus. There may be the odor of garlic on the breath, and a metallic taste in the patient's mouth. Cyanosis, hypotension, tachycardia, and ventricular arrhythmias may develop. Neuropathy usually occurs late (approximately 1–2 weeks) after ingestion, or may become most intense during this time period. Severe volume depletion and acute renal tubular necrosis may occur, with death resulting from circulatory failure. Symptoms of poisoning with arsine gas usually manifest approximately 2–24 hours after exposure and may initially include nausea and vomiting, headache, anorexia, and paresthesias. Hematemesis and abdominal pain are also common, and acute renal failure, cardiac damage, anemia and hemolysis, or pulmonary edema may also occur. The diagnosis of chronic intoxication is usually difficult and should be considered in patients with a combination of GI symptomatology; neuropathy; and cutaneous, cardiovascular, and renal disturbances.

Analysis of urine, hair, and nails, using ion emission spectroscopy, is important for the diagnosis of chronic arsenic poisoning. Treatment of acute poisoning includes removal of residual arsenic by gastric lavage or emesis, and treatment with dimercaprol, or British anti-lewisite (BAL), which combines with arsenic through its sulfhydryl groups to produce cyclic water-soluble complexes. However, the inherent toxicity of this compound limits its therapeutic usefulness. Less toxic derivatives of BAL are available, such as 2,3-dithioerythritol, which is less toxic in cell culture, while showing greater efficacy than BAL at rescuing arsenical-poisoned cells in culture (Boyd, 1989). In severe poisoning, hemodialysis can be used to remove the arsenic–dimercaprol complexes.

Mercury

Mercury compounds exist in four different forms with different toxicologic potential: elemental or metallic (Hg^o); mercurous (Hg^+); mercuric (Hg^{2+}); and alkyl mercury (i.e., organomercurials). Elemental mercury is poorly absorbed from the GI tract if mucosal integrity is preserved, and shows no toxic effect unless it is converted to the divalent form. This may occur slowly by oxidation–reduction with water and chloride ion if a GI site for mercury stasis exists, but this is uncommon. Significant poisoning occurs

with elemental mercury when it is inhaled or absorbed through the skin. It can pass through the blood–brain barrier, and can accumulate in the CNS, where oxidation produces mercuric ion; thus, primarily pulmonary and CNS toxicities are produced.

Of the two inorganic salts of mercury, mercurous (Hg^+) salts are poorly soluble and thus poorly absorbed. However, the mercuric (Hg^{2+}) salt is readily soluble and is readily absorbed after oral ingestion or inhalation. Severe inflammation of the mouth as well as other GI symptoms can result. The kidney is also a preferred site of accumulation of inorganic mercuric compounds, where acute renal tubular and glomerular damage can ensue. Both elemental mercury and the inorganic mercury compounds are excreted mainly in urine.

In contrast to elemental and inorganic mercury, organic mercury compounds, containing alkyl, aryl, and alkoxyalkyl moieties, are environmental pollutants. These compounds contain at least one covalent mercury–carbon bond. Both the alkoxyalkyl and aryl mercurial compounds undergo metabolic breakdown and biotransformation to produce inorganic mercury, which toxicologically acts and manifests intoxication as would the above-mentioned inorganic mercury compounds. In contrast, the mercury–carbon bonds that occur within the methyl and ethyl forms are extremely stable and produce greater toxicity than the aryl and the alkoxyalkyl forms. The alkyl forms are more lipid soluble, pass readily through biological membranes and, on ingestion, show generally greater absorption into the body. Their major chemical effect is on the CNS, and they show a biological half-life of 70–90 days. Because bile is the major route of excretion, methyl-mercury can be reabsorbed into the blood, via the enterohepatic system, accounting, in part, for its extended half-life. The major mechanism of action of mercury poisoning is through covalent bonding with protein sulfhydryl groups, producing widespread and nonspecific enzyme dysfunction, inactivation, and denaturation.

Mercury, depending on its form, may cause systemic toxicity or local skin and mucous membrane lesions. Both organic and elemental mercury can cause CNS effects, whereas GI symptomatology primarily occurs with inorganic salts. Elemental mercury may also produce severe pulmonary reactions.

In general, acute toxicity, with elemental, inorganic, or most organic forms, can be diagnosed from 24-hour urine levels. Blood levels may rise rapidly after acute exposure, but fall rapidly and may not reflect total body burden. In contrast, because the short-chain alkyl organic mercuric compounds are mainly excreted in the bile, blood levels are better indicators of tissue levels and significant acute exposure. Hair analysis for mercury may help identify chronic mercury exposure.

Treatment includes gastric lavage or emesis to remove the ingested poison as well as the use of dimercaprol and succimer. However, in methyl- and alkyl-mercury poisoning, dimercaprol is contraindicated because it has been found to increase the concentration of these compounds in the brain (Bryson, 1989). In these cases, treatment is symptomatic, although new agents are being evaluated clinically.

Iron

Acute iron poisoning is common in young children and is usually the result of ingestion of iron-containing products. Although ferric ions from food are usually reduced to ferrous ions and absorbed in the stomach, the large and small bowel can rapidly absorb toxic amounts (> 30 mg/kg) of elemental iron. Once absorbed into the body, iron removal is difficult. Large doses of iron are thought to cause acute mucosal cell damage, and significant absorption of iron occurs once the binding capacity of transferrin is exceeded. Unbound iron in the serum causes toxicity by hepatic cell damage, shock, and production of lactic acidosis. The hepatotoxicity seems to be dose related, occurs within 1–2 days of ingestion, and has been associated with levels equal to or greater than 1700 µg/dL (Tenenbein, 2001).

Vomiting appears to be an early manifestation of iron intoxication, along with severe gastroenteritis, melena, abdominal pain, and hematemesis. This occurs up to 6 hours after ingestion. For up to the next 10 hours, the patient may appear to improve. This is deceptive because manifestations of systemic toxicity (cyanosis, convulsions, shock, coagulopathy, renal and hepatic failure) may occur, producing death. Both patients who develop severe systemic symptomatology and those who do not may develop late complications, including GI obstructions or strictures.

Definitive diagnosis is made with measurements of serum iron concentration and the total iron-binding capacity (TIBC) of transferrin. In addition to supportive treatment, emesis or gastric lavage is used to prevent iron absorption. Chelation therapy with deferoxamine is also utilized if the acute intoxication is severe.

Lead

Both organic and inorganic compounds of lead may be highly toxic, with their most serious effects occurring on the central and peripheral nervous systems. Absorption may occur by either inhalation or ingestion. If greater than 0.5 mg of lead is absorbed per day, lead accumulation and toxicity are believed to occur, whereas 0.5 g of absorbed lead is considered a fatal dose. However, acute toxicity is uncommon and is generally observed in patients who have been exposed to high concentrations of lead dusts. Lead poisoning is seen in children in large cities who consume lead in the form of paint (pica). Acute manifestations are primarily CNS symptoms (encephalopathy, convulsions, stupor), and GI symptomatology such as colic. Chronic toxicity with lead accumulating in blood, soft tissues, and bone is more common. The largest body compartment of lead is bone, which contains approximately 96% of the total body burden. The half-life of lead in bone is 32 years, and bone may act as a reservoir for endogenous intoxication. Chronic toxicity may be manifested by a wide range of systemic effects, including general malaise, weight loss, anorexia, constipation; lead encephalopathy exhibited by malaise with apathy, drowsiness, stupor, and seizures; peripheral neuropathy with wrist drop or foot drop; and lead nephrosis with albuminuria, hematuria, and pyuria and anemia (hypochromic, micro- or normocytic) with basophilic stippling, the latter finding often a strong clue.

In addition, lead-induced pathologic changes may occur at even low levels of lead exposure. Needleman and Gatsonis (1990) reviewed 24 studies of childhood lead exposure to provide statistical evidence that low doses of lead may produce an intellectual deficit in children. Schwartz and colleagues (1990) examined lead-induced anemia in children 1–5 years of age, using a cross-sectional epidemiologic study. They found a relationship between age, blood lead level, and hematocrit such that younger children had an increased risk of anemia at lower blood levels than children only a few years older. It thus appears that lead may produce deleterious effects, especially in children, at low levels of exposure. Generally, serum lead levels greater than or equal to 10 µg/dL indicate excessive lead absorption in children, while concentrations greater than 25 µg/dL indicates consideration of chelation therapy in the child. The Centers for Disease Control (CDC) recommend universal screening of children, beginning at 6 months of age (Klaassen, 2001; Bernard, 2003).

Organolead compounds such as tetraethyl and tetramethyl lead are lipid soluble and, like the organomercurials discussed previously, produce their major toxic effects on the CNS. Lead encephalopathy may occur early in the onset of intoxication, and does not correlate well with blood lead concentrations. Hyperactive deep tendon reflexes, intention tremor, abnormal jaw jerk, and abnormalities of stance and gait are the most consistently observed neurologic manifestations of organolead toxicity.

Lead appears to interact with thiol, carboxylic, and phosphate groups to form stable complexes with enzymes and proteins (Bryson, 1989). This is particularly well known for heme synthesis, in which lead blocks the action of delta-aminolevulinic acid (ALA) synthetase, delta-ALA dehydratase (ALAD), coproporphyrinogen decarboxylase, and ferrochetalase, producing anemia. These disruptions in heme synthesis allow for objective testing for inorganic lead exposure. Increased amounts of ALA in urine, decreased ALAD activity in red blood cells, increased amounts of free erythrocyte protoporphyrin, and elevated amounts of zinc protoporphyrin are found with inorganic lead poisoning. The assay for zinc protoporphyrin is a particularly simple fluorometric one that is widely used and is an excellent screening test. The most sensitive screening test for organolead poisoning is decreased ALAD activity in urine because changes in the activities of other enzymes and in the levels of the products of heme synthesis are not consistent. Although whole blood lead concentrations are a reliable indicator of recent lead exposure, the short half-life of circulating lead in blood makes estimates of total body burden unreliable. However, use of in vivo X-ray fluorescence of bone allows determination of cumulative lead burden (Kosnett, 1994). Treatment of poisoning includes supportive therapy as well as removal of soluble lead compounds by gastric lavage. Dilute magnesium sulfate or sodium sulfate solutions are commonly used. In addition, chelating agents such as dimercaprol, calcium disodium edetate, and succimer may be utilized, if necessary.

Quantitation of Lead in Serum. Lead levels in serum may be determined directly using either atomic absorption spectroscopy or a newer, more readily accessible method, called *anode* stripping voltammetry. In the latter method, a voltaic cell is set up such that the anode consists of a mercury-coated graphite rod. When a negative potential is applied to this anode, cationic metals, such as lead, 'plate out' in their metallic forms on the anode. The applied voltage is then stopped. Since there is an excess of electrons on the anode, current will flow to the cathode. Each of the metals plated on the anode will therefore become

oxidized back to their respective ionic forms (i.e., be stripped from the anode). The metals with lowest oxidation potentials will strip first. Each metal will strip from the anode in the order of oxidation potential, recorded as the half-wave potential, which is a constant for a given metal. The total current associated with the stripping of each metal is proportional to the concentration of that metal.

Organophosphates and Carbamates

The *organophosphates* are esters of phosphoric acid or thiophosphoric acid, whereas the *carbamates* are synthetic derivatives of carbamic acid. Although these are two distinctly different types of compounds, they both interfere with neurotransmission and are widely used as pesticides in agriculture. Both compounds inhibit the enzyme acetylcholinesterase (AChE), which normally hydrolyzes the neurotransmitter acetylcholine (ACh) after ACh has effected an action potential and has been released from its receptor site. Both compounds produce inhibition by reacting with the active site of AChE. This occurs by phosphorylation with the organophosphates to produce a relatively stable phosphate ester bond; and by carbamoylation with the carbamates to form a more labile, and hence more easily reversible, carbamate ester bond. Both compounds thus cause accumulation of ACh at neuronal synapses and myoneural junctions to produce toxicity.

ACh is an important neurotransmitter in both the peripheral and central nervous systems. It is located at a number of different synapses in the CNS, at the ganglionic synapses between the sympathetic and parasympathetic pre- and postganglionic fibers, at the junctions between parasympathetic postganglionic fibers and effector organs, and at the junctions between somatic motor neurons and skeletal muscle cells. Thus, signs and symptoms of organophosphate poisoning include parasympathetic manifestations such as salivation, lacrimation, urination, and defecation (SLUD); pupillary constriction; bradycardia; and bronchoconstriction, which may predominate at low-dose poisoning. Autonomic ganglionic and somatic motor manifestations (such as muscular weakness, twitching, areflexia, tachycardia, and hypertension) and CNS manifestations (such as confusion, slurred speech, ataxia, convulsions, and respiratory and/or cardiovascular center depression) may predominate in severe intoxication. Death usually results from respiratory failure as a result of a combination of central depression, bronchospasm, excessive bronchial secretions, and respiratory muscle paralysis.

It should be noted that morbidity and mortality due to carbamate poisoning is less severe, since carbamates do not penetrate the CNS as effectively as organophosphates, and central cholinergic effects are thus minimal. In addition, the much greater lability of the carbamate ester bond allows for spontaneous reactivation of AChE. This, in turn, decreases the slope of the toxicity dose–response curve, as compared with the curve for organophosphates, such that small increments in carbamate dose are less likely to produce severe increases in toxicity.

In addition to acute poisoning, organophosphates may produce an intermediate syndrome occurring 1–4 days after poisoning, and/or delayed neurotoxicity usually occurring 2–5 weeks after acute exposure. The former syndrome develops after acute cholinergic crisis and appears to involve cranial nerve palsies, proximal limb weakness, and respiratory paralysis with the patient requiring ventilatory support (Senanayake, 1987, 1998). In contrast, delayed neurotoxicity, which is not seen with all organophosphate compounds, appears to be due to neurotoxic esterase inhibition and usually produces a distal and symmetric sensorimotor polyneuropathy of the extremities (Davies, 1987; Tafuri, 1987).

Diagnosis of organophosphate poisoning depends on a history of exposure shortly before the onset of illness, signs and symptoms of diffuse parasympathetic stimulation, and laboratory confirmation of exposure by measurement of erythrocyte acetylcholinesterase and plasma pseudo-cholinesterase activities. Whereas AChE is found primarily in nervous tissue and erythrocytes, pseudocholinesterase is found in plasma. The latter enzyme is much more nonspecific in its action than AChE, in that in addition to hydrolysis of ACh, pseudocholinesterase can hydrolyze many other natural and synthetic esters. Both activities may be decreased, and both activities can be measured in the laboratory. However, only inhibition of AChE is considered specific for organophosphate poisoning because a number of conditions may produce a low plasma pseudocholinesterase level (Tafuri, 1987). Thus, the latter measurement is more sensitive but less specific than the red blood cell cholinesterase level for organophosphate poisoning. Generally, levels 30–50% of normal indicate exposure, and toxic manifestations occur with greater than 50% inhibition; however, symptoms may not appear until levels are 20% or less of normal. In actuality, confirmation of poisoning, rather than diagnosis, occurs by laboratory determinations. Because baseline values of cholinesterase levels prior to exposure are unlikely to be available, sequential postexposure cholinesterase determinations appear to be the best way to confirm organophosphate poisoning (Coye, 1987).

Treatment of acute poisoning includes respiratory support, if necessary, decontamination of the patient, and gastric lavage or emesis. In the presence of symptoms, atropine is given to ameliorate excessive parasympathetic stimulation by competitively blocking the action of ACh at muscarinic receptors. Pralidoxime is also given as a specific antidote for organophosphate poisoning. If pralidoxime is given within 24–48 hours of exposure, it may reactivate phosphorylated cholinesterase by removal of the covalently bound phosphate group from the enzyme's active site. However, this time period is variable, and utilization of pralidoxime after 48 hours may be indicated (Clark, 2002; Howland, 2002). Chronic poisoning is usually treated by avoidance of further exposure until cholinesterase levels become normal.

References

General References

Bryson PD (ed): Comprehensive Review in Toxicology. Rockville, Aspen Publishers, 1989.

Goldfrank LR, Flomenbaum NE, Lewin NA, et al: (eds): Goldfrank's Toxicologic Emergencies, 7th ed. New York, McGraw-Hill, 2002.

O'Neil MJ, Smith A, Heckelman PE, et al: (eds): The Merck Index: An Encyclopedia of Chemicals, Drugs, and Biologicals, 13th ed. Whitehouse Station, Merck and Co, 2001.

Sweetman SC, Blake PS, McGlashan JM, et al: (eds): Martindale: The Complete Drug Reference, 33rd ed. London, The Pharmaceutical Press, 2002.

Basic Techniques for Detecting Drugs

Boone CM, Ensing K: Is capillary electrophoresis a method of choice for systematic toxicological analysis? Clin Chem Lab Med 2003; 41:773–781.

Davis IM, Bousquet RW, Childs PS: Gas chromatography/mass spectroscopy in clinical and forensic toxicology. In Service Training and Continuing Education, Vol 10, No 12. Washington, DC, American Association for Clinical Pathology, 1989, pp 7–21.

Engelhardt H: One century of liquid chromatography: From Tswett's columns to modern high speed and high performance separations. J Chromatogr B 2004; 800: 3–6.
This is an excellent overview of the development and history of liquid chromatography in the 20th century, describing early successes of 'adsorption biochemical analysis' as well as the recent modern revolution in analysis.

Marquet P: Progress of liquid chromatography–mass spectrometry in clinical and forensic toxicology. Ther Drug Monit 2002; 24:255–276.

Maurer HH: Liquid chromatography–mass spectrometry in forensic and clinical toxicology. J Chromatogr B 1998; 713:3–25.

Niessen WMA: Progress in liquid chromatography–mass spectrometry instrumentation and its impact on high-throughput screening. J Chromatogr A 2003; 1000:413–436.

Niessen WMA, Tinke AP: Liquid chromatography–mass spectrometry: general principles and instrumentation. J Chromatogr A 1995; 703:37–57.

Petersen JR, Okordudu AO, Mohammad A, Payne DA: Capillary electrophoresis and its application in the clinical laboratory. Clin Chim Acta 2003; 330:1–30.

Pincus MR, Rendell M: General quantitative treatment for the binding of divalent antibodies to antigens immobilized on a solid phase. Proc Natl Acad Sci USA 1981; 78:5924–5927.

Rodbard D, Ruder HJ, Vaitukaitis J, et al: Mathematical analysis of kinetics of radioligand assays: Improved sensitivity obtained by delayed addition of labeled ligand. J Clin Endocrinol Metab 1971; 33:343–355.

Shihabi ZK: Applications of Capillary Electrophoresis in the Clinical Laboratory, Check Sample, Vol. 33. Clinical Chemistry No. CC 94-4 (CC-242). Chicago, American Society of Clinical Pathologists, 1993.

Tagliaro F, Turrina S, Pisi P, et al: Determination of illicit and/or abused drugs and compounds of forensic interest in biosamples by capillary electrophoretic/electrokinetic methods. J Chromatogr B 1998; 713:27–49.

Drugs of Abuse

Azmitia EC, Murphy RB, Whitaker-Azmitia PM: MDMA (ecstasy) effects on cultured serotonergic neurons: Evidence for Ca²⁺-dependent toxicity linked to release. Brain Res 1990; 510:97–103.

Bayorh MA, Zokowska-Grojec Z, Palkovits M, et al: Effect of phencyclidine (PCP) on blood pressure and catecholamine levels in discrete brain nuclei. Brain Res 1984; 321:315–318.

Bell J, Seres V, Bowron P, et al: The use of serum methadone levels in patients receiving methadone maintenance. Clin Pharmacol Ther 1988; 43:623–629.

Cami J, Farre, M: Drug addiction. N Engl J Med 2003; 349:975–986.
This is a discussion of drug addiction and the various factors involved in drug abuse, the molecular mechanism of action of various drugs, and the neurobiology and neuroadaptation of drug addiction.

DeCresce RP, Mazura AC, Lifshitz MS, Tilson JE: Drug Testing in the Workplace. Chicago, American Society of Clinical Pathology Press, 1989.

Fraser AD: Use and abuse of the benzodiazepines. Ther Drug Monit 1998; 20:481–489.

Frishman WH, Del Vecchio A, Sanal S, Ismail A: Cardiovascular manifestations of substance abuse Part 1: Cocaine. Heart Disease 2003; 5:187–201.

Gianoulakis C: Endogenous opioids and addiction to alcohol and other drugs of abuse. Curr Topics Med Chem 2004; 4:39–50.

Gill JR, Hayes JA, deSouza IS, et al: Ecstasy (MDMA) deaths in New York City: A case series and review of the literature. J Forensic Sci 2002; 47:121–126.

Hollander JE, Hoffman RS: Cocaine. In Goldfrank LR, Flomenbaum NE, Lewin NA, et al: (eds): Goldfrank's Toxicologic Emergencies, 7th ed. New York, McGraw-Hill, 2002, pp 1004–1019.

Hurd YL, Kehr J, Ungerstedt U: In vivo microdialysis as a technique to monitor drug transport: Correlation of extracellular cocaine levels and dopamine outflow in the rat brain. J Neurochem 1988; 51:1314–1316.

Iversen L: Cannabis and the brain. Brain 2003; 126:1252–1270.

Johanson CE, Fischman MW: The pharmacology of cocaine related to its abuse. Pharmacol Rev 1989; 41:3–52.

Lange RA, Hillis LD: Cardiovascular complications of cocaine use. N Engl J Med 2001; 345:351–358.

Lange RA, Cigarroc RO, Yancy CW, et al: Cocaine-induced coronary artery vasoconstriction. N Engl J Med 1989; 321:1557–1562.

Martin BR, Sim-Selley LJ, Selley DE: Signaling pathways involved in the development of cannabinoid tolerance. Trends Pharmacol Sci 2004; 25:325–330.

Murphy RB, Pincus MR, Beinfeld MC, et al: Enkephalin is a competitive antagonist of cholecystokinin in the gastrointestinal tract, as predicted from prior conformational analysis. J Protein Chem 1992; 11:723–729.

Pincus MR, Carty RP, Chen JM, et al: On the biologically active structures of cholecystokinin, little gastrin and enkephalin in the gastrointestinal system and in brain. Proc Natl Acad Sci USA 1987; 84:4821–4825.

Poklis A: Analytic/forensic toxicology. In Klaassen CD (ed): Casarett and Doull's Toxicology: The Basic Science of Poisons, 6th ed. New York, McGraw-Hill, 2001, pp 1089–1108.

Schuster DI, Ehrlich GK, Murphy RB: Purification and partial amino acid sequence of a 28 kDa cyclophilin-like component of the rat liver sigma receptor. Life Sci 1994; 55:PL151–156.

Snyder SH and Pasternak GE: Historical review: Opioid receptors. Trends Pharmacol Sci 2003; 24:198–205.
Early molecular biology of opioid receptors is historically reviewed including receptor localization, identification, and cloning.

Tseng LF: Evidence for epsilon-opioid receptor-mediated beta-endorphin-induced analgesia. Trends Pharmacol Sci 2001; 22:623–630.

Tso PH, Wong YH: Molecular basis of opioid dependence: Role of signal regulation by G-proteins. Clin Exp Pharm Phys 2003; 30:307–316.

Therapeutic Drugs

Asconape JJ: Some common issues in the use of antiepileptic drugs. Semin Neurol 2002; 22:27–39.

Bazil CW, Pedley TA: Advances in the medical treatment of epilepsy. Annu Rev Med 1998; 49:135–162.

Braun F, Lort T, Ringe B: Update of current immunosuppressive drugs used in clinical organ transplantation. Transpl Int 1998; 11:77–81.

Brodtkorb E: Antiepileptic drug treatment: Clinical considerations and concerns. Progr Brain Res 1998; 116:395–406.

Burns MJ: The pharmacology and toxicology of atypical antipsychotic agents. J Toxicol Clin Toxicol 2001; 39:1–14.

Dancey JE: Clinical development of mammalian target of rapamycin inhibitors. Hematol Oncol Clin N Am 2002; 16:1101–1114.

Drosos AA: Newer immunosuppressive drugs: Their potential role in rheumatoid arthritis therapy. Drugs 2002; 62:891–907.

Dunn CJ, Wagstaff AJ, Perry CM, et al: Cyclosporin: An updated review of the pharmacokinetic properties, clinical efficacy and tolerability of a microemulsion-based formulation (Neoral) in organ transplantation. Drugs 2001; 61:1957–2016.

Gerson B (ed): Therapeutic drug monitoring I: Pharmacokinetics, technology, and methodology. Clin Lab Med 1987a; 7:267–492.

Gerson B (ed): Therapeutic drug monitoring II: Patient care and applications. Clin Lab Med 1987b; 7:499–714.

Grem JL, de Carvalho M, Wittes RE, Allegra CJ: Chemotherapy: The properties and uses of single agents: Methotrexate. In Macdonald JS, Haller DG, Mayer RJ (eds): Manual of Oncologic Therapeutics, 3rd ed. Philadelphia, JB Lippincott Co, 1995, p 108.

Hardman JG, Limbird LE, Gilman AG: Goodman & Gilman's The Pharmacological Basis of Therapeutics, 10th ed. New York, McGraw-Hill, 2001.

Hess AD, Esa AH, Colombani PM: Mechanisms of action of cyclosporine: Effect on cells of the immune system and on subcellular events in T cell activation. Transplant Proc 1988; 20(Suppl 2):29–40.

Hojo M, Morimoto T, Maluccio M, et al: Cyclosporine induces cancer progression by a cell-autonomous mechanism. Nature 1999; 397:530–534.

Howanitz PJ, Howanitz JH: Therapeutic drug monitoring and toxicology. In Henry JB (ed): Clinical Diagnosis and Management by Laboratory Methods, 17th ed. Philadelphia, WB Saunders, 1984, pp 362 and 370.

Ingelman-Sundberg M: Pharmacogenetics of cytochrome P450 and its applications in drug therapy: The past, present and future. Trends Pharmacol Sci 2004; 25:193–200.
An overview of cytochrome P450 pharmacogenetics, its clinical relevance, and possible future benefit for maximizing effective drug therapy.

Isoniemi H: New trends in maintenance immunosuppression. Ann Chir Gynaecol 1997; 86:164–170.

Kahan BD: Pharmacokinetics and pharmacodynamics of cyclosporine. Transplant Proc 1989; 21(Suppl 1):9–15.

Kronbach T, Fischer V, Meyer VA: Cyclosporine metabolism in human liver: Identification of a cytochrome P-450 III gene family as the major cyclosporine-metabolizing enzyme explains interactions of cyclosporine with other drugs. Clin Pharmacol Ther 1988; 43:630–635.

McEvoy GK, Miller J, Litvak K (eds): American Hospital Formulary Service Drug Information 2004. Bethesda, MD, American Society of Health-System Pharmacists, 2004.

Miller BW, Brennan DC: Clinical experience with Neoral (cyclosporine for microemulsion) in renal transplantation. Today's Therapeutic Trends 1998; 16:73–86.

Mueller XM: Drug immunosuppression therapy for adult heart transplantation. Part 1: Immune response to allograft and mechanism of action of immunosuppressants. Ann Thorac Surg 2004; 77:354–362.

Opie, LH, Gersh, BJ: Drugs for the Heart, 5th ed. Philadelphia, WB Saunders, 2001.

Pesce AJ, Rashkin M, Kotagal U: Standards of laboratory practice: theophylline and caffeine monitoring. National Academy of Clinical Biochemistry. Clin Chem 1998; 44:1124–1128.

Phiel CJ, Klein PS: Molecular targets of lithium action. Annu Rev Pharmacol Toxicol 2001; 41:789–813.

Philip AT, Gerson B: Toxicology and adverse effects of drugs used for immunosuppression in organ transplantation. Clin Lab Med 1998; 18:755–765.

Roenigk Jr. HH, Auerbach R, Maibach HI, et al: Methotrexate in psoriasis: Consensus conference. J Am Acad Dermatol 1998; 38:478–485.

Scott LJ, McKeage K, Keam SJ, Plosker GL: Tacrolimus: A further update of its use in the management of organ transplantation. Drugs 2003; 63:1247–1297.

Slattery JT, Risler LJ: Therapeutic monitoring of busulfan in hematopoietic stem cell transplantation. Ther Drug Monit 1998; 20:543–549.

Sunheimer R, Capaldo G, Kashanian F, et al: Serum analyte pattern characteristic of fulminant hepatic failure. Ann Clin Lab Sci 1994; 24:101–109.

Sztajnkrycer MD: Valproic acid toxicity: Overview and management. J Toxicol Clin Toxicol 2002; 40:789–801.

Tugwell P, Bennett K, Gent M: Methotrexate in rheumatoid arthritis: Indications, contraindications, efficacy, and safety. Ann Intern Med 1987a; 107:358–366.

Tugwell P, Bennett K, Gent M: Position paper: Methotrexate in rheumatoid arthritis. Ann Intern Med 1987b; 107:418–419.

Tugwell P, Pincus T, Yocum D, et al: Combination therapy with cyclosporine and methotrexate in severe rheumatoid arthritis. N Engl J Med 1995; 333:137–141.

Uetrecht JP: Mechanism of drug-induced lupus. Chem Res Toxicol 1988; 1:133–143.

Valdes R, Jortani SA, Gheorghiade M: Standards of laboratory practice: Cardiac drug monitoring. National Academy of Clinical Biochemistry. Clin Chem 1998; 44:1096–1109.

Warner A, Privitera M, Bates D: Standards of laboratory practice: Antiepileptic drug monitoring. National Academy of Clinical Biochemistry. Clin Chem 1998; 44:1085–1095.

White S, Wong SHY: Standards of laboratory practice: Analgesic drug monitoring. National Academy of Clinical Biochemistry. Clin Chem 1998; 44:1110–1123.

Yaari Y, Selzer ME, Pincus JH: Phenytoin: Mechanism of its anticonvulsant action. Ann Neurol 1986; 20:171–184.

Toxins and Poisons

Clark RF: Insecticides: Organic phosphorus compounds and carbamates. In Goldfrank LR, Flomenbaum NE, Lewin NA, et al: (eds): Goldfrank's Toxicologic Emergencies, 7th ed. New York, McGraw-Hill, 2002, pp 1346–1360.

Bernard SM: Should the Centers for Disease Control and Prevention's childhood lead poisoning intervention level be lowered? Am J Public Health 2003; 93:1253–1260.

Boyd VL, Harbell JW, O'Connor RJ, et al: 2,3-Dithioerythritol, a possible new arsenic antidote. Chem Res Toxicol 1989; 2:301–306.

Brandt-Rauf PW, Pincus MR: Molecular markers of carcinogenesis. Pharmacol Ther 1998; 77:135–148.

Caraco Y: Genetic determinants of drug responsiveness and drug interactions. Ther Drug Monit 1998; 20:517–524.

Coye MJ, Barnett PG, Midtling JE, et al: Clinical confirmation of organophosphate poisoning by serial cholinesterase analyses. Arch Intern Med 1987; 147:438–442.

Davies JE: Changing profile of pesticide poisoning. N Engl J Med 1987; 316:807–808.

De Vivo I, Marion MJ, Smith SJ, et al: Mutant c-K-ras-p21 in chemical carcinogenesis in humans exposed to vinyl chloride. Cancer Causes Control 1994; 5:273–278.

Howland MA, Aaron CK: Antidotes in depth: Pralidoxime. In Goldfrank LR, Flomenbaum NE, Lewin NA, et al. (eds): Goldfrank's Toxicologic Emergencies, 7th ed. New York, McGraw-Hill, 2002, pp 1361–1365.

Klaassen CD (ed): Casarett and Doull's Toxicology: The Basic Science of Poisons, 6th ed. New York, McGraw-Hill, 2001.

Kosnett MJ, Becker CE, Osterloh JD, et al: Factors influencing bone lead concentration in a suburban community assessed by non-invasive K x-ray fluorescence. JAMA 1994; 271:197–203.

Needleman HL, Gatsonis CA: Low-level lead exposure and the IQ of children: A meta-analysis of modern studies. JAMA 1990; 263:673–678.

Perera FP, Hemminki K, Young TL, et al: Detection of polycyclic aromatic hydrocarbon–DNA adducts in white blood cells of foundry workers. Cancer Res 1988; 48: 2288–2291.

Peto J: Cancer epidemiology in the last century and the next decade. Nature 2001; 411:390–395.
Reviews the effective use of cancer epidemiology in the 20th century for identification of various causes of cancer in humans.

Pincus, MR, Friedman, FK: Oncoproteins in the diagnosis of human malignancies. Molecular Diagnostics 2003; 1:23–38.

Santella R, Hatch M, Pirastu R, et al: Carcinogen evaluation: In vitro testing, in vivo testing, and epidemiology. Semin Occupational Med 1987; 2:245–255.

Schwartz J, Landrigan PJ, Baker EL Jr, et al: Lead-induced anemia: Dose–response relationships and evidence for a threshold. Am J Public Health 1990; 80:165–168.

Senanayake N: Organophosphorus insecticide poisoning. Ceylon Med J 1998; 43:22–29.
This is an excellent update on acute and chronic organophosphorus poisoning and the pathophysiology and behavioral effects of poisoning.

Senanayake N, Karalliedde L: Neurotoxic effects of organophosphorus insecticides: An intermediate syndrome. N Engl J Med 1987; 316:761–763.

Tafuri J, Roberts J: Organophosphate poisoning. Ann Emerg Med 1987; 16:193–202.

Tenenbein, M: Hepatotoxicity in acute iron poisoning. J Toxicol Clin Toxicol 2001; 39:721–726.

CHAPTER 24

Evaluation of Endocrine Function

Helena A. Guber MD, Amal F. Farag MD, James Lo PhD, James Sharp MD

KEY POINTS

• The endocrine system is a finely integrated system whereby the hypothalamus, pituitary, and target glands continually communicate through feedback inhibition and stimulation, to control all aspects of metabolism, growth and reproduction. By understanding this interplay, and carefully manipulating these systems via provocative and suppressive stimuli, it is possible to characterize an underlying abnormality and provide directed treatment.

• Prolactin levels can be elevated due to a variety of pharmacologic and physiologic stimuli; however, values greater than 200 ng/mL are almost always associated with the presence of a pituitary tumor.

• The initial screen for someone suspected of having acromegaly should be a serum IGF-1.

• It is often unnecessary to perform provocative stimulation tests to document growth hormone deficiency in patients with either a known history of pituitary disease or in those with evidence of three or more pituitary hormone deficiencies.

• Provided the hypothalamic–pituitary–thyroid axis is intact, the ultrasensitive TSH test is the best method for detecting clinically significant thyroid dysfunction.

• Whenever measuring thyroglobulin as a tumor marker for thyroid cancer, always check a simultaneous sample for thyroglobulin antibodies.

• The chromatographic measurement of plasma free metanephrines and normetanephrines is the best screening test for pheochromocytoma. The patient should avoid caffeine, alcohol and acetaminophen, monoamine oxidase inhibitors and tricyclic antidepressants for at least 5 days before testing.

• It is frequently unnecessary to perform an ACTH stimulation test in critically ill patients. A random cortisol of greater than 25 μg/dl (700 nmol/L) during stress makes it highly unlikely that the patient is adrenally insufficient.

• The measurement of day 2–3 FSH is a good indicator of follicular reserve, a day 21–22 progesterone is used to assess whether cycles are ovulatory.

Pituitary Gland

The endocrine system is a finely tuned servo-system, whereby the hypothalamus, pituitary and various endocrine glands communicate through an intricate scheme of feedback inhibition and stimulation. In the classic sense, a hormone is defined as a substance that acts at a site distant from its place of origin. Under the rubric of hormones we now include moieties that act in an autocrine (act directly upon themselves), paracrine (act adjacent to the cells of origin) and intracrine (act within the cells of origin without ever exiting the cells) fashion. It is through this intimate interplay of signals that the endocrine system serves to control metabolism, growth, fertility and responses to stress.

The pituitary gland, also known as the hypophysis, is located within the confines of the sella turcica; it is connected by the infundibular stalk to the median eminence of the hypothalamus. It is divided into an anterior lobe (adenohypophysis) and a posterior lobe (neurohypophysis). It weighs about 0.6 grams and measures about 12 mm in transverse and 8 mm in anteroposterior diameter. The anterior pituitary possesses five distinct hormone synthesizing and secreting populations of cells. These cell groups include somatotrophs which secrete growth hormone (GH), lactotrophs which secrete prolactin (PRL), thyrotrophs which secrete thyroid-stimulating hormone (TSH), gonadotrophs which secrete the α- and β-subunits of follicle-stimulating hormone (FSH) and luteinizing hormone (LH) and corticotrophs which secrete pro-opiomelanocortin (POMC). POMC is cleaved within the pituitary to form adrenocorticotropin (ACTH) and β-lipotropin (β-LPH). The hypothalamus communicates with the anterior pituitary by secreting its own set of trophic hormones that are specific for each of the cell populations. (Fig. 24-1) These trophic hormones travel along the infundibular stalk to the adenohypophysis through a system of portal vessels.

In contrast to the anterior pituitary the posterior pituitary does not synthesize hormones, the hormones that it secretes, arginine vasopressin (AVP) (also known as antidiuretic hormone [ADH]) and oxytocin are synthesized in the paraventricular and supraoptic nuclei of the hypothalamus, transported along axons and stored in the nerve terminals that end in the neurohypophysis. A summary of the different hormones secreted by the pituitary can be found in Table 24-1.

Abnormalities of pituitary function fall within two broad categories, those of hormonal excess and those of hormonal deficiency. Hormonal excess usually occurs as the result of clonal expansion of a distinct population of cells; however, it can result from an increase in trophic hormones from either the hypothalamus or ectopic sites. The causes of hormonal deficiency are more varied (Table 24-2) and can result in the deficiency of one or more hormones, often with a continued and progressive loss of other hormones with time.

Pituitary Tumors

Pituitary tumors are classified as either microadenomas (< 1 cm in greatest diameter and confined to the sella) or macroadenomas (≥ 1 cm in greatest diameter). They are further subcategorized into secretory and nonsecretory varieties (Table 24-3). All tumors have the potential to grow; in doing so they can compress the optic chiasm resulting in visual field defects, of which bitemporal hemianopia is the most frequent presentation. Invasion into the cavernous sinus can lead to compression of cranial nerves III, IV, VI, V_1, V_2 and the intracavernous portion of the internal carotid artery. It can also lead to hydrocephalus due to obstruction of the third ventricle. Aside from the oversecretion of a particular hormone and extension into

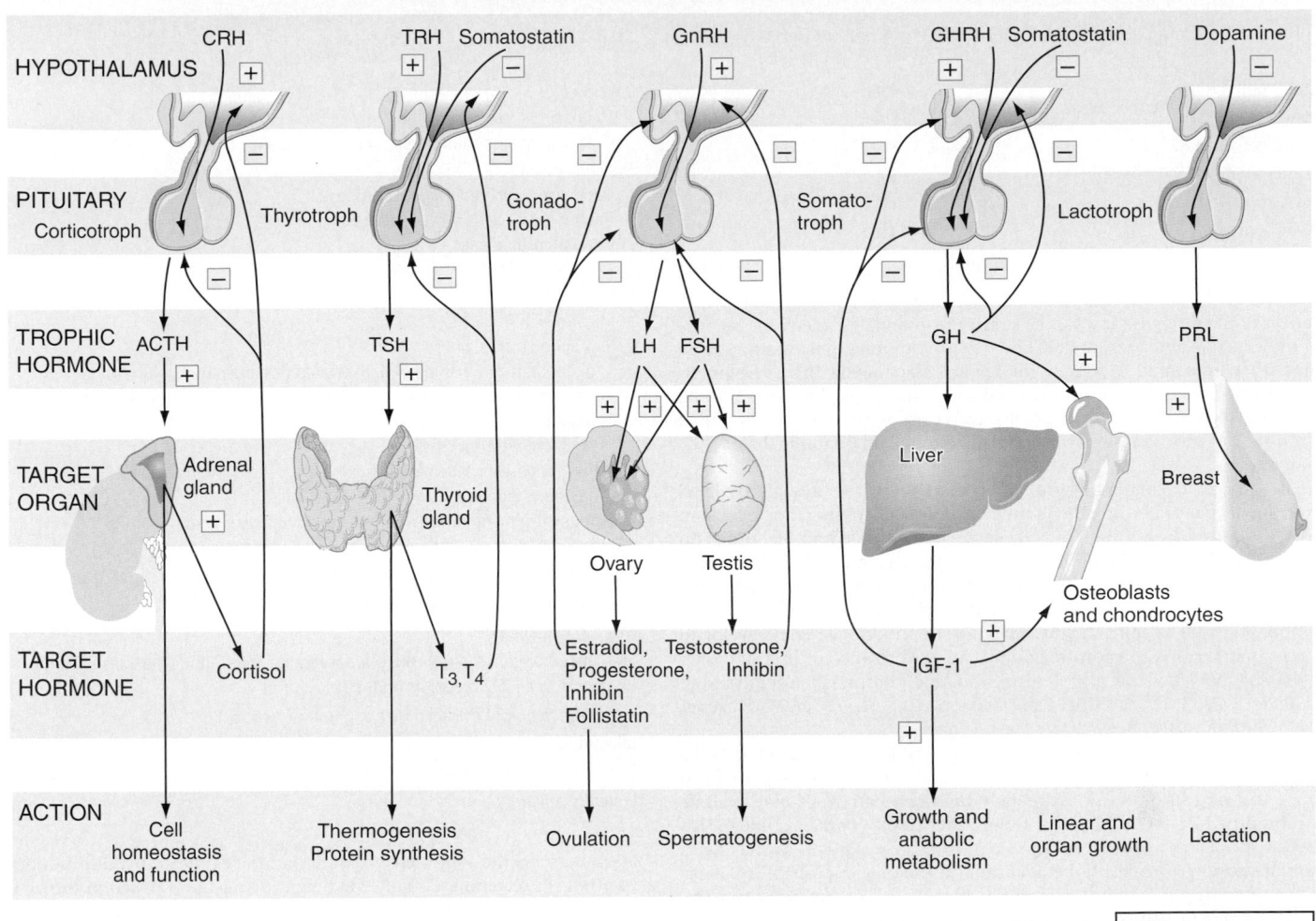

	Stimulation
+	Stimulation
−	Suppression

Figure 24–1 The hypothalamic–pituitary–target organ axis. (Redrawn from Melmed S, Kleinberg D: Anterior Pituitary. *In* Larsen PR, Kronenberg HM, Melmed S, et al, eds: Williams Textbook of Endocrinology. 10th edn. Phildelphia: Saunders; 2003:181 with permission.)

Table 24–1 Hormones of the Pituitary

Anterior pituitary – adenohypophysis

Growth hormone (somatotropin) (GH)

Thyroid-stimulating hormone (thyrotropin) (TSH)

Gonadotropins:
  Follicle-stimulating hormone (FSH)
  Luteinizing hormone (LH)

Pro-opiomelanocortin (POMC)
  Adrenocorticotropin (ACTH)
  β-Lipotropin

Prolactin (PRL)

Posterior pituitary – neurohypophysis

Arginine vasopressin (AVP) = antidiuretic hormone (ADH)

Oxytocin

Table 24–2 Causes of Pituitary Hormonal Deficiency

Pituitary neoplasm:
  Pituitary adenoma
  Craniopharyngioma
  Metastases or rarely primary carcinoma
Iatrogenic:
  Radiation
  Hypophysectomy
  Stalk resection
Granulomatous disease:
  Sarcoidosis
Infection:
  Tuberculosis
  Syphilis
  Fungi
Hemorrhage and infarction:
  Postpartum necrosis (Sheehan's syndrome)
  Head trauma
  Apoplexy
Aneurysms of the internal carotid artery
Autoimmune lymphocytic hypophysitis
Hemochromatosis
Primary hypothalamic disorders:
  Tumor
  Granulomas
Idiopathic or genetic deficiencies of hormones within the pituitary or hypothalamus

surrounding regions, these tumors can also cause hormonal deficiency due to compression of other cell lineages within the pituitary.

Prolactin

Prolactin is a polypeptide produced by the lactotrophs of the pituitary; it is responsible for the initiation and maintenance of lactation. Its secretion is normally kept at low levels by the inhibitory actions of dopamine produced by the hypothalamus. As with several pituitary hormones, prolactin is secreted in a circadian fashion, with the highest levels being attained during sleep and a nadir occurring between 10 a.m. and noon (Sassin, 1972). Prolactin is secreted in a pulsatile fashion, the amplitude and frequency of which not only varies throughout the day, but is also impacted upon by a

Table 24-3 Relative Frequency of Occurrence of Pituitary Tumors

Lactotroph (PRL)	30%
Somatotroph (GH)	15%
Combined GH/PRL	8%
Corticotroph (ACTH)	15%
Thyrotroph (TRH)	1%
Pleurihormonal	4%
Nonfunctioning	27%

Table 24-4 Causes of Hyperprolactinemia

Physiologic:
 Sleep, stress, postprandially, pain
 Coitus, pregnancy, nipple stimulation or nursing
Systemic disorders:
 Chest wall or thoracic spinal cord lesions
 Primary or secondary hypothyroidism
 Adrenal insufficiency
 Chronic renal failure
 Cirrhosis
Medications:
 Psychiatric medications:
  phenothiazines, haloperidol, thioxanthines, buspirone, olanzapine, risperidone, domperidone, monoamine oxidase inhibitors, fluoxetine, amitriptylene
 Metoclopramide
 Antihypertensives: labetolol, α-methyldopa, reserpine, verapamil
 Cimetidine, ranitidine
 Estrogens, oral contraceptives, oral contraceptive withdrawal
 Opiates: heroin, methadone, morphine, apomorphine
Prolactin-secreting pituitary tumor: prolactinoma, acromegaly
Macroadenoma (compressing the pituitary stalk)
Macroprolactinemia
Pressure on or transection of the pituitary stalk – interrupting the transmission of dopamine to the D2 receptors on the lactotrophs
Ectopic secretion of prolactin by nonpituitary tumors
Idiopathic
Polycystic ovarian disease
Epileptic seizures

variety of physiologic stimuli (i.e., stress, postprandially, exercise). Because of these factors and a serum half-life of 26–47 minutes, it is recommended that when screening a patient for hyperprolactinemia three specimens be obtained at 20- to 30-minute intervals. These samples can either be analyzed separately and their results averaged, or alternatively, an equal aliquot from each sample can be pooled into one final sample that is then analyzed.

The major circulating form of prolactin is the nonglycosylated monomer. A number of other forms can occur including 'big' prolactin and macroprolactin ('big, big' prolactin), considered to be prolactin coupled with immunoglobulin (Yazigi, 1997; Conner, 1998). Because these forms all react with immunoassays they can result in falsely high PRL results in patients in whom a pathological elevation of PRL is not supported by CT or MRI. Various analytical methods have been developed to eliminate this confusion, including the performance of immunoassay following polyethylene glycol extraction and centrifugal ultrafiltration. (Amadori, 2003; Diver, 2001; Fahie-Wilson, 2003; Toldy, 2003; Prazeres, 2003; Suliman, 2003)

In some instances of prolactinoma, the values of prolactin may be extremely elevated. Because usually only a single dilution is performed when assaying for prolactin, extremely high concentrations may saturate the binding sites resulting in a falsely low result (Barkan, 1998). This 'hook' effect may result in misdiagnosing the patient as having a nonfunctioning chromophobe adenoma. If the pretest probability of the patient having a macroprolactinoma is high, it is recommended that the serum sample be subjected to at least a 1 : 100 dilution.

Prolactin acts on breast tissue, where in the setting of estrogen priming, it stimulates lactation. Prolactin also acts at the hypothalamus to inhibit the secretion of gonadotropin-releasing hormone (GnRH). Inhibition of GnRH results in a decrease in the release of LH and FSH from the anterior pituitary. In females, this leads to a decrease in estrogen and progesterone synthesis and secretion by the ovaries and a failure of ovarian follicular maturation (ovulation). In males, a deficiency of FSH and LH causes a decrease in testicular production and synthesis of testosterone and a halt in spermatogenesis. In addition there is some suggestion that hyperprolactinemia may also stimulate adrenal androgen production as well as have an effect on immune responsiveness (Lobo, 1980; Walker, 1993).

The reference value for serum prolactin is 1–25 ng/mL (1–25 µg/L) for women and 1–20 ng/mL (1–20 µg/L) for men. The higher prolactin levels seen in females begins post-puberty and are presumably due to the stimulatory effect of estrogen (Eastman, 1996). During pregnancy there is a progressive rise in serum prolactin with levels reportedly reaching as high as 500 ng/mL by the third trimester (Rigg, 1977). This is largely due to an increase in number of prolactin-secreting cells and can be associated with a doubling or even greater increase in pituitary gland size (Scheithauer, 1990). Prolactin levels fall back to baseline about 3 weeks postpartum in women who are not breastfeeding. In nursing mothers basal prolactin levels remain moderately elevated and with episodic bursts in secretion in response to suckling.

Prolactin levels are increased by many physiologic and pathologic factors as well as by a wide variety of medications (Table 24–4). Elevations in prolactin resulting from physiologic and pharmacologic stimuli rarely exceed 200 ng/mL.

Prolactin deficiency can be seen with pituitary necrosis or infarction and in some cases of pseudohypoparathyroidism. In women with complete prolactin deficiency, menstrual disorders and infertility have been found (Kauppila, 1997). It is prolactin excess that is associated with clinical pathology. Hyperprolactinemia leads to inhibition of GnRH secretion, which typically manifests as sexual dysfunction and infertility in both men and women. Women may present with luteal phase abnormalities, oligomenorrhea or frank amenorrhea, with or without galactorrhea. Men will present with hypoandrogenemia, decreased libido and impotence.

Pituitary adenomas are an important cause of hyperprolactinemia; however, any sella or parasellar process that compresses the pituitary stalk

and interrupts the tonic delivery of dopamine can lead to a disinhibition of prolactin secretion. Usually the height of elevation of serum prolactin levels correlates with the likelihood of the presence of a pituitary tumor, with levels of prolactin in excess of 200 ng/mL almost always signifying the presence of a prolactinoma (Frantz, 1998; Freda, 1999; Kleinberg, 1977). Unlike other functioning pituitary tumors, the degree of elevation of prolactin correlates fairly well with the size of the tumor.

Hyperprolactinemia exists in 20–40% of patients with acromegaly; this is due either to the presence of a mixed tumor (containing both lactotrophs and somatotrophs) or to interference with the normally active, prolactin-inhibitory mechanisms (e.g., interruption of dopamine delivery owing to stalk compression by a tumor, resulting in disinhibition of prolactin secretion). Another important cause of hyperprolactinemia is hypothyroidism. Thyrotropin-releasing hormone (TRH) not only stimulates TSH secretion but it also stimulates prolactin secretion as well, thus explaining the mild hyperprolactinemia seen in both primary (thyroid) and secondary (pituitary) hypothyroidism. Treatment with thyroid hormone replacement will usually return the prolactin back to normal. Rarely, hyperprolactinemia may be caused by ectopic hormone production.

It is important to evaluate all patients discovered to have an abnormally elevated prolactin. Thyroid-function tests (free thyroxine [FT$_4$] and TSH) are always indicated to rule out hypothyroidism. Since hyperprolactinemia can be found in upwards of 40% of cases of acromegaly, it is appropriate to measure insulin-like growth factor (IGF-1) discussed below. Other hormones that may be assayed include FSH, LH, testosterone, estradiol and if clinically indicated, tests of adrenal axis function. All patients should undergo either CT or MRI of the sella, with and without contrast. MRI provides better contrast and anatomic detail and is better for visualizing microadenomas. Formal visual field examination is also a key monitoring tool in managing patients with pituitary tumors and should be done at least yearly in patients with stable disease.

Growth Hormone

Growth hormone (GH) is synthesized, stored and secreted by the somatotrophs of the pituitary in response to the secretion of growth hormone-releasing hormone (GHRH) by the hypothalamus. Somatostatin, also produced by the hypothalamus, inhibits GH release. Although evidence exists for the direct action of GH on long bone growth in children, the majority of its anabolic and metabolic actions are mediated indirectly through an intermediary, insulin-like growth factor I (IGF-I) (also called somatomedin C). IGF-I is synthesized in the liver and in certain target

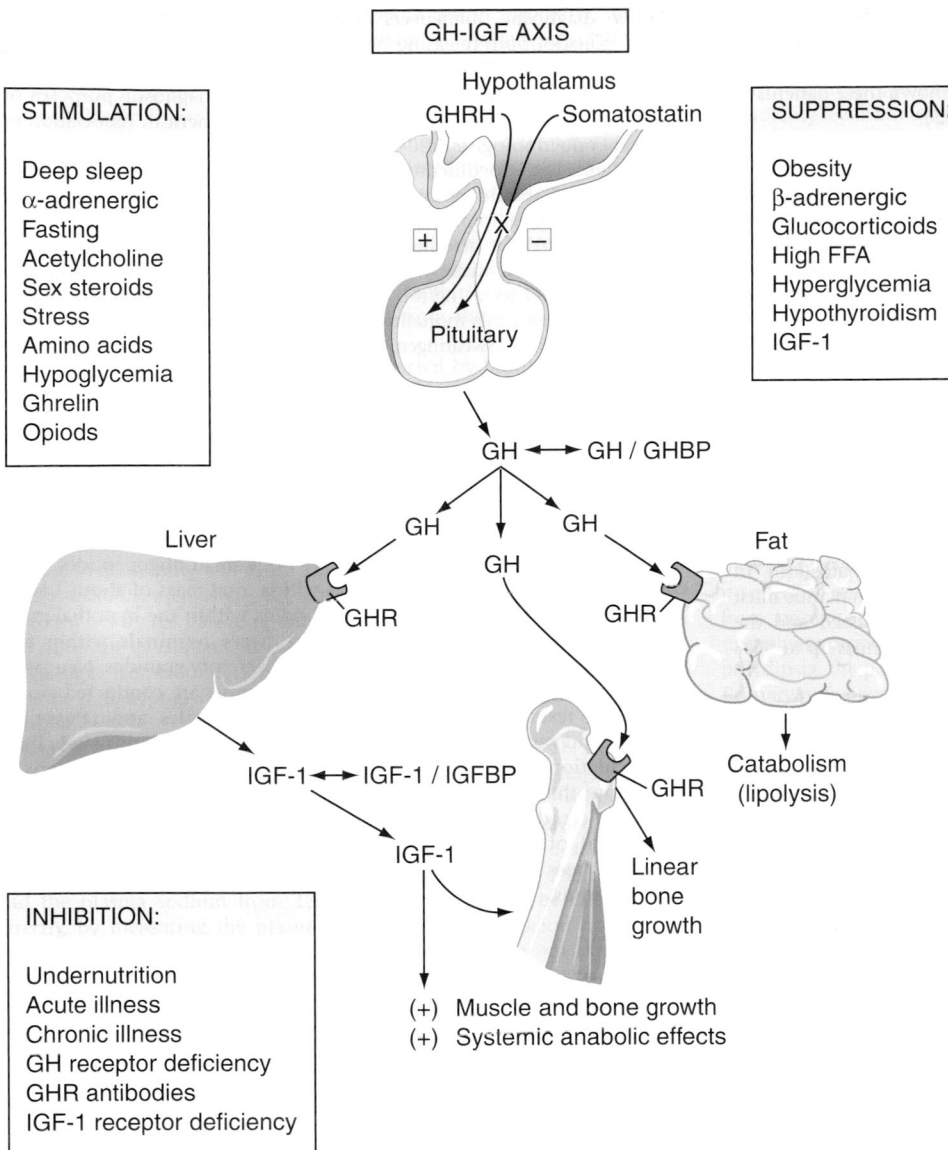

GH-IGF AXIS

Hypothalamus

GHRH — Somatostatin

Pituitary

STIMULATION:

Deep sleep
α-adrenergic
Fasting
Acetylcholine
Sex steroids
Stress
Amino acids
Hypoglycemia
Ghrelin
Opiods

SUPPRESSION:

Obesity
β-adrenergic
Glucocorticoids
High FFA
Hyperglycemia
Hypothyroidism
IGF-1

GH ↔ GH / GHBP

Liver

GH GHR

Fat

GH GHR

Catabolism (lipolysis)

IGF-1 ↔ IGF-1 / IGFBP

IGF-1

GHR

Linear bone growth

INHIBITION:

Undernutrition
Acute illness
Chronic illness
GH receptor deficiency
GHR antibodies
IGF-1 receptor deficiency

(+) Muscle and bone growth
(+) Systemic anabolic effects

Figure 24–2 Hypothalamic–pituitary–growth hormone axis. Feedback loop influencing GH–IGF-1 secretion and action. GHRH = growth hormone-releasing hormone; GH = growth hormone; GHBP = growth hormone-binding protein; GHR = growth hormone receptor; IGF-1 = insulin-like growth hormone 1 (somatomedin C); IGFBP = insulin-like growth hormone-binding protein; FFA = free fatty acids. (After Melmed S, Kleinberg D: Anterior pituitary. *In* Larsen PR, Kronenberg HM, Melmed S, Polonsky KS (eds): Williams Textbook of Endocrinology, 10th ed. Philadelphia: Saunders; 2003:221 with permission.)

tissues, in response to stimulation by GH. IGF-I circulates in the blood complexed to IGF-binding proteins (IGF-BP); IGF-BP3 is the predominant circulating species. As with all hormones, it is the free, unbound form that is biologically active. Similarly to somatostatin, IGF-1 negatively feeds back on the pituitary to inhibit GH secretion.

GH is secreted in a pulsatile fashion; the frequency and amplitude of the peaks are greatest during puberty, exhibiting a steady decline with increasing age (Casanueva, 1992). Since up to 70% of GH secretion occurs during stage 4 (slow wave) sleep, it has been suggested that the age-related decline in stage 4 sleep may account for the decline in GH seen with aging (Van Cauter, 1998, 2000). In addition to GHRH and somatostatin, several other factors regularly mediate GH secretion (Fig. 24–2). Major stress (i.e., surgery, sepsis), fasting, sex steroids, chronic malnutrition, apomorphine, levodopa and high-protein meals all stimulate GH secretion. Women tend to have higher GH levels than men, perhaps due to estrogen sensitization of the hypothalamus to other GH stimuli (Eastman, 1996).

Serum GH is undetectable for most of the day in healthy, nonstressed individuals. This fact along with the episodic nature of GH secretion makes a single sampling difficult to interpret. As a result, the diagnosis of GH deficiency is made using GH measurements following pharmacologic stimulation, and GH excess is confirmed by failure of GH suppression following an oral glucose load. GH is commonly measured by chemi-luminescent immunoassay.

Growth Hormone Deficiency

Idiopathic growth hormone deficiency is the most common cause of GH deficiency (GHD) in children, whereas pituitary adenoma is the most common cause in adult-onset GHD. There is no simple, reproducible method for determining abnormal GH secretory patterns. In healthy

individuals, 70–80% of GH results are below 1 ng/mL (< 1 g/L), but secretory peaks typically reach 20–40 ng/mL (20–40 g/L) (Baumann, 1987). Thus, in a child with decreased growth velocity, a low or nondetectable GH does not necessarily indicate GHD. Similar to GH, IGF-I declines with aging. IGF-1 is more diagnostically useful in patients younger than age 40; however, it is still not sensitive enough to be used as a stand-alone test to make the diagnosis of GHD (Almeretti, 2003).

Manipulation of the endocrine system through stimulation and suppression of the various axes is often required for diagnosing conditions of hormonal deficiency and surfeit. In this vein, GHD is diagnosed by showing a failure of GH to increase adequately in response to pharmacologic stimulation. The insulin tolerance test (ITT) has long been considered the 'gold standard' for diagnosing GHD; however it is most unpleasant for the patient, requires the attendance of a physician throughout the testing period and is contraindicated in those with a history of seizures or, cardiac or cerebrovascular disease. Failure of GH to rise above 5 ng/mL in adults and above 10 ng/mL in children is considered to be abnormal. In subjects unable to undergo ITT or in those needing a second confirmatory test, arginine stimulation alone or in combination with GHRH is usually the next step. Combination testing with GHRH plus arginine is preferred, as many normal adults will fail stimulation with arginine alone (Biller, 2002). A failure of GH to rise above 4.1 carries a sensitivity of 95% and specificity of 91% in diagnosing GH deficiency (Biller, 2002). Other methods to assess for GHD include: 24-hour or night-time monitoring of GH and provocative tests using clonidine, L-dopa, or glucagon (following priming with propranolol). All of these tests carry significant individual variability and have not been systematically studied; they are used mainly in the pediatric population (Rose, 1988). The same normal ranges hold for these tests as described for the ITT. There

Table 24-5 Water-Deprivation Test for Diagnosing and Classifying Diabetes Insipidus

In those with mild polyuria, the patient may be instructed to withhold all fluid intake from 10 p.m. onward. For those with more severe polyuria (8–10 L/day), water deprivation should be started early in the morning under close observation

1. During testing the patient is forbidden to take in anything by mouth
2. Obtain the following baseline parameters: urine vol and osmolality (Uosm), plasma osmolality (Posm) and plasma sodium (P_{Na}). Also record the weight and blood pressure (BP)/pulse (P) seated and standing.
3. Urine and plasma are collected hourly for Uvol, Uosm, Posm. Wt, BP, P are also recorded. Also, record requests for fluid.
4. When either: the Uosm has plateaued (e.g. hourly increase of < 30 mOsm/kg for 3 consecutive hours) or body wt has decreased by 3–5% or the patient develops a > 20 mm/Hg drop in systolic BP — obtain samples for Uvol, Uosm, Posm, P_{Na} and AVP (plasma).
5. Administer 1 μg of desmopressin i.v. or i.m., or 5 μg of aqueous vasopressin (AVP) s.c. Uosm, urine output and plasma osmolality are recorded at 30, 60 and 120 min after the injection. The highest Uosm value is used to evaluate the patient's response to AVP.

Precautions

When possible discontinue any medications that can influence ADH secretion. Observe for hypotension and nausea which may stimulate ADH secretion. The patient should not be permitted to smoke during the test

Interpretation

Normal	Final Uosm before AVP challenge is higher than Posm. Following AVP challenge, the Uosm is less than 10% higher than the maximal Uosm achieved with water restriction alone
Neurogenic DI	Final Uosm before AVP challenge is less than Posm. Following AVP administration there is a greater than 50% increase in Uosm
Nephrogenic DI	Final Uosm before AVP challenge is less than Posm. Following AVP administration there is a less than 10% increase in Uosm
Partial central DI	Uosm may be higher than Posm following dehydration; however, there is only a 10–50% increase in Uosm following the administration of AVP
Partial nephrogenic DI	Uosm may be higher than Posm following dehydration; however, there is a greater than 10% increase in Uosm following the administration of AVP

Plotting the basal and post-dehydration Uosm and plasma ADH on the nomograms from Zerbe & Robertson will permit further distinction between partial nephrogenic DI, partial central DI and primary polydipsia (Figs 24–3 and 24–4)

Uosm = urine osmolality; Posm = plasma osmolity

Table 24-6 Tests in the Differential Diagnosis of Disorders of Water Homeostasis

Disorder	Baseline			After 12-hour fluid restriction			Urine osmolality post-AVP challenge
	Serum Na+ and osmolality	Urine Na+ and osmolality	Serum ADH	Serum Na+ and osmolality	Urine Na+ and osmolality	Serum ADH	
Normal control	N	N	N	N	High	High	Same
SIADH	Low	N–High	High	Low-N	High	High	
Neurogenic DI	N–High	Low	Low	High	Low–N	Low	Increased
Nephrogenic DI	N–High	Low	N–High	High	Low–N	High	Same
Psychogenic polydipsia	Low–N	Low	Low	N	N–High	N–High	Same

SIADH = Syndrome of inappropriate antidiuretic hormone secretion; DI = diabetes insipidus; ADH = antidiuretic hormone; AVP = arginine vasopressin; N = normal.

Syndrome of Inappropriate Secretion of ADH (SIADH)

The syndrome of inappropriate secretion of ADH (SIADH) is characterized by a euvolemic hypo-osmolar hyponatremia, associated with a hyperosmolar urine (the result of a continued inappropriate natriuresis). By definition, SIADH cannot be diagnosed until nonosmotic stimuli for ADH secretion and other pathologies that interfere with free water clearance have been excluded (Vistorina, 2002). Physiologic triggers of ADH secretion include nausea, pregnancy, hypoglycemia, intracranial hypertension, mechanical ventilation and hypoxia. Hypothyroidism and glucocorticoid deficiency cause a decrease in free water clearance leading to a dilutional hyponatremia. Mineralocorticoid deficiency can lead to hyponatremia due to increased renal sodium loss. It is therefore extremely important to test for deficiencies of these axes and to institute appropriate hormonal replacement therapy before making a diagnosis of SIADH. Other confounding factors that can hamper the diagnosis of SIADH include renal disease, cardiac disease and medications such as diuretics. In these situations, one can cautiously perform a water load test (Table 24–8). In the absence of medications or other conditions that may impair diuresis, a failure to excrete 80–90% of the administered water load within 4 hours and suppress the Uosm to < 100 mOsm/kg is consistent with the diagnosis of SIADH.

In the right clinical setting, the diagnosis of SIADH can often confidently be made based upon serum and urine electrolyte determinations alone. A spot urine Na+ < 30 mEq/L can distinguish those with hyponatremia due to volume depletion, from those with SIADH, in whom the urine Na+ > 30 mEq/L (Chung, 1987). In contrast, differentiating the patient with euvolemia and SIADH from one with hypovolemia and

concomitant renal salt wasting (e.g., salt-losing nephropathy, diuretic use) can be much more difficult. In addition to hyponatremia, both have a spot U_{Na^+} > 30 mEq/L and a fractional excretion of Na+ > 1. The fractional excretion of sodium (FE_{Na} [%]) is calculated as:

$$\frac{U_{[Na^+]} \times P_{[Cr]}}{P_{[Na^+]} \times U_{[Cr]}} \times 100 \qquad (24–2)$$

where $U_{[Na^+]}$ = urine sodium concentration; $P_{[Na^+]}$ = plasma sodium concentration; $U_{[Cr]}$ = urine creatinine concentration; $P_{[Cr]}$ = plasma creatinine concentration.

One way to differentiate between the two is to administer 1 L of 0.9% NaCl intravenously over 24 hours for 2 days. A rise of serum Na+ by more than 5 mEq/L is suggestive of hypovolemia. In SIADH there is either no change or an increase of less than 5 mEq/L. Alternatively, fluid restriction to 600–800 mL/day for 2–3 days will lead to improvement in hyponatremia in SIADH but not in renal salt-wasting (Table 24–6).

The etiology for renal salt-wasting in SIADH is twofold. At the onset of the disease, there is volume expansion, which inhibits the renin–aldosterone axis and also leads to greater delivery of sodium to the distal tubules. Continued sodium loss is due to secretion of atrial natiuretic protein (Kamoi, 1990)

Because of hyperfiltration and the local actions of ADH on the renal V2 receptor, SIADH is one of the two states in which some of the lowest uric acid levels occur; the other is pregnancy. In SIADH the serum levels of ADH may be variably increased, usually out of proportion to Posm; however, approximately 20% of cases meeting the physiologic diagnosis of

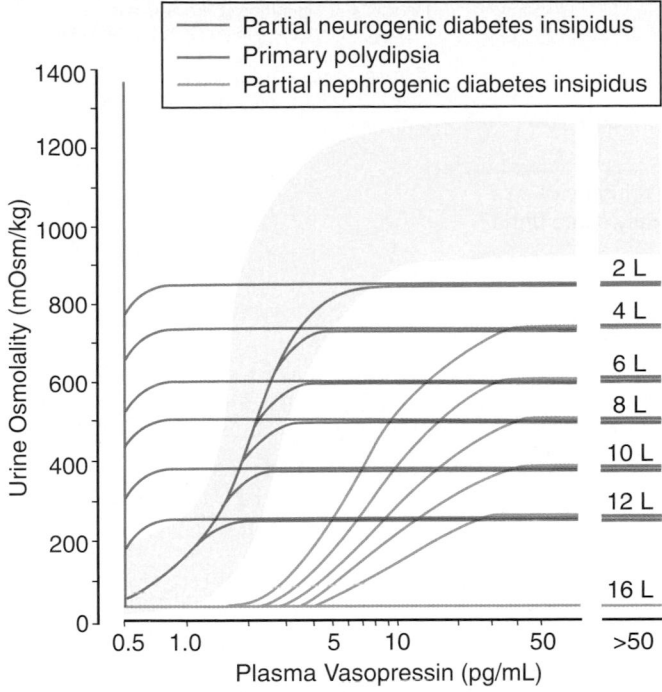

Figure 24–3 The relationship between urine osmolality and plasma vasopressin (ADH) in patients with polyuria of diverse etiologies and severity. Each of the three categories of polyuria is described by its own family of sigmoid curves of differing heights. The differences in height within a family reflect differences in maximum concentrating capacity due to 'washout' of the medullary concentration gradient. They are proportional to the severity of the polyuria (indicated in liters per day at the right end of each plateau). The normal response is depicted in yellow. The three categories of polyuria differ principally in the ascending portion of the dose–response curve. In patients with partial neurogenic diabetes insipidus, the curve lies to the left of normal, reflecting increased sensitivity to the antidiuretic effects of very low concentrations of plasma ADH. In contrast, in patients with partial nephrogenic diabetes insipidus, the curve lies to the right of normal, reflecting decreased sensitivity to ADH. In primary polydipsia, the relationship of Uosm to ADH remains relatively normal. (Redrawn from Bichet DG: Diabetes Insipides and Vasopressin. *In* Moore WT, Eastman RC, eds: Diagnostic Endocrinology, 2nd edn. St. Louis: Mosby; 1996:158, with permission.)

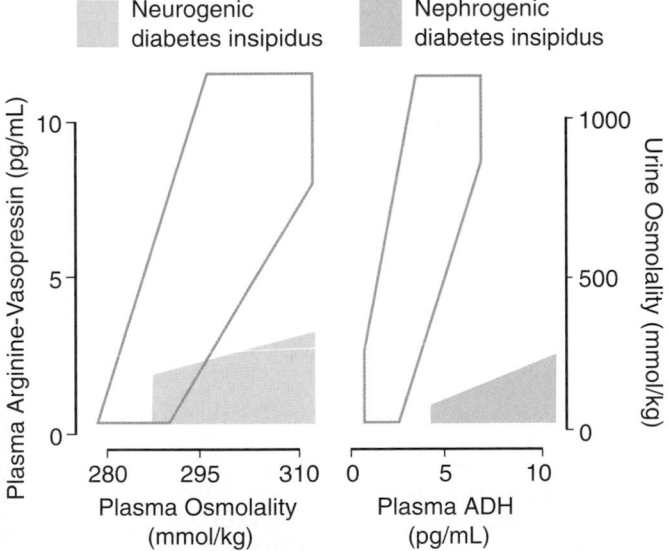

Figure 24–4 *Left:* Relationship between plasma arginine vasopressin (ADH) and plasma osmolality during the infusion of hypertonic saline. Patients with primary polydipsia and nephrogenic diabetes insipidus have values within the normal range (open area) in contrast to patients with neurogenic diabetes insipidus, who show a subnormal plasma ADH response to a rise in osmolality (pink). *Right:* Relationship between urine osmolality and plasma ADH during dehydration and water loading. Patients with primary polydipsia and neurogenic diabetes have values within the normal range (open area) in contrast to patients with nephrogenic diabetes insipidus, who have hypotonic urine despite high plasma ADH (green). (Redrawn from Bichet DG: Diabetes Insipides and Vasopressin. *In* Moore TW, Eastman RC, eds: Diagnostic Endocrinology, 2nd edn. St. Louis: Mosby; 1996:168, with permission.)

Table 24–7 Causes of Diabetes Insipidus

Central

Primary:
  Familial
  Idiopathic
Acquired:
  Tumors – craniopharyngioma, pituitary tumors, metastases (i.e., lung, breast), Rathke's cleft cyst, nonlymphocytic leukemia
  Granulomatous disorders – sarcoidosis, Langerhans' cell histiocytosis, Wegener's granulomatosis
  Traumatic – head trauma, surgery
  Infectious – tuberculosis, meningitis, encephalitis
  Vascular – cerebral aneurysm, sickle cell, Shehan's syndrome
  Drugs – alcohol, diphenylhydantoin, chlorpromazine and α-adrenergic agonists
  Other – lymphocytic hypophysitis, hypoxic encephalopathy

Nephrogenic

Hereditary:
  Mutation in the V2 receptor
  Mutation in the aquaporin gene
Acquired:
  Drugs – lithium, phenytoin, demeclocycline, vinblastine, cisplatinum, propoxyphene, colchicine, gentamicin, amphotericin, ethanol, atrial natriuretic hormone, norepinephrine, methoxyflurane anesthetics, furosemide
  Electrolyte disorders – hypercalcemia, hypokalemia
  Systemic illnesses – sickle cell, multiple myeloma, amyloidosis, sarcoidosis, Sjögren's syndrome, polycystic kidney disease
  Other – low-protein diet, post-obstructive uropathy

Table 24–8 Water Load Test

1 Baseline: the patient must be euvolemic and have a serum Na$^+$ between 125–150 mmol/L and Posm > 275 mOsm/kg

2 The patient is given 20 mL of water per kilogram of body weight (max. = 1500 mL) to drink over 30 minutes

3 With the patient maintained in the recumbent position, urine output is collected every hour for the next 5 hours. Record the volume and osmolality of each specimen

Interpretation

Normals	Excrete 80–90% of the administered water load within 4 hours and suppress the Uosm to < 100 mOsm/kg
SIADH	Failure to meet these criteria in the absence of medications or other conditions that may impair diuresis is consistent with the diagnosis of SIADH

SIADH will not have detectable levels of ADH (Zerbe, 1980). This may be due to insensitivity of the assay to low levels of ADH, an increased renal sensitivity to ADH, or perhaps the presence of another hormone with antidiuretic activity (Kamoi, 1997).

The diagnosis of SIADH is largely a diagnosis of exclusion, having ruled out other causes for hyponatremia (Fig. 24–5). It most often occurs as a manifestation of the paraneoplastic syndrome; however, it may also occur in central nervous system (CNS) trauma or infection, lung disease or from medications (vinca alkaloids, tricyclic antidepressants, serotonin receptor uptake inhibitors [SSRIs]) (Table 24–9).

Thyroid Gland

The normal thyroid gland weighs about 15–25 grams. It is divided into lobules that are each composed of 20–40 follicles separated by highly vascular connective tissue. The follicles are ring-shaped structures, in which a single cell band of follicular cells surrounds a central hub containing colloid, thyroid hormone, thyroglobulin (Tg) and a variety of other glycoproteins. The follicles are the site of thyroid hormone synthesis and storage. The thyroid gland also contains parafollicular or C-cells, which are responsible for the synthesis and secretion of calcitonin, a hormone important in calcium metabolism.

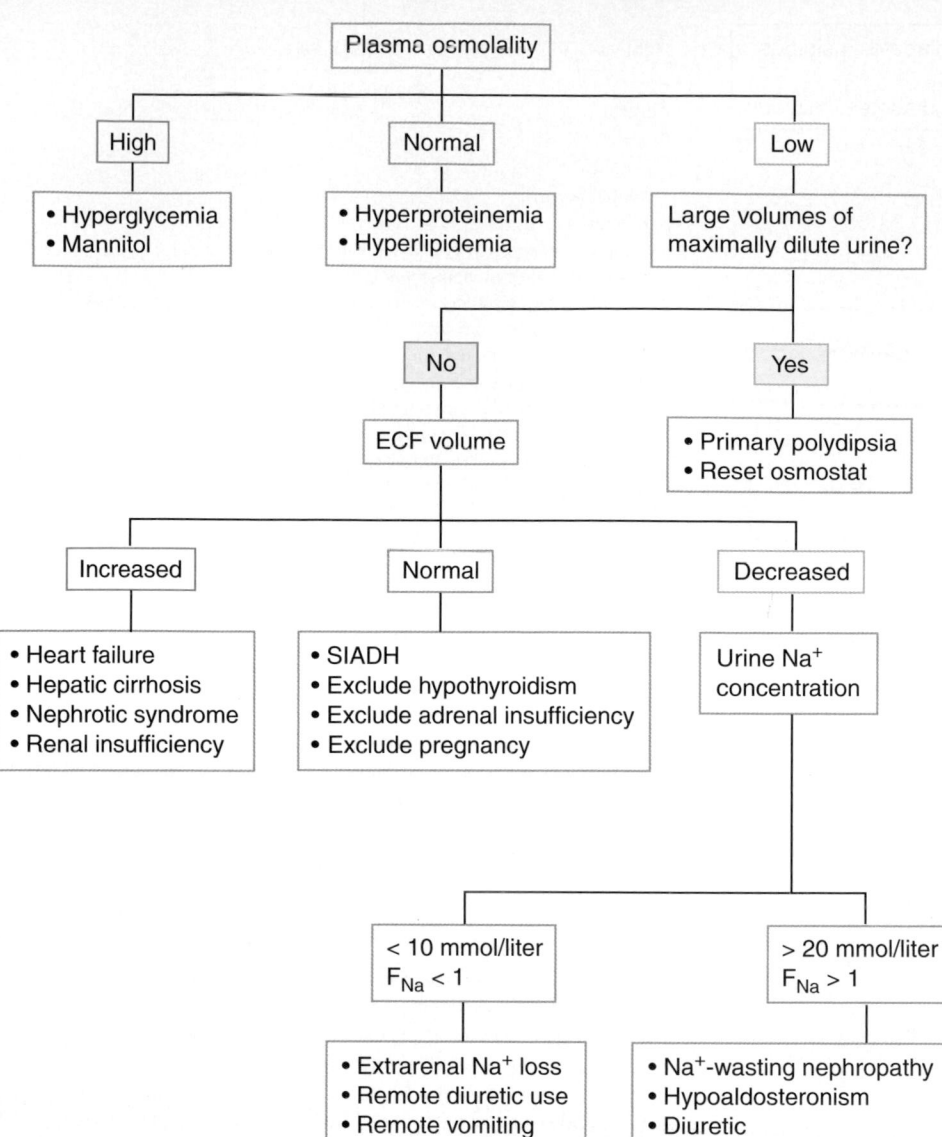

Figure 24–5 Algorithm for the evaluation of hyponatremia. (After Singer GG: Fluid and electrolyte management. *In* Carey CF, Lee HH, Woeltje KF (eds): The Washington Manual of Medical Therapeutics, 29th ed. Philadelphia, Lippincott-Raven, 1998, p 44 with permission.)

An intact hypothalamic–pituitary–thyroid (HPT) axis and a ready source of iodide are required for normal thyroid hormone synthesis. The hypothalamus secretes thyrotropin-releasing hormone (TRH), which in turn stimulates the thyrotrophs of the anterior pituitary to secrete thyroid-stimulating hormone (TSH, thyrotropin). As implied by the name, TSH stimulates thyroid hormone synthesis and secretion by the thyroid gland. Thyroid hormone acts peripherally to mediate numerous metabolic activities; it also negatively feeds back on the hypothalamus and pituitary to maintain thyroid hormone concentrations within narrow limits.

Under TSH stimulation, iodine enters the follicular cells as inorganic iodide and is transformed into thyroid hormones, thyroxine (T_4) and 3,5,3'-triiodothyronine (T_3) through a series of metabolic steps. The sequence of events as depicted in Figure 24–6 can be broken down into: (1) active transport of iodide into the cell; (2) iodination of the tyrosyl residues on Tg; (3) coupling of iodotyrosine molecules within Tg to form T_4 and T_3; (4) proteolysis of Tg with release of free iodotyrosine, T_4 and T_3, and secretion of iodothyronine into the circulation; (5) deiodination of iodotyrosines within the thyroid and reuse of liberated iodide; and (6) deiodination of T_4 to T_3.

One hundred percent of circulating T_4 is of thyroidal origin whereas only 20% of T_3 is of thyroidal origin; 80% is produced enzymatically in nonthyroidal tissues by 5'-monodeiodination of T_4 (Lum, 1984). Approximately 110 nmol (85 μg) of T_4 and 10 nmol (8.5 μg) of T_3 are produced daily by the thyroid. The thyroid hormones circulate attached to plasma proteins. About 70% of T_4 is bound to thyroxine-binding globulin (TBG), 20% to transthyretin (formerly called binding prealbumin) and 10% to albumin. While most of the circulating T_3 is bound to TBG, it does so with a tenfold reduced affinity as compared with that of T_4 (Braverman, 2000;

Robbins, 1996). A small percentage of T_4 and T_3 remains unbound to protein, with about 0.03% of T_4 and 0.3% of T_3 arising by peripheral deiodination, with the liver and kidney having an important role in this transformation. As with other hormones, it is the free component that is metabolically active.

Table 24–9 Causes of SIADH

CNS disease:
  Neoplasm, infection, trauma, cerebrovascular accident

Neoplasm:
  Oat cell carcinoma and adenocarcinoma of the lung, pancreatic cancer, lymphoma

Pulmonary infection:
  TB, pneumonia, positive-pressure ventilation

Idiopathic

Medications:
  Oral hypoglycemics – chlorpropamide, tolbutamide
  Antineoplastics – vincristine, cyclophosphamide
  Diuretics – hydrochlorothiazide
  Psychotropics – amitriptyline, phenothiazines, selective serotonin reuptake inhibitors (SSRIs), monoamine oxidase inhibitors
  Other – morphine, barbiturates, clofibrate, nicotine, acetylcholine, anesthetic agents, β-adrenergic stimulants, metoclopramide, desmopressin

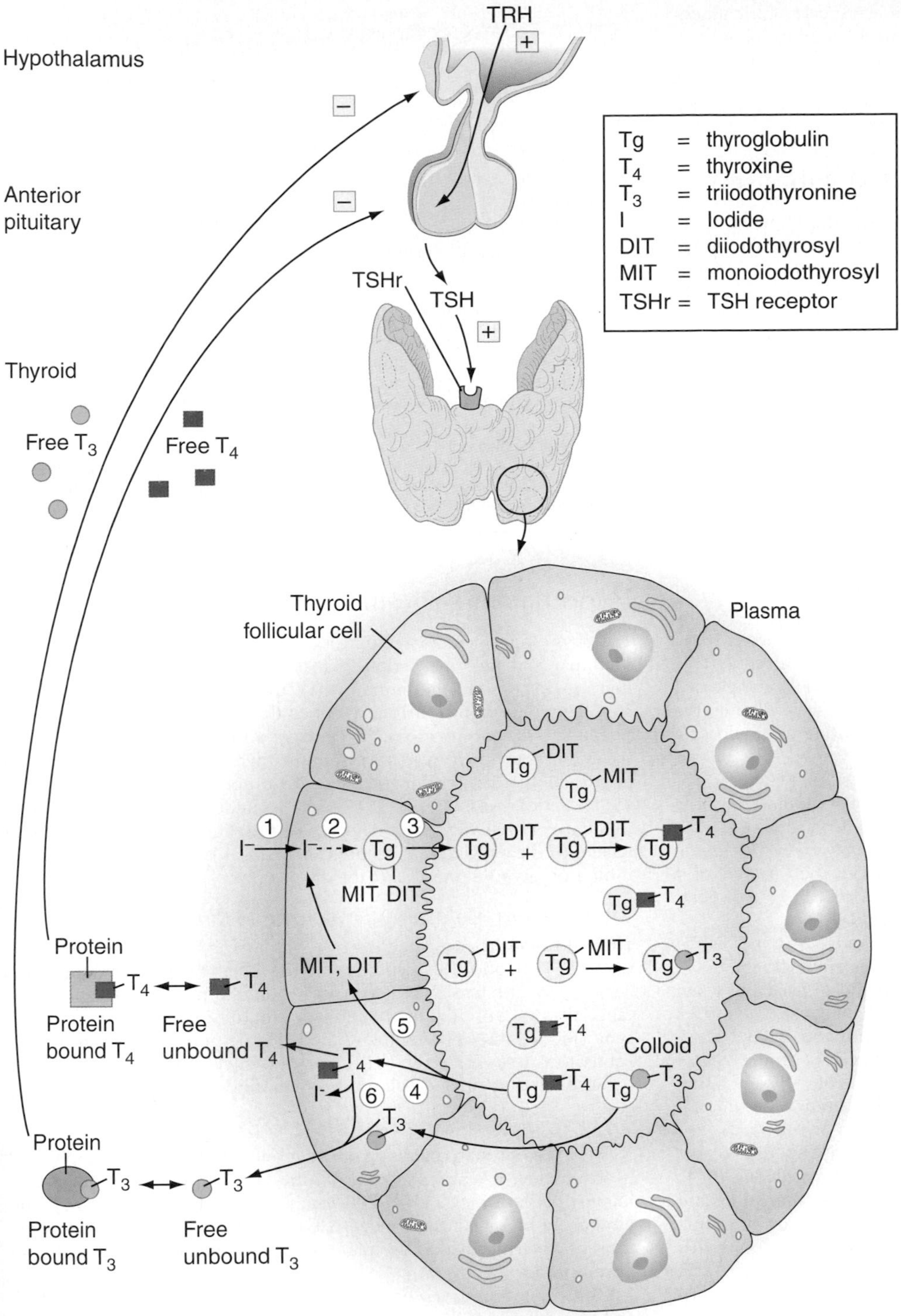

Figure 24–6 Hypothalamic–pituitary–thyroid axis and thyroid hormone synthesis. The steps for thyroid hormone synthesis and release are described in further detail in the text.

Tg	=	thyroglobulin
T_4	=	thyroxine
T_3	=	triiodothyronine
I	=	Iodide
DIT	=	diiodothyrosyl
MIT	=	monoiodothyrosyl
TSHr	=	TSH receptor

Thyroid disease may be classified into hyperthyroidism, hypothyroidism and euthyroidism. Signs and symptoms of hyperthyroidism include heat intolerance, tachycardia, weight loss, weakness, emotional lability and tremor. The most common clinical syndrome associated with hyperthyroidism is Graves' disease caused by circulating antibodies to the TSH receptor. Other disorders that lead to hyperthyroidism include toxic adenoma and rarely, TSH-secreting pituitary tumors and thyroid carcinoma.

Hypothyroidism results in hoarseness, cold sensitivity, dry skin, constipation, bradycardia and muscle weakness. Myxedema coma is an advanced stage of thyroid hormone deficiency characterized by progressive stupor, hypothermia and hypoventilation. Failure of the thyroid itself to secrete an adequate amount of thyroid hormone is called primary hypothyroidism and is most commonly iatrogenic in origin, the result of either ablation with radioactive iodine or surgery to treat hyperthyroidism. Secondary hypothyroidism occurs when TSH secretion is decreased as a result of a pituitary disorder. Tertiary hypothyroidism is the result of hypothalamic dysfunction.

Thyroid diseases such as goiter, thyroid adenoma and thyroid carcinoma typically occur in individuals who are euthyroid. The development of more sensitive assays permits the diagnosis of subclinical hyper- and hypothyroidism: these patients appear clinically euthyroid; however, their TSH values are respectively either suppressed or elevated. A number of clinical situations can lead to difficulties in the interpretation of thyroid function tests: the presence of abnormal protein-binding proteins (either congenital or drug induced), alterations in thyroid hormone metabolism as seen in those hospitalized with acute psychiatric illness, or those on medications that either affect thyroid hormone binding or the HPT axis directly. The most important and most common problem with thyroid function tests probably occurs in those patients with various illnesses that do not directly involve the thyroid, so-called nonthyroidal illness.

Thyroid Hormone Synthesis and Metabolism

Iodine is a major component of thyroid hormone; the main source of iodine is dietary intake. Deiodination of organic iodine containing moieties within the gland serves as another source. Inorganic iodide is transported into the follicular cell by the sodium–iodide symporter (NIS) located in the basolateral membrane (Chambard, 1983). TSH modulates NIS activity: an increase in TSH secretion augments the uptake of iodide into the follicular cell. Iodide transport into the thyroid gland is also influenced by the serum iodide level; iodide deficiency increases pump activity and iodide excess inhibits iodide uptake.

Thyroglobulin is a glycoprotein synthesized by the rough endoplasmic reticulum in the basal and perinuclear regions of the follicular cell. It is acted upon by the Golgi apparatus in the apical portion of the follicular cell, where its tyrosyl residues are iodinated leading to the formation of mono- and diiodotyrosyls (MIT and DIT). Tg is then transferred into the colloid for storage (Vassart, 1973a; Roth, 1985). This transformation of thyroglobulin into thyroid hormone requires two separate oxidative reactions both catalyzed by thyroid peroxidase (TPO), the binding of iodide to Tg tyrosyl residues to form the iodotyrosyls MIT and DIT, and the subsequent coupling of MIT and DIT to produce T_4 and T_3. (Deme, 1976; Bjorkman, 1981). T_4 is formed by the coupling of two molecules of DIT; T_3 results from the union of one MIT and one DIT. T_4 and T_3 are released from Tg via lysosomal degradation. They are then secreted into the circulation at the basal membrane. All these reactions are under the control of TSH.

About half of all T_4 is monodeiodinated in the 5' position to form T_3 3, 5, 3' triiodothyronine about 40% undergoes deiodination of the inner ring of T_4 to form reverse T_3 (rT_3 3, 3', 5' triiodothyronine). The formation of rT_3, the third major circulating form of thyroid hormone, is catalyzed by the enzyme 5-deiodinase. Reverse T_3 has no biologic activity, has a short half-life of 4 hours, circulates bound to TBG and its formation is considered a disposal pathway in the peripheral metabolism of T_4 (LoPresti, 1989).

The intake of iodide influences the DIT to MIT ratio in Tg. DIT is the preferential iodotyrosine formed, thus when there is abundant iodide, T_4 is the predominant form of hormone synthesized and secreted, but when iodide sources are diminished, MIT is produced in greater quantities leading to more T_3 formation and release. In addition, the thyroid gland has a 5'-deiodinase that converts T_4 to T_3. This process is under the control of TSH so that T_3 secretion is enhanced during periods of TSH stimulation (i.e., primary hypothyroidism and cases with TSH-stimulating immunoglobulin [TSI]) (Ishii, 1983).

The monodeiodination of T_4 to T_3 and rT_3 accounts for 70% of the peripheral metabolism of T_4 (LoPresti, 1989), the remainder of T_4 metabolism occurs by conjugation of T_4 to sulfate, deamination and decarboxylation to form the acetic acid analog tetrac, and by ether link cleavage (Engler, 1989) (Table 24–10). T_3 but not rT_3 can be conjugated with sulfate to form T_3-sulfate and can be converted to its acetic acid analog, triac (Engler, 1989). The enzymes responsible for these reactions are the phenolsulfotransferases which are present in many tissues throughout the body and the L-aminotransferase located in the liver, respectively (Engler, 1984).

Protein-bound thyroid hormones do not enter cells and are considered to be biologically inert and function as storage reservoirs for circulating thyroid hormones. In contrast, the minute levels of free hormone fractions readily enter cells by specific membrane transport mechanism to exert their biological effects. These effects are mediated by T_3 receptors located in the nucleus of the cell.

Four isoforms of the T_3 receptors have been described: α_1, α_2, β_1 and β_2 (Brent, 1991). α_1 and β_1 receptors are present in most tissues. Binding of T_3 to them promotes thyroid hormone action, presumably by increasing mRNA and protein synthesis. The β_2 receptor is unique to the pituitary and is central in the negative-feedback regulation of TSH by thyroid hormone. The α_2 receptor is inhibitory and acts as a negative regulator of thyroid hormone action.

Mutations in the β receptors, which diminish the ability of T_3 to bind to the nucleus, have been described in the syndrome of thyroid hormone resistance. Individuals with this syndrome have growth and mental retardation of varying degrees as well as hypothyroidism (Refetoff, 1991).

Table 24–10 Metabolic Dynamics of T_4 and T_3

	T_4	T_3
Production rate (nmol/day)	110	50
Fraction of circulating hormone of thyroid origin	100%	20%*
Serum concentration		
Total (nmol/L)	100	1.8
Free (pmol/L)	20	5
Fraction of total hormone in free form	0.0002	0.003
Half-life (days)	~ 7	0.75
Relative metabolic potency	0.3	1.0

* 80% of circulating T_3 comes from the peripheral deiodination of T_4. To convert total T_4 from nmol/L to μg/dL or free T_4 from pmol/L to ng/dL divide by 12.87. To convert total T_3 from nmol/L to ng/dL or free T_3 from pmol/L to pg/dL, multiply by 65.1.

After Larsen PR, Davies TF, Schlumberger MJ, Hay ID: Thyroid physiology and diagnostic evaluation of patients with thyroid disorders. *In* Larsen PR, Kronenberg HM, Melmed S, Polonsky KS (eds): Williams Textbook of Endocrinology, 10th ed. Philadelphia, Saunders, 2003, p 342.

Hypothalamic–Pituitary–Thyroid (HPT) Axis

The physiologic regulators responsible for integrating the function of the thyroid gland and the periphery include the hypothalamic hormone, thyrotropin-releasing hormone (TRH); the pituitary hormone, thyroid-stimulating hormone (TSH) also termed thyrotropin; and the serum free-T_4 and free-T_3 concentrations. TRH enhances TSH synthesis, stimulates the secretion of any preformed TSH from the thyrotrophs and modulates the bioactivity of TSH, resulting in the secretion of bioactive TSH (Shupnik, 1986; Beck-Peccos, 1985). TRH itself is under the negative-feedback influence of circulating thyroid hormones (TRH mRNA levels are inversely related to the circulating T_3 values (Kakucska, 1992). The same feedback inhibition occurs at the level of the thyrotrophs.

Thyrotropin-Releasing Hormone (TRH)

Thyroid hormones regulate their own production by feedback inhibition to both TRH and TSH synthesis in the hypothalamus and pituitary, respectively. TRH acts also on the production of other pituitary hormones, especially prolactin. Leptin plays a significant role in the regulation of TRH gene (Bjobeck, 2004) affecting the individual's appetite for food intake. Laboratory tests for serum TRH are not useful for thyroid disorders because it is difficult to develop a specific antibody.

Thyroid-Stimulating Hormone (TSH)

TSH is a glycoprotein consisting of two mono-covalently linked alpha and beta subunits. The alpha-subunit has the same amino acid sequences as luteinizing hormone (LH), follicle-stimulating hormones (FSH) and human chorionic gonadotropin (HCG). It is the beta-subunit that carries the specific information to the binding receptors for expression of hormonal activities.

The radioimmunoassay for measuring TSH was first developed by Odell and colleagues in 1965. By the mid-1980s a 'sensitive' immunometric TSH method using either monoclonal or polyclonal antibodies was developed which had an improved sensitivity to 0.1–0.2 mU/L. A third-generation nonisotopic immunometric TSH assay using a chemiluminescent label was developed in the 1990s; this is the assay method which is currently in common use. Its sensitivity was reduced to about 0.005 mU/L, which is 100 times more sensitive than the most 'sensitive' TSH assay and 1000 times more sensitive than radioimmunoassay methods. Although a fourth-generation TSH assay has recently been developed with a sensitivity of 0.0004 mU/L, in addition to it not being widely available the third-generation assays provide sufficient sensitivity for the vast majority of clinical applications. The American Thyroid Association (ATA) recommendations state that third-generation assays should be able to quantitate TSH in the 0.010–0.020 mU/L range on an interassay basis with a coefficient of variation of 20% or less. In reporting assay results the ATA recommends using functional sensitivity, defined as the point at which the interassay precision has a coefficient of variation equal to or less than 20% (Spencer, 1996).

Owing to improvements in the sensitivity of the TSH assay, this test alone can identify virtually all instances of hyperthyroidism and hypothyroidism, except when there is damage to the hypothalamus or

Table 24–11 Characterization of Thyroid Disorders According to Results of Thyroid Function Tests

Disorder	TSH	T_4	T_3	FT_4	Tg	TBG	rT_3	ATPO	ATG	TBII	TSI	TBA
Primary hypothyroidism	↑	↓	N or ↓	↓	N or ↓	N	↓	N or ↑	N or ↑	N or ↑	n	n or ↑
Transient neonatal hypothyroidism	↑	↓	↓	↓	N or ↓	N	↓	N	N	↑	n	↑
Hashimoto thyroiditis hypothyroidism	↑	N or ↓	N or ↓	N or ↓	N or ↓	N	↓	↑	↑	n or ↑	n	n or ↑
Graves' disease	↓	↑	↑	↑	↑	N	↑	↑	↑	↑	↑	n or ↑
Neonatal Graves' disease	↓	↑	↑	↑	↑	N	↑	n or ↑	n or ↑	↑	↑	n or ↑
TSH deficiency	N or ↓	↓	↓	↓	↓	N	↓	n	n	n	n	n
Thyroid dishormonogenesis	↑	↓	↓	↓	N, ↓ or ↑	N	↑	n	n	n	n	n
Thyroid hormone resistance	N or ↑	↑	↑	↑	↑	N	↑	n	n	n	n	n
TSH-dependent hyperthyroidism	↑	↑	↑	↑	↑	N	↑	n	n	n	n	n
T_4 protein-binding abnormalities*	N	V	V	N	N	V+	V	n	n	n	n	n
Nonthyroidal illness	V	N or ↓	↓	V	N	N	N or ↑	n	n	n	n	n
Subacute thyroiditis†	↓ or ↑	↑ or ↓	↑ or ↓	↑ or ↓	↑ or ↓	N	↑ or ↓	n	n	n	n	n

TSH = thyroid-stimulating hormone; T_4 = thyroxine; T_3 = triiodothyronine; FT_4 = free thyroxine; Tg = thyroglobulin; TBG = thyroxine-binding globulin; rT_3 = reverse T3; ATPO = antithyroid peroxidase; ATG = antithyroglobulin; TBII = TSH-binding inhibiting immunoglobulin; TSI = thyroid-stimulating immunoglobulin; TBA = TSH receptor-blocking antibody; N = normal; n = negative; V = variable.

* The spectrum of binding protein abnormalities includes increased or decreased TBG binding, increased or decreased transthyretin binding, and ↑ albumin binding.

† Subacute thyroiditis involves a transient period of hyperthyroidism followed by a transient hypothyroid state.

After Fisher DA (ed): Disorders of Thyroid Function, online version of the Quest Diagnostic Manual, 3rd ed. p 268.

pituitary, thyroid hormone resistance, or interference with normal functioning of the HPT axis due to medication. TSH results within the reference interval usually exclude thyroid dysfunction and help distinguish the profound TSH suppression typical of severe Graves' thyrotoxicosis (TSH < 0.01 mIU/L) from the modest degrees of TSH suppression (0.01–0.1 mIU/L) observed with mild (subclinical) primary hyperthyroidism and some cases of nonthyroidal illness. Of note, as assay sensitivity has improved, the normal range has not changed, remaining between approximately 0.5–5.0 mIU/L in most laboratories. However, the serum TSH concentration detected in patients with severe thyrotoxicosis has been lower with each successive improvement in the TSH assays: using a fourth generation assay, the serum TSH is < 0.004 mIU/L in patients with severe hyperthyroidism. Hyperthyroid patients have suppressed TSH values, with the exception of those few individuals who have hyperthyroidism caused by a TSH-producing tumor or other diseases such as pituitary resistance to thyroid hormone. Subclinical hyperthyroidism is defined by the presence of a low TSH with normal levels of T_4 and T_3 (Table 24–11).

In most individuals with hypothyroidism, serum TSH results are clearly elevated, but results may be inappropriately normal for the level of T_4 and T_3 in those with pituitary and hypothalamic disorders. The term subclinical hypothyroidism is used to describe patients with elevated TSH concentration but with normal levels of T_4, T_3 and free thyroxine (FT_4). An important cause for both increased and decreased TSH results is nonthyroidal illness (NTI). Patients with NTI tend to have low TSH results during their acute illness, then TSH rises to within or above the reference range with resolution of the underlying illness, ultimately returning to the normal once the acute illness has resolved. The situation is complicated because medications, including glucagons, opioids, glucocorticoids and dopamine suppress TSH. The sensitive TSH assays are helpful in the evaluation of thyroid hormone treatment for both replacement therapy and suppressive therapy.

Despite the clinical sensitivity of TSH, a TSH-centered strategy has two primary limitations. First, it assumes that hypothalamic–pituitary function is intact and normal. Second, it assumes that the patient is stable (i.e., the patient had no recent therapy for hyper- or hypothyroidism) (Wardle, 2001). If either of these criteria is not met, the serum TSH result can be misleading (Table 24–11). In these instances, to confirm the presence of thyroid dysfunction, in addition to measuring TSH, measurement of free T_4 (FT_4) with or without total T_4 may prove helpful. Serum Free T_3 along with serum TSH measurements are appropriate in patients suspected of hyperthyroidism as they may have T_3 thyrotoxicosis, which is characteristically associated with a normal to low-normal T_4.

Thyroxine

After release from its thyroid follicles, thyroxine will bind to various proteins in the blood (thyroid-binding globulin, albumin, thyretin). Thyroxine can be measured by immunoassay after separating the hormone from his carrier protein. The reference range is 5–12.5 μg/dL in adults with slightly lower results for certain pediatric age groups. Although TSH is the most important test of thyroid function, thyroxine measurements are often used along with TSH and can be important in interpreting TSH results. The combination of a low T_4 and an increased TSH is indicative of primary hypothyroidism, whereas an elevated T_4 and T_3 along with a decreased TSH are characteristic of primary hyperthyroidism. Hyperthyroidism, however, has been reported in patients with an elevated serum T_4 but with serum T_3 levels within the reference range or low. This so-called T_4 thyrotoxicosis can occur in patients with iodine-induced thyrotoxicosis, patients on beta-blockers, amiodarone or large doses of steroids, and in thyrotoxic patients with NTI. A suppressed TSH level associated with a normal to normal-low T_4 and a high T_3 characterizes T_3 thyrotoxicosis. This is more common in a toxic nodule (Table 24–11).

Severe nonthyroidal illness is associated with low T_4 as well as low T_3, this so-called low T_4 and T_3 syndrome (an adaptive response to reduce metabolic demands and conserve protein stores (LoPresti, 1995)) and is associated with a poor prognosis (Chopra, 1997). It is thought to arise from a maladjusted central inhibition of hypothalamic-releasing hormone (TRH) (Van den Berghe, 1998; 2000) (Fig. 24–7).

Euthyroid hyperthyroxinemia is distinguished by the presence of an increased serum T_4 level in association with a normal TSH, in an otherwise euthyroid individual. This entity has a variety of causes including increased binding proteins as may be seen with certain drugs (e.g., estrogen) or medical conditions (e.g., liver disease). It is also seen in patients who are acutely hospitalized for psychiatric illness and in patients with familial dysalbuminemia. When medications or other factors cause an increased protein binding, there is a consequent increase in the serum total T_4 level; conversely, a decrease in binding capacity leads to a decrease in serum total T_4. These perturbations do not have any physiologic effect, as it is the free hormone, not the protein-bound component that is bioactive. In these situations, free T_4 correlates better with thyroid functional status than does serum total T_4.

Table 24–13 Urinary Iodine Excretion and Iodine Deficiency

Urinary Iodine Excretion µg/L	> 100	50–99	20–49	< 20
degree of deficiency*	none	mild	moderate	severe
Goiter prevalence	< 5%	5–19.9%	2–29.9%	> 30%

* IDD Newsletter Aug 1999; 15:33–48.

From Demers LM, Spencer CA (eds): NACB Laboratory Support for the Diagnosis and Monitoring of Thyroid Disease. 2003, p 75.

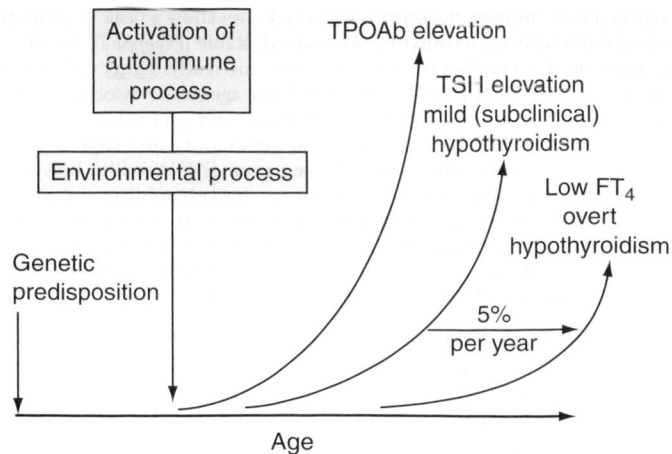

Figure 24–8 Depiction of the evolution of primary hypothyroidism of autoimmune etiology. (From Demers LM, Spencer CA: NACB: Laboratory support for the diagnosis and monitoring of thyroid disease, 2003, p 47.)

USA (Delange, 1995; Dunn, 1998). Since most of the ingested iodine is excreted in the urine, measurement of urinary iodine excretion (UI) provides an accurate estimate of dietary iodine intake (Dunn, 1998). The excretion of UI is expressed as µg of iodine per volume (pg/dL) of urine. The suggested ranges for UI excretion are shown in Table 24–13.

Screening Programs for Detection of Neonatal Hypothyroidism

The prevalence of hypothyroidism in newborns is estimated from 1 in 3000–5000. It is higher in certain ethnic groups and increased in iodine-deficient regions worldwide. Early detection of hypothyroidism in the neonatal period is critical to eliminate the severe mental retardation associated with thyroid hormone deficiency. Measuring T_4 and TSH is used for screening, which is performed using dry blood spots or cord serum. The detection rate depends on the tests used and timing of specimen collection. Measurement of only T_4 carries a high false-positive rate, necessitating recall of a large number of infants for retesting. Causes of false-positive results include low T_4 levels, which occur in both premature infants and those with congenital absence of TBG. Screening with only T_4 may miss infants with compensated or partial thyroid insufficiency. As about 15% of infants with primary thyroid disorders have compensated hypothyroidism (normal serum T_4 levels in association with elevated TSH), an elevated TSH is the most sensitive test for the diagnosis of congenital hypothyroidism. However, false-positive results are occasionally seen as, for example, in premature or severely stressed infants. In addition, by screening with TSH alone, those infants with hypothalamic or pituitary disease will be missed. Very-low-birth-weight infants should be retested at 2 and 4–6 weeks to detect late-onset transient hypothyroidism (Frank, 1996). For newborns, if the initial TSH value is < 10 mIU/L, no further action need be taken; if it lies in the 10–20 mIU/L range, then a repeat test needs to be performed in 2–6 weeks. Finally, if the initial blood spot TSH > 20 mIU/L, endocrinological evaluation is necessary to make the diagnosis of hypothyroidism.

Nonthyroidal Illness (NTI)

Seriously ill patients can have abnormal thyroid tests even without underlying thyroid pathology (DeGroot, 1992; Kaptein, 1996). A rapid decline in both the total and free T_3 typically develops in the setting of severe illness (e.g., myocardial infarction, sepsis) (Piketty, 1996). As the severity of the illness increases the serum total T_4 falls because of T_4-binding protein disruption by inhibitors in the circulation (Wartofsky, 1982; Docter, 1993; Wilcox, 1994). Patients with NTI whose T_4 levels drop below 2 ng/dL carry an exceptionally poor prognosis. The alterations in thyroid function tests seen during NTI are termed the 'euthyroid sick syndrome' or 'low T_4 syndrome.' Figure 24–7 shows the spectrum of changes in the thyroid tests as they relate to the severity and the stage of the illness. Patients with nonthyroidal illness (NTI) tend to have low or low-normal TSH, normal or low-normal T_4 but very low T_3 during their acute illness, then TSH rises to within normal or above normal with resolution of the underlying illness and finally returns to the normal range (Faber, 1987). This situation can be complicated if certain drugs are used for that illness, e.g., glucagon, dopamine and high doses of corticosteroids suppress TSH and can mask hypothyroid status during their use (Brabant, 1989; Samuels, 1997; Kaptein, 1980; Skamene, 1984).

In uremia, there is accumulation of indoleacetic acid, which will interfere with thyroid hormone binding (Iitaka, 1998).

Physiologic Variables

For practical purposes, variables such as age, gender, race, season, phase of menstrual cycle, cigarette smoking, exercise, fasting or phlebotomy-induced stasis have minor effects on the thyroid function tests in ambulatory adults (Hollowell, 2002). Studies have suggested that each individual has a genetically determined FT_4 set-point (Meikle, 1988; Andersen, 2002), any deviation from this set-point will be sensed by the

pituitary and cause reciprocal change in TSH secretion. In the early stages of developing thyroid dysfunction, a serum TSH abnormality will precede the development of an abnormal FT_4 because TSH responds exponentially to subtle FT_4 changes as shown in Figure 24–8.

Despite the wider serum TSH variability seen in older individuals, there appears to be no justification for using a widened or age-adjusted reference range. This conservative approach is justified by reports that mildly suppressed or elevated TSH is associated with increased cardiovascular morbidity and mortality (Sawin, 1991; Parle, 2001). In children, the hypothalamic–pituitary–thyroid axis undergoes progressive maturation and modulation; there is a continuous decline of the TSH/FT_4 ratio from the time of mid-gestation until after puberty (Nilson, 1993; Adams, 1995; Lu, 1999; Zurakowski, 1999; Fisher, 2000a,b) and as a result, higher TSH concentrations are typically seen in children.

During pregnancy, estrogen production increases progressively elevating the TBG concentration, resulting in an increase in the total T_4 and T_3 reference range to approximately 1.5 times the nonpregnancy upper reference level by 16 weeks of gestation (Weeke, 1982; Pedersen, 1993; Nohr, 2000). Although TBG excess leads to an increase in both serum total thyroxine (T_4) and triiodothyronine (T_3) concentrations, the serum free T_4 and T_3 concentrations remain unchanged.

Serum HCG, which has structural similarity to TSH, has weak thyroid-stimulating activity (Talbot, 2001). The increase in HCG soon after fertilization results in a small increase in free T_4 and T_3 concentrations, usually within the normal reference range. These changes result in a fall in serum TSH during the first trimester; a subnormal serum TSH may be seen in about 20% of mothers who have normal pregnancies (Glinoer, 1990, 1997; Panesar, 2001). The peak rise in HCG and nadir of TSH occur together at about 10–12 weeks of gestation. In 2% of pregnancies, the increase in FT_4 reaches supranormal levels and, if prolonged, may lead to a syndrome entitled 'gestational transient thyrotoxicosis' (GTT), characterized by more pronounced symptoms and signs of thyrotoxicosis. This condition is frequently associated with first trimester hyperemesis gravidarum (Goodwin 1992, Hershman 1999).

Medications and Thyroid Function Tests

Drugs can cause both in vitro and in vivo effects on thyroid tests. This can lead to the misinterpretation of test results, inaccurate diagnoses and further unnecessary tests (Surks, 1995; Kailajarvi, 2000). Estrogen-induced TBG elevation causes abnormally high total T_4 and total T_3, but has no effect on TSH or free T_4 and free T_3. Glucocorticoids in large doses can suppress TSH and decrease the conversion of T_4 to T_3 (Samuels, 1997; Kaptein, 1980). Dopamine suppresses TSH and can temper the expected rise in TSH in hospitalized patients with primary hypothyroidism (Kaptein, 1980). Propranolol suppresses the conversion of T_4 to T_3 (this is one of the reasons it is used in the treatment of thyrotoxicosis).

Iodide, found in iodide-containing contrast media used in CT scans and coronary angiography, or in solution to sterilize skin, and radiopaque dyes can cause both hyper- and hypothyroidism in susceptible patients (Meurisse, 2000). Iodine-containing drugs such as amiodarone (used as an antiarrhythmic agent) have complex effects on thyroid function and can cause either hypothyroidism (10% of patients) or hyperthyroidism (1–2%) in susceptible individuals with positive antibodies (TPOAb) (Martino, 1987, 2001; Daniels, 2001; Harjai, 1997; Caron, 1995).

Lithium inhibits thyroid hormone synthesis and release and can cause hypothyroidism in about 15–50% of patients, especially those patients with positive TPOAb (Lazarus, 1998; Kusalic, 1999; Oakley, 2000). The mechanism of lithium action is similar to that of iodide. Lithium is concentrated by the thyroid and inhibits thyroidal iodine uptake. It also inhibits iodotyrosine coupling, alters thyroglobulin structure, and inhibits thyroid hormone secretion. The latter effect is critical to the development of hypothyroidism and goiter (Lazaraus, 1998).

Drugs such as phenytoin, carbamazepine, and furosemide competitively inhibit thyroid binding to serum proteins in vitro and will cause an artifactual increase in free T_4 and reduction in total T_4 and free T_4 index. Therapeutic doses of phenytoin can also induce acceleration of T_4 disposal and perhaps also directly suppress TSH centrally, all of these mechanisms being responsible for the reduced T_4 (Surks, 1995). Heparin can stimulate in vitro lipoprotein lipase and liberate free fatty acids which inhibit T_4 binding to serum proteins and falsely elevate free T_4 (Mendel, 1987).

Medications such as phenobarbital, phenytoin, rifampin and carbamazepine increase the rate of thyroid hormone clearance by increasing the deiodination of T_4 and T_3. Hypothyroid patients treated with any of these medications need to have their hormone levels monitored closely, as an increase in levothyroxine (L-T_4) dose may be required. In turn, changes in thyroid hormone status affect the clearance of many medications, including those listed above (e.g., hyperthyroidism can lead to increased clearance of phenobarbital, hypothyroidism to decreased clearance). Owing to these various alterations in thyroid hormone parameters, the best indicator of thyroid status is the measurement of TSH along with the FT_4. For those with pituitary disease or on dilantin, T_4 by equilibrium dialysis should be used.

Somatostatin or its analog octreotide, which is used to treat acromegaly (Itoh, 1988) and dopamine (Kaptein, 1980) both inhibit TSH synthesis to undetectable levels in patients with severe NTI.

Thyroid Illness

Hyperthyroid patients may present with one or all of the following signs and symptoms: weight loss, sweating, heat intolerance, palpitations, insomnia, increased bowel movement, tremors, infertility or amenorrhea. They have suppressed TSH values with the exception of those few individuals who have secondary hyperthyroidism caused by TSH-producing pituitary tumors, or other rare disorders such as pituitary resistance to thyroid hormones. Subclinical hyperthyroidism is defined as low TSH ($< 0.1 \mu IU/mL$) with levels of T_4 and T_3 within the reference values without any signs or symptoms of hyperthyroidism (Ross, 1991). Detection of subclinical hyperthyroidism is particularly important in patients who are over 60 as they have increased risk of atrial fibrillation, increased cardiovascular mortality (Sawin, 1994) and osteoporosis. Minimal thyroid hormone excess can cause atrial fibrillation and stimulate osteoclastic activity in bone, causing osteoporosis.

Patients with primary hypothyroidism can present with one or all of the following signs and symptoms: cold intolerance, constipation, water retention, hypercholesterolemia, depression, pretibial myxedema, periorbital edema and elevated TSH with low T_4 and T_3. TSH is low in patients with secondary hypothyroidism caused by pituitary or hypothalamic disorders. Patients with subclinical hypothyroidism have elevated TSH levels ($> 4.5 \mu U/mL$) but both T_4 and T_3 are within the reference range. In 2004, the 13-member expert panel led by Surks published their findings in the January issue of *JAMA* and recommended TSH reference limits of 0.4–$4.5 \mu U/mL$ and that patients with TSH ranges from 4.5–$10 mU/L$ not be routinely treated. The 2002 AACE guidelines (American Association of Clinical Endocrinologists, 2002) recommend treatment of those with TSH $> 10 \mu U/mL$ or those with goiter and positive TPOAb whose TSH is between 4.5–$10 \mu U/mL$. TPOAb measurement is useful for establishing the presence of autoimmunity; those with elevated antibodies have a greater probability of developing overt thyroid failure.

Screening for thyroid disease

The American Thyroid Association guidelines recommend screening at age 35 and every 5 years thereafter (Ladenson, 2000). This appears to be a cost-effective strategy, especially for women (Parle, 2001) and the elderly (Ladenson, 2000; Vanderpump, 1995; Parle 2001). Hashimoto's thyroiditis is an autoimmune disease of the thyroid caused when sensitized T lymphocytes and/or autoantibodies bind to cell membrane causing cell lysis and inflammatory reaction resulting in cellular damage. This is associated with high TSH and positive TPOAb and is encountered with increasing prevalence with increasing age (Vanderpump, 1995). The incidence of low TSH is also increased in the elderly (Vanderpump, 1995).

There is mounting evidence to indicate that a persistent TSH abnormality may lead to major risks if left untreated. One study reported a higher cardiovascular mortality rate in patients with chronically low TSH

(Parle, 1991), and there are numerous reports that indicate that mild hypothyroidism in early pregnancy increases fetal loss and impairs the IQ of the offspring (Pop, 1995, 1999; Haddow, 1999). It is important to always confirm any TSH abnormality in a fresh specimen drawn 3 weeks later before making the diagnosis of mild abnormalities.

Uses of L-Thyroxine (L-T_4)

An average replacement dose is $1.6 \mu g/kg$ body weight/day for adults, up to $4.0 \mu g/kg$ body weight/day for children and lower doses for older individuals ($1.0 \mu g/kg$ body weight/day) (Sawin, 1983; Davis, 1984). The initial dose and the optimal time needed to establish the full replacement dose is dependent upon the age, weight and cardiac status of each patient. The requirement might increase during pregnancy and in postmenopausal women starting hormonal replacement (Arafah, 2001). A serum TSH between 0.5–$2.0 \mu U/mL$ is the therapeutic goal level for L-T_4 replacement in primary hypothyroidism. A serum FT_4 concentration in the upper third of the reference interval is the therapeutic target in central hypothyroidism.

TSH should be used to monitor patients receiving thyroid hormone replacement therapy as well as those treated with hormone to suppress malignant thyroid diseases (Spencer, 1990). Both TSH and FT_4 should be used to monitor hypothyroid patients suspected of intermittent noncompliance. At least 6 weeks is needed before retesting TSH following a change in the dose of L-T_4. Annual TSH measurement is recommended in patients on a steady dose of T_4. If FT_4 is being assayed patients should withhold their levothyroxine dose the day of the test, as serum FT_4 will be increased (about 13%) above baseline for 9 hours after ingesting the last dose (Ain, 1993); the TSH, however, is unlikely to be affected. Ideally, L-T_4 should be taken before meals, at the same time every day and at least 4 hours from any other medications or vitamins/dietary supplements.

L-T_4 is used to suppress TSH in patients with well-differentiated thyroid carcinoma for which thyrotropin is considered a trophic factor (Dulgeroff, 1994). It is recommended to use a TSH target of 0.05–$0.1 \mu U/mL$ for low-risk patients and a TSH value of $< 0.1 \mu U/mL$ for high-risk patients. If the thyroglobulin level is undetectable and there is no evidence of recurrence 5–10 years after thyroidectomy, the dose of L-T_4 can be reduced to give low-normal TSH values $< 0.4 \mu U/mL$.

Calcitonin

Medullary thyroid carcinoma (MTC) originates from the C cells of the thyroid. It accounts for 5–8% of thyroid cancers and 0.57% of thyroid nodules (Pacini, 1994).

25% of MTC are hereditary (multiple endocrine neoplasia types 2A and 2B) (Cobin, 2001; Brandi, 2001; Dunn, 1994) These are autosomal dominant inherited multiglandular syndromes. An important, recurring MTC genetic mutation was found to be located on the chromosome sub-band 10q11.2 (Mulligan, 1993; Hofstra, 1994).

The C-cell secretes calcitonin. An elevated level of calcitonin in circulating blood indicates the presence of MTC. Mature calcitonin results from post-translational modification of a larger 141-amino-acid precursor (preprocalcitonin) within the parafollicular C-cells. Preprocalcitonin undergoes cleavage of a single peptide to form procalcitonin; the latter has 116 amino acid residues. The immature calcitonin peptide consisting of 33 amino acids is located centrally within the procalcitonin molecule. The mature, active, 32-amino-acid calcitonin is produced from immature calcitonin by the enzyme peptidylglycine-amidating mono-oxidase (PAM). Measurement of calcitonin is done by two-site immunometric assays using monoclonal antibodies: one recognizes the N-terminal region and the other the C-terminal region). This method is more sensitive and more specific (van Heyningen, 1994; Becker, 1996; Motte, 1988). The cutoff level in healthy adults is about 10 ng/L.

Serum calcitonin measurements are used as tumor marker for detecting residual thyroid tissue or metastasis in patients with MTC. It should be measured prior to and 6 months after surgery. The presence of residual tissue or a recurrence of MTC can only be ruled out if both basal and post-pentagastrin- or calcium-stimulated calcitonin are undetectable. Provocative stimuli, such as calcium and pentagastrin (Pg) or omeprazole have been used to detect C-cell abnormalities, as they increase calcitonin level at all stages of MTC (Wells, 1978; Gagel, 1996; Wion-Barbot, 1997; Barbot, 1994; Erdogan, 1997; Vieira, 2002; Vitale, 2002).

In the pentagastrin stimulation test for the diagnosis of MTC, an intravenous infusion of Pg ($0.5 \mu/kg$ body weight) is given over 5 seconds; blood samples are collected at baseline, 1, 2, 5 and 10 minutes after starting the infusion. Interpretations of results are summarized in Table 24–14.

In the calcium stimulation test, intravenous injection of $2.5 mg/kg$ of calcium gluconate is given over 30 seconds, and blood samples are then collected at baseline, 1, 2 and 5 minutes. An increase in the plasma calcitonin

Table 24–14 Interpretation of the Pentagastrin (Pg) Test

Peak Calcitonin (CT) ng/L (pg/mL)	Interpretation
< 10	Normal (80% of adults)
> 30 but < 50	5% of normal adults
> 50 but < 100	Possible MTC or other thyroid pathology
> 100	Probable MTC
Basal or post-Pg CT value > 10 pg/mL	C-cell pathology or residual tissue in MEN 2 patients and MTC patients after surgery

MTC = medullary thyroid cancer; MEN 2 = multiple endocrine neoplasia 2.
From Demers LM, Spencer CA (eds): NACB Laboratory Support for the Diagnosis and Monitoring of Thyroid Disease. 2003, p 69.

Table 24–15 Conditions in which Calcitonin may be Elevated Other than MTC

Neuroendocrine tumors	Small cell lung cancer, intestinal and bronchial carcinoid, all neuroendocrine tumors
Benign C-cell hyperplasia (HCC)	Autoimmune thyroid disease, differentiated thyroid cancer
Other diseases	Kidney disease, hypergastrinemia, hypercalcemia

From Demers LM, Spencer CA (eds): NACB Laboratory Support for the Diagnosis and Monitoring of Thyroid Disease. 2003, p 70.

level above 100 ng/L is an indication of C-cell hyperplasia. The calcium infusion test has been reported to be less sensitive than the Pg test for the diagnosis of MTC, but if combined with the Pg test it enhances the sensitivity of the Pg test (Wells, 1978).

Calcitonin may also be elevated in other conditions unrelated to thyroid neoplastic conditions as summarized in Table 24–15.

Adrenal Gland

The adrenal glands are pyramidal structures located above each kidney, each weighing approximately 4–6 grams. Anatomically, the adrenal is divided into two distinct parts, the medulla (inner layer) and the cortex (outer layer). The medulla, which is of neural crest origin (ectoderm), stores and secretes catecholamines. The cortex is of mesenchymal origin and is further divided into three zones: the outermost zona glomerulosa, which produces mineralocorticoids; the zona fasciculata, which is responsible for glucocorticoid production; and the inner zona reticularis, which synthesizes androgens. The cortex comprises about 80–90% of the adrenal gland. The glands have a very rich arterial supply that forms a subcapsular plexus and empties into a central vein. By weight they have the highest perfusion of blood per gram of tissue, a feature that assures rapid dissemination of their hormones throughout the body in response to stress.

Hormones of the Adrenal Medulla

The adrenal medulla is part of the sympathoadrenal axis. Being of neural crest origin, it possesses the capability of synthesizing catecholamines through the process of amine precursor uptake and decarboxylation (APUD). The initial and rate-limiting step in catecholamine synthesis is the conversion of tyrosine to 3,4-dihydroxyphenylalanine (dopa) by the enzyme tyrosine hydoxylase (TH). Through a series of steps L-dopa is subsequently converted to dopamine (D), norepinephrine (NE) and epinephrine (E) (Fig. 24–9). Epinephrine is almost exclusively produced and secreted by the adrenal medulla, where the ratio of NE : E is about 1 to 4. However, since all three catecholamines are also synthesized within the central and sympathetic nervous systems, the peripheral NE : E ratio is more like 9 to 1.

The catecholamines are metabolized by either catechol-*O*-methyltransferase (COMT) or monoamine oxidase (MAO). COMT converts dopamine (D) to methoxytyramine, epinephrine (E) to metanephrine (MN) and norepinephrine (NE) to normetanephrine (NMN), all of which in turn can be oxidized to vanillylmandelic acid (VMA) by MAO. MAO can also convert E and NE to 3,4-dihydroxymandelic acid, which is acted upon by COMT to form VMA. 3-Methoxy-4-hydroxyphenylacetic acid (homovanillic acid [HVA]) is the final product of dopamine metabolism.

Pheochromocytoma

Pheochromocytomas are rare catecholamine-producing tumors, with an incidence of about 500–1600 per year (Pacak, 2001a). They account for < 1% of all secondary causes for hypertension. Although 90% of pheochromocytomas are benign, they are almost invariably lethal if not diagnosed and properly treated (Pacak, 2001a). Approximately 90% of the tumors arise within the adrenal medulla and 10–15% are of extra-adrenal origin (paraganglioma). The majority of pheochromocytomas are sporadic; however, 10–20% are familial, occurring as part of the multiple endocrine neoplasia type 2A or 2B (MEN-2A, MEN-2B), von Hippel–Lindau (VHL) disease, neurofibromatosis type 1 (NF-1) or familial paraganglioma. The hereditary forms tend to present at a younger age, and the tumors are usually intra-adrenal and bilateral. Genetic testing should be performed when the diagnosis of pheochromocytoma is made in individuals younger than age 50; the choice of genetic testing is guided by the patient's medical and family history.

Sustained or paroxysmal hypertension is the most common manifestation of this disease and is present in about 90% of patients. Remarkably, 10% of patients are normotensive. More than 90% will present with paroxysmal attacks characterized by at least two out of the three of the following symptoms: headaches associated with palpitations and diaphoresis (Sheps, 1994). Other symptoms include orthostatic hypotension, labile blood pressure, excessive sweating, anxiety, nervousness, weight loss, fatigue, pallor and tremor. These symptoms can last from a few seconds to several hours, with the interval between attacks being highly variable, from several times a day to once every few months. Indications for screening for pheochromocytoma are listed in Table 24–16.

There is great debate as to which test is the best for diagnosing pheochromocytoma. With improvement in assay technique, evidence has come to support the chromatographic measurement of the plasma free metanephrine and normetanephrine levels as the initial test. The diagnosis of pheochromocytoma is made if the plasma concentration of either free metanephrine or normetanephrine is about four times the upper reference limit. Further testing is required in patients with high levels that are less than four times the upper reference limit (Sheps, 1994; Eisenhofer, 2004a,b).

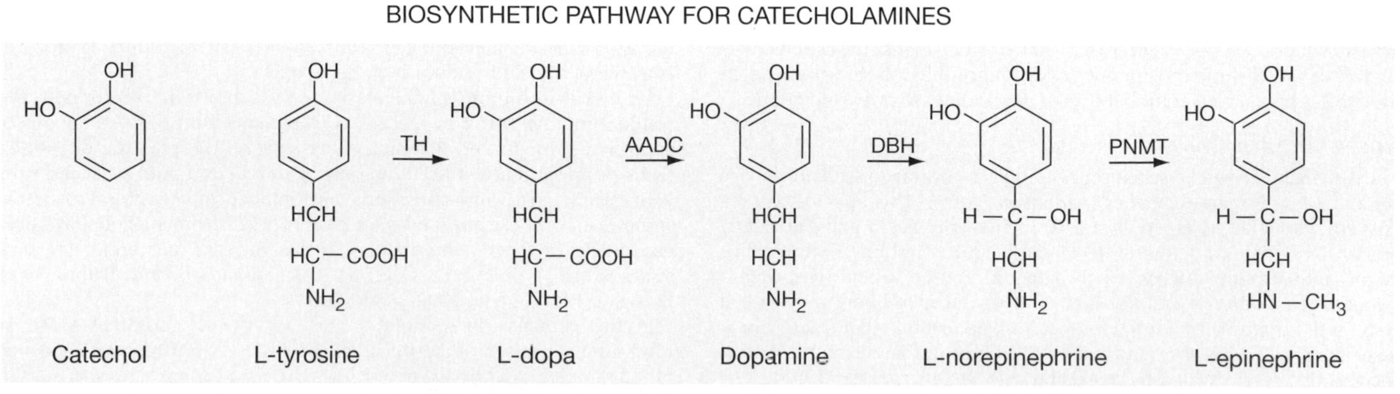

BIOSYNTHETIC PATHWAY FOR CATECHOLAMINES

Figure 24–9 Catecholamines: biosynthetic pathway. The rate-limiting step is the conversion of L-tyrosine to L-3-4-dihydroxyphenylalanine (L-dopa) through the actions of tyrosine hydroxylase. AADC = aromatic L-amino acid decarboxylase; DBH = dopamine β-hydroxylase; PNMT = phenylethanolamine *N*-methyltransferase; TH = tyrosine hydroxylase. (Redrawn from Dluhy RG, Lawrence JE, Williams GH: Endocrine hypertension. *In* Larsen PR, Kronenberg HM, Melmed S, Polansky KS (eds): Williams Textbook of Endocrinology, 10th ed. Philadelphia, WB Saunders, 2003, p 555 with permission.)

Table 24–16 Indications for Screening for Pheochromocytoma

1 Hypertension with episodic features suggestive of pheochromocytoma
2 Refractory hypertension
3 Prominent lability of blood pressure
4 Severe pressor response during anesthesia, parturition, surgery or angiography
5 Unexplained hypotension due to anesthesia, surgery or pregnancy
6 Family history of pheochromocytoma, MEN-2A or -2B, VHL disease, neurofibromatosis
7 Incidentally discovered adrenal mass
8 Idiopathic dilated cardiomyopathy
9 Spells or attacks occurring during exertion, twisting and turning of the torso, straining, coitus, or micturition

After Dluhy RG, Lawrence JE, Williams G: Endocrine hypertension. *In* Larsen PR, Kronenberg HM, Melmed S, Polonsky KS (eds): Williams Textbook of Endocrinology, 10th ed. Philadelphia: WB Saunders, 2003, p 557.

Table 24–17 Sensitivity and Specificity of Hormone Levels for Diagnosing Pheochromocytoma

	Sensitivity		Specificity	
	Hereditary	Sporadic	Hereditary	Sporadic
Plasma				
Free metanephrines	97%	99%	96%	82%
Catecholamines	69%	92%	89%	72%
Urine				
Fractionated metanephrines	96%	97%	82%	45%
Catecholamines	79%	91%	96%	75%
Total metanephrines	60%	88%	97%	89%
Vanillylmandelic acid	46%	77%	99%	86%

After Pacak, 2004; Lenders, 2002.

In centers where this assay is not available, the initial test should be the chromatographic measurement of a 24-hour urine collection for normetanephrine, metanephrine, fractionated free catecholamines (epinephrine, norepinephrine, dopamine) and creatinine (Eisenhofer, 2004a,b; Lenders, 2002). Metanephrine is the most sensitive and specific of these metabolites (Heron, 1996). The diagnosis of pheochromocytoma can also be made by measuring plasma catecholamines; however, since their half-life is short and they are secreted episodically, it is only of use if the sample is collected during a paroxysm. Values from either the 24-h urine collection or plasma catecholamines that are two to three times the upper limit of normal are usually diagnostic of pheochromocytoma.

When dealing with 'sporadic' pheochromocytoma the choice and interpretation of diagnostic tests depends on the pretest level of suspicion for disease. In these settings, the 24-h urinary metanephrine and catecholamine measurements provide clinically acceptable sensitivity and significantly better specificity than fractionated plasma free metanephrine values (Sawka, 2003). Because of the difficulties in collecting a complete 24-h urine sample from pediatric patients, fractionated plasma free metanephrines should be considered the biochemical test of choice in that population (Weise, 2002) (Table 24–17).

There are a number of factors that cause false-positive test results, either by stimulating catecholamine secretion and/or by interfering with the assay (Table 24–18). When assaying for plasma free metanephrines patients should abstain from caffeinated beverages and alcohol for 24 hours before testing. They should also avoid acetaminophen, tricyclic antidepressants, phenoxybenzamine, α-agonists (e.g., aldomet) and monoamine oxidase inhibitors for at least 5 days prior to testing (Lenders, 1995). When testing for catecholamines in addition to metanephrines, the patient should also avoid nicotine, sympathomimetics (theophylline, pseudoephedrine), α-agonists (e.g., albuterol) and levodopa/carbidopa. If antihypertensive medications are needed, angiotensin-converting enzyme inhibitors (ACEI), angiotensin receptor blockers and selective α$_1$-adrenoceptor blockers (e.g., prazocin) can be used without fear of causing false-positive results (Eisenhofer, 2003).

Table 24–18 Effects of Medications on Testing for Pheochromocytoma

	Plasma				Urine			
Medication class	NMN	NE	MN	E	NMN	NE	MN	E
Tricyclics	+	+	−	−	+	+	−	−
Phenoxybenzamine	+	+	−	−	+	+	−	−
Buspirone	−	−	−	−	−	+	−	−
α-Adrenergic blockers	−	−	−	−	−	+	−	−
β-Adrenoceptor blockers	−	−	+	−	+	+	+	+
Calcium channel blockers	−	+	−	−	−	+	−	+
Sympathomimetics	+	+	−	−	+	+	−	−

* Diuretics, angiotensin-converting enzyme inhibitors and angiotensin II receptor blockers have little influence on the frequency of false-positive results.

NMN = normetanephrine; NE = norepinephrine; MN = metanephrines; E = epinephrine.

After Eisenhofer, 2003.

Although urinary catecholamine levels may be elevated in renal insufficiency and renal failure, the measurement of plasma free metanephrines can be used to reliably diagnose pheochromocytoma in both these conditions (Eisenhofer, 2004b). Stressors such as an acute MI, congestive heart failure, surgery and acute cerebrovascular accident are all associated with elevated levels of catecholamines. In these situations one can either treat empirically and test once the patient has stabilized, or use other diagnostic tests including imaging studies. Plasma normetanephrine concentrations increase with age, and as a result elderly patients are particularly susceptible to having false-positive tests; the use of fractionated urinary metanephrines and catecholamines may be more suitable for this population (Sawka, 2003).

Plasma levels of normetanephrine less than 112 ng/liter (0.61 nmol/liter) and of metanephrine less than 61 ng/liter (0.31 nmol/liter) virtually exclude pheochromocytoma so that no immediate further testing for the tumor should be necessary. With plasma concentrations of normetanephrine above 400 ng/liter (2.19 nmol/liter) or metanephrine above 236 ng/liter (1.20 nmol/liter), the probability of pheochromocytoma is so high that the immediate task is to locate the tumor (Eisenhofer, 2003).

More often than not, test results return as equivocal, requiring the need for confirmatory tests such as the clonidine suppression test, glucagon stimulation test or the measurement of urinary fractionated catecholamines. Clonidine is a centrally acting α-adrenergic agonist; it suppresses catecholamine release from the nervous system but has no effect on its release by the tumor (Bravo, 1981). In those with pheochromocytoma clonidine fails to adequately suppress plasma levels of norepinephrine. The clonidine suppression test is indicated only if the plasma catecholamines are greater than 1000 pg/mL (5.9 nmol/L). It is unreliable in those with normal or mildly elevated plasma catecholamines (Taylor, 1986; Elliott, 1988; Sjoberg, 1992). Eisenhofer et al. have shown that measuring plasma normetanephrines pre- and post-clonidine increases the sensitivity and specificity of this test, especially in those who only have modest elevations of norepinephrine (Eisenhofer, 2003). The glucagon stimulation test can lead to dangerous rises in blood pressure and is rarely used. It should only be performed in patients whose blood pressure is well controlled, and a physician must be present throughout the test. A rise in plasma norepinephrine to greater than threefold or greater than 2000 pg/mL is diagnostic of pheochromocytoma (Table 24–19). The proposed mechanism of action would be the stimulation of glucagon-sensitive adenylate cyclase receptors expressed on these tumors.

Unless the history is compelling or the patient falls into one of the categories of genetically inherited disorders, it is often unnecessary to repeat testing in those with slightly positive results.

Chromogranin A (CgA) is a protein that is stored and secreted along with the catecholamines from the adrenal medulla and the sympathetic nervous system. Although it is elevated in more than 80% of pheochromocytomas, it is not specific for this disorder, being secreted by other chromaffin tissues (Hsiao, 1991). CgA was initially thought to be useful in the diagnosis of pheochromocytoma, since medications typically used to treat it had no impact on CgA secretion or measurement. Despite a relatively high sensitivity of 86%, it has poor diagnostic specificity. This is, in large part, due to the fact that the kidneys play a major role in the clearance of CgA from the circulation so that even mild degrees of renal impairment (e.g., creatinine clearance [CrCl] < 80 mg/mL/min) can lead to significant

Table 24–19 Pharmacologic Tests for Diagnosing Pheochromocytoma

Clonidine suppression test

Indications	Patients with hypertension and clinical findings or family history that is highly suggestive of pheochromocytoma and the catecholamines are elevated but not to the extent that is diagnostic of pheochromocytoma
Interpretation	*Normal:* decrease in NE to below normal or a > 50% decline from baseline. A decrease in normetanephrines to below normal or a 40% decline from baseline *Pheochromocytoma:* failure of NE to drop below normal or decrease by more than 50% from baseline. Failure of normetanephrines to drop below normal or decrease by more than 40% from baseline

Glucagon stimulation test

Indications	When clinical findings or family history are highly suggestive of pheochromocytoma but blood pressure is normal and catecholamines are only modestly elevated
Interpretation	*Pheochromocytoma:* A threefold or greater increase in plasma NE or a rise in the level to > 2000 pg/mL

increases in serum concentration of CgA (Bravo, 2003). Among hypertensive patients with creatinine clearance less than 80 mL/min, the overall sensitivity, specificity, accuracy, and positive and negative predictive values of serum CgA dropped to 85%, 50%, 59%, 38%, and 90%, respectively. However, when combined with elevated plasma catecholamines in patients with creatinine clearance at least 80 mL/min, the diagnostic specificity and positive predictive values improved to 98% and 97%, respectively (Canale, 1994). Its major use is in the postoperative monitoring for recurrence of these tumors.

Testing procedures. For the 24-hour urine collections, creatinine is measured to verify the adequacy of the collection. To preserve the specimen adequately, the urine should be collected in a container into which 25 mL of 6 N HCl has been added.

Plasma catecholamines are collected following an overnight fast (water permitted). The patient is placed in a reclining position in a quiet environment and a heparin lock is inserted intravenously. After 20–30 minutes, blood is collected in a prechilled EDTA lavender top tube. The whole blood sample should be kept in ice-water until centrifuged (preferably at 4°C). Separation of plasma should take place within 2 hours of phlebotomy; the sample should then be frozen immediately.

Both urine and plasma specimens should be analyzed using high-performance liquid chromatography with tandem mass spectrometry, as this technique greatly eliminates problems caused by interfering substances (Taylor, 2002). For the urine metabolites it is important to use age-appropriate references ranges when interpreting the results. It is also important to be aware that reference ranges can not only vary widely from one laboratory to another but even within the same laboratory, as newer methodologies replace less-sensitive assays.

Additional Follow-Up Testing. Once the diagnosis is confirmed biochemically, the tumor should be localized by either computed tomography (CT) scan or magnetic resonance imaging (MRI) of the adrenals. If that is negative, imaging studies of the abdomen, chest and pelvis should be performed. CT has greater sensitivity, while MRI has greater specificity. MRI is superior to CT in detecting extra-adrenal lesions and has the advantage of not requiring ionizing radiation or needing ionic contrast.

If a tumor cannot be located by either CT or MRI, or if metastatic disease is suspected, scanning with ^{131}I or ^{123}I labeled meta-iodobenzyl-guanidine (MIBG) should be performed. Octreoscanning and positron emission tomography are reserved for when the other techniques have failed.

Following successful tumor resection, the prognosis is generally excellent. Urinary metanephrines should be retested several weeks after surgery to ensure that the resection was complete, and measured periodically thereafter as an early marker of disease recurrence (Werbel, 1995).

An algorithm to evaluate pheochromocytoma has been proposed by Eisenhoffer (Eisenhofer, 2003) (Fig. 24–10).

Neuroblastoma

Similarly to pheochromocytoma, neuroblastoma is of neural crest origin, arising within the adrenals or the sympathetic chain. It is the second most common solid malignant tumor in childhood, usually occurring before the age of 3. Symptoms relate primarily to tumor mass rather than to hypertension, which is often mild or absent. At the time of diagnosis, 70%

of cases will have distant metastases. About 90% of patients have elevated urinary homovanillic acid (HVA) levels at the time of diagnosis, whereas almost 75% of patients have increased urinary VMA levels (Tuchman, 1985). Both tests should be ordered when screening for the disease. In healthy children, at least up until the age of about 15, urinary VMA and metanephrines tend to be higher (per milligram of creatinine) and more variable than in adults. Urinary metanephrines also can be elevated in neuroblastoma patients, but are not a sensitive measure of residual tumor. Urinary HVA also is increased in familial dysautonomia (Riley-Day syndrome) and some pheochromocytoma patients.

Hormones of the Adrenal Cortex

The adrenal cortex is composed of three distinct zones; the outermost is the zona glomerulosa, followed by the intermediate zona fasciculata that surrounds the innermost zona reticularis. In the broadest terms, each zone is responsible for the synthesis and secretion of a unique set of hormones: the zona glomerulosa – mineralocorticoids (aldosterone); the zona fasciculata – glucocorticoids (cortisol); and the zona reticularis – sex steroids (dehydroepiandrosterone sulfate [DHEAS] and androgens). However, under certain pathologic and physiologic conditions these distinctions become blurred.

Mineralocorticoid axis

The chief mineralocorticoid is aldosterone, which promotes the reabsorption of sodium and water by the kidney to help maintain blood pressure and tonicity. Expression of the enzyme CYP11B2 (aldosterone synthetase) within the glomerulosa is site specific; as a result, the synthesis of aldosterone and its intermediary 18-hydroxylated metabolites are restricted to the zona glomerulosa. The precursor molecules to aldosterone, 11-deoxycorticosterone (DOC) and 11-deoxycortisol similarly possess mineralocorticoid activity. However, unlike aldosterone they can be synthesized within the zona fasciculata as well as in the zona glomerulosa, which explains the hypertension and electrolyte disturbances seen in some forms of congenital adrenal hyperplasia. Although aldosterone will respond to acute changes in ACTH, it is mainly under the control of the renin–angiotensin system.

The zona fasciculata which makes up 75% of the cortex, is responsible for the synthesis and secretion of the glucocorticoids and to a lesser extent androgens and estrogens. The glucocorticoids are 21-carbon steroid compounds with a hydroxyl group on carbon 17, hence the synonym 17-hydroxycorticosteroids. Cortisol is the key glucocorticoid, regulating its own secretion through negative feedback on the hypothalamic–pituitary–adrenal (HPA) axis, inhibiting ACTH release from the pituitary and corticotropin-releasing hormone (CRH) from the hypothalamus. Both CRH and AVP (ADH) are produced by the parvocellular neurons of the paraventricular nuclei of the hypothalamus. ACTH secretion is stimulated by CRH and, to a much lesser extent, by AVP. ACTH in turn stimulates cortisol production by the adrenals. Cortisol is needed in times of stress to maintain blood pressure, blood sugar and prevent shock. Although cortisol is the most important glucocorticoid, corticosterone, which is a hormone of the mineralocorticoid pathway, also possesses glucocorticoid activity.

Androgens and estrogens are produced by the zona reticularis. The androgens are 18-carbon steroids with saturated A rings, in contrast to the estrogens, which are 17-carbon steroids with unsaturated A rings.

The functions of these hormones are summarized in Table 24–20.

Congenital Disorders of Adrenal Cortical Enzyme Deficiencies

The hormones of the adrenal cortex are steroid derivatives, synthesized from LDL cholesterol. LDL is delivered to the adrenals and taken up by the LDL receptors. Steroid acute regulatory protein (StAR) then shuttles it across the mitochondrial membrane where is begins its journey down the steroidogenic pathway (Fig. 24–11). The enzymes that catalyze these synthetic reactions are of four general types: hydroxylases, dehydrogenases, desmolases and isomerases. Because most of the inborn errors of metabolism affecting steroid hormone synthesis in the adrenal cortex involve deficiencies of hydroxylases, they constitute the most clinically important group of enzymes.

At least eight different metabolic defects in the synthesis of cortisol and aldosterone have been described, each characterized by a deficiency of a specific adrenal enzyme. The vast majority of these enzymatic deficiencies are inherited as an autosomal recessive trait with variable degrees of penetrance. Those enzymatic defects that uniquely affect the biosynthesis of cortisol are grouped together under the rubric of congenital adrenal hyperplasia (CAH). These five enzymes are: $P450_{scc}$ (defect in StAR), 3β-hydroxysteroid dehydrogenase, 21-hydroxylase, 11-hydroxylase and 17-hydroxylase. CRH and ACTH synthesis and secretion are normally under

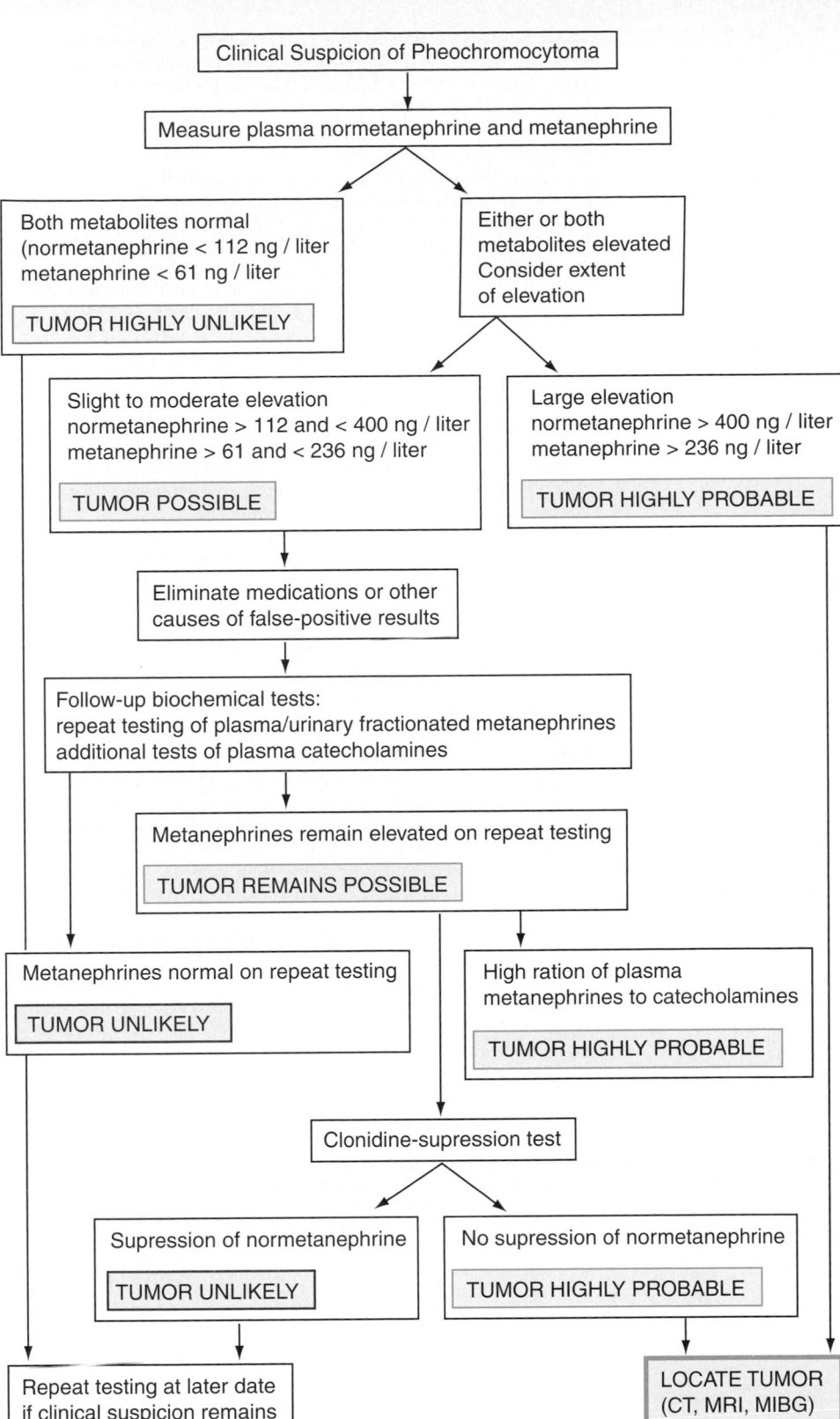

Figure 24–10 Algorithm for the evaluation of pheochromocytoma. MIBG = ^{131}I-meta-iodobenzylguanidine. (Redrawn from Eisenhofer G, Goldstein DS, Walther MM, et al: Biochemical diagnosis of pheochromocytoma: How to distinguish true- from false-positive test results. J Clin Endocrinol Metab 2003; 88(6):2656–2666 with permission.)

the negative-feedback control of cortisol. In CAH, defects in the enzymes necessary for cortisol production lead to cortisol deficiency; cortisol deficiency results in a disinhibition of the negative feedback on CRH and ACTH production. As a consequence, CRH and ACTH levels rise, inducing adrenal hyperplasia and a forward push in steroidogenesis, as the body tries to compensate and normalize cortisol production. Not only does this result in a build-up of hormonal precursors directly preceding the enzymatic defect, but it also causes a massive shunting of these precursors down the remaining functional pathways. The clinical manifestations of CAH are heterogeneous, depending upon the severity and location of the enzymatic defects, which hormones are deficient and which are produced in excess. Symptoms range from shock, salt wasting, anomalous sexual

development in infancy to hirsutism and infertility in the adult. Sometimes, as in partial enzymatic deficiencies of cortisol synthesis, near-adequate hormone synthesis is possible if hypersecretion of ACTH is able to stimulate adrenal hyperplasia to compensate for the deficiency. The clinical manifestations of various adrenal cortical enzyme deficiencies and their associated laboratory findings are summarized in Table 24–21.

The diagnosis is made by measuring the various serum hormone levels and assessing which steroids are produced in excess, and which are deficient, and by calculating the precursor/product ratio and comparing these results to the age- and sex-matched normative data. Since levels of hormones distal to the block (product hormones) may be elevated as a result of peripheral conversion of the markedly elevated precursor

Table 24–20 Physiologic Effects of Steroids

Representative hormone	Biological effects
Cortisol (as a representative glucocorticoid)	Protein nitrogen catabolism increased
	Gluconeogenesis
	Increased blood glucose concentration
	Decreased glucose tolerance
	Increased liver glycogen
	Increased liver glycogenolysis
	Decreased peripheral uptake and utilization of glucose
	Decreased synthesis of acid-sulfated mucopolysaccharides
	Fat synthesis and redistribution
	Cellular or tissue effects
	Anti-inflammatory
	Dissolution of lymphoid tissue
	Lymphopenia
	Eosinopenia
	Increased erythropoiesis
	Alteration of cellular permeability, especially decreased membrane permeability to water
	Increased gastric (HCl and pepsin) secretion
Aldosterone (as a representative mineralocorticoid)	Electrolyte regulation
	Sodium (Na$^+$) retention
	Potassium (K$^+$) excretion
	Retention of water and expansion of extracellular fluid volume
	Increases in blood pressure
Androgens (as representative sex hormones)	Protein nitrogen anabolism
	Growth and maturation – osseous and muscular
	Body hair (pubic and axillary)

hormones, the use of precursor/product ratios is important in avoiding misdiagnosis due to misleading elevation of product hormones (Levine, 2002). If hormone levels return as borderline but the clinical suspicion for CAH remains high, the steroid levels should be re-measured 60 minutes following the intravenous administration of 0.25 mg of ACTH. ACTH drives steroidogenesis forward, accentuating the block. When there is a proband, the diagnosis can be more accurately determined by genotyping.

CAH is categorized according to the severity of disease into classic (neonatal, severe) and nonclassic (late-onset, cryptogenic) forms. The classic form is further subdivided into salt-losing and non-salt-losing (simple virilizing) variants.

21-Hydroxylase Deficiency

The enzyme 21-hydroxylase (also referred to as CYP21, CYP21A2, P450$_{c21}$) is located within the mitochondrial endoplasmic reticulum. It is the most common cause of CAH, occurring in about 95% of all cases. Screening of newborns using capillary heel blood on paper filter disks has identified this disorder in about 1 in 14 000 persons in North America, and as high as 1 in 300 in the Yupik Eskimos of Alaska (Pang 1988, 1982) The classic form is detected in about 1 in 16 000 life births and the nonclassic is seen in about 0.2 % of the general white population, but can be as high as 1–2% in those of Eastern European Jewish ancestry (Therrell, 2001; Speiser, 1985).

21-OH catalyzes the conversion of 17-hydroxyprogesterone (17-OHP) to 11-deoxycortisol (compound S), and progesterone to 11-deoxycorticosterone (DOC). Thus, 21-OH deficiency leads to elevated levels of the steroid precursors 17-OHP and pregnanetriol in the urine and 17-OHP in the serum. These precursors are shunted toward the pathway leading to excess androstenedione and testosterone production (Fig. 24–12). Clinical presentation often correlates with the severity of enzymatic dysfunction. The classic variety presents in the newborn period or early childhood with adrenal insufficiency and virilization, with or without salt-wasting. The nonclassic form presents in late childhood as early adrenarche or in young adulthood as hirsutism, amenorrhea and infertility. The presentation in women is very similar to that of polycystic ovarian disease. Males may develop precocious puberty, adrenal rests within the testes and infertility.

A close functional relationship exists between the adrenal cortex and the adrenal medulla. Dysplasia of the medulla and catecholamine hyposecretion have been described in classic 21-OH deficiency. In a study of 38 children with classic (CYP21A2) disease, levels of plasma epinephrine and metanephrine and urinary epinephrine were 40–80% lower in affected individuals than in normals (Merke, 2000). In another study, those with classic (CYP21A2) disease showed a significantly decreased catecholamine response to exercise that was unaffected by the administration of stress doses of glucocorticoids (Weise, 2004). It has been suggested that the degree of medullary impairment may be a biomarker for CAH severity (Merke, 2002).

Diagnosis. Prenatal diagnosis is important because suppressive treatment with steroids can abrogate the development of virilization of the female fetus. Diagnosis is made either by measuring the level of 17-OHP in amniotic fluid or by genotyping cells obtained by chorionic villous sampling. The genes responsible for 21-OH deficiency, *CYP21* (CYP21A2) and *CYP21P* (CYP21A) are located on chromosome 6. Of these two homologous genes only *CYP21* is active, deleterious mutations within

Table 24–21 Congenital Adrenal Hyperplasia: Clinical and Biochemical Features

Feature	21-Hydoxylase deficiency	11β-Hydroxylase deficiency	17β-Hydroxylase deficiency	3β-Hydroxysteroid deficiency	Lipoid hyperplasia	Aldosterone synthase deficiency
Defective gene	CYP21	CYP11B1	CYP17	HSD3B2	StAR	CYP11B2
Incidence	1:15 000	1 : 100 000	Rare	Rare	Rare	Rare
Ambiguous genitalia	+ (Female)	+ (Female)	+ (Male) Absent puberty (female)	+ (Male) Mild in female	+ (Male) Absent puberty (female)	Normal
Acute adrenal insufficiency	+	Rare	No	+	++	Salt wasting only
Laboratory findings	↑ plasma 17-OHP and pregnanetriol Greatly ↑ urinary pregnanetriol and 17-KS	↑ serum DOC and 11-deoxycortisol ↑ urinary 17-OHCS and 17-KS	↑ serum DOC, 18-OH DOC, B and 18-OHB	↑ serum 17OH-pregnenolone, pregnenolone and DHEA ↑ urinary 17-KS ↑ Δ5/Δ4 serum and urinary steroids	All serum and plasma steroids are decreased	↑ serum B, 11-DOC and 18-OHB
Glucocorticoids	↓	↓	↓	↓	↓	Normal
Mineralocorticoids	↓	↑	↑	↓	↓	↓
Androgens	↑	↑	↓	↓ male, ↑ female	↓	Normal

B = corticosterone; 18-OHB = 18-hydroxycorticosterone; DOC = 11-deoxycorticosterone; 17-KS = 17-ketosteroids; 17-OHP = 17α-hydroxyprogesterone; 17-OHCS = 17-hydroxycorticosteroids; DHEA = dehydroepiandrosterone.

After Stewart PM: The adrenal cortex. *In* Larsen PR, Kronenberg HM, Melmed S, Polonsky KS (eds): Williams Textbook of Endocrinology, 10th ed. Philadelphia, Saunders, 2003, p 533.

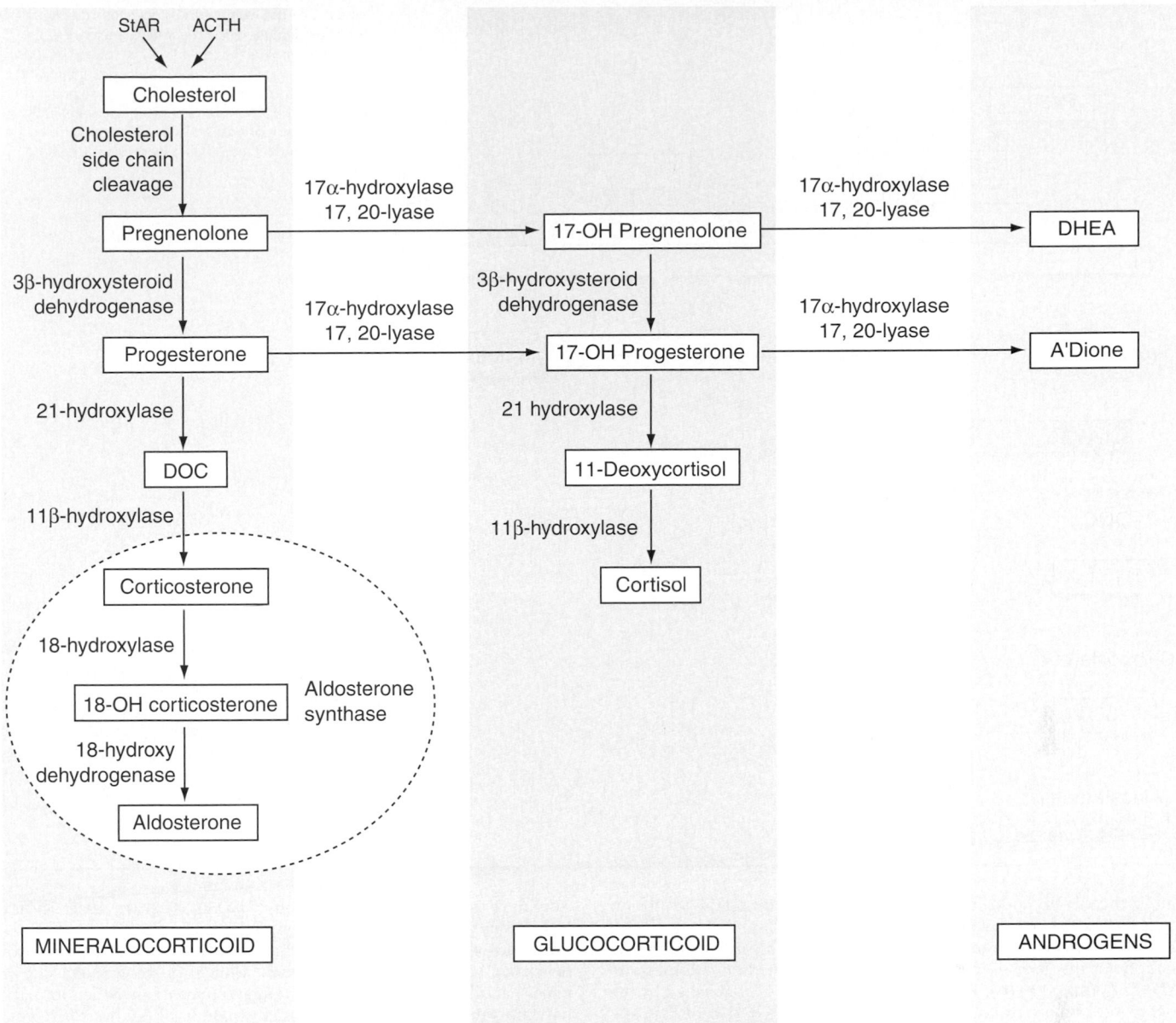

Figure 24–11 Steroidogeneic pathways of the adrenal cortex. The adrenal steroids are categorized according to mineralocorticoid, glucocorticoid or androgenic activity. StAR = steroid acute regulatory protein; ACTH = adrenocorticotropin; A'dione = androstenedione; DHEA = dihydroepiandosterone; DOC = deoxycorticosterone. The chemical structures for these steroids are shown in Fig. 25–1 in the succeeding chapter.

CYP21P interfere with normal gene expression. These mutations can be identified by polymerase chain reaction (PCR) and Southern blotting on chorionic villus samples (New, 1995; White, 1994a).

Neonatal screening, which is now mandatory in many states, is performed by measuring 17-OHP or by genotyping blood that has been obtained from a heelstick and collected on filter paper. Aside from genotyping being the most definitive test for diagnosing CAH, the fact that the genotype correlates fairly well with disease severity means that it can also be used as a prognostic tool (Nordenstrom, 1999).

In the newborn with salt wasting, unstimulated 17-OHP levels are typically > 8000 ng/dL, rising to 100 000 ng/dL (3000 nmol/L) following the administration of ACTH. Levels in the simple virilizing variant range from 10 000–30 000 ng/dL (300–1000 nmol/L). Those with nonclassic disease typically have 17-OHP levels ranging from 1500–10 000 ng/dL (50–300 nmol/L) (New, 1983). It is of note that randomly drawn hormone levels may be normal in those with nonclassic disease; therefore it is important to test during the early morning. If the results are equivocal, the diagnosis can be confirmed by comparing serum 17-OHP levels before and 60 minutes after the administration of 0.25 mg ACTH (Cortrosyn). ACTH acts to stimulate steroidogenesis, serving to dramatically increase the bottleneck at the site of the enzymatic block, resulting in a dramatic increase in precursors, in this case, 17-OHP. Post-ACTH 17-OHP values < 330 g/dL are normal, 330–1000 ng/dL indicate heterozygote carrier, and levels > 2000 ng/dL are diagnostic for nonclassic CAH. If a proband is

available, genotyping is superior to these older biochemical tests in identifying heterozygotes (Honour, 1993).

The goal of glucocorticoid and mineralocorticoid replacement therapy in children is the attainment of normal growth, weight, pubertal development, and optimization of final adult height. On the other hand, the major treatment goals in adults are a lessening of signs of virilization and a resumption of fertility. The objective of mineralocorticoid replacement is to normalize the plasma renin activity. The aim of glucocorticoid replacement is to keep the 17-OHP level partially suppressed to between 100–1000 ng/dL (3–30 nmol/L) and the ACTH under 100 ng/L, thereby preventing shunting toward testosterone synthesis, and normalizing levels of androstenedione and testosterone. Normalization of 17-OHP should not be attempted, since this requires supraphysiologic levels of glucocorticoids and may result in Cushing's syndrome (Speiser, 2003).

11β-Hydroxylase (11-OH) Deficiency

The second most common enzyme deficiency of the adrenal cortex, accounting for about 7% of all cases of CAH, is the 11β-hydroxylase (11-OH) deficiency. A defect in this enzyme blocks the final conversion of 11-deoxycortisol to cortisol and DOC to corticosterone. As with 21-OH deficiency, there is a compensatory increase in ACTH secretion leading to adrenal hyperplasia and a mass action shunting of precursor steroids toward testosterone synthesis, resulting in signs of virilization. This block also results in the accumulation of DOC; DOC's mineralocorticoid activity

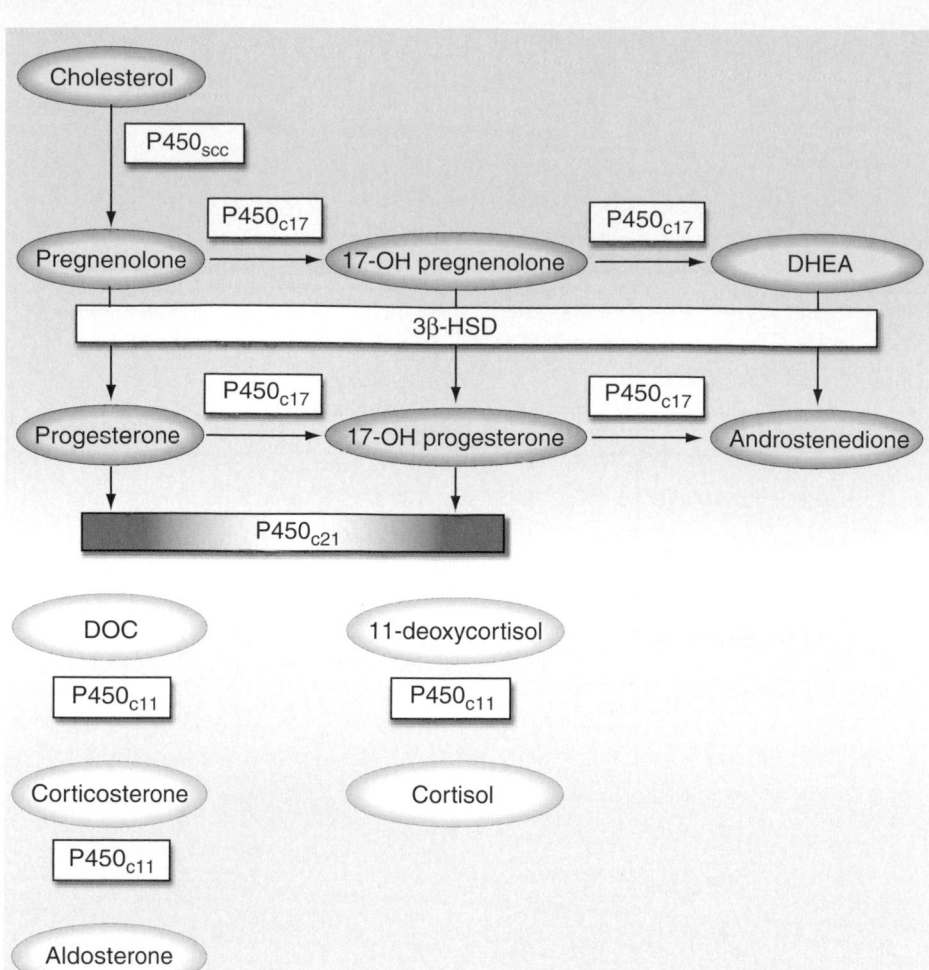

Figure 24–12 Defective steroidogenesis due to 21-hydroxylase deficiency. The relative increase in the hormones proximal to the block is depicted by the more intense color. The more severe the enzymatic defect the greater the concentration of the precursor hormones. DHEA = dihydroepiandrosterone; DOC = 11-deoxycorticosterone; P459 SCC = cytochrome P450-dependent side chain clearage enzyme.

leads to the development of hypertension and hypokalemia, similar to what is seen with hyperaldosteronism (Fig. 24–13).

11-OH deficiency is an autosomal recessive disorder caused by mutations of the genes *CYP11B1* and *CYP11B2*, located on chromosome 8q21-q22 (White, 1994b). Diagnosis in the neonate is established by the presence of a high basal and a high ACTH-stimulated 11-deoxycortisol. They will also have elevated concentrations of urinary tetrahydro-11-deoxycortisol in the urine. During childhood and in young adults the diagnosis of 11-OH deficiency is made by the presence of elevated early-morning and ACTH-stimulated serum levels of 11-deoxycortisol that are more than three times the upper limit for age-matched normals. Levels of DOC and adrenal androgens (androstenedione, dehydroepiandrosterone and dehydroepiandrosterone sulfate) are also elevated. Plasma renin activity and aldosterone are often suppressed due to elevations of DOC, which causes salt and water retention. Unlike the heterozygotes with 21-OH deficiency, those with 11-OH deficiency often fail to show a rise in precursors following ACTH-stimulation (Pang, 1980). However, an exuberant response has been seen in those who had hirsutism (Gabrilove, 1965).

Prenatal diagnosis of 11β-hydroxylase (11-OH) deficiency is made by measuring levels of tetrahydro-11-deoxycortisol (THS) in the maternal urine or amniotic fluid. These levels begin to rise in the first trimester. In addition to THS, there is also an elevation of levels of 11-deoxycortisol and the THS to tetrahydrocortisol plus tetrahydrocortisone ratio (Rosler, 1988).

Treatment is the replacement of glucocorticoids, causing normalization of DOC and plasma renin activity.

3β-Hydroxysteroid Dehydrogenase (3β-HSD) Deficiency

3β-Hydroxysteroid dehydrogenase (3β-HSD), which catalyzes the second enzymatic step in steroidogenesis, is coded by two genes, *HSD3BI* and *HSD3BII*. *HSD3BII* is expressed in the adrenals and gonads; *HSD3BI* is expressed in placenta, skin and other peripheral tissues and usually remains intact in CAH. A defect in 3β-HSD leads to a block in the conversion of Δ-5 steroids (pregnenolone, 17-OH pregnenolone, and dihydroepiandrosterone) to Δ-4 steroids (progesterone, 17-OHP, androstenedione), resulting in an increase in circulating levels of Δ-5

steroids (Fig. 24–14). However, because *HSD3BI* is usually intact, levels of the Δ-4 steroids may be normal or even elevated.

Patients with classic disease will have manifestations of glucocorticoid deficiency, with or without the accompaniment of salt wasting. Affected males have incomplete masculinization and females are either normal or have ambiguous genitalia. A late-onset variant has been described which is associated with features typical of PCOS such as hirsutism, oligomenorrhea and infertility (Pang, 1985).

Previous criteria for the diagnosis of 3β-HSD deficiency examined the basal and ACTH-stimulated Δ-4 to Δ-5 steroid ratios, 17-OH-pregnenolone (17-OHP) to cortisol, and levels of pregnenolone, 17-OH-pregnenolone and dehydroepiandrosterone in urine and blood. The standard for diagnosing this disorder has been recently revised to correlate more closely with genotypic studies. The ACTH-stimulated Δ-5-17 P levels, and Δ-5-17 P to cortisol ratios have been shown to be the best indices for definitively diagnosing 3β-HSD deficiency (Lutfallah, 2002). Applicability of these new criteria to patients with the nonclassic variant is still debatable.

Treatment consists of glucocorticoid and mineralocorticoid as well as sex steroids in accordance with normal growth and development.

17-Hydroxylase Deficiency

17-hydroxylase (CYP17, $P450_{c17}$), is expressed in both the adrenals and gonads and encodes two enzymes, 17α-hydroxylase and 17,20-lyase. 17α-Hydroxylase catalyzes the conversion of pregnenolone and progesterone to their respective 17-OH derivatives. 17,20-Lyase converts 17-OH pregnenolone to dihydroepiandrosterone (DHEA) and 17-OH progesterone to androstenedione. CYP17 deficiency blocks the conversion of pregnenolone and progesterone to the 17-hydroxy derivatives, causing shunting from testosterone and cortisol synthesis to aldosterone (Fig. 24–15). Accordingly these patients develop hypertension and hypokalemic alkalosis in association with incomplete masculinization (in the male) and decreased testosterone and cortisol levels. 17-OH deficiency is diagnosed by demonstrating high DOC, pregnenolone and progesterone levels, along with decreased urinary 17-ketosteroids and 17-hydroxycorticosteroids. The gene associated with this condition (*CYP17*), has been located on chromosome 10q, the same gene as 17,20-desmolase (Kater, 1994).

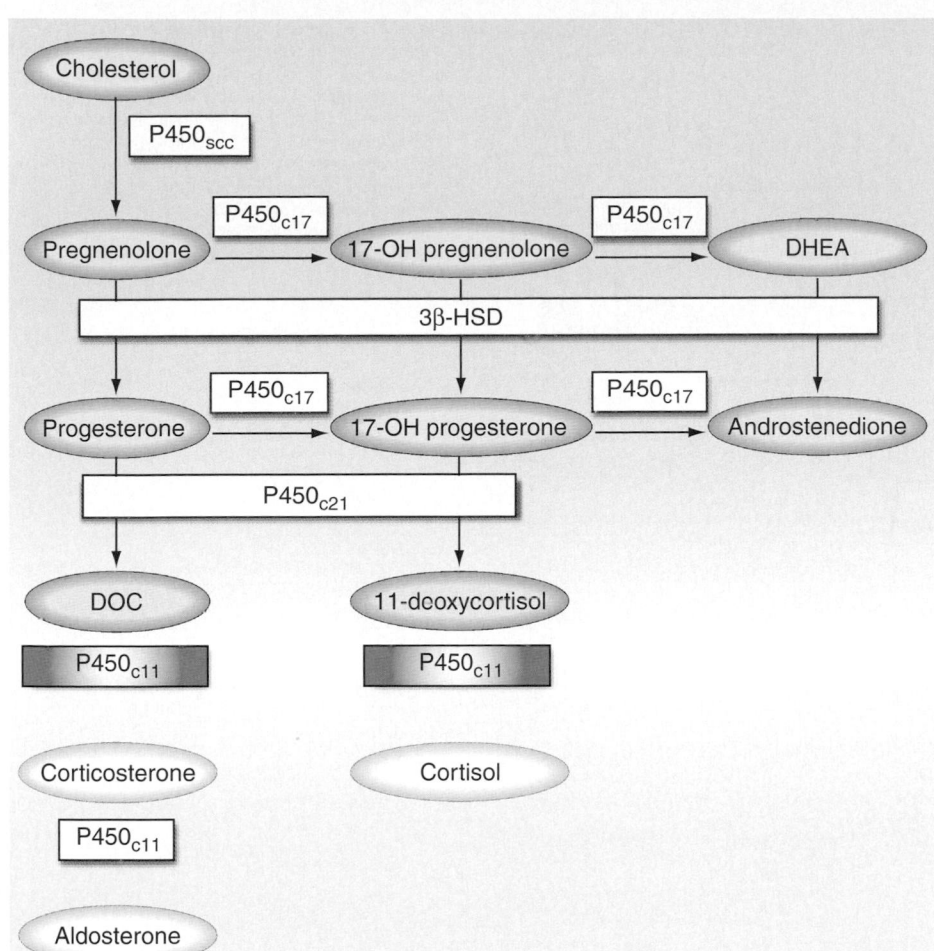

Figure 24–13 Defective steroidogenesis due to 11β-hydroxylase deficiency. The relative increase in the hormones proximal to the block is depicted by the more intense color. The more severe the enzymatic defect the greater the concentration of the precursor hormones. High levels of 11-deoxycorticosterone (DOC) created by the block produce a state of mineralocorticoid excess. DHEA = dihydroepiandrosterone; P459 SCC = cytochrome P450-dependent side chain clearage enzyme.

Congenital Lipoid Adrenal Hyperplasia

Congenital lipoid adrenal hyperplasia (lipoid CAH) is the most severe form of CAH in which the synthesis of all gonadal and adrenal cortical steroids is markedly impaired. Lipoid CAH may be caused by a defect in either the steroidogenic acute regulatory protein (StAR) or the P450$_{scc}$ (Fujieda, 2003). StAR, located on chromosome 8p11, controls the rate-limiting step in steroidogenesis. It is responsible for the shuttling of cholesterol from the outer to the inner mitochondrial membrane. 20,22-Desmolase (CYP11A1, P450$_{scc}$ [scc = side chain cleavage]) converts cholesterol to pregnenolone (Fig. 24–16). Pathologically, the adrenal cortex shows marked accumulation of cholesterol and other lipids, which is the primary distinguishing feature from congenital adrenal hypoplasia.

The presentation of this extremely rare disorder is that of severe adrenal insufficiency with hypotension, salt wasting, and feminization of external genitalia in males. Occasionally, females may not present until the onset of puberty. Diagnosis is made by the presence of extremely low cortisol and aldosterone concentrations, elevated ACTH and plasma renin activity.

Aldosterone Synthetase Deficiency (CYP11B2)

Aldosterone synthetase (CYP11B2) is the final step in the steroid synthetic pathway leading to the production of aldosterone. It stimulates a multistep process, the 11-hydroxylation of DOC to corticosterone, the 18-hydroxylation of corticosterone to 18-hydroxycorticosterone and finally the 18-dehydrogenation to aldosterone. Isolated enzyme deficiency leads to salt wasting, hyperkalemia and metabolic acidosis. This condition may be diagnosed by demonstrating the presence of metabolites of corticosterone and 11-deoxycorticosterone in the urine, elevated serum DOC and deficiency of corticosterone, 18-hydroxycorticosterone or aldosterone in the serum.

Cortisol and the Glucocorticoids

The adrenal cortex secretes cortisol in response to ACTH, a diurnal rhythm and stress. ACTH, synthesized in the adenohypophysis, is formed from the cleavage of a much larger precursor molecule: pro-opiomelanocortin (POMC). In addition to ACTH, cleavage of POMC releases β-lipotropin (β-LPH), which in turn is cleaved to yield γ-LPH and β-endorphin. Within the

ACTH sequence are α-MSH and the corticotropin-like intermediate lobe protein (CLIP). Endorphins, which act on neurons in the brain, comprise a distinct peptidergic system related to pain perception. Although β-endorphin is secreted in parallel with ACTH, the significance of this remains unknown.

ACTH consists of 39 amino acid residues, of which residues 1–24 at the amino-terminal possess full hormonal activity. Occasionally POMC is incompletely processed; this leads to the formation of other forms of ACTH that usually have little biologic activity although they may retain immunoreactivity. These forms may predominate in malignant conditions such as ectopic production by primary or metastatic lung cancer, and in some patients with Nelson's syndrome, a disorder characterized by the occurrence of a pituitary tumor and skin hyperpigmentation following bilateral adrenalectomy. Defects in POMC cleavage enzymes may also be responsible for the formation of rare forms of isolated ACTH deficiency (Nussey, 1993).

ACTH is secreted in response to several factors, of which corticotropin-releasing hormone (CRH) and arginine-vasopressin (AVP) are the most important. Among the other moieties reported to stimulate ACTH secretion are atrial natriuretic factor (ANF), angiotensin II, interleukin-6 (IL-6), interleukin-1 (IL-1) and tumor necrosis factor-alpha (TNFα) (Rivier, 1983; Chrousos, 1998).

CRH is released in a circadian pattern and in response to physiologic stimuli such as stress and hypoglycemia. Synthetic forms of CRH are used in testing anterior pituitary reserves of ACTH by comparing plasma ACTH or cortisol before and 1 hour after CRH stimulation (Grodum, 1993). This test is useful in distinguishing between lesions affecting the hypothalamus, pituitary and adrenal glands (Fukata, 1993). If the lesion is in the hypothalamus, after a time delay, ACTH levels rise following CRH administration. If it is in the pituitary, there is no significant ACTH response. If there is primary adrenal insufficiency, administration of CRH causes a further rise in an already elevated ACTH level, but there is little or no rise in the level of cortisol.

The hypothalamic–pituitary–adrenal (HPA) axis consists of various feedback loops that control cortisol synthesis and secretion. When plasma cortisol increases, it suppresses the release of ACTH, CRH and AVP, which

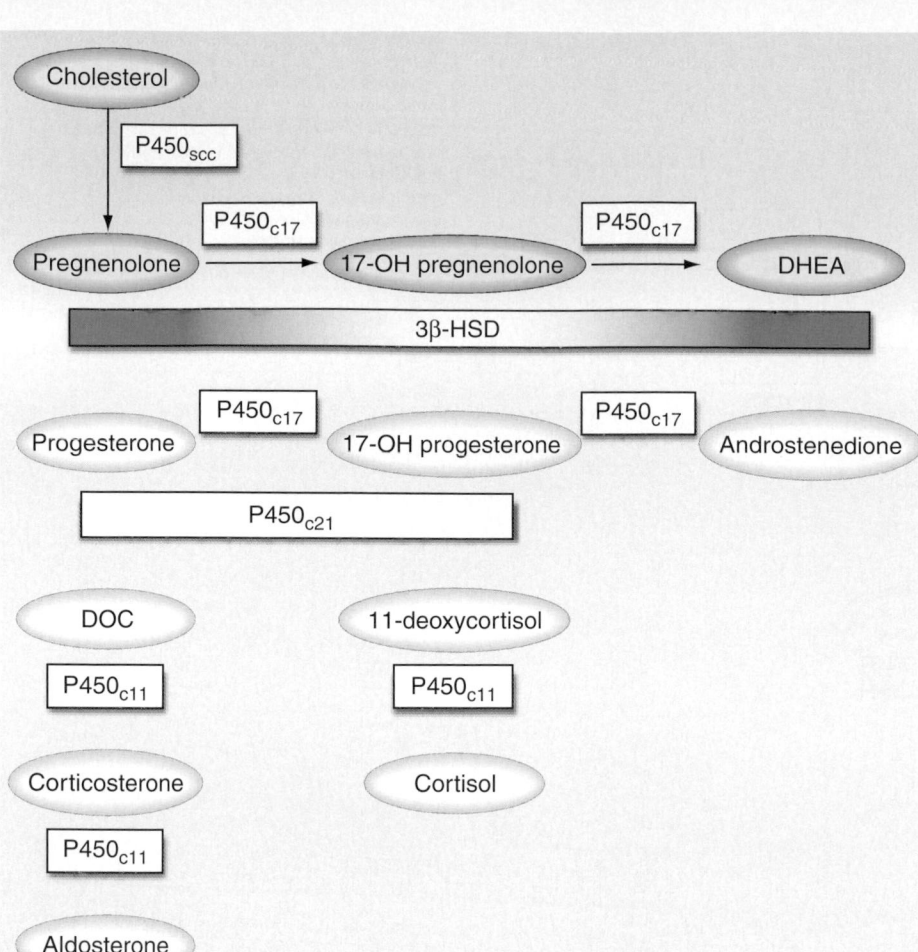

Figure 24–14 Defective steroidogenesis due to 3β-hydroxysteroid dehydrogenase deficiency. The relative increase in the hormones proximal to the block is depicted by the more intense color. The more severe the enzymatic defect the greater the concentration of the precursor hormones. 17α-hydroxyprogesterone levels may be elevated due to peripheral conversion of 17α-hydroxy pregnenolone. DHEA = dihydroepiandrosterone; DOC = 11-deoxycorticosterone; P459 SCC = cytochrome P450-dependent side chain clearage enzyme.

in turn leads to a lowering of the cortisol level. Conversely, when serum cortisol reaches a nadir, the pituitary responds by increasing ACTH production, resulting in stimulation of cortisol formation. By this mechanism, ACTH and cortisol control the concentration of each other within a very narrow range, and a small change in one results in a concomitant change in the other. When the adrenal is unable to respond to ACTH because of damage or disease, cortisol levels are low and ACTH levels are high. In those conditions in which the pituitary is destroyed, ACTH is not formed and cortisol levels are consequently low. Damage to the hypothalamus is also associated with low ACTH and cortisol levels; testing with CRH may permit the distinction between these two entities. If the HPA axis is interrupted by the administration of large amounts of exogenous glucocorticoids, they will have an inhibitory effect on the hypothalamus and pituitary, suppressing CRH and ACTH secretion. If this suppression continues over a period of weeks, the pituitary may become persistently suppressed and lead to atrophy of the adrenals. As a result, the HPA axis becomes unable to secrete cortisol in times of stress.

The second influence on plasma cortisol levels is the diurnal pattern, which is due to the circadian pattern of ACTH release. Major increases in secretion occur between 0400 and 0800 hours, followed by a decrease in ACTH during the rest of the day. In subjects with a normal sleep–wake cycle, the lowest ACTH concentrations are found shortly after midnight. Sudden changes in sleep–wake patterns have little effect on the diurnal pattern but permanent changes in daily sleep habits result in a gradual change in diurnal secretory patterns. Superimposed on the circadian periodicity is an ultradian rhythm of 10–18 secretory bursts per 24 hours (Horrocks, 1990).

The third important influence on cortisol secretion is stress. Stimuli such as surgical trauma, pyrogens, hypoglycemia and hemorrhage are capable of bringing about an acute increase in ACTH and cortisol secretion. This response to stress may be absent or decreased in magnitude in patients in whom large doses of steroids have been administered for some time. The initiation of any stress response is dependent upon an intact nervous system. For example, trauma normally results in the acute release of ACTH and cortisol; however, in patients with spinal cord transections, which interrupt the normal transmission of neurologic stimuli, the same trauma applied to an extremity will not elicit any ACTH or cortisol response. There is evidence that the stress response of cortisol is mediated through excitatory and inhibitory inputs that become integrated at the level of the hypothalamus and modulate CRH secretion. Cortisol levels also rise after meals, especially those high in protein and also in depression (Linkowski, 1987).

Most disorders of cortisol secretion can be classified by the patterns of response of the following three hormones to suppression and stimulation: ACTH, plasma cortisol and urinary free cortisol (Snow, 1992).

Laboratory Measurement of ACTH

Plasma ACTH is measured using either a two-site radioimmunometric assay (RIA) or an immunochemiluminometric assay. To prevent degradation of ACTH, it is best to collect the sample in a prechilled EDTA (ethylenediamine tetraacetic acid) (lavender top) tube. The specimen should be kept in an ice bath and should be processed as soon as possible. Following centrifugation in a refrigerated centrifuge, the specimen should be separated, transferred to a plastic tube and kept frozen at −20°C until time of analysis. The normal reference range is 2–12 pmol/L (9–52 pg/mL) at 7–10 a.m. Plasma ACTH is a useful tool for distinguishing primary (adrenal) from secondary (pituitary) or tertiary (hypothalamic) adrenal insufficiency. In primary adrenal insufficiency, low cortisol concentrations are found along with increased ACTH levels. In secondary or tertiary adrenal insufficiency both ACTH and cortisol are expected to be low. ACTH levels best discriminate between healthy individuals and those with adrenal insufficiency when specimens for ACTH are collected between 8 a.m. and 10 a.m.

ACTH is less useful in diseases of cortisol excess. Up to 50% of the patients may have normal ACTH levels in Cushing's disease. Although the values tend to run higher (> 20 pmol/L [> 90 pg/mL]) in Cushing's syndrome due to ectopic ACTH production, the values overlap with those seen in Cushing's disease in 30% of cases (Findling, 1992). Because of the normal diurnal variation in ACTH and cortisol secretion, measurement of these values during their expected nadir, from 11 p.m. to 1 a.m., is helpful in confirming the diagnosing of ACTH-dependent Cushing's. An elevated midnight ACTH of greater than 5 pmol/L (23 pg/mL) in the face of an elevated serum cortisol confirms the diagnosis of ACTH-dependent Cushing's. Those patients with ectopic ACTH-secreting tumors charac-

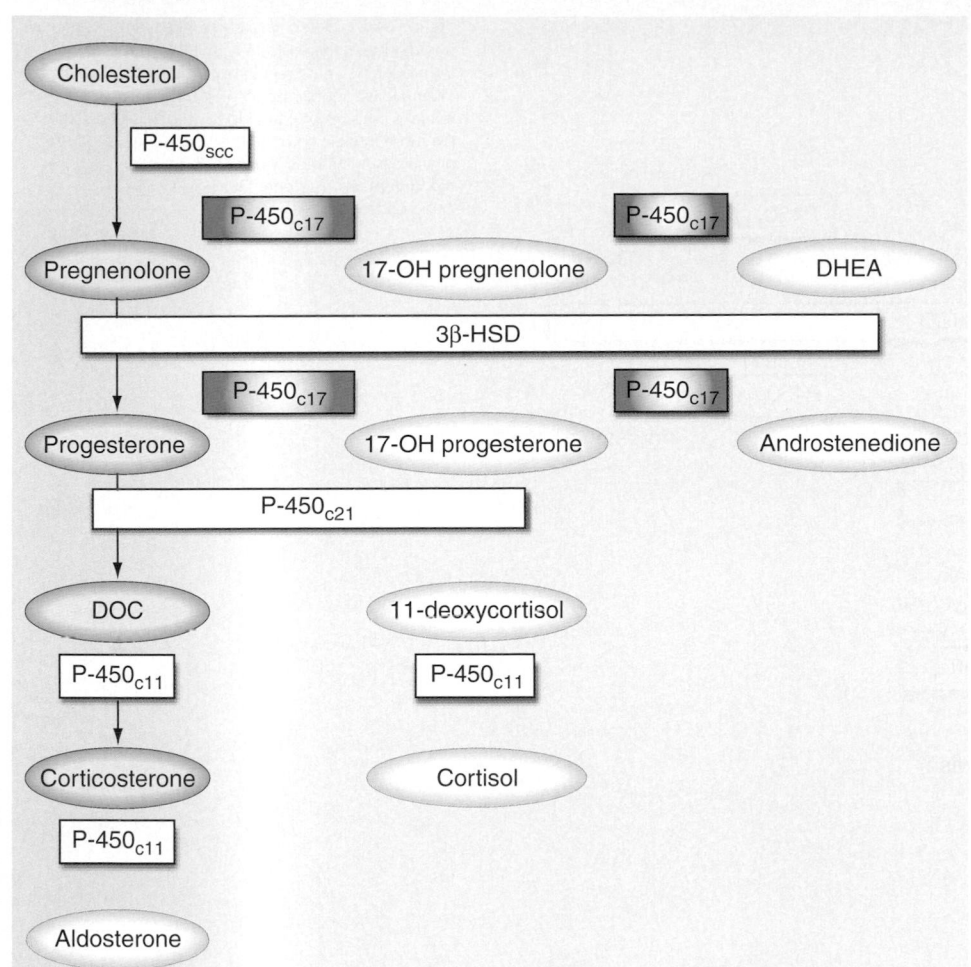

Figure 24–15 Defective steroidogenesis due to 17-hydroxylase deficiency. The relative increase in the hormones proximal to the block is depicted by the more intense color. The more severe the enzymatic defect the greater the concentration of the precursor hormones. High levels of 11-deoxycorticosterone (DOC) and corticosterone created by the block produce a state of mineralocorticoid excess. DHEA = dihydroepiandrosterone; P459 SCC = cytochrome P450-dependent side chain clearage enzyme.

teristically have markedly elevated plasma ACTH (usually > 200 pg/mL) and an elevated serum cortisol. Measurement of ACTH by plasma extraction, which detects ACTH precursors and fragments, may be useful in distinguishing patients with cancer-related syndromes or ACTH-secreting tumors from those with Cushing's disease, as the former entities are more likely to produce these other forms of ACTH (White, 1993). ACTH-secreting neoplasms may be occult, creating diagnostic difficulties; in this instance ACTH measurements using selective venous sampling has proven useful in the localization of the lesion.

In patients with increased levels of circulating glucocorticoids due to adrenal adenomas or carcinomas, ACTH secretion is inhibited; hence, circulating ACTH levels are low or undetectable. In patients with pituitary-induced adrenal hyperplasia, plasma ACTH may be at or above the upper reference interval at 9 a.m., but fail to show the expected fall after midnight. Another use of ACTH assays is in the determination of adequacy of cortisol replacement in congenital adrenal hyperplasia. When replacement therapy is optimal, ACTH values are similar to those seen in a reference population.

Plasma Corticotropin-Releasing Hormone (CRH)

Corticotropin-releasing hormone measurements are performed by liquid chromatography and tandem mass spectrometry and remain largely a research tool.

CRH circulates in one of two forms, either free or bound to CRH-binding protein. The level of CRH-binding protein increases during pregnancy. CRH is increased in patients with Cushing's syndrome due to ectopic production of CRH. The reference range for plasma CRH in men and nonpregnant women is < 34 pg/mL. The normative range varies throughout pregnancy: first trimester < 40 pg/mL; second trimester < 153 pg/mL; and third trimester < 847 pg/mL (Goland, 1986).

Serum Cortisol Measurements

About 90% of circulating cortisol is bound to serum protein, of which 10–20% is loosely bound to albumin and the remainder bound to the glycoprotein transcortin (cortisol-binding globulin [CBG]). The remaining 10% of circulating cortisol is the unbound, free hormone. It is believed that only free cortisol is active and that the protein-bound fraction is metabolically inert, probably serving as a reservoir for free cortisol. Protein binding also may protect cortisol from deactivation by the liver or filtration by the kidney.

One of the earliest and simplest methods used to determine serum cortisol was a fluorometric assay developed by Nelson & Samuels, which was based upon a technique first developed by Porter & Silber (Nelson, 1952; Porter, 1950). A more specific method for cortisol estimation is immunoassay. Advantages include small specimen volume and rapid turnaround time. Some of the antibodies that are used show a large degree of cross-reactivity with other steroids such as 11-deoxycortisol, deoxycorticosterone and synthetic steroids such as dexamethasone. Although cross-reactivity does not pose a problem with baseline testing, in stimulatory and suppressive maneuvers such as metyrapone or dexamethasone suppression, this can lead to spuriously high measurements. With deterioration of renal function, various steroids and their glucuronides accumulate in the blood. Because of their structure, conjugates may cross-react with some cortisol antibodies, producing an interference that can be of the same magnitude as the actual cortisol concentration. In CAH, high concentrations of cortisol precursors occur in the serum because of an enzyme defect. Because these precursors cross-react with assay antibodies, spurious elevations of cortisol are found; the degree of interference varies with the assay used and cannot be easily predicted. Nonisotopic immunoassay methods using organometallic tracers, fluorescence polarization and enzyme immunoassay techniques have also been developed for cortisol determinations (Bacarese-Hamilton, 1992; Lentjes, 1993; Philomin, 1994). The major disadvantage of cortisol assays continues to be lack of specificity.

The measurement of cortisol by RIA and chemiluminescent immunometric techniques has largely been supplanted by high-performance liquid chromatography (HPLC) with tandem mass spectrometry, which appears to offer the ultimate in specificity. Most HPLC systems for cortisol measurements use reverse-phase liquid chromatography with ultraviolet detection (Volin, 1992). This method is both highly sensitive and free from many of the sources of interference encountered in immunoassays (Samaan, 1993).

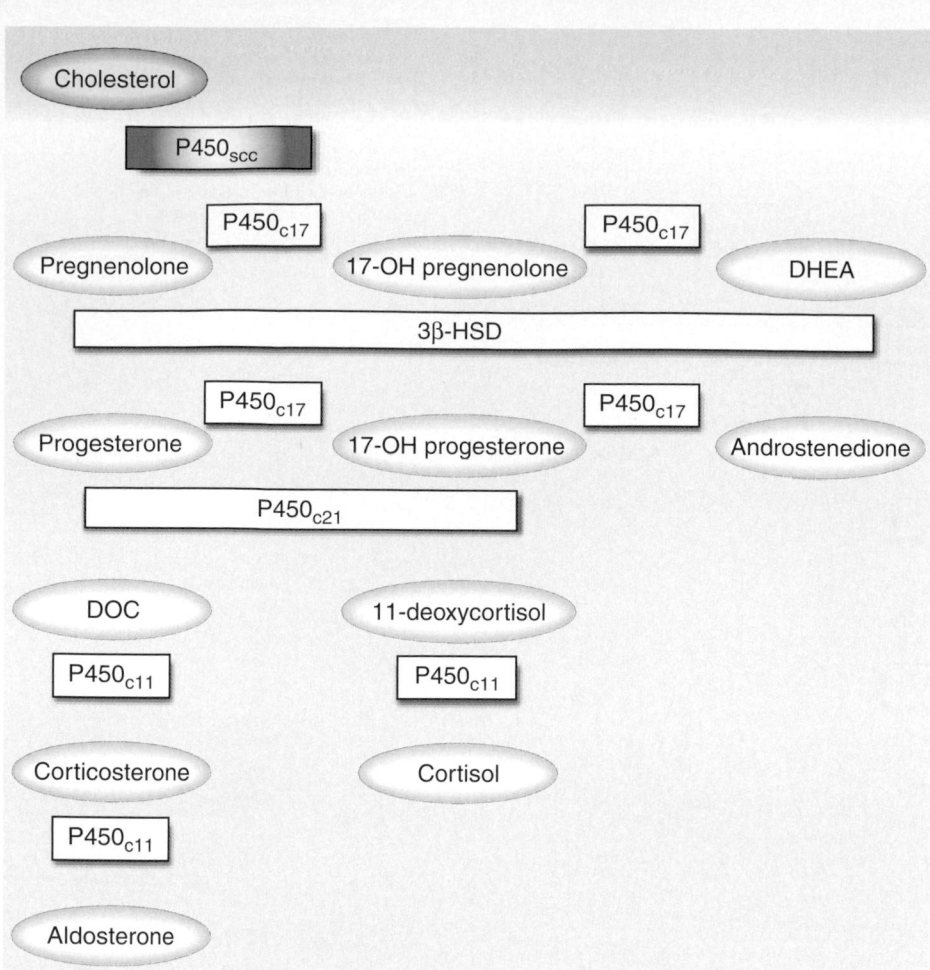

Figure 24–16 Defective steroidogenesis in congenital lipoid adrenal hyperplasia is due to a defect in either steroidogenic acute regulatory protein (StAR) or side chain cleavage enzyme ($P450_{scc}$). The relative increase in the hormones proximal to the block is depicted by the more intense color. In this disorder the synthesis of all classes of steroids is defective. DHEA = dihydroepiandrosterone; DOC = 11-deoxycorticosterone.

Serum cortisol is collected in a no additive (red top) tube. Reference values for serum cortisol for men and women roughly range from 5–25 μg/dL (140–690 nmol/L) at 8 a.m. to 10 a.m., dropping to about 3–12 μg/dL (80–330 nmol/L) by 4 p.m. Because of wide swings in basal cortisol levels resulting from its diurnal and ultridian pattern of secretion, serum cortisol assays are most useful when evaluated in the context of dynamic manipulation (i.e. adrenal stimulation or suppression).

Salivary cortisol

Up to 30% of urinary free cortisol and dexamethasone suppression screening tests may return an incorrect result. Recent studies have shown that the use of a midnight salivary cortisol (MSC) is a viable alternative.

One study compared the sensitivity for the detection of Cushing's syndrome by nighttime salivary cortisol levels with that of simultaneous inpatient serum cortisol levels and urine glucocorticoid excretion. It was found that the salivary cortisol measurements worked as well as plasma measurements and better than urine glucocorticoid excretion. The authors concluded that the measurement of bedtime salivary cortisol was a practical and accurate screening test for the diagnosis of Cushing's syndrome (Papanicolaou, 2002). Another study compared the diagnostic performance of midnight salivary cortisol (MSC) measurement with that of midnight serum cortisol (MNC) and urinary free cortisol (UFC) in differentiating 41 patients with Cushing's syndrome from 33 with pseudo-Cushing states, 199 with simple obesity, and 27 healthy normal weight volunteers. In the whole study population, no statistically significant differences in terms of sensitivity, specificity, diagnostic accuracy, and predictive values were observed among tests. In particular, the overall diagnostic accuracy for MSC, was similar to those of UFC and MNC (Putignano, 2003).

Urinary Free Cortisol (UFC) Measurements

Only 1% of the total adrenal secretion appears in the urine as cortisol, but it is this fraction that provides a valuable aid in the diagnosis of adrenal disease. In the kidney, glomerular filtration of free cortisol is followed by passive tubular reabsorption without a demonstrable reabsorption maximum. Urine collected over 24 hours is the best specimen to submit because it provides an integrated profile of total cortisol secretion. The urine should also be assayed for creatinine to ensure that an adequate specimen has been submitted. The reliability of the test may be further improved by submitting urine collected over 2 or 3 days because day-to-day fluctuations in cortisol excretion are known to occur.

At serum cortisol levels of about 20–25 μg/dL (the upper 8 a.m. reference value), the binding capacity of transcortin is exceeded; this leads to a very rapid and disproportionate increase in the unbound fraction compared with the total serum cortisol. For example, a doubling of the cortisol from 20 to 40 μg/dL results in at least a fivefold increase in the unbound cortisol in serum. At these levels, free cortisol clearance by the kidneys is directly proportional to the unbound serum cortisol concentration and leads to a steep rise in cortisol clearance. Thus, when urinary free cortisol excretion rather than serum cortisol is used, it is easier to discriminate patients with adrenal hyperfunction from a reference population.

Urinary free cortisol levels are unaffected by alterations in hepatic metabolism of cortisol. Although total cortisol production and urinary 17-hydroxycorticosteroids (17-OHCS) may be increased, the serum cortisol and urinary free cortisol remain within the reference interval. Because the renal clearance of cortisol is dependent on normal kidney function, it is not surprising that patients with renal disease may have low urinary values. UFC is unreliable when the creatinine clearance (CrCl) is < 20 mL/min, and is of reduced reliability when the CrCl is < 60 mL/min (Chan, 2004). Increased serum concentration of transcortin during pregnancy and with estrogen therapy result in increased serum cortisol levels. This increase is not reflected by an elevation of cortisol metabolites in urine, but urinary free cortisol may be increased. Conditions in which spuriously elevated levels occur include starvation, use of topical steroids and perhaps hydration in the form of water loading.

Method. HPLC with mass spectrometry is considered the current reference method for measuring urinary free cortisol (UFC); it has a diagnostic sensitivity of 100% and specificity of 98% for distinguishing patients with Cushing's syndrome from normal individuals (Rudd, 1985). Prior assays (like RIA) were less specific with a tendency to overestimate the amount of cortisol present. When measuring free cortisol in the urine by RIA, reference intervals have been found to vary with patient gender (men had higher reference intervals than women), the use of extraction procedure and the RIA test kit (Lamb, 1994).

The normal range varies according to the assay technique used; however, values that are four times the upper reference limit are diagnostic for Cushing's syndrome. A low urinary free cortisol value is suggestive of adrenal hypofunction; however, because there is great overlap with the normal reference interval, this test is not used for making the diagnosis of adrenal insufficiency.

Hypercortisolism: Cushing's Syndrome

Cushing's syndrome is a group of clinical and metabolic disorders characterized by adrenocortical hyperfunction; it is associated with excess production of glucocorticoids, or glucocorticoids and androgens. Patients with severe forms of the syndrome are easily recognizable when the disorder is florid. In less severely afflicted individuals, the vague signs and symptoms that occur may not be easily recognized as caused by hypercortisolism. Although many patients with ectopic ACTH-producing tumors have elevated ACTH and glucocorticoids because of the rapid growth of these tumors, the patients' demise may occur before the clinical signs of the syndrome appear.

Laboratory findings in Cushing's syndrome are (1) excessive and persistent production of cortisol measured as elevated serum cortisol, urinary free cortisol or 17-OHCS, (2) loss of circadian rhythm of ACTH and cortisol, (3) loss of suppression of cortisol production by administration of the synthetic glucocorticoid dexamethasone, and (4) hyperglycemia. Of the clinical findings that suggest Cushing's syndrome, the most common are central obesity, hypertension and hirsutism.

Cushing's disease is a state of glucocorticoid excess resulting from an ACTH-secreting pituitary adenoma. Cushing's syndrome is a more global term that encompasses a wide variety of entities associated with hypercortisolemia. The evaluation of a patient suspected of having Cushing's syndrome is best divided into two phases. The first phase is the actual documentation of hypercortisolism, the second is the identification of the pathophysiologic process behind the hypercortisolism. Cushing's syndrome is most commonly iatrogenic in origin; however, it may also be due to ectopic production of CRH or ACTH by a tumor or due to a primary adrenal malignancy. Adrenal Cushing's syndrome is a disorder of excess autonomous production of cortisol by the adrenals resulting in suppression of the hypothalamic–pituitary axis. Adrenal Cushing's (adenoma or carcinoma) accounts for less than 20% of the cases, whereas pituitary Cushing's accounts for about 68%, and ectopic production of ACTH outside the pituitary–adrenal axis is the cause of about 12% of cases (Orth, 1995). Because the treatment and prognosis differ depending on of the cause, it is important that a specific diagnosis be reached.

Tests used for the Diagnosis of Cushing's Syndrome (Fig. 24–17)

Screening tests. There are three screening tests used in the evaluation of a patient suspected of having Cushing's syndrome, the 24-hour urinary free cortisol, the overnight dexamethasone suppression test and either the plasma or salivary midnight cortisol level. Each has its own merits and drawbacks.

The 24-hour urinary free cortisol is a reflection of the unbound circulating cortisol that is freely filtered by the glomerulus. Unlike serum cortisol, it is unaffected by the level of circulating CBG. HPLC or gas chromatography coupled with mass spectrometry provides the best specificity for measuring urinary free cortisol. The upper range of normal with these methods is 110–138 nmol/24 h (40–50 µg/h) (Raff, 2003). The creatinine should be measured in all collections to ensure the adequacy of the specimen. Urinary cortisol excretion is decreased when the glomerular filtration rate is < 30 mL/min, and may thus be normal despite the presence of excessive cortisol production (Arnaldi, 2003). Values greater than four times the upper limit of normal are diagnostic of Cushing's syndrome. However, 10–15% of patients with Cushing's syndrome will have at least one in four 24-hour urine collections for free cortisol return as normal (Nieman, 1990). If cortisol excretion is normal but the clinical suspicion is high, either repeat the study or use a different screening method. Milder elevations can be seen in pseudo-Cushing's and during normal pregnancy. Pseudo-Cushing's is an entity characterized by HPA axis overactivity but without true Cushing's syndrome. It has been described in depression, anxiety disorders, alcoholism and morbid obesity.

The overnight dexamethasone suppression test is a much simpler test to perform. The patient takes 1 mg of dexamethasone orally between the hours of 11 p.m. and 12 midnight. The plasma cortisol is drawn the following morning between 8 a.m. and 9 a.m. The original criterion for an abnormal response was the failure to suppress the morning cortisol level

to < 5 µg/dL (138 nmol/L); however, this has been revised downward to < 1.8 µg/dL (50 nmol/L) (Arnaldi, 2003; Findling, 1999). Failure to suppress could be due to Cushing's syndrome or pseudo-Cushing's; it may even occur in some patients who are normal. The false-positive rate can be as high as 30%, occurring for a variety of reasons: the medication was taken too early; the patient was on phenobarbital, dilantin or other medication known to accelerate the metabolism of dexamethasone; malabsorption; alcoholism; or morbid obesity. Pregnancy and drugs such as estrogen, which increase serum transcortin, the cortisol-binding protein, may also result in elevated cortisol levels. Because of these and possibly other factors, about 1% of healthy individuals, 13% of obese patients, and 25% of hospitalized and chronically ill patients show false-positive overnight dexamethasone suppression tests. False-negative results, on the other hand, occur in less than 2% of patients.

The late night (11 p.m.) salivary cortisol is a simple test that carries high diagnostic sensitivity and specificity. The patient can collect the sample at home. There are two methods for collecting the sample: the patient can chew on a cotton tube for 2–3 minutes and then place the cotton tube into a plastic tube; or alternatively they can expectorate directly into a test tube. The sample is then mailed to the reference laboratory; since salivary cortisol is very stable there is little concern about degradation during transport. The sample is analyzed using enzyme-linked immunosorbent assay (EIA) or radioimmunoassay (RIA), the normative values vary according to the reference laboratory.

Confirmatory Tests for the Diagnosis of Cushing's Syndrome. A positive screen for Cushing's syndrome is followed by confirmatory testing with either a midnight plasma cortisol or low-dose dexamethasone suppression test (DST) performed alone or with the administration of CRH.

The midnight plasma cortisol requires hospital admission for at least 48 hours, insertion of a line for i.v. access prior to 10 p.m., the patient to be sleeping at the time of the blood draw and availability of staff to draw the blood at midnight. A midnight plasma cortisol greater than 7.5 µg/dL (207 nmol/L) is diagnostic of Cushing's; this has a 100% specificity for normals and those with pseudo-Cushing's (Papanicolaou, 1998). More recently, several authorities have suggested using 1.8 µg/dL (50 nmol/L) as the cutoff for normal. This value carries a very high degree of sensitivity (Newell-Price, 1995).

The low-dose (2-day 2 mg) dexamethasone suppression test (DST) requires the collection of two baseline 24-hour urines for urinary free cortisol (UFC). The patient is then given 0.5 mg dexamethasone orally every 6 hours for the next 2 days. On day two of dexamethasone another 24 h urine is collected for UFC. A normal response is a decrease in UFC to less than 10 µg (27 nmol) per 24 hours on the second day of dexamethasone. This has a sensitivity of 97–100% for discriminating Cushing's syndrome from normals (Newell-Price, 1998). Instead of measuring UFC, serum cortisol can be measured at 9 a.m. and at 48 hours following the first dose of dexamethasone. In this case a normal response consists of the plasma cortisol suppressing to less than 1.8 µg/dL (50 nmol/L), which has a sensitivity and specificity of more than 95% (Newell-Price, 1998). Performance of the DST with CRH has been purported to better distinguish Cushing's syndrome from pseudo-Cushing's (Yanovski, 1993).

Tests for Defining the Cause of Cushing's. Once the diagnosis of Cushing's syndrome is established, the next step is to determine its cause. Cushing's is categorized as being either ACTH-dependent or ACTH-independent; this is accomplished by either measuring the plasma ACTH, or performing a high-dose DST or a CRH stimulation test (Table 24–22).

ACTH-independent Cushing's syndrome results from autonomous production of cortisol; which would feedback on the hypothalamus and pituitary and cause suppression of CRH and ACTH secretion. The technique for measuring plasma ACTH has been described previously. Values below the level of detection or below 10 pg/mL (2 pmol/L) at 9 a.m. with a concomitantly elevated cortisol support an ACTH-independent cause for Cushing's syndrome. Plasma levels greater than 20 pg/mL (4 pmol/L) in the face of hypercortisolism are strongly suggestive of an ACTH-dependent cause. A CRH stimulation test with measurement of ACTH is indicated for values between 10–20 pg/mL (2–4 pmol/L) (Orth, 1995). Although patients with ectopic ACTH production tend to have markedly elevated ACTH levels, there is great overlap with the levels seen in Cushing's disease; therefore it cannot reliably be used to distinguish between these entities.

The high-dose (two-day 8 mg) dexamethasone suppression test is useful for distinguishing Cushing's disease from adrenal or ectopic Cushing's. It is of note that neuroendocrine tumors such as bronchial carcinoid may also suppress on high-dose dexamethasone. For the high-dose DST a baseline 24-hour urine for UFC is collected. Beginning on day 1, the patient receives 2 mg of dexamethasone orally every 6 hours for 48 hours; urine for UFC is collected on day 1 and on day 2. As an alternative to

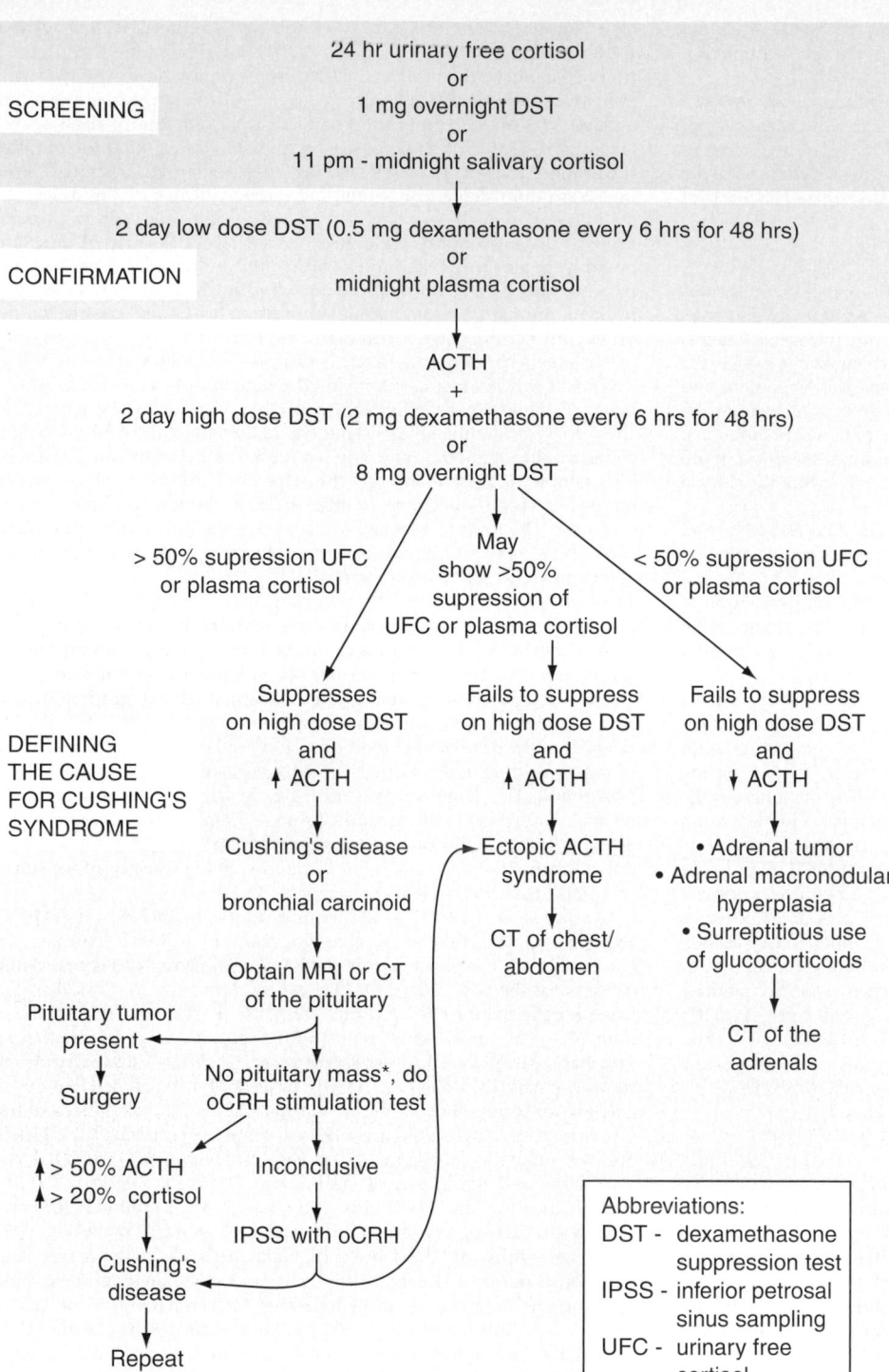

Figure 24–17 Algorithm for the evaluation of Cushing's syndrome. All screening tests must be followed by a confirmatory test. ACTH = adrenocorticotropic hormone; oCRH = ovine corticotropin-releasing hormone.

SCREENING

24 hr urinary free cortisol
or
1 mg overnight DST
or
11 pm - midnight salivary cortisol

CONFIRMATION

2 day low dose DST (0.5 mg dexamethasone every 6 hrs for 48 hrs)
or
midnight plasma cortisol

ACTH
+
2 day high dose DST (2 mg dexamethasone every 6 hrs for 48 hrs)
or
8 mg overnight DST

> 50% supression UFC or plasma cortisol

May show >50% supression of UFC or plasma cortisol

< 50% supression UFC or plasma cortisol

DEFINING THE CAUSE FOR CUSHING'S SYNDROME

Suppresses on high dose DST and ↑ ACTH

Fails to suppress on high dose DST and ↑ ACTH

Fails to suppress on high dose DST and ↓ ACTH

Cushing's disease or bronchial carcinoid

Ectopic ACTH syndrome

• Adrenal tumor
• Adrenal macronodular hyperplasia
• Surreptitious use of glucocorticoids

Obtain MRI or CT of the pituitary

CT of chest/ abdomen

CT of the adrenals

Pituitary tumor present

Surgery

No pituitary mass*, do oCRH stimulation test

↑ > 50% ACTH
↑ > 20% cortisol

Inconclusive

Cushing's disease

IPSS with oCRH

Repeat radiologic studies

Abbreviations:
DST -   dexamethasone suppression test
IPSS - inferior petrosal sinus sampling
UFC -   urinary free cortisol

* If there is no pituitary mass, obtain a chest x-ray and chest CT to rule out bronchial carcinoid before proceeding to IPSS

measuring UFC, plasma cortisol can be collected before, during and after dexamethasone. Suppression of either UFC or plasma cortisol by 50% or more from baseline is diagnostic of Cushing's disease. Most patients with adrenal adenomas, carcinomas, or ectopic ACTH syndromes do not show suppression. This test has a sensitivity and specificity of 60–85%; the greater the degree of suppression, the greater the specificity.

The 8-mg overnight dexamethasone suppression test has been reported by several authors to share similar sensitivity and specificity to the high-dose DST (Dicheck, 1994). An 8-a.m. plasma cortisol is obtained and 8 mg of dexamethasone is administered orally at 11 p.m.. An 8-a.m. plasma cortisol is obtained the next morning. Reduction of cortisol to less than 5 µg/dL is strongly supportive of Cushing's disease (Fig. 24–17).

Most pituitary tumors and a few ectopic ACTH-secreting tumors will respond to CRH stimulation with an increase in plasma ACTH and

cortisol, whereas there is little response in those with adrenal-Cushing's. For the CRH stimulation test two basal plasma cortisol and ACTH levels are collected about 5 minutes apart, then 1 µg/kg of body weight or a single dose of 100 µg of synthetic ovine CRH (oCRH) is injected intravenously. Blood is sampled every 15 minutes for 1–2 hours for cortisol and ACTH. Normal subjects will show a rise in ACTH and cortisol (approximately 15–20%), with those with Cushing's disease typically showing a greater than 50% rise in ACTH and greater than 20% rise in cortisol above baseline (Stewart, 2003; Kaye, 1990; Newell-Price, 2002). Ovine CRH is superior to human CRH in distinguishing among the different causes of Cushing's syndrome (Nieman, 1989). Vasopressin stimulates ACTH release through the V3 receptors in the anterior pituitary. Administration of 10 units of vasopressin intramuscularly normally causes a doubling of ACTH levels and an increase in serum cortisol of 150 µg/L

Table 24–22 Differential Diagnosis of Hormonal Values Seen in Cushing's Syndrome

Cause	Plasma ACTH	Plasma cortisol (PM)	High dose or overnight dexamethasone suppression
Pituitary-dependent	N – slightly ↑	↑	Yes
Adrenal disease	↓ – undetectable	↑	No
Ectopic Cushing's*	↑↑↑	↑↑	Usually no
Pseudo-Cushing's	N – slightly ↑	N – ↑	Usually yes

* ACTH levels may overlap with values seen in pituitary dependent disease.
N = normal.

over baseline. This offers no advantage over testing with CRH. It may prove useful, however, in differentiating Cushing's disease from pseudo-Cushing's syndrome and in the postoperative assessment of Cushing's disease (Newell-Price, 2002).

In rare instances it may be necessary to use selective sampling of the inferior petrosal sinus blood to document that the pituitary is the source of excess ACTH. This invasive, technically difficult procedure carries a relatively high cost and complication rate and should only be performed at a center well experienced with this technique. The ACTH concentration in the petrosal sinus blood should exceed twice that of peripheral venous blood to ensure a diagnostic sensitivity and specificity of 100% (Orth, 1995). In those with ectopic production the ratio is usually less than 1.4 : 1. Use of CRH during sampling increases the sensitivity and specificity.

Since the incidence of 'incidentaloma' of the adrenals and pituitary has been reported to be as high as 10%, imaging studies should only be performed after the hormonal diagnosis of Cushing's disease or syndrome has been made. In Cushing's disease, visualization of the sella is performed either by MRI or CT, with and without contrast. For adrenal-Cushing's the test of choice is CT of the abdomen; for ectopic disease CT of the chest may also be needed.

Pseudo-Cushing's Syndrome

Excess activity of the hypothalamic–pituitary axis similar to that seen in pituitary Cushing's syndrome has been demonstrated in some patients with alcoholism, major depression and obesity. Resolution of the underlying problem results in normalization of the HPA axis. These patients may not suppress on a low-dose DST and may have elevated UFC. Depressed patients who fail to suppress cortisol secretion in response to dexamethasone also show an impaired ACTH response to exogenous CRH, but will usually retain a normal cortisol response (Thalen, 1993; Gold, 1986). A single serum cortisol above 7.5 µg/dL at midnight has been shown to discriminate Cushing's syndrome from pseudo-Cushing's with 100% specificity (Papanicolaou, 1998). A more definitive test for distinguishing between these two entities is the combined dexamethasone–oCRH test. oCRH is infused 2 hours after a low-dose dexamethasone test. A plasma cortisol concentration greater than 38 nmol/L measured at 15 min following the administration of oCRH correctly identifies all cases of Cushing's syndrome and all cases of pseudo-Cushing's, with a specificity, sensitivity and diagnostic accuracy of 100% (Yanovski, 1993).

Adrenal Insufficiency

Adrenal insufficiency is categorized according to the key site of dysfunction within the HPA axis: primary (adrenal); secondary (pituitary); and tertiary (hypothalamic). A major distinction between primary adrenal insufficiency and either of the central causes is that primary disease is associated with mineralocorticoid deficiency. In the western world, primary adrenal insufficiency, also known as Addison's disease, is most commonly due to autoimmune adrenalitis (70–90% of all cases), other causes include tuberculosis (most common cause worldwide), granulomatous disorders, metastatic disease, hemorrhage, HIV-AIDS and infection. The most common cause of central adrenal insufficiency is HPA axis suppression due to prolonged treatment with pharmacologic doses of steroids.

Tests for the Diagnosis of Adrenal Insufficiency.

Basal Hormone Measurements. An 8 a.m. to 9 a.m. plasma cortisol of < 3 µg/dL (83 nmol/L) is indicative of adrenal insufficiency and obviates the need for further testing. Although most patients with hypocortisolism have low serum cortisol levels, a level drawn during a time of stress that falls within the reference range does not exclude the diagnosis. Rather, it may support this diagnosis, because a suboptimal cortisol level may have risen into the reference interval in response to a very high ACTH level induced by stress. A random cortisol of > 25 µg/dL (700 nmol/L) during stress makes it unlikely that the patient is adrenally insufficient (Burke, 1985).

ACTH Stimulation Test. The most convenient procedure for studying patients suspected of having hypocortisolism is the ACTH stimulation test. The test, which can be performed at any time of day, consists of drawing a baseline serum cortisol and then administering 250 µg of Cosyntropin (commercially available ACTH analogue) intravenously or intramuscularly. Serum for cortisol is again collected at 30 and 60 minutes following Cosyntropin. A normal response is a cortisol level of greater than 18–20 µg/dL (500–550 nmol/L) at either time point (Burke, 1985; Speckart, 1971). Drawing an ACTH level at baseline may help in distinguishing primary adrenal insufficiency (associated with an elevated ACTH usually greater than 50–100 pg/mL) from secondary or tertiary forms (which would have a low ACTH level < 10 pg/mL) (Oelkers, 1992) (refer to Laboratory Measurement of ACTH, p. 350). The aldosterone response to ACTH may also help in making this distinction; a failure of aldosterone to increase by more than 4 ng/dL over baseline suggests primary adrenal dysfunction.

Steroids should never be withheld from a critically ill patient suspected of having adrenal insufficiency. A random sample for cortisol and ACTH should be drawn and treatment initiated with dexamethasone, which does not interfere with the cortisol assay. Formal testing should take place as soon as possible, within 72 hours, before HPA axis suppression occurs from steroid treatment.

Several studies have supported the use of a 1-µg dose of ACTH instead of the full 250-µg dose for diagnosing adrenal insufficiency. The premise is that the massively supraphysiologic dose of 250 µg will cause those with partial adrenal insufficiency to mount a normal response, and that these individuals would fail to show an adequate rise in cortisol in response to a 1-µg test dose. This procedure has not gained wide acceptance nor has the normal range been standardized.

The insulin tolerance test (ITT) has long been considered the gold standard for assessing the HPA axis. Unlike the ACTH stimulation test, the ITT assesses the integrity of the entire HPA axis. If the HPA axis is intact, the insulin-induced hypoglycemia stimulates the hypothalamus and pituitary to secrete CRH and ACTH respectively, which in turn leads to a rise in cortisol. This test, is contraindicated in individuals with ischemic heart disease, the elderly (> age 70) and those with a history of seizures. Patients highly suspected of having central adrenal insufficiency (i.e., prior pituitary surgery or radiation therapy) should receive a lower dose (0.05 U/kg) of insulin. Glucose and cortisol are measured at baseline and then 15, 30, 45, 60, 90 and 120 minutes following insulin administration. In order for the test to be valid. Adequate hypoglycemia must be attained (signs and symptoms of hypoglycemia and a glucose of < 40 mg/dL (2.2 mmol/L)). A normal response is a rise in the cortisol level to greater than or equal to 18 µg/L or 20 µg/L at any time during the test (Burke, 1985; Grinspoon, 1994; Nelson, 1978). The cortisol response to hypoglycemia can reliably be predicted by the response to acute ACTH stimulation, a safer, cheaper and quicker test (Stewart, 2003). The ITT is mainly used as a second-line measure to further evaluate those patients who had a borderline response to the ACTH stimulation test.

In the days before the commercial availability of a reliable assay to measure ACTH, it was common to perform a prolonged ACTH stimulation test (ACTH infusion over a 2-day period) to distinguish central from primary adrenal insufficiency. In other hormone systems, lack of stimulation normally leads to an upregulation of the end-organ receptors; however, the adrenals downregulate their ACTH receptors in response to a lack of stimulation. A short ACTH stimulation test would typically produce an inadequate response. By priming the system with prolonged exposure to Cortrosyn, those with hypothalamic disease display a delayed but normal rise in cortisol.

Overnight Metyrapone Test. Metyrapone has also been used to assess the integrity of the HPA axis. Metyrapone inhibits 11β-hydroxylase, preventing the conversion of 11-deoxycortisol (compound S) to cortisol. Under normal circumstances the metyrapone-induced drop in cortisol is detected at the level of the hypothalamus and pituitary, a compensatory increase in CRH and ACTH secretion occurs stimulating steroidogenesis, leading to a build-up of 11-deoxycortisol, the hormone preceding the block. Patients with central adrenal insufficiency fail to increase CRH and/or ACTH, steroidogenesis is not stimulated and the 11-deoxycortisol fails to increase. 30 mg/kg metyrapone is administered orally at midnight; blood for cortisol and 11-deoxycortisol is collected the following morning at 8 a.m. A rise of the 11-deoxycortisol to greater than 7 µg/dL (200 nmol/L) is normal (Grinspoon, 1994; Fiad, 1994). An abnormal response is defined by an 11-deoxycortisol less than 7 µg/dL accompanied by a cortisol less than 5 µg/dL. This test should be performed with caution as it may provoke an addisonian crisis in those with central hypocortisolism.

II

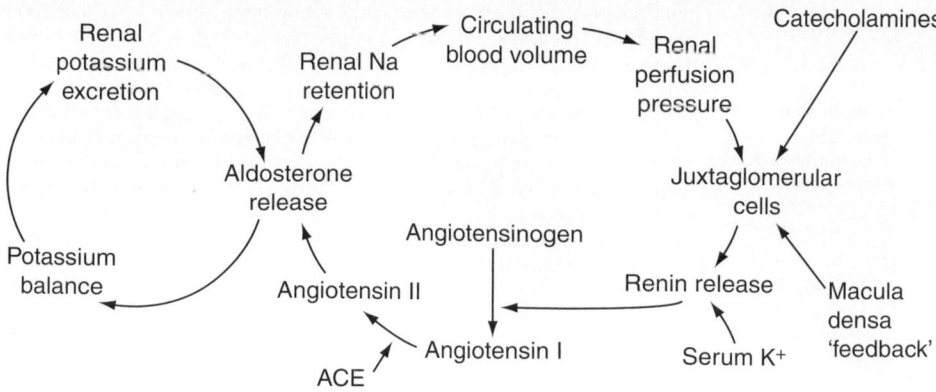

Figure 24–18 Renin–aldosterone axis. Elevated K+ inhibits renin secretion but has a stimulatory effect on aldosterone. Catecholaminergic influence is variable, beta-adrenergic activity stimulates and alpha-adrenergic activity inhibits renin secretion from the juxtaglomerular cells. (Redrawn from Braunwald E, Fauci AD, Kasper D, et al. (eds): Harrisons Principles of Internal Medicine, 15th ed. New York, McGraw-Hill, 2001, p 2087.)

Corticotropin-Releasing Hormone (CRH) Test. The ovine corticotropin-releasing hormone (oCRH) test can be used not only to diagnose hypocortisolism, but to localize the site of damage (Schutte, 1984). It is a safe test; however, it is expensive. After blood is drawn for baseline ACTH and cortisol, 100 µg oCRH is administered intravenously. Blood is then collected for cortisol and ACTH every 15 minutes for 60–90 minutes. Normal response: cortisol > 20 µg/dL. Basal ACTH levels and their change in response oCRH are used to localize the site of pathology. Plasma corticotropin usually peaks at 15–30 minutes; the cortisol usually peaks at around 30–40 minutes post-oCRH injection (Oelkers, 1996).

Antibodies against 21-hydroxylase antigen should be assayed in those whose Addison's disease (primary adrenal insufficiency) does not have an obvious explanation. Positive antibodies confirm autoimmune adrenalitis; these patients should be screened and monitored for the development of other autoimmune disorders.

The use of steroids for the treatment of many malignant and immunologic disorders is a common iatrogenic cause of adrenal insufficiency. The degree of adrenal suppression is dependent on the specific glucocorticoid dose, duration, frequency, and route of administration. To assess adrenal function in a patient being tapered off exogenous steroids, the morning glucocorticoid dose is omitted and the 8 a.m. cortisol level is measured. If it is greater then 10 µg/dL, routine supplementation of steroids can be ended. Because the adrenal cortex lags behind the pituitary in recovery from steroid suppression, complete adrenal recovery can also be demonstrated by an appropriate rise in serum cortisol following an 8 a.m. cosyntropin infusion.

Renin–Aldosterone Axis

At least 20 million people in the United States have hypertension, with 90–98% of the cases classified as essential hypertension. The mortality and morbidity from associated myocardial, cerebrovascular, and renal complications necessitate aggressive treatment of this disorder. Investigation into the etiology of hypertension revealed the importance of the renin–angiotensin–aldosterone system, not only in the origin and persistence of hypertension but also as a guide to its treatment. The role of the renin–aldosterone axis is to maintain blood pressure within normal limits by sensing the plasma volume, salt balance and renal perfusion pressure and then adjusting it.

Renin is a proteolytic enzyme, which although formed by other tissues throughout the body, is mainly formed and stored by juxtaglomerular (JG) cells within the macula densa of the kidney. Renin is synthesized from a larger precursor protein, prorenin (big renin) and converted to its active form within the JG cells. Renin's release into the circulation occurs in response to a variety of triggers: a drop in renal hydrostatic pressure, hyponatremia, hyperkalemia, a decrease in catecholamines, angiotensin II or atrial natriuretic hormone. There are several isoenzymes of renin. Their release is regulated by cAMP. Renin acts on angiotensinogen (renin substrate), an α_2-globulin formed by the liver, converting angiotensinogen to angiotensin I. Angiotensin I is in turn converted into angiotensin II, by angiotensin-converting enzyme (ACE). ACE is found in the pulmonary and vascular endothelium as well as in cell membranes of the kidney, heart and brain (Brewster, 2004). It is believed that angiotensin II is the peptide responsible for the physiologic effects on target tissue. Angiotensin II not only stimulates the release of aldosterone, but it is also a very potent vasoconstrictor, stimulates the release of catecholamines from the adrenals, norepinephrine from the sympathetic nervous system and stimulates the release of vasopressin. The octapeptide angiotensin II is further split to a heptapeptide, angiotensin III, or angiotensin I may be changed directly to angiotensin III without being converted to angiotensin II. Although there is still speculation

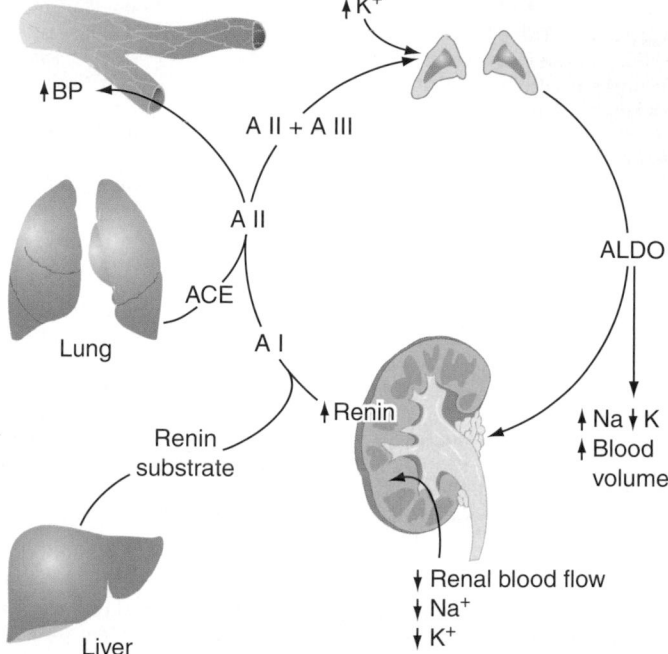

Figure 24–19 The normal renin–angiotensin–aldosterone axis. Renin, secreted by the kidney, cleaves angiotensin I from renin substrate (angiotensinogen), produced by the liver. Angiotensin I is converted to angiotensin II by angiotensin-converting enzyme (ACE), mainly in the lung. Angiotensin II increases peripheral vascular resistance and together with angiotensin III, stimulates aldosterone secretion, which results in sodium retention and increased plasma volume. (Adapted from Stewart PM: The Adrenal Cortex. *In*: Larsen PR, Kronenberg HM, Melmed S, Polansky KS (eds): Williams Textbook of Endocrinology, 10th edn. Philadelphia: WB Saunders, 2003: p. 499.)

about the functions of angiotensin III, it appears to modulate aldosterone secretion. The active angiotensins are rapidly cleared by various aminopeptidases (angiotensinases) within the circulation and during transit through tissues. These relationships are shown in Figure 24–18.

Renin, through its product, angiotensin II, directly stimulates the synthesis and secretion of aldosterone by the adrenal zona glomerulosa. Renin release, the rate-limiting step in the renin–aldosterone axis, is dependent on changes in effective plasma volume, which, in turn, are dependent on tubular reabsorption of sodium by the kidney. Low plasma volume and low serum sodium stimulate the secretion of renin, resulting in aldosterone release, which in turn causes sodium retention with an increase in plasma volume, blood pressure and potassium loss. Conversely, an increase in effective blood volume or acute elevation in blood pressure results in low renin, low angiotensin, low aldosterone and subsequent sodium loss. In contradistinction to aldosterone, renin secretion is inhibited by hyperkalemia (Fig. 24–19).

Aldosterone (and glucocorticoids) act at the mineralocorticoid receptor located in the cells lining the collecting ducts of the kidney to cause reabsorption of sodium, leading to an increase in intravascular volume. Aldosterone also causes renal potassium loss. Studies have suggested a role for aldosterone in the development and perpetuation of vasculopathy; it has been shown to stimulate genes for collagen synthesis, tissue growth factors, inflammatory factors and plasminogen activator inhibitor type 1 (Brilla, 1994; Schunkert, 1997; Luft, 2002; Rocha, 2000; Brown, 2000).

Table 24–23 Causes for Hypertension Associated with High Levels of Plasma Renin

Renin-secreting tumor	Cushing's syndrome
Malignant accelerated hypertension	Iatrogenic
Renovascular hypertension	Volume-depleting agents
Major arterial lesions	Vasodilating agents
Segmental lesions	Glucocorticoids
Chronic renal failure	Estrogens
End stage	
Transplant rejection	

The synthesis of aldosterone is restricted to the zona glomerulosa; here the enzyme aldosterone synthetase converts corticosterone to aldosterone. The major stimuli for aldosterone secretion are angiotensin II and hyperkalemia. ACTH is a much weaker stimulus. Somatostatin, atrial natriuretic hormone, dopamine and heparin directly inhibit aldosterone synthesis. Cortisol circulates at a much higher concentration than aldosterone, and although it binds with equal affinity to the mineralocorticoid receptor, it does not normally function as a major mineralocorticoid. The reason is that the enzyme 11β-hydroxysteroid dehydrogenase II (11-HSD-2, also known as CYP11B2), expressed by the mineralocorticoid target cells in the collecting tubules, acts to converts cortisol to cortisone, an inactive metabolite.

Renin and Hypertension

The work of Laragh has indicated that essential hypertension can be classified on the basis of renin measurements as high, low, or normal renin and that drug selection can be based on this classification (Laragh, 1972; Laragh, 1993). About 15% of patients with essential hypertension have high-renin hypertension. Hyper-reninemia resulting from renal parenchymal disease or renal vasculopathy, leads to increased aldosterone production and the subsequent retention of sodium and enhanced potassium excretion. Patients with this condition are hypervolemic, intensely vasoconstrictive, and more prone to ischemic injury. Renin profiling has shown renin to be an independent risk factor for myocardial infarction. Even if the pressures are controlled by antihypertensives, if they do not address plasma renin activity, such patients fare worse than people with lower renin levels (Alderman, 1991). The increased aldosterone (secondary aldosteronism) may contribute significantly to the symptoms and course of high-renin hypertension. Some of the causes of high-renin hypertension are listed in Table 24–23.

Renin-secreting tumors are an extremely rare finding and can be difficult to diagnose. They can be benign or malignant, renal or extrarenal. The most common location is in the juxtaglomerular apparatus. A young patient with markedly elevated plasma renin activity, hyperaldosteronism, and hypokalemia in the absence of a renovascular lesion typifies the classic clinical presentation (Corvol, 1994). Malignant hypertension is also associated with high plasma renin activity and aldosterone. When such patients are given medications which interrupt the renin-aldo axis, such as angiotensin converting enzyme inhibitors (ACEI), the blood pressure often normalizes. In renal vascular hypertension, the renin and aldosterone levels are also elevated. However, in contradistinction to malignant hypertension, treatment with ACEs usually results in a further deterioration of renal function. Patients suspected of having renal artery stenosis should undergo further testing, e.g. Captopril induced renogram, renal duplex ultrasound or MR angiography A positive test leads to renal vein angiograms and catheterization for selective blood sampling. In unilateral renal disease, both plasma renin and aldosterone are elevated. Asymmetry in the renin levels obtained during renal vein catheterization offers one of the best measurements to judge the likelihood of blood pressure response to corrective surgery. When the ratio of plasma renin in the renal vein of the affected side to nonaffected side is at least 1.5 : 1, surgery may lead to improvement. With suppression of renin release from the nonaffected side, renal vein renin levels approximating those found in blood specimens obtained from the inferior vena cava also indicate probable success of curative surgery. However, almost 40% of these patients have peripheral blood plasma renin activity that is within the reference interval (Streeten, 1979). Consequently, peripheral plasma renin is a poor predictor of response to surgery. Renin secretion can be found in lung cancers, hepatic hamartoma, and other unusual conditions (Anderson, 1989).

When there is an acceleration of hypertension, renin is usually markedly increased; however, with chronic renal failure, almost any renin level can be expected. A small number of hypertensive patients on dialysis have intractable, accelerated hypertension. In those patients in whom dialysis

Table 24–24 Causes of Hypertension Associated with Low Levels of Plasma Renin

'Primary' excess of mineralocorticoids

Primary aldosteronism

Pseudoprimary (idiopathic) aldosteronism

Glucocorticoid-suppressible aldosteronism

11-Deoxycorticosterone excess (CAH due 11β-hydroxylase deficiency)

18-Hydroxy-11-deoxycorticosterone excess

Adrenal carcinoma (excess mineralocorticoids and/or glucocorticoids)

'Secondary' excess of mineralocorticoids

Licorice ingestion

Excess sodium intake

Hyporenin hypoaldosteronism:
Longstanding essential hypertension
Diabetes mellitus

cannot control the hypertension, markedly elevated plasma renin levels can be lowered by nephrectomy, or in the case of renal artery stenosis, angioplasty or revascularization (Sonkodi, 1990; Tullis, 1999; Whitehouse, 1981). ACEI can be used to mitigate the rise in aldosterone. In those renal transplant patients with rejection, elevated plasma renin may be indicative of renal ischemia. Systemic hypertension occurs in patients with Cushing's syndrome. Some of these patients have increased plasma renin and renin substrate. Other Cushing's syndrome patients have hypokalemia associated with the secretion of a minor mineralocorticoid (such as DOC or corticosterone) that causes hypertension (Krakoff, 1975). In still other patients, severely elevated cortisol levels overwhelm the capacity of 11-hydroxysteroid dehydrogenase (11-HSD) to convert cortisol to cortisone, leading to a picture of excess mineralocorticoid activity with suppressed plasma renin activity. Other causes of high-renin hypertension include treatment with medications such as diuretics, vasodilators or other antihypertensives. Hormonal agents such as glucocorticoids; as well as some estrogen-containing oral contraceptives have been found to increase renin substrate activity.

Although plasma renin activity, aldosterone, and urinary sodium excretion may be normal in 60% of hypertensive patients, evidence has accumulated that indicates that renin–angiotensin plays a significant part in normal-renin hypertension. The response of many hypertensive patients with normal renin to angiotensin converting enzyme inhibitors or angiotensin II antagonists (saralasin) has implicated renin and angiotensin II in sustaining hypertension in these patients. Moreover, Ames showed that once the blood pressure was increased by angiotensin infusion, it could be maintained with only one-fifth of the original dose (Ames, 1965).

It was found that low-renin essential hypertension, which involves chronic expansion of plasma and extracellular fluid volume, is characterized by aldosterone oversecretion and responds to diuretic therapy. At least 25% of patients with essential hypertension are found to have low-renin hypertension. Most investigators have characterized this state as hyporesponsive, meaning that low-renin-hypertensive patients fail to respond as well as healthy subjects do with upright posture, sodium restriction, diuretics, vasodilators, or a combination of these. Atrial natriuretic peptide may be elevated in these patients, along with an exaggerated response of aldosterone to renin (Sergev, 1990). Renin suppression increases with age, and appears to be more common in women, and in the black population.

Listed in Table 24–24 are a group of syndromes associated with low levels of plasma renin. These have been divided into a subgroup that is of adrenal origin (primary) and a subgroup that is nonadrenal or secondary in origin. Primary aldosteronism is uncommon compared with renin hypertension. It is characterized by (1) systolic and diastolic hypertension caused by oversecretion of aldosterone by an adrenal adenoma (aldosterone-producing adenoma [APA]) or hyperplasia (idiopathic hyperaldosteronism [IHA]), (2) low renin or a high aldosterone/renin ratio (> 50), (3) renal potassium wasting and (4) sodium retention. Several potential screening tests to detect primary aldosteronism and to separate unilateral aldosterone-producing adenomas from other causes of primary aldosteronism have been used. Low-salt diet (< 2 g/day), stress, upright posture, and diuretics all increase plasma aldosterone, whereas a high-salt diet and lying in a supine position suppress aldosterone secretion in healthy subjects. Combinations of these maneuvers have been used in the diagnosis of excessive aldosterone secretion; however, they do not reliably distinguish APA from IHA. When healthy subjects are placed on a high-salt diet and lie in the supine position, they suppress their plasma aldosterone levels to less than 10 ng/dL (278 pmol/L).

Primary Hyperaldosteronism – Screening and Confirmation Tests

The algorithm proposed by Blumenfeld for evaluating hypertensive patients suspected of having primary hyperaldosteronism is to initially measure the serum potassium (Blumenfeld, 1994). If it is less than 3.6 mmol/L, then plasma renin activity is measured. A plasma renin activity of < 1.0 ng/mL/h leads to a 24-hour urine collection for aldosterone and potassium excretion. The findings of a 24-hour urinary potassium greater than 30 mEq/24 h in the face of hypokalemia and an aldosterone greater than 15 μg/24 h, leads to localization of adrenal pathology.

Although patients with primary hyperaldosteronism classically present with either spontaneous or easily provokable hypokalemia, many will in fact have serum potassium levels that are within the normal range. Thus, the preferred screening test is a plasma aldosterone concentration/plasma renin activity (PAC/PRA) ratio, PAC expressed in ng/dL and PRA in ng/mL/h. This is performed after having the patient remain upright for at least 2 hours, and ideally with the patient having been off spironolactone and eplerenone for 4–6 weeks and off all other antihypertensives for at least 2 weeks. Similarly, hypokalemia should be corrected, and the patient should not be on a sodium-restricted diet. A PAC/PRA ratio of greater than 30 is suggestive of primary hyperaldosteronism, a value of greater than 50 is virtually diagnostic (Blumenfeld, 1994; Weinberger, 1993). It is of note that the lower limit of normal for the PRA assay varies by laboratory; therefore the diagnosis is only supported when both the PAC/PRA ratio and the PAC are elevated.

The diagnosis of primary hyperaldosteronism is confirmed by performing a saline suppression test. This can be accomplished by either infusing 2 liters of 0.9% saline over 4 hours, or by administering sodium chloride tablets 10–12 g daily for 3 days. A plasma aldosterone at the end of the 4-hour infusion of greater than 5 ng/dL (140 pmol/L) confirms the diagnosis – some authors support using a cutoff of greater than 10 ng/dL (280 pmol/L). On the last day of oral sodium administration a 24 h urine is collected for aldosterone, creatinine (to assess for adequacy of the collection) and sodium (> 200 mEq/day confirms adequate sodium intake). An aldosterone collected of greater than 10 μg/24 h (28 nmol/24 h) following 3 days of sodium loading also confirms the diagnosis (Bravo, 1983, 1994; Holland, 1984).

Differentiating Among the Different Causes of Primary Hyperaldosteronism

The aldosterone-producing adenoma (APA) differs from idiopathic hyperaldosteronism due to adrenal hyperplasia (IHA) by more extreme blood pressures, greater potassium wasting and higher atrial natriuretic peptide levels. There also tends to be higher urinary and serum levels of 18-oxocortisol, 18-hydroxycortisol (serum > 300 ng/dL) and 18-hydroxycorticosterone (serum > 100 ng/dL). A positive postural stimulation test (plasma aldosterone: ambulating < 130% of supine) has a moderate sensitivity and specificity for adenoma but not for hyperplasia. Once the diagnosis of primary hyperaldosteronism is confirmed, the next step is to image the adrenals either by CT or MRI, looking for bilateral hyperplasia or a unilateral hypodense adenoma. The specificity of imaging to correctly categorize the patients as having APA versus IHA varies from 67–84% (Doppmann, 1992; Gleason, 1993; Harpe, 1999; Magill, 2001). Removal of the adenoma is curative in 35% of cases and leads to improvement in another 55% (Blumenfeld, 1994). Hyperplasia is not always bilateral. Surgery can cure or improve the hypertension in patients with unilateral disease. For those in whom the disease is bilateral, medical treatment with drugs such as spironolactone leads to improvement in 76% of cases.

Bilateral adrenal vein sampling is technically demanding and entails risk; however, as performed by an experienced radiologist it is the gold standard for distinguishing adenoma from hyperplasia. An intravenous infusion of ACTH at 50 μg per hour is started 30 minutes prior to sampling and continued throughout the procedure; this serves to accentuate the difference between the right and the left adrenals in instances of adenoma. Samples for aldosterone and cortisol are obtained from each adrenal vein and from the periphery. Measurement of cortisol ensures the samples are taken from the adrenal veins; the cortisol levels should show a < 20% difference between both adrenals. The adrenal vein aldosterone/cortisol (A/C) ratio is higher than the peripheral A/C on the side with adenoma. An A/C ratio of > 1 bilaterally indicates hyperplasia. The PAC is usually at least fivefold higher on the side with the adenoma; no gradient is seen in hyperplasia (Doppmann, 1996). Several studies have shown a discrepancy between radiologic findings and surgical findings in up to a third of all cases; however, criteria as to which patients should be referred for venous sampling remain to be clearly defined.

Given the increased prevalence (5–10%) of adrenal incidentalomas (nonfunctioning adrenal tumors) with increasing age, some authorities have recommended the use of adrenal vein sampling for those patients

Table 24–25 Differentiating the Various Causes of Hyperaldosteronism

Disorder	Aldosterone	Renin	Serum K⁺
Primary hyperaldosteronism	↑	↓	↓
Renin-secreting tumor	↑	↑	↓ – N
Dexamethasone-suppressible hyperaldosteronism	↑	↓	↓
Renovascular hypertension	N – ↑	N – ↑	↓ – N
Bartter's syndrome	↑	↑	↓
Diuretics, congestive heart failure, cirrhosis, nephrotic syndrome	↑	↑	N – ↓

N = normal.

with hyperaldosteronism who are older than age 40 with the finding of a unilateral hypodense adrenal nodule > 1 cm on CT scan (Young, 1999). Based on the findings of large prospective studies, others have suggested that this technique's major strength may be in evaluating those patients with a high probability of AHA but with either normal findings or bilateral nodular disease on CT. Again, it should be stressed that this test is technically difficult and even in the best of hands is only successful in approximately 92–96% of cases (Young, 1999; Radin, 1992; Doppman, 1992).

Renin may be suppressed by the ingestion of licorice (which has a high content of glycyrrhizic acid), chewing tobacco and excessive sodium intake. It is also suppressed in the syndrome of hyporenin hypoaldosteronism which is most commonly seen in patients with diabetes mellitus and renal disease. Secondary aldosteronism results from nonadrenal disease, in which both adrenal glands are stimulated (Table 24–25). Typically, these patients are not hypertensive. Such conditions as nephrosis, cirrhosis, and heart failure are usual causes. In all of these conditions, both renin and aldosterone are increased. The response of the renin–aldosterone system in pregnancy is especially complex; there appear to be increased renin, renin substrate, angiotensin II, and aldosterone.

Families with glucocorticoid-remediable aldosteronism have well-documented mendelian inheritance (Kurtz, 1993; Lifton, 1992). This dominantly inherited disorder characterized by hyperaldosteronism, hyporeninemia and hypertension is the result of the aldosterone synthetase (CYP18) being translocated onto the ACTH-sensitive promoter sequence of the 11β-hydroxylase (CYP11B) gene within the zona fasciculata. Thus, aldosterone synthesis is stimulated by ACTH. Diagnosis is confirmed by normalization of aldosterone following 4–6 weeks of steroid suppression.

Liddle syndrome is another rare autosomal dominant disorder; it is characterized by hypertension and hypokalemia with low PRA and PAC. The defect is due to a mutation in the sodium channel within the renal collecting ducts, leading to enhanced sodium reabsorption and increased potassium secretion.

Aldosterone Measurements

An isolated aldosterone measurement with no attention to patient preparation is of little clinical value. Even when time of sampling, posture, and dietary sodium and potassium are controlled, it is difficult to discriminate with certainty between primary aldosteronism and other forms of hypertension by using plasma aldosterone measurements alone. Assays are performed on plasma using extraction to remove aldosterone from plasma proteins followed by chromatography and RIA. Urine is assayed using acid hydrolysis, extraction and RIA. Normative values exist for different age groups, posture and sodium intake (Table 24–26).

Renin Measurements

There are important technical differences in the determination of renin using current methodologies. Renin measurements are of two types: plasma renin activity (PRA) and direct renin assay. The PRA is a bioassay wherein a plasma specimen containing renin is allowed to react with its substrate, angiotensinogen; after a specified period of time, the reaction is terminated and measurement of generated angiotensin I is made by RIA. For the estimation of plasma renin activity (PRA), the endogenous substrate is not eliminated. Therefore, the rate of generation of angiotensin I is influenced by both the concentration of endogenous renin and its substrate. This type of assay is the most widely used method for the determination of renin. Comparison of results among laboratories is not

Table 24–26 Differentiating the Various Causes of Hypoaldosteronism

Disorder	Aldosterone	Renin	Serum K+
Addison's disease	↓	↑	↑
Cushing's syndrome	↓	↓	N or ↓
Liddle's syndrome	↓	↓	↓
Hyporenin hypoaldosteronism	↓	↓	↑
Apparent mineralocorticoid excess	↓	↓	↓
Isolated hypoaldosteronism	↓	↑	↑

N = normal.

possible because of procedural differences such as variations of pH, ionic strength, the length of the assay, the angiotensinase inhibitor, lack of a specific reference preparation and the conditions under which the specimen was obtained. In addition, literature on renin assays reveals confusion regarding units of measurements employed, and even when an attempt is made to express the many arbitrary units in the same terms (nanograms of angiotensin liberated per milliliter per hour), there are wide ranges reported for human plasma renin activity in reference populations.

When measuring renin concentration rather than PRA, the effect of substrate is eliminated. The direct renin assay utilizes an antibody directed to the renin molecule itself. The sample is then analyzed using either immunochemiluminescence (ICMA) or RIA techniques.

Assays of PRA and plasma renin concentration provide similar information, except in a few clinical situations. With oral contraceptive administration, plasma renin concentration remains within the reference interval, whereas PRA increases owing to the increase in substrate. Other procedures such as freezing, thawing, and acidification have been found to convert prorenin to renin and thereby increase values in plasma renin concentration assays.

Because renin release is controlled by many physiologic and pharmacologic variables, it is extremely important to know the conditions under which the blood specimen was obtained. Such conditions as upright posture, the administration of diuretics, or low-sodium diets are potent stimuli of renin release and should be adequately controlled prior to the measurement of plasma renin. Renin also appears to be extremely labile, so that the variables involved in specimen processing should be vigorously controlled. Blood should be drawn into an iced ethylenediamine tetraacetic acid (EDTA) tube, which inactivates the enzymes (e.g., angiotensinases), centrifuged at 4°C, and the plasma should be separated promptly from the cells, frozen immediately and kept frozen until ready to be analyzed; with this technique the specimen is stable for several months at −20°C.

The direct measurement of renin substrate, angiotensin I, or angiotensin II is not used widely in clinical practice because of tedious extraction or concentration steps as well as difficulty in eliminating formation or degradation of these compounds by proteases and other enzymes involved in the renin system. Although angiotensin-converting enzyme (ACE) levels can be easily measured, they are of little use in the diagnosis of hypertensive disorders.

References

Adams LM, Emery JR, Clark SJ, et al: Reference ranges for new thyroid function tests in premature infants. J Pediatr 1995; 126:122–127.

Ain KB, Pucino F, Shiver T, et al: Thyroid hormone levels affected by time of blood sampling in thyroxine-treated patients. Thyroid 1993; 3:81–85.

Alderman MH, Hadavan S, Oor WI, et al: Association of the renin–sodium profile with the risk of myocardial infarction in patients with hypertension. N Engl J Med 1991; 324:1098.

Almeretti G, Corneli G, Baldelli R, et al: Diagnostic reliability of a single IGF-I measurement in 237 adults with total anterior hypopituitarism and severe GH deficiency. Clin Endocrinol (Oxf) 2003; 59(1):56–61.

Amadori P, Dilberis C, Marcolla A, et al: Macroprolactinemia: predictability on clinical basis and detection by PEG precipitation with two different immunometric methods. J Endocrinol Invest 2003; 26(2):148–156.

American Association of Clinical Endocrinologists: Medical Guidelines for Clinical Practice for the Evaluation and Treatment of Hyperthyroidism and Hypothyroidism. Endocr Pract 2002; 8(6):457–469.
An excellent reference for the diagnosis and treatment of commonly seen thyroid disorders, created by a consensus panel of experts in the field.

American Association of Clinical Endocrinologists: Medical Guidelines for Clinical Practice for the Diagnosis and Treatment of Acromegaly. Endocrine Practice 2004; 10(3): 213–225.
An excellent reference for the diagnosis and treatment of acromegaly, created by a consensus panel of experts in the field of acromegaly

Ames RP, Borkpwski AJ, Sicinski AM, et al: Prolonged infusion of angiotensin II and norepinephrine and blood pressure, electrolyte balance, aldosterone and cortisol secretion in normal man and in cirrhosis with ascites. J Clin Invest 1965; 44:1171.

Andersen S, Pedersen KM, Bruun NH, Laurberg P: Narrow individual variations in serum T4 and T3 in normal subjects: a clue to the understanding of subclinical thyroid disease. J Clin Endocrinol Metab 2002; 87:1068–1072.

Anderson PW, Macaulay L, Do S, et al: Extrarenal renin-secreting tumors: Insights into hypertension and ovarian renin production. Medicine 1989; 68:257.

Arafah BM: Estrogen therapy may necessitate and increase in thyroxine dose for hypothyroidism. N Engl J Med 2001; 344:1743–1749.

Arnaldi G, Angeli A, Atkinson AB, et al: Diagnosis and complications of Cushing's syndrome: A consensus statement. J Clin Endocrinol Metab 2003; 88:5593–5602.

Ayus JC, Arieff AI: Glycine induced hypo-osmolar hyponatremia. Arch Intern Med 1997; 157(2):223–226.

Bacarese-Hamilton T, Cattini R, Shandley C, et al: A fully automated enzyme immunoassay for the measurement of cortisol in biologic fluids. Eur J Clin Chem Clin Biochem 1992; 30:531.

Ballabio M, Posyyachinda M, Ekins RP: Pregnancy-induced changes in thyroid function: role of human chorionic gonadotropin as a putative regulator of maternal thyroid. J Clin Endocrinol Metab 1991; 73:824.

Barbot N, Calmettes C, Schuffenecker I, et al: Pentagastrin stimulation test and early diagnosis of medullary carcinoma using an immunoradiometric assay of calcitonin: comparison with genetic screening in hereditary medullary thyroid carcinoma. J Clin Endocrinol Metab 1994; 78:114–120.

Barkan A: Acromegaly, diagnosis and therapy. Endocrinol Metab Clin North Am 1989; 18:277–310.

Barkan AL, Chandler WF: Giant pituitary prolactinoma with falsely low serum prolactin: the pitfall of the 'high-dose hook effect': case report. Neurosurgery 1998; 42:913–915.

Baumann G: Acromegaly. Endocrinol Metab Clin North Am 1987; 16:685–703.

Beck-Peccos P, Amr S, Menezes-Ferreira M, et al: Decreased receptor binding of biologically inactive thyrotropin in central hypothyroidism: effect of treatment with thyrotropin releasing hormone. N Engl J Med 1985; 312:1085–1089.

Becker KL, Nylen FS, Cohen R, Snider RH: Calcitonin: structure, molecular biology and actions. *In* Beleziakin JP, Raisz LE, Rodan GA (eds): Principle of Bone Biology. San Diego, Academic Press, 1996, pp 471–474.

Bigos R, Ridgeway E, et al: Spectrum pituitary alterations with mild and severe thyroid impairment. J Clin Endocrinol Metab 1978; 46:317.

Biller BMK, Samuels MH, Zagar A, et al: Sensitivity and specificity of six tests for the diagnosis of adult GH deficiency. J Clin Endocrinol Metab 2002; 87:2067–2079.

Bitton RN, Wexler CI: Free triiodothyronine toxicosis: a distinct entity. Am J Med 1990; 88:531–533.

Bjorkman U, Ekholm R, Denef J-F: Cytochemical localization of hydrogen peroxidase in isolated thyroid follicle. J Utrastruct Res 1981; 71:105–115.

Blumenfeld JD, Sealey JE, Schussel Y, et al: Diagnosis and treatment of primary hyperaldosteronism. Ann Intern Med 1994; 121:877–885.

Brabant A, Brabant G, Schuermeyer T, et al: The role of glucocorticoids in the regulation of thyrotropin. Acta Endocrinol 1989; 121:95–100.

Brandi ML, Gagel RJ, Angeli A, et al: Consensus guidelines for diagnosis and therapy of MEN type 1 and type 2. J Clin Endocrinol Metab 2001; 86:5658–5671.

Braverman LE, Utiger RD (eds): Werner and Ingbar's 'The Thyroid.' A Fundamental and Clinical Test. Philadelphia, Lippincott-Raven, 2000.

Bravo EL: Primary aldosteronism. Endocrinol Metab Clin North Am 1994; 23:271.

Bravo EL, Tagle R: Pheochromocytoma: State-of-the-art and future prospects. Endocr Rev 2003 24(4):539–553.

Bravo EL, Tarazi RC, Fouad FM, et al: Clonidine-suppression: a useful aid in the diagnosis of pheochromocytoma. N Engl J Med 1981; 305:623.

Bravo EL, Tarazi RC, Dustan HP, et al: The changing clinical spectrum of primary aldosteronism. Am J Med 1983; 74:641–651.

Brent GA, Moore DD, Larsen PR: Thyroid hormone regulation of gene expression. Ann Rev Physiol 1991; 53:17–35.

Brewster UC, Perazella MA: The renin–angiotensin–aldosterone system and the kidney: Effects on kidney disease. Am J Med 2004; 116:263–272.

Brilla CG, Zhou G, Matsubara L, et al: Collagen metabolism in cultured adult rat cardiac fibroblasts: response to angiotensin I and aldosterone. J Mol Cell Cardiol 1994; 26:809–820.

Brown NJ, Kim KS, Chen YQ, et al: Synergistic effect of adrenal steroids and angiotensin II on plasminogen activator inhibitor-1 production. J Clin Endocrinol Metab 2000; 85:336–344.

Burke CW: Adrenal insufficiency. Clin Endocrinol Metab 1985; 14(4):947–976.

Canale MP, Bravo EL: Diagnostic specificity of serum chromogranin-A for pheochromocytoma in patients with renal dysfunction. J Clin Endocrinol Metab 1994; 78:1139–1144.

Caron P: Effect of amiodarone on thyroid function. Press Med 1995; 24:1747–1751.

Casanueva FF: Physiology of growth hormone secretion and action. Endocrinol Metab Clin North Am 1992; 21:483–517.

Chan JL, Lit LC, Law FL, et al: Diminished free cortisol excretion in patients with moderate and severe renal impairment. Clin Chem 2004; 50:757–759.

Chiovato L, Bassi P, Santini F, et al: Antibodies producing compliment-mediated thyroid toxicity in patients with atrophic or goiterous autoimmune thyroiditis. J Clin Endocrinol Metab 1993; 77:1700–1705.

Chopra I: Euthyroid sick syndrome: is it a misnomer? J Clin Endocrinol Metab 1997; 82:329–334.

Chrousos GP: The hypothalamic–pituitary–adrenal axis and immune mediated inflammation. N Engl J Med 1998; 332;1351–1362.

Chung HM, Kluge R, Schrier RW, Anderson RJ: Clinical assessment of extracellular fluid volume in hyponatremia. Am J Med 1987; 83:905–908.

Cobin RH, Gharib H, Bergman DA, et al: AACE/AAES medical/surgical guidelines for clinical practice: Management of thyroid carcinoma. Endocrine Pract 2001; 7:203–220.

Conner P, Fried G: Hyperprolactinemia: etiology, diagnosis and treatment alternatives. Acta Obstet Gynecol Scand 1998; 77:249–262.

Corvol P, Pinet F, Plouin PF, et al: Renin-secreting tumors. Endocrinol Metab Clin North Am 1994; 23:255.

Daniels GH: Amiodarone-induced thyrotoxicosis. J Clin Endocrinol Metab 2001; 86:3–8.

Davies T, Roti E, et al: Thyroid controversy: Stimulating antibodies. J Clin Endocrinol Metab 1998; 83: 3777–3780.

Davis FB, LaMantia RS, Spaulding FW, et al: Estimation of a physiologic replacement dose of levothyroxine in elderly patients with hypothyroidism. Arch Int Med 1984; 144:1752–1754.

De Bellis A, Bizzarro A, Amoresano Paglionico V, et al: Detection of vasopressin cell antibodies in some patients with autoimmune endocrine diseases without overt diabetes insipidus. Clin Endocrinol (Oxf) 1994; 40:173–177.

De Bellis A, Colao A, Di Salle F, et al: A longitudinal study of plasma vasopressin cell antibodies, posterior pituitary function and magnetic resonance imaging evaluations in subclinical autoimmune central diabetes insipidus. J Clin Endocrinol Metab 1999; 84:3047–3051.

De Brabandere VI, Hou P, Stockl D, et al: Isotope dilution-liquid chromatography/electrospray ionization-tandem mass spectrometry for the determination of serum thyroxine as a potential reference method. Rapid Commun Mass Spectrom 1998; 12:1099–1103.

DeGroot LJ, Major G: Admission screening by thyroid function tests in an acute general care teaching hospital. Amer J Med 1992; 93:558–564.

Delange F: Correction of iodine deficiency: benefits and possible side effects. Eur J Endocrinol 1995; 132:542–543.

Deme D, Pommier J, Nunez J: Kinetics of thyroglobulin iodination of hormone synthesis catalyzed thyroid peroxidase. Role of iodide in the coupling reaction. Eur J Biochem 1976; 70:435–440.

Demers LM, Spencer CA: NACB: Laboratory support for the diagnosis and monitoring of thyroid disease, 2003, pp 1–78.
Excellent compilation of the latest recommendations on the diagnosis and monitoring of thyroid disease.

Dicheck HL, Nieman LK, Oldfield EH, et al: A comparison of the standard high-dose dexamethasone suppression test and the overnight 8 mg dexamethasone suppression test for the diagnosis of Cushing's syndrome. J Clin Endocrinol Metab 1994; 78:418–422.

Dimaraki EV, Jaffe CA, DeMott-Friberg R, et al: Acromegaly with apparently normal GH secretion: Implications for diagnosis and follow-up. J Clin Endocrinol Metab 2002; 87:3537–3542.

Diver MJ, Ewins DL, Worth RC, et al: An unusual form of big, big (macro) prolactin in a pregnant patient. Clin Chem 2001; 47(2):346–348.

Docter R, Van Toor H, Krenning EP, et al: Free thyroxine assessed with three assays in sera of patients with nonthyroidal illness and of subjects with abnormal concentrations of thyroxine-binding proteins. Clin Chem 1993; 39:1668–1674.

Doppmann JL, Gill JR Jr: Hyperaldosteronism: sampling the renal veins. Radiology 1996; 198:309–312.

Doppmann JL, Gill JR Jr, Miller DL, et al: Distinction between hyperaldosteronism due to bilateral adrenal hyperplasia and unilateral aldosteronoma: reliability of CT. Radiology 1992; 184:677–682.

Dulgeroff AJ, Hershman JM. Medical therapy for differentiated thyroid carcinoma. Endocrinol Rev 1994; 15:500–515.

Dunn JT: What happens to our iodine? J Clin Endocrinol Metab 1998; 83:3398–3400.

Dunn JT: When is thyroid nodule a sporadic medullary carcinoma? J Clin Endocrinol Metab 1994; 78:824–825.

Eastman RC, Merriman GR, Moore WT, Tanjuatco AJP: Acromegaly, hyperprolactinemia, gonadotropin-secreting tumors and hypopituitarism. In Moore WT, Eastman RC (eds): Diagnostic Endocrinology, 2nd edition. St. Louis, Mosby-Year Book, 1996, p 73.

Eddy RL, Gilliland PF, Ibarra JD, et al: Human growth hormone release: comparison of provocative test procedures. Am J Med 1974 56: 179.

Eisenhofer G, Pacak K: Diagnosis of pheochromocytoma. In Harrison's Principles of Internal Medicine. McGraw-Hill. Online. Available: http://www.accessmedicine.com/, 2004a.

Eisenhofer G, Goldstein DS, Walther, et al: Biochemical diagnosis of pheochromocytoma: how to distinguish true from false-positive test results. J Clin Endocrinol Metab 2003, 88:2656–2666.

Eisenhofer G, Lenders JW, Pacak K: Biochemical diagnosis of pheochromocytoma. Front Horm Res 2004b; 31:76–106.

Elliott W, Murphy MB: Reduced specificity of the clonidine suppression test in patients with normal plasma catecholamine levels. Am J Med 1988; 84:419–424.

Engler D, Burger AG: The deiodination of the iodothyronines and their derivatives in man. Endocrine Rev 1984; 5:151–184.

Erdogan MF, Gullu S, Baskal N, et al: Omeprazole: calcitonin stimulation test for the diagnosis follow-up and family screening in medullary carcinoma of the thyroid gland. Ann Surg 1997; 188:139–141.

Ericsson UB, Tegler L, Lennquist S, et al: Serum thyroglobulin in differentiated thyroid carcinoma. Acta Chir Scand 1984; 150:367–375.

Ezzat S: Acromegaly. Endocrinol Metab Clin North Am 1997; 26:703–723.

Faber J, Kirkegaard C, Rasmussen B, et al: Pituitary–thyroid axis in critical illness. J Clin Endocrinol Metab 1987; 65:315–320.

Fahie-Wilson M: In hyperprolactinemia, testing for macroprolactin is essential. Clin Chem 2003; 49(9):1434–1436.

Fiad TM, Kirby JM, Cunningham SK, McKenna TJ: The overnight single-dose metyrapone test is a simple and reliable index of the hypothalamic–pituitary axis. Clin Endocrinol (Oxf) 1994; 40:603–609.

Findling JW: Clinical application of a new immunoradiometric assay for ACTH. Endocrinologist 1992; 2:360–365.

Findling JW, Raff H: Newer diagnostic techniques and problems in Cushing's disease. Endocrinol Metab Clin North Am 1999; 28:191–210.

Fisher DA, Nelson JC, Carlton EI, Wilcox RB: Maturation of human hypothalamic–pituitary–thyroid function control. Thyroid 2000a; 10:229–234.

Fisher DA, Schoen EJ, La Franchi S, et al: The hypothalamic–pituitary–thyroid negative feedback control axis in children with treated congenital hypothyroidism. J Clin Endocrinol Metab 2000b; 85:2722–2727.

Frank J, Faix J, Hermos RJ, et al: Thyroid function in very low birth weight infants: effects on neonatal hypothyroidism screening. J Pediatr 1996; 128:548–554.

Frantz AG: Hyperprolactinemia. In Collu R, Brown GM, Van Loon GR (eds): Clinical Neuroendocrinology, Boston, Blackwell Scientific Publications, 1998, pp 311–332.

Freda PU, Wardlaw SL: Clinical Review 110: Diagnosis and treatment of pituitary tumors. J Clin Endocrinol Metab 1999; 84(11):3859–3866.

Freda PU, Post KD, Powell JS, Wardlaw SL: Evaluation of disease status with sensitive measures of growth hormone secretion in 60 post-operative patients with acromegaly. J Clin Endocrinol Metab 1998; 83:3808–3816.

Fuchs AR, Fuchs F, Husslein P: Oxytocin receptors and human parturition: A dual role for oxytocin in the initiation of labor. Science 1982; 215:1396.

Fujieda K, Okuhara K, Abe S, et al: Molecular pathogenesis of lipoid adrenal hyperplasia and adrenal hypoplasia congenita. J Steroid Biochem Mol Biol 2003; 85(2–5):483–489.

Fukata J, Shimizu N, Imura H, et al: Human corticotrophin-releasing hormone test in patients with hypothalamo-pituitary–adrenocortical disorders. Endocrinol J 1993: 40:597.

Gabrilove JL, Sharma DC, Dorfman RI: Adrenocortical 11-β-hydroxylase deficiency and virilism first manifest in an adult woman. N Engl J Med 1965; 272:1189–1194.

Gagel RF: The abnormal pentagastrin test. Clin Endocrinol 1996; 44:221–222.

Gleason PE, Weinberger MG, Pratt JH, et al: Evaluation of diagnostic tests in the differential diagnosis of primary aldosteronism: unilateral adenoma versus bilateral micronodular hyperplasia. J Urol 1993; 150:1365–1368.

Glinoer D: The regulation of thyroid function in pregnancy: pathways of endocrine adaptation from physiology to pathology. Endocrinol Rev 1997; 18:404–433.

Glinoer D, De Nayer P, Bourdoux P, et al: Regulation of maternal thyroid function during pregnancy. J Clin Endocrinol Metab 1990; 71:276–287.

Goland RS, Wardlaw SL, Stark RI, et al: High levels of corticotropin-releasing hormone immunoactivity in maternal and fetal plasma during pregnancy. J Clin Endocrinol Metab 1986; 63:1199–1203.

Gold PW, Loriaux L, Roy A, et al: Responses to corticotrophin-releasing hormone in the hypercortisolism of depression and Cushing's disease. N Eng J Med 1986; 314(21):1329–1335.

Goodwin TM, Monotoro M, Mestman JH, et al: The role of chorionic gonadotropin in transient hyperthyroidism of hyperemesis gravidarum. J Clin Endocrinol Metab 1992; 75:1333–1337.

Grinspoon SK, Biller BMK: Laboratory assessment of adrenal insufficiency. J Clin Endocrinol Metab 1994; 79:923–931.

Grodum E, Petersen PH, Hangaard J, et al: Biological description of the cortisol response to corticotrophin releasing hormone (CRH) stimulation. An optimization and simplification of the test. Ups J Med Sci 1993; 98:311.

Guo J, Jaume JC, Rapoport B, et al: Recombinant thyroid peroxidase-specific Fab converted to immunoglobulin G (IgG) molecules: evidence for thyroid cell damage IgG, but not IgG$_4$ autoantibodies. J Clin Endocrinol Metab 1997; 82:925–931.

Haddow JE, Palomaki GE, Allan WC, et al: Maternal thyroid deficiency during pregnancy and subsequent neuropsychological development of the child. N Engl J Med 1999; 341:549–555.

Hahn RG: Natriuresis and 'dilutional' hyponatremia after infusion of glycine 1.5%. J Clin Anesth 2001; 13:167–174.

Harjai KJ, Licata AA: Effects of amiodarone on thyroid function. Ann Intern Med 1997; 126:63–73.

Harpe R, Ferrett CG, McKnight JA, et al: Accuracy of CT scanning and adrenal vein sampling in the pre-operative localization of aldosterone-secreting adrenal adenomas. Q J Med 1999; 92:643–650.

Hartman MC, Crowe BJ, Biller BM, et al: Which patients do not require a GH stimulation test for the diagnosis of adult GH deficiency. J Clin Endocrinol Metab 2002; 87:477–485.

Hay ID, Bayer MF, Kaplan MM, et al: American Thyroid Association assessment of current free thyroid hormone and thyrotropin measurements and guidelines for future clinical assays. Clin Chem 1991; 37:2002–2008.

Heithorn R, Hauffa BP, Reinwein D: Thyroid antibodies in children of mothers with autoimmune thyroid disorder. Eur J Pediatr 1999; 158:24–28.

Heron E, Chatellier G, Billaud E, et al: The urinary metanephrine-to-creatinine ratio for the diagnosis of pheochromocytoma. Ann Intern Med 1996; 125:300–303.

Hershman JM: Human chorionic gonadotropin and the thyroid: hyperemesis gravidarum and trophoblastic tumors. Thyroid 1999; 9:653–657.

Hillier TA, Abbott RD, Barrett EJ: Hyponatremia: Evaluating the correction factor for hyperglycemia. Am J Med 1999; 106:399–403.

Hofstra RM, Landsvater RM, Ceccherini I, et al: A mutation in the RET proto-oncogene associated with multiple endocrine neoplasia type 2B and sporadic medullary thyroid carcinoma. Nature 1994; 367:375–376.

Holdaway IM, Rajasoorya RC, Gamble GD: Factors influencing mortality in acromegaly. J Clin Endocrinol Metab 2004; 89:667–674.

Holland OB, Brown H, Kuhnert L, et al: Further evaluation of saline infusion for the diagnosis of primary aldosteronism. Hypertension 1984; 6:717–723.

Hollowell JG, Staehling NW, Hannon WH, et al: Serum TSH, T(4), and thyroid antibodies in the United States population (1988 to 1994): National Health and Nutrition Examination Survey (NHANES III). J Clin Endocrinol 2002; Metab 87:489–499.

Holtzman EJ, Ausiello DA: Nephrogenic diabetes insipidus: Causes revealed. Hosp Pract (Off ed) 1994; 29(3):89–93, 97–98, 103–104.

Honour JW, Rumsby G: Problems in diagnosis and management of congenital adrenal hyperplasia due to 21-hydroxylase deficiency. J Steroid Biochem Mol Biol 1993; 45:69.

Horrocks PM, Jones AF, Ratcliffe WA, et al: Patterns of ACTH and cortisol pulsatility over twenty four hours in normal males and females. Clin Endocrinol 1990; 32:127–134.

Hsiao RJ, Parmer RJ, Takiyyuddin MM, et al: Chromogranin A storage and secretion: Sensitivity and specificity for the diagnosis of pheochromocytoma. Medicine (Baltimore) 1991; 70:33–45.

Iitaka M, Kawasaki S, Sakurai S, et al: Serum substances that interfere with thyroid hormone assays in patients with chronic renal failure. Clin Endocrinol 1998; 48:739–746.

Ishii H, Inada M, Tanaka K, et al: Induction of outer and inner ring monodeiodinases in human thyroid gland by thyrotropin. J Clin Endocrinol Metab 1983; 57:500–505.

Itoh S, Tanaka K, Kimagae M, et al: Effect of subcutaneous injection of a long acting analogue of somatostatin (SMS 201-995) on plasma thyroid stimulating hormone in normal human objects. Life Sci 1988; 42:2691–2699.

Jenkins JS, Nussey SS: The role of oxytocin: present concepts. Clin Endocrinol (Oxf) 1991; 34:515–525.

Johnson AM, Eagles JM: Lithium associated clinical hypothyroidism: prevalence and risk factors. Br J Psychiatry 1999; 175:336–339.

Kailajarvi M, Takala T, Gronroos P, et al: Reminders of drug effects on laboratory test results. Clin Chem 2000; 64:1395–1400.

Kakucska I, Rand W, Lechan RM: Thyrotropin-releasing hormone gene expression in hypothalamic paraventricular nucleus is dependent upon feedback regulation by both triiodothyronine and thyroxine. Endocrinology 1992; 130:2845–2850.

Kamoi K: Syndrome of inappropriate antidiuresis without involving inappropriate secretion of vasopressin in an elderly woman: Effect of intravenous administration of the nonpeptide vasopressin V2 receptor antagonist OPC-31260. Nephron 1997; 76:111–115.

Kamoi K, Ebe T, Kobayashi O, et al: Atrial natriuretic peptide in patients with the syndrome of inappropriate antidiuretic hormone secretion and with diabetes insipidus. J Clin Endocrinol Metab 1990; 70:1385–1390.

Kaptein EM: Thyroid hormone metabolism and thyroid diseases in chronic renal failure. Endocrinol Rev 1996; 17:45–63.

Kaptein EM, Spencer CA, Kamiel MB, Nicoloff JT: Prolonged dopamine administration and thyroid hormone economy in normal and critically ill subjects. J Clin Endocrinol Metab 1980; 51:387–393.

Kater CE, Biglieri EG: Disorders of steroid 17 alpha-hydroxylase deficiency. Endocrinol Metab Clin North Am 1994; 23:341.

Kauppila A: Isolated prolactin deficiency. Curr Ther Endocrinol Metab 1997; 6:31–33.

Kaye TB, Crapo L: The Cushings syndrome: an update on diagnostic tests. Ann Intern Med 1990; 112:434–444.

Kleinberg DL, Noel GL, Frantz AG: Galactorrhea: a study of 235 cases, including 48 with pituitary tumors. N Engl J Med 1977; 296(11):589–600.

Krakoff L, Nicolis G, Amsel B: Pathogenesis of hypertension in Cushing's syndrome. Am J Med 1975; 58:216.

Kumar S, Berl T: Sodium. Lancet 1998; 352:220–228.

Kurtz TW, Spence MA; Genetics of essential hypertension. Am J Med 1993; 94:77.

Kusalic M, Engelsmann F: Effect of lithium and maintenance therapy on thyroid and parathyroid function. J Psych Neurosci 1999; 24:227–233.

Ladenson PW, Singer PA, Ain KB, et al: American Thyroid Association Guidelines of detection of thyroid dysfunction. Arch Intern Med 2000; 160:1573–1575.

Lamb EJ, Noonan KA, Burrin JM: Urine-free cortisol excretion: Evidence of sex-dependence. Ann Clin Biochem 1994; 31:455.

Langsteger W: Clinical aspect and diagnosis of thyroid hormone transport protein anomalies. Curr Top Pathol 1997; 91:129–161.

Laragh JH: Renin profiling for the diagnosis, risk assessment and the treatment of hypertension. Kidney Int 1993; 44:1163.

Laragh JH, Baer L, Brunner HR, et al: Renin, angiotensin and aldosterone system in pathogenesis and management of hypertensive vascular disease. Am J Med 1972; 52:633.

Lazarus JG: The effects of lithium therapy on thyroid and thyrotropin-releasing hormone. Thyroid 1998; 8:909–913.

Lenders JW, Keiser HR, Goldstein DS, et al: Plasma metanephrines in the diagnosis of pheochromocytoma. Ann Int Med 1995; 123:101–109.

Lenders JW, Pacak K, Walther MM, et al: Biochemical diagnosis of pheochromocytoma: which test is best? JAMA 2002; 287:1427–1434.

Lentjes EG, Romijn F, Massen RJ, et al: Free cortisol in serum assayed by temperature-controlled ultra-filtration before fluorescence polarization immunoassay. Clin Chem 1993; 39:2518.

Levine LS: Congenital adrenal hyperplasia. In Lavin N (ed): Manual of Endocrinology and Metabolism, 3rd ed, Philadelphia, Lippincott, Williams and Wilkins, 2002, pp 147–162.

Lifton RP, Dluhy RG, Powers M: A chimaeric 11 beta-hydroxylase/aldosterone synthase gene causes glucocorticoid-remediable aldosteronism and human hypertension. Nature 1992; 355(6357):262–265.

Lindheimer MD, Davison JM: Osmoregulation, the secretion of arginine vasopressin and its metabolism during pregnancy. Eur J Endocrinol 1995; 132:133–143.

Linkowski P, Medlwicz J, Kerlhofs M, et al: 24-hr profiles of adrenocorticotropin, cortisol and growth hormone in major depressive illness: effect of anti-depressant treatment. J Clin Endocrinol Metab 1987; 65:141–152.

Lobo RA, Kletzky OA, Kaptein EM, et al: Prolactin modulation of dehydroepiandrosterone sulfate secretion. Am J Obstet Gynecol 1980; 138:632.

LoPresti JS, Eigen A, Kaptein E, et al: Alterations in 3,3',5'-triiodothyronine metabolism in response to propylthiouracil, dexamethasone and thyroxine administration in man. J Clin Invest 1989; 84:1650–1656.

LoPresti JS, Nicoloff JT: Non-thyroidal illness in endocrinology, 3rd edn. Philadelphia: WB Saunders, 1995: 665–675.

Lu FL, Yau KI, Tsai KS, et al: Longitudinal study of serum free thyroxine and thyrotropin levels by chemiluminescent immunoassay during infancy.

Taiwan Erh K'o I Hseh Hui Tsa Chih 1999; 40:225–227.

Luft FC: Proinflammatory effects of angiotensin II and endothelin: targets for progression of cardiovascular and renal disease. Curr Opin Nephrol Hypertens 2002; 11:59–66.

Lum SM, Nicoloff JT: Peripheral tissue mechanism for maintenance of serum triiodothyronine values in a thyroxine-deficient state in man. J Clin Invest 1984; 73:570–575.

Lutfallah C, Wang W, Mason JI, et al: Newly proposed hormonal criteria via genotypic proof for type II 3-β-hydroxysteroid dehydrogenase deficiency. J Clin Endocrinol Metab 2002 87(6):2611–2622.

McLeod JF, Kovacs L, Gaskill MB, et al: Familial neurohypophyseal diabetes insipidus associated with a signal peptide mutation. J Clin Endocrinol Metab 1993; 77:599A–599G.

Maghnie M, Cosi G, Genovese E, et al: Central diabetes insipidus in children and young adults. N Engl J Med 2000; 343:998–1007.

Magill SB, Raff H, Shaker JL, et al: Comparison of adrenal vein sampling and computed tomography in the differentiation of primary aldosteronism. J Clin Endocrinol Metab 2001; 86:1066–1071.

Martino E, Aghini-Lombardi F, Mariotti S, et al: Amiodarone: a common source of iodine-induced thyrotoxicosis. Horm Res 1987; 26:158–171.

Martino F, Bartalena L, Bogazzi F, Braverman LE: The effects of amiodarone on the thyroid. Endoc Rev 2001; 22:240–254.

Masrorakos G, Weber JS, Magiakou MA, et al: Hypothalamic–pituitary–adrenal axis and stimulation of systemic vasopressin secretion by recombinant interleukin-6 in humans: potential implications for the syndrome of inappropriate vasopressin secretion. J Clin Endocrinol Metabol 1994; 79:934–939.

Meikle AW, Stringham JD, Woodward MG, Nelson JC: Hereditary and environmental influences on the variation of thyroid hormones in normal male twins. J Clin Endocrinol Metab 1988; 66(3):588–592.

Mendel CM, Frost PH, Kunitake ST, Cabalieri RR: Mechanism of the heparin-induced increase in the concentration of free thyroxine in plasma. J Clin Endocrinol Metab 1987 65:1259–1264

Merke DP, Bornstein SR, Avila NA, Chrousos GP: Future directions in the study and management of congenital adrenal hyperplasia due to 21-hydroxylase deficiency. Intern Med 2002; 136:320–334.

Merke DP, Chrousos GP, Eisenhofer G, et al: Adrenomedullary dysplasia and hypofunction in patients with classic 21-hydroxylase deficiency. N Engl J Med 2000; 343:1362–1368.

Meurisse M, Gollogly MM, Degauque C, et al: Iatrogenic thyrotoxicosis: causal circumstances, pathophysiology and principles of treatment – review of the literature. World J Surg 2000; 24:1377–1385.

Mevorach RA, Bogaert GA, Kogan BA: Urine concentration and enuresis in healthy pre-school children. Arch Pediatr Adolesc Med 1995; 149(3):259–262.

Motte P, Vauzelle P, Garder P, et al: Construction and clinical validation of a sensitive and specific assay for mature calcitonin using monoclonal anti-peptide antibodies. Clin Chim Acta 1988; 174:35–54.

Mulligan LM, Kwok JB, Healey CS, et al: Germ-line mutations of the RET proto-oncogene in multiple endocrine neoplasia type 2A. Nature 1993; 363:458–460.

Nelson DH, Samuels LT: A method for the determination of 17-hydroxycorticosteroids in blood: 17-Hydroxycorticosterone in the peripheral circulation. J Clin Endocrinol Metab 1952; 12:519–526.

Nelson JC, Tindall DJ: A comparison of the adrenal responses to hypoglycemia, metyrapone and ACTH. Am J Med Sci 1978; 275:165–172.

Nelson JC, Wilcox RB: Analytical performance of free and total thyroxine assays. Clin Chem 1996; 42:146–154.

Nelson JC, Clark SJ, Borut DL, et al: Age-related changes in serum free thyroxine during childhood and adolescence. J Pediatr 1993; 123:899–905.

New MI: Steroid 21-hydroxylase deficiency (congenital adrenal hyperplasia). Am J Med 1995; 98:2S–8S.

New MI, Lorenzen F, Lerner AJ, et al: Genotyping steroid 21-hydroxylase deficiency: hormonal reference data. J Clin Endocrinol Metab 1983; 57:320–326.

Newell-Price J, Morris DG, Drake WM, et al: Optimal response criteria for the human CRH test in the differential diagnosis of ACTH-dependent Cushing's syndrome. J Clin Endocrinol Metab 2002; 87:1640–1645.

Newell-Price J, Trainer P, Besse M, Grossman A: The diagnosis and differential diagnosis of Cushing's syndrome and pseudo-Cushing's states. Endocr Rev 1998; 19:647–672.

Newell-Price J, Trainer PJ, Perry LA, et al: Single sleeping mid-night cortisol has 100% sensitivity for the diagnosis of Cushing's syndrome. Clin Endocrinol 1995; 43:545–550.

Nieman LK, Cutler GB Jr: The sensitivity of the urine free cortisol measurement as a screening test for Cushing's syndrome (abstract). In Programs and Abstracts of the Endocrine Society 72nd Annual Meeting, Atlanta, GA. Endocrine Soc, 1990, p 822.

Nieman LK, Cutler GB Jr, Oldfield EH, et al: The ovine corticotrophin-releasing hormone (CRH) stimulation test is superior to the human CRH stimulation test for the diagnosis of Cushing's disease. J Clin Endocrinol Metab 1989; 69:165–159.

Nilson JC, Clarke SJ, Borat DI, et al. Age related changes in serum free thyroxine during childhood and adolesence. J Pediatr 1993; 123:899–905.

Nohr SB, Jorgensen A, Pedersen KM, Laurberg P. Postpartum thyroid dysfunction in pregnant thyroid peroxidase antibody-positive women living in an area with mild to moderate iodine deficiency: Is iodine supplementation safe? J Clin Endocrinol Metab 2000; 85:3191–198.

Nordenstrom A, Thilen A, Hadenfeldt L, et al: Genotyping is a valuable diagnostic complement to neonatal screening for congenital adrenal hyperplasia due to steroid 21-hydroxylase deficiency. J Clin Endocrinol Metab 1999; 84:1505.

Nussey SS, Soo SC, Gibson S, et al: Isolated congenital ACTH deficiency: A cleavage enzyme defect? Clin Endocrinol 1993; 39:381.

Oakley PW, Dawson AH, Whyte IM: Lithium: Thyroid effects and altered renal handling. Clin Toxicol 2000; 38:333–337.

Oelkers W: Adrenal Insufficiency. N Eng J Med 1996; 335(16):1206–1212.

Oelkers W, Diederich S, Bahr V: Diagnosis and therapy surveillance in Addison's disease: Rapid adrenocorticotropin (ACTH) test and measurement of plasma ACTH, renin activity and aldosterone. J Clin Endocrinol Metab 1992; 75:259–264.

Orme SM, McNally RJ, Cartwright RA, Belchetz PE: Mortality and cancer incidence in acromegaly: a retrospective cohort study. United Kingdom Acromegaly Study Group. J Clin Endocrinol Metab 1998; 83:2730–2734.

Orth DN: Cushing's syndrome. N Engl J Med 1995; 332:791.

Pacak K, Chrousos GP, Koch CA, et al: Pheochromocytoma: progress in diagnosis, therapy and genetics. In Margioris A, Chrousos GP (eds): Adrenal Disorders, Vol 1. Totawa, Humana Press, 2001a pp 479–523.

Pacak K, Eisenhofer G, Carrasquillo JA, et al: 6-[^{18}F] fluorodopamine positron emission tomography (PET) scanning for diagnostic localization of pheochromocytoma. Hypertension 2001b 38:6–8.

Pacak K, Eisenhofer G, Ilias I: Diagnostic imaging of pheochromocytoma. Front Horm Res 2004; 31:76–106.

Pacini F, Fontanelli M, Fugazzola L, et al: Routine measurement of serum calcitonin in nodular thyroid diseases allows the preoperative diagnosis of unsuspected sporadic medullary thyroid carcinoma. J Clin Endocrinol Metab 1994; 78:826–829.

Panesar NS, Li CY, Rogers MS: Reference intervals for thyroid hormones in pregnant Chinese women. Ann Clin Biochem 2001; 38:329–332.

Pang S, Lerner AJ, Stoner E: Late-onset adrenal steroid 3-β-hydroxysteroid dehydrogenase deficiency. I.

A cause of hirsutism in pubertal and postpubertal women. J Clin Endocrinol Metab 1985; 60:428–439.

Pang S, Levine LS, Lorenzen F, et al: Hormonal studies in obligate heterozygotes and siblings of patients with 11-β-hydroxylase deficiency congenital adrenal hyperplasia. J Clin Endocrinol Metab 1980; 50:586–589.

Pang S, Murphey W, Levine LS, et al: A pilot newborn screening for congenital adrenal hyperplasia in Alaska. J Clin Endocrinol Metab 1982; 55:413–420.

Pang SY, Wallace MA, Hofman L: Worldwide experience in newborn screening for classical congenital adrenal hyperplasia due to 21-hydroxylase deficiency. Pediatrics 1988; 81:866–874.

Papanicolaou DA, Mullen N, Kyrou I, Nieman L: Nighttime salivary cortisol: A useful test for the diagnosis of Cushing's syndrome. J Clin Endocrinol Metab 2002; 87:4515–4521.

Papanicolaou DA, Yanovski JA, Cutler GB Jr, et al: A single mid-night serum cortisol measurement distinguishes Cushing's disease from pseudo-Cushing state. J Clin Endocrinol Metab 1998; 83:1163–1167.

Parle JV, Masisonneuve P, Sheppard MC, et al: Prediction of all-cause and cardiovascular mortality in elderly people from one low serum thyrotropin result: a 10-year study. Lancet 2001; 358:861–865.

Pedersen KM, Laurberg P, Iversen E, et al: Amelioration of some pregnancy associated variation in thyroid function by iodine supplementation. J Clin Endocrinol Metab 1993; 77:1078–1083.

Philomin V, Vassieres A, Jaouen G: New applications of carbonylmetalloimmunoassay (CMIA): A non-radioisotopic approach to cortisol assay. J Immuno Methods 1994; 171:201.

Piketty ML, D'Herbomez M, Le Guillouzic D, et al: Clinical comparison of three labeled-antibody immunoassays of free triiodothyronine. Clin Chem 1996; 42:933–941.

Pop VJ, De Vries E, Van Baar AL, et al: Maternal thyroid peroxidase antibodies during pregnancy: a marker of impaired child development? J Clin Endocrinol Metab 1995; 80:3561–3566.

Pop VJ, Kuijpens JL, van Baar Al, et al: Low maternal free thyroxine concentrations during pregnancy are associated with impaired psychomotor development in infancy. Clin Endocrinol 1999; 50:147–148.

Porter CC, Silber RH: A quantitative color reaction for cortisone and related 17,21-dihydroxy-20-ketosteroids. J Biol Chem 1950; 185:201–207.

Prazeres S, Santos MA, Ferreira HG, Sobrinho LG: A practical method for the detection of macroprolactinaemia using ultrafiltration. Clin Endocrinol (Oxf) 2003; 58(6):686–690.

Putignano P, Toja P, Dubini A, et al: Midnight salivary cortisol versus urinary free and midnight serum cortisol as screening tests for Cushing's syndrome. J Clin Endocrinol Metab 2003; 88:4153–4157.

Radetti G, Persani L, Moroder W, et al: Transplacental passage of anti-thyroid auto-antibodies in a pregnant woman with auto-immune thyroid disease. Prenat diagn 1999; 19:468–471.

Radin DR, Manoogian C, Nadler JL: Diagnosis of primary hyperaldosteronism: Importance of correlating CT findings with endocrinologic studies. AJR Am J Roentgenol 1992; 158:553.

Raff H, Findling JW: A physiologic approach to diagnosis of the Cushing syndrome. Ann Intern Med 2003; 138:980–991.

Rajasoorya C, Holdaway IM, Wrightson P, et al: Determinants of clinical outcome and survival in acromegaly. Clin Endocrinol (Oxf) 1994; 41:95–102.

Refetoff S: Thyroid hormone resistance syndrome. In The Thyroid, 6th ed. Philadelphia, JB Lippincott, 1991.

Reihman DH, Farber MO, Heath DA: Effect of hypoxemia on sodium and water excretion in chronic obstructive lung disease. Am J Med 1985; 78:87–94.

Rigg LA, Lein A, Yen SSC: Pattern of increase in circulating prolactin levels during human gestation. Am J Obstet Gynecol 1977; 129:454–456.

Rivier C, Vale W: Effect of angiotensin II on ACTH release in vivo: role of corticotrophin-releasing factor. Regul Pept 1983; 7:253–258.

Robbins J: Thyroid hormone transport protein and the physiology of hormone binding. In Gray CH, James VHT (eds): Hormones in Blood. London, Academic Press, 1996, pp 96–110.

Robertson GL: The use of vasopressin assays in physiology and pathophysiology. Semin Nephrol 1994; 14(4):368–383.

Rocha R, Steir CT, Kifor I, et al: Aldosterone: a mediator of myocardial necrosis and renal arteriopathy. Endocrinology 2000; 141:3871–3878.

Rose S, Ross J, et al: The advantage of measuring stimulated as compared with spontaneous growth hormone levels in the diagnosis of growth hormone deficiency. N Engl J Med 1988; 319:201–207.

Rosler A, Weshler N, Leiberman E, et al: 11 Beta-hydroxylase deficiency congenital adrenal hyperplasia: update of prenatal diagnosis. J Clin Endocrinol Metab 1988; 66:830–838.

Ross DS: Subclinical hyperthyroidism. In Braverman LE, Utiger RD (eds): Werner and Jngbar's The Thyroid: a Fundamental and Clinical Text, 6th ed. Philadelphia, JB Lippincott, 1991, pp 1249–1255.

Roth J, Taatjes D, Lucocq J, et al: Demonstration of an extensive trans-tubular network continuous with the Golgi apparatus stack that may function in glycosylation. Cell 1985; 43:287–295.

Rudd BT: Measurement of urine 17-oxogenic steroids, 17-hydroxycorticosteroids, and 17-oxosteroids has been superseded by better tests. Br Med J 1985; 291:805.

Samaan GJ, Porquet D, Demelier JF, et al: Determination of cortisol and associated glucocorticoids in serum and urine by an automated liquid chromatographic assay. Clin Biochem 1993; 26:153.

Samuels MH, Veldhuis JD, Henry PM, et al: Pathophysiology of pulsatile and copulsatile release of thyroid-stimulating hormone, and alpha subunit. J Clin Endocrinol Metab 1990; 71:425.

Sapin R, Schliener JL, Kaltenbach G, et al: Determination of free triiodothyronine by six different methods in patients with non-thyroid illness and in patients treated with amiodarone. Ann Clin Biochem 1993; 32:314–324.

Sassin JF, Frantz AG, Weitzman ED, Kapen S. Human prolactin: 24-hour pattern with increased release during sleep. Science 1972; 177:120–1207.

Sawin CT, Geller A, Kaplan MM, et al: Low serum thyrotropin (thyroid stimulating hormone) in older persons with hyperthyroidism. Arch Intern Med 1991; 151:165–168.

Sawin CT, Geller A, Wolf PA, et al: Low serum thyrotropin concentrations as risk factor for atrial fibrillation in older persons. N Engl J Med 1994; 331:1249–1252.

Sawin CT, Herman T, Molitch ME, et al: Aging and the thyroid: decreased requirement for thyroid hormone in older hypothyroid patients. Am J Med 1983; 75:206–209.

Sawka AM, Jaeschke R, Singh RJ, Young WF Jr: A comparison of biochemical tests for pheochromocytoma: Measurement of fractionated plasma metanephrines compared with the combination of 24-hour urinary metanephrines and catecholamines. J Clin Endocrinol Metab 2003; 88:553–558.

Scheithauer BW, Sano T, Kovacs KT, et al: The pituitary gland in pregnancy: A clinicopathologic and immunohistochemical study of 69 cases. Mayo Clin Proc 1990; 65:461–474.

Schlumberger MCP, Fragu P, Lumbroso J, et al: Circulating thyrotropin and thyroid hormones in patients with metastases of differentiated thyroid carcinoma: Relationship to serum thyrotropin levels. J Clin Endocrinol Metab 1980; 51:513–519.

Schunkert H, Hense HW, Muscholl M, et al: Associations between circulating components of the renin–angiotensin–aldosterone system and left ventricular mass. Heart 1997; 77:24–31.

Schutte HM, Chrousos GP, Avergerinos P, et al: The corticotrophin-releasing hormone stimulation test: a possible aid in the evaluation of patients with adrenal insufficiency. J Clin Endocrinol Metab 1984; 58:1064–1067.

Sergev O, Racz K, Varga I, et al: Atrial natriuretic peptide in normal and low renin essential hypertension. Kidney Int 1990 30:S107–S108.

Sheps SG, Jiang NS, Klee GG, et al: Recent developments in the diagnosis and treatment of pheochromocytoma. Endo Rev 1994; 15:356–368.

Shupnik MA, Greenspan SL, Ridgway EC: Transcriptional regulation of thyrotropin subunit genes by thyrotropin-releasing hormone and dopamine pituitary cell cultures. J Biol Chem 1986; 261:12675–12679.

Sjoberg RJ, Simcic KJ, Kidd GS: The clonidine suppression test for pheochromocytoma. A review of its utility and pitfalls. Arch Int Med 1992; 152:1193–1197.

Skamene A, Patel YC. Infusion of graded concentrations of somatostatin in man: pharmaco-kinetics and differential inhibitory effects on pituitary and islet hormones. Clin Endocrinol 1984; 20:555–564.

Snow K, Jiang N, Kao PC, et al: Biochemical evolution of adrenal dysfunction: The laboratory perspective. Mayo Clin Proc 1992; 67:1055.

Sonkodi S, Abraham G, Mohacsi G: Effects of nephrectomy on hypertension, renin activity and total renal function in patients with chronic renal artery occlusion. J Hum Hypertens 1990; 4(3):277–279.

Speckart PF, Nicoloff JT, Bethune JE: Screening for adrenocortical insufficiency with Cosyntropin (synthetic ACTH). Arch Intern Med 1971; 128:761–763.

Speiser PW, White P: Congenital adrenal hyperplasia. N Engl J Med 2003; 349:776–788.

Speiser PW, Dupont B, Rubinstein P, et al: High frequency of nonclassical steroid 21-hydroxylase deficiency. Am J Hum Genet 1985; 37:650–667.

Spencer CA: Clinical evaluation of free T4 techniques. J Endocrinol Invest 1986; 9:57–66.

Spencer CA, Nicoloff JT: Serum TSH measurement: A 1990 status report. Thyroid Today 1990; 13:1–12.

Spencer CA, Wang CC: Thyroglobulin measurement: Techniques, clinical benefits and pitfalls. Endocrinol Metab Clin N Amer 1995; 24:841–863.

Spencer CA, LoPresti JS, Fatema S, Nicoloff JT: Detection of residual and recurrent differentiated thyroid carcinoma by serum thyroglobulin measurement. Thyroid 1999; 9·435 441.

Spencer CA, LoPresti JS, Patel A, et al: Applications of new chemiluminometric thyrotropin assay to subnormal measurements. J Clin Endocrinol Metab 1990; 70:453–460.

Spencer CA, Takeuchi M, Kazarosyan M: Current status and performance goals for serum thyroglobulin (TSH) assays. Clin Chem 1996; 42:140–145.

Stewart PM: The adrenal cortex. In Larsen PR, Kronenberg HM, Melmed S, Polonsky KS (eds): Williams Textbook of Endocrinology, 10th ed. Philadelphia, Saunders, 2003, pp 491–551.
One of the best written and most respected general endocrine reference textbooks; the chapter on the adrenals is concise, lucid, and well referenced.

Streeten DHP, Tomycz N, Anderson GH: Reliability of screening methods for the diagnosis of primary aldosteronism. Ann J Med 1979; 67:403.

Suliman AM, Smith TP, Gibney J, McKenna TJ: Frequent misdiagnosis and mismanagement of hyperprolactinemia in patients before the introduction of macroprolactin screening: Application of a new strict laboratory definition of macroprolactinemia. Clin Chem 2003; 49(9):1504–1509.

Surks MI, Chopra IJ, Maraish CN, et al: American Thyroid Association guidelines for use of laboratory tests in thyroid disorders. JAMA 1990; 263:1529–1532.

Surks MI, Sievert R. Drugs and thyroid function. N Engl J Med 1995; 333:1688–1694.

Swearingen B, Barker FG II, Katznelson L, et al: Long-term mortality after transphenoidal surgery and adjunctive therapy for acromegaly. J Clin Endocrinol Metab 1998; 83:3419–3426.

Talbot JA, Lambert A, Anobile CJ, et al: The nature of human chorionic gonadotrophin glycoforms in gestational thyrotoxicosis. Clin Encrinol 2001; 55:33–39.

Taylor HC, Mayes D, Anton AH: Clonidine suppression test for pheochromocytoma: Examples of misleading results. J Clin Endocrinol Metab 1986; 63:238–242.

Taylor RL, Singh RJ: Validation of liquid chromatography–tandem mass spectrometry method for analysis of urinary conjugated metanephrine and normetanephrine for screening of pheochromocytoma. Clin Chem 2002; 48:533–539.

Thalen BE, Kjellman BF, Ljunggren JG, et al: Release of corticotrophin after administration of corticotrophin releasing hormone in depressed patients in relation to the dexamethasone suppression test. Acta Psychiatr Scand 1993; 87:133.

Therrell BL: Newborn screening for congenital adrenal hyperplasia. Endocrinol Metab Clin North Am 2001; 21:245–291.

Toldy E, Locsei Z, Szabolcs I, et al: Macroprolactinemia: the consequences of a laboratory pitfall. Endocrine 2003; 22(3): 267–273.

Trainer P: Editorial: Acromegaly – consensus, what consensus? J Clin Endocrinol Metab 2002; 87(8):3534–3536.

Tuchman M, Morris C, et al: Value of random urinary homovanillic acid levels in the diagnosis and management of patients with neuroblastoma. Comparison of 24-hour urine collections. Pediatrics 1985; 75:324–328.

Tullis MJ, Caps MT, Zierler RE: Blood pressure, antihypertensive medication and atherosclerotic renal artery stenosis. Am J Kidney Dis 1999; 33(4):675–681.

Utiger R: Decreased extrathyroidal triiodothyronine production and nonthyroidal illness: Benefits or harm? Am J Med 1980; 69:807–810.

Van Cauter E: Slow wave sleep and release of growth hormone. JAMA 2000; 284:2717–2718.

Van Cauter E, Plat L, Copinschi G: Interrelations between sleep and the somatotropic axis. Sleep 21:553–566.

Van den Berghe G, De Zegher F, Bouillon R: Acute and prolonged critical illness as different neuroendocrine paradigms. J Clin Endocrinol Metab 1998; 83:1827–1834.

Van den Berghe G: Novel insights into the neuroendocrinology of critical illness. Eur J Endocrinol 2000; 143:1–3.

Van Heyningen V: One gene – four syndromes. Nature 1994; 367:319–20.

Vanderpump MPJ, Tunbridge WMG, French JM, et al: The incidence of thyroid disorders in the community: a twenty year follow up of the Whickham survey. Clin Endocrinol 1995; 43:55–68.

Vassart G, Dumont JE: Identification of polysomes synthesizing thyroglobulin. Eur J Biochem 1973a; 32(2):322–330.

Vassart G, Brocas H, Nokin P, Dumont JE: Translation in *Xenopus* oocytes of thyroglobulin mRNA isolated by poly(U)-Sepharose affinity chromatography. Biochim Biophys Acta 1973b; 324(4):575–580.

Vieira AEF, Mello MP, Elias LLK, et al: Molecular and biochemical screening for the diagnosis and management of medullary thyroid carcinoma in multiple endocrine neoplasia type 2A. Horm Metab Res 2002; 34:202–206.

Vistorina WM, Rydstedt LL, Sowers JR: Clinical disorders of vasopressin. In Lavin N (ed): Manual of Endocrinology and Metabolism, 3rd ed. Philadelphia, Lippincott, Williams and Wilkins, 2002, pp 68–82.

Vitale G, Ciccarelli A, Caraglia M, et al: Comparison of two provocative tests for calcitonin in medullary thyroid carcinoma: omeprazole vs pentagastrin. Clin Chem 2002; 48(9):1505–1510.

Volin P: Simultaneous determination of serum cortisol and cortisone by reversed-phase liquid chromatography with ultraviolet detection. J Chromatogr 1992; 584:147.

Walker SE, Allen SH, McMurray RW: Prolactin and autoimmune disease. Trends Endocrinol Metab 1993; 4:47–151.

Wardle CA, Fraser WD, Squire CR: Pitfalls in the use of thyrotropin concentration as a first-line thyroid-function test. Lancet 2001; 357:1013–1014.

Wartofsky L, Burman KD: Alterations in thyroid function in patients with systemic illness: the 'euthyroid sick syndrome'. Endocrinol Rev 1982; 3:164–217.

Weeke J, Dybkjaer L, Granlie K, et al: A longitudinal study of serum TSH and total and free iodothyronines during normal pregnancy. Acta Endocrinol 1982; 101:531–57.

Weinberger MH, Fineberg NS: The diagnosis of primary aldosteronism and separation of two major subtypes. Arch Intern Med 1993; 153:2125.

Weise M, Drinkard B, Mehlinger SL, et al: Stress dose of hydrocortisone is not beneficial in patients with classic congenital adrenal hyperplasia undergoing short-term, high-intensity exercise. J Clin Endocrinol Metab 2004; 89:3679.

Weise M, Merke DP, Pacak K, et al: Utility of plasma free metanephrines for detecting childhood pheochromocytoma. J Clin Endocrinol Metab 2002; 87:1955–1960.

Wells SA, Baylin SB, Linehan W, et al: Provocative agents and the diagnosis of medullary carcinoma of the thyroid gland. Ann Surg 1978; 188:139–141.

Werbel SS, Ober KP: Pheochromocytoma. Update on diagnosis, localization and management. Med Clin North Am 1995; 79(1):131–153.

White MC, Clark AJL: The cellular and molecular basis of the ectopic ACTH syndrome. Clin Endocrinol 1993; 39:131.

White PC, Curnow KM, Pascoe L: Disorders of steroid 11-beta-hydroxylase isoenzymes. Endocr Rev 1994b; 15:421–438.

White PC, Tusie-Lina MT, New MI, et al: Mutations in steroid 21-hydroxylase (CYP21). Hum Mutat 1994a; 3:373.

Whitehouse WM Jr, Kazmers A, Zelenock GB: Chronic total renal artery occlusion: effects of treatment of secondary hypertension and renal function. Surgery 1981; 89(6):753–763.

Wilcox RB, Nelson JC, Tomei RT: Heterogeneity in affinities of serum proteins for thyroxine among patients with non-thyroidal illness as indicated by the serum free thyroxine response to serum dilution. Eur J Endocrinol 1994; 131:9–13.

Willie S, Aili M, Harris A, et al: Plasma and urinary levels of vasopressin in enuretic and non-enuretic children. Scand J Urol Nephrol 1994; 28:119–122.

Wion-Barbot N, Schuffenecker I, Niccoli P, et al: Results of the calcitonin stimulation test in normal volunteers compared with genetically unaffected members of MEN 2A and familial medullary thyroid carcinoma families. Ann Endocrinol 1997; 58:302–308

Yanovski JA, Cutler GB Jr, Chrousos GP, Nieman LK: Corticotropin-releasing hormone stimulation following low-dose dexamethasone administration. A new test to distinguish Cushing's syndrome from pseudo-Cushing's states. JAMA 1993; 269:2232–2238.

Yazigi R, Quinero C, et al: Prolactin disorders. Fertil Steril 1997; 7:215–225.

Yokoyama Y, Ueda T, Irahara M, et al: Release of oxytocin and prolactin during breast massage and suckling in puerperal women. Eur J Obstet Gynecol Reprod Biol 1994; 53:17–20.

Young WF Jr: Primary aldosteronism: A common and curable form of hypertension. Cardiol Rev 1999; 7(4):207–214.

Yuasa H, Ito M, Nagasaki H, et al: Glu-47, which forms a salt bridge between neurophysin II and arginine vasopressin is deleted in patients with familial central diabetes insipidus. J Clin Endocrinol Metab 1993; 77:600–604.

Zerbe RL, Robertson GL: Vasopressin function in the syndrome of inappropriate antidiuresis. Ann Rev Med 1980; 31:315–327.

Zerbe RL, Robertson GL: Osmotic and nonosmotic regulation of thirst and vasopressin secretion. In Maxwell MH, Kleeman CR, Narins RG (eds): Clinical disorders of fluid and electrolyte metabolism, 4th ed, New York, McGraw-Hill, 1987.

Zerbe RL, Robertson GL: A comparison of plasma vasopressin measurements with a standard indirect test in the differential diagnosis of polyuria. New Eng J Med 1981; 304:1539–1546.

Zurakowski D, Di Canzio J, Majzoub JA: Pediatric reference intervals for serum thyroxine, triiodothyronine, thyrotropin and free thyroxine. Clin Chem 1999; 45:1087–1091.

II

CHAPTER 25

Reproductive Function and Pregnancy

Robert A. Webster PhD

KEY POINTS

- Reproductive function and pregnancy are regulated by the complex interaction of a variety of hormones, synthesized and secreted by the testis (testosterone), ovary (estradiol and progesterone), pituitary (FSH and LH), hypothalamus (GnRH), and placenta (HCG, estrogens, and progesterone).

- Laboratory evaluation of reproductive function in the male typically begins with semen analysis. If the results are normal, further evaluation may be unnecessary. If the results are abnormal, then serum hormone measurements are important, particularly of testosterone, FSH, and LH.

- Reproductive dysfunction in the female is often indicated by amenorrhea and/or infertility. Laboratory evaluation, as in the male, involves serum hormone measurements, particularly of HCG, PRL, TSH, FT_4, FSH, LH, and androgens.

- Infertility can be treated by several assisted reproductive technologies (ARTs). These involve a variety of clinical manipulations, all of which are directed at externally controlling as much of the reproductive process as possible in order to achieve pregnancy and bring it to term. Laboratory monitoring of serum hormone levels (estradiol, progesterone, and HCG) plays an important role in these protocols.

- Early pregnancy is monitored by measuring serum HCG concentrations and determining that the pattern of dramatic increase during the first trimester is as expected.

- The risk for the most common birth defects, neural tube defects (NTDs) and Down syndrome (DS), is determined during the early second trimester by screening of maternal serum for levels of AFP, HCG, and unconjugated estriol (uE3).

- Fetal hemolytic disease (erythroblastosis fetalis) is monitored by spectrophotometrically estimating the level of bilirubin in amniotic fluid.

- The status of fetal lung maturation is estimated from the evaluation of pulmonary surfactant in amniotic fluid. This can be accomplished by several methods, including determination of (1) the lecithin/sphingomyelin ratio (L/S) and phosphatidyl glycerol (PG) by chromatography or (2) the microviscosity by fluorescence polarization.

- Toxemia of pregnancy, or pre-eclampsia, is characterized by hypertension and proteinuria, and consequently can be monitored by urine protein measurements.

- Premature rupture of membranes can be evaluated by immunoassay of fetal fibronectin in amniotic fluid.

Normal Physiology

Normal reproductive function is mediated by a variety of hormones synthesized and secreted by the gonads (testes and ovaries), adrenals, pituitary, hypothalamus, and placenta. In addition, peripheral nonglandular tissues can contribute to hormone synthesis. Paracrine and autocrine mediators are also involved, but in almost all cases their exact roles are not well understood.

Sex Steroids

The testes and ovaries synthesize sex steroids (androgens and estrogens) from cholesterol via the same initial pathway used in the adrenal glands to synthesize mineralcorticoids, glucocorticoids, and androgens (Fig. 25-1). The specific hormone secreted by an endocrine gland depends upon the presence and relative activities of various enzymes in the steroid pathway. Whereas the adrenal synthesizes androgens like dehydroepiandrosterone (DHEA), DHEA-sulfate (DHEAS), and androstenedione, the testis metabolizes these steroids primarily to testosterone. The ovary converts testosterone to estradiol, and androstenedione to estrone. Peripheral tissues (including those targeted by androgens) reduce testosterone to dihydrotestosterone (DHT). Since DHT is two to three times more potent than testosterone, this process yields an enhanced or activated androgenic effect. Peripheral tissues, such as liver, also hydroxylate estradiol to estriol, a metabolite with only one-hundredth the estrogenic potency of its precursor. Thus, this conversion is an inactivation process. During pregnancy, estriol is synthesized via a different pathway, and it may play a different role than estradiol (see below). Peripheral tissues also convert adrenal androgens to testosterone and androgens to estrone and estradiol, the latter occurring in adipose tissue. Estrone is about one-tenth as potent as estradiol. Note that although progesterone serves as an intermediate in the synthesis of all the other steroid hormones, it also functions as a sex steroid in its own right in females.

As with any hormone, the sex steroids act at tissue sites distant from their sites of synthesis and secretion. Once in the blood, most of the hydrophobic sex steroids become reversibly and noncovalently bound to

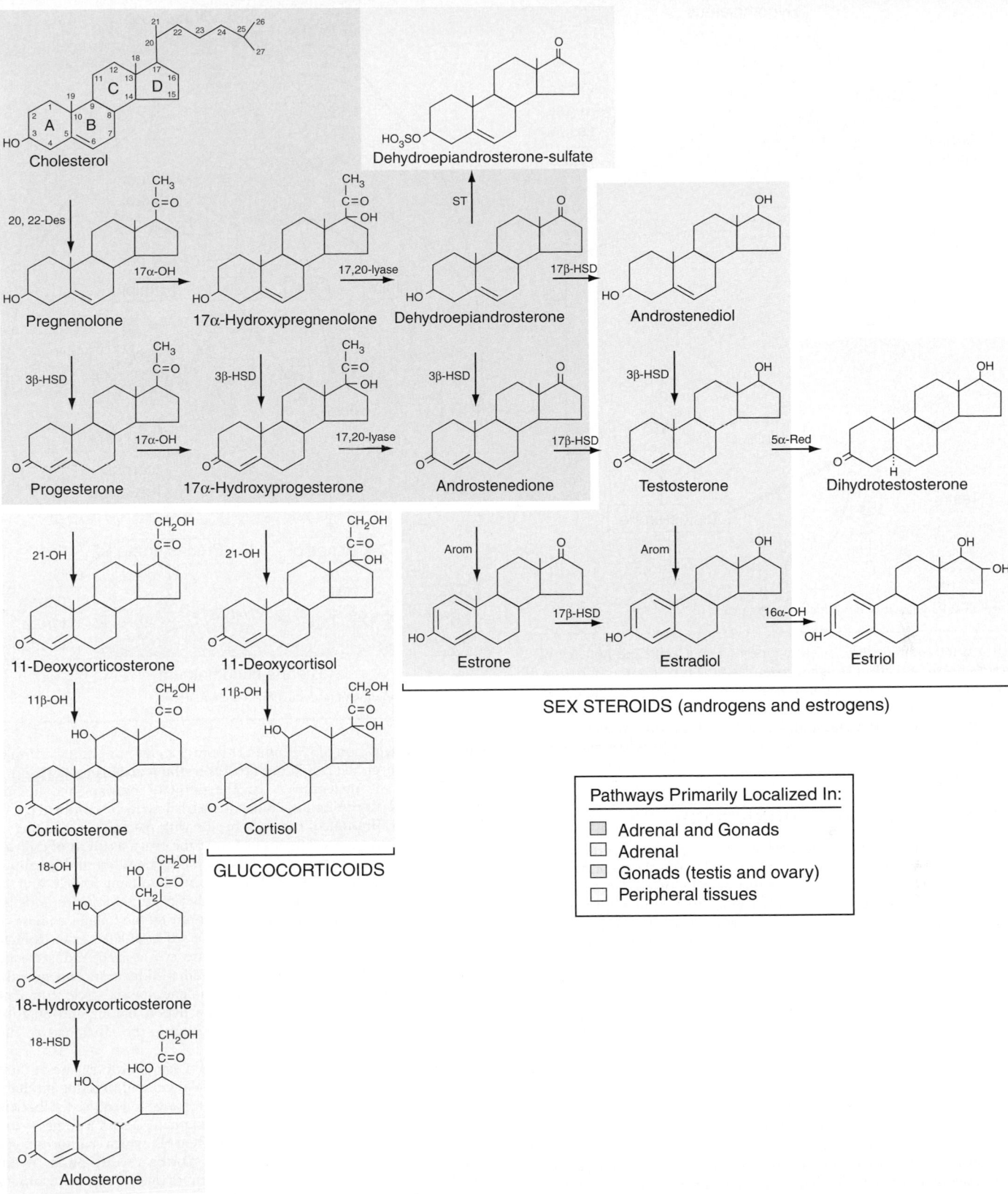

Figure 25–1 Steroid hormone synthesis. Enzyme abbreviations: 20,22-Des = 20,22 desmolase; 3β-HSD = 3β-hydroxysteroid dehydrogenase; 21-OH = 21-hydroxylase; 11β-OH = 11β-hydroxylase; 18-OH = 18-hydroxylase; 18-HSD = 18-hydroxysteroid dehydrogenase; 17α-OH = 17α-hydroxylase; 17β-HSD = 17β-hydroxysteroid dehydrogenase; ST = sulfotransferase; Arom = aromatase; 5α-Red = 5α-reductase; 16α-OH = 16α-hydroxylase.

plasma proteins. This interaction includes low-affinity, nonspecific binding to hydrophobic sites on albumin and high-affinity binding to specific transport proteins that are synthesized by the liver. Sex hormone-binding globulin (SHBG) transports androgens and estrogens, while corticosteroid-binding globulin (CBG) transports progesterone (as well as glucocorticoids). In blood, only about 1–2% of the sex steroids are free

(unbound). About half of the remainder is bound to SHBG or CBG, and about half is bound to albumin. Only the free fraction is biologically active, since only the free hormone can exit the vascular system (by diffusion) and interact with target cells.

Each steroid binds with high affinity to specific receptor proteins that activate or inactivate genes in the target cell. Thus, the same hormone can

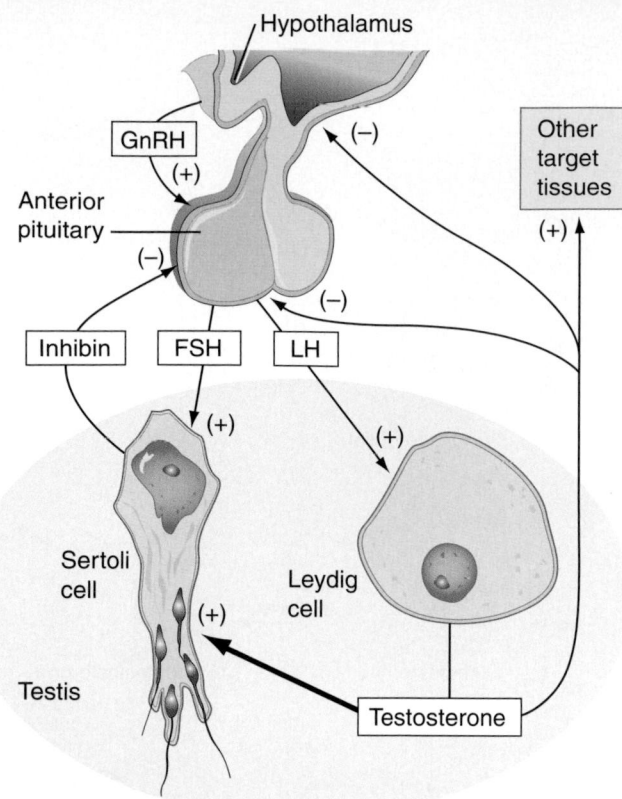

Figure 25–2 Regulation of reproduction in the male.

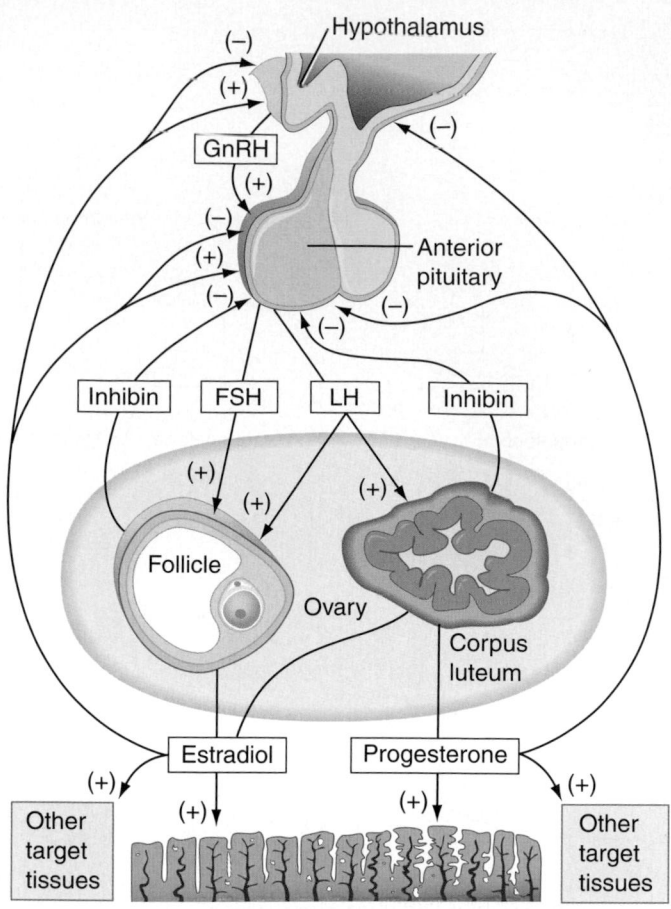

Figure 25-3 Regulation of reproduction in the female.

elicit a different response in each type of target cell. The potency of a steroid's hormonal effect (e.g. androgenic effect) is primarily a function of its affinity for the specific receptor protein and the affinity of that complex for the chromatin acceptor sites. Thus DHT is a more potent androgen than testosterone. DHEA and androstenedione bind only weakly, if at all, to the androgen receptor; hence their androgenic effect is low, and most if not all their androgenic activity derives from their peripheral conversion to testosterone.

Regulation of Male Reproduction

Figure 25–2 summarizes the regulation of reproduction in the human male. Gonadotropin-releasing hormone (GnRH) is a decapeptide that is synthesized and secreted by neuroendocrine cells of the hypothalamus, primarily in the arcuate nucleus. GnRH binds to specific cell membrane receptors on gonadotrophs in the anterior pituitary, resulting in the synthesis and secretion of two protein hormones, follicle-stimulating hormone (FSH) and luteinizing hormone (LH), both named for their effects in females. Both FSH and LH are similar to thyroid-stimulating hormone (TSH), in that all three consist of two subunits and all share the same α-subunit. Each has a different β-subunit, however, which thus confers their functional specificity.

The seminiferous tubules of the testis contain cells in various stages of spermatogenesis (spermatogonia, spermatocytes, spermatids) along with Sertoli cells and Leydig cells. FSH induces Sertoli cells to synthesize and secrete androgen-binding protein (ABP) into the lumen of the seminiferous tubule, and this maintains the high testosterone concentration required for normal spermatogenesis. LH induces Leydig cells to synthesize testosterone; some enters the general circulation and is transported to other target tissues, such as skeletal muscle, where it has an anabolic effect. Some is also transported to the hypothalamus and anterior pituitary, where the testosterone has a negative-feedback effect – that is, it decreases the synthesis and secretion of GnRH, FSH, and LH, and this decreases testosterone synthesis by Leydig cells.

Sertoli cells also synthesize and secrete another protein hormone, inhibin. It interacts with gonadotrophs in the anterior pituitary, where it has a negative feedback effect: it decreases the synthesis and secretion of FSH, but not LH. The exact role of inhibin in the regulatory process is not understood.

Regulation of Female Reproduction

Figure 25–3 summarizes the regulation of reproduction in the human female. As in the male, GnRH from the hypothalamus increases the synthesis and secretion of FSH and LH from the anterior pituitary. Unlike the male, however, the regulatory process in the female is cyclical and is referred to as the menstrual cycle. The pituitary, ovarian, and uterine changes that occur during the 28-day menstrual cycle are summarized in Figure 25–4. As illustrated, the cycle begins with menses, or shedding of uterine endometrium. During this period in the ovary, a cohort of follicles is 'recruited' to begin further growth and development. From this cohort, one follicle (usually) is 'selected' to be the dominant follicle and to continue growth and development. The other recruited follicles undergo regression, or atresia. These processes occur during the follicular phase of the ovarian cycle, primarily as a result of the action of FSH. As the follicle grows, increasing amounts of estradiol are synthesized and secreted. Estradiol restores the endometrium via cell proliferation and growth; hence the proliferative phase of the uterine endometrial cycle. Estradiol also has a negative-feedback effect on the hypothalamus and anterior pituitary, causing a decline in FSH levels during the latter part of the follicular phase.

Near the end of the follicular phase, when estradiol levels are at their highest, its feedback effect on the hypothalamus and anterior pituitary switches to positive. The mechanism for this change to positive feedback is not understood. Its effect, however, is dramatic. It causes a surge in the secretion of GnRH, FSH, and particularly LH, which culminates in ovulation. The oocyte enters the oviduct. Owing to disruption of the follicle, estradiol synthesis and secretion drop dramatically. The disrupted follicle begins to differentiate into the corpus luteum: thus begins the luteal phase of the ovarian cycle. The corpus luteum synthesizes estradiol *and* progesterone as a result of the action of LH. The combination of the two steroids acts on the uterine endometrium to cause development of numerous exocrine glands, producing the secretory phase of the uterine endometrial cycle. This phase prepares the endometrium for implantation, should fertilization and early development occur. LH levels decline gradually during the luteal phase, indicating restoration of negative-feedback regulation of the hypothalamus and anterior pituitary by estradiol and progesterone.

As in the male, inhibin has a selective negative-feedback effect on FSH. In the female, however, there are two different forms. One is synthesized and secreted by the developing follicles (inhibin B), and the other is from

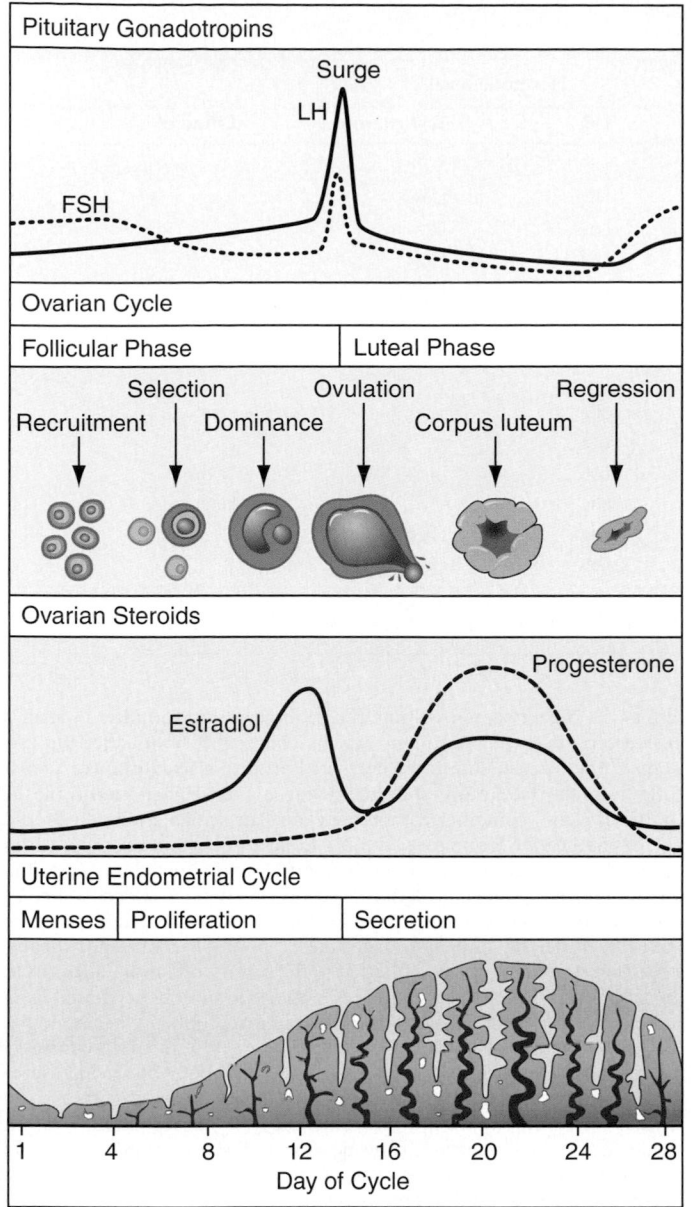

Figure 25-4 Pituitary, ovarian, and uterine changes during the human menstrual cycle.

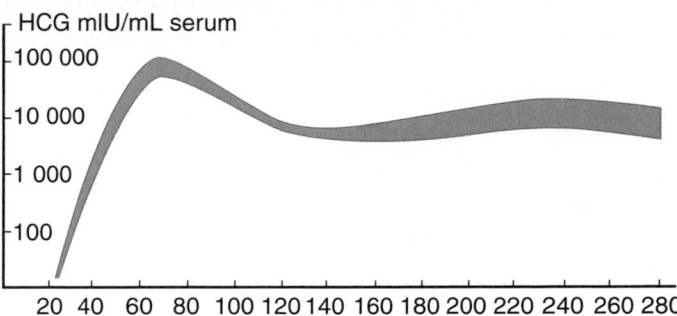

Figure 25-5 Serum HCG levels during normal pregnancy. (After Lau, HL: Testing for pregnancy. *In* Hagerstown, MD: Practice of Medicine, Vol II. Harper & Row, 1975, Ch 29; and Braunstein GD, Rasor J, Adler D, Danzer H, Wade ME: Am J Obstet Gynecol 1976; 126:678.)

During the first trimester of pregnancy, HCG increases from < 5 mIU/mL serum to > 100 000 mIU/mL (Fig. 25–5). This increase is responsible for the similarly dramatic increases in the levels of estradiol and progesterone. By the end of the first trimester, however, HCG levels begin to decline significantly. Estradiol and progesterone continue to increase, because by this time the placenta has assumed most steroid synthesis, including significant amounts of estrone and estriol. Unlike HCG, these steroid levels increase as placental mass grows. Steroid intermediates from the fetal adrenal gland and fetal liver also contribute to this process. For example, estriol is not synthesized by hydroxylation of estradiol (Fig. 25–1), but rather by conversion from fetal 16-hydroxy-DHEAS; this is why maternal estriol measurements were historically used to assess fetal well-being in late pregnancy (Carr, 2004). The estrogenic potency of estriol is only about one-hundredth that of estradiol and only one-tenth that of estrone. However, estriol promotes uteroplacental blood flow as potently as other estrogens and this may be the reason for its dramatic increase during the last two trimesters (Resnik, 1974).

Another hormone synthesized in large quantities by the placenta during the last two trimesters is human placental lactogen (HPL). It is structurally similar to both prolactin and growth hormone, and has both lactogenic and growth-promoting activities, although both are relatively weak. In addition, HPL is an insulin antagonist and thus may play a role in maternal glucose utilization. However, its exact role is unclear since apparently normal pregnancies have been described in which HPL is not detectable in maternal blood or placenta (Sideri, 1983). Unlike HCG, the increase in HPL also parallels the steady increase in placental mass (Carr, 2004).

The placenta also synthesizes inhibin. Whereas gonadal (testicular and ovarian) inhibin functions as an endocrine inhibitor of pituitary FSH secretion, placental inhibin may function as a paracrine or autocrine inhibitor of placental HCG secretion (Mesiano, 2004). Its exact regulatory role, however, has not been elucidated.

Parturition is the process by which the fetus is expelled from internal environment of the maternal uterus to the external environment. This occurs as a result of a change in the activity of the uterine myometrium (smooth muscle), from irregular, long-lasting, low-frequency contractions to regular, high-intensity, high-frequency contractions. The initiation of this process in humans is not well understood, and seems to differ from that of other mammals. For example, progesterone inhibits uterine contractions during gestation, and in most other mammals the onset of parturition is preceded by a significant decrease in maternal plasma progesterone; in humans, however, this does not occur. A 'parturition cascade' has been postulated for humans that involves multiple and redundant endocrine, paracrine, and autocrine mediators. These mediators are thought to include: fetal cortisol and DHEAS; placental estriol, oxytocin, prostaglandins, and corticotropin-releasing hormone; and maternal oxytocin. The effects of these mediators may also be modulated by changes in their receptor levels (Norwitz, 2004).

Parturition is followed by lactation. Initial development of the mammary gland occurs at puberty, when estradiol causes growth and branching of the ducts, and progesterone causes formation of the alveoli. Similarly, during pregnancy, the high concentrations of estrogens and progesterone cause further branching of the ducts and growth of the alveoli. The secretory capability of the alveolar epithelial cells is induced by prolactin, which increases during pregnancy, and by HPL. At parturition, the decrease in estrogen and progesterone eliminates their inhibitory effect on milk secretion, which still requires prolactin. Milk

the corpus luteum (inhibin A) (Welt, 1999). Again, the exact regulatory roles they play are not understood.

In an infertile cycle, the corpus luteum begins to regress near the end of the luteal phase. This results in a decrease in estradiol and progesterone synthesis and secretion. Since these steroids are required for maintenance of the secretory endometrium, it begins to deteriorate and is ultimately shed during menstruation. With the drop in estradiol and progesterone, their negative feedback effects decrease, and FSH and LH rise to begin another cycle.

Pregnancy

If the oocyte is fertilized during its transit down the oviduct, it develops into a multicellular blastocyst by the time it reaches the uterus. Around the time of implantation (about 9 days after ovulation), and before the corpus luteum begins to regress, *increasing* amounts of an LH-like hormone, human chorionic gonadotropin (HCG), are found in maternal blood. HCG is synthesized and secreted by the trophoblast cells of the developing placenta. It is a dimeric protein hormone that has the same α-subunit as LH, FSH, and TSH, but a different β-subunit. The β-subunit of HCG is very similar to that of LH, but larger. Hence, HCG can interact with the LH receptors on luteal cells. This interaction prevents regression of the corpus luteum and allows it to continue synthesis and secretion of estradiol and progesterone, both of which are required for appropriate maintenance of the uterine endometrium throughout pregnancy.

II

Table 25–1 Changes in Reproductive Hormone Levels in Different Disease States

| Disease state | | Hormone level | | | |
Classification	Example	FSH	LH	Testosterone	Estradiol
Male					
Primary deficiency	Klinefelter's syndrome	High	High	Low	–
Secondary deficiency	Panhypopituitarism	Low	Low	Low	–
Primary excess	Testicular tumor	Low	Low	High	–
Secondary excess	Precocious puberty	High	High	High	–
Other	Seminiferous tubule failure	High	Normal	Normal	–
Other	Partial androgen insensitivity	Normal	High	High	–
Female					
Primary deficiency	Menopause	High	High	–	Low
Secondary deficiency	Sheehan's syndrome	Low	Low	–	Low
Primary excess	Feminizing ovarian tumor	Low	Low	–	High
Secondary excess	Gonadotropin-producing tumor (rare)	High	High	–	High
Other	Polycystic ovarian syndrome	Normal	High	High	–
Other	Masculinizing ovarian tumor	Low	Low	High	–

After Nickel KL: The gonads. *In* Kaplan LA, Pesce AJ (eds): Clinical Chemistry – Theory, Analysis, and Correlation, 3rd ed, St Louis, Mosby, 1996, pp. 892–911, with permission.

ejection, however, requires oxytocin, acting as part of a neuroendocrine reflex. This reflex is initiated by the suckling stimulus, which generates nerve impulses that travel from the nipple to the hypothalamus. There they cause secretion of oxytocin from neuroendocrine cells in the posterior pituitary. The oxytocin travels to the mammary gland, where it stimulates the contraction of smooth muscle cells surrounding the alveoli, causing milk ejection. Prolactin also participates in this neuroendocrine reflex, in that the nerve impulses reaching the hypothalamus also inhibit the synthesis and secretion of dopamine, which functions as a prolactin release-inhibiting hormone. This then promotes the release of prolactin from the anterior pituitary, which then also travels to the mammary gland, where it stimulates milk secretion, to replace that lost by ejection. As long as lactation continues, plasma prolactin concentrations remain elevated. This postpartum hyperprolactinemia causes postpartum amenorrhea due to interference with the normal regulation by GnRH of FSH and LH secretion. Although this hypogonadotropic state will prevent pregnancy, it is not considered a reliable means of contraception, particularly in modern societies where breastfeeding is variable.

Laboratory Evaluation of Reproductive Function

Table 25–1 describes laboratory findings in various male and female reproductive disease states typically categorized according to (1) hormone deficiency or excess and (2) primary (gonad) or secondary (pituitary) dysfunction. In primary disease states, gonadal steroid levels are inversely related to pituitary gonadotropin levels, whereas in secondary disease states, they are directly related (e.g. both high or both low). These changes occur because gonadal steroids provide negative feedback to gonadotropins. For example, in primary ovarian failure, the decrease in estradiol reduces its negative-feedback effect on the hypothalamic–pituitary axis, resulting in increases in FSH and LH.

Male Evaluation

The evaluation of reproductive dysfunction in the male usually begins with semen analysis, since it is a cost-effective and relatively simple procedure. In addition, if the results are normal, further evaluation is often unnecessary. If semen analysis is abnormal, then hormone analyses are performed.

Semen Analysis. In addition to its use in the evaluation of reproductive dysfunction, particularly infertility, semen analysis is also used to select donors for therapeutic insemination and to monitor the success of surgical procedures, such as varicocelectomy and vasectomy. Semen analysis consists of microscopic and macroscopic components, and the latter includes measuring physical (e.g. volume) and chemical (e.g. pH) properties. Useful guides and references for the procedure are available (Gilbert, 1992; Mortimer, 1994; Tomlinson, 1999; World Health Organization, 1999).

Sample Collection. The patient should be instructed to collect semen after 3 days of sexual abstinence. Longer periods of abstinence usually result in a higher semen volume but reduced sperm motility. In such a case, a second semen specimen may be collected 2 hours after the first sample. The bladder should be evacuated prior to ejaculation. For semen collection, the laboratory should provide a pre-weighed sterile plastic (polypropylene) container with a screw top. The semen specimen should be delivered to the laboratory within 1 hour of collection and kept warm during transportation. A post-ejaculate urine sample may be collected at this time if retrograde ejaculation is suspected. Two specimens collected within 2- to 3-week intervals should be used for evaluation, and if they are markedly different, additional specimens should be collected. Ideally, semen specimens should be collected in the privacy of a room adjacent to the laboratory, because some samples require sperm to be separated from seminal plasma as soon as possible. Assisted reproductive technologies (ARTs – see below), such as in vitro fertilization (IVF), require that motile sperm be isolated from seminal plasma within 1 hour of ejaculation to protect sperm from the inhibitory effects of seminal plasma on fertilization. Semen should be obtained by masturbation, and if circumstances preclude such collection, special Silastic condoms should be made available for semen collection with intercourse. Incomplete semen specimens should not be analyzed.

Macroscopic Examination should be performed after liquefaction, which usually occurs in less than 20 minutes at room temperature. Failure to liquefy may indicate inadequate prostate secretion. Semen should be thoroughly mixed before examination, and its viscosity recorded. The volume of ejaculate can be measured by weighing the collection cup before and after specimen collection. The appearance of a yellow hue in a semen specimen is associated with pyospermia, and a rust color with small bleedings in the seminal vesicle. The pH ranges from 7.2–7.8, but may be 8.0 or above due to acute infection in the prostate, seminal vesicle, or epididymis. The pH will be 7.0 or lower if there is contamination with urine, an obstruction in the ejaculatory ducts, or when the specimen consists of mainly prostatic fluid.

Microscopic Examination should be performed to obtain estimates of sperm concentration, motility, and agglutination. Other cellular elements such as polygonal cells of the urethral tract and 'round cells' such as spermatogenic cells and leukocytes can also be observed when sperm are counted in a hemocytometer. Since sperm motility and velocity are temperature dependent, these parameters must be assessed on a microscope with a warm stage. Typically, 8 μL of semen (of normal viscosity) placed under a 22 × 22-mm glass coverslip will yield a wet preparation that is 16.5 μm deep. Alternatively, 4 μL of sample added to disposable slides with two wells (used with thick glass coverslips) produces a 20-μm deep preparation. A hemocytometer or microchamber may be used for the sperm count. At least four different fields in each of the two specimen aliquots should be counted and the mean of the eight separate readings recorded. Total sperm count is then calculated by multiplying the dilution factor (normal concentration range 20–50 million/mL) by its volume (normal range 2–5 mL). Motility (normal range 50% or above) is expressed as the percentage of sperm that move. In addition, forward movement is graded. Sperm moving rapidly in a straight line with little yaw and lateral movement are Grade 4, or if they move more slowly, Grade 3. Grade 2 sperm move even more slowly and with substantial yaw. Grade 1 sperm have no forward progression. Zero progression denotes absence of any motility. If motility is less than 50%, a viability stain of eosin Y with nigrosin as a counterstain is done. In brightfield microscopy, dead sperm will stain red, whereas live sperm will exclude the dye and appear unstained. In samples with no visible sperm, such as post-vasectomy semen, the entire sample should be centrifuged, and the pellet examined for intact or damaged sperm fragments. The analysis should be repeated in 4–6 months.

Agglutination occurs when motile sperm stick to each other in an orientation that is reproducible within a given specimen, such as head to head, tail-to-tail, mid-piece to mid-piece, or mixed ways depending on the specificity of sperm antibodies. Agglutination suggests an immunologic cause of infertility and a description of the type of agglutination should be recorded. This can usually be distinguished from clumping due to bacterial infection or tissue debris, which typically involves nonspecific orientation of the sperm.

Round cells should be differentiated into two classes, immature germ cells with a single or double highly condensed nucleus with a relatively large area of cytoplasm; and polymorphonuclear leukocytes, which are smaller than the germ cells and have a lower nuclear/cytoplasmic ratio. Peroxidase staining specifically identifies the polymorphonuclear leukocytes in the presence of lymphocytes and other cells that normally occur in semen. Bacterial contamination should be noted, as should the presence or absence of epithelial cells. If no sperm are seen in association with a low semen volume, a fructose test should be performed to confirm the presence of fluid from the seminal vesicle, and the same test should be performed on post-ejaculate urine to rule out retrograde ejaculation. However, the significance of a fructose test result has declined over the years because of the availability of more direct diagnostic tools such as transrectal ultrasonography.

Sperm morphology can predict fertility (Ombelet, 1997). Typically, > 50% of the sperm in a semen specimen should exhibit normal morphology. Morphologically abnormal sperm usually have multiple defects, and the average number of defects per sperm, designated as the teratozoospermic index, is a significant predictor of sperm function both in vivo and in vitro. Wide variability in the size of the acrosomal cap is the most obvious characteristic of abnormal sperm. An acrosomal cap less than one-third of the head surface is considered abnormal, as are retention of a cytoplasmic droplet of more than half of the head size and a tail less than 45 μm long. Of particular note is the direct relationship between acrosome size and the frequency of fertilization or pregnancy. Computer-mediated morphology screening is particularly useful in samples with very low numbers of normal sperm where they may otherwise remain undetected.

Immunologic Tests. Sperm antibody binding to head or tail antigens is considered specific for immunologic infertility. The antibodies are usually of the IgA or IgG classes, and rarely IgM class; IgA antibodies are the most clinically significant. Current methods detect sperm-bound antibodies by direct or indirect mixed agglutination reaction (MAR) tests for IgG and IgA or by immunobead assay, which detects all classes but with varying sensitivity. Both tests require motile sperm. The direct MAR test can be performed on fresh semen and the result can be read within a few minutes with a light microscope. Semen is mixed with latex particles coated with nonspecific human IgG and then monospecific antisera to human IgG is added. The anti-IgG bridges the sperm-bound IgG, if present, and particle-bound IgG, to form mixed agglutinates. In the absence of sperm-bound IgG, the anti-IgG only agglutinates the latex particles. Under light microscopy the localized binding of the particles identifies the antibody as being specific to head, tail, or any other region of the sperm structure. An indirect test can also be done with this reagent to detect the presence of sperm antibody in semen, cervical mucus, or serum.

The immunobead assay can detect all three immunoglobulin classes when beads are coated with monospecific antisera to each class. Therefore, sperm are washed to remove all free immunoglobulin before the beads are added. An indirect assay can also be designed with this reagent. The test is best read under phase microscopy. Increased risk of men developing sperm antibody is associated with vasectomy, repeat infections, obstruction of the ducts, cryptorchidism, varicocele, testicular biopsy, trauma, torsion, cancer, and genetic predisposition (Gilbert, 1992). In women, sperm antibody is usually associated with intense mucosal inflammation of the genital tract.

Genital tract infections (Part VII – Medical Microbiology) may have significant adverse effects on male and female fertility. For example, *Escherichia coli* can cause sperm agglutination and immobilization, and the adherence of *E. coli* to sperm is mediated by mannose and mannose-binding cell surface structures present on both cell types (Wolff, 1993; Sarkar, 1974). Special precaution should be taken in collecting a semen specimen for bacteria or yeast detection, in order to eliminate the possibility of external sources of contamination. Seminal plasma cultures may help diagnose male accessory gland infection, particularly of the prostate. If the concentration of bacteria exceeds 1000 colony-forming units per milliliter, the colonies should be identified and tested for antibiotic sensitivity.

Accessory Glands. Seminal vesicle, prostate, and epididymis function can be evaluated by analyzing unique constituents of each. Prostate secretions, for example, are acidic and contain acid phosphatase. Seminal fluid that is more alkaline than normal (pH > 8.0) and has reduced acid phosphatase suggests prostate dysfunction. Fructose is a measure of seminal vesicle secretory function. In azoospermia caused by the congenital absence of vasa deferentia, a low fructose level may indicate an associated dysgenesis of the seminal vesicles. Ejaculatory duct obstruction, or agenesis of the vasa deferentia and seminal vesicles, may result in the production of semen with low volume, low pH, lack of coagulation, and absence of characteristic semen odor. Neutral α-glucosidase originates solely from the epididymis, and its measurement is of diagnostic value for distal ductal obstruction when considered with hormonal and testicular findings.

Image Analysis. Routine semen evaluation can be carried out by an automated image analysis system that uses sperm head movement to derive the magnitude of various swimming parameters. However, human sperm are extremely heterogeneous with respect to morphology, swimming characteristics, and sperm DNA content. Thus there is no reference to evaluate specimens as normal or abnormal, fertile or infertile. Hence, semen evaluation by manual methods performed by trained technical staff remains a standard practice of andrology laboratories.

Hormone Analysis. If multiple semen analyses demonstrate azoospermia (no sperm), oligospermia (< 20 million sperm per mL), or other abnormality, then hormone analyses are performed to help identify the specific dysfunction. An example of a diagnostic algorithm is shown in Figure 25–6.

Decreased testosterone accompanied by increased LH and FSH indicates primary testicular failure. This can be either an acquired or genetic disease (Klinefelter's syndrome). Decreased testosterone accompanied by decreased or inappropriately normal LH and FSH indicates hypothalamic–pituitary disease, resulting in secondary testicular failure. When LH and FSH levels are normal, secondary disease can be confirmed with an HCG stimulation test. HCG interacts with LH receptors, and in the male such interaction stimulates Leydig cells, if they are normal, to synthesize and secrete testosterone. Thus, administration of HCG should cause an increase in serum testosterone in secondary testicular failure, but not in primary testicular failure.

If hypothalamic–pituitary disease is suspected, then prolactin (PRL) should also be measured. Hyperprolactinemia interferes with the normal regulation of FSH and LH secretion by GnRH; and prolactinomas are the most common type of pituitary tumor. However, if prolactin is elevated, primary hypothyroidism must be excluded as a possible cause. In primary hypothyroidism, thyroid-stimulating hormone (TSH) and thyrotropin-releasing hormone (TRH) are elevated. Although the function of TRH is to stimulate the synthesis and secretion of TSH, TRH also stimulates the synthesis and secretion of prolactin. Thus, an elevated TSH suggests that primary hypothyroidism is the cause of the hyperprolactinemia, whereas a normal TSH suggests that a prolactinoma is the cause. If the latter were the case, then imaging techniques would be used to further evaluate the hypothalamic–pituitary axis.

If *normal testosterone*, LH, and FSH levels accompany oligospermia or azoospermia, then seminal fluid fructose should be evaluated. Its absence suggests the congenital absence of vasa deferentia and seminal vesicles. Its presence suggests either ductal obstruction or spermatogenic failure, which can be distinguished using testicular biopsy. Oligospermia accompanied by normal testosterone and LH with increased FSH suggests seminiferous tubule failure. The increase in FSH is likely due to reduced negative-feedback inhibition by decreased Sertoli cell inhibin. *Increased testosterone* and LH with normal FSH suggest either primary hyperthyroidism or partial androgen insensitivity, which can be distinguished by measuring TSH. In these conditions, the differential effect on LH and FSH is again likely due to the selective effect of inhibin on FSH.

In evaluation protocols such as that shown in Figure 25–6, it is becoming more common to measure not just total testosterone, but also free and/or bioavailable testosterone. The latter represents the sum of the free testosterone plus that bound weakly to albumin. The remaining testosterone is bound tightly to SHBG. Free or bioavailable testosterone

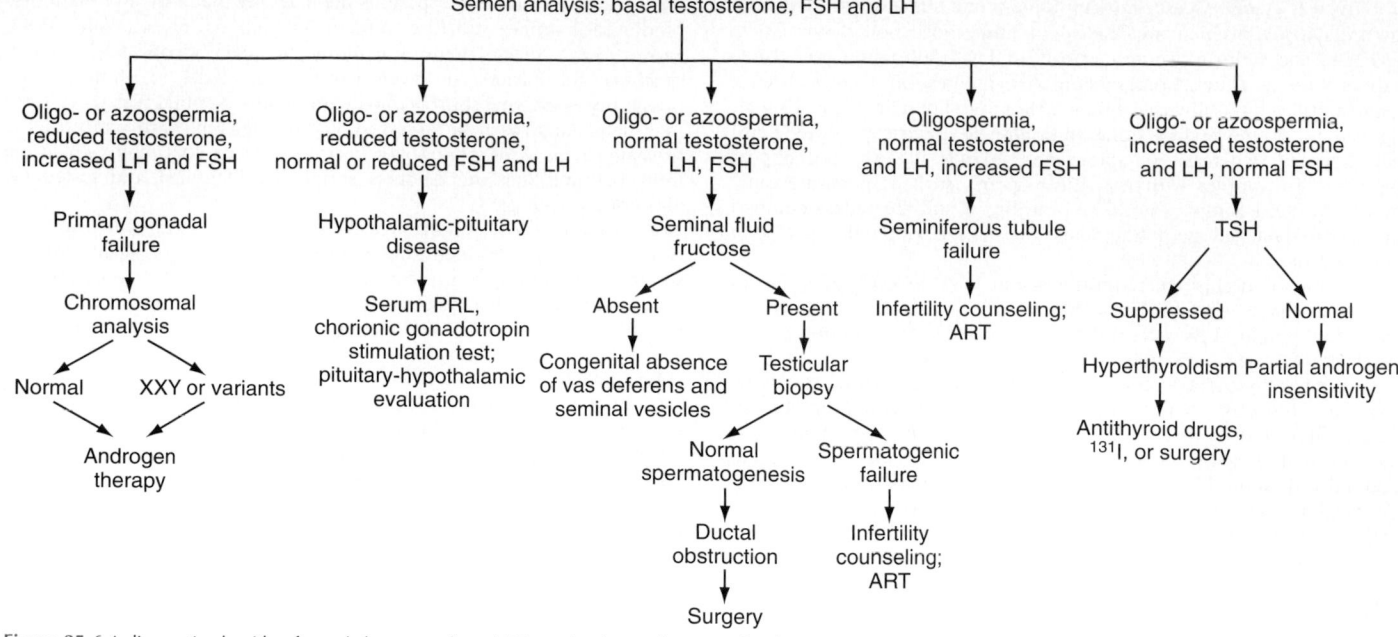

Figure 25-6 A diagnostic algorithm for male hypogonadism. ART = assisted reproductive technology; PRL = prolactin. (After Braunstein GD: Testes. *In* Greenspan FS, Gardner DG (eds): Basic and Clinical Endocrinology, 7th ed. New York, Lange Medical Books/McGraw-Hill, 2004, pp 478–510, with permission.)

more accurately represents the biologically active hormone in conditions where the concentration of SHBG is altered. For example, SHBG levels are increased with decreased testosterone, increased estrogen, hyperthyroidism, and liver disease; whereas they are decreased with increased testosterone, hypothyroidism, and acromegaly. Thus, if SHBG is high, total testosterone may be normal, but the free or bioavailable hormone may be low. Conversely, if SHBG is low, total testosterone may be normal, but free or bioavailable hormone may be high (Ismail, 1986). Methods for measuring total testosterone are readily available on automated immunoassay analyzers, but methods for measuring free and bioavailable testosterone are much more labor intensive. Consequently, free and bioavailable testosterone analyses are usually performed in a reference laboratory. The same considerations apply to testosterone measurements in females (see below).

Gynecomastia, or breast development in males, is thought to be due to a relative imbalance of androgen (decreased) and estrogen (increased) acting at the mammary gland. The decrease in androgen action can be due to either a concentration deficiency and/or a receptor deficiency (insensitivity). The condition is not uncommon during the neonatal and pubertal periods. A variety of other causes have been identified, including endocrine abnormalities, tumors, systemic diseases, and many drugs. Discontinuing or changing medications can exclude drug-induced disease, and liver or kidney disease can be identified through biochemical blood screens. Measuring serum testosterone, estradiol, LH, HCG, prolactin, and TSH can identify an endocrine abnormality or hormone-secreting tumor. Results from these tests together with imaging methods can help differentiate among the following as possible causes of gynecomastia: primary or secondary testicular failure, hyperthyroidism, androgen resistance, prolactinoma, testicular or extratesticular germ cell tumor, Leydig or Sertoli cell tumor, or adrenal tumor (Braunstein, 2004).

Female Evaluation

Amenorrhea can be defined as the absence of menstrual flow. In patients who have not exhibited menses by age 16, this is often due to a genetic and/or anatomic abnormality. In such cases, however, an endocrine abnormality is still a possible cause, and the presence or absence of secondary sexual characteristics (e.g. breast development) is an important indicator in the evaluation. An endocrine abnormality is a more likely cause in patients who have a history of menstruation, but who have not experienced menses for > 3 months. A stepwise approach to evaluating amenorrhea (Fig. 25–7) is based on measuring HCG, PRL, TSH, free thyroxine (FT_4), FSH, LH, and androgen levels and assessing estrogen status. *Step 1:* HCG is measured to exclude pregnancy. Although a result > 5 mIU/mL is typically indicative of pregnancy, an elevated result can also be obtained with trophoblastic disease or an HCG-secreting tumor. *Step 2:* PRL, TSH, and FT_4 are measured to exclude a prolactinoma and thyroid

disease. Increased prolactin accompanied by normal TSH and FT_4 results suggests a prolactinoma, which would be further evaluated by imaging techniques. Hyperprolactinemia, however, can also be caused by primary hypothyroidism, as indicated by high TSH and low FT_4 (see Male Evaluation). The mechanism by which increased prolactin causes amenorrhea is the same as that discussed previously for postpartum amenorrhea in females and for hypogonadism in males. Low TSH and FT_4 suggest secondary hypothyroidism, in which case the patient should be evaluated for panhypopituitarism, a deficiency of all anterior pituitary hormones. Hyperthyroidism (increased FT_4) can also be associated with amenorrhea. *Step 3:* If HCG, PRL, TSH, and FT_4 are all normal, then endogenous estrogen status is evaluated with the progestin withdrawal test. Progestin is administered either orally for 5–7 days or by one intramuscular injection (progestin dissolved in oil). The presence of withdrawal bleeding within 7 days after treatment indicates (1) that the outflow tract is intact and (2) that sufficient estrogen was present at the outset to stimulate endometrial growth. If withdrawal bleeding is absent, the genital tract should be evaluated using imaging techniques and, *Step 4,* serum FSH and LH levels should be determined. Elevated FSH and LH indicate primary ovarian failure, whereas low or inappropriately normal FSH and LH indicate secondary ovarian failure. The latter is of hypothalamic–pituitary origin and can result from a variety of clinical disorders, including Sheehan's syndrome, eating disorders, weight loss, and stress. If withdrawal bleeding is present, then, *Step 5,* serum androgens are measured. Elevated testosterone indicates either an ovarian tumor or polycystic ovarian syndrome (PCOS). The latter is a clinical entity often associated with enlarged ovaries and infertility, as well as amenorrhea. Increased DHEAS suggests an adrenal tumor. 17-OH progesterone is an androgen precursor (Fig. 25–1), and an increase in serum levels can indicate congenital or adult-onset adrenal hyperplasia, due to 21-hydroxylase deficiency. The above abnormalities may be accompanied by hirsutism, i.e. male pattern of hair growth in females. The tests in Step 5 can also be used to evaluate hirsutism when it is the primary clinical presentation.

Since amenorrhea or oligomenorrhea is often associated with infertility (Lobo, 1997), the latter can be evaluated by the same type of diagnostic algorithm as that shown in Figure 25–7. Infertility can occur, however, with apparently normal menstruation. This occurs with luteal phase deficiency, in which maturation of the secretory endometrium is delayed so that implantation of the blastocyst does not occur. In many cases, but not all, such an 'out-of-phase' endometrium can be demonstrated by histological evaluation of an endometrial biopsy from the late luteal phase. The mechanism for this condition is unknown, but may involve abnormal follicular development, ovulation, and/or luteal function, resulting in suboptimal synthesis and secretion of estradiol and/or progesterone. A variety of clinical causes have been identified, including certain medications, systemic disease states, and endocrine abnormalities.

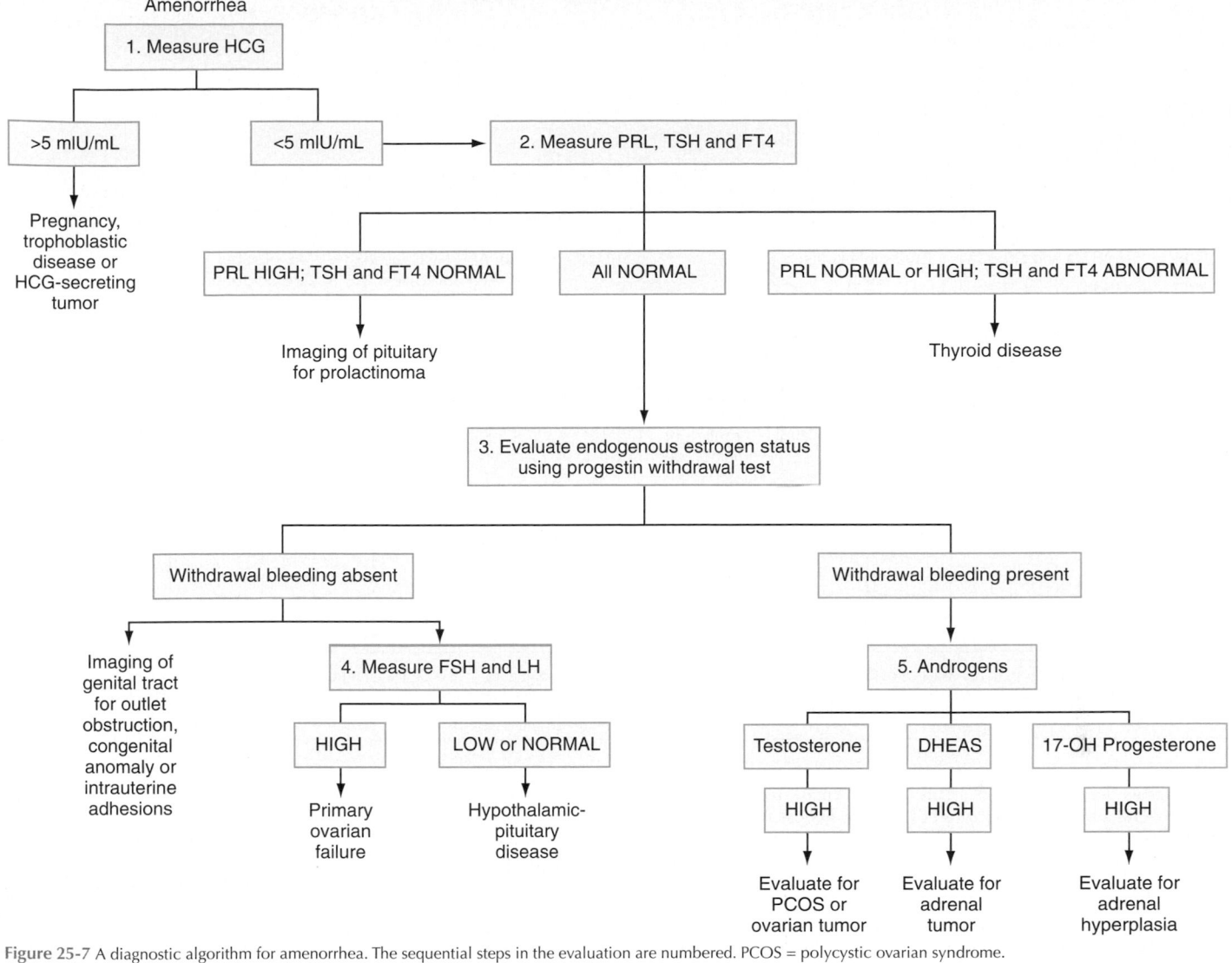

Figure 25-7 A diagnostic algorithm for amenorrhea. The sequential steps in the evaluation are numbered. PCOS = polycystic ovarian syndrome.

In addition to an 'out-of-phase' endometrial biopsy, diagnosis has been based upon either low serum progesterone during the luteal phase or a shortened luteal phase. The latter is determined by careful monitoring of basal body temperature during the menstrual cycle, since it increases with increasing progesterone and decreases with decreasing progesterone (Strauss, 2004).

Assisted Reproductive Technology (ART)

A couple is considered infertile if they fail to conceive after 6 months of unprotected intercourse. Initial treatments can include artificial insemination with washed and concentrated sperm and/or ovulation induction with clomiphene citrate. If these are unsuccessful, then one of several ARTs may be attempted. ARTs involve not only ovulation induction, but also oocyte retrieval and other manipulations that are performed to control as much of the reproductive process as possible in order to achieve pregnancy and bring it to term. Much of this external control requires significant monitoring utilizing laboratory analyses.

Indications for ART treatment include andrologic, immunologic, and idiopathic infertility, as well as tubal disease and endometriosis. It is not uncommon for several causes of infertility to be present in one couple. ART can also be applied in infertile couples requiring oocyte donation. The latter involves two distinct groups of patients: (1) females without gonadal function due to gonadal dysgenesis, premature menopause (which may occur spontaneously, or after surgical castration or castration induced by chemo- or radiotherapy) or resistant-ovary syndrome, and (2) women with functional ovaries but who do not wish to use their own oocytes to become pregnant because of the risk of transmitting chromosomal abnormalities to the offspring (e.g., if there is a history of autosomal dominant disease or X-linked disease, or when both partners are carriers of an autosomal recessive disease) (Van Steirteghem, 1992; Pados, 1994).

A typical ART protocol has three basic components: administration of medications, performance of clinical procedures, and monitoring (Trounson, 2000). Initially a GnRH analog (Lupron) may be given to suppress normal FSH and LH synthesis and secretion, although this is not always necessary. The next step is to stimulate follicular growth using a human menopausal gonadotropin (HMG) preparation, which will have either FSH and LH activity or predominantly FSH activity, depending on the specific material used. Unlike a normal reproductive cycle in which typically only one dominant follicle matures, in an ART cycle multiple follicles undergo growth and maturation. The number of follicles and their increase in size are monitored by regular ultrasound analysis. The function of the developing follicles is monitored by sequential serum estradiol measurements. When sufficient follicular maturation is achieved, based upon ultrasound and estradiol analyses, a bolus of HCG is administered. This HCG functions as a surrogate LH surge, and the HCG interacts with follicular LH receptors to initiate the process of ovulation. This process is not allowed to progress to completion. Ovulation would normally occur approximately 48 hours after HCG administration. Therefore, 12 hours prior to induced ovulation, the oocytes are 'retrieved' from the stimulated follicles. Each oocyte is then mixed with sperm. Depending on the type of ART used, the gametes are either transferred immediately to the fallopian tube or they are incubated together for up to 48 hours and the resulting zygotes or embryos are transferred to the fallopian tube or uterus.

Oocyte retrieval disrupts the follicles, as does normal ovulation, and as a consequence, estradiol levels drop immediately afterwards. As the follicles differentiate into corpora lutea, however, estradiol levels rebound and

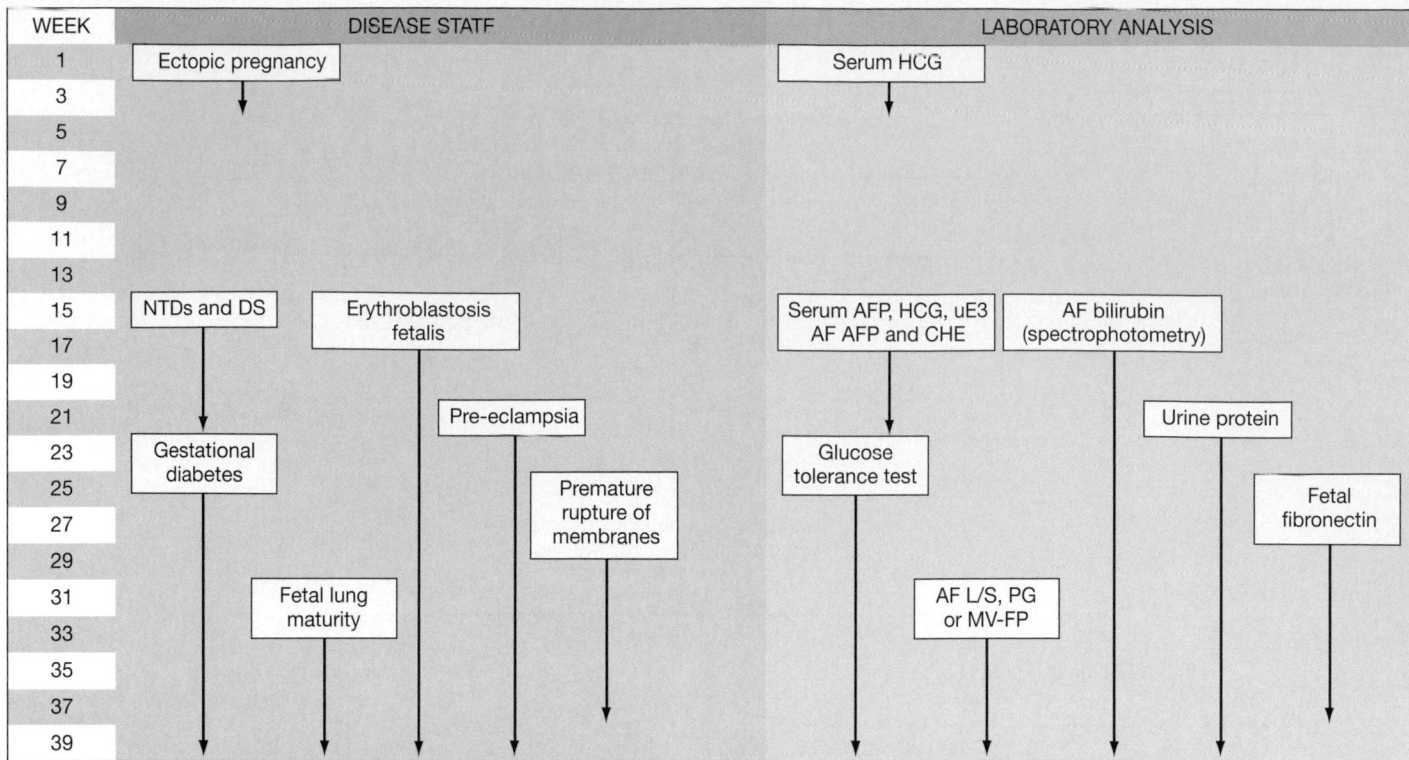

Figure 25-8 Approximate gestational weeks for laboratory evaluation of major disease states in pregnancy (when clinically indicated). AF = amniotic fluid; AFP = α-fetoprotein; AChE = acetylcholinesterase; DS = Down syndrome; HCG = human chorionic gonadotropin; L/S = lecithin/sphingomyelin ratio; MV-FP = microviscosity by fluorescence polarization; NTDs = neural tube defects; PG = phosphatidyl glycerol; uE3 = unconjugated estriol.

serum progesterone increases. This process may require 'boosting,' however, with additional injections of HCG (lower dose than that used for oocyte retrieval) and/or injections of progesterone. As in a normal cycle, estradiol plus progesterone are required to prepare the uterine endometrium for implantation. Therefore serum levels of the two steroids are monitored after transfer. Serum HCG measurements begin about 10 days after transfer to determine if pregnancy has been achieved. About 20 days after transfer, ultrasound examination can be used to confirm the presence of a gestational sac.

Laboratory Evaluation of Pregnancy

On a patient's first visit to an obstetrician, ideally early in the first trimester, a number of clinical laboratory tests are routinely ordered to identify disorders that can be treated or prevented (Willet, 1994). Simple, inexpensive blood and urine tests are carried out for anemia, red cell alloimmunization, and suspected viral or bacterial infections. Sometimes, the clinical history, physical examination, or test results indicate additional studies for genetic disease, disorders of coagulation or thrombosis, causes of spontaneous abortion, and other conditions. The laboratory procedures used routinely to monitor pregnancy are summarized in Figure 25–8.

HCG and Early Pregnancy

Elevated HCG in maternal serum and urine are both reliable indicators of pregnancy. Immunometric ('sandwich') assays are used for both. Currently most serum assays measure both the free β-subunit and intact HCG (α-plus β-subunit), utilizing two different antibodies directed at different epitopes on the β-subunit. These assays can quantify HCG as low as 1–2 mIU/mL. Typically, urine assays use one antibody directed at the β-subunit and the other directed at the α-subunit, allowing these assays to measure intact HCG and fragments that appear in urine. Serum HCG increases above the reference interval (typically 4–6 mIU/mL) by implantation, 6–12 (mean, 9.1) days after ovulation (Wilcox, 1999). Urine HCG levels are commonly measured by qualitative immunoassay test kits with detection limits of approximately 20 mIU/mL. These methods can detect elevated urine HCG 2–3 days later than the serum methods. Qualitative assays meant for home use have detection limits of

about 50 mIU/mL, and thus can detect elevated urine levels several days later, or shortly after the first missed menses.

Serum HCG increases dramatically during the first trimester, reaching a peak at about 10 weeks of gestation (Fig. 25–5). Throughout pregnancy, intact HCG is the predominant form present. However, a small quantity of free β-subunit is present in the first trimester. Free α-subunit appears in the second trimester and steadily increases in the last trimester (Ozturk, 1987).

If serum HCG levels continue to rise beyond 10 weeks, then a trophoblastic tumor should be considered. Other types of tumors, particularly germ cell tumors of the testes, also produce HCG. Tumor production often includes significant amounts of free β-subunit, in addition to intact HCG. The use of HCG as a tumor marker is discussed more fully in Chapter 75. Quantitative HCG results are indicated when a patient presents with early gestational vaginal bleeding or abdominal pain that may suggest the presence of ectopic pregnancy or spontaneous abortion. A simple protocol using only ultrasound and quantitative HCG examinations provides for more accurate diagnosis and sound management than clinical judgment alone (Koh, 1997). Since HCG concentrations rise quickly in early normal pregnancy, serial measurements can be used to ensure that there is an intrauterine implantation. A doubling of HCG in 2–3 days provides greater than 80% probability of intrauterine implantation of the fertilized ovum. When HCG concentrations exceed 1500–2000 μIU/mL, an intrauterine gestational sac becomes visible on ultrasound examination in a normal pregnancy. Absence of a sac or presence of an adnexal mass indicates a possible ectopic pregnancy. Furthermore, a failure to double the serum HCG suggests a loss of pregnancy.

Estradiol and progesterone measurements may provide additional information. Low serum progesterone (< 15 ng/mL) or estradiol (< 200 ng/mL) indicates a blighted ovum with 90% likelihood. If HCG is less than 1000 mIU/mL in a patient with vaginal bleeding, a progesterone concentration of less than 5 ng/mL is 94% predictive of an abnormal pregnancy.

Medical intervention using intramuscular methotrexate for unruptured ectopic pregnancy is less costly than surgery, may be a less complicated procedure, and may improve the patient's future fertility. Cases may be selected for methotrexate treatment by using ultrasound to ascertain a tubal implantation and differentiate it from an interstitial one for which methotrexate is not indicated. Ultrasound also ensures a small volume (< 3 cm) of conceptual tissue with absent fetal heart motion. A serum progesterone decrease to concentrations of less than 1.5 ng/mL may be a better predictor of resolution because HCG concentrations do not decline as rapidly after surgery (and may sometimes increase) (Saraj, 1998).

The laboratory can provide tests to help determine why an early pregnancy aborted spontaneously. For example, in recurrent abortion, the antiphospholipid syndrome may be identified by the presence of anticardiolipin and specific phospholipid antibodies in the first trimester. If termination occurs in the second trimester, a test for fetal cells in maternal blood may detect a large fetomaternal hemorrhage.

Neural Tube Defects

Screening for fetal structural defects using maternal serum biochemical markers has become routine obstetric practice. Screening programs were initiated to detect neural tube defects (NTDs) by finding increased α-fetoprotein (AFP) concentrations in maternal serum. Importantly, folic acid supplementation has been found to reduce the recurrence risk of NTDs by as much as 70% in women who have had a previously affected child (ACOG, 1993).

NTDs comprise some of the most common, severe congenital malformations (Botto, 1999). They occur when there is failure of the neural plate and its coverings to fuse properly by the 27th day after conception. Anencephaly involves absence of the calvarium, cranial vault, and cerebral hemispheres and is lethal before or shortly after birth. Spina bifida most commonly presents as a lumbar (or cervical) meningomyelocele, with herniation of meninges, spinal cord, and nerve roots. The severity of complications such as paralysis or muscle weakness, fecal and/or urinary incontinence, and intellectual impairment are at least partly dependent on the vertebral level and extent of spina bifida, which may be open (referring to whether the defect is completely uncovered or covered only by a very thin membrane) or closed (covered by skin or a thick membrane). Approximately 80% of spina bifida defects are open. The distinction is important, since maternal serum screening will detect *only* open defects.

The incidence of NTDs in the United States is 1–2 per 1000 pregnancies. The frequency in some populations (e.g., northern Ireland) is as high as 6–8 per 1000. Racial and ethnic backgrounds appear to influence the incidence. Caucasians in the US have an average occurrence of 1.6 per 1000 compared to African Americans with an incidence of 0.9 per 1000 (Myrianthopoulos, 1987).

NTDs are sporadic in 90% of cases and represent isolated defects with a multifactorial etiology, involving both genetic and nongenetic factors. However, there is an increased risk of recurrence in families. For example, when a couple has had one offspring with an NTD, the risk in each subsequent pregnancy for any type of NTD increases to approximately 1–3% (Toriello, 1983).

Although NTDs are typically isolated defects, it is important that a full evaluation of an affected fetus or infant be performed in order to rule out other disorders that may be associated with a different prognosis and/or different recurrence risk. Fetuses with certain chromosome anomalies may present with NTDs; a few single-gene disorders also produce NTDs. Acquired conditions, such as the amniotic band syndrome, may result in these defects but are not associated with increased recurrence risk. Teratogenic exposure, such as maternal valproate ingestion, is associated with increased risk for NTDs. Women with insulin-dependent diabetes mellitus (IDDM) also have a three- to fivefold increased risk for NTDs over the general population (ACOG, 1993).

NTD screening consists of measuring serum AFP concentrations in maternal blood, typically utilizing an immunoassay on an automated analyzer. AFP is the most abundant protein in fetal serum throughout fetal development. Liver AFP production is constant through approximately 30 weeks' gestation and then decreases. The AFP concentration in fetal serum is maximal at approximately 3 mg/mL by 12–14 weeks' gestation and declines throughout the rest of pregnancy. AFP levels continue to decline following birth, and by 1 year the serum AFP concentration is approximately 1 ng/mL, a level that persists throughout adult life. AFP diffuses across the amniotic membranes, producing a concentration in amniotic fluid (AF) that is approximately 100-fold less than in fetal serum. AFAFP peaks at 13–14 weeks and then decreases in the second trimester by about 10% per week. Small amounts of AFP are also transferred across the placenta from fetal serum and across the amniotic membranes from the AF to maternal serum (MS), where concentrations of AFP are nearly 1000-fold less than in AF. In the second trimester, when maternal screening is performed, MSAFP levels *increase* approximately 15% per gestational week. This MSAFP increase, while AF levels are decreasing, is due to combined changes in transfer to MS and maternal clearance (Ashwood, 1999).

The association of an increased MSAFP level with open fetal NTDs was first reported in 1974 (Brock, 1974). The AFP is elevated because fetal serum, from exposed neural membranes and blood vessels, leaks into AF. There is a subsequent transudation of AFP from AF to MS. Since AFP is exclusively fetal in origin, AFAFP can be used as a marker to detect NTDs. The increased AFP levels in AF are also reflected, although to a lesser extent, in MS. This measurable increase forms the basis of mid-trimester MSAFP screening for open NTDs (UK Collaborative Study, 1977).

MS screening is based on the comparison of serum AFP levels from pregnant women in the mid-trimester of pregnancy to median AFP values from women with normal fetuses at comparable gestational ages. These comparisons are subsequently expressed as multiples of the median (MoM). Median values are based on data from the reference population that is screened. Expressing patient results as MoMs normalizes the values, allows for direct comparison of results between laboratories, and avoids variation based on procedural differences.

Clinical factors that must be considered when calculating patient-specific results (Ashwood, 1999) include the following:

1. *Maternal weight:* MSAFP concentration decreases with increasing maternal weight. While the fetus itself produces a constant amount of AFP, the maternal blood volume will vary according to the weight of the mother. Failure to adjust for maternal weight causes increases in both the false-positive and false-negative results and affects the sensitivity and specificity of the test (Johnson, 1990a). Laboratories routinely adjust the MSAFP MoM for maternal weight. Similar mathematical corrections are also applied to HCG and unconjugated estriol MoM calculations for Down syndrome (see below).

2. *Race:* Although the reasons are not known, African American women have MSAFP values that are approximately 10–15% higher than Caucasian women (Johnson, 1990b). It is necessary to mathematically correct for this difference or to correct by comparing African American patients to normal median values generated from that reference population.

3. *Insulin-dependent diabetes mellitus (IDDM):* MSAFP levels in otherwise normal women with IDDM are approximately 20% lower than in the general population; therefore, the MoM values must be adjusted upward to adjust for this phenomenon. This is typically accomplished by multiplying the initial MoM value by a factor, using a mathematical constant to increase the initial MoM result.

4. *Multiple gestation:* Multiple gestation (e.g., twins) will yield higher MSAFP levels, since each fetus contributes its own AFP to the maternal blood. The MSAFP level is approximately proportional to the number of fetuses, and the effect can be factored into the laboratory calculation and interpretation of the results. Screening for fetal defects is not as reliable as for single pregnancies, since one cannot determine the individual AFP contributions of each fetus. Therefore, the NTD detection rate is lower for multiple pregnancies than for single ones. The same principle applies to MoM adjustments for HCG and unconjugated estriol when performing multiple marker analysis for Down syndrome (see below).

5. *Gestational age determination:* In order to establish a valid MoM value, a reliable estimate of gestational age is essential. The most common reason for abnormal MS screening results is incorrect estimation of gestational age. Typically, laboratories follow specific protocols based on the information obtained from the obstetric care provider in order to determine the most reliable gestational age. If pregnancy is initially dated using ultrasound, the sensitivity and specificity of screening is accurate (Wald, 1994); however, ultrasound information is frequently not available at the time of MS screening. Pregnancies with positive screening results that originally were dated by using the last menstrual period should have the gestational age verified by ultrasound. If the two estimated gestational ages differ by a defined amount (laboratory protocols vary, but usually by more than 9 days), then the results are recalculated based on the ultrasound results.

The goal of any maternal serum-screening program is to identify those women at sufficient risk for a fetal disorder to warrant further evaluation and follow-up. MSAFP levels are used as a major screening tool to identify those women considered at high risk for open NTDs. MSAFP values from pregnancies with open NTDs are increased (median value of 7 MoM with anencephaly and 4 MoM with open spina bifida). It is important to point out that MSAFP testing is a *screening* rather than a diagnostic tool and cannot discriminate all affected pregnancies from all unaffected pregnancies. Programs have been established, therefore, to identify individuals at sufficiently high risk to warrant further diagnostic evaluation.

A screening cutoff is established by choosing a MoM value that maximizes the detection rate for NTDs but maintains an acceptably low false-positive rate. Depending on the laboratory, cutoffs range from 2.0–2.5 MoM, such that the detection rate (sensitivity) for open spina bifida is 75–85% (much higher for anencephaly), while the false-positive rate ranges from 2–4%.

Although MSAFP screening programs were originally established to detect fetal NTDs, any open fetal defect that allows fetal serum to leak into surrounding AF or that increases protein loss in fetal urine may also result in elevated MSAFP levels. Open ventral wall defects (gastroschisis and omphalocele) may be detected by elevated AFP levels. Congenital nephrosis, an autosomal recessive disease, can present with very high MSAFP and AFAFP levels because of the abnormal fetal kidney function. Also, fetal skin anomalies may allow fetal serous fluid to leak into the AF and result in elevated MSAFP levels.

Placental abnormalities can result in elevated MSAFP levels, because of compromise in the fetomaternal membranes or placental structure. Elevated MSAFP levels that are not explained by a genetic or congenital problem are frequently associated with obstetric complications during pregnancy, including threatened abortion, low birth weight, pre-eclampsia, and oligohydramnios (Burton, 1988).

If MSAFP screening suggests an increased risk for a NTD, but ultrasound results are normal, a patient may elect to undergo amniocentesis. AFP can then be measured in AF. Due in part to the much higher concentration of AFP in AF than in MS (see above), AFAFP is a better predictor of NTDs. Laboratories that analyze AFAFP levels should also measure AF acetylcholinesterase (AChE) in any sample that has elevated AFP levels (> 2.0 MoM). As discussed in Chapter 20 on enzymology, AChE is an enzyme that is only derived from neural tissue and consequently present in very high concentration in cerebrospinal fluid (CSF). Therefore, it can be used as a sensitive and specific marker for open NTDs. In addition, it can discriminate NTDs from other fetal defects with increased AFP, and rule out false-positive AFP results.

Down Syndrome

MSAFP screening programs were initiated to identify pregnancies at increased risk for NTDs. Subsequently, an association was described between *low* MSAFP values and fetal Down syndrome (DS) (Merkatz, 1984). Using an MSAFP value and age to evaluate women at increased risk for having a fetus with DS, the detection rate is doubled when compared to maternal age screening alone, but this is not considered a sufficiently sensitive or specific screening protocol. Several other maternal serum markers have now been shown to demonstrate altered concentrations with fetal DS. The two analytes most frequently assayed in the second trimester in conjunction with MSAFP are unconjugated estriol (uE3) and HCG (Palomaki, 1997). Like MSAFP, uE3 levels in the second trimester are *decreased* in pregnancies with DS by a similar order of magnitude to that seen with MSAFP. HCG, in contrast, is *increased* in affected pregnancies. In fact, HCG is the single best discriminator of the three serum measurements in separating affected and unaffected pregnancies, with the median MoM level at approximately 2.0 in affected pregnancies. A patient-specific risk for DS may be calculated using all three markers (MSAFP, uE3, and HCG) in combination with maternal age (Ashwood, 1999). The detection rate (sensitivity) of this screening method is approximately 60%, with a false-positive rate of approximately 5% (Palomaki, 1996). Figure 25–9 outlines a protocol for simultaneous DS and NTD screening. More recently, inhibin A has been incorporated as a fourth marker in MS screening for DS by some laboratories. As occurs with HCG, inhibin A is *increased* in DS pregnancies. It is estimated that adding inhibin A analysis to the current three-marker protocol increases the detection rate of DS to nearly 75% with a 5% false-positive rate (Haddow, 1998).

Erythroblastosis Fetalis

Severe hemolytic disease in a fetus is marked by anemia accompanied by normoblastic hyperplasia (erythroblastosis), and may be followed by congestive heart failure (hydrops) and intrauterine death. The role of transfusion medicine in the management of immunized (sensitized) Rh_0-negative mothers is reviewed in Chapter 35.

Hemoglobin, released by hemolysis, is catabolized to unconjugated bilirubin. A fetus with hemolytic disease does not develop hyperbilirubinemia or become jaundiced, however, because the placenta normally removes the bilirubin. Concomitantly, some of the bilirubin appears in the AF, and monitoring the AF bilirubin concentration by spectrophotometry (Liley's test) provides a means of determining the degree and progression of hemolytic disease.

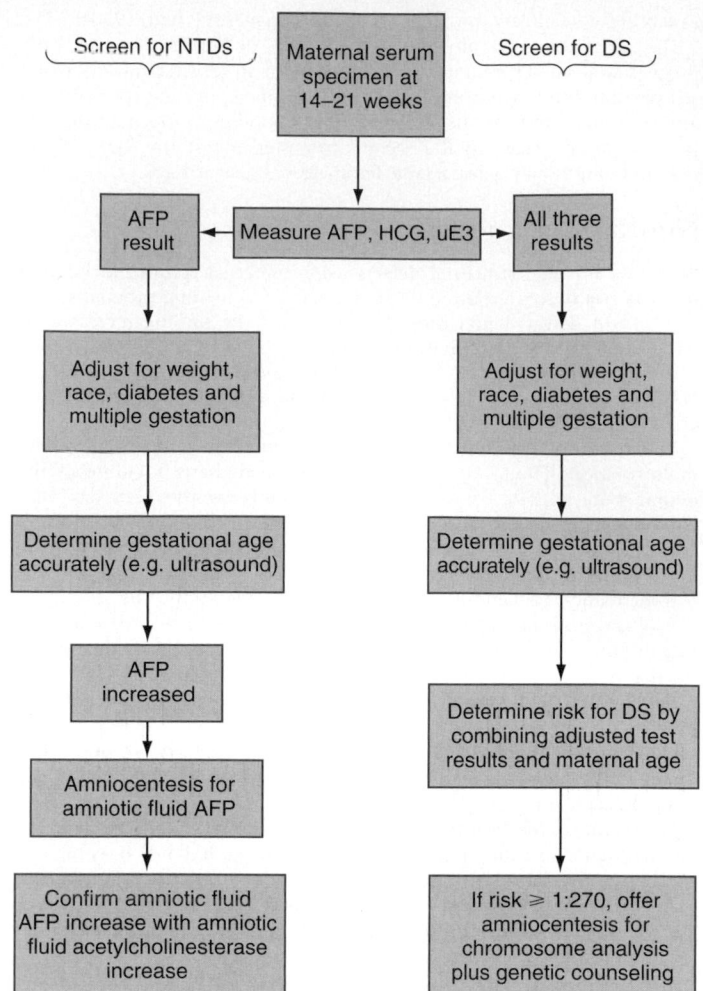

Figure 25-9 A diagnostic algorithm for the simultaneous screening of fetuses for neural tube defects (NTDs) and Down syndrome (DS).

Bilirubin absorbs light maximally at a wavelength of 450 nm and imparts a yellow color to AF. The latter is both maternal and fetal in origin so that pigmentation will not discriminate between a hemolytic process in the mother and one in the child. In erythroblastosis, severity of anemia (or hemolytic rate) correlates with the net absorbance of light at 450 nm. Bilirubin is bound to albumin, its concentration is dependent on the protein's turnover, and its concentration in AF does not change rapidly. If a previous pregnancy's outcome was fetal death from erythroblastosis, the AF from the current pregnancy should be initially sampled at about 10 weeks prior to the gestational week of the death of the prior fetus. Spectrophotometry of aspirated fluid is most accurate after 26–28 weeks. Prior to that time, mild fetal anemia may be monitored by antibody titers or, possibly, by the maximal flow velocity of the umbilical vein as shown by ultrasound (Iskaros, 1998). Severe anemia can be detected by determining peak systolic blood velocity in the middle cerebral artery (Mari, 2000).

A specimen of AF (5 mL) is collected, protected from light, and centrifuged or filtered. Light absorbance of the fluid is plotted continuously between wavelengths 350 nm and 700 nm. The resulting spectrophotometric curve can be used to (1) determine whether or not the fluid contains bilirubin and/or other pigmented products of hemolysis, and (2) quantify the bilirubin pigment that is present.

The initial curve may plot wavelength (abscissa) against total absorbance (ordinate) on linear coordinates. The 'actual' absorbance at 450 nm is observed from the original (linear) plot. The pigment curve is then transformed to a straight line by transferring the two absorbance values observed at 365 nm and 550 nm to semilog scale graph paper (the y-axis is logarithmic). These two points are well above and below the 450 nm absorbance peak of bilirubin pigment so that a straight line drawn between them represents the background absorbance of the unpigmented fluid itself. The 'expected' absorbance at 450 nm is then recorded from the straight line drawn on the log plot. The difference between actual and expected absorbance values is the calculated 'net' absorbance at 450 nm.

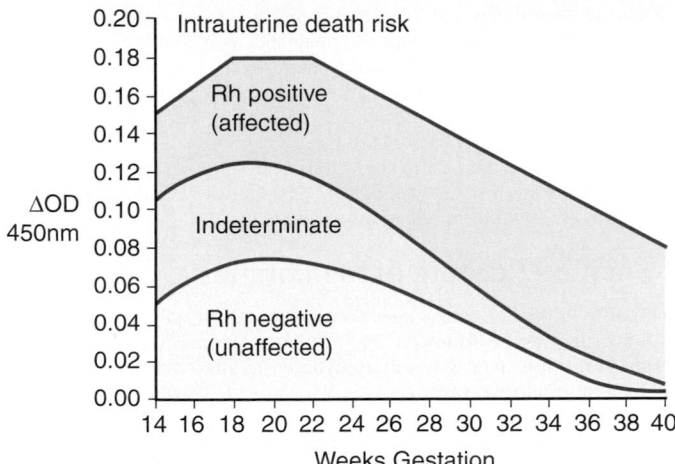

Figure 25-10 Graph for interpretation of net absorbance at 450 nm of amniotic fluid. Four zones are indicative of relative level of fetal hemolytic disease. (From Queenan JT, Tomai TP, Ural SH, et al: Deviation in amniotic fluid optical density (OD) at a wavelength of 450 nm in Rh-immunized pregnancies from 14–40 weeks' gestation: A proposal for clinical management. Am J Obstet Gynecol 168:1370 1376, 1993, with permission.)

This value is then corrected for hemoglobin interference, since hemoglobin also absorbs at 450 nm. To compute the correction for hemoglobin, the absorbance of the specimen at 410 nm (at which wavelength hemoglobin but not bilirubin absorbs) is determined. The 'expected' 410-nm absorbance is subtracted from this value. The absorbance of hemoglobin at 450 nm is 5% of its absorbance at 410 nm; thus the net hemoglobin absorbance value at 410 nm is then multiplied by 0.05 and is subtracted from the net 450 nm absorbance. The net absorbance is recorded on a Liley graph, which denotes weeks of gestation on the linear abscissa and net absorbance on the log scale ordinate (Ashwood, 1999).

Net absorbance at 450 nm decreases as the duration of an unaffected pregnancy increases after 28 weeks. (Prior to 26 weeks, background absorbance is relatively constant.) Decreasing absorbance reflects fluid dilution by fetal urine and accounts for the negative slopes of lines demarcating Liley's prediction zones (lower = zone 1, mid = zone 2, upper = zone 3) for mild, moderate, and severe hemolysis, respectively. The greater is the net absorbance at 450 nm, the greater is the hemolysis. Although Liley's method originally applied only to the third trimester of pregnancy, data have been presented showing use of the technique can be extended through the second trimester (Queenan, 1993), when AF specimens may also be obtained for evaluation of NTDs and/or DS (Figure 25–10).

Serial testing (every 14 days or less) is common practice and allows one to trend net absorbance values. High and increasing values may indicate the need for more frequent AF analyses, early delivery, or cordocentesis with fetal hematocrit determination and, if necessary, intrauterine transfusion (Queenan, 1993). Trends are usually unidirectional, either paralleling the negatively sloped lines on Liley's graph or showing a positive slope. The slopes of trend lines may change in some cases, sometimes dramatically. For example, when early net absorbance values are in the midzone, net absorbance may increase sharply if hemolysis worsens. After 30 weeks' gestation, the Liley test result is usually combined with an assessment of fetal lung maturity: amniotic pigment and surfactant analyses both assist with the clinical decision of whether or not to induce delivery (see below).

Liley test results must be interpreted by an experienced physician who can integrate clinical findings, history, blood bank information, and other laboratory data. Maternal and fetal acid–base imbalances can alter AF pH and shift the wavelengths of pigment absorbance maxima. Pigments that may be present other than bilirubin (as discussed above), methemalbumin, and meconium. Each produces a characteristic spectrophotometric effect. Blood contamination (with interference by hemolysis) is encountered frequently. Less often, in vivo maternal jaundice or hemolysis can cause misinterpretation. The presence of fetal red cells in AF indicates worsening of anemia by blood loss, or may explain a rise in maternal antibody titer (anamnestic response to a new fetomaternal hemorrhage), development of new antibodies, and subsequent increase in the net absorbance of AF at 450 nm. Meconium staining of AF is a sign of fetal distress. Exposure of AF to light, maternal use of steroids, markedly increased AF hemoglobin concentration, and

poor calibration of a spectrophotometer may each cause inaccurate net absorbance measurements.

Attempts at amniocentesis occasionally result in an aspirate that is not AF. Fetal ascites, the AF of a twin, amniotic cyst contents, and (most commonly) maternal urine may be mistakenly submitted as AF. A spectrophotometric tracing of maternal urine is similar to a curve of normal AF, except that the curve is of greater negative slope. Maternal urine contains urea nitrogen in a concentration of about 300 mg/dL and creatinine of greater than 10 mg/dL. In AF, urea nitrogen concentration is usually about 30 mg/dL and creatinine is less than 3.5 mg/dL. Precautionary creatinine or urea nitrogen measurements of AF can be carried out to distinguish AF from urine. Use of dipsticks to detect protein and glucose in AF are less useful because either material may be present in both AF and urine of pregnant women. It should be noted that the presence of fetal hemoglobin can interfere with many creatinine methods.

Blood is visibly evident even when diluted by AF a thousandfold (v : v). Bloody taps occur in 2–3% of early amniocentesis aspirates and 20% in late ones. The presence of blood may interfere with tests for net absorbance, surfactant, and others. Sometimes the blood is of fetal origin, raising the possibilities of subsequent fetal anemia and primary or anamnestic alloimmunization.

Gestational Diabetes

Any glucose intolerance in a pregnant woman is termed gestational diabetes (see Ch. 16), regardless of the state of glucose tolerance antepartum or postpartum. The prompt diagnosis and treatment of gestational diabetes may help to avoid maternal pre-eclampsia as well as fetal death after 32 weeks and neonatal macrosomia (abnormally large body size), hypoglycemia, polycythemia, or jaundice.

Fetal Lung Maturity

Fetal lung maturation is marked by production of a detergent-like material, surfactant, which forms a film on the alveolar surfaces. The presence of surfactant reduces surface tension at the lung's tissue–air interface. Surfactant decreases the work of breathing by reducing resistance to lung expansion during inspiration and preventing alveolar collapse during expiration. Deficiency of surfactant produces respiratory distress syndrome (RDS), a disorder that results in hypoxia, acidemia, and vascular protein transudation into alveolar air spaces (hyaline membrane disease).

Prior to 35 weeks' gestation, the major component of surfactant is α-palmitic β-myristic lecithin. After that time, dipalmitic lecithin predominates and phosphatidyl glycerol (PG) appears about a week later. PG increases until term and maintains alveolar stability. Minor phospholipid components of surfactant include phosphatidyl inositol, phosphatidyl ethanolamine, phosphatidyl serine, and sphingomyelins.

The lung maturation process occurs rapidly (1–2 days). Since sphingomyelin (S) concentration in AF is constant during the third trimester, it serves as a reference material against which surfactant lecithin (L) can be compared. Measurement of an L/S ratio (see below) avoids problems associated with variability in chemical extraction and inaccuracy in estimates of absolute concentration per AF volume.

Although exogenous surfactant is available for prophylaxis and therapy in newborn RDS, the disease may be avoidable in some cases by delaying delivery until fetal lungs have matured or by medicating the mother to induce production of surfactant in her fetus. Fetal surfactant production may be evaluated using tests of AF samples. Prior to delivery, fetal respiratory motions cause surfactant to diffuse from the unexpanded lungs through the fluid-containing bronchial tree and into the amniotic space. AF surfactant can be monitored during the third trimester. Surfactant analysis is important in managing the disorders associated with RDS: preterm labor, premature rupture of membranes, maternal diabetes, chronic maternal hypertension, fetal growth retardation, alloimmune hemolytic disease, and early delivery by cesarean section.

Surfactant in AF may be measured by either physical or chemical means. The great number of procedures available suggests that none is ideal in predicting RDS or its absence. A method's clinical usefulness is related to simplicity, availability over 24 hours, turnaround time, low cost, and clinical accuracy. The reference method remains the L/S ratio, which is determined by thin-layer chromatography, but microviscosity tests (fluorescence polarization) provide inexpensive, accurate, and popular methods. A bedside 'click' test, in which microscopic observations of surfactant-induced rhythmic changes in bubble size, has been advocated (Osborn, 1998).

The L/S ratio test was the first practical chemical test to assess fetal pulmonary status (Gluck, 1971) and remains the reference test. Commercial kits are available for L/S determinations. Following extraction and purification with solvents, AF surfactant lipids are chromatographed on thin-layer silica (see Chs 4 and 23 on principles of instrumentation and toxicology and therapeutic drug monitoring, respectively). The phospholipids are made visible by heat charring or staining. Densitometric quantification determines the L/S ratio. L/S ratios > 2.0 usually indicate maturity; ratios of 1.5–2.0 borderline maturity: and ratios < 1.5 immaturity. Sensitivities and specificities ranging between 80–85% have been reported for the test. Some believe the test is unsatisfactory in diabetic women, in whose neonates RDS can occur when L/S ratios are greater than 2.0 (Dubin, 1992). The presence of phosphatidyl glycerol on the thin-layer chromatogram of an L/S ratio > 2.0 indicates fetal pulmonary maturity with virtual certainty in any patient.

The L/S ratio test method is slow, labor intense, and insensitive, and pre-analytical variables affect accuracy. One variable is dilution by fluid secretions (e.g., when AF is aspirated from the vagina instead of by amniocentesis). Analytical error results from overcentrifugation (speed and time), blood contamination (hemolysis), and the imprecision of thin-layer chromatography. Meconium interferes because it can prevent clear separation of lecithin and sphingomyelin.

Rapid tests for PG have been developed because chromatography is cumbersome and often unavailable when needed (e.g., nights, weekends). A rapid latex agglutination method for PG is available and can screen for pulmonary maturity. If immature or equivocal results are observed, the chromatographic method is indicated (Ashwood, 1992). Glycerol contamination (lubricant) may interfere with PG analyses.

Microviscosity of AF correlates with the reference L/S ratio test results in clinical studies and can be measured by fluorescence polarization. A fluorescent dye is mixed with AF, in which the dye interacts with both surfactant and albumin. The greater the concentration of surfactant, relative to a constant concentration of albumin, the lower the viscosity. The degree of fluorescence polarization is inversely related to surfactant concentration and its lower viscosity. The method may give erroneous results for concentrated AF specimens (e.g., in fetal urinary tract obstruction) and for specimens containing visible amounts of blood. AF samples are prepared by filtration to avoid loss of surfactant caused by centrifugation. An automated fluorescence polarization commercial assay instrument (Abbott Laboratories, Abbott Park, IL) is used widely, is rapid, and appears accurate in most clinical situations (Bender, 1994).

Toxemia of Pregnancy (Pre-eclampsia)

Pre-eclampsia is a late-gestational disease (> 20 weeks) characterized by hypertension with proteinuria of greater than 0.3 g/L in a 24-hour urine specimen or greater than 1.0 g/L in a random specimen. Pre-eclampsia affects about 1 in 10 pregnant women and is more frequent in first pregnancies, diabetics, multiple gestations, and women who have experienced it in previous pregnancies.

Pre-eclampsia may be preventable by oral administration of salicylates or calcium, but laboratory monitoring, other than urinalysis, is usually not required in mild disease. Severe or convulsive disease (eclampsia) requires active intervention and monitoring.

Toxemia of pregnancy can mimic other disorders including hypertension, renal or hepatic disease, systemic lupus erythematosus, idiopathic thrombocytopenic purpura, microangiopathic anemias, and especially thrombotic thrombocytopenic purpura. The latter rarely presents late in pregnancy but, unlike pre-eclampsia, it persists after delivery.

The proteinuria of toxemia is of a glomerular type (mostly albumin) and the urine sediment contains hyaline and finely granular casts. It does not contain bacteria, red cells, or waxy or broad casts. The urine protein is monitored to determine the progress or control of the illness. Creatinine clearance is decreased to less than 130 mL/min (see Ch. 14).

The blood usually shows thrombocytopenia and a relative erythrocytosis because plasma volume does not increase, as it should in normal gestation. There are mild-to-moderate increases in urea (> 15 mg/dL) and creatinine (> 0.8 mg/dL) and a marked increase in uric acid. Lactate dehydrogenase (LD) is increased primarily because of hepatic disease (mostly LD_5). Sometimes because of hemolysis (e.g., in the HELLP syndrome – *h*emolysis, *e*levated *l*iver enzymes and *l*ow *p*latelets), there is increased LD_1 and LD_2. Alanine aminotransferase is usually twice normal, bilirubin is mildly increased (> 1.2 mg/dL), and the D-dimer is increased. Urine calcium excretion may be decreased (< 12 mg/dL/24 h) and this finding may precede clinical toxemia.

Delivery terminates toxemia so that labor may be therapeutically induced if disease is severe and the pregnancy is beyond 36 weeks, or if there is evidence of fetal pulmonary maturity (see above). Prior to 36 weeks, the pre-eclamptic patient is treated by bed rest. Hepatic and renal function tests are usually monitored daily along with platelet counts, blood smears, and quantitative D-dimer.

Worsening pre-eclampsia is characterized by oliguria (< 400 mL/24 h), severe thrombocytopenia (platelets < 50 000/μL), increasing serum creatinine, and total LD of greater than 1000 U/L.

Premature Rupture of Membranes

Premature rupture of membranes occurs when AF escapes before the onset of labor. It may be followed by a variety of complications including chorioamnionitis, fetal pulmonary hypoplasia, placental abruption, and neonatal respiratory distress.

AF constitutes part of the posterior vaginal fluid pool and identification of the amniotic component is optimally carried out within 2 hours of membrane rupture. Unlike vaginal secretions whose pH is acidic (pH of 4.5–5.5), AF is alkaline with pH of 7.0–7.5. The vaginal pool aspirate of a gravida with watery discharge can be tested with nitrazine paper to estimate pH visually. A positive test is indicated by a blue color and a negative one by a yellow-green color. The cervical plug must not contaminate the aspirate. There are 5% false positives related to presence of blood, mucus, semen, alkaline urine, or soap. False negatives are less likely (1%), but may be seen with membrane rupture that occurred more than 24 hours earlier or if sampling was inadequate. The nitrazine test is usually performed at the bedside and is said to have an overall accuracy of about 90% in the absence of bloody show, vaginal discharge, or prolonged membrane rupture (Friedman, 1969).

An aliquot of the aspirated fluid can also be applied to a glass microscope slide, dried for 5 minutes and examined microscopically for a 'fern' pattern, which indicates the presence of AF in the vaginal fluid pool. False-positive ferning occurs in less than 2% of cases and is associated with the presence of blood, urine, or cervical mucus. False-negatives occur in less than 5%.

Fetal fibronectin is a chorionic trophoblast protein that normally accumulates in the virtual space between the placenta and the uterine decidua. If fetal fibronectin is increased in maternal plasma or AF or cervicovaginal secretions between 22–34 weeks' gestation, it denotes loss of integrity of the fetal membranes as a result of infection, pre-eclampsia, or premature rupture. False positives (< 5%) may be related to recent sexual intercourse.

When membranes are intact, but there is an increase in fetal fibronectin in vaginal fluid (> 0.05 μg/mL), premature labor is likely (Ascarelli, 1997). In such cases, there is a 25-fold increase in relative risk of delivery within 7 days among women with symptoms of preterm labor between 24–34 weeks' gestation. The fibronectin test appears to have value in singleton and twin pregnancies, but not in prolonged (> 42 weeks) pregnancies. An immunoassay for fetal fibronectin is commercially available (Adeza Biomedical Corp., Sunnyvale, CA).

Fetal Asphyxia

Although newborns are not usually adversely affected by acidosis until blood pH is less than 7.10, an acidemia with pH less than 7.20 has been used as an obstetric action limit to prevent hypoxic neurologic damage. At delivery, fetal blood pH is determined in a capillary blood sample collected from the skin of the presenting part (e.g., scalp). Blood collection is often difficult and samples may be rejected by the laboratory because of insufficient volume, contamination with air bubbles, and clotting. Repeated sampling is usual and offers the advantages of demonstrating a trend in values and of detecting some spurious results. Maternal acid–base imbalance can affect fetal blood pH and cause misinterpretation. The technical problems, low predictive value for neurologic damage, and low compliance with practice guidelines (Skelton, 1997) have raised doubts about the value of fetal scalp pH measurements.

In routine deliveries, a segment of clamped umbilical cord may be removed and stored until the neonatal condition is assessed at 5 minutes. If the infant appears clinically stable and vigorous, and the Apgar score is 'satisfactory', the cord sample is discarded. If there is a clinical reason for obtaining blood gas analyses, an umbilical artery (the vein, if necessary) may be sampled and submitted for analysis (ACOG Committee, 1994). The benefit of blood gas measurement is that a base deficit can be determined so that respiratory and metabolic components of acidosis can be assessed.

Other Evaluations

Infections During Pregnancy. Viral, bacterial, and parasitic infections can have a significant impact on the mother, fetus, or both. Important examples are human immunodeficiency virus (HIV), hepatitis virus (A, B, and C), rubella virus, varicella virus, parvovirus B19, cytomegalovirus (CMV), *Chlamydia trachomatis*, group B streptococcus (GBS), *Neisseria gonorrhoeae*, syphilis, tuberculosis, toxoplasmosis, and malaria. These are discussed in Part VII.

Hematological and Coagulation Disorders. Various disorders can have a negative effect on the mother, fetus, or both, including maternal anemias (nutritional, sickle cell), maternal and fetal thrombocytopenias (idiopathic thrombocytopenic purpura, fetal alloimmune thrombocytopenia, thrombotic thrombocytopenic purpura), maternal coagulopathies (acute disseminated intravascular coagulation, von Willebrand's disease), and maternal thrombophilias. These are described in Parts IV and V.

References

American College of Obstetrics and Gynecology: Committee Opinion No. 120: Folic Acid for the Prevention of Recurrent Neural Tube Defects. Washington, DC, ACOG, 1993.

American College of Obstetrics and Gynecology: Committee Opinion No. 138: Utility of Umbilical Cord Blood Acid–Base Assessment. Washington, DC, ACOG, 1994.

Ascarelli MH, Morrison JC: Use of fetal fibronectin in clinical practice. Obstet Gynecol Surv 1997; 52:S1–S12.

Ashwood E: Evaluating health and maturation of the unborn; the role of the clinical laboratory. Clin Chem 1992; 38:1529.

Ashwood ER: Clinical chemistry of pregnancy. *In* Burtis CA, Ashwood ER (eds): Tietz Textbook of Clinical Chemistry, 3rd ed. Philadelphia, WB Saunders, 1999.

Includes detailed descriptions of (1) calculation of risk for neural tube defects and Down syndrome from maternal serum screening results and (2) amniotic fluid spectrophotometry of bilirubin for erythroblastosis fetalis (Liley's test).

Bender TM, Stone LR, Amenta JS: Diagnostic power of lecithin/sphingomyelin ratio and fluorescence polarization assays for respiratory distress syndrome compared by relative operating characteristic curves. Clin Chem 1994; 40:541.

Botto LD, Moore CA, Khoury MJ, et al: Neural-tube defects. N Engl J Med 1999; 241:1509–1518.

Braunstein GD: Testes. In Greenspan FS, Gardner DG (eds): Basic and Clinical Endocrinology, 7th ed. New York, Lange Medical Books/McGraw-Hill, 2004, pp 478–510.

Brock DJ, Bolton AE, Scringeour RA: Prenatal diagnosis of spina bifida and anencephaly through maternal plasma α-fetoprotein. Lancet 1974; i:767–769.

Burton BK: Outcome of pregnancy in patients with unexplained elevated or low levels of maternal serum α-fetoprotein. Obstet Gynecol 1988; 72:709–713.

Carr BR, Rehman KS: Fertilization, implantation, and endocrinology of pregnancy. *In* Griffin JE, Ojeda SR (eds): Textbook of Endocrine Physiology, 5th ed. New York, Oxford University Press, 2004, pp 249–273.

Dubin S: Assessment of fetal lung maturity by laboratory methods. Clin Lab Med 1992; 12:603.

Friedman ML, McElin TW: Diagnosis of ruptured fetal membranes: Clinical study and review of the literature. Am J Obstet Gynecol 1969; 104:544–550.

Gilbert BR, Cooper GW, Goldstein M: Semen analysis in the evaluation of male factor subfertility. AUA Update Series 1992; 11:250–255.

Gluck L, Kulovich MV, Borer R, et al: Diagnosis of the respiratory distress syndrome by amniocentesis. Am J Obstet Gynecol 1971; 109:440–445.

Haddow JE, Palomaki GE, Knight GJ, et al: Second trimester screening for Down's syndrome using maternal serum dimeric inhibin A. J Med Screen 1998; 5:115–119.

Iskaros J, Kingdom J, Morrison JJ, et al: Prospective non-invasive monitoring of pregnancies complicated by red cell alloimmunization. Ultrasound Obstet Gynecol 1998; 11: 432–437.

Ismail AA, Astley P, Burr WA, et al: The role of testosterone measurement in the investigation of androgen disorders. Ann Clin Biochem 1986; 23:113–134.

Johnson AM, Palomaki GE, Haddow JE: The effect of adjusting maternal serum α-fetoprotein levels for maternal weight in pregnancies with fetal open spina bifida. A United States Collaborative Study. Am J Obstet Gynecol 1990a; 163:9–11.

Johnson AM, Palomaki GE, Haddow JE: Maternal serum α-fetoprotein levels in pregnancies among black and white women with fetal open spina bifida. A United States Collaborative Study. Am J Obstet Gynecol 1990b; 162:328–331.

Koh GH, Yeo GS: Diagnosis of ectopic pregnancy – why we need a protocol. Singapore Med J 1997; 38:369–374.

Lobo RA, Mishell DR, Paulson RJ, et al: (eds): Mishell's Textbook of Infertility, Contraception, and Reproductive Endocrinology, 4th ed. Malden, MA, Blackwell Science, 1997.

General reference for clinical evaluation of reproductive function in the female.

Mari G: Noninvasive diagnosis by Doppler ultrasonography of fetal anemia due to maternal red-cell alloimmunization. N Engl J Med 2000; 342:9–14.

Merkatz IR, Nitowsky HM, Macri JN, et al: An association between low maternal serum α-fetoprotein and fetal chromosomal abnormalities. Am J Obstet Gynecol 1984; 148:886–894.

Mesiano S, Jaffe RB: The endocrinology of human pregnancy and fetal-placental neuroendocrine development. *In* Strauss JF, Barbieri RL (eds): Yen and Jaffe's Reproductive Endocrinology, 5th ed. Philadelphia, Elsevier Saunders, 2004, pp 327–366.

Mortimer D: Practical Laboratory Andrology. New York, Oxford University Press, 1994.

Descriptive guide and reference for clinical evaluation of reproductive function in the male.

Myrianthopoulos NC, Melnick M: Studies in neural tube defects. 1. Epidemiology and etiologic aspects. Am J Med Genet 1987; 26:783–796.

Norwitz ER: Endocrine diseases of pregnancy. *In* Strauss JF, Barbieri RL (eds): Yen and Jaffe's Reproductive Endocrinology, 5th ed. Philadelphia, Elsevier Saunders, 2004, pp 735–785.

Ombelet W, Bosmans E, Janssen M, et al: Semen parameters in a fertile versus subfertile population: A need for a change in the interpretation of semen testing. Hum Reprod 1997; 12:987–993.

Osborn DA, Lockley C, Jeffery HE, et al: Interobserver reliability of the click test: A rapid bedside test to determine surfactant function. J Paediatr Child Health 1998; 34:544–547.

Ozturk M, Bellet D, Manil L, et al: Physiological studies of human chorionic gonadotropin (hCG), αhCG, and βhCG as measured by specific monoclonal immunoradiometric assays. Endocrinology 1987; 120:549–558.

Pados G, Camus M, Van Steirteghem A: The evolution and outcome of pregnancies from oocyte donation. Hum Reprod 1994; 9:538–542.

Palomaki GE, Knight GJ, McCarthy JE, et al: Maternal serum screening for Down's syndrome in the United States: A 1995 survey. Am J Obstet Gynecol 1997; 176:1046–1051.

Palomaki GE, Never LM, Haddow JE: Can reliable Down's syndrome detection rates be determined from prenatal screening intervention trials? J Med Screen 1996; 3:12–17.

Queenan JT, Tomai TP, Ural SH, et al: Deviation in amniotic fluid optical density at a wavelength of 450 nm in Rh-immunized pregnancies from 14–40 weeks gestation: A proposal for clinical management. Am J Obstet Gynecol 1993; 168:1370–1376.

Resnik R, Killam AP, Battaglia FC, et al: The stimulation of uterine blood flow by various estrogens. Endocrinology 1974; 94:1192.

Saraj AJ, Wilcox JH, Najmabadi S, et al: Resolution of hormonal markers of ectopic gestation: A randomized trial comparing single-dose intramuscular methotrexate with salpingostomy. Obstet Gynecol 1998; 92:989–994.

Sarkar S, Jones OW, Shioura N: Constancy in human sperm DNA content. Proc Natl Acad Sci USA 1974; 71:3512–3516.

Sideri M, De Virgiliis G, Guidobono F, et al: Immunologically undetectable human placental lactogen in a normal pregnancy. Br J Obstet Gynaecol 1983; 90:771.

Skelton AK, Madan MP, Thompson WD, et al: Utilization patterns of cord blood gas analysis. Obstet Gynecol 1997; 90:538–541.

Strauss JF, Barbieri RL (eds): Yen and Jaffe's Reproductive Endocrinology, 5th ed. Philadelphia, Elsevier Saunders, 2004.

Comprehensive reference for all aspects of reproductive function and pregnancy.

Strauss JF, Lessey BA: The structure, function, and evaluation of the female reproductive tract. *In* Strauss JF, Barbieri RL (eds): Yen and Jaffe's Reproductive Endocrinology, 5th ed. Philadelphia, Elsevier Saunders, 2004, pp 255–305.

Tomlinson MJ, Effrossini K, Barratt CR: The diagnostic and prognostic value of traditional semen parameters. J Androl 1999; 20: 588–593.

Toriello HV, Higgins JV: Occurrence of neural tube defects among first-, second-, and third-degree relatives of probands: Results of a United States study. Am J Med Genet 1983; 15:601–606.

Trounson AO, Gardner DK: Handbook of In Vitro Fertilization, 2nd ed. Boca Raton, CRC Press, 2000.

General reference for assisted reproductive technologies (ARTs).

UK Collaborative Study on α-Fetoprotein in Relation to Neural Tube Defects. Maternal serum α-fetoprotein measurement in antenatal screening for anencephaly and spina bifida in early pregnancy. Lancet 1977; i:1323–1332.

Van Steirteghem AC, Pados G, Devroey P: Oocyte donation for genetic indications. Reprod Fertil Dev 1992; 4:681–688.

Wald NJ, Kennard A, Smith D: First trimester biochemical screening for Down's syndrome. Ann Med 1994; 26:23–29.

Welt CK, McNicholl DJ, Taylor AE, et al: Female reproductive aging is marked by decreased secretion of dimeric inhibin. J Clin Endocrinol Metab 1999; 84:105–111.

Wilcox A, Baird DD, Weinberg CR: Time of implantation of the conceptus and loss of pregnancy. N Engl J Med 1999; 340: 1796–1799.

II

Willett GD (ed): Laboratory Testing in Ob/Gyn. Boston, Blackwell Scientific Publications, 1994.
Comprehensive and concise summary of laboratory evaluation of the female.

Wolff H, Panhans A, Stolz W, et al: Adherence of *Escherichia coli* to sperm: A mannose mediated phenomenon leading to agglutination of sperm and *E. coli*. Fertil Steril 1993; 60:154–158.

World Health Organization: WHO Laboratory Manual for the Examination of Human Semen and Sperm Cervical Mucus Interaction. London, Cambridge University Press, 1999.

CHAPTER 26
Vitamins and Trace Elements

Martin J. Salwen MD

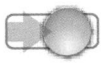

KEY POINTS

- Very small amounts of vitamins and trace elements are needed to satisfy metabolic requirements.

- Vitamins are essential organic substances that the body cannot synthesize, or does not sufficiently synthesize. This is species specific. Vitamins may function variously as enzymatic cofactors, antioxidants, or like hormones, and are active in energy metabolism, protein metabolism, blood cell maturation, and bone formation. Vitamins are unrelated chemically and have different physiological activities and food sources.

- Vitamins may be single chemicals (e.g., ascorbic acid), or include a family of closely related compounds (e.g., vitamins A, D, E, K, and cobalamine). They may be classified according to water or lipid solubility which affects absorption and transport, storage, toxicity, excretion, and the disease conditions that cause deficiencies even when there is sufficient nutritional intake.

- To assess both dietary intake and body stores requires different test strategies for diagnosis of deficiency or toxicity. Deficiencies are especially important at the age extremes of life and in malnutrition of whatever cause. Often, a therapeutic trial of the nutrient considered deficient is the most reliable approach to diagnosis and treatment.

- Essential trace elements have specific metabolic functions that cannot be replaced by other minerals.

- Deficiencies of trace elements may result from insufficient ingestion because: soil, water, or plants in the region are inadequate in a specific element; other dietary substances interfere with absorption; protein needed for absorption or metabolism is lacking; or there is inadequate supplementation in a patient receiving total parenteral nutrition.

- Trace elements have structural, signal transduction, and catalytic functions. Some are components of metalloenzymes, or function as enzyme cofactors, provide electron and oxygen transport, or are active in the maintenance of macromolecule conformation.

- To avoid contamination, trace elements must be analyzed with considerable care since they are widely distributed in the environment and are present, in very minute concentration, in body fluids and tissues. Thus, techniques must be sensitive enough to analyze concentrations of μg/L or even ng/L.

- Trace element concentrations in body fluids correlate poorly with the amount in body stores. Serum levels are unreliable because of the influence of unrelated conditions. There are no particularly good assays for trace element dietary status. Test results need be interpreted with caution.

- The only definitive test of human trace element deficiency is assessment of the clinical response to controlled supplementation with the element considered deficient.

- The intake required to cause toxicity is very variable for the different trace elements.

Vitamins and trace elements are a collection of heterogeneous dietary ingredients necessary for health and survival. They are collectively described as micronutrients because of the very small amounts required to satisfy their diverse physiological roles, and their functions are as varied as their compositions (Mason, 1996). The almost two dozen essential nutrients are unrelated organic catalysts and elements that are not endogenously synthesized (Rubin, 2005). Deficiency and toxicity states are often insidious for both, and may be attributable to an inappropriate intake or to defective utilization. Deficiencies are most often due to malnutrition (McLaren, 1994). Initially the interest was in the prevention of deficiency diseases and elucidation of the biochemical roles of these micronutrients as coenzymes and cofactors. Research in the assessment of vitamin and trace element nutriture has further identified their many other important functions such as antioxidant activity, hormone-like stimulation and their regulatory roles (Machlin, 1992).

Dietary reference intake (DRI) is an umbrella term that includes reference values or estimates of the dietary level of each essential nutrient. DRI was introduced by the Food and Nutrition Board, Institute of Medicine of the National Academy of Sciences (Institute of Medicine, 1997, 1998, 2000, 2002) and provides four dietary reference values, primarily intended for nutritionists (Barr, 2002). *Recommended dietary allowance* (RDA) is the average daily dietary amount sufficient for the nutrient requirements of most (97–98%) healthy people categorized by age, gender, and physiological need. The RDA is derived from the *estimated average requirement* (EAR), the average daily nutrient intake level estimated to meet the requirements of half the healthy individuals in a particular life stage and gender group. The *adequate intake* (AI) is an estimate of average recommended daily intake value when the RDA cannot be determined. The *tolerable upper intake level* (UL) is the highest level of daily nutrient intake that is likely to pose no risk of adverse health effects for almost all individuals in the general population (Institute of Medicine, 1998). As intake increases above the UL, the potential risk of adverse effects increases.

Micronutrients have been invested with a magical aura. There is a widespread misguided belief that 'megadoses' can provide that cure-all elixir. Perhaps this is an awareness of the extraordinary physiological prowess of minute quantities of these ingestants. However, they also pose a hazard. Although safe within the tolerable upper intake level (UL) (Institute of Medicine, 1998), there is the risk of toxic overdose.

Several groups of people warrant selective micronutrient supplementation. These include: pregnant women, neonates and infants; the aged; patients receiving long-term parenteral nutrition or hyperalimentation; and those with altered nutritional or metabolic states. Poverty and food faddism are continued causes of deficiencies. For the general population, with only rare exceptions, vitamin and trace element supplementation is not required and is unnecessary and even wasteful, because of their ubiquitous distribution and ready availability from a variety of sources.

This section will review the micronutrients that include vitamins and the essential trace mineral elements. The 13 vitamins are outlined in Table 26–1, with their functions and deficient and toxic states summarized, and the 10 essential trace mineral elements are similarly presented in Table 26–4, with their functions and the effects of deficiency and toxicity summarized.

Table 26–1 Vitamins: Functions, Deficiency Syndromes, and Toxicity

Vitamins	Functions	Deficiency syndromes	Toxicity
Water soluble			
Ascorbate (vitamin C)	Many redox reactions, hydroxylation of collagen	Scurvy	Chronic megadoses of 10–150 times the RDA (1–15 g), cramps, diarrhea, nausea, kidney stones. Megadoses, body accelerates the drug metabolism. Can produce scurvy if megadoses abruptly stop
Biotin	Cofactor in carboxylation reactions	Rare. Caused by lack of biotin in total parenteral nutrition. Also, avidin in raw egg whites binds biotin in gut, preventing absorption. Dermatitis, glossitis, hair loss, anorexia, depression, and hypercholesterolemia	No known toxicity
Cobalamine (vitamin B_{12})	Folate metabolism and DNA synthesis, maintenance of myelinization of spinal tracts	Megaloblastic anemia, peripheral neuropathy	No appreciable toxicity
Folate	Transfer and use 1-carbon units in DNA and amino acid synthesis	Megaloblastic anemia, neural tube defects	Teratogenic effect in rodent model. No adverse effects at high oral doses
Niacin (nicotinic acid)	Incorporated into NAD and NAD phosphate, redox reactions	Pellegra: dementia, dermatitis, diarrhea	Excess preformed niacin and nicotinic acid cause vascular dilation, 'flushing'; hepatotoxic
Thiamine (vitamin B_1)	As pyrophosphate, is coenzyme in decarboxylation reactions	Dry (neuromuscular) and wet (cardiac failure) beriberi, Wernicke–Korsakoff syndrome	Only when given parenterally. Headache, muscle weakness, cardiac arrhythmia, convulsions
Pantothenic acid (vitamin B_3)	Incorporated in coenzyme A	No syndrome recognized	Very high doses: diarrhea
Pyridoxine (vitamin B_6)	Derivatives are coenzymes in many intermediary reactions; amino acid, phospholipid and glycogen metabolism	Chelosis, glossitis, dermatitis, peripheral neuropathy, convulsions	Long-term megadose supplementation causes ataxia, and sensory neuropathy. The UL is 100 mg/day
Riboflavin (vitamin B_2)	Converted to flavin coenzymes, cofactor for many enzymes in intermediary metabolism	Ariboflavinosis, cheilosis, angular stomatitis, glossitis, dermatitis, corneal vascularization	Toxicity to riboflavin has not been reported. Absorption limited normally
Fat soluble			
Vitamin A (retinol)	A component of retinal rod pigment. Role in vision in dim light, growth; reproduction; maintenance of resistance to infection	Squamous metaplasia, especially glandular, follicular hyperkeratosis; xerophthalmia; night blindness; reproductive disorders; vulnerability to infection	Livers of polar bears and large animals have very high levels of vitamin A Acute: can cause drowsiness, headache, vomiting, stupor, skin pealing, and papilledema Chronic: teratogenic, osteoporosis, hepatotoxicity Carotenoids in excess: distinct orange-yellow skin color
Vitamin D (cholecalciferol)	Promotes absorption of calcium and phosphorus; mineralization of bones and teeth	Rickets in children; osteomalacia in adults Hypocalcemia, tetany	High intake of vitamin D: hypercalcemia and hypercalciuria, toxicity above UL of 50 µg. Bone demineralization, constipation, muscle weakness, renal calculi
Vitamin E (tocopherol)	Antioxidant, scavenges free radicals; cellular respiration, primarily in muscle, RBC integrity	Spinocerebellar degeneration, ataxia	Mild GI distress, nausea; coagulopathies in patients receiving anticonvulsants
Vitamin K (phytomenadione)	Cofactor of procoagulants – hepatic factors II (prothrombin), VII and X, protein C and protein S	Defective clotting, bleeding disorder	Foods containing vitamin K cause no toxicity problems. Excess amounts of vitamin K may decrease clotting time

Data from Berdanier, 1998; Combs, 1998; Eastwood, 2003; Grodner, 2004; Kane, 2005; Katz, 2001.

Vitamins

Vitamins are organic molecules that are required in microgram to milligram amounts for health, growth, and reproduction (McCormick, 1994). Except for vitamin D, the body depends completely on the dietary intake for vitamins, although there is some enteric bacterial production of vitamin K, nicotinic acid, riboflavin, biotin, cobalamine, and folic acid (Eastwood, 2003; Grodner, 2004). However, these syntheses occur mostly in the colon and are not nutritionally significant since the vitamins produced are poorly absorbed. The lack of each vitamin results in a clearly definable metabolic deficit. This is species specific, since there are differences in the synthesizing capabilities of different species. Many lower animals can produce their own ascorbic acid. Humans, however, cannot synthesize ascorbic acid, for example, and require ascorbate to prevent scurvy (Combs, 1998).

Vitamins may be classified according to their properties, such as function, nutritional source, or their solubility in water. See Table 26–1: *Vitamins: Functions, Deficiency Syndromes, and Toxicity*. In this discussion, vitamins are divided into two groups based on solubility. Solubility affects the absorption and transport. Water-soluble vitamins are easily absorbed, which allows for minimal storage. However, deficiencies can develop quickly, within weeks (Grodner, 2004). Thiamine, riboflavin, niacin, pyridoxine, cobalamine, vitamin C, folate, pantothenic acid, and biotin are water soluble. Vitamins A, D, E, and K are considered water insoluble or fat soluble, and depend upon normal lipid digestion and micellar solubilization for absorption, such as the presence of bile. Malabsorption of fat may result in deficiencies of the fat-soluble vitamins despite an adequate dietary intake.

Vitamins are in almost all foods, but no one food group is a good source for all vitamins (Grodner, 2004). See Table 26–2: 'Vitamins: RDA, Food

Table 26–2 Vitamins: RDA, Food Sources, and Analysis of Body Levels

Vitamins	RDA	Food sources	Laboratory assessment for subclinical deficiency states:
Water soluble			
Ascorbic acid (vitamin C)	M: 90 mg F: 75 mg Smokers: 125 mg	Fruits and vegetables: citrus fruits, red and green peppers, strawberries, tomatoes, broccoli, potatoes, green leafy vegetables	Fasting specimen required. S-ascorbic acid; deficiency < 11.4 µmol/L. WBC-ascorbic acid by HPLC, reflects tissue stores. Preparation and assay difficult. < 11.4 nmol/10^8 cells associated with scurvy; 24-h U-ascorbic acid; reflects recent dietary intake Vitamin C load test U
Biotin	AI: 30 µg	Liver, kidneys, peanut butter, egg yolks, yeast	Microbiological assay
Cobalamine (vitamin B_{12})	M/F: 2.4 µg	Meat, fish, poultry, eggs, and dairy products	S-vitamin B_{12} by RIA: deficiency < 74–59 pmol/L U-methylmalonic acid

Folate	M/F:400 µg
	Pregnancy: 600 µg
	Lactation: 500 µg
		Leafy green vegetables, legumes, cereals, some fruits and juices	Hemolysis interferes: RBC-folate; S-folate
			S-methyltetrahydrofolate reflects recent intake, not stores. Cutoff point, negative folate balance < 6.8 nmol/L
			Polyglutamate forms of folate present reflect body folate stores.
			Folate (nmol/L):
			   depleted < 368
			   deficient < 322
			   anemia < 227
			U-formiminoglutamic acid (FIGLU)
			Histidine load test U

Niacin (nicotinic acid)	Niacin equivalent (NE) = 1 mg niacin or 60 mg tryptophan M: 16 mg NE/day F: 14 mg NE/day	Protein-containing foods are good sources for both niacin and tryptophan. Meats, poultry, fish, legumes, enriched cereals, milk, coffee and tea	Ratio of RBC-nicotinamide adenine dinucleotide (NAD) and NADP nucleotide: < 1 may indicate risk of niacin deficiency Ratio of 2-pyridone (40–60%) and N′-methyl nicotinamide (20–30%): deficiency of niacin when ratio < 1
Pantothenic acid	AI 5 mg	Whole grain cereals, legumes, meat, fish, poultry	Whole blood-pantothenic acid: inadequate intake <100 µg/dL 24-h U-pantothenic acid: abnormally low < 1 mg/day

Pyridoxine (vitamin B_6)	M/F: 1.3 mg	Whole grains, cereals, legumes, chicken, fish, pork, and eggs	P-pyridoxal-5′-phosphate, cation exchange HPLC, assay by fluorometry.
			B_6 status:
			   > 30 nmol/L adequate
			   ≥ 0.8 acceptable
			   < 0.5 marginal or inadequate
			RBC-aminotransferases, reflect long-term pyridoxine status; ALT more sensitive to B_6 deficiency than AST
			U-4-pyridoxic acid, dietary intake of B_6
			U-xanthenuric acid, tryptophan metabolite
			Tryptophan load test U

Riboflavin (vitamin B_2)	M: 1.3 mg F: 1.1 mg Riboflavin destroyed by light	Milk, enriched grains, broccoli, asparagus, dark leafy greens, whole grains, enriched breads, cereals. Also dairy products, meats, fish, poultry, and eggs	RBC-glutathione reductase, expressed as ratio of assays with and without flavin adenine dinucleotide 24-h U-riboflavin measures recent intake, not body stores, nonspecific; varies with physical activity
Thiamine (vitamin B_1)	M: 1.2 mg F: 1.1 mg	Whole or enriched grains, flour, lean pork, legumes, seeds and nuts	RBC-transketolase activity, expressed as ratio of assays with and without thiamine pyrophosphate 24-h U-thiamine measures recent dietary intake, not body stores
Fat soluble			
Vitamin A (retinol)	Retinol activity equivalents = RAE M: 900 µg RAE F: 700 µg RAE	Natural preformed vitamin A only in fat of animal-related foods: whole milk, butter, liver, egg yolks, and fatty fish. Carotenoids are found in deep green, yellow, and orange fruits and vegetables: broccoli, cantaloupe, sweet potato, carrots, tomatoes, spinach	Hemolysis interferes Liver retinol stores: S-retinol, insensitive test Dose response: S-retinol and dehydroretinol by HPLC 4–6 h after oral 3,4-didehydroretinyl acetate (100 µg/kg); more sensitive index of marginal retinol status than S-retinol Relative dose response (RDR): retinol-binding protein (RBP), index of retinol, low specificity. In Vitamin A deficiency RBP accumulates in liver as apo-RBP (RBP not bound to retinol). After retinol dose, retinol binds to apo-RBP in liver; holo-RBP (RBP bound to retinol) released from liver causing increased S-retinol. Blood sample at baseline and 5 h after oral vitamin A. Calculate RDR (%): > 14–20%, marginal vitamin A status S-carotenoids indicate current intake of carotenoids Rapid dark adaptation (RDA) for night blindness

Vitamin D	AI M/F: 5 µg
	Ages:
	51–70 years 10 µg
	> 70 years 15 µg
		Butter, egg yolks, liver, and fatty fish. Vitamin D-fortified milk Sunlight exposure converts precursor to active vitamin D	S-25-hydroxy vitamin D:
			   deficiency < 3 nmol/L
			   toxicity: > 500 nmol/L
			separate S-25(OH)-D by HPLC, assay by CPBA, indicates total endogenous and exogenous vitamin D, reflects vitamin D content of liver

II

Table 26–2 Vitamins: RDA, Food Sources, and Analysis of Body Levels (*cont'd*)

Vitamins	RDA	Food sources	Laboratory assessment for subclinical deficiency states
Vitamin E (tocopherol)	α-Tocopherol equivalents = a-TE M/F: 15 mg a-TE	Vegetable oils, corn, soy, safflower. Whole grains, seeds, nuts, wheat germ, green leafy vegetables	Ratio S-tocopherol to S-lipids: reverse phase HPLC with high-sensitivity fluorescence detector; levels correlate with S-cholesterol; deficiency when ratio < 0.6 mg total tocopherol/g serum lipids
Vitamin K	AI M: 120 μg F: 90 μg	Vitamin K synthesized by bacteria in jejunum and ileum; dietary intake is still required. Dark green leafy vegetables	Prothrombin time

M = male; F = female; P = plasma; RBC = red blood cell (erythrocyte): S = serum; U = urine; WBC = white blood cell (leukocyte); HPLC; high-performance liquid chromatography; CPBP competitive protein binding assay.

Data from Grodner, 2004; Gibson, 2002; Brewster, 1996; McCormick, 1994.

Sources, and Analysis of Body Levels'. The vitamin B complex includes: thiamine, riboflavin, niacin, pyridoxine, and cobalamine. Cobalamine is only present in animal products, which include meat, especially liver, milk, cheese, eggs, and other animal proteins. All of the other members of the vitamin B complex are found in leafy green vegetables, milk, and liver. Vitamin A and niacin have precursor substances that can be converted to the active vitamin form in humans. Vitamin K and biotin are produced by the gut microflora, but in insufficient quantities to sustain metabolism. Niacin and vitamin D can be made in the human body. Both thiamine and biotin have natural antagonists (Williams, 2002).

Deficiencies are particularly important at the extremes of life and are a concern for the developing fetus and infant, and for the aged (Seymour, 2000). Deficiencies are also frequent for those with protein–energy malnutrition in developing nations. In developed countries, the conditions resulting in vitamin deficiencies include decreased intake, absorption, or production. Decreased intake characteristically occurs in patients suffering from alcoholism (thiamine); small bowel disease (folate and the fat-soluble vitamins, A, D, E, and K); vegans (vitamin D, cobalamine); and the elderly (vitamin D, folate). Conditions resulting in decreased absorption are liver and biliary tract disease (vitamins A, D, E, K); and ileal disease or resection (cobalamine). Conditions causing decreased production are renal disease (vitamin D); and drugs such as methotrexate (folate). Deficiencies also occur in those with long-term chronic disease such as acquired immunodeficiency syndrome (AIDS). The assessment of body stores and the chronic nutritional state for the micronutrients continues to present difficulties. Tests often indicate only the recent nutritional intake. A therapeutic trial of the nutrient considered deficient is often the easiest and most reliable approach. Specific diagnostic strategies are helpful (Feldman, 1994; Gibson, 2002). See Table 26–2.

Toxicity rarely results from excessive dietary intake. Toxicity is usually due to overdoses of vitamin supplements. Single large doses of the water-soluble vitamins are rarely toxic, because they are rapidly excreted, but repeated doses can cause toxicity. Vitamin A has a toxic potential greater than that for the other hypervitaminoses, although the actual incidence is low. Intakes as low as 25 times the RDA are considered potentially toxic for vitamin A. Carotenoids have a low toxicity. Vitamin D is the other vitamin with a relatively high potential for toxicity. Intakes of about 50 times the RDA have been reported as toxic in humans. Children have been particularly sensitive when large doses of vitamin D were used for prophylaxis or treatment of rickets, and hypervitaminosis D has been exacerbated by high intakes of calcium and phosphorus (Combs, 1998).

Water-Soluble Vitamins

Thiamine (Vitamin B₁). Thiamine pyrophosphate (TPP) is an essential cofactor of enzymes involved in carbohydrate and amino acid intermediary metabolism, and is important in brain function. Good sources include yeast, legumes, enriched grain products and pork. Early signs of deficiency include anorexia, weight loss, muscle weakness, apathy, confusion, and irritability. Later consequences include edema and high-output cardiac failure (wet beriberi), polyneuropathy with depressed reflexes, paresthesias, weakness and muscle atrophy (dry beriberi), and psychosis (Wernicke–Korsakoff syndrome) characterized by dementia, ataxia, and ophthalmoplegia. Lesions of the mamillary bodies and the area that abuts the third ventricle are distinctive findings (Rubin, 2005). The infantile form occurs in infants that are breastfed for months, without supplementation. Cardiac failure in young infants may be sudden and rapidly fatal. Alcohol abuse in adults is often associated with deficiency,

perhaps because alcohol interferes with thiamine uptake and metabolism. Thiamine deficiency is also seen in those with poor nutrition. No toxicity is described from high oral doses. Antithiamine factors are present in betel, tea, and some foods. In the United States all bread and flour are enriched with thiamine. There is a significant loss of thiamine when foods are cooked in water, because it is unstable at high temperatures. Thiamine is produced in the colon by normal enteric bacteria, but the contribution is apparently slight. Thiamine is absorbed throughout the small intestine, and is bound to albumin in the plasma. At high thiamine intakes, the excess is excreted in the urine (Kohlmeier, 2003). Red blood cell transketolase activity with or without TPP added is a useful test for assessing thiamine deficiency. Heparinized whole blood is required, and the test is best run on a fresh specimen (Truswell, 2002a). The most reliable test for thiamine deficiency is the response to the parenteral administration of thiamine (Rubin, 2005).

Riboflavin (Vitamin B₂) normally forms two coenzymes, flavin mononucleotide and flavin adenine dinucleotide. These have an important role in electron transport in several oxidative systems. Dietary sources include milk and dairy products, meat, poultry, fish, and green vegetables. Bread and cereals are fortified with riboflavin. Absorption is mostly in the jejunum. In humans, riboflavin is so prevalent in the diet, that deficiency severe enough to cause marked debilities is not known. Mild riboflavin deficiencies are probably commonplace. Deficiency frequently occurs in association with lack of thiamine and/or niacin (Guyton, 1997). With prolonged deficiency, there is cracking and swelling of the lips (cheilosis), cracking and inflammation of the angles of the mouth (angular stomatitis), deep-red smooth tongue (glossitis, atrophy), a greasy scaling of the cheeks and the areas behind the ears (seborrheic dermatitis), and normocytic anemia (Kohlmeier, 2003). Interstitial keratitis of the cornea is the most troubling lesion. It results in corneal opacification and ulceration (Rubin, 2005). Deficiencies during infancy and childhood impair growth. There is little danger of toxicity, since excess riboflavin is rapidly lost. A 24-h urine collection will indicate the recent riboflavin intake (Kohlmeier, 2003).

Niacin (Nicotinic acid) has a major role in the formation of nicotinamide adenine dinucleotide (NAD) and its phosphate NADP, which are important in intermediary metabolism and a large number of oxidation–reduction reactions. Animal proteins are foods high in tryptophan, such as meat, eggs, and milk. They are good sources for endogenously synthesized niacin. Urine is the main excretory path for niacin metabolites. Niacin is in many grains. Deficiency causes pellagra, which is now uncommon, but seen these days in malnourished alcoholics and in food faddists who do not eat sufficient protein, are tryptophan deficient, and are not taking exogenous niacin. Malabsorption of tryptophan, as seen in Hartnup disease, or the carcinoid syndrome, where the tryptophan is consumed to make serotonin, may produce mild symptoms of pellagra. Pyridoxine and riboflavin deficiencies increase the requirement for niacin, because they are both cofactors and are required for the synthesis of niacin. Corn is a poor source of tryptophan, and the niacin in corn is bound and poorly available. Pellagra is prevalent in areas where corn (maize) is the staple food, as in certain parts of Africa (Guyton, 1997).

Pellagra is characterized by dermatitis, diarrhea, dementia and, if untreated, death. There is a scaly dermatitis of those areas exposed to light or to pressure, such as the knees and elbows. The hands show a rough scaly dermatitis with a glove-like distribution, and a pattern of hyperkeratosis, vascularization, and chronic inflammation. Similar lesions are seen in the mouth and vaginal mucous membranes (Rubin, 2005). Excessive intake of niacin causes flushing (burning and itching of the face, chest, and arms) and gastric irritation. Liver damage may result from continued, very high doses, which have been used as a cholesterol-lowering drug.

Pyridoxine (Vitamin B$_6$) is a coenzyme and participates in more than 100 transamination, decarboxylation, and other reactions, including the initial step of porphyrin synthesis, glycogen mobilization, amino acid transsulfuration, and neurotransmitter synthesis. Good food sources include fortified cereals, organs meats, muscle foods, potatoes, and fruits other than citrus. Cooking results in leaching of the pyridoxine into the discard water. Urine is the major excretory pathway. Deficiencies are usually seen with other vitamin or protein deficiency, and occur in alcoholics. Deficiency of pyridoxine is uncommon, and may cause a microcytic hypochromic anemia where the iron stores are saturated, epileptic seizures, EEG abnormalities, depression, confusion, seborrheic dermatitis, and possibly platelet and clotting abnormalities. Several inborn errors of amino acid metabolism respond to very high doses of pyridoxine. Homocysteinuria, where there is an increased risk of cardiovascular disease, responds to supplements of folate, cobalamine, and sometimes pyridoxine.

Biochemical tests (Truswell, 2002)
- Measurement of plasma pyridoxal 5′-phosphate (PLP). This is the major coenzyme form in the body and the primary form of circulating vitamin B$_6$ in plasma. Normal > 30 nmol/L indicates adequate status in adult.
- Urinary 24-h ↓ pyridoxic acid. Level reflects recent dietary intake of vitamin B$_6$. It varies with age, sex, and pregnancy. More than 0.8 mg/day is acceptable vitamin B$_6$ status.
- Urinary xanthurenic acid after a tryptophan (or methionine) oral load is an indirect measure of functional vitamin B$_6$ deficiency.
- Activity of erythrocyte alanine aminotransferase (RBC-ALT), with and without in vitro PLP. RBC-ALT is diminished in deficiency.

Excessive Intake. Very high doses of pyridoxine (> 100 mg/day in adults) may cause a peripheral sensory neuropathy, and possibly skin lesions (Kohlmeier, 2003).

Cobalamine (Vitamin B$_{12}$) contains cobalt; the structure is complex and only synthesized by bacteria. It is produced by colonic bacteria, but not absorbed. Cobalamine performs many metabolic functions as a hydrogen acceptor coenzyme. Its most significant function is to act as a coenzyme for reducing ribonucleotides to deoxyribonucleotides, a step in the formation of genes. The two main functions of cobalamine are the promotion of growth, and the promotion of red blood cell maturation. Inadequate dietary intake is not the usual cause of cobalamine deficiency. Most common is malabsorption due to either atrophy of the gastric mucosa so that there is inadequate intrinsic factor, or disease of the terminal ileum. Cobalamine deficiency causes megaloblastic anemia in which the erythrocytes fail to mature properly. Demyelination of the large nerve fibers of the spinal cord, especially the posterior and lateral columns, also occurs. The demyelination causes loss of sensation and motor power in the lower limbs. Normal body stores are sufficient to last for 3–6 years. Sources are liver, shellfish, fish, meat eggs, milk, cheeses, and yogurt. Vegans are at risk of a cobalamine deficiency (Eastwood, 2003). Plasma cobalamine < 80 pg/mL indicates a cobalamine deficiency. Elevated serum or urinary methylmalonate and raised plasma homocysteine indicate that the cobalamine is low. The Schilling test measures absorption of cobalamine, with and without intrinsic factor, tested on different days (West, 2002). Cobalamine has extremely low toxicity and doses as large as 3 mg/day are tolerated without toxic effect. The average dietary intake of cobalamine is less than 1 µg/day (Eastwood, 2003).

Ascorbate (Vitamin C) is a powerful reducing agent that is involved in many oxidation–reduction reactions and the transfer of protons. Ascorbate participates in the synthesis of chondroitin sulfate and in the formation of the hydroxyproline of collagen. It has an important role in wound healing, the biosynthesis of some neurotransmitters, and immune function (Rubin, 2005). It is essential for gums, arteries, and other soft tissues, and bone (collagen synthesis), for brain and nerve function (neurotransmitter and hormone synthesis); also for nutrient metabolism (especially iron, protein, and fat), and for antioxidant defense and free radical scavenging (directly and by vitamin E activation). Ascorbate is in high concentration in leukocytes, adrenal gland, pituitary, and brain. Food sources are citrus fruits, berries, tomatoes, and many fruits and vegetables. Prolonged storage and overcooking cause significant vitamin loss. The RDA is 90 mg/day for men and 75 mg/day for women. Deficiency causes scurvy, with symptoms of bleeding gums, if there are teeth, painful swollen joints, poor wound healing, confusion, fatigue, and diminished immune function. Scurvy, now mostly seen in alcoholics, and in the aged poor living alone. The symptoms of scurvy have been described since antiquity. The disease was widespread among sailors in the 16th to 18th centuries,

and the typical pattern was that of having bleeding gums, painful, swollen joints, and muscle weakness. Onset was within months of the start of a voyage. British expeditions had devastating losses of men due to scurvy. The carnage prompted the Admiralty to seek a cure and in 1747 James Lind, a Scottish surgeon, performed a clinical nutrition experiment on board ship, testing six different diet supplements given to six pairs of scorbutic sailors. Oranges and lemons cured scurvy, which he described in his 1753 *Treatise of The Scurvy* (Jacob, 1994). He believed that scurvy was caused by dampness and crowding. Only subsequently was it understood that scurvy was due to ascorbate deficiency. Excessive intake of 2000 mg or more daily may cause gastric and intestinal irritation, cause kidney stones, and interfere with copper metabolism. Unlike other vertebrates, humans are not able to complete the synthesis of ascorbate (Kohlmeier, 2003). Testing to assess ascorbate status can be done using serum or leukocytes. Both correlate well with dietary intake. Urine assays tend to reflect recent dietary intake (Skeaff, 2002).

Folate is the generic name for compounds related to folic acid (pteroylglutamic acid). Its most important function is the synthesis of purines and pyrimidines, which are required for deoxyribonucleic acid formation (Guyton, 1997). It is also important for the maturation of erythrocytes. It is widely available from plants and to a lesser extent, organ meats. More than half of the folate content of food is lost during cooking. Deficiency results in a megaloblastic anemia and leukopenia. In pregnancy, fetal neural tube defects are associated with low folate levels, and periconceptual supplementation markedly reduced the incidence (Wildman, 2000).

Pantothenic acid is part of coenzyme A (CoA) and of acyl carrier protein (ACP). Both are carriers of acyl groups. Acetyl-CoA is involved in the tricarboxylic acid cycle, and CoA in the synthesis of lipids. It is transported in erythrocytes as CoA. The highest tissue concentrations are found in liver, adrenals, kidneys, brain, heart, and testes. CoA and ACP are metabolized to free pantothenic acid and excreted in the urine. Urine levels indicate dietary intake and range from 2–7 mg/day. Pantothenic acid is widely present in foods, and dietary deficiency only occurs in severe malnutrition with other nutrient deficiencies. The 'burning feet syndrome' that was seen in malnourished prisoners of war during World War II responded to large doses of Ca-pantothenate (Truswell, 2002a).

Biotin is a coenzyme for several carboxylase enzymes: pyruvate carboxylase (provides oxaloacetate for tricarboxylic acid cycle), acetyl CoA (coenzyme A) carboxylase (fatty acid synthesis). Biotin deficiency is rare, since it is widely distributed in foods, and large intestine bacterial production supplements the dietary intake. Avidin, an antivitamin, is found in uncooked egg white, and can produce a deficiency of biotin when large amounts are ingested, because avidin binds biotin in the gut, preventing absorption. Biotin deficiency in humans has resulted from the failure to include biotin in total parenteral nutrition and is characterized by a scaly dermatitis, glossitis, hair loss, anorexia, depression, and hypercholesterolemia (Truswell, 2002a).

Fat-Soluble Vitamins

Vitamin A (Retinol). Vitamin A activity is obtained from two compound classes: preformed vitamin A, retinol and related compounds, and the precursors β-carotene and related carotenoids. The latter are the provitamin and are found in yellow and red vegetable pigments that are abundant in vegetables and some fruits. Retinol is essential for vision at low light intensities, synthesis of 'active sulfate', and reproduction. Functions in which retinoic acid also participates include cellular differentiation, involvement in morphogenesis; synthesis of glycoproteins; gene expression; immunity; growth; and prevention of cancer and heart disease (Truswell, 2002b). Vitamin A is needed to maintain certain specialized cell membranes; for skeletal maturation; to participate in forming the light-sensitive rods of the retina; and in the structure of cell membranes. Vitamin A deficiency is unusual in developed countries, but continues to be a frequent cause of blindness due to corneal damage in the poorer regions of the world, particularly parts of Africa, the Middle East, and Southeast Asia. Retinol is in high concentration in fish livers, and leafy, green vegetables are a rich source of carotene (Rubin, 2005). Hippocrates (466–377 BCE) wrote that liver could cure night blindness (West, 2002). Vitamin A deficiency is seen where the diet has lacked dairy produce and vegetables for a long time, or in malabsorption syndromes (Eastwood, 2003). Deficiency results in squamous metaplasia and, as a result, the sweat and tear ducts are blocked by squamous debris. The epithelia of the trachea, bronchi, renal pelvis, pancreatic ducts, uterus, and salivary glands are often affected. The earliest sign of vitamin A deficiency is vision loss in dim light (night blindness). Toxicity is usually produced by excessive vitamin A supplements, especially in children. Vitamin A toxicity occurred in explorers who ate polar bear livers, which have an exceptionally high concentration of vitamin A. In toxicity the liver and spleen are enlarged with lipid-laden macrophages. Vitamin A is in the hepatocytes and prolonged toxicity causes cirrhosis. Headache, hyperexcitability, and bone pain are early symptoms. The lesions are mostly reversible, early in the course, upon discontinuation of the excessive dosing. High doses of synthetic derivatives of retinoic acid are teratogenic. Excessive carotene is benign and causes a jaundice-like discoloration of the skin (Rubin, 2005).

Vitamin D. Ultraviolet light exposure of the skin converts naturally occurring 7-dehydrocholesterol to cholecalciferol or vitamin D_3. Because the body can produce vitamin D, some have termed this a hormone. It is a vitamin for those who are mostly indoors, especially in northern latitudes, as well as those whose clothing completely covers their skin, blocking sunlight. Cholecalciferol is diet-derived from animal sources, particularly fish liver and oils. Ergocalciferol, or vitamin D_2, which is of equal potency in humans, is derived from its provitamin ergosterol, which occurs in fungi and plants and is the major synthetic form used to fortify milk and margarine. Both vitamins D_2 and D_3 require hydroxylation to the active form, which occurs in the liver and kidney. Vitamin D promotes absorption of calcium and phosphate from the small intestine (DeLuca, 1992; Truswell, 2002b). Deficiency results from an inadequate diet; insufficient sunlight reaching the skin; inadequate absorption as occurs in fat malabsorption syndromes; or failure of conversion to the active metabolite, because of chronic hepatic or renal disease. In children before the epiphyses have closed, the bone lesion syndrome is called rickets; in the adult, osteomalacia. The incidence has declined with the addition of ergosterol to milk and other foods (Rubin, 2005). The major function of vitamin D is the homeostasis of Ca^{2+} and phosphate, regulating intestinal adsorption, bone mineralization and mobilization, and renal excretion (Combs, 1998). Hypervitaminosis D is often due to the ingestion of excessive vitamin D preparations. The abnormal conversion of active metabolites occurs sometimes in sarcoidosis. Hypervitaminosis D causes hypercalcemia. Early symptoms are weakness and headache. The sequelae of hypercalcemia include hypercalciuria, nephrocalcinosis, nephrolithiasis, and ectopic calcification of blood vessels, heart and lungs (Rubin, 2005). Overexposure to ultraviolet light will result in sunburn of the skin, but will not cause hypervitaminosis D. Plasma calcium and phosphate fall in vitamin D deficiency and plasma alkaline phosphatase (bone isoenzyme) is increased in rickets and osteomalacia. The most direct way of determining vitamin D status is by an assay of plasma 25(OH)D (Truswell, 2002b).

Vitamin E (Tocopherol) is a fat-soluble antioxidant, or free radical scavenger that inactivates oxygen free radicals. There are eight naturally occurring forms. Vitamin E is the only known lipid-soluble antioxidant in plasma and red blood cell membranes. Corn and soy beans are rich in vitamin E. Deficiency is very uncommon, but may occur as a result of malabsorption, in total parenteral nutrition or in premature infants. The clinical findings in deficiencies have been inconsistent, with reports of ataxia and lost reflexes. There is no known toxicity (Eastwood, 2003).

Vitamin K (Phytomenadione) is involved in the activation of important proteins in blood coagulation, prothrombin (II), factor VII, factor IX, and factor X, as well as protein C and protein S. Deficiency of the factors listed can result in defective clotting and a bleeding disorder. Prothrombin time functionally monitors the vitamin K activity. Vitamin K occurs in two forms: K_1 is present in fresh green vegetables (e.g. broccoli, cabbage, and spinach) and beef liver; K_2 is produced by intestinal bacteria. Dietary deficiency is uncommon. It does occur in fat malabsorption as in sprue and biliary obstruction. Also, antibiotic sterilization of the intestinal flora may result in vitamin K deficiency.

Trace Elements

Trace mineral elements are metals, except selenium and the halogens, fluoride, and iodine. Individually, they are in tissue concentrations of < 1 µg/g of wet tissue (Kane, 2005) and constitute < 0.01% of the dry body weight (Gibson, 1990; Taylor, 1996). They are referred to as trace elements because quantitation with the then available analytical methods was not possible (O'Dell, 1997). Essential trace elements are those that result in an impairment of normal health, function, or development, when there is a deficiency which is corrected when supplemented with physiological levels of that element (Mertz, 1981a; Gibson, 1990), and have specific in vivo metabolic functions that cannot be effectively replaced by other similar elements (Milne, 1994).

The various essential trace elements were discovered by several different means. Deficiencies of some of these elements were found in areas where

Table 26–3 Classification of Trace Mineral Elements

Essential in humans and animals	Essential in some animals and possibly in humans	Possibly essential in some animals	Not essential
Chromium	Arsenic	Bromine	Aluminum
Cobalt	Boron	Cadmium	Antimony
Copper	Lithium	Lead	Bismuth
Fluorine	Nickel	Strontium	Germanium
Iodine	Silicon	Tin	Mercury
Iron	Vanadium		Selenium
Manganese			Silver
Molybdenum			Thalium
Selenium			Titanium
Zinc			

After Gibson, 1990; O'Dell, 1997.

the soil, water, or plants were inadequate in a specific element, such as iodine, fluorine, cobalt, or copper. Deficiencies were also identified when essential elements became biologically unavailable because of interference from other dietary ingestants, such as the zinc deficiency, seen especially in males in the Middle East and in Hispanics in Denver, from eating unleavened bread high in phytate, which is compounded by the high fiber content and low meat intake of their diets (Wildman, 2000), and the anemia of zinc-induced copper deficiency (Milne, 1994). Other deficiencies were caused by a mutation resulting in the lack of a protein needed to absorb or metabolize the element. The symptoms of still other deficiencies were identified in patients whose diets lacked a necessary element or in those on total parenteral nutrition not supplemented with an essential trace element (O'Dell, 1997).

Ten trace mineral elements have been generally recognized as essential in humans – see Table 26–3: 'Classification of Trace Mineral Elements'. Only copper, iodine, iron, selenium, and zinc are associated with well-characterized deficiency states (Kane, 2005). A necessary biochemical role has not been conclusively demonstrated for chromium, fluorine, or manganese, although signs of deficiency have been described (Mertz, 1981b). It is difficult to create a deficiency model, because of the ubiquitous distribution of these elements in the environment and food supply, which frequently causes contamination of the testing system, and because only minute amounts are needed to support physiologic processes. It remains uncertain whether other trace mineral elements are essential in animals and humans. Some authors have concluded that arsenic, boron, lithium, nickel, silicon, and vanadium, which have been shown to have an essential biochemical role in some animal species, are presumptively essential in humans as well (Milne, 1994).

The roles of the trace mineral elements include structural, signal transduction, and especially catalytic properties – see Table 26–4: 'Function, Deficiency, and Toxicity of Essential Trace Mineral Elements'. Some of the trace mineral elements are components of metalloenzymes, function as enzyme cofactors, provide electron and oxygen transport, are active in the maintenance of macromolecule conformation, or vitamin and hormonal activity. These trace minerals are avidly accumulated by cells under the control of several families of proteins (Finney, 2003). Normally, homeostasis of these elements is tightly controlled. Only some of the biochemical mechanisms of the clinical effects of trace element deficiencies have been determined (Mertz, 1981b).

Deficiencies of trace elements are usually due to nutritional deficiency; inadequate supplementation in total parenteral nutrition; or a disease state in which there is insufficient intestinal absorption, or increased excretion or utilization. Deficiencies can also be due to interaction between trace elements (e.g., zinc and copper) and with other nutrients (e.g., zinc and vitamin A) interfering with absorption or adversely affecting metabolic utilization. Large amounts of dietary zinc interfere with intestinal copper absorption and result in copper deficiency and anemia (Milne, 1994; Willis, 2005).

Genetic defects in trace element metabolism include Menkes' kinky hair syndrome (copper), congenital atransferrinemia (iron), acrodermatitis enteropathica (zinc), and xanthine and sulfite oxidase deficiencies (molybdenum) (Gibson, 1990).

Trace elements must be analyzed with considerable care since they are widely distributed in the environment (e.g. water, air) and biological

Table 26–4 Function, Deficiency and Toxicity of Essential Trace Mineral Elements

Element	Function/enzyme component	Effects of deficiency	Effects of toxicity
Chromium	Potentiates insulin action, glucose and lipid metabolism, Cr(III) low toxicity, poorly absorbed Component of glucose tolerance factor	No method to determine deficiency in humans; impaired glucose tolerance in type 2 diabetes, insulin resistance, hyperglycemia, peripheral neuropathy, hyperlipidemia	Cr(VI) toxic, oxidative damage, skin ulcers, contact dermatitis, asthma, renal and hepatic necrosis, lung cancer
Cobalt	Hemoglobin synthesis Component of vitamin B_{12}	Cobalt deficiency, as such, not in humans; symptoms due to lack of vitamin B_{12}: anemia, anorexia, growth depression	Cardiomyopathy, heart failure, goiter, hypothyroidism; warm sensation, vomiting, diarrhea
Copper	Cellular respiration, neurotransmitter regulator, oxidation reaction, electron transport, collagen synthesis, development of vascular and skeletal structures and CNS, antioxidant Component of CuZnSOD, metallothionein, cytochrome c, tyrosinase, dopamine β-hydroxylase, lysyl oxidase	*Menkes' kinky hair syndrome:* X-linked; congenital failure of Cu absorption; abnormal collagen crosslinking, muscle weakness, iron-refractory hypochromic anemia, leukopenia, neurological defects, hypopigmentation. In prematurity: bone fractures, skeletal defects Occurs in malnourished children and premature infants not supplemented	Relatively nontoxic *Wilson's disease:* autosomal recessive; failure to excrete Cu in bile; excess Cu in liver, kidneys, brain, eyes; hepatic necrosis, hypertension, Kayser–Fleischer rings in eyes; Cu interferes with absorption of iron and zinc
Fluorine	Prevents tooth decay	Increased dental caries	Mottled enamel, fluorosis
Iodine	Component of thyroid hormone	Goiter, hypothyroidism, cretinism in infants, myxedema in adults	Goiter, thyrotoxicosis

Iron	Oxygen transport, respiration, amino acids and free radical metabolism, lipids, oxidative phosphorylation
	Component of hemoglobin, metalloenzymes, vitamin A
		Hypochromic microcytic anemia, glossitis, angular stomatitis, cheilosis, koilonychia
		Blood loss or inadequate iron intake; iron deficiency anemia: < 7 g/100 mL blood
			Hemochromatosis:
			    genetic, primary, autosomal recessive
			    acquired, secondary, iron overload
			iron deposition in liver, pancreas, heart and skin

Manganese	Bone and connective tissue Component of metalloenzymes: hydrolases, oxidoreductases, and lipases, pyruvate caboxylase, superoxide dismutase, and arginase	Not well-defined in humans; skeletal and cartilage defects	Least toxic of trace elements Psychiatric disorders: memory, speech, hallucinations; syndrome resembles Parkinson's and Wilson's diseases
Molybdenum	DNA metabolism, essential for uric acid production Component of sulfite and xanthine oxidase	Naturally occurring deficiency not known; growth depression, hypercuprinemia, defective keratin formation, goiter, cretinism	Anemia, goiter, thyrotoxicosis, hypouricemia, hyperoxypurinemia
Selenium	Protects against oxidative damage of lipid, gene expression, thyroxin deiodinase Component of glutathione peroxidase	*Keshan disease:* cardiomyopathy, cardiomegaly, heart failure, cataracts, osteoarthritis in children, myopathy, discolored/thickened nails, impaired growth	Hair and nail loss, selenosis, tooth decay, neuropathy, liver failure, garlic odor on breath
Zinc	Protein synthesis, zinc finger proteins – gene expression, immunity, needed for normal skin, bones and hair Component of metallothionein, ~ 300 enzymes	*Acrodermatitis enteropathica*; causes cardiomyopathy in children In children, low height, hypogeusia, growth retardation, infertility, immune deficits, delayed wound healing, glossitis, seborrheic-like dermatitis, osteoporosis	Relatively nontoxic, nausea, vomiting and GI irritation, causes copper deficiency

After Fausto da Silva, 1991; Alcock, 1996; Kane, 2005.

devices (e.g. needles, syringes, stoppers) and thus can readily contaminate a sample (McNeely, 1986). Special collection and handling are necessary. Clean room techniques and ultra-pure reagents must be used. Reference materials and strict quality control are requisite with each assay run to assure analytical accuracy. It is especially important that trained technical personnel perform the testing (Mertz, 1975; Veillo, 1986). Improved materials are now available for collection, processing, and analysis of trace elements that reduce contamination. These include trace element-free syringes, evacuated tubes with fitted siliconized needles, acid-washed glassware, and standard reference materials with certified values (Casey, 1983; Gibson, 1990).

The major advances in understanding and managing the dynamics of trace mineral elements during the past two decades have been achieved by the extraordinary precision and sensitivity of the improved analytical instruments. Atomic absorption spectrometry (AAS) is the most widely used instrument for clinical trace element analysis in biological samples. Graphite furnace AAS (GFAAS) has improved the limit of quantitation

(LOQ) to parts per billion (ppb, µg/L) and permits the simultaneous measurement of multiple elements. Zeeman effect background correction improves the element signal measurement when testing in complex specimens such as serum, plasma or blood, and other specimen handling enhancements have further improved sensitivity and precision. Flame AAS (FAAS) has a LOQ of parts per million (ppm, mg/L). Atomic emission spectrometry (AES) consists of flame AES and plasma source emission spectrometry, which measures photon output rather than photon absorption as in AAS. The emission line(s) of the excited electrons are measured. The LOQ is ppm (mg/L). The sample in neutron activation analysis (NAA) is irradiated with low-energy neutrons for the production of radioactive nuclides. In NAA there is excitation of the atomic nucleus, so that the trace element is determined independently of its physical or chemical state. The newly formed radionuclide emits X- or γ-rays. The LOQ is ppb (µg/L) to parts per trillion (ppt, ng/L) with multi-element detection, but with a limited dynamic range. This technique is especially suited for in

Table 26–5 Properties of Essential Trace Mineral Elements

Element	Tissue distribution	Body content	Transport (Reference value)	Excretion
Chromium	Spleen, heart	4–6 mg Cr (III)	Transferrin-P 0.15 µg/mL Cr (0.12–2.1 µg/L)	Urine 100–200 ng/day
Cobalt	Muscle, liver, fat	1.1 mg	Albumin (0.11–0.45 µg/L)	Urine 80%
Copper	Muscle and liver Liver 30–50 µg/g dry; 50–70% of body Cu	50–80 mg (1.2–2.5 µg/g fat-free tissue)	Ceruloplasmin 60–95%, albumin, transcuperin (Cu-S: 70–140 µg/dL AAS)	Feces includes bile and unabsorbed dietary Cu
Iodine	Thyroid: 70–80% of total body I in thyroxin bound to thyroglobulin	15–20 mg (11–15 mg in thyroid)	Thyroxine-binding protein, 80% thyroxine-binding prealbumin (transthyretin)	Urine 100–150 µg/day
Iron	RBC Hb 400–600 mg/L, liver, spleen, bone marrow 25%, myoglobin	4–5 g (3/4 in Hb) 50 mg/kg 2.5 g in RBCs	Transferrin-P (2–2.5 g/L) Ferritin-S 1 µg/L = 10 mg tissue iron stores Hemosiderin 1 g iron	Bile 84 µg/kg, blood loss, menses, GI mucosal cells
Manganese	Liver, bone, pancreas	12–20 mg	(Mn-blood: 200 nmol/L)	Bile and intestinal secretions
Molybdenum	Liver, kidney, bone, adrenal	Blood 30–700 nmol/L	RBC protein, α_1-macroglobulin (S: 8–34 µg/L)	Urine 90%, bile 10%
Selenium	Liver, kidney, muscle	15 mg	Protein [Se-P: 7–30 µg/dL]	Urine 60%, feces 40%
Zinc	Muscle 60%, bone 30%, liver, prostate, semen	1.2–2.3 g	Albumin 60–70%, α_2-macroglobulin (Zn-P: 11–22 µmol/L)	Feces, gut secretions, GI mucosal cells

P = plasma; S = serum; AAS = atomic absorption spectrometry.

Data from: Fausto da Silva, 1991; Milne, 1994; O'Dell, 1997; Kohlmeier 2003.

vitro trace element determination in biologic matrices. In instrumental neutron activation analysis (INAA) there is direct measurement of the emitted X or γ radiation. Inductively coupled plasma–mass spectroscopy (ICP-MS) is a highly sensitive and specific method for the measurement of multiple trace elements in a single run over an especially broad dynamic range with low background interference and LOQs of ppb (µg/L) to ppt (ng/L). An internal standard is used for enhanced precision (Milne, 1994; Chan, 1998a).

An assessment of trace element status requires a measurement of either the concentration in accessible tissues (hair, nails) and body fluids (serum, urine), or the activity of a trace element-dependent enzyme. There are no particularly good indicators for the determination of trace element dietary status because of the poor correlation with total body stores. The only definitive test of human trace mineral element deficiency is the clinical response to controlled supplementation with the element of concern followed by evaluation of improvement of an impaired function (Milne, 1994; Eastwood, 2003). Combination testing yields a more reliable interpretation, especially when the findings are concordant. The interpretation of plasma or serum levels can be deceptive because of the response to stress or when there is expansion of the blood volume or a decrease in serum albumin as occurs, for example, in the third trimester of pregnancy. Also, hemolysis interferes with assays. Serum zinc, copper, manganese, chromium, and molybdenum levels are not reliable for assessing nutritional status or dietary intake because the results do not reflect body stores. Both serum and urine concentrations indicate recent dietary intake. See Table 26–5: 'Properties of Essential Trace Mineral Elements'.

Hair and nail clippings need be collected with care and washed to avoid surface contamination.

Trace element assays in blood, serum, or urine, usually reflect the current nutriture. The first morning void urine is less affected by recent dietary intake. Load tests measure the change in urine concentration following a loading dose of the mineral element. When tissue levels are low, the deficiency will cause retention of the element. Similarly, tolerance tests measure the change in plasma concentration following a challenge dose. Usually the dose is in the pharmacological range rather than the physiological level normally experienced. Hair, fingernail or toenail analyses provide a retrospective window or an assessment of chronic exposure for the period of hair or nail growth (Gibson, 2002). Because of the risk of environmental contamination, hair and nail clippings are of limited use in determining dietary intake or body status, except when reduced (Eastwood, 2003).

'All substances are poisons … dose differentiates a poison.' Paracelsus (1493–1541)

Toxicity is never a question of presence, only the amount. Each of the essential and nonessential trace mineral elements can be toxic when present in high concentrations. A poison is too much of anything. Toxicity is quite variable for the different trace elements. Some have a high toxicity. The toxic effects of selenium are produced by intake of only 10 times the nutritional requirement. In contrast, chromium toxicity has never been reported after oral pharmacological doses (Gibson, 1990).

Copper (Cu)

Copper is the third most abundant trace element in the human body, following zinc and iron. It is a very effective cation in reactions which involve electron transfer and binding to organic molecules (Samman, 2002).

Biochemistry. Copper is involved in electron transport and oxidation reactions and is essential for cellular respiration, neurotransmitter regulation, collagen synthesis, nutrient metabolism, especially iron, and as an antioxidant against free radicals (Kohlmeier, 2003).

Copper is present in all living cells (Marston, 1952) and functions mostly as a component of the cuproenzymes and copper-containing proteins. Copper-containing plasma amine oxidases catabolize some active amines such as tyramine, histidine, and polyamines, and inactivate the catecholamines (norepinephrine, tyramine, dopamine, and serotonin). Another cuproenzyme, *lysyl oxidase* helps collagen proteins crosslink into larger fibers. Also, copper is a component of *cytochrome c oxidase*, which catalyzes the cellular utilization of oxygen (Wildman, 2000). Extracellular *superoxide dismutase* is in high concentration in the lungs, thyroid, and uterus. Copper/zinc dismutases are in the cytosol of most cells, especially brain, thyroid, liver, pituitary, and erythrocytes. Both dismutases scavenge and reduce superoxide radicals. Copper-containing proteins include ceruloplasmin, albumin, and transcuperin, which transport copper; metallothionein, which sequesters and stores copper; and clotting factor V (Chan, 1998)

Dietary Sources. Rich sources of copper include liver, shellfish, chocolate, nuts, and seeds. Copper pipes or vessels do not increase the copper content of water unless exposed to acids (Kohlmeier, 2003). The average daily copper intake of American adults is about 1.6 mg in males and 1.2 mg in females. Adults should get at least 0.9 mg/day (Institute of

Medicine, 2002). Smoking, strenuous exercise, infections and injuries, increase the need for copper.

Metabolism. Copper absorption occurs in the stomach and especially in the small intestine (Wapnir, 1998). Bile adds about 5 mg/day to the ingested copper. Absorption is decreased by excessive zinc or iron intake. Too much copper may cause iron deficiency. Histidine, as well as gluconate and citrate, enhance copper absorption (Wildman, 2000). Ascorbate decreases copper absorption by reducing Cu^{2+} to Cu^+ (Kohlmeier, 2003).

Newly absorbed copper is transported bound to albumin and transcuperin and rapidly cleared from the blood circulation by the liver. When copper re-enters the circulation, it is as ceruloplasmin, which transports 65–90% of the plasma copper, and metallothionein and other copper-containing proteins. Ceruloplasmin is not a transporter protein since the copper is not exchangeable (Eastwood, 2003). Metallochaperones are specific binding proteins which provide targeted intracellular copper transport to shuttle copper for metabolic needs (Kohlmeier, 2003). Excess copper is bound to thionein, decreasing the potential for copper toxicity (Wildman, 2000). Free copper ions are a source of oxygen free radicals, and intracellular free copper is kept at a very low concentration.

Excretion is primarily in the feces, which includes unabsorbed dietary copper, and biliary and gastrointestinal secretions, although small amounts are also lost in sweat, urine and saliva.

Testing. The total copper in an adult human is 50–80 mg of copper, mainly concentrated in muscle and liver. The liver has the highest copper concentration, averaging between 30–50 µg/g dry tissue. Reference ranges for serum copper concentration are age and sex dependent and are higher in pregnancy. There is diurnal variation with peak values in the morning. Ranges are: for women, 49–184 µg/dL (7.7–29.0 µmol/L); for men, 59–118 µg/dL (9.3–18.6 µmol/L) by ICP-MS (Chan, 1998b). The most widely used clinical analytical method is flame AAS. Serum or plasma copper levels are insensitive for the diagnosis of copper deficiency and are decreased only in severe deficiency (Gibson, 2002). Lower concentrations may indicate depleted copper stores. However, circulating copper levels are affected by factors unrelated to nutrition. Pregnancy, infections, inflammatory conditions, stress, or oral contraception, increase the circulating copper level. Corticosteroids and corticotropin lower the circulating copper level (Jacob, 1993). Reduced serum proteins due to nephrosis, malabsorption, or malnutrition cause the serum copper to be low, without reflecting inadequate liver copper stores. Ceruloplasmin, a copper-containing protein, is a useful indicator of copper status. It is an α_2-globulin acute phase reactant. Ceruloplasmin is sensitive to the same factors that affect plasma copper and may be measured immunochemically or by its oxidase activity (Milne, 1994). It is increased in patients with infections, neoplasms, pregnancy, and hormonal contraception (Kohlmeier, 2003). Measurement of erythrocyte superoxide dismutase is useful for assessing copper status. The activity is reduced in copper-deficient states.

Genetic diseases. Menkes' syndrome and Wilson's disease are genetic defects in copper metabolism. *Menkes' syndrome* is a rare X-linked recessive congenital defect of copper absorption that usually has a clinical onset by 3 months of age. There is poor mental development, failure to keratinize hair, skeletal problems, and degenerative changes in the aorta. The brittle hair is kinky or twisted, and there is poor skin and hair pigmentation, hypothermia, and seizures. Hair resembles that of wool from sheep that graze in pastures lacking copper. The affected infants are copper deficient and there is decreased serum and liver copper. RBC copper is normal (Wildman, 2000).

Wilson's disease (hepatolenticular degeneration) is an autosomal recessive disease that results from impaired biliary copper excretion. It presents in children and young adults, between ages 6–40 years. Excess copper is deposited in the liver, and the basal nuclei of the brain, causing sclerosis, and there are abnormalities of kidney, cornea and brain. Most often the presenting disease pattern is that of acute, chronic or fulminant hepatitis. Symptoms include neurological disorders, cirrhosis of the liver, and Kayser–Fleischer rings due to the deposition of copper in the corneas. Urinary copper is increased to > 100 µg/24 h, and serum ceruloplasmin is usually decreased. Clinical severity of the disease correlates poorly with the ceruloplasmin level, since ceruloplasmin may be normal or increased in response to hepatic inflammation. Serum copper is generally decreased because of the low ceruloplasmin and serum copper levels are not useful diagnostically. Serum ceruloplasmin < 20 mg/dL with increased hepatic copper of > 250 µg/g dry weight is diagnostic. Chelation is an effective treatment in promoting excretion of the copper (Milne, 1994).

Deficiency is unlikely except in people with either rare genetic disorders or experiencing prolonged malnutrition or starvation. Deficiencies have been observed in premature babies, malnourished infants and adults; long-term hyperalimentation with infusates deficient in copper; patients with sickle cell disease receiving zinc therapy; and those treated with copper-chelating agents like penicillamine (Milne, 1994). Reduced copper levels have been found in elderly patients with femoral neck fractures (Conlan, 1990). Symptoms of copper deficiency include hypochromic anemia, ataxia, neutropenia, osteoporosis and bone and joint abnormalities, decreased skin pigmentation, and neurological abnormalities. Body stores last only a few weeks when intake is low.

Copper toxicity has not been reported from food intake. Doses in excess of 10 mg/day cause nausea, vomiting, abdominal cramps, diarrhea, and can cause liver injury, especially in infants. Acute poisoning may present with hemolysis, and brain and hepatic cellular damage (Eastwood, 2003). Higher doses can cause coma and death. Excess supplements or ingestion of contaminated water are the usual sources. Ingestion of fungicides containing copper sulfate or industrial exposure sometimes cause acute copper poisoning (Williams, 1982).

Zinc (Zn)

Zinc is second to iron as the most abundant trace element in the body. It is the most common catalytic metal ion in the cytoplasm of cells. Total body stores of zinc in adult women are 1.5 g and in men 2.5 g, which is distributed in all tissues. It is almost entirely intracellular (King, 1994). Most zinc is in skeletal muscle (~ 60%) and bone (~ 30%) (Wildman, 2000). It is a cofactor for almost 300 enzymes, and is involved in almost all aspects of metabolism. Zinc is important in protein and nucleic acid synthesis, and essential for gene activation (Kohlmeier, 2003) and for the synthesis and action of insulin (Samman, 2002). Zinc is only present in the divalent state in biological systems and oxidation–reduction functions are not possible. Important zinc-containing metalloenzymes are carbonic anhydrase, alkaline phosphatase, RNA, and DNA polymerases, reverse transcriptase, thymidine kinase, carboxypeptidases, alcohol dehydrogenase, and superoxide dismutase (SOD).

Dietary Sources. Zinc is ubiquitous in food. Oysters are especially rich in zinc. Other shellfish and meats are also good sources. Plants have much lower concentrations. Phytate from whole grains and some vegetables interfere with zinc absorption (Kohlmeier, 2003). The estimated average requirement to maintain adequate stores is 8 mg/day for women eating a mixed diet and 11 mg/day for men (Institute of Medicine, 2002). Vegetarians and pregnant or nursing woman need slightly more. Zinc is excreted primarily by the intestine.

Metabolism. Zinc is mainly absorbed from the duodenum although some is absorbed in the small intestine. Some zinc enters the intestinal lumen with pancreatic secretions. Intraluminal digestion by proteases, DNAses, and RNAses frees zinc so that complexes with histidine, cysteine, and nucleotides are formed that improve absorption. Phytate reduces absorption. High dietary calcium and low protein will also reduce zinc absorption (Samman, 2003). Metallothionein regulates zinc transfer into the portal blood. In blood, the zinc is bound to albumin and α_2-macroglobulin, with zinc blood concentrations of 10–17 µmol/L.

Muscle and bones, which contain most of the body's zinc stores, have a slow turnover, with a half-life of 300 days (Wastney, 2000). The half-life of the metallothionein-bound zinc in the liver is about 2 weeks; it can be readily mobilized and cover for an insufficient dietary intake. However, the liver pool is small, and contains less than 170 mg. Zinc deficiency can become functionally significant within a week (Miller, 1994).

Almost all blood zinc is complexed to the large proteins, albumin or α_2-macroglobulin, so that there is little zinc in the glomerular filtrate. Urine losses are about 0.5 mg/day (Kohlmeier, 2003). About 1 mg/day is lost in sweat, skin, and hair. Fecal losses, which include diet and endogenous secretions, can be less than 1 mg/day (Sian, 1996). Each ejaculate contains about 0.5 mg, probably from prostatic secretions.

Inadequate zinc impairs DNA replication, food digestion and absorption, taste and appetite, growth and wound healing, synaptic transmission, gene expression, response to oxidant stress, immune function, and other functions.

Zinc fingers are looped sequence-specific DNA-binding proteins that act as transcriptional mediators for nucleic acids. Zinc chelates with cysteine and/or histidine, which binds to a specific DNA region and controls gene expression or repression primarily through targeting promoter regions of the genes (Wildman, 2000).

Deficiency. Zinc deficiency is common in patients with diabetes mellitus, alcohol abuse, and malabsorption syndromes, and liver and kidney diseases. Symptoms are general because of the many enzymes and tissues affected. In severe deficiencies there is hypogonadism, dwarfism, deformed bones, poor wound healing, abnormal hair and nails, loss of taste, gastrointestinal disturbances, poor chylomicron formation, CNS abnormalities, immunodeficiencies, and malabsorption. Zinc deficiency may cause teratogenicity during pregnancy, with congenital malformations, fetal dysmaturity, prematurity, neural tube defects, and spina bifida (Chan, 1998).

Nutritional zinc deficiency is fairly prevalent despite the wide availability of zinc in foods. Zinc deficiency produces a syndrome of growth retardation, male hypogonadism, skin changes, mental lethargy, hepatosplenomegaly, iron deficiency anemia, and geophagia (eating clay). It has been encountered in mostly male children in Iran and Egypt as a result of a low-zinc diet with a high-fiber content that decreases the available zinc for absorption. Zinc deficiency has also been reported from Turkey, Portugal, Morocco, and Yugoslavia (Milne, 1994). In some areas of the Middle East, people frequently eat unleavened bread that is high in phytate. Yeast contains phytase. However, the recipe for the dough of the unleavened bread does not include yeast. The high fiber content and low meat and low protein intake in this population result in zinc deficiency. They respond well to dietary zinc sulfate supplementation (Eastwood, 2003). Growth failure, reduced taste acuity, and hypogonadism in young adults in New York and Tennessee and in school children in Colorado have been ascribed to zinc deficiency (Milne, 1994). Zinc deficiency has also been reported in old age, pregnancy, lactation, steatorrhea, extensive burns, renal disease, and diuretic and antimetabolite therapies. Zinc deficiency in alcoholics and in cirrhosis will show low serum zinc concentrations and demonstrate increased urinary excretion (Eastwood, 2003; Prasad, 1982).

Acrodermatitis enteropathica is a rare autosomal recessive disorder with impaired intestinal absorption and transport of zinc. Symptoms include hyperpigmented skin lesions, pustular and bullous dermatitis, alopecia, growth retardation, diarrhea, secondary infection, irritability, lethargy, and depression. Plasma or serum zinc is below 40 µg/mL. Oral zinc therapy results in rapid and complete remission (Chan, 1998b).

A case of zinc deficiency, called 'acquired acrodermatitis enteropathica,' has been reported in a 41-year-old woman, with alcohol abuse and type 1 diabetes mellitus, complicated by retinopathy, nephropathy, and end-stage renal disease. There was a 5-month history of alopecia, brittle scalp hair, diarrhea, angular cheilitis, and a pruritic, scaly erythematous eruption involving the extremities, perineum and buttocks. A skin biopsy disclosed confluent parakeratosis with absence of the granular layer. Serum zinc levels were markedly reduced at 0.35 µg/mL (5.4 µmol/L) (normal: 0.66–1.10 µg/mL [10.1–16.8 µmol/L]). Oral zinc sulfate resolved her diarrhea, and her skin eruption cleared and hair began to regrow (Wang, 2005).

Zinc toxicity is rare in humans. Animals given high levels of supplementation manifest dysphagia. The other effects, like weight loss, are attributed to reduced food intake.

Inhalation of zinc oxide fumes is the most common cause of metal fume fever. Symptoms are of a flu-like illness with onset 4–6 hours after exposure to the fumes. Fatigue, chills, myalgias, cough, dyspnea, leukocytosis, thirst, metallic taste, and salivation characterize this self-limited illness, with resolution of symptoms in 36 hours.

Testing. There is no single test that is definitive for the status of zinc stores. There are two groups of tests: analysis of zinc in a body tissue or body fluid, such as plasma, serum, blood cells or urine; and testing a zinc-dependent function, such as taste acuity or the measurement of the activity of zinc-containing enzymes. In most instances, the assays will show a decrease with zinc deficiency. Test results need to be interpreted with caution, because the levels may be affected by unrelated conditions. There is diurnal variation of zinc levels. Zinc levels decrease after meals and are elevated after fasting. Albumin levels significantly affect the circulating zinc level. Also, many steroids, including adrenocortical and gonadal, depress the zinc level. Erythrocyte levels are 10 times that of serum, and hemolysis is a serious problem affecting the usefulness of the results.

Flame atomic absorption spectrometry (FAAS) is the method of choice for clinical testing for zinc in body fluids. Inductively coupled plasma–mass spectrometry (ICP-MS) is the reference testing method used for zinc testing in serum or plasma.

The plasma level reference value for zinc is 70–120 µg/dL (10.7–18.4 µmol/L), of which a third is bound to α_2-macroglobulin and the rest to albumin: 10–20% of the blood zinc is in the plasma. The remainder is associated with carbonic anhydrase in the erythrocytes. Hemolysis must be avoided. Fasting morning levels of zinc below 70 µg/dL (10.7 µmol/L) suggest marginal deficiency. Serum zinc values are 5–10% higher than plasma values. Zinc levels are lower when there is nonfasting, infection, inflammation, steroid administration, pregnancy, or hypoalbuminemia.

Zinc in erythrocytes and hair gives a long-term assessment of body zinc status. Lowered hair zinc has been demonstrated in several different zinc-deficient conditions. Care must be taken to avoid environmental contamination, and to sample hair grown during the condition under study, and not in the prior time period (Milne, 1994). Urinary zinc excretion reference values are 0.15–1.00 mg/day (2.3–15.3 µmol/day). Urinary zinc excretion is usually decreased in zinc deficiency. In some conditions associated with zinc deficiency, such as cirrhosis, severe alcoholism, sickle cell anemia, postsurgical periods, and total parenteral nutrition, increased urinary zinc excretion is often present (Jacob, 1993).

Hyperzincemia is a familial disorder that results in elevated serum zinc levels, but does not cause any apparent toxicity. Zinc overdoses that result in similar plasma zinc levels have been known to be fatal (Wildman, 2000).

References

Alcock NW: Trace elements. *In* Kaplan LA, Pesce AJ (eds): Clinical Chemistry, 3rd ed. St Louis, Mosby, 1996, pp 746–759.

Barr SI, Murphy SP, Poos MI: Interpreting and using the dietary references intakes in dietary assessment of individuals and groups, Am Diet Assoc 2002; 102:780–788.

Berdanier CD: CRC Desk Reference for Nutrition. Boca Raton, CRC Press, 1998.

Brewster MA: Vitamins. *In* Kaplan LA, Pesce AJ (eds): Clinical Chemistry, 3rd ed. St Louis, Mosby, 1996, pp 760–792.

Casey CE, Robinson MF: Some aspects of nutritional trace element research. *In* Siegel H (ed): Metal Ions in Biological Systems, Vol 16. New York, Marcel Dekker, 1983, pp 1–26.

Chan S, Gerson B, Reitz RE, Sadjadi S: Technical and clinical aspects of spectrophotometric analysis of trace elements in clinical samples. *In* Gerson B (ed): Clinics in Laboratory Medicine 1998a; 18(4):615–629.

Chan S, Gerson B, Subramaniam S: The role of copper, molybdenum, selenium, and zinc in nutrition and health. Clinics in Laboratory Medicine 1998b; 18(4):673–685.

Combs, GF Jr: The Vitamins, 2nd ed. San Diego, Academic Press, 1998.

Conlan D, Korula R, Tallentire D: Serum copper levels in elderly patients with femoral-neck fractures. Age Ageing 1990; 19:212–214.

DeLuca HF: New concepts of vitamin D function. *In* Sauberlich HE, Machlin LJ (eds): Beyond Deficiency. Ann N Y Acad Sci 1992; 669:59–69.

Eastwood M: Principles of Human Nutrition, 2nd ed. Oxford, Blackwell, 2003.

Fausto da Silva JJR, Williams RJP: The Biological Chemistry of the Elements. Oxford, Clarendon Press, 1991.

Feldman EB: Assessment of nutritional status. *In* Noe DA, Rock RC (eds): Laboratory Medicine. Baltimore, Williams & Wilkins, 1994.

Finney LA, O'Halloran TV: Transition metal speciation in the cell: Insights from the chemistry of metal ion receptors. Science 2003; 300:931–936.

Gibson R: Determining nutritional status. *In* Mann J, Truswell AS (eds): Essentials of Human Nutrition, 2nd edition. Oxford, Oxford University Press, 2002, 467–497.

Gibson RS: Principles of Nutritional Assessment. Oxford, Oxford University Press, 1990.

Grodner M, Long S, DeYoung S: Foundations and Clinical Applications of Nutrition, 3rd ed. St Louis, Mosby, 2004.

Guyton AC, Hall JE: Human Physiology and Mechanisms of Disease, 6th edition. Philadelphia, WB Saunders, 1997.

Institute of Medicine: Dietary Reference Intakes for Calcium, Phosphorus, Magnesium, Vitamin D, and Fluoride. Washington, DC, National Academy Press, 1997.

Institute of Medicine: Dietary Reference Intakes for Thiamin, Riboflavin, Niacin, Vitamin B6, Folate, Vitamin B12, Pantothenic Acid, Biotin, and Choline. Washington, DC, National Academy Press, 1998.

Institute of Medicine: Dietary Reference Intakes for Vitamin C, Vitamin E, Selenium, and Carotenoids,. Washington, DC, National Academy Press, 2000.

Institute of Medicine: Dietary Reference Intakes for Vitamin A, Vitamin K, Arsenic, Boron, Chromium, Copper, Iodine, Iron, Manganese, Molybdenum, Nickel, Silicon, Vanadium, and Zinc (Micronutrients). Washington, DC, National Academy Press, 2002.

Jacob RA: Vitamin C. *In* Shils ME, Olsen JA, Shike M: Modern Nutrition in Health and Disease, 8th ed. Philadelphia, Lea & Febiger, 1994, pp 432–448.

Jacob RA, Milne DB: Biochemical Assessment of Vitamins and Trace Metals. Labbe RF (ed): Clinics in Laboratory Medicine 1993; 13(2):371–385.

Kane AB, Kumar V: Environmental and nutritional pathology. In Kumar V, Abbas AK, Fausto N (eds): Robbins and Cotran Pathologic Basis of Disease, 7th ed. Philadelphia, Saunders, 2005, pp 415–468.

Katz DL: Nutrition in Clinical Practice. Philadelphia, Lippincott Williams & Wilkins, 2001.

King JC, Keen CL: Zinc. *In*: Shils ME, Olsen JA, Shike M (eds): Modern Nutrition in Health and Disease, 8th edn. Malvern, PA: Lea & Febiger, 1994; 214–230.

Kohlmeier M: Nutrient Metabolism. San Diego, Academic Press, 2003.

This text provides a systematic presentation of the metabolism of the vitamins and trace elements, with masterful integration of the vast subject of nutritional metabolism and biochemistry, in the context of normal human physiology. Extensive current references are provided.

McCormick DB, Greene HL: Vitamins. *In* Burtis CA, Ashwood ER (eds): Tietz Textbook of Clinical Chemistry, 2nd ed. Philadelphia, WB Saunders, 1994, pp 1275–1316.

Machlin LJ: Introduction. *In* Sauberlich HE, Machlin LJ (eds): Beyond Deficiency. Ann N Y Acad Sci 1992; 669:1–6.

McLaren DC: Clinical manifestations of human vitamin and mineral disorders: A résumé. *In* Shils ME, Olsen JA, Shike M: Modern Nutrition in Health and Disease, 8th ed. Philadelphia, Lea & Febiger, 1994, pp 909–923.

McNeely MDD: Nutrition, vitamins, and trace elements. *In* Gornall AG (ed): Applied Biochemistry of Clinical Disorders, 2nd ed. Philadelphia, Lippincott, 1986, pp 487–501.

Mann J, Truswell AS (eds): Essentials of Human Nutrition, 2nd ed. Oxford, Oxford University Press, 2002.

The trace elements and vitamins with a focus on deficiencies, toxicity, and biochemical testing, and an appendix assessing numerous standard and newly introduced static and dynamic biochemical tests, and load and tolerance tests, the findings, utility and their interpretability.

Marston HR: Cobalt, copper and molybdenum in the nutrition of animals and plants. Physiol Rev 1952; 32:153–157.

Mason JB: Consequences of altered micronutrient status. *In* Bennett JC, Plum F (eds): Cecil Textbook of Medicine, 20th ed. Philadelphia, WB Saunders, 1996, pp 1144–1154.

Mertz W: Trace-element nutrition in health and disease: Contributions and problems of analysis. Clin Chem 1975; 21:468–475.

Mertz W: The essential trace elements. Science 1981a; 213(4514):1332–1338.

Mertz W: The scientific and practical importance of trace elements. Philos Trans R Soc Lond B Biol Sci 1981b; 294:9–18.

Milne DB: Trace elements. *In* Burtis CA, Ashwood ER (eds): Tietz Textbook of Clinical Chemistry, 2nd ed. Philadelphia, WB Saunders, 1994, pp 1317–1353.

O'Dell BL, Sunde RA: Handbook of Nutritionally Essential Mineral Elements. New York, Marcel Dekker, 1997.

Prasad AS: Clinical and biochemical spectrum of zinc deficiency in human subjects. *In* Prasad AS (ed): Clinical, Biochemical, and Nutritional Aspects of Trace Elements. New York, NY, Alan R Liss, 1982, pp 3–62.

Rubin E, Strayer DS: Environmental and nutritional pathology. *In* Rubin E, Gorstein F, Rubin R, et al: (eds): Rubin's Pathology: Clinicopathologic Foundations of Medicine, 4th ed. Philadelphia, Lippincott, Williams & Wilkins, 2005, pp 312–355.

Samman S: Trace elements. *In* Mann J, Truswell AS (eds): Essentials of Human Nutrition, 2nd ed. Oxford, Oxford University Press, 2002, pp 159–188.

Seymour CA: Trace metal disorders. *In* Ledingham JGG, Warrell DA (eds): Concise Oxford Textbook of Medicine. Oxford, Oxford University Press, 2000, pp 710–718.

Sian L, Mingyan X, Miller LV, et al: Zinc absorption and intestinal losses of endogenous zinc in young Chinese women with marginal zinc intakes. Am J Clin Nutr 1996; 63:348–353.

Sies H, Stahl W, Sundquist AR: Antioxidant functions of vitamins. *In* Sauberlich HE, Machlin LJ (eds): Beyond Deficiency, Ann N Y Acad Sci 1992; 669:7–20.

Skeaff M: Vitamin C and E. *In* Mann J, Truswell AS (eds): Essentials of Human Nutrition, 2nd ed. Oxford, Oxford University Press, 2002, pp 231–247.

Taylor A: Detection and monitoring of disorders of essential trace elements. Ann Clin Biochem 1996; 33: 486–510.

The findings in deficiencies of essential trace elements due to metabolic disorders, with descriptions of the clinical disorders, the clinical signs and test results for the assessment of trace element status, the findings, interpretability and utility of the data; nonoccupational disorders associated with accumulation of essential trace elements; protocols for testing in genetic, therapeutic, and disease states, including nonanalytical factors affecting interpretation and analytical techniques.

Truswell S: Vitamins D and K. In Mann J, Truswell AS (eds): Essentials of Human Nutrition, 2nd ed. Oxford, Oxford University Press, 2002b, pp 249–258.

Truswell S, Milne R: The B vitamins. *In* Mann J, Truswell AS (eds): Essentials of Human Nutrition, 2nd ed. Oxford, Oxford University Press, 2002a, pp 209–230.

Veillon C: Trace element analysis of biological samples. Anal Chem 1986; 58:851A–866A.

Wang LC, Bushey S: Acquired acrodermatitis enteropathica. N Engl J Med 2005; 352:1121.

Wapnir RA: Copper absorption and bioavailability. Am J Clin Nutr (Suppl) 1998; 67:1054S–1060S.

Wastney ME, House WA, Barnes RM, et al: Kinetics of zinc metabolism: variation with diet, genetics and disease. J Nutr 2000; 130(5S Suppl): 1355S–1359S.

West CE: Vitamin A and carotenoids. *In* Mann J, Truswell AS (eds): Essentials of Human Nutrition, 2nd edition. Oxford, Oxford University Press, 2002, pp 188–207.

Wildman REC, Medeiros DM: Advanced Human Nutrition. Boca Raton, CRC Press, 2000.

Presents the biochemistry and physiology of the vitamins and the essential trace elements including tables of functions, tissue content and excretion, deficiency and toxicity symptoms, and the food sources with their micronutrient content.

Williams DM: Clinical significance of copper deficiency and toxicity in the world population. *In* Prasad AS (ed): Clinical, Biochemical, and Nutritional Aspects of Trace Elements. New York, Alan R Liss, 1982, pp 277–299.

Williams P: Food toxicity and safety. *In* Mann J, Truswell AS (eds): Essentials of Human Nutrition, 2nd edition. Oxford, Oxford University Press, 2002, pp 416–432.

Willis MS, Monaghan SA, Miller ML, et al: Zinc-induced copper deficiency. Am J Clin Pathol 2005; 123:125–131.

II

PART III

Urine and Other Body Fluids

Edited by

Richard A. McPherson MD, Gregory A. Threatte MD,
Matthew R. Pincus MD PhD, Mark S. Lifshitz MD

Basic Examination of Urine

Richard A McPherson, MD, Jonathan Ben-Ezra, MD Shourong Zhao, MD

KEY POINTS

• Many different diseases can display abnormalities in the urine. Therefore, examination of the urine is an important laboratory function.

• Basic urinalysis consists of gross examination of the urine, and a dipstick analysis for blood, white cells, sugar, and other substances. The dipstick may be read either manually or by an automated instrument.

• A microscopic analysis of urine may be necessary in many cases. This is to detect cellular elements, casts, and crystals. Each of these items can be caused by several different disease states.

• Although microscopic examination of the urine is usually performed manually, there are several automated instruments that can perform this analysis.

• Red blood cells within the urine can come from any point along the urinary tract. Dysmorphic red blood cells are often a sign of glomerular disease.

• The first voided morning urine, because it is the most concentrated, is often the best specimen for analysis. Some procedures may require a 12- or 24-hour urine sample.

• Specific gravity and osmolality measurements reflect the concentrating ability of the kidneys. After a period of dehydration, the osmolality should be three to four times that of plasma.

• Proteinuria of over 4 g/day is seen in the nephrotic syndrome. Although nephrotic syndrome is usually seen in primary renal disease, it can occasionally be seen in a systemic disease which affects the kidneys.

• Ketonuria can be seen in diabetics. It can also be seen in other states, such as febrile illnesses and cachexia.

• The dipstick nitrite and leukocyte esterase tests are used to help diagnose urinary tract infections. Positive results should be confirmed by microscopic analysis of the urine.

• Urinary calculi are most commonly formed from calcium. Work-up of habitual stone formers should include both analysis of the urine and of the stone.

A significant amount of information can be obtained through the examination of urine. Careful examination enables the detection of disease processes intrinsic to the urinary system, both functional (physiologic) and structural (anatomic). The progression or regression of various lesions can also be monitored with only minimal distress to the patient. Furthermore, systemic disease processes, such as endocrine or metabolic abnormalities, can be detected through the recognition of abnormal amounts of disease-specific metabolites excreted in the urine. Laboratory urine tests will continue to play an essential role in clinical medicine.

The purpose of this chapter is to highlight the pertinent information that can be provided by the most common urine tests. Two main types of urinalysis are currently performed. These include (1) the dipstick (reagent strip) urinalysis, which is commonly performed in screening laboratories, physician offices, and as patient home testing; and (2) the basic (routine) urinalysis, which adds a microscopic examination of urine sediment to the reagent strip urinalysis. These examinations utilize various laboratory disciplines, particularly chemistry and microscopy. In addition to these front line diagnostic procedures, new technologies including immunocytochemistry, molecular diagnostics, DNA ploidy, and cell cycle analysis are constantly evolving to provide additional diagnostic and prognostic information. Urine microbiology studies, crucial to the diagnosis of infectious pathogens of the urinary tract, are addressed elsewhere in this text. It is important to remember that each of these modalities has a certain clinical utility, and Table 27–1 lists the benefits of commonly ordered urine laboratory examinations.

Dipstick urinalysis provides information about multiple physiochemical properties of urine. Used predominantly in screening, dipstick testing requires less sophisticated training of personnel, and results are obtainable in only a few minutes. It has been shown that in certain situations, particularly when evaluating patients with signs or symptoms that prompt a urinalysis for the detection of blood or infection, urinalysis dipsticks can be substituted for a full routine urinalysis, with urine microscopy reserved for patients with discordance between clinical presentation and dipstick results (Jou, 1998). The routine urinalysis consists of two major components: (1) physicochemical determinations (appearance, specific gravity, and reagent strip measurements), and (2) a brightfield or phase contrast microscopic examination of urine sediment for evidence of hematuria, pyuria, casts (cylindruria), and crystalluria. The latter examination is typically more time consuming and necessitates expertise in microscopy for an accurate interpretation; however, instrumentation is now available that automates routine urinalysis partially or completely. Cytopathologic urine sediment examination also requires special training, and is the mainstay for diagnosis and follow-up of urinary tract neoplasms, as well as some non-neoplastic conditions, particularly renal allograft rejection.

We present in detail the pertinent components of the routine urinalysis. The various methodologies are briefly reviewed including sample preparation, reagent strip reactions, confirmatory testing, and microscopic methods. Major emphasis is given to clinicopathologic correlation relating to the laboratory findings obtained from these urine tests.

III

Table 27–1 Benefits of Common Urine Laboratory Tests

Type of test	Aims	Clinical utility			
		Screen	Diagnosis	Monitor	Prognosis
Urine chemistry (reagent strip)	Glucosuria Proteinuria Hematuria Leukocyturia Infection	+++	±	+	+
Wet urinalysis (routine)	Diabetes Proteinuria Hematuria Leukocyturia Infections Cylindruria Crystalluria	++++	++	++	+
Urine microbiology	Infections	++	++++	++	+
Urine cytology (conventional)	Cancer Inflammation Viral infections	+	++	+	–
Cytodiagnostic urinalysis	Glomerular and renal tubular disorders LUT disorders Nonbacterial infections Lithiasis	+	++++	+++	++
Image cytometry and DNA analysis	Urothelial cancer	–	++	+++	+++
Flow cytometry	Urothelial cancer	–	+	+++	++

LUT = Lower urinary tract.

From Schumann GB, Schumann JL, Marcussen N: Cytodiagnostic Urinalysis of Renal and Lower Urinary Tract Disorders. New York, Igaku-Shoin Medical Publishers, 1995, with permission.

Urine Formation

In the normal adult, approximately 1200 mL of blood perfuses the kidneys each minute, which accounts for about 25% of the cardiac output. The glomeruli (normally numbering at least 1 million per kidney) receive blood through afferent arterioles, and an ultrafiltrate of the plasma passes through each glomerulus into Bowman's space. From here the filtrate is passed through the tubules and collecting ducts where reabsorption or secretion of various substances and the concentration of urine can occur. Ultimately, the original glomerular filtrate volume of about 180 L in 24 hours is reduced to about 1–2 L, depending on the status of hydration. This urine formed in the kidneys passes from the collecting ducts into the renal pelvis, ureters, bladder, and urethra to be voided.

The kidneys take part in several regulatory functions. Through glomerular filtration and tubular secretion, numerous waste products are eliminated from the body, including nitrogenous products of protein catabolism, and both organic and inorganic acids and bases. Fluid, electrolytes (including sodium, potassium, calcium, and magnesium), and acid–base status are regulated in homeostasis. Furthermore, the kidneys provide important hormonal regulation with erythropoietin and renin production, as well as vitamin D activation. Any derangement of these functions by renal or systemic disease can be reflected as chemically or cytologically altered urine.

Components of Basic (Routine) Urinalysis

The basic (routine) urinalysis consists of four parts: specimen evaluation, gross/physical examination, chemical screening, and sediment examination.

Specimen Evaluation

Before one proceeds with any examination, the urine specimen must be evaluated in terms of its acceptability. Considerations include proper labeling, proper specimen for the requested examination, proper preservative, visible signs of contamination, and whether any transportation delays may have caused significant deterioration. Each laboratory should have written and enforced guidelines for the acceptance or rejection of specimens. A properly labeled specimen must have the patient's full name, and the date and time of collection. Additional information may be required by the institution, but these three essentials constitute minimum labeling requirements.

The first voided morning urine, which is the most concentrated, is best for routine urinalysis. At times, a catheterized specimen or suprapubic collected urine specimen is received. If a single specimen is submitted for multiple measurements, bacteriologic examination should be done first, provided that the urine has been properly collected. With pediatric patients and persons in acute renal failure, only a small volume of urine may be available for processing, and in such cases, a notation should be made and the measurements most pertinent to the diagnosis should be performed first. For quantitative measurements, timed (12- or 24-hour) urinary collection is preferred to random specimens.

Gross/Physical Examination

Appearance

Some of the more important changes in the gross appearance of urine are described in this section. A comprehensive list is provided in Table 27–2.

Color

The yellow color of urine is due largely to the pigment urochrome, excretion of which is generally proportional to the metabolic rate. It is increased during fever, thyrotoxicosis, and starvation. Small amounts of urobilins and uroerythrin (pink pigment) also contribute to urine coloration. In normal individuals, both pale and dark yellow urine can be produced, and these differences are rough indicators of hydration and urine concentration. Pale urine, typically of low specific gravity, is excreted following high fluid intake, while darker urine is seen when fluids are withheld. Note that pale urine of high specific gravity may be found in diabetes mellitus. For color changes of urine in pediatric patients, see Cone (1968). Table 27–3 lists the urine color changes associated with commonly used drugs.

Red Urine. The most common abnormal color is red or red-brown. When seen in females, menstrual flow contamination should be considered. Hematuria (presence of red blood cells, [RBCs]), hemoglobinuria, and myoglobinuria may produce pink, red, or red-brown coloration. All three of these conditions are easily detectable on reagent strip testing; however, further evaluation is necessary for absolute differentiation (see later under Blood, Hemoglobin, Hemosiderin, and Myoglobin in Urine).

In the porphyrias, urine coloration is variable. It is usually red in congenital erythropoietic porphyria and porphyria cutanea tarda, while in lead porphyrinuria the urine color is generally normal. In acute intermittent hepatic porphyria, it is normal but darkens on standing. Red urine also may be associated with the use of drugs and dyes in diagnostic tests; for example, phenolsulfonphthalein, which is sometimes used in assessing renal function, will cause a red color in alkaline urine. Patients with an unstable hemoglobin may produce urine with red-brown color that does not give a positive indication of hemoglobin or bilirubin. The pigment is probably a dipyrrole or bilifuscin. An innocuous red urine associated with ingestion of beets is seen in genetically susceptible persons.

Yellow-Brown or Green-Brown Urine. Yellow-brown or green-brown urine is generally associated with bile pigments, chiefly bilirubin. On shaking the urine specimen, a yellow foam may be seen, which distinguishes bilirubin from a normal, dark, concentrated urine, which will have white foam. In severe obstructive jaundice, the urine may be dark green.

Orange-Red or Orange-Brown Urine. Excreted urobilinogen is colorless, but is converted in the presence of light and low pH to urobilin, which is dark yellow to orange. Urobilin will not color the foam on shaking, and in this way may be confused with a concentrated normal urine; reagent strip testing would be confirmatory in this situation.

Dark Brown or Black Urine. Acid urine containing hemoglobin will darken on standing due to the formation of methemoglobin. 'Cola-colored' urine may be seen with rhabdomyolysis (Keverline, 1998) and in some patients taking L-dopa. Rarer causes of dark brown urine are

Table 27–2 Appearance and Color of Urine

Appearance	Cause	Remarks
Colorless	Very dilute urine	Polyuria, diabetes insipidus
Cloudy	Phosphates, carbonates	Soluble in dilute acetic acid
	Urates, uric acid	Dissolve at 60°C and in alkali
	Leukocytes	Insoluble in dilute acetic acid
	Red cells ('smoky')	Lyse in dilute acetic acid
	Bacteria, yeasts	Insoluble in dilute acetic acid
	Spermatozoa	Insoluble in dilute acetic acid
	Prostatic fluid	
	Mucin, mucous threads	May be flocculent
	Calculi, 'gravel'	Phosphates, oxalates
	Clumps, pus, tissue	
	Fecal contamination	Rectovesical fistula
	Radiographic dye	In acid urine
Milky	Many neutrophils (pyuria)	Insoluble in dilute acetic acid
	Fat	
	Lipiduria, opalescent	Nephrosis, crush injury – soluble in ether
	Chyluria, milky	Lymphatic obstruction – soluble in ether
	Emulsified paraffin	Vaginal creams
Yellow	Acriflavine	Green fluorescence
Yellow-orange	Concentrated urine	Dehydration, fever
	Urobilin in excess	No yellow foam
	Bilirubin	Yellow foam if sufficient bilirubin
Yellow-green	Bilirubin–biliverdin	Yellow foam
Yellow-brown	Bilirubin–biliverdin	'Beer' brown, yellow foam
Red	Hemoglobin	Positive ⎫
	Erythrocytes	Positive ⎬ reagent strip for blood
	Myoglobin	Positive ⎭
	Porphyrin	May be colorless
	Fuscin, aniline dye	Foods, candy
	Beets	Yellow alkaline, genetic
	Menstrual contamination	Clots, mucus
Red-purple	Porphyrins	May be colorless
Red brown	Erythrocytes	
	Hemoglobin on standing	
	Methemoglobin	Acid pH
	Myoglobin	Muscle injury
	Bilifuscin (dipyrrole)	Result of unstable hemoglobin
Brown-black	Methemoglobin	Blood, acid pH
	Homogentisic acid	On standing, alkaline; alkaptonuria
	Melanin	On standing, rare
Blue-green	Indicans	Small intestine infections
	Pseudomonas infections	
	Chlorophyll	Mouth deodorants

Table 27–3 Urine Color Changes with Commonly Used Drugs*

Drug	Color
Alcohol, ethyl	Pale, diuresis
Anthraquinone laxatives (senna, cascara)	Reddish, alkaline: yellow-brown, acid
Chlorzoxazone (Paraflex) (muscle relaxant)	Red
Deferoxamine mesylate (Desferal) (chelates iron)	Red
Ethoxazene (Serenium) (urinary analgesic)	Orange, red
Fluorescein sodium (given i.v.)	Yellow
Furazolidone (Furoxone) (Tricofuron) (an antibacterial, antiprotozoal nitrofuran)	Brown
Indigo carmine dye (renal function, cytoscopy)	Blue
Iron sorbitol (Jectofer) (possibly other iron compounds forming iron sulfide in urine)	Brown on standing
Levodopa (L-dopa) (for parkinsonism)	Red then brown, alkaline
Mepacrine (Atabrine) (antimalarial) (intestinal worms, *Giardia*)	Yellow
Methocarbamol (Robaxin) (muscle relaxant)	Green-brown
Methyldopa (Aldomet) (antihypertensive)	Darkens; if oxidizing agents present, red to brown
Methylene blue (used to delineate fistulas)	Blue, blue-green
Metronidazole (Flagyl) (for *Trichomonas* infection, amebiasis, *Giardia*)	Darkening, reddish brown
Nitrofurantoin (Furadantin) (antibacterial)	Brown-yellow
Phenazopyridine (Pyridium) (urinary analgesic), also compounded with sulfonamides (Azo Gantrisin, etc.)	Orange-red, acid pH
Phenindione (Hedulin) (anticoagulant) (important to distinguish from hematuria)	Orange, alkaline; color disappears on acidifying
Phenol poisoning	Brown; oxidized to quinones (green)
Phenolphthalein (purgative)	Red-purple, alkaline pH
Phenolsulfonphthalein (also sulfobromophthalein)	Pink-red, alkaline pH
Rifampin (Rifadin, Rimactane) (tuberculosis therapy)	Bright orange-red
Riboflavin (multivitamins)	Bright yellow
Sulfasalazine (Azulfidine) for ulcerative colitis	Orange-yellow, alkaline pH

* Other commonly used drugs have been noted to produce color change once or occasionally: amitriptyline (Elavil) – blue-green; phenothiazines – red; triamterene (Dyrenium) – pale blue (blue fluorescence in acid urine). An extensive list may be found in Young et al: Clin Chem 1975; 21:379.

III

homogentisic acid (alkaptonuria) and melanin. Urine containing homogentisic acid will darken more rapidly when alkaline.

Clarity (Character)

Urine is normally clear, and the presence of particulate material in an unspun specimen warrants further investigation. The differential diagnosis for cloudy urine is broad, and includes several nonpathologic entities. Turbidity may simply be due to the precipitation of crystals or nonpathologic salts referred to as amorphous. Phosphate, ammonium urate, and carbonate can precipitate in alkaline urine; these redissolve when acetic acid is added. Uric acid and urates cause a white, pink, or orange cloud in acid urine and redissolve on warming to 60°C.

Cloudy urine can be attributed to the presence of various cellular elements. Leukocytes may form a white cloud similar to that caused by phosphates, but the cloud remains after acidification. Likewise, bacterial growth may cause a uniform opalescence that is not removed by acidification or by filtration, and it has been suggested that turbidimetric assessment using a double-beam turbidimeter may be useful for urine infection screening (Livsey, 1995). Turbidity may also be due to RBCs, epithelial cells, spermatozoa, or prostatic fluid. Prostatic fluid normally contains a few leukocytes and other formed elements.

Miscellaneous etiologies for cloudy urine include mucus from the lower urinary tract or genital tract, blood clots, menstrual discharge, and other particulate material such as pieces of tissue, small calculi, clumps of pus, and fecal material. Fecal material in urine may occur with a fistulous connection between the colon or rectum and bladder. Contamination with powders or with antiseptics that become opaque with water (phenols) will also cause a turbid urine.

Chyluria. This is a rare condition in which the urine contains lymph. It is associated with obstruction to lymph flow and rupture of lymphatic vessels into the renal pelvis, ureters, bladder, or urethra. Although parasitic infection with *Wuchereria bancrofti* (filariasis) is the prevailing etiology (Cortvriend, 1998), abdominal lymph node enlargement and tumors have also been associated with chyluria. Even with filariasis, this condition is rare.

The appearance of the urine varies with the amount of lymph present, ranging from clear to opalescent or milky. Clots may form, and if sufficient lymph is present, the urine may layer with the chylomicrons on top and fibrin and cells beneath. Chylomicrons may not be apparent microscopically unless they have coalesced as microglobules. This fatty material can be extracted from urine using an equal volume of ether or chloroform. Urine phosphates, in contradistinction, will not clear with this method.

Pseudochyluria occurs with the use of paraffin-based vaginal creams for the treatment of *Candida* infections.

Lipiduria. Fat globules appear in the urine most often with the nephrotic syndrome; these are neutral fats (triglycerides) and cholesterol. Lipiduria can also be present in patients who have sustained skeletal trauma with fractures to major long bones or the pelvis. Presumably, the source of lipid is exposed fatty marrow. Keep in mind that in addition to these endogenous lipids, oily contaminants such as paraffin may float on the urine surface as well. Microscopic examination of the urine may be required to classify fatty materials as Oil Red O positive droplets or cholesterol esters with polarization.

Odor

Urine normally will have a faint, aromatic odor of undetermined source. Specimens with extensive bacterial overgrowth can be recognized by an ammoniacal, fetid odor. Additionally, ingestion of asparagus or thymol produces distinctive odors in urine.

Characteristic urine odors associated with amino acid disorders include the following:

Isovaleric acidemia and glutaric acidemia	Sweaty feet
Maple syrup urine disease (MSUD)	Maple syrup
Methionine malabsorption	Cabbage, hops
Phenylketonuria	Mousy
Trimethylaminuria	Rotting fish
Tyrosinemia	Rancid

Lack of odor in urine from patients with acute renal failure suggests acute tubular necrosis rather than prerenal failure.

Urine Volume

Under ordinary conditions, the main determinant of urine volume is water intake. The average adult produces from 600–2000 mL of urine per day, with night urine generally not in excess of 400 mL. In pregnancy, the usual diurnal variation may be reversed. Young children, compared to adults, may excrete about three to four times as much urine per kilogram of body weight. Measurement of the urine output during timed intervals may be valuable in clinical diagnosis.

Increases in Urine Volume

Production of more than 2000 mL of urine in 24 hours is termed polyuria; nocturia is excretion of more than 500 mL of urine at night with a specific gravity of less than 1.018. In general, high volumes of urine tend to result in a low specific gravity.

Excessive intake of water (polydipsia) will result in polyuria, as will consumption of certain drugs with a diuretic effect, such as caffeine, alcohol, thiazides, and other diuretics. Intravenous solutions may increase the urine output. Increased salt intake and high-protein diets will also require more water for excretion.

Pathologic states that result in excess renal fluid loss/urine excretion can be divided into three groups:

Defective Hormonal Regulation of Volume Homeostasis. Diabetes insipidus can be due to either a deficiency (central/pituitary variety) of or renal unresponsiveness (nephrogenic) to antidiuretic hormone. In either situation, there is excessive thirst and water intake, together with marked polyuria and nocturia. Up to 15 L of urine per day may be produced.

Defective Renal Salt/Water Absorption. This can be due to the administration of diuretic agents, or an abnormality of the renal tubules, resulting in sodium wasting or impairment of the countercurrent mechanism. In progressive chronic renal failure, functioning renal tissue is diminished and the ability to concentrate urine is gradually lost. To excrete the daily renal water and solute load, an increase in urine volume per residual nephron results, and the urine eventually becomes iso-osmotic with the plasma ultrafiltrate.

Osmotic Diuresis. In diabetes mellitus with hyperglycemia there is an excessive amount of glucose excreted, causing a solute diuresis.

Decreases in Urine Volume

Oliguria is the excretion of less than 500 mL of urine per 24 hours, and anuria is the near complete suppression of urine formation. Water deprivation will cause a decrease in urine volume even before signs of dehydration appear. Oliguria can be rather abrupt in onset, as with acute renal failure, or due to a chronic progressive renal disease. In either case, retention of nitrogenous waste products (azotemia) can occur (see Chap. 14).

The causes of acute renal failure are classically categorized as follows.

Prerenal. Loss of intravascular volume may result from hemorrhage, or from dehydration associated with prolonged diarrhea, vomiting, excess sweating, or severe burns. So-called third spacing is the shifting of intravascular fluids to extracellular spaces. Additionally, conditions such as congestive heart failure, sepsis, anaphylaxis, or renal artery embolic occlusion may result in a decrease of renal blood flow.

Postrenal. Bilateral hydronephrosis, resulting from high-grade or longstanding obstruction of the urinary tract, may be associated with a marked decrease in urine flow and even anuria. This can occur with prostatic hyperplasia and carcinoma. Bilateral ureteral obstruction due to stones, clots, and sloughed tissue, and urethral obstruction due to stricture or valves are other forms of obstruction. The anuria associated with sulfonamide therapy and dehydration is due to obstruction caused by the precipitation of crystals in the renal tubules when the urinary pH is acidic.

Renal Parenchymal Disease. This should be considered only after other pre- and postrenal causes of oliguria have been ruled out. The list of conditions is extensive and includes various vascular disorders, acute glomerulonephritis, interstitial nephritis, and acute tubular necrosis (ATN). A common cause of ATN is renal ischemia due to either heart failure or hypotension. Numerous nephrotoxic agents may produce ATN, including several antibiotics, mercury, cadmium, carbon tetrachloride, and glycerol. Other etiologies include hemoglobinuria and myoglobinuria, associated with hemolysis and muscle damage, respectively, as well as excessive amounts of intratubular proteins or crystals.

Chronic renal failure, a progressive and irreversible loss of renal function, results from several disease entities. These include hypertensive and diabetes-associated nephrosclerosis, chronic glomerulonephritis, polycystic kidney disease, and other urologic disorders. Urinary specific gravity is low and proteinuria, casts, and renal cells may be evident. Pyelonephritis or interstitial nephritis will cause predominantly tubular dysfunction with polyuria early in the disease, but later oliguria of chronic renal failure supervenes.

Specific Gravity and Osmolality

The volume of excreted urine and the concentration of its solutes are varied by the kidney to maintain the homeostasis of body fluid and electrolytes. Specific gravity and osmolality measurements reflect the relative degree of concentration or dilution of a urine specimen. This in turn aids in evaluating the concentrating and diluting abilities of the kidneys. Both of these indices, as well as urine color, have been found to be reliable indicators of hydration status (Armstrong, 1998).

The specific gravity of a specimen indicates the relative proportion of dissolved solid components to total volume of the specimen; in other words, it reflects the density of the specimen. Osmolality, on the other hand, indicates the number of particles of solute per unit of solution. Larger particles, such as proteins and sugars, tend to elevate the specific gravity more than smaller electrolytes. In critical circumstances, the measurement of osmolality of urine (and plasma) is preferred to the measurement of specific gravity.

Specific Gravity

Urea (20%), sodium chloride (25%), sulfate, and phosphate contribute most of the specific gravity of normal urine. Normal adults with adequate fluid intake will produce urine of specific gravity 1.016–1.022 over a 24-hour period; however, normal kidneys have the ability to produce urine with specific gravity that ranges from 1.003–1.035. If a random specimen of urine has a specific gravity of 1.023 or more, concentrating ability can be considered normal. Minimum specific gravity after a standard water load should be less than 1.007.

Urines of low specific gravity are called hyposthenuric, the specific gravity being less than 1.007. In diabetes insipidus, loss of concentrating ability (as described above) results in large volumes of urine being produced with specific gravity as low as 1.001 (specific gravity of water is 1.000). Prolonged excretion of urine with low specific gravity can also be seen with various renal abnormalities including pyelonephritis and glomerulonephritis. High specific gravity can be seen after excess water loss/dehydration, adrenal insufficiency, hepatic disease, or congestive heart failure. When there is little or no variability between several specimens from a patient, and the specific gravity is fixed at about 1.010, this is known as isosthenuric. This finding is indicative of severe renal damage in which there is disruption of both concentrating and diluting abilities.

Methods. Several methods are available to measure specific gravity – reagent strip, refractometer, urinometer, and the falling drop method.

Reagent Strip. This is an indirect method for measuring specific gravity. The reagent area has three main ingredients present: polyelectrolyte, indicator substance, and buffer. The principle of this methodology is based on the pK_a change of the pretreated polyelectrolytes in relation to ionic concentration of the urine. When the ionic concentration is high, the pK_a is decreased, as is the pH. The indicator substance then changes color relative to ionic concentration and this is translated to specific gravity values. This method is not affected by high amounts of glucose, protein, or radiographic contrast material, all of which tend to elevate the specific gravity readings obtained from refractometers and urinometers, described below.

Refractometer. This is also an indirect method. The refractive index of a solution is related to the content of dissolved solids present. The index is the ratio of the velocity of light in air to the velocity of light in a solution. It varies directly with the proportion of particles in solution and, therefore, with the specific gravity.

The clinical refractometer is a device that requires only a few drops of urine (unlike the 15 mL of urine necessary with the urinometer). Although the refractometer measures refractive index of a solution, the scale used is valid only for urine and cannot be used to indicate the specific gravity of salt or sugar solutions. This should be kept in mind if salt solutions are to be used for calibration. Special graphs or tables are required to convert refractive index scale numbers to solute concentration in aqueous solutions if this should be required (American Optical Catalog Number 10403). The specific gravity reading on the refractometer is generally slightly lower than a urinometer reading on the same urine specimen by about 0.002.

Procedure.
A temperature-compensated hand model is available. The instrument is temperature compensated between 60° and 100°F. It is damaged by heat above 150°F and by immersion of the eyepiece and focusing ring in water. It should read zero with distilled water; the zero reading can be reset if necessary by breaking the seal over the setscrew, turning it with a small screwdriver, and resealing. Always check calibration daily. Copper sulfate solution can be adjusted to monitor a high specific gravity level as an additional check.

To make a specific gravity determination of urine, clean the surfaces of the cover and prism with a drop of distilled water and a damp cloth and allow it to dry. Close the cover. Hold horizontally and apply a drop of urine at the notched bottom of the cover so that it flows over the prism surface by capillary action. Point the instrument toward a light source at an angle that gives optimal contrast. Rotate the eyepiece until the scale is in focus. Read directly on the specific gravity scale the sharp dividing line between light and dark contrast. The entire procedure should be repeated with a second drop of urine from the same sample.

Urinometer. This is a hydrometer adapted to directly measure the specific gravity of urine at room temperature. It should be checked each day by measuring the specific gravity of distilled water. If the urinometer does not give a reading of 1.000, an appropriate correction must be applied to all readings taken with that urinometer. The accuracy of a urinometer may be further checked with solutions of known specific gravity.

Because temperature influences the specific gravity, urine samples should be allowed to come to room temperature before a reading is made, or a correction of 0.001 should be made for each 3°C above or below the calibration temperature indicated on the urinometer. Corrections must also be made for protein or glucose present; subtract 0.003 for every 1 g/dL of protein and 0.004 for every 1 g/dL of glucose.

Procedure.
The urinometer vessel is filled three fourths full with urine (minimum volume required is about 15 mL). The urinometer is inserted with a spinning motion to make sure that it is floating freely. (When reading the urinometer, be sure that it is not touching the sides or the bottom of the cylinder. Avoid surface bubbles, which obscure the meniscus.) Read the bottom of the meniscus.

Falling Drop Method. This is a direct method for measuring specific gravity. It is more accurate then the refractometer, and more precise then the urinometer. This method utilizes a specially designed column filled with water-immiscible oil. A measured drop of urine is introduced into the column, and as this drop falls, it encounters two beams of light; breaking the first beam starts a timer, while breaking the second turns it off. The falling time is measured electronically and expressed as a specific gravity (Free, 1996).

Osmolality
The normal adult with a normal fluid intake will produce a urine of about 500–850 mOsm/kg water. The normal kidney is able to produce a urine osmolality in the range of 800–1400 mOsm/kg water in dehydration, and a minimal osmolality of 40–80 mOsm/kg water during water diuresis. After a period of dehydration, the osmolality of the urine should be three to four times that of the plasma (e.g., with a plasma osmolality of 285 mOsm/kg water, the urine osmolality should be at least 855 mOsm/kg water).

Methods. The freezing point depression method is commonly employed. A solution containing 1 osmol or 1000 mOsm/kg water depresses the freezing point 1.86°C below the freezing point of water. For method, see Chapter 4.

Table 27–4 Recommendations for reagent strips

Storage

Protect from moisture and excessive heat.

Store in cool, dry area but not in a refrigerator.

Check for discoloration with each use; discoloration may indicate loss of reactivity.

Do not use discolored strips or tablets.

Keep container tightly stoppered.

Check manufacturer's directions with each new lot number for changes in procedure.

Testing

Test urine as soon as possible after receipt.

Remove only enough strips for immediate use; recap tightly.

Test a well-mixed, unspun urine sample.

Urine samples must be at room temperature before testing.

Do not touch the test area with fingers.

Do not use reagent strips in the presence of volatile acids or alkaline fumes.

Dip reagent strip into urine briefly – no longer than 1 second.

Drain excess urine off – run edge of strip along rim of tube or blot edge on absorbent paper.

Do not allow reagents to run together.

Do not lay reagent strip directly on workbench surface.

Follow exact timing recommendations for each chemical test.

Hold reagent strip close to the color chart and read under good lighting.

Know sources of error, sensitivity, and specificity of each test on the reagent strip.

Think! Make correlations between patient history and individual test, then follow through.

Chemical Screening

Reagent strips are the primary methodology for the chemical examination of urine. Although easily used, they represent multiple complex, state-of-the-art chemical reactions. Table 27–4 lists recommendations for both the storage and the use of reagent strips. Although the reading of the strips has traditionally been done manually, there are now automated instruments, such as the Bayer Atlas, that will aspirate a precise amount of urine, deposit it on the dipstick, and read the chemical reactions on the reagent strip by reflectance (Lyon, 2003; Penders, 2002). These systems provide excellent reproducibility of results, and are not prone to some of the inconsistencies which occur when human hands try to time the reactions, and human eyes attempt to discriminate different shades of color reactions.

It should be noted that reagent strip methods are changed periodically, sensitivities and color reactions altered, and new measurements added. Manufacturers supply tables of common interfering substances, and these should be consulted. Interference with ascorbic acid and drugs producing colored urines such as phenazopyridine (Pyridium) and other azo compounds, and methylthioninium chloride (methylene blue) may be encountered. More detailed information on drug interference is listed in Young (1990).

The chemical measures most commonly found on reagent strips will be discussed first, with less commonly measured chemical parameters following. A discussion on the clinical application of each analyte will precede reagent strip and other methodologies. Confirmatory methods will be included when available and necessary.

Urine pH
The kidneys and lungs normally work in concert to maintain acid–base equilibrium. The lung excretes carbon dioxide, whereas the renal contribution is that of reclaiming and generating bicarbonate, and secreting ammonium ions. The proximal renal tubule is responsible for the bulk of the bicarbonate reabsorption/generation, and the distal tubule provides the remaining function.

The tubular cells exchange hydrogen ions for sodium of the glomerular filtrate. The metabolic activity of the body produces nonvolatile acids, principally sulfuric, phosphoric, and hydrochloric acids, but also small amounts of pyruvic, lactic, and citric acids and ketone bodies. These are excreted by the glomerulus as salts (sodium, potassium, calcium, and ammonium salts) and, together with ammonia produced by the proximal tubules, can then go on to trap secreted hydrogen ions for elimination in the urine (see Ch. 14).

Normal pH

The average adult on a normal diet excretes about 50–100 mEq of hydrogen ions in 24 hours to produce urine of about pH 6. In healthy individuals, urine pH may vary from 4.6–8.

Acid Urine

Acid urine may be produced by a diet high in meat protein and with some fruits such as cranberries. During the mild respiratory acidosis of sleep, a more acid urine may be formed. Also, therapeutic acidification of the urine by various pharmacologic agents, including ammonium chloride, methionine, and methenamine mandelate, is used in the treatment of some calculi. This would include phosphate and calcium carbonate stones, which tend to develop in alkaline urines.

In acid–base disturbances, the pH of the urine reflects attempts at compensation by the kidneys. Patients with metabolic or respiratory acidosis should produce acid urine with increased titratable acidity and ammonium ion concentration. In diabetic ketoacidosis, large amounts of hydrogen ions are excreted, much of it as ammonium ion. In potassium depletion such as in hypokalemic alkalosis of prolonged vomiting or in hypercorticism, or with prolonged use of diuretics, there may be paradoxical aciduria with slightly acid urine in the presence of a metabolic alkalosis.

Alkaline Urine

Alkaline urine may be induced by use of a diet high in certain fruits and vegetables, especially citrus fruits. The urine tends to become less acid following a meal (the so-called alkaline tide). This was long believed to be a urinary compensation for gastric acid secretion; however, recent studies do not support this view (Johnson, 1995). Sodium bicarbonate, potassium citrate, and acetazolamide may be used to induce alkaline urine in the treatment of some calculi, particularly those composed of uric acid, cystine, or calcium oxalate. These agents may also be used in some urinary tract infections (the antibiotics neomycin, kanamycin, and streptomycin are more active in alkaline urine), in sulfonamide therapy, and in the treatment of salicylate poisoning.

The capacity to exchange hydrogen ion for cation and the formation of ammonia is decreased when tubular function is impaired. In classic renal tubular acidosis, glomerular filtration is normal but the distal tubular ability to form ammonia and exchange hydrogen ions for cations is defective. Systemic acidosis results. The urine is relatively alkaline, and the pH cannot be lowered below 6–6.5, even with the administration of an acid-loading substance. Additionally, titratable acidity and the concentration of ammonium are decreased (Singh, 1995). In proximal renal tubular acidosis there is bicarbonate wasting. This can also be found in Fanconi's syndrome.

In metabolic alkalosis, an alkaline urine with higher levels of urinary bicarbonate is produced and ammonia production is decreased. The kidney may produce urine with a pH as high as 7.8. In respiratory alkalosis, an alkaline urine is produced that is associated with increased excretion of bicarbonate.

Methods

Reagent Strip. Indicators methyl red and bromothymol blue give a range of orange, green, and blue colors as the pH rises, permitting estimation of pH values to within half a unit within the range of 5–9. It should be read immediately, but time is not critical. Care should be taken not to have excessively wet strips where acid buffer from the protein patch runs into the pH patch, causing it to become orange.

Measurement of urine pH and acidity must always be made on freshly voided specimens. If precise measurements are required, the container should be filled in order to minimize the amount of dead space and the urine covered tightly. The container should be kept cold, preferably on ice, but not frozen. On standing, the pH tends to rise because of loss of carbon dioxide and because bacterial growth produces ammonia from urea.

pH Electrode. Although the estimate of the pH obtainable by indicator strip is usually sufficient, in patients with disturbances of acid–base balance, urinary pH may be accurately measured with a pH meter with a glass electrode. Because the pH meter may tend to drift, it must be standardized with three buffers of known pH immediately prior to use. After standardization, spray the electrodes with distilled water, clean, and dry with tissue. Immerse the electrode in the urine sample, and report the pH of urine at the temperature of measurement.

Titratable Acidity of Urine. The pH of the urine is largely dependent on the amount of mono- and dibasic phosphate present. Titratable acidity is measured by titrating an aliquot of 24-hour urine (collected on ice) with 0.1 N NaOH with pH 7.4 as an end point. This measurement may be used together with urinary ammonia determination in patients with chronic acidosis of obscure origin. Normal titratable acidity is in the range of 200–500 mL 0.1 N NaOH (or 6 mL 0.1 N NaOH per kg body weight) or 20–40 mEq/24 h. This procedure can be found in previous editions of this book (Henry, 1996).

Protein in Urine

Normally, up to 150 mg of protein is excreted in the urine daily, with the average urine protein concentration varying from 2–10 mg/dL, depending on urine volume. Anderson has demonstrated more than 200 urinary proteins, derived both from plasma and the urinary tract (Anderson, 1979). About one third is albumin, and the remaining plasma proteins include small globulins, including α-, β-, and γ-globulins. Plasma proteins with molecular weight less than 50 000–60 000 pass through the glomerular basement membrane and are normally reabsorbed by proximal tubular cells. Albumin, molecular weight 69 000, is apparently filtered but only in very small amounts. Retinol binding, β_2-microglobulin, immunoglobulin light chains, and lysozyme are excreted in small amounts. Tamm–Horsfall glycoprotein (uromucoid), secreted by distal tubular cells and cells of the ascending loop of Henle, constitutes about one third or more of the total normal protein loss. Immunoglobulin A (IgA) in secretions of the urinary tract, enzymes and proteins from tubular epithelial cells, other desquamated cells, and leukocytes also contribute to urine protein.

Detection of an abnormal amount of protein in urine is an important indicator of renal disease because protein has a very low maximal tubular rate (Tm) of reabsorption; increased filtration of protein quickly saturates the reabsorptive mechanism. Screening methods are routinely used to differentiate normal protein excretion from abnormal, and therefore should not detect less than about 8–10 mg/dL in a normal adult with a normal rate of urine flow. The reagent strip method is sensitive to albumin; the acid precipitation methods detect all proteins and will therefore indicate the presence of globulins, as well as albumin. It should be noted that a very dilute random urine specimen may have a falsely low protein value. Because a positive result for protein is significant, it should be confirmed by a second method and on repeated specimens. Depending on the history and examination, confirmatory measurements for elevated protein should be accompanied by the evaluation of renal function, examination of the urine sediment, and urine culture.

Functional proteinuria is usually less than 0.5 g/day, and can be seen in various situations in which dehydration contributes to the level of protein measured in urine. With strenuous exercise, a mixture of high- and low-molecular-weight proteins appears in the urine, and many casts, both hyaline and granular, can be seen. Functional proteinuria may also accompany congestive heart failure, cold exposure, and fever. In any event, the proteinuria resolves with appropriate treatment or rest within 2–3 days.

Intermittent, transient proteinuria can occasionally be seen in patients with a normal history, physical examination, and otherwise normal renal function. Except for the occasional proteinuria, urinalysis is also normal. These patients are typically followed every 6 months to check for hypertension or other abnormalities, and the overall prognosis is good. A transient proteinuria may also occur in normal pregnancy, but any proteinuria in pregnancy is an important finding and requires investigation. Persistent proteinuria of 1–2 g/day in an asymptomatic person, or when accompanied by hematuria, has a poorer prognosis than intermittent (transient) or postural proteinuria.

Postural Proteinuria

Postural proteinuria (orthostatic) occurs in 3–5% of apparently healthy young adults. In this condition, proteinuria is found during the day but not at night when a recumbent position is assumed. Persistent proteinuria may develop in some of these healthy subjects at a later date, and renal biopsies have shown abnormalities of the glomerulus in a few cases (Robinson, 1961). Proteinuria is apparently related to an exaggerated lordotic position and may result from renal congestion or ischemia. The total daily excretion of protein rarely exceeds 1 g, and in most instances, no other evidence of renal disease develops.

To evaluate the possibility of postural proteinuria, the patient is instructed to empty his or her bladder upon going to bed in the evening. Immediately upon rising in the morning, the patient voids and saves this specimen. After 2 hours of standing and walking about, the patient voids again and saves the specimen. The two urine specimens are assessed for protein, and if the first is negative and the second positive, the patient may have postural proteinuria. Frequent examination of the patient should be made to re-evaluate this condition.

Proteinuria in the Elderly

The incidence of significant proteinuria found on urinalysis in the elderly population is substantially increased when compared with patients below age 60. It has been estimated that the elderly population in general has a three- to fourfold greater incidence of glomerulonephritis, approximately one quarter of those affected having a minimal change-like disorder that may respond to steroid therapy. Occult malignancies in this population may also give rise to membranous glomerulonephritis, with resultant proteinuria (Threatte, 1986).

Proteinuria Quantification

More useful information for diagnosis of kidney disease and for following response to treatment is obtained by quantitatively analyzing the amount of protein excreted over a 24-hour period. It should be noted that the accuracy of measurements of any quantitative urine determination depends on the adequacy and completeness of the urine collection. Erroneous results are often related to collection problems. Repeat measurements may be needed to decide whether the proteinuria is intermittent or persistent.

Heavy Proteinuria (> 4 g/day). Heavy protein loss is characteristically seen with the nephrotic syndrome. Classically, a low serum albumin level, generalized edema, and increased serum lipids (cholesterol, triglycerides, and phosphatides) accompany this disorder. Lipoproteins, low density and very low density, are increased in serum, whereas high density lipoprotein, a smaller molecule, has been demonstrated in the urine (de Mendoza, 1976). It has been suggested that loss of lipoprotein lipase in urine contributes to the rise of serum lipid levels. γ-Globulin is also lost in the urine and this may contribute to a susceptibility to bacterial infections commonly found in nephrotic patients. When lipid is lost in urine, many granular casts, fatty casts, and fat-filled renal tubular epithelial cells (oval fat bodies) are found in the sediment. Cholesterol ester droplets may be demonstrable by polarization.

Nephrotic syndrome is principally associated with glomerular dysfunction/damage due to (1) primary renal diseases, including idiopathic disease and (2) systemic diseases with renal involvement. Transient or mechanical causes include severe congestive heart failure, constrictive pericarditis, and renal vein thrombosis. The last as a consequence of the nephrotic syndrome because of losses of anticlotting factors in urine and elevation of serum fibrinogen. In children, a common cause of nephrotic syndrome is minimal change disease (also known as nil lesion), a steroid-responsive glomerular disorder. Acute, rapidly progressive, and chronic glomerulonephritis are causes of heavy proteinuria, and may be accompanied by urinary erythrocytes or erythrocyte casts. Diabetes mellitus and lupus erythematosus are systemic diseases that frequently cause glomerular injury and heavy proteinuria. Urine sediment may be 'telescoped,' that is, display all kinds of cells and casts in lupus nephritis or with a hypersensitivity reaction. Malaria, malignant hypertension, toxemia of pregnancy, heavy metals (gold, mercury), drugs (penicillamine), neoplasia in general, amyloidosis, sickle cell disease, renal transplant rejection, and rarely primary antiphospholipid syndrome (Levy, 1998) are additional causes of heavy proteinuria.

Moderate Proteinuria (1.0–4.0 g/day). Moderate proteinuria may be found in the vast majority of renal diseases, including those mentioned above, as well as nephrosclerosis, multiple myeloma, and toxic nephropathies. Also included are degenerative, malignant, and inflammatory conditions of the lower urinary tract, including irritative conditions such as the presence of calculi.

Minimal Proteinuria (< 1.0 g/day). Minimal proteinuria may be noted in chronic pyelonephritis, in which case it may be intermittent, and in relatively inactive phases of glomerular diseases. It is also seen with nephrosclerosis, chronic interstitial nephritis, congenital diseases such as polycystic disease and medullary cystic disease, and renal tubular diseases. In tubular diseases, the urinary sediment is usually not abnormal, but erythrocytes, leukocytes, and tubular cells may be seen with interstitial nephritis. Significant sediment findings may, however, sometimes accompany trace protein results. Minimal proteinuria is also present in postural proteinurias and transient proteinuria.

Qualitative Categories of Proteinuria

The detection of the types of protein present in urine requires electrophoretic separation of urine proteins. Based on these and on clinical findings, proteinuria may be separated into a glomerular pattern and tubular pattern, indicating which part of the nephron is primarily involved. However, these anatomic entities tend to merge as disease progresses.

Glomerular Pattern. Glomerular disease causes proteinuria, which may be heavy (> 3–4 g/day). A loss or reduction of the fixed negative charge on the glomerular basement membrane allows albumin to permeate into Bowman's space in large quantities, more than can be reabsorbed by the proximal tubular cells. When serum albumin is lost in urine, other proteins of similar size or charge are also lost (e.g., antithrombin, transferrin, prealbumin, α_1-acid glycoprotein, α_1-antitrypsin). Because tubular function

may still be normal, very small plasma proteins are largely reabsorbed. Large proteins, in contradistinction, are not seen in urine while the glomerulus is still selective (e.g., α_2-macroglobulin and β-lipoprotein). As larger proteins appear, the proteinuria is less selective, indicating greater damage to the glomerulus (e.g., with membranous nephropathy and proliferative glomerulonephritis).

Tubular Pattern. This is associated with loss of a small amount of urinary protein that would otherwise be largely reabsorbed. These proteins are usually of low molecular weight (e.g., α_1-microglobulin, β-globulins such as β_2-microglobulin, light chain immunoglobulins, and lysozyme), usually without a clear predilection for albumin-sized molecules. By radioimmunoassay, β_2-microglobulin excretion has been measured in microgram amounts in urine as an indication of tubular damage; its normal excretion is about 100 µg/day. A tubular pattern proteinuria occurs with renal tubular diseases such as Fanconi's syndrome, cystinosis, Wilson's disease, and pyelonephritis, and with renal transplantation rejection. The amount of proteinuria is typically lower than that seen with glomerular diseases, and is about 1–2 g/day. Tubular proteinuria may be missed by the reagent strip test because of the absence or very low amounts of albumin, but may be detected by an acid precipitation method.

Overflow Proteinuria. Overflow proteinuria is due to the overflow of excess levels of a protein in the circulation, and can be seen with hemoglobin, myoglobin, or immunoglobulin loss into the urine. These proteins are not initially associated with glomerular or tubular diseases, but may themselves cause renal damage. Myoglobin may cause acute tubular necrosis (see under Myoglobin). Hemoglobin in low amounts is not thought to be toxic unless hypovolemia is present.

Bence Jones Proteinuria. Bence Jones proteinuria is associated with multiple myeloma, macroglobulinemia, and malignant lymphomas. The incidence of Bence Jones proteinuria in multiple myeloma has been estimated as 50–80%; however, its demonstration depends greatly on the technique used. Bence Jones protein may be missed altogether if only a reagent strip test for protein is used. Electrophoresis and immunofixation electrophoresis (IFE) methods are the best detection and quantification methods.

Excretion of Bence Jones protein in large amounts, sometimes several grams in 24 hours, causes the tubular cells to deteriorate because of the high levels of protein reabsorbed. Inclusions may form in the cells, and desquamated cells may form casts in the tubular lumen. Casts also form from immunoglobulin and Tamm–Horsfall protein mixtures. With renal failure, less protein is reabsorbed and more Bence Jones protein and other proteins appear in the urine. The damaged kidney is sometimes called a myeloma kidney, and the nephrotic syndrome may follow.

Microalbuminuria. Microalbuminuria is the presence of albumin in urine above the normal level but below the detectable range of conventional urine dipstick methods. Several authors have suggested that these lower urine albumin levels ranging from 20–200 mg/L (or an approximate rate of excretion of 20–200 µg/min) are an indicator of early and possibly reversible glomerular damage (Mogensen, 1984; Viberti, 1982). In diabetic patients, microalbuminuria is associated with a four- to sixfold increase in cardiovascular mortality, and is an independent risk factor for renal mortality (Zelmanovitz, 1998; Bakris, 1996). It is also more prevalent in hypertensive subjects (Gerber, 1998). Various methodologies have been introduced, including immunologic test systems and dye-binding chemical test strips, both of which will be discussed below.

Methods

Several screening methods and quantitative methods are available for the analysis of protein in urine. Because a positive screening test may have serious implications, it is important to be able to confirm results by a second, different method. Common screening tests include the qualitative/semiquantitative colorimetric reagent strip test, as well as precipitation-based testing (see Table 27–5).

Accurate results are obtained with reagent strips only when albumin is increased. Because of the lack of sensitivity of the reagent strip to globulins, it may be necessary to use an acid precipitation method for screening purposes. This will depend on the patient population and the diseases being screened. Reagent strips do have the advantage of avoiding false-positive reactions with organic iodides, such as those used for X-ray contrast and tolbutamides or other drugs.

Most other qualitative screening methods rely on protein precipitation (e.g., with heat and acetic acid, with nitric acid, and with sulfosalicylic [SSA] and trichloroacetic acids). These methods will precipitate globulins as well as albumin. In practice, negative reagent strips with positive SSA methodology in urine specimens are attributable to X-ray dye, to

Table 27–5 Screening Test for Detection of Proteinuria

Urine constituents or condition	Reagent strip	Acid precipitation
Highly buffered alkaline urine	May cause FP	May cause FN
Drug metabolites	No effect	May cause FP
Radiocontrast media	No effect	May cause FP
Turbidity	No effect	May cause FP
Quarternary ammonium groups or chlorhexidine	May cause FP	No effect

FP = false positive; FN = false negative.

penicillins, and rarely to an isolated increase in globulins. Sulfosalicylic and trichloroacetic acids are used to precipitate protein in the cold and are used as a convenient screening method. The sensitivity may be as low as 0.25 mg/dL, depending on the technique used.

Reagent Strip. This method takes advantage of the protein-error of pH indicators. Because proteins carry a charge at physiologic pH, their presence will elicit a pH change. The reagent strip is impregnated with tetrabromphenol blue buffered to an acid pH of 3, or tetrachlorophenol-tetrabromosulfophthalein. In the absence of protein the strip is yellow; 30–60 seconds following urine application, variable shades of green develop depending on the type and concentration of protein present. Results may be read in a 'plus' system as negative, trace, and 1+ to 4+. Most methods will detect 5–20 mg of albumin per deciliter.

As stated above, reagent strips tend to be more sensitive to albumin than to globulins, Bence Jones protein, or mucoprotein. 'Trace' results may be seen with physiologic normal excretion of protein in concentrated urine specimens from healthy individuals. High salt levels will lower results. Exceptionally alkaline and/or highly buffered urine samples may give positive results in the absence of significant proteinuria (e.g., with a patient on alkaline medication or with bacterial contamination). False-positive results can occur with quaternary ammonium compounds, amidoamines in fabric softeners, chlorhexidine, and with excessive leaching of the acid buffer of the test strip by excessive wetting. The method is unaffected by urine turbidity, radiographic media, and most drugs or their metabolites.

Sulfosalicylic Acid Method – Qualitative.

This method depends on formation of a precipitate for determination of the presence of protein.

Procedure. Specimens should be centrifuged, and a clear supernatant used. To approximately 3 mL of supernatant urine in a clean test tube, aliquot an equal amount of 3% SSA. Invert to mix. Let stand exactly 10 minutes. Invert again twice. Using ordinary room light (not a lamp), observe the degree of turbidity and/or precipitation and grade the results according to the following descriptions:

Negative – no turbidity (~ 5 mg/dL or less)
Trace – perceptible turbidity (~ 20 mg/dL)
1+ – Distinct turbidity, but no discrete granulation (~ 50 mg/dL)
2+ – Turbidity with granulation, but no flocculation (~ 200 mg/dL)
3+ – Turbidity with granulation and flocculation (~ 500 mg/dL)
4+ – Clumps of precipitated protein, or solid precipitate (~ 1.0 g/dL or more).

This method will detect about 5–10 mg/dL. Albumin, globulins, glyco-proteins, and Bence Jones proteins are all detected. High levels of detergents may decrease the result. When radiographic dye is present, SSA precipitate will increase on standing and typical crystals are seen on the microscopic examination of the precipitate. In this situation, another urine specimen from the patient should be assayed. However, the effects of the radiographic media may persist up to 3 days. A reagent strip test may be substituted, or the heat and acetic acid method may be used. In the acetic acid method, radiographic contrast media will clear with heat, whereas protein will increase.

Quantitative Protein Determinations and Confirmatory Methods.
Quantitative measurements of urine protein are typically adaptations of one of the various precipitation methods, or are colorimetric in nature. SSA and trichloroacetic acid (TCA) are commonly used as precipitants; the resultant turbidity can be measured by a photometer or nephelometer. If a visual interpretation is performed, a set of gelled commercial standards that correspond to 10, 20, 30, 40, 50, 75, and 100 mg/dL may be used, with results reported in milligrams per deciliter as opposed to the 'plus' method of screening precipitation tests. With SSA, the turbidity produced with albumin is 2.4 times that produced with globulin, and polypeptides,

glycoproteins, and Bence Jones proteins are also precipitated with this method. Of historic note, Exton's reagent contains sulfosalicylic acid, sodium sulfate, and an indicator – bromphenol blue. TCA, in contradistinction, will cause γ-globulin to be precipitated with greater turbidity than albumin; however, the difference is not marked.

More precise measurements suitable for smaller amounts of protein are available, and in these methods, a TCA precipitate is dissolved in sodium hydroxide and measured by use of the biuret reaction. The quantitative TCA-biuret method is tedious but gives good precision. A color correction blank is used. For a comparison of biuret methods with the SSA turbidity method, see Lizana (1977).

Several dye-binding colorimetric methods are available to quantitate urine protein. These include Coomassie blue, Ponceau S, and benzethonium chloride turbidity methods (McElderry, 1982). Pyrogallol Red-Molybdate will also react with protein to form a bluish purple complex that absorbs at 600 nm.

Methods used to quantitate urinary protein have not been satisfactory. Participants in the College of American Pathologists' (CAP) proficiency testing surveys will be aware that the mean values reported vary twofold between methods, with the SSA method producing high values. Precision is poor, with the SSA turbidimetric method showing the poorest coefficient of variation. The TCA-biuret, Coomassie blue, and TCA turbidity methods show closer agreement and about half the coefficient of variation of the SSA method. Problems arise from nonstandardized methods. With turbidity methods, these include different acid concentrations and timing, and variation in the protein standard.

Microalbuminuria Determination Methods. Very small amounts of proteins, such as albumin and β$_2$-microglobulin, are measured by immunologic means using antibodies to the proteins, nephelometric methods, or radioimmunoassay. The Micral II test strip (Boehringer Mannheim, Indianapolis, IN) is an immunologic test system that gives an almost immediate, reliable semiquantitative determination of low urine albumin concentrations (Kutter, 1998). Oxytetracycline may interfere with this method, causing higher readings. There is no interference with pH. A newer method, the Clinitek microalbumin (Bayer Diagnostics, Tarrytown, NY), is a highly sensitive dye-binding method. It also has the further advantage of an additional test pad for the simultaneous measurement of creatinine concentration. This method is not absolutely specific for albumin, for the dye compound also reacts with Tamm–Horsfall mucoprotein.

Bence Jones Proteinuria Determination Methods. The best method for detection of Bence Jones protein in urine is by protein electrophoresis. The traditional electrophoretic procedure employs the Amido black stain on a 200-fold concentrated urine. Newer methods, performed on less concentrated urine, including a modified Coomassie brilliant blue stain, are comparably sensitive and specific (Wong, 1997). The presence of Bence Jones globulin or clonal production of immunoglobulin is indicated by a single sharp peak in the globulin region on protein electrophoresis. Bence Jones globulin represents either the κ or λ immunoglobulin light chain.

Bence Jones protein precipitates at temperatures between 40° and 60°C, and redissolves near 100°C. Other methods depend on precipitation in the cold with salts, ammonium sulfate, and acids. In the presence of marked Bence Jones proteinuria, most methods yield positive results. When only a small amount of Bence Jones protein is present or when other globulins are present, results may be doubtful. False-positive reactions are seen when other globulins are precipitated by acetic acid in the heat precipitation method. A false-negative reaction may occur if the Bence Jones protein is too concentrated and the precipitate does not redissolve on boiling.

Glucose and Other Sugars in Urine

Various sugars may be found in the urine under certain circumstances, both pathologic and physiologic. These include glucose, fructose, galactose, lactose, maltose, pentose, and sucrose. Glucose is by far the most common, and will be discussed below.

Glucose

The presence of detectable amounts of glucose in urine is termed glycosuria, and this condition occurs whenever the glucose level in the blood surpasses the renal tubule capacity for reabsorption. Glucose may appear in the urine at different blood glucose levels, and there is not always a concomitant hyperglycemia. Glomerular blood flow, tubular reabsorption rate, and urine flow also will influence its appearance. When hyperglycemia is present, however, glycosuria usually occurs when the blood level is more than 180–200 mg/dL. Glycosuria may be seen in several different conditions described below.

Diabetes Mellitus. Although hyperglycemia alone is not necessarily indicative of diabetes mellitus, the appearance of glucose in the urine necessitates further work-up. When glycosuria is present, it is typically accompanied by polyuria and thirst. Inadequate carbohydrate utilization in these patients results in elevated ketone levels in the blood and urine due to increased fat metabolism.

For diabetics, the advantage of a urine method over a blood test for glucose is that it is painless and inexpensive. Urine glucose measurements are most useful for well-controlled diabetics who do not have to make frequent adjustments in their insulin/hypoglycemic agents. In insulin-dependent diabetes, a negative urine measurement could correspond to a wide range of serum glucose levels: this is attributed to a great variation in renal threshold for glucose in diabetic patients. Therefore, urine measurements may be misleading, and home blood glucose monitoring is preferred.

Monitoring for glycosuria in diabetic patients is not without problems. Reagent strips may be difficult to interpret at the 1 g/dL (1%) and 2 g/dL (2%) glucose levels, and copper reduction tests or newer, more sensitive reagent strips may be more efficacious. With the Clinitest tablet method, diabetic patients are able to estimate reducing substance levels in urine to about 10 g/dL, using one drop of specimen rather than two or five drops. In some clinics, the 24-hour urine glucose measurement is found to be useful for monitoring patients. It represents a defined longer time period, and with blood levels of glycated hemoglobin, it contributes to the regular overall long-term management of the disease.

Several studies have looked at the usefulness of urine dipstick testing for glycosuria as a screening method for diabetes, and the results have been mixed. Bullimore (1997) concentrated on patients over 50 years old in a general practice setting, and found this method to be practical and effective, whereas Friderichsen (1997) came to an opposing conclusion. He suggests that if diabetes screening is carried out in general practice, blood glucose measurements should be utilized for patients in selected risk groups. Routine dipstick glucose analysis can identify gravidas at increased risk for gestational diabetes (Gribble, 1995).

Other Causes of Glycosuria. Glycosuria with concomitant hyperglycemia is seen in several endocrine disorders (see Table 16–3). These include pituitary and adrenal disorders such as acromegaly, Cushing's syndrome, hyperadrenocorticism, functioning α- or β-cell pancreatic tumors, hyperthyroidism, and pheochromocytoma. Pancreatic disease with loss of functioning islet cells is also associated with glycosuria – for example, carcinoma, pancreatitis, and cystic fibrosis.

Numerous other causes of glycosuria with hyperglycemia have been recognized. These include central nervous system (CNS) disorders, including brain tumor or hemorrhage, hypothalamic disease, and asphyxia. Disturbances of metabolism associated with burns, infection, fractures, myocardial infarction, and uremia, as well as liver disease, glycogen storage diseases, obesity, and feeding after starvation may all be associated with glycosuria, as are certain drugs (e.g., thiazides, corticosteroids and adrenocorticotropic hormone [ACTH], and birth control pills).

In pregnancy, there is an increase in glomerular filtration rate and all of the filtered glucose may not be reabsorbed. In this situation, glycosuria may appear at relatively low blood glucose levels. Persistent, or greater than trace amounts, of glycosuria should be investigated. In some patients, diabetes occurs only during pregnancy. Glucose tolerance may also be decreased in the aged, especially when the patients have a poor intake of carbohydrate, but this is not necessarily accompanied by glycosuria.

Glycosuria without hyperglycemia is usually associated with renal tubular dysfunction. True inherited renal glycosuria is uncommon; it is associated with reduced glucose reabsorption. In renal tubular transport diseases, glycosuria may be accompanied by impairment of reabsorption of water, amino acid, bicarbonate, phosphate, and sodium, a pattern seen in Fanconi's syndrome. Galactosemia, cystinosis, lead poisoning, and myeloma are further examples of conditions associated with renal tubular dysfunction and possible glycosuria.

Other Sugars in Urine

Small amounts of disaccharides are normally excreted in the urine – about 50 mg in 24 hours. With intestinal diseases such as severe sprue or acute enteritis, the level may rise to 250 mg or more. Fructose, galactose, lactose, maltose, and L-xylulose are found in urine in patients with inherited metabolic disorders (Scriver, 1989). If an inherited disorder is suspected, the sugar may be identified by thin-layer chromatography. Qualitative confirmatory tests are generally not satisfactory for sugars.

Fructose. Fructose appears in urine in association with inherited enzyme deficiencies that cause benign essential fructosuria and serious fructose intolerance associated with severe vomiting and liver and kidney disease. Fructosuria may also be seen with parenteral feedings that include fructose. Urinary fructose can also be used as a marker of sucrose intake in dietary intervention studies (Luceri, 1996).

Galactose. Galactose is found in the urine in genetic disorders of galactose metabolism associated with a deficiency of galactose-1-phosphate uridyl transferase or galactokinase. In these diseases, galactose derived from dietary lactose is not converted to glucose, and early detection followed by dietary restriction may control the disease.

Lactose. Lactose may appear in the urine late in normal pregnancy or during lactation. In lactose intolerance, high levels of sugars accumulate in the gut, and lactose will be absorbed and excreted unchanged in the urine.

Pentose. Pentosuria may follow the ingestion of large amounts of fruits, causing the excretion of L-xylulose and L-arabinose in amounts up to 0.1 g/day. It may also be seen with certain drug therapies and with benign essential pentosuria.

Sucrose. Sucrose may appear in the urine after the ingestion of very large amounts of sucrose. Sucrase deficiency is associated with intestinal diseases such as sprue in the same manner as lactase deficiency. Sucrose intolerance is an inherited disorder associated with sucrase and α-dextrinase (isomaltase) deficiencies. Symptoms are similar to those seen with lactase deficiency and occur in the first few weeks of life when sweetened food is ingested. Tolerance may develop, but sucrose may have to be avoided permanently. Factitious sucrosuria may create a high-specific-gravity urine with negative glucose oxidase and negative copper reduction tests.

Methods

Reagent Strip. This method is based on a specific glucose oxidase and peroxidase method, a double sequential enzyme reaction; reagent strips differ only in the chromogen used. The method is specific for glucose. It does not react with lactose, galactose, fructose, or reducing metabolites of drugs. The reagent strips may be used for semiquantitative results, and results should be reported as approximate grams per deciliter. Combination glucose and ketone reagent strips not only detect ketonuria, they also help detect suppression of the glucose reaction by ketones seen with some reagent strips.

False-positive readings may be produced by strongly oxidizing cleaning agents in the urine container. Low specific gravity may falsely elevate results. Sodium fluoride used as a preservative will cause false-negative readings, as can a high specific gravity and occasionally ascorbic acid. Glycolytic enzymes from cells and bacteria will reduce glucose levels in urine on standing; prompt refrigeration or testing is essential.

Chemistry

$$Glucose + O_2 \xrightarrow{\text{Glucose oxidase}} Gluconic\ acid + H_2O_2$$

$$H_2O_2 + Chromogen \xrightarrow{\text{peroxidase}} Oxidized\ chromogen + H_2O$$

The chromogens utilized in some common dipstick tests include the following:

Clinistix – o-toluidine chromogen. Color changes from pink to purple. This formulation detects 100 mg/dL of glucose and is more sensitive to interfering substances such as ascorbic acid than the following.

Multistix – potassium iodide chromogen. Color changes from blue to brown at 30 seconds.

Chemstrip – an aminopropyl-carbazol chromogen. Color changes from yellow to orange-brown at 60 seconds.

Copper Reduction Tests. As a screening test, the glucose oxidase method will not detect increased levels of galactose or other sugars in urine. It is therefore important that a copper reduction method be used, especially for young pediatric patients. This method will detect sufficient quantities of any reducing substances in the urine, including reducing sugars such as lactose, fructose, galactose, maltose, and the pentoses. In those instances when the copper method is positive and the glucose oxidase method is negative, glycosuria is ruled out; but before investigating for other sugars, the clinical findings and drug history should be evaluated. Although the copper reduction method will detect nonglucose reducing sugars, the yield for these sugars is extremely low.

Normal neonatal infants during the first 10–14 days of life may excrete urine giving a positive reaction due to glucose, galactose, fructose, and lactose. Normal pregnant and postpartum women may also give positive reactions due to the presence of lactose.

Of the copper reduction methods used for screening purposes, the qualitative Benedict method is more sensitive to reducing substances in urine than the single-tablet (Clinitest) copper reduction method. Many substances in urine, metabolites, or drug-related metabolites will influence urinary sugar methods (Table 27–6). Strong reducing substances such as ascorbic acid, gentisic acid, or homogentisic acid may inhibit the enzyme method while contributing to the positivity of the copper reduction method. The tablet method is not affected as much as the Benedict method. Very large doses of ascorbic acid do not affect the two-drop copper reduction method. Drugs will give false-positive or unusual colors

CHAPTER: **27** Basic Examination of Urine

Table 27–6 Reactions of Substances to Test for Glucosuria

Constituent	Glucose oxidase reagent strip	Copper reduction tablet test
Glucose	Positive	Positive
Sugars other than glucose		
Fructose		
Galactose		
Lactose	No effect	Positive
Maltose		
Pentose		
Sucrose		
Ketones (large amounts)	May depress color	No effect
Creatine	No effect	May cause false positive
Uric acid		
Homogentisic acid (alkaptonuria)	No effect	Positive
Drugs*		
Ascorbic acid (large amounts)	May delay color	Trace positive
Cephalosporins (Keflin), etc.	No effect	Positive, brown color
L-Dopa (large)	False negative	No effect
Nalidixic acid glucuronide	No effect	Positive
Probenecid	No effect	Positive
Pyridium	Orange color may affect result	
Salicylate (large)	May lower reading	No effect
X-ray dye (diatrizoates)	No effect	Black color
Contaminants		
Hydrogen peroxide	False positive	May inhibit positive test
Hypochlorite (bleach)	False positive	
Sodium fluoride	False negative	No effect

* Other drugs implicated in copper reduction are amino acids, caronamide, chloral, chloroform, chloramphenicol. formaldehyde, hippuric acid, isoniazid, thiazides, oxytetracycline, p-aminosalicylic acid, penicillin, phenols, streptomycin, phenothiazine, and sulfonamides.

Data from Caraway (1962), Wirth (1965), Young (1975).

with Clinitest, especially the cephalosporins and radiographic media. Although large doses of ascorbic acid do not affect the two-drop Clinitest for sugars (i.e., do not cause false-positive results), delay may occur in color development with the glucose oxidase method.

Chemistry. Copper sulfate, sodium hydroxide, sodium carbonate, and citric acid are incorporated into each Clinitest tablet. Copper sulfate reacts with reducing substances in the urine, converting cupric sulfate to cuprous oxide. Based on Benedict's copper reduction reaction,

$$Cu^{2+} \xrightarrow{\text{Hot alkaline solution}} Cu^+$$

$$Cu^+ + OH^- \longrightarrow CuOH \text{ (yellow)}$$

$$2CuOH \xrightarrow{\text{Heat}} Cu_2O \text{ (red)} + H_2O$$

Heat is caused by the reaction of sodium hydroxide with water and citric acid.

Procedure. Clinitest reagent tablets will detect 250 mg of reducing substance per deciliter of urine. Both a five-drop and a two-drop Clinitest method can be used, and corresponding color charts are available (Belmonte, 1967). The two-drop method was developed in response to a so-called pass-through phenomenon that may occur if more than 2 g/dL of sugar is present in the urine. In the pass-through phenomenon, the solution that results after addition of the Clinitest tablet goes through the entire range of colors and back to a dark greenish brown. This final color does not compare with any section of the color chart; however, it corresponds most closely to a significantly lower result. It is important to observe the entire reaction and for 15 seconds after boiling inside the tube has stopped so that the reversion to a different color is not missed and a falsely low result reported.

Five-Drop Method.

Place five drops of urine in a dry test tube and add 10 drops of water. Add one Clinitest tablet by easing it into the tube without touching it – it

contains strong alkali. Watch while boiling takes place, but do not shake or touch the bottom of the tube – it is hot. Wait for 15 seconds after boiling stops, then shake the tube gently, and immediately compare the color of the solution with the color scale. Results correspond to the following approximate concentrations: negative; 0.25 g/dL; 0.5 g/dL; 0.75 g/dL; 1.0 g/dL; 2.0 g/dL; pass-through. It is important to watch the solution carefully while it is boiling. If the solution passes through orange to a dark shade of greenish brown, it indicates that more than 2 g/dL sugar is present, and this should be recorded as greater than 2 g/dL without reference to the color scale. Urine samples showing this pass-through phenomenon should be retested with the two-drop method.

Two-Drop Method.

Place two drops of urine in a test tube and add 10 drops of water. Add one Clinitest tablet. Watch while boiling takes place, but do not shake. Wait 15 seconds after the boiling stops, then shake the tube gently and compare the color of the solution with the color scale supplied for the two-drop method. The pass-through phenomenon may also occur with the two-drop method with large concentrations of sugar, over 5 g/dL. Report results as 1 g/dL, 2 g/dL, 3 g/dL, 5 g/dL, and more than 5 g/dL if a pass-through reaction occurs. Negative or low-level results should have the five-drop method performed.

Precautions. Observe the precautions in the literature supplied with the Clinitest tablets. The bottle must be kept tightly closed at all times to prevent absorption of moisture and kept away from direct heat and sunlight in a cool, dry place. The tablets normally have a spotted bluish white color. If not stored properly, they will absorb moisture or deteriorate from heat, turning dark blue or brown. In this condition, they will not give reliable results. They are also available individually packaged in aluminum foil to help prevent this absorption of moisture. Although more expensive, such packaging is useful when a limited number of measurements are performed.

Additional Tests for Sugars. As stated above, the copper reduction method will detect the majority of nonglucose sugars that might be present in urine, apart from sucrose, which is not a reducing sugar. It does not, however, differentiate between these sugars, therefore necessitating more complicated testing. Additional confirmatory testing will be discussed below.

Fructose. Fructose is identified by thin-layer chromatography. A qualitative measurement, a resorcinol test, is useful. Fructose will also reduce Benedict's reagent at low temperatures.

Galactose. Thin-layer chromatography is used to identify galactose in urine. However, the disease is usually identified by erythrocyte enzyme assay when suspected.

Lactose. Lactose is identified by thin-layer chromatography or a qualitative lactose test, such as described below.

Procedure.

To 15 mL urine in a test tube, add 3 g lead acetate. Shake and filter. Boil filtrate, add 2 mL concentrated NH_4OH, and boil. Lactose will cause the formation of a brick-red solution and then a red precipitate with clear supernatant.

Pentose. At concentrations of 250–300 mg/dL, L-xylulose will reduce Benedict's qualitative reagent at 50°C (water bath) within 10 minutes or at room temperature in several hours. Generally, the pentoses are identified by thin-layer chromatography.

Sucrose. Sucrose will ferment yeast and can be separated by chromatography but needs to be stained with a substance not dependent on reducing properties.

Ketones in Urine

Whenever there is a defect in carbohydrate metabolism or absorption or an inadequate amount of carbohydrate in the diet, the body compensates by metabolizing increasing amounts of fatty acids. When this increase is large, ketone bodies, the products of incomplete fat metabolism, begin to appear in the blood and are consequently excreted in the urine. In ketonuria, the three ketone bodies present in the urine are acetoacetic (diacetic) acid (20%), acetone (2%), and 3-hydroxybutyrate (about 78%). Acetone is formed nonreversibly from acetoacetic acid; β-hydroxybutyric acid (3-hydroxybutyrate) forms reversibly from acetoacetic acid.

$$\text{Acetoacetic acid} \xrightarrow{-CO_2} \text{Acetone}$$

$$\text{Acetoacetic acid} \underset{-2H}{\overset{+2H}{\rightleftarrows}} \text{3-Hydroxybutyrate}$$

Depending on the methods used, total ketone bodies (as acetone) can range as high as 17–42 mg/dL. According to Killander (1962), up to 2 mg acetoacetic acid per deciliter is normal. Ketonemia and ketonuria are commonly seen in uncontrolled diabetes mellitus, as well as several other conditions to be discussed below.

Diabetic Ketonuria

Ketonuria implies the presence of ketoacidosis (ketosis) and may provide a warning of impending coma. Up to 50 mg of acetoacetic acid per deciliter may be present without clinical evidence of ketosis. Type 1 diabetic patients are more prone to episodes of ketosis, often associated with infection, stress, or other problems in management. Whereas there are large amounts of ketones and glucose in urine in diabetic ketoacidosis, ketonuria is not found with the hyperosmolar hyperglycemic coma sometimes occurring in type 2 diabetics.

Nondiabetic Ketonuria

In infants and children, ketonuria commonly occurs in a variety of conditions, such as acute febrile diseases and toxic states accompanied by vomiting or diarrhea. Inherited metabolic disease should be suspected when there is severe persistent neonatal ketosis. Ketonuria may be present in hyperemesis of pregnancy, in cachexia, and following anesthesia. In these cases, ketonuria is likely related to increased tissue (especially fat) catabolism in the face of limited food intake. In pregnancy, a normal patient may have a low fasting blood glucose level and mild ketonuria. Occasionally ketonuria is seen following exposure to cold or severe exercise, or with a low-carbohydrate diet for weight reduction.

Lactic Acidosis

Lactic acidosis may coexist with many conditions including shock, diabetes mellitus, renal failure, liver disease, infections, and in response to certain drugs, especially phenformin and salicylate poisoning. Acetoacetate and 3-hydroxybutyrate may both be highly elevated, although usually the butyrate is high and acetoacetate low. Under these circumstances, ketonuria may not be detected by the usual nitroprusside test.

Methods

Because acetone, acetoacetic acid, and 3-hydroxybutyrate are all present in the urine with ketonuria, methods that indicate the presence of any one of these three ketone bodies are generally satisfactory to detect this condition. Commonly used nitroprusside strip and tablet tests based on the Rothera method detect acetoacetic acid and acetone. Different methods measure acetoacetic acid alone, or both acetone and acetoacetic acid. Ferric chloride (Gerhardt's test) detects acetoacetic acid. These methods do not measure 3-hydroxybutyrate, the predominant ketone body.

In urine and plasma, reagent strips and tablets react to 10 mg of acetoacetic acid per deciliter and are less sensitive to acetone. The blood level of ketone bodies may be estimated by the urine ketone dipstick at the bedside. This is especially helpful in determining the severity of ketosis in the treatment of diabetic acidosis.

When a patient is being followed with qualitative determinations of acetone and acetoacetic acid, repeated reports of marked elevations would not reflect the change that is actually taking place. In such an instance, semiquantitative results can be obtained with either the reagent strip or Rothera's tablet test by measuring several dilutions of each specimen.

Problems can occur with false-negative results because of unstable reagents and labile ketones. Bacterial action will cause loss of acetoacetic acid, which can happen in vivo as well as in vitro. Acetone is lost at room temperature but not if kept in a closed container in a refrigerator. Refrigerated samples should be brought to room temperature for testing. Preservatives do not prevent decay of ketones. If results are unexpected, fresh reagents, checked against known positive and negative controls, should be used.

Reagent Strip. This method is based on a nitroprusside (sodium nitroferricyanide) reaction for ketones. Different formulations are available. Reagent strips without alkali react to acetoacetic acid and not to acetone. With large (3+) results, urine may be diluted and remeasured, reporting a 'moderate' result and the dilution factor.

Chemstrip reagent strips contains sodium nitroferricyanide and glycine, which react with acetoacetic acid and acetone in an alkaline medium to form a violet dye. A positive result is indicated by a color change from beige to violet, which is read at 60 seconds. The method detects about 10 mg/dL of acetoacetic acid and 70 mg/dL of acetone, and the sensitivity and reaction of the reagent strip are similar to those of the tablet (Acetest), described below.

Multistix contains buffers and sodium nitroferricyanide, which react with acetoacetic acid, producing a pink-maroon color in 15 seconds. The reagent area detects 5–10 mg acetoacetic acid per deciliter of urine. It does not react with acetone.

Reagent strips correlate only moderately well with quantitative acetoacetate in plasma and poorly with total blood ketones. Color reactions (false positives) occur after the use of phthaleins (BSP or PSP dyes) or in the presence of extremely large amounts of phenylketones, and

the preservative 8-hydroxyquinoline, or L-dopa metabolites. Acetylcysteine (aerosol) produces a strong red color. The antihypertensive drugs methyldopa and captopril give positive results. False-negative results occur because of loss of reagent reactivity.

Nitroprusside Tablet Test. A tablet test method may be useful if the urine has an interfering color. These tablets are very sensitive to humidity and will deteriorate if not stored properly. The Acetest tablet contains sodium nitroprusside, glycine, and a strongly alkaline buffer. It can be used to assay whole blood, plasma, serum, or urine.

Acetest will detect 5–10 mg of acetoacetic acid per deciliter of urine and 20–25 mg acetone per deciliter of urine. Like the reagent strips, it does not react with 3-hydroxybutyrate. It will give positive results with L-dopa and large amounts of phenylketones and with BSP and PSP dyes, which react with the alkali in the tablets.

Procedure. Place the tablet on a clean surface, preferably a piece of white paper. Place one drop of urine, serum, plasma, or whole blood on the tablet. For urine measurements, compare the color of the tablet with a color chart at 30 seconds. For serum or plasma measurements, compare color of tablet with color chart at 2 minutes. For whole blood measurements, remove clotted blood from tablet and compare color of tablet with color chart, 10 minutes after application of the specimen.

If acetone and acetoacetic acid are present, the tablet will show a color varying from lavender to deep purple. Report the results as negative, small, moderate, or large. If large, a dilution may be made. Report these analyses in a form such as this: undiluted 'large,' 1 : 2 dilution 'large,' 1 : 4 dilution 'moderate,' etc.

Other Tests for Ketones. The Gerhardt ferric chloride test has been used for many years as a measurement for acetoacetic acid. However, ferric chloride methods are not very specific and the sensitivity is low, about 25–50 mg/dL. The ferric chloride method gives positive results with salicylate and L-dopa. The test tube nitroprusside method of Rothera is sensitive to acetoacetic acid, about 1–5 mg/dL, and to acetone with a sensitivity of 10–25 mg/dL.

Blood, Hemoglobin, Hemosiderin, and Myoglobin in Urine

The presence of an abnormal number of blood cells in urine is known as hematuria, whereas the term hemoglobinuria refers to the presence of free hemoglobin in solution in urine. Hematuria is relatively common, hemoglobinuria uncommon, and myoglobinuria rare.

Hematuria

Although asymptomatic microscopic hematuria may be detected by dipstick testing in up to 16% of screening populations (Rockall, 1997), many serious diseases of the urinary tract release red blood cells into the urine. A retrospective investigation of microscopic hematuria by renal biopsy disclosed several histopathologic findings including membranous nephropathy, IgA nephropathy, non-IgA mesangioproliferative glomerulonephritis, focal glomerulosclerosis, and mild glomerular abnormalities. More than 15% of patients in this study showed normal histology (McGregor, 1998). Hematuria can occur with disease (neoplastic and non-neoplastic) or trauma (including calculi) anywhere in the kidneys or urinary tract, as well as with bleeding disorders and anticoagulant usage, and with the use of other drugs such as cyclophosphamide. A rare case of giant cell arteritis presenting with fever and hematuria has been reported (Govil, 1998). Hematuria may also be seen in healthy persons undertaking excessive exercise (marathon runners) in whom bleeding originates from the bladder mucosa.

Because of the diagnostic importance of small amounts of hematuria and because of the tendency of erythrocytes to undergo lysis in urine, a screening test for hemoglobin is a useful adjunct to the microscopic examination of the sediment. In fact, some studies suggest reagent strip hemoglobin screening may be more sensitive than urine microscopy in detecting hematuria (Ooi, 1998). However, a common problem with the method is the inhibition of the hemoglobin reagent strip by interfering substances, commonly ascorbic acid, and this problem emphasizes the need for a routine microscopic examination in order to screen for hematuria. A positive test for hemoglobin with a normal urinary sediment suggests that a fresh urine sample should be examined for erythrocytes, since an alkaline pH or urine specific gravity of less than 1.010 may cause lysis of erythrocytes.

Hemoglobinuria

Any cause of hemolysis has the potential of causing hemoglobinuria, but the presence of hemoglobinuria indicates significant intravascular hemolysis as opposed to extravascular hemolysis. Hemoglobin binds to plasma haptoglobin, and free hemoglobin will pass through the

CHAPTER: 27   Basic Examination of Urine

Table 27–7 Some causes of hemolysis and hemoglobinuria

Erythrocyte trauma	Prosthetic cardiac valves (especially aortic)
	Ostium primum repair with patch causing turbulence
	Extensive burns
	Severe exercise
	Marching
	Severe trauma to muscle and other vascular tissues
Organisms	Malaria
	Bartonella
	Clostridium welchii toxin
	Brown recluse spider bite
Erythrocyte enzyme deficiencies	Glucose-6-phosphate dehydrogenase subjects in the following situations: exposure to oxidant drugs (acetanilid, sulfamethoxazole, nitrofurantoin), antimalarials (primaquine, etc.), fava beans (*Vicia fava*) in susceptible groups, with diabetic acidosis, and with infections
Unstable hemoglobin diseases	With exposure to oxidant drugs
Immune-mediated (see Chs 31 and 35)	Hemolytic uremic syndrome
	Thrombotic thrombocytopenic purpura
	Incompatible blood transfusions
	Warm antibodies (autoimmune – transient after infection, drug-induced)
	Cold antibodies
	IgM – viral anti-i mycoplasma anti-I
	IgG – paroxysmal, Donath–Landsteiner anti-P
	Membrane sensitivity, complement-mediated (paroxysmal nocturnal hemoglobinuria)
	Drugs
	Acting as haptens (penicillins)
	Immune complex (quinidine, phenacetin)
	α-Methyldopa
Normal subjects	Oxidative hemolysis due to drugs, large doses or exposure to naphthalene (mothballs), some sulfonamides, sulfones, nitrofurantoin

Table 27–8 Urine and plasma findings with intravascular hemolysis

Test	Moderate hemolysis	Marked hemolysis
Urine		
Bilirubin (conjugated)	Absent	Absent
Urobilinogen	Normal or elevated	Elevated
Hemoglobin	Absent	Present
Hemosiderin	Absent	Present (late)
Plasma		
Bilirubin (conjugated)	Elevated	Elevated
Haptoglobin	Decreased	Absent
Hemoglobin	Elevated	Elevated (marked)

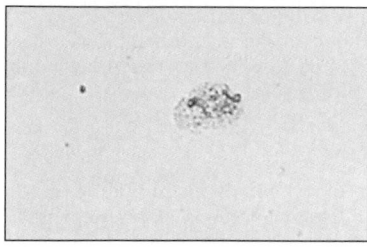

Figure 27–1 Renal tubular epithelial cell (unstained) containing brown pigment, iron (× 260).

glomerulus as αβ dimers (MW, 32 000), once this binding capacity is saturated. Some hemoglobin is reabsorbed by proximal tubular cells, and the remaining hemoglobin is excreted.

Hemoglobinuria may follow severe exertion in which there is direct trauma to small blood vessels, and many other causes of acute erythrocyte lysis are summarized in Table 27–7. Plasma appears pink at levels of about 50 mg/dL of hemoglobin, and with marked hemolysis, plasma levels may reach 1 g/dL. The plasma hemoglobin level is more often increased in severe acquired hemolytic anemias than in hereditary hemolytic anemias. However, moderately elevated levels occur with sickle cell disease and homozygous thalassemias. Note that unstable hemoglobins can cause a brown-pigmented urine; this is thought to be due to a dipyrrole or bilifuscin, and there is no reaction with the reagent strip test for heme. A comparison of expected urine and plasma findings with moderate and marked hemolysis is shown in Table 27–8.

Hemosiderin in Urine

Free hemoglobin is readily filtered by the glomeruli, and can be subsequently reabsorbed by proximal tubular cells where it can be catabolized into ferritin and hemosiderin. Hemosiderin will be present 2–3 days after an acute hemolytic episode that caused hemoglobinuria. At this time the reagent strip method for hemoglobin is often negative, however hemosiderin can be found as yellow-brown granules that are free or in epithelial cells and occasionally in casts (Fig. 27–1). Hemosiderin also appears in the urine sediment in diseases with a true siderosis of kidney parenchyma (hemochromatosis). Although the existence of hemosiderinuria indicates a chronic hemolytic state, its presence is rarely needed to make the diagnosis of hemolysis; other tests, such as serum bilirubin, lactate dehydrogenase, and haptoglobin levels will usually point to the correct diagnosis.

Because of the intermittent presence of hemosiderinuria, urinary iron levels may be quantitated to establish the presence of chronic intravascular hemolysis. Normal urinary iron excretion is about 0.1 mg/day, and it is increased with hemochromatosis and in association with erythrocytes traumatized by prosthetic heart valves. Urinary iron levels are normal with pernicious anemia and in hereditary spherocytosis.

Myoglobinuria

When there is acute destruction of muscle fibers (rhabdomyolysis) as with trauma, myoglobin is released, rapidly cleared from blood, and excreted in the urine as a red-brown pigment. Free myoglobin, a monomer with molecular weight of 17 000, is excreted quickly, whereas the hemoglobin–haptoglobin complex is more slowly removed. Myoglobinuria has been seen following a number of strenuous exercises, such as marathon running and karate. Other less common conditions associated with sustained or recurrent myoglobinuria include dermatomyositis (Rose, 1996), defects of muscle phosphofructokinase and adenosine monophosphate deaminase (Bruno, 1998), and mitochondrial trifunctional protein deficiency (Miyajima, 1997).

The diagnosis of rhabdomyolysis and myoglobinuria is usually made from the history and other laboratory findings as follows. Typically, the patient has muscle tenderness or cramps and voids red-brown urine within a day or two after exertion. The reagent strip urine test for hemoglobin is markedly positive, and protein and a few red blood cells are present. Serum is clear and has a markedly elevated creatine kinase (CK), aldolase, and a normal haptoglobin level. Serum creatinine may be increased. The urine usually clears in 2–3 days and the serum CK level declines. The serum measurements and history help distinguish myoglobinuria from hemoglobinuria.

The distinction between hematuria, hemoglobinuria and myoglobinuria may be difficult to make on examination of the urine. In all three cases, the urine can be dark red to brown, and some erythrocytes are seen in the sediment (to a much greater degree with hematuria). The reagent strip test for blood is also positive in all three cases. If serum can be examined, it will often be pink with hemoglobinemia but a normal color with myoglobinemia because this pigment is cleared so rapidly. Accurate quantitative measurement of urine myoglobin can also be performed by immunoassay; although there may be some slight interference by hemoglobin, this is an excellent way to detect and quantify the presence of myoglobinuria (Loun, 1996). See Table 27–9, comparing hemoglobinuria, myoglobinuria, and hematuria.

Methods

Reagent Strip for Heme Compounds (Hemoglobin, Myoglobin). This method is based on the liberation of oxygen from peroxide in the reagent strip by the peroxidase-like activity of heme in free hemoglobin, lysed erythrocytes, or myoglobin. Intact erythrocytes are lysed on the strip, causing the hemoglobin to react. Therefore, well-mixed urine must be tested, as intact erythrocytes may be missed if only supernatant urine is used. The reagent area is impregnated with a buffered mixture of an organic peroxide and the chromogen tetramethylbenzidine.

$$H_2O_2 + \text{Chromogen} \xrightarrow{\text{Heme peroxidase activity}} \text{Oxidized chromogen (color change)} + H_2O$$

Table 27–9 Differentiation of Hematuria, Hemoglobinuria, and Myoglobinuria

Condition	Plasma findings	Urine findings

Hematuria	Color – normal	Color – normal, smoky, pink, red, brown
		Erythrocytes – many
		  Renal – red blood cell casts
		  Protein – marked increase
		  Lower urinary tract – no casts
		  Protein – present or absent

Hemoglobinuria	Color – pink (early) Haptoglobin – low	Color – pink, red, brown Erythrocytes – occasional Pigment casts – occasional Protein – present or absent Hemosiderin – late
Myoglobinuria	Color – normal Haptoglobin – normal Creatine kinase – marked increase Aldolase – increased	Color – red, brown Erythrocytes – occasional Dense brown casts – occasional Protein – present or absent

Heme catalyzes the oxidation of tetramethylbenzidine to produce a green color. The strip is read at 60 seconds following sample application.

Multistix and Chemstrip detect 0.05–0.3 mg hemoglobin per deciliter urine. Note that 0.3 mg hemoglobin per deciliter is equivalent to that from 10 lysed erythrocytes per microliter. Normal erythrocytes contain approximately 30 pg of hemoglobin per cell.

Sensitivity is reduced in urine specimens with high specific gravity, in which erythrocyte lysis may not occur, and also when protein levels are high. Ascorbic acid in large concentrations may cause a false-negative result, as can formalin when used as a urine preservative. The presence of nitrite in large amounts will delay the reaction. Oxidizing contaminants such as hypochlorites (bleach) or iodine from skin-cleansing preparations may produce false-positive results. Microbial peroxidase, associated with urinary tract infection, potentially causes a false-positive reading.

Other Tests for Hemoglobin and Myoglobin. Qualitative tests have been generally unsatisfactory in separating myoglobin and hemoglobin, and both conditions may be present following crush injuries. Hemoglobin and myoglobin can be bound to proteins in urine, and this contributes to the difficulty of separating them by salt precipitation or acetate electrophoresis. The salt precipitation method of Blondheim (1958) is described below.

Qualitative Test for Myoglobin

1. Use a fresh urine specimen. Observe the color. Characteristically, urine with myoglobinuria is red when fresh and turns brown on standing, but some myoglobin may be present without color change. Myoglobin is less stable at an acid pH. Neutralize and refrigerate specimen pending testing.
2. Mix 1 mL of urine and 3 mL of 3% sulfosalicylic acid to assay for protein. If the pigment is precipitated, it is a protein. Filter. If the filtrate is a normal color, no abnormal nonprotein pigment is present. (*Note*: The heat and acetic acid test does not precipitate myoglobin or hemoglobin.)
3. To 5 mL of urine in a test tube, add 2.8 g of ammonium sulfate. Dissolve by mixing. The urine is now 80% saturated with ammonium sulfate. This is optimal for precipitation of hemoglobin. Filter or centrifuge. If the supernatant shows a normal color, the precipitated pigment is hemoglobin. If the supernatant fluid is colored, this is presumptive evidence of myoglobin.

This precipitation test has been largely replaced with specific immunoassays for myoglobin.

Capillary electrophoresis has been shown to successfully separate urinary hemoglobin from myoglobin based on differing electrophoretic mobility (Shihabi, 1995).

Detection of Hemosiderin in Urine. The Prussian blue reaction is used to demonstrate iron in hemosiderin (Fig. 27–2). A dry smear and alternative wet preparation are described below.

Dry Procedure. When stained with Prussian blue reagent, hemosiderin appears as blue granules, 1–3 µm, singly or in groups, in renal tubular epithelial cells, as amorphous sediment, or as blue granules in casts. An iron stain used for the detection of siderocytes in blood or bone marrow is also suitable. Urine is collected in an iron-free glass container, overnight. Let stand for 2 hours. Decant three fourths of it and centrifuge the remainder. Make a smear(s) of the sediment and allow to air dry. (*Note*: All

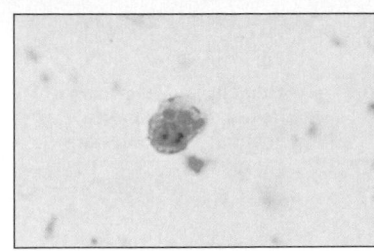

Figure 27–2 Renal tubular epithelial cell positive with Prussian blue stain, hemosiderin (×260).

glassware, slides, coverslips, etc., should be iron free. Water should be demineralized.)

Reagents.

The Prussian blue reagent is made fresh.

Prussian blue stain: Add concentrated HCl to an aliquot of the potassium ferrocyanide solution (20% in demineralized water) until a white precipitate forms that remains stable on shaking. Filter through No. 5 filter paper.

Working counterstain: Dilute 1 mL safranin O stain (0.5 g in 100 mL distilled water) to 50 mL with phosphate buffer (pH 6.4–4.7).

Procedure

1. Fix the smear in methyl alcohol for 10 minutes.
2. Rinse with iron-free water (demineralized) and air dry.
3. Stain with Prussian blue reagent for 30 minutes.
4. Wash gently for at least 4 minutes with iron-free water and air dry.
5. Counterstain with safranin O for 1–5 minutes.
6. Rinse with iron-free water. Air dry.
7. Mount coverslip.

Wet Procedure

1. Centrifuge a complete morning specimen or random urine sample for 5 minutes and pool the sediment. Examine several drops of sediment microscopically, searching for coarse yellow-brown granules, especially within renal tubular epithelial cells or casts.
2. If such granules are seen, suspend the rest of the sediment in a fresh mixture of 5 mL of 2% potassium ferrocyanide solution and 5 mL of 1% hydrochloric acid (HCl) and allow to stand for 10 minutes.
3. Centrifuge, and discard the supernatant. Examine the sediment microscopically. Coarse granules of hemosiderin appear blue in this preparation in cells, casts, and amorphous material. If granules do not stain, re-examine after 30 minutes (occasionally the reaction is delayed).

Bilirubin in Urine

Bilirubin is a breakdown product of hemoglobin that is formed in the reticuloendothelial cells of the spleen, liver, and bone marrow. It is initially carried in the blood linked to albumin; this unconjugated bilirubin (or indirect bilirubin) is water insoluble and therefore unable to pass through the glomerular barrier of the kidney. Unconjugated bilirubin is transported to the liver where it is conjugated with glucuronic acid to form bilirubin glucuronide. This conjugated form of bilirubin (direct bilirubin) is water soluble and able to pass through the glomerulus of the kidney into the urine. Conjugated bilirubin is normally excreted in the bile into the duodenum, and normal adult urine contains only 0.02 mg of bilirubin per deciliter. This small amount is not detected by the usual testing methods. Excretion of bilirubin is enhanced by alkalosis.

Conjugated bilirubin appearing in urine generally indicates that there is excess conjugated bilirubin in the bloodstream. This can occur when there is either (1) obstruction to bile outflow from the liver (intra- or extrahepatic), or (2) hepatocellular disease with resultant inability of hepatocytes to sufficiently excrete conjugated bilirubin into the bile. For example, bilirubinuria may be present when intracanalicular pressure rises secondary to periportal inflammation, fibrosis, or hepatocyte swelling. Gallstones in the common bile duct or carcinoma of the head of the pancreas are possible sources of extrahepatic biliary obstruction leading to bilirubinuria. Bilirubinuria is often seen with acute viral hepatitis or drug-induced cholestasis prior to the appearance of jaundice, and it typically accompanies jaundice of acute alcoholic hepatitis. In persons exposed to potentially hepatotoxic drugs or toxins, a positive test for bilirubinuria may be an early indication of cholestasis or liver damage. In congenital hyperbilirubinemias, bilirubin will appear in the urine in the Dubin–Johnson and the Rotor types, and is not present with Gilbert's disease or Crigler–Najjar disease.

Bilirubinuria is associated with yellow-brown to greenish brown urine that may have a yellow foam, elevated serum bilirubin (conjugated), jaundice, and pale-colored feces. These acholic stools are so called because

Table 27–10 Urine and Fecal Findings in Jaundice

Finding	Normal	Obstruction to bile flow	Hemolysis, hemolytic anemia	Liver damage, hepatitis, cholestasis
Urinary bilirubin	Absent	Increased, dark urine	Absent	Increased early
Urinary urobilinogen	Present	Neoplasm – low or absent; gallstones – variable	Increased	Decreased early; increased late
Fecal color	Dark	Pale; intermittent with gallstones in common bile duct; persistent with neoplasm in duct or pancreas	Dark	Pale early and dark late in hepatitis; pale with cholestasis

of the absence of bilirubin-derived pigment. A positive test for urinary bilirubin with a negative test for urobilinogen in urine is indicative of intra- or extrahepatic biliary obstruction. This test is valuable in the differential diagnosis of jaundice, since bilirubinuria is not found with hemolytic jaundice. Table 27–10 summarizes the typical urine and fecal findings in jaundice of various etiologies.

Methods

Reagent Strip. The test is based on the coupling reaction of bilirubin with a diazonium salt in acid medium. When this method is used, normal urine contains no detectable bilirubin. Specific tests differ in the diazonium salt utilized. Multistix uses diazotized 2,4-dichloroaniline as the diazo salt, with a color change from cream-buff to tan at 20 seconds. This system will detect 0.8 mg per deciliter urine; however, the color change may be difficult to read. Chemstrip uses 2,6-dichlorobenzene-diazonium tetrafluoroborate, and the color changes from pink to violet at 30–60 seconds. This test detects 0.5 mg per deciliter urine.

Urine must be fresh because bilirubin glucuronide in urine quickly hydrolyzes to less reactive free bilirubin. Oxidation of bilirubin in specimens that have stood too long, especially when exposed to light, will result in false-negative findings. Large amounts of ascorbic acid and nitrite can also lower bilirubin results. Metabolites of drugs such as phenazopyridine (Pyridium) give a reddish color at the low pH of the strip and mask the result. Rifampin and large amounts of chlorpromazine metabolites may cause false positives, whereas salicylates do not interfere. Urobilinogen does not affect the result.

Confirmatory Bilirubin Tests. The diazo test method, in which bilirubin is coupled to *p*-nitrobenzene diazonium *p*-toluene sulfonate to form a blue or purple color (in the form of a tablet or reagent strip), is commonly used. The reagent strip test is much less reactive to the free bilirubin than is the tablet test, so that a difference in results becomes more apparent as the urine ages. Another test employs a ferric chloride reagent to oxidize bilirubin to a green biliverdin. The diazo tablet method is described below.

Diazo Tablet Method. Tablets contain *p*-nitrobenzene diazonium *p*-toluene, as well as sulfosalicylic acid and sodium bicarbonate. The later substances provide an acid medium for the reaction and an effervescent mixture that will ensure the solution of a portion of the tablet when water is added. (Ictotest kit, including absorbent mats and reagent tablets, is available through Bayer Corporation, Tarrytown, NY.)

Note: Reagent tablets are hygroscopic, and they should be protected from moisture or high humidity. The tablets are packed in a brown bottle, since prolonged direct exposure to strong light results in decomposition of the stabilized diazonium compound. Prolonged exposure of several weeks to temperatures of 100°F or more may also result in deterioration of the tablets. A brown discoloration indicates deterioration, and when each new bottle is opened, tablets should be checked for positive and negative reactions.

Procedure

1. Place 10 drops of specimen on an asbestos–cellulose mat provided with the kit. Bilirubin, if present, will be adsorbed onto the mat surface.
2. Place a reagent tablet on the moistened area of the mat.
3. Place one drop of water onto the tablet. Wait 5 seconds, then place a second drop so that the water runs off the tablet onto the mat. If bilirubin is present, there will be a coupling of bilirubin with *p*-nitrobenzene diazonium *p*-toluene sulfonate from the tablet, as

shown by the formation of a blue to purple color within 30 seconds. The tablet should be moved to reveal the purple color. A pink or red color is negative.

The diazo test reacts positively to bilirubin in amounts as low as 0.05–0.1 mg per deciliter. There is no purple reaction with urobilin or other pigments, although high levels of urobilin or indican give a red color. Azo compounds cause an atypical color (e.g., Pyridium). Rifampin may also interfere. Chlorpromazine metabolites in large amounts produce a purple color, and the metabolites of the anti-inflammatory drugs mefenamic and flufenamic acid cause false-positive results.

Wash-Through Tablet Method. When false-positive reactions are suspected (e.g., with chlorpromazine), the contaminant can be diluted out with water in the mat.

Procedure.

Prepare duplicate mats with 10 drops of urine on each. Add 10 drops of water to one mat. Place a reagent tablet on each mat and then two drops of water onto each tablet. Bilirubin, if present, is adsorbed into the mat fibers and will appear the same on each mat; an interfering substance produces a light color or no color on the mat with the extra water.

Urobilinogen in Urine

Conjugated bilirubin from the liver eventually reaches the duodenum, complexed with cholesterol, bile salts, and phospholipids within the bile. The conjugated bilirubin is not absorbed from the small intestine, but instead passes on into the colon, where resident bacteria hydrolyze the conjugate. The free bilirubin is then reduced to urobilinogen, mesobilirubinogen, and stercobilinogen. Up to 50% of the urobilinogen is reabsorbed into the portal circulation and re-excreted, unconjugated, into the bile. The vast majority of remaining urobilinogen is excreted in feces as colored urobilins or stercobilin, which are formed after further removal of hydrogen. A small amount is excreted in the urine.

Urobilinogen represents a group of closely related tetrapyrrole compounds, and because a mixture of substances is actually measured, the term 'units' is frequently used instead of the more precise milligrams-per-deciliter terminology. These are roughly equivalent. Normal output of urobilinogen in the urine is 0.5–2.5 mg or units/24 h. These substances are colorless and labile, as opposed to the urobilins, the oxidation products of urobilinogen that impart yellow-orange color to normal urine. Output of urobilinogen is increased in alkaline urine; the level is decreased in acid urine.

Whenever the liver is unable to efficiently remove the reabsorbed urobilinogen from the portal circulation, more urobilinogen than normal is routed through the kidney and hence excreted in the urine. This can occur when there is hepatocellular damage due to viral hepatitis, drugs, or toxic substances, or in some cases of cirrhosis. With congestive heart failure, liver congestion prevents effective urobilinogen handling, and re-excretion into the bile is impaired. If there is an infection, such as cholangitis associated with obstruction, large amounts of urobilinogen are excreted in urine together with bilirubin.

In contradistinction, an excess of urobilinogen in urine together with absent bilirubin is typically associated with hemolysis. This can be seen following acute lysis of erythrocytes, as well as with the destruction of erythrocyte precursors in the bone marrow with megaloblastic anemias. There is also an increased urobilinogen accompanying bleeding into tissues and the subsequent formation of excess bilirubin. These jaundiced patients have dark-colored stools because excess urobilinogen is also excreted into the feces. Urinary urobilinogen may be increased when there is fever, associated with dehydration and concentrated urine.

Persistent absence of urinary urobilinogen occurs with complete obstruction of the outflow of bile into the intestine, accompanied by pale stools. Broad-spectrum antibiotics, which suppress the normal intestinal flora, may prevent the conversion of bilirubin to urobilinogen, and therefore reduce its excretion in feces and urine.

The brown pigment mesobilifuscin is a dipyrrole that normally contributes to fecal and urine color. It does not react with tests for blood or bilirubin. Although it is not derived from bilirubin as is urobilinogen, it is likely a by-product of heme synthesis. Its excess causes a dark brown urine that can be seen with homozygous β-thalassemia or whenever Heinz bodies form in erythrocytes (e.g., with the unstable hemoglobins).

Methods

Reagent Strip. Testing is based on either the Ehrlich aldehyde reaction or the formation of a red azo dye from a diazonium compound.

Multistix utilizes the former method; its test area is impregnated with an acid buffer solution and *p*-dimethylaminobenzaldehyde, which produces a reddish brown color with urobilinogen. Color varies from light yellow to shades of red-brown, and values from 0.2–1 mg per deciliter are considered normal. This test methodology is not specific for urobilinogen and will detect substances known to react with the Ehrlich reagent including porphobilinogen, *p*-aminosalicylic acid metabolites, sulfonamides, procaine, 5-hydroxyindoleacetic acid, indole, and methyldopa (Aldomet). It is not a reliable method for the detection of porphobilinogen.

The Chemstrip urobilinogen test area is impregnated with 4-methoxybenzene-diazonium-tetrafluoroborate, which couples with urobilinogen in an acid medium to form a red azo dye. Results are read at 10–30 seconds, and the test can detect approximately 0.4 mg/dL. This test is specific for urobilinogen, unlike the Ehrlich reagent-based methodologies.

A freshly voided sample is best for testing, given that urobilinogen is quite labile and will potentially form nonreactive urobilin in acid urine. Both reagent strips are affected by the metabolites of drugs such as phenazopyridine (Pyridium), which colors the urine orange-red in an acid medium, and other compounds such as Azo-Gantrisin. These may mask the reaction with urobilinogen or give a false-positive result. Bilirubin and blood do not usually affect the test, but bilirubin may occasionally cause a green color.

Other Urobilinogen and Porphobilinogen Tests. Qualitative testing for urobilinogen and porphobilinogen may be performed when reagent strip testing indicates more than 1 mg/dL of Ehrlich-reacting substance present in the urine (see later under Porphyrins, for more information on these testing modalities).

Quantitative tests for urobilinogen in urine are seldom performed. Consult Henry (1979) for a 2-hour quantitative urobilinogen method and Davidsohn (1974) or Schwartz (1944) for 24-hour quantitation. For quantitative comparative purposes in the same patient, a 2-hour test is used in which urine is collected from 2–4 p.m. after lunch. This period after the meal coincides with heightened excretion of urobilinogen, as the pH of the urine is more nearly neutral. Other 2-hour periods may be tested for comparison.

Indirect Tests for Urinary Tract Infection

It is not uncommon for significant urinary tract infections to be present in patients who do not experience typical symptomatology. Given that these infections if untreated can cause severe renal damage, many physicians are finding it prudent to request tests for bacteriuria in high-risk individuals. These would include patients who are elderly, pregnant, or diabetic, and those with a previous history of urinary tract infections. The two most commonly utilized testing modalities for indirect assessment of bacteriuria and leukocyturia are the reagent strip nitrite and leukocyte esterase, respectively. These tests are discussed below. An immunochromatographic test strip for the measurement of urinary lactoferrin may also prove to be useful for the rapid diagnosis of urinary tract infection (Arao, 1999). The microscopic urinalysis serves as a rapid confirmatory test for the presence of leukocytes and bacteria, with bacteriologic culture remaining the 'gold standard' for detecting bacteriuria.

Nitrite
Many bacteria that are urinary tract pathogens are able to reduce nitrate to nitrite, and thus will generate a positive urine nitrite test when present in significant numbers ($> 10^5$–10^6/mL bladder urine). Common organisms include *Escherichia coli*, *Klebsiella*, *Enterobacter*, *Proteus*, *Staphylococcus*, and *Pseudomonas* species; *Enterococcus* is unable to reduce nitrate to nitrite. If the nitrite test is positive, a culture should be considered, provided that the specimen was properly collected and stored prior to testing. A first morning clean-voided midstream specimen is best.

According to Kunin (1975), self-administered repeated nitrite tests (three tests) in a small group of patients revealed about 70% overall positive results when compared with cultures. When only *E. coli* was present, bacteriuria detected by a positive nitrite test in any of the three first morning specimens showed 93% agreement with culture results. There were no significant false-positive nitrite results in his large test group. Other authors report more disappointing results with nitrite dipstick screening for urinary tract infections, particularly in hospital inpatients (Zaman, 1998).

Methods. The test depends on the conversion of nitrate to nitrite by bacterial action in the urine. Because it typically requires overnight (minimum of 4 hours) bladder incubation for the infecting bacterial population to convert urinary nitrate to nitrite, a first morning specimen is best. A positive result is indication for culture, unless the specimen has been improperly stored after collection, allowing contaminant bacterial growth.

Reagent Strip. The nitrite testing area of Multistix is impregnated with *p*-arsanilic acid, which forms a diazonium salt when it reacts with nitrite present in the urine. This compound is then able to couple with benzoquinoline to form a pink azo dye. This method detects 0.075 mg of

nitrite per deciliter in solution and is read at 40 seconds. Chemstrip contains a benzoquinoline and sulfanilamide, which produce a pink azo dye with nitrite at 30 seconds, and is able to detect 0.05 mg of nitrite per deciliter. Note that pink spots or edges are interpreted as negative.

False-positive results most commonly occur with poorly collected/stored specimens due to contaminants and postcollection bacterial proliferation. False positives may also be produced by medications that color the urine red or turn red in an acid medium (e.g., phenazopyridine).

False-negative nitrite results may be due to ascorbic acid, urobilinogen, or low pH (< 6). Random specimens collected during the day, and urine from patients with draining catheters, do not show good correlation between the nitrite test and significant bacteriuria, presumably because of the time required for the chemical reduction to nitrite in the bladder urine. Additionally, some false-negative results occur because some nitrate-reducing organisms form compounds other than nitrite, such as ammonia, nitric and nitrous oxide, hydroxylamine, and nitrogen, and will therefore give a negative nitrite test result. Lack of dietary nitrate may also produce false-negative results, even when a significant number of organisms are present.

Leukocyte esterase
Extracts of human neutrophil azurophilic (primary) granules contain up to 10 proteins showing esterolytic activity, and this esterase activity is commonly used as a marker for these cells. Because neutrophils and other cells are labile in urine, leukocyte esterase activity can be indicative of remnants of cells that are not visible microscopically.

The presence of significant numbers of neutrophils in the urine suggests urinary tract infection; however, difficulty has arisen in determining suitable cutoff points for normal and abnormal numbers of these cells. Because quantitative counts are so low, precision is poor. Positive leukocyte esterase results correlate with 'significant' numbers of neutrophils, either intact or lysed, and with the use of a chamber count of about 10 neutrophils/μL of fresh urine as a cutoff point, the number of false-negative and false-positive results is low. Likewise, using a concentrated (10 : 1) urine sediment and a cytocentrifuged stained preparation, a negative reagent strip test is associated with fewer than 100 neutrophils in 10 high-power fields (hpf) (450×). The leukocyte esterase test may also be useful in the work-up of suspect urethritis in male patients, and has a high negative predictive value in this diagnostic setting (Bowden, 1998).

Methods
Reagent Strip. The test is similar in principle to the naphthol chloroacetate reaction used for granulocyte esterase detection in hematology. Neutrophilic esterases catalyze the hydrolysis of esters to produce their respective alcohols and acids. For example, Multistix utilizes 3-hydroxy-5-phenyl-pyyrole-*N*-tosyl-L-alanine ester as a substrate, which reacts in the presence of leukocyte esterase to form pyrrole alcohol. The alcohol then reacts with a diazonium salt to produce a purple color. The intensity of the color produced is proportional to the amount of enzyme present, which is related to the number of neutrophils present.

Cells originating from the urinary tract (i.e., urothelium) and erythrocytes do not contribute to the esterase level. Elevated urine specific gravity, protein, and glucose may all decrease test results, as can the presence of boric acid and certain antibiotics such as tetracycline, cephalexin, and cephalothin. Very large amounts of ascorbic acid may inhibit the reaction.

Contamination of urine with vaginal fluid may give positive results, and large numbers of squamous epithelial cells and bacteria would be seen on microscopic evaluation. Also, *Trichomonas* and eosinophils may represent alternative cellular sources of esterases causing false-positive results. Oxidizing agents and formalin may give false-positive colors, and nitrofurantoin and other strong colors may affect color interpretation.

Miscellaneous Chemical Screening Tests
Ascorbic Acid
Large quantities of ascorbic acid may occasionally be found in the urine of individuals taking therapeutic doses of vitamin C or other preparations containing abundant ascorbic acid. Because of its reducing properties, ascorbic acid may inhibit several reagent strip reactions (i.e., glucose, blood, bilirubin, nitrite, and leukocyte esterase). Reagent strips from various manufacturers differ in their susceptibility to this substance, and suspicious results should be investigated. For example, when the microscopic examination of urine sediment shows more than two erythrocytes per high power field but heme is not detected by the reagent strip method, it may be useful to check for the presence of ascorbic acid.

Urine tests for ascorbic acid have also been used as an indication of adequate ascorbic acid therapy. With the usual western diet, 2–10 mg/dL is excreted daily, while after ingestion of large amounts of ascorbic acid, levels in urine may rise to 200 mg/dL. Oxalate and sulfate are the metabolites of ascorbic acid, and with ingestion of large quantities (1 g or more per day), oxalate stones may form in susceptible persons.

Methods. Several manufacturers have developed reagent strip methods for detecting ascorbic acid, discussed below. Gas chromatographic/mass spectrometric measurement is a more accurate quantitative method (Deutsch, 1997).

Reagent Strip. The ascorbic acid testing area of C-Stix reagent strips is impregnated with phosphomolybdates buffered in an acid medium. The phosphomolybdates are reduced by ascorbic acid to molybdenum blue, and this test detects 5 mg/dL of ascorbic acid in urine after 10 seconds. Gentisic acid and L-dopa may cause false-positive results.

Stix reagent strips are not as sensitive as C-Stix; they can detect about 25 mg/dL of ascorbic acid at 60 seconds. The reagent in Stix is methylene green, which is reduced to its colorless form with ascorbic acid. Neutral red provides a background color, and the overall color changes from blue to purple at levels of 150 mg/dL. This same testing method is also incorporated into Multistix multiple reagent strips. Large amounts of bilirubin and pH greater than 7.5 interfere with the color. False-positive results are not seen with urates, salicylates, gentisic acid, or creatinine.

5-Hydroxyindoleacetic Acid

Serotonin (5-hydroxytryptamine) is produced by the argentaffin cells of the intestines from tryptophan, and is carried in the blood by platelets. Carcinoid tumors (argentaffinoma) can produce excessive amounts of serotonin, especially when metastatic. Characteristic symptoms include intestinal and vasomotor disturbances, and bronchoconstriction; edema, right-sided valvular heart disease, and neurologic symptoms may also be present.

Although serotonin in the urine can be analyzed directly by high-performance liquid chromatographic methods (Panholzer, 1999), screening tests that detect the serotonin metabolite 5-hydroxyindoleacetic acid in the urine are more commonly used. The quantitative method is more sensitive, since it eliminates the interfering keto acids and indoleacetic acid. The normal excretion of 5-hydroxyindoleacetic acid in 24 hours is 1–5 mg.

Screening Test. A random urine specimen is usually sufficient for screening purposes; if a 24-hour collection is made, it should be acidified with HCl. Boric acid may also be used as a preservative. Patients should be instructed not to take any drugs for 72 hours before the test; phenothiazines, acetanilid drugs, and mephenesin, a muscle relaxant, will interfere with this test.

The principle of the test is based on the development of a purple color specific for 5-hydroxyindoles with nitrous acid and 1-nitroso-2-naphthol. Ethylene dichloride is used to remove interfering chromogens. For procedure, see Henry (1984).

Melanin

Normal melanocytes convert tyrosine to dihydroxyphenylalanine (DOPA), then to dopaquinone, and by oxidative steps to melanin. The enzyme tyrosinase is required for the first conversion step, and is found in specific organelles in melanocytes called melanosomes. Its formation is increased by melanin-stimulating hormone. Melanosomes with pigment are normally transferred from melanocytes to skin and mucous membrane cells. Enlarged melanosomes are found in some neoplastic cells (e.g., nevus, melanoma).

An increased urinary excretion of melanin metabolites occurs as malignant melanoma metastasizes, although it is unusual to find dark-colored urine in these patients, even when the specimen stands at room temperature for 24 hours. These urinary melanogens include indoles, catechols, and catecholamines. DOPA does not appear in large amounts in urine from melanotic patients.

There is no simple specific test for melanuria. Screening tests for melanin should be made on fresh specimens of urine and include tests based on nonspecific color reactions produced with ferric chloride, Ehrlich's aldehyde reagent, and nitroferricyanide. Procedures for the ferric chloride and nitroferricyanide tests for melanin can be found in Henry (1984).

A column cation-exchange chromatographic method allows detection of melanin metabolites in urine. Another approach is to measure DOPA oxidase levels in urine. The enzyme is increased in the urine of patients with melanoma and is markedly increased with liver metastases.

Rarely, cells containing melanin pigment are seen in urine sediment when there is melanuria with pigment uptake by renal tubular cells, and when there is metastatic melanoma to the bladder. A ferrous ion uptake stain can be used to color the melanin in cells dark blue.

Porphyrins

The porphyrias are a group of diseases resulting from defects in the synthesis of heme. These are inherited enzyme deficiencies in which the enzyme substrate is usually excreted in excess in urine and/or feces. During the acute porphyric attack, high levels of porphobilinogen are excreted, but between attacks levels of porphobilinogen may be increased or normal. The patterns of excretion of the various porphyrins vary with the different diseases, and together with the clinical findings helps establish the diagnosis.

The porphyrins are excreted in most of the porphyrias and in lead poisoning. Additionally, porphyrin metabolism may be abnormal in patients with established human immunodeficiency virus (HIV) infection, particularly when there is a concomitant hepatitis C virus infection (O'Connor, 1996).

Skin photosensitivity and cutaneous lesions frequently accompany high levels of porphyrins. The one entity without skin lesions is acute intermittent porphyria. In patients presenting with neurologic disease and acute abdominal pain – the hepatic group – there is increased production and excretion of δ-aminolevulinic acid (ALA) and porphobilinogen during the acute porphyric attack. This is likely due to increased activity of ALA synthase and subsequent increased production of the precursors. Exacerbations of the hepatic diseases are precipitated by drugs known to induce liver enzyme activity (e.g., barbiturates and certain steroids).

Methods. In patients suspected of having an acute porphyric attack, porphobilinogen is sought in urine specimens. The Watson–Schwartz test is used to separate causes of a positive Ehrlich-reacting test and to give an indication of large amounts of urobilinogen or the presence of porphobilinogen. A positive result for porphobilinogen in the Watson–Schwartz test can be further confirmed by the Hoesch test, since the former may show false-positive results for porphobilinogen as a result of drugs such as methyldopa. When a qualitative porphobilinogen test is specifically requested or a known porphyric patient is being followed, the simpler Hoesch test may be used instead of the Watson–Schwartz test.

Urine specimens for urobilinogen or porphobilinogen must be fresh. If the testing will be delayed, the pH should be adjusted to near neutral (pH 7) and the specimen stored in a refrigerator, where it is stable for about 1 week. Urine may darken if the patient has porphyria, especially if left at room temperature.

Watson–Schwartz Test. The Ehrlich's aldehyde reaction and Watson–Schwartz tests are based on solubility differences between urobilinogen and porphobilinogen. Urobilinogen can be extracted by chloroform and/or butanol, whereas porphobilinogen will remain in an aqueous phase.

Procedure

1. To 2.5 mL fresh urine, add 2.5 mL Ehrlich's reagent and mix.
2. Add 5 mL saturated sodium acetate and mix. Check with pH paper to confirm that the solution is in the pH range of 4–5. Adjust pH if necessary.
3. Add 5 mL of chloroform; insert a stopper and shake vigorously for 1 minute. Permit the phases to separate.
4. Examine the upper (aqueous) phase. If the color is absent, consider the result of the screening test to be negative and stop.
5. If color is present, separate the upper (aqueous) phase and add 5 mL of butanol. Insert a stopper and shake vigorously for 1 minute. Allow phases to separate.
6. A 'pink to rose red' color in the lower aqueous layer indicates a positive result and suggests a concentration of porphobilinogen that is several times normal. A color in the upper butanol layer indicates an increase in urobilinogen concentration (Fig. 27–3).

Hoesch's Test. The Hoesch test is based on the inverse Ehrlich's reaction (i.e., of maintaining an acid solution by adding a small urine volume to a relatively large reagent volume), eliminating the problem of urobilinogen reactivity. The sensitivity is similar to that of the Watson–Schwartz test, but the reaction is for porphobilinogen. This test will detect about 20–100 mg/L of porphobilinogen, and urobilinogen in amounts up to 200 mg/L does not give a positive result (red color). A yellow color may be caused by urea.

The urorosein urinary pigment related to indoleacetic acid will produce a positive Hoesch test (in response to strong HCl), and the rose color may be confused with a positive porphobilinogen result. Some of the false-positive problems may be excluded by testing the specimen with concentrated HCl (6 mol/L) separately in conjunction with the Hoesch test. Urine from a patient having an acute porphyric attack may be dark red in color, necessitating a 1 : 10 dilution with water prior to testing.

The Watson–Schwartz test detects greater than 6 mg/L and the Hoesch test greater than 11 mg/L of porphobilinogen. The Watson–Schwartz test is more sensitive than the Hoesch test for porphobilinogen, and may yield a positive result between attacks of acute intermittent porphyria. Large doses

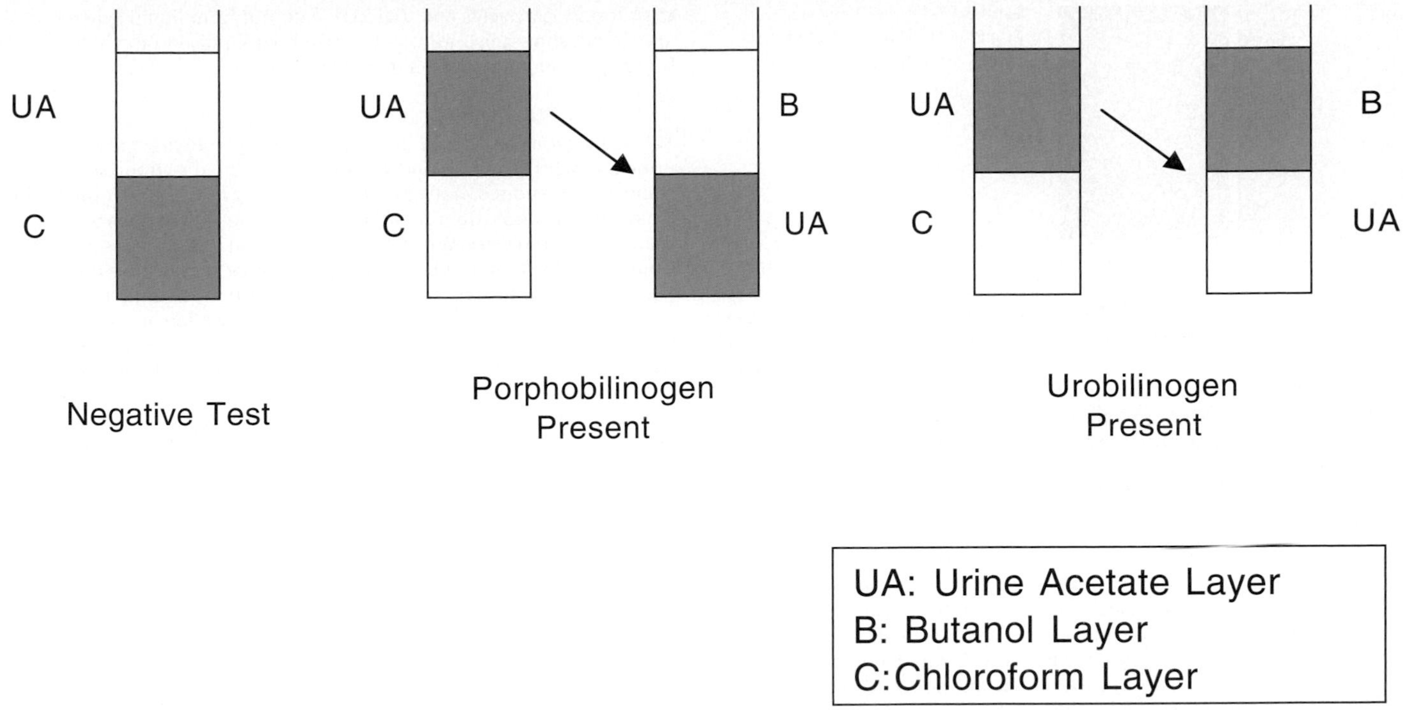

Figure 27–3 Watson–Schwartz Test. Interpretation of screening method for urine urobilinogen and porphobilinogen.

UA: Urine Acetate Layer
B: Butanol Layer
C: Chloroform Layer

of methyldopa (Aldomet) gave positive results, as did indoles in some patients with intestinal ileus, and the drug phenazopyridine (Pyridium), which becomes orange with HCl. A quantitative porphobilinogen test is necessary if either the Watson–Schwartz test or the Hoesch test result is questionable; this situation may arise because of the instability of porphobilinogen.

Alternative urine screening tests for porphobilinogen have been described. These include a micellar electrokinetic capillary chromatographic method (Luo, 1996), as well as a semiquantitative kit in which urine is pretreated with ion-exchange resin and the color of the Ehrlich–porphobilinogen adduct is compared to a set of standards (Deacon, 1998).

Uroporphyrin and coproporphyrin can be detected by fluorescence. An orange-red fluorescence is seen if a positive specimen is placed near an ultraviolet light source.

Fluorescence Screening Procedure for Porphyrin. In this method, the urine is acidified and the extracted porphyrin exposed to ultraviolet light.

1. Place 5 mL urine in a stoppered glass centrifuge tube. Add 3 mL of a mixture of one part glacial acetic acid with four parts of ethyl acetate.
2. Shake and allow to separate. Centrifuging will accelerate the separation.
3. Using a Wood's lamp, observe the upper layer for fluorescence. Inspect the tube in a dark room with ultraviolet reflected light. A lavender to violet color indicates the presence of porphyrins; pink to red fluorescence indicates higher levels of porphyrin. Pale blue with no pink color is negative. Normal urine may fluoresce blue.

To increase the sensitivity of the test and remove interfering drug metabolites, transfer the upper layer to a glass tube and acidify with 0.5 mL of 3 M HCl (25 mL concentrated HCl diluted to 100 mL with water). Shake. Porphyrins are extracted into the lower aqueous layer and will give a red-orange fluorescence.

An alternative screening method utilizes an anion exchange resin column. Porphyrins are adsorbed, eluted, and exposed to fluorescent light. This method removes interfering substances and is similar in principle to the quantitative method for total porphyrins and for coproporphyrin and uroporphyrin.

Screening tests together with the clinical findings will indicate whether quantitative tests should be done. The latter are usually performed by reference or research laboratories.

Urine specimens for quantitative porphobilinogen should be kept at a near neutral pH (between 6 and 7) and protected from light. Frozen specimens are fairly stable, although ALA is more stable if the urine is acidic. If the urine is to be tested for both substances, the near neutral pH is preferred and the urine aliquot is frozen. These substances are quantitated by eluting from different columns and reacting with Ehrlich's reagent. A micellar electrokinetic capillary chromatographic method has been described that allows separation of ALA and porphobilinogen (Luo, 1996).

Urine specimens for quantitative porphyrins are collected in a dark container containing 5 g sodium carbonate for a 24-hour specimen to give a concentration of 0.1% sodium carbonate or to produce urine of neutral pH. Coproporphyrin and uroporphyrin can be separated by thin-layer chromatography or by extraction and fluorometry and quantitated using ion-exchange columns. Additional methods include the Bio-Rad (porphyrin) column test, spectrophotometry (Zuijderhoudt, 1998), capillary electrophoresis (Chiang, 1997), fast atom bombardment mass spectrometry (Luo, 1997), and laser desorption/ionization time-of-flight mass spectrometry (Jones, 1995).

Fecal porphyrins can be qualitatively estimated using extraction and ultraviolet (UV) light, or quantitated. In some porphyrias, erythrocytes may show fluorescence when an unstained blood smear is examined microscopically. The nucleated bone marrow erythrocytes give greater fluorescence.

Examination of Urine Sediment

Microscopic examination of urine, in conjunction with dipstick chemical analysis, aids in the detection of renal and urinary tract disease processes. With microscopy, one can detect those cellular and noncellular elements of urine that do not give distinct chemical reactions. Microscopy can also serve as a confirmatory test in some circumstances (e.g., erythrocytes, leukocytes, and bacteria).

In order to perform a microscopic evaluation of urine with competence, one must be knowledgeable of numerous morphologic entities (e.g., organisms, hematopoietic and epithelial cells, crystals, and casts). Also, microscopists must be aware of the clinical relevance of urine findings as well as the common chemical abnormalities associated with microscopic interpretations. Discrepancies should be investigated before a report is issued.

Centrifuged urine sediment should contain all the insoluble materials (commonly referred to as formed elements) that have accumulated in the urine following glomerular filtration and during passage of fluid through the renal tubules and lower urinary tract. Cellular elements are from two sources: (1) desquamated/spontaneously exfoliated epithelial lining cells of the kidney and lower urinary tract, and (2) cells of hematogenous origin (leukocytes and erythrocytes). Cellular and noncellular casts may be seen; these are formed in the renal tubules and collecting ducts. Crystals may also be present, of variable clinicopathologic significance. Organisms (bacteria, fungi, viral inclusion cells, parasites) and neoplastic cells represent elements that are typically foreign to urine, and when detected, necessitate further investigation.

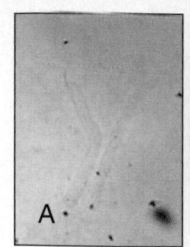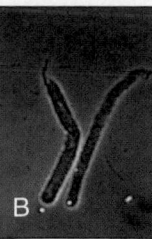

Figure 27–4 *A*, Hyaline casts. Brightfield (×100). *B*, Hyaline casts. Phase-contrast microscopy (×100).

'Normal' or reference values for formed elements will vary from one laboratory to another because of (1) the variation in concentration of random urine specimens, and (2) the different methods used to concentrate the sediment by centrifugation. There is no specific standardized procedure. Individual laboratories have established their own reference values, often in conjunction with the nephrologists and nephropathologists.

Methods for Examining Urine Sediment

In general, randomly collected urine specimens are satisfactory for microscopic evaluation; however, it is recommended that examination take place when the sample is fresh, particularly if no preservative has been added. Cells and casts begin to lyse within 2 hours of collection. Refrigeration (2–8°C) helps prevent the lysis of pathologic entities; however, this may increase the precipitation of various amorphous and crystalline materials. Midstream collection is recommended for females to reduce contamination from vaginal elements.

Brightfield Microscopy

Although brightfield microscopy can be performed to a limited extent on unstained urine preparations, the identification of leukocytes, histiocytes, epithelial cells, and cellular casts may be difficult. Subdued light is more effective in delineating the more translucent structures of the urine such as hyaline casts, crystals, and mucous threads. A crystal-violet safranin stain is commonly used to aid in the delineation of the formed elements in urine.

Supravital Stain Reagents

Solution I:	Crystal violet	3.0 g
	Ethyl alcohol (95%)	20.0 mL
	Ammonium oxalate	0.8 g
Solution II:	Safranin O	1.0 g
	Ethyl alcohol (95%)	40.0 mL
	Distilled water	400.0 mL

Three parts of solution I and 97 parts of solution II are mixed and filtered. The mixture should be clarified by filtering every 2 weeks and discarded after 3 months. Separately, solutions I and II can be kept indefinitely at room temperature.

Several commercially available staining reagents are available. A 2% solution of methylene blue and toluidine blue may also be used as a simple, quick supravital stain.

Procedure. Add one or two drops of stain to approximately 1 mL of concentrated urine sediment. Mix with a pipet and place a drop of this suspension on a slide and coverslip.

Phase-Contrast Microscopy

Phase-contrast microscopy is beneficial for the detection of more translucent formed elements of the urinary sediment, notably casts that may escape detection using ordinary brightfield microscopy. Phase-contrast microscopy has the advantage of hardening the outlines of even the most transparent formed elements, making detection simple (Fig. 27–4*A* and *B*). Scanning time is decreased and the yield increased. Several microscopes have been designed to allow the operator to perform either brightfield or phase-contrast examinations, depending on which objectives or condensors are utilized.

Polarized Microscopy

This is used to distinguish crystals and fibers from cellular or protein cast material. Lipid droplets or spherocrystals containing cholesterol esters are anisotropic in polarized light, show up brightly against a dark field, and form Maltese crosses with crossed polars. Visible evidence of anisotropy depends on the orientation of the crystal in the field; not all will be seen. If a red retardation plate is inserted, the cholesterol droplet will show typical blue and yellow quadrants against a red background. Starch granules will have a similar appearance when polarized but are much larger. Crystals, hair, and clothing fibers also show up brightly, but do not exhibit Maltese

cross forms. Fatty acids and triglyceride do not form liquid spherocrystals and do not show anisotropy, but glycosphingolipids in Fabry's disease are birefringent and may be seen in urinary sediments.

Quantitative Counts

The hemocytometer is used in many labs for quantifying the elements of urine sediment. The cells and casts from undiluted well-mixed urine are counted and reported as the number of cells per microliter. Normal values for neutrophils vary from 5–30/µL according to different workers; upper limits for erythrocytes vary from 3–20/µL and casts as few as 1–2/µL. Counting cells from an unspun sample of urine in a hemocytometer has advantages over the examination of cytocentrifuged spun urine. These include a decrease in variability caused by centrifugation and suspension, a fixed volume of urine for examination, and a marked visual field for accurate counting. Kesson (1978) provided evidence that chamber counts on centrifuged urine sediments are more reliable in predicting renal functional abnormalities than is a conventional method using cells per high power field. Recovery of cells may vary depending on centrifuge speed, specific gravity, and pH.

Microscopic Components in Urine Sediment

Cells

Erythrocytes

Under high power, unstained erythrocytes (RBCs) appear as pale biconcave disks that may vary somewhat in size but are usually about 7 µm in diameter. If the specimen is not fresh when it is examined, erythrocytes may appear as faint, colorless circles or 'shadow cells,' because the hemoglobin may dissolve out. They may become crenated in hypertonic urine and appear as small, rough cells with crinkled edges. In dilute urine, the cells will swell and rapidly lyse, releasing hemoglobin and leaving only empty cell membranes referred to as 'ghost cells.'

On occasion, erythrocytes may be confused with oil droplets or yeast cells. Oil droplets, however, exhibit a greater variation in size and are highly refractile, and yeast cells usually show budding. If identification is difficult, two preparations may be made and a few drops of acetic acid added to one. Erythrocytes are lysed in the acidified preparation.

Erythrocytes are found in small numbers (0–2 cells/hpf) in normal urine; more then 3 cells/hpf is considered abnormal. The presence of increased numbers of erythrocytes in the urine may indicate a variety of urinary tract and systemic conditions. These include: (1) renal disease – glomerulonephritis, lupus nephritis, interstitial nephritis associated with drug reactions, calculus, tumor, acute infection, tuberculosis, infarction, renal vein thrombosis, trauma (including renal biopsy), hydronephrosis, polycystic kidney, and occasionally acute tubular necrosis and malignant nephrosclerosis; (2) lower urinary tract disease – acute and chronic infection, calculus, tumor, stricture, and hemorrhagic cystitis following cyclophosphamide therapy; (3) extrarenal disease – acute appendicitis, salpingitis, diverticulitis, acute febrile episodes, malaria, subacute bacterial endocarditis, polyarteritis nodosa, malignant hypertension, blood dyscrasias, scurvy, and tumors of the colon, rectum, and pelvis; (4) toxic reactions due to drugs, such as sulfonamides, salicylates, methenamine, and anticoagulant therapy; and (5) physiologic causes, including exercise. When increased numbers of erythrocytes are found in the urine in conjunction with erythrocyte casts, bleeding may be assumed to be renal in origin.

Dysmorphic Erythrocytes. Numerous studies have concentrated on the variable morphology of urinary erythrocytes, attempting to localize the site of origin of hematuria. Red blood cells with cellular protrusions or fragmentation are termed dysmorphic (Fig. 27–5), and some authors have suggested that their presence in urine samples is strongly suggestive of renal glomerular bleeding (Fracchia, 1995). Others have not found dysmorphic morphology reliable in predicting primary renal hematuria (Favaro, 1997; Ward, 1998). The so-called 'G$_1$ cell,' which has a doughnut shape with one or more membrane blebs, may be more specific than dysmorphic cells for diagnosing glomerular hematuria (Dinda, 1997). Another study describes immunocytochemical staining of urinary erythrocytes with Tamm–Horsfall protein in renal hematuria, and this appears to be even more reliable than cellular morphology in terms of separating renal from nonrenal sources of erythrocytes (Fukuzaki, 1996). Normal persons may also have a mixture of distorted and undistorted erythrocytes in urine.

Leukocytes

Neutrophils. The polymorphonuclear leukocyte (neutrophil) is the predominant type of leukocyte (white blood cell [WBC]) that appears in the

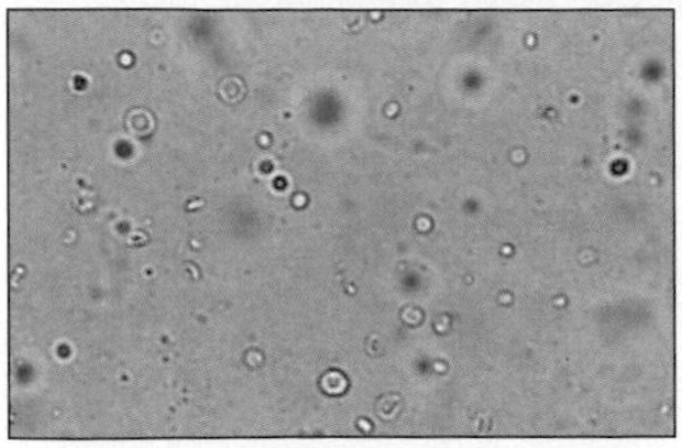

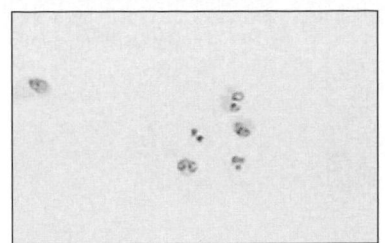

Figure 27–5 Dysmorphic erythrocytes (× 160).

Figure 27–7 Eosinophils (× 500).

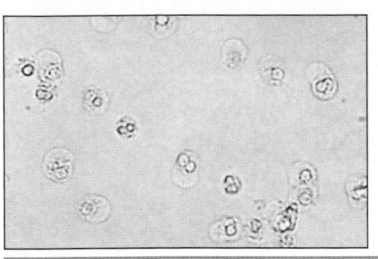

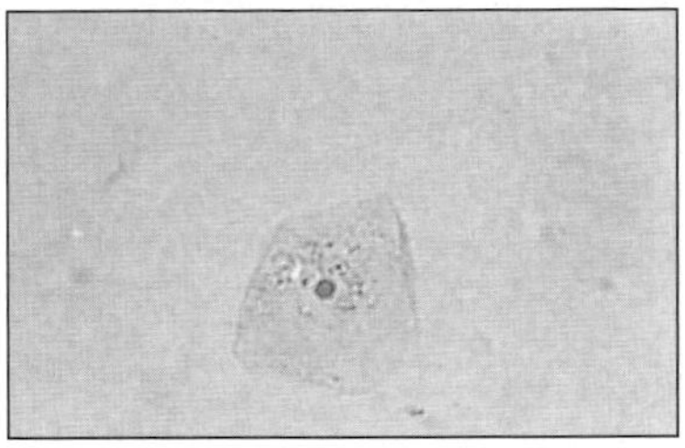

Figure 27–6 Neutrophils with dilute acetic acid (× 100).

Figure 27–8 Squamous epithelial cell. Pyridium stained (× 200).

urine. Under high power, these cells appear as granular spheres about 12 µm in diameter with multilobated nuclei. Nuclear segments may sometimes appear as small, round, discrete nuclei. When cellular degeneration has begun, nuclear detail may be lost, and neutrophils may then become difficult to distinguish from renal tubular epithelial cells. Dilute acetic acid may enhance nuclear detail so that definition may still be possible (Fig. 27–6). Ultimately, however, with continued degeneration, neutrophilic nuclear segments fuse, making distinction from mononuclear cells difficult or impossible. Supravital staining may also be helpful in emphasizing nuclear detail. With crystal-violet safranin, neutrophilic nuclei appear reddish purple and cytoplasmic granules violet. The peroxidase cytochemical reaction is also useful in distinguishing neutrophils from tubular cells.

In dilute or hypotonic urine, neutrophils swell and their cytoplasmic granules exhibit brownian movement. Because of the refractility of the moving granules, neutrophils in this setting are known as 'glitter' cells. These cells stain poorly with supravital stains, and will show loss of nuclear segmentation. The leukocyte esterase reagent strip is valuable in the confirmation of pyuria in hypotonic urine specimens.

Additionally, leukocytes are rapidly lysed in hypotonic or alkaline urine. Approximately 50% are lost following 2–3 hours of standing at room temperature. This necessitates prompt examination of the urinary sediment following collection.

Pyuria. Typically less than 5 leukocytes/hpf are seen in normal urine, although females will not uncommonly have somewhat higher quantities present. Increased numbers of leukocytes (principally neutrophils) in the urine is termed pyuria, and indicates the presence of infection or inflammation in the urinary tract. When accompanied by leukocyte casts or mixed leukocyte–epithelial cell casts, increased urinary leukocytes are considered to be renal in origin.

Infection, either bacterial or nonbacterial, may be centered in the renal parenchyma (pyelonephritis), or may be localized as cystitis, prostatitis, urethritis, or balanitis. In women, the acute urethral syndrome (dysuria–pyuria syndrome) is regularly associated with greater than 8 neutrophils/µL in clean-catch urine specimens; however, bacterial colony counts are lower than expected. *Chlamydia trachomatis* as well as staphylococci and coliforms are causative agents. Urinary neutrophil counts greater than 30 cells/hpf suggest acute infection, and repeated sterile cultures in this setting may indicate tuberculosis or a nephritis. Gross pyuria may reflect rupture of a renal or urinary tract abscess. It should be noted that the common finding of leukocytes in urine is not as reliable an indication of urinary tract infection as the detection of bacteriuria by Gram's stain or culture of a fresh midstream specimen.

Increased leukocytes may be found in a variety of other urinary tract diseases including glomerulonephritis, systemic lupus erythematosus (SLE), and interstitial nephritis. Calculous disease at any level may give rise to increased numbers of urinary leukocytes because of either stasis-induced ascending infection or localized mucosal inflammatory response. Bladder tumors, as well as a variety of acute or chronic localized inflammatory processes, may also cause leukocytes to be increased in the urine. Urine leukocytes may also be transiently increased during fevers and following strenuous exercise.

Eosinophils. These cells are not normally seen in urine, and the finding of more than 1% eosinophils among the leukocyte population present is considered significant (Fig. 27–7). Evaluation of a concentrated stained urine is necessary to properly evaluate urine for the presence of eosinophils. A cytocentrifuge preparation with Wright's, Diff-Quik, or Papanicolaou stain is commonly used, and the Hansel secretion stain (methylene blue and eosin-Y in methanol, Libe Labs, Florissant, MO) has also been shown to be an excellent stain for recognition of eosinophiluria. Appropriately stained, bilobed eosinophils may be noted in patients with tubulointerstitial disease associated with hypersensitivity to drugs such as penicillin and its analogues. The cellular pattern in allergic interstitial nephritis typically also includes many erythrocytes and some renal tubular epithelial cells. Eosinophiluria is also seen in other acute disorders of the genitourinary tract, with small numbers seen in urinary tract infections and renal transplant rejections.

Lymphocytes and Mononuclear Leukocytes. Small lymphocytes are normally present in urine, and along with histiocytes are more easily differentiated in stained smears. When mononuclear cells (histiocytes, lymphocytes, or plasma cells) constitute 30% or more of a differential count, chronic inflammation is indicated. Many small lymphocytes may be found in urine during renal transplant rejection. Plasma cells and atypical lymphocytes should be noted when present, and further investigation is warranted.

Epithelial Cells

Squamous Epithelial Cells. These cells are the most frequent epithelial cell seen in normal urine, and likewise the least significant. The distal one third of the urethra is lined by squamous epithelial cells, and in the urine these cells are large and flat, with abundant cytoplasm and small round central nuclei (Fig. 27–8). Their margins are often folded. When stained with crystal-violet safranin, nuclei are purple and cytoplasm pink to violet. Many of the squamous cells present in female urine may be derived from the vagina or vulva.

Transitional (Urothelial) Epithelial Cells. Transitional epithelial cells line the urinary tract from the renal pelvis to the lower third of the urethra. These cells are smaller than squamous cells, their size ranging from 40–200 µm. They are round or pear shaped, with a round centrally located nucleus. Occasional binucleate forms may be seen. When stained, transitional cells have dark blue nuclei with variable amounts of pale blue cytoplasm (Fig. 27–9). Another helpful clue to the proper identification of transitional cells is a characteristic 'endo–ecto cytoplasmic' rim.

A few urothelial cells are present in normal urine, reflecting normal desquamation; like squamous cells, they are rarely of pathologic significance. The exception is the presence of large clumps or sheets of transitional cells in the absence of instrumentation (i.e. catheterization). This situation necessitates cytologic examination with the Papanicolaou stain to evaluate for possible transitional cell carcinoma.

Renal Tubular Epithelial Cells. These are the most significant types of epithelial cells found in urine because the finding of an increased number indicates tubular damage (Figs 27–10 and 27–11). Small numbers of tubular cells may be seen in normal urine, reflecting the normal sloughing of aging cells. They may be present in somewhat larger numbers in the urine of normal newborns.

The Papanicolaou stain has been shown to be especially useful in distinguishing renal tubular cells from other mononuclear cells in urine. Renal epithelial cells from the proximal and distal convoluted tubules occur singly and are large (14–60 µm), oblong cells with characteristic

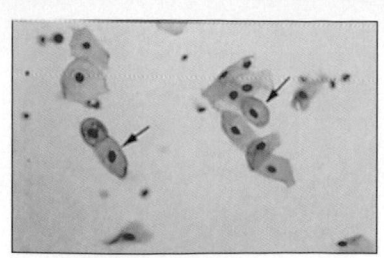

Figure 27–9 Transitional epithelial cells. Papanicolaou stained (×430).

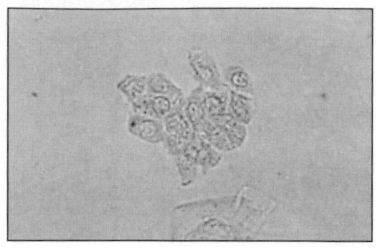

Figure 27–10 Renal tubular epithelial cells (×200).

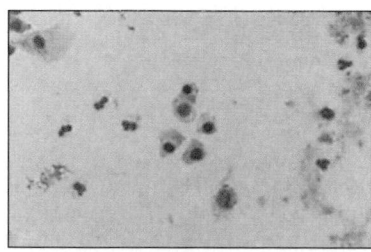

Figure 27–11 Renal tubular epithelial cells and neutrophils. Papanicolaou stained (×430).

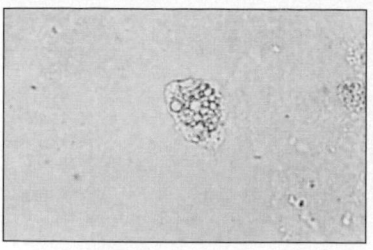

Figure 27–12 Oval fat body (×160).

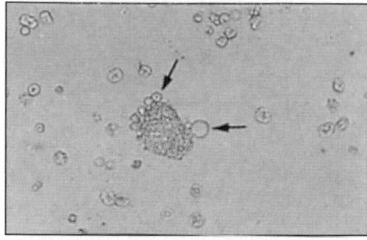

Figure 27–13 Oval fat body with attached fat droplets. Brightfield (×160).

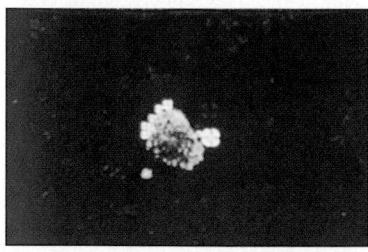

Figure 27–14 Oval fat body with attached fat droplets. Polarized (×160).

coarsely granular eosinophilic cytoplasm. Nuclei may be multiple but are small with dense chromatin and rare nucleoli. Increased numbers of proximal and distal convoluted renal epithelial cells are seen in cases of acute tubular necrosis and certain drug or heavy metal toxicity.

Epithelial cells from the collecting ducts measure 12–20 µm and are identified by their characteristic cuboidal or polygonal shape and large, usually slightly eccentric nucleus. Cytoplasmic properties include a basophilic endo–ecto cytoplasmic rim commonly found in transitional epithelial cells. Increased numbers of collecting duct epithelial cells are found in renal transplant rejection, acute tubular necrosis (diuretic phase), and other ischemic injuries to the kidney. They may also be found in increased numbers in malignant nephrosclerosis as well as in cases of acute glomerulonephritis accompanied by tubular damage. Ingestion of various drugs and chemicals may cause significant tubular desquamation. Collecting duct tubular cells are easily found in the urine following salicylate intoxication.

Renal epithelial fragments of collecting duct origin have been described. Three or more renal cells of collecting duct origin constitute a renal epithelial fragment and indicate a more severe form of renal tubular injury with basement membrane disruption. Renal epithelial fragments are indicative of ischemic necrosis and are usually found accompanying varying degrees of renal tubular injury and pathologic casts. Proximal and distal convoluted tubular cells are not found in fragment form. Proper identification of renal epithelial fragments is essential, not only in the diagnosis of a more severe form of renal tubular injury but also in avoiding a false-positive diagnosis of low-grade transitional cell carcinoma.

Lipids in Renal Tubular Epithelial Cells. Oval fat bodies are tubular cells that have absorbed lipoproteins with cholesterol and triglycerides leaked from nephrotic glomeruli (Fig. 27–12). Oval fat bodies therefore constitute one form of lipiduria. Lipids may also appear in the urine as free fatty droplets, or within histiocytes as ingested material. The presence of any or all of these lipid forms accompanied by marked proteinuria is characteristic of the nephrotic syndrome.

Positive identification of lipid is required before reporting lipiduria. When free or incorporated droplets contain large amounts of cholesterol, they exhibit Maltese cross formation under polarized light (Figs 27–13 and 27–14). When they contain large amounts of triglycerides, fat stains (Oil Red O or Sudan III) are required for positive lipid identification.

Pigment in Renal Tubular Epithelial Cells. With hemoglobinuria or myoglobinuria, heme pigment is absorbed into the cells and converted to hemosiderin. The iron-laden cells are desquamated and found in the urine sediment. The cytoplasmic granules appear yellow-brown and stain for iron with Prussian blue. These cells may also be incorporated into casts (Figs 27–1 and 27–2).

Melanin granules are absorbed into the tubular cells in rare cases of melanuria. The desquamated pigmented cells may be demonstrated in the sediment. Pigmented tumor cells are also found when there are melanoma metastases to the bladder.

Bilirubin pigment colors all of the elements of the sediment, including renal tubular epithelial cells and casts. Note that urobilin does not color cells and casts.

Casts

Casts are the only formed elements of urine that have the kidney as their sole site of origin. Tamm–Horsfall protein is the glycoprotein secreted by the thick part of the ascending loop of Henle (and possibly the distal tubule), which constitutes about one third of the total urinary protein in normal individuals. It is generally held that Tamm–Horsfall protein forms the matrix of all casts. The protein forms a meshwork of fibrils that can potentially trap any elements present in the tubular filtrate including cells, cell fragments, or granular material.

Casts can be quite variable in their appearance, size, shape, and stability. Perhaps this variability is one factor in the apparent low precision for cast identification in some laboratories (Yoo, 1995; Rasoulpour, 1996). The width of a cast depends on the size of the tubule in which it was formed. Broad casts are seen in dilated tubules or with stasis in collecting ducts. Thin casts occur in tubules compressed by swollen interstitial tissue or because of disintegration. Casts may be short and stubby, or long and convoluted. The latter variety appears when there is diuresis after urinary stasis. Casts typically have parallel sides and blunt ends, but with age they may begin to disintegrate and show thinning and irregularities. Fibrils may separate, causing a frayed appearance. Tails and tapering ends can be seen, and these disintegrating forms are referred to as cylindroids.

In the normal person, very few casts are seen in the urinary sediment. In kidney diseases, they may appear in large numbers and in many forms. Increased numbers of casts usually indicate that kidney disease is widespread and that many nephrons are involved. Large numbers of casts may also be seen in healthy persons after strenuous exercise accompanied by proteinuria.

Cast formation increases with lower pH, increased ionic concentration, and when there is stasis or obstruction of the nephron by cells or cell debris. It is also increased when larger than normal amounts of plasma proteins enter the tubules. Usually the protein in excess is albumin, but globulins such as the Bence Jones immunoglobulin cause cast formation, as do hemoglobin and myoglobin. The plasma proteins possibly react or

Table 27–11 Classification of casts

Matrix
    Hyaline – variable size
    Waxy – often broad in use
Inclusions
    Granules – proteins, cell debris
    Fat globules – triglycerides, cholesterol esters
    Hemosiderin granules
    Crystals – uncommon
    Melanin granules – rare
Pigments
    Hemoglobin, myoglobin, bilirubin, drugs
Cells
    Erythrocytes and red blood cell remnants
    Leukocytes – neutrophils, lymphocytes, monocytes, and histiocytes
    Renal tubular epithelial cells
    Mixed cells – erythrocytes, neutrophils, and renal tubular cells
    Bacteria

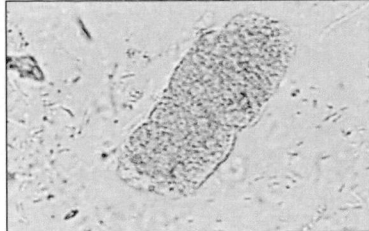

Figure 27–16 Fine granular cast becoming waxy (× 200).

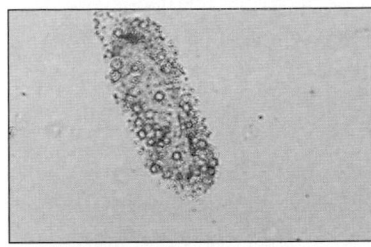

Figure 27–17 Erythrocyte cast (× 200).

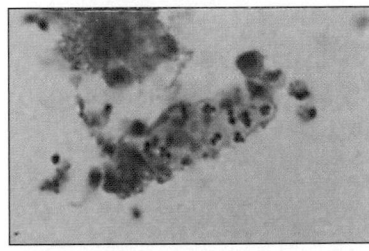

Figure 27–18 Leukocyte cast. Papanicolaou stained (× 200).

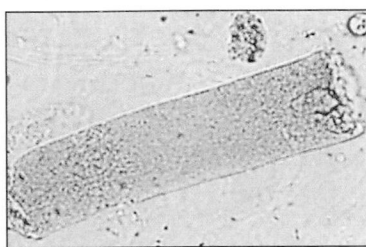

Figure 27–15 Waxy cast (× 200).

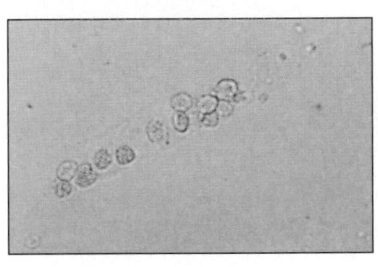

Figure 27–19 Cellular cast (× 200).

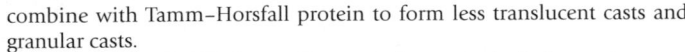

combine with Tamm–Horsfall protein to form less translucent casts and granular casts.

Casts may be classified according to their matrix, inclusions, pigments, and cells present, as shown in Table 27–11. A detailed discussion, including clinical significance, follows.

Cast Matrix

Hyaline Casts. These are the most frequently observed casts, consisting almost entirely of Tamm–Horsfall protein; zero to two hyaline casts per low power field (lpf) is considered normal. Hyaline casts are translucent with brightfield microscopy, pink with supravital staining, and are more easily visualized with phase-contrast microscopy (Fig. 27–4A and B). Increased numbers are seen with renal diseases and transiently with exercise, heat exposure, dehydration, fever, congestive heart failure, and diuretic therapy.

Waxy Casts. With chronic renal diseases, some casts become denser in appearance and are known as waxy. These differ from hyaline casts in that they are easily visualized because of their high refractive index. With brightfield microscopy, waxy casts are homogeneously smooth in appearance with sharp margins, blunted ends, and cracks or convolutions frequently seen along the lateral margins, indicating a measure of brittleness (Fig. 27–15).

Waxy casts are commonly associated with tubular inflammation and degeneration. They are observed most frequently in patients with chronic renal failure. They are also found during acute and chronic renal allograft rejection. Early waxy casts are believed by some investigators to reflect the final phase of dissolution of the fine granules of granular casts (Fig. 27–16). Because time is required for granules to undergo lysis, waxy casts imply localized nephron obstruction and oliguria. When waxy casts are unusually broad, they are known as renal failure casts. These casts imply advanced tubular atrophy and/or dilation, in turn reflecting end-stage renal disease and extreme stasis of urine flow.

Cellular Casts

Erythrocyte (Red Blood Cell) Casts. Finding these casts in the urine is quite significant because they are an indication of bleeding within the nephron. Glomerular damage allows erythrocytes to escape into the tubule, and if there is concomitant proteinuria and conditions are optimal for cast formation, red cell casts form in the distal nephron. In urine, these casts appear yellow under the low-power objectives. A prerequisite for the identification of an erythrocyte cast is that red blood cell outlines be sharply defined in at least part of the cast (Fig. 27–17). The amount of matrix material that may be visible ranges from scant to a prominent delicate hyaline matrix with only one or two red cells visible. These casts are better visualized with phase-contrast microscopy or with supravital staining, in which case the erythrocytes are colorless or lavender in a pink matrix. With prolonged stasis, red cell casts may degenerate and appear in the urine as reddish brown, coarsely granular hemoglobin (blood) casts.

Pathologic disorders in which erythrocyte casts appear in the sediment include many acute glomerulonephritides, IgA nephropathy, lupus nephritis, subacute bacterial endocarditis, and renal infarction. Rarely, tubulointerstitial disease may allow transtubular entry of erythrocytes with subsequent incorporation into a cast. This may occur in severe pyelonephritis. Additionally, the appearance of erythrocyte and leukocyte casts has been found to coincide with renal relapse in patients with SLE (Herbert, 1995).

Leukocyte (White Blood Cell) Casts. White blood cell casts are refractile, exhibit granules, and frequently multilobated nuclei will be visible (Fig. 27–18) unless disintegration has begun. Phase-contrast microscopy may be helpful in delineating nuclear segmentation. Supravital stains also enhance their visualization.

Leukocytes usually enter tubular lumina from the interstitium, and for the most part leukocyte casts (Fig. 27–19) reflect tubulointerstitial disease with neutrophilic exudates and interstitial inflammation. The most common disease of this category is pyelonephritis. Leukocyte casts may also be present in glomerular disease owing to the chemotactic effect of complement. They are also seen with interstitial nephritis, lupus nephritis, and even in the nephrotic syndrome.

Renal Tubular Epithelial Cell Casts. Renal tubular epithelial cell casts may be quite difficult to distinguish from leukocyte casts, particularly in unstained preparations viewed with brightfield microscopy. Supravital staining, phase-contrast microscopy, and Papanicolaou staining (Figs 27–19 and 27–20) are helpful in delineating between these two cast types. The

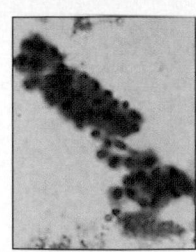

Figure 27–20 Renal tubular epithelial cell cast. Papanicolaou stained (×430).

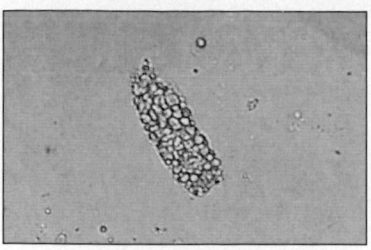

Figure 27–24 Fatty cast. Brightfield, nonpolarized (×160).

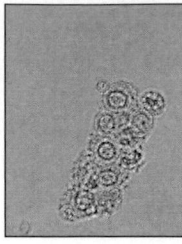

Figure 27–21 Mixed (leukocyte and renal epithelial tubular cell) cast (×200).

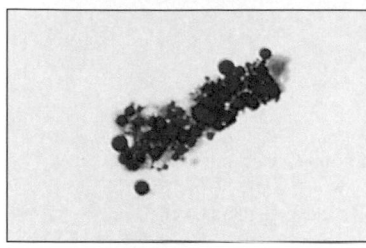

Figure 27–25 Fatty cast. Positive Oil Red O (×200).

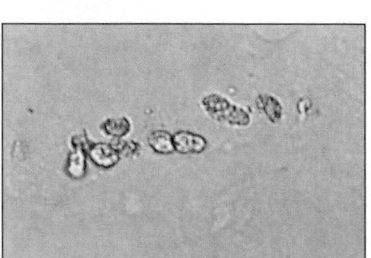

Figure 27–22 Cellular cast (×200).

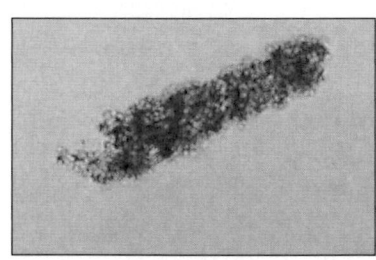

Figure 27–26 Hemoglobin cast (×200).

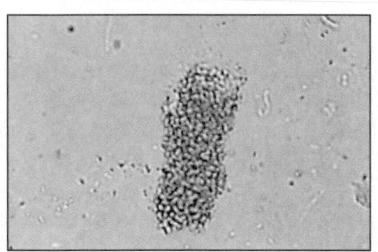

Figure 27–23 Granular cast (×200).

most reliable distinguishing characteristic of renal tubular cells is their singular round nuclei.

Renal tubular epithelial cell casts are seen in urine with acute tubular necrosis, viral disease (e.g., cytomegalovirus disease), or exposure to a variety of drugs. Heavy metal poisoning, ethylene glycol, and salicylate intoxication may cause tubular cells and casts to appear in the urine. In transplant units, these cells and casts constitute one of the more reliable criteria for detecting acute allograft rejection after the third postoperative day.

Mixed Cellular Casts. Not infrequently, two distinct cell types may be present within a single cast. This has been referred to as a mixed cast, and examples might include leukocyte/renal, erythrocyte/leukocyte, and eosinophil/renal (Fig. 27–21). When the cell types cannot be established with certainty, the resulting cast is known as a cellular cast (Fig. 27–22). Some inferences as to cell type may be drawn from the dominant population of free cells in the surrounding sediment.

Inclusion Casts

Granular Casts. Granular casts are fairly common, and may appear in both pathologic and nonpathologic conditions (Fig. 27–23). Granules may be small or large, and may originate from plasma protein aggregates that pass into the tubules from damaged glomeruli, as well as from cellular remnants of leukocytes, erythrocytes, or damaged renal tubular cells. Fine salt precipitates and lysosomes may also be granular components. Protein aggregates include fibrinogen, immune complexes, and globulins With prolonged stasis, large granules in casts may become smaller, and there appears to be no advantage to separating kinds of granular casts.

Granular casts appear with glomerular and tubular diseases but are also a feature of tubulointerstitial disease and renal allograft rejection. They may accompany pyelonephritis, viral infections, and chronic lead poisoning. Coarsely granular casts occur, with hematuria, in cases of renal papillary necrosis. It is possible that some fine granules represent calcium

phosphate precipitants in hyperparathyroidism. Granular casts may also be seen following periods of extreme stress or strenuous exercise.

Fatty Casts. Fatty material is incorporated into the cast matrix from lipid-laden renal tubular cells. These are commonly seen when there is heavy proteinuria and are a feature of nephrotic syndrome (Figs 27–24 and 27–25).

Crystal Casts. Casts containing urates, calcium oxalate, and sulfonamides (sulfamethoxazole) are occasionally seen. A matrix is visible in a true crystal cast, and the crystals may polarize. These casts indicate deposition of crystals in the tubule or collecting duct. Hematuria, possibly related to tubular damage, regularly accompanies crystal casts. These casts should be carefully distinguished from clumps of crystals forming at room or refrigerator temperatures.

Pigmented Casts

Hemoglobin (Blood) Casts. Hemoglobin casts typically appear yellow to red, although sometimes the color is quite pale (Fig. 27–26). Most often hemoglobin casts, also known as blood casts, are seen with erythrocyte casts and glomerular disease. Less commonly, they are seen with tubular bleeding and rarely with hemoglobinuria.

Hemosiderin Casts. Hemosiderin granules in casts derive from pigment-laden renal tubular cells.

Myoglobin Casts. These casts are red-brown in color and occur with myoglobinuria following acute muscle damage. These may be associated with acute renal failure.

Bilirubin and Other Drug Casts. Bilirubin is seen in urine when there is obstructive jaundice, and will color casts a deep yellow brown. Drugs, such as phenazopyridine (Pyridium), cause a bright yellow to orange color in acid urine and will color casts and cells.

Broad Casts

Broad casts are defined as those with a diameter two to six times that of normal casts. They indicate tubular dilation and/or stasis in the distal collecting duct. All types of casts may occur in broad forms, and they are typically seen in individuals with chronic renal failure. They portend a poor prognosis.

Other Miscellaneous Casts or Cast-Like Structures

Bacteria may become embedded in cast matrices, and on supravital staining, they appear dark purple with a pale pink matrix. Mucous threads are commonly confused with casts. However, these are larger, long, and ribbon-like, with poorly defined edges and pointed or split ends, in contradistinction to casts that tend to have well-defined edges and blunt ends.

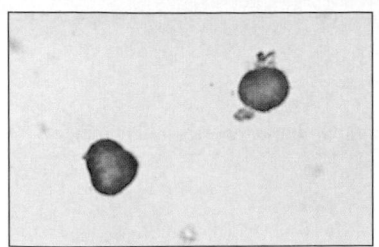

Figure 27–27 Acid urates (×160).

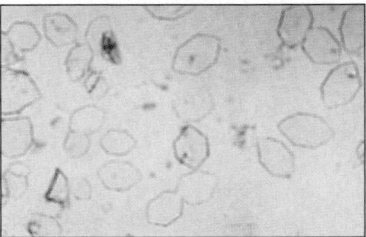

Figure 27–29 Large uric acid plate, laminated (×160).

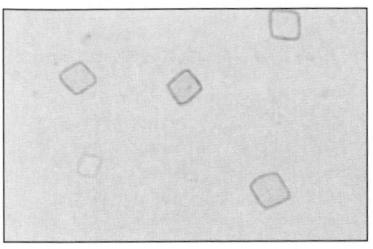

Figure 27–28 Uric acid crystals (×160).

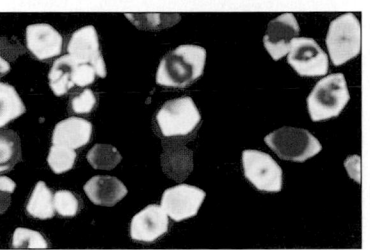

Figure 27–30 Hexagonal uric acid crystals. Brightfield (×50).

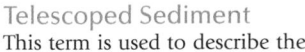

Figure 27–31 Hexagonal uric acid crystals. Polarized (×50).

Telescoped Sediment

This term is used to describe the simultaneous occurrence of elements of glomerulonephritis as well as those of the nephrotic syndrome in the same urine specimen. A telescoped sediment might therefore include red cells, red cell casts, cellular casts, broad waxy casts, lipid droplets, oval fat bodies, and fatty casts. Such sediment may be found in collagen vascular disease (notably lupus nephritis) and subacute bacterial endocarditis.

Crystals

Crystals form by the precipitation of urinary salts when alterations in multiple factors affect their solubilities. These include changes in pH, temperature, and concentration. The precipitates can appear in the urine in the form of either true crystals or amorphous material. The majority of crystal formation takes place in refrigerated specimens and those allowed to sit at room temperature for several hours. In vivo, increased solute concentration is typically responsible for crystal formation.

Although the majority of crystals in the urine are of limited clinical significance, proper identification is essential so as not to miss the relatively few abnormal crystals that are associated with various pathologic conditions. Knowledge of urine pH is a valuable aid in crystal identification because it is the pH that determines which chemical will precipitate. Many of the commonly seen crystals have characteristic morphologies; however, variability does exist, sometimes leading to confusion between pathologic and nonpathologic crystal structures. For the purposes of separating the abnormal from more commonly occurring 'nuisance' crystals, a summary of crystal morphology is presented (Table 27–12).

Crystals Found in Normal Acid Urine

Amorphous Urates (Calcium, Magnesium, Sodium, and Potassium Urates). Amorphous urates will precipitate upon standing in concentrated urine of a slightly acid pH. When large amounts are present, the urine sediment may appear pink-orange to reddish brown on macroscopic examination; this appearance has been referred to as 'brick dust.' Microscopically, this amorphous material appears as yellow-brown small granules that can form clumps and adhere to fibers and mucous threads. Amorphous urates will convert to uric acid crystals with acidification with acetic acid, and dissolve with heat (60°C) and with dilute alkali.

Crystalline Urates (Sodium, Potassium, and Ammonium). These biurates and acid urates form small brown spheres (Fig. 27–27) or colorless needles in slightly acid urine. The spheres may cluster in pairs and triplets. Like amorphous urates, these crystalline forms will slowly revert to uric acid plates on acidification with acetic acid.

Crystalline Uric Acid. Uric acid crystals occur at low pH (5–5.5) and are seen in a variety of shapes including rhombic or four-sided flat plates, prisms, oval forms with pointed ends (lemon shaped), wedges, rosettes, and irregular plates (Figs 27–28 and 27–29). The majority are colored, typically yellow or reddish brown. Rarely they are colorless and hexagonal-shaped, resembling cystine (Fig. 27–30). Unlike cystine, they show birefringence with polarized light (Fig. 27–31).

Large numbers of uric acid crystals and urates may reflect increased nucleoprotein turnover, especially during chemotherapy of leukemias or lymphoma. Increased quantities may be seen with Lesch–Nyhan syndrome, and they may provide circumstantial evidence for the nature of

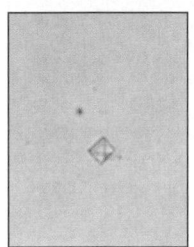

Figure 27–32 Calcium oxalate crystals (×200).

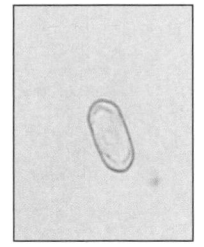

Figure 27–33 Calcium oxalate. Unusual oval form (×200).

small stones lodged in the ureters, especially when radiolucent and found in conjunction with raised serum uric acid levels. They may also herald the urate nephropathy of gout.

Calcium Oxalates. Dihydrates may appear at pH 6 or in neutral urine. Their classic form is that of a small, colorless, octahedron that resembles an envelope (Fig. 27–32). Dumbbell shapes and ovoid forms may occur (Fig. 27–33). Longer forms occur in calcium oxalate monohydrate. Oxalate crystals are insoluble in acetic acid.

Oxalate crystals in large numbers may reflect severe chronic renal disease or ethylene glycol or methoxyflurane toxicity. Oxaluria has come into prominence as a reflection of the increased absorption of oxalates from food following small bowel diseases and resection, notably for Crohn's disease. Oxaluria may also be present in genetically susceptible persons following large doses of ascorbic acid.

Crystals Found in Normal Alkaline Urine

Amorphous Phosphates (Calcium and Magnesium). Like amorphous urates, amorphous phosphates have a granular appearance microscopically; unlike the former they tend to be colorless and will produce a fine or lacy white precipitate macroscopically. Clumps or

Table 27–12 Characteristics of Amorphous and Crystalline Urinary Sediments

Substance	Description	Acid	Neutral	Alkaline	Solubility characteristics and comments
		Urine pH where found			
Ampicillin	Uncommon – from high dose; colorless; long prisms that form clusters, sheaves	+	–	–	
Bilirubin	Reddish brown; amorphous needles, rhombic plates, or cubes; may color uric acid crystals	+	–	–	Soluble in alkali, acid, acetone, and chloroform
Cholesterol	Rare; colorless; flat plate with corner notch; accompanies fatty casts and oval fat bodies	+	+	–	Very soluble in chloroform, ether, and hot alcohol
Calcium carbonate	Colorless; small granules in pairs, fours; spheres; rarely needles	–	+	+	Soluble in acetic acid with effervescence
Calcium oxalate	Dihydrate – common; colorless; small refractile octahedron Monohydrate – uncommon; dumbbell and ovoid rectangle	+	+	–	Soluble in dilute HCl
Cystine	Colorless; hexagonal plates, often laminated; rapidly destroyed by bacteria; may be confused with uric acid, but cystine is soluble in dilute hydrochloric acid	+	–	–	Soluble in alkali (especially ammonia) and dilute HCl; insoluble in boiling water, acetic acid, alcohol, ether; apply cyanide–nitroprusside reaction
Hematin	Small, biconvex 'whetstone' seen with hemoglobinuria	+	–	–	
Hemosiderin	Golden brown; granules in clumps, in cells, casts	+	+	–	Blue with Prussian blue
Hippuric acid	Rare; colorless, needles, rhombic plates and four-sided prisms; distinguish from phosphates	+	+	+	Soluble with hot water and alkali; insoluble in acetic acid
Indigotin	Rare; blue; amorphous or small crystals; colors other crystals	+	+	+	Very soluble in chloroform; soluble in ether; insoluble in acetone
Phosphates					
Amorphous phosphate (magnesium, calcium)	Colorless; fine, granular precipitate	–	+	+	Insoluble with heat; soluble with acetic acid, dilute HCl
Calcium hydrogen phosphate	Less common; colorless, star-shaped or long, thin prisms or needles; form rosettes	sl	+	sl	Slightly soluble in dilute acetic acid, soluble in dilute HCl
Triple phosphate (ammonium, magnesium)	Common form: colorless; three- to six-sided prisms, 'coffin lids' Less often: flat, fern leaf form, sheets, flakes	–	+	+	Soluble in dilute acetic acid
Radiographic media (meglumine diatrizoate)	Intravenous: colorless; thin, rhombic plates, some with notch, resemble cholesterol plates; elongated crystals Retrograde: colorless; long, pointed crystals	+	–	–	Soluble in 10% NaOH: insoluble in ether and chloroform; high specific gravity in urine: polarizes with interference colors
Sulfonamides					
Acetylsulfadiazine	Wheat sheaves with eccentric binding	+	–	–	
Acetylsulfamethoxazole	Brown; dense spheres or irregular divided spheres	+	–	–	
Sulfadiazine	Brown; dense globules	+	–	–	Soluble in acetone
Tyrosine	Rare; colorless or yellow, appears black with focusing; fine silky needles in sheaves or rosettes	+	–	–	Soluble in alkali, dilute mineral acid, relatively heat soluble; insoluble in alcohol, ether
Urates					
Amorphous (calcium, magnesium, sodium, potassium)	Common; colorless to yellow-brown; amorphous, granular precipitate	+	+	–	Soluble in dilute alkali; soluble at 60°C or lower; change to uric acid crystal with concentrated HCl or acetic acid
Monosodium urate	Colorless; needles or amorphous precipitate	+	–	–	
Urates (sodium, potassium, ammonium)	Brown; small, spherical; clusters resemble biurates	sl	+	–	Soluble at 60°C; change to uric acid with glacial acetic acid
Ammonium biurate	Common in 'old' urine; dark yellow or brown; spheres or 'thorn apples' (spheres with horns)	–	+	+	Soluble at 60°C with acetic acid; soluble strong alkali; change to uric acid with concentrated hydrochloric or acetic acid
Uric acid	Common; yellow, red-brown. brown; large variety of shapes – rhombic, four-sided plates, rosettes, 'whetstones' lemon shapes; rarely, colorless hexagonals	+	–	–	Soluble in alkali: insoluble in alcohol and acids; polarizes with interference colors
Xanthine	Rare; colorless; small, rhombic plates	+	+	–	Soluble in alkali; soluble with heat; insoluble in acetic acid

sl = Slight.

masses can often be seen by light microscopy (Fig. 27–34). Large amounts of this material may precipitate out upon prolonged standing at room temperature or in a refrigerator.

Calcium and magnesium monohydrogen phosphates are the least soluble in alkaline urine, although the dihydrogen phosphates may be soluble at a similar pH. Phosphates, in general, will dissolve in acids such as dilute hydrochloric and nitric acids and vary in solubility in acetic acid. They do not dissolve in dilute sodium hydroxide solutions or alcohol.

Crystalline Phosphates. Triple phosphate (ammonium magnesium phosphate) crystals are one of the most easily identified urine crystal, although they commonly show a variation in size. They are colorless, three- to six-sided prisms with oblique ends referred to as coffin lids (Fig. 27–35).

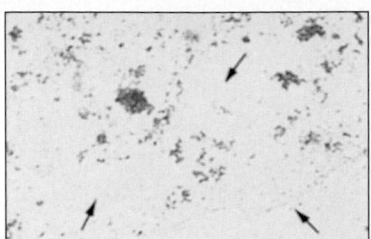

Figure 27–34 Calcium phosphate (large clear plate). Almost amorphous phosphates (×64).

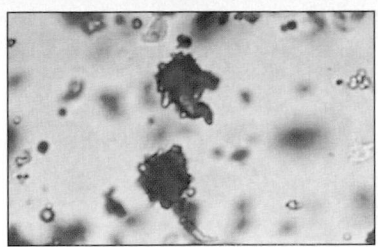

Figure 27–37 Ammonium biurate (×160).

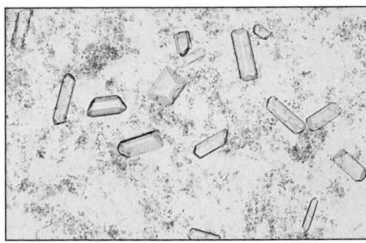

Figure 27–35 Triple phosphate (×50).

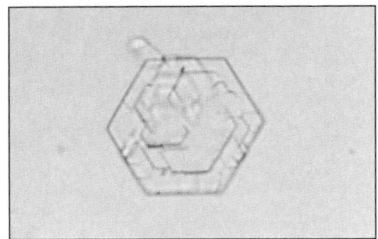

Figure 27–38 Cystine (hexagonal, laminated) (×200).

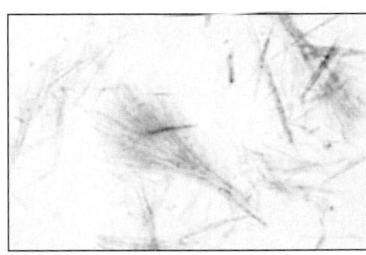

Figure 27–36 Calcium phosphate (fine sheaves) (×160).

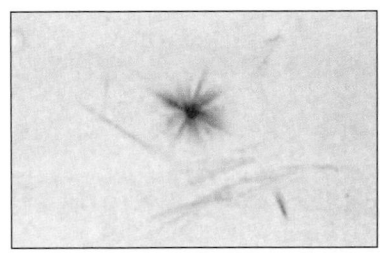

Figure 27–39 Tyrosine crystals (×160).

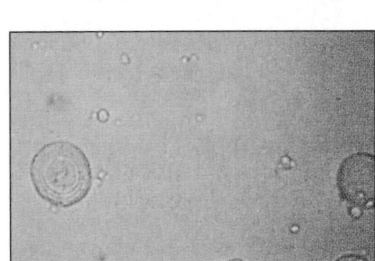

Figure 27–40 Leucine crystals (×160).

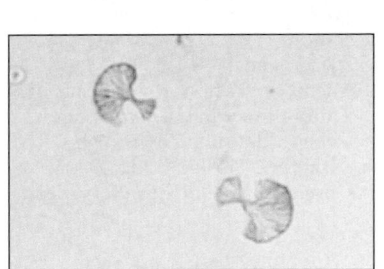

Figure 27–41 Sulfadiazine (×160).

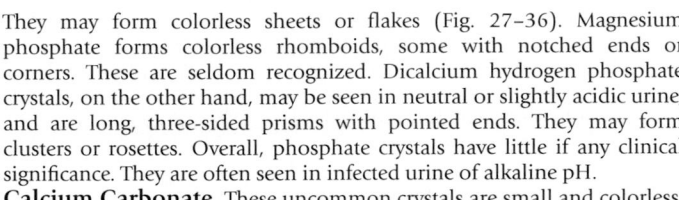

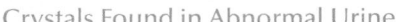

They may form colorless sheets or flakes (Fig. 27–36). Magnesium phosphate forms colorless rhomboids, some with notched ends or corners. These are seldom recognized. Dicalcium hydrogen phosphate crystals, on the other hand, may be seen in neutral or slightly acidic urine, and are long, three-sided prisms with pointed ends. They may form clusters or rosettes. Overall, phosphate crystals have little if any clinical significance. They are often seen in infected urine of alkaline pH.

Calcium Carbonate. These uncommon crystals are small and colorless, with dumbbell or spherical shapes. They may form pairs, fours, or clumps. They are distinguished from other crystals/amorphous material by their production of carbon dioxide in the presence of acetic acid.

Ammonium Biurate. Like the typical urate crystals, ammonium biurate crystals have a yellow-brown color and appear as spheres with radial or concentric striations and irregular projections or thorns (Fig. 27–37). Referred to as thorn apples, they may also be seen in neutral and occasionally in slightly acid urine. They dissolve with heat at 60°C and with acetic acid, reappearing as typical uric acid crystals after about 20 minutes.

Crystals Found in Abnormal Urine

Cystine. Cystine crystals are colorless, refractile, hexagonal plates (Fig. 27–38), which appear in acid urine. They are soluble in water at pH less than 2 or greater than 8, and they may be confused with hexagonal forms of uric acid (Fig. 27–30). Whereas uric acid crystals polarize (Fig. 27–31), thin cystine crystals do not, although thick laminated forms may polarize. Furthermore, both cystine and uric acid are soluble in ammonia water, but cystine will also dissolve in dilute hydrochloric acid and uric acid will not.

Cystine crystals are among the most important crystals identified in urine sediment. They occur in patients with cystinuria and may be associated with cystine calculi. Confirmatory testing is by the cyanide–nitroprusside reaction (see later under Cystinuria).

Tyrosine. In acidic urine, tyrosine forms fine silky needles that may be arranged in sheaves or clumps, especially after refrigeration. These may be colorless or yellow, appearing black as the microscope is focused (Fig. 27–39). They are soluble in alkali (ammonia and potassium hydroxide) and in dilute hydrochloric acid; they are not soluble in alcohol or ether.

These crystals are quite uncommon. They are less soluble than leucine, and are therefore more often precipitated in urine (see later under Tyrosinuria). Tyrosine and leucine crystals are occasionally seen in the urine of patients with severe liver disease (see later under Urinary Screening for Inherited Metabolic Diseases).

Leucine. These crystals are also rare, appearing as yellow, oily-appearing spheres with radial and concentric striations (Fig. 27–40). They are soluble in both acids and alkalis. Leucine and tyrosine crystals may occur together; leucine may be precipitated with tyrosine crystals if alcohol is added to the urine.

Sulfonamide (Sulfadiazine) Crystals. These crystals may be seen in urine of acid pH, and may take on various morphologies, depending on the form of drug involved. They may be seen as yellow-brown sheaves of wheat with central bindings, striated sheaves with eccentric bindings (Fig. 27–41), rosettes, arrowheads, petals, needles, and round forms with radial striations. They are occasionally colorless. Confirmatory testing is by the diazo reaction. High-performance liquid chromatographic and colorimetric methods have also been described (Simo-Alfonso, 1995; Mount, 1996).

With the advent of soluble sulfonamides, sulfa crystals are not as frequently found in urine, especially when the urine is examined at 37°C. Prior to this, these crystals could be seen in the urine of patients on sulfonamide therapy who were inadequately hydrated. This could result in renal tubular damage if there was crystal formation within the nephron. Currently, sulfamethoxazole (Bactrim, Septra) is seen with some regularity.

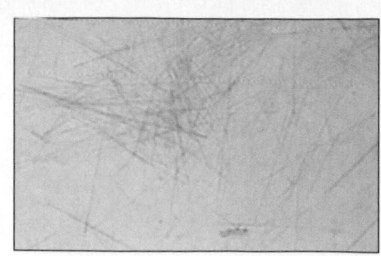

Figure 27–42 Ampicillin (× 160).

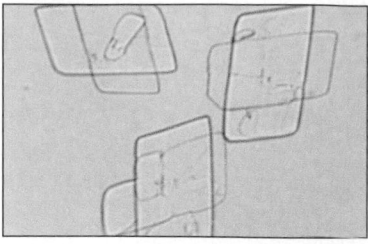

Figure 27–43 Renografin (meglumine diatrizoate). Brightfield (× 160).

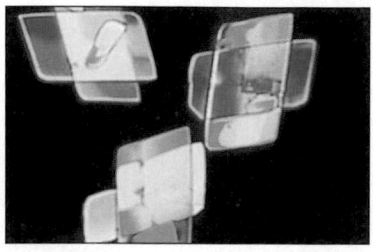

Figure 27–44 Renografin (meglumine diatrizoate). Polarized (× 160).

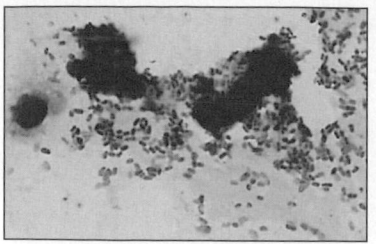

Figure 27–45 Bacteria (× 200).

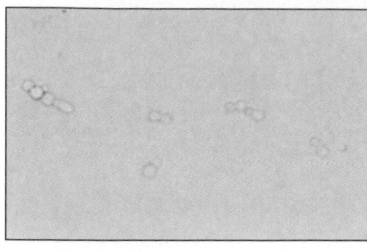

Figure 27–46 *Candida*. Budding yeasts (× 200).

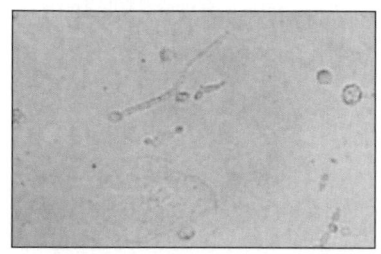

Figure 27–47 *Candida*. Pseudohyphae (× 160).

Ampicillin (High Dosage). Ampicillin may crystallize in the urine under conditions of high dosage. These crystals appear in urine of acid pH as long, fine colorless structures (Fig. 27–42). They may form coarse sheaves after refrigeration.

Radiographic Media (Meglumine Diatrizoate). Urinary crystals follow radiographic examinations using diatrizoate dyes. They may be found in urine of acid pH shortly after intravenous radiographic studies (particularly if the patient has not been well hydrated), appearing as flat, clear, colorless notched rhombic plates or longer, slender rectangles. They are easily polarized, showing interference colors (Figs 27–43 and 27–44). They may also be seen after retrograde cystograms as long, colorless needles, forming clusters after refrigeration. The presence of radiographic crystals should correlate with a high specific gravity (> 1.040).

Other Drugs. One must always remember to check the patient's drug therapy when unusual crystals are found in the urine. Several drugs have been reported to cause crystalluria when administered in high-dosage schedules or following overdose. Examples include high-dosage 6-mercaptopurine therapy, primidone overdosage, and dihydroxyadenine from massive blood transfusion.

Abnormal Cells and Other Formed Elements

Tumor Cells. Malignant tumor cells exfoliated from the renal pelvis, ureter, bladder wall, and urethra are best identified using cytologic techniques. Myeloma cells have also been noted in urine, both with and without apparent renal involvement. For a comprehensive discussion of disease types and cytologic morphologies, the reader is directed to standard urinary cytology references (Bibbo, 1997).

Viral Inclusion Cells. Epithelial cells containing inclusion bodies may be found in the urine sediment in various viral infections involving the urinary tract. Syncytial giant cells containing eosinophilic, intranuclear inclusion are seen in patients during herpetic infections. In children or immunosuppressed patients with cytomegalovirus infection, the affected cells are enlarged and contain basophilic intranuclear inclusion and/or cytoplasmic bodies. Polyomavirus-infected cells contain dense, basophilic, homogeneous intranuclear inclusions that often completely fill the nucleus. Cytologic techniques are far more sensitive in detecting all of the aforementioned viral cytopathic effects.

Platelets. These have been demonstrated in urine. Up to 30 000/μL have been demonstrated by phase-contrast microscopy and confirmed by electron microscopy in the urine of patients with hemolytic-uremic syndrome.

Bacteria. Finding bacteria in urine may or may not be significant, depending on the method of urine collection and how soon after

collection of the specimen the examination takes place. If bacteria are identified with Gram's stain in an uncentrifuged urine specimen under an oil-immersion lens, it suggests that more than 100 000 organisms/mL are present (i.e. significant bacteriuria). Most commonly, rod-shaped bacteria are seen, since the enteric organisms are the causative agents in the majority of urinary tract infections (Fig. 27–45). Leukocytes will usually be seen in the sediment as well.

Acid-fast bacilli may be seen in urine sediment, but because the urethral flora may contain nonpathogenic acid-fast organisms, the presence of *Tuberculosis* in urine must be substantiated by culture and/or polymerase chain reaction (PCR) methodology.

Fungi. Yeasts (most commonly *Candida* species) may be causative agents in urinary tract infection (e.g., in diabetes mellitus), but yeasts are also common contaminants from the skin, female genital tract, and the air. On microscopic examination, they may be confused with erythrocytes; the presence of budding helps to identify them as yeast cells (Fig. 27–46). Pseudohyphae of *Candida* are occasionally found (Fig. 27–47).

Parasites. Parasites and parasitic ova may be seen in urine sediments as a result of fecal or vaginal contamination. When noted, repeat examination should be performed on a fresh, clean-voided urine specimen. Although *Trichomonas vaginalis* may be present in urine as a result of vaginal contamination, urethral or bladder infection can occur and, when suspected, the protozoa should be searched for immediately in a wet preparation of the sediment. Motility of the organism is helpful in making the appropriate identification. In patients with schistosomiasis due to *Schistosoma haematobium*, typical ova are shed directly into the urine accompanied by erythrocytes from the urinary bladder. Amebae are rarely seen in the urine; these may reach the bladder from lymphatics or more likely from fecal contamination of the urethra. The pathogenic *Entamoeba histolytica* is usually accompanied by erythrocytes and leukocytes.

Contaminants and Artifacts

Partly digested muscle fibers or vegetable cells may be found when there is fecal contamination (Fig. 27–48). Spermatozoa are occasionally present, and pollen grains contaminate specimens seasonally (Fig. 27–49). Fibers from many different sources may be seen, including cotton, hair, wood fibers from applicator sticks, and synthetic fibers from disposable diapers. Unlike casts, these fibers polarize brightly.

Starch granules from surgical gloves are the most common contaminants of urine and other body fluids. Microscopically, they appear bright and faintly striated with an irregular outline and central depression (Fig. 27–50). With crossed polarizing filters, starch granules exhibit a typical Maltese cross pattern, and because of their large size (several times

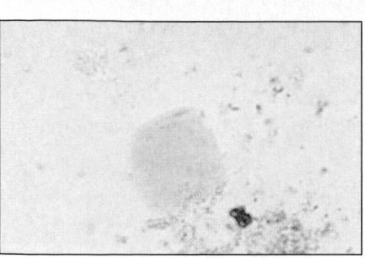

Figure 27–48 Muscle fiber (×200).

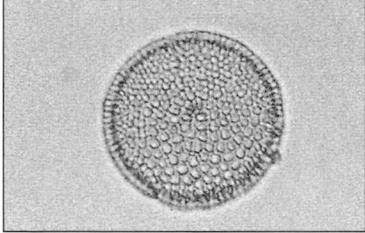

Figure 27–49 Pollen grain (×160).

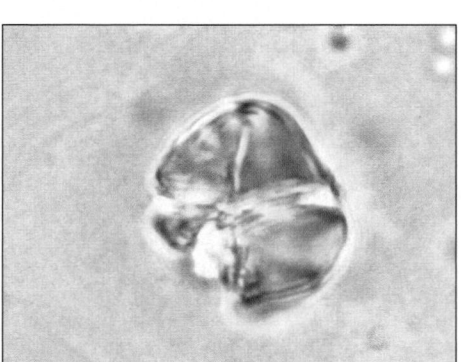

Figure 27–50 Starch granule (×160).

7. Comment on:
   a. Squamous and transitional cells if present in large numbers or as fragments (transitional cells).
   b. Bacteria, yeast, and microorganisms. Bacteriuria detectable on low power should be reported as at least 2+.
   c. Crystals (quantitated under low power). Presence of abnormal crystals should be confirmed chemically and correlated with the patient history.
   d. Large amounts of mucus.
8. The authors recommend confirming the following results with cytopathologic examination or specific chemical tests (crystals):
   a. More than two renal epithelial cells/hpf
   b. Pathologic casts
   c. Atypical mononuclear cells, particularly urothelial cells
   d. Tissue fragments
   e. Pathologic crystals

Review entire report, including physical, chemical, and microscopic data, and correlate with available clinical information. Discrepancies should be resolved before releasing report. Normal values for the procedure: 0–10 RBCs/hpf, 0–10 WBCs/hpf, 0–2 hyaline casts/lpf. Values will vary, depending on standardized system used.

The routine urinalysis is a helpful diagnostic tool in the work-up and follow-up of various urinary system disorders. Table 27–13 summarizes the macroscopic, reagent strip, and microscopic findings typical for the most commonly encountered entities.

Automated Urinalysis

Several instruments have been developed to partially or completely automate routine urinalysis. In addition to enhancing work flow, automation can also standardize some aspects of manual urinalysis. Most of these instruments can be interfaced with laboratory information systems, facilitating reporting and result retrieval.

Several instruments are available to automate either the macroscopic/chemical analysis or the microscopic portions of the routine urinalysis. For example, fully automated urine chemistry reagent strip analyzers from several manufacturers are equipped to perform automatic pipetting or test strip dipping, as well as carry out photometric measurements of the reagent strip fields.

The IRIS Urinalysis work stations combine several automated subsystems to perform a complete urinalysis. Specific gravity is measured by a mass gravity meter, urine chemistries are measured by a standard reflectance spectrophotometer, and microscopic analysis is facilitated with an automated intelligent microscopy system. No centrifugation is involved, and the handling of the specimen is minimal. A touch-sensitive video screen eliminates keyboard entry. In the analysis, the urine specimen is poured into the instrument's entry port over a urine chemistry reagent strip. This reagent strip is then placed in the reflectance photometer reader platform. The urine chemistries are automatically timed, read, and collated by the internal computer. A portion of the specimen is diverted to the harmonic oscillator mass gravity meter for specific gravity determination and the rest of the specimen is then stained and passed into a laminar flow chamber where the formed elements are detected and imaged by a video camera mounted to a microscope and a stroboscopic lamp that allows stop–motion images. Images of cells, casts, crystals, yeast, and bacteria found in the sediment are then sorted by size and presented to the operator on the touch-sensitive screen for identification. Because the volume of the laminar flow chamber is known, the images can be counted and related to a volume of urine with a precision that exceeds that which can be obtained with a centrifuged specimen, glass slide, and coverslip. The system can remove the need for microscopic analysis in most cases (Hughes, 2003). The computer then consolidates the report for printing or transmission to the laboratory information system (LIS).

The IRIS system bases its analysis on cell image analysis. Another way to analyze urinary cells and casts is by flow cytometry. These analyzers typically stain the DNA and membranes of the formed elements in native urine, pass the sample as a laminar flow through a laser beam, and measure the light scatter, fluorescence, and impedance. The UF-100 (Sysmex) analyzes urine by flow cytometry, and gives quantitative results for red and white blood cells, epithelial cells, casts, and bacteria (Fig. 27–51). It can detect yeast, crystals, dysmorphic red blood cells and pathologic casts (Fig. 27–52) in the urine (Ben-Ezra, 1998; Ottinger, 2003). This technology may be useful in decreasing the number of urine specimens requiring routine microscopy (Fenili, 1998). Normal values are fewer than 20 RBCs/μL, fewer than 25 WBCs/μL, and fewer than 2000 bacteria/μL. Similar to the microscopic examination of urine on unspun specimens, the automated systems are not prone to the artifacts that characterize examination of spun urine sediment.

larger than an erythrocyte), they are not likely to be confused with cholesterol droplets. Oil droplets from catheter lubricants may be confused with cells, especially red cells. Lipid material from vaginal creams also forms droplets in urine and may form large amorphous aggregates.

Methods for Urinalysis

Basic (Routine) Urinalysis Procedure

1. Pour 10–15 mL of a well-mixed urine specimen into a graduated disposable centrifuge tube. Perform physical examination and reagent strip chemical evaluations. Centrifuge at 450 *g* for 5 minutes.
2. Carefully remove and save the supernatant. The final volume used to resuspend the sediment may vary with the standardized system used but should remain a constant within any given laboratory. Use a disposable pipet, specialized tube, or pipet system to concentrate the sediment.
3. Gently resuspend the sediment in the remaining supernatant, and add one drop of supravital stain if desired. Using an appropriate pipet, load/charge the examination chamber of a standardized slide. Allow the urine to settle for 30–60 seconds.
4. Examine with low- and high-power objectives. Subdued light or phase-contrast illumination will be required to detect sediment entities with a low refractive index. The fine focus should be varied continuously while scanning. Systematically progress around the entire examination chamber, being careful to examine along the edges for casts.
5. Count the number of casts in at least 10 lpf, average, and report the number of casts per lpf. A reasonable range may be used in reporting (e.g., 0–2, 2–5, 5–10). Use high power to identify casts by type. Casts will not be missed if phase-contrast microscopy is used (see Fig. 27–4*A* and *B*).
6. Identify and count erythrocytes, leukocytes, and renal epithelial cells using the high-power objective. Count at least 10 hpf, average, and report as cells/hpf. A reasonable range may be used for reporting.

Table 27–13 Various Urinary System Diseases and Corresponding Urinalysis Abnormalities

Diseases	Macroscopic urinalysis	Microscopic urinalysis
Acute glomerulonephritis	Gross hematuria 'Smoky' turbidity Proteinuria	Erythrocyte and blood casts Epithelial casts Hyaline and granular casts Waxy casts Neutrophils Erythrocytes
Chronic glomerulonephritis	Hematuria Proteinuria	Granular and waxy casts Occasional blood casts Erythrocytes Leukocytes Epithelial casts Lipid droplets
Acute pyelonephritis	Turbid Occasional odor Occasional proteinuria	Numerous neutrophils (many in clumps) Few lymphocytes and histiocytes Leukocyte casts Epithelial casts Renal epithelial cells Erythrocytes Granular and waxy casts Bacteria
Chronic pyelonephritis	Occasional proteinuria	Leukocytes Broad waxy casts Granular and epithelial casts Occasional leukocyte cast Bacteria Erythrocytes
Nephrotic syndrome	Proteinuria Fat droplets	Fatty and waxy casts Cellular and granular casts Oval fat bodies and/or vacuolated renal epithelial cells occurring singly or as cellular clusters
Acute tubular necrosis	Hematuria Occasional proteinuria	Necrotic or degenerated renal epithelial cells Neutrophils and erythrocytes Granular and epithelial casts Waxy casts Broad casts Epithelial tissue fragments
Cystitis	Hematuria	Numerous leukocytes Erythrocytes Transitional epithelial cells occurring singly or as fragments Histiocytes and giant cells Bacteria Absence of casts
Dysuria–pyuria syndrome	Slightly turbid	Numerous leukocytes, bacteria Erythrocytes No casts
Acute renal allograft rejection (lower nephrosis)	Hematuria Occasional proteinuria	Renal epithelial cells Lymphocytes and plasma cells Neutrophils Renal epithelial casts Renal epithelial fragments Granular, bloody, and waxy casts
Urinary tract neoplasia	Hematuria	Atypical mononuclear cells with enlarged, irregular hyperchromatic nuclei and sometimes containing prominent nucleoli that

Table 27–13 Various Urinary System Diseases and Corresponding Urinalysis Abnormalities (cont'd)

Diseases	Macroscopic urinalysis	Microscopic urinalysis
		occur singly or as tissue fragments Neutrophils Erythrocytes Transitional epithelial cells
Viral infection	Hematuria Occasional proteinuria	Enlarged mononuclear cells and/or multinucleated cells with prominent intranuclear and/or cytoplasmic inclusions Neutrophils Lymphocytes and plasma cells Erythrocytes

Special Testing and Monitoring Techniques

Urinary Calculi

Nephrolithiasis is a common condition affecting nearly 5 in 1000 persons. It is a heterogeneous disorder, with stones developing from a wide variety of metabolic or environmental disturbances. Although the majority of studies have concentrated on nonorganic components, many stones have been found to be associated with an organic matrix containing lipids and protein, suggesting the involvement of cellular membranes in the nucleation of crystals (Khan, 1996). One study showed that antisera raised against these stone matrix proteins had cross-reactivity between proteins isolated from different stones irrespective of their mineral composition (Siddiqui, 1998). Many stone patients have also been found to show elevation of interleukin-6 (IL-6), which may in the future be useful as a potential marker for stone disease (Rhee, 1998).

Upper (renal) stones are common in western industrialized countries, whereas bladder stones are uncommon. The passage of stones down the ureter produces renal colic, which is characterized by severe pain in the flank radiating to the groin. Hematuria frequently accompanies stone passage. If stones obstruct the pelvis of the kidney or ureter, hydronephrosis can result, and infection is a common consequence. Recurrences are frequent, but with appropriate identification of the stones and the risk factors associated with them, stone formation may be greatly reduced.

Calcium oxalate or a mixture of oxalate and calcium phosphate is often found in stones (~ 80%). Mixed calcium phosphate, magnesium ammonium phosphate, and uric acid are the next most common constituents (3–10% each), and these are followed by cystine stones (1–2%). Carbonate, which is frequently detected in chemical analysis, probably results from adsorption of carbon dioxide to the calcium phosphate crystal. Males are more often affected with calcium stones than females, and children are not often affected with calcium stones.

Calcium oxalate precipitates at an acid or neutral pH, and calcium phosphate – hydroxyapatite $Ca_{10}(PO)_6(OH)_2$ – forms calculi at the normal urinary pH of 6.0–6.5. Uric acid, which is not very soluble, will crystallize at a low pH (5.3) and form stones. Magnesium ammonium phosphate (struvite) forms stones at alkaline pH, where the ammonium level is high. These tend to form in the pelvis of the kidney but apparently are not attached to papillae, as are the calcium stones. They may, however, develop on pre-existing nuclei when there is infection from organisms such as *Proteus* causing alkalization of the urine. Struvite stones may become large, forming casts of the kidney pelvis and showing staghorns. Mixed stones may form when calcium or uric acid crystals (or stones) cause obstruction followed by infection and the subsequent deposition of ammonium salts.

Hypercalciuria and Calcium Stones

Calcium homeostasis is maintained by parathyroid hormone (PTH) and 1,25-dihydroxycholecalciferol ($1,25(OH)_2D$). Both affect bone resorption by osteoclasts. PTH causes a diminution of phosphorus reabsorption and an increase in calcium reabsorption by renal tubular cells. It also causes increased synthesis of $1,25(OH)_2D$, which acts upon the small intestinal mucosa, causing increased absorption of calcium and phosphorus. Low serum ionized calcium levels cause increased PTH secretion, and low serum phosphorus stimulates $1,25(OH)_2D$ synthesis.

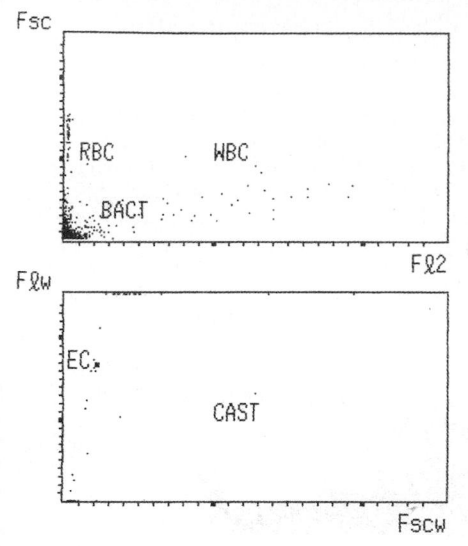

RBC	9.8	[/µL]	1.8[/HPF]
HBC	4.2	[/µL]	0.8[/HPF]
EC	4.1	[/µL]	0.7[/HPF]
CAST	0.00	[/µL]	0.00[/LPF]
BACT	607.5	[/µL]	—

Path.CAST · · · · · X'TAL
SRC · · · · · · · · · SPERM
YLC

RBC-Info.

OB/Hb · · · · · · · · PRO
L.Est. · · · · · · · NIT

Figure 27–51 Printout from UF-100 automated urine analyzer, showing normal urine. Note the lack of RBCs, WBCs, bacteria, and casts.

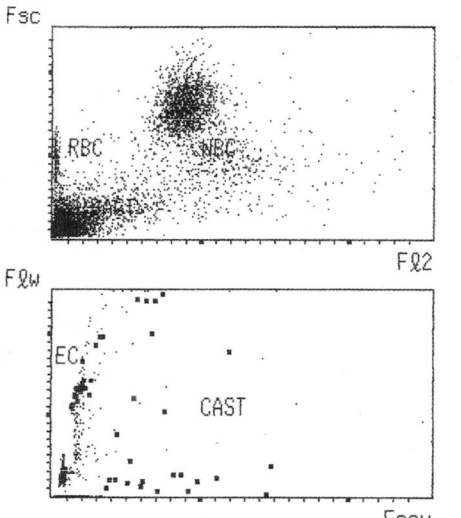

RBC	226.8	[/µL]	40.8[/HPF]
HBC	766.1	[/µL]	137.9[/HPF]
EC	27.0	[/µL]	4.9[/HPF]
CAST	3.07	[/µL]	8.90[/LPF]
BACT	12500.4	[/µL]	5+

Path.CAST ▉ · · · · · X'TAL
SRC · · · · · · · · · SPERM
YLC

RBC-Info. · · · · Dysmorphic ?

OB/Hb · · · · · · · · PRO
L.Est. · · · · · · · NIT

Figure 27–52 Printout from UF-100 automated urine analyzer, showing abnormal urine. Compare with Figure 27–51. Note the sizable number of RBCs, WBCs, bacteria, and casts.

About 40% of patients with calcium stones will have hypercalciuria, defined as a daily urinary excretion of calcium in excess of 0.1 mmol/kg (Houillier, 1998). Increased calcium in urine may result from an increase in intestinal calcium absorption, a lack of appropriate renal tubular reabsorption of calcium, resorption or loss of calcium from bone, or a combination of these factors. In a few instances of hypercalciuria, an underlying disease process can be identified. In most cases, however, it is primary, or idiopathic hypercalciuria (IH). Although the exact mechanism of hypercalciuria is still unknown in this disorder, it most likely includes a combination of factors, including those listed above. Three hypotheses to account for IH pathophysiology have been proposed. These include possible defects in the fatty acid content of cell membranes, an increased expression of the vitamin D or calcium receptors of the 25-hydroxyvitamin D_1 α-hydroxylase, or a disease of monocytes (Bataille, 1998).

Excess loss of calcium in urine and the possibility of stone formation may be secondary to a variety of other conditions. For instance, hypercalciuria may occur with increased absorption of calcium from the gut. This may occur when there is excessive loss of phosphorus from the kidney and low serum phosphorus levels, and when there is increased serum $1,25(OH)_2D$ with normal serum phosphorus levels. Increased resorption of bone may occur with immobilization of the skeleton, rapidly progressive bone disease, thyrotoxicosis, and Cushing's disease, leading to hypercalciuria. Calcium may be lost from bone as a result of osteolytic tumors, as well as in the presence of renal disease such as distal renal tubular acidosis and medullary sponge kidney. Sarcoidosis, vitamin D excess, and furosemide may also cause renal hypercalciuria.

About 5–10% of calcium stones are associated with primary hyperparathyroidism. In this disorder, increased mineral turnover in bone and hypercalcemia are important causes of hypercalciuria. Affected patients often present with stone symptoms, and there may be calcium phosphate deposits in the renal tissue, cornea, and other organs.

Dietary hypercalciuria is an uncommon cause of calcium stones; it is associated with a large calcium intake, of the order of 3–4 g/day, together with a high protein intake. About 800 mg/day is the normal recommended adult intake.

As stated previously, calcium oxalate stones are the most common. They may form with excess oxalate and uric acid in the urine, the latter sometimes providing a nidus for stone formation. Newly formed calcium oxalate aggregates are about 20–25 µm in diameter, much smaller than the outlet of the collecting ducts. Adherence to the epithelial surface apparently allows stones to continue growth rather than be excreted. Calcium phosphate stone formation is favored by a less acid urine as seen in renal tubular acidosis, with infection, and in persons consuming large amounts of alkali. These stones are also seen in primary hyperparathyroidism, although the urine is in the normal pH range. In a patient exposed to heat and dehydration, these may contribute to a rise in urinary solute levels, followed by crystallization and stone formation.

Hyperoxaluria

The majority of calcium stones (70–80%) contain oxalate. Some of the oxalate in urine is dietary in origin from beverages (tea, cocoa, coffee, cola), vegetables (beans, rhubarb, spinach), nuts, berries, and citrus fruits. Oxalate is also derived from ascorbic acid.

The gastrointestinal system plays an important role in oxalate homeostasis. Oxalate absorption increases when calcium and magnesium intake decreases. Disorders of the small bowel such as Crohn's disease, ileal resection, and intestinal bypass surgery may result in excessive oxalate absorption, with subsequent excretion in the urine. Malabsorption with steatorrhea causes loss of calcium as soaps, and malabsorption with increased bile salts remaining in the gut is thought to promote oxalate absorption in the colon. Additionally, absence of *Oxalobacter formigenes* from the intestinal tract of patients with cystic fibrosis appears to lead to increased absorption of oxalate, thereby increasing the risk of hyperoxaluria (Sidhu, 1998).

Other causes of hyperoxaluria include pyridoxine deficiency and primary hyperoxaluria. The latter is a rare inherited autosomal recessive disease with oxoglutarate carboligase deficiency. There is systemic oxalosis and renal failure in young adulthood. Renal transplantation and large doses of pyridoxine or nicotinamide have been tried for the treatment of these patients.

Hyperuricuria

Excessive excretion of uric acid may be due to excessive dietary intake of purines (liver, dried beans, some fish, meat) or various disease processes. Endogenous uric acid production is increased in gout, glycogen storage diseases, Lesch–Nyhan syndrome, many leukemias, and treated tumors with associated cell necrosis. Chemotherapy and irradiation can lead to an increased breakdown of tumor cells (nucleotide/purine forms uric acid), which may cause acute renal failure secondary to tubular and ureteral obstruction by masses of uric acid crystals.

In gout, about 20% of patients form stones, most of which are pure uric acid or mixed uric acid and calcium. Heat, dehydration, and unusually acid urine contribute to stone formation. Gouty nephropathy occurs with sodium urate deposits in the medulla even when stones are not present, and masses of crystals may cause obstruction of terminal collecting ducts in the kidney. Uricosuric drugs cause potential problems with massive uric acid output in the first 3–4 days of treatment.

Normally, about one third of the uric acid formed is degraded by bacteria in the colon. Absence of bacteria or intestinal diversions may cause increased absorption of uric acid from the gut. Because ileostomy patients lose large amounts of alkaline fluid from the intestine, they excrete concentrated acidic urine and are likely to produce uric acid stones.

The average uric acid excretion by adults is 500–600 mg/24 h. Solute concentration as well as pH appears to be important in the solubility of uric acid and urate. Uric acid, a weak acid, forms free insoluble, undissociated uric acid and a urate (which is more soluble with some sodium and potassium present) at pH 5.5. The amount of free uric acid present in urine will decrease as the pH rises, and at pH 7 uric acid is more soluble as urate. With high salt concentrations the urate becomes less soluble. If the urine volume is low, solubility of uric acid at acid pH will be exceeded.

Whereas large quantities of uric acid crystals are regularly seen in urinary sediment, uric acid stone formation is not common. Uric acid crystals form a sludge that may obstruct the nephron without forming a stone. On the other hand, uric acid and sodium acid urate crystals are found as nuclei for calcium stones. Most normal persons with a pH of 6 have urine saturated with uric acid but do not form stones. Further acidity or dehydration is apparently required to engender stone formation.

Cystine Stones

Cystine stones form in patients with an inherited amino acid transport disorder (see later under Cystinuria). Cystine, ornithine, lysine, and arginine are subsequently excreted in large amounts in the urine. Of these, only cystine forms crystals and stones. Cystine does not become soluble until the urine pH is 7.4, and stones form over a range of normal urinary pH. Heterozygous carriers for the disease will have increased amounts of cystine in urine but do not form stones; homozygotes are stone formers. A 24-hour quantitative urine cystine measurement is needed to detect the potential stone formers and should always be done when cystine crystals are found in random specimens.

Rare Calculi

Calculi containing sulfonamides have been described, and silica calculi have been reported in patients ingesting silica gel over a long period of time. Triamterene (Dyazide, Dyrenium), a relatively insoluble diuretic, may contribute to stone formation. It can form 1- to 2-mm mustard-colored stones, giving a bright blue fluorescence when dissolved in butanol and with exposure to ultraviolet light. Rare adenine stones have been described in children with an inherited enzyme deficiency disorder and hyperuricemia. Xanthine stones are uncommon and may be associated with a genetic disorder with an absence of xanthine oxidase.

Laboratory Tests Used to Investigate Stone Formers

Urine Examinations

1. Routine urinalysis, qualitative test for cystine, and urine culture. Hematuria is a constant finding when stones are present, even when they are asymptomatic. Proteinuria is usually not a feature of calculous disease, but with renal tubular damage there may be increased excretion of low-molecular-weight plasma proteins such as β_2-microglobulin, and some albumin. Erythrocyte casts are usually not found, and other casts are unusual. Leukocytes are increased when infection is present, and the reagent strip nitrite and leukocyte esterase may be elevated. Multiple clusters of nonmalignant transitional cells may be found in urine of patients with calculous disease and may be helpful in the diagnosis of unsuspected calculi.

2. Twenty-four hour urine specimen: Sodium, calcium, phosphorus, uric acid, oxalate, and creatinine clearance. Supersaturation values from 24-hour urine collections have been shown to accurately reflect stone compositions (Asplin, 1998). Some authors suggest that spot urine samples are sufficient for the metabolic evaluation of stone formers, although due to day-to-day variation, three samples should be obtained to overcome the doubtful significance of a single result (Strohmaier, 1997).

3. Urine pH determination on a fresh specimen is important in determining the kinds of crystals likely to be precipitated; for example, uric acid with low pH (5–5.5), and triple phosphate with alkaline urine.

Serum Chemistry

Appropriate tests include calcium, phosphorus, uric acid, and electrolytes.

Stone Analysis

Calculi may be of various sizes, commonly described as sand, gravel, or stone. The physical characteristics of the various calculi rarely will suffice for their identification, but a few points are worth noting. Uric acid and urate stones are typically yellow to brownish red and are moderately hard. Phosphate stones are usually pale and friable. Calcium oxalate stones are very hard, often of a dark color, and typically have a rough surface. Cystine stones are yellow-brown and feel somewhat greasy.

Several methods are available for the analysis of calculi, such as optical crystallography, X-ray diffraction, and infrared spectroscopy. Electron beam analysis and mass spectroscopy are also used. A simplified method for analysis of renal calculi is presented by Farrington (1980). A quantitative method for five of eight frequently measured substances has been described using available clinical chemistry methods: calcium, phosphorus, magnesium, ammonium, and uric acid. Cystine, oxalate, and carbonate are detected by qualitative means and interpreted with the quantitative results to characterize the stones. Most laboratories send calculi specimens out to more specialized laboratories for chemical analysis, where both chemical and specialized tests should be used for determining the composition of the stones.

Method for gross examination of calculi

1. Wash the stone(s) free from blood, mucus, preservation solution, and so forth. Place stones in a beaker, cover with several thicknesses of gauze held firmly in place with rubber bands, and wash under cold running water. Drain, remove gauze carefully, and dry beaker and stones in an oven. Rinse tiny stones with water from a squeeze bottle (not running water).

2. Record the dimension of the stone.

3. Describe briefly the color and texture of the stone's exterior surface. The stone may be photographed for record purposes.

4. Cut, saw, or break the stone so as to examine the interior. Note whether there is a foreign body that may have acted as a nucleus for its formation. Describe the color and texture of the interior and layers, if present.

5. Reduce small stones to a fine powder by pulverizing with a mortar and pestle.

6. If possible, where there is a very large stone, it may be advisable to make separate analyses of layers that appear to have different constituents.

Because most small calculi consist of calcium oxalate, the best way to analyze them is to put all available powder in one test tube. (If the stone is very tiny, it may be placed directly in the test tube and crushed with a spatula.) Reagents used for the chemical determination of rare stones may be found in an earlier edition of this book (Henry, 1996). It is important to have known positive material to test the reagents.

Radiologic Examination

Asymptomatic stones are sometimes found. The majority of stones are radiopaque except pure uric acid and the rare xanthine; cystine stones are opaque because of their sulfur content.

Urinary Screening for Inherited Metabolic Diseases

Urine has been used for many years to screen for metabolic diseases, particularly those resulting from a genetic predisposition. In many of these diseases, either an abnormal metabolite or a larger than normal amount of a normal metabolite is excreted in the urine. Since these conditions are uncommon, their symptoms often nonspecific, and some may be treatable if early diagnosis is confirmed, blood and urine should be analyzed using techniques that are highly selective and sensitive. Numerous inborn errors of metabolism have been identified, and this section will describe only some of the more common disease entities.

Aminoacidurias

The excretion of one or more amino acids in the urine may be due to either a block in a major metabolic pathway (overflow type) or a deficiency in renal tubular function (renal type). Phenylketonuria is an example of overflow aminoaciduria in which an enzyme substrate and other metabolites in the pathway accumulate, causing increased body fluid levels and increased substrate excretion in urine. Unlike the overflow type diseases, the renal type aminoacidurias do not have high levels of the amino acid in the blood because the primary defect is in the renal tubular reabsorption mechanism. An example of renal transport aminoaciduria is cystinuria.

Phenylketonuria. Phenylketonuria is an autosomal recessive inherited disorder in which there is absence of the enzyme phenylalanine hydroxylase. Both sexes are affected equally, with an incidence of about 1 in 11 000. Allelic heterogeneity can be quite extensive, particularly in the United States (Guldberg, 1996). Mental retardation is the major clinical finding, and dietary restriction of phenylalanine has proven efficacious in these patients.

Because it is not converted to tyrosine in this disorder, phenylalanine and other normal metabolites accumulate in abnormal amounts. Plasma phenylalanine and phenylpyruvic acid levels are elevated; urinary phenylpyruvic acid (highest), phenylacetic acid, and phenylalanine are increased. Urinary indoleacetic acid and other indoles arising from altered tryptophan metabolism and indican (an indole) are also increased. The excretion of 5-hydroxyindoleacetic acid is diminished, paralleling the low level of serum 5-hydroxytryptamine. The urine and sweat of these patients has a characteristic mousy/musty odor due to phenylacetic acid.

Methods. Phenistix reagent strips contain ferric ammonium sulfate, magnesium sulfate, and cyclohexylsulfamic acid. At 30 seconds following immersion into urine, the color of the test area is compared with the color chart provided. A positive test result is a gray to gray-green color. The test detects 5–10 mg/dL. Salicylates and metabolites of phenothiazine derivatives may cause a pink to purple color. Ion-exchange high-performance liquid chromatography (HPLC) has been found suitable for quantitative confirmatory testing of abnormal specimens (Reilly, 1998).

Alkaptonuria. Normally, phenylalanine and tyrosine are metabolized to homogentisic acid (dihydroxyphenylacetic acid), which is then oxidized to maleylacetoacetic acid. In alkaptonuria, the enzyme homogentisic acid oxidase (HAO) is deficient, and homogentisic acid is excreted in urine in large quantities. The urine characteristically turns brown-black on standing or with alkaline pH. Patients with alkaptonuria develop dark blue to black pigmentation in cartilage and connective tissue, and frequently the disease is not diagnosed until arthritis has already developed.

Methods. Screening methods include the ferric chloride and silver nitrate tests. A transient, dark blue color is seen as two drops of 10% ferric chloride solution are added to about 2 mL urine containing homogentisic acid. The silver nitrate test involves adding 4 mL of 3% silver nitrate to 0.5 mL urine, mixing, and then adding several drops of 10% NH_4OH. Homogentisic acid will cause a black color to develop. Confirmatory methods include paper or thin-layer chromatography, and capillary electrophoresis. These methods should distinguish homogentisic acid from gentisic acid, an aspirin metabolite.

Tyrosinuria. Tyrosinemia with tyrosinuria occurs when there is abnormal metabolism of tyrosine derived from the diet or from phenylalanine. This may be part of a generalized amino acid disorder associated with liver disease, or may represent one of the various genetic disorders involving tyrosine metabolism. Tyrosine crystals may appear in the urine as fine, silky crystals scattered singly or aggregated to form sheaves. They appear brown to black, precipitate at an acid pH, and are soluble in alkali. Small quantities of tyrosine may appear in the urine of normal individuals.

Transitory hypertyrosinemia may occur in low-birth-weight and premature infants as a benign condition. Typically, these infants are asymptomatic, and there is no liver or renal disease present. The elevated tyrosine levels may on occasion be accompanied by transiently elevated phenylalanine levels. Tyrosine and the phenolic acids, *p*-hydroxyphenyllactic and *p*-hydroxyphenylpyruvic acid, are excreted in larger than normal amounts in the urine. The nature of the enzymatic defect has not been well characterized, and the tyrosine level of these patients usually returns to normal within a few weeks to months.

Type I hereditary tyrosinemia (tyrosinosis) is an autosomal recessive disorder characterized by defects in fumarylacetoacetate hydrolase and maleylacetoacetate hydrolase. Succinylacetoacetone and succinylacetone accumulate and inhibit renal function, various hepatic enzymes, and porphobilinogen synthetase. Patients may experience liver failure, renal dysfunction, rickets, and acute intermittent porphyria-like symptoms. Hepatoma is a late complication. Generalized aminoaciduria, phosphaturia, glycosuria, and uricosuria may occur. A low-tyrosine/phenylalanine diet is the mainstay of therapy.

Type II tyrosinemia (Richner–Hanhart syndrome) is an autosomal recessive inherited deficiency of tyrosine aminotransferase. Patients will have tyrosinemia, tyrosinuria, and increased urinary phenolic acids. The metabolism of other amino acids, renal function, and hepatic function are otherwise normal. Erosions of the cornea, soles, and palms are common, and mental retardation sometimes occurs. Therapy centers on a low-tyrosine/phenylalanine diet.

Methods. The nitrosonaphthol test for tyrosine is a nonspecific screening method and should be confirmed by chromatography or quantitative serum assay of tyrosine. Tyrosine and tyramine form soluble red complexes with nitrosonaphthol.

Maple Syrup Urine Disease. MSUD is one of a group of diseases associated with abnormal branched chain amino acid metabolism. These include hypervalinemia, isovaleric acidemia causing 'sweaty feet' odor, and other rare diseases. Several different clinical forms of MSUD have been described, together with various sites of biochemical derangement. The classic type of MSUD, inherited as an autosomal recessive trait, is marked by severe neonatal vomiting, seizures, stupor, irregular respirations, and often hypoglycemia. Left untreated, these patients become rapidly comatose and die. Leucine, isoleucine, valine, and their corresponding keto acids are elevated in the plasma and excreted in the urine. Deficient decarboxylases and other enzymes are thought to prevent the conversion of the keto acids to fatty acids. Intermittent, intermediate, thiamine-responsive, and dihydrolipoyl dehydrogenase (E3) deficiency forms of MSUD have also been described (Holmes, 1997).

The urine of patients with MSUD has an odor resembling maple syrup, caramelized sugar, or curry, the source of which is not certain. The urinary keto acids are demonstrable by the first week of life.

Methods. The dinitrophenylhydrazine screening test indicates the presence of α-keto acids in the urine. Insoluble hydrazones form from the reaction of carbonyl groups with dinitrophenylhydrazine. A positive result is seen with MSUD and possibly in phenylketonuria (phenylpyruvic acid), histidinemia (imidazole pyruvic acid), and methionine malabsorption (oasthouse syndrome). The test is positive with ketonuria due to other inherited diseases and other causes. A preliminary screening test for ketones should be performed.

Procedure

1. Reagent and control (ketoglutaric acid, 25 mg in 100 mL normal urine) should be at room temperature.
2. Add 10 drops of reagent (100 mg of 2,4-dinitrophenylhydrazine in 100 mL of 2 N HCl) to 1 mL of clear urine.
3. Within 10 minutes, a yellow or chalky white precipitate indicates a positive reaction. It should be the same as or greater than the control precipitate.

Gas or thin-layer chromatographic analysis or nuclear magnetic resonance (NMR) spectroscopy of the urine may be used for confirmatory methods (Holmes, 1997).

Cystinuria. Cystinuria is a common amino acid disorder that occurs equally in both sexes, with an incidence estimated at about 1 per 10 000 (homozygous) and in larger numbers for heterozygotes. In mass screening programs for infants, the homozygous form is detected at about the same rate as phenylketonuria. The defective transport of cystine by the epithelial cells of the renal tubules and gut is transmitted as an autosomal recessive

III

trait. The basic defect is not known. Although large amounts of the dibasic acids, ornithine, lysine, and arginine, are also excreted in this disease, cystine is the only one that crystallizes out, with stone formation as a clinical manifestation.

Cystinosis, a recessively inherited disorder of unknown cause, is characterized by intracellular cystine crystal deposition within lysosomes. Crystals may accumulate in the kidney, eye, bone marrow, and spleen. In the severe form of this disorder, there is photophobia, renal failure, rickets, and growth failure. With renal tubular involvement, Fanconi's syndrome develops and there is a generalized aminoaciduria and glucosuria. Benign and intermediate varieties of cystinosis have been described. Unlike cystinuria, the cystine loss in cystinosis parallels the loss of other amino acids in the urine.

Urinary cystine is sometimes detected in patients with various renal tubular diseases. Cystine is excreted with other amino acids in Wilson's disease, Lowe's disease, and with the aminoaciduria of Hartnup's disease.

Methods. Examine a first morning urine specimen for colorless, hexagonal crystals of cystine. Cystine may not always crystallize in a concentrated urine although present in large amounts.

The cyanide–nitroprusside test used for the qualitative determination of urine cystine is Brand's modification of the Legal nitroprusside reaction. Cystine is reduced to cysteine by sodium cyanide, and the free sulfhydryl groups then react with nitroprusside to produce a red-purple color. Cysteine, cystine, homocystine, and ketones (dark red) all will give positive reactions. The qualitative test separates normal, heterozygote, and homozygote ranges of excretion. The lower limit of the test was 35–60 µmol of cystine per mole of creatinine, and this corresponded to the heterozygote range. Homozygous stone formers usually excrete more than 300 mg/g creatinine and are also detected by this test.

Procedure

1. Place 3–5 mL urine in a test tube and add 2.0 mL sodium cyanide solution (5 g/dL water) and allow to stand for 10 minutes. Timing is important. Treat a control solution in the same way. For a positive control, use 5 mg cystine dissolved in 10 mL 0.1 N HCl, diluted to 100 mL with normal urine.
2. Add fresh, aqueous sodium nitroprusside solution (5 g/dL) dropwise (about five drops), and mix.
3. Read immediately as positive or negative. A stable red-purple color will develop with cystine. 'Trace' results may also be reported. A concentrated normal specimen could give a weakly positive 'trace' result.

Further identification and quantification of cystine may be accomplished by thin-layer or quantitative ion-exchange chromatography, or high-voltage electrophoresis.

Homocystinuria. The classic form of homocystinuria is due to deficiency of cystathionine β-synthase, which catalyzes the formation of cystathionine from homocystine and serine in the methionine pathway. Homocysteine is rapidly oxidized to homocystine, which accumulates along with methionine and is excreted in the urine. Children with this disease may have seizures, thromboses, mental retardation, arachnodactyly, and kyphoscoliosis. Connective tissue manifestations are thought to result from accumulation of the intermediate homocysteine, which interferes with collagen crosslinking.

Urine for testing must be fresh because homocystine is labile. The cyanide nitroprusside test, described above, is positive. Quantitative chemical analysis reveals high levels of homocystine, methionine, and cysteine-homocysteine disulfide. Urine levels are monitored to follow the effects of the methionine-restricted diet used to treat this disease.

Additional Urine Testing Modalities

A latex agglutination nephelometric immunoassay has been developed to measure urinary basic fetoprotein (BFP). Levels of this substance may be elevated with ureter stones, infection, and prostate and bladder cancers, making BFP a nonspecific marker of inflammation or tumor (Itoh, 1998).

The urine Trinder spot test, performed by emergency room physicians, is a sensitive screen for salicylates.

Rendl et al. describe a semiquantitative rapid urinary iodide test, suitable for epidemiologic surveys of iodine deficiency, particularly in developing countries (Rendl, 1998).

Lastly, a monoclonal antibody assay for the detection of free urinary pyridinium crosslinks can help to identify bone resorption in patients with osteoporosis, hyperthyroidism, hyperparathyroidism, and Paget's disease of bone (Gomez, 1996).

Cytopathologic examination of the urine is commonly performed to detect malignancies. There are now ELISA and FISH tests to detect carcinoma of the urinary bladder. These tests are discussed in more detail in Chapter 75.

References

Anderson NG, Anderson NL, Tollaksen SL: Proteins of human urine. I. Concentration and analysis by two-dimensional electrophoresis. Clin Chem 1979; 25:119.

Arao S, Matsuura S, Nonomura M, et al: Measurement of urinary lactoferrin as a marker of urinary tract infection. J Clin Microbiol 1999; 37:553–557.

Armstrong LE, Soto JA, Hacker FT Jr, et al: Urinary indices during dehydration, exercise, and rehydration. Int J Sport Nutr 1998; 8:345–355.

Asplin J, Parks J, Lingeman J, et al: Supersaturation and stone composition in a network of dispersed treatment sites. J Urol 1998; 159:1821–1825.

Bakris DL: Microalbuminuria: Prognostic implications. Curr Opin Nephrol Hypertens 1996; 5:219–223.

Bataille P, Fardellone P, Ghazali A, et al: Pathophysiology and treatment of idiopathic hypercalciuria. Curr Opin Rheumatol 1998; 10:373–388.

Belmonte MM, Sarkozy E, Harpur E: Urine sugar determination by the two drop Clinitest method. Diabetes 1967; 16:557.

Ben-Ezra J, Bork L, McPherson RA: Evaluation of the Sysmex UF-100 automated urinalysis analyzer. Clin Chem 1998; 44: 92–95.
In this study, the authors compare the Sysmex UF-100 automated urinalysis analyzer with manual microscopy. The UF-100 showed good correlation with microscopy for detection of cellular elements and casts in the urine.

Bibbo M (ed): Comprehensive Cytopathology, 2nd ed. Philadelphia, WB Saunders Company, 1997.

Blondheim SH, Margoliash E, Shafur E: A simple test for myohemoglobinuria (myoglobinuria). JAMA 1958; 167:453.

Bowden FJ: Reappraising the value of urine leukocyte esterase testing in the age of nucleic acid amplification. Sex Transm Dis 1998; 25:322–326.

Bruno C, Minetti C, Shanske S, et al: Combined defects of muscle phosphofructokinase and AMP deaminase in a child with myoglobinuria. Neurology 1998; 50:296–298.

Bullimore SP, Keyworth C: Finding diabetes – a method of screening in general practice. Br J Gen Pract 1997; 47:371–374.

Chiang SC, Li SF: Separation of porphyrins by capillary electrophoresis in fused-silica and ethylene vinyl acetate copolymer capillaries with visible absorbance detection. Biomed Chromatogr 1997; 11:366–370.

Cone TE Jr: Diagnosis and treatment: Some syndromes, diseases and conditions associated with abnormal coloration of the urine or diaper. Pediatrics 1968; 41:654.

Cortvriend J, Van Nuffel J, Van den Bosch H, et al: Non-parasitic chyluria: A case report and review of the literature. Acta Urol Belg 1998; 66:11–15.

Davidsohn I, Henry JB (eds): Todd-Sanford Clinical Diagnosis by Laboratory Methods, 15th ed. Philadelphia, WB Saunders Company, 1974.

de Mendoza SG, Kashyap ML, Chen CY, et al: High density lipoproteinuria in nephrotic syndrome. Metabolism 1976; 25:1143.

Deacon AC, Peters TJ: Identification of acute porphyria: Evaluation of a commercial screening test for urinary porphobilinogen. Ann Clin Biochem 1998; 35:726–732.

Deutsch JC: Gas chromatographic/mass spectrometric measurement of ascorbic acid and analysis of ascorbic acid degradation in solution. Methods Enzymol 1997; 279:13–24.

Dinda AK, Saxena S, Guleria S, et al: Diagnosis of glomerular haematuria: Role of dysmorphic red cell, G1 cell, and bright-field microscopy. Scand J Clin Lab Invest 1997; 57:203–208.
This study shows that the presence of dysmorphic red blood cells in the urine has excellent sensitivity (82%) and specificity (100%) in the diagnosis of glomerular disease.

Farrington CJ, Liddy ML, Chalmers AH: A simplified sensitive method for analysis of renal calculi. Am J Clin Pathol 1980; 73:96.

Favaro S, Bonfante L, D'Angelo A, et al: Is the red cell morphology really useful to detect the source of hematuria? Am J Nephrol 1997; 17:172–175.

Fenili D, Pirovano B: The automation of sediment urinalysis using a new urine flow cytometer (UF-100). Clin Chem Lab Med 1998; 36:909–917.

Fracchia JA, Motta J, Miller LS, et al: Evaluation of asymptomatic microhematuria. Urology 1995; 46:484–489.

Free HM (ed): Modern Urine Chemistry. New York, Bayer Corporation, 1996.

Friderichsen B, Maunsbach M: Glycosuric tests should not be employed in population screening for NIDDM. J Public Health Med 1997; 19:55–60.

Fukuzaki A, Kaneto H, Ikeda S, et al: Determining the origin of hematuria by immunocytochemical staining of erythrocytes in urine for Tamm–Horsfall protein. J Urol 1996; 155:248–251.

Gerber LM, Johnson K, Alderman MH: Assessment of a new dipstick test in the screening for microalbuminuria in patients with hypertension. Am J Hypertens 1998; 11:1321–1327.
The authors examined the applicability of a urine dipstick method in detecting microalbuminuria. Specificity with this test was 90%, with a negative predictive value of 93–97%. Comparison between random and 24-hour urines showed good correlation.

Gomez B Jr, Ardakani S, Evans BJ, et al: Monoclonal antibody assay for free pyridinium cross-links. Clin Chem 1996; 42:1168–1175.

Govil YK, Sabanathan K, Scott D: Giant cell arteritis presenting as renal vasculitis. Postgrad Med J 1998; 74:170–171.

Gribble RK, Meier PR, Berg RL: The value of urine screening for glucose at each prenatal visit. Obstet Gynecol 1995; 86:405–410.

Guldberg P, Levy HL, Hanley WB, et al: Phenylalanine hydroxylase gene mutations in the United States: Report from the Maternal PKU Collaborative Study. Am J Hum Genet 1996; 59:84–94.

Henry JB (ed): Clinical Diagnosis and Management by Laboratory Methods, 16th ed. Philadelphia, WB Saunders Company, 1979.

Henry JB (ed): Clinical Diagnosis and Management by Laboratory Methods, 17th ed. Philadelphia, WB Saunders Company, 1984.

Henry JB (ed): Clinical Diagnosis and Management by Laboratory Methods, 19th ed. Philadelphia, WB Saunders Company, 1996.

Herbert LA, Dillon JJ, Middendorf DF, et al: Relationship between appearance of urinary red blood cell/white blood cell casts and the onset of renal relapse in systemic lupus erythematosus. Am J Kidney Dis 1995; 26:432–438.

Holmes E, Foxall PJ, Spraul M, et al: 750 MHz 1H NMR spectroscopy characterization of the complex metabolic pattern of urine from patients with inborn errors of metabolism: 2-hydroxyglutaric aciduria and maple syrup urine disease. J Pharm Biomed Anal 1997; 15:1647–1659.

Houillier P, Boulanger H: Hypercalciuria. Rev Prat 1998; 48:1213–1217.

Hughes C, Roebuck MJ: Evaluation of the IRIS 939 UDx flow microscope as a screening system for urinary tract infection. J Clin Pathol 2003; 56:844–859.

Itoh Y, Sakabe K, Kawai T: Basic fetoprotein in normal and pathologic urine. Ren Fail 1998; 20:239–241.

Johnson CD, Mole DR, Pestridge A: Post prandial alkaline tide: Does it exist? Digestion 1995; 56:100–106.

Jones RM, Lamb JH, Lim CK: Urinary porphyrin profiles by laser desorption/ionization time-of-flight mass spectrometry without the use of classical matrices. Rapid Commun Mass Spectrom 1995; 9:921–923.

Jou WW, Powers RD: Utility of dipstick urinalysis as a guide to management of adults with suspected infection or hematuria. South Med J 1998; 91:266–269.

Kesson AM, Talbolt JM, Gyory AZ: Microscopic examination of urine. Lancet 1978; 2:809.

Keverline JP: Recurrent rhabdomyolysis associated with influenza-like illness in a weight-lifter. J Sports Med Phys Fitness 1998; 38:177–179.

Khan SR, Atmani F, Glenton P, et al: Lipids and membranes in the organic matrix of urinary calcific crystals and stones. Calcif Tissue Int 1996; 59:357–365.

Killander J, Sjolin S, Zaar B: Rapid tests for ketonuria. Scand J Clin Lab Invest 1962; 14:311.

Kunin CM, Degroot JE: Self-screening for significant bacteriuria. JAMA 1975; 231:1349.

Kutter D: A chemical test strip to determine low concentrations of albumin and creatinine in urine. Lab Med 1998; 29:769–772.

Levy Y, George J, Ziporen L, et al: Massive proteinuria as a main manifestation of primary antiphospholipid syndrome. Pathobiology 1998; 66:49–52.

Livsey SA: Turbidimetric urine screening. Br J Biomed Sci 1995; 52:71–73.

Lizana J, Brito M, Davis MR: Assessment of five quantitative methods for determination of total proteins in urine. Clin Biochem 1977; 10:89.

Loun B, Astles R, Copeland KR, Sedor FA: Adaptation of a quantitative immunoassay for urine myoglobin. Predictor in detecting renal dysfunction. Am J Clin Pathol 1996; 105:479–486.

Luceri C, Caderni G, Lodovici M, et al: Urinary excretion of sucrose and fructose as a predictor of sucrose intake in dietary intervention studies. Cancer Epidemiol Biomarkers Prev 1996; 5:167–171.

Luo JL, Deka J, Lim CK: Determination of 5-aminolaevulinic acid dehydratase activity in erythrocytes and porphobilinogen in urine by micellar electrokinetic capillary chromatography. J Chromatogr A 1996; 722:353–357.

Luo J, Lamb JH, Lim CK: Analysis of urinary and faecal porphyrin excretion patterns in human porphyrias by fast atom bombardment mass spectrometry. J Pharm Biomed Anal 1997; 15:1289–1294.

Lyon ME, Ball CL, Lyon AW, Walpole E, Church DL: A preliminary evaluation of the interaction between urine specific gravity and leukocyte esterase results using Bayer Multistix and the Clinitek 500. Clin Biochem 2003; 36: 579–581.

McElderry LA, Tarbit I, Cassells-Smith AJ: Six methods for urinary protein compared. Clin Chem 1982; 28:356.

McGregor DO, Lynn KL, Bailey RR, et al: Clinical audit of the use of renal biopsy in the management of isolated microscopic hematuria. Clin Nephrol 1998; 49:345–348.

Miyajima H, Orii KE, Shindo Y, et al: Mitochondrial trifunctional protein deficiency associated with recurrent myoglobinuria in adolescence. Neurology 1997; 49:833–837.

Mogensen CE: Microalbuminuria predicts clinical proteinuria and early mortality in maturity-onset diabetes. N Engl J Med 1984; 310:356.

Mount DL, Green MD, Zucker JR, et al: Field detection of sulfonamides in urine: The development of a new and sensitive test. Am J Trop Med Hyg 1996; 55:250–253.

O'Connor WJ, Murphy M, Darby C, et al: Porphyrin abnormalities in acquired immunodeficiency syndrome. Arch Dermatol 1996; 132:1443–1447.

Ooi SB, Kour NW, Mahadev A: Haematuria in the diagnosis of urinary calculi. Ann Acad Med Singapore 1998; 27:210–214.

Ottinger C, Huber AR: Quantitative urine particle analysis: integrative approach for the optimal combination of automation with UF-100 and microscopic review with KOVA cell chamber. Clin Chem 2003; 617–623.

Panholzer TJ, Beyer J, Lichtwald K: Coupled-column liquid chromatographic analysis of catecholamines, serotonin, and metabolites in human urine. Clin Chem 1999; 45:262–268.

Penders J, Fiers T, Delanghe JR: Quantitative evaluation of urinalysis test strips. Clin Chem 2002; 48:2236–2241.

Rasoulpour M, Banco L, Laut JM, et al: Inability of community-based laboratories to identify pathological casts in urine samples. Arch Pediatr Adolesc Med 1996; 150:1201–1204.

Reilly AA, Bellisario R, Pass KA: Multivariate discrimination for phenylketonuria (PKU) and non-PKU hyperphenylalaninemia after analysis of newborns' dried blood-spot specimens for six amino acids by ion-exchange chromatography. Clin Chem 1998; 44:317–326.

Rendl J, Bier D, Groh T, et al: Rapid urinary iodide test. J Clin Endocrinol Metab 1998; 83:1007–1012.

Rhee E, Santiago L, Park E, et al: Urinary IL-6 is elevated in patients with urolithiasis. J Urol 1998; 160:2284–2288.

Robinson RR, Glover SN, Phillippi PJ, et al: Fixed and reproducible orthostatic proteinuria. Am J Pathol 1961; 39:291.

Rockall AG, Newman-Sanders AP, al-Kutoubi MA, et al: Haematuria. Postgrad Med J 1997; 73:129–136.

This is a review article on hematuria from a clinical perspective. It proposes a rational algorithm for the laboratory and clinical work-up of patients with hematuria.

Rose MR, Kissel JT, Bickley LS, et al: Sustained myoglobinuria: The presenting manifestation of dermatomyositis. Neurology 1996; 47:199–123.

Schwartz S, Shorov V, Watson CJ: Studies of urobilinogen. IV. Quantitative determination of urobilinogen by means of Evelyn photoelectric colorimeter. Am J Clin Pathol 1944; 14:598.

Scriver CR, Beaudet AL, Sly WS, Valle D: Metabolic Basis of Inherited Diseases, 6th ed. New York, McGraw-Hill, 1989.

Shihabi ZK: Myoglobinuria detection by capillary electrophoresis. J Chromatogr B Biomed Appl 1995; 669:53–58.

Siddiqui AA, Sultana T, Buchholz NP, et al: Proteins in renal stones and urine of stone formers. Urol Res 1998; 26:383–388.

Sidhu H, Hoppe B, Hesse A, et al: Absence of Oxalobacter formigenes in cystic fibrosis patients: A risk factor for hyperoxaluria. Lancet 1998; 352:1026–1029.

Simo-Alfonso EF, Ramis-Ramos G, Garcia-Alvarez-Coque MC, et al: Determination of sulphonamides in human urine by azo dye precolumn derivatization and micellar liquid chromatography. J Chromatogr B Biomed Appl 1995; 670:183–187.

Singh PP, Pendse AK, Ahmed A, et al: A study of recurrent stone formers with special reference to renal tubular acidosis. Urol Res 1995; 23:201–203.

Strohmaier WL, Hoelz KJ, Bichler KH: Spot urine samples for the metabolic evaluation of urolithiasis patients. Eur Urol 1997; 32:294–300.

This study describes the clinical and laboratory work-up of urolithiasis patients. Spot urines were equally as informative as 24-hour urines in the evaluation of these patients.

Threatte GA: Laboratory evaluation of renal function in the elderly. In Michelis MF, Davis BB, Preuss HG (eds): Geriatric Nephrology, Vol I. New York, Field, Rich and Associates, Inc, 1986, pp 18–21.

Viberti GC, Jarrett RJ, Mahmud U, et al: Microalbuminuria as a predictor of clinical nephropathy in insulin-dependent diabetes mellitus. Lancet 1982; 1:1430.

Ward JF, Kaplan GW, Mevorach R, et al: Refined microscopic urinalysis for red blood cell morphology in the evaluation of asymptomatic microscopic hematuria in a pediatric population. J Urol 1998; 160:1492–1495.

Wong WK, Wieringa GE, Stec Z, et al: A comparison of three procedures for the detection of Bence-Jones proteinuria. Ann Clin Biochem 1997; 34:371–374.

Yoo YM, Tatsumi N, Kirihigashi K, et al: Inaccuracy and inefficiency of urinary sediment analysis. Osaka City Med J 1995; 41:41–48.

In this study, the authors examined the laboratory characteristics of manual urine microscopy. Counts of cellular elements, but not casts, showed good reproducibility, even by inexperienced technologists. Most of the casts found were nonpathologic hyaline casts.

Young DS: Effects of drugs on clinical laboratory tests. Washington, DC, AACC Press, 1990.

Zaman Z, Borremans A, Varhaegen J, et al: Disappointing dipstick screening for urinary tract infection in hospital inpatients. J Clin Pathol 1998; 51:471–472.

Zelmanovitz T, Gross JL, Oliveira J, et al: Proteinuria is still useful for the screening and diagnosis of overt diabetic nephropathy. Diabetes Care 1998; 21:1076–1079.

Zuijderhoudt FM, Dorresteijn-de Bok J: Comparison of the Bio-Rad Porphyrin Column Test with a simple spectrophotometric test for total urine porphyrin concentration. Ann Clin Biochem 1998; 35:418–421.

CHAPTER 28

Cerebrospinal, Synovial, and Serous Body Fluids

Joseph A. Knight MD, Carl R. Kjeldsberg MD

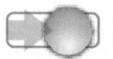

KEY POINTS

• The etiologic cause of fluid accumulation in various body cavities (i.e., joints, chest, abdomen) is critical for proper treatment of these disorders.

• Appropriate laboratory examination of these fluids is therefore critical for the diagnosis of numerous diseases (i.e., bacterial, viral and fungal infections; distinction between various arthritides; primary [i.e., mesothelioma] and metastatic malignancies; among others).

• Accurate test interpretation depends on appropriate specimen collection, turnaround time, physician/laboratory communication, and reliable reference values.

Cerebrospinal Fluid

In adults, approximately 500 mL of cerebrospinal fluid (CSF) is produced each day (0.3–0.4 mL/min). The total adult volume varies from 90–150 mL, about 25 mL of which is in the ventricles and the remainder in the subarachnoid space. In neonates, the volume varies from 10–60 mL. Thus, the total CSF volume is replaced every 5–7 hours (Wood, 1980). An estimated 70% of CSF is derived by ultrafiltration and secretion through the choroid plexuses. The ventricular ependymal lining and cerebral subarachnoid space account for the remainder. CSF leaves the ventricular system through the medial and lateral foramina, flowing over the brain and spinal cord surfaces within the subarachnoid space. CSF resorption occurs at the arachnoid villi, predominantly along the superior sagittal sinus.

The CSF has several major functions: (a) it provides physical support since the 1500 g brain weighs about 50 g when suspended in CSF; (b) it confers a protective effect against sudden changes in acute venous (respiratory and postural) and arterial blood pressure or impact pressure; (c) it provides an excretory waste function since the brain has no lymphatic system; (d) it is the pathway whereby hypothalamus releasing factors are transported to the cells of the median eminence; and (e) it maintains central nervous system ionic homeostasis.

The concept of the blood–brain barrier (BBB) is derived from dye-exclusion (tryphan blue) studies. It consists of two morphologically distinct components: a unique capillary endothelium held together by intercellular tight junctions, and the choroid plexus, where a single layer of specialized choroidal ependyma cells connected by tight junctions overlies fenestrated capillaries. The CSF ionic components (e.g., H^+, K^+, Ca^{2+}, Mg^{2+}, bicarbonate, etc.) are tightly regulated by specific transport systems, whereas glucose, urea, and creatinine diffuse freely but require 2 or more hours to equilibrate. Proteins cross by passive diffusion at a rate dependent on the plasma-to-CSF concentration gradient and inversely proportional to their molecular weight and hydrodynamic volume (Fishman, 1992). Thus, the BBB maintains the relative homeostasis of the central nervous system environment during acute perturbations of plasma components.

Specimen Collection and Opening Pressure

Cerebrospinal fluid may be obtained by lumbar, cisternal, or lateral cervical puncture or through ventricular cannulas or shunts. Details of the performance of lumber puncture are described elsewhere (Herndon, 1989; Ward, 1992). Respiratory compromise may occur in infants if the head is flexed (Ward, 1992).

A manometer should be attached prior to fluid removal to record the opening pressure. CSF pressure varies with postural changes, blood pressure, venous return, Valsalva maneuvers, and factors that alter cerebral blood flow. The normal opening adult pressure is 90–180 mm of water in the lateral decubitus position with the legs and neck in a neutral position.

It may be slightly higher if the patient is sitting up and varies up to 10 mm with respiration. However, the pressure may be as high as 250 mm of water in obese patients. In infants and young children the normal range is 10–100 mm of water, attaining the adult range by age 6–8 years (Fishman, 1992). Opening pressures above 250 mmH₂O are diagnostic of intracranial hypertension which may be due to meningitis, intracranial hemorrhage, and tumors (Seehusen, 2003). If the opening pressure is greater than 200 mmH₂O in a relaxed patient, no more than 2.0 mL should be withdrawn.

Idiopathic intracranial hypertension is most commonly seen in obese women during their childbearing years. When an elevated opening pressure is noted, CSF must be removed slowly and the pressure carefully monitored. Additional CSF should not be removed if the pressure reaches 50% of the opening pressure (Conly, 1983).

Elevated pressures may be present in patients who are tense or straining and in those with congestive heart failure, meningitis, superior vena cava syndrome, thrombosis of the venous sinuses, cerebral edema, mass lesions, hypo-osmolality, or conditions inhibiting CSF absorption. Opening pressure elevation may be the only abnormality in cryptococcal meningitis and pseudotumor cerebri (Hayward, 1987). Decreased CSF pressure may be present in spinal–subarachnoid block, dehydration, circulatory collapse, and CSF leakage. A significant pressure drop after removal of 1–2 mL suggests herniation or spinal block above the puncture site and no further fluid should be withdrawn.

Up to 20 mL of CSF may normally be removed. However, the clinician should not only be aware of the quantity of CSF required for the requested tests to ensure that a sufficient sample is submitted, but also provide an appropriate clinical history to the laboratory. The sample site (i.e., lumbar, cisternal, etc.) should be noted since cytologic and chemical parameters vary at different sites. The necessity for a simultaneous serum glucose should also be considered. This is best obtained 2–4 hours before lumbar puncture because of the delay in serum–CSF equilibrium.

The CSF specimen is usually divided into three serially collected sterile tubes: tube 1 for chemistry and immunology studies; tube 2 for microbiologic examination; and tube 3 for cell count and differential. An additional tube may be inserted in the No. 3 position for cytology if a malignancy is suspected. However, under certain conditions some variations are critical. For example, if tube 1 is hemorrhagic due to a traumatic puncture, it should not be used when protein studies are the most important aspect of the analysis (i.e., suspected multiple sclerosis). Indeed, tube 3 should be examined for the major purpose of the CSF collection. Perhaps the only definite statement one can make is that tube 1 should never be used for microbiology since it may be contaminated with skin bacteria. If questions arise, communication between the laboratory and clinician is critical prior to CSF analysis.

Glass tubes should be avoided since cell adhesion to glass affects the cell count and differential. Specimens should be delivered to the laboratory and processed quickly to minimize cellular degradation, which begins within 1 hour of collection. Refrigeration is contraindicated for culture specimens because fastidious organisms (e.g., *Haemophilus influenzae* and *Neisseria meningitidis*) will not survive.

Indications and Recommended Tests

Indications for lumbar puncture can be divided into four major disease categories: meningeal infection, subarachnoid hemorrhage, primary or metastatic malignancy, and demyelinating diseases (American College of Physicians, 1986). Identification of infectious meningitis, particularly bacterial, is the most important indication for CSF examination (Table 28–1). Recommended laboratory tests are directed toward identification of these disorders (Table 28–2). CSF examination for other diseases is generally less helpful but often provides supportive evidence of a clinical diagnosis or helps to rule out other diseases. Limited routine studies followed by retrospective ordering of the more focused tests (as needed) on the stored specimen has been advocated as a way of improving test efficiency (Albright, 1988).

Gross Examination

Normal CSF is crystal clear and colorless and has a viscosity similar to that of water. Abnormal CSF may appear cloudy, frankly purulent, or pigment tinged. Turbidity or cloudiness begins to appear with leukocyte (WBC) counts over 200 cells/μL or red cell (RBC) counts of 400/μL. However, grossly bloody fluids have RBC counts greater than 6000/μL. Microorganisms (bacteria, fungi, amebas), radiographic contrast material, aspirated epidural fat, and a protein level greater than 150 mg/dL (1.5 g/L) may also produce varying degrees of cloudiness. Experienced observers

Table 28–1 Diseases Detected by Laboratory Examination of CSF

High sensitivity, high specificity

Bacterial, tuberculous, and fungal meningitis

High sensitivity, moderate specificity

Viral meningitis

Subarachnoid hemorrhage

Multiple sclerosis

Central nervous system syphilis

Infectious polyneuritis

Paraspinal abscess

Moderate sensitivity, high specificity

Meningeal malignancy

Moderate sensitivity, moderate specificity

Intracranial hemorrhage

Viral encephalitis

Subdural hematoma

Sensitivity is the ability of a test to detect disease when it is present; specificity is the ability of a test to exclude disease when it is not present.

From American College of Physicians, Health and Public Policy Committee: The diagnostic spinal tap. Ann Intern Med 1986; 104:880, with permission.

Table 28–2 Recommended CSF Laboratory Tests

Routine

Opening CSF pressure

Total cell count (WBC and RBC)

Differential cell count (stained smear)

Glucose (CSF/plasma ratio)

Total protein

Useful under certain conditions

Cultures (bacteria, fungi, viruses, *Mycobacterium tuberculosis*)

Gram stain, acid-fast stain

Fungal and bacterial antigens

Enzymes (LD, ADA, CK-BB)

Lactate

Polymerase chain reaction (TB, viruses)

Cytology

Electrophoresis (protein, immunofixation)

Proteins (C-reactive, 14-3-3, tau, beta-amyloid, transferrin)

VDRL test for syphilis

Fibrin-derivative D-dimer

Tuberculostearic acid

CSF = cerebrospinal fluid; TB = tuberculosis; VDRL = Venereal Disease Research Laboratories; LD = lactate dehydrogenase; ADA = adenosine deaminase; CK-BB = creatine kinase-BB.

Modified from Kjeldsberg CR, Knight JA: Body Fluids: Laboratory Examination of Amniotic, Cerebrospinal, Seminal, Serous, and Synovial Fluids, 3rd ed. © American Society for Clinical Pathology, Chicago, 1993, with permission.

III

may be able to detect cell counts of less than 50 cells/μL with the unaided eye by observing for Tyndall's effect (Simon, 1978). Here, direct sunlight directed on the tube at a 90-degree angle from the observer will impart a 'sparkling' or 'snowy' appearance as suspended particles scatter the light.

Clot formation may be present in patients with traumatic taps, complete spinal block (Froin's syndrome), or suppurative or tuberculous meningitis. It is not seen in patients with subarachnoid hemorrhage. Fine surface pellicles may be observed after refrigeration for 12–24 hours. Clots may interfere with cell count accuracy by entrapping inflammatory cells.

Viscous CSF may be encountered in patients with metastatic mucin-producing adenocarcinomas, cryptococcal meningitis due to capsular polysaccharide, or liquid nucleus pulposus resulting from needle injury to the annulus fibrosus.

CHAPTER: 28 Cerebrospinal, Synovial, and Serous Body Fluids

Table 28–3 Xanthochromia and Associated Diseases/Disorders

CSF supernatant color	Associated diseases/disorders
Pink	RBC lysis/hemoglobin breakdown products
Yellow	RBC lysis/hemoglobin breakdown products
	Hyperbilirubinemia
	CSF protein > 150 mg/dL (1.5 g/L)
Orange	RBC lysis/hemoglobin breakdown products
	Hypervitaminosis A (carotenoids)
Yellow-green	Hyperbilirubinemia (biliverdin)
Brown	Meningeal metastatic melanoma

Table 28–4 CSF Reference Values for Differential Cytocentrifuge Counts

Cell type	Adults (%)	Neonates (%)
Lymphocytes	62 ± 34	20 ± 18
Monocytes	36 ± 20	72 ± 22
Neutrophils	2 ± 5	3 ± 5
Histiocytes	Rare	5 ± 4
Ependymal cells	Rare	Rare
Eosinophils	Rare	Rare

Pink-red CSF usually indicates the presence of blood and is grossly bloody when the RBC count exceeds 6000/μL. It may originate from a subarachnoid hemorrhage, intracerebral hemorrhage, cerebral infarct, or a traumatic spinal tap.

Xanthochromia. Xanthochromia commonly refers to a pale pink to yellow color in the supernatant of centrifuged CSF, although other colors may be present (Table 28–3). To detect xanthochromia, the CSF should be centrifuged and the supernatant fluid compared with a tube of distilled water. Xanthochromic CSF is pink, orange, or yellow owing to RBC lysis and hemoglobin breakdown. Pale pink to orange xanthochromia from released oxyhemoglobin is usually detected by lumbar puncture performed 2–4 hours after the onset of subarachnoid hemorrhage, although it may take as long as 12 hours. Peak intensity occurs in about 24–36 hours and then gradually disappears over the next 4–8 days. Yellow xanthochromia is derived from bilirubin. It develops about 12 hours after a subarachnoid bleed and peaks at 2–4 days, but may persist for 2–4 weeks.

Visible CSF xanthochromia may also be due to the following: (1) oxyhemoglobin resulting from artifactual red cell lysis caused by detergent contamination of the needle or collecting tube or a delay of more than 1 hour without refrigeration before examination; (2) bilirubin (bilirhachia) in jaundiced patients; (3) CSF protein levels over 150 mg/dL, which are also present in bloody traumatic taps (over 100 000 RBCs/μL) or in pathologic states such as complete spinal block, polyneuritis, and meningitis; (4) Merthiolate disinfectant contamination; (5) carotenoids (orange) in people with dietary hypercarotenemia (i.e., hypervitaminosis A); (6) melanin (brownish) from meningeal metastatic melanoma; and (7) rifampin therapy (red-orange).

Although spectral absorbance scans provide an objective record of xanthochromia, careful gross CSF inspection has comparable sensitivity (Britton, 1983). Spectrophotometry can also help to differentiate hemoglobin-derived substances from other xanthochromic pigments with different maximal absorption peaks.

Differential Diagnosis of Bloody CSF. A traumatic tap occurs in about 20% of lumbar punctures. Distinction of a traumatic puncture from pathologic hemorrhage is, therefore, of vital importance. Although the presence of crenated RBCs is not useful, the following observations may be helpful in distinguishing the two forms of bleeding.

1. In a traumatic tap, the hemorrhagic fluid usually clears between the first and third collected tubes, but remains relatively uniform in subarachnoid hemorrhage.
2. Xanthochromia, microscopic evidence of erythrophagocytosis, or hemosiderin-laden macrophages indicate a subarachnoid bleed in the absence of a prior traumatic tap. RBC lysis begins as early as 1–2 hours after a traumatic tap. Thus, rapid evaluation is necessary to avoid false-positive results.
3. A commercially available latex agglutination immunoassay test for crosslinked fibrin derivative D-dimer is specific for fibrin degradation and is negative in traumatic taps (Lang, 1990). However, false-positive results might be expected in disseminated intravascular coagulation, fibrinolysis, or trauma from repeated lumbar punctures.

Microscopic Examination

Total Cell Count. Cell counts are performed on undiluted CSF in a manual counting chamber. Automated leukocyte and erythrocyte counting has been described (Talstad, 1984), but precision is poor in the low counts normally encountered in CSF. The inherent precision of manual counts is also limited. For example, using 18 large squares (1 mm² each) in a Fuchs–Rosenthal type chamber with a depth of 0.2 mm, a total volume of 3.6 μL (18 × 0.2 μL/square) is examined. With 5 cells/μL, a total of 18 cells is counted. The coefficient of variation (CV), defined as 100

divided by the square root of the number of cells counted, is 24%; ± 2 CV is about 48%. A Neubauer hemocytometer with nine 1 mm² squares with a depth of 0.1 mm has a CV of 45% (+ 90% for 2 CV) with the same cell concentration. More recently, automated flow cytometry of CSF, using the UF-100 flow cytometer, was found to yield rapid and reliable WBC and RBC counts (Van Acker, 2001).

The normal leukocyte cell count in adults is 0–5 cells/μL. It is higher in neonates, ranging from 0–30 cells/μL, with the upper limit of normal decreasing to adult values by adolescence. No RBCs should be present in normal CSF. If numerous (except a traumatic tap), a pathologic process is probable (e.g., trauma, malignancy, infarct, hemorrhage). Although red cell counts have limited diagnostic value, they may give a useful approximation of the true CSF white blood count (WBC) or total protein in the presence of a traumatic puncture by correcting for leukocytes or protein introduced by the traumatic puncture. To be valid, all measurements (WBC, RBC, protein) must be performed on the same tube. This procedure also assumes that the blood is derived exclusively from the traumatic tap. The corrected WBC count is:

$$WBC_{corr} = WBC_{obs} - WBC_{added}$$

where:

$$WBC_{added} = WBC_{BLD} \times RBC_{CSF}/RBC_{BLD}$$

and:

WBC_{obs} = CSF leukocyte count
WBC_{added} = leukocytes added to CSF by traumatic tap
WBC_{BLD} = peripheral blood leukocyte count
RBC_{CSF} = CSF erythrocyte count
RBC_{BLD} = peripheral blood erythrocyte count.

An analogous formula may be used to correct for 'added total protein' (TP):

$$TP_{added} = [TP_{serum} \times (1 - HCT)] \times RBC_{CSF}/RBC_{BLD}$$

In the presence of a normal peripheral blood RBC count and serum protein, these corrections amount to about 1 WBC for every 700 RBCs and 8 mg/dL protein for every 10 000 RBC/μL. This latter RBC correction factor is reasonably accurate as long as the peripheral WBC count is not extremely high or low. Moreover, the accuracy of these corrections is limited by the precision of the CSF RBC count, which can significantly limit its value.

An observed-to-expected (added) WBC count ratio greater than 10 has a sensitivity of 88% and a specificity of 90% for bacterial meningitis. When the predicted WBC is below the observed count, the probability of bacterial meningitis appears to be low (Mayefsky, 1987; Bonadio, 1990).

Differential Cell Count. Suggested differential count reference ranges are presented in Table 28–4. A differential performed in a counting chamber is unsatisfactory because the low cell numbers have poor precision, and identifying the cell type beyond granulocytes and 'mononuclears' is difficult in a wet preparation. Direct smears of the centrifuged CSF sediment are also subject to significant error from cellular distortion and fragmentation.

The *cytocentrifuge* is rapid, requires minimal training, and allows Wright's staining of air-dried cytospins. Indeed, it is the recommended method for differential cell counts in all body fluids (Rabinovitch, 1994). Cell yield and preservation are better than with simple centrifugation. From 30–50 cells can be concentrated from 0.5 mL of 'normal' CSF. Variable artifactual distortions may be seen, but they are minimized when the specimen is fresh, albumin is added to the specimen (2 drops of 22% bovine serum albumin), and the cell concentration is adjusted to about 300 WBC/L prior to centrifugation (Kjeldsberg, 1993).

Filtration and sedimentation methods are too cumbersome for routine use. Filtration does, however, allow concentration of large volumes of CSF for cytologic examination or culture, while retaining the fluid filtrate for additional studies.

In adults, a normal CSF contains a small number of *lymphocytes* and *monocytes* in an approximate 70 : 30 ratio (Fig. 28–1). A higher proportion of monocytes is present in young children in whom up to 80% may be

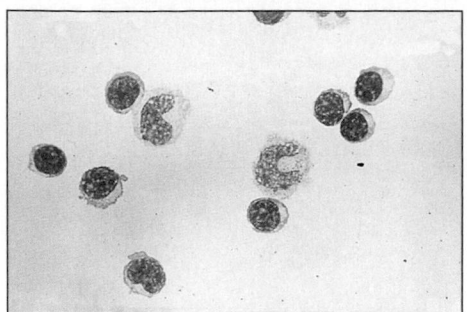

Figure 28–1 CSF cytology (lymphocyte to monocyte distribution ratio 70 : 30).

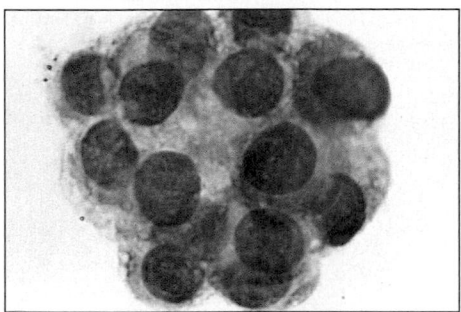

Figure 28–2 Choroid plexus cells in CSF.

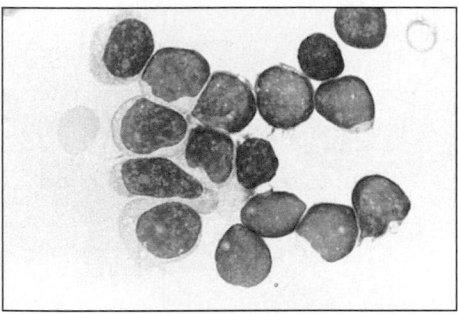

Figure 28–3 Cluster of blast-like cells in CSF from premature newborn. (From Kjeldsberg CR, Knight JA: Body Fluids: Laboratory Examination of Amniotic, Cerebrospinal, Seminal, Serous and Synovial Fluids, 3rd ed. © American Society for Clinical Pathology, Chicago, 1993, with permission.)

Table 28–5 Causes of Increased CSF Neutrophils

Meningitis
  Bacterial meningitis
  Early viral meningoencephalitis
  Early tuberculous meningitis
  Early mycotic meningitis
  Amebic encephalomyelitis
Other infections
  Cerebral abscess
  Subdural empyema
  AIDS-related CMV radiculopathy
Following seizures
Following CNS hemorrhage
  Subarachnoid
  Intracerebral
Following CNS infarct
Reaction to repeated lumbar punctures
Injection of foreign material in subarachnoid space (e.g., methotrexate, contrast media)
Metastatic tumor in contact with CSF

CNS = central nervous system; CSF = cerebrospinal fluid; CMV = cytomegalovirus.

Table 28–6 Causes of CSF Lymphocytosis

Meningitis
  Viral meningitis
  Tuberculous meningitis
  Fungal meningitis
  Syphilitic meningoencephalitis
  Leptospiral meningitis
  Bacterial due to uncommon organisms
  Early bacterial meningitis where leukocyte counts are relatively low
  Parasitic infestations (e.g., cysticercosis, trichinosis, toxoplasmosis)
  Aseptic meningitis due to septic focus adjacent to meninges
Degenerative disorders
  Subacute sclerosing panencephalitis
  Multiple sclerosis
  Drug abuse encephalopathy
  Guillain–Barré syndrome
  Acute disseminated encephalomyelitis
Other inflammatory disorders
  Handl syndrome (headache with neurologic deficits and CSF lymphocytosis)
  Sarcoidosis
  Polyneuritis
  CNS periarteritis

CSF = cerebrospinal fluid; CNS = central nervous system.

III

normal (Pappu, 1982). Erythrocytes due to minor traumatic bleeding are commonly seen, especially in infants. Small numbers of neutrophils (PMNs) may also be seen in 'normal' CSF specimens, most likely as a result of minor hemorrhage (Hayward, 1988) and improved cell concentration methods. No general consensus regarding an upper limit of normal for PMNs has been established. We accept up to 7% neutrophils with a normal WBC count. Over 60% neutrophils has been reported in high-risk neonates without meningitis (Rodriguez, 1990). The number of PMNs may be decreased by as much as 68% within the first 2 hours after lumbar puncture owing to cell lysis (Steele, 1986).

Traumatic puncture may result in the presence of bone marrow cells, cartilage cells, squamous cells, ganglion cells, and soft tissue elements. In addition, ependymal and choroid plexus cells may rarely be seen (Fig. 28–2). Moreover, blast-like primitive cell clusters, most likely of germinal matrix origin, are sometimes found in premature infants with intraventricular hemorrhage (Fig. 28–3).

Increased CSF *neutrophils* occur in numerous conditions (Table 28–5). In early bacterial meningitis, the proportion of PMNs usually exceeds 60%. However, in about one-quarter of cases of early viral meningitis the proportion of PMNs also exceeds 60%. Viral-induced neutrophilia usually changes to a lymphocytic pleocytosis within 2–3 days. A total PMN count of over 1180 cells/μL (or more than 2000 WBC/μL) has a 99% predictive value for bacterial meningitis (Spanos, 1989). Persistent neutrophilic meningitis (over 1 week) may be noninfectious or due to less common pathogens such as *Nocardia, Actinomyces, Aspergillus,* and the zygomycetes (Peacock, 1984).

Increased CSF *lymphocytes* have been reported in various diseases/disorders (Table 28–6). Lymphocytosis (> 50%) is not uncommon in early acute bacterial meningitis when the CSF leukocyte count is under 1000/μL (Powers, 1985). Atypical reactive lymphoplasmacytoid and immunoblastic variants may be present. Blast-like lymphocytes may be seen admixed with small and large lymphocytes in the CSF of neonates.

Plasma cells, not normally present in CSF, may appear in a variety of inflammatory conditions (Table 28–7) along with large and small lymphocytes and in association with malignant brain tumors (Fishman, 1992). Multiple myeloma may also rarely involve the meninges (Oda, 1991).

Although *eosinophils* are rarely present in normal CSF, they may be increased in a variety of CNS conditions (Table 28–8). For example, eosinophilia is frequently mild (1–4%) in a general inflammatory response, but in children with malfunctioning ventricular shunts, it may be marked (Fig. 28–4). A suggested criterion for eosinophilic meningitis is 10% eosinophils (Kuberski, 1981); parasitic invasion of the CNS is the most common cause worldwide. *Coccidioides immitis* is a significant cause of CSF eosinophilia in endemic regions of the United States (Ragland, 1993).

Increased CSF *monocytes* lack diagnostic specificity and are usually part of a 'mixed cell reaction' that includes neutrophils, lymphocytes, and plasma cells. This pattern is seen in tuberculous and fungal meningitis,

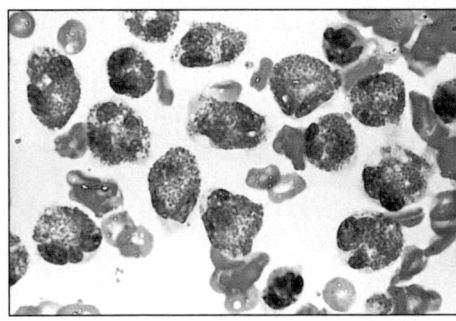

CHAPTER: 28 Cerebrospinal, Synovial, and Serous Body Fluids

Table 28–7 Causes of CSF Plasmacytosis

Acute viral infections
Guillain–Barré syndrome
Multiple sclerosis
Parasitic CNS infestations
Sarcoidosis
Subacute sclerosing panencephalitis
Syphilitic meningoencephalitis
Tuberculous meningitis

CSF = cerebrospinal fluid; CNS = central nervous system.

Table 28–8 Causes of CSF Eosinophilic Pleocytosis

Commonly associated with

Acute polyneuritis
CNS reaction to foreign material (drugs, shunts)
Fungal infections
Idiopathic eosinophilic meningitis
Idiopathic hypereosinophilic syndrome
Parasitic infections

Infrequently associated with

Bacterial meningitis
Leukemia/lymphoma
Myeloproliferative disorders
Neurosarcoidosis
Primary brain tumors
Tuberculous meningoencephalitis
Viral meningitis

CSF = cerebrospinal fluid; CNS = central nervous system.

Modified with permission from Kjeldsberg CR, Knight JA: Body Fluids: Laboratory Examination of Amniotic, Cerebrospinal, Seminal, Serous and Synovial Fluids, 3rd ed. © American Society for Clinical Pathology, Chicago, 1993.

Figure 28–4 Eosinophils in CSF from a child with malfunctioning ventricular shunt.

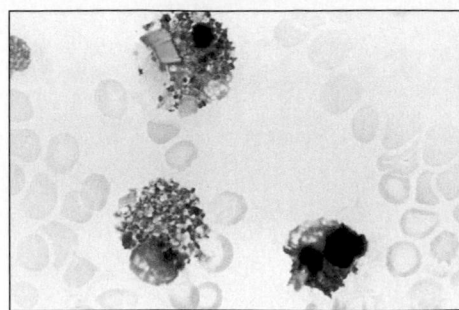

Figure 28–5 Hemosiderin-laden macrophages (siderophages) from the CSF of a patient with subarachnoid hemorrhage. Hemosiderin crystals (golden-yellow) are also present. (From Kjeldsberg CR, Knight JA: Body Fluids: Laboratory Examination of Amniotic, Cerebrospinal, Seminal, Serous and Synovial Fluids, 3rd ed. © American Society for Clinical Pathology, Chicago, 1993, with permission.)

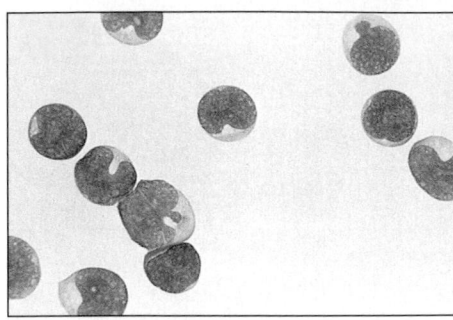

Figure 28–6 Acute lymphoblastic leukemia in CSF. Note uniformity of the blast cells.

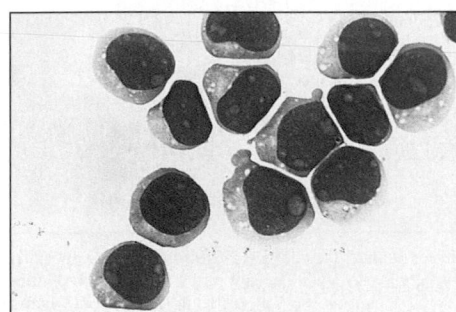

Figure 28–7 Acute myeloblastic leukemia in CSF.

chronic bacterial meningitis (i.e., *Listeria monocytogenes* and others), leptospiral meningitis, ruptured brain abscess, *Toxoplasma* meningitis and amebic encephalomeningitis. A mixed cell pattern without neutrophils is characteristic of viral and syphilitic meningoencephalitis. *Macrophages* with phagocytosed erythrocytes (*erythrophages*) appear from 12–48 hours following a subarachnoid hemorrhage or traumatic tap. Hemosiderin-laden macrophages (*siderophages*) appear after about 48 hours and may persist for weeks (Fig. 28–5). Brownish yellow or red hematoidin crystals may form after a few days.

Cerebrospinal fluid examination for tumor cells has moderate sensitivity and high specificity (97–98%) (Marton, 1986). Sensitivity depends on the type of tumor. CSF examination of leukemic patients has the highest sensitivity (about 70%), followed by metastatic carcinoma (20–60%) and primary CNS malignancies (30%). Sensitivity may be optimized by using filtration methods with larger fluid volumes or by performing serial punctures in patients in whom a tumor is strongly suspected.

Leukemic involvement of the meninges is more frequent in patients with acute lymphoblastic leukemia (Fig. 28–6) than in those with acute myeloblastic leukemia (Fig. 28–7); both are significantly more common

than CNS involvement in the chronic leukemias. A leukocyte count over 5 cells/μL with unequivocal lymphoblasts in cytocentrifuged preparations is commonly accepted as evidence of CSF involvement. The incidence of CNS relapse in children with lymphoblasts but cell counts less than 6 cells/μL appears to be low and is not significantly different from cases in which no blasts are identified (Odom, 1990; Gilchrist, 1994; Tubergen, 1994).

Non-Hodgkin's lymphomas involving the leptomeninges are usually high-grade tumors (lymphoblastic, large cell immunoblastic, and Burkitt lymphomas) (Fig. 28–8); low-grade lymphomas and Hodgkin's lymphoma are significantly less common (Bigner, 1992; Walts, 1992). T cells predominate in normal and inflammatory conditions, whereas most lymphomas, especially those occurring in immunocompromised hosts, are of B cell lineage. Lymphoblastic lymphoma, the most common T cell lymphoma, can be detected by terminal deoxynucleotidyl transferase (TdT) stain.

The polymerase chain reaction (PCR) and multiparameter flow cytometry can increase sensitivity of lymphoma detection (Rhodes, 1996; Finn, 1998). However, their clinical utility for daily practice has yet to be proven in long-term prospective studies.

Amebae, fungi (especially *Cryptococcus neoformans*), and *Toxoplasma gondii* organisms may be present on cytocentrifuge specimens, but may be difficult to recognize without confirmatory stains.

Chemical Analysis

Reference values for lumbar cerebrospinal fluid in adults are listed in Table 28–9.

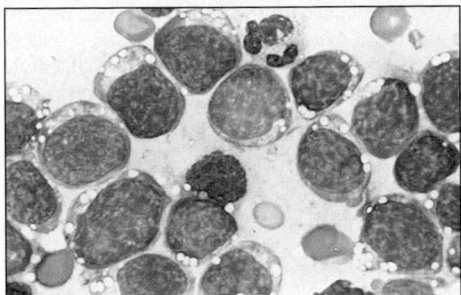

Figure 28–8 Burkitt's lymphoma in CSF. The cells are characterized by blue cytoplasm with vacuoles and slightly clumped chromatin pattern. (From Kjeldsberg CR, Knight JA: Body Fluids: Laboratory Examination of Amniotic, Cerebrospinal, Seminal, Serous and Synovial Fluids, 3rd ed. © American Society for Clinical Pathology, Chicago, 1993, with permission.)

Table 28–9 Adult Lumbar CSF Reference Values

Analyte	Conventional units	SI units
Protein	15–45 mg/dL	0.15–0.45 g/L
Prealbumin	2–7%	
Albumin	56–76%	
Alpha-1-globulin	2–7%	
Alpha-2-globulin	4–12%	
Beta-globulin	8–18%	
Gamma-globulin	3–12%	
Electrolytes		
Osmolality	280–300 mOsm/L	280–300 mmol/L
Sodium	135–150 mEq/L	135–150 mmol/L
Potassium	2.6–3.0 mEq/L	2.6–3.0 mmol/L
Chloride	115–130 mEq/L	115–130 mmol/L
Carbon dioxide	20–25 mEq/L	20–25 mmol/L
Calcium	2.0–2.8 mEq/L	1.0–1.4 mmol/L
Magnesium	2.4–3.0 mEq/L	1.2–1.5 mmol/L
Lactate	10–22 mg/dL	1.1–2.4 mmol/L
pH		
Lumbar fluid	7.28–7.32	
Cisternal fluid	7.32–7.34	
P_{CO_2}		
Lumbar fluid	44–50 mmHg	
Cisternal fluid	40–46 mmHg	
P_{O_2}	40–44 mmHg	
Other constituents		
Ammonia	10–35 µg/dL	6–20 µmol/L
Glutamine	5–20 mg/dL	0.3–1.4 mmol/L
Creatinine	0.6–1.2 mg/dL	45–92 µmol/L
Glucose	50–80 mg/dL	2.8–4.4 mmol/L
Iron	1–2 µg/dL	0.2–0.4 µmol/L
Phosphorus	1.2–2.0 mg/dL	0.4–0.7 mmol/L
Total lipid	1–2 mg/dL	0.01–0.02 g/L
Urea	6–16 mg/dL	2.0–5.7 mmol/L
Urate	0.5–3.0 mg/dL	30–180 µmol/L
Zinc	2–6 µg/dL	0.3–0.9 µmol/L

Proteins.

Total Protein. Over 80% of the CSF protein content is derived from blood plasma, in concentrations of less than 1% of the plasma level (Table 28–10).

Prealbumin (transthyretin), transferrin, and small quantities of nerve tissue-specific proteins are the major qualitative differences that normally exist between CSF and plasma proteins. Although some authors have argued against routine measurement of total protein (American College of Physicians, 1986), it is the most common abnormality found in CSF. Thus, an increased CSF protein serves as a useful, albeit nonspecific, indicator of meningeal or CNS disease.

Reference values.

CSF total protein reference values vary considerably between laboratories owing to differences in methodology, instrumentation, and type of reference standard used (College of American Pathologists CSF Chemistry Survey, Set M-B, 1991*; Gerbaut, 1986). CSF protein levels of 15–45 mg/dL have long been accepted as the 'normal' reference range

Table 28–10 Mean Concentrations of Plasma and CSF Proteins

Protein	CSF (mg/L)	Plasma/CSF ratio
Prealbumin	17.3	14
Albumin	155.0	236
Transferrin	14.4	142
Ceruloplasmin	1.0	366
IgG	12.3	802
IgA	1.3	1346
Alpha-2-microglobulin	2.0	1111
Fibrinogen	0.6	4940
IgM	0.6	1167
Beta-lipoprotein	0.6	6213

CSF = cerebrospinal fluid.

Adapted from Felgenhauer K: Klin Wochenschr 1974; 52:1158, with permission.

(Silverman, 1994). Using the classic Lowry method, the reported adult range was 24.1–48.5 mg/dL (Tibbling, 1977). Others reported a reference range of 14–49 mg/dL using a trichloroacetic acid-ponceau-S method (Breebaart, 1978) and were 22.3–50.3 mg/dL with a biuret method (Ahonen, 1978). Reference levels were also compared using three different methods: (a) a modified biuret technique; (b) Dupont aca method in which protein was precipitated and then reacted with trichloroacetic acid; and (c) a Kodak Ektachem colorimetric slide technique (Lott, 1989). All three methods gave similar, although significantly higher, levels than those previously reported (i.e., 14–62 mg/dL; 16–61 mg/dL; and 12–60 mg/dL, respectively).

While there have been reported discrepancies in both gender and those over age 60 years, the differences are probably not significant. However, infants have significantly higher CSF protein levels than older children and adults. Thus, a mean level of 90 mg/dL for term infants and 115 mg/dL for preterm infants were reported; the upper levels were 150 mg/dL and 170 mg/dL, respectively (Sarff, 1976). Similarly, others recently noted that the CSF protein concentration fell rapidly from birth to 6 months of age (mean levels, 108 mg/dL to 40 mg/dL), plateaued between 3 and 10 years (mean, 32 mg/dL) and then rose slightly from 10–16 years (mean, 41 mg/dL) (Biou, 2000).

Elevated CSF protein levels may be caused by increased permeability of the blood–brain barrier, decreased resorption at the arachnoid villi, mechanical obstruction of CSF flow due to spinal block above the puncture site, or an increase in intrathecal immunoglobulin synthesis. Common conditions associated with elevated lumbar CSF protein values (over 65 mg/dL) are summarized in Table 28–11.

Low lumbar CSF total protein levels (< 20 mg/dL) normally occur in some young children between 6 months and 2 years of age and in patients with conditions associated with increased CSF turnover. These include the following: (a) removal of large CSF volumes; (b) CSF leaks induced by trauma or lumbar puncture; (c) increased intracranial pressure, probably due to an increased rate of protein resorption by the arachnoid villi; and (d) hyperthyroidism (Fishman, 1992).

Protein electrophoresis of concentrated normal CSF reveals two distinct differences from serum: a prominent transthyretin (prealbumin) band and two transferrin bands. Transthyretin is relatively high because of its dual synthesis by the liver and choroid plexus. The second transferrin band, referred to as beta-2-transferrin or tau protein, migrates more slowly than its serum equivalent owing to cerebral neuraminidase digestion of sialic acid residues.

Methodology.

Turbidimetric methods, commonly based on trichloroacetic acid (TCA) or sulfosalicylic acid (SSA) and sodium sulfate for protein precipitation, are popular because they are simple, rapid, and require no special instrumentation. However, they are temperature sensitive and require much larger specimen volumes (about 0.5 mL). Moreover, some methods are prone to significant variation from changes in the albumin/globulin ratio (Schriever, 1965). A false protein elevation may be observed using TCA methods in the presence of methotrexate (Kasper, 1988). Benzethonium chloride or benzalkonium chloride have been used as precipitating agents in automated and micromethods (Luxton, 1989; Shephard, 1992).

College of American Pathologists, 325 Waukegan Road, Northfield, IL.

Table 28–11 Conditions Associated with Increased CSF Total Protein

Traumatic spinal puncture
Increased blood–CSF permeability
  Arachnoiditis (e.g., following methotrexate therapy)
  Meningitis (bacterial, viral, fungal, tuberculous)
  Hemorrhage (subarachnoid, intracerebral)
  Endocrine/metabolic disorders
    Milk–alkali syndrome with hypercalcemia
    Diabetic neuropathy
    Hereditary neuropathies and myelopathies
    Decreased endocrine function (thyroid, parathyroid)
    Other disorders (uremia, dehydration)
Drug toxicity
  Ethanol, phenothiazines, phenytoin
CSF circulation defects
  Mechanical obstruction (tumor, abscess, herniated disk)
  Loculated CSF effusion
Increased IgG synthesis
  Neurosyphilis, multiple sclerosis
  Subacute sclerosing panencephalitis
Increased IgG synthesis and blood–CSF permeability
  Guillain–Barré syndrome
  Collagen vascular diseases (e.g., lupus, periarteritis)
  Chronic inflammatory demyelinating polyradiculopathy

CSF = cerebrospinal fluid.

Colorimetric methods include the Lowry method, dye-binding, methods using Coomassie brilliant blue (CBB) or Ponceau S, and the modified biuret method. The CBB method is rapid, highly sensitive, and can be used with small sample sizes. Immunologic methods measure specific proteins, require only 25–50 µL of CSF, and are relatively simple to perform once conditions and reagents have been standardized. Automated methods are also commonly used and usually show good correlation with the standard methods (Lott, 1989).

Albumin and IgG Measurements. The permeability of the blood–brain barrier may be assessed by immunochemical quantification of the CSF albumin-to-serum albumin ratio in grams per deciliter (g/dL). The normal ratio of 1 : 230 (Tourtellotte, 1985) yields an unwieldy decimal of 0.004, which prompted the use of the *CSF/serum albumin index*, which is arbitrarily calculated as follows:

$$\text{CSF/Serum Albumin Index} = \frac{\text{CSF albumin (mg/dL)}}{\text{Serum albumin (g/dL)}} \qquad (28\text{–}1)$$

An index value less than 9 is consistent with an intact barrier. Slight impairment is considered with index values of 9–14, moderate impairment with values of 14–30, and severe impairment at values greater than 30 (Silverman, 1994). The index is slightly elevated in infants up to 6 months of age, reflecting the immaturity of the blood–brain barrier, and increases gradually after age 40 years. A traumatic tap invalidates the index calculation.

Increased intrathecal IgG synthesis is reflected by an increase in the CSF/serum IgG ratio:

$$\text{CSF/Serum IgG Ratio} = \frac{\text{CSF IgG (mg/dL)}}{\text{Serum IgG (g/dL)}} \qquad (28\text{–}2)$$

The normal ratio is 1/390 or 0.003 (Tourtellotte, 1985). Like the albumin index, the CSF/serum IgG index may be obtained by using milligrams per deciliter for the CSF IgG value. The CSF/serum IgG index normal range is 3.0–8.7.

The *CSF/serum IgG index* can be elevated by intrathecal IgG synthesis or increased plasma IgG cross-over from breakdown of the blood–brain barrier. Immunoglobulin derived from plasma cross-over may be corrected by dividing the CSF/serum IgG index by the CSF/albumin index to yield the CSF IgG index.

$$\text{CSF IgG Index} = \frac{\text{CSF IgG (mg/dL)/Serum IgG (g/dL)}}{\text{CSF albumin (mg/dL)/Serum albumin (g/dL)}} \qquad (28\text{–}3)$$

or

$$\text{CSF IgG Index} = \frac{\text{CSF IgG (mg/dL)} \times \text{Serum albumin (g/dL)}}{\text{Serum IgG (g/dL)} \times \text{CSF albumin (mg/dL)}} \qquad (28\text{–}4)$$

The normal reference range for the IgG index varies, reflecting variations in the determination of the four index components. A reasonable normal upper limit is 0.8 (Souverijn, 1989). However, each laboratory should determine its own critical ratio.

The *IgG synthesis rate* is calculated by an empirical formula (Tourtellotte, 1985):

$$\text{IgG synthesis rate (mg/day)} = [(\text{CSF IgG} - \text{Serum IgG/369}) - \qquad (28\text{–}5)$$
$$(\text{CSF albumin} - \text{Serum albumin/230}) \times (\text{Serum IgG/Serum albumin}) \times 0.43] \times 5 \text{ dL/day}$$

All protein concentrations are expressed in milligrams per deciliter. The first bracketed term represents the difference between the measured CSF IgG and the IgG expected from diffusion across a normal blood–brain barrier; 369 is the normal serum/CSF ratio. The second bracketed term represents the difference between measured CSF albumin and expected albumin if the blood–brain barrier is intact; 230 is the normal serum/CSF albumin ratio. The CSF albumin excess is multiplied by the IgG/albumin ratio and the molecular weight ratio of IgG to albumin (0.43) to correct for changes in CSF IgG due to increased barrier permeability. The number 5 converts the result from a concentration to a daily amount, assuming an average daily CSF production of 500 mL (i.e., 5 dL). The formula does not consider variations in CSF production or immunoglobulin consumption. It assumes that the IgG/albumin ratio remains constant over various degrees of blood–brain barrier impairment, a concept that may lead to variable error (Lefvert, 1985). The normal reference interval for the synthesis rate is -9.9 to $+3.3$ mg/day. Values greater than 8.0 mg/day indicate an increased rate (Silverman, 1994).

The percentage of CSF IgG is normally 3–5% of total CSF protein, but in multiple sclerosis (MS) the concentration approaches that of plasma (15–18%) (Hersey, 1980). The CSF IgG index and IgG synthesis rate have a sensitivity of 90% in patients with definite MS, but the sensitivity is lower in patients with possible MS in whom accuracy is most needed (Marton, 1986). In addition, the specificity for MS is only moderate because increased intrathecal IgG synthesis occurs in many other inflammatory neurologic diseases.

The immunoglobulin index and synthesis rate calculations may also be applied to IgM, IgA, immunoglobulin light chains, and specific antibodies to infectious microorganisms. For example, increased synthesis of IgM and free kappa light chains have been suggested as markers for MS (Rudick, 1989; Lolli, 1991).

Electrophoretic Techniques. Although the diagnosis of multiple sclerosis (MS) is ultimately a clinical one, there have been significant advances in laboratory testing for this disorder. CSF total protein is increased in less than 50% of patients with MS. Indeed, if the CSF protein exceeds 100 mg/dL, the patient probably does not have MS. However, the gammaglobulin fraction, as determined by CSF electrophoresis, is often increased in MS. Thus, the CSF total protein/gammaglobulin ratio exceeds 0.12 in about 65% of cases (Johnson, 1977). Using *electroimmunodiffusion*, a CSF IgG/albumin ratio greater than 0.25 is present in about 75% of cases (Tourtellotte, 1971). Furthermore, levels greater than the mean CSF IgG index + 3 S.D. are present in 80–85% of MS cases. However, this upper reference level varies significantly between laboratories and 0.58, 0.66, and 0.77 have been reported as cutoff values (Tibbling, 1977; Olsson, 1976, Markowitz, 1983, respectively). Therefore, laboratories should establish their own reference values.

High-resolution agarose gel electrophoresis of concentrated CSF from patients with MS often shows discrete populations of IgG, the *oligoclonal bands*. Although these discrete IgG populations are normally absent, two or more bands are necessary to support the diagnosis of MS; a single band is not considered a positive result. Using this technique, oligoclonal bands have been reported in 83–94% of patients with definite MS, 40–60% of those with probable MS, and 20–30% of possible MS cases. However, they are also frequently present in patients with subacute sclerosing panencephalitis, various viral CNS infections, neurosyphilis, neuroborreliosis, cryptococcal meningitis, Guillain–Barré syndrome, transverse myelitis, meningeal carcinomatosis, glioblastoma multiforme, Burkitt's lymphoma, chronic relapsing polyneuropathy, Behçet's disease, cysticercosis, and trypanosomiasis, among others (Trotter, 1989; Chalmers, 1990; Fishman 1992; Hall, 1992). Subsequent studies indicate that agarose gel electrophoresis sensitivity for MS is less than previously reported (see below).

Oligoclonal light chains (both kappa and lambda) are present in about 90% of MS patients (Gallo, 1989; Sindic, 1991). They have also occasionally been identified in the CSF of those who are negative for IgG oligoclonal bands. However, because of their uncommon occurrence in the absence of IgG and cost-ineffectiveness, as well as the ready availability of magnetic resonance imaging, it is unlikely this technique will become common.

Table 28–12 CSF Proteins and Central Nervous System Diseases

Protein	Major diseases/disorders
Alpha-2-macroglobulin	Subdural hemorrhage, bacterial meningitis
Beta-amyloid and tau proteins	Alzheimer's disease
Beta-2-microglobulin	Leukemia/lymphoma, Behçet's syndrome
C-reactive protein	Bacterial and viral meningitis
Fibronectin	Lymphoblastic leukemia, AIDS, meningitis
Methemoglobin	Mild subarachnoid/subdural hemorrhage
Myelin basic protein	Multiple sclerosis, tumors, others
Protein 14-3-3	Creutzfeldt–Jakob disease
Transferrin	CSF leakage (otorrhea, rhinorrhea)

Coomassie brilliant blue (CBB) or paragon violet stains can resolve oligoclonal bands in only 5 µg of IgG (Silverman, 1994). However, *silver staining* is 20–50 times more sensitive than CBB and can be used on unconcentrated CSF. Importantly, these electrophoretic techniques must be simultaneously carried out on the patient's serum to be certain that a polyclonal gammopathy is not present (e.g., liver disease, systemic lupus, rheumatoid arthritis, chronic granulomatous disease) since these disorders may be accompanied by immunoglobulin diffusion into the CSF and yield false-positive results.

Immunofixation electrophoresis (IFE) is more sensitive than agarose gel electrophoresis and does not require CSF concentration (Cawley, 1976). A subsequent study reported a sensitivity of 74% using this technique compared with 57% for agarose gel electrophoresis (Cavuoti, 1998). More recently, using a semiautomated immunofixation-peroxidase technique, the sensitivity was 83% and the specificity was 79% in patients with clinically definite MS (Richard, 2002). However, IFE provides fewer bands than *isoelectric focusing and Ig immunoblotting* (IgG-IEF). Moreover, the bands by IFE tend to be more diffuse.

In 1994, a consensus report concluded that IgG-IEF is the most sensitive method for the detection of oligoclonal bands (Andersson, 1994). In support of this, a recent study showed that IgG-IEF detected 100% of definite MS but only about 50% were positive by agarose electrophoresis (Lunding, 2000). Others detected 91% of MS cases but only 68% with agarose (Seres, 1998). Similarly, a semiautomated IgG-IEF technique identified 90% of MS cases compared with 60% for agarose electrophoresis (Fortini, 2003). Nevertheless, a 2002 survey found that 90% of the 235 laboratories performing CSF analysis for oligoclonal bands used agarose electrophoresis; fewer than 10% used IEF (College of American Pathologists, 2002).

In summary, the diagnosis of MS, as with many other neurologic disorders, is ultimately a clinical one based on neurologic history and physical examination. Nevertheless, advanced laboratory results such as elevated IgG indices and the presence of oligoclonal bands, as well as neuroimaging techniques, have proven to be invaluable in the diagnosis of MS.

Other CSF Proteins. Approximately 300 different proteins have been identified in CSF using two-dimensional electrophoresis, the first dimension being isoelectric focusing and the second polyacrylamide gel in the presence of sodium dodecyl sulfate (Harrington, 1986). Using this technique, four abnormal proteins were identified in patients with Creutzfeldt–Jacob (C-J) disease. Two of these proteins (molecular mass about 40 kilodaltons (kDa) each) were also present in some, but not all, patients with herpes simplex encephalitis, Parkinson's disease, Guillain–Barré syndrome and schizophrenia. They were not present in various other neurologic disorders nor in 100 normal CSF control specimens. However, these and two other proteins (molecular masses about 26 and 29 kDa) were present in all cases of C-J disease and in 5 of 10 cases of herpes simplex encephalitis. Neither of these latter proteins were present in any other neurologic disease or the controls.

An increased concentration of various specific CSF proteins has been associated with several central nervous system diseases (Table 28–12).

Myelin Basic Protein (MBP). MBP, a component of the myelin nerve sheath, is released during demyelination as a result of various neurologic disorders, especially MS. Thus, MBP has been shown to positively correlate with CSF leukocyte count, intrathecal IgG synthesis, and the CSF/serum albumin concentration quotient (Sellebjerg, 1998). These results support the use of MBP in CSF as a surrogate disease marker during acute MS exacerbations. Others found that analysis of antibody against MBP in patients with a clinically isolated syndrome is a rapid and precise method in predicting early conversion to clinically definite MS (Berger, 2003). However, increased CSF levels have also been reported in Guillain–Barré

syndrome, lupus erythematosus, subacute sclerosing panencephalitis, various brain tumors, and following CNS irradiation and chemotherapy (Brooks, 1989; Mahoney, 1984). Its measurement has also been proposed as a prognostic marker in patients with serious head injury (Noseworthy, 1985).

Alpha-2-macroglobulin (A2M). Except for a small amount transported across the blood–brain barrier (BBB) in pinocytic vesicles, A2M is normally excluded from the CSF because of its large size. The number of these vesicles is increased in certain polyneuropathies, resulting in an increased CSF A2M level. Significant elevation reflects subdural hemorrhage or breakdown of the BBB, as occurs in bacterial meningitis. A2M measurement alone, or in relationship with albumin and IgG, may assist in the evaluation of neurologic disorders, increased CSF protein, and the rapid differentiation between bacterial and aseptic meningitis (Meucci, 1993; Kanoh, 1997).

Beta-2-microglobulin (B2M). This protein is part of the HLA class I molecule on the surface of all nucleated cells. CSF levels above 1.8 mg/L are associated with leptomeningeal leukemia and lymphoma but are not highly specific (Weller, 1992) in that they have a maximal positive predictive value of 78% in cases with a positive cytology (Jeffrey, 1990). B2M was also recently shown to be a marker of neuro-Behçet's syndrome (Kawai, 2000). Moreover, viral infections, including HIV-1, other inflammatory conditions and various malignancies have also been associated with elevated levels. However, the measurement of B2M remains primarily investigational.

C-Reactive Protein (CRP). Early studies indicated that CSF CRP is useful in differentiating viral (aseptic) meningitis from bacterial meningitis (Corral, 1981; Abramson, 1985; Stearman, 1994). Others reported that CSF CRP is a more useful screening test for viral versus bacterial meningitis, especially in children (Sormunen, 1999). A meta-analysis of CRP studies since 1980 suggested that a normal CSF or serum CRP has a high probability in ruling out bacterial meningitis (i.e., negative predictive value about 97%) (Gerdes, 1998). Moreover, a recent study not only found increased CSF CRP levels in bacterial meningitis, but that the levels were significantly higher in patients with Gram-negative bacterial meningitis than in those with Gram-positive bacterial meningitis (Rajs, 2002).

Fibronectin. This large glycoprotein (molecular mass about 420 kDa) is normally present in essentially all tissues and body fluids. Its primary function is in cell adhesion and phagocytosis (Ruoslahti, 1981). Thus, cell adhesion allows leukocytes to adhere to and pass through the vascular endothelia and migrate to the inflammatory site.

In children with acute lymphoblastic leukemia, elevated CSF fibronectin levels are associated with a poor prognosis, presumably due to leukemic involvement of the central nervous system (Rautonen, 1989). Significant CSF elevations have also been reported in Burkitt's lymphoma (Rajantie, 1989), some metastatic solid tumors, astrocytomas, and bacterial meningitis (Weller, 1990; Torre, 1991). Decreased levels have been reported in viral meningitis and AIDS dementia complex (Torre, 1991; 1993).

Beta-Amyloid Protein 42 and Tau Protein. The diagnosis of Alzheimer's disease (AD) is based on the presence of dementia and a specific clinical profile (i.e., from medical history, clinical examination) suggestive of AD together with the exclusion of other causes of dementia. Pathologically, the disease is characterized by the presence of neurofibrillary tangles and amyloid plaques.

Recent studies indicate that the measurement of biochemical markers increases the diagnostic accuracy, especially early in the course of the disease when clinical symptoms are mild and vague and overlap with cognitive changes that accompany aging and ischemic dementia. Thus, increased CSF levels of microtubule-associated tau protein and decreased levels of beta-amyloid protein ending at amino acid 42 have been shown to significantly increase the accuracy of AD diagnosis (Andreasen, 2001; Riemenschneider, 2002; Sunderland, 2003). Indeed, the predictive value for early AD is greater than 90% (Andreasen, 2001). Others found that the calculated ratio of phosphorylated tau protein to beta-amyloid peptide is superior to either measure alone (Maddalena, 2003). The results were as follows: distinguishing patients with AD from healthy controls (sensitivity, 96%; specificity, 97%); AD from subjects with non-AD dementia (sensitivity, 80%; specificity, 73%); and AD from subjects with other neurologic disorders (sensitivity, 80%; specificity, 89%).

Protein 14-3-3. The transmissible spongiform encephalopathies constitute a group of uniformly fatal neurodegenerative diseases. Of these, Creutzfeldt–Jakob disease (CJD) is the major spongiform disease in humans. Two proteins, designated 130 and 131, have been detected in low concentrations in CSF from CJD patients. These proteins have the same amino acid sequence as protein 14-3-3 (Hsich, 1996). Moreover, in patients with dementia, a positive immunoassay for the 14-3-3 protein in CSF strongly supported a diagnosis of CJD. In a subsequent study of patients with suspected CJD, the sensitivity of the 14-3-3 protein determined by immunoassay was 97% and the specificity was 87% (Lemstra, 2000). False-positive results were primarily seen in patients with stroke and meningoencephalitis.

Others, using a modified Western blot technique, reported a 94.7% positive predictive value and 92.4% negative predictive value for CJD (Zerr, 1998). False-positive results from a single CSF analysis were seen in patients with herpes simplex encephalitis, atypical encephalitis, metastatic lung cancer, and hypoxic brain damage.

Transferrin and CSF Leakage. Cerebrospinal fluid leakage usually presents as otorrhea or rhinorrhea following head trauma, in some cases beginning months to years after the injury. Recurrent meningitis is a serious complication making accurate identification of the leaking fluid very important. In this regard, protein and glucose measurements are too nonspecific to be of value. Transferrin, an iron-binding glycoprotein with a molecular mass of about 77 kDa, is synthesized primarily in the liver. However, two transferrin isoforms are present in the CSF; the major isoform (beta-1-transferrin) is present in all body fluids. The second isoform (beta-2-transferrin), present only in the central nervous system, is produced in the central nervous system by the catalytic conversion of beta-1-transferrin by neuraminidase. Immunofixation electrophoresis readily identifies both isoforms.

Protein electrophoresis with transferrin immunofixation is a noninvasive, rapid, and inexpensive test of high sensitivity and specificity that requires as little as 0.1 mL of fluid (Ryall, 1992; Normansell, 1994). Several reports have demonstrated the value of this technique in the diagnosis of CSF otorrhea and rhinorrhea, conditions in which both isoforms are readily identified (Irjala, 1979; Rouah, 1987; Zaret, 1992). Others stressed the importance of beta-2-transferrin identification in both CSF and inner ear perilymphatic leakage, as well as possible sources of error due to the presence of a transferrin allelic variant (Skedros, 1993a,b; Sloman, 1993).

Methemoglobin and Bilirubin. Although most cases of subarachnoid and intracerebral hemorrhage are readily identified by computed tomography (CT), patients with mild subarachnoid hemorrhage, small subdural or cerebral hematomas, blood seepage from an aneurysm or neoplasm, and from small cerebral infarcts are often not identified by this technique. In these cases, CSF spectrophotometric analysis has been shown to detect methemoglobin in colorless CSF ($< 0.3 \, \mu mol/L$) (Trbojevic-Cepe, 1992). However, an increase in CSF bilirubin is now recognized as the key finding supporting the diagnosis of subarachnoid hemorrhage (UK National External Quality Assessment Scheme for Immunochemistry Working Group, 2003). Thus, a single net bilirubin absorbance cutoff point of > 0.007 absorbance units is recommended in the decision tree for interpretation and reporting of results.

Glucose. Derived from blood glucose, fasting CSF glucose levels are normally 50–80 mg/dL (2.8–4.4 mmol/L), about 60% of plasma values. Results should be compared with plasma levels, ideally following a 4-hour fast, for adequate clinical interpretation. The normal CSF/plasma glucose ratio varies from 0.3–0.9 with fluctuations of blood levels because of the lag in CSF glucose equilibration time.

CSF values below 40 mg/dL (2.2 mmol/L) or ratios below 0.3 are considered to be abnormal. Hypoglycorrhachia is a characteristic finding of bacterial, tuberculous, and fungal meningitis. However, sensitivity can be as low as 55% for bacterial meningitis (Hayward, 1987), so a normal level does not exclude these conditions. Some cases of viral meningoencephalitis also have low glucose levels, but generally not to the degree seen in bacterial meningitis. Meningeal involvement by a malignant tumor, sarcoidosis, cysticercosis, trichinosis, ameba (*Naegleria*), acute syphilitic meningitis, intrathecal administration of radioiodinated serum albumin, subarachnoid hemorrhage, symptomatic hypoglycemia, and rheumatoid meningitis may also produce low CSF glucose levels (Fishman, 1992).

Decreased CSF glucose results from increased anaerobic glycolysis in brain tissue and leukocytes and impaired transport into the CSF. Bacteria are usually present in insufficient quantities to be a major contributor. CSF glucose levels normalize before protein levels and cell counts during recovery from meningitis, making it a useful parameter in assessing response to treatment.

Increased CSF glucose is of no clinical significance, reflecting increased blood glucose levels within 2 hours of lumbar puncture. A traumatic tap may also cause a spurious increase in CSF glucose.

Lactate. CSF and blood lactate levels are largely independent of each other. The reference interval for older children and adults is 9.0–26 mg/dL (1.0–2.9 mmol/L) (Knight, 1981). Newborns have higher levels, ranging from about 10–60 mg/dL (1.1–6.7 mmol/L) for the first 2 days, and 10–40 mg/dL (1.1–4.4 mmol/L) for days 3 to 10 (McGuinness, 1983).

Elevated CSF lactate levels reflect CNS anaerobic metabolism due to tissue hypoxia.

Lactate measurement has been used as an adjunctive test in differentiating viral meningitis from bacterial, mycoplasma, fungal, and tuberculous meningitis in which routine parameters yield equivocal results. In patients with viral meningitis, lactate levels are usually below 25 mg/dL (2.8 mmol/L) and almost always less than 35 mg/dL (3.9 mmol/L), whereas bacterial meningitis typically has levels above 35 mg/dL (Bailey, 1990; Cameron, 1993). Using 30–36 mg/dL as the cutoff value for bacterial meningitis, the sensitivity and specificity are about 80% and 90%, respectively. Viral meningitis, partially treated bacterial meningitis, and tuberculous meningitis often have intermediate lactate levels that overlap each other, limiting the use of lactate measurements in this differential diagnosis.

Persistently elevated ventricular CSF lactate levels are associated with a poor prognosis in patients with severe head injury (DeSalles, 1986).

F2-isoprostanes. F2-isoprostanes are increased in diseased regions of the brain in patients with Alzheimer's disease (AD) (Pratico, 1998). Compared with age-matched controls, CSF F2-isoprostanes are also elevated in patients with probable AD (Montine, 1999). Therefore, in conjunction with CSF tau and beta-amyloid protein, the measurement of CSF F2-isoprostanes appear to enhance the accuracy of the laboratory diagnosis of AD (Montine, 2001).

Enzymes. A wide variety of enzymes derived from brain tissue, blood, or cellular elements have been described in the CSF. Although CSF enzyme assays are not commonly used in the diagnosis of CNS diseases, there are diseases/disorders whereby they may prove useful.

Adenosine deaminase (ADA). ADA catalyzes the irreversible hydrolytic deamination of adenosine to produce inosine. Since ADA is particularly abundant in T lymphocytes, which are increased in tuberculosis, its measurement has been recommended in the diagnosis of pleural, peritoneal, and meningeal tuberculosis. Moreover, higher ADA levels are present in tuberculous infections than in viral, bacterial, and malignant diseases (Blake, 1982; Mann, 1982). More recently, ADA levels greater than 15 U/L were found to be a strong indication of tuberculous meningitis since nontuberculous meningitis consistently had levels less than 15 U/L (Choi, 2002). However, ADA has limited utility in HIV-associated neurologic disorders (Corral, 2004).

Creatine kinase (CK). Brain tissue is rich in CK since it participates in maintaining an adequate supply of adenosine triphosphate. Increased CSF CK activity has been reported in numerous CNS disorders including hydrocephalus, cerebral infarction, various primary brain tumors, and subarachnoid hemorrhage, among others (Savory, 1979). In patients with head trauma, CSF CK levels correlate directly with the severity of the concussion (Florez, 1976).

CSF CK-MM and CK-MB are not normally present and when identified, they are due to blood contamination (CK-MM) and an equilibrium between CK-BB and CK-MM to produce CK-MB. Since the CK-BB isoenzyme comprises about 90% of brain CK activity and mitochondrial CK (CKmt) the other 10%, CK isoenzyme measurements are more specific for CNS disorders than total CK (Chandler, 1984).

CSF CK-BB is increased about 6 hours following an ischemic or anoxic insult. Global brain ischemia following respiratory or cardiac arrest results in diffuse cerebral injury with peak CK-BB levels in about 48 hours (Chandler, 1986). Here, CSF CK-BB activity less than 5 U/L (upper normal level) indicates minimal neurologic damage; 5–20 U/L indicates mild to moderate CNS injury; and levels between 21–50 U/L are commonly correlated with death. Death occurs in essentially all patients with levels above 50 U/L.

Increased CSF CK-BB levels are also associated with the outcome following a subarachnoid hemorrhage (Coplin, 1999). Here, a CK-BB level greater than 40 U/L increased the chance of an unfavorable early or late outcome to 100%. The death rate was 13% when the CSF CK-BB level was less than 40 U/L.

Lactate dehydrogenase (LD). LD activity is high in brain tissue with a predominance of the electrophoretically fast-moving isoenzyme fractions LD1 and LD2. A total LD activity of 40 U/L is a reasonable upper limit of normal for adults and 70 U/L for neonates (Donald, 1986; Engelke, 1986). LD is useful in differentiating a traumatic tap from intracranial hemorrhage since a current traumatic tap with intact RBCs does not significantly elevate the LD level (Engelke, 1986). The sensitivity and specificity are about 70–85% depending on the cutoff value. As with lactate, LD activity is also significantly higher in bacterial meningitis than in aseptic meningitis (Donald, 1986; Engelke, 1986). Using a cutoff of 40 U/L, the sensitivity is about 86% and the specificity about 93%.

Total CSF LD levels are also increased in patients with CNS leukemia, lymphoma, metastatic carcinoma, bacterial meningitis, and subarachnoid hemorrhage (Kjeldsberg, 1993). CSF LD isoenzymes have been shown to add considerable specificity in the evaluation of various metastatic brain tumors (Fleisher, 1981). Thus, the LD5 to total LD ratio is increased (i.e., above 10–15%) in patients with leptomeningeal metastases from carcinoma of the breast, lung, and malignant melanoma. Isoenzyme analysis also shows a distinct pattern in young children with infantile spasms (Nussinovitch, 2003a) and febrile convulsions (Nussinovitch, 2003b). Compared with controls, both disorders are characterized by decreased LD1, increased LD2 and LD3, and no changes in LD4 and LD5.

Computed tomography (CT) is of limited value in estimating the recovery potential and neurologic outcome during the early stages of ischemic brain injury. However, compared with controls (mean LD, 11.2 U/L), patients with an early stroke had a mean level of 40.9 U/L; those with a transient ischemic attack (TIA) had a mean value of 11.8 U/L (Lampl, 1990). Moreover, in patients with hypoxic brain injury an increased LD level 72 hours following resuscitation indicates a poor prognosis (Karkela, 1992).

Lysozyme. Lysozyme (muramidase) catalyzes the depolymerization of mucopolysaccharides. Since the enzyme is particularly rich in neutrophil and macrophage lysosomes, its activity is very low in normal CSF. However, CSF lysozyme activity is significantly increased in patients with both bacterial and tuberculous meningitis. Thus, discriminant analysis demonstrated that 97% of patients with bacterial meningitis had increased lysozyme levels (Ribeiro, 1992). Others found that patients with tuberculous meningitis had significantly higher CSF lysozyme levels than those with bacterial meningitis, partially treated bacterial meningitis, and controls (Mishra, 2003). The diagnostic sensitivity and specificity for tuberculous meningitis were 93.7% and 84.1%, respectively. Increased levels are also present in cerebral atrophy, various CNS tumors, multiple sclerosis, intracranial hemorrhage, and epilepsy (Kjeldsberg, 1993).

Ammonia, Amines, and Amino Acids. CSF ammonia levels vary from 30–50% of the blood values. Elevated levels are generally proportional to the degree of existing hepatic encephalopathy, but are difficult to quantify. Moreover, since hepatic encephalopathy generally correlates with blood ammonia levels, the measurement of CSF ammonia has little, if any, clinical value. However, cerebral glutamine, synthesized from ammonia and glutamic acid, serves as the means for CNS ammonia removal. Thus, CSF glutamine levels reflect the concentration of brain ammonia. Glutamine reference intervals are method dependent; the upper reference level is about 20 mg/dL. Values over 35 mg/dL are usually associated with hepatic encephalopathy (Fishman, 1992). Elevated CSF glutamine levels have also been reported in patients with encephalopathy secondary to hypercapnia and sepsis (Mizock, 1989).

A major etiologic theory of schizophrenia involves dopamine. The cornerstone for this theory lies with the fact that neuroleptic drugs which block dopamine receptors are effective in the treatment of this disorder. Thus, it has been reported that CSF levels of homovanilic acid (HVA), a metabolite of the biogenic amines, is related to the severity of schizophrenic psychosis (Maas, 1997). However, HVA concentration varied as a function of psychosis rather than being related to the diagnosis of schizophrenia per se. Others reported decreased CSF levels of 5-hydroxyindoleacetic acid (5-HIAA), a metabolite of serotonin, in schizophrenic patients with suicidal behavior (Cooper, 1992). This report adds further support for a possible relationship between suicide and CNS serotonin metabolism.

Although free CSF amino acids are relatively high in infants less than 30 days of age, their concentration is further increased in those with febrile convulsions and bacterial meningitis. Gamma-aminobutyric acid (GABA), a major inhibitory brain transmitter, is significantly decreased in basal ganglia neurons, and very low or undetectable in the CSF of patients with Alzheimer's disease and Huntington's disease (Achar, 1976; Dubowitz, 1992). In addition, CSF GABA was detected in all patients with migraine attacks, but not in those with tension headaches or the control group without headaches (Welch, 1975). Conversely, infants with startle disease, a rare inherited autosomal dominant disorder characterized by either seizures or the so-called 'stiff baby syndrome,' have significantly decreased CSF GABA levels (Dubowitz, 1992; Berthier, 1994).

Electrolytes and Acid–Base Balance. There are no clinically useful indications for the measurement of CSF sodium, potassium, chloride, calcium or magnesium. Measurement of CSF pH, P_{CO_2}, and bicarbonate are also not practical for patient care (Fishman, 1992).

Tumor Markers. Numerous studies have shown that various tumor markers are increased in the CSF of patients with both primary and metastatic tumors. However, the value of most of these tests in routine clinical practice has not been established.

Carcinoembryonic antigen (CEA). CEA is an oncofetal protein produced by a variety of carcinomas. An early study found increased CEA levels in 44% of patients with metastatic brain tumors (Suzuki, 1980). Others reported that

Table 28–13 Typical Lumbar CSF Findings in Meningitis

Test	Bacterial	Viral	Fungal	Tuberculous
Opening pressure	Elevated	Usually normal	Variable	Variable
Leukocyte count	≥1000/μL	<100/μL	Variable	Variable
Cell differential	Mainly neutrophils*	Mainly lymphocytes†	Mainly lymphocytes	Mainly lymphocytes
Protein	Mild–marked increase	Normal–mild increase	Increased	Increased
Glucose	Usually ≤40 mg/dL	Normal	Decreased	Decreased: may be <45 mg/dL
CSF-to-serum glucose ratio	Normal–marked decrease	Usually normal	Low	Low
Lactic acid	Mild–marked increase	Normal–mild increase	Mild–moderate increase	Mild–moderate increase

* Lymphocytosis present in about 10% of cases.
† Neutrophils may predominate early in disease.

Data from Arevalo, 1989; Body, 1987; Fishman, 1992; Tang, 1988; Wubbel, 1998; Zunt, 1999.

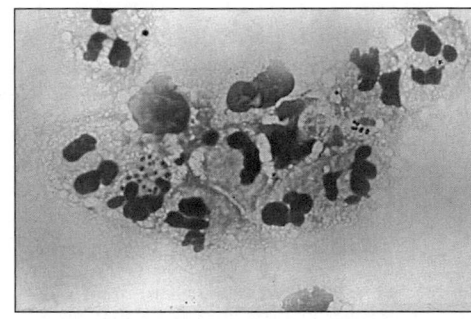

Figure 28–9 CSF Gram stain showing Gram-negative diplococci characteristic of *N. meningitidis.*

CSF levels of CEA have a sensitivity of only about 31%, although the specificity is about 90% for detecting metastatic carcinoma of the leptomeninges (Klee, 1986; Twijnstra, 1986). More recently, CSF levels of CEA in patients with benign, primary malignant, and metastatic brain tumors were 0.31 ng/mL, 0.92 ng/mL, and 6.3 ng/mL, respectively (Batabyal, 2003).

Other oncofetal proteins include *human chorionic gonadotropin* (HCG), produced by choriocarcinoma and malignant germ cell tumors with a trophoblastic component, and *alpha-fetoprotein,* a glycoprotein produced by yolk sac elements of germ cell tumors. The results of a recent study concluded that both beta-HCG and alpha-fetoprotein may be useful in the diagnosis and monitoring of the response to therapy in patients with CNS germ cell tumors (Seregni, 2002).

Elevation of CSF *ferritin* is a sensitive indicator of CNS malignancy but has very low specificity since it is also increased in patients with inflammatory neurologic diseases (Zandman-Goddard, 1986).

Microbiological Examination

A thorough and prompt examination of cerebrospinal fluid is essential for the diagnosis of CNS infection because an inaccurate or delayed report may result in significant mortality or morbidity. Although changes in opening pressure, total cell and differential counts, total protein, and glucose suggest an infectious etiology (Table 28–13), Gram stain and culture are critical for a definitive diagnosis.

Bacterial Meningitis. The most common agents of bacterial meningitis are group B streptococcus (neonates), *Neisseria meningitidis* (3 months and older) (Fig. 28–9), *Streptococcus pneumoniae* (3 months and older), *Escherichia coli* and other Gram-negative bacilli (newborn to 1 month), *Haemophilus influenzae* (3 months to 18 years) and *Listeria monocytogenes* (neonates, elderly, alcoholics, and immunosuppressed) (Graves, 1989;

Wenger, 1990). *H. influenzae*, once the most common bacterial cause of meningitis in young children, has decreased dramatically from widespread use of *H. influenzae* type b vaccine. Cerebrospinal fluid shunts, head trauma, and neurosurgery place patients at risk for CNS infections from *Staphylococcus* species, aerobic Gram-negative bacilli, and *Propionibacterium* species.

The Gram stain remains an accurate, rapid method to diagnose CNS infections. All specimens should be concentrated by centrifugation before Gram stain and culture. Depending upon the type of infecting microorganism and its concentration in the cerebrospinal fluid, Gram stain sensitivity ranges from 60–90% with the greatest sensitivity corresponding to higher concentrations of bacteria (about 10^5 colony-forming units/mL). For example, the sensitivity of the Gram stain for detecting *Listeria monocytogenes* and Gram-negative bacilli is 50% or less (Greenlee, 1990). For patients with many polymorphonuclear leukocytes but no organisms seen on Gram stain, the more sensitive acridine orange stain may be helpful. Cultures have a sensitivity of 80–90%, but are about 30% less in partially treated cases (Greenlee, 1990).

Although standard culture-based methods remain the mainstay for diagnosis, the Binax NOW® *Streptococcus pneumoniae* antigen test, an immunochromatographic membrane assay that detects the presence of the C polysaccharide cell-wall antigen common to all pneumococcal serotypes, has proven a valuable tool for the rapid diagnosis of pneumococcal meningitis from cerebrospinal fluid. Latex agglutination bacterial antigen tests (BAT) performed on CSF to detect *H. influenzae, N. meningitidis, S. pneumoniae*, and beta-hemolytic group-B streptococcus historically were used as an adjunct to Gram stain and culture; however, the sensitivity is approximately the same as the Gram stain and a negative test does not rule out the diagnosis of bacterial meningitis. Perhaps the best application of latex agglutination antigen tests is in partially treated, community-acquired meningitis that is negative for microorganisms by Gram stain (Perkins, 1995; Wilson, 1997). Urine reagent strips have also been used for characterizing bacterial meningitis (Moosa, 1995). Although they are not used in well-staffed laboratories, they may be useful in small facilities where microscopy and culture are unavailable.

The *limulus lysate assay* is a very sensitive test for the presence of endotoxin, a product of most Gram-negative bacteria. It is particularly useful as a rapid test in the newborn where early diagnosis and treatment are critical. However, since endotoxin is ubiquitous and contamination widespread, adequate precautions must be taken. Despite its great sensitivity, the test has never become popular in clinical laboratories. Rather, it has been primarily used to ensure that solutions used for parenteral nutrition are sterile.

Recent studies indicate that the use of the polymerase chain reaction (PCR) and sequencing of 16S ribosomal RNA in CSF is very useful in the diagnosis of bacterial meningitis (Schuurman, 2004). Compared with bacterial culture, the assay showed a sensitivity of 86%, a specificity of 97%, a positive predictive value of 80%, and a negative predictive value of 98%. Nucleic acid amplification tests may also be helpful for patients already receiving antimicrobial therapy or for detecting more fastidious pathogens such as *N. meningitidis* (Seward, 2000; Porritt, 2000; Baethgen, 2003).

Spirochetal Meningitis. The incidence of neurosyphilis has increased in recent years, primarily in patients with HIV infection. In one report, 44% of patients with neurosyphilis had AIDS (Flood, 1998). Unfortunately, the remaining patients who may have had HIV infection without AIDS were not studied.

The diagnosis of CNS infection in patients with syphilis relies primarily on CSF parameters and serologic testing. Abnormalities in CSF protein and cell counts are common in syphilitic meningitis, although they are nonspecific. CSF serologic testing to diagnose neurosyphilis is difficult. The standard nontreponemal test performed on CSF is the VDRL (Venereal Disease Research Laboratory). If there are few erythrocytes contaminating the CSF, the VDRL specificity is high, but its sensitivity is only 50–60% (Davis, 1989). Treponemal tests, such as the treponemal antibody absorption (FTA-ABS), are both sensitive and specific for syphilis; however, their use on CSF for neurosyphilis is controversial. The CSF FTA-ABS is highly sensitive, but false-positive results may occur. Moreover, in the absence of CSF abnormalities or clinical suspicion, it should not be used as a screening test. Thus, the following generalizations have been proposed (Davis, 1989): (1) a nonreactive serum FTA-ABS test rules out neurosyphilis; (2) a reactive serum FTA-ABS test with a nonreactive CSF FTA-ABS test essentially rules out neurosyphilis; (3) a reactive CSF VDRL test makes a diagnosis of neurosyphilis likely; and (4) a reactive CSF FTA-ABS test may indicate active neurosyphilis, asymptomatic neurosyphilis, treated neurosyphilis, or a false-positive reaction.

Viral Meningitis. Enteroviruses (echoviruses, Coxsackieviruses, polio-viruses) are responsible for up to 80% of meningitis cases, with a seasonal peak in late summer. Indeed, echoviruses 9 (E9) and 30 (E30) have been mainly responsible for the recent increase in cases of aseptic meningitis (Morbidity and Mortality Weekly Report, 2003). Most patients present with a CSF pleocytosis and although neutrophils may be observed early in the infection, patients soon develop a predominance of lymphocytes.

Prior to molecular diagnostic testing, meningitis was a diagnosis of exclusion since the sensitivity of viral cultures can be exceedingly low. Thus, in an early study a specific etiologic diagnosis by viral cultures varied from 72% for enteroviruses to 5% for herpes simplex virus (HSV) (Marton, 1986).

Reverse transcriptase polymerase chain reaction (RT-PCR) is significantly more sensitive than cell culture (Dumler, 1999; Hausfater, 2004). Arguably, it has evolved as the 'gold standard' for the diagnosis of viral meningitis secondary to enterovirus, herpes simplex virus, cytomegalovirus, and varicella zoster virus. Importantly, for patients with arbovirus-associated meningitis, acute and convalescent sera and CSF remain the cornerstone for diagnosis. The results of a commercially available reverse transcription (RT)-PCR assay (Penter RT-PCR test), compared with cell culture and an in-house RT-PCR assay, showed the following: 52% were positive by cell culture; 76% were positive by the inhouse RT-PCR assay; and 80% were positive by the commercial RT-PCR test (Jacques, 2003). Moreover, RT-PCR is equally sensitive to the reference RT-PCR and both are significantly more sensitive for the rapid diagnosis of entero- and rhinovirus infections (Kares, 2004). The use of RT-PCR may also result in significant cost savings by shortening hospital stays and eliminating unnecessary diagnostic and therapeutic interventions (Ramers, 2000).

PCR amplification of HSV-2 DNA in CSF may be useful in the early diagnosis of HSV encephalitis, having shown excellent correlation with brain biopsy (Lakeman, 1995). False negatives might occur in very early infections and bloody taps. Since PCR may become negative 1–14 days following symptom onset, serum and CSF serologies for HSV antibody may be useful in conjunction with PCR.

Human Immunodeficiency Virus (HIV). A wide variety of CSF abnormalities may be found in HIV-positive patients with or without neurologic disease including lymphocytic pleocytosis, elevated IgG indexes, and oligoclonal bands (Chalmers, 1990; Hall, 1992). Identifying opportunistic infections is the most important indication for examining the CSF. Serious fungal infections may exist in the presence of little or no CSF parameter abnormalities.

Fungal Meningitis. Cryptococcus is the most frequently isolated fungal pathogen from CSF. India ink or nigrosin stains for cryptococcus capsular halos have a sensitivity of about 25%, increasing to 53% with multiple lumbar punctures (Marton, 1986). Detection of cryptococcal antigen from sera or CSF using latex agglutination has higher sensitivity, ranging from 60–95%. False negatives due to a prozone effect or low concentration of polysaccharide antigen may occur. Early disease, intraparenchymal infection, infection with nonencapsulated *Cryptococcus neoformans* variants and immune complexes (corrected with pronase treatment) may also produce false negatives. Conversely, sera or CSF from patients with rheumatoid factor or *Trichosporon beigelii* infections may be falsely positive. If clinical suspicion for dimorphic or filamentous fungi is high, large volumes of CSF (approximately 15–20 mL) are optimal for culture to improve recovery of fungal organisms.

Tuberculous Meningitis. Abnormal CSF with elevated protein and lymphocytic predominance are the hallmark features of tuberculous meningitis. The sensitivity of CSF acid-fast stains for the diagnosis of tuberculous meningitis is highly variable, ranging from 10–12% (Greenlee, 1990) to greater than 50% (Thwaites, 2004). Large volumes of CSF, often from multiple lumbar punctures, are recommended to improve the sensitivity of both acid-fast stain and culture (Marton, 1986).

PCR nucleic acid amplification for detecting *Mycobacterium tuberculosis* DNA-specific sequences shows great promise in the rapid and accurate diagnosis of tuberculous meningitis (Lin, 1995; Desai, 2002). However, a negative PCR result does not exclude the diagnosis of tuberculous meningitis. Indeed, if a high clinical suspicion remains, empiric therapy should be initiated.

DOT enzyme linked immunosorbent assay (DOT ELISA) has been standardized to detect tuberculosis antigens and antibodies against *M. tuberculosis* in CSF. Using this technique, a positive reaction was present in 86% of cases with suspected tuberculous meningitis (Kashyap, 2003). Only 5% of patients with other disorders, mainly pyogenic meningitis, were positive.

Other tests have also been shown to be useful in some cases of tuberculous meningitis. For example, ligase chain reaction amplification is reportedly a rapid method for the early diagnosis of tuberculous meningitis (Rajo, 2002). Here, the sensitivity, specificity, positive predictive value and negative predictive value were 55.5%, 100%, 100%, and 92.9%, respectively.

Table 28–14 Synovial Fluid Findings by Disease Category

		Category			
Finding	Normal	Group I Noninflammatory	Group II Inflammatory	Group III Infectious	Group IV Hemorrhagic
Clarity	Transparent	Transparent	Transparent/opaque	Opaque	Opaque
Color	Clear to pale yellow	Xanthochromic	Xanthochromic to white/bloody	White	Red-brown or xanthochromic
WBCs/mL	0–150	< 3000	3000–75 000	50 000–200 000	50–10 000
PMNs (%)	< 25	< 30	> 50	> 90	< 50
RBCs	No	No	No	Yes	Yes
Glucose (blood/SF difference mg/dL)	0–10 (0–0.56 mmol/L)	0–10 (0–0.56 mmol/L)	0–40 (0–2.2 mmol/L)	20–100 (1.11–5.5 mmol/L)	0–20 (0–1.11 mmol/L)

WBCs = white blood cells; PMNs = polymorphonuclear cells, neutrophils; RBCs = red blood cells; SF = synovial fluid.

Modified from Kjeldsberg CR, Knight JA: Body Fluids: Laboratory Examination of Amniotic, Cerebrospinal, Seminal, Serous and Synovial Fluids, 3rd ed. Copyright © American Society for Clinical Pathology, Chicago, 1993, with permission.

Moreover, adenosine deaminase (ADA) levels are significantly higher in tuberculous meningitis than in other types of meningitis and CNS disorders (Pettersson, 1991). Indeed, a level greater than 15 U/L is a strong indicator of tuberculous meningitis (Choi, 2002).

Primary Amebic Meningoencephalitis (PAM). This rare disease is caused by the free-living ameba *Naegleria fowleri* or *Acanthamoeba* species. *Naegleria* is more likely to cause an acute inflammatory response with a neutrophilic pleocytosis, decreased glucose level, an elevated protein concentration, and the presence of erythrocytes. Gram stain is always negative. *Acanthamoeba* more often produces a granulomatous meningitis. Motile *Naegleria* trophozoites may be visualized by light or phase-contrast microscopy in direct wet mounts, allowing rapid diagnosis. Intact and degenerating organisms may be identified on Wright's or Giemsa-stained cytospins, but must be distinguished from macrophages (dos Santos, 1970; Benson, 1985). Acridine orange stain is useful to differentiate ameba (brick red) from leukocytes (bright green).

Synovial Fluid

Synovium refers to the tissue lining synovial tendon sheaths, bursae, and diarthrodial joints except for the articular surface. It is composed of one to three cell layers that form a discontinuous surface overlying fatty, fibrous, or periosteal joint tissue.

Synovial fluid (synovia, SF) is an imperfect ultrafiltrate of blood plasma combined with hyaluronic acid produced by the synovial cells. Small ions and molecules (e.g., Na^+, K^+, glucose, urea, etc.) readily pass into the joint space and are, therefore, similar in concentration to plasma, while large molecules are absent or present in trace amounts. Resorption of synovial molecules is by the lymphatics and is not size dependent. SF acts as a lubricant and adhesive, and provides nutrients for the avascular articular cartilage.

Examination of the synovial fluid is essential to distinguish infectious from noninfectious arthritis. Results from gross and microscopic examination of synovial fluid have traditionally been divided into 'reaction types,' as depicted in Table 28–14. These groupings are largely descriptive and there is considerable overlap between them. Except for Gram stain, culture, and crystal examination, synovial fluid parameters can be nonspecific and must be integrated into the clinical context.

Noninflammatory effusions (Group I) typically have leukocyte counts less than 3000/µL, with a minority of neutrophils. Osteoarthritis, traumatic arthritis, neuropathic osteoarthropathy, pigmented villonodular synovitis, and early rheumatic fever usually present with little inflammatory response. Early rheumatoid arthritis, early bacterial infections, and viral arthritis may also present as noninflammatory effusions.

Inflammatory effusions (Group II) have leukocyte counts between 3000 and 75 000, with neutrophils accounting for over 50% of the population. Rheumatoid arthritis, systemic lupus erythematosus (SLE), Reiter's syndrome, rheumatic fever, acute crystal-induced arthritis, arthritis associated with inflammatory bowel disease, psoriatic arthritis, and fat droplet synovitis are examples of this reaction group.

Purulent (infectious) effusions (Group III) typically have leukocyte counts greater than 50 000, of which 90% or more are neutrophils. Bacterial, fungal, and tuberculous joint infections constitute this group.

Hemorrhagic effusions (Group IV) may be seen in association with traumatic arthritis, pigmented villonodular synovitis, synovial hemangioma, neuropathic osteoarthropathy, joint prostheses, and hematologic disorders (hemophilia, thrombocytopenia, anticoagulant therapy, sickle cell disease or trait, myeloproliferative syndrome).

Specimen Collection

Joint fluid aspiration (arthrocentesis) should be confined to patients with an undiagnosed effusion or a significant clinical change related to a known effusion (Pal, 1999). It should be performed by an experienced operator using good sterile technique. Caution is necessary to avoid aspirating a sterile joint in someone with bacteremia, or through a cutaneous or periarticular soft tissue infection into a sterile joint. Large joints such as the knee normally contain no more than 4.0 mL of synovia, so small sample size is common unless an effusion is present.

Synovial fluid must be collected with sterile, disposable needles and plastic syringes to avoid contamination by birefringent particulates. The syringe may be heparinized with 25 U of sodium heparin/mL of SF in routine arthrocentesis. Oxalate, lithium heparin, and powdered ethylenediaminetetraacetic acid (EDTA) anticoagulants should be avoided because they form crystal artifacts that may be misleading during the microscopic examination. Prior to aspiration, turn or manipulate the joint to ensure mixing of its contents.

The specimen should ideally be separated into three parts: 3–10 mL into a sterile heparinized tube or syringe for microbiological studies; 2–5 mL in an anticoagulant tube (sodium heparin or liquid EDTA) for microscopic examination; and about 5 mL into a plain (no anticoagulant) tube for chemical analysis (normal synovial fluid does not clot since fibrinogen is absent). Heparin concentrations greater than 125 U/mL have an inhibitory effect on some pathogenic bacteria (Rosett, 1980). Specimens for culture should, therefore, be at least 1–2 mL in volume if they are submitted in green top heparin tubes (Becton Dickinson, Rutherford, NJ) containing 143 U/tube of heparin, or submitted in recapped syringes after removing the needle and excess air.

'Dry taps' may still have fluid within the needle, which may be sufficient for the most critical tests. Such specimens should be submitted with the needle still on the syringe, its tip stuck into a sterile cork. Good communication with the laboratory is crucial to the appropriate processing of such specimens.

Recommended Tests

The laboratory examination of synovial fluid is of major importance in the differential diagnosis of joint disease, especially in crystal-induced and infectious arthritis. When either is suspected, arthrocentesis and a systematic examination of the synovial fluid are imperative, and when examination is carried out properly it is usually diagnostic. In other joint diseases a specific diagnosis may not be possible. Nevertheless, fluid examination is still important if only to rule out infectious arthritis, which is a critical diagnosis to make since a joint may be irreversibly damaged within a couple of days if not properly treated. This is especially true when *Staphylococcus aureus* is the infectious organism. Therefore, routine tests should be directed toward the diagnosis of these two disorders (Table 28–15). Although other tests are not of practical value for routine use, they may provide important diagnostic information under certain circumstances.

It is critical that these tests be performed well because they can provide highly specific diagnostic information. However, a major problem in the

Table 28–15 Recommended Synovial Fluid Tests

Routine tests

Gross examination (color, clarity)
Total and differential leukocyte counts
Gram's stain and bacterial culture (aerobic and anaerobic)
Crystal examination with polarizing microscope and compensator

Useful tests in certain circumstances

Fungal and acid-fast stains and cultures
PCR for bacterial and mycobacterial DNA
Serum–synovial fluid glucose differential
Lactate and other organic acids
Complement
Enzymes
Uric acid

PCR = polymerase chain reaction; DNA = deoxyribonucleic acid.

Modified from Kjeldsberg CR, Knight JA: Body Fluids: Laboratory Examination of Amniotic, Cerebrospinal, Seminal, Serous and Synovial Fluids, 3rd ed. Copyright © American Society for Clinical Pathology, Chicago, 1993, with permission.

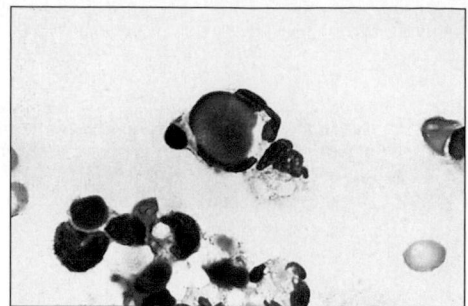

Figure 28–10 LE cell in the synovial fluid from a patient with systemic lupus erythematosus.

laboratory examination of synovial fluid is that, in contrast to CSF and amniotic fluid, in most laboratories there is no consensus as to what constitutes a 'routine' analysis (Hasselbacher, 1987). Moreover, quality performance is not consistent, in part due to the fact that the average laboratory examines only one to two synovial fluids each month (Hasselbacher, 1987; Rabinovitch, 1994).

Gross Examination

Total volume should be recorded at the bedside, especially if the sample is to be divided for submission to different laboratory sections.

Color should be evaluated in a clear glass tube against a white background. Normal SF is colorless but is often pale yellow due to diapedesis of a few RBCs associated with even mild trauma. Noninflammatory and inflammatory disorders are usually straw- to yellow-colored (xanthochromia). Septic fluid may be yellow, brown, or green depending on the chromogens produced by the offending organism and the host response, including the presence of WBCs and RBCs.

A *traumatic tap* produces an uneven distribution of blood during arthrocentesis or streaking in the syringe. Although pale yellow xanthochromia is difficult to distinguish from normal, a red-brown color following centrifugation is good evidence of pathologic hemarthrosis.

Clarity relates to the number and type of particles within the synovia. Since normal SF is transparent, newsprint is easily read through the tube. Although translucent fluid obscures details, black and white areas can be distinguished, while opaque fluid completely obscures the background.

Leukocytes are most commonly responsible for changes in clarity. However, very large numbers of crystals may produce an opaque, milky opalescent fluid without leukocytes. A shimmering, oily-appearing specimen suggests an abundance of cholesterol crystals which may grossly resemble pus.

Increased turbidity is less often due to concentrations of fibrin, free-floating 'rice bodies' (fragments of degenerating proliferative synovial cells or microinfarcted synovium), metal and plastic particles from patients with joint prostheses, or cartilage fragments in osteoarthritis. A 'ground pepper' appearance from pigmented cartilage fragments may be the result of a metabolic disorder (i.e., ochronosis).

Microscopic Examination

Total Cell Count. Total leukocyte counts should be performed promptly to avoid degenerative cell loss, which begins as soon as 1 hour following arthrocentesis. Tubes must be inverted before sampling to ensure uniform mixing. Cell counts are usually performed in a standard hemocytometer. Automated cell counters may be used, but they risk clogging the machine aperture or obtaining spuriously high cell counts from non-WBC particles (e.g., crystals and fat globules), especially in multichannel machines. A wet-prep slide count of 0–2 leukocytes per high-power field (hpf) (averaged over 10 fields) predicts less than 1300 WBCs by cell count (Clayburne, 1992).

Leukocyte counts greater than 10 000/μL, and often greater than 50 000/μL, are characteristic of crystal-induced arthritis (e.g., gout,

pseudogout), chronic inflammatory arthritis (e.g., rheumatoid arthritis, systemic lupus erythematosus, ankylosing spondylitis, and others), and septic arthritis (Kjeldsberg, 1993). Osteoarthritis, osteochondritis dissicans, trauma, and synovioma usually have total WBC counts less than 10 000/μL.

Leukocyte counts over 50 000/μL require dilution, which should be done with saline, not acetic acid, to avoid mucin clot formation and cell clumping. Highly viscous synovial fluid should be incubated with hyaluronidase before counting, especially if automated counters are used.

Erythrocytes should be routinely counted unless it is an obvious traumatic tap. If a large number of red cells interferes with the leukocyte count, they may be lysed by dilution with 0.3 normal saline or 1% saponin in saline.

The upper reference level for SF leukocytes is 150–200/μL (Kjeldsberg, 1993). Elevated cell counts are used to help divide findings into different disease categories, but are nonspecific for any particular disease because of extensive overlap.

Differential Leukocyte Count. Cytospin preparations are preferred over smears from centrifuged SF because the cell morphology is significantly better. Treatment with hyaluronidase may be necessary to produce thin smears in viscous specimens.

Neutrophils normally account for about 20% of SF leukocytes. Neutrophils generally exceed 50% in urate gout, pseudogout, and rheumatoid arthritis (RA); they most often exceed 75% in acute bacterial arthritis. Using 75% as a cutoff, the sensitivity for an inflammatory process is about 75% and the specificity is 92% (Shmerling, 1990). These cells frequently exhibit degenerative changes and may contain bacteria, crystals, lipid droplets, vacuoles, or dark blue to black granular inclusions (ragocytes, RA cells) which are similar to toxic granulation occasionally seen in peripheral blood smears. The presence of ragocytes in patients with RA may indicate a poorer outcome (Davis, 1988).

LE (lupus erythematosus) cells, not uncommonly present in patients with lupus arthritis, are most often neutrophils which have phagocytosed the nuclei of degenerating cells (Fig. 28–10). However, LE cells are not pathognomonic for systemic lupus erythrematosus since they have also been identified in the synovial fluid of RA patients (Hunder, 1970).

Lymphocytes, normally constituting about 15% of the SF cells, are prominent in early RA and other collagen disorders, and chronic infections. Reactive forms, including immunoblasts, are also occasionally present.

Monocytes and *macrophages* are the most common cells present in normal SF, accounting for approximately 65% of the cell count. Monocytosis may be self-limited in viral arthritis or serum sickness, or more chronic in systemic lupus erythematosus (SLE) or undifferentiated connective tissue disorders. Reiter's cells, originally believed to be specific for Reiter's syndrome, are macrophages containing degenerating neutrophils (Fig. 28–11).

Eosinophilia, defined as over 2% of the leukocyte count, has been reported in rheumatoid arthritis, rheumatic fever, metastatic carcinoma, Lyme disease, parasitic infections, chronic urticaria, angioedema, following arthrography (allergic reaction to dye), and irradiation (Podell, 1980; Kay, 1988).

Synovial cells have no pathologic significance. They appear similar to mesothelial cells and may be difficult to distinguish from monocytes and macrophages.

Lipid bodies are associated with trauma, aseptic necrosis, and RA. These droplets often form Maltese crosses under polarized light, can be associated with a leukocyte response, and may cause spurious elevations of the automated WBC count (Wise, 1987).

Crystal Examination. Crystals in synovial fluid lead to acute inflammation with increased WBC counts and a neutrophil-predominant infiltrate. Crystal identification, especially if intracellularly in neutrophils or macrophages, is pathognomonic for a crystal-induced arthritis (Judkins, 1997).

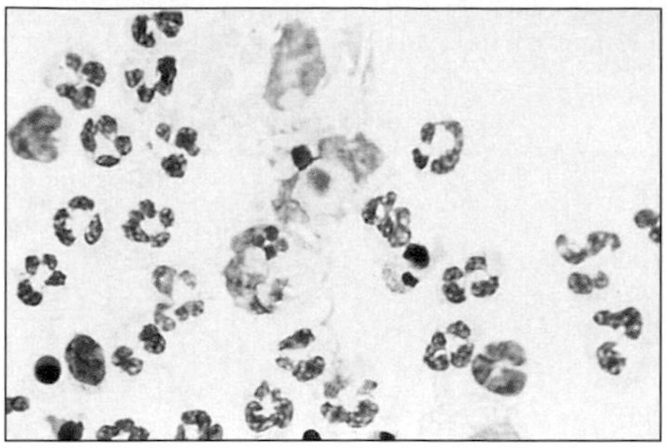

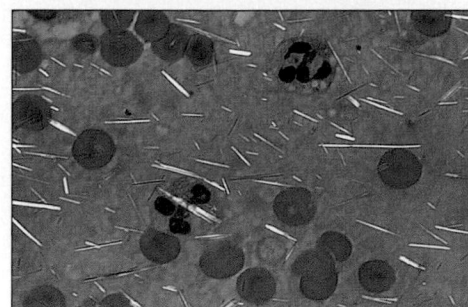

Figure 28–11 Reiter's cells in the synovial fluid from a patient with Reiter's syndrome.

Figure 28–12 Monosodium urate crystals under polarized light from a patient with urate gout.

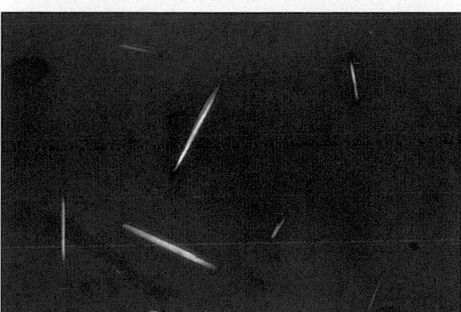

Figure 28–13 Monosodium urate crystals in synovial fluid. Compensated polarized light. (From Kjeldsberg CR, Knight JA: Body Fluids: Laboratory Examination of Amniotic, Cerebrospinal, Seminal, Serous and Synovial Fluids, 3rd ed. © American Society for Clinical Pathology, Chicago, 1993, with permission.)

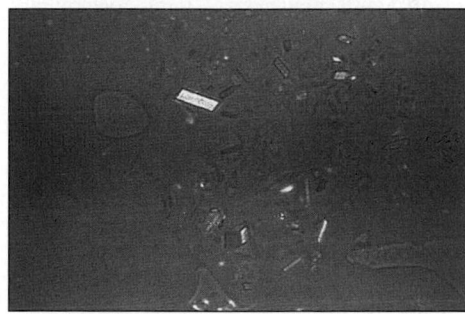

Figure 28–14 Calcium pyrophosphate dihydrate crystals in synovial fluid from a patient with pseudogout. Compensated polarized light. (From Kjeldsberg CR, Knight JA: Body Fluids: Laboratory Examination of Amniotic, Cerebrospinal, Seminal, Serous and Synovial Fluids, 3rd ed. © American Society for Clinical Pathology, Chicago, 1993, with permission.)

Gout refers to the process of crystal deposition in articular tissue. Common usage typically implies urate gout, and an inflammatory response to crystal deposition is referred to as gouty arthritis. The most common types of endogenous crystals responsible for gouty arthritis are *monosodium urate monohydrate* (urate gout), *calcium pyrophosphate dihydrate* (pyrophosphate gout, chondrocalcinosis, or 'pseudogout'), apatite and other *basic calcium phosphates* (BCP; apatite gout), *calcium oxalate* (oxalate gout), and *lipids* (lipid gout).

Except for BCP, all of the above crystals can be detected by polarized light microscopy. A high-quality polarizing microscope with first-order red plate compensator should be used. The *polarizer* filter is placed directly above the light source. The *analyzer* (another polarizing filter) is placed between the specimen slide and microscope oculars, oriented 90 degrees from the polarizer to produce a dark background The *compensator* is placed between the polarizer and analyzer, usually oriented 45 degrees (halfway) between the planes of the two polarizing filters.

Initial examination should be performed on a wet preparation using polarized light. Phase-contrast microscopy enhances crystal detection. The slide and coverslip must be cleaned and carefully dried immediately prior to use to avoid birefringent dust particulate artifacts. The coverslip edges are sealed with nail polish, which retards but does not prevent evaporation. The coverslip edge is used to find the proper plane of focus. However, crystals in this location should be ignored because they are most likely artifacts. Most crystals are scanned with a 10× objective and evaluated with at least a 40× objective, concentrating especially on cellular areas. Complete examination requires 100× oil immersion, however, because apparently negative fluids on scanning may contain a large population of small crystals (Gatter, 1991). Aligning the crystals' orientation to the compensator by rotating the microscope stage or the compensator facilitates recognition and identification. Crystal morphology, the extinction angle, strength and sign of any birefringence (i.e., the ability to refract light and split the incident light into two rays; a fast ray and a slow ray), are noted. Nevertheless, the sensitivity and specificity of polarized microscopy for crystals is only 78% and 79% respectively, for monosodium urate (Hasselbacher, 1987) and 12% and 67% for calcium pyrophosphate dihydrate (McGill, 1991). However, repeat examination following 24 hours of refrigeration at 4°C may result in a significant increase in the number of crystal-positive fluids (Yuan, 2003).

The Diff Quik staining method may be a reliable alternative to polarized microscopy. The overall specificity, sensitivity, and accuracy were respectively 87.5%, 94.4%, and 91.9%. The overall positive predictive value was 92.7%; the negative predictive value was 90.3% (Selvi, 2001). Moreover, other more sophisticated and reliable methods, such as X-ray crystallography and Fourier transform infrared spectroscopy, have been described for identifying and characterizing crystals in biologic specimens (Rosenthal, 2001).

Monosodium urate (MSU) crystals appear as needle-shaped rods 5–20 μm long, but may be only 1–2 μm in length or, rarely, appear as rounded spherolites. They are strongly birefringent (Fig. 28–12): yellow when oriented parallel to the compensator, blue with perpendicular orientation (negative birefringence or elongation) (Fig. 28–13). A control slide of MSU crystals should always be used for comparison. Alternatively, betamethasone, a steroid that appears as a strongly negative birefringent rod, can be used to prepare a reference slide for the polarizing microscope (Judkins, 1997).

MSU crystals are found in 90% of acute urate gout and about 75% of patients between attacks. Intracellular MSU crystals are characteristic of acute urate gout. They may occasionally be observed as a result of inflammation in septic arthritis (McCarty, 1988).

Calcium pyrophosphate dihydrate (CPPD) crystals are found in a group of conditions collectively known as CPPD crystal deposition disease. These crystals appear as rhomboids, rods, or rectangles 1–20 μm in length. CPPD crystals are weakly birefringent with positive elongation (blue when aligned with compensator axis; Fig. 28–14). Many are too small to polarize the light, making them difficult to detect without phase-contrast microscopy. Extinction is incomplete and occurs between 20–30 degrees from the angle of the polarizer and analyzer (oblique or inclined extinction).

CPPD crystals are associated with degenerative arthritis and in arthritides associated with hypomagnesemia, hemochromatosis, hyperparathyroidism, and hypothyroidism (Jones, 1992).

Calcium hydroxyapatite and the other BCP crystals are typically too small and nonbirefringent (isotropic) to see with light microscopy unless they are clumped into 1- to 50-μm spherical microaggregates. *Alizarin red S dye* may be used to stain these and other calcium-containing crystals (Lazcano, 1993). At present, identification of BCP crystals is not important for diagnosis, prognosis, or as a guide in treatment.

Calcium oxalate dihydrate crystals are 5- to 30-μm bipyramidal octahedral 'envelopes' with variable birefringence and positive elongation. They are seen in arthropathy associated with chronic renal dialysis and primary oxalosis, a rare inborn error of metabolism. The monohydrate form is birefringent but nondescript in shape.

Lipid crystals are 1- to 20-μm spheres with a Maltese cross appearance and positive birefringence under compensated polarized light. They have been implicated as a cause of acute arthritis (McCarty, 1988).

Crystalline corticosteroids from intra-articular injection may have an appearance similar to MSU or CPPD crystals and persist up to a month

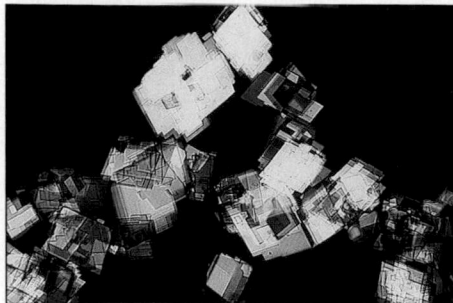

Figure 28–15 Cholesterol crystals in synovial fluid. Polarized light.

Table 28–16 Reference Intervals for Synovial Fluid Constituents		
Constituent	**Synovial fluid**	**Plasma**
Total protein	1–3 g/dL	6–8 g/dL
Albumin	55–70%	50–65%
Alpha-1-globulin	6–8%	3–5%
Alpha-2-globulin	5–7%	7–13%
Beta-globulin	8–10%	8–14%
Gamma-globulin	10–14%	12–22%
Hyaluronic acid	0.3–0.4 g/dL	
Glucose	70–110 mg/dL	70–110 mg/dL
Uric acid	2–8 mg/dL	2–8 mg/dL
Lactate	9–29 mg/dL	9–29 mg/dL

Modified from Kjeldsberg CR, Knight JA: Body Fluids: Laboratory Examination of Amniotic, Cerebrospinal, Seminal, Serous and Synovial Fluids, 3rd ed. Copyright © American Society for Clinical Pathology, Chicago, IL, 1993, with permission.

following injection. Most often they have blunt, jagged edges without clear crystal structure because they are prepared by grinding up larger crystalline forms. Triamcinolone hexacetonide is negatively birefringent but most others show positive birefringence.

Cholesterol crystals typically appear as irregular birefringent plates often with notched corners (Fig. 28–15). In chronic effusions (e.g., tuberculous arthritis, RA, SLE), needle- or rhomboid-shaped crystals similar to MSU or CPPD may be present (Ettlinger, 1979). Very small (1–5 microns) irregular, rod- and needle-shaped cholesterol crystals identified by X-ray diffraction analysis and by ultrastructural studies, have been identified in osteoarthritis effusions (Fam, 1981). Cholesterol crystals are ethanol and ether soluble and are not phagocytosed by leukocytes. Moreover, if the crystals are cholesterol, quantitative analysis should show that the SF level exceeds the plasma level.

Glove powder introduced during joint surgery appears as round, strongly birefringent particles 5–30 µm in diameter with a Maltese cross appearance when polarized.

A variety of other crystals or particulates may be present in synovial fluid. These include monoclonal immunoglobulin crystals or cryoglobulins, Charcot–Leyden crystals, amyloid fragments, cartilage fragments, collagen fibrils and fibrin strands, hematoidin crystals from prior hemorrhage, crystals from certain anticoagulants, nail polish, prosthetic fragments, and dust particles (Gatter, 1991).

Chemical Analysis

Chemical analyses of SF generally offer only supportive information to the routine tests. High viscosity may be remedied by dilution with normal saline, sonication, or hyaluronidase treatment. Reference intervals for the more important chemical analytes are shown in Table 28–16.

Mucin Clot Test. Addition of acetic acid to SF precipitates hyaluronate into a mucin clot, which may be graded as good, fair, or poor. A fair to poor mucin clot test reflects dilution and depolymerization of hyaluronic acid, a nonspecific finding of several inflammatory arthritides. Although of historic interest, the mucin clot test has minimal clinical utility (Baker, 1991).

Glucose. Proper interpretation of SF glucose values requires comparison with serum levels, ideally preceded by a fast of 8 hours to allow glucose to equilibrate across the synovial membrane. The serum–synovia differential is less than 10 mg/dL in normal and many noninflammatory conditions. In septic arthritis, this difference ranges from 20–60 mg/dL, but overlaps significantly with other inflammatory conditions, thereby limiting its clinical usefulness. Using a cutoff value of 75 mg/dL, the sensitivity of low glucose for detecting an inflammatory joint disease is only 20%; the specificity is 84% (Shmerling, 1990).

In vitro glycolysis by large numbers of leukocytes may falsely reduce SF glucose values unless testing is performed within 1 hour of collection. However, tubes containing sodium fluoride, an inhibitor of glycolysis, prevent the loss of glucose.

Protein. The mean normal protein concentration is 1.38 g/dL in living volunteers (Weinburger, 1989); it is 1.88 g/dL in cadavers. This difference most likely represents method variations. A reliable reference interval is 1.0–3.0 g/dL. With increasing inflammation, larger proteins (e.g., fibrinogen) enter the synovial space. Spontaneous clot formation may be detected in non-anticoagulated specimen tubes (fibrin clot test). Measurement of SF protein is very nonspecific; the sensitivity is about 52% and the specificity 56% for inflammatory disorders. The total protein level is not generally useful in patient diagnosis, treatment, or outcome (Shmerling, 1990).

Enzymes. Numerous enzymes have been studied in SF, including lactate dehydrogenase, aspartate aminotransferase, adenosine deaminase, acid and alkaline phosphatase, and lysozyme among others (Kjeldsberg, 1993). *Lactate dehydrogenase* is elevated in RA, gout, failed arthroplasties, and

infectious arthritis. This increase most likely reflects the neutrophil infiltrate. Elevated *acid phosphatase* may have negative prognostic value in RA, but is not specific (Luukkainen, 1989). Although enzyme analysis of SF is currently not clinically relevant, the measurement of various hydrolases may have significant predictive value in joint prognosis, especially RA.

Organic Acids. When compared with nonseptic monoarticular arthritis, SF *lactic acid* levels are usually increased in patients with septic arthritis (Kjeldsberg, 1993). Levels significantly greater than 30 mg/dL (3.7 mmol/L) are commonly associated with septic arthritis due to Gram-positive cocci and Gram-negative bacilli. Thus, the measurement of SF lactate may provide rapid provisional evidence for infection in specimens with negative Gram stains, a common occurrence especially with Gram-negative bacilli. However, normal or intermediate levels neither rule in nor rule out infection. Moreover, gonococcal arthritis is notorious for having normal SF lactate levels (Curtis, 1983).

Using gas–liquid chromatography, the presence of other organic acids not normally present in SF (e.g., *n-valeric, n-hexanoic*, and *succinic acids*) may be very helpful in differentiating septic from nonseptic arthritis (Brook, 1980; Borenstein, 1982).

Uric Acid. Synovial fluid uric acid levels generally, albeit not always, parallel serum levels in gout and noninflammatory arthropathies. An exception is inflammatory joint disorders other than gout, where SF urate levels may be significantly lower than in the paired serum (Beutler, 1996). It provides little clinical value in synovial fluid analysis except in some cases where gout is suspected but crystals are not identified (Reeves, 1965). Increased SF uric acid levels in these cases support a diagnosis of gout.

Lipids. In contrast to plasma, normal synovial fluid contains extremely low concentrations of lipids. Synovial fluid lipid abnormalities include (1) rare cholesterol-rich pseudochylous effusions typically associated with chronic RA; (2) lipid droplets, usually the result of trauma; and (3) extremely rare chylous effusions seen in association with RA, systemic lupus erythematosus (SLE), filariasis, pancreatitis, and trauma (Wise, 1987). These diseases can usually be differentiated clinically and by gross and microscopic examination; quantification of lipids currently has no clinical value in joint fluid analysis except in cases where cholesterol crystals may resemble MSU or CPPD. In these cases, a cholesterol level that exceeds the plasma level supports the presence of cholesterol crystals.

Immunologic Studies

Rheumatoid factor (RF) is found in synovia of about 60% of RA patients, usually at a titer equal to or slightly lower than the serum titer. *Antinuclear antibodies* (ANA) are found in the SF of about 70% of patients with SLE and 20% of patients with RA. Neither is specific enough for practical use. SF *complement* levels, normally about 10% of serum levels, increase to 40–70% of serum activity with inflammation, proportional to the increase of protein exudation. Complement consumption in SLE and RA in particular, results in levels less than 30% of serum complement. Complement is also decreased in some cases of bacterial and crystal-induced arthritis, so measurement is impractical for routine diagnosis.

Microbiological Examination

Immediate transportation of joint fluid and good communication of clinical suspicions to the laboratory are extremely important in the rapid identification of an infectious agent.

Septic arthritis may be acute or chronic, and Gram stain and culture should be performed as part of the routine synovial fluid evaluation. Gram stain sensitivity varies from about 75% for staphylococcal infections, 50% for most Gram-negative organisms, to less than 25% for gonococcal (GC) infections (Goldenberg, 1985).

Culture sensitivity ranges from 75–95% for nongonococcal joint infections in patients who have not received antibiotics. For patients with gonorrhea, the sensitivity is only 10–50% (Shmerling, 1994).

Although not in routine practice, the use of polymerase chain reaction with universal primers to detect bacterial DNA may prove useful particularly for the more fastidious, uncultivable pathogens (e.g., *Borrelia burgdorferi*, *Chlamydia* sp., *Mycoplasma* sp.) (Nocton, 1994; Li, 1996). Viruses are often associated with acute infectious arthritis and depending upon the putative virus, serology, viral culture and detection of viral DNA by nucleic acid amplification should be performed.

Depending upon the clinical history, infectious arthritis may be associated with particular exposures and their associated pathogens. Arthritis develops in approximately 60% of patients with Lyme disease resulting from exposure to ticks infected with *Borrelia burgdorferi* (Golightly, 1993). The PCR test for detecting *B. burgdorferi* DNA in synovial fluid is positive in 96% of untreated cases (Nocton, 1994; Exner, 2003).

In patients with a travel history or outdoor occupations, synovial fluid/tissue should be examined for fungal pathogens by KOH/calcofluor white stain and cultured on selective fungal media. For example, a patient with a recent travel history to Arizona may present with a monoarticular arthritis secondary to *Coccidioides immitis*. Patients with a chronic arthritis and risk factors for *Mycobacterium tuberculosis* or nontuberculous infections should undergo a synovial biopsy.

Ziehl–Neelsen or Kinyoun stains for acid-fast organisms have a sensitivity of about 20%. Cultures for *M. tuberculosis* are positive in about 80% of proven cases. Since conventional culture methods for *M. tuberculosis* are often very time-consuming, applying PCR for the detection of *M. tuberculosis* is a novel and promising technique for more rapid diagnosis. Synovial biopsy is recommended for suspected tuberculous arthritis to provide a more rapid diagnosis (Verettas, 2003; Titov, 2004).

Pleural Fluid

The pleural cavity is a potential space lined by mesothelium of the visceral and parietal pleura. The pleural cavity normally contains a small amount of fluid that facilitates movement of the two membranes against each other. This fluid is a plasma filtrate derived from capillaries of the parietal pleura. It is produced continuously at a rate dependent on capillary hydrostatic pressure, plasma oncotic pressure, and capillary permeability. Pleural fluid is reabsorbed through the lymphatics and venules of the visceral pleura.

An accumulation of fluid is called an effusion, which results from an imbalance of fluid production and reabsorption. This fluid accumulation in the pleural, pericardial, and peritoneal cavities is known as a *serous effusion*.

Specimen Collection

Thoracentesis is indicated for any undiagnosed pleural effusion or for therapeutic purposes in patients with massive symptomatic effusions. However, serous fluids are frequently neither collected, handled, or tested for in a completely satisfactory manner. Indeed, this improper collection/handling and often undertesting or inappropriate testing is more common than with other body fluids. The laboratory often receives a large syringe or vacuum bottle which must then be circulated through the various laboratory sections. Moreover, a large blood or fibrin clot may be present due to inadequate anticoagulation or mixing.

Except for an EDTA tube for total and differential cells counts, the specimen should be collected in heparinized tubes to avoid clotting. Aliquots for aerobic and anaerobic bacterial cultures are best inoculated into blood culture media at the bedside. If malignancy, fungal infection, or mycobacterial infection is suspected, all remaining fluid (100 mL or more) should be submitted to maximize yield of stains and culture. Since serous effusions are more forgiving than CSF in maintaining cellular integrity, fresh specimens for cytology may be stored up to 48 hours in the refrigerator with satisfactory results. For pH measurements, the fluid should be collected anaerobically in a heparinized syringe and submitted to the laboratory on ice. Grossly purulent specimens do not require pH measurement and may clog the analyzer.

Transudates and Exudates

It has long been recognized that the initial classification of a pleural fluid as a *transudate* or an *exudate* greatly simplifies the process of arriving at a correct final diagnosis. Moreover, it determines whether further testing is needed.

Transudates are usually bilateral owing to systemic conditions leading to increased capillary hydrostatic pressure or decreased plasma oncotic pressure (Table 28–17). Malignant effusions may infrequently be transudative due to a simultaneous confounding clinical condition such as congestive heart failure (Ashchi, 1998). Exudates are more often unilateral, associated with localized disorders that increase vascular permeability or interfere with lymphatic resorption (Table 28–17).

Recommended Tests

The evaluation of serous body fluids (pleural, pericardial, peritoneal) is directed first toward differentiating transudative from exudative effusions. Transudates generally require no further work-up. However, the fluid should be retained for 7–10 days in case further testing is needed. To separate the two, several chemical parameters have been proposed, although none are 100% accurate (Table 28–18).

Classical teaching stressed that exudates and transudates can be distinguished on the basis of total protein concentrations above (exudates) or below (transudates) 3.0 g/dL. However, using total protein alone misclassifies both exudates and transudates by about 30% (Melsom, 1979). It is now well accepted that test combinations increase sensitivity (any positive parameter indicates an exudate), improve accuracy, and are the basis for the well-established Light's criteria (Light, 1972). Accordingly, an exudate meets one or more of the following criteria: (1) pleural fluid/serum protein ratio greater than 0.5; (2) pleural fluid/serum lactate dehydrogenase (LD) ratio greater than 0.6; and (3) pleural fluid LD level

---

Table 28–17 Classification of Pleural Effusions

Transudates: increased hydrostatic pressure or decreased plasma oncotic pressure

Congestive heart failure

Hepatic cirrhosis

Hypoproteinemia (e.g., nephrotic syndrome)

Exudates: increased capillary permeability or decreased lymphatic resorption

Infections
  Bacterial pneumonia
  Tuberculosis, other granulomatous diseases (e.g., sarcoidosis, histoplasmosis, etc.)
  Viral or mycoplasma pneumonia
Neoplasms
  Bronchogenic carcinoma
  Metastatic carcinoma
  Lymphoma
  Mesothelioma (increased hyaluronate content of effusion fluid)
  Pulmonary infarct (may be associated with hemorrhagic effusion)
Noninfectious inflammatory disease involving pleura
  Rheumatoid disease (low pleural fluid glucose in most cases)
  Systemic lupus erythematosus (LE cells are occasionally present)

Fluid from extrapleural sources

Pancreatitis (elevated amylase activity in effusion fluid)

Ruptured esophagus (elevated amylase activity and low pH)

Urinothorax (elevated creatinine and low pH)

Table 28–18 Laboratory Criteria for Pleural Fluid Exudate

Pleural fluid/serum protein ratio	≥ 0.50
Pleural fluid/serum LD ratio	≥ 0.60
Pleural fluid LD	≥ 2/3 upper limit of normal serum LD
Pleural fluid cholesterol	> 45 mg/dL
Pleural fluid/serum cholesterol ratio	≥ 0.30
Serum–pleural fluid albumin gradient	≤ 1.2 g/dL
Pleural fluid/serum bilirubin ratio	≥ 0.60

LD = lactate dehydrogenase.

III

Table 28–19 Pleural Effusion: Recommended Tests

Routine tests
Gross examination
Pleural fluid/serum protein ratio
Pleural fluid/serum LD ratio
Examination of Romanowski-stained smear (malignant cells, LE cells)

Useful tests in most patients
Stains and cultures for microorganisms
Cytology

Useful tests in selected cases
Pleural fluid cholesterol
Pleural fluid/serum cholesterol ratio
Albumin gradient
pH
Lactate
Enzymes (ADA, amylase, LD)
Interferon-gamma
C-reactive protein
Lipid analysis
Tumor markers
Immunologic studies
Tuberculostearic acid
Pleural biopsy

ADA = adenosine deaminase; LD = lactate dehydrogenase.

Modified from Kjeldsberg CR, Knight JA: Body Fluids: Laboratory Examination of Amniotic, Cerebrospinal, Seminal, Serous and Synovial Fluids, 3rd ed. Copyright © American Society for Clinical Pathology, Chicago, 1993, with permission.

Table 28–20 Characteristic Features of Chylous and Pseudochylous Effusions

Feature	Chylous	Pseudochylous
Onset	Sudden	Gradual
Appearance	Milky-white, or yellow to bloody	Milky or greenish, metallic sheen
Microscopic examination	Lymphocytosis	Mixed cellular reaction, cholesterol crystals
Triglycerides*†	≥ 110 mg/dL (≥ 1.24 mmol/L)	< 50 mg/dL (< 0.56 mol/L)
Lipoprotein electrophoresis	Chylomicrons present	Chylomicrons absent

* Values in parentheses are SI units.

† Triglyceride levels between 50 mg/dL and 110 mg/dL are equivocal and require electrophoresis to confirm chylothorax.

Modified from Kjeldsberg CR, Knight JA. Body Fluids: Laboratory Examination of Amniotic, Cerebrospinal, Seminal, Serous and Synovial Fluids, 3rd ed. Copyright © American Society for Clinical Pathology, Chicago, IL, 1993, with permission.

greater than two-thirds of the serum upper limit of normal. The sensitivity and specificity are about 98% and 80%, respectively.

Several subsequent reports support Light's criteria as the most reliable method to differentiate transudates from exudates (Peterman, 1984; Burgess, 1995; Gazquez, 1998; Assi, 1998).

Several alternative measurements have been proposed to differentiate exudates from transudates. Testing for total cholesterol, the albumin gradient, or a combination of LD and total cholesterol may discriminate effusions with equivocal Light's criteria results. For example, the albumin gradient is recommended to confirm a clinical transudate misclassified as an exudate by Light's criteria (Light, 1997). That is, a serum albumin level greater than 1.2 g/dL higher than the pleural fluid level indicates the fluid is a transudate (Burgess, 1995). In many such cases the patient is being diuresed. Other test combinations have equaled but not surpassed the performance of Light's criteria.

Some tests, such as the combination of pleural fluid LD and cholesterol, may be more convenient and cost-effective by avoiding the need for simultaneous blood tests (Costa, 1995). Bilirubin measurement is not a strong discriminator of effusions (Heffner, 1997).

Further analysis of exudates is directed toward ruling out malignancy and infection. Cytology and appropriate bacterial stains and cultures are the most useful tests in this regard. Moreover, since pleural fluid DNA levels are significantly increased in exudates, quantitative analysis may be an effective new method to evaluate the etiologic causes of serous effusions (Chan, 2003). The recommended tests for the evaluation of pleural effusions are summarized in Table 28–19. The type of tests ordered and interpretation of test results should always be correlated with the clinical findings and differential diagnosis. Total leukocyte, differential, and red cell counts are of limited use in the evaluation of serous effusions.

Gross Examination

Transudates are typically clear, pale yellow to straw-colored, odorless, and do not clot. Approximately 15% of transudates are blood tinged. A bloody pleural effusion (hematocrit >1%) suggests trauma, malignancy, or pulmonary infarction (Jay, 1986). A traumatic tap is suggested by uneven blood distribution, fluid clearing with continued aspiration, or formation of small blood clots. A pleural fluid hematocrit greater than 50% of the blood hematocrit is good evidence for a hemothorax (Light, 1995).

Exudates may grossly resemble transudates, but most show variable degrees of cloudiness or turbidity, and often clot if not heparinized. A fecalent odor may be detected in anaerobic infections. Turbid, milky, and/or bloody specimens should be centrifuged and the supernatant examined. If the supernatant is clear, the turbidity is most likely due to cellular elements or debris. If the turbidity persists after centrifugation, a chylous or pseudochylous effusion is likely.

True chylous effusions are produced by leakage from the thoracic duct from obstruction by lymphoma, carcinoma, or traumatic disruption. A creamy top layer of chylomicrons may form in the specimen on standing. Idiopathic congenital chylothorax is the most common form of pleural effusion in the newborn.

Pseudochylous or chyliform effusions may have a milky, greenish, or 'gold paint' appearance. They accumulate gradually through the breakdown of cellular lipids in longstanding effusions such as rheumatoid pleuritis, tuberculosis, or myxedema. Features that distinguish true chylous from pseudochylous effusions are summarized in Table 28–20.

Microscopic Examination

Cell Counts. Leukocyte counts are unreliable in separating transudates (< 1000/μL) from exudates (> 1000/μL). Although red cell counts above 100 000/μL are highly suggestive of malignancy, trauma, or pulmonary infarction, they have little practical value.

Differential Leukocyte Count and Cytology. Examination should be performed on a stained smear, preferably prepared by cytocentrifugation and an air-dried Romanowski's stain. Indeed, examination by the hematology laboratory can be highly effective in the detection of malignant cells, especially hematologic malignancies (Kendall, 1997). Filtration or automated concentration methods with Papanicolaou stain may also be used, especially if there is concern for cell loss.

Cytologic analysis will establish the diagnosis for metastatic carcinoma in 70% or more cases when both smears and cell blocks are examined (Light, 2002). However, the sensitivity is significantly less efficient if the patient has a mesothelioma (10%), squamous cell carcinoma (20%), lymphoma (25–50%), or sarcoma (25%). Preparation of cell blocks is unnecessary except for effusions in which malignancy is an important consideration (Jonasson, 1990).

Mesothelial cells are common in pleural fluids from inflammatory processes (Fig. 28–16). They are, however, conspicuously scarce in patients with tuberculous pleurisy, empyema, and rheumatoid pleuritis, and in patients who have had pleurodesis. Fibrin deposition and fibrosis occurring in these conditions prevent mesothelial cell exfoliation. Well-differentiated carcinoma cells may be easily recognized (Fig. 28–17) or they may be highly undifferentiated (Fig. 28–18). A panel of immunocytochemical stains may be necessary for confirmation.

Neutrophils predominate in pleural fluid from patients with pleural inflammation (Table 28–21). Over 10% of transudates will also have a predominance of neutrophils, but this has no clinical significance.

Lymphocytes predominate in the disorders summarized in Table 28–21. Most are small, but medium, large, and reactive (transformed) variants may be seen. Nucleoli and nuclear cleaving are more prominent in effusions than in the peripheral blood. *Plasma cells* may also be observed. Lymphocytosis associated with transudates is of no clinical significance.

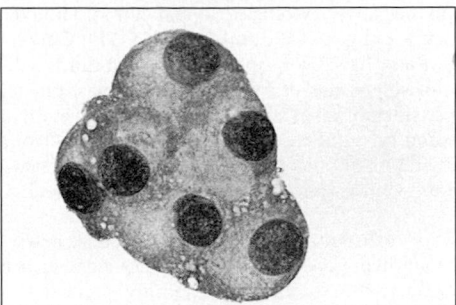

Figure 28–16 Mesothelial cells in pleural fluid.

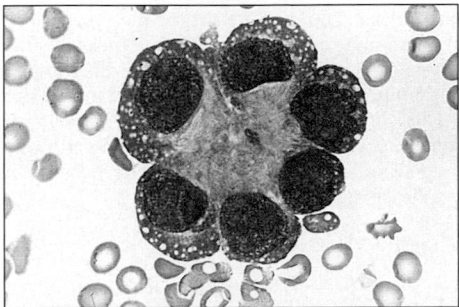

Figure 28–17 Well-differentiated breast carcinoma cells in pleural fluid.

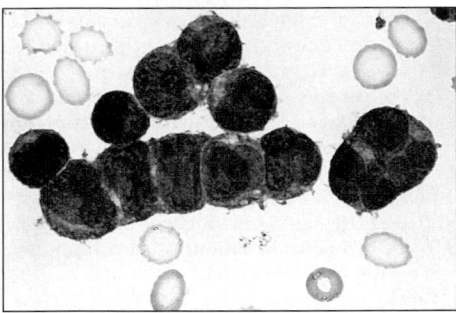

Figure 28–18 Undifferentiated oat cell carcinoma of lung showing typical molding of nuclei.

Table 28–21 Cellular Differential of Pleural Effusions
Neutrophilia (>50%)
Bacterial pneumonia (parapneumonic effusion)
Pulmonary infarction
Pancreatitis
Subphrenic abscess
Early tuberculosis
Transudates (over 10%)
Lymphocytosis (> 50%)
Tuberculosis (mesothelial cells are rare)
Viral infection
Malignancy
True chylothorax
Rheumatoid pleuritis
Systemic lupus erythematosus
Uremic effusions
Transudates (approximately 30%)
Eosinophilia (> 10%)
Pneumothorax (air in pleural space)
Trauma
Pulmonary infarction
Congestive heart failure
Infection (especially parasitic, fungal)
Hypersensitivity syndromes
Drug reaction
Rheumatologic diseases
Hodgkin's disease
Idiopathic

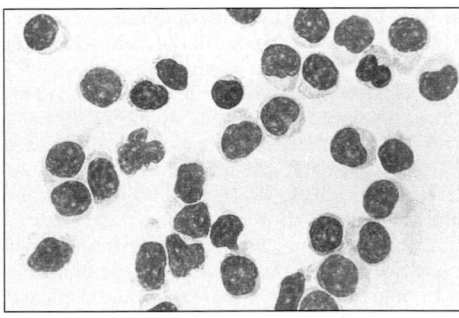

Figure 28–19 Pleural effusion in patient with non-Hodgkin's lymphoma, small lymphocytic type. (From Kjeldsberg CR, Knight JA: Body Fluids: Laboratory Examination of Amniotic, Cerebrospinal, Seminal, Serous and Synovial Fluids, 3rd ed. © American Society for Clinical Pathology, Chicago, 1993, with permission.)

Non-Hodgkin's lymphomas or chronic lymphocytic leukemia (CLL) may be difficult to distinguish from benign lymphocyte-rich serous effusions (Fig. 28–19).

Immunophenotyping by flow cytometry or immunocytochemistry, in conjunction with cellular morphology, is usually helpful for making a correct diagnosis. The relative proportions of T cells, B cells, and light chains are, by themselves, not definitive for separating benign from malignant exudates (Ibrahim, 1989).

An eosinophilic effusion is one having 10% or more *eosinophils*. The most common causes are related to the presence of air or blood in the pleural cavity (Table 28–21). Most of these are exudates; however, in about 35% of patients the etiology is unknown (Adelman, 1984). Though not of much assistance in diagnosing the cause of an effusion, eosinophilia appears to be independently associated with longer survival (Rubins, 1996). A small number of *mast cells* or *basophils* often accompany eosinophils. Eosinophil-derived *Charcot–Leyden crystals* may also be seen.

Chemical Analysis

Protein. The measurement of pleural fluid total protein or albumin has little clinical value except when combined with other parameters to differentiate exudates from transudates. Protein electrophoresis shows a pattern similar to serum except for a higher proportion of albumin; it has little value for differential diagnosis (Light, 1995).

Glucose. The glucose level of normal pleural fluid, transudates, and most exudates is similar to serum levels. Decreased pleural fluid glucose, accepted as a level below 60 mg/dL (3.33 mmol/L) or a pleural fluid/serum glucose ratio less than 0.5, is most consistent and dramatic in rheumatoid pleuritis and grossly purulent parapneumonic exudates (Sahn, 1982). Low pleural fluid glucose may also be present in malignancy, tuberculosis, nonpurulent bacterial infections, lupus pleuritis, and esophageal rupture.

Lactate. Pleural fluid lactate levels can be a useful adjunct in the rapid diagnosis of infectious pleuritis. Levels are significantly higher in bacterial and tuberculous pleural infections than in other pleural effusions. Moderate elevations are generally observed in malignant effusions (Brook, 1980). Values greater than 90 mg/dL (10 mmol/L) have a positive predictive value for infectious pleuritis of 94% and a negative predictive value of 100% (Gastrin, 1988).

Enzymes. *Amylase* elevations above the serum level (usually 1.5–2.0 or more times greater) indicate the presence of pancreatitis, esophageal rupture, or malignant effusion (Light, 1973). Elevated amylase derived from esophageal rupture or malignancy is the salivary isoform, which differentiates it from pancreatic amylase (Kramer, 1989).

Pleural fluid *lactate dehydrogenase* (LD) levels rise in proportion to the degree of inflammation. In addition to its use in separating exudates from transudates, declining LD levels during the course of an effusion indicate that the inflammatory process is resolving. Conversely, increasing levels indicate a worsening condition requiring aggressive work-up or treatment. LD isoenzyme analysis may be helpful in diagnosing problematic exudates, but is not routinely recommended (Lossos, 1997).

Adenosine deaminase (ADA), which is particularly rich in T lymphocytes, is significantly increased in tuberculous pleuritis. At a level of 50 U/L, the sensitivity, specificity, positive predictive value, negative predictive value, and efficiency for tuberculosis are 91%, 81%, 84%, 89%, and 86%, respectively (Burgess, 1996). When the lymphocyte/neutrophil ratio is 0.75 or greater, the percentages are 88%, 95%, 95%, 88%, and 92%, respectively. ADA levels of 40 U/L or greater are present in about 99.6% of patients with verified tuberculous pleuritis (Lee, 2001). However, in patients with lymphocyte-rich pleural fluids from nontuberculous causes, ADA levels less than 40 U/L are present in 97.1% of cases.

Interferon-gamma (INF-gamma). Pleural fluid INF-gamma levels are significantly increased in pleural fluid of patients with tuberculous pleuritis. The sensitivity of levels 3.7 IU/L or greater is 99% and the specificity is 98% (Villena, 1996a). The test sensitivity does not differ in HIV-positive and HIV-negative patients. Only about 20% of patients with effusions due to hematologic malignancies have INF-gamma levels slightly above 3.7 IU/L (Villena, 2003a).

pH. Pleural fluid pH measurement has the highest diagnostic accuracy in assessing the prognosis of parapneumonic (pneumonia-related) effusions (Heffner, 1995). A parapneumonic exudate with a pH greater than 7.30 generally resolves with medical therapy alone. A pH less than 7.20 indicates a complicated parapneumonic effusion (loculated or associated with empyema) requiring surgical drainage.

Patients with borderline complicated exudates (pH 7.20–7.30) may be closely watched with repeat measurements. A concomitant pleural glucose level below 60 mg/dL (3.33 mmol/L), however, strongly suggests impending empyema. Rheumatoid pleuritis and malignant effusions with a poor response to pleurodesis also have pH values below 7.20 and a low glucose level (Rodriquez-Panadero, 1989). A pH below 6.0 is characteristic of *esophageal rupture*, although the pH in severe empyema may also be 6.0 or less (Good, 1980).

Urinothorax, a collection of urine presumably produced by lymphatic drainage of perirenal accumulations into the pleural cavity, is also associated with a pleural fluid pH less than 7.30. These effusions are transudative because of their low protein content, smell of urine, and have a creatinine level greater than in simultaneously drawn serum (Miller, 1988).

Lipids. Some serous effusions appear to be chylous (i.e., a milky appearance) but are not (pseudochylous) whereas others may not look chylous but are. Although pseudochylous fluids may be partially due to increased leukocytes and necrotic debris, they are primarily due to the presence of increased lecithin–globulin complexes. A true chylous effusion has chylomicrons at the origin on lipoprotein electrophoresis. Lipid measurements are also helpful in identifying chylous effusions (Staats, 1980). Thus, pleural fluid triglyceride levels above 110 mg/dL indicate a chylous effusion; values between 60–110 mg/dL (0.68–1.24 mmol/L) are less certain and require lipoprotein electrophoresis to confirm a chylothorax. Nonchylous and pseudochylous effusions generally have triglyceride levels below 50 mg/dL (0.56 mmol/L) and no chylomicrons on electrophoresis (Table 28–20).

Cholesterol measurements may be useful in separating transudates from exudates, especially when there is a question regarding Light's criteria. A total cholesterol value of 54 mg/dL or more and a pleural fluid/serum cholesterol ratio of 0.32 or higher each have sensitivity and specificity values similar to Light's criteria (Suay, 1995). Elevated levels and the presence of cholesterol crystals may be seen with pleural effusions that have been present for several years.

C-Reactive Protein (CRP). Pleural fluid CRP is often a clinically useful screening test for organ disease, index of disease activity, and measure of response to therapy (Castano, 1992). Pleural fluid CRP levels > 30 mg/L reportedly have a sensitivity of 93.7%, specificity of 76.5%, and a positive predictive values of 98.4% in parapneumonic infections (Turay, 2000). The mean CRP values are about 90 mg/L in parapneumonic infections compared with 26 mg/L and 23 mg/L for tuberculous and malignant effusions, respectively.

Tuberculostearic Acid (TSA, 10-Methyloctadecanoic acid). TSA was first isolated from the bacillus *Mycobacterium tuberculosis*. This fatty acid is a structural component of mycobacteria and is not normally present in human tissue. Using gas chromatography/mass spectroscopy, TSA was measured in sputum, bronchial washings, and pleural fluid from patients with pulmonary tuberculosis (Muranishi, 1990). Here, pleural fluid TSA was identified in 24 of 32 (75%) patients with active tuberculosis; bronchial washings were positive for TSA in 15 of 22 cases. In patients with other pulmonary disorders, only 4 of 46 pleural fluids and 3 of 69 bronchial washings had detectable levels. A later smaller study reported the following for pleural fluid TSA: sensitivity, 54%, specificity, 80%, positive predictive value, 75%, negative predictive value, 61%, and efficacy, 66% (Yorgancioglu, 1996).

Tumor Markers. Although not recommended as a routine test, various tumor markers are often a useful adjunct in enigmatic noninflammatory exudates with negative cytology. Several tumor markers, especially carcinoembryonic antigen (CEA), CA 15-3, CA 549, CA 72-4 and CYFRA 21-1, among others, have been studied in pleural fluids. CEA is probably the most useful single marker for adenocarcinomas, but reported cutoff values vary considerably. The sensitivity of CEA for malignant effusions varies depending on tumor origin and is about 50% overall. Although complicated parapneumonic effusions may result in elevated CEA levels (Garcia-Pachon, 1997), they are usually not a problem to distinguish clinically.

A combination of tumor markers increases the accuracy of diagnosis. Thus, a combination of CEA, CA 15-3, and CA 72-4 had an accuracy of 90% with 78% sensitivity, 95% specificity, 88% positive predictive value, and 91% negative predictive value (Villena, 1996b). Similarly, CA 15-3 and CEA combined had an accuracy of 87% (Romero, 1996); a combination of CA 549, CEA, and CA 15-3 had a sensitivity of 65%, specificity 99%, and accuracy 85% (Villena, 2003b). The use of the cytokeratin 19 fragment (CYFRA 21-1) may also be useful in combination with other tumor markers.

Other tumor markers may also be useful in the diagnosis of unexplained effusions. For example, a marked increase in pleural fluid prostate-specific antigen (PSA) led to the correct diagnosis of a patient with metastatic prostate cancer who presented with severe anemia, peripheral edema, and pleural and pericardial effusions that were negative by cytologic examination (Chin, 1999).

Immunologic Studies

Approximately 5% of patients with rheumatoid arthritis (RA) and 50% with systemic lupus erythematosus (SLE) develop pleural effusions sometime during the course of their disease.

Rheumatoid factor (RF) is commonly present in pleural effusions associated with seropositive RA. Although a pleural fluid titer of 1 : 320 or greater in a patient with known RA is reasonable evidence of rheumatic pleuritis (Halla, 1980), elevated RF titers up to 1 : 1280 have been identified in 41% of patients with bacterial pneumonia, 20% of patients with malignant effusions, and 14% of patients with tuberculosis, making a routine test for RF of little value (Levine, 1968).

Antinuclear antibody (ANA) titers may be useful in the diagnosis of effusions due to lupus pleuritis; the sensitivity is about 85% using a cutoff titer of 1 : 160 (Good, 1983). The specificity is not high, however, because elevated ANA titers also occur in various other conditions. Thus, pleural fluid ANA titers are not clinically useful.

Decreased *complement* levels (CH50 < 10 U/mL or C4 level below 10×10^{-5} U/g protein) are present in most patients with rheumatoid or lupus pleuritis (Hunder, 1972; Halla, 1980). However, complement measurements are not highly specific and are of little value for routine diagnosis, although they may be helpful in the diagnosis of otherwise enigmatic effusions.

Microbiological Examination

Bacteria most commonly associated with parapneumonic effusions are *Staphylococcus aureus*, *Streptococcus pneumoniae*, beta-hemolytic group A streptococci, gamma-streptococci, and some Gram-negative bacilli. Anaerobic bacteria are isolated in a significant proportion of cases, so both anaerobic and aerobic cultures should be performed. The sensitivity of the Gram stain is approximately 50% (Ferrer, 1999).

For patients with suspected *M. tuberculosis*, direct staining of tuberculous effusions for acid-fast bacteria has a sensitivity of 20–30%; positive cultures are found in 50–70% of cases (Baer, 2001). Pleural biopsy yields the highest culture sensitivity (50–75%) and may provide a rapid presumptive diagnosis of tuberculosis by histopathologic demonstration of granulomas or acid-fast bacteria. Combining culture and acid-fast stains with pleural biopsy increases the sensitivity to about 95% (Jay, 1986).

Adenosine deaminase (ADA) can provide rapid chemical evidence for tuberculous effusions independent of HIV status (Burgess, 1996; Riantawan, 1999; Lee, 2001). Although the ADA-2 isoenzyme form is elaborated by activated lymphocytes in tuberculosis, only mild elevations occur in lymphocyte-rich pleural effusions from nontuberculous causes. However, the relatively low prevalence of tuberculous pleurisy in North America anticipates a lower positive predictive value rate compared to the excellent results reported in the Asian and European literature where tuberculosis is more common. Moreover, the colorimetric Giusti method by which most ADA data were derived is, unfortunately, not widely available in the United States (Roth, 1999).

Pleural fluid interferon-gamma is also significantly increased in tuberculous pleuritis and may be helpful in some cases since it is independent of HIV status and only modestly increased in about 20% of hematologic malignancies (Villena, 2003).

Table 28–22 Etiology of Pericardial Effusions	
Idiopathic (most often viral)	Renal failure
Infection	Hemorrhage
Bacteria	Trauma
Tuberculosis	Anticoagulant therapy
Fungi	Leakage of aortic aneurysm
Viruses	Autoimmune disorders
AIDS-related (usually viral)	Hypothyroidism
Neoplasm	Rheumatoid arthritis
Metastatic carcinoma	Systemic lupus erythematosus
Lymphoma	Inflammatory bowel disease
Drugs	Wegener's granulomatosis
Hydralazine	Acute myocardial infarction
Procainamide	Radiation therapy
Phenytoin	

AIDS = acquired immunodeficiency syndrome.

Pericardial Fluid

From 10–50 mL of fluid is normally present in the pericardial space, produced by a transudative process similar to pleural fluid. Pericardial effusions are most often caused by viral infection, enterovirus being the most common. They may also develop as a result of bacterial, tuberculous or fungal infections, autoimmune disorders, renal failure, myocardial infarction, mediastinal injury, the effects of various drugs, or may be idiopathic (Table 28–22). HIV-infected patients commonly have asymptomatic pericardial effusions, which may become large in more advanced disease (Silva-Cardosa, 1999). Many of the recommended laboratory tests described for pleural fluid also pertain to pericardial effusions (Table 28–19).

Specimen Collection

Pericardial effusions of unknown etiology or large effusions with signs of cardiac tamponade are generally submitted for laboratory examination. Fluid is obtained either by pericardiotomy following limited thoracotomy, or by pericardiocentesis (sterile needle aspiration).

Normal pericardial fluid is pale yellow and clear. Large effusions (> 350 mL) are most often caused by malignancy or uremia, or are idiopathic. In HIV-associated cardiac tamponade, 45% are idiopathic while tuberculous and bacterial effusions each account for about 20% of cases (Chen, 1999). Infection or malignancy typically produces turbid effusions, whereas effusions due to uremia are usually clear and straw-colored. These and several other disorders may produce hemorrhagic effusions.

Blood-like fluid obtained by pericardiocentesis might represent a hemorrhagic effusion or inadvertent aspiration of blood from the heart. Blood obtained from the heart chamber will have a hematocrit comparable to peripheral blood, and blood gas analysis yields results similar to venous or arterial blood. In contrast, the hematocrit of a hemorrhagic effusion is usually lower than that of the peripheral blood. The pH and P_{O_2} are lower and the P_{CO_2} is higher than in venous or arterial blood (Mann, 1978). Blood from a cardiac puncture clots but a hemorrhagic effusion usually does not.

A milky appearance suggests the presence of a chylous or pseudochylous effusion. Identification and differentiation of these effusions are discussed under Pleural Fluid.

Gross Examination

The *postpericardiotomy syndrome* is a fairly common but nonspecific complication of cardiac surgery (or other cardiac damage) that develops days to weeks following the initial injury. It is hallmarked by the development of fever, pleuritic chest pain, and other signs of pleural, pericardial and less often, lung inflammation. Exudative pleural effusions develop in over 80% of the cases. These are often serosanguinous to hemorrhagic and typically have a pH greater than 7.4 and a normal glucose level (Stelzner, 1983). There are no specific tests for diagnosing this syndrome. Diagnosis, therefore, remains one of clinical exclusion. Although the etiology is uncertain, the time course, presence of antimyocardial antibodies, and response to anti-inflammatory therapy suggests an immune-mediated process. Increased levels of antimyocardial antibodies relative to serum, decreased complement levels and immune complexes, have been documented in pleural fluid from a single patient with the syndrome (Kim, 1996).

Exudates and Transudates

Until recently, the criteria for differentiating exudates from transudates had not been carefully studied in pericardial effusions. According to Light's criteria, a pleural exudate has one or more of the following: pleural fluid/serum protein ratio > 0.5; pleural fluid/serum lactate dehydrogenase (LD) ratio > 0.6; and a pleural fluid LD level > 200 U/L. Using Light's criteria for pericardial fluid has now been shown to be the most reliable diagnostic tool for identifying pericardial exudates and transudates (Burgess, 2002a).

Routine testing of pericardial effusions should probably be limited to cell count, glucose, total protein, LD, bacterial culture, and cytology (Meyers, 1997). Other more specific tests are appropriate for diseases of high clinical suspicion.

Microscopic Examination

The hematocrit and red cell count document the presence of a hemorrhagic effusion, but are of limited value for differential diagnosis. Total leukocyte counts over 10 000/μL suggest bacterial, tuberculous, or malignant pericarditis. However, low counts may also be encountered in these conditions, limiting the value of this measurement (Agner, 1979). Although formal leukocyte differentials add little diagnostic information, a stained smear should always be examined.

Cytologic identification of malignant cells is usually not difficult. Metastatic carcinoma of the lung and breast are most frequently observed in malignant pericardial effusions. Cytology has a sensitivity of 95% and a specificity of 100% (Meyers, 1997).

Chemical Analysis

Chemical parameters for the diagnosis of pericardial effusions have not been studied to the same extent as in other body fluids. Although pericardial effusions are very similar to pleural fluids, routine application of these tests requires further studies to fully appreciate their diagnostic importance.

Protein. A value greater than 3.0 g/dL has a sensitivity of 97% for exudative effusions, but a specificity of only 22% which significantly limits its usefulness. Thus, total protein has no discriminating power in pericardial diagnosis (Meyers, 1997).

Glucose. Pericardial glucose levels less than 60 mg/dL have a diagnostic accuracy of only 36% in identifying pericardial exudates (Meyers, 1997). Values less than 40 mg/dL (< 2.22 mmol/L) are common in bacterial, tuberculous, rheumatic, or malignant effusions.

pH. Pericardial fluid pH may be markedly decreased (< 7.10) in rheumatic or purulent pericarditis. Malignancy, uremia, tuberculosis, and idiopathic disorders may have moderate decreases in the range of 7.20–7.30 (Kindig, 1983).

Lipids. Separation of true chylous from pseudochylous effusions may be facilitated by triglyceride and cholesterol measurements, as well as lipoprotein electrophoresis for chylomicrons (Table 28–20). See Lipids section in Pleural Fluids for further details in the diagnosis of chylous effusions.

Enzymes. A pericardial fluid *lactate dehydrogenase* (LD) level greater than 200 U/L has been suggested as a cutoff for pericardial exudates (Burgess, 2002a). Moreover, the measurement of LD and creatine kinase in postmortem pericardial fluid within 48 hours of death may be useful in establishing acute myocardial injury in cases where such injury is suspected but cannot be established by the usual histologic methods (Luna, 1982; Stewart, 1984). Pericardial fluid levels of CK-MB, myoglobin, and troponin I in postmortem pericardial fluid are also significantly increased in patients with myocardial injury (Perez-Carceles, 2004).

Adenosine deaminase (ADA) activity is a useful adjunctive test for tuberculous pericarditis in suspicious cases with negative acid-fast stains. The median ADA level in tuberculous pericarditis is significantly higher than in other pathologic effusions (Burgess, 2002b). Using a cutoff of 30 U/L, the sensitivity was 94%, specificity 68%, and positive predictive value 80%. Using a cutoff of 40 U/L, the sensitivity and specificity were 93% and 97%, respectively (Koh, 1994).

Interferon-gamma (INF-gamma). Increased INF-gamma levels have been reported in tuberculous serous effusions, including tuberculous pericarditis (Burgess, 2002b). Here, the INF-gamma level was greater than 1000 pg/L, which was significantly higher than in effusions from other pathologic conditions. A cutoff value of 200 pg/L resulted in a sensitivity and specificity of 100% for the diagnosis of tuberculous pericarditis.

Polymerase Chain Reaction (PCR). PCR is a sensitive technique and may be more specific than adenosine deaminase in the diagnosis of tuberculous pericarditis (Lee, 2002). However, a negative test does not rule

CHAPTER: 28 Cerebrospinal, Synovial, and Serous Body Fluids

Table 28–23 Etiology of Peritoneal Effusions

Transudates: increased hydrostatic pressure or decreased plasma oncotic pressure

Congestive heart failure

Hepatic cirrhosis

Hypoproteinemia (e.g., nephrotic syndrome)

Exudates: increased capillary permeability or decreased lymphatic resorption

Infections
   Primary bacterial peritonitis
   Secondary bacterial peritonitis (e.g., appendicitis, bowel rupture)
   Tuberculosis

Neoplasms
   Hepatoma
   Lymphoma
   Mesothelioma
   Metastatic carcinoma
   Ovarian carcinoma
   Prostate cancer

Trauma

Pancreatitis

Bile peritonitis (e.g., ruptured gallbladder)

Chylous effusion

Damage to or obstruction of thoracic duct (e.g., trauma, lymphoma, carcinoma, tuberculosis and other granulomas [e.g., sarcoidosis, histoplasmosis, etc.], parasitic infestation)

out tuberculous pericarditis since some pericardial fluids from patients with large tuberculous effusions may not contain *M. tuberculosis*.

Immunologic Studies

A negative antinuclear antibodies (ANA) test makes the diagnosis of lupus serositis highly unlikely. Conversely, high ANA titers in pericardial effusions lack specificity, even when they are as high as 1 : 5120 (Leventhal, 1990; Wang, 2000). If a high ANA titer is unexplained, malignancy should be considered.

Microbiological Examination

The sensitivity of the Gram stain and culture for bacterial pericarditis is similar to other serous body fluids (i.e., about 50% and 80%, respectively). Important aerobic bacteria include *S. aureus*, *S. pneumoniae*, *S. pyogenes*, beta-hemolytic group A streptococcus, and Gram-negative bacilli. Although infectious pericarditis due to anaerobic bacteria is not uncommon, the bacteria are often not recognized due to inconsistent methods used for their isolation and identification (Brook, 2002). The major anaerobic organisms are the *Bacteroides fragilis* group, anaerobic streptococci, *Clostridium* species, *Fusobacterium* species, and *Bifidobacterium* species.

Diagnosis of a specific etiologic agent in viral pericarditis is difficult because the viruses (e.g., Coxsackieviruses, influenza virus, mumps) are rarely isolated from pericardial fluid. Obtaining acute and convalescent sera for antibody response to suspected viral pathogens may help support the diagnosis (Bellinger, 1987). Viral infection probably accounts for most idiopathic HIV-associated pericardial effusions.

The sensitivity of acid-fast stains and culture for tuberculous pericarditis is about 50% (Agner, 1979). PCR is a sensitive technique and may be more specific than the use of adenosine deaminase in the diagnosis of tuberculous pericarditis (Lee, 2002). However, a negative test does not exclude the diagnosis of tuberculous pericarditis.

Peritoneal Fluid

Ascites is the pathologic accumulation of excess fluid in the peritoneal cavity. Up to 50 mL of fluid is normally present in this mesothelial-lined space. As with pleural and pericardial fluids, it is produced as an ultrafiltrate of plasma dependent on vascular permeability, and hydrostatic and oncotic Starling forces.

Transudates and Exudates

Common causes of peritoneal effusions are listed in Table 28–23. The laboratory criteria for classifying ascitic fluid as a transudate or exudate are not as well defined as they are for pleural and pericardial fluids. For example, infected or malignancy-related samples are not uncommonly reported with protein concentrations in the transudative range (i.e., < 3.0 g/dL), and many patients with cirrhotic or heart failure ascites have protein values in the exudative range (> 3.0 g/dL) (Runyon, 1992).

The *serum–ascites albumin gradient*, defined as the serum albumin concentration minus the ascitic fluid albumin concentration, is widely considered as the most reliable method to differentiate peritoneal transudates from exudates (Runyon, 1992). Ascites caused by portal hypertension has a gradient of at least 1.1 g/dL (> 11 g/L; transudate), whereas ascites produced by other causes has a gradient less than 1.1 g/dL (exudate) (Runyon, 1992). Indeed, the diagnostic accuracy was 98% for the serum–ascites albumin gradient compared with only 52–80% for four other markers: ascitic fluid total protein; ascites/serum total protein ratio; ascitic fluid LD concentration; and ascites/serum LD ratio (Akriviadis, 1996).

An ascitic fluid to serum bilirubin ratio of 0.6 or greater is also significantly associated with exudates (Elis, 1998). Indeed, the accuracies of the bilirubin ratio, the serum–ascites albumin gradient, and Light's criteria were 81.5%, 84%, and 80.2%, respectively. Others suggested that if both the ascitic fluid LDH is > 130 U/L and the ascitic fluid to serum total protein ratio is > 0.4, the fluid should be regarded as an exudate (Paramothayan, 2002).

Although the serum–ascites albumin gradient is probably the best single method to differentiate an ascitic exudate from a transudate, other methods compare favorably. Nevertheless, there are no ideal biochemical markers that allows complete discrimination between ascitic fluid exudates and transudates.

Specimen Collection

Paracentesis. Diagnostic paracentesis is performed in most patients with new ascites, or if there is a change in the clinical picture of a patient with ascites, such as rapid fluid accumulation or fever development. A minimum of 30 mL is needed for complete evaluation. If possible, at least 100 mL should be provided for cytologic examination. Samples for cell counts should be placed in an EDTA-anticoagulated venipuncture tube. Culture specimens should include blood culture bottles that have been inoculated at the bedside with ascitic fluid (10 mL per culture bottle).

Diagnostic Peritoneal Lavage (DPL). This procedure is no longer recommended as a routine technique for the evaluation of abdominal trauma. Concerns of oversensitivity and nonspecificity, and improvements in noninvasive diagnostic procedures such as computed tomography and ultrasound, have limited its common use to (1) rapid screening for significant abdominal hemorrhage and (2) evaluation of hollow viscus injuries.

A catheter is placed through a small incision into the abdominal cavity. If less than 15 mL of gross blood can be aspirated, DPL is performed by infusing 1.0 L of saline or Ringer's solution (20 mg/kg in children) and retrieving the fluid by gravity drainage. At least 600 mL should be recovered to avoid falsely low counts (Sullivan, 1997). The catheter is sometimes left in place so DPL may be repeated in 2–3 hours if initial results are negative or indeterminate.

Commonly accepted criteria for DPL interpretation after trauma are shown in Table 28–24. The positive predictive value is only 23% for an isolated (no other abnormal criteria) leukocyte count of 500/μL or greater (Soyka, 1990).

The conventional DPL criteria may be unreliable in detecting hollow viscus injury when blood is present from a simultaneous solid-organ injury not requiring surgical repair, resulting in unnecessary exploratory laparotomies. Suggested modifications of DPL criteria to adjust for this source of bleeding include either of the following: (a) a WBC count greater than or equal to the red blood cell (RBC) count divided by 150 where RBC is $10 \times 10^4/mm^3$ or greater (Otomo, 1998); or (b) a cell count ratio greater than 1.0 (Fang, 1998). The cell count ratio is defined as the ratio between WBC/RBC counts in the lavage fluid divided by the WBC/RBC ratio in the peripheral blood. These new criteria have a reported specificity of 97% for hollow organ injury, especially if DPL is performed at least 3 hours following injury.

Other applications of DPL include the evaluation of patients with suspected acute peritonitis or pancreatitis. For example, a WBC count in the lavage fluid of 200 cells/mm³ was associated with a 99% probability of acute peritonitis (Larson, 1992).

Peritoneal Dialysis. Dialysate fluid from renal patients undergoing chronic ambulatory peritoneal dialysis should be submitted to the laboratory to check for infection.

Table 28–24 Criteria for Evaluation of Peritoneal Lavage

Positive result

Aspiration of > 15 mL gross blood on catheter placement

Grossly bloody lavage fluid

RBC > 100 000/µL after blunt trauma

RBC > 50 000/µL after penetrating trauma

WBC > 500/µL

Amylase > 110 U/dL

Indeterminate result

Small amount of gross blood on catheter placement

RBC 50 000–100 000/µL after blunt trauma

RBC 1000–50 000/µL after penetrating trauma

WBC 100–500/µL

Negative result

RBC < 50 000/µL after blunt trauma

RBC < 1000/µL after penetrating trauma

WBC < 100/µL

RBC = red blood cell count: WBC = white blood cell count.

Modified from Feied CF: Diagnostic peritoneal lavage. Postgrad Med 1989; 85:40, with permission.

Table 28–25 Recommended Tests in Peritoneal Effusion

Useful in most patients

Gross examination

Cytology

Stains and culture for microorganisms

Serum–ascites albumin concentration gradient

Useful in selected disorders

Total leukocyte and differential cell counts

RBC count (lavage)

Bilirubin

Creatinine/urea nitrogen

Enzymes (ADA, ALP, amylase, LD, telomerase)

Lactate

Cholesterol (malignant ascites)

Fibronectin

Tumor markers (CEA, PSA, CA 19-9, CA 15-3, CA-125)

Immunocytology/flow cytometry

Tuberculostearic acid

RBC = red blood cell; CEA = carcinoembryonic antigen; PSA = prostate-specific antigen; ALP = alkaline phosphatase; ADA = adenosine deaminase; LD = lactate dehydrogenase.

Modified from Kjeldsberg CR, Knight, JA: Body Fluids: Laboratory Examination of Amniotic, Cerebrospinal, Seminal, Serous and Synovial Fluids. 3rd ed. Copyright © American Society for Clinical Pathology, Chicago, IL, 1993, with permission.

Peritoneal Washings. This procedure is performed intraoperatively to document early intra-abdominal spread of gynecologic and gastric carcinomas. Samples are generally sent for cytologic examination only.

Recommended Tests

The most important tests for the evaluation of ascitic fluid are listed in Table 28–25. Relative importance varies depending on the type of sample and clinical findings. For example, RBC and WBC counts are more important than cytology or the serum–ascites albumin gradient in the evaluation of the abdominal effects of trauma. Gross examination provides immediate information in the clinical and laboratory triage.

Gross Examination

Whereas transudates are generally pale yellow and clear, exudates are cloudy or turbid due to the presence of leukocytes, tumor cells, or increased protein

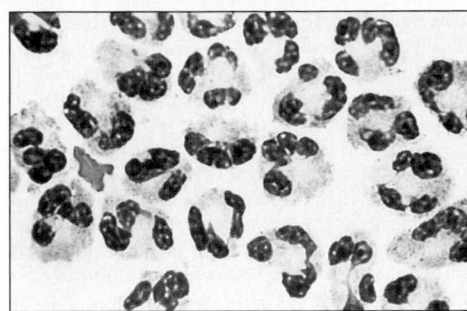

Figure 28–20 Neutrophils in a patient with bacterial peritonitis.

levels. The presence of food particles, foreign material, or green-yellow bile staining in a DPL specimen suggests perforation of the gastrointestinal or biliary tract. Acute pancreatitis and cholecystitis may also cause greenish discoloration.

Blood-tinged or grossly bloody fluid must be distinguished from a traumatic tap in which the blood usually clears with continued paracentesis. As little as 15 mL of blood per liter of fluid produces a bright red opaque color such that newsprint cannot be read through the lavage tubing. In most cases, the ability to read newsprint through the tubing results in a negative DPL. Opaque specimens require cell counts because newsprint readability is lost well below the 100 000 RBCs/µL criterion for a positive DPL (Bellows, 1998). Bloody ascites is also seen in malignancy and tuberculosis.

Milky fluid that does not clear with centrifugation suggests a chylous or pseudochylous effusion. True chylous peritoneal effusions are significantly less common than chylous pleural fluids. They are caused by disruption or blockage of lymphatic flow by trauma, lymphoma, carcinoma, tuberculosis or other granulomatous diseases (e.g., sarcoidosis), hepatic cirrhosis, adhesions, or parasitic infestation. Differentiation of true chylous and pseudochylous effusions is discussed under Pleural Fluid, Gross Examination.

Microscopic Examination

The total leukocyte count is useful in distinguishing ascites due to uncomplicated cirrhosis from spontaneous bacterial peritonitis (SBP), which is caused by migration of bacteria from the intestine into the ascitic fluid. Approximately 90% of patients with SBP will have leukocyte counts greater than 500/µL, over 50% of which are neutrophils (Fig. 28–20) (Runyon, 1984; Stewart, 1986).

The ascitic fluid total neutrophil count is the preferred method for the diagnosis of SBP. Cutoff values of 250 and 500 neutrophils/µL have been recommended, with a diagnostic accuracy of about 94% for 500 neutrophils/µL and about 90% for 250 neutrophils/µL (Stassen, 1986; Albillos, 1990).

Cell counts, total protein, and albumin gradient values vary with fluid shifts associated with ascites formation and resolution. For example, diuresis may cause the WBC count to increase from 300/µL to 1000/µL or more. When obtained by DPL, a leukocyte count of 200/µL or more is reported to be associated with a 99% probability for acute peritonitis (Alverdy, 1988; Larson, 1992).

Eosinophilia (> 10%) is most commonly associated with the chronic inflammatory process associated with chronic peritoneal dialysis. It has also been reported in congestive heart failure, vasculitis, lymphoma, and ruptured hydatid cyst.

Cytology has an overall sensitivity of 40–65% for malignant ascites. However, peritoneal carcinomatosis accounts for only about two-thirds of malignant effusions; cytology has a sensitivity of over 95% when confined to these cases (Runyon, 1988). Immunocytochemical stains are useful in characterizing atypical cells in equivocal cases.

Chemical Analysis

Protein.

The serum–ascites albumin gradient is superior to total protein content in differentiating cirrhosis from other causes of peritoneal effusion (Runyon, 1992). Spontaneous bacterial peritonitis is commonly associated with low total protein (< 3.0 g/dL) and a high serum–ascites albumin gradient (> 1.1 g/dL), making total protein measurements of little value in this disorder. Extracellular fluid shifts associated with ascites formation and resorption also cause variations in protein content.

Glucose. Early reports indicated that peritoneal fluid glucose levels of 50 mg/dL or less are present in 30–60% of cases of tuberculous peritonitis and about 50% of patients with abdominal carcinomatosis (Polak, 1973; Brown, 1976). However, a more recent study found decreased glucose levels in most cases of tuberculous ascites (Bansal, 1998). Nevertheless, glucose measurements are of little value since the sensitivity and specificity are generally too low to be of practical value.

Enzymes. *Amylase* activity in normal peritoneal fluid is similar to plasma levels. A level greater than three times the plasma value is good evidence of pancreas-related ascites, including acute pancreatitis and pancreatic pseudocyst (Runyon, 1987a). Amylase is not recommended in the routine evaluation of ascites, however, because the prevalence of pancreatic ascites is low. Retrospective amylase measurement on a stored specimen is indicated if initial studies are not diagnostic. However, amylase levels in peritoneal lavage fluid may be valuable in patients following blunt and penetrating abdominal trauma (McAnena, 1991). Here, amylase levels greater than or equal to 20 U/L had a sensitivity of 87%, a specificity of 75%, and a positive predictive value of 46% for significant intra-abdominal injury. In these cases, laparotomy should be considered. Gastroduodenal perforation, acute mesenteric vein thrombosis, intestinal strangulation, or necrosis may also produce elevated amylase levels. Although various nonpancreatic malignancies may rarely produce amylase elevations, isoenzyme evaluation usually identifies the salivary isoform in these latter cases (Kosches, 1989).

Elevated *alkaline phosphatase* (ALP) levels greater than 10 U/L in diagnostic peritoneal lavage fluid are very useful in predicting hollow visceral injury in patients who would otherwise not undergo laparotomy (specificity 99.8%, sensitivity 94.7%) (Jaffin, 1993). Ascitic fluid ALP measurements may also be helpful in the differentiation of primary bacterial peritonitis from secondary bacterial peritonitis due to bowel perforation. Secondary peritonitis has significantly higher mean ALP levels than spontaneous bacterial peritonitis (SBP). Thus, ALP levels > 240 U/L were present in 92% of patients with secondary peritonitis versus 12% for SBP (Wu, 2001). The sensitivity and specificity for differentiating secondary peritonitis from SBP were 92% and 88%, respectively.

Lactate dehydrogenase (LD) activity is often increased in malignant effusions (Gerbes, 1991). An ascitic fluid/serum LD ratio greater than 0.6 has a reported sensitivity of 80% (Boyer, 1978). Combined measurement of ascitic fluid LD and cholesterol totally discriminated peritoneal carcinomatosis from cirrhosis and hepatocarcinoma-related ascites (Castaldo, 1994; Halperin, 1999). Although both serum and peritoneal fluid LD levels are significantly higher in patients with ovarian cancer than with benign ovarian tumors or other gynecological malignancies, peritoneal fluid LD has higher diagnostic sensitivity (87%) and diagnostic accuracy (90%) than serum LD (60% and 77%, respectively) (Schneider, 1997). LD has also been used for the early diagnosis of spontaneous bacterial peritonitis in which it has a diagnostic accuracy of about 74% using an ascitic fluid/serum ratio cutoff of 0.4 (Lee, 1987).

The presence of *telomerase* is a specific discriminatory marker in malignant ascites (Tangkijvanich, 1999). Thus, telomerase activity was detected in 81% of malignant peritoneal effusions with a sensitivity of 76% and specificity of 95.7%.

Adenosine deaminase (ADA) is commonly used in endemic areas to identify patients with tuberculous peritonitis (Burgess, 2001). Using ROC curves and a cutoff value of 30 U/L, the sensitivity and specificity were 94% and 92%, respectively. Using a cutoff value of 33 U/L, the sensitivity, specificity, positive and negative predictive values, and overall diagnostic accuracy for diagnosing tuberculous peritonitis were 100%, 96.6%, 95%, 100%, and 98%, respectively (Dwivedi, 1990).

Fibronectin. Using a cutoff value of 85 µg/mL (85 mg/L), fibronectin was more reliable in differentiating malignant from sterile ascites (diagnostic accuracy, 79%) than were total protein, LD, gamma-glutamyltransferase, pH, amylase, triglycerides, leukocyte count, and cytologic examination (Colli, 1986). In a subsequent study using a cutoff of 94.6 µg/mL, the sensitivity, specificity, positive accuracy, negative accuracy, and overall diagnostic accuracy in the diagnosis of malignant ascites was 100%, 95%, 93.8%, 100%, and 97.1%, respectively (Sood, 1997).

Lactate. Ascitic fluid lactate has been used with pH measurements to differentiate SBP from uncomplicated ascites. Sensitivity and specificity are approximately 90% using a cutoff of 40 mg/dL (4.44 mmol/L), with a positive predictive value of 62% (Stassen, 1986). Although not as accurate as leukocyte counts, the high specificity of lactate in hepatic ascites suggests that it has some value in the diagnosis of SBP in otherwise equivocal cases. Malignant and tuberculous ascites are also associated with elevated lactate levels.

Patients with hollow viscous perforation, gangrenous intestine, peritonitis, or intra-abdominal abscess have a peritoneal fluid minus plasma lactate level of at least 13.5 mg/dL (1.5 mmol/L), which reportedly separates these patients completely from those with other conditions producing acute abdominal problems (DeLaurier, 1994). Additional studies are necessary to determine the utility of measuring ascitic fluid lactate in surgical decision making.

Creatinine and Urea. Measurement of creatinine and urea nitrogen is useful to differentiate between peritoneal fluid and urine. Elevated peritoneal fluid urea nitrogen and creatinine, in association with elevated serum urea but normal serum creatinine (due to back-diffusion of urea), suggest urinary bladder rupture.

Bilirubin. The mean (± SD) ascitic fluid bilirubin concentration in various types of ascites was reported as 0.7 ± 0.8 mg/dL and the mean ascitic fluid/serum bilirubin ratio was 0.38 ± 0.44 (Runyon, 1987b). An ascitic fluid bilirubin greater than 6.0 mg/dL and an ascitic fluid/serum bilirubin ratio over 1.0 suggests choleperitoneum from a ruptured gallbladder. A ratio of 0.6 or greater has been advocated as an additional marker for an exudative process, though its accuracy is not as high as the serum–ascites albumin gradient (Elis, 1998).

pH. Ascitic fluid pH may be helpful in the diagnosis of SBP in patients with cirrhotic ascites, especially if it is used in conjunction with the leukocyte count (Attali, 1986; Stassen, 1986). A pH less than 7.32 or a blood–ascitic fluid pH difference of more than 0.1 has a reported sensitivity and specificity of about 90% for SBP, the pH differential being slightly more accurate. Peritoneal fluid pH appears useless in detecting SBP, however, in the absence of neutrophils (Runyon, 1991). Patients with an ascitic fluid pH of less than 7.15 have a poor prognosis (Attali, 1986). Low pH is also found in patients with malignant and pancreatic ascites and tuberculous peritonitis.

Cholesterol. The ascitic fluid cholesterol level is a moderately useful index in separating malignant ascites (> 45–48 mg/dL) from cirrhotic ascites (Mortensen, 1988; Castaldo, 1994). The sensitivity and specificity average just over 90% using a cutoff value of 45–48 mg/dL (1.2 mmol/L). Thus, using a cutoff value of 48 mg/dL, the sensitivity, specificity, positive and negative predictive value, and overall diagnostic accuracy for differentiating malignant from nonmalignant ascites were reported as 96.5%, 96.6%, 93.3%, 98.3%, and 96.6%, respectively (Garg, 1993).

Interleukin-8 (IL-8). IL-8, a cytokine produced by a variety of cells in response to stimuli such as bacterial lipopolysaccharide, is significantly higher in spontaneous bacterial peritonitis compared with sterile ascites (Martinez-Bru, 1999). Using a cutoff value of 100 ng/L, the sensitivity and specificity were both 100% in cirrhotic patients.

Tuberculostearic Acid (TSA; 10-Methyloctadecanoic Acid). As noted in the Pleural Fluid section, TSA was detected in pleural fluid in 75% of patients with pulmonary tuberculosis using gas chromatography/mass spectroscopy (Muranishi, 1990). Using quantitative chemical ionization gas chromatography/mass spectrometry, the measurement of TSA is also a valuable technique to identify tuberculous peritonitis, as well as tuberculous meningitis (spinal fluid) and pneumonia (pleural fluid) (Brooks, 1998).

Tumor Markers. Because of their reportedly low sensitivity and specificity, the measurement of tumor markers is generally considered to be of little value. They are often useful, however, in selected cases such as in following a patient's response to therapy and in the early detection of tumor recurrence. They may also be very useful in cases where cytology is negative but suspicion of malignant ascites is high. Indeed, the poor sensitivity of cytological examinations is disappointing, being positive in only 40% (35 of 89 patients) of malignant cases while tumor markers were positive in 80% (Cascinu, 1997). Moreover, excluding small cell lung and renal cancers where specific tumor markers are lacking, tumor markers (i.e., CEA, CA 19-9, CA 15-3, PSA) in ascitic fluid for other carcinomas were positive in 97% of cases. These tumor markers, as well as alpha-fetoprotein, were also found to be very specific (over 90%) for serous fluid malignancies, although their sensitivities were low (19–38%) (Sari, 2001). The measurement of *prostate-specific antigen (PSA)* may also be a valuable marker for the diagnosis of malignant effusions due to prostate cancer (Appalaneni, 2004).

Carcinoembryonic antigen (CEA) has a sensitivity of only 40–50% and a specificity of about 90% using a cutoff value of 3.0 ng/mL (Mezger, 1988). Using a 5 mg/mL cutoff, the specificity is about 97% (Gulyas, 2001). Elevated CEA levels in peritoneal washings suggest a poor prognosis in gastric carcinoma (Irinoda, 1998).

Ascitic fluid *CA-125* is elevated to some degree in a variety of nonmalignant conditions. Indeed, cardiovascular and chronic liver disease may be the most frequent diagnoses in patients with increased CA-125 levels (Miralles, 2003), thereby supporting the general opinion that CA-125 lacks adequate specificity as a marker for malignancy. However, extremely high levels are more likely to be caused by epithelial carcinomas of the ovary, fallopian tubes, or endometrium.

The sensitivity for ovarian carcinoma depends on the tumor's stage (range 40–95%) and histologic subtype (mucinous adenocarcinomas have lower values) (Molina, 1998).

DNA ploidy analysis by flow cytometry or image analysis might provide useful complementary diagnostic information in cases with equivocal cytology results when the malignant cells carry an aneuploid karyotype. Image analysis appears to be more practical than flow cytometry when the tumor cells are scarce (Rijken, 1991).

Microbiological Examination

Primary peritonitis occurs at any age and is associated in children with nephrotic syndrome and in adults with cirrhotic liver disease. Spontaneous bacterial peritonitis (SBP) occurs in patients with ascites in the absence of recognized secondary causes such as bowel perforation or intra-abdominal abscess. The bacteria in SBP are most often normal intestinal flora and over 92% are monomicrobial. Aerobic Gram-negative bacilli (e.g., *E. coli* and *Klebsiella pneumoniae*) are responsible for two-thirds or more of all cases (Gilbert, 1995), followed by *S. pneumoniae, Enterococcus* sp., and rarely anaerobes. The Gram stain has a sensitivity of 25% in SBP (Lee, 1987) and routine cultures are positive in only about 50% of cases (Castellote, 1990). Inoculation of blood culture bottles at the bedside and concentration of large volumes of fluid can improve sensitivity, but up to 35% of infected patients may still have negative ascitic fluid cultures (Marshall, 1988).

Ascitic fluid total neutrophil count is the preferred method for the diagnosis of SBP (see under Microscopic Examination). However, as noted above, in difficult cases several analytes may be useful in differentiating SBP from secondary bacterial or tuberculous peritonitis. More recently, the polymerase chain reaction (PCR) has been successfully used in the detection of bacterial DNA in culture-negative ascitic fluid (Such, 2002).

The sensitivity of acid-fast stains for *M. tuberculosis* is no more than 20–30% and cultures have a sensitivity of only 50–70% (Reimer, 1985). Application of PCR to detect *M. tuberculosis* DNA has been studied, but a negative result does not exclude the diagnosis (Schwake, 2003). In a patient with a high clinical suspicion for tuberculous peritonitis, laparoscopic examination with biopsy may be indicated.

Selected References

Fishman RA: Cerebrospinal Fluid in Diseases of the Nervous System, 2nd ed. Philadelphia, WB Saunders, 1992.

Hasselbacher P: Variation in synovial fluid analysis by hospital laboratories. Arthritis Rheumatism 1987; 30:637.

Kjeldsberg CR, Knight JA: Body Fluids: Laboratory Examination of Amniotic, Cerebrospinal, Seminal, Serous, and Synovial Fluids, 3rd ed. American Society of Clinical Pathologists, Chicago, IL, 1993.

Light RW: Pleural effusions. N Engl J Med 2002; 346:1971.

Runyon BA, Montano AA, Evangelos A, et al: The serum–ascites albumin gradient is superior to the exudate–transudate concept in the differential diagnosis of ascites. Ann Intern Med 1992; 117:215.

References

Abramson JS, Hampton KD, Babu S, et al: The use of C-reactive protein from cerebrospinal fluid for differentiating meningitis from other central nervous system diseases. J Infect Dis 1985; 151:854.

Achar VS, Welch KM, Chabi, et al: Cerebrospinal fluid gamma-aminobutyric acid in neurologic disease. Neurology 1976; 26:777.

Adelman M, Albelda S, Gottlieb J, et al: Diagnostic utility of pleural fluid eosinophilia. Am J Med 1984; 77:915.

Agner RC, Gallis HA: Pericarditis. Differential diagnosis considerations. Arch Intern Med 1979; 139:407.

Ahonen A, Myllyla W, Hokkanen E: Measurement of reference values for certain proteins in cerebrospinal fluid. Acta Neurol Scand 1978; 57:358.

Akriviadis EA, Kapnias D, Hadjigavriel M, et al: Serum/ascites albumin gradient: its value as a rational approach to the differential diagnosis of ascites. Scand J Gastroenterol 1996; 31:814.

Albillos A, Cuervas-Mons V, Millan L, et al: Ascitic fluid polymorphonuclear cell count and serum to ascites albumin gradient in the diagnosis of bacterial peritonitis. Gastroenterology 1990; 98:134.

Albright RE, Christenson RH, Habig RL, et al: Cerebrospinal fluid (CSF) TRAP: A method to improve CSF laboratory efficiency. Am J Clin Pathol 1988; 90:707.

Alverdy JC, Saunders J, Chamberlin WH, et al: Diagnostic peritoneal lavage in intra-abdominal sepsis. Am Surg 1988; 54:456.

American College of Physicians: The diagnostic spinal tap. Ann Intern Med 1986; 104:880.

Andersson M, Alvarez-Cermeno J, Bernardi G, et al: Cerebrospinal fluid in the diagnosis of multiple sclerosis: A consensus report. J Neurol Neurosurg Psychiatry 1994; 57:897.

Andreasen N, Minthon L, Davidsson P, et al: Evaluation of CSF-tau and CSF-Abeta42 as diagnostic markers for Alzheimer disease in clinical practice. Arch Neurol 2001; 58:373.

Appalaneni V, Yellinedi S, Baumann MA: Diagnosis of malignant ascites in prostate cancer by measurement of prostate specific antigen. Am J Med Sci 2004; 327:262.

Arevalo CE, Barnes PF, Duda M, Leedom JM: Cerebrospinal fluid cell counts and chemistries in bacterial meningitis. South Med J 1989; 82:1122.

Ashchi M, Golish J, Eng P, et al: Transudative malignant pleural effusions: Prevalence and mechanisms. South Med J 1998; 91:23.

Assi Z, Caruso JL, Herndon J, Patz EF Jr: Cytologically proved malignant pleural effusions: Distribution of transudates and exudates. Chest 1998; 113:1302.

Attali P, Turner K, Pelleteir G, et al: pH of ascitic fluid: Diagnostic and prognostic value in cirrhotic and noncirrhotic patients. Gastroenterology 1986; 90:1255.

Baer KE, Smith GP: Serous body cavity fluid examination. Lab Med 2001; 32:85.

Baethgen LF, Moraes C, Weidlich L, et al: Direct-test PCR for detection of meningococcal DNA and its serogroup characterization: Standardization and adaptation for use in a public health laboratory. J Med Microbiol 2003; 52:793.

Bailey EM, Domenico P, Cunha BA: Bacterial or viral meningitis? Measuring lactate in CSF can help you know quickly. Postgrad Med 1990; 88:217.

Baker DG: Chemistry, serology and immunology. *In* Gatter RA, Schumacher HR (eds): A Practical Handbook of Joint Fluid Analysis, 2nd ed. Philadelphia, Lea & Febiger 1991, p 70.

Bansal S, Kaur K, Bansal AK: Diagnosing ascitic etiology on a biochemical basis. Hepatogastroenterology 1998; 45:1673.

Batabyal SK, Ghosh B, Sengupta S, et al: Cerebrospinal fluid and serum carcinoembryonic antigen in brain tumors. Neoplasma 2003; 50:377.

Bellinger RL, Vacek JL: A review of pericarditis. 2. Specific pericardial disorders. Postgrad Med 1987; 82:105.

Bellows CF, Salomone JP, Nakamura SK, et al: What's black and white and red (read) all over? The bedside interpretation of diagnostic peritoneal lavage fluid. Am Surg 1998; 64:112.

Benson RL, Ansbacher L, Hutchison RE, et al: Cerebrospinal fluid centrifuge analysis in primary amebic meningoencephalitis due to *Naegleria fowleri*. Arch Pathol Lab Med 1985; 109:668.

Berger T, Rubner P, Schautzer F, et al: Antimyelin antibodies as a predictor of clinically definite multiple sclerosis after a first demyelinating event. N Engl J Med 2003; 349:139.

Berthier M, Bonneau D, Desbordes JM, et al: Possible involvement of a gamma-hydroxybutyric acid receptor in startle disease. Acta Paediatr 1994; 83:678.

Beutler AM, Keenan GE, Soloway S, et al: Soluble urate in sera and synovial fluids from patients with different joint disorders. Clin Exp Rheumatol 1996; 14:249.

Bigner SH: Cerebrospinal fluid (CSF) cytology: Current status and diagnostic applications. J Neuropathol Exp Neurol 1992; 51:235.

Biou D, Benoist J-F, Huong CN-TX, et al: Cerebrospinal fluid protein concentrations in children: Age-related values in patients without disorders of the central nervous system. Clin Chem 2000; 46:399.

Blake J, Berman P: The use of adenosine deaminase in the diagnosis of tuberculosis. S Afr Med J 1982; 62:19.

Body BA, Oneson RH, Herold DA: Use of cerebrospinal fluid lactic acid concentration in the diagnosis of fungal meningitis. Ann Clin Lab Sci 1987; 17:429.

Bonadio WA, Smith DS, Goddard S, et al: Distinguishing cerebrospinal fluid abnormalities in children with bacterial meningitis and traumatic lumbar puncture. J Infect Dis 1990; 162:251.

Borenstein DG, Gibbs CA, Jacobs RP: Gas-liquid chromatographic analysis of synovial fluid. Arthritis Rheum 1982; 25:947.

Boyer TD, Kahn AM, Telfer BR: Diagnostic value of ascitic fluid lactic dehydrogenase, protein, and WBC levels. Arch Intern Med 1978; 138:1103.

Breebaart K, Becker H, Jongebloed FA: Investigation of reference values of components of cerebrospinal fluid. J Clin Chem Clin Biochem 1978; 16:561.

Britton C, Hultman E, Murray V, et al: The diagnostic accuracy of CSF analyses in stroke. Acta Med Scand 1983; 214:3.

Brook I: Pericarditis due to anaerobic bacteria. Cardiology 2002; 97:55.

Brook I, Reza MJ, Bricknell SK, et al: Abnormalities in synovial fluid of patients with septic arthritis detected by gas-liquid chromatography. Ann Rheum Dis 1980; 39:168.

Brooks BR: Nonimmunoglobulin proteins in human cerebrospinal fluid. *In* Herndon RM, Brumback RA (eds): Cerebrospinal Fluid. Boston, Kluwer Academic Publishers, 1989, p 167.

Brooks JB, Syriopoulou V, Butler WR, et al: Development of a quantitative chemical ionization gas chromatography–mass spectrometry method to detect tuberculostearic acid in body fluids. J Chromatogr B Biomed Sci Appl 1998; 712:1.

Brown KD, An ND: Tuberculous peritonitis. Am J Gastroenterol 1976; 66:277.

Burgess LJ, Maritz FJ, Taljaard JJ: Comparative analysis of the biochemical parameters used to distinguish between pleural transudates and exudates. Chest 1995; 107:1604.

Burgess LJ, Maritz FJ, LeRoux I, Taljaard JJ. Combined use of pleural adenosine deaminase with lymphocyte/neutrophil ratio. Increased specificity for the diagnosis of tuberculous pleurisy. Chest 1996; 109:414.

III

CHAPTER: **28** Cerebrospinal, Synovial, and Serous Body Fluids

Burgess LJ, Swanepoel CG, Taljaard JJ: The use of adenosine deaminase as a diagnostic tool for peritoneal tuberculosis. Tuberculosis 2001; 8:243.

Burgess LJ, Reuter H, Taljaard JJ, Doubell AF: Role of biochemical tests in the diagnosis of large pericardial effusions. Chest 2002a; 121,495.

Burgess LJ, Reuter H, Carstens ME, et al: The use of adenosine deaminase and interferon-gamma as diagnostic tools for tuberculous pericarditis. Chest 2002b; 122:900.

Cameron PD, Boyce JM, Ansari BM: Cerebrospinal fluid lactate in meningitis and meningococcaemia. J Infect 1993; 26:245.

Cascinu S, Del Ferro E, Barbanti I, et al: Tumor markers in the diagnosis of malignant serous effusions. Am J Clin Oncol 1997; 20:247.

Castaldo G, Oriani G, Cimino L, et al: Total discrimination of peritoneal malignant ascites from cirrhosis and heptocarcinoma-associated ascites by assays of ascitic cholesterol and lactate dehydrogenase. Clin Chem 1994; 40:478.

Castano VJL, Amores AC: Use of pleural fluid C-reactive protein in laboratory diagnosis of pleural effusions. Eur J Med 1992; 1:201.

Castellote J, Xiol X, Verdaguer R, et al: Comparison of two ascitic fluid culture methods in cirrhotic patients with spontaneous bacterial peritonitis. Am J Gastroenterol 1990; 85:1605.

Cavuoti D, Baskin L, Jialal I: Detection of oligoclonal bands in cerebrospinal fluid by immunofixation electrophoresis. Am J Clin Pathol 1998; 109:585.

Cawley LP, Minard BJ, Tourtellotte WW, et al: Immunofixation electrophoresis techniques applied to identification of proteins in serum and cerebrospinal fluid. Clin Chem 1976; 22:1262.

Chalmers AC, Aprill BS, Shephard H: Cerebrospinal fluid and human immuno-deficiency virus: Findings in healthy, asymptomatic, seropositive men. Arch Intern Med 1990; 150:1538.

Chan MHM, Chow KM, Chan ATC, et al. Quantitative analysis of pleural fluid cell-free DNA as a tool for the classification of pleural effusions. Clin Chem 2003; 49:740.

Chandler WL, Clayson KJ, Longstreth WT Jr, et al: Creatine kinase isoenzymes in human cerebrospinal fluid and brain. Clin Chem 1984; 30:1801.

Chandler WL, Clayson KJ, Longstreth WT Jr, et al: Mitochondrial and BB isoenzymes of creatine kinase in cerebrospinal fluid from patients with hypoxic-ischemic brain damage. Am J Clin Pathol 1986; 86:533.

Chen Y, Brennessel D, Walters J, et al: Human immunodeficiency virus-associated pericardial effusions: Report of 40 cases and review of the literature. Am Heart J 1999; 137:516.

Chin NW, Sinay LJ, Taylor J, et al: Metastatic prostate cancer presenting as pleural and pericardial effusions. Fed Pract 1999; 16:19.

Choi SH, Kim YS, Bae IG, et al. The possible role of cerebrospinal fluid adenosine deaminase activity in the diagnosis of tuberculous meningitis in adults. Clin Neurol Neurosurg 2002; 104:10.

Clayburne G, Baker DG, Schumacher HR: Estimated synovial fluid leukocyte numbers on wet drop preparations as a potential substitute for actual leukocyte counts. J Rheumatol 1992; 19:60.

College of American Pathologists: Cerebrospinal Fluid Survey M-B: Participant Summary Report. Northfield, IL: College of American Pathologists, 2002.

Colli A, Buccino G, Cocciolo M, et al: Diagnostic accuracy of fibronectin in the differential diagnosis of ascites. Cancer 1986; 58:2489.

Conly JM, Ronald AR: Cerebrospinal fluid as a diagnostic body fluid. Am J Med 1983; 75:102.

Cooper SJ, Kelly CB, King DJ: 5-Hydroxyindoleacetic acid in cerebrospinal fluid and prediction of suicidal behaviour in schizophrenia. Lancet 1992; 340:940.

Coplin WM, Longstreth WT Jr, Lam AM, et al: Cerebrospinal fluid creatine kinase-BB isoenzyme activity and outcome after subarachnoid hemorrhage. Arch Neurol 1999; 56:1348.

Corral CJ, Pepple JM, Moxon ER, Hughes WT: C-reactive protein in spinal fluid of children with meningitis. J Pediatr 1981; 99:365.

Corral I, Quereda C, Navas E, et al: Adenosine deaminase activity in cerebrospinal fluid of HIV-infected patients: Limited value for diagnosis of tuberculous meningitis. Eur J Clin Microbiol Infect Dis 2004; 23:471.

Costa M, Quiroga T, Cruz E. Measurement of pleural fluid cholesterol and lactate dehydrogenase. A simple and accurate set of indicators for separating exudates from transudates. Chest 1995; 108:1260.

Curtis GDW, Newman RJ, Slack MPE: Synovial fluid lactate and the diagnosis of septic arthritis. J Infect 1983; 6:239.

Davis LE, Schmitt JW: Clinical significance of cerebrospinal fluid tests for neurosyphilis. Ann Neurol 1989; 25:50.

Davis MJ, Denton J, Freemont AJ, Holt PJ: Comparison of serial synovial fluid cytology in rheumatoid arthritis: Delineation of subgroups with prognostic implications. Ann Rheum Dis 1988; 47:559.

DeLaurier GA, Ivey RK, Johnson RH: Peritoneal fluid lactate and diagnostic dilemmas in acute abdominal disease. Am J Surg 1994; 167:302.

Desai MM, Pal RB: Polymerase chain reaction for the rapid diagnosis of tuberculous meningitis. Indian J Med Sci 2002; 56:546.

DeSalles AAF, Kontos HA, Becker DP, et al: Prognostic significance of ventricular CSF lactic acidosis in severe head injury. J Neurosurg 1986; 65:615.

Donald PR, Malan C: Cerebrospinal fluid lactate and lactate dehydrogenase activity in the rapid diagnosis of bacterial meningitis. S Afr Med J 1986; 69:39.

dos Santos JGN: Fetal primary amebic meningoencephalitis: A retrospective study in Richmond, Virginia. Am J Clin Pathol 1970; 54:737.

Dubowitz LM, Bouza H, Hird MF, Jaeken J: Low cerebrospinal fluid concentration of free gamma-aminobutyric acid in startle disease. Lancet 1992; 340:80.

Dumler JS, Valsamakis A: Molecular diagnosis for existing and emerging infections. Complementary tools for a new era of clinical microbiology. Am J Clin Pathol 1999; 112:533.

Dwivedi M, Misra SP, Misra V, Kamar R: Value of adenosine deaminase estimation in the diagnosis of tuberculous ascites. Am J Gastroenterol 1990; 85:1123.

Elis A, Meisel S, Tishler T, et al: Ascitic fluid serum bilirubin concentration ratio for the classification of transudates or exudates. Am J Gastroenterol 1998; 93:401.

Engelke S, Bridgers S, Saldanha RL, et al: Cerebrospinal fluid lactate dehydrogenase in neonatal intracranial hemorrhage. Am J Med Sci 1986; 291:391.

Ettlinger RE, Hunder GC: Synovial effusions containing cholesterol crystals. Mayo Clin Proc 1979; 54:366.

Exner MM, Lewinski MA: Isolation and detection of Borrelia burgdorferi DNA from cerebral spinal fluid, synovial fluid, blood, urine, and ticks using the Roche MagNA Pure system and real-time PCR. Diagn Microbiol Infect Dis 2003; 2003;46:235.

Fam AG, Pritzker KP, Cheng PT, Little AH: Cholesterol crystals in osteoarthritic joint effusions. J Rheumatol 1981; 8:273.

Fang J-F, Chen R-J, Lin B-C: Cell count ratio: New criterion of diagnostic peritoneal lavage for detection of hollow organ perforation. J Trauma 1998; 45:540.

Ferrer A, Osset J, Alegre J, et al: Prospective clinical and microbiological study of pleural effusions. Eur J Clin Microbiol Infect Dis 1999; 18:237.

Finn WG, Peterson LC, James C, et al: Enhanced detection of malignant lymphoma in cerebrospinal fluid by multiparameter flow cytometry. Am J Clin Pathol 1998; 110:341.

Fishman RA: Cerebrospinal Fluid in Diseases of the Nervous System, 2nd ed. Philadelphia, WB Saunders, 1992.

Fleisher M, Wasserstrom WRT, Schold SC, et al: Lactic dehydrogenase isoenzymes in the cerebrospinal fluid of patients with systemic cancer. Cancer 1981; 47:2654.

Flood J, Weinstock HS, Guroy M, et al: Neurosyphilis during the AIDS epidemic, San Francisco, 1985–1992. J Infect Dis 1998; 177:931.

Florez G, Cabeza A, Gonzalez JM, et al: Changes in serum and cerebrospinal fluid enzyme activity after head injury. Acta Neurochir 1976; 35:3.

Fortini AS, Sanders EL, Weinshenker BG, Katzmann JA: Cerebrospinal fluid oligoclonal bands in the diagnosis of multiple sclerosis. Am J Clin Pathol 2003; 120:672.

Gallo P, Tavolato B, Bergenbrant S, Siden A: Immunoglobulin light chain patterns in the cerebrospinal fluid: A study with special reference to the occurrence of free light chains in cerebrospinal fluid with and without oligoclonal immunoglobulin G. J Neurol Sci 1989; 94:241.

Garcia-Pachon E, Padilla-Navas I, Dosda ME, et al: Elevated level of carcinoembryonic antigen in nonmalignant pleural effusions. Chest 1997; 111:643.

Garg R, Sood A, Arora S, et al: Ascitic fluid cholesterol in differential diagnosis of ascites. J Assoc Physicians India 1993; 41:644.

Gastrin B, Lovestad A: Diagnostic significance of pleural fluid lactate concentration in pleural and pulmonary disease. Scand J Infect Dis 1988; 20:85:.

Gatter RA, Schumacher HR: A Practical Handbook of Joint Fluid Analysis, 2nd ed. Philadelphia, Lee & Febiger, 1991.

Gazquez I, Porcel JM, Vives M, et al. Comparative analysis of Light's criteria and other biochemical parameters for distinguishing transudates from exudates. Resp Med 1998; 92:762.

Gerbaut L, Macart M: Is standardization more important than methodology for assay of total protein in cerebrospinal fluid? Clin Chem 1986; 32:353.

Gerbes AL, Jungst D, Xie Y, et al: Ascitic fluid analysis for the differentiation of malignancy-related and nonmalignant ascites. Cancer 1991; 68:1808.

Gerdes LU, Jorgensen PE, Nexo E, Wang P: C-reactive protein and bacterial meningitis: a meta-analysis. Scand J Clin Lab Invest 1998; 58:383.

Gilbert JA, Kamath PS: Spontaneous bacterial peritonitis: An update. Mayo Clin Proc 1995; 70:365.

Gilchrist GS, Tubergen DG, Sather HN, et al: Low numbers of CSF blasts at diagnosis do not predict for the development of CNS leukemia in children with intermediate-risk acute lymphoblastic leukemia. A Childrens Cancer Group report. J Clin Oncol 1994; 12:2594.

Goldenberg DL, Reed JL: Bacterial arthritis. N Engl J Med 764; 1985; 312:.

Golightly MG: Laboratory considerations in the diagnosis and management of lyme borreliosis. Am J Clin Pathol 1993; 99:168.

Good JT, Taryle DA, Maulitz RM, et al: The diagnostic value of pleural fluid pH. Chest 1980; 78:55.

Good JT, King TE, Antony VB, et al: Lupus pleuritis. Chest 1983; 84:714.

Graves M: Cerebrospinal fluid infections. In Herndon RM, Brumback RA (eds): The Cerebrospinal Fluid. Boston, Kluwer Academic Publishers, 1989, p 143.

Greenlee JE: Approach to diagnosis of meningitis. Cerebrospinal fluid examination. Infect Dis Clin North Am 1990; 4:583.

Gulyas M, Kaposi AD, Elek G, et al: Value of carcinoembryonic antigen (CEA) and cholesterol assays of ascitic fluid in cases of inconclusive cytology. J Clin Pathol 2001; 54:831.

Hall CD, Snyder CR, Robertson KR, et al: Cerebrospinal fluid analysis in human immunodeficiency virus infection. Ann Clin Lab Sci 1992; 22:139.

Halla JT, Schrohenloher RE, Volankis JE: Immune complexes and other laboratory features of pleural effusions. Ann Intern Med 1980; 92:748.

Halperin R, Hadas E, Bukovsky I, Schneider D: Peritoneal fluid analysis in the differentiation of ovarian cancer and benign ovarian tumor. Eur J Gynecol Oncol 1999; 20:40.

Harrington MG, Merrill CR, Asher DM, et al: Abnormal proteins in the cerebrospinal fluid of patients with Creutzfeldt–Jacob disease. N Engl J Med 1986; 315:279.

Hasselbacher P: Variation in synovial fluid analysis by hospital laboratories. Arthritis Rheum 1987; 30:637.

Hausfater P, Fillet AM, Rozenberg F, et al: Prevalence of viral infection markers by polymerase chain reaction amplification and interferon-alpha measurements among patients undergoing lumbar puncture in an emergency department. J Med Virol 2004; 73:137.

Hayward RA, Oye RK: Are polymorphonuclear leukocytes an abnormal finding in cerebrospinal fluid? Results from 225 normal cerebrospinal fluid specimens. Arch Intern Med 1988; 148:1623.

Hayward RA, Shapiro MF, Oye RK: Laboratory testing on cerebrospinal fluid: A reappraisal. Lancet 1987; 1:8523.

Heffner JE, Brown LK, Barbieri C, DeLeo JM.: Pleural fluid chemical analysis in parapneumonic effusions. A meta-analysis. Am J Respir Crit Care Med 1995; 151:1700.

Heffner JE, Brown LK, Barbieri CA: Diagnostic value of tests that discriminate between exudative and transudative pleural effusions. Primary Study Investigators. Chest 1997; 111:970.

Herndon RM, Brumback RA (eds): The Cerebrospinal Fluid. Boston, Kluwer Academic Publishers, 1989.

Hersey LA, Trotter JL: The use and abuse of the cerebrospinal fluid IgG profile in the adult: A practical evaluation. Ann Neurol 1980; 8:126.

Hsich G, Kenney K, Gibbs CJ, et al: The 14-3-3 protein in cerebrospinal fluid as a marker for transmissible spongiform encephalopathies. N Engl J Med 1996; 335:924.

Hunder GG, Pierre RV: In vivo LE cell formation in synovial fluid. Arthritis Rheum 1970; 13:448.

Hunder GG, McDuffie FC, Hepper NGG: Pleural fluid complement activity in systemic lupus erythematosus and rheumatoid arthritis. Ann Intern Med 1972; 76:357.

Ibrahim RE, Teich D, Smith ER, et al: Flow cytometric surface light chain analysis of lymphocyte-rich effusions. Cancer 1989; 63:2024.

Irinoda T, Terashima M, Takagane A, et al: Carcinoembryonic antigen level in peritoneal washing is prognostic factor in patients with gastric cancer. Oncol Rep 1998; 5:661.

Irjala K, Suorpaa J, Laurent B: Identification of CSF leakage by immunofixation. Arch Otolaryngol 1979; 105:447.

Jacques J, Carquin J, Brodard V, et al: New reverse transcription-PCR assay for rapid and sensitive detection of enterovirus genomes in cerebrospinal fluid specimens of patients with aseptic meningitis. J Clin Microbiol 2003; 41:5726.

Jaffin JH, Ochsner MG, Cole FJ, et al: Alkaline phosphatase levels in diagnostic peritoneal lavage as a predictor of hollow visceral injury. J Trauma 1993; 34:829.

Jay SJ: Pleural effusions. II: Definitive evaluation of the exudate. Postgrad Med 1986; 80:181.

Jeffrey GM, Frampton CM, Legge HM, et al: Cerebrospinal fluid β₂-microglobulin levels in meningeal involvement by malignancy. Pathology 1990; 22:20.

Johnson KP, Nelson BJ: Multiple sclerosis: diagnostic usefulness of cerebrospinal fluid. Ann Neurol 1977; 2:425.

Jonasson JG, Ducatman BS, Wang HH: The cell block for body cavity fluids: Do the results justify the cost? Mod Pathol 1990; 3:667.

Jones AC, Chuck AJ, Arie EA, et al: Diseases associated with calcium pyrophosphate deposition disease. Semin Arthritis Rheum 1992; 22:188.

Judkins SW, Cornbleet PJ: Synovial fluid crystal analysis. Lab Med 1997; 28:774.

Kanoh Y, Ohtani H: Levels of interleukin-6, CRP and alpha 2 macroglobulin in cerebrospinal fluid (CSF) and serum as indicators of blood–CSF barrier damage. Biochem Mol Biol Int 1997; 43:269.

Kares S, Lonnrot M, Vuorinen P, et al: Real-time PCR for rapid diagnosis of entero- and rhinovirus infections using LightCycler. J Clin Virol 2004; 29:99.

Karkela J, Pasanen M, Kaukinen S, et al: Evaluation of hypoxic brain injury with spinal fluid enzymes, lactate, and pyruvate. Crit Care Med 1992; 20:378.

Kashyap RS, Kainthla RP, Biswas SK, et al: Rapid diagnosis of tuberculous meningitis using simple DOT ELISA method. Med Sci Monit 2003; 9:123.

Kasper LM, Moorehead WR, Oel TO, et al: An alternative method assaying cerebrospinal fluid protein in the presence of methotrexate. Clin Chem 1988; 34:2091.

Kawai M, Hirohata S: Cerebrospinal fluid beta(2)-microglobulin in neuro-Behçet's syndrome. J Neurol Sci 2000; 179:132.

Kay J, Eichenfield AH, Athreya BH, et al: Synovial fluid eosinophilia in Lyme disease. Arthritis Rheum 1988; 31:1384.

Kendall B, Dunn C, Solanki P. A comparison of the effectiveness of malignancy detection in body fluid examination by the cytopathology and hematology laboratories. Clin Pathol Lab Med 1997; 121:976.

Kim S, Sahn SA: Postcardiac injury syndrome. An immunologic pleural fluid analysis. Chest 1996; 109:570.

Kindig JR, Goodman MR: Clinical utility of pericardial fluid pH determination. Am J Med 1983; 75:1077.

Kjeldsberg CR, Knight JA: Body Fluids: Laboratory Examination of Amniotic, Cerebrospinal, Seminal, Serous and Synovial Fluids. 3rd ed. Chicago, American Society of Clinical Pathologists Press, 1993.

Klee GG, Tallman RD, Goellner JR, et al: Elevation of carcinoembryonic antigen in cerebrospinal fluid among patients with meningeal carcinomatosis. Mayo Clin Proc 1986; 61:9.

Knight JA, Dudek SM, Haymond RE: Early (chemical) diagnosis of bacterial meningitis – cerebrospinal fluid glucose, lactate, and lactate dehydrogenase compared. Clin Chem 1981; 27:1431.

Koh KK, Kim EJ, Cho CH, et al: Adenosine deaminase and carcinoembryonic antigen in pericardial effusion diagnosis, especially in suspected tuberculous pericarditis. Circulation 1994; 89:2728.

Kosches DS, Sosnowik D, Lendvai S, et al: Unusual anodic migrating isoamylase differentiates selected malignant from nonmalignant ascites. J Clin Gastroenterol 1989; 11:43.

Kramer MR, Saldana MJ, Cepero RJ, et al: High amylase levels in neoplasm-related pleural effusion. Ann Intern Med 1989; 110:567.

Kuberski T: Eosinophils in cerebrospinal fluid: Criteria for eosinophilic meningitis. Hawaii Med J 1981; 40:97.

Lakeman FD, Whitley RJ: Diagnosis of herpes simplex encephalitis: Application of polymerase chain reaction to cerebrospinal fluid from brain-biopsied patients and correlation with disease. National Institute of Allergy and Infectious Diseases Collaborative Antiviral Study Group. J Infect Dis 1995; 171:857.

Lampl Y, Paniri Y, Eshel Y, et al: Cerebrospinal fluid lactate dehydrogenase levels in early stroke and transient ischemic attacks. Stroke 1990; 21:854.

Lang DT, Berberian LB, Lee S, et al: Rapid differentiation of subarachnoid hemorrhage from traumatic lumbar puncture using the D-dimer assay. Am J Clin Pathol 1990; 91:403.

Larson FA, Haller CC, Delcore R, Thomas JH. Diagnostic peritoneal lavage in acute peritonitis. Am J Surgery 1992; 164:449..

Lazcano O, Li CY, Pierre RV, et al: Clinical utility of the Alizarin Red S stain on permanent preparations to detect calcium-containing compounds in synovial fluid. Am J Clin Pathol 1993; 99:90.

Lee HH, Carlson RW, Bull DM: Early diagnosis of spontaneous bacterial peritonitis. Values of ascitic fluid variables. Infection 1987; 15:232.

Lee J-H, Lee CW, Lee S-G, et al: Comparison of polymerase chain reaction with adenosine deaminase activity in pericardial fluid for the diagnosis of tuberculous pericarditis. Am J Med 2002; 113:519.

Lee YCG, Rogers JT, Rodriguez RM, et al: Adenosine deaminase levels in nontuberculous lymphocytic pleural effusions. Chest 2001; 120:356.

Lefvert AK, Link H: IgG production within the central nervous system: A critical review of proposed formulae. Ann Neurol 1985; 17:13.

Lemstra AW, van Meegen MT, Vreyling JP, et al: 14-3-3 testing in diagnosing Creutzfeldt–Jakob disease: A prospective study in 112 patients. Neurol 2000; 55:514.

Leventhal LJ, DeMarco DM, Zurier RB: Antinuclear antibody in pericardial fluid from a patient with primary cardiac lymphoma. Arch Intern Med 1990; 150:1113.

Levine H, Szanto M, Grieble HG, et al: Rheumatoid factor in nonrheumatoid pleural effusions. Ann Intern Med 1968; 69:487.

Li F, Bulbul R, Schumacher HRJ, et al: Molecular detection of bacterial DNA in venereal-associated arthritis. Arthritis Rheum 1996; 39:950.

Light RW: Pleural Diseases, 3rd ed. Baltimore, Williams & Wilkins, 1995.

Light RW: Diagnostic principles in pleural disease. Eur Respir J 1997; 10:476.

Light RW: Pleural effusion. N Engl J Med 2002; 346:1971.

Light RW, Ball WC Jr: Glucose and amylase in pleural effusions. JAMA 1973; 225:257.

Light RW, MacGregor MI, Luchsinger PC, et al: Pleural effusions: The diagnostic separation of transudates and exudates. Ann Intern Med 1972; 77:507.

Lin JJ, Harn HJ, Hsu YD, et al: Rapid diagnosis of tuberculous meningitis by polymerase chain reaction assay of cerebrospinal fluid. J Neurol 1995; 242:147.

Lolli F, Siracusa G, Amato MP, et al: Intrathecal synthesis of free immunoglobulin light chains and IgM in initial multiple sclerosis. Acta Neurol Scand 1991; 83:239.

Lossos IS, Breuer R, Intrator O, et al: Differential diagnosis of pleural effusion by lactate dehydrogenase isoenzyme analysis. Chest 1997; 111:648.

Lott JA, Warren P: Estimation of reference intervals for total protein in cerebrospinal fluid. Clin Chem 1989; 35:1766.

Luna A, Villanueva E, Castellano M, Jimenez G: The determination of CK, LDH and its isoenzymes in pericardial fluid and its application to the post-mortem diagnosis of myocardial infarction. Forensic Sci Int 1982; 19:85.

Lunding J, Midgard R, Vedeler CA: Oligoclonal bands in cerebrospinal fluid: A comparative study of isoelectric focusing, agarose gel electrophoresis and IgG index. Acta Neurol Scand 2000; 102:322.

Luukkainen R, Kaarela K, Huhtala H, et al: Prognostic significance of synovial fluid analysis in rheumatoid arthritis. Ann Med 1989; 21:269.

Luxton RW, Patel P, Keir G, et al: A micro-method for measuring total protein in cerebrospinal fluid by using benzethonium chloride in microliter plate wells. Clin Chem 1989; 35:1731.

Maas JW, Bowden CL, Miller AL, et al: Schizophrenia, pyschosis, and cerebrospinal fluid homovanillic acid concentrations. Schizophr Bull 1997; 23:147.

McAnena OJ, Marx JA, Moore EE: Peritoneal lavage enzyme determinations following blunt and penetrating abdominal trauma. J Trauma 1991; 31:1161.

McCarty DJ: Crystal identification in human synovial fluids. Rheum Disease Clin North Am 1988; 14:253.

McGill NW, York H. Reproducibility of synovial fluid examination for crystals. Aust NZ J Med 1991; 34:710.

III

McGuinness GA, Weisz SC, Bell WE: CSF lactate levels in neonates. Am J Dis Child 1983; 137:48.

Maddalena A, Papassotiropoulos A, Muller-Tillmanns B, et al: Biochemical diagnosis of Alzheimer disease by measuring the cerebrospinal fluid ratio of phosphorylated tau protein to β-amyloid peptide42. Arch Neurol 2003; 60:1202.

Mahoney DH Jr., Fernbach DJ, Glaze DG, et al: Elevated myelin basic protein levels in cerebrospinal fluid of children with acute lymphoblastic leukemia. J Clin Oncol 1984; 2:58.

Mann AD, Millen JE, Glauser FL: Bloody pericardial fluid. The value of blood gas measurements. JAMA 1978; 239:2151.

Mann AD, Macfarlane CM, Verburg CJ, et al: The bromide partition test and CSF adenosine deaminase activity in the diagnosis of tuberculous meningitis in children. S Afr Med J 1982; 62:432.

Markowitz H, Kokmen E: Neurologic diseases and the cerebrospinal fluid immunoglobulin profile. Mayo Clin Proc 1983; 58:273.

Marshall JB: Finding the cause of ascites. The importance of accurate fluid analysis. Postgrad Med 1988; 83:189.

Martinez-Bru C, Gomez C, Cortes M, et al: Ascitic fluid interleukin-8 to distinguish spontaneous bacterial peritonitis and sterile ascites in cirrhotic patients. Clin Chem 1999; 45:2027.

Marton KI, Gean AD: The spinal tap: A new look at an old test. Ann Intern Med 1986; 104:840.

Mayefsky JH, Roughmann KJ: Determination of leukocytosis in traumatic spinal tap specimens. Am J Med 1987; 82:1175.

Melsom RD: Diagnostic reliability of pleural fluid protein estimation. J Royal Soc Med 1979; 72:823.

Mezger J, Permanetter W, Georges AL, et al: Tumour associated antigens in diagnosis of serous effusions. J Clin Pathol 1988; 41:633.

Meucci G, Rossi G, Bertini R, et al: Laser nephelometric evaluation of albumin, IgG and alpha2-macroglobulin: Applications to the study of alterations of the blood–brain barrier. J Neurol Sci 1993; 118:73.

Meyers DG, Meyers RE, Prendergast TW: The usefulness of diagnostic tests on pericardial fluid. Chest 1997; 111:1213.

Miller KS, Wooten S, Sahn SA: Urinothorax: A cause of low pH transudative pleural effusions. Am J Med 1988; 85:448.

Miralles C, Orea M, Espana P, et al: Cancer antigen 125 associated with multiple benign and malignant pathologies. Ann Surg Oncol 2003; 10:150.

Mishra OP, Batra P, Ali Z, et al: Cerebrospinal fluid lysozyme level for the diagnosis of tuberculous meningitis in children. J Trop Pediatr 2003; 49:13.

Mizock BA, Rackow EC, Burke GS: Elevated cerebrospinal fluid glutamine in septic encephalopathy. J Clin Gastroenterol 1989; 11:362.

Molina R, Filella X, Jo J, et al: CA 125 in biological fluids. Int J Biol Markers 1998; 13:224.

Morbidity and Mortality Weekly Report: Outbreaks of aseptic meningitis associated with echoviruses 9 and 30 and preliminary surveillance reports on enterovirus activity – United States, 2003. JAMA 2003; 290:1444.

Mortensen PB, Kristensen SD, Bloch A, et al: Diagnostic value of ascitic fluid cholesterol levels in the prediction of malignancy. Scand J Gastroenterol 1988; 23:1085.

Montine TJ, Beal MF, Cudkowicz ME, et al: Increased cerebrospinal fluid F2-isoprostane concentration in probable Alzheimer's disease. Neurology 1999; 52:562.

Montine TJ, Kaye JA, Montine KS, et al: Cerebrospinal fluid Abeta42, tau, and F2-isoprostane concentrations in patients with Alzheimer disease, other dementias, and in age-matched controls. Arch Pathol Lab Med 2001; 125:510.

Moosa AA, Quortum HA, Ibrahim MD: Rapid diagnosis of bacterial meningitis with reagent strips. Lancet 1995; 345:1290.

Muranishi H, Nakashima M, Isobe R, et al: Measurement of tuberculostearic acid in sputa, pleural effusions, and bronchial washings. A clinical evaluation for diagnosis of pulmonary tuberculosis. Diagn Microbiol Infect Dis 1990; 13:235.

Nocton JJ, Dressler F, Rutledge RJ, et al: Detection of Borrelia burgdorferi DNA by polymerase chain reaction in synovial fluid from patients with lyme arthritis. N Engl J Med 1994; 330:229.

Normansell DE, Stacy EK, Booker CF, et al: Detection of beta-2-transferrin in otorrhea and rhinorrhea in a routine clinical laboratory setting. Clin Diagn Lab Immunol 1994; 1:68.

Noseworthy TW, Anderson BJ, Noseworthy AF, et al: Cerebrospinal fluid myelin basic protein as a prognostic marker in patients with head injury. Crit Care Med 1985; 13:743.

Nussinovitch M, Harel D, Eidlitz-Markus T, et al: Lactic dehydrogenase isoenzyme in cerebrospinal fluid of children with infantile spasms. Eur Neurol 2003a; 49:231.

Nussinovitch M, Avitzur Y, Finkelstein Y, et al: Lactic dehydrogenase isoenzyme in cerebrospinal fluid of children with febrile convulsions. Acta Paediatr 2003b; 92:186.

Oda K, Egawa H, Okuhara T, et al: Meningeal involvement in Bence Jones multiple myeloma. Cancer 1991; 67:1900.

Odom LF, Wilson H, Cullen J, et al: Significance of blasts in low-cell count cerebrospinal fluid specimens from children with acute lymphoblastic leukemia. Cancer 1990; 66:1748.

Olsson JE, Pettersson BL: A comparison between agar gel electrophoresis and CSF serum quotients of IgG and albumin in neurological disease. Acta Neurol Scand 1976; 53:308.

Otomo Y, Henmi H, Mashiko K, et al: New diagnostic peritoneal lavage criteria for diagnosis of intestinal injury. J Trauma 1998; 44:991.

Pal B, Nash J, Oppenheim B, et al: Is routine synovial fluid analysis necessary? Lessons and recommendations from an audit. Rheumatol Int 1999; 18:181.

Pappu ID, Purolit DM, Levkoff AH: CSF cytology in the neonate. Am J Dis Child 1982; 136:297.

Paramothayan NS, Barron J: New criteria for the differentiation between transudates and exudates. J Clin Pathol 2002; 55:69.

Peacock JEJ, McGinnis MR, Cohen MS: Persistent neutrophilic meningitis: Report of four cases and review of the literature. Medicine 1984; 63:379.

Perez-Carceles MD, Noguera J, Jimenez JL, et al: Diagnostic efficacy of biochemical markers in diagnosis postmortem of ischaemic heart disease. Forensic Sci Int 2004; 142:1.

Perkins MD, Mirrett S, Reller LB: Rapid bacterial antigen detection is not clinically useful. J Clin Microbiol 1995; 33:1486.

Peterman TA, Speicher CE: Evaluating pleural effusions: A two-stage laboratory approach. JAMA 1984; 252:1051.

Pettersson T, Klockars M, Weber TH, et al: Diagnostic value of cerebrospinal fluid adenosine deaminase determination. Scand J Infect Dis 1991; 23:97.

Podell TE, Ault M, Sullam P, et al: Synovial fluid eosinophilia. Arthritis Rheum 1980; 23:1060.

Polak M, Torres Da Costa AC: Diagnostic value of the estimation of glucose in ascitic fluid. Digestion 1973; 8:347.

Porritt RJ, Mercer JL, Munro R: Detection and serogroup determination of Neisseria meningitidis in CSF by polymerase chain reaction (PCR). Pathology 2000; 32:42.

Powers W: Cerebrospinal fluid lymphocytosis in acute bacterial meningitis. Am J Med 1985; 79:216.

Pratico D, Lee VM, Trojanowski JQ, et al: Increased F2-isoprostanes in Alzheimer's disease: Evidence for enhanced lipid peroxidation in vivo. FASEB J 1998; 12:1777.

Rabinovitch A, Cornbleet PJ: Body fluid microscopy in US laboratories. Data from two College of American Pathologists surveys, with practice recommendations. Arch Pathol Lab Med 1994; 118:13.

Ragland SA, Arsura E, Ismail Y, et al: Eosinophilic pleocytosis in coccidioidal meningitis: Frequency and significance. Am J Med 1993; 95:254.

Rajantie J, Koskiniemi M, Siimes MA, et al: CSF fibronectin concentration in Burkitt's lymphoma: An early marker for CNS involvement. Eur J Haematol 1989; 42:313.

Rajo MC, Perez Del Molina ML, Lado Lado FL, et al: Rapid diagnosis of tuberculous meningitis by ligase chain reaction amplification. Scand J Infect Dis 2002; 34:14.

Rajs G, Finzi-Yeheskel Z, Rajs A, Mayer M: C-reactive protein concentrations in cerebral spinal fluid in gram-positive and gram-negative bacterial meningitis. Clin Chem 2002; 48:591.

Ramers C, Billman G, Hartin M, et al: Impact of a diagnostic cerebrospinal fluid enterovirus polymerase chain reaction test on patient management. JAMA 2000; 283:2680.

Rautonen J, Koskiniemi M, Siimes MA, et al: Elevated cerebrospinal fluid fibronectin concentration indicates poor prognosis in children with acute lymphoblastic leukemia. Int J Cancer 1989; 43:32.

Reeves B: Significance of joint fluid uric acid levels in gout. Ann Rheum Dis 1965; 24:569.

Reimer LG: Approach to the analysis of body fluids for the detection of infection. Clin Lab Med 1985; 5:209.

Rhodes CH, Glantz MJ, Glantz L, et al: A comparison of polymerase chain reaction of cerebrospinal fluid and conventional cytology in the diagnosis of lymphomatous meningitis. Cancer 1996; 77:543.

Riantawan P, Chaowalit P, Wongsangiem M, et al: Diagnostic value of pleural fluid adenosine deaminase in tuberculous pleuritis with reference to HIV coinfection and a Baysian analysis. Chest 1999; 116:97.

Ribeiro MA, Kimura RT, Irulegui I, et al: Cerebrospinal fluid levels of lysozyme, IgM and C-reactive protein in the identification of bacterial meningitis. J Trop Med Hyg 1992; 95:87.

Richard S, Miossec V, Moreau J-F, et al: Detection of oligoclonal immunoglobulins in cerebrospinal fluid by an immunofixation-peroxidase method. Clin Chem 2002; 48:167.

Riemenschneider M, Lautenschlager N, Wagenpfeil S, et al: Cerebrospinal fluid tau and beta-amyloid 42 proteins identify Alzheimer disease in subjects with mild cognitive impairment. Arch Neurol 2002; 59:1729.

Rijken A, Dekker A, Taylor S, et al: Diagnostic value of DNA analysis in effusions by flow cytometry and image analysis. A prospective study on 102 patients as compared with cytologic examination. Am J Clin Pathol 1991; 95:6.

Rodriguez AF, Kaplan SL, Mason EO Jr: Cerebrospinal fluid values in the very low birth weight infant. J Pediatr 1990; 116:971.

Rodriquez-Panadero F, Mejias JL: Low glucose and pH levels in malignant pleural effusions. Am Rev Respir Dis 1989; 139:663.

Romero S, Fernandez C, Arriero JM, et al: CEA, CA 15-3 and CYFRA 21-1 in serum and pleural fluid of patients with pleural effusions. Eur Respir J 1996; 9:17.

Rosenthal AK, Mandel N: Identification of crystals in synovial fluids and joint tissues. Curr Rheumatol Rep 2001; 3:11.

Rosett W, Hodges GR: Antimicrobial activity of heparin. J Clin Microbiol 1980; 11:30.

Roth BJ: Searching for tuberculosis in the pleural space. Chest 1999; 116:3.

Rouah E, Rogers BB, Buffone GJ: Transferrin analysis by immunofixation as an aid in the diagnosis of cerebrospinal fluid otorrhea. Arch Pathol Lab Med 1987; 111:756.

Rubins JB, Rubins HB: Etiology and prognostic significance of eosinophilic effusions. A prospective study. Chest 1996; 110:1271.

Rudick RA, French CA, Breton D, et al: Relative diagnostic value of cerebrospinal fluid kappa chains in MS, comparison with other immunoglobulin tests. Neurology 1989; 39:964.

Runyon BA: Amylase levels in ascitic fluid. J Clin Gastroenterol 1987a; 9:172.

Runyon BA: Ascitic fluid bilirubin concentration as a key to choleperitoneum. J Clin Gastroenterol 1987b; 9:543.

Runyon BA, Antillon MR: Ascitic fluid pH and lactate: Insensitive and nonspecific tests in detecting ascitic fluid infection. Hepatology 1991; 13:929.

Runyon BA, Hoefs JC: Ascitic fluid analysis in the differentiation of spontaneous bacterial peritonitis from gastrointestinal tract perforation into ascitic fluid. Hepatology 1984; 4:447.

Runyon BA, Hoefs JC, Morgan TR: Ascitic fluid analysis in malignancy-related ascites. Hepatology 1988; 8:1104.

Runyon BA, Montano AA, Evangelos A, et al: The serum-ascites albumin gradient is superior to the exudate–transudate concept in the differential diagnosis of ascites. Ann Intern Med 1992; 117:215.

Ruoslahti E, Engvall E, Hayman EG: Fibronectin: current concepts of its structure and function. Coll Res 1981; 1:95.

Ryall RG, Peacock MK, Simpson DA: Usefulness of beta 2-transferrin assay in the detection of cerebrospinal fluid leaks following head injury. J Neurosurg 1992; 77:737.

Sahn SA: The differential diagnosis of pleural effusions. West J Med 1982; 137:99.

Sarff LD, Platt LH, McCracken GH Jr: Cerebrospinal fluid evaluation in neonates: Comparison of high risk infants with and without meningitis. J Pediatrics 1976; 88:473.

Sari R, Yildirim B, Sevinc A, et al: The importance of serum and ascites fluid alpha-fetoprotein, carcinoembryonic antigen, CA 19-9, and CA 15-3 levels in differential diagnosis of ascites etiology. Hepatogastroenterology 2001; 48:1616.

Savory J, Brody JP: Measurement and diagnostic value of cerebrospinal fluid enzymes. Ann Clin Lab Sci 1979; 9:68.

Schneider D, Halperin R, Langer R, et al: Peritoneal fluid lactate dehydrogenase in ovarian cancer. Gynecol Oncol 1997; 66:399.

Schriever H, Gambino SR: Protein turbidity produced by trichloroacetic acid and sulfosalicylic acid at varying temperatures and varying ratios of albumin and globulin. Am J Clin Pathol 1965; 44:667.

Schuurman T, de Boer RF, Kooistra-Smid AMD, van Zwet AA: Prospective study of use of PCR amplification and sequencing of 16S ribosomal DNA from cerebrospinal fluid for diagnosis of bacterial meningitis in a clinical setting. J Clin Microbiol 2004; 42:734.

Schwake L, von Herbay A, Junghanss T, et al: Peritoneal tuberculosis with negative polymerase chain reaction results: Report of two cases. Scand J Gastroenterol 2003; 38:221.

Seehusen DA, Reeves MM, Fomin DA: Cerebrospinal fluid analysis. Am Family Phys 2003; 68:1103.

Sellebjerg F, Christiansen M, Nielsen PM, Frederiksen JL: Cerebrospinal fluid measures of disease activity in patients with multiple sclerosis. Mult Scler 1998; 4:475.

Selvi E, Manganelli S, Catenaccio M, et al: Diff Quik staining method for detection and identification of monosodium urate and calcium pyrophosphate crystals in synovial fluids. Ann Rheum Dis 2001; 60:194.

Seregni E, Massimino M, Nerini Molteni S, et al: Serum and cerebrospinal fluid human chorionic gonadotropin (hCG) and alpha-fetoprotein (AFP) in intracranial germ cell tumors. Int J Biol Markers 2002; 17:112.

Seres E, Bencsik K, Rajda C, et al: Diagnostic studies of cerebrospinal fluid in patients with multiple sclerosis [In Hungarian]. Orv Hetil 1998; 139:1905.

Seward RJ, Towner KJ: Evaluation of a PCR-immunoassay technique for detection of Neisseria meningitidis in cerebrospinal fluid and peripheral blood. J Med Microbiol 2000; 49:451.

Shephard MD, Whiting MJ: Nephelometric determination of total protein in cerebrospinal fluid and urine using benzalkonium chloride as precipitation reagent. Ann Clin Biochem 1992; 29:411.

Shmerling RH: Synovial fluid analysis. A critical reappraisal. Rheum Dis Clin North Am 1994; 20:503.

Shmerling RH, Delbanco TL, Tosteson ANA, et al. Synovial fluid tests. What should be ordered? JAMA 1990; 264:1009.

Silva-Cardosa J, Moura B, Martins L, et al: Pericardial involvement in human immunodeficiency virus infection. Chest 1999; 115:418.

Silverman LM, Christenson RH: Amino acids and proteins. In Burtis CA, Ashwood ER (eds): Tietz Textbook of Clinical Chemistry, 2nd ed. Philadelphia, WB Saunders, 1994, p 625.

Simon RP, Abele JS: Spinal-fluid pleocytosis estimated by the Tyndall effect. Ann Intern Med 1978; 89:75.

Sindie CJ, Laterte EC: Oligoclonal free kappa and lambda bands in the cerebrospinal fluid. J Neuroimmunol 1991; 33:63.

Skedros DG, Cass SP, Hirsh BE, Kelly RH: Beta-2-transferrin assay in clinical management of cerebral spinal fluid and perilymphatic fluid leaks. J Otolaryngol 1993a; 22:341.

Skedros DG, Cass SP, Hirsh BE, Kelly RH: Sources of error in the use of beta-2 transferrin analysis for diagnosing perilymphatic and cerebral spinal fluid leaks. Otolaryngol Head Neck Surg 1993b; 109:861.

Sloman AJ, Kelly RH: Transferrin allelic variants may cause false positives in the detection of cerebrospinal fluid fistulae. Clin Chem 1993; 39:1444.

Sood A, Moudgil A, Sood N, et al: Role of fibronectin in diagnosis of malignant ascites. J Assoc Physicians India 1997; 45:283.

Sormunen P, Kallio MJ, Kilpi T, Peltola H: C-reactive protein is useful in distinguishing Gram stain-negative bacterial meningitis from viral meningitis in children. J Pediatr 1999; 134:725.

Souverijn JHM, Smit WG, Peet R, et al: Intrathecal Ig synthesis: Its detection by isoelectric focusing and IgG index. J Neurol Sci 1989; 93:211.

Soyka JM, Martin M, Sloan EP, et al: Diagnostic peritoneal lavage: Is an isolated WBC count > 500/mm^3 predictive of intra-abdominal injury requiring celiotomy in blunt trauma patients? J Trauma 1990; 30:874.

Spanos A, Harrell FEJ, Durack DT: Differential diagnosis of acute meningitis: An analysis of the predictive value of initial observations. JAMA 1989; 262:2700.

Staats BA, Ellefson RD, Budahn LL, et al: The lipoprotein profile of chylous and non-chylous pleural effusions. Mayo Clin Proc 1980; 55:700.

Stassen WN, McCullough AJ, Bacon BR, et al: Immediate diagnostic criteria for bacterial infection of ascitic fluid. Gastroenterology 1986; 90:1247.

Stearman M, Southgate HJ: The use of cytokine and C-reactive protein measurements in cerebrospinal fluid during acute infective meningitis. Ann Clin Biochem 1994; 31:255.

Steele RW, Marmer DJ, O'Brien MD, et al: Leukocyte survival in cerebrospinal fluid. J Clin Microbiol 1986; 23:965.

Stelzner TJ, King TEJ, Antony VB, et al: The pleuropulmonary manifestations of the postcardiac injury syndrome. Chest 1983; 84:383.

Stewart RV, Zumwalt RE, Hirsch CS, Kaplan L: Postmortem diagnosis of myocardial disease by enzyme analysis of pericardial fluid. Am J Clin Pathol 1984; 82:411.

Stewart RJ, Gupta RK, Purdie GI, et al: Fine catheter aspiration cytology of peritoneal cavity improves decision-making about difficult cases of acute abdominal pain. Lancet 1986; 2:1414.

Suay VG, Moragon EM, Viedma EC, et al: Pleural cholesterol in differentiating transudates and exudates. Respiration 1995; 62:57.

Such J, Frances R, Munoz C, et al: Detection and identification of bacterial DNA in patients with cirrhosis and culture-negative nonneutrocytic ascites. Hepatology 2002; 36:135.

Sullivan KR, Nelson MJ, Tandberg D: Incremental analysis of diagnostic peritoneal lavage fluid in adult abdominal trauma. Am J Emerg Med 1997; 15:277.

Sunderland T, Linker G, Mirza N, et al: Decreased beta-amyloid1-42 and increased tau levels in cerebrospinal fluid of patients with Alzheimer disease. JAMA 2003; 289:2094.

Suzuki Y, Tanaka R: Carcinoembryonic antigen in patients with intracranial tumors. J Neurosurg 1980; 53:355.

Talstad I: Electronic counting of spinal fluid cells. Am J Clin Pathol 1984; 81:506.

Tang LM: Serial lactate determinations in tuberculous meningitis. Scand J Infect Dis 1988; 20:81.

Tangkijvanich P, Tresukolos D, Sanpatamukul P, et al: Telomerase assay for differentiating between malignancy-related and nonmalignant ascites. Clin Cancer Res 1999; 5:2470.

Thwaites GE, Chau TT, Farrar JJ: Improving the bacteriological diagnosis of tuberculous meningitis. J Clin Microbiol 2004; 42:378.

Tibbling G, Link H, Ohman S: Principles of albumin and IgG analyses in neurological disorders, I: Establishment of reference values. Scand J Clin Lab Invest 1977; 37:385.

Titov AG, Vyshnevskaya EB, Mazurenko SI, et al: Use of polymerase chain reaction to diagnose tuberculous arthritis from joint tissues and synovial fluid. Arch Pathol Lab Med 2004; 128:205.

Torre D, Zeroli C, Issi M, et al: Cerebrospinal fluid concentration of fibronectin in meningitis. J Clin Pathol 1991; 44:783.

Torre D, Zeroli C, Ferrario G, et al: Cerebrospinal fluid concentration of fibronectin in HIV-1 infection and central nervous system disorders. J Clin Pathol 1993; 46:1039.

Tourtellotte WW, Tavolato B, Parker JA, et al. Cerebrospinal fluid electroimmunodiffusion. Arch Neurol 1971; 25:345.

Tourtellotte WW, Staugaitis SM, Walsh MJ, et al: The basis of intra-blood–brain barrier IgG synthesis. Ann Neurol 1985; 17:21.

Trbojevic-Cepe M, Vogrinc Z, Brinar V. Diagnostic significance of methemoglobin determination in colorless cerebrospinal fluid. Clin Chem 1992; 38:1401.

Trotter JL, Rust RS: Human cerebrospinal fluid immunology. In Herndon RM, Brumback RA (eds): The Cerebrospinal Fluid. Boston, Kluwer Academic Publishers, 1989, p 179.

Tubergen DG, Cullen JW, Boyett JM, et al: Blasts in CSF with a normal cell count do not justify alteration of therapy for acute lymphoblastic leukemia in remission: A Childrens Cancer Group study. J Clin Oncol 1994; 12:273.

Turay UY, Yildirim Z, Turkoz Y, et al: Use of pleural fluid C-reactive protein in diagnosis of pleural effusions. Respir Med 2000; 94:432.

Twijnstra A, Nooyen WJ, van Zanten AP, et al: Cerebrospinal fluid carcinoembryonic antigen in patients with metastatic and nonmetastatic neurological diseases. Arch Neurol 1986; 43:269.

UK National External Quality Assessment Scheme for Immunochemistry Working Group. National guidelines for the analysis of cerebrospinal fluid for bilirubin in suspected subarachnoid hemorrhage. Ann Clin Biochem 2003; 40:481.

Van Acker JT, Delanghe JR, Langlois MR, et al: Automated flow cytometric analysis of cerebrospinal fluid. Clin Chem 2001; 47:556.

Verettas D, Kazakos C, Tilkeridis C, et al: Polymerase chain reaction for the detection of Mycobacterium tuberculosis in synovial fluid, tissue samples, bone marrow aspirate and peripheral blood. Acta Orthop Belg 2003; 69:396.

Villena V, Lopez-Encuentra A, Echave-Sustaeta J, et al: Interferon-gamma in 388 immunocompromised and immunocompetent patients for diagnosing pleural tuberculosis. Eur Respir J 1996a; 9:2635.

Villena V, Lopez-Encuentra A, Echave-Sustaeta J, et al: Diagnostic value of CA 72-4, carcinoembryonic antigen, CA 15-3, and CA 19-9 assay of pleural

III

fluid. A study of 207 patients. Cancer 1996b; 78:736.

Villena V, Lopez-Encuentra A, Pozo F, et al: Interferon gamma levels in pleural fluid for the diagnosis of tuberculosis. Am J Med 2003a; 115:365.

Villena V, Lopez-Encuentra A, Echave-Sustaeta J, et al: Diagnostic value of CA 549 in pleural fluid. Comparison with CEA, CA 15-3 and CA 72-4. Lung Cancer 2003b; 40:289.

Walts AE: Cerebrospinal fluid cytology: Selected issues. Diagn Cytopathol 1992; 8:394.

Wang DY, Yang PC, Yu WL, et al: Serial antinuclear antibodies titre in pleural and pericardial fluid. Eur Respir J 2000; 15:1106.

Ward E, Gushurst CA: Uses and techniques of pediatric lumbar puncture. Am J Dis Child 1992; 146:1160.

Weinburger A, Simkin PA: Plasma proteins in synovial fluids of normal human joints. Semin Arthritis Rheum 1989; 19:66.

Welch KM, Chabi E, Bartosh K, et al: Cerebrospinal fluid gamma aminobutyric acid level in migraine. Br Med J 1975; 30:516.

Weller M, Sommer N, Stevens A, et al: Increased intrathecal synthesis of fibronectin in bacterial and carcinomatous meningitis. Acta Neurol Scand 1990; 82:138.

Weller M, Stevens A, Sommer N, et al: Humoral CSF parameters in the differential diagnosis of hematologic CNS neoplasia. Acta Neurol Scand 1992; 86:129.

Wenger JD, Hightower AW, Broome CV, et al: Bacterial meningitis in the United States: Report of a multistate surveillance study, 1986. J Infect Dis 1990; 162:1316.

Wilson ML. Clinically relevant, cost-effective clinical microbiology: Strategies to decrease unnecessary testing. Am J Pathol 1997; 107:154.

Wise CM, White RE, Agudelo CA: Synovial fluid lipid abnormalities in various disease states: Review and classification. Semin Arthritis Rheum 1987; 16:222.

Wood JH: Neurobiology of CSF. New York, Plenum Press, 1980.

Wu SS, Lin OS, Chen YY, et al: Ascitic fluid carcinoembryonic antigen and alkaline phosphatase levels for the differentiation of primary from secondary bacterial peritonitis with intestinal perforation. J Hepatol 2001; 34:215.

Wubbel L, McCracken GH Jr: Management of bacterial meningitis: 1998. Pediatr Rev 1998; 19:78.

Yorgancioglu A, Akin M, Dereli S, et al: The diagnostic value of tuberculostearic acid in tuberculous pleural effusions. Monaldi Arch Chest Dis 1996; 51:108.

Yuan S, Bien C, Wener MH, et al: Repeat examination of synovial fluid for crystals: Is it useful? Clin Chem 2003; 49: 1562.

Zandman-Goddard G, Matzner Y, Konijn AM, et al: Cerebrospinal fluid ferritin in malignant CNS involvement. Cancer 1986; 58:1146.

Zaret DL, Morrison N, Gullbranson R, Keren DF: Immunofixation to quantify beta-2-transferrin in cerebrospinal fluid from skull injury. Clin Chem 1992; 38:1909.

Zerr I, Bodemer M, Gefeller O, et al: Detection of 14-3-3 protein in the cerebrospinal fluid supports the diagnosis of Creutzfeldt–Jakob disease. Ann Neurol 1998; 43:32.

Zunt JR, Marra CM: Cerebrospinal fluid testing for the diagnosis of central nervous system infection. Neurol Clin 1999; 17:675.

PART IV

Hematology

Edited by

Robert E. Hutchison MD, Richard A. McPherson MD

CHAPTER 29

Basic Examination of Blood and Bone Marrow

Neerja Vajpayee MD, Susan S. Graham MS, Sylva Bem MD

KEY POINTS

• Assessment of erythrocyte, leukocyte and platelet counts from manual and automated particle counters is central to the diagnosis and management of hematological diseases.

• With few exceptions, manual methods have been replaced by automated hematology analyzers. The selection of analyzers is varied and voluminous enough to meet the needs of any hematology laboratory setting.

• Hematology automation combined with sophisticated algorithms for data interpretation has made dramatic improvements in the utility of automated analyzers in patient care. Newer instrumentation has progressed far beyond the screening tool of the past.

• Examination of peripheral blood and bone marrow smear/biopsy represents the cornerstone of hematological diagnosis. The bone marrow examination provides a semiquantitative and qualitative assessment of the state of hematopoiesis, and aids in diagnosis of several hereditary and acquired benign and malignant diseases.

Hematology includes the study of blood cells and coagulation. It encompasses analyses of the concentration, structure, and function of cells in blood; their precursors in the bone marrow; chemical constituents of plasma or serum intimately linked with blood cell structure and function; and function of platelets and proteins involved in blood coagulation. Advancement of molecular biological techniques and their increased use in hematology has led to detection of several genetic mutations underlying the altered structure and function of cells and proteins that result in hematological diseases.

Hematology Principles and Procedures

Hemoglobin

Hemoglobin (Hb), the main component of the red blood cell (RBC), is a conjugated protein that serves as the vehicle for the transportation of oxygen (O_2) and carbon dioxide (CO_2). When fully saturated, each gram of hemoglobin holds 1.34 mL of oxygen. The red cell mass of the adult contains approximately 600 g of hemoglobin, capable of carrying 800 mL of oxygen. A molecule of hemoglobin consists of two pairs of polypeptide chains ('globins') and four prosthetic heme groups, each containing one atom of ferrous iron. Each heme group is precisely located in a pocket or fold of one of the polypeptide chains. Located near the surface of the molecule, the heme reversibly combines with one molecule of oxygen or

carbon dioxide. The main function of hemoglobin is to transport oxygen from the lungs, where oxygen tension is high, to the tissues, where it is low. At an oxygen tension of 100 mmHg in the pulmonary capillaries, 95–98% of the hemoglobin is combined with oxygen. In the tissues, where the oxygen tension may be as low as 20 mmHg, the oxygen readily dissociates from hemoglobin; in this instance, less than 30% of the oxygen would remain combined with hemoglobin.

Reduced Hb is hemoglobin with iron unassociated with oxygen. When each heme group is associated with one molecule of oxygen, the hemoglobin is referred to as oxyhemoglobin (HbO_2). In both Hb and HbO_2, iron remains in the ferrous state. When iron is oxidized to the ferric state, methemoglobin (hemiglobin; Hi) is formed, and the molecule loses its capacity to carry oxygen or carbon dioxide.

Anemia is a decrease below normal of the hemoglobin concentration, erythrocyte count, or hematocrit. It is a very common condition and is frequently a complication of other diseases. Clinical diagnosis of anemia or of high hemoglobin based on estimation of the color of the skin and of visible mucous membranes is highly unreliable. The correct estimation of hemoglobin is important and is one of the routine tests performed on practically every patient.

Hemoglobin Derivatives

Hemiglobin (Methemoglobin [Hi])

Methemoglobin is a derivative of hemoglobin in which the ferrous iron is *oxidized* to the ferric state, resulting in the inability of Hi to combine reversibly with oxygen. The polypeptide chains are not altered. A normal individual has up to 1.5% methemoglobin. Methemoglobinemia will cause chocolate brown discoloration of blood, cyanosis and functional 'anemia' if present in high enough concentration. Cyanosis becomes obvious at a concentration of about 1.5 g Hi/dL (i.e., 10% of hemoglobin). Comparable degrees of cyanosis will be caused by 5 g Hb per deciliter of blood, 1.5 g Hi per deciliter of blood, and 0.5 g SHb per deciliter of blood. The degree of cyanosis, however, is not necessarily correlated with the concentration of Hi. A small amount of Hi is always being formed but is reduced by enzyme systems within the erythrocyte. The most important is the NADH-dependent methemoglobin reductase system (NADH-cytochrome-b_5 reductase). Others, which may function mainly as reserve systems, are ascorbic acid, reduced glutathione, and NADPH-methemoglobin reductase. The latter requires a natural cofactor or an auto-oxidizable dye such as methylene blue for activity.

Methemoglobinemia, an increased amount of Hi in the erythrocytes, results from either an increased production of Hi or decreased NADH-cytochrome-b_5 reductase activity, and may be hereditary or acquired (Jaffé, 1989). The hereditary form is divided into two major categories. In the first, methemoglobinemia is due to a decrease in the capacity of the erythrocyte to reduce the Hi that is constantly being formed back to Hb. This is most often due to *NADH-cytochrome-b₅ reductase deficiency*, which is inherited as an autosomal recessive characteristic. The homozygote has methemoglobin levels of 10–50% and is cyanotic. Only occasionally is polycythemia present as a compensating mechanism. Hemiglobin concentrations of 10–25% may give no apparent symptoms; levels of 35–50% result in mild symptoms, such as exertional dyspnea and headaches; and levels exceeding 70% are probably lethal. Therapy with ascorbic acid or methylthioninium chloride (methylene blue) in this form of hereditary methemoglobinemia will reduce the level of Hi, the latter apparently by activation of the NADPH-methemoglobin reductase system. Heterozygotes have intermediate levels of NADH-cytochrome-b₅ reductase activity and normal blood levels of Hi. They may become cyanotic because of methemoglobinemia after exposure to oxidizing chemicals or drugs in amounts that will not affect normal individuals.

In the second major category of hereditary methemoglobinemia, the reducing systems within the erythrocyte are intact, but the structure of the hemoglobin molecule itself is abnormal. A genetically determined alteration in the amino acid composition of either α- or β-globin chains may form a hemoglobin molecule that has an enhanced tendency toward oxidation and a decreased propensity of the methemoglobin formed to be reduced back to hemoglobin. Their principal consequence is asymptomatic cyanosis as a result of methemoglobinemia; they are designated as various forms of *hemoglobin M (Hb M)*. In six of the seven Hb M variants, tyrosine is substituted for histidine in the heme pocket of the proximal or distal globin chain. Nagai (1995) showed by spectroscopy that a considerable proportion of the mutant subunits of Hb M Saskatoon and Hb M Boston stay in the fully reduced form under circulation conditions. They are inherited as autosomal dominant traits (Lukens, 2004). Methylthioninium chloride (methylene blue) therapy in these individuals is without effect, and treatment is not necessary.

Most cases of methemoglobinemia are classified as secondary or acquired, due mainly to exposure to drugs and chemicals that cause increased formation of hemiglobin. Chemicals or drugs that directly oxidize HbO₂ to Hi include nitrites, nitrates, chlorates, and quinones. Other substances, which are aromatic amino and nitro compounds, probably act indirectly through a metabolite, since they do not cause Hi formation in vitro. These include acetanilid, phenacetin, sulfonamides, and aniline dyes. Ferrous sulfate may produce methemoglobinemia after ingestion of very large doses. Levels of drugs or chemicals that would not cause significant methemoglobinemia in a normal individual may do so in someone with a mild reduction in NADH-cytochrome-b₅ reductase activity that, under ordinary circumstances, is not cyanotic. Such individuals are newborn infants and persons heterozygous for NADH-cytochrome-b₅ reductase deficiency (Bunn, 1986). Hemiglobin is reduced back to Hb by the erythrocyte enzyme systems. It can also be reduced (slowly) by the administration of reducing agents, such as ascorbic acid or sulfhydryl compounds (glutathione, cysteine); these, as well as methylthioninium chloride (methylene blue), are of value in cases of hereditary NADH-cytochrome-b₅ reductase deficiency. In cases of acquired or toxic methemoglobinemia, methylthioninium chloride is of great value; its rapid action is not based on its own reduction capacity but on its acceleration of the normally slow NADPH-methemoglobin reductase pathway. Hemiglobin can combine reversibly with various chemicals (e.g., cyanides, sulfides, peroxides, fluorides, and azides). Because of the strong affinity of Hi for cyanide, the therapy of cyanide poisoning is to administer nitrites to form Hi, which then combines with the cyanide. Thus, the free cyanide (which is extremely poisonous to the cellular respiratory enzymes) becomes less toxic when changed to HiCN.

Hemiglobin is quantitated by spectrophotometry. If Hi is elevated, drugs or toxic substances must first be eliminated as a cause. Congenital methemoglobinemia due to NADH-cytochrome-b₅ reductase deficiency is determined by assay of the enzyme. An abnormal hemoglobin (Hb M) may also be responsible for methemoglobinemia noted at birth or in the first few months of life.

Sulfhemoglobin

Sulfhemoglobin is a mixture of oxidized, partially denatured forms of hemoglobin that form during oxidative hemolysis (Jandl, 1996). During oxidation of hemoglobin, sulfur (from some source, which may vary) is incorporated into heme rings of hemoglobin, resulting in a green hemochrome. Further oxidation usually results in the denaturation and precipitation of hemoglobin as Heinz bodies (Fig. 29–1). Sulfhemoglobin cannot transport oxygen, but it can combine with carbon monoxide (CO) to form carboxysulfhemoglobin. Unlike methemoglobin, sulfhemoglobin cannot be reduced back to hemoglobin, and it remains in the cells until they break down. The blood is mauve-lavender in sulfhemoglobinemia. Sulfhemoglobin has been reported in patients receiving treatment with

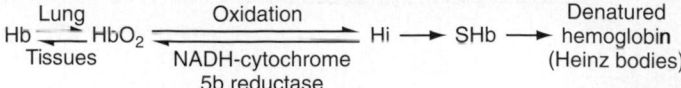

Figure 29–1 Simplified concept of oxidation of hemoglobin (Hb) to methemoglobin (Hi) as proposed by Jandl (1996). Reversible binding and release of oxygen occur in lungs and tissues; oxidation of ferrous ions and formation of hemoglobin are reversible in the red cell to a limited extent; continued oxidation leads to irreversible conformational changes and sulfhemoglobin; still further oxidation results in denaturation of the hemoglobin and precipitation within the erythrocyte as Heinz bodies.

sulfonamides or aromatic amine drugs (phenacetin, acetanilid), as well as in patients with severe constipation, in cases of bacteremia due to *Clostridium perfringens* and in a condition known as enterogenous cyanosis. The concentration of sulfhemoglobin in vivo normally is less than 1%, and in these conditions seldom exceeds 10% of the total hemoglobin. It results in cyanosis and is usually asymptomatic. The reason some patients develop methemoglobinemia, some sulfhemoglobinemia, and others Heinz bodies and hemolysis is not well understood. Sulfhemoglobin is quantitated by spectrophotometry.

Carboxyhemoglobin (HbCO)

Endogenous CO produced in the degradation of heme to bilirubin normally accounts for about 0.5% carboxyhemoglobin in the blood, and is increased in hemolytic anemia. Hemoglobin has the capacity to combine with carbon monoxide with an affinity 210 times greater than for oxygen. Carbon monoxide will bind with hemoglobin even if its concentration in the air is extremely low (e.g., 0.02–0.04%). In those cases, HbCO will build up until typical symptoms of poisoning appear. HbCO cannot bind and carry oxygen. Furthermore, increasing concentrations of HbCO shift the Hb–oxygen dissociation curve increasingly to the left, thus adding to the anoxia. If a patient poisoned with carbon monoxide receives pure oxygen, the conversion of HbCO to HbO₂ is greatly enhanced. HbCO is light sensitive and has a typical, brilliant, cherry red color.

Acute carbon monoxide poisoning is well known. It produces tissue hypoxia as a result of decreased oxygen transport. Chronic poisoning, a result of prolonged exposure to small amounts of carbon monoxide, is less well recognized but is of increasing importance. The chief sources of the gas are gasoline motors, illuminating gas, gas heaters, defective stoves, and the smoking of tobacco. Exposure to carbon monoxide is thus one of the hazards of modern civilization. The gas has even been found in the air of busy streets of large cities in sufficient concentration to cause mild symptoms in persons such as traffic police officers who are exposed to it over long periods of time. Chronic exposure through tobacco smoking may lead to chronic elevation of HbCO and an associated left shift in the oxygen dissociation curve; smokers tend to have higher hematocrits than nonsmokers and may have polycythemia. Healthy persons exposed to various concentrations of the gas for an hour do not experience definite symptoms (headache, dizziness, muscular weakness, and nausea) unless the concentration of the gas in the blood reaches 20–30% of saturation; however, it appears that in chronic poisoning, especially in children, serious symptoms may occur with lower concentrations. HbCO may be quantitated by differential spectrophotometry or by gas chromatography.

Determining the Concentration of Hemoglobin

The cyanmethemoglobin (hemiglobincyanide; HiCN) method has the advantage of convenience and a readily available, stable standard solution.

Hemiglobincyanide (HiCN) Method

Principle. Blood is diluted in a solution of potassium ferricyanide and potassium cyanide. The potassium ferricyanide oxidizes hemoglobin to hemiglobin (Hi; methemoglobin), and potassium cyanide provides cyanide ions (CN⁻) to form HiCN, which has a broad absorption maximum at a wavelength of 540 nm (Fig. 29–2, Table 29–1). The absorbance of the solution is measured in a spectrophotometer at 540 nm and compared with that of a standard HiCN solution.

Reagent. The diluent is detergent-modified Drabkin reagent:

0.20 g	Potassium ferricyanide (K₃Fe(CN)₆)
0.05 g	Potassium cyanide (KCN)
0.14 g	Dihydrogen potassium phosphate (anhydrous) (KH₂PO₄)

Non-ionic detergent – e.g.,

0.5 mL	Sterox S.E. (Harleco), *or*
1.0 mL	Triton X-100 (Rohm and Haas)

Distilled water to 1000 mL

The solution should be clear and pale yellow, have a pH of 7.0–7.4, and give a reading of zero when measured in the photometer at 540 nm against a water blank.

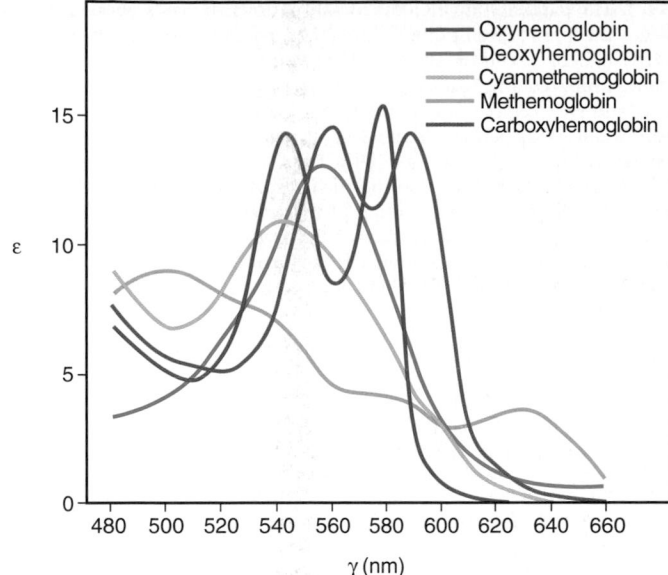

Figure 29–2 Absorption spectra of oxyhemoglobin (HbO₂), deoxyhemoglobin (Hb), methemoglobin (hemiglobin [Hi]), and cyanmethemoglobin (hemiglobincyanide [HiCN]). (Morris MW, Skrodzki Z, Nelson DA. Zeta sedimentation ratio (ZSR), a replacement for the erythrocyte sedimentation rate (ESR). *Am J Clin Patnol* 1975; 64:254–6. © 1975 American Society for Clinical Pathology.)

Table 29–1 Nomenclature and Absorption Maxima of Hemoglobins

Term	Symbol	Absorption peak 1 λ	ε	Absorption peak 2 λ	ε	Absorption peak 3 λ	ε
Hemoglobin	Hb	431	(140)	555	(13.04)		
Oxyhemoglobin	HbO₂	415	(131)	542	(14.37)	577	(15.37)
Carboxyhemoglobin	HbCO	420	(192)	539	(14.36)	568.5	(14.31)
Hemiglobin (methemoglobin)	Hi	406	(162)	500	(9.04)	630	(3.70)
Hemiglobincyanide (cyanmet Hb)	HiCN	421	(122.5)	540	(10.99)		

The wavelength (λ) in nanometers for each maximum is followed by the extinction coefficient (ε) placed in parentheses.

After van Assendelft OW, 1970.

Substituting dihydrogen potassium phosphate, KHP₂PO₄, in this reagent for sodium bicarbonate, NaHCO₃, in the original Drabkin reagent shortens the time needed for complete conversion of Hb to HiCN from 10 minutes to 3 minutes. The detergent enhances lysis of erythrocytes and decreases turbidity from protein precipitation.

Care must be taken with KCN in the preparation of the Drabkin solution, as salts or solutions of cyanide are poisonous. The diluent itself contains only 50 mg KCN per liter, less than the lethal dose for a 70-kg person. However, because HCN is released by acidification, exposure of the diluent to acid must be avoided. Disposal of reagents and samples in running water in the sink is advised. The diluent keeps well in a dark bottle at room temperature, but should be prepared fresh periodically.

Method. Twenty microliters of blood is added to 5.0 mL of diluent (1 : 251), mixed well, and allowed to stand at room temperature for at least 3 minutes (Dacie, 1991). The absorbance is measured, against the reagent blank, in the photoelectric colorimeter at 540 nm or with an appropriate filter. A vial of HiCN standard is then opened and the absorbance measured, at room temperature, in the same instrument in a similar fashion. The test sample must be analyzed within a few hours of dilution. The standard must be kept in the dark when not in use and discarded at the end of the day.

Hb (g/dL) = [A⁵⁴⁰ test sample/A⁵⁴⁰ standard] × [Concentration of standard (mg/dL)/100 mg/g] × 251

It is usually convenient to calibrate the photometer to be used for hemoglobinometry by preparing a standard curve or table that will relate absorbance to Hb concentration in grams per deciliter. The absorbance of fresh HiCN standard is measured against a reagent blank. Absorbance

readings are made of fresh HiCN standard and of dilutions of this standard in the reagent (1 in 2, 1 in 3, and 1 in 4) against a reagent blank. Hb values in grams per deciliter are calculated for each solution as described previously. When the absorbance readings are plotted on linear graph paper as the ordinates against Hb concentration as the abscissa, the points should describe a straight line that passes through the origin. An advantage of the HiCN method is that most forms of hemoglobin (Hb, HbO₂, Hi, and HbCO, but not SHb) are measured.

The test sample can be directly compared with the HiCN standard, and the readings can be made at the convenience of the operator because of the stability of the diluted samples. Increased absorbance not due to hemoglobin may be caused by turbidity due to abnormal plasma proteins, hyperlipemia, large numbers of leukocytes (counts > 30 × 10⁹/L), or fatty droplets, any of which may lead to increased light scattering and apparent absorbance.

Errors in Hemoglobinometry

The sources of error may be those of the sample, the method, the equipment, or the operator.

Errors Inherent in the Sample. Improper venipuncture technique may introduce hemoconcentration, which will make hemoglobin concentration and cell counts too high. Improper technique in fingerstick or capillary sampling can produce errors in either direction.

Errors Inherent in the Method. The HiCN method is the method of choice. The use of HiCN standard for calibration of the instrument and for the test itself eliminates a major source of error. The broad absorption band of HiCN in the region of 540 nm makes it convenient to use it both in filter-type photometers and in narrow-band spectrophotometers. With the exception of SHb, all other varieties of hemoglobin are converted to HiCN.

Errors Inherent in the Equipment. The accuracy of equipment is not uniform. A good grade of pipet with a guaranteed accuracy of greater than 99% is desirable. Calibration of pipets will lessen errors. Significant error can be introduced by the use of unmatched cuvets; therefore, flow-through cuvets are preferred. The wavelength settings, the filters, and the meter readings require checking. The photometer must be calibrated in the laboratory before its initial use and must be rechecked frequently to reduce the method's error to 2% (± CV).

Operator's Errors. Human errors can be reduced by good training, understanding the clinical significance of the test and the necessity for a dependable method, adherence to oral and written instructions, and familiarity with the equipment and with the sources of error. Errors increase with fatigue and tend to be greater near the end of the day. A technologist who is patient and critical by nature and by training and who is interested in the work is less prone to make errors.

The preceding discussion applies to manual techniques of hemoglobinometry. Automated equipment is widely used and eliminates most errors.

Spectrophotometric Identification of Hemoglobins

The various hemoglobins have characteristic absorption spectra, which can be determined easily with a spectrophotometer. The useful absorbance maxima are given in Table 29–1. The maxima for Hi vary considerably with pH. The maxima given in the two right-hand columns are useful for distinguishing among these forms of hemoglobin. The absorbance between 405–435 nm (the Soret band) is considerably greater and may be used when small concentrations of hemoglobin are to be measured.

Hematocrit (Packed Cell Volume)

The hematocrit of a sample of blood is the ratio of the volume of erythrocytes to that of the whole blood. It is expressed either as a percentage (conventional) or as a decimal fraction (SI units). The units (L/L) are implied. Dried heparin and ethylenediaminetetraacetic acid (EDTA) are satisfactory anticoagulants. Before taking a sample from a tube of venous blood for a hematological determination, it is important to mix the blood thoroughly. If the tube has been standing, this requires at least 60 inversions of the tube, or 2 minutes on a mechanical rotator; less than this leads to unacceptable deterioration in precision (Fairbanks, 1971). The number of inversions required to achieve homogeneity of a specimen depends on the dimensions of the container. Standard 10–14 × 75-mm tubes, containing 5 mL of blood and an air bubble comprising at least 20% of the tube volume, require at least eight inversions (NCCLS, 1993). The venous hematocrit agrees closely with the hematocrit obtained from a skin puncture; both are greater than the total body hematocrit. The hematocrit may be measured directly by centrifugation with macromethods or micromethods, or indirectly as the product of the mean corpuscular volume (MCV) times RBC count in automated instruments. In blood kept at room temperature, swelling of erythrocytes between 6 and 24 hours raises the hematocrit and MCV. Cell counts and indices are stable for 24 hours at 4°C (Brittin, 1969).

The Wintrobe macromethod hematocrit employs centrifugation of blood in a thick-walled glass tube with a uniform internal bore and a flattened bottom. It is no longer used.

Gross Examination

Hematocrit determination is performed by centrifugation. Inspection of the specimen after spinning may furnish valuable information. The relative heights of the red cell column, buffy coat, and plasma column should be noted. The buffy coat is the red-gray layer between the red cells and plasma; it includes platelets and leukocytes.

An orange or green color of the plasma suggests increased bilirubin, and pink or red suggests hemoglobinemia. Poor technique in collecting the blood specimen is the most frequent cause of hemolysis. If the specimens are not obtained within an hour or two after a fat-rich meal, cloudy plasma may point to nephrosis or certain abnormal hyperglobulinemias, especially cryoglobulinemia.

Hematocrit Measurement by Micromethod

Equipment

A capillary hematocrit tube about 7 cm long with a uniform bore of about 1 mm is used. For blood collection directly from a skin puncture, heparinized capillary tubes are available.

Procedure

The microhematocrit tube is filled by capillary attraction, from either a free-flowing puncture wound or a well-mixed venous sample. The capillary tube should be filled to at least 5 cm. The empty end is sealed with modeling clay. The filled tube is placed in the radial grooves of the microhematocrit centrifuge head with the sealed end away from the center. Place the bottom of the tube against the rubber gasket to prevent breakage. Centrifugation for 5 minutes at 10 000–12 000 g is satisfactory unless the hematocrit exceeds 50%; in that case, an additional 5 minutes' centrifugation should be employed in order to ensure minimal plasma trapping. The capillary tubes are not graduated. The length of the blood column, including the plasma, and of the red cell column alone must be measured in each case with a millimeter rule and a magnifying lens or with one of several commercially available measuring devices. The instructions of the manufacturer must be followed.

Interpretation of Results

Typical reference values for adult males are 0.41–0.51 L and for females, 0.36–0.45 L. A value below an individual's normal or below the reference interval for age and sex indicates anemia, and a higher value, polycythemia. The hematocrit reflects the concentration of red cells, not the total red cell mass. The hematocrit is low in hydremia of pregnancy, but the total number of circulating red cells is not reduced. The hematocrit may be normal or even high in shock accompanied by hemoconcentration, though the total red cell mass may be considerably decreased owing to blood loss. The hematocrit is unreliable as an estimate of anemia immediately after a loss of blood or immediately following transfusions.

Sources of Error

Centrifugation. Adequate duration and speed of centrifugation are essential for a correct hematocrit. The red cells must be packed so that additional centrifugation does not further reduce the packed cell volume. In the course of centrifugation, a small proportion of the leukocytes, platelets, and plasma are trapped between the red cells. The error resulting from the former is, as a rule, quite insignificant. The amount of trapped plasma is larger in high hematocrits than in low hematocrits. Trapped plasma accounts for about 1–3% of the red cell column in normal blood (about 0.014 in a hematocrit of 0.47), slightly more in macrocytic anemia, spherocytosis, and hypochromic anemia (Dacie, 1991). Even greater amounts of trapped plasma occur in the hematocrits of patients with sickle cell anemia and vary depending on the degree of sickling and consequent rigidity of the cells. In using the microhematocrit as a reference method for calibrating automated instruments, correction for trapped plasma is recommended (ICSH, 1980).

Sample. Posture, muscular activity, and prolonged tourniquet-stasis can cause the same order of changes in hematocrit and cell concentrations as they do for nonfilterable soluble constituents. Unique to the hematocrit is the error due to excess EDTA (inadequate blood for a fixed amount of EDTA): the hematocrit will be falsely low as a result of cell shrinkage, but the hemoglobin and cell counts will not be affected. There is no uniformity as to which EDTA salt is used for anticoagulation (O'Broin,

1997). The tripotassium (K_3-EDTA) salt shrinks red cells about 2% and lowers the packed cell volume compared to the dipotassium salt (K_2-EDTA) (Koepke, 1989). Also, since K_3-EDTA is a liquid, the measured hemoglobin, red and white cell counts are decreased 1–2%. Although the ICSH and NCCLS recommend the K_2-EDTA salt (powder), the K_3-EDTA is more often used, perhaps because of its increased miscibility and fewer instances of specimen clotting (Geller, 1996).

Other Errors. Technical errors include failure to mix the blood adequately before sampling, improper reading of the level of cells and plasma, and inclusion of the buffy coat as part of the erythrocyte volume. With good technique the precision of the hematocrit, expressed as ± 2 CV (coefficient of variation) is ± 1%. With low hematocrit values, the CV is greater because of reading error.

Erythrocyte Indices

Wintrobe introduced calculations for determining the size, content, and Hb concentration of red cells; these erythrocyte indices have been useful in the morphologic characterization of anemias. They may be calculated from the red cell count, hemoglobin concentration, and hematocrit.

Mean Cell Volume (MCV)

The MCV is the average volume of red cells and is calculated from the hematocrit and the red cell count. MCV = Hct × 1000/RBC (in millions per µL), expressed in femtoliters or cubic micrometers. If the hematocrit = 0.45 and the red cell count = 5×10^{12}/L, 1 L will contain 5×10^{12} red cells, which occupy a volume of 0.45 L.

The MCV = 0.45 L/5×10^{12} = 90×10^{-15} L

One femtoliter (fL) = 10^{-15} L = 1 cubic micrometer (μm^3).

Mean Cell Hemoglobin (MCH)

The MCH is the content (weight) of Hb of the average red cell; it is calculated from the Hb concentration and the red cell count.

MCH = Hb (in g/L)/RBC (in millions/µL)

The value is expressed in picograms. If the Hb = 15 g/dL and the red cell count is 5×10^{12}/L, 1 L contains 150 g of Hb distributed in 5×10^{12} cells.

MCH = 150/(5×10^{12}) = 30×10^{-12} (pg)

One picogram (pg) = 10^{-12} g

Mean Cell Hemoglobin Concentration (MCHC)

The MCHC is the average concentration of Hb in a given volume of packed red cells. It is calculated from the Hb concentration and the hematocrit.

MCHC = Hb (in g/dL)/Hct, expressed in g/dL

If the Hb = 15 g/dL and the Hct = 0.45, the

MCHC = 15 g/dL/0.45 = 33.3 g/dL

Discussion

Indices are determined in the electrical impedance instruments somewhat differently. The MCV is derived from the mean height of the voltage pulses formed during the red cell count, and the Hb is measured by optical density of HiCN. The other three values are calculated as follows:

Hct = MCV × RBC; MCH = Hb/RBC; MCHC = (Hb/Hct) × 100

The reference values for the indices will depend on whether they are determined from the centrifuged hematocrit or the cell counters. The values in normal individuals will be similar if both are corrected for trapped plasma. However, because of increased trapped plasma in hypochromic anemias and sickle cell anemia, the MCHC calculated from the microhematocrit will be significantly lower than the MCHC derived from the electrical impedance counters.

The 95% reference intervals for normal adults are as follows: MCV = 80–96 fL; MCH = 27–33 pg; and MCHC = 33–36 g/dL (Ryan, 2001a). In a healthy person, there is very little variation, no more than ± 1 unit in any of the indices. Deviations from the reference value for an individual or outside the reference intervals for normal persons are useful particularly in characterizing morphologic types of anemia.

In *microcytic anemias,* the indices may be as low as an MCV of 50 fL, an MCH of 15 pg, and an MCHC of 22 g/dL; rarely do any become lower.

In *macrocytic anemias,* the values may be as high as an MCV of 150 fL and an MCH of 50 pg, but the MCHC is normal or decreased (Dacie, 1991). The MCHC typically increases only in spherocytosis, and rarely is over 38 g/dL.

Manual Blood Cell Counts

Counts of erythrocytes, leukocytes, and platelets are each expressed as concentrations – cells per unit volume of blood. The unit of volume was expressed as cubic millimeters (mm^3) because of the linear dimensions of the hemocytometer (cell counting) chamber.

$$1 \ mm^3 = 1.00003 \ \mu L$$

Although there is no consistency in the literature in the use of traditional/conventional units versus Système International d'Unites (SI) units, the International Committee for Standardization in Hematology recommends that the unit of volume be the liter (SI units) as on the right in the following examples:

Erythrocytes:

$5.00 \times 10^6/mm^3 = 5.00 \times 10^6/\mu L$ (conventional) $= 5.00 \times 10^{12}/L$ (SI units)

Leukocytes:

$7.0 \times 10^3/mm^3 = 7.0 \times 10^3/\mu L$ (conventional) $= 7.0 \times 10^9/L$ (SI units)

Platelets:

$300 \times 10^3/mm^3 = 300 \times 10^3/\mu L$ (conventional) $= 300 \times 10^9/L$ (SI units)

Except for some platelet counts and low leukocyte counts, the hemocytometer is no longer used for routine blood cell counting. Yet it is still necessary for the technologist to be able to use this method effectively and to know its limitations. Any cell counting procedure includes three steps: dilution of the blood; sampling the diluted suspension into a measured volume; and counting the cells in that volume.

Erythrocyte Counts

Manual

Combining a microcapillary tube with a plastic vial containing a premeasured volume of diluent, the Unopette (Becton-Dickinson, Franklin Lakes, NJ) is a valuable system for manual dilutions. After the capillary tube is filled, it is pushed into the container and the sample is washed out by squeezing the soft plastic vial. This system is especially convenient for microsampling. Unopettes are available with diluents for counts of RBCs, white blood cells (WBCs), platelets, eosinophils, and reticulocytes.

Semiautomated Methods

Instruments are available for precise and convenient diluting, which both aspirate the sample and wash it out with the diluent. The dilutor should perform a 1 : 250 or 1 : 500 dilution with a coefficient of variation of less than 1%.

Manual Reticulocyte Counts

Principle

Reticulocytes are immature non-nucleated red cells that contain ribonucleic acid (RNA) and continue to synthesize hemoglobin after loss of the nucleus. When blood is briefly incubated in a solution of new methylene blue or brilliant cresyl blue, the RNA is precipitated as a dye–ribonucleoprotein complex. Microscopically, the complex appears as a dark blue network (reticulum or filamentous strand) or at least two dark blue granules that allow reticulocytes to be identified and enumerated (ICSH, 1998). A proposed reference method for reticulocyte counting based on the determination of the reticulocyte/red cell ratio has been published (ICSH, 1998), expanding on the 1994 ICSH red cell count reference method.

Reagent. One percent new methylene blue in a diluent of citrate-saline (one part 30 g/L sodium citrate plus four parts 9 g/L sodium chloride).

Controls. Although commercial controls are available, Ebrahim (1996) describes a method requiring about 2 hours that produces a multilevel control that is stable for several months. Hypotonic dialysis of RBCs in the presence of RNA followed by a short period of hypertonic dialysis to reseal the pores of the RBC membrane results in about 20% of the RBCs as 'synthetic reticulocytes' with various amounts of encapsulated RNA.

Procedure

Three drops each of reagent and blood are mixed in a test tube, incubated 15 minutes at room temperature, and remixed. Two wedge films are made on glass slides and air dried.

Viewed microscopically with an oil-immersion lens, reticulocytes are pale blue and contain dark blue reticular or granular material, and red cells stain pale blue or blue-green. The percentage of reticulocytes is determined in at least 1000 red cells. A Miller disk inserted in the eyepiece allows rapid estimation of large numbers of red cells by imposing two squares (one square is nine times the area of the other) onto the field of view (Brecher, 1950). Reticulocytes are counted in the large square and red cells in the small square in successive microscopic fields until at least 300 red cells are counted. This provides an estimate of reticulocytes among at least 2700 red cells, as follows:

Reticulocytes (percent) = [No. reticulocytes in large squares/(No. red cells in small squares × 9)] × 100

The absolute reticulocyte count is determined by multiplying the reticulocyte percentage by the red cell count.

Reference Values

Normal adults have a reticulocyte count of 0.5–1.5% or 24–$84 \times 10^9/L$. In newborn infants, the percentage is 2.5–6.5%; this falls to the adult range by the end of the second week of life.

Interpretation

Because reticulocytes are immature red cells that lose their RNA a day or so after reaching the blood from the marrow, a reticulocyte count provides an estimate of the rate of red cell production. An absolute reticulocyte count or reticulocyte production index is more helpful than the percentage (see Ch. 30).

Sources of Variation

Because such a small number of actual reticulocytes are counted, the sampling error in the manual reticulocyte count is relatively large. The 95% confidence limits may be expressed as follows:

$$R \pm 2\sqrt{[R(100 - R)/N]}$$

where R is the reticulocyte count in percent and N is the number of erythrocytes examined. This means that if only 1000 erythrocytes are evaluated, the 95% confidence limits for a 1% count are 0.4–1.6%; for a 5% count, 3.6–6.4%; and for a 10% count, 8.1–11.9%.

Leukocyte Counts

Specimen Collection. EDTA should be used; heparin is unsatisfactory as an anticoagulant

Hemocytometer Method (Manual Method)

Although this method is only occasionally used in leukocyte counting, the technologist should be able to perform it:

1. as a check on the validity of electronic methods for calibration purposes
2. as a check on the validity of electronic counts in patients with profound leukopenia or thrombocytopenia
3. for blood specimens with platelet counting interference (i.e., very microcytic RBCs), and
4. as a back-up method.

It is also commonly used as a method for counting cells in cerebrospinal fluid (CSF).

Counting Chamber. The hemocytometer is a thick glass slide with inscribed platforms of known area and precisely controlled depth under the coverslip. Counting chambers and cover glasses should be rinsed in lukewarm water immediately after use; wiped with a clean, lint-free cloth; and allowed to air dry. The surfaces must not be touched with gauze or linen because these materials may scratch the ruled areas.

Diluting Fluid. The diluting fluid lyses the erythrocytes so that they will not obscure the leukocytes. The fluid must be refrigerated and filtered frequently to remove yeasts and molds.

Procedure

1. Well-mixed blood is diluted 1 : 20 in diluting fluid and the vial rotated for about 5 minutes. The chamber is loaded with just enough fluid to fill the space beneath the cover glass.
2. The cells are permitted to settle for several minutes, and the chamber is surveyed with the low-power objective to verify uniform cell distribution.
3. Counting is performed. The condenser diaphragm of the microscope is partially closed to make the leukocytes stand out clearly under a low-power (10×) objective lens. The leukocytes are counted in each of the four large (1 mm^2) corner squares (A, B, C, and D in Fig. 29–3). A total of eight large corner squares from two sides of a chamber are counted.
4. Each large square encloses a volume of 1/10 mm^3, and the dilution is 1 : 20. A general formula is as follows:

Leukocyte count (cells/mm^3) = $(cc/lsc) \times d \times 10$

where cc is the total number of cells counted, d is the dilution factor, 10 is the factor transforming value over one large square (1/10 mm^3) to the volume in mm^3, and lsc is the number of large squares counted. In leukopenia, with a total count below 2500, the blood is diluted 1 : 10. In leukocytosis, the dilution may be 1 : 100 or even 1 : 200.

Sources of Error. Errors may be due to the nature of the sample, to the operator's technique, and to inaccurate equipment. Errors that are inherent in the distribution of cells in the counting volume are called 'field' errors and can be minimized only by counting more cells.

Hemocytometer leukocyte counts show a CV of about 6.5% for normal and increased counts, and about 15% in leukopenic blood. Utilizing

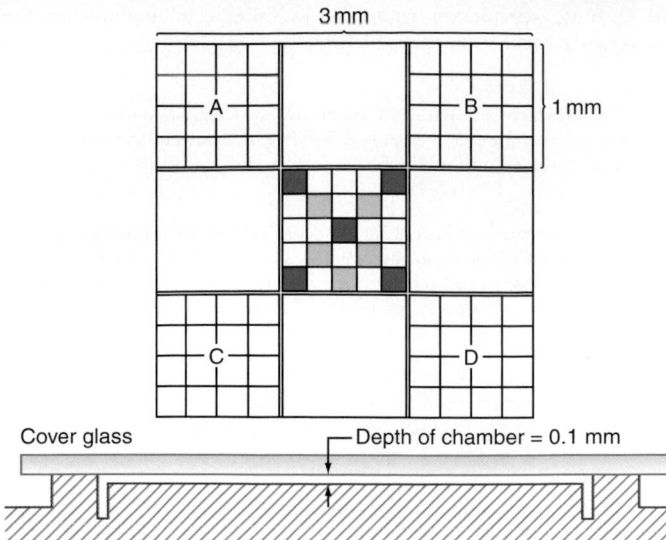

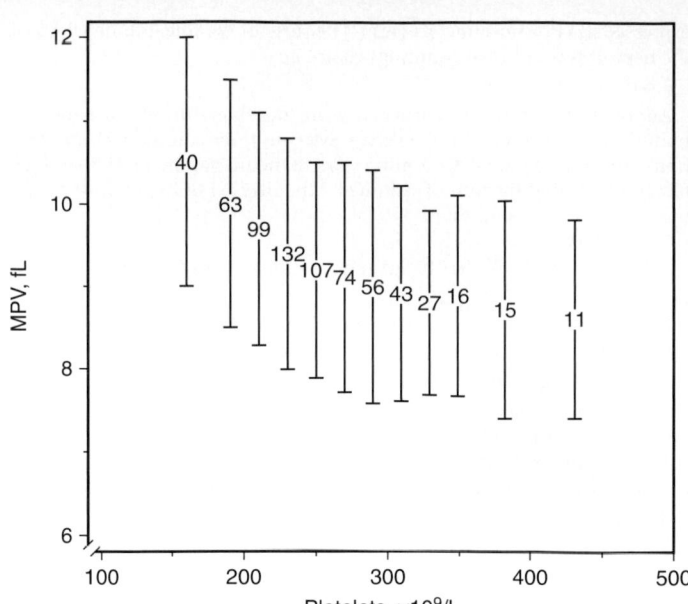

Figure 29–3 The upper figure is a diagram of the improved Neubauer ruling; this is etched on the surface of each side of the hemocytometer. The large corner squares, A, B, C, and D, are used for leukocyte counts. The five blue squares in the center are used for red cell counts or for platelet counts, and the 10 green plus blue squares for platelet counts. Actually, each of the 25 squares within the central sq mm has within it 16 smaller squares for convenience in counting. The lower figure is a side view of the chamber with the cover glass in place.

Figure 29–4 Mean platelet volume related to platelet count in 683 normal subjects. Each group is shown as mean (number) 2 SD (bar) of subjects grouped by platelet counts of 128–179, 180–199, 200–219, 220–239, 240–259, 260–279, 280–299, 300–319, 320–339, 340–359, 360–403, 404–462 × 10⁹/L. The number of the mean position is the number of subjects in the group (Bessman, 1981).

electronic counters, on the other hand, results in CVs of approximately 1–3%.

Errors Due to the Nature of the Sample. Partial coagulation of the venous blood causes changes in the distribution of the cells and/or decrease of their number. Failure to mix the blood thoroughly and immediately before dilution introduces an error, which depends on the degree of sedimentation.

Operator's Errors. Errors caused by faulty technique may occur during dilution, when the chamber is loaded, and when the cells are counted.

Errors Due to Equipment. Equipment errors can be diminished by using pipets and hemocytometers which are certified by the US Bureau of Standards.

Inherent or Field Errors. Even in a perfectly mixed sample, variation occurs in the number of suspended cells that are distributed in a given volume (i.e., come to rest over a given square). This 'error of the field' is the minimal error. Another error is the 'error of the chamber,' which includes variations in separate fillings of a given chamber, and in sizes of different chambers. Still another is the 'error of the pipet,' which includes variations in filling a given pipet, and in the sizes of different pipets. In performing a WBC count, if 200 cells are counted using two chambers and one pipet, the CV = 9.1%, corresponding to 95% confidence limits of ± 18.2% (twice the CV). Using four chambers and two pipets and counting twice as many cells reduces the 95% confidence limits to ± 12.8%. This relatively large percentage error is of little practical consequence because of the physiologic variation of the leukocyte count.

Nucleated Red Cells. Nucleated red blood cells (NRBCs) will be counted and cannot be distinguished from leukocytes with the magnification used. If their number is high as seen on the stained smear, a correction should be made according to the following formula:

True leukocyte count = (Total count × 100)/(100 + No. of NRBCs)

where the No. of NRBCs = the number of nucleated red cells that are counted during the enumeration of 100 leukocytes in the differential count.

Example. The blood smear shows 25 nucleated red cells per 100 leukocytes. The total nucleated cell count is 10 000.

True leukocyte count = 10 000 × 100/125 = 8000/μL (8.0 × 10⁹/L)

Reference value. In the total leukocyte count, no distinction is made among the six normal cell types (neutrophils and bands, lymphocytes, monocytes, eosinophils, and basophils). The reference interval for adults is 4.5–11.0 × 10⁹/L.

Platelet Counts

Platelets are thin disks, 2–4 μm in diameter and 5–7 fL in volume (in citrated blood). They function in hemostasis, in maintaining vascular integrity, and in the process of blood coagulation.

In EDTA-blood, the mean platelet volume (MPV) increases with time up to 1 hour in vitro, is relatively stable between 1–3 hours, and then increases further with time. Change from a discoid to a spherical shape accounts for this increase in apparent volume in EDTA compared with citrate (Rowan, 1982). For reproducible results, platelet volume measurements obtained with multichannel instruments should be made between 1–3 hours after the blood is drawn. The frequency distribution of platelet volumes in an individual is log normal. There is, however, a nonlinear, inverse relationship between the MPV and the platelet count within normal individuals (Fig. 29–4). Therefore, reference values for the MPV appear to vary with the platelet count (Bessman, 1981). The MPV is generally increased in hyperthyroidism (Ford, 1988) and myeloproliferative disease (Small, 1981). Platelets are more difficult to count, because they are small (must be distinguished from debris) and have a tendency to adhere to glass, any foreign body, and particularly to one another. It is often possible to recognize a significant decrease in the number of platelets by a careful inspection of stained films. With capillary blood, films must be made evenly and very quickly after the blood is obtained in order to avoid clumping and to minimize the decrease due to adhesion of platelets to the margins of the injured vessels. A better estimate is possible by examining stained films made from venous blood with EDTA as an anticoagulant (EDTA-blood), in which platelets are evenly distributed and where clumping normally does not occur. The visual method of choice employs the phase-contrast microscope. This is the reference method. Laboratories performing over five platelet counts per day can justify electronic platelet counting; both the voltage pulse counting and the electro-optical counting systems are satisfactory.

Hemocytometer Method – Phase-Contrast Microscope

Specimen. Venous blood is collected with EDTA as the anticoagulant. Blood from skin puncture wounds gives more variable results, but is satisfactory if the blood is flowing freely and if only the first few drops are used.

Diluent Solution. One percent ammonium oxalate is mixed in distilled water. The stock bottle is kept in the refrigerator. The amount needed for the day is filtered before use and the unused portion discarded at end of day.

Procedure

1. Well-mixed blood is diluted 1 : 100 in diluting fluid, and the vial containing the suspension is rotated on a mechanical mixer for 10–15 minutes.
2. The hemocytometer is filled in the usual fashion, using a separate capillary tube for each side.
3. The chamber is covered with a Petri dish for 15 minutes to allow settling of the platelets in one optical plane. A piece of wet cotton or filter paper is left beneath the dish to prevent evaporation.
4. The platelets appear round or oval and frequently have one or more dendritic processes. Their internal granular structure and a purple

sheen allow the platelets to be distinguished from debris, which is often refractile. Ghosts of the red cells that have been lysed by the ammonium oxalate are seen in the background.

5. Platelets are counted in 10 small squares (the black squares in Fig. 29–3), five on each side of the chamber. If the total number of platelets counted is fewer than 100, more small squares are counted until at least 100 platelets have been recorded; 10 squares per side (black plus shaded squares; see Fig. 29–3) or all 25 squares in the large central square on each side of the hemocytometer, if necessary. If the total number of platelets in all 50 of these small squares is fewer than 50, the count should be repeated with a 1 : 20 or 1 : 10 dilution of blood.

Calculation. Each of the 25 small squares defines a volume of $1/250\,\mu L$ ($1/25\,mm^2$ area × $1/10$ mm depth): the platelet count (per μL) = (Number of cells counted/Number of squares counted) × Dilution × 250.

By adjusting the number of squares so that at least 100 platelets are counted, the field error (the statistical error due to counting a limited number of platelets in the chamber) can be kept in the same range for low platelet counts as for high platelet counts. It has been shown that the CV due to combined field, pipet, and chamber errors is about 11% when at least 100 platelets are counted and 15% when 40 platelets are counted.

Platelet counts tend to be the least reproducible of the blood cell counts, and the technologist must be vigilant to ensure their accuracy. This includes the readiness to confirm suspicious or abnormal results with a freshly drawn sample. Whenever the platelet count is in question, such as with an instrument flag, the blood film (prepared from EDTA-blood) must be checked to corroborate the count and to detect abnormalities in platelets or other blood elements that may give a false value. Further, due to the low number of platelets counted in the manual method, and the high degree of imprecision with severe thrombocytopenia (CV > 15%), 7×10^9 platelets/L is the lowest count that should be reported from manual quantitation (Hanseler, 1996).

Sources of Error. Blood in EDTA is satisfactory for 5 hours after collection at 20°C and for 24 hours at 4°C, provided that no difficulty was encountered in collection. Platelet clumps present in the chamber imply a maldistribution and negate the reliability of the count; a new sample of blood must be collected. The causes of platelet clumping are likely to be initiation of platelet aggregation and clotting before the blood reaches the anticoagulant; imperfect venipuncture; delay in the anticoagulant contacting the blood; or, in skin puncture technique, delay in sampling. Capillary blood gives similar mean values, but errors are about twice those with venous blood, probably because the platelet level varies in successive drops of blood from the skin puncture wound.

Falsely Elevated Counts. Fragments of leukocyte cytoplasm that are sometimes numerous in leukemias may falsely elevate the count. The phase-contrast hemocytometer method must be employed in these cases with a correction made based on the ratio of fragments to platelets determined from the blood film.

Falsely low counts. These can occur if platelets adhere to neutrophils (platelet satellitism) or if there is platelet clumping due to agglutinins (Lombarts, 1988), spontaneous aggregation, or incipient clotting due to faulty blood collection. The first two of these phenomena appear to depend on EDTA (Dacie, 1991). The reported incidence of EDTA-induced in vitro platelet clumping and pseudothrombocytopenia has ranged from 0.1% (Bartels, 1997) to 2% (Lippi, 1990). Alterations in the platelet histograms or quantitative cutoff measures derived from them should be used to screen for pseudothrombocytopenia (Bartels, 1997).

Variation in automated platelet count

There are standard guidelines with each instrument that mandate performing manual platelet counts below and above the established reference ranges. For example, an automated platelet count below 30×10^9/L using Technicon HP81 should be replaced by the manual procedure (Hanseler, 1996).

Comparing the ADVIA 120 to Coulter STKS, Stanworth (1999) showed that in some cases of thrombocytopenia due to peripheral consumption, the ADVIA gave higher platelet counts and the blood film showed some large platelets. Further study with platelet-specific monoclonal antibodies such as CD61 will likely determine which is the more correct count. Cantero (1996) showed that visibly turbid plasma in blood specimens resulted in on average a 47% increase in platelet count with the Technicon H P83.

Reference values for platelet counts are $150–450 \times 10^9$/L. The reference values for MPV are approximately 6.5–12 fL in adults.

Reticulated Platelets

Reticulated platelets are those newly released circulating platelets that have residual RNA. Reticulated platelet counts are an estimate of thrombopoiesis

(Rapi, 1998), analogous to a reticulocyte count's use as an estimate of erythropoiesis. Matic (1998) describes an optimized flow cytometric analysis method after incubating whole blood with thiazole orange, which has a 3000-fold increase in fluorescence after binding to RNA. Phycoerythrin-labeled antibodies directed against GPIb on the surface of the platelet are also in the incubation mixture to distinguish platelets from other cells or debris. Recombinant human erythropoietin seems to improve platelet function in uremia not only through correction of the anemia, but also by increasing young platelets, detected as reticulated platelets (Tassies, 1998). Significantly lower median levels of reticulated platelets in frequent plateletpheresis donors than in new donors suggests that repeat platelet donation might lead to a relative exhaustion of thrombopoiesis (Stohlawetz, 1998). Depending on the conditions of the measurement, published normal values for reticulated platelets vary tremendously from 3–20% (Matic, 1998).

Increased reticulated platelet values have been reported in idiopathic thrombocytopenic purpura (Koike, 1998; Saxton, 1998), and hyperthyroidism (Stiegler, 1998). In neonates younger than 30 weeks' gestation the reticulated platelet count was about twice that seen in full-term infants (Peterec, 1996). Bone marrow recovery after chemotherapy for acute myeloid leukemia (AML) showed an increase in reticulated platelets after about day 20 (Stohlawetz, 1999). *Decreased* reticulated platelet values have been reported in association with aplasia and liver cirrhosis (Koike, 1998; Saxton, 1998).

Electronic Counting

Due to the relatively low cost, reduced time (for labor and results), and increased accuracy of the automated analyzers, semiautomated instruments are rarely used in clinical practice these days. Speed of performance, elimination of visual fatigue of the technician, and improved precision are decisive advantages of the electronic cell counter over the hemocytometer/manual methods of performing blood cell counts. The electronic counting instruments are discussed in more detail below under Instrument Technology.

Physiologic Variation

Physiologic Variation in Erythrocytes

Changes in red cell values are greatest during the first few weeks of life (Fig. 29–5). At the time of birth, as much as 100–125 mL of placental blood may be added to the newborn if tying the cord is postponed until its pulsation ceases. In a study of newborns whose cords had been clamped late, the average capillary red cell counts were 0.4×10^{12}/L higher 1 hour after and 0.8×10^{12}/L higher 24 hours after birth compared with newborns whose cords had been clamped early. Capillary blood (obtained by skin puncture) gives higher RBC and Hb values than venous blood (cord). The differences may amount to about 0.5×10^{12} RBC/L and 3 g Hb/dL. The slowing of capillary circulation and the resulting loss of fluid may be the responsible factor. Examination of venous blood furnishes more consistent results than examination of capillary blood.

In the full-term infant, nucleated red cells average about 0.5×10^9/L. The normoblast count declines to about 200/μL at 24 hours, 25/μL at 48 hours, and less than 5/μL at 72 hours. By 7 days, it is rare to find circulating normoblasts (Barone, 1999).

The normal *reticulocyte count* at birth ranges from 3–7% during the first 48 hours, during which time it rises slightly. After the second day, it falls rather rapidly to 1–3% by the seventh day of life. Hemoglobin concentration in capillary blood during the first day of life averages 19.0 g/dL, with 95% of normal values falling between 14.6–23.4 g/dL. In cord blood the average is 16.8 g/dL, with 95% of normal between 13.5–20 g/dL. There is frequently an initial increase in the hemoglobin level of venous blood at the end of 24 hours compared with that of cord blood. At the end of the first week, the level is about the same as in cord blood and it does not begin to fall until after the second week. During the first 2 weeks, the lower limit of normal is 14.5 g/dL for capillary blood and 13.0 g/dL for venous blood. The hematocrit in capillary blood on the first day of life averages 0.61, with 95% of normal values between 0.46–0.76. In cord blood, the average is 0.53. The changes during the first few weeks parallel the hemoglobin concentration. The Hb and Hct are highest at birth but fall rather steeply in the first days and weeks of life to a minimum at 2 months of age, at which time the lower limit of the 95% reference values and the mean value for the Hb are 9.4 and 11.2 g/dL, and for the Hct are 0.28 and 0.35, respectively. After the age of 4 months, the lower limit for the Hb is 11.2 g/dL and the Hct is 0.32; the values rise gradually until about age 5 years, and somewhat more steeply in boys than in girls thereafter (Shannon, 1996). The normal MCV at birth ranges from

IV

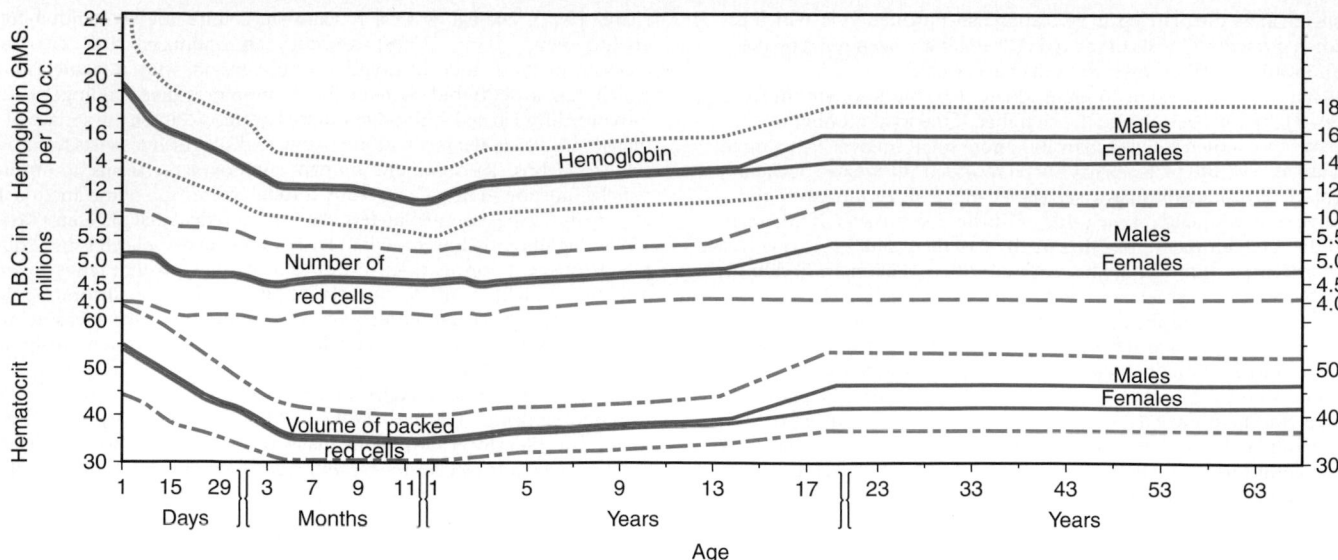

Figure 29–5 Values for hemoglobin, hematocrit (volume of packed red cells), and red cell counts from birth to old age. Mean values are heavy lines. Reference interval for hemoglobin is indicated by dotted lines, for red cell counts by interrupted lines, and for hematocrit by dotted interrupted lines. The scales on the ordinate are similar so that relative changes in hemoglobin, red cell count, and hematocrit are apparent on inspection. The scale for age, however, is progressively altered (Wintrobe, 1974).

104–118 fL, compared with the adult reference interval of 80–96 fL. Because the RBC does not fall to the degree that the Hb and Hct do, the MCV decreases abruptly, then gradually, during the first few months of life. The lowest value is reached at about 1 year. In studies in which iron deficiency and thalassemia are excluded, the lower reference limit (95% reference values) for the MCV gradually rises between the ages of 1 year and 15 years – in boys from 70 to 76 fL, and in girls from 70 to 78 fL (Shannon, 1996). Reference intervals for red blood cell values in sexually mature adults are given in Table 29-2. The indices are similar in males and females, but the Hb is 1–2 g/dL higher in males, with commensurate increments in Hct and RBCs (Fig. 29-5). This is believed to be mainly the effects of androgen in stimulating erythropoietin production and its effect on the marrow. In older men, the Hb tends to fall and in older women the Hb tends to fall to a lesser degree (in some studies) or even rise slightly (in other studies). In older individuals, therefore, the sex difference is less than 1 g Hb/dL (Dacie, 1991). Posture and muscular activity change the concentration of the formed elements. The Hb, Hct, and RBC increase by several percent when the change from recumbency to standing is made, and strenuous muscular activity causes a further increase, presumably owing primarily to loss of plasma water. Diurnal variation that is not related to exercise or to analytical variation also occurs. The Hb is highest in the morning, falls during the day, and is lowest in the evening, with a mean difference of 8–9% (Dacie, 1991).

In persons living at a higher altitude, the Hb, Hct, and RBC are elevated over what they would be at sea level. The difference is about 1 g Hb/dL at 2 km altitude and 2 g Hb/dL at 3 km. Increased erythropoiesis is secondary to anoxic stimulation of erythropoietin production. People who are smokers also tend to have a mild erythrocytosis.

Physiologic Variation in Leukocytes

The total white cell count at birth and during the first 24 hours varies within wide limits. Neutrophils are the predominant cell, varying from $6–28 \times 10^9/L$; about 15% of these are band forms (Altman, 1974), and a few myelocytes are present. Neutrophils drop to about $5 \times 10^9/L$ during the first week and remain at about the same level thereafter. Lymphocytes are about $5.5 \times 10^9/L$ at birth, and change little during the first week. They become the predominant cell, on the average, after the first week of life and remain so until about age 7, when neutrophils again predominate. The upper limit of the 95% reference interval for lymphocytes at age 6 months is 13.5, at 1 year 10.5, at 2 years 9.5, at 6 years 7.0, and at 12 years $6.0 \times 10^9/L$. For neutrophils at the same ages, the values are 8.5, 8.5, 8.5, 8.0, and $8.0 \times 10^9/L$, respectively, all somewhat higher than those for adults (see Table 29-3).

Diurnal variation has been recognized in the neutrophil count, with highest levels in the afternoon and lowest levels in the morning at rest. Exercise produces leukocytosis, which includes an increased neutrophil concentration as a result of a shift of cells from marginal to circulating granulocyte pool. Increased lymphocyte drainage into the blood also appears to contribute to the total increase. Both the average and the lower reference values for neutrophil concentration in the black population are

Table 29-2 Typical Blood Cell Values in a Normal Population of Young Adults

	Men	Women
White cell count ($\times 10^9/L$ blood)	7.8 (4.4–11.3)	
Red cell count ($\times 10^{12}/L$ blood)	5.21 (4.52–5.90)	4.60 (4.10–5.10)
Hemoglobin (g/dL blood)	15.7 (14.0–17.5)	13.8 (12.3–15.3)
Hematocrit (percent)	46 (41.5–50.4)	40.2 (35.9–44.6)
Mean cell volume (fL/red cell)	88.0 (80.0–96.1)	
Mean cell hemoglobin (pg/red cell)	30.4 (27.5–33.2)	
Mean cell hemoglobin concentration (g/dL RBC)	34.4 (33.4–35.5)	
Red cell distribution width (CV, percent)	13.1 (11.6–14.6)	
Platelet count ($\times 10^9/L$ blood)	311 (172–450)	

The mean and reference internal (normal range) are given. Because the distribution curves may be nongaussian, the reference interval is the nonparametric central 95% confidence interval. Results are based on 426 normal adult men and 212 normal adult women. Studies were performed on the Coulter model S-Plus IV (Morris, 1975).

lower than in the white; this difference must be taken into account in assessing neutropenia. Cigarette smokers have higher average leukocyte counts than nonsmokers. The increase is greatest (about 30%) in heavy smokers who inhale, and affects neutrophils, lymphocytes, and monocytes.

There appear to be mild changes during the menstrual cycle. Neutrophils and monocytes fall and eosinophils tend to rise during menstruation. Basophils have been reported to fall during ovulation. The availability of precise automated leukocyte analyzers provides the potential for investigating physiologic sources of variation that have been obscured by the statistical error in traditional microscopic differential counts (Statland, 1978).

Physiologic Variation in Platelets

The average platelet count is slightly lower at birth than in older children and adults, and may vary from $84–478 \times 10^9/L$ (Barone, 1999). After the first week of life, the reference intervals are those of the adult. In women, the platelet count may fall at the time of menstruation. Women have higher platelet (and WBC and neutrophil) counts than men, and Africans (and less so Afro-Caribbeans) have lower platelet, WBC, and neutrophil

Table 29-3 Normal Leukocyte Count, Differential Count, and Hemoglobin Concentration at Various Ages

Age	Leukocytes*								Hemoglobin (g/dL blood)
	Total leukocytes	Total neutrophils	Band neutrophils	Segmented neutrophils	Eosinophils	Basophils	Lymphocytes	Monocytes	
12 months	11.4 (6.0–17.5)	3.5 (1.5–8.5) *31*	0.35 *3.1*	3.2 (1.0–8.5) *28*	0.30 (0.05–0.70) *2.6*	0.05 (0–0.20) *0.4*	7.0 (4.0–10.5) *61*	0.55 (0.05–1.1) *4.8*	12.6 (11.1–14.1)
4 years	9.1 (5.5–15.5)	3.8 (1.5–8.5) *42*	0.27 (0–1.0) *3.0*	3.5 (1.5–7.5) *39*	0.25 (0.02–0.65) *2.8*	0.05 (0–0.2) *0.6*	4.5 (2.0–8.0) *50*	0.45 (0–0.8) *5.0*	12.7 (11.2–14.3)
6 years	8.5 (5.0–14.5)	4.3 (1.5–8.0) *51*	0.25 (0–1.0) *3.0*	4.0 (1.5–7.0) *48*	0.23 (0–0.65) *2.7*	0.05 (0–0.2) *0.6*	3.5 (1.50–7.0) *42*	0.40 (0–0.8) *4.7*	13.0 (11.4–14.5)
10 years	8.1 (4.5–13.5)	4.4 (1.8–8.0) *54*	0.24 (0–1.0) *3.0*	4.2 (1.8–7.0) *51*	0.20 (0–0.60) *2.4*	0.04 (0–0.2) *0.5*	3.1 (1.5–6.5) *38*	0.35 (0–0.8) *4.3*	13.4 (11.8–15.0)
21 years	7.4 (4.5–11.0)	4.4 (1.8–7.7) *59*	0.22 (0–0.7) *3.0*	4.2 (1.8–7.0) *56*	0.20 (0–0.45) *2.7*	0.04 (0–0.2) *0.5*	2.5 (1.0–4.8) *34*	0.30 (0–0.8) *4.0*	15.5 (13.5–17.5) 13.8 (12.0–15.6)

* Values are expressed as mean (95% reference) values. For leukocytes and differential count cell types, the units are cells $\times 10^9/\mu L$; the numbers in italic type are mean percentages.

Source: For leukocyte and differential count (Altman, 1961); For hemoglobin concentrations (Dalman, 1987).

counts than Caucasians (Bain, 1996). Reported mean (95% reference ranges) for platelet counts were 218 (143–332) for Caucasian men and 183 (115–290) for African men versus 246 (169–358) for Caucasian women and 207 (125–342) for African women. Tsang (1998), for Australians west of Sydney and aged 49 or more, lists 247 (128–365) for mean platelet counts for men and 275 (147–403) for women.

Erythrocyte Sedimentation Rate

Erythrocyte sedimentation rate (ESR) is a useful, but nonspecific marker of underlying inflammation. More recently, high-sensitivity C-reactive protein and other inflammatory markers have been used to detect or monitor disease, particularly cardiovascular disease and metabolic syndrome (Rifai, 2005; Pearson, 2003). When well-mixed venous blood is placed in a vertical tube, erythrocytes will tend to fall toward the bottom. The length of fall of the top of the column of erythrocytes in a given interval of time is called the erythrocyte sedimentation rate (ESR). Several factors are involved.

Plasma Factors

An accelerated ESR is favored by elevated levels of fibrinogen and, to a lesser extent, α_2-, β-, and γ-globulins. These asymmetric protein molecules have a greater effect than other proteins in decreasing the negative charge of erythrocytes (zeta potential) that tends to keep them apart. The decreased zeta potential promotes the formation of rouleaux, which sediment more rapidly than single cells. Removal of fibrinogen by defibrination lowers the ESR. There is no absolute correlation between the ESR and any of the plasma protein fractions. Albumin and lecithin retard sedimentation, and cholesterol accelerates the ESR.

Red Cell Factors

Anemia increases the ESR, because the change in the erythrocyte plasma ratio favors rouleau formation, independently of changes in the concentration of the plasma proteins. By any method of measurement, the ESR is most sensitive to altered plasma proteins in the hematocrit range of 0.30–0.40 (Bull, 1975). The sedimentation rate is directly proportional to the weight of the cell aggregate and inversely proportional to the surface area. Microcytes sediment slower than macrocytes, which have decreased surface area/volume ratios. Rouleaux also have a decreased surface area/volume ratio and accelerate the ESR. Red cells with an abnormal or irregular shape, such as sickle cells or spherocytes, hinder rouleaux formation and lower the ESR.

Stages in the ESR

Three stages can be observed: (1) In the initial 10 minutes, there is little sedimentation as rouleaux form. (2) For about 40 minutes, settling occurs at a constant rate. (3) Sedimentation slows in the final 10 minutes as cells pack at the bottom of the tube.

Methods

Westergren Method

Because of its simplicity, the Westergren method is widely used. The ICSH (1993) has recommended it as the reference method utilizing undiluted whole blood. The ICSH states that the patient's hematocrit should not exceed 35% because reproducibility of sedimentation may be poorer in narrow tubes. A formula to convert between diluted blood ESR and undiluted is: Diluted blood ESR = (Undiluted ESR × 0.86) − 12.

Equipment. The Westergren tube is a straight pipet 30 cm long, 2.55 mm in internal diameter, and calibrated in millimeters from 0–200. It holds about 1 mL. The Westergren rack is also used, with levelers as needed for a vertical tube position.

Reagent. A 0.105 molar solution (range, 0.10–0.136) of sodium citrate is used as the anticoagulant–diluent solution (31 g of $Na_3C_6H_5O_7 \bullet H_2O$ added to 1 L of distilled water in a sterile glass bottle). This is filtered and kept refrigerated without preservatives.

Procedure

1. Two milliliters of whole blood is added to 0.5 mL of sodium citrate and mixed by inversion.
2. A Westergren pipet is filled to the 0 mark and placed exactly vertical in the rack at room temperature without vibration or exposure to direct sunlight.
3. After exactly 60 minutes, the distance from the 0 mark to the top of the column of red cells is recorded in millimeters as the ESR value. If the demarcation between plasma and red cell column is hazy, the level is taken where the full density is first apparent.

Modified Westergren Method

A modification of the Westergren method produces the same results but employs blood anticoagulated with EDTA rather than with citrate. This is more convenient, since it allows the ESR to be performed from the same tube of blood as is used for other hematological studies. Two milliliters of well-mixed EDTA-blood is diluted either with 0.5 mL of 3.8% sodium citrate or with 0.5 mL of 0.85% sodium chloride. Undiluted blood anticoagulated with EDTA gives poor precision (ICSH, 1977). The ESR gradually increases with age. Westergren's original upper limits of normal (10 mm/h for men and 20 mm/h for women) appear to be too low. According to studies of Böttiger (1967) and Zauber (1987), upper limits of reference values for the Westergren method should be as follows:

	Men	Women
Below age 50 years	15 mm/h	20 mm/h
Above age 50 years	20 mm/h	30 mm/h
Above age 85 years	30 mm/h	42 mm/h

Smith (1994) states that the rise in ESR with age likely reflects higher disease prevalence in the elderly and therefore for practical purposes it may be advisable to use the standard normal range in elderly patients.

Sources of Error

If the concentration of the anticoagulant is higher than recommended, the ESR may be elevated. Sodium citrate or EDTA does not affect the rate of sedimentation if used in the proper concentration. Heparin, however, alters the membrane zeta potential and cannot be used as an anticoagulant. It can also increase the ESR when used as a medication in vivo (Penchas, 1978). Bubbles left in the tube when it is filled will affect the ESR. Hemolysis may modify the sedimentation. The cleanliness of the tube is important. Tilting the tube accelerates the ESR. The red cells

IV

aggregate along the lower side while the plasma rises along the upper side. Consequently, the retarding influence of the rising plasma is less effective. An angle of even 3 degrees from the vertical may accelerate the ESR by as much as 30%. Plastic ESR pipets have slightly higher (1–2 mm/h) values than glass (Schneiderka, 1997).

Temperature should be within the range of 20–25°C. Lower or higher temperatures in some cases alter the ESR. If the blood has been kept refrigerated, it should be permitted to reach room temperature and be mixed by inversion a minimum of eight times before the test is performed. The test should be set up within 2 hours after the blood sample is obtained (or 12 hours if EDTA is used as the anticoagulant and the blood is kept at 4°C); otherwise, some samples with elevated ESRs will be falsely low (Morris, 1975). On standing, erythrocytes tend to become spherical and less readily form rouleaux.

There is no effective method for correcting for anemia in the Westergren method, as there is in the Wintrobe method.

VES-MATIC 20 Instrument

The VES-MATIC 20 instrument is a bench top analyzer designed to measure the erythrocyte sedimentation rate (ESR) in 20 blood samples (Plebani, 1998; Caswell, 1991). It is completely automated. The blood is collected in the special cuvets, and carefully mixed by the instrument; the samples are then left to sediment for a certain period. The 18-degree slant of the tubes with respect to the vertical axis causes an acceleration of the sedimentation, allowing results comparable to those of Westergren at the first hour to be obtained in only 25 minutes, while those comparable to Westergren at the second hour require only 45 minutes. The optoelectric sensors automatically read the erythrocyte sedimentation level. The data are elaborated and then printed or visualized on the display.

Micro-ESR Method

This method has more utility in pediatric patients. Barrett (1980) described a micro-ESR method using 0.2 mL blood to fill a plastic disposable tube 230 mm long with a 1-mm internal bore. Capillary blood values correlated well with venous blood micro-ESR and Westergren ESR values. Kumar (1994) refers to a micro-ESR (mESR) that utilizes whole blood to completely fill a 75-mm heparinized microhematocrit capillary tube.

Application

The ESR is one of the oldest laboratory tests still in use. Although some of its usefulness has decreased as more specific methods of evaluating disease (such as C-reactive protein [CRP]) have been developed (Zlonis, 1993), new clinical applications are being reported (Saadeh, 1998). Recently, the ESR has been reported to be of clinical significance in sickle cell disease (low value in absence of painful crisis, moderately increased 1 week into crisis); osteomyelitis (elevated, helpful in following therapy); stroke (ESR of ≥28 mm/h has poorer prognosis); prostate cancer (ESR ≥37 mm/h has higher incidence of disease progression and death), and coronary artery disease (ESR > 22 mm/h in white men had high risk of CAD) (Saadeh, 1998). In pregnancy, the ESR increases moderately, beginning at the tenth to twelfth week, and returns to normal about 1 month postpartum. The ESR tends to be markedly elevated in monoclonal blood protein disorders such as multiple myeloma or macroglobulinemia, in severe polyclonal hyperglobulinemias due to inflammatory disease, and in hyperfibrinogenemias.

Moderate elevations are common in active inflammatory disease such as rheumatoid arthritis, chronic infections, collagen disease, and neoplastic disease. The ESR has little diagnostic value in these disorders, but can be useful in monitoring disease activity. It is simpler than measurement of serum proteins, which has tended to replace the ESR. Because the test is often normal in patients with neoplasms, connective tissue disease, and infections, a normal ESR cannot be used to exclude these diagnostic possibilities. In patients with known cancer, however, when the value exceeds 100 mm/h, metastases are usually present (Sox, 1986). The ESR is of little value in screening asymptomatic patients for disease; history and physical examination will usually disclose the cause of an elevated ESR (Sox, 1986). The ESR is useful and is indicated in establishing the diagnosis and in monitoring polymyalgia rheumatica and temporal arteritis where the rate typically exceeds 90 mm/h (Zlonis, 1993). Emergency physicians continue to use the ESR in evaluating temporal arteritis, septic arthritis, pelvic inflammatory disease, and appendicitis (Olshaker, 1997). Freeman (1997) urges immediate quick ESR estimation if giant cell arteritis is clinically indicated, as a delay of even a few hours in starting steroid therapy may result in irreversible visual failure. Harrow (1999) concludes that an ESR of 5 mm or less at 30 minutes correctly identifies the majority of patients with normal ESR without misclassifying elevated ESRs.

In Hodgkin's disease, the ESR may be a very useful prognostic blood measurement in the absence of systemic ('B') symptoms (fever, weight

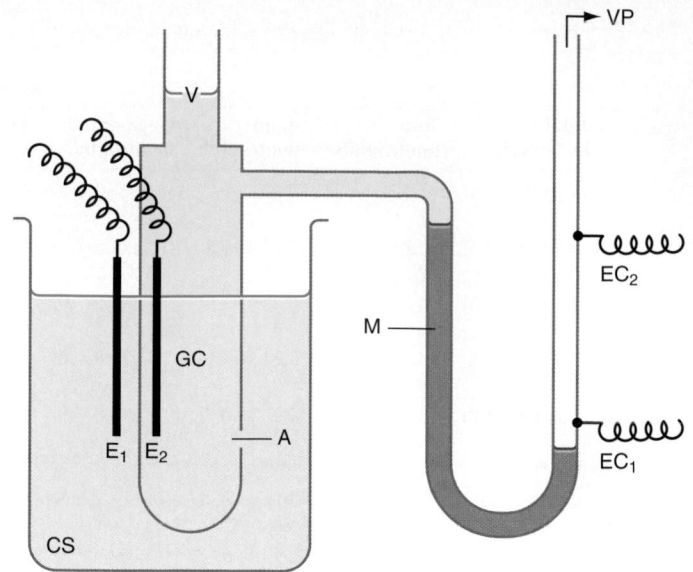

Figure 29–6 Schematic diagram of particle counter in which changes in electrical resistance are counted as voltage pulses. CS = cell suspension; GC = glass cylinder; A = aperture; E_1 and E_2 = platinum electrodes; V = value; M = mercury column; EC_1 and EC_2 = electrical contacts; VP = vacuum pump. (Diagram adapted from Ackerman, 1972).

loss, night sweats). In one study (Vaughan Hudson, 1987), one-third of asymptomatic patients had both an ESR of less than 10 mm/h and an excellent survival rate regardless of age, stage, or histopathology. The asymptomatic patients with an ESR of 60 mm/h or greater had a survival rate as poor as those with systemic symptoms.

Iversen (1996) reported that 70% of renal cell carcinoma patients had an increased ESR, which had been significantly rising for up to 6 years before diagnosis. They argue for a systematic graphing and baseline determination of the ESR over time, which shows a marked elevation in ESR 1 year prior to diagnosis. Such a trend of increasing ESR should lead to further investigation, such as a renal ultrasound, which may then lead to curative nephrectomy before metastases occur.

Instrument Technology

The multichannel instruments used in the modern laboratory for performing cell counts are based on the principles of electric impedance, light scattering, radiofrequency conductivity and/or cytochemistry (Ward, 2000). The principles of these techniques are discussed in the following section.

Electrical Impedance

Cells passing through an aperture through which a current is flowing cause changes in electrical resistance that are counted as voltage pulses. This principle, illustrated in Figure 29–6, is used in instruments marketed by Coulter (LH 700, GEN•S, HmX, A•T, etc.; Beckman Coulter, Inc., Brea, CA); Sysmex (XE-2100, XT 2000i, HST-N, etc.; Sysmex America, Inc., Mundelein, IL); Abbott (Cell-Dyn 3500, 3700, 4000, etc.; Abbott Diagnostics, Santa Clara, CA); ABX (Micros 60, Pentra 60, Pentra 120, Pentra 120 Retic, etc.; ABX Diagnostics, Inc., Irvine, CA), and others. An accurately diluted suspension of blood (CS) is made in an isotonic conductive solution that preserves the cell shape. The instrument has a glass cylinder (GC) that can be filled with the conducting fluid and has within it an electrode (E_2) and an aperture (A) of 100 µm diameter in its wall. Just outside the glass cylinder is another electrode (E_1). The cylinder is connected to a U-shaped glass tube that is partly filled with mercury (M) and that has two electrical contacts (EC_1 and EC_2). The glass cylinder is immersed in the suspension of cells to be counted (CS) and is filled with conductive solution and closed by a valve (V). A current now flows through the aperture between E_1 and E_2. As mercury moves up the tube, the cell suspension is drawn through the aperture into the cylinder. Each cell that passes through the aperture displaces an equal volume of conductive fluid, increasing the electrical resistance and creating a voltage pulse, because its resistance is much greater than that of the conductive solution. The pulses, which are proportional in height to the volume of the cells, are counted. This is the Coulter principle.

In the simplest system, the counting mechanism is started when the mercury contacts EC_1 and stopped when it contacts EC_2; during this time the cells are counted in a volume of suspension exactly equal to the volume of the glass tubing between contact wires EC_1 and EC_2. If two or more cells

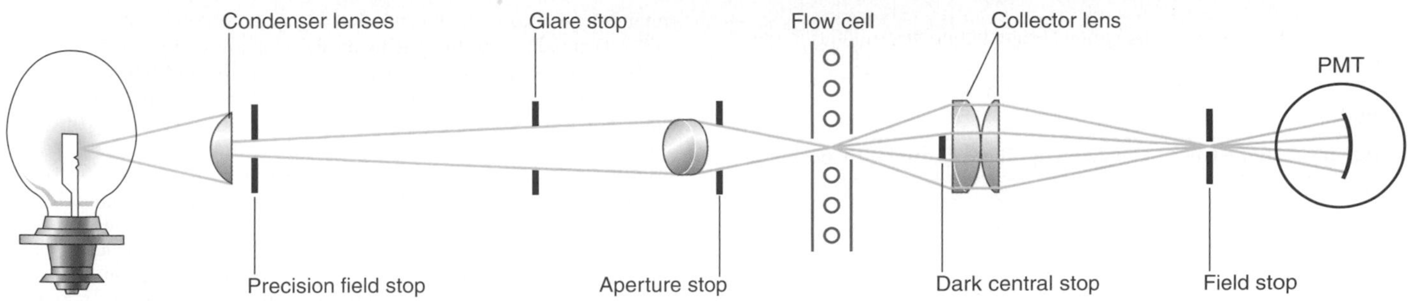

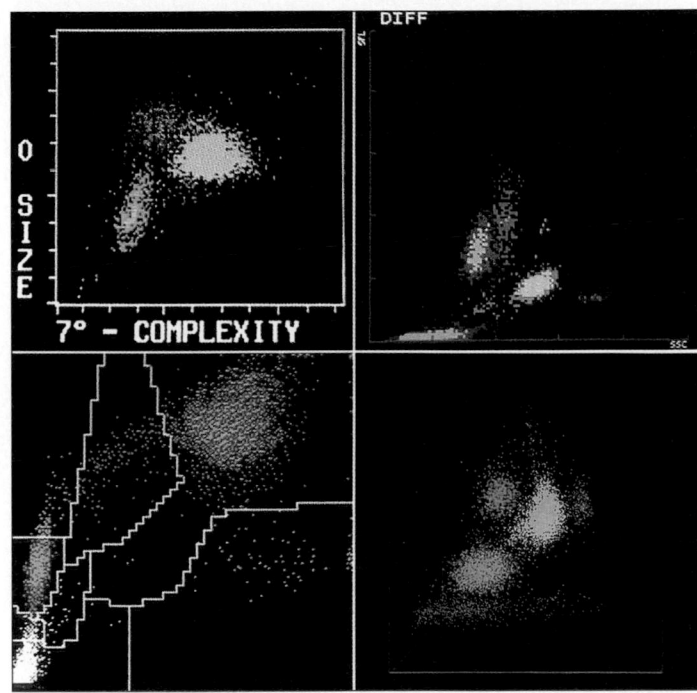

Figure 29–7 Schematic diagram of the electro-optical cell counter. Light is focused on the flow cell. Only light scattered by a cell reaches the photomultiplier tube (PMT), which converts to an electrical pulse. (From Mansberg HP: Adv Automated Anal 1970; 1:213, with permission. Reprinted courtesy of Technicon Instrument Corporation, Tarrytown, NY.)

enter the aperture simultaneously, they will be counted as one pulse; this produces a coincidence error for which corrections are now automatically made by analyzers. A threshold setting or pulse discriminator allows the exclusion of pulses below an adjustable height on certain counters. On others, a second threshold also excludes the counting of pulses *above* a certain height. One therefore counts only the cells in the 'window' between the two settings. Systematically changing each threshold by given increments, one can determine a frequency distribution of relative cell volumes. Such cell size distributions can be automatically plotted and are valuable in the study of red cells, white cells, or platelets when two or more changing populations of cells are present. This is the basis for determination of the blood cell histograms, which are now routinely produced by the multichannel hematology analyzers.

Radiofrequency Conductivity
Conductivity is determined using a high-frequency electromagnetic probe that provides information on the cells' internal constituents (chemical composition, nuclear characteristics, and granular constituents) by permeating the lipid layer of a cell's membrane. Conductivity is especially helpful in differentiating between cells of like size such as small lymphocytes and basophils (Burns, 1992; Bentley, 1993). This principle is utilized in instruments marketed by Coulter (LH 700, GEN∑•S, HmX, A•T, etc.; Beckman Coulter, Inc., Brea, CA) and Sysmex (XE-2100, XT 2000i, HST-N, etc.; Sysmex America, Inc., Mundelein, IL).

Light Scattering
In the electro-optical analyzers (Fig. 29–7), a light-sensitive detector measures light scattering. All major multichannel analyzers now employ optical methodology, at least to some extent. The size of the pulse detected is proportional to the size of the particle (WBC, RBC, or platelet). While the precision of the instruments employing optical methodology is equivalent to that of systems utilizing electrical impedance, some systems employ a combination of the two methods in order to supply an internal comparison. Forward angle scatter of a laser-generated monochromatic light determines cell surface characteristics, morphology, and granulation. Measurement of light scatter at multiple angles allows for enhanced differentiation of cell types. For example, in the Abbott Cell Dyn, four simultaneous light scattering measurements are made on each white cell. Zero-degree forward angle is primarily affected by and thus determines cell size. Ten-degree light scatter is an indicator of cell structure or complexity and is especially helpful to resolve basophils and separate all cell populations. Ninety-degree light scatter separates granulated cells and is termed *lobularity*. Depolarized 90-degree light scattering resolves eosinophils due to their large crystalline *granularity*. Abnormal cells can have distinctive locations in the size versus complexity scatterplot and help to determine WBC suspect flags (Cornbleet, 1992) such as for blasts, variant lymphs, bands, and immature granulocytes. Fluorescent DNA dyes are used in the Abbott automated hematology systems to enumerate nucleated RBCs and identify populations of atypical lymphocytes and nonviable WBCs. Adaptive gating technology permits better separation of overlapping clusters of cell types. Suspect flags are generated when the distinction cannot be clearly delineated, as is often the case in the presence of abnormal WBC populations or interfering substances.

Cytochemistry
A methodology unique to the Bayer automated hematology series (Bayer Diagnostics, Tarrytown, NY) is the use of a cytochemical reaction to determine the peroxidase activity of white blood cells. The mean peroxidase index (MPXI), a measure of neutrophil-staining intensity, is determined for each specimen. The relative positivity seen in neutrophils, eosinophils, and monocytes is used in conjunction with data derived from

Figure 29–8 WBC scattergrams/cytograms. *Top left:* Abbott CELL-DYN 4000 WBC scatterplot, light scatter vs. volume. *Top right:* Sysmex XT 2000i, WBC scattergram, side-scattered light vs. side fluorescence. *Bottom left:* Bayer Advia 120, WBC peroxidase cytogram. *Bottom right:* Coulter LH 750, WBC scattergram, light scatter vs. volume.

light scatter to determine the WBC differential (Simson, 1986). ABX Diagnostics utilizes a cytochemical reagent which fixes the WBCs in their native state and subsequently stains their intracellular and plasmic membranes with chlorazol black E (Clinical Case Studies: Interpretation Guide for ABX 5-Part Diff Hematology Analyzers, ABX Horiba Diagnostics).

Reporting/Flagging
Each instrumentation system combines the data generated by these methodologies in their own configuration to provide a five- or six-part WBC differential along with RBC morphology and platelet parameters (Fig. 29–8). The principles of measurement specific to selected systems are detailed in Table 29–4. Data generated by the instrument that is not acceptable based on instrument- or user-defined criteria are flagged to alert the technologist that reporting the sample requires further investigation. Extreme care must be taken when defining these criteria, as the addition of each lessens the advantage provided by automating the process. The best configurations are developed with the patient population in mind. In addition, follow-up should be tailored to minimize the extended time necessary to derive the correct result.

Sources of Error
Table 29–5 lists the various causes of erroneous results obtained from the automated cell counters.

Automated Reticulocyte Counting
Many of the same principles applied in the determination of the WBC differential may be utilized to determine reticulocyte counts, resulting in

Table 29-4 Principles Used by Various Multichannel Instruments in the Clinical Laboratory

	Method			
Instrument	**Impedance**	**Conductivity**	**Light Scatter**	**Cytochemistry**
Abbott	×	×	×	
ABX	×		×	×
Bayer			×	×
Coulter	×	×	×	
Sysmex	×	×	×	

Table 29–5 Potential Causes of Erroneous Results With Automated Cell Counters

Parameter	Causes of spurious increase	Causes of spurious decrease
WBC	Cryoglobulin, cryofibrinogen Heparin Monoclonal proteins Nucleated red cells Platelet clumping Unlysed red cells	Clotting Smudge cells Uremia plus Immunosuppressants
RBC	Cryoglobulin, cryofibrinogen Giant platelets High WBC (> 50 000/μL)	Autoagglutination Clotting Hemolysis (in vitro) Microcytic red cells
Hemoglobin	Carboxyhemoglobin (> 10%) Cryoglobulin, cryofibrinogen Hemolysis (in vitro) Heparin High WBC (> 50 000/μL) Hyperbilirubinemia Lipemia Monoclonal proteins	Clotting Sulfhemoglobin (?)
Hematocrit (automated)	Cryoglobulin, cryofibrinogen Giant platelets High WBC (> 50 000/μL) Hyperglycemia (> 600 mg/dL)	Autoagglutination Clotting Hemolysis (in vitro) Microcytic red cells
Hematocrit (microhematocrit)	Hyponatremia Plasma trapping	Excess EDTA Hemolysis (in vitro) Hypernatremia
MCV	Autoagglutination High WBC (> 50 000/μL) Hyperglycemia Reduced red cell deformability	Cryoglobulin, Cryofibrinogen Giant platelets Hemolysis (in vitro) Microcytic red cells Swollen red cells
MCH	High WBC (> 50 000/μL) Spuriously high Hb Spuriously low RBC	Spuriously low Hb Spuriously high RBC
MCHC	Autoagglutination Clotting Hemolysis (in vitro) Hemolysis (in vivo) Spuriously high Hb Spuriously low Hct	High WBC (> 50 000/μL) Spuriously low Hb Spuriously high Hct
Platelets	Cryoglobulin, cryofibrinogen Hemolysis (in vitro and in vivo) Microcytic red cells Red cell inclusions White cell fragments	Clotting Giant platelets Heparin Platelet clumping Platelet satellitosis

From Cornbleet J, 1983.

enhanced precision and increased accuracy in routine practice (Metzger, 1987). Depending on the specific model of analyzer, this process may be semi- or fully automated. All methods rely on the addition of a stain or dye to detect the RNA content of the RBC. Such stains include new methylene blue (NMB), oxazine, auramine O, polymethine and thiazole orange. The methods of detection include impedance, light scatter, absorption, and fluorescence intensity. Reticulocyte fractions are separated based on the RNA content with the more immature cells containing the highest amount of reticulum. The immature reticulocyte fraction (IRF) quantitatively describes the youngest reticulocytes with the greatest staining intensity. This parameter allows early detection of an increased erythropoietic response, important in determining the response of the bone marrow recovering from chemotherapy or transplant or in response to erythropoietin therapy. It may also be used in conjunction with the absolute reticulocyte count to classify anemias (Davis, 1994, 1996; d'Onofrio, 1996).

Blood Film Examination

Microscopic examination of the blood spread on a glass slide or coverslip yields useful information regarding all the formed elements of the blood. The process of making thin blood film causes mechanical trauma to the cells. Also the cells flatten on the glass during drying, and the fixation and staining involve exposure to methanol and water. Some artifacts are inevitably introduced but these can be minimized by good technique.

Examination of Wet Preparations

It is sometimes advantageous to examine fresh blood under the microscope to avoid artifacts of fixation or staining. This is readily accomplished by sealing a small drop of blood diluted with isotonic sodium chloride beneath a coverslip on a glass slide. Buffered glutaraldehyde will preserve the cells for re-examination at a later time. Petroleum jelly or xipamide (Aquaphor) may be used to seal the edges of the coverslip to the slide. Wet preparations are employed to detect sickling, and spherocytes may be readily detected in this manner. Wet preparations may be examined to make sure the erythrocyte abnormalities seen on fixed films are not artifacts of drying or staining.

Making and Staining Blood Films

Examination of the blood film is an important part of the hematological evaluation. The reliability of the information obtained depends heavily on well-made and well-stained films that are systematically examined. Blood films should be prepared immediately if possible. Three methods of making films are described: the two-slide or wedge method, the cover glass method, and the spinner method.

Wedge Method

Place a drop of blood 2–3 mm in diameter about 1 cm from the end of a clean, dust-free slide that is on a flat surface. With the thumb and forefinger of the right hand, hold the end of a second (spreader) slide against the surface of the first slide at an angle of 30–45 degrees and draw it back to contact the drop of blood. Allow the blood to spread and form the angle between the two slides. Push the 'spreader slide' at a moderate speed forward until all the blood has been spread into a moderately thin film. The spreader slide should be clean, dry, and slightly narrower than the first slide so that the edges can be easily examined with the microscope.

The slides should be rapidly air dried by waving the slides or with an electric fan. The thickness of the film can be adjusted by changing the angle of the spreader slide or the speed of spreading, or by using a smaller or larger drop of blood. At a given speed, increasing the angle of the spreader slide will increase the thickness of the film. At a given angle, increasing the speed with which the spreader slide is pushed will also increase the thickness of the film. The film should not cover the entire surface of the slide. In a good film, there is a thick portion and a thin portion and a gradual transition from one to the other. The film should have a smooth, even appearance and be free from ridges, waves, or holes. The edge of the spreader must be absolutely smooth. If it is rough, the film has ragged tails containing many leukocytes. In films of optimal thickness, there is some overlap of red cells in much of the film but even distribution and separation of red cells toward the thin tail. The faster the film is air-dried, the better the spreading of the individual cells on the slide. Slow drying (e.g., in humid weather) results in contraction artifacts of the cells. The slide may be labeled by writing the identification with a lead pencil on the frosted end or directly on the thicker end of the blood film.

Cover Glass Method

No. 1 or $1^{1}/_{2}$ cover glasses 22 mm square are recommended.

Touch a cover glass to the top of a small drop of blood without touching the skin and place it, blood side down, crosswise on another cover glass so that the corners appear as an eight-pointed star. If the drop is not too large and if the cover glasses are perfectly clean, the blood will spread out evenly and quickly in a thin layer between the two surfaces. Just as it stops spreading, pull the cover glasses quickly but firmly apart on a plane parallel to their surfaces. The blood usually is much more evenly spread on one of the cover glasses than it is on the other. Cover glasses should be placed film side up on clean paper and allowed to dry in the air, or they may be inserted back to back in slits made in a cardboard box. Films from venous blood may be prepared similarly with a drop of blood on a coverslip and proceeding as described.

Spinner Method

Blood films that combine the advantages of easy handling of the wedge slide and uniform distribution of cells of the cover glass preparation may be made with special types of centrifuges known as spinners (Rogers, 1973). The spinner slide produces a uniform blood film, in which all cells are separated (a monolayer) and randomly distributed. White cells can be easily identified at any spot in the film. On a wedge smear there is a disproportion of monocytes at the tip of the feather edge, of neutrophils just in from the feather edge, and of both at the lateral edges of the film (Rogers, 1973). This is of little practical significance, but it does result in slightly lower monocyte counts in wedge films.

Blood Stains

The aniline dyes used in blood work are of two general classes: basic dyes, such as methylene blue; and acid dyes, such as eosin. Nuclei and certain other structures in the blood are stained by the basic dyes and, hence, are called basophilic. Structures that take up only acid dyes are called acidophilic, or eosinophilic. Other structures stained by a combination of the two are called neutrophilic.

Polychrome methylene blue and eosin stains are the outgrowth of the original time-consuming Romanowsky's method and are widely used. They stain differentially most normal and abnormal structures in the blood. The thiazine's basic components consist of methylene blue (tetramethylthionine) and, in varying proportions, its analogues produced by oxidative demethylation: azure B (trimethylthionine); azure A (asymmetric dimethylthionine); symmetric dimethylthionine; and azure C (monomethylthionine) (Lillie, 1977). The acidic component, eosin, is derived from a xanthene skeleton. Most Romanowsky's stains are dissolved in methyl alcohol and combine fixation with staining. Among the best known methods are Giemsa and Wright's stains.

Wright's Stain

This is a methyl alcoholic solution of eosin and a complex mixture of thiazines, including methylene blue (usually 50–75%), azure B (10–25%), and other derivatives (Lubrano, 1977). Wright's stain certified by the Biological Stain Commission is commercially available as a solution ready for use or as a powder. The buffer solution (pH 6.4) contains primary (monobasic) potassium phosphate (KH_2PO_4), anhydrous 6.63 g; secondary (dibasic) sodium phosphate (Na_2HPO_4), anhydrous 2.56 g; and distilled water to make 1 L. A more alkaline buffer (pH 6.7) may be prepared by using 5.13 g of the potassium salt and 4.12{ts}g of the sodium salt.

Procedure

1. To prevent the plasma background of the film from staining blue, blood films should be stained within a few hours of preparation or fixed if they must be kept without staining.
2. Fixation and staining may be accomplished by immersion of the slides in reagent-filled jars or by covering horizontally supported slides or coverslips with the reagents. In the latter method, covering the film with copious stain avoids evaporation, which leads to precipitation.
3. Fixation is for 1–2 minutes with absolute methanol.
4. The slide is next exposed to undiluted stain solution for 2 minutes. Then, without removing the stain from the horizontal slide, an equal amount of buffer is carefully added, and mixed by blowing gently.
5. The stain is flushed from the horizontal slide with water. Washing for more than 30 seconds reduces the blue staining. The back of the slide is cleaned with gauze.
6. The slide is allowed to air-dry in a tilted position.
7. Cover glasses are mounted film side down on a slide with Canada balsam or other mounting medium.

Films stained well with Wright's stain have a pink color when viewed with the naked eye. Under low power, the cells should be evenly

distributed. The red cells are pink, not lemon yellow or red. There should be a minimum of precipitate. The color of the film should be uniform. The blood cells should be free from artifacts, such as vacuoles. The nuclei of leukocytes are purple, the chromatin and parachromatin clearly differentiated, and the cytoplasmic neutrophilic granules tan in color. The eosinophilic granules are red-orange and each distinctly discernible. The basophil has dark purple granules. Platelets have dark lilac granules. Bacteria (if present) are blue. The cytoplasm of lymphocytes is generally light blue; that of the monocytes has a faint blue-gray tinge. Malarial parasites have sky-blue cytoplasm and red-purple chromatin. The colors are prone to fade if the preparation is mounted in a poor quality of balsam or exposed to the light.

Staining Problems

Excessively Blue Stain. Thick films, prolonged staining time, inadequate washing, or too high an alkalinity of stain or diluent tends to cause excessive basophilia. In such films, the erythrocytes appear blue or green, the nuclear chromatin is deep blue to black, and the granules of the neutrophils are deeply overstained and appear large and prominent. The granules of the eosinophils are blue or gray. Staining for a shorter time or using less stain and more diluent may correct the problem. If these steps are ineffective, the buffer may be too alkaline and a new one with a lower pH should be prepared.

Excessively Pink Stain. Insufficient staining, prolonged washing time, mounting the coverslips before they are dry, or too high an acidity of the stain or buffer may cause excessive acidophilia. In such films, the erythrocytes are bright red or orange, the nuclear chromatin is pale blue, and the granules of the eosinophils are sparkling brilliant red. One of the causes of the increased acidity is exposure of the stain or buffer to acid fumes. The problem may be a low pH of the buffer, or it may be the methyl alcohol, which is prone to develop formic acid as a result of oxidation on standing.

Other Staining Problems. Inadequately stained red cells, nuclei, or eosinophilic granules may be due to understaining or excessive washing. Prolonging the staining or reducing the washing may solve the problem.

Precipitate on the film may be due to unclean slides; drying during the period of staining; inadequate washing of the slide at the end of the staining period, especially failure to hold the slide horizontally during initial washing; inadequate filtration of the stain; or permitting dust to settle on the slide or smear.

Other Stains

Besides Wright's stain, Romanowsky-type stains include a number of others: Giemsa, Leishman's, Jenner's, May–Grünwald, MacNeal's, and various combinations. Some have been particularly recommended for certain purposes, such as Geimsa stain for excellence in staining malarial parasites and protozoa.

Reference Method

Studies have demonstrated the ability of the combination of just two dyes – azure B and eosin Y – to give the full range of colors provided by ideal Romanowsky's staining of blood and marrow cells. This is the reference method for Romanowsky's staining (ICSH, 1984a).

Automated Slide Stainer

Automated slide stainers are being used in several laboratories for routine hematology and microbiology slides. The stainer is a compact instrument with microprocessor control for flexibility in staining applications. Several slides can be stained uniformly in minutes. Typically any automated stainer has several user-definable programs to choose from. Staining problems are encountered even with the use of automatic stainers and must be dealt with on an individual basis.

Erythrocytes

In the blood from a healthy person, the erythrocytes, when not crowded together, appear as circular, homogeneous disks of nearly uniform size, ranging from 6–8 µm in diameter (Fig. 29–9). However, even in normal blood, individual cells may be as small as 5.5 µm and as large as 9.5 µm. The center of each is somewhat paler than the periphery. In disease, erythrocytes vary in their hemoglobin content, size, shape, staining properties, and structure.

Color

Hemoglobin Content

The depth of staining furnishes a rough guide to the amount of hemoglobin in red cells, and the terms normochromic, hypochromic, and hyperchromic are used to describe this feature of red cells. *Normochromic*

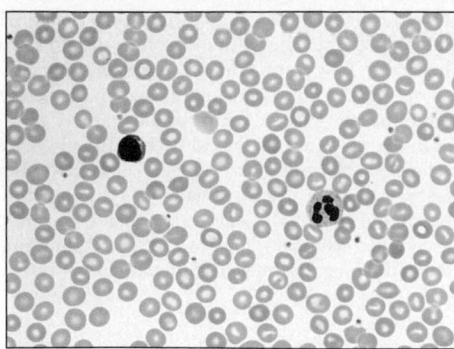

Figure 29–9 Normal peripheral smear. Erythrocytes appear as circular, homogeneous disks of nearly uniform size, ranging from 6–8 μm in diameter, with central pallor not exceeding more than one-third of the cell. On an average the red cells are approximately the same size as the nucleus of a small lymphocyte (× 500).

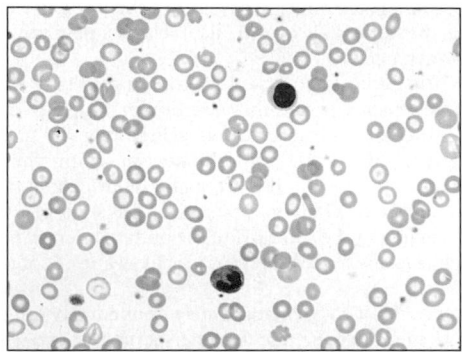

Figure 29–10 Microcytic hypochromic red cells in iron deficiency anemia. Red cells are hypochromic – the amount of hemoglobin per cell is decreased and the central pale area becomes larger (more than one third) (× 500).

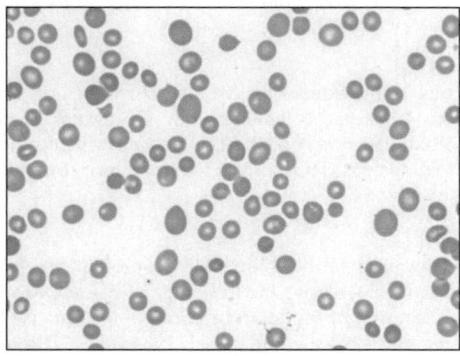

Figure 29–11 Macrocytes. Red cells are larger and thicker, stain deeply and lack central pallor (× 500).

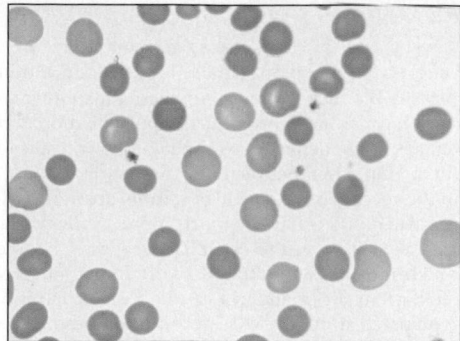

Figure 29–12 Hereditary spherocytosis. Spherocytes are nearly perfectly round in shape, smaller than normal red cells and lack central pallor (hyperchromic) (× 1000).

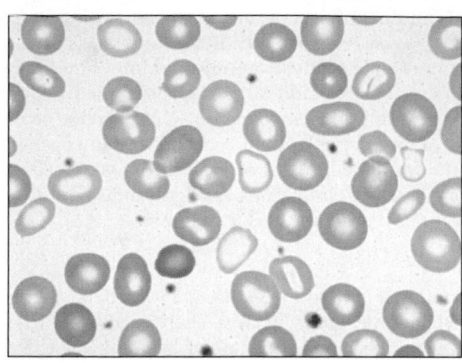

Figure 29–13 Dimorphic anemia. Anisocytosis and anisochromia characterized by presence of microcytic hypochromic cells, normocytic cells and few macrocytes (× 1000).

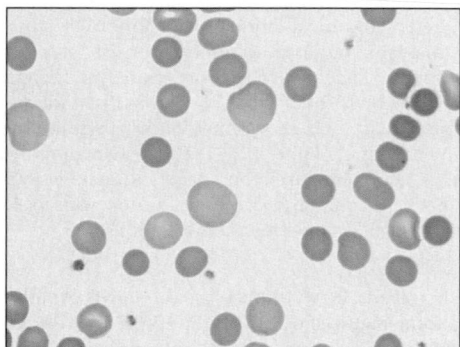

Figure 29–14 Polychromatophilia. Polychromatophilic red cells are young red cells, larger than the mature red cells, lack central pallor and appear slightly basophilic on Wright's stain. These are called reticulocytes when stained supravitally with brilliant cresyl blue (× 1000).

refers to normal intensity of staining (Fig. 29-9). When the amount of hemoglobin is diminished, the central pale area becomes larger and paler. This is known as *hypochromia*. The MCH and MCHC are usually decreased (Fig. 29-10). In megaloblastic anemia, because the red cells are larger and hence thicker, many stain deeply and have less central pallor (Fig. 29-11). These cells are *hyperchromic* because they have an increased MCH, but the MCHC is normal. In hereditary spherocytosis (Fig. 29-12), the cells are also hyperchromic; though the MCH is normal, the MCHC is usually increased because of a reduced surface/volume ratio. The presence of hypochromic cells and normochromic cells in the same film is called *anisochromia* or, sometimes, a dimorphic anemia (Fig. 29-13). This is characteristic of sideroblastic anemias, but also is found some weeks after iron therapy for iron deficiency anemia or in a hypochromic anemia after transfusion with normal cells.

Polychromatophilia

A blue-gray tint to the red cells (polychromatophilia or polychromasia) is a combination of the affinity of hemoglobin for acid stains and the affinity of RNA for basic stains. The presence of residual RNA in the red cell indicates that it is a young red cell that has been in the blood 1–2 days. These cells are larger than the mature red cells and may lack the central pallor (Fig. 29-14). Young cells with residual RNA are polychromatophilic red cells on air-dried films stained with Wright's stain but are reticulocytes when stained supravitally with brilliant cresyl blue. Therefore, increased polychromasia implies reticulocytosis; it is most marked in hemolysis and in acute blood loss.

Size

The red cells may be abnormally small, or *microcytes* (Fig. 29-10); abnormally large, or *macrocytes* (Fig. 29-11), or show abnormal variation in size (*anisocytosis*) (Fig. 29-13). Anisocytosis is a feature of most anemias; when it is marked in degree, both macrocytes and microcytes are usually present. In analyzing causes of anemia, the terms *microcytic* and *macrocytic* have most meaning when considered as cell volume rather than cell diameter. The mean cell volume is measured directly on a multichannel analyzer. We perceive the diameter directly from the blood film and infer volume (and the hemoglobin content) from it. Thus, the red cells in Figure 29-10 are microcytic; because they are hypochromic, they are thinner than normal and the diameter is not decreased proportionately to the volume. Also, the mean cell volume in the blood of the patient with spherocytosis (Fig. 29-12) is in the normal range; though many of the cells have a small diameter, their volume is not decreased because they are thicker than normal.

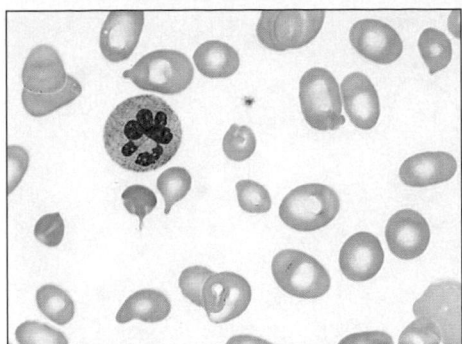

Figure 29–15 Poikilocytosis. Variation in shape of red cells. Abnormally shaped cells including oval, pear-shaped, and other irregularly shaped cells (× 1000).

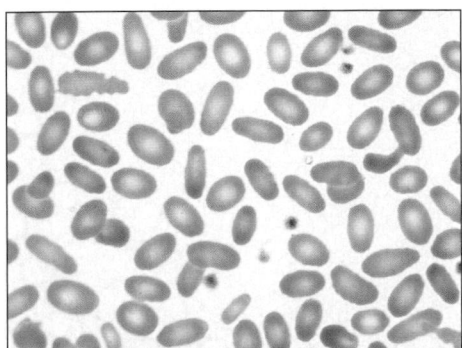

Figure 29–16 Hereditary elliptocytosis. The majority of the cells are elliptocytes. They are also seen in a normal person's blood, but usually are less than 10% of cells. They are also common in iron deficiency anemia, myelofibrosis, megaloblastic anemia and sickle cell anemia (× 1000).

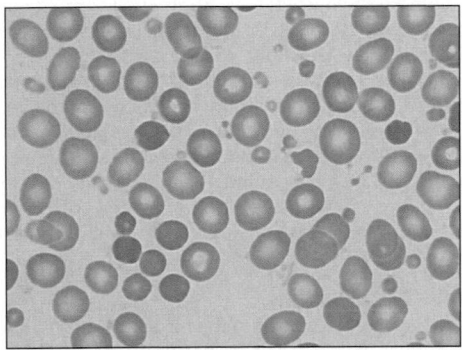

Figure 29–17 Thermal injury. Tiny bits of membrane (in excess of hemoglobin) are removed from the red cell surface, leading to formation of spherocytes (× 1000).

Shape

Variation in shape is called *poikilocytosis*. Any abnormally shaped cell is a poikilocyte. Oval, pear-shaped, teardrop-shaped, saddle-shaped, helmet-shaped, and irregularly shaped cells may be seen in a single case of anemia such as megaloblastic anemia (Fig. 29–15).

Elliptocytes are most abundant in hereditary elliptocytosis (Fig. 29–16), in which the majority of the cells are elliptical; this is a dominant condition that is only occasionally associated with hemolytic anemia. Elliptocytes are seen in normal persons' blood, but number less than 10% of the cells. They are more common, however, in iron deficiency anemia (Fig. 29–10), myelofibrosis with myeloid metaplasia, megaloblastic anemias and sickle cell anemia.

Spherocytes are nearly spherical erythrocytes in contradistinction to normal biconcave disks. Their diameter is smaller than normal. They lack the central pale area or have a smaller, often eccentric, pale area (because the cell is thicker and can come to rest somewhat tilted instead of perfectly flattened on the slide). They are found in hereditary spherocytosis (HS) (Fig. 29–12); in some cases of autoimmune hemolytic anemia (AHA) and in some conditions in which there has been a direct physical or chemical injury to the cells, such as from heat (Fig. 29–17). In each of these three instances, tiny bits of membrane (in excess of hemoglobin) are removed

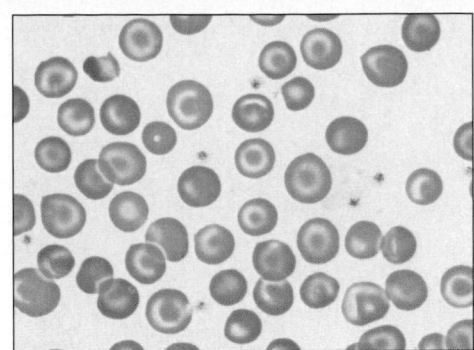

Figure 29–18 Target cells. Red cells with thin membrane, peripheral rim of hemoglobin and dark, central, hemoglobin-containing area. They are frequently seen in hemoglobin C disease, in hypochromic anemias and in liver disease (× 1000).

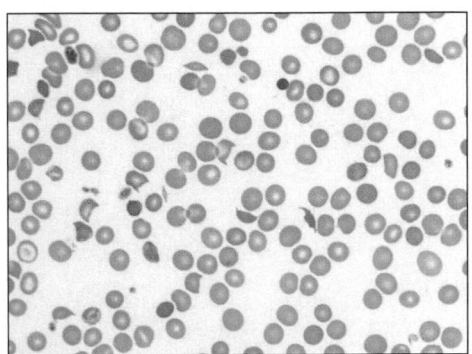

Figure 29–19 Schistocytes. Presence of cell fragments is indicative of hemolysis. Schistocytes can be seen in several conditions including microangiopathic hemolytic anemia, megaloblastic anemia, burns and disseminated intravascular coagulation (× 500).

from the adult red cells, leaving the cell with a decreased surface/volume ratio. In HS and AHA, this occurs in the reticuloendothelial system; in other instances (e.g., the patient with body burns) this may occur intravascularly.

Target cells are erythrocytes that are thinner than normal (leptocytes) and when stained show a peripheral rim of hemoglobin with a dark, central, hemoglobin-containing area. They are found in obstructive jaundice (Fig. 29–18), in which there appears to be an augmentation of the cell surface membrane; in the postsplenectomy state, in which there is a lack of normal reduction of surface membrane as the cell ages; in any hypochromic anemia, especially thalassemia; and in hemoglobin C disease.

Schistocytes (cell fragments) indicate the presence of hemolysis, whether in megaloblastic anemia, severe burns (Fig. 29–17), or microangiopathic hemolytic anemia (Fig. 29–19). The latter process is associated with either small blood vessel disease or fibrin in small blood vessels and results in intravascular fragmentation; particularly characteristic are helmet cells and triangularly shaped cells. Burr cells are irregularly contracted red cells with prominent spicules and are seen in the same process; however, this term is used differently by different hematologists, and therefore leads to confusion.

Acanthocytes are irregularly spiculated red cells in which the ends of the spicules are bulbous and rounded (Fig. 29–20); they are seen in abetalipoproteinemia, hereditary or acquired, and certain cases of liver disease. *Crenated cells* or echinocytes (Fig. 29–21) are regularly contracted cells that may commonly occur as an artifact during preparation of films, or may be due to hyperosmolarity, or to the discocyte–echinocyte transformation. In vivo, the latter may be associated with decreased red cell adenosine triphosphate (ATP) as a result of any of several causes. Artifacts resembling crenated cells consisting of tiny pits or bubbles indenting the red cells (Fig. 29–22) may be caused by a small amount of water contaminating the Wright's stain (or absolute methanol, if this is used first as a fixative).

Structure

Basophilic Stippling (Punctate Basophilia)

This is characterized by the presence, within the erythrocyte, of irregular basophilic granules, which vary from fine to coarse (Fig. 29–23). They stain deep blue with Wright's stain. The erythrocyte containing them may stain normally in other respects, or it may exhibit polychromatophilia. Fine

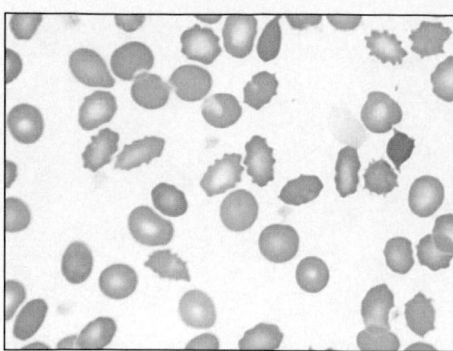

Figure 29–20 Acanthocytes. Irregularly spiculated cells with bulbous and rounded ends, frequently seen in abetalipoproteinemia, or certain cases of liver disease (×1000).

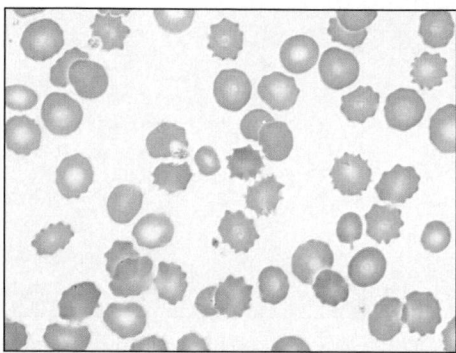

Figure 29–21 Echinocytes. Regularly contracted cells with sharp ends; may occur as an artifact during film preparation or due to hyperosmolarity or decreased ATP due to several causes (×1000).

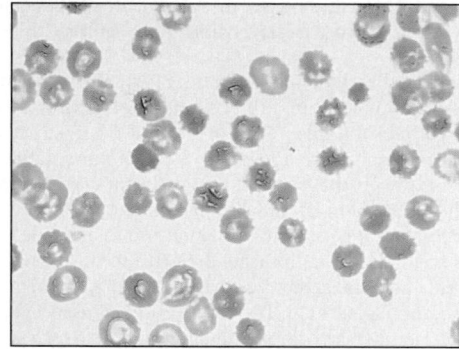

Figure 29–22 Artifact. Tiny pits or bubbles in the red cells. They can be caused by a small amount of water contaminating the Wright's stain or insufficient slide drying (×500).

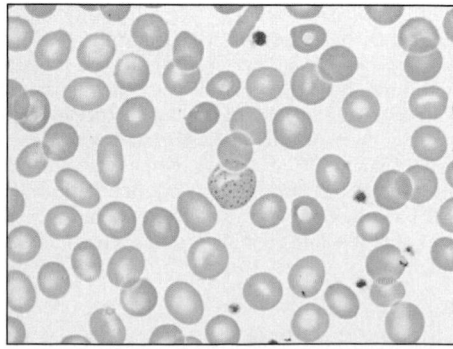

Figure 29–23 Basophilic stippling. Presence of irregular basophilic granules either fine or coarse; commonly seen in increased red cell production. Coarse stippling is usually seen in lead poisoning, or other anemias due to impaired hemoglobin synthesis, such as megaloblastic anemia (×1000).

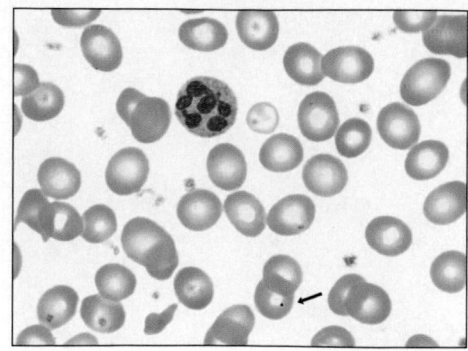

Figure 29–24 Howell–Jolly bodies. Smooth round remnants of nuclear chromatin. Seen in post-splenectomy states, hemolytic and megaloblastic anemias (a hypersegmented neutrophil is also seen) (×1000).

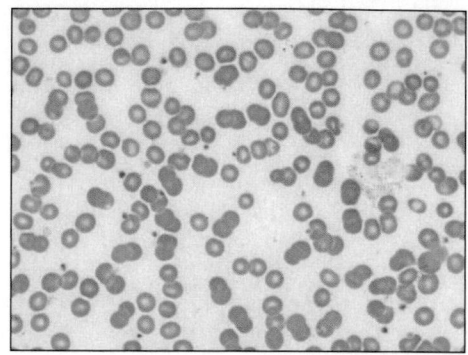

Figure 29–25 Rouleaux formation. Alignment of red cells one upon another so that they resemble a stack of coins. It is usually caused by elevated plasma fibrinogen or globulins (×500).

stippling is commonly seen when there is increased polychromatophilia and, therefore, with increased production of red cells. Coarse stippling may be seen in lead poisoning or other diseases with impaired hemoglobin synthesis, in megaloblastic anemia, and in other forms of severe anemia; it is attributed to an abnormal instability of the RNA in the young cell. Red cells with inorganic iron-containing granules (as demonstrated by stains for iron) are called *siderocytes*. Sometimes these granules stain with Wright's stain; if so, they are called *Pappenheimer bodies*. In contrast to basophilic stippling, Pappenheimer bodies are few in number in a given red cell and are rarely seen in the peripheral blood except after splenectomy.

Howell–Jolly Bodies

These particles are smooth, round remnants of nuclear chromatin. Single Howell–Jolly bodies may be seen in megaloblastic anemia (Fig. 29–24), hemolytic anemia, and after splenectomy. Multiple Howell–Jolly bodies in a single cell usually indicate megaloblastic anemia or some other form of abnormal erythropoiesis.

Cabot Rings

These are ring-shaped, figure-of-eight, or loop-shaped structures. Occasionally they are formed by double or several concentric lines. They are observed rarely in erythrocytes in pernicious anemia, lead poisoning, and certain other disorders of erythropoiesis. They stain red or reddish purple with Wright's stain and have no internal structure. The rings are probably microtubules remaining from a mitotic spindle (Bessis, 1977). They are interpreted as evidence of abnormal erythropoiesis.

Malarial Stippling

Fine granules may appear in erythrocytes that harbor *Plasmodium vivax*. With Wright's stain, the minute granules, 'Schüffner's granules,' stain purplish red. They are sometimes so numerous that they almost hide the parasites. These red cells are, as a rule, larger than normal.

Rouleaux Formation

This is the alignment of red cells one upon another so that they resemble stacks of coins. On air-dried films, rouleaux appear as in Figure 29–25. Elevated plasma fibrinogen or globulins cause rouleaux to form and also promote an increase in the erythrocyte sedimentation rate. Rouleaux formation is especially marked in paraproteinemia (monoclonal gammopathy). *Agglutination*, or clumping, of red cells is more surely

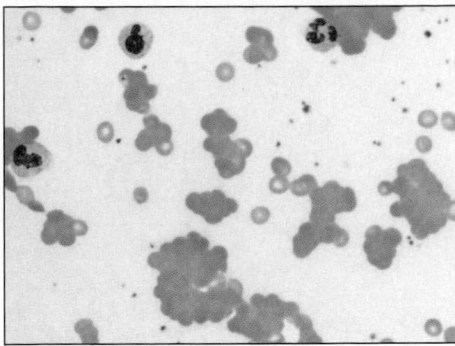

Figure 29–26 Agglutination. Clumping of red cells, which is more irregular than the linear rouleaux formation. It is caused by cold agglutinins (× 500).

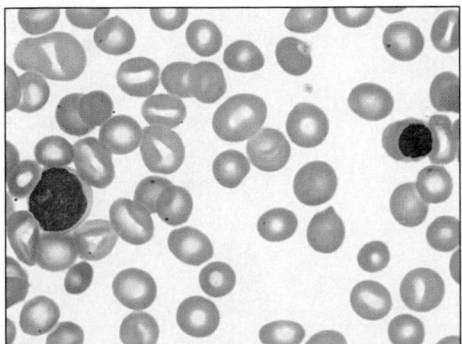

Figure 29–27 Nucleated red cells/normoblast. Precursors of mature red cells, normoblasts are usually present only in the bone marrow. Their presence in blood is usually associated with increased red cell production or infiltrative bone marrow disorders (× 1000).

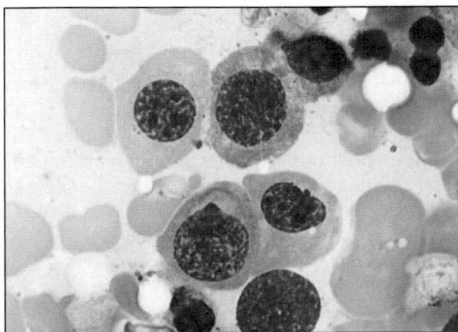

Figure 29–28 Megaloblast. Large nucleated red cell with abnormal 'open' nuclear chromatin. They are frequently seen in the bone marrow in myelodysplastic syndromes or other megaloblastic anemias. Occasionally these can also be seen in the peripheral blood (× 1000).

separated from rouleaux in wet preparations, and on air-dried films tends to show more irregular and round clumps than the linear rouleaux. Cold agglutinins are responsible for this appearance (Fig. 29–26).

Nucleated Red Cells

In contrast to erythrocytes of lower vertebrates and to most mammalian cells, the mammalian erythrocyte lacks a nucleus. Nucleated red cells (normoblasts, Figs 29–27 and 29–48) are precursors of the non-nucleated mature red cells in the blood. In the human, normoblasts are normally present only in the bone marrow. The stages in their production (see Ch. 30) from the earliest to the latest are the pronormoblast, basophilic normoblast, polychromatophilic normoblast, and orthochromatic normoblast. In general, nucleated red cells that might appear in the blood in disease are polychromatic normoblasts. In some, however, the cytoplasm is so basophilic that it is difficult to recognize the cell as erythroid except by the character of the nucleus; intensely staining chromatin, and sharp separation of chromatin from parachromatin. Such erythroid cells are often mistaken for lymphocytes, an error that usually can be prevented by careful observation of the nucleus. The megaloblast (Fig. 29–28) is a distinct, nucleated erythroid cell, not merely a larger normoblast. It is characterized by large size and abnormal 'open' nuclear

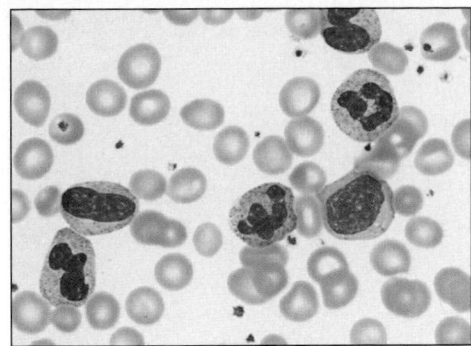

Figure 29–29 Leukemoid reaction. Left-shifted neutrophilic series with neutrophils, bands and myelocytes. The neutrophils also show coarse toxic granulation (× 1000).

Table 29–6 Conditions Associated with Leukoerythroblastosis

0.63	0.26	Solid tumors and lymphomas
	0.24	Myeloproliferative disorders, including chronic myeloid leukemia (CML)
	0.13	Acute leukemias
0.37	0.03	Benign hematologic conditions
	0.08	Hemolysis
	0.26	Miscellaneous, including blood loss

Proportions are based on a series of 215 cases discovered in a study of 50 277 blood film examinations in a 6-month period, a proportion of 0.004.

Data are from Weick JK, Hagedorn AB, Linman JW: Leukoerythroblastosis: Diagnostic and prognostic significance. Mayo Clin Proc 1974; 49:110.

chromatin pattern. Cells of this series are not found in normal marrow but are characteristically present in the marrow and sometimes the blood of patients with pernicious anemia or other megaloblastic anemias.

Significance of Nucleated Red Cells
Normoblasts are present normally only in the blood of the fetus and of very young infants. In the healthy adult, they are confined to the bone marrow and appear in the circulating blood only in disease, in which their presence usually denotes an extreme demand made on the marrow, extramedullary hematopoiesis, or marrow replacement. Large numbers of circulating nucleated red cells are particularly found in hemolytic disease of the newborn (erythroblastosis fetalis) and thalassemia major.

Leukoerythroblastotic Reaction
The presence of normoblasts and immature cells of the neutrophilic series in the blood is known as a leukoerythroblastotic reaction (Fig. 29–29). This often indicates space-occupying disturbances of the marrow, such as myelofibrosis with myeloid metaplasia, metastatic carcinoma, leukemias, multiple myeloma, Gaucher's disease, and others. Nonetheless, in the study of Weick (1974), over a third of the patients with a leukoerythroblastotic reaction did not have malignant or potentially malignant disease (Table 29–6). In patients with metastatic malignancy, a leukoerythroblastotic reaction is good evidence for marrow involvement by tumor.

Leukocytes on Peripheral Blood Smear Examination

Before evaluating leukocytes on the Romanowsky's-stained blood film, one should first determine that the film is well made, the distribution of the cells is uniform, and the staining of cells is satisfactory. One first scans the counting area of the slide and, in wedge films, the lateral and feather edges, where monocytes, neutrophils, and large abnormal cells (if present) tend to be disproportionately represented. With coverslip preparations this uneven distribution is less likely to occur. Suspicious cells are detected at 100× magnification, and confirmed at high power. Because nucleated red cells, macrophages, immature granulocytes, immature lymphoid cells, megakaryocytes, and abnormal cells are not normally found in blood, they should be recorded if present.

While scanning under low power, it is advisable to estimate the leukocyte count from the film. Even though it is a crude approximation, it sometimes enables one to detect errors in total count. One then proceeds to determine the percentage distribution of the different types of

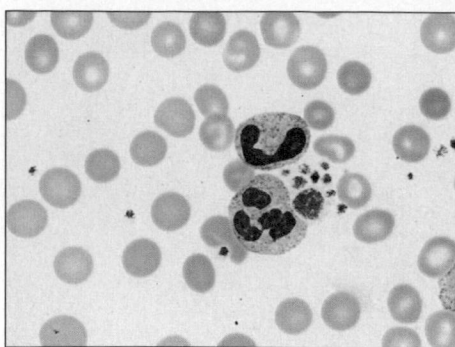

Figure 29–30 Neutrophil and band form. Neutrophil and band form depicting separation of nuclear lobes in the mature neutrophil vs. horseshoe-shaped nucleus in the band form. A giant platelet is also seen (× 1000).

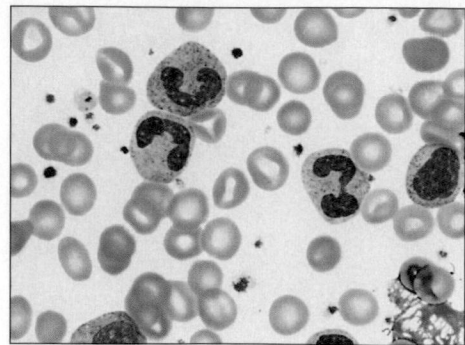

Figure 29–31 Neutrophilic granules. Cytoplasmic granules in myelocytes and mature neutrophils (× 1000).

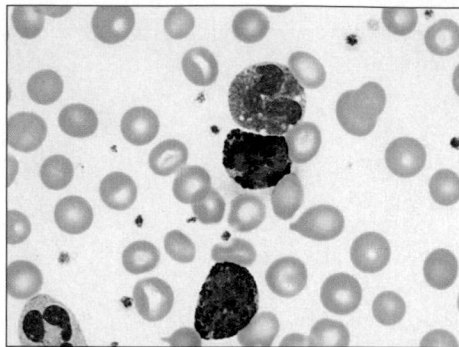

Figure 29–32 Basophil (below), eosinophil (above). Eosinophilic granules are coarser and bigger and often do not overlie the nucleus, unlike the basophil, which has large deeply basophilic granules often obscuring nuclear details (× 1000).

leukocytes, which is known as the differential leukocyte count. In patients with leukopenia it may be necessary to concentrate the leukocytes by centrifuging blood anticoagulated with EDTA and preparing films from the top layer of the packed cells. This buffy coat contains primarily leukocytes and platelets. In the crenellation technique of counting, the field of view is moved from side to side across the width of the slide in the 'counting area,' just behind the feather edge, where the red cells are separated from one another and are free of artifacts. As each leukocyte is encountered, it is classified, until 100, 200, 500, or 1000 leukocytes have been counted. The greater the number of cells counted, the greater the precision but for practical reasons 100-cell counts are usually made. A record of the count may be kept by using a mechanical or electronic tabulator. Leukocytes that cannot be classified should be placed together in an unidentified group. In some conditions, notably leukemia, there may be many of these unidentified leukocytes. During the differential leukocyte counting procedure, the morphology of erythrocytes and platelets is examined and the number of platelets is estimated. The absolute concentration of each variety of leukocyte is its percentage times the total leukocyte count. An increase in absolute concentration is an absolute increase; an increase in percentage only is a relative increase. Reference intervals are more useful if given as absolute concentrations rather than percentages (Table 29–3).

Leukocytes Normally Present in Blood

Neutrophil (Polymorphonuclear Neutrophilic Leukocyte; Segmented Neutrophilic Granulocyte)

Neutrophils average 12 μm in diameter; they are smaller than monocytes and eosinophils and slightly larger than basophils. The nucleus stains deeply; it is irregular and often assumes shapes comparable to such letters as E, Z, and S. What appear to be separate nuclei normally are segments of nuclear material connected by delicate filaments.

A filament has length but no breadth as one focuses up and down. A *segmented neutrophil* (Figs 29–30 and 29–49) has at least two of its lobes separated by a filament. A *band neutrophil* (Figs 29–30 and 29–49) has either a strand of nuclear material thicker than a filament connecting the lobes, or a U-shaped nucleus of uniform thickness. The nucleus in both types of neutrophils has coarse blocks of chromatin and rather sharply defined parachromatin spaces. If, because of overlapping of nuclear material, it is not possible to be certain whether or not a filament is present, the cell should be placed in the segmented category (Mathy, 1974). The number of lobes in normal neutrophils ranges from two to five, with a median of three. The cytoplasm itself is colorless, has tiny granules (0.2–0.3 μm) that stain tan to pink with Wright's stain. About two-thirds of these are specific granules and one-third azurophil granules. With light microscopy the two types of granules often cannot be distinguished in the mature cell (Fig. 29–31). Segmented neutrophils average 56% of leukocytes; reference intervals are $1.8-7.0 \times 10^9/L$ in white adults but have a lower limit of about $1.1 \times 10^9/L$ in black adults. Band neutrophils average 3% of leukocytes; the upper reference value is about $0.7 \times 10^9/L$ in white people and slightly lower in black people (using the preceding definition and counting 100 cells in the differential) (Table 29–3).

Normally, about 10–30% of the segmented neutrophils have two lobes, 40–50% have three lobes, 10–20% four, and no more than 5% have five lobes. A 'shift to the left' occurs when there are increased bands and less mature neutrophils in the blood, as well as a lower average number of lobes in segmented cells (Figs 29–29 and 29–31).

Neutrophil production and physiology are discussed in subsequent chapters. Neutrophilia or neutrophilic leukocytosis is an increase in the absolute count, and neutropenia is a decrease.

Eosinophil (Eosinophilic Granulocyte)

Eosinophils average 13 μm in diameter. The structure of these cells is similar to that of the polymorphonuclear neutrophils, with the striking difference that, instead of the neutrophilic granules, their cytoplasm contains larger round or oval granules having a strong affinity for acid stains (Fig. 29–32). They are easily recognized by the size and color of the granules, which stain bright red with eosin. The cytoplasm is colorless. The nucleus stains somewhat less deeply than that of the neutrophils and usually has two connected segments (lobes), rarely more than three. Eosinophils average 3% of the leukocytes in adults, and the upper reference value is $0.6 \times 10^9/L$ when calculated from the differential count. If allergic individuals are excluded, the upper limit is probably $0.35 \times 10^9/L$ or 350/μL. The lower reference value is probably 40/μL; a decrease in eosinophils (eosinopenia) can be detected only by counting large numbers of cells as in direct hemocytometer counts (Dacie, 1991) or with a flow cytometer automated differential counter.

Basophil (Basophilic Granulocyte)

In general, basophils resemble neutrophils, except that the nucleus is less segmented (usually merely indented or partially lobulated) and granules are larger and have a strong affinity for basic stains (Figs 29–32 and 29–33). In some basophils, most of the granules may be missing because they are soluble in water, leaving vacuoles or openings in the cytoplasm. The granules then are a mauve color. In a well-stained film the granules are deep purple, and the nucleus is somewhat paler and is often nearly hidden by the granules, so that its form is difficult to distinguish. Unevenly stained granules of basophils may be ring shaped and resemble *Histoplasma capsulatum* or protozoa.

Basophils are the least numerous of the leukocytes in normal blood and average 0.5%. The 95% reference values for adults are $0-0.2 \times 10^9/L$ when derived from the differential count.

Monocyte

The monocyte is the largest cell of normal blood (Fig. 29–34). It generally is about two to three times the diameter of an erythrocyte (14–20 μm), although smaller monocytes sometimes are encountered. It contains a single nucleus, which is partially lobulated, deeply indented, or horseshoe shaped. Occasionally, the nucleus of a monocyte may appear round or oval. The cytoplasm is abundant. The nuclear chromatin often appears to

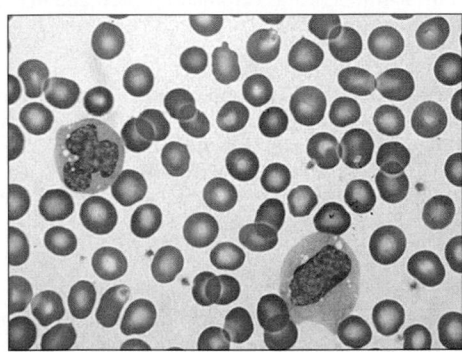

Figure 29–33 Basophil (center), neutrophilic myelocyte and band (left). The granules in the basophil are much bigger and coarser compared to the fine azurophilic granules of the neutrophil and precursors (× 1000).

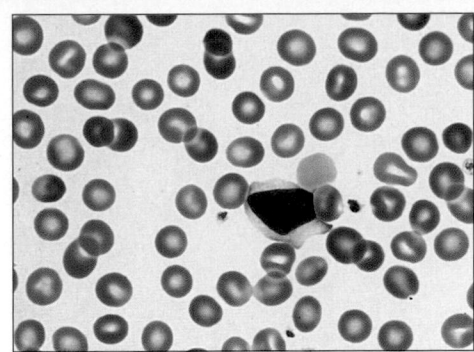

Figure 29–35 Lymphocyte. This is a benign reactive lymphocyte with moderately abundant pale gray cytoplasm hugging the surrounding red cells and distinct separation of chromatin/parachromatin (× 1000).

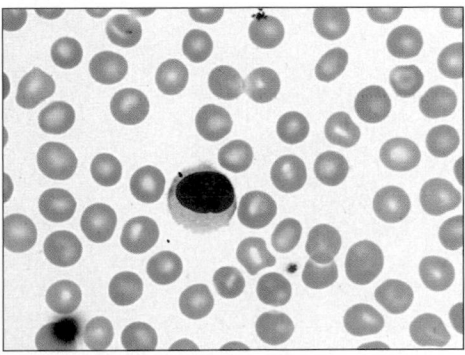

Figure 29–34 Monocyte. Of the normal blood cells, the monocyte is the largest and has the most delicate nuclear chromatin pattern. There is moderate amount of light gray cytoplasm with fine granularity and vacuolation (× 500).

Figure 29–36 Reactive large lymphocyte with moderately abundant gray-blue cytoplasm (× 1000).

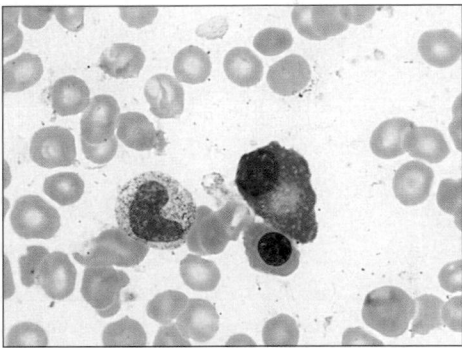

Figure 29–37 Plasma cell. Eccentric round nucleus with clumped nuclear chromatin and moderate amount of basophilic cytoplasm with prominent nuclear hof (× 1000).

IV

be in fine, parallel strands separated by sharply defined parachromatin. The nucleus stains less densely than that of other leukocytes. The cytoplasm is blue-gray and has a ground glass appearance and often contains fine red to purple granules that are less distinct and smaller than the granules of neutrophils. Occasionally, blue granules may be seen. When the monocyte transforms into a macrophage, it becomes larger (20–40 μm); the nucleus may become oval and the chromatin more reticular or dispersed, so that nucleoli may be visible. A perinuclear clear zone (Golgi) may be evident. The fine red or azurophil granules are variable in number or may have disappeared. The more abundant cytoplasm tends to be irregular at the cell margins and to contain vacuoles. These are phagocytic vacuoles, which may contain ingested red cells, debris, pigment, or bacteria. Evidence of phagocytosis in monocytes or the presence of macrophages in directly made blood films is pathologic and often indicates the presence of active infection.

Monocytes average 4% of leukocytes, and the reference interval for adults is approximately $0–0.8 \times 10^9$/L, depending on the method of performing the differential count (Table 29–3).

Lymphocyte

Lymphocytes are mononuclear cells without specific cytoplasmic granules. Small lymphocytes are about the size of an erythrocyte or slightly larger (6–10 μm) (Fig. 29–9). The typical lymphocyte has a single, sharply defined nucleus containing heavy blocks of chromatin. The chromatin stains dark blue with Wright's stain, whereas the parachromatin stands out as lighter-stained streaks; at the periphery of the nucleus, the chromatin is condensed. Characteristically, there is a gradual transition or smudging between the chromatin and the parachromatin. The nucleus is generally round but is sometimes indented at one side. The cytoplasm stains pale blue except for a clear perinuclear zone. Larger lymphocytes (Figs 29–35 and 29–36), 12–15 μm in diameter, with less densely staining nuclei and more abundant cytoplasm, are frequently found, especially in the blood of children, and may be difficult to distinguish from monocytes. The misshapen, indented cytoplasmic margins of lymphocytes are due to pressure of neighboring cells. In the cytoplasm of about one-third of the large lymphocytes, a few round, red-purple granules are present. They are larger than the granules of neutrophilic leukocytes. There is a continuous spectrum of sizes between small and large lymphocytes and, indeed, there can be a transition from small to large to blast forms as well as the reverse. It is not meaningful to classify small lymphocytes and large lymphocytes

separately. The presence of a significant proportion of atypical lymphocytes and blast forms (nonleukemic lymphoblast, reticular lymphocytes) must be noted; these indicate transformation of lymphoid cells as a response to antigenic stimulation. Plasma cells have abundant blue cytoplasm, often with light streaks or vacuoles, an eccentric round nucleus, and a well-defined clear (Golgi) zone adjacent to the nucleus (Fig. 29–37). The nucleus of the plasma cell has heavily clumped chromatin, which is sharply defined from the parachromatin, and often arranged in a radial or wheel-like pattern. Plasma cells are not present normally in blood.

Lymphocytes average 34% of all leukocytes, and range from $1.5–4 \times 10^9$/L in adults. The lymphocytes and their derivatives, the plasma cells, operate in the immune defenses of the body.

Artifacts

Broken Cells

Damaged or broken leukocytes (Figs 29–38 and 29–39) constitute a small proportion of the nucleated cells in normal blood. Bare nuclei from ruptured cells (Figs 29–40 and 29–41) vary from fairly well-preserved nuclei without cytoplasm to smudged nuclear material, sometimes with strands arranged in a coarse network, the so-called basket cells. They probably represent fragile cells, usually lymphocytes that have been broken in preparing the film. They are apt to be numerous when there is

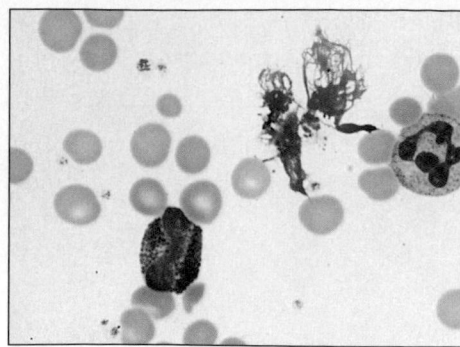

Figure 29–38 Broken cell. A broken cell of the myeloid series with ruptured cell membrane and disintegration of cytoplasmic contents (× 1000).

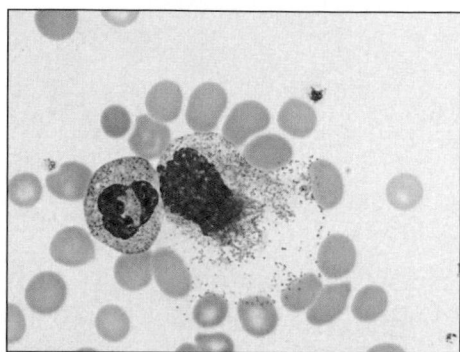

Figure 29–39 Ruptured cell. Ruptured/disintegrating leukocyte (× 1000).

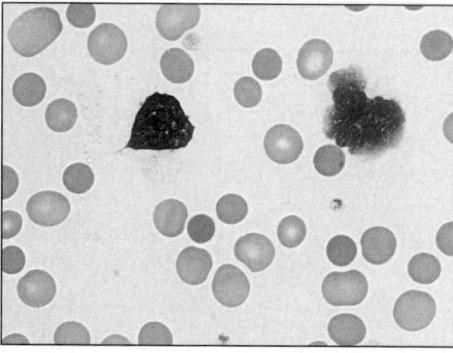

Figure 29–40 Smudge cell. Nuclear remnant from a damaged/broken white cell (× 1000).

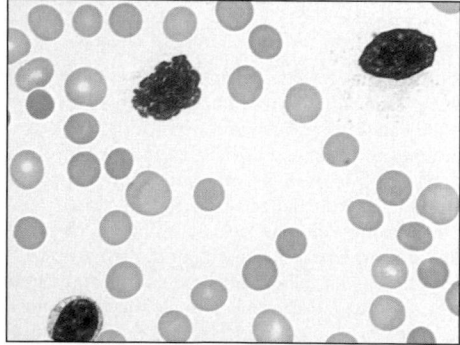

Figure 29–41 Basket cells (× 1000).

an atypical lymphocytosis, in chronic lymphocytic leukemia, and in acute leukemias.

Degenerative Changes

As EDTA-blood ages in the test tube, changes in leukocyte morphology begin to take place (Sacker, 1975). The degree of change varies among cells and in different individuals. Within a half hour the nuclei of neutrophils may begin to swell, with some loss of chromatin structure. Cytoplasmic vacuoles appear especially in monocytes and neutrophils. Nuclear lobulation appears in mononuclear cells; deep clefts may cause the nucleus to resemble a cloverleaf (radial segmentation of the nuclei; Rieder cells). Finally, loss of the cytoplasm and a smudged nucleus may be all that remains of the cell (Fig. 29–40). Degenerative changes occur more rapidly in oxalated blood than in EDTA-blood. They arise more rapidly with increasing concentrations of EDTA, such as occur when evacuated blood collection tubes are incompletely filled.

Contracted Cells

In the thicker part of wedge films, drying is slow. Obvious changes in the film are rouleaux of the erythrocytes and shrinkage of the leukocytes. Because the leukocytes are contracted and heavily stained, mononuclear cells are difficult to distinguish. Optimal cell identification is usually impossible in these areas.

Endothelial Cells

Endothelial cells from the lining of the blood vessel may appear in the first drop of blood from a fingerstick specimen or, rarely, in venous blood. They have an immature reticular chromatin pattern and may be mistaken for histiocytes or for tumor cells.

Radial segmentation of the nuclei

Use of oxalated blood results in the appearance of abnormal segmentation of the nuclei of leukocytes on the blood film. This segmentation differs from that of the granulocytes in that the lobes appear to radiate from a single point, giving a cloverleaf or a cartwheel picture. Extensive changes can occur within an hour or two in oxalated blood. Less extensive changes occur with other anticoagulants, including EDTA.

Vacuolation

Vacuoles may develop in the nucleus and cytoplasm of leukocytes, especially monocytes and neutrophils from blood anticoagulated with EDTA. Vacuoles may be associated with swelling of the nuclei and loss of granules from the cytoplasm.

'Pseudophagocytosis'

Occasionally a small lymphocyte or more often an erythrocyte will lie atop a granulocyte or a monocyte and thus appear to have been ingested. The true position of such cells can be suspected because they will come into sharp focus in a plane above that of the larger cell.

Sources of Error in the Differential Leukocyte Count

Even in perfectly made blood films, the differential count is subject to the same errors of random distribution. For interpretation of day-to-day or slide-to-slide differences in the same patient, it is helpful to know how much of the variation is ascribable to chance alone Table 29–7 gives 95% confidence limits for different percentages of cells in differential counts performed, classifying a total of 100–10 000 leukocytes. In comparing the percentages from two separate counts, if one number lies outside the confidence limits of the other, it is probable that the difference is significant (i.e., not due to chance). Thus, on the basis of a 100-cell differential count, if the monocytes were 5% one day and 10% the next, it is probable that the difference is due solely to sampling error. Although the difference could be real, one cannot be sure because of the small number of cells counted. If, on the other hand, the differential count totaled 500 cells, the difference between 5% and 10% is significant; one can be reasonably certain (with a 5% chance of being wrong) that the difference is a real one and not due to chance alone. Of course, this is a minimal estimate of the error involved in differential counts, since it does not include mechanical errors (due to variations in collecting the blood samples, inadequate mixing, irregularities in distribution depending on the type and quality of the blood films, and poor staining) or errors in cell identification, which depend on the judgment and experience of the observer. Meticulous technique as well as accurate and consistent cell classification are therefore required. The physician who interprets the results must be aware of the possible sources of error, especially the error due to chance in the distribution of cells. Table 29–3 shows the distribution of the various types of leukocytes in the blood of normal persons. Absolute concentrations are given, as these have considerably greater significance than percentages alone.

Automated Differential Leukocyte Counting

Because the differential leukocyte count is nonspecific, nonprecise, error-prone, usually labor intensive, expensive to perform, and of limited clinical significance as a screening test, some investigators suggested that it may be prudent to discontinue use of the differential count as an inpatient screening test for adults (Connelly, 1982). Automation of the differential count eliminates some of the detractions. Ideally, requirements for the

Table 29-7 Ninety-Five Percent Confidence Limits for Various Percentages of Blood Cells of a Given Type as Determined by Differential Counts*

a	n = 100	n = 200	n = 500	n = 1000	n = 10 000
0	0.0–3.6	0.0–1.8	0.0–0.7	0.0–0.4	0.0–0.1
1	0.0–5.4	0.1–3.6	0.3–2.3	0.5–1.8	0.8–1.3
2	0.0–7.0	0.6–5.0	1.0–3.6	1.2–3.1	1.7–2.3
3	0.6–8.5	1.1–6.4	1.7–4.9	2.0–4.3	2.6–3.4
4	1.1–9.9	1.7–7.7	2.5–6.1	2.9–5.4	3.6–4.5
5	1.6–11.3	2.4–9.0	3.3–7.3	3.7–6.5	4.5–5.5
6	2.2–12.6	3.1–10.2	4.1–8.5	4.6–7.7	5.5–6.5
7	2.9–13.9	3.9–11.5	4.9–9.6	5.5–8.8	6.5–7.6
8	3.5–15.2	4.6–12.7	5.8–10.7	6.4–9.9	7.4–8.6
9	4.2–16.4	5.4–13.9	6.6–11.9	7.3–10.9	8.4–9.6
10	4.9–17.6	6.2–15.0	7.5–13.0	8.2–12.0	9.4–10.7
15	8.6–23.5	10.4–20.7	12.0–18.4	12.8–17.4	14.3–15.8
20	12.7–29.2	14.7–26.2	16.6–23.8	17.6–22.6	19.2–20.8
25	16.9–34.7	19.2–31.6	21.3–29.0	22.3–27.8	24.1 25.9
30	21.2–40.0	23.7–36.9	26.0–34.2	27.2–32.9	29.1–31.0
35	25.7–45.2	28.4–42.0	30.8–39.4	32.0–38.0	34.0–36.0
40	30.3–50.3	33.2–47.1	35.7–44.4	36.9–43.1	39.0–41.0
45	35.0–55.3	38.0–52.2	40.6–49.5	41.9–48.1	44.0–46.0
50	39.8–60.2	42.9–57.1	45.5–54.5	46.9–53.1	49.0–51.0
55	44.7–65.0	47.8–62.0	50.5–59.4	51.9–58.1	54.0–56.0
60	49.7–69.7	52.9–66.8	55.6–64.3	56.9–63.1	59.0–61.0
65	54.8–74.3	58.0–71.6	60.6–69.2	62.0–68.0	64.0–66.0
70	60.0–78.8	63.1–76.3	65.8–74.0	67.1–72.8	69.0–70.9
75	65.3–83.1	68.4–80.8	71.0–78.7	72.2–77.7	74.1–75.9
80	70.8–87.3	73.8–85.3	76.2–83.4	77.4–82.4	79.2–80.8
85	76.5–91.4	79.3–89.6	81.6–88.0	82.6–87.2	84.2–85.7
90	82.4–95.1	85.0–93.8	87.0–92.5	88.0–91.8	89.3–90.6
91	83.6–95.8	86.1–94.6	88.1–93.4	89.1–92.7	90.4–91.6
92	84.8–96.5	87.3–95.4	89.3–94.2	90.1–93.6	91.4–92.6
93	86.1–97.1	88.5–96.1	90.4–95.1	91.2–94.5	92.4–93.5
94	87.4–97.8	89.8–96.9	91.5–95.9	92.3–95.4	93.5–94.5
95	88.7–98.4	91.0–97.6	92.7–96.7	93.5–96.3	94.5–95.5
96	90.1–98.9	92.3–98.3	93.9–97.5	94.6–97.1	95.5–96.4
97	91.5–99.4	93.6–98.9	95.1–98.3	95.7–98.0	96.6–97.4
98	93.0–99.9	95.0–99.4	96.4–99.0	96.9–98.8	97.7–98.3
99	94.6–99.9	96.4–99.9	97.7–99.7	98.2–99.5	98.7–99.2
100	96.4–100.0	98.2–100.0	99.3–100.0	99.6–100.0	99.9–100.0

* n is the number of cells counted; a, the observed percentage of cells of the given type. The limits for n = 100, 200, 500, and 1000 are exact; for n = 10 000, they have been determined with Freeman and Tukey's approximation as described in the Geigy tables.

Courtesy of Prof CL Rümke (1985).

automated differential leukocyte counting system should include the following:

1. The distribution of cells analyzed should be identical with that in the blood.
2. All leukocytes usually found in blood diseases should be accurately identified, or detected and 'flagged' in some way.
3. The speed of the process should enable a large number of cells to be counted in order to minimize statistical error, and
4. The instrument should be cost-effective (Bentley, 1977).

The impedance counters and flow cytometer systems and their differential counts are discussed earlier under Instrument Technology.

The automated systems have the advantage of rapidly analyzing larger numbers of cells and significantly reducing the statistical error of counting.

The disadvantages are that the categories of cells are not completely consonant with those with which we are familiar on Romanowsky's-stained films. An 'unclassified' category is difficult to interpret. When an abnormal result occurs, a film must be made and examined. Because of concern regarding the instrument flags, each laboratory should devise a

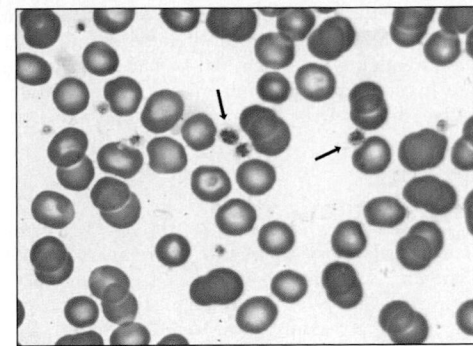

Figure 29–42 Platelet. Platelets are round to oval 2–4 μm in diameter and separated from one another (× 1000).

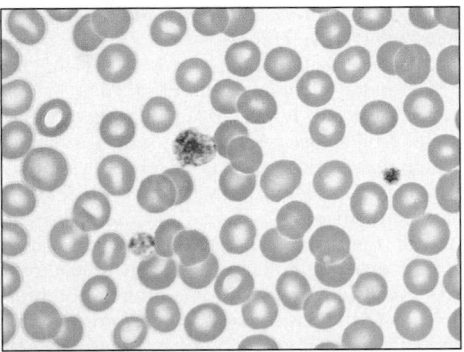

Figure 29–43 Platelet/giant platelet. Platelets show fine granularity and an occasional larger (giant) form is noted (× 1000).

policy for blood film examination and visual counting when indicated. Camden (1993) provides guiding questions to be asked in selecting a new hematology analyzer for your laboratory. The International Committee for Standardization in Hematology (1984b) also published a protocol for evaluation of automated blood cell counters.

Digital Image Processing

A uniformly made and stained blood film is placed on a motor-driven microscope stage. A computer controls scanning the slide and stopping it when leukocyte(s) are in the field. The optical details (e.g., nuclear and cytoplasmic size, density, shape, and color) are recorded by a television camera, analyzed by computer, and converted to digital form; these characteristics are compared with a memory bank of such characteristics for the different cell types. If the pattern fits that of a normal cell type, it is identified as such; otherwise, it is classified as other or unknown. The coordinates of the unknown cells are kept by the instrument and relocated at the end of the count so that the technologist can classify them (Lapen, 1982; Parthenis, 1992; Mukherjee, 2004).

Platelets on Peripheral Blood Smear Examination

In films made from EDTA-blood and stained with Romanowsky's stains, platelets are round or oval, 2–4 μm in diameter, and separated from one another (Fig. 29–42). The platelet count may be estimated from such films. On the average, if the platelet count is normal, about one platelet is found per 10–30 red cells. At 1000× magnification, this is equivalent to about 7–20 platelets per oil immersion field in the areas where red cell morphology is optimal (Fig. 29–43). Platelets contain fine purple granules that usually fill the cytoplasm. Occasionally, granules are concentrated in the center (the 'granulomere') and surrounded by a pale cytoplasm (the 'hyalomere'); these are probably activated platelets, the appearance resulting from contraction of the microtubular band. A few platelets may have a decreased concentration of granules (hypogranular platelets). In EDTA-blood from normal individuals, the fraction of platelets that exceed 3 μm in diameter and the fraction of platelets that are hypogranular are both less than 5% if the films are made at 10 minutes or 60 minutes after the blood is drawn. If films are made immediately or at 3 hours after blood drawing, the fraction of large platelets and the fraction of hypogranular or activated platelets are increased (Zeigler, 1978). These artifacts make it necessary to standardize time of film preparation when evaluating platelet size from films. In patients with immune thrombocytopenia, large platelets/giant platelets (Fig. 29–30) are increased in number. They are also increased in patients with the rare Bernard–Soulier syndrome and in patients with myelophthisis or myeloproliferative syndromes; in the latter, the platelets are frequently hypogranular or have a distinct granulomere and hyalomere. In blood films made from skin puncture wounds, platelets assume irregular shapes with sharp projections and tend to clump together.

Bone Marrow Examination

Marrow aspiration and biopsy can be carried out as an office procedure on ambulatory patients with minimal risk. It compares favorably with ordinary venipuncture and is less traumatizing than a lumbar puncture. As for any other special procedure, however, the clinical indications for marrow examination should be clear. In each instance the physician should have in mind some reasonable prediction of its result and consequent benefit to the patient. Without exception, the peripheral blood should be examined carefully first. It is a relatively uncommon circumstance to find hematological disease in the bone marrow without evidence of it in the peripheral blood.

It is estimated that the weight of the marrow in the adult is 1300–1500 g. The marrow can undergo complete transformation in a few days and occasionally even in a few hours. As a rule, this rapid transformation involves the whole organ, as evidenced by the fact that a small sample represented by a biopsy or aspiration is usually fairly representative of the whole marrow. This conclusion is in accord with results of studies of biopsy samples simultaneously removed from several sites. According to these observations, the various sites chosen for removal of marrow for studies are in most instances equally good. Consequently, the difficulty of access, the risks involved, the ease of obtaining a good biopsy specimen, and the discomfort to the patient are the main reasons for selection of a site in the particular patient. Within a given site, the cellular distribution may vary with apparently hyperplastic or hypoplastic areas. This is particularly the case immediately below the cortex. Occasionally, the failure to obtain quantitatively or qualitatively adequate material in one site may be followed by success in another location. Also, the need for repeated aspirations or biopsies may indicate the use of several different sites. We regard the posterior iliac crest as the preferred site. The large marrow space allows both aspiration and biopsy to be performed with ease at one time. The techniques of marrow aspiration and biopsy have been adequately reviewed (Hyun, 1988).

Preparation of the Aspirate and Biopsy Section

Marrow Films. Delay, no matter how brief, is undesirable. Films can be made in a manner similar to that for ordinary blood counts. Gray particles of marrow are visible with the naked eye. They are the best material for the preparation of good films and serve as landmarks for the microscopic examination of stained smears.

Direct Films. A drop of marrow is placed on a slide a short distance away from one end. A film 3–5 cm long is made with a spreader, not wider than 2 cm, dragging the particles behind but not *squashing* them. A trail of cells is left behind each particle.

Imprints. Marrow particles can also be used for preparation of imprints. One or more visible particles are picked up with a capillary pipet, the broken end of a wooden applicator, or a toothpick and transferred immediately to a slide and made to stick to it by a gentle smearing motion. The slide is air dried rapidly by waving and then is stained.

Crush Preparations. Marrow particles in a small drop of aspirate may be placed on a slide near one end. Another slide is carefully placed over the first. Slight pressure is exerted to crush the particles, and the slides are separated by pulling them apart in a direction parallel to their surfaces. All films should be dried rapidly by whipping them through the air or by exposing them to a fan. As the aspirated material is being spread, the appearance of fat as irregular holes in the films gives assurance that marrow and not just blood has been obtained.

Special studies. A sterile anticoagulated sample containing viable unfixed cells in single cell suspension is the best substrate for nearly all special studies that are likely to be required on a marrow sample. Specifically, flow cytometry is best performed on an EDTA or heparin anticoagulated aspirate specimen, which is stable for at least 24 hours at room temperature. For cytogenetic or cell culture analysis, anticoagulated marrow should be added to tissue culture medium and analyzed as soon as possible to maintain optimal cell viability. Cytogenetic specimens are generally not adversely affected by overnight incubation. DNA is relatively stable and can be extracted and analyzed from paraffin-embedded tissue sections. However, RT-PCR assays, involving amplification of cDNA

prepared from cellular messenger RNA, are often needed for molecular diagnosis of translocations associated with leukemia and lymphoma. Messenger RNA has a variable half-life in an intact cell and is degraded rapidly (of the order of seconds to minutes) in a cell lysate by ubiquitous RNAses. For maximal mRNA recovery cell suspensions, mostly buffy coat or mononuclear cell preparations should be lysed in an appropriate RNAse-inhibitor containing buffer as soon as possible after sampling. EDTA is the preferred anticoagulant, as heparin can interfere with some molecular assays (Ryan, 2001b).

Histologic Sections. The needle biopsy and the clotted marrow particles (fragments) are fixed in Zenker's acetic solution (5% glacial acetic acid; 95% Zenker's) for 6–18 hours, or in B-5 fixative for 1–2 hours (Hyun, 1988). Excessive time in either fixative makes the tissue brittle. While these fixatives, particularly B-5, provide the best histology, they contain toxic mercuric chloride and are gradually being replaced by fixatives such as zinc formalin and other preparations. The tissue is processed routinely for embedding in paraffin, cut at 4 μm, and stained routinely with hematoxylin and eosin (H&E). Giemsa and periodic acid–Schiff (PAS) stains are frequently useful. Embedding the tissue in plastic material allows thinner sections to be examined and better survival of protein structure so that enzyme histochemistry and immunocytochemistry are practical for identification of cell lineages.

Sections provide the best estimate of cellularity and a picture of marrow architecture but are somewhat inferior for the study of cytologic details. Another disadvantage is that particles adequate for histological sections are not always obtained, especially in conditions in which the diagnosis depends on marrow evidence (e.g., myelofibrosis or metastatic cancer).

Staining Marrow Preparations

Romanowsky's Stain. Marrow films should be stained with a Romanowsky's stain (e.g., Wright–Giemsa) in a manner similar to that for blood films. A longer staining time may be necessary for marrows with greater cellularity. Several special stains may be performed on peripheral blood smears, bone marrow aspirate and touch imprint smears and bone marrow biopsy sections besides the usual Romanowsky and hematoxylin and eosin stains. These include the cytochemical stains (myeloperoxidase, Sudan black B, naphthol As-D chloroacetate esterase, nonspecific esterases, acid phosphatases, leukocyte alkaline phosphatase, periodic acid–Schiff stain, toluidine blue and iron stain) and immunocytochemical stains depending upon the disease and preliminary morphological examination of the smear and/or section (Perkins, 2004). The procedure for the iron stain is discussed in this chapter. The relevance of other stains is mentioned in the subsequent chapters along with the respective diseases.

Perls' Test for Iron

Procedure. One film containing marrow particles is fixed for 10 minutes in formalin vapor, immersed for 10 minutes in a freshly prepared solution that contains 0.5% potassium ferrocyanide and 0.75% hydrochloric acid, rinsed, dried, and counterstained with Nuclear Fast Red.

Interpretation. The Prussian blue reaction is produced when hemosiderin or ferritin is present; iron in hemoglobin is not stained. Report as negative or 1+ to 5+. Storage iron, which is contained in macrophages, can be evaluated only in the marrow particles on the film. In adults, 2+ is normal, 3+ slightly increased, 4+ moderately increased, and 5+ markedly increased. Storage iron in the marrow is located in macrophages. Normally, a small number of blue granules are seen. In iron deficiency, blue-staining granules are absent or extremely rare. Storage iron is increased in most other anemias, infections, hemochromatosis, hemosiderosis, hepatic cirrhosis, uremia, and cancer, and after repeated transfusions. Sideroblasts (Fig. 29–44) are normoblasts that contain one or more particles of stainable iron. Normally, from 20–60% of the late normoblasts are sideroblasts; in the remainder, no blue granules can be detected. The percentage of sideroblasts is decreased in iron deficiency anemia (in which storage iron is decreased) and also in the common anemias associated with infection, rheumatoid arthritis, and neoplastic disease (in which storage iron is normal or increased). The number of sideroblasts is increased when erythropoiesis is impaired for other reasons; it is roughly proportional to the degree of saturation of transferrin. The Prussian blue reaction can also be performed on slides previously stained with a Romanowsky's stain to identify sideroblasts or to determine whether iron is present in other cells of interest. Further, iron stain is also used to evaluate for presence of abnormal sideroblasts and ring sideroblasts (Fig. 29–45) seen in various hematological diseases.

Sections. Routine H&E stains are satisfactory for most purposes. Romanowsky's stains can be used to good advantage with fixed material. Iron stains are best performed on films that contain particulate marrow tissue. They are less sensitive in sections of marrow

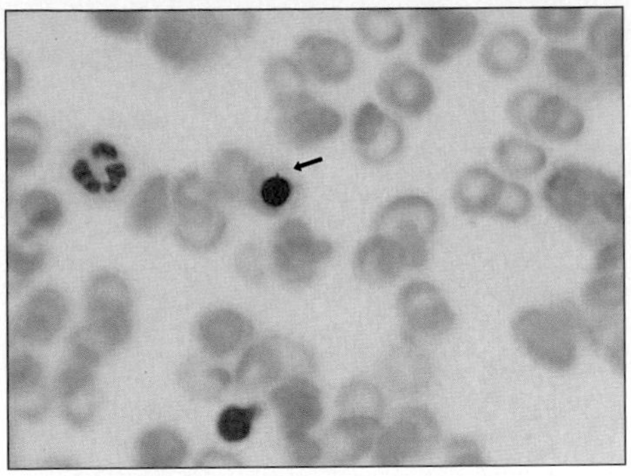

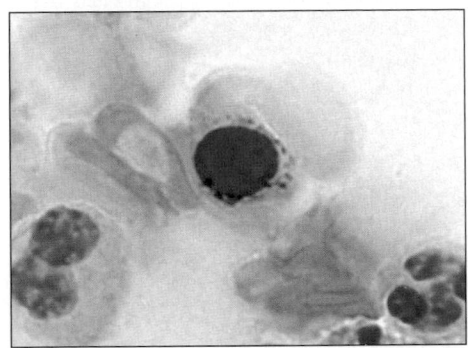

Figure 29–44 Normal sideroblast. Single iron granule seen in the cytoplasm of a maturing normoblast. Identification requires high magnification and bright illumination, focusing up and down (×1000).

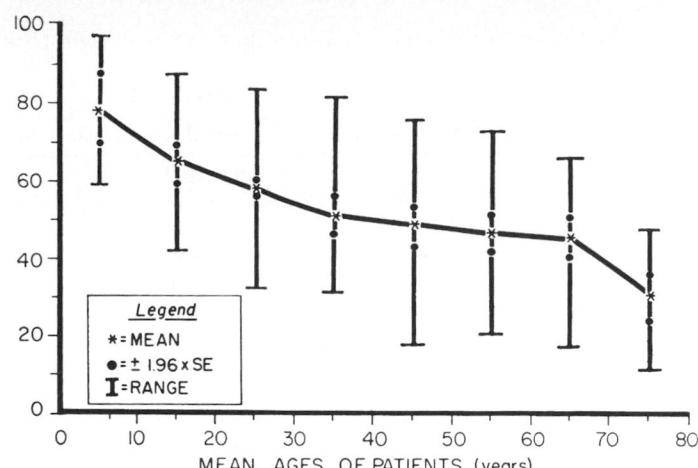

Figure 29–46 Marrow cellularity in hematologically normal individuals. Percent cellularity on the ordinate, versus age, grouped by decade, on the abscissa. (From Hartsock RJ, Smith EB, Petty CS. Am J Clin Pathol 1965; 43:326, with permission.)

Figure 29–45 Ring sideroblast. Siderotic granules forming a perinuclear ring spanning more than half of the nuclear diameter (Prussian blue stain × 1000).

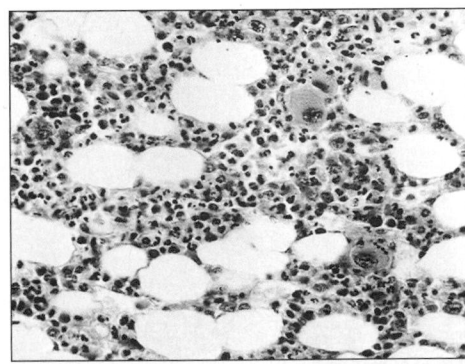

Figure 29–47 Marrow biopsy (× 1470). Cellularity here is between 60–70%, which is normal for an adult. Three megakaryocytes are present, which is normal for this size of field. Granulocyte maturation appears normal, with all stages present. Very few normoblasts are noted. (Normoblasts have intensely staining nuclei and tend to occur in clusters.) The myeloid/erythroid (M/E) ratio is higher than 4 : 1, indicating erythroid hypoplasia. No other abnormalities are noted.

because some iron is lost in processing and a lesser thickness of tissue is examined in sections.

Examination of Marrow

It is desirable to establish a routine procedure in order to obtain the maximum information from examination of the marrow.

Peripheral Blood

The complete blood cell count, including platelet count and reticulocyte count, should be performed on the day of the marrow study and the results incorporated in the report. The pathologist or hematologist who examines the marrow should also carefully examine the blood film as previously described and incorporate the observations in the marrow report.

Cellularity of the Marrow

The marrow cellularity is expressed as the ratio of the volume of hematopoietic cells to the total volume of the marrow space (cells plus fat and other stromal elements). Cellularity varies with the age of the subject and the site. For example, at age 50 years, the average cellularity in the vertebrae is 75%; sternum, 60%; iliac crest, 50%; and rib, 30%. Normal cellularity of the iliac bone at different ages has been well defined by Hartsock (1965), as summarized in Figure 29–46. If the percentage is increased for the patient's age, the marrow is hypercellular, or hyperplastic; if decreased, the marrow is hypocellular, or hypoplastic. Marrow cellularity is best judged by histological sections of biopsy or aspirated particles (Fig. 29–47) but should be also estimated from the particles that are present in marrow films. This is done by comparing the areas occupied by fat spaces and by nucleated cells in the particles as well as the density of nucleated cells in the 'tail' or fallout of the particles. Comparison of films and sections on each marrow specimen will enable the observer to estimate cellularity reasonably well from films, a skill that is useful in the instances when sectioned material is unavailable.

Distribution of Cells

The distribution of the various cell types can be ascertained in two ways. First, one scans several slides under low, then high magnification; and, on the basis of previous experience, one estimates the number and distribution of cells. Second, one actually makes a differential count of 300–1000 cells and calculates the percentage of each type of cell. A combination of both methods is preferred. The second of these methods, careful differential counting, is an essential part of training in this work, without which accuracy in the first method may be difficult to achieve. The differential count also affords an objective record from which future changes may be measured.

One first scans the marrow films under low power (100× or 200× magnification), looking for irregularities in cell distribution, the number of megakaryocytes, and the presence of abnormal cells. Then one selects areas on the films where marrow cells are both undiluted with blood cells and separated and spread out sufficiently to allow optimal identification. These areas are usually just behind marrow particles on the direct films, or near the particles on the crushed films. The differential count is performed at 400× or 1000× magnification. Examples of reference intervals for differential counts of the marrow at selected different ages are given in Table 29–8.

Changes in the marrow cell distribution are most dramatic in the first month of life, during which a predominance of granulocytic cells at birth changes to a predominance of lymphocytes. This predominance of lymphocytes characterizes the bone marrow during infancy. A small proportion of 'immature' or transitional lymphoid cells (fine nuclear chromatin, high nuclear/cytoplasmic ratio, small to intermediate cell size) is normally present; it may be that these cells include stem cells and progenitor cells. These cells probably include cells designated as 'hematogones'; they may be increased in iron deficiency anemia, immune thrombocytopenic purpura, and other disorders, especially in infancy. Normoblasts fall after birth; rise to a maximum at 2 months; then fall to a stable, relatively low level by 4 months and remain there during most of infancy. The myeloid/erythroid (M/E) ratio is the ratio of total granulocytes to total normoblasts. In newborns and infancy, it is somewhat higher than in later childhood or adult life (Table 29–8). In adults, the range is broad, varying from about 1.2 : 1 to 4 : 1. Both the differential count and the M/E ratio are relative values and must be interpreted with respect to the cellularity

Table 29-8 Differential Cell Counts of Bone Marrow in Percent of Total Nucleated Cells

Cell types	Rosse (1977)			Mauer (1969)	Jandl (1987)
	Birth (Mean, SD)	1 Month (Mean, SD)	18 Months (Mean, SD)	Childhood (Mean, Range)	Adult (Mean, Range)
Normoblasts, total	14.48 ± 7.24	8.04 ± 5.00	8.21 ± 3.71	23.1	21.5 (14.2–30.4)
Pronormoblasts	0.02 ± 0.06	0.10 ± 0.14	0.08 ± 0.13	0.5 (0.0–1.5)	0.6 (0.2–1.4)
Basophilic n.	0.24 ± 0.25	0.34 ± 0.33	0.50 ± 0.34	1.7 (0.2–4.8)	2.0 (0.7–3.7)
polychromatophilic n.	13.06 ± 6.78	6.90 ± 4.45	6.97 ± 3.56	18.2 (4.8–34.0)	12.4 (12.2–24.2)
Orthochromatic n.	0.69 ± 0.73	0.54 ± 1.88	0.44 ± 0.49	2.7 (0.0–7.8)	6.5 (2.0–22.7)
Neutrophils, total	60.37 ± 8.66	32.35 ± 7.68	36.06 ± 7.40	57.1	56.0 (45.1–66.5)
Myeloblasts	0.31 ± 0.31	0.62 ± 0.50	0.06 ± 0.08	1.2 (0.0–3.2)	1.0 (0.5–1.8)
Promyelocytes	0.79 ± 0.91	0.76 ± 0.65	0.64 ± 0.59	1.4 (0.0–4.0)	3.4 (2.6-4.6)
Myelocytes	3.95 ± 2.93	2.50 ± 1.48	2.49 ± 1.39	18.3 (8.5–29.7)	11.9 (8.1–16.9)
Metamyelocytes	19.37 ± 4.84	11.30 ± 3.59	12.42 ± 4.15	23.3 (14.0–34.2)	18.0 (9.8–25.3)
Bands	28.89 ± 7.56	14.10 ± 4.63	14.20 ± 5.23		11.0 (8.5–20.8)
Segmented	7.37 ± 4.64	3.64 ± 2.97	6.31 ± 3.91	12.9 (4.5–29.0)	10.7 (8.0–16.0)
Eosinophils	2.70 ± 1.27	2.61 ± 1.40	2.70 ± 2.16	3.6 (1.0–9.0)	3.2 (1.2–6.2)
Basophils	0.12 ± 0.20	0.07 ± 0.16	0.10 ± 0.12	0.06 (0.0–0.8)	<0.1 (0.0–0.2)
Lymphocytes, total	15.6	49.0	45.5	16.0 (4.8–35.8)	15.8 (10.8–22.7)
Transitional	1.18 ± 1.13	1.95 ± 0.94	1.99 ± 1.00		
Small	14.42 ± 5.54	47.05 ± 9.24	43.55 ± 8.56		
Plasma cells	0.00 ± 0.02	0.02 ± 0.06	0.06 ± 0.08	0.4 (0.2–0.6)	1.8 (0.2–2.2)
Monocytes	0.88 ± 0.85	1.01 ± 0.89	2.12 ± 1.59		1.8 (0.2–2.8)
Megakaryocytes	0.06 ± 0.15	0.05 ± 0.09	0.07 ± 0.12		< 1.0 (0.0–0.2)
Reticulum cells					0.3 (0.0–0.5)
M/E ratio	4.2	4.0	4.4	2.9 (1.2–5.2)	2.5 (1.2–5.0)

Data are from Rosse, 1977; Mauer, 1969; and Jandl, 1987.

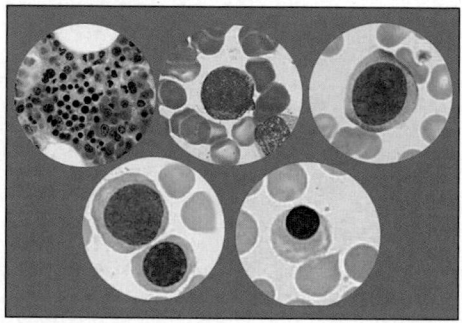

Figure 29–48 Normal erythroid maturation. Various stages of normoblastic erythroid maturation (× 1000).

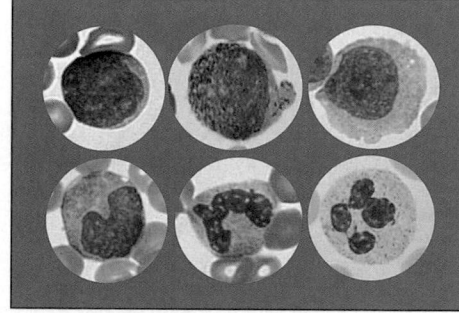

Figure 29–49 Normal myeloid (neutrophilic) maturation. Various stages of normal myeloid maturation from the blast to the mature neutrophil.

or with respect to other evidence that one of the systems is normal. An *increased* M/E ratio (e.g., 6 : 1) may be found in infection, chronic myelogenous leukemia, or erythroid hypoplasia. A *decreased* M/E ratio (i.e., <1.2 : 1) may mean a depression of leukopoiesis or a normoblastic hyperplasia, depending on the marrow cellularity. The number of megakaryocytes is estimated more reliably in sections than in marrow films. In scanning areas of films with good cellularity under low power (100×), an average of one to three megakaryocytes should be found in each field in a normal marrow.

Maturation

While examining the cells during the differential count, one should evaluate whether maturation is normal (Figs 29–48 and 29–49) – that is, whether nuclear and cytoplasmic development is in balance. Impaired cytoplasmic maturation in normoblasts, for example, occurs when hemoglobin synthesis is impaired; impaired nuclear maturation occurs in megaloblastic anemias. Bizarre or dysplastic maturation occurs as a result of certain drugs, in some leukemias, and in dysmyelopoietic syndromes.

Presence of Rare Cell Types or Abnormal Cells

In scanning the marrow, one looks for the presence of rare or unexpected cell types.

Tissue mast cells (Fig. 29–50) are normally very infrequent. They are increased in number in aplastic or refractory anemias, and in lymphoproliferative disorders.

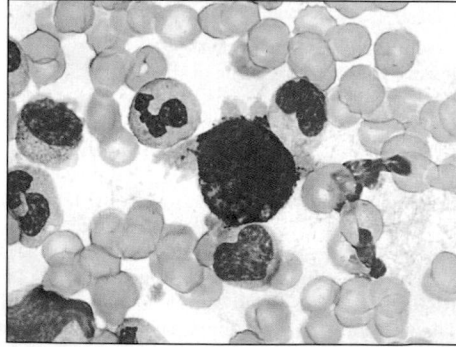

Figure 29–50 Tissue mast cell. Mast cells contain numerous dense dark-purple cytoplasmic granules that can completely cover the round nucleus (× 1000).

Osteoblasts (Fig. 29–51) are cells that synthesize the collagen matrix of bone. Osteoclasts are cells that resorb bone and are thought to result from the fusion of histiocytes. Both cell types are normally present in small numbers in the aspirates of infants and children. They are uncommonly seen in adult marrow, except when bone destruction or repair is occurring, as in hyperparathyroidism, Paget's disease, metastatic tumor, or a recent biopsy at the same site.

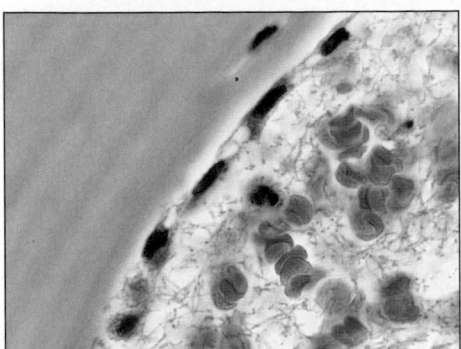

Figure 29–51 Osteoblast. Frequently found in pediatric patients, osteoblasts line the bone trabeculae. In smears they appear as cells with eccentrically placed nuclei, resembling plasma cells, but the cytoplasmic clearing is more centrally located and not in the Golgi area like in plasma cells (× 1000).

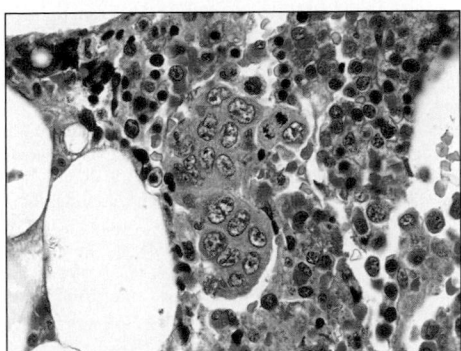

Figure 29–52 Metastatic tumor. Bone marrow biopsy with islands of metastatic gastric adenocarcinoma (× 1000).

Osteoblasts are large cells with a single eccentric nucleus that has reticular chromatin and a prominent nucleolus. The cytoplasm is moderately basophilic; a large pale Golgi zone is separated from the nucleus, rather than abutting it as in plasma cells. Osteoblasts are often present in clusters and may be confused with immature plasma cells or myeloma cells. Osteoclasts are large, multinucleated cells up to 100 µm diameter that may be mistaken for megakaryocytes. They have multiple nuclei that are separate (not joined as in megakaryocytes). The chromatin is reticular, and a prominent nucleolus is usually present. The cytoplasm may be basophilic but usually has pink-purple granules that resemble megakaryocyte granules. Coarse fragments of purple-staining material are often present. Clusters of *metastatic neoplastic cells* (Fig. 29–52) may be found in one or more marrow films of patients with metastatic tumor in the bone sampled; they may be found in biopsy sections and not in films; in both; or, less commonly, in one or more films and not the biopsy. Some metastatic neoplastic cells resemble myeloblasts or other primitive blasts. The clue to recognizing them is that they almost always appear in clusters or clumps of cells; this is not true of hematopoietic blast cells.

Evaluation of the Biopsy Specimen

Histologic sections allow better estimates of the marrow cellularity and the number of megakaryocytes than do marrow films (Fig. 29–47). In good histologic preparations, the cell distribution and maturation abnormalities can be quite reliably determined. In addition to more reliable detection of the presence of lymphomas or metastatic tumor, the histologic pattern can often be diagnostic of the type of neoplasm. Other focal lesions not found in films include granulomas, abscesses, and vascular lesions. In some conditions, such as myelofibrosis and hairy cell leukemia, the bone marrow cannot be aspirated, and biopsy is necessary to establish a diagnosis. Trabeculae should always be examined in order to detect bone abnormalities. Osteosclerosis with thickened bone trabeculae may accompany myelofibrosis or be congenital. In osteoporosis the bone trabeculae are thin. Osteomalacia is characterized by a recognizable osteoid seam. Osteitis fibrosa occurs in hyperparathyroidism and is characterized by irregular osteoclastic bone resorption, endosteal fibrosis, and some osteoblastic activity in areas of bone regeneration. Irregularly widened trabeculae with a 'mosaic' pattern are typical findings in Paget's disease of bone.

Interpretation

The summary of the marrow report includes an estimate of cellularity, an estimate of the number of megakaryocytes, the M/E ratio, statements about any cytologic or maturation abnormalities, an estimate of the storage iron and proportion of sideroblasts, and statements about any other abnormal findings present. A summary of the abnormalities in the blood cell counts and morphology is also made. An *interpretation* of the observed findings is made, which of course includes a diagnosis if this is possible. In making such an interpretation, one should include an integration of the marrow and blood observations with clinical findings and other laboratory data. Alterations in blood and marrow cells are discussed with reference to the diseases and disorders considered in subsequent chapters.

Indications for Marrow Study

In microcytic anemias, evaluation of the iron stores and sideroblasts allows categorization of the anemia (i.e., iron deficiency, anemia of chronic disease, sideroblastic).

In macrocytic anemias, marrow examination will confirm whether the process is megaloblastic or not; there are some cases in which the changes in the blood are minimal, yet the marrow is megaloblastic. In normocytic anemias (or macrocytic anemias) without an increased reticulocyte production index, the marrow is evaluated for quantitative or qualitative abnormalities in erythropoiesis (e.g., pure red cell aplasia or myelodysplasia).

In neutropenia, thrombocytopenia, or pancytopenia, marrow study is helpful in assessing the presence and normality of the precursor cells in each series. This enables one to assess the probabilities of decreased production, impaired maturation, or increased destruction as the mechanism of the disorder. In cytopenias, marrow examination sometimes will reveal the presence of leukemia or other hematological neoplasia.

In immunoglobulin abnormalities, the diagnosis of plasma cell myeloma or macroglobulinemia may be confirmed if infiltrations of abnormal plasma cells or lymphocytes are present. Marrow examination is essential for the diagnosis and classification of acute leukemia. It is frequently performed to assist in the diagnosis and staging of other neoplasms including lymphomas and metastatic tumors, and to assess response to therapy of hematological disorders. If the marrow cannot be aspirated ('dry tap'), biopsy is essential. Marrow biopsy should also be performed if there are blood changes suggesting myelofibrosis with myeloid metaplasia, or if granulomatous disease or metastatic tumor is suspected.

References

Ackerman P: Electronic Instrumentation in the Clinical Laboratory. Boston, Little, Brown and Co., 1972, p 140.

Altman PL, Dittmer DS (eds): Blood and Other Body Fluids. Washington, DC, Federation of American Societies for Experimental Biology, 1961.

Altman PL, Dittmer DS: Biology Data Book, Vol III, 2nd ed. Bethesda, MD, Federation of American Societies for Experimental Biology 1974, p 1856.

Bain BJ: Ethnic and sex differences in the total and differential white count and platelet count. J Clin Pathol 1996; 49:664–666.

Barone, MA: Lab values. *In* McMillan JA, Deangelis CD, Feigin RD, et al: (eds):Oski's Pediatrics, Principles and Practice, 3rd ed. Lippincott, Williams & Wilkins, 1999, p 2224.

Barrett BA, Hill PI: A micromethod for the erythrocyte sedimentation rate suitable for use on venous or capillary blood. J Clin Pathol 1980; 33:1118.

Bartels PC, Schoorl M, Lombarts AJ: Screening for EDTA-dependent deviations in platelet counts and abnormalities in platelet distribution histograms in pseudothrombocytopenia. Scand J Clin Lab Invest 1997; 57:629–636.

Bentley SA, Lewis SM: Automated differential leukocyte counting: The present state of the art. Br J Haematol 1977; 35:481–485.

Bentley SA, Johnson A, Bishop CA: A parallel evaluation of four automated hematology analyzers. Am J Clin Pathol 1993; 100:626–632.

Bessis M: Blood Smears Reinterpreted, translated by G Brecher. New York, Springer-Verlag 1977, p 60.

Bessman JD, Williams LJ, Gilmer PR Jr: Mean platelet volume. The inverse relation of platelet size and count in normal subjects, and an artifact of other particles. Am J Clin Pathol 1981; 76:289–293.

Böttiger LE, Svedberg CA: Normal erythrocyte sedimentation rate and age. Br Med J 1967; 2:85–87.

Brecher G, Schneiderman M: A time-saving device for the counting of reticulocytes. Am J Clin Pathol 1950; 20:1079–1093.

Brittin GM, Brecher G, Johnson CA, et al: Stability of blood in commonly used anticoagulants. Use of refrigerated blood for quality control of the Coulter Counter Model S. Am J Clin Pathol 1969; 52:690–694.

Bull BS: Is a standard ESR possible? Lab Med 1975; 6:31.

Bunn HF, Forget BG: Hemoglobin: Molecular, Genetic and Clinical Aspects. Philadelphia, WB Saunders Company, 1986, p 623.

Bunn HF, Forget BG, Ranney HM: Human Hemoglobins. Philadelphia, WB Saunders Company, 1977, p 2.

Burns ER, Lampasso J, Kowatch N, et al: Performance characteristics of state-of-the-art hematology analyzers. Clin Lab Sci 1992; 5:181–185.

Camden TL: How to select the ideal hematology analyzer. Med Lab Obs 1993; 25:29–33.

Cantero M, Conejo JR, Jimenez A: Interference from lipemia in cell count by hematology analyzers. Clin Chem 1996; 42:987–988.

Caswell M, Stuart J: Assessment of Diesse Ves-matic automated system for measuring erythrocyte sedimentation rate. J Clin Pathol 1991; 44:946–949.

Connelly DP, McClain MP, Crowson TW, et al: The use of the differential leukocyte count for inpatient case finding. Hum Pathol 1982; 13:294–300.

Cornbleet J: Spurious results from automated hematology cell analyzers. Lab Med 1983; 14:509.

Extremely useful reference for analysis of spurious results obtained from automated cell counters. It discusses reasons for spurious results with each parameter in a nicely tabulated format.

Cornbleet PJ, Myrick D, Judkins S, et al: Evaluation of the Cell-Dyn 3000 differential. Am J Clin Pathol 1992; 98:603–614.

Dacie JV, Lewis SM: Practical Haematology, 7th ed. Edinburgh, Churchill Livingstone, 1991, p 33.

Dalman PR: Developmental changes in red blood cell production and function. In Rudolph AM, Hoffman JIE (eds): Pediatrics, 18th ed. Norwalk, CT, Appleton & Lange, 1987, pp 1011–1012.

Davis BH: Immature reticulocyte fraction (IRF): by any name, a useful clinical parameter of erythropoietic activity. Lab Hematol 1996; 2:2–8.

Davis BH, Bigelow NC: Automated reticulocyte analysis. Clinical practice and associated new parameters. Hematol Oncol Clin North Am 1994; 8: 617–630.

d'Onofrio G, Tichelli A, Foures C, et al: Indicators of haematopoietic recovery after bone marrow transplantation: The role of reticulocyte measurements. Clin Lab Haematol 1996 18:45–53.

Ebrahim A, Ryan WL: Encapsulation of ribonucleic acid in human red cells for use as a reticulocyte quality control material for flow cytometric analysis. Cytometry 1996; 25:156–163.

Fairbanks VF, Fahey JL, Beutler E: Clinical Disorders of Iron Metabolism, 2nd ed. New York, Grune & Stratton, 1971, p 178.

Ford HC, Toomath RJ, Carter JM, et al: Mean platelet volume is increased in hyperthyroidism. Am J Hematol 1988; 27:190–193.

Freeman AG: Is the erythrocyte sedimentation rate outdated? J R Soc Med 1997; 90:179–180.

Geller A: Vacutainer systems. Franklin Lakes, NJ, Becton Dickinson, 1996.

Hanseler E, Fehr J, Keller H: Estimation of the lower limits of manual and automated platelet counting. Am J Clin Pathol 1996; 105:782–787.

Harrow C, Singer AJ, Thode HC: Facilitating the use of the erythrocyte sedimentation rate in the emergency department. Acad Emerg Med 1999; 6:658–660.

Hartsock RJ, Smith EB, Petty CS: Normal variations with aging of the amount of hematopoietic tissue in bone marrow from the anterior iliac crest. Am J Clin Pathol 1965; 43:326–331.

Hyun BH, Gulati GL, Ashton JK: Bone marrow examination: Techniques and interpretation. Hematol Oncol Clin North Am 1988; 2:513–523.

International Committee for Standardization in Haematology (ICSH): Recommendation for measurement of erythrocyte sedimentation rate of human blood. Am J Clin Pathol 1977; 68:505.

International Committee for Standardization in Haematology (ICSH): Expert Panel on Blood Cell Sizing: Recommendation for reference method for determination of packed cell volume of blood. J Clin Pathol 1980; 33:1–7.

International Committee for Standardization in Haematology (ICSH): ICSH reference method for staining of blood and bone marrow films by azure B

and eosin Y (Romanowsky stain). Br J Haematol 1984a; 57:707–710.

International Committee for Standardization in Haematology (ICSH): Protocol for evaluation of automated blood cell counters. Clin Lab Haematol 1984b; 6:69–84.

This protocol evaluates automated blood cell counters to assess the performance, advantages and limitations of such instruments.

International Council for Standardization in Haematology (Expert Panel on Blood Rheology): ICSH recommendations for measurement of erythrocyte sedimentation rate. J Clin Pathol 1993; 46:198–203.

International Committee for Standardization in Haematology: Reference method for the enumeration of erythrocytes and leucocytes. Clin Lab Haematol 1994; 20: 77–79.

International Council for Standardization in Hematology, Expert Panel on Cytometry: Proposed reference method for reticulocyte counting based on the determination of the reticulocyte to red cell ratio. Clin Lab Haematol 1998; 20:77–79.

Iversen OH, Roger M, Solberg HE, et al: Rising erythrocyte sedimentation rate during several years before diagnosis can be a predictive factor in 70% of renal cell carcinoma patients. The benefit of knowing subject-based reference values. J Int Med 1996; 240:133–141.

Jaffé ER, Hultquist DE: Cytochrome b_5 reductase deficiency and enzymopenic hereditary methemoglobinemia. In Scriver CR, Beaudet AL, et al: (eds): The Metabolic Basis of Inherited Disease, 6th ed. New York, McGraw-Hill, 1989.

Jandl JH: Blood: Textbook of Hematology, 1st ed. Boston, Little, Brown & Co, 1987.

Jandl JH: Blood: Textbook of Hematology, 2nd ed. Boston, Little, Brown & Co, 1996, p 505.

Koepke JA, van Assendelft OW, Bull BS: Standardisation of EDTA anticoagulation for blood counting procedures. Lab Medica 1989; 5:15–17.

Koike Y, Yoneyama A, Shirai J: Evaluation of thrombopoiesis in thrombocytopenic disorders by simultaneous measurement of reticulated platelets of whole blood and serum thrombopoietin concentrations. Thromb Haemost 1998; 79:1106–1110.

Kumar V, Singhi S: Predictors of serious bacterial infection in infants up to 8 weeks of age. Ind Peds 1994; 32:171–180.

Lapen D: A standardized differential stain for hematology. Cytometry 1982; 2:309–315.

Lillie RD (ed): HJ Conn's Biological Stains, 9th ed. Baltimore, Williams & Wilkins, 1977, p 416.

Lippi U, Schinella M, Nicoli M: EDTA-induced platelet aggregation can be avoided by a new anticoagulant also suitable for complete blood count. Haematology 1990; 75:38–41.

Lombarts AJ, deKieviet W: Recognition and prevention of pseudothrombocytopenia and concomitant pseudoleukocytosis. Am J Clin Pathol 1988; 89:634–639.

Lubrano GJ, Dean WW, Heinsohn HG, et al: The analysis of some commercial dyes and Romanowsky stains by high-performance liquid chromatography. Stain Technol 1977 52:13–23.

Lukens JN: Hemoglobins associated with cyanosis: Methemoglobinemia and low affinity hemoglobins. In Wintrobe's Clinical Hematology, 11th ed. Philadelphia, Lippincott, Williams & Wilkins, 2004, p 1487.

Mathy KA, Koepke JA: The clinical usefulness of segmented vs. stab neutrophil criteria for differential leukocyte counts. Am J Clin Pathol 1974; 61:947–958.

Matic GB, Chapman ES, Zaiss M: Whole blood analysis of reticulated platelets: Improvements of detection and assay stability. Cytometry 1998; 34:229–234.

Mauer AM: Pediatric Hematology, New York, McGraw-Hill, 1969.

Metzger DK, Charache S: Flow cytometric reticulocyte counting with thioflavin T in a clinical hematology

laboratory. Arch Pathol Lab Med 1987; 111:540–544.

Morris MW, Skrodzki Z, Nelson DA: Zeta sedimentation ratio (ZSR), a replacement for the erythrocyte sedimentation rate (ESR). Am J Clin Pathol 1975 164:254–256.

Mukherjee DP, Ray N, Acton ST: Level set analysis for leukocyte detection and tracking. IEEE Trans Image Process 2004; 13:562–572.

Nagai M, Mawatari K: Studies of the oxidation states of hemoglobin M Boston and hemoglobin M Saskatoon in blood by EPR spectroscopy. Biochem Biophys Res Commun 1995; 210:483–490.

NCCLS: Methods for the Erythrocyte Sedimentation Rate Test, 3rd ed. Candidate standard for approval. NCCLS document H2-A3. Villanova, PA, NCCLS, 1993.

O'Broin S, Kelleher B, O'Connor G: Uniformity of anticoagulation for full blood counting. Clin Lab Haematol 1997; 19:159–160.

Olshaker JS, Jerrard DA: The erythrocyte sedimentation rate. Clinical laboratory in emergency medicine. J Emerg Med 1997; 15:869–874.

Parthenis K, Metaxaki-Kossionides C: Blood analysis using black and white digital images. J Biomed Eng 1992; 14:287–292.

Pearson TA, Mensah GA, Alexander RW, et al: Markers of inflammation and cardiovascular disease: Application to clinical and public health practice: A statement for health care professionals from The Centers for Disease Control and Prevention and the American Heart Association. Circulation 2003; 107:499–511.

Penchas S: Heparin and the ESR. Arch Intern Med 1978; 138:1865–1866.

Perkins SL: Examination of the blood and bone marrow. In Wintrobe's Clinical Hematology, 11th ed. Philadelphia, Lippincott. Williams & Wilkins, 2004, pp 3–21.

Comprehensive review of blood and bone marrow examination including detailed discussion of various ancillary studies which can be done for establishing the diagnosis of hematological diseases.

Peterec SM, Brennan SA, Rinder HM: Reticulated platelet values in normal and thrombocytopenic neonates. J Pediatr 1996; 129:269–274.

Plebani M, DeToni S, Sanzari MC, et al: The TEST 1 automated system. A new method for measuring erythrocyte sedimentation rate. Am J Clin Pathol 1998; 110:334–340.

Rapi S, Ermini A, Bartolini L: Reticulocytes and reticulated platelets: Simultaneous measurement in whole blood by flow cytometry. Clin Chem Lab 1998; Med 36:211–214.

Rifai N: High-sensitivity C-reactive protein: A useful marker for cardiovascular disease risk predication and the metabolic syndrome. Clin Chem 2005; 51:504–505.

Rogers CH: Blood sample preparation for automated differential systems. Am J Med Technol 1973; 39:435–442.

Rosse C, Kraemer MJ, Dillon TL, et al: Bone marrow cell populations of normal infants; the predominance of lymphocytes. J Lab Clin Med, 1977; 89(6):1225–1240.

Rowan RM, Fraser C: Platelet size distribution analysis. In van Assendelft OW, England JM (eds): Advances in Hematological Methods: The Blood Count. Boca Raton, FL, CRC Press 1982, p 125.

Rümke CL: The imprecision of the ratio of two percentages observed in differential white blood cell counts: A warning. Blood Cells 1985; 11:137–140.

Ryan DH: Examination of the blood: In Williams Hematology, 6th ed. New York, McGraw Hill, 2001a, pp 9–14.

Ryan DH: Examination of the marrow: In Williams Hematology, 6th ed. New York, McGraw Hill, 2001b, pp 17–24.

Extensive review of bone marrow examination including discussion of marrow aspiration technique.

Saadeh C: The erythrocyte sedimentation rate: Old and new clinical applications. South Med J 1998; 91:220–225.

Sacker LS: Specimen collection. *In* Lewis SM, Coster JF (eds): Quality Control in Haematology. New York, Academic Press, 1975, p 211.

Saxton BR, Blanchette VW, Butchart S: Reticulated platelet counts in the diagnosis of acute immune thrombocytopenic purpura. J Pediatr Hematol Oncol 1998; 20:44–48.

Schneiderka P, Dohnal L, Shachova J: Erythrocyte sedimentation rate in glass and plastic pipettes. Sb Lek 1997; 98:301–315.

Shannon K, Pearson HA: Blood and blood forming tissues. *In* Rudolph CD, Rudolph AM, Hostetter MK, et al: (eds): Rudolph's Pediatrics, 21st ed. New York, McGraw Hill Companies, 2002, p 1521.

Simson E (ed): Proceedings of the Technicon H-1 Hematology Symposium. Tarrytown, NY, Technicon Instruments Inc, 1986.

Small BM, Bettigole RE: Diagnosis of myeloproliferative disease by analysis of platelet volume distribution. Am J Clin Pathol 1981; 76:685–691.

Smith EM, Samadian S: Use of the erythrocyte sedimentation rate in the elderly. Br J Hosp Med 1994; 51:394–397.

Sox HC Jr, Liang MH: The erythrocyte sedimentation rate. Guidelines for rational use. Ann Intern Med 1986; 104:515–523.

Stanworth SJ, Denton K, Monteath J: Automated counting of platelets on the Bayer ADVIA 120. Clin Lab Haematol 1999; 21:113–117.

Statland BE, Winkel P, Harris SC, et al: Evaluation of biologic sources of variation of leukocyte counts and other hematologic quantities using very precise automated analyzers. Am J Clin Pathol 1978; 69:48.

Stiegler G, Stohlawetz P, Brugger S: Elevated numbers of reticulated platelets in hyperthyroidism: Direct evidence for an increase of thrombopoiesis. Br J Haematol 1998; 101:656–658.

Stohlawetz P, Stiegler G, Jilma B: Measurement of the levels of reticulated platelets after plateletpheresis to monitor activity of thrombopoiesis. Transfusion 1998; 38:454–458.

Stohlawetz P, Stiegler P, Knobl P: The rise of reticulated platelets after intensive chemotherapy for AML reduces the need for platelet transfusions. Ann Hematol 1999; 78:271–273.

Tassies D, Reverter JC, Cases A: Effect of recombinant human erythropoietin treatment on circulating reticulated platelets in uremic patients: Associations with early improvement in platelet function. Am J Hematol 1998; 59:105–109.

Tsang CW, Lazarus R, Smith W: Hematological indices in an older population sample: Derivation of healthy reference values. Clin Chem 1998; 44:96–101.

Vaughan Hudson B, Maclennan KA, Bennett MH, et al: Systemic disturbance in Hodgkin's disease and its relation to histopathology and prognosis. Clin Radiol 1987; 38:257.

van Assendelft OW: Spectrophotometry of Haemoglobin Derivatives. Assen, The Netherlands, Royal Van Gorcum Ltd, 1970.

Ward P: The CBC at the turn of the millennium: an overview. Clin Chem 2000; 46:1215–1220. *This review article effectively summarizes current methodologies utilized by automated hematology analyzers. It also offers comments on advantages and limitations of selected CBC and differential parameters.*

Weick JK, Hagedorn AB, Linman JW: Leukoerythroblastosis: Diagnostic and prognostic significance. Mayo Clin Proc 1974; 49:110–113.

Wintrobe MM: Clinical Hematology, 7th ed. Philadelphia, Lea & Febiger, 1974.

Zauber NP, Zauber AG: Hematologic data of healthy very old people. JAMA 1987; 257:2181–2184.

Zeigler Z, Murphy S, Gardner FH: Microscopic platelet size and morphology in various hematologic disorders. Blood, 1978; 51:479–486.

Zlonis M: The mystique of the erythrocyte sedimentation rate. A reappraisal of one of the oldest laboratory tests still in use. Clin Lab Med 1993; 13:787–800.

IV

CHAPTER 30

Hematopoiesis

Sharad Mathur MD, Katherine Schexneider MD, Robert E. Hutchison MD

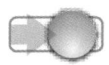

KEY POINTS

• Hematopoietic tissue arises in the bone marrow from stem cells that differentiate into granulocytes, monocytes, lymphocytes, megakaryocytes and erythroid cells.

• Differentiation and maturation of hematopoietic cells are influenced by soluble factors including growth factors and cytokines, by interaction with the bone marrow stroma, and are mediated partly through interaction of adhesion molecules.

• The primary function of erythrocytes is delivery of oxygen from lungs to tissues. This is dependent on the particular properties and adequate production of hemoglobin, and is regulated by oxygen tension in the kidneys where erythropoietin is produced.

• Inherited or acquired abnormalities of heme-biosynthesis, known as 'porphyrias' because of abnormal accumulation of porphyrins and metabolites, primarily affect the nervous system.

• Neutrophils and monocytes are derived from a common progenitor cell under the influence of growth factors, and are the major phagocytic cells. They, and the other granulocytic cells (eosinophils, basophils and mast cells) respond to soluble factors, eliminate microorganisms and modulate immunity.

• Megakaryocytes, stimulated by thrombopoietin, give rise to platelets and thus effect primary hemostasis.

• Lymphocytes arise in thymus and peripheral lymphoid tissue as well as in bone marrow. They are made up of complex populations of genetically distinct individual B cells, T cells, NK cells and related subtypes. These interact with other cells, secrete soluble factors including principally cytokines and immunoglobulins, and effect both humoral and cellular immunity.

Stem Cells

In postnatal life in humans, erythrocytes, granulocytes, monocytes, and platelets are normally produced only in the bone marrow. Lymphocytes are produced in the secondary lymphoid organs, as well as in the bone marrow and thymus gland.

Most bone marrow cells are morphologically recognizable precursors of granulocytes or erythrocytes with smaller numbers of platelet precursors (megakaryocytes), lymphocytes, monocytes, macrophages, stromal cells (endothelial cells, fibroblasts, osteoblasts, and osteoclasts), eosinophils, plasma cells, basophils, mast cells, and blasts. The latter includes hematopoietic stem cells (HSC), which are capable of self-renewal and differentiation; and progenitors, which differentiate along a specific pathway.

Hematopoietic Stem Cells and Progenitors

Pleuripotential hematopoietic stem cells give rise to common myeloid progenitors and common lymphoid progenitors (Akashi, 2000; Kondo, 1997). Common myeloid progenitors give rise to granulocyte/macrophage lineage-restricted progenitors and megakaryocyte/erythrocyte lineage-restricted progenitors. These cells subsequently generate lineage-committed progenitors for the production of granulocytes, macrophages, platelets and erythrocytes. Common lymphoid progenitors give rise to B lymphocytes, T lymphocytes, and natural killer cells. While HSCs can give rise to all types of blood cells, successive levels of progenitors have a more limited differentiating capability. Likewise, the capacity for self-renewal is progressively lost and terminally differentiated cells cannot divide.

Human HSCs express CD34 but lack the major histocompatibility complex (MHC) class II antigen, HLA-DR (Quesenberry, 2001). CD34 is a glycoprotein that is encoded on chromosome 1q and is expressed by hematopoietic stem cells as well as early progenitor cells. These cells also express high levels of multidrug-resistant (MDR1) protein and lack lineage commitment markers such as CD38, CD33, thy-1, and CD71. These earliest known precursor cells constitute less than 1% of bone marrow cells, and have the morphology of blasts. HSCs also occur in small numbers in the peripheral blood and are increased with administration of growth factors and/or some chemotherapeutic agents, allowing the use of peripheral blood as well as bone marrow to obtain stem cells used for bone marrow transplantation (Siena, 1989). Lineage commitment can be recognized by additional expression of CD38 antigen along with other

Table 30–1 Lineage-Specific Markers

Erythroid-CD71
Myeloid-CD33
B-lymphoid-CD10
T-lymphoid-CD7/CD5

antigens such as CD71 for erythroid, CD33 for myeloid, CD10 for B-lymphoid, and CD7/CD5 for T-lymphoid differentiation (Table 30–1) (Terstappen, 1991). Selection and differentiation with progressively narrower lineage-restriction are influenced by local effects in the bone marrow microenvironment and humoral factors and probably involves MHC class II molecule interactions.

Based on in vitro culture studies and colony assays, multiple levels of progenitors with progressively limited differentiating capability are identified (Coulombel, 2004). The earliest myeloid progenitor is the colony-forming unit-granulocyte, erythrocyte, macrophage, megakaryocyte (CFU-GEMM) cell that expresses CD34 and CD33. Under the influence of different growth factors and cytokines, CFU-GEMM cells develop into colony-forming unit-granulocyte-macrophage (CFU-GM) cells and colony-forming unit-megakaryocyte-erythroid (CFU-MegE) cells. CFU-GM cells differentiate into colony-forming unit-granulocyte (CFU-G) cells, precursors of neutrophils, and colony-forming unit-macrophage (CFU-M) cells, precursors of monocytes, macrophages, and dendritic cells (Fig. 30–1). CFU-MegE cells give rise to burst-forming unit-erythrocyte (BFU-E) cells (and subsequently colony-forming unit-erythrocyte (CFU-E) cells) and colony-forming unit-megakaryocyte (CFU-Meg) cells. Progenitors committed to development of eosinophils, basophils, and mast cells are also described (colony-forming unit-eosinophil (CFU-Eo) cells, colony-forming unit-basophil (CFU-Baso) cells, and colony-forming unit-mastocyte (CFU-Mast) cells). The hematopoietic stem cell also gives rise to osteoclasts, which are part of the monocytic and phagocytic system. In addition, there is also evidence that HSCs can transdifferentiate into nonhematopoietic cells (Zubair, 2002).

Hematopoietic Growth Factors

Soluble or membrane-bound biochemical factors contributing to control of hematopoiesis include hematopoietic growth factors and interleukins.

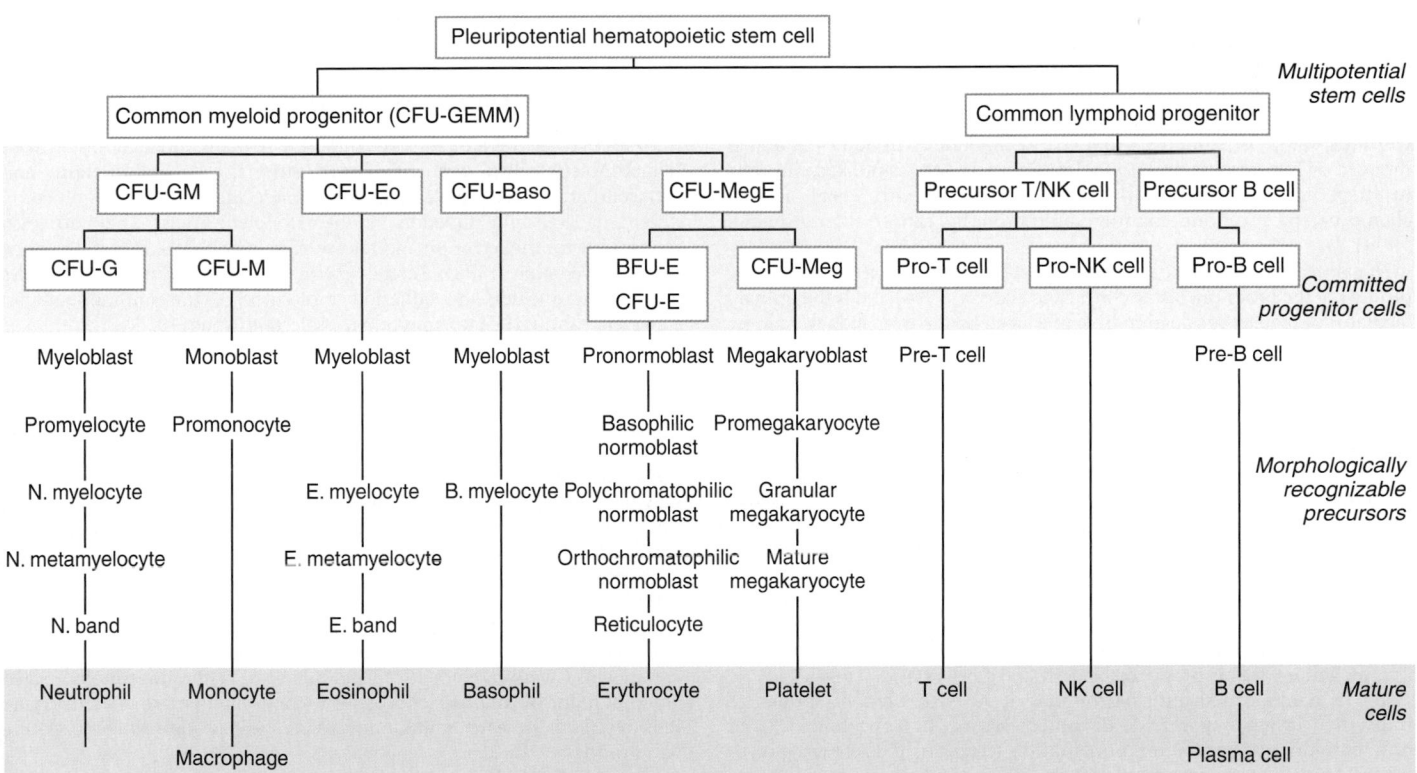

Figure 30–1 Hypothetical scheme of hematopoiesis. CFU-GEMM = colony-forming unit-granulocyte/erythrocyte/macrophage/megakaryocyte; CFU-GM = colony-forming unit-granulocyte/macrophage; CFU-G = colony-forming unit-granulocyte; CFU-M = colony-forming unit-macrophage; CFU-Eo = colony-forming unit-eosinophil; CFU-Baso = colony-forming unit-basophil; CFU-MegE = colony-forming unit-megakaryocyte/erythroid; BFU-F = burst-forming unit-erythrocyte; CFU-E = colony-forming unit-erythrocyte; CFU-Meg = colony-forming unit-megakaryocyte; N. = neutrophil; E. = eosinophil; B. = basophil.

They consist of acidic glycoproteins, which are functionally diverse but structurally conserved (Kaushansky, 1993). They regulate the proliferation and differentiation of hematopoietic precursor cells and facilitate the function of mature blood cells. Hematopoietic growth factors may act locally near the site at which they are produced or they may circulate in the blood. They act at low concentrations, are produced by many different kinds of cells, and usually affect more than one lineage (Quesenberry, 2001). They often act synergistically with other growth factors and may act on neoplastic cells as well as normal cells. Growth factors also tend to enhance membrane integrity and prevent apoptosis.

Genes associated with hematopoietic growth factors have been identified, cloned, and sequenced. Their products have been generated by recombinant DNA methods. Molecular structures are frequently predicted using computer models from sequence data as well as analyzed directly by crystallography and magnetic resonance spectroscopy. Pure molecules are utilized experimentally and several are now used therapeutically as drugs. The rapid growth in knowledge of hematopoietic growth factors and the complexity of their activities defies simple summation. Factors chiefly involved in hematopoiesis are briefly noted here.

Granulocyte/macrophage colony-stimulating factor (GM-CSF) is a pan-myeloid growth factor, stimulating erythroid, granulocyte, monocyte, megakaryocyte, and eosinophil progenitors, resulting primarily in increases of neutrophils, monocytes, and eosinophils, and in activation of phagocytic function. It is a 14- to 35-kDa glycoprotein encoded on the long arm of chromosome 5. GM-CSF is utilized clinically to combat neutropenia in patients receiving chemotherapy and in those undergoing bone marrow transplantation (Mertelsmann, 1993). Myeloid hyperplasia may result in the bone marrow in these settings.

Granulocyte colony-stimulating factor (G-CSF) stimulates granulocyte production and functional activation. It is an 18-kDa protein encoded on the long arm of chromosome 17 (Bagby, 1991). G-CSF is frequently used to treat neutropenia and may induce less toxicity than GM-CSF (Root, 1999). It is also the growth factor most commonly used to mobilize CD34+ stem cells in the peripheral blood (Hübel, 2003).

Monocyte/macrophage colony-stimulating factor (M-CSF) (also known as colony-stimulating factor-1 [CSF-1]) stimulates monocyte–macrophage production and activity. It consists of two species of glycoprotein (40–50 and 70–90 kDa) that are encoded on the long arm of chromosome 5 (Bagby, 1991). CSF-1 induces macrophage production of interleukin (IL)-1. The CSF-1 receptor is the product of the FMS gene and acts as a tyrosine kinase to mediate cell activation.

Erythropoietin (EPO) stimulates proliferation, growth, and differentiation of erythroid precursors, resulting in increased erythrocyte counts, and may have a minor effect on megakaryocytes. EPO has a dominant effect on CFU-E, pronormoblasts, and basophilic normoblasts. Maximal BFU-E stimulation requires other growth factors such as IL-3 and GM-CSF. EPO, an 18-kDa protein (34–39 kDa when glycosylated) encoded on the long arm of chromosome 7, is primarily produced in the kidney in adult life and is induced by hypoxia (Bagby, 1991). Recombinant EPO is utilized clinically to treat anemia, particularly that associated with renal failure, chemotherapy, or bone marrow infiltration by cancer (Mertelsmann, 1993).

Thrombopoietin (TPO) is a 35-kDa polypeptide that is a ligand for the product of the proto-oncogene c-mpl (Kaushansky, 1994) and is the primary regulator of platelet production. It is produced by the liver, kidney, marrow stroma, and other tissues and stimulates both the production and differentiation of megakaryocytic precursor cells (Kaushansky, 2003). It is essential for the full maturation of megakaryocytes and enhances platelet production. It is used to speed the recovery of blood platelets after cytoreductive therapies.

IL-3 is a multipotential colony-stimulating factor that has activities analogous to GM-CSF but occurs at an earlier level. The 14- to 28-kDa protein is encoded near the GM-CSF gene on the long arm of chromosome 5, and is closely linked to the genes for GM-CSF, IL-4, and IL-5. IL-3 is produced by T cells, endothelial cells, fibroblasts, macrophages, and mast cells. It activates indirectly by stimulating other cytokines (Bagby, 1991).

IL-5 activates cytotoxic T cells, induces immunoglobulin secretion, and stimulates eosinophils. It is a 50- to 60-kDa product of the long arm of chromosome 5 that is produced by activated T cells (Jandl, 1996).

IL-6 is a broad activating factor that appears to exert its influences indirectly through synergy with other factors. IL-6 facilitates B cell differentiation, promotes immunoglobulin secretion, and acts as a growth factor for malignant plasma cells (Teoh, 1997). It functions along with IL-3 to increase replication of myeloid precursors, synergizes with IL-2 and IL-4, and stimulates platelet production. It is a 26-kDa product of the short arm of chromosome 7 (Jandl, 1996) and is secreted by T cells, macrophages, and fibroblasts.

IL-9 is a T cell growth factor and mast cell-activating factor that also has effects in stimulating erythroid and myeloid proliferation. It is a 30- to 40-kDa glycoprotein encoded on chromosome 5 (Quesniaux, 1992).

IL-11 promotes formation of antigen-specific immunoglobulin-secreting B cells and synergizes with IL-3 to stimulate megakaryocyte production and pleuripotential stem cell proliferation. IL-11 synergizes with IL-4 to promote stem cell proliferation. It is a 23-kDa glycoprotein encoded on the long arm of chromosome 19 (Quesniaux, 1992).

Kit ligand (KL) is the ligand for the tyrosine kinase receptor *c-kit* and has been referred to as 'stem cell factor' or 'steel factor.' It synergizes with most other growth factors including GM-CSF and IL-3 to stimulate myeloid, erythroid, and lymphoid progenitors (Quesniaux, 1992). The KL receptor is encoded on chromosome 4, whereas KL or steel factor is mapped to chromosome 12 (Broudy, 1997). KL stimulates the growth, viability, and adhesion of primitive progenitor cells, erythroid precursors (BFU-E, CFU-E), myeloid precursors (CFU-GM), megakaryocytic precursors (CFU-Meg), and mast cells. It also stimulates the growth of B cells, T cells, NK cells, and dendritic cells (Lyman, 1998).

Flt-3 ligand (FL) stimulates primitive progenitor cells, often in synergy with KL. Similarly to the KL receptor, the FL receptor is also a tyrosine kinase. It acts synergistically with other growth factors to stimulate T cells, B cells, NK cells, and dendritic cells. In contrast to KL, FL does not stimulate mast cells (Lyman, 1998).

Other regulators of HSCs include tumor necrosis factor (TNF)-α and transforming growth factor (TGF)-β. HSCs express receptors of the notch and Wnt families, and these cytokine pathways are also likely important in self-renewal and differentiation (Ohishi, 2003; Sauvageau, 2004).

HSCs and the earliest myeloid progenitors (CFU-GEMM) require KL, FL, IL-3, and IL-6 for duplication and differentiation into committed progenitors. Further development of myeloid progenitors (CFU-G and CFU-M) requires G-CSF and M-CSF in addition to GM-CSF and IL-3. G-CSF is primarily responsible for neutrophil differentiation, M-CSF for monocyte/macrophage differentiation, IL-5 for eosinophil differentiation, IL-3 and KL for basophil differentiation, and KL for mast cell differentiation. Development of the earliest erythroid progenitor (BFU-E) is independent of EPO, but subsequent differentiation into CFU-E needs EPO in addition to other growth factors such as GM-CSF, IL-3, and KL. EPO is solely responsible for further maturation of the erythroid lineage. Megakaryocyte development is dependent on TPO, in concert with IL-3, IL-6, IL-11, and KL.

Laboratory assays are available for most hematopoietic growth factors and cytokines, and are helpful in the diagnostic work-up of a wide variety of diseases. Disease states caused by selective deficiency of a growth factor, such as anemia of renal failure due to low EPO levels, can be treated by administration of recombinant protein.

Adhesion Molecules in Hematopoiesis

Adhesion molecules are required to modulate many interactions between hematopoietic cells and growth factors, stromal cells, endothelium, and extracellular matrix. These cell-surface molecules influence induction, differentiation, and function of hematopoietic cells. They are also responsible for the retention and release of hematopoietic cells in the bone marrow (Verfaillie, 1998). Several major families of adhesion molecules exist. These include the adhesion molecules of the immunoglobulin supergene family, the integrins, and the selectins (Long, 1992).

Another group of adhesion molecules includes the mucin-like molecules and represents a family of glycoproteins expressed on tissues of the hematopoietic system. These sialomucins have been found on progenitor cells, including stem cells that possess the antigens CD34, CD43, CD45RA, P selectin glycoprotein ligand-1 (PSGL-1), and CD164 (Verfaillie, 1998). Functional studies demonstrate that CD164 molecules may have a major role in the adhesion of hematopoietic progenitor cells to the bone marrow stromal cells and may be potent signaling molecules with the capacity to suppress hematopoietic cell proliferation (Zannettino, 1998).

Many extracellular matrix components interact with receptors on hematopoietic cells. These include fibronectin, thrombospondin, hyaluronic acid, hemonectin, laminin, and heparin sulfate. Receptors for some of these are known. CD44, receptor for hyaluronic acid, is an antigenically related group of inducible cell-surface proteins variably expressed on all leukocytes. It is required for early granulopoiesis as well as trafficking of mature lymphocytes.

Another class of compounds, the chemokines, are important in regulating blood cell trafficking and homing. The chemokine CXCL12 (SDF-1a) is expressed by bone marrow stromal cells and microvascular endothelium. HSCs express CXCR4, the receptor for CXCL12. The interaction of CXCL12 and CXCR4 is involved in HSC engraftment. GM-

CSF-induced mobilization of HSCs is likely due to reduction in CXCL12 and CXCR4 activity (Campbell, 2003).

Hematopoietic Tissues

Embryonic and Fetal Hematopoiesis

Beginning in the first month of prenatal life, the first blood cells arise outside the embryo in the mesenchyme of the yolk sac as *blood islands*. These cells are predominantly *primitive erythroblasts*, which are large and megaloblastic, are formed intravascularly, and retain their nuclei. At the sixth week, hematopoiesis begins in the liver, and this becomes the major hematopoietic organ of early and midfetal life. *Definitive erythroblasts*, which become non-nucleated red cells, are formed extravascularly in the liver, and granulopoiesis and megakaryocytes are present to a lesser degree. In the middle part of fetal life, the spleen and to a lesser extent lymph nodes have a minor role in hematopoiesis, but the liver continues to dominate. In the latter half of fetal life, the bone marrow becomes progressively more important as a site of blood cell production. As this occurs, the liver's role diminishes.

Postnatal Hematopoiesis

Shortly after birth, hematopoiesis in the liver ceases and the marrow is the only site for the production of erythrocytes, granulocytes, and platelets. Hematopoietic stem cells and committed progenitor cells are maintained in the marrow. Lymphocytes (of the B cell type) continue to be produced in the marrow, as well as in the secondary lymphoid organs, whereas T lymphocytes are produced in the thymus and also in the secondary lymphoid organs (see Lymphocytes).

At birth, the total marrow space is occupied by active hematopoietic (red) marrow. As body growth progresses and marrow space increases during infancy, only part of that space is needed for hematopoiesis; the remaining space is occupied by fat cells. Later in childhood, only the flat bones (the skull, vertebrae, thoracic cage, shoulder, and pelvis) and the proximal parts of the long bones of the upper and lower limbs are sites of blood cell formation. The remaining marrow space is fatty or yellow marrow that can be replaced by hematopoietic cells if continuous, intensive stimulation exists.

The marrow circulation is closed – that is, arterioles deriving from central longitudinal arteries (i.e., in long bones) connect directly with broad venous sinuses that anastomose and eventually empty into central longitudinal veins. The flattened endothelium of the sinuses is partially covered by adventitial reticular cells, a form of fibroblast that elaborates argentophilic reticulin fibers. These reticular cells and fibers form the supporting meshwork of the marrow stroma, where the hematopoietic cells reside. The reticular cells are but minimally phagocytic; they may swell and take up water, may become fat cells, and possibly may induce hematopoietic stem cells to become committed progenitor cells. After proliferation and maturation have occurred in the marrow stroma, blood cells gain entrance to the blood through or between the endothelial cells of the sinus wall. This requires displacement of adventitial cells. Stromal mesenchymal cells and sinusoidal endothelial cells produce a variety of cytokines and chemokines involved in hematopoiesis.

Erythrocyte Production

The erythrocyte is a vehicle for the transport of hemoglobin, which is produced in precursor cells of the erythrocytes, the normoblasts. The function of hemoglobin is the transport of oxygen and carbon dioxide. The erythrocyte is also metabolically capable of keeping hemoglobin in a functional state.

Normoblastic Maturation

The earliest recognizable erythroid precursor is the *pronormoblast* (Fig. 30–2). At about 20 μm diameter, it is the largest of the erythroid precursors. The nucleus has a fine, uniform chromatin pattern that is somewhat more distinct and more intensely stained than that of the myeloblast. The nuclear membrane is prominent. One or more prominent nucleoli are present. The cytoplasm has a heterogeneous quality and is moderate in amount and basophilia; no granules are present. The pronormoblast undergoes mitosis and forms two basophilic normoblasts.

The *basophilic normoblast* (Fig. 30–3) is somewhat smaller and has slightly coarser chromatin that stains intensely; the chromatin may be partially clumped and the pattern may suggest a wheel with broad spokes.

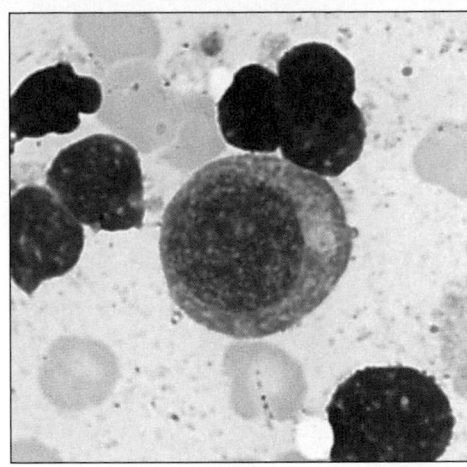

Figure 30–2 Pronormoblast with a large round nucleus, fine chromatin, and basophilic cytoplasm (Wright–Giemsa, ×250).

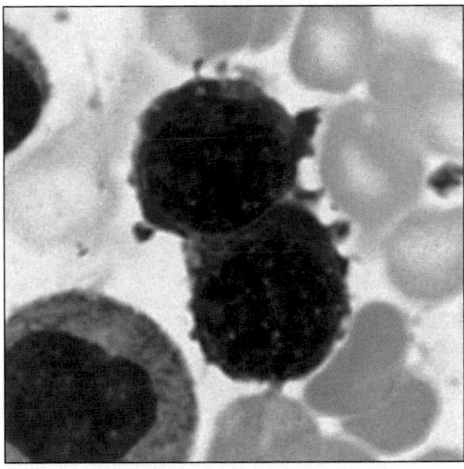

Figure 30–3 Basophilic normoblasts with chromatin condensation and deeply basophilic cytoplasm (Wright–Giemsa, ×250).

The parachromatin (the nonchromatin part of the nucleus) is distinct and stains pink. Nucleoli are present but not often visible. The nuclear/cytoplasmic (N/C) ratio is moderate; about one-fourth of the total cell area appears to be cytoplasm. The cytoplasm is deeply basophilic, owing to the abundance of RNA; much of this is evident as polyribosomes in electron micrographs. The cell borders of early normoblasts frequently appear irregular, owing to the presence of pseudopodia.

After mitosis of the basophilic normoblast, evidence of continuing hemoglobin production becomes visible in the cytoplasm of the two daughter cells as polychromasia – that is, mixtures of the red-staining of hemoglobin with the blue of RNA in varying shades of gray. This cell is the *polychromatophilic normoblast* (Fig. 30–4), which is slightly smaller than the basophilic normoblast. The nucleus occupies about half of the area of the cell, stains intensely, and has moderately condensed chromatin that is sharply distinct from the pink parachromatin. The polychromatophilic normoblast undergoes one or two mitotic divisions.

After the last mitosis, the nucleus becomes small and dense (pyknotic) and the *orthochromatic normoblast* stage is reached (Fig. 30–5). Mitosis is no longer possible. The cell is smaller than the polychromatophilic normoblast and has a lower N/C ratio. The cytoplasm contains more abundant hemoglobin and fewer polyribosomes and remains slightly polychromatophilic.

Finally, accompanied by cytoplasmic contractions and undulations, the nucleus and a small rim of cytoplasm are ejected from the orthochromatic normoblast, forming the *reticulocyte* (Fig. 30–6). On air-dried films with Romanowsky-type stains, the reticulocyte is polychromatophilic as a result of the retention of RNA.

In the marrow, developing erythroid cells are usually in contact with macrophages in what are termed 'erythroblastic islands' (Fig. 30–7). These erythroblastic islands are usually broken up when aspirated marrow is spread on slides, but fragments of macrophage cytoplasm may sometimes be seen attached to the separated normoblasts, especially on Prussian blue-stained films.

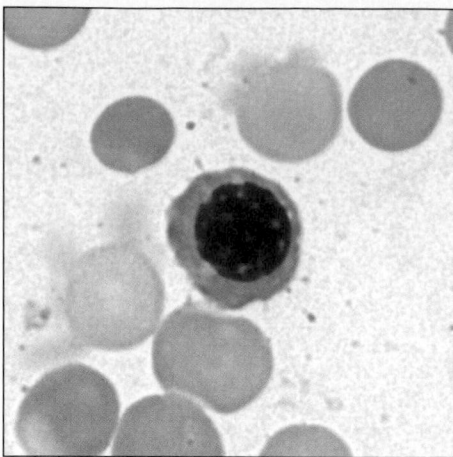

Figure 30–4 Polychromatophilic normoblast with light blue cytoplasm due to accumulation of hemoglobin (Wright–Giemsa, ×250).

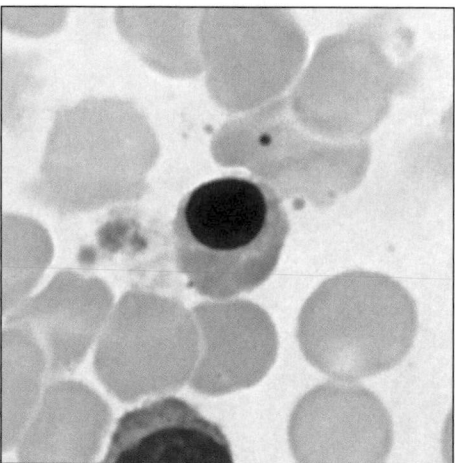

Figure 30–5 Orthochromatic normoblast with pyknotic nucleus and pink-gray cytoplasm (Wright–Giemsa, ×250).

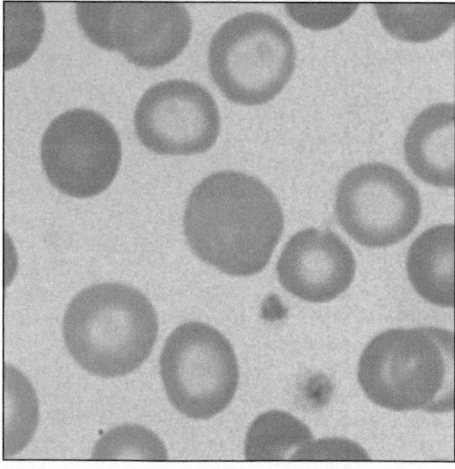

Figure 30–6 Reticulocyte (polychromatophilic erythrocyte) with pink-gray cytoplasm due to residual RNA (Wright–Giemsa, ×250).

During proliferation and maturation, iron is transferred from plasma transferrin into the cells in the normoblastic series. The pronormoblast and basophilic normoblast have the highest content of RNA, which begins to decline in the polychromatophilic normoblasts as hemoglobin increases in amount. Synthesis of RNA gradually decreases in each stage through the orthochromatic normoblasts. When the nucleus is no longer present (in the reticulocyte), RNA synthesis ceases, yet the RNA already present remains for a few days, and protein and heme synthesis continue in the reticulocyte until the cell loses its RNA and mitochondria.

During this maturation process, three or four mitotic divisions occur in a period of 3 days, resulting in the potential production of 16 reticulocytes

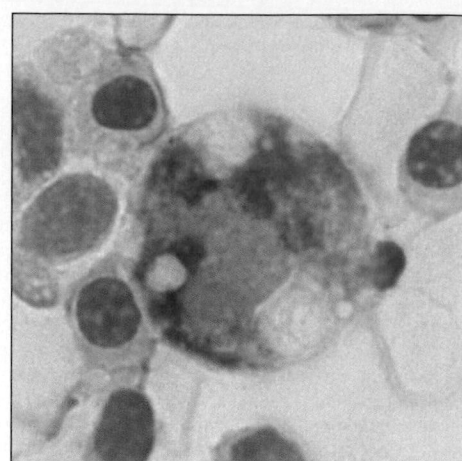

Figure 30–7 Siderophage with associated normoblasts (part of an erythroblastic island) in the bone marrow (Prussian blue, ×250).

from each pronormoblast. The reticulocytes are larger than mature red cells and remain in the marrow stroma for 1–2 days before being released into the blood.

In the marrow the reticulocytes are about equal in number to the nucleated erythrocytes and slightly greater in number than the reticulocytes in the circulating blood. If sufficiently severe hypoxia is present, this marrow pool of reticulocytes can be released. This approximately doubles the number of circulating reticulocytes.

Normally, reticulocytes remain as such, slowly synthesizing hemoglobin, for 2–3 days in the marrow and 1 day in the blood. Residual ribosomes, mitochondria, and other organelles are then removed, and the mature erythrocytes circulate for about 120 days. During this time they gradually age, certain enzymatic activities diminish, and they are finally destroyed within phagocytic cells of the reticuloendothelial system.

Megaloblastic Maturation

Abnormal maturation of erythroid precursors that occurs in vitamin B_{12} deficiency or folic acid deficiency is known as megaloblastic maturation, and the abnormal erythroid cells are called *megaloblasts*. Because of impaired ability of the cells to synthesize DNA, the intermitotic and mitotic phases are prolonged. This results in enlarged cells, with nuclear maturation lagging behind cytoplasmic maturation (nuclear–cytoplasmic dissociation). The nuclear chromatin pattern is more delicate and more 'open,' with prominent parachromatin. Karyorrhexis, or breaking up of the nucleus, and Howell–Jolly bodies are frequently noted. Megaloblastic development parallels normoblastic maturation; the stages of promegaloblast, basophilic megaloblast, polychromatophilic megaloblast, and orthochromatic megaloblast may be recognized.

Regulation of Erythrocyte Production

The number of erythrocytes in the blood may be regulated by changing the rate of production. The rate of erythrocyte destruction does not vary appreciably in normal individuals. Increased production of erythrocytes occurs when oxygen transport to the tissues is impaired, as in anemia, in cardiac or pulmonary disorders, and in the low oxygen tension of high altitudes. Erythrocyte production decreases when an individual is hypertransfused or exposed to high oxygen tension.

Oxygen affinity of hemoglobin is modulated by the concentration of phosphates, in particular 2,3-diphosphoglycerate (2,3-DPG) in the red cell. These phosphates combine with the β-chains of reduced hemoglobin and diminish its affinity for oxygen (Fig. 30–8). In areas of tissue hypoxia, as oxygen moves from hemoglobin into the tissues, the amount of reduced hemoglobin in the red cells increases, binding more 2,3-DPG, further reducing its oxygen affinity so that more oxygen can be delivered to the tissues. If hypoxia persists, depletion of free 2,3-DPG leads to increased glycolysis, production of more 2,3-DPG, and a persistently lower oxygen affinity of the hemoglobin.

Tissue hypoxia induces formation of EPO via production of the transcriptional factor hypoxia-inducible factor-1 (HIF-1). HIF-1 is a heterodimer consisting of alpha and beta subunits, of which the alpha subunit is regulated by hypoxia. Under conditions of normal oxygen tension, HIF-1α undergoes proteosomal degradation, but it is stable under hypoxic conditions. EPO effects the production of more red cells in the bone

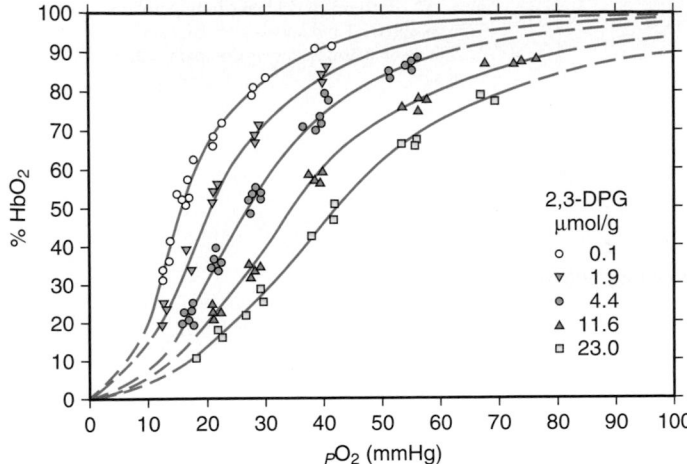

Figure 30–8 Oxygen dissociation curves of hemoglobin at different concentrations of 2,3-diphosphoglycerate (DPG). The curve is sigmoidal and shifts to the right with increasing concentrations of 2,3-DPG; this results in decreased affinity of hemoglobin for oxygen and increased delivery of oxygen to the tissues. (Reprinted from Oxygen Affinity of Hemoglobin and Red Cell Acid Base Status, Duhm J, p. 583, Copyright 1972, with permission from Elsevier.)

2,3-DPG
μmol/g
○ 0.1
▽ 1.9
◉ 4.4
▲ 11.6
□ 23.0

Hippel–Lindau protein is involved in HIF-1α degradation). This results in elevation of EPO levels and an autosomal recessive form of hereditary polycythemia known as Chuvash polycythemia (Gordeuk, 2004).

Measurement of EPO is accomplished by in vitro immunologic methods utilizing serum or plasma, with ethylenediamenetetraacetic acid (EDTA) plasma providing greater sensitivity (Lindstedt, 1998). Elevated levels are detected in patients with secondary polycythemia and in aplastic anemia. Decreased levels below the normal range are found in normal individuals after transfusion and in primary polycythemia (polycythemia vera). However, considerable overlap exists and normal EPO levels may be found in both primary and secondary polycythemia (Spivak, 2002). Anti-EPO antibodies have been described in pure red-cell aplasia and systemic lupus erythematosus (Casadevall, 1996; Schett, 2001); these may interfere with immunoassays for EPO and may contribute to anemia.

Synthesis of Hemoglobin

Heme Synthesis. Heme synthesis occurs in most cells of the body, except the mature erythrocytes, but most abundantly in the erythroid precursors. Succinylcoenzyme A condenses with glycine to form the unstable intermediate α-amino β-ketoadipic acid, which is readily decarboxylated to δ-aminolevulinic acid (ALA) (Fig. 30–9). This condensation requires pyridoxal phosphate (vitamin B_6) and occurs in mitochondria.

ALA is excreted normally in small amounts in the urine, but in certain abnormalities of heme synthesis (e.g., lead poisoning) excretion is increased. Two molecules of ALA condense to form the monopyrrole, porphobilinogen, catalyzed by the enzyme ALA-dehydrase. Porphobilinogen is also normally excreted in small amounts in the urine. Markedly elevated amounts appear in the urine in acute intermittent porphyria, and are easily detected by a color reaction with Ehrlich's aldehyde reagent.

Four molecules of porphobilinogen react to form uroporphyrinogen III or I (Fig. 30–10). The type III isomer is converted, by way of copro-porphyrinogen III and protoporphyrinogen, to protoporphyrin. In certain

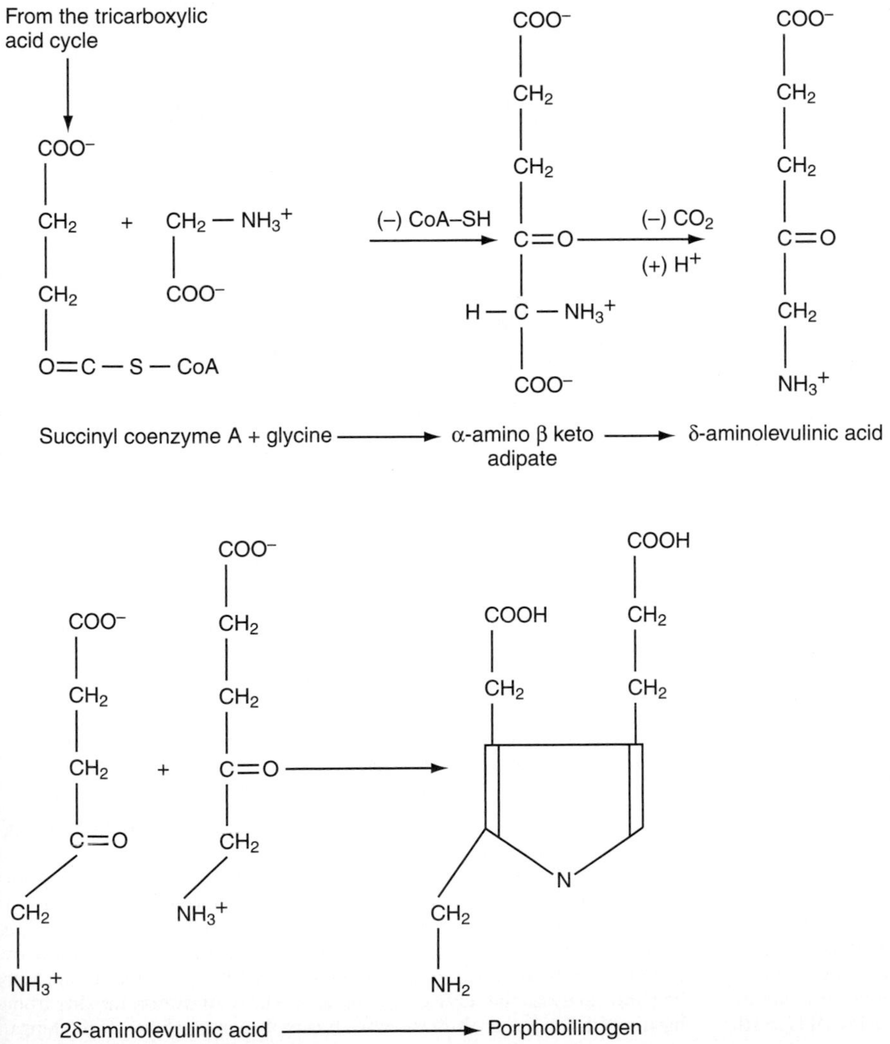

marrow. It acts by inducing committed progenitor cells (CFU-E and BFU-E) in the marrow to proliferate and differentiate into pronormoblasts, by shortening the generation time of normoblasts, and by promoting early release of reticulocytes into the blood. The result is increased numbers of marrow normoblasts in a normal ratio of cell types, a condition known as normoblastic hyperplasia. Increased cellular expression of HIF-1α can result from a 598C→T mutation in the von Hippel–Lindau gene (the von

Figure 30–9 Formation of porphobilinogen from succinylcoenzyme A and glycine. (From Leavell BS: Fundamentals of Clinical Hematology, 4th ed. Philadelphia, WB Saunders Company, 1976, with permission.)

From the tricarboxylic acid cycle

Succinyl coenzyme A + glycine ⟶ α-amino β keto adipate ⟶ δ-aminolevulinic acid

2δ-aminolevulinic acid ⟶ Porphobilinogen

IV

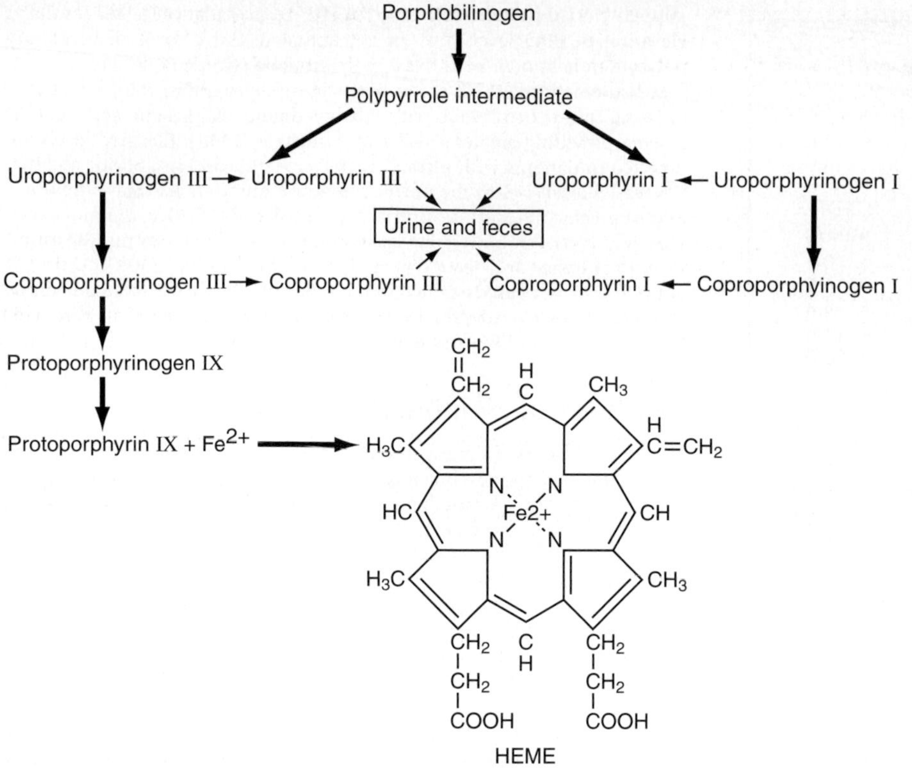

Porphobilinogen

↓

Polypyrrole intermediate

Uroporphyrinogen III → Uroporphyrin III   Uroporphyrin I ← Uroporphyrinogen I

Urine and feces

Coproporphyrinogen III → Coproporphyrin III   Coproporphyrin I ← Coproporphyinogen I

Protoporphyrinogen IX

↓

Protoporphyrin IX + Fe^{2+} ⟶ (heme structure)

HEME

Figure 30–10 Formation of heme from porphobilinogen. (From Leavell BS: Fundamentals of Clinical Hematology, 4th ed. Philadelphia, WB Saunders Company, 1976, with permission.)

diseases when this pathway is partially blocked, the type I isomers of uroporphyrinogen and coproporphyrinogen are formed and their oxidized excretion products, uroporphyrin I and coproporphyrin I, are increased in amount.

Protoporphyrin is normally found in mature erythrocytes. In lead poisoning and in iron deficiency, levels of free erythrocyte protoporphyrin (FEP) are increased. Iron is inserted into protoporphyrin by the mitochondrial enzyme ferrochelatase to form the finished heme moiety.

Other abnormalities of heme synthesis (the porphyries) are discussed later in this chapter.

Globin Synthesis. Globin synthesis occurs in the cytoplasm of the normoblast and reticulocyte. The polypeptide chains are manufactured on the ribosomes. Specific small soluble RNA (sRNA) molecules determine the placement of each amino acid according to the code in the messenger RNA (mRNA). Progressive growth of the polypeptide chain begins at the amino end. This process of protein synthesis occurs on ribosomes clustered into polyribosomes, which are held together by the mRNA. Because the reticulocyte can synthesize hemoglobin for at least 2 days after loss of its nucleus, it appears that the mRNA for hemoglobin is quite stable. The polypeptide chains released from the ribosomes are folded into their three-dimensional configurations spontaneously.

Control of hemoglobin synthesis is exerted primarily through the action of heme. Increased heme inhibits further heme synthesis by inhibiting the activity and synthesis of ALA synthase. Heme also promotes globin synthesis, mainly at the site of chain initiation, the interaction of ribosomes with mRNA.

Structure and Function of Hemoglobin

In each hemoglobin (Hb) molecule, one heme group is inserted into a hydrophobic pocket of one folded polypeptide chain (Bunn, 1986). Normal adult HbA consists of four heme groups and four polypeptide chains (two α-chains and two β-chains), which form a roughly globular hemoglobin molecule (Fig. 30–11). The ferrous iron atoms have six coordination bonds – four to the pyrrole nitrogens of heme, one to the imidazole nitrogen of histidine of the globin chain (87-α or 92-β), and one that is reversibly bound to oxygen. As the oxygen partial pressure increases, the four heme groups sequentially bind one molecule of oxygen each. In the process, a change in the overall configuration of the hemoglobin molecule occurs, which favors the additional binding of oxygen.

The sigmoid-shaped oxygen dissociation curve of hemoglobin reflects this increasing affinity for oxygen with increasing partial pressure of oxygen in the lungs (Fig. 30–8). In the tissues, the conversion of oxygenated Hb to Hb, the decreasing pH and increasing temperature produced by metabolic processes, and the binding of more 2,3-DPG to Hb

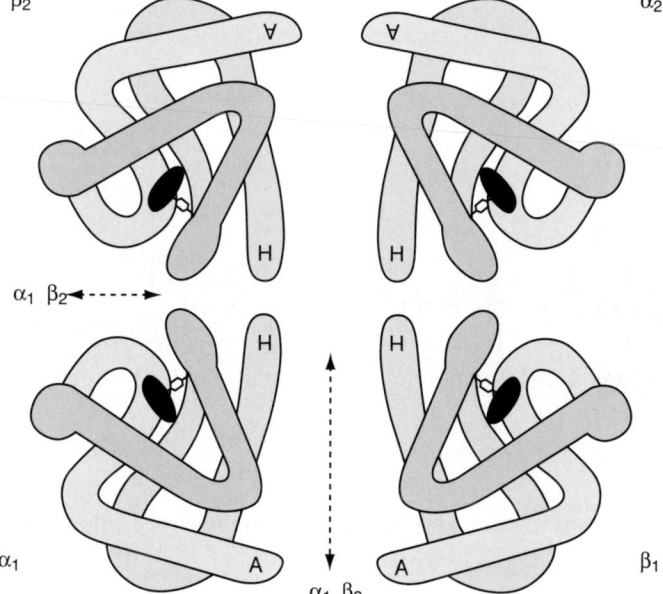

Figure 30–11 The hemoglobin molecule (tetramer, molecular weight 64 500 Da). The heme group for each monomeric polypeptide chain is depicted as a black disk, connected to an imidazole group of histidine, and located near the surface of the molecule in a 'pocket' formed by the polypeptide chain. The letters A and H designate alphahelix segments of each polypeptide chain: A is the amino-terminal segment, and H is the carboxy-terminal segment. The four monomers are separated in this drawing, but actually make contact along a relatively large area ($\alpha_1\beta_1$) which is thought to be the relatively fixed or stabilizing contact area, and a smaller ($\alpha_1\beta_2$) area thought to be the functional contact area, where movement occurs during oxygenation and deoxygenation, changing the molecular configuration. (Redrawn from White JM, Dacie JV: Prog Hematol 1971; 7:69, with permission.)

result in a shift of the Hb–oxygen dissociation curve to the right, favoring the release of oxygen from hemoglobin.

Carbon dioxide (CO_2) is transported in erythrocytes as well as in plasma. A small part of red cell CO_2 is dissolved and is bound to amino groups of hemoglobin as carbamino-CO_2, but most is in the bicarbonate form. The enzyme carbonic anhydrase catalyzes the transformation of carbon dioxide to bicarbonate in the red cell while in the tissue capillary bed and catalyzes the reverse reaction (the release of carbon dioxide from bicarbonate) in the erythrocyte when it is in the capillary bed of the lungs.

Erythrocyte Destruction

The erythrocyte gradually undergoes metabolic changes over the course of its 120-day life span, at which time the less viable senescent cell is removed from the circulation. Certain glycolytic enzymes diminish in activity as the cell ages. Older red cells have a smaller surface area and an increased mean cell hemoglobin concentration (MCHC) compared with younger cells. Furthermore, aged red cells lose sialic acid from their membranes, exposing an asialoglycophorin. This senescent antigen is recognized and an autoantibody is synthesized by the host. After the binding of the autoantibody, the senescent cell is removed from the circulation by the reticuloendothelial system, primarily within the spleen. About 3 million cells are normally removed from the blood per second without any demonstrable histologic evidence of erythrophagocytosis.

In some pathologic states, the reticuloendothelial system removes younger sensitized or abnormal red cells at a rapid rate. Subsequently, erythrophagocytosis is often evident. In autoimmune hemolytic anemia, the reticuloendothelial system removes red cells following the binding of autoantibodies or complement to reticulocytes and young red cells. In other pathologic states, red cells are removed because of structural defects that interfere with their normal passage through microcirculation of the reticuloendothelial system.

Degradation of Hemoglobin

After removal of the red cell from the circulation, hemoglobin is broken down within the macrophages of the reticuloendothelial system into its three constituents – iron, protoporphyrin, and globin. The iron goes into storage and may be completely reutilized. The globin may be degraded and returned to the amino acid pool of the body. In contrast, the protoporphyrin ring is split, converted to bilirubin, and excreted from the body.

In the macrophage, the protoporphyrin ring is cleaved by a heme oxidase enzyme at the α-methene bridge, yielding 1 mol of carbon monoxide (CO) and 1 mol of biliverdin. The CO appears in the blood as HbCO and is eventually exhaled. Biliverdin is reduced to bilirubin in the macrophage, and bilirubin is transported to the liver by plasma albumin. It is removed from the plasma by the liver cell, conjugated mainly with glucuronide, and excreted in the bile. In the intestine, reduction by bacteria occurs, and bilirubin is transformed into urobilinogen, mesobilirubinogen, and stercobilinogen, compounds that are collectively designated urobilinogens.

Estimation of exhaled CO, HbCO, or fecal urobilinogen can be used as measures of hemoglobin breakdown. When production of red cells is diminished and the level of circulating hemoglobin is low, as in aplastic anemia, urobilinogen excretion is reduced. When destruction of erythrocytes is increased, as in hemolytic anemia, all three are increased in amount.

In normal humans, about 80–90% of the excreted bile pigment measured as fecal urobilinogen is derived from breakdown of senescent erythrocytes that have lived 100–120 days. However, about 10–20% of the pigment is excreted within the first few days. This early labeled bile pigment comes from nonhemoglobin heme formed in the liver, as well as from the breakdown of newly formed hemoglobin in the bone marrow. Much of the latter may represent hemoglobin from the pieces of cytoplasm of the orthochromatic normoblast that are lost during the process of nuclear extrusion.

In certain hematologic diseases, notably thalassemia, megaloblastic anemia, refractory anemia, and erythropoietic porphyria, this early labeled bile pigment fraction may be markedly increased. This intramedullary destruction of hemoglobin, which never appears in circulating erythrocytes, is known as *ineffective erythropoiesis*.

Erythrokinetics

The balance between delivery of erythrocytes to the blood and removal of erythrocytes from the blood results in a relatively constant hemoglobin mass in the circulation. Anemia occurs when the removal of erythrocytes from the blood is increased and cannot be compensated for by increased production, or when the delivery of erythrocytes to the blood is decreased, or when both processes exist together.

When anemia develops, tissue hypoxia leads to elevated levels of erythropoietin in the plasma. Resultant normoblastic hyperplasia produces more erythrocytes for delivery to the circulation. The marrow in a normal individual is capable of six to eight times the normal output of erythrocytes with extreme stimulation. This capacity must be compared with the output actually attained when one is evaluating the marrow response of a given patient.

Measurements that assess *effective erythropoiesis* (production and delivery of erythrocytes to the circulation), *ineffective erythropoiesis*, and destruction of erythrocytes may be necessary to determine the mechanism and the cause of anemia.

Measurements of Total Production of Erythrocytes or Hemoglobin

The *total mass of erythropoietic cells* in the body cannot be easily measured. An estimate is made by examining a sample of bone marrow from a normally active site and determining the cellularity and the percentage of total nucleated cells that are erythropoietic (see Bone Marrow Examination, Ch. 29). When marrow activity increases, usually the additional hematopoietic cells replace the fat in the red marrow sites before extension occurs into the yellow marrow of the long bones. One assumes that the sample is representative of the marrow as a whole, an assumption that usually is valid.

The *plasma iron turnover* is calculated from the serum iron level and the rate of removal of injected radioactive iron from the plasma. About 25–30% of the iron is not used in erythropoiesis and is primarily taken up by the liver. The remaining 70–75% is taken up by erythropoietic cells and is therefore a measure of total erythropoiesis, both effective and ineffective.

Measurements of Total Destruction of Erythrocytes or Hemoglobin

Determination of *fecal urobilinogen* is an estimate of the total excretion of bile pigments – the breakdown products of heme. This measurement includes pigment derived from hemoglobin formed and destroyed in the marrow without ever reaching the circulating erythrocytes. Limitations include diminished conversion of bilirubin to urobilinogen because of oral administration of broad-spectrum antibiotics, and failure of pigment to reach the intestine in obstructive jaundice.

A portion (up to 50%) of the excreted urobilinogen is reabsorbed into the portal circulation and re-excreted into the bile, without conjugation, by the liver. Only a small amount is normally excreted in the urine. Increased urinary urobilinogen is seen with severe liver disease as well as in conditions associated with increased heme catabolism that overwhelm the metabolic capacity of the liver. Thus, hepatocellular damage, cirrhosis, hepatic congestion due to congestive heart failure, obstructive liver disease, cholangitis, hemolytic anemia, and ineffective erythropoiesis are all associated with elevation of urinary urobilinogen.

Measurements of Effective Production of Erythrocytes

Reticulocyte Count. Because the RNA of the reticulocyte disappears about a day after its entry into the blood, enumeration of reticulocytes will be a measure of the number of cells being delivered by the marrow to the blood each day – that is, a measure of effective erythropoiesis. The absolute reticulocyte count is calculated by multiplying the reticulocyte percentage by the erythrocyte count. To give a meaningful expression of erythropoiesis, the absolute reticulocyte count, or some estimate of it, and not simply the percentage, must be used. The normal absolute reticulocyte count is approximately 50×10^9/L, or 1% of circulating erythrocytes. Because the normal maturation time for reticulocytes in the blood is 1 day, production of reticulocytes is 50×10^9/L/day.

A second consideration is an adjustment for increased maturation time of reticulocytes in the blood as a result of accelerated release from the marrow, an effect of erythropoietin. The need for this is recognized by the presence of large, polychromatic cells or nucleated red cells in the blood film, indicating a shift of excessively immature reticulocytes from the marrow into the blood. To avoid an overestimate of daily erythrocyte production, a correction factor is used based on estimated maturation time of reticulocytes in the blood. This varies inversely with hematocrit as follows (Hillman, 1996):

Hematocrit (%)	Reticulocyte Maturation Time (days)
45	1.0
35	1.5
25	2.0
15	2.5

If a patient has a Hct of 0.25, a red count of 2.89×10^{12}/L, and a reticulocyte count of 7%, he will have an absolute reticulocyte count of

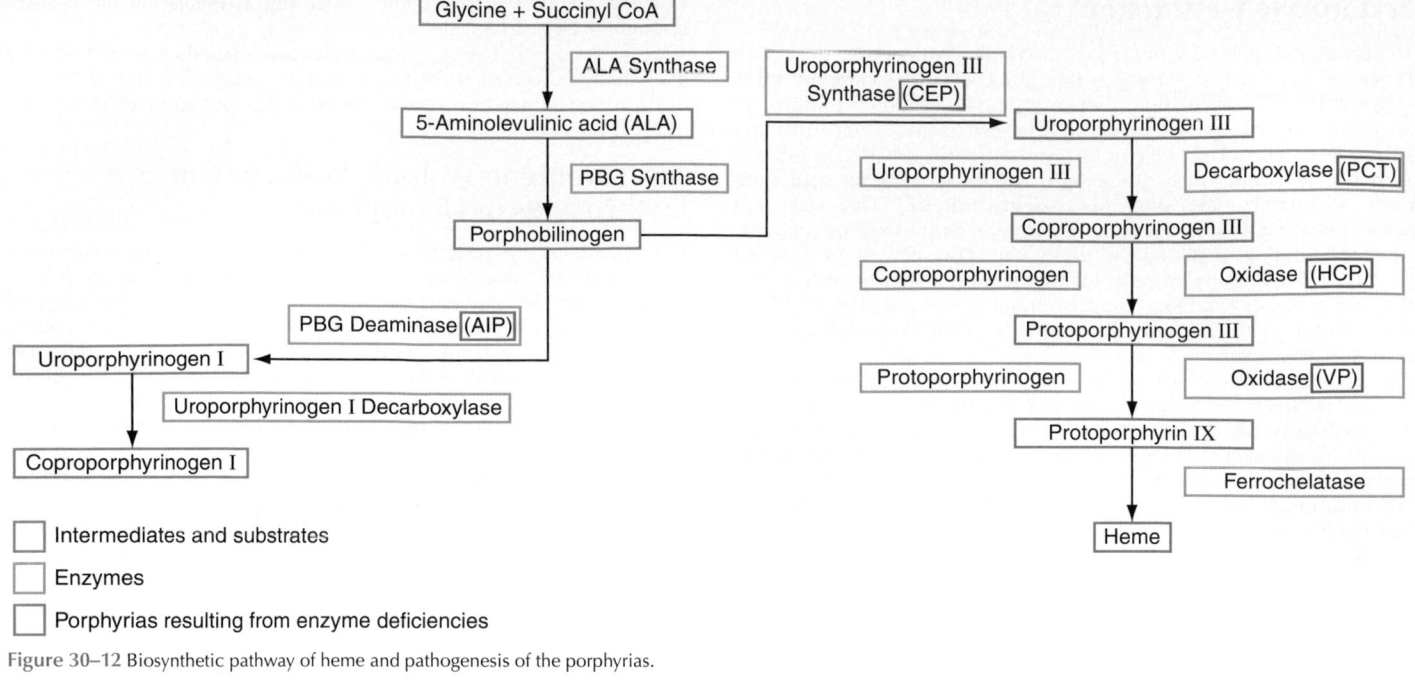

Figure 30–12 Biosynthetic pathway of heme and pathogenesis of the porphyrias.

202×10^9/L. Because the average normal absolute reticulocyte count is 50×10^9/L, the patient has:

$(202 \times 10^9$/L$)/(50 \times 10^9$/L$)$

or four times as many reticulocytes as normal. However, this must be corrected for the increased maturation time: $4 \times \frac{1}{2} = 2$. Therefore, two times as many reticulocytes are entering the blood per day as in a normal individual – that is, the red cell production is two times normal.

If only the hematocrit is available, the same correction can be made as follows:

Correction for anemia:
Patient's reticulocyte count (7%)/Normal reticulocyte count (1%) × Patient's Hct (0.25)/Normal Hct (0.45) = 4
Correction for shift:
Corrected reticulocyte index (4) × 1/Maturation time (2) = 2

These corrections are necessary in order to assess the degree of red cell production in response to anemia.

A normal individual with a normal supply of iron can increase red cell production by two times normal within a week if the hematocrit drops to 0.35, or to three times the normal if the hematocrit drops to 0.25. Only if there is a parenteral supply of iron (such as in hemolysis) can the maximal red cell production of six to eight times normal be achieved.

If an appropriate marrow response to anemia has not been reached in 1–2 weeks, some impairment of red cell production exists.

The *erythrocyte utilization of iron* is a measure of the amount of an injected dose of iron that appears in the hemoglobin of circulating erythrocytes. It is derived from the plasma iron turnover and the percentage of radioactive iron that has been injected and that appears in the circulating erythrocytes after 2 weeks, assuming that none of the newly formed cells have been destroyed in that time interval. This, too, is a measure of effective erythropoiesis.

Measurements of Effective Survival of Erythrocytes in Blood

The *erythrocyte survival* can be determined by removing a sample of blood, labeling the erythrocytes with chromium-51 (^{51}Cr), inactivating the excess ^{51}Cr remaining in the plasma, and reinjecting the labeled erythrocytes into the patient. The ^{51}Cr is bound to the β-chain of the hemoglobin molecule and for the most part is not released until the red cell is removed from the circulation and the hemoglobin is degraded. Measurements of radioactivity in the red cells are made at 2 hours or 24 hours (the zero time, or 100% level) and at 1- to 3-day intervals until over 50% of the activity has disappeared. The results are usually expressed as the ^{51}Cr half-survival time. The normal range is 28–38 days. (The reason it is not 60 days is that ^{51}Cr is eluted from the hemoglobin at the rate of about 1% per day.) If the production of erythrocytes equals destruction (i.e., if a steady state exists), the erythrocyte survival is also a measure of effective production of erythrocytes.

Summary

Total erythropoiesis refers to the total production of hemoglobin or red cells; effective erythropoiesis refers to production of hemoglobin or red cells that reach the circulation; and ineffective erythropoiesis refers to production of hemoglobin or red cells that never reach the circulating blood. These concepts of the *erythrokinetic* approach to the study of anemia are useful, especially in anemias that defy easy classification.

The Porphyrias

Physiology

Heme biosynthesis is an essential pathway that occurs in all metabolically active cells containing mitochondria and is most prominent in bone marrow and liver. The erythroid marrow is the major heme-forming tissue in the body, producing 85% of the daily heme requirement. Heme complexed with globin is preserved in circulating red blood cells for approximately 120 days, whereas heme produced in liver for cytochromes and enzymes is subject to much more rapid turnover, measurable in hours. A brief sequence of the heme biosynthesis pathway, with the disease states associated with specific enzymes deficiencies along the pathway, is shown in Figure 30–12.

Porphyrins are compounds composed of four pyrrole rings connected by methene bridges, differentiated by substituents found in the eight peripheral positions. The arrangement of four nitrogen atoms in the center of the porphyrin ring enables porphyrins to chelate various metal ions, such as iron, or in disease states, zinc. The biosynthetic intermediates between porphobilinogen (PBG) and protoporphyrin are not porphyrins but rather their reduced forms, the porphyrinogens. They are colorless, nonfluorescent compounds readily converted to porphyrins by weak oxidizing agents, such as air in the presence of light.

Analytic Techniques

Several analytic techniques are employed to diagnose and classify the porphyrias and to monitor known patients presenting with recurrent attacks. We preface this discussion by emphasizing that the porphyrias are rare, usually inherited, disorders and that a family history, thorough past medical history, and a history of present illness including probing for exacerbating factors, are all critical adjuncts to the laboratory evaluation of patients. In the appropriate context, a new patient presenting with an acute neurovisceral

Table 30–2 Key Features of the Major Porphyrias

Porphyria	Inheritance	Enzyme deficiency	Excess metabolites	Clinical features	Exacerbating factors
Acute intermittent porphyria	Autosomal dominant	PBG deaminase	PBG(U) ALA(U) Darkened urine on standing	Abdominal pain; psychiatric symptoms	Steroid hormones
Congenital erythropoietic porphyria	Autosomal recessive	Uroporphyrinogen I synthase, and/or UPG III cosynthase	UP(U) CP(U) UP(E) Red, fluorescent pigment in urine	Photosensitivity; red urine, teeth; hemolysis	Sunlight
Hereditary coproporphyria	Autosomal dominant	Coproporphyrinogen oxidase	CP III (F, U) PBG(U) ALA(U) Red, fluorescent pigment in urine	Photosensitivity	Stress
Variegate porphyria	Autosomal dominant	Protoporphyrinogen oxidase	PBG(U) ALA(U) UP(U, F) CP(U, F) Red, fluorescent pigment in urine	Photosensitivity	Stress
Porphyria cutanea tarda	Autosomal dominant Acquired	Uroporphyrinogen decarboxylase	UP I (U) UP III (U) Acid induces pink fluorescence	Photosensitivity	Alcohol, hepatic injury, iron overload

PBG = porphobilinogen; ALA = aminolevulinic acid; UPG = uroporphyrinogen; UP = uroporphyrin; CP = coproporphyrin; U = urine; F = feces.
E = erythrocyte

attack may be screened with a urine porphobilinogen (PBG) level. This is reliably increased, often to greater than 10 times the upper reference limit, during attacks in the acute porphyrias – acute intermittent porphyria (AIP), variegate porphyria (VP), hereditary coproporphyria (HCP), and the rare δ-aminolevulinic acid dehydratase deficiency which is not further discussed in this chapter (Deacon, 2001). Historically, the most widely used screening procedure for PBG has been the Watson–Schwartz test. However, this test has been shown to have insufficient sensitivity for routine screening. Chromatography is the methodology in current practice in many laboratories.

If the screening tests for PBG and/or aminolevulinic acid (ALA) are positive, then classification of the acute porphyria should be made. High-performance liquid chromatography (HPLC) can separate individual porphyrins; this, combined with measurement of total fecal porphyrins, reliably distinguishes between AIP and HCP (Deacon, 2001). VP may be diagnosed by measurement of fecal and urine metabolites, and also by the fluorescence emission peak of 624–627 nm, which is unique among the porphyrias (Poh-Fitzpatrick, 1980). Beyond routine analysis of fecal and urine metabolites, one may consider plasma fluorescence scanning, as it offers reasonable sensitivity in the work-up of VP (Hift, 2004). Enzyme assays have not been widely used in the diagnosis of porphyrias because of technical difficulties and ambiguous results, except for the assay for PBG deaminase in diagnosing AIP. DNA analysis for specific mutations is useful in families, but the multitude of mutations limits its use as a screening tool. A key exception exists with VP, where the R59W mutation is prevalent (Sandberg, 2004).

The porphyrias comprise a group of inherited and acquired disorders of heme biosynthesis due to a deficiency of a specific enzyme in the biosynthetic pathway, culminating in the excess production and increased excretion of precursors formed in the steps prior to the enzyme defect. The porphyrias are classified as acute (AIP, HCP, VP) and nonacute or cutaneous (hereditary coproporphyria and porphyria cutanea tarda). The clinical manifestations of an acute attack are characterized by dysfunction of the central, peripheral, and autonomic nervous systems. The pathogenesis of the neuropathy in affected persons can be explained by accumulation of porphyrins and their precursors (ALA and PBG are neurotoxic), deficiency of heme in neural tissues, depletion of essential substrates, and accumulation of abnormal products derived from other pathways. The central features of the major porphyrias are summarized in Table 30–2 and discussed below.

Acute Intermittent Porphyria (AIP)

AIP is the most common acute and probably the most common inherited porphyria (Chemmanur, 2004). It is inherited in an autosomal dominant

fashion with incomplete penetrance, making family studies more challenging. PBG deaminase deficiency has been demonstrated in all examined tissues. Diagnosis rests on demonstration of elevated levels of ALA and PBG in urine during acute attacks (with PBG greater in amount than ALA), with the PBG enzyme assay, and if the mutation is known in another family member, by DNA analysis. The acute patient typically presents with colicky abdominal pain, nausea and vomiting, mental confusion, tachycardia and, in half, a motor neuropathy (Chemmanur, 2004). As noted above, it is at this point that urine metabolite levels can aid in the diagnosis. Frequently, patients have metabolite levels at or near the reference range during quiescent periods. Characteristically, the urine of AIP patients turns dark red upon exposure to air and light as PBG is oxidized to a porphyrin spontaneously. Unlike the other porphyrias discussed here, AIP lacks cutaneous manifestations. Prevention is the mainstay of management, with avoidance of particular drugs (barbiturates and sulfonamides among many others), hormonal changes and fasting. Specifically, a low-carbohydrate diet may trigger an attack. In a time when such diets are popular with the general public, clinicians may wish to caution all acute porphyria patients on the risks these diets carry.

Hereditary Coproporphyria (HCP)

Also inherited in an autosomal dominant fashion with incomplete penetrance, HCP is less common than AIP. It is due to a deficiency of coproporphyrinogen oxidase. Clinically, HCP resembles a milder form of AIP with its neurovisceral attacks, but cutaneous manifestations are seen in roughly a third of patients (Chemmanur, 2004). Fecal coproporphyrinogen III is excreted both during and between attacks, while ALA and PBG are seen in urine during an acute crisis. ALA excretion usually exceeds that of PBG, and this, coupled with the cutaneous findings (if present) help differentiate HCP from AIP. Prevention, including sunscreen, is central to management.

Variegate Porphyria (VP)

Like AIP and HCP, VP is inherited as an autosomal dominant disorder with low penetrance. It is sometimes referred to as South African porphyria due to its prevalence in the white population in this region. Patients have approximately 50% activity of protoporphyrinogen oxidase. Thus, they excrete fecal protoporphyrins and coproporphyrins and urine ALA, PBG and coproporphyrins. Induction of hepatic ALA synthase I by precipitating factors, such as barbiturates, oral contraceptives or a low-

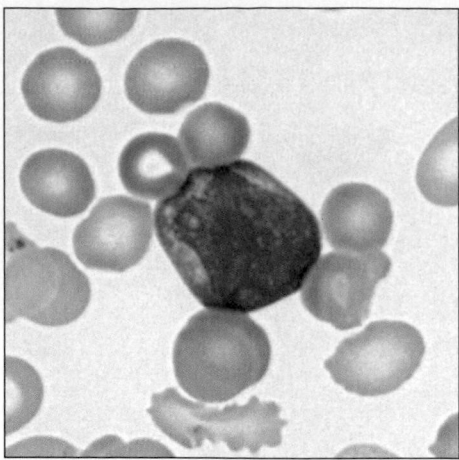

Figure 30–13 Myeloblast with high N/C ratio, fine chromatin, visible nucleoli, and basophilic cytoplasm (Wright–Giemsa, ×250).

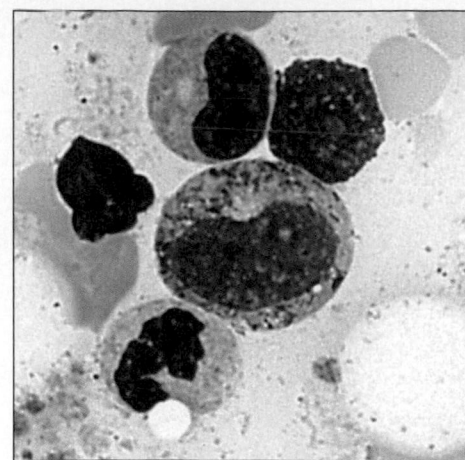

Figure 30–14 Promyelocyte (center) with azurophilic granules in the cytoplasm; the nuclear chromatin is still fine. A metamyelocyte and a segmented neutrophil are also seen (Wright–Giemsa, ×250).

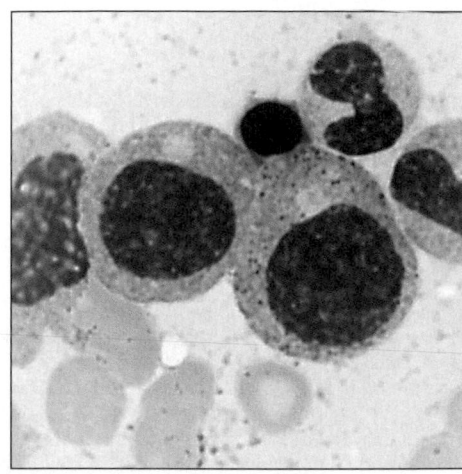

Figure 30–15 Myelocytes have secondary granules in the cytoplasm and show condensation of nuclear chromatin. Persistent primary granules are seen in early myelocytes (center-right) and are lost as myelocytes mature. A band neutrophil and orthochromatic normoblast are also seen (Wright–Giemsa, ×250).

carbohydrate diet, specifically results in the increased ALA and PBG seen during acute attacks (Chemmanur, 2004). Cutaneous manifestations in the form of erosions or bullae following trauma to sun-exposed skin are seen at a younger age than is observed with porphyria cutanea tarda. Diagnosis is made by conventional measurements of metabolites, family history and DNA analysis. Avoidance of triggering factors remains the major approach to patient care.

Congenital Erythropoietic Porphyria (CEP)

CEP is distinct from the other porphyrias discussed, both in its inheritance (it is a recessive disorder) and its severity. Patients present shortly after birth with red-pigmented urine, hemolytic anemia and severe cutaneous photosensitivity. Erythrodontia is striking and may be a useful clue if the diagnosis has not already been made. The deficient enzyme is uroporphyrinogen III synthase, and ALA synthase activity is increased. Coproporphyrin I and uroporphyrin I are present in urine. The prognosis for CEP is significantly worse than for the other porphyrias, with death occurring at an early age in many cases.

Porphyria Cutanea Tarda (PCT)

PCT is the most common of the porphyrias in the US, and is usually acquired rather than inherited in dominant fashion. The deficient enzyme is uroporphyrinogen decarboxylase (UROD), and researchers have postulated the presence of an inhibitor of UROD, possibly secondary to iron and metabolites of uroporphyrinogen. Interestingly, patients with hemochromatosis are at increased risk for acquired PCT (Chemmanur, 2004). Patients present with cutaneous findings alone, and these are due to mild trauma to sun-exposed areas, not simple photosensitivity. Diagnostic laboratory findings include increased uroporphyrins with smaller increases in urine coproporphyrins. Exacerbating factors, such as alcohol, an inducer of hepatic ALA synthase I, and estrogens, should be avoided. Additional management strategies involve phlebotomy to reduce the hepatic iron load, chloroquine to complex porphyrins for urinary excretion, and sunscreen (Chemmanur, 2004).

Neutrophils

The common progenitor cell for neutrophils and monocytes (CFU-GM) divides and gives rise to the progenitor cells for granulocytes (CFU-G) and for monocytes (CFU-M). CFU-G and CFU-M cells give rise to myeloblasts and monoblasts, respectively, under stimulation of colony-stimulating factors for granulocytes and monocytes (see Fig. 30–1).

Morphology of Neutrophil Precursors

The *myeloblast* (Fig. 30–13) is a cell about 15 μm in diameter with a moderately high N/C ratio; a large oval to quadrangular nucleus; very fine, uniform chromatin pattern; delicate nuclear membrane; and two to five nucleoli. The cytoplasm is pale, clear blue, and without granules. The appearance of azurophilic (primary) granules (~ 0.5 μm diameter) heralds the earliest promyelocyte (Fig. 30–14) and indicates that the cell is to be a neutrophil. The *promyelocyte* stage encompasses the entire period of production of azurophilic granules. The promyelocyte is slightly larger

than the myeloblast. The nuclear chromatin begins to condense, and the nucleoli are less obvious. The cytoplasm is basophilic and is filled by more and more azurophilic granules. The *neutrophil myelocyte* stage begins with the appearance of specific neutrophil (secondary) granules, at first only in the Golgi region; as more specific granules develop, they spread throughout the cytoplasm (Fig. 30–15). With successive mitoses, the number of azurophilic granules (whose production has ceased at the end of the promyelocyte stage) is diminished. The early neutrophil myelocyte, therefore, has a rather fine, dispersed nuclear chromatin pattern, many azurophilic granules, and few specific granules. The late neutrophil myelocyte has a somewhat more condensed chromatin pattern, a cytoplasm well filled with specific granules, and rather few azurophilic granules. The myelocyte is the latest stage capable of cell division. The next stage, the *neutrophil metamyelocyte*, is distinguished by an indented, kidney-shaped nucleus with more condensed chromatin (Fig. 30–16). From this stage on, changes in the cytoplasm are insignificant. In the *band neutrophil* (stab form), the nucleus has more condensed chromatin and a rather uniform elongated shape (Fig. 30–17). Partial constriction of the nucleus occurs in the band stage, until a fine filament (length but no breadth) is formed between two of the lobes, at which point the cell is classified as a *segmented neutrophil* (Fig. 30–18).

During development and maturation, neutrophilic precursors express various cell-surface markers that can be used for immunophenotypic recognition. Myeloblasts express the HSC marker CD34 as well as HLA-DR and myeloid lineage specific markers CD13, CD33, CD15, and CD117. Mature neutrophils express CD13, CD15, CD16, and CD11b, but lose HLA-DR and CD33.

The mature human neutrophil has twice as many specific granules as azurophilic granules (Table 30–3). The azurophilic granules (formed in the promyelocyte stage) contain lysosomal enzymes (e.g., acid hydrolases:

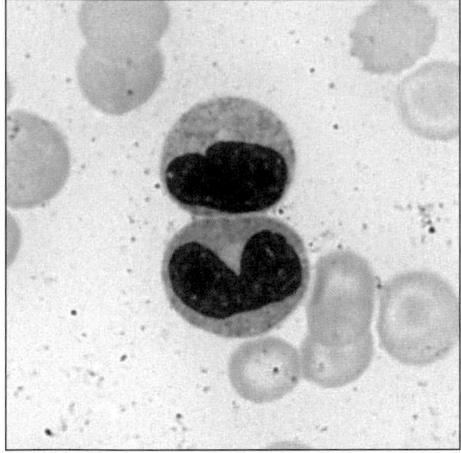

Figure 30–16 Metamyelocytes show nuclear indentation and increased chromatin clumping (Wright–Giemsa, ×250).

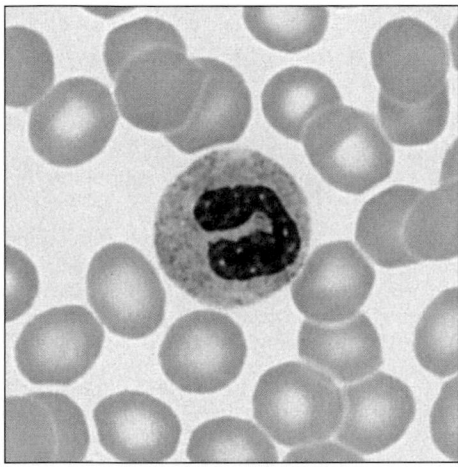

Figure 30–17 Band neutrophil with mature nucleus with clumped chromatin but without segmentation (Wright–Giemsa, ×250).

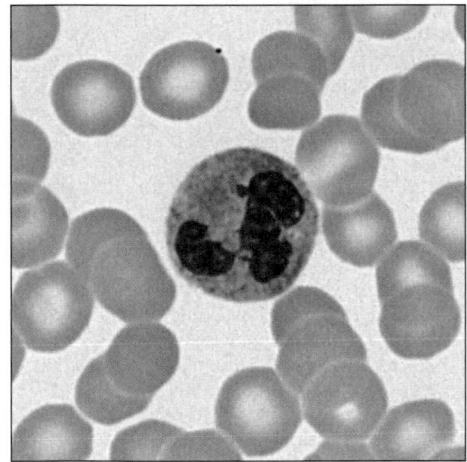

Figure 30–18 Segmented neutrophil with multiple nuclear lobes joined by fine chromatin filaments (Wright–Giemsa, ×250).

acid phosphatase, β-glucuronidase), myeloperoxidase, elastase, arylsulfatase, and cationic antibacterial proteins, along with other enzymes and proteins. The specific granules (formed in the myelocyte stage) contain lysozyme, lactoferrin, collagenase, plasminogen activator, aminopeptidase, and vitamin B$_{12}$-binding protein, as well as other enzymes and proteins. Tertiary granules, similar in size to the specific granules, contain gelatinase. Alkaline phosphatase is located in yet another type of cytoplasmic organelle lighter in density than specific granules. These organelles first appear during the late myelocyte stage.

Table 30–3 Neutrophil Constituents and Functions

Azurophilic granules (formed in promyelocyte stage)

Lysosomal enzymes: acid hydrolases, acid phosphatase, beta-glucuronidase

Myeloperoxidase

Elastase

Arylsulfatase

Cationic antibacterial proteins

Specific granules (formed in myelocyte stage)

Lysozyme

Lactoferrin

Collagenase

Plasminogen activator

Aminopeptidase

Tertiary granules

Gelatinase

Cytoplasmic organelles

Alkaline phosphatase

Neutrophil functions

Phagocytosis

Bactericidal activity

Distribution and Kinetics

For each neutrophil in the blood vessels, about 16 precursors are present in the marrow. From the time of differentiation into a myeloblast, through about five mitotic divisions (three of which occur at the myelocyte stage), it takes about 14 days until the progeny of that cell reach the blood. The last 6–7 days are spent in the maturation and storage pool. When a neutrophil enters the blood, it moves readily between a circulating granulocyte pool (CGP), which is sampled in the leukocyte count, and a marginal granulocyte pool (MGP), which is not, but is either marginated along vessel walls or sequestered in capillary beds. In less than a day after it arrives, the neutrophil emigrates from the circulation in a random manner and enters the tissues. From there, if not utilized in an inflammatory exudate, neutrophils leave the body within a few days via secretions in bronchi, saliva, gastrointestinal tract, and urine, or they are destroyed by the reticuloendothelial system.

Function

Neutrophils are able to move in a zigzag manner, but their motion changes to a straight line path if a chemotactic attractant or factor (e.g., a bacterium coated with certain components of complement) is within a certain distance. Neutrophils express chemokine receptors CXCR1 and CXCR2, which are responsible for neutrophil migration in response to chemokines. Neutrophils also have receptors for the Fc portion of IgG as well as for complement (C3) and bind and phagocytose the coated particle. Phagocytosis occurs, with the formation of a phagocytic vacuole that contains the ingested particle; accompanying this process is an increase in metabolic activity and energy production. Specific granules, followed shortly by azurophilic granules, empty their contents into the phagocytic vacuoles, a process known as degranulation. Bactericidal activity occurs within the vacuole, mediated by H$_2$O$_2$, superoxide anion (O$_2^-$), myeloperoxidase, and a halide ion generating the free halogen, or by other enzymatic activity. Other substances can act as chemotactic factors too. The C5a fragment is a chemotactic factor and is also an anaphylatoxin that causes smooth muscle contraction. Substances liberated by bacteria and metabolic products of arachidonic acid may also act as chemotactic factors for neutrophils. Neutrophils are thus important in defense against infectious disease. If their enzymes are activated and released outside the cell, neutrophils can cause tissue necrosis, tissue injury, and inflammation.

Eosinophils

Eosinophils are produced in the bone marrow. In vitro culture studies show that there is a separate eosinophilic committed progenitor cell (CFU-Eo) in the marrow that is distinct from the CFU-GM, CFU-G, and CFU-M. Three growth factors (GM-CSF, IL-3, IL-5) produced by T lymphocytes influence eosinophil development. IL-5 promotes terminal maturation, functional activation, and prevention of apoptosis of eosinophils.

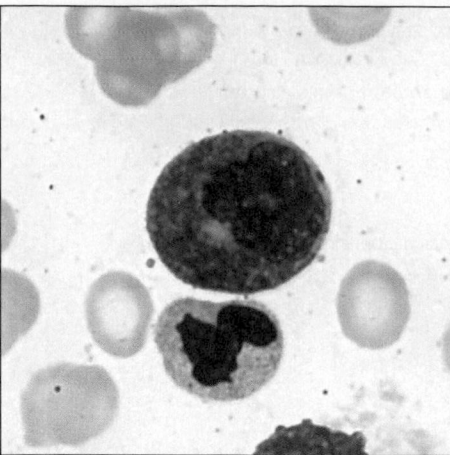

Figure 30–19 Eosinophil myelocyte with ovoid nucleus and eosinophilic secondary granules in the cytoplasm. A segmented neutrophil is also seen (Wright–Giemsa, ×250).

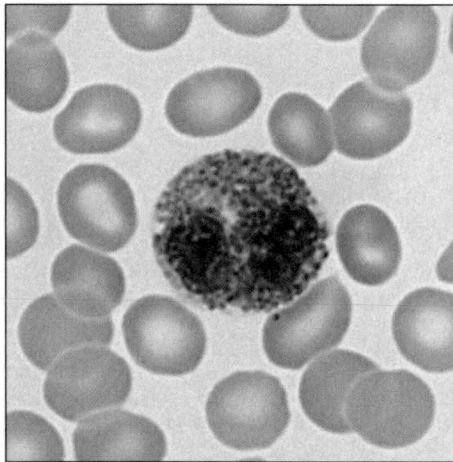

Figure 30–20 Mature eosinophil with bilobed nucleus and large eosinophilic cytoplasmic granules (Wright–Giemsa, ×250).

Morphology of Eosinophil Precursors

The cell that is the precursor for the earliest recognizable eosinophil, the eosinophil myelocyte, is presumably a distinctive myeloblast. However, it is morphologically indistinguishable from that which gives rise to neutrophils and monocytes or to basophils (Figs 30–1 and 30–13). In the early eosinophil myelocyte, the granules are large and take the basophilic stain. As the cell matures, the granules appear olive-green and finally the characteristic red-orange color (Figs 30–19 and 30–20). Nuclear maturation is similar to that of the neutrophil. Eosinophils are slightly larger than neutrophils and have fewer nuclear lobes. Mature eosinophils express CD16 and CD32.

Electron micrographs of eosinophils show characteristic granules that have a dense crystalloid core in a less dense matrix. Immature granules, appearing in the myelocyte, at first have no crystalloids but develop them as maturation proceeds. Mature granules are of two types: the larger granule (0.5–1.5 μm in largest diameter) with a dense crystalloid, and a smaller granule (0.1–0.5 μm diameter) without a crystalloid. The smaller granules appear later during maturation, after the myelocyte stage.

Eosinophil-specific granules (Table 30–4) contain major basic protein (MBP) in the crystalloid core; MBP is toxic to parasites and cells, neutralizes heparin, and induces histamine release from basophils. Granule constituents in the matrix include acid hydrolases, peroxidase, phospholipase, and cathepsin. The specific granules also contain eosinophil cationic protein (ECP), eosinophil-derived neurotoxin (EDN), and eosinophil protein X (EPX). ECP shortens coagulation time and alters fibrinolysis; it also inhibits lymphocyte proliferation and is a potent neurotoxin. EDN and EPX are strong neurotoxins (Gleich, 1986). The smaller granules contain arylsulfatase; both granule types contain peroxidase and acid phosphatase. Eosinophil peroxidase is different from the type of peroxidase present in neutrophils and monocytes; also, eosinophils contain no alkaline phosphatase or muramidase. Eosinophils

Table 30–4 Eosinophil Constituents and Functions

Eosinophil-specific granules

Larger granules
   Major basic protein
   Acid hydrolases
   Peroxidase
   Phospholipase
   Cathepsin
   Eosinophil cationic protein
   Eosinophil-derived neurotoxin
   Eosinophil protein X
Smaller granules
   Arylsulfatase
   Peroxidase
   Acid phosphatase

Eosinophil functions

Anthelmintic activity – major basic protein, eosinophilic cationic protein, peroxidase

Phagocytosis

Allergic response

Dampen inflammatory reactions

secrete IL-1, IL-3, IL-6, IL-8, TNF-α, and GM-CSF. TNF-α appears to be the cause of fibrosis in Hodgkin's disease (Roberts, 1999).

Distribution and Kinetics

The kinetics of eosinophils are similar to those of neutrophils. They are stored in the bone marrow for several days after going through the various maturational stages. The half-life in the blood is approximately 18 hours before entering the tissues where they survive for at least 6 days. Eosinophils in the tissues, however, are at least 100 times as numerous as the total number of eosinophils in the blood; they are located primarily in skin, lung, and gastrointestinal tract (i.e., the epithelial barriers to the outside world).

Function

Eosinophils act as phagocytes and modulate inflammatory responses (Table 30–4). Eosinophils leave the blood when adrenal corticosteroid hormones increase. They proliferate in response to immunologic stimuli and this proliferative response is mediated, at least with some antigens, by T lymphocytes, monocytes, and mast cells. Eosinophils destroy helminths by generating potent oxidants and releasing cationic proteins. Eosinophils participate in some inflammatory conditions, particularly allergic reactions, asthma, and certain myocardial diseases (Gleich, 1986). Although eosinophils phagocytose foreign particles and antigen–antibody complexes, this is not their only activity. Another major function of eosinophils is to dampen hypersensitivity and inflammatory reactions. There is evidence that eosinophils modulate reactions that occur when tissue mast cells and basophils degranulate. Eosinophils express the chemokine receptor CCR3. Among the chemotactic factors that attract eosinophils, eosinophil chemotactic factor of anaphylaxis (ECF-A) is present in basophils and mast cells; also, eosinophils contain substances that inactivate factors released by mast cells and basophils, such as histamine, slow-reacting substances of anaphylaxis, and platelet-activating factor (PAF).

When there is an intense or prolonged eosinophilic inflammatory reaction, there is often the formation of Charcot–Leyden crystals. These hexagonal bipyramidal crystals are composed of lysophospholipase localized in the cytoplasm of eosinophils (Jandl, 1996).

Basophils and Mast Cells

There is no evidence for basophil development in the in vitro colonies containing neutrophils and monocytes or eosinophils. It is appears that basophils develop from a separate committed progenitor cell that has been derived from the hematopoietic stem cell.

Morphology

Basophils develop from a cell resembling a myeloblast. The first recognizable stage is a *basophil myelocyte*, with the appearance of the specific basophil

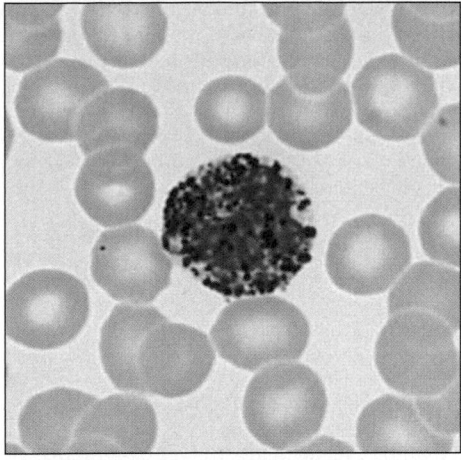

Figure 30–21 Mature basophil with large dark red-purple basophilic granules that partially obscure the nucleus (Wright–Giemsa, ×250).

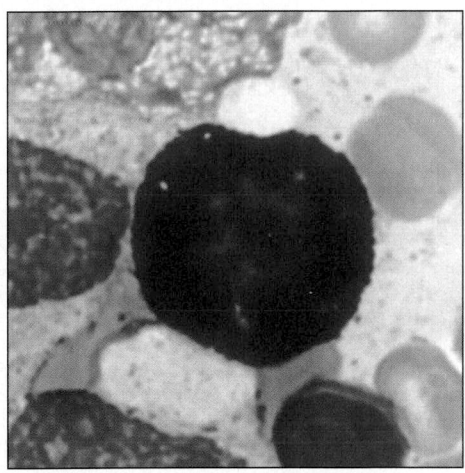

Figure 30–22 Bone marrow mast cell shows numerous uniform purple granules in the cytoplasm that partially obscure the nucleus (Wright–Giemsa, ×250).

granules. These granules (about 0.2–1 μm in diameter) are larger than the azurophilic granules of the promyelocyte and often are irregular in shape. As the cell matures, the granules become more metachromatic (red-purple) because of increasing acid mucopolysaccharide (heparin) content. During maturation, cytoplasmic RNA decreases, and the nucleus partially segments. Because of incomplete nuclear segmentation, stages analogous to the neutrophil are not readily identified. In mature basophils, the nucleus has condensed but smudged chromatin and the background cytoplasm lacks basophilia (residual RNA) (Fig. 30–21). Mature basophils express CD32.

In contrast, *tissue mast cells* are connective tissue cells of mesenchymal origin that contain metachromatic cytoplasmic granules. They are widely distributed throughout the body, including bone marrow, thymus, and spleen, but they do not normally appear in blood. On Romanowsky-stained films (Fig. 30–22) they are usually larger than basophils and have a low N/C ratio and a round or oval reticular nucleus that is usually obscured by abundant red-purple granules. The granules are smaller, more round and regular, and less soluble than basophil granules. The cytoplasmic granules are often spindle-shaped rather than round.

Distribution and Kinetics

Basophils have a life span similar to eosinophils. The maturation time in the marrow is approximately 7 days. Basophils circulate in the blood and are not normally found in tissues, in contrast to mast cells, which can spend 9–18 months in connective tissue (Jandl, 1996). GM-CSF, IL-3, and IL-5 influence basophil production. However, IL-3 is the principal growth factor for basophilic growth, whereas *c-kit* ligand enhances the number and activation state of mast cells (Lyman, 1998).

Function

With regard to circulating numbers, basophils respond to adrenal corticosteroids in similar fashion to eosinophils. Basophil granules

Table 30–5 Basophil Constituents and Functions

Basophil-specific granules
Histamine
Heparin
Peroxidase
Eosinophilic chemotactic factor-A
Other cellular constituents
Slow-reacting substance of anaphylaxis
Platelet-activating factor
Basophil functions
Immediate hypersensitivity reactions
Some delayed hypersensitivity reactions

contain histamine, heparin, and peroxidase (Table 30–5). Basophils synthesize and store histamine and ECF-A. They synthesize and release slow-reacting substance of anaphylaxis (SRS-A) and probably PAF at the time of stimulation, but do not store them. Basophils lack hydrolytic enzymes such as alkaline and acid phosphatase, at least in cytochemically demonstrable amounts. Glycogen is abundant outside the granules. Though ultrastructurally different, mast cells have similar cytochemical characteristics except for the presence of proteolytic enzymes and serotonin, which basophils lack. In tissues the two cell types appear to function in a similar manner.

Basophils (as well as mast cells) appear to be involved in immediate hypersensitivity reactions, such as allergic asthma. IgE binds readily to basophil and mast cell membranes. When specific antigen reacts with the membrane-bound IgE, degranulation occurs with the release of mediators of immediate hypersensitivity (e.g., histamine, SRS-A, PAF, heparin, and ECF-A). The latter leads to the accumulation of eosinophils, which contain substances that tend to counteract these mediators. Basophils are also involved in some delayed hypersensitivity reactions, 'cutaneous basophil hypersensitivity,' such as contact allergies, in which they appear to undergo a different type of degranulation response.

Monocytes and Macrophages

Monocytes share the same committed progenitor cell as neutrophils, the CFU-GM (see Fig. 30–1).

Morphology

In normal marrow, it is not possible morphologically to distinguish the 'monoblast' from the myeloblast. The earliest recognizable cell in this series is the *promonocyte*, which is 15–20 μm in diameter, somewhat larger than the myeloblast. The N/C ratio is moderate, and the nucleus may be oval or indented with a fine uniform or slightly streaked chromatin pattern and two to five nucleoli. The cytoplasm is basophilic with a ground-glass appearance and a variable number of fine azurophilic granules (Fig. 30–23). The *monocyte*, which is present in both blood and marrow, is only slightly smaller; it has a moderate to low N/C ratio and an indented or lobed nucleus with a fine-streaked, only slightly condensed, delicate chromatin pattern. Nucleoli are indistinct or obscured. The cytoplasm is opaque, more gray than blue, and contains an abundance of fine azurophilic granules (Fig. 30–24).

Macrophages are the tissue component of the monocyte system and arise from emigrated blood monocytes. Macrophages are larger than monocytes and measure 15–80 μm in diameter. They have irregular cell membranes, often with blebs and pseudopodia. The N/C ratio is high with an oblong and/or indented nucleus. Although macrophages are located in virtually all tissues of the body, the greatest number is in the bowel, liver, bone marrow, and spleen.

In promonocytes, monocytes, and macrophages, the granules (Table 30–6) contain acid hydrolase, arylsulfatase, nonspecific esterase, and peroxidase. There may be more than one type of granule. As the cell matures, peroxidase activity diminishes and acid phosphatase, arylsulfatase, and nonspecific esterase activity increases. The enzyme activity is in the rough endoplasmic reticulum, Golgi zone, coated vesicles, and digestive vacuoles, suggesting that in the macrophage the coated vesicles are a second form of primary lysosome that shuttles hydrolytic enzymes from the Golgi to the digestive vacuoles.

In addition to these enzymes, monocytes and macrophages possess numerous surface receptors and surface antigens. Monocytes and

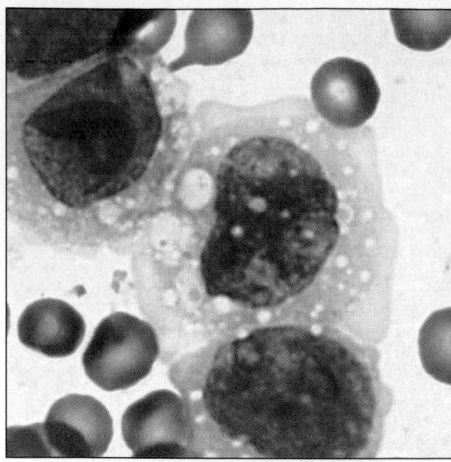

Figure 30–23 Promonocytes have fine nuclear chromatin, often with visible folds and basophilic cytoplasm that may contain vacuoles (Wright–Giemsa, ×250).

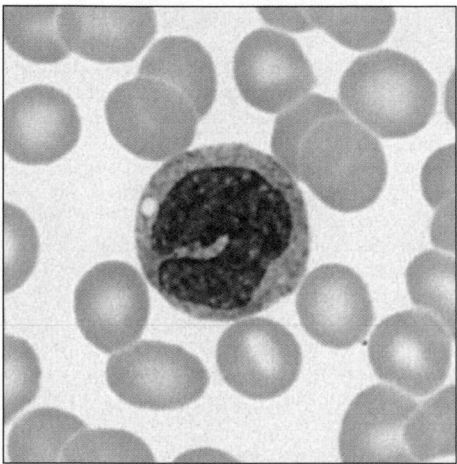

Figure 30–24 Mature monocyte with an indented nucleus, delicate chromatin, basophilic cytoplasm and fine azurophilic granules (Wright–Giemsa, ×250).

Table 30–6 Monocyte/Macrophage Constituents and Functions

Granule and other constituents

Acid hydrolase

Arylsulfatase

Nonspecific esterase

Peroxidase

Acid phosphatase

Monocyte/macrophage functions

Phagocytosis – bacteria, cellular debris, senescent cells

Antigen processing

Cell-mediated immunity – antibody-dependent cellular cytotoxicity

Synthesis of bioactive molecules

macrophages possess class I (HLA-A, B, C) antigens and class II (HLA-DR, DP, DQ) gene complex molecules. The CD4 T cell antigen (molecule) is not only present on T-helper cells but also present on monocytes and macrophages. Since the CD4 molecule acts as a receptor for the human immunodeficiency virus type-1 (HIV-1), the virus infects monocytes and macrophages along with T-helper cells. Monocytes and macrophages express CD11 (CD11a, b, c) antigens, markers that define surface adhesion glycoproteins. CD14, CD64, and CD68 antigens are also present on monocytes and macrophages. These surface molecules are often used to identify the lineage of mononuclear cells in hematology and lymphoid malignancies.

Distribution and Kinetics

After promonocytes are formed, they respond to M-CSF and undergo two or three mitotic divisions in a period of about 50–60 hours before being released into the blood. Under conditions of increased demand, the cycle time can shorten, with earlier release of more immature cells into the blood. Blood monocytes are distributed in a circulating monocyte pool and a marginal monocyte pool, in a ratio of 1 : 3.5. Once monocytes enter the blood, they leave randomly with a half-time of 8.4 hours; this time period is shortened in splenomegaly or acute infection, and may be prolonged in monocytosis. After monocytes leave the blood, they spend several months, perhaps longer, as tissue macrophages.

Function

The monocyte is formed in the marrow, transported by the blood, and migrates into the tissues, where it transforms into a histiocyte or macrophage to spend the majority of its life span. The blood monocytes and tissue macrophages make up a mononuclear phagocyte system (reticuloendothelial system).

The mononuclear phagocyte system has an important role in defense against microorganisms, including mycobacteria, fungi, bacteria, protozoa, and viruses (Table 30–6). The cells are motile and respond to chemotactic factors (complement components as well as lymphokines and γ-interferon from activated T lymphocytes); they become immobilized by migration-inhibition factor from activated lymphocytes. They engage in phagocytosis, a process that is enhanced if the particle is coated by IgG or complement for which the macrophages have membrane receptors. After phagocytosis, they kill ingested microorganisms.

These mononuclear phagocytes are an integral part of both humoral and cell-mediated immunity. They handle or process antigens, providing contact of the antigen (or antigenic information) with lymphocytes. They also respond to various lymphokines and monokines and act as effector (e.g., cytotoxic) cells in the cell-mediated immune response. Monocytes and macrophages function in antibody-dependent cellular cytotoxicity. They have the ability to kill a variety of malignant cells (Weinberg, 2004) by promoting both cytostasis and cytolysis. Some of the ability of macrophages to destroy malignant cells may be attributed to the production of hydrogen peroxide (H_2O_2), nitrous oxide (NO) and reactive oxygen intermediates.

Macrophages remove and process senescent cells and debris through phagocytosis and digestion: for example, erythrocytes, leukocytes, and megakaryocyte nuclei are removed by macrophages in the marrow; inhaled particulate material is removed by alveolar macrophages in the lungs.

Macrophages may be 'activated' by either specific factors (e.g., cytophilic antibody) or nonspecific factors (e.g., in response to phagocytosed material). Activation results in enlargement of the cell and enhanced metabolism, phagocytosis, microbicidal activity, cytotoxicity, secretion of cytolytic proteins (including TNF-α), and the like.

Macrophages synthesize and secrete a large number of biologically active molecules, including enzymes, complement components, binding proteins, coagulation factors, cytokines and growth factors, chemotactic factors, angiogenesis factors, and bioactive lipids. This system, therefore, has multiple functions that include host defense, control of hematopoiesis, and policing of the environment within the body (Johnston, 1988).

Megakaryocytes

Platelets originate from polyploid megakaryocytes, the largest of all hematopoietic cells, which number less than 1% of the total nucleated marrow cells. Megakaryocytes arise from the multipotential hematopoietic stem cell, and then from a committed progenitor cell, the CFU-Meg (see Fig. 30–1). Megakaryocyte proliferation is largely regulated by thrombopoietin. Additional growth factors including kit-ligand, IL-3, IL-6, and IL-11 support megakaryocytic development in the presence of thrombopoietin (Kaushansky, 1995). Serum thrombopoietin levels are generally inversely proportional to platelet count; however, levels are elevated in liver disease and inflammatory states, probably through hepatocyte or marrow stromal cell responses (Kaushansky, 2003).

Morphology

Committed progenitor cells are not morphologically distinguishable from lymphocytes. Megakaryocyte development is characterized by endomitosis, nuclear division without cytoplasmic division, which results in ploidies varying from 2N to 64N. Most are 8N and 16N, with smaller numbers on either side. Nuclear lobes do not correlate precisely with ploidy. Nuclear chromatin is intensely staining, rather dispersed early, more compact and dense later. Nucleoli are small at all stages of megakaryocyte development.

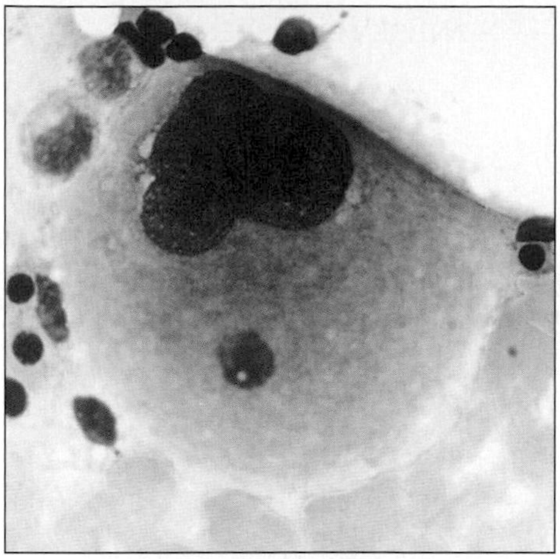

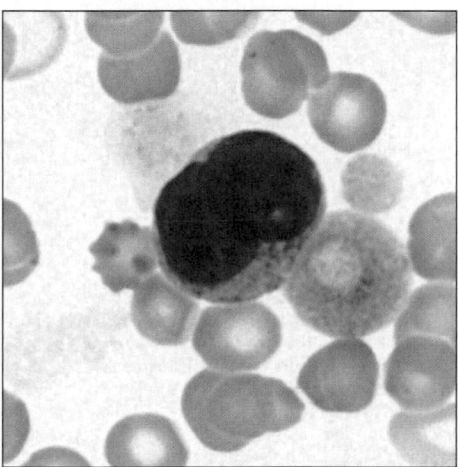

Figure 30–25 Megakaryocyte with a large, lobated nucleus and abundant granular cytoplasm (Wright–Giemsa, ×250).

Figure 30–26 Dwarf megakaryocyte with bilobed nucleus and scant granular cytoplasm; a few giant platelets are also seen. These cells are most often associated with myeloproliferative or myelodysplastic disorders (Wright–Giemsa, ×250).

The earliest recognizable *megakaryoblast* has overlapping nuclear lobes and a small amount of basophilic cytoplasm. During the course of maturation, nuclear lobes increase and spread out and red-pink granules become visible, first in the center of the cell. In the *mature megakaryocyte*, the nucleus is more compact, basophilia has disappeared, and the granules are clustered into small aggregates (Fig. 30–25).

The formation of individual platelets is a complex process. Megakaryocytes develop invaginated surface membranes (demarcation membranes) that provide a membrane reserve for proplatelet formation (Italiano, 2003). Proplatelets are pseudopodial extensions of megakaryocytes that progressively branch and thin out. Microtubular action is important in the formation of proplatelets and in bringing granule and organelle constituents into the proplatelets. Platelets are formed at the ends of proplatelets and released by microtubular action (Hartwig, 2003).

Megakaryocytes in Blood

Whole megakaryocytes or fragments may occasionally be found in normal blood films. If buffy coat films are examined, they are consistently present. Megakaryocyte fragments in blood films may be as small as lymphocytes and are recognized by the deeply stained chromatin (with a sharper chromatin–parachromatin separation than in lymphocyte nuclei) and by fragments of attached megakaryocyte cytoplasm. They are found more frequently than normal in myelophthisic processes, myeloproliferative disorders, or after stress or injury to the marrow.

Dwarf or micromegakaryocytes (Fig. 30–26) show evidence of abnormal megakaryopoiesis: agranular cytoplasm with hyaloplasmic zones or pseudopods; and association with large atypical platelets having similar cytoplasmic characteristics. These abnormal dwarf megakaryocytes are rarely found in any condition except myeloproliferative or myelodysplastic disorders.

Distribution and Kinetics

The maturation time for megakaryocytes in the marrow is about 5 days in humans. Platelets are released into the marrow sinuses over a period of several hours (Hartwig, 2003), and the megakaryocyte nuclei are phagocytosed by macrophages. Newly released platelets appear larger, more active metabolically, and more effective hemostatically. Platelets circulate at a stable concentration that averages $275 \times 10^9/L$. At any one time, about two-thirds of the total platelets are in the circulation, and the remaining third are present in the spleen. In asplenic individuals, all platelets are circulating. In diseases characterized by splenic enlargement, 80–90% of platelets may be sequestered in the spleen, resulting in a decreased concentration of circulating platelets (thrombocytopenia).

Platelets survive 8–11 days in the circulation. Some platelets are utilized in maintaining vascular integrity and in plugging small vascular injuries (random loss), and others are removed by the mononuclear phagocytic system when they become senescent.

Function

Platelets normally function in (1) maintaining the integrity of blood vessels; and (2) forming hemostatic plugs to stop blood loss from injured vessels, and, in the process, promoting coagulation of plasma factors.

Lymphocytes

Primary lymphoid tissue

During fetal life, lymphocyte precursors originate in the bone marrow and undergo antigen-independent lineage commitment. Maturation and selection of T cells occur primarily in the thymus, and of B cells, in the marrow and peripheral lymphoid organs (Denning, 1988; Bertoli, 1988). The T cell population is largely self-renewable following thymic involution. B cells are only capable of limited self-renewal. They are dependent on recruitment from marrow stem cells to replenish programmed B cells and plasma cells that are incapable of self-renewal (Jandl, 1996). Although the maturation of natural killer (NK) cells is not completely understood, data indicate a common T/NK precursor cell (Spits, 1995). While NK cell differentiation can occur in the thymus, it is likely that the bone marrow is the main site for NK cell development.

B Cell Development: Bone Marrow (Table 30–7). A distinct organ, the bursa of Fabricius, is present in birds and serves as the primary site of B cell development. In the human, a bursal equivalent exists in the liver during the eighth or ninth week of gestation, and later is found in the bone marrow after the hematopoietic stem cells have populated that organ. During adult life, generation of B cells occurs in the bone marrow.

B cell differentiation can be divided conveniently into two stages (Cooper, 1987). The initial stage of B cell differentiation involves the antigen-independent generation of diversity through rearrangement of the immunoglobulin heavy and light chain genes. The second stage is regulated by antigen triggering, T cell interaction, macrophages, and various growth factors (Fig. 30–27). This stage occurs predominantly in the secondary lymphoid organs.

A progenitor cell gives rise to the first recognizable B cell in man and mammals. This cell in humans is the pro-B (progenitor) cell that is characterized by receptor CD19 and TdT, but contains no cytoplasmic or surface bound immunoglobulin (Hagman, 1994). Differentiation of pro-B cells requires immunoglobulin gene rearrangement. The pre-B cell is characterized by the presence of intracytoplasmic μ heavy chains without any surface-bound immunoglobulin ($sIg^- c\mu^+$). It also contains HLA-DR antigens, CD19, CD79a, and other surface markers. Humoral proteins influence pre-B cell differentiation.

Table 30–7 Key Cell Surface Markers in Lymphocyte Development

Cell name	CD markers
Progenitor B cell	CD19, TdT, CD79a, HLA-DR
Pre-B cell	CD19, TdT, CD10, CD20, cytoplasmic μ
Naive mature B cell	CD19, CD20, Bcl-2, surface IgM
Centroblasts	CD19, CD20, CD10, Bcl-6
Mature B cells (peripheral blood)	CD19, CD20, CD21, CD22, CD24, CD38
Plasma cells	CD38, CD138, cytoplasmic Ig

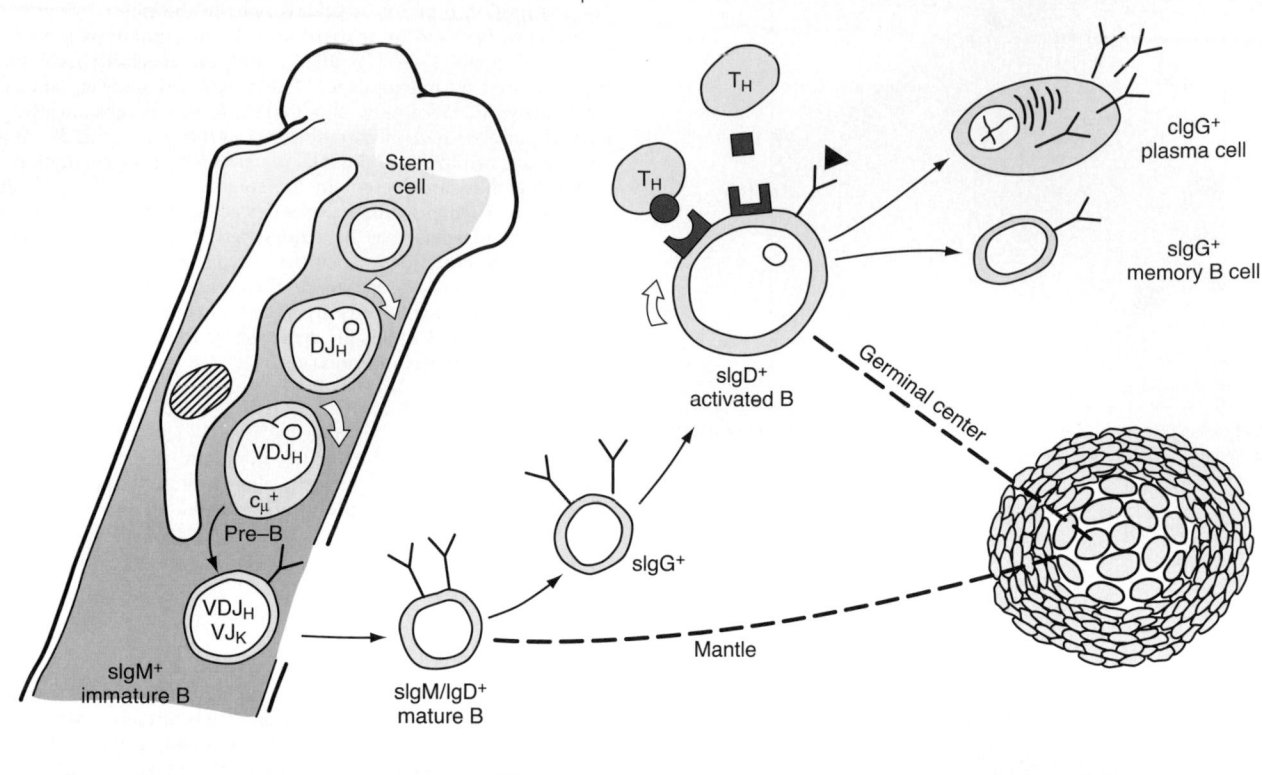

Bone marrow | Blood | Follicle

Figure 30–27 Differentiation of pre-B cells into B cells occurs independently of antigen, whereas the proliferation and terminal differentiation of B cells are antigen driven. Hematopoietic stem cells with stromal cell help give rise to pre-B cells. These proliferate (open arrow denotes cell cycling), rearrange DJ and VDJ gene segments, then express μ chains in cytoplasm ($c\mu^+$). A small, resting pre-B cell (not shown) with rearranged VJk gene assembles a complete IgM$_k$ molecule, becoming an immature B cell and leaving the bone marrow. Expression of sIgD marks entry of the cell into the mature, resting phase (or G_0) characteristic of most blood and mantle zone B cells. Switching an alternative isotype (IgG in this case) may occur before encounter with antigen or afterwards. Antigen triggers the resting B cell to enlarge (in G_1 phase of the cell cycle) and present processed antigen and DR to the antigen-specific T cell receptor–T_3 complex. T-helper cells (T_H) secrete growth factors that bind to newly expressed receptor, further enhancing proliferation (S and M phases) in germinal centers. The activated B cell can be induced to differentiate into plasma cells, which secrete their abundant cytoplasmic IgG. Alternatively, it can become a memory B cell with refined specificity poised to deliver an anamnestic immune response on its next encounter with antigen. (From Bertoli LF, Burrows PD: Normal B-lineage cells: Their differentiation and identification. Clin Lab Med 1988; 8:15, with permission.)

In becoming a pre-B cell, a lymphoid stem cell undergoes *DJ* and *VDJ* gene segment rearrangement to form a functional *V* gene for the μ heavy chain (Fig. 30–28). A productive heavy chain gene rearrangement is then followed by a rearrangement of the *VJ* gene segment of the light chain. Rearrangement of the κ light chain gene on chromosome 2 occurs first. If the κ rearrangements at both loci are nonproductive, rearrangement of the λ light chain gene on chromosome 22 follows. The controls exerted during pre-B cell development allow only one productive *VH* and *VL* gene to emerge, limiting each B cell to one unique antibody structure (Bertoli, 1988). The combination of the μ heavy chain and κ or λ light chain allows the pre-B cell to generate an intact immunoglobulin molecule and express surface IgM. Isotype switching (changing from IgM/IgD to IgG1, etc.) and constant heavy gene deletions occur in pre-B cells and more differentiated B cells. The switching of μ cells to $\gamma1$ or $\alpha2$ cells occurs by the formation of a DNA loop in which all intervening constant heavy genes are deleted (Fig. 30–29). IgD can be coexpressed with IgM through alternative RNA processing.

Pre-B cells give rise to naive mature B cells that characteristically express surface-bound immunoglobulin. These cells are present in primary lymphoid follicles, in follicular mantle zones, and in the circulation. In addition to IgD and IgM, these cells often express CD5 and are positive for Bcl-2.

In the second stage of differentiation, naive B cells interact with antigen and undergo transformation in the presence of T cells and macrophages. This process occurs in the germinal center. The B cells transform into blastic cells (centroblasts) that express Bcl-6 and CD10. Rapid division and expansion of B cell clones occurs in an attempt to identify cells with immunoglobulin that provides the best fit for the stimulating antigen. Antigenic specificity is further refined through the process of somatic mutation in the variable region gene. Centroblasts give rise to centrocytes, which are cleaved follicle center cells. These cells express the modified immunoglobulin (following somatic mutation). Cells with lower affinity for the antigen are destroyed through apoptosis (cells in the germinal center do not express Bcl-2; therefore, they can undergo apoptosis).

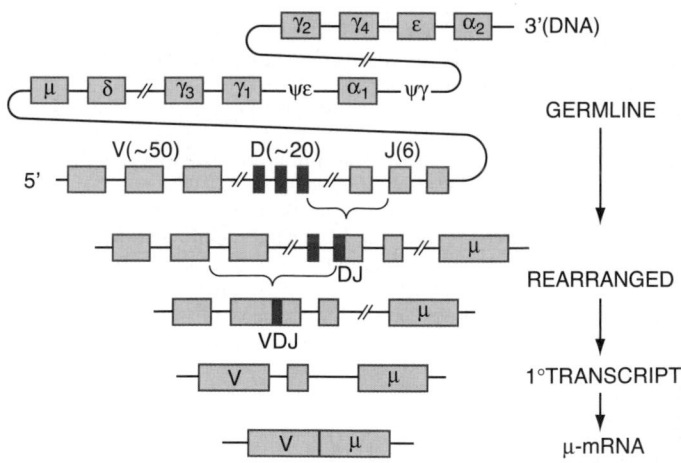

Figure 30–28 Generation of a functional Ig gene requires DNA rearrangement. In the germline and in somatic nonlymphoid cells, V, D, and J gene segments are widely separated in the DNA of chromosome 14. A cell committed to the B lineage first undergoes D to J rearrangement, juxtaposing the D and J segments, and deleting intervening DNA sequences. This is followed by V to DJ rearrangement, generating a complete VDJ exon. The primary RNA transcript is processed to yield a contiguous V (VDJ) mRNA. (From Bertoli LF, Burrows PD: Normal B-lineage cells: Their differentiation and identification. Clin Lab Med, 1988; 8:15, with permission.)

Surviving centrocytes differentiate into either plasma cells that produce circulating immunoglobulin, or memory B cells that provide rapid humoral response the next time the same antigen is encountered. Memory B cells are present in the marginal zone of the follicle.

The state of immunoglobulin genes is, therefore, a good indicator of the developmental stage of B cells. The presence of immunoglobulin gene

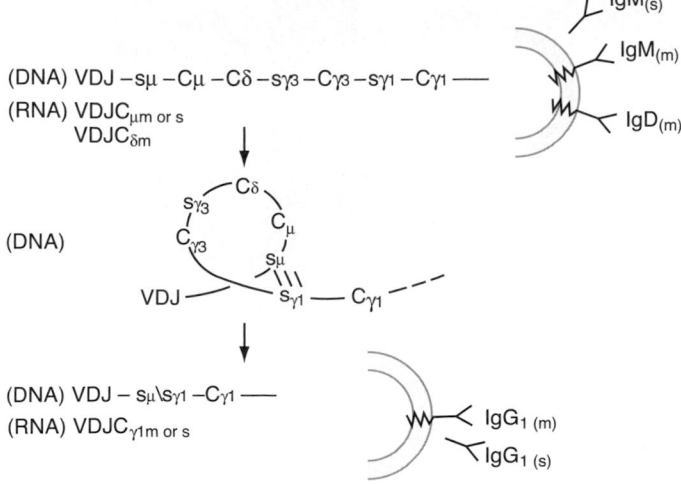

(DNA) VDJ – sμ – Cμ – Cδ – sγ3 – Cγ3 – sγ1 – Cγ1 ——

(RNA) VDJC$_{\mu m \text{ or } s}$
VDJC$_{\delta m}$

(DNA)

(DNA) VDJ – sμ\sγ1 – Cγ1 ——

(RNA) VDJC$_{\gamma 1m \text{ or } s}$

IgM$_{(s)}$
IgM$_{(m)}$
IgD$_{(m)}$

IgG$_1$ $_{(m)}$
IgG$_1$ $_{(s)}$

Figure 30–29 Alternative strategies for expression of non-IgM isotypes. IgD can be coexpressed with IgM by alternative processing of a primary RNA transcript of VDJ-Cμ-Cδ to yield μ membrane (m), μ secretory (s), and δ$_m$ RNAs. The production of IgG, IgA, or IgE isotypes involves DNA rearrangement. During the switch from IgM to IgG, for example, intrachromosomal recombination between homologous switch (s) regions results in deletions of C$_\mu$, C$_\delta$, and C$_{\gamma 3}$ so that C$_{\gamma 1}$ is now the first C gene 3′ of the VDJ exon. Thus, the same variable region is expressed with a different constant region. (From Bertoli LF, Burrows PD: Normal B-lineage cells: Their differentiation and identification. Clin Lab Med 1988; 8:15, with permission.)

Table 30–8 Summary of T Cell Maturation

Stage	Maturation events	Cell surface markers
Pro-T cell	Migration from marrow to thymic cortex	CD2, CD44
α/β Pre-T cell	Migration from thymic cortex to medulla, elimination of self-recognizing T cells, α/β TCR rearrangement (for T cells destined for either the helper or suppressor subset)	TdT, CD1, CD2, CD3, CD4, CD5, CD7, CD8
γ/δ Pre-T cell	Migration from thymic cortex to medulla, elimination of self-recognizing T cells, γ/δ TCR rearrangement (for T cells destined for the cytotoxic subset)	TdT, CD1, CD2, CD3, CD7
Mature T cell	Loss of ability to make TdT, circulation in peripheral blood as helper, suppressor or cytotoxic subset	Helper T: CD2, CD3, CD4, CD5, CD7 Suppressor T: CD2, CD3, CD5, CD7, CD8 Cytotoxic T: CD2, CD3, CD7

rearrangement identifies primitive B cells. Somatic mutations resulting in variable region sequences that are different from germline sequences identify a B cell that has been stimulated by antigen. Germinal center B cells can be distinguished from post-germinal center B cells by the presence of intraclonal diversity in the former due to ongoing somatic mutations.

In the peripheral blood, approximately 6–15% of B cells express surface-bound IgM (90% of these coexpress IgD), 1–3% IgG, and 0.5–2% IgA. Mature B cells express receptors for Fc portions of Ig isotypes, C3b and C3d fragments of complement, interferon, and IL-4. Mature B cells also express CD19, CD20, CD21, CD22, CD24, and CD38.

Plasma cells are characterized by abundant cytoplasmic immunoglobulin, reflecting the immunoglobulin commitment of the activated B cell. At this stage, Fc and C3 receptors, HLA-DR antigen, and surface-bound immunoglobulin are greatly reduced, but the cells express CD38 and CD138. Thus, the lymphocytes bearing sIg give rise to cells committed to the synthesis of IgM, IgG, and IgA.

T Cell Development: Thymus (Table 30–8). The microenvironment of the thymus is necessary for the differentiation of T cells. The human thymus has two parts – the cortex and the medulla. The cortex is subdivided into two portions, the subcapsular cortex and the inner cortex, and is populated predominantly by small lymphocytes with a few scattered epithelial cells. Fibrous septa extend from the capsule to the medullary region. The medulla is composed mostly of epithelial cells with a small component of lymphocytes. In the medulla, Hassall's corpuscles, small islands of partially hyalinized epithelial cells, are present.

Pro-T cells migrate from the bone marrow or fetal liver to the thymus where they are processed into functionally mature T cells for circulation in the blood and to the peripheral or secondary lymphoid tissues. The earliest T cells in the thymus express CD2 and CD44 (Schattner, 2001). Subsequently these cells express CD25 and CD3. The T cell receptor (TCR) genes are organized in a similar manner to immunoglobulin genes. They possess V, D, J, and C regions and undergo rearrangement during early T cell maturation. In addition to the heterodimeric glycoproteins (α/β or γ/δ), the TCR/CD3 complex also consists of additional subunits; CD3-ε, -ξ and -η (Blumberg, 1990). The TCR recognizes foreign peptides held in an association with self-MHC molecules. The TCRs of CD4+ α/β T cells recognize nonself peptides held in the groove of class II MHC molecules, while TCRs of CD8+ α/β T cells recognize nonself polypeptides bound to the class I molecules (MacLennan, 1999).

The maturation of T cells is complex, however; at least three stages with multiple intermediate substages have been defined (Paraskevas, 2004b). In the first stage, pro-T cells migrate from either the bone marrow or the fetal liver to the cortex of the thymus. In the second stage, pro-T cells migrate first from the subcapsular cortex to the inner cortex and then to the thymic medulla (Table 30–8). During this time, T cells with the ability to recognize foreign antigens are retained, while T cells with the ability to recognize self-antigens are eliminated.

In early T cell development, the gamma and beta chain genes rearrange simultaneously, with TCR commitment dependent on expression of surrogate alpha chain and development of a pre-TCR (Haks, 1998; Kang, 2001). Thymic α/β T cells first coexpress both CD4 and CD8, with subsequent downregulation of one or the other. In the thymic medulla, the pre-T cells lose the ability to make TdT as they convert to mature T cells (third stage) and then circulate in the blood and peripheral lymphoid tissues.

The majority of post-thymic (peripheral) T cells express α/β TCR, while a small minority do not, but rather express γ/δ chains. NK cells express only ε chains with cytoplasmic CD3. Mature T cells are of at least three types. The T-helper cells possess α/β TCR chains and express CD2, CD3, CD4, CD5, and CD7 cell markers. T-suppressor/cytotoxic cells have α/β TCR chains and express CD2, CD3, CD5, CD7, and CD8 cell markers. Mature T cells with γ/δ TCR chains exhibit CD2, CD3, and CD7, lack CD4 and CD8 and seem to function as another population of cytotoxic cells (Paraskevas, 2004b).

Antigen-independent development of T cells is controlled by interaction with thymic epithelial cells and thymic fibroblasts as well as by the influences of cytokines, growth factors, and thymic hormones. IL-1, IL-2, IL-3, IL-4, IL-7, and KL are critical in the growth and differentiation of thymic lymphocytes. Thymic hormones produced by thymic epithelial cells also induce T cell function.

In the T-zone area of the peripheral lymphoid system, the T cell antigen-dependent pathway occurs through the binding of the TCRs to antigen peptides associated with appropriate MHC I and MHC II molecules on macrophages or interdigitating dendritic cells (IDCs). This results in the release of IL-1 by the activated macrophages, which in turn leads to the formation of IL-2 receptors on T cells and the subsequent synthesis and release of IL-2 by these activated T cells. In this activation process many other cytokines (including IL-4, IL-6, IL-10, TNF, and interferon) are released and appropriate cytokine receptors are upregulated. These events result in the activation and maturation of T-helper cells, T-suppressor cells, T-cytotoxic cells, and other immunoregulatory cells. This activation process not only increases the number of antigen-specific T cells, but also alters the immunophenotype and changes the expression of certain adhesion molecules on T cells. For example, LFA-1 (a heterodimer formed from CD11a and CD18) and VLA-4 (a heterodimer of CD29 and CD49d, CD44, and CD2) are upregulated, while L-selectin (CD62L) is downregulated (MacLennan, 1999). Changes in the expression of adhesion markers allow for the proper circulation of T cells in the body.

Natural Killer (NK) cell: Bone Marrow. Immunophenotypic and functional data suggest that NK cells and T cells have a close developmental relationship. The expression of CD3 proteins has been found in human fetal NK cells. Thus, it is likely that NK cells and T cells have a common precursor cell. Although NK cells can develop in the thymus, the thymic environment is not required for NK cell differentiation. In fact, it seems most likely that

IV

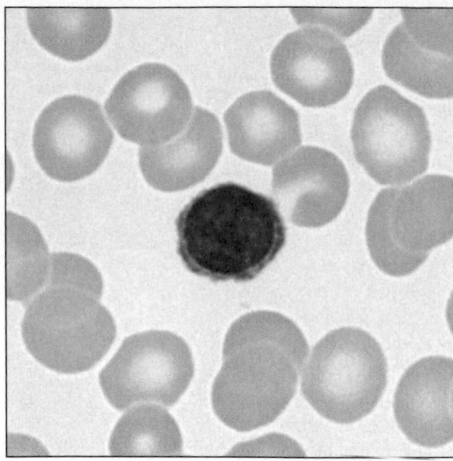

Figure 30–30 Small lymphocyte with high N/C ratio, condensed chromatin, and scant basophilic cytoplasm (Wright–Giemsa, ×250).

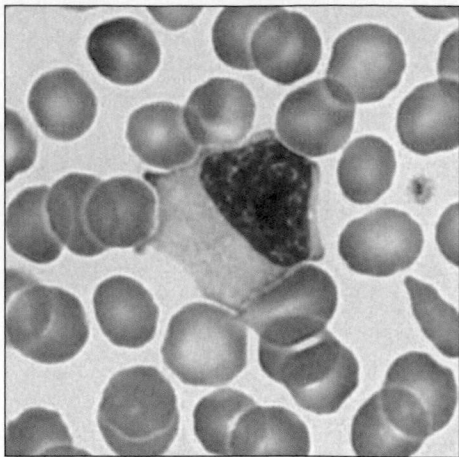

Figure 30–31 Atypical lymphocyte with large nucleus, finer chromatin, and abundant basophilic cytoplasm scalloping around adjacent red blood cells (Wright–Giemsa, ×250).

the bone marrow is the main site for NK cell differentiation (Spits, 1995). Fetal NK cells possess CD3γ, δ, ε and CD28, while adult NK cells express CD2, CD3ξ, CD7, CD8α, CD16, and CD56. KL, IL-7, and IL-2 are critical in the development of NK cells (Spits, 1995). NK cells proliferate in the presence of IL-2, and their activity can be augmented by exposure to γ-interferon. NK cells appear to be targeted against virus-infected cells unable to signal cytotoxic T cells (usually as a result of low expression of class I MHC molecules). Since NK cells possess the Fc portion of IgG, they participate in antibody-dependent cell lysis (MacLennan, 1999).

Secondary Lymphoid Tissue

In late fetal and postnatal life, lymphocytes are produced in the secondary lymphoid tissue: spleen, lymph nodes, and intestine. Lymphocytes of the secondary lymphoid organs are progeny from stem cells that have been influenced by primary lymphoid organs. The secondary lymphoid organs are thus composed of a mixture of B cells and T cells. Lymphopoiesis in secondary lymphoid organs depends solely on antigenic stimulation. B cells and T cells tend to localize in anatomically distinct parts of the lymphoid tissues where proliferation can take place.

Lymphocyte Function and Physiology

T cells and their progeny function in cell-mediated immunity, which includes delayed hypersensitivity, graft rejection, graft-versus-host reactions, defense against intracellular organisms (such as tubercle bacillus and brucella), and defense against neoplasms. B cells and their progeny perform in humoral immunity, or the production of antibodies, either as a lymphocyte or after transformation into a plasma cell.

The majority of the circulating lymphocytes are T cells that have a life span of months to years. The B cells are a minor population (10–20% of the lymphocytes), probably have a short life span measured in days (with the exception of memory B cells), and are distinguished by the presence of considerable immunoglobulin on their surface membrane.

Lymphocytes circulate in the blood and home to appropriate lymphoid organs. During fetal development, lymphocytes migrate from the fetal liver to bone marrow or thymus. Later, pro-T cells migrate from the bone marrow to the thymus while immature B cells home to secondary lymphoid tissues. After thymic processing, virgin T cells also home to specific areas in the peripheral lymphoid tissues. The circulation of lymphocytes is regulated by multiple cell-surface adhesion molecules and chemokines including the integrins, selectins, and leukocyte (L) selectin. The circulation and homing of lymphocytes is a very complex, multistep phenomenon reviewed elsewhere (Springer, 1994; Paraskevas, 2004a). However, in the postcapillary venule of lymphoid tissue, the lymphocyte travels from the blood through the endothelium and into the lymphoid tissue, where it may stay or percolate through and return to the blood via the thoracic duct lymph. Small lymphocytes (Fig. 30–30) have little cytoplasm and, in electron micrographs, few organelles and relatively little RNA. After antigenic stimulation, small lymphocytes (B cells or T cells, depending on the nature of the antigen) become activated, increase their RNA synthesis, and undergo blast transformation. On Romanowsky-stained films, these blasts are large cells (15–25 μm) with abundant, rather deep blue cytoplasm, a large reticular nucleus with uniform chromatin,

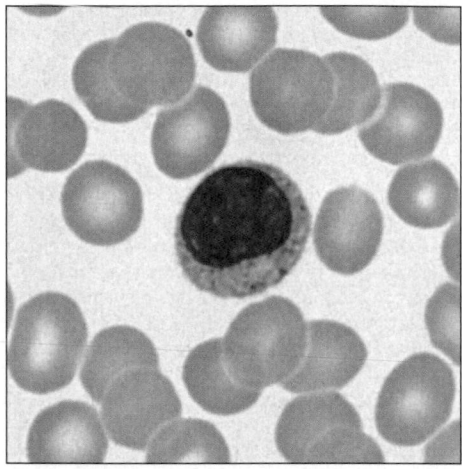

Figure 30–32 Large granular lymphocyte with azurophilic cytoplasmic granules (Wright–Giemsa, ×250).

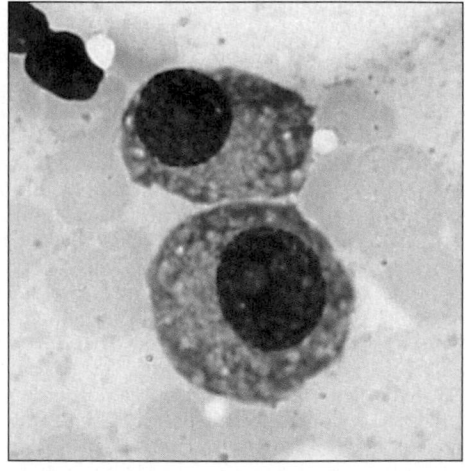

Figure 30–33 Plasma cells with abundant basophilic cytoplasm, eccentric nucleus, and perinuclear clear Golgi zone (Wright–Giemsa, ×250).

and prominent nucleoli. This cell is called the *reticular lymphocyte* (nonleukemic lymphoblast; 'immunoblast'). If the blasts are derived from B cells, the new lymphocytes function in the production of antibodies (B cells, plasma cells); if the blasts are derived from T cells, the progeny act in the cellular immune response. The latter is mediated by several soluble factors produced by the activated T cell, including IL-2, which induces the proliferation of T cells; IL-3, which is a multipotential colony-stimulating factor; IL-4, which promotes the proliferation of B cells; IL-5, which enhances the proliferation of eosinophils as well as B cells; IL-6, which promotes differentiation of B cells; lymphotoxin, which is directly toxic to cells; and migratory inhibitory factor, which promotes adherence of macrophages and keeps them at the site. Atypical lymphocytes (Fig. 30-31) are seen in certain viral infection like infectious mononucleosis. These cells have large nuclei with fine chromatin and more abundant cytoplasm that often scallops around adjacent red blood cells. Large granular lymphocytes (Fig. 30-32) contain azurophilic granules in their cytoplasm; these cells most often represent cytotoxic T cells or natural killer cells.

Plasma cells have abundant blue cytoplasm, often with light streaks or vacuoles, an eccentric round nucleus, and a well-defined clear (Golgi) zone adjacent to the nucleus. The nucleus of the plasma cell has heavily clumped chromatin, which is sharply defined from the parachromatin and often arranged in a radial or wheel-like pattern (Fig. 30-33).

References

Akashi K, Traver D, Miyamoto T, Weissman IL: A clonogenic common myeloid progenitor that gives rise to all myeloid lineages. Nature 2000; 404:193-197.

Bagby GC, Segal GM: Growth factors and control of hematopoiesis. In Hoffman R, Berry EJ, Shattil SJ, et al (eds): Hematology, Basic Principles and Practice. New York, Churchill Livingstone, 1991, p 97.

Bertoli LF, Burrows PD: Normal B-lineage cells: Their differentiation and identification. Clin Lab Med 1988; 8:15-30.

Blumberg RS, Ley S, Sancho J, et al: Structure of the T cell antigen receptor: Evidence for two CD3 epsilon subunits in the T cell receptor-CD3 complex. Proc Natl Acad Sci USA 1990; 87:7220-7224.

Broudy VC: Stem cell factor and hematopoiesis. Blood 1997; 90:1345-1364.

Bunn HF, Forget BG: Hemoglobin: Molecular, Genetic and Clinical Aspects. Philadelphia, WB Saunders Company, 1986, p 13.

Campbell KJ, Kim CH, Butcher EC: Chemokines in the systemic organization of immunity. Immunol Rev 2003; 195:58-71.

Casadevall N, Dupuy E, Molho-Sabatier P, et al: Autoantibodies against erythropoietin in a patient with pure red-cell aplasia. N Engl J Med 1996; 334:630-633.

Chemmanur AT, Bonovsky HL: Hepatic porphyries: diagnosis and management. Clin Liver Dis 2004; 4:807-838.

Cooper MD: Current concepts. B lymphocytes: Normal development and function. N Engl J Med 1987; 317:1452-1456.

Coulombel L: Identification of hematopoietic stem/progenitor cells: strength and drawbacks of functional assays. Oncogene 2004; 23:7210-7222.

Deacon AC, Elder GH: Best Practice No 165: front line tests for the investigation of suspected porphyria. J Clin Pathol 2001; 54:500-507.

Denning SM, Haynes BF: Differentiation of human T cells. Clin Lab Med 1988; 8:1-14.

Gleich GJ, Adolphson CR: The eosinophilic leukocyte: Structure and function. Adv Immunol 1986; 39:177-253.

Gordeuk VR, Sergueeva AI, Miasnikova GY, et al: Congenital disorder of oxygen sensing: association of the homozygous Chuvash polycythemia VHL mutation with thrombosis and vascular abnormalities but not tumors. Blood 2004; 103:3924-3932.

Hagman J, Grosschedl R: Regulation of gene expression at early stages of B-cell differentiation. Curr Opin Immunol 1994; 6:222-230.

Haks MC, Krimpenfort P, Borst J, Kruisbeek AM: The CD3gamma chain is essential for development of both the TCRalphabeta and TCRgammadelta lineages. EMBO J 1998; 17:1871-1882.

Hartwig J, Italiano J: The birth of the platelet. J Thromb Haemost 2003; 1:1580-1586.

Hift RJ, Davidson BP, van der Hooft C, et al: Plasma fluorescence scanning and fecal porphyrin analysis for the diagnosis of variegate porphyria: precise determination of sensitivity and specificity with detection of protoporphyrinogen oxidase mutations as a reference standard. Clin Chem 2004; 50:915-923.

Hillman RS, Finch CA: Red Cell Manual, 7th ed. Philadelphia, FA Davis, 1996, p 58.

Updated classic work illustrating the morphology of red blood cells, with descriptions of red cell disorders and with pathophysiology, diagnosis and treatment of anemias.

Hübel K, Engert A: Clinical applications of granulocyte colony-stimulating factor: an update and summary. Ann Hematol 2003; 82:207-213.

Italiano JE, Shivdasani A: Megakaryocytes and beyond: the birth of platelets. J Thomb Haemost 2003; 1:1174-1182.

Jandl JH: Blood cell formation. In Jandl JH (ed): Blood: Textbook of Hematology, 2nd ed. Boston, Little, Brown, 1996.

Johnston RB Jr: Current concepts: Immunology. Monocytes and macrophages. N Engl J Med 1988; 318:747-752.

Kang J, Volkmann A, Raulet DH: Evidence that gammadelta versus alphabeta T cell fate determination is initiated independently of T cell receptor signaling. J Exp Med 2001; 193:689-698.

Kaushansky K: Thrombopoietin: The primary regulator of platelet production. Blood 1995; 86:419-431.

Kaushansky K: Thrombopoietin: a tool for understanding thrombopoiesis. J Thromb Haemost 2003; 1:1587.

A review of the effects of the primary hormonal regulator of platelet production and the underlying mechanisms through which it works.

Kaushansky K, Karplus PA: Hematopoietic growth factors: Understanding functional diversity in structural terms. Blood 1993; 82:3229-3240.

Kaushansky K, Lok S, Holly RD, et al: Promotion of megakaryocyte progenitor expansion and differentiation by the c-Mpl ligand thrombopoietin. Nature 1994; 369:568-571.

Kondo M, Weissman IL, Akashi K: Identification of clonogenic common lymphoid progenitors in mouse bone marrow. Cell 1997; 91:661-672.

Lindstedt G, Lundberg PA: Are current methods of measurement of erythropoietin (EPO) in human plasma or serum adequate for the diagnosis of polycythaemia vera and the assessment of EPO deficiency? Scand J Clin Lab Invest 1998; 58:441-458.

Long MW: Blood cell cytoadhesion molecules. Exp Hematol 1992; 20:288-301.

Lyman SD, Jacobsen SEW: c-Kit ligand and Flt3 ligand: Stem/progenitor cell factors with overlapping yet distinctive activities. Blood 1998; 91:1101-1134.

MacLennan ICM, Drayson MT: Normal lymphocytes and non-neoplastic lymphocyte disorders. In Hoffbrand AV, Lewis SM, Tuddenham EGD (eds): Postgraduate Haematology, 4th ed. Oxford, Butterworth Heinemann, 1999, p 267.

Mertelsmann R: Hematopoietic cytokines: From biology and pathophysiology to clinical application. Leukemia 1993; (Suppl 2): S168-S177.

Ohishi K, Katayama N, Shiku H, et al: Notch signalling in hematopoiesis. Semin Cell Dev Biol 2003; 14:143-150.

Paraskevas F: The lymphatic system. In Foerster J, Lukens J, Rogers GM, et al (eds): Wintrobe's Clinical Hematology, 11th ed. Baltimore, Williams & Wilkins, 2004a, p 409-438.

Paraskevas F: T lymphocytes and NK cells. In Foerster J, Lukens J, Rogers GM, et al (eds): Wintrobe's Clinical Hematology, 11th ed. Baltimore, Williams & Wilkins, 2004b, p 475-526.

Poh-Fitzpatrick MB. A plasma porphyrin fluorescence marker for variegate porphyria. Arch Dermatol 1980; 116:543-547.

Quesenberry PJ, Colvin GA: Hematopoietic stem cells, progenitor cells, and cytokines. In Beutler E, Lichtman M, Coller B, et al (eds): Williams Hematology, 6th ed. New York, McGraw-Hill, 2001, pp 153-176.

Quesniaux VFJ: Interleukins 9, 10, 11, and 12 and kit ligand: A brief overview. Res Immunol 1992; 143:385-400.

Roberts PJ, Linch DC, Webb DKH: Phagocytes. In Hoffbrand AV, Lewis SM, Tuddenham EGD (eds): Postgraduate Haematology, 4th ed, Oxford, Butterworth Heinemann, 1999, p 235.

Root RK, Dale DC: Granulocyte colony-stimulating factor and granulocyte-macrophage colony-stimulating factor: Comparisons and potential for use in the treatment of infections in nonneutropenic patients. J Infect Dis 179 1999; (Suppl 2):S342-S352.

Sandberg S, Elder GH. Diagnosing acute porphyries. Clin Chem 2004; 50:803-805.

Sauvageau G, Iscove NN, Humphries RK: In vitro and in vivo expansion of hematopoietic stem cells. Oncogene 2004; 23:7223-7232.

Schattner EJ, Casali P: The immune system: structure and function. In Knowles DM (ed): Neoplastic hematopathology, 2nd ed. Philadelphia, Lippincott Williams & Wilkins, 2001, p 43-92.

Comprehensive and authoritative review of the human immune system.

Schett G, Firbas U, Füreder W, et al: Decreased serum erythropoietin and its relation to anti-erythropoietin antibodies in anaemia of systemic lupus erythematosus. Rheumatology 2001; 40:424-431.

Siena S, Bregni M, Brando B, et al: Circulation of CD34+ hematopoietic stem cells in the peripheral blood of high-dose cyclophosphamide-treated patients: Enhancement by intravenous recombinant human granulocyte-macrophage colony-stimulating factor. Blood 1989; 74:1905-1914.

Spits H, Lanier L, Phillips JH: Development of human T and natural killer cells. Blood 1995; 85:2654-2670.

Spivak JL: Polycythemia vera: myths, mechanisms, and management. Blood 2002; 100:4272-4290.

Springer TA: Traffic signals for lymphocyte recirculation and leukocyte emigration: The multistep paradigm. Cell 1994; 76:301-314.

Teoh G, Anderson KC: Interaction of tumor and host cells with adhesion and extracellular matrix molecules in the development of multiple myeloma. Hematol Oncol Clin North Am 1997; 11:27-42.

Terstappen LW, Huang S, Safford M, et al: Sequential generations of hematopoietic colonies derived from single nonlineage-committed CD34+CD38- progenitor cells. Blood 1991; 77:1218-1227.

Verfaillie CM: Adhesion receptors as regulators of the hematopoietic process. Blood 1998; 92:2609-2612.

Weinberg JB: Mononuclear phagocytes. In Foerster J, Lukens J, Rogers GM, et al (eds): Wintrobe's Clinical Hematology, 11th ed. Baltimore, Williams & Wilkins, 2004, p 349-386.

Zannettino ACW, Buhring HJ, Niutta S, et al: The sialomucin CD164 (MGC-24v) is an adhesive glycoprotein expressed by human hematopoietic progenitors and bone marrow stromal cells that serves as a potent negative regulator of hematopoiesis. Blood 1998; 92:2613-2628.

Zubair AC, Silberstein L, Ritz J: Adult hematopoietic stem cell plasticity. Transfusion 2002; 42:1096-1101.

IV

M. Tarek Elghetany MD, Katalin Banki MD

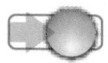

KEY POINTS
• Anemia may result from bone marrow production defect or shortened red cell survival.

• Hemolytic anemia may be caused by extrinsic factors, usually acquired, such as chemical agents or antibodies, or intrinsic factors, usually inherited, such as disorders of the red cell membrane, enzymes, or hemoglobinopathy.

• Stem cell disorders, such as inherited and acquired aplastic anemia, and paroxysmal nocturnal hemoglobinuria usually affect more than one cell line.

• Non-bone marrow diseases, such as endocrine, renal, and inflammatory disorders, significantly influence bone marrow function.

• For the initial assessment of anemia, a complete blood count, a peripheral blood smear, and a reticulocytic count need to be examined.

Anemias

Anemia is considered to be present if the hemoglobin (Hb) concentration or the hematocrit (Hct) is below the lower limit of the 95% reference interval for the individual's age, sex, and geographic location (altitude) (Table 31–1). This means that 2.5% of normal individuals will be classified as anemic. Conversely, an individual whose hemoglobin falls within the reference intervals for age and sex yet significantly below his or her own reference values should be considered anemic.

Anemia may be absolute, when there is decreased red blood cell (RBC) mass, or relative, when associated with a higher plasma volume. Causes of absolute anemia fall into two major pathophysiologic categories: impaired red cell production and increased erythrocyte destruction or loss in excess of the ability of the marrow to replace these losses. Several authors have included posthemorrhagic anemia in the latter category (Hillman, 1996; Erslev, 2001b). The presence of anemia may be a sign of an underlying disorder whose cause should be identified, since correction may be very important to the individual. Relative anemia may occur with pregnancy, macroglobulinemia, and post-flight astronauts.

Anemia also may be classified by red cell morphology as macrocytic, normocytic, or microcytic, an approach that is useful in differential diagnosis (see later discussion). Both the pathophysiologic and morphologic classifications should be understood. Some anemias have more than one pathogenetic mechanism and go through more than one morphologic stage (e.g., blood loss anemia).

Clinical signs and symptoms result from the diminished delivery of oxygen to the tissues and, therefore, are related to the lowered hemoglobin concentration and blood volume, and dependent on the rate of these changes. Modifying factors are compensatory adjustments in the cardiac output, the respiratory rate, and the oxygen affinity of hemoglobin. When anemia develops slowly in a patient who is not otherwise severely ill, hemoglobin concentrations as low as 6 g/dL may develop without producing any discomfort or physical signs as long as the patient is at rest.

In general, the anemic patient complains of easy fatigability and dyspnea on exertion, and often of faintness, vertigo, palpitation, and headache. The more common physical findings are pallor, a rapid bounding pulse, low blood pressure, slight fever, some dependent edema, and systolic murmurs. In addition to these general signs and symptoms, certain clinical findings are characteristic of the specific type of anemia.

Impaired Production – Iron Deficiency Anemia

Iron Metabolism (Fairbanks, 2001b)

Iron is an essential component of hemoglobin, of myoglobin (in muscle cells), and of certain enzymes (in most body cells). The major 'pools' of iron in the body are illustrated in Figure 31–1. Two-thirds or more of the body's total iron is in the erythron (normoblasts and erythrocytes); each milliliter of red cells contains about 1 mg of iron. Storage iron is present in macrophages of the reticuloendothelial system in two forms: ferritin and hemosiderin. Ferritin is a water-soluble complex of ferric salt and a protein, apoferritin. Apoferritin has a molecular weight of approximately 450 000 Da and consists of 24 subunits with a variable ratio of H (heavy) and L (light) types. Apoferritin forms a shell around a crystalline core of predominately ferric oxyhydroxide (FeOOH). The genes for the H and L subunits have been located on chromosomes 11 and 19, respectively. Hemosiderin is water-insoluble and consists mostly of aggregates of ferric oxyhydroxide core crystals with partially or completely degraded protein shell. Protein degradation usually occurs in lysosomes. Most of the iron utilized in hemoglobin synthesis is that recently released from degraded Hb in macrophages and transported to the normoblasts by plasma transferrin (a β-globulin, molecular weight 80 000 Da, gene located on chromosome 3). Each molecule of apotransferrin binds two atoms of ferric iron. Subsequently, transferrin binds to transferrin receptors (CD71) on the cell membrane of erythroid precursors, reticulocytes, and most body cells. The transferrin–transferrin receptor complex is rapidly internalized, iron is released, and apotransferrin returns to the circulation and binds more iron.

Very little iron is lost from the body, and this mainly from loss of cells in the gastrointestinal (GI) tract and to a lesser extent from the skin and in the urine. The iron excreted in women averages more than that in men because of menstrual blood loss. About 1 mg is lost each day, while for menstruating females iron loss is about 2 mg/day. Iron balance is maintained by control of absorption. In the United States, dietary iron averages 15 mg/day with 7% absorption in men, and 11 mg/day in women with 13% absorption. Absorption can be increased in iron deficiency, but only to about 20% of ingested iron in meat-containing diets, and less in vegetarian diets (Hillman, 1996). Absorption takes place largely in the

Table 31–1 Reference Values Below Which Anemia is Considered to Exist at Sea Level

Age (years)	Hb (g/dL)
Both sexes	
1–2	11
3–5	11.2
6–11	11.8
Females	
12–15	11.9
16–69	12
≥70	11.8
Males	
12–15	12.6
16–19	13.6
20–49	13.7
50–69	13.3
≥70	12.4

From Looker, 1997.

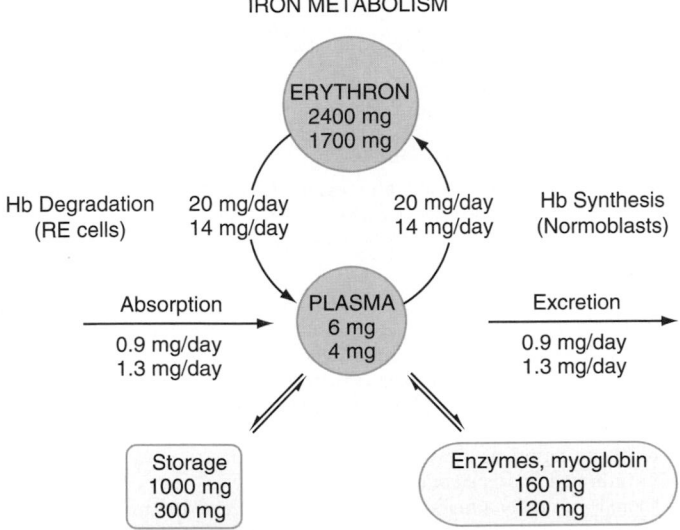

IRON METABOLISM

Figure 31–1 Scheme of iron metabolism. The upper figure in each position is average for an 80-kg man; the lower figure is for a 65-kg woman. (Data from Hillman & Finch, 1974.) The plasma iron, bound largely to transferrin, is central in this scheme. It completely turns over several times a day in supplying iron for heme synthesis. Each day, about 1/120 of the total circulating red cells are destroyed and the same number of new red cells are delivered to the blood. That proportion of the total erythron iron enters the plasma from the site of Hb degradation, the macrophages of the reticuloendothelial (RE) system, and travels (bound to transferrin) to the normoblasts in the marrow. Storage iron largely resides also in the macrophages of the RE system. Absorbed iron enters the plasma pool, bound to transferrin. Excreted iron is largely from loss of cells.

small intestine, most efficiently in the duodenum and upper jejunum. Heme iron is absorbed more efficiently than inorganic iron. Iron absorption is facilitated by ascorbate and citrate while inhibited by phytates and tannins. Acid production by the stomach lowers the pH in the duodenum, thus enhancing the solubility and uptake of nonheme ferric iron. Although the mechanism of iron entry into mucosal cells of the upper gastrointestinal tract remains largely unknown, more than one pathway seems to be in place, including an independent mechanism for heme absorption. Recent studies suggest the presence of an iron transport channel called divalent metal transporter (DMT), which is regulated by iron regulatory proteins. DMT-1 regulates iron transport from intestinal surface to inside the cell. This process is aided by the recently discovered duodenal cytochrome b, which reduces iron to the ferrous form. The transport of iron from intestinal cells to plasma involves another transport system, which includes ferroportin-1 and hephaestin (Brissot, 2004). Ferroportin-1 is located at the basolateral membrane of apical enterocytes and it functions as a transport protein delivering iron to the plasma. Hephaestin, named after the Greek god *Hephaestus*, who forged iron, has a ferroxidase activity that contributes to iron transport by transforming iron

to the ferric form to enable its uptake by circulating apotransferrin. Ceruloplasmin also has ferroxidase activity and is involved as well in the release of iron from the cells. Another recently identified 25-amino-acid antimicrobial peptide, hepcidin, has been shown to play a major role in iron homoeostasis, possibly through a hormonal effect. Hepcidin appears to control GI iron absorption and the release of iron from macrophages. It has been shown that decreased hepcidin expression was associated with increased iron absorption and its release from macrophages. The relationship with the hemochromatosis gene, *HFE*, remains unclear although early studies suggest that *HFE* controls hepcidin expression (Brugnara, 2003; Brissot, 2004).

In the plasma, the total iron averages 110 μg/dL (19.7 μmol/L). The great majority of this is bound to the transferrin, which has a capacity to bind 330 μg of iron per deciliter (or 59.1 μmol/L) and therefore is about one-third saturated. A very small amount of iron in plasma is in ferritin. Plasma (or serum) ferritin averages about 100 μg/L in men (less in women: about 50 μg/L).

Iron Deficiency Anemia

When iron loss exceeds iron intake for a time long enough to deplete the body's iron stores, insufficient iron is available for normal hemoglobin production. When well developed, iron deficiency is characterized by a hypochromic microcytic anemia.

Iron deficiency results only when there is an increased need for iron (e.g., during rapid growth in infancy and childhood or during pregnancy) or when excessive loss of blood has reduced the body's reserves of iron (e.g., following repeated hemorrhages, excessive menstruation, or multiple pregnancies).

Iron deficiency is probably the most common cause of anemia on the planet, affecting at least one-third of the world's population (Fairbanks, 2001a). Children between the ages of 6–24 months are particularly susceptible. It is caused by insufficient dietary iron to meet the needs of rapid growth. After the first 4–6 months of life, the iron stores present from birth have been exhausted, and the infant depends on dietary iron. An infant maintained on milk and carbohydrates without supplements of iron-containing foods is likely to develop an iron deficiency anemia, the 'milk anemia' of infancy. In a recent study in the US, iron deficiency anemia was reported in 3% of toddlers aged 1–2 years and in 2–5% of adolescent girls and women of childbearing age (Looker, 1997). Defective absorption of iron and eventual iron deficiency anemia occur after total gastrectomy or even subtotal gastrectomy. Prolonged treatment of peptic ulcers and acid reflux by H₂ blockers and acid pump blockers may cause defective iron absorption. Except for the sprue syndrome, other causes of malabsorption of iron are extremely rare. Since iron deficiency increases the rate of absorption of both iron and lead, lead intoxication may accompany iron deficiency.

If an adult male had absolutely no iron intake or absorption (which would be extremely unlikely), his body iron stores of 1000 mg would last for 3–4 years before he would even begin to become iron deficient. Therefore, almost all cases of iron deficiency anemia in adult males are due to chronic blood loss.

The sequence of events in developing iron deficiency anemia is usually as follows (Hillman, 1996): When blood loss exceeds absorption, a negative iron balance exists. Iron is mobilized from stores, storage iron decreases, plasma ferritin decreases, iron absorption increases, and plasma iron-binding capacity (transferrin) increases. This stage is known as *iron depletion*. After iron stores are depleted, the plasma iron concentration falls, saturation of transferrin falls below 15%, and the percentage of sideroblasts decreases in the marrow. As a result of lack of iron for heme synthesis, red cell protoporphyrin increases. This second stage is *iron deficient erythropoiesis*; anemia may not yet be present. The third stage is *iron deficiency anemia*; in addition to the above abnormalities, anemia is detectable. The anemia is at first normochromic and normocytic, gradually becomes microcytic, and finally microcytic and hypochromic.

Clinical Features. Clinical findings may be due to the underlying cause of the blood loss itself, to the general manifestations of anemia (see previous discussion), or to iron deficiency. Those that are probably attributable to lack of tissue iron include paresthesia, such as numbness and tingling; atrophy of epithelium of the tongue with burning or soreness; fissures or ulcers at the corners of the mouth (angular stomatitis); chronic gastritis, which leads to decreased gastric secretions but few symptoms; 'pica,' which is the craving to eat unusual substances such as dirt or ice; concave or spoon-shaped nails (koilonychia); and difficulty swallowing owing to 'webs' of tissue or partial strictures at the junction of the esophagus and hypopharynx. The latter two findings are relatively uncommon. Splenomegaly may occur but is quite uncommon.

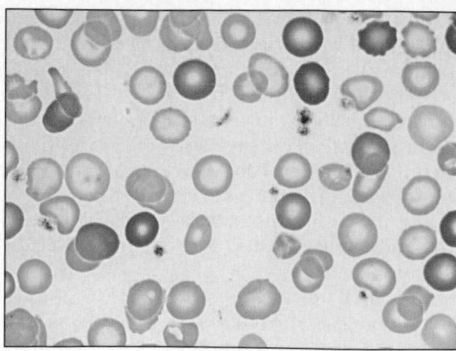

Figure 31–2 Iron deficiency anemia, post-transfusion. The cells are pale with an enlarged central pallor, in sharp contrast to the transfused normochromic cells.

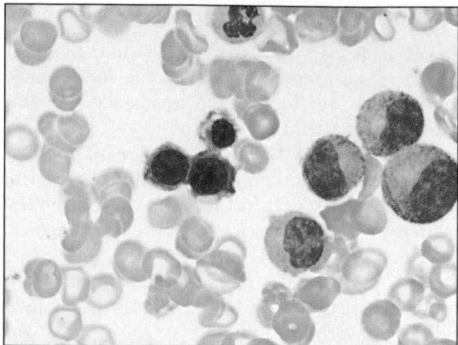

Figure 31–3 Marrow film, iron deficiency anemia. The three normoblasts have irregular margins and irregular clear spaces, reflecting lack of hemoglobin synthesis (i.e., defective cytoplasmic maturation).

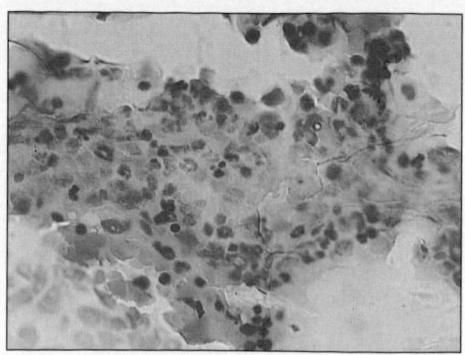

Figure 31–4 Marrow film, Prussian blue reaction. Depleted iron stores: no blue-green staining iron is visible. On a scale of 0 to 5+, the iron is normal from 1+ to 3+ for women and from 2+ to 3+ for men.

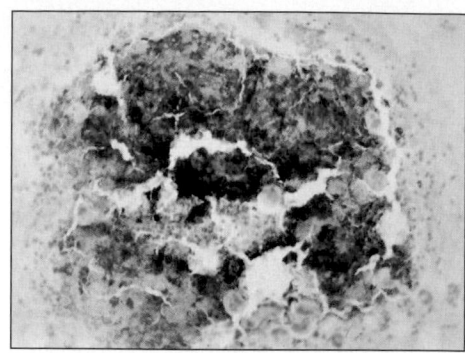

Figure 31–5 Marrow film, Prussian blue reaction. On a scale of 0 to 5+, the amount of storage iron is judged at 5+, which is markedly increased.

Laboratory Features

Blood. In early iron deficiency anemia, the stained blood film often shows normochromic normocytic erythrocytes (Hillman, 1996). In later stages, the picture is one of microcytosis, anisocytosis, poikilocytosis (including elliptical and elongated cells), and varying degrees of hypochromia. The plasma membranes of iron-deficient cells are abnormally stiff and this abnormality contributes to the development of poikilocytes, particularly elongated hypochromic elliptocytes (pencil cells). Anisocytosis may be identified by automated blood counters as increased red cell distribution width (RDW). This finding, however, proved not specific for iron deficiency anemia (Fairbanks, 2001a). Reticulocytes are usually decreased in absolute numbers except following iron therapy. The mean corpuscular volume (MCV) is low, and the Hb and Hct are relatively lower than the erythrocyte count. Osmotic fragility may be decreased because the red cells are thinner than normal (see Figs 29–10 and 31–2).

The leukocyte count is normal or slightly lowered. Granulocytopenia and a small number of hypersegmented neutrophils may be present. Megaloblastic changes in severe iron deficiency may be related to decreased activity of the enzyme ribonucleotide reductase, which contains an essential nonheme iron atom (Beck, 1991). However, the detection of hypersegmented neutrophils should raise the suspicion for a mild folate deficiency, which may become more overt after iron therapy (Dallman, 1993). Platelets may be increased, whether the lack of iron is due to blood loss or dietary deficiency, but tend to be decreased in severe anemia.

Marrow. Normoblastic hyperplasia occurs early, but in later stages the limiting effect of severe iron deficiency restricts erythropoiesis to the basal level. The normoblasts are smaller than normal, deficient in the amount of hemoglobin in the cytoplasm, and irregular in shape with frayed margins (Fig. 31–3). Giant neutrophil bands or metamyelocytes, if present, are rarely due to iron deficiency per se; usually they indicate an associated cobalamin or folate deficiency (see later under Megaloblastic Anemia). Iron stains should be performed routinely (Figs 31–4 and 31–5). *Storage iron* is absent, unless iron has recently been administered in some form. The proportion of normoblasts that are *sideroblasts* is decreased (< 20%); this proportion is usually about the same as the percent saturation of transferrin (or total iron-binding capacity [TIBC]) and is a measure of iron delivery to the normoblasts.

Serum Iron. The reference interval is 50–160 μg/dL (9–29 μmol/L) in adults. The level is lower in iron deficiency but also in infections and the anemia of chronic disease.

Serum Iron-Binding Capacity. The reference interval for adults is 250–400 μg/dL (45–72 μmol/L). In iron deficiency anemia, the serum TIBC is increased. It is normal or decreased in the anemia of chronic disease. If chronic infection coexists with chronic blood loss, the TIBC may not be increased, even though the patient is iron deficient.

Percent Saturation of TIBC. The ratio of serum iron to TIBC is the percent saturation of the TIBC. Normally this is 20–55%; values below 15% indicate iron deficient erythropoiesis.

There is normally a marked diurnal variation in serum iron by as much as 30%, with highest values in the morning and lowest values late in the day. Consequently, fasting morning blood specimens are preferred for the diagnosis of iron deficiency. The TIBC remains relatively constant in a normal individual. Pregnancy and oral contraceptives increase TIBC.

Serum iron is usually higher in the first 90 days of life, then it dips to a somewhat lower reference interval for the second month of life and the value gradually increases with age until it reached the adult range approximately at the age of 15 years (Ritchie, 2002b; Soldin, 2004). On the other hand, the TIBC gradually rises with age until it reaches values that are comparable to those of adults at the age of 15 years (Soldin, 2004). Similarly, percent saturation in children is less than in adults and it reaches the adult value at the age of 15–18 years (Ritchie, 2002b).

Serum Ferritin. In adults, the reference values are 12–300 μg/L, with higher values in men than in women. Serum ferritin appears to be in equilibrium with tissue ferritin and is a good reflection of storage iron in normal subjects and in most disorders. The equivalence of 1 μg/L of serum ferritin with 8–10 mg storage iron has been suggested. In patients with some hepatocellular diseases, malignancies, and inflammatory diseases, serum ferritin is a disproportionately high estimate of storage iron because serum ferritin is an acute phase reactant. In such disorders, iron deficiency anemia may exist with a normal serum ferritin concentration. In the presence of inflammation, persons with a serum ferritin level of less than 50–60 μg/L are likely to respond to iron therapy (Fairbanks, 2001a). A *low* value, 12 μg/L, indicates low iron stores; falsely low values mimicking iron deficiency have not been found.

In infancy and childhood, between the ages of 6 months and 15 years, the reference interval for serum ferritin is somewhat lower than in early infancy or adult life (Soldin, 2004). In men, serum ferritin gradually rises between the ages of 18–30 years, whereas in women it does not. However, postmenopausal women have a much higher ferritin level than premenopausal women and it is comparable to that in men (Van den Bosch, 2001). Serum ferritin levels do not display diurnal variation.

Erythrocyte Porphyrins. Because heme is formed by insertion of iron into protoporphyrin IX, the latter is increased in iron deficient erythropoiesis, whether owing to iron deficiency or anemia of chronic disease. It is also increased in lead poisoning and in some cases of sideroblastic anemia but is normal in thalassemia. Zinc usually becomes attached to protoporphyrin forming zinc protoporphyrin (ZPP). A relatively simple micromethod measuring ZPP in whole blood has been shown to be useful in distinguishing microcytosis due to iron deficiency from that due to β-thalassemia minor (Labbé, 2004). The normal reference interval was 10–99 μg/dL of erythrocytes; in iron deficiency, the erythrocyte porphyrins became elevated before the development of anemia and may be one of the earliest indicators of iron deficiency (Labbé, 2004).

Serum Transferrin Receptors. Transferrin receptors (TRs) also exist in a soluble form in the circulation. Serum TRs (STRs) are produced by shedding of membrane TRs during erythrocyte maturation. STRs vary with the rate of erythropoiesis. Patients with aplastic anemia have lower than normal levels of STRs, while patients with autoimmune hemolytic anemia have higher values. Iron deficiency anemia is associated with increased serum levels of TRs probably as a result of increased membrane TRs synthesis and expression secondary to iron starvation (Fairbanks, 2001a). STRs are usually not increased in anemia of chronic disease although patients with rheumatoid arthritis have been found to have increased STRs in the absence of iron deficiency (Fairbanks, 2001a; Brugnara, 2003).

Serum Transferrin to Serum Ferritin Ratio (R/F Ratio). The R/F ratio has been suggested as a new approach to estimate total body iron stores. Yet the R/F ratio continued to have a limited value in individuals with inflammation or liver diseases (Brugnara, 2003).

Reticulocyte Hemoglobin Content. Some automated hematology analyzers may offer an assay of hemoglobin content within reticulocytes (CHr; in pg/cell). Earlier studies suggest that this parameter may be best applied in children. However, further studies are needed before it becomes a routine parameter for assessment of iron status (Fairbanks, 2001a; Brugnara, 2003).

Differential Diagnosis. Anemia due to iron deficiency usually must be distinguished from other microcytic or hypochromic anemias. These include the thalassemia traits, longstanding anemia of chronic disease, and the sideroblastic anemias (see later discussions of these entities). Bone marrow storage iron and serum ferritin will be decreased in iron deficiency and normal or elevated in all others. In *thalassemia trait,* the ZPP is normal, serum iron is normal, and the condition is present in family members. In β-thalassemia trait, Hb A$_2$ and sometimes Hb F are increased. Indeed, the Hb A$_2$ is often decreased in iron deficiency. In *anemia of chronic diseases* (chronic infection, rheumatoid arthritis, or neoplastic disease), although the serum iron is low, as in iron deficiency, the TIBC is low or normal. In the *sideroblastic anemias,* which include chronic lead poisoning, the serum iron and percent TIBC saturation are increased, and pathologic 'ring' sideroblasts are present in the marrow.

Management. The first principle in therapy is that the underlying cause be identified and corrected. Ferrous iron is given orally, about 200 mg/day, in three doses between meals. This will provide 40–60 mg of absorbed iron per day, which, with the iron produced by turnover of senescent red cells, will be sufficient to increase production to two or three times normal (Hillman, 1996). The reticulocyte count will reach a maximum at 5–10 days then gradually decrease toward normal. Monitoring the hemoglobin is best; Hb should increase by 0.1–0.2 g/dL/day after the fifth day and by at least 2 g/dL for each of the subsequent 3 weeks. After the hemoglobin has returned to normal, iron therapy should be continued for at least 2 months in order to replenish storage iron.

Impaired Production – Megaloblastic Anemia

Macrocytosis with Normoblastic Marrow

Macrocytic anemias that are not megaloblastic may be due to early release of erythrocytes from the marrow, so-called shift reticulocytes. This may occur in response to acute blood loss, hemolysis, bone marrow infiltration, and high level of erythropoietin associated with bone marrow failure diseases such as aplastic anemia, refractory anemia, and Diamond–Blackfan anemia. Nonmegaloblastic macrocytosis is also found in hypothyroidism, in individuals with an excessive alcohol intake, and in liver disease (Hillman, 1996).

Megaloblastic Anemia

Blood. Macrocytic anemias associated with megaloblastosis differ from nonmegaloblastic macrocytic anemia in that macro-ovalocytes and giant hypersegmented neutrophils are present in the blood (Figs 29–11, 31–6,

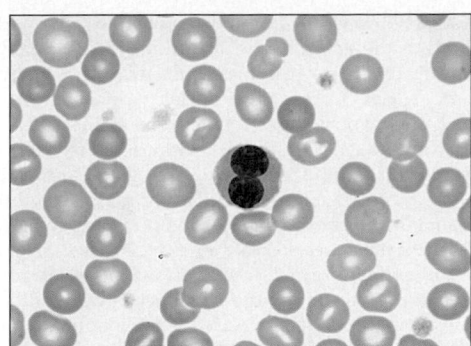

Figure 31–6 Blood film, megaloblastic anemia. Macrocytosis and a circulating megaloblast with abnormal, binucleated nucleus and open chromatin.

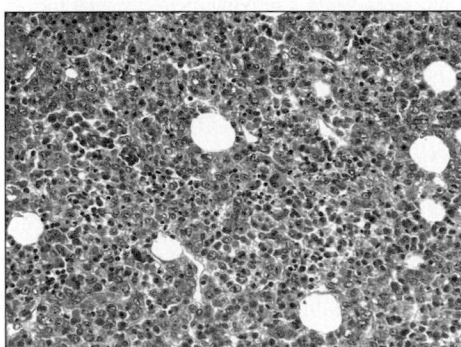

Figure 31–7 Hypercellular marrow in megaloblastic anemia. The cellularity is over 95%.

and 29–15). Pancytopenia is the rule. The anemia is macrocytic with an elevated MCV and is characterized by macro-ovalocytes and often extreme degrees of anisocytosis and poikilocytosis. Microcytes and dacrocytes are common. Basophilic stippling, multiple Howell–Jolly bodies, nucleated red cells with karyorrhexis, and even megaloblasts may be seen. Leukopenia is present. Granulocytes have increased numbers of lobes, presumably a result of abnormal nuclear maturation. Five lobes in more than 5% of the neutrophils constitutes hypersegmentation (Herbert, 1985), as do any neutrophils with six or more lobes. Thrombocytopenia is usually encountered and, on rare occasions, is sufficiently severe to be responsible for bleeding. It is worth noting that significant morphologic changes may occur in the blood in the absence of anemia and also that neurologic symptoms may be present in the absence of anemia.

Marrow. Megaloblastic anemia is characterized by enlargement of all rapidly proliferating cells of the body, including marrow cells. The major abnormality is the diminished capacity for deoxyribonucleic acid (DNA) synthesis. The cells have both a prolonged intermitotic resting phase and a block early in mitosis. The number of mitotic figures is increased. Ribonucleic acid (RNA) synthesis is less impeded than is DNA synthesis; hence, cytoplasmic maturation and growth continue, accounting for enlargement of the cells. The delicate chromatin and the prominent parachromatin result in a distinctly more 'open' chromatin pattern than is seen in the erythroid precursors (Figs 29–28 and 31–6). The nuclei undergo karyorrhexis readily, and multiple Howell–Jolly bodies may be present. There are usually more cells analogous to the pronormoblast and basophilic normoblast (i.e., the promegaloblast and basophilic megaloblast) than are seen in normal erythropoiesis. This has sometimes been termed 'maturation arrest,' or nuclear–cytoplasmic asynchrony. Giant polychromatic megaloblasts are especially distinctive. The same general features are seen in the other cell lines. In the granulocytic series, the cells are larger, with retarded nuclear maturation and large cytoplasmic mass; often the specific granules themselves are distinctly larger. The chromatin pattern is less condensed (more 'open'), and as a result the nucleus appears to stain poorly. Abnormally contorted nuclear configurations are common. The giant metamyelocyte is the most characteristic of the abnormal granulocytes. Megakaryocytes, too, are large and have separated nuclear lobes or nuclear fragments.

The bone marrow is hyperplastic (Fig. 31–7). The fat is replaced, and red marrow extends into the long bones. The number of erythroid precursors (megaloblasts) is increased, and the myeloid/erythroid ratio is decreased. If the megaloblastic process is incompletely developed, or if the patient has been inadequately treated, the findings may be only partial. Because they persist longer, the granulocytic alterations are especially helpful in assessing recently treated megaloblastic anemia. The marrow findings result from the effects of impaired nucleic acid synthesis, leading to megaloblastosis and hypoxic stress, giving rise to increased numbers of erythroid cells. If the patient is transfused with packed red cells, the number of erythroid precursors diminishes but the cytologic abnormalities persist.

Erythrokinetics. In megaloblastic anemias, the mass of erythroid tissue is increased, plasma iron turnover is rapid, and urine and fecal urobilinogen are increased. These measures indicate an *increase of total erythropoiesis* that may be up to three times normal. Decreased rate of appearance of iron in the Hb of circulating erythrocytes and reticulocytopenia indicate *ineffective erythropoiesis*. In addition to increased destruction of the defective erythroid precursors in the marrow, survival of circulating erythrocytes is short, indicating hemolysis. Indirect serum bilirubin is increased, serum iron is increased, endogenous carbon monoxide production is increased, and serum lactate dehydrogenase is usually greatly elevated. Serum muramidase may be elevated, implying ineffective granulocytopoiesis.

Megaloblastic anemia is nearly always due to cobalamin or folic acid deficiency. The findings described are similar for either.

Cobalamin (Vitamin B$_{12}$) Metabolism

Vitamin B$_{12}$ (cyanocobalamin) has a molecular weight of 1355 Da. The molecule's two major parts are (1) a 'planar group' (the corrin nucleus), a ring structure surrounding a cobalt atom; and (2) a 'nucleotide' group, which consists of the base, 5,6-dimethylbenzimidazole, and a phosphorylated ribose esterified with 1-amino, 2-propanol. A cyanide group is in coordinate linkage with the trivalent cobalt. Different forms of vitamin B$_{12}$ result from replacement of the cyanide by hydroxy, adenosyl, or methyl groups; generically, these are termed *cobalamins*.

Cobalamin is the only vitamin exclusively synthesized by micro-organisms. It is found in practically all animal tissues. It is stored primarily in the liver in the form of adenosylcobalamin. The human liver contains approximately 1 μg/g of liver. Cobalamin is initially bound to R binders (cobalamin-binding proteins with *R*apid electrophoretic mobility) present in saliva or food, released by trypsin digestion, and is then bound by other R binders at the acid pH of the stomach. On entering the duodenum, cobalamin is released by pancreatic enzymes to finally bind to gastric intrinsic factor (IF), a 44-kDa glycoprotein produced in the parietal cells of the stomach. The gene for IF is located on chromosome 11. This cobalamin–IF complex, which is very resistant to digestion, then adheres to specific receptor sites on the epithelial cells of the ileum, at which sites the cobalamin is absorbed. A recent study indicates that the cobalamin–IF receptor is a combination of two proteins: a 460-kDa called cubilin and a 45- to 50-kDa protein called amnionless. Both proteins are also present in renal tubules. Mutation of either of the two genes can produce megaloblastic anemia with proteinuria, also known as Imerslund–Gräsbeck syndrome (Fyfe, 2004). The concentration of the receptor in the ileum increases progressively until it reaches its maximum near the terminal ileum. The cobalamin–IF complex is taken into the cell, where cobalamin is released and the IF is destroyed. The receptor recycles to the surface of the cell (Babior, 2001a).

Cobalamin is transported in the plasma as methylcobalamin, bound to a group of proteins named transcobalamin II (TC II) and haptocorrins (variously called TC I, TC III, R binder, cobalophilin (see below). Ninety percent of newly absorbed cobalamin is bound to TC II, which serves as the chief transport protein, rapidly delivering the vitamin to the liver, hematopoietic cells, and other dividing cells. Some cobalamin binds to haptocorrins, which prevents its loss from the plasma; this cobalamin is a passive reservoir in equilibrium with body stores in the liver but not taken up by other body cells. The reference values for plasma cobalamin depend on the method of assay, but commonly are 200–900 ng/L (150–670 pmol/L). One-third of the binding sites on transcobalamins are normally occupied: 70–90% of the plasma cobalamin is bound to haptocorrins, mostly TC I; this is very slowly cleared from the plasma. The remainder is bound to TC II, which remains only about 5% saturated; much of newly absorbed cobalamin bound to TC II is removed from the plasma during the first few hours, but a small fraction remains bound for several weeks.

The relative importance of the transcobalamins is illustrated by the clinical effects of congenital deficiency. Lack of TC II results in severe megaloblastic anemia in infancy; yet the serum cobalamin level is normal. Lack of TC I is not accompanied by anemia or megaloblastosis; yet the serum cobalamin level is decreased (Babior, 2001b).

TC I and III are R-type proteins. TC III is probably an isoprotein of TC I, which is unsaturated with cobalamin and thus less charged. Much of the serum TC III is released from granulocytes during blood clotting in vitro;

TC III does not appear to bind significant amounts of plasma cobalamin under normal conditions. Haptocorrins (TC I and III) may arise from granulocytes, salivary glands, and liver, as well as from other tissues. Elevation of TC I and III accounts for the elevation of total cobalamin-binding proteins in myeloproliferative diseases. TC II is also synthesized by a variety of cells including renal cells, enterocytes, and hepatocytes. TC II acts as an acute phase reactant and its levels are increased in inflammatory and infectious conditions (Carmel, 1999).

The daily requirement for cobalamin is in the range of 2–5 μg/day. The body's stores of 2–5 mg will last for several years if intake is cut off, as is the case if total gastrectomy is performed (Beck, 1991).

Cobalamin Deficiency

Although the true prevalence of cobalamin deficiency in the general population is unknown, it increases with age. Approximately 15% of adults older than 65 years have laboratory findings of vitamin B$_{12}$ deficiency. The widespread use of proton-pump inhibitors to control gastric secretion is becoming a contributing factor (Oh, 2003). Cobalamin deficiency is produced by any of several mechanisms which are not always exclusive of each other and involve inadequate intake and reduced absorption.

Inadequate Intake

A dietary deficiency is an *extremely rare* cause of megaloblastic anemia in the US, and is seen only in persons who completely abstain from animal food, including milk and eggs. Only strict vegetarians are known to develop this form of cobalamin deficiency.

Defective Production of Intrinsic Factor

This is the most common cause of cobalamin deficiency.

Pernicious anemia

Pernicious anemia (PA) is a 'conditioned' nutritional deficiency of cobalamin that is caused by a failure of the gastric mucosa to secrete intrinsic factor. This abnormality is genetically determined but usually is not manifested until late in life; less than 10% of cases occur under age 40. Modern surveys indicate that PA is as common in black people as in Caucasian people (Carmel, 1999).

Clinical Features. The disorder is equally common in males and females. Symptoms of *anemia* and the combination of skin pallor and jaundice giving a lemon-yellow appearance of the skin are often present. The tongue may be sore, smooth, and pale (atrophic glossitis) or red and raw (acute glossitis). *Gastrointestinal symptoms* may be prominent and include episodic abdominal pain, constipation, and diarrhea. Diffuse and irregular degeneration of the white matter of the *central nervous system* (CNS) characteristically involves the posterior and lateral columns of the spinal cord (subacute combined degeneration) and sometimes other sites. Symmetric sensations of 'pins and needles' of the distal extremities, numbness and tingling, loss of position sensation (difficulty with balance and gait), and loss of vibratory sensation (perhaps the most constant sign) are indicative of peripheral neuropathy and posterior column lesions. Lateral column involvement gives rise to weakness, spasticity, and increased deep tendon reflexes. Sometimes, the brain may be affected, and the patient shows irritability, emotional instability, or a change in personality. Neuropsychiatric disorders may be associated with cobalamin deficiency even without accompanying hematologic manifestations (Lindenbaum, 1988). The mechanism of CNS defects in cobalamin deficiency may be related to defective methyl group metabolism (Babior, 2001b).

Gastric Findings. Atrophic gastritis of varying degree is found in most adults with PA, and gastric atrophy involving all coats of the wall in the remainder. IF and hydrochloric acid (HCl) are secreted by gastric parietal cells in the human; in adult PA, IF secretion is absent and almost always there is histamine-refractory achylia and achlorhydria – a decreased volume of gastric juice and lack of HCl secretion.

Immune Abnormalities. Autoantibodies have been found in the serum of patients with pernicious anemia (Babior, 2001b). *Antiparietal cell antibodies* react with gastric parietal cells and are present in over 90% of patients. These parietal cell antibodies are also present in patients with chronic gastritis, such as that associated with iron deficiency, and in some patients with thyroiditis and myxedema; they are also present in 4–5% of age-matched healthy individuals. When these antibodies are chronically injected into rats, they decrease gastric HCl, IF, and pepsin secretion and produce gastric atrophy. The major antigen to which these antibodies are produced is the acid-producing enzyme H$^+$-K$^+$-ATPase, a 92-kDa protein present on the luminal membrane of parietal cells. The antiparietal cell antibodies are probably not directly linked to the pathogenesis of PA since the target antigen is not easily accessible to these antibodies. However, PA is likely caused by CD4+ T cells recognizing the H$^+$–K$^+$-ATPase (Babior, 2001b).

Another type of autoantibody is directed against intrinsic factor. *Anti-intrinsic factor antibodies* occur in the serum, saliva, and gastric juice of about 75% of patients with PA. Two types of anti-IF antibodies occur: 'blocking' antibodies, which block the binding of cobalamin to IF, and 'binding' antibodies, which bind to the cobalamin–IF complex and prevent the complex from binding to receptors in the ileum. Although these antibodies can cause some functional impairment in vivo, it is not clear whether the antibodies are the cause or an effect of the disease. IF antibodies in the absence of PA occur in a small percentage of individuals with hyperthyroidism (Graves' disease) and similarly in persons with insulin-dependent diabetes.

Family studies in patients with pernicious anemia have shown an increased incidence of the disease in relatives, and many relatives have achlorhydria and partial defects of cobalamin absorption. Relatives of patients with pernicious anemia also have a higher incidence of gastric parietal cell antibodies and of thyroid antibodies than normal.

It is possible that adult pernicious anemia is a genetically determined autoimmune gastritis. However, the relationship of the gastric lesion to the antibodies remains unclear.

Pernicious Anemia in Children

Two forms of PA in children exist. *Congenital pernicious anemia* usually appears early in the second year of life. IF secretion is either lacking or the secreted IF is functionally defective, but acid secretion and the appearance of the gastric mucosa are normal. Antibodies to parietal cells and to IF are absent. *Juvenile pernicious anemia* occurs usually in older children and is like that of adults, with gastric atrophy, achlorhydria, and serum antibody to IF and parietal cells, although the latter may be absent in a subset of patients (Rosenblatt, 1999).

Gastrectomy

Surgical removal of the stomach (total or even subtotal occasionally) will remove the source of intrinsic factor. This will lead to megaloblastic anemia after the body's stores of cobalamin have been exhausted, in 3–6 years, if cobalamin therapy has not been given. Frequently, the anemia is in partly due to iron deficiency.

Defective Absorption of Cobalamin

Malabsorption Syndromes. Celiac disease, tropical sprue, resection of the small bowel, or inflammatory disease of the small bowel may be associated with multiple defects of absorption, including other vitamins. Folic acid deficiency (absorbed principally in the upper small bowel) is more commonly seen than cobalamin deficiency (absorbed principally in the lower small bowel) in diseases leading to malabsorption. The reason for this is probably the lesser time necessary for depletion of body stores of folic acid.

The Imerslund–Gräsbeck syndrome is an autosomal recessively inherited defect in the intestinal absorption of cobalamin, in the presence of normal intrinsic factor. In many patients, proteinuria of the tubular type is also found. As mentioned earlier, the syndrome is caused by a defect in the cubilin/amnionless receptor (Fyfe, 2004).

Lack of Availability of Cobalamin. In certain countries, infestation with the fish tapeworm *Diphyllobothrium latum* is common enough that cobalamin deficiency may occur occasionally when it is present. The worm successfully competes with the host for the ingested cobalamin. Most common in Finland, it is rarely seen in the US.

Bacteria in a blind loop of intestine may also preferentially utilize ingested cobalamin to the detriment of the host.

Vitamin B$_{12}$ or folate deficiency may exert indirect cardiovascular effects. Both deficiencies are associated with hyperhomocystinemia, which is an independent factor for atherosclerosis and vascular thrombosis (Oh, 2003).

Diagnosis of Cobalamin Deficiency

Recognition of megaloblastic anemia indicates the likelihood of cobalamin deficiency or folic acid deficiency. In addition, evidence of neurologic involvement favors cobalamin deficiency. This diagnosis can be established by one of four methods.

Therapeutic Trial. With the patient on a diet low in cobalamin and folate, a parenteral physiologic dose of cobalamin (10 µg/day) is given. Optimal hematologic response indicates deficiency, and consists of reticulocytosis beginning on the third or fourth day and reaching a peak on the seventh day. Erythropoiesis becomes normoblastic by 2 days, and leukopoiesis becomes normal by 12–14 days. Within a week, leukocyte and platelet counts have returned to normal and the hemoglobin concentration begins to rise.

Serum Cobalamin Assay. This is the usual method of detecting a cobalamin-deficient state. Microbiological assay of serum cobalamin employs an organism (e.g., *Euglena gracilis*) that requires cobalamin for growth. Although the microbiological method is precise and reliable, it requires at least 48 hours of incubation and is subject to the inhibitory effect of antibiotics. Radioisotopic dilution and chemiluminescence assays are more rapid and widely used and give results comparable with those of the *Euglena* assay, provided that the binding protein is specific for biologically active cobalamin; a standardized intrinsic factor preparation is most satisfactory. However, these methods may produce false normal values in approximately 10% of patients with cobalamin deficiency (Zittoun, 1999).

Reference values are 200–900 ng/L. In megaloblastic anemia due to cobalamin deficiency, serum cobalamin is usually less than 100 ng/L. Individuals with folate deficiency and mild cobalamin deficiency and who are pregnant have borderline values between 100–200 ng/L. Patients with HIV infection often have low serum cobalamin levels in the absence of clinical manifestations (Ward, 2002). Spuriously normal cobalamin levels have been recorded in patients with cobalamin deficiency associated with overgrowth of intestinal bacteria, which produce biochemically inert B$_{12}$ analogues (Ward, 2002). Measurement of TC II-bound cobalamin (holotranscobalamin II) may provide additional information, since its levels fall below the normal range long before total serum cobalamin does and probably represent a state of negative cobalamin balance (Zittoun, 1999). However, its clinical utility has been limited (Ward, 2002).

Methylmalonic Acid and Homocysteine Assays. Because a cobalamin coenzyme is essential for the isomerization of methylmalonate to succinate, urine excretion of increased amounts of methylmalonate is found in cobalamin deficiency. Provided that the rare inborn error of metabolism methylmalonic aciduria is not present, this is a sensitive test for cobalamin deficiency, but it is not usually necessary for the diagnosis. In addition, plasma levels of methylmalonic acid and homocysteine are increased as well. Following several weeks of therapy, their plasma concentration returns to normal. Plasma levels of these metabolites should be interpreted with caution in patients with chronic renal failure because of the tendency of these metabolites to accumulate (Zittoun, 1999).

Deoxyuridine Suppression Test. This measures the ability of marrow cells in vitro to utilize deoxyuridine in DNA synthesis. Normally, in marrow cells the major source of thymidine for DNA is by de novo synthesis from deoxyuridine, which requires intact cobalamin and folate enzymes; therefore, less than 10% of added tritium-labeled thymidine (^{3}H-Tdr) is incorporated into DNA. In megaloblastic marrows due to cobalamin or folate deficiency, deoxyuridine cannot be efficiently converted to thymidine, and more ^{3}H-Tdr is taken up into DNA. An abnormal deoxyuridine suppression test indicates either cobalamin or folate deficiency. This test is very sensitive and produces abnormal results before anemia or macrocytosis is observed (Zittoun, 1999). A lymphocyte microdeoxyuridine suppression test (Herbert, 1985) requires only 1 mL of blood, making this diagnostic modality available to infants and children.

Detecting the Cause of Cobalamin Deficiency

Clinical history is useful in suggesting whether cobalamin or folate deficiency is the cause of megaloblastic anemia. Clinical associations of pernicious anemia include a family history of PA in one-third of patients, certain endocrine deficiencies (thyroid disease, diabetes mellitus, hypothyroidism, Addison's disease), and certain immune disorders (immune thrombocytopenic purpura, autoimmune hemolytic anemia, and acquired hypogammaglobulinemia). Cobalamin deficiency is likely in strict vegetarians, and in patients with paresthesias, neuropathy, or a previous gastrectomy.

In cobalamin-deficient patients, it is important to demonstrate a lack of IF. To do so, the ability of the patient to absorb an oral dose of radioactive cobalamin may be measured. The usual method is the Schilling test, which measures radioactivity in a 24-hour sample of urine. Two hours after oral administration of 0.5–2.0 µg of radioactive cobalamin, a large 'flushing' dose of nonlabeled cobalamin is given parenterally. Normal individuals will excrete over 7% of a 1-µg dose of ingested cobalamin in the urine in 24 hours, whereas patients lacking IF excrete less. If the excretion is low, the test must be repeated using the same procedure except that hog IF is given orally along with the labeled cobalamin. If the 24-hour excretion is normal, the low value in the first part was due to IF deficiency. If the excretion remains abnormal in the second part of the procedure, an explanation for malabsorption of cobalamin on the basis of intestinal disease must be sought. The validity of the results depends on good renal function and an accurate urine collection. The Schilling test will be abnormal in PA even after the patient is treated with cobalamin and is in remission. Some patients may absorb vitamin B_{12} in water (as given in the original Schilling test) but fail to absorb vitamin B_{12} bound to protein in food. A modification of the Schilling test is being introduced to include protein-bound B_{12} using egg yolk or chicken serum (Zittoun, 1999).

Other tests that will establish the diagnosis of PA are direct assay of IF, demonstrating it to be deficient in gastric juice. The combination of megaloblastic anemia, decreased serum cobalamin, and serum antibodies to IF is essentially diagnostic of PA, obviating the need for the Schilling test (Lindenbaum, 1983).

Folic Acid Metabolism

Folic acid or pteroylmonoglutamic acid contains three parts: pteridine, *p*-aminobenzoate, and L-glutamic acid (Beck, 1991). In nature, folic acid occurs mainly as less soluble polyglutamates, with multiple glutamic acid residues attached to one another. Folic acid is present in a wide variety of foods, such as eggs, milk, leafy vegetables, yeast, liver, and fruits, and also is formed by intestinal bacteria. Folates are extremely thermolabile and prolonged cooking (> 15 minutes) in large quantities of water in the absence of reducing agents destroys folate.

Conjugase enzymes in bile and intestine hydrolyze the polyglutamates prior to absorption, which is rapid and occurs in the proximal jejunum, mostly by a carrier-mediated mechanism. In the plasma, one-third of the folate is free, while two-thirds is nonspecifically and loosely bound to serum proteins. A small amount of folate is specifically bound to folate-binding proteins, the physiologic significance of which is unclear (Babior, 2001a). Folate is rapidly removed from plasma to cells and tissues for utilization. The principal form of folate in serum, erythrocytes, and liver is 5-methyltetrahydrofolate (5-methyl-FH$_4$); the liver is the chief storage site. Intracellular folates exist primarily as polyglutamates. There is a significant enterohepatic circulation and bile contains 2–10 times the folate concentration of normal serum. The minimal daily requirement is about 50 μg of pteroylmonoglutamate or 400 μg of total folate; a typical reference interval for serum folate is 5–21 μg/L (11–48 nmol/L) and for red cell folate 150–600 μg/L (340–1360 nmol/L) of red blood cells.

The Folate–Cobalamin Relationship

The anemia of cobalamin deficiency is partially corrected by folate even in the absence of cobalamin supplementation while the reverse is not true. Therefore, some of the megaloblastic manifestations in cobalamin deficiency are actually caused by abnormalities in folate metabolism (Babior, 2001b). The most accepted theory for their interrelationship is the methylfolate trap theory. This theory is based on the observation that the methyl form of tetrahydrofolate (FH$_4$) would leak out of cells unless conjugated to form polyglutamates. Methyl FH$_4$ is a poor substrate for the conjugating enzyme. Cobalamin is essential for the process of conversion of methyl FH$_4$ to FH$_4$. Accumulation of methyl FH$_4$ is followed by its leakage out of the cells (Babior, 2001a).

Folic Acid Deficiency (Babior, 2001b)

Inadequate Intake of Folate

Evolution of Laboratory Abnormalities. Herbert delineated the sequence of events in the onset of folate-deficient megaloblastic anemia. After a folate-deficient diet was initiated, the various abnormalities were established as follows: 3 weeks, low serum folate; 5 weeks, hypersegmented neutrophils in bone marrow; 7 weeks, hypersegmented neutrophils in peripheral blood, with bone marrow showing increased and abnormal mitoses and basophilic intermediate megaloblasts; 10 weeks, bone marrow showing some large metamyelocytes and polychromatophilic intermediate megaloblasts; 13 weeks, high excretion of formiminoglutamic acid (FIGLU) in urine; 17 weeks, low erythrocyte folate; 18 weeks, macro-ovalocytosis of erythrocytes with many large metamyelocytes in bone marrow; 19 weeks, overtly megaloblastic bone marrow; 20 weeks, anemia (Herbert, 1985).

At this time, changes in the intestinal epithelium had not yet appeared. Therefore, in the human, with no dietary intake of folic acid, anemia will appear in 3–6 months. The peripheral blood and bone marrow features of megaloblastic anemia due to folic acid deficiency are similar to those of cobalamin deficiency; however, leukopenia and thrombocytopenia are less constant. Folic acid deficiency has usually been found in association with some complicating factor.

Nutritional Folate Deficiency. Megaloblastic anemia due to lack of folate is most commonly associated with insufficient dietary intake. The usual diet does not contain much above the minimal requirements, and body stores in the adult are sufficient for only about 3 months' needs. Dietary folate deficiency is especially common in the tropics and in India, and even in those locations it is usually associated with increased demand

for folate in pregnancy, rapid growth in infancy, infection, or hemolytic anemia. Elderly persons on inadequate diets in the US may develop folate-deficient megaloblastic anemia.

Folate deficiency in infancy is uncommon in the US. Human milk or fresh cow's milk contains sufficient folate, but heated milk, powdered milk, and goat's milk do not. If the infant's milk lacks folate, if the diet is low in ascorbic acid, or if infection or diarrhea is a problem, megaloblastic anemia may occur.

Megaloblastic anemia in pregnancy is not uncommon, because of the fetal requirements for folate. The mother's plasma folate level gradually falls during pregnancy, and at birth the plasma level in the newborn averages five times that of the mother. Megaloblastic anemia is more frequent in multipara, may be precipitated by infection, and is usually due to folate deficiency rather than cobalamin deficiency. Pregnant women should receive, in addition to iron, folic acid supplements. Recent studies indicate that folate supplementation for pregnant women reduces the risk for giving birth to babies with neural tube defects.

Liver Disease. Liver disease associated with alcoholism may lead to folate-deficient megaloblastic anemia because of the grossly inadequate diet of the alcoholic and because the liver is the major site for folate storage and metabolism (Zittoun, 1999). With an adequate dietary folic acid intake, however, the anemia that is found with liver disease is macrocytic and normoblastic, not megaloblastic.

Defective Absorption of Folate

Defective absorption of folic acid occurs in association with malabsorption syndromes discussed previously and in the blind-loop syndrome, in which bacteria preferentially utilize folate.

Nontropical sprue, or adult celiac disease, is an important cause of malabsorption in adults or children that is related to dietary gluten (wheat protein). Included among the signs of malabsorption may be megaloblastic anemia due to folic acid deficiency (Beck, 1991). Jejunal biopsy shows villous atrophy. The folate deficiency as well as the malabsorption responds to a gluten-free diet. Folic acid therapy (parenteral) corrects the folate deficiency but not the general malabsorption.

Tropical sprue is a poorly understood malabsorptive disorder that is common in the Caribbean, India, and Southeast Asia. Evidence of malabsorption includes megaloblastic anemia due to folate deficiency. Treatment with folic acid brings considerable improvement in the general malabsorption as well as the anemia, but antimicrobial treatment is recommended in addition.

Megaloblastic anemia or decreased serum and red cell folate without anemia has been associated with the long-term use of anticonvulsant drugs, phenytoin, phenobarbital, and primidone. The problem appears to be a drug-induced malabsorption of pteroylpolyglutamate. Oral contraceptives cause malabsorption of folate in a small proportion of women, owing to impaired deconjugation of pteroylpolyglutamate (Beck, 1991).

Increased Requirement for Folate

The increased need in pregnancy and in infants (multiple birth) has been mentioned. Increased cell turnover that occurs in neoplasia and in the markedly stimulated hematopoiesis of hemolytic anemias may result in megaloblastic erythropoiesis. The basis for this is increased need for a marginal supply of folate.

Inadequate Utilization of Folate

Inadequate utilization of folic acid is relatively rare. Folic acid antagonists, such as methotrexate, block folic acid metabolism and because of this are used in therapy of some malignant neoplasms. In addition to inhibiting the growth of the tumor, they will also induce megaloblastic hematopoiesis.

In addition to the previously mentioned nutritional problem in alcoholics, *alcohol* may exert a direct effect in suppressing hematopoiesis by blocking metabolism of folate. In addition, alcohol can interfere with folate absorption and folate enterohepatic circulation. Plasma homocysteine is usually elevated in alcoholics (Zittoun, 1999).

Diagnosis of Folate Deficiency

Folic acid deficiency or cobalamin deficiency is suspected when the blood and bone marrow show findings characteristic of megaloblastic anemia; usually serum folate and cobalamin levels are then determined.

Serum and Red Cell Folate. A microbiological assay for folic acid activity employing *Lactobacillus casei* is a reliable method for the definitive diagnosis (Beck, 1991). Radioisotopic and chemiluminescence methods employing different folate binders are widely used because of rapidity and greater convenience. Although the correlation with the microbiological assay is generally good, discrepancies seem to be frequent and, on the basis of other data, tend to be resolved in favor of the microbiological

Table 31–2 Correlation of Vitamin B$_{12}$ and Folate Levels With Clinical Status: Three Laboratory Tests Needed to Separate Four Clinical Situations

Clinical situation	Serum vitamin B$_{12}$ (pg/mL)	Serum folate (ng/mL)	Red cell folate (ng/mL)
Normal*	Normal (200–900)	Normal (5–16), indeterminate (3–5), or low (< 3)	Normal (> 150)
Vitamin B$_{12}$ deficiency	Low (< 100)	Normal (5–16) or high (> 16)	Low (< 150)
Folic acid deficiency	Normal	Low	Low
Deficiency of both	Low	Low	Low

* Normal includes transient states of negative folate balance.

assay. False-normal red cell folate levels have been reported in 16–40% of patients identified by microbiological assays (Zittoun, 1999). Unlike serum folate (which is entirely 5-methyltetrahydrofolate), red cell folates are a heterogeneous mixture of different forms with varying polyglutamate chain lengths, which pose challenges to nonmicrobiological assays.

The serum folate level is decreased (< 3 µg/L) in megaloblastic anemia due to folate deficiency but is usually normal or increased in cobalamin deficiency. A low serum folate level precedes decrease of red cell or tissue folate; it indicates a negative folate balance but does not by itself indicate tissue folate deficiency. In cobalamin deficiency, serum folate is decreased in 10% of cases, increased in 20%, and normal in the remainder (Tietz, 1990).

The red cell folate is a better test of body folate stores and is decreased in megaloblastic anemia due to folate deficiency. In cobalamin deficiency, however, red cell folate is low in almost two-thirds of cases, so this needs to be excluded before regarding a low red cell folate as proof of severe folate deficiency. Therefore, three measurements are often useful in distinguishing between deficiencies of folic acid and cobalamin (Table 31–2).

Urinary Formiminoglutamic Acid. Folic acid coenzymes are required for the conversion of FIGLU to glutamic acid in the catabolism of histidine. When oral histidine is given, FIGLU will appear in increased amounts in the urine if folate deficiency is present. The test is useful in patients with megaloblastic anemia due to antifolate drugs; these patients have normal serum folate levels but greatly decreased tissue coenzyme levels (Beck, 1991).

Therapeutic Trial. The therapeutic trial remains an excellent way to discriminate between folic acid and vitamin B$_{12}$ deficiency. Physiologic doses of folic acid (parenteral, 50–200 µg/day) will allow an adequate reticulocyte response in patients with folic acid deficiency, but not in cobalamin deficiency. On the other hand, the usual therapeutic doses of folic acid (5–15 mg/day) or larger doses of cobalamin (500–1000 µg) may induce a partial response in a patient with megaloblastic anemia due to the other deficiency.

Deoxyuridine Suppression Test. See earlier discussion.

Plasma Homocysteine Assay. As with cobalamin deficiency, total plasma homocysteine is increased in approximately 75% of patients with folate deficiency. The level of methylmalonic acid is normal (Zittoun, 1999).

Acute Megaloblastic Anemia

Acute megaloblastic anemia may develop over the course of only a few days. The most common cause has been related to nitrous oxide (N$_2$O) anesthesia. N$_2$O rapidly destroys methylcobalamin causing a rapidly progressive megaloblastic anemia. Acute folate deficiency may occur in some patients in intensive care units because of a combination of factors (decreased intake, total parenteral nutrition, dialysis, surgery, sepsis, medications). Serum folate may be normal (Babior, 2001b).

Therapy for Megaloblastic Anemia

Although it may be necessary to treat severely anemic patients with both vitamins, it is usually possible to determine which deficiency is the cause and treat only with the deficient vitamin.

The maximal reticulocyte response occurs in 7 days. Within 4–6 hours after the initial therapy (if parenteral), the marrow shows decreased early megaloblasts and the appearance of pronormoblasts. Within 2–4 days, the marrow is predominantly normoblastic. Granulocytic abnormalities

return to normal more slowly, and hypersegmented neutrophils disappear from the blood only after 12–14 days.

PA is treated parenterally with 1000 µg of cyanocobalamin daily for 2 weeks, then weekly until the hematocrit is normal, and then monthly for the lifetime of the patient (Babior, 2001b). High concentrations of oral cobalamin, i.e., 1000 µg per day, force absorption of some cobalamin through an alternative system. Some reports recommend the use of oral cobalamin therapy instead of injections (Oh, 2003).

In folate deficiency, oral therapy is generally used at a dosage of 1–2 mg/day. Cobalamin deficiency must be excluded, and corrected if present, to avoid the occurrence of neuropathies of cobalamin deficiency. Supplemental dietary folic acid during pregnancy is reported to reduce the incidence of neural tube defects in the baby.

Other Defects of Nucleoprotein Synthesis

Other defects of nucleoprotein synthesis may lead to megaloblastic anemias that do not respond to cobalamin or folic acid.

Congenital Defects. Orotic aciduria is a very rare autosomal recessive condition in which certain enzymes required for pyrimidine synthesis are absent. The findings are excessive urinary excretion of orotic acid, failure of normal growth and development, and megaloblastic anemia that is refractory to cobalamin and folate but that responds to uridine.

Inborn defects in enzymes involved in folate metabolism, including methyltetrahydrofolate reductase and glutamate formiminotransferase deficiencies, have also been described.

Synthetic Inhibitors. Synthetic inhibitors of purine synthesis (6-mercaptopurine, tioguanine, azathioprine), of pyrimidine synthesis (5-fluorouracil), or of deoxyribonucleotide synthesis (cytosine arabinoside or hydroxycarbamide [hydroxyurea]) are used in chemotherapy for neoplasia and may concomitantly produce megaloblastosis.

Refractory Anemias. Anemias that are megaloblastic and that fail to respond to cobalamin or folic acid are considered with the myelodysplastic syndromes (see Ch. 32). The megaloblastic changes are usually atypical and do not include the characteristic granulocytic features, but other dysplastic changes are present.

Impaired Production – Other

Anemia of Chronic Diseases (Means, 2003)

The term anemia of chronic disease (ACD) designates an anemia syndrome typically found in patients with chronic infections, inflammatory or neoplastic disorders, which is characterized by reduced reticulocyte response accompanied by low serum iron despite adequate iron stores. ACD occurs in approximately 50% of hospitalized patients, as identified by laboratory studies. ACD has also been observed in acute trauma and critical care patients.

The erythrocytes are usually normocytic and normochromic, although in 20–50% of patients the anemia is microcytic and hypochromic. Anisocytosis and poikilocytosis are slight. The reticulocyte count is usually not elevated. Leukocytes and platelets are not distinctively altered, except by the causative disease.

The marrow is normocellular or minimally hypocellular or hypercellular, and the cell distribution is not greatly disturbed. The normoblasts may have frayed hypochromic cytoplasm, and the appearance of hemoglobin in the cells may be delayed (as in iron deficiency anemia). Sideroblasts are decreased, but storage iron is normal or increased.

The serum iron concentration is characteristically decreased, the TIBC is decreased or normal (in contrast to iron deficiency anemia, in which the TIBC is elevated), and the percent saturation is decreased. Erythrocyte protoporphyrin and serum ferritin are elevated.

The most important pathogenetic mechanism of ACD is the presence of high levels of cytokines, which may result in decreased red cell survival, altered iron metabolism, direct inhibition of hematopoiesis, and decreased erythropoietin secretion. Tumor necrosis factor-α (TNF-α) plays a significant role in inflammation and immune response. TNF-α levels are increased in patients with cancer, rheumatoid arthritis, infections, and the acquired immunodeficiency syndrome (AIDS). In vitro inhibition of human erythroid colony formation (BFU-E and CFU-E) by TNF-α has been reported. Similarly, an inhibitory action of interleukin-1 (IL-1) and interferon-γ (IFN-γ) on erythropoiesis has been implicated. Ceramide, a product of cytokine-induced enzymatic hydrolysis of cell membrane sphingomyelin, plays a role as a messenger in the inhibitory effects of IFN-γ (Means, 2003).

Erythropoietin (EPO) levels, although above normal, have been disproportionate to the degree of anemia, indicating relative EPO deficiency in anemia of chronic disease. Inhibitory effects of cytokines on EPO synthesis sites such as renal and liver cells have been suggested. The relative deficiency of EPO induces neocytolysis, i.e., selective hemolysis of the youngest red blood cells. Thus, a mild hemolytic event usually accompanies ACD (Trial, 2001).

Recently, hepcidin has been shown to be elevated in ACD through induction by IL-6. This elevation may provide a key mechanism to increased storage iron and its defective release from stores in ACD (Brugnara, 2003).

The anemia usually fails to respond to iron therapy. However, patients treated with EPO have shown improvement.

Anemia of Renal Insufficiency

A normocytic normochromic anemia is commonly encountered in patients with chronic renal failure (CRF). The correlation between the severity of the anemia and the degree of elevation of the blood urea nitrogen (BUN) is positive but not strictly linear. When creatinine clearance falls below 20 mL/min, the hematocrit is usually below 0.30 (Caro, 2001).

Several factors are often involved in the anemia of chronic renal failure. Decreased production of EPO by the damaged kidney is probably the important factor in most cases in which the BUN exceeds 100 mg/dL. Both ineffective erythropoiesis and impaired ability of the marrow to respond to EPO appear to be present in some degree.

Inhibitors of erythropoiesis have been demonstrated in the plasma of patients with chronic renal failure. The nature of these inhibitory factors is not known; however, parathyroid hormone and spermine have been implicated as inhibitors of erythropoiesis. Recent studies indicate the presence of a high level of inflammatory cytokines, such as IL-1, IL-4, IL-6, and TNF-α in patients with CRF. As discussed under Anemia of Chronic Diseases, these cytokines exert a bone marrow suppressive effect and probably contribute to the development of anemia (Stenvinkel, 2003).

Hemolysis is a significant feature in many cases of chronic renal failure. There appears to be an extracorpuscular factor in uremic plasma that has a detrimental effect on red cell metabolism and results in morphologically deformed cells (echinocytes and spiculated red cells). Numerous irregularly contracted and fragmented cells are seen in the hemolytic uremic syndrome and in malignant hypertension as a result of traumatic damage incurred by the red cells in traversing the damaged small blood vessels. Changes in red cell membrane adenosine triphosphatase (ATPase) and transketolase may render the red cells more sensitive to oxidant drugs or chemicals.

In addition, bleeding is a common problem in chronic renal disease, probably owing either to thrombocytopenia, in some patients, or to platelet functional defects, which are present in most patients. Anemia due to iron deficiency from blood loss should always be suspected. Folic acid deficiency may be a problem in patients in a dialysis program, since folic acid is readily moved into the dialysis bath.

Anemia in Liver Disease

Chronic posthemorrhagic anemia; hypoplastic anemia secondary to viral-induced marrow suppression; folate-deficient megaloblastic anemia due to poor nutrition in alcoholic cirrhosis; and acquired hemolytic anemias associated with either Coombs'-positive red cells, congestive splenomegaly, or lipid disturbances may occur in liver disease (Gallagher, 2001). Iron deficiency anemia is the most common, occurring in approximately 50% of patients, followed by hypersplenism in approximately 25% of patients (Ozatli, 2000). Interferon (INF)-α and ribavarin (Rbv) are common therapies for hepatitis C infection. Rbv induces suppression of erythropoiesis, possibly through downregulation of erythropoietin receptors. In addition, Rbv can cause a dose-dependent hemolytic anemia. INF-α can produce anemia through suppression of hematopoietic progenitor cell proliferation and induction of apoptosis of erythroid progenitor cells (Dieterich, 2003).

In addition to these, there is an anemia associated with liver disease that is characterized by shortened red cell survival and relatively inadequate red cell production. It is exaggerated by an increased blood volume that appears to correlate with the degree of portal hypertension. The red cells are normocytic or macrocytic (thin macrocytes). Frequently, target cells are present, especially in obstructive jaundice; these have increased surface membrane with increased cholesterol and lecithin content. However, the phospholipid/cholesterol ratio is normal. Reticulocytes may be slightly increased, and platelets may be normal or decreased. The bone marrow may be slightly hypercellular, and erythropoiesis is macronormoblastic rather than megaloblastic. Changes in leukocytes, such as are present in megaloblastic anemias, are not seen, and this type of anemia does not respond to cobalamin (vitamin B$_{12}$) or folic acid. The anemia is of unknown origin.

A small proportion of patients with severe cirrhosis have a hemolytic anemia associated with 'spur cells,' which are red cells with thorny projections similar to acanthocytes. As with target cells, the spur cells are secondary to lipid abnormalities in the plasma; they have increased surface membrane with increased cholesterol but normal phospholipid content in the membrane. The increased membrane cholesterol tends to associate with the outer membrane leaflet making it more rigid. The spleen attempts to remodel the membrane resulting in characteristic membrane projections (Gallagher, 2001).

Anemia in Endocrine Disease

Uncomplicated anemia in hypothyroidism is mild to moderate; it is normochromic and normocytic without reticulocytosis and with normal red cell survival. It reflects a decreased marrow production due to a smaller tissue oxygen requirement and subsequent reduced erythropoietin secretion. Because plasma volume is decreased in hypothyroidism, the apparent degree of anemia may not be proportional to the decrease in red cell mass. Hypothyroidism may, of course, be complicated by iron deficiency anemia, particularly in females, due to menorrhagia. Macrocytosis is frequently observed. Although the incidence of pernicious anemia in patients with hypothyroidism may be increased, most cases of macrocytosis are due to folate deficiency (Erslev, 2001a).

In adrenal cortical hormone deficiency, there is a mild normochromic normocytic anemia. The etiology is unclear, but the anemia is corrected by hormone replacement.

Deficient testosterone secretion in men results in a decrease in red cell production of 1–2 g Hb/dL (to a value comparable with that in women). This appears to be due to the effect of androgens on EPO secretion and also through enhancing EPO action on the marrow.

Pituitary deficiency also causes anemia. It tends to result in a greater depression of hemoglobin concentration because of the effect on multiple endocrine glands and possibly the loss of growth hormone effect.

A small number of patients with hyperparathyroidism have a normocytic, normochromic anemia. Earlier studies suggested that the parathyroid hormone may suppress normal erythropoiesis. More recent studies failed to support this theory. The anemia of hyperparathyroidism is likely related to marrow fibrosis or decreased erythropoietin secretion secondary to renal calcification (Erslev, 2001a).

Anemia Associated with Bone Marrow Infiltration (Myelophthisic Anemia)

This anemia is associated with marrow replacement by (or involvement with) metastatic carcinoma, multiple myeloma, leukemia, lymphoma, lipidoses or storage disease, and certain other conditions.

Normochromic and normocytic (occasionally macrocytic) anemia of varying severity is present. Reticulocytes are often increased, and the number of normoblasts is usually out of proportion to the severity of the anemia. The leukocyte count is normal or reduced (occasionally elevated), and immature neutrophils and even myeloblasts may be found. Platelets are normal or decreased, and bizarre, atypical platelets can sometimes be seen.

Examination of the marrow will usually reveal the condition responsible for this reaction. Mechanical crowding out of the hematopoietic tissue by the pathologic process has been assumed but not proved and probably is not the usual cause. Often the amount of erythropoietic tissue in the marrow as determined by morphologic and kinetic studies is normal or increased. The mechanism described earlier under Anemia of Chronic Diseases may often play a role, but the reason for the outpouring of immature cells into the blood is not clear.

In addition to myelophthisic anemias, circulating normoblasts and immature neutrophils can also be seen in hemolytic anemias, severe anemias due to other causes, severe infections, and congestive heart failure, but usually the normoblasts are not as numerous.

The *leukoerythroblastotic reaction* associated with myelophthisic anemias cannot always be distinguished from the blood picture of myelosclerosis with myeloid metaplasia (MMM), which is one of the myeloproliferative disorders. In MMM, enlargement of the spleen and liver is almost always found. In the blood film, more severe red cell abnormalities, leukocytosis, myeloblasts and immature granulocytes of all varieties (not just neutrophils), increased basophils, more atypical platelets, more numerous megakaryocyte fragments, and dwarf megakaryocytes are all findings more characteristic of MMM than of a leukoerythroblastotic reaction of some other cause. Examination of the bone marrow by a needle biopsy or surgical biopsy is necessary to differentiate MMM from myelophthisic anemias.

Aplastic Anemia

The term aplastic anemia (AA) usually refers to pancytopenia associated with a severe reduction in the amount of hematopoietic tissue that results in deficient production of blood cells. The marrow, though hypocellular, may have patchy areas of normocellularity or even hypercellularity. The diagnosis of *severe aplastic anemia* is made in pancytopenic patients when at least two of the following three peripheral blood values – granulocytes less than $0.5 \times 10^9/\text{L}$, platelets less than $20 \times 10^9/\text{L}$, or reticulocytes less than $40\,000/\mu\text{L}$ or 1% (corrected for hematocrit) – are present and the bone marrow is less than 30% cellular (Camitta, 1982). The term *very severe aplastic anemia* is used when granulocytes are less than $0.2 \times 10^9/\text{L}$ (Young, 2002). Otherwise, the aplastic anemia would be classified as moderate. The incidence of AA is 2–5 per million per year based on retrospective studies although industrialized countries may have a higher incidence (Shadduck, 2001).

Clinical Features. The clinical course may be acute and fulminating, with profound pancytopenia and a rapid progression to death, or the disorder may have an insidious onset and a chronic course. The symptoms and signs depend on the degree of the deficiencies: bleeding from thrombocytopenia, infection from neutropenia, and signs and symptoms of anemia. As a rule, splenomegaly and lymphadenopathy are absent. Bleeding is the most common presentation of AA, occurring in approximately 40% of patients (Young, 2000). Bleeding usually manifests as easy bruisability, gum bleeds, and episodic nosebleeds. Less than 5% of patients present with infection.

Etiology. Aplastic anemias are of diverse etiology. Since 1980, in approximately 70% of cases no specific etiologic agent could be correlated with the disease; such cases are considered idiopathic. Drug- and chemical-related aplastic anemias account for 11–20%, and those associated with infectious hepatitis account for 2–9% of cases (Young, 2000).

Pathogenesis. Hematopoietic failure may occur at any level in the differentiation of bone marrow precursor cells. There may be insufficient stem cells assayed as long-term culture-initiating cells, or insufficient committed stem cells (progenitor cells). The CD34+ cells in the bone marrow, which contain most of the stem cells and committed progenitor cells, are markedly decreased in patients with AA. Although in theory, AA could result from defective marrow microenvironment, these defects do not appear to be causative for most patients (Young, 2002).

The mechanism of AA is suggested to fall under two main categories: direct damage and immune-mediated destruction of marrow cells. Direct damage to the hematopoietic stem and progenitor cells could be caused by a known agent, such as cytotoxic drugs, irradiation and viruses, or unknown agent that in some way alters the ability of the cell to proliferate or differentiate. Immune-mediated destruction of stem and progenitor cell compartments results from cytotoxic lymphocyte activation, cytokine production, and specific cell elimination. Recent studies favor immune-mediated mechanism for AA and suggest that chemical and viral antigens may initiate the destructive immune process (Young, 2002). In fact, acquired AA is being viewed now as an immune-mediated syndrome.

Prognosis. Complications are due to infection, bleeding, and problems of iron overload from repeated transfusions. The prognosis appears to depend on the severity of marrow damage. However, the initial blood count and response to therapy during the first few months of treatment are important prognostic factors (Young, 2000). In a series of 101 patients treated by conventional methods (Williams, 1978), 25% of patients died within 4 months of the onset of symptoms, 50% died within 12 months, and 71% within 5 years. Those who died within 4 months had significantly lower reticulocyte, neutrophil, and platelet counts; a lower percentage of myeloid cells in the marrow; and a shorter interval between onset of symptoms and visit to the physician (Lynch, 1975). Other factors that correlated with a poor prognosis included male gender, but not age of the patient or etiology of the aplasia (Williams, 1978). Yet, the age of the patient usually influences the decision of which therapy the patient should receive. In some survivors, partial recovery is common. With the introduction of modern treatment protocols by immunosuppressive therapy and bone marrow transplantation, long-term survival rates of more than 60% are reported. The survivors have much higher risk of developing myelodysplastic syndrome, paroxysmal nocturnal hemoglobinuria, and acute leukemia (Young, 2002).

Management. Treatment includes bone marrow transplantation for patients with severe disease under 50 years of age if there is an HLA-matched donor. Children and young adults have a much higher survival probability compared to older adults (Young, 2002). Immune suppression using antilymphocyte globulin, ciclosporin, and corticosteroids may induce hematologic remission in some patients. Androgens appear to be least helpful in the stimulation of any residual marrow. Supportive care must be used with caution. Certainly, appropriate antibiotics should be used to combat infections; however, the risk for sensitization should be considered with the administration of blood products. Single-donor platelets or platelets from HLA-matched donors are preferred (Alter, 1998).

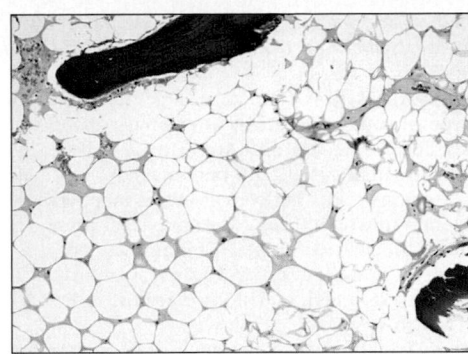

Figure 31–8 Section of hypocellular marrow, aplastic anemia. The cellularity is less than 5%.

Idiopathic Aplastic Anemia

In patients with pancytopenia and a hypocellular marrow, a search should be made for evidence of significant exposure to radiation, drugs, and chemicals of known or possible propensity to injure the marrow so that further exposure can be eliminated. Nevertheless, in approximately 70% of the cases of aplastic anemia, no suspected causal relationship to toxic agents can be found, and it is these that are designated as idiopathic.

The symptoms and signs do not differ, but the onset is commonly more insidious than in toxic or hypersensitive aplastic anemias.

Blood. The red cells are usually normal to increased in size with varying degrees of anisocytosis and poikilocytosis, particularly oval macrocytes. Macrocytosis may be a prominent feature, particularly in response to high levels of erythropoietin. The red cell distribution width (RDW) may be increased, even without transfusion (Elghetany, 1997). Polychromasia, stippling, and normoblasts are most often conspicuously absent. Leukopenia with marked decrease in granulocytes and a relative lymphocytosis are observed. In severe leukopenia, there is often also an absolute lymphocytopenia. Neutrophil granules may be larger than normal and may stain dark red (unlike the 'toxic' granules found in infections), and the neutrophil alkaline phosphatase may be elevated. However, neutrophil left shift is not seen in the absence of infection (Elghetany, 1997). Thrombocytopenia is part of the picture. The serum iron is usually increased. The serum cobalamin and folate levels are usually normal. Although an occasional patient is hypogammaglobulinemic, most patients have normal levels of serum immunoglobulins.

Bone Marrow. In most cases, the aspirate consists of red cells, lymphocytes, some plasma cells, mast cells, and fatty particles. Marrow sections will show fatty tissue with inconspicuous fibrosis and islands of lymphocytes and plasma cells (Fig. 31–8). Though focal areas of predominantly erythroid normocellularity or hypercellularity (hot spots) may sometimes be present, the overall cellularity is decreased. Storage iron is increased.

Erythrokinetics. The increased serum iron concentration is a valuable early sign of erythroid hypoplasia and reflects the decreased plasma iron turnover. In addition, the erythrocyte utilization of iron is decreased. Both effective and total erythropoiesis, therefore, are decreased in aplastic anemia.

Aplastic Anemia Associated with Chemical or Physical Agents

Toxic Aplastic Anemias. A number of physical and chemical agents produce marrow damage in all humans and animals exposed to a sufficient dose. Examples are ionizing radiation; mustard compounds; benzene; and antineoplastic agents such as busulfan, urethane, and antimetabolites. Benzene is less of a problem than in the past due to reduction in exposure.

Ionizing Radiation. The effects depend on the radiosensitivity of the cells and the capacity of the cells to regenerate, as well as the survival rate of the cells in the blood. Erythroid cells are most sensitive, granulocytes have intermediate sensitivity, and the megakaryocytes are the least sensitive of the three. Stromal cells are relatively insensitive.

After acute exposure to radiation, the reticulocyte count falls, but the red cells decline slowly because of their long survival. Within the first few hours, there is a neutrophilic leukocytosis due to a shift from marginal and probably marrow storage pools. A fall in lymphocytes occurs after the first day and is responsible for the early leukopenia, since lymphocytes are sensitive to irradiation and are directly killed. After 5 days or so, granulocytes begin to fall. The platelets decrease later. Platelets are often the last to return to normal in the recovery phase. Chronic exposure to low-dose irradiation, including localized radiation for ankylosing spondylitis, is associated with delayed increased risk for aplastic anemia (Shadduck, 2001).

Hypersensitive Aplastic Anemias. A large number of drugs produce marrow damage in some individuals after single or repeated exposures. Effects are not dose related as they are in toxic aplasia. Agents include antimicrobial drugs (Salvarsan, chloramphenicol, sulfonamides, chlortetracycline, streptomycin), anticonvulsants (mephenytoin, trimethadione), analgesics (phenylbutazone), antithyroid drugs (carbimazole), antihistaminics (tripelennamine), H_2-histamine receptor antagonists (cimetidine), insecticides (DDT), and other chemicals – some known (gold compounds, quinacrine, chlorpromazine, hair dyes, bismuth, mercury) and others unknown.

Chloramphenicol is an important drug in this category. This antibiotic was considered to be the most common cause of AA at the peak of its use, which began in 1949. Reactions of the marrow to chloramphenicol are of two types, which are possibly unrelated (Alter, 1998).

In about half the patients who receive chloramphenicol, increased serum iron, reticulocytopenia with anemia, neutropenia, and thrombocytopenia are found. The marrow may show decreased erythroid cells and vacuolization of primitive erythroid and granulocyte precursors. These changes are dose related, time dependent, and reversible.

In a very small proportion of persons receiving chloramphenicol, an irreversible aplastic anemia develops that may be fatal. The pancytopenia occurs 3 weeks to 5 months from the last dosage. No relationship has been established between the reversible erythropoietic lesion and the development of aplastic anemia; it may be that individual susceptibility is responsible for the latter. For this reason, it is essential that restraint be employed in using the drug, because monitoring its administration with blood cell counts is not an effective preventive measure.

Aplastic Anemia Associated with Other Disease

Infection. Viral infections are frequently associated with limited marrow suppression, typically neutropenia and less commonly thrombocytopenia. Marrow aplasia has been described as a rare sequela to viral hepatitis, occurring a few months after onset when the hepatitis is resolving. It is estimated at less than 0.07% of hepatitis cases in children and 2% of patients with non-A, non-B hepatitis. Most cases are seronegative for hepatitis A, B, C, and G with only rare cases of A or B types. These patients are usually males and under age 20; the prognosis is usually grave and bone marrow transplantation is considered early in the course of the disease (Young, 2002). Parvovirus has been associated with transient erythroid aplastic crisis in patients with chronic hemolytic disorders (Young, 2002). Human immunodeficiency virus (HIV) and Epstein–Barr virus may also cause hematopoietic depression. The mechanism of virus-induced bone marrow failure may be related to direct cytotoxicity, or more likely immune-mediated mechanisms secondary to molecular mimicry, antigen spread, and danger signals caused by the infection (Young, 2002).

Paroxysmal Nocturnal Hemoglobinuria. This rare hemolytic process (see later discussion) may be followed by aplastic anemia. Usually in paroxysmal nocturnal hemoglobinuria (PNH) a variable degree of marrow hypofunction coexists. Curiously, in some patients who present with aplastic anemia, the red cell defect of PNH may be present or may appear during the course of the disease. According to Lewis (1967), about 15% of patients with aplastic anemia have a demonstrable PNH red cell defect, with or without clinical hemolysis. However, with recent introduction of more sensitive techniques, such as flow cytometry, as high as 40% of patients with AA may have some surface marker evidence of PNH, particularly early during the course of the disease. The clonal expansion of PNH cells may have immunologic background as evidenced by the strong association of HLA-DR2 and PNH (Young, 2002).

Pregnancy. Pregnancy occurring in a patient with acquired aplastic anemia may make the pancytopenia more severe. Occasionally, however, aplastic anemia occurs during pregnancy and remits following delivery. In some such cases, aplasia recurs during a second pregnancy. The infants may be anemic, thrombocytopenic, or leukopenic (Fleming, 1968). Survival rates for AA in pregnancy have been relatively high for the mother (83%) and baby (75%). Hemorrhage is the most common cause of death in these patients (Young, 2000).

Thymoma. Although thymomas are usually associated with pure red cell aplasias, other bone marrow elements may also become depressed. Pancytopenia, often with hypoplastic bone marrow, occurs in rare cases with thymoma. Aplastic anemia may occur as a late complication after the treatment of thymoma (Ritchie, 2002a)

Immunologic Diseases. AA occurs in approximately 10% of cases of eosinophilic fasciitis. The prognosis of AA in this setting is usually poor. AA may be associated with systemic lupus erythematosus (SLE) and rheumatoid arthritis (RA), although the role of drug therapy in the pathogenesis of AA has been considered (Young, 2000). AA may also complicate multiple sclerosis, congenital immunodeficiency syndromes, and immune thyroid disease.

Inherited Aplastic Anemia

The term *inherited aplastic anemia* designates individuals with a congenital or genetic predisposition to chronic bone marrow failure, which may be associated with other congenital anomalies. Between 30–35% of childhood AA cases are inherited. In a study of 134 children with AA, 40 patients were diagnosed with inherited aplastic anemia, 26 had Fanconi's anemia (FA), 10 had familial aplastic anemia without classic signs of Fanconi's anemia, and four presented with amegakaryocytic thrombocytopenia that later developed into complete aplasia (Alter, 1998).

Fanconi's Anemia. FA is an autosomal recessive disorder with a carrier frequency of 1/300 in the US and Europe (Alter, 2002). Often more than one member of a family is affected. The pancytopenia becomes obvious after infancy and usually significant by the eighth year of life. The anemia is usually normochromic and may be macrocytic; increased levels of fetal hemoglobin (Hb F) and i antigen may be observed; the marrow is generally hypocellular. Developmental anomalies are present and may include hyperpigmentation, short stature, hypogonadism, malformations of the extremities (e.g., aplasia of the radius and abnormalities of the thumbs), microcephaly, and malformation of other organs (e.g., heart and kidneys). Chromosomal defects consisting of random breaks and rearrangements characteristically are present in blood lymphocytes as well as in marrow cells. Chromosomal breakage becomes more evident when the cultured cells are challenged with alkylating and DNA cross-linking agents such as mitomycin C and diepoxybutane. A breakthrough in investigating FA evolved from the observation that hybrid cells from FA and normal cells resulted in correction of the abnormal chromosome fragility, a process known as complementation. More than 10 complementation groups have been distinguished to date. The most common is complementation group A (FANCA), which occurs in approximately 70% of FA patients. Several FA proteins form a nuclear complex that is involved in chromosomal stability (Alter, 2002). The predicted median survival in FA is 19 years. Patients with FA are at a higher risk of developing leukemia and nonhematologic tumors, particularly in the liver, with an overall incidence of neoplasia of 15% (Alter, 1998).

Other Inherited Aplastic Anemia. A few children present with bleeding manifestations secondary to amegakaryocytic thrombocytopenia. As their disease progresses, they develop a pancytopenia and a hypocellular marrow. Chromosome breakage studies are usually normal. The mode of inheritance is autosomal recessive. The molecular defect is related to mutation in the gene for thrombopoietin receptor, *c-mpl*, which maps to 1p35 (Alter, 2002).

Pancytopenia and hypoplastic anemia may develop in a subset of patients with other familial disorders. Some patients with dyskeratosis congenita (reticulated hyperpigmentation of skin, dystrophic nails, and mucous membrane leukoplakia), and Shwachman–Diamond syndrome (exocrine pancreatic insufficiency and neutropenia) develop aplastic anemia during the course of their disease (Alter, 2002).

Pure Red Cell Aplasia

Transitory Arrest of Erythropoiesis (Transient Aplastic Crises)

This may occur during the course of a hemolytic anemia (often preceded by an infection), and the combination of aplasia and hemolysis becomes a life-threatening situation. Red cell production may occasionally cease during or following rather minor infections in normal children or adults, at which time the marrow will show absence of all but a few of the most immature erythroid precursors. Aplastic episodes in chronic hemolytic anemias often appear to be due to parvovirus B19 infection. This virus inhibits erythropoiesis by infecting mature erythroid progenitor cells (CFU-E). The morphologic hallmark of the disease is the presence of scattered giant pronormoblasts in the bone marrow aspirate with marked reduction in the more mature erythroid precursors. Nuclear inclusion may be difficult to identify in the Wright's stain. The aplastic crises resulting from parvovirus infection are transient, with erythroid marrow recovery in 1–2 weeks after onset (Erslev, 2001c).

Transient Erythroblastopenia of Childhood

Transient erythroblastopenia of childhood (TEC) occurs in previously healthy children, usually under the age of 8 years, with most cases between 1–3 years of age. It is characterized by a moderate to severe normocytic anemia, severe reticulocytopenia, transient neutropenia (20%), and increased platelet counts (60% of patients). Macrocytosis is usually observed during recovery owing to the effect of reticulocytes. A history of a viral infection within the previous 3 months is frequently elicited. The bone marrow is generally normocellular and shows virtual absence of erythroid precursors, except for a few early forms. The patients recover within 1 or 2 months without therapy. The pathogenesis appears to involve humoral inhibition of erythropoiesis or decreased stem cells in many of the patients who have been studied, but parvovirus has not been proven to be the cause of TEC (Alter, 2002).

Congenital Red Cell Aplasia (Diamond–Blackfan Anemia; Congenital Hypoplastic Anemia)

This is a rare, congenital red cell aplasia that usually becomes obvious during the first year of life but may occur as late as 6 years of age. The severe anemia is normochromic and slightly macrocytic; reticulocyte level is low; leukocytes are normal or slightly decreased; platelets are normal or increased; and the marrow usually shows a reduction in all developing erythroid cells, but normal granulocytic and megakaryocytic cell lines. In a small number of cases, residual erythroid precursors are detected. These precursors are mostly pronormoblasts. Hemoglobin F is elevated (5% to 25%) to a degree not expected for the patient's age, and the antigen i is often present. Red cell adenosine deaminase (ADA) is usually increased. These findings contrast with TEC. In the anemic phase of the latter, the red cells are normocytic, the Hb F is normal, the antigen i is absent, and red cell enzymes are at a lower level (characteristic of an older cell population) (Alter, 1998).

The defect appears to be in the erythroid-committed progenitor cells. CFU-Es and BFU-Es are decreased in the marrow, and BFU-Es, which normally circulate, are absent or decreased in the blood. In addition, these progenitor cells exhibit an acceleration in programmed cell death (apoptosis) and fail to respond in in vitro culture systems to normal T cells and to usual levels of EPO, suggesting a qualitative defect. A mutation in RPS19 gene was detected in 25% of patients. This gene encodes a ribosomal protein subunit of nucleolar localization (Alter, 2002).

About 75% of patients respond at least partially to corticosteroids, and the overall long-term survival is about 65%, though many patients require long-term steroid use (Alter, 1998).

Acquired Pure Red Cell Aplasia.

In middle-aged adults, selective failure of red cell production occurs rarely. Reticulocytopenia and a cellular marrow devoid of all but the most primitive erythroid precursors are characteristic. Leukocyte and platelet production is normal. About half of the reported cases have been associated with thymoma, usually a noninvasive spindle cell type. However, only 5–10% of patients with thymoma have the anemia. Remission of the anemia occurs in about one-fourth of the cases following surgical removal of the thymoma. Chronic acquired red cell aplasia has also been associated with other conditions, such as drugs, collagen vascular disorders, lymphoproliferative disorders of granular lymphocytes, or other disorders with immunologic aberrations. Most of these anemias appear to be part of a spectrum of autoimmune cytopenias in which the target cells are either erythroid stem cells or normoblasts. In some patients, antibodies that react with these cells have been identified. Corticosteroids and immunosuppressive drugs have been used as therapy, but less than half the patients achieve satisfactory remission (Erslev, 2001c).

Sideroblastic Anemia

Sideroblastic anemia is characterized by hypochromic, often microcytic, red cells in the blood usually mixed with normochromic cells, so that the appearance is dimorphic (Fig. 29–13). The serum iron concentration is increased, the TIBC is decreased, and the percent saturation of the iron-binding protein is greatly elevated. The marrow shows markedly increased storage iron (Fig. 31–5), erythroid hyperplasia with evidence of defective hemoglobinization, and increased numbers of sideroblasts. In addition, there are increased numbers of siderotic granules per cell, and granules surround the nucleus (with most authors requiring at least one-third of the circumference) forming 'ring sideroblasts' (Koc, 1998) (Fig. 32–17). In the latter, iron loading of mitochondria is seen by electron microscopy. These findings are associated with defective synthesis of heme, which may be due to any of several possible enzyme defects. Occasionally, megaloblast-like changes are seen in the erythroid cells, but changes typical of cobalamin or folate deficiency are not seen in granulocytes unless folate deficiency coexists.

Hereditary Sideroblastic Anemias

Hereditary sideroblastic anemias include several modes of inheritance (i.e., X-linked, autosomal dominant, and autosomal recessive). The X-linked forms generally exhibit low levels of δ-aminolevulinic acid synthase (ALAS) enzyme. This occurs in males and may not appear until adolescence. It is rare, but a few well-documented family studies exist. In

contrast to acquired sideroblastic anemia, the ring sideroblast abnormality is usually found in late, nondividing erythroblasts (Bottomley, 1982). The gene for ALAS-2 isoenzyme (erythroid ALAS) has been localized to the X chromosome, and a point mutation of this gene (Xp11.21) seems to occur in the majority of X-linked sideroblastic anemia (Koc, 1998). Mutations of the ALAS-2 gene may result in enzyme low affinity for pyridoxal phosphate, structural instability, abnormal catalytic site, or increased susceptibility to mitochondrial proteases. The degree of anemia improves with pyridoxine supplementation when the mutation disrupts the catalytic association between the enzyme and pyridoxal phosphate (Alcindor, 2002). Hereditary sideroblastic anemias may be due to a defect in the mitochondria, i.e. mitochondrial cytopathy. Most of these disorders are produced by deletions in the mitochondrial genome, which may be as much as 30% of the entire mitochondrial genome (Alcindor, 2002). These rare diseases are usually associated with systemic manifestations such as Pearson's syndrome (pancreatic insufficiency, vacuolation of bone marrow cells, ring sideroblasts and a variable degree of marrow failure).

Acquired Sideroblastic Anemias

Acquired Idiopathic Sideroblastic Anemia. When other causes of sideroblastic anemia cannot be identified, the term primary or idiopathic is applied. Acquired idiopathic sideroblastic anemia (AISA) is more common, has its onset in later adult life, and is seen in either sex. AISA is generally considered to constitute a subgroup of the myelodysplastic syndromes (refractory anemia with ring sideroblasts [RARS]) (Jaffe, 2001; see also Ch. 32). The dimorphic anemia has both hypochromic-microcytic and macrocytic red blood cells, and the MCV is usually high (Fig. 29–15). At least 15% of erythroblasts (early and late forms) in bone marrow are ring sideroblasts. Other manifestation of dysplasia in the erythroid cell line may be seen. Dysplastic features may involve myeloid and megakaryocytic cell lines as well. There is growing evidence that AISA may be caused by mutations of mitochondrial DNA (Gattermann, 1997).

Secondary (Drug- or Toxin-Induced) Sideroblastic Anemia

This form of sideroblastic anemia is secondary to some agent that interferes with heme synthesis; recognition is important because hematologic improvement occurs if the agent is removed.

The *antituberculosis drugs* isoniazid, cycloserine, and pyrazinamide cause sideroblastic abnormalities in some patients on long-term therapy.

Lead poisoning is an important member of this group because environmental exposure to lead is usually unrecognized and needs to be detected. Lead interferes with heme synthesis by blocking the enzymes ALA synthase, ALA dehydratase, and heme synthase. These blocks are only partial and of different degree; ALA and coproporphyrin are increased in the urine. *Chloramphenicol* also results in ring sideroblast formation, probably by inhibiting mitochondrial protein synthesis. *Copper deficiency or zinc overload* can produce sideroblastic anemia, vacuolated marrow cells, and neutropenia. Large quantities of ingested zinc interfere with copper absorption and produce manifestations of copper deficiency. Copper chelators in large doses, such as penicillamine, can produce sideroblastic anemia.

Ethanol-induced anemia is perhaps the most common of the reversible sideroblastic anemias. Folate deficiency, hypomagnesemia, and hypokalemia are concomitant findings. After withdrawal of alcohol intake, the abnormal sideroblasts usually disappear within a few days.

Primary pyridoxine deficiency, often associated with malnutrition, is occasionally associated with sideroblastic anemia. However, other manifestations, such as peripheral neuropathy and dermatitis, dominate the clinical presentation. Sideroblastic anemia as the sole manifestation of pyridoxine deficiency has not been reported in humans although it occurs in animals (Alcindor, 2002).

Refractory Anemia

There is an ill-defined group of chronic anemias usually occurring in individuals over the age of 50. Normocytic or macrocytic anemia, reticulocytopenia, often pancytopenia, and a hypercellular marrow showing erythroid hyperplasia with a variable degree of dyserythropoiesis are present. Often the patient has been treated with cobalamin, folic acid, and iron without response. The process is usually unremitting, and in a small proportion of cases develops additional dysplastic changes in marrow cells and increased blast cells and evolves into an acute leukemia. Refractory anemias, therefore, are considered one of the myelodysplastic syndromes (see Ch. 32).

Congenital Dyserythropoietic Anemias (CDA)

Congenital dyserythropoietic anemias (CDAs) represent a family of inherited refractory anemias characterized by ineffective erythropoiesis and marrow erythroid multinuclearity.

At least three types have thus far been separated on the basis of marrow and serologic findings (Heimpel, 2004). CDA-I has megaloblastic changes with some binuclearity in approximately 5% of marrow erythroblasts, internuclear chromatin bridges, and a macrocytic anemia. Some cases have an abnormality in the *CDAN1* gene located on the long arm of chromosome 15 (Heimpel, 2004). CDA-II is more common than the others and shows binuclearity and multinuclearity of 10–40% of erythroid precursors with pluripolar mitoses and karyorrhexis. The anemia is normocytic. CDA-II is distinguished from the others because it has a positive acidified serum test (with some, but not all normal sera) and a negative sucrose hemolysis test. It is known as hereditary erythroblastic multinuclearity with positive acidified serum test (HEM-PAS). The red cells have an antigen not present on normal or PNH cells, and about one-third of normal sera contain the corresponding immunoglobulin M (IgM) antibody. In addition, red cells in CDA-II react strongly with anti-i and anti-I. Electron microscopy demonstrates an excess of endoplasmic reticulum parallel to the cell membrane, which gives the appearance of a double membrane in late erythroblasts and some erythrocytes. CDA-II is thought to be related to abnormal membrane glycosylation. CDA-III has giant erythroid precursors, with more pronounced multinuclearity (gigantoblasts) in 10–40% of erythroid precursors, and a macrocytic anemia. In contrast to CDA-I and CDA-II, which are autosomal recessive, CDA-III has autosomal dominant inheritance. A putative gene for CDA-III has been recently localized on chromosome 15 near the *CDAN1* gene (Heimpel, 2004). Other variants have also been described in a small number of families.

Blood Loss Anemia

Acute Posthemorrhagic Anemia

Blood may be lost from the circulation externally or internally into a tissue space or body cavity. If blood is lost over a short period of time in amounts sufficient to cause anemia, *acute posthemorrhagic anemia* occurs. Normal healthy individuals are able to compensate for rapid blood loss of up to 20% of the circulating blood volume with few symptoms (Hillman, 1996). After a single episode of excessive bleeding, the major manifestations are those due to depletion of blood volume (hypovolemia). After a day or so, blood volume is returned to previous levels by movement of fluid into the circulation, and anemia becomes evident.

The earliest hematologic change is a transient fall in the platelet count, which may rise to elevated levels within an hour. The next development is a moderate neutrophilic leukocytosis with a shift to the left; a maximum leukocyte count of $10–35 \times 10^9/L$ may occur in 2–5 hours. The Hb and Hct do not fall immediately, but only slowly as tissue fluids move into the circulation to compensate for the lost blood volume. The fall in Hb and Hct may not reveal the full extent of the red cell loss until 2–3 days after the hemorrhage.

The anemia that develops at first is normochromic and normocytic, with a normal MCV and mean cell hemoglobin concentration (MCHC) and only minimal anisocytosis and poikilocytosis. Increased erythropoietin secretion stimulates erythroid proliferation in the marrow, and reticulocytes begin to reach the circulation in 3–5 days, reaching a maximum by 10 days or so. During this period, transient macrocytosis (increased MCV), increased polychromasia, and normoblasts may appear in the blood. It takes about 2–4 days after the blood loss for the leukocyte count to return to normal, and about 2 weeks for the morphologic changes to disappear. Return of red cell values is slower.

Chronic Posthemorrhagic Anemia

If blood is lost in small amounts over an extended period of time, both the clinical and hematologic features that characterize acute posthemorrhagic anemia are lacking. Regeneration of red cells occurs at a slower rate.

The reticulocyte count may be normal or slightly increased. Significant anemia does not usually develop until after storage iron is depleted; the anemia, therefore, is one of iron deficiency (q.v.). The anemia is at first normochromic and normocytic, and gradually the newly formed red cells become microcytic, then hypochromic. The leukocyte count is normal or slightly decreased, owing to neutropenia. Platelets are commonly increased, and only later, in severe iron deficiency, are they likely to be decreased.

The cause of blood loss must be identified, for it is toward this that definitive treatment must be directed.

Hemolysis – General

Anemias that are due primarily to increased red cell destruction are *hemolytic anemias*. A shortened red cell survival, therefore, proves that hemolysis is present; this measurement is usually unnecessary in practice.

Hemolytic anemias may be due to a defect of the red cell itself, an *intrinsic hemolytic anemia*: these are usually hereditary, and are commonly grouped as *membrane, metabolic,* or *hemoglobin* defects. Alternatively, the hemolysis may be due to a factor outside the red cell and acting upon it, an *extrinsic hemolytic anemia*: these are almost always acquired. The terms *intravascular hemolysis* and *extravascular hemolysis* refer to the *site* of the destruction of the red cell: within the circulating blood or outside it, respectively.

Erythrocyte Survival Studies. A shortened red cell survival defines hemolysis. If the hemolytic process is moderate or severe, the following studies will suffice to show that hemolysis is present. If the hemolytic process is mild or obscure, red cell survival studies may be necessary.

Radioactive chromium (^{51}Cr) is convenient and widely used. Labeled chromate is added to a blood sample in vitro and binds to β-chains of hemoglobin. The chromated red cells are injected intravenously and their disappearance is measured by counting blood, which is sampled every 1–2 days for 10–14 days. Residual activity is an index of the intravascular life span of the labeled red cells. Because ^{51}Cr emits γ-rays, external scanning can detect sites of red cell destruction.

The erythrocyte lifespan is usually expressed as the period during which one-half of the radioactivity remains in the blood (the $T_{\frac{1}{2}}$ ^{51}Cr; see Fig. 31–9). Chromium normally elutes from the red cells at a rate of 1% per day. Thus, the half-life of the ^{51}Cr-labeled erythrocytes in normal individuals is 25–32 days instead of 60 days. Blood loss, change in hematocrit, and recent blood transfusions significantly complicate the interpretation of survival data; therefore, a steady state is necessary for usable results.

In autoimmune hemolytic anemias, the slope of red cell survival produces a straight line when plotted on semilogarithmic paper (Fig. 31–9). In other hemolytic anemias, two cell populations may exist. In these situations, the survival curve may be composed of an initial steep slope followed by a flatter component (Fig. 31–10). This type of curve has been seen in hereditary enzyme-deficiency hemolytic anemias, sickle cell anemia, and PNH (Dacie, 1991).

Hemoglobin Destruction

Laboratory findings differ, depending on the site of blood destruction, the amount of destroyed blood, and the rate of destruction. If the destruction is *intravascular* and the quantity of destroyed blood is large, free hemoglobin and methemalbumin will be present in the plasma (hemoglobinemia and methemalbuminemia). The urine may contain free hemoglobin and also hemosiderin.

Free hemoglobin readily dissociates into αβ dimers ($α_2β_2 \rightarrow 2αβ$). These are bound to haptoglobin, an $α_2$-globulin, and the hemoglobin–haptoglobin complex is rapidly removed from the circulation and catabolized by the liver parenchymal cells. This process prevents hemoglobin from appearing in the urine. However, when the plasma hemoglobin level exceeds 50–200 mg/dL (8–31 µmol/L), which is the capacity of haptoglobin to bind hemoglobin, the free αβ dimers of hemoglobin readily pass through the glomerulus of the kidney. Part of the hemoglobin is then absorbed by the proximal tubular cells, where the hemoglobin iron is converted to hemosiderin. When these tubular cells are later shed into the urine, *hemosiderinuria* results. If the amount of hemoglobin in the tubular lumen exceeds the capacity of the tubular cell to absorb it, it reaches the urine (*hemoglobinuria*). In the process, it may be oxidized to methemoglobin (hemiglobin). Plasma hemoglobin not bound to haptoglobin or removed by the kidney is oxidized to hemiglobin. The oxidized heme groups (hemin) are bound to *hemopexin*, a β-globulin, and the complex is rapidly cleared by the hepatic parenchymal cells. If hemopexin is depleted, hemin groups bind to albumin, forming methemalbumin. Once hemopexin again becomes available, it removes the hemin groups from albumin for hepatic clearance (Hillman, 1996).

Lactate dehydrogenase (LD) is released from red cells and is increased in serum in hemolysis, especially in intravascular hemolysis; it is cleared more slowly than is hemoglobin. If the upper reference value is 207 IU/L, the LD in hemolytic anemia may be increased as much as 800 IU/L. In megaloblastic anemia, associated with marked ineffective erythropoiesis, the LD is greatly increased to several thousand units. Serum LD is also increased in other forms of cellular injury. In hemolytic anemias, there is reversal of the LD isoenzyme pattern with LD_1 exceeding LD_2.

The normal plasma hemoglobin level is 0.5–5 mg/dL (0.08–0.78 µmol/L). A rise to 10 mg/dL imparts to the plasma a yellow to orange color. With further increase, the color becomes pink. Levels up to 25–30 mg/dL are common in hemolytic anemia. Higher levels usually indicate intravascular hemolysis and are seen in hemolytic transfusion reactions and in paroxysmal cold and nocturnal hemoglobinurias.

If hemolysis is primarily *extravascular*, no hemoglobinemia, hemoglobinuria, or hemosiderinuria is present. Hemolysis is detected by

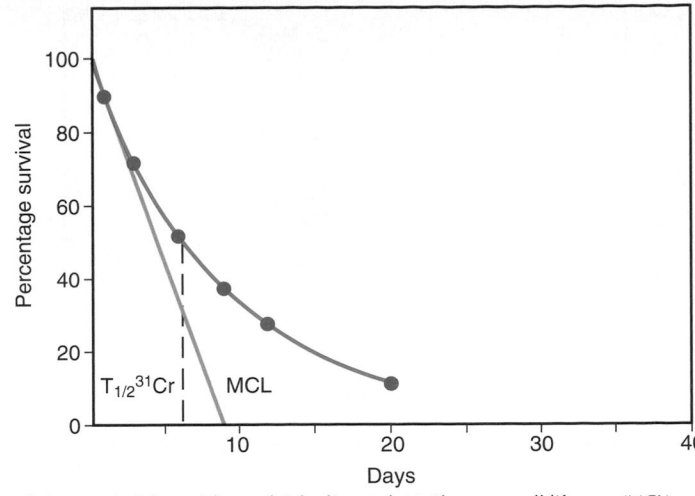

Figure 31–9 Results of ^{51}Cr erythrocyte survival curve in patients with autoimmune hemolytic anemia (left, semi-log and right, linear plots). The mean cell life span (MCL) was 9–10 days and is recorded at a period when 37% of cells are still circulating. The time of 50% survival ($T_{\frac{1}{2}}$Cr) was 6–7 days. (From Dacie, 1991, p 386 with permission.)

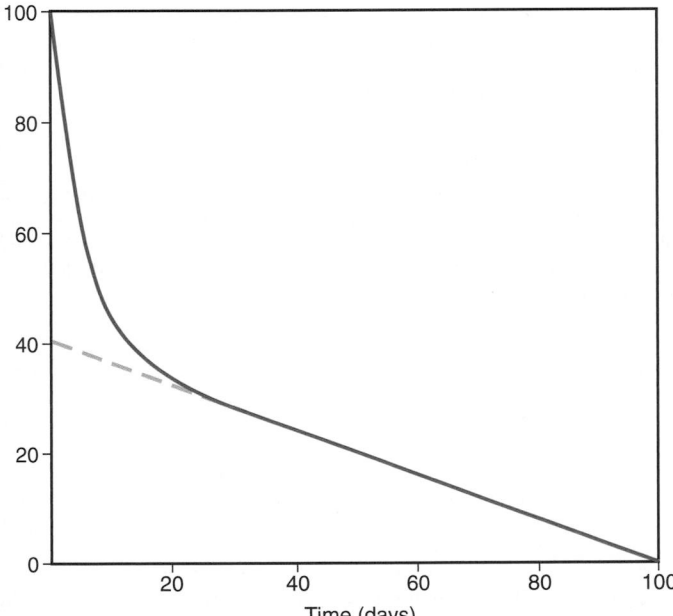

Figure 31–10 Results of ^{51}Cr erythrocyte survival curve in a patient with hemolytic anemia containing two cell populations. The percent survival is on the ordinate. By extrapolating the flatter curve to time 0, it can be estimated that 40% of the cells have a mean life span of 100 days. Sixty percent of cells have a mean life span of 5 days. (From Bentley SA, 1977.)

measuring an increase in one of the products of heme catabolism (see Ch. 30).

1. An increase in carbon monoxide (CO) expired (a research technique), or in the blood carboxyhemoglobin level.
2. An increase in indirect-reacting serum bilirubin; because this is bound to albumin, it will not appear in the urine.
3. An increase in urine urobilinogen or, more consistently, in fecal urobilinogen.

The normal urobilinogen in a 24-hour specimen is 0.5–4 mg (0.8–6.75 μmol) in urine and 40–280 mg (0.068–0.470 mmol) in the stool. Following excessive hemolysis, it may increase to 5–200 mg in the urine and to 300–400 mg in the stool. The examination of feces is more dependable than examination of the urine because it may show an increase when the urine shows none. It may show an increase even when the serum bilirubin concentration is not raised because the normal liver can remove large amounts of (indirectly reacting) bilirubin and of reabsorbed urobilinogen from the blood.

Hemolytic anemia is characterized also by increased red cell production. Because of the availability of maximal amounts of iron for hemoglobin formation, red cell production reaches the maximal degree possible (about eight times normal) in severe chronic hemolytic anemia, if complicating factors such as folate deficiency do not intervene. If red cell

destruction exceeds the capacity of the marrow to replace red cells at the same rate, hemolytic anemia occurs. With less severe hemolysis, the marrow may be able to produce enough red cells so that anemia does not occur; this is called compensated hemolysis.

Sudden worsening of the degree of anemia may occur in chronic hemolytic anemias and be due to either of two basic mechanisms. Occasionally, episodes of bone marrow failure (transient arrest of erythropoiesis; see earlier discussion) characterized by erythroid hypoplasia and reticulocytopenia may upset the equilibrium between production and destruction of red cells. In most instances, these *aplastic crises* are probably due to parvoviral infection (Young, 1984). On the other hand, an increased rate of red cell destruction may occur, associated with infection or other illness that increases splenic size. This is not associated with erythroid aplasia, and is called a *hemolytic crisis*.

Blood Film. The anemia is normocytic or macrocytic. Macrocytosis is due to the presence of immature red cells, which are larger than normocytes. Polychromasia is usually prominent; it may be excessively basophilic and normoblasts may be present, both of which indicate a 'shift' of marrow reticulocytes into the blood. Other red cell abnormalities may give a clue to the nature of the hemolytic process. Spherocytes suggest hereditary spherocytosis or autoimmune hemolysis (Fig. 29–12); schistocytes imply traumatic hemolytic anemia (see Fig. 29–19); sickle cells, target cells, or crystals suggest a hemoglobinopathy. When hemolytic anemia is acute, increased numbers and younger forms of leukocytes and platelets are often released from the marrow together with erythrocytes. The result is leukocytosis with a 'shift to the left' and thrombocytosis with both normal and giant platelets.

Bone Marrow. Normoblastic hyperplasia is present and may be striking in degree. Storage iron is usually increased and sideroblasts are normal or increased in number, reflecting the abundance of available iron for hemoglobin synthesis.

Hemolysis – Membrane Disorders

Hereditary Spherocytosis

Hereditary spherocytosis (HS) affects 1 in 5000 of the population, occurring predominantly in those of Northern European ancestry. It is characterized by spherocytic red cells that are intrinsically defective, splenomegaly, and familial occurrence (most often autosomal dominant). In about 15–30% of cases, however, neither parent is affected. The hemolytic process is variable in severity and is corrected by splenectomy, though the spherocytosis remains.

The laboratory findings are those of a chronic extravascular hemolytic process: evidence of increased pigment catabolism, erythroid hyperplasia, and reticulocytosis. The direct antiglobulin test is negative. The red cells characteristically have increased osmotic fragility. On the blood film, spherocytes have a smaller diameter and are more intensely stained than normal cells. They have decreased or absent central pallor; if present, the pallor may be eccentric (Fig. 29–12). The MCV is normal and the MCHC is often increased, reflecting a decrease in cell surface.

Osmotic Fragility Test. Red cells are suspended in a series of tubes containing hypotonic solutions of NaCl varying from 0.9–0.0%,

IV

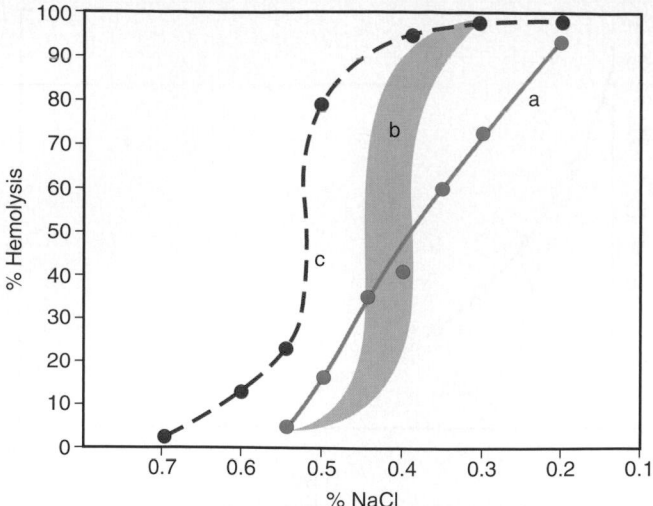

Figure 31–11 Erythrocyte osmotic fragility. *a*, Thalassemia, showing a small fraction of cells with increased fragility (lower left) and a larger fraction of cells with decreased fragility (upper right). *b*, Normal curves fall in shaded area. *c*, Hereditary spherocytosis, showing increased osmotic fragility.

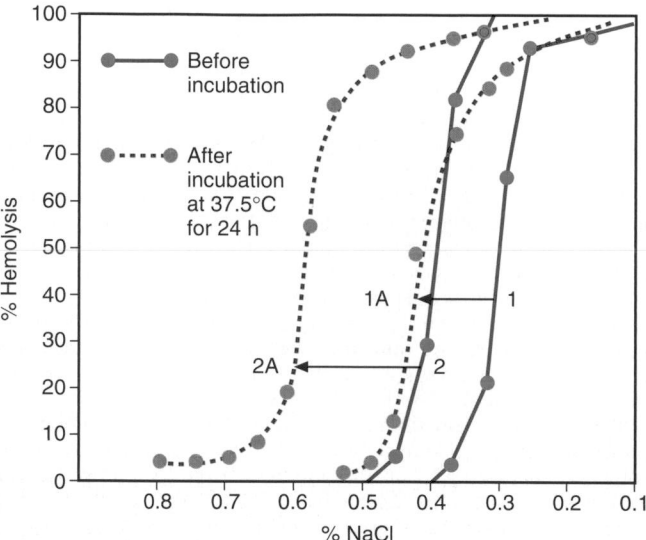

Figure 31–12 The effect of incubation on erythrocyte osmotic fragility. The change in the osmotic fragility curve from 'before incubation' to 'after incubation' is illustrated for normal blood (1 → 1A), and blood from a patient with hereditary spherocytosis (2 → 2A). Blood in hereditary spherocytosis characteristically shows a greater increase in fragility with incubation than does normal blood or even blood of acquired spherocytosis (e.g., autoimmune hemolytic anemia).

incubated at room temperature for 30 minutes, and centrifuged. The percent hemolysis in the supernatant solutions is measured and plotted for each NaCl concentration. Cells that are more spherical, with a decreased surface/volume ratio, have a limited capacity to expand in hypotonic solutions and lyse at a higher concentration of NaCl than do normal biconcave red cells. They are said to have increased osmotic fragility. Conversely, cells that are hypochromic and flatter have a greater capacity to expand in hypotonic solutions, lyse at a lower concentration than do normal cells, and are said to have decreased osmotic fragility (Fig. 31–11).

The osmotic fragility of freshly drawn blood is usually increased in HS, but may be normal in mildly affected patients. In blood that is incubated at 37°C for 24 hours before performing the test, the osmotic fragility is almost always increased (Fig. 31–12).

The increased osmotic fragility of freshly drawn blood is characteristic but not specific; it may occur in acquired spherocytic anemias. A greater difference in median fragility (after incubation from before incubation) occurs in HS cells than in control normal cells; this is an important diagnostic feature in HS. A tail of very fragile cells conditioned by the spleen is usually seen. The tail usually disappears after splenectomy. Cells with increased surface/volume ratio are osmotic resistant. These cells are seen in iron deficiency, thalassemia, liver disease, and reticulocytosis.

Autohemolysis Test. Sterile, defibrinated blood is incubated at 37°C for 48 hours (Dacie, 1991). During this time, red cells undergo a complex series of changes, lose membrane, and become more spherocytic. In normal blood, without added glucose, the amount of autohemolysis at 48 hours is 0.2–2.0%. In normal blood, incubated with added glucose, the amount of autohemolysis is less: 0–0.9%.

In HS, autohemolysis is virtually always increased; with glucose, the lysis is diminished to a variable extent. Rarely, patients with strong clinical and laboratory evidence for HS will have normal incubated osmotic fragility. In these patients, the abnormal autohemolysis test is useful in confirming a diagnosis of HS (Fukagawa, 1979).

The erythrocytes are abnormally permeable to sodium, and there is no defect in energy metabolism, which is, in fact, increased. The increased metabolic activity has been explained as an attempt to compensate for a membrane defect that leaks cations, with degenerative changes and the loss of cell membrane accelerated by the metabolic and physical stress of passage through the spleen.

The genetic defects in HS are heterogeneous but affect the skeletal proteins of the red cell membrane. HS can be divided into the following pathogenetic categories: (1) isolated partial deficiency of spectrin; (2) combined partial deficiency of spectrin and ankyrin; (3) partial deficiency of band 3 protein; (4) deficiency of protein 4.2; and (5) other less common defects. Most of these abnormalities are related to the synthesis of abnormal protein, mostly through point mutations or frameshift (Gallagher, 2000). The loss of surface area in HS is probably related to separation and loss of membrane lipid bilayer from the skeleton. Recent studies suggest that normal spectrin density is required for normal cohesion between the lipid bilayer and membrane skeleton (Mohandas, 1993).

Hereditary Elliptocytosis

This autosomal dominant condition probably includes more than one genetic variant. In the US population, the prevalence is approximately 3–5 per 10 000. It is more common in individuals of African and Mediterranean ancestry. All cases of hereditary elliptocytosis (HE) are associated with weakening of the membrane skeleton and defective association of proteins that hold the skeleton together (Gallagher, 2000). On the basis of red cell morphology, HE can be divided into three groups: (1) common HE (including hereditary pyropoikilocytosis [HPP]), with elliptocytes that may be rod shaped; (2) spherocytic HE; and (3) Southeast Asian ovalocytosis. The most commonly defined abnormality appears to be a defect in spectrin resulting in impaired association of spectrin dimers into spectrin tetramers and spectrin oligomers. Other abnormalities include a defect in protein 4.1 and deficiency of glycophorin C. HPP is associated with two abnormalities: a mutation in spectrin that disrupts spectrin heterodimer self-association and a partial deficiency of spectrin that results in decreased spectrin/band 3 ratio.

Common HE. Most persons with the common form of HE (~ 90% of cases) are nonanemic; a minority of this group (perhaps 10–20%) have mild hemolysis. Nonhypochromic elliptocytes are abundant in the blood film, numbering over 25% (see Fig. 29–16), whereas in normal individuals less than 5% of the red cells are elliptical, although an earlier report describes a normal percentage of 15% (Gallagher, 2000). The deformity is increased in sealed, moist preparations.

In a subgroup of common HE, especially in black families, affected neonates transiently have moderate poikilocytosis, red cell fragmentation, and budding, with hemolytic anemia; during the first year of life, hemolysis declines and typical HE emerges. The worsening of hemolysis in the neonatal period has been attributed to the presence of fetal hemoglobin, which binds poorly to 2,3-diphosphoglycerate (2,3-DPG). Higher levels of the latter exert a destabilizing effect on spectrin-protein 4.1–actin interaction (Gallagher, 2000).

Hereditary Pyropoikilocytosis. HPP is a severe congenital hemolytic anemia, which is characterized by microcytosis, striking micropoikilocytosis and fragmentation, and autosomal recessive inheritance. HPP represents a subtype of common HE. It occurs primarily in black people. In contrast to normal red cells, which show budding and fragmentation when heated to 49°C, HPP red cells fragment at 45–46°C.

Spherocytic HE. This subgroup accounts for 10% of cases. A mild to moderate hemolytic anemia and splenomegaly are present, with both elliptocytes and spherocytes, and abnormal osmotic fragility and autohemolysis tests. Poikilocytes and fragments are usually absent. The molecular basis of this subtype is unknown.

Southeast Asian Ovalocytosis. This subgroup occurs with high frequencies (20–30%) in certain populations of the Far East, particularly Malaysia. Hemolysis is usually absent or mild. The erythrocytes are less elongated and some have the appearance of stomatocytic ovalocytes. Many cells contain one or two transverse ridges or a longitudinal slit. This condition is associated with increased resistance to malaria. The underlying defect is related to a mutation in band 3 (Mohandas, 1993; Gallagher, 2000).

Hereditary Stomatocytosis (Hereditary Hydrocytosis)

This is a rare, autosomally transmitted disorder. Heterozygotic individuals have no anemia, and 1–25% stomatocytes in the blood film. In presumed homozygotic individuals, about one-third of the red cells are stomatocytes, and there is a mild to moderate hemolytic anemia. The membrane abnormality results in increased permeability of the membrane to Na^+ and K^+ (and therefore water), resulting in hydrated, macrocytic red cells. The MCV may be as high as 150 fL. The osmotic fragility and autohemolysis are increased. Although the exact membrane defect is not known, several reports indicate the absence of a membrane protein called stomatin located in the band 7 region (Gallagher, 2000).

Paroxysmal Nocturnal Hemoglobinuria

PNH is an acquired clonal stem cell disorder characterized by the production of abnormal erythrocytes, granulocytes, and platelets (Beutler, 1999; Johnson, 2002). The red cell defect renders them more susceptible to complement-mediated intravascular lysis. Three types of erythrocytes have been described according to their in vitro sensitivity: type I with normal sensitivity, type II with medium sensitivity (three to five times the normal) and type III with extreme sensitivity (15–25 times the normal). Several complement defense proteins are decreased or absent in PNH. These proteins include: decay accelerating factor (DAF, CD55), membrane inhibitor of reactive lysis (MIRL, CD59), and C8-binding protein (homologous restriction factor). DAF is a glycoprotein that antagonizes the convertase complexes of complement. MIRL is a protein that controls the membrane attack complex, C5b-9. Other proteins that are deficient in PNH include CD58 (leukocyte function antigen 3), CD14 (endotoxin-binding protein receptor), CD24, and CD16a (Fcγ receptor). Membrane-associated enzymes such as acetyl cholinesterase and leukocyte alkaline phosphatase may be deficient as well. Recent work indicates that deficient proteins and enzymes are attached to the cell membrane by a common glycolipid anchor called glycosylphosphatidyl inositol (GPI). Deficiency of GPI results in secondary deficiency of the attached proteins. Therefore, PNH can be redefined as partial or complete lack of GPI-linked proteins on a population of cells of the hematopoietic system (Johnson, 2002).

PNH is a rare disease with an estimated annual incidence of 4 per million (Johnson, 2002). The disease is characterized by chronic intravascular hemolysis with or without obvious hemoglobinuria. Hemosiderinuria is, however, almost constantly present. Typical nocturnal or sleep-related hemoglobinuria is present in less than 25% of patients. Bouts of hemolysis could be initiated by infection, surgery, whole blood transfusion, injection of contrast dyes, or even severe exercise.

The blood usually shows a normocytic anemia with a reticulocytosis that is often less than expected for the degree of anemia. Hypochromic microcytic anemia is not uncommon, however, and is due to loss of iron in the urine. Neutropenia occurs in three-fifths and thrombocytopenia in two-thirds of patients at some time during the course of disease, so that pancytopenia is common. The direct antiglobulin test is usually negative.

The marrow may be hypercellular with erythroid hyperplasia, but it may be hypocellular. In some patients, marrow failure may occur during the course of PNH; in others, aplastic anemia is the initial diagnosis, with signs of PNH manifesting simultaneously or later. As mentioned earlier, approximately 40% of patients with AA have evidence of PNH clones at diagnosis (Young, 2002).

Thrombotic complications are common, occurring in approximately 20% of patients and represent a major cause of mortality. Thrombosis commonly occurs in hepatic, cerebral, and abdominal veins. The absence of CD59 on platelets results in externalization of phosphatidylserine, a site for prothrombinase complexes and thus increases the propensity for thrombosis. The disease may undergo partial remissions and exacerbations. In over half of patients, both the proportion of abnormal cells and the clinical severity decrease with time. In approximately 3–5% of PNH patients the disease progresses to acute leukemia.

Sucrose Hemolysis Test. This test should be performed whenever the diagnosis of PNH is considered, also in hypoplastic anemias, and in any hemolytic anemia of obscure origin (Hartmann, 1970). The principle of the test is that sucrose provides a medium of low ionic strength that promotes the binding of complement to the red cells. In PNH, a proportion of the red cells are abnormally sensitive to complement-mediated lysis. Suspicious results can be seen in some other hematologic diseases, especially megaloblastic anemia and autoimmune hemolytic anemia. False-negative results occur if the serum lacks complement

Table 31–3 Acidified Serum Test

	1	2	3	4	5	6	7
Fresh normal serum		0.5	0.5			0.5	0.5
Patient's serum			0.5				
Heat-inactivated normal serum				0.5			0.5
0.2 N HCl		0.05	0.05	0.05		0.05	0.05
50% patient's red cells	0.05	0.05	0.05	0.05			
50% normal red cells					0.05	0.05	0.05
Pattern of lysis in positive test	Trace	+++	+	–	–	–	–

Modified from Dacie, 1991, p 261.

activity. A simpler screening test, called the sugar water test, applies the same principle of mixing blood with sugar and observing for hemolysis.

Acidified Serum Test (Ham Test).

Definitive diagnosis of PNH used to depend on a positive acidified serum test (Ham, 1939; Dacie, 1991). In acidified serum, complement is activated by the alternative pathway, binds to red cells, and lyses the abnormal PNH cells that are unusually susceptible to complement. The patient's washed red cells are mixed with ABO-compatible normal serum (fresh or properly stored) and acid; after an hour's incubation at 37°C, the PNH cells are lysed, as indicated in Table 31–3. The patient's own serum may or may not result in lysis, depending on residual complement, and the other tubes provide controls.

In PNH, usually 10–50% of the cells are lysed. If lysis also occurs with heat-inactivated serum, the test is not positive, as spherocytic or antibody-sensitized cells may be responsible. A positive acidified serum test occurs in congenital dyserythropoietic anemia, type II (CDA-II) or HEM-PAS (see earlier discussion). In this situation, however, lysis does not occur with the patient's own serum, and only with about 30% of normal sera. Also, the sugar water screening test is negative in CDA-II.

Flow cytometry using immunofluorescent staining of red cells with a monoclonal antibody against deficient proteins such as CD55, CD58, and CD59 is gradually becoming the standard method of diagnosing PNH. Granulocytes provide excellent diagnostic targets for flow cytometry.

The gene responsible for PNH phenotype has been identified on the X chromosome and designated phosphatidyl inositol glycan A or *PIG-A* . More than 120 somatic mutations of the *PIG-A* gene have been described.

Hemoglobin Disorders

There are two main groups of inherited disorders of hemoglobins: (1) structural variants, with defects in the structure of and (2) thalassemias, with defects in the synthesis of a globin chain. There is an overlap between these groups; 44 structural variants also have a thalassemic phenotype with decreased synthesis, and hence, level of the abnormal globin chain. Hereditary persistence of fetal hemoglobin (HPFH) is related to the thalassemias, although the phenotype is not clearly thalassemic. The majority of thalassemia involves α- or β-globin chains. δ-, γ- and εγδβ-thalassemias are known, but clinically less significant.

Normal Hemoglobins

The heme group is identical in all hemoglobins. The protein part of the molecule is a tetramer, made up of two dimers; each dimer contains an α-like and a β-like globin. From the combination of two α-like and four β-like globins three distinct hemoglobins are found postnatally in normal individuals, and there are three additional embryonic hemoglobins, present only in the first 3 months of gestation (Fig. 31–13).

Hb A ($\alpha_2\beta_2$). Hemoglobin A is the major normal adult hemoglobin, comprising about 97% of the total. It consists of two identical α-chains, each with 141 amino acids; and two identical β-chains, with 146 amino acids each. Each chain is linked with one heme group. The molecule is ellipsoidal, with the four heme groups at the surface of the molecule, where they function by combining reversibly with oxygen.

Hb F ($\alpha_2\gamma_2$). Hemoglobin F is the major hemoglobin of the fetus and the newborn infant. The increased oxygen affinity of fetal blood versus adult blood is due to its lower affinity for 2,3-diphosphoglycerate (DPG). The two α-chains are identical to those of Hb A, while the two γ-chains, with 146 amino acid residues, differ from β-chains. In normal individuals, Hb F has two types of γ-chains, which differ by one amino acid, having either

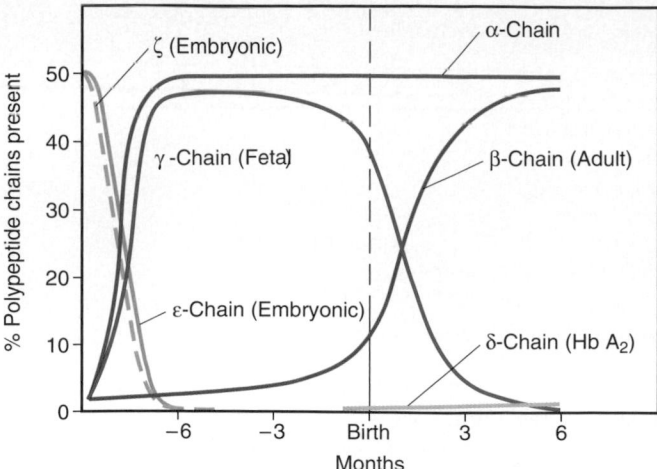

Figure 31–13 Relative proportions of polypeptide chains of hemoglobin present during fetal and neonatal life. (From Bunn, 1977.)

CHAPTER: 31 Erythrocytic Disorders

alanine ($^A\gamma$) or glycine ($^G\gamma$) at position 136. The ratio of $^G\gamma$ to $^A\gamma$ chains changes from 3 : 1 at birth to 2 : 3 by age 12 months (Weatherall, 2001). There is a common polymorphism of the $^A\gamma$ gene, in which threonine replaces isoleucine at position 75. This Hb F variant is called Hb F Sardinia and is without functional abnormalities.

During fetal life, Hb F predominates, as γ-chain production is high. β-chain production begins before the twentieth week of prenatal life, so that Hb A is 10% of the total between 20–35 weeks and 15–40% at the time of birth. After birth, smaller amounts of Hb F are produced; by 6 months Hb F is usually less than 8% and by 12 months it is less than 5% in about 90% of infants. Between 12–24 months of age, Hb F is usually less than 3%, but varies from 3–10% in about 20% of infants. After the age of 2 years, Hb F is normally less than 2% in children. Only traces of Hb F (< 1.0%) are found in adults. This switch from γ-globin to β-globin is much delayed in sickle cell patients, who might not reach their stable Hb F level until adolescence (Huisman, 1980). A similar delay in decline in Hb F is also seen in thalassemia trait (Schroter, 1981). During fetal life, all red cells produce and contain Hb F, whereas in adults only 3–5% do so (Weatherall, 2001). The Hb F-containing cells (F cells) may increase in number when reactivation of Hb F synthesis occurs in normal pregnancy and in some disorders of erythropoiesis, particularly chronic bone marrow failure syndromes. Approximately 10% of total hemoglobin is a negatively charged variant of Hb F, designated Hb F_1, owing to post-translational acetylation of the amino-terminal ends of the γ-chains.

Elevated Hb F is found in a few hemoglobinopathies, in β- and $\delta\beta$-thalassemias, and in hereditary persistence of fetal hemoglobin (HPFH). In certain acquired hematopoietic disorders, the Hb F level may also be elevated. These include megaloblastic anemia, myelofibrosis, aplastic anemia, paroxysmal nocturnal hemoglobinuria, refractory anemias, leukemias, and solid tumors (up to 5–10%). In the second trimester of pregnancy there could be a slight increase and, in hydatidiform moles, a more significant increase, up to 6%. The highest levels of Hb F are found in juvenile chronic myeloid leukemia, Fanconi anemia and erythroleukemia (30–50%).

Hb A_2 ($\alpha_2\delta_2$). Hemoglobin A_2 accounts for 1.5–3.5% of normal adult hemoglobin. Its two α-chains are the same as in Hb A; its two δ-chains differ from β-chains in only 10 of their 146 amino acids. Less efficient transcription of the δ-globin gene compared to the β-gene is the result of differences in the promoter area (Delvoye, 1993; Tang, 1997) and the

second intron (Kosche, 1985). δ-Chain synthesis begins late in fetal life. The level of Hb A_2 gradually increases during the first year of life, at which time the adult level is reached.

Increased Hb A_2 is seen almost exclusively in β-thalassemias. It rarely reaches 6% and never more than 12%. Hb A_2 is occasionally increased in hyperthyroidism and megaloblastic anemia and it has been reported to be increased in sickle cell trait (Whitten, 1981) and sickle cell disease, but the increase is only modest and the level stays below 4.5%. It may be decreased in iron deficiency anemia and α-thalassemia. If an individual with β-thalassemia trait has concomitant severe iron deficiency, the increase in Hb A_2 might be dampened down and appear equivocal; in these instances, retesting should be performed after the iron deficiency is corrected. Because of its developmental delay, Hb A_2 might not be useful in diagnosing β-thalassemia trait in young infants.

Embryonic Hemoglobins. The zeta (ζ) chain is the embryonic analogue of the α-chain and may combine with epsilon (ε) chains to form Hb Gower-1 ($\zeta_2\varepsilon_2$) or with γ-chains to form Hb Portland ($\zeta_2\gamma_2$). The ε-chain is the embryonic counterpart of the γ, β, and δ-chains and combines with α-chains to form Hb Gower-2 ($\alpha_2\varepsilon_2$). Hb Gower-1, Hb Portland, and Hb Gower-2 are the embryonic hemoglobins and are found in normal human embryos and fetuses with a gestational age of less than 3 months.

The Globin Gene Clusters. Globin synthesis is controlled by two separate gene clusters. The ζ gene and two α genes (α-like globins) together with nonfunctioning pseudogenes are on chromosome 16. Genes for the ε, δ, β and the two γ-chains (β-like globins) and two pseudogenes are located on chromosome 11 (Fig. 31–14). Note that there are two functioning α genes on a haploid chromosome (balanced by only one β gene). The different globin genes evolved from a common ancestor by gene duplication. There is considerable polymorphism of regulatory sequences within these clusters, accounting for normal variations and wide phenotypic differences in hemoglobinopathy and thalassemia syndromes.

Glycosylated Hemoglobins. The term glycation or glycosylation implies the linkage of a sugar to a protein. Approximately 5% of Hb A undergoes post-translational glycosylation resulting in linkage of sugars to serine, asparagine, and hydroxylysine residues. The glycosylated hemoglobins have been designated Hb A_{Ia} (< 1%), Hb A_{Ib} (< 2%), and Hb A_{Ic} (3%). Glycosylation of hemoglobin increases linearly over the 120-day life span of the red cell. Hb A_{Ic} contains a molecule of glucose attached nonenzymatically by a ketoamine linkage to the amino-terminal amino group of each β-chain. Hb A_{Ic} is elevated two- to threefold in patients with diabetes mellitus. The measurement of Hb A_{Ic} has been used as an index of metabolic control of diabetes during the preceding 2–3 months (Bunn, 1994). Hb A_{Ic} may be falsely decreased in conditions associated with rapid red cell turnover, such as hemolytic anemia.

Laboratory Investigation of Hemoglobinopathies and Thalassemias

Current recommendations include CBC by a modern cell counter with accurate MCV, RBC, MCH and MCHC values, Hb H test, ferritin, HPLC for Hb A_2 and Hb F measurement and detection of Hb variants, followed by alkaline and acid electrophoresis when a variant is found and additional studies (Sickledex) as necessary (Clarke, 2000).

Cation-Exchange HPLC. Numerous automated systems have been developed in the last 20 years and HPLC is now the method of choice for initial screening of hemoglobin variants and to separate and determine percentages of hemoglobin A, hemoglobin A_2, and hemoglobin F (Wilson, 1983). A cation-exchange HPLC system, Bio-Rad Variant by Bio-Rad Laboratories, emerged as the leading commercial kit. Resolution of this system is claimed to be similar to that of isoelectric focusing, and data

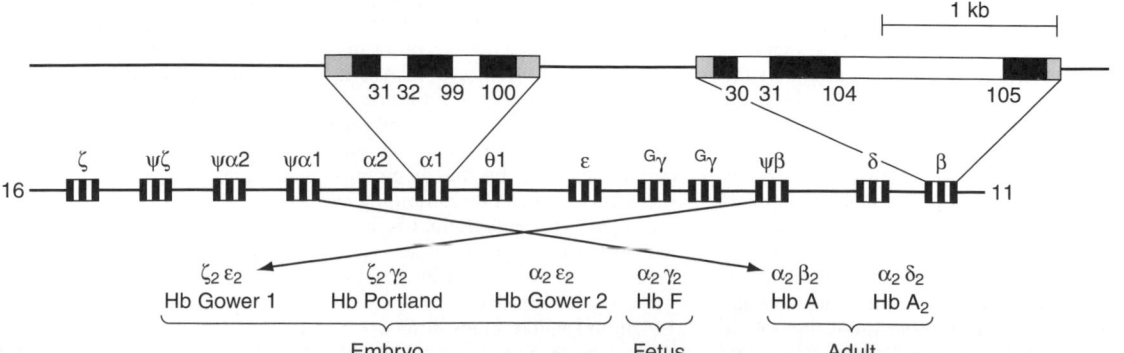

Figure 31–14 The α- and β-globin gene clusters on chromosome 16 and 11, respectively. In the extended α- and β-globin genes the introns are shaded dark, the 5' and 3' noncoding regions are green, and the exons are unshaded. (From Weatherall DJ, Clegg JB: The Thalassaemia Syndromes, 4th edn. Oxford, Blackwell Scientific Publications, 2001. By permission.)

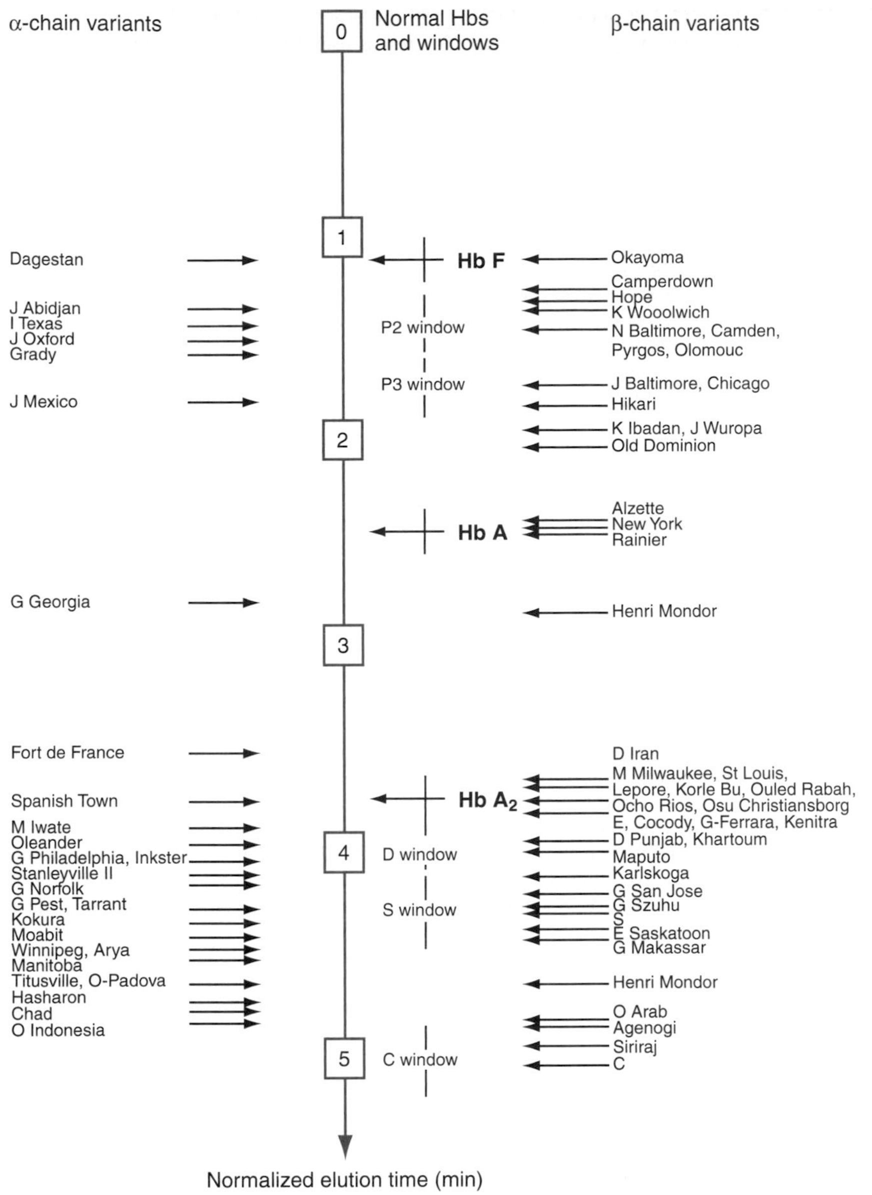

α-chain variants | Normal Hbs and windows | β-chain variants

Figure 31–15 Elution times of 74 hemoglobins. Elution times were normalized to a reference value of 3.8 minutes for Hb A₂. Cation-exchange HPLC separation by the Bio-Rad Variant system, using the β Thalassemia Short program. (From Riou, 1997.)

0

1 — Hb F

Dagestan →
Okayoma ←
Camperdown ←
Hope ←
K Wooolwich ←
N Baltimore, Camden, Pyrgos, Olomouc ←

P2 window

J Abidjan →
I Texas →
J Oxford →
Grady →

P3 window

J Mexico →
J Baltimore, Chicago ←
Hikari ←
K Ibadan, J Wuropa ←
Old Dominion ←

2

Hb A
Alzette ←
New York ←
Rainier ←

G Georgia →
Henri Mondor ←

3

Fort de France →
D Iran ←
M Milwaukee, St Louis, ←
Lepore, Korle Bu, Ouled Rabah, ←
Ocho Rios, Osu Christiansborg ←

Spanish Town → Hb A₂
E, Cocody, G-Ferrara, Kenitra ←

M Iwate →
Oleander →
D Punjab, Khartoum ←

G Philadelphia, Inkster →
Maputo ←

4 — D window

Stanleyville II →
Karlskoga ←

G Norfolk →
G San Jose ←

G Pest, Tarrant →
G Szuhu ←

S window

Kokura →
S ←

Moabit →
E Saskatoon ←

Winnipeg, Arya →
G Makassar ←

Manitoba →
Titusville, O-Padova →
Henri Mondor ←

Hasharon →
Chad →
O Arab ←
Agenogi ←

O Indonesia →
Siriraj ←

5 — C window
C ←

Normalized elution time (min)

banks of retention times are available (Figs 31–15 and 31–16) (Riou, 1997; Globin Gene Server). Variants detected by HPLC are confirmed by an alternative technique, such as electrophoresis.

Hemoglobin Electrophoresis and Isoelectric Focusing.

Hemoglobin molecules in an alkaline solution have a net negative charge and move toward the anode in an electrophoretic system. A practical method for routine hemoglobin electrophoresis is cellulose acetate at alkaline pH (Briere, 1965). It is rapid and reproducible and separates hemoglobins S, F, C, A, and A₂ (Figs 31–17 and 31–18). Quantification of the major bands is easily accomplished. Those with an electrophoretic mobility greater than that of Hb A at pH 8.6 are known as the 'fast hemoglobins'; these include, in the order of increasing mobility, hemoglobins K, J, Bart's, N, I and H. Hemoglobins A₂, C, E and O Arab at the slow end are unresolved from each other, as are S, D, G, and Lepore. Citrate agar electrophoresis at an acid pH (Milner, 1975) provides ready separation of hemoglobins that migrate together on cellulose acetate: S from D and G, and C from E and O (Fig. 31–19). Isoelectric focusing separates hemoglobins based on their isoelectric point along a pH gradient with a high resolution (Fig. 31–20). Capillary isoelectric focusing is a rapidly developing automated system with a performance similar to that of HPLC (Mario, 1997).

Alkali Denaturation Test for Hb F. Fetal hemoglobin resists alkali denaturation; adult hemoglobin does not (Singer, 1951). A hemolysate is alkalinized and then neutralized, and the denatured adult hemoglobin is precipitated by ammonium sulfate. A filtrate will then contain only alkali-resistant hemoglobin, which is measured and expressed as a percentage of the total. The modification of Betke (1959) is reliable for Hb F less than 15%, but underestimates Hb F at higher levels. The reference interval is 0.2–1.0% for adults. This method has been largely replaced by HPLC estimation of Hb F.

Acid Elution Slide Test for F Cells. The modification of the original method of Kleihauer and Betke by Shepard (1962) is useful for analyzing the distribution of Hb F among red cells. Hemoglobins other than Hb F are eluted from the red cells on an air-dried blood film by a citric acid–phosphate buffer (pH 3.3). Only Hb F remains in the fixed red cells, and the distribution can be determined after staining. In normal adults, almost all red cells appear as ghosts; 1–5% of red cells contain residual hemoglobin (Hb F).

In most types of HPFH, the Hb F is distributed evenly among red cells (pancellular distribution). In all other conditions, such as thalassemia or a hemoglobinopathy, and in the less common Swiss-type HPFH the distribution of the Hb F is heterogeneous or uneven among red cells (heterocellular distribution). Flow cytometry is also used to detect F cells.

Hb A₂ Quantitation. Hemoglobin A₂ quantitation is challenging for two reasons: (1) its level is low with a narrow range and only modest increase in disease, requiring a high degree of precision, and (2) hemoglobin variants with similar charge or retention time interfere with its estimation. Several laboratory methods of varying accuracy and precision are being used. Cation-exchange HPLC (Head, 2004), microcolumn chromatography (Steinberg, 1991) and cellulose acetate electrophoresis with elution are considered to be sufficiently precise. Densitometry of electrophoretic bands on cellulose acetate membrane is unreliable (Schmidt, 1975). Increasingly, cation-exchange HPLC is the method of choice, which also provides accurate measurement of Hb F along with separation of hemoglobin variants. In the presence of Hb S, however, its level is falsely elevated, because Hb S adducts have similar retention times (Suh, 1996).

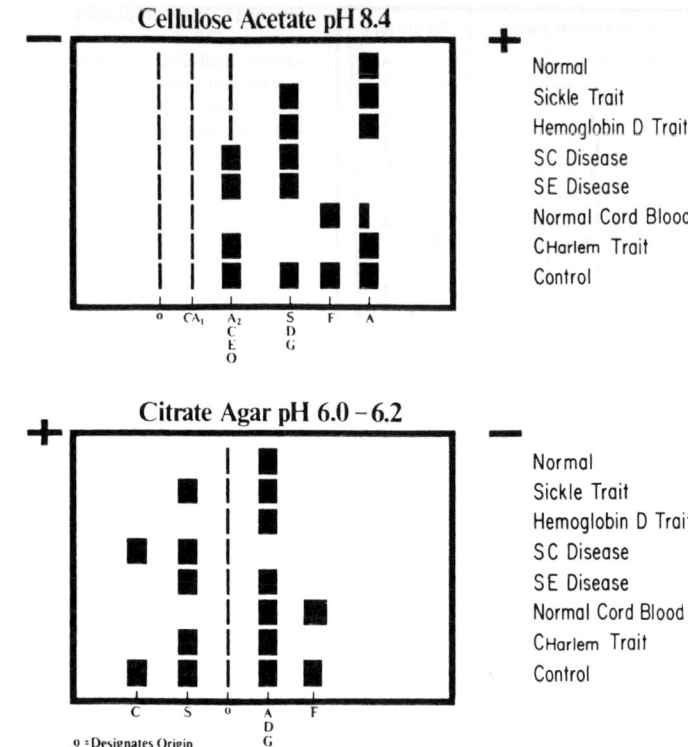

Figure 31–19 Hemoglobin electrophoresis. Comparison of various hemoglobin samples on cellulose acetate (at pH 8.4) and citrate agar (at pH 6), showing relative mobilities. The control is a composite sample. The relative amounts of hemoglobin are not necessarily proportional to the size of the band. (Redrawn from Schmidt RM, Brosious EF: Basic Laboratory Methods of Hemoglobinopathy Detection, 6th edn. Atlanta, U.S. Department of Health, Education and Welfare, Centers for Disease Control, [HEW Publ. No. (CDC) 77-8266] 1976.)

when flying at very high altitude in unpressurized airplanes. Slightly increased incidence of hematuria, impaired ability to concentrate urine and bacteriuria in women, have been reported. Sickle cell trait confers protection to children from the lethal effects of falciparum malaria, which accounts for the major distribution of Hb S in central Africa.

The stained blood film appears normal, except perhaps for a few target cells. Blood cell counts are normal. The sickle cell preparation is positive, and almost all the red cells eventually sickle. The solubility test is positive.

Hemoglobin separation shows 60% Hb A, 40% Hb S, normal Hb F, normal to slightly increased Hb A_2, up to 4.5%.

The proportion of Hb S is decreased in the presence of α-thalassemia; Hb S is less than 35% when one α-gene is deleted, and less than 29% when two genes are lost (Head, 2004). In the latter, cells are hypochromic and microcytic. Since 27% of African Americans carry the α^+-thalassemia gene, it is not surprising that this diagnostic dilemma is quite common. Hb S may also be diminished in iron and folate deficiency.

Sickle Cell Disease (HB SS)

Homozygous Hb S disease is a serious chronic hemolytic anemia, first manifested in early childhood and often fatal before the age of 30 years. With modern medical care many patients live longer, but the median age of death in the US is still only in the 40s. Hemoglobin S is found mostly in the black population; 1 of every 600 black persons in the US has sickle cell anemia (Steinberg, 1999).

In hemoglobin S, (β6 glu→val) the glutamic acid in the sixth position on the β-chain is replaced by valine. Hemoglobin S is freely soluble when fully oxygenated; when oxygen is removed, Hb S polymerizes, with formation of tactoids (fluid crystals) that are rigid and deform the cell into the shape that gave the cell its name. A strong interaction between the side chain of β6 valine and the hydrophobic pocket of β85 phenylalanine and 88 leucine of another Hb S molecule is probably the basis of polymer formation. In homozygous Hb S disease, sickling occurs at physiologic oxygen tensions, and the rigidity of the red cells is responsible for the hemolysis as well as for most of the complications. These irreversibly sickled cells result from membrane reorganization during repeated episodes of sickling and unsickling in addition to cell dehydration that markedly reduces cellular deformability (Mohandas, 1993). Sickle cells contain high calcium levels, which stimulate potassium and water loss

Table 31–4 Functional Classification of Hemoglobin Variants

I. Homozygous: Hemoglobin polymorphisms: the variants that are most common

Hb S	$\alpha_2\beta_2^{6\,Val}$	Severe hemolytic anemia: sickling
Hb C	$\alpha_2\beta_2^{6\,Lys}$	Mild hemolytic anemia
Hb D Punjab	$\alpha_2\beta_2^{121\,Gln}$	No anemia
Hb E	$\alpha_2\beta_2^{26\,Lys}$	Mild microcytic anemia

II. Heterozygous: Hemoglobin variants causing functional aberrations or hemolytic anemia in the heterozygous state

A. Hemoglobins associated with methemoglobinemia and cyanosis

Hb M Boston $\alpha_2^{58\,Tyr}\beta_2$
Hb M Iwate $\alpha_2^{87\,Tyr}\beta_2$
Hb M Saskatoon $\alpha_2\beta_2^{63\,Tyr}$
Hb M Milwaukee $\alpha_2\beta_2^{67\,Glu}$
Hb M Hyde Park $\alpha_2\beta_2^{92\,Tyr}$
Hb FM Osaka $\alpha_2\gamma_2^{63\,Tyr}$
Hb FM Fort Ripley $\alpha_2\gamma_2^{92\,Tyr}$

B. Hemoglobins associated with altered oxygen affinity

1. Increased affinity and polycythemia

Hb Chesapeake $\alpha_2^{92\,Leu}\beta_2$
Hb J Capetown $\alpha_2^{92\,Gln}\beta_2$
Hb Malmo $\alpha_2\beta_2^{97\,Gln}$
Hb Yakima $\alpha_2\beta_2^{99\,His}$
Hb Kempsey $\alpha_2\beta_2^{99\,Asn}$
Hb Y psi (Ypsilanti) $\alpha_2\beta_2^{99\,Tyr}$
Hb Hiroshima $\alpha_2\beta_2^{146\,Asp}$
Hb Rainier $\alpha_2\beta_2^{145\,Cys}$
Hb Bethesda $\alpha_2\beta_2^{145\,His}$

2. Decreased affinity – may have mild anemia or cyanosis

Hb Kansas $\alpha_2\beta_2^{102\,Thr}$
Hb Titusville $\alpha_2^{94\,Asn}\beta_2$
Hb Providence $\alpha_2\beta_2^{82\,Asn}$
Hb Agenogi $\alpha_2\beta_2^{90\,Lys}$
Hb Beth Israel $\alpha_2\beta_2^{102\,Ser}$
Hb Yoshizuka $\alpha_2\beta_2^{108\,Asp}$

C. Unstable hemoglobins

1. Hb may precipitate as Heinz bodies after splenectomy: 'congenital Heinz body anemia'

a. Severe hemolysis: no improvement after splenectomy

Hb Bibba $\alpha_2^{136\,Pro}\beta_2$
Hb Hammersmith $\alpha_2\beta_2^{42\,Ser}$
Hb Bristol $\alpha_2\beta_2^{67\,Asp}$
Hb Olmsted $\alpha_2\beta_2^{141\,Arg}$

b. Severe hemolysis: improvement after splenectomy

Hb Torino $\alpha_2^{43\,Val}\beta_2$
Hb Ann Arbor $\alpha_2^{80\,Arg}\beta_2$
Hb Genova $\alpha_2\beta_2^{28\,Pro}$
Hb Shepherd's Bush $\alpha_2\beta_2^{74\,Asp}$
Hb Koln $\alpha_2\beta_2^{98\,Met}$
Hb Wein $\alpha_2\beta_2^{130\,Asp}$

c. Mild hemolysis: intermittent exacerbations

Hb L-Ferrara $\alpha_2^{47\,Gly}\beta_2$
Hb Hasharon $\alpha_2^{47\,His}\beta_2$
Hb Leiden $\alpha_2\beta_2^{6\,or\,7}$ (Glu deleted)
Hb Freiburg $\alpha_2\beta_2^{23}$ (Val deleted)
Hb Seattle $\alpha_2\beta_2^{70\,Asp}$
Hb Louisville $\alpha_2\beta_2^{42\,Leu}$
Hb Zurich $\alpha_2\beta_2^{63\,Arg}$
Hb Gun Hill $\alpha_2\beta_2^{91-97}$ (5 a. a. deleted)

d. No disease

Hb Etobicoke $\alpha_2^{84\,Arg}\beta_2$
Hb Dakar $\alpha_2^{112\,Gln}\beta_2$
Hb Sogn $\alpha_2\beta_2^{14\,Arg}$
Hb Tacoma $\alpha_2\beta_2^{30\,Ser}$

2. Tetramers of normal chains: appear in thalassemias

Hb Bart's γ_4
Hb H β_4
Hb α_4

Modified, in part, from Winslow, 1983, pp 2281–2317.

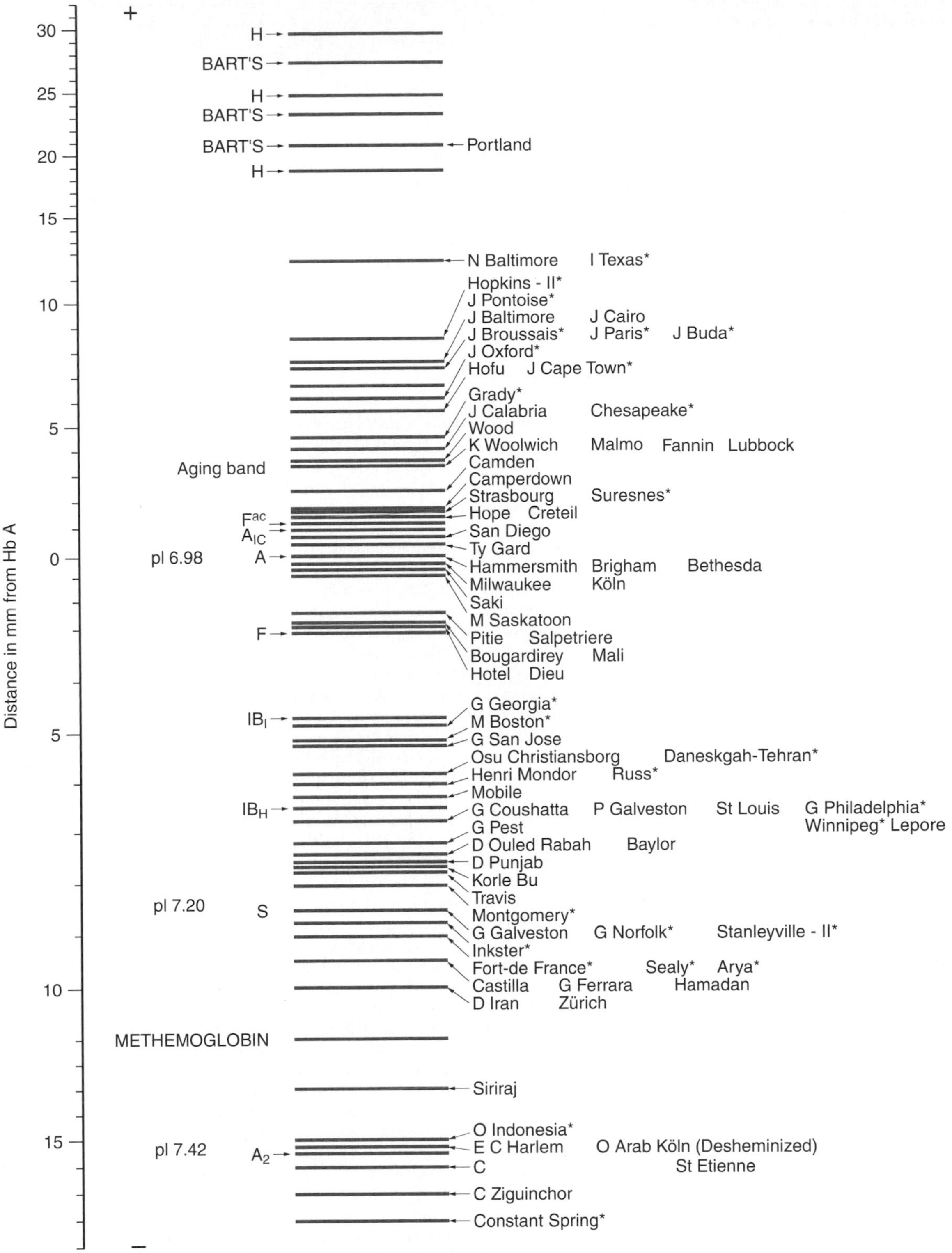

Figure 31–20 Comparison of 57 hemoglobin variants by isoelectric focusing. Asterisk denotes α-chain variants. (Reprinted from J Chromatogr Biomed Appl, Vol. 227, Bassett P, Braconnier F, Rosa J, An update on electrophoretic and chromatographic methods in the diagnosis of hemoglobinopatries, pp 267–304, Copyright 1982, with permission from Elsevier.)

Distance in mm from Hb A

+

30 — H →
— BART'S →
25 — H →
— BART'S →
20 — BART'S → ← Portland
— H →
15

— N Baltimore   I Texas*
    Hopkins - II*
    J Pontoise*
10 — J Baltimore   J Cairo
    J Broussais*   J Paris*   J Buda*
    J Oxford*
    Hofu   J Cape Town*
    Grady*
5 — J Calabria   Chesapeake*
    Wood
    K Woolwich   Malmo   Fannin   Lubbock
    Camden
Aging band   Camperdown
    Strasbourg   Suresnes*
Fac →   Hope   Creteil
AIc →   San Diego
pI 6.98   A →   Ty Gard
0   Hammersmith   Brigham   Bethesda
    Milwaukee   Köln
    Saki
    M Saskatoon
F →   Pitie   Salpetriere
    Bougardirey   Mali
    Hotel   Dieu

    G Georgia*
IBI →   M Boston*
5   G San Jose
    Osu Christiansborg   Daneskgah-Tehran*
    Henri Mondor   Russ*
    Mobile
IBH →   G Coushatta   P Galveston   St Louis   G Philadelphia*
    G Pest   Winnipeg* Lepore
    D Ouled Rabah   Baylor
    D Punjab
    Korle Bu
    Travis
pI 7.20   S   Montgomery*
    G Galveston   G Norfolk*   Stanleyville - II*
    Inkster*
    Fort-de France*   Sealy*   Arya*
10   Castilla   G Ferrara   Hamadan
    D Iran   Zürich

METHEMOGLOBIN

← Siriraj

    O Indonesia*
15   pI 7.42   A2 →   E C Harlem   O Arab Köln (Desheminized)
    C   St Etienne
    ← C Ziguinchor
    ← Constant Spring*

−

IV

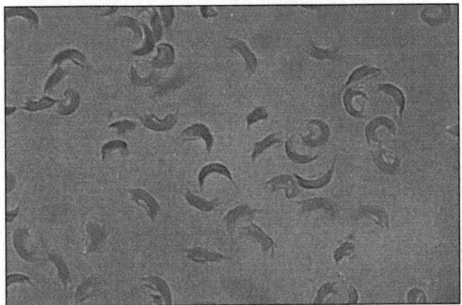

Figure 31–21 Sickle cell preparation, in sodium metabisulfate; sickle cell anemia. Even in sickle cell trait, all cells eventually sickle.

(Gardos effect) and exaggerate cell dehydration (Weatherall, 1999). The hemolytic component is mostly extracellular and is caused by clustering of band 3 of the cell membrane, with the consequence of increased IgG binding and recognition by macrophages. Integrins ($\alpha_4\beta_1$) on the sickle cell surface attach to fibronectin and adhesion molecules expressed on endothelial cells; this is enhanced by inflammatory cytokines, von Willebrand factor and platelet activation and together these interactions cause vaso-occlusion.

Complications. In early childhood, bilateral painful swelling of the dorsa of the hands or feet occurs as a result of sickling and capillary stasis; this is known as the *hand–foot syndrome* or sickle cell dactylitis. It lasts about 2 weeks, is accompanied by changes of periostitis as observed by X-ray, and does not occur after the age of 4.

The spleen is central to three complications: A *sequestration crisis* refers to sudden pooling of blood and rapid enlargement of the spleen, resulting in hypovolemic shock. This may occur in early childhood when

Table 31–5 Prevalence of Common Hemoglobin Disorders among African Americans

	(%)
Traits	
Silent α-thalassemia (αα/–α)	24
Hb AS	8.6
α-thalassemia trait (–α/–α)	5.7
Hb AC	2.4
β-thalassemia trait	1.5
HPFH	0.1
Hbs D and G	0.026
All others	0.3
Sickling disorders	
Hb SS	0.16
Hb S/C	0.13
Hb S/thal	0.06
Hb S/HPFH	0.004
Other disorders	
Hb CC	0.02
Hb C/β-thalassemia	0.02
Homozygous β-thalassemia	0.005

Data from Schneider, 1976, Pierce, 1977, and Motulsky, 1973.

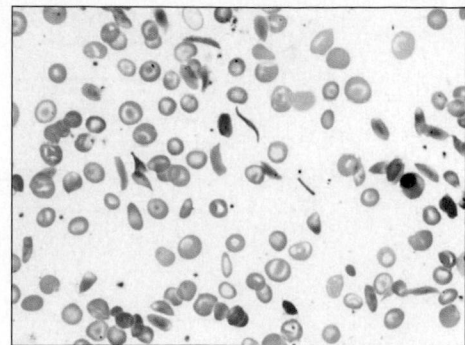

Figure 31–22 Blood film, sickle cell anemia. The erythrocytes are far from one another, suggesting a severe anemia. Numerous pointed sickle cells and target cells are present. Close to the nucleated red blood cell, elliptical cells are seen. These cells have a dense center, instead of the usual central pallor, suggesting that they are incipient sickle cells. (× 500)

splenomegaly is present and is often preceded by infection. *Functional asplenia* (Pearson, 1969) consists of inadequate antibody responses under some conditions and an impaired ability of the reticuloendothelial system to clear bacteria and particulate material from the blood, probably owing to reticuloendothelial blockade. This may partly explain the increased risk of infection in children with the disease. Salmonellal and pneumococcal infections are unusually prevalent in children with sickle cell anemia. Vaso-occlusive episodes result in progressive infarction, fibrosis, and contraction of the spleen – so-called *autosplenectomy*. Though splenomegaly is present in childhood, a small fibrotic remnant is the rule in the adult.

From early childhood, patients cannot produce a concentrated urine, apparently as a result of anoxic damage in the medullae of the kidneys. Hematuria as a result of papillary necrosis is common. Renal insufficiency occurs in 5–20% of adults (Steinberg, 1999).

Vaso-occlusive crises are debilitating episodes of abdominal and bone or joint pain, accompanied by fever, which are probably due to plugging of small blood vessels by masses of sickled cells. Bone necrosis occurs in 10–50% of patients and may be a focus for salmonellal osteomyelitis. Acute chest syndrome represents episodes of acute chest pain often associated with a new infiltrate in the chest film. Approximately 40% of patients experience at least one episode of acute chest syndrome. Although an infectious etiology has been suspected in earlier studies, fat embolism is now considered to play a major role in this syndrome. The various complications as a result of recurring vaso-occlusive crises involve many body organs (Steinberg, 1999).

Aplastic crises can occasionally afflict any patient with chronic hemolytic anemia. A temporary failure of red cell production that would not be noticed in a person with a normal red cell life span will cause a serious fall in hemoglobin concentration in hemolytic anemia. This may be a result of infection, particularly parvovirus B19, exposure to toxic drugs, or folic acid deficiency; sometimes no cause can be found. *Hemolytic crises* due to a further increase in hemolysis are rare.

Diagnosis. The anemia is normochromic and normocytic; polychromasia is increased and nucleated red blood cells are present. Sickle cells are almost always found in the stained smear (Fig. 31–22). Target cells are numerous, and Howell–Jolly and Pappenheimer bodies are regularly seen in older children and adults as a result of asplenia. The microhematocrit as an estimate of degree of anemia is unreliable because of excessive plasma trapping. Neutrophilia and thrombocytosis are usual. The marrow shows normoblastic hyperplasia.

No Hb A is found if the patient has not been transfused recently; over 80% of the hemoglobin is Hb S, 1– 20% Hb F, and 2–4.5% Hb A$_2$ (Wrightstone, 1974). The fetal hemoglobin is distributed unevenly among the red cells. Hb S and several D and G hemoglobins have the same electrophoretic mobility at alkaline pH, but of these, only Hb S gives a positive sickling test.

Hemoglobin SC Disease. The frequency of Hb SC disease is almost the same as that of Hb SS disease in African American. It causes a mild

hemolytic anemia. Crises are less frequent and less painful than in sickle cell anemia. The onset is usually in childhood, but it might be undetected until later in life. The life expectancy is only modestly shortened. The body habitus is normal or stocky in contrast to the asthenic features in sickle cell anemia. Splenomegaly might be the only finding by physical examination. Fatigue, dyspnea on effort, frequent upper respiratory infections, attacks of mild jaundice, and arthralgias are seen. Constant hip and low back pain may be present with aseptic necrosis of the head of the femur. Hematuria from renal medullary infarction and splenic infarcts has been described. In pregnancy, crises are more frequent and there is an increase in thrombotic tendency, which can cause massive thromboembolism and sudden death following childbirth. There is a higher incidence of retinopathy in Hb SC disease than in SS disease.

Anemia varies from moderate to very mild and is normochromic–normocytic. Anisocytosis and poikilocytosis are mild to severe, and target cells are numerous – up to 85% of the erythrocytes. Plump and angulated sickled cells are often present on the film. The sickling test is positive. Hb S is 50% and Hb C is slightly less. Hb F is usually under 2%. The proportions of hemoglobins are the same in patients with coexistent α-thalassemia (Steinberg, 1983).

Hb S/β-Thalassemia. This is the third most common sickling disorder after Hb SS and Hb SC in African Americans, and the most common one in people from the Mediterranean. It usually runs a milder course in black people, (usually S/β$^+$-thalassemia), but causes a severe sickling disorder with manifestations similar to those of sickle cell anemia in people of Italian, Turkish, or Greek descent.

In Hb S/β^0-thalassemia, Hb A is absent; Hb S is 75–90%, Hb F 5–20% and Hb A$_2$ 4–6%. This disorder clinically and hematologically resembles sickle cell disease, except for the spleen, which remains enlarged after childhood and into adult life. The main difference is that in Hb S/β^0-thalassemia, the MCV and MCH are decreased and the Hb A$_2$ might be significantly increased. Family study is often necessary for a clear distinction (Lehmann, 1977; Wrightstone, 1974). On the blood smear, pronounced microcytosis, variable hypochromia, and many target cells are present. As a consequence of reduced cellular hemoglobin, Hb S polymers are formed more slowly and fewer sickled cells are present on the smear.

In Hb S/β$^+$-thalassemia, Hb A is 15–30%; Hb S is over 50%; Hb F is 1–20%; and Hb A$_2$ is 4–6%. Though these individuals clinically may resemble those with sickle trait (Hb AS), in S/β$^+$-thalassemia the amount of Hb S always exceeds Hb A, while in Hb AS, Hb A always exceeds Hb S.

Hb SS/α-Thalassemia. Thirty to forty percent of patients with sickle cell anemia are heterozygous and 2–3% are homozygous for α$^+$-thalassemia (Higgs, 1982). MCV (83 fL in heterozygotes and 72 fL homozygotes) and MCH are decreased. Hemoglobin level is higher and reticulocyte count is significantly lower, as compared to sickle cell anemia. On the smear, sickled cells are uncommon similarly to Hb S/β^0-thalassemia. Although the anemia is less severe, the vaso-occlusive disease is not, and some studies even show increased morbidity and mortality. As described earlier, δ-chains successfully compete with the positively charged β^S-chains for limited amount of α-chains, and Hb A$_2$ levels increase. Hematologically this cannot be separated from Hb S/β^0-thalassemia (Table 31–6). Whenever microcytosis and increased Hb A$_2$ are present in sickle cell anemia, family or molecular studies are to be done to differentiate these entities.

Hemoglobin SD Disease (Hb S/D-Los Angeles). SD disease simulates but is less severe than sickle cell anemia, and thus may also resemble SC disease. It is occasionally seen in the African-American population. On routine (alkaline) electrophoresis, the pattern is

Table 31–6 Differential Diagnosis of Sickle Cell/Thalassemia Syndromes

Genotype	Clinical expression	Hb	MCV	Hb F	Hb A_2	Hb A
SS	Severe	7–8	85–95	2–20	2–4	
S/β^0-thal	Moderate to severe	8–10	65–75	5–20	4–6	
SS/α-thal	Moderate to severe	8–10	70–85	2–20	3–5	
S/HPFH	Asymptomatic to mild	13–14	75–85	20–30	1–3	
S/β^+-thal	Mild to moderate	11–12	70–80	1–13	3–6	10–30

Modified from Bunn, 1986 and Steinberg, 2001.

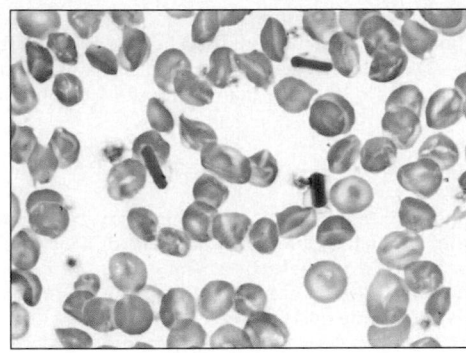

Figure 31–23 Hemoglobin C disease, after splenectomy. Prior to splenectomy the only morphologic abnormality was the presence of target cells. After splenectomy, Howell–Jolly bodies and hemoglobin crystals, such as that in the center, were present. Note that almost all of the hemoglobin in this particular cell is in the dark bar, and the membrane is still visible. Some such crystals are distinctly hexagonal. ($\times$1000)

indistinguishable from sickle cell anemia because Hb S and Hb D cannot be separated. Agar gel electrophoresis at pH 6.2 will separate Hb S and Hb D.

Hb S/O Arab. Compound heterozygotes of Hb S and Hb O Arab (β121 glu→lys) have a severe sickling disorder. Hb O Arab is found in black and Arabic people. Hb E and a few other, less frequent β variants also cause sickling disorders with Hb S. Coexistence of an α-chain variant and sickle cell trait does not cause a sickling disorder.

Other Common β-Chain Variants

Hb C Trait. (β6 glu→lys) Hemoglobin C is prevalent in West Africans and in about 2–3% of black people. The heterozygous state (Hb AC) is asymptomatic, without anemia, with normal MCV and normal red cell life span. The MCHC might be slightly elevated. Target cells are present on blood film. Hb C makes up about 40% of the total hemoglobin. When microcytosis is present, it is usually caused by coexistent α-thalassemia and Hb C is reduced to 38%, 32% and 24% in patients with three, two and one α-gene, respectively (Huisman, 1977).

Hb C Disease. Homozygous Hb C disease is a mild hemolytic anemia with splenomegaly that is often asymptomatic but occasionally results in jaundice and abdominal discomfort. Life expectancy is normal. In the US, 0.02% of black people have Hb C disease (Schneider, 1976). Reticulocytosis is low for the degree of anemia. The anemia is largely a consequence of low oxygen affinity of Hb C (Bunn, 1986) and should not be treated. The MCV is normal or decreased, and the MCHC is normal or increased. Numerous target cells with an admixture of microspherocytes and minimal polychromasia are seen in the blood. Osmotic fragility is biphasic, with both increased and decreased fragility, but is not used in the diagnosis today. Hexagonal or rod-shaped crystals may be seen in erythrocytes in the stained smear, especially after splenectomy or after slow drying of the smear (Fig. 31–23). As opposed to Hb S, crystals of Hb C tend to melt at low P_{O_2} and do not cause vaso-occlusive disease. The red cells are dehydrated (causing the increased MCHC), owing to loss of cations and water as a result of interaction of the abnormal hemoglobin with the red cell membrane. As a consequence, the cells are more rigid and less deformable than normal, increasing their likelihood of being trapped and destroyed in the spleen. Hb F is elevated at 2–4% and Hb A_2, when measured by HPLC, might be slightly increased; the remainder of hemoglobin is Hb C.

Hb C/β^+-Thalassemia. This occurs mainly in black people, in whom it tends to result in little disability, except for anemia in pregnancy. Red cell indices are typical of β-thalassemia trait but there is anisocytosis and 20–50% target cells. There is usually between 65–80% Hb C, 16–30% Hb A and 2–5% Hb F.

Hb C/β^0-Thalassemia. People of Mediterranean extraction usually have a moderately severe hemolytic anemia with β^0 or a severe β^+ genotype. This combination is extremely rare in the African population. Hb C/β^0-thalassemia may be difficult to distinguish from Hb C disease since Hb A is absent in both and there is an overlap in Hbs A_2 and F levels. Hb A_2 is elevated to about twice the normal and Hb F is elevated at 3–10%.

Hb D Los Angeles (Punjab) (β 121 glu→gln). This constitutes the most common D-variant in African Americans (< 0.02%). In the Punjab region of India heterozygosity reaches 3% (Bunn, 1986). Homozygotes have normal red cell indices, no evidence of hemolysis and 95% Hb D with normal Hbs F and A_2 (Bunn, 1986). Double heterozygotes for Hb D Punjab/β^0-thalassemia have a mild hemolytic anemia with thalassemic red cell indices and increased Hbs F and A_2.

The significance of Hb D Punjab is that compound heterozygosity with Hb S produces a moderately severe sickling disorder (see Hb SD Disease above). Other, less frequent D hemoglobins (D Iran, D Ibadan) and G hemoglobins do not cause sickling, a major difference for genetic counseling. D and G hemoglobins migrate with Hb S on alkaline electrophoresis, but are separated from S at acidic pH, migrating with Hb

A. It is more difficult to separate them from each other. Careful analysis of isoelectric focusing and HPLC are helpful in most cases.

Hb G Philadelphia (α 68asn→lys). This is the most common α-chain variant in black people (Schneider, 1976). Almost invariably, the linked α-gene is deleted ($-\alpha^G$). Simple heterozygotes ($-\alpha^G/\alpha\alpha$) have 30% Hb G and normal red cell indices, but double heterozygotes with α-gene deletion on the other chromosome as well ($-\alpha^G/-\alpha$) have 45% Hb G and a thalassemia trait phenotype. As with other α-chain variants, a minor hemoglobin, a combination of α^G with δ, is present close to Hb A_2 and helps to differentiate Hb G Philadelphia from β-chain variant G and D hemoglobins.

Hb E (β 26 glu→lys). This is probably the most prevalent hemoglobin variant worldwide and the third most common in the US, behind S and C. It is found primarily in Southeast Asia, especially in people of Thai and Burmese extraction, but is also found in black people and white people. Hb E is associated with a β-thalassemia phenotype as well as with a structurally abnormal globin chain. The mutation that causes amino acid substitution also activates a cryptic splice site that competes with the normal RNA splice donor site, and the normally processed RNA is decreased. In the laboratory, Hb E can be demonstrated to be unstable. It precipitates abnormally in the heat denaturation test and with isopropanol, yet this has no in vivo significance; the red cell survival is normal (Fairbanks, 1980).

Hb E Trait (Hb AE). Hb AE is asymptomatic, with borderline microcytosis (MCV = 84 ± 5) and no anemia. Hb A is 65–70% of the total hemoglobin, Hb E is 30%, and Hb F is normal. Coexistence of one α-thalassemia gene does not change any of the above parameters and can be proven only by DNA analysis. If two or three α-thalassemia genes are also present, the proportion of Hb E decreases to 21% and 14%, respectively. The proportion of Hb E is also significantly lower in iron deficiency.

Hemoglobin E Disease. This is also asymptomatic; it resembles a thalassemia trait, with microcytosis (average MCV = 70 fL), erythrocytosis, normal MCHC and slight anemia. Thus, Hb E behaves as an extremely mild thalassemia. The reticulocyte count is normal, but there are 20–80% target cells on the blood film. Hb E accounts for over 90% of the hemoglobin, with Hb F from 1–10% and no Hb A.

Hb E/β-Thalassemia. In sharp contrast with hemoglobin E disease, this is a severe condition. It is one of the most important thalassemia syndromes, most common in Southeast Asia. There is marked clinical variability; rarely, there are very few symptoms, but the usual picture is that of thalassemia intermedia or thalassemia major. Most of the thalassemia alleles are of the β^0 or severe β^+ variety. Ineffective erythropoiesis, a consequence of excess α-globins, red cell indices, red cell morphology and the clinical manifestations are quite similar to those in homozygous β-thalassemia. Hemoglobins E, F and A_2 are present. Hb F shows extreme variation, from 5–85%; the mean Hb F is 42% and Hb E is 58% (Steinberg, 2001).

Disorders of Hemoglobin Function and Stability

A number of amino acid substitutions occur in the heme pocket, where they either increase the stability of the methemoglobin form (Hb M) or alter the affinity of the heme for oxygen; the latter usually alters the stability of the molecule as well. Other substitutions affect the $\alpha\beta$ contact sites; these also can change stability and oxygen affinity of the molecule (Bunn, 1994).

IV

These functionally significant hemoglobinopathies are heterozygous; usually the concentration of the abnormal hemoglobin is less than 50%. Generally, the hemoglobins with abnormal α-chains form a smaller proportion of the total (10–25%) than do those with abnormal β-chains (35–50%).

Hemoglobins Associated with High Oxygen Affinity and Polycythemia

Eighty-six abnormal hemoglobins with high oxygen affinity that are associated with familial erythrocytosis are known today (Globin Gene Server). Some are listed in Table 31–4. The oxygen dissociation curve is shifted to the left. The P_{50}, the partial pressure of oxygen at which hemoglobin is 50% saturated, is decreased. Under physiologic conditions, the normal P_{50} of whole blood is 26 mmHg; in this disorder, it has ranged from 5–23 mmHg. Because the hemoglobin has high affinity for oxygen, the tissues are relatively hypoxic at any given P_{O_2}, resulting in increased erythropoietin production and polycythemia. These disorders are autosomal dominant; only heterozygotes have been described. The hemoglobin concentration has ranged from 15–23.8 g/dL. Measurement of oxygen affinity is required to establish the diagnosis (Bunn, 1986). Because the amino acid substitution is inside the molecule, often the abnormal hemoglobin is indistinguishable from Hb A on electrophoresis or HPLC.

Hemoglobin Chesapeake. An α-chain abnormality associated with mild asymptomatic polycythemia in a Caucasian family was first described in 1966 (Clegg). The features were similar to those of benign familial polycythemia. The abnormal hemoglobin, accounting for about 30% of the total, had an increased affinity for oxygen that resulted in significantly elevated hematocrit levels.

Hemoglobins Associated with Low Oxygen Affinity

There are far fewer variants with decreased oxygen affinity (see Table 31–4; Bunn, 1986). The hemoglobin–oxygen dissociation curve is shifted to the right (increased P_{50}). These individuals have mild 'anemia,' as they can unload more oxygen to the tissues and they simply do not need that much hemoglobin. A handful of variants with markedly decreased affinity are associated with cyanosis. In these, oxygen uptake is impaired in the lung and the level of deoxyhemoglobin is more than 5 g/dL, causing cyanosis. These patients have a slate gray color of their skin and mucous membranes. They have no anemia. Many of the unstable hemoglobins also have decreased oxygen affinity; however, the hemolytic state dominates the clinical picture.

Hemoglobin Kansas. This low-affinity hemoglobin, described in a Caucasian boy, had just the opposite property from Hb Chesapeake. The clinical features were cyanosis since infancy, normal arterial oxygen tension, and reduced oxygen saturation. Electrophoresis after conversion to methemoglobin allowed separation from Hb A (Reissman, 1961).

M Hemoglobins: Pseudocyanosis

Nine abnormal hemoglobins are associated with clinical methemoglobinemia and cyanosis that do not respond to methylthioninium chloride (methylene blue) (Globin Gene Server; Bunn, 1994). The color is similar to cyanosis, a brownish color, caused by methemoglobin. The common feature is that all have an amino acid substitution at or near the heme group, so that methemoglobin is unusually stable, and reduction to ferrous heme and hence reversible binding of oxygen are prevented. Methemoglobin constitutes no more than 3% of the total hemoglobin in normal humans.

Cyanosis from birth is seen in Hb M disease with α-chain abnormalities, or in fetal Hb M (Hb FM Osaka). In the latter, cyanosis will disappear after the γ-chains have been replaced by β-chains by 6 months of age. Cyanosis does not appear until nearly 6 months of age in Hb M variants with β-chain abnormalities, for the same reason (Bunn, 1994). The cyanosis is, of course, not associated with enzyme abnormalities in the red cell, toxic drugs, or cyanotic heart disease, conditions that must be considered in the differential diagnosis. Patients usually have no other symptoms.

All Hb M disorders thus far discovered have been in heterozygotes, probably because homozygosity is lethal. Some types of Hb M will not separate from Hb A on alkaline electrophoresis. If the hemolysate is first converted to methemoglobin, the Hb M will migrate differently from normal methemoglobin at pH 7.1. The absorption spectra of the eluted Hb M, which may be distinctive, can be compared with that of normal methemoglobin (Bunn, 1994).

Unstable Hemoglobins (Bunn, 1998)

Over 100 hemoglobin variants have been described in which the hemoglobin precipitates within the red cell as Heinz bodies. Some are listed in Table 31–4. About 75% of the abnormalities are β-chain. Rare unstable hemoglobins such as Hb F Poole are related to unstable γ-chain variants. Amino acid substitution or deletion renders the Hb molecule

unstable. Precipitated Hb attaches to the cell membrane and shortens its survival; the cells are inflexible. Heinz bodies are removed by the spleen and the further damaged cells have a shortened survival. The oxygen affinity is usually abnormal and may be increased or decreased. Some of these unstable hemoglobins cause 'congenital Heinz body hemolytic anemias.'

All patients have been heterozygous. The clinical features have shown considerable variation, from severe hemolytic anemia in the first year of life (e.g., Hb Hammersmith, Hb Bristol) to a very mild chronic hemolytic anemia (e.g., Hb Louisville, Hb Hasharon) that may be exacerbated by drugs (e.g., Hb Zurich). A few unstable hemoglobins have been discovered incidentally in clinically normal individuals (e.g., Hb Tacoma, Hb Sogn).

Jaundice and splenomegaly are common, as in other hemolytic anemias. More distinctive in some cases is the excretion of darkly pigmented urine (only during hemolytic crises in mild variants). The urine pigment appears to be dipyrrole, probably a breakdown product of heme molecules after separation from globin (Dacie, 1991). Cyanosis is present in some patients and is due to methemoglobinuria and sulfhemoglobinemia or to low oxygen affinity.

The anemia is normocytic and normochromic to hypochromic, the latter because of the removal of precipitated hemoglobin from aging red cells by the macrophages of the spleen and other reticuloendothelial organs. Prominent basophilic stippling, probably related to excessive clumping of ribosomes, is a common feature. Occasional 'bite cells' may be seen. Patients with relatively high hemoglobin concentrations in the steady state usually have hemoglobin variants with a high oxygen affinity and an unexpectedly high reticulocyte count (e.g., Hb Köln, Hb Gun Hill). On the other hand, patients with rather low hemoglobin concentrations may be relatively asymptomatic if their hemoglobin has a low oxygen affinity; their reticulocyte counts are unexpectedly low for the hemoglobin concentration (e.g., Hb Hammersmith). Heinz bodies are rarely seen in circulating red cells before splenectomy, though sometimes they may be generated by incubating the red cells with brilliant cresyl blue or new methylene blue. After splenectomy, Heinz bodies are readily demonstrable in a large proportion of cells; the blood film shows irregularly contracted cells and basophilic stippling that may be pronounced.

In splenectomized patients, the Heinz bodies may interfere with hemoglobin determinations and with electronic platelet and white cell counts. Before measuring the absorbance of the hemolysate, it should be centrifuged to remove the Heinz bodies. Platelet and leukocyte counts should be performed by visual methods. Hemoglobin electrophoresis is normal in about one-fourth of patients. Hb A_2 may be elevated in β-chain variants because of the loss of the abnormal hemoglobin from the cells, and this phenotype may resemble thalassemia intermedia. Hb F may be increased to a level of 10–15%. The key laboratory determinations are the heat instability and isopropanol precipitation tests.

Heat Instability Test. Most unstable hemoglobins precipitate more rapidly than normal hemoglobins when incubated at 50°C (Dacie, 1991). Both normal and unstable hemoglobins precipitate more rapidly in Tris-buffer than in phosphate buffers. In a hemolysate in Tris-buffer, an easily visible precipitate forms within an hour if an unstable hemoglobin is present; the control sample is clear or slightly cloudy. Slight precipitation is equivocal; the test should be repeated and the isopropanol precipitation test performed as well. Precipitates accounting for 10–40% of the total Hb are found in unstable hemoglobin disorders.

Isopropanol Precipitation Test. A relatively nonpolar solvent weakens the internal bonds of hemoglobin and decreases its stability (Carrell, 1972). An unstable hemoglobin precipitates within 20 minutes in the nonpolar solvent isopropanol, whereas a normal hemolysate remains clear for 30–40 minutes. False-positive results occur with high levels of Hb F.

Thalassemias

In thalassemias globin chains, usually of normal structure, are produced at a decreased rate. β-Thalassemia refers to decreased production of β-chains; α-thalassemia, δβ-, δ-, and γδβ-thalassemias refer to reduced synthesis of the respective polypeptide chains. As a result, there is an overall deficit of hemoglobin tetramers in the red cells and the MCV and MCH are reduced. However, it is not the lack of the affected globin chain, but the accumulation of the unaffected one, that causes hemolysis (in α-thalassemia) and ineffective hematopoiesis (primarily in β-thalassemia) in the severe forms of the disease.

Thalassemias occur predominantly in persons of Mediterranean, African, and Asian ancestry as, similarly to hemoglobin variants or G6PD deficiency, thalassemia genes are under selective pressure by malaria. In Greece and Southern Italy the prevalence of β-thalassemia is around 10% and that of α-thalassemia is 5%. Twenty-five to thirty percent of black people

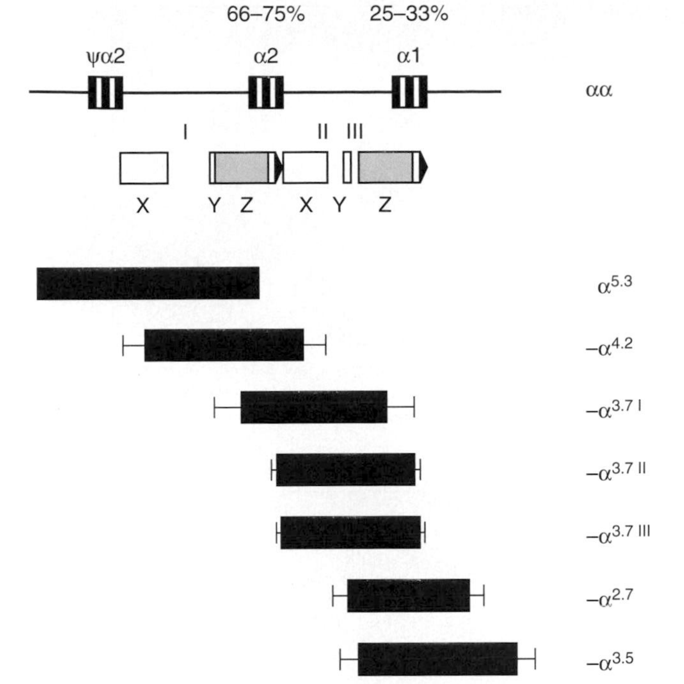

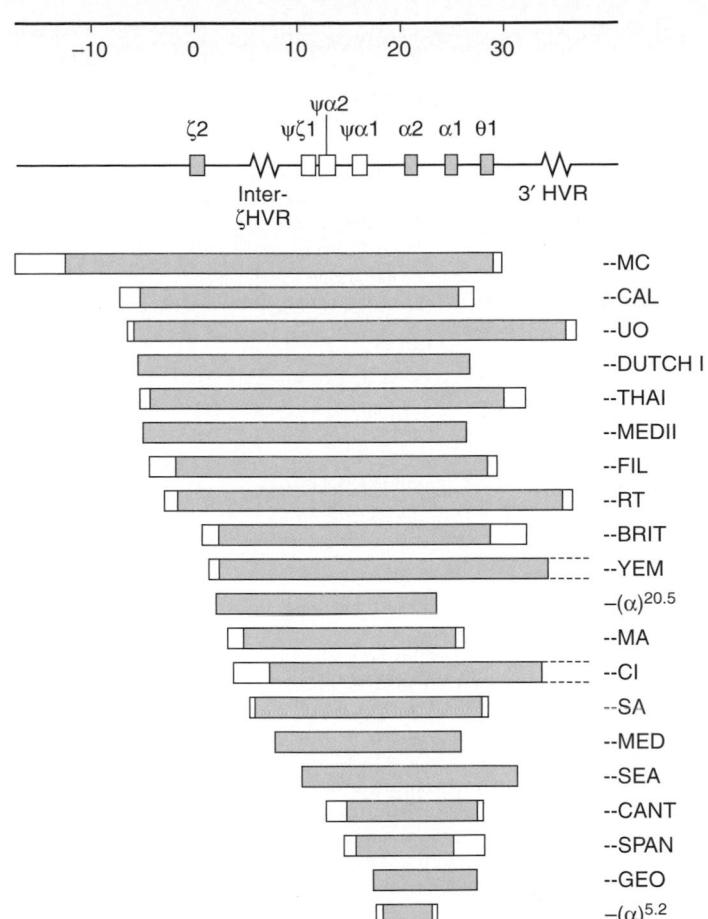

Figure 31–24 Deletions that cause α⁺-thalassemia. The homologous boxes (X, Y, and Z) are interrupted by nonhomologous segments (I, II, and III). Black bars show the extent of each deletion and thin bars show the breakpoint areas. In each case, only one α-gene is deleted.

Figure 31–25 Large deletions of the α-gene complex cause α⁰-thalassemia. No α-chain synthesis is directed from the chromosome. MED (Mediterranean) and SEA (South-East Asian) deletions are the most frequent.

and 20% of Thai people carry an α-thalassemia gene. Because structural variants and thalassemias occur in the same population, a wide variety of diseases emerge from their interactions.

Several classifications are used. The clinical classification defines thalassemia major, a severe and transfusion-dependent form; thalassemia intermedia with less severe symptoms; and thalassemia minor (carrier state or trait), without clinical symptoms, but with hematological abnormalities. The genetic classification is based on the gene(s) affected by the mutation, heterozygous/homozygous state, absent/reduced rate of globin synthesis, etc. Finally, specific mutations cause well-defined syndromes and can be used for classification.

Molecular Defects

In β-thalassemia, there is considerable heterogeneity in the molecular defects. One hundred ninety-seven different mutations have been identified as the cause of β-thalassemia. Most are associated with single base substitutions that produce defects in promoter activity, RNA processing/splicing, or translation, resulting in decreased or unstable mRNA. Large deletions are uncommon. In rare structural variants, the production of highly unstable β-chains results in the phenotype of β-thalassemia (Bunn, 1998). Despite this diversity 20 common mutations account for 80% of β-thalassemia alleles in the world population (Weatherall, 1999). In β⁰-thalassemia, β-chain synthesis is absent on the affected chromosome. mRNA is absent, or may be present, but nonfunctional. In β⁺-thalassemia, β-globin chains are present but reduced in quantity because the molecular defects have resulted in the production of unstable or decreased amounts of mRNA.

In δβ⁰-thalassemia, large deletions involve the δβ or ᴬγδβ gene complex. As a result, no Hb A or Hb A₂ synthesis is supported from the affected chromosome, but the γ is gene upregulated and Hb F production is increased. Lepore hemoglobins have δβ fusion globins that are the result of unequal crossover between δ- and β-globin genes during meiosis.

The α-thalassemias are generally due to gene deletion of various lengths. There are two α-globin genes on each chromosome 16, surrounded by two highly homologous duplication units, each containing three homologous segments (Z, X and Y). Unequal crossing over between the Z segments produces a chromosome with one α gene ($-\alpha^{3.7}$), and one with three ($\alpha\alpha\alpha$). Similar nonreciprocal crossing over between X boxes causes another common deletion ($-\alpha^{4.2}$) (Fig. 31–24). This recombination has a high probability and chromosomes with missing or extra α genes are found in every civilization; nonetheless, only the thalassemic alleles became frequent in certain populations, under pressure from malaria. These defects, affecting only one of the genes, are called α⁺-thalassemia. The heterozygous genotype can be written ($-\alpha/\alpha\alpha$). Nondeletion defects are less common ($\alpha^T\alpha/\alpha\alpha$). α⁰-Thalassemia determinant results from

deletion of both α-globin genes on the chromosome (Fig. 31–25), which therefore directs no α-chain synthesis ($--/\alpha\alpha$).

Hb Constant Spring is due to an abnormal termination codon in an α-globin gene that results in an elongated α-chain with 31 extra amino acids. Because of marked reduction in the mRNA stability, clinical phenotype of α-thalassemia is seen (Orkin, 1998).

β-Thalassemias

The clinical and hemoglobin findings in the β-thalassemias are summarized in Tables 31–7 and 31–8. The disorders are very heterogeneous, phenotypically as well as at the level of the molecular defects. The terms thalassemia major, thalassemia intermedia, and thalassemia minor refer to clinical severity and are not genetic designations.

Homozygous β-Thalassemia (Thalassemia Major; Cooley's Anemia). With an absence (β⁰) or a marked decrease (β⁺) in β-chain production, there is an excess of α chains. Aggregates of α-chains are unstable and precipitate in the normoblast or red cell and damage the cells. Excess α-chains and their degradation products, heme, hemin, and iron, which serve as foci for the generation of reactive oxygen species, result in the partial oxidation of band 4.1 and a reduced spectrin/band 3 ratio in red

Table 31–7 β-Thalassemias and their Associated Biochemical and Molecular Defects

	Typical DNA defect	β-chain	δ-chain	γ-chain	Hb F distribution	α : Non-α-globin imbalance
β⁺-Thalassemia	Mutation	↓	+	+	Heterocellular	+++
β⁰-Thalassemia	Mutation	0	+	+	Heterocellular	++++
δβ-Thalassemia	Deletion	0	0	+++	Heterocellular	++
HPFH	Deletion	0 or ↓	0	++++	Pancellular	+

Modified from Forget, 1982.

Table 31–8 Major Categories of β-Thalassemia Syndromes

Syndrome	Genotype	Clinical features	Hemoglobin pattern
Homozygous states:			
β⁺-thalassemia	β⁺/β⁺	Thalassemia major or intermedia	↓↓ Hb A, ↑↑ Hb F, variable Hb A₂
β⁰-thalassemia	β⁰/β⁰	Thalassemia major	> 95% Hb F, rest Hb A₂
δβ⁰-thalassemia	δβ⁰/δβ⁰	Thalassemia intermedia	100% Hb F
Hb Lepore	Lepore/Lepore	Thalassemia major	85% Hb F, 15% Hb Lepore
Heterozygous states:			
β⁺-thalassemia	β⁺/β	Thalassemia minor	Hb A, ↑ Hb A₂, ±↑ Hb F
β⁰-thalassemia	β⁰/β	Thalassemia minor	Hb A, ↑ Hb A₂, ±↑ Hb F
δβ⁰-thalassemia	δβ⁰/δβ	Thalassemia minor	Hb A, 5–20% Hb F, ±↓ Hb A₂
Hb Lepore	Lepore/β	Thalassemia minor	Hb A, ↑ Hb F, ↓ Hb A₂, 10% Hb Lepore

Modified from Orkin, 1976.

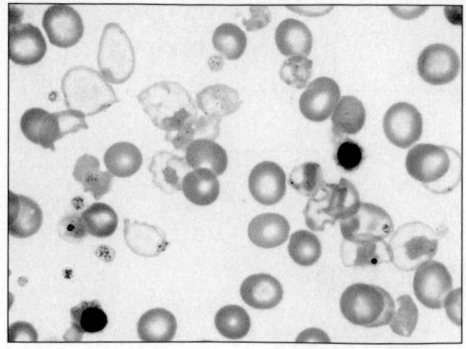

Figure 31–26 Homozygous β-thalassemia. A few cells contain hardly any hemoglobin and the hemoglobin is often precipitated at the membrane. Bizarre target cells, Howell–Jolly bodies and poorly hemoglobinized nucleated red blood cells are seen.

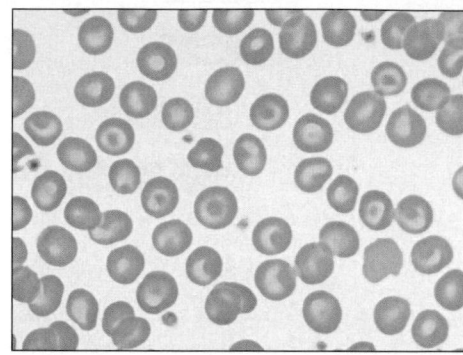

Figure 31–27 β-Thalassemia trait. Hypochromic, microcytic red blood cells with frequent targeting. Mild anemia.

blood cell precursors. Precipitates and cells are removed, causing ineffective erythropoiesis and a severe hemolytic anemia. Furthermore, clustering of band 3 in the membrane may be followed by opsonization with autologous IgG and complement and removal by macrophages (Weatherall, 1999).

Clinical findings include jaundice and splenomegaly, which become evident early in childhood. Prominent frontal bones, cheekbones, and jaws impart a mongoloid appearance. These changes and the X-ray findings of thinned cortex of the long and flat bones and thickening of the skull with osteoporosis ('hair-on-end' appearance) reflect the extreme bone marrow hyperplasia. Growth is stunted and puberty is delayed. Most patients require regular transfusions and develop problems due to iron loading. Iron overload commonly develops, and the major cause of death is cardiac failure due to myocardial siderosis by the end of the third decade.

Unlike most hemolytic diseases, the anemia is hypochromic and microcytic. Extreme poikilocytosis with bizarre shapes, target cells, ovalocytosis, Cabot rings, Howell–Jolly bodies, nuclear fragments, siderocytes, anisochromia, anisocytosis, and often extreme normoblastosis are present (Fig. 31–26). Poikilocytosis is more striking in patients with intact spleens; normoblastosis is more severe after splenectomy. Normoblasts have hypochromic cytoplasm and, especially after splenectomy, aggregates of densely staining hemoglobin, which probably represent precipitated α-chains. Incubation of the blood with methyl violet stains these precipitates in both red cells and normoblasts. The reticulocyte count is less elevated than expected for the degree of anemia because of destruction of erythroid precursors in the marrow. Osmotic resistance of the red cells, serum iron, and indirect-reacting bilirubin are increased.

In the marrow, marked normoblastic hyperplasia is present. Many late normoblasts show inclusion bodies as in the blood. Intramedullary destruction of hemoglobin (ineffective erythropoiesis) is markedly increased in thalassemia major. Gaucher-like cells are present. Storage iron and sideroblasts are increased.

In β⁰-thalassemia, Hb A is absent, Hb F is as high as 98%, and Hb A₂ is about 2%. In β⁺-thalassemias (Mediterranean), Hb F is 60–95%, with Hb A present. Although Hb A₂ may or may not be increased, the ratio of A₂ to A is always increased. In black people with β⁺-thalassemia, the clinical features are less severe (thalassemia intermedia) and transfusion is usually unnecessary; Hb F is 20–40%, Hb A₂ is 2–5%, and the rest is Hb A (Table 31–8).

Heterozygous β-Thalassemia (β-Thalassemia Trait; Thalassemia Minor; Cooley's Trait). This is caused by either β⁰-thalassemia gene with absent or β⁺-thalassemia gene with reduced β-globin chain synthesis. There are usually no symptoms or abnormal physical signs. The only clinical presentation might be a refractory anemia of pregnancy (Weatherall, 2001).

Most β-thalassemia heterozygotes have a mild anemia, but occasionally the Hct and Hb might be normal. Those of African origin have higher hemoglobin levels than people from the Mediterranean region, reflecting their milder genotype. Characteristically, the RBC is elevated (5–7 M/μL), the MCH is low (usually less than 22 pg), and the MCV is low (between 55–70 fL). The MCHC is sometimes low but often normal. The reticulocyte count is twice the normal value. On stained films, the cells have a moderate degree of microcytosis, hypochromia, anisocytosis and poikilocytosis; target cells and basophilic stippling are often, but not always, present (Fig. 31–27). Osmotic fragility is decreased. In the marrow there is mild normoblastic hyperplasia with ragged cytoplasmic borders, a sign of defective hemoglobinization.

Hb A₂ is elevated in the 3.5–7% range; Hb F is slightly elevated (1–3%) in about half of the cases. In the few cases where Hb F exceeds 4%, it is likely that a gene for HPFH is also present (Mazza, 1976). The relatively rare deletional forms tend to have higher levels of Hb F (up to 9%) and in a few families, in which the deletion included the promoter region, Hb F was found to be unusually high (up to 14%) (Weatherall, 2001). In infants there is a slower than normal decline in Hb F level and the adult steady-state level is not reached until adolescence. This is a particularly important consideration in double heterozygosity for β-thalassemia and Hb S, when Hb F level is used to predict prognosis.

In a few cases both Hb A₂ and F are normal. These are difficult to distinguish from α-thalassemia trait, and only molecular studies might be definitive. Studies indicate that the bulk of these cases results from the co-inheritance of both β and δ-thalassemia (Weatherall, 1994), either in trans or in cis to the β-thalassemia gene. In other patients with normal hemoglobin pattern, there are only minimal hematologic changes (the 'silent' β-thalassemia gene), and only a more severe β-thalassemia syndrome in a family member suggests the presence of a very mild β-thalassemia gene.

Iron studies are little different from normal (Weatherall, 2001), although iron deficiency often complicates thalassemia trait in childhood and during pregnancy. In severe iron deficiency the level of Hb A₂ may fall into the normal range, thus obscuring the diagnosis of β-thalassemia trait, but this is unusual. Most often, although the level of A₂ falls, it remains elevated above the normal range (Weatherall, 2001). Nevertheless, when iron deficiency is present, repeat measurement of Hb A₂ is recommended after replenishment of iron.

The differential diagnosis between iron deficiency and β- or α-thalassemia trait can be difficult. Increase in RBC in the presence of decreased MCV is the hallmark of thalassemia trait. An MCV/RBC ratio < 13 suggests thalassemia trait; a ratio > 13 is more consistent with iron deficiency, but this or other formulas are not conclusive enough for diagnosis.

(δβ)⁰-Thalassemia. This used to be called F thalassemia, a helpful name, as you have to think of it when there are thalassemic indices and significantly increased level of Hb F. β- and δ-chains are not produced, but this is nearly, though not completely, compensated by an increased output of γ-chains. The heterozygous state is similar to a mild β-thalassemia trait, except that Hb A₂ is not increased, or is even slightly reduced (mean level is 2.4%), and Hb F is significantly increased (5.4–20%). In the homozygous state, hemoglobin consists of only Hb F.

Clinically, (δβ)⁰-thalassemia behaves as a mild form β-thalassemia. In the heterozygous state the hemoglobin is normal or slightly reduced, the MCH is between 21–26 pg and the MCV is 65–79 fL. There are no clinical symptoms. Homozygotes have a mild form of thalassemia intermedia with a hemoglobin level of 10–13 g/dL, mildly thalassemic red cell indices and only minimal hepatosplenomegaly. It is most common in the Mediterranean population. The mild phenotype is the result of increased production of γ-chains, which compensates to some degree for the lack of β-chains.

The molecular defect is a long deletion involving the β and δ and, often, also the ᴬγ gene. There are 21 different deletions described (Globin Gene Server), but the hematological findings are essentially the same. When the ᴬγ gene is also deleted, the accurate nomenclature is (ᴬγδβ)⁰-thalassemia; homozygotes have a somewhat more severe phenotype.

(δβ)⁺-Thalassemia: Lepore Hemoglobins. In the Lepore hemoglobins an abnormal δβ fusion chain is produced, a result of chromosome crossing-over and fusion of genetic material at the δβ genes. No δ- and β-chain synthesis is directed from the affected chromosome. Because Hb F production is only slightly increased and the composite δβ-chain is synthesized at a very slow rate, it results in a thalassemic phenotype. The hematological abnormalities are similar to those seen in β⁰-thalassemia. Hb Lepore migrates slightly faster than Hb S on alkaline electrophoresis and usually constitutes about 10% of the total hemoglobin in the heterozygotes, while Hb A₂ averages 2% and Hb F is 2–3% (Efremov, 1978). In homozygotes, Hb Lepore is 10–15% and the rest is Hb F. Different Hb Lepores have been described depending on the point of fusion, but they behave quite similarly. This is a much more severe thalassemia gene than the (δβ)⁰ form and causes transfusion-dependent thalassemia major in the homozygous state.

Hereditary Persistence of Fetal Hemoglobin (HPFH)

A group of conditions with persistence of fetal hemoglobin production beyond infancy, but without significant hematologic abnormalities is known as HPFH. It is found in about 0.1% of African Americans. HPFH is closely related to β- and δβ-thalassemias, with which it forms a continuous spectrum. At one end of the spectrum, there is minimal γ-chain production and no compensation for deficiency of β-chains in β-thalassemia, while at the other end Hb F production is up and almost entirely compensates for the deficit in HPFH (Weatherall, 2001).

As a result, at least in heterozygotes, there is no clear evidence of thalassemia (except maybe borderline microcytosis in a few cases) and this serves as a criterion in diagnosis. In clinical practice, a patient with significantly elevated Hb F and reduced Hb A₂ is suspected to have HPFH if red cell indices are normal, but is diagnosed with δβ⁰-thalassemia if the indices are thalassemic. Nevertheless, there is a slight α/non-α chain imbalance and HPFH is considered a mild form of δβ⁰-thalassemia.

Deletional HPFH. In the six deletional forms the δβ gene complex is deleted. The black and Ghanaian forms are the most common, but Indian, Italian and Southeast-Asian forms are also well documented. Homozygotes have slightly microcytic, hypochromic red cells, but no anemia. Hb F is 100%; no Hb A or Hb A₂ is present. The hematocrit can even be high, a result of high oxygen affinity of Hb F. In the heterozygote, no hematologic abnormalities are found. Hb F is 15–30%, and Hb A₂ is 1–2.1%. Hb F is homogeneously (evenly) distributed among the red cells (pancellular). This is in contrast to β- or δβ-thalassemia, in which the distribution is heterocellular.

Hb Kenya. This is a hemoglobin analogous to the Lepore hemoglobins which is associated with an HPFH phenotype. It contains a ᴬγβ fusion gene. In the heterozygote, Hb Kenya is around 10%, F 7% and A₂ is reduced.

Nondeletional HPFH. There is mutation in the promoter region of one of the γ-genes, resulting in increased synthesis of Hb F. The output from the δ and β genes in cis is reduced. Levels of Hb F ranges from 3–31% in the different forms, Hb A₂ is invariably low and the red cell indices are close to normal. There are two particulars to keep in mind. First, β-chain synthesis is not absent from the affected chromosome and compound heterozygotes of this form of HPFH and Hb C or S on the other chromosome do have Hb A (around 30%). The hemoglobin composition is similar to that seen in Hb S/β⁺-thalassemia, except Hb A₂ is reduced. Second, it is not rare to find it together with an α-thalassemia gene, which is highly prevalent in African-Americans.

Heterocellular or Swiss type HPFHs has less Hb F, ranging from 2–10%. The genetic background is varied and often poorly understood, but the

Table 31–9 α-Thalassemia Syndromes

Syndrome	Defective genes	Genotype	Clinical features	Newborn	After first year
Hydrops fetalis	4	—/—	Fetal or neonatal death with severe anemia	Hb Bart's >80% Hb H, Hb Portland	
Hb H disease	3	—/–α (—/αα^CS)	Chronic hemolytic anemia	Hb Bart's 20–40% (Hb CS)	Hb H 5–30% (Hb CS 2–3%)
Thalassemia minor	2	—/αα –α/–α α^Tα/–α	Asymptomatic, mild anemia, thalassemic indices	Hb Bart's 5–10%	None
Silent carrier	1	–α/αα (αα/αα^CS)	No clinical or hematologic abnormality	Hb Bart's ±1–2% (Hb CS)	None (Hb CS 1%)

Modified from Wintrobe, 1981.

uneven distribution of Hb F separates this group. When inherited with a β variant or thalassemia, the result is an unusually high level of Hb F (Weatherall, 2001).

α-Thalassemias

α-Thalassemia is probably the most common single gene disorder in humans. Its distribution is largely limited to tropical and subtropical regions of Asia and Africa and the Mediterranean (Higgs, 1989), where it reaches extremely high frequencies.

There are two α-globin genes on each chromosome 16. α-Thalassemias are classified according to the total output from these two linked α-globin genes. In α⁰-thalassemia both genes are inactive (—/), while in α⁺-thalassemia only one gene is defective, due either to deletion (–α/)or, less frequently, to mutation (α^Tα/). Nondeletional forms usually result in less globin output from the linked α-gene and more severe phenotypes. Rarely, the chromosome has a deletion and a separate mutation (α^T–/). Previously, α⁰ and α⁺ were called α-thalassemia 1 and 2. This was rather confusing, as the milder defect with one affected gene was called α-thalassemia 2 and the more severe genotype with two defective genes α-thalassemia 1. Alternatively, these terms were also used to describe clinical phenotypes.

Unlike the extremely unstable α-chains in β-thalassemia, excess β- and γ-chains can form stable tetramers, hemoglobin H (β₄) and Bart's (γ₄). These precipitate in the aging red cells and, through interaction with the cell membrane, cause hemolysis. This is mostly a hemolytic anemia, whereas in β-thalassemia ineffective erythropoiesis predominates.

α-Thalassemia Syndromes

Four α-thalassemia syndromes result from the combination of these genotypes (Bunn, 1986), which roughly correspond to a loss of 4, 3, 2, or 1 genes from the normal complement (αα/αα) (see Table 31–9). In the following discussion, nondeletion forms are not always depicted separately, for sake of simplicity.

Hemoglobin Bart's Hydrops Fetalis (—/—). Complete absence of α-chains is incompatible with life. Infants are stillborn with severe edema, marked anemia, and marked hepatosplenomegaly. The blood shows marked anisocytosis, poikilocytosis, microcytosis, and erythroblastosis. ABO or Rh incompatibility is absent. Because of the absence of α-chains, no Hb A or Hb F is present. Large quantities of Hb Bart's (γ₄), a variable amount of Hb Portland and traces of Hb H (β₄) are present; all of these migrate faster than Hb A on alkaline electrophoresis. Hb Bart's is functionally useless for oxygen transfer, causing extreme intrauterine hypoxia.

Hemoglobin H Disease (–α/—). Three of the four α-genes are absent. There is a chronic hemolytic anemia with the clinical picture of thalassemia intermedia in a minority of cases, though the severity varies and most patients do well. Hb H disease is very common in Southeast Asia, but is also seen in the Mediterranean and the Middle East; it is very rare, however, in black people, as α⁰-thalassemia is uncommon in this group. Splenomegaly and sometimes hepatomegaly are present. Hemoglobin values average 3 g/dL less than in age- and sex-matched controls.

IV

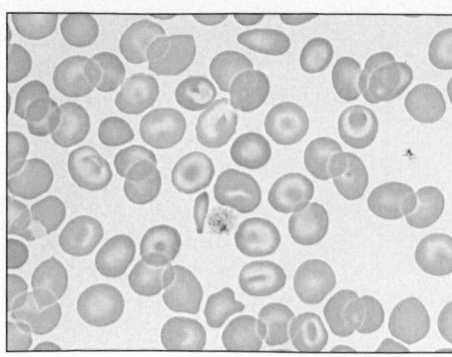

Figure 31–28 Hemoglobin H disease. Mild anemia and target cells.

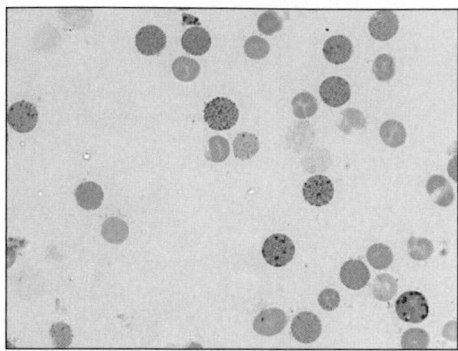

Figure 31–29 Hemoglobin H preparation. Film made after incubation of blood with brilliant cresyl blue. Several red cells contain multiple small pale blue inclusions.

Transfusion is rarely needed. Anemia may become more severe during pregnancy but the hemoglobin rarely falls below 7 g/dL. The MCV (60–70 fL) and MCH (17–21 pg) are decreased (Higgs, 1989) and RBC is increased (6–6.2 M/μL). The blood film shows hypochromia, basophilic stippling, and anisopoikilocytosis with target cells (Fig. 31–28). Reticulocytes range from 4–5%.

Hemoglobin electrophoresis shows a rapidly migrating band of Hb H (β_4) accounting for approximately 9% (from 1–40%) of the hemoglobin, and the slightly less rapidly migrating Hb Bart's in half of the cases. Hb H can be precipitated in vitro and lost from the hemolysate by careless handling or prolonged storage. In old hemolysates a series of bands migrates as Hb H. Hb Bart's is alkali resistant and may be measured with Hb F (which is not increased in Hb H disease). The percentage of Hb Bart's is 2–40% at birth; it gradually falls thereafter averaging 4.8%, but the level in adults is quite variable. As in other α-thalassemia syndromes, there is more Hb Bart's at birth, than Hb H in adult life. Hb A_2 is diminished.

Hemoglobin H Preparation. Vital staining of the blood with an oxidizing dye such as brilliant cresyl blue induces inclusion bodies (Hb H precipitates) in many of the red cells. During incubation of two parts of blood in one of 1% brilliant cresyl blue stain, the unstable Hb H (β_4) gradually precipitates as multiple small pale blue inclusions uniformly distributed on the red cell membrane (Fig. 31–29) (Jones, 1981). Hb H inclusions must be distinguished from (1) the granules and reticular networks in reticulocytes, which are darker blue in color; and (2) preformed Heinz bodies, which are larger, also darker blue, and often attached to the membrane. After 20 minutes of incubation at room temperature, Hb H inclusions are present in at least half of the red cells in Hb H disease, and in a very rare red cell in α-thalassemia trait. The larger, single Heinz bodies may be found after splenectomy in Hb H disease.

α-Thalassemia Trait (Heterozygous α°-Thalassemia (—/αα) or Homozygous α⁺-Thalassemia (−α/−α)). Absence of two α-genes results in clinical features similar to β-thalassemia minor with very mild anemia and thalassemic indices with MCV ranging from 65–75 fL (Higgs, 1989). The α-chain/β-chain synthesis ratio is decreased (~ 0.6). Diagnosis is best made by finding 5–10% Hb Bart's in cord blood; normally, only trace amounts (< 0.5%) are found. In adults, Hb Bart is undetectable and hemoglobin studies are perfectly normal, except that Hb A_2 might be reduced. Hb H inclusions are found in α⁰-thalassemia, but rarely in heterozygous or homozygous α⁺-thalassemia, and only in a very small percentage of red cells, if exhaustively sought after (Wasi, 1974) and if the sample is enriched for Hb H-containing red cells (Jones, 1981). Otherwise, no evidence of hemoglobin imbalance is detectable by standard techniques, and the diagnosis is one of excluding iron deficiency, anemia of chronic disease, and β-thalassemia. In contrast to β-thalassemia, Hb F is normal and Hb A_2 is normal or decreased. This condition is absolutely benign and most patients are diagnosed on routine screening. The hematological findings are identical in the two distinct genotypes found in different populations: (—/αα), common in Southeast Asia and the Mediterranean and exceedingly rare in black people; and (−α/−α), most common in those of African descent.

Silent Carrier α-Thalassemia (Heterozygous α⁺-Thalassemia, (αα/−α). In this condition, one of four α-globin genes is absent. The hematologic findings are normal, except the MCV might be slightly reduced with a mean value of 81 fL and a range of 75–85 fL and the MCH might be minimally decreased; many times, however, the red cell indices are perfectly normal. During the neonatal period, heterozygous α⁺-thalassemia can be diagnosed by a raised level of Hb Bart (1–2%) in the cord blood. Hb Bart disappears by the age of 6 months and the diagnosis can only be made by molecular or globin chain synthesis studies. Since only 40% of newborns with the α⁺-thalassemia genotype have detectable Hb Bart in their cord blood (Higgs, 1982), failure to detect Hb Bart's in the newborn does not rule out silent carrier α-thalassemia, and newborn screening should not be used to rule out this entity.

From large studies comparing hematological findings of different genotypes it became apparent that there is a continuum between normal, silent carrier and α-thalassemia trait. Since there is no clear separation between one- and two-gene defects, some authors group these together as milder α-thalassemia phenotypes. None of the α-thalassemia genes or their combinations can be identified with certainty without molecular studies.

Hemoglobin Constant Spring ($\alpha^{CS}\alpha$/). Hb Constant Spring is due to an abnormal termination codon in an α-gene that results in an elongated α-chain with 31 extra amino acids. It is far the most common of the elongated α-chain variants. Because of marked reduction in the mRNA stability, the clinical phenotype of α-thalassemia is seen (Orkin, 1998). Similarly to other nondeletional α⁺-thalassemia genes, it causes a more severe phenotype. The homozygous state appears as an asymptomatic, mild hemolytic anemia, with a hemoglobin level of 9–11 g/dL. The red cell indices are unusual for thalassemia: the MCV is normal (88 fL) and the RBC is low (3.9 M/μL). Hemoglobin consists of 5–8% Hb CS, normal Hb A_2, trace amounts of Hb Bart's, and the rest Hb A (Weatherall, 1994). Heterozygotes have a silent carrier phenotype with no hematologic abnormality and about 1% Hb CS. The abnormal Hb migrates more slowly than Hb A_2 at alkaline pH and is easily missed. Hb CS is common in Southeast Asia, where it is found in about 50% of cases of Hb H disease ($\alpha^{CS}\alpha$/—).

Screening and Prenatal Diagnosis of Hemoglobin Disorders

In populations where there is a significant incidence of severe forms of thalassemia or sickle cell anemia, women should be screened early in pregnancy for thalassemia and the sickle cell trait (Weatherall, 1985, 1994; Alter, 1988). If both parents are carriers, prevention of severe disease is possible through genetic counseling and offering prenatal diagnosis with the option of therapeutic abortion. In high-frequency regions screening of school children or premarital counseling has been implemented. Initial tests include MCV (< 80 fL), MCH (< 27 pg) and HPLC to estimate Hb A_2 (> 3.5%) and to detect common hemoglobin variants (cutoff values are in parenthesis). In prenatal diagnosis, fetal DNA analysis of chorionic villi replaced fetal blood analysis by the early 1990s.

Hemolysis – Metabolic Disorders

Deficient enzyme activity in the erythrocyte may result in abnormalities that lead to premature destruction and hemolytic anemia; these disorders are usually inherited. However, interference with or oxidative stress on erythrocyte metabolism can sometimes result in hemolysis in individuals who have normal erythrocytes.

Erythrocyte Metabolism. The mature red cell lacks mitochondria and, therefore, lacks oxidative phosphorylation and Krebs cycle activity. Energy production is mainly glycolytic, 90% of which occurs through the Embden–Meyerhof pathway, as glucose goes to lactic acid with the net production of 2 mol of ATP (Fig. 31–30). ATP is needed for the energy-requiring reactions in the cell: for active cation transport across the membrane, for maintaining membrane deformability, and for preserving the cell's biconcave shape. Glucose uptake by red cells is independent of insulin. Approximately 90% of glucose is consumed in the glycolytic pathway, while 10% is utilized in the pentose phosphate pathway (hexose monophosphate [HMP] shunt). One step of the glycolytic pathway replenishes NADH, which plays a major role in protecting hemoglobin

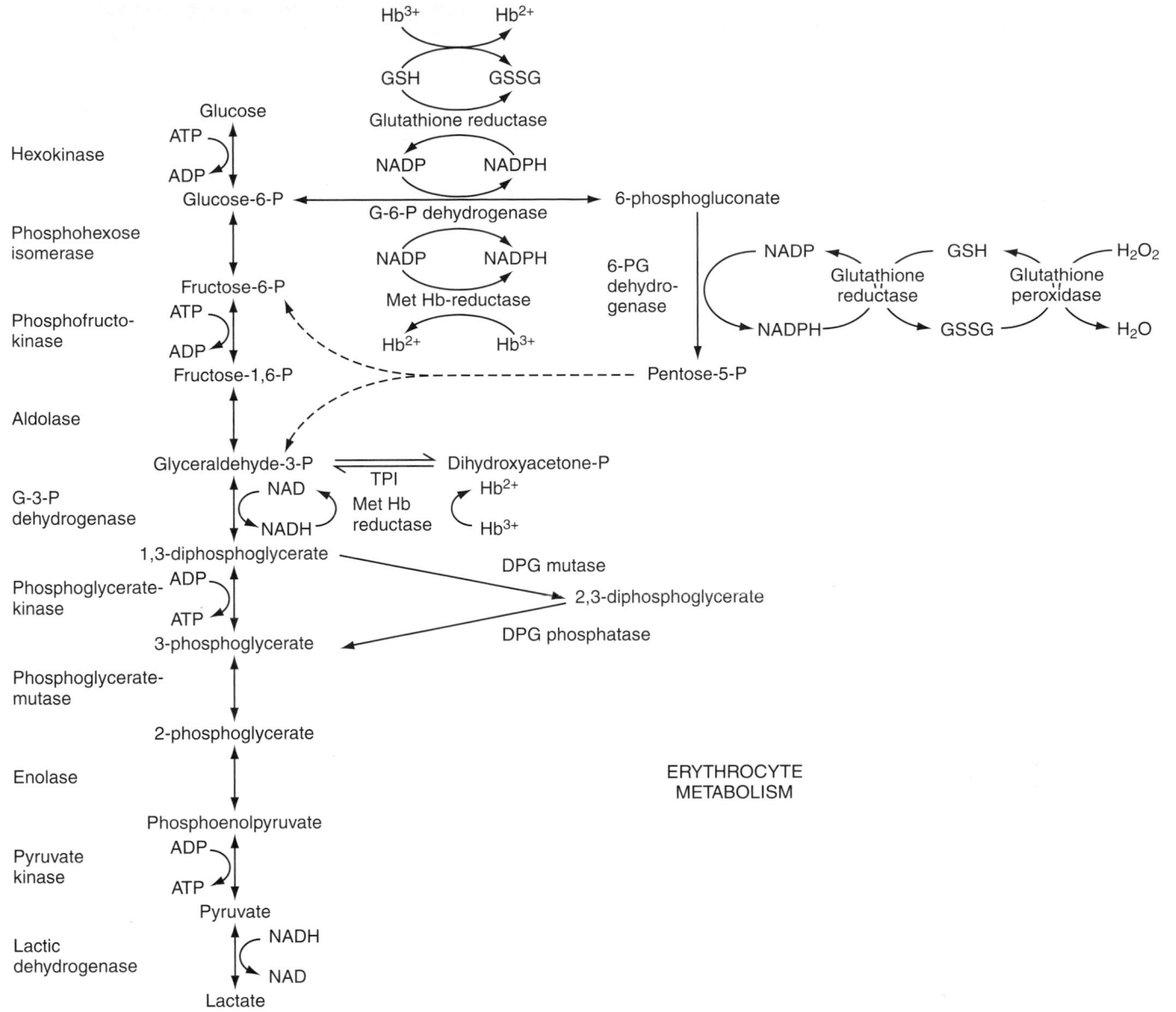

Figure 31–30 Erythrocyte metabolism is discussed in the text. Normally, most hemiglobin (methemoglobin, Hb³⁺) is reduced to hemoglobin (Hb²⁺) by nicotinamide adenine dinucleotide-linked methemoglobin reductase (NAD, Met Hb reductase). NADP-linked methemoglobin reductase requires methylene blue for activation and is more effective in drug-induced methemoglobinemia than the normal cell mechanism. (GSH = reduced glutathione; GSSG = oxidized glutathione.) (Reproduced with permission of the McGraw-Hill Companies.)

from oxidative stress. Most of the hemiglobin (methemoglobin) produced in the normal cell (about 3% of the total per day) is reduced by NAD-linked Met Hb reductase. The HMP shunt generates NADPH in the first two steps, through the enzymes G6PD and 6-phosphogluconate. NADPH production is linked to glutathione reduction and, through this mechanism, to preservation of vital enzymes and hemoglobin from oxidation. Small amounts of oxidized hemoglobin (methemoglobin) are reduced by GSH. The activity of the HMP shunt increases when the cell is exposed to an oxidant drug, probably as a result of increased NADP production. If an enzyme in this pathway lacks activity, GSH cannot be produced and hemoglobin will be oxidized by the oxidant stress. Oxidation in the red cells is mediated by high-energy derivatives of oxygen referred to collectively as activated oxygen (Prchal, 2000). Oxidized globin chains denature and precipitate as Heinz bodies, which adhere to the membrane, inducing rigidity and a tendency to lyse. Moderate enzyme deficiencies in this pathway (e.g., in G6PD) may not be associated with anemia under normal conditions; however, an acute hemolytic episode occurs if the cells are challenged by oxidant stress (e.g., drugs, infection).

Deficiencies in the Embden–Meyerhof pathway result in impaired ATP generation and a chronic hemolytic anemia. The mechanism of the red cell destruction here is less clear. Heinz bodies are not formed. A lack of cell deformability and impaired cation pumping are important in the hemolytic process. However, ATP deficiency is difficult to demonstrate in many patients, and other disorders associated with more severe ATP deficiency are not associated with significant hemolysis (Prchal, 2000).

The Rapoport–Luebering shunt provides for the conversion of 1,3-diphosphoglycerate (1,3-DPG) to 2,3-DPG instead of directly to 3-phosphoglycerate (3-PG) (Fig. 31–30). If this shunt is operating, generation of 2 mol of ATP (per mole of glucose) is bypassed; the result is no net energy production in glycolysis. However, 2,3-DPG combines with the β-chain of hemoglobin and decreases the affinity of hemoglobin for oxygen. At a given partial pressure of oxygen, therefore, increased 2,3-DPG allows more oxygen to leave hemoglobin and go to the tissues; the oxygen dissociation curve is shifted to the right. Increased activity of this shunt is apparently stimulated by hypoxia.

Glucose-6-Phosphate Dehydrogenase Deficiency. About 10% of male African Americans who were given the antimalarial drug primaquine during the Korean War developed a self-limited, acute hemolytic anemia (Beutler, 1994; Prchal, 2000). The relationship between antimalarial drugs and hemolysis had been observed earlier in the 1920s (Beutler, 1999). Only the older red cells were destroyed, and it was eventually determined that the deficiency in the susceptible red cells was in G6PD. Reticulocytes have five times higher enzyme activity than the oldest erythrocyte population (Prchal, 2000). It has since been found that G6PD deficiency is widespread throughout the world. Among white people, the highest incidence is in Kurdish Jewish people; the deficiency is common in the Middle East, Mediterranean countries, and in Asian people.

Because G6PD is determined by a gene on the X chromosome, full expression of the deficiency is found in the male hemizygote. Partial

Hemolytic Uremic Syndrome (HUS).

HUS occurs most commonly in infants less than 2 years of age and is often preceded by an infection associated with diarrhea. It is likely that some of these cases are due to one of several serotypes of *Escherichia coli* that produce a verotoxin (named for its toxicity against African green monkey kidney [vero] cells). Infection with *Shigella dysenteriae* and occasionally other microbes can also cause HUS in children and adults. Shiga toxin is encoded by *S. dysenteriae*. Shiga toxins 1 and 2 can be present in several *E. coli* serotypes, the most common is *E. coli* 0157:H7. Shiga toxins cause bloody diarrhea, then enter the circulation and travel in the plasma on the surface of platelets or monocytes (Moake, 2002). Recent studies suggest that these toxins become attached to glomerular capillary endothelium and other renal epithelial cells. Shiga toxins together with locally secreted cytokines cause the release of unusually large multimers of von Willebrand factor, which promote platelet aggregation in renal vasculature (Moake, 2002). Hemolytic anemia with schistocytes (owing to interaction of red cells with microvascular thrombotic lesions), variable thrombocytopenia, and uremia are the cardinal features. Death formerly occurred in almost half the cases; the renal pathology has included acute glomerulonephritis and thrombotic and necrotic vascular lesions associated with patchy, bilateral renal cortical necrosis. With supportive therapy, including transfusions and dialysis, some investigators have reported mortality reduced to 5–15%. Nonetheless, minor to major renal impairment has been reported in approximately 50% of patients. A familial variant of HUS has been reported in association with familial deficiency of factor H, which is a component of complement. These patients have a much higher mortality rate (Moake, 2002).

Thrombotic Thrombocytopenic Purpura (TTP).

TTP may occur at any age but has a peak incidence in the third decade; it occurs more often in females than in males. The annual incidence is 3.7 cases per 100 000 (Ahmed, 2002). The triad of clinical manifestations present in most patients includes hemolytic anemia, thrombocytopenia, and neurologic symptoms; in addition, fever and renal diseases are often present, which constitutes the classic pentad. Pathologically, microvascular occlusive lesions with hyaline thrombi and endothelial proliferation are widespread throughout the body. Until 1997, the etiology was unknown. Different theories included endothelial injury by oxidant stress, antiendothelial antibodies, anti-CD36 (glycoprotein IV located on microvasculature) antibodies, platelet aggregating factors, and release of large von Willebrand factor (vWF) multimers into the plasma. In 1996, a protease that cleaves vWF subunits was identified in normal plasma. In 1997 and the following years, several reports indicated deficient vWF-cleaving protease in patients with TTP due to either low enzyme levels (in familial cases) or the presence of IgG enzyme inhibitor (in nonfamilial cases). These observations were confirmed with further studies, which showed normal levels of vWF-cleaving protease in HUS (Moake, 2004). The enzyme has been further characterized as number 13 in a family of 19 distinct ADAMTS-type enzymes identified to date (*a* disintegrin *a*nd *m*etalloprotease with eight *t*hrombospondin-1-like domains). Therefore, the vWF-cleaving metalloprotease is now being referred to as ADAMTS13 (Moake, 2004). In the absence of vWF-cleaving protease, ultra-large vWF multimers secreted by endothelial cells would not be processed normally. These highly adhesive multimers may induce platelet clumping in the microcirculation under shear stress resulting in the clinical manifestation of TTP. The disease is acute, and until the 1980s was fatal in well over half of the cases. With the therapy of plasma exchange by plasmapheresis and plasma transfusions (in addition to platelet inhibitors), the remission rate has improved and long-term survival now approaches 90% (Moake, 2004).

Pre-eclampsia/Eclampsia.

Pre-eclampsia and eclampsia are microangiopathic disorders occurring with pregnancy and sharing some features of HUS or TTP. Approximately 4–39% of patients with severe pre-eclampsia develop HELLP syndrome: *h*emolysis, *e*levated *l*iver enzymes and *l*ow *p*latelet count. The syndrome becomes manifest usually during the third trimester although some patients may develop it during the postpartum period. Most patients recover within a few days after delivery. A small subset of patients develop severe persistent multisystem disease that requires plasma exchange (McMinn, 2001).

Infectious Agents

Destruction of erythrocytes by plasmodia is responsible for the anemia in malaria. This is supported by the observation that the osmotic and mechanical fragility of parasitized erythrocytes is increased. Inhibition of marrow activity may be an additional factor. Fulminant hemoglobinuria (Blackwater fever) is a complication of *P. falciparum* malaria.

Oroya fever, a frequently fatal disease that occurs in Peru, is characterized by a hemolytic anemia and leukocytosis. *Bartonella bacilliformis* is the responsible agent.

Table 31–11 Classification of Immune Hemolytic Anemias

Autoimmune hemolytic anemias

Associated with warm antibodies

Associated with cold antibodies

Combined warm and cold antibodies

Alloimmune hemolytic anemias

Transfusion associated hemolytic anemia

Hemolytic disease of newborn
  Rh incompatibility
  ABO incompatibility

Drug-induced hemolytic anemia

Drug adsorption

Autoantibody induction

Neoantigen formation

Babesiosis, a protozoan infection transmitted by ticks from rodents or cattle, is associated with hemolysis; parasites may be seen in red cells in Romanowsky's-stained blood films.

Hemolytic anemia with cold agglutinins may complicate mycoplasmal pneumonia and infectious mononucleosis. This is due to the effect of antibody on the red cells.

Hemolytic anemia of varying severity is frequent in some bacterial infections. A notable example is *Clostridium perfringens* septicemia following septic abortion or biliary tract surgery, which may be accompanied by a dramatic and life-threatening hemolytic crisis.

Immune Hemolytic Anemias

Immune hemolytic anemias are disorders in which erythrocyte survival is reduced because of the deposition of immunoglobulin and/or complement on the red cell membrane. The immune hemolytic anemias can be grouped according to the presence of autoantibodies, alloantibodies, or drug-related antibodies (Table 31–11).

Autoimmune Hemolytic Anemia. The autoimmune hemolytic anemias (AIHAs) are due to an altered immune response resulting in the production of antibody against the host's own erythrocytes, with subsequent hemolysis. The incidence of AIHA is estimated at 10–30 cases per 1 million population (Gehrs, 2002). The AIHAs can be classified according to serologic or clinical characteristics (Table 31–12). Some AIHAs are mediated by antibodies with maximum binding affinity at 37°C, and other AIHAs are mediated by antibodies with their maximum binding affinity at 4°C. In addition, AIHAs could be viewed according to their association with other disorders. In a study of 1834 patients, approximately 40% of cases of AIHA have been associated with an underlying disease, while the remainder were idiopathic (Sokol, 1992). Lymphoproliferative disorders account for approximately half of the cases of both warm and cold AIHA (Gehrs, 2002).

Etiology and Pathophysiology. The cause of the production of autoantibody in patients with AIHA is unknown. However, several mechanisms have been suggested. Autoimmune antibodies, particularly cold-reacting antibodies, are sometimes produced following an infection. This is typically seen with the elaboration of anti-I in patients with *Mycoplasma pneumoniae* infections and anti-i in patients with infectious mononucleosis. The cold agglutinins of anti-I and anti-i specificity are strikingly similar to one another in the structure of antigen-binding sites. These antibodies react with antibodies that also identify the product of the VH4-34 gene segment in B cells. It has been hypothesized that infections can cause the production of antibodies of a population of B cells utilizing this gene segment. These antibodies will also have cold agglutinins activity against the I/i antigens (Rosse, 2004).

The amount of antibody, its avidity for the erythrocyte autoantigen, and its ability to fix complement are significant variables. Opsonization of red cells can destroy them in the circulation (intravascular hemolysis) or cause their accelerated removal from the circulation by tissue macrophages (extravascular hemolysis). The major sites for these macrophages are the spleen, and to a lesser extent the liver (Gehrs, 2002).

The development of AIHA in patients with lymphoproliferative disorders or with autoimmune disorders may relate to some abnormality with B cells, T cells, macrophages, or the interaction among these cells. Perhaps loss of T cell suppressor function could result in unrestrained production of red cell antibody by B cells. This hypothesis is strengthened by the observation that methyldopa, a drug known to cause the development

Table 31–12 Autoimmune Hemolytic Anemia (AIHA)*

Condition	Warm AIHA	Cold AIHA CHAD	Cold AIHA PCH	Mixed AIHA
Idiopathic	282 (23)	194 (16)	5 (< 1)	47 (4)
Drug-induced disorders	184 (15)	0	0	2 (< 1)
Neoplasia	165 (14)	81 (7)	0 (0)	26 (2)
Non-Hodgkin's lymphoma	27	25	0	8
Chronic lymphocytic leukemia	65	4	0	8
Hodgkin's lymphoma	11	7	0	5
Carcinomas	37	30	0	4
Miscellaneous	25	15	0	1
Infections	9 (< 1)	76 (6)	14 (1)	2 (< 1)
Pneumonia–mycoplasma	0	21	0	0
Viral pneumonia	2	19	0	0
Infectious mononucleosis	0	11	1	0
Miscellaneous	7	25	13	2
Collagen diseases	30 (2)	15 (1)	0 (0)	20 (2)
Systemic lupus erythematosus	7	4	0	16
Rheumatoid arthritis	21	6	0	4
Others	2	5	0	0
Miscellaneous disorders	45 (4)	20 (2)	0	6 (< 1)
Totals	715 (58)	386 (32)	19 (2)	103 (8)

* Numbers in parentheses are percentages.

CHAD = cold hemagglutinin disease; PCH = paroxysmal cold hemoglobinuria.

Modified from Sokol, 1985.

of anti-red cell antibodies, inhibits the activation of suppressor T lymphocytes (Gehrs, 2002).

In AIHA associated with warm-type antibody, there is IgG coating of erythrocytes with or without complement fixation. Clearance of red cells occurs mostly in the spleen. In the absence of complement fixation, it appears that the Fc portion of the red cell-bound IgG immunoglobulin interacts with the Fc receptor present on the membrane of splenic macrophages located along the cords of Billroth. Thus, sensitized erythrocytes are retained, phagocytosed, or fragmented by splenic macrophages during their passage through the spleen.

In AIHA associated with the production of cold-type autoantibody, the erythrocytes are usually coated with IgM immunoglobulin. Under these circumstances, the fixation of complement frequently occurs. In paroxysmal cold hemoglobinuria, the offending antibody is an IgG immunoglobulin that fixes complement. If the entire complement sequence is activated, there may be intravascular hemolysis. This phenomenon may occur in cases of cold hemagglutinin disease as well as in paroxysmal cold hemoglobinuria. If complement activation fails to proceed to completion but is halted at an intermediate stage, intravascular lysis of the erythrocytes may not occur. However, extravascular hemolysis can still continue. In this situation, sensitized cells with C3b on the membrane are bound in the liver by the interaction of C3b and its receptors on Kupffer's cells. Erythrocytes may be phagocytosed entirely or portions of the cells may be removed, resulting in fragmentation and spherocyte formation.

Approximately 7% of patients with AIHA satisfy diagnostic criteria for both warm and cold autoantibodies (Sokol, 1992). In these cases, IgG and C3d sensitize the erythrocytes. The serum contains IgM cold autohemagglutinins (optimally reactive at 4°C, but with a high thermal amplitude at 37°C) and IgG warm autoantibodies.

AIHA Associated with Warm Antibody. The warm antibody type of AIHA is slightly more frequent in females than in males and is most likely to occur in individuals 40 years or older. The clinical signs and symptoms frequently are those of an underlying disorder. However, in individuals with idiopathic AIHA, the patient may have noted the presence of a mild upper respiratory tract infection just prior to the onset of hemolysis. As the disorder progresses, there may be weakness, dizziness, and fever. Jaundice can be a presenting complaint. Pregnancy carries a fivefold risk of developing autoantibodies compared to control population (Gehrs, 2002).

Laboratory findings include the presence of a moderate to severe anemia. The neutrophil count may be increased. In a small proportion of cases, thrombocytopenia can exist. The peripheral film frequently shows spherocytosis, red cell fragmentation, polychromasia, and a few normoblasts. Reticulocyte percentage is high in approximately 50% of patients and is often associated with increased MCV. The lack of reticulocytosis should not keep one from making a diagnosis of AIHA. The bone marrow exhibits normoblastic erythroid hyperplasia, sometimes with mild megaloblastic changes.

There is usually a decrease in serum haptoglobin and an increase in unconjugated bilirubin and LD. The osmotic fragility and autohemolysis test can be either normal or abnormal.

The direct and indirect antiglobulin tests indicate the presence of erythrocyte antibodies. The specificity of the autoantibodies is usually directed against antigens of the Rh system, membrane protein band 3 and band 4.1, and glycophorin A. However, activity against U, LW, Kell, jk^a, and Fy^a antigens may also occur. The warm antibody is most likely an IgG immunoglobulin with subclass IgG1 and less frequently with IgG3. When either IgG2 or IgG4 is present on the red cells alone, there is no associated hemolytic reaction (Packman, 2001a). Occasionally the antibody may be an IgA immunoglobulin and rarely an IgM immunoglobulin. Complement may be detected on the erythrocyte membrane in slightly over half of the cases.

In some cases, sensitized red cells contain less immunoglobulin than can be detected using commercially prepared antiglobulins, which are normally sensitive to 250–500 molecules of IgG per red cell (Gilliland, 1976). Under these circumstances, the autoantibody can at times be detected with an antiglobulin consumption test.

The clinical course of AIHA associated with warm antibody is characterized by periods of remissions and relapse. In secondary AIHA, the course and prognosis are related to the nature of the underlying disorder. In idiopathic AIHA, the complications of the hemolytic disorder may be severe and lead to the demise of the patient.

AIHA Associated with Cold Antibody. AIHA associated with cold antibody can be mediated by an IgM immunoglobulin and less frequently by an IgG immunoglobulin. The IgM autoantibody is associated with a syndrome known as cold agglutinin disease, whereas the IgG autoantibody is seen with paroxysmal cold hemoglobinuria.

Cold Agglutinin Disease.

Cold agglutinin disease occurs in individuals usually over the age of 50 years and in females more often than in males. In some cases, cold agglutinin disease is associated with a lymphoproliferative disorder or infection (especially with *Mycoplasma pneumoniae* or infectious mononucleosis). Cases unassociated with an underlying disorder are listed as idiopathic. Virtually all sera from healthy individuals contain low-titer cold agglutinins, regarded as benign or harmless and are polyclonal. The postinfectious cold agglutinins are usually polyclonal. By contrast, monoclonal cold agglutinins are generally pathogenetic and may arise from B cell lymphoma (Gehrs, 2002). Cold agglutinin disease represents approximately 20% of AIHA.

Symptoms and signs vary widely. Some individuals may complain of acrocyanosis or Raynaud's phenomenon. Others will have episodes of hemolysis following exposure to cold.

The laboratory findings usually indicate an anemia. Spherocytes and polychromatophilic erythrocytes are present to a variable degree in the blood film. There may be marked red cell agglutination, which should be differentiated from rouleaux formation (see Figs 29–25 and 29–26). A mild leukocytosis can exist. Red cell agglutination may interfere with automated hematology counts, particularly MCHC, which tends to be high.

The cold antibody is usually an IgM immunoglobulin with anti-I, or less frequently anti-i, specificity. Rarely do other specificities exist. In the chronic idiopathic form of cold agglutinin disease, the antibody tends to be monoclonal IgM, *k* with anti-I specificity (Gehrs, 2002). The autoantibody is also capable of fixing complement. When the titer of cold antibody is very high, the thermal range of antibody activity may extend up to 37°C. The direct antiglobulin test is positive only if the reagents contain anticomplement activity. Thus, one usually observes a positive antiglobulin reaction with the broad-spectrum and non-γ-reagents but no agglutination with only the γ-reagent. On cold exposure and antibody binding to red cells, the complement may be activated to the stage of C3b, which adheres to the red cells after entering the systemic circulation. In the hepatic circulation, macrophages carry specific receptors for C3b. However, cells usually escape hepatic destruction.

Paroxysmal Cold Hemoglobinuria.

Paroxysmal cold hemoglobinuria is a very rare disorder that can occur in an individual of any age. Females are as frequently involved as males.

IV

Table 31–14 Laboratory Features in Microcytic Hypochromic Anemias

| | Serum iron | Serum TIBC | % Saturation | Marrow | | Serum ferritin | ZPP | Hb A₂ | Hb F |
				% Sideroblasts	Iron stores				
Iron deficiency	↓	↑	↓	↓	↓	↓	↑	N–↓	N
β-Thalassemia trait	N (↑)	N	N	N	N–↑	N–↑	N	↑	N–↑
Anemia of chronic disease	↓	N–↓	↓	↓	N–↑	N–↑	↑	N	N
Sideroblastic anemia	↑	↓	↑	↑	↑	↑	↑ (↓)	N	N–↑

TIBC = total iron-binding capacity; ZPP = zinc protoporphyrins; ↓ = decreased; N = normal; ↑ = increased.

examinations to perform are hemoglobin electrophoresis and determination of Hb A₂ and Hb F. Family studies are often necessary.

Sideroblastic anemias include idiopathic refractory sideroblastic anemias, which are part of the myelodysplastic syndromes (see Ch. 32), as well as anemias that occur after therapy with certain drugs (e.g., isoniazid) or in chronic lead poisoning. Coarse basophilic stippling is common in this group of anemias.

Table 31–14 summarizes some laboratory distinctions within the microcytic anemias.

Normocytic and Normochromic Anemias (Normal MCV)

This large group of anemias has many causes. A useful approach is evaluation of the erythrokinetics in a given patient (see Ch. 30). Often, the reticulocyte production index (RPI) and examination of the bone marrow will suffice. The RPI is the simplest measure of effective erythropoiesis.

Optimal Marrow Response: Reticulocyte Production Index Greater than Two. If the output of reticulocytes has exceeded two times normal, as determined by the absolute reticulocyte count or RPI, it can be assumed that the marrow has reached an optimal response. The cause for the anemia is then either *acute blood loss* or *hemolysis*. If blood loss cannot be proved, evidence that hemolysis is in fact present must be sought.

Erythroid hyperplasia of the marrow, serum bilirubin, and urine or fecal urobilinogen will indicate whether erythropoietic activity and destruction are increased. Red cell survival determination may be needed to prove hemolysis in some cases. Low serum haptoglobin and high LD point to hemolysis, but a normal level does not exclude it. None of these measurements will specify whether hemolysis is intravascular or extravascular, but elevated plasma hemoglobin, hemoglobinuria, and hemosiderinuria indicate intravascular hemolysis.

Once it is determined that excessive hemolysis is occurring, the type of hemolytic mechanism must be ascertained.

Direct Antiglobulin (Coombs') Test. If the direct antiglobulin reaction is *positive* using broad-spectrum reagents, tests to determine the presence of IgG, IgM, or complement on the red cells should be undertaken. If immunoglobulin is present on the red cells, tests for antibody specificity, cold agglutinins, Donath–Landsteiner antibody, and serum protein electrophoresis may help to define the process.

If the direct antiglobulin reaction is *negative*, the examinations performed next will depend on the clinical findings and the results of the measurements already made.

If hereditary spherocytosis is suspected, osmotic fragility before and after 24-hour incubation at 37°C and family studies will be necessary.

If a nonspherocytic congenital hemolytic anemia is suspected, screening for G6PD and PK deficiencies, hemoglobin electrophoresis, and a sickle cell test will be helpful. If these are negative, the heat instability test, isopropanol solubility test, and autohemolysis test should be considered.

If thalassemia seems likely, determinations of Hb A₂ and Hb F and perhaps looking for Hb H inclusions are appropriate. Thalassemias are usually microcytic and hypochromic anemias; β-thalassemia major, β-thalassemia intermedia, and hemoglobin H disease are hemolytic disorders and may have an increased RPI.

If drug-induced hemolysis is suspected, a test for Heinz bodies, screening test for G6PD and, if possible, tests for a drug-dependent autoantibody are indicated.

If the nature of the hemolytic anemia is obscure, a flow cytometry test for PNH should be performed.

Inadequate Marrow Response: Reticulocyte Production Index Less than Two. The mechanism of the anemia may be ineffective erythropoiesis. Conditions with the greatest degree of ineffective erythropoiesis appear in other categories (e.g., megaloblastic anemia and thalassemia), but some idiopathic refractory anemias have a hyperplastic bone marrow and impaired delivery of the cells to the blood. In some of these, abnormalities in erythroid precursors suggestive of megaloblastic change may be present, but the granulocytic and megakaryocytic changes usually seen in megaloblastic anemia are lacking.

A low reticulocyte count may indicate decreased production caused by inadequate stimulation of the marrow. Chronic renal disease may result in impaired production of erythropoietin. Certain endocrinopathies, such as hypopituitarism or hypothyroidism, may result in regulation of hemoglobin production at a lower level as a result of decreased tissue need for oxygen.

A large group of normochromic anemias associated with various chronic diseases form a heterogeneous group characterized by failure of the marrow to meet the need of a slightly decreased red cell survival. Some of these are anemia of chronic disorders associated with infection, cancer, or rheumatoid arthritis and have the defect in iron metabolism noted previously under the hypochromic microcytic anemias.

Inability of the marrow to respond to erythropoietin may be due to damage to the marrow by drugs or toxic chemicals, to unknown causes, or to infiltration of the marrow by neoplastic cells or fibrous tissue.

In those conditions with low reticulocyte counts in which the marrow is not effectively producing erythrocytes, it is usually helpful to examine the bone marrow. Other studies to determine the underlying disease process can then proceed according to the marrow picture, the assessment of erythrokinetics, and the clinical findings.

Polycythemia

Polycythemia (erythrocytosis) is classically defined as an elevated hematocrit level above the normal range. In clinical setting polycythemia exists when hemoglobin and red cell count are increased reflecting an elevation of the total red cell volume (Maran, 2004).

Absolute polycythemia refers to an increase in the total red cell mass in the body; in *relative polycythemia*, the total red cell mass is normal, but the hematocrit is elevated because the plasma volume is decreased. Polycythemia may be classified as in Table 31–15. Some classifications are based on erythropoietin response (Cazzola, 2004) while others are based on the underlying mechanism, i.e., primary or secondary, and congenital or acquired (Gordeuk, 2005).

Relative Polycythemia

Relative polycythemia refers to an increase in hematocrit or red cell count as a result of decreased plasma volume; total red cell mass is not increased. This occurs in acute dehydration (e.g., in severe diarrhea or burns), and in patients on diuretic therapy.

In *spurious polycythemia* (apparent polycythemia, Gaisböck's syndrome), the red cell mass is often high normal and the plasma volume is low normal; these patients have been regarded as an extreme of the normal physiologic state. Almost all are men, have a high incidence of tobacco smoking, and tend to be obese and to have hypertension. Sleep apnea and diuretics may be contributory factors. Serum erythropoietin level is normal (Cazzola, 2004).

Absolute Polycythemia

Appropriately Increased Erythropoietin Production Due to Hypoxia

Arterial Oxygen Unsaturation. Lack of oxygen reaching the blood for whatever reason results in arterial unsaturation, impaired oxygen delivery to the tissues, increased production of erythropoietin, erythroid hyperplasia in the marrow, and resultant erythrocytosis. The red cell mass

Table 31–15 Pathophysiological Classification of Polycythemia

Relative polycythemia

1. Diminished plasma volume: dehydration; shock
2. Spurious polycythemia (stress polycythemia; Gaisböck's syndrome)

Absolute polycythemia

1. Secondary polycythemia with appropriately increased erythropoietin production
   a. Decreased oxygen loading: hypoxia, high altitude; pulmonary disease; cyanotic heart disease; carboxyhemoglobinemia; methemoglobinemia; Hb M
   b. Decreased oxygen unloading: high oxygen affinity hemoglobinopathy, biphosphoglycerate deficiency
2. Secondary polycythemia with inappropriately increased erythropoietin production
   a. Neoplasms: Wilms' tumor, renal carcinoma; cerebellar hemangioma; hepatoma
   b. Localized tissue hypoxia: polycystic kidney; renal artery stenosis
   c. Post-renal transplant
   d. Acute hepatitis
3. Genetic polycythemia
   a. Primary familial congenital polycythemia (mutated Epo receptor)
   b. Chuvash polycythemia (mutated *VHL* gene)
4. Primary marrow disorders
   a. Polycythemia vera

Modified from Cazzola, 2004.

is increased. As a response to the hypoxia, the red cell 2,3-DPG and the P_{50} are increased. In contrast to polycythemia vera, there is usually no leukocytosis or thrombocytosis, and the neutrophil alkaline phosphatase is normal. Arterial oxygen unsaturation may be the cause of polycythemia in persons living at high altitudes; in patients with chronic pulmonary disease and a block in diffusion of oxygen into the blood; in cyanotic heart disease in which there is right-to-left shunt; and in caroboxy-hemoglobinemia mostly related to cigarette smoking. In case of carbon monoxide poisoning, hypoxia is caused by two mechanisms: direct reduction of oxygen saturation and interference with oxygen release from hemoglobin (Landaw, 1990).

High Oxygen Affinity Hemoglobinopathy. Another cause of tissue hypoxia is the presence of a structurally abnormal hemoglobin that has a high affinity for oxygen (Prchal, 2003) (see earlier under Disorders of Hemoglobin Function and Stability). As in other functional hemo-globinopathies, the disorder occurs in the heterozygote. More than 100 hemoglobin mutations associated with increased oxygen affinity have been identified (Prchal, 2003). The abnormal hemoglobin releases less oxygen to the tissues than does normal hemoglobin at the same Po_2; the oxygen dissociation curve is shifted to the left, and the P_{50} is decreased. The red cell 2,3-DPG is not increased. As in arterial oxygen unsaturation, there is increased erythropoietin production and erythrocytosis. It must be emphasized that routine hemoglobin electrophoresis often does not detect these hemoglobin variants because the amino acid substitution is at one of the $\alpha\beta$ contact sites or near the heme pocket. A low P_{50} therefore is presumptive evidence for a hemoglobinopathy. Some high-affinity hemoglobins associated with polycythemia are unstable; in these instances, the heat instability test is positive.

Other causes of altered oxygen affinity include deficiency of red cell enzyme 2,3-DPG and hemoglobin M (Gordeuk, 2005).

Inappropriate Erythropoietin Production

Neoplasms. Neoplasms, either benign or malignant, have been associated with polycythemia. Renal neoplasms account for the majority. In almost all cases, erythrocytosis has disappeared after resection of the tumor. The mechanism is not clear. Some of these neoplasms have been shown to contain, and presumably produce, erythropoietin (e.g., cerebellar hemangioma, renal cell carcinoma, Wilms' tumor, some hepatomas).

Renal Disorders. In other neoplasms or growths (e.g., renal cysts, hydronephrosis, ovarian carcinoma, some hepatomas), it appears that the mass impinging on the kidney induces increased renal production of erythropoietin as a result of increased pressure or local hypoxia within the kidney. Renal artery stenosis is also associated with polycythemia. Post-transplant erythrocytosis occurs in 10–20% of renal transplant recipients.

The therapeutic effects of angiotensin-converting enzyme inhibitors in this condition suggest a role for angiotensin II in regulating erythropoiesis (Prchal, 2003).

Familial Polycythemia. The most common familial polycythemia is due to the presence of a *high oxygen affinity hemoglobin*, which is inherited as an autosomal dominant trait. Congenital polycythemia may be due to a defect in the hypoxia-sensing mechanism, which relies on the transcription factor hypoxia inducible factor-1 (HIF-1) and the von Hippel–Lindau protein (pVHL). Hypoxia results in increased levels of HIF-1, which provides transcription regulation of the erythropoietin gene (*EPO*). The α-subunit is the active component of HIF-1 and is degraded by pVHL. von Hippel–Lindau syndrome is an autosomal dominant disorder associated with mutations in the *VHL* gene. These mutations result in increased levels of HIF-1α and increased levels of erythropoietin (Prchal, 2003; Gordeuk, 2005). Chuvash polycythemia is an autosomal recessive congenital polycythemia that is endemic in the Chuvash population of the Russian federation. It has been reported to be associated with a high mortality rate due to thrombotic and hemorrhagic complications.

Congenital polycythemia may occur secondary to a defect in the erythropoietin receptor while having a normal hypoxia sensing mechanism. Primary familial and congenital polycythemia (PFCP) is an autosomal dominant disorder present at birth. PFCP is associated with low serum erythropoietin level and in vitro hypersensitivity of erythroid progenitors to erythropoietin. Although mutations in the erythropoietin receptor gene (*EPOR*) with resulting truncated receptor have been described in PFCP, the exact mechanism of polycythemia is unclear (Prchal, 2003; Gordeuk, 2005). As mentioned earlier, marked decrease in red cell 2,3-DPG associated with *deficiency of 2,3-DPG mutase* activity results in polycythemia and appears to be inherited as an autosomal recessive condition.

Polycythemia Vera

Polycythemia vera is a panmyelosis – that is, a condition in which excessive proliferation occurs in megakaryocytes and granulocytes as well as in erythrocytes. It is manifested by erythrocytosis, leukocytosis, and thrombocytosis of varying degree. The etiology is unknown. Polycythemia vera is discussed with the myeloproliferative disorders.

Measurement of Erythrocyte and Plasma Volume

The diagnosis of absolute polycythemia depends on reliable measurements of erythrocyte and plasma volumes. The erythrocyte and plasma volumes are measured by the use of radioactive isotopic tracers and the dilution principle. The most commonly employed tracers are ^{51}Cr in the form of sodium chromate bound to erythrocytes for measurement of erythrocyte volume. ^{125}I or ^{131}Iodine is bound to albumin and can be used to measure plasma volume.

For detailed description of measurement of red cell and plasma volume, see the report of the International Committee for Standardization in Haematology (1980).

Erythrocyte Volume. In brief, blood is collected from the patient and the erythrocytes are labeled with ^{51}Cr. The chromated erythrocytes are washed in saline. An aliquot of the ^{51}Cr erythrocytes diluted in saline is injected intravenously into the patient. After a period of equilibration, usually 10–20 minutes, a sample of blood is withdrawn from the opposite arm. In cases in which the equilibration time is likely to be prolonged (as in splenomegaly, heart failure, or shock), another sample should be withdrawn 60 minutes after injection.

Radioactivity of each sample is recorded by a scintillation counter. The erythrocyte volume (EV) is calculated using the formula

$$EV \text{ (mL)} = I \text{ (cpm)}/C \text{ (cpm/mL)}$$

where $I =$ total injected radioactivity (counts/min)

C = radioactivity in erythrocytes after mixing is complete (counts/min/mL of erythrocytes).

Plasma Volume. Approximately 20 mL of blood is withdrawn from a patient. After centrifugation, the plasma is removed and radioiodine labeled albumin is added. After mixing, the labeled plasma is injected intravenously into the patient. At 10, 20, and 30 minutes following the injection, 5 mL of blood is removed and the radioactivity is counted in a well-type scintillation counter. The radioactivity at zero time (P_0) is determined by plotting the three points on semilogarithmic graph paper and extrapolating to zero time. A standard is prepared by diluting an aliquot of the radioiodine-labeled albumin with saline containing a small amount of detergent.

The plasma volume (PV) is calculated using the formula:

$$PV \text{ (mL)} = S \text{ (cpm/mL)} \times D \times V \text{ (mL)}/P_0 \text{ (cpm/mL)}$$

IV

Table 31–16 Clinical Effect of Variable Relationship Between Red Cell Volume and Plasma Volume

Red cell volume	Plasma volume	Cause	Effect
Normal	High	Pregnancy Cirrhosis Nephritis Congestive cardiac failure	Pseudoanemia
Normal	Low	Stress Peripheral circulatory failure Dehydration Edema Prolonged bed rest	Pseudopolycythemia
Low	Normal	Anemia	Accurate reflection of degree of anemia
Low	High	Anemia	Anemia less severe than indicated by blood count
Low	Low	Hemorrhage Severe anemia (when hematocrit < 0.2)	Anemia more severe than indicated by blood count
High	Normal to low	Polycythemia	Accurate reflection of polycythemia or polycythemia less severe than apparent
High	High	Polycythemia (when hematocrit > 0.5)	Polycythemia more severe than apparent
Normal or high even	High	Marked splenomegaly	Pseudoanemia

From Dacie, 1975.

where

S = counting rate of standard (counts/min/mL)
D = dilution of diluted standard solution
V = volume of radioiodine-labeled albumin solution injected
P_0 = counting rate of plasma sample corrected to zero time (counts/min/mL).

Interpretation. The normal erythrocyte volume for men is 20–36 mL/kg, and for women it is 19–31 mL/kg. The plasma volume for men is 25–43 mL/kg; for women, 28–45 mL/kg. In newborns and premature infants, the red cell volume and plasma volume in milliliters per kilogram are higher than in adults.

Patients with polycythemia have red cell volumes exceeding 36 mL/kg for men and 32 mL/kg for women. Changes in erythrocyte volume and plasma volume in a variety of conditions are recorded in Table 31–16.

References

Ahmed S, Siddiqui RK, Siddiqui AK, et al: HIV associated thrombotic microangiopathy. Postgrad Med J 2002; 78:520–525.

Alcindor T, Bridges KR: Sideroblastic anaemias. Br J Haematol 2002; 116:733–743.

Alter BP: Prenatal diagnosis: General introduction, methodology, and review. Hemoglobin 1988; 12:763–772.

Alter BP: Bone marrow failure syndromes in children. Pediatr Clin North Am 2002; 49:973–988.

Alter BP, Young NS: The bone marrow failure syndromes. In Nathan DG, Orkin SH (eds): Nathan, Oski's Hematology of Infancy and Childhood, 5th ed. Philadelphia, WB Saunders Company, 1998, p 237.

Babior BM: Metabolic aspects of folic acid and cobalamine. In Beutler E, Lichtman MA, Coller BS, et al: (eds): Williams Hematology, 6th ed. New York, McGraw-Hill, 2001a, p 305.

Babior BM: The megaloblastic anemia. In Beutler E, Lichtman MA, Coller BS, et al: (eds): Williams Hematology, 6th ed. New York, McGraw-Hill, 2001b, p 425.

Baier JE, Poehlau D: Is alpha-methyldopa-type autoimmune hemolytic anemia mediated by interferon-gamma? Ann Hematol 1994; 69:249–251.

Basset P, Braconnier F, Rosa J: An update on electrophoretic and chromatographic methods in the diagnosis of hemoglobinopathies. J Chromatogr Biomed Appl 1982; 227:267–304.

Beck WS (ed): Hematology, 5th ed. Cambridge, MA, The MIT Press, 1991.

Bentley SA Red cell survival studies reinterpreted. Clin Haematol 1977; 6:601–623.

Betke K, Martl HR, Schlicht I. Estimation of small percentages of foetal haemoglobin. Nature 1959; 184:1877–1878.

Beutler E: Hemolytic Anemia in Disorders of Red Cell Metabolism, New York, Plenum Medical Book Company, 1978.

Beutler E: Red cell enzyme defects as nondiseases and as diseases. Blood 1979a; 54:1–7.

Beutler E: Red Cell Metabolism: A Manual of Biochemical Methods, 3rd ed. Orlando, FL, Grune & Stratton, 1984.

Beutler E: The molecular biology of enzymes and erythrocyte metabolisms. In Stamatoyannopoulos G, Nienhuis AW, Majerus PW, Varmus H (eds): The Molecular Basis of Blood Diseases, 2nd ed. Philadelphia, WB Saunders Company, 1994, p 331.

Beutler E, Luzzatto L: Hemolytic anemia. Semin Hematol 1999; 36:38–47.

Beutler E, Blume KG, Kaplan JC, et al: International committee for standardization in haematology: Recommended screening test for glucose-6-phosphate dehydrogenase (G-6-PD) deficiency. Br J Haematol 1979b; 43:465–467.

Bottomley SS: Sideroblastic anaemia. Clin Haematol 1982; 11:389–409.

Briere RO, Golias T, Batsakis JG: Rapid qualitative and quantitative hemoglobin fractionation. Cellulose acetate electrophoresis. Am J Clin Pathol 1965; 44:695–701.

Brissot P, Troadec MB, Loreal O: The clinical relevance of new insights in iron transport and metabolism. Curr Hematol Rep 2004; 3:107–115.

A comprehensive update about iron transport including the proposed role of hepcidin.

Brugnara C: Iron deficiency and erythropoiesis: New diagnostic approaches. Clin Chem 2003; 49:1573–1578.

Bunn HF: Sickle hemoglobin and other hemoglobin mutants. In Stamatoyannopoulos G, Nienhuis AW, Majerus PW, Varmus H (eds): The Molecular Basis of Blood Diseases, 2nd ed. Philadelphia, WB Saunders Company, 1994, p 207.

Bunn HF: Human Hemoglobins; Normal and abnormal. In Nathan DG, Orkin SH (ed): Nathan, Oski's Hematology of Infancy and Childhood, 5th ed. Philadelphia, WB Saunders Company, 1998, p 729.

Bunn HF, Forget BG: Hemoglobin: Molecular, Genetic and Clinical Aspects. Philadelphia, WB Saunders Company, 1986.

This classic book provides elegant description of major hemoglobinopathies and includes essential clues to differential diagnosis in a concise manner.

Bunn HF, Forget BG, Ranney HM: Human Hemoglobins. Philadelphia, WB Saunders Company, 1977

Camitta BM, Storb R, Thomas ED: Aplastic anemia (second of two parts): Pathogenesis, diagnosis, treatment, and prognosis. N Engl J Med 1982; 306:712–718.

Carmel R: Ethnic and racial factors in cobalamin metabolism and its disorders. Semin Hematol 1999; 36:88–100.

Caro J, Erslev AJ: Anemia of chronic renal failure. In Beutler E, Lichtman MA, Coller BS, et al: (eds): Williams Hematology, 6th ed. New York, McGraw-Hill, 2001, p 399.

Carrell RW, Kay R: A simple method for the detection of unstable haemoglobins. Br J Haematol 1972; 23:615–619.

Cazzola M: Serum erythropoietin concentration as a diagnostic tool for polycythemia vera. Haematologica 2004; 89:1159–1160.

Clarke GM, Higgins TN: Laboratory investigation of hemoglobinopathies and thalassemias: Review and update. Clin Chem 2000; 46:1284–1290.

Clegg JB, Naughton MA, Weatherball DJ: Abnormal human haemoglobins. separation and characterization of the alpha and beta chains by chromatography, and the determination of two new variants, HB Chesapeak and HB J (Bangkok). J Mol Biol 1966; 19:91–108.

Dacie JV, Lewis SM: Practical Haematology, 5th ed. Edinburgh, Churchill Livingstone, 1975.

Dacie JV, Lewis SM: Practical Haematology, 7th ed. Edinburgh, Churchill Livingstone, 1991.

Dallman PR, Yip R, Oski FA: Iron deficiency and related nutritional anemias. In Nathan DG, Oski FA (eds): Hematology of Infancy and Childhood, 4th ed. Philadelphia, WB Saunders Company, 1993, p 413.

Delvoye NL, Destroismaisons NM, Wall LA: Activation of the beta-globin promoter by the locus control region correlates with binding of a novel factor to the CAAT box in murine erythroleukemia cells but not in K562 cells. Mol Cell Biol 1993; 13:6969–6983.

Dieterich DT, Spivak JL: Hematologic disorders associated with hepatitis C virus infection and their management. Clin Infect Dis 2003; 37:533–541.

Donath J, Landsteiner K: Uber paroxysmale Haemoglobinurie. Munch Med Wschr 1904; 51:1590.

Efremov GD, Mladenovski B, Petkov G, et al: Lepore hemoglobinopathy in Yugoslavia. New Istanbul Contrib Clin Sci 1978; 12:211–232.

Elghetany MT, Hudnall SD, Gardner FH: Peripheral blood picture in primary hypocellular refractory anemia and idiopathic acquired aplastic anemia: An additional tool for differential diagnosis. Haematologica 1997; 82:21–24.

Erslev AJ: Anemia of endocrine disorders. In Beutler E, Lichtman MA, Coller BS, et al: (eds): Williams Hematology, 6th ed. New York, McGraw-Hill, 2001a, p 407.

Erslev AJ: Clinical manifestations and classification of erythrocyte disorders. In Beutler E, Lichtman MA, Coller BS, et al: (eds): Williams Hematology, 6th ed. New York, McGraw-Hill, 2001b, p 369.

Erslev AJ: Pure red cell aplasia. In Beutler E, Lichtman MA, Coller BS, et al: (eds): Williams Hematology, 6th ed. New York, McGraw-Hill, 2001c, p 391.

Erslev AJ: Traumatic cardiac hemolytic anemia. In Beutler E, Lichtman MA, Coller BS, et al: (eds): Williams Hematology, 6th ed. New York, McGraw-Hill, 2001d, p 619.

Fairbanks V, Beutler E: Iron deficiency. In Beutler E, Lichtman MA, Coller BS, et al: (eds): Williams Hematology, 6th ed. New York, McGraw-Hill, 2001a, p 447.

Fairbanks V, Beutler E: Iron metabolism. In Beutler E, Lichtman MA, Coller BS, et al: (eds): Williams Hematology, 6th ed. New York, McGraw-Hill, 2001b, p 295.

Fairbanks VF, Fernandez MN: The identification of metabolic errors associated with hemolytic anemia. JAMA 1969; 208:316–320.

Fairbanks VF, Oliveros R, Brandabur JH, et al.: Homozygous hemoglobin E mimics beta-thalassemia minor without anemia or hemolysis: hematologic, functional, and biosynthetic studies of first North American cases. Am J Hematol 1980; 8:109–121.

Fleming AF: Hypoplastic anaemia in pregnancy. J Obstet Gynaecol Br Commonw 1968; 75:138–141.

Forget BG: Molecular studies of genetic disorders affecting the expression of the human β-globin gene: A model system for the analysis of inborn errors of metabolism. Recent Prog Horm Res 1982; 38:257–277.

Fukagawa N, Friedman S, Gill FM, et al: Hereditary spherocytosis with normal osmotic fragility after incubation. Is the autohemolysis test really obsolete? JAMA 1979; 242:63–64.

Fyfe JC, Madsen M, Hojrup P, et al: The functional cobalamin (vitamin B12)-intrinsic factor receptor is a novel complex of cubilin and amnionless. Blood 2004; 103:1573–1579.

The first article to investigate the mechanism of Imerslund–Gräsbeck syndrome.

Gallagher PG: Acanthocytosis, stomatocytosis, and related disorders. In Beutler E, Lichtman MA, Coller BS, et al: (eds): Williams Hematology, 6th ed. New York, McGraw-Hill, 2001, p 519.

Gallagher PG, Jarolim P: Red cell membrane disorders. In Hoffman R, Benz EJ, Shattil SJ, et al: (eds): Hematology Basic Principles and Practice, 3rd ed. Philadelphia, Churchill Livingstone, 2000, p 576.

Garratty G: Review: Drug-induced immune hemolytic anemia – the last decade. Immunohematol 2004; 20:138–146.

A detailed review about the prevalence and mechanism of cephalosporin-induced hemolytic anemia.

Gattermann N, Retzlaff S, Wang YL, et al: Heteroplasmic point mutations of mitochondrial DNA affecting subunit I of cytochrome c oxidase in two patients with acquired idiopathic sideroblastic anemia. Blood 1997; 90:4961–4972.

Gehrs BC, Friedberg RC: Autoimmune hemolytic anemia. Am J Hematol 2002; 69:258.

Gilliland BC: Coombs-negative immune hemolytic anemia. Semin Hematol 1976; 13:267–275.

Globin Gene Server: Online. Available: http://globin.cse.psu.edu/

An up-to-date interactive database of Hb variants and thalassemias

Gordeuk VR, Stockton DW, Prchal JT: Congenital polycythemias/erythrocytoses. Haematologica 2005; 90:109–116.

Ham TH: Studies on the destruction of red blood cells. I. Chronic hemolytic anemia with paroxysmal nocturnal hemoglobinuria: An investigation of the mechanism of hemolysis, with observations on five cases. Arch Intern Med 1939; 64:1271.

Hartmann RC, Jenkins DE Jr, Arnold AB: Diagnostic specificity of sucrose hemolysis test for paroxysmal nocturnal hemoglobinuria. Blood 1970; 35:462–475.

Head CE, Conroy M, Jarvis M, et al.: Some observations on the measurement of haemoglobin A2 and S percentages by high performance liquid chromatography in the presence and absence of alpha thalassaemia. J Clin Pathol 2004; 57:276–280.

Heimpel H: Congenital dyserythropoietic anemias: Epidemiology, clinical significance, and progress in understanding their pathogenesis. Ann Hematol 2004; 83(10):613–621.

Herbert V: Megaloblastic anemias. Lab Invest 1985; 52:3–19.

Higgs DR, Aldridge BE, Lamb J, et al: The interaction of alpha-thalassemia and homozygous sickle-cell disease. N Engl J Med 1982; 306:1441–1446.

Higgs DR, Vickers MA, Wilkie AO, et al: A review of the molecular genetics of the human alpha-globin gene cluster. Blood 1989; 73:1081–1104.

Hillman RS, Finch CA: Red Cell Manual, 4th ed. Philadelphia, FA Davis, 1974.

Hillman RS, Finch CA: Red Cell Manual, 7th ed. Philadelphia, FA Davis, 1996.

Huisman TH: Trimodality in the percentages of beta chain variants in heterozygotes: The effect of the number of active HB alpha structural loci. Hemoglobin 1977; 1:349–382.

Huisman TH: The human fetal hemoglobins. Tex Rep Biol Med 1980; 40:29–42.

Huisman THJ: The Hemoglobinopathies. Methods in Hematology, Vol 15. Edinburgh, Churchill Livingstone, 1986.

Huisman, A: Syllabus of Human Hemoglobin Variants, 2nd ed. Augusta, GA, The Sickle Cell Anemia Foundation, 1998.

International Committee for Standardization in Haematology: Recommended methods for measurement of red-cell and plasma volume. J Nucl Med 1980; 21:793.

Jacob HS, Jandl JH: A simple visual screening test for glucose-6-phosphate dehydrogenase deficiency employing ascorbate and cyanide. N Engl J Med 1966; 274:1162–1167.

Jaffe ES, Harris NL, Stein H, Vardiman JW (eds): World Health Organization Classification of Tumors. Pathology and Genetics of Tumours of Haematopoietic and Lymphoid Tissues. Lyon, IARC Press, 2001, p 63.

Johnson RJ, Hillmen P: Paroxysmal nocturnal haemoglobinuria: Nature's gene therapy? Mol Pathol 2002; 55:145–152.

Jones JA, Broszeit HK, LeCrone CN, et al: An improved method for detection of red cell hemoglobin H inclusions. Am J Med Technol 1981; 47:94–96.

Koc S, Harris JW: Sideroblastic anemias: Variations on imprecision in diagnostic criteria, proposal for an extended classification of sideroblastic anemias. Am J Hematol 1998; 57:1–6.

Kosche KA, Dobkin C, Bank A: DNA sequences regulating human beta globin gene expression. Nucleic Acids Res 1985; 13:7781–7793.

Labbé RF, Dewanji A: Iron assessment tests: Transferrin receptor vis-a-vis zinc protoporphyrin. Clin Biochem 2004; 37:165–174.

Landaw SA: Polycythemia vera and other polycythemic states. Clin Lab Med 1990; 10:857–871.

Lehmann H, Huntsman RG, Casey R, et al: Erythrocyte disorders, anemias related to abnormal globin. In Williams WJ, Beutler E, Erslev AJ, Rundles RW (eds): Hematology, 2nd ed. New York, McGraw-Hill, 1977, p 494.

Lewis SM, Dacie JV: The aplastic anaemia–paroxysmal nocturnal haemoglobinuria syndrome. Br J Haematol 1967; 13:236–251.

Lindenbaum J: Status of laboratory testing in the diagnosis of megaloblastic anemia. Blood 1983; 61:624–627.

Lindenbaum J, Healton EB, Savage DG, et al: Neuropsychiatric disorders caused by cobalamin deficiency in the absence of anemia or macrocytosis. N Engl J Med 1988; 318:1720–1728.

Looker AC, Dallman PR, Carroll MD, et al: Prevalence of iron deficiency in the United States. JAMA 1997; 277:973–976.

Lynch RE, Williams DM, Reading JC, et al: The prognosis in aplastic anemia. Blood 1975; 45:517–528.

McMinn JR, George JN: Evaluation of women with clinically suspected thrombotic thrombocytopenic purpura–hemolytic uremic syndrome during pregnancy. J Clin Apheresis 2001; 16:202–209.

Maran J, Prchal J: Polycythemia and oxygen sensing. Pathol Biol (Paris) 2004; 52:280–284.

Mario N, Baudin B, Aussel C, et al: Capillary isoelectric focusing and high-performance cation-exchange chromatography compared for qualitative and quantitative analysis of hemoglobin variants. Clin Chem 1997; 43:2137–2142.

Mazza U, Saglio G, Cappio FC, et al: Clinical and haematological data in 254 cases of beta-thalassaemia trait in Italy. Br J Haematol 1976; 33:91–99.

Means RT Jr: Recent developments in the anemia of chronic disease. Curr Hematol Rep 2003; 2:116–121.

Milner PF, Gooden HM: Rapid citrate-agar electrophoresis in routine screening for hemoglobinopathies using a simple hemolysate. Am J Clin Pathol 1975; 64:58–64.

Miwa S: Pyruvate kinase deficiency and other enzymopathies of the Embden–Meyerhof pathway. Clin Haematol 1981; 10:57–80.

Moake JL: Thrombotic microangiopathies. N Engl J Med 2002; 347:589–600.

An excellent review of pathophysiologic mechanisms, clinical presentation, and management of thrombotic microangiopathy. The accompanying figures are exceptionally well designed and simple.

Moake JL: Idiopathic thrombotic thrombocytopenic purpura. Hematology 2004; 408 (The annual meeting of the American Society of Hematology, San Diego, December 2004).

Mohandas N, Chasis JA: Red blood cell deformability, membrane material properties and shape: Regulation by transmembrane, skeletal and cytosolic proteins and lipids. Semin Hematol 1993; 30:171–192.

Motulsky AG: Frequency of sickling disorders in US Blacks. N Engl J Med 1973; 288:31–33.

Oh R, Brown DL: Vitamin B12 deficiency. Am Fam Physician 2003; 67:979–986.

Old J: Haemoglobinopathies. Prenat Diagn 1996; 16:1181–1186.

Old JM: DNA-based diagnosis of hemoglobin disorders. In Steinberg MH, Forget BG, Higgs DR and Nagel RL (eds): Disorders of Hemoglobin, Cambridge, Cambridge University Press, 2001, p 941.

Orkin SH, Nathan DG: The thalassemias. N Engl J Med 1976; 295:710–714.

Orkin SH, Nathan DG: The thalassemias. In Nathan DG, Orkin SH (eds): Nathan, Oski's Hematology of Infancy and Childhood, 5th ed. Philadelphia, WB Saunders Company, 1998, p 811.

Ozatli D, Koksal AS, Haznedaroglu IC, et al: Erythrocytes: Anemias in chronic liver diseases. Hematol 2000; 5:69–76.

Packman CH: Acquired hemolytic anemia due to warm reacting antibodies. In Beutler E, Lichtman MA, Coller BS, et al: (eds): Williams Hematology, 6th ed. New York, McGraw-Hill, 2001a, p 639.

Packman CH: Drug related immune hemolytic anemia. In Beutler E, Lichtman MA, Coller BS, et al: (eds): Williams Hematology, 6th ed. New York, McGraw-Hill, 2001b, p 657.

Paglia DE, Valentine WN: Haemolytic anaemia associated with disorders of the purine and pyrimidine salvage pathways. Clin Haematol 1981; 10:81–98.

Pearson HA, Spencer RP, Cornelius EA: Functional asplenia in sickle-cell anemia. N Engl J Med 1969; 281:923–926.

Pierce HI, Sumiko KK, Sofroniadou K, et al: Frequencies of thalassemia in American Blacks. Blood 1977; 49:981–986.

Prchal JT: Classification and molecular biology of polycythemias (erythrocytoses) and thrombocytosis. Hematol Oncol Clin North Am 2003; 17(5):1151–1158.

Prchal JT, Gregg XT: Red cell enzymopathies. In Hoffman R, Benz EJ, Shattil SJ, et al: (eds): Hematology Basic Principles and Practice, 3rd ed. Philadelphia, Churchill Livingstone, 2000, p 561.

Ramasethu J, Luban NLC: Alloimmune hemolytic anemia of the newborn. In Beutler E, Lichtman MA, Coller BS, et al: (eds): Williams Hematology, 6th ed. New York, McGraw-Hill, 2001, p 665.

Reissman KR, Ruth WE, Nomura TA: A human hemoglobin with lowered oxygen affinity and impaired heme–heme interactions. J Clin Invest 1961; 40:1826.

Riou J, Godart C, Hurtrel D, et al: Cation-exchange HPLC evaluated for presumptive identification of hemoglobin variants. Clin Chem 1997; 43:34–39.

Ritchie DS, Underhill C, Grigg AP: Aplastic anemia as a late complication of thymoma in remission. Eur J Haematol 2002a; 68:389–391.

Ritchie RF, Palomaki GE, Neveux LM, et al: Reference distributions for serum iron and transferrin saturation: A practical, simple, and clinically relevant approach in a large cohort. J Clin Lab Anal 2002b; 16:237–245.

Rosenblatt DS, Whitehead VM: Cobalamin and folate deficiency: Acquired and hereditary disorders in children. Semin Hematol 1999; 36:19–34.

Rosse WF: Cold-induced immune hemolytic anemia. Hematology 2004; 58 (The annual meeting of the American Society of Hematology, San Diego, December 2004).

Schmidt RM, Brosious EF: Basic Laboratory Methods of Hemoglobinopathy Detection, 6th ed. Atlanta, US Department of Health, Education and Welfare, Centers for Disease Control, [HEW Publ. No. (CDC) 77-8266], 1976.

Schmidt RM, Rucknagel DL, Necheles TF: Comparison of methodologies for thalassemia screening by HB A$_2$ quantitation. J Lab Clin Med 1975; 86:873–882.

Schneider RG, Hightower B, Hosty TS, et al: Abnormal hemoglobins in a quarter million people. Blood 1976; 48:629–637.

Schroter W, Nafz C: Diagnostic significance of hemoglobin F and A$_2$ levels in homo- and heterozygous beta-thalassemia during infancy. Helv Paediatr Acta 1981; 36:519–525.

Shadduck RK: Aplastic anemia. In Beutler E, Lichtman MA, Coller BS, et al: (eds): Williams Hematology, 6th ed. New York, McGraw-Hill, 2001, p 375.

Shepard MK, Weatherall DJ, Conley CL: Semi-quantitative estimation of the distribution of fetal hemoglobin in red cell populations. Bull Johns Hopkins Hosp 1962; 110:293–310.

Shulman IA, Branch DR, Nelson JM, et al: Autoimmune hemolytic anemia with both cold and warm autoantibodies. JAMA 1985; 253:1746–1748.

Singer K, Chernoff AI, Singer L: Studies on abnormal hemoglobins. I. Their demonstration in sickle cell anemia and other hematologic disorders by means of alkali denaturation. Blood 1951; 6:413–428.

Sokol RJ, Hewitt S: Autoimmune hemolysis: A critical review. Crit Rev Oncol Hematol 1985; 4:125–154.

Sokol RJ, Booker DJ, Stamps R: The pathology of autoimmune haemolytic anaemia. J Clin Pathol 1992; 45:1047–1052.

Soldin OP, Bierbower LH, Choi JJ, et al: Serum iron, ferritin, transferrin, total iron binding capacity, hs-CRP, LDL cholesterol and magnesium in children; new reference intervals using the Dade dimension clinical chemistry system. Clin Chim Acta 2004; 342:211–217.

Steinberg MH: Management of sickle cell disease. N Engl J Med 1999; 340:1021–1030.

Steinberg MH, Adams JG 3rd: Hemoglobin A$_2$: Origin, evolution, and aftermath. Blood 1991; 78:2165–2177.

Steinberg MH, Coleman MB, Adams JG, et al: The effects of alpha-thalassaemia in HbSC disease. Br J Haematol 1983; 55:487–492.

Steinberg MH, Forget BG, Higgs DR, Nagel, RL: Disorders of Hemoglobins 1st ed. Cambridge, Cambridge University Press, 2001.

Comprehensive reference book on the disorders of hemoglobin; detailed account of hemoglobin variants.

Stenvinkel P: Anaemia and inflammation: What are the implications for the nephrologist? Nephrol Dial Transplant 2003; 18:17–22.

Suh DD, Krauss JS, Bures K: Influence of hemoglobin S adducts on hemoglobin A$_2$ quantification by HPLC. Clin Chem 1996; 42:1113–1114.

Tang DC, Ebb D, Hardison RC, et al: Restoration of the CCAAT box or insertion of the CACCC motif activates [corrected] delta-globin gene expression. Blood 1997; 90:421–427.

Tietz NW (ed): Clinical Guide to Laboratory Tests, 2nd ed. Philadelphia, WB Saunders Company, 1990.

Trial J, Rice L, Alfrey CP: Erythropoietin withdrawal alters interactions between young red blood cells, splenic endothelial cells, and macrophages: An in vitro model of neocytolysis. J Investig Med 2001; 49:335–345.

Valentine WN: The Stratton lecture. Hemolytic anemia and inborn errors of metabolism. Blood 1979; 54:549–559.

Van den Bosch G, Van den Bossche J, Wagner C, et al: Determination of iron metabolism-related reference values in a healthy adult population. Clin Chem 2001; 47:1465–1467.

Ward PC: Modern approaches to the investigation of vitamin B12 deficiency. Clin Lab Med 2002; 22:435–445.

Wasi P, Na-Nakorn S, Pootrakul S-N: The alpha-thalassemias. Clin Haematol 1974; 3:383.

Weatherall DJ: Prenatal diagnosis of inherited blood diseases. Clin Haematol 1985; 14:747–774.

Weatherall DJ: The thalassemias. In Stamatoyannapoulos G, Niehuis AW, Majerus PW, Varmus H (eds): The Molecular Basis of Blood Disease, 2nd ed. Philadelphia, WB Saunders Company, 1994, p 157.

Weatherall DJ, Clegg JB: Genetic disorders of hemoglobin. Semin Hematol 1999; 36:24–37.

Weatherall DJ, Clegg JB: The Thalassaemia Syndromes, 4th ed. Oxford, Blackwell Scientific Publications, 2001.

A complete study of thalassemias and their interaction with variant hemoglobins.

Whitten WJ, Rucknagel DL: The proportion of Hb A2 is higher in sickle cell trait than in normal homozygotes. Hemoglobin 1981; 5:371–378.

Williams DM, Lynch RE, Cartwright GE: Prognostic factors in aplastic anaemia. Clin Haematol 1978; 7:467–474.

Wilson JB, Headlee ME, Huisman TH: A new high-performance liquid chromatographic procedure for the separation and quantitation of various hemoglobin variants in adults and newborn babies. J Lab Clin Med 1983; 102:174–186.

Winslow RM, Anderson WF: The hemoglobinopathies. In Stanbury JB, Wyngaarden JB, Fredrickson DS, et al: (eds): The Metabolic Basis of Inherited Disease, 5th ed. New York, McGraw-Hill, 1983, pp 2281–2317.

Wintrobe MM, Lee GR, Boggs DR, et al: Clinical Hematology, 8th ed. Philadelphia, Lea & Febiger, 1981.

Wrightstone RN, Huisman TH: On the levels of hemoglobins F and A$_2$ in sickle-cell anemia and some related disorders. Am J Clin Pathol 1974; 61:375–381.

Young N, Mortimer P: Viruses and bone marrow failure. Blood 1984; 63:729–737.

Young NS: Acquired aplastic anemia. Ann Intern Med 2002; 136:534–546.

This article highlights the most recent thoughts in the immunologic mechanism of aplastic anemia with a short discussion of its relationship to myelodysplastic syndrome and paroxysmal nocturnal hemoglobinuria.

Young NS, Maciejewski JP: Aplastic anemia. In Hoffman R, Benz EJ, Shattil SJ, et al: (eds): Hematology Basic Principles and Practice, 3rd ed. Philadelphia, Churchill Livingstone, 2000, p 297.

Zittoun J, Zittoun R: Modern clinical testing strategies in cobalamin and folate deficiency. Semin Hematol 1999; 36:35–46.

Leukocytic Disorders

Robert E. Hutchison MD, Naif Z. Abraham Jr MD PhD

KEY POINTS

• Leukocytes are regulated by complex homeostatic mechanisms which direct their response to infection and inflammation.

• Leukocytosis often reflects an underlying abnormality, while leukopenia, especially neutropenia, places a patient at risk for infection.

• Hematopoietic neoplasms have been categorized by a World Health Organization classification according to cell of origin, cytogenetic and molecular abnormalities, immunophenotype and clinical features.

• Acute leukemias are rapidly progressing neoplasms of precursor myeloid or lymphoid cell origin. Understanding of biology is associated with improvements in therapy.

• Chronic myeloproliferative disorders and myelodysplastic syndromes are heterogeneous disorders of differentiated myeloid cells. They are often initially indolent but ultimately progress.

• Non-Hodgkin lymphomas most often arise from mature B cells. They are pathologically and clinically heterogeneous. T cell lymphomas are less common, also heterogeneous, and often difficult to treat successfully.

• Hodgkin lymphoma is now considered a neoplasm of defective B cells. Much of its pathology is due to an associated inflammatory milieu.

Leukocytes

Leukocytes, or white blood cells, are found within the bone marrow (BM), the peripheral blood, and the tissues. Leukocytes are among the essential elements of the hematopoietic–lymphoreticular–immune system, which functions to protect the human body from non-self cells (infection) and altered-self cells (cancer). The overall system is extraordinarily complex and exquisitely integrated throughout (healthy) life. Various alterations, which we are beginning to understand at the molecular level, may lead to neoplastic or non-neoplastic disease. Normal leukocyte development is reviewed in Chapter 30; however, to understand some of these disease processes, we will briefly summarize main aspects of phagocytic leukocytes, the vascular pathway used in their movement and migration, the immune leukocytes, and apoptosis or 'programmed cell death.'

Let's begin with the hematopoietic system and the phagocytic leukocytes, the neutrophils, monocytes, eosinophils, and basophils. In adults, these cells are formed in the bone marrow, are released into the peripheral blood, and then can move into the tissues as needed. Complex molecular control and signaling is needed along every point of this journey, from differentiation, maturation, and commitment, to cell death by either apoptosis or necrosis. Hematopoietic cells develop in a complex bone marrow microenvironment, or stroma, containing fat cells and myofibroblasts as well as plasma cells, lymphocytes, and macrophages. There is a constant molecular balance involving cell adhesion molecules (CAM), proteases, and cytokines – small receptor-binding proteins generated by various cells that serve as autocrine or paracrine signals (Table 32–1). The net effect of these interactions directs ultimate cellular outcome.

In the marrow, granulocytic, monocyte/macrophage, and dendritic cell maturation result from an interplay of positive and negative cytokine stimulations by granulocyte colony-stimulating factor (G-CSF), granulocyte/macrophage colony stimulating factor (GM-CSF), interleukin (IL)-3, IL-4, and IL-5 on stem cells and myeloid progenitor cells (Martinez-Moczygemba, 2003). Mobilization of neutrophils, as in infection, will produce peripheral neutrophilia with immature forms (left shift), as well as increase in neutrophil production. Cytokines activate precursor cell surface receptors (e.g., G-CSF-receptors) and increase proliferation as needed. Other chemokines, such as IL-8, may also cause increased production; both IL-8 and neutrophil gelatinase B may be involved in release of leukocytes from marrow sinuses (van Eeden, 2000; Starckx, 2002).

Once released into the peripheral blood, molecular interactions with endothelial cells direct leukocytes to their ultimate destination. Selectins are transmembrane glycoprotein CAMs that are found on leukocytes (i.e., L-selectin) and activated endothelium (i.e., E- and P-selectins), are involved in leukocyte adhesion to endothelium and possibly function as signaling molecules (Patel, 2002).

As leukocytes travel in vascular lumens, they interact with endothelial integrin ligands or receptors. These integrins are instrumental in binding leukocytes and allowing them to pass across the endothelium (Alon, 2002). It is important to understand that the vasculature of normal (as well as 'abnormal') tissues is not uniform at the molecular level. It is highly specialized to the specific region or organ of the body such that the endothelial cells contain tissue- or organ-specific molecules on their luminal surfaces (Ruoslahti, 2000). This provides one mechanism whereby specific leukocyte trafficking or homing can occur.

Once the leukocyte has arrived at the intended site (e.g., infection), the leukocyte and endothelial cell interact at the molecular level such that the leukocyte can either migrate through the endothelial cell (transcytosis) or between the intercellular junctions. The junctional adhesion molecule (JAM) family of adhesion proteins is expressed by endothelial cells, epithelial cells, and blood cells and appears to play a significant role in blood cell migration or diapedesis across the endothelial barrier (Luscinskas, 2002).

IV

Table 32–1 Characteristics of Key Cell Signaling Biomolecules

Biomolecule	Target	Function
G-CSF	Myeloid bone marrow precursors	Increase proliferation and development of neutrophils
L-selectins	Endothelial cell integrin receptors	Bind leukocytes to endothelial cells to facilitate adhesion and diapedesis
Chemokines	Leukocytes via chemokine receptors	Direct migration and activation of leukocytes via cytokine chemoattractant properties
Fas/CD95 ligand (membrane protein)	*Fas*/CD95 (membrane receptor)	Apoptosis via death-inducing complex
Caspases	Protein substrates	Apoptosis via enzymatic cascades
Bcl-2 antiapoptotic protein family (Bcl-2, Bcl-xL)	Mitochondrial outer membrane (MOM), nuclear membrane, endoplasmic reticulum	Decreases cell sensitivity to apoptosis
Bcl-2 pro-apoptotic protein family (Bax, Bok, Bak)	MOM, nuclear membrane, endoplasmic reticulum	Increases cell sensitivity to apoptosis

Additional leukocyte migration and positioning occurs through chemotactic cytokines or chemokines, which rapidly attract leukocytes and provide multiple levels of migration control (Moser, 2004). Chemokines are varied and are produced by blood and tissue cells (Rot, 2004). Leukocyte chemokine receptors mediate directional migration through a concentration gradient, allowing sequential migration of leukocytes to multiple chemoattractants; this is based on multiple chemoattractant receptors and overlapping patterns of receptors on leukocyte subsets allowing 'multistep navigation' (Foxman, 1997). Chemokines are classified into functional subfamilies as 'inflammatory,' 'lymphoid/homeostatic' or 'dual.' The former type attracts mainly neutrophils (infection, inflammation, tumor). Lymphoid/homeostatic chemokines maintain hemostasis and are involved in immune responses and surveillance, and in hematopoiesis in the bone marrow. Dual-function chemokines appear to be involved in both types of function (Sallusto, 2000; Moser, 2004). In addition to leukocyte trafficking and recruitment, biological functions include lymphoid organ development, wound healing, angiogenesis, and (pathologic) metastasis (Rossi, 2000; Romagnani, 2004).

The immune leukocytes include lymphocytes, plasma cells, and dendritic cells. Lymphocytes can be divided into T cells, B cells, natural killer (NK) cells and killer (K) cells, and are usually distinguished on the basis of cell surface molecules that have been given CD or cluster of differentiation numbers. Plasma cells are antibody-secreting cells that develop from B cells. Dendritic cells are phagocytic cells that are present in different organs of the body and stimulate an immune response by processing and presenting antigen (Banchereau, 2000; Lipscomb, 2002). Natural killer and killer cells may also be described as large granular lymphocytes (LGL cells) based on their morphology with Romanowsky stains. NK cells recognize antigen naturally or nonimmunologically – activation is not needed for activity. K cells, however, utilize antibody bound to target cells for binding and cytotoxicity (antibody-dependent cell-mediated cytolysis).

Apoptosis (programmed cell death) is an active and controlled breakdown of a cell due to an internal cellular program, in contrast to necrosis, which is inflammatory and passive, and causes cell death by factors external to the cell. Apoptosis produces recognizable features, including cell shrinkage, nuclear condensation and fragmentation, and phagocytosis of cell remnants. It is involved in regulation of steady-state levels of cells undergoing proliferation.

Two fairly well defined pathways, an 'intrinsic' and an 'extrinsic' death program, have been identified (Schultz, 2003; Martin, 2004). The intrinsic pathway involves mitochondrial participation in the process and appears to be initiated by various forms of cell stress and cell damage. The mitochondrial outer membrane (MOM) becomes permeable, allowing for the release of cytochrome c. This, in turn, promotes activation of procaspase-9 within the apoptosome complex (an oligomer of apoptotic protease-activating factor-1 or APAF-1, normally present as an inactive monomer in the cytoplasm of the cell), leading to apoptosis. The release of other mitochondrial apoptotic proteins such as endonuclease G and apoptosis-inducing factor may also contribute to cell death (Saelens, 2004).

Modulation of MOM permeability occurs through the Bcl-2 protein family. Bcl-2 is a 25-kDa oncoprotein, normally located on chromosome segment 18q21. In addition to mitochondria, Bcl-2 appears to be located on nuclear membrane and endoplasmic reticulum (see Schinzel, 2004). Bcl-2 and related protein Bcl-xL are antiapoptotic and inhibit mitochondrial permeability and thus cytochrome-c protein release and APAF-1 activation. Bax, Bok, and Bak are examples of one type of Bcl-2 *pro-apoptotic* protein family, termed BH123 proteins. BH123 proteins show 3 (out of 4) areas of *Bcl-2* protein structural *homology* (termed BH1, BH2, and BH3) to Bcl-2 (Petros, 2004). These proteins, when activated, stimulate protein release by permeabilization of MOM. Activation of the BH123 proteins occurs via a second type of Bcl-2 pro-apoptotic family protein termed BH3-only proteins, which are a family of proteins that share protein structural homology to Bcl-2 at only the BH3 domain of Bcl-2. The BH3-only proteins include Bad, Bid, Bim, and others.

Caspases (cysteine proteinases with specificity for aspartate residues) play a central role in this process and are initially present within the cell as inactive precursors. Once caspases are activated via release of cytochrome c, a cascade of enzymatic cleavage of additional cellular substrates ensues, causing either activation or inactivation of these substrates. This leads to an orderly disassembly of the cell via the destruction of numerous cellular targets and apoptotic cell death (Green, 2003; Martin, 2004; Orrenius, 2004). It should be noted that both caspase-dependent and caspase-independent pathways for cell death are activated by mitochondrial proteins (Saelens, 2004). Endoplasmic reticulum (ER), the cytoplasmic organelle responsible for protein synthesis and correct protein folding and assembly, may also be an initiation site for a caspase cascade and initiation of apoptosis following ER stress (Szegezdi, 2003; Rao, 2004). A family of inhibitor of apoptosis proteins (IAP), can block apoptosis by inhibiting the caspase activation pathways.

Death receptors (DRs) are one subset of the tumor necrosis factor (TNF) family of receptors and transmit apoptotic signals via the *extrinsic* pathway. *Fas*/CD95 and TNF receptor-1 (TNFR1) are two known death receptors. They are bound by extracellular agonists or TNF ligands of the TNF superfamily (e.g., TNF-alpha, and FAS/CD95 ligand) to initiate the cascade. These ligands may be either soluble or membrane-bound. The DR transmits a signal through the cell membrane via a cytoplasmic portion of the receptor termed the death domain. This is a protein-interaction domain that when activated, initiates a series of protein interactions with additional adapter proteins such as Fas-associated death domain (FADD) protein, ultimately producing a death-inducing signaling complex (DISC) incorporating specific caspase molecules. This triggers a cascade of activation of additional caspase molecules (in addition to other proteases such as granzymes, cathepsins, and calpains) and leads to apoptotic cell death (Green, 2003; Ivanovska, 2004; Jiang, 2004).

Fas can also activate nuclear factor (NF)-kappaB, an ubiquitously expressed transcription factor normally found in an inactive state within the cell cytoplasm. This factor appears to be involved in apoptotic gene regulation as well as regulation of a number of immune and inflammatory processes (Aggarwal, 2004; McDonald, 2004). NF-kappaB may also function as a tumor promoter in inflammation-associated cancer (Pikarsky, 2004).

As can be imagined, apoptosis is critical for homeostasis in the body, and appears to play a role in numerous pathological states (cancer, degenerative disease, persistent infection, autoimmune disease). In B and T cell development, it eliminates cells with either nonfunctional B or T cell receptors, autoreactive or self-destructive B or T cell receptors, as well as regulating activation of these cells with respect to the duration and magnitude of an inflammatory response (Marsden, 2003; Ivanovska, 2004). Apoptosis also plays a critical role in granulocyte development, by increasing their relatively short life span at the site of infection or by downregulating the inflammatory response once the inciting agent has been negated. Apoptosis also prevents the release of enzymes and other inflammatory mediators from senescent granulocytes into surrounding healthy tissue, preventing tissue destruction.

Non-Neoplastic Disorders

Currently, laboratory examination of leukocytes occurs as part of the automated complete blood count (CBC) for almost every patient. The concentration of all the white cells, also known as the total leukocyte count or white blood cell (WBC) count, as well as the relative and absolute concentrations of the neutrophilic granulocytes, lymphocytes, monocytes, eosinophils, and basophils are determined and compared to normal values for the patient's age and sex. Usually the absolute concentrations (i.e., the product of the WBC count and the percentage of the respective cell series, such as lymphocytes or neutrophils) are of most value in

Table 32–2 Key Causes of Neutrophilia

Acute inflammatory — collagen vascular, vasculitis
Acute infectious — bacterial, some viral, fungal, parasitic
Drugs, toxins, metabolic — corticosteroids, growth factors, uremia, ketoacidosis
Tissue necrosis — burns, trauma, MI, RBC hemolysis
Physiologic — stress, exercise, smoking pregnancy
Neoplastic — carcinomas, sarcomas, myeloproliferative disorders

determining abnormalities. Abnormal results from the automated count are 'flagged' and are then reviewed by a skilled laboratory technologist.

These abnormalities include *leukocytosis*, which is an increase in the total WBC (white blood cell) count above the upper limit of normal for age and sex, and *leukopenia*, which is a decrease in the total WBC count below the lower limit of normal for age and sex. Additional quantitative study of leukocytes includes the relative and absolute concentrations of the various forms of white cells (the differential count). An increase in the absolute concentration of cells in each series is termed *neutrophilia* (neutrophilic leukocytosis), *lymphocytosis*, *monocytosis*, *eosinophilia* (eosinophilic leukocytosis), and *basophilia* (basophilic leukocytosis). A decrease in the absolute concentration is termed *neutropenia*, *lymphopenia* or *lymphocytopenia*, *monocytopenia*, *eosinopenia*, and *basopenia*. Abnormalities may occur in both neoplastic conditions (e.g. leukemia or marrow infiltration by metastatic tumor) and non-neoplastic conditions (e.g. infection, drug effect or nutritional deficiency). Increase in any cell type may be clinically important, but decrease is usually significant only for neutrophils. Usually an isolated monocytopenia, eosinopenia or basopenia identified in a CBC is not considered a significant abnormality. Qualitative study of leukocytes includes structural abnormalities in cytoplasm and nucleus and functional abnormalities as well.

One purpose of the examination of leukocytes is to help in establishing a diagnosis. Occasionally this alone may furnish a specific diagnosis – for example, in leukemia. More frequently, this examination is more helpful diagnostically when interpreted with other clinical or laboratory data – for example, in acute appendicitis, infectious mononucleosis, or another type of infection. Another purpose is to help in establishing a prognosis. For example, leukopenia in acute appendicitis or pneumonia is considered prognostically unfavorable.

Finally, study of the leukocytes is helpful in following the course of disease. For example, toxic effects of radiotherapy and chemotherapy may be recognized, and recovery monitored, by examination of leukocytes.

Granulocytic and Monocytic Disorders

Neutrophilia

Neutrophilic leukocytosis or neutrophilia refers to an absolute concentration of neutrophils in the blood above normal for age. The normal reference interval (established for each laboratory separately) is approximately $1.8-7.0 \times 10^3/\mu L$ for adults, with a slightly wider range ($1.0-8.5 \times 10^3/\mu L$) in young children. Key causes of neutrophilia are listed in Table 32–2.

Mechanisms. The primary factors influencing the neutrophil count are (1) the rate of inflow of cells from the bone marrow (mitosis/proliferation, maturation/storage and release); (2) the proportion of neutrophils in the marginal (cells adhering to vessel walls) granulocyte pool (MGP) and the circulating (nonadhering cells) granulocyte pool (CGP) of the blood – MGP and CGP are approximately equal in size and in equilibrium in health; and (3) the rate of outflow of neutrophils from the blood (migration from and through vessels into tissue, both randomly and at sites of inflammation, infection, etc.).

Physiologic leukocytosis is produced by factors or situations that are not related to underlying tissue pathology. Severe exercise, hypoxia, stress, or the injection of epinephrine will result in a decrease in the MGP and a corresponding increase in the CGP, resulting in a 'pseudoneutrophilia' (i.e., no change in total blood granulocyte pool or TBGP). This simple redistribution of cells between the CGP and MGP, also known as demargination, is the release and detachment of leukocytes from molecular receptors on vessel luminal walls. This may be, in part, due to epinephrine-induced activation of β-receptors on endothelial cells, releasing cyclic adenosine monophosphate (cAMP), which ultimately alters or modulates the properties and characteristics of cell surface adhesion molecules and increases the release of neutrophils (as well as other leukocytes) into the circulation (Gabriel, 1998; Heine, 2001; Shephard, 2003).

Stress of greater severity or injection of endotoxin, corticosteroids, or etiocholanolone also results in an increased inflow of cells to the blood from the marrow maturation/storage pool. Interleukin-6, an important regulator of the acute phase response, appears to play a significant role in both the demargination of circulating cells (initial wave of circulating neutrophils) and the release of neutrophils from the marrow (second wave of circulating neutrophilic granulocytes) (Suwa, 2000). As a result, the mitotic pool appears to be increased to replenish the maturation/storage pool from which more mature cells exit into the TBGP, and both MGP and CGP are enlarged. A 'greater' neutrophilia is possible in this situation because of the additional egress of cells from the maturation/storage pool (in addition to demargination), and immature cells, such as band neutrophils and metamyelocytes, are likely to be present (Suwa, 2000).

As mentioned above, neutrophilia may be produced by corticosteroids, which increase release of neutrophils from the marrow, decrease the egress of neutrophils from the blood, and increase demargination.

Pathologic leukocytosis is an increased WBC count that occurs as a result of disease, and usually is a response to tissue damage. This leukocytosis is most often a neutrophilia.

In addition to the random loss of neutrophils from the circulation in various body secretions, neutrophils leave the blood by ameboid movement when attracted to a focus of inflammation in tissues, presumably responding to a multitude of chemotactic molecules and gradients. It is from the MGP that the neutrophils leave the blood, pass between capillary endothelial cells, and reach the tissues.

In acute infection, increased margination of neutrophils and outflow from blood to tissues would lead to neutropenia were there not a flow of neutrophils from the marrow storage compartment into the blood. Because the latter overcompensates, the result is a neutrophilia. Usually, production and storage compartments then increase in the marrow and are able to sustain the increased CGP (neutrophilia) and MGP in the face of the increased flow of neutrophils from the blood into the inflammatory site. In these instances, the marrow will show granulocytic hyperplasia (increased myeloid to erythroid [M : E] ratio and increased cellularity), with maturation intact. An increase in immature peripheral blood granulocytes is usually present, often termed 'shift to the left.'

If the demand for neutrophils is extremely great, as in severe infection, there may be depletion of the marrow storage pool and a decreased CGP (neutropenia) and MGP, because the supply of cells is insufficient for the demand. In these instances, the marrow will show increased numbers of early neutrophil precursors, through the myelocyte stage, but decreased numbers of metamyelocytes, bands, and neutrophils.

Determinants. Certain host factors modify the degree of neutrophilic response. Children respond more intensely than adults. The degree of neutrophilia may be impaired by the same factors that impair erythrocyte production (iron, folate, or cobalamin deficiency) or by marrow failure due to other causes. Imperfectly defined factors that enable the body to localize an infection may play a role: the more localized the process, the more pronounced the neutrophilia.

Other factors modifying the neutrophilic response are due more to the microorganism than to the host. Pyogenic bacteria, especially, induce neutrophilia. Within limits, the more virulent the agent, the higher the neutrophil count. When the infection is overwhelming, however, there is apt to be a neutropenia and a greater shift to the left.

Treatment of infections with antibiotics may modify the leukocytic response to infection. Steroid therapy, though causing neutrophilia, tends to impair the host response to infection, probably because of diminished movement of neutrophils into the tissues and increased lysosomal stability.

Neutrophilia is occasionally seen in patients with solid tumors, particularly large-cell carcinomas of the lung. The neutrophilia is secondary to several factors including response to tissue necrosis and underlying infection as well as to the production of myeloid growth factors (Peterson, 1993). Neutrophilia can also be seen with gastrointestinal and hepatic tumors, Hodgkin lymphoma (HL), renal cell carcinoma and metastatic bone marrow disease (Hernandez, 2002; Blay, 1997). A recent study (Ruka, 2001) analyzing hematological alterations in patients with histologically confirmed sarcomas found that a number of blood alterations including neutrophilia, monocytosis, thrombocytosis and lymphocytopenia correlated strongly with elevated levels of various circulating cytokines and soluble cytokine receptor levels detected in the peripheral blood. It is thought that cytokine production by tumor cells is responsible for these hematological changes.

Neutropenia

Neutropenia is a reduction of the absolute neutrophil count (ANC) below $\sim 1.5-2 \times 10^9/L$ for white people and below $\sim 1.2-1.3 \times 10^9/L$ for black

IV

CHAPTER: 32 Leukocytic Disorders

Table 32–3 Key Causes of Neutropenia (brief partial list)

Drugs — cancer chemotherapy, chloramphenicol, sulfas/other antibiotics, phenothiazines, benzodiazepine, antithyroids, anticonvulsants, quinine, quinidine, indometacin, procainamide, thiazides

Radiation

Toxins — alcohol, benzene compounds

Intrinsic defects — Fanconi's, Kostmann's, cyclic neutropenia, Chédiak–Higashi

Immune-mediated — collagen vascular disorders, RA, AIDS

Hematologic — megaloblastic anemia, myelodysplasia, marrow failure, marrow replacement

Infectious — any overwhelming infection

Others — starvation, hypersplenism

people. Remember that the ANC is the product of the WBC count and the percentage of neutrophils and bands that have been enumerated in the WBC differential count. The term *agranulocytosis* has been used for severe neutropenia, usually $< 0.5 \times 10^9$/L; this can also be associated with depletion of eosinophils and basophils as well. The term severe chronic neutropenia (SCN) refers to patients with ANC $< 0.5 \times 10^9$/L for months or years, usually with diseases that primarily cause neutropenia in the absence of other cytopenias (Dale, 2002a). If the neutrophil count is less than 1×10^9/L, the risk of infection is considerably increased over normal, and if the neutrophil count is less than 0.5×10^9/L, the risk of infection is greater still.

The mechanisms by which neutropenia occurs include (1) decreased flow of neutrophils from marrow into blood as a result of either lack of production or ineffective production (i.e., a proliferation or maturation defect); (2) increased removal of neutrophils from the blood (survival defect); (3) altered distribution between CGP and MGP; or (4) combinations of these mechanisms. Neutropenias are not so neatly classified as anemias. It should be noted that drugs induce neutropenia through several mechanisms and are a very important consideration in any differential diagnosis of leukopenia. Causes and conditions associated with neutropenia are shown in Table 32–3.

The list in Table 32–3 is not exhaustive; let us discuss a few of these conditions in further detail.

Drugs (Bhatt, 2004; Andres, 2004) are an important cause of neutropenia, may act in different ways, and may affect either progenitor or mature cell populations. Drugs are the most common cause of acute neutropenia ('agranulocytosis') and will typically show a lack of granulocytic cells in the marrow. In some patients, however, a pronounced progenitor hyperplasia may be present, sometimes termed 'maturation arrest' or 'promyelocytic hyperplasia.'

Drugs may initiate immune-mediated actions of destruction via immune complex formation (quinidine) or complement-mediated cell lysis (propylthiouracil). Some drugs, including penicillin, aminopyrine, and gold, act as haptens. Inhibition of granulopoiesis or myeloid toxicity occurs with chemotherapeutic agents, chlorpromazine and others. These effects tend to be dose dependent and reversible. Important and limiting side effects of cancer chemotherapy are severe neutropenia with its risk of infection, as well as severe thrombocytopenia with risk of bleeding; anemia is more readily controlled with transfusion.

Radiation damages, alters, and destroys bone marrow progenitor and stem cells as well as marrow stromal elements. Radiation type, dose, and duration are all factors that determine the extent of bone marrow damage, such as aplasia or hypoplasia. Radiation affects and alters or damages a number of molecular targets, including DNA structure, gene translation and transcription, and apoptotic and other signaling pathways both within and between cells. Lymphocytes are most sensitive and are directly killed by exposure. The lymphocyte count correlates with, and has been used to assess dose and severity of exposure (Dainiak, 2002). In addition, other hematopoietic precursors undergoing mitosis are very sensitive to injury and death.

Intrinsic defects or constitutional disorders associated with neutropenia usually present at birth or early infancy and are rare. Those due to myeloid hypoplasia or a proliferation defect include Fanconi's anemia, Kostmann's syndrome, Schwachman–Diamond syndrome, and cyclic neutropenia. Those that are due to a maturation defect include myelokathexis and Chédiak–Higashi syndrome.

Fanconi's anemia (FA) is an inherited bone marrow failure syndrome that usually occurs in childhood and rarely presents in adulthood. This condition is heterogeneous in its clinical manifestations, but was classically defined by aplastic anemia and congenital physical malformations. The

aplastic anemia of FA patients appears to be indistinguishable from acquired aplasia. FA patients are also susceptible to hematopoietic and certain solid organ malignancies. Diagnosis is made by cytogenetic analysis looking for chromosome breakage after exposure to either diepoxybutane or mitomycin C.

As can be imagined from the variation in clinical presentations and manifestations of this syndrome, the underlying molecular pathology is complex. Currently, at least 11 FA genetic subtypes exist and 7 FA genes have been cloned. One gene, FANCD1, is actually BRCA2, which, like BRCA1, is a DNA repair gene that appears to be a putative breast and ovarian cancer susceptibility gene identified in certain families with an inherited predisposition to breast and ovarian cancer. These genes probably function as tumor suppressor genes and appear to be involved in the molecular pathway(s) responsible for the disruption of DNA repair in FA (Tischkowitz, 2004; Levitus, 2004). The mechanism of pathogenesis, however, remains to be elucidated.

Kostmann's syndrome, originally termed 'infantile genetic agranulocytosis,' is a rare severe (ANC usually $< 200/\mu$L) congenital neutropenia appearing in early infancy. Initially identified as showing an autosomal recessive pattern of inheritance, both sporadic and autosomal dominant cases also occur. The marrow usually shows the presence of early granulocytes (promyelocyte/myelocyte arrest) but few maturing forms are seen; neutrophil survival is normal. Although the underlying genetic defect in myeloid precursor cells is not entirely elucidated, mutations in the gene (ELA2) encoding neutrophil elastase appear to be present in most patients. These mutations may be responsible for the untimely initiation of apoptosis in myelocytes, producing their premature destruction, and interrupting the normal cycle of maturation. There may be, in addition, other underlying molecular/genetic changes producing DNA mutations and genome instability, which contribute to initiation and progression of this disease (Christensen, 2004; Zeidler, 2002).

Patients with cyclic neutropenia typically present with recurrent episodes of symptomatic infection (fatigue, mouth ulcers, cervical lymphadenopathy, fever) due to cyclic episodes of severe neutropenia. The latter is due to the periodicity or cycling of neutrophil production. The disease usually presents in childhood, but may present in adulthood. Typically, oscillations of neutrophil and monocyte levels (between near normal levels and very low levels) occur over an approximately 21-day period. Mutations in ELA2, the gene for neutrophil elastase, have been identified in many patients (Dale, 2002b). This appears to be responsible for selective apoptotic death of neutrophil progenitors, a mechanism similar to that seen in Kostmann's syndrome, as discussed above.

Chronic familial neutropenia or benign familial neutropenia refers to a lower than 'normal' neutrophil count found in some ethnic populations. It is an incidental and clinically stable finding with no predisposition to infection, and is considered a genetic variation.

It is important to note that the two most common causes of congenital neutropenia are neutropenia of pregnancy-induced hypertension (PIH – most common) and overwhelming bacterial infection. Typical signs of infection including a granulocytic left shift, toxic granulation, and Döhle bodies accompany the latter, while these changes are not seen in PIH. Neither usually continues beyond the first week of life, and other causes should be searched for in infants with persistent neutropenia (Christensen, 2004).

Patients with congenital or primary immunodeficiency diseases may exhibit some degree of neutropenia. Males with X-linked agammaglobulinemia (XLA) are often neutropenic, and XLA should be considered in the differential diagnosis of chronic neutropenia in an infant. An abnormal nonreceptor tyrosine kinase, involved in signal transduction and differentiation of hematopoietic cells, appears to be involved. This is due to various mutations in the gene Btk (Bruton's or B lymphocyte tyrosine kinase) on the long arm of the X chromosome (q22). Other congenital syndromes having a prominent association with neutropenia include selective IgA deficiency, common variable immunodeficiency, and hyper IgM syndrome (Cham, 2002).

Certain autoimmune diseases can also be associated with chronic neutropenia. Both rheumatoid arthritis (RA) and systemic lupus erythematosus (SLE) show this association (Starkebaum, 2002). The combination of chronic neutropenia and RA is termed Felty's syndrome (FS) and patients will develop symptoms due to both RA (e.g., subcutaneous nodules, contractures, erythema, warmth, tenderness, symmetric involvement of large and small joints, musculoskeletal pain) and chronic neutropenia (symptoms of recurrent bacterial and fungal infections). Many of these cases are associated with large granular lymphocyte (LGL) leukemia.

SLE may present with multisystemic involvement, making presenting symptoms highly variable. Organ systems frequently affected include the skin, kidney, bone marrow, central nervous system (CNS), and symmetric involvement of joints. Again, the pathophysiology is complex; alterations in neutrophil proliferation and survival with neutropenia due, at least in part, to immune-mediated destruction, occur in both SLE and FS, and with increased neutrophil apoptosis also occurring in SLE (Starkebaum, 2002).

Primary autoimmune myelofibrosis (Bass, 2001; Pullarkat, 2003; Rizzi, 2004) is a relatively rare, but recently described clinicopathologic entity in patients who do not have SLE or another well-defined autoimmune disease. Although this entity is still being defined, patients present with chronic peripheral blood cytopenias, bone marrow fibrosis with variable marrow cellularity and bone marrow lymphoid aggregates in the absence of other disorders that typically cause myelofibrosis. These include primary marrow hematological neoplasia, infection, metastatic cancer, or osteopathy such as Paget's disease or hyperparathyroidism. Prognosis of these patients appears to be very good with corticosteroid therapy.

Isolated neutropenia or agranulocytosis is fairly uncommon in adults. When a myelophthisic process, such as metastatic carcinoma, disseminated tuberculosis, or Gaucher's disease, infiltrates the bone marrow, the damage is not limited to granulopoiesis but affects normoblasts and megakaryocytes as well. Because of the short life span of granulocytes, however, neutropenia is the earliest recognizable effect in the blood. It may take weeks before damage to the erythropoietic tissue becomes manifest because of the usually long life span of erythrocytes. Platelets have a rather short life span but, on the other hand, megakaryocytes are more resistant to damage.

Neutropenia due to increased ineffective granulocytopoiesis occurs in megaloblastic anemias and with drugs that have an antifolate effect. In these conditions, there is usually an associated anemia and thrombocytopenia. The marrow is usually hyperplastic. In megaloblastic anemia due to nutritional deficiency, drug-induced suppression of DNA synthesis, or an inborn error of metabolism, asynchronous nuclear/cytoplasmic maturation (megaloblastic change or megaloblastosis) is identified in marrow progenitor cells. Ineffective granulocytopoiesis may also occur in myelodysplasia, discussed in the section on neoplastic disorders.

In starvation, cellularity tends to be decreased, and a morphologic marrow change termed serous fat atrophy or gelatinous transformation of the bone marrow is present. This change shows a loss of hematopoietic cells within the marrow stroma replaced by small or shrunken fat cells expanded by an intercellular, homogeneous, eosinophilic material. Bone marrow hypocellularity is typically seen with advanced disease. Neutropenia with bone marrow hypoplasia can be associated with a decrease in plasma or serum lysozyme (muramidase).

Transient neutropenia may occur early in some infections, followed by leukocytosis once the marrow production catches up with the demand. As previously noted, in severe, extensive bacterial infection, neutropenia with a shift to the left may be due to inability of marrow production to keep up with the peripheral utilization. Some bacterial infections, notably brucellosis and *Salmonella* infections, are prone to be associated with neutropenia; they may have some depressing effect on the marrow as well. Patients with viral infections such as measles and rubella have neutropenia for several days after appearance of the rash; this is probably due in part to increased utilization. Other acute viral infections, such as hepatitis, infectious mononucleosis, and influenza, may also cause acute neutropenia. Lymphocytosis is present and persists after the neutropenia subsides.

The neutropenia of hypersplenism has been attributed to selective removal of neutrophils by the spleen. It is associated with neutrophilic hyperplasia of the marrow and is corrected by splenectomy. Splenomegaly due to many causes may result in shortened neutrophil survival and neutropenia; these include congestive splenomegaly, Felty's syndrome, Gaucher's disease, and lymphoma. In some cases of Felty's syndrome (neutropenia and splenomegaly in rheumatoid arthritis), there may be a neutrophil-specific antibody involved. Ramirez et al. (2004) recently showed enhanced apoptosis in patients with cirrhosis and ascites, which appeared to be dependent upon elevated activity levels of caspase-3 in these patients. These patients are prone to neutropenia and infection, and, in the past, this was largely attributed to hypersplenism with increased splenic clearance of neutrophils. However, these recent findings suggest other mechanisms, at least in part, may also be contributory.

Pseudoneutropenia may be caused by increased margination of neutrophils in some individuals, without a decrease in the total granulocyte count. Rather than showing an equal distribution between MGP and CGP, an increased proportion of neutrophils appears to be present in the MGP. Small doses of endotoxin will cause a shift of neutrophils into the MGP from the CGP, giving an apparent neutropenia, prior to causing a leukocytosis. In animals, anesthetic agents such as ether will cause the same kind of pseudoneutropenia.

Table 32–4 Morphologic Alterations in Neutrophils

Toxic granulation — azurophilic cytoplasmic granules seen in severe infections, other toxic conditions and reactive conditions

Cytoplasmic vacuoles — seen in infection, indicating phagocytosis

Döhle bodies — pale blue, oval cytoplasmic remnants of ribosomes seen in infections and other toxic conditions

May–Hegglin anomaly — rare autosomal dominant condition with pale blue cytoplasmic ribosomal inclusions *resembling* Döhle bodies

Alder–Reilly anomaly — prominent azurophilic granulation not related to infection

Pelger–Huët anomaly — bilobed or rounded nuclei with pince-nez shape

Chédiak–Higashi syndrome — autosomal recessive disorder with giant granules, likely representing giant fused lysosomes, and abnormal leukocyte function

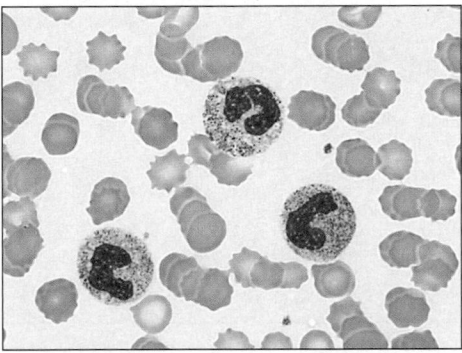

Figure 32–1 A neutrophil with toxic granulation is pictured, along with two bands. Basophilic inclusions (Döhle bodies) are present as well (× 1000).

Morphologic Alterations in Neutrophils

In addition to quantitative changes, qualitative morphologic alterations also occur in neutrophils. Some of these, such as toxic granules or cytoplasmic vacuoles, are acquired and disappear after the stimulus that provoked them is gone. Others are hereditary and persist through life, with or without functional impairment. These are well illustrated and reviewed by Brunning (1970) and more recently by Kroft (2002).

It should be noted that disorders of leukocyte function may exist without any structural abnormality detectable with the usual modes of morphologic examination.

Toxic Granulation (Table 32–4). Toxic granules are dark blue to purple cytoplasmic granules in the metamyelocyte, band, or neutrophil stage. They are peroxidase-positive and may be numerous or few in number; there may be less peroxidase activity in toxic than in normal neutrophils. Toxic granulation is found in infections or other toxic conditions, but may also be seen in noninfectious reactive conditions (Fig. 32–1).

Normally, neutrophil granules are tan to pink in color in neutrophil metamyelocytes, bands, and mature forms. Even the nonspecific or azurophil granules that are dark blue in the promyelocyte stage normally lose their basophilia in the mature neutrophil, where they constitute about one-third of the granules in the human. Toxic granules are azurophil granules that have retained their basophilic staining reaction by lack of maturation, or that have developed increased basophilia in the mature neutrophil. In addition, perhaps skipped divisions during the development of the neutrophil may result in a greater proportion of the granules being of the azurophil type. Increased basophilia of azurophil granules simulating toxic granules may occur in normal cells with prolonged staining time or decreased pH of the staining reaction.

Cytoplasmic vacuoles are also signs of toxic change if films are made from fresh blood free of anticoagulant to eliminate the possibility of degeneration artifacts. Toxic vacuolization appears to be greater than 90% specific for infection, and when present with toxic granulation, Döhle inclusion bodies, or a left shift, appear to be very predictive of systemic infection (Kroft, 2002). Vacuoles or irregular depletion of granules implies that phagocytosis has occurred (Fig. 32–2).

Döhle Inclusion Bodies. These are small, oval inclusions in the peripheral cytoplasm of polymorphonuclear neutrophils, which stain pale blue with Wright stain (Fig. 32–1). They are remnants of free ribosomes or rough-surfaced endoplasmic reticulum persisting from an earlier stage of

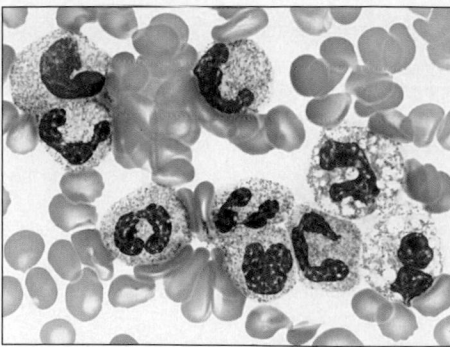

Figure 32–2 Leukemoid toxic neutrophilia with left shift and toxic vacuolization (×1000).

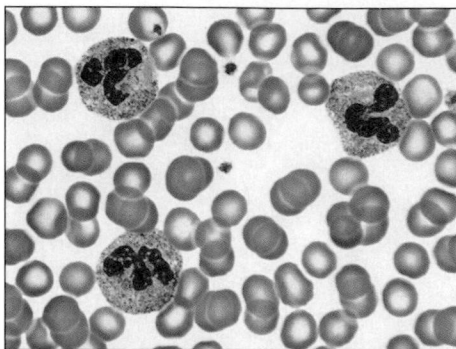

Figure 32–3 May–Hegglin anomaly, showing Döhle-like inclusions (×1000).

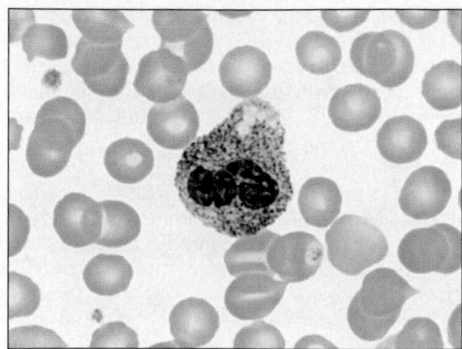

Figure 32–4 The Alder–Reilly anomaly may be found in healthy individuals, or in mucopolysaccharidoses, in which granules are metachromatic (×1000).

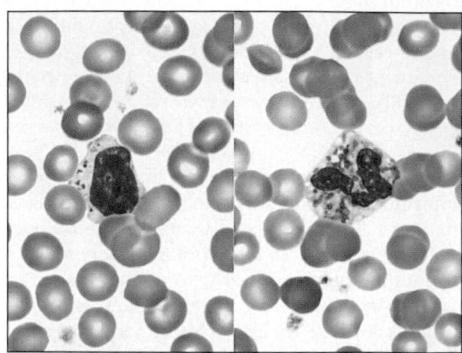

Figure 32–5 Genetic mucopolysaccharidoses often show abnormal lymphocyte granules with surrounding halos. In these cells from the same blood film, neutrophils showed similar change (×1000).

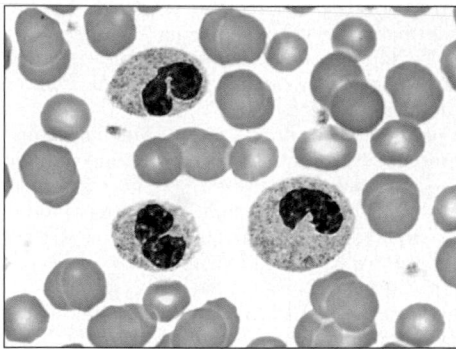

Figure 32–6 Inherited Pelger–Huët anomaly (×1000).

development. Originally, Döhle bodies were described as being especially prominent in scarlet fever, but they may be seen in many other infectious diseases, in burns, in aplastic anemia, and following administration of toxic agents. They may accompany toxic granulation in the neutrophil. With the light microscope, Döhle bodies resemble the inclusions seen in the May–Hegglin anomaly. Another toxic change in the neutrophil is the occasional appearance of several sharp or blunt spicules extending out from the nucleus.

May–Hegglin Anomaly. This is a rare autosomal dominant condition involving the nonmuscle myosin heavy chain 9 gene (*MYH9*) linked to chromosome 22q12-13 (Kelley, 2000; Martignetti, 2000; Seri, 2000). The mutations appear to alter the assembly and stability of myosin and may be responsible for the underlying pathophysiology and changes seen in leukocyte and platelet structure and function. It appears that at the molecular level various mutations in *MYH9* are, at least partially, responsible for a phenotypic spectrum of illness. This spectrum appears to include May–Hegglin anomaly, and Sebastian, Fechtner, and Epstein platelet syndromes (Heath, 2001; Seri, 2003). This spectrum may be phenotypically modified by aberrant fibulin-1 gene expression, which also may be responsible for the clinical variability of disease (Toren, 2003). Fibulin-1 is a gene encoding for a secreted glycoprotein present in the basal membrane of many organs.

Although clinically variable, this anomaly is characterized by the presence of pale blue inclusions resembling Döhle bodies in neutrophils, by giant platelets and, in some persons, by thrombocytopenia (Fig. 32–3). The inclusions are larger and more prominent than the Döhle bodies found in infections. They have been described in eosinophils, basophils, and monocytes as well as in neutrophils (Brunning, 1970). The blue staining of the inclusions can be abolished by prior treatment of the cells with ribonuclease. With electron microscopy, the appearance of the inclusions differs from that of Döhle bodies (composed of parallel strands of rough endoplasmic reticulum), suggesting structural alterations in RNA and ribosomes (So, 2003). Granulocyte function is normal.

Alder–Reilly Anomaly. Dense, prominent, larger than normal azurophilic granulation in all white blood cells was described by Alder in 1939 (Fig. 32–4). In neutrophils it may resemble toxic granulation, but it is unrelated to infection and is not transient. In 1941, Reilly described similar granulocytes in some but not all patients with gargoylism; Hurler's syndrome or, more generally, the genetic mucopolysaccharidoses (Reilly, 1941). Other observations have shown that the heavy granulation in neutrophils can occur either as a feature of the genetic mucopolysaccharidoses or independently in otherwise healthy persons (Brunning, 1970).

Occurring more often than the Alder–Reilly anomaly in the genetic mucopolysaccharidoses is a metachromatic inclusion in the lymphocytes surrounded by a clear space (Fig. 32–5). Macrophages in the marrow frequently contain similar granulation. This group of disorders is inherited and is characterized by deficiencies or derangement in various lysosomal enzymes required for degrading mucopolysaccharides. The result is abnormal deposition and storage of mucopolysaccharides in multiple organs. Skeletal abnormalities are prominent.

Pelger–Huët Anomaly. This hereditary, autosomal dominant condition involves failure of normal segmentation of granulocytic nuclei. Most nuclei are bilobed and rounded, with a characteristic spectacle or pince-nez shape (Fig. 32–6). The chromatin is quite coarse, and these are not normal young band forms. When a large number of band-like neutrophils appear in the differential count in a patient without infection or other cause, careful analysis of the blood films of the patient and of family members will occasionally establish the presence of the Pelger–Huët anomaly. The cells are functionally normal.

A similar appearing, acquired disorder of nuclear segmentation in granulocytes may be found in cases of granulocytic leukemia, myelodysplastic and some myeloproliferative disorders, some infections, and after exposure to certain drugs (Brunning, 1970); this is called the pseudo-Pelger–Huët anomaly. In addition to the band forms and neutrophils with only two segments, mature cells with round, nonsegmented nuclei and coarse chromatin are common. In contrast to the congenital Pelger–Huët

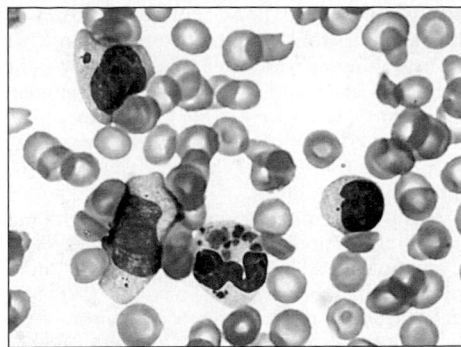

Figure 32–7 Chédiak–Higashi neutrophil and lymphocytes with large granules (×1000).

anomaly, ring-shaped and other abnormal nuclei may be seen, and the cytoplasm is usually hypogranular.

Chédiak–Higashi Syndrome. Partial oculocutaneous albinism, photophobia, immune deficiency, abnormally large granules in leukocytes and other granule-containing cells, neurologic defects, and frequent pyogenic infections characterize this rare, autosomal recessive disorder (Introne, 1999). An accelerated lymphoma-like phase occurs, with lymphadenopathy, hepatosplenomegaly, and pancytopenia; lymphoid infiltrates are widespread, and death ensues at an early age. Granulocytes, monocytes, and lymphocytes contain giant granules (Fig. 32–7), which appear to be abnormal lysosomes. The pathogenesis of this disorder is linked to an abnormality of granule maturation causing an enlargement and apparent fusion of granules and vesicles (such as lysosomes, melanosomes, and platelet dense granules) in all cell types. Leukocyte functional abnormalities exist. Although the mechanism is not fully elucidated, a mouse genetic model *beige*, currently under study, has revealed a mutation in the gene *CHS/beige* coding for the CHS1 or Lyst protein. The *LYST* (*ly*sosomal *t*rafficking regulator) gene appears to be involved in regulation of vesicular size, trafficking, and intracellular movement such that vesicular migration and release are abnormal (Ward, 2002).

'Myelokathexis' applies to peripheral neutropenia with the presence of bone marrow neutrophils. WHIM (*w*arts, *h*ypogammaglobulinemia, *i*nfection, and *m*yelokathexis) syndrome is a rare, autosomal dominant disease of leukocyte trafficking involving chromosome 2q21. The disease appears to be due to mutations in the chemokine receptor gene *CXCR4* and altered leukocyte response to its functional ligand CXCL12. Hematologic changes include severe peripheral neutropenia with lymphopenia also common, but with granulocytic hyperplasia of the bone marrow (Gorlin, 2000; Hernandez, 2003; Gulino, 2003, 2004).

Functional Disorders of Neutrophils

Inherited and acquired disorders affecting neutrophils and other leukocytes may result in abnormal function and consequent susceptibility to infections. Deficiencies of humoral factors (antibodies, components of complement) may result in defective chemotaxis or opsonization. As described above, some inherited disorders, such as the May-Hegglin, Alder–Reilly, and Pelger–Huët anomalies have altered morphologic appearances, but apparently normal granulocytic function. Other inherited conditions, such as the Chédiak–Higashi syndrome and specific granule deficiency (SGD), display both altered morphology and function. Inherited conditions such as chronic granulomatous disease (CGD), myeloperoxidase deficiency (MYD), and leukocyte adhesion deficiency (LAD) exhibit functional disorders with essentially normal morphology on Wright's- and Giemsa-stained films.

Chronic granulomatous disease (Lakshman, 2001; Vignais, 2002; Heyworth, 2003; Jurkowska, 2004) is a rare, primary immunodeficiency affecting neutrophils, eosinophils, macrophages, and monocytes, and results from the inability of these phagocytic cells to kill intracellular microorganisms. Patients present with recurrent bacterial and fungal infections (skin, liver, mouth, lymph nodes). These lead to chronic granulomatous lesions (a hallmark of the disease) that may, in turn, obstruct vital organ systems, and ultimately lead to death. Symptoms occur early in life, and both autosomal recessive (~66%) and X-linked (~33%) modes of inheritance are known.

Disease etiology is due to genetic defects in any one of the membrane-bound or cytoplasmic components of NADPH oxidase. This enzyme complex is not assembled and thus inactive in the resting cell but, with cell stimulation, the membrane and cytoplasmic components come together and are assembled into the active NADPH oxidase–protein complex, which can begin functioning. Once assembled, this enzyme is responsible for production of superoxide anion ($NADPH + 2O_2 \rightarrow 2O^-_2 + NADP^+ + H^+$), as well as hydrogen peroxide and hypochlorous acid, molecular mediators of microbial cell death. The production of these highly reactive oxygen free radical species is often referred to as the 'respiratory burst' indicating the increased oxygen consumption that occurs with NADPH oxidase activation. Thus, any defect in this enzyme, which either prohibits or significantly reduces its activity, will allow intracellular microorganisms to remain viable, and ultimately spread (by cell mobility and seeding of adjacent tissue) producing recurrent infection and granulomatous disease. Global gene expression profiling studies (Kobayashi, 2004) suggest that both an increase in proinflammatory activity and defective neutrophil apoptosis may be also be involved.

Myeloperoxidase (MPO) is present in neutrophils (in azurophil/primary granules) and monocytes (in lysosomes), but is not present in promonocytes and tissue macrophages. MPO catalyzes the cellular production of hypochlorite (ClO^-) or hypochlorous ($HOCl$) acid ($H_2O_2 + Cl^- \rightarrow H_2O + ClO^-$). HOCl is a strong oxidant normally involved in the destruction of intracellular microorganisms as well as possibly tumor cells (Hoy, 2002). Although a single gene encodes MPO, the translation product undergoes a number of complex modification reactions, including insertion of heme, to produce the final active enzyme molecule (Nauseef, 2004).

Primary MYD is a congenital disorder that is not uncommon and that is easily identifiable with automated cell counters incorporating measurement of MPO activity in the differential count. Secondary MYD, which can be transient and corrected with treatment of the underlying disease, may occur secondary to conditions such as myeloid neoplasms, drugs, severe infectious diseases, diabetes mellitus, and pregnancy (Lanza, 1998). Primary MYD may be either total or partial, and in general, does not show an increased frequency of infection in most individuals (Lanza, 1998; Lakshman, 2001; Suzuki, 2004), although an increase has been reported in a recent study (Kutter, 2000).

Human eosinophilic peroxidase is closely related structurally to MPO, but is found within the granules of eosinophils and is encoded by a different gene. Deficiency is thought to be extremely rare, is unrelated to MYD, may show autosomal recessive inheritance, and appears to be without clinical symptoms (Nakagawa, 2001).

Patients with an extremely rare condition, specific granule deficiency (SGD), present with multiple bacterial infections, atypical bilobed nuclei within neutrophils, and a lack of secondary/specific cytoplasmic granules within neutrophils on Wright stained peripheral blood films. SGD also affects eosinophils. In addition to granule deficiencies and impaired bactericidal activity, neutrophils are defective in chemotaxis, receptor upregulation, and disaggregation. A mutation in a myeloid specific transcription factor gene (CCAAT/*e*nhancer *b*inding *p*rotein-*e*psilon or *C/EBPe*) appears to play a role in this disease (Rosenberg, 1993; Gombart, 2001; Khanna-Gupta, 2001).

Since proper neutrophil function is dependent upon cell–cell adhesion via the integrins, it is not surprising that leukocyte adhesion deficiency (LAD) diseases exist. Integrins are essentially nonadhesive surface molecules in circulating leukocytes, which upon proper stimulation, become adhesive or develop increased binding properties for their specific ligands. This appears to occur via either conformational change in the integrin molecule structure and/or clustering of increased numbers of molecules on the cell surface. Ultimately, defective leukocyte adhesion and migration occur, resulting clinically in recurrent infection and leukocytosis.

Three types of leukocyte adhesion deficiencies have been described (Bunting, 2002; Gabius, 2002; McDowall, 2003; Etzioni, 2004). In LAD I, a mutation in the β_2 subunit (of CD18) produces a lack of normal expression of the integrin causing either its absence or dysfunction at the cell surface. Recurrent severe infections, neutrophilia with severe infection, and delayed separation of the umbilical cord are seen. LAD II is due to a mutation affecting fucose transport leading to the impaired expression of selectin ligands on leukocytes (CD15a or sialyl Lewis X) as well as other cells. Neutrophilia (with and without infection) and developmental abnormalities occur. In LAD III, CD18 and CD15a are normally expressed on leukocytes. Instead, there seems to be a defect in integrin activation (via endothelial chemokines) due to mutation in leukocyte-expressed G-protein-coupled receptors (GPCRs). If binding between leukocyte GPCRs and endothelial expressed chemokines does not occur, integrin activation, and leukocyte adhesion cannot occur. Recurrent severe infections, neutrophilia with infection, and bleeding tendencies occur. The latter is seen because platelet GPIIbβ3 integrins are not activated. Some forms of LAD can be diagnosed by flow cytometry, by revealing the lack of expression of CD18 or CD15a on neutrophils (Roos, 2001).

IV

Table 32–5 Key Causes of Eosinophilia

Allergic — urticaria, hay fever, asthma

Inflammatory — eosinophilic fasciitis, Churg–Strauss syndrome

Parasitic — trichinosis, filariasis, schistosomiasis

Nonparasitic infections — systemic fungal, scarlet fever, chlamydial pneumonia of infancy

Respiratory — pulmonary eosinophilic syndromes (Loeffler's, tropical pulmonary eosinophilia), Churg–Strauss syndrome

Neoplastic — CML, Hodgkin lymphoma, T cell lymphomas

Idiopathic hypereosinophilic syndromes — affecting heart, liver, spleen, CNS, other organs

Others — certain drugs, hematologic and visceral malignancies, GI inflammatory diseases, sarcoidosis, Wiskott–Aldrich

Eosinophilia

Eosinophilia exists if blood eosinophils exceed $\sim 0.35 \times 10^9/L$ when large numbers of cells are counted, as with automated instruments or direct chamber counts; or $\sim 0.5 \times 10^9/L$ when the count is calculated from the 100- or 200-cell differential and the total leukocyte count. Eosinophilia is typically associated with allergic processes (the most common cause in ambulatory outpatients in North America) (Brigden, 1999) and parasitic infections; both are common secondary or reactive types of eosinophilia. Classically, the major function of eosinophils appeared to be the release of granule contents or reactive oxygen species generated by the cell membrane to damage the target organism or offending cell (Shurin, 1988). At present, eosinophil function appears more complex, in that additional functions with immunoregulatory and proinflammatory signaling roles also appear to exist. Thus, the eosinophil appears to be capable of acting as both an effector and/or a regulatory cell.

Similar factors influence the eosinophil count as described above for the neutrophil count. These factors are (1) mitosis/proliferation, maturation/storage, and release in, and from, the bone marrow; (2) the rate of outflow of eosinophils from the blood (rolling, tethering, adhesion, and migration); (3) trafficking of eosinophils to specific sites of accumulation; and (4) the survival and rate of eosinophil destruction in the tissues. Eosinophil production is stimulated by IL-5, migration is influenced by the chemokine eotaxin, and the two factors interact in producing eosinophilia (Palframan, 1998). Causes and conditions associated with eosinophilia are shown in Table 32–5.

Distinction of causes of secondary eosinophilia is somewhat arbitrary and there is extensive overlap between conditions. It may be more important to distinguish between reactive eosinophilia, that due to clonal processes (such as acute myeloid leukemia), and idiopathic eosinophilia with evidence of organ involvement, though there is also overlap among these as well.

Eosinophilic leukemias usually have increased proportions of myeloblasts and eosinophilic myelocytes, and the presence of an abnormal karyotype or other evidence of a myeloproliferative disorder suggests eosinophilia arising from a leukemic clone, while eosinophilia arising in lymphoid leukemias is likely reactive (Bain, 1996). Eosinophilia is usually present in chronic myeloid leukemia (CML) and some cases present with marked eosinophilia as the primary feature. (Gotlib, 2003). Chronic eosinophilic leukemia is distinct from CML and shows different but varied cytogenetic abnormalities (Bain, 2004).

A number of hematologic neoplasias may be accompanied by eosinophilia, such as acute leukemia, systemic mast cell disease, plasma cell dyscrasias, myelodysplastic and myeloproliferative diseases. It may also occur with a primary neoplasm originating in another organ, such as lung, soft tissue, or colon. Rare case reports are present in the literature associating an eosinophilic leukemoid reaction with metastatic melanoma (Oakley, 1998), malignant fibrous histiocytoma (MFH) (Melhem, 1993), and lung carcinoma (Varindani, 1982). It appears that abnormalities in cytokine expression and regulation are responsible, at least in part, for this reaction. A granulocytic leukemoid reaction was present in one patient with MFH (Melhem, 1993).

Eosinophilia is often a prominent component in tissue affected by Hodgkin lymphoma and extensive involvement has been reported to impart an adverse prognosis (von Wasielewski, 2003). Tissue and blood eosinophilia is also seen in T cell lymphomas and may similarly be a negative prognostic feature (Tancrede-Bohin, 2004). Eosinophilia is sometimes prominent in acute lymphoblastic leukemia, particularly those with t(5,14)(q31;q32) (Bain, 2001a).

Hypersensitivity, allergic reactions and atopic conditions such as bronchial asthma and seasonal rhinitis (hay fever) are characterized by eosinophilia. These immune reactions are mediated by immunoglobulin E (IgE), which results in mast cell and basophil degranulation with the release of a chemotactic factor for eosinophils. Eosinophils are found in the blood, marrow, and sputum (in bronchial asthma), and in nasal and conjunctival discharges (in hay fever). Blood eosinophilia is usually only mild or moderate $(0.4–1.0 \times 10^9/L)$.

In asthma, absolute eosinophil counts have been useful in management because the level of eosinophils positively correlates with pulmonary performance, indicates the adequacy of steroid therapy, and may indicate the presence of complicating infections.

Skin disorders include a number of heterogeneous disorders, some with known etiology, others unknown or idiopathic, showing local cutaneous infiltrates with eosinophils (and typically other types of inflammatory cells). Some are commonly associated with peripheral eosinophilia and others are not (Christophers, 2000). Atopic dermatitis and eczema are often accompanied by blood eosinophilia, especially in children. In pemphigus, eosinophilia is characteristic. Eosinophilia is frequently associated with acute urticarial reactions but is uncommon in chronic urticaria. In any case, it is important to recognize that the recruitment of eosinophils is dependent upon the proper interaction of chemokines (IL5) and their receptor molecules as well as their interaction with specific subset lymphocyte populations (T-helper type 2 (Th2) lymphocytes) in these cutaneous responses and conditions.

Moderate to severe peripheral blood eosinophilia is most commonly associated with infection by helminths (parasitic worms including nematodes, trematodes, cestodes). This is the commonest cause of eosinophilia in the world (Brigden, 1999). Eosinophilia is more pronounced if tissues are invaded (e.g., trichinosis) than when parasites inhabit the lumen of a viscus (e.g., tapeworm). Some parasites, such as *Taenia solium* (cysticercosis) produce little inflammatory response while alive, but trigger an inflammatory response upon degeneration of the organism. Other parasites, such as *Trichinella spiralis* (trichinosis) incite peripheral eosinophilia upon larval invasion of the muscles and encystment. Note that the absence of eosinophilia does not exclude a parasitic infection (Schulte, 2002).

In trichinosis, eosinophil levels begin to rise in the blood within days after infection. The peak of the eosinophilia is during the third or fourth week. Eosinophilia may be absent, however, in severe infestation with trichinae.

Leukocytosis and eosinophilia extending over months are seen in toxocariasis or visceral larva migrans. Migrating larvae of either the dog (*Toxocara canis*) or cat (*T. cati*) nematode cause this infestation. In this condition, pulmonary lesions (Löffler's syndrome or simple eosinophilic pneumonia) may be present; an immune hypersensitivity reaction to the nematode *Ascaris lumbricoides* has been classically associated with Löffler's syndrome.

Another parasitic infestation with eosinophilia is creeping eruption (cutaneous larva migrans) caused by larvae of the dog (*Ancylostoma braziliense*) or cat (*A. caninum*) hookworm. Eosinophilia in these infections is T cell dependent (Basten, 1970) and, as indicated earlier, dependent upon multiple chemokine and chemotactic molecules and receptors and intercellular interactions.

Eosinophilia of various degrees is seen in some infectious diseases. In scarlet fever, eosinophilia is commonly associated with the cutaneous rash, which is probably allergic in nature. Chorea may be associated with eosinophilia, but other forms of rheumatic fever are not.

Eosinophilic pneumonias with acute presentations typically include simple pulmonary eosinophilia or *Löffler's* syndrome, parasitic infections, drug-induced eosinophilic pneumonias, and idiopathic acute eosinophilic pneumonia. A number of pulmonary eosinophilic syndromes with more chronic presentations also exist. Other classification schemes divide eosinophilic pneumonia into idiopathic (of unknown cause) and secondary (infection, drug, immunologic and/or systemic disease) pneumonia.

Löffler's syndrome (simple eosinophilic pneumonia) affects all age groups and is characterized by repeated, transient pulmonary exudates accompanied by fever and clinical symptoms of bronchitis, often producing sputum that contains eosinophils. The syndrome resolves in a few weeks. It may be caused by a variety of exposures including certain drugs, inhaled antigens, or helminth (see above) infestation. The latter occurs during periods of dissemination or migration when the parasites pass from the blood into the alveoli of the lung. *Löffler's* syndrome may also be idiopathic.

Many drugs are associated with blood or pulmonary eosinophilia and pulmonary infiltrates. Symptoms may be mild, or more severe, leading to fulminant respiratory failure. However, the prognosis is favorable in most

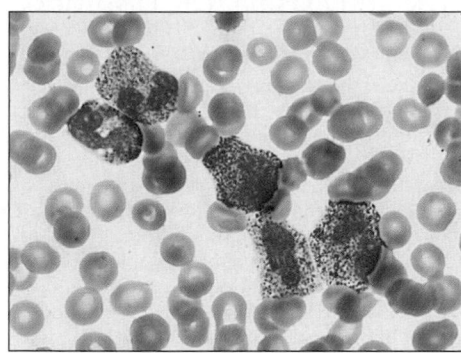

Figure 32–8 Marked eosinophilia of unknown cause, suggesting hypereosinophilic syndrome, peripheral blood (× 1000).

cases, with resolution of the disease occurring with elimination of the offending drug. Thus, a careful drug history is critical for diagnosis in these patients. Implicated drugs include: pilocarpine, physostigmine, digitalis, *p*-aminosalicylic acid, sulfonamides, chlorpromazine, phenytoin, some antidiabetic drugs, some anticancer agents, and many others. A common mechanism for the production of eosinophilia has not been identified. It is important to remember that patients with kidney and/or liver disease have a higher incidence of drug reaction, including eosinophilia, than patients without these conditions.

Tropical pulmonary eosinophilia is a syndrome of paroxysmal cough and bronchospasm associated with marked eosinophilia. It is found mainly in India, Africa, Southeast Asia, and the South Pacific. However, it may be seen in any racial group living in an endemic area. *Wuchereria bancrofti* (a parasite of humans that inhabits the lymphatics) is the most common and widely distributed cause of this disease. Very high titers of serum IgG and IgE levels against microfilarial antigens are present. The disease is probably a hyperimmune reaction caused by microfilariae, which may be found occasionally in lung or lymph node biopsy specimens, but not usually in blood. Response to the antifilarial drug diethylcarbamazine is curative.

Persistent high levels of eosinophils for long periods of time, no evidence of known causes of eosinophilia, and signs and symptoms of organ damage and injury are criteria for inclusion of patients in idiopathic hypereosinophilic syndrome (HES) (Fig. 32–8). HES appears to be a heterogeneous syndrome composed of a number of different disorders of varying severity. Although the pathogenesis of HES is not entirely understood, dysregulation of intra- or intercellular molecular communication(s) appears to be involved, at least in some forms of HES. This dysregulation leads to persistently activated eosinophils which release eosinophil granule proteins and enzymes, lipid mediators, and cytokines, chemokines, and growth factors; this not only produces tissue damage and injury, but also sets up an 'autocrine loop' that continually activates cells and continues to produce eosinophil degranulation causing further cell and tissue damage. Some forms appear to be T cell mediated, involving a subset of Th-2 type lymphocytes. At least two distinct forms of hematologic variants appear to exist: the myeloid variant and the lymphoid variant, differing in clinical presentation, long-term behavior, and risk for malignant transformation (Brito-Babapulle, 2003; Roufosse, 2003). Clonal populations of eosinophils have been found in some patients with HES (Chang, 1999). In other patients with HES, abnormal clonal populations of T cells have been identified; these clonal populations may be precursors of malignancy (Simon, 1999).

The organ most consistently affected in HES is the heart, with mural thrombi formation, myocarditis, endocardial and myocardial fibrosis, constrictive pericarditis, and fibroplastic endocarditis (Brito-Babapulle, 2003). Hepatosplenomegaly is common. Other organ systems may be involved and include the CNS and retina, lungs, skin, gastrointestinal (GI) tract, and kidney.

There are occasional reports of persistent eosinophilia occurring in families in the absence of any known cause. This condition is known as 'familial' or 'constitutional' eosinophilia and appears to be benign (Naiman, 1964). The exact prevalence of 'familial' eosinophilia is unknown.

Basophilia

Basophilia is an increase of the absolute basophil count above 0.2×10^9/L. Causes of basophilia are listed in Table 32–6. Reactive basophilia is an uncommon finding overall. Basophilia is seen most frequently in hypersensitivity and allergic reactions, chronic myeloid leukemia (Fig. 32–9), myeloid metaplasia (extramedullary myelopoiesis), and polycythemia vera.

Table 32–6 Key Causes of Basophilia

Myeloproliferative disease
Allergic — food, drugs, foreign proteins
Infectious — variola, varicella
Chronic hemolytic anemia — especially post-splenectomy
Inflammatory — collagen vascular diseases, ulcerative colitis

Figure 32–9 Marked basophilia, and an eosinophil, in a patient with Philadelphia chromosome positivity (× 1000). Courtesy of Robin Abaya, MD.

Table 32–7 Key Causes of Monocytosis

Infectious — tuberculosis, subacute bacterial endocarditis, syphilis, protozoan, rickettsial
Recovery from neutropenia
Hematologic — leukemias, myeloproliferative disorders, lymphomas, multiple myeloma
Inflammatory — collagen vascular diseases, chronic ulcerative colitis, sprue, myositis, polyarteritis, temporal arteritis
Others — solid tumors, immune thrombocytopenic purpura, sarcoidosis

Relative basophilia may be transient following irradiation. Basophilia may be present in hypothyroidism and chronic hemolytic anemia and following splenectomy.

Monocytosis

Monocytosis is an increase of monocytes above the upper reference value, usually 1.0×10^9/L. The most common causes are recovery from neutropenia and indolent infections. Causes and associations of monocytosis are shown in Table 32–7.

Monocytosis is present during the recovery stage from acute infections and from agranulocytosis, in which it is considered a favorable sign. Monocytosis may be present in subacute bacterial endocarditis. In this condition, monocytes may show phagocytosis of other blood cells, red blood cells, and leukocytes. It may be present in mycotic, rickettsial, protozoal, and viral infections.

Infectious disease, however, is an uncommon cause of monocytosis. In a study of 160 successive cases of absolute monocytosis (Maldonado, 1965), over half (85) were associated with *hematologic disease*. These included acute monocytic and granulocytic leukemias; lymphoma (HL most frequently); multiple myeloma; and myeloproliferative disorders.

Monocytopenia

Monocytopenia is a decrease in circulating monocytes below the lower reference value of 0.2×10^9/L. Few studies have dealt with monocytopenia, because of (1) the large number of cells that must be counted in a differential in order to obtain reliable counts; (2) the distributional bias of wedge blood film for monocytes compared with the spinner-made blood film; and (3) the unavailability, until fairly recently, of automation allowing large numbers of cells to be counted routinely.

During therapy with prednisone, monocytes fall during the first few hours after the first dose, but return to above original levels by 12 hours. Monocytopenia has also been observed in hairy cell leukemia. Monocytopenia is uncommon as an isolated finding.

IV

Table 32–8 Key Causes of Lymphocytosis

Infectious — many viral, pertussis, tuberculosis, toxoplasmosis, rickettsial
Chronic inflammatory — ulcerative colitis, Crohn's
Immune mediated — drug sensitivity, vasculitis, graft rejection, Graves', Sjögren's
Hematologic — ALL, CLL, lymphoma
Stress — acute, transient

Lymphocytic and Plasmacytic Disorders

Lymphocytes in Normal Individuals

In normal individuals, the absolute numbers of lymphocytes and T cells are highest in young children. The percentage of lymphocytes in the blood is normally up to about 50% for the first 5 years. During the first decade of life, the absolute lymphocyte count and the absolute number of T cells decrease but remain higher than observed in the adult. By the time of adolescence, the absolute lymphocyte count and the absolute number of T cells have leveled off to values observed throughout adulthood. The absolute number of B lymphocytes remains stable during all stages of life (Davey, 1977; Perkins, 2004). In adolescence and adulthood, lymphocytes constitute about 20–40% of all leukocytes or 1.5–4.0 × 10⁹ cells/L.

There is some disagreement regarding the absolute number of lymphocytes and number of T cells in aged individuals. Although some studies (Diaz-Jouanen, 1975) indicate that there is a decrease in total lymphocyte count and T cell numbers, other investigators find no significant change in total lymphocytes or T cells in aged individuals (Davey, 1977; Weksler, 1974). The normal CD4 : CD8 ratio is between 1.0 and 3.4, but we have seen values as high as 12 in reactive conditions. In the neonate, the number of total T cells and CD8+ T cells may be similar or decreased compared to adults, whereas CD4+ T cells may be similar or increased (De Waele, 1988).

Lymphocytosis

Lymphocytosis is an increase in the number of lymphocytes in the peripheral blood; the reference intervals are ∼ 1.5–4.0 × 10⁹/L in the adult and ∼ 1.5–8.8 × 10⁹/L in the child. Relative lymphocytosis (an increase in the percentage of lymphocytes) is present in various conditions and is especially prominent in disorders with neutropenia. Lymphocytosis is unusual in acute bacterial infections, but is commonly associated with viral infections (EBV, hepatitis) (Table 32–8).

Acute Infectious Lymphocytosis

Acute infectious lymphocytosis (AIL) is a contagious condition characterized by lymphocytosis and occurring mainly in children. The incubation period is 12–21 days. Antibody and viral studies have indicated a relationship between infectious lymphocytosis and Coxsackievirus A, Coxsackievirus B6, echoviruses, and adenovirus type 12. No association has been noted with Epstein–Barr virus (EBV), cytomegalovirus, or herpesvirus. The disease has variable systemic manifestations, from mild and nonspecific to more marked symptoms such as vomiting, fever, abdominal discomfort, signs suggesting involvement of the nervous system, cutaneous rashes, upper respiratory infections, and diarrhea. Leukocytosis (20–50 × 10⁹/L, occasionally > 100 × 10⁹/L) precedes the clinical manifestations.

In AIL, from 60–95% of blood leukocytes are small mature lymphocytes and are probably of T cell origin (Cassuto, 1977). In contrast to infectious mononucleosis, atypical lymphocytes are uncommon. There is usually eosinophilia. The lymphocytosis usually lasts 3–5 weeks, sometimes longer. Other blood changes are unusual. The marrow has no characteristic changes; an increased percentage of lymphocytes has been observed but is probably an artifact as a result of admixture of peripheral blood. Lymph node enlargement is rare and minimal when present. The spleen and liver are rarely, if ever, enlarged. Lymph node biopsy may show reactive follicular hyperplasia but no characteristic changes. In some cases there has been an increase of white cells in the cerebrospinal fluid (CSF), with about 40% lymphocytes.

A chronic form of infectious lymphocytosis in children also occurs. The leukocyte count is 10–25 × 10⁹/L, with 60–80% lymphocytes of normal appearance. Slight eosinophilia, monocytosis, and plasmacytosis are also present. As a rule, the children have enlargement of tonsils, lymph nodes, and spleen and a history of recurrent upper respiratory infections. The marrow shows no abnormalities.

Pertussis

Whooping cough (pertussis), though reduced by routine immunization, still occurs in unimmunized children, and is most severe in infants. It also occurs in adults with immunity reduced since childhood vaccination. The etiologic agent is *Bordetella pertussis*, a highly infectious agent that produces an inflammatory reaction of the entire respiratory tract. The incubation period is approximately 6–20 days, and the first symptoms are those of a head cold. Later, the patient develops paroxysms of coughing productive of thick sputum. The paroxysms typically end with a 'whooping' sound, due to deep inspiration, giving the disease its descriptive name. There is frequently pain over the trachea and bronchi. The disease typically lasts 6–12 weeks.

Patients frequently develop significant lymphocytosis with counts higher than 30 × 10⁹/L recorded. The lymphocytes are small, mature T cells with a normal CD4 : CD8 ratio (Hudnall, 2000). The lymphocyte count is highest during the first 3 weeks of the illness, and then decreases during the fourth and subsequent weeks (Lagergren, 1963). The lymphocytosis is at least partially due to the release of lymphocytosis-promoting factor (LPF) or pertussis toxin from the organism. This factor(s) may cause a transient increased mobilization of lymphocytes from lymphoid organs followed by inhibition of recirculation of lymphocytes from blood into the lymph flow. Thus, the lymphocytosis is due to a redistribution of lymphocytes into the peripheral circulation without increased lymphopoiesis (Rai, 1971; Spangrude, 1985). At the molecular level, this absolute lymphocytosis appears to be due, at least in part, to the absence of L-selectin on many circulating lymphocytes (Hudnall, 2000). This seems reasonable since L-selectin is an endothelial adhesion and lymph node homing receptor, and an absence of this surface molecule would essentially prevent circulating lymphocytes from finding their 'home' in most lymph nodes. They would remain in the circulation for longer time periods and cause an increase in number (lymphocytosis) in the blood. The exact mechanism of loss of L-selectin from the lymphocyte cell surface is not presently known.

Chronic Lymphocytosis/Persistent Polyclonal B Cell Lymphocytosis

Persistent reactive lymphocytosis is an uncommon event in adults and significant lymphocytosis should raise the suspicion of neoplastic disease, such as chronic lymphocyte leukemia. Coexistence of neutropenia or classic Felty's syndrome suggests large granular lymphocyte (LGL) leukemia. Often tissue biopsy and/or immunophenotyping of peripheral blood will point towards a specific disease or diagnosis. Mononucleosis or lymphocytosis due to other viruses occasionally presents in later life, however.

A rare condition, persistent polyclonal lymphocytosis, has been reported in adults, predominantly in female smokers, and in the postsplenectomy state (Himmelmann, 2001). Persistent polyclonal B cell lymphocytosis appears to be a benign polyclonal B cell proliferation, showing binucleated atypical lymphocytes in the peripheral blood. Polyclonal serum IgM is usually increased. The majority (65–85% vs. 15–20% in normals) of the peripheral B cells appear to be IgM+/IgD+/CD27+ memory B cells (Loembe, 2002). Occasional bcl-2/Ig gene rearrangements (t(14;18) commonly associated with follicular lymphoma) have been found (Delage, 1997). Although the cause is unknown, dysregulation of Fas-mediated apoptosis and the CD40 survival pathways appear to be involved (Loembe, 2001; Roussel, 2003).

Retrovirus-Associated Diseases and Conditions

Human T lymphotropic virus type 1 (HTLV-1), discovered in 1980 by Poiesz and Gallo, is a retrovirus associated with adult T cell leukemia/lymphoma (ATL) (Poiesz, 1980). It is endemic in areas of Japan, the Caribbean basin, and the southeastern United States. HTLV-2, a second human retrovirus, was found in a patient with hairy cell leukemia (Kalyanaraman, 1982). A third human retrovirus, human immuno-deficiency virus type I (HIV-1), was recognized and confirmed as the cause of acquired immunodeficiency syndrome (AIDS – discussed further below) over the next 2 years. Later, in 1985, a second but distinct type of human immunodeficiency virus (HIV-2) was identified.

HIV-1 infects both monocyte/macrophages and T cells (both essential cells for normal immune system function), using cell surface chemokine receptors (CCR5 on the former and CXCR4 on the latter); infection ultimately causes a progressive loss of CD4+ lymphocytes, disrupts normal immune function, and produces immunodeficiency and disease. Disease not only includes many different types of infections, but also an increase in neoplastic disease, including lymphomas. At present, it appears that HIV-1 plays an indirect role (through immune dysregulation and not by direct induction) in the development of these lymphomas (Knowles, 2003). HTLV-1 and -2 also infect and transform T cells: primarily CD4+ cells with HTLV-1 and CD8+ cells with HTLV-2. HTLV-1 immortalizes CD4+ lymphoblasts in some patients, producing ATL. Although HTLV-2

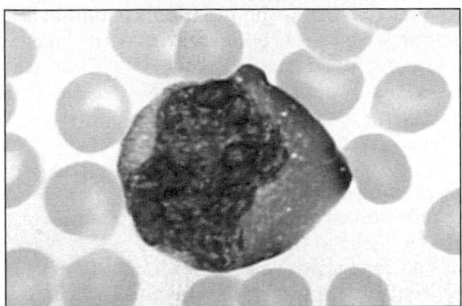

Figure 32–10 Infectious mononucleosis, showing a large activated lymphoid cell in the blood (× 1000).

was originally identified in a patient with hairy cell leukemia, a definitive link between HTLV-2 infection and human disease does not currently exist.

Several cases have now been reported of a transient T cell lymphocytosis in patients infected with HTLV-1 (Kinoshita, 1985; Ehrlich, 1988). In most patients, the disorder is characterized by few clinical symptoms consisting of fever, limited lymphadenopathy, and occasional skin rash. The peripheral blood lymphocyte count is usually less than $20 \times 10^9/L$; however, 10–40% of these lymphocytes are immature forms. In most of these cases, the lymphocytosis is monoclonal and, therefore, leukemic. Although some patients with this infection progress to ATL, most (90–95%) of patients with antibodies against HTLV-1 are symptom free. While most individuals exhibit only a viral-like syndrome, others manifest a chronic progressive leukemia, and still others develop tropical spastic paraparesis (Davey, 1991). ATL typically develops decades after initial infection, and thus is usually seen in older patients.

Infectious Mononucleosis (IM) and Epstein–Barr Virus (EBV) Infection

IM is usually a self-limited infectious disease characterized by sore throat, prolonged malaise, atypical lymphocytosis with presence of large transformed lymphocytes (Fig. 32–10), lymphadenopathy (most often posterior cervical), and often splenomegaly. In immunocompromised patients, EBV is associated with benign B cell hyperplasia, malignant lymphoma, and post-transplantation lymphoproliferative disease (Thompson, 2004; Hess, 2004).

Etiology and Pathophysiology. IM is a disorder secondary to an infection with the EBV (human herpesvirus 4). When the primary infection occurs in healthy individuals during early childhood, the disease often goes unnoticed. However, when the infection involves healthy adolescent individuals or adults, the resultant disorder is the IM syndrome. In most cases, the virus gains entry into the body through the oropharyngeal epithelial and lymphoid tissues, and the virus appears to infect both tissues. The virus attaches to C3d complement receptors (CD21) on B lymphoid cells and enters into the cells. The Epstein–Barr virus then stimulates DNA synthesis in these B cells and induces the formation of several new antigens, including the viral capsid antigen (VCA), the membrane antigen (MA), early antigen (EA), both diffuse (EA-D) and restricted (EA-R) subtypes, Epstein–Barr nuclear antigens (EBNA), and the lymphocyte-detected membrane antigen (LYDMA) (Harrington, 1988). Thus, the earliest phase of this disease is characterized by an infection of B cells that proliferate, develop neo-antigens, circulate, stimulate an immune response, and synthesize immunoglobulin (Sixbey, 1984). VCA, EA, and EBNA are the viral proteins most important for serodiagnosis in immunocompetent patients (see Hess, 2004). Clinical and laboratory features are summarized in Table 32–9.

Typically, the humoral immune response is characterized by the rise in titer of IgG and IgM viral capsid antibodies during the incubation and early prodrome periods. The titer of IgM capsid antibody starts to fall during the second and third weeks of illness and then diminishes to undetectable levels within the following several months. The IgG viral capsid antibody decreases during convalescence but remains detectable for life. Approximately 2–3 weeks after the onset of illness, the Epstein–Barr virus antibodies against the early antigens appear and then decline over the succeeding 2 months. The titer of the Epstein–Barr virus nuclear antigen antibodies rises during the later portion of convalescence and is apparently detectable throughout life.

The cellular immune response in IM is characterized by a proliferation and activation of T cells usually during the second week of illness in response to the EBV-induced B cell infection and activation. Because these activated T cells are mostly from the cytotoxic/suppressor cell

Table 32–9 Summary of Features of Infectious Mononucleosis in Immunocompetent Patients

Pathophysiology

Epstein–Barr virus (HHV-4)

Virus enters through oropharyngeal epithelial and lymphoid cells

Virus attaches to CD21 on B cells

Viral antigens – viral capsid antigen (VCA), early antigen (EA), Epstein–Barr nuclear antigen (EBNA) – are produced and elicit antibody production

Humoral immune response

IgM against VCA rises during incubation and prodrome, falls over few weeks–months

IgG against VCA rises during incubation, decreases during convalescence, remains detectable for life

Antibodies to EA rise 2–3 weeks after onset of illness, then fall

Antibodies to EBNA rise during convalescence, detectable for life

Cellular immune response

T cells activated during 2nd week of illness

CD8-positive cytotoxic T cells kill infected B cells

NK cells kill infected B cells

Some resting memory B cells remain latently infected

Clinical features

2- to 5-week incubation period

Vague onset of symptoms

Fever, sore throat, lymphadenopathy

Adolescents, young adults more often symptomatic than younger children

Laboratory features

Leukocytosis with absolute lymphocytosis and atypical lymphocytes

Transient monocytosis

Relative and absolute neutropenia early on

Mild thrombocytopenia in half of cases

Hemolytic anemia in 1–3% of cases, often with anti-I specificity

Elevated transaminases in 85–100% of cases, but clinical jaundice rare

Spot test is simple, rapid, specific, based on agglutination of horse RBCs

Heterophil antibody test is based on differential absorption of IM-specific HA by beef RBC stroma and guinea pig kidney

subpopulation, there is a marked suppression and destruction of EBV-infected B cells. Indeed, most of the atypical lymphocytes observed in the peripheral blood of patients with IM during the second week of illness possess the CD8 antigen. These cytotoxic/suppressor T cells kill infected B cells and diminish the polyclonal antibody production induced by the Epstein–Barr virus. In addition to the T-cytotoxic cells, the activity of natural killer (NK) cells has a profound effect on limiting the proliferation of the EBV-infected B cells in patients with IM (Purtilo, 1981). It is also likely that EBV-infected B cells are destroyed, at least in part, through the mechanism of antibody-dependent cellular cytotoxicity, a process requiring the presence of both cytotoxic cells and antibody. This process of B cell proliferation followed by the inhibitory and destructive effects of EBV-directed antibody production, as well as T cell and NK cell cytotoxic effects, occurs within the patient's peripheral blood, bone marrow, lymphoid tissues and, perhaps to a limited degree, all tissues of the body.

Ultimately, most immunocompetent individuals have serologic evidence of past EBV infection (infection occurs in over 90% of normal adults worldwide). EBV has the capacity to not only infect cells (many of which are destroyed by an intact immune system) but to produce a latent infection in resting memory B cells, and in some cases, produce transformation of lymphocytes to malignant lymphoma (Kuppers, 2003; Thorley-Lawson, 2004). However, the majority of latently infected individuals show no disease manifestations throughout their lifetimes.

The resting memory B cells can act as a reservoir of EBV, since viral antigens (easily recognized by an intact immune system) are not expressed on the lymphocyte surface. In this model of EBV infection, mechanisms of viral persistence and transformation appear to be dependent on the interaction between the stage of maturation of the infected lymphocyte and the genetic expression of different groups (or 'programs') of viral proteins within the infected lymphocyte (Kuppers, 2003; Thorley-Lawson, 2004). In addition, different types of EBV-associated tumors (such as African Burkitt lymphoma [BL], nasopharyngeal carcinoma, B cell lymphoproliferative disease or post-transplant lymphoproliferative disease in immunocompromised individuals, and HL) also appear to exhibit different groups of viral protein expression (Wong, 2002).

Clinical Features. IM has been observed in patients from 3 months to 70 years of age but is most common in adolescents and young adults. A 2- to 5-week incubation period prior to symptoms usually occurs. The onset is vague, indefinite, and similar to the onset of other infectious diseases. Patients usually have fever, sore throat with ulcerative pharyngitis, and lymphadenopathy.

Complications. Of the rare anemias associated with IM, hemolytic anemia is the most common, occurring in 1–3% of cases. The cause now appears to be related to the anti-I antibody produced frequently in this disease.

Mild thrombocytopenia occurs in about half the cases, but the platelet count is not often less than 100×10^9/L. Thrombocytopenic purpura with hemorrhagic complications is exceedingly rare. Splenic rupture may also occur. Neutropenia, pancytopenia, and hemophagocytic syndrome may rarely occur and be fatal (Mroczek, 1987). Two rare conditions resulting from EBV infection in healthy individuals are chronic active EBV infection (CAEBV) and EBV hemophagocytic syndrome (EBVHS). Both conditions show high morbidity and mortality and appear to be related to ectopic EBV infection in T cells and natural killer cells, in contrast to the usual B cell infection that commonly occurs in IM (Kasahara, 2002).

Abnormal liver function tests indicative of hepatitis occur in 85–100% of patients with IM. Clinical jaundice is rare, but cases have been reported in which jaundice and acute pharyngitis were the only clinical manifestations of IM, with positive hematologic and serologic findings. Although uncommon, complications may also involve the nervous system, heart, kidney, and lungs.

Approximately one-third of patients with IM carry β-hemolytic streptococci in the pharynx. Thus, one should give attention to strict clinical, hematologic, and serologic criteria in distinguishing IM from streptococcal pharyngitis.

Hematologic Features. Leukocytes are increased, usually ranging from $12–25 \times 10^9$/L. Rarely, counts as high as 80×10^9/L have been recorded. The leukocytosis is usually due to lymphocytosis (60–90%) composed of a variety of atypical lymphocytes. The total leukocyte count, as a rule, returns to normal within 3 weeks. The atypical lymphocytes have nuclear alterations and an increase in the amount and basophilia of cytoplasm.

Lymphocytes include 'monocytoid' lymphocytes which likely correspond to immunoblasts in lymph nodes (Fig. 32–10). Other atypical lymphocytes, which are more numerous, include plasmacytoid lymphocytes and those with small nuclei but abundant cytoplasm.

Often the number of monocytes rises transiently. The term *mononucleosis* refers to an increase of lymphocytes and not monocytes.

The cytologic alterations are not pathognomonic of IM. Similar cells are found in a variety of disorders, including cytomegalovirus mononucleosis, toxoplasmosis, and infectious hepatitis, and usually to a lesser extent in viral pneumonia, varicella, mumps, and viral exanthemas of children.

Neutrophils are relatively and absolutely decreased in most cases during the first week of illness. During this time, there may be a shift to the left, with an increase of band cells and metamyelocytes. Toxic granules and Döhle bodies may be seen. The eosinophils are within normal limits.

The bone marrow from patients with IM usually shows an increased cellularity. There are an increased number of lymphocytes, macrophages, plasma cells, megakaryocytes, and erythroid cells. The neutrophilic series appears decreased. About half of the cases may have collections of mononuclear cells forming loose granulomas.

Serologic Findings in Immunocompetent Patients

Heterophil Antibody. Paul (1932) first described the presence of sheep cell agglutinins in the sera of patients with IM. Sheep cell agglutinins are not, however, specific for IM and can be present in other disorders.

Davidsohn (1937) demonstrated that the heterophil antibodies in patients with IM are absorbed by beef erythrocytes, in contrast to heterophil antibodies present in other disorders. The latter are absorbed by the Forssman's antigen such as that found in guinea pig kidney. The differential absorption test (Paul–Bunnell–Davidsohn test) is highly specific for IM (Davidsohn, 1969).

The spot test for IM (Lee, 1968) is based on the principle that horse erythrocytes are more sensitive than sheep erythrocytes in testing for IM. A positive test for IM shows agglutination of horse erythrocytes by serum absorbed with guinea pig kidney but not by serum absorbed with beef erythrocyte stroma. The spot test has proved to be a simple, rapid, highly specific, and sensitive test for the heterophil antibodies of IM. False-positive tests occur, but are very rare. The spot test is still in use, as well as other similarly performing immunoassays and latex-based detection tests for heterophil antibody (Rogers, 1999). False-negative tests occur

particularly in young children who produce heterophil antibodies (IgM) in limited amounts. In heterophil-negative IM, the diagnosis may be substantiated by assay for antibody to EBV.

As previously mentioned, several antibodies are produced by the host in response to a variety of Epstein–Barr virus antigens (see Table 32–9). Antibody to the viral capsid antigen arises within the first 2 weeks of the onset. This antibody, measured by an immunofluorescent or other method, is used for determining exposure to EBV. Assaying for the presence of EBV antibody is usually limited to the few cases of heterophil-negative IM.

In addition to heterophil and EBV antibodies, patients with IM frequently produce antibodies to a wide variety of antigens. Antibodies against human erythrocytes, leukocytes, and platelets have been described. Patients with IM have an increased frequency of cold agglutinins. Positive tests to rheumatoid factor and antinuclear factor have been reported.

In immunocompromised patients, serologic tests are of limited value, and direct detection methods are considered more reliable. Determination of EBV viral load by polymerase chain reaction (PCR) appears, at present, to be one of the better tests for this patient population (Hess, 2004).

Differential Diagnosis. The clinical, hematologic, and serologic features of IM permit an accurate diagnosis to be made in over 90% of the cases. When the heterophil test is negative, one must consider several possibilities. The patient could still have EBV antibody-positive but heterophil-negative IM. Cytomegalovirus infection, however, is the most common cause of heterophil-negative mononucleosis. Other possibilities include toxoplasmosis, infectious hepatitis, human herpesvirus 6, human immunodeficiency virus types 1 and 2, and ingestion of drugs (*p*-aminosalicylic acid, phenytoin [Dilantin], and diaminodiphenylsulfone) (see Tsaparas, 2000 and Taylor, 2003).

Course. Classic IM is a benign disorder, and complications occur in less than 5% of patients. The disorder usually resolves in 3–4 weeks. Fatalities are extremely rare, but tend to occur in members of the same family (Purtilo, 1979). Further studies indicate that the affected individuals frequently suffer from X-linked lymphoproliferative disease (XLP). This group of immunosuppressed individuals possesses a rare, familial, fatal form of combined immunodeficiency, apparently involving both B and T cells. All untreated patients die by approximately 40 years of age. EBV infection can produce any one of three severe complications in XLP: fulminant IM, life-threatening lymphoproliferative diseases and B cell lymphoma, and dysgammaglobulinemia. Although classically associated with EBV infection, XLP can occur in patients seronegative for EBV. XLP has been mapped to human chromosome Xq24-25, which codes for a cell surface receptor present on T and NK cells, but not B cells. An uncontrolled cytotoxic T cell response is thought to be responsible for liver necrosis and bone marrow failure, ultimately causing death (Thompson, 2004). In addition to XLP, EBV-associated lymphoproliferative disorders can occur in individuals with congenital and acquired immunodeficiencies.

Cytomegalovirus Infection

Some individuals infected with cytomegalovirus develop a syndrome similar to infectious mononucleosis. This disorder can occur following massive blood transfusions (post-transfusion mononucleosis) or spontaneously in previously healthy individuals (cytomegalovirus mononucleosis). The patient has fever, chills, profound malaise, and myalgia. There may be a sore throat (but not exudative pharyngitis) and lymphadenopathy. Occasionally splenomegaly is found, but hepatomegaly does not occur. Commonly involved systems in immunocompromised patients are the CNS, GI, and pulmonary systems, although disease may be found in almost any organ system.

Leukocytosis is characteristic with absolute lymphocytosis. Usually 20% or more of the leukocytes are atypical lymphocytes. Bone marrow aspirates have shown an increased number of normal lymphocytes and atypical lymphocytes. Abnormal liver function test results are the most frequent abnormal laboratory finding (Wreghitt, 2003). In a small percentage of patients, there may be an increased titer of cold agglutinins, rheumatoid factor, and antinuclear antibodies. There is no rise in heterophil, Epstein–Barr virus, or *Toxoplasma gondii* antibodies. The diagnosis is usually made by isolating the cytomegalovirus from urine, saliva, blood or tissue biopsy, or by serology.

Toxoplasmosis

Toxoplasma gondii, a protozoan parasite, can produce, in the young and old, a disease (toxoplasmosis) similar to infectious mononucleosis. Diagnosis is critical in congenitally infected fetuses and newborns, women infected during pregnancy, immunocompromised patients, and patients with chorioretinitis (Remington, 2004).

Only a small proportion (~ 10%) of immunocompetent individuals are symptomatic. These patients typically present with lymphadenopathy,

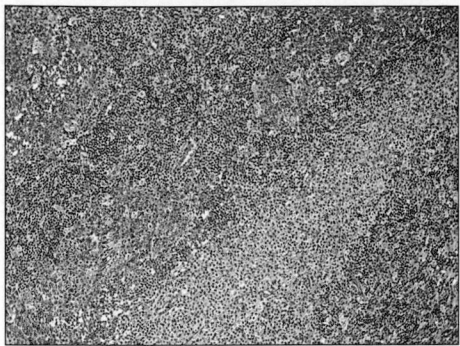

Figure 32–11 Toxoplasmosis lymphadenitis shows follicular hyperplasia with monocytoid B cell hyperplasia (lower right-center) and scattered individual and aggregates of histiocytes, often impinging on the germinal center/mantle zone border (×200).

commonly cervical. Some patients may also show fever, headache, sore throat, hepatosplenomegaly, chorioretinitis, and an increased number of atypical lymphocytes in the peripheral blood. In immunocompromised patients, disease commonly involves the CNS and eyes, but may also involve the lungs, and heart.

The histopathology of lymph nodes is usually distinctive, with scattered epithelioid histiocytes which often blur the germinal center/mantle zone border, and with sinus monocytoid B cell hyperplasia (Fig. 32–11). Morphology correlates closely with elevated *Toxoplasma* antibody titers (Dorfman, 1973). Bone marrow biopsy specimens have no specific pathologic lesion.

The diagnosis is established by demonstrating an elevation of *Toxoplasma* antibodies in immunocompetent patients. In immunocompromised patients, serological tests are not sensitive, and direct detection of the organism from blood, body fluids, or in tissue is necessary for definitive diagnosis.

Lymphocytopenia

Lymphocytopenia is present when the absolute lymphocyte count is below ~ 1.0×10^9/L in adults and below ~ 2.0×10^9/L in children. Normally, about 80% of circulating peripheral blood lymphocytes are CD3+ T cells, and the majority (~ 65%) of these cells are CD4+ helper T cells. A number of immunologic deficiency disorders that are genetically determined have lymphocytopenia along with various other immunologic defects of either humoral or cell-mediated immunity. Lymphocytopenia in these disorders is due to impaired lymphopoiesis. Increased levels of adrenocortical hormones, the administration of chemotherapeutic drugs, or irradiation will result in lymphocytopenia. Impaired drainage of the intestinal lymphatics with loss of lymphocytes into the intestines owing to a number of causes has been implicated as a mechanism for lymphocytopenia. In advanced cases of non-Hodgkin and Hodgkin lymphomas as well as in terminal cases of carcinoma, lymphocytopenia is often observed. Causes and conditions associated with lymphocytopenia include those in Table 32–10.

Acquired Immunodeficiency Syndrome

Acquired immunodeficiency syndrome (AIDS) is usually a progressively fatal infectious disorder with characteristic clinical, hematologic, and serologic abnormalities.

Etiology. AIDS is a disorder secondary to an infection with the human immunodeficiency viruses 1 (HIV-1) and 2 (HIV-2), RNA retroviruses that are cytotropic for CD4+ T cells and for macrophages. Viral entry into a cell is not by the interaction with the CD4 receptor alone; in addition, expression of chemokine co-receptors is essential for virus entry into cells and also determines target cell tropism (Starr-Spires, 2002). Other cell types, such as monocytes, macrophages, and CNS microglial cells also coexpress these receptors and can support viral replication. HIV is responsible for both direct killing of infected cells and indirect killing of neighboring cells, utilizing both apoptotic-dependent and apoptotic-independent mechanisms of cell destruction (Badley, 2003).

HIV infection is spread by contamination with secretions, excretions, blood, and tissues that contain the virus. Because of the cytotropic effect of the AIDS viruses for CD4+ cells, there is a marked decrease in the number of T-helper cells and an imbalance in T-suppressor/cytotoxic cells in the blood and the lymphoid tissues of the body. As a result, a profound cellular immune depression occurs characterized by infections with a variety of opportunistic organisms. Initially, B cells are not involved and immunoglobulin levels are normal or increased. However, as the disease

Table 32–10 Key Causes of Lymphopenia
Destructive — radiation, chemotherapy, corticosteroids
Debilitative — starvation, aplastic anemia, terminal cancer, collagen vascular disease, renal failure
Infectious — viral hepatitis, influenza, typhoid fever, TB
AIDS associated — HIV cytopathic effect, nutritional imbalance, drug effect
Congenital immunodeficiency — Wiskott–Aldrich
Abnormal lymphatic circulation — intestinal lymphangiectasia, obstruction, thoracic duct drainage/rupture, CHF

progresses, there is an increased frequency of malignancy in these patients. AIDS-associated cancers include Kaposi's sarcoma, non-HL, and cervical cancer (all AIDS-defining cancers), as well as HL and anogenital cancers (Mbulaiteye, 2003; Bellan, 2003). Although the etiology of these malignancies is undoubtedly multifactorial, recent studies suggest that HIV may possess oncogenic potential (De Falco, 2003; Lazzi, 2002). In addition, the function of monocytes and NK cells is abnormal.

Hematologic Features. The most common hematologic abnormality in patients with AIDS is anemia of chronic disease and lymphopenia (80–85% of cases), particularly of the T-helper/inducer (CD4) subset. Thrombocytopenia occurs in approximately 30% of cases, and neutropenia in 40%, often with a left shift; the former is often immune mediated (Hoxie, 1995).

The peripheral blood film usually displays atypical lymphocytes that have a plasmacytoid appearance. Monocytes are often large with a fine nuclear chromatin and cytoplasmic vacuoles. Immune-mediated anemia, thrombocytopenia, and neutropenia have also been described in AIDS.

The bone marrow is usually normocellular to hypercellular (Castella, 1985). There are often increased numbers of immature myeloid precursor cells, macrophages laden with iron, and plasma cells. There are defects in bone marrow progenitor cells such as colony-forming unit-granulocyte, monocyte (CFU-GM); colony-forming unit-granulocyte, erythrocyte, monocyte, megakaryocyte pluripotential stem cell (CFU-GEMM); colony-forming unit-megakaryocyte (CFU-MK); and burst-forming unit-erythrocyte (BFU-E). Many drugs used to treat AIDS and its infectious complications are also myelosuppressive. It is important to remember that the suppression of the marrow is, in many patients, multifactorial, resulting from an interaction of direct HIV cytopathic effect, dysregulation of the immune system and of apoptosis, possible complicating infection and/or nutritional imbalance, and drug effect. The most clinically valuable information of bone marrow biopsy is usually the identification of either infection or malignancy in the marrow.

Functional Disorders of Lymphocytes

Functional disorders of lymphocytes can be inherited or acquired. The immune deficiency may be due to a disorder of maturation or function of monocytes and antigen-presenting cells, B cells, T cells, stem cells, suppressor cells, or a combination. These may cause either antibody production defects or a combination of antibody production and T cell function defects. Acquired disorders may be due to malnutrition, infection, or malignancy as well as any insult that may significantly perturb immune regulation and cellular communication. Acquired functional abnormalities of lymphocytes are frequently observed in lymphoid malignancies. For example, decreased B cell function is observed in chronic lymphocytic leukemia, in which two-thirds of the patients have hypogammaglobulinemia. In multiple myeloma, there is a diminished synthesis of normal immunoglobulin in the presence of high levels of paraprotein.

Diminished T cell activity has been described in patients with HL, sarcoidosis, and leprosy. In HL, the diminished T cell activity may be the result of the suppressive effects of monocytes. In autoimmune diseases, a loss of suppressor T cells has been observed.

In severe malnutrition and in patients with terminal malignancies, there is diminished humoral and cell-mediated immunity.

The diagnosis of functional disorders of lymphocytes requires the use of skin tests, enumeration of B and T cells and their subsets, measurement of serum immunoglobulin and antibodies, and a variety of in vitro lymphocyte assays that record their response to mitogens and antigens. Molecular testing, including cytogenetic and fluorescent in situ hybridization (FISH) analysis, flow cytometry, and polymerase chain reaction, may be required for definitive diagnosis. A thorough history and physical examination should always precede any testing. It is probably best to begin a workup with less expensive and easily obtainable tests.

IV

Table 32–11 Key Causes of Plasmacytosis

Viral — infectious mononucleosis, measles, rubella, HIV
Bacterial — tuberculosis, syphilis, streptococcus, staphylococcus
Parasitic — malaria, trichinosis
Inflammatory — SLE, RA, inflammatory bowel disease, alcoholic liver disease
Neoplastic — plasma cell leukemia, myeloma, CLL
Immune stimulation — immune complex disease (serum sickness), drug sensitivity, transfusion
Trauma

Plasmacytosis

Plasma cells are not normally present in circulating blood. They are increased in a variety of chronic infections, in allergic states, in the presence of neoplasms, and in other conditions in which the serum γ-globulin concentration is elevated. Plasma cells have also been recorded in the blood of patients with viral disorders, including rubella, measles, chickenpox, and mumps. They are moderately increased in cutaneous exanthemas, infectious mononucleosis, syphilis, subacute bacterial endocarditis, sarcoidosis, and collagen diseases. Rarely, bacterial sepsis may show a peripheral plasmacytosis mimicking plasma cell leukemia (Shtalrid, 2003). Their increase is usually linked with an increase in lymphocytes, monocytes, and eosinophils. Causes and conditions associated with plasmacytosis include those illustrated (Table 32–11).

In the marrow, an average of 1–2% of plasma cells are present in adults. An increase beyond 4% is significant; lower values are found in children. Increases of up to 20% of plasma cells may be found in a variety of conditions other than multiple myeloma, including metastatic carcinoma, chronic granulomatous infections, conditions linked with hypersensitivity, and following administration of cytotoxic drugs. They are often increased in aplastic anemia, but this is probably just a relative increase. On the other hand, they are decreased or absent in agammaglobulinemia.

Leukemoid Reactions

A leukemoid reaction is an excessive leukocytic response in the peripheral blood. It includes leukocytosis of $50 \times 10^9/L$ or higher with a shift to the left; lower counts, even below normal, with considerable numbers of immature granulocytes; and similar quantitative or qualitative changes in lymphocytes or monocytes. Depending on the predominant cell, leukemoid reactions may be neutrophilic, eosinophilic, lymphocytic, or monocytic. No clear explanation for these apparent temporary aberrations in normal regulatory control mechanisms is yet available, although in some instances they appear to be due to an elevation of cytokines or granulocyte colony-stimulating factor by tumor (Melhem, 1993; Nara, 2003; Nimieri, 2003). The reactions are irregular in degree, even when associated with the same inciting agent.

Neutrophilic Leukemoid Reactions

Excessive neutrophilia may occur in many situations, including hemolysis, hemorrhage, malignancy with bone involvement, HL, myelofibrosis, infections (especially tuberculosis), severe burns, eclampsia, and certain intoxications.

Examination of the blood is usually more helpful than marrow examination. Leukemoid reactions lack the characteristic differential count that is seen in chronic myelogenous leukemia (CML), including the myelocyte 'peak,' eosinophilia, and basophilia (Fig. 32–12).

Eosinophilic Leukemoid Reactions

Cells as immature as eosinophilic myelocytes rarely appear in the blood in reactive eosinophilia, in which the leukocyte count may exceed $50 \times 10^9/L$ (Fig. 32–8). Eosinophilic leukemoid reactions usually occur in children and usually are caused by parasitic infections. As with granulocytic leukemoid reactions, some eosinophilic leukemoid reactions have been associated with tumor (Oakley, 1998; Melhem, 1993).

Erythroblastosis and Leukoerythroblastosis

In patients with or without anemia, circulating normoblasts frequently are accompanied by a neutrophilic leukemoid reaction; this, then, is a *leukoerythroblastotic reaction*. A moderate anemia with normoblasts in the peripheral blood is fairly common in metastatic carcinoma involving bone marrow. Leukoerythroblastosis may also be associated with marrow infection and/or fibrosis, and may be seen in benign conditions such as GI bleeding and hemolytic anemia (Weick, 1974).

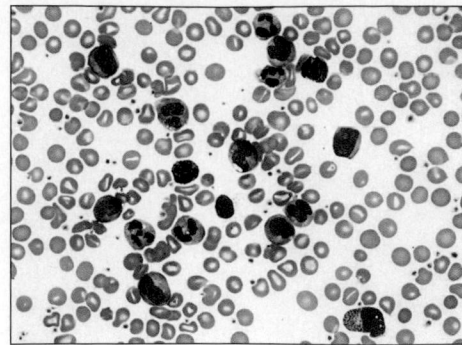

Figure 32–12 Chronic myeloid leukemia with increased segmented neutrophils, myelocytes, basophils and an occasional blast (× 500).

Lymphocytic Leukemoid Reactions

Extremely high counts of normal-appearing lymphocytes may occur in infectious lymphocytosis and in pertussis (see above). When atypical lymphocytes are strikingly increased or immature (which may occur in conditions such as infectious mononucleosis), the distinction from leukemia may be difficult.

Examination of the marrow *may be* useful, since lymphocytes are minimally increased, if at all, in most leukemoid reactions in contrast to leukemia. Flow cytometric studies of peripheral blood and/or bone marrow would reveal a nonclonal population of lymphocytes with a normal combination of cell surface markers in benign proliferations.

Neoplastic Disorders Primarily Involving Leukocytes

Overview of Hematopoietic Neoplasms

Hematopoietic neoplasms constitute a diversity of disorders which have in common their derivation from hematopoietic stem cells of the bone marrow or lymphoid organs and which are known or assumed to be clonal processes arising due to genetic errors. Given the diversity and regulatory complexity of hematopoietic cells, it is not surprising that neoplasms involving these tissues are also quite diverse, differing in predominant cells within a neoplasm, degree of differentiation, rates of proliferation and apoptosis, clinical features and response to therapy. Diagnosis and classification of hematopoietic tumors has changed with our understanding of disease. In the 19th century, 'leukemia' referred to the white or pale color of blood, which contained increased leukocytes compared to red corpuscles, neither of which could be microscopically seen in detail without differential staining. 'Chlorosis' and 'chloroma' referred to the grossly greenish tinge of granulocytic cells. 'Lymphoma,' first used by Virchow, referred to tumors of the lymph glands.

After the development of Romanowsky stains (such as Wright–Giemsa), and later hematoxylin and eosin (H&E), as well as improvements in microscopes, hematopoietic tumors could be classified by morphology, clinical features and the location of the abnormal proliferations. Hematopoietic tumors were referred to as leukemias when they primarily involved the blood and bone marrow, and lymphomas or sarcomas when they primarily involved the soft tissue. 'Acute' referred to diseases with aggressive clinical courses and 'chronic' to those which progressed more slowly. Morphologic subtyping based on predominant cell types progressed into the 1950s and 1960s with development of cytochemical stains to differentiate subtypes of myeloid cells and some lymphoid cells (such as hairy cell leukemia).

From about 1970 on, an explosion of knowledge and new technology has occurred which provides many new tools for understanding these tumors. These include the discovery of B cells, T cells and other immunologic compartments, monoclonal antibodies and leukocyte differentiation antigens, cytogenetic karyotyping, immunoglobulin and T cell gene rearrangements, PCR, nucleic acid arrays and most recently proteomic assays. Many, though certainly not all, hematopoietic tumors can now be characterized at the level of the genetic abnormality and the resultant intracellular pathway perturbations. This offers tremendous opportunity to develop therapies targeted to the specific abnormalities. Examples include chronic myeloid leukemia, with a t(9;22)(q34;q11) *BCR/ABL* translocation and resultant abnormal tyrosine kinase, which has been targeted with the drug Gleevec (imatinib mesylate) (Druker, 2004)

Table 32–12 Key Features of the Major Myeloproliferative and Myelodysplastic/Myeloproliferative Disease

Disorder	Demographics	Laboratory features, morphology	Cytogenetics	Prognosis
CML	Middle-aged; occasionally any age	WBC > $50 \times 10^3/\mu L$, spectrum of maturation of granulocytic cells, myelocyte peak, basophilia, anemia, low NAP	t(9;22)(q34;q11) *BCR-ABL*	Chronic phase ~ 5 years. ?effect of Gleevec®. Eventual blast crisis worse prognosis
PV	Middle-aged, M > F	RBC > $6 \times 10^6/\mu L$, Hb > 18.5 g/dL in males, > 16.5 g/dL in females, increased platelet count, moderate neutrophilia	May be present, but *may not* be t(9;22)	10–20 years
CIM	Typically over 50 years.	Leukoerythroblastic anemia, moderately increased WBC with left shift, normal–decreased platelets with atypical morphology. Fibrotic BM with atypical megakaryocytes and RBC and granulocyte precursors	+8, +9, del(20q), del(13q), del(1p) and others are seen in 80% of patients, often herald conversion to AML or CML. *May not* be t(9;22).	5 years median survival
ET	5th decade (M = F), second peak in 30s (F > M)	Platelets > $\times 10^3$, abnormal morphology. BM with large, multilobular, clustered megakaryocytes	del(13q22), +8, +9 seen in 5–10% of cases. *May not* be t(9;22).	Stable for many years (most cases)
CMML	Median 65–75 years, M > F	Monocytosis > $1 \times 10^3/\mu L$ for 3 months, cytopenias, dysplasias in myeloid lineage in BM, < 20% blasts + promonocytes in BM	+8, −7, 12p abnormalities in 20–40% of cases. *May not* be t(9;22).	20–30 months with progression to AML in 15–30%
JMML	Under 3 years, M > F	Monocytosis > $1 \times 10^3/\mu L$, WBC > $10 \times 10^3/\mu L$, left shifted granulocytes, increased Hb F	Monosomy 7, *May not* be t(9;22).	Poor. Possible benefit from BMT

CML = chronic myeloid leukemia; PV = polycythemia vera; CIM = chronic idiopathic myelofibrosis; ET = essential thrombocythemia; CMML = chronic myelomonocytic leukemia; JMML = juvenile myelomonocytic leukemia; BM = bone marrow; NAP – neutrophil alkaline phosphatase; BMT = bone marrow transplant.

and acute promyelocytic leukemia with t(15;17)(q22;q12) *PML/RARα* and an abnormal receptor for retinoic acid, which responds to all-*trans* retinoic acid.

Classification of leukemias and, particularly, lymphomas became confusing in the 1970s and 1980s as knowledge progressed. The French–American–British (FAB) Cooperative Group developed consensus criteria for leukemias and myelodysplastic syndromes (Bennett, 1976, 1982), while lymphoma classification varied internationally. In North America, the standard lymphoma classification became the National Cancer Institute (NCI) Working Formulation for Clinical Usage (Non-Hodgkin's Lymphoma Pathologic Classification Project, 1982) and in Europe, the updated Kiel Classification (Stansfeld, 1988). These were synthesized in the Revised European American Lymphoma Classification (Harris, 1995). Most recently, hematopathologists and oncologists recognize that uniform diagnostic criteria are essential for all hematopoietic neoplasms. The current global classification of hematopoietic tumors sponsored by the World Health Organization (WHO) (Jaffe, 2001a) recognizes the predominance of the abnormal biology of each tumor, and utilizes a combination of diagnostic techniques, varying with each tumor, to arrive at the diagnosis. Morphology, immunophenotype, cytogenetics and molecular genetics are all utilized, and cytochemical assays are used in some cases. Many of the tumors may present as leukemias or soft-tissue tumors (lymphomas), and these terms remain descriptively useful. The WHO classification also utilizes a two-tiered approach for acute myeloid leukemias, which recognizes that in many areas of the world molecular and cytogenetic testing is not available and, where it is, it is not always productive. For such cases (acute myelogenous leukemia [AML], not otherwise classified), morphologic criteria are based on the earlier FAB classification.

Chronic Myeloproliferative Diseases

The chronic myeloproliferative disorders recognized by the WHO are chronic myeloid leukemia (CML), chronic neutrophilic leukemia (CNL), chronic eosinophilic leukemia/hypereosinophilic syndrome, polycythemia vera (PV), chronic idiopathic myelofibrosis, and essential thrombocythemia (ET) (Vardiman, 2001a). These are clonal proliferations of a pluripotential stem cell that can differentiate along granulocytic, erythroid, and megakaryocytic lines (Adamson, 1976; Fialkow, 1977). Each has a chronic course that may terminate as acute leukemia, myelofibrosis, or a coagulopathy, but only one, CML, has a consistently recurrent genetic abnormality (Nowell, 1960). Key features of the major disorders are summarized in Table 32–12.

Chronic Myelogenous Leukemia
Clinical Features. CML occurs in young and middle-aged adults. The age-specific incidence, however, increases markedly after 50 years of age.

The onset is insidious and the disorder may be discovered accidentally on a routine blood test. The patient may have symptoms of anemia and weight loss or simply may complain of malaise. The spleen enlarges progressively, and the patient begins to lose weight and have fever and night sweats associated with increased metabolism as a result of granulocyte turnover. The discomfort associated with an enlarged spleen may bring the patient to the doctor. Infarcts in the spleen may produce left upper quadrant pain. Excessive bleeding or bruising may occur in the later stages of the disease. Lymphadenopathy, though often present, is rarely prominent (Cortes, 2004).

Laboratory Features.
Blood. The leukocyte count is usually over $50 \times 10^9/L$ and may exceed $300 \times 10^9/L$. The differential count is characteristic. There is a complete spectrum of granulocytic cells, from a few myeloblasts to mature neutrophils, with myelocytes and neutrophils exceeding the other cell types (Savage, 1997). This bimodal distribution helps to exclude other myeloproliferative disorders and reactive leukocytosis (Fig. 32–12). Myeloblasts are less than 10% of the cells. The relative percentage of neutrophil myelocytes increases as the total leukocyte count increases. Basophilia is consistently present and eosinophilia is almost always noted, along with the presence of eosinophil myelocytes. Monocytes are also absolutely increased in most patients.

Normocytic anemia is present in the majority of patients at diagnosis and a few normoblasts can usually be found. Thrombocytosis is present in over half while less than 15% have thrombocytopenia.

Marrow. The marrow is markedly hypercellular, primarily as a result of granulocytic proliferation, with all stages represented. Eosinophil and basophil precursors are usually increased. Normoblasts tend to be relatively decreased. Frequently, the marrow cannot be aspirated because of the density of cellularity or (especially later in the disease) because of increased reticulin, which can be demonstrated on marrow biopsy. Macrophages laden with blue pigment (sea-blue histiocytes) or macrophages indistinguishable from Gaucher's cells are found in some patients.

It is well to remember that even a typical bone marrow is not diagnostic of CML. On the other hand, the diagnosis can be made from the peripheral blood film in most cases.

Neutrophil Alkaline Phosphatase. The neutrophil alkaline phosphatase (NAP) is greatly reduced or absent in over 90% of patients with CML. It is greatly elevated in polycythemia vera; elevated, normal, or low in idiopathic myelofibrosis; and normal or elevated in leukemoid reactions. During remission of CML with a normal-appearing blood picture, in most cases, the NAP continues to be low; in about one-third of patients, it returns to normal. The NAP increases in the accelerated and blastic phases of the disease. It may also increase in response to infection as it does in normal individuals.

Cytogenetic Abnormalities. In over 95% of patients with typical CML, cultured cells from the blood or bone marrow possess the cytogenetic abnormality t(9;22)(q34;q11), involving the *ABL1* gene on the long arm of chromosome 9 and the *BCR* gene on the long arm of chromosome 22. An abnormally small chromosome formed by this translocation is called the Philadelphia (Ph') chromosome (Nowell, 1960). The *BCR–ABL1* gene fusion results in a novel RNA transcript and subsequently a protein growth factor with tyrosine kinase activity, which is higher than normal protein 145 coded for by *ABL1*. Variant translocations involving additional genes and cryptic translocations requiring molecular detection occur. Most translocations involve a *BCR* breakpoint at the major breakpoint region (M-BCR) with resultant p210 protein, and an occasional breakpoint at the mu region results in a p230 protein with associated prominent neutrophilic maturation. Minor breakpoint region (m-BCR) translocations with resultant p190 protein are usually associated with acute lymphoblastic leukemia (ALL), but rare m-BCR translocations in CML are associated with increased monocytosis, and small amounts of p190 may be found in standard CML (Vardiman, 2001b).

Other Findings. Serum cobalamin and transcobalamins are usually increased considerably, as a result of increased transcobalamin I, and are thought to reflect the size of the total blood granulocyte pool. Serum muramidase (lysozyme) is also increased.

Course. Treatment with either busulfan or hydroxycarbamide (hydroxyurea) in the past usually controlled the disease in the chronic phase, but without hematologic bone marrow remission or clearing of the Ph' chromosome. Improved results have been obtained with recombinant interferon-alpha or allogeneic transplant (Silver, 1999). A synthetic protein kinase inhibitor, STI-571 (imatinib mesylate; Gleevec), specifically targets the BCR-ABL protein, and is the most promising current therapy. This treatment results in frequent clinical remission, though relapses occur and long-term survival benefits are not yet known (Angstreich, 2004).

Except for those cases cured by transplantation, the disease changes after a variable period, depending partly on therapy, into a more aggressive or accelerated phase (Cortes, 2003). This is characterized by one or more features of progressive myeloproliferation: increased blood or marrow blasts of 10–19%; peripheral blood basophilia > 20%; persistent thrombocytopenia unrelated to therapy < 100×10^9/L; thrombocytosis > 1000×10^9/L; increasing leukocytosis and splenomegaly unresponsive to therapy; or cytogenetic clonal evolution. Granulocytic dysplasia, increased small dysplastic megakaryocytes and reticulin fibrosis are also suggestive.

Blast phase is essentially a progression to acute leukemia and is defined by > 20% blasts in the blood or bone marrow, large aggregates of blasts in the marrow or in extramedullary locations. Blast lineage is myeloid in 70% of cases and may include any myeloid cell types (neutrophilic, eosinophilic, basophilic, monocytic, erythroid or megakaryocytic) though Auer rods are rarely found. In approximately one-third of cases, however, the appearance is that of ALL (Rosenthal, 1977). Usually these are of precursor B-lineage, with expression of terminal deoxyribonucleotidyl transferase (TdT), CD34, CD19, CD10 but negative surface Ig. Occasional cases are precursor T-lineage with TdT, CD3, cytoplasmic CD3 (cCD3) and CD7. Myeloid antigens are often coexpressed and bilineal myeloid/lymphoid cases are rarely found. Blast transformation appears because of secondary genetic changes involving p53, retinoblastoma (Rb) and other genes (Calabretta, 2004).

Chronic Neutrophilic Leukemia

Chronic neutrophilic leukemia is a rare myeloproliferative disorder characterized by persistent and unexplained neutrophilia of > 25×10^9/L mature granulocytes resembling reactive neutrophilia (Elliot, 2001; Imbert, 2001a). It typically affects older adults, presents with splenomegaly and sometimes hepatomegaly, often with mucocutaneous bleeding, pruritus or gout. There may be a left shift with bands present and toxic granulation. Bone marrow findings are hypercellularity with granulocytic hyperplasia showing a myeloid : erythroid ratio of up to 20 : 1 and predominance of mature neutrophils to myelocytes. Erythroid cellularity and megakaryocytes may be increased, but dysplasia is not present. Cytogenetics are usually (90%) normal, with some cases showing abnormalities including +8, +9, del(20q), and del(11q). Cases with variant Ph'-positive chromosome and neutrophilia are considered CML.

Because there is not a genetic marker for this disease, it is likely that many of these are reactive processes due to occult malignancy or other causes of inflammation. Multiple myeloma has most often been implicated, but other neoplasms may induce marked neutrophilia with or without marrow involvement.

Chronic Eosinophilic Leukemia and Hypereosinophilic Syndrome

Chronic eosinophilic leukemia (CEL) is a clonal proliferation of eosinophils with chronic increase in the blood and often organ damage due to tissue infiltration. The blood contains > 1.5×10^9/L mostly mature eosinophils and often increased but fewer than 20% blasts in the blood or marrow. If blasts are not increased and there is no evidence of monoclonality, the term hypereosinophilic syndrome (HES) is recommended (Fig. 32–8). Causes of reactive eosinophilia must be ruled out.

Some cases of CEL have clonal cytogenetic abnormalities; +8, i(17q) or 8p11 translocations including t(8;13)(p11;q12), t(8;9)(p11;q32-34) and t(6;8)(q27;p11). The 8p11 translocation may also occur in AML, precursor B- or precursor T-ALL. The clinical outcome of CEL and HES is usually indolent with 5-year survival of about 80% (Bain, 2001a).

Polycythemia Vera (PV)

Polycythemia vera is a clonal stem cell proliferation affecting primarily the erythroid series, characterized by excessive proliferation of erythroid and also usually granulocytic and megakaryocytic elements in the marrow (panmyelosis). This is reflected in the blood in an absolute increase in the red cell mass, leukocytosis, and thrombocytosis. Serum and urine erythropoietin are decreased. The production of erythrocytes is autonomous with 'endogenous erythroid colonies' (EEC) growing in vitro without erythropoietin, but it does respond to erythropoietin when the patient has become anemic through blood loss (Pierre, 2001). Pathology may be related to decreased expression of the thrombopoietin receptor, c-Mpl (Kaushansky, 2003) and overexpression of the polycythemia rubra vera-1 messenger RNA (Pahl, 2004). There is initially a proliferative phase and eventually a spent phase with anemia, marrow fibrosis, increased splenomegaly and extramedullary hematopoiesis.

Clinical Features. The disease is slightly more frequent in men than in women. It usually begins in middle age. Affected patients exhibit ruddy cyanosis, and splenomegaly is present in two-thirds. Thrombotic or hemorrhagic phenomena occur in about half of patients, and thrombosis is most common (Chomienne, 2004). Myocardial infarction, cerebral thrombosis, splenic or pulmonary infarcts, and thrombophlebitis account for the most frequent thrombotic episodes; upper gastrointestinal bleeding, often from peptic ulcer, is the most common bleeding problem. Pruritus, especially after bathing, is common.

Laboratory Features

Blood. Erythrocytes exceed $6–12 \times 10^{12}$/L, and the hemoglobin is > 18.5 g/dL (males) or > 16.5 g/dL (females). The mean cell volume (MCV), mean cell hemoglobin (MCH), and mean cell hemoglobin concentration (MCHC) are normal or low. The erythrocytes become hypochromic and microcytic if chronic blood loss has occurred. Macrocytes, polychromatic cells, and normoblasts may be found but are not a prominent feature of the disease. Red cell production is increased. Red cell destruction is normal during the period of erythrocytosis; later in the disease, as splenomegaly develops, the red cell survival diminishes. The total blood volume is increased, primarily because of the increased red cell mass, though the plasma volume may also be elevated to a lesser degree. Blood viscosity is high, and it may be difficult to prepare good blood films. The erythrocyte sedimentation rate (ESR) is reduced.

The platelet count is increased in about two-thirds of patients, often to levels exceeding 1000×10^9/L. In 80% of untreated patients, functional platelet abnormalities are present (Gilbert, 1975) with decreased aggregation in response to ADP and epinephrine. Functional defects may be related to decreased expression of c-Mpl on platelets (Moliterno, 1998), though there is an increase in megakaryocytes (Bock, 2004). There is no consistent abnormality of secondary hemostasis.

Moderate neutrophilic leukocytosis in the range of $10–30 \times 10^9$/L is common. Immature granulocytes are seen in about one-half of cases, and basophils are often absolutely increased. The NAP is markedly elevated in 80% of patients. Serum transcobalamins and serum muramidase are usually elevated.

The arterial oxygen saturation is normal. Hyperuricemia appears in many patients with PV as a result of the increased nucleic acid metabolism, and in some patients, secondary gout or renal uric acid stones occur.

Marrow. The marrow is moderately to markedly hypercellular, with prominent normoblastic erythroid hyperplasia in panmyelosis. Megakaryocytes show increase and clustering of variable small and large megakaryocytes associated with increase of dilated sinuses (Michiels, 1997) and frequently cluster around sinusoids (Pierre, 2001) (Fig. 32–13). Increased reticulin is often present and storage iron is decreased or absent in 95% of cases.

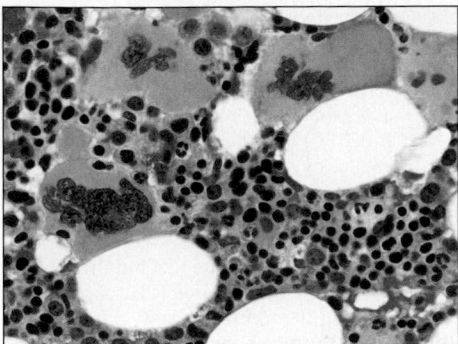

Figure 32–13 Bone marrow biopsy in polycythemia vera shows panmyelosis with normoblastic hyperplasia (× 500).

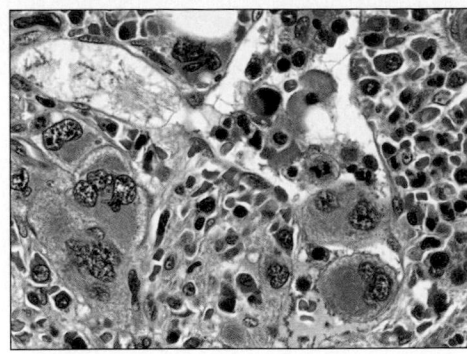

Figure 32–14 Bone marrow biopsy in chronic idiopathic myelofibrosis, with increased spacing between cells suggesting fibrosis and intrasinusoidal hematopoiesis (× 500).

Diagnosis. Criteria of the WHO (Pierre, 2001) for the diagnosis of polycythemia vera are as follows:

1. Elevated RBC mass > 25% above mean normal, or Hb > 18.5 (males) or 16.5 (females) g/dL
2. No cause of secondary erythrocytosis, including familial erythrocytosis, and no elevation of erythropoietin (EPO) due to: hypoxia (arterial P_{O_2} < 92%), high oxygen affinity hemoglobin, truncated EPO receptor or inappropriate EPO production by tumor.

Both of the above must be present as well as any one of splenomegaly, clonal genetic abnormality other than *BCR/ABL*, or endogenous colony formation in vitro; or any two of thrombocytosis (> 400×10^9/L), leukocytosis (> 12×10^9/L), bone marrow biopsy showing panmyelosis with prominent erythroid and megakaryocytic proliferation, or low serum erythropoietin.

Polycythemia vera is a chronic disease; patients usually live 10–20 years under good control. Phlebotomy, chlorambucil, radioactive phosphorus (^{32}P), and hydroxycarbamide (hydroxyurea) have been used to control the manifestations of the disease.

In about 20–40% of patients, the spent or post-polycythemic phase occurs with progressive anemia, gradual splenic enlargement, and further elevation of the leukocyte count, with more immature granulocytes and more circulating nucleated red cells. Many erythrocytes become oval, and teardrop cells (dacrocytes) become prominent. Bone marrow aspiration becomes impossible because of myelofibrosis; and splenomegaly increases, owing to extramedullary hematopoiesis. The manifestations at this stage of the disease are indistinguishable from those of myelofibrosis with myeloid metaplasia. Another late complication of polycythemia vera is acute leukemia or myelodysplastic syndrome (MDS) (Landaw, 1986). There is a slight increase, 2–3%, in patients treated with phlebotomy alone, and greater (10%) in those treated with cytotoxic agents.

Chronic Idiopathic Myelofibrosis (CIM)

There have been many names for this disorder, including myelofibrosis with myeloid metaplasia, agnogenic myeloid metaplasia, primary myelofibrosis, myelosclerosis with myeloid metaplasia, myeloid megakaryocytic hepatosplenomegaly, aleukemic myelosis, essential megakaryocytic granulocytic metaplasia (EMGM), and many others. It is well named but not well understood.

This is a chronic, progressive clonal panmyelosis characterized by megakaryocytic and often granulocytic hyperplasia with varying degrees of reactive fibrosis of the marrow and extramedullary hematopoiesis (Thiele, 2001a). There is typically leukoerythroblastic anemia with marked red cell abnormalities, circulating normoblasts, immature granulocytes, and atypical platelets. CIM is an uncommon disease with an incidence one-third that of CML. It occurs typically in persons over the age of 50 and has an insidious onset, with weight loss, anemia, and abdominal discomfort due to the large spleen. Often the liver is enlarged as well, and the patient may be slightly jaundiced. X-ray shows patchy osteosclerosis in up to half of patients, but osteoporosis may be seen also.

A prefibrotic stage in 20–30% of cases is characterized by mild normocytic anemia with poikilocytosis including dacrocytes, nucleated RBCs, thrombocytosis and mild leukocytosis with some immature forms. The marrow is hypercellular and contains abnormal megakaryocytes, which cluster around sinuses and trabeculae. The histopathology of the bone marrow is dominated by atypical, enlarged and immature megakaryocytes with cloud-like immature nuclei (Michiels, 1999), and also small megakaryocytes. Fibrosis may be minimal initially. Intrasinusoidal hematopoiesis is often present (Fig. 32–14).

Characteristic findings of presentation in fibrotic stage include moderate normochromic, normocytic anemia (often with some hypochromic cells and basophilic stippling), moderate anisocytosis, and marked poikilocytosis including prominent teardrop forms (dacrocytes) and elliptocytes. Normoblasts are often increased out of proportion to the degree of anemia with slight reticulocytosis. The anemia may have a complicated origin, with components of marrow failure, ineffective erythropoiesis, and hemolysis. Splenomegaly due to extramedullary hematopoiesis is typical.

The leukocyte count is moderately increased; immature neutrophils and occasionally myeloblasts are present. Basophils are often increased. Platelets are normal or decreased in number (rarely increased) and often atypical with distinct clear 'zones.' Micromegakaryocytes the size of lymphocytes with both nucleus and cytoplasm or small megakaryoblasts may usually be found if searched for; on rare occasions, they are present in considerable numbers.

In vitro blood cell culture shows increased colonies (CFU-GM) similar to in CML. Serum GM-CSF is high, serum uric acid is frequently increased and cobalamin is normal or elevated.

It is usually impossible to aspirate marrow, and biopsy is necessary. The marrow is fibrotic, with residual islands of atypical megakaryocytes, erythroid, and granulocytic precursors. The fibrosis is of loose connective tissue with scanty collagen, but reticulin fibers are abundant. Foci of osteoid and/or new bone formation in endophytic plaques (Thiele, 2001b) may be found, and bony trabeculae may be irregularly thickened (myelosclerosis). The marrow may show a mixture of hyperplasia and fibrosis in one sample or may vary in different sites of the body. Megakaryocytes with abnormal nuclei cluster or form sheets which may be found in sinuses with other marrow precursors. Extramedullary hematopoiesis is found in the spleen and liver.

Biology. While the proliferating megakaryocytes are neoplastic, the stromal proliferation is reactive due to inappropriate release of megakaryocyte/platelet-derived growth factors, including platelet-derived growth factor (PDGF), transforming growth factor (TGF)-beta, basic fibroblast growth factor (bFGF) and calmodulin (Reilly, 1998).

Chromosomal studies show absence of *BCR/ABL*, but often variable changes also seen in other myeloproliferative and myelodysplastic disorders; +8, +9, del(20q), del(13q) and del(1p). Eighty percent of patients acquire nonspecific chromosomal alterations whose appearance frequently reflects a conversion to AML or CML.

Course. The natural course is increasing fibrosis with progressive anemia and enlargement of the spleen. Hemolysis frequently becomes an increasing element in the anemia and infections may be a serious problem. Portal hypertension occurs in 10–20% of cases and may result in bleeding esophageal varices. Hypertension may be due to portal vein thrombosis or intrahepatic obstruction as a result of myeloid metaplasia coupled with increased portal blood flow.

Androgen preparations, corticosteroids, and erythropoietin are helpful in control of anemia (Tefferi, 2003). The median survival has been about 5 years, considerably less than that of polycythemia vera; however, some patients live longer and in those the terminal event is frequently an acute leukemia. Recent therapeutic advances with durable remission of cytopenias have been reported with thalidomide and prednisone (Mesa, 2004).

Occasionally, patients exhibit cytopenias and marrow fibrosis due to other causes, some of which may show favorable response to specific therapies. These include metastatic tumors, primary hematopoietic tumors such as hairy cell leukemia or plasma cell dyscrasia (Meerkin, 1994), damage from radiation, and rarely autoimmune myelofibrosis

IV

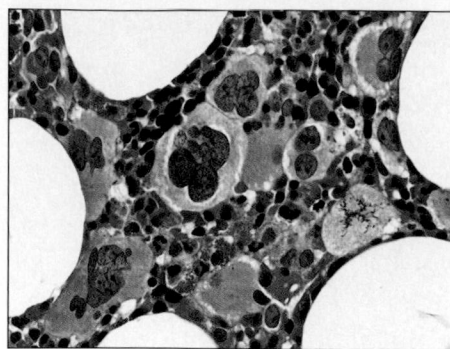

Figure 32–15 Bone marrow biopsy in essential thrombocythemia (ET), with increased and clustered megakaryocytes (× 500).

(Hasselbalch, 1987; Pullarkat, 2003). Malnourished children with vitamin D deficiency (rickets) sometimes show myelofibrosis. A role of solvents in myelofibrosis has been postulated (Brandt, 1987) but is not clear or well documented; neither is it known whether solvent-associated cases are neoplastic or secondary myelofibrosis. Benzene has been most suspected and is a known inducer of AML at threshold levels of exposure. General environmental exposure appears much lower than likely to be associated with hematologic malignancies (Duarte-Davidson, 2001). Peritrabecular marrow fibrosis occurs in primary hyperparathyroidism or secondary hyperparathyroidism of chronic renal failure.

Essential Thrombocythemia (ET)

Thrombocythemia is a clonal myeloproliferative disorder primarily affecting the megakaryocytic lineage with principal manifestation of sustained thrombocytosis. It most often occurs in the fifth decade, with equal sex distribution, with a second peak of incidence in females in their 30s (Imbert, 2001b).

Clinical Features. Patients often (50%) present with asymptomatic thrombocytosis, but up to half of patients present with hemorrhage or thrombosis. The latter occurs as arterial or venous thrombosis or as microvascular occlusion resulting in transient ischemic attacks (TIA) or digital ischemia. Characteristic recurrent, spontaneous mucosal hemorrhages are most common in the GI tract or upper airway. Hemorrhages are occasionally preceded or accompanied by thrombosis. Mild splenomegaly occurs in 50% of cases.

Laboratory features

Blood. The most striking feature is the marked increase in platelets ($> 600 \times 10^9$/L; usually $> 1000 \times 10^9$/L), often with abnormal and giant forms and usually accompanied by fragments of megakaryocytes. Neutrophilic leukocytosis is sometimes present. Hypochromic microcytic anemia due to chronic blood loss is present in many cases. Platelet function defects in thrombocythemia are frequently demonstrable. The most typical finding is decreased aggregation in response to epinephrine.

Marrow. The marrow shows increased and enlarged megakaryocytes with mature cytoplasm and multilobulated nuclei and a tendency to cluster in a normal or only slightly hypercellular bone marrow (Michiels, 1999) (Fig. 32–15). Megakaryocyte nuclei are not described as atypical but often are distinctive and resemble other MPDs. Erythroid proliferation may be present secondary to blood loss. Biopsy features may be indistinguishable from those of PV, but usually with less erythroid prominence. Splenic extramedullary hematopoiesis may be present.

Cultured marrow typically shows in vitro spontaneous colony formation of megakaryocytes and also erythroid colonies (Niittyvuopio, 2004). Abnormal (decreased) labeling of bone marrow for the thrombopoietin (TPO) receptor c-Mpl may aid in separating ET from reactive thrombocytosis (Gale, 2003).

Diagnosis. Criteria of the WHO for the diagnosis of thrombocythemia are as follows (Imbert, 2001b):

1. Sustained platelet count $> 600 \times 10^9$/L
2. Bone marrow biopsy showing proliferation of mainly megakaryocytes with enlarged mature nuclei.

The following must be excluded:

- Hemoglobin less than 18.5 (males) and 16.5 (females) g/dL or normal red cell mass.
- Stainable iron in marrow, normal ferritin, or normal MCV.
- No evidence of CML; no Philadelphia chromosome or *BCR/ABL*.
- No evidence of myelofibrosis; collagen fibrosis of marrow absent and minimal or absent reticulin fibrosis.
- No known cause for reactive thrombocytosis; neoplasm, inflammation or infection, or history of splenectomy.

Genetics. There is no known specific genetic abnormality. *BCR/ABL* translocations must be ruled out to exclude CML. Ph'-positive thrombocytosis is likely an early form of CML, and differs morphologically by lack of the characteristic large clustered megakaryocytes (Michiels, 2004). Occasional cases (5–10%) show del(13q22), +8 or +9 (Imbert, 2001b). Other abnormalities such as del(5q) or abnormalities of 3q21q26.2 suggest MDS with thrombocytosis.

Most cases are stable for many years, but a small proportion may merge into other chronic myeloproliferative disorders or, rarely, develop into acute leukemia. Historically, alkylating agents and radiophosphorus have been used to treat essential thrombocythemia, but these were complicated by secondary leukemias. Hydroxycarbamide (hydroxyurea) has been more recently used, but it too has leukemogenic potential. Anagrelide is currently in use and is considered more safe and reliable (Silverstein, 1999). Development of erythrocytosis with increased red cell mass raises the possibility of polycythemia vera, and there is some crossover between the two entities. Endogenous erythroid colony (EEC) formation may provide early identification of cases at risk for PV (Griesshammer, 2004). Fibrosis rarely occurs.

Chronic Myeloproliferative Disease, Unclassifiable (CMPD, U)

These are disorders with features of MPD but which do not meet criteria for a specific entity or have intermediate features (Thiele, 2001b). Examples of CMPD, U include pre-fibrotic CIM, pre-polycythemic PV and post-polycythemic PV (without prior diagnosis), and cases with features of MPD but presenting with some dysplasia or increased blasts. *BCR/ABL* and other specific cytogenetic abnormalities are absent. This category overlaps with myelodysplastic/myeloproliferative disease, unclassifiable. Often, with follow-up, characteristic findings develop which allow definite diagnosis (Bain, 2001b).

Myelodysplastic and Myelodysplastic/Myeloproliferative Diseases

Myeloproliferative diseases are, in general, disorders in which proliferation of hematopoietic cells outpaces apoptosis, and cellular elements in the blood are increased while the morphology of hematopoiesis is near normal. Myelodysplastic diseases or syndromes (MDS) are disorders in which apoptosis predominates, there is ineffective hematopoiesis and cytopenias occur (Greenberg, 1998; List, 2004). The myelodysplastic/myeloproliferative disorders show features of both, with variable increases in cells as well as cytopenias and morphologic dysplasia (Vardiman, 2001c). These include chronic myelomonocytic leukemia (CMML), atypical CML (aCML), juvenile chronic myelomonocytic leukemia (JCMML), and unclassifiable forms. CMML and JMML are included in Table 32–12.

MDS occur primarily in persons over age 50 and usually present as an anemia refractory to hematinics, with or without neutropenia and thrombocytopenia. Liver, spleen, or lymph nodes are not usually enlarged. The marrow is hypercellular with abnormal maturation in one or more of the three hematopoietic cell lines, and blast cells are often increased. This group of disorders has also been called dysmyelopoietic syndromes or 'preleukemias' because of the high proportion of cases that ultimately progress to overt acute leukemia. The FAB Cooperative Group (Bennett, 1976, 1982) described and classified these disorders, and their nomenclature remains useful with certain modification, per the WHO classification (Brunning, 2001a). A scoring system for predicting survival and risk of acute leukemic transformation has been developed based on percentage of blasts, cytogenetics, and extent of cytopenias (Greenberg, 1997). In general, blast count greater than 5% elevates risk, > 10% increases risk more; complex chromosomal abnormalities or chromosome 7 abnormalities are high risk; del(5q), isolated del(2q), -Y and normal cytogenetics are low risk; other cytogenetic findings are intermediate risk; and more than one cytopenia increases risk.

Types of Abnormal Cellular Maturation

Dyserythropoiesis resembles megaloblastic change and includes nuclear fragmentation or karyorrhexis, multinuclearity, nuclear budding or bridging, basophilic stippling, and ring sideroblasts (Bennett, 1986). These features may also be seen in toxicity due to drugs, chemotherapy, heavy metals, alcohol and other toxins (Brunning, 2001a) (Figs 32–16 and 32–17). Erythroid cells may be decreased or increased in number. Erythrocytic abnormalities in the blood film include presence of oval macrocytes, anisochromasia, basophilic stippling, dacrocytes, and reticulocytopenia.

Dysgranulopoiesis includes nuclear/cytoplasmic asynchrony, hypogranulation, nuclear hyposegmentation with increased chromatin conden-

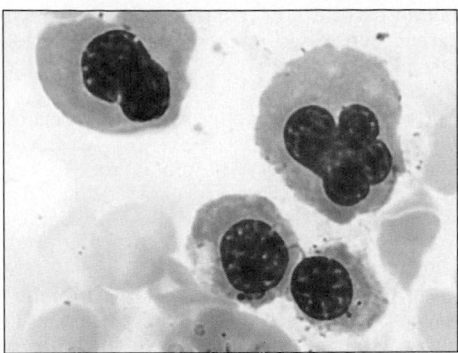

Figure 32–16 Drug-induced dyserythropoiesis, with irregular nuclear lobation in the cells above right, compared to two relatively normal normoblasts (× 1000).

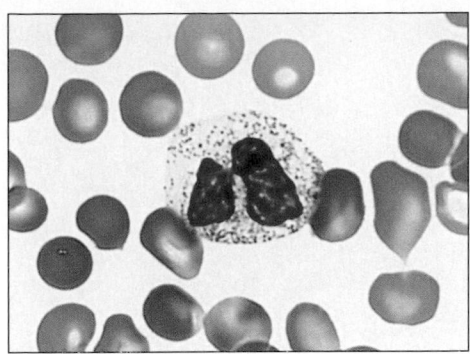

Figure 32–18 Pseudo Pelger–Huët neutrophil (× 1000).

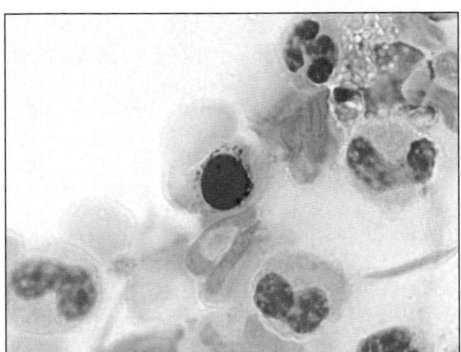

Figure 32–17 A ring sideroblast is present in the center of the field (× 1000).

Myelodysplastic/Myeloproliferative Diseases (see Table 32–12)

Chronic Myelomonocytic Leukemia. CMML is a clonal stem cell disorder in which the predominant feature is persistent monocytosis ($> 1 \times 10^9$/L for more than 3 months) for which other causes have been excluded (Vardiman, 2001d). Typically, cytopenias are present in the blood (anemia, thrombocytopenia, and/or neutropenia) but neutrophilia with morphologic abnormalities also occurs. There is absence of a Philadelphia chromosome or *BCR/ABL*, dysplasia of one or more myeloid lineage, and fewer than 20% blasts plus promonocytes in the marrow (Fig. 32–21). The marrow also shows monocytosis and often has increased promonocytes, which may be distinguished from abnormal myelocytes by nonspecific esterase (alpha naphthyl acetate or alpha naphthyl butyrate esterase) staining or strong labeling with antilysozyme or CD68. Eosinophilia or basophilia may be present, and there are frequently plasmacytoid-appearing monocytes. When eosinophils exceed 1.5×10^9/L, the WHO recommends the subcategory of CMML with eosinophilia.

In CMML and also in the acute myeloid leukemias with monocytic differentiation, promonocytes are considered equivalent to blasts and are included with them to determine the blast percentage. Promonocytes are monocytic precursors which have recognizable monocyte morphology but with immature chromatin and finely convoluted or cerebriform nuclei (Fig. 32–22). Blast percentages typically are < 5% in the blood and < 10% in the marrow, and such cases are referred to as CMML-1. The subcategory CMML-2 refers to cases with 5–19% blasts in the blood, 10–19% in the marrow or when Auer rods are present. This indicates aggressive disease with likely impending transformation to acute leukemia.

sation, occasionally abnormal large azurophilic granules, inappropriately prominent nucleoli or other abnormalities. Neutrophil precursors and monocytes often resemble one another. Neutrophils with mature chromatin but decreased granulation and bilobed or unilobed nuclei resemble the cells of Pelger–Huët anomaly and are termed 'pseudo Pelger–Huët' cells (Figs 32–18 and 32–19).

Dysmegakaryocytopoiesis includes large megakaryocytes with unsegmented nuclei, micromegakaryocytes, and megakaryocytes with two or more small, unconnected nuclei (Fig. 32–20). Megakaryocytes may be decreased in number. In the blood film, giant hypogranular platelets are frequent and micromegakaryocytes are seen rarely.

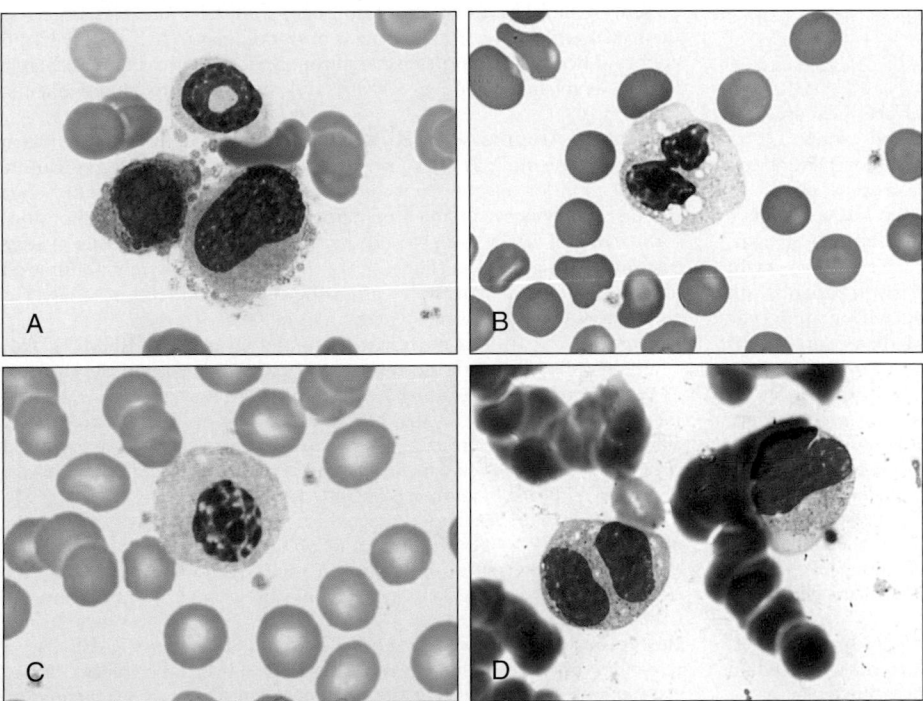

Figure 32–19 Other forms of neutrophil dysplasia.
A, Ring neutrophil along with dysplastic erythroid and megakaryocytic cells in the marrow (× 1000).
B, Pelger–Huët neutrophil resembling a monocyte (× 1000). *C*, Mononuclear Pelger–Huët cell (× 1000).
D, Large irregularly lobated and granulated neutrophil precursors (× 1000).

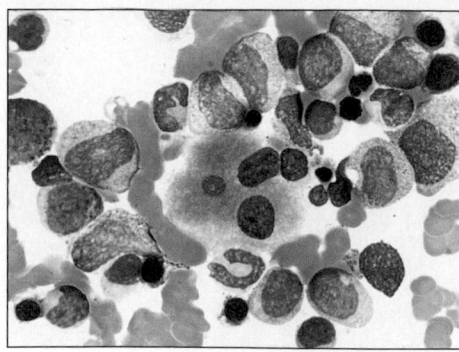

Figure 32–20 A dysplastic megakaryocyte showing unconnected nuclear lobes. Mononuclear forms are also frequent in myelodysplasia (× 500).

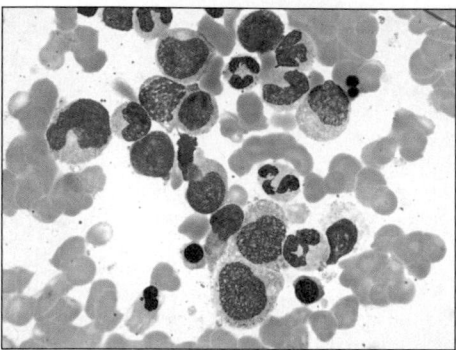

Figure 32–21 This case of chronic myelomonocytic leukemia (CMML) shows moderate trilineage dysplasia and monocytosis (× 500).

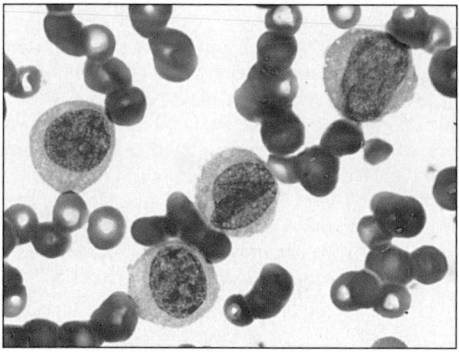

Figure 32–22 Promonocyte (center) shows immature chromatin and finely convoluted nuclear folds in comparison to monoblasts.

The immunophenotype is CD13/CD33+; variable CD14/CD68/CD64/CD4-positive. Plasmacytoid monocytes may be seen and express CD14, CD43, CD56, CD68 and CD4, with variable CD2/CD5. Cytogenetic abnormalities in 20–40% of cases include +8, −7/del, and abnormalities of 12p.

CMML occurs most often at older age (median 65–75 years) with a male predominance. Symptoms are usually those related to cytopenias (fatigue, infection or bleeding) or hypermetabolic state (fever, weight loss, night sweats). Hepatosplenomegaly may be present particularly in patients with elevated WBC. Lymphadenopathy may be associated with granulocytic sarcoma and evolution to acute leukemia. Median survival is 20–30 months with progression to AML in 15–30%.

Atypical Chronic Myeloid Leukemia (aCML). This disease shows myelodysplastic and myeloproliferative features, a predominant component of increased neutrophils and precursors with dysplastic features, and dysplasia of other cell lines (Vardiman, 2001e). Ph' chromosome or BCR/ABL is absent. These cases have previously been considered along with CML or CMML, but are Ph' chromosome and BCR/ABL negative and, while monocytosis is often present, it is less prominent than neutrophilia. The marrow is hypercellular with variable features of each lineage. A variant, 'syndrome of abnormal chromatin clumping,' shows exaggerated chromatin condensation as well as other dysplastic features.

Cytogenetics show +8, +13, del(20q), i(17q) or del(12p) in up to 80%. aCML occurs in later years and has a generally poor outcome with median survival of 20 months and a 25–40% transformation to acute leukemia.

Criteria for diagnosis of aCML (Vardiman, 2001e):
- Leukocytosis due to increased mature and immature neutrophils.
- Prominent dysgranulopoiesis.
- No Ph' chromosome or BCR/ABL.
- Neutrophil precursors (promyelocytes, myelocytes, metamyelocytes) > 10% of WBCs.
- No or minimal absolute monocytosis; monocytes < 10% of WBCs.
- Hypercellular marrow with granulocytic proliferation and granulocytic dysplasia, with or without dysplasia of erythroid and/or megakaryocytic lineages.
- Fewer than 20% blasts in blood or marrow.

Juvenile Myelomonocytic Leukemia (JMML). This is a clonal disorder of predominantly granulocytic and monocytic lineages, with dysplasia in these and frequently other lineages, occurring in children or young adolescents (Luna-Fineman, 1999; Vardiman, 2001e). It has been previously referred to as Ph'-negative CML, CMML or monosomy 7 syndrome (in some cases). The occurrence is 1.3 cases per million children under 14 years, and most cases are less than 3 years of age, with a 2 : 1 male predominance. The prognosis is poor and death is usually due to organ failure from leukemic infiltrates, though some patients benefit from bone marrow transplant.

Criteria for diagnosis of JMML (Vardiman, 2001f):
- Peripheral blood monocytosis > 1×10^9/L.
- Absence of Ph' chromosome or BCR/ABL.
- Plus two of the following:
  – Hemoglobin F increased for age
  – Immature granulocytes in the blood
  – WBC > 10×10^9/L
  – Clonal chromosomal abnormality (including monosomy 7)
  – GM-CSF hypersensitivity of myeloid progenitors in vitro.

Myelodysplastic/Myeloproliferative Disease, Unclassifiable

This category of the WHO classification is used for those cases with features of myelodysplastic disease but with the addition of prominent myeloproliferative features including thrombocytosis > 600×10^9/L with megakaryocytic hyperplasia or WBC > 13×10^9/L, with or without splenomegaly, no previous CMPD or MDS and absence of a chromosomal abnormality specific to another disease (BCR/ABL, del(5q), t(3;3)(q21;q26), inv(3)(q21;q26) (Bain, 2001b). A provisional entity of refractory anemia with ringed sideroblasts (RARS) associated with marked thrombocytosis is included in this category.

Myelodysplastic Syndromes (Brunning, 2001b,c,d,e,f,g) (Table 32–13)

Refractory Anemia (RA). This clonal disorder involves primarily the erythroid lineage with ineffective erythropoiesis but without increased blasts. Anemia with reticulocytopenia and abnormal erythrocytes are the presenting findings. Abnormal granulocytes are rare, and blasts are less than 1% in the blood. The marrow is normocellular to hypercellular with erythroid hyperplasia and/or dyserythropoiesis and fewer than 5% blasts. Survival is relatively good (> 5 years) and progression to acute leukemia (AL) low (6%).

Refractory Anemia with Ring Sideroblasts (RARS). In RARS, in addition to the findings of RA, ring sideroblasts are present and constitute 15% or more of marrow erythroid precursors. These are nucleated RBC precursors in which stainable iron particles (iron-encrusted mitochondria) form a ring of 10 or more closely associated with and encircling at least one-third of the nucleus (Fig. 32–17). Defective cytoplasmic maturation and anisochromic erythrocytes are associated abnormalities. Survival is similar to RA, with a lower progression to AL (< 2%).

Refractory Cytopenia with Multilineage Dysplasia (RCMD). This is a clonal disorder with bicytopenias or pancytopenia and dysplasia of 10% or more of the precursors of two or more lineages. Blasts are not increased, with < 1% in the blood and < 5% in the marrow. Ring sideroblasts may be present, but when they exceed 15% of erythroid precursors, the case is classified as Refractory Cytopenia with Multilineage Dysplasia and Ring Sideroblasts (RCMD-RS).

In contrast with RA and RARS, which infrequently show cytogenetic abnormalities (< 10%), RCMD and RCMD-RS show them in up to 50%. These include trisomy 8, monosomy 7, del(7q), monosomy 5, del(5q), del(20q) and complex karyotypes. Survival is ~33 months, and AL conversion 11%.

Refractory Anemia with Excess Blasts (RAEB-1 and RAEB-2). In refractory anemia with excess blasts-1 (RAEB-1), the blood shows cytopenia in two or three of the cell lines, and less than 5% circulating

Table 32–13 Key Features of the Major Myelodysplastic Syndromes

Disorder	Demographics	Laboratory features, morphology	Cytogenetics	Prognosis
Refractory anemia (RA)	Over age 50	PB with anemia, reticulocytopenia, blasts < 1%. BM with erythroid hyperplasia and/or dyspoiesis, < 5% blasts.	Rare abnormalities	Good, > 5 years; 6% progress to AML
Refractory anemia with ringed sideroblasts (RARS)	Over age 50	Similar to RA, ≥ 15% ringed sideroblasts in BM	Rare abnormalities	Good, > 5 years, with ≤ 2% to AML
Refractory cytopenia with multilineage dysplasia (RCMD)	Over age 50	PB with cytopenias of ≥ 2 cell lines, < 1% blasts, < 1 × 10⁹/L monocytes. BM with dysplasia of ≥ 10% of precursors of ≥ 2 cell lines, < 5% blasts.	+8, −7, del(7q), −5, others in up to 50%	33 months, 11% to AML
Refractory anemia with excess blasts (RAEB)	Over age 50	RAEB-1: PB with cytopenias of ≥ 2 cell lines, < 5% blasts, < 1 × 10⁹/L monocytes. BM with hypercellularity, dyspoiesis, 5–9% blasts without Auer rods	+8, −5, del(5q), −7, del(7q), del(20q)	RAEB-1: < 2 years with 25% to AML
		RAEB-2: Similar to RAEB-1, but also PB with > 5% blasts, or 10–19% BM blasts, or Auer rods		RAEB-2: < 2 years with 33% to AML
5q- Syndrome	Middle-aged–older females	PB with thrombocytosis, < 5% blasts. BM with increased, hypolobated megakaryocytes, < 5% blasts	5q- is sole abnormality	Good

PB = peripheral blood; BM = bone marrow.

blasts. The marrow is hypercellular, with variable erythroid or granulocytic hyperplasia. Dyspoietic changes are present in all three cell lines, and 5–9% of the marrow cells are blasts. Less than 5% blasts are present in the blood and no Auer rods are found. Clusters of 5–8 blasts and promyelocytes in the marrow interstitium are frequently seen on sections and are referred to as abnormal localization of immature precursors (ALIP). These should be noted on pathology reports as they may indicate more aggressive disease. Hypocellular marrow is seen in a minority of cases (10–15%). These may be difficult to interpret, as the patients are often older, with decreased cellularity to begin with, and because marrow stress in hypoplastic anemia often causes some dysplasia. A diagnosis of MDS should be made cautiously when the marrow is hypoplastic.

RAEB-2 has findings similar to those of RAEB-1, but with any of the following: (1) greater than 5% blasts in the blood, (2) 10–19% blasts in the marrow, or (3) the presence of Auer rods. Cytogenetic abnormalities include +8, −5, del(5q), −7, del(7q) and del(20q). Survival is usually less than 2 years in RAEB-1 or -2 with either progressive marrow failure and cytopenias or progression to AL in 25% for RAEB-1 and 33% for RAEB-2.

Myelodysplastic Syndrome, Unclassified

The myelodysplastic syndrome unclassified category is used when the clinical and hematologic findings of myelodysplasia exist, but without specific features to allow placement in one of the other categories. Patients usually have neutropenia or thrombocytopenia with a hypercellular bone marrow and dysplasia of granulocytic or megakaryocytic lineage. There are less than 5% blasts in the bone marrow and they are not increased in the blood.

Myelodysplastic Syndrome Associated with Isolated Del(5q) Abnormality; 5q- Syndrome

This clonal abnormality has features similar to RA, but with increased megakaryocytes in the marrow, usually including hypolobated forms, and peripheral thrombocytosis. Blasts are less than 5% in the marrow and blood; lymphoid aggregates are often present. The sole cytogenetic abnormality is del(5q) between bands 5q31 and 5q33. It usually occurs in middle age or older women and carries a favorable prognosis.

Acute Myeloid Leukemias

Acute myeloid leukemia (AML) is the most common form of acute leukemia (AL) during the first few months of life, but during childhood and adolescence constitutes approximately one-third of AL. In the middle and later years of life it becomes the most frequent AL, with a median age of 60, and an occurrence of 10/100 000 per year in those over 60 years. Viruses, radiation, cytotoxic chemotherapy, benzene and smoking have been linked to increased incidence, but most cases are not known to be associated with such factors.

Table 32–14 Clinical and Laboratory Features of AML

Affects all ages, but increases with older age (> 60 years)
May resemble acute infection at presentation
Requires 20% blasts in blood or marrow for diagnosis
Key myeloid antigens are myeloperoxidase, CD13, CD33, CD117
Recurrent cytogenetic abnormalities characterize certain subtypes
Classification made by morphology, cytogenetics, cytochemistry, flow cytometry

The onset often resembles acute infection and includes signs of granulocytic insufficiency, with ulcerations of mucous membranes (especially of the mouth and throat) and fever. Enlargement of lymph nodes, spleen, and liver is not pronounced. Marked prostration and general malaise may be present. In untreated cases, the course is rapidly progressive.

AML classification currently utilizes a multilayered approach which recognizes recurrent acquired cytogenetic abnormalities associated with specific types, history of predisposing factors (prior cytotoxic therapy), association with MDS or related abnormalities, and a morphologic stratification for those for which none of these can be appreciated. This approach requires, or at least encourages, attempts to define the morphology, cytogenetics and immunophenotype of each case. With advances in molecular cytogenetics and fluorescence in-situ hybridization, and widespread adoption of these and other techniques, it is likely that most cases will eventually be categorized by their genetic abnormalities. Knowledge of these changes is particularly important because therapies may be targeted to the biochemical pathways or even nucleic acid perturbations involved (Gilliland, 2004).

The French–American–British (FAB) Cooperative Group published proposals in 1976 for the classification of acute leukemias (Bennett, 1976) and subsequent revised criteria for the classification of ALL (Bennett, 1981) and AML (Bennett, 1985a,b) based on morphology of cells in Romanowsky-stained blood and marrow films and certain supplemental cytochemical reactions or serum lysozyme levels (see Tables 32–14 and 32–15). These criteria have been superseded by the current WHO classification (Brunning, 2001h), but basic morphologic tenets remain and FAB criteria are the basis for subtyping AML, not otherwise classified.

The diagnosis of AML requires the presence of 20% blasts in the marrow or blood. Myeloblasts generally have central nuclei with fine, uncondensed chromatin and often prominent nucleoli (usually three to five) but have variable cytoplasm and may have some cytoplasmic granules. Primitive myeloblasts are identified by monoclonal antibodies against myeloid-associated antigens (MPO, CD13, CD33, CD117). More mature myeloblasts can also be identified by cytochemical reactions with

Table 32–15 Key Features of the Major Acute Myeloid Leukemias (AML)

Category	Cell morphology	Cell surface markers	Cytogenetics	Prognosis
AML with t(8;21)	Large blasts, with abundant basophilic cytoplasm, Auer rods, dysplasia, abnormal granules, maturing granulocytes	CD 13, 33,117, CD19, CD34	t(8;21)(q22;q22) *AML1/ETO*	More favorable than AML without recurrent genetic abnormality
AML with inv(16)	Blasts with both monocytic and neutrophilic differentiation, increased eosinophils/immature eosinophils	CD 13, 33, 14, 4, 64	inv(16)(p13;q22) or t(16;16)(p13;q22)	Superior to other AML
Acute promyelocytic leukemia	Promyelocytes with azurophilic granules, Auer rods	CD 13, 33 CD2±, DR–	t(15;17)(q22;q12) *PML/RARα* Variants all involve 17q12	Good if responsive to ATRA
AML with 11q23	Variable. Monocytic differentiation seen in t(9;11)	CD 13, 33, 34, ± 56, 57. CD 14, 4, 36 with monocytic differentiation	t(9;11)(p22;q23), others	Less favorable than other AML
AML, therapy related	Multilineage dysplasia, RS, increased basophils	CD 13, 33, 34, ± 56, 57	11q23 abnormality seen with topoisomerase II inhibitor-associated AML	Median survival < 3 years
AML, not otherwise categorized				
AML, minimally differentiated	M0 in FAB. Myeloblasts, < 3% positive for SBB, MPO or ANA	CD 13, 33, 117 in ≥ 20% of blasts	Nonspecific/not available	Poor
AML without maturation	M1 in FAB. Myeloblasts ≥ 90% of nonerythroids in BM, ≥ 3% positive for SBB or MPO	CD 13, 33, 117	Nonspecific/not available	Poor
AML with maturation	M2 in FAB. Same as for AML with t(8;21)	CD 13, 33, 117	Nonspecific/not available	Variable. Less favorable than AML with t(8;21)
Acute myelomonocytic leukemia	M4 in FAB. Monocytic cells 20–79%, granulocytic 30–80% of nonerythroids	CD 13, 33, 14, 4, 11b, 11c, 64, 36, 68	Nonspecific/not available	Variable. Less favorable than AML with inv(16)
Acute monoblastic/ monocytic	M5 in FAB. ≥ 80% of nonerythroids are monoblasts (M5a) or show monocytic diff (M5b)	CD 13, 33, 117, 14, 4, 11b, 11c, 64, 68, 36	t(8;16)(p1l; p13) seen in some acute monocytic leukemia cases Nonspecific/not available	Poor
Erythroleukemia	M6 in FAB. ≥ 50% erythroblasts and ≥ 20% myeloblasts in nonerythroids. Pure erythroleukemia without myeloid blasts is rare	Glycophorin A, Hb A in erythroid blasts; CD 13, 33, 117 in myeloblasts	Nonspecific	Poor
Acute megakaryoblastic leukemia	Polymorphic megakaryoblasts, may simulate lymphoblasts. PB may show megakaryocytic fragments	CD 41, 61, 36, often CD 13, 33	Nonspecific in adults. Infants may show t(1;22)(p13;q13)	Poor, especially with t(1;22)

ATRA = all-*trans* retinoic acid; PB = peripheral blood.

granulocyte-associated enzymes using myeloperoxidase (MPO), Sudan black B (SBB), and ASD-chloroacetate esterase (CAE) assays, though flow cytometric assays are gradually replacing these. Monoblasts are frequently large with abundant cytoplasm, diffuse chromatin and often prominent nucleoli. Monoblasts are characterized by strong reaction with alpha-naphthyl acetate esterase (ANA), which is inhibited in monocytes by sodium fluoride as well as by alpha-naphthyl butyrate esterase (ANB), or antibodies including antilysozyme, CD68, CD64 and CD36. For cases with monocytic differentiation, promonocytes are considered equivalent to blasts (Fig. 32–22). Promonocytes are immature recognizable monocytes with some chromatin condensation but with fine nuclear convolutions. Abnormal promyelocytes are also considered blast equivalents for the diagnosis of acute promyelocytic leukemia. Megakaryoblasts are identified by antibodies against platelet-associated antigens or electron microscopy for platelet peroxidase.

Initial assessment for suspected AML is based on a 500-cell count of the marrow aspirate. First, it is necessary to calculate the percentage of erythroid precursor cells. The diagnosis of AML-erythroleukemia is established when more than 50% of the bone marrow cells are erythroid precursors and when myeloblasts represent more than 20% of the remaining nonerythroid (NE) cells, i.e. nucleated cells not including erythroid precursors, lymphocytes, or plasma cells. The diagnosis of myelodysplastic syndrome is suggested when less than 20% of the nonerythroid cells are myeloblasts, and dysplastic alterations are present. Once the diagnosis of AML has been made, only nonerythroid cells should be considered in the differential count for the further assignment of the subtypes.

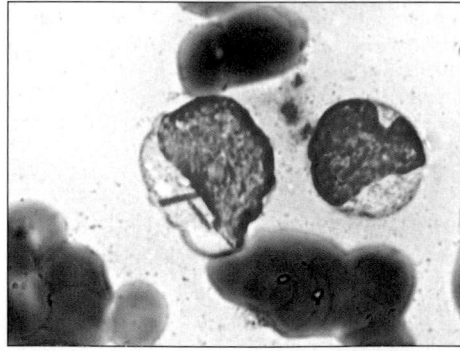

Figure 32–23 Auer rods vary from prominent, as in this cell, to thin and delicate.

A helpful finding in the diagnosis of AML is the presence of Auer rods, eosinophilic rod-like cytoplasmic inclusions derived from myeloperoxidase-positive primary granules. Phi bodies, which appear as strings of eosinophilic bead-like granules, are derived from catalase-positive microperoxisomes and are seen in larger numbers in AML and also MDS (Cardullo, 1981). They are not, however, generally given the same diagnostic import as Auer rods. With Romanowsky stains, Auer rods are linear or spindle-shaped, red-purple inclusions in myeloblasts or promyelocytes (Fig. 32–23). Less commonly, they may be seen in more

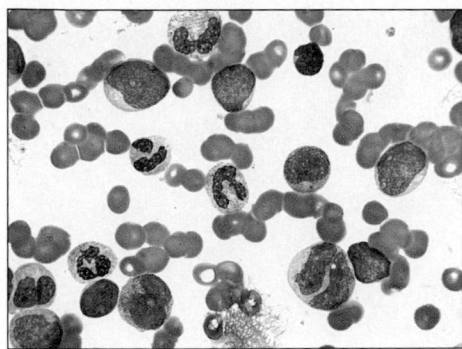

Figure 32–24 This case of AML with t(8;21) shows granulocyte maturation with abnormal granulation and bilobed precursors (×500).

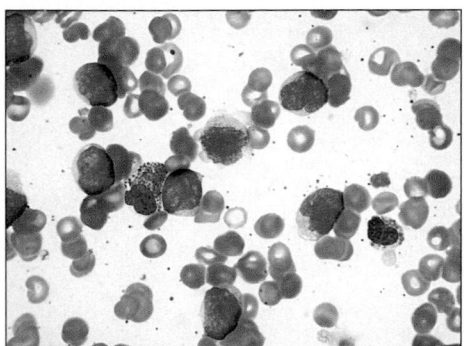

Figure 32–25 AML with inv16 shows myelomonocytic differentiation with eosinophilia. (Two eosinophils are present in this view.)

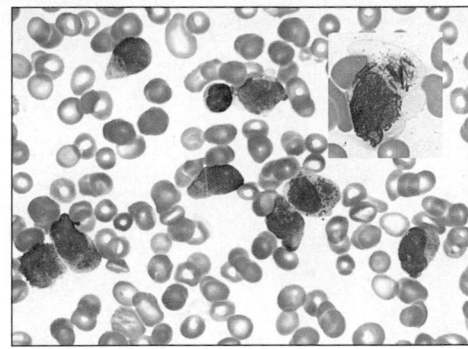

Figure 32–26 Acute promyelocytic leukemia with t(15;17) shows predominantly abnormal promyelocytes (×500). Inset: Abnormal promyelocytes with bundles of Auer rods are known as 'faggot cells' from their resemblance to bundles of firewood, or faggots (×1000).

mature neutrophils (in AML with t(8;21)). Auer rods are derivatives of azurophilic granules and stain positively for SBB, MPO, CAE, and acid phosphatase. Auer rods can be found in any of the subtypes of AML, but they are especially associated with those with granulocytic differentiation.

The main categories of AML in the WHO Classification are (1) AML with recurrent cytogenetic abnormalities; (2) AML with multilineage dysplasia; (3) AML, therapy related; and (4) AML, not otherwise categorized (subclassified by morphology and immunophenotype).

Acute Leukemia with Recurrent Genetic Abnormalities

AML with t(8;21)(q22;q22), AML1/ETO (Brunning, 2001i). The morphology usually corresponds to acute myeloid leukemia with neutrophilic maturation and these represent 5–12% of AML with predominance in young patients. Blasts are 20% or more in the marrow (or blood) and maturing neutrophilic precursors constitute more than 10% of marrow nucleated cells (not including nucleated red blood cells [NRBCs], lymphocytes and plasma cells). There are characteristic but variable morphologic findings: large blasts with abundant basophilic cytoplasm; maturing neutrophil precursors with peripheral cytoplasmic basophilia; frequent Auer rods, often long, sharp and tapered and sometimes present in myelocytes and mature forms up to segmented neutrophils; abnormal granulation including giant Chédiak–Higashi-like or secondary granules or homogeneous waxy-appearing secondary granulation; and nuclear dysplasia with bilobed nuclei which may be widely separated (Fig. 32–24). Monocytosis is not prominent and monocytes are less than 20% of the marrow. The immunophenotype is distinctive with frequent variable coexpression of CD19 and CD34 along with myeloid markers, and sometimes CD56.

Occasional cases of AML with t(8;21) show monocytic differentiation, only slight neutrophilic differentiation, less than 20% blasts or present with granulocytic sarcoma. The outcome of AML with t(8;21) is generally more favorable than from AML without recurrent genetic abnormalities or with MDS-associated abnormalities.

AML with inv(16)(p13q22) or t(16;16)(p13;q22), CBFβ/MYH11. These correspond to acute myelomonocytic leukemia with abnormal eosinophils (Bitter, 1984). The occurrence and outcome are similar to AML with t(8;21). These cases show > 20% blasts in marrow and/or blood with differentiation to both monocytic and neutrophilic lineages (> 20% each). There are characteristically increased eosinophils (Fig. 32–25) including those with large basophilic granules (as in eosinophil promyelocytes) and often weak cytoplasmic positivity for chloroacetate esterase. This type is associated with the chromosomal abnormality inv(16)(p13q22) or its variant t(16;16)(p13;q22) with fusion of the CBFB gene on 16q and MYH11 on 16p and variable resultant chimeric mRNAs (because of differing breakpoints) and a BCGB-MYH11 fusion protein. The prognosis is superior to other AML and either reverse transcriptase polymerase chain reaction (RT-PCR) or FISH are useful for diagnosis, particularly when the eosinophils are few or not apparent.

The immunophenotype typically shows both granulocytic (CD13, CD33, MPO) and monocytic (CD14, CD4, CD64, CD36, CD11, CD11b and lysozyme) markers, sometimes with CD2 coexpression.

Acute Promyelocytic Leukemia (APL) with t(15;17)(q22;q12), PML/RARA and Variants. Promyelocytes instead of myeloblasts predominate in the marrow in hypergranular promyelocytic leukemia (M3) (McKenna, 1982) (Fig. 32–26). Azurophilic granules are abundant and intensely stained. Auer rods are found in almost all cases, and frequently are multiple (10 or more) in a given cell (Fig. 32–26). Hemorrhagic complications are frequent due to disseminated intravascular coagulation (DIC) apparently initiated by procoagulant material from leukemic cell granules.

The characteristic chromosomal abnormality t(15;17)(q22;q21) shows fusion of the retinoid acid receptor gene-alpha (RARA) on chromosome 17 with the PML gene on chromosome 15. The RARA–PML fusion gene is transcribed as a chimeric mRNA. The leukemia usually responds to therapy with all-trans retinoic acid (ATRA), which is usually given in addition to chemotherapy, and the prognosis is better than for other AML. The molecular genetic abnormality may be detected in the laboratory by cytogenetics, RT-PCR or FISH. Achievement of remission often occurs as a slow 'maturation' process rather than therapy-induced aplasia followed by remission seen in treatment of other acute leukemias.

Variant translocations include t(11;17)(q23;q21), t(5;17)(q32;q12), and t(11;17)(q13;q21). Some variants, such as t(11;17)(q23;q21), do not respond to ATRA.

Hypogranular or microgranular variants of M3 (M3V) occur in which cytoplasmic granules appear sparse with light microscopy and numerous, but smaller, by electron microscopy (Golomb, 1980; Bennett, 1980). Nuclei of most leukemic cells are bilobed or reniform, and confusion with an atypical monocytic leukemia is frequent. The cytochemical staining reactions are somewhat less positive than in the hypergranular M3. Auer rods, single or multiple, and typical hypergranular promyelocytes are found in variable numbers, and there appears to be a spectrum between typical and hypogranular types. The WBC may be high.

In APL the majority of leukemic cells stain for MPO, SBB, and CAE. In approximately 25% of the cases, more than 20% of the leukemic cells stain strongly and diffusely for ANA; however, these leukemic cells do not exhibit any immunophenotypic characteristics of monocytes. Clinically, these cases behave similarly to other cases of acute promyelocytic leukemia.

AML with 11q23 (MLL) Abnormalities. The 11q23 abnormalities are present in a more diverse group of leukemias than are other recurrent genetic abnormalities. Chromosome band 11q23 abnormalities, which involve the MLL gene, are not specific for AML, but are also found in ALL, mixed lineage leukemias, and occasionally in lymphomas. The most common translocation in AML involving this region is t(9;11)(p22;q23). Others include t(6;11)(q27;q23), t(10;11)(p12;q23), t(11;17)(q23;q21), and t(11;19)(q23;p13) (Caligiuri, 1997). Most cases of t(9;11) show monocytic differentiation (monoblastic or myelomonocytic) (Fig. 32–27). In general, the prognosis of AML with 11q23 abnormalities is less favorable than for other AML with standard chemotherapy, but there is evidence that

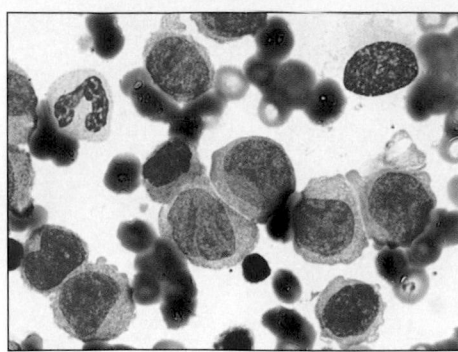

Figure 32–27 AML with monocytic differentiation and 11q23 abnormality (× 1000).

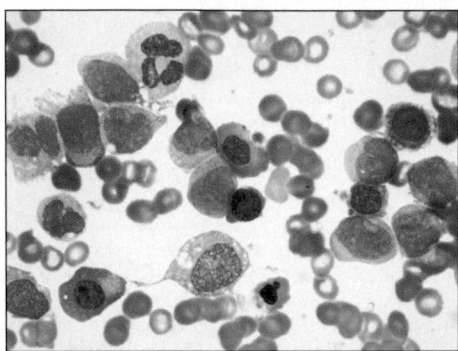

Figure 32–28 AML with multilineage dysplasia showing dysgranulopoiesis and dyserythropoiesis (× 1000).

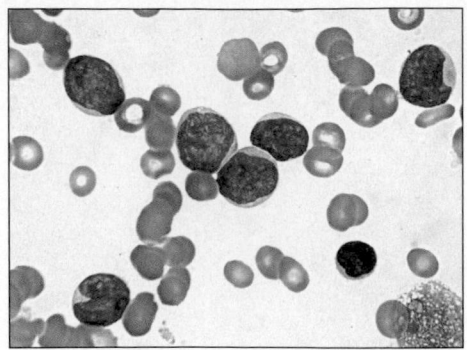

Figure 32–29 AML, minimally differentiated resembles ALL and requires immunophenotyping for diagnosis (× 500).

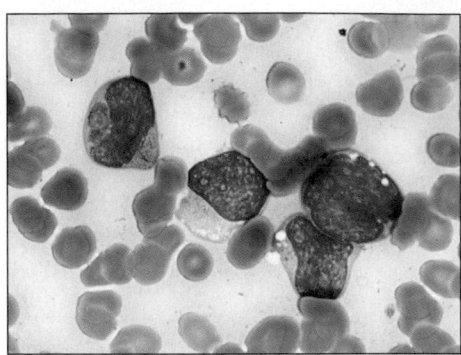

Figure 32–30 AML without maturation shows blasts with less than 10% maturing neutrophils. Auer rods are present in the cell at upper left.

children with t(9;11) respond similarly to patients without 11q23 abnormalities (Martinez-Climent, 1999).

Acute Myeloid Leukemia with Multilineage Dysplasia (Brunning, 2001j)

These leukemias either arise from MDS or occur de novo, but share features with MDS. They typically occur in older people and have a poor prognosis. They are characterized by 20% or more blasts in blood and/or marrow as well as dysplasia in > 50% of cells of at least two lineages. Cases of erythroleukemia (see below for criteria) and > 50% dysplasia of either granulocytes or megakaryocytes are also classified as AML with multilineage dysplasia. Dysplastic features are similar to MDS of various types (Fig. 32–28).

Cytogenetic abnormalities, also seen in MDS, include: 3q-, −5, −7, 7q-, +8, +9, 11q-, 12p-, −18, +19, 20q-, +21, t(1;7), t(2;11), abnormalities of 3q26 (associated with thrombocytosis) and complex karyotypes. The immunophenotype often includes primitive blasts with myeloid phenotype and CD34 expression, CD56 and/or CD7.

Acute Myeloid Leukemia and MDS, Therapy Related (Brunning, 2001k)

These disorders are related to prior cytotoxic chemotherapy or radiation, and are divided into two types; those related to alkylating agents or radiation, and those secondary to topoisomerase inhibitors.

Alkylating Agent-Related AML/MDS. These are related to mutagenic effects of alkylating agents (including chlorambucil, cyclophosphamide, thiotepa and busulfan) or radiation. They usually occur 5–6 years post-exposure and most often present as MDS. Refractory cytopenia with multilineage dysplasia, with or without ring sideroblasts, is most common, followed by RAEB-1 or -2. Ring sideroblasts occur in two-thirds of cases (> 15% ring sideroblasts occur in one-third), and increased basophils are common, though Auer rods are infrequent. Cytogenetic features are similar to MDS and AML with multilineage dysplasia. Response to therapy and outcome are poor.

Topoisomerase II Inhibitor-Related AML. Previous chemotherapy with topoisomerase II inhibitors (including epipodophyllotoxins etoposide and teniposide, and doxorubicin) is also associated with secondary leukemia, either ALL or AML, but different cytogenetic abnormalities are typically involved: 11q23 (MLL) abnormalities including t(9;11), t(11;19) and t(6;11), and also t(3;21), t(8;21), inv(16), or t(15;17). The latency period following therapy is also shorter, median less than 3 years. These most often show monoblastic or myelomonocytic morphology. Response to therapy is possibly similar to that of de novo AML.

Acute Myeloid Leukemia not Otherwise Classified (Brunning, 2001l)

These cases do not fulfill criteria for the previous categories, or cytogenetic studies were unsuccessful or could not be performed. The categorization is similar to French–American–British (FAB) Cooperative Group criteria.

Acute Myeloblastic Leukemia, Minimally Differentiated. In acute myeloblastic leukemia, minimally differentiated, myeloblasts display less than 3% positivity with SBB, MPO, or ANA (Bennett, 1991). When examined for myeloid and lymphoid markers using either flow cytometry or immunocytochemistry, however, at least 20% of the blasts exhibit myeloid-associated antigens (CD13, CD33, CD117 and/or MPO). Stem cell antigens CD34, CD38, HLA-DR and TdT are often expressed while lineage-specific lymphoid markers cCD3, cCD20 and cCD79a are absent. Some primitive markers often associated with lymphoid lineage including CD2, CD7 and CD19 are not lineage specific and sometimes expressed (Fig. 32–29).

Acute Myeloblastic Leukemia without Maturation (M1). In this category, myeloblasts represent at least 90% of the nonerythroid cells in the bone marrow (Bennett, 1985a,b) and at least 3% of the blasts label with either MPO or SBB. Positive staining for CAE is sometimes also present but is less sensitive. CD13, CD33, CD117 and/or MPO antigens are usually detectable as well as other less specific markers. CD3, CD20 and CD79a are usually absent (Fig. 32–30).

Acute Myeloblastic Leukemia with Maturation. Myeloblasts represent 20% (per WHO) to 89% of the total marrow cells, granulocytes from promyelocytes to neutrophils are greater than 10% of the nonerythroid cells, and monocytes and their precursor cells are less than 20% (Fig. 32–31). The majority of blasts stain with MPO, SBB, and CAE.

Cases with t(8;21)(q22;q22) are categorized as AML with recurrent cytogenetic abnormality t(8;21).

Acute Myelomonocytic Leukemia. In acute myelomonocytic leukemia, myeloblasts constitute more than 20% of the total marrow cells. The sum of the monoblasts, promonocytes, and monocytes is more than 20% but is less than 80% of the nonerythroid cells. The cells of the granulocytic series (myeloblasts, promyelocytes, myelocytes, and other more mature forms) also represent 20–80% of the nonerythroid cells (Fig. 32–32). Peripheral blood monocytosis (> 5 × 10⁹/L) is usually present.

In myelomonocytic leukemia there is variable staining of the leukemic cells with myeloperoxidase, SBB, CAE, and periodic acid–Schiff (PAS). In most cases, leukemic cells exhibit diffuse and intense staining with ANA and

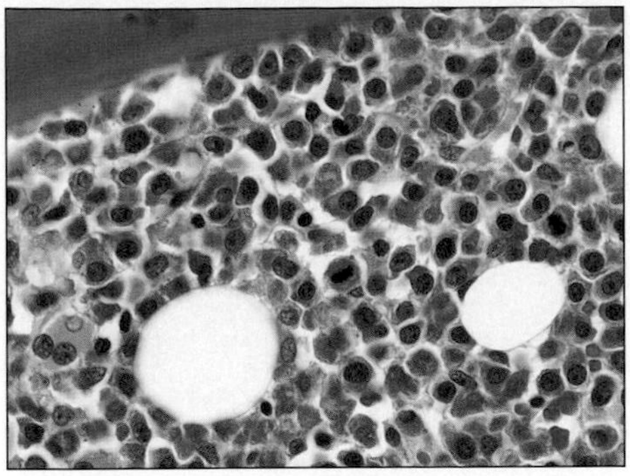

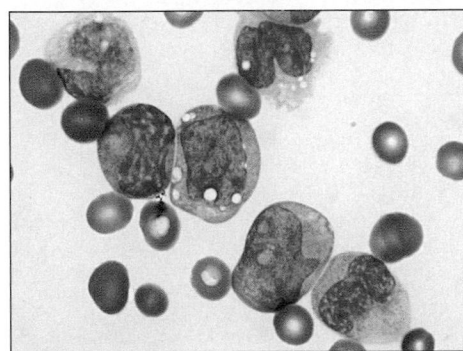

Figure 32–31 AML with maturation shows maturing granulocytic cells on this biopsy (× 200).

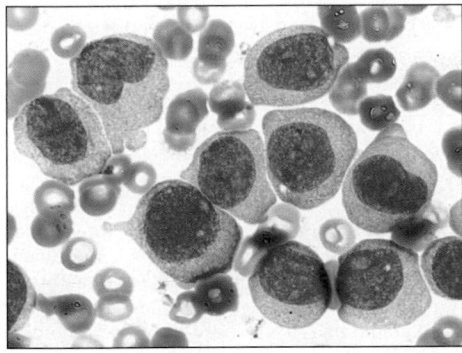

Figure 32–32 Acute myelomonocytic leukemia shows blasts and dual differentiation to granulocytes and monocytes (× 1000). Acute monocytic leukemia shows monoblasts and maturing monocytes. Promonocytes are counted as blasts, and show finely convoluted nuclei (× 1000).

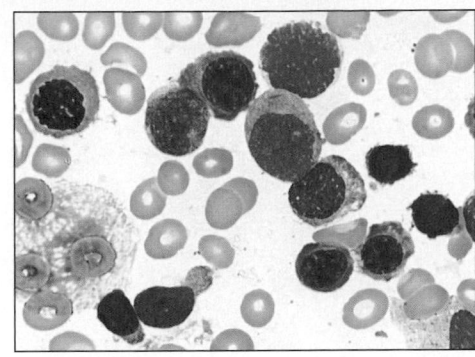

Figure 32–34 Erythroleukemia, erythroid/myeloid, shows predominance of erythroid precursors with myeloblasts constituting 20% or more of nonerythroid cells. An Auer rod is seen in the blast at upper center (× 1000).

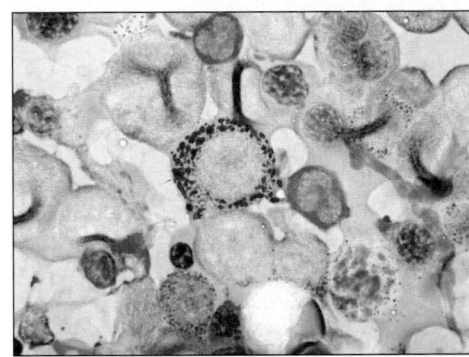

Figure 32–35 Coarse PAS-positive granules are often seen in erythroid precursors in erythroleukemia (× 1000).

Figure 32–33 Acute monoblastic leukemia shows predominantly monoblasts (× 1000).

ANB. In some cases, these nonspecific esterases cannot be demonstrated and the diagnosis may be made on the Romanowsky stains and/or immunophenotyping.

Immunologic markers are variable but usually show myeloid antigens CD13 and/or CD33 as well as variable expression of monocytic markers CD14, CD4, CD11b, CD11c, CD64, CD36, CD68 and lysozyme. Some pure myeloblasts may be present including those with CD34 and CD117 expression and a second population of variably mature monocytes. Cases with recurrent cytogenetic abnormalities are categorized separately.

Acute Monoblastic and Acute Monocytic Leukemia. In this disorder, 80% or more of the marrow nonerythroid cells are monoblasts, promonocytes, or monocytes (Figs 32–22 and 32–33). Two subtypes are recognized. The monoblastic subtype is characterized by large blasts accounting for 80% or more of the marrow monocytic cells. The monocytic subtype has fewer monoblasts (< 80% of the marrow monocytic cells) and more promonocytes and monocytes (Bennett, 1985a). In both, ANA and ANB label the leukemic cells diffusely and intensely (80% or more of leukemic cells). Occasional cases fail to show nonspecific esterases and the diagnosis is made from Romanowsky stains and/or immunophenotypic techniques. Antilysozyme and CD68 are particularly useful on slides. Both myeloid and monocytic markers are frequently expressed, as in acute myelomonocytic leukemia. The

translocation t(8;16)(p11;p13) has been associated with AML-M5 (or M4) with erythrophagocytosis.

Erythroleukemia. The diagnosis of erythroleukemia is made when more than 50% of the nucleated cells of the bone marrow are erythroblasts and 20% or more of the nonerythroid cells are myeloblasts. In most cases, termed erythroleukemia (erythroid/myeloid), there is a mixture of variable proportions of erythroid precursors and myeloblasts (sometimes abnormal monocytic and megakaryocytic elements are present as well) (Fig. 32–34).

Very rarely there is virtually no granulocytic involvement in the neoplastic process and primitive erythroblasts predominate. This has been known as *erythremic myelosis* and is now known as pure erythroid leukemia. Morphologic abnormalities of the erythroblasts are often pronounced with atypical megaloblastic features, bizarre nuclear shapes, and multinucleated giant forms. The cytoplasm may contain pseudopods and/or vacuoles, particularly in the pro- and basophilic erythroblasts.

In some cases, the erythroid cells may show strong cytoplasmic PAS positivity (Fig. 32–35). This is granular in early erythroid precursors and diffuse in later stages. Erythroid precursors are PAS-negative in normal individuals and in most diseases, including nutritional megaloblastic anemia. They are sometimes positive, however, in iron deficiency anemia, thalassemia, and refractory anemia with ring sideroblasts. In erythroleukemia, myeloblasts usually stain with SBB, MPO, and CAE. A nonspecific esterase-positive monocytic component may also be present. Neoplastic erythroid precursors are also sometimes positive for the ANA and ANB (Hayhoe, 1984).

Acute Megakaryoblastic Leukemia. The diagnosis of acute megakaryoblastic leukemia, like other forms of acute myeloid leukemia requires ≥ 20% blasts in the marrow. Megakaryoblasts are very polymorphic; some blasts simulate lymphoblasts while others are larger and have pseudopods or stringy cytoplasmic projections. The cytoplasm is usually light blue and may or may not possess granules (Fig. 32–36). The nuclei often have one to three nucleoli. Micromegakaryocytes may be present and are not counted as blasts.

The blasts are cytochemically undifferentiated. They do not stain with SBB, MPO, CAE, or ANB. ANA is, however, usually positive in a focal cytoplasmic pattern (Fig. 32–37). The PAS reaction shows diffuse and peripheral granular (often in large blocks) staining.

Megakaryocytic lineage is most often (Bennett, 1985b) demonstrated by immunophenotyping using monoclonal antibodies against platelet glycoproteins Ib (CD41) or IIb/IIIa (CD61) (Erber, 1987). Blasts are often

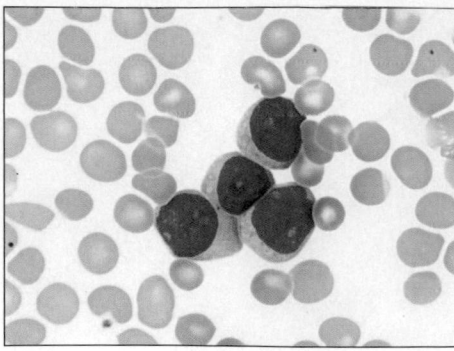

Figure 32–36 Blasts sometimes cluster in acute megakaryocytic leukemia (× 1000).

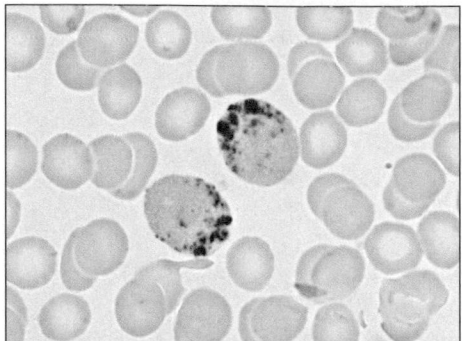

Figure 32–37 ANA-positive granules in megakaryoblasts.

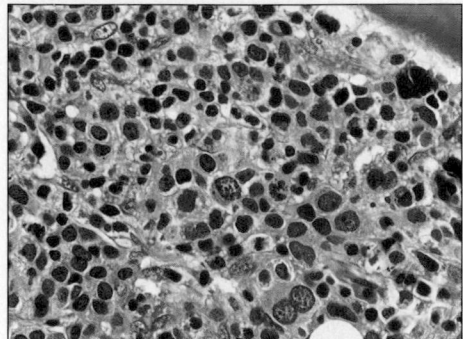

Figure 32–38 Acute panmyelosis with myelofibrosis shows involvement of all three myeloid lineages, with fibrosis (× 200).

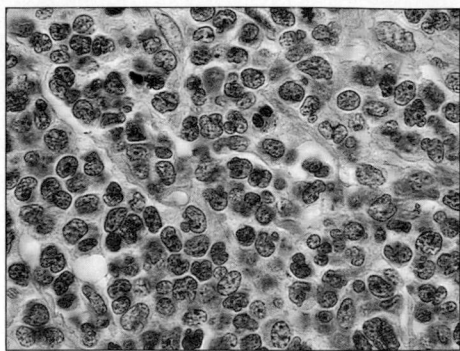

Figure 32–39 Granulocytic sarcoma, in this case presenting in the skin, resembles lymphoma but with large blastic or monocytoid cells. Eosinophils or precursors are frequently present (× 500).

also positive for myeloid antigens CD13 and CD33, and characteristically for CD36. Care must be taken to differentiate this disease from AML with minimal differentiation by flow cytometry, which may show artifactual positivity for platelet markers due to adherence of platelets to blasts, and this can be done by immunochemical examination of cytospins. Truly positive cells show membrane and/or cytoplasmic labeling rather than adherent platelets.

In the peripheral blood, there is usually pancytopenia with marked leukopenia and anemia. Megakaryocytic fragments are sometimes present in the blood. The bone marrow shows variable and sometimes pronounced myelofibrosis, often resulting in futile attempts at obtaining marrow aspirate films.

Clumping of blasts may simulate metastatic tumor such as neuroblastoma or small cell carcinoma. Infants with t(1;22)(p13;q13) often show marrow infiltration mimicking neuroblastoma.

Young children (1–4 years of age) with Down syndrome (trisomy 21) have an increased incidence of megakaryoblastic leukemia which may be transient and spontaneously remit in 1–3 months. Subsequent transient or persistent relapses may occur. The blasts also tend to show erythroid features, indicating derivation from a multipotential erythroid/megakaryocytic precursor (Zipursky, 1992). These patients often respond well to therapy but tolerate intensive therapy less well than others (Gamis, 2004).

Acute Basophilic Leukemia. Acute basophilic leukemia is a rare form of AML in which the blastic cells differentiate along the basophil lineage. The peripheral blood usually demonstrates anemia and thrombocytopenia with leukocytosis. The bone marrow is infiltrated by blastic cells simulating lymphoblasts or myeloblasts. Blasts are generally negative for Sudan black B and myeloperoxidase. There may be an increase in mature basophils or in blasts staining with toluidine blue. The diagnosis historically rests on the identification of blasts with basophilic granules by ultrastructural methods (Brunning, 1994).

Acute Panmyelosis with Myelofibrosis. This is a rare form of acute leukemia with panmyeloid proliferation and marrow fibrosis. There is typically pancytopenia. Red blood cells show minimal poikilocytosis but dysplastic features in myeloid cells are often seen, and also atypical platelets.

The bone marrow sample frequently shows a dry tap and on biopsy, clusters of blasts, late erythroid precursors and dysplastic megakaryocytes are seen in a variably fibrotic background (Fig. 32–38). This is differentiated from acute megakaryoblastic leukemia by involvement of all three myeloid lineages, rather than only the megakaryocytic.

Granulocytic Sarcoma. This neoplasm has also been called myeloblastic sarcoma, extramedullary myeloid cell tumor, and chloroma. It represents a localized tumor of myeloblasts or monoblasts infiltrating extramedullary sites (Fig. 32–39). These tumors have been reported to occur in the skin, lymph nodes, nasopharyngeal and upper respiratory tract tissues, breast, ovary, bone, perineural and epidural structures, the eye and other orbital structures, and a variety of soft tissues (Neiman, 1981). Granulocytic sarcomas have been reported in 3–8% of autopsied cases of chronic myelogenous leukemia and may precede the occurrence of acute myeloid leukemia in < 1% of cases (Muss, 1973).

Granulocytic sarcomas may occur at any age. Three clinical settings are found: (1) no known disease; (2) a known myeloproliferative disorder, and (3) acute myeloid leukemia (Neiman, 1981). The diagnosis depends on recognizing the nature of the primitive cells that can often be mistaken for solid tumors including non-HLs, amelanotic melanomas, or undifferentiated carcinoma (Hutchison, 1990). The diagnosis is facilitated by making touch imprint preparations of cut sections of the tumor and staining them with Romanowsky stains, by cytochemical reactions, and by immunophenotyping. Anti-MPO and CD68 are particularly useful for granulocytic or monocytic lineage in paraffin sections.

Acute Leukemias of Ambiguous Lineage (Brunning, 2001m)

Some cases of acute leukemia have features that are indeterminate between lymphoid and myeloid lineage, or have features of more than one lineage. This is a controversial area of difficult-to-classify leukemia. Many leukemias which appear to be of defined lineage have one or more immunologic markers which are aberrant, or show lineage infidelity. A single such marker is usually insignificant. ALL with myeloid markers respond similarly to other ALL, and lymphoid markers in AML are also clinically important mostly if they help define a subtype, such as CD19 expression in AML with t(8;21). CD117 has been proposed as a good indicator of myeloid lineage (Bene, 1998). For cases that are truly ambiguous, a scoring system has been accepted by the WHO classification (Table 32–16) (Anon, 1998).

Ambiguous acute leukemias fall into several categories as explained below: **Undifferentiated Acute Leukemia.** These are rare acute leukemias in which the predominant cells are blast forms that cannot be classified using morphologic, cytochemical, ultrastructural, immunologic, or DNA analytical methods (Raghavachar, 1986; Sobol, 1988). CD34, CD38, HLA-DR are frequently expressed and CD7 and TdT may be. These may have abnormalities of chromosomes 13, 12, or region 5q (Cuneo, 1996).

Table 32–16 Scoring System for Markers of Acute Leukemia Lineage

Score	B-lymphoid	T-lymphoid	Myeloid
2	CytCD79a	CD3(m/cyt)	MPO
	Cyt IgM	Anti-TCR	
	CytCD22		
1	CD19	CD2	CD117
	CD20	CD5	CD13
	CD10	CD8	CD33
		CD10	CD65
0.5	TdT	TdT	CD14
	CD24	CD7	CD15
		CD1a	CD64

Myeloid lineage (AML-M0) = myeloid score ≥ 4 and lymphoid score ≤ 3[*]
Lymphoid lineage (T or B) = lymphoid score ≥ 4 and myeloid score ≤ [*]
Biphenotypic lineage = T or B lymphoid and myeloid score each > 2 (but < 4)[†]

[*] Thalhammer-Scherrer R, Mitterbauer G, Simonistsch I, et al: The immunophenotype of 325 adult acute leukemias. Am J Clin Pathol 2002; 117:380–389.
[†] EGIL (European Group for the Immunological Classification of Leukaemias): The value of c-kit in the diagnosis of biphenotypic acute leukemia. Leukemia 1998; 12:2038.

Bilineal Acute Leukemia. In these rare disorders there are blasts cells of more than one distinct hematopoietic lineage, including myeloid and lymphoid or B and T cell lineage.

Biphenotypic Leukemia. These cases show one population of leukemic cells with multiple lineage expression (mixed lineage). This term is reserved for those cases with multiple lineage-specific markers of more than one lineage. Cases have been identified in both pediatric and adult patients (Sobol, 1987; Stass, 1986; Cheson, 1990).

Both bilineal and biphenotypic leukemias have frequent cytogenetic abnormalities. The Philadelphia chromosome is associated with cases showing a CD10+ precursor B lymphoblastic component, and t(4;11)(q21;q23) or other 11q23 abnormality with CD10-negative precursor B lineage and monocytic lineage. Rearranged immunoglobulin heavy chain (IgH) and T cell receptor (TCR) genes are frequent, but are not specific and may be found in other AML (Adriaansen, 1991).

Precursor (Lymphoblastic) B and T Cell Neoplasms

Historically, lymphoid leukemias and lymphomas have been classified separately. Leukemias are hematopoietic malignancies primarily involving bone marrow and blood and have been most extensively categorized by the FAB group. Lymphomas are those primarily involving lymphoid organs or other soft tissues and have been subject to numerous classification schemes that evolved rapidly because of advances in immunology, oncology, and genetics. Since publication of the Revised European–American Lymphoma (REAL) classification (Harris, 1994), lymphoid leukemias and lymphomas have been classified by the biologic features of the disease rather than the anatomic distribution, and generally provide an international consensus in classification (Berard, 1997). The WHO classification focuses on cytogenetic and molecular findings whenever possible (Brunning, 2001n,o).

Precursor B Lymphoblastic Leukemia/Lymphoblastic Lymphoma

Clinical Features. This category of malignancy most often presents as leukemia and is the prototype of acute lymphoblastic leukemia (ALL). The other major type of ALL is precursor T lymphoblastic, which is less common and tends to present as lymphoma or concurrently as both leukemia and lymphoma. ALL is generally thought of as a clinical entity which is pathologically subtyped, and warrants some general discussion.

Acute lymphoblastic leukemia is the most common malignancy of children and adolescents. There are 3000–4000 new cases per year in the US, two-thirds of which are children. The evolution of treatment with combination chemotherapy, CNS treatment, and intensified therapy for high-risk categories has led to cure rates of nearly 80% in children. In adults, only 30–40% are cured, due in part to higher frequency of adverse genetic abnormalities (Pui, 2004). Adult ALL incidence increases in middle to older age, similarly to genetically high-risk AML. Individuals with

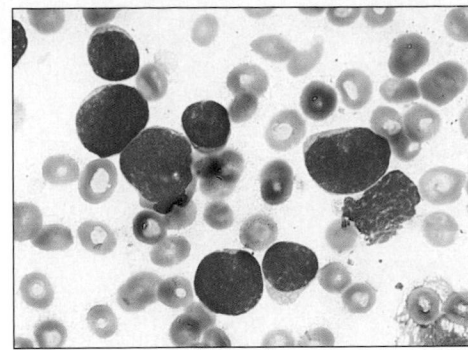

Figure 32–40 Precursor B ALL, with small to medium size blasts and lack of conspicuous nucleoli (× 1000).

this disorder often present with symptoms of fatigue, fever, and bleeding. Generalized lymphadenopathy, splenomegaly, and hepatomegaly are common findings. Because the leukemic cells infiltrate many tissues of the body, other symptoms may occur. Leg pain can be associated with periosteal infiltrates; and headaches, nausea, and vomiting with meningeal leukemia. A rapid onset of unconsciousness may indicate subarachnoid hemorrhage.

Presentation is occasionally in skin, bone and/or lymph node without bone marrow involvement (< 25% blasts in the marrow). These cases are referred to as lymphoma. They most often occur in young people (< 18 years) and show overlapping features with precursor B-ALL, with TdT, B-lineage markers and frequent additional 21q chromosome material (Maitra, 2001). Morphology in tissue sections shows diffuse infiltrations of small cells (nuclei smaller than histiocyte nuclei) with diffuse chromatin, inconspicuous nucleoli, scant cytoplasm, high mitotic rate, and frequently a 'starry-sky' pattern of admixed histiocytes (indicating high apoptotic rate).

Anemia is present in precursor B-ALL if clinical manifestations are fully developed. It is usually normocytic. Frequently, nucleated red cells are present. Thrombocytopenia of moderate to marked degree is the rule. The leukocyte count is occasionally very high (> 100×10^9/L), often is slightly elevated, but is perhaps most frequently normal or decreased. The predominant cell is the lymphoblast.

Marrow. By the time the patient is symptomatic, the hematopoietic cells and fat are usually replaced by a diffuse infiltration of lymphoblasts. Blast percentage is usually greater than 50%. Predominance of small blasts with high nuclear to cytoplasmic (N/C) ratios and inconspicuous nucleoli (L1 type in the FAB classification) is most common in childhood ALL (Fig. 32–40). Chromatin is diffuse in some cells but may also show variable condensation, and blasts may be difficult to distinguish from the normal lymphocytes of young children. Larger blasts with more abundant cytoplasm, prominent nucleoli and often irregular nuclei (FAB L2) also occur and tend to predominate in adult ALL.

The blasts are negative for SBB, peroxidase, and naphthol ASD CAE. Azurophilic granules may be present, but they are SBB and peroxidase negative. In other cases, ALL blasts may exhibit some SBB reactivity, but peroxidase is negative.

Blasts characteristically express TdT, cytoplasmic CD22 and CD79a, CD19 and HLA-DR. CD10 (common ALL antigen) is expressed in many. Variable expression is seen for CD34. Cytoplasmic mu immunoglobulin heavy chain (cyt-mu) indicates a slightly more mature state, but surface immunoglobulin is negative. Myeloid-associated antigens CD13, CD33, or CD15 may be expressed.

Cytogenetics. Cytogenetic findings are increasingly important in diagnosis and prognostication in ALL, and have been previously reviewed (Brunning, 2001n, Mrozek, 2004). The translocation t(12;21)(p12;q22) occurs in approximately 25% of precursor B lymphoblastic leukemia, correlates with high density CD10 and HLA-DR expression with negative CD9 and CD20, and is associated with good prognosis. The TEL gene at 12p12 is fused with the AML1 gene at 21q22 with a resultant fusion protein. The abnormality is difficult to detect by karyotyping, but can be detected by RT-PCR analysis for the chimeric mRNA or by FISH.

The Ph' chromosome, t(9;22) with production of a fusion BCR–ABL, occurs in about 30% of adult (20% detected at karyotyping) and 6% of childhood ALL. The t(9;22) is the most frequent adult ALL translocation and is associated with poor prognosis. Two types are found: that identical to CML involving the bcr region of BCR with resultant p210 kd fusion protein, occurring in half of adult Ph'-positive ALL, and another with breakpoint upstream of bcr and producing a smaller chimeric message

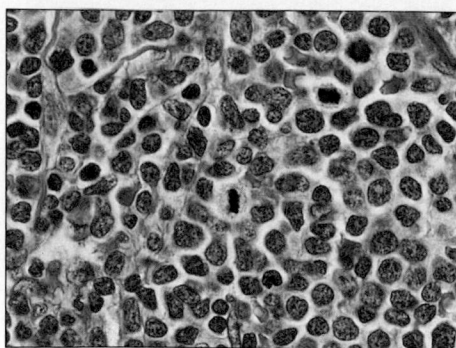

Figure 32–41 Precursor T lymphoblastic lymphoma (× 500).

and p190 kD protein. The latter occurs in most childhood Ph'-positive cases. Ph'-positive ALL is most often precursor B cell lineage, but also may present with biphenotypic myeloid differentiation.

Abnormalities of the *MLL* gene at chromosome region 11q23 are seen in 5–7% of ALL (Le Beau, 2000) as well as in AML. ALL with t(4;11)(q21;q23) is associated with poor prognosis, high WBC count and immature B-lineage phenotype with lack of CD10. It is most common in infants, and many cases of ALL with this abnormality are biphenotypic. t(11;19)(q23;p13.3) is the next most frequent *MLL* abnormality in ALL, but also occurs in AML-M5. Overall, 11q23 (*MLL*) abnormalities, with the possible exception of t(9;11) in AML, confer poor prognosis.

Another translocation, t(1;19)(q23;p13), and variants, is associated with pre-B cell ALL (with cytoplasmic mu Ig). It involves the *E2A* gene at 19p13, which encodes transcription factors, and *PBX* at 1q23. This has also been associated with decreased response to therapy.

Hyperdiploidy has been long recognized as a favorable prognostic factor in childhood ALL. Patients with greater than 50 chromosomes have improved prognosis and those with greater than 56 have even better outlook. These patients usually have precursor B-lineage ALL.

Approximately 80% of children with precursor B-ALL are cured. Favorable factors are age 5–10 years, hyperdiploidy (best, 54–62 with trisomy 4, 10, and/or 17), t(12;21), and normal or low WBC. Poor risk factors are age less than 1 year, t(9;22) and t(4;11).

Precursor T Lymphoblastic Leukemia/Lymphoblastic Lymphoma (T-LBL)

Precursor T lymphoblastic leukemia, which accounts for 10–20% of cases of ALL, occurs predominantly in boys, who tend to be slightly older than children with precursor B lymphoblastic ALL. Patients with T-lineage ALL often have a high leukocyte count and mediastinal involvement. Blast morphology is heterogeneous, similar to B-ALL, and immunophenotyping is required for diagnosis. The immunophenotype reflects thymic T cells which have a distinct maturation pattern (Reinherz, 1980) and the blasts show varying maturity. Most cases exhibit TdT, CD7 and cytoplasmic CD3 with variable CD1a, CD2 and CD5. Some cases, of early thymic phenotype, lack CD4 or CD8 but most (midcortical thymic phenotype, particularly in lymphoma presentation) coexpress CD4 and CD8. In late cortical thymic phenotype, CD4 or CD8 alone may be present, and in these TdT and/or CD1a are particularly helpful for diagnosis. Myeloid markers such as CD13, CD33 and/or CD117 may be present, and CD79a may be present occasionally.

Presentation as lymphoma often shows a more mature thymic phenotype than leukemic presentation (Crist, 1988). These are relatively common lymphomas of adolescents and young adults (one-third of pediatric NHLs) and also occur later in life. They typically present in the mediastinum and/or peripheral lymph nodes, and pleural effusions are common. Airway compromise or superior vena cava syndrome is frequently present, resulting in emergent need for therapy and limiting diagnostic procedures.

Morphology. T-LBL usually shows diffuse tissue involvement by blasts with nuclei smaller than those of histiocytes or reactive endothelial cells, (Fig. 32–41) though some show nuclei similar in size to Burkitt lymphoma (BL). Chromatin is usually finely dispersed to slightly clumped, but rarely as much as Burkitt. Mitotic rates are high and there is often a 'starry sky' pattern similar to Burkitt. Neoplastic cells sometimes show selective T-zone involvement of lymph nodes and/or a leukemia-like infiltration pattern in soft tissue.

The differential diagnosis of T-LBL in young patients is primarily between it, BL and occasionally large B cell lymphoma (LBCL). Mediastinal location favors T-LBL over BL, but not LBCL. In adults, the differential diagnosis also includes blastoid and blastic variants of mantle

cell lymphoma. Granulocytic sarcoma is also in the differential in any age group. Expression of TdT and lineage-specific T cell markers without B or myeloid markers is usually diagnostic.

Genetics. T cell receptor genes are frequently rearranged, but Ig heavy chain genes may also be rearranged (Brunning, 2001o). Patients with T cell ALL frequently show translocations of alpha and delta T cell receptor loci at 14q11.2, the beta locus at 7q35, or gamma locus at 7p14-15, usually with genes encoding transcription factors. Partner genes include *MYC* (8q24.1), *TAL1* (1p32), *RBTN1* (11p15), *RBTN2* (11p13), *HOX11* (10q24) and *LCK* (1p34.3-35). *TAL1* regulatory gene deletions occur in 25% of cases and del(9p) involving *CDKN2* is also frequent (Mrozek, 2004).

Mature B Cell Neoplasms

These constitute the most numerous and possibly most diverse group of hematopoietic neoplasms. The overall rates vary from 1.2/100 000 population/year in China to 15/100 000 in the US. There is geographic variation in mature lymphoma/leukemia with follicular and diffuse large B cell predominating in western developed countries, constituting 50% of NHL, and myeloma is also common (Harris, 2001a). T/NK diseases are more frequent in Asia than in the western countries. The cells affected in mature B cell malignancies are those making up the humoral immune system, which is itself very complex and includes innumerable clones of B lymphocytes with genetically distinct immunoglobulin gene rearrangements. They exist at many states of maturation and are both influenced by and affect many regulatory pathways. The normal cells and the tumors are influenced by immune status and perturbations, viruses, other microorganisms and antigenic stimuli. There is tremendous variation in the growth rates and aggressiveness of tumors in this large group, corresponding to high proliferative rates of some cells and quiescence of others. There is also a correspondingly variable tendency toward apoptosis which influences response to antineoplastic therapies. Clinical behaviors relate to clonal escape from regulation, to the balance of proliferation and apoptosis, and modulation by therapy. Features of major categories are shown in Table 32–17.

Chronic Lymphocytic Leukemia/Small Lymphocytic Lymphoma (CLL/SLL)

This is a clonal proliferation of small B lymphocytes involving bone marrow, blood and lymph nodes. It is common, usually indolent at least initially, but difficult if not impossible to cure (Muller-Hermelink, 2001). Cases with predominant involvement in the marrow and blood are traditionally called CLL while lymphomas are called SLL, but the current concept is that they are a single entity. The majority of cases are leukemic and constitute 90% of chronic lymphoid leukemias in the US and Europe. It is rare under the age of 40; most cases occur over the age of 60 and it is more than twice as common in men as in women. The onset is insidious and the disease is commonly discovered by chance during the investigation of another problem. Most patients are > 50 years.

The tumors show diffuse infiltrates of small mature lymphocytes with clumped chromatin and scant to moderate cytoplasm (Fig. 32–42). Admixed prolymphocytes and proliferation centers (containing increased prolymphocytes and lymphocytes with increased cytoplasm) are characteristic. Mitotic rates are very low.

CLL/SLL shows a characteristic phenotype of monoclonal B cells (CD19/CD20/CD79a) with dim surface Ig (single light chain with IgM or IgM and IgD), coexpression of usual T cell marker CD5 and expression of CD23. CD22, CD10 and cyclin D1 are negative. This pattern is very useful to distinguish CLL/SLL from mantle cell, follicular, and marginal zone lymphomas. Bcl-6 is negative and bcl-2 variable.

Ig heavy and (monotypic) light chain genes are rearranged. Trisomy 12 is present in 20% of cases, del(13q14) in 50%, del(11q22-23) and/or mutations in this region in 20%, del(17p13) at the *p53* locus in 10% and del(6q21) in 5%. Cytogenetic abnormalities may indicate poorer prognosis. These abnormalities cannot often be detected by karyotype since CLL cells do not grow well in culture, but are detectable by FISH probes.

The leukocyte count is usually between 30–200 × 10⁹/L. In the typical type of CLL, 90% or more of the cells are small lymphocytes that are monotonously similar in appearance and usually look normal. Nuclear chromatin may be coarsely condensed and more sharply separated by parachromatin than in normal lymphocytes or, in some cases, the chromatin is less condensed than normal. Sometimes nucleoli are evident in many of the lymphocytes. Size variation is minimal. Cytoplasm is of slight to moderate amount. Less than 10% of lymphocytes are prolymphocytes or reticular lymphocytes (transformed lymphocytes).

Often there is neither anemia nor thrombocytopenia at the time of diagnosis. Anemia due to impaired production does develop as the

Table 32–17 Key Features of the Major Mature B Cell Neoplasms

Lymphoma	Demographics, clinical and laboratory presentation	Morphology	Cell surface markers Positive	Negative	Cytogenetics
CLL/SLL	M > F, over 60 years. Insidious onset of fatigue, lymphadenopathy. WBC > 30K, anemia, thrombocytopenia, occasionally AIHA	Monomorphic, small lymphocytes with slight–moderate cytoplasm, condensed chromatin	CD5, 19, 20, 23, 79a, dim sIg	CD10, 22, Bcl-6	+12, del(13q14), del(11q22-23), Ig rearrangement
B cell PLL	M >> F, mean age 65 years. Massive splenomegaly, minimal lymphadenopathy, WBC > 100K	Prolymphocytes ≥55% with large vesicular nucleus, condensed chromatin, moderate cytoplasm	CD19, 20, bright sIg	Often CD5, 23 negative	del(11q23), del(13q14), Ig rearrangement
Hairy cell leukemia	M > F, median age 50 years. Insidious onset with splenomegaly, monocytopenia	Medium-sized cells with round–oval nuclei, reticular chromatin, frayed cytoplasmic borders	CD 19, 20, 22, 79a, 103, 25, 11c	CD5, 10, 23	Ig rearrangement
Lymphoplasmacytic lymphoma	M ≈ F, mean age 63. BM, nodal and splenic involvement, and frequent IgM paraprotein with hyperviscosity (WM) causing decreased visual acuity, risk for CVA, neuropathies	Plasmacytoid lymphocytes and plasma cells with PAS-positive inclusions (Dutcher bodies)	CD19, 20, 22, 38, 79a, bright sIgM, cIgM	CD5, 10, 23	t(9;14)(p13;q32)
Alpha heavy chain disease	Younger adults in poorer Mediterranean communities with malabsorption, diarrhea	Lymphoplasmacytic infiltrate of intestinal mucosa	NA	NA	NA
MALT lymphoma	F > M, median age 61. Indolent course involving stomach, other GI sites. Associated with antecedent autoimmune disease (SS, Hashimoto's) or *H. pylori* infection	Lymphoepithelial lesions with small lymphocytes, centrocytes, monocytoid lymphocytes and reactive germinal centers	CD19, 20, 22, 79a, sIg, bcl-2	CD5, 10, 23, bcl-6	+3, t(11;18)(q21;q21)
Follicular lymphoma	F > M, median age 59 years. Peripheral lymphadenopathy dominates, with central adenopathy, BM and splenic involvement frequent	Follicle-like structures with small, cleaved lymphocytes and varying numbers of larger centroblasts which allow for cytologic grading	CD19, 20, 22, 23, 79a, 10, bcl-2, bcl-6	CD5, 43	t(14;18)(q32;q21)
Mantle cell lymphoma	M > F, median age 60 years. Lymphadenopathy, marked splenomegaly, BM involvement. Aggressive course	Atrophic germinal centers, prominent mantle zones, monomorphic cells with small–medium nuclei	CD19, 20, 22, 5, 43, bcl-2, cyclin D1	CD10, 23, bcl-6	t(11;14)(q13;q32)
Diffuse large B cell lymphoma	M > F, all ages, associated with HIV. Nodal and extranodal sites, CNS. Aggressive course	Diffuse infiltrate of variably large B cells, sometimes with centroblastic or immunoblastic morphology	CDCd19, 20, 22, 79a, sIg. Occasionally CD30 (anaplastic variant)	CD5 (usually), 23	t(14;18) in 20–30%, 3q27 abnormality in up to 30%, complex abnormality
Mediastinal large B cell lymphoma	F > M, young–middle-aged adults. Airway compression, superior vena cava syndrome	Sclerotic lesions with clear, multilobated or RS-like cells	CD45, 19, 20	CD5, 10	Ig rearrangement
Primary effusion lymphoma	Rare, associated with HHV-8 in immunosuppressed, younger male homosexuals. Pleural effusion	Immunoblastic or anaplastic cells	CD19, 20, 79a, often CD30, 38, 138	sIg, cIg	Ig, occasionally TCR rearrangement
Burkitt lymphoma	1. Endemic: children in Africa, jaw mass, M > F 2. Sporadic: children–young adults, worldwide, M > F, abdominal organs 3. Immunodeficiency-associated: HIV patients	Uniform cells with round–oval nuclei, multiple nucleoli, high mitotic rate	CD19, 2, 20, 79a, sIg, often CD10	TdT	t(8;14)(q24;q32)

WM = Waldenström's macroglobulinemia; PAS = periodic acid–Schiff; SS = Sjögren's syndrome; RS = Reed–Sternberg.

marrow is replaced by leukemic cells. In addition, erythrocyte life span in some patients with CLL may be reduced. This is especially true when there is marked splenomegaly. Autoimmune hemolytic anemia develops in about 10% of patients. Thrombocytopenia is often slight and occasionally becomes severe as the disease progresses, so that hemorrhagic manifestations appear. Thrombocytopenia is usually due to hypoproliferation but may also be secondary to an immune process or splenic sequestration. Patchy, nodular, or interstitial involvement of the bone marrow by neoplastic lymphocytes is associated with a relatively good outcome. A diffuse infiltrate of the bone marrow, however, usually correlates with a poor

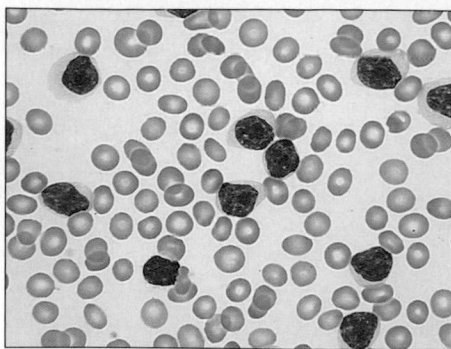

Figure 32–42 B cell chronic lymphocytic leukemia (×1000).

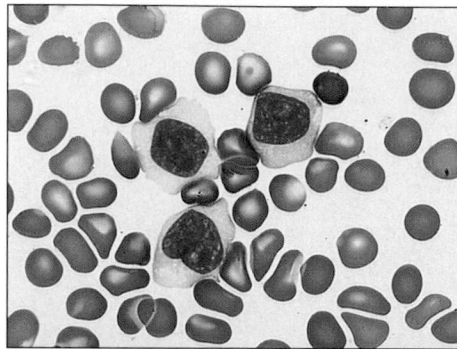

Figure 32–43 B cell prolymphocytic leukemia typically shows high WBC, large lymphocytes with moderately abundant cytoplasm and prominent nucleoli, though variability exists (×1000).

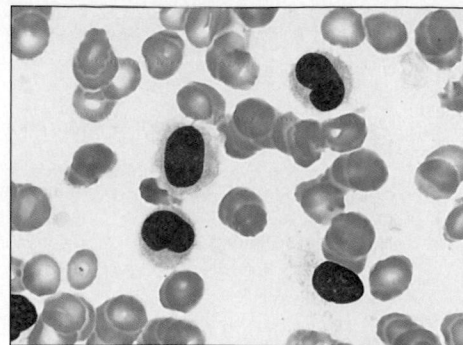

Figure 32–44 Hairy cell leukemia shows lymphoid cells with foamy cytoplasm and cytoplasmic projections, and oval or indented nuclei with reticular chromatin (×1000).

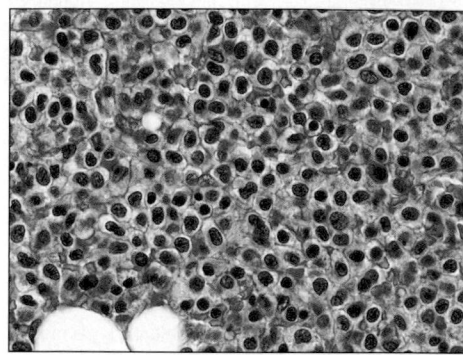

Figure 32–45 Hairy cell leukemia in a bone marrow biopsy shows small nuclei with moderate cytoplasm and distinct cytoplasmic boundaries (×500).

prognosis and/or advanced disease (Bartl, 1982a, Montserrat, 1987). An increased proportion of prolymphocytes (between 10–55%) has been referred to as mixed CLL/PLL and may correlate with aggressive disease (Bennett, 1989; Melo, 1987). Expression of markers CD38 or ZAP-70 and p53 abnormalities have been investigated for possible prognostic value, but results are inconclusive (Kim, 2004; Mainou-Fowler, 2004). Anemia, B-symptoms and International Prognostic Index (IPI) may provide the best prognostic information (Nola, 2004). The median survival for patients with CLL is about 7 years, but recent therapy such as fludarabine shows promise for better survival.

B Cell Prolymphocytic Leukemia

Prolymphocytic leukemia was originally described as a variant of CLL (Galton, 1974). The male : female ratio is 6.5 : 1 and the mean age is 65 years. PLL is characterized by a very marked lymphocytosis (usually greater than $100 \times 10^3/\mu L$), massive splenomegaly, moderate hepatomegaly, and inconspicuous lymphadenopathy. The malignant lymphoid cells have a large vesicular nucleolus, condensed nuclear chromatin, and moderate amount of cytoplasm (Fig. 32–43). More than 55% of blood leukemic cells are prolymphocytes. Immunophenotype varies from SLL/CLL by bright surface Ig (monoclonal IgM with or without IgD), lack of CD5 in two-thirds of cases, usually lack of CD23 and presence of FMC-7. Abnormalities of p53 are frequent and deletions at 11q23 and 13q14 occur. Prolymphocytic leukemia is usually less responsive to treatment than CLL in general, and has a poorer prognosis (Catovsky, 2001a).

Hairy Cell Leukemia

Bouroncle (1958) initially described this disorder, which is clinically variable in its manifestations. Hairy cell leukemia (HCL) occurs more frequently in males than in females. The mean age of afflicted patients is 50 years. It has an insidious onset and is characterized by proliferation of the abnormal cells in the reticuloendothelial organs and blood. Splenomegaly is the predominant physical finding (Foucar, 2001).

Pancytopenia or depression of only two cell lines is the usual finding, with variable numbers of hairy cells. Monocytopenia is characteristic and hairy cells are usually infrequent in the blood, though they may result in leukocytosis. In the majority of cases, bone marrow aspiration is difficult. Marrow biopsy shows a marrow that varies in cellularity, often having both hypocellular and hypercellular areas and reticulin fibrosis. Hypocellular cases of HCL occur and mimic aplastic anemia.

Morphologically, the cells are medium sized (10–20 μm diameter), with round to oval nuclei, though many are notched, dumbbell or bean

shaped. The chromatin pattern is usually uniformly reticular, and nucleoli are small and inconspicuous. In some cells, chromatin is more condensed, resembling that of a lymphocyte. The cytoplasm is moderate in amount, light blue-gray and exhibiting numerous hair-like projections and frayed borders, most prominent on electron micrographs (Fig. 32–44).

In marrow sections, the cells with small central nuclei, abundant cytoplasm and reticulin fibrosis produce a characteristic fried-egg appearance which may, however, resemble erythroid islands when involvement is not extensive (Fig. 32–45). Chromatin is usually more delicate and nuclei more irregular than in erythroid precursors. In small or poorly preserved biopsies, HCL may be mistaken for large B cell lymphoma.

Splenectomy specimens are usually diagnostic with red pulp infiltrates of cells similar to those in the marrow. In addition, the cells tend to line splenic sinuses, obliterating the endothelium and producing red cell 'lakes' which lack visible endothelium. Lymph nodes may show paracortical infiltrates and liver may show sinus infiltration.

Cytochemically, these cells contain acid phosphatase, which is resistant to inhibition by tartrate (tartrate resistant acid phosphatase – TRAP); this is in contrast to the isoenzymes of acid phosphatase present in other hemic cells (Yam, 1971).

Immunophenotype is mature B cell (CD19, CD20, CD22, CD79a, DBA.44, surface membrane immunoglobulin [SMIg]) with expression of hairy cell-associated markers CD103, CD25, CD11c and FMC-7. Cyclin D1 is often expressed. Cells are negative for CD5, CD10 and CD23. Antibodies to annexin A1 (ANXA1) may also prove to be useful (Falini, 2004). Immunoglobulin heavy and light chain genes are rearranged, with somatic mutation of V gene regions. No specific genetic abnormalities are yet described.

The clinical course is usually chronic, but may be acute or subacute. The median survival is between 5–6 years. Traditionally, splenectomy has offered significant benefit to many patients. Treatment with alpha-interferon provided the first chemotherapy remissions, but 2'-deoxycoformycin and 2-chlordeoxyadenosine now produce more durable remissions.

Hairy Cell Variants

Most cases of 'hairy cell variant' are described as lymphoproliferative disorders resembling HCL but with high WBC and presence of prominent nucleoli (Sainati, 1990). These have morphology and clinical features intermediate between HCL and PLL (Fig. 32–46). Response to

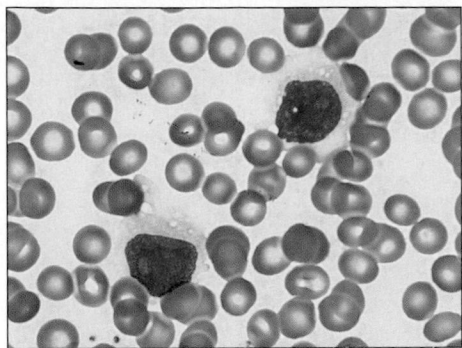

Figure 32–46 Hairy cell leukemia variant shows morphology intermediate between usual HCL and PLL.

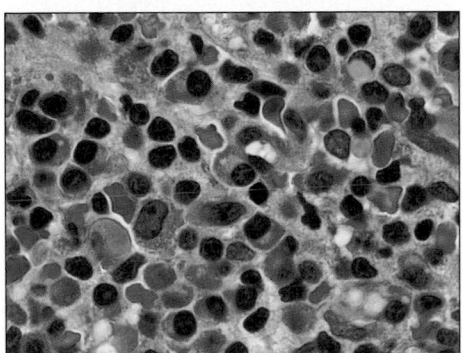

Figure 32–47 Lymphoplasmacytic lymphoma involving the marrow, with associated Waldenström's macroglobulinemia. Lymphocytes, plasma cells, plasmacytoid lymphocytes and a rare Dutcher body (upper right) (× 1000).

chemotherapy is poor but the clinical course is chronic, and remission may be attained with splenectomy. TRAP and CD103 are variable and CD25 is usually negative. A very rare form of variant HCL has been described, mostly in Japanese patients, and is referred to as 'Japanese variant' (Machii, 1993). This disorder shows slightly more prominent nucleoli than typical HCL, but less so than prolymphocytoid variants, also variable CD103 and TRAP, negative CD25 and usually lack of surface Ig (Wu, 2000; Yamaguchi, 1996). It shows clonal rearrangement of Ig genes and must be distinguished from polyclonal B cell lymphocytosis with similar morphology (Machii, 1997).

Lymphoplasmacytic Lymphoma (LPL)/Waldenström's Macroglobulinemia

Lymphoplasmacytic lymphoma is a term derived from the Kiel Classification (Stansfeld, 1988) for tumors that were known previously in North America as small lymphocytic lymphoma (or chronic lymphocytic leukemia) with plasmacytoid differentiation. These tumors differ, however, by the presence of plasmacytoid lymphocytes and plasma cells, secretion of a monoclonal IgM paraprotein, and lack of CD expression. They usually involve bone marrow, lymph nodes and spleen (Fig. 32–47).

Lymph nodes show diffuse infiltrates of lymphocytes, plasmacytoid lymphocytes and plasma cells. Proliferation centers are not present, and monocytoid B cells are not seen. The infiltrate may be paracortical with sparing of sinuses. PAS-positive inclusions are often seen in the cytoplasm and Golgi-centered inclusions frequently invaginate into the nucleus of the lymphoid cells, forming 'Dutcher bodies.' Tissue mast cells are frequently increased.

The bone marrow usually shows nodular and/or diffuse interstitial infiltrates of similar cells. Blood involvement may be present, but with lower WBC than CLL.

The immunophenotype shows B cell markers CD19, CD20, CD22, CD79a with bright surface and cytoplasmic IgM (occasionally IgG or IgA) but not IgD, and monoclonal kappa or lambda light chain. It differs from CLL by absence of CD5 and bright Ig expression. CD10 and CD23 are also negative, CD38 is positive and CD43 is variable.

Ig heavy and light chain genes are clonally rearranged and there is somatic mutation of variable regions, consistent with a post-antigen selection (post-germinal center) state of maturation and differing from CLL (Berger, 2001). Lymphoma with translocation t(9;14)(p13;q32) involving the PAX-5 gene at 9p13, which encodes B cell-specific activator

protein (BSAP), is most often lymphoplasmacytic (Offit, 1992; Iida, 1999).

A polymorphic morphologic variant with more aggressive course was described in the Kiel classification (Lennert, 1975) but is not recognized as a subtype by the WHO. Del6q21 is reported as the most frequent recurring abnormality in LPL, particularly with polymorphic morphology, and −8 as well as other abnormalities are sporadically reported (Schop, 2003; Mansoor, 2001).

The term Waldenström's macroglobulinemia refers to the clinical syndrome of monoclonal IgM paraprotein (> 3 g/dL) with symptomatic hyperviscosity and/or cryoglobulinemia. It has a peak incidence between ages 60–70. Symptoms of increased viscosity include visual disturbances, neurologic symptoms, impaired kidney function, and congestive heart failure. Hemorrhagic phenomena may occur due to interference of complexes with platelets and clotting factors. Cryoglobulinemia occurs somewhat more frequently than with myeloma and often results in Raynaud's phenomenon.

Normochromic, normocytic anemia is sometimes associated with thrombocytopenia or pancytopenia. Relative or slight absolute lymphocytosis is usually found. Marked rouleau formation is present on the blood film, and the sedimentation rate is usually extremely rapid, although it may be low if macrocryoglobulins are present and the test is carried out at a lower temperature. The anemia is occasionally hemolytic with a positive Coombs' test.

Serum globulin is usually markedly increased. The *relative serum viscosity* may be simply measured using an Ostwald viscometer. The average time for descent of the serum at room temperature is expressed as a ratio to that of distilled water. The normal range is 1.4–1.8. It is considerably elevated in most patients with macroglobulinemia. Symptoms of hyperviscosity appear in most patients when the relative serum viscosity is between 6–8, though the threshold varies among patients. The paraprotein is identified by *immunoelectrophoresis*. Light chain proteinuria occurs in about 10% of patients.

Many cases previously placed in this category are now felt to represent low-grade lymphoma of mucosal-associated lymphoid tissue (MALT) lymphoma with plasmacytoid expression. There is no definite biologic marker to separate the two, but MALT lymphomas typically involve epithelial organs, and macroglobulinemia is not the presenting feature. Many cases of cryoglobulinemia due to lymphoplasmacytic lymphoma and MALT lymphoma are associated with hepatitis C virus (Sansonno, 1996).

Gamma Heavy Chain Disease

A small number of patients produce and excrete heavy chain fragments without associated light chains. Some of these proteins show structural mutations. The classification of associated lymphoproliferative disorders is somewhat ambiguous. The WHO categorizes gamma heavy chain disease both with LPL and myeloma (Berger, 2001); mu and alpha heavy chain disease with myeloma (Grogan, 2001).

Gamma heavy chain disease (HCD) is a lymphoproliferative disorder characterized by secretion of a truncated gamma chain without light chain binding sites. It presents with lymphadenopathy, hepatosplenomegaly, fever, and propensity to infections. Anemia is constantly present, often with leukopenia and thrombocytopenia. Atypical lymphocytes or plasma cells are frequently present in the blood, and a few cases have terminated in plasma cell leukemia. The marrow is usually abnormal, with increased plasma cells, lymphocytes and eosinophils. A rather broad serum protein 'spike' has been found in the βγ region in most patients, accompanied by hypogammaglobulinemia. The diagnosis is made by showing that the protein reacts on immunoelectrophoresis with antisera to gamma chains but not to light chains. The protein is also found in the urine in varying amounts, though concentration techniques may be necessary to demonstrate it.

Alpha Heavy Chain Disease

Alpha heavy chain disease appears to be more common than gamma-HCD, and involves a younger age group. The uniform clinical pattern in most patients is malabsorption and diarrhea accompanying a massive lymphoplasmacytic infiltration of intestinal mucosa, or a histiocytic lymphoma of the intestine. In a few patients, the respiratory tract has been involved instead. Bone marrow and other lymphoid organs have not been involved. Usually, routine protein electrophoresis is negative, but small amounts of alpha-chain may be detected in the serum and sometimes in the urine with immunoelectrophoresis. The abnormal protein does not contain light chains. It is most common in Mediterranean areas and is associated with poor living conditions in low socioeconomic groups. Similar to MALT lymphoma, many cases may initiate an infectious antigen-driven proliferation. It has also been referred to as Mediterranean abdominal lymphoma and immunoproliferative small intestinal disease (IPSID).

IV

The few patients who have been described with mu heavy chain disease have had chronic lymphocytic leukemia with vacuolated plasma cells in the marrow. Routine serum electrophoresis showed only hypogammaglobulinemia. The mu heavy chain was detected by serum immunoelectrophoresis; it was not found in the urine. In most patients, however, the urine contained kappa light chain in large amounts (Franklin, 1975).

Multiple Myeloma

Multiple myeloma is a neoplastic proliferation of plasma cells, primarily occurring in the bone marrow. Though plasma cells also proliferate in lymph nodes and spleen, these organs are rarely enlarged (Grogan, 2001).

Multiple myeloma is rare under age 40. The mean age at the time of diagnosis is 62 years with an equal sex distribution. Bone pain is the most common symptom, and pathologic fractures are frequent. Neurologic symptoms may be prominent from encroachment of tumor that has broken through the bony cortex on spinal nerves or spinal cord. Bone destruction leads to calcium mobilization, with increase of calcium in the serum and metastatic calcification. The growth of myeloma cells in the marrow produces multiple tumors, which appear on X-ray as multiple punched-out osteoporotic lesions; occasionally the growth is diffuse and appears as diffuse osteoporosis. A propensity to infection is common because of impaired production of antibodies. There may be an association of plasma cell disorders with human herpesvirus type 8 (HHV-8).

There is usually a normochromic, normocytic anemia and normoblasts may be present in the blood. The leukocyte count is slightly decreased, normal, or slightly increased. Myeloid left shift occasionally to the myeloblast may be found. The platelet count is usually normal, but may be decreased. The most striking feature of the blood film is the marked degree of rouleau formation.

The bone marrow shows the presence of plasma cells or myeloma cells, varying from less than 1% to over 90%, depending on the degree of involvement in the site of the marrow aspirated. Diagnosis of myeloma and its variants is based on both pathology and clinical findings, including serum monoclonal immunoglobulin and radiologic evidence of lytic bone lesions (Durie, 2003; Grogan, 2001) (Table 32–18). Lytic bone lesions are associated with increased osteoclastic activity, hypercalcemia and neurologic changes. This may be related to activity of the receptor activator for NF kappaB (RANK) ligand (Sezer, 2003) and has stimulated interest in its receptor, osteoprotegerin (OPG).

Cytologically, the cells may be indistinguishable from normal plasma cells, but they usually show abnormal chromatin, such as less clumping of nuclear chromatin, large nucleoli, lack of perinuclear clear zone, lighter blue cytoplasm, or varying degrees of anaplasia (Fig. 32–48). Immature, plasmablastic and anaplastic variants are described.

Serum globulin is usually increased, often strikingly so. This increase is responsible for the tendency toward rouleau formation and an elevated ESR. Serum protein electrophoresis usually shows an M-spot, a homogeneous band in the gamma- or beta-region; less commonly, there is hypogammaglobulinemia (when only light chains are produced by the neoplastic plasma cells). Immunoelectrophoresis indicates that the monoclonal protein is IgG in over half the cases, IgA in about one-fifth, IgD in less than 1%, and IgE very rarely. Roughly 5% of myeloma proteins are cryoglobulins – that is, proteins that precipitate from cooled serum and redissolve on warming. Some tumors secrete free monoclonal light chains (Bence Jones protein) in addition to the whole immunoglobulin molecule, and in about one-quarter, only light chains are produced. Hypogammaglobulinemia is found in the latter group because light chains are filtered through the renal glomerulus, leaving little or none in the serum, in addition to the fact that immunoglobulin production by the nonmalignant plasma cells is greatly reduced. If renal damage has occurred, albumin and whole immunoglobulin molecules are also found in the urine. Excretion of light chains sometimes results in obstruction and loss of nephrons, and the so-called myeloma kidney. Renal insufficiency is common and is the presenting feature of multiple myeloma in some cases. Amyloidosis, which is present in about 10–15% of cases of multiple myeloma, may be a factor in the renal failure.

Median survival after diagnosis of multiple myeloma is approximately 3 years. In almost 5% of patients, acute leukemia develops (usually myelomonocytic). This may be preceded by sideroblastic anemia.

Monoclonal Gammopathy of Undetermined Significance

Monoclonal gammopathy of undetermined significance is the term utilized when a monoclonal serum immunoglobulin is present but there is no detectable myeloma. Most (75%) are IgG, with smaller proportions

Table 32–18 Diagnostic Criteria for Plasma Cell Myeloma and for Monoclonal Gammopathy of Undetermined Significance (MGUS), Indolent and Smoldering Myeloma

Major criteria for plasma cell myeloma	Minor criteria for plasma cell myeloma
A. Marrow plasmacytosis (> 30%)	1. Marrow plasmacytosis (10–30%)
B. Plasmacytoma on biopsy	2. M-component: present but less than for C
C. M-component	3. Lytic bone lesions
Serum: IgG > 3.5 g/dL, IgA > 2 g/dL	4. Reduced normal immunoglobulins (< 50% normal):
Urine: > 1 g/24 h of Bence-Jones (BJ) protein	IgG < 600 mg/dL, IgA < 100 mg/dL, IgM < 50 mg/dL

Myeloma

One major and one minor criterion or three minor criteria which must include 1 and 2, in symptomatic patient

MGUS

M-component present, but less than myeloma levels

Marrow plasmacytosis < 10%

No lytic bone lesions

No myeloma-related symptoms

Smoldering myeloma

Same as MGUS except:

Serum M-component at myelomas levels

Marrow plasmacytosis 10–30%

Indolent myelomas

Same as myeloma except:

M-component: IgG < 7 g/dL, IgA < 5 g/dL

Rare bone lesions (≤ 3 lytic lesions), without compression fractures

Normal hemoglobin, serum calcium and creatinine

No infections

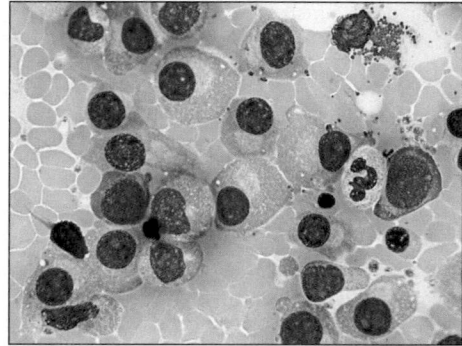

Figure 32–48 Myeloma in the bone marrow showing large plasma cells with nucleoli (× 1000).

of IgM (15%) and IgA (10%). Twenty-five percent progress to myeloma over a 20-year follow-up (Grogan, 2001). There is a monoclonal Ig (M-component) of < 3.5 g/dL IgG or < 2 g/dL IgA, or < 1 g/dL urine light chain (Bence Jones protein) (Table 32–18).

Smoldering and Indolent Myeloma

Smoldering myeloma shows 30% or more plasma cells in the marrow, > 3.5 g/dL IgG or > 2 g/dL IgA, or > 1 g/dL urine light chain (Bence Jones protein), but no lytic lesions and no myeloma symptoms including anemia, renal insufficiency or hypercalcemia.

Indolent myeloma is similar but with up to three lytic bone lesions, up to 7 g/dL IgG or 5 g/dL IgA.

Plasma Cell Leukemia

Often in multiple myeloma a few plasma cells are found in the peripheral blood. Only in the rare instances of myeloma in which large numbers of plasma cells circulate (either > 20% of blood leukocytes or > 2 × 10⁹/L) is the term plasma cell leukemia used (Fig. 32–49). Patients with plasma cell

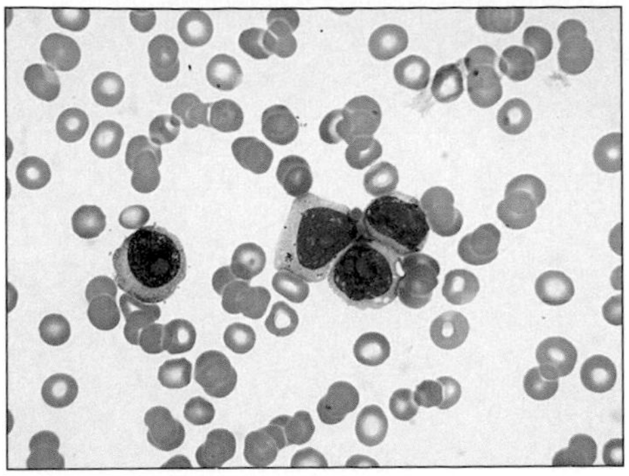

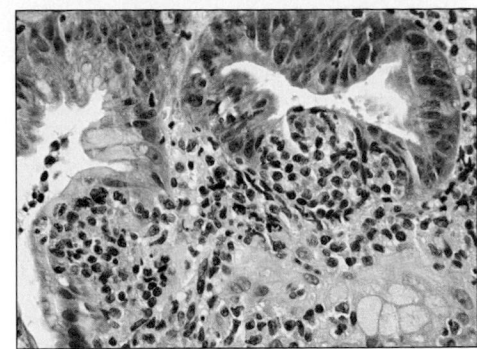

Figure 32–49 Plasma cell leukemia with cells resembling immunoblasts (×1000).

Figure 32–50 MALT lymphoma with nests in lymphocytes in gastric epithelium (×500).

leukemia tend to have tissue infiltration, advanced stage disease, and poor survival (Woodruff, 1978).

The immunophenotype of neoplastic plasma cells varies slightly from normal plasma cells and can be utilized for flow cytometric detection. CD19 and CD20 are usually absent or dim (CD19 is present on normal plasma cells) and CD56 is usually expressed in myeloma, but not in plasma cell leukemia. CD38 and CD138 are expressed. Monoclonal cytoplasmic immunoglobulin is present and occasionally surface Ig as well. CD45 is variable. When utilizing flow cytometry, plasma cells can be identified for gating by coexpression of CD38 and CD138, with subsequent analysis of CD56. CD56 strongly positive plasma cells are presumptively neoplastic, and usually show monoclonal cytoplasmic kappa or lambda. Immunohistochemical labeling or mRNA in-situ hybridization of bone marrow sections for kappa and lambda usually identifies monoclonal plasma cells.

Cytogenetic studies were hampered in the past by lack of mitoses in these terminally differentiated plasma cells. Panels of FISH assays, however, frequently show abnormalities (Cady, 2004). Monosomy or partial deletion of 13q14 occurs in 15–40%, del(17)(p13) (*p53* gene) in 25%. The latter, as well as del(7q) (multidrug resistance) are likely adverse features. Gains of chromosomes 3, 5, 7, 9, 11, 15, and 19, and losses of 8, 13, 14 and X are common, and t(11;14)(q13;q32) may be present with resultant cyclin D1 overexpression.

Solitary plasmacytomas occurring in bone are treated with radiation but have a high incidence of progression to myeloma, with occasional solitary recurrence. Extramedullary solitary plasmacytomas occur in GI tract, bladder, CNS, breast, thyroid, testis, parotid gland, lymph nodes or skin, and are also irradiated. They recur in one-quarter of patients but progress to myeloma in only about 15%.

Primary amyloidosis is an uncommon presentation of plasma cell neoplasms of various types and results from abnormal polymerization of immunoglobulin into beta-pleated sheets in connective tissue. It may be detected by homogeneous pink staining of thickened blood vessels in abdominal fat, bone marrow, rectum or other tissues, using Congo Red stain with characteristic apple-green birefringence under polarized light. It may involve the heart with subsequent congestive failure, liver with hepatomegaly, kidney with nephrotic syndrome or renal failure, nerves with sensory/motor loss and other organs.

Non-amyloid immunoglobulin deposition may result in organ dysfunction in rare disorders known as light chain deposition disease (LCDD) or heavy chain deposition disease (HCDD) (Grogan, 2001).

Marginal Zone B Cell Lymphomas

Marginal zone lymphomas are clonal B cell disorders previously included under the terminology of SLL (Isaacson, 2001a,b,c,d). They differ both clinically and immunologically from SLL and include several types, which share relatively slow clinical courses and presence of variable numbers of small lymphocytes with abundant cytoplasm, centrocytes (small cells with irregular nuclei), and plasma cells. Many arise in mucosal-associated lymphoid tissue (MALT) of the GI tract, salivary glands, lungs, and other epithelial organs. Others arise in the splenic marginal zones and some may be primary in lymph nodes.

Extranodal Marginal Zone B Cell Lymphoma of Mucosal-Associated Lymphoid Tissue (MALT)

Extranodal marginal zone B cell lymphoma of mucosal-associated lymphoid tissue (MALT) is an indolent lymphoma of mucosal tissue including stomach, other GI tract, bronchi, salivary glands, thyroid, skin and other areas. MALT lymphoma of the stomach is in many cases an antigen-driven clonal

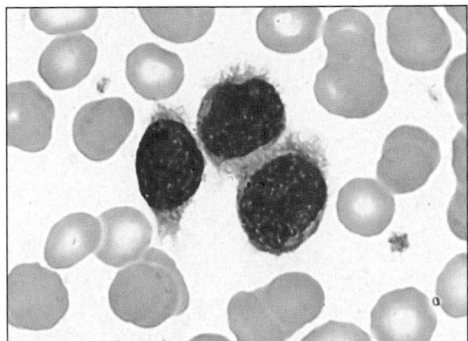

Figure 32–51 Villous lymphocytes.

B cell proliferation related to infection by *Helicobacter pylori*, which is also associated with gastric ulcers, and early cases may respond to antibacterial therapy. Other patients have autoimmune disorders such as Sjögren's syndrome or Hashimoto's thyroiditis. The terminology of MALT lymphomas refers only to those of predominantly small cells, although large cell and other aggressive lymphomas also may arise in the same tissues.

Gastric or other mucosa is infiltrated by small lymphocytes that form clusters within the epithelium referred to as lymphoepithelial lesions (Fig. 32–50). Submucosa contains diffuse infiltrates of small lymphocytes, centrocytes, monocytoid lymphocytes, and plasma cells. Germinal centers, apparently reactive to the entire process, are usually present. Plasma cells are often abundant at the periphery of the lesions and generally are monoclonal.

The immunophenotype is B cell (CD19, CD20, CD22, CD79a) with surface Ig. CD5, CD10, bcl-6 and usually CD23 are negative. Bcl-2 is frequently positive, as are marginal zone and dendritic cell-associated markers CD21 and CD35, and CD43 is variable (Isaacson, 2001b).

Immunoglobulin genes are clonally rearranged with somatic mutations of V regions. Trisomy 3 is present in 60% and t(11;18)(q21;q21), involving the apoptosis inhibiting gene *API2* with MLT at 18q21, in 25–50%. t(1;14)(p22;q32) and t(14;18)(q32;q21) are also described, with activation of NF-kappaB-mediated antiapoptotic pathways (Gascoyne, 2003).

Splenic Marginal Zone Lymphoma (SMZL)

This is a disorder with many clinical, laboratory, and morphologic features similar to HCL, and features similar to SLL/CLL (Isaacson, 2001d). It has been referred to as splenic lymphoma with circulating villous lymphocytes. The disease is more common in men than in women. Patients are often in their seventh decade of life and present with splenomegaly. In contrast to HCL, the leukocyte count is elevated. Some patients (~1/3) show a small monoclonal gammopathy, usually IgM. The neoplastic cells are of medium size with clumped chromatin, moderately basophilic cytoplasm, and short cytoplasmic villi, often with a polar distribution (Fig. 32–51). The bone marrow may demonstrate patchy infiltrates or massive involvement. Neoplastic cells may circulate in the blood even in the absence of marrow involvement.

In the spleen, the neoplastic infiltrate expands from the white pulp into the red pulp. The tumor arises from splenic marginal zones, which in reactive processes are seen as an outer zone of pale lymphocytes with moderately abundant cytoplasm surrounding the white pulp and

IV

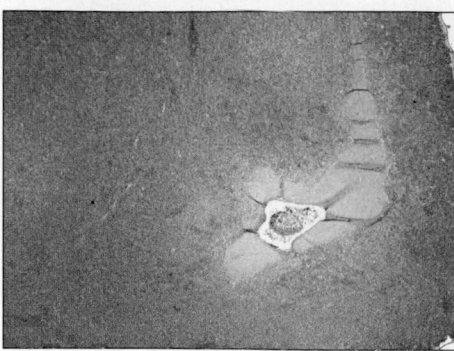

Figure 32–52 Splenic marginal zone lymphoma showing mild white pulp expansion and patchy red pulp involvement (×100).

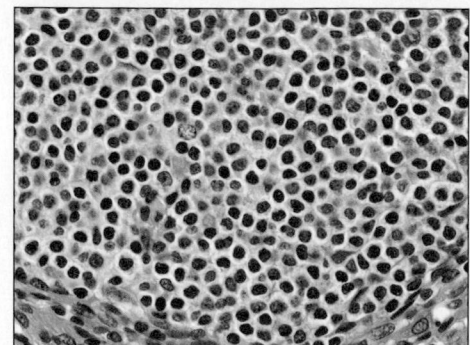

Figure 32–54 Nodal marginal zone lymphoma showing a nodule of monocytoid B cells (×200).

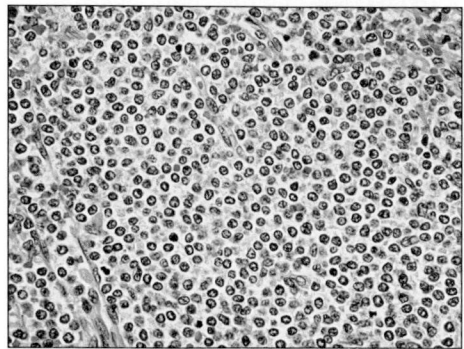

Figure 32–53 Higher-power view of splenic red pulp involvement by monocytoid splenic marginal zone cells in splenic marginal zone lymphoma (×200).

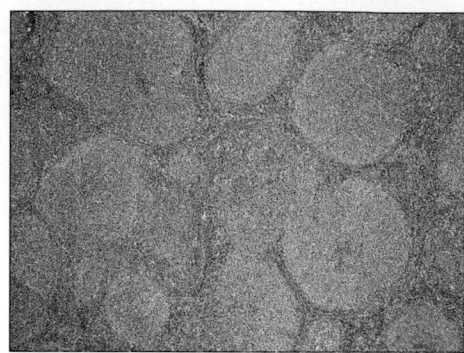

Figure 32–55 Low-power view of follicular lymphoma, recapitulating lymph node germinal centers (×200).

imparting a target-like appearance. In some cases, reactive follicles with germinal centers are present and an expanded marginal zone surrounds the white pulp and involves the red pulp. Marginal zone hyperplasia may mimic this disorder. Other cases show predominantly red pulp involvement (Figs 32–52 and 32–53). Red cell lakes are not present. Lymph nodes are not characteristically involved. The tartrate-resistant acid phosphatase (TRAP) stain is usually negative, although positive reactions have been recorded.

The immunophenotype is mature B cell with surface IgM and IgD (similar to SLL/CLL), CD20 and CD79 are positive. CD5, CD10, CD23, cyclin D1, CD103 and CD43 are characteristically negative.

Immunoglobulin genes are clonally rearranged with somatic mutations. Translocation at 7q21-32 is noted in 40% of cases, but trisomy 3 and t(11;18) seen in extranodal marginal zone lymphomas of MALT are unusual (Dogan, 2003). Bcl-2 is variable, typically expressed according to some studies (Pawade, 1995) but not others (Menendez, 2004). Hepatitis C may play a role in the pathogenesis in some cases (Iannitto, 2004; Kelaidi, 2004; Weng, 2003).

SMZL is indolent but has shown poor response to therapy. New approaches utilizing chemotherapy combined with anti-CD20 therapy appear promising (Arcaini, 2004).

Nodal Marginal Zone Lymphoma

These have been called 'monocytoid B cell lymphoma' and may resemble either nodal involvement by MALT lymphoma or splenic marginal zone lymphoma (Fig. 32–54). The rarity of this tumor (1.8% of lymphoid neoplasms) and the presence of unsuspected extranodal involvement in up to one-third of cases (Isaacson, 2001c) raises the possibility that it is not distinct from other forms of MZL.

The immunophenotype is similar to MALT or SMZL, with surface Ig (IgM/IgD, IgM, less often IgA or IgG), B cell markers (CD19, CD20, CD22, CD79a), expression of CD23, variable CD43, and absence of CD5 or CD10. Bcl-2 is expressed in a majority of cases and survivin overexpressed in about 50%, suggesting activation of antiapoptotic pathways. Nodal MZL is heterogeneous at the molecular and immunohistochemical levels (Camacho, 2003). Ig heavy and (monotypic) light chain genes are rearranged. Trisomy 3 and t(1;18) are infrequent.

Follicular Lymphoma

Follicular lymphoma (FL) is a group of related lymphomas of germinal center-derived B cells. Morphologic distinction between the subgroups is

based on the number of centroblasts in the neoplastic follicles (Nathwani, 2001).

The overall morphologic pattern (Fig. 32–55) is recapitulation of lymph node follicles, but with limited diversity of cell type and lack of proliferation of other lymph node structures. The tumors generally show crowded follicles of more than usual uniformity, lacking distinct mantles and with little intervening paracortex, and lacking normal germinal center 'tingible body' macrophages and polarization. Most often, small irregular cells (small cleaved cells or centrocytes) predominate with variable numbers of admixed large cells (large cleaved and noncleaved cells or centroblasts). There may be diffuse infiltrates as well. The term 'follicular' indicates a greater than 75% follicular pattern; 'follicular and diffuse' refers to cases that are 25–75% follicular; and 'diffuse' refers to cases with less than 25% follicular pattern (see Table 32–19).

Cytologic grading is based on the average number of centroblasts (CB) per high-power field (hpf) within neoplastic follicles (Figs 32–56 and 32–57). A hpf is defined as that with a 40× lens and an ocular with an 18 mm field of view. Using a 40× lens with a 20 mm 10× ocular requires a downward adjustment of a factor of 1.2, while a 50× lens with a 22 mm 10× ocular, often used in wet hematology, provides a nearly equivalent field of view, albeit with higher resolution.

Marginal zone or monocytoid B cell differentiation occurs in up to 10% of cases. It usually appears around follicles and in interfollicular areas and resembles a composite lymphoma. FL shows an immunophenotype of mature B cells with bright monoclonal surface Ig, CD19, CD20, CD22, CD23, CD79a and CD10 expression. Bcl-2 (cytoplasmic) and bcl-6 (nuclear) are both usually expressed, which help separate FL from reactive hyperplasia (bcl-2-negative/bcl-6-positive) and other lymphomas not of germinal center cell (GCC) derivation (bcl-6-negative). CD5 and CD43 are typically absent.

IgH is clonally rearranged along with a light chain Ig gene and there is t(14;18)(q32;q21) with juxtaposition of IgH and *BCL-2*. Bcl-2 protein is inappropriately expressed and subsequent inhibition of apoptosis is considered a primary pathogenic mechanism of FL. Standard PCR assays are relatively insensitive for IgH and t(14;18) because only 75% of IgH breakpoints are in the major breakpoint region (MBR) or minor cluster region (mcr) targeted by standard primers. Quantitative real-time PCR and FISH assays provide improved sensitivity (Jiang, 2002; Jenner, 2002). Other abnormalities may be seen including a variant Bcl-2 rearrangement, t(2;18)(p12;q21), 6q23-36 abnormalities and deletions/abnormalities of 9p or 17p13 involving *TP53* (both associated with large cell

Table 32–19 Follicular Lymphoma: Grading and Variants

Grading	Definition
Grade 1	0–5 centroblasts per hpf*
Grade 2	6–15 centroblasts per hpf*
Grade 3	> 15 centroblasts per hpf*
3a	Centrocytes present
3b	Solid sheets of centroblasts

Reporting of pattern	Proportion follicular
Follicular	> 75%
Follicular and diffuse	25–75%†
Focally follicular	< 25%†

Follicular lymphoma: variants	
Diffuse follicle center lymphoma	
Grade 1	0–5 centroblasts/hpf*
Grade 2	6–15 centroblasts/hpf*
Cutaneous follicle center lymphoma	

* hpf = high-power field of 0.159 mm² (40× objective, 18-mm field of view ocular; count 10 hpf and divide by 10).

If using a 10-mm field of view ocular, count 8 hpf and divide by 10, or count 10 hpf and divide by 12 to get the number of centroblasts/0.159 mm² hpf.

If using a 22-mm field of view ocular, count 7 hpf and divide by 10, or count 10 hpf and divide by 15 to get the number of centroblasts/0.159 mm² hpf.

† Give approximate % in report.

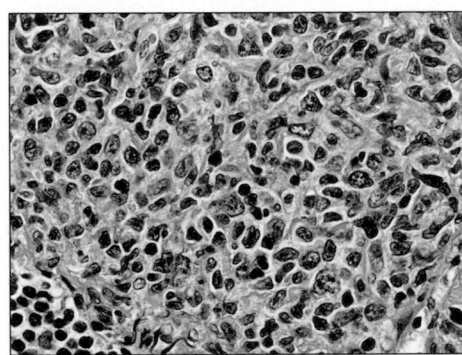

Figure 32–56 Follicular lymphoma, grade 2, showing centrocytes with 5–15 centroblasts per high-power field (hpf). Grade 1 shows < 5 centroblasts per hpf.

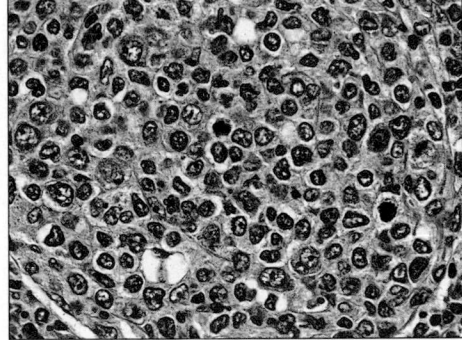

Figure 32–57 Follicular lymphoma, grade 3a, shows centrocytes with > 15 centroblasts per hpf (× 500).

transformation), rearrangements or mutations of *BCL-6* at 3q27, and abnormalities of X, 1, 2, 4, 5, 7, 12, 13, and 18 (Nathwani, 2001).

Prognosis is variable, with grade 1 and 2 disease generally showing an indolent course but lack of cure. Grade 3 is more aggressive but likely more curable. Attempts to identify patients requiring aggressive therapy has led to a follicular lymphoma international prognostic index (FLIPI) (Solal-Celigny, 2004) based on age, stage, hemoglobin, number of nodal areas involved and LDH, which appears to be valid at least for FL in first relapse (Montoto, 2004).

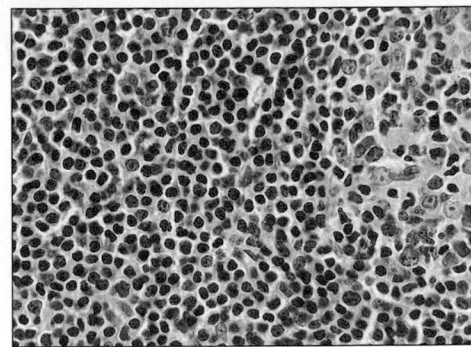

Figure 32–58 Mantle cell lymphoma, showing an expanded mantle around residual germinal center.

Diffuse Follicle Center (Centre) Lymphoma

Diffuse follicle center (centre) lymphoma is essentially a diffuse transformation of grade 1 or 2 FL. Diagnosis requires phenotyping to rule out mantle cell or marginal zone lymphoma, and includes previous categories of diffuse small cleaved cell, centrocytic diffuse, diffuse mixed small cleaved and large cell and centrocytic/centroblastic diffuse. The current nomenclature is 'follicular lymphoma, grade 1 (or 2), predominantly diffuse.'

Diffuse large B cell lymphoma (DLBCL) is considered by WHO authors to be a different entity even when it arises in FL (Nathwani, 2001). In these situations, two diagnoses are recommended, such as 'follicular lymphoma, grade 3/3 (75%), with diffuse large B cell lymphoma (25%),' when the DLBCL occupies 25% of the sampled tumor. Leukemic involvement by FL may also occur and is known as 'lymphosarcoma cell leukemia.' Flow cytometry is helpful to distinguish between that, CLL, and leukemic mantle cell or marginal zone lymphomas.

Mantle Cell Lymphoma

Since the REAL classification was published, it has become recognized that mantle cell lymphoma (MCL) is a dangerous form of lymphoma that combines refractoriness to therapy with an aggressive clinical course, and poor survival (ILSG, 1997). Refractoriness is likely due in part to strong expression of Bcl-2 also seen in normal mantle cells, follicular lymphomas and some other leukemias, lymphomas, and solid tumors (Korsmeyer, 1999). Bcl-2 inhibits apoptotic pathways exploited by many chemotherapies.

The tumor usually shows a diffuse or sometimes mantle zone pattern (Swerdlow, 2001). In the mantle zone pattern, atrophic germinal centers are often seen in the center of nodules, and these may also be seen as occasional small naked follicles within a diffuse infiltrate. Nuclei are small to medium size with clumped to moderately dispersed chromatin and a moderately increased mitotic rate. Nuclear membranes are typically slightly irregular with occasional small round and cleaved nuclei also present. Scattered histiocytes with lightly eosinophilic cytoplasm are often present. A blastic or 'blastoid' variant shows slightly larger nuclei with blast-like chromatin and higher mitotic rate simulating lymphoblastic lymphoma (Fig. 32–58).

These are monoclonal (monotypic surface IgM and IgD) B cells (CD19, CD20, CD22) with characteristic coexpression of CD5 (and CD43) and absence of CD23. Bcl-2 and cyclin-D1 are expressed while bcl-6 and CD10 are negative. Rare cases occur without CD5 expression (Liu, 2002).

Immunoglobulin heavy and (monotypic) light chain genes are rearranged. The majority of cases have t(11;14)(q13;q32) involving the Ig heavy chain gene and *bcl-1* with overexpression of *PRAD-1* which encodes cyclin-D1. In diagnostic laboratories, many cases do not show demonstrable *bcl-1* translocation by PCR and cyclin-D1 expression may not be detected for technical reasons. FISH assay, which may be performed from fresh cell suspensions, nuclei extracted from paraffin or, in some cases, thin sections from paraffin blocks, is usually confirmatory. Complex karyotype is often seen in advanced or blastoid cases and secondary 8q24 abnormalities are associated with blastic/blastoid morphology and leukemic presentation (Au, 2002; Hao, 2002; Viswanatha, 2000). *BCL-2* rearrangements are absent.

Diffuse Large B Cell Lymphoma

DLBCL is a simplified category which includes a variety of morphologies, all of which share diffuse pattern, large cells and mature B cell phenotype (Gatter, 2001a). It occurs in both nodal and extranodal sites, and at all ages. It is frequent in immunosuppressed patients, often in association with EBV, and is the most common lymphoma of the CNS. The various

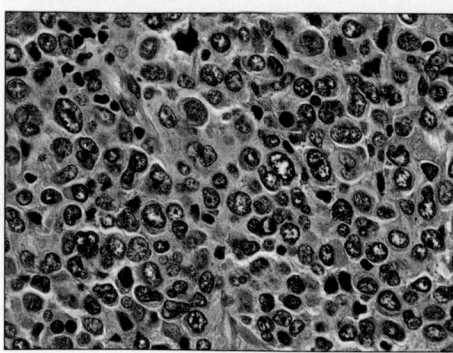

Figure 32–59 Diffuse large B cell lymphoma with centroblasts and admixed centrocytes (× 500).

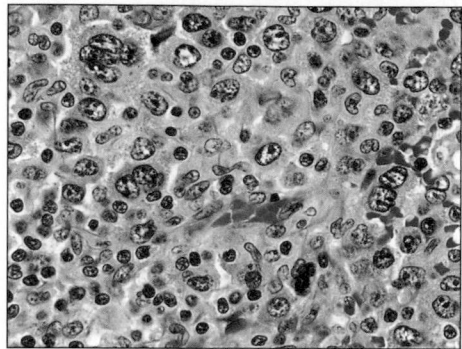

Figure 32–60 Diffuse large B cell lymphoma, with polymorphism and Reed–Sternberg-like cells (× 1000).

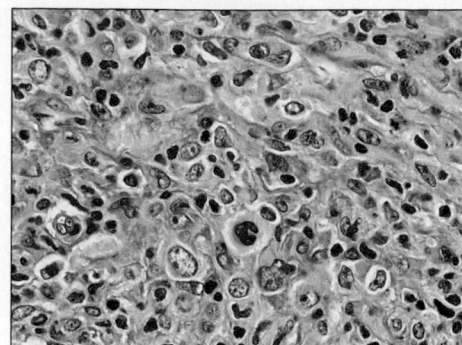

Figure 32–61 Mediastinal large B cell lymphoma with sclerosis (× 500).

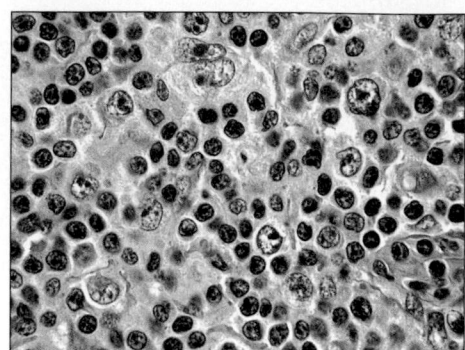

Figure 32–62 T cell and histiocyte-rich large B cell lymphoma resembles lymphocyte predominant Hodgkin lymphoma, but the majority of small cells are T cells (× 500).

morphologies are mimicked by peripheral T cell lymphomas, and phenotyping is required for diagnosis.

DLBCL presents with diffuse infiltration by large B cells (nuclei larger than histiocyte or endothelial cell nuclei) with variable morphology. They may be centroblasts and/or centrocytes with scant cytoplasm and multiple nucleoli (*centroblastic* morphologic variant) (Fig. 32–59). Some cases show plasmacytoid immunoblasts with large nuclei, one (or more) prominent nucleoli, and abundant amphophilic cytoplasm that may be eccentric (*immunoblastic* variant). *Plasmablastic lymphoma* resembles this variant, but expresses plasma cell antigens CD38 and CD138, occurs primarily in the oral cavity of HIV patients, and is associated with EBV. It has an aggressive behavior. Other cases of DLBCL show polymorphic cell morphology with large and small cells, and Reed–Sternberg-like giant cells (*anaplastic* variant) (Fig. 32–60). Still others occasionally show large cells with clear cytoplasm.

Neoplastic cells show surface Ig, sometimes cytoplasmic Ig, and B cell markers (CD19, CD20, CD22, CD79a). CD30 is occasionally present in variable numbers of cells. CD20 expression by immunohistochemistry (IHC) is usually very helpful in paraffin-section diagnosis, as flow cytometry may be hampered for technical reasons by the large cell size.

In DLBLC, Ig heavy and (monotypic) light chain genes are rearranged. *Bcl-2* and/or *bcl-6* abnormalities and protein expression are frequent (Skinnider, 1999; Capello, 2000).

Diffuse large B cell lymphomas with expression of full length ALK protein resemble T cell anaplastic large cell lymphoma (ALCL) in morphology and expression of CD30 and ALK, but lack t(2;5) and NPM-ALK fusion protein. A very rare variant of ALCL, with clathrin gene involvement (CLTL-ALK), shows B cell derivation with expression of CD79a but absent CD20.

Gene array studies have separated DLBCL into at least four major expression groups; GCC-like, activated B cell (ABC)-like, type 3, and mediastinal large B cell lymphoma (Rosenwald, 2002, 2003; Savage, 2003). Of the first three, GCC-like shows better response to therapy than ABC or type 3. *BCL-2* and *BCL-6* are in the gene cluster of GCC-like tumors, and may be surrogates for this category. In the GCC category, cases with t(14;18) show lower proliferation but do not differ in outcome by treatment (Iqbal, 2004). Bcl-2 protein is associated with resistance to apoptosis and chemotherapy, but that may be overcome with humanized monoclonal anti-CD20 (Mounier, 2003).

Mediastinal (Thymic) Large B Cell Lymphoma

Mediastinal (thymic) large B cell lymphoma (MLBCL) often appears in young adulthood to middle age and is more frequent in women.

Histology is variable, but diffuse or compartmentalizing sclerosis is frequent, and clear cells, multilobated cells, or Reed–Sternberg-like cells may be present (Fig. 32–61). Symptoms are often related to the location, with airway compression or superior vena cava syndrome, and often local invasion and local recurrence after therapy. CD45, CD19 and CD20 are expressed, but not CD5 or CD10 (Banks, 2001a). CD30 is expressed in some cases but not with the phenotype of classical HL. Ig genes are clonally rearranged; IgV and Bcl-6 gene hypermutations are consistent with GCC cell derivation but occur similarly to normal thymic B cells (Csernus, 2004). Gene expression array analysis shows MLBCL to be similar to classical HL (Savage, 2003). A majority of patients respond to standard CHOP chemotherapy, but long-term survival may be better with more aggressive approaches (Andreopoulou, 2004; Zinzani, 2002).

T Cell/Histiocyte Rich Large B Cell Lymphoma

T cell/histiocyte rich large B cell lymphoma (TCHRLBCL) variant is very difficult to distinguish from lymphocyte predominant HL (LPHL), but the distinction is important as this is a usually aggressive tumor which presents with advanced stage, while LPHL is often localized, indolent and requires less therapy. TCHRLBCL exhibits a diffuse infiltrate of large B cells which may appear as centroblasts or immunoblasts or resemble lymphocyte and histiocytic (L&H) cells of LPHL, and include Reed–Sternberg-like cells (Fig. 32–62). Large B cells constitute 10% or less of total cells, while T cells constitute the majority. The phenotype is similar to LPHL, with CD20, CD79a, and EMA positivity. J-chain, Oct-2 and Bob-1 are also expressed. Surface/cytoplasmic Ig, if monoclonal, is somewhat helpful, but LPHL is also now considered a clonal B cell disease. The primary distinctions are the diffuse infiltrate, T cell background, lack of CD3/CD57 rosettes around neoplastic cells in a nodular B cell background as seen in nodular LPHL, and advanced-stage presentation.

Intravascular Large B Cell Lymphoma

Intravascular large B cell lymphoma is a rare tumor which is largely restricted to the intravascular lumina of small vessels (Gatter, 2001b). It is very aggressive, widely disseminated at diagnosis, and often undiagnosed until autopsy. The findings are often hemorrhage, thrombosis and/or necrosis of tissues throughout the body, with tumor only inconspicuously present in the small vessels. B cell markers are expressed (CD19, CD20, CD22, D79a) and CD5 in some. Clonal Ig gene rearrangements are present with somatic hypermutation consistent with post-GCC derivation (Kanda, 2001). Rare T cell cases are described (Merchant, 2003). Vascular

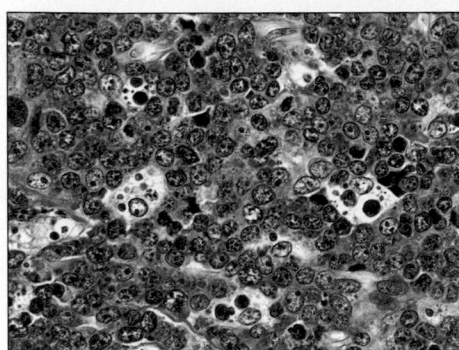

Figure 32–63 Burkitt lymphoma (× 500).

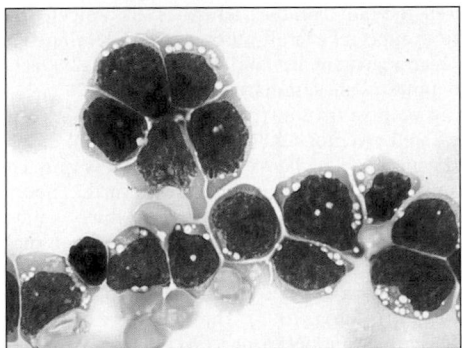

Figure 32–64 Burkitt lymphoma cytology (× 1000).

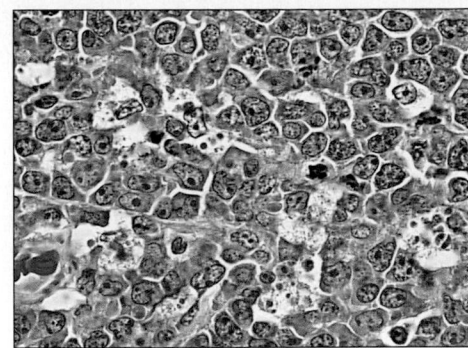

Figure 32–65 Atypical Burkitt, or Burkitt-like lymphoma, with moderate pleomorphism and increased number of prominent nucleoli (× 500).

show lack of surface membrane immunoglobulin (SMIg) or expression of TdT, and these require cytogenetic confirmation. Burkitt leukemia/lymphomas show very high proliferative rates and rapid disease progression. While they are rapidly fatal if untreated, recent results of therapy in pediatric patients have shown long-term survival of better than 90% (Patte, 2001). Outcome in adults has also improved, but long-term survival is less than in children (50–70%) (Kasamon, 2004; Blum, 2004).

Burkitt leukemia/lymphoma shows characteristic cytogenetic abnormalities consisting of translocation of c-myc on chromosome region 8q24 to one of the immunoglobulin genes (heavy chain-14q32, kappa –2q11, or lambda 22q11) to give t(8;14), t(2;8), or t(8;22). Most cases show t(8;14)(q24;q32). C-myc promotes both proliferation and apoptosis (Le Beau, 2000), and presumably causes uncontrolled proliferation of immunoglobulin-bearing B cells. These cells are sensitive to chemotherapy, however.

Atypical Burkitt Lymphoma (aBL)

Cases of lymphoma occur with histologic and clinical features intermediate between Burkitt and large B cell lymphoma. The histology is similar to BL, except that there is generally more pleomorphism with presence of large cells (up to 25%) as well as medium size cells and with greater irregularity of nuclei and more prominent nucleoli than typical Burkitt (Fig. 32–65). Cytoplasm is usually less distinct than in BL.

Previously called Burkitt-like or non-Burkitt lymphoma, some cases were found to have bcl-2 and not c-myc abnormalities (Yano, 1992). The REAL classification placed most cases with this histology in the category of diffuse large B cell lymphoma.

In children, the clinical presentation of aBL is similar to Burkitt (Hutchison, 1989) though cytogenetic studies do not show c-myc translocations (Lones, 2004). In adults, bcl-2 along with c-myc translocations have been identified in some patients and are adverse features (MacPherson, 1999).

The term atypical BL is used for those tumors with intermediate histology, a proliferation rate of nearly 100% by Ki-67 (Mib-1) immunohistochemistry, and/or demonstration of myc translocation (Diebold, 2001).

In a child with a rapidly growing tumor and presentation similar to Burkitt (such as ileocecal or other abdominal site, extranodal site with effusions, endocrine or gonadal sites, etc.) these are treated as BL (Cairo, 2003). Fixation and other technical artifacts blur the morphologic distinction and classification shows greater interobserver variation than other pediatric lymphomas (Lones, 2000).

In adults, children with slower growing tumors, tumors with 90–95% proliferation rates or those with complex karyotypes, the classification becomes murky. The trend in treatment of large B cell lymphoma in young people is to use therapies designed for BL (Patte, 2001) In adults, they are often treated as DLBCL. There may be a role for more aggressive therapy, but that generally means increased morbidity, so it is controversial and generally not utilized. Aggressive pediatric regimens have been successfully tested in adults with BL (Nicola, 2004).

Lymphomatoid Granulomatosis (LG)

LG is an angiocentric lymphoproliferative disorder involving the lung and/or other sites including brain, kidney, liver, skin, upper respiratory tract, and GI tract (Katzenstein, 1979). It is considered to be an EBV-driven B cell neoplasm with a prominent reactive T cell component, sometimes in a setting of immunosuppression (Wilson, 1996; Katzenstein, 1990). It has histologic features similar to NK/T cell lymphoma of nasal type (Jaffe, 2001b).

adhesion molecules CD29 (beta 1 integrin) and CD54 (ICAM-1) have been reported absent (Ponzoni, 2000).

Primary Effusion Lymphoma (Body Cavity Based Lymphoma)

This is another rare tumor presenting in serous effusions but without tumors. Cytology is usually immunoblastic or anaplastic. It is associated with the Kaposi's sarcoma virus human herpesvirus-8 (HHV-8) in immunodeficient patients. Tumor cells label as B cells and have Ig rearrangements, though T cell varieties have been reported. EBV can usually be detected using in situ hybridization (ISH) for EBV-encoded ribonucleotide (EBER), but EBV-latent membrane protein-1 (LMP) is absent by immunohistochemistry (Banks, 2001b). The pathogenesis may be related to viral activation of the alternative NF-kappaB pathway (Matta, 2004).

Burkitt Lymphoma

Burkitt lymphoma (BL) was first described in the jaws of African children by Dennis Burkitt in 1958 (Burkitt, 1958). It was first defined as a distinct tumor entity by the WHO in 1968 (Berard, 1985) and remains so in the current WHO classification (Diebold, 2001). It represents approximately one-third of pediatric NHL, but also occurs in adults. Several epidemiologic types of BL exist. The prototype is 'endemic' BL, which occurs predominately in children in Africa and other equatorial regions and is associated with EBV. 'Sporadic' BL occurs worldwide in children and adults and is not usually associated with EBV. Patients with HIV or other immune suppression often have EBV-related BL which is, however, different from the endemic form at the molecular level. BL is a very proliferative tumor that grows very rapidly.

The tumor shows a diffuse infiltrate with pushing borders of medium-sized relatively uniform cells with round to oval nuclei containing three to five moderately prominent nucleoli in relatively clear parachromatin (Fig. 32–63). Cytoplasm is moderate, basophilic, and tends to square off between adjacent cells. Lipid-laden cytoplasmic vacuoles are seen in imprints (Fig. 32–64). There are both high mitotic and high apoptotic rates and a prominent pattern of 'starry sky' macrophages. In most cases, the histology is distinctive, but there is some overlap with both DLBCL and occasionally lymphoblastic lymphoma.

Burkitt leukemia/lymphoma exhibits leukemic cells with moderately clumped chromatin and basophilic vacuolated cytoplasm (Fig. 32–63) and with surface immunoglobulin restricted to one light chain. Typically they show lack of TdT, presence of B cell antigens CD19, CD22, CD20, CD79a, often CD10, and expression of monoclonal surface Ig. Rare cases

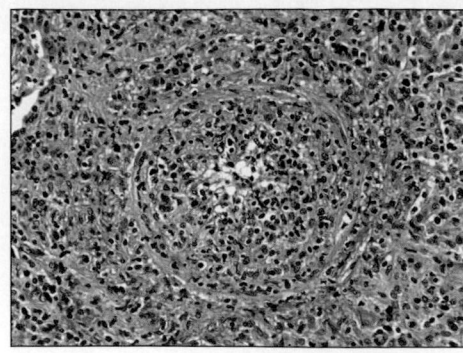

Figure 32–66 Lymphomatoid granulomatosis, showing a polymorphous angiodestructive pulmonary infiltrate (×200). Courtesy of Dr. Anna-Luise Katzenstein.

Grading is related to the number of clonal EBV-positive lymphocytes. Grade I lesions are polymorphic with only occasional large cells. Grade II is mixed with large pleomorphic cells in a mixed inflammatory background. Grade III is essentially diffuse large B cell lymphoma.

Outcome is variable, with waxing and waning, sometimes spontaneous remissions, and often progression to pulmonary failure in a median of 2 years. Appropriate therapy is related to grade. Grade III lesions are treated with systemic chemotherapy, while grades I and II may be treated with alpha-interferon.

T Cell and Natural Killer Cell Neoplasms

T cell and NK cell lymphomas and leukemias are a diverse group of neoplasms which are uncommon to rare compared to B cell lymphomas. While they comprise only about 12% of lymphomas overall, an approximately equal number of categories is recognized by the WHO. Most of these are typified by clonal rearrangement of genes encoding CD3, the T cell receptor complex which is an antigen receptor of the immunoglobulin supergene family, though true NK cell neoplasms do not show clonal rearrangement by clinical tests (Jaffe, 2001c). Features of major T/NK neoplasms are summarized in Table 32–20.

The majority of post-thymic (peripheral) T cells express alpha-beta chains of the T cell receptor (TCR), while a small minority do not, but rather express gamma-delta chains. NK cells express only epsilon chains with cytoplasmic CD3. T cell clonality studies in the laboratory usually focus on gamma-delta receptor rearrangement which is present in all or most T cells. This is because in early T cell development, the gamma and beta chain genes rearrange simultaneously, with TCR commitment dependent on expression of surrogate alpha chain and development of a pre-TCR (Haks, 1998; Kang, 2001). The repertoire of significant gamma gene 'families' is much smaller (four to six) than beta families, and TCR-gamma PCR assay is far more efficient for routine use than is TCR-beta PCR, which requires approximately 25 different primer sets (Shadrach, 2004). TCR-gamma PCR is also effective with DNA extracted from formalin and has largely replaced Southern blot analysis of TCR beta. Flow cytometry assays using antibodies for each TCR V beta family is also useful and rapid, but requires a large number of antibodies, and RT-

Presentation is usually cough, dyspnea and chest pain with constitutional symptoms including fever, malaise, weight loss, GI symptoms, myalgias and neurologic symptoms. Bilateral mid to lower lung nodules are most commonly seen, often with nodules in the brain, kidney, skin and subcutaneous tissue.

Histology shows an angiocentric and angiodestructive infiltrate of polymorphic lymphocytes, plasma cells, immunoblasts and histiocytes, with inconspicuous neutrophils and eosinophils and without well-formed granulomas. Fibrinoid necrosis of vessels is often seen (Fig. 32–66), as is tissue infarction.

Immunophenotyping shows variable numbers of CD79a, usually CD20-positive B cells with EBV LMP-1 expression, variable CD30 expression and lack of CD15. EBER is generally positive in some studies (Myers, 1995). The majority of background cells are reactive T cells with CD4 predominance. Higher-grade lesions (with more B cells) show clonal rearrangement of the IgH receptor genes. T cell receptor genes are not clonally rearranged.

Table 32–20 Key Features of the Major Mature T and NK Cell Neoplasms

Lymphoma	Demographics, clinical and laboratory presentation	Morphology	Cell Surface Markers Positive	Cell Surface Markers Negative	Gene Rearrangements
T cell PLL	M > F, median age 69 years. Lymphocytosis > 100 × 10³, anemia, thrombocytopenia, HSM, skin lesions	Prolymphocyte with prominent nucleoli, perinuclear chromatin, abundant cytoplasm	CD7; CD4 (60%), CD4/8 (25%), CD8 (15%)		TCRα-β, inv(14)(q11;q32)
LGL leukemia	Median age 63. Neutropenia causing infections, anemia, mild lymphocytosis, LGL > 2 × 10³	Moderately sized cell with condensed chromatin, abundant pale blue cytoplasm, azurophilic granules	CD3, 8, 57, TCRα-β Some variants are CD4+ or CD4/8+ or CD4/8–	CD4	TCRγ, β
Aggressive NK cell leukemia	Asian teens–young adults. Constitutional symptoms, HSM, variable WBC	Variable, may resemble LGL cells or appear blastic	cCD3ε, 2, 56	sCD3, 57	Clonal episomal EBV, del(6)(q21;q25)
Adult T cell leukemia-lymphoma	Associated with HTLV-1, frequent in Japan, Caribbean, central Africa. Acute variant with skin, lymph node involvement, hypercalcemia	Moderately large, blastic cells with convoluted nuclei (floret cells), agranular, basophilic cytoplasm	CD 2, 3, 5, 25, often CD30	CD4, 7	TCR genes
Extranodal NK/T cell lymphoma, nasal type	M > F, Latin America and Asia. Massive nasopharyngeal destruction. EBV associated	Polymorphic lymphoid cells, often angiocentric or angioinvasive, with mucosal ulceration	CD2, 56, cCD3ε	CD4, 8, 5, 16, 56	Clonal episomal EBV
Mycosis fungoides/Sézary syndrome (SS)	M > F, middle-age–older. Dermatitis progressing to ulcerated lesions. PB blood involvement in SS	Dermal band-like infiltrates of lymphocytes with cerebriform nuclei, microabscesses	CD2, 3, 4	CD7, 8	TCR genes
Primary cutaneous CD30-positive	M > F, adults–elderly. Limited to skin lesions	Polymorphic lymphoid cells, some anaplastic	CD4, 30	Often CD2, 3, 5	TCR genes ALK-negative
Anaplastic large cell lymphoma	M ≈ F, teens, young adults. Peripheral, abdominal adenopathy, extranodal and BM involvement, frequent B symptoms	Pleomorphic large cells, wreath-like nuclei, multiple nucleoli, abundant cytoplasm	CD30 (cytoplasmic and Golgi), CD2, 4	CD3, 5, 7, EBV	t(2;5)(p23;q35) Other variants involve 2p23

PLL = prolymphocytic leukemia; HSM = hepatosplenomegaly; LGL = large granular lymphocyte; EBV = Epstein–Barr virus; PB = peripheral blood ; BM = bone marrow.

PCR for V beta family transcripts may be utilized (Langerak, 2001; Morice, 2004).

Mature alpha-beta T cells express CD2, CD3, CD5, CD7 and either CD4 or CD8. They are negative for TdT and CD1. Normal resting lymphoid tissue usually shows a CD4 : CD8 ratio of two to one. Differentiation to one or the other in the thymus involves activation or silencing of CD4 or CD8 from CD4+CD8+ cells, but is poorly understood (Yasutomo, 2000). Primarily mature CD4 cells proliferate in the post-thymic environment (Foa, 1980). The CD4 : CD8 ratio drops in acute inflammation and rises to often high levels in recovery and chronic inflammation, so that these are not good markers of clonality. Peripheral T cell neoplasms often lose expression of a normal pan-T cell antigen such as CD7 and show predominance of CD4 or CD8 (Knowles, 1989). Care must be taken to distinguish abnormal alpha-beta T cells from normal NK cells.

Gamma-delta T cells typically are doubly negative for CD4 and CD8 and also often CD5-negative, with CD2 expression and show a maturation sequence of CD7. Since they are usually only 1–2% of normal T cells, increase in these cells is a suspicious finding of itself. NK cells are highly variable in expression of pan-T cell antigens CD2 and CD7, often CD5-negative, typically express CD16 (a low-affinity Fc receptor also found on monocytes and granulocytes), with variable CD56 and CD57. CD3 is detectable in the cytoplasm with polyclonal antibodies but is also present on the surface in some NK neoplasms. Cytotoxic granule constituents TIA-1, granzyme-B and perforin are usually present in NK cells and cytotoxic T cells.

T-Prolymphocytic Leukemia

T-prolymphocytic leukemia is an uncommon disorder with a median age of 69 years, and the disease is slightly more frequent in males than in females. Patients present with a marked lymphocytosis ($> 100 \times 10^9$/L), anemia, and thrombocytopenia. In most cases, the neoplastic cell is a prolymphocyte with a prominent 'punched-out' nucleolus showing distinct perinucleolar chromatin and moderately abundant cytoplasm. In approximately 20% of patients, however, the lymphocytes lack distinctive features and do not possess a prominent nucleolus. Hepatosplenomegaly, lymphadenopathy and skin involvement are common (Catovsky, 2001b).

The immunophenotype is most often CD4+ peripheral T cell (60%), with CD4/CD8 coexpression in 25% and CD8+ in 15%. CD7 is strong and surface CD3 weak.

There is clonal TCR alpha-beta (and gamma-delta) rearrangement. 80% show inv(14)(q11;q32) and 10% t(14;14)(q11;q32) involving TCR alpha-beta locus and oncogenes TCL1 and TCL1b. Chromosome 8 abnormalities t(8;8)(p11-12;q12) or trisomy 8q are seen in 70%, and other abnormalities include t(X;14)(q28;q11) and deletions at 11q23.

T-prolymphocytic leukemia is a rapidly progressive malignancy with survival usually less than 1 year. Recent progress has been made with new therapies including CAMPATH-1H (Dearden, 2001; Cao, 2003).

Large Granular Lymphocyte (LGL) Leukemia

The median age of these patients is 63 years. Sixty to seventy percent of patients are symptomatic with recurrent infections due to neutropenia. Anemia or rheumatoid arthritis are also common (Lamy, 2003). Lymphocytosis is usually mild (up to 20×10^3/μL) and lymphocyte number may be normal. LGL cells are usually at least 2×10^3/μL (Chan, 2001a). Chronic neutropenia is frequent, splenomegaly may be present, and there may be anemia and/or thrombocytopenia. Large granular lymphocytes are at least relatively increased and show moderate size with abundant light blue cytoplasm and condensed chromatin. Azurophilic cytoplasmic granules vary in number and size (Fig. 32–67). The bone marrow exhibits a moderate interstitial infiltrate of granulated lymphocytes. Erythroid and myeloid elements may be normal or hypoplastic in occasional cases. The spleen typically shows red pulp infiltrates.

The common variant is CD3/CD8/CD57/TCR alpha-beta+; CD4-negative. Uncommon variants express CD4 (Lima, 2003), dually express CD4 and CD8, show doubly negative CD4/CD8, and/or have variable expression of CD57 and CD56. Cases reactive with CD3 and CD56 tend to behave aggressively (Gentile, 1994). Cases of LGL leukemia following renal transplant have been seen (Gentile, 1998) and those of donor origin following bone marrow transplant (Au, 2003). Benign LGL lymphocytosis following bone marrow transplant is likely related to the early emergence of LGL cells (Niederwieser, 1987).

TCR gamma gene rearrangement is usually clonal by PCR and TCR beta is usually rearranged. While a single clonal band usually confirms a suspicious diagnosis, PCR assays may show a dominant clone emerging from an oligoclonal population of autoimmune disorder. This, along with a typically indolent course, makes cases with low WBC very difficult to

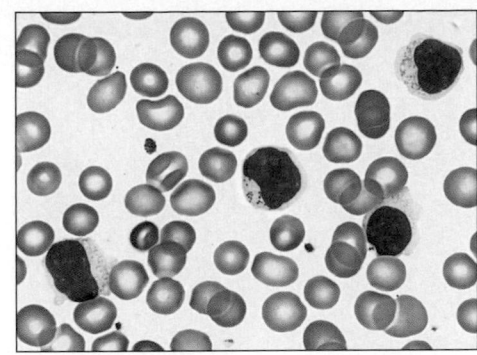

Figure 32–67 Large granular lymphocyte leukemia (× 1000).

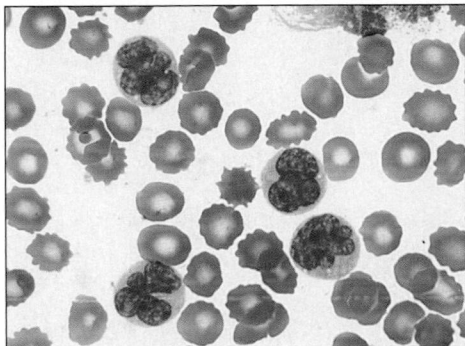

Figure 32–68 NK leukemia in an adult, with floret cells resembling adult T cell leukemia.

diagnose. Low-dose methotrexate, ciclosporin, or cyclophosphamide often induce long-lasting remission (Lamy, 2003).

Aggressive NK Cell Leukemia

This is a rare aggressive leukemia of NK cells associated with EBV and usually occurring in Asian teens and young adults. It usually presents with constitutional symptoms. The WBC is variable, hepatosplenomegaly is common, and it sometimes shows lymphadenopathy, hepatosplenomegaly, coagulopathy, hemophagocytic syndrome and/or multiorgan failure (Chan, 2001b).

Morphology of leukemic cells is variable, sometimes resembling LGL leukemia, sometimes showing larger lymphoid cells with condensed chromatin and basophilic cytoplasm, and sometimes showing blastic or transformed cells.

The immunophenotype is surface CD3-negative, cytoplasmic CD3 epsilon/CD2/CD56-positive, and expression of cytotoxic molecules (TIA-1, granzyme-B, and/or perforin). CD16 is variable and CD57 negative.

TCR genes are not rearranged. Clonality may be established by detecting clonal episomal EBV (analyzing tandem repeats by Southern blot), or finding clonal cytogenetic abnormalities such as del(6)(q21;q25).

Indolent NK cell proliferation also occurs and is characterized by adult onset, lack of constitutional symptoms, lack of EBV, and a CD57+ phenotype (along with CD2, CD16 and CD56, with negative surface CD3) (Fig. 32–68).

Adult T Cell Leukemia-Lymphoma (ATLL)

ATLL is a highly variable but often clinically aggressive T cell leukemia/lymphoma associated with HTLV-1 retrovirus infection (Poiesz, 1980). It is most endemic in southwestern Japan but also in the Caribbean basin, the southeastern US, and central Africa. Transmission of HTLV-1 may occur vertically (from mother to child), or through sexual contact, intravenous drug abuse, or blood transfusion. Only a minority of individuals infected with HTLV-1 (2.5%) develop ATLL and it is typically after a latent period of many years. Acute infection results in a flu-like syndrome.

The *acute variant* typically shows leukemia, skin involvement, generalized lymphadenopathy, lytic bone lesions and hypercalcemia. The blood film demonstrates anemia and thrombocytopenia with the presence in blood and marrow of moderately large blastic cells with convoluted or clover-leafed nuclei and condensed chromatin ('floret cells'). Nucleoli are small or absent and the cytoplasm is agranular and basophilic. Admixed blast-like cells are present. Marrow involvement is often patchy with

IV

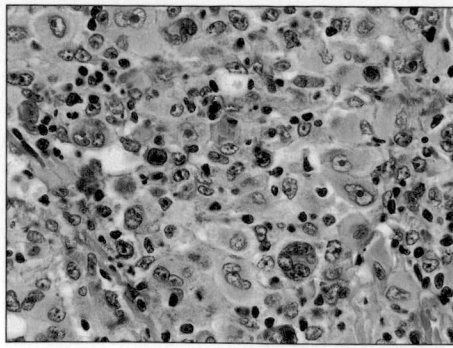

Figure 32–69 Adult T cell leukemia/lymphoma, with anaplastic features (× 500).

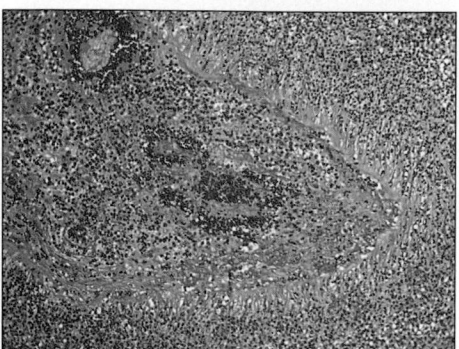

Figure 32–70 Nasal/nasal-like T/NK lymphoma, showing angioinvasion and destruction (× 200).

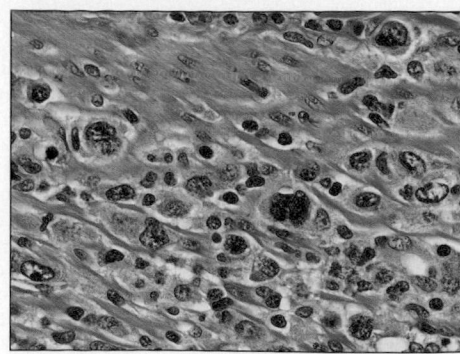

Figure 32–71 Enteropathy-associated T cell lymphoma infiltrating the muscularis of the small bowel (× 500).

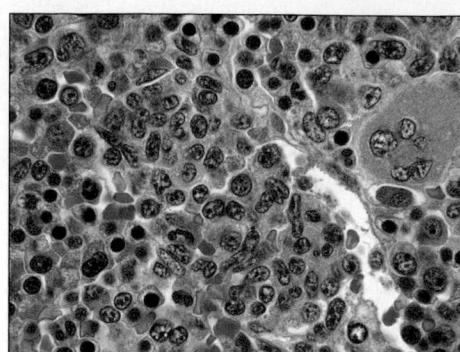

Figure 32–72 Hepatosplenic T cell lymphoma showing intrasinusoidal involvement of the bone marrow (× 500).

increased osteoclastic activity. Skin lesions resemble mycosis fungoides including presence of Pautrier's microabscesses, but often with more pleomorphic cells.

Lymph nodes in acute or *lymphomatous variant* show highly variable morphology, often with features and diversity reminiscent of anaplastic large cell lymphoma (Kikuchi, 2001). Histology may resemble common ALCL, small cell variant, HL or typical large cell lymphoma (Fig. 32–69).

The *chronic variant* often resembles mycosis fungoides and the *smoldering variant* shows low-level leukemic involvement with < 5% circulating neoplastic cells. Clonal integration of HTLV-1 is an invariable finding and essentially diagnostic (Yamaguchi, 2002), but it should be noted that HTLV-1 infection is chronic and these patients may have other hematologic diseases just as do other people.

The immunophenotype of ATLL is CD2/CD3/CD5/CD25-positive, usually CD4+ and CD7-negative. CD30 is often positive but ALK is negative. Cytotoxic markers are negative. TCR genes are clonally rearranged. Occasional patients with smoldering disease show a Hodgkin-like lymphoproliferative disorder of EBV-infected B cells with CD30 and CD15 expression, likely related to chronic immunosuppression. It may be noted that both HTLV-1 and EBV are potent inducers of CD30.

Extranodal NK/T Cell Lymphoma, Nasal Type

These lymphomas have been referred to as lethal midline granuloma, polymorphic reticulosis and angiocentric T cell lymphoma. They are extranodal lymphomas usually of NK cell derivation which are associated with EBV and most common in Asia and Latin America. They typically involve nasopharynx, palate, skin, GI tract, testes or other sites. The hemophagocytic syndrome is sometimes associated (Chan, 2001c).

The histology shows diffuse infiltrates of lymphoid cells of varying, often polymorphic cytology, from small lymphocytes to large cells, immunoblasts and/or anaplastic cells. There are typically mucosal ulcerations and areas showing an angiocentric and angioinvasive pattern (Fig. 32–70) with fibrinoid necrosis of vessels and associated infarction-like necrosis.

Immunophenotype is usually CD2/CD56-positive, with cCD3 epsilon and expression of cytotoxic molecules. CD43, CD45Ro, HLA-DR, CD25, CD95 and FAS ligand are also expressed, but CD4, CD8, CD5, CD16 and CD57 are negative.

TCR alpha-beta and gamma-delta and IgH genes are germ line, but clonal episomal EBV is present. EBER ISH is positive. Del(6)(q21;q25) is occasionally described. Prognosis is variable.

Enteropathy-Type T Cell Lymphoma

This is a clonal T cell malignancy of intraepithelial T cells. It is associated with celiac disease, but patients often present simultaneously with malabsorption and lymphoma (Isaacson, 2001a). It usually occurs in the jejunum or ileum, with other locations in or outside of the GI tract reported.

Morphology shows variable small, medium to large size neoplastic cells, often with pale to eosinophilic cytoplasm and eccentric angulated nuclei. In some cases, the cytology is similar to anaplastic large cell lymphoma with wreath-like multinucleation and horseshoe nuclei (Fig. 32–71). Other cases have bland-appearing small lymphocytes. Histiocytes and eosinophils are often abundant.

The phenotype is CD3, CD7, CD103-positive, CD8 variable, CD4-negative, often with double-negative CD4/CD8. Small cell variants are CD8/CD56-positive. Cytotoxic molecules are expressed. TCR genes are clonally rearranged and patients with celiac disease typically have HLA DQA1*0501 and DQB1*0201. This is usually an aggressive disease.

Hepatosplenic T Cell Lymphoma

This is a rare neoplasm, usually of gamma-delta T cells, which shows sinusoidal infiltration of spleen, liver and bone marrow. It is most common in adolescent or young adult males. Patients present with massive splenomegaly, hepatomegaly, pronounced thrombocytopenia and sometimes leukocytosis and anemia (Jaffe, 2001d).

Histology shows diffuse splenic red pulp involvement by small to medium size lymphoid cells with slightly dispersed chromatin and moderate cytoplasm. Liver shows similar cells in sinuses. Diagnosis is best made in the bone marrow with presence of a characteristic infiltration of sinuses but otherwise intact architecture and hematopoiesis (Fig. 32–72). Immunophenotyping of sections is extremely helpful because of inconspicuous morphology on H&E.

The immunophenotype is CD3 and TIA-1-positive, with double-negative CD4 and CD8, negative CD5, granzyme B and perforin (Belhadj, 2003). TCR delta1 antibodies are positive and TCR alpha-beta negative, though some cases of alpha-beta type occur.

TCR gamma PCR is positive, and TCR beta occasionally positive. Most cases are EBV-negative, but EBV-positive cases occur (Taguchi, 2004). Isochromosome 7q is usually described, with occasional trisomy 8. The disease is aggressive, with early responses to therapy but usual relapse and progression. There are no data from clinical trials.

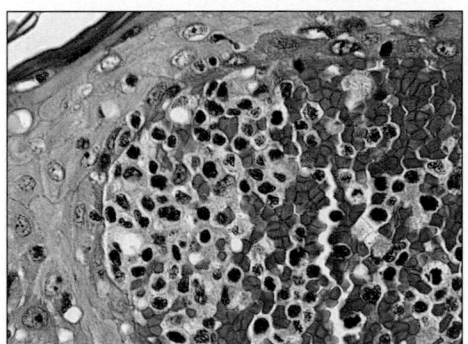

Figure 32–73 Subcutaneous panniculitis-like T cell lymphoma (× 500).

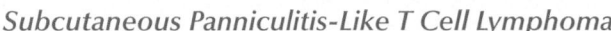

Figure 32–74 Cutaneous T cell lymphoma, showing a large Pautrier's microabscess (× 20).

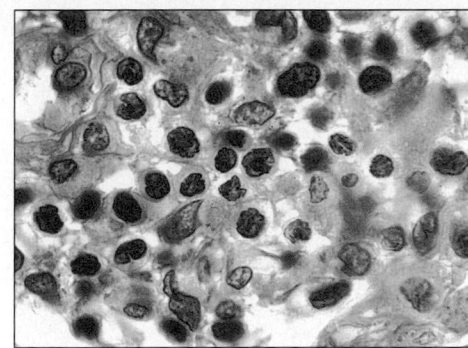

Figure 32–75 Neoplastic lymphocytes with convoluted nuclei in mycosis fungoides (× 1000).

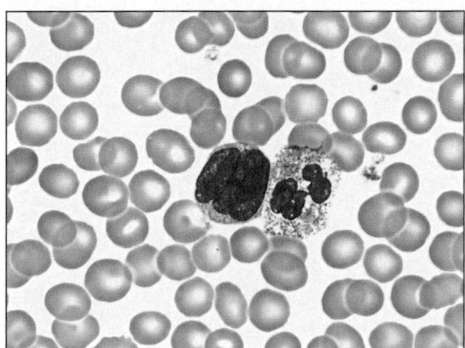

Figure 32–76 Sézary cell in the blood along with a neutrophil (× 1000).

Subcutaneous Panniculitis-Like T Cell Lymphoma

This neoplasm of cytotoxic T cells usually occurs as multiple nodules in the subcutaneous fat of the trunk or extremities and mimics benign panniculitis. The overlying epidermis and dermis are not involved but the septae of subcutaneous adipose are infiltrated. The lymphoid infiltrate is polymorphic and may be deceptively bland though some large cells are usually present (Fig. 32–73). There is rimming of fat cells by lymphocytes and usually vascular involvement with areas of necrosis and histiocytic infiltrates. Acute inflammatory cells are not typically present as they are in benign panniculitis, and multinucleated giant cells are usually not seen.

The immunophenotype is usually mature CD8+ T cell with expression of granzyme B, perforin and TIA-1, with a genotype of clonal alpha-beta T cell type (Go, 2004). Twenty-five percent are gamma-delta T cell with double-negative CD4/CD8 and expression of CD56 (Jaffe, 2001e).

The disease is typically aggressive, and hemophagocytic syndrome is seen in about 37%. Median survival is approximately 27 months, but long-term remissions may be obtained with anthracycline-based therapy (Go, 2004).

Blastic NK Cell Lymphoma

This is another rare tumor of NK derivation but blastic morphology which presents in the skin or rarely nasal cavity of middle-aged to older individuals and may involve lymph nodes, bone marrow or soft tissue (Chan, 2001d).

Morphology shows diffuse dermal and/or soft tissue infiltrates of medium-sized blasts. Rosettes may be seen. The phenotype is CD4, CD56 and CD43-positive; CD3, CD2, CD7 and usually CD68-negative. Myeloid markers myeloperoxidase and CD33 are negative, TdT and CD34 variably expressed, and TCR genes are not rearranged. CD99 is reported positive (Shapiro, 2003). The disease resembles lymphoblastic lymphoma or granulocytic sarcoma and is aggressive.

Mycosis Fungoides and Sézary Syndrome

Mycosis fungoides occurs twice as frequently in men as in women. It usually affects individuals in their middle to late years.

The disorder first appears as an eczematoid, psoriasiform, or nonspecific exfoliative dermatitis. The lesions tend to form plaques and then tumors that often ulcerate. Some patients develop generalized erythroderma.

Biopsies of the skin reveal band-like lymphocytic infiltrates in the dermis (Fig. 32–69), often with admixed histiocytes and occasional eosinophils (Ralfiaer, 2001b). T cells with irregular nuclei (Fig. 32–74) show single cell infiltration of the epidermis and often form clusters known as Pautrier's abscesses (Fig. 32–75). These are usually accompanied by parakeratosis and acanthosis, typically with minimal or no spongiosis, and elongation of rete pegs. The nuclei of at least a portion of neoplastic cells typically have a cerebriform appearance. The extent of the cutaneous infiltrate is not always directly correlated with severity of disease. Communication with the dermatologist or other treating physician is important and even subtle changes in a clinically suspicious patient taken seriously.

Phenotype is usually mature T cell with CD8 expression and lack of CD7, but this is not usually conclusive. TCR genes are clonally rearranged and PCR analysis of formalin-fixed biopsy tissue should be attempted in suspicious cases.

In advanced stages of the disease, neoplastic cells infiltrate the lymph nodes, liver, spleen, and other organs. Early nodal involvement (category I) shows dermatopathic changes with scattered atypical cerebriform lymphocytes. Category II shows partial nodal effacement and category III shows diffuse involvement.

Rare atypical mononuclear cells with cerebriform nuclei (Sézary cells) may be present in the peripheral blood (Fig. 32–76). Lymphocytosis with these cells (especially in the erythremic patient) is called *Sézary syndrome*.

The disorder may follow a prolonged chronic course. However, following lymph node infiltration, the disease becomes more progressive, and death, usually due to infection, occurs within 2 years.

Therapy is topical in early cases. More advanced disease has been treated with PUVA, retinoids, alpha-interferon and, more recently, alemtuzumab (Campath) (Pichardo, 2004).

Primary Cutaneous CD30-Positive T Cell Lymphoproliferative Disorder

This category in the WHO classification includes primary cutaneous anaplastic large cell lymphoma (ALK-negative), lymphomatoid papulosis and borderline lesions (Ralfkiaer, 2001a). These disorders share the features of dermal infiltrates of polymorphic lymphoid cells including a variable proportion of anaplastic or Reed–Sternberg-like cells with expression of CD30, and typically relapsing/remitting clinical course.

Cutaneous ALCL resembles systemic ALCL (Fig. 32–77) except that it is indolent, does not exhibit detectable ALK expression or genetic translocations. Lymphomatoid papulosis has been considered a variant of pityriasis lichenoides et varioliformis acuta (PLEVA), with an inverted vase-like lymphoid infiltrate containing variable numbers of CD30-positive large cells. It has been associated with HL in a number of instances.

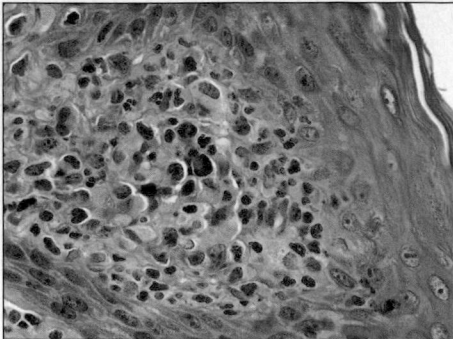

Figure 32–77 Cutaneous ALCL (× 1000).

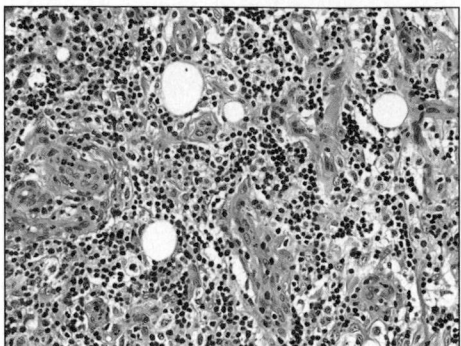

Figure 32–78 Angioimmunoblastic lymphoma showing arborizing vessels and lymphoid infiltrate infiltrating fat. In other areas of this case, plasma cells and immunoblasts are present. Clear cells are also frequently present (× 200).

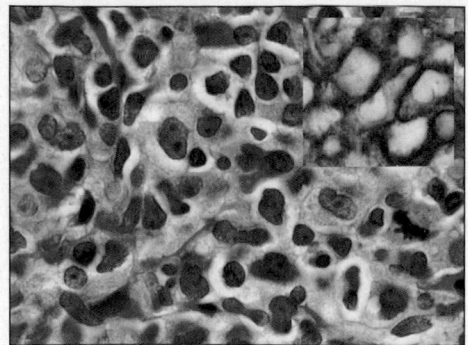

Figure 32–79 Peripheral T/NK cell lymphoma, unspecified; CD3 expression is seen in inset (× 1000).

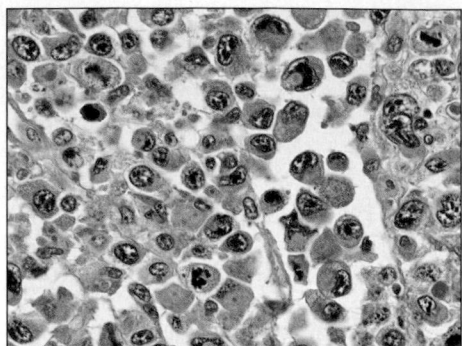

Figure 32–80 Anaplastic large cell lymphoma in an adolescent (× 500).

Both disorders share the phenotype of CD4-positive mature T cells with variable loss of pan-T cell antigens, expression of cytotoxic molecules and strong CD30 expression. ALK is negative. TCR genes are clonally rearranged. Atypical regressing histiocytosis is an older term used for both disorders.

Angioimmunoblastic T Cell Lymphoma

This disorder has been termed angioimmunoblastic lymphadenopathy with dysproteinemia (AILD), and abnormal immune response. It is a clonal T cell lymphoma that presents with constitutional symptoms and polyclonal hypergammaglobulinemia. While once thought to be initially a reactive process with a spectrum of progression to lymphoma, it is now felt to be neoplastic from the onset.

Histology shows paracortical lymph node hyperplasia with depletion of lymphocytes, increased plasma cells and prominent high endothelial postcapillary venules with PAS-positive hyalinization and 'burned-out' residual follicles (Fig. 32–78). Clusters of lymphocytes with small nuclei but moderately abundant clear cytoplasm are usually present and increase in prominence with progression. The immunophenotype is mature T cell with CD4 predominance, polyclonal plasma cells and prominent dendritic cells near vessels detected by CD21/CD23.

TCR genes are usually rearranged and IgH genes are also rearranged in a minority of cases containing EBV, presumably as a secondary event to immunosuppression. Trisomy 3, 5 or an additional X chromosome has been described. The disease is aggressive, and infectious complications are common (Jaffe, 2001f).

Peripheral T/NK Cell Lymphoma, Unspecified

These neoplasms are characteristically diverse and may consist of sheets of large cells (Fig. 32–79), paracortical lymph node expansion by mixed small and large cells, clear cells, predominantly small cells, and cases with striking pleomorphism resembling ALCL or HL. Abnormal patterns of T-antigen expression are helpful for diagnosis. Pan-T cell antigens (CD3, CD2, CD5, CD7) are usually present in some combination, but one or more are often aberrantly not expressed. CD4+ cases are more frequent than CD8+, but both double-positive and double-negative cases also occur (Ralfkiaer, 2001c). In paraffin sections, CD3, CD45Ro, and CD43 are helpful if positive, but the latter two are also present in myeloid tumors and some B cell lymphomas. CD68 is also rarely expressed.

T zone variant of PTCL, unspecified, shows paracortical expansion with preserved GCC. The cytomorphology is variable with small and medium

size cells, lymphocytes, plasma cells, endothelial hyperplasia and sometimes clusters of clear cells and/or cells resembling those in Hodgkin lymphoma.

The lymphoepithelioid variant, formerly known as Lennert's lymphoma, exhibits clusters of epithelioid histiocytes.

These tumors are typically aggressive and often belie their sometimes bland or reactive appearance. Clonal rearrangement of TCR genes is essential for confident diagnosis.

Anaplastic Large Cell Lymphoma

ALCL was first recognized relatively recently as NHL reactive with the Hodgkin-associated antibody Ki-1 (anti-CD30) (Stein, 1985). Primary ALCL is most common in adolescents and young adults and comprises about 10–15% of pediatric lymphomas. Cases in young people were likely overlooked previous to routine immunophenotyping, and retrospective review shows that about half of pediatric large cell lymphomas have been of T cell phenotype with 'polymorphic immunoblastic' morphology, which is now associated with ALCL (Hutchison, 1991). In addition, the morphology is variable and not of itself diagnostic, and a variety of 'secondary' ALCLs (including progressions of other lymphomas, post-transplant tumors, and EBV- and HTLV-1-associated lymphomas) also express CD30.

Primary ALCL appears associated with chromosomal abnormalities involving chromosome region 2p23 such as t(2;5)(p23;q35) in which the gene for a tyrosine kinase anaplastic lymphoma kinase is fused to that of the nucleolar shuttle protein nucleophosmin, with a resultant NPM-ALK fusion protein, which is highly expressed (Morris, 1994). The terms ALKoma and ALK lymphoma have been proposed (Benharroch, 1998). Variant genetic abnormalities involving ALK also occur, usually with ALK overexpression (Falini, 1999). Secondary ALCL and primary cutaneous ALCL are usually ALK-negative. The clinical implications of primary or secondary ALCL are not yet fully elucidated.

ALCL usually shows diffuse infiltrates or aggregates of large, sometimes pleomorphic cells with abundant cytoplasm and indented or horseshoe-shaped nuclei and sometimes wreath-like multilobated nuclei (Fig. 32–80). Lymph node sinus and superficial paracortical involvement are common, cohesive sheets of tumor cells often simulate carcinoma, and some cases show a polymorphic Hodgkin-like pattern. True Reed–Sternberg cells are not seen. Histologic variants include small cell and lymphohistiocytic types, but these also express ALK and show similar phenotype otherwise.

Essentially all exhibit CD30. Most primary cases in young people express ALK, which is usually both nuclear and cytoplasmic, but is only cytoplasmic in some genetic variants. Slightly more than half show

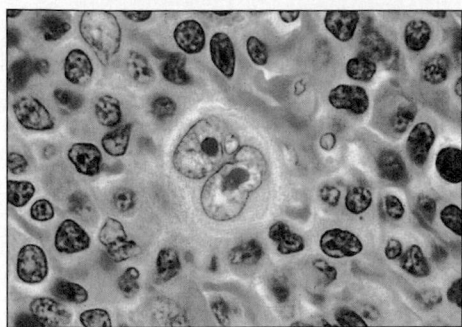

Figure 32–81 A Reed–Sternberg cell in a case of mixed cellularity Hodgkin lymphoma (× 1000).

peripheral T cell phenotype by IHC, but with variable expression of CD3, CD43, and CD45Ro. There is also variable expression of CD45, CD25, and EMA. CD68 or CD15 is only occasionally expressed. T cell surface marker-negative cases have been referred to as 'null,' but recent evidence suggests that while up to 90% show TCR rearrangements, there is typical defective expression of TCR (Delsol, 2001; Bonzheim, 2004).

CD56 expression occurs and is related to adverse prognosis (Suzuki, 2000). Cytotoxic granules with labeling by marker TIA-1 are also described (Felgar, 1999). Signal transducer and activator of transcription 3 (STAT3) is often overexpressed, with activation of antiapoptotic pathways and increased expression of bcl-2, bcl-xl, survivin and others, and decreased caspase-mediated apoptosis (Amin, 2004). Survivin expression in about half of cases is possibly associated with adverse outcome (Schlette, 2004). Abnormal apoptotic signaling may offer future therapeutic targets. ALCL differs from HL in that ALK expression abrogates CD30 induction of NF-kappaB whereas CD30 activates NF kappa B in HL (Horie, 2004).

The majority exhibit t(2;5)(p23;q35), but variants are also seen including: t(1;2)(q25;p23) involving TPM3 which encodes a tropomyosin; inv(2)(p23;q35) involving ATIC; and t(2;3)(p23;q35) involving TFG (TRAK fused gene). These all show cytoplasmic without nuclear ALK. Other partner genes include TPM4, CLTC, MSN, ALO17 and MYH9 (Lamant, 2003). Those with CLTC-ALK have been identified as large B cell lymphoma (CD20-negative, CD79a+) each with IgH rearrangement and also TCR rearrangements in one. They show granular cytoplasmic staining with ALK. Cytogenetics showed t(2;17)(p23;q23) (De Paepe,

2003). Rare cases of B cell ALCL, with or without ALK, are classified by the WHO with LBCL.

Hodgkin Lymphoma

The nomenclature of HL, formerly called Hodgkin's disease, is little changed from that of the Rye conference (Lukes, 1966). The hallmark of HL is the Hodgkin Reed–Sternberg (HRS vs. RS) cell, which is a large binucleated, multinucleated or mononuclear (Hodgkin) cell with each nucleus bearing a very large inclusion-like nucleolus (Fig. 32–81). These neoplastic cells appear in an immunoproliferative background containing variable numbers of lymphocytes, histiocytes, eosinophils and plasma cells. Degenerating 'mummified' neoplastic cells are also often present. Mixed cellularity, nodular sclerosis, lymphocyte-depleted and lymphocyte-rich classical subtypes have similar biology and are all referred to as 'classical' HL (Stein, 2001a). Nodular lymphocyte predominant (NLPHL) HL appears to be a different entity.

The most common phenotype of HRS cells in classical HL is expression of CD30, CD15, and fascin with absence of CD45 and T cell markers. B cell-associated markers CD20 and/or CD79 are expressed in a minority of cases (< 30%) and are usually focal and weak. Occasional cases show strong CD20 expression. B cell transcription factors Oct2 and Bob.1 are absent, as is immunoglobulin J chain. Light chain immunoglobulin antibodies may show generalized cytoplasmic labeling. Standard Ig and TCR gene rearrangement studies are negative in classical HL, but sequencing of amplified single cell IgH genes suggest that most cases of HL are derived from clonal B lymphocytes (Stein, 1999). EBV is associated with a substantial portion of cases of classical HL (Herbst, 1992).

HL may occur from early childhood to old age. Increased frequency is noted between 15–35 years and after age 50. Males predominate, especially in childhood; disease in females under age 30 is usually nodular sclerosis in type (Table 32–21).

Nodular Lymphocytic Predominant HL

The histology of NLPHL is of effacement of lymph node architecture by a nodular infiltrate of small B cells with an associated follicular dendritic network and scattered or clustered large cells referred to as L&H cells, after the original Lukes and Butler terminology of lymphocytic and histiocytic HL. Nodularity may be vague. L&H cells are quite variable in cytology from case to case, although they are usually more uniform within a case. The appearance most often described is that exhibiting large nuclei with vesicular chromatin, moderately prominent nucleoli, and convoluted

Table 32–21 Key Features of Hodgkin Lymphomas

Lymphoma	Demographics, clinical presentation	Morphology	Cell surface markers	Prognosis
Nodular, lymphocyte predominant	M > F, 30–50 years, with peripheral lymphadenopathy	L&H cells with large, convoluted nuclei, vesicular chromatin, prominent nucleoli (popcorn cells) loosely aggregated in nodules	CD45, 20, 22, 79a; bcl-6	Good for stages I, II. Poor for advanced-stage disease
Nodular sclerosis	M = F, < 30 years with mediastinal mass, occasionally spleen or lung involvement. 40% have B symptoms. Most patients present with stage II disease	Broad bands of collagen, nodules of lymphoid tissue with 'lacunar cells' showing abundant pale cytoplasm. Classic HRS cells rare	CD15, 30	Fair–good
Mixed cellularity	M > F, median age 37 years. Peripheral lymphadenopathy common, ± spleen, BM. B symptoms common. Patients often stage III or IV	Classic HRS cells with large, mono-, bi- or multinucleation, prominent nucleoli found in mixture of lymphocytes, plasma cells, eosinophils, histiocytes	CD15, 30	Fair–good
Lymphocyte depletion	M > F, median age 37 years. May present as acute febrile illness with pancytopenia, BM, visceral organ involvement, B symptoms, advanced stage common. Associated with HIV	Classic HRS cells common with paucity of background lymphocytes. Pleomorphic HRS cells mimic a sarcoma	CD15, 30	Fair–good stage for stage when compared to other CHL. HIV patients have more aggressive course
Lymphocyte rich classical	M > F, older age. Peripheral lymphadenopathy. B symptoms rare. Most patients with stage I or II disease	Scattered classic HRS cells among numerous small lymphocytes. Nodular growth pattern	CD15, 30	Good

L&H = lymphocyte and histiocytic; HRS = Hodgkin Reed–Sternberg; BM = bone marrow; CHL = classical Hodgkin lymphoma.

IV

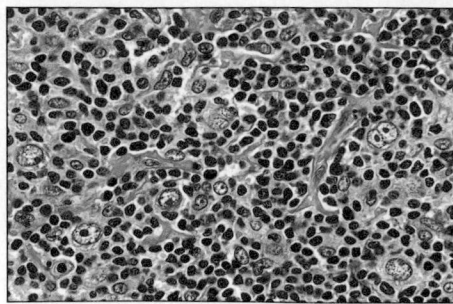

Figure 32–82 Lymphocyte predominant Hodgkin lymphoma, with L&H cells showing round rather than popcorn nuclei (× 500).

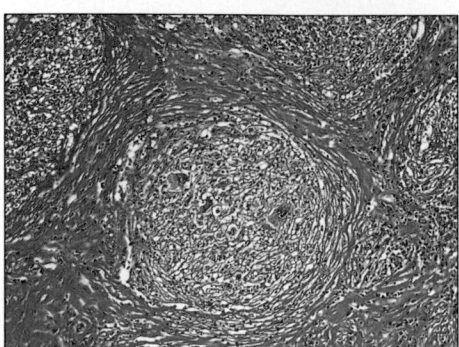

Figure 32–83 Dense fibrosis in a case of nodular sclerosis Hodgkin lymphoma (× 200).

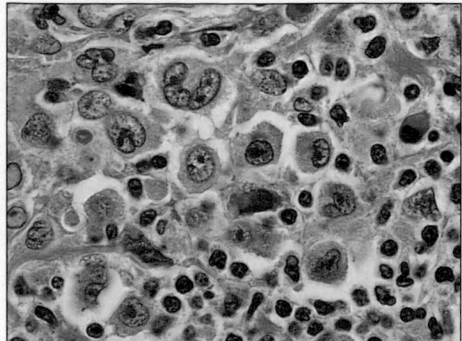

Figure 32–84 A cluster of HRS cells in a nodule of nodular sclerosis Hodgkin lymphoma (× 500).

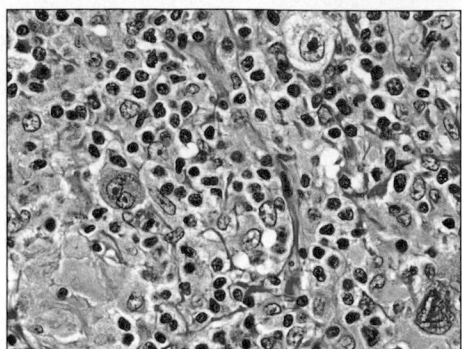

Figure 32–85 Scattered Hodgkin Reed–Sternberg cells in mixed cellularity Hodgkin lymphoma (× 500).

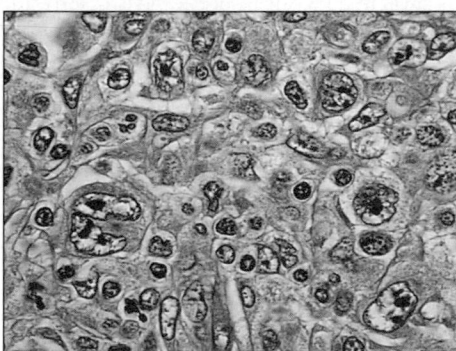

Figure 32–86 Lymphocyte depleted Hodgkin lymphoma shows predominance of neoplastic cells with few lymphocytes (× 500).

nuclei resembling popcorn ('popcorn cells'). Cytoplasm is moderate in amount and clear, retracted or slightly eosinophilic. Probably more often the neoplastic cells show round to oval nuclei with distinct eosinophilic or basophilic nucleoli, but less prominent than in HRS cells (Fig. 32–82). With experience, these cells become quite distinctive. Occasional HRS cells may be seen, but are not always present, and rarely predominate. Their phenotype, however, is different from classic HRS cells. L&H cells are usually loosely aggregated in the centers of nodules but are scattered elsewhere.

The phenotype of L&H cells is mature B cell, expressing CD45, CD20, CD22, CD79a, bcl-6, BOB.1, Oct-2, CD75 and usually J-chain. CD30 is absent or weak and EMA is frequently expressed. The nodules are composed of mostly B cells but with abundant admixed CD3 and CD3/CD57-positive T cells which tend to form rosettes around L&H cells. These are not always present, but are diagnostically helpful when they are. Nodules contain a follicular dendritic network which may be illuminated by CD21, CD35 or CD23 antibodies (Pileri, 2002). Cytoplasmic Ig is present but does not appear clonal even though B cells have been proven to be monoclonal by single cell PCR (Stein, 2001b).

IgH is clonally rearranged by sensitive assays in the research setting, but this is usually not detectable in routine clinical laboratory settings. L&H cells are of germinal center or post-germinal center derivation with somatic mutations of Ig genes which are ongoing in about half of studied cases (Braeuninger, 1997; Pileri, 2002).

Progressive transformation of lymph node germinal centers (PTGC) has been described as a precursor lesion to NLPHL, but there is no proven relationship. Most cases of PTGC do not lead to lymphoma.

Nodular Sclerosis (NS)

This is characterized by broad bands of collagen separating nodules of lymphoid tissue and the presence of 'lacunar cells,' which are large atypical histiocytes with abundant pale cytoplasm (Figs 32–83 and 32–84). Classic Reed–Sternberg cells are variable in number. Fibrosis may be inconspicuous in early lesions, but neoplastic cell clustering is usually present.

NS HL is graded on the basis of the number of neoplastic cells. When sheets of neoplastic cells are present in 25% or more of nodules, the tumor is designated grade 2. This is frequently associated with necrosis, and has been termed syncytial variant. The NS variety of HL is common, often presenting as a mediastinal mass in a young woman.

Mixed Cellularity (MC)

MC shows a diffuse polymorphic infiltrate of lymphocytes, plasma cells, eosinophils, histiocytes, and Reed–Sternberg cells, which are sometimes

quite numerous (Fig. 32–85). Necrosis and disorderly fibrosis may be present. This subtype is less common in young people than is NS, and is the most frequent subtype with EBV involvement.

Lymphocyte Depletion (LD)

This type is uncommon, often presents at older age, and may be associated with diffuse fibrosis. Neoplastic cells predominate and lymphocytes are relatively diminished compared to other forms of HL (Fig. 32–86). It is sometimes associated with an acute febrile illness accompanied by pancytopenia and lymphocytopenia. There may be a paucity of peripheral lymphadenopathy, though some patients have a generalized enlargement of lymph nodes. Bone marrow involvement is common, but lymphocytosis and thrombocytosis, often seen in other types of HL, are usually absent (Neiman, 1973).

Normocytic anemia is seen in about 50% of HL cases. Leukocyte and platelet counts are variable and eosinophilia may be present. The blood and marrow findings as well as many of the histologic features appear to be manifestations of host responses to the disease. Immunologic studies in HL have shown that cell-mediated immunity is defective when extensive disease is present.

Clinical staging defines *Stage I disease* as limited to lymph nodes in one anatomic region or two contiguous regions on one side of the diaphragm. *Stage II disease* involves more than two contiguous regions or two noncontiguous regions on one side of the diaphragm. *Stage III disease* is present on both sides of the diaphragm but is confined to lymphoid tissue. *Stage IV disease* involves bone marrow or any other organ, in addition to lymphoid tissue. The incidence of bone marrow involvement in untreated cases of HL is approximately 10% (Bartl, 1982b). All stages are additionally classified as 'A' if systemic symptoms are absent, 'B' if they are present. An aggressive approach to the management of HL has resulted in improved survival with many cures, especially in young patients.

Immunodeficiency-Associated Lymphoproliferative Disorders

Lymphomas and uncontrolled polyclonal lymphoid proliferations occur with increased frequency in patients with immune dysfunction. These dysfunctional states fall in three main categories; primary (congenital) immune deficiency states, HIV infection and iatrogenic immunodeficiency, particularly due to post-transplant immunosuppression but also due to prolonged immunosuppressive therapy for other reasons.

Most of these are B cell lymphoproliferative disorders associated with infection or reactivation of EBV or other virus and include large B cell lymphoma and variants, Burkitt lymphoma and polymorphic B cell hyperplasia. Hodgkin and peripheral T cell lymphomas occur rarely.

Primary immune deficiencies are each rare disorders and include Wiskott–Aldrich syndrome (WAS), ataxia telangiectasia (AT), common variable immunodeficiency syndrome (CVID), severe combined immuno-deficiency (SCID), X-linked immunoproliferative disorder (XLP), Nijmegan breakage syndrome (NBS), hyper-IgM syndrome, and autoimmune lymphoproliferative syndrome (ALPS) (Borisch, 2001).

ALPS involves inherited mutations of the FAS gene, which blocks apoptosis. This involves different mutations of varying effect, may be more common than previously thought and show an adult onset in some cases (Oren, 2002). Hyper-IgM syndrome results from mutations in CD40 ligand with inhibition of T/B cell interaction and B cell maturation. AT and NBS are abnormalities of DNA repair. WAS is a syndrome of thrombocytopenia, skin rash and recurrent infections which is fatal but curable by allogeneic bone marrow transplantation.

Fatal EBV infectious mononucleosis is a common occurrence in XLP and SCID. Large B cell lymphomas are the most common tumors in most primary immunodeficiencies, and lymphomatoid granulomatosis is increased in WAS.

HIV-Associated Lymphomas

Inadequately treated HIV shows a markedly increased incidence of high-grade B cell lymphomas associated with EBV (Knowles, 1988; Raphael, 2001). These are primarily Burkitt, atypical Burkitt and large B cell lymphoma. HIV-associated BL is similar to endemic Burkitt with EBV association and *c-myc* translocation but with different breakpoints (Haluska, 1989). BL with plasmacytoid differentiation is unique to HIV. MALT lymphomas occur even in children with HIV; HL and NK lymphomas occur rarely. Primary effusion lymphomas in HIV are due to KHSV/HHV-8 infection and are associated with Kaposi sarcoma and multicentric Castleman's disease. The incidence of HIV-associated lymphomas has dropped substantially in developed nations since the introduction of highly active antiretroviral therapy (HAART).

Post-Transplant Lymphoproliferative Disorders (PTLD)

These are also EBV associated, due to chronic infection and/or reactivation (Collins, 2002). PTLD are composed of a unique spectrum of lymphoproliferative disorders, which have been divided into morphologic categories (Harris, 2001b). In many cases, these tumors regress when immunosuppressive therapy is reduced, but this is unpredictable.

Plasmacytic hyperplasia (PH) is composed of numerous plasma cells and scattered immunoblasts. Infectious mononucleosis-like PTLD shows paracortical expansion of lymph nodes with increased immunoblasts. Both are early or low-grade lesions with a slow progression.

Polymorphic PTLD shows increased immunoblasts and plasma cells in a lymphoid background. Monomorphic PTLD is essentially diffuse lymphoma, usually large B cell. A Hodgkin-like PTLD is likely to be a large B cell lymphoma with Hodgkin-like features, previously called polymorphic immunoblastic in the Working Formulation (Fig. 32–87). Monomorphic T cell lymphomas also occur rarely.

A disorder similar to PTLD also may occur with chronic immuno-suppression for other reasons. The most prominent is use of methotrexate in the treatment of rheumatoid arthritis (Harris, 2001c).

Histiocytic and Dendritic Cell Neoplasms

These are rare disorders that affect lymph nodes and soft tissues, and occasionally the bone marrow (Jaffe, 2001g).

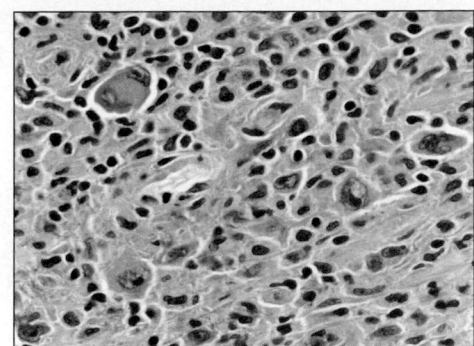

Figure 32–87 Large B cell lymphoma (anaplastic subtype) arising in polymorphic PTLD, in the GI tract (×500).

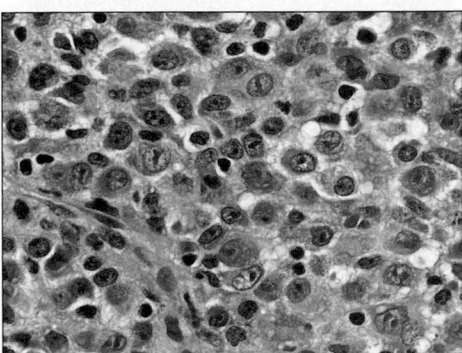

Figure 32–88 Histiocytic sarcoma in a child. This case showed expression of monocytic markers and enzymes, lack of lymphoid markers and lack of lymphoid gene rearrangements (×500).

Histiocytic sarcoma, also known as true histiocytic lymphoma, is a malignant tumor of noncirculating cells of monocyte macrophage lineage (Weiss, 2001a). The differential diagnosis includes monocytic leukemia and large B or peripheral T cell lymphoma. It resembles a large cell lymphoma or histiocytic sarcoma of monocytic lineage (Fig. 32–88). Tumor cells show nuclear features of malignancy. These label with CD68, lysozyme, alpha-1-antitrypsin and antichymotrypsin, and others label with other monocyte macrophage markers (i.e. CD64, CD14). Some hemophagocytosis may be seen.

Hemophagocytic Syndromes

These are often mistaken for histiocytic malignancy. They present with hepatosplenomegaly, fever and other constitutional symptoms, cytopenias and infiltrates of macrophages in involved organs including bone marrow with hemophagocytosis primarily of red blood cells (Fig. 32–89). Hemophagocytosis may be difficult to identify in occasional otherwise usual cases. These are usually associated with recent viral infection, EBV or CMV, but familial hemophagocytic syndromes also occur.

The cause of the disorder is often cryptic, but there is frequently an aggressive course. Approximately 60% of patients succumb within 2 months (Chen, 2004; Karras, 2004), but some patients respond to immune therapy.

Langerhans' Histiocytosis

Langerhans' cell histiocytosis (LCH) is a neoplastic proliferation of Langerhans' cells, which are dendritic cells normally found primarily in the skin (Weiss, 2001b). It presents in a variety of ways, including unifocal disease, usually in the bone or occasionally lymph node, skin or lung of an adolescent or young adult. These have been termed eosinophilic granuloma. Multifocal unisystem disease usually involves bone of children with frequent spread to adjacent soft tissues, also known as Hand–Schuler–Christian disease. Skull involvement may lead to diabetes insipidus, tooth loss or exophthalmos. Multiple lung lesions may be seen in adults. Multifocal multisystem disease, Letterer–Siwe disease, occurs in infants. It is an aggressive disease with fever, skin rash, hepatosplenomegaly, lymphadenopathy, bone involvement and pancytopenia.

Histologically, the disease consists of infiltrates of Langerhans' cells. They resemble benign histiocytes but have a coffee-bean shaped nucleus with a linear central groove (Fig. 32–90). Variable numbers of eosinophils and lymphocytes are usually present. The infiltrates form nodules in bone, involve upper dermis of the skin, and may involve lymph node sinuses

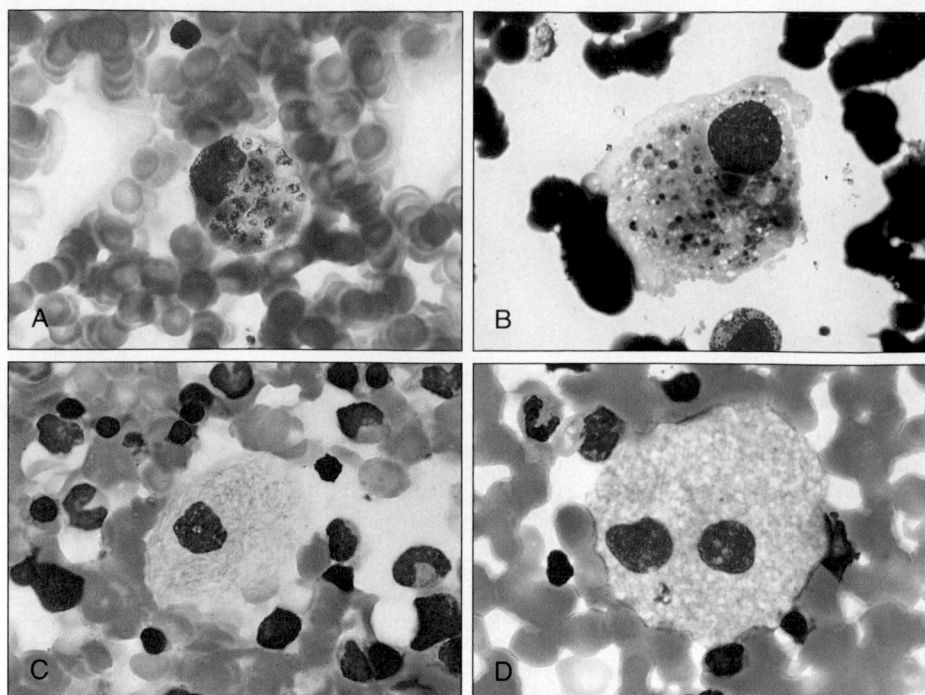

Figure 32–89 *A*, Histiocytic hyperplasia occurring in infection-associated hemophagocytic syndrome; this macrophage contains platelets as well as erythrocytes (× 1000). Compare with: *B*, a histiocyte containing cell debris in a patient with HIV (× 1000); *C*, an abnormal macrophage in Gaucher's disease (× 1000); and *D*, one in Niemann–Pick disease (× 1000).

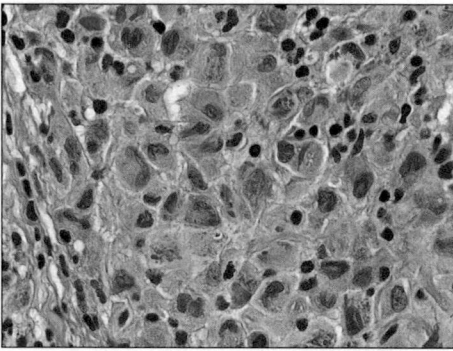

Figure 32–90 Langerhans' cell histiocytosis, showing typical nuclear folding and grooves (× 500).

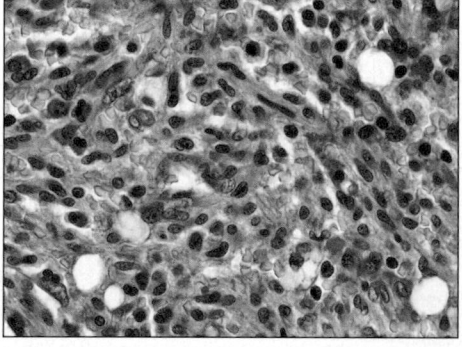

Figure 32–91 Mastocytosis in the bone marrow, presenting after treatment for acute myeloid leukemia (× 500).

and splenic red pulp. Giant cells are sometimes present but differ from multinucleated histiocytes (as in juvenile xanthogranuloma) by the presence of characteristic nuclei.

Immunophenotyping shows reactivity for CD1a and S-100 protein, and may be weakly reactive with CD45 and CD68, but are negative for T and B cell-specific antibodies and follicular dendritic markers CD21 and CD35. Electron microscopy remains useful in some cases due to characteristic Birbeck granules, which are pentalaminar racket-shaped structures pathognomonic of Langerhans' cells.

Outcome is largely dependent on extent of organ involvement, with localized disease showing a high rate of event-free survival, but extensive disease showing only a variable response to chemotherapy. Pulmonary disease in adults may remit spontaneously on cessation of smoking.

A cytologically malignant form of LCH has been termed Langerhans' cell sarcoma (Weiss, 2001c). These usually present with multiorgan disease, high mitotic rate and aggressive behavior.

Interdigitating Dendritic Cell Sarcoma/Tumor (IDCS)

This is a rare tumor of lymph node paracortical interdigitating dendritic cells (Weiss, 2001d). It has the gross and microscopic appearance of a sarcoma, tan in color, with a firm lobulated appearance, sometimes with hemorrhage or necrosis, and microscopic fascicles, whorls and/or storiform pattern. Lymphocytes are scattered throughout and plump epithelioid cells may be present. Atypia is variable.

Immunophenotyping is essential to diagnosis. The tumor cells are positive for S-100, with variable weak positivity for CD45 and monocyte markers CD68 and lysozyme. CD1a, CD21 and CD35 are negative. Other myeloid, B and T cell markers, EMA and CD30 are also negative. Background lymphocytes are reactive T cells. Prognosis is variable.

Follicular Dendritic Cell Sarcoma/Tumor (FDCS)

This is another rare dendritic cell tumor derived from follicular dendritic cells, which are phenotypically different than IDCS (Weiss, 2001e). Involvement is usually cervical lymph nodes, with axillary, mediastinal, mesenteric and retroperitoneal node involvement also described. Microscopically, they show fascicles, storiform pattern and/or complete (360°) whorls.

The immunophenotype shows positivity for CD21, CD23 and CD35, with variable S-100 and CD68, negative CD1a, occasional CD45 and CD20. Other myeloid, T and B cell markers, cytokeratins and HMB-45 are negative. CD117 is also negative (Hornick, 2002).

These tumors are indolent, with frequent good response to simple resection.

Dendritic Cell Sarcoma, Not Otherwise Specified

Dendritic cell sarcomas which do not fall into the above specific categories are termed DCS, not otherwise specified (Weiss, 2001f). They are also called indeterminate cell sarcoma, and express CD1a and S-100 without Birbeck granules.

Mast Cell Disease

Mast cell disease (mastocytosis) is an often enigmatic neoplastic proliferation of mast cells involving skin, bone marrow, lymph nodes, and/or spleen (Valent, 2001a,b). Symptoms are complex and arise from secretion of vasoactive amines including histamine and serotonin as well as from mass effects. Urticaria with pigmentation is common with skin involvement and is referred to as *urticaria pigmentosa*. Systemic mastocytosis presents with variable constitutional symptoms, skin disorder including urticaria,

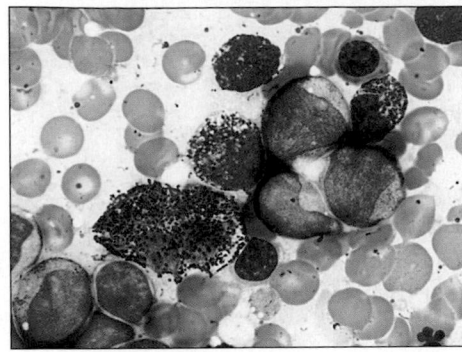

Figure 32–92 Acute leukemia with early mast cell disease, prior to therapy (earlier specimen from case shown in Fig. 32–91) (×1000).

are found in involved organs, often with associated fibrosis. Mast cells normally are mononuclear cells with central nuclei, clumped chromatin and dense basophilic granules. They are frequently difficult to identify, however, as mast cell granules are not well preserved in fixed tissue and cells may appear like bland clear cells, histiocytes, fibroblasts or others.

Mast cells may be identified in tissue using Giemsa or toluidine blue stains. Mast cell tryptase is the most specific marker, but cells also express CD117 as well as CD45, CD33, CD68, CD2 and CD25. Mast cells lack myeloperoxidase but often express chloroacetate esterase.

Bone marrow involvement is sometimes difficult to identify, with paratrabecular and perivascular aggregates of increased lymphocytes, eosinophils, neutrophils, mast cells and fibroblasts. Patterns of involvement are highly variable and biopsy is most helpful. Mast cells are frequently increased in hematologic neoplasms and are most apparent around bone marrow particles on aspirate smears. In addition, systemic mastocytosis sometimes presents with simultaneous acute leukemia and is only detected after treatment of the acute process (Figs 32–91 and 32–92). Leukemia of mast cells also occurs.

A spectrum of disorders of mastocytosis has been described (Valent, 2001a,b). The outcome is highly variable, with cutaneous disease usually indolent. In children, it usually regresses. Systemic disease without skin involvement is more aggressive than with skin disease, and mast cell leukemia and sarcoma are highly aggressive.

pruritus and dermatographism, symptoms of systemic histamine release, bone pain, arthralgia and fractures, splenomegaly, hepatomegaly or lymphadenopathy.

Mastocytosis is likely due to mutations of the receptor for stem cell factor, KIT, with CD117 expression. Morphologically, increased mast cells

References

Adamson JW, Fialkow PJ, Murphy S, et al: Polycythemia vera: Stem-cell and probable clonal origin of the disease. N Engl J Med 1976: 295:913–916.

Adriaansen HJ, Soeting PW, Wolvers-Tettero IL, et al: Immunoglobulin and T-cell receptor gene rearrangements in acute non-lymphocytic leukemias. Analysis of 54 cases and a review of the literature. Leukemia 1991; 5:744–751.

Aggarwal BB: Nuclear factor-kappaB: The enemy within. Cancer Cell 2004; 6:203–208.

Alder A: Uber konstitutionell bedingte Granulations-veranderungen den Leukocyten. Arch Klin Med 1939; 138:372–378.

Alon R, Feigelson S: From rolling to arrest on blood vessels: Leukocyte tap dancing on endothelial integrin ligands and chemokines at sub-second contacts. Semin Immunol 2002; 14:93–104.

Amin HM, McDonnell TJ, Ma Y, et al: Selective inhibition of STAT3 induces apoptosis and G(1) cell cycle arrest in ALK-positive anaplastic large cell lymphoma. Oncogene 2004; 23:5426–5434.

Andreopoulou E, Pectasides D, Dimopoulos MA, et al: Primary mediastinal large B-cell lymphoma: Clinical study of a distinct clinical entity and treatment outcome in 20 patients: Review of the literature. Am J Clin Oncol 2004; 27:312–316.

Andres E, Noel E, Kurtz JE, et al: Life-threatening idiosyncratic drug-induced agranulocytosis in elderly patients. Drugs Aging 2004; 21:427–435.

Angstreich GR, Smith BD, Jones RJ: Treatment options for chronic myeloid leukemia: Imatinib versus interferon versus allogeneic transplant. Curr Opin Oncol 2004; 16:95–99.

Anon: The value of c-kit in the diagnosis of biphenotypic acute leukemia. EGIL 1998; 12:2038.

Arcaini L, Orlandi E, Scotti M, et al: Combination of rituximab, cyclophosphamide, and vincristine induces complete hematologic remission of splenic marginal zone lymphoma. Clin Lymphoma 2004; 4:250–252.

Au WY, Gascoyne RD, Viswanatha DS, et al: Cytogenetic analysis in mantle cell lymphoma: A review of 214 cases. Leuk Lymphoma 2002; 43:783–791.

Au WY, Lam CC, Lie AK, et al: T-cell large granular lymphocyte leukemia of donor origin after allogeneic bone marrow transplantation. Am J Clin Pathol 2003; 120:626–630.

Badley AD, Roumier T, Lum JJ, et al: Mitochondrion-mediated apoptosis in HIV-1 infection. Trends Pharmacol Sci 2003; 24:298–305.

Bain BJ: Eosinophilic leukaemias and the idiopathic hypereosinophilic syndrome. Br J Haematol 1996; 95:2–9.

Bain BJ: Relationship between idiopathic hypereosinophilic syndrome, eosinophilic leukaemia, and systemic mastocytosis. Am J Hematol 2004; 77:82–85.

Bain B, Pierre R, Imbert M, et al: Chronic eosinophilic leukaemia and the hypereosinophilic syndrome. In Jaffe ES, Harris NL, Stein H, et al: (eds): World Health Organization Classification of Tumours. Pathology and Genetics of Tumours of Haematopoietic and Lymphoid Tissues. Lyon, IARC Press, 2001a, pp 29–31.

Bain B, Vardiman JW, Imbert M, et al: Myelodysplastic/myeloproliferative disease, unclassifiable. In Jaffe ES, Harris NL, Stein H, et al: (eds): World Health Organization Classification of Tumours. Pathology and Genetics of Tumours of Haematopoietic and Lymphoid Tissues. Lyon, IARC Press, 2001b, pp 58–59.

Banchereau J, Briere F, Caux C, et al: Immunobiology of dendritic cells. Annu Rev Immunol 2000; 18:767–811.

Banks PM, Warnke RA: Mediastinal (thymic) large B-cell lymphoma. In Jaffe ES, Harris NL, Stein H, et al: (eds): World Health Organization Classification of Tumours. Pathology and Genetics of Tumours of Haematopoietic and Lymphoid Tissues. Lyon, IARC Press, 2001a, pp 175–176.

Banks PM, Warnke RA: Primary effusion lymphoma. In Jaffe ES, Harris NL, Stein H, et al: (eds): World Health Organization Classification of Tumours. Pathology and Genetics of Tumours of Haematopoietic and Lymphoid Tissues. Lyon, IARC Press, 2001b, pp 179–180.

Bartl R, Frisch B, Burkhardt R, et al: Assessment of marrow trephine in relation to staging in chronic lymphocytic leukaemia. Br J Haematol 1982a; 51(1):1–15.

Bartl R, Frisch B, Burkhardt R, et al: Assessment of bone marrow histology in Hodgkin's disease: Correlation with clinical factors. Br J Haematol 1982b; 51(3):345–360.

Bass RD, Pullarkat V, Feinstein DI, et al: Pathology of autoimmune myelofibrosis. A report of three cases and a review of the literature. Am J Clin Pathol 2001; 116:211–216.

Basten A, Beeson PB: Mechanism of eosinophilia. II. Role of the lymphocyte. J Exp Med 1970; 131:1288–1305.

Belhadj K, Reyes F, Farcet JP, et al: Hepatosplenic gammadelta T-cell lymphoma is a rare clinicopathologic entity with poor outcome: Report on a series of 21 patients. Blood 2003; 102:4261–4269.

Bellan C, De Falco G, Lazzi S, et al: Pathologic aspects of AIDS malignancies. Oncogene 2003; 22:6639–6645.

Bene MC, Bernier M, Casasnovas RO, et al: The reliability and specificity of c-kit for the diagnosis of acute myeloid leukemias and undifferentiated leukemias. The European Group for the Immunological Classification of Leukemias (EGIL). Blood 1998; 92:596–599.

Benharroch D, Meguerian-Bedoyan Z, Lamant L, et al: ALK-positive lymphoma: A single disease with a broad spectrum of morphology. Blood 1998; 91:2076–2084.

Bennett JM: Classification of the myelodysplastic syndromes. Clin Haematol 1986; 15:909–923.

Bennett JM, Catovsky D, Daniel MT, et al: Proposals for the classification of the acute leukaemias. French–American–British (FAB) Cooperative Group. Br J Haematol 1976; 33:451–458.

Bennett JM, Catovsky D, Daniel MT, et al: A variant form of hypergranular promyelocytic leukaemia (M3). Br J Haematol 1980; 44:169–170.

Bennett JM, Catovsky D, Daniel MT, et al: The morphological classification of acute lymphoblastic leukaemia: Concordance among observers and clinical correlations. Br J Haematol 1981; 47:553–561.

Bennett JM, Catovsky D, Daniel MT, et al: Proposals for the classification of the myelodysplastic syndromes. Br J Haematol 1982; 51:189–199.

Bennett JM, Catovsky D, Daniel MT, et al: Proposed revised criteria for the classification of acute myeloid leukemia. A report of the French–American–British Cooperative Group. Ann Intern Med 1985a; 103:620–625.

Bennett JM, Catovsky D, Daniel MT, et al: Criteria for the diagnosis of acute leukemia of megakaryocyte lineage (M7). A report of the French–American–British Cooperative Group. Ann Intern Med 1985b; 103:460–462.

Bennett JM, Catovsky D, Daniel MT, et al: Proposals for the classification of chronic (mature) B and T lymphoid leukaemias. French–American–British (FAB) Cooperative Group. J Clin Pathol 1989; 42:567–584.

Bennett JM, Catovsky D, Daniel MT, et al: Proposal for the recognition of minimally differentiated acute myeloid leukemia (AML-MO). Br J Haematol 1991; 78:325–329.

Berard CW: Morphological definition of Burkitt's tumour: Historical review and present status. IARC Sci Publ 1985; 60:31–35.

Berard CW, Hutchison RE: The problem of classifying lymphomas: An orderly prescription for progress. Ann Oncol 1997; 8:3–9.

Berger F, Isaacson PG, Piris MA, et al: Lymphoplasmacytic lymphoma/Waldenstrom macroglobulinemia. In Jaffe ES, Harris NL, Stein H, et al: (eds): World Health Organization

Classification of Tumours. Pathology and Genetics of Tumours of Haematopoietic and Lymphoid Tissues. Lyon, IARC Press, 2001, pp 132–134.

Bhatt V, Saleem A: Review: Drug-induced neutropenia – pathophysiology, clinical features, and management. Annals of Clin & Lab Sci 2004; 34:131–137.

This is a recent review of the mechanisms of action, clinical features, diagnosis, and management of drug-induced neutropenia, including the use of filgrastim and pegfilgrastim in patients undergoing chemotherapy.

Bitter MA, Le Beau MM, Larson RA, et al: A morphologic and cytochemical study of acute myelomonocytic leukemia with abnormal marrow eosinophils associated with inv(16)(p13q22). Am J Clin Pathol 1984; 81:733–741.

Blay JY, Rossi JF, Wijdenes J, et al: Role of interleukin-6 in the paraneoplastic inflammatory syndrome associated with renal-cell carcinoma. Int J Cancer 1997; 72:424–430.

Blum KA, Lozanski G, Byrd JC: Adult Burkitt leukemia and lymphoma. Blood 2004; 104:3009–3020.

Bock O, Schlue J, Mengel M, et al: Thrombopoietin receptor (Mpl) expression by megakaryocytes in myeloproliferative disorders. J Pathol 2004; 203:609–615.

Bonzheim I, Geissinger E, Roth S, et al: Anaplastic large cell lymphomas lack the expression of T-cell receptor molecules or molecules of proximal T-cell receptor signaling. Blood 2004; 104:3358–3360.

Borisch B, Raphael M, Swerdlow SH, et al: Lymphoproliferative diseases associated with primary immune disorders. In Jaffe ES, Harris NL, Stein H, et al: (eds): World Health Organization Classification of Tumours. Pathology and Genetics of Tumours of Haematopoietic and Lymphoid Tissues. Lyon, IARC Press, 2001, pp 257–259.

Bouroncle BA, Wiseman BK, Doan CA: Leukemic reticuloendotheliosis. Blood 1958; 13:609–630.

Braeuninger A, Kuppers R, Strickler JG, et al: Hodgkin and Reed–Sternberg cells in lymphocyte predominant Hodgkin disease represent clonal populations of germinal center-derived tumor B cells. Proc Natl Acad Sci USA 1997; 94:9337–9342.

Brandt L: Leukaemia and lymphoma risks derived from solvents. Med Oncol Tumor Pharmacother 1987; 4:199–205.

Brigden ML: A practical workup for eosinophilia. You can investigate the most likely causes right in your office. Postgrad Med 1999; 105:193–210.

Brito-Babapulle F: The eosinophilias, including the idiopathic hypereosinophilic syndrome. Br J Haematol 2003; 121:203–223.

Brunning RD: Morphologic alterations in nucleated blood and marrow cells in genetic disorders. Hum Pathol 1970; 1:99.

Brunning RD, McKenna RW: Atlas of Tumor Pathology. Tumors of the Bone Marrow. Armed Forces Institute of Pathology, 1994.

Brunning RD, Bennett JM, Flandrin G, et al: Myelodysplastic syndromes: Introduction. In Jaffe ES, Harris NL, Stein H, et al: (eds): World Health Organization Classification of Tumours. Pathology and Genetics of Tumours of Haematopoietic and Lymphoid Tissues. Lyon, IARC Press, 2001a, pp 63–67.

Brunning RD, Bennett JM, Flandrin G, et al: Refractory anaemia. In Jaffe ES, Harris NL, Stein H, et al (eds): World Health Organization Classification of Tumours. Pathology and Genetics of Tumours of Haemaltopoietic and Lymphoid Tissues. Lyon, IARC Press, 2001b, p.68.

Brunning RD, Bennett JM, Flandrin G, et al: Refractory anaemia with ringed sideroblasts. In Jaffe ES, Harris NL, Stein H, et al: (eds): World Health Organization Classification of Tumours. Pathology and Genetics of Tumours of Haematopoietic and Lymphoid Tissues. Lyon, IARC Press, 2001c, p 69.

Brunning RD, Bennett JM, Flandrin G, et al: Refractory cytopenia with multilineage dysplasia. In Jaffe ES, Harris NL, Stein H, et al: (eds): World Health Organization Classification of Tumours. Pathology and Genetics of Tumours of

Haematopoietic and Lymphoid Tissues. Lyon, IARC Press, 2001d, p 70.

Brunning RD, Bennett JM, Flandrin G, et al: Refractory anaemia with excess blasts. In Jaffe ES, Harris NL, Stein H, et al: (eds): World Health Organization Classification of Tumours. Pathology and Genetics of Tumours of Haematopoietic and Lymphoid Tissues. Lyon, IARC Press, 2001e, p 71.

Brunning RD, Bennett JM, Flandrin G, et al: Myelodysplastic syndrome, unclassifiable. In Jaffe ES, Harris NL, Stein H, et al: (eds): World Health Organization Classification of Tumours. Pathology and Genetics of Tumours of Haematopoietic and Lymphoid Tissues. Lyon, IARC Press, 2001f, p 72.

Brunning RD, Bennett JM, Flandrin G, et al: Myelodysplastic syndrome associated with isolated del(5q) chromosome abnormality ('5q-syndrome'). In Jaffe ES, Harris NL, Stein H, et al: (eds): World Health Organization Classification of Tumours. Pathology and Genetics of Tumours of Haematopoietic and Lymphoid Tissues. Lyon, IARC Press, 2001g, p 73.

Brunning RD, Matutes E, Harris NL, et al: Acute myeloid leukaemia: Introduction. In Jaffe ES, Harris NL, Stein H, et al: (eds): World Health Organization Classification of Tumours. Pathology and Genetics of Tumours of Haematopoietic and Lymphoid Tissues. Lyon, IARC Press, 2001h, pp 77–80.

Brunning RD, Matutes E, Flandrin G, et al: Acute myeloid leukaemia with recurrent genetic abnormalities. In Jaffe ES, Harris NL, Stein H, et al: (eds): World Health Organization Classification of Tumours. Pathology and Genetics of Tumours of Haematopoietic and Lymphoid Tissues. Lyon, IARC Press, 2001i, pp 81–87.

Brunning RD, Matutes E, Harris NL, et al: Acute myeloid leukaemia with multilineage dysplasia. In Jaffe ES, Harris NL, Stein H, et al: (eds): World Health Organization Classification of Tumours. Pathology and Genetics of Tumours of Haematopoietic and Lymphoid Tissues. Lyon, IARC Press, 2001j, pp 88–89.

Brunning RD, Matutes E, Flandrin G, et al: Acute myeloid leukaemias and myelodysplastic syndromes, therapy related. In Jaffe ES, Harris NL, Stein H, et al: (eds): World Health Organization Classification of Tumours. Pathology and Genetics of Tumours of Haematopoietic and Lymphoid Tissues. Lyon, IARC Press, 2001k, pp 89–91.

Brunning RD, Matutes E, Flandrin G, et al: Acute myeloid leukaemia not otherwise categorised. In Jaffe ES, Harris NL, Stein H, et al: (eds): World Health Organization Classification of Tumours. Pathology and Genetics of Tumours of Haematopoietic and Lymphoid Tissues. Lyon, IARC Press, 2001l, pp 91–105.

Brunning RD, Matutes E, Borowitz M, et al: Acute leukaemias of ambiguous lineage. In Jaffe ES, Harris NL, Stein H, et al: (eds): World Health Organization Classification of Tumours. Pathology and Genetics of Tumours of Haematopoietic and Lymphoid Tissues. Lyon, IARC Press, 2001m, pp 106–107.

Brunning RD, Borowitz M, Matutes E, et al: Precursor B lymphoblastic leukaemia/lymphoblastic lymphoma (precursor B-cell acute lymphoblastic leukaemia). In Jaffe ES, Harris NL, Stein H, et al: (eds): World Health Organization Classification of Tumours. Pathology and Genetics of Tumours of Haematopoietic and Lymphoid Tissues. Lyon, IARC Press, 2001n, pp 111–114.

Brunning RD, Borowitz M, Matutes E, et al: Precursor T lymphoblastic leukaemia/lymphoblastic lymphoma (precursor T-cell acute lymphoblastic leukaemia). In Jaffe ES, Harris NL, Stein H, et al: (eds): World Health Organization Classification of Tumours. Pathology and Genetics of Tumours of Haematopoietic and Lymphoid Tissues. Lyon, IARC Press, 2001o, pp 115–117.

Bunting M, Harris ES, McIntyre TM, et al: Leukocyte adhesion deficiency syndromes: Adhesion and tethering defects involving beta 2 integrins and selectin ligands. Curr Opin Hematol 2002; 9:30–35.

Burkitt D: A sarcoma involving the jaws in African children. Br J Surg 1958; 46:218–223.

Cady FM, Muto DN, Ciabeterri G, et al: Utility of interphase FISH panels for routine clinical cytogenetic evaluation of chronic lymphocytic leukemia and multiple myeloma. J Assoc Genet Technol 2004; 30:77–81.

Cairo MS, Sposto R, Perkins SL, et al: Burkitt's and Burkitt-like lymphoma in children and adolescents: A review of the Children's Cancer Group experience. Br J Haematol 2003; 120:660–670.

Calabretta B, Perrotti D: The biology of CML blast crisis. Blood 2004; 103:4010–4022.

Caligiuri MA, Strout MP, Gilliland DG: Molecular biology of acute myeloid leukemia. Semin Oncol 1997; 24:32–44.

Camacho FI, Algara P, Mollejo M, et al: Nodal marginal zone lymphoma: A heterogeneous tumor: A comprehensive analysis of a series of 27 cases. Am J Surg Pathol 2003; 27:762–771.

Capello D, Vitolo U, Pasqualucci L, et al: Distribution and pattern of BCL-6 mutations throughout the spectrum of B-cell neoplasia. Blood 2000; 95:651–659.

Cardullo L de S, Morilla R, Catovsky D: Significance of phi bodies in acute leukaemia. J Clin Pathol 1981; 34:153–157.

Cassuto JP, Schneider M, Bourg M, et al: Acute infectious lymphocytosis as a T-cell lymphoproliferative syndrome. Br Med J 1977; 2:1331–1332.

Castella A, Croxson TS, Mildvan D, et al: The bone marrow in AIDS. A histologic, hematologic, and microbiologic study. Am J Clin Pathol 1985; 84:425–432.

Catovsky D, Montserrat E, Muller-Hermelink HK, et al: B-cell prolymphocytic leukaemia. In Jaffe ES, Harris NL, Stein H, et al: (eds): World Health Organization Classification of Tumours. Pathology and Genetics of Tumours of Haematopoietic and Lymphoid Tissues. Lyon, IARC Press, 2001a, pp 131–132.

Catovsky D, Ralfkiaer E, Muller-Hermelink HK: T-cell prolymphocytic leukaemia. In Jaffe ES, Harris NL, Stein H, et al: (eds): World Health Organization Classification of Tumours. Pathology and Genetics of Tumours of Haematopoietic and Lymphoid Tissues. Lyon, IARC Press, 2001b, pp 195–196.

Cham B, Bonilla MA, Winkelstein J: Neutropenia associated with primary immunodeficiency syndromes. Semin Hematol 2002; 39:107–112.

Chan JKC, Jaffe ES, Ralfkiaer E: Extranodal NK/T-cell lymphoma, nasal type. In Jaffe ES, Harris NL, Stein H, et al: (eds): World Health Organization Classification of Tumours. Pathology and Genetics of Tumours of Haematopoietic and Lymphoid Tissues. Lyon, IARC Press, 2001a, pp 204–207.

Chan JKC, Jaffe ES, Ralfkiaer E: Blastic NK-cell lymphoma. In Jaffe ES, Harris NL, Stein H, et al: (eds): World Health Organization Classification of Tumours. Pathology and Genetics of Tumours of Haematopoietic and Lymphoid Tissues. Lyon, IARC Press, 2001b, pp 214–215.

Chan JKC, Wong KF, Jaffe ES, et al: Aggressive NK-cell leukaemia. In Jaffe ES, Harris NL, Stein H, et al: (eds): World Health Organization Classification of Tumours. Pathology and Genetics of Tumours of Haematopoietic and Lymphoid Tissues. Lyon, IARC Press, 2001c, pp 198–200.

Chan WC, Catovsky D, Foucar K, et al: T-cell large granular lymphocyte leukaemia. In Jaffe ES, Harris NL, Stein H, et al: (eds): World Health Organization Classification of Tumours. Pathology and Genetics of Tumours of Haematopoietic and Lymphoid Tissues. Lyon, IARC Press, 2001d, pp 197–198.

Chang HW, Leong KH, Koh DR, et al: Clonality of isolated eosinophils in the hypereosinophilic syndrome. Blood 1999; 93:1651–1657.

Chen CJ, Huang YC, Jaing TH, et al: Hemophagocytic syndrome: A review of 18 pediatric cases. J Microbiol Immunol Infect 2004; 37:157–163.

Cheson BD, Cassileth PA, Head DR, et al: Report of the national cancer institute-sponsored workshop on definitions of diagnosis and response in acute myeloid leukemia. J Clin Oncol 1990; 8:813–819.

Chomienne C, Rain JD, Briere J, et al: Risk of leukemic transformation in PV and ET patients. Pathol Biol (Paris) 2004; 52:289–293.

Christensen RD, Calhoun DA: Congenital neutropenia. Clin Perinatol 2004; 31:29–38.

Christophers E: Eosinophilic diseases of the skin. Chem Immunol 2000; 76:230–243.

Collins CM, Medveczky PG: Genetic requirements for the episomal maintenance of oncogenic herpesvirus genomes. Adv Cancer Res 2002; 84:155–174.

Cortes J: Natural history and staging of chronic myelogenous leukemia. Hematol Oncol Clin North Am 2004; 18:569–584.

Cortes J, Kantarjian H: Advanced-phase chronic myeloid leukemia. Semin Hematol 2003; 40:79–86.

Crist WM, Shuster JJ, Falletta J, et al: Clinical features and outcome in childhood T-cell leukemia-lymphoma according to stage of thymocyte differentiation: A Pediatric Oncology Group study. Blood 1988; 72:1891–1897.

Csernus B, Timar B, Fulop Z, et al: Mutational analysis of IgVH and BCL-6 genes suggests thymic B-cells origin of mediastinal (thymic) B-cell lymphoma. Leuk Lymphoma 2004; 45:2105–2110.

Cuneo A, Ferrant A, Michaux JL, et al: Cytogenetic and clinicobiological features of acute leukemia with stem cell phenotype: Study of nine cases. Cancer Genet Cytogenet 1996; 92:31–36.

Dainiak N: Hematologic consequences of exposure to ionizing radiation. Exp Hematol 2002; 30:513–528.
This article reviews common forms of ionizing radiation, including measurement, as well as dose response for normal marrow elements, effects on cells at the cellular level, and clinical effects of exposure.

Dale DC: Introduction: Severe chronic neutropenia. Semin Hematol 2002a; 39:73–74.

Dale DC, Bolyard AA, Aprikyan A: Cyclic neutropenia. Semin Hematol 2002b; 39:89–94.

Davey FR, Huntington S: Age-related variation in lymphocyte subpopulations. Gerontology 1977; 23:381–389.

Davey FR, Hutchison RE: Pathology and immunology of adult T-cell leukemia/lymphoma. Curr Opin Oncol 1991; 3:13–20.

Davidsohn I: Serologic diagnosis of infectious mononucleosis. JAMA 1937; 108:289.

Davidsohn I, Lee CL: The clinical serology of infectious mononucleosis. In Carter RL, Penman HG (eds): Infectious Mononucleosis. Oxford, Blackwell Scientific Publications, 1969.

De Falco G, Bellan C, Lazzi S, et al: Interaction between HIV-1 Tat and pRb2/p130: A possible mechanism in the pathogenesis of AIDS-related neoplasms. Oncogene 2003; 22:6214–6219.

De Paepe P, Baens M, van Krieken H, et al: ALK activation by the CLTC-ALK fusion is a recurrent event in large B-cell lymphoma. Blood 2003; 102:2638–2641.

De Waele M, Foulon W, Renmans W, et al: Hematologic values and lymphocyte subsets in fetal blood. Am J Clin Pathol 1988; 89:742–746.

Dearden CE, Matutes E, Cazin B, et al: High remission rate in T-cell prolymphocytic leukemia with CAMPATH-1H. Blood 2001; 98:1721–1726.

Delage R, Roy J, Jacques L, et al: Multiple bcl-2/Ig gene rearrangements in persistent polyclonal B-cell lymphocytosis. Br J Haematol 1997; 97:589–595.

Delsol G, Ralfkiaer E, Stein H, et al: Anaplastic large cell lymphoma. In Jaffe ES, Harris NL, Stein H, et al: (eds): World Health Organization Classification of Tumours. Pathology and Genetics of Tumours of Haematopoietic and Lymphoid Tissues. Lyon, IARC Press, 2001, pp 230–235.

Diaz-Jouanen E, Strickland RG, Williams RC: Studies of human lymphocytes in the newborn and the aged. Am J Med 1975; 58:620–628.

Diebold J, Jaffe ES, Raphael M, et al: Burkitt lymphoma. In Jaffe ES, Harris NL, Stein H, et al: (eds): World Health Organization Classification of Tumours. Pathology and Genetics of Tumours of Haematopoietic and Lymphoid Tissues. Lyon, IARC Press, 2001, pp 181–184.

Dogan A, Isaacson PG: Splenic marginal zone lymphoma. Semin Diagn Pathol 2003; 20:121–127.

Dorfman RF, Remington JS: Value of lymph-node biopsy in the diagnosis of acute acquired toxoplasmosis. N Engl J Med 1973; 289:878–881.

Druker BJ: Imatinib as a paradigm of targeted therapies. Adv Cancer Res 2004; 91:1–30.

Duarte-Davidson R, Courage C, Rushton L, et al: Benzene in the environment: An assessment of the potential risks to the health of the population. Occup Environ Med 2001; 58:2–13.

Durie BG, Kyle RA, Belch A, et al: Myeloma management guidelines: A consensus report from the scientific advisors of the international myeloma foundation. Hematol J 2003; 4:379–398.

Ehrlich GD, Han T, Bettigole R, et al: Human T-lymphotropic virus type I-associated benign transient immature T-cell lymphocytosis. Am J Hematol 1988; 27:49–55.

Elliott MA, Dewald GW, Tefferi A, et al: Chronic neutrophilic leukemia (CNL): A clinical, pathologic and cytogenetic study. Leukemia 2001; 15:35–40.

Erber WN, Breton-Gorius J, Villeval JL, et al: Detection of cells of megakaryocyte lineage in haematological malignancies by immuno-alkaline phosphatase labelling cell smears with a panel of monoclonal antibodies. Br J Haematol 1987; 65:87–94.

Etzioni A, Alon R: Leukocyte adhesion deficiency III: A group of integrin activation defects in hematopoietic lineage cells. Curr Opin Allergy Clin Immunol 2004; 4:485–490.

Falini B, Pulford K, Pucciarini A, et al: Lymphomas expressing ALK fusion protein(s) other than NPM-ALK. Blood 1999; 94:3509–3515.

Falini B, Tiacci E, Liso A, et al: Simple diagnostic assay for hairy cell leukaemia by immunocytochemical detection of annexin A1 (ANXA1). Lancet 2004; 363:1869–1871.

Felgar RE, Salhany KE, Macon WR, et al: The expression of TIA-1+ cytolytic-type granules and other cytolytic lymphocyte-associated markers in CD30+ anaplastic large cell lymphomas (ALCL): Correlation with morphology, immunophenotype, ultrastructure, and clinical features. Hum Pathol 1999; 30:228–236.

Fialkow PJ, Jacobson RJ, Papayannopoulou T: Chronic myelocytic leukemia: Clonal origin in a stem cell common to the granulocyte, erythrocyte, platelet and monocyte/macrophage. Am J Med 1977; 63:125–130.

Foa R, Lauria F, Catovsky D: Evidence that T colony formation is a property of T mu (helper) lymphocytes. Clin Exp Immunol 1980; 42:152–155.

Foucar K, Catovsky D: Hairy cell leukaemia. In Jaffe ES, Harris NL, Stein H, et al: (eds): World Health Organization Classification of Tumours. Pathology and Genetics of Tumours of Haematopoietic and Lymphoid Tissues. Lyon, IARC Press, 2001, pp 138–141.

Foxman EF, Campbell JJ, Butcher EC: Multistep navigation and the combinatorial control of leukocyte chemotaxis. J Cell Biol 1997; 139:1349–1360.

Franklin EC: Mu-chain disease. Arch Intern Med 1975; 135:71–72.

Gabius HJ, Andre S, Kaltner H, et al: The sugar code: Functional lectinomics. Biochim Biophys Acta 2002; 1572:165–177.

Gabriel HH, Kindermann W: Adhesion molecules during immune response to exercise. Can J Physiol Pharmacol 1998; 76:512–523.

Gale RE: Pathogenic markers in essential thrombocythemia. Curr Hematol Rep 2003; 2:242–247.

Galton DA, Goldman JM, Wiltshaw E, et al: Prolymphocytic leukaemia. Br J Haematol 1974; 27:7–23.

Gamis AS: Acute myeloid leukemia and Down syndrome evolution of modern therapy-state of the art review. Pediatr Blood Cancer, 2004.

Gascoyne RD: Molecular pathogenesis of mucosal-associated lymphoid tissue (MALT) lymphoma. Leuk Lymphoma 2003; 44:S13–20.

Gatter KC, Warnke RA: Diffuse large B-cell lymphoma. In Jaffe ES, Harris NL, Stein H, et al: (eds): World Health Organization Classification of Tumours. Pathology and Genetics of Tumours of Haematopoietic and Lymphoid Tissues. Lyon, IARC Press, 2001a, pp 171–174.

Gatter KC, Warnke RA: Intravascular large B-cell lymphoma. In Jaffe ES, Harris NL, Stein H, et al: (eds): World Health Organization Classification of Tumours. Pathology and Genetics of Tumours of Haematopoietic and Lymphoid Tissues. Lyon, IARC Press, 2001b, pp 177–178.

Gentile TC, Hadlock KG, Uner AH, et al: Large granular lymphocyte leukaemia occurring after renal transplantation. Br J Haematol 1998; 101:507–512.

Gentile TC, Uner AH, Hutchison RE, et al: CD3+, CD56+ aggressive variant of large granular lymphocyte leukemia. Blood 1994; 84:2315–2321.

Gilbert HS, Ornstein L: Basophil counting with a new staining method using alcian blue. Blood 1975; 46:279–286.

Gilliland DG, Jordan CT, Felix CA. The molecular basis of leukemia. Hematology (Am Soc Hematol Educ Program) 2004; 80–97.
This paper describes the molecular genetics of adult and pediatric leukemias and relates recent findings to current and future therapies.

Go RS, Wester SM: Immunophenotypic and molecular features, clinical outcomes, treatments, and prognostic factors associated with subcutaneous panniculitis-like T-cell lymphoma: A systematic analysis of 156 patients reported in the literature. Cancer 2004; 101:1404–1413.

Golomb HM, Rowley JD, Vardiman JW, et al: 'Microgranular' acute promyelocytic leukemia: A distinct clinical, ultrastructural, and cytogenetic entity. Blood 1980; 55:253–259.

Gombart AF, Shiohara M, Kwok SH, et al: Neutrophil-specific granule deficiency: Homozygous recessive inheritance of a frameshift mutation in the gene encoding transcription factor CCAAT/enhancer binding protein-epsilon. Blood 2001; 97:2561–2567.

Gorlin RJ, Gelb B, Diaz GA, et al: WHIM syndrome, an autosomal dominant disorder: Clinical, hematological, and molecular studies. Am J Med Genet 2000; 91:368–376.

Gotlib V, Darji J, Bloomfield K, et al: Eosinophilic variant of chronic myeloid leukemia with vascular complications. Leuk Lymphoma 2003; 44:1609–1613.

Green DR: Overview: Apoptotic signaling pathways in the immune system. Immunol Rev 2003; 193:5–9.

Greenberg P, Cox C, Le Beau MM, et al: International scoring system for evaluating prognosis in myelodysplastic syndromes. Blood 1997; 89:2079–2088.

Greenberg PL: Apoptosis and its role in the myelodysplastic syndromes: Implications for disease natural history and treatment. Leuk Res 1998; 22:1123–1136.

Griesshammer M, Klippel S, Strunck E, et al: PRV-1 mRNA expression discriminates two types of essential thrombocythemia. Ann Hematol 2004; 83:364–370.

Grogan TM, Van Camp B, Kyle RA, et al: Plasma cell neoplasms. In Jaffe ES, Harris NL, Stein H, et al: (eds): World Health Organization Classification of Tumours. Pathology and Genetics of Tumours of Haematopoietic and Lymphoid Tissues. Lyon, IARC Press, 2001, pp 142–156.

Gulino AV: WHIM syndrome: A genetic disorder of leukocyte trafficking. Curr Opin Allergy Clin Immunol 2003 3:443–450.

Gulino AV, Moratto D, Sozzani S, et al: Altered leukocyte response to CXCL12 in patients with warts, hypogammaglobulinemia, infections, myelokathexis (WHIM) syndrome. Blood 2004; 104:444–452.

Haks MC, Krimpenfort P, Borst J, et al: The CD3gamma chain is essential for development of both the TCRalphabeta and TCRgammadelta lineages. EMBO J 1998; 17:1871–1882.

Haluska FG, Russo G, Kant J, et al: Molecular resemblance of an AIDS-associated lymphoma and endemic Burkitt lymphomas: Implications for their pathogenesis. Proc Natl Acad Sci USA 1989; 86:8907–8911.

Hao S, Sanger W, Onciu M, et al: Mantle cell lymphoma with 8q24 chromosomal abnormalities: A report of 5 cases with blastoid features. Mod Pathol 2002; 15:1266–1272.

Harrington DS, Weisenburger DD, Purtilo DT: Epstein–Barr virus-associated lymphoproliferative lesions. Clin Lab Med 1988; 8:97–118.

Harris NL: Mature B-cell neoplasms: Introduction. In Jaffe ES, Harris NL, Stein H, et al: (eds): World Health Organization Classification of Tumours. Pathology and Genetics of Tumours of Haematopoietic and Lymphoid Tissues. Lyon, IARC Press, 2001a, pp 121–126.

Harris NL, Swerdlow SH: Methotrexate-associated lymphoproliferative disorders. In Jaffe ES, Harris NL, Stein H, et al: (eds): World Health Organization Classification of Tumours. Pathology and Genetics of Tumours of Haematopoietic and Lymphoid Tissues. Lyon, IARC Press, 2001b, pp 270–271.

Harris NL, Jaffe ES, Stein H, et al: A revised European–American classification of lymphoid neoplasms: A proposal from the International Lymphoma Study Group. Blood 1994; 84:1361–1392.

Harris NL, Jaffe ES, Stein H, et al: Lymphoma classification proposal: Clarification. Blood 1995; 85:857–860.

Harris NL, Swerdlow SH, Frizzera G, et al: Post-transplant lymphoproliferative disorders. In Jaffe ES, Harris NL, Stein H, et al: (eds): World Health Organization Classification of Tumours. Pathology and Genetics of Tumours of Haematopoietic and Lymphoid Tissues. Lyon, IARC Press, 2001c, pp 264–269.

Hasselbalch H, Jans H, Nielsen PL: A distinct subtype of idiopathic myelofibrosis with bone marrow features mimicking hairy cell leukemia: Evidence of an autoimmune pathogenesis. Am J Hematol 1987; 25:225–229.

Hayhoe FG: Cytochemistry of the acute leukaemias. Histochem J 1984; 16:1051–1059.

Heath KE, Campos-Barros A, Toren A, et al: Nonmuscle myosin heavy chain IIA mutations define a spectrum of autosomal dominant macrothrombocytopenias: May–Hegglin anomaly and Fechtner, Sebastian, Epstein, and Alport-like syndromes. Am J Hum Genet 2001; 69:1033–1045.

Heine G, Gabriel H, Weindler J, et al: Painful regional anaesthesia induces an immunological stress reaction: The model of retrobulbar anaesthesia. Eur J Anaesthesiol 2001; 18:505–510.

Herbst H, Pallesen G, Weiss LM, et al: Hodgkin's disease and Epstein–Barr virus. Ann Oncol 1992; 3:27–30.

Hernandez AM: Peripheral blood manifestations of lymphoma and solid tumors. Clin Lab Med 2002; 22:215–253.

This article describes the correlation of findings identified on peripheral blood films in patients with various types of lymphoid leukemia and lymphoma, including morphology of various lymphoma cells in the circulating blood during disease.

Hernandez PA, Gorlin RJ, Lukens JN, et al: Mutations in the chemokine receptor gene CXCR4 are associated with WHIM syndrome, a combined immunodeficiency disease. Nat Genet 2003; 34:70–74.

Hess RD: Routine Epstein–Barr virus diagnostics from the laboratory perspective: Still challenging after 35 years. J Clin Microbiol 2004; 42:3381–3387.

Heyworth PG, Cross AR, Curnutte JT: Chronic granulomatous disease. Curr Opin Immunol 2003; 15:578–584.

Himmelmann A, Gautschi O, Nawrath M, et al: Persistent polyclonal B-cell lymphocytosis is an expansion of functional IgD(+)CD27(+) memory B cells. Br J Haematol 2001; 114:400–405.

Horie R, Watanabe M, Ishida T, et al: The NPM-ALK oncoprotein abrogates CD30 signaling and constitutive NF-kappaB activation in anaplastic large cell lymphoma. Cancer Cell 2004; 5:353–364.

Hornick JL, Fletcher CD: Immunohistochemical staining for KIT (CD117) in soft tissue sarcomas is very limited in distribution. Am J Clin Pathol 2002; 117:188–193.

Hoxie JA: Hematologic manifestations of AIDS. In Hoffman R, Benz EJ, Shattil SJ (eds): Hematology. Basic Principles and Practice. New York, Churchill Livingstone, 1995.

Hoy A, Leininger-Muller B, Kutter D, et al: Growing significance of myeloperoxidase in non-infectious diseases. Clin Chem Lab Med 2002; 40:2–8.

Hudnall SD, Molina CP: Marked increase in L-selectin-negative T cells in neonatal pertussis. The lymphocytosis explained? Am J Clin Pathol 2000; 114:35–40.

Hutchison RE, Fairclough DL, Holt H, et al: Clinical significance of histology and immunophenotype in childhood diffuse large cell lymphoma. Am J Clin Pathol 1991; 95:787–793.

Hutchison RE, Kurec AS, Davey FR: Granulocytic sarcoma. Clin Lab Med 1990; 10:889–901.

Hutchison RE, Murphy SB, Fairclough DL, et al: Diffuse small noncleaved cell lymphoma in children, Burkitt's versus non-Burkitt's types. Results from the Pediatric Oncology Group and St. Jude Children's Research Hospital. Cancer 1989; 64:23–28.

Iannitto E, Ambrosetti A, Ammatuna E, et al: Splenic marginal zone lymphoma with or without villous lymphocytes. Hematologic findings and outcomes in a series of 57 patients. Cancer 2004; 101:2050–2057.

Iida S, Rao PH, Ueda R, et al: Chromosomal rearrangement of the PAX-5 locus in lymphoplasmacytic lymphoma with t(9;14)(p13;q32). Leuk Lymphoma 1999; 34:25–33.

ILSG – The Non-Hodgkin's Lymphoma Classification Project: A clinical evaluation of the International Lymphoma Study Group classification of non-Hodgkin's lymphoma. Blood 1997; 89:3909–3918.

Imbert M, Bain B, Pierre R, et al: Chronic neutrophilic leukaemia. In Jaffe ES, Harris NL, Stein H, et al: (eds): World Health Organization Classification of Tumours. Pathology and Genetics of Tumours of Haematopoietic and Lymphoid Tissues. Lyon, IARC Press, 2001a, pp 27–28.

Imbert M, Pierre R, Thiele J, et al: Essential thrombocythaemia. In Jaffe ES, Harris NL, Stein H, et al: (eds): World Health Organization Classification of Tumours. Pathology and Genetics of Tumours of Haematopoietic and Lymphoid Tissues. Lyon, IARC Press, 2001b, pp 39–41.

Introne W, Boissy RE, Gahl WA: Clinical, molecular, and cell biological aspects of Chediak–Higashi syndrome. Mol Genet Metab 1999; 68:283–303.

Iqbal J, Sanger WG, Horsman DE, et al: BCL2 translocation defines a unique tumor subset within the germinal center B-cell-like diffuse large B-cell lymphoma. Am J Pathol 2004; 165:159–166.

Isaacson P, Wright D, Ralfkiaer E, et al: Enteropathy-type T-cell lymphoma. In Jaffe ES, Harris NL, Stein H, et al: (eds): World Health Organization Classification of Tumours. Pathology and Genetics of Tumours of Haematopoietic and Lymphoid Tissues. Lyon, IARC Press, 2001a, pp 208–209.

Isaacson PG, Muller-Hermelink HK, Piris MA, et al: Extranodal marginal zone B-cell lymphoma of mucosa-associated lymphoid tissue (MALT lymphoma). In Jaffe ES, Harris NL, Stein H, et al: (eds): World Health Organization Classification of Tumours. Pathology and Genetics of Tumours of Haematopoietic and Lymphoid Tissues. Lyon, Press, IARC Press, 2001b, pp 157–160.

Isaacson PG, Nathwani BN, Piris MA, et al: Nodal marginal zone B-cell lymphoma. In Jaffe ES, Harris NL, Stein H, et al: (eds): World Health Organization Classification of Tumours. Pathology and Genetics of Tumours of Haematopoietic and Lymphoid Tissues. Lyon, IARC Press, 2001c, p 161.

Isaacson PG, Piris MA, Catovsky D, et al: Splenic marginal zone lymphoma. In Jaffe ES, Harris NL, Stein H, et al: (eds): World Health Organization Classification of Tumours. Pathology and Genetics of Tumours of Haematopoietic and Lymphoid Tissues. Lyon, IARC Press, 2001d, pp 135–137.

Ivanovska I, Galonek HL, Hildeman DA, Hardwick JM: Regulation of cell death in the lymphoid system by Bcl-2 family proteins. Acta Haematol 2004; 11:42–55.

Jaffe ES: Histiocytic and dendritic cell neoplasms: Introduction. In Jaffe ES, Harris NL, Stein H, et al: (eds): World Health Organization Classification of Tumours. Pathology and Genetics of Tumours of Haematopoietic and Lymphoid Tissues. Lyon, IARC Press, 2001b, pp 275–277.

Jaffe ES, Ralfkiaer E: Mature T-cell and NK-cell neoplasma: Introduction. In Jaffe ES, Harris NL, Stein H, et al: (eds): World Health Organization Classification of Tumours. Pathology and Genetics of Tumours of Haematopoietic and Lymphoid Tissues. Lyon, IARC Press, 2001c, pp 191–194.

Jaffe ES, Ralfkiaer E: Hepatosplenic T-cell lymphoma. In Jaffe ES, Harris NL, Stein H, et al: (eds): World Health Organization Classification of Tumours. Pathology and Genetics of Tumours of Haematopoietic and Lymphoid Tissues. Lyon, IARC Press, 2001d, pp 210–211.

Jaffe ES, Ralfkiaer E: Subcutaneous panniculitis-like T-cell lymphoma. In Jaffe ES, Harris NL, Stein H, et al: (eds): World Health Organization Classification of Tumours. Pathology and Genetics of Tumours of Haematopoietic and Lymphoid Tissues. Lyon, IARC Press, 2001e, pp 212–213.

Jaffe ES, Ralfkiaer E: Angioimmunoblastic T-cell lymphoma. In Jaffe ES, Harris NL, Stein H, et al: (eds): World Health Organization Classification of Tumours. Pathology and Genetics of Tumours of Haematopoietic and Lymphoid Tissues. Lyon, IARC Press, 2001f, pp 225–226.

Jaffe ES, Wilson WH: Lymphomatoid granulomatosis. In Jaffe ES, Harris NL, Stein H, et al: (eds): World Health Organization Classification of Tumours. Pathology and Genetics of Tumours of Haematopoietic and Lymphoid Tissues. Lyon, IARC Press, 2001g, pp 185–187.

Jaffe ES, Harris NL, Stein H, et al: (eds): World Health Organization Classification of Tumours. Pathology and Genetics of Tumours of Haematopoietic and Lymphoid Tissues, 3rd ed. Lyon, International Agency for Research on Cancer, 2001a.

This provides a comprehensive and uniform classification of hematopoietic neoplasms. It was commissioned by the WHO through the major organizations of hematopathology, with clinical input from cooperative groups and cancer centers and is intended to provide the standard diagnositic criteria for worldwide use. It also provides a comprehensive review of the state of knowledge of hematopoietic neoplasms through the 20th century.

Jenner MJ, Summers KE, Norton AJ, et al: JH probe real-time quantitative polymerase chain reaction assay for bcl-2/IgH rearrangements. Br J Haematol 2002; 118:550–558.

Jiang F, Lin F, Price R, et al: Rapid detection of IgH/BCL2 rearrangement in follicular lymphoma by interphase fluorescence in situ hybridization with bacterial artificial chromosome probes. J Mol Diagn 2002; 4:144–149.

Jiang X, Wang X: Cytochrome C-mediated apoptosis. Annu Rev Biochem 2004; 73:87–106.

Jurkowska M, Bernatowska E, Bal J: Genetic and biochemical background of chronic granulomatous disease. Arch Immunol Ther Exp (Warsz) 2004; 52:113–120.

Kalyanaraman VS, Sarngadharan MG, Robert-Guroff M, et al: A new subtype of human T-cell leukemia virus (HTLV-II) associated with a T-cell variant of hairy cell leukemia. Science 1982; 218:571–573.

Kanda M, Suzumiya J, Ohshima K, et al: Analysis of the immunoglobulin heavy chain gene variable region of intravascular large B-cell lymphoma. Virchows Arch 2001; 439:540–546.

Kang J, Volkmann A, Raulet DH: Evidence that gammadelta versus alphabeta T cell fate determination is initiated independently of T cell receptor signaling. J Exp Med 2001; 193:689–698.

Karras A, Thervet E, Legendre C, et al: Hemophagocytic syndrome in renal transplant recipients: Report of 17 cases and review of literature. Transplantation 2004; 77:238–243.

Kasahara Y, Yachie A: Cell type specific infection of Epstein–Barr virus (EBV) in EBV-associated hemophagocytic lymphohistiocytosis and chronic active EBV infection. Crit Rev Oncol Hematol 2002; 44:283–294.

Kasamon YL, Swinnen LJ: Treatment advances in adult Burkitt lymphoma and leukemia. Curr Opin Oncol 2004; 16:429–435.

Katzenstein AL, Peiper SC: Detection of Epstein–Barr virus genomes in lymphomatoid granulomatosis: Analysis of 29 cases by the polymerase chain reaction technique. Mod Pathol 1990; 3:435–441.

Katzenstein AL, Carrington CB, Liebow AA: Lymphomatoid granulomatosis: A clinicopathologic study of 152 cases. Cancer 1979; 43:360–373.

Kaushansky K: Etiology of the myeloproliferative disorders: The role of thrombopoietin. Semin Hematol 2003; 40:6–9.

Kelaidi C, Rollot F, Park S, et al: Response to antiviral treatment in hepatitis C virus-associated marginal zone lymphomas. Leukemia 2004; 18:1711–1716.

Kelley MJ, Jawien W, Ortel TL, et al: Mutation of MYH9, encoding non-muscle myosin heavy chain A, in May–Hegglin anomaly. Nat Genet 2000; 26:106–108.

Khanna-Gupta A, Zibello T, Sun H, et al: C/EBP epsilon mediates myeloid differentiation and is regulated by the CCAAT displacement protein (CDP/cut). Proc Natl Acad Sci USA 2001; 98:8000–8005.

Kikuchi M, Jaffe ES, Ralfkiaer E: Adult T-cell leukaemia/lymphoma. In Jaffe ES, Harris NL, Stein H, et al (eds): World Health Organization Classification of Tumours. Pathology and Genetics of Tumours of Haematopoietic and Lymphoid Tissues. Lyon, IARC Press, 2001, pp 200–203.

Kim SZ, Chow KU, Kukoc-Zivojnov N, et al: Expression of ZAP-70 protein correlates with disease stage in chronic lymphocytic leukemia and is associated with, but not generally restricted to, non-mutated Ig VH status. Leuk Lymphoma 2004; 45:2037–2045.

Kinoshita K, Amagasaki T, Ikeda S, et al: Preleukemic state of adult T cell leukemia: Abnormal T lymphocytosis induced by human adult T cell leukemia-lymphoma virus. Blood 1985; 66:120–127.

Knowles DM: Immunophenotypic and antigen receptor gene rearrangement analysis in T cell neoplasia. Am J Pathol 1989; 134:761–785.

Knowles DM: Etiology and pathogenesis of AIDS-related non-Hodgkin's lymphoma. Hematol Oncol Clin North Am 2003; 17:785–820.

Knowles DM, Chamulak GA, Subar M, et al: Lymphoid neoplasia associated with the acquired immunodeficiency syndrome (AIDS). The New York University Medical Center experience with 105 patients (1981–1986). Ann Intern Med 1988; 108:744–753.

Kobayashi SD, Voyich JM, Braughton KR, et al: Gene expression profiling provides insight into the pathophysiology of chronic granulomatous disease. J Immunol 2004; 172:636–643.

Korsmeyer SJ: BCL-2 gene family and the regulation of programmed cell death. Cancer Res 1999; 59:1693s–1700s.

Kroft SH: Infectious diseases manifested in the peripheral blood. Clin Lab Med 2002; 22:253–277.
A review of both nonspecific hematopoietic changes in the peripheral blood during infection as well as findings for the few diseases in which peripheral blood film review plays a primary diagnostic role.

Kuppers R: B cells under influence: Transformation of B cells by Epstein–Barr virus. Nat Rev Immunol 2003; 3:801–812.

Kutter D, Devaquet P, Vanderstocken G, et al: Consequences of total and subtotal myeloperoxidase deficiency: Risk or benefit? Acta Haematol 2000; 104:10–15.

Lagergren J: The white blood cell count and the erythrocyte sedimentation rate in pertussis. Acta Paediatr 1963; 52:405–409.

Lakshman R, Finn A: Neutrophil disorders and their management. J Clin Pathol 2001; 54:7–19.

Lamant L, Gascoyne RD, Duplantier MM, et al: Non-muscle myosin heavy chain (MYH9): A new partner fused to ALK in anaplastic large cell lymphoma. Genes Chromosomes Cancer 2003; 37:427–432.

Lamy T, Loughran TP, Jr: Clinical features of large granular lymphocyte leukemia. Semin Hematol 2003; 40:185–195.

Landaw SA: Acute leukemia in polycythemia vera. Semin Hematol 1986; 23:156–165.

Langerak AW, van Den Beemd R, Wolvers-Tettero IL, et al: Molecular and flow cytometric analysis of the Vbeta repertoire for clonality assessment in mature TCRalphabeta T-cell proliferations. Blood 2001; 98:165–173.

Lanza F: Clinical manifestation of myeloperoxidase deficiency. J Mol Med 1998; 76:676–681.

Lazzi S, Bellan C, De Falco G, et al: Expression of RB2/p130 tumor-suppressor gene in AIDS-related non-Hodgkin's lymphomas: Implications for disease pathogenesis. Hum Pathol 2002; 33:723–731.

Le Beau MM, Larson RA: Cytogenetics and neoplasia. In Hoffman R, Benz EJ, Shattil SJ (eds): Hematology. Basic Principles and Practice. New York, Churchill Livingstone, 2000, p 848.

Lee CL, Davidsohn I, Panczyszyn O: Horse agglutinins in infectious mononucleosis. II. The spot test. Am J Clin Pathol 1968; 49:12–18.

Lennert K, Stein H, Kaiserling E: Cytological and functional criteria for the classification of malignant lymphomata. Br J Cancer 1975; 31:29–43.

Levitus M, Rooimans MA, Steltenpool J, et al: Heterogeneity in Fanconi anemia: Evidence for 2 new genetic subtypes. Blood 2004; 103:2498–2503.

Lima M, Almeida J, Dos Anjos Teixeira M, et al: TCRalphabeta+/CD4+ large granular lymphocytosis: A new clonal T-cell lymphoproliferative disorder. Am J Pathol 2003; 163:763–771.

Lipscomb MF, Masten BJ: Dendritic cells: Immune regulators in health and disease. Physiol Rev 2002; 82:97–130.

List AF, Vardiman J, Issa JP, Dewitte TM: Myelodysplastic syndromes. Hematology (Am Soc Hematol Educ Program). 2004; 297–317.
This overview of myelodysplastic syndromes covers the spectrum from microscopic diagnosis to laboratory science and the translation of recent findings into therapeutic strategies.

Liu Z, Dong HY, Gorczyca W, et al: CD5-mantle cell lymphoma. Am J Clin Pathol 2002; 118:216–224.

Loembe MM, Lamoureux J, Deslauriers N, et al: Lack of CD40-dependent B-cell proliferation in B lymphocytes isolated from patients with persistent polyclonal B-cell lymphocytosis. Br J Haematol 2001; 113:699–705.

Loembe MM, Neron S, Delage R, et al: Analysis of expressed V(H) genes in persistent polyclonal B cell lymphocytosis reveals absence of selection in CD27+IgM+IgD+ memory B cells. Eur J Immunol 2002; 32:3678–3688.

Lones MA, Auperin A, Raphael M, et al: Mature B-cell lymphoma/leukemia in children and adolescents: Intergroup pathologist consensus with the revised European–American lymphoma classification. Ann Oncol 2000; 11:47–51.

Lones MA, Sanger WG, Le Beau MM, et al: Chromosome abnormalities may correlate with prognosis in Burkitt/Burkitt-like lymphomas of children and adolescents: A report from Children's Cancer Group study CCG-E08. J Pediatr Hematol Oncol 2004; 26:169–178.

Lukes RJ, Carver LL, Hall TC: Hodgkin's disease, report of nomenclature committee. Cancer Res 1966; 26:1311.

Luna-Fineman S, Shannon KM, Atwater SK, et al: Myelodysplastic and myeloproliferative disorders of childhood: A study of 167 patients. Blood 1999; 93:459–466.

Luscinskas FW, Ma S, Nusrat A, et al: Leukocyte transendothelial migration: A junctional affair. Semin Immunol 2002; 14:105–113.

McDonald PP: Transcriptional regulation in neutrophils: Teaching old cells new tricks. Adv Immunol 2004; 82:1–48.

McDowall A, Inwald D, Leitinger B, et al: A novel form of integrin dysfunction involving beta1, beta2, and beta3 integrins. J Clin Invest 2003; 111:51–60.

Machii T, Tokumine Y, Inoue R, et al: Predominance of a distinct subtype of hairy cell leukemia in Japan. Leukemia 1993; 7:181–186.

Machii T, Yamaguchi M, Inoue R, et al: Polyclonal B-cell lymphocytosis with features resembling hairy cell leukemia-Japanese variant. Blood 1997; 89:2008–2014.

McKenna RW, Parkin J, Bloomfield CD, et al: Acute promyelocytic leukaemia: A study of 39 cases with identification of a hyperbasophilic microgranular variant. Br J Haematol 1982; 50:201–214.

MacPherson N, Lesack D, Klasa R, et al: Small noncleaved, non-Burkitt's (Burkitt-like) lymphoma: Cytogenetics predict outcome and reflect clinical presentation. J Clin Oncol 1999; 17:1558–1567.

Mainou-Fowler T, Dignum HM, Proctor SJ, et al: The prognostic value of CD38 expression and its quantification in B cell chronic lymphocytic leukemia (B-CLL). Leuk Lymphoma 2004; 45:455–462.

Maitra A, McKenna RW, Weinberg AG, et al: Precursor B-cell lymphoblastic lymphoma. A study of nine cases lacking blood and bone marrow involvement and review of the literature. Am J Clin Pathol 2001; 115:868–875.

Maldonado JE, Hanlon DG: Monocytosis: A current appraisal. Mayo Clin Proc 1965; 40:248–259.

Mansoor A, Medeiros LJ, Weber DM, et al: Cytogenetic findings in lymphoplasmacytic lymphoma/Waldenstrom macroglobulinemia. Chromosomal abnormalities are associated with the polymorphous subtype and an aggressive clinical course. Am J Clin Pathol 2001; 116:543–549.

Marsden VS, Strasser A: Control of apoptosis in the immune system: Bcl-2, BH3-only proteins and more. Annu Rev Immunol 2003; 21:71–105.

Martignetti JA, Heath KE, Harris J, et al: The gene for May–Hegglin anomaly localizes to a <1-mb region on chromosome 22q12.3-13.1. Am J Hum Genet 2000; 66:1449–1454.

Martin DA, Elkon KB: Mechanisms of apoptosis. Rheum Dis Clin North Am 2004; 30:441–454.

Martinez-Climent JA, Garcia-Conde J: Chromosomal rearrangements in childhood acute myeloid leukemia and myelodysplastic syndromes. J Pediatr Hematol Oncol 1999; 21:91–102.

Martinez-Moczygemba M, Huston DP: Biology of common beta receptor-signaling cytokines: IL-3, IL-5, and GM-CSF. J Allergy Clin Immunol 2003; 112:653–666.

Matta H, Chaudhary PM: Activation of alternative NF-kappa B pathway by human herpes virus 8-encoded Fas-associated death domain-like IL-1 beta-converting enzyme inhibitory protein (vFLIP). Proc Natl Acad Sci USA 2004; 101:9399–9404.

Mbulaiteye SM, Parkin DM, Rabkin CS: Epidemiology of AIDS-related malignancies: an international perspective. Hematol Oncol Clin North Am 2003; 17:673–696.

IV

Meerkin D, Ashkenazi Y, Gottschalk-Sabag S, et al: Plasma cell dyscrasia with marrow fibrosis. A reversible syndrome mimicking agnogenic myeloid metaplasia. Cancer 1994; 73:625–628.

Melhem MF, Meisler AI, Saito R, et al: Cytokines in inflammatory malignant fibrous histiocytoma presenting with leukemoid reaction. Blood 1993; 82:2038–2044.

Melo JV, Catovsky D, Gregory WM, et al: The relationship between chronic lymphocytic leukaemia and prolymphocytic leukaemia. IV. Analysis of survival and prognostic features. Br J Haematol 1987; 65:23–29.

Menendez P, Vargas A, Bueno C, et al: Quantitative analysis of bcl-2 expression in normal and leukemic human B-cell differentiation. Leukemia 2004; 18:491–498.

Merchant SH, Viswanatha DS, Zumwalt RE, et al: Epstein–Barr virus-associated intravascular large T-cell lymphoma presenting as acute renal failure in a patient with acquired immune deficiency syndrome. Hum Pathol 2003; 34:950–954.

Mesa RA, Elliott MA, Schroeder G, et al: Durable responses to thalidomide-based drug therapy for myelofibrosis with myeloid metaplasia. Mayo Clin Proc 2004; 79:883–889.

Michiels JJ, Juvonen E: Proposal for revised diagnostic criteria of essential thrombocythemia and polycythemia vera by the Thrombocythemia Vera Study Group. Semin Thromb Hemost 1997; 23:339–347.

Michiels JJ, Berneman Z, Schroyens W, et al: Philadelphia (Ph) chromosome-positive thrombocythemia without features of chronic myeloid leukemia in peripheral blood: Natural history and diagnostic differentiation from Ph-negative essential thrombocythemia. Ann Hematol 2004; 83:504–512.

Michiels JJ, Kutti J, Stark P, et al: Diagnosis, pathogenesis and treatment of the myeloproliferative disorders essential thrombocythemia, polycythemia vera and essential megakaryocytic granulocytic metaplasia and myelofibrosis. Neth J Med 1999; 54:46–62.

Moliterno AR, Siebel KE, Sun AY, et al: A novel thrombopoietin signaling defect in polycythemia vera platelets. Stem Cells 1998; 16:185–192.

Montoto S, Lopez-Guillermo A, Altes A, et al: Predictive value of follicular lymphoma international prognostic index (FLIPI) in patients with follicular lymphoma at first progression. Ann Oncol 2004; 15:1484–1489.

Montserrat E, Rozman C: Bone marrow biopsy in chronic lymphocytic leukemia: A review of its prognostic importance. Blood Cells 1987; 12:315–326.

Morice WG, Kimlinger T, Katzmann JA, et al: Flow cytometric assessment of TCR-Vbeta expression in the evaluation of peripheral blood involvement by T-cell lymphoproliferative disorders: A comparison with conventional T-cell immunophenotyping and molecular genetic techniques. Am J Clin Pathol 2004; 121:373–383.

Morris SW, Kirstein MN, Valentine MB, et al: Fusion of a kinase gene, ALK, to a nucleolar protein gene, NPM, in non-Hodgkin's lymphoma. Science 1994; 263:1281–1284.

Moser B, Wolf M, Walz A, et al: Chemokines: Multiple levels of leukocyte migration control. Trends Immunol 2004; 25:75–84.

Mounier N, Briere J, Gisselbrecht C, et al: Rituximab plus CHOP (R-CHOP) overcomes bcl-2-associated resistance to chemotherapy in elderly patients with diffuse large B-cell lymphoma (DLBCL). Blood 2003; 101:4279–4284.

Mroczek EC, Weisenburger DD, Grierson HL, et al: Fatal infectious mononucleosis and virus-associated hemophagocytic syndrome. Arch Pathol Lab Med 1987; 111:530–535.

Mrozek K, Heerema NA, Bloomfield CD: Cytogenetics in acute leukemia. Blood Rev 2004; 18:115–136.

Muller-Hermelink HK, Catovsky D, Montserrat E, et al: Chronic lymphocytic leukaemia/small lymphocytic lymphoma. In Jaffe ES, Harris NL, Stein H, et al: (eds): World Health Organization Classification of Tumours. Pathology and Genetics of Tumours of Haematopoietic and Lymphoid Tissues. Lyon, IARC Press, 2001, pp 127–130.

Muss HB, Moloney WC: Chloroma and other myeloblastic tumors. Blood 1973; 42:721–728.

Myers JL, Kurtin PJ, Katzenstein AL, et al: Lymphomatoid granulomatosis. Evidence of immunophenotypic diversity and relationship to Epstein–Barr virus infection. Am J Surg Pathol 1995; 19:1300–1312.

Naiman JL, Oski FA, Allen FH Jr, et al: Hereditary eosinophilia: Report of a family and review of the literature. Am J Hum Genet 1964; 16:195–203.

Nakagawa T, Ikemoto T, Takeuchi T, et al: Eosinophilic peroxidase deficiency: Identification of a point mutation (D648N) and prediction of structural changes. Hum Mutat 2001; 17:235–236.

Nara T, Hayakawa A, Ikeuchi A, et al: Granulocyte colony-stimulating factor-producing cutaneous angiosarcoma with leukaemoid reaction arising on a burn scar. Br J Dermatol 2003; 149:1273–1275.

Nathwani BN, Harris NL, Weisenburger D, et al: Follicular lymphoma. In Jaffe ES, Harris NL, Stein H, et al: (eds): World Health Organization Classification of Tumours. Pathology and Genetics of Tumours of Haematopoietic and Lymphoid Tissues. Lyon, IARC Press, 2001, pp 162–167.

Nauseef WM: Lessons from MPO deficiency about functionally important structural features. Jpn J Infect Dis 2004; 57:S4–5.

Neiman RS, Barcos M, Berard C, et al: Granulocytic sarcoma: A clinicopathologic study of 61 biopsied cases. Cancer 1981; 48:1426–1437.

Neiman RS, Rosen PJ, Lukes RJ: Lymphocyte-depletion Hodgkin's disease. A clinicopathological entity. N Engl J Med 1973; 288:751–755.

Nicola MD, Carlo-Stella C, Mariotti J, et al: High response rate and manageable toxicity with an intensive, short-term chemotherapy programme for Burkitt's lymphoma in adults. Br J Haematol 2004; 126:815–820.

Niederwieser D, Gastl G, Rumpold H, et al: Rapid reappearance of large granular lymphocytes (LGL) with concomitant reconstitution of natural killer (NK) activity after human bone marrow transplantation (BMT). Br J Haematol 1987; 65:301–305.

Niittyvuopio R, Juvonen E, Kekomaki R, et al: The predictive value of megakaryocytic and erythroid colony formation and platelet function tests on the risk of thromboembolic and bleeding complications in essential thrombocythaemia. Eur J Haematol 2004; 72:245–251.

Nimieri HS, Makoni SN, Madziwa FH, et al: Leukemoid reaction response to chemotherapy and radiotherapy in a patient with cervical carcinoma. Ann Hematol 2003; 82:316–317.

Nola M, Pavletic SZ, Weisenburger DD, et al: Prognostic factors influencing survival in patients with B-cell small lymphocytic lymphoma. Am J Hematol 2004; 77:31–35.

Non-Hodgkin's Lymphoma Pathologic Classification Project: National cancer institute-sponsored study of classifications of non-Hodgkin's lymphoma. Cancer 1982; 49:2112–2135.

Nowell PC, Hungerford DA: A minute chromosome in human chronic granulocytic leukemia. Science 1960; 132:1497–1500.

Oakley SP, Garsia RJ, Coates AS: Eosinophilic leukaemoid reaction and interleukin-5 in metastatic melanoma. Med J Aust 1998; 169:501.

Offit K, Parsa NZ, Filippa D, et al: t(9;14)(p13;q32) denotes a subset of low-grade non-Hodgkin's lymphoma with plasmacytoid differentiation. Blood 1992; 80:2594–2599.

Oren H, Ozkal S, Gulen H, et al: Autoimmune lymphoproliferative syndrome. Report of two cases and review of the literature. Ann Hematol 2002; 81:651–653.

Orrenius S: Mitochondrial regulation of apoptotic cell death. Toxicol Lett 2004; 149:19–23.

Pahl HL: Diagnostic approaches to polycythemia vera in 2004. Expert Rev Mol Diagn 2004; 4:495–502.

Palframan RT, Collins PD, Williams TJ, et al: Eotaxin induces a rapid release of eosinophils and their progenitors from the bone marrow. Blood 1998; 91:2240–2248.

Patel KD, Cuvelier SL, Wiehler S: Selectins: Critical mediators of leukocyte recruitment. Semin Immunol 2002; 14:73–81.

Patte C, Auperin A, Michon J, et al: The Societe Francaise d'Oncologie Pediatrique LMB89 protocol: Highly effective multiagent chemotherapy tailored to the tumor burden and initial response in 561 unselected children with B-cell lymphomas and L3 leukemia. Blood 2001; 97:3370–3379.

Paul JR, Bunnell WW: The presence of heterophile antibodies in infectious mononucleosis. Am J Med Sci 1932; 183:90.

Pawade J, Wilkins BS, Wright DH: Low-grade B-cell lymphomas of the splenic marginal zone: A clinicopathological and immunohistochemical study of 14 cases. Histopathology 1995; 27:129–137.

Perkins SL: Appendix A. Normal blood and bone marrow values in humans. Table A. Leukocyte count and differential count reference values in children. In Greer JP, Foerster J, Lukens JN, et al: (eds): Wintrobe's Clinical Hematology, 11th ed. Philadelphia, Lippincott, Williams & Wilkins, 2004, p. 2702.

Peterson L, Hrisinko MA: Benign lymphocytosis and reactive neutrophilia. Laboratory features provide diagnostic clues. Clin Lab Med, 1993; 13:863–877.

Petros AM, Olejniczak ET, Fesik SW: Structural biology of the bcl-2 family of proteins. Biochim Biophys Acta 2004; 1644:83–94.

Pichardo DA, Querfeld C, Guitart J, et al: Cutaneous T-cell lymphoma: A paradigm for biological therapies. Leuk Lymphoma 2004; 45:1755–1765.

Pierre R, Imbert M, Thiele J, et al: Polycythaemia vera. In Jaffe ES, Harris NL, Stein H, et al: (eds): World Health Organization Classification of Tumours. Pathology and Genetics of Tumours of Haematopoietic and Lymphoid Tissues. Lyon, IARC Press, 2001, pp 32–34.

Pikarsky E, Porat RM, Stein I, et al: NF-kappaB functions as a tumour promoter in inflammation-associated cancer. Nature 2004; 431:461–466.

Pileri SA, Ascani S, Leoncini L, et al: Hodgkin's lymphoma: The pathologist's viewpoint. J Clin Pathol 2002; 55:162–176.

Poiesz BJ, Ruscetti FW, Gazdar AF, et al: Detection and isolation of type C retrovirus particles from fresh and cultured lymphocytes of a patient with cutaneous T-cell lymphoma. Proc Natl Acad Sci USA 1980; 77:7415–7419.

Ponzoni M, Arrigoni G, Gould VE, et al: Lack of CD 29 (beta1 integrin) and CD 54 (ICAM-1) adhesion molecules in intravascular lymphomatosis. Hum Pathol 2000; 31:220–226.

Pui CH, Relling MV, Downing JR: Acute lymphoblastic leukemia. N Engl J Med 2004; 350:1535–1548.
This review describes the molecular genetic alterations, prognostic factors, molecular epidemiology and pharmacogenetics of pediatric and adult acute lymphoblastic leukemia.

Pullarkat V, Bass RD, Gong JZ, et al: Primary autoimmune myelofibrosis: Definition of a distinct clinicopathologic syndrome. Am J Hematol 2003; 72:8–12.

Purtilo DT: Immunopathology of the X-linked lymphoproliferative syndrome. Haematol Blood Transfus 1981; 26:207–214.

Purtilo DT, Paquin L, DeFlorio D, et al: Immunodiagnosis and immunopathogenesis of the X-linked recessive lymphoproliferative syndrome. Semin Hematol 1979; 16:309–343.

Raghavachar A, Bartram CR, Ganser A, et al: Acute undifferentiated leukemia: Implications for cellular origin and clonality suggested by analysis of surface markers and immunoglobulin gene rearrangement. Blood 1986; 68:658–662.

Rai KR, Chanana AD, Cronkite EP, et al: Studies on lymphocytes 18. Mechanism of lymphocytosis induced by supernatant fluids of *Bordetella pertussis* cultures. Blood 1971; 38:49–59.

Ralfkiaer E, Jaffe ES: Mycosis fungoides and Sezary syndrome. *In* Jaffe ES, Harris NL, Stein H, et al: (eds): World Health Organization Classification of Tumours. Pathology and Genetics of Tumours of Haematopoietic and Lymphoid Tissues. Lyon, IARC Press, 2001b, pp 216–220.

Ralfkiaer E, Delsol G, Willemze R, et al: Primary cutaneous CD30-positive T-cell lymphoproliferative disorders. *In* Jaffe ES, Harris NL, Stein H, et al: (eds): World Health Organization Classification of Tumours. Pathology and Genetics of Tumours of Haematopoietic and Lymphoid Tissues. Lyon, IARC Press, 2001a, pp 221–224.

Ralfkiaer E, Muller-Hermelink HK, Jaffe ES: Peripheral T-cell lymphoma, unspecified. *In* Jaffe ES, Harris NL, Stein H, et al: (eds): World Health Organization Classification of Tumours. Pathology and Genetics of Tumours of Haematopoietic and Lymphoid Tissues. Lyon, IARC Press, 2001c, pp 227–229.

Ramirez MJ, Titos E, Claria J, et al: Increased apoptosis dependent on caspase-3 activity in polymorphonuclear leukocytes from patients with cirrhosis and ascites. J Hepatol 2004; 41:44–48.

Rao RV, Ellerby HM, Bredesen DE: Coupling endoplasmic reticulum stress to the cell death program. Cell Death Differ 2004; 11:372–380.

Raphael M, Borisch B, Jaffe ES: Lymphomas associated with infection by the human immune deficiency virus (HIV). *In* Jaffe ES, Harris NL, Stein H, et al: (eds): World Health Organization Classification of Tumours. Pathology and Genetics of Tumours of Haematopoietic and Lymphoid Tissues. Lyon, IARC Press, 2001, pp 260–263.

Reilly JT: Pathogenesis and management of idiopathic myelofibrosis. Baillières Clin Haematol 1998; 11:751–767.

Reilly WA: The granules in the leukocytes in gargoylism. Am J Dis Child 1941; 62:482.

Reinherz EL, Kung PC, Goldstein G, et al. Discrete stages of human intrathymic differentiation: Analysis of normal thymocytes and leukemic lymphoblasts of T-cell lineage. Proc Natl Acad Sci USA 1980; 77:1588–1592.

Remington JS, Thulliez P, Montoya JG: Recent developments for diagnosis of toxoplasmosis. J Clin Microbiol 2004; 42:941–945.

Rizzi R, Pastore D, Liso A, et al: Autoimmune myelofibrosis: Report of three cases and review of the literature. Leuk Lymphoma 2004; 45:561–566.

Rogers R, Windust A, Gregory J: Evaluation of a novel dry latex preparation for demonstration of infectious mononucleosis heterophile antibody in comparison with three established tests. J Clin Microbiol 1999; 37:95–98.

Romagnani P, Lasagni L, Annunziato F, et al: CXC chemokines: The regulatory link between inflammation and angiogenesis. Trends Immunol 2004; 25:201–209.

Roos D, Law SKA: Hematologically important mutations: Leukocyte adhesion deficiency. Blood Cells Mol Dis 2001; 27:1000–1004.

Rosenberg HF, Gallin JI: Neutrophil-specific granule deficiency includes eosinophils. Blood 1993; 82:268–273.

Rosenthal S, Canellos GP, DeVita VT Jr, et al: Characteristics of blast crisis in chronic granulocytic leukemia. Blood 1977; 49:705–714.

Rosenwald A, Wright G, Chan WC, et al: The use of molecular profiling to predict survival after chemotherapy for diffuse large-B-cell lymphoma. N Engl J Med 2002; 346:1937–1947.

Rosenwald A, Wright G, Leroy K, et al: Molecular diagnosis of primary mediastinal B cell lymphoma identifies a clinically favorable subgroup of diffuse large B cell lymphoma related to Hodgkin lymphoma. J Exp Med 2003; 198:851–862.

Rossi D, Zlotnik A: The biology of chemokines and their receptors. Annu Rev Immunol 2000; 18:217–242.

Rot A, von Andrian UH: Chemokines in innate and adaptive host defense: Basic chemokinese grammar for immune cells. Annu Rev Immunol 2004; 22:891–928.

This recent article presents an overview of chemokine communication and signaling mechanisms in immunity.

Roufosse F, Cogan E, Goldman M: The hypereosinophilic syndrome revisited. Annu Rev Med 2003; 54:169–184.

Roussel M, Roue G, Sola B, et al: Dysfunction of the Fas apoptotic signaling pathway in persistent polyclonal B-cell lymphocytosis. Haematologica 2003; 88:239–240.

Ruka W, Rutkowski P, Kaminska J, et al: Alterations of routine blood tests in adult patients with soft tissue sarcomas: Relationships to cytokine serum levels and prognostic significance. Ann Oncol 2001; 12:1423–1432.

Ruoslahti E, Rajotte D: An address system in the vasculature of normal tissues and tumors. Annu Rev Immunol 2000; 18:813–827.

Saelens X, Festjens N, Vande Walle L, et al: Toxic proteins released from mitochondria in cell death. Oncogene 2004; 23:2861–2874.

Sainati L, Matutes E, Mulligan S, et al: A variant form of hairy cell leukemia resistant to alpha-interferon: Clinical and phenotypic characteristics of 17 patients. Blood 1990; 76:157–162.

Sallusto F, Mackay CR, Lanzavecchia A: The role of chemokine receptors in primary, effector, and memory immune responses. Annu Rev Immunol 2000; 18:593–620.

Sansonno D, De Vita S, Cornacchiulo V, et al: Detection and distribution of hepatitis C virus-related proteins in lymph nodes of patients with type II mixed cryoglobulinemia and neoplastic or non-neoplastic lymphoproliferation. Blood 1996; 88:4638–4645.

Savage DG, Szydlo RM, Goldman JM: Clinical features at diagnosis in 430 patients with chronic myeloid leukaemia seen at a referral centre over a 16-year period. Br J Haematol 1997; 96:111–116.

Savage KJ, Monti S, Kutok JL, et al: The molecular signature of mediastinal large B-cell lymphoma differs from that of other diffuse large B-cell lymphomas and shares features with classical Hodgkin lymphoma. Blood 2003; 102:3871–3879.

Schinzel A, Kaufmann T, Borner C: Bcl-2 family members: Integrators of survival and death signals in physiology and pathology. Biochim Biophys Acta 2004; 1644:95–105.

Schlette EJ, Medeiros LJ, Goy A, et al: Survivin expression predicts poorer prognosis in anaplastic large-cell lymphoma. J Clin Oncol 2004; 22:1682–1688.

Schop RF, Fonseca R: Genetics and cytogenetics of Waldenstrom's macroglobulinemia. Semin Oncol 2003; 30:142–145.

Schulte C, Krebs B, Jelinek T, et al: Diagnostic significance of blood eosinophilia in returning travelers. Clin Infect Dis 2002; 34:407–411.

Schultz DR, Harrington WJ Jr: Apoptosis: Programmed cell death at a molecular level. Semin Arthritis Rheum 2003; 32:345–369.

This article reviews mechanisms and regulatory and effector proteins of the extrinsic and intrinsic apoptotic pathways, and includes a glossary of terms in the appendix.

Seri M, Cusano R, Gangarossa S, et al: Mutations in MYH9 result in the May–Hegglin anomaly, and Fechtner and Sebastian syndromes. The May–Hegglin/Fechtner Syndrome Consortium. Nat Genet 2000; 26:103–105.

Seri M, Pecci A, Di Bari F, et al: MYH9-related disease: May–Hegglin anomaly, Sebastian syndrome, Fechtner syndrome, and Epstein syndrome are not distinct entities but represent a variable expression of a single illness. Medicine (Baltimore) 2003; 82:203–215.

Sezer O, Heider U, Zavrski I, et al: RANK ligand and osteoprotegerin in myeloma bone disease. Blood 2003; 101:2094–2098.

Shadrach B, Warshawsky I: A comparison of multiplex and monoplex T-cell receptor gamma PCR. Diagn Mol Pathol 2004; 13:127–134.

Shapiro M, Wasik MA, Junkins-Hopkins JM, et al: Complete remission in advanced blastic NK-cell lymphoma/leukemia in elderly patients using the hyper-CVAD regimen. Am J Hematol 2003; 74:46–51.

Shephard RJ: Adhesion molecules, catecholamines and leucocyte redistribution during and following exercise. Sports Med 2003; 33:261–284.

Shtalrid M, Shvidel L, Vorst E: Polyclonal reactive peripheral blood plasmacytosis mimicking plasma cell leukemia in a patient with staphylococcal sepsis. Leuk Lymphoma 2003; 44:379–380.

Shurin SB: Pathologic states associated with activation of eosinophils and with eosinophilia. Hematol Oncol Clin North Am 1988; 2:171–179.

Silver RT, Woolf SH, Hehlmann R, et al: An evidence-based analysis of the effect of busulfan, hydroxyurea, interferon, and allogeneic bone marrow transplantation in treating the chronic phase of chronic myeloid leukemia: Developed for the American Society of Hematology. Blood 1999; 94:1517–1536.

Silverstein MN, Tefferi A: Treatment of essential thrombocythemia with anagrelide. Semin Hematol 1999; 36:23–25.

Simon HU, Plotz SG, Dummer R, et al: Abnormal clones of T cells producing interleukin-5 in idiopathic eosinophilia. N Engl J Med 1999; 341:1112–1120.

Sixbey JW, Nedrud JG, Raab-Traub N, et al: Epstein–Barr virus replication in oropharyngeal epithelial cells. N Engl J Med 1984; 310:1225–1230.

Skinnider BF, Horsman DE, Dupuis B, et al: Bcl-6 and bcl-2 protein expression in diffuse large B-cell lymphoma and follicular lymphoma: Correlation with 3q27 and 18q21 chromosomal abnormalities. Hum Pathol 1999; 30:803–808.

So CC, Wong KF: May–Hegglin anomaly. Br J Haematol 2003; 120:373.

Sobol RE, Bloomfield CD, Royston I: Immunophenotyping in the diagnosis and classification of acute lymphoblastic leukemia. Clin Lab Med 1988; 8:151–162.

Sobol RE, Mick R, Royston I, et al: Clinical importance of myeloid antigen expression in adult acute lymphoblastic leukemia. N Engl J Med 1987; 316:1111–1117.

Solal-Celigny P, Roy P, Colombat P, et al: Follicular lymphoma international prognostic index. Blood 2004; 104:1258–1265.

Spangrude GJ, Sacchi F, Hill HR, et al: Inhibition of lymphocyte and neutrophil chemotaxis by pertussis toxin. J Immunol 1985; 135:4135–4143.

Stansfeld AG, Diebold J, Noel H, et al: Updated Kiel classification for lymphomas. Lancet 1988; 1:292–293.

Starckx S, Van den Steen PE, Wuyts A, et al: Neutrophil gelatinase B and chemokines in leukocytosis and stem cell mobilization. Leuk Lymphoma 2002; 43:233–241.

Starkebaum G: Chronic neutropenia associated with autoimmune disease. Semin Hematol 2002; 39:121–127.

Starr-Spires LD, Collman RG: HIV-1 entry and entry inhibitors as therapeutic agents. Clin Lab Med 2002; 22:681–701.

Stass SA, Mirro J, Jr: Lineage heterogeneity in acute leukaemia: Acute mixed-lineage leukaemia and lineage switch. Clin Haematol 1986; 15:811–827.

Stein H, Hummel M: Cellular origin and clonality of classic Hodgkin's lymphoma: Immunophenotypic and molecular studies. Semin Hematol 1999; 36:233–241.

Stein H, Delsol G, Pileri S, et al: Classical Hodgkin lymphoma. *In* Jaffe ES, Harris NL, Stein H, et al: (eds): World Health Organization Classification of Tumours. Pathology and Genetics of Tumours of Haematopoietic and Lymphoid Tissues. Lyon, IARC Press, 2001a, pp 244–253.

Stein H, Delsol G, Pileri S, et al: Nodular lymphocyte predominant Hodgkin lymphoma. *In* Jaffe ES, Harris NL, Stein H, et al: (eds): World Health Organization Classification of Tumours. Pathology

IV

and Genetics of Tumours of Haematopoietic and Lymphoid Tissues. Lyon, IARC Press, 2001b, pp 240–243.

Stein H, Mason DY, Gerdes J, et al: The expression of the Hodgkin's disease associated antigen ki-1 in reactive and neoplastic lymphoid tissue: Evidence that Reed–Sternberg cells and histiocytic malignancies are derived from activated lymphoid cells. Blood 1985; 66:848–858.

Suwa T, Hogg JC, English D, et al: Interleukin-6 induces demargination of intravascular neutrophils and shortens their transit in marrow. Am J Physiol Heart Circ Physiol 2000; 279:H2954–60.

Suzuki K, Muso E, Nauseef WM: Contribution of peroxidases in host-defense, diseases and cellular functions. Jpn J Infect Dis 2004; 57:S1–2.

Suzuki R, Kagami Y, Takeuchi K, et al: Prognostic significance of CD56 expression for ALK-positive and ALK-negative anaplastic large-cell lymphoma of T/null cell phenotype. Blood 2000; 96:2993–3000.

Swerdlow SH, Berger F, Isaacson PG, et al: Mantle cell lymphoma. In Jaffe ES, Harris NL, Stein H, et al: (eds): World Health Organization Classification of Tumours. Pathology and Genetics of Tumours of Haematopoietic and Lymphoid Tissues. Lyon, IARC Press, 2001, pp 168–170.

Szegezdi E, Fitzgerald U, Samali A: Caspase-12 and ER-stress-mediated apoptosis: The story so far. Ann N Y Acad Sci 2003; 1010:186–194.

Taguchi A, Miyazaki M, Sakuragi S, et al: Gamma/delta T cell lymphoma. Intern Med 2004; 43:120–125.

Tancrede-Bohin E, Ionescu MA, de La Salmoniere P, et al: Prognostic value of blood eosinophilia in primary cutaneous T-cell lymphomas. Arch Dermatol 2004; 140:1057–1061.

Taylor GH: Cytomegalovirus. Am Fam Physician 2003; 67:519–524.

Tefferi A: The forgotten myeloproliferative disorder: Myeloid metaplasia. Oncologist 2003; 8:225–231.

Thalhammer-Scherrer R, Mitterbauer G, Simonitsch I, et al: The immunophenotype of 325 adult acute leukemias. Am J Clin Pathol 2002; 117:380–389.

Thiele J, Imbert M, Pierre R, et al: Chronic myeloproliferative disease, unclassifiable. In Jaffe ES, Harris NL, Stein H, et al: (eds): World Health Organization Classification of Tumours. Pathology and Genetics of Tumours of Haematopoietic and Lymphoid Tissues. Lyon, IARC Press, 2001a, pp 42–44.

Thiele J, Pierre R, Imbert M, et al: Chronic idiopathic myelofibrosis. In Jaffe ES, Harris NL, Stein H, et al: (eds): World Health Organization Classification of Tumours. Pathology and Genetics of Tumours of Haematopoietic and Lymphoid Tissues. Lyon, IARC Press, 2001b, pp 35–38.

Thompson MP, Kurzrock R: Epstein–Barr virus and cancer. Clin Cancer Res 2004; 10:803–821.

Thorley-Lawson DA, Gross A: Persistence of the Epstein–Barr virus and the origins of associated lymphomas. N Engl J Med 2004; 350:1328–1337.

Tischkowitz M, Dokal I: Fanconi anaemia and leukaemia – clinical and molecular aspects. Br J Haematol 2004; 126:176–191.

Toren A, Rozenfeld-Granot G, Heath KE, et al: MYH9 spectrum of autosomal-dominant giant platelet syndromes: Unexpected association with fibulin-1 variant-D inactivation. Am J Hematol 2003; 74:254–262.

Tsaparas YF, Brigden ML, Mathias R, et al: Proportion positive for Epstein–Barr virus, cytomegalovirus, human herpesvirus 6, toxoplasma, and human immunodeficiency virus types 1 and 2 in heterophile-negative patients with an absolute lymphocytosis or an instrument-generated atypical lymphocyte flag. Arch Pathol Lab Med 2000; 124:1324–1330.

Valent P, Horny HP, Escribano L, et al: Diagnostic criteria and classification of mastocytosis: A consensus proposal. Leuk Res 2001a; 25:603–625.

Valent P, Horny HP, Li CY, et al: Mastocytosis. In Jaffe ES, Harris NL, Stein H, et al: (eds): World Health Organization Classification of Tumours. Pathology and Genetics of Tumours of Haematopoietic and Lymphoid Tissues. Lyon, IARC Press, 2001b, pp 293–302.

van Eeden SF, Terashima T: Interleukin 8 (IL-8) and the release of leukocytes from the bone marrow. Leuk Lymphoma 2000; 37:259–271.

Vardiman JW: Myelodysplastic/myeloproliferative diseases: Introduction. In Jaffe ES, Harris NL, Stein H, et al: (eds): World Health Organization Classification of Tumours. Pathology and Genetics of Tumours of Haematopoietic and Lymphoid Tissues. Lyon, IARC Press, 2001a, pp 47–48.

Vardiman JW, Brunning RD, Harris NL: Chronic myeloproliferative diseases. In Jaffe ES, Harris NL, Stein H, et al: (eds): World Health Organization Classification of Tumours. Pathology and Genetics of Tumours of Haematopoietic and Lymphoid Tissues. Lyon, IARC Press, 2001b, pp 15–17.

Vardiman JW, Imbert M, Pierre R, et al: Atypical chronic myeloid leukaemia. In Jaffe ES, Harris NL, Stein H, et al: (eds): World Health Organization Classification of Tumours. Pathology and Genetics of Tumours of Haematopoietic and Lymphoid Tissues. Lyon, IARC Press, 2001c, pp 53–54.

Vardiman JW, Pierre R, Bain B, et al: Chronic myelomonocytic leukaemia. In Jaffe ES, Harris NL, Stein H, et al: (eds): World Health Organization Classification of Tumours. Pathology and Genetics of Tumours of Haematopoietic and Lymphoid Tissues. Lyon, IARC Press, 2001d, pp 49–52.

Vardiman JW, Pierre R, Imbert M, et al: Juvenile myelomonocytic leukaemia. In Jaffe ES, Harris NL, Stein H, et al: (eds): World Health Organization Classification of Tumours. Pathology and Genetics of Tumours of Haematopoietic and Lymphoid Tissues. Lyon, IARC Press, 2001e, pp 55–57.

Vardiman JW, Pierre R, Thiele J, et al: Chronic myelogenous leukaemia. In Jaffe ES, Harris NL, Stein H, et al: (eds): World Health Organization Classification of Tumours. Pathology and Genetics of Tumours of Haematopoietic and Lymphoid Tissues. Lyon, IARC Press, 2001f, pp 20–26.

Varindani MK, Pitchumoni CS, Lucariello RJ: Eosinophilic leukemoid reaction in pulmonary carcinoma. N Y State J Med 1982; 82:347–348.

Vignais PV: The superoxide-generating NADPH oxidase: Structural aspects and activation mechanism. Cell Mol Life Sci 2002; 59:1428–1459.

Viswanatha DS, Foucar K, Berry BR, et al: Blastic mantle cell leukemia: An unusual presentation of blastic mantle cell lymphoma. Mod Pathol 2000; 13:825–833.

von Wasielewski S, Franklin J, Fischer R, et al: Nodular sclerosing Hodgkin disease: New grading predicts prognosis in intermediate and advanced stages. Blood 2003; 101:4063–4069.

Ward DM, Shiflett SL, Kaplan J: Chediak–Higashi syndrome: A clinical and molecular view of a rare lysosomal storage disorder. Curr Mol Med 2002; 2:469–477.

Weick JK, Hagedorn AB, Linman JW: Leukoerythroblastosis. Diagnostic and prognostic significance. Mayo Clin Proc 1974; 49:110–113.

Weiss LM, Grogan TM, Muller-Hermelink HK, et al: Histiocytic sarcoma. In Jaffe ES, Harris NL, Stein H, et al: (eds): World Health Organization Classification of Tumours. Pathology and Genetics of Tumours of Haematopoietic and Lymphoid Tissues. Lyon, IARC Press, 2001a, pp 278–279.

Weiss LM, Grogan TM, Muller-Hermelink HK, et al: Langerhans cell histiocytosis. In Jaffe ES, Harris NL, Stein H, et al: (eds): World Health Organization Classification of Tumours. Pathology and Genetics of Tumours of Haematopoietic and Lymphoid Tissues. Lyon, IARC Press, 2001b, pp 280–282.

Weiss LM, Grogan TM, Muller-Hermelink HK, et al: Interdigitating dendritic cell sarcoma/tumour. In Jaffe ES, Harris NL, Stein H, et al: (eds): World Health Organization Classification of Tumours. Pathology and Genetics of Tumours of Haematopoietic and Lymphoid Tissues. Lyon, IARC Press, 2001c, pp 284–285.

Weiss LM, Grogan TM, Muller-Hermelink HK, et al: Follicular dendritic cell sarcoma/tumour. In Jaffe ES, Harris NL, Stein H, et al: (eds): World Health Organization Classification of Tumours. Pathology and Genetics of Tumours of Haematopoietic and Lymphoid Tissues. Lyon, IARC Press, 2001d, pp 286–288.

Weiss LM, Grogan TM, Muller-Hermelink HK, et al: Dendritic cell sarcoma, not otherwise specified. In Jaffe ES, Harris NL, Stein H, et al: (eds): World Health Organization Classification of Tumours. Pathology and Genetics of Tumours of Haematopoietic and Lymphoid Tissues. Lyon, IARC Press, 2001e, p 289.

Weiss LM, Grogan TM, Pileri SA, et al: Langerhans cell sarcoma. In Jaffe ES, Harris NL, Stein H, et al: (eds): World Health Organization Classification of Tumours. Pathology and Genetics of Tumours of Haematopoietic and Lymphoid Tissues. Lyon, IARC Press, 2001f, p 283.

Weksler ME, Hutteroth TH: Impaired lymphocyte function in aged humans. J Clin Invest 1974; 53:99–104.

Weng WK, Levy S: Hepatitis C virus (HCV) and lymphomagenesis. Leuk Lymphoma 2003; 44:1113–1120.

Wilson WH, Kingma DW, Raffeld M, et al: Association of lymphomatoid granulomatosis with Epstein–Barr viral infection of B lymphocytes and response to interferon-alpha 2b. Blood 1996; 87:4531–4537.

Wong M, Pagano JS, Schiller JT, et al: New associations of human papillomavirus, Simian virus 40, and Epstein–Barr virus with human cancer. J Natl Cancer Inst 2002; 94:1832–1836.

Woodruff RK, Malpas JS, Paxton AM, et al: Plasma cell leukemia (PCL): A report on 15 patients. Blood 1978; 52:839–845.

Wreghitt TG, Teare EL, Sule O, et al: Cytomegalovirus infection in immunocompetent patients. Clin Infect Dis 2003; 37:1603–1606.

Wu ML, Kwaan HC, Goolsby CL: Atypical hairy cell leukemia. Arch Pathol Lab Med 2000; 124:1710–1713.

Yam LT, Li CY, Lam KW: Tartrate-resistant acid phosphatase isoenzyme in the reticulum cells of leukemic reticuloendotheliosis. N Engl J Med 1971; 284:357–360.

Yamaguchi K, Watanabe T: Human T lymphotropic virus type-I and adult T-cell leukemia in Japan. Int J Hematol 2002; 76:240–245.

Yamaguchi M, Machii T, Shibayama H, et al: Immunophenotypic features and configuration of immunoglobulin genes in hairy cell leukemia – Japanese variant. Leukemia 1996; 10:1390–1394.

Yano T, van Krieken JH, Magrath IT, et al: Histogenetic correlations between subcategories of small noncleaved cell lymphomas. Blood 1992; 79:1282–1290.

Yasutomo K, Doyle C, Miele L, et al: The duration of antigen receptor signalling determines CD4+ versus CD8+ T-cell lineage fate. Nature 2000; 404:506–510.

Zeidler C, Welte K: Kostmann syndrome and severe congenital neutropenia. Semin Hematol 2002; 39:82–88.

Zinzani PL, Stefoni V, Tani M, et al: MACOP-B regimen followed by involved-field radiation therapy in early-stage aggressive non-Hodgkin's lymphoma patients: 14-year update results. Leuk Lymphoma 2001; 42:989–995.

Zipursky A, Poon A, Doyle J: Leukemia in Down syndrome: A review. Pediatr Hematol Oncol 1992; 9:139–149.

CHAPTER 33

The Flow Cytometric Evaluation of Hematopoietic Neoplasia

Brent L. Wood MD PhD, Michael J. Borowitz MD PhD

KEY POINTS

- Flow cytometry is a powerful, rapid and cost-effective technique for the identification and monitoring of hematopoietic neoplasms.

- Successful implementation of flow cytometry requires careful attention to details of instrument and reagent performance.

- Normal hematopoietic cells are characterized by a reproducible gain and loss of antigen expression with maturation.

- Hematopoietic neoplasms show deviation from the normal patterns of antigen expression, allowing for their diagnosis and classification.

- The flow cytometric detection of residual disease following therapy allows for the monitoring of therapeutic response.

Introduction

The diagnosis, classification and post-therapeutic monitoring of hematopoietic neoplasms has greatly benefited from the widespread application of immunophenotypic studies over the past two decades. The subdivision of hematopoietic neoplasms by their correspondence to normal hematopoietic lineages and stages of differentiation is a basic tenet of current classification systems, e.g., the World Health Organization (WHO) classification (Jaffe, 2001). This information is largely provided by immunophenotyping and has resulted in the incorporation of immunophenotypic data into the definition of many hematopoietic neoplasms to the extent that certain diagnoses cannot be confidently made without immunophenotypic studies.

Flow cytometry is a rapid and convenient technique for generating immunophenotypic data. The ability to perform multiparametric analysis on an individual cellular basis is a unique feature of the technique and offers distinct advantages over competing immunophenotypic methods such as immunohistochemistry. Guidelines for the use of flow cytometry for the immunophenotyping of leukemic cells in the clinical laboratory have been published (NCCLS, 1998), and an NIH-sponsored consensus conference on the flow cytometric analysis of leukemia and lymphoma was convened in 1995 to attempt standardization of clinical practice (US–Canadian Consensus, 1997). Despite these efforts, considerable heterogeneity exists in the clinical application of this technique to the evaluation of leukemia and lymphoma, and this lack of standardization represents a significant challenge to the ability to consistently provide high quality results.

Medical indications for performing flow cytometry in a clinical setting currently can be divided into four basic areas:

1. The diagnosis and classification of hematopoietic neoplasms. The ability to accurately identify abnormal subpopulations of cells, assign lineage and determine maturational stage adds improved reproducibility to the diagnosis of hematopoietic neoplasms, particularly for chronic lymphoproliferative disorders and acute leukemias. Flow cytometry is widely used for this purpose.

2. Assessment of biologic parameters associated with prognosis. The expression of specific molecules at the time of diagnosis has been associated with long-term clinical outcome and can be easily assessed by flow cytometry. An example is the expression of CD38 or Zap-70 in chronic lymphocytic leukemia where the increased expression of either has been associated with poor long-term survival (Damle, 1999; Crespo, 2003).

3. Detection of antigens used as therapeutic targets. A variety of immunologic reagents are now available for therapeutic use that specifically target antigens expressed by hematopoietic neoplasms, e.g., CD20, CD52, CD33, etc. Confirming the expression of the antigen of interest by the tumor is a necessary prerequisite for use of these expensive therapies.

4. Detection of residual neoplastic cells following therapy. The ability of flow cytometry to routinely identify and quantitate the presence of abnormal hematopoietic cells with a sensitivity of 0.01% is increasingly being used as a surrogate measure of response to therapy and impending relapse (Campana, 2003).

Technical Considerations

Instrumentation

The basic principle of flow cytometry relies on the injection of a monodisperse suspension of particles (cells) into the center of a flowing stream of fluid (sheath) that then passes through a small quartz capillary tube at a constant velocity (Shapiro, 2003). The sheath fluid serves to maintain the particles in the center of the flowing stream where they may be illuminated by one or more focused light sources, typically lasers. The light scattered by the particles is collected by detectors positioned at a variety of angles around the capillary to give information about the cross-sectional area, and hence size (low angle or forward scatter) or complexity/granularity (high angle or side scatter) of each individual particle as it transits the capillary. In addition, if fluorescent molecules or fluorochromes are attached to the particles, they may be excited by the incident light, giving rise to fluorescent emission that can be collected by the use of additional detectors and optical filters (Fig. 33–1). The net result is a multiparametric analysis of each individual particle with the number of parameters evaluated dependent on the number of fluorescent molecules used and the complexity of instrument design.

Optimization and standardization of instrument performance is critical for the success of any flow cytometric study, but is of particular importance in the analysis of hematopoietic neoplasms because of the wide range of signal intensities that must be detected. The preferred approach is to define a set of instrument conditions that allow for optimal instrument performance and to perform daily quality control of the instrument to consistently achieve that level of performance. Adherence to a consistent and fixed level of instrument performance greatly simplifies quality control and provides reproducible data for subsequent interpretation. Daily assessment of the fluorescence intensity and coefficient of variation

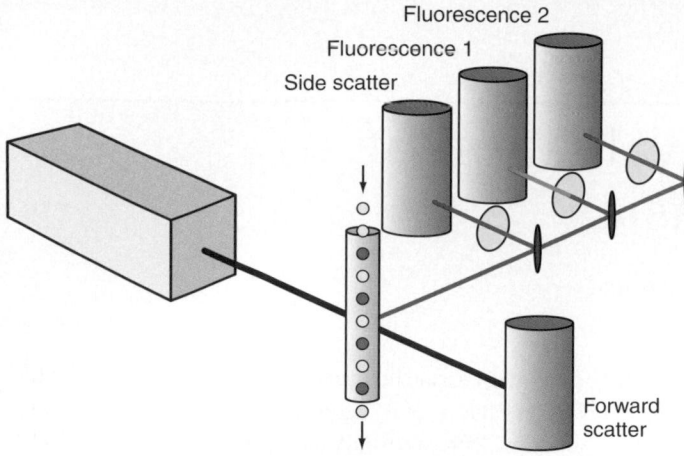

Figure 33–1 Schematic of a flow cytometer. A flowing stream of particles (center) is illuminated by a laser (left) and the resulting low angle (forward scatter) or right angle (side scatter) light scatter collected by appropriately positioned detectors. In addition, fluorescent molecules attached to the particles may be excited by the laser light and the resulting emission routed through a series of optical mirrors and filters to the appropriate detectors (fluorescence 1 and fluorescence 2).

(CV), using particles having stable, moderately bright fluorescence and assessment of instrument noise using nonfluorescent particles, is the cornerstone of instrument quality control.

There are relatively few instrument variables over which the operator has control on a flow cytometer, principally: detection threshold, detector gain, rate of sample flow, and for some multilaser instruments, laser delay time. The detection threshold or discriminator is associated with a single parameter and is the value that must be achieved for the system to recognize that a particle has passed through the capillary to initiate signal processing. Typically, forward scatter is used to identify particles having a size greater than some desired value, e.g. cells equal to or larger than lymphocytes. Of particular importance is the gain or voltage supplied to each detector, commonly a photomultiplier tube, as this has a direct impact on the ability to separate signals of interest from background instrument noise (signal-to-noise ratio). The voltage applied to each detector should be adjusted to optimize the signal-to-noise ratio and allow the detection of the weakest required signals for each detector. This often results in negative cellular populations being positioned such that they completely occupy the lowest decade of a logarithmic scale. Finally, for instruments having multiple lasers that intersect the capillary stream at different points (spatially separated lasers), a parameter must be supplied

to allow synchronization of signal processing to account for the different times at which a single particle encounters each laser as it transits through the capillary. This laser delay time should be adjusted to maximize signal intensity for each laser. It should be noted that the laser delay time is highly dependent on the transit time of the particle through the capillary and so requires a stable fluidic system to remain constant, a problem historically on certain instruments.

The rate at which the sample is introduced or aspirated through the system can be controlled by the operator, but is limited by two factors: the rate at which the instrument electronics can process the signals that are generated, and sample concentration. If particles pass through the instrument more rapidly than they can be processed by the electronics, the data for a subset of the particles will be lost while another subset will show unusual and undesirable artifacts, typically a variable loss of signal intensity over a wide range. It is critically important to select a sample aspiration rate and concentration appropriate to the instrument to be used. One additional phenomenon related to sample concentration is termed coincidence, the simultaneous presence of more than one particle in the laser resulting in a single recorded event having composite characteristics of the particles involved. Coincidence can represent a significant problem for rare event detection and can be minimized using methods for doublet discrimination during analysis, techniques beyond the scope of this chapter.

Reagents

The identification of cellular characteristics beyond those provided by light scatter measurements commonly utilizes fluorochromes that either directly interact with cellular structures such as DNA or interact indirectly through conjugation to antibodies. Each fluorochrome has a unique excitation and emission spectrum that partly determines the performance characteristics of the reagent and dictates which fluorochromes may be used simultaneously (Fig. 33–2). In an effort to increase the number of usable simultaneous fluorochromes possible from a single excitation source, tandem fluorochromes have been devised, e.g., PE-Cy5, that rely on excitation of a primary fluorochrome (PE) that transfers its energy to a secondary fluorochrome (Cy5) providing the predominant fluorochrome emission at a longer wavelength. Tandem fluorochromes are required for high-level multicolor flow cytometry, but have more complex emission spectra as well as decreased fluorochrome stability under some circumstances. The other important fluorochrome characteristic, the intensity of emission, is related to the relative efficiency of excitation by the light sources utilized and the quantum efficiency of the fluorochrome itself (Fig. 33–3). Differences in emission intensity directly correlate with differences in detection sensitivity and are a key consideration in the design of reagent panels, as discussed later.

The use of multiple simultaneous fluorochromes, i.e., multicolor flow cytometry, is required for the analysis of leukemia and lymphoma with

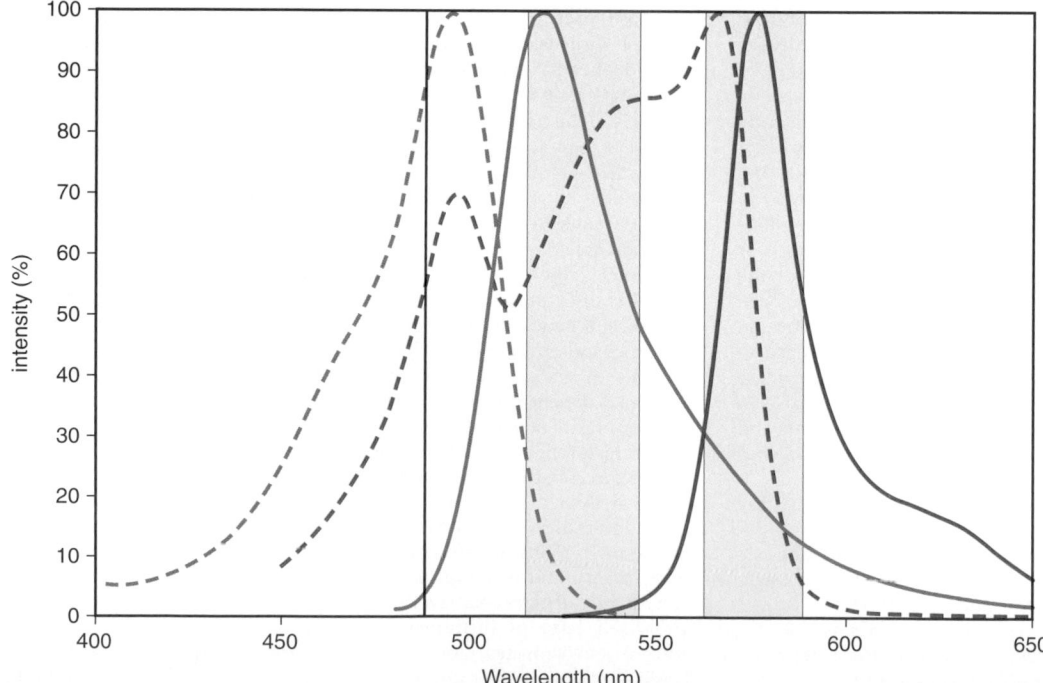

Figure 33–2 Fluorochrome emission spectra. Each fluorescent molecule possesses a characteristic absorption (dotted line) and emission spectrum (solid line) whose wavelength maxima are spectrally separated, the degree of separation termed the Stokes shift. Although a small amount of the fluorescein emission occurs at the same wavelength as phycoerythrin, the fluorescence emission of fluorescein (green) can be separated from that of phycoerythrin (orange) using appropriate optical filters (shaded areas). The 488 nm laser commonly used to excite each of these fluorochromes is indicated by a blue line.

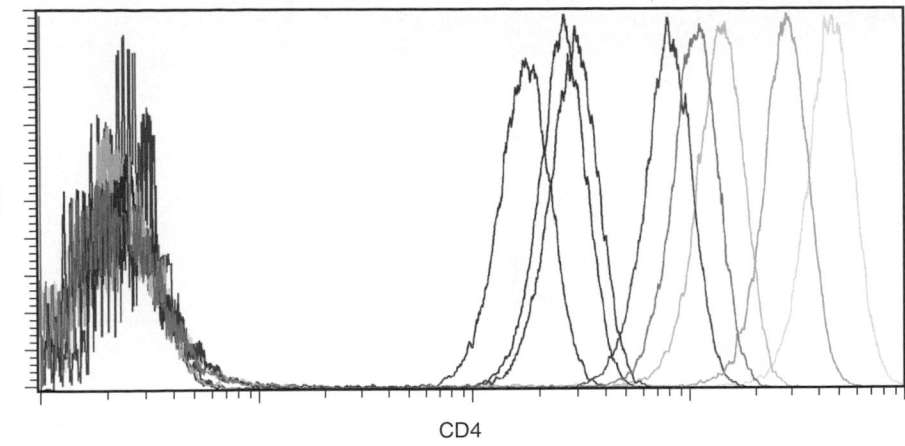

Figure 33–3 Comparison of fluorochrome emission intensity. Fluorochromes are characterized by differences in relative intensity of emission that are important to take into account to achieve optimal sensitivity. The relative fluorescence intensity for CD4 expression on lymphocytes is pictured for fluorescein (FITC) (blue), phycoerythrin (PE) (green), PE-Texas Red (orange), PE-Cy5 (yellow), PerCP-Cy5.5 (red), PE-Cy7 (light blue), allophycocyanin (APC) (magenta) and APC-Cy7 (purple). The actual intensities observed are dependent on the clone of antibody used, ratio of fluorochrome to protein in the antibody conjugate, method of specimen preparation, instrument performance characteristics, and method of instrument setup.

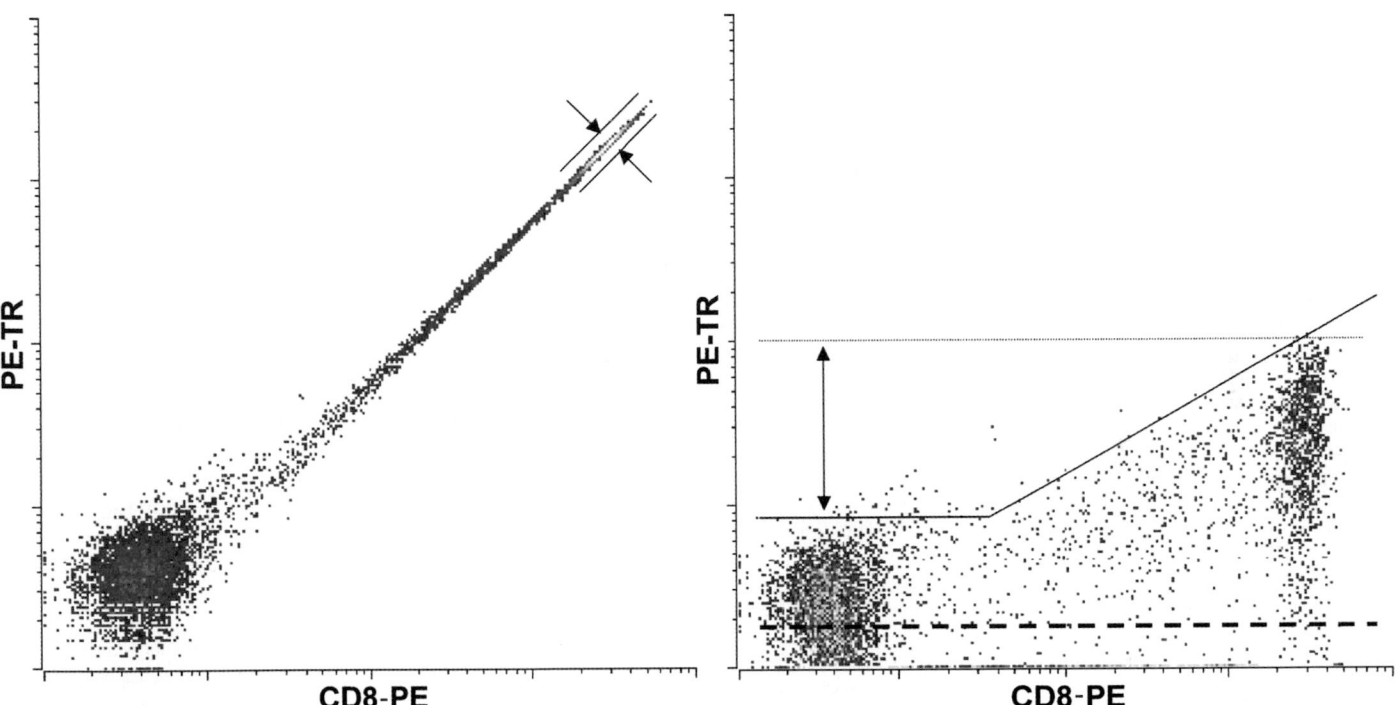

Figure 33–4 Compensation. The fluorescence emission of lymphocytes labeled with CD8-PE appears in both the PE and PE-Texas Red detectors because of the emission of PE in both regions of the spectrum examined by these detectors. Note that no PE-Texas Red conjugated antibody is used in this experiment. Without compensation applied (left), cells expressing abundant CD8 show bright signals for both PE and PE-Texas Red with a width to the population (arrows) due to measurement errors inherent in the method. Once compensation is correctly applied (right), the centers of the positive and negative populations have the same low-level of PE-Texas red emission (dotted line) with many events lying on the horizontal axis. However, the PE-positive population shows a much broader degree of apparent PE-Texas Red background fluorescence than the PE-negative population (solid line and arrow), If a PE-Texas Red conjugated antibody had been used, CD8-positive cells might have been erroneously interpreted as doubly positive, but this apparent 'positivity' is a direct result of measurement errors and logarithmic data display. The practical result is that the sensitivity for the detection of low-level PE-Texas Red is compromised in the presence of bright PE fluorescence.

three being the minimum number recommended under current consensus guidelines (US–Canadian Consensus, 1997). Since most fluorochromes have overlapping emission spectra, determination of the fluorescence due to a specific fluorochrome in a single detector requires subtraction of the portion of the signals contributed by each of the other fluorochromes in the sample, a process termed compensation. The appropriate amount of each signal to subtract, i.e., compensation coefficient, may be represented by an n by n matrix where n is the number of fluorochromes. Consequently, as the number of fluorochromes used increases, the number of compensation coefficients that must be determined increases geometrically and software rapidly becomes required to do this process correctly. To determine the compensation coefficients, a series of samples singly labeled with each fluorochrome are evaluated with the positive population as bright as the brightest signal one plans to evaluate. Since the spectral characteristics of the tandem fluorochromes can vary significantly between lots and manufacturers, separate compensation controls are often required for each lot and conjugate of these reagents. Software, either on the instrument or on offline computers, is used to analyze the resulting data and calculate compensation coefficients.

While the process of determining and correctly applying compensation is now made simple through software, the use of multiple fluorochromes can result in significant display artifacts that reflect compromised low-level detection sensitivity (Roederer, 2001). This is particularly a problem when one attempts to detect low-level signals in the presence of brightly overlapping fluorochrome emissions. Understanding the impact of compensation-related effects is the single most difficult aspect of multicolor flow cytometry and the least understood by most users. The implications of overlapping fluorochrome emission have direct consequences for panel design and data interpretation (Fig. 33–4). When compensation settings are not appropriate for the reagents used, artifacts arise that can lead to both the misattribution of low-level positivity and the inability to recognize the presence of subpopulations (Fig. 33–5). The use of software compensation provides a nondestructive method for data collection and allows for the adjustment of compensation settings following acquisition, supplying a way to correct for inadvertent compensation errors.

Antibodies are an integral part of the immunophenotypic evaluation of leukemia and lymphoma. It is important to determine the correct amount of each antibody to use by evaluating a series of samples labeled with

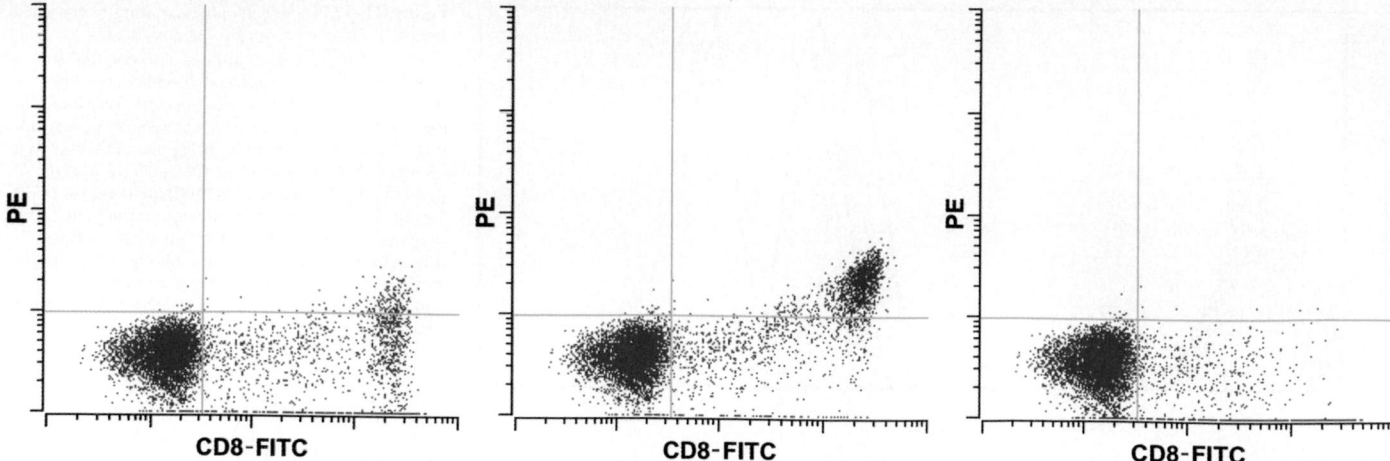

Figure 33–5 Inappropriate compensation. The fluorescence emission of lymphocytes singly labeled with CD8-FITC shows minimal apparent PE fluorescence when 8% of the FITC signal is subtracted from the PE signal, i.e. appropriate compensation (left). If the degree of compensation is decreased to 7.2% (center), the CD8-positive population appears to express low PE and could be misinterpreted as immunophenotypic aberrancy depending on the PE antibody included. Note the lack of symmetry and pointed end of the positive population as a clue to the inaccurate compensation. If the compensation is increased to 8.8%, the positive population is compressed on the X-axis and appears not to exist.

different concentrations of antibodies, i.e., titering (Stewart, 2000). The object of titering is to maximize the signal-to-noise ratio by providing as bright a signal as possible on positive populations while maintaining a low level of background nonspecific binding. For high-specificity antibodies used for cell surface labeling, one should be able to achieve saturation, a consistent intensity on positive populations at higher antibody concentrations, without significant increases in background on negative populations. The inability to do so indicates a poor quality antibody. For intracellular labeling, saturation is typically not achieved because of relatively high levels of nonspecific antibody binding by intracellular constituents, generally a linear function of antibody concentration, and optimization of signal-to-noise by titering becomes critical for adequate reagent performance (Jacobberger 2000).

Panel Design

The pairing of reagents with appropriate fluorochromes is a key factor in assuring appropriate signal intensity and detection sensitivity. The following four steps can aid in the construction of appropriate reagent panels.

1. Determine the purpose for each potential combination of reagents. Each reagent combination should have a clearly defined objective or should not be further pursued.
2. Select a group of cellular targets. The selected group of targets or antigens should be able to successfully address the purpose of the reagent combination and should be relatively independent of fluorochrome or availability of commercial conjugates. The reagent combination should be the minimum needed to answer the question being asked. There are a variety of ways in which antibodies are commonly combined for use in the identification of abnormal hematopoietic populations, but these generally fall into one of the categories outlined in Table 33–1.
3. Assign a fluorochrome to each target. The basic principle is that highly expressed antigens should be coupled with dim fluorochromes and dimly expressed antigens should be coupled with bright fluorochromes. This principle provides reasonable signal intensities and avoids compensation problems due to excessively bright fluorescence. Commercial availability often limits choice of fluorochromes, though most companies offer custom conjugation services that can provide reagents that might be better suited to a particular purpose than those more generally available.
4. Test reagent combinations. The reagent combination must be empirically tested to assure that signal intensities are as expected, low level sensitivity is appropriate where important, and unexpected interactions between reagents do not occur. A sample prepared with all reagents of interest should be compared with the same sample prepared with a series of preparations each lacking one of the component reagents (fluorescence-minus-one controls) as well as with a second series containing each single reagent independently (single-stained controls). Unexpected changes in intensity of one or more reagents indicate potential problems with the reagent combination.

Table 33–1 Reagent Panel Design Strategies for the Detection of Hematopoietic Neoplasms

Principle	Example implementation
At least one reagent for population identification	CD45 for general cell type Lineage associated antigen for specific cell lineage, e.g., CD19 for B cells
Multiple antigens of same lineage and maturational stage to identify inappropriate expression levels	Use of CD2, CD3, CD4, CD5, CD7 or CD8 simultaneously to evaluate mature T cells
Multiple antigens of same lineage but different maturational stages to identify normal maturation and dyssynchronous expression	Use of CD13 and CD16 simultaneously to demonstrate neutrophilic maturation
Separation of different cell lineages	Use of CD11b and CD15 simultaneously to separate monocytic and neutrophilic maturation
Demonstration of clonality	Use of kappa and lambda in combination with a B cell lineage reagent, e.g., CD19
Identify frankly aberrant antigen expression	Use of T or NK cell associated antigens such as CD7 or CD56 in combination with CD34

Specimen Handling and Sample Preparation

Any specimen from whom a single cell suspension can be generated is suitable for flow cytometric immunophenotyping, including peripheral blood, bone marrow, lymph node, etc. Blood and bone marrow may be anticoagulated with EDTA, heparin or acid citrate dextrose (ACD), with heparin generally preferred due to improved stability with specimen age. Tissue specimens are best transported and stored in tissue culture media, such as RPMI 1640, and a single cell suspension generated by mechanical dissociation using either scalpel and forceps, needle and syringe, or wire screen mesh (Braylan, 1989) followed by filtration through fine gauge wire mesh to remove aggregates. Specimens of all types are commonly stored at room temperature prior to preparation, although refrigeration will retard degradation when preparation must be delayed.

Analysis of white blood cells in peripheral blood or bone marrow requires erythrocyte removal for efficient evaluation. Density-gradient centrifugation, e.g., ficoll-hypaque, was historically used for this purpose, but results in the selective loss of cellular subpopulations and gives relatively poor recovery on bone marrow specimens. Erythrocyte lysis using ammonium chloride or a variety of commercial preparations has become the standard technique for sample preparation in clinical laboratories (Carter, 1992). Currently recommended methods involve the

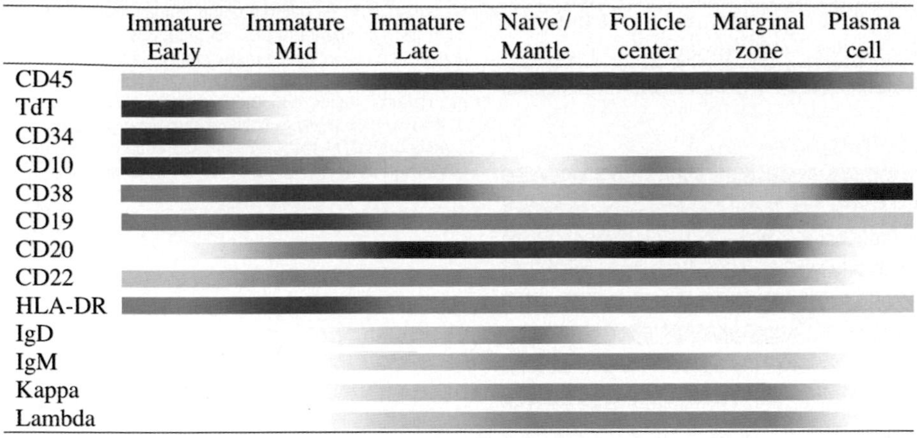

	Immature Early	Immature Mid	Immature Late	Naive / Mantle	Follicle center	Marginal zone	Plasma cell
CD45							
TdT							
CD34							
CD10							
CD38							
CD19							
CD20							
CD22							
HLA-DR							
IgD							
IgM							
Kappa							
Lambda							

Figure 33–6 B cell differentiation. The intensity of antigen expression throughout B cell maturation is depicted for antigens commonly used in the clinical laboratory. Normal mature B cells express either kappa or lambda light chains, never both. Darker color represents a higher level of antigen expression.

addition of antibodies to an aliquot of blood or marrow, followed by erythrocyte lysis, and washing with a buffered salt solution such as phosphate buffered saline (PBS) to remove cell debris, the lysing reagent, and unbound antibody. Inclusion of a small amount of formaldehyde (0.25–0.5%) either with the lysing reagent or following washing is a convenient way to stabilize both antibody binding and specimen stability. When analysis of light chain expression on B cells is required, serum immunoglobulin must be removed by repeated washing prior to antibody addition. Once prepared, samples should be acquired on the instrument as soon as reasonably possible to avoid sample and fluorochrome degradation, although fixation and refrigerated storage will delay degradation.

Data Acquisition

As the prepared sample is evaluated on the flow cytometer, it is important to collect enough events to allow detection of the population of interest. For populations that represent a large percentage of the total, relatively few events need to be acquired, while infrequent populations require the acquisition of larger numbers of events. Since in the evaluation of hematopoietic neoplasms one rarely knows what the likely population frequency will be for a given sample, it is most convenient to acquire a fixed number of total events that ensures the desired minimum level of sensitivity. For example, if a sensitivity of 0.1% is desired and 50 events are determined to be adequate for confident population identification, then 50 000 total white blood cell events will need to be acquired. The acquisition of fewer events will compromise the ability to detect low frequency populations, an important consideration when evaluating for residual disease following therapy and a situation where acquisition of a larger number of events is often desirable.

Instrument carryover between samples becomes a significant concern when evaluating for the presence of small abnormal populations. Most commercial instruments have a manufacturer's specification for carryover of roughly 1%, a relatively high level when one is looking for infrequent populations. To minimize carryover, a small amount of water should be run between each aliquot of sample acquired until background returns to an acceptably low level. Failure to do so will result in the sporadic appearance of populations having unexpected immunophenotypes that can be mistaken for neoplastic disease.

Interpretive Considerations

The identification of hematopoietic neoplasia by immunophenotyping relies on the principle that neoplastic cells express patterns of antigen expression that are distinctly different from those of their normal counterparts. Antigen expression in normal cells is a tightly regulated process resulting in a characteristic pattern of antigen acquisition and loss with maturation that is cell lineage specific. Neoplastic cells commonly show nonrandom alterations in antigen expression that include:

1. Gain of antigens not normally expressed by cell type or lineage.
2. Abnormally increased or decreased levels of expression (intensities) of antigens normally expressed by cell type or lineage, including the complete loss of normal antigens in some instances.
3. Asynchronous antigen expression, i.e., expression of antigens normally expressed by the cell type or lineage, but at an inappropriate time during maturation.
4. Abnormally homogeneous expression of one or more antigens by a population that normally exhibits more heterogeneous expression.

The consequence is that the immunophenotypic identification of hematopoietic neoplasia rests on a thorough knowledge of the normal patterns of antigens expressed by hematopoietic cells.

Normal Patterns of Antigen Expression

All hematopoietic cells arise from hematopoietic stem cells, a quiescent cell population that possesses long-term regenerative potential and is present at a low frequency in the bone marrow. The stem cell population in humans can be identified if a sufficient number of cells is evaluated and shows expression of bright CD34, CD133, intermediate CD45, dim to absent CD38, variable CD90 and dim expression of CD123, CD117, HLA-DR, CD13 and CD33. Maturation toward lineage-committed progenitors is accompanied by a slight decrease in CD34 and CD45, loss of CD133 and CD90, and an increase in CD38 and HLA-DR. Further maturation along each lineage occurs in the bone marrow until mature, functional, albeit naive progeny are released into the peripheral blood. The one exception is T cells whose earliest precursors migrate to the thymus where maturation to functional forms occurs. The patterns of antigenic change with maturation for the B cell, T cell, neutrophilic, monocytic and erythroid lineages have been elucidated by multiple investigators (Wood, 2004; Lucio, 1999; McClanahan, 1999; Almasri, 1998; Ginaldi, 1996b; Hoffkes, 1996; Harada, 1993; Inghirami, 1990; Terstappen, 1990a,b,c; 1992b; Loken, 1987, 1988) and a summary for each lineage is presented in Figures 33–6 through 33–10, respectively.

Abnormal Patterns of Antigenic Expression in Hematopoietic Neoplasia

Most hematopoietic neoplasms have abnormal immunophenotypes that are characteristic enough to allow their detection, even at relatively low levels of involvement. In some cases, the immunophenotype is characteristic enough to allow classification using immunophenotypic data alone. However, within each group there is sufficient variability that correct diagnosis relies on recognition of the overall immunophenotypic pattern and not the expression of individual antigens or the rigid application of immunophenotypic profiles. The following discussion emphasizes general immunophenotypic principles useful for the diagnosis and classification of hematopoietic neoplasia, as a complete discussion of the antigenic abnormalities seen in each subtype of disease is beyond the scope of this chapter.

Acute Leukemia
Diagnosis and Classification
The diagnosis of acute leukemia relies on the enumeration of the percentage of blasts in the peripheral blood or bone marrow; the current criterion in the WHO classification for the diagnosis of acute leukemia is greater than 20% blasts (Jaffe, 2001). In flow cytometry, the identification of blasts relies on the demonstration of the expression of immature antigens by a population having appropriate CD45 expression and light scatter characteristics. Although it is the overall immunophenotype that allows identification of blasts, antigens commonly used for blast identification include CD34, CD117, CD133 and terminal deoxynucleotidyl transferase (TdT). White blood cells express CD45 at distinct levels of intensity characteristic of both lineage and stage of differentiation that when used in conjunction with orthogonal light scatter (side scatter)

IV

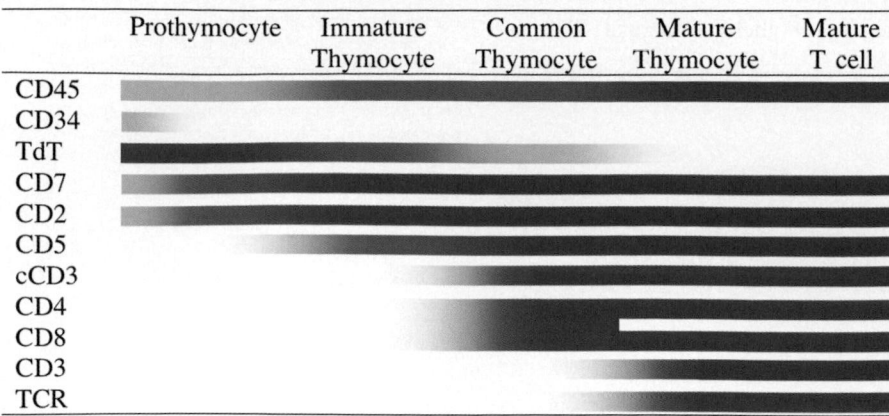

Figure 33–7 T cell differentiation. The intensity of antigen expression throughout T cell maturation is depicted for antigens commonly used in the clinical laboratory. T cell maturation occurs largely in the thymus, and most maturational stages will not be seen outside of that organ. At the common thymocyte stage, the immature T cells express both CD4 and CD8 with subsequent stages showing expression of one or the other but not both. Darker color represents a higher level of antigen expression.

	Prothymocyte	Immature Thymocyte	Common Thymocyte	Mature Thymocyte	Mature T cell
CD45					
CD34					
TdT					
CD7					
CD2					
CD5					
cCD3					
CD4					
CD8					
CD3					
TCR					

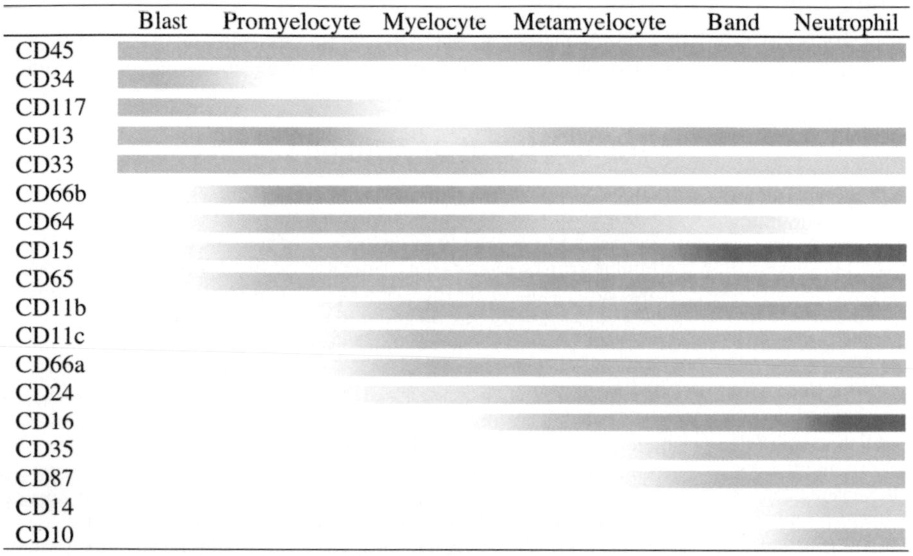

Figure 33–8 Neutrophil differentiation. The intensity of antigen expression throughout neutrophil maturation is depicted for antigens commonly used in the clinical laboratory. Darker color represents a higher level of antigen expression.

	Blast	Promyelocyte	Myelocyte	Metamyelocyte	Band	Neutrophil
CD45						
CD34						
CD117						
CD13						
CD33						
CD66b						
CD64						
CD15						
CD65						
CD11b						
CD11c						
CD66a						
CD24						
CD16						
CD35						
CD87						
CD14						
CD10						

	Blast	Promonocyte	Monocyte
CD45			
CD34			
CD13			
CD33			
HLA-DR			
CD64			
CD15			
CD11b			
CD36			
CD4			
CD14			
CD16			

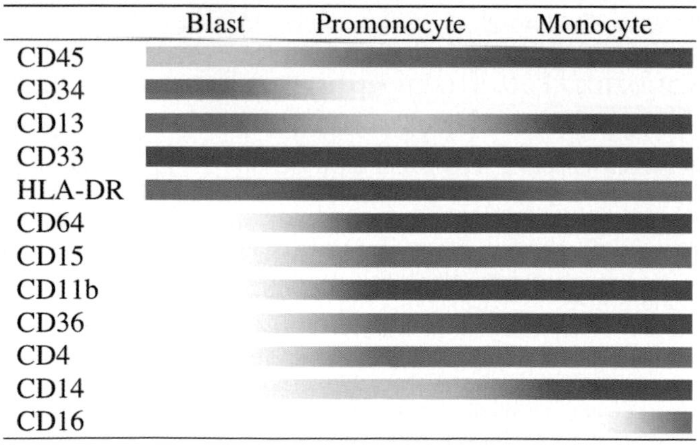

Figure 33–9 Monocyte differentiation. The intensity of antigen expression throughout monocyte maturation is depicted for antigens commonly used in the clinical laboratory. Darker color represents a higher level of antigen expression.

allows delineation of the basic white blood cell populations (Borowitz, 1993; Stelzer, 1993) (Fig. 33–11). This technique is particularly useful for the identification of blasts given their expression of intermediate CD45 and low side scatter, and CD45 vs. side scatter analysis has become standard practice in the clinical laboratory for this purpose.

While flow cytometry is excellent at identifying and enumerating blasts, there are two issues that suggest caution in utilizing flow cytometric blast percentages for making an initial diagnosis of acute leukemia. First, the blast percentage obtained from bone marrow specimens is often inaccurate due to a combination of peripheral blood dilution (artifactual decrease) and partial lysis of nucleated erythroid precursors during specimen processing (artifactual increase). Second, blasts identified by immunophenotyping do not always directly correspond to blasts as identified by morphology. This is true because leukemic populations, like normal populations, consist of a maturational continuum and there is not perfect concordance between specific antigenic changes and the arbitrary morphologic changes that distinguish blasts from more differentiated cells. Moreover, in some types of leukemia, early neutrophilic (promyelocytes) and monocytic (promonocytes) precursors are intentionally included in morphologic

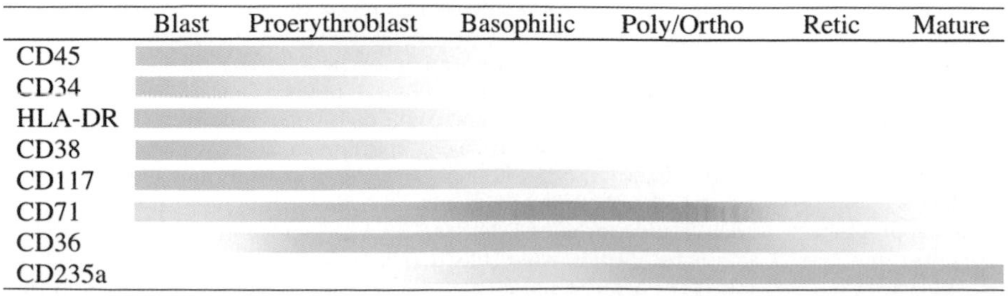

	Blast	Proerythroblast	Basophilic	Poly/Ortho	Retic	Mature
CD45						
CD34						
HLA-DR						
CD38						
CD117						
CD71						
CD36						
CD235a						

Figure 33–10 Erythroid differentiation. The intensity of antigen expression throughout erythrocyte maturation is depicted for antigens commonly used in the clinical laboratory. Darker color represents a higher level of antigen expression.

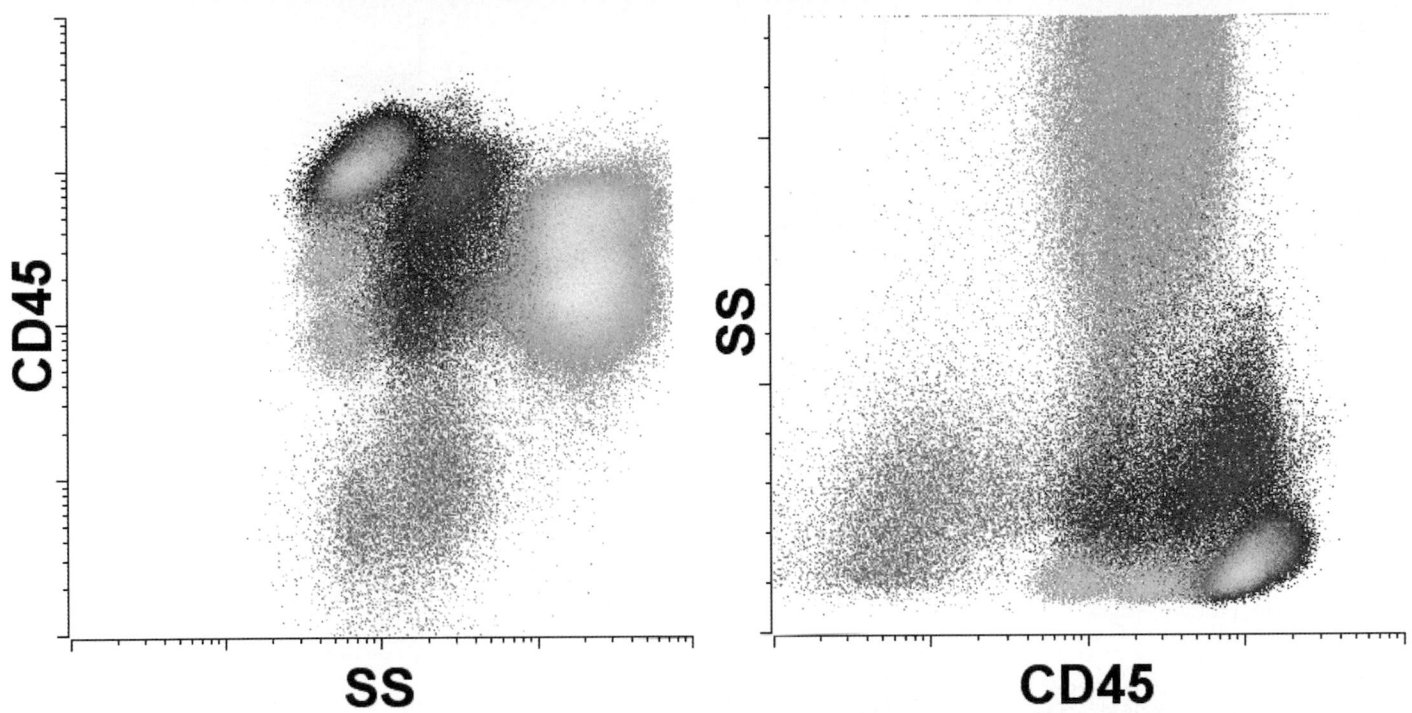

Figure 33–11 CD45 vs. side scatter. The display of CD45 vs. side scatter is increasingly used in the clinical laboratory as a starting point for the identification of white blood cell populations. The data are commonly displayed with side scatter on a logarithmic (left) or linear (right) scale. Major white cell populations colored are lymphocytes (blue), B cells (light blue), monocytes (purple), maturing neutrophils (green), blasts (red), basophils (dark purple) and maturing erythrocytes (orange).

blast counts. Nevertheless, if one pays attention to these limitations the diagnosis of acute leukemia can generally be correctly suggested.

While in most cases of acute leukemia the diagnosis (i.e., the recognition of the presence of 20% blasts) is made by morphology, flow cytometry can be extremely useful in excluding a diagnosis of acute leukemia when the marrow is populated by cells that may mimic acute leukemia. A common situation in which this can occur is in the presence of increased normal B cell precursors that may resemble primitive lymphoblasts morphologically, especially in suboptimal specimens. While these cells superficially resemble leukemic precursor-B lymphoblasts immunophenotypically, multiparameter flow cytometry can readily distinguish these normal immature precursors (hematogones) from acute leukemia (McKenna, 2001; Lucio 1999; Weir, 1999). Additionally, some non-hematolymphoid tumors such as small cell carcinoma or pediatric small round cell tumors can resemble leukemic blasts on smears but are readily distinguished from leukemic blasts by flow cytometry where they appear as CD45-negative cells lacking specific markers of B cell, T cell or myeloid lineage, often with higher side scatter than might be expected for a cell with so little cytoplasm (Chang, 2003).

The major role for flow cytometry in acute leukemia is classification. Classification is largely a matter of lineage assignment and correlation with normal maturational stage. The determination of lineage in particular is a decision of major therapeutic importance with a primary distinction being whether the leukemia is of myeloid or lymphoid lineage. The immunophenotypic characteristics of acute myeloid leukemia (Orfao, 2004; Weir, 2001; Khalidi, 1998; Macedo, 1995a,b; Bradstock, 1994; Reading, 1993; Terstappen, 1992a) and acute lymphoblastic leukemia (Weir, 1999; Khalidi, 1999; Farahat, 1995) and their similarities to normal populations have been well described in numerous publications. In general, it is the overall pattern of antigen expression rather than expression of any single antigen that allows determination of lineage. This is in part due to the lack of lineage specificity of many antigens commonly used for immunophenotyping. As a rule, the more closely an antigen is expressed at the level commonly seen in cells of that lineage, the more likely it accurately reflects lineage differentiation; for example dim expression of the B cell antigen CD19 has relatively poor lineage specificity, as it may be seen in acute myeloid leukemia, while brighter and more uniform CD19 expression at the level seen on normal B cells is more typical of precursor B cell lymphoblastic leukemia. A subset of cytoplasmic antigens are the most lineage-restricted antigens currently known and are used to arbitrate lineage assignment in cases

Table 33–2 Antigens Used for Lineage Assignment in Acute Leukemia

	AML	ALL – B cell	ALL – T cell
Definitive	Cytoplasmic MPO	Cytoplasmic CD79a Cytoplasmic CD22	Cytoplasmic CD3 Surface CD3
Strongly associated	CD117	CD19 CD10 – bright	CD7 – bright
Moderately associated	CD13 CD33	TdT – moderate to bright	CD5 CD2

where the surface immunophenotype is unclear. Table 33–2 lists antigens commonly used for lineage assignment. In rare cases, the leukemic cells may show differentiation along more than one lineage (Matutes, 1997; Bene, 1995; Hanson, 1993), most commonly either myeloid and B cell or myeloid and T cell, as evidence of the stem cell nature of these forms of acute leukemia. If a single blast population shows such differentiation it is commonly termed biphenotypic acute leukemia while if two abnormal blast populations are present, each having a distinct and different lineage, it is termed bilineal acute leukemia. Examples of immunophenotypic patterns seen in acute leukemia are provided in Figures 33–12 through 33–15.

Prognostic Factors

While there have been several reports about the prognostic significance of particular surface markers in both acute lymphoid and myeloid leukemia (Schabath, 2003), for the most part these have not stood the test of time, and currently do not have a significant impact on therapy. One reason for this is that the presence of recurrent cytogenetic abnormalities in acute leukemia is now recognized as an important prognostic feature having therapeutic implications; these are now an integral part of the WHO classification of acute leukemia. In many cases, the underlying cytogenetic abnormality is associated with characteristic immunophenotypic features that aid in suggesting an appropriate classification (Hrusak, 2002; Porwit-MacDonald, 1996; Orfao, 1999); with few exceptions, once cytogenetic abnormalities are accounted for, immunophenotype is no longer prognostic. However, some markers, such as CD56 expression in AML with t(8;21) (Baer, 1997), have been associated with adverse prognosis within that cytogenetically defined leukemia. A summary of phenotypic features

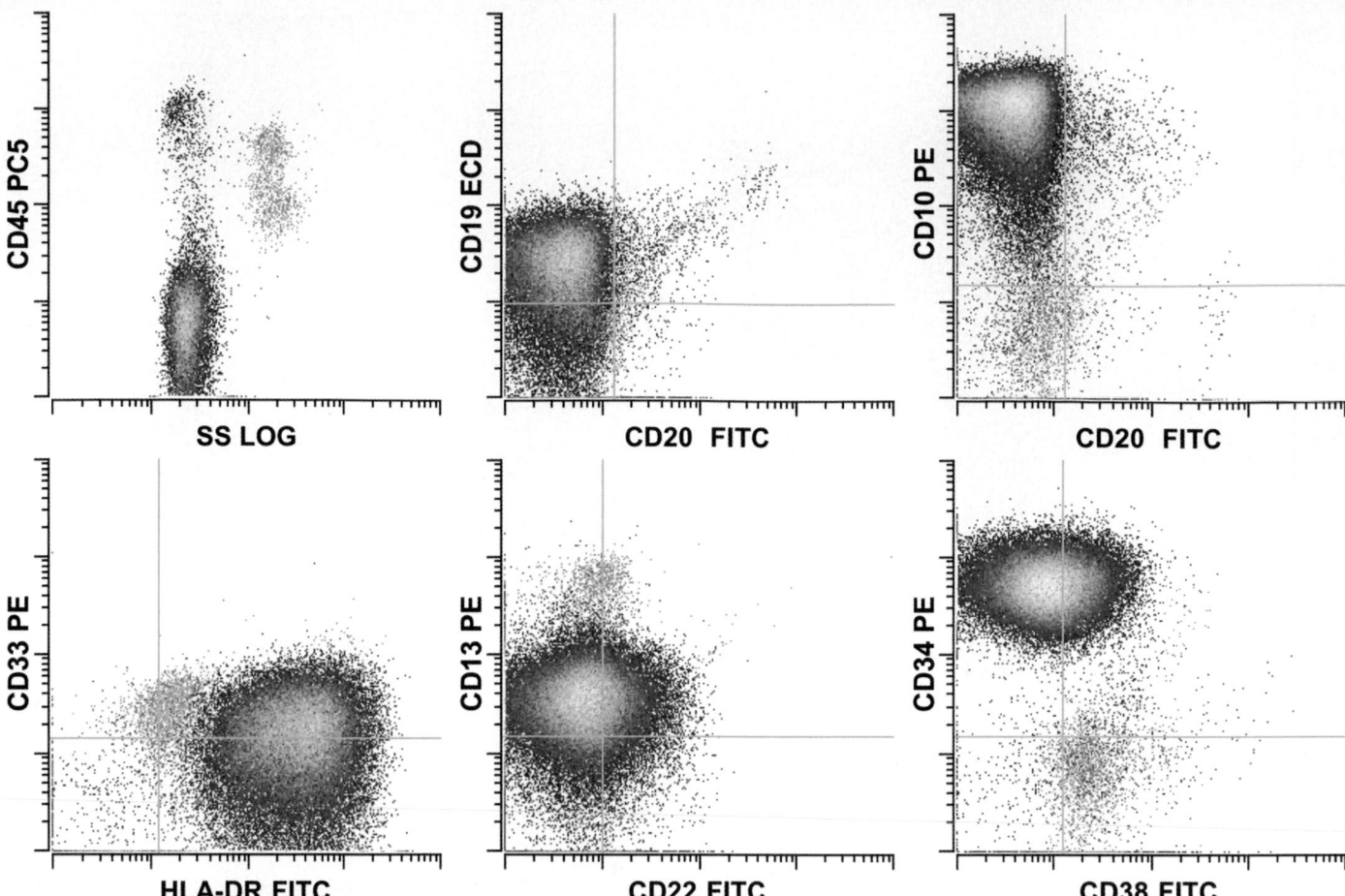

Figure 33–12 Precursor B cell lymphoblastic leukemia/lymphoma (acute lymphoblastic leukemia). The neoplastic cell population (red) in comparison with normal immature B cells shows abnormal expression of B cell associated antigens CD19 (dim), CD22 (very dim) and CD10 (bright) along with aberrant expression of CD45 (absent), CD34 (bright) and CD38 (dim). In addition, the low level expression of myeloid associated antigens CD13 and CD33 is seen, a feature frequently seen in this disorder and not suggesting myeloid differentiation by itself. The cells have low side scatter, as is typical of lymphoid blasts.

Table 33–3 Association of Immunophenotype with Cytogenetic Abnormalities in Acute Leukemia

	Immunophenotype
Acute myeloid leukemia	
t(15;17)	HLA-DR negative, CD15 low to absent, CD33 bright, CD34 low to absent
t(8;21)	CD34 bright, CD56 positive, CD19 dim, TdT positive, CD15 positive
Acute lymphoblastic leukemia	
t(12;21) (by FISH)	CD10 positive, CD20 low to negative, CD9 low to negative
MLL, e.g., t(4;11)	CD10 negative, CD15 positive

associated with cytogenetic or molecular abnormalities is provided in Table 33–3.

Therapeutic Targets

In AML, the most commonly used therapeutic targeting antibody is anti-CD33 (gemtuzumab ozogamicin) CD33 is expressed in the great majority of cases of AML, and though it is sometimes of low density, this does not appear to affect the utility of antibody therapy (Linenberger, 2005). Relatively little is known about the role of monitoring changes in CD33 expression. In ALL, there have not to date been many studies using therapeutic monoclonal antibodies, although anti-CD22 (epratuzumab) and CD52 (alemtuzamab) are now used in some clinical trials. The near

ubiquitous expression of CD22 in B precursor ALL limits the role of flow cytometry in determining eligibility for such trials.

Residual Disease Monitoring in Acute Leukemia

Many of the large number of antibodies that can be used to help classify acute leukemia are not, in and of themselves, essential for determination of lineage. However, a larger panel of antibodies, properly selected, can be very useful to identify specific differences between the leukemic population and background normal elements, thereby enhancing the ability to use flow cytometry to detect minimal residual disease. Thus, the purpose of flow cytometric immunophenotyping in acute leukemia at diagnosis goes beyond simple assignment of lineage and extends to the description of a 'signature immunophenotype' characteristic of that leukemia, knowledge of which is useful in assessing follow-up samples (Vidriales, 2003; Campana, 2003). An important caveat is that immunophenotypic changes between diagnostic samples and persistent or recurrent disease are frequently observed, particularly for acute myeloid leukemia (Voskova, 2004; Baer, 2001). Accordingly, it is necessary that one monitor more than one antigenic pattern and not expect exactly the same immunophenotype seen at diagnosis to persist following therapy. Examples of particularly informative combinations useful for detecting aberrant expression of antigens in minimal residual disease are shown in Table 33–4. The detection of minimal residual disease in acute leukemia has been demonstrated to be correlated with risk of relapse and overall survival for both acute myeloid leukemia (Feller, 2004; San Miguel, 2001) and acute lymphoblastic leukemia (Dworzak, 2002; Coustan-Smith, 2000), and is increasingly used to guide therapeutic decision-making.

Lymphoma

Diagnosis and Classification

As with leukemia, flow cytometry can contribute both to the diagnosis and to the classification of lymphoma. The immunophenotypic diagnosis of

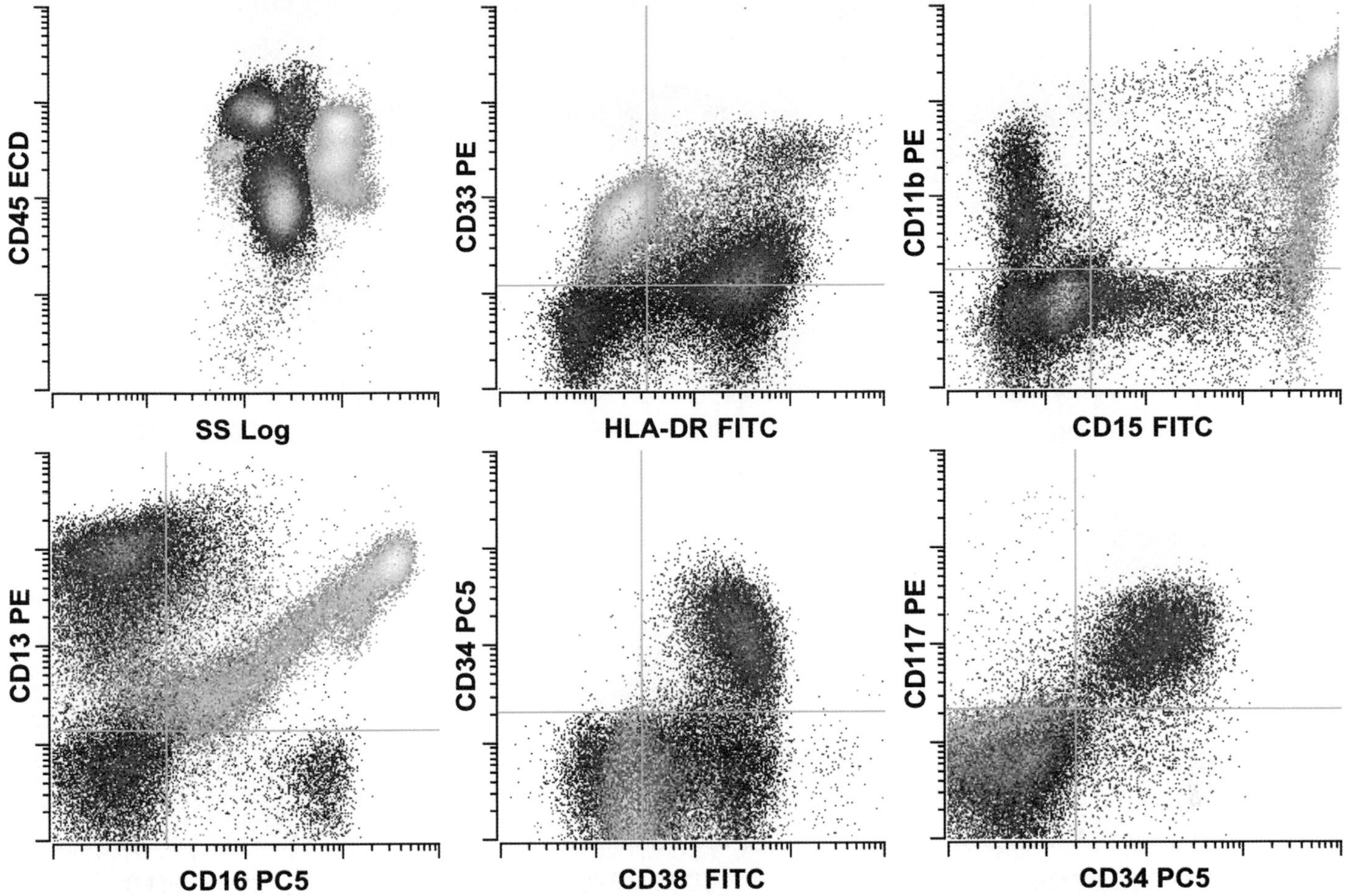

Figure 33–13 Acute myeloid leukemia with differentiation. The neoplastic cell population consists of blasts (red) showing abnormal expression of the myeloid associated antigens CD33 (dim), CD13 (bright) and CD15 (dim partial) in association with immature antigens CD34 and CD117. The blasts do not express more mature neutrophilic antigens CD11b or CD16 and are typical of the relatively immature forms seen in many cases of acute myeloid leukemia. There are background maturing granulocytes (green) that are normal and not part of the leukemic population

Table 33–4 Four-Color Antibody Combinations Useful for Minimal Residual Disease Detection

Acute myeloid leukemia	Acute lymphoblastic leukemia – B cell
CD34/CD33/HLA-DR/CD45	CD20/CD10/CD19/CD45
CD34/CD117/CD33/CD45	CD9/CD34/CD19/CD45
CD15/CD117/CD33/CD34	CD58/CD10/CD38/CD19
CD15/CD13/CD33/CD34	CD38/CD10/CD34/CD19
HLA-DR/CD117/CD33/CD34	CD20/CD10/CD19/CD34
Chronic lymphocytic leukemia	**Acute lymphoblastic leukemia – T cell**
CD20/CD79a/CD19/CD5	TdT/CD5/CD3/CD7

Antibody combinations from Vidriales, 2003, Weir, 1999, and Rawstron, 2001.

lymphoma relies on the identification of an expanded population of abnormal mature lymphocytes. By far and away, the most common way in which such an expansion is assessed by flow cytometry is through the demonstration of light chain restriction in B cell proliferations. As with all neoplastic cells, neoplastic lymphocytes arise from a single precursor that undergoes clonal expansion. However, unlike most cells, each lymphocyte normally expresses one of a series of polymorphic molecules on its surface that provides a unique identity, and in the case of B cells this identifying molecule is immunoglobulin. Because individual immunoglobulin molecules contain one of two forms of light chain, either kappa or lambda, reagents directed against light chains can be used as markers of clonality for B cells (Braylan, 1993; Fukushima, 1996; Geary, 1993).

In the case of T cell proliferations, the T cell receptor genetic locus is more complex, but the use of a larger series of reagents directed against the beta-chain families of the T cell receptor can be used to demonstrate clonality for T cells (Lima, 2001; Morice, 2004). The use of reagents directed against killer-inhibitory receptors (KIR antigens) has even been suggested to allow demonstration of NK cell clonality (Morice, 2003). The assumption behind all of these assays is that clonality equates with malignancy. While clonality is a necessary consequence of neoplasia, clonal expansion is also a normal and necessary component of the immune response following antigenic stimulation, so the demonstration of clonality by itself it is not entirely sufficient for the diagnosis of lymphoma.

It is increasingly recognized that a subset of otherwise normal individuals may contain small clonal populations of lymphocytes, best documented in the case of B cells (Chen, 2004; Kussick, 2004; Rawstron, 2002). Unlike in acute leukemia, well-defined numerical criteria as to the degree of involvement by a clonal population necessary for diagnosis have not been developed. Thus, it is not clear whether these clonal populations represent an early subclinical stage of disease, a precursor population without the full complement of genetic abnormalities required for neoplasia, or an incidental finding of no clinical consequence. Consequently, it is necessary that flow cytometric findings suggesting lymphoma are put in both a morphologic and clinical context before a definitive diagnosis of lymphoma is made.

In addition to light chain restriction, or restricted T beta receptor gene usage, lymphomas, like leukemias show alterations in antigen expression that deviate from normal maturation. In many cases these alterations also provide evidence for neoplasia. Moreover, specific alterations are seen in specific types of lymphoma, thereby permitting classification as well as diagnosis in many cases, for example increased expression of the T cell antigen CD5 in either chronic lymphocytic leukemia or mantle cell lymphoma (Matutes, 1994a; Tworek, 1998). Alteration in the intensity of immunoglobulin expression is also a common abnormality in B cell lymphoma and can be useful even when immunoglobulin expression

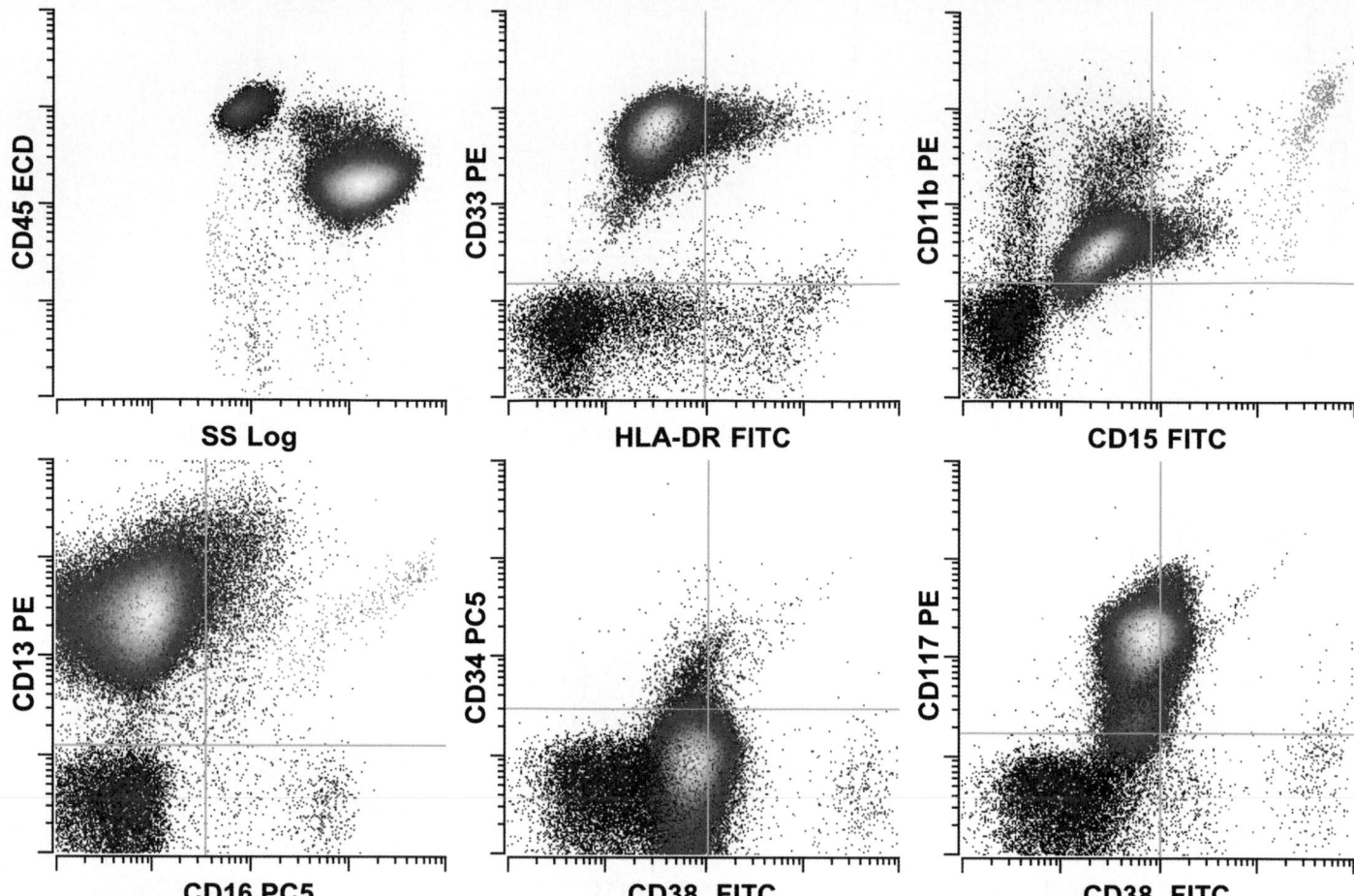

Figure 33–14 Acute promyelocytic leukemia. The neoplastic cell population consists of promyelocytes (red) showing abnormal expression of the myeloid associated antigens CD33 (bright) and CD13 (intermediate) with high side scatter indicating abundant cytoplasmic granularity. The population lacks expression of CD34 and HLA-DR, antigens commonly present on true myeloid blasts, and retains expression of CD117 as is seen on a subset of normal promyelocytes. However, in contrast to normal promyelocytes, the abnormal cells lack significant expression of CD15, a characteristic and common abnormality in this disorder.

is entirely absent (Li, 2002). Similarly, T cell lymphoma often shows alterations in the expression of one or more T cell antigens (Picker, 1987; Ginaldi, 1996a). However, special care must be taken in interpreting small populations of phenotypically abnormal T cells especially in unusual sites, because a large number of reactive conditions can be associated with expansions of populations that are not commonly seen in normal blood or lymph nodes (McClanahan, 1999).

An even more powerful method to diagnose lymphoma is to combine the detection of clonality with the ability to identify alterations in antigen intensity through multicolor flow cytometry. For instance, coupling the identification of follicle center B cells using CD19 and CD10 with the detection of kappa and lambda light chains in a four-color analysis allows one to identify the presence of light chain restriction specifically within the follicle center B cell population, greatly increasing both the specificity and sensitivity of the analysis. Examples of immunophenotypic patterns seen in lymphoma are provided in Figures 33–16 through 33–20. One important limitation of this type of analysis is the current inability to routinely identify Hodgkin lymphoma or T cell-rich B cell lymphoma, the common theme being difficulty detecting neoplasms composed of relatively rare, large atypical cells.

The classification of lymphoma relies on the recognition of specific patterns of antigenic expression that are similar to some normal maturational stage, yet deviate sufficiently to allow the identification of the abnormal population. Among B cell lymphoma there are two entities that can be both diagnosed and classified with a high degree of confidence based on immunophenotypic data alone: chronic lymphocytic leukemia/small lymphocytic lymphoma (CLL/SLL) and hairy cell leukemia. CLL/SLL is characterized by the coexpression of CD5 by the abnormal B cells, a decreased intensity of clonal light chain expression, decreased expression of a variety of mature B cell antigens including CD20, CD22 and CD79b, and presence of the activation antigen CD23 without significant FMC7, an activation epitope of CD20 (Serke, 2001)

(Fig. 33–16). This constellation of immunophenotypic findings is diagnostic for CLL/SLL (Matutes, 1994a; Tworek, 1998). The only other B cell neoplasm that consistently expresses CD5 is mantle cell lymphoma, a more aggressive lymphoma that is important to distinguish from CLL/SLL. In contrast to CLL/SLL, mantle cell lymphoma shows relatively bright expression of mature B cell antigens such as CD20 and CD79b, expresses clonal immunoglobulin at a relatively normal to high level, and expresses FMC7 without significant CD23 (Fig. 33–17). Although mantle cell lymphoma can generally be readily distinguished from CLL/SLL, because some other low-grade lymphoproliferative disorders can occasionally express CD5 and mimic the mantle cell phenotype, a definitive diagnosis requires either FISH demonstrating t(11;14) or overexpression of cyclin D1 by immunohistochemistry. These other rare CD5-positive B cell neoplasms cannot be distinguished by their immunophenotypic criteria and a combination of clinical history, morphology and cytogenetic abnormalities is often required to reach a correct classification.

Hairy cell leukemia is characterized by the increased expression of a variety of B cell antigens including CD19, CD20 and CD22, clonal surface light chain restriction, markedly increased expression of the cell adhesion molecules CD11c and CD103, and expression of the alpha-chain of the interleukin-2 receptor, CD25 (Fig. 33–18) (Matutes, 1994b; Robbins, 1994). In addition, the cells exhibit a variable degree of increased side scatter due to the abundant cytoplasm they possess, often giving the cells light scatter characteristics similar to those of monocytes. This finding, in combination with the monocytopenia that is common in this disorder, is a frequent cause for false-negative results, particularly when one relies on relatively tight gates to identify the lymphocyte population either by light scatter parameters alone or with CD45 vs. side scatter.

Another immunophenotypic finding which aids in the classification of B cell lymphoma is expression of CD10, an antigen present on immature B

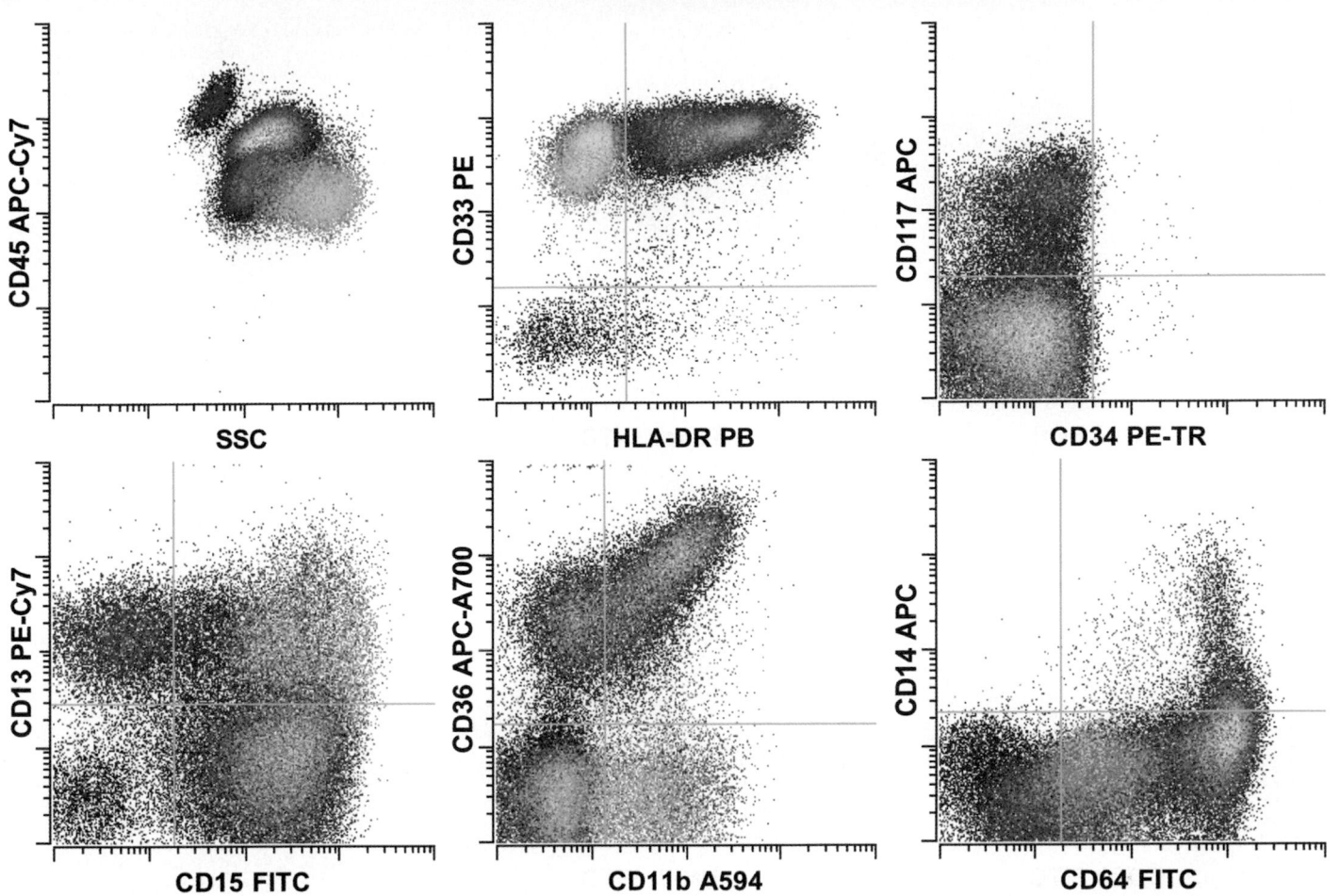

Figure 33–15 Acute myelomonocytic leukemia. The neoplastic cells consist of a relatively small population of blasts (red) with a larger population of cells showing monocytic differentiation (violet). The blasts show abnormal expression of CD33 (bright), CD13 (intermediate), HLA-DR (intermediate) and CD117 (intermediate) without CD34. The monocytic differentiation is reflected in the acquisition of early monocyte antigens CD64 (bright), and CD36 (intermediate to bright) along with other more mature myelomonocytic antigens CD15 (intermediate) and CD11b (low to intermediate) without significant acquisition of the mature monocyte antigen CD14 (absent) or marked gain in the expression of CD45 as is seen in mature monocytes. This finding suggests differentiation to the promonocyte stage, a population usually included in morphologic blast counts. In addition, a lesser degree of neutrophilic differentiation (green) is present.

cells and on normal mature B cells as they transit through the follicle center. Among B cell lymphomas, CD10 is expressed on the majority of cases of follicular lymphoma (Almasri, 1998) (Fig. 33–19), a significant subset of large B cell lymphomas, and on Burkitt lymphoma, in each of these cases indicating origin from the follicle center. In follicular lymphoma, the expression of CD10 is often coupled with decrease in CD19 intensity (Yang, 2005) that differs from the normal somewhat higher level of CD19 seen in normal germinal center B cells. Demonstration of bcl-2 overexpression by the CD10-positive B cell population can be quite useful in confirming neoplasia (Cook, 2003), particularly in cases lacking surface light chain expression, and reflects the presence of an underlying t(14;18) characteristic of follicular lymphoma. While CD10 positivity alone does not allow definitive classification, its presence significantly reduces the possible entities that must be considered, with morphology generally being required to allow definitive classification.

The role of immunophenotyping in the classification of T cell lymphoma is less well described, although certain associations have been noted that require larger studies for validation. As a general rule, the majority of T cell lymphomas are composed of CD4-positive T cells and exhibit abnormal patterns of antigenic expression. In angioimmunoblastic T cell lymphoma, the abnormal T cells are CD4-positive and commonly show loss or decreased expression of surface CD3 (Serke, 2000) with abnormal coexpression of CD10 (Attygalle, 2002) (Fig. 33–20). In mycosis fungoides/Sézary syndrome the abnormal T cells are also typically CD4-positive and can show a variety of immunophenotypic abnormalities commonly including alterations in the intensity of CD3 and CD4, and the decreased expression or loss of CD7 (Bogen, 1996; Lima, 2003). However, CD7 is normally variably expressed on CD4-positive T cells; decreased expression is associated with a normal memory immunophenotype, and expanded subpopulations with this immunophenotype may be seen in a variety of reactive conditions

including inflammatory skin lesions (Murphy, 2002). Consequently, the demonstration of a loss of CD7 by itself does not allow definitive classification nor a definitive diagnosis of lymphoma and generally requires the presence of additional antigenic abnormalities to be informative. The expression of CD30 in combination with an aberrant pattern of T cell antigen expression can be useful in the identification of anaplastic large cell lymphoma (Juco, 2003). Finally, large granular lymphoproliferative disorder (large granular lymphocytic leukemia) is generally characterized by a clonal expansion of CD8-positive T cells having variably decreased expression of CD5 or CD7 and the expression of NK cell-associated antigens such as CD57, CD56 or CD16 (Richards, 1995). However, similar clonal expansions may be seen in a wide variety of non-neoplastic conditions and knowledge of the clinical context is required for an understanding of the clinical significance.

Prognostic Factors

As noted above, flow cytometry is widely used to assess markers of prognostic significance in CLL, including CD38 (Damle, 1999) and ZAP70 (Crespo, 2003). Although these assays are widely available, there are problems with interpretation of results. The distribution of CD38 on CLL cells is often continuous, not discrete, and arbitrary criteria have been used to distinguish positive from negative cases. This problem is even greater in the case of ZAP70 assessment, where expression is often very dim, and where questions have been raised about the best method to determine positivity. Nonetheless, the majority of cases are either clearly positive or clearly negative for each of these markers and many papers, using varying techniques, have demonstrated their prognostic significance. However, a certain number of cases with borderline positivity are best considered as indeterminate for expression. To date there are no prognostic markers in other types of lymphoma that are as well established as those in CLL/SLL.

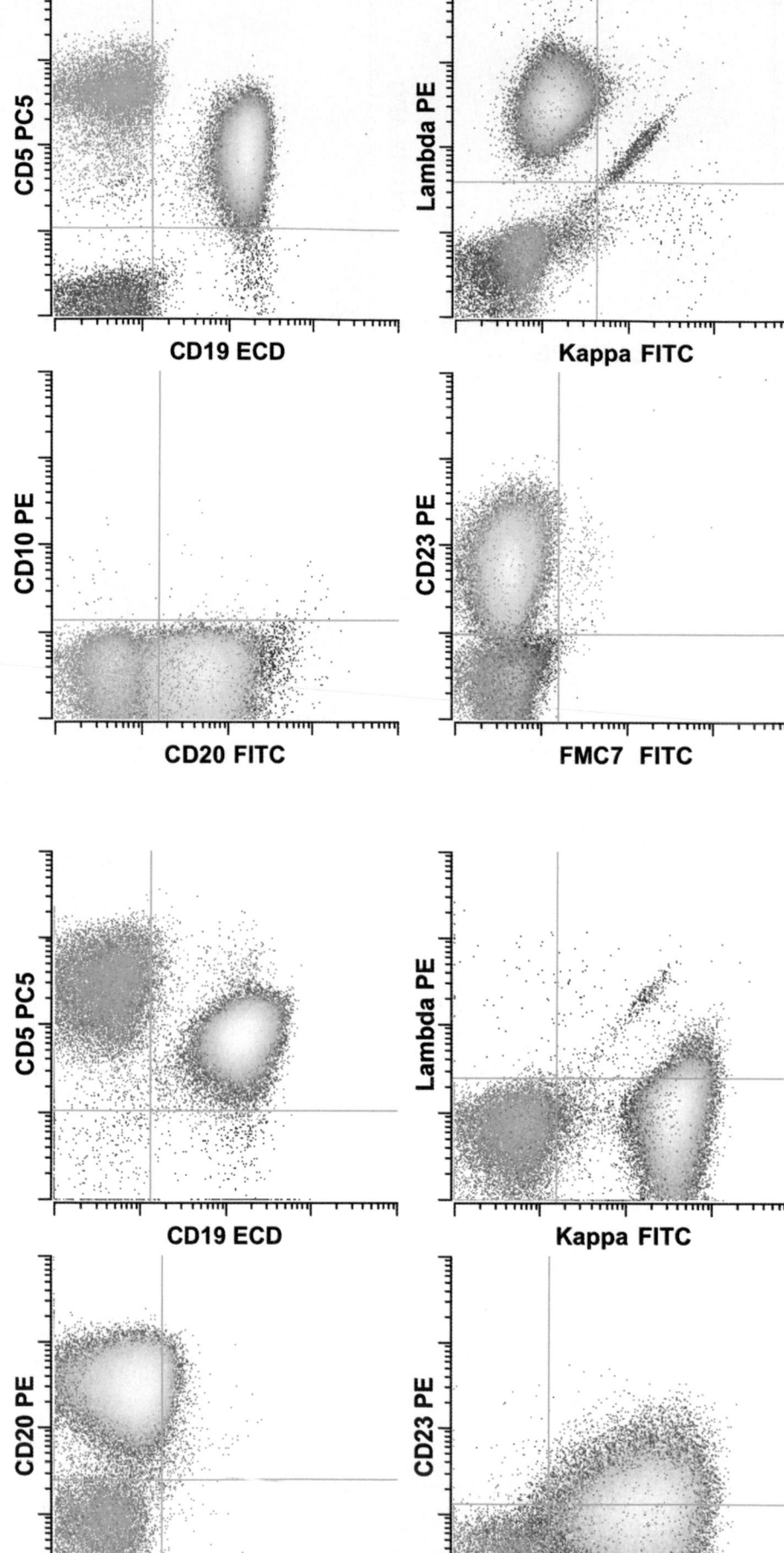

Figure 33–16 Chronic lymphocytic leukemia/small lymphocytic lymphoma. The neoplastic B cell population (gold) shows abnormal expression of the B cell antigens CD19 (intermediate) and CD20 (low) with surface lambda light chain expression (low), coexpression of CD5 and CD23 (intermediate). The combination of CD5 coexpression, low-level light chain restriction, low-level CD20 and CD23 without FMC7 is diagnostic for this particular disorder. The important differential is with mantle cell lymphoma (see Fig. 33–17).

Figure 33–17 Mantle cell lymphoma. The neoplastic B cell population (gold) shows expression of B cell antigens CD19 (intermediate), CD20 (intermediate) and kappa light chain restriction (bright) along with coexpression of CD5 (intermediate) and FMC7 (intermediate) with only low CD23. The overall pattern of antigen expression differs from that seen in CLL/SLL (see Fig. 33–16) and suggests mantle cell lymphoma. Definitive diagnosis would require demonstration of t(11;14) by FISH or cyclin D1 overexpression by immunohistochemistry.

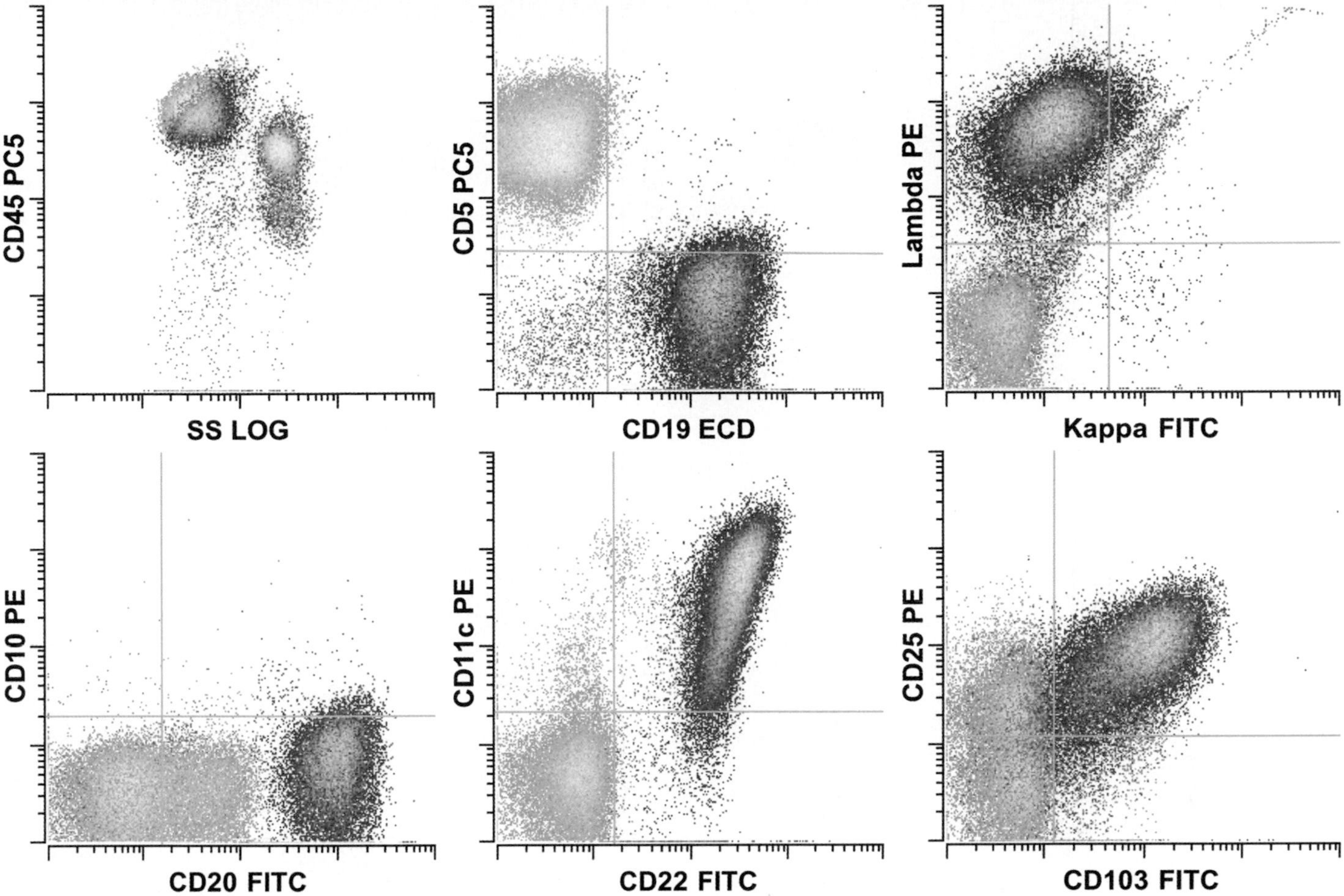

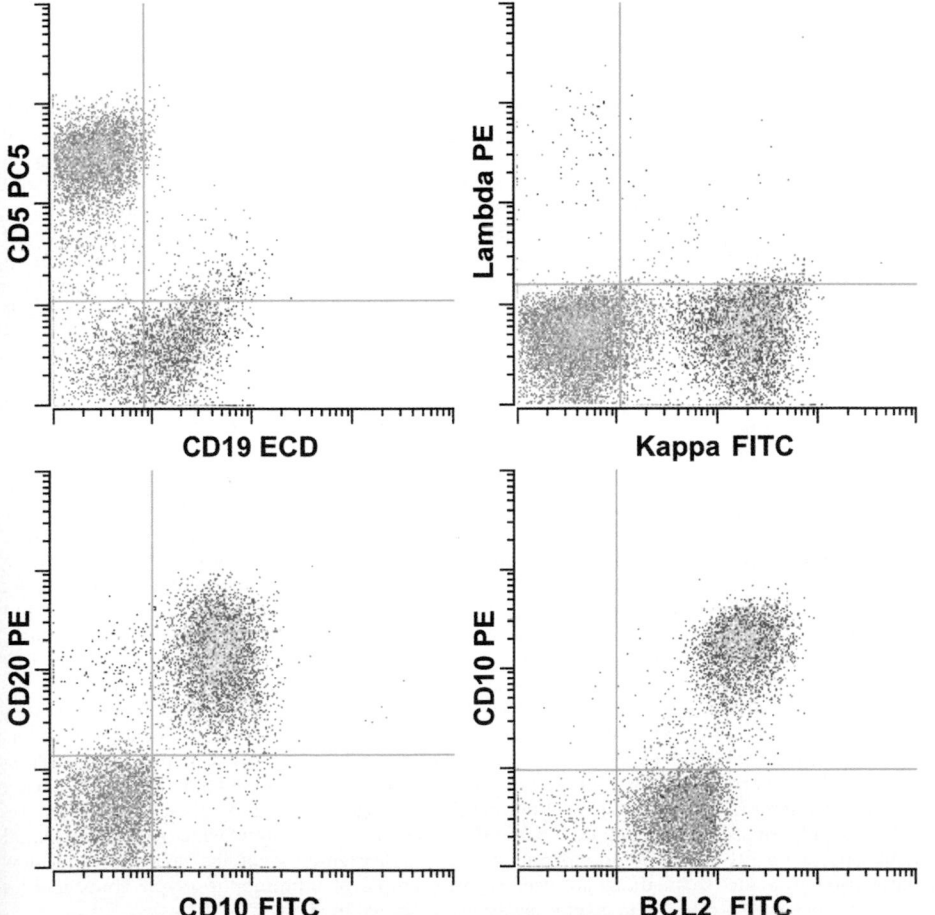

Figure 33–18 Hairy cell leukemia. The neoplastic B cell population (red) shows expression of B cell antigens CD19 (intermediate), CD20 (bright), CD22 (bright) and surface lambda light chain restriction (intermediate) with aberrant expression of the adhesion molecules CD11c (variably bright) and CD103 (intermediate), and CD25 (intermediate). This immunophenotype is diagnostic for hairy cell leukemia. Note the absence of monocytes by CD45 vs. side scatter, a characteristic finding in hairy cell leukemia.

Figure 33–19 Follicular lymphoma. The neoplastic B cell population (gold) shows abnormal expression of the B cell antigens CD19 (dim), CD20 (intermediate) and surface kappa light chain restriction (intermediate) with coexpression of the follicle center associated antigen CD10 (intermediate). In addition, the neoplasm shows the overexpression of cytoplasmic Bcl-2 due to the presence of the t(14;18) characteristic of follicular lymphoma. Overexpression of Bcl-2 is not by itself diagnostic of follicular lymphoma, but its combined expression with CD10 is much more specific, as normal CD10-positive follicular B cells would be expected to be negative.

IV

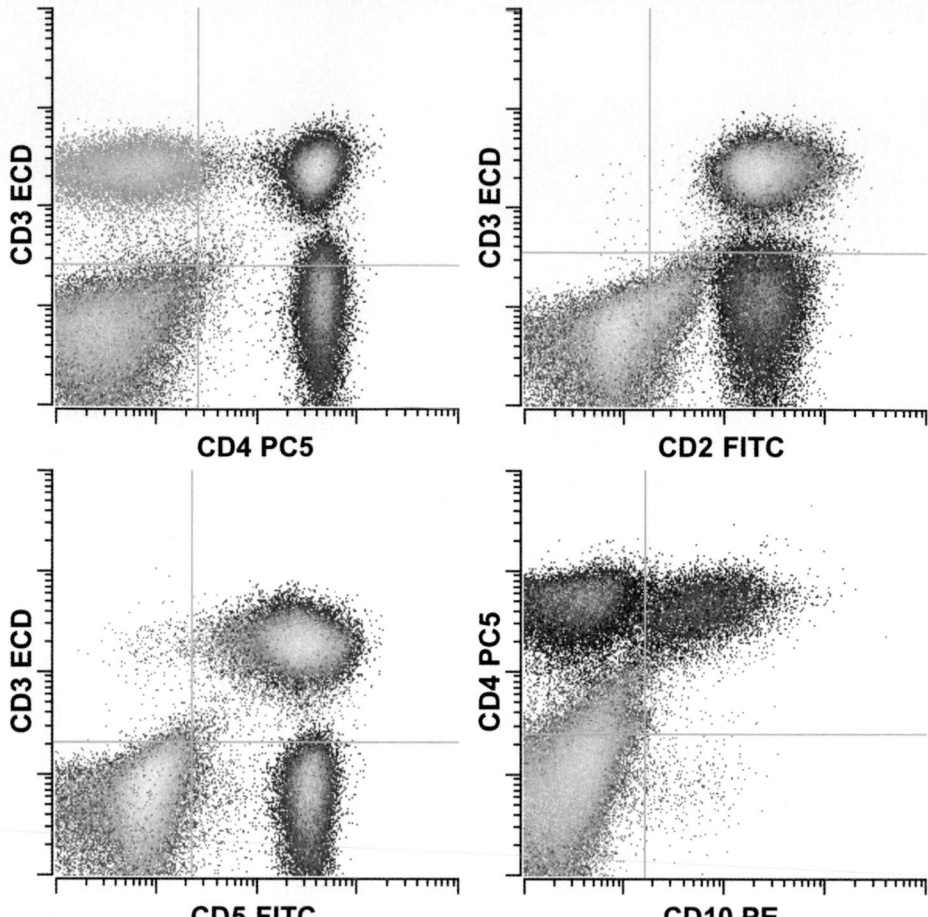

Figure 33–20 Angioimmunoblastic T cell lymphoma. The neoplastic T cell population (blue) shows expression of the T cell associated antigens CD2 (intermediate) and CD5 (intermediate) along with the helper T cell antigen CD4, but without surface CD3. In addition, the neoplastic cells coexpress CD10. The composite immunophenotype is characteristic of that seen in angioimmunoblastic T cell lymphoma.

Therapeutic Targets

The most widely used therapeutic antibody is anti-CD20 (rituxamab). Determination of CD20 expression is essential to establish the suitability of this therapy, though it is expressed by the great majority of B cell lymphomas. Following therapy, B cells may persist but show loss of CD20 expression. Assessment of samples with more than one B cell marker, such as the combination of CD19 and CD20, is helpful in demonstrating the presence of residual B cells lacking CD20. Anti-CD52 (alemtuzamab) is occasionally used to treat cases of refractory lymphoma; because of the side effects associated with this therapy documentation of expression is important, though the great majority of lymphomas will express CD52.

Minimal Residual Disease Detection

Detecting low levels of involvement can be important in accurately staging patients with lymphoma (Douglas, 1999). This is particularly applicable to studies of bone marrow, where detection of small populations of light-chain restricted B cells can be seen in cases in which morphology is either negative or equivocal. (Stacchini, 2003; Sanchez, 2002; Palacio, 2001; Duggan, 2000), although the cost-effectiveness of this approach has been questioned (Hanson, 1999). Similarly, the peripheral blood may be evaluated for lymphoma to aid in the timing or advisability of stem cell collection and the resulting harvested stem cell product may be tested for the presence of residual lymphoma to minimize the amount of tumor reinfused in patients undergoing bone marrow transplantation. In addition, as in acute leukemia, minimal residual disease studies have been employed in patients with chronic lymphocytic leukemia and have demonstrated an association between the presence of residual disease following therapy and both event-free and overall survival (Moreton, 2005; Rawstron, 2001). In these cases, methods to demonstrate clonal populations of light-chain restricted B cells are not as sensitive as methods that rely on the presence of small phenotypically aberrant populations using principles similar to those used in acute leukemia.

Plasma Cell Neoplasms

Plasma cell neoplasms are generally not difficult to identify by flow cytometry (Ruiz-Arguelles, 1994; Ocqueteau, 1998). The expression of bright CD38 and/or CD138 is used to identify the plasma cell population with common abnormalities being decreased CD45, decreased CD19 and abnormal coexpression of CD56 or CD117 in combination with the identification of cytoplasmic light chain restriction. An example of immunophenotypic abnormalities seen in plasma cell neoplasms is presented in Figure 33–21. It is important to recognize that flow cytometric analysis typically underestimates the percentage of plasma cells present in a specimen, sometimes dramatically, possibly due to plasma cell aggregation and apoptosis,

Myelodysplastic Syndromes and Myeloproliferative Disorders

The same principles used to identify other hematopoietic neoplasms can be used to identify myelodysplastic syndromes and myeloproliferative disorders (Kussick, 2003a,b; Wells, 2003; Elghetany, 1998). Abnormalities in antigen expression can be identified on myeloid blasts, maturing neutrophils and maturing monocytes with common abnormalities being alterations in the intensity of expression of CD34, CD117, HLA-DR and aberrant expression of antigens such as CD7 or CD56 on myeloid blasts, abnormal patterns of CD13 and CD16 expression and decreased side scatter on maturing neutrophils, and aberrant CD56 expression on maturing monocytes (Kussick, 2003b; Wells, 2003). Similar abnormalities in addition to basophilia may be identified in myeloproliferative disorders (Kussick, 2003a), although this has been less well studied. While abnormalities can be demonstrated in essentially all cases having cytogenetic abnormalities, low-grade myelodysplasia predominantly affecting the erythroid lineage as well as polycythemia vera and essential thrombocythemia are not consistently identified currently and new methods are needed. An example of immunophenotypic abnormalities seen in myelodysplasia is presented in Figure 33–22.

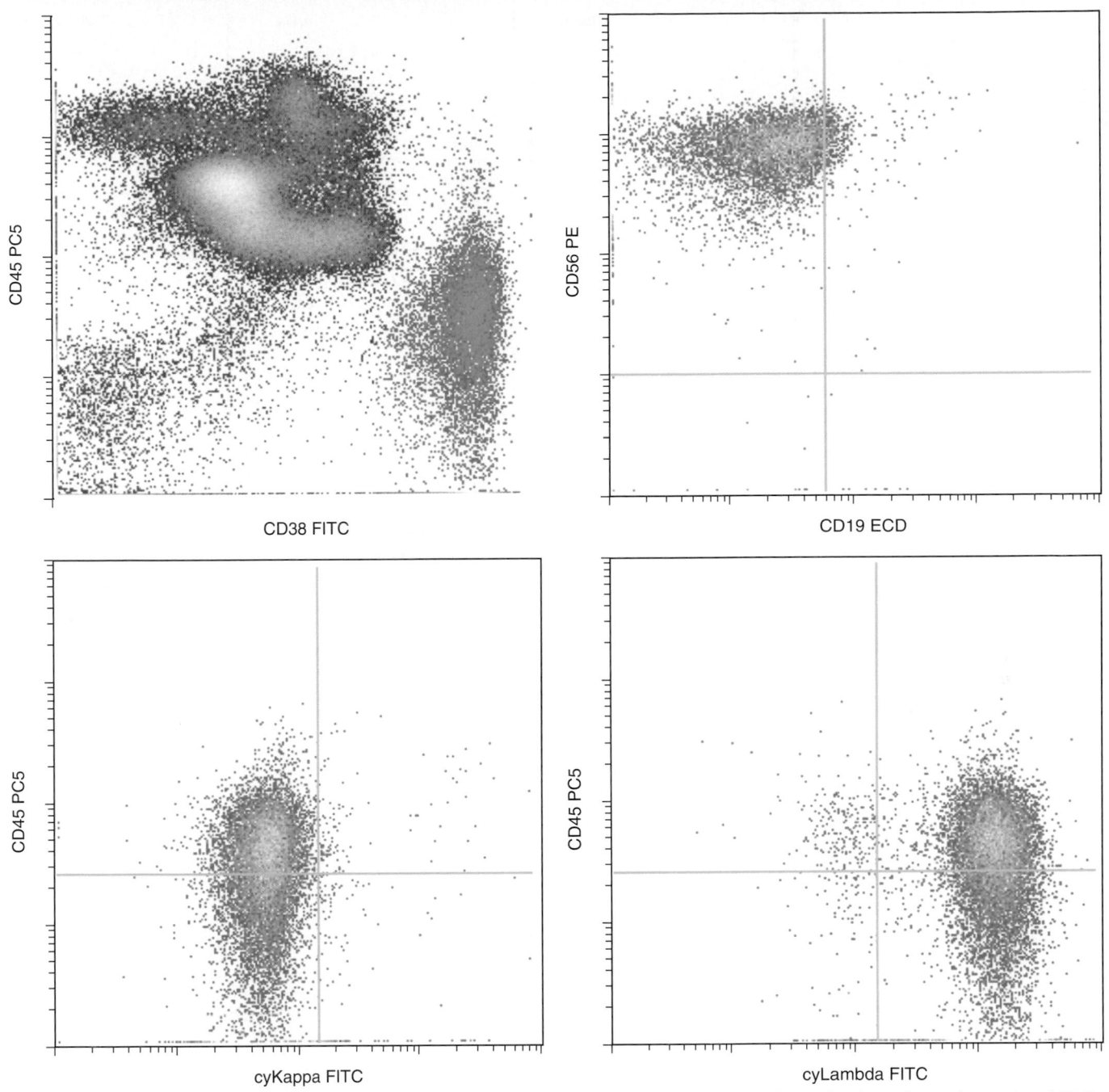

Figure 33–21 Plasma cell neoplasm. The neoplastic plasma cell population (green) is identified by the bright expression of CD38, but shows abnormal expression of CD45 (low), CD19 (absent) and cytoplasmic lambda light chain restriction with aberrant expression of CD56 (bright). This immunophenotype is characteristic of that seen in a variety of plasma cell neoplasms including multiple myeloma, plasmacytoma and monoclonal gammopathy of uncertain significance (MGUS). Definitive classification requires clinical and laboratory correlation.

Paroxysmal Nocturnal Hemoglobinuria

Certain non-neoplastic hematopoietic disorders can be diagnosed using the same principles used to identify hematopoietic neoplasms. Paroxysmal nocturnal hemoglobinuria (PNH) is an acquired clonal stem cell disorder characterized by the loss of a variety of cell surface proteins on all progeny of the hematopoietic stem cell, including erythrocytes, neutrophils, monocytes, lymphocytes and platelets. The loss of these proteins is the result of mutation of a key enzyme required for the synthesis of the glycosyl-phosphatidyl-inositol (GPI) linkage used to attach these proteins to the cell surface. Detection of the loss of GPI-linked proteins is readily accomplished by flow cytometry (Richards, 2000) and serves as the principal diagnostic method for this disorder. For clinical testing, it is recommended that at least two GPI-linked antigens be evaluated on at least two different cell lineages, commonly evaluated antigens being CD55 and CD59 on both erythrocytes and white blood cells, CD14 on monocytes and CD66b on granulocytes. Platelets and lymphocytes are generally not evaluated. Another reagent increasingly used for the diagnosis of PNH is the fluorescent derivative of a mutant form of the bacterial toxin, aerolysin, which binds specifically to the GPI-linkage and can identify GPI-deficient cells with a high degree of sensitivity and specificity (Brodsky, 2000).

Summary

Flow cytometry is a powerful, rapid and cost-effective technique for the identification and monitoring of hematopoietic neoplasms. Successful implementation requires careful attention to instrument and reagent performance, as well as a strong working knowledge of normal patterns of antigenic expression on hematopoietic cells.

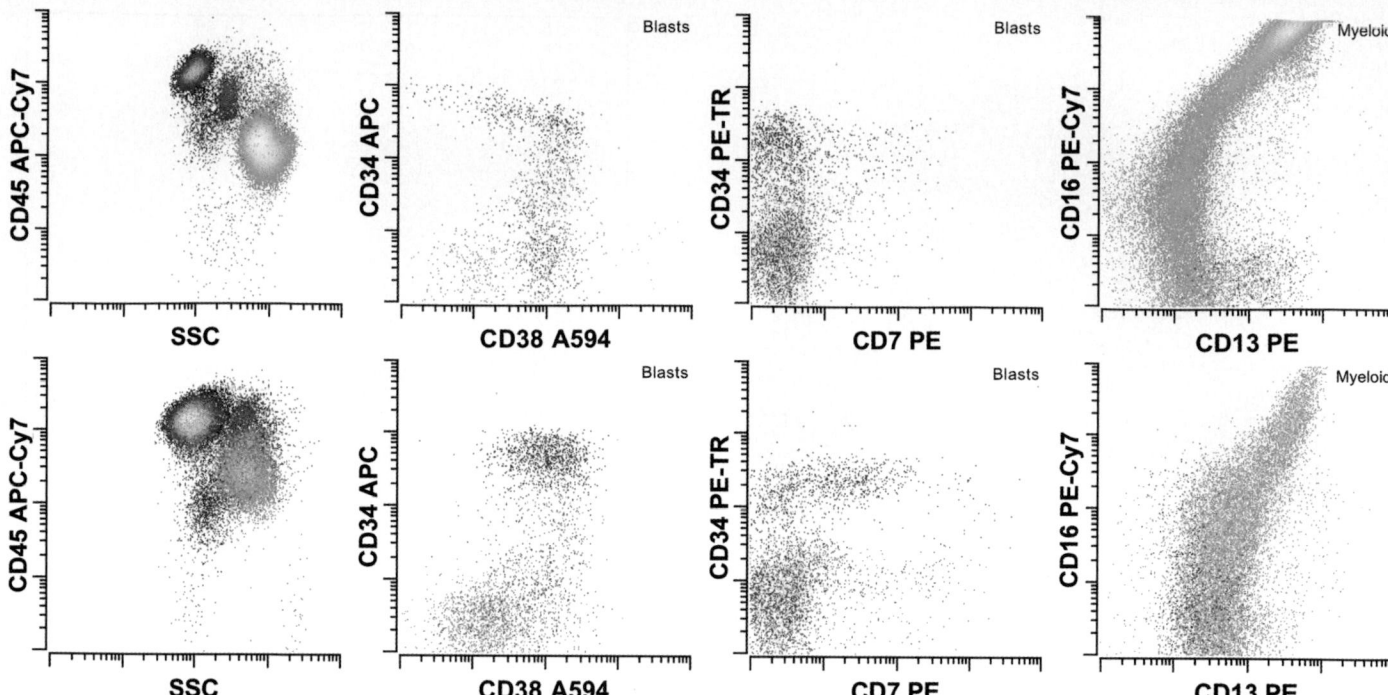

Figure 33–22 Myelodysplasia. A sample from a patient with low-grade myelodysplasia (lower row) is compared with a normal bone marrow (upper row). Abnormalities commonly seen in myelodysplasia include neutrophil hypogranularity as indicated by decreased side scatter (left), decreased CD45 expression by the blasts (red, left), homogeneity of the myeloid blasts (red, left center), acquisition of lymphoid associated antigens (CD2, CD5, CD7 or CD56) by myeloid blasts (right center) and abnormal patterns of myelomonocytic maturation such as abnormal CD13 and CD16 on maturing neutrophilic forms (right). The decreased side scatter is best noted by comparing the relative positions of the neutrophils (green) and monocytes (magenta). It is the combined presence of these abnormalities that suggests the presence of a myeloid stem cell disorder, such as myelodysplasia.

References

Almasri NM, Iturraspe JA, Braylan RC: CD10 expression in follicular lymphoma and large cell lymphoma is different from that of reactive lymph node follicles. Arch Pathol Lab Med 1998; 122(6):539–544.

Attygalle A, Al-Jehani R, Diss TC, et al: Neoplastic T cells in angioimmunoblastic T-cell lymphoma express CD10. Blood 2002; 99(2):627–633.

Baer MR, Stewart CC, Lawrence D, et al: Expression of the neural cell adhesion molecule CD56 is associated with short remission duration and survival in acute myeloid leukemia with t(8;21)(q22;q22). Blood 1997; 90:1643–1648.

Baer MR, Stewart CC, Dodge RK, et al: High frequency of immunophenotype changes in acute myeloid leukemia at relapse: implications for residual disease detection (Cancer and Leukemia Group B Study 8361). Blood 2001; 97(11):3574–3580.

Bene MC, Castoldi G, Knapp W, et al: Proposals for the immunological classification of acute leukemias. European Group for the Immunological Characterization of Leukemias (EGIL). Leukemia 1995; 9(10):1783–1786.

Bogen SA, Pelley D, Charif M, et al: Immunophenotypic identification of Sezary cells in peripheral blood. Am J Clin Pathol 1996; 106(6):739–748.

Borowitz MJ, Guenther KL, Shults KE, et al: Immunophenotyping of acute leukemia by flow cytometric analysis. Use of CD45 and right-angle light scatter to gate on leukemic blasts in three-color analysis. Am J Clin Pathol 1993; 100(5):534–540.

Bradstock K, Matthews J, Benson E, et al: Prognostic value of immunophenotyping in acute myeloid leukemia. Australian Leukaemia Study Group. Blood 1994; 84(4):1220–1225.

Braylan RC, Benson NA: Flow cytometric analysis of lymphomas. Arch Pathol Lab Med 1989; 113(6):627–633.

Braylan RC, Benson NA, Iturraspe J: Analysis of lymphomas by flow cytometry. Current and emerging strategies. Ann N Y Acad Sci 1993; 677:364–378.

Brodsky RA, Mukhina GL, Li S, et al: Improved detection and characterization of paroxysmal nocturnal hemoglobinuria using fluorescent aerolysin. Am J Clin Pathol 2000; 114(3):459–466.

Campana D: Determination of minimal residual disease in leukemia patients. British Journal of Haematology 2003; 121:823–838.

Carter PH, Resto-Ruiz S, Washington GC, et al: Flow cytometric analysis of whole blood lysis, three anticoagulants, and five cell preparations. Cytometry 1992; 13(1):68–74.

Chang A, Benda PM, Wood BL, et al: Lineage-specific identification of nonhematopoietic neoplasms by flow cytometry. Am J Clin Pathol 2003; 119(5):643–655.

Chen W, Asplund SL, McKenna RW, et al: Characterization of incidentally identified minute clonal B-lymphocyte populations in peripheral blood and bone marrow. Am J Clin Pathol 2004; 122(4):588–595.

Cook JR, Craig FE, Swerdlow SH: bcl-2 expression by multicolor flow cytometric analysis assists in the diagnosis of follicular lymphoma in lymph node and bone marrow. Am J Clin Pathol 2003; 119(1):145–151.

Coustan-Smith E, Sancho J, Hancock ML, et al: Clinical importance of minimal residual disease in childhood acute lymphoblastic leukemia. Blood 2000; 96:2691–2696.

Crespo M, Bosch F, Villamor N, et al: ZAP-70 expression as a surrogate for immunoglobulin-variable-region mutations in chronic lymphocytic leukemia. New England Journal of Medicine 2003; 348(18):1764–1775.

Damle RN, Wasil T, Fais F, et al: Ig V gene mutation status and CD38 expression as novel prognostic indicators in chronic lymphocytic leukemia. Blood 1999; 94(6):1840–1847.

Douglas VK, Gordon LI, Goolsby CL, et al: Lymphoid aggregates in bone marrow mimic residual lymphoma after rituximab therapy for non-Hodgkin lymphoma. Am J Clin Pathol 1999; 112(6):844–853.

Duggan PR, Easton D, Luider J, et al: Bone marrow staging of patients with non-Hodgkin lymphoma by flow cytometry: correlation with morphology. Cancer 2000; 88(4):894–899.

Dworzak MN, Froschl G, Printz D et al: Prognostic significance and modalities of flow cytometric minimal residual disease detection in childhood acute lymphoblastic leukemia. Blood 2002; 99:1952–1958.

Elghetany MT: Surface marker abnormalities in myelodysplastic syndromes. Haematologica 1998; 83(12):1104–1115.

Farahat N, Lens D, Zomas A, et al: Quantitative flow cytometry can distinguish between normal and leukaemic B-cell precursors. Br J Haematol 1995; 91(3):640–646.

Feller N, van der Pol MA, van Stijn A, et al: MRD parameters using immunophenotypic detection methods are highly reliable in predicting survival in acute myeloid leukaemia. Leukemia 2004; 18(8):1380–1390.

Fukushima PI, Nguyen PK, O'Grady P, et al: Flow cytometric analysis of kappa and lambda light chain expression in evaluation of specimens for B-cell neoplasia. Cytometry 1996; 26(4):243–252.

Geary WA, Frierson HF, Innes DJ, et al: Quantitative criteria for clonality in the diagnosis of B-cell non-Hodgkin's lymphoma by flow cytometry. Mod Pathol 1993; 6(2):155–161.

Ginaldi L, Matutes E, Farahat N, et al: Differential expression of CD3 and CD7 in T-cell malignancies: a quantitative study by flow cytometry. Br J Haematol 1996a; 93(4):921–927.

Ginaldi L, Farahat N, Matutes E, et al: Differential expression of T cell antigens in normal peripheral blood lymphocytes: a quantitative analysis by flow cytometry. J Clin Pathol 1996b; 49(7):539–544.

Hanson CA, Abaza M, Sheldon S, et al: Biphenotypic leukaemia: immunophenotypic and cytogenetic analysis. Br J Haematol 1993; 84(1):49–60.

Hanson CA, Kurtin PJ, Katzmann JA, et al: Immunophenotypic analysis of peripheral blood and bone marrow in the staging of B-cell malignant lymphoma. Blood 1999; 94(11):3889–3896.

Harada H, Kawano MM, Huang N, et al: Phenotypic difference of normal plasma cells from mature myeloma cells. Blood 1993; 81(10):2658–2663.

Hoffkes HG, Schmidtke G, Uppenkamp M, et al: Multiparametric immunophenotyping of B cells in peripheral blood of healthy adults by flow cytometry. Clin Diagn Lab Immunol 1996; 3(1):30–36.

Hrusak O, Porwit-MacDonald A: Antigen expression patterns reflecting genotype of acute leukemias. Leukemia 2002; 16:1233–1258.

Inghirami G, Zhu BY, Chess L, et al: Flow cytometric and immunohistochemical characterization of the gamma/delta T-lymphocyte population in normal human lymphoid tissue and peripheral blood. Am J Pathol 1990; 136(2):357–367.

Jacobberger JW: Flow cytometric analysis of intracellular protein epitopes. In Stewart C, Nicholson JKA (eds): Immunophenotyping, 1st ed. New York, Wiley-Liss, 2000, pp 361–406.

Jaffe ES, Harris NL, Stein H, Vardiman JW (eds): World Health Organization Classification of Tumours. Pathology and Genetics of Tumours of Hematopoietic and Lymphoid Tissues, 1st ed. Lyon, IARC Press, 2001.
A definitive and well-illustrated text expounding the most modern and comprehensive classification of human hematopoietic disease achieved through international consensus.

Juco J, Holden JT, Mann KP, et al: Immunophenotypic analysis of anaplastic large cell lymphoma by flow cytometry. Am J Clin Pathol 2003; 119(2):205–212.

Khalidi HS, Medeiros LJ, Chang KL, et al: The immunophenotype of adult acute myeloid leukemia: high frequency of lymphoid antigen expression and comparison of immunophenotype, French–American–British classification, and karyotypic abnormalities. Am J Clin Pathol 1998; 109(2):211–220.

Khalidi HS, Chang KL, Medeiros LJ, et al: Acute lymphoblastic leukemia. Survey of immunophenotype, French–American–British classification, frequency of myeloid antigen expression, and karyotypic abnormalities in 210 pediatric and adult cases. Am J Clin Pathol 1999; 111(4):467–476.

Kussick SJ, Wood BL: Four-color flow cytometry identifies virtually all cytogenetically abnormal bone marrow samples in the workup of non-CML myeloproliferative disorders. Am J Clin Pathol 2003a; 120(6):854–865.

Kussick SJ, Wood BL: 4 color flow cytometry to identify abnormal myeloid populations. Arch Pathol Lab Med 2003b; 127:1140–1147.

Kussick SJ, Kalnoski M, Braziel RM, et al: Prominent clonal B-cell populations identified by flow cytometry in histologically reactive lymphoid proliferations. Am J Clin Pathol 2004; 121(4):464–472.

Li S, Eshleman JR, Borowitz MJ: Lack of surface immunoglobulin light chain expression by flow cytometric immunophenotyping can help diagnose peripheral B-cell lymphoma. Am J Clin Pathol 2002; 118(2):229–234.

Lima M, Almeida J, Santos AH, et al: Immunophenotypic analysis of the TCR-Vbeta repertoire in 98 persistent expansions of CD3(+)/TCR-alphabeta(+) large granular lymphocytes: utility in assessing clonality and insights into the pathogenesis of the disease. Am J Pathol 2001; 159(5):1861–1868.

Lima M, Almeida J, dos Anjos Teixeira M, et al: Utility of flow cytometry immunophenotyping and DNA ploidy studies for diagnosis and characterization of blood involvement in CD4+ Sezary's syndrome. Haematologica 2003; 88(8):874–887.

Linenberger ML: CD33-directed therapy with gemtuzumab ozogamicin in acute myeloid leukemia: progress in understanding cytotoxicity and potential mechanisms of drug resistance. Leukemia 2005; 9(2):176–182.

Loken MR, Shah VO, Dattilio KL, et al: Flow cytometric analysis of human bone marrow. II. Normal B lymphocyte development. Blood 1987; 70(5):1316–1324.

Loken MR, Shah VO, Hollander Z, et al: Flow cytometric analysis of normal B lymphoid development. Pathol Immunopathol Res 1988; 7(5):357–370.

Lucio P, Parreira A, van den Beemd MW, et al: Flow cytometric analysis of normal B cell differentiation: a frame of reference for the detection of minimal residual disease in precursor-B-ALL. Leukemia 1999; 13(3):419–427.

Macedo A, Orfao A, Vidriales MB, et al: Characterization of aberrant phenotypes in acute myeloblastic leukemia. Ann Hematol 1995a; 70(4):189–194.

Macedo A, Orfao A, Gonzalez M, et al: Immunological detection of blast cell subpopulations in acute myeloblastic leukemia at diagnosis: implications for minimal residual disease studies. Leukemia 1995b; 9(6):993–998.

McClanahan J, Fukushima PI, Stetler-Stevenson M: Increased peripheral blood gamma delta T-cells in patients with lymphoid neoplasia: A diagnostic dilemma in flow cytometry. Cytometry 1999; 38(6):280–285.

McKenna RW, Washington LT, Aquino DB, et al: Immunophenotypic analysis of hematogones (B-lymphocyte precursors) in 662 consecutive bone marrow specimens by 4-color flow cytometry. Blood 2001; 98(8):2498–2507.

Matutes E, Owusu-Ankomah K, Morilla R, et al: Immunological profile of B-cell disorders and proposal of a scoring system for the diagnosis of CLL. Leukemia 1994a; 8(10):1640–1645.

Matutes E, Morilla R, Owusu-Ankomah K, et al: The immunophenotype of hairy cell leukemia (HCL). Proposal for a scoring system to distinguish HCL from B-cell disorders with hairy or villous lymphocytes. Leuk Lymphoma 1994b; 14 Suppl 1:57–61.

Matutes E, Morilla R, Farahat N, et al: Definition of acute biphenotypic leukemia. Haematologica 1997; 82(1):64–66.

Moreton P, Kennedy B, Lucas G, et al: Eradication of minimal residual disease in B-cell chronic lymphocytic leukemia after alemtuzumab therapy is associated with prolonged survival. J Clin Oncol 2005; 23:1–9.

Morice WG, Kurtin PJ, Leibson PJ, et al: Demonstration of aberrant T-cell and natural killer-cell antigen expression in all cases of granular lymphocytic leukaemia. Br J Haem 2003; 120:1026–1036.

Morice WG, Kimlinger T, Katzmann JA, et al: Flow cytometric assessment of TCR-Vbeta expression in the evaluation of peripheral blood involvement by T-cell lymphoproliferative disorders: a comparison with conventional T-cell immunophenotyping and molecular genetic techniques. Am J Clin Pathol 2004; 121(3):373–383.

Murphy M, Fullen D, Carlson JA: Low CD7 expression in benign and malignant cutaneous lymphocytic infiltrates: experience with an antibody reactive with paraffin-embedded tissue. Am J Dermatopathol 2002; 24(1):6–16.

National Committee for Clinical Laboratory Standards. Clinical applications of flow cytometry: immunophenotyping of leukemic cells; approved guideline. NCCLS Document H43-A, Vol 18, No 8, 1998.
Useful reference document on technical issues related to the clinical performance of flow cytometry for leukemia and lymphoma.

Ocqueteau M, Orfao A, Almeida J, et al: Immunophenotypic characterization of plasma cells from monoclonal gammopathy of undetermined significance patients. Implications for the differential diagnosis between MGUS and multiple myeloma. Am J Pathol 1998; 152(6):1655–1665.

Orfao A, Chillon MC, Bortoluci AM, et al: The flow cytometric pattern of CD34, CD15 and CD13 expression in acute myeloblastic leukemia is highly characteristic of the presence of PML-RAR alpha gene rearrangements. Haematologica 1999; 84(5):405–412.

Orfao A, Ortuno F, de Santiago M, et al: Immunophenotyping of acute leukemias and myelodysplastic syndromes. Cytometry A 2004; 58:62–71.

Palacio C, Acebedo G, Navarrete M, et al: Flow cytometry in the bone marrow evaluation of follicular and diffuse large B-cell lymphomas. Haematologica 2001; 86(9):934–940.

Picker LJ, Weiss LM, Medeiros LJ, et al: Immunophenotypic criteria for the diagnosis of non-Hodgkin's lymphoma. Am J Pathol 1987; 128:181–201.

Porwit-MacDonald A, Janossy G, Ivory K, et al: Leukemia-associated changes identified by quantitative flow cytometry. IV. CD34 overexpression in acute myelogenous leukemia M2 with t(8;21). Blood 1996; 87(3):1162–1169.

Rawstron AC, Kennedy B, Evans PA, et al: Quantitation of minimal disease levels in chronic lymphocytic leukemia using a sensitive flow cytometric assay improves the prediction of outcome and can be used to optimize therapy. Blood 2001; 98(1):29–35.

Rawstron AC, Green MJ, Kuzmicki A, et al: Monoclonal B lymphocytes with the characteristics of 'indolent' chronic lymphocytic leukemia are present in 3.5% of adults with normal blood counts. Blood 2002; 100(2):635–639.

Reading CL, Estey EH, Huh YO, et al: Expression of unusual immunophenotype combinations in acute myelogenous leukemia. Blood 1993; 81(11):3083–3090.

Richards SJ, Short M, Scott CS: Clonal CD3+CD8+ large granular lymphocyte (LGL)/NK-associated (NKa) expansions: primary malignancies or secondary reactive phenomena? Leuk Lymphoma 1995; 17(3–4):303–311.

Richards SJ, Rawstron AC, Hillmen P: Application of flow cytometry to the diagnosis of paroxysmal nocturnal hemoglobinuria. Cytometry 2000; 42(4):223–233.

Robbins BA, Ellison DJ, Spinosa JC, et al: Diagnostic application of two-color flow cytometry in 161 cases of hairy cell leukemia. Blood 1994; 82(4):1277–1287.

Roederer M: Spectral compensation for flow cytometry: visualization artifacts, limitations, and caveats. Cytometry 2001; 45:194–205.

Ruiz-Arguelles GJ, San Miguel JF: Cell surface markers in multiple myeloma. Mayo Clin Proc 1994; 69(7):684–690.

Sanchez ML, Almeida J, Vidriales B et al: Incidence of phenotypic aberrations in a series of 467 patients with B chronic lymphoproliferative disorders: basis for the design of specific four-color stainings to be used for minimal residual disease investigation. Leukemia 2002; 16(8):1460–1469.

IV

San Miguel JF, Vidriales MB, Lopez-Berges C, et al: Early immunophenotypical evaluation of minimal residual disease in acute myeloid leukemia identifies different patient risk groups and may contribute to postinduction treatment stratification. Blood 2001; 98(6):1746–1751.

Schabath R, Ratei R, Ludwig WD: The prognostic significance of antigen expression in leukaemia. Best Pract Res Clin Haematol 2003; 16(4):613–628.

Serke S, van Lessen A, Hummel M, et al: Circulating CD4+ T lymphocytes with intracellular but no surface CD3 antigen in five of seven patients consecutively diagnosed with angioimmunoblastic T-cell lymphoma. Cytometry 2000; 42(3):180–187.

Serke S, Schwaner I, Yordanova M, et al: Monoclonal antibody FMC7 detects a conformational epitope on the CD20 molecule: evidence from phenotyping after rituxan therapy and transfectant cell analyses. Cytometry 2001; 46(2):98–104.

Shapiro HM: Practical Flow Cytometry, 4th ed. New York, Wiley-Liss, 2003.

The definitive exposition of technical issues related to flow cytometry.

Stacchini A, Demurtas A, Godio L, et al: Flow cytometry in the bone marrow staging of mature B-cell neoplasms. Cytometry B Clin Cytom 2003; 54(1):10–18.

Stelzer GT, Shults KE, Loken MR: CD45 gating for routine flow cytometric analysis of human bone marrow specimens. Ann N Y Acad Sci 1993; 677:265–280.

Stewart CC, Mayers GL: Kinetics of antibody binding to cells. *In* Stewart C, Nicholson JKA (eds): Immunophenotyping, 1st ed. New York, Wiley-Liss, 2000, pp 1–22.

The entire volume is an excellent, modern general reference on the use of immunophenotyping in a variety of settings.

Terstappen LW, Loken MR: Myeloid cell differentiation in normal bone marrow and acute myeloid leukemia assessed by multi-dimensional flow cytometry. Anal Cell Pathol 1990b; 2(4):229–240.

Terstappen LW, Johnsen S, Segers-Nolten IM, et al: Identification and characterization of plasma cells in normal human bone marrow by high-resolution flow cytometry. Blood 1990a; 76(9):1739–1747.

Terstappen LW, Hollander Z, Meiners H, et al: Quantitative comparison of myeloid antigens on five lineages of mature peripheral blood cells. J Leukoc Biol 1990c; 48(2):138–148.

Terstappen LW, Safford M, Konemann S, et al: Flow cytometric characterization of acute myeloid leukemia. Part II. Phenotypic heterogeneity at diagnosis. Leukemia 1992a; 6(1):70–80.

Terstappen LW, Huang S, Picker LJ: Flow cytometric assessment of human T-cell differentiation in thymus and bone marrow. Blood 1992b; 79(3):666–677.

Tworek JA, Singleton TP, Schnitzer B, et al: Flow cytometric and immunohistochemical analysis of small lymphocytic lymphoma, mantle cell lymphoma, and plasmacytoid small lymphocytic lymphoma. Am J Clin Pathol 1998; 110(5):582–589.

US–Canadian Consensus recommendations on the immunophenotypic analysis of hematologic neoplasia by cytometry. Bethesda, Maryland, November 16–17, 1995. Cytometry 1997; 30(5):213–274.

Comprehensive description of consensus guidelines for the practical performance of clinical flow cytometry for the diagnosis of leukemia and lymphoma.

Vidriales M, San Miguel JF, Orfao A, et al: Minimal residual disease monitoring by flow cytometry. Best Pract Res Clin Haem 2003; 16:599–612.

Voskova D, Schoch C, Schnittger S, et al: Stability of leukemia-associated aberrant immunophenotypes in patients with acute myeloid leukemia between diagnosis and relapse: comparison with cytomorphologic, cytogenetic, and molecular genetic findings. Cytometry B Clin Cytom 2004; 62B(1):25–38.

Weir EG, Cowan K, LeBeau P, et al: A limited antibody panel can distinguish B-precursor acute lymphoblastic leukemia from normal B precursors with four color flow cytometry: implications for residual disease detection. Leukemia 1999; 13(4):558–567.

Weir EG, Borowitz MJ: Flow cytometry in the diagnosis of acute leukemia. Semin Hematol 2001; 38:124–138.

Wells DA, Benesch M, Loken MR, et al: Myeloid and monocytic dyspoiesis as determined flow cytometric scoring in myelodysplastic syndrome correlates with the IPSS and with outcome after hematopoietic stem cell transplantation. Blood 2003; 102:394–403.

Wood BL: Multicolor immunophenotyping: human immune system hematopoiesis. Methods Cell Biol 2004; 75:559–576.

Yang W, Agrawal N, Patel J, et al: Diminished expression of CD19 in B-cell lymphomas. Cytometry B Clin Cytom 2005; 63(1):28–35.

CHAPTER: 33   The Flow Cytometric Evaluation of Hematopoietic Neoplasia

CHAPTER 34

Immunohematology

Wendy V. Beadling MS MT(ASCP)SBB, Laura Cooling MD MS

KEY POINTS

• Blood group antigens play a variety of physiological roles as membrane structures involved in maintaining erythrocyte cytoskeleton integrity, as well as in membrane transport, cell signaling, immune complement regulation, and as receptors/modulators of disease.

• The ABO histo-blood group antigens are widely expressed throughout the body and are the single most important blood group for selection and transfusion of blood products as well as a major consideration in solid organ and bone marrow transplantation.

• The recipient immune response to exposure to foreign red cell antigens through transfusion or pregnancy may include antibody production and complement activation resulting in hemolysis (e.g., transfusion reaction; hemolytic disease of the newborn [HDN]).

• Pretransfusion and perinatal blood testing are performed to prevent transfusion reactions and HDN, and must include the key serologic evaluations of ABO and Rh antigen typing, antibody detection/identification, and crossmatching.

• Antihuman globulin reagents as used in either direct or indirect testing are integral to virtually all red cell antibody detection and identification techniques.

• Patients with complex serologic problems such as antibodies to high-frequency antigens and autoantibodies may require utilization of a variety of special immunohematologic studies (enzymes, adsorption, elution) to provide compatible blood for transfusion.

Basic Immunohematologic Concepts

The term *immunohematology* refers to the serologic, genetic, biochemical, and molecular study of antigens associated with membrane structures on the cellular constituents of the blood, and immunologic properties and reactions of all blood components and constituents. Fundamental discoveries in the area of immunohematology have played an integral role in the development of *transfusion medicine*, which represents a branch of clinical pathology involving the transfusion of blood, its components, and its derivatives (see Ch. 35). In this integrated relationship, immunohematologists perform a variety of serologic laboratory examinations, evaluate and interpret the reactions observed, and provide selected advanced investigations to aid in the study of the pathogenesis, diagnosis, prevention, and management of immunization associated with transfusion, pregnancy and organ transplantation. Immunogenetics has assumed an increasing role, superseding immunohematologic methods employed in the resolution of parentage problems. Over the years, research in the field of immunohematology has contributed significantly to the fundamental understanding of human genetics and immunology, the elucidation of cell membrane structure and function, and has been applied in the areas of anthropology and forensic science. Hemapheresis has facilitated and enhanced tissue banking and targeted therapies with preparation and modification of blood components/derivatives.

Blood Group Antigens

The term *blood group* refers not only to genetically encoded erythrocyte antigen systems but also to the immunologic diversity expressed by other

IV

blood constituents including leukocytes, platelets, and plasma. Blood constituent antigens that are produced by alleles at a single gene locus or by a group of closely linked loci constitute a blood group antigen *system*. Most blood group genes, with a few exceptions, are located on the autosomal chromosomes and are inherited following Mendelian rules of inheritance, leading to their application as useful genetic markers. The majority of blood group alleles demonstrate codominance as well, meaning that genetic heterozygotes at a particular locus will express both gene products.

Many membrane-associated structures of blood cells and constituents of plasma may be defined as *antigens* because they have the capability of reacting with a complementary antibody or cell receptor. The majority of these antigens are also *immunogens*, since they are able to elicit an antibody-mediated immunologic response if introduced as a foreign substance into a responsive host. Each antigen may have a variety of different epitopes or specific antigenic determinants. Epitopes are discrete, immunologically active regions of the antigen, whose molecular configuration confers the ability to interact with specific lymphocyte membrane receptors or secreted complementary antibody. In the process of antigenic stimulation, many cells are involved with recognition of the various epitopes contained within a complex antigen.

Immunogenicity

The ability of an antigen to elicit an immune response is known as its immunogenicity. The immunogenicity of an antigen is determined not only by certain innate characteristics of the antigen itself but also by the host's genetically determined immune responsiveness. Characteristics of antigens that determine their immunogenicity include the degree of foreignness; molecular size and configuration, which may change with temperature, pH, and ionic environment; and antigenic complexity as measured by the number of available epitopes or antigenic determinants.

Blood group antigens vary greatly in their ability to elicit an immune response. The A, B, and D (Rh$_o$) antigens are certainly the most immunogenic, and thus all blood transfused must be matched for these antigens between the blood donor and the recipient. Approximately 50–75% of D-negative individuals would produce anti-D if transfused with only one unit of D-positive blood. After the D antigen, K is the next most immunogenic, followed by Fy^a and common Rh antigens, based on the frequency with which their corresponding antibodies are encountered. Using the same criteria, other common blood group antigens such as Fy^b, Jk^a, Jk^b, and s are much less immunogenic. The relative immunogenicities of some clinically important red cell antigens are listed in Table 34–1.

Chemical Characteristics

The chemical composition, complexity and molecular size of an antigen determine most of its physical and biological properties, including immunogenicity. As a general rule, pure polysaccharides are not immunogenic except in certain species such as humans and mice (Virella, 2001). Also, pure lipid and nucleic acids are not immunogenic, but can be antigenic, since they can serve as haptens. Haptens are well-defined chemical groupings that are too small to be immunogenic by themselves but can induce an antibody response when attached to a carrier protein.

Although pure protein may be immunogenic, the most potent immunogens are usually complex macromolecular glycoproteins and lipoproteins. Thus, it is not surprising that red blood cell (RBC) antigens are glycoproteins, lipoproteins, and glycolipids. Experiments with peptide chain polymers have shown that aromatic amino acids, such as tyrosine and phenylalanine, can contribute significantly to overall immunogenicity (Virella, 2001). In glycoproteins, immunogenicity may also be influenced by the extent of branching in the polysaccharide side chains. Whereas the immunogenicity of an antigen relates to the total complex molecular structure, the areas where antigen combines with specific antibody (i.e., the epitopes) are usually limited to one or a few simple structures (terminal sugars, amino acids) exposed on the exterior, mobile surface of the molecule (Roitt, 2001). These are often referred to as immunodominant structures because they determine the specificity and optimal binding energy of antigen–antibody interactions.

Antigen Density

The number of antigenic sites on a foreign substance, whether a complex molecule or cell, will contribute to the strength and end result of an immunologic response. Studies of blood group antigens have demonstrated that antigen density contributes to the efficiency of antibody binding and extent of complement activation, thus determining the likelihood of RBC hemolysis.

Various techniques have been used over the years to determine the number of copies of specific blood group antigens on the RBC membrane.

Table 34–1 Relative Immunogenicity of Selected Clinically Important Blood Group Antigens*

Antigen	Relative potency	Antigen	Relative potency
D	0.70	K	0.10
C	0.041	E	0.0338
k	0.030	e	0.0112
Fy^a	0.0046	C	0.0022
Jk^a	0.0014	S	0.0008
Jk^b	0.0006	s	0.0006

* These figures represent the approximate percentage of persons negative for a specific antigen who, if transfused with one unit of corresponding antigen-positive blood, would develop antibodies to that specific antigen. When relative potency of K antigen is 0.1 as estimated by Kornstad (1958), the relative potency of other blood groups can be estimated as shown by Mollison (1993).

Table 34–2 Number of Membrane Sites for Selected Native Erythrocyte Antigens Estimated by Radioimmunoassay*

Antigen	Phenotype	Number of antigenic sites	Antigen	Phenotype	Number of antigenic sites
A	A$_1$ adult	$810-1170 \times 10^3$	D	DCce	$9.9-14.6 \times 10^3$
	newborn	$250-370 \times 10^3$		Dce	$12-20 \times 10^3$
	A$_2$ adult	$240-290 \times 10^3$		DcEe	$14-16.6 \times 10^3$
	newborn	140×10^3		DCe	$14.5-19.3 \times 10^3$
	A$_1$B adult	$460-850 \times 10^3$		DcE	$15.5-33.3 \times 10^3$
	newborn	220×10^3		DCcEe	$23-21 \times 10^3$
	A$_2$B adult	140×103		D – –	$110-202 \times 10^3$
B	B adult	750×10^3		weak D (D^u)	$0.8-3 \times 10^3$
	A$_1$B adult	430×10^3	c	c+C–	$70-85 \times 10^3$
I	I+	500×10^3		c+C+	$37-53 \times 10^3$
K	K+k–	6.1×10^3	e	e+E–	$18.2-24.4 \times 10^3$
	K+k+	3.5×10^3		e+E+	$13.4-14.5 \times 10^3$
			E	e-E+	$0.45-25.6 \times 10^3$

* Figures taken from Mollison (1993).

Historically, radioimmunoassay (RIA) (Hughes-Jones, 1971), enzyme-linked immunosorbent assay (ELISA) (Caren, 1982), and electron microscopy using ferritin-labeled anti-immunoglobulin (Masouredis, 1980) have been used to indirectly calculate the number of antigen sites on RBC membranes. More recently, flow cytometry has been used to quantitate and analyze RBC antigen distribution for a number of blood group systems (Nance, 1988). Table 34–2 lists the estimated densities of common RBC antigens.

Blood Group Antibodies

Immunoglobulins and Antigen Binding

Immunoglobulins are protein molecules that are produced in response to antigenic stimulation and that demonstrate specific antibody activity. To understand antibodies, one must first be familiar with immunoglobulin structure and function. Information on immunoglobulins that is relevant to blood banking is summarized in Tables 34–3 and 34–4.

The specificity of an antibody is determined by the hypervariable or complementarity-determining regions of an immunoglobulin molecule. There are three hypervariable regions in each of the light and heavy chains that comprise the immunoglobulin molecule (Roitt, 2001). Amino acid sequence heterogeneity in the hypervariable regions, which allows for variation in the configuration of the peptide chains in the variable loops, determines the combining specificity for each antibody. The combining site of an antibody, where it is in physical contact with an antigenic determinant or epitope, is called the *paratope*. For simple, linear antigens (sequential epitopes), the combining site may be in contact with five or six amino acids or hexose units. In the case of a globular protein antigen, as many as 16 amino acids of what is generally a discontinuous or conformational epitope may be in contact with the antibody-combining site (Roitt, 2001).

Table 34-3 Important Properties of Human Immunoglobulin (Ig) Classes

	IgG	IgM	IgA	IgD	IgE
Heavy chain isotype	γ	μ	α	δ	ε
Light chains	K or λ	K or λ	K or λ	K or λ	K or λ
No. of four-peptide units	1	5	1–2	1	1
Valency (Ag binding)	2	5(10)*	2–4	2	2
Development in immune response	Late primary, secondary	Early primary			
Half-life in vivo (days)	21	10	6	3	2
Serum concentration (mg/mL)	8–16	0.5–2	1.4–4	0–0.04	Trace
Percentage of total serum Ig	80	6	13	0–1	
Extravascular distribution	Tissue	Fluids	Secretions		Secretions
Inactivated by sulfhydryl reagents	–	++++	±		
Crosses placenta	Yes	No	No	No	No
Induces agglutination	+	++++	++		
Fixes complement	++ (classical)	+++ (classical)	+ (alternative)	–	–
Binding to Fcγ receptors	+++	–	+	–	+

* Valency of 10 is only observed with very small haptens.
Data from Roitt (2001).

Table 34–4 Some Known Properties of the Four Immunoglobulin G Subclasses

Subclasses of IgG	IgG1	IgG2	IgG3	IgG4
Heavy chain subclass	γ1	γ2	γ3	γ4
Allotypic markers	a, x, f, z	N	b0, b1, b3, g, s, t, etc.	4a, 4b (isoallotypes)
Half-life in vivo (days)	21	21	7	21
Relative serum concentration (%)	64–70	23–28	4–7	3–4
Placental transfer	++	±	++	++
Complement fixation	+++	++	++++	±
Macrophage binding	+++	+	+++	±
Binding to staph A protein	Yes	Yes	No	Yes
Antibodies showing subclass restriction	Anti-Rh	Anti-dextrans		Anti-AHF

Data from Roitt (2001).

Binding involves formation of multiple noncovalent bonds between the antigen and amino acids of the paratope. The attractive forces between antigen and antibody, which include electrostatic and van der Waal's forces, hydrogen bonds, and hydrophobic interactions, become significant when the distance between the interacting groups is small. As a result, the better the physical fit between epitope and paratope, the higher the overall binding energy and the greater the affinity of the resulting reaction between antibody and antigen (Roitt, 2001).

Blood Group Alloantibodies and Autoantibodies

The majority of clinically significant blood group antibodies fall into the IgG or IgM immunoglobulin classes with occasional IgA forms found among autoantibodies and against antigens in certain blood group systems. Blood group antibodies are usually classified as (1) alloantibody, which reacts with a foreign antigen not present on the patient's own erythrocytes, or as (2) autoantibody, which reacts with an antigen on the patient's own cells. RBC autoantibodies are discussed later in this chapter.

Some alloantibodies to erythrocyte antigens are called 'naturally occurring' – that is, the antigenic stimulus is unknown. Naturally occurring antibodies may appear regularly in the serum of persons who lack the corresponding antigen, such as in the ABO blood group system. Other naturally occurring antibodies are produced only in a small subset of individuals.

Most blood group alloantibodies are produced as the result of immunization to foreign erythrocyte antigens either by exposure through transfusion of blood components or through pregnancy, usually at the time of delivery. It is the presence of such alloantibodies to RBCs that necessitates the selection of specific antigen-negative components for transfusion. Identification of alloantibodies and selection of compatible blood components remains the most important function of a transfusion medicine service.

The Complement System and Blood Banking

Complement plays a key role in the pathophysiology of hemolysis because of its involvement in the sensitization and destruction of either transfused RBCs by alloantibody or destruction of autologous RBCs by autoantibody. Complement is also important in immunohematologic testing.

Role of Complement in Erythrocyte Destruction

Antibody binding to RBC antigens is the most common reason for complement activation on the RBC membrane in vivo. Complement may also be activated on RBCs via a carrier/hapten antibody complex such as penicillin-coated RBCs and antipenicillin antibodies. Complement components may also be attached to the membrane via a nonspecific mechanism induced by certain drugs or when erythrocytes are 'innocent bystanders' in another immune reaction.

RBC–antibody complexes usually activate complement by the classical pathway. However, the mode of destruction and extent of RBC hemolysis depends primarily on the class of immunoglobulin involved and the activity of an individual's reticuloendothelial (RE) system.

Intravascular Hemolysis. Intravascular RBC hemolysis is usually caused by antibodies directed against the ABO antigens. Rarely, other IgM blood group antibodies, as well as some IgG antibodies that are potent activators of complement (e.g., antibodies of the Kidd blood group system), can induce intravascular hemolysis. Intravascular lysis occurs when large amounts of complement are rapidly activated resulting in complete activation of the complement cascade with assembly of the terminal membrane-attack complex (C5b6789). This complex polymerizes to form pores in the RBC membrane so that extracellular fluid enters the cell, causing it to swell and burst by osmotic lysis.

Extravascular Hemolysis. IgG antibodies cause the majority of extravascular hemolysis via the RE system, which removes complement-coated RBCs. When IgG antibodies bind RBCs and activate complement, complement regulatory proteins generally stop the activation process at the C3/C4 level. RBC-bound C3b is degraded to iC3b, which is enzymatically inactive, by factor I and factor H. iC3b is further degraded to C3c and C3dg by factor I and CR1, a cofactor and C3b/C4b receptor (Freedman, 1994) (Fig. 34–1). Decay accelerating factor (DAF) also participates by inhibiting C3 convertase (C4b2b) formation, as well as promoting C3 convertase degradation. On RBCs, CR1 and DAF carry the Knops and Cromer blood group antigens, respectively.

Initially, C3b/iC3b-coated RBCs are rapidly sequestered in the liver by monocytes and macrophages, which have receptors for C3b (Table 34–5). Although phagocytic cells also have receptors for C4b, the role, if any, of C4b in immune hemolysis of erythrocytes is not defined (Freedman, 1994). A portion of the RBCs sequestered in the liver are immobilized and destroyed by phagocytosis with a half-life of about 2 minutes (Mollison, 1993). Within 15–20 minutes, however, destruction slows and many of the cells escape extravascular destruction through the action of the complement regulatory protein, factor I, as previously described. C3dg, the iC3b fragment produced by factor I cleavage, remains attached to RBCs, but has no enzymatic or opsonic properties. As a result, sequestered C3dg-coated RBCs are released back into the circulation and survive normally (Fig. 34–1). In the circulation, C3dg is cleaved, leaving C3d attached to the RBC membrane.

In the absence of complement activation, IgG-coated RBCs are removed by phagocytic cells via Fcγ receptors. Although phagocytosis is not complement dependent, Mollison (1989) demonstrated that RBCs coated with both IgG and complement tend to show accelerated removal by the liver, whereas RBCs coated only with IgG tend to be destroyed more slowly in the spleen, displaying a linear pattern of removal with a minimum half-life of 20 minutes. Theoretically, RBCs coated only with IgG antibody could also be the targets of antibody-dependent cellular cytotoxicity mechanisms (Mollison, 1993), because natural killer cells possess Fcγ receptors.

IV

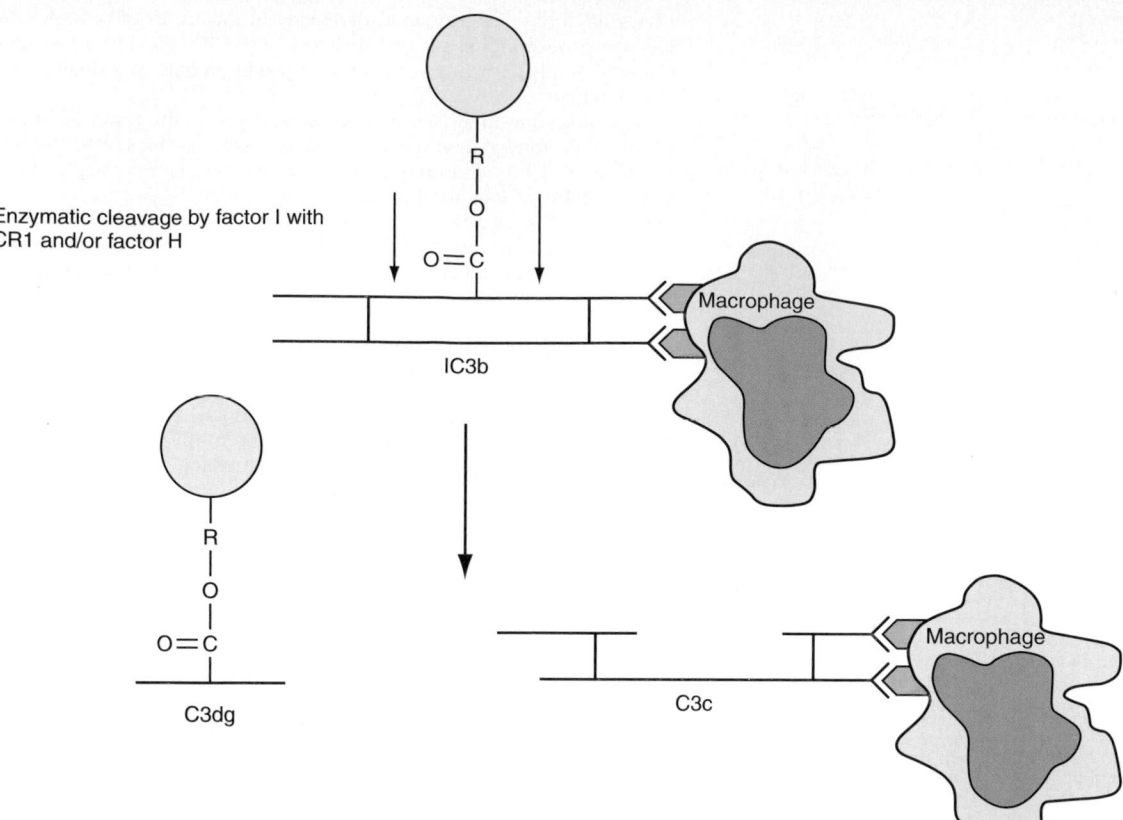

Enzymatic cleavage by factor I with CR1 and/or factor H

Macrophage

IC3b

C3dg

C3c

Macrophage

Table 34–5 Complement Receptors on Human Cells

Receptor	Ligand	Distribution
CR1 (CD35)	C3b, C4b	Erythrocytes, neutrophils, monocytes, macrophages, B lymphocytes, follicular dendritic cells
CR2 (CD21)	C3d, C3dg, iC3b	B cells
CR3 (CD11b/CD18)*	iC3b	Monocytes, macrophages, neutrophils, natural killer cells
CR4 (CD11c/CD18)*	iC3b	

* Members of the integrin receptor family.

Erythrocyte Antigens and Antibodies

Over 700 erythrocyte antigens have been reported in the literature and have been organized into 29 blood group systems by the International Society of Blood Transfusion (ISBT) (Table 34–6). Many described erythrocyte antigens are high-frequency or public antigens expressed by most donors (> 90–99%), whereas others are extremely rare (private antigens). In the following section, we review the more common RBC antigens and antibodies encountered on the transfusion service. Table 34–7 summarizes several commonly encountered RBC alloantibodies according to their immunoglobulin class, serologic phase of detection, clinical significance, and statistics on finding compatible blood.

ABO Blood Group System (ISBT No. 001 and 018)

Originally discovered in 1900, the ABO blood group system is the single most important blood group for the selection and transfusion of blood. Histo-blood group antigens, ABO epitopes are found on many tissues and body fluids including RBCs, platelets, and endothelial cells (Issitt, 1998). Because ABO antigens are so widely expressed, ABO antigens are also a major consideration in solid organ and bone marrow transplantation.

The ABO blood group system consists of three antigens, A, B and H, and four phenotypes: group A, B, AB, and O. A and B are autosomal codominant antigens (ISTB No. 001) and are expressed on group A, B, and

AB red cells, respectively. In contrast, the group O phenotype is an autosomal recessive phenotype, reflecting the absence of a functional *ABO* gene. Group O individuals express the H antigen (ISBT No. 018), the biosynthetic precursor of both A and B antigens (Fig. 34–2). Group O is the most frequent ABO phenotype in most populations tested, particularly among Native Americans. Expression of ABO antigens on RBCs is usually accompanied by the presence of naturally occurring antibodies against the missing antithetical antigen(s). Table 34–8 shows the serologic reactions and frequencies of the four major ABO phenotypes.

Null and weak phenotypes

The ABO system also contains several phenotypes associated with weakened, anomalous, or a complete absence of ABO antigen expression. The most common ABO subtypes encountered in the blood bank are A_1 and A_2 (Table 34–9). A_1 donors are distinguished from A_2 donors by the agglutination of A_1 RBCs by *Dolichos biflorus*. A comparison of A_1 and A_2 red cells indicates both quantitative and qualitative differences in A antigen expression between the two. The ABO system contains additional weak A and weak B phenotypes. The serologic characteristics of some weak group A, B, and O subtypes are shown in Table 34–10.

Anomalous ABO expression can be either inherited (cis-AB, B[A]) or acquired (acquired B). In the cis-AB phenotype, A and B antigens are synthesized by the same enzyme and are inherited as a single, autosomal dominant allele. Likewise, the B(A) phenotype, an autosomal dominant phenotype characterized by trace A antigen expression on group B RBCs, is due to synthesis of A antigen by the B-gene enzyme. The acquired B phenotype, on the other hand, is an acquired enzymatic modification of group A_1 red cells in vivo. The acquired B phenotype usually occurs in the setting of bacterial infection or cancer and reflects enzymatic deacetylation of group A antigen to form a B-like antigen on RBCs. The *cis*-AB, B(A), and acquired B phenotypes are usually detected because of discrepancies in ABO typing (Issitt, 1998).

Bombay and *para*-Bombay are two rare null phenotypes characterized by an absence of all ABH antigens on RBCs. In the classic Bombay phenotype (Oh), neither AB nor H antigens are present on RBCs or in secretions. *Para*-Bombay also shows little or no ABH antigens on RBCs, sometimes accompanied by normal expression of ABH antigens in secretions and body fluids.

Biochemistry

The ABO antigens are carbohydrate antigens and, therefore, represent a post-translation modification of glycoproteins and glycolipids. On RBC

Table 34–6 Terminology for Blood Group System Genes and Gene Products

Traditional nomenclature		ISBT nomenclature		ISGN nomenclature		Gene product name
Name	Symbol	Symbol	Number	Gene	Chromosome	
ABO	ABO	ABO	001	*ABO*	9q34.1	α1,3-*N*-acetylgalactosaminyltransferase (A antigen)
						α1,3-galactosyltransferase (B antigen)
MNS	MNSs	MNS	002	*GYPA*	4q28.2	Glycophorin A
				GYPB		Glycophorin B
				GYPE		Glycophorin E
P	P_1	P_1	003	*α4GalT1*	22q13	α1,4-galactosyltransferase (P^k, P_1 antigens)
Rh	Rh	RHD	004	*RHD*	1p36.1	RhD protein
		RHCE		*RHCE*		RhCE protein
Lutheran	Lu	LU	005	*LU*	19q13.2	Lutheran glycoprotein, B-CAM
Kell	K	KEL	006	*KEL*	7q33	Kell glycoprotein
Lewis	Le	LE	007	*FUT3*	19p13.3	α-3/4-fucosyltransferase
Duffy	Fy	FY	008	*DARC*	1q22	Duffy associated receptor cytokine glycoprotein
Kidd	Jk	JK	009	*SLC14A1*	18q11	Urea transporter (HUT11)
Diego	Di	DI	010	*SLC4A1*	17q12	Anion exchanger 1 (AE1, Band 3)
Yt	Yt	YT	011	*ACHE*	7q22	Acetylcholinesterase
Xg	Xg	XG	012	*XG*	Xp22.3	Xg glycoprotein
Scianna	Sc	SC	013	*HERMAP*	1p34	Human erythroid membrane associated protein
Dombrock	Do	DO	014	*ART4*	12p13.2	ADP-ribosyltransferase
Colton	Co	CO	015	*AQP1*	7p14	Aquaporin 1 (CHIP)
Landsteiner–Wiener	LW	LW	016	*LW*	19p13.3	LW glycoprotein
Chido/Rodgers	Ch/Rg	CH/RG	017	*C4A, C4B*	6p21.3	C4A, C4B complement glycoproteins
Hh	Hh	H	018	*FUT1*	19q13.3	α1,2-fucosyltransferase
Kx	Kx	XK	019	*XK*	Xp21.1	Kx glycoprotein
Gerbich	Ge	GE	020	*GYPC*	2q14	Glycophorin C and glycophorin D
Cromer	Cromer	CROM	021	*DAF*	1q32	CD55 (decay-accelerating factor)
Knops	Kn	KN	022	*CR1*	1q32	CD35 (complement receptor 1)
Indian	In	IN	023	*CD44*	11p13	CD44
Ok	Ok	OK	024	*CD147*	19p13.3	CD147, extracellular matrix metalloproteinase inducer
Raph	Raph	MER2	025	*MER2*	11p15.5	Not defined
John Milton Hagen	JMH	*JMH*	026	*SEMA-L*	15q22.3	Semaphorin CD108
I	I	I	027	*IGnT*	6p24	β1,6-*N*-acetylglucosaminyltransferase
Globoside	Gb4	GLOB	028	*β3GalT3*	3q25	β1,3-*N*-acetylgalactosaminyltransferase
GIL	GIL	GIL	029	*AQP3*	9p13	Aquaglyceroporin

After Garratty (2000); Daniels (2002); and Reid (2004a).

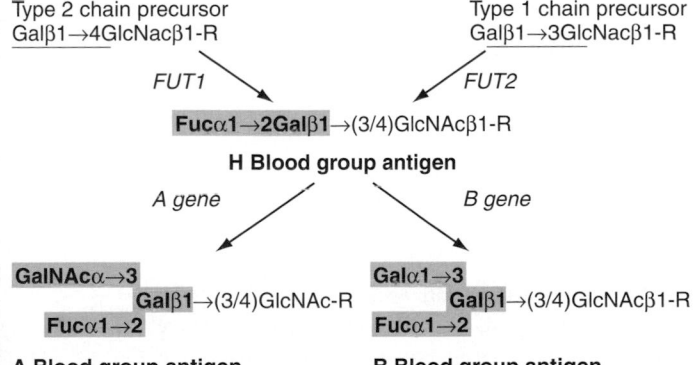

Figure 34–2 Synthesis of type 1 and type 2 chain H and AB antigens. Type 1 chain and type 2 chain precursors (underlined) are fucosylated by *FUT1* and *FUT2* fucosyltransferases to form H antigen. H antigen then serves as a substrate for *A* and *B* glycosyltransferases. The terminal carbohydrate epitopes denoting blood group H, A, and B antigens are highlighted in amber. Fuc = fucose; Gal = galactose; GalNAc = *N*-acetylgalactosamine; R = other oligosaccharide.

glycoproteins and polylactosaminylceramides, ABO antigens are usually expressed on type 2 chain oligosaccharides, characterized by repeating lactosaminyl (Galβ 1-4GlcNAcβ 1-3)$_n$ motifs (Fig. 34–2). On glycosphingolipids, ABO antigens can be expressed on multiple (type 1, 2, 3, and 4 chain) oligosaccharide precursors. ABH antigens expressed on RBC

glycoproteins and most glycosphingolipids (type 2, 3, and 4 chain) are of RBC origin. In contrast, type 1 chain ABO antigens are synthesized by gastrointestinal mucosa, secreted into plasma, and passively adsorbed onto red cell membranes. Synthesis of type 1 chain ABO antigens is linked to the Lewis blood group system.

The first step in the synthesis of ABH antigens is the synthesis of the H or group O antigen, the immediate biosynthetic precursor of both A and B antigens. The H antigen is formed by the addition of fucose (Fuc), in an α 1-2 linkage, to a terminal galactose. This reaction is catalyzed by two different enzymes, depending on whether the fucose is being added to a type 1 or type 2 chain oligosaccharide acceptor. Fucosyltransferase type 1 (*FUT1*), the product of the H or *FUT1* gene, catalyzes the formation of type 2 chain H antigen. In contrast, fucosyltransferase type 2 (*FUT2*), the product of the *Secretor* gene, catalyzes the transfer of fucose to type 1 chain precursors to form type 1 chain H or Le^d antigen (Lowe, 1994). Inactivating mutations in *FUT1* are responsible for the Bombay and *para*-Bombay phenotype (Kelly, 1994). Bombay and *para*-Bombay nonsecretors also have inactivating mutations in *FUT2* (Lowe, 1994; Daniels, 2002).

Once H antigen is formed, it can serve as a substrate for *A* gene and *B* gene glycosyltransferases. The A antigen is formed by *A*-gene glycosyltransferase, which adds an *N*-acetylgalactosamine (GalNAc), in an α 1-3 linkage, to the subterminal galactose of H antigen. Likewise, the B antigen is formed by the addition of an α 1-3 galactose (Gal) to the same galactose by the *B*-gene glycosyltransferase. Biochemically, the A and B antigen are very similar, only differing by the presence of an *N*-acetyl group. It is fascinating that such a minor chemical modification should have such profound immunologic consequences. The removal of the *N*-acetyl group on A antigen by

CHAPTER: 34 Immunohematology

Table 34–7 Serologic Characteristics and Clinical Significance of Red Cell Alloantibodies

Antibody	Usual Ig class	Most common phase of reactivity			Clinical significance		Approximate % of compatible donors	
		Sal	Alb	AGT	HTR	HDN	White	Black
D	IgG	Few	X	X	Yes	Yes	15	8
C	IgG		X	X	Yes	Yes	30	68
E	IgG	Few	X	X	Yes	Yes	70	98
c	IgG		X	X	Yes	Yes	20	1
e	IgG		X	X	Yes	Yes	2	2
C^w	IgG/IgM	Some	X	X	Yes	Yes	98	100
K	IgG	Rare		X	Yes	Yes	91	97
k	IgG		X		Yes	Yes	0.2	0.1
Kp^a	IgG	Rare		X	Yes	Yes	98	99.9
Kp^b	IgG		X		Yes	Yes	< 0.1	0.1
Js^a	IgG		X		Yes	Yes	> 99.9	81
Js^b	IgG		X		Yes	Yes	< 0.1	1
Fy^a	IgG		X		Yes	Yes	34	90
Fy^b	IgG		X		Yes	Yes	17	77
Jk^a	IgG		X		Yes	Yes	23	9
Jk^b	IgG		X		Yes	Yes	28	5
M*	IgM	X			Few	Yes	22	30
N	IgM	X			Rare	Rare	28	26
S	IgG/IgM		Some	X	Yes	Yes	45	69
s	IgG			X	Yes	Yes	11	3
U	IgG			X	Yes	Yes	0	1
Lu^{a†}	IgM	X			?	Yes	92	96
Lu^{b†}	IgG			X	Yes	Mild	< 0.1	< 0.1
P$_1$‡	IgM	X	Some		Rare	No	21	6
P	IgM	X	Some	Some	Probable	Yes	< 0.1	0.1
PP$_1$P^{k†}	IgG/IgM	X	Some	Some	Probable	Yes	< 0.1	0.1
Le^{a‡}	IgM	X	Some		Yes	No	78	77
Le^{b‡}	IgM	X			Yes	No	28	45
I	IgM	X	Few		Rare	No	< 0.1	< 0.1
i	IgM	X	Few		?	No	< 0.1	< 0.1

* Most examples of anti-M also have a small but significant IgG component

† Exhibits characteristic mixed field agglutination pattern.

‡ May occasionally show in vitro hemolysis.

Table 34–8 Routine ABO Grouping Results and Phenotype Frequencies

Cells against known antisera		Serum against red cells of known phenotype		Interpretation	Frequencies (%) in US population			
Anti-A	Anti-B	A	B		White	Black	Native American	Asian
−	−	+	+	O	45	49	79	40
+	−	−	+	A	40	27	16	28
−	+	+	−	B	11	20	4	27
+	+	−	−	AB	4	4	< 1	5

Composite figures calculated from Mourant (1976).

circulating deacetylase enzymes is responsible for the acquired B phenotype (Issitt, 1998)

Molecular Biology

The genes for the synthesis of AB and H antigens have been cloned. Both *FUT1* (*H* gene) and *FUT2* (*Se* gene) are located together on chromosome 19q13.3 and reflect a gene duplication (Lowe, 1994). FUT1 is a 365-amino-acid, type II transmembrane glycoprotein, composed of a large, 240-amino-acid, carboxy-terminal catalytic domain, which is anchored within the Golgi lumen by a short transmembrane and cytosolic domain.

Table 34–9 Differentiating Characteristics of the A$_1$ and A$_2$ Subgroups

Group	A$_1$	A$_2$
Quantitative differences		
Reaction with diluted anti-A	++++	++
No. of antigen sites: Adult	1 000 000	250 000
Newborn	310 000	140 000
Quantitative differences		
Reaction with *Dolichos biflorus* (anti-A$_1$) lectin	++++	0
Anti-A$_1$ in serum	No	1–8%
Biochemistry/molecular differences		
Glycolipid erythrocyte variants containing antigens	A^a, A^b, A^c, A^d (linear and complex branched chains)	A^a, A^b (linear chains only)
N-acetyl-galactosaminyltransferase activity	Normal activity Optimal at pH 6	Decreased activity Optimal at pH 7
Gene	Consensus A101 allele	Pro156>Leu, 1059-101delC Frameshift + 21 extra amino acids

Table 34–10 Serologic Differentiation of the ABO Groups

Phenotype	Red cells with anti-					Serum with red cells			Substances in saliva of secretors	Level of transferase in serum	Antigen sites per RBC × 10³
	A	A₁	B	A, B	H	A₁	B	O			
A¹	++++	++++	0	++++	0/+	0	++++	0	A, H	Normal (optimal activity at pH 6.0)	810–1170
A_int	++++	++	0	++++	++	0	++++	0	A, H		
A₂	++++	0	0	++++	+++	*	++++	0	A, H	Decreased (optimal activity at pH 7.0)	240–1290
A₃	++^mf	0	0	++^mf	+++	*	++++	0	A, H	Low	30
A_x	0/±	0	0	++	++++	+†	++++	0	H	Very low	4
A_m	0‡	0	0	0	++++	0	++++	0	A, H	Low (A₁ or A₂ enzyme may be present)	0.2–1.9
B	0	0	++++	++++	++	++++	0	0	B, H	Normal	750
B₃	0	0	++^mf	++^mf	+++	++++	0	0	B, H	Low	
O	0	0	0	0	++++	++++	++++	0	H	Normal	1700
O_h	0	0	0	0	0	++++	++++	++++	None§ (classic Bombay)	Normal	

* May have anti-A₁ in serum.

† A_x subgroups usually have anti-A₁ but not always.

‡ A antigen specificity demonstrated only after adsorption–elution procedures.

§ Bombay secretors (para-Bombay) have been reported.

mf = mixed field (minor population of agglutinates).

Table 34–11 Key Amino Acids in Distinguishing A, B and Hybrid Glycosyltransferases*

RBC phenotype	Amino acid number of A/B glycosyltransferase					Gene type†
	176	234	235	266	268	
A	Arg	Pro	Gly	Leu	Gly	AAAA
B	Gly	Pro	**Ser**	**Met**	**Ala**	BBBB
Cis-AB	Arg	Pro	Gly	Leu	**Ala**	AAAB
Cis-AB^Taipei	Arg	Pro	Gly	**Met**	Gly	AABA
Cis-AB	**Gly**	Pro	**Ser**	Leu	**Ala**	BBAB
B(A)	**Gly**	Pro	Gly	**Met**	**Ala**	BABB
B(A)	**Gly**	**Ala**	**Ser**	**Met**	**Ala**	BBBB
O03	Arg	Pro	Gly	Leu	**Arg‡**	AAAX

* Modified from Reid (2004b); Daniels (2002). Amino acids that differ from the A101 (A₁ type) consensus allele are highlighted in bold.

† Gene type refers to amino acid positions 176, 235, 266, and 268. These four positions differ between A (AAAA) and B alleles. Amino acids at 235, 266 and 268 strongly influence substrate specificity. Hybrid glycosyltransferases have amino acids matching both A and B consensus alleles at these positions.

‡ O03 allele (historically O²), associated with a group O phenotype, possesses an inactivating missense mutation at amino acid 268.

More then 20 mutant *FUT1* alleles have been described (Issitt, 1998; Fernandez-Mateos, 1998).

The *ABO* gene locus is located on chromosome 9q34 and encodes the A and B glycosyltransferases (Yamamoto, 1995). The gene is large, spanning 18 kb, and contains seven exons. The product of the *ABO* gene is a 41-kDa, 353-amino-acid type II transmembrane glycoprotein. A comparison of A and B enzymes shows nearly 98% identity, differing by four key amino acids at residues 176, 235, 266, and 268 (Table 34–11). Amino acid 268 is absolutely critical in determining the activity and substrate specificity (UDP-GalNAc vs. UDP-Gal) of the enzyme. Substrate specificity is also influenced by amino acid residues 235 and 266. The polymorphism at residue 176 is not biologically significant (Yamamoto, 1990).

The cloning and sequencing of the *ABO* gene locus has also uncovered the molecular basis of group O and ABO subtypes. Over 20 group O alleles are known, although two deletion mutants (O¹, O^1var) are the most common and the ancestral genes for most group O alleles (Roubinet, 2004). Interestingly, the O² allele (O03) found in many Europeans, contains a single missense mutation at amino acid residue 268 (Table 34–11) (Yamamoto, 1995).

Several ABO subtypes are also the result of mutations at the *ABO* gene locus. Two mutations are associated with the A² allele: A Pro156>Leu substitution and a single nucleotide deletion (nucleotide 1060). The latter results in the translation of an additional 21 amino acids at the carboxy-terminus of the enzyme and is responsible for the decreased enzyme activity, altered isoelectric point, and restricted substrate specificity of the A₂ glycosyltransferase (Yamamoto, 1995). Similarly, the A^el allele is characterized by a nucleotide insertion, leading to a frameshift mutation (amino acid 269) and translation of 37 additional amino acids (Olsson, 1995). The frameshift mutation in the A^el allele may be particularly deleterious because of its immediate proximity to amino acid residue 268. Single point mutations appear to be responsible for the decreased enzyme activity of A³, A^x, A^finn, A^end, B³, B^x, and B^v alleles (Yamamoto, 1995; Olsson, 2001). In contrast, the *cis*-AB and B(A) alleles, which can synthesize both A and B antigens, are molecular chimeras with characteristics of both the A¹ and B gene consensus alleles (Table 34–11) (Yamamoto, 1995).

ABO Antibodies

Antibodies against ABO antigens are the most important antibodies in transfusion medicine. In general, ABO antibodies are naturally occurring. It is believed the immune stimulus for the formation of ABO antibodies may be exposure to ABH-like substances found in nature (e.g., bacterial polysaccharides). ABO antibodies are weak or absent in the sera of newborns until 3–6 months of age. Adult levels of ABO antibodies are reached by 5–10 years of age and decrease only slightly with advancing age (Auf der Maur, 1993). Anti-A,B is found exclusively in group O individuals and appears to recognize an epitope common to both A and B antigens. Prior to the development of anti-A and anti-B monoclonal antibody typing reagents, anti-A,B was useful in identifying A_x and weak B subgroups.

In general, ABO antibodies are detected as room temperature, saline agglutinins with optimal reactivity at 4°C (Table 34–7). Most naturally occurring ABO antibodies are of IgM isotype, although IgA and IgG antibodies with ABO specificity are also present (Rieben, 1991). ABO IgG antibodies, reactive at 37°C, can also occur following immune stimulation by transfusion or pregnancy. These antibodies are generally of higher titer and less readily neutralized by soluble blood group substances. ABO antibodies can fix complement and can cause hemolysis in vivo and in vitro.

Clinically, ABO antibodies are a cause of hemolytic transfusion reactions and hemolytic disease of the newborn (HDN). ABO antibodies are also a cause of acute rejection in solid organ transplantation. As a result, solid organ transplants should be ABO compatible with the recipient's sera. In ABO-incompatible bone marrow transplantation, ABO antibodies can result in hemolysis and a delay in erythroid and megakaryocyte engraftment (Worel, 2003).

IV

Anti-A₁. Anti-A₁ is a naturally occurring antibody found in the sera of some A₂, A₂B, Aₓ, and A₃ individuals. Anti-A₁ hemagglutinates A₁ RBCs, but not A₂ and other weak RBC phenotypes. Although uncommon, anti-A₁ has been implicated in transfusion reactions and solid organ rejection.

Anti-H. Anti-H is usually a benign, naturally occurring antibody in the sera of A₁ and A₁B nonsecretors. Anti-H reacts most strongly with group O erythrocytes, followed by A₂, A₂B, B, A₁ and A₁B (refer to Table 34–48 below). Because H antigen is present to some degree on all RBCs, anti-H is an autoantibody in most individuals. In contrast, alloanti-H is a clinically significant alloantibody in Bombay (O$_h$) and para-Bombay individuals. Because all RBCs express some H antigen, finding compatible RBCs can be extremely difficult in these patients.

Biological Role

The biological role of ABH antigens is still not known. Depression of A and B antigen expression can occur in malignancy and is often associated with increased metastatic potential. Furthermore, multiple studies have linked specific ABO types with a higher incidence of many diseases, including autoimmune, neoplastic, and infectious disorders. For a complete review of ABH and human disease, the reader is referred to Issitt (1998) and Garratty (1994a).

MNSs Blood Group System (ISBT No. 002)

Discovered in 1927, the MNSs blood group was the second blood group system identified after ABO. Today, the MNSs blood group system consists of over 43 antigens of which only four (M/N and S/s) are commonly encountered in the clinical setting. As shown in Table 34–12, the M and N antigens are fairly evenly distributed in both black people and white people, with approximately 25% of donors homozygous for either M or N antigen. In contrast, the S antigen is nearly twice as frequent in white people (57%) than in black people (30%). In a minority (< 1%) of black people, an S–s– or null phenotype can be observed. Like Rh antigens, the MNSs blood group antigens are expressed only on RBCs. There are approximately one million M/N and 170–250 thousand S/s epitopes per RBC.

Null Phenotypes

There are three major null phenotypes in the MNSs system, U–, Mᵏ and En (a–). The U– phenotype is the most common and is observed exclusively in black people. In S–s–U– individuals, there is a loss or recombination of glycophorin B which carries the S/s and U antigens. Recombinant glycophorin B, such as the Henshaw phenotype, can react weakly with some examples of human anti-U and are known as U variants (S–s–Uᵛᵃʳ). The En (a–) phenotype is an M–N– phenotype due to loss of glycophorin A, which carries M, N and En (a) antigens. The MᵏMᵏ phenotype lacks all MNSs antigens due to deletion of both glycophorins A and B.

Table 34–12 Phenotypes of the MNSs System

Glycophorin A antigens			Glycophorin B antigens				Phenotype	Phenotype frequencies (%)	
M	N	En (a)	'N'	S	s	U		White	Black
+	0	+					M+N−	28	26
+	+	+					M+N+	50	44
0	+	+					M−N+	22	30
			+	+	0	+	S+s−U+	11	3
			+	+	+	+	S+s+U+	44	28
			+	0	+	+	S−s+U+	45	69
Null phenotypes									
0	0	0	+	+/0	+/0	+	En (a–)	Rare	Rare
0	0	0	0	0	0	0	MᵏMᵏ	Rare	Rare
			0	0	0	0	S−s−U−	Rare	< 1
			0	0	0	wk+	S−s−Uᵛᵃʳ (23% Henshaw+)	Rare	< 1

Biochemistry

The M/N antigens reside on glycophorin A, a major RBC membrane glycoprotein. In the membrane, glycophorin A is present as a dimer, usually in association with band 3, the erythrocyte anion exchanger (AE1). Structurally, glycophorin A is a 31-kDa, 131-amino-acid, type 1 glycoprotein composed of a large, 72-amino-acid extracellular domain, a transmembrane domain, and a short cytoplasmic tail (Fig. 34–3). The molecule is heavily glycosylated, possessing 15 O-linked and one N-linked carbohydrate side chains. The O-linked glycans consist of mono- (17%), di- (78%), and trisialo-oligosaccharides (5%), linked to either a serine or threonine residue. Because of the large number of sialylated O-linked glycans on glycophorin A, nearly 60% and 50% of the total molecular weight is carbohydrate and sialic acid, respectively. Not surprisingly, glycophorin A is the major sialomucin on RBCs and contributes significantly to the overall negative charge or zeta potential. The M and N antigens reside on the extreme amino-terminus of glycophorin A (Huang, 1995).

The S/s and U antigens reside on glycophorin B, a related RBC glycoprotein (Fig. 34–3). Glycophorin B is a 20-kDa, 72-amino-acid glycoprotein composed of a large, extracellular N-terminal domain containing 11 O-linked glycans. Although glycophorin B shares considerable homology with glycophorin A at the amino-terminus, glycophorin B is smaller, lacking

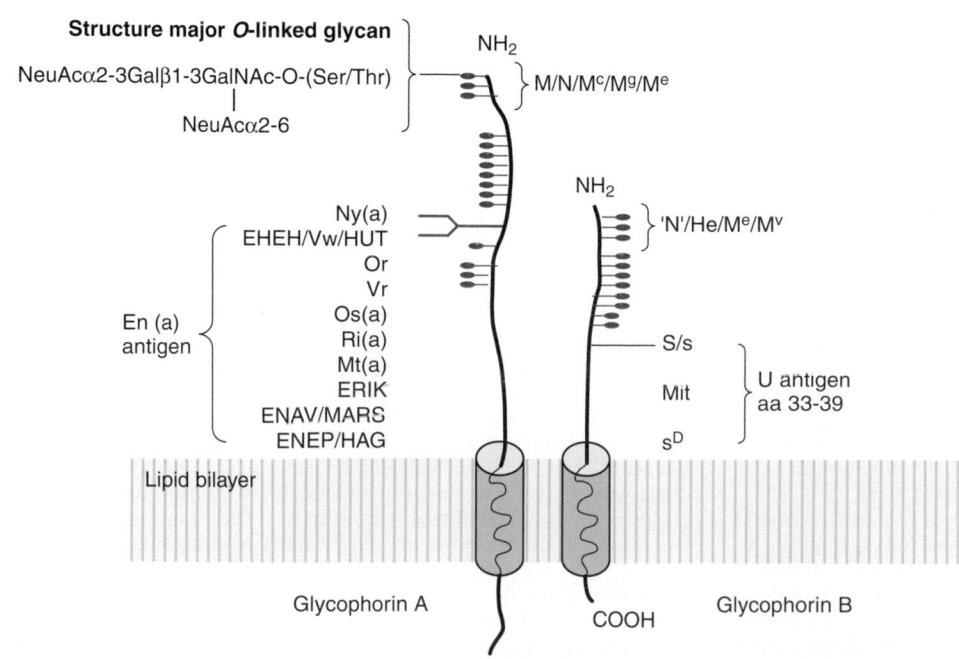

Structure major *O*-linked glycan

NeuAcα2-3Galβ1-3GalNAc-O-(Ser/Thr)
  |
  NeuAcα2-6

M/N/Mᶜ/Mᵍ/Mᵉ

'N'/He/Mᵉ/Mᵛ

En (a) antigen:
Ny(a)
EHEH/Vw/HUT
Or
Vr
Os(a)
Ri(a)
Mt(a)
ERIK
ENAV/MARS
ENEP/HAG

S/s
Mit
sᴰ
U antigen aa 33–39

Lipid bilayer

Glycophorin A
Glycophorin B
COOH
COOH

Figure 34–3 Glycophorin A and B. Glycophorin A and glycophorin B possess 11–15 O-linked glycans (—•), consisting predominantly of a disialotetrasaccharide (78%), along the amino-terminal half of the extracellular domain. Glycophorin A also possesses a single, biattenary N-glycan, indicated by a branched structure. The single transmembrane domain for both molecules is indicated by a solid amber cylinder. The allelic antigens, M and N, reside at the extreme amino-terminus of glycophorin A and differ by only two amino acids at residues 1 and 5. The N antigen is also present at the amino-terminus of glycophorin B and is designated 'N' antigen. The S/s antigens are located at amino acid 29 of glycophorin B. The locations of high- and low-incidence antigens are shown. The En (a) and U antigens involve large stretches of protein near the lipid bilayer and are missing in deletion and recombinant glycophorins.

both an *N*-glycan and a cytoplasmic tail. In the membrane, glycophorin B appears to be closely associated with the Rh immune complex. The S/s epitope is located at amino acid 29 (Issitt, 1998).

Molecular Biology

The genes for glycophorin A (*GYPA*) and B (*GYPB*) reside on chromosome 4q28-q31 as part of a 330-kb gene cluster encoding glycophorins A, B, and E (5′-A-B-E-3′). Studies indicate that glycophorin B and E arose from glycophorin A by gene duplication and nonhomologous recombination. Like many erythroid-specific genes, the promoter region contains consensus sequences for Sp1 and GATA-1 (Rahuel, 1994). The greater stability of glycophorin A mRNA (> 24 hours) over glycophorin B mRNA (< 17 hours) may explain the greater numbers of glycophorin A on RBCs (Rahuel, 1994).

The biochemical nature of the MNSs antigens has long been known. The M and N antigens lie at the extreme amino-terminus of glycophorin A (amino acids 1 through 5) and include both protein and carbohydrate as part of the immune epitope. It is amino acid differences at positions 1 and 5, however, that define the M/N antigens (Table 34–13). Not surprisingly, several low-incidence M and N antigen variants are the result of different amino acid substitutions (M^g, M^c) and/or altered expression of *O*-linked glycans (M_1, Tm, Can). In addition to glycophorin A, the N antigen is also expressed on the extreme amino-terminus of glycophorin B. The latter is referred to as the 'N' antigen to distinguish it from N antigen on glycophorin A (Issitt, 1998).

Glycophorin A also possesses several high-incidence antigens, including En(a) and ENEP. The En (a–) phenotype is the result of recombination between *GYPA* and *GYPB* genes to form a Lepore-type A-B hybrid (exons A1-B2-B5) lacking most of *GYPA*. The M^k allele, which is also M–N– En (a–), is characterized by a large deletion of *GYPA* and *GYPB* resulting in a nonfunctional *GYPA-E* hybrid. Loss of glycophorin A can coincide with loss of Wr^b expression, an antigen on band 3. It is believed that Wr^b requires an electrostatic interaction between a glutamic acid (Glu658) on band 3 and the ENEP antigen on glycophorin A (Poole, 1999).

Unlike the complexity of the M/N antigens, the S/s antigen is a single amino acid polymorphism on glycophorin B (Met29 Thr). The U antigen is a high-incidence antigen involving amino acids 33–39 on glycophorin B. Loss of glycophorin S-s-U antigens can be observed with M^k and other recombinant GYPB alleles such as Henshaw. It is estimated that 90% Henshaw+ RBC are U– or U^{var} and account for 23% of all S–s–U– patients.

Recombination and gene conversion events are also responsible for several rare MNSs antigens in the Miltenberger system. The Hil, SAT, and Miltenberger class V and XI antigens are glycophorin A-B Lepore-type hybrids, whereas St^a and Dantu are glycophorin B-A or anti-Lepore hybrids. Like Henshaw+ phenotype, other Miltenberger antigens are the consequence of gene conversion where segments of one glycophorin are inserted into the other to form glycophorin B-A-B and A-B-A hybrids (Reid, 2004b).

MNSs Antibodies

Anti-M and -N

Antibodies against M and N antigens are naturally occurring antibodies of IgM isotype, usually detected as room-temperature saline agglutinins (Table 34–7). Anti-M and anti-N may show dosage, reacting more weakly with heterozygous (M/N) cells than with homozygous (M/M or N/N) cells. Because the M and N antigens reside on glycophorin A, the reactivity of anti-M and anti-N is destroyed by pretreatment of RBCs with proteolytic enzymes or neuraminidase. Some examples of anti-M and anti-N can be enhanced by acidification of serum to pH 6.5, use of an albumin diluent, or preincubation of RBCs in a glucose-containing solution.

Clinically, anti-M is a commonly encountered antibody in the blood bank. In contrast, anti-N is distinctly uncommon, despite the fact that 25% of patients are negative for N antigen (M homozygous). The rarity of anti-N is due to the presence of 'N' antigen on glycophorin B. When observed, anti-N is usually an autoantibody, reacting with both N and 'N' antigens. An autoanti-N (anti-N_f) is reported in hemodialysis patients. Formaldehyde used to sterilize dialysis equipment reportedly reacts with the terminal leucine on N and 'N' antigens, creating a neoantigen (Issitt, 1998). In general, anti-M and anti-N are clinically insignificant antibodies and only rarely cause hemolytic transfusion reactions or HDN. In contrast, potent hemolytic anti-N alloantibodies are observed in patients lacking glycophorin B (S–s–U–). In these patients, severe hemolytic transfusion reactions and HDN are known following exposure to N+ RBCs.

Anti-S, -s and -U

Unlike anti-M and anti-N, antibodies against S, s, and U antigens are always clinically significant (Table 34–7). All are antibodies of IgG isotype, reactive at 37°C, arising from immune stimulation. Some examples of anti-S and anti-s show dosage. Enzymatic modification of RBCs with proteases, but not neuraminidase, can decrease the reactivity of some anti-S and anti-s. The reactivity of anti-U is resistant to proteolytic digestion. Anti-S, -s and -U are a cause of hemolytic transfusion reactions and HDN.

Biological Role

Despite the prevalence of glycophorin A and B on RBCs, their biological role is still unknown: Their absence is not associated with any known hematologic or pathologic sequelae. Glycophorin A and B may play a role in *Plasmodium falciparum* infections. *P. falciparum* can adhere to RBCs via sialic acid, which is highly expressed on glycophorins. Glycophorin-deficient phenotypes, such as En (a–), are relatively resistant to *P. falciparum* in vitro. Similar results can be obtained after neuraminidase treatment of RBCs (Garratty, 1994a).

P Blood Group System (ISBT No. 003 and 028)

The P blood group system consists of three major blood group antigens; P^k, P, and P_1. Like the Lewis system (see below), the P blood group antigens are glycosphingolipids, consisting of an antigenically active carbohydrate moiety covalently linked to a ceramide lipid tail. P^k and P antigens are high-frequency antigens on most donor RBCs (> 99.9%). RBCs are particularly rich in P antigen, which makes up nearly 6% of the total RBC lipid (van Deenen, 1974). P^k and P antigens are also expressed on nonerythroid cells including lymphocytes, platelets, plasma, kidney, lung, heart, endothelium, placenta, uroepithelium, fibroblasts, and synovium (Cooling, 1995, 1998; Spitalnik, 1995). In contrast, the P_1 antigen is uniquely expressed on RBCs (Cooling, 1998). Approximately 79% of white and 94% of black donors express P_1 on their RBCs (Table 34–14). P_1 expression is variable between individuals and can be lost with in vitro storage.

Null/Weak Phenotypes

Several P blood group phenotypes have been described (Table 34–14). The P_1 and P_2 phenotypes account for > 99% donors. Both possess P^k and P antigens and differ only in the expression of the P_1 antigen. Three, autosomal recessive null phenotypes have been identified, as well as weak variants (Issitt, 1998; Kundu 1978, 1980). The molecular basis for the null phenotypes has been elucidated (Hellberg, 2002; Steffensen, 2000). There is an association between the P^k variant and LKE-negative phenotype in some donors (Cooling, 2001, 2003a). Because they lack P antigen, p and P^k individuals are resistant to parvovirus B19 (Brown, 1994).

Biochemistry

The synthesis of the P^k, P, and P_1 antigens proceeds from the stepwise addition of sugars to lactosylceramide, a ceramide dihexose (CDH) (Fig. 34–4). The first step is the synthesis of the P^k antigen, the ultimate precursor of all globo-type glycosphingolipids. To make P^k antigen, Gb_3 synthase (α4GalT1) adds a galactose, in an α1-4 linkage, to CDH. The P^k antigen can then serve as a substrate for Gb_4 synthase (β3GalT3). In some cells, including RBCs, the P antigen is further elongated to form additional, globo-family antigens such as Luke (LKE), Forssman and type 4 chain ABH antigens (globo-ABH).

Unlike P^k and P antigens, the P_1 antigen is not a globo-glycosphingolipid but is a member of the neolacto-family (type 2 chain glycosphingolipids). In P_1 individuals, a terminal α1,4 galactose is added to paragloboside to form P_1. The P_1 antigen is not expressed on RBC glycoproteins despite the presence of multiple type 2 chain precursors (polylactosamine) on *N*-linked glycans (Yang, 1994).

Molecular Biology

The genes responsible for P^k, P_1 and P have been cloned. P^k and P_1 antigens are synthesized by α4GalT1, an α1,4 galactosyltransferase (Steffensen, 2000; Iwamura, 2003). The *α4GalT1* gene resides on chromosome 22q13 and is organized into two exons, of which only one (exon 2) encodes the enzyme. The α4GalT1 enzyme is a 353-amino-acid type II glycoprotein containing two *N*-glycosylation sites and five cysteine residues. Like many galactosyltransferases, it possesses a DXD motif or UDP-Gal binding site. Several missense and frameshift mutations (insertions and deletions) in the enzyme catalytic domain have been identified among p individuals (Steffensen, 2000; Koda, 2002). The absence of P_1 antigen in P_2 individuals may involve mutations in the α4GalT1 promoter. Studies of P_2 donors have shown homozygosity for an allele containing an insertion (-551C-500) and a single nucleotide substitution (T-160>C) in the 5′ upstream region (Iwamura, 2003). Although no significant differences in promoter activity could be demonstrated in reporter assays, it is

Table 34–13 MNSs Blood Group Antigens

High frequency		Frequency	Glycophorin*	Amino acid change (high→low)	Frequency	Low frequency	
ISBT	Name					Name	ISBT
MNS1	M	78%	GPA	**Ser**^{1}-Ser-Thr-Thr-**Gly**^{5}			
MNS2	N	72%	GPA	**Leu**^{1}-Ser-Thr-Thr-**Glu**^{5}			
MNS4	s	89–93%	GPB	Thr29>Met	31–55%	S	MNS3
MNS5	U	≥ 99%	GPB	Amino acids 33–39		He	MNS6
			B-A^M-B	**Trp**^{1}-Ser-Thr-Thr-**Gly**^{5}	3–7% black people		
			B-A-B/A-B-A	Mutant GYP: exons A2- Bψ^3	Rare	Mi^a	MNS7
			GPA	**Ser**^{1}-Ser-Thr-Thr-**Glu**^{5}	Rare	M^c	MNS8
MNS40	ENEH	100%	GPA	Thr28>Met	Rare	Vw	MNS9
			GPA	Thr28>Lys	Rare	HUT	MNS19
			B-A-B	Mutant GYPB: pseudoexon 3	6–9% Asian people	Mur	MNS10
			GPA	**Leu**^{1}-Ser-Thr-**Asn**^{4}-**Glu**^{5}	Rare	M^g	MNS11
			GPA	Ser47>Tyr	Rare	Vr	MNS12
MNS13	M^e	78%	GPA/GP:He	Gly^5 of GPA and Henshaw+			
			GPA	Thr58>Ile	1% Thai people	Mt^a	MNS14
			B-A	Mutant GYP: exons B2-A2/A4	2% Asian people	St^a	MNS15
			GPA	Glu55>Lys	Rare	Rl^a	MNS16
			Unknown	Unknown	Rare	Cl^a	MNS17
			GPA	Asp27>Glu	Rare	Ny^a	MNS18
			A-B/A-B-A	Mutant GYP: exons A3-B4	6% Chinese people	Hil	MNS20
			GPB	**Leu**^{1}-Ser-**Ser**-Thr-Glu^5	Rare	M^v	MNS21
			Unknown		Rare	Far	MNS22
			GPB	Pro39>Arg	Rare	s^D	MNS23
			GPB	Arg35>His	Rare	Mit	MNS24
			B^s-A	Mutant GYP: exons B4-A5	0.5% black people	Dantu	MNS25
			GPA	Arg49>Thr	0.7% Thai people	Hop	MNS26
MNS29	ENKT	100%	GPA	Arg49>Thr; Tyr52>Ser	Rare	Nob	MNS27
MNS28	En (a–)	100%	GPA	GPA molecule			
MNS30	'N'	> 99%	GYB	**Leu**^{1}-Ser-Thr-Thr-**Glu**^{5}			
			GPA	Arg31>Trp	Rare	Or	MNS31
			A-B-A	Mutant GYP: Asn45	0.4% Danish people	DANE	MNS32
			A-B^S	Mutant GYP: exons A3-B4, S+	Rare	TSEN	MNS33
			A-B/B-A-B	Mutant GYP: exons A3-B4	6% Chinese people	MINY	MNS34
			B-A-B/A-ψB-A	Mutant GP: anti-Mur+HUT	6% Chinese people	MUT	MNS35
			A-B	Mutant GYP: exons A4-B5	Rare	SAT	MNS36
			GPA	Gly59>Arg	Rare	ERIK	MNS37
			GPA	Pro54>Ser	Rare	Os^a	MNS38
MNS39	ENEP	100%	GPA	Ala65>Pro	Rare	HAG	MNS41
MNS42	ENAV	100%	GPA	Glu63>Lys	15% Native American people	MARS	MNS43

* Glycophorin A (GPA), glycophorin B (GPB) or hybrid, recombinant glycophorins containing elements of GPA and GPB. ψB refers to GPB pseudoexons.
After Daniels (2002) and Reid (2004).

Table 34–14 P Blood Group System

RBC phenotype	RBC antigens	Possible antibodies	Molecular basis		Frequencies (%)	
			α4GalT1	β3GalT3	White	Black
P_1	P^k, P, P_1	None	Normal	Normal	79	94
P_2	P^k, P	Anti-P_1	ins-551C, -160C*	Normal	21	6
Null phenotypes						
P_1^k	↑P^k, P_1	Anti-P	Normal	Null allele[+]	Rare	Rare
P_2^k	↑P^k	Anti-P, anti-P_1	ins-551C, -160C*	Null allele[+]	Rare	Rare
p	None	Anti-P^k, P, P_1 (Tja)	Null allele[‡]	Normal	Rare	Rare
Weak phenotypes						
Variant P^k	↑P^k, ↓P	Anti-P	Unknown	Unknown	Rare	Rare
Weak P	↓P^k, ↓P	None	Unknown	Unknown	Rare	Rare

* Homozygosity for an allele carrying an insertion (ins-551C-550) and a missense mutation (A-160>G) in the α4GalT1 promoter has been linked to a P_2 phenotype. The α4GalT1 opening reading frame encodes a functional enzyme (Iwamura, 2003; Steffensen, 2000).

[+] Multiple inactivating mutations have been identified in β3GalT3 open reading frame associated with the P^k phenotype (Hellberg, 2002).

[‡] Multiple inactivating mutations have been identified in α4GalT1 open reading frame associated with the p phenotype (Steffensen, 2000; Koda, 2002).

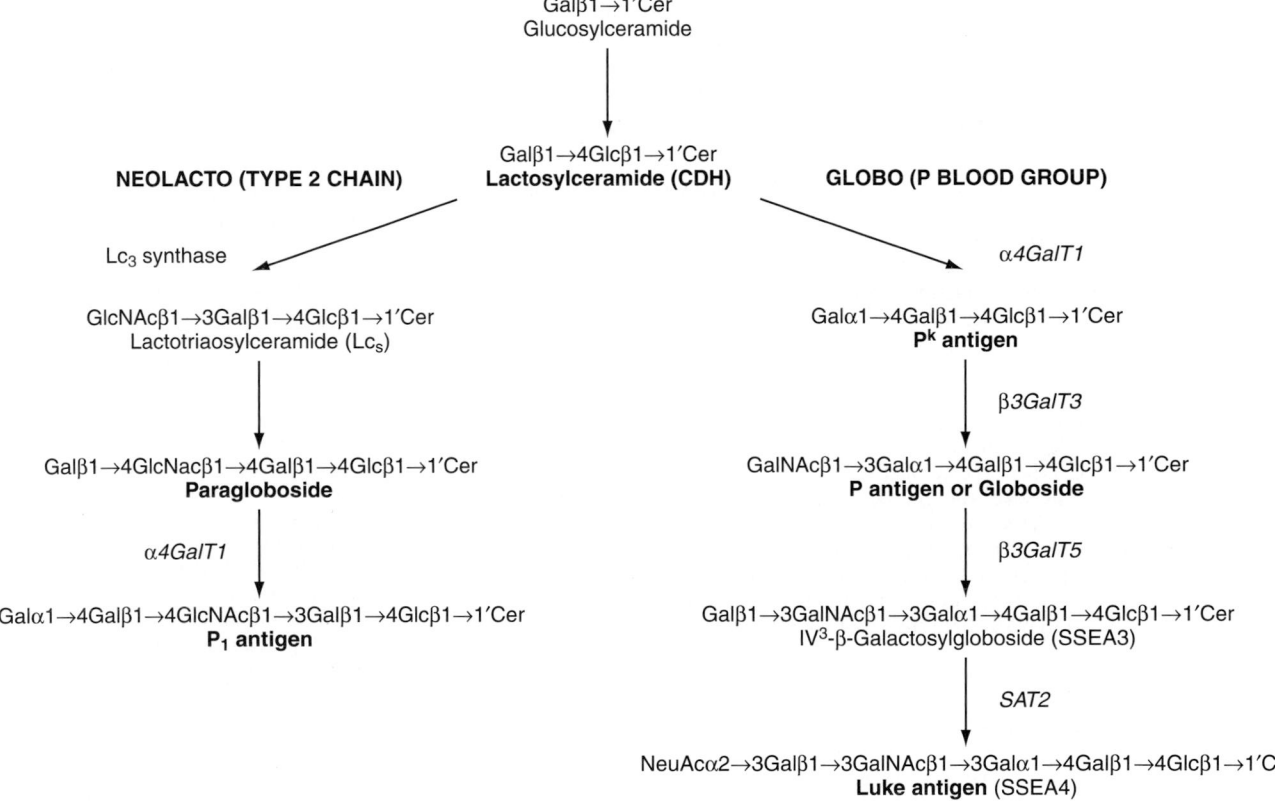

Figure 34–4 Synthesis of P blood group antigens. Cer = ceramide; Gal = galactose; GalNAc = N-acetylgalactosamine; Glc = glucose; GlcNAc = N-acetylglucosamine; SSEA = stage-specific embryonic antigen; NeuAc = acetylneuraminic acid.

hypothesized that decreased α4GalT1 transcription is the basis for the P_2 phenotype.

Globoside or P antigen, a β1,3 N-acetylgalactosaminyltransferase, is the product of β3GalT3 (Okajima, 2000). The gene resides on chromosome 3q25 and contains six exons although only exon 6 encodes the enzyme. A member of the β1,3 galactosyltransferase family, β3GalT3 possesses seven conserved domains common to most β1,3 galactosyltransferases as well as a DXD motif. Of four P^k individuals studied to date, two missense (Glu266>Ala, Gly271>Arg), nonsense (C102>Tstop), and frameshift (ins537A) mutations were identified (Hellberg, 2002). In mice, the absence of β3GalT3 is lethal (Vollrath, 2001).

From Figure 34–4, it is now clear how different P blood group phenotypes arise. Because nearly all people inherit both α4GalT1 and β3GalT3, both P^k and P antigens are synthesized on RBCs (P_2 phenotype). The P_1 antigen is absent on those individuals whose α4GalT1 allele possesses mutations in the promoter. The rare P^k phenotype lacks a functional β3GalT3 gene, resulting in an absence of P antigen and an accumulation of CDH and P^k. Likewise, the p phenotype lacks a functional α4GalT1 gene resulting in an absence of P_1 and all globo-glycolipids. As a result, there is increased synthesis of 'p' antigen or sialoparagloboside (SPG; NeuAcα 2-3Galβ 1-4GlcNAcβ 1-3Galβ 1-4Glcβ 1-1Cer) on p RBCs due to a compensatory increase in neolactoglycolipid synthesis. The P^k variant and weak P phenotypes described by Kundu (1980, 1978) are hypothesized to reflect decreased expression/activity in β3GalT3 and α4GalT1, respectively.

P Blood Group Antibodies
Anti-P_1

Clinically, the most common antibody observed is anti-P_1, which is detected in one-quarter to two-thirds of P_2 donors (Issitt, 1998). Anti-P_1 is a naturally occurring antibody of IgM isotype and is often detected as a weak, room-temperature agglutinin. Rare examples of anti-P_1 are reactive at 37°C or show in vitro hemolysis. Because P_1 expression varies in strength between individuals, anti-P_1 may not react with all P_1-positive cells tested. Anti-P_1 can bind complement and may be detected in the indirect antiglobulin test (IAT) if polyspecific antihuman globulin (AHG) is used. Antibody reactivity can be eliminated by prewarming sera or by the addition of soluble P_1 substance from hydatid cyst fluid, earthworms and bird eggs. Anti-P_1 titers are often elevated in patients with hydatid cyst disease, fascioliasis (liver fluke), and in bird fanciers (Issit, 1998). Some examples of anti-P_1 have I blood group specificity (anti-IP_1).

In general, anti-P_1 is not clinically significant and its presence rarely requires transfusion of antigen-negative blood. The exception is patients with an anti-P_1 showing in vitro hemolysis. Because of the risk of immediate and delayed hemolytic transfusion reactions, these patients should receive P_1-negative (P_2), crossmatch-compatible units. Anti-P_1 is not a cause of HDN.

Alloanti-PP_1P^k

Anti-PP_1P^k (historically known as anti-Tj^a) is a separable mixture of anti-P, anti-P_1, and anti-P^k in the sera of p individuals. These antibodies are naturally occurring and may be IgM only or IgM plus IgG (IgG3). Because anti-PP_1P^k antibodies are potent hemolysins, these patients can only be transfused with p RBCs. In women, anti-PP_1P^k and anti-P are associated with HDN and spontaneous abortion. Early and frequent plasmapheresis has been used with therapeutic success in alloimmunized pregnant women of the p and P^k phenotypes (Spitalnik, 1995).

Alloanti-P

Anti-P is also a naturally occurring, IgM alloantibody in the serum of P^k (and p) individuals. It is a potent hemolysin and can cause in vivo hemolysis following transfusion of P-positive (P_1 and P_2) RBCs. Anti-P is a cause of HDN and is associated with spontaneous abortions.

Auto-Anti-P (Donath–Landsteiner)

An autoantibody with anti-P specificity is seen in patients with paroxysmal cold hemoglobinuria (PCH), a clinical syndrome in children following viral infection. In PCH, autoanti-P is an IgG, biphasic hemolysin capable of binding RBCs at colder temperatures, followed by intravascular hemolysis at body temperature. This characteristic can be demonstrated in vitro in the Donath–Landsteiner test. See full description in later sections on immunohematologic methods.

Biological Role

Unlike many antigens, the physiologic role of the P blood group antigens is not known. There is some evidence that the P^k antigen may be associated with the α-interferon and MHC class II receptors (Ghislain, 1994; George, 2001) and may modulate cell signaling via lipid rafts (Kovbasnjuk, 2001). The P blood group antigens may also play a role in cellular differentiation and neoplasia. The P^k and P antigens are differentially expressed during embryogenesis, hematopoiesis and intestinal mucosa differentiation (Jacewicz, 1995; Cooling, 2003b). The P^k antigen is a marker of apoptosis in germinal center B cells, Burkitt lymphoma and lymphoblastic leukemia (Mangeney, 1991).

Several P blood group antigens are receptors for microbial pathogens. The P blood group antigen is the receptor for parvovirus B19, a single-stranded DNA virus associated with multiple clinical sequelae including aplastic crises (Brown, 1994; Cooling, 1995). The P_1 and P^k antigens are receptors for shiga toxin, produced by *Shigella dysenteriae* and enterohemorrhagic *Escherichia coli* (EHEC) strains. In addition to gastroenteritis, EHEC infection is the most common cause of community-acquired hemolytic uremic syndrome, probably reflecting toxin binding to P^k antigen on glomerular vascular endothelium and platelets (Boyce, 1995; Cooling, 1998; Karpman, 2001). P, P^k, and Luke blood group antigens on uroepithelium are cell receptors for P-fimbriae, a bacterial adhesin and colonization factor expressed on uropathogenic *E. coli* strains. The P^k antigen also serves as a receptor for *Streptococcus suis* and *Pseudomonas aeruginosa* (Spitalnik, 1995).

Rh Blood Group System (ISBT No. 004)

The first and most clinically important characterization of the Rh system antigens came when Landsteiner and Wiener (1940) published studies of animal experiments involving the immunization of guinea pigs and rabbits with rhesus monkey RBCs. The resulting antiserum agglutinated 85% of human RBCs, and the antigen defined was called the Rh (rhesus) factor. This anti-Rh was later reported to have the same specificity as antibodies studied earlier by Levine and Stetson (1939) that were responsible for hemolytic disease of the newborn (HDN). Interestingly, the anti-Rh developed by Landsteiner and Wiener was later shown to recognize a different blood group antigen, named LW for its discoverers.

Table 35–15 Comparison of Wiener, Fisher–Race, and Rosenfield Nomenclatures for Antigens of the Rh Blood Group System

Wiener	Fisher–Race	Rosenfield
Rh_o	D	RH1
rh′	C	RH2
rh″	E	RH3
hr′	c	RH4
hr″	e	RH5

Table 34–16 Wiener and Fisher–Race Nomenclatures for the Rh Haplotypes and their Population Frequencies*

Wiener	Fisher–Race[†]	Frequencies in US population			
		White	Black	Native American	Asian
R^0	Dce	0.04	0.44	0.02	0.03
R^1	DCe	0.42	0.17	0.44	0.70
R^2	DcE	0.14	0.11	0.34	0.21
R^z	DCE	0.00	0.00	0.06	0.01
r	dce	0.37	0.26	0.11	0.03
r′	dCe	0.02	0.02	0.02	0.02
r″	dcE	0.01	0.00	0.01	0.00
r^y	dCE	0.00	0.00	0.00	0.00

* Composite figures calculated from Mourant (1976).

[†] In Fisher–Race nomenclature, 'd' indicates the lack of D antigen.

Today, the Rh system is probably the most complex red cell antigen system in humans, encompassing some 50 antigens, many phenotypic variants, and complex etiologic relationships. Hence, the following review is basic and highlights the most current information. For a detailed, historical review of the Rh system, readers should consult Issitt (1998) and Daniels (2002).

Theories of Rh Inheritance and Classification System

Using five basic antisera, anti-D, anti-C, anti-E, anti-c, and anti-e, Wiener identified five different factors or antigens (Table 34–15) that, from population and family studies, appeared to be inherited as two complexes of up to three factors each. There were eight possible combinations of three-factor complexes if one included 'd' as designating the lack of D, because no anti-d had ever been demonstrated. Wiener proposed a single-locus inheritance system with eight alternative common alleles coding for two Rh *agglutinogens*, capable of expressing up to three different antigenic determinants. Wiener's nomenclature for the eight different genes and allelic frequencies are listed in Tables 34–16 and 34–17.

Fisher and Race later proposed a different inheritance theory and nomenclature system based on genetic evidence of the antithetical or allelic nature of the C/c and the E/e antigens (Race, 1948). These investigators proposed a system of three closely linked loci or subloci on each chromosome, which were inherited as a block of genes (haplotype). They also introduced the DCE nomenclature to name the alleles, including the use of 'd' to designate the lack of D locus (Table 34–15). Rosenfeld proposed a numerical system of naming the antigens in 1962, because the increasing number of Rh antigens rendered an alphabetical notation impractical (Table 34–18). It was also appreciated that this nomenclature contained no inferences as to the genetic inheritance of the antigens.

Biochemistry

Tremendous progress has been made in deciphering the biochemistry and molecular biology of the Rh blood group system. It is now clear that Rh consists of three integral membrane proteins: RHD, RHCE, and Rh-associated glycoprotein (RHAG). RHD and RHCE are highly homologous proteins, differing by approximately 30 amino acids. Both are 30-kDa, 416-amino-acid multipass proteins containing 12 transmembrane domains, six extracellular loops, and a cytoplasmic amino- and carboxy-terminus (Fig. 34–5). Both proteins possess two to three molecules of palmitate (C16 fatty acid) covalently linked to transmembrane cysteine residues. Palmitoylation of Rh proteins may help maintain the phospholipid asymmetry of the RBC membrane (Avent, 1999).

Table 34–17 Frequencies of Common Rh Phenotypes*

D	C	c	E	e	Rh	DCE	Rh	DCE	White	Black	Native American	Asian
+	+	+	+	+	Rh₁Rh₂	DCcEe	R^1R^2	DCe/DcE	0.1176 (89%)	0.0374 (100%)	0.2992 (89%)	0.294 (97%)
							R₁r″	DCe/dcE	0.0084 (6%)		0.0088 (3%)	
							r^1R^2	dCe/DcE	0.0056 (5%)		0.0135 (4%)	0.0084 (2.8%)
							rR^z	dce/DCE		0.0132 (4%)	0.0006 (0.2%)	
+	+	+	−	+	Rh₁rh	DCce	R^1R^0	DCe/Dce	0.0168 (5%)	0.1495 (63%)	0.0176 (15%)	0.042 (50%)
							R^1r	DCe/dce	0.3108 (95%)	0.0884 (37%)	0.0968 (85%)	0.042 (50%)
+	−	+	+	+	Rh₂rh	DcEe	R^2R^0	DcE/Dce	0.0112 (10%)	0.0968 (63%)	0.0136 (15%)	0.0126 (50%)
							R^2r	DcE/dce	0.1035 (90%)	0.0572 (37%)	0.0748 (85%)	0.0126 (50%)
+	+	−	−	+	Rh₁Rh₁	DCe	R^1R^1	DCe/DCe	0.176 (91%)	0.029 (81%)	0.194 (92%)	0.490 (93%)
							R^1r^1	DCe/dCe	0.017 (9%)	0.007 (19%)	0.017 (8%)	0.028 (7%)
+	+	−	+	+	Rh₁Rh$_z$	DCEe	R^1R^z	DCe/DCE		0.053 (100%)		
+	−	+	+	−	Rh₂Rh₂	DcE	R^2R^2	DcE/DcE	0.02 (88%)	0.012 (100%)	0.116 (94%)	0.044 (100%)
							R₂r″	DcE/dcE	0.003 (12%)		0.007 (6%)	
+	+	+	+	−	Rh₂Rh$_z$	DCcE	R^2R^z	DcE/DCE			0.041 (100%)	
+	−	+	−	+	Rh₀Rh₀	Dce	R^0R^0	Dce/Dce	0.0016 (5%)	0.1936 (46%)	0.0004 (8%)	0.0009 (33%)
							R^0r	Dce/dce	0.0296 (95%)	0.2286 (54%)	0.0044 (92%)	0.0018 (67%)
−	−	+	−	+	rhrh	dce	rr	dce/dce	0.1369 (100%)	0.0676 (100%)	0.0121 (100%)	0.0009 (100%)
−	+	+	−	+	rh′rh	dCce	rr′	dce/dCe	0.0055 (100%)	0.0014 (100%)	0.0044 (100%)	0.0012 (100%)
−	−	+	+	+	rh″rh	dcEe	rr″	dce/dcE	0.0028 (100%)		0.0022 (100%)	

* Estimated from haplotype frequencies (p, q from Table 34–16) using p2 for homozygotes and 2pq for heterozygotes.

† + = positive; − = negative.

‡ (%) = percentage of genotypes within a given phenotype.

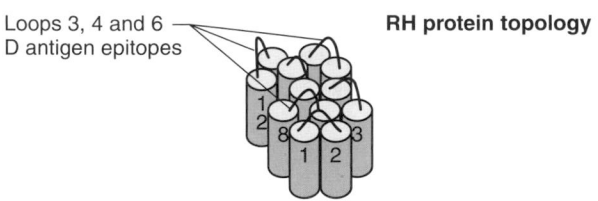

RH protein topology

Loops 3, 4 and 6
D antigen epitopes

RHCE protein

C^w/Mar
C^x
RH26
C/c/G
RH35
E^w
hr^s
E/e
V
Hr
VS
Cys16
(C, RH53)
Crawford
Hr^B

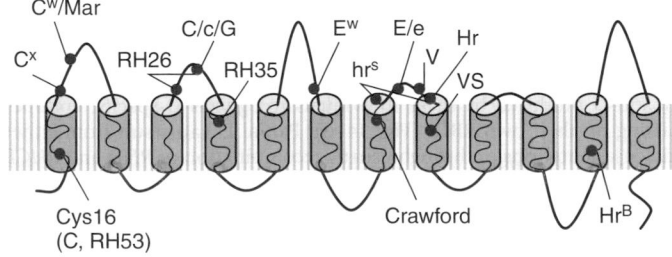

RHD protein

RhD antigen (loops 3,4,6)

Tar G
3   4   6
Hr^B

Weak D mutations (o)

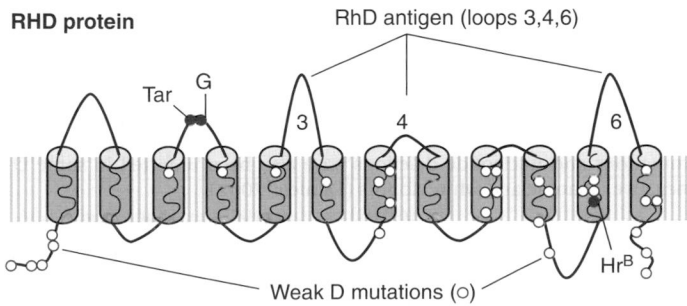

Figure 34–5 RH proteins. Both RHD and RHCE proteins are multipass protein with 12 transmembrane domains, indicated by solid amber cylinders. The location of Rh antigens denoted by single amino acid polymorphisms is denoted (●). The RhD epitope is a complex antigen involving structures on the third, fourth and sixth extracellular loops. Missense mutations in RHD, leading to weak D expression, are indicated by open circles (o).

RHAG is a 45- to 70-kDa multipass glycoprotein, evolutionarily related to RhD and RhCcEe glycoproteins. RHAG is a 409-amino-acid glycoprotein with 12 transmembrane domains and a single, large *N*-linked carbohydrate side chain on the first extracellular loop. Overall, there are approximately 170 000 molecules each of RH and RHAG proteins per RBC. RHD, RHCE, and RHAG are erythroid-specific proteins (Avent, 1999).

In the RBC membrane, RHD, RHCE, and RHAG proteins exist as part of an Rh immune complex, composed of two molecules of Rh (RHD and RHCE) and two molecules of RHAG (Eyers, 1994). The importance of RHAG for the expression and correct assembly of Rh proteins cannot be understated. In the absence of functional RHAG protein, neither RHD nor RHCE proteins will be expressed (Rh₍null₎ and Rh₍mod₎ phenotypes). In addition to RHAG, Rh proteins may be topologically associated with CD47, the LW glycoprotein (ICAM4), DARC or Duffy glycoprotein, band 3, and glycophorin B. At least two non-Rh antigens, Fy⁵ and U, may require noncovalent interactions between Rh, DARC glycoprotein (Fy⁵) and glycophorin B (U), respectively (Ridgwell, 1994).

Molecular Biology

The genes for RHD (*RHD*) and RHCE (*RHCE*) proteins span 65 kb on chromosome 1p34-36.1 and share nearly 92% sequence identity. The two genes are separated by only 30 kb and have opposite orientations, facing each other at their 3′ ends (Fig. 34–6). The RHD gene is also flanked by two homologous sequences known as rhesus boxes. The RHAG gene (*RHAG*) resides on chromosome 6p11.1 and shares 36% homology with the *RHD* and *RHCE* genes. All three genes possess 10 exons and at least one GATA-1 consensus sequence in the promoter region (Iwamoto, 1998; Cherif-Zahar, 1994). It is believed that *RHAG* and *RH* genes arose by gene duplication 250–350 million years ago. A second gene duplication 8–11 million years ago resulted in the ce and D alleles (cDe or R⁰ haplotype). The remaining *RHCe* alleles are believed to be the product of point mutations, recombination, and gene conversion of the *RHD* and *RHCE* genes (Avent, 1999).

D Antigen

The cloning of *RHD* and *RHCE* genes opened the door to understanding the complex immunology of many Rh antigens and phenotypes. The D antigen, the most immunogenic of all the Rh antigens, resides on the RHD protein. Current evidence suggests that D is a highly complex antigen, depending on both specific amino acids and the tertiary structure of the RHD protein itself. At present, nine 'D-specific' amino acids (Met169, Met170, Ile172, Phe223, Ala226, Glu233, Asp350, Ala353, and Gly354) have been identified as functional D epitopes. The nine amino acids lie

IV

Rh$_{null}$ Phenotype

Rh$_{null}$ erythrocytes lack all Rh antigens, due to an apparent absence of RHD and RHCE proteins. In addition, Rh$_{null}$ erythrocytes lack the high-frequency antigens Fy^5 and LW and may have markedly decreased expression of S/s and U antigens. The absence of these non-Rh antigens reflects the complex topologic association of Duffy, LW, and glycophorin B proteins with Rh proteins on RBC membranes.

Extremely rare (< 1 in 6 million), Rh$_{null}$ cells have abnormalities in RBC morphology (spherocytes, stomatocytes), water content, cell volume, cation fluxes, and phospholipid asymmetry. Rh$_{null}$ cells show increased osmotic fragility and a shortened circulating half-life, often accompanied by a mild hemolytic anemia (Rh deficiency syndrome). Because Rh$_{null}$ individuals can become sensitized to multiple Rh antigens, including high-frequency antigens, transfusion support can be quite difficult. Some alloimmunized Rh$_{null}$ individuals can produce anti-RH29, which reacts with all RBCs except Rh$_{null}$.

The Rh$_{null}$ phenotype can arise from two, distinct genetic backgrounds – regulator and amorph. The Rh$_{null}$-amorph type is the result of nonsense mutations in the RHCE gene in D-negative people. Because of the absence of RHD and RHCE proteins, Rh$_{null}$-amorph RBCs have reduced (but not absent) expression of RHAG protein (Daniels, 2002). The Rh$_{null}$ regulator type arises from mutations in RHAG (Reid, 2004b).

Rh$_{mod}$ Phenotype

Mutations in *RHAG* are also observed in the Rh$_{mod}$ phenotype. Rh$_{mod}$ RBCs have markedly decreased RH and RHAG expression, detectable only by careful adsorption and elution studies. Like Rh$_{null}$ individuals, persons with Rh$_{mod}$ may have laboratory evidence of Rh deficiency syndrome with a mild hemolytic anemia. Three Rh$_{mod}$ samples have been studied, each containing a single, different missense mutation in the *RHAG* gene (Reid, 2004b).

Rh Antibodies

Antibodies against Rh antigens are routinely encountered in the blood bank (see Table 34–7). D is the most immunogenic Rh antigen, followed by c, E, C, and e (Harmening, 1999). In general, antibodies against Rh antigens are the result of immune stimulation by either transfusion or pregnancy. Exceptions are some examples of anti-C^w and anti-E, which can be naturally occurring. Most antibodies against Rh antigens are of IgG isotype (IgG1 and IgG3), although rare examples of IgM and IgA are known. Anti-Rh antibodies are reactive at 37°C and are usually detected in the AHG phase of testing. The reactivity of anti-Rh antibodies can be enhanced with enzyme-treated RBCs.

Clinically, antibodies against Rh are associated with hemolytic transfusion reactions. However, because Rh antibodies do not fix complement, incompatible RBCs are almost always cleared through extravascular destruction. To prevent sensitization to the D antigen, Rh-negative patients should be transfused with Rh-negative RBCs. This is particularly true for young girls and women of childbearing age. For transfusion in alloimmunized patients, RBC units should be negative for the Rh antigen of interest and crossmatch compatible with the recipient's serum through the AHG phase of testing. One possible exception may be R^{1}R^1 (CDe/CDe) patients who have developed anti-E alloantibodies. Because these patients are at increased risk of delayed hemolytic transfusion reactions due to the subsequent development of anti-c, many blood bankers advocate transfusing only R^{1}R^1 units to R^{1}R^1 patients (Shirey, 1994).

Antibodies against Rh antigens are also a major cause of HDN. All Rh-negative women should receive Rh immune globulin (IgG anti-D) prophylactically in midpregnancy, following an invasive procedure (i.e., amniocentesis), and immediately after delivery to prevent alloimmunization. Rh immune globulin prophylaxis is also recommended in women with partial D phenotypes since these women can be at risk for D alloimmunization (Ansart-Pirenne, 2004). Rh immune globulin may also be given following transfusion of RhD+ platelet concentrates or after accidental transfusion of RhD+ RBCs. In the latter, Rh immune globulin is given after two-volume RBC exchange with RhD-negative RBCs (Nester, 2004) Administration of one vial of Rh immune globulin is recommended for every 30 mL of whole blood or 15 mL packed RBCs transfused. Rh immune globulin should be given within 72 hours of exposure in order to prevent active immunization. Rh immune globulin is not given to Rh-negative women who are already immunized to D antigen (i.e., have anti-D).

It is also recommended to give Rh immune globulin to Rh-negative women with anti-G alloantibodies. As stated earlier, anti-G behaves as an anti-C + anti-D due to recognition of a Ser103 or C-type antigen on both RHD and RHCE proteins. In general, HDN secondary to anti-G or anti-C +

anti-G is mild when compared to HDN due to anti-D. However, because these women may still become immunized to D-specific epitopes on the RHD protein, many blood bankers advocate giving Rh immune globulin to Rh-negative women with anti-G antibodies (Shirey, 1997). Separation of anti-G from a true anti-C + anti-D is very laborious, requiring sequential adsorption and elution (Yesus, 1985). One clue suggesting the presence of anti-G is an anti-C titer at least fourfold higher then anti-D (Shirey, 1997). It is not necessary, however, to separate anti-G from anti-C + anti-D for routine transfusion. With very rare exceptions, RBCs negative for D and C antigens are also negative for G antigen.

Biological Role

The specific physiologic function of the Rh proteins is still unknown; however, there is a strong belief that Rh proteins may constitute a membrane transporter. The Rh proteins are homologous with ammonium transporters of the Mep/Amt family. In addition, Rh-like homologs have been discovered in invertebrate life forms such as the nematode worm *Caenorhabditis elegans* and a marine sponge, *Geodia cydonium* (Avent, 1999).

Lutheran Blood Group System (ISBT No. 005)

The Lutheran (Lu) blood group system contains 18 antigens including four pairs of allelic antigens and 10 high-incidence antigens. Lutheran is a minor constituent of RBC membranes, averaging only 2000–5000 molecules per cell, and can vary in strength between donors (Issitt, 1998). Even in a single individual, there is considerable heterogeneity in Lutheran expression, with only 40–50% of red cells positive for Lutheran antigens by flow cytometry (El Nemer, 1998). Lutheran antigens are ubiquitously expressed on human tissues. In addition to RBCs, Lutheran glycoprotein is expressed by colon, small intestine, ovary, testis, prostate, thymus, spleen, pancreas, kidney, skeletal muscle, liver, lung, placenta, brain, heart, and bone marrow (Rahuel, 1996).

Null/Weak Phenotypes

Three distinct Lu$_{null}$ phenotypes, with distinct patterns of inheritance, are known: autosomal recessive, autosomal dominant (In(Lu)) and X-linked recessive (Table 34–19). The autosomal recessive phenotype is characterized by a complete absence of all Lutheran antigens on RBCs. As a consequence, these individuals can make an alloantibody to Lutheran glycoprotein (anti-Lu3) which reacts with all Lu-positive RBCs.

The autosomal dominant and X-linked recessive forms are characterized by very weak Lutheran expression, often detected only after adsorption and elution. In(Lu) RBCs, the autosomal dominant Lu$_{null}$ phenotype, occurs in 1 : 3000 individuals and are identified by weak expression of Lutheran and other glycosylated antigens (P$_1$, i, Indian/CD44 antigens) and enhanced expression of CDw75 (Daniels, 2002). The X-linked form

Table 34–19 Phenotypes of the Lutheran System

Reactions with anti-			Phenotype	Frequency (%) US population		Comments
Lu^a	Lu^b	Lu-3		Caucasian	Black	
+	0	+	Lu (a+b−)	0.1	0.1	
+	+	+	Lu (a+b+)	7	5	
0	+	+	Lu (a−b+)	93	95	
Null phenotypes (Lu$_{null}$)						
0	0	0	Lu (a−b−)	Very rare	Very rare	Autosomal recessive Normal CD44, i/I, CD75 Make an anti-Lu-3
0/W*	0/w*	w*	Lu (a−b−)	Very rare	Very rare	In (Lu), autosomal dominant ↓CD44, I/i; ↑CD75
0/W*	0/w*	w*	Lu (a−b−)	Very rare	Very rare	X-linked recessive (XS2) Absent CD75

* Weak Lu antigens detected only by adsorption and elution techniques.

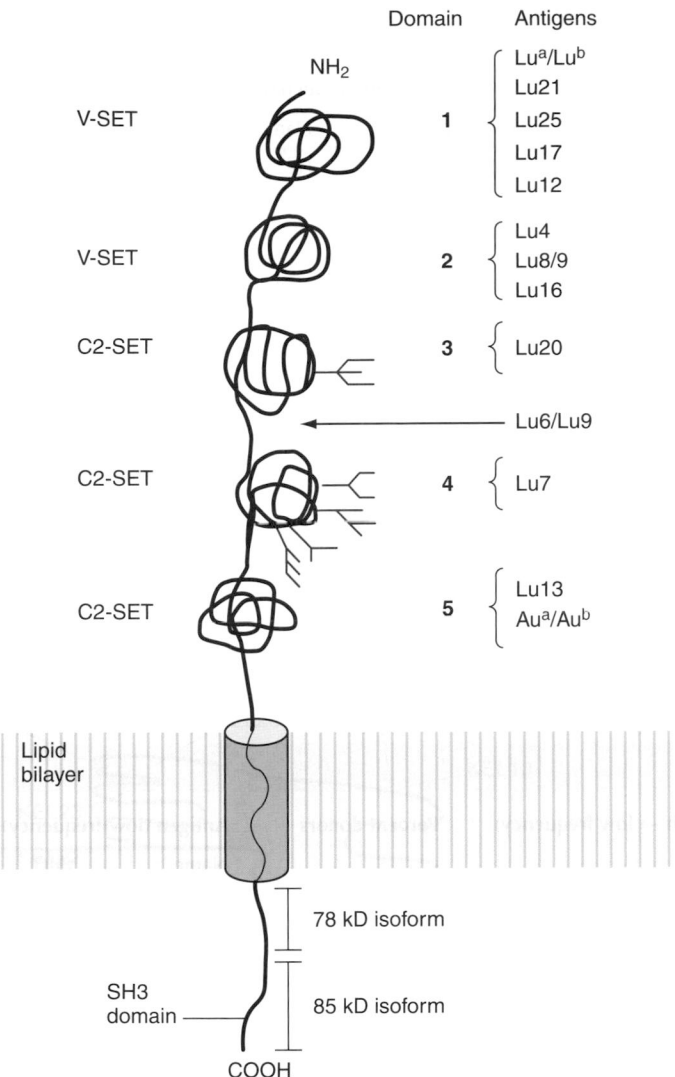

Figure 34–7 Lutheran glycoprotein. The Lutheran antigens reside on one of five immunoglobulin domains (V, C2-like). The transmembrane domain is indicated by a solid amber cylinder. The length of the cytoplasmic domain can vary from 19 amino acids (78-kDa form) to 59 amino acids (85-kDa isoform). The latter also possesses a consensus-binding motif for Src protein (SH3 domain).

In the figure, labels include: NH₂, Domain, Antigens, V-SET, C2-SET, Lipid bilayer, 78 kD isoform, 85 kD isoform, SH3 domain, COOH. Domain 1: Luᵃ/Luᵇ, Lu21, Lu25, Lu17, Lu12. Domain 2: Lu4, Lu8/9, Lu16. Domain 3: Lu20. Lu6/Lu9. Domain 4: Lu7. Domain 5: Lu13, Auᵃ/Auᵇ.

responsible for the 78-kD minor isoform (El Nemer, 1997; Rahuel, 1996). Although no TATA or CAAT boxes are present in the 5′ flanking or promoter region of the gene, it does possess consensus sequences for several *cis*-regulatory elements including the ubiquitous Sp1, AP2, EGR-1, Ets, and GATA-1, an erythroid transcription binding protein (El Nemer, 1997).

The molecular basis for most Lutheran antigens are now known (Table 34–20). Most are the result of single nucleotide polymorphisms (Crew, 2003; Daniels, 2002). In contrast, the molecular basis for the Lu_null phenotypes is still relatively unknown. The autosomal recessive, true Lu_null phenotype arises from inheritance of two silent amorph (*Lu*) alleles (Cartron, 1998). The genes responsible for the autosomal dominant In(Lu) and X-linked recessive (XS2) have not been identified or cloned. It is hypothesized that the genes represent inhibitors, capable of suppressing or downregulating LU gene transcription.

Lutheran Antibodies

In general, Lutheran antibodies are not clinically significant and are only rarely associated with HDN and hemolytic transfusion reactions. Anti-Luᵃ is the most common Lutheran alloantibody encountered in the blood bank and is often an IgM, room-temperature agglutinin. Because not all RBCs express detectable Lu antigens (El Nemer, 1998), anti-Luᵃ can display mixed field agglutination. Anti-Luᵇ is a relatively rare, IgG antibody that is typically detected in the IAT. Reactivity of anti-Luᵃ, Luᵇ and other Lutheran antibodies can be inhibited by pretreatment of RBCs with chymotrypsin, trypsin, AET and DTT.

Biological Role

Biologically, Lutheran is a high-affinity receptor for laminin, a basement membrane protein involved in cell differentiation, adhesion, migration, and proliferation. Overexpression of LU glycoprotein in ovarian carcinoma and other cancers is hypothesized to facilitate tumor cell adhesion and metastasis (Rahuel, 1996). In sickle cell patients, increased Lutheran expression on reticulocytes and sickle cells may contribute to the pathophysiology of vaso-occlusive crises. Patients with sickle cell disease have indirect evidence of chronic vascular injury with shedding of microvascular endothelial cells and exposure of vascular basement membrane (Solovey, 1997). In these patients, increased exposure of laminin on the thrombotic subendothelium, coupled with increased expression of laminin receptor on reticulocytes and sickle cells, may promote red cell adhesion and circulatory stasis (El Nemer, 1998; Parsons, 2001). Because Lutheran is expressed late in erythroid differentiation, it does not appear to play a role in adhesion to bone marrow extracellular matrix (El Nemer, 1998). It may, however, be involved in the migration of erythrocytes out of the bone marrow (Southcott, 1999). Recent evidence showing an interaction between Lu/B-CAM and spectrin raise the possibility that Lu may also function in cell signaling (Kroviarski, 2004).

Kell and Kx Blood Group Systems (ISBT No. 006 and 019)

First identified in 1945, the Kell blood group system currently consists of 24 high- and low-frequency antigens (Table 34–21). Eleven Kell antigens belong to five sets of allelic antigens, whereas the remainder are predominantly high-incidence antigens (> 99% population). Many low-incidence Kell antigens (K, Jsᵃ, Ulᵃ, Kpᵃ, Kpᶜ) show distinct racial differences. The Kell antigen is found on RBCs, erythroid and megakaryocyte progenitors, skeletal muscle and testis. RBCs express approximately 2000–6000 copies of Kell protein per cell (Issitt, 1998).

Null and Weak Phenotypes

K₀K₀ is an autosomal recessive, true null phenotype that completely lacks all Kell antigens (Table 34–22). As a consequence, these individuals can make an alloantibody to the Kell glycoprotein (anti-Ku). Unlike McLeod RBCs (see below), K₀K₀ RBCs have enhanced expression of Kx antigen, present on the XK protein. A K₀K₀ RBC can be produced in the laboratory by treating Kell-positive RBCs with sulfhydryl-reducing agents.

Kell antigens are significantly depressed/absent on McLeod RBCs, an X-linked recessive phenotype characterized by the absence of XK protein on RBCs (Kx antigen, XK1; ISBT 019), acanthocytes and neuromuscular disorders. Because McLeod individuals lack XK and Kell proteins, these individuals can make alloantibodies directed against both proteins. As a consequence, McLeod individuals are incompatible with both Kell-positive and K₀K₀ RBCs. Depressed Kell expression is also observed in K_mod and Gerbich-negative RBCs, two autosomal recessive phenotypes. Like the K₀K₀ phenotype, some Kell_mod individuals have increased Kx (KEL15) expression and can develop an anti-KEL5 (anti-Ku) following

has weakened Lutheran, enhanced i and CDw75 and normal P₁, i and CD44 expression. Because both In(Lu) and X-linked recessive Lu_null phenotypes express some Lutheran antigen on RBCs and other tissues, neither is associated with the development of anti-Lu3 (Rao, 1995). In(Lu) RBCs can display subtle abnormalities including increased poikilocytosis and increased hemolysis during in vitro storage (Ballas, 1992).

Biochemistry

The Lutheran antigens reside on two, isomeric type 1 glycoproteins, Lu-glycoprotein (85 kD) and epithelial cancer antigen (B-CAM, 78 kD) (Parsons, 1987). The 85-kD glycoprotein is the predominant isoform found on RBCs and normal tissues. Members of the immunoglobulin superfamily, the 78- and 85-kD glycoproteins share a common, large (518-amino-acid) extracellular domain with five immunoglobulin regions and five potential N-glycosylation sites (Fig. 34–7). Three immunoglobulin domains are of the constant-region-2 (C2) type, whereas the remaining two are variable-region (V) domains. The 7-kD difference between the 78-kD and 85-kD isoforms reflects the length of the COOH-terminal cytoplasmic tail. In addition to its longer length, the cytoplasmic domain of the 85-kD isoform possesses an SH3 motif, a potential binding site for Src protein. The cytoplasmic domain also interacts with spectrin, a cytoskeletal protein (Kroviarski, 2004). Because it is a highly folded protein, stabilized by disulfide bonds, Lutheran is destroyed by sulfhydryl-reducing agents and many proteases.

Molecular Biology

The gene for Lutheran (*LU*) resides on chromosome 19q13.2-13.3. It is a 12.5-kb gene containing 15 exons: Alternate splicing of exon 13 is protein, also serves as a substrate for casein kinase 2 (Carbonnet, 1998). Kell has been shown to cleave endothelin-3, a potent vasoconstrictor and mitogen that is involve in migration of neural crest cells and the enteric nervous system (Lee, 1999).

In contrast to Kell, the absence of XK protein is strongly associated with several abnormal clinical and laboratory findings. McLeod RBC have shortened survival, decreased permeability to water, and abnormal morphology (acanthocytes). The McLeod syndrome, characterized by both hematologic and neuromuscular abnormalities, typically presents with areflexia, dystonia and choreiform movements late in life. Late-onset muscular dystrophy and cardiomyopathy can also be seen. Both the hematologic and neuromuscular defects in McLeod patients are believed to result from the absence of XK protein on red cells, brain, heart, and skeletal muscle (Ho, 1994). It is interesting that the Huntington's disease gene, another neurodegenerative disorder, is located near the XK gene on the X chromosome (Issit, 1998).

The McLeod phenotype can also be associated with chronic granulomatous disease (CGD), a functional neutrophil defect resulting in severe, recurrent, life-threatening bacterial infections. In two-thirds of patients, GCD results from a deletion or mutation of the cytochrome b gene (CYBB) on the X chromosome. Because of the proximity of the CYBB and XK genes on the X chromosome, approximately 7% of patients with X-linked GCD also express a McLeod phenotype (Curnutte, 1995).

Lewis Blood Group System (ISBT No. 007)

The Lewis blood group system primarily consists of two antigens, Lewis[a] (Le[a]) and Lewis[b] (Le[b]). Four additional antigens (Le[ab], Le[bH], ALe[b], BLe[b]) reflect the influence of ABO on Lewis synthesis and antigenicity. On RBCs, the Lewis antigens reside on glycosphingolipids, composed of a Lewis-active carbohydrate head group linked to a ceramide (N-acyl sphingosine) lipid tail. Unlike most RBC antigens, the Lewis antigens are not of erythroid origin. Lewis antigens are synthesized in the gastrointestinal tract and passively adsorbed onto RBCs from a soluble pool of secreted Lewis substance in plasma. Tissues and fluids expressing Lewis include plasma, saliva, RBCs, platelets, lymphocytes, endothelium, uroepithelium, and bowel mucosa. In some tissues, Lewis antigens are expressed on glycosphingolipids, glycoproteins, and mucins (Hauser, 1995; Issitt, 1998).

Three Lewis phenotypes are observed in adults, Le (a+b−), Le (a−b+) and Le (a−b−): The Le (a+b+) is only rarely observed, usually on RBCs of very young children and some individuals of Polynesian, Japanese, or Taiwanese ancestry (Issitt, 1998). As shown in Table 34–23, the Le (a−b−) phenotype is five times more common in black people than in white people. The Le (a−b−) phenotype is also increased in neonates due to developmentally delayed expression of the Lewis and Secretor genes. By 5 years of age, most children will express adult levels of Lewis antigens on their RBCs. The amount of Lewis antigen on RBCs is also influenced by

Table 34–23 The Lewis Blood Group System

Phenotype	Frequencies (%) in US adults		Possible genotype		ABH and Lewis substances in saliva and plasma		
	White	Black	Le Gene	Se Gene	Group O	Group A	Group B
Le (a+b−)	22	23	Le/Le or Le/le	se/se	Le[a]	Le[a]	Le[a]
Le (a−b+)	72	55	Le/Le or Le/le	Se/Se or Se/se	Type 1 H	Type 1 H and A	Type 1 H and B
					Le[a], Le[b]	Le[a], Le[b], ALe[b]	Le[a], Le[b], BLe[b]
Le (a−b−)	6	22	le/le	Se/se	Type 1 H	Type 1 H and A	Type 1 H and B
			le/le	se/se	Type 1 chain precursor (Le[c])	Type 1 chain precursor (Le[c])	Type 1 chain precursor (Le[c])

ABO type. Le (a−b+) RBCs from group O donors appear to have more Le[b] then A[1] and B cells. As will be discussed below, group A[1] and B donors can convert Le[b] to ALe[b] and BLe[b], respectively (Issitt, 1998).

Biochemistry

Although biosynthetically related to each other, the Le[a] and Le[b] antigens are not allelic antigens. They represent the complex interaction of two distinct glycosyltransferases, fucosyltransferase type II (FUT2) and fucosyltransferase type III (FUT3). FUT3 is the product of the Lewis gene (Le/FUT3) and is an α 1-3/4 fucosyltransferase. FUT2, the product of the Secretor gene (Se), is an α 1-2 fucosyltransferase related to the H-gene. How Le, Se, and ABO genes interact to yield the different combinations of RBC and plasma phenotypes are shown in Table 34–23 and Figure 34–9.

The precursor molecule for Lewis and related antigens is a type 1 chain precursor, historically known as the Le[c] antigen. In Le (a+b−) donors, FUT3 or Lewis adds an α 1-4 linked fucose to Le[c] to form the Le[a] antigen. Because these donors lack the Se/FUT2 gene (se/se), no type 1 chain H (Le[d]) is made. As a result, only Le[a] antigen is present in plasma, saliva, and RBCs.

The Le (a−b+) red cell phenotype results from the inheritance of both Le and Se genes. FUT3 still converts a small amount of type 1 chain precursor to Le[a] antigen. However, most Le[c] substance is converted to type 1 chain H or Le[d] by FUT2 (Fig. 34–9). FUT3 subsequently adds a second fucose to form Le[b] antigen (Lowe, 1994). In group A and B persons, type 1 chain H is further modified by the A/B glycosyltransferase to form type 1 chain A and B antigens. Like type 1 chain H and Le[c] antigens, these molecules can

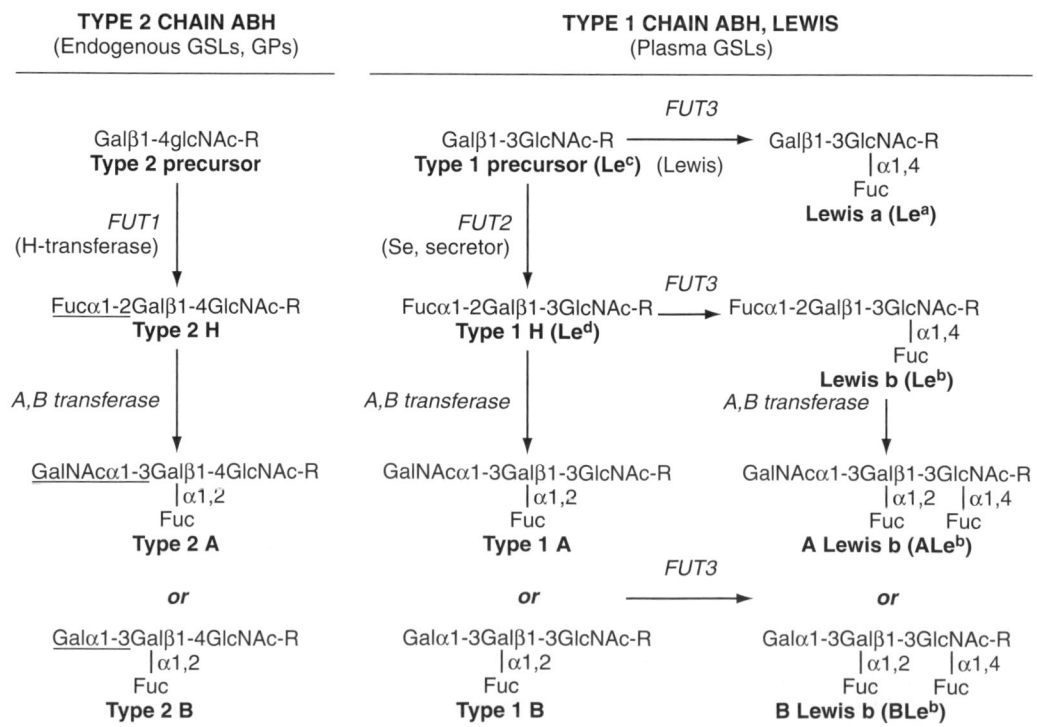

TYPE 2 CHAIN ABH (Endogenous GSLs, GPs)

Galβ1-4glcNAc-R
Type 2 precursor

↓ *FUT1* (H-transferase)

Fucα1-2Galβ1-4GlcNAc-R
Type 2 H

↓ *A,B transferase*

GalNAcα1-3Galβ1-4GlcNAc-R
|α1,2
Fuc
Type 2 A

or

Galα1-3Galβ1-4GlcNAc-R
|α1,2
Fuc
Type 2 B

TYPE 1 CHAIN ABH, LEWIS (Plasma GSLs)

Galβ1-3GlcNAc-R   —*FUT3*→   Galβ1-3GlcNAc-R
Type 1 precursor (Le[c]) (Lewis) |α1,4
                                               Fuc
                                          Lewis a (Le[a])

↓ *FUT2* (Se, secretor)

Fucα1-2Galβ1-3GlcNAc-R —*FUT3*→ Fucα1-2Galβ1-3GlcNAc-R
Type 1 H (Le[d]) |α1,4
                                            Fuc
                                       Lewis b (Le[b])

↓ *A,B transferase*   ↓ *A,B transferase*

GalNAcα1-3Galβ1-3GlcNAc-R   GalNAcα1-3Galβ1-3GlcNAc-R
|α1,2 |α1,2 |α1,4
Fuc   Fuc   Fuc
Type 1 A   **A Lewis b (ALe[b])**

or   —*FUT3*→   *or*

Galα1-3Galβ1-3GlcNAc-R   Galα1-3Galβ1-3GlcNAc-R
|α1,2 |α1,2 |α1,4
Fuc   Fuc   Fuc
Type 1 B   **B Lewis b (BLe[b])**

Figure 34–9 Synthesis of Lewis and type 1 chain ABH antigens. R = ceramide; Fuc = fucose; Gal = galactose; GalNAc = N-acetylgalactosamine; Glc = glucose; GlcNAc = N-acetylglucosamine; Le = Lewis.

Table 34-24 Phenotype Frequencies in the Duffy System

Reactions with anti-			RBC Phenotype	White people		Black people	
Fy^a	Fy^b	Fy3		Frequency*	Genotypes†	Frequency*	Genotypes*
+	−	+	Fy (a+b−)	17	FY*A/FY*A	9	FY*A/FY*A FY*A/FY*Fy
+	+	+	Fy (a+b+)	49	FY*A/FY*B	1	FY*A/FY*B
−	+	+	Fy (a−b+)	34	FY*B/FY*B	22	FY*B/FY*B FY*B/FY**Fy
−	−	−	Fy (a−b−)	Very rare	FY*amorph	68	FY*Fy/FY*Fy
+/−	w	w	Fy (a+b^w) Fy (a−b^w)	<0.1%	FY*A/FY*X FY*X	Very rare	FY*A/FY*X FY*X FY*X/FY*Fy

* Frequency (%) US population.

† Abbreviations: *FY*A* = *Fy^a* allele; *FY*B* = *Fy^b* allele; *FY*Fy* = *FY*B* allele carrying a *GATA-1* promoter mutation; *FY*X* = *FY*B* gene containing either missense or *Sp1* promoter mutation with weak *Fy^b* expression; *FY*amorph* = silent *FY* gene containing disruptive mutations (deletion, frameshift, nonsense). See accompanying text.

serve as substrates for FUT3 to form ALe^b and BLe^b (Fig. 34–9). In group A$_1$ donors, ALe^b is the major Le^b antigen found in plasma (Lindstrom, 1992).

The Le (a–b–) red cell phenotype occurs in individuals who lack the *Le/FUT3* gene. Individuals who are negative for both *Le* and *Se* alleles (*le/le, se/se*) are unable to synthesize either Le^a antigen or type 1 chain H antigens. As a result, only type 1 chain precursor or Le^c antigen is present in secretions and plasma. In contrast, individuals who inherit at least one *Se* allele can express type 1 chain glycolipids with ABH activity.

Molecular Biology

The *FUT3* or Lewis gene resides on chromosome 19p13.3 near two other α 1-3 fucosyltransferase genes, *FUT5* and *FUT6*. All three α 1-3 fucosyltransferases are highly homologous, consistent with gene duplication (Weston, 1992). The gene encodes a 361-amino-acid type II glycoprotein with both α 1-3 (Le^a) and α 1-4 (Le^X) fucosyltransferase activity. *FUT3* is highly expressed in colon, stomach, small intestine, lung, and kidney, with weaker expression in salivary gland, bladder, uterus, and liver. *FUT6* is coexpressed with *FUT3* in most tissues (Cameron, 1995).

The Le (a–b–) or null phenotype arises from inactivating mutations in *FUT3*. Over 10 missense mutations in the *FUT3* gene have been identified, with most *FUT3* null alleles possessing at least two mutations (Daniels, 2002; Reid, 2004b). The Lewis weak (Le^w) phenotype, characterized by a Le (a–b–) RBC phenotype and the presence of Lewis-active substance in saliva, is due to a single missense mutation in the transmembrane domain (T59>G). The latter has normal enzyme activity but decreased Golgi retention (Mollicone, 1994).

The *FUT2* (*Se*) gene resides on chromosome 19q13.3 as part of a 100-kb gene cluster that includes the *H* gene (*FUT1*) and *Sec1*, an inactive *FUT2*-like pseudogene (Kelly, 1995). Multiple null alleles have been reported, with distinct geographic and ethnic distributions. Most null alleles are the result of nonsense mutations (Daniels, 2002). The partial secretor phenotype has been linked to an Ile129>Phe mutation (Yu, 1995).

Lewis Antibodies

Like ABO, antibodies against Le^a and Le^b antigens are naturally occurring IgM antibodies (Table 34–7). Most examples are detected as room temperature agglutinins; however, some examples are reactive in the IAT. Although uncommon, some examples demonstrate in vitro hemolysis. Because Le^a and Le^b are glycosphingolipids, antibody reactivity can be enhanced by pretreatment of RBCs with enzymes. Antibody reactivity is neutralized by the addition of commercially available soluble Lewis substance or plasma containing the soluble Lewis antigen of interest. Anti-Le^b can be observed in individuals of either Le (a+b–) and Le (a–b–) phenotype, whereas anti-Le^a is only observed in Le (a–b–) individuals. Anti-Le^a is not observed in the Le (a–b+) phenotype, since these individuals synthesize a small amount of Le^a. Interestingly, some Le (a–b+) women can transiently become phenotypically Le (b–), with the development of anti-Le^b, during pregnancy. Some examples of anti-Le^b can demonstrate ABH specificity (anti-Le^{bH}, anti-Le^b, anti-Le^b), reacting more strongly with Le^b-positive RBCs of specific ABO types.

Anti-Lewis antibodies are seldom clinically significant. They are not associated with HDN and only rarely associated with hemolytic transfusion reactions. There is speculation they could play a role in renal graft rejection in black, Le (a–b–) individuals (Spitalnik, 1984). For transfusion, patients with anti-Lewis antibodies reactive only at room temperature may be safely transfused with crossmatch-compatible RBCs.

In contrast, examples of anti-Le^a or anti-Le^b that are hemolytic in vitro should receive antigen-negative, crossmatch-compatible RBCs. If antigen-negative blood is not available, the infusion of plasma, containing the soluble Lewis antigen of interest, may be helpful in neutralizing or inhibiting circulating antibody prior to RBC transfusion (Mollison, 1993).

Biological Role

The Lewis blood group antigens play an important role in disease. *Helicobacter pylori*, a causative agent of gastritis and ulcers, binds H, Le^b, and Le^y antigens via recognition of a terminal Fucα1-2Gal epitope (Boren, 1993). The latter appears to explain the increased incidence of ulcers and stomach cancer among blood group O and secretors. A Lewis null and/or nonsecretor phenotype has also been linked with a higher incidence of recurrent candida vaginitis and urinary tract infections (Sheinfeld, 1989; Hilton, 1995). A Le (a–b–) phenotype is associated with an increased incidence of heart disease (Ellison, 1999). Aberrant expression of sialyl-Le^a occurs in many gastrointestinal and uroepithelial cell cancers and may contribute to tumor metastasis. Sialyl-Le^a is a ligand for the endothelial adhesion molecule E-selectin and may mediate tumor cell–endothelium interactions (Takada, 1993). Sialyl-Le^a is also the epitope for the tumor marker CA 19-9, a useful serologic marker for monitoring patients with gastrointestinal and other malignancies.

Duffy Blood Group System (ISBT No. 008)

The Duffy (Fy) blood group system was discovered in 1951 and contains five to six antigens, Fy^a, Fy^b, Fy3, Fy5, and Fy6. Fy^a and Fy^b are autosomal codominant antigens whereas Fy3, Fy5, and Fy6 are high-incidence antigens present on all RBCs except the Duffy null phenotype. The Fy4 antigen, originally described on Fy (a–b–) RBCs, is now thought to be a distinct, unrelated antigen. Fy^a and Fy^b antigens are common antigens in white people whereas the Duffy null or Fy (a–b–) phenotype is the predominant phenotype in black people (Table 34–24). Fy^x, characterized by extremely low Fy^b expression, is somewhat rare. In addition to RBCs, the Duffy antigens are expressed on cerebellar Purkinje's cells and postcapillary venule endothelial cells. There are also reports of Duffy antigens on endothelial cells of renal glomeruli, vasa recta, thyroid and pulmonary capillaries, alveolar type 1 squamous cells, and epithelial cells of renal collecting tubules (Chaudhuri, 1997; Hadley, 1997). RBCs possess approximately 12 000–14 000 copies of Fy glycoprotein (DARC) per cell (Daniels, 2002).

Biochemistry

The Duffy antigens reside on DARC or Duffy antigen receptor for chemokines (Fig. 34–10). The latter is a 338-amino-acid, integral membrane glycoprotein, containing a 62-amino-acid extracellular amino-terminus, seven transmembrane domains, and an intracellular carboxy-terminus rich in serine and threonine residues. The amino-terminal domain possesses three *N*-glycosylation sites and is linked to the third extracellular loop by a disulfide bond to form a hepatohelical structure. A second disulfide bond exists between the first and second extracellular loops. The Fy^a, Fy^b, and Fy6 antigens reside on the amino-terminal domain of DARC and are sensitive to proteolytic cleavage. The amino-terminal domain is also the binding site for *Plasmodium vivax* and plays a role in chemokine binding. The high-incidence antigen, Fy3, is believed to reside on the third extracellular loop (Hadley, 1997; Wasniowska, 2004).

IV

CHAPTER: 34 Immunohematology

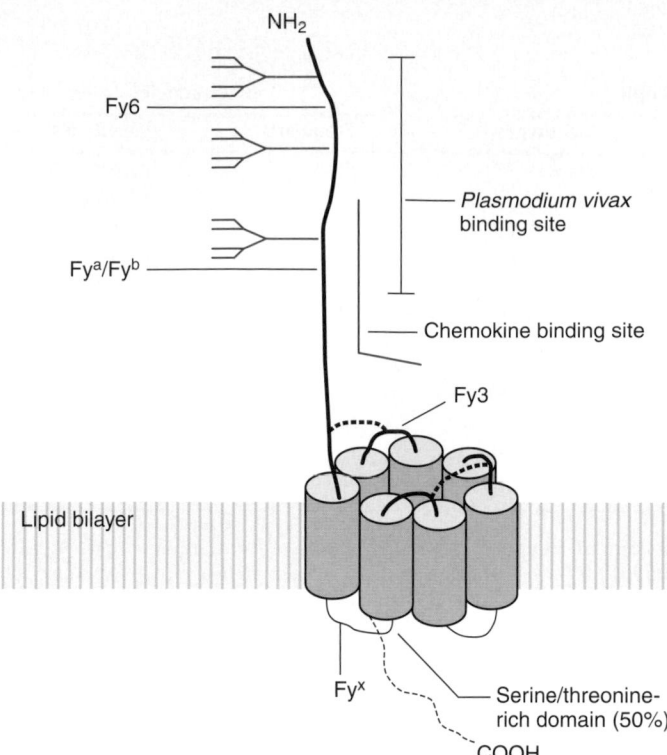

Figure 34–10 Duffy glycoprotein or DARC (*duffy antigen receptor for chemokine molecule*). DARC contains a 62-amino-acid, extracellular amino-terminal domain and seven transmembrane domains, indicated by solid amber cylinders. A disulfide bond exists between the amino-terminal domain and the third extracellular loop. A second disulfide bond exists between the first and second extracellular loops. Three *N*-glycosylation sites are indicated by branched structures. The sites of the Fy3, Fy6, and Fyª/Fyᵇ antigens are indicated by arrows. The binding site for *Plasmodium vivax* exists between amino acids 8 and 44 and includes the Fy6 and Fyª/Fyᵇ antigens. The chemokine-binding site lies in a cleft between the amino-terminal domain and the third extracellular loop. The mutation leading to the Fyˣ phenotype, characterized by weak Fyᵇ expression, is present in the first cytoplasmic loop.

Molecular Biology

Located on chromosome 1q22-23, the Duffy gene (*FY*) is a 1014-bp gene containing two exons, a small upstream exon encoding the first seven amino acids, and a second exon encoding the rest of the molecule (Hadley, 1997). The promoter region contains consensus sequences for multiple *cis*-regulatory elements including AP-1, Sp1, and GATA-1, an erythroid transcription activator binding protein that controls transcription of DARC in erythroid cells (Iwamoto, 1996). Phylogenetic studies indicate that *Fy*B* is the ancestral gene of human and nonhuman primates (Li, 1997). Genetic studies have identified four Duffy alleles: *FY*A*, *FY*B*, *FY*Fy*, and *FY*X* responsible for the Fyª, Fyᵇ, Fy null, and Fyˣ phenotypes, respectively (Table 34–24). The codominant alleles, *FY*A* and *FY*B*, differ by a single amino acid (Asp42Gly; G131A). The Fyˣ phenotype (*FY*X*), characterized by extremely weak Fyᵇ expression, arises from an Arg89>Cys substitution in the first cytoplasmic loop, leading to protein instability (Tournamille, 1998; Yazdanbakhsh, 2000).

Two distinct mechanisms are responsible for the Fy null or Fy (a–b–) phenotype. In white people and others, the *FY* gene is disrupted (*FY*amorph*), leading to a complete absence of DARC on all tissues (Daniels, 2002). As a result, these individuals can make alloantibodies to all Duffy antigens, including high-incidence antigens (Fy3, Fy5). In contrast, black Fy (a–b–) individuals are homozygous for *FY*Fy*, a *FY*B*-like allele that possess a point mutation in the *FY* gene promoter that abrogates the consensus binding site for GATA-1. The latter is an erythroid transcription binding factor that regulates the expression of *FY* and other genes in RBCs (Iwamoto, 1996; Moulds, 1998). As a result, *FY* transcription is absent in RBCs but is present in endothelial and epithelial cells, which utilize other promoter enhancer elements. Because Fyᵇ is expressed on nonerythroid cells, black Fy (a–b–) individuals do not make anti-Fyᵇ and only rarely make anti-Fy3.

Duffy Antibodies

Antibodies against Fyª, Fyᵇ, and other Duffy antigens are clinically significant and are associated with HDN, immediate and delayed

Table 34–25 Phenotypes of the Kidd System

Reactions with anti-			Phenotype	Frequency (%) US population		Comments
Jkª	Jkᵇ	Jk3		Caucasian	Black	
+	0	+	Jk (a+b–)	28	57	Autosomal codominant
+	+	+	Jk (a+b+)	49	34	Sensitive 2 M urea
0	+	+	Jk (a–b+)	23	9	
Null phenotypes (Jk_null)						
0	0	0	Jk (a–b–)	Very rare	Very rare	Autosomal recessive Resistant 2 M urea
0/w*	0/w*	w*	Jk (a–b–)	–	–	In (Jk), autosomal dominant Rare, Japanese only Partially resistant 2 M urea

* Weak Jk antigens detected only by adsorption and elution techniques.

hemolytic transfusion reactions. They are usually of IgG isotype, reactive at 37°C and are only detected in the IAT. Antibodies against Fyª, Fyᵇ, and Fy6 antigens, which reside on the long amino-terminal domain of DARC, can be inhibited by prior protease digestion of RBCs. In contrast, Fy5 and Fy3 antigens are relatively resistant to protease digestion. Antibodies against Duffy antigens can demonstrate dosage.

Clinically, anti-Fyª is the most common alloantibody encountered and can be observed in Fy (a–) individuals of all races. Anti-Fyᵇ is relatively uncommon and observed primarily in nonblack people. Alloantibodies against the high-incidence antigens Fy3 and Fy5 are rare, occurring predominantly in white, Fy null individuals. Anti-Fy3 behaves like an anti-Fyª⁺ᵇ, reacting with all Duffy-positive RBC. Anti-Fy5 also reacts like an anti-Fyª⁺ᵇ but requires the presence of Rh antigens for reactivity. Anti-Fy6 has not been observed clinically, but is the epitope for an anti-Duffy monoclonal antibody (Daniels, 2002).

Biological Role

DARC is a chemokine-binding protein, capable of binding several inflammatory chemokines from the C-X-C and C-C families (Gardner, 2004), including interleukin-8, RANTES, and MCP-1 (Fig. 34–10). DARC does not transmit an intracellular signal upon binding chemokines, but may facilitate leukocyte recruitment to sites of inflammation by establishing a chemokine gradient and transporting chemokines across activated endothelium (Lee, 2003a). In mice, DARC acts as a chemokine sink, helping to maintain circulating chemokine concentrations (Fukuma, 2003). In humans, there is no clinical syndrome associated with a Fy null phenotype; however, DARC and a Fy null phenotype may contribute to poor graft survival following renal transplantation (Akalin, 2003; Segerer, 2003). The DARC binding site for chemokines lies in a cleft involving the amino-terminal domain and the third extracellular loop (Fig. 34–10).

DARC is also the receptor for *P. vivax*, which binds DARC near the Fy⁶ epitope. Reticulocytes from Fy null individuals are resistant to *P. vivax* infection, providing a selective advantage to populations living in malaria endemic areas. The latter likely explains the prevalence of the Fy null phenotype among black people.

Kidd Blood Group System (ISBT No. 009)

The Kidd blood group system consists of two allelic antigens, Jkª and Jkᵇ. Inheritance is autosomal codominant with three predominant phenotypes (Table 34–25). A fourth phenotype, Jk_null or Jk (a–b–), is very rare except among Polynesians (≤ 1%) and Finns. In addition to RBCs, Kidd antigens are expressed along descending vasa recta endothelial cells of the renal medulla. There is also evidence to suggest low-level, constitutive expression of Kidd on heart, skeletal muscle, colon, small intestine, thymus, brain, pancreas, spleen, prostate, bladder, and liver (Olives, 1996). There are 14 000 Kidd epitopes per human RBC (Lucien, 2002).

Null Phenotypes

Jk_null is autosomal recessive, reflecting homozygosity for a *JK*Jk* or amorph allele (Table 34–25). In(Jk) is a second Jk_null phenotype that is characterized by very weak Kidd expression. Like In(Lu), the In(Jk) phenotype is autosomal dominant due to a suppressor gene at a distant, unrelated locus. Interestingly, Jk_null RBCs are resistant to lysis by 2 M urea,

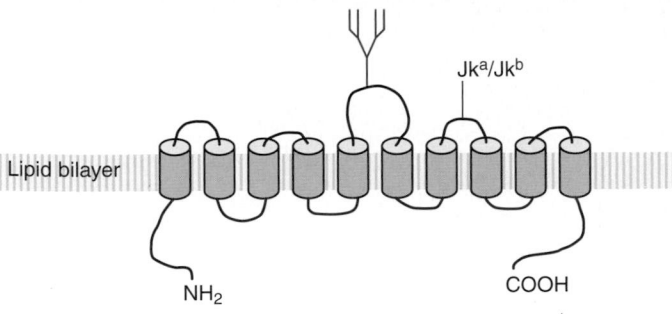

Jk^a/Jk^b

Lipid bilayer

NH₂   COOH

Figure 34–11 The Kidd/urea transporter glycoprotein. The site of Jk^a/Jk^b polymorphism at residue 280 is indicated by a solid line. The *N*-glycosylation site is indicated by a branched structure on the third extracellular loop. The 10 transmembrane domains are represented by amber cylinders.

a lytic agent used by some automated hematology analyzers. In(Jk) RBCs have intermediate resistance to urea (Issitt, 1998).

Biochemistry

The apparent resistance to urea by Jk$_{null}$ RBCs became clear with cloning and isolation of the human erythroid urea transporter (UT-B). The latter is a 43- to 45-kDa multipass glycoprotein, which shares 60% homology with the vasopressin-sensitive urea transporter of rabbits (UT2) and humans (HUT2, UT-A) (Lucien, 1998). The molecule is a 391-amino-acid protein with 10 transmembrane domains and a cytosolic amino- and carboxy-terminus (Fig. 34–11). A single *N*-glycan is present on the third extracellular loop (Asn222) and expresses ABO antigens (Lucien, 2002). The Jk^a/Jk^b antigens reside on the fourth extracellular loop at amino acid 280. The third extracellular loop may play a key role in urea transport.

Molecular Biology

The Kidd glycoprotein is encoded by a 30-kb gene (*JK*, *SLC14A1*, *UT-B*) on chromosome 18q12-21. This is the same location as the human HUT2/UT-A urea transporter (61% homology), suggesting that the two genes arose by gene duplication. The JK gene is organized over 11 exons, although only exons 4–11 encode the mature protein (Lucien, 1998). Like many blood group genes, the promoter region contains a GATA-1 consensus sequence as well as other *cis*-regulatory elements (AP-2, AP-3, NF-ATp, Sp1, Ets-1). A single base-pair transition (G823A) is the molecular basis of the Jk^a/Jk^b polymorphism, resulting in an Asp280 (Jk^a) or Asn280 (Jk^b) (Lucien, 2002). In the autosomal recessive Jk$_{null}$ phenotype, five distinct inactivating mutations have been identified, including splice site, nonsense and missense mutations (Daniels, 2002). The etiology of the In(Jk) phenotype is unknown.

Kidd Antibodies

Clinically, anti-Jk or Kidd antibodies are a common cause of hemolytic transfusion reactions, accounting for nearly one-quarter of all delayed hemolytic transfusion reactions and 75% of those with true hemolytic sequelae (Ness, 1990). They are usually of IgG1 or IgG3 isotype and are capable of activating complement (Table 34–7). Antibody reactivity can be enhanced with enzyme-treated RBCs and by the presence of complement. An anti-Jk^3, which reacts with all RBCs except Jk$_{null}$, is observed in Jk$_{null}$ individuals (Table 34–25).

Anti-Jk antibodies can be difficult to detect or identify in the blood bank. Anti-Jk antibodies are often low titer with weak avidity and can display dosage in vitro. Furthermore, anti-Jk antibodies are frequently transient, disappearing rapidly after immune stimulation. As a consequence, patients previously sensitized to Kidd antigens may be negative for anti-Jk antibodies in later blood samples. Following transfusion of 'crossmatch-compatible,' Jk-positive RBCs, sensitized patients can mount a brisk anamnestic antibody response with rapid and extensive in vivo hemolysis as RBCs are cleared by extravascular and intravascular hemolysis. Although uncommon, anti-Jk can cause a mild HDN.

Biological Role

Biologically, JK/UT-B functions in the facilitated transport of urea. In kidney, transport of urea by JK/UT-B on vasa recta endothelial cells is thought to help stabilize osmotic gradients in the renal medulla during the concentration of urine. On RBCs, JK/UT-B may help preserve the osmotic stability of RBCs as they pass through the kidney. Although Jk$_{null}$ individuals exhibit a slightly decreased capacity to concentrate urine, the absence of JK/UT-B is not associated with a clinical syndrome. It is likely that other mechanisms exist to compensate or reduplicate the function of JK/UT-B on tissues (Lucien, 1998).

Table 34-26 Diego Blood Group Antigens

Antigen (high-frequency)	Percent donors	Amino acid change* (high → low frequency)	Percent donors	Antigen (low-frequency)
Di^b	> 99.9%	Pro854>Leu	Very rare[†]	Di^a
Wr^b	99%	Glu658>Lys	1%	Wr^a
		Val557>Met	< 0.1%	Wd^a
		Pro548>Leu	< 0.1%	Rb^a
		Thr552>Ile	< 0.1%	WARR
		Arg432>Trp	< 0.1%	ELO
		Gly565>Ala	< 0.1%	Wu
		Asn569>Lys	< 0.1%	Bp^a
		Arg656>His	< 0.1%	Mo^a
		Arg656>Cys	< 0.1%	Hg^a
		Tyr555>His	< 0.1%	Vg^a
		Lys551>Asn	< 0.1%	Tr^a
		Arg646>Gln	< 0.1%	Sw^a
		Glu429>Asp	< 0.1%	NFLD
		Pro566>Ser	< 0.1%	Jn^a
		Pro566>Ala	< 0.1%	KREP
		Pro561>Ser	< 0.1%	BOW
		Glu480>Lys	< 0.1%	Fr^a
		Arg646>Trp	< 0.1%	SWI

* Referenced in Jarolim et al. (1998); Issitt (1998); Reid (2004b).

† Di^a antigen has a much higher incidence among North and South American Indians, Asian people, and people of Mongolian ancestry (e.g., Eastern Poland).

Diego Blood Group System (ISBT No. 010)

The Diego blood group system consists of 21 antigens, including four sets of allelic antigens (Table 34–26). Nineteen antigens are rare, low-incidence antigens present on less then 1% of donors. In general, there are no apparent racial differences in the expression of most Diego antigens except Di^a. Initially described in 1955, Di^a antigen is rare in all populations except those of Mongolian ancestry, Asian people, and native South American Indians. In some South American Indian populations, the frequency of Di^a can reach 50% (Issitt, 1998). In addition to RBCs, Diego antigens are expressed by human kidney along the collecting ducts (Tanner, 1993). There are one million copies of Diego glycoprotein (AE1) per RBC.

Biochemistry

The Diego blood group system resides on band 3, also known as anion exchange protein 1 (AE1). AE1 is a 100-kDa, 991-amino-acid glycoprotein containing two functionally distinct domains, a large 40-kDa amino-terminal cytoplasmic domain and a transmembrane domain comprising the carboxy-terminal half of the molecule (Fig. 34–12). On RBCs, AE1 is an oligomer, usually existing as either a dimer or tetramer through the formation of intramolecular disulfide bonds. The amino-terminal cytoplasmic domain binds several key cytoskeletal proteins (band 4.1, band 4.2, and ankyrin) and three glycolytic enzymes; glutaraldehyde-3-phosphate dehydrogenase (G3PD), aldolase, and phosphofructokinase (PFK). Binding of hemochromes or denatured hemoglobin to the extreme amino-terminus of AE1 is believed to play a role in Heinz body formation. There is also an apparent, noncovalent association of AE1 with glycophorin A on RBC membranes (Low, 1986).

The remainder of AE1 is membrane associated, containing 12–14 transmembrane domains, which constitute the carboxy-terminal half of the molecule. Whereas the amino-terminal domain is involved in membrane stability, the carboxy-terminal domain functions as an anion transporter, facilitating transfusion of Cl$^-$ and HCO$_3^-$ anions across the cell membrane (Tanner, 1993). The carboxy-terminal, transmembrane domain is also the site of all the Diego antigens described to date. There is also a single *N*-glycosylation site, which displays a massive, highly branched, polylactosaminoglycan with both ABO and I blood group activity (Fukuda, 1984). It is estimated that nearly half of all ABO epitopes on RBCs are associated with AE1.

Molecular Biology

AE1 is the product of a 20-exon, 17-kb gene (*SLC4A1*) on chromosome 17 (17qter). The cloning of the AE1 gene was invaluable in assigning several

IV

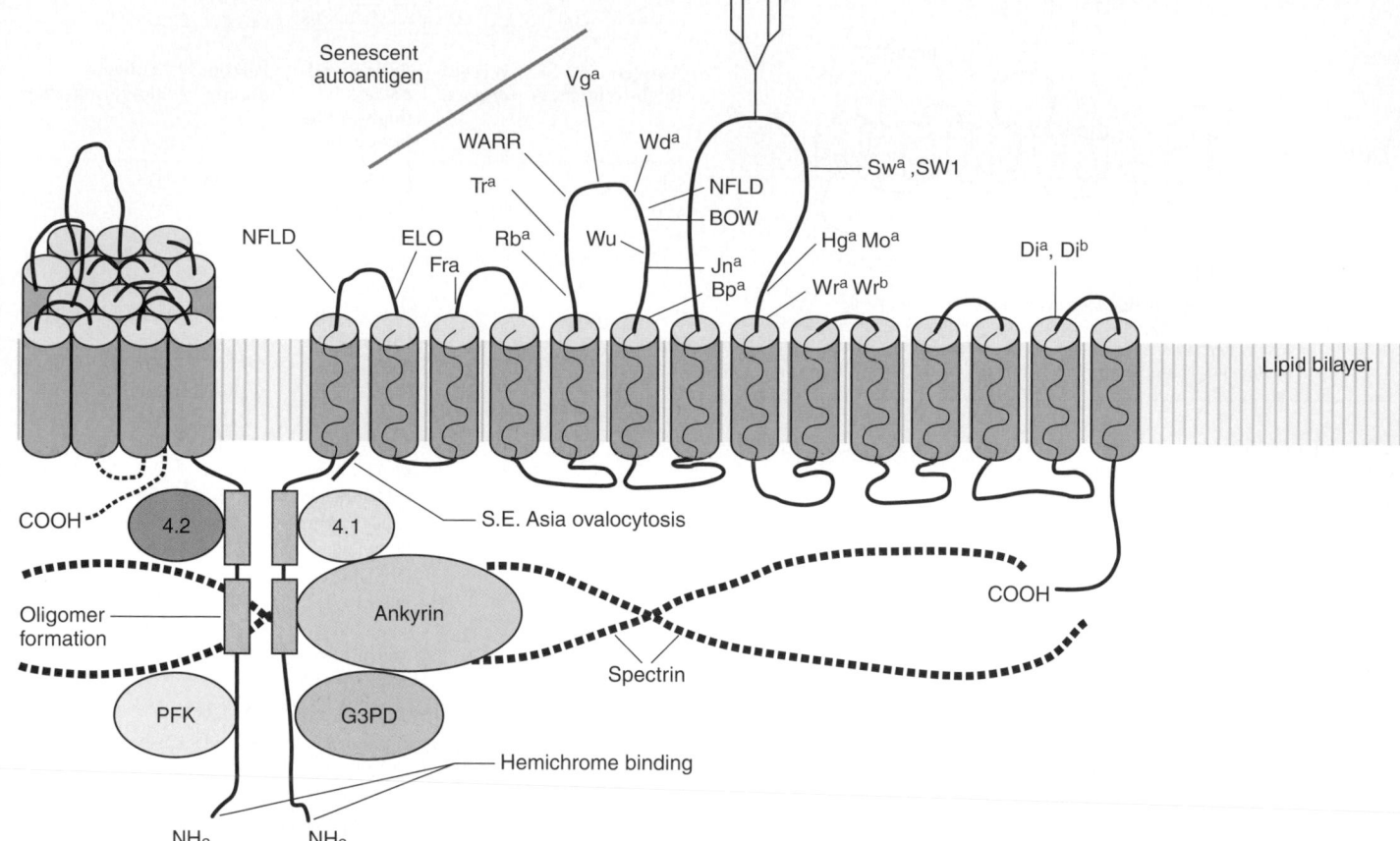

Figure 34–12 Structure of anion exchange protein AE1 (band 3). AE1 is a multipass glycoprotein with 14 transmembrane domains, indicated by solid amber cylinders. The Diego blood group antigens reside along the extracellular loops and are indicated by solid lines. The AE1 senescent autoantigen is on the third extracellular loop between Rb^a and Vg^a antigens. The massive N-glycan is shown by a branched structure on the fourth extracellular loop. The large cytoplasmic domain has binding sites for cytoskeletal proteins 4.2, 4.1, and ankyrin as well as the glycolytic enzymes phosphofructokinase (PFK) and glutaraldehyde-3-phosphate dehydrogenase (G3PD). In the red cell membrane, AE1 exists as oligomers (dimers, tetramers) linked by interchain disulfide bonds along the amino-terminal cytoplasmic domain (solid rectangles). An 8-amino-acid deletion at the boundary of the amino-terminal cytoplasmic domain and first transmembrane domain is responsible for Southeast Asia ovalocytosis (SAO).

orphan antigens to the Diego system. Like so many blood group antigens, every Diego antigen identified to date is the result of a point mutation, leading to an amino acid polymorphism, in the translated protein (Table 34–26, Fig. 34–12). Most of these amino acid polymorphisms occur among nonconserved amino acid residues, based on a comparison of AE1 with the sequences of other anion transporters (Jarolim, 1998; Reid, 2004b). The Diego system also contains two examples of allelic, low-incidence antigens: Mo^a/Hg^a and Jn^a/KREP. In each case, two distinct amino acid substitutions at the same amino acid residue lead to different alloantigens. A similar example exists in the Kell system (Kp^a, Kp^b, and Kp^c).

The most interesting Diego antigen, however, is Wr^b. As stated earlier, AE1 is topically associated with glycophorin A in the RBC membrane. RBCs lacking glycophorin A (En (a–) phenotype) are phenotypically Wr (a–b–), implying that Wr^b is on glycophorin A. Available evidence now suggests that Wr^b is formed by an electrostatic interaction between glycophorin A and a glutamic acid (Glu658) on AE1. Which specific amino acid on glycophorin A is critical to Wr^b formation is still a matter of debate, but clearly part of the Wr^b epitope involves amino acids on glycophorin A (see Fig. 34–8) (Poole, 1999).

Diego Antibodies

Antibodies against Diego blood group antigens can be either immune stimulated or naturally occurring. Antibodies against Di^a, Di^b, Wr^b, and ELO are usually immune stimulated. These antibodies are of IgG isotype and are detected in the AHG phase of testing. Anti-Di^a, Di^b, and Wr^b can be associated with decreased red cell survival, hemolytic transfusion reactions and HDN. Anti-Wr^b is also associated with autoimmune hemolytic anemia (Issitt, 1998).

In contrast, antibodies against the majority of other Diego antigens are usually naturally occurring, room temperature, saline agglutinins. Anti-Wr^a is particularly common, occurring in 1 in 100 donors. Antibodies against Wd^a and WARR are also fairly common, with anti-WARR reported in 13–18% of donors (Issitt, 1998).

Biological Role

Functionally, AE1 plays a critical role in gas transport and acid–base equilibrium. To facilitate the removal of CO_2, RBCs hydrate CO_2 via carbonic anhydrous to form bicarbonate ion (HCO_3^-) which is readily soluble in plasma. As the level of intracellular HCO_3^- rises, RBCs exchange HCO_3^- ions for Cl^- in plasma (the Cl^- shift or Hamburger shift). This process is mediated by AE1 as RBCs pass through capillaries and small capillary venules. Because of the high copy number of AE1 on the RBC membrane, anion exchange is 90% complete within 0.4–0.5 second. In the kidney, AE1 is expressed along the basolateral membrane of type A intercalated cells of renal collecting ducts, where it functions in acid secretion and bicarbonate readsorption (Tanner, 1993). Given the physiologic importance of AE1, it is not surprising that no Diego null phenotype has been described to date.

AE1 also plays a role in the RBC cytoskeleton (Fig. 34–12). The long, amino-terminal half of the molecule binds several peripheral proteins involved in the stability of the RBC membrane. AE1 tetramers bind ankyrin, protein 4.2 and protein 4.1, which help to anchor and stabilize the RBC membrane to the underlying cytoskeleton (Tanner, 1993). AE1 protein may also serve as a senescent autoantigen, marking old RBCs for removal by the reticuloendothelial system. As RBCs age, they bind an increasing amount of immunoglobulin and complement C3. At least one 'senescent' autoantigen on RBCs is located on AE1, between amino acids 538 and 554 (between Rb^a and Vg^a antigens; Fig. 34–12) (Kay, 1994).

Cartwright Blood Group System (ISBT No. 011)

Discovered in 1956, the Cartwright (Yt) blood group system consists of two autosomal codominant antigens, Yt^a and Yt^b. Yt^a is a high-incidence antigen expressed by 99.8% of Caucasian donors. The incidence of Yt^b varies by race, ranging from 0% in Japanese to 24–26% in the Mideast (Issitt, 1998). Yt antigens are missing on PNH III RBCs, which are devoid of all glycophosphoinositol (GPI)-linked glycoproteins. In addition to RBCs, Cartwright antigens are expressed on neural synapses and

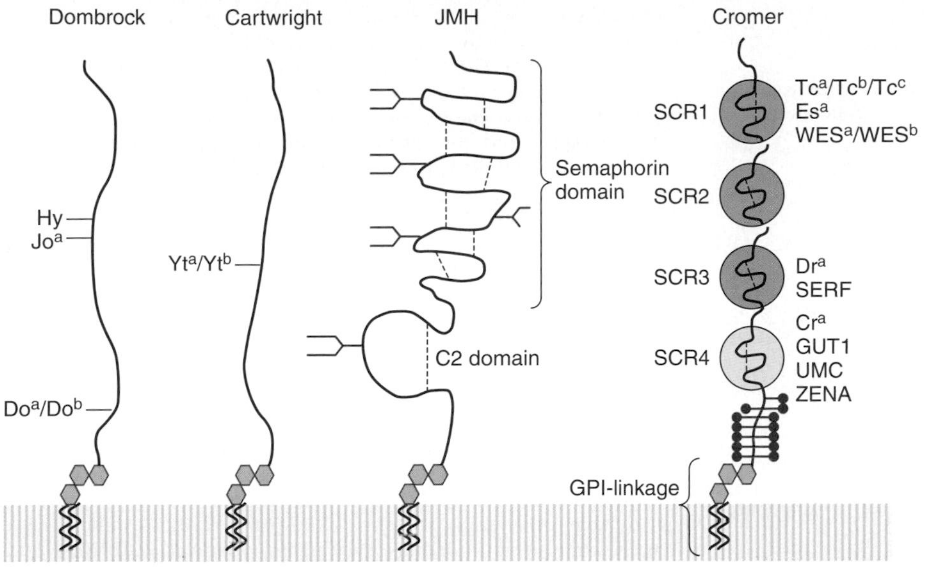

Figure 34–13 Blood group antigens on glycophosphoinositol-linked glycoproteins.

neuromuscular junctions (Masson, 1994). There are 7000–10 000 molecules of Yt glycoprotein per RBC.

Biochemistry

The Cartwright antigens are located on acetylcholinesterase (ACHE), a β-carboxyesterase responsible for degradation of the neurotransmitter acetylcholine. Several different molecular forms of acetylcholinesterase have been isolated, including large heteromeric forms composed of several catalytic subunits covalently linked to collagen. On RBCs, acetylcholinesterase is expressed as a palmitoylated, glycophosphoinositol (GPI)-linked glycoprotein (Fig. 34–13) (Li, 1991). Human erythrocyte acetylcholinesterase is unique in the palmitoylation or covalent linkage of a palmitic fatty acid to the inositol ring, which renders the molecule resistant to phospholipase C. In RBC membranes, ACHE usually exists as a 160-kD dimer and possess both *N*- and *O*-linked glycans.

Molecular Biology

The gene for acetylcholinesterase (*ACHE*) possesses four exons, spanning 4.5–4.7 kb, on chromosome 7q22. Alternate splicing of exon 3 is responsible for the GPI-linked form of acetylcholinesterase observed in RBCs (Li, 1991). The Yt^a and Yt^b antigens represent a single amino acid polymorphism at residue 322, where His322 is Yt^a and Asn322 is Yt^b (Bartels, 1993). The Yt^a/Yt^b polymorphism is not located near the catalytic site of the enzyme and has no effect on enzyme activity (Masson, 1994).

Cartwright Antibodies

In general, anti-Yt^a and Yt^b are clinically benign, although shortened red cell survival and even delayed hemolytic transfusion reactions have been reported. Neither antibody is associated with HDN (Issitt, 1998). Anti-Yt^a and anti-Yt^b are of IgG isotype, arising from immune stimulation, and are usually detected in the IAT. Despite the high incidence of Yt^a in the general population, anti-Yt^a is more common than anti-Yt^b, suggesting that Yt^a is the more immunogenic antigen.

Biological Role

Acetylcholinesterase is a critical enzyme required for the rapid degradation of acetylcholine on postsynaptic membranes of nerves and muscles. The role of acetylcholinesterase on RBCs is unknown.

Xg Blood Group System (ISBT No. 012)

The Xg blood group system contains a single antigen, Xg^a. As a result, only two phenotypes are known; Xg^a-positive and Xg^a-negative. Because the Xg^a antigen is encoded by a gene on the X chromosome, the incidence of the Xg^a-positive phenotype is higher among women. Among Caucasians, approximately 89% of women and 66% of men are Xg^a-positive. Similar results have been found in other ethnic populations (Byrne, 2004). Xg appears to be specific for RBCs. There are approximately 9000 molecules of Xg^a per RBC (Reid, 2004b).

Biochemistry and Molecular Biology

The Xg^a antigen is located on a 24- to 29-kDa, 180-amino-acid glycoprotein named XG protein. A type 1 glycoprotein, XG protein possesses a large, 117-amino-acid, amino-terminal extracellular domain, a single transmembrane domain, and a short, carboxy-terminal cytoplasmic tail. Of 11 potential *O*-glycosylation sites, only three appear to be glycosylated. The protein is encoded by a 2.4-kb gene (*XG*) located on the X chromosome at the pseudoautosomal boundary/X-specific boundary (pAB1X).

In the RBC membrane, the XG protein may be topologically associated with a second protein, MIC2 or CD99. The latter is a 32.5-kDa glycoprotein biochemically similar to XG protein. Evidence suggesting a near-neighbor relationship of the XG and MIC2 proteins includes MIC2 inhibition of anti-Xg^a antibodies and co-immunoprecipitation of MIC2 by anti-Xg^a. And finally, high MIC2 expression is observed on Xg^a-positive, but not Xg^a-negative, erythrocytes (Daniels, 2002).

Xg^a Antibodies

Anti-Xg^a is not associated with either hemolytic transfusion reactions or HDN (Byrne, 2004). Anti-Xg^a may be immune stimulated or naturally occurring. Most examples are of IgG isotype, including some capable of activating complement. Because of differences in Xg^a-positive phenotype between men and women, most examples (> 85%) of anti-Xg^a are observed in men.

Scianna Blood Group System (ISBT No. 013)

The Scianna (Sc) blood group system (Table 34–27) contains four antigens, Sc1, Sc2, Sc3, and Rd (Radin) (Wagner, 2003). Sc1 and Sc2 are antithetical antigens; Sc3 is a high-incidence antigen present on all RBCs except Sc$_{null}$ (1–, –2, –3); Rd is a low-incidence antigen; Scianna appears to be specific for RBCs and erythropoietic tissues.

Biochemistry

Scianna antigens reside on *e*rythrocyte *m*embrane-*a*ssociated *p*rotein (ERMAP), a 60–68 kD, 446-amino-acid glycoprotein. Like Lutheran, Ok and LW proteins, ERMAP is a member of the immunoglobulin superfamily. The molecule is a type 1 single-pass transmembrane protein possessing a single IgV domain and a large cytoplasmic domain that is likely involved in signal transduction. The latter possess both SH3 and B30.2 domains as well as multiple phosphorylation sequences for protein kinase C, tyrosine kinase and casein kinase II (Su, 2001). Three Scianna antigens are located in the extracellular domain near the IgV domain. The molecule possesses several cysteine residues and is sensitive to sulfhydryl-reducing agents.

Molecular Biology

The *ERMAP* gene resides on chromosome 1p34 and consists of 11 exons spanning 19 kb. Sc1, Sc2 and Rd are the result of single amino acid polymorphisms (Table 34–27). Of one Sc$_{null}$ studied to date, there was a deletion and frameshift mutation (307del2), leading to a truncated, nonfunctional molecule (Wagner, 2003).

Scianna Antibodies

Anti-Scianna antibodies are rare and generally benign. They are usually of IgG isotype with some examples binding complement. Most examples are immune stimulated; however, naturally occurring anti-Sc2 antibodies are

Table 34–27 Phenotypes of the Scianna System

Reactions with anti-Sc				Phenotype	Amino acid	Frequency (%) population*
Sc1	Sc2	Sc3	Rd			
+	0	+	0	Sc (1, –2)	Gly57	99%
+	+	+	0	Sc (1, 2)		0.7%
0	+	+	0	Sc (–1, 2)	Arg57	< 0.01%
0	0	0	0	Sc (–1, –2, –3) or Sc null	307del2	Rare
0/+	0/+	+	+	Rd+	Pro60>Ala	< 0.01%

* From Issitt (1998).

Table 34–28 Phenotypes of the Dombrock System

Reactions with anti-Dombrock antibodies					Phenotype	Amino acid change	Frequency (%) population		Comments
Doa	Dob	Gya	Hy	Joa			White	Black	
+	0	+	+	+	Do (a+b–)	Asn265	18	11	
+	+	+	+	+	Do (a+b+)		49	44	
0	+	+	+	+	Do (a–b+)	Asp265	33	45	
Null/weak phenotypes									
0	0	0	0	0	Do$_{null}$ or Gy(a–)	Loss exon 2*	Rare	Rare	Associated with PNH III†
0	w	w	0	0/+	Hy–	Gly108>Val	0	Rare	
w	0/w	+	w	0	Jo (a–)	Thr350>Ile	0	Rare	

* Loss of exon 2 has been associated with splice-site, frameshift and nonsense mutations (Reid, 2003a).
† PNH III RBCs lack GPI-linked glycoproteins, including Dombrock antigens, CD55 and CD59.

known. The antigens are relatively resistant to enzymes but can be weakened with DTT and AET. They are not a cause of transfusion reactions. Anti-Rd and anti-Sc2 have been associated with HDN. Autoantibodies against Sc1 and Sc3 antigens have been associated with warm autoimmune hemolytic anemia (Issitt, 1998).

Biological Role

The biological role of ERMAP is unknown although its structure suggests it may play a role in RBC adhesion and signaling. The IgV domain possesses a C1q recognition sequence that may mediate adhesion between marrow macrophages and erythroblasts in erythroid islands. Because ERMAP shares homology with the B7 family of proteins (CD80, CD86) and neural autoantigens, there is speculation that ERMAP could be involved in immune recognition and autoimmune anemia (Su, 2001).

Dombrock Blood Group System (ISBT No. 014)

The Dombrock blood group system contains five antigens; Doa (DO1), Dob (DO2), Gya (DO3), Hy (DO4), and Joa (DO5). Doa and Dob are autosomal codominant antigens expressed by 67% and 82% of white donors, respectively (Table 34–28). Gya, Hy, and Joa are high-incidence antigens found on virtually all donors (> 99.9%). In addition to RBCs, Dombrock mRNA has been identified in fetal liver and spleen (Gubin, 2000).

Null/Weak Phenotypes

The Do$_{null}$ or Gy (a–) phenotype is a rare, autosomal recessive phenotype (Table 34–28). An acquired Do$_{null}$ phenotype can be observed in paroxysmal nocturnal hemoglobinuria type III (PNH-III). A hematopoietic stem cell disorder, PNH III is characterized by chronic hemolysis due to an absence of all GPI-linked glycoproteins, including decay-accelerating factor (DAF/Cromer blood group) and Dombrock.

Biochemistry

Dombrock antigens reside on an ADP-ribosyltransferase, which catalyzes the transfer of ADP-ribose from NAD to a protein acceptor. The cloned

molecule is a 47- to 58-kD, 314-amino-acid glycoprotein that is anchored into the RBC membrane via a glycophosphoinositol glycolipid tail (GPI-linked, Fig. 34–13). The molecule has five potential N-glycosylation sites, two myristoylation sites and five cysteine residues (Gubin, 2000; Daniels, 2002). As a consequence, Dombrock can be destroyed by disulfide reducing agents and phosphatidylinositol phospholipase C (PI-PLC), which cleaves GPI-linked proteins (Gubin, 2000).

Molecular Biology

The gene for Dombrock (DO, ART4) spans 14 kb on chromosome 12p13.2-12.1. The gene consists of three exons although exon 2 encodes over 70% of the translated protein and includes all five Dombrock antigens. Doa, Dob, Joa and Hy are the result of a single amino acid polymorphism (Table 34–28). The Do$_{null}$ or Gy (a–) phenotype is the result of mutations that abolish exon 2 (Reid, 2003a).

Dombrock Antibodies

Anti-Dombrock antibodies can be clinically significant although many examples are benign. They are commonly found in mixtures of alloantibodies and can be difficult to identify. Anti-Dombrock antibodies are capable of causing shortened RBC survival, acute and delayed hemolytic transfusion reactions. They are not associated with HDN. Anti-Dombrock antibodies are usually of IgG isotype, arising from immune stimulation by transfusion or pregnancy. Antibody reactivity can be enhanced by use of papain- or ficin-treated RBCs. Conversely, antibody reactivity is reduced or abolished by treatment of red cells with sulfhydryl-reducing agents (DTT, AET), trypsin, chymotrypsin, and pronase.

Biological Role

Although Dombrock is an ADP-ribosyltransferase, no enzyme activity has been reported on RBC membranes (Reid, 2003a). There is also no known clinical syndrome associated with a Do$_{null}$ phenotype. It has been hypothesized that Dombrock may play a role in clearing circulating NAD+ and/or post-translational modification of proteins (Reid, 2003a). Dombrock may also contribute to integrin-mediated cell adhesion via an RGD motif at the Dob antigen: the RGD motif is abolished in the Doa phenotype.

Colton Blood Group System (ISBT No. 015)

The Colton blood group system was initially identified in 1967 and consists of two, autosomal codominant antigens, Coa and Cob. Coa is a high-incidence antigen present on 99.7% of donors. Cob is expressed by less then 11% of donors, only 0.3% being Co (a–b+). Although very rare, a Co (a–b–) or null phenotype is reported. In addition to RBCs, Colton antigens are expressed on renal proximal tubules, thin descending limb of Henle, renal vasa recta endothelium, choroid plexus, ciliary body, microvessels, gallbladder, placenta, and some epithelial cells (Ma, 1998). There are 120 000–160 000 molecules of Colton glycoprotein per RBC.

Biochemistry

The Colton blood group antigens reside on aquaporin 1 (AQP-1) or CHIP (channel-forming integral protein), a water-selective membrane channel (Fig. 34–14). Cloned in 1991, AQP-1 is a 269-amino-acid, multipass integral membrane protein containing six transmembrane domains. Crystallographic studies suggest that the first intracellular and third extracellular loops fold back into the plasma membrane, overlapping at two Asp-Pro-Ala (NPA) sequences to form a water channel. There is a single N-glycosylation site (Asn42), capable of expressing ABH antigens, in the first extracellular loop near the Colton blood group epitope (residue 45). The latter is variably glycosylated in vivo, leading to a spectrum of AQP-1 glycoforms, ranging from 40–60 kDa (Agre, 1994). In RBC membranes, AQP-1 exists as a 'homotetramer,' a square array of AQP-1 monomers, which may help stabilize the structure and functional integrity of individual monomers (Knepper, 1994).

Molecular Biology

AQP-1 is a 17-kb gene on chromosome 7p14. The gene has four exons and both TATA and Sp1 consensus sequences in the promoter region (Moon, 1993). The Coa and Cob antigens are the result of an A314T polymorphism, leading to either an Ala45 (Coa) or Val45 (Cob) (Smith, 1994). Several different inactivating mutations of the AQP-1 gene are associated with the Colton null phenotype, including deletion of exon 1, frameshift and missense mutations. An acquired Colton null phenotype is also reported in rare patients with monosomy 7 and congenital dyserythropoietic anemia (Agre, 1994).

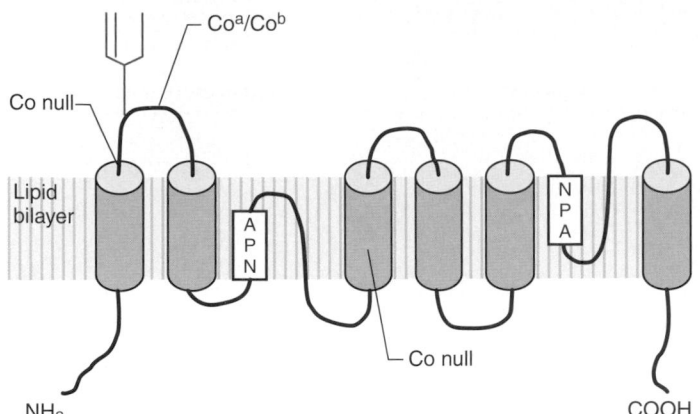

Figure 34–14 Structure of aquaporin-1 (AQP-1, CHIP). AQP-1 is a multipass protein containing six transmembrane domains, indicated by solid amber cylinders. The first cytoplasmic and third extracellular loop fold back into the lipid bilayer, overlapping at two Asp-Pro-Ala (NPA) motifs, to form a water channel. The N-glycosylation site is indicated by a branched structure on the first extracellular loop. The Co^a/Co^b polymorphism at amino acid 45 is indicated by a solid line. The sites of two mutations leading to a Colton null phenotype are also shown.

Colton Antibodies

Anti-Colton antibodies can be clinically significant, associated with shortened RBC survival, hemolytic transfusion reactions and HDN (Table 34–7). Antibodies to Co^a and Co^b are usually of IgG isotype, resulting from immune stimulation by either transfusion or pregnancy. Some examples of anti-Co^a and anti-Co^b are reported to bind complement. Anti-Colton antibodies are detectable in the AHG phase of testing and are enhanced with protease-treated RBC. Colton null individuals can also make an anti-Co3 (anti-Co^{a+b}), an alloantibody that reacts equally well with Co (a+b−) and Co (a−b+) RBCs (Issitt, 1998).

Biological Role

Biologically, AQP-1 is a major molecular water channel on RBCs and facilitates the concentration of urine in kidney (Ma, 1998). Despite its importance in water regulation, Colton-null individuals show little or no adverse clinical effects. Colton-null RBCs appear morphologically normal in appearance and number, although mild decreases in RBC life span is reported (Mathai, 1996). The absence of any clinically significant hematologic sequelae in Colton-null individuals is most likely due to the presence of a second aquaporin, AQP-3. A glycerol and, perhaps, urea transporter, AQP-3 (GIL blood group) is moderately permeable to water and appears to account for the residual water permeability on Colton null RBCs (Roudier, 1998).

LW Blood Group System (ISBT No. 016)

Named in honor of its discoverers, the LW or Landsteiner–Wiener blood group system is most important for its role in the history of the Rh blood group system. Landsteiner and Wiener originally developed antibodies against the LW antigens by immunizing rabbits with rhesus monkey red cells. The resulting 'anti-Rh' antibodies were initially believed to recognize the RhD antigen; however, later investigators proved that the antibodies developed by Landsteiner and Wiener recognized a non-Rh (LW) antigen.

The LW blood group system consists of two allelic antigens, LW^a and LW^b. LW^a is a high-frequency antigen (99% of white donors). Expression of LW antigen is dependent on RhD protein expression, with the highest expression observed on Rh-positive red cells. LW antigens are absent from Rh_{null} erythrocytes. An LW (a−b−) or null phenotype can also be seen in very rare individuals who are homozygous for a silent LW allele. The LW antigen is expressed on RBCs and placenta. There are approximately 3600–5000 molecules of LW glycoprotein per RBC (Issitt, 1998).

Biochemistry

The LW antigens reside on intracellular adhesion molecule type 4 (ICAM-4, CD242), a 40- to 47-kD type 1 glycoprotein. A member of the immunoglobulin superfamily, ICAM consists of two extracellular C2-like domains, a single transmembrane domain and a short cytoplasmic tail. There are four N-glycosylation sites and evidence of O-glycosylation. The molecule has three disulfide bonds and is sensitive to reducing agents such as DTT (Reid, 2004b).

Molecular Biology

The ICAM4 gene resides on chromosome 19p13. The LW^a and LW^b antigens arise from a single nucleotide polymorphism (A308G), leading to either a Gln70 (LW^a) or Arg70 (LW^b). Of two LW-null individuals studied, one possessed a 10-bp deletion in the coding sequence (Hermand, 1995).

LW Antibodies

Clinically benign, anti-LW antibodies are not a cause of hemolytic transfusion reactions or HDN. They are usually of IgG isotype and detected in the IAT. Antibody activity can be reduced by EDTA and pretreatment of RBCs with sulfhydryl-reducing agents (DTT, AET). In addition to anti-LW^a and -LW^b, LW null individuals can make an anti-LW^{ab}, which reacts with both LW (a+b−) and LW (a−b+) erythrocytes.

Biological Role

LW glycoprotein is a potential counter-receptor for the β_2-integrin protein Mac1 (CD11b/CD18) and LFA-1 (CD11a/CD18). It is hypothesized that the LW glycoprotein may participate in adhesive interactions during early erythroid development. LW expression is elevated in sickle cell patients and may be involved in microvascular occlusion (Reid, 2004b). LW glycoprotein may also be involved in red cell senescence by binding to Mac1 receptors on splenic macrophages (Issitt, 1998).

Chido/Rodgers Blood Group System (ISBT No. 017)

The Chido/Rodgers (Ch/Rg) blood group system contains 10 antigens, including two pairs of antithetical antigens and three conformational antigens. The latter require coexpression of two, spatially distinct Ch/Rg antigens that together generate a third, conformational antigen (Table 34–29). Most Ch/Rg antigens are high-incidence antigens (> 90%). Like the Lewis blood group antigens, Ch/Rg antigens are of plasma origin and are passively adsorbed onto RBC membranes. Ch/Rg are weakly expressed on cord RBCs and some glycophorin A deficient RBCs (Issitt, 1998).

Biochemistry/Molecular Biology

Chido/Rodgers antigens are antigenic determinants on the C4d fragment of the C4 complement molecule. C4 is the product of two, highly homologous genes (99% identity), C4A and C4B, on chromosome 6p21.3 near the HLA locus. At present, there are over fifty C4 alleles identified, including null alleles, making the genetics of this system quite difficult. Each gene spans approximately 22 kb and is organized into 41 exons. Four amino acids in exon 26 are responsible for distinguishing C4A from C4B. Most Chido/Rodgers antigens are determined by amino acid polymorphisms encoded in exons 25 and 28 (Giles, 1988). In general, Chido antigens are on C4B and Rodgers antigens are on C4A although examples of C4B expressing Rodgers antigens (and vice versa) are known (Giles 1987, 1988). On protein electrophoresis, C4A migrates faster then C4B.

Chido/Rodgers Antibodies

Antibodies against Ch/Rg antigens do not cause hemolytic transfusion reactions or HDN. There are rare reports of anaphylaxis following transfusion of plasma and platelets (Westhoff, 1992). Anti-Ch/Rg antibodies are of IgG isotype and are usually detected with AHG. Antibody reactivity can be enhanced by incubating RBCs in a low ionic sucrose solution. Antibody reactivity can be inhibited by plasma or by treatment of RBCs with proteases (Reid, 2004b).

Biological Role

C4 deficiency is associated with autoimmune disorders and susceptibility to bacterial meningitis. Specific C4 allotypes have been linked to several autoimmune disorders including rheumatoid arthritis and Graves' disease.

Gerbich Blood Group System (ISBT No. 020)

The Gerbich (Ge) blood group system contains seven antigens: three high-frequency (> 99%; Table 34–30) and four low-frequency antigens. The Gerbich glycoproteins (GPC/D; Fig. 34–15) are on fetal and adult RBCs, platelets, kidney and fetal liver. There are between 180 000–250 000 molecules of Gerbich per RBC (Reid, 2004b).

Null/Weak Phenotypes

There are three autosomal-recessive phenotypes associated with the loss of high-incidence Gerbich antigens; Yus (Ge −2,3,4), Gerbich (Ge −2, −3,4) and Leach (Ge −2, −3, −4). Gerbich antigens are decreased in patients with hereditary elliptocytosis due to protein 4.1 deficiency (Daniels, 2002).

Table 34–29 Chido/Rodgers Blood Group Antigens

Chido (Ch) antigens		Name	Frequency*	Amino acid	Frequency*	Name	Rodgers (Rg) antigens	
CH/RG3†	CH/RG1	Ch1	96%	Arg1191 Leu / Ala1188 Val	98%	Rg1	CH/RG11	CH/RG12†
		Ch3	93%	Conformational epitope	95%	Rg2		
	CH/RG6	Ch6	96%	Ser1157 Asn	95%	Rg3	CH/RG13	
CH/RG7†		WH	Rare	Conformational epitope (Ch6+Rg1)				
CH/RG2†	CH/RG4	Ch4	96%	His1106 Asp / Ile1105 Leu / Ser1102 Lys / Leu1101 Pro				
		Ch2	91%	Conformational epitope (Ch4+Ch5)				
	CH/RG5	Ch5	94%	Gly1054 Asp				

* Calculated from Giles (1987) and Issitt (1998).

† Conformational epitopes require the presence of two Ch/Rg antigenic determinants.

Table 34–30 Gerbich Blood Group Antigens

High frequency		Frequency	GP*	Amino acid change (high → low)	Frequency	Low frequency	
ISBT	Name					Name	ISBT
GE2	Ge2	>99%	GPD	N' terminus			
GE3	Ge3	>99%	GPC	aa 43–50			
			GPD	aa 22–29			
GE4	Ge4	>99%	GPC	N-terminus			
GE5	Webb	>99%	GPC	Ser8>Asn	Rare	(Webb–)	
			GPC+D	Duplication of exon 3	2% black people 1.5% Finnish people	Ls^a	GE6
GE7	An^a	>99%	GPD	Ser2>Ala	0.01%	(An^a–)	
GE8	Dh^a	>99%	GPC	Leu14>Ala	<0.01%	(Dh^a–)	
Gerbich null phenotypes†							
			GPC	Deletion exon 2	Rare	Yus	(Ge–2,3,4)
			GPC	Deletion exon 3	10–50% Melanesian people	Gerbich	(Ge–2,–3,4)
			GPC	Deletion exons 3+4	Rare	Leach	(Ge–2,–3,–4)

* Glycophorin C (GPC) or glycophorin D (GPD).

† Yus and Gerbich phenotypes are the result of mutant GPC alleles. No GPD is found in Yus, Gerbich or Leach phenotypes.

Biochemistry

Gerbich antigens are expressed on two biosynthetically related type 1 glycoproteins, glycophorin C (GPC; Fig. 34–15) and glycophorin D (GPD). GPC is a 40-kD, 128-amino-acid glycoprotein bearing one N-linked and 12 O-linked glycans. GPD is a 107-amino-acid variant, lacking 21 amino acids at the amino-terminus (Reid, 2004b). The cytoplasmic domain interacts with several cytoskeletal proteins, including spectrin, protein 4.1 and p55.

Molecular Biology

GPC and GPD are the products of a single gene, *GYPC*, on chromosome 2q14-121. The gene spans 13.5 kb and is organized into four exons. Exons 1–3 encode the extracellular domain: exon 4 is responsible for the transmembrane domain and cytoplasmic tail. The promoter region contains classical CCAC and TATA sequences, as well as transcription factor binding sites for Sp1, GATA-1 and NF-E6. GPD is the product of leaky translation at a downstream, alternative AUG residue (Met22).

As shown in Table 34–30, the high-frequency antigens Ge2 and Ge4 are the NH$_2$-termini of GPD and GPC, respectively. Ge3 is encoded by exon 3 and is shared by both molecules. With the exception of Ls^a, low-frequency Ge antigens are the result of single amino acid polymorphisms. The Gerbich null or Leach phenotype results from deletion of exons 3 and 4. As a result, no GPC or GPD protein is expressed (Fig. 34–15). The Yus and Gerbich phenotypes are deletion mutants characterized by variant GPC synthesis and a complete loss of GPD synthesis. As a result, Yus and Gerbich can express high-incidence antigens present on GPC (Ge3, Ge4) but not GPD (Ge2).

Gerbich Antibodies

Anti-Gerbich antibodies are usually, but not always, clinically significant. There are reports of shortened RBC survival and delayed hemolysis following transfusion of Gerbich-incompatible RBCs. There is one report of severe HDN. Autoantibodies against Gerbich antigens have been associated with severe autoimmune hemolytic anemia (Reid, 2004b).

Anti-Gerbich antibodies can be of IgM or IgG isotype. Most are immune-stimulated although naturally occurring anti-Ge are known. They may be detected at room temperature and are enhanced by AHG. Gerbich antigens are resistant to chymotrypsin but are sensitive to other proteases (trypsin, pronase).

Biological Role

Like Diego/Band 3, GPC/GPD help anchor the membrane to the underlying cytoskeleton. In patients with protein 4.1 deficiency and hereditary elliptocytosis, GPC/GPD are decreased (75% normal). Likewise, the Ge null (Leach) phenotype is associated with marked elliptocytosis due to reduced membrane stability and deformability (Daniels, 2002). Because they are rich in sialic acid, GPC and GPD can bind influenza virus. GPC and GPD may bind *P. falciparum*.

Cromer Blood Group System (ISBT No. 021)

The Cromer system (Cr/CROM) contains 13 antigens, including five antithetical antigens and 10 high-incidence antigens (Table 34–31). Cromer antigens are present on decay accelerating factor (DAF, CD55),

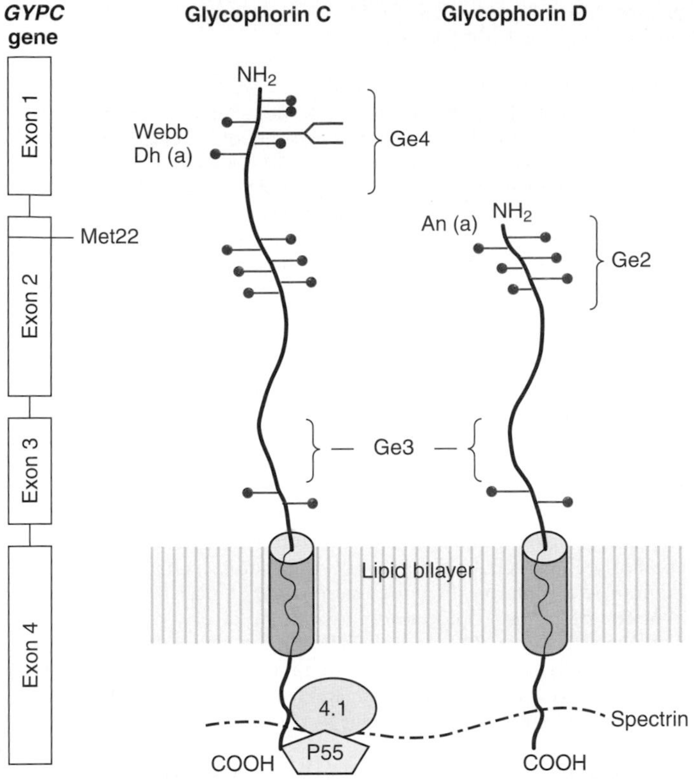

Figure 34–15

GYPC gene | **Glycophorin C** | **Glycophorin D**

Exon 1
Exon 2
Exon 3
Exon 4

NH₂
Webb
Dh (a)
} Ge4
Met22
An (a) NH₂
} Ge2
{ — Ge3 — {
Lipid bilayer
4.1
P55
Spectrin
COOH
COOH

Figure 34–15 Gerbich antigens on glycophorin C and glycophorin D. *O*-linked (—•) and *N*-linked glycans are shown. Also shown is the relationship of the *GYPC* gene to both proteins. Glycophorin D is the result of alternative translation at Met22 in exon 2. Deletions of different exons are responsible for the three Gerbich null phenotypes. Glycophorin C and D may interact with spectrin, protein 4.1 and p55 of the cytoskeleton.

Table 34–31 Cromer Blood Group Antigens

High-frequency antigens			Amino acid change (high → low)	Low-frequency antigens		
ISBT	Name	Frequency		Frequency	Name	ISBT
CROM1	Crᵃ	>99%	Ala193>Pro	Rare		
CROM2	Tcᵃ	>99%	Arg18>Leu	6% black people 0% white people	Tcᵇ	CROM3
			Arg18>Pro	Rare	Tcᶜ	CROM4
CROM5	Drᵃ	>99%	Ser165>Leu	Rare		
CROM6	Esᵃ	>99%	Ile46>Asn	Rare		
CROM7	IFC	>99%	Heterogeneous	Rare	Inab	
CROM9	Wesᵇ	>99%	Leu48>Arg	2% black people <0.5% white people	Wesᵃ*	CROM8
CROM10	UMC	>99%	Thr216>Met	Rare		
CROM11	GUT1	>99%	Arg206>His	Rare		
CROM12	SERF	>99%	Pro182>Leu	Rare		
CROM13	ZENA	>99%	His208>Gln	Rare		

* Because of their proximity, Wesᵃ weakens Esᵃ expression.

which is widely expressed on tissues and in secretions. DAF has been identified on all hematopoietic cells, vascular endothelium, gastrointestinal and genitourinary epithelium, brain and body fluids (Storry, 2002). Cromer is expressed on cord RBCs.

Null/Weak Phenotypes

Inab or Cromer null phenotype is a rare autosomal recessive phenotype, characterized by a complete absence of all Cromer antigens, but normal expression of CD59 and other glycosyl phosphoinositol (GPI)-linked

Table 34–32 Knops Blood Group Antigens

High frequency		Frequency	Amino acid change (high → low)	Frequency	Low frequency	
ISBT	Name				Name	ISBT
KN1	Knᵃ	99%	Val1561>Met	4% white people	Knᵇ	KN2
KN3	Mcᵃ	99%	Lys1590>Glu	45% black people	Mcᵇ	KN6
KN4	Sl1 (Slᵃ)	98% white people 52% black people	Arg1601>Gly	Black people only	Sl2 (Vil)	KN7
	Sl4*	100% black people 96% white people	Ser1610>Thr	4% white people	Sl5*	
KN8	Sl3†		Arg1601+Ser1610			
KN5	Ykᵃ	92% white people 98% black people	Unknown			

* Sl4 and Sl5 are theoretical antigens not formally added to the Knops family at this time.

† Sl3 is a conformational antigen that requires the presence of both Sl1 (Arg1601) and 'Sl4' (Ser1610)

glycoproteins. Many individuals with the Inab phenotype suffer from chronic gastrointestinal disorders, particularly a chronic protein-losing gastroenteropathy. CD55/Cromer is also missing on PNH III RBCs, which lack all GPI-linked glycoproteins. Weak Cromer expression (40% normal) is observed in the Dr(a−) phenotype.

Biochemistry

CD55/DAF is a highly glycosylated, 381-amino-acid, 70-kD GPI-linked glycoprotein (Fig. 34–13). The extracellular domain consists of four short consensus repeat (SCR) domains, capable of binding complement components (C3b/C4b), followed by a 70-amino-acid stretch rich in *O*-linked glycans (50% serine/threonine). Each SCR domain contains four highly conserved cysteine residues, resulting in two intrachain disulfide bonds/SCR. As a consequence, DAF is sensitive to sulfhydryl-reducing agents. The molecule contains a single *N*-glycosylation site near SCR1 (Medof, 1987).

Molecular Biology

The *DAF* gene spans 40 kb on chromosome 1q32 and is organized into 11 exons. Most Cromer antigens reflect single amino acid polymorphisms (Table 34–31) (Storry, 2002; Reid, 2003b, 2004a). The Inab phenotype is the result of either nonsense or splice site mutations. The etiology of the Dr(a−) phenotype is quite interesting. A single amino acid polymorphism (596C>T) leads to both a Ser165>Leu polymorphism and an alternative splice site. In Dr(a−) individuals, two mRNA species are observed, encoding a truncated mutated protein arising from alternate splicing (major transcript) and the full DAF bearing the Leu165 polymorphism (minor transcript). Dr(a−) RBC have weakened expression of DAF and all Cromer antigens (Storry, 2002).

Cromer Antibodies

The clinical significance of anti-Cr antibodies is variable. In some individuals, anti-Cr antibodies are associated with decreased RBC survival and hemolytic transfusion reactions. Cromer antibodies do not cause HDN owing to adsorption of antibodies by DAF on trophoblast epithelium (Storry, 2002; Daniels, 2002).

Anti-Cromer antibodies are usually of IgG isotype, arising from immune stimulation. They are detected in the IAT and can give weak, variable results (high-titer, low-avidity antibodies). Anti-Cromer can be inhibited by plasma, urine and platelet concentrates. Antibody reactivity is highly sensitive to pretreatment of RBCs with chymotrypsin and pronase, but not other proteases. Cromer antigens are weakened, but not destroyed, by AET and DTT.

Biological Role

CD55/DAF protects cells from complement, by promoting the decay of two C3 convertases, C4b2a and C3bBb (Lindahl, 2000). CD55 is also

IV

receptor for uropathogenic and intestinal *E. coli* strains bearing Afa/Dr and X adhesins, echovirus and Coxsackie B virus.

Knops Blood Group System (ISBT No. 022)

The Knops blood group contains 7–10 antigens, including six antithetical antigens (Table 34–32). Several Knops antigens (Kn^b, Mc^a, Sl^a) are racially segregated. Knops antigens are present on adult and cord RBCs, neutrophils, B lymphocytes and dendritic cells (Reid, 2004b). Knops can vary in strength between individuals, with approximately 1% of donors showing extremely weak Knops expression (10% normal, Helgeson phenotype).

Biochemistry

Knops resides on complement receptor 1 (CR1, CD35), a 220-kD glycoprotein (Moulds, 2001). The extracellular domain consists of 30 short consensus repeats (SCR), arranged into four long homologous regions (LHR) that are capable of binding C4b and C3b. The molecule also possesses six to eight *N*-glycosylation sites.

Molecular Biology

The *CR1* gene resides on chromosome 1q32. There are four CR1 alleles (CR*1-4), of which CR1*1 is the most common (Daniels, 2002). Variation in CR1 strength and copy number appears to be genetically determined. To date, all Knops antigens arise from amino acid polymorphisms (Table 34–31; Moulds, 2001, 2002, 2004). KN4/7 (Sl/Vil) antigens may be expanded to include five antigens, reflecting the influence of a second amino acid polymorphism (Ser1610>Ser) and a conformational antigen (Sl3) that requires Sl1 and Sl4 coexpression (Moulds, 2002).

Knops Antibodies

Knops antibodies are clinically insignificant. Knops-incompatible RBCs have normal survival following transfusion. Knops antibodies are of IgG isotype, arising from immune stimulation, and are usually only detected with AHG. Historically classified as an HTLA (high-titer, low-avidity) antibody, Knops antibodies are notoriously difficult to work with because of their low avidity, biologic variation in Knops expression, antigen degradation and the presence of additional alloantibody specificities. Knops antigens are resistant to proteases but are weakened by sulfhydryl-reducing agents (AET, DTT).

Biological Role

A complement regulatory protein, CR1 can bind C3b/C4b immune complexes, promoting their degradation by factor 1. CR1 also enhances phagocytosis of C3b/C4b-coated particles and could play a role in *Leishmania*, *Legionella* and *Mycobacteria* infections (Daniels, 2002). CR1 also binds *P. falciparum* with rosette formation – a clinical finding associated with severe malaria. Because Sl(a–) RBCs show reduced *P. falciparum* binding and rosetting, it was hypothesized that the Sl(a)/Sl2 phenotype, which is present in 70% of African black people, may provide protection against severe malaria. A recent study, however, found no correlation among Sl1/Sl2 phenotype, malaria infection or disease severity (Zimmerman, 2003). Despite the latter, the extremely high incidence of the Sl(a–) or Sl2 phenotype in Africa suggests a past selective advantage for the Sl(a–) phenotype in this population.

Indian Blood Group System (ISBT No. 023)

The Indian (In) blood group contains two autosomal codominant antigens, In^a (IN1) and In^b (IN2). In^b is a high-frequency allele (99% white people) whereas In^a is relatively rare except among Indian (4%) and Arab populations (11–12%). AnWj is another high-incidence antigen that is believed to belong to the Indian blood group. Indian antigens are carried by the CD44 glycoprotein and are widely expressed on all hematopoietic cells, epithelial cells and neural tissue. There are approximately 6 000–10 000 CD44 molecules per RBC (Byrne 2004; Reid, 2004b).

Null/Weak Phenotypes

Indian antigens, including AnWj, are depressed on In(Lu) RBCs. In and AnWj are transiently depressed on cord RBCs during pregnancy and autoimmune hemolytic anemia due to autoanti-AnWj (Daniels, 2002).

Biochemistry

Indian antigens are present on CD44, an ubiquitous glycoprotein on many cell membranes. CD44 is heterogeneous between tissues due to tissue-specific differences in mRNA processing and glycosylation. In RBCs, CD44 is an 80- to 85-kD, 341-amino-acid type 1 glycoprotein bearing a large, heavily glycosylated extracellular domain containing six cysteine residues, six *N*-glycans, three chondroitin sulfate and several *O*-linked glycans. Like Diego/Band 3, CD44 can bind the cytoskeletal proteins, protein 4.1 and ankyrin (Daniels, 2002).

Molecular Biology

CD44 resides on chromosome 11p13. The gene spans 50 kb and contains 20 exons, which are able to generate an array of spliceform variants. In RBCs, CD44 is encoded by exons 1–5, 16, 17, 18 and 20. A single amino acid polymorphism is responsible for the In^a (Pro46) and In^b (Arg46) antigens. The etiology of the AnWj antigen is unknown.

Indian Antibodies

Antibodies against both Indian and AnWj antigens can be clinically significant, with shortened RBC survival and transfusion reactions. They are not associated with HDN. Autoimmune anemia due to autoanti-AnWj has been reported. Anti-Indian antibodies are usually of IgG isotype, arising from immune stimulation. They can present as saline agglutinins and are enhanced by AHG. In^a and In^b antigens, but not AnWj, are destroyed by proteases and AET. Anti-Indian antibodies are also inhibited by plasma, which contains soluble CD44.

Biologic Role

CD44 is a major adhesion molecule on leukocytes. CD44 binds a spectrum of extracellular matrix proteins, including collagen, fibronectin, laminin and hyaluron. In bone marrow, CD44 may participate in the adhesion of erythroid progenitors to stromal fibroblasts. In leukocytes, CD44 may facilitate WBC–endothelial adhesion, helping to localize WBC to sites of inflammation. CD44 has been implicated in tumor metastasis, wound remodeling, and embryonic differentiation. AnWj/CD44 is also a receptor for *Haemophilus influenzae*.

OK Blood Group System (ISBT No. 024)

The OK system contains a single high-frequency antigen, Ok^a (> 99% donors). The Ok^a glycoprotein is present on RBCs, WBCs and hematopoietic progenitors. Ok^a resides on CD147, a 35- to 68-kD, 251-amino-acid *N*-linked glycoprotein. A member of the immunoglobulin superfamily, CD147 possesses an IgC2 and IgV domain. The gene for CD147 resides on chromosome 19pter. The Ok(a–) phenotype arises from a Glu92>Lys mutation (Daniels, 2002). CD147 is a leukocyte-activation-associated protein and may participate in cell adhesion, tumorigenesis and wound healing via stimulation of enzymes required for remodeling of the extracellular matrix (Daniels, 2002).

Anti-Ok^a is rare and described only in Japan. Anti-Ok^a is of IgG isotype, arising from immune stimulation, and is associated with shortened RBC survival following transfusion of Ok^a-incompatible RBCs. The Ok^a antigen is resistant to enzymes, sialidases and sulfhydryl-reducing agents.

RAPH Blood Group System (ISBT No. 025)

The Raph blood group system contains a single antigen, RAPH or MER2. RAPH is expressed by 92% donors and can vary in strength. Raph is present on CD34+ cells, fibroblasts and RBCs. There is a progressive decrease in RAPH/MER2 expression with increasing erythroid maturation. RAPH is expressed on MER2, a 40-kD protein encoded by a gene on chromosome 11p15. The antigen is sensitive to most proteases except ficin. Three examples of anti-MER2 are known. All were of IgG isotype, arising from transfusion and pregnancy. Two examples fixed complement. There are no reports of hemolytic transfusion reactions or HDN due to anti-RAPH.

JMH Blood Group System (ISBT No. 026)

The JMH (John Milton Hagen) system contains a single, high-incidence antigen, JMH (> 99% donors). In addition to RBCs, JMH is found on lymphocytes, activated macrophages, thymus, brain, respiratory epithelium, placenta, testes and spleen (Reid, 2004b).

Biochemistry and Molecular Biology

JMH is carried on CD108 (SEMA-L), a semaphorin family glycoprotein (Fig. 34–13). The protein is a 666-amino-acid protein composed of a large 500-amino-acid sema domain, a C2-type immunoglobulin domain, five *N*-glycosylation and six myristoylation sites. The molecule is anchored into the cell membrane by a glycophosphoinositol tail (GPI-linked) and is absent on PNH III RBCs. The molecule contains 19 cysteine residues and is sensitive to sulfhydryl-reducing agents. The gene for *SEMA-L* is on chromosome 15q22.

JMH Antibodies

Anti-JMH antibodies do not cause hemolytic transfusion reactions or HDN, although shortened RBC survival has been documented. The antibodies are

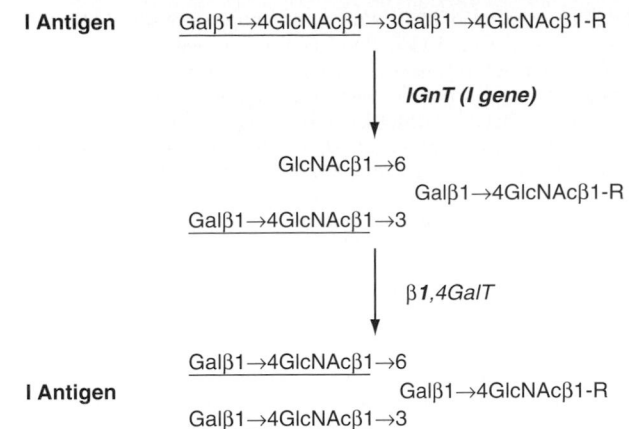

I Antigen Galβ1→4GlcNAcβ1→3Galβ1→4GlcNAcβ1-R

IGnT (I gene)

GlcNAcβ1→6

Galβ1→4GlcNAcβ1-R

Galβ1→4GlcNAcβ1→3

β1,4GalT

Galβ1→4GlcNAcβ1→6

I Antigen Galβ1→4GlcNAcβ1-R

Galβ1→4GlcNAcβ1→3

Figure 34–16 Structure of blood group I and i antigens. The immunologically active terminal lactosaminyl epitopes are underlined. I antigen synthesis requires the action of IGnT, a β1-6-N-acetylglucosaminyltransferase. Gal = galactose; GlcNAc = N-acetylgalactosamine; R = other oligosaccharide.

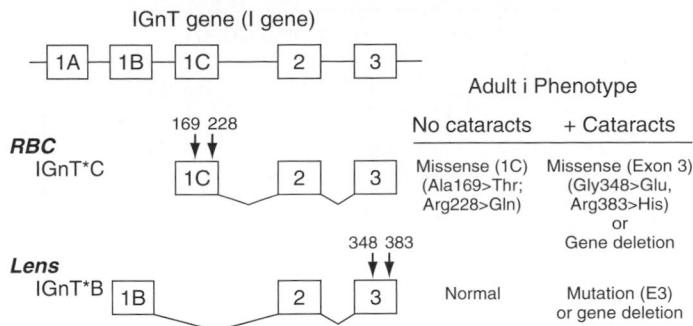

Figure 34–17 The I gene, showing three different exon 1. In human RBCs and lens, a different IGnT mRNA is translated, based on which exon 1 is utilized. Mutations in I gene can result in an adult i phenotype and cataracts. In Europeans, mutations are usually only in exon 1C and affect I antigen synthesis in RBCs. In Asia, adult i phenotype involves either gene deletion or mutations in exon 3. As a result, there is a loss of IGnT activity in all tissues.

of IgG isotype and can be naturally occurring. The JMH antigen is sensitive to proteases and DTT.

Biological Role

This is unknown. Semaphorin proteins are implicated in cell signaling.

I Blood Group System (ISBT No. 027)

The I blood group system contains two biosynthetically related antigens, I and i. The biosynthetic precursor to I antigen, the i antigen is on cord cells, because of developmental delays in the enzyme responsible for I antigen synthesis. By 18 months of age, i decreases and I increases to levels observed on adult RBCs (Hakomori, 1981). Both antigens are ubiquitously expressed on glycolipids and glycoproteins of all cell types.

Null Phenotype

The i_{adult} phenotype is a rare, autosomal recessive phenotype found in 0.01–0.03% donors. In Asia, the i_{adult} phenotype can be associated with congenital cataracts. Elevated i antigen is also observed on cord RBCs, reticulocytes, and in stressed erythropoiesis such as in PNH (Navenot, 1997). Elevated i antigen, with chronic hemolysis, is also observed in HEMPAS, a congenital dyserythropoietic anemia. Increased i antigen in HEMPAS disease is the direct result of defects in glycosylation (Fukuda, 1990).

Biochemistry

Type 2 chain oligosaccharides, both i and I antigens terminate in a Galβ1-4GlcNAc or lactosaminyl epitope, and differ only in complexity and multivalency. As shown in Figure 34–16, the i antigen is a linear oligosaccharide. The I antigen is derived from i antigen by the action of β1-6 N-acetylglucosaminyltransferase, a first step in the synthesis of large, branched multivalent complex polylactosamines (Fig. 34–16). Both i and I can be further modified by other glycosyltransferases to yield ABH, Le^x and related antigens.

Molecular Biology

The I antigen, a β1-6 glucosaminyltransferase, is the product of IGnT. The gene spans approximately 100 kb on chromosome 6p34. The gene contains five exons, including three tissue-specific exon 1 (Fig. 34–17). As a consequence, three different IGnT spliceforms are possible, depending on which exon 1 is utilized (Inaba, 2003). IGnT*C, composed of exons 1C, 2 and 3, is found in RBCs. IGnT*B is synthesized in the human lens (Yu, 2003).

Both the i_{adult} phenotype and congenital cataracts have been linked to mutations in IGnT. In white i_{adult} individuals without cataracts, mutations have been found in exon 1C (nt 505, 683), leading to a loss of IGnT*C activity in RBCs (Inaba, 2003). In contrast, i_{adult} with cataracts is characterized by either missense mutations in exon 3 (nt 1049, 1154) or a major deletion of the IGnT gene. As a result, there is a loss of IGnT*C and IGnT*B activity in RBC and lens, respectively (Yu, 2003). The loss of IGnT*B activity in lens is believed to underlie the formation of cataracts.

Anti-I and i Antibodies

Anti-I and anti-i are antibodies of IgM isotype, reactive at room temperature (Table 34–7). Autoantibodies to I are relatively common and are usually low-titered cold agglutinins. Some anti-I can have IH specificity, reacting stronger with group O and A2 RBC (refer to Table 34–48 below). Although generally benign, hemolysis secondary to high-titered anti-I is observed in cold autoimmune hemolytic anemia (CAD). CAD can occur in the setting of malignancy and infection, particularly *Mycoplasma pneumoniae*. These antibodies display a wide thermal amplitude, often agglutinating RBCs at temperatures of 30–34°C. In contrast, alloanti-I is relatively rare and found as a naturally occurring antibody in i_{adult} individuals. Anti-i is also uncommon but has been reported in infectious mononucleosis and alcoholic cirrhosis.

GIL Blood Group System (ISBT No. 029)

The GIL blood group system contains one high-incidence antigen, GIL (100% donors). The GIL protein is highly expressed on RBCs, kidney, small intestine, stomach, colon, spleen, eye and respiratory tract (Reid, 2004b).

Biochemistry

GIL is carried by aquaglyceroporin (AQP3), a member of the MIP family of water channels. Like Colton (AQP1), AQP3 is a 46-kD multi-pass protein containing six transmembrane domains and a single N-glycosylation site. The molecule is present in the cell membrane as dimers, trimers and tetramers (Daniels, 2002).

Molecular Biology

The AQP3 gene spans 6 kb on chromosome 9p13 and is organized into six exons. The GIL-negative phenotype is the result of splice site and frameshift mutations in AQP3.

GIL Antibodies

Anti-GIL is associated with hemolytic transfusion reactions. There are no reports of clinical HDN due to anti-GIL despite a positive direct antiglobulin test (DAT). Anti-GIL is usually of IgG isotype, reactive at 37°C and enhanced with AHG. The antigen is resistant to proteases, sialidases and DTT.

Biological Role

AQP3/Gil is a membrane water channel capable of transporting urea and glycerol. See Colton blood group system.

Immunohematology Tests and Procedures

Basic Principles – Hemagglutination

Specific hemagglutination is the single most important in vitro immunologic reaction in blood banking because it is the end-point of almost all test systems designed to detect RBC antigens and antibodies. The hemagglutination process actually occurs in two stages. The first stage, often referred to as RBC sensitization, is simply the combination of paratope and epitope in a reversible reaction that follows the law of mass action and has an associated equilibrium constant. Antigen and antibody are held together by noncovalent attractions. In stage two, multiple RBCs with bound antibody form a stable latticework through antigen–antibody bridges formed between adjacent cells. This latticework is the basis of all visible agglutination reactions.

Formation of the latticework during the second stage of hemagglutination is naturally impeded by the fact that RBCs in solution normally repel each

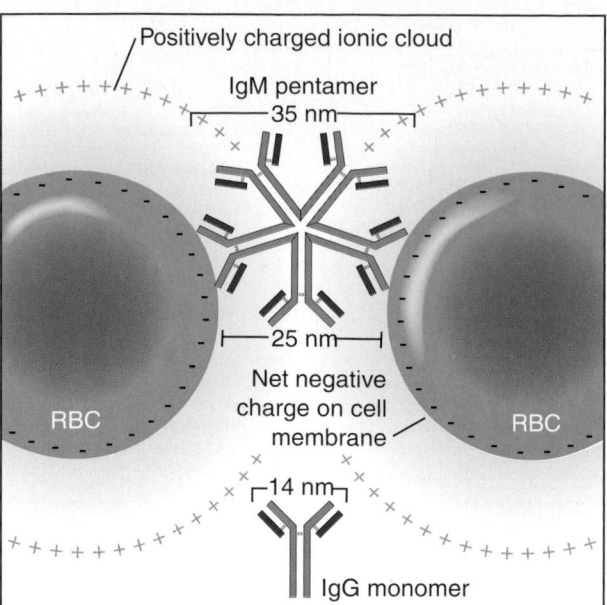

Figure 34–18 Erythrocytes are kept apart in an ionic medium by the zeta potential which in turn influences the agglutinating capacity of IgG and IgM.

other. This is due to the net negative charge of the RBC membrane created by sialic acid. If RBCs are suspended in an ionic medium such as normal saline, cations arrange themselves around each cell to form an 'ionic cloud.' Cations closest to the cell membrane are firmly bound and move with the RBC, while the outer cations move freely. The difference in charge at the surface between the inner and outer cation layers, called the surface of shear, creates an electrical potential named the zeta potential (Fig. 34–18). The zeta potential keeps RBCs in solution about 25 nm apart (Lewis, 1999). Another factor that may be important in keeping RBCs apart is the water of hydration. Proponents of this theory suggest that the hydrophilic polar heads of lipid molecules making up the outer cell membrane bilayer attract water molecules. The water thus creates a surface tension that helps to keep the cells apart.

One situation whereby the natural influence of the zeta potential to keep RBCs apart is circumvented is the phenomenon of rouleaux formation or 'pseudoagglutination.' Patients with multiple myeloma, Waldenström's macroglobulinemia, and hyperviscosity syndromes have high concentrations of abnormal serum proteins that change the net surface charge on the RBC membrane. The cells thus cluster together in clumps that resemble macroscopic hemagglutination. Plasma expanders, such as dextran and hydroxyethyl starch, as well as some intravenous X-ray contrast materials can also cause rouleaux formation. Rouleaux can be differentiated from true agglutination by direct microscopy: (1) by the classical 'stacked-coin' formation in rouleaux and (2) by the loss of rouleaux after washing and resuspension in saline. Nonspecific agglutination can also be seen in cord blood samples contaminated with Wharton's jelly. The presence of hyaluronic acid and albumin in cord blood is responsible for this problem.

Factors Affecting Specific Hemagglutination

The extent of RBC sensitization and the facilitation of the second stage latticework formation are influenced firstly by inherent characteristics of the specific antigens and antibodies involved. In most immuno-hematology procedures, IgM antibodies can facilitate the second stage of hemagglutination because of their large diameter (35 nm), which allows them to span the distance between two adjacent RBCs in solution (Fig. 34–18). Because of their innate agglutinating ability, IgM antibodies are frequently referred to as direct agglutinins. Most IgG antibodies, on the other hand, are considerably smaller (14 nm) and are unable to induce visible agglutination without the assistance of secondary enhancing reagents. Thus, IgG antibodies are commonly referred to as indirect agglutinins.

The density and accessibility of specific antigens on the RBC membrane are also critical in second-stage latticework formation. This can be illustrated by comparing the ABO and Rh antigens. There are approximately 1 million ABO antigens per RBC, displayed on the large, extramembranous glycoproteins. Because of their high density and easy accessibility, ABO antibodies can readily bind exposed ABO antigens and agglutinate RBCs. In contrast, Rh antigens average only 10 000–30 000 sites per cell and, as multipass integral membrane proteins, are considered intramembranous. As a consequence, Rh antigens are less easily agglutinated by Rh antisera.

In another example of the influence of antigen density, RBCs that are homozygous for a particular blood group gene will often give stronger reactions than heterozygous cells. This is because homozygotes express twice as many copies, or a double dose, of the antigen per cell. In immuno-hematologic testing this phenomenon is frequently referred to as dosage.

Secondarily to inherent antigen and antibody characteristics, the first and second stages of the hemagglutination reaction may also be influenced by manipulating various physical and/or chemical parameters of the reaction environment. An outline of how these various parameters may be controlled is shown in Table 34–33.

Grading of Hemagglutination Reactions

Hemagglutination in blood bank testing is observed and graded according to the strength of the reaction. Hemolysis is considered the strongest positive reaction that can occur and indicates the presence of a potent, complement-fixing antibody. After incubating recipient serum and reagent RBCs, the serum should first be examined for hemolysis prior to resuspending the cell button. When reading for agglutination, the tube should be shaken, using a gentle wrist action, until all cells are dislodged. This is most easily accomplished by holding the tube at a sharp angle so that the fluid 'cuts' across the cell button such that the cells can be easily resuspended. When cells no longer adhere to the tube, it should be tilted back and forth gently until an even suspension of cells (or agglutination) is observed. Proper illumination with a concave mirror is an invaluable aid for macroscopic reading. By placing the tube about 2.5 inches above a 3-inch concave mirror, aggregates can be differentiated easily from the free cells by looking at the mirror, not at the tube.

Table 34–34 lists two protocols for evaluating the strength of agglutination using numerical grading and/or scoring. Figure 34–19 illustrates the appearance of different agglutination grades. Although the agglutination grade gives an approximate idea regarding the potency or strength of a particular antibody, the scoring method is much more useful in semiquantitative procedures, particularly when used in conjunction with titration to compare the relative antibody strengths of two different sera.

The Antihuman Globulin Test

Even with use of enhancement media, such as albumin or enzymes, and the final step of centrifugation, many IgG antibodies are still not able to directly produce detectable hemagglutination. To visualize reactions by these antibodies, antihuman globulin (AHG) reagents, which contain specific antibodies to human immunoglobulins or complement components, must be utilized. The antibodies in AHG sera act as bridges between RBCs already sensitized with antibody or complement to produce the characteristic latticework of second-stage hemagglutination (see Fig. 34–20). This is the basis of the antihuman globulin test.

The antihuman globulin test is also called the Coombs' test in honor of one of the investigators who first developed the test for laboratory use (Coombs, 1945), although the principle was actually described much earlier in 1908 by Moreschi (Simpson, 1999). When the test is used to detect antibodies or complement bound to RBCs in vivo, it is called the direct antiglobulin test (DAT). When the test is used to detect the reaction of antibody and RBCs in vitro after an appropriate incubation phase, it is called the indirect antiglobulin test (IAT).

Antihuman Globulin Reagents and Procedures

Various preparations of antihuman globulin sera are available for blood bank testing depending on the application (direct or indirect) for which it is being utilized and whether one wishes to detect RBC sensitization by IgG, complement components, or both.

Polyspecific Reagents

Polyclonal, polyspecific AHG reagents are produced by hyperimmunizing animals, usually rabbits, with purified immunoglobulin or complement to produce high-titered, high-avidity, IgG antibodies. For a given batch of reagent, the animal sera are harvested, pooled, adsorbed to remove heterophil agglutinins, and then titrated to ascertain the dilution necessary for optimal reactivity in routine use. Conventional polyspecific (also called broad-spectrum) AHG contains polyclonal IgG antibodies to the spectrum of human IgG subclasses and the C3 complement cleavage products, C3b and C3d. Some anti-C4b and anti-C4d activity may also be present. However, most manufacturers adsorb out anti-C4 activity from their polyspecific AHG reagents because it has been shown that in vitro complement activation by clinically insignificant cold agglutinins results in much more C4d binding than C3d (Mollison, 1993). Excluding anti-C4 activity thus reduces the number of false positives in both DAT and IAT testing using polyspecific reagents. Because immunization against IgG will

Table 34–33 Factors Affecting the Hemagglutination Reaction

Reaction parameter	Effect	Manipulation
Temperature	Influences the equilibrium constant and/or reaction rate depending on the class of antibody involved	Decreasing the temperature to 24°C or even to 4°C enhances the reaction of IgM antibodies Prewarming or maintaining a reaction temperature of 37°C provides the optimum temperature for detection of IgG antibodies, while preventing most IgM antibodies from reacting
Incubation time	Different ag/ab reactions reach equilibrium over different time periods	Increasing the time of incubation in a given test system may enhance the detection of a weakly reactive antibody
pH	At a pH range of 6.5–7.5, chemical groups on ag and ab are oppositely charged, providing optimal ionic forces of attraction for most blood group antibodies	Changing the pH affects the equilibrium constant for selected antibodies that may react preferentially in a more acidic environment – e.g., anti-M and anti-Pr
Ionic strength	In an isotonic saline medium, sodium cations and chloride anions cluster around erythrocyte ag and blood group ab, respectively, acting to neutralize ag/ab attractive forces	LISS (low ionic strength solutions) – addition of LISS reduces the shielding effect on oppositely charged ab and ag, thus increasing the rate of reaction and the equilibrium constant for red cell sensitization
Antibody concentration	Can affect first and second stage agglutination by influencing the number of antibody molecules attached to each erythrocyte	Increasing the serum to cell concentration increases the rate and/or affects the equilibrium constant of red cell sensitization by IgG antibodies. May help to induce second stage agglutination by IgM antibodies PEG (polyethylene glycol) – addition of this large space-occupying molecule effectively increases the relative concentration of ag and ab respective to the volume of the reaction, greatly increasing the rate of reaction. Is used only in AHG testing to detect IgG antibodies
Zeta potential	Causes red cells to repel each other in solution. If the zeta potential can be reduced or the red cells brought together by physical means, second stage agglutination of sensitized red cells can be facilitated	Centrifugation – forcing cells closer together facilitates latticework formation Enzymes – cleave sialic acid residues to lower the zeta potential and also improve accessibility of certain blood group antigens Albumin – reduces zeta potential and/or water of hydration to allow red cells to approach each other more closely Polybrene/protamine – provide an excess of cations that neutralize the repulsive force between red cells, producing both nonspecific aggregation and antibody-mediated latticework formation. The final addition of sodium citrate disperses nonspecific aggregates, while specific ag/ab agglutinates remain

ag = antigen; ab = antibody; AHG = antihuman globulin.

Table 34–34 Grading of Hemagglutination

Grade	Appearance	Score
H	Hemolysis – presence of free hemoglobin in the serum	10
4+	One solid aggregate	10
3+	Several medium to large aggregates	8
2+	Many small to medium aggregates with a clear background	5
1+	Many small aggregates with a turbid background	3
+ or w	Few small aggregates with many unagglutinated cells	2
$\pm^m$ or $+^m$	Aggregates visible only under microscopic magnification	1
0	Negative – absence of aggregates; all cells unagglutinated	0
mf	Mixed field agglutination – presence of minor population of agglutinated cells superimposed on a negative background	NA
R	Rouleaux – nonspecific aggregation appearing like a stack of coins; disappears with addition of saline	NA

also produce anti-light chain antibodies in a polyclonal response, one should remember that polyclonal antiglobulin sera may cross-react with IgA or IgM light chains unless the manufacturer specifies that the anti-IgG component is heavy chain specific.

At present, the most commonly used polyspecific AHG reagents consist of rabbit polyclonal anti-IgG blended with murine monoclonal antibodies to C3b and C3d complement components. There is also a polyspecific reagent available derived exclusively from murine monoclonal antibodies to IgG, C3b and C3d. The activity of anti-IgG and anti-complement in polyspecific antisera, whether polyclonal or monoclonal, will vary somewhat among different manufacturers and between lots produced by the same manufacturer. However, all AHG sera must contain levels of anti-IgG and anti-C3d activity that meet or exceed the reference standards of the Food and Drug Administration (FDA) (21CFR660.52; Code of Federal Regulations, 2001b).

Monospecific Reagents

Commercially available FDA-licensed monospecific reagents include anti-IgG, anti-C3b+C3d, and anti-C3d. Monospecific anti-IgG or anti-complement may also be polyclonal or monoclonal in origin. For monoclonal anti-IgG, manufacturers must blend monoclonals against a variety of IgG epitopes or select a clone with specificity for an epitope common to all variants of IgG to ensure that the spectrum of human IgG subclasses will react with their reagent. With polyclonal monospecific anti-IgG, again one should keep in mind that it may contain anti-light chain activity unless the manufacturer labels it as heavy chain specific.

Production of murine monoclonal blends of monospecific anti-complement has allowed manufacturers to develop reagents containing quantities of purified anti-C3b and C3d of known potency that are less likely to give false-positive results due to other anti-complement activities found in polyclonal reagents (Simpson, 1999).

Choosing Which AHG Reagent to Use

The direct antiglobulin test or DAT is an important diagnostic serologic technique used for the detection of antibody-mediated complement activation on RBC membranes in vivo. Thus, polyspecific AHG reagents containing both anti-IgG and anti-complement activity are typically used for initial DAT evaluation. This is especially important when the DAT is being performed to aid in the diagnosis of cold autoimmune hemolytic anemia and some forms of drug-induced hemolytic anemia where complement may be the only evidence of immune-mediated hemolysis. Circulating red cells that have been involved in activation of the complement cascade will have mostly C3d on the surface as the result of complement regulatory protein degradation of C3b (Fig. 34–1). Therefore, polyspecific AHG sera used in DAT testing must contain anti-C3d reactivity at minimum and usually contain some anti-C3b reactivity, as well.

The indirect antiglobulin test or IAT is used for detection of in vitro antibody binding to RBCs, regardless of the antibody's ability to fix complement. It is unclear whether polyspecific AHG, which contains anti-complement reactivity, improves serum antibody detection by the IAT. There are rare reports of antibodies that were detected only by their ability to bind

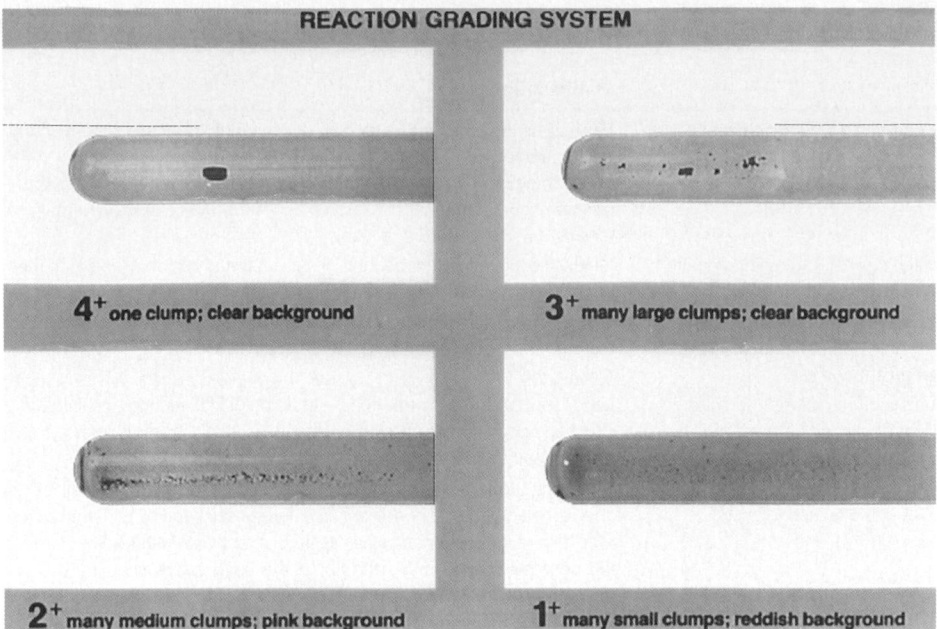

REACTION GRADING SYSTEM

4$^+$ one clump; clear background

3$^+$ many large clumps; clear background

2$^+$ many medium clumps; pink background

1$^+$ many small clumps; reddish background

Figure 34–19 Agglutination grading system showing macroscopic hemagglutination reactions.

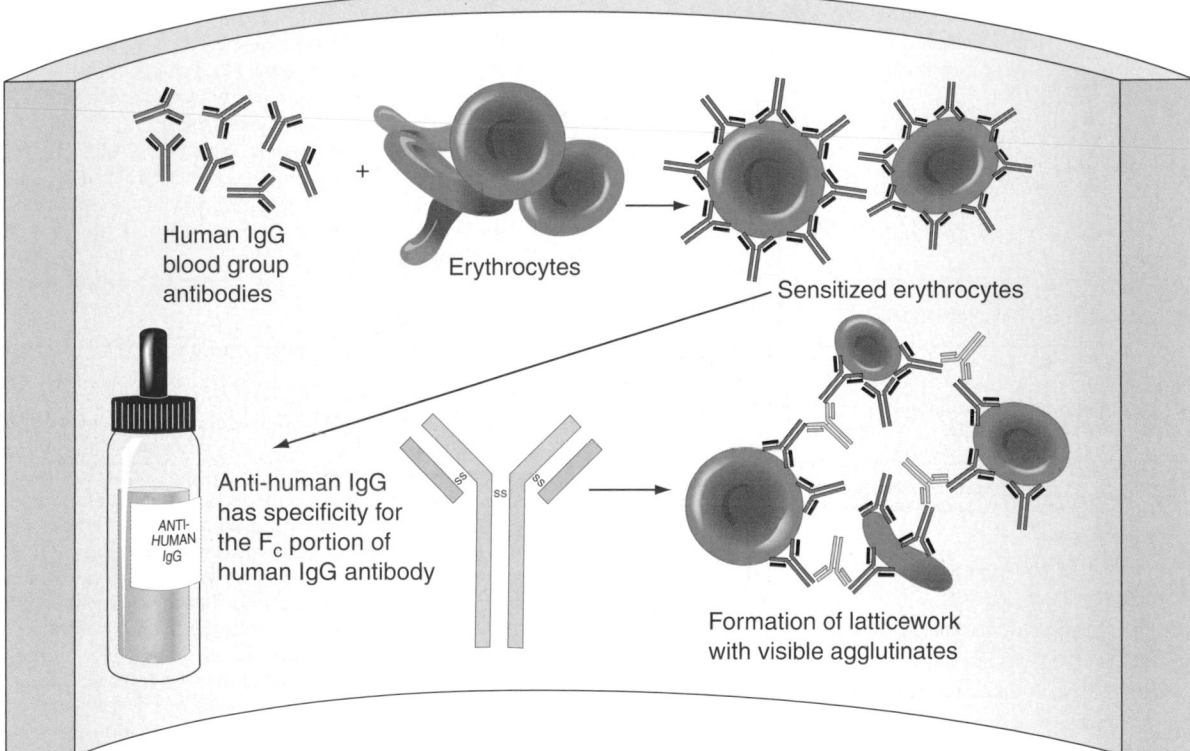

Human IgG blood group antibodies

+ Erythrocytes

Sensitized erythrocytes

Anti-human IgG has specificity for the F$_c$ portion of human IgG antibody

ANTI-HUMAN IgG

Formation of latticework with visible agglutinates

Figure 34–20 Antihuman globulin antibodies form a bridge between adjacent erythrocytes sensitized with human IgG or complement components.

complement in vitro and would have been missed using monospecific anti-IgG reagents (Brecher, 2002). One possible advantage of using polyspecific AHG containing anti-complement activity is that the reactions in the IAT often are stronger than those seen with monospecific anti-IgG alone (Wright, 1979). However, many laboratories choose to use monospecific anti-IgG in antibody detection and identification tests and in crossmatch procedures, because use of this reagent will avoid detection of complement activation by clinically insignificant cold-reactive autoagglutinins or alloantibodies.

Table 34–35 compares the various applications for the DAT and IAT techniques. Antiglobulin testing may be performed using test tubes, capillary tubes, microtiter plates, or gel microtube techniques (see later section on Compatibility Testing). These procedures may be semiautomated or fully automated, particularly in facilities that perform large-volume testing, such as blood collection centers. Unless otherwise specified, procedures referred to in this chapter employ tube testing. The American Association of Blood Banks *Technical Manual* (Brecher, 2002),

Methods in Immunohematology (Judd, 1994), and *Immunohematology Methods* (Mallory, 1993) are excellent general references for most common procedures as well as more specialized techniques.

Quality Control of the Antihuman Globulin Test

In order to standardize antiglobulin sera, and to confirm true-negative antiglobulin reactions, two types of quality control RBCs are normally used: those coated with IgG and those coated with C3b and/or C3d. To sensitize RBCs with IgG, Rh antibodies are usually used. RBCs coated with C3b are prepared by incubation of whole blood in either a low-ionic-strength sucrose medium or with human anti-Le^a or anti-I. C3d-coated RBCs are prepared by incubating C3b-coated cells with fresh serum or trypsin to split C3b→C3d. IgG or complement-coated control cells should give a 1+ to 2+ reaction (Fig. 34–19) when tested with anti-IgG or anti-C3b+C3d.

Quality control cells for the antiglobulin test are referred to as check cells, Coombs' control cells, and sensitized cells. In a true-negative test,

Table 34–35 Applications for the Direct and Indirect Antiglobulin Techniques

	Applications	Purpose	What is detected
Direct antiglobulin test	Investigation of HTR	To detect circulating donor red cells that are sensitized with recipient antibody. A positive DAT is the first immunohematologic evidence of a hemolytic reaction after transfusion	DAT positive due to IgG and/or C3d depending on the antibodies responsible
	Diagnosis of HDN	To detect maternal antibodies that have crossed the placenta to sensitize fetal red cells	DAT almost always positive due to IgG; occasionally C3d if ABO antibodies involved
	Diagnosis of AIHA	To detect autoantibody sensitizing a patient's own red cells	Warm autoantibodies: DAT almost always positive due to IgG Cold autoantibodies: DAT may be due to C3d only
	Investigation of drug-induced hemolysis	To detect anti-drug/red cell antibodies and/or subsequent activation of the complement system	DAT may be positive due to IgG, C3d, or both depending on the mechanism involved (see later under Investigation of Autoimmune Hemolytic Anemia)
Indirect antiglobulin test	Antibody detection (or antibody screen)	To detect clinically significant IgG alloantibodies in the recipient	Recipient IgG antibodies bound to reagent screening cells*
	Antibody identification	To specifically identify those antibodies detected by reagent screening cells or by donor red cells	Recipient IgG antibodies bound to reagent cells from a panel of 10–12 donors*
	Crossmatching	To detect antibodies that may have been missed by the antibody screen because of absence of the corresponding antigen or presence of a dosing antibody	Recipient IgG antibodies bound to donor red cells*
	Red cell antigen typing	To type patient or donor red cells for antigens that can be detected by IgG antisera reactive only by the AGT. A common example of this would be the weak D test	Specific binding of reagent IgG antibodies to red cells positive for the corresponding antigen

HTR = hemolytic transfusion reaction; HDN = hemolytic disease of the newborn; AIHA = autoimmune hemolytic anemia; AGT = antihuman globulin test.

* If complement is fixed in vitro, it may be detected if polyspecific antiglobulin is used.

free active antiglobulin reagent should remain. Control cells, sensitized with IgG and/or C3, are added to all negative tests and centrifuged. Hemagglutination of check cells confirms both the presence and reactivity of the AHG reagent, thus validating a negative test result. If the control cells fail to agglutinate in any tube, the tests must be repeated because they are invalid and may have yielded false-negative results. False-negative tests can occur for a variety of reasons and are listed in Table 34–36.

Sensitivity of the Antihuman Globulin Test
Although the antiglobulin test is extremely sensitive, a negative test by no means excludes the possible presence of antibodies on RBCs. It is estimated that 200–500 IgG or C3 molecules bound per cell are required for detection by antiglobulin antibodies (Brecher, 2002); a smaller number of molecules bound per erythrocyte will give a negative reaction. Also, AHG sera may possess greater activity against some subclasses of IgG than against others; consequently, certain antihuman globulin sera may produce negative results with RBCs coated by a particular IgG subclass.

Compatibility Testing

The term compatibility testing has historically been used synonymously with the serologic crossmatch test. In its broader context, however, compatibility testing is an entire quality process composed of many procedures designed to provide the safest blood product possible for the recipient of a transfusion. These procedures include proper record-keeping, accurate donor and recipient identification, as well as the actual serologic testing of the recipient specimen prior to transfusion. Outlined in the following sections and in Table 34–37 are the steps in compatibility testing required by the AABB *Standards for Blood Banks and Transfusion Services* (Silva, 2004), referred to henceforth as the AABB *Standards*.

Specimen Requirements
Recipient Sample Identification
Proper identification of patient blood samples and donor units is absolutely essential in blood banking. Recipient blood specimens must be labeled by the phlebotomist at the bedside directly from information on the patient's wristband. If the patient's wristband is not attached for any reason, signed confirmation of the patient's identity by nursing staff should be obtained before the blood is drawn. The recipient's blood specimen label should be legible and should include at least the patient's full name, hospital identification number, and specimen collection date,

and it should be securely attached to the specimen tube when it is accepted by blood bank personnel. Unlabeled or improperly labeled blood specimens are unacceptable under any circumstances. During testing, all test tubes or other types of aliquot or reaction containers must also be accurately identified directly from the label on the recipient sample.

Each pretransfusion blood sample should be accompanied by an appropriate order or requisition, containing at least the patient's full name and hospital identification number. The signature or initials of the phlebotomist should be on the requisition, as the test requisition will remain as a permanent record of that particular specimen collection. Upon specimen receipt, the label on the tube must be compared with the information on the requisition for any discrepancies. If there is any doubt as to the proper identity of the sample, a redraw must be obtained.

Type of Sample
Traditionally, serum has been the preferred specimen for compatibility testing, although plasma is increasingly used due to newer testing technologies (e.g., gel test). Problems with plasma in conventional antiglobulin techniques are primarily technical: formation of small fibrin clots during testing may trap RBCs and resemble agglutination; fibrin may also trap serum and cause neutralization of AHG reagent if not removed before washing. Rouleaux formation may be enhanced in plasma if fibrinogen levels are high. If serum is used, blood samples should be collected in siliconized plain tubes without serum separator gel.

Appearance
Some blood bank laboratories have policies in place to reject grossly hemolyzed recipient blood samples as unacceptable for pretransfusion testing unless there is no other choice. Using serum that is already hemolyzed may mask antibody-induced hemolysis that would ordinarily be detectable in antibody screening tests. Lipemia may rarely cause difficulty in evaluating agglutination results, although lipemia is not usually a cause for rejection of a pretransfusion sample.

Age of Sample
According to AABB *Standards*, if a patient has been pregnant or transfused within the preceding 3 months, or if the history is uncertain or unavailable, all crossmatching and red cell transfusions from any given sample must be completed within 72 hours of when the pretransfusion blood sample was drawn. Requiring a new pretransfusion sample every 72 hours on previously transfused or pregnant individuals ensures that the sample being tested is fairly representative of the patient's current immune status.

Table 34–36 Basic Procedures for Direct and Indirect Antiglobulin Testing by Tube Method

Procedure		Reasons for invalid reactions in antiglobulin testing	
		False positive	**False negative**
Direct antiglobulin test (DAT)	1. Prepare a 3–5% suspension in normal saline of the red cells to be tested 2. Add 1 drop of red cell suspension to a tube and wash three to four times with saline 3. Blot the tube after the last wash 4. Add 2 drops of polyspecific AHG (anti-IgG +anti-complement) 5. Centrifuge and examine for agglutination* 6 Add check cells to all negative tubes (see Quality Control of the Antihuman Globulin Test)	Over-centrifugation Direct agglutination by strong cold agglutinins Over-incubation with enzyme-treated cells Improper use of PEG or polycation enhancement reagents Inadequate resuspension of cell button Rouleaux formation‡	AHG reagent failure† Failure to add AHG reagents† Improper or inadequate washing† Delayed washing (elution of weakly attached antibody) Serum/cell ratio too low Failure to add test serum or enhancement reagents Under-centrifugation Resuspension of cell button too vigorous
	Note: For DAT, blood samples should be collected in EDTA to prevent fixation of complement in vitro by clinically insignificant cold autoagglutinins	Dirty glassware Small fibrin clots may trap cells and mimic agglutination	
Indirect antiglobulin test (IAT)	1. Place one drop of each 3–5% red cell suspension to be tested in a tube (e.g., donor cells, reagent screening cells) 2. Add 2–3 drops of patient serum or the recommended number of drops of commercially prepared antisera to each tube 3. Add recommended number of drops of enhancement media such as LISS or albumin if indicated 4. Incubate at 37°C for the time period indicated for the assay being performed (from 15–60 minutes) 5. If part of the procedure, centrifuge and examine serum for hemolysis and the cells for agglutination 6. Whether step 5 is performed or not, continue by washing the tube(s) three to four times with normal saline 7. Blot tubes dry after the last wash 8. Add 2 drops of antiglobulin sera (either poly or monospecific anti-IgG) to all tubes 9. Centrifuge and examine for agglutination* 10. Add check cells to all negative tubes	Cells with a positive DAT will yield false-positive results in any indirect antiglobulin test	

* Protocol may include optional microscopic examination to confirm macroscopically negative tests.
† Will be detected by use of Coombs' control cells
‡ Rouleaux will cause false-positive results in indirect tests read after 37°C incubation.

Table 34–37 Required Steps in Pretransfusion Compatibility Testing*

Phlebotomy/recipient identification	Phlebotomist must positively identify the recipient and recipient's blood sample • Transfusion request and labeled patient blood sample must contain at least two pieces of independent identifying information for that patient (e.g., name, hospital number, date of birth) • Phlebotomist must sign either sample label or requisition • Transfusion service will ensure that identifying information on the requisition and sample label is in agreement
Recipient testing	Perform ABO and Rh typing on recipient's blood specimen – red cell and serum testing are required Review previous records for comparison with current typing results and also for information regarding presence of previously detected clinically significant antibodies Test recipient's serum or plasma to detect clinically significant antibodies • Method must include 37°C incubation with conversion to antihuman globulin or validated equivalent technique
Donor testing	Confirm ABO and Rh type on donor red cell units as required • Confirmation testing for ABO group required on all units (serum testing not required) • Comfirmation of Rh type required only on those units labeled as Rh negative
Crossmatch	Select ABO and Rh compatible red cell components for transfusion Perform serologic or electronic crossmatch of red cell components • Full antiglobulin crossmatch required if current antibody screen is positive or the patient has a known history of clinically significant antibodies
Labeling	Label all red cell products or other components with the recipient's identifying information • Label must contain at least two independent patient identifiers, donor unit number and compatibility test results, if performed

* Requirements paraphrased from Brecher (2002) – see *AABB Standards* (Silva, 2004) for specific wording.

Sample Storage

AABB *Standards* also require that all pretransfusion samples must be stored at 1–6°C for at least 7 days after testing is completed, along with at least one representative segment from each of the donor units crossmatched on the recipient. The purpose of this is to ensure that repeat or additional testing of the donor or patient may be performed later if the patient experiences a delayed hemolytic reaction or other adverse effect of transfusion.

Documentation and Record-Keeping

General Considerations

All blood banks must have a manual or computerized system of record-keeping that contains the results or outcomes of all tests and activities carried out in the blood bank. Records must be complete and retrievable within a reasonable time frame. Transfer or dissemination of information from any records regarding patients must conform to requirements of the institution's confidentiality policies in accordance with federal and state laws and regulations. Records must be preserved for different periods of time depending on federal, state, and accrediting agency requirements.

Documentation of the entire compatibility testing process must include records of patient identification, order entry, individual special transfusion needs, date and time of testing, results of patient testing, identity of the technologist who performed the testing, and blood component issue. A computerized system is ideal for capturing this information and enables rapid and easy retrieval of these data for a given patient, including records of ABO and Rh type, antibody problems, transfusion history, and requirements for special types of blood products. From a more global perspective, computerized retrieval of data for groups of patients also greatly enhances the monitoring of blood product utilization within the facility including blood ordering and transfusion practices of physicians.

Results and interpretation of all patient testing should be documented on appropriate manual worksheets or entered into the computer immediately upon observation of the results. In a manual record-keeping system, all forms should be filled out with ink, not pencil. If results must be changed on manual worksheets, original results must not be obliterated; a single line should be placed through them and the new results initialed by the technologist making the change. A continuously updated list of initials used by all personnel working in the blood bank on all shifts must be part of the permanent blood bank records. Changes to computerized results must also be completely documented as part of the computerized result record with ability to track both the original and corrected data (Brecher, 2002).

Check of Previous Records

Manual or computerized records must be checked for previous results on a given patient when a new sample is received. ABO and Rh tests on the current specimen should be checked against previous results, if available, to help verify that the specimen was collected from the correct individual. Information on any unexpected antibodies identified previously is also extremely important, since the titer of an antibody may fall to levels that cannot be detected by antibody screening procedures. If a clinically significant antibody was previously identified, the patient must receive RBCs negative for the corresponding antigen (antigen-negative) even if current tests for antibody detection are negative.

ABO Grouping

Antisera and reagent RBCs for ABO grouping are well standardized and readily available commercially. Most blood bank laboratories use monoclonal reagent antisera derived from antibodies produced by hybridoma cell lines, although a few (Shulman, 2001) still use polyclonal ABO typing reagents manufactured from pools of high-titered human antibodies. ABO grouping consists of two parts commonly referred to as red cell grouping (forward type) and serum grouping (back type). In forward grouping, a 3–5% RBC suspension is tested with commercially prepared anti-A and anti-B to test for antigens on the RBC membrane. In reverse grouping, patient or donor serum is tested against reagent cells of known A_1 and B phenotype to test for the expected ABO antibodies in the patient's serum (see Table 34–8). ABO grouping is carried out at room temperature with only an immediate-spin centrifugation step required to promote a macroscopic agglutination reaction.

ABO Grouping of Donors

The collecting facility is required to ABO type all donors by RBC and serum ABO grouping methods. The transfusion service, or other laboratory responsible for compatibility testing, must confirm the ABO group of all units of RBCs or whole blood received. RBC grouping is performed from an integral segment attached to each donor unit. For units labeled as group O, anti-A,B alone may be used for donor confirmatory testing since only group O RBCs will fail to hemagglutinate with anti-A,B.

ABO Grouping of Recipients

Every pretransfusion patient blood specimen must also be tested for ABO group. Both RBC and serum grouping are required for the initial ABO testing of all patient samples, and the results of RBC and serum testing should agree with each other (Table 34–8) before any results are reported and blood is transfused.

Some blood banks routinely include the use of anti-A,B in the RBC grouping procedure. However, this reagent does not usually yield any additional useful information except for the detection of the A_x or B_x subgroups. Anti-A,B is also frequently used as a convenient reagent for use in repeat testing to confirm initial typing of a group O patient.

ABO Grouping Discrepancies

Interpretation of ABO blood grouping results is generally straightforward. In the event that the results of RBC and serum grouping do not agree, the testing is repeated to rule out any clerical or technical error. If results are unchanged, a discrepancy is present that may be due to problems with either the patient's serum or cells.

In contrast to RBC grouping, in which reactions are usually strong and clear cut, the reactions of serum grouping may vary greatly in strength. An extended period of incubation at room temperature or incubation at 4°C may be required to demonstrate the presence of weak serum ABO agglutinins (Table 34–10). Group O cells may also used in serum testing to confirm the suspected presence of an unexpected room-temperature reactive alloantibody. If anti-A_1 is suspected in the serum of an A subgroup phenotype, A_2 and O cells may be tested in the serum grouping to confirm the presence of anti-A_1.

Anti-A_1 typing reagent can be useful in red cell testing to confirm a suspected A subgroup phenotype (Table 34–10). To confirm and classify weak ABO subgroups and rare ABO phenotypes, special techniques such as adsorption–elution, secretor studies, or tests for serum A, B, or H transferases may be necessary. The observance of weak mixed field reactions (minor population of agglutinates) can also be informative.

Table 34–38 lists some of the many reasons for ABO discrepancies. Brecher (2002) and Harmening (1999) review a more complete description of these problems and the protocols for resolution. If a blood transfusion is needed emergently, and an ABO discrepancy occurs that cannot be resolved in a timely manner, group O packed RBCs, AB fresh frozen plasma, or both may be given. However, it is important to be certain that sufficient pretransfusion blood specimen is obtained from the patient so that the work-up may be continued. In some cases, it may be necessary to send a pretransfusion specimen to a reference laboratory for further evaluation.

RH Typing

Several types of antisera are available for detection of the RhD antigen. Today, the most commonly utilized anti-D typing reagent in tube testing is a saline-reactive, low-protein, monoclonal/polyclonal blend containing murine monoclonal IgM anti-D for immediate direct agglutination of D-positive red cells, and human polyclonal IgG anti-D necessary for weak D (formerly called D^u) testing. Also available is a reagent blend of monoclonal IgM and monoclonal IgG anti-D from human/murine heterohybridoma lines suitable for both direct and subsequent weak D testing of RBCs.

Prior to the availability of monoclonal blended reagents, most routine D typing was performed using rapid tube anti-D made from pooled human sera and containing high-molecular-weight protein additives that enhanced the direct agglutinating capability of human IgG anti-D. However, due to the high protein concentration in these rapid tube reagents, spontaneous, false-positive aggregation can be observed in patients with abnormal serum proteins, or whose RBCs are heavily sensitized with autoantibody. As a control, manufacturers of high-protein Rh typing sera recommend running a parallel diluent control containing no antibody, to detect false-positive reactions. For saline-reactive Rh typing reagents in use today, a concurrent negative reaction with anti-A or anti-B is a sufficient negative control. However, patients who appear to be AB, Rh-positive should be retyped for D simultaneously with anti-D and an inert control reagent such as 6–8% bovine albumin.

Direct typing for the D antigen is carried out at room temperature by the immediate spin technique, after mixing one drop of saline-washed 3–5% RBC suspension and one drop of commercial anti-D. If weak D testing is necessary, RBCs are tested by the IAT with an IgG anti-D. A parallel test with a negative diluent control is always included for the weak D test.

RH Typing of Donors

As required by the AABB *Standards*, all whole blood donor units are tested by the collecting facility for the D antigen by direct agglutination methods. A test for weak D phenotype is performed on all donor units giving a negative result by routine D typing tests. If either routine D testing or weak D testing is positive, the unit label shall read Rh-positive. The transfusion service must reconfirm the D type of all RBC units labeled Rh-negative by testing red cells from an integral attached segment by a direct anti-D agglutination method. Repeat testing of donor units by the transfusion service for weak D is not required by the AABB *Standards*.

Table 34–38 Some Causes of ABO Grouping Discrepancies

	Problems with red cell testing	Problems with serum testing
Unexpected positive reactions	Acquired B antigen associated with colon and gastric cancers, intestinal obstructions	Rouleaux-forming proteins present, e.g., plasma expanders, monoclonal gamma globulins
	Cord cells contaminated with Wharton's jelly	Room-temperature alloantibody present, e.g., anti-M, N, P_1
	Autoagglutination caused by cold autoantibodies	Cold autoagglutinin present, e.g., anti-I, IH
	Cells heavily coated with warm autoantibody	Passively acquired ABO antibodies
	Polyagglutination	Subgroup of A with anti-A_1 in serum
	Acriflavine antibody (against dye used in anti-B)	cis-AB with weak anti-B in serum
	Genetic chimerism*	
	Bone marrow transplants*	
	Administration of red cells outside ABO group*	
Unexpected negative reactions	A or B subgroups	Age of patient (elderly, newborn)
	Antigen depression due to leukemia or other disease state	Hypogammaglobulinemia
	High levels of soluble blood group substances associated with pseudomucinous ovarian cyst	Immunosuppression
		Genetic chimerism

* Look for mixed field appearance of reactions with reagent antisera.

RH Typing of Recipients

Every pretransfusion recipient blood specimen must be tested for the D antigen by direct typing. Indirect testing for weak D in recipients is not necessary: patients who fail to agglutinate after direct agglutination are typed as Rh-negative. Some blood banks do perform weak D testing for prenatal specimens; however, more recent data shows that many donors typing as weak D possess a partial D phenotype and are at risk for RhD alloimmunization. Erythrocyte typing for the C, c, E, and e antigens of the Rh system is not be performed routinely but may be done to determine the most probable Rh genotype in the evaluation of antibody problems and parentage studies.

Antibody Detection

All specimens submitted for pretransfusion testing must be screened for clinically significant antibodies in the recipient serum (antibody screen). Because clinically significant antibodies typically react at body temperature, most laboratories omit room temperature incubation entirely. AABB *Standards* require that the method used must incorporate incubation at physiologic or body temperature (37°C) followed by conversion to the IAT. If a method other than the IAT is used, it must have documented and validated equivalent sensitivity in its ability to detect clinically significant antibodies (Brecher, 2002). A variety of different antibody screening protocols, utilizing different technologies, are in use today. Currently, none of the available technologies is capable of detecting all RBC antibodies.

Reagent Red Blood Cells

Reagent RBCs or screening cells used for the detection and identification of antibodies in a patient's serum are usually obtained from commercial manufacturers. AABB *Standards* require that antibody detection in recipients shall be performed using reagent cells that are not pooled. Typically, antibody screening cells consist of two to three group O reagent cells selected from different donors of known phenotype. Sets of cells are prepared so that all antigens to the most commonly encountered blood group antibodies are represented and must include C, c, D, E, e, Fy^a, Fy^b, Jk^a, Jk^b, K, k, Le^a, Le^b, P_1, M, N, S and s antigens. An 'antigram' that lists the blood group antigenic makeup of each cell (Fig. 34–21) accompanies each lot of screening RBCs. When possible, cells that are homozygous for selected antigens are used, which increases the likelihood of detecting weak or dosing antibodies. A three-cell screening panel ensures homozygosity for more antigens such as Jk^a, Jk^b, Fy^a, Fy^b, S, and s, against which the corresponding antibodies are likely to exhibit dosage, but it is also more expensive to buy and use. Several studies (Cordle, 1990; Hoeltge, 1995; Judd, 1997) have shown that use of three red blood samples for antibody detection rarely reveals a clinically significant antibody not detected by a two-cell screening procedure.

Antibody Detection Protocols

Tube Tests

In conventional test tube methods, one volume 3–5% screening reagent cells and two volumes patient serum (giving an average volume/volume

ratio of serum to cells of approximately 50 : 1) are incubated at 37°C with an enhancement medium for the time specified by the manufacturer, centrifuged, and examined for hemolysis or agglutination. The screening cells are then washed three to four times with saline, and AHG reagent is added for final detection of IgG alloantibodies.

Because different blood group antibodies commonly show characteristic reaction patterns by IAT technique (Table 34–7), close examination at different phases of testing in this conventional protocol may yield helpful information in evaluating cases where the screen is positive:

- Direct agglutination of the cells in albumin or LISS after 37°C incubation frequently indicates the presence of an Rh antibody.
- IgM antibodies possessing a wide thermal range, such as anti-I, anti-P_1, and Lewis antibodies, may show reactions in albumin or LISS. However, these reactions generally become much weaker after conversion to the IAT.
- With rare exceptions, in vitro hemolysis of reagent cells after 37°C indicates the presence of Lewis, Kidd, Ii, P, PP_1P^k, or Vel antibodies.
- The vast majority of IgG antibodies, with the exception of Rh, will not be detected until after washing and conversion to the IAT.
- Reaction of the different screening cells in multiple phases or with varying strengths usually indicates that more than one antibody is present.

Column Agglutination Technologies

An alternative methodology for alloantibody detection, which is increasing in use by many transfusion services, is column agglutination technology, first described by Lapierre et al. in 1990. This technology utilizes the differential migration of RBC agglutinates through a small microtube containing a dextran acrylamide, size exclusion gel column. With the ID-Microtyping System (ID-MTS) available commercially in the United States (Ortho-Clinical Diagnostics; Raritan, NJ), gel antiglobulin tests are performed in a plastic card approximately 5 × 7 cm in dimension and holding six microtubes. Anti-IgG is incorporated into the gel column matrix, and precisely measured volumes of screening reagent RBCs (0.8% suspension in LISS) and plasma are incubated at 37°C in the reaction chamber above the column matrix. With six microtubes per card, a two-cell screen for three different patients can be performed in one gel card.

Following incubation, the plastic cards are centrifuged under carefully controlled conditions. IgG-coated RBCs agglutinate as they come into contact with the AHG reagent in the matrix and are trapped. Reaction strength and size determine the migration of the agglutinates, ranging from the largest (4+) agglutinates at the top, with migration of weaker, smaller agglutinates further into the gel column (Fig. 34–22). Unagglutinated RBCs pass easily through the column and are found as a pellet at the bottom. Because the plasma or serum remains in the reaction chamber above the matrix, repeated washing steps and addition of control cells to check the activity of the AHG reagent are unnecessary. The end-point hemagglutination reactions are very stable, allowing the cards to be kept for supervisory review of questionable reactions. The cards can be photocopied or digitally photographed and downloaded as permanent laboratory data.

In addition to antibody detection, anti-IgG gel cards can be used for antibody identification and crossmatching. For direct antiglobulin testing, either anti-IgG or polyspecific anti-IgG + C3d cards are available. There are

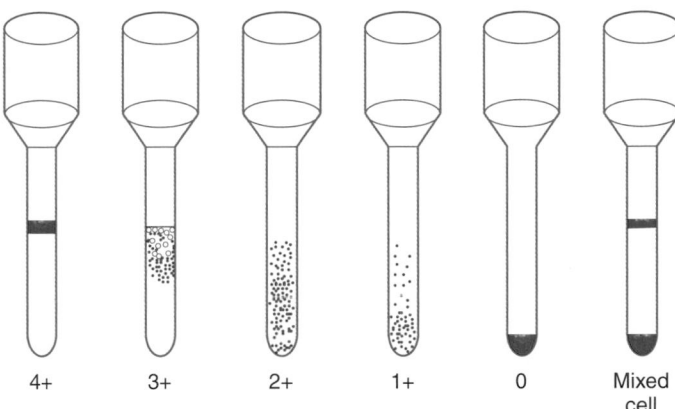

VIAL	Donor	Rh								MNSs				P	Lewis		Lutheran		Kell				Duffy		Kidd		Sex linked
		D	C	E	c	e	f	Cw	V	M	N	S	s	P1	Lea	Leb	Lua	Lub	K	k	Kpa	Jsa	Fya	Fyb	Jka	Jkb	Xga
I	R1R1	0	0	0	+	+	+	0	0	+	0	+	0	+	+	0	0	+	0	+	0	0	+	+	+	0	+
II	R2R2	0	0	0	+	+	+	0	0	+	+	0	+	+	0	+	0	+	+	+	0	0	0	+	0	+	+

Figure 34–21 The 'antigram' accompanying each lot of reagent screening red blood cells.

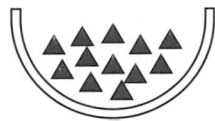

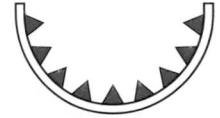
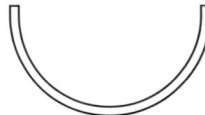

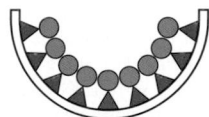
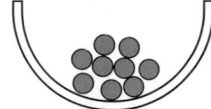

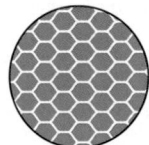
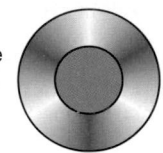

Figure 34–22 Appearance of reactions patterns and grading for gel or column agglutination technology.

Figure 34–23 Principle of solid phase adherence technology with appearance of positive and negative reactions.

also cards for ABO/Rh typing with gel columns incorporating anti-A, anti-B, and anti-D for RBC typing, and two neutral gel columns for ABO serum grouping, in which 0.8% suspensions of reagent A1 and B cells are mixed with patient serum.

In the development of the column agglutination technology, it proved to have an equivalent, if not improved, sensitivity over standard LISS tube testing for antibody detection (Lapierre, 1990). In practice, gel testing actually offers a number of other advantages over conventional tube procedures. With current personnel shortages and the need to have cross-trained, generally less experienced laboratory technologists working in the blood bank, there has been a quest for a number of years for more standardized serologic blood bank testing with a less subjective end point than manual resuspension and reading of agglutination used in conventional tube tests. Column agglutination technology has contributed greatly to standardization of the IAT with aspects that include precise preparation of RBC suspensions, measured reagent delivery volumes, and a reliable, stable agglutination end point. Elimination of repetitive washing steps, manual macroscopic and/or microscopic readings, and addition of antibody-coated control cells allows busy technologists to more effectively utilize their time in performing multiple tasks. In addition, testing can be automated (ProVue™, Ortho Diagnostics, NJ), permitting high-throughput testing, electronic interpretations and validation, and digital documentation of results.

In a retrospective, 12-month study performed to compare the first 6 months before and after implementation of the ID-MTS in a blood bank laboratory that previously used a conventional LISS IAT, repeat antibody screen testing due to ambiguous result interpretation and/or check cells having failed went from a rate of nearly 3% with LISS to just slightly over 0.50% using the gel test (Armstrong, unpublished data). The study also demonstrated a marked reduction using the gel method in the detection and evaluation of clinically insignificant cold antibodies. In reviewing the total distribution of antibody specificities identified in the 6 months before and after gel implementation, clinically insignificant antibodies (anti-Lea, -Leb, -P1, -Sda, -I/HI) accounted for 56% of all antibody work-ups using standard LISS tube testing; in the 6 months after gel implementation, this percentage dropped to 16%. A final finding of this study was that elimination of the many manipulations inherent in conventional LISS tube tests resulted in a significant savings in 'hands-on' time. Although a formal process analysis was not undertaken, time studies on type and screen, full antiglobulin crossmatch, and antibody identification indicated a marked impact on workflow that would have even greater significance when performing batched testing.

Solid Phase Adherence Tests

Another alternative to tube tests for alloantibody detection is indirect solid-phase adherence test systems. In this application, reagent RBCs are bound to the bottom of microplate wells. Serum and an enhancement reagent are added and incubated at 37°C, allowing for alloantibody to bind to the solid phase. After washing to remove unbound serum globulins, indicator RBCs coated with antihuman IgG are added and the plates are centrifuged. If there has been a reaction between the reagent cells and serum alloantibody, the antiglobulin-coated indicator cells will bind and cover the bottom surface of the well, whereas a discrete button in the bottom of the well indicates a negative reaction (Fig. 34–23). Wells may be read manually or with an automated reading device. As with column agglutination, positive reactions are very stable so that the plate may be covered, stored at 2–8°C, and read or re-read up to 2 days later.

Direct solid-phase test systems are also available for applications such as ABO and Rh typing of red cells. For these tests, microplate wells are coated with the appropriate antibodies. Test cells are added, incubated and the plates are then centrifuged. For positive reactions, the RBCs adhere to the entire bottom surface of the antibody-coated well, while negative reactions result in a tightly packed cell button in the bottom of the well. Instrumentation is available for automated and semi-automated testing using solid phase technology.

Antibody Identification

When red cell alloantibodies are detected in the serum of a prospective blood recipient, as indicated by a positive antibody screen, the antibody must be identified so that antigen-negative blood can be provided for transfusion, if required. Antibody identification is accomplished by first testing an extended panel of reagent RBCs of known phenotype against

Table 34–39 Simple Panel Example

Cells in a panel	Known antigenic composition					Test serum	
	D	**C**	**c**	**E**	**e**	**Y**	**Z**
No. 1	+	+	+	0	0	+	0
No. 2	+	+	0	+	+	+	+
No. 3	+	0	+	0	+	+	0
No. 4	0	0	+	0	+	0	0
No. 5	0	0	+	0	+	0	0
No. 6	0	+	0	+	+	0	+

Table 34–40 Probability Values Based on Fisher's Exact Method

Total number of cells tested	Antigen-positive cells that react with antibody	Antigen-negative cells that do not react with antibody	p value
5	3	2	0.100
6	4	2	0.067
6	3	3	0.050
7	5	2	0.048
7	4	3	0.029
8	6	2	0.036
8	5	3	0.018
8	4	4	0.014
9	7	2	0.028
9	6	3	0.012
10	8	2	0.022
10	7	3	0.008
10	6	4	0.005
10	5	5	0.004

the recipient's serum by the IAT technique. An autocontrol is always included as part of testing to help differentiate whether autoantibody, alloantibody or both are present. The immunohematologist then compares the pattern of positive and negative serum reactions to the antigen phenotype pattern on the printed worksheet that accompanies each panel, to find a match.

Interpreting the Results of Antibody Identification

Table 34–39 shows a greatly simplified example of how one would compare the pattern of serum reactivity to the antigen phenotype on each panel red cell to find a match. Serum Y reacts with cells No. 1 through 3, which are positive for the D antigen, but does not react with cells No. 4 through 6, which are negative for the D antigen; thus, the pattern of positive and negative serum reactions matches the phenotype pattern for the D antigen, and therefore serum Y appears to contain anti-D. Similarly, the pattern of reactivity for serum Z matches the phenotype pattern for the E antigen, and thus serum Z appears to contain anti-E. However, before such identification can be conclusively stated, one must evaluate the chance that serum Z is reacting by coincidence with an antigen other than E that is present on the two E-positive cells and is absent from the four E-negative cells, leading to an erroneous conclusion. The same possibility must be considered for the probable anti-D in serum Y. In antibody identification, therefore, one must be sure that enough cells of differing antigenic composition are tested to definitively identify a single antibody or combination of antibodies in a given serum.

Fisher's exact method has traditionally been used to statistically calculate the probability that a single antibody has been correctly identified within a confidence interval of 95% (i.e., the probability that the same results would be obtained by random chance because of a different antibody is 1 in 20). This method compares the number of positive and negative results with the number of cells tested that express or lack the corresponding antigen and with the total number of cells tested (Race, 1975).

Table 34–40 lists the probability values calculated by Fisher's exact method that are achieved with differing combinations of positive and negative cells in the total number tested. It can be seen that a p value of 0.05 can be achieved with a minimum of 6 cells – 3 cells being positive for an antigen reacting with the antibody and 3 cells negative for the antigen failing to react with the antibody. Most manufacturers supply reagent cell panels with 10–11 cells with at least one of the combinations of positive and negative cells from Table 34–40 for most of the antigens to which unexpected antibodies are commonly encountered. Consequently, most simple antibody identifications are valid at a p value considerably less than 0.05 except in cases where there are antibodies to low- or high-frequency antigens or when there are multiple antibodies in the same serum. In these situations, additional cells may have to be tested from other panels to achieve identification within the 95% confidence interval.

Figure 34–24 shows the results of a panel tested against patient serum with a conventional tube antiglobulin testing method and examined for agglutination both after the 37°C incubation phase and finally after the addition of antihuman globulin. In a quick overview of the panel results, an immunohematologist will at once notice that there is agglutination with different cells after centrifugation in both phases of the test, indicating the probable presence of multiple antibodies. Following is an outline of the strategy used in evaluating antibody identification results.

1. The autocontrol is negative indicating that the serum reactivity is most probably due to alloantibodies. However, if the autocontrol were positive, it is important that DAT testing be performed to confirm or rule out prior in vivo sensitization of the patient's cells. The DAT should be examined closely for the appearance of mixed field agglutination. In recently transfused patients, attachment of alloantibody to a minor population of transfused donor RBCs causes classic mixed field agglutination and is frequently the first sign of a developing immune response that may result in a delayed hemolytic transfusion reaction.

2. The first step that is performed by many immunohematologists in evaluating antibody identification results is to *rule out* those antibodies where the serum has failed to react with a cell known to carry the corresponding antigen. Although not required, whenever possible it is best to rule out antibodies based on lack of reactivity with cells demonstrating the homozygous form of an antigen, so as not to erroneously rule out weakly reactive antibodies that show dosage. Using the homozygous 'rule of thumb' for ruling out antibodies, cells No. 3, 5, 6, and 7 are not reactive with the serum and may be used to rule out anti-D, anti-C, anti-c, anti-e, anti-M, anti-N, anti-s, anti-P_1, anti-Lu^b, anti-k, anti-Fy^b, anti-Jk^a, anti-Jk^b. Expression of the antigens f, V, Le^a, Le^b, and Xg^a cannot be characterized as homozygous due to the mechanisms of their inheritance, but because at least one of the four cells above are positive for these antigens, and the serum did not react with them, the corresponding antibodies may be eliminated from consideration.

3. Because of reactions seen in different phases and demonstrating different agglutination strengths, at least two antibodies are likely present in the serum:

   • Cells No. 4 and 10 show direct agglutination in the 37°C phase followed by stronger agglutination in the AHG phase, which is very typical of Rh system antibodies. These are the only two cells on the panel positive for the E antigen, which has not been ruled out. Thus, it is likely that anti-E is one of the antibodies involved.

   • Cells No. 2 and 8 show very strong agglutination in the AHG phase only. Examining the antigens across the top of the panel that have not been ruled out, one sees the phenotype of the panel cells for the K antigen fits the serum reactivity of these two cells. Thus, it is likely that anti-K is a second antibody involved.

   • The remaining serum reactions with cells No. 1, 9, and 11 cannot be explained by either anti-E or anti-K, but could be explained by anti-Fy^a, because all three of these cells are positive for the Fy^a antigen, and Fy^a has not been ruled out.

4. Anti-S should be ruled out by testing another cell positive in the homozygous state for S antigen that at the same time is negative for Fy^a, K, and E antigens.

5. Antibodies to low-frequency antigens such as C^w, Lu^a, Kp^a, and Js^a may be ruled out by testing appropriate cells if available. Alternatively, antibodies to low-frequency antigens may not be ruled out by many blood banks; instead the antiglobulin crossmatch would be used to detect any potential incompatibility between donor cells and the theoretical presence of one or more of these antibodies in the patient's serum.

6. Ruling out of additional antibodies may also sometimes be accomplished by typing the patient's cells for selected antigens. This is particularly helpful when a patient's serum contains multiple antibodies, and the reagent cell resources available to the blood bank are limited. If one of the antibodies that must be ruled out in a mixture of antibodies is anti-Jk^b, for example, the patient's cells may be typed for the Jk^b antigen with specific antisera. If the patient

Name: *John Doe*

Hospital Number: *0001234.56*

Rh phenotype		D	C	E	c	e	f	Cw	V	M	N	S	s	P₁	Leᵃ	Leᵇ	Luᵃ	Luᵇ	K	k	Kpᵃ	Jsᵃ	Fyᵃ	Fyᵇ	Jkᵃ	Jkᵇ	Xgᵃ	Vial	37C	AHG	CC
				Rh							**MNSs**			**P**	**Lewis**		**Lutheran**		**Kell***				**Duffy**		**Kidd**			**Vial**			
1	rr	0	0	0	+	+	+	0	0	+	0	+	0	+	+	0	0	+	0	+	0	0	+	+	+	0	+	1	0		1
2	rr	0	0	0	+	+	+	0	0	+	+	0	+	+	0	+	0	+	+	+	0	0	0	+	0	+	+	2	0		3
3	r′r	0	0	0	+	+	+	0	0	+	0	+	+	+	0	+	0	+	0	+	0	0	0	+	0	+	0	3	0	0	2
4	r″r	0	0	+	+	+	+	0	0	+	+	+	+	0	0	+	+	+	0	+	0	0	0	+	0	+	0	4	1	2	
5	rr	0	0	0	+	+	+	0	0	0	+	+	+	+	0	+	0	+	0	+	0	0	0	+	0	+	+	5	0	0	2
6	R₀r	+	0	0	+	+	+	0	+	+	+	0	+	+	0	0	0	+	0	+	0	0	0	0	+	0	0	6	0	0	2
7	R₁R₁	+	+	0	0	+	0	0	0	+	0	+	0	0	+	0	0	+	0	+	0	0	0	+	+	0	0	7	0	0	2
8	R₁R₁	+	+	0	0	+	0	0	0	+	+	+	+	0	+	0	0	+	+	+	0	0	+	0	0	+	+	8	0		3
9	R₁R₁ʷ	+	+	0	0	+	0	+	0	+	+	0	+	+	0	+	0	+	0	+	0	0	+	+	+	+	+	9	0		1
10	R₂R₂	+	0	+	+	0	0	0	0	+	+	0	+	+	+	0	0	+	0	+	+	0	+	0	0	+	+	10	1	2	
11	rr	0	0	0	+	+	+	0	0	0	+	0	+	+	0	+	+	+	0	+	+	0	0	+	+	+	0	11	0		1
																												Auto	0	0	2

AHG = antihuman globulin
CC = Coombs' control cells
* Unless otherwise specified, it is understood that all cells are positive for the high frequency antigens Kpᵇ and Jsᵇ

Figure 34–24 A typical panel worksheet showing an example of antibody identification results.

expresses the Jkᵇ antigen, then the presence of an alloantibody to Jkᵇ can be conclusively eliminated.

7. On the panel in Figure 34–24, there are at least 3 cells negative for all three antigens – Fyᵃ, K, and E – that do not react with the serum. However, to conclusively identify all three antibodies within the 95% confidence interval, there must also be three separate cells positive only for Fyᵃ antigen, three positive only for K antigen, and three positive only for E antigen that do react with the serum. Thus, anti-Fyᵃ can be identified with confidence; however, two more cells positive for K antigen and one more cell positive for E antigen must be tested with the serum to conclusively identify the presence of anti-K and anti-E.

8. If antibody identification is being performed for the first time on a particular patient, it is common practice to also type patient RBCs for the antigens to which he or she has developed antibodies, as a confirmation of the identification made. The patient's RBCs should lack the antigens corresponding to the antibodies present.

Crossmatching

For many years, prior to administration of whole blood or red cell components, a major serologic crossmatch was required prior to the transfusion of whole blood or packed RBCs. This protocol required a 37°C incubation followed by conversion to the IAT, just as in antibody detection tests. However, in 1984, this requirement was eliminated by the AABB *Standards* as long as (1) the current antibody screen on the patient is completely negative and (2) there is no past history of clinically significant antibodies. Currently, for patients who meet these criteria, only a procedure designed to detect ABO incompatibility need be used. This may consist of a serologic immediate spin procedure or an electronic crossmatch as described in more detail below.

Immediate Spin Serologic Crossmatch

The serologic test to detect ABO incompatibility commonly consists of an immediate spin protocol employing a 3–5% saline suspension of donor RBCs prepared from an integral segment taken from the selected donor unit. Cells are usually washed once to remove any anticoagulant or plasma protein that could interfere with the testing. A drop of donor cell suspension is mixed with recipient serum, centrifuged immediately, and examined for hemolysis and/or agglutination. This procedure has come to be known as the abbreviated or immediate-spin crossmatch.

Use of the immediate-spin crossmatch procedure in clinical settings has shown it to be a safe and cost-effective alternative to the antiglobulin crossmatch (Cordle, 1990; Judd, 1988; Shulman, 1990), though there are reports of this technique failing to detect ABO incompatibility when recipient ABO antibodies are of low titer or when donor cells belong to a weak ABO subgroup (Berry-Dortch, 1985; Shulman, 1987). Rare false-

negative results can occur due to a prozone effect in Group O/Group A major incompatibility, particularly if there is a delay in centrifugation (Judd, 1988). The prozone/delay apparently allows for the fixation of C1 complement on RBC membranes, which sterically hinders hemagglutination. Suspension of donor cells in EDTA-saline eliminates this problem by chelating calcium necessary for formation of the C1 complement complex. In addition to false negatives, the immediate-spin crossmatch can cause false-positive results due to rouleaux, cold-reactive antibodies, and fibrin – all of which may result in delay of issuing the blood for transfusion. In a survey of pretransfusion practices throughout the US conducted from January 1995 to January 1996 (Maffei, 1998), slightly more than half of the 1047 hospitals responding to a question on routine crossmatching protocols reported using the immediate-spin crossmatch for patients with no clinically significant antibodies.

Electronic Crossmatch

In 1994 Butch et al. first reported on a proposed standard operating procedure that would replace the immediate-spin serologic crossmatch with a computer or 'electronic crossmatch' or EXM. This has been advocated for some time by those who argue that the immediate-spin serologic crossmatch will occasionally fail in its ultimate purpose to identify ABO incompatibilities between a recipient and an incompatible donor unit chosen erroneously for crossmatch. Proponents of the electronic crossmatch state that the best way to ensure compatibility is to reduce the human error factor that would allow the wrong units to be crossmatched in the first place by assigning final verification of ABO compatibility between donor and recipient to a computer system (Judd, 1991). This would also eliminate time-consuming investigation of false-positive serologic reactions.

Similarly to the use of the immediate-spin crossmatch, the electronic crossmatch may be used only for patients who have no currently detected clinically significant antibodies or any history of alloantibodies. The EXM is permissible provided that specific testing criteria are met and extensive validation of the blood bank information system has been performed to meet current AABB *Standards* and FDA requirements as outlined in a 1997 FDA internal document (Judd, 2002). The FDA requirement that facilities wishing to implement the EXM submit a request for variance to the Code of Federal Regulations for Compatibility Testing (21CFR606.151; 2001a) has been eliminated. Table 34–41 summarizes the AABB *Standards* requirements.

Critical elements required in computer validation for the EXM (Judd, 1998) include updated hardware, instrumentation interfaces, historical records checks, reaction interpretation algorithms, prevention functions and warnings for ABO assignment/release, and personnel competency assessment. Because the safety of this procedure will be only as good as the electronic information that is entered and stored in the system, maximal

Table 34–41 Requirements for Implementation of the Electronic Crossmatch*

Computer system has been validated on-site to ensure that only ABO-compatible red cell components are selected for transfusion

There have been at least two determinations of the recipient's ABO group, one of which is from the current sample

The donor unit blood type has been confirmed serologically from an integrally attached segment

The system contains the following data items:

Donor unit number

Component name

ABO/Rh type of component

Interpretation of donor confirmatory test results

Two unique identifiers for recipient

Recipient's ABO group/Rh type

Recipient's current antibody screen results[†]

A method exists to verify the correct entry of data prior to release of components

The software contains logic to warn user of discrepancies between donor unit labeling and confirmatory test results, or of ABO incompatibilities between the recipient and the donor unit

---

* Requirements paraphrased from Brecher (2002) – see *AABB Standards* (Silva, 2004) for specific wording.

[†] The electronic crossmatch can be used only if current antibody detection tests on the recipient are negative and there is no known history of clinically significant blood group antibodies.

---

use of bar codes to identify both donors and patients should be implemented. After extensive experience with electronic crossmatching at the University of Michigan, Judd (1998) recommends that bar-coded patient identification be mandatory, both at the time of sample collection and prior to transfusion, and that pretransfusion specimen labels be generated at the bedside from the bar code on the patient identification wristband.

In the survey of US pretransfusion practices cited earlier (Maffei, 1998), 1% of the 1047 responding hospitals reported using the electronic crossmatch. Outside of the US, several countries, including Sweden, Denmark, Australia, and Hong Kong, have published reports on their experience with electronic crossmatching (Chan, 1996; Cox, 1997; Säfwenberg, 1997).

Antiglobulin Crossmatch

As mentioned previously, if the pretransfusion antibody screen detects a clinically significant antibody, or a check of patient records indicates that such antibodies have been detected previously, a major crossmatch between the recipient serum and donor red cells must be performed by the antiglobulin method used routinely by a given laboratory. Optimally, red cell units for transfusion should also be phenotyped with commercially available antisera of known potency to demonstrate the lack of antigens to which the patient has formed antibodies.

A full antiglobulin procedure may also be chosen for all crossmatching at the discretion of a given blood bank laboratory. For patients with a negative antibody screen, the full crossmatch may rarely detect alloantibodies to low-frequency antigens not present on the screening cells (e.g., Kp[a], Wr[a]). In addition, antibody detection tests could theoretically fail due to the presence of an antibody displaying dosage, deterioration of antigen from the reagent cells during storage, or because of technical error. However, reports in the literature surveying the experience of various institutions that have eliminated the antiglobulin crossmatch (except in instances where it is required) show the predictive value of routinely performing an antiglobulin crossmatch is minimal. The actual incidence of missing a *clinically significant* antibody is very low – less than 0.05% (Mintz, 1982; Cordle, 1990). A multicenter study involving 1.3 million immediate-spin crossmatches demonstrated an observed risk of acute hemolytic reaction of only 0.0004% using the immediate-spin crossmatch technique (Shulman, 1990).

Compatibility Testing In Emergencies

In urgent situations, blood may need to be released for transfusion prior to the completion of compatibility tests, or even before a patient blood specimen is available. If the ABO and Rh types of the patient are not known, group O-negative packed RBCs are released. If a blood specimen is available, and there is time to perform ABO and Rh typing, type-specific

blood may be released. All units are conspicuously labeled to indicate they are uncrossmatched and that the patient's serum has not been screened for unexpected antibodies. In these situations, the patient's physician *must* sign a release form stating that the clinical situation warrants the release of uncrossmatched blood. In such cases, the antibody screen is promptly completed, and crossmatches are performed by the laboratory's protocol. In the event of a positive screen or incompatible crossmatch, the physician should be notified immediately of any antibodies or incompatibility detected.

Massive transfusion occurs when the number of emergently transfused RBCs equals or exceeds the patient's blood volume in a relatively short time frame (< 24 hours). Under these circumstances, many blood banks initiate a massive transfusion policy that permits switching to an immediate-spin crossmatch, even in patients with known RBC alloantibodies. In these instances, serum antibody is typically diluted and undetectable in vitro due to the large volume of blood and fluids transfused. Most protocols for massive transfusion return to the use of the routine crossmatch procedure within 24 hours of when the patient is stabilized. Transfusion of antigen-positive units could result in an increase of antibody titer and lead to a delayed hemolytic transfusion reaction in patients with alloantibodies.

Preoperative Crossmatch Protocols

Studies on the safety and efficacy of the antiglobulin antibody detection protocol (Boral, 1977; Mintz, 1982; Cordle, 1990; Heddle, 1992), show that at least 99% of clinically significant antibodies will be detected by a standard two-cell antibody screen. In reality, a two-cell screen is greater than 99% effective in preventing incompatible transfusions, based on the actual occurrence of common alloantibodies and antigen frequencies in the general population (Boral, 1977). As a result of these reports, most transfusion services have adopted a type and screen-only protocol for surgical procedures that do not routinely require transfusion. The type and screen protocol, when used in conjunction with preoperative blood ordering guidelines (maximum surgical blood order schedule: Friedman, 1976; Henry, 1977), allows for much more efficient blood inventory management and reduction in the C/T (crossmatch/transfusion) ratio. For elective surgical procedures that do not routinely require transfusion, only a type and antibody screen is ordered. Blood orders for elective surgical procedures requiring transfusion are set at a level that reflects actual usage patterns for a given operative procedure at a particular institution. For blood ordering guidelines to be successful, they should come under periodic review and revision as new surgical procedures are adopted and techniques are refined.

The preoperative type and screen protocol requires no further serologic work as long as the patient's antibody screen is negative and there is no known history of clinically significant antibodies. If a patient unexpectedly requires transfusion during surgery, ABO and Rh compatible units are selected, and an immediate-spin crossmatch or EXM may be performed. If no ABO incompatibility is detected, the blood can be safely released to the operating room with a minimal turnaround time.

If the preoperative antibody screen is positive or previous records indicate a known clinically significant antibody, standard operating procedures should specify a minimum number of antigen-negative units that would be held by the blood bank for use by the patient during surgery. These units must be crossmatched with the patient's serum using a full antiglobulin crossmatch procedure prior to transfusion.

Special Antibody Identification Techniques

Patients who have undergone repeated transfusions may respond by forming multiple unexpected blood group antibodies. Autoantibodies and alloantibodies to high-frequency antigens will react with all cells tested, including all RBCs used for antibody identification, making it extremely difficult to detect other underlying alloantibodies. When complicated problems such as these are encountered, special techniques are required to resolve the problem and find compatible units for transfusion. Special techniques used in antibody identification frequently involve: (1) an attempt to eliminate selected antibody reactivity that is interfering with identification of other specificities in the same serum or (2) an effort to enhance or more clearly characterize the reactivity of an antibody that thus far has escaped definitive identification. Some of these techniques are outlined below as well as in Tables 34–42 and 34–43. The reader is also referred to the American Association of Blood Banks *Technical Manual* (Brecher, 2002), *Applied Blood Group Serology* (Issitt, 1998), *Methods in Immunohematology* (Judd, 1994), and *Immunohematology Methods* (Mallory, 1993) as excellent references for most common procedures in addition to more specialized techniques.

Table 34–42 Special Techniques in Antibody Identification: Serum Procedures

	Procedure	Application/effect
Hemagglutination inhibition	Inhibit antibody reactivity by mixing serum with a specific soluble antigen source in parallel with a dilution control; retest against known antigen-positive cells	Confirm specificity by neutralizing the following antibodies: anti-P_1, anti-Le^a and Le^b, anti-Sd^a, anti-ABH; anti-I; anti-Ch/Rg. May also allow for easier identification of other antibodies in a mixture
Serum adsorption	Adsorb serum antibodies with autologous cells, selected allogeneic cells, or rabbit erythrocyte stroma (REST) at appropriate temperature for reactivity of antibody	Physically removes broadly reactive autoantibodies or alloantibodies from serum by reacting with absorbing cells to allow for detection of underlying IgG antibodies – particularly useful in cases of WAIHA. May be combined with elution in complicated cases involving identification of multiple antibodies
Sulfhydryl reagents	Pretreat serum with sulfhydryl reagents such as 2-ME or DTT	Destroys pentameric structure of agglutinating IgM antibodies, effectively bypassing cold reactive auto- and alloantibodies to allow for detection of underlying IgG alloantibodies
Titration	Prepare serial twofold dilutions of serum and test against antigen-positive indicator cell	• Aids in identification of HTLA antibodies (titer of 1 : 64 or greater) • Used to measure increase in production of IgG antibodies during pregnancy • May rarely be useful in identifying alloantibodies of a higher titer present with a warm autoantibody
Prewarming	Keep all test components (test tubes, cells, serum, saline) at 37°C prior to testing; use monospecific anti-IgG AHG reagents	Bypasses reactivity of cold auto- or alloagglutinins of limited titer and thermal amplitude – prevents direct agglutination of test cells and/or in vitro complement activation in antibody detection and identification tests
Saline replacement	For tests in which patient or test red cells are suspended in serum and are suspected to have formed rouleaux, the serum is removed and replaced with equal volume of saline	Useful in obtaining valid results in ABO serum grouping or evaluating the presence of apparent agglutination when examining screening cells after 37°C incubation and centrifugation. Pseudoagglutination due to rouleaux will be dispersed by removal of the offending proteins and addition of a high ionic strength medium.

* See also Table 34–33 for effects of antibody concentration, pH, incubation time, etc.

Table 34–43 Special Antibody Identification Techniques: Red Cell Procedures

	Procedure	Application/effect
Enzyme treatment	Two-stage procedure (preferred): Incubate test red cells with enzyme solution at 37°C; wash cells thoroughly to remove enzyme completely and retest cells with serum being investigated	• Eliminates some antibody reactivity by destroying corresponding antigen structures – MNS, Duffy, Ch/Rg; may be easier to pick out different specificities in a serum containing multiple antibodies • Enhances sensitization, agglutination, and/or hemolysis by other antibodies – Rh, Kidd, many IgM blood group antibodies; may allow for easier identification of weakly reactive antibodies
AET/DTT	Pretreat test red cells with AET or DTT; wash away reagent and retest cells with serum being investigated	Effectively creates Kell 'null' cells for use in identifying alloantibodies in a mixture containing antibody to a high-frequency antigen in the Kell system
Elution	Remove and recover antibody from red cells by techniques such as glycine acid, organic solvents	Concentrates antibody that was coating red cells into a solution suitable for further identification procedures. Used in investigating positive DAT in cases of HDN, HTR, autoimmune hemolytic anemias
Chloroquine diphosphate	Washed packed red cells are incubated in a 1 : 4 ratio with chloroquine at room temperature. Reagent is removed by multiple saline washes	Dissociates IgG from patient red cells with a positive DAT so that they may be typed with blood grouping reagents that require an indirect antiglobulin technique. Only anti-IgG should be used as the AHG reagent, as complement proteins are not dissociated with chloroquine
ZZAP	For adsorption purposes, aliquots of washed, packed red cells are incubated with ZZAP at 37°C. Cells are then washed with large volumes of saline to remove ZZAP. The combination of DTT and enzymes destroys coating IgG autoantibodies	• Removal of autoantibodies from the patient cells provides free antigen sites for adsorption of autoantibody from the serum • ZZAP also can be used to destroy Kell, Cartwright, Gerbich, Dombrock system antigens
Dispersal of IgM-mediated autoagglutination	Incubate cell suspension with sulfhydryl reagents or wash cells multiple times with 37°C saline	Dissociation of cold autoagglutination permits valid ABO red cell typing and may aid in evaluating DAT results
Lectin typing	Reagents commonly derived from plant seeds are used to test for the presence or absence of a specific blood group antigen on the red cell membrane – used in place of an antibody reagent	Useful in typing for specific antigens such as A_1, H, and N and in classifying different polyagglutinable red cell conditions
Cell separation techniques	Washed cells from the patient are centrifuged in microhematocrit tubes, and the top 5 mm containing the lightest cells are harvested Differential agglutination may be performed based on known differences in antigen phenotype between donor and recipient	Useful in the following: • Phenotyping of autologous cells in recently transfused individuals • Evaluating whether a DHTR may be evolving in a patient with autoimmune hemolytic anemia • Estimating survival of transfused cells

IV

Table 34–44 Sources of Soluble Antigens for Hemagglutination Inhibition

Soluble substance	Source
ABH	Secretor saliva
Le^a, Le^b	Secretor saliva
P$_1$	Hydatid cyst fluid or pigeon eggs
Sd^a	Human or guinea pig urine
Ch^a, Rg^a	Plasma from Ch/Rg (+) individuals
I	Human milk

Serum Procedures to Eliminate Antibody Reactivity

Hemagglutination Inhibition

Hemagglutination inhibition is used to neutralize selected blood group antibodies with their corresponding antigen found in soluble form in human saliva, serum, or other body fluids, as well as in substances in nature (see Table 34–44). The identity of a suspected antibody is confirmed if it no longer agglutinates antigen-positive reagent cells after addition of soluble antigen. Hemagglutination inhibition may be particularly useful when working with a serum specimen containing multiple specificities. The principle of hemagglutination inhibition is also used to determine the secretor status of individuals with weak ABO subgroups (Table 34–10).

Antibody Adsorption

Adsorption is a process used to physically remove antibodies from sera. The adsorption procedure may be performed using washed and/or enzyme-treated autologous RBCs, phenotypically matched allogeneic cells, cells selected to be positive for a specific combination of blood group antigens or red blood cell stroma. The incubation temperature and times used in the adsorption process depend on the immunoglobulin class and thermal range of the antibodies being adsorbed. In general, using a low antibody : cell ratio will increase adsorption efficiency.

Adsorption using allogeneic cells is helpful in separating multiple alloantibodies in a complex mixture (differential adsorption) or in eliminating the reactivity of an alloantibody to a high-frequency antigen. In patients with autoantibodies, adsorption with autologous RBCs, phenotypically matched cells, and rabbit erythrocyte stroma (REST) is often used to selectively remove warm and cold reactive autoantibodies, respectively. Removal of autoantibodies is necessary to identify any potential underlying alloantibodies the patient may have (see later under Investigation of Autoimmune Hemolytic Anemia and also Figure 34–25).

Thiol Reagents

Sulfhydryl compounds such as 2-mercaptoethanol (2-ME) or dithiothreitol (DTT) cleave disulfide bonds and are frequently used to inactivate the agglutinating capacity of IgM antibodies by cleaving intersubunit disulfide bonds, as well as bonds linking IgM subunits to the J chain (Mollison, 1993), thus destroying the pentameric structure of the IgM molecule. These reagents are useful in investigating the presence of clinically significant IgG alloantibodies in a serum that contains broadly agglutinating IgM cold autoantibodies. They can also be used to dissociate autoagglutination caused by these cold antibodies that may interfere with ABO/Rh typing and DAT testing. In prenatal studies, sulfhydryl reagents are frequently utilized to evaluate a serum containing an antibody such as anti-M that commonly has both an IgM and IgG component. By destroying the agglutinating anti-M, the serum can be tested for IgG anti-M that is capable of crossing the placenta to cause HDN.

Serum Antibody Titration

Serum titration is a method used to semiquantitatively determine the amount of antibody present in a given serum. Serial two-fold dilutions of serum are prepared and then tested with RBCs possessing the corresponding antigen. Each dilution is read for macroscopic agglutination, and the titer of the antibody is expressed as the reciprocal of the highest serum dilution that gives macroscopic agglutination.

Antibody titration is used in the presumptive identification of HTLA (high-titer, low-avidity) antibodies. Most antibodies (excluding HTLA) that initially give weak (± or ±^{m}) reactions in IAT tests will seldom react at dilutions of greater then 1:2. In contrast, HTLA antibodies characteristically give the same weak (± or ±^{m}) reactions at multiple serum dilutions, often reacting at dilutions equal to or greater than 1:64. If such an antibody is suspected, a titration is performed to demonstrate that the weakly reactive antibody is still reactive at a high dilution, thus allowing

Table 34–45 Effect on Antigen Expression/Antibody Reactivity by Enzyme* Treatment of Test Cells

Effect	Antigens
Destroyed	Fy^a, Fy^b
	M, N
	HTLA- Ch/Rg, JMH
	Pr
	Xg^a
Variable	Lu^a, Lu^b
	S, s
Enhanced	ABH
	I/i
	Jk^a, Jk^b
	Le^a, Le^b
	P
	Rh
Usually unaffected	Kell

* Using ficin or papain.
Data from Issitt (1998), Brecher (2002).

its classification as an HTLA. These antibodies are often directed against Ch/Rg, JMH and Knops antigens.

In prenatal studies, clinically significant IgG alloantibodies capable of causing HDN are titrated periodically in the maternal serum during pregnancy. An increasing titer usually indicates that fetal cells possess the corresponding antigen and are stimulating the mother to produce more antibody, thus providing valuable information to the physician regarding how the pregnancy should be managed.

Special Red Cell Procedures for Antibody Identification

Reagent or patient RBCs can be modified in various ways by the immunohematologist to either abolish or enhance the reactivity of corresponding antibodies. Patient cells are also subjected to procedures designed to remove antibody that has bound in vivo so that the antibody may be recovered and identified and/or provide RBCs for further testing.

Destruction of Red Cell Antigens

Available reagents for treating RBCs for the purpose of destroying certain blood group antigens include various proteolytic enzymes (e.g., papain, ficin), neuraminidase (removes sialic acid), ZZAP (a combination of a protease and sulfhydryl reagent), aminoethylisothiouronium bromide (AET) and DTT. In a serum containing multiple alloantibodies, selective pretreatment of RBCs with enzymes can destroy specific antigens, eliminating specific alloantibody reactivity. Enzymes are also thought to remove the water of hydration and decrease the zeta potential, allowing RBCs to more closely approach each other. As a result, they can enhance the reactivity of a weak, potentially significant antibody and facilitate its identification. Table 34–45 lists antibodies whose reactivity will be enhanced or eliminated by enzyme treatment of test RBCs. Note, AET and DTT can be used to create RBCs negative for all antigens of the Kell blood group system (except Kx); these reagents may also destroy certain antigens reacting with HTLA antibodies.

Antibody Elution

Elution is the process used to remove antibodies bound to RBCs in vivo, as indicated by a positive DAT. Elution is commonly used to concentrate and solubilize antibodies from RBCs for subsequent identification studies. The elution of an antibody with known blood group and/or drug specificity can be diagnostic in the evaluation of acute and delayed hemolytic transfusion reactions, HDN, autoimmune hemolytic anemia, and immune hemolytic anemia induced by medication.

Elution may be accomplished by a variety of methods that alter or reverse the forces of attraction that hold the antigen and antibody together. Various methods involve adding heat, disrupting antigen structure by exposing the RBC membrane to freezing and thawing, organic solvents, and altering the pH to dissociate RBC–antibody complexes. All methods require numerous washes prior to elution to remove any serum containing unbound antibody. To ensure the complete removal of serum antibody, the saline from the last wash must be tested against appropriate cells to detect any residual unbound antibody. The last wash control should show an absence of antibody reactivity before the elution procedure is performed. Optimally, eluates should be tested on the same day they are prepared but may be stored at −20°C or lower if there is a delay in testing. Table 34–46 lists some of the common elution methods and their applications. For a more comprehensive listing and specific descriptions of elution procedures, see Mallory (1993).

Removal of Antibody From Red Cells to Facilitate Antigen Typing

Many antisera used for RBC antigen typing require the IAT technique. As a result, RBC samples with a positive DAT cannot be used for antigen typing since these cells are already coated with IgG antibody and will yield a false-positive result. Most elution methods that remove blood group antibodies from the surface of erythrocytes destroy either the cells or the antigens. However, treatment of antibody-coated RBCs with chloroquine diphosphate dissociates antibody while leaving the antigens relatively intact (Edwards, 1982). Glycine/EDTA can also be used under carefully controlled conditions to dissociate IgG from RBCs, but overtreatment with this reagent can cause irreversible damage to the RBC membrane. After chloroquine or glycine treatment, RBCs can be antigen typed with antihuman globulin reactive antisera. Please note that glycine/EDTA-treated cells cannot be typed for Kell system antigens, as they are destroyed.

Care should be exercised when interpreting antigen typing results with chloroquine-treated cells. There are reports that Rh antigens, and possibly other blood group antigens, can be weakened, resulting in false-negative reactions. Saline-reactive antisera, including monoclonal grouping reagents, should not be used with chloroquine-treated cells (Gamma Biologicals Inc., 2001). For either chloroquine or glycine/EDTA, it is prudent to treat known antigen-positive cells in parallel as a control. Only monospecific anti-IgG should be used in the IAT because complement components are not dissociated by chloroquine from DAT-positive RBCs.

Red Blood Cell Typing With Lectin Reagents

Lectin typing reagents contain proteins that will recognize specific carbohydrates on the RBC membrane, causing direct hemagglutination. Lectin reagents are usually derived from plant seeds, but these receptor proteins are also found in some invertebrate animals and lower vertebrates. Because the potency of lectin reagents may vary with the preparation, each lot should be standardized before use. Although many lectins have been described, only a few have been found useful in blood banking (Bird, 1988). Sources for selected lectin reagents and their applications are listed in Table 34–47.

Separation of Autologous From Transfused Red Cells

In transfused patients, it may be necessary to separate autologous from transfused cells. Autologous RBC for antigen typing may be necessary in a transfused patient with multiple alloantibodies, a warm autoantibody and possible alloantibodies, or an antibody to a high-incidence antigen. The

ability to perform a DAT, and possibly even elution, on separated autologous and/or transfused cells can help evaluate whether a recently transfused individual with a warm autoimmune hemolytic anemia (WAIHA) is developing a delayed hemolytic transfusion reaction (DHTR) due to new alloantibodies. In rare cases, DAT testing on separated autologous RBCs may be required to differentiate a WAIHA from a DHTR involving a high-incidence antigen. In a final application, one could roughly estimate the proportion of surviving, transfused RBCs when a DHTR is suspected.

Two basic techniques for separating autologous from transfused RBCs are differential agglutination and density separation using centrifugation. In the first technique, antibodies are used to agglutinate only one

Table 34–46 Antibody Elution Techniques

Method	Principle*	Application
Heat	Addition of heat changes equilibrium constant of antigen–antibody reaction and antibodies are released	• Recovery of ABO antibodies in cases of ABO HDN • Gentle heat elution (at 45°C) may be useful for removing antibody from cells that is causing false-positive direct hemagglutination tests
Freeze–thaw	Damage to the red cell membrane by hemolysis alters complementary fit between antigen and antibody	Recovery of ABO antibodies in cases of ABO HDN
Acid (e.g., digitonin acid, glycine acid/EDTA)	At an acid pH, antigen and antibody become negatively charged and repulse each other	• Good recovery of most IgG blood group antibodies (may be less sensitive for Kidd) • Glycine/EDTA also used to dissociate antibody but leave red cells intact for phenotyping
Organic solvents (e.g., chloroform, xylene, ether)	Disrupts lipid bilayer of red cell membrane, altering complementary fit and/or reversing selected attractive forces between antigen and antibody	High yield recovery of most IgG blood group antibodies

* Issitt (1998).

Table 34–47 Lectins Useful in Immunohematologic Testing

Lectin	Activity inhibited by	Serologic specificity	Application
Ulex europaeus	α-L-fucose	Anti-H	Secretor status testing, classification of weak A subgroups, investigation of possible Bombay phenotype
Vicia graminea	O-linked N blood group tetrasaccharides (galactose [β 1,3] N-acetyl-galactosamine)	Anti-N	Red cell antigen typing
Griffonia simplicifolia I*	α-D-galactose	Anti-B, Tn	Red cell antigen typing Investigation of acquired B/polyagglutination
Dolichos biflorus	Terminal α-N-acetyl-D-galactosamine	Anti-A, Tn, Cad	Classification of A subgroups, investigation of polyagglutination
Griffonia simplicifolia II*	α- or β-N-acetyl-D-glucosamine	Anti-Tk	Confirmation of Tk polyagglutination
Helix pomatia	α-N-acetyl-D-galactosamine	Anti-A, Tn, Cad	Gives distinctive mixed field reaction with VA polyagglutination
Arachis hypogaea	β-D-galactose	Anti-T, Tk, Th, Tx	Investigation of polyagglutination
Glycine soja (max)	α-N-acetyl-D-galactosamine	Anti-T, Tn	
Leonurus cardiaca	α-N-acetyl-D-galactosamine	Anti-Cad specific at appropriate dilution	
Salvia sclerea	α-N-acetyl-D-galactosamine	Anti-Tn specific	
Salvia horminum	α-N-acetyl-D-galactosamine	Anti-Tn, Cad (separable)	
Vicia cretia	Galactose (β 1,3) N-acetyl-galactosamine	Anti-T, Th	

* Formerly known as *Bandeiraea simplicifolia* I and II.

population of cells, based on known antigenic differences between recipient and donor. Unagglutinated cells are physically removed from the agglutinates and sequentially reacted with more antisera until no more agglutinates are formed. In the second technique, washed packed RBCs are centrifuged in multiple sealed microhematocrit tubes. Transfused cells are older, smaller, and denser than newly formed autologous cells (reticulocytes) and will spin toward the bottom of the tube. After centrifugation, the top 5 mm of each tube is cut away, and the cells are harvested from these small segments. These sections will contain the larger and lighter autologous cells. This method will be effective only if the patient is producing normal or high numbers of reticulocytes.

Molecular Typing

A patient's phenotype can also be determined by molecular typing of genomic DNA. This is particularly useful in transfused patients with multiple/complex antibody problems, including autoantibodies and alloantibodies to high-incidence antigens. Primers for amplification and restriction fragment length polymorphisms are available in several immunohematology reference texts (Reid, 2004b). At present, patient samples for genotyping are sent to a few established reference laboratories. Rapid advances in high-throughput DNA typing may permit complete genetic typing of patients in the future.

Investigation of Autoimmune Hemolytic Anemia

Autoantibodies, in general, are produced by an individual's own immune system against self or an antigen that is present in that same individual. Although produced against self-antigens, these antibodies typically react with the same antigen found in other normal individuals. If the antibodies produced are against blood cell constituents, the pathologic result could be hemolytic anemia, thrombocytopenia, or leukopenia. In many cases, these autoantibodies cause no demonstrable clinical symptoms.

The DAT is integral to the diagnosis of autoimmune hemolytic anemia (AIHA), because it can confirm the presence of antibody that has attached in vivo to the patient's own red cells. The DAT can help differentiate AIHA from congenital anemias caused by abnormalities in RBC cytoskeleton, enzymes, or hemoglobin. The DAT may be positive due to IgG and/or complement components, depending on the class or subclass of autoantibody involved. A positive DAT by itself, however, does not mean an individual has AIHA. Approximately 8% of hospitalized patients have a positive DAT without any signs of hemolysis (Petz, 1993). In patients with suspected AIHA, the antibody screen may also be positive due to free autoantibody in the serum.

Autoantibodies are categorized as cold (usually IgM) or warm (usually IgG), based on the temperature of in vitro reactivity in the IAT. In some cases, patients may have mixed type AIHA with both cold and warm reactive autoantibodies. The causative antibodies of these categories of anemias will be described here; additional information regarding the etiology and pathophysiology of AIHA is covered in another chapter.

Warm Autoimmune Hemolytic Anemia (WAIHA)

Individuals with warm reactive autoantibodies account for approximately 70–80% of the cases of AIHA, having an overall incidence of about 1 in 50 000 to 1 in 80 000 (Issitt, 1998). Warm autoimmune hemolytic anemia (WAIHA) may be classified as either primary or idiopathic (of unknown etiology), or secondary. Secondary WAIHA is often observed in autoimmune diseases (frequently systemic lupus erythematosus), lymphoproliferative disorders and following viral infections. With the advent of improved diagnostic procedures, the percentage of WAIHA classified as idiopathic has dropped to about 30% of cases (Issitt, 1998). Patients with warm autoantibodies and a positive DAT will not all present with symptomatic anemia, but may exist in a chronic compensated state for some time before progressing to overt anemia.

Serologic Characteristics

Causative antibodies in WAIHA are usually IgG and polyclonal in nature, showing optimal in vitro reactivity at 37°C. The vast majority of warm autoantibodies that are in the serum and/or recovered in eluates from the patients' RBCs, can be demonstrated only by use of IAT technique.

Warm autoantibodies will be demonstrated on the patient's RBCs in about 80% of cases of WAIHA. The DAT profiles in several large studies show that 40–50% are due to IgG only, 45–60% are IgG and complement, and 0–15% are complement only (Issitt, 1998). In those instances where the DAT is negative, the use of more sensitive techniques, such as radioisotope or enzyme-labeled direct antiglobulin testing, can demonstrate low levels of IgG or, less frequently, IgM and IgA on the RBCs (Englefriet, 1992).

Immunoglobulin subclass studies in WAIHA indicate that causative antibodies are predominantly IgG1 and/or IgG3. Despite the ability of these subclasses to activate complement, immune destruction of the patient's autologous cells occurs largely through the spleen and liver via extravascular pathways. Patients whose RBCs are coated with IgG3 antibodies are more likely to show overt anemia, apparently because of the greater capacity of IgG3 for binding to Fc receptors on macrophages (Englefriet, 1992). A more recent study shows that the presence of multiple IgG subclasses, rather than a single subclass, has a synergistic effect on the severity of hemolysis (Fabijanska-Mitek, 1997).

In general, warm autoantibodies display a broad specificity, reacting with all normal RBCs. Many broadly reactive antibodies can show Rh specificity, failing to react with Rh_{null} RBCs. On occasion, autoantibodies will demonstrate a single Rh specificity such as anti-e (most frequently) or anti-c. Warm autoantibody specificities have also been reported to include those in the Kell, Kidd, MNSs, and ABO blood group systems, as well as anti-Vel and anti-LW. Relatively few individuals with WAIHA will show a single simple specificity (Issitt, 1998).

Occasionally, an autoantibody will mimic a single alloantibody specificity, but further testing shows that the antibody can be adsorbed to exhaustion with either antigen-positive or antigen-negative cells. These mimicking antibodies can occur in patients either positive or negative for the corresponding antigen, and the autoantibody may or may not be reactive in vitro (except by adsorption–elution studies), with the patient's own cells (Issitt, 1998).

Serologic Testing Beyond the DAT

Transfusion is usually avoided for as long as possible in patients with WAIHA. If transfusion is necessary, it is important to characterize the autoantibody and exclude the presence of RBC alloantibodies. Typical investigation strategies should always include adsorption of the serum, followed by antibody detection and identification on the adsorbed serum. Subsequent testing can also be performed on eluted antibody, although it seldom yields further useful information *unless* the serum is nonreactive.

Autoadsorption. Because a strong, broadly reactive serum autoantibody can mask the presence of significant alloantibodies, adsorption studies should be performed in these patients. Autoadsorption using autologous cells can be performed on patients who have not been recently transfused (within the last 3 months). For patients who have a strong positive DAT, autologous cells should be treated with ZZAP (Branch, 1982) prior to adsorption. ZZAP contains DTT, which reduces disulfide bonds in the IgG autoantibodies coating the RBCs. This destabilizes the immunoglobulin structure, rendering the autoantibodies susceptible to digestion by cysteine-activated papain, the second component of ZZAP. By stripping bound autoantibody from cells, ZZAP treatment increases the adsorptive capacity of autologous RBCs (see Fig. 34–25). If the serum contains a high concentration of autoantibody, multiple, sequential autoadsorptions may be necessary to remove all autoantibody activity. If available in sufficient quantity, autoadsorbed serum should be used to perform crossmatching, particularly if antibody detection studies reveal presence of underlying alloantibodies.

If the patient has had recent RBC transfusions, and the patient's red cell phenotype is known, adsorption may be performed using allogeneic cells of the same phenotype as the patient. Alternatively, if the patient's RBC phenotype is unknown, differential adsorptions may be performed on three separate aliquots of the patient's serum with different red cell samples of R_1, R_2, and rr phenotypes. One of the red cell samples should lack Jk^a and one should lack Jk^b (Brecher, 2002). ZZAP treatment of the adsorbing cells will effectively destroy Fy^a, Fy^b, all Kell system antigens, and the M, N, S, and s antigens, thereby conferring on the adsorbing cell samples the capacity to remove autoantibody activity while preserving potential alloantibodies in the serum. The different aliquots of serum are then tested against cells of known phenotype to detect and/or identify alloantibody specificity.

Elution. In the majority of cases of WAIHA, an eluate of the patient's cells will demonstrate the same broadly reactive antibody seen in serum. In the rare instances where the serum is only weakly reactive or negative, an eluate may concentrate the warm autoantibody to facilitate identification and evaluation of its spectrum of reactivity. If the eluate is nonreactive with normal reagent RBCs, the presence of drug-induced autoantibodies should be investigated (see below).

Cold Autoimmune Hemolytic Anemia (CAIHA)

Cold autoantibodies may be detected in the serum of many normal individuals if tested under the right conditions. However, the majority of these antibodies are benign cold agglutinins that show optimal reactivity at 4°C and little or no reactivity at 37°C. Cold agglutinins are more often

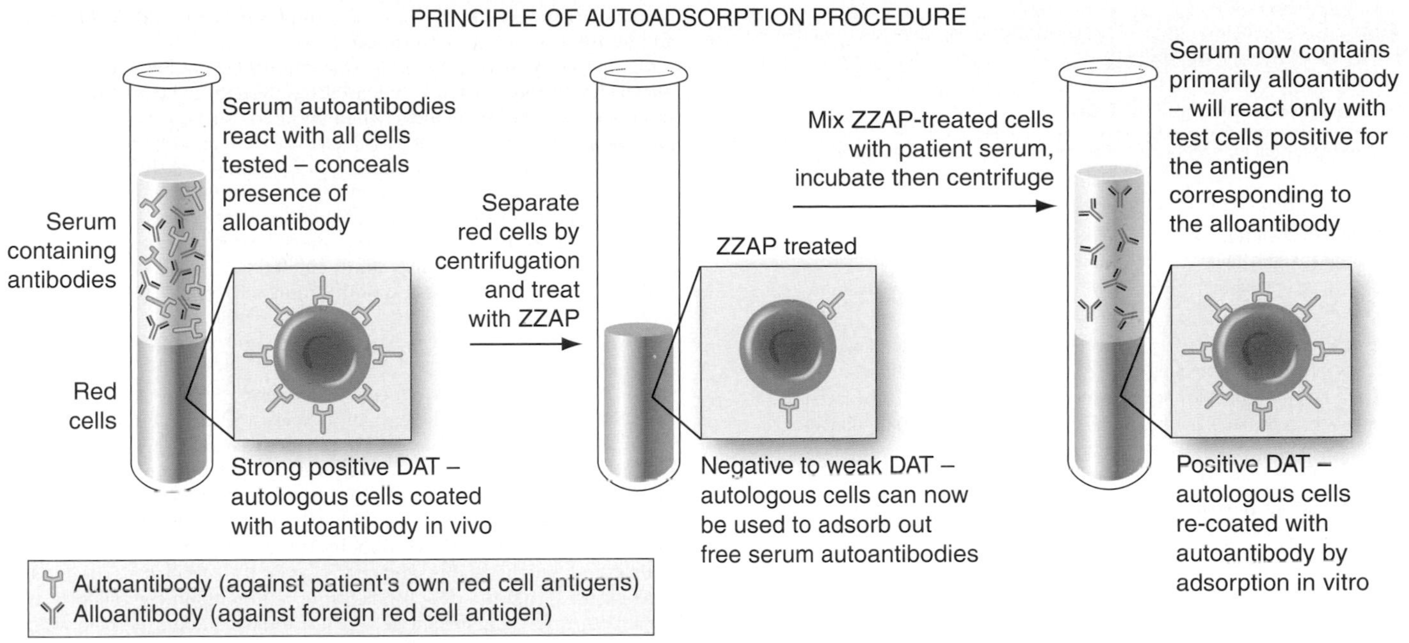

Serum containing antibodies

Red cells

Serum autoantibodies react with all cells tested – conceals presence of alloantibody

Strong positive DAT – autologous cells coated with autoantibody in vivo

Separate red cells by centrifugation and treat with ZZAP

ZZAP treated

Negative to weak DAT – autologous cells can now be used to adsorb out free serum autoantibodies

Mix ZZAP-treated cells with patient serum, incubate then centrifuge

Serum now contains primarily alloantibody – will react only with test cells positive for the antigen corresponding to the alloantibody

Positive DAT – autologous cells re-coated with autoantibody by adsorption in vitro

⊤ Autoantibody (against patient's own red cell antigens)
⊤ Alloantibody (against foreign red cell antigen)

Figure 34–25 Autoadsorption procedure used to evaluate whether underlying alloantibodies are present in a patient with autoimmune hemolytic anemia.

Table 34–48 Differentiating Characteristics of Cold Red Cell Autoagglutinins

Antibody specificity	Clinical significance	IAT antibody screen[*]	Ig class	Relative reaction strengths with selected red cells at room temperature[†]				
				O_{adult}	O_{cord}	$A_{1\ adult}$	$A_{2\ adult}$	Autologous
I	Acute CHD associated with *Mycoplasma pneumoniae* with antibody titers > 1000 at 4°C	Pos	IgM	3+	w+	3+	3+	3+
i	Acute CHD associated with mononucleosis	Pos	IgM	w+	3+	w+	w+	Weaker than O_{cord}
Pr	Rare cause of CHD[‡]	Pos	Reported cases of IgM, IgA, IgG	3+	3+	3+	3+	3+
P	PCH associated with certain viral infections in children	Neg	IgG[§]	Negative in routine agglutination tests; autoanti-P is a biphasic hemolysin (Donath–Landsteiner antibody)				
H	Benign except as alloantibody in Bombay phenotype	Weak to neg	IgM	3+	3+	1+	2+	0 to w+
IH	Benign	Weak to neg	IgM	3+	1+	1+	2+	0 to w+

[*] Antigen expression: O_{adult} (I+ i– H+^{s}); O_{cord} (I– i+ H+^{s}); A_1 (I+ i – H+^{w}); A_2 (I+ i – H+).

[†] Reagent cells showing agglutination in 37°C phase may be much weaker after conversion to IAT.

[‡] May be differentiated from anti-I by enzymes or increasing pH – anti-Pr reactivity is decreased by both techniques.

[§] Autoanti-P is the only pathologic cold autoantibody known to be routinely of the IgG class to IAT.

IV

than not a nuisance that may interfere with ABO/Rh typing, antibody detection and crossmatching using polyspecific AHG. Although usually ignored as clinically insignificant, cold agglutinins may become pathologic by virtue of expanded thermal amplitude and a significant increase in titer, frequently in association with certain disease states. Direct antiglobulin testing along with serum titration and characterization of thermal amplitude are the most important serologic tests in evaluating a possible diagnosis of CAIHA. Table 34–48 outlines some of the serologic differentiating characteristics of various cold agglutinating autoantibodies, both pathologic and benign.

Cold Hemagglutinin Disease (CHD)

Cold hemagglutinin disease (CHD) accounts for about 20% of total cases of AIHA (Issitt, 1998). As with WAIHA, CHD may be idiopathic or secondary, particularly after infections by certain bacteria or viruses. Anti-I is the most frequent autoantibody in idiopathic CHD. It is also the cause of an acute-onset, secondary CHD following *Mycoplasma pneumoniae* infections. In contrast to the low-titered anti-I cold agglutinins found in normal sera (usually less than 1 : 64 when tested at 4°C), anti-I in CHD is often of very high titer, with ranges of 1 : 10 000 to 1 : 1 000 000 (Prasad, 1993). The antibody also has an expanded thermal amplitude, reacting

with RBCs at temperatures in the range of 30–34°C in vitro, especially in tests with albumin-suspended RBCs (Issitt, 1998). The DAT is typically positive with polyspecific and anti-C3 reagents.

In vivo hemolysis is the result of antibody binding to a patient's RBCs in the peripheral vessels of the extremities, which are cooler (32°C and lower). As the cells recirculate to the body core and warm to 37°C, complement is activated and cells are destroyed. Hemolysis of cells may occur intravascularly, but according to Garratty (1994b), occurs more commonly via extravascular (C3b) pathways by macrophages in the reticuloendothelial system. Hemolysis may be chronic or episodic, depending on the thermal range of the antibody, and may be triggered by exposure to cold temperatures.

Because anti-I reacts broadly with virtually all adult RBCs, the antibody can cause great difficulty in compatibility testing. As with warm autoantibodies, one of the primary concerns is to detect and identify any potential underlying IgG alloantibodies. Techniques to circumvent the autoanti-I in serum testing may include prewarming, cold autoadsorption, adsorption with rabbit erythrocyte stroma (REST), or treatment of the serum with sulfhydryl reagents such as DTT or 2-ME (see section on Special Antibody Identification Techniques).

Anti-i is a second antibody that has been implicated in CAIHA, detected most frequently as an IgM cold autoantibody in patients with infectious

Table 34–49 Selected Drugs Associated With a Positive DAT and/or Hemolysis Due to Drug-Induced Autoantibodies

Reported mechanism	Drug
Drug-independent autoantibody induction	Chlorpromazine, ibuprofen, levodopa, mefenamic acid, methyldopa, nomifensine, procainamide, tolmetin
Drug dependent (drug adsorption – high affinity binding to cell membrane)	Penicillin, carbenicillin, cephalothin, second- and third-generation cephalosporins, erythromycin, methicillin, naficillin, tolbutamide
Drug dependent (immune complex – low affinity binding to cell membrane but efficient complement activation)	Acetaminophen, antihistamines, second- and third-generation cephalosporins, chlorpromazine, isoniazid, phenacetin, quinidine, quinine, rifampin, stibophen, streptomycin, sulfonylurea derivatives, tetracycline
Nonimmunologic protein adsorption	Cephalothin, cisplatin, suramin

Data derived from Brecher (2002).

mononucleosis and certain lymphoproliferative disorders. Monoclonal forms of anti-i may be seen in the latter. Perhaps 10–20% of patients with infectious mononucleosis will have significant cold agglutinin titers, but few go on to actually develop CHD due to anti-i (Prasad, 1993).

Finally, anti-Pr antibodies (originally called anti-Sp) are an infrequent cause of CHD. Anti-Pr specificities may initially react like anti-I, but may be differentiated by their equally strong reactions with cord and adult RBCs (Table 34–48). In addition, anti-Pr is nonreactive with enzyme-treated red cells, whereas anti-I is enhanced by enzyme treatment. Anti-Pr in patients with CHD is usually monoclonal and may be IgG, IgM, or IgA (Issitt, 1998).

Paroxysmal Cold Hemoglobinuria

Paroxysmal cold hemoglobinuria, or PCH, is an autoimmune hemolytic syndrome often seen in children following infection by mumps, chickenpox, measles, and other viruses. Historically, PCH was also seen in syphilitic patients. Autoanti-P, also known as the Donath–Landsteiner (DL) antibody, is the causative antibody in PCH. It is an IgG, biphasic autohemolysin capable of binding to RBCs at cold temperatures and causing intravascular hemolysis of those cells at body temperature (Table 34–48). This characteristic can be demonstrated in vitro by the diagnostic Donath–Landsteiner procedure to aid in the confirmation of PCH. In this test, three sets of tubes containing patient serum and group O cells are incubated, one at 4°C followed by 37°C, one only at 4°C, and one only at 37°C. If the first set shows hemolysis, but the other two do not, this indicates the presence of the biphasic hemolysin characteristic of PCH. The Donath–Landsteiner test requires that a fresh blood sample be used to ensure that an adequate supply of complement is available, because complement is relatively unstable and deteriorates during storage. It is also important not to draw the blood into an anticoagulant such as EDTA because chelation of calcium ions will prevent complement activation and thus in vitro hemolysis.

Because the autoantibody in PCH rarely reacts above 4°C in vitro, routine antibody detection tests are usually negative and crossmatches are compatible. Patient RBCs sensitized by the DL antibody will most commonly give a positive DAT due to C3 only and usually only during or right after an episode of hemolysis (Prasad, 1993). Because the antibody dissociates easily from RBCs during washing, the DAT is usually negative with anti-IgG. IgG may be detected, however, if the cells are washed with cold saline and tested with cold anti-IgG reagent (Brecher, 2002).

Positive Direct Antiglobulin Tests and Hemolytic Anemia Induced by Medication

A number of therapeutic drugs are known to induce a positive DAT, and in some cases can cause an acquired hemolytic anemia (see Table 34–49). It is also well documented that a positive DAT may be produced in patients receiving high-dose intravenous gammaglobulin therapy owing to passively acquired specific blood group antibodies as well as nonspecific binding to RBCs by IgG dimers and aggregates in the gammaglobulin preparation (Knezevic-Maramica, 2003). Traditionally, there have been four mechanisms proposed to explain drug-associated hemolytic anemia:

induction of autoantibody, immune complex formation, drug adsorption, and nonspecific protein adsorption.

More recently, a unifying model (Salama, 1992) has been suggested that may be applicable to many different drugs thought to be operating via the mechanisms mentioned above. The hypothesis suggests that the immune process is initiated by a primary interaction between RBCs and the drug or its metabolites, even though the drug may be only loosely bound to RBCs in vivo. This provides the composite determinants (or neoantigen) necessary for production of drug-dependent antibodies, as in the drug adsorption and immune complex mechanisms, or drug-independent autoantibodies that recognize subtle alterations in the RBC membrane. For a more complete discussion of this topic see Garratty (1994b).

Stimulation of Red Cell Autoantibody Production – Drug Independent

About 20% of hypertensive patients who receive methyldopa (Aldomet) for more than 3–6 months will eventually develop a positive DAT, but only 0.8% will develop a hemolytic anemia (Petz, 1993). The DAT gradually becomes negative after stopping methyldopa treatment, although it may take months to more than 2 years. Serologically, autoantibodies eluted from RBCs, or free in the serum, are indistinguishable from autoantibodies found in patients with WAIHA. The antibodies are usually of the IgG class, with both κ and λ light chains, and many show Rh specificity. One possible mechanism is that the drug binds to the cell membrane and subtly alters the structure, forming neoantigens that stimulate autoantibody formation. About 10% of patients with Parkinson's disease receiving L-dopa, a closely related drug, also develop RBC autoantibodies, but these rarely result in overt hemolysis (Petz, 1993).

Drug-Dependent Autoantibodies

Penicillin-type Antibodies (Drug Adsorption Mechanism). About 3% of patients receiving large doses of penicillin intravenously ($> 10 \times 10^6$ IU/day) develop a positive DAT, although only a few of these patients will have hemolytic anemia (Garratty, 1993). Breakdown products of benzyl penicillin exhibit a high binding affinity for the RBC membrane, which results in the formation of haptenic benzylpenicilloyl (BPO) determinants. Certain patients can form high-titered antibodies against penicillin metabolites and to a lesser extent, red cell membrane components. The resulting antibody–drug–RBC complex yields a positive DAT with anti-IgG. The DAT becomes negative again within days to several weeks after discontinuing penicillin. Both the patient's serum and eluates prepared from patient's RBCs, usually react only with penicillin-coated RBCs in in vitro testing.

Penicillin antibodies may be IgM or IgG. IgM antibodies are very common if a sensitive method is used for detection. Those antibodies associated with immune hemolytic anemia are usually of IgG isotype (Garratty, 1993). Hemolysis is usually through extravascular destruction mediated by cells of the RE system, although rare cases of complement-mediated intravascular hemolysis have been reported. Several cases of acquired hemolytic anemia have also been reported in association with the first-generation cephalosporin, cephalothin, and later-generation cephalosporins in a mechanism similar to that of penicillin.

Drug/Cell Membrane Antibodies (Immune Complex). A wide variety of drugs may cause hemolytic anemia via the so-called immune complex mechanism (Table 34–49). In the unifying concept, these drugs loosely bind to the RBC membrane with subsequent formation of antibodies reacting with both drug and membrane components. The cell–drug–antibody complex may then stimulate activation of the complement cascade. Drugs acting by this mechanism most often are associated with episodes of acute intravascular hemolysis with hemoglobinemia and hemoglobinuria that may prove fatal (Petz, 1993). The DAT in these cases is usually positive with anti-C3d only. The antibodies implicated may be IgM or IgG (Brecher, 2002). They can only be detected in test systems where serum/eluate, test cells, and free drug are all present simultaneously. Although the mechanism leading to antibody production may be similar to that of so-called drug adsorption, the drugs in this category are classified separately primarily by the DAT result (C3d+) and characteristic severe intravascular hemolysis.

Nonimmunologic Adsorption of Serum Proteins. Patients taking high-dose cephalothin (6–14 g/day) for prolonged periods have been reported to develop a positive DAT, with a frequency ranging widely from 3–81% (Garratty, 1993). Hemolysis is rarely, if ever, associated with the phenomenon (Brecher, 2002). It was subsequently shown that RBCs exposed to cephalothin in vitro are able to nonspecifically adsorb plasma and serum proteins (albumin, immunoglobulins, complement). These proteins can be detected by polyspecific AHG sera in the DAT. It has been hypothesized that the adsorption occurs because of a change in erythrocyte membrane properties induced by cephalothin and other drugs.

References

Agre P, Smith BL, Baumgarten R, et al: Human red cell aquaporin CHIP. Expression during normal fetal development and in a novel form of congenital dyserythropoietic anemia. J Clin Invest 1994; 94:1050–1058.

Akalin E, Neylan JF: The influence of Duffy blood group on renal allograft outcome in African Americans. Transplantation 2003; 75:1496–1500.

Ansart-Pirenne H, Asso-Bonnet M, Le Pennec P-Y, et al: RhD variants in Caucasians: consequences for checking clinically relevant alleles. Transfusion 2004; 44:1282–1286.

Auf der Maur C, Hodel M, Nydegger UE, Rieben R: Age dependency of ABO histo-blood group antibodies: Reexamination of an old dogma. Transfusion 1993; 33:915–918.

Avent ND: The rhesus blood group system: Insights from recent advances in molecular biology. Transfus Med Rev 1999; 13:245–266.

Ballas SK, Marcolina MJ, Crawford MN: In vitro storage and in vivo survival studies of red cells from persons with the In(Lu) gene. Transfusion 1992; 32:607–611.

Bartels CF, Zelinski T, Lockridge O: Mutation at codon 322 in the human acetylcholinesterase (ACHE) gene accounts for YT blood group polymorphism. Am J Hum Genet 1993; 52:928–936.

Berry-Dortch S, Woodside CH, Boral LI: Limitations of the immediate spin crossmatch when used for detecting ABO incompatibility. Transfusion 1985; 25:176–178.

Bird GWG: Lectins: A hundred years. Immunohematology 1988; 4:45–48.

Boral LI, Henry JB: The type and screen: A safe alternative and supplement in selected surgical procedures. Transfusion 1977; 17:163–168.

Boren T, Falk P, Roth KA, et al: Attachment of *Helicobacter pylori* to human gastric epithelium mediated by blood group antigens. Science 1993; 262:1892–1895.

Boyce TG, Swerdlow DL, Griffin PM: *Escherichia coli* O157:H7 and the hemolytic-uremic syndrome. N Engl J Med 1995; 333:364–367.

Branch DR, Petz LD: A new reagent (ZZAP) having multiple applications in immunohematology. Am J Clin Pathol 1982; 78:161–167.

Brecher M (ed): Technical Manual, 14th ed. Bethesda, MD, American Association of Blood Banks, 2002.
Techniques and policies for the collection, processing, testing and dispensing of blood components.

Brown KE, Hibbs FR, Gallinella G, et al: Resistance to parvovirus B19 infection due to a lack of virus receptor (erythrocyte P antigen). New Eng J Med 1994; 330:1192–1196.

Butch SH, Judd WJ, Steiner EA, et al: Electronic verification of donor–recipient compatibility: The computer crossmatch. Transfusion 1994; 34:105–109.

Byrne KM, Byrne PC: Review: other blood group systems–Diego, Yt, Xg, Scianna, Dombrock, Colton, Landsteiner–Wiener, and Indian. Immunohematology 2004; 20:50–58.

Cameron HS, Szczepaniak D, Weston BW: Expression of human chromosome 19p α (1,3) fucosyltransferase genes in normal tissues. J Biol Chem 1995; 270:20112–20122.

Caren LD, Bellavance R, Grumet FC: Demonstration of gene dosage effects on antigens in the Duffy, Ss and Rh systems using an enzyme-linked immunosorbent assay. Transfusion 1982; 22:475–478.

Carbonnet F, Hattab C, Cartron J-P, Bertrand O: Kell and Kx, two disulfide-linked proteins of the human erythrocyte membrane are phosphorylated in vivo. Biochem Biophys Res Commun 1998; 247:569–575.

Cartron JP, Bailly P, Le Van Kim C, et al: Insights into the structure and function of membrane polypeptides carrying blood group antigens. Vox Sang 1998; 74:29–64.

Chan A, Chan JC, Wong LY et al: From maximum surgical blood ordering schedule to unlimited computer crossmatching: evolution of blood transfusion for surgical patients at a tertiary hospital in Hong Kong. Transf Med 1996; 6:121–124.

Chaudhuri A, Nielsen S, Elkjaer ML, et al: Detection of Duffy antigens in the plasma membranes and caveolae of vascular endothelial and epithelial cells of noneryythroid organs. Blood 1997; 89:701–712.

Cherif-Zahar B, Le Van Kim C, Rouillac C, et al: Organization of the gene (RHCE) encoding the blood group RhCcEe antigens and characterization of the promoter region. Genomics 1994; 19:68–74.

Code of Federal Regulations: Title 21 – Food and Drugs, Part 606, Subpart H-Laboratory Controls. Washington, DC, US Government Printing Office, 2001a.

Code of Federal Regulations: Title 21 – Food and Drugs, Part 660, Subpart F – Anti-human globulin. Washington, DC, US Government Printing Office, 2001b.

Cooling LL, Kelly K: Inverse expression of P^k and Luke blood group antigens on human RBCs. Transfusion 2001; 41:898–907.

Cooling LLW, Koerner TAW, Naides SS: Multiple glycosphingolipids determine the tissue tropism of parvovirus B19: J Infect Dis 1995; 172:1198–1205.

Cooling LLW, Walker KE, Gille T, Koerner TAW: Shiga toxin binds human platelets via globotriaosylceramide (P^k antigen) and a novel platelet glycosphingolipid. Infect Immun 1998; 66:4355–4366.

Cooling L, Hwang D, Gu Y: Globoside synthase can regulate Pk and LKE expression on human RBC: evidence for the P^k-variant phenotype among some LKE-weak and LKE-negative donors [abstract]. Transfusion 2003a; 43:SP194.

Cooling LLW, Zhang D-S, Naides SJ, Koerner TAW: Glycosphingolipid expression in acute nonlymphocytic leukemia: common expression of shiga toxin and parvovirus B19 receptors on early myeloblasts. Blood 2003b; 101:711–721.

Coombs RRA, Mourant AE, Race RR: A new test for the detection of weak and incomplete Rh agglutinins. Br J Exp Pathol 1945; 26:255–266.

Cordle DG, Strauss RG, Snyder EL, et al: Safety and cost containment data that advocate abbreviated pretransfusion testing. Am J Clin Pathol 1990; 94:428–431.

Cox C, Enno S, Deveridge S, et al: Remote electronic blood release system. Transfusion 1997; 37:960–964.

Crew VK, Green C, Daniels G: Molecular bases of the antigens of the Lutheran blood group system. Transfusion 2003; 43:1729–1737.

Curnutte J, Bemiller L: Chronic granulomatous disease with McLeod phenotype: An uncommon occurrence [abstract]. Transfusion 1995; 35:S239 1995.

Daniels G: Human Blood Groups, 2nd ed. Oxford, UK, Blackwell Science, 2002.
Summarizes each blood group system including serology, biochemistry, and molecular basis for the major blood group antigen systems.

Edwards JM, Moulds JJ, Judd WJ: Chloroquine dissociation of antigen–antibody complexes: A new technique for typing red blood cells with a positive direct antiglobulin test. Transfusion 1982; 22:59–61.

El Nemer W, Rahuel C, Colin Y, et al: Organization of the human LU gene and molecular basis of the Lu^a/Lu^b blood group polymorphism. Blood 1997; 89:4608–4616.

El Nemer W, Gane P, Colin Y, et al: The Lutheran blood group glycoproteins, the erythroid receptors for laminin, are adhesion molecules. J Biol Chem 1998; 273:16686–16693.

Ellison RC, Zhang Y, Myers RH, et al: Lewis blood group phenotype as an independent risk factor for coronary heart disease (The NHLBI Family Heart Study). Am J Cardiol 1999; 83:345–348.

Englefriet CP, Overbeeke MAM, von dem Borne AFG: Autoimmune hemolytic anemia. Semin Hematol 1992; 29:3–12.

Eyers SAC, Ridgwell K, Mawby WJ, Tanner MJA: Topology and organization of human Rh (rhesus) blood group related polypeptides. J Biol Chem 1994; 269:6417–6423.

Fabijanska-Mitek J, Lopienska H, Zupanska B: Gel test application for IgG subclass detection in auto-immune haemolytic anaemia. Vox Sang 1997; 72:233–237.

Fernandez-Mateos P, Cailleau A, Henry S, et al: Point mutations and deletion responsible for the Bombay H null and the Reunion H weak blood groups. Vox Sang 1998; 75:37–46.

Freedman J, Semple JW: Complement in transfusion medicine. *In* Garraty G (ed): Immunobiology of Transfusion Medicine. New York, Marcel Dekker, 1994, pp 403–434.

Friedman BA, Oberman HA, Chadwick AR, et al: The maximum surgical blood order schedule and surgical blood use in the United States. Transfusion 1976; 16:380–387.
The historical standard for the design, use and implementation of the MSBOS for blood ordering.

Fukuda M: HEMPAS disease: Genetic defect of glycosylation. Glycobiology 1990; 1:9–15.

Fukuda M, Dell A, Oates JE, Fukuda MN: Structure of branched lactosaminoglycan, the carbohydrate moiety of band 3 isolated from adult human erythrocytes. J Biol Chem 1984; 259:8260–8273.

Fukuma N, Akimitsu N, Hamamoto H, et al: A role of the Duffy antigen for the maintenance of plasma chemokine concentrations. Biochem Biophys Res Comm 2003; 303:137–139.

Gamma Biologicals, Inc: Gamma-Quin chloroquine diphosphate solution for removal of red-cell-bound immunoglobulin – directions for use. Houston, TX, Gamma Biologicals, Inc., 2001.

Gardner L, Patterson AM, Ashton BA, et al: The human Duffy antigen binds selected inflammatory but not homeostatic chemokines. Biochem Biophys Res Comm 2004; 321:306–312.

Garratty G: Immune cytopenia associated with antibiotics. Transfus Med Rev 1993; 7:255–267.

Garratty G: Do blood groups have a biological role? *In* Garraty G (ed): Immunobiology of Transfusion Medicine. New York, Marcel Dekker, 1994a, pp 201–255.

Garratty G: Review: Immune hemolytic anemia and/or positive direct antiglobulin tests caused by drugs. Immunohematology 1994b; 10:41–50.

Garratty G, Issitt PD, Lublin DM, et al: Terminology for blood group antigens and genes – historical origins and guidelines in the new millennium. Transfusion 2000; 40:L477–489.

George T, Boyd B, Price M, et al: MHC class II proteins contain a potential binding site for the verotoxin receptor glycolipid CD77. Cell Mol Biol 2001; 47:1179–1185.

Ghislain J, Lingwood CA, Fish EN: Evidence for glycosphingolipid modification of the type 1 IFN receptor. J Immunol 1994; 153:3655–3663.

Giles CM: Three Chido determinants detected on the B5Rg+ allotype of human C4: their expression in Ch-typed donors and families. Human Immunol 1987; 18:111–112.

Giles CM, Uring-Lambert B, Goetz J, et al: Antigenic determinants expressed by human C4 allotypes; a study of 325 families provides evidence for the structural antigenic model. Immunogenetics 1988; 27:442–448.

Gubin AN, Njoroge JM, Wojda U, et al: Identification of the Dombrock blood group glycoprotein as a polymorphic member of the ADP-ribosyltransferase gene family. Blood 2000; 96:2621–2627.

Hadley TJ, Peiper SC: From malaria to chemokine receptor: The emerging physiologic role of the Duffy blood group antigen. Blood 1997; 89:3077–3091.

Hakomori S: Blood group ABH and Ii antigens of human erythrocytes: Chemistry, polymorphism, and their developmental change. Semin Hematol 1981; 18:39–62.

Harmening DM, Firestone D: The ABO blood group system. *In* Harmening DM (ed): Modern Blood

Banking and Transfusion Practices, 4th ed. Philadelphia, FA Davis, 1999, pp. 90–125.

Hauser R: Le^a and Le^b tissue glycosphingolipids. Transfusion 1995; 35:577–581.

Heddle NM, O'Hoski P, Singer J, et al: A prospective study to determine the safety of omitting the antiglobulin crossmatch from pretransfusion testing. Br J Haematol 1992; 81:579–584.

Hellberg A, Poole J, Olsson ML: Molecular basis of the globoside-deficient P^k blood group phenotype. J Biol Chem 2002; 277:29455–29459.

Henry JB, Mintz PD, Webb W: Optimal blood ordering for elective surgery. JAMA 1977; 237:451.

Hermand P, Gane P, Mattei MG, et al: Molecular basis and expression of the LW^a/LW^b blood group polymorphism. Blood 1995; 86:1590–1594.

Hilton E, Chandrasekaran V, Rindos P, Isenberg HD: Association of recurrent candidal vaginitis with inheritance of Lewis blood group antigens. J Infect Dis 1995; 172:1616–1619.

Ho M, Chelly J, Carter N, et al: Isolation of the gene for McLeod syndrome that encodes a novel membrane transport protein. Cell 1994; 77:869–880.

Hoeltge GA, Domen RE, Rybicki LA, et al: Multiple red cell transfusions and alloimmunization. Arch Pathol Lab Med 1995; 119:42–45.

Huang CH, Blumenfeld O: MNSs blood groups and major glycophorins. In Carton JP, Rouger P (eds): Blood Cell Biochemistry, Vol 6: Molecular Basis of Human Blood Group Antigens. New York, Plenum Press, 1995, pp. 153–188.

Hughes-Jones NC, Gardner B, Lincoln P: Observations of the number of available c, D, e, and E antigen sites on red cells. Vox Sang 1971; 21:210–216.

Inaba M, Hiruma T, Togayachi A, et al: A novel I-branching β1,6-N-acetylglucosaminyltransferase involved in human blood group I antigen expression. Blood 2003; 101:2870–2876.

Issitt PD, Anstee DJ: Applied Blood Group Serology, 4th ed. Durham, NC, Montgomery Scientific Publications, 1998.

A comprehensive text detailing the history, serology, disease associations and possible biologic role of blood group antigens and antibodies.

Iwamura K, Furukawa K, Uchikawa M, et al: The blood group P$_1$ synthase gene is identical to the Gb3/CD77 synthase gene. J Biol Chem 2003; 278:44429–44438.

Iwamoto S, Li J, Sugimoto N, et al: Characterization of the Duffy gene promoter: Evidence for tissue-specific abolishment of expression in Fy(a-b-) of black individuals. Biochem Biophys Res Commun 1996; 222:852–859.

Iwamoto S, Omi T, Yamasaki M, et al: Identification of 5′ flanking sequence of RH50 gene and the core region for erythroid-specific expression. Biochem Biophys Res Commun 1998; 243:233–240.

Jacewicz MS, Acheson DWK, Mobassaleh M, et al: Maturational regulation of globotriaosylceramide, the shiga-like toxin 1 receptor, in cultured human gut epithelial cells. J Clin Invest 1995; 96:1328–1335.

Jarolim P, Rubin HL, Storry J, Reid ME: Characterization of seven low incidence blood group antigens carried by erythrocyte band 3 protein. Blood 1998; 92:4836–4843.

Judd WJ: Are there better ways than the crossmatch to demonstrate ABO incompatibility? Transfusion 1991; 31:192–194.

Judd WJ: Methods in Immunohematology, 2nd ed. Durham, NC, Montgomery Scientific Publications, 1994.

Judd WJ: Testing for unexpected red cell antibodies – two or three reagent red cell samples. Immunohematology 1997 13:90–92.

Judd WJ: Requirements for the electronic crossmatch. Vox Sang 1998; 74:409–417.

Summarizes the federal regulations, computer requirements and implementation issues for the electronic crossmatch.

Judd WJ: Red blood cell immunology and compatibility testing. In Simon TL, Dzik WH, Snyder EL (eds): Rossi's Principles of Transfusion

Medicine, 3rd ed. Philadelphia, Lippincott, Williams & Wilkins, 2002, pp 69–88.

Judd WJ, Walter WJ, Steiner EA: Clinical and laboratory findings on two patients with naturally occurring anti-Kell agglutinins. Transfusion 1981; 21:184–188.

Judd WJ, Steiner EA, O'Donnell DB, et al: Discrepancies in reverse ABO typing due to prozone: How safe is the immediate-spin crossmatch? Transfusion 1988; 28:334–338.

Karpman D, Papdopoulou D, Nilsson K, et al: Platelet activation by shiga toxin and circulatory factors as a pathogenetic mechanism in the hemolytic uremic syndrome. Blood 2001; 97:3100–3108.

Kay MMB: Cellular and molecular biology of senescent antigen. In Garratty G (ed): Immunobiology of Transfusion Medicine. New York, Marcel Dekker, 1994, pp 173–198.

Kelly RJ, Ernst LK, Larsen RD, et al: Molecular basis for H blood group deficiency in Bombay (Oh) and para-Bombay individuals. Proc Natl Acad Sci USA 1994; 91:5843–5847.

Kelly RJ, Rouquier S, Giorgi D, et al: Sequence and expression of a candidate for the human secretor blood group α (1,2) fucosyltransferase gene (FUT2). J Biol Chem 1995; 270:4640–4649.

Knepper MA: The aquaporin family of molecular water channels. Proc Natl Acad Sci USA 1994; 91:6255–6258.

Knezevic-Maramica I, Kruskall MS: Intravenous immune globulins: an update for clinicians. Transfusion 2003; 43:1460–1480.

Koda Y, Soejima M, Sato H, et al: Three-base deletion and one-base insertion of the α(1,4)galactosyltransferase gene responsible for the p phenotype. Transfusion 2002; 42:48–51.

Kornstad L, Heisto H: The frequency of formation of Kell antibodies in recipients of Kell-positive blood. In Proceedings of the 6th Congress of the European Society of Haematology Copenhagen, 1958, pp 754–758.

Kovbasnjuk O, Edidin M, Donowitz M: Role of lipid rafts in shiga toxin 1 interaction with the apical surface of Caco-2 cells. J Cell Science 2001; 114:4025–4031.

Kroviarski Y, El Nemer W, Gane P, et al: Direct interaction between the Lu/B-CAM adhesion glycoproteins and erythroid spectrin. Br J Haematol 2004; 126:255–264.

Kundu SK, Steane SM, Bloom JEC, Marcus DM: Abnormal glycolipid composition of erythrocytes with a weak P antigen. Vox Sang 1978; 35:160–167.

Kundu SK, Evans A, Rizvi J, et al: A new P^k phenotype in the P blood group system. J Immunol 1980; 7:431–439.

Landsteiner K, Wiener AS: An agglutinable factor in human blood recognized by immune sera for rhesus blood. Proc Soc Exp Biol Med 1940; 43:223–224.

Lapierre Y, Rigal D, Adam J, et al: The gel test: A new way to detect red cell antigen–antibody reactions. Transfusion 1990; 30:109–113.

Lee JS, Frevert CW, Wurfel MM, et al: Duffy antigen facilitates movement of chemokine across the endothelium in vitro and promotes neutrophil transmigration in vitro and in vivo. J Immunol 2003a; 170:5244–5251.

Lee S: Molecular basis of Kell blood group. Vox Sang 1997; 73:1–11.

Lee S, Lin M, Mele A, et al: Proteolytic processing of big endothelin-3 by the Kell blood group protein. Blood 1999; 94:1440–1450.

Lee S, Russo DCW, Reid ME, Redman CM: Mutations that diminish expression of Kell surface protein and lead to the Kmod RBC phenotype. Transfusion 2003b; 43:1121–1125.

Levine P, Stetson RE: An unusual case of intragroup agglutination. JAMA 1939; 113:126.

Lewis VN, Martin S: Fundamentals of immunology for blood bankers. In Harmening DM (ed): Modern Blood Banking and Transfusion Practices, 4th ed. Philadelphia, FA Davis, 1999, pp 36–70.

Li J, Iwamoto S, Sugimoto N, et al: Dinucleotide repeat in the 3′ flanking region provides a clue to the molecular evolution of the Duffy gene. Hum Genet 1997; 99:573–577.

Li Y, Camp S, Rachinsky TL, et al: The gene structure of mammalian acetylcholinesterase. J Biol Chem 1991; 266:23083–23090.

Lindahl G, Sjobring U, Johnsson E: Human complement regulators: a major target for pathogenic microorganisms. Curr Opin Immunol 2000; 12:44–51.

Lindstrom K, Breimer ME, Jovall P-A, et al: Non-acid glycosphingolipid expression in plasma of an A$_1$ Le(a–b+) secretor human individual: Identification of an ALe^b heptaglycosylceramide as major blood group component. J Biochem 1992; 111:337–345.

Low PS: Structure and function of the cytoplasmic domain for band 3: Center of erythrocyte membrane–peripheral protein interactions. Biochim Biophys Acta 1986; 864:145–167.

Lowe JB: Carbohydrate-associated blood group antigens: The ABO, H/Se, and Lewis loci. In Garratty G (ed): Immunobiology of Transfusion Medicine. New York, Marcel Dekker, 1994, pp 3–36.

Lucien N, Sidoux-Walter F, Olives B, et al: Characterization of the gene encoding the human Kidd blood group/urea transporter protein. J Biol Chem 1998; 273:12973–12980.

Lucien N, Sidoux-Walter F, Roudier N, et al: Antigenic and functional properties of the human red blood cell urea transporter hUT-B1. J Biol Chem 2002; 277:34101–34108.

Ma T, Yang B, Gillespie AN, et al: Severely impaired urinary concentrating ability in transgenic mice lacking aquaporin-1 water channels. J Biol Chem 1998; 273:4296–4299.

Maffei LM, Johnson ST, Shulman IA, Steiner EA: Survey on pretransfusion testing. Transfusion 1998; 38:343–349.

Mallory D (ed): Immunohematology Methods, 1st ed. Rockville, MD, The American National Red Cross, 1993.

Mangeney M, Richard Y, Coulaud D, et al: CD77: An antigen of germinal center B cells entering apoptosis. Eur J Immunol 1991; 21:1131–1140.

Masouredis SP, Sudora E, Mahan L, et al: Quantitative immunoferritin microassay of Fy^a, Fy^b, Jk^a, V and Di^b antigen site numbers on human red cells. Blood 1980; 56:969–977.

Masson P, Froment MT, Sorenson RC, et al: Mutation His322Asn in human acetylcholinesterase does not alter electrophoretic and catalytic properties of the erythrocyte enzyme. Blood 1994; 83:3003–3005.

Mathai JC, Mori S, Smith BL, et al: Functional analysis of aquaporin-1 deficient red cells. J Biol Chem 1996; 271:1309–1313.

Medof ME, Lublin DM, Holers VN, et al: Cloning and characterization of cDNAs encoding the complete sequence of decay-accelerating factor of human complement. Proc Natl Acad Sci USA 1987; 84:2007–2011.

Mintz PD, Haines AL, Sullivan MF: Incompatible crossmatch following nonreactive antibody detection test: Frequency and cause. Transfusion 1982; 22:107–110.

Mollicone R, Reguigne I, Kelly RJ, et al: Molecular basis for Lewis α (1,3/4)-fucosyltransferase gene deficiency (FUT3) found in Lewis-negative Indonesian pedigrees. J Biol Chem 1994; 269:20987–20994.

Mollison PL: Further observations on the patterns of clearance of incompatible red cells. Transfusion 1989; 39:347–354.

Mollison PL, Englefriet CP, Contreras M: Blood Transfusion in Clinical Medicine, 9th ed. Oxford, Blackwell Scientific Publications, 1993.

Moon C, Preston GM, Griffin CA, et al: The human aquaporin-CHIP gene. J Biol Chem 1993; 268:15772–15778.

Moulds JM, Hayes S, Wells TD: DNA analysis of Duffy genes in American blacks. Vox Sang 1998; 74:248–252.

Moulds JM, Zimmerman PA, Doumbo OK, et al: Molecular identification of Knops blood group polymorphisms found in long homologous region D of complement receptor 1. Blood 2001; 97:2879–2885.

Moulds JM, Zimmerman PA, Doumbo OK, et al: Expansion of the Knops blood group system and subdivision of Sl^a. Transfusion 2002; 42:251–256.

Moulds JM, Doumbo TO, Lyke DKE, et al: Identification of the Kn^a/Kn^b polymorphism and a method for Knops genotyping. Transfusion 2004; 44:164–169.

Mourant AE, Kopec AC, Domaniewska-Sobczak K: The Distribution of the Human Blood Groups and Other Biochemical Polymorphisms, 2nd ed. Oxford, Oxford University Press, 1976.

Nance ST: Applications of flow cytometry in blood transfusion science. In Moore SB (ed): Progress in Immunohematology. Arlington, VA, American Association of Blood Banks, 1988, pp 1–30.

Navenot JM, Muller JY, Blanchard D: Expression of blood group i antigen and fetal hemoglobin in paroxysmal nocturnal hemoglobinuria. Transfusion 1997; 37:291–297.

Ness PM, Shirey RS, Thomas SK, et al: The differentiation of delayed serologic and delayed hemolytic transfusion reactions: Incidence, long-term serologic findings, and clinical significance. Transfusion 1990; 30:688–693.

Nester TA, Rumsey DM, Howell CC, et al: Prevention of immunization to D+ red blood cells with red blood cell exchange and intravenous RH immune globulin. Transfusion 2004; 44:1720–1723.

Okajima T, Nakamura Y, Uchikawa M, et al: Expression cloning of human globoside synthase cDNAs. J Biol Chem 2000; 275:40498–40503.

Olives B, Martial S, Mattei M-G, et al: Molecular characterization of a new urea transporter in the human kidney. FEBS Lett 1996; 386:156–160.

Olsson ML, Thuresson B, Chester MA: An A^{el} allele-specific nucleotide insertion at the blood group ABO locus and its detection using a sequence specific polymerase chain reaction. Biochem Biophys Res Commun 1995; 216:642–647.

Olsson ML, Irshaid NM, Maaf-Hosseini B, et al: Genomic analysis of clinical samples with serologic ABO blood grouping discrepancies: identification of 15 novel A and B subgroup alleles. Blood 2001; 98:1585–1593.

Parsons SF, Mallinson G, Judson PA, et al: Evidence that the Lu^b blood group antigen is located on red cell membrane glycoproteins of 85 and 78 kd. Transfusion 1987; 27:61–63.

Parsons SF, Lee G, Spring FA, et al: Lutheran blood group and its newly characterized mouse homologue specifically bind α5 chain-containing human laminin with high affinity. Blood 2001; 97:312–320.

Petz LD: Drug-induced autoimmune hemolytic anemia. Transfus Med Rev 1993; 8:242–254.

Poole J, Banks J, Bruce LJ, et al: Glycophorin A mutation Ala65→Pro gives rise to a novel pair of MNS alleles ENEP (MNS39) and HAG (MNS41) and altered Wr^b expression: Direct evidence for GPA/band 3 interaction necessary for normal Wr^b expression. Transfus Med 1999; 9:167–174.

Prasad AS: Acquired hemolytic anemias. In Bick RL (ed): Hematology: Clinical and Laboratory Practice, 1st ed, Vol I. St Louis, Mosby, 1993, pp 391–407.

Race RR: The Rh genotypes and Fisher's theory. Blood 1948; 3:27–42.

Race RR, Sanger R: Blood Groups in Man, 6th ed. Oxford, Blackwell Scientific Publications, 1975.

Rahuel C, Elouet J-F, Cartron J-P: Post-transcriptional regulation of the cell surface expression of glycophorins A, B, and E. J Biol Chem 1994; 269:32752–32758.

Rahuel C, Le Van Kim C, Mattei MG, et al: A unique gene encodes spliceoforms of the B-cell adhesion molecule cell surface glycoprotein of epithelial cancer and of the Lutheran blood group glycoprotein. Blood 1996; 88:1865–1872.

Rao N, Telen MJ: Lutheran antigens, Lutheran regulatory genes and Lutheran regulatory gene targets. In Cartron JP, Rouger P (eds): Blood Cell Biochemistry, Vol 6: Molecular Basis of Human Blood Group Antigens. New York, Plenum Press, 1995, pp 281–297.

Reid ME: The Dombrock blood group system: a review. Transfusion 2003a; 43:107–114.

Reid RE, Lomas-Francis C: The Blood Group Antigen Facts Book, 2nd ed. San Diego, CA, Elsevier Academic Press, 2004b.

A succinct listing of the required serologic and molecular testing for each blood group antibody and antigen.

Reid ME, Hue-Roye K, Powell V, et al: ZENA: A new high prevalence Cromer blood group antigen [abstract]. Transfusion 2004a; 44S:26A.

Reid ME, Storry JR, Hue-Roye K, et al: SERF: A new high prevalence antigen in the Cromer blood group system [abstract]. Transfusion 2003b; 43S:6A.

Ridgwell K, Eyers SAC, Mawby W, et al: Studies on the glycoprotein associated with Rh (rhesus) blood group antigen expression in the human red blood cell membrane. J Biol Chem 1994; 269:6410–6416.

Rieben R, Buchs JP, Fluckiger E, Nydegger UE: Antibodies to histo-blood group substances A and B: Agglutination titers, Ig class, and IgG subclasses in healthy persons of different age categories. Transfusion 1991; 31:607–615.

Roitt I, Delves PJ: Roitt's Essential Immunology, 10th ed. Oxford; Malden, MA: Blackwell Science Ltd., 2001.

Roudier N, Verbavatz J-M, Maurel C, et al: Evidence for the presence of aquaporin-3 in human red blood cells. J Biol Chem 1998; 273:8407–8412.

Roubinet F, Despiau S, Calafell F, et al: Evolution of the O alleles of the human ABO blood group gene. Transfusion 2004; 44:707–715.

Russo D, Redman C, Lee S: Association of XK and Kell blood group proteins. J Biol Chem 1998; 273:13950–13956.

Russo DCW, Lee S, Reid ME, Redman CM: Point mutations causing the McLeod phenotype. Transfusion 2002; 42:287–293.

Säfwenberg J, Högman CF, Cassemar B: Computerized delivery control – a useful and safe complement to the type and screen compatibility testing. Vox Sang 1997; 72:162–168.

Salama A, Mueller-Eckhardt C: Immune-mediated blood cell dyscrasias related to drugs. Semin Hematol 1992; 29:54–63.

Segerer S, Bohmig GA, Exner M, et al: When renal allografts turn DARC: Transplantation 2003; 75:1030–1034.

Sheinfeld J, Schaeffer AJ, Cordon-Cardo C, et al: Association of the Lewis blood group phenotype with recurrent urinary tract infections in women. N Engl J Med 1989; 320:773–777.

Shirey RS, Edwards RE, Ness PM: The risk of alloimmunization to c (Rh4) in R$_1$R$_1$ patients who present with anti-E. Transfusion 1994; 34:756–758.

Shirey RS, Mirabella DC, Lumadue JA, Ness PM: Differentiation of anti-D, -C, and -G: Clinical relevance in alloimmunized pregnancies. Transfusion 1997; 37:493–496.

Shulman IA: The risk of an overt hemolytic transfusion reaction following the use of an immediate spin crossmatch. Arch Pathol Lab Med 1990; 114:412–414.

Shulman IA, Nelson JM, Lam HT, et al: Additional limitations of the immediate spin crossmatch to detect ABO incompatibility [Letter]. Am J Clin Pathol 1987; 87:677.

Shulman IA, Downes KA, Sazama K, et al: Pretransfusion compatibility testing for red blood cell administration. Curr Opin Hematol 2001; 8:397–404.

Silva MA (Committee chair): Standards for Blood Banks and Transfusion Services, 23rd ed. Bethesda, MD, American Association of Blood Banks, 2004.

Regulatory standards governing the collection, testing, processing, dispensing, transfusing and tracking of blood components.

Simpson PP, Hall PE: The antiglobulin test. In Harmening DM (ed): Modern Blood Banking and Transfusion Practices, 4th ed. Philadelphia, FA Davis, 1999, pp 71–78.

Smith BL, Preston GM, Spring FA, et al: Human red cell aquaporin CHIP. Molecular characterization of ABH and Colton blood group antigens. J Clin Invest 1994; 94:1043–1049.

Solovey A, Lin Y, Browne P, et al: Circulating activated endothelial cells in sickle cell anemia. N Engl J Med 1997; 337:1584–1590.

Southcott MJ, Tanner MJ, Anstee DJ: The expression of human blood group antigens during erythropoiesis in a cell culture system. Blood 1999; 93:4425–4435.

Spitalnik PF, Spitalnik SL: The P blood group system: Biochemical, serological and clinical aspects. Transfus Med Rev 1995 9:110–122.

Spitalnik S, Pfaff W, Cowles J, et al: Correlation of humoral immunity to Lewis blood group antigens with renal transplant rejection. Transplant 1984; 37:265–268.

Steffensen R, Carlier K, Wiels J, et al: Cloning and expression of the histo-blood group P^k UDP-galactose: Galβ1-4Glcβ1-1Cer α1,4 galactosyltransferase. J Biol Chem 2000; 275:16723–16729.

Storry JR, Reid ME: The Cromer blood group system: a review. Immunohematology 2002 18:95–103.

Su YY, Gordon CT, Ye TZ, et al: Human ERMAP: An erythroid adhesion/receptor transmembrane protein. Blood Cells Mol and Dis 2001 27:938–949.

Takada A, Ohmori K, Yoneda T, et al: Contribution of carbohydrate antigens sialyl Lewis A and sialyl Lewis X to adhesion of human cancer cells to vascular endothelium. Cancer Res 1993; 53:354–561.

Tanner MJA: Molecular and cellular biology of the erythrocyte anion exchanger (AE1). Semin Hematol 1993; 30:34–57.

Tournamille C, Kim CLV, Gane P, et al: Arg89Cys substitution results in very low membrane expression of the Duffy antigen/receptor for chemokines in Fy^x individuals. Blood 1998; 92:2147–2156.

Van Deenen LLM, de Grier J: Lipids of the red cell membrane. In Surgenor DM (ed): The Red Cell Membrane, 2nd ed. New York, Academic Press, 1974, pp 147–156.

Vaughan JI, Manning M, Warwick RM, et al: Inhibition of erythroid progenitor cells by anti-Kell antibodies in fetal alloimmune anemia. N Engl J Med 1998; 338:798–803.

Virella G, Bierer BE: The induction of an immune response: antigens, lymphocytes, and accessory cells. In Virella G (ed): Medical Immunology, 5th ed. New York, Marcel Dekker, Inc., 2001, pp 51–76.

Vollrath B, Fitzgerald KJ, Leder P: A murine homologue of the Drosophila brainiac gene shows homology to glycosyltransferases and is required for preimplantation development of the mouse. Mol Cell Biol 2001; 21:5688–5697.

Wagner FF, Flegel WA: Review: the molecular basis of the Rh blood group phenotypes. Immunohematology 2004; 20:23–36.

Wagner FF, Gassner C, Muller TH, et al: Molecular basis of weak D phenotypes. Blood 1999; 93:385–393 1999.

Wagner T, Bernascher G, Geissler K: Inhibition of megakaryocytopoiesis by Kell-related antibodies [letter]. New Engl J Med 2000; 343:72.

Wagner FF, Poole J, Flegel WA: Scianna antigens including Rd are expressed by ERMAP. Blood 2003; 101:752–757.

Wasniowska K, Lisowska E, Halverson GR, et al: The Fy^a, Fy6 and Fy3 epitopes of the Duffy blood group system recognized by new monoclonal antibodies: identification of a linear Fy3 epitope. Br J Haematol 2004; 124:118–122.

Westhoff CM, Siperd BD, Wylie DE, Toalson LD: Severe anaphylactic reactions following transfusions of platelets to a patient with anti-Ch. Transfusion 1992; 32:576–579.

Weston BW, Nair RP, Larsen RD, Lowe JB: Isolation of a novel human α (1,3) fucosyltransferase gene and molecular comparison to the human Lewis blood group α (1,3/4) fucosyltransferase gene. J Biol Chem 1992; 267:4152–4160.

Worel N, Kalhs P, Keil F, et al. ABO mismatch increases transplant-related morbidity and mortality in patients given nonmyeloablative allogeneic HPC transplantation. Transfusion 2003; 43:1153–1161.

Wright MS, Issitt PD: Anticomplement and the indirect antiglobulin test. Transfusion 1979; 19:688–694.

Yamamoto FI: Molecular genetics of the ABO histo-blood group system. Vox Sang 1995; 69:1–7.

Yamamoto FI, Hakomori SI: Sugar-nucleotide donor specificity of histo-blood group A and B transferases is based on amino acid substitutions. J Biol Chem 1990; 265:19257–19262.

Yang Z, Bergstrom J, Karlsson K-A: Glycoproteins with Galα 1-4Gal are absent from human erythrocyte membranes, indicating that glycolipids are the sole carriers of P blood group activities. J Biol Chem 1994; 269:14620–14624.

Yazdanbakhsh K, Rios M, Storry JR, et al: Molecular mechanisms that lead to reduced expression of Duffy antigens. Transfusion 2000; 40:310–320.

Yesus YW, Akhter JE: Hemolytic disease of the newborn due to anti-C and anti-G masquerading as anti-D. Am J Clin Pathol 1985; 84:769–772.

Yu L-C, Yang Y-H, Broadberry RE, et al: Correlation of a missense mutation in the human secretor α 1,2-fucosyltransferase gene with the Lewis (a+b+) phenotype: A potential molecular basis for the weak secretor allele (Se^w). Biochem J 1995; 312:329–332.

Yu L-C, Twu Y-C, Cou M-L, et al: The molecular genetics of the human I locus and molecular background explain the partial association of the adult I phenotype with congenital cataracts. Blood 2003; 101:2081–2092.

Zimmerman PA, Fitness J, Moulds JM, et al: CR1 Knops blood group alleles are not associated with severe malaria in the Gambia. Genes Immunity 2003; 4:368–373.

CHAPTER 35

Transfusion Medicine

Robertson D. Davenport MD, Paul D. Mintz MD

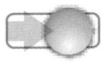

KEY POINTS
• Criteria for blood donor eligibility are established by the FDA to minimize risks to both the donor and transfusion recipient.

• Blood components (red blood cells, platelet concentrates, fresh frozen plasma, cryoprecipitate) are manufactured and stored in a manner to minimize functional loss of desired constituents.

• Leukocyte reduction of blood components reduces alloimmunization to HLA antigens, CMV transmission, and febrile reactions. Irradiation of blood components can prevent graft-vs.-host disease.

• Accurate identification of the pretransfusion blood sample and the intended recipient is the most important step in preventing acute hemolytic transfusion reactions.

• Restrictive red cell transfusion (hemoglobin target 7–9 g/dl) is associated with improved survival in critically ill patients less than 55 years old or with lower APACHE II scores.

• Platelet transfusion is generally indicated for microvascular bleeding, platelet count < 10 000/mL, or platelet count < 50 000/mL prior to an invasive procedure.

• Failure to respond to platelet transfusion may be due to immune causes (HLA or platelet-specific antibodies), nonimmune clinical causes (bleeding, splenomegaly, DIC, medications), or product-specific causes (ABO incompatibility, age of component).

• Plasma transfusion is generally indicated for coagulation factor deficiency, DIC, dilutional coagulopathy, urgent coumadin reversal, and TTP.

• Potentially severe adverse effects of transfusion include hemolytic reactions, allergic reactions, transfusion-related acute lung injury, bacterial contamination, and graft-vs.-host disease.

• Current risks of transfusion-transmitted HIV or hepatitis are very low, but the risks of other transfusion-transmitted diseases (CMV, parvovirus B-19, West Nile virus) may be significant in some populations.

Background

Transfusion medicine (TM) is a multidisciplinary specialty encompassing all aspects of blood donation, blood component preparation, blood cell serology, and blood transfusion therapy. The term blood banking has largely been superseded by transfusion medicine to emphasize the importance of patient care and clinical outcomes.

Operationally, transfusion medicine is divided between blood centers and transfusion services. Blood centers recruit and collect blood from donors, and manufacture and distribute blood components. Transfusion services perform pretransfusion compatibility testing, select and issue blood components for patients, and provide medical support for blood transfusion. Most hospital transfusion services do not collect their own blood, but rather rely on regional blood centers.

Blood centers and transfusion services (collectively known as blood establishments) are regulated by the Food and Drug Administration (FDA). All blood establishments must be registered with the FDA, and blood centers that manufacture blood components must be licensed. Criteria for the acceptability of blood donors, performance of pretransfusion testing, manufacture of blood components, donor infectious disease testing, and evaluation and reporting of adverse events associated with transfusion are all defined by the FDA. Blood establishments are subject to periodic unannounced inspections by the FDA. Compliance with federal regulations is an essential aspect of transfusion medicine. In addition, professional organizations such as AABB, the College of American Pathologists (CAP), and the Joint Commission on the Accreditation of Healthcare Organizations (JCAHO)

IV

have accreditation standards for transfusion services, and conduct voluntary peer inspections.

Blood Collection

Approximately 60% of the adult US population is eligible to donate blood, although only about 5% actually do so annually. Approximately 15 million units of whole blood and red blood cells are collected annually in the US. Virtually all donors are voluntary and noncompensated. The average blood donor is a college-educated male, between the ages of 30 and 50, who is married and has above average income. However, donations among women and minority groups are increasing. As the utilization of blood components increases and donor eligibility requirements are tightened, efforts to recruit additional donors will be critical to assure an adequate blood supply.

Donor criteria are established for the protection of the blood donor and the transfusion recipient. Current (2006) donor qualification criteria are listed in Table 35–1. Criteria for donor protection include a minimum age of 17 years, a minimum weight of 110 pounds, normal vital signs, a minimum hemoglobin concentration, and a specified donation interval. Criteria for the protection of the recipient include history or risk factors for infectious disease transmission (hepatitis, HIV, malaria, and others), risk of bacteremia, ingestion of certain medications, and history of malignancy. Blood centers are required to maintain a registry of deferred donors and each donor must be checked against this registry prior to any donation. The donor is typically given the opportunity to confidentially indicate that his donation should not be used for transfusion (self-exclusion). Finally, every donation must be tested for infectious disease markers as defined by FDA regulations. Current (2006) donor testing requirements are indicated in Table 35–2.

Blood must be collected in a manner to minimize the risk of bacterial contamination. The skin at the venipuncture site must be prepared with an antibacterial scrub. Whole blood is collected into sterilized bag sets containing anticoagulant and attached satellite bags to facilitate component manufacture in a closed system. The rate of blood flow must be sufficient to prevent clot formation during phlebotomy. The volume of blood withdrawn is less than 10% of the donor's expected blood volume. Typically, whole blood donations are either 450 or 500 mL.

Blood components can also be collected by apheresis. The advantage of apheresis donation is that a greater volume of the desired components may be obtained from a single donation. The most common use of the apheresis donation is the collection of platelets (commonly called single donor platelets). Plasma may also be collected, typically concurrently with platelets. Apheresis donation allows for the collection of two units of red blood cells from suitable donors. Leukocytes may also be collected by apheresis. This is most commonly utilized for the collection of hematopoietic progenitor cells for either autologous or allogeneic transplantation. Granulocytes or mononuclear cells may be collected by apheresis for special applications.

Autologous donation is the collection of blood from a patient in advance of scheduled surgery for transfusion during or after the procedure to compensate for expected blood loss. Autologous transfusion prevents the transmission of blood-borne pathogens from allogeneic donors, and is desired by some patients. It is not completely free of risk, however, particularly that of bacterial contamination. Whether or not autologous transfusion actually decreases the need for allogeneic transfusion or improves patient outcome is controversial. Benefit in either reducing allogeneic blood exposure or improving outcome has not been shown in controlled prospective randomized trials. Candidates for autologous donation must not have underlying disease that would put them at risk from this procedure. They must not be significantly anemic; although a lower hemoglobin level than allowed for allogeneic donation may be acceptable. They must not be at risk for bacteremia, since the most serious adverse consequence of autologous transfusion is bacterial contamination. Patients with heart disease, particularly aortic stenosis, may be unable to tolerate phlebotomy. Pregnancy does not itself constitute a contraindication to autologous donation; however, the value of autologous donation except in certain high-risk situations such as *placenta previa* is minimal. Autologous donations can occur more frequently than allogeneic donations. Typically, two or three units may be collected several weeks before surgery. Optimally, there should be sufficient time from donation to surgery to allow for recovery of a substantial portion of the collected red cell mass. This may require iron supplementation. Erythropoietin stimulation has been used as an adjunct to autologous donation.

Some patients desire to select donors for themselves (directed or designated donation) rather than receiving blood from the community blood supply. This provides some patients with the perception of greater safety, although there is no evidence that directed donation reduces the risk of transfusion-transmitted disease. Directed donors must meet all criteria for allogeneic blood donation. In addition, directed donors must be compatible with the intended recipient. There are certain situations in which directed donation is contraindicated. Donation of any plasma-

Table 35–1 Requirements of Allogeneic Donor Qualification

Category	Criteria
Age	At least 17 years
Whole blood volume collected	Maximum of 10.5 mL/kg
Donation interval	8 weeks after whole blood donation
	16 weeks after two-unit red cell collection
	4 weeks after infrequent apheresis
	At least 2 days after plasma, platelet, or leukocyte apheresis
Blood pressure	≤180 mmHg systolic
	≤100 mmHg diastolic
Pulse	50–100 beats per minute, without pathologic irregularities
	< 50 acceptable if an otherwise healthy athlete
Temperature	≤37.5°C orally
Hemoglobin	≥12.5 g/dL
Drug therapy	Finasteride, isotretinoin – defer 1 month after last dose
	Dutasteride – defer 6 months after last dose
	Acitretin – defer 3 years after last dose
	Etretinate – defer indefinitely
	Ingestion of medications that irreversibly inhibit platelet function (aspirin) within 36 hours of donation precludes use of donor as sole source of platelets
General medical history	Free of major organ disease, cancer, abnormal bleeding tendency
Pregnancy	Defer for 6 months
Recipient of blood transfusion or tissue transplant	Defer for 12 months
	Family history of CJD or recipient of dura mater or human pituitary growth hormone – defer indefinitely
Vaccinations and immunizations	Recipient of toxoid, synthetic or killed viral, bacterial, or other vaccine – no deferral
	Recipient of life attenuated viral or bacterial vaccine – 2- or 4-week deferral
	Smallpox vaccine – refer to current FDA guidance
	Hepatitis B immune globulin and unlicensed vaccines – 12-month deferral
Infectious diseases – indefinite deferral	Viral hepatitis after 11th birthday
	Positive test for hepatitis B surface antigen
	Repeat reactive test for anti-HBc on more than one occasion
	Clinical or laboratory evidence of HCV, HTLV, or HIV infection by current FDA regulations
	Previous donation associated with hepatitis, HIV, or HTLV transmission
	History of babesiosis or Chagas' disease
	Stigma of parenteral drug use
	Injection of nonprescription drugs
	Risk of vCJD according to current FDA guidelines
Infectious diseases – 12-month deferral	Mucous membrane exposure to blood
	Nonsterile skin or needle penetration
	Sexual contact with an individual with a confirmed positive test for hepatitis B surface antigen
	Sexual contact with an individual with viral hepatitis
	Sexual contact with an individual with HIV infection or at higher risk for HIV infection
	Incarceration in a correctional institution for more than 72 consecutive hours
	History of syphilis or gonorrhea
West Nile virus	Defer according to current FDA guidance
Malaria	Confirmed diagnosis – defer for 3 years after becoming asymptomatic
	Travel to or residence in an endemic area as defined by the CDC – defer according to FDA guidance

Table 35–2 Donor Infectious Disease Testing

Hepatitis B surface antigen

Hepatitis B core antibody (enzyme immunoassay, EIA)

Hepatitis C virus antibody (enzyme immunoassay, EIA)

HIV-1 and HIV-2 antibodies (enzyme immunoassay, EIA)

HTLV-I and HTLV-II antibodies (enzyme immunoassay, EIA)

Serologic test for syphilis

Hepatitis C RNA (nucleic acid test)

HIV RNA (nucleic acid test)

West Nile virus DNA (nucleic acid test, in evaluation)

Hepatitis B virus DNA (nucleic acid test, in evaluation)

containing blood component from a mother to her child is particularly problematic because the formation of HLA antibodies to fetal antigens is common in pregnancy, and transfusion of such antibodies can precipitate transfusion-related acute lung injury (see below). Transfusions from close relatives should be avoided in recipients of hematopoietic progenitor cell transplants, because of the risk of immunization to HLA and other histocompatibility antigens, which may endanger graft survival. There are rare circumstances under which directed donation may be desirable. These include rare blood group compatibility requirements and the limitation of donor exposures for patients with long-term expected transfusion requirements such as aplastic anemia. In cases of neonatal alloimmune thrombocytopenia, collection of maternal platelets may be the best way of providing compatible antigen-negative platelets. In the past, donor-specific transfusion was utilized in kidney transplantation. However, with current immunosuppressive regimens, the value of donor-specific transfusion in prolonging renal graft survival is questionable.

Adverse effects of donations may occur. Up to 36% of donors interviewed 3 weeks after donation report some adverse effect, mostly minor such as arm bruise or soreness (Newman, 2003). More serious adverse effects such as vasovagal symptoms occur in about 5% and nausea and vomiting in about 1%. Repeat donors are less likely to have reactions than first-time donors. Smaller donors are at greater risk of post-donation syncope. Most syncope reactions occur shortly after donation. However, delayed reactions can occur, and if the donor is at work or driving these can be very serious. Very rarely, arterial puncture or nerve injury can occur (Newman, 1996, 2001). Seizures following blood donation have been reported, although it is unlikely that there is a causal relationship (Krumholz, 1995). Some highly apprehensive donors hyperventilate, leading to respiratory alkalosis and tetany. This can usually be managed easily by having the donor breathe into a paper bag.

Personnel at a collection site should be prepared to treat donor reactions. Vasovagal syncope can usually be managed easily by placing the donor into a supine position and applying a cold compress to the forehead. It is rare that intravenous fluids are required. A physician should be available to donor site personnel for consultation, and there should be availability of emergency medical support if necessary. Vasovagal reactions can be minimized by prior hydration of the donor, or by caffeine (Sauer, 1999).

Blood Component Manufacture

Whole blood donations are commonly manufactured into components. This facilitates the treatment of different patients with requirements for red blood cells, plasma proteins, or platelets. The goals of component manufacture are to maintain viability and function, and to prevent detrimental changes or contamination of the desired constituents.

Red Blood Cells

Red blood cells (RBC) are prepared from whole blood by centrifugation and removal of plasma. The most commonly used anticoagulant-preservative solution for RBC is CPDA-1. This is supplemented with dextrose and adenine to preserve red cell ATP levels. RBC in CPDA-1 may be stored for up to 35 days at 1–6°C. RBC may also have an additive solution containing glucose and other substrates added during manufacture. Such additive solutions permit a longer storage period (42 days) and have a lower hematocrit. During storage, red cells undergo senescence changes similar to aging in vivo, such that a portion of transfused red cells are rapidly cleared by the spleen. The maximum allowable storage time for RBC is defined by the requirement for recovery of 70% of transfused cells 24 hours after transfusion. Leakage of intracellular potassium occurs during red cell

storage. The potassium concentration in the supernatant of RBC can reach levels of 76 mmol/L, which may appear alarmingly high. However, the total amount of potassium in a unit of RBC at outdate is small compared to daily physiologic requirements, and hyperkalemia following transfusion is rare except in special circumstances (see below). Red cells lose intracellular 2,3-DPG during storage resulting in a shift of the hemoglobin–oxygen disassociation curve to the left. Thus, shortly after transfusion, stored red cells have relatively high oxygen affinity. Normal levels of 2,3-DPG are restored within 24 hours of transfusion. The shift in oxygen association with storage is rarely clinically significant.

Plasma

Plasma may be stored in the liquid state at 1–6°C, or maybe frozen for extended preservation. In the liquid state at refrigerator temperatures there is a loss of labile clotting factors, particularly factor VIII and factor V. Fresh frozen plasma (FFP) is separated from the red blood cells and placed at −18°C within 8 hours of collection. FFP may be stored for up to 1 year at −18°C or lower. Prior to transfusion, FFP is thawed at 37°C, and must be transfused within 24 hours. Thawed plasma not used within 24 hours may be relabeled as 'Plasma.' Thawed plasma can be kept at refrigerator temperatures for up to 5 days and still maintain adequate levels of factors V and VIII (Downes, 2001).

Cryoprecipitated Antihemophilic Factor

Cryoprecipitated antihemophilic factor (cryoprecipitate or cryo) is the cold insoluble portion of plasma remaining after FFP has been thawed at refrigerator temperatures. It contains approximately 50% of the factor VIII and 20–40% of the fibrinogen present in the original plasma unit. Cryo also contains von Willebrand factor (vWF) and factor XIII. FDA regulations require that a unit of cryoprecipitate contain at least 80 IU of factor VIII, although most blood centers achieve higher levels routinely. A unit of cryoprecipitate contains approximately 250 mg of fibrinogen, but testing for the fibrinogen content is not required. Cryoprecipitated antihemophilic factor was a major advance in the treatment of hemophilia A prior to development of safe purified clotting factor concentrates. Currently, cryo is used mainly as a source of fibrinogen.

Platelet Concentrates

Platelet concentrates (PC) are prepared from whole blood by centrifugation of platelet-rich plasma and expressing the platelet-poor plasma. Platelet concentrates must contain at least 5.5×10^{10} platelets per unit. They are stored at room temperature (20–24°C) because platelets stored at refrigerator temperatures (1–6°C) have greatly diminished post-transfusion survival. Current FDA regulations allow PC to be stored for up to 5 days with continuous gentle agitation. At the end of the storage, the pH of the PC must be 6.0 or higher. Platelet concentrates typically contain a small amount of red cells, which is visibly apparent, and can cause alloimmunization to red cell antigens. Platelet concentrates contain 30–50 mL of plasma. It is typically necessary to pool five or more PC in order to obtain a therapeutic dose for a typical adult patient.

Platelet concentrates prepared by apheresis (Platelets, Pheresis; or single donor platelets) are stored and handled in the same manner as platelet concentrates prepared from whole blood. Each apheresis platelet unit should contain a minimum of 3.0×10^{11} platelets. It is possible to collect two platelet units in a single apheresis session from some donors. One apheresis platelet unit will typically provide a therapeutic dose for an adult patient.

Leukocyte Components

Granulocytes can be prepared by apheresis. Granulocytes may be stored at room temperature for up to 24 hours. However, after even brief in vitro storage granulocytes may have reduced ability to circulate and migrate to areas of inflammation (McCullough, 1983). It is desirable that they be transfused as soon as possible after collection. Donor stimulation with granulocyte colony-stimulating factor (G-CSF) is usually necessary to obtain a sufficient number of granulocytes to be a therapeutic dose for an adult patient (Heuft, 2002). Granulocyte units contain a substantial amount of red blood cells and must be ABO compatible with the recipient.

Mononuclear cells collected by apheresis can be a source of hematopoietic progenitor cells (HPCs) for autologous or allergenic transplantation. The number of circulating HPCs can be increased by growth factor (G-CSF or GM-CSF) stimulation. Autologous HPCs for transplantation in patients with lymphoma or hematologic malignancies are typically collected when the bone marrow is recovering from chemotherapy, because there are relatively high numbers of circulating stem cells at that time. HPCs may be stored frozen after addition of a cryoprotective agent, such as DMSO, for an extended period of time. After thawing at 37°C, HPCs should be transfused as soon as possible. Mononuclear cells can also be used as a source of lymphocytes for induction of graft-vs.-tumor effect, known as donor lymphocyte infusion (DLI) (Gilleece, 2003).

Leukocyte-Reduced Blood Components

Leukocytes present in blood components, particularly RBC and PC, may cause adverse effects. Such untoward effects include febrile nonhemolytic transfusion reactions, immunization to leukocyte (particularly HLA) antigens with subsequent refractoriness to platelet transfusions, transmission of leukocyte-associated viruses, and graft-versus-host disease. To minimize most of these adverse impacts, many blood centers and transfusion services have instituted the use of leukocyte-reduced components for all transfusions (universal leukocyte reduction). It must be noted that leukocyte reduction has not been shown to reduce post-transfusion graft-vs.-host disease and is not used for this purpose. In order to be considered leukocyte-reduced, blood components must be prepared by a method known to reduce the total number of residual leukocytes to less than 5×10^6 per unit for RBC and less than 8.3×10^5 for whole-blood derived PC (Fridey, 2003).

Leukocyte reduction is typically accomplished by filtration, either at the time of component manufacture (prestorage leukocyte reduction) or at the time of transfusion (poststorage leukocyte reduction). Both methods are effective for removing leukocytes. However, prestorage leukocyte reduction has the advantage of preventing accumulation of leukocyte-derived biologic response modifiers, particularly cytokines, which may cause adverse reactions (Heddle, 1999). In addition, filtration at the time of manufacture allows for better process control. Certain apheresis devices can reliably produce platelet concentrates containing less than 1×10^6 leukocytes. There are subtle differences in the distribution of leukocyte subsets between such components and those produced by filtration (Pennington, 2001). These differences, however, are unlikely to be clinically significant.

Leukocyte reduction failures may occur during filtration of blood from donors with sickle trait. Such filtration failures are due to hemoglobin S polymerization in an environment of low oxygen tension and high osmolality (Beard, 2004). Leukocyte reduction is not an effective means of preventing graft-vs.-host disease (Hayashi, 1993). Clearly, granulocytes and hematopoietic progenitor cells cannot be leukocyte reduced.

Special Components

Cryoprecipitate-reduced plasma (cryopoor plasma) is the supernatant remaining from the production of cryoprecipitate. It is relatively deficient in high-molecular-weight forms of von Willebrand factor while retaining normal levels of the vWF-cleaving metalloprotease (Blackall, 2001). For these reasons, cryoprecipitate-reduced plasma is an attractive alternative to FFP for the treatment of patients with thrombotic thrombocytopenia purpura. There is, however, at present no definitive evidence that plasma exchange with cryoprecipitate-reduced plasma results in improved patient outcome.

Red blood cells can be stored in the frozen state after addition of a cryoprotective agent, such as glycerol. Frozen RBC can be stored in mechanical freezers or liquid nitrogen for up to 10 years. Frozen units are thawed rapidly at 37°C. The cryoprotective agent must be removed by progressive addition of washing solutions with decreasing osmolality. Failure to properly deglycerolize frozen RBC can result in hemolysis. Cryopreservation and deglycerolization of sickle trait red cells by standard methods can result in the formation of a jelly-like mass. This can be overcome by using a modified process (Meryman, 1976). After deglycerolization, red cells can be stored for up to 1 day at 1–6°C if processed by an open method, or up to 14 days if processed by a closed method. The main use of frozen RBC is to maintain an inventory of rare antigen-negative units.

RBC and PC can be washed to remove plasma proteins and electrolytes. Washing can be accomplished by either manual or automated methods. There can be substantial loss of cells during the washing process. In addition, washing of platelets can result in clumping and activation with reduced viability (Pineda, 1989). Because this is an open process, washed red cells may be stored for 24 hours at refrigerator temperatures, and washed platelets must be transfused within 4 hours of preparation. The main use of washed components is the prevention of severe allergic reactions. Washing is not an effective means of leukocyte reduction.

Transfusion-associated graft-vs.-host disease (TA-GVHD) can be prevented by irradiation of components containing viable lymphocytes (RBC, PC, granulocytes, and nonfrozen plasma). This can be accomplished by exposure to either gamma rays or X-rays. The minimum dose should be 25 Gy delivered to the center of the blood container and no less than 15 Gy to the periphery. Irradiation causes chromosomal damage, which prevents replication of transfused lymphocytes in the recipient. However, irradiated cells are immunogenic. Thus, irradiation is not equivalent to leukocyte reduction. Irradiation also causes damage to red cell membranes with increased potassium leakage and decreased post-transfusion survival (Moroff, 1999). Irradiated red cells must have the outdate shortened to no more than 28 days from the date of irradiation. Platelets appear to sustain minimal damage from irradiation, and so their expiration date need not be altered (Sweeney, 1994). Clearly, hematopoietic progenitor cells must not be irradiated. Irradiation is not sufficient to prevent transmission of viral infections, including cytomegalovirus, or bacterial contamination.

Pathogen Reduction

Although great progress has been made in reducing the risks of transfusion-transmitted diseases, some risk remains. In addition, there is the possibility that a new transmissible disease may emerge as a threat to blood safety. For these reasons, strategies to inactivate contaminating microorganisms (pathogen reduction) are presently under active development. Blood derivatives such as albumin, coagulation factor concentrates, and immunoglobulins are commonly treated by a variety of methods including heat and solvent-detergent, which are highly effective against viruses including human immunodeficiency virus (HIV), hepatitis B virus (HBV), and hepatitis C virus (HCV). The solvent-detergent treatment process disrupts the lipid envelope of viruses such as HIV, HBV, and HCV. However, it is ineffective against nonlipid-enveloped viruses. In addition, it destroys cell membranes and so is not applicable to cellular blood components. Solvent-detergent treated plasma is available in Europe and is licensed by the FDA, although it is not presently available in the US. Solvent-detergent treated plasma contains predictable levels of all coagulation factors, and is effective in the treatment of thrombotic thrombocytopenic purpura (TTP) (Horowitz, 1992; Moake, 1994). It may, however, contain reduced levels of protein S, and has been associated with thrombotic complications (Doyle, 2003).

Psoralen compounds intercalate between bases of RNA and DNA, and when exposed to UV light form covalent crosslinks that prevent replication. Psoralen treatment is highly effective against viruses, bacteria, and protozoans (Lin, 2004). A psoralen treatment method for platelet concentrates has been shown to be safe and effective in a randomized trial (McCullough, 2004). The treatment process does result in a statistically significant, and possibly clinically significant, reduction in post-transfusion platelet recovery. Because psoralen treatment requires exposure to light, its applicability to red blood cells is limited. An alternative approach to pathogen reduction is the use of a polyamine that reacts specifically with guanine in nucleic acids (Inactine™). This forms an adduct that disrupts nucleic acid replication. This technique has also been shown to be highly effective against many viruses, bacteria, and protozoans (Zavizion, 2003; Lazo, 2002). While each of these techniques is promising, there remain questions of toxicity and immunogenicity.

Selection of Blood Components

Blood components must be serologically compatible with the recipient. ABO compatibility is the primary consideration. Transfused red cells must be compatible with recipient antibodies, and transfused plasma must be compatible with recipient red cells. Therefore, whole blood must be of identical ABO type to the recipient. Red blood cells contain a limited amount of plasma, and need to be compatible but not necessarily identical with ABO of type of the recipient. Similarly, plasma and platelet concentrates contain few, if any, red cells. ABO compatible blood component selection is summarized in Table 35–3. Red blood cells must also be negative for clinically significant antigens when transfused to alloimmunized recipients. It is highly desirable to transfuse only Rh-negative red cells to Rh-negative recipients, because there is approximately a 30% risk of immunization to Rh(D) (Frohn, 2003). This is particularly important for women of childbearing potential, because of the risk of hemolytic disease of the newborn in subsequent pregnancies.

Special considerations apply to recipients of ABO incompatible hematopoietic progenitor cell transplants. During the course of transplantation, such individuals will change their blood type. Transfused red cells should be compatible with both donor and recipient isohemagglutinins, and transfused plasma-containing components should be compatible with both donor and recipient red cells. Thus, the optimal choice for such a patient will depend on current and expected future typing results.

Table 35–3 ABO Compatibility

Donor type	Recipient type			
	O	**A**	**B**	**AB**
O	R	R	R	R
	P			
A		R		R
	P	P		
B			R	R
	P		P	
AB				R
	P	P	P	R

R = red cells are compatible; P = plasma-containing components (platelets, FFP) are compatible.

Red Blood Cells

The primary consideration in selection of RBC is serologic compatibility for the prevention of hemolytic transfusion reactions. Since the post-transfusion survival of red cells is inversely related to length of storage, it is desirable to select fresh (typically less than 10 days old) units in situations where it is particularly desirable to limit the number of transfusions, such as intrauterine and neonatal transfusion. For large volume transfusions of pediatric patients (such as exchange transfusion or cardiac surgery) it may be desirable to select hemoglobin S-negative (sickle-negative) units. It is also preferable to select sickle-negative red cells for transfusion to patients with sickle cell disease, because the presence of hemoglobin S in donor red cells may complicate monitoring the effectiveness of transfusion therapy. It has, however, never been shown that red cell transfusion from asymptomatic sickle trait donors is deleterious, and in some cases such as rare blood requirements, the use of a sickle trait donor may be the only option. Heavily transfused patients, particularly those with sickle cell disease, are at risk of alloimmunization and hemolytic transfusion reactions (Vichinsky, 1990). Such patients may benefit from prophylactic administration of antigen-matched red cells, particularly Rh and Kell (Ambruso, 1987; Castellino, 1999).

Exchange transfusion of the neonate with hemolytic disease of the newborn is a special case. In this situation, both antigen-negative red cells and plasma (for oncotic pressure and bilirubin binding capacity) are needed. Red cells must be compatible with the maternal antibodies, including ABO antibodies. Reconstituted whole blood, prepared by combining RBC and compatible FFP to a desired hematocrit (typically 50%), is commonly used, although whole blood may be used if available.

Platelets

Major ABO compatibility is less of an issue in platelet transfusion than in red cell transfusion. ABO antigens are expressed weakly on platelets. ABO incompatible platelet transfusions may result in lower post-transfusion survival, although this is usually not clinically significant. Transfusion of isohemagglutinins contained in the plasma of apheresis platelets from donors with high-titer anti-A or anti-B can cause an acute hemolytic reaction (Larsson, 2000). Therefore, if non-ABO-identical platelets must be transfused, overriding consideration is typically given to plasma compatibility with the recipient. Some centers will screen apheresis platelets to ensure that high-titer incompatible anti-A or anti-B (e.g., < 1 : 200 reactivity at immediate spin) is not transfused.

Failure to achieve an expected platelet count increment after platelet transfusion on two or more occasions is commonly considered refractoriness. The failure to respond with an appropriate increase in platelet count after transfusion (platelet refractoriness) may be due to immune causes (HLA or platelet-specific antibodies), nonimmune clinical causes (bleeding, splenomegaly, DIC, medications), product-specific causes (ABO incompatibility; older products give lower increments), or the fact that some donors' platelets store poorly. A poor increment following a single platelet transfusion must not be presumed to be due to alloimmunization. The refractoriness is often multifactorial and changes with the patient's underlying condition and therapy. HLA antibodies are the most common cause of immune-mediated platelet refractoriness. HLA class I antigens are expressed on platelets, and class I antibodies are common in patients who have been previously pregnant or transfused with non-leukocyte-reduced blood components. Leukocyte reduction has

been shown to effectively prevent both alloimmunization and platelet refractoriness in previously unexposed patients with leukemia (Trial to Reduce Alloimmunization to Platelets Study Group, 1997). Antibodies to platelet specific antigens are a relatively rare cause of platelet refractoriness. There are several effective strategies for selection of platelets for the alloimmunized refractory recipient. The use of crossmatch-compatible platelets is usually the first line (O'Connell, 1990). If the patient's HLA antibody specificities can be defined, it may be possible to select antigen-negative donors (Petz, 2000). Donors matched for HLA class I antigens may be selected. However, owing to constraints of donor availability, finding optimal matches may be very difficult. Even with a large donor base, many 'HLA-matched' transfusions are mismatched for at least one antigen (Dahlke, 1984).

Pretransfusion Testing

The most critical step in pretransfusion testing is proper collection and identification of the recipient blood sample. The most common cause of an acute hemolytic transfusion reaction is misidentification of the sample or patient (Sazama, 1990; Linden, 2000). Each transfusion service must develop and implement policies and procedures for patient identification and specimen collection. The pretransfusion samples should be labeled at the time of phlebotomy by comparison with the patient's permanent identifier (typically a wristband). The label should contain at least two unique identifiers, such as patient name and hospital registration number. The date of sample collection and identity of the phlebotomist must also be documented. In emergency situations when the patient's identity is unknown, there must be a unique identifier assigned. This identifier must remain with the patient throughout the course of transfusion even if the patient is subsequently identified. There must be policies and procedures for management of patients with confidential or alias names.

Samples for pretransfusion testing should be collected no more than 3 days before transfusion, unless it is known that the patient has not been pregnant or transfused within the preceding 3 months. The common practice of patient admission on the same day as elective surgery presents special challenges. In this setting, pretransfusion samples may be collected during a preceding outpatient visit. One option is to require such patients to wear an identification wristband, although many patients find this undesirable. Another alternative is to assign a unique number to the pretransfusion specimen and affix this number to an identification form that the patient must provide on the day of surgery (Butch, 1994). Pretransfusion samples must be retained until at least 7 days after each transfusion. Typically, transfusion services retain pretransfusion samples for a fixed time, such as 56 days.

Routine pretransfusion testing consists of ABO and Rh(D) typing, and screening for unexpected red cell antibodies. If the antibody screen is positive, antibody identification tests should be performed. The results of current testing should be compared to records of the previous testing, if available. Clinically significant red cell antibodies may become undetectable over time, but may cause delayed hemolytic reactions owing to an anamnestic response. Therefore, a history of a clinically significant red cell antibody should be honored by providing only antigen-negative red cells for transfusion. Any discrepancy in current testing or disagreement with previous records must be resolved before pretransfusion testing can be concluded.

Some patients present particular challenges in pretransfusion testing. Newborns typically have weak or absent isohemagglutinins. Expected ABO antibodies may not be present until 6 months of age. Recently transfused patients may show a mixture of circulating red cells, if they have not received ABO-identical units. Unexpected red cell antibodies can be acquired passively from transfusion of platelet concentrates or immunoglobulins. Some patients may lack expected isohemagglutinins because of disease or immunosuppressive therapy. Recipients of allogeneic HPC transplants may have complex and variable typing results, which necessitate conclusion of a 'declared' blood type. In urgent situations when the blood type cannot be concluded, selection of group O red cells and group AB plasma is usually safe. If antibody identification tests cannot be completed, a medical judgment must be made regarding the urgency of transfusion and risks of incompatibility. It may be desirable to issue red cells lacking antigen specificities that cannot be excluded, if available. The occurrence of a weakly expressed Rh(D) antigen may complicate pretransfusion testing.

The final step of pretransfusion compatibility testing is the crossmatch. The purpose of the crossmatch is a final check of ABO compatibility and, to a lesser extent, detection of unidentified antibodies. A major crossmatch is performed between the recipient's serum or plasma and donor red cells.

A minor crossmatch, between recipient red cells and donor or plasma, is usually unnecessary. In the absence of unexpected red cell antibodies, a crossmatch can be performed by direct agglutination ('immediate spin') for detection of ABO incompatibility. When unexpected red cell antibodies are present, the crossmatch should be performed by antiglobulin technique. For antibodies judged to be clinically significant, antigen-negative cells are selected for crossmatch. An alternative for assurance of ABO compatibility is the so-called computer crossmatch. This is applicable when at least two determinations of the recipient's ABO group have been made, at least one on a current sample, and there are no unexpected antibodies (Butch, 1997). A validated computer system can then assure that issued blood complements are ABO compatible. The presence of red cell autoantibodies presents a special problem. In this setting, it is essential that alloantibodies be excluded. Typically, the crossmatch will be positive. Many transfusion services have a policy of issuing 'least reactive' units, although the value of this policy has been called into question (Petz, 2003).

In urgent situations, emergency release of blood complements before completion of compatibility testing may be indicated. The goals of emergency release are to provide red cells for oxygen-carrying capacity and plasma for coagulation factor content to a rapidly bleeding patient. ABO compatibility is the first priority (see above discussion of component selection). Antibodies to other blood group antigens typically do not cause acute hemolytic reactions, and are therefore of lower priority. However, when there is a history of prior antibodies, or antibody identification tests are partially complete, it may be preferable to select antigen-negative RBC, if available. Finally, documentation of the medical order for emergency release of blood components should be obtained, usually after the fact.

Transfusion Administration

The transfusion service is responsible for developing and implementing policies and procedures for the administration of blood components. A physician's order is required to prepare, dispense, and administer blood components. Optimally, venous access should be established prior to issuing a blood component. The selection of location and type of access depends on the volume, timing, and expected duration of transfusion therapy. Peripheral access with an 18-gauge needle or catheter is typically sufficient. Smaller catheters may be used; however, high-pressure flow through a small lumen may cause hemolysis (de la Roche, 1993). Central venous access is desirable for high-volume administration or long-term therapy.

Prior to administration of a transfusion, accurate identification of the component and intended recipient is essential. This process should include at least two unique identifiers, such as name and registration number, and comparison to a permanent identifier, such as a wristband. Additionally, the unit identifier on the blood container should be checked against the associated documentation (transfusion form or attached tag). The ABO and Rh type on the unit label must agree with the associated documentation, and compatibility with the patient's recorded blood type should be verified. The expiration time and date of the blood component should be verified as acceptable. Many institutions require two qualified individuals to perform the identity check before transfusion. The physician's order and patient's consent for transfusion should also be verified.

All blood components must be administered through a filter intended to retain clots and particles, typically 170–260 μm pore size. Administration sets should contain a drip chamber, attached compatible intravenous solution, and a means of controlling the flow rate. During surgery, it is routine practice to add a microaggregate filter through which the blood component flows first. This decreases the metabolic burden placed on the recipient to process aggregates of fibrin and cellular debris that accumulate during storage, and helps to preserve the patency of the intravascular line. Care should be taken to avoid admixture of the blood components with incompatible i.v. solutions. Normal saline is the preferred solution for all transfusions. Calcium-containing solutions should be avoided as these may precipitate clotting. RBC should not be administered with 5% dextrose as this may cause hemolysis. Medications should not be added to blood components. Leukocyte reduction filters may be used for the transfusion of RBC or PC to reduce the incidence of febrile transfusion reactions, HLA alloimmunization, or CMV transmission. The appropriate filter must be selected for the blood component, since clogging or filter failure may occur if improperly used.

It may be desirable to administer refrigerated blood components (RBC or plasma) through a blood-warming device. Transfusion of cold components faster than 100 mL per minute for 30 minutes may increase the risk of cardiac arrest (Boyan, 1963). Blood-warming devices should

Table 35–4 Red Cell Transfusion Guidelines

Symptomatic anemia in a euvolemic patient

Acute blood loss of < 15% of estimated blood volume

Preoperative Hb < 9.0 g/dL with expected blood loss > 500 mL

Hb < 7.0 g/dL in a critically ill patient

Hb < 8.0 g/dL in a patient with an acute coronary syndrome

Hb < 10.0 g/dL with uremic or thrombocytopenic bleeding

Sickle cell disease:

    Acute sequestration: Hb < 5.0 g/dL or decrease of 20% from baseline

    Acute chest syndrome: Target Hb = 10 g/dL, HbS fraction < 30%

    Stroke prophylaxis: Target HbS fraction < 30%

    General anesthesia: Target Hb = 10.0 g/dL, HbS fraction < 60%

have a visible thermometer and audible alarm to avoid exceeding temperature limits. Blood components should never be warmed by use of tap water, conventional microwave ovens, or any other nonapproved warming device.

The desirable rate of administration depends on the patient's blood volume, cardiac status, and hemodynamic state. Except for urgent resuscitation, the transfusion should be started slowly (approximately 2 mL/min for the first 15 minutes). The patient should be carefully observed for the first 15 minutes of infusion, since severe reactions such as hemolysis, anaphylaxis, or sepsis may manifest after a small volume has entered the circulation. Subsequently, the administration rate may be increased. In general, it is desirable to complete a red cell transfusion within 2 hours and a platelet or plasma transfusion within 30–60 minutes. Any transfusion should be completed within 4 hours of initiation. Patients at risk of volume overload may require slower administration. If the total administration time exceeds 4 hours, smaller volume blood components should be provided. When high flow rates are required, such as in some resuscitation or surgical situations, a pressure infusion device may be used. When using such devices, care must be taken to avoid mechanical hemolysis or air embolism. During transfusion, the patient's vital signs should be checked at regular intervals, and any suspected reaction should prompt interruption of the transfusion and immediate investigation.

Blood Component Therapy

All transfusion decisions are clinical judgments that should be made taking into account clinical and laboratory data. There are no absolute indications, and few contraindications, to blood transfusion.

Red Cell Transfusion

Red blood cells provide oxygen-carrying capacity. Red cell transfusion may be used to treat acute or chronic anemia. A patient's ability to tolerate anemia depends upon the degree of anemia, physiologic adaptive mechanisms, and cardiac or respiratory disease. Normal physiologic adaptations to anemia include increased cardiac output, redistribution of blood flow, increased oxygen extraction, and increased red cell 2,3-DPG resulting in rightward shift of the oxygen–hemoglobin dissociation curve. General guidelines for red cell transfusion are summarized in Table 35–4. Symptomatic anemia, regardless of hemoglobin concentration, in a euvolemic patient is an indication for transfusion. Symptoms of anemia include fatigue, tachycardia, tachypnea, dyspnea on exertion, postural hypotension, and impaired mentation. Anemia may precipitate angina in patients with coronary artery disease. Generally, acute blood loss of greater than 15% of a patient's blood volume may be an indication for red cell transfusion. Studies of post-surgical morbidity in patients who refused blood transfusion have indicated that for patients with a preoperative hemoglobin of at least 6 g/dL, without underlying coronary artery disease, and sustaining operative blood loss of less than 2 g/dL of hemoglobin; there is little relationship between mortality and degree of preoperative anemia (Carson, 1996). Mortality increases with preoperative hemoglobin levels below 6 g/dL (Spence, 1990). However, with a hemoglobin loss of 2–4 g/dL, perioperative mortality increases with preoperative hemoglobin levels below 10 g/dL. This risk is magnified by the presence of cardiovascular disease (angina, myocardial infarction, congestive heart failure, or peripheral vascular disease). One study of patients undergoing elective operations demonstrated no mortality despite hemoglobin levels as low as 6 g/dL provided the blood loss was less than 500 mL (Carson, 1988).

The Transfusion Requirements in Critical Care (TRICC) study has been the largest randomized prospective trial to date comparing restrictive and liberal transfusion strategies (Hebert, 1999). The TRICC trial enrolled 838 critically ill patients with hemoglobin level < 9.0 g/dL. The subjects were randomized to receive either liberal or restrictive transfusion regimens. The liberal regimen was a transfusion trigger of 10 g/dL with a target of 10–12 g/dL. The restrictive regimen was a transfusion trigger of 7.0 g/dL with a target of 7.0–9.0 g/dL. The primary result was no statistically significant difference in 30-day mortality, although there was a trend favoring lower mortality in the restrictive strategy group (18.7% vs. 23.3%, p = 0.11). Cardiac events, primarily pulmonary edema and myocardial infarction, occurred more frequently in the liberal than the restrictive transfusion group (21.0% vs. 13.2%, p < 0.001). Subgroup analysis showed lower mortality in the restrictive strategy group among patients with lower disease severity measured by Acute Physiology and Chronic Health Evaluation (APACHE II) scores (8.7% vs. 16.1%, p = 0.03) and among patients younger than 55 years of age (5.77% vs. 13.07%, p = 0.02). Thus, it appears that many critically ill adult patients can tolerate hemoglobin levels less than 10 g/dL.

Whether the results of the TRICC trial are generalizable to patients with acute coronary syndromes is open to debate. A large retrospective cohort study of patients > 65 years of age with acute myocardial infarction has examined the association between admission hemoglobin and 30-day mortality (Wu, 2001). This showed a clear relationship between increasing mortality and lower initial hemoglobin. Furthermore, among patients who received transfusion, there was a lower adjusted odds of 30-day mortality when the admission hematocrit was less than 33%, whereas there were higher odds of death for transfused patients with admission hematocrit > 36%, after adjustment for clinical factors, medication used, and predictors of transfusion. These results suggested that red cell transfusion may result in lower short-term mortality among elderly patients with acute myocardial infarction who survived at least 2 days, if the hematocrit on admission is 30% or lower. However, inherent drawbacks of the retrospective study design, such as survivor bias, limit the conclusions that can be drawn from this study. An analysis of transfusion effect on 30-day mortality in patients with acute coronary syndromes presented somewhat different results (Rao, 2004). This was a reanalysis of three interventional drug trials with the primary outcome measure being 30-day mortality. Ten percent of subjects in the study were transfused. The transfused subjects were more likely to have comorbidities, including a higher Killip class, than nontransfused subjects. The cumulative mortality among transfused subjects was greater than in nontransfused subjects (p < 0.001). For subjects with a nadir hematocrit of 20%, there was no statistically significant difference in odds of death between transfused and nontransfused individuals.

Transfusion of the patient with sickle cell disease (SCD) presents unique challenges. The indications for transfusion are to augment oxygen-carrying capacity in severe anemia, and to improve microvascular circulation by decreasing the proportion of sickle red cells. Oxygen delivery in SCD is a balance between oxygen-carrying capacity and blood viscosity. Optimal oxygen delivery is usually achieved when the post-transfusion hematocrit is about 30% (Schmalzer, 1987). There are no universally accepted laboratory parameters for transfusion in SCD. Hb values of less than 5 g/dL, or an acute drop of 20% from baseline during an acute illness, are general indications for red cell transfusion. Acute splenic sequestration can produce sudden hypovolemia and cardiovascular collapse, necessitating prompt transfusion. In this setting, the rise in Hb following transfusion may be greater than expected because of release of sequestered red cells. Careful monitoring is essential to avoid overtransfusion (Powell, 1992). Acute chest syndrome may be life threatening. Prompt transfusion may prevent progression to respiratory failure (Mallouh, 1988). Exchange transfusion with a goal of achieving Hb S level of 30% or less and hematocrit of 30% is a typical approach. Chronic transfusion therapy can reduce the risk of stroke in SCD. In children, transfusion with the goal of maintaining Hb S levels below 30% can reduce the risk of stroke (Adams, 1998). How long a chronic transfusion regimen must be maintained is an open question. Termination, even after several years of therapy, can result in reversion to high risk of stroke (Adams, 2004). Prior to general anesthesia, transfusion is indicated to achieve a Hb of 10 g/dL and Hb S level of approximately 60% (Vichinsky, 1995). In uncomplicated pregnancy, prophylactic red cell transfusion is not beneficial. However, transfusion may be indicated in high-risk pregnancy or when there is a history of previous fetal loss (Seoud, 1994).

In autoimmune hemolytic anemia, transfusion may be indicated if there are cardiac or neurologic symptoms. Most patients with autoimmune hemolytic anemia tolerate transfusion of incompatible red cells, if alloantibodies have been excluded (Salama, 1992). Transfused red cells are usually not cleared any more rapidly than the patient's own red cells. Importantly, a necessary red cell transfusion must never be withheld because of crossmatch incompatibility. It is far more dangerous not to give such a transfusion to a patient with autoimmune hemolytic anemia than it is to provide it.

Red cell transfusion may be beneficial in bleeding associated with uremia. There is an inverse relationship between hematocrit and bleeding time in patients with chronic renal failure. Transfusion to a Hb of 10 g/dL may be beneficial in the bleeding uremic patient (Fernandez, 1985).

Transfusion of one unit of red blood cells to an adult patient can usually be expected to raise the Hb by 1 g/dL and the hematocrit by 3%. However, the expected hematocrit increase may range from about 2–9% depending on the patient's vascular volume (Gorlin, 2000).

Table 35–5 Platelet Transfusion Guidelines

Thrombocytopenia due to decreased production
    Stable patent: Platelet count < 10 000/µL
    Fever: Platelet count < 20 000/µL
    Bleeding, invasive procedure or surgery: Platelet count < 40 000–50 000/µL
    Retinal or CNS bleeding: platelet count < 100 000/µL
Microvascular bleeding due to platelet dysfunction

Platelet Transfusion

Platelet transfusion is indicated for prevention or treatment of hemorrhage due to thrombocytopenia or platelet dysfunction, as summarized in Table 35–5. Prophylactic transfusion is indicated when the platelet count is less than 5000/µL. For stable patients undergoing chemotherapy, a prophylactic platelet transfusion threshold of 10 000/µL is often used (Rebulla, 1997). The goal of prophylactic therapy is to achieve platelet counts above 25 000/µL (Schlossberg, 2003). If the patient is febrile, a threshold for prophylactic transfusion of 20 000/µL is typically used. For bleeding patients, or for those undergoing an invasive procedure, including endoscopy, or surgery, the goal of platelet transfusion therapy is to achieve sustained levels above 40 000–50 000/µL (British Committee for Standards in Haematology, Blood Transfusion Task Force, 2003). This usually ensures hemostasis, though it may take longer than normal to achieve. For this reason, for patients experiencing bleeding in critical spaces, such as the retina or central nervous system, a target of 100 000/µL is the standard of practice, as this level typically ensures no abnormal delay in hemostasis. In bleeding associated with platelet dysfunction, or thrombocytopenic bleeding associated with coagulopathy, there is no single transfusion threshold, and therapy must be guided by the patient's clinical condition. Cardiopulmonary bypass may result in a transient acquired platelet dysfunction that may manifest as microvascular bleeding. The platelet count is not usually a useful indicator in such situations. Prophylactic platelet transfusion in routine cardiopulmonary bypass is not indicated.

The platelet transfusion is relatively contraindicated in immune thrombocytopenic purpura (ITP). In this setting, post-transfusion platelet survival is extremely brief and platelet transfusion is only indicated if there is severe hemorrhage. Clearly transfusion in the setting of intravascular platelet consumption should be undertaken with great caution. Platelet transfusion in heparin-induced thrombocytopenia or thrombotic thrombocytopenic purpura can be deleterious (Harkness, 1981; Gordon, 1987).

Transfusion of one apheresis platelet unit, or equivalent pool of whole-blood-derived platelet concentrates, can typically be expected to raise the platelet count of an adult by 20 000–40 000/µL. As a practical matter, it can be estimated that approximately one hour post-transfusion the blood platelet count should increase by 8000–10 000/µL for each 1×10^{11} platelets transfused for each square meter of body surface area (Strauss, 1995). However, there are many reasons why this increment may not be achieved. Consumption or bleeding, splenomegaly, platelet antibodies, and drugs are all causes of a poor response to platelet transfusion. Drugs that can cause an inadequate platelet increment include antibiotics, heparin, antiplatelet agents (clopidogrel, tirofiban), quinidine, and antithymocyte globulin, and many others. In assessing platelet transfusion effectiveness, it is useful to take into account dose and body size by calculating the corrected count increment (CCI).

$$CCI = \frac{\text{Platelet count increment} \times \text{BSA}}{\text{Number of platelets transfused } (\times 10^{11})}$$

BSA = body surface area (m^2).
    Example:
Pretransfusion platelet count = 8000/µL
Post-transfusion platelet count = 36 000/µL
BSA = 1.5 m^2

CHAPTER: 35 Transfusion Medicine

Table 35–6 Plasma Transfusion Guidelines

Coagulation factor deficiency, factor concentrate unavailable
Dilutional coagulopathy
Hemorrhage in liver disease
Disseminated intravascular coagulation (DIC)
Coumadin reversal
Thrombotic thrombocytopenic purpura (TTP)

Table 35–7 Cryoprecipitate Transfusion Guidelines

Factor VIII deficiency, factor concentrate unavailable
von Willebrand disease, factor concentrate unavailable
Hypofibrinogenemia
Factor XIII deficiency
Uremic bleeding (DDAVP preferred)
Topical fibrin sealant (commercial product preferred)

Platelet dose = 3.0×10^{11}

$$CCI = \frac{24\,000 \times 1.5}{3} = 12\,000$$

A CCI > 7500 at 1 hour or a CCI > 4500 at 24 hours generally indicates a successful transfusion. Obtaining a platelet count within 1 hour of completing the transfusion may be helpful to distinguish immune from nonimmune causes of platelet refractoriness. Typically, immune refractoriness will result in an inadequate platelet increment when measured at 1 hour. Typical nonimmune refractoriness will manifest as an adequate CCI at 1 hour, but shortened survival time so that the platelet count by 24 hours may be back to baseline. It must be appreciated that the CCI does not indicate that an adequate platelet count has been achieved. It only indicates the adequacy of a platelet count increment in relation to the number of platelets transfused.

Plasma Transfusion

Guidelines for plasma transfusion are summarized in Table 35–6. Plasma may be used to replace any plasma protein deficiency. Purified protein concentrates, such as factor VIII, albumin, or immunoglobulin, are preferable for replacement of specific deficiencies since these are highly purified, standardized, and carry extremely low risk of infectious disease transmission. Plasma is most commonly used for replacement of coagulation factor deficiencies when no factor concentrate is available. Multifactorial deficiencies are common in liver disease, massive bleeding, multiorgan system failure, and warfarin therapy. The degree to which factor deficiency may contribute to bleeding in such cases is controversial. Standard coagulation tests such as the prothrombin time (PT) and activated partial thromboplastin time (aPTT) are commonly used to assess the need for plasma transfusion; however, these tests are poorly predictive of bleeding risk. In general, if the PT and aPTT are less than 1.5 times the midpoint of the reference range, there is no benefit to be obtained from plasma transfusion. If the INR is used, in general there is no benefit from plasma transfusion if it is less than 1.5; although for nervous system and retinal hemorrhage, plasma may be reasonably used unless the INR is less than 1.3. For maximal hemostatic effect, plasma should be transfused immediately before an invasive procedure. For the bleeding patient, plasma transfusion may need to be repeated every 3–4 hours to maintain adequate coagulation factor levels. In general, a dose of 10–20 mL per kilogram is necessary to achieve a hemostatic effect. Plasma is the preferred choice for rapid reversal of warfarin, although factor IX complex concentrate is also effective (Boulis, 1999). Plasma is a source of vWF protease activity, which may be deficient in thrombotic thrombocytopenic purpura.

Cryoprecipitate Transfusion

General guidelines for the transfusion of cryoprecipitate are summarized in Table 35–7. Cryo can be used for factor VIII or vWF replacement. High purity or recombinant factor concentrates, however, are better alternatives. Cryo is a good source of fibrinogen and factor XIII. Most patients with hypofibrinogenemia also have deficiencies of other coagulation factors and are better treated with FFP. There is some evidence that cryo may be effective in the treatment of uremic bleeding, possibly by providing high-molecular-weight forms of the vWF (Triulzi, 1990). DDAVP is a preferred therapy for this situation, however. DDAVP may become ineffective after repeated short-term use; at which point, cryo transfusion could be initiated. Cryo, when mixed with calcium and thrombin, can be used to make a topical fibrin sealant for surgery, although more concentrated, virally-inactivated commercial products are available. Each unit of cryoprecipitate can be assumed to contain at least 80 units of factor VIII activity and 250 mg of fibrinogen, although the actual content is variable.

Massive Transfusion

Massive transfusion, usually defined as replacement of one blood volume within 24 hours, necessitates a systematic approach. Large-volume blood loss is often due to trauma, but also occurs in gastrointestinal hemorrhage (particularly with chronic liver disease), ruptured aortic aneurysms, and some surgical procedures such as liver transplantation. No single massive transfusion protocol will be optimal for all patients, although establishing an institutional policy is helpful since these cases can become chaotic. Special attention should be paid to patient and sample identification to avoid transfusion errors.

The priorities in transfusion management of massive bleeding are the prevention or treatment of hypovolemic shock, maintenance of adequate oxygen-carrying capacity, maintenance of oncotic pressure, correction or prevention of coagulopathy, and avoidance of adverse effects of transfusion. Initial patient evaluation should include pertinent medical history (especially liver, kidney, cardiovascular, and hematologic diseases), history of previous transfusions or pretransfusion testing problems, examination for microvascular bleeding, complete blood count (CBC), and coagulation profile (PT, aPTT, fibrinogen). Note that in hypovolemia, the CBC will underestimate blood loss. A sample for pretransfusion testing should be obtained and processed as soon as possible. Initial resuscitation is usually with crystalloid fluids. Red cell transfusion should be considered if there is greater than 15% loss of estimated blood volume (about 1000 mL in a typical adult) with ongoing bleeding. RBC transfusions should be fully crossmatched if possible; however, the patient should not suffer adversely for want of serologically compatible RBC. Transfusion can be started with group O uncrossmatched RBC. If the patient's Rh type is unknown, Rh(D)-negative RBC are preferable, especially for females with child-bearing potential.

Coagulopathies may occur during massive transfusion because of dilution, consumption, or dysfunction. During resuscitation with RBC and fluids, measured factor levels and platelet counts are often higher than would be expected on a purely dilutional basis (Counts, 1979; Murray, 1995) with considerable variation between patients. Consumptive coagulopathies occur with DIC, burns, brain injury, hyperthermia, and sepsis. These usually manifest by prolonged PT and aPTT, lower than expected fibrinogen and platelet count, and the presence of fibrin degradation products or D-dimers. Platelet or coagulation factor dysfunction can occur in hypothermia, acidosis, liver disease, or renal failure. There is no single established protocol for plasma or platelet transfusion in massive bleeding. However, plasma is typically given if the PT or aPTT is greater than 1.5 times the reference range, and platelets are typically given for counts less than 50 000. It may be prudent to reserve platelet transfusion until after surgical control of major bleeding has been obtained, since it is likely to be ineffective during rapid blood loss. Cryoprecipitate may be given if the fibrinogen is less then 100 mg/dL, but, hypofibrinogenemia is usually accompanied by deficiency of other factors, so plasma is often a better choice. Therapy is best guided by frequent assessment of coagulation parameters.

Complications of massive transfusion include hypothermia, hypo-calcemia, and acid–base disorders. Hypothermia can be avoided by use of high-flow warming devices. When the transfusion rate exceeds about 100 mL/min there may be a clinically significant drop in ionized calcium due to accumulation of citrate, and calcium supplementation may be indicated. Liver disease, hypotension, and hypothermia may exacerbate hypocalcemia. Monitoring the corrected QT interval is useful. Measurement of total calcium will not accurately indicate the level of ionized calcium. During rapid transfusion of RBC, a modest decrease in arterial pH may be seen (Vretzakis, 2000) while metabolic alkalosis is common after massive transfusion because of metabolism of citrate.

Neonatal and Pediatric Transfusion

Neonates particularly receive RBC transfusions because of anemia of prematurity, hemolytic disease of the newborn (HDN), or iatrogenic blood loss. The unique physiology of the neonatal period and relative fragility of the developing brain vasculature necessitate some differences from the approach to older children or adults. Guidelines for neonatal

Table 35–8 Guidelines for Neonatal Transfusion

RBC transfusion

Hematocrit < 20% with symptomatic anemia

Hematocrit < 30% with supplemental O_2 < 35% or mechanical ventilation with MAP < 6 cmH$_2$O

Hematocrit < 35% with supplemental O_2 > 35% or mechanical ventilation with MAP > 6 cmH$_2$O

Hematocrit < 45% with cyanotic congenital heart disease or extracorporeal oxygenation

Plasma transfusion

Coagulation factor deficiency, factor concentrate unavailable

Disseminated intravascular coagulation (DIC)

Platelet transfusion

Platelet count < 30 000/μL in term infant with platelet production failure

Platelet count < 50 000/μL in stable premature infant

Platelet count < 100 000/μL unstable premature infant

Adapted from Roseff 2002

transfusion are summarized in Table 35–8. RBC transfusion of 15 mL/kg will typically increase the hemoglobin by 2–3 g/dL, and platelet transfusion of 10 mL/kg will typically increase the platelet count by 40 000–50 000/μL. For large-volume transfusion, as in exchange transfusion or cardiac surgery, selection of fresh RBC (typically < 10 days old) may be indicated. However, with transfusion of 15 mL/kg, most infants tolerate transfusion of RBC stored until outdate without adverse effects (Strauss, 1996). For a premature infant with an expected ongoing transfusion requirement, use of aliquots of a single unit until outdate can significantly reduce donor exposures. Premature and low-birth-weight infants are at greater risk of CMV infection and graft-vs.-host disease (see below).

Exchange transfusion of the neonate for hyperbilirubinemia is usually indicated if the total bilirubin is greater than 25 mg/dL. Relating the total bilirubin to hours since birth is predictive of kernicterus risk (Bhutani, 1999). A two-blood volume exchange is typically used, which can be expected to reduce the total bilirubin by 25% and the fetal red cell mass by about 70%. Whole blood or RBC reconstituted with compatible plasma to hematocrit of 45% can be used.

Transfusion Reactions

Transfusion reactions are a diverse group of adverse reactions to transfusion that usually present during or shortly after transfusion. The work-up and treatment of a transfusion reaction must be predicated on the clinical picture, especially in atypical cases. If a transfusion reaction occurs while a transfusion is in progress, the transfusion should be stopped immediately and the i.v. line should be kept open with saline. It is important to recognize that the unit a patient is reacting to is not necessarily the one that is being infused. All suspected transfusion reactions should be reported to the blood bank or transfusion service.

Febrile Nonhemolytic Reactions

A febrile transfusion reaction is defined as a rise in temperature of 1°C or greater, possibly accompanied by chills or rigors. Symptoms usually occur during the transfusion but may be delayed for up to 1 hour after the procedure has been completed. A patient who is hypothermic at the start of a transfusion and then manifests an expected temperature rise to normal, without symptoms, is not having a febrile reaction. In some patients, it may be impossible to distinguish between a febrile transfusion reaction and disease-related fever.

It is important to rule out a hemolytic transfusion reaction or bacterial contamination of the unit. Antipyretics, such as acetaminophen (325–500 mg) can be administered. Antipyretics are not necessarily required, as the fever of nonhemolytic transfusion reactions is self-limited and usually resolves within 2–3 hours. Diphenhydramine (50–100 mg) is commonly administered in this setting but probably has no effect on the course of febrile reactions.

There is controversy as to whether the transfusion can be restarted after a reaction has been diagnosed and the patient has been treated. The principal argument in favor of restarting the transfusion is the reduction in the number of donor exposures, especially if pooled platelet concentrates are involved (Oberman, 1994). Arguments against restarting the transfusion include the possibility that the patient may have a continued febrile reaction to the unit, and, if a hemolytic reaction or bacterial contamination has not been definitely excluded, a severe reaction may ensue (Widmann, 1994). The decision to restart the transfusion should be driven by the clinical condition of the patient and the results of transfusion reaction testing.

Premedication with antipyretics is often used to prevent febrile reactions, although the efficacy of premedication has not been established. A randomized, placebo-controlled trial failed to show prevention of febrile reactions by acetaminophen and diphenhydramine, but the number of subjects may have been insufficient to demonstrate a relatively small difference (Wang, 2002).

Some, but not all, studies have shown a reduction in the incidence of febrile reactions since the introduction of universal leukocyte reduction (Ibojie, 2002; Dzik, 2002; Uhlmann, 2001). It is clear, though, that leukocyte reduction does not prevent all febrile reactions. Febrile reactions also have been attributed to the accumulation of pyrogenic cytokines in units during storage (Muylle, 1993). These biologic mediators are produced primarily by leukocytes. Febrile reactions to platelet transfusion can be reduced by using platelet concentrates less than 4 days old (Kelley, 2000). Filtration at the time of transfusion will not remove pyrogenic cytokines from blood units, although it may remove other cytokines and activated complement components (Snyder, 1996). The use of prestorage leukocyte reduction has been shown to reduce the generation of cytokines in stored platelets and red cells, and may be more effective than poststorage leukocyte reduction in preventing febrile reactions (Federowicz, 1995). Accumulated cytokines can be removed by either plasma reduction or the washing of cellular blood components (Heddle, 1994). Plasma removal appears to be equivalent to prestorage leukocyte reduction in prevention of febrile reactions (Heddle, 2002). Plasma removal will not prevent all febrile reactions.

Allergic Reactions

Mild allergic reactions to transfusion are commonplace. They may occur with any type of blood component, including autologous RBC (Domen, 2003). Presenting symptoms include pruritus, urticaria, erythema, and cutaneous flushing. About 10% of allergic reactions have pulmonary signs and symptoms, but not cutaneous involvement. Gastrointestinal involvement may include nausea, vomiting, abdominal pain, and diarrhea.

Should an allergic reaction occur, the transfusion should be discontinued and i.v. access maintained. If there is upper airway involvement, prompt intubation may be necessary. Oxygen should be administered if there is dyspnea or evidence of desaturation. Mild allergic reactions usually will respond to i.v. antihistaminics such as diphenhydramine (50–100 mg). More severe reactions may require epinephrine. In mild cutaneous reactions, the transfusion usually can be restarted after treatment without a recurrence or worsening of the symptoms. In more serious reactions, particularly if there is airway involvement, restarting the transfusion is not advisable.

With the exceptions of IgA and haptoglobin deficiency, the specific antigen to which the patient is reacting cannot usually be identified. Premedication with an antihistaminic, such as diphenhydramine, 25–50 mg, administered orally or i.v., may prevent mild allergic reactions. Steroids such as methylprednisolone (125 mg) may help patients who manifest repeated allergic reactions, although the efficacy of steroids has not been proven.

Patients who have had repeated or significant allergic reactions may benefit from the concentration of cellular blood components through the removal of most of the plasma or by the washing of red cells and platelets. However, the routine use of washed components for patients with cutaneous allergic reactions is unwarranted.

Severe Allergic (Anaphylactic) Reactions

In addition to the signs of typical milder allergic reactions, anaphylactic or anaphylactoid reactions manifest cardiovascular instability, including hypotension, tachycardia, loss of consciousness, cardiac arrhythmia, shock, and cardiac arrest. Respiratory involvement with dyspnea or stridor may be more pronounced than is seen usually in typical allergic reactions.

If an anaphylactic reaction occurs, the transfusion should be discontinued and i.v. access maintained. Supportive care, including intubation, oxygen, i.v. fluids, and placement of the patient in the Trendelenburg position, should be instituted promptly. Epinephrine should be available immediately. For hypotension unresponsive to supportive measures or for significant bronchospasm, subcutaneous epinephrine 0.3–0.5 mg (0.3–0.5 mL of a

IV

1 : 1000 solution) can be given. This dose can be repeated every 20–30 minutes for up to three doses. Alternatively, 0.5 mg of epinephrine may be given i.v. (5 mL of a 1 : 10 000 solution) and repeated every 5–10 minutes for refractory hypotension.

An antihistamine such as diphenhydramine, 50–100 mg, can be given i.v., particularly when there are cutaneous manifestations such as urticaria. Aminophylline (6 mg/kg loading dose) may be useful when there is bronchospasm. Steroids are probably not effective in the acute situation, but if symptoms persist, a drug such as hydrocortisone (500 mg) may be given.

Patients with IgA deficiency who develop anti-IgA can have anaphylactic reactions (Vyas, 1969). Patients who have significant allergic reactions should be evaluated for their quantitative IgA levels. Recent transfusion may elevate serum IgA levels falsely. However, if IgA deficiency has been established, anti-IgA testing should be done, usually by a reference laboratory. IgA-deficient plasma can be obtained from rare donor registries, if necessary. Red cells and platelets can be washed to remove sufficient amounts of IgA to prevent reactions.

Patients with haptoglobin deficiency can have similar anaphylactic transfusion reactions due to IgG or IgE antihaptoglobin (Shimada, 2002). Haptoglobin deficiency is rare in North American populations, but is more common than IgA deficiency among Japanese patients suffering anaphylactic reactions.

Acute Hemolytic Reactions

Acute hemolytic transfusion reactions (AHTRs), by definition, present within 24 hours of transfusion. Intravascular hemolysis is much more common in acute hemolytic reactions than is extravascular hemolysis. The presenting signs include fever and chills, nausea, vomiting, pain, dyspnea, tachycardia, hypotension, bleeding, and hemoglobinuria. Fever may be the initial sign of an AHTR. Therefore, any increase in temperature of 1°C or greater should result in a red cell transfusion being stopped and a laboratory evaluation initiated. Renal failure is a later complication. Pain during an AHTR has been reported as localizing to the flanks, back, abdomen, chest, head, and infusion site. A subjective feeling of distress is reported sometimes. Unexpected bleeding may be due to disseminated intravascular coagulation (DIC). During surgery, hypotension and excessive bleeding may be the only signs of an AHTR. Both may be attributed to other causes; therefore, physicians must be mindful of the possibility of a hemolytic reaction in this circumstance.

Laboratory findings in AHTRs include hemoglobinemia, hemoglobinuria, elevated lactate dehydrogenase, hyperbilirubinemia, and low haptoglobin. The blood urea nitrogen and creatinine will be elevated if renal failure has occurred. The direct antiglobulin test (DAT) may show positive results with a mixed-field pattern if transfused incompatible red cells are present in the circulation. Red cell antibody identification studies may or may not show positive results, depending on the specificity of the antibody involved and the amount of antibody in the serum. ABO incompatibility owing to a clerical error is the most common cause of AHTRs.

In the event of an acute hemolytic reaction, the transfusion should be discontinued and i.v. access maintained. The identity of the patient and the unit or units of RBCs should be reconfirmed, and other units of RBCs that have been dispensed for the patient should be located and quarantined. The reaction must be reported to the blood bank promptly. If a misidentification is discovered, there may be another patient (e.g., with a similar name) who may also be at risk of receiving incompatible blood.

The treatment of an AHTR must be guided by the clinical response of the patient. Patients who have minimal symptoms may be managed best by careful observation. However, in severe reactions, early vigorous intervention may be lifesaving. It bears repeating that the severity of AHTRs is related directly to the volume of incompatible blood transfused. Thus, early recognition, discontinuation of the transfusion, and prevention of the transfusion of additional incompatible units are the essential first steps of treatment. Initial attention must be paid to cardiovascular support. If hypotension is present, fluid resuscitation and pressor support may be indicated. Care should be taken to avoid fluid overload, however, especially in patients with impaired cardiac or renal function.

Because the load of incompatible red cells in the circulation dictates the severity and course of AHTRs, an exchange transfusion with antigen-negative blood may be considered. Again, the decision to perform an exchange transfusion must be guided by the clinical response of the patient. It is not appropriate to expose a patient to the added risk of infectious disease if the hemolytic process is well tolerated. With ABO incompatibility, however, an exchange transfusion may greatly reduce the chance of morbidity or death.

Because renal failure is a significant problem in some patients, attention should be given to prevention. Early treatment of hypotension and DIC are the most important interventions to limit the extent of possible renal impairment. Maintenance of urine output with i.v. fluids and diuretics, mannitol or furosemide, early in the course of the reaction has been used successfully. Hydration with normal saline and 5% dextrose (1 : 1 ratio) at a rate of 3000 mL/m² per day and administration of sodium bicarbonate to maintain the urine pH above 7.0 have been recommended (Nussbaumer, 1995). Infusion of an initial dose of 20% mannitol 100 mL/m² given over 30–60 minutes followed by 30 mL/m² per hour for the next 12 hours has also been recommended (Slavc, 1992). However, if oliguria in the face of euvolemia is present, fluid loading may be contraindicated.

Further transfusion of red cells should be avoided until the cause of the reaction has been established. Foremost, however, no patient should be allowed to exsanguinate for lack of serologically compatible blood. Group O RBC lacking other known clinically significant antigens to which the patient currently has an antibody should be obtained, if possible. The results of serologic tests performed up to this point must be considered, and clinical judgment exercised. While the focus of attention in most AHTRs is on red cells, care should be taken to avoid the transfusion of plasma or platelets that may aggravate hemolysis, especially when ABO incompatibility is a possible cause. Undue haste in both serologic evaluation and decision-making must be avoided because human errors are committed most often under pressure.

Delayed Hemolytic Reactions

By definition, delayed hemolytic transfusion reactions (DHTRs) occur at least 24 hours after transfusion of the offending unit. The time from transfusion to diagnosis of a DHTR is quite variable. Most patients present within the first 2 weeks after receiving the transfusion. However, clinical DHTR may be recognized more than 6 weeks later. Almost all DHTRs are due to an anamnestic response to a red cell antigen to which the patient has previously made an antibody, the concentration of which was too low to detect in pretransfusion testing. Rarely, a DHTR may be due to primary alloimmunization to a red cell antigen. Typically, hemolysis is extravascular, but intravascular hemolysis may occur also. Fortunately, these reactions tend to be much less severe than AHTRs; accordingly, they may be overlooked. Some patients will present with only unexpected anemia. Other clinical signs include fever or chills, jaundice, pain, or dyspnea. Rarely renal failure may ensue. In patients with sickle cell disease, DHTRs may precipitate a sickle crisis (Mintz, 1986).

Laboratory findings in DHTRs include anemia, elevated lactate dehydrogenase, hyperbilirubinemia, low haptoglobin, leukocytosis, the presence of a new red cell antibody, and a positive reaction on a DAT. The degree of hyperbilirubinemia will depend on the rate and amount of hemolysis as well as on liver function. Typically, unconjugated bilirubin levels are elevated during active hemolysis. Depressed haptoglobin levels do not necessarily indicate intravascular hemolysis as they may be seen with extravascular hemolysis as well.

Many patients tolerate DHTRs well and may need only to be followed carefully. Generally, fluid loading and diuresis are not indicated unless there is active intravascular hemolysis. Complications, such as renal failure or sickle crisis, should be treated as such. If there is a large burden of antigen-positive red cells, an exchange transfusion should be considered. In general, transfusion should be avoided until the causative antibody can be identified and antigen-negative units obtained. However, as with AHTRs, a patient should not be allowed to have significant morbidity from anemia for the lack of serologically compatible blood. The selection of red cells for transfusion needs to be based on the results of serologic testing and good communication between the medical director of the blood bank and the patient's physician.

Because extravascular hemolysis is similar to AIHA, in which high-dose intravenous immunoglobulin (IVIG) infusion may be useful, IVIG may be considered in the treatment of DHTRs also. A single dose of IVIG, 400 mg/kg, infused within 24 hours of transfusion, has been used successfully to prevent transfusion reactions in alloimmunized patients for whom compatible blood could not be obtained (Kohan, 1994). Five patients so treated had sustained increases in hematocrit. No transfusion reaction developed in any of the cases.

Bacterial Contamination of Blood Components

The clinical presentation of a transfusion reaction caused by bacterially contaminated blood components is usually dramatic. The onset of symptoms in most cases is during the transfusion or shortly after it; delayed presentation of more than 1 day has rarely been reported with contaminated platelet transfusions. Fever, chills, hypotension, shock, nausea, and vomiting are the most commonly reported symptoms (Perez,

2001; Kuehnert, 2001). Dyspnea, pain, and diarrhea may occur also. High fever or hypotension during or shortly after transfusion are particular clues that a contaminated unit may have been transfused. The clinical complications due to bacterial contamination are significant, often resulting in shock, renal failure, DIC, and death. The mortality rate is high and depends on the type of component involved, the identity and amount of the causative organism, and the clinical condition of the patient. Patient factors associated with clinical reactions include thrombocytopenia and pancytopenia. Risk factors for fatality include contamination by Gram-negative rods, greater patient age, smaller volume of component transfused, and younger age of stored platelet concentrate. The latter two factors most likely reflect greater numbers of organisms in the component. The organism involved depends on the type and storage of the blood component. RBC have been found to contain *Acinetobacter, Escherichia, Staphylococcus, Yersinia* and *Pseudomonas* species. Gram-positive cocci such as *Staphylococcus* and *Streptococcus*, Gram-negative rods such as *Acinetobacter, Klebsiella, Salmonella, Escherichia*, and *Serratia*, and Gram-positive rods such as *Propionibacterium* have been reported in platelet concentrates (Andreu, 2002; Kuehnert, 2001). Some transfusion services culture for bacteria all platelet concentrates that have caused a febrile transfusion reaction, since, if a red cell concentrate exists from the same donation, it can be withdrawn.

Usually, treatment must be initiated before the causative organism has been identified. If a reaction occurs, the transfusion should be discontinued, the unit with its associated tubing should be removed, and any other blood bags that have been recently transfused should be recovered. Supportive care of circulation and respiration should be initiated as required. Antibiotic therapy initially should include broad-spectrum coverage such as a β-lactam and an aminoglycoside until microbiological stains or cultures indicate the causative organism.

Methods for limiting bacterial contamination include culture, inspection of platelet concentrates for 'swirling,' and measurement of oxygen consumption (AuBuchon, 2002; Wagner, 1996; Ortolano, 2003). Some studies have found that the use of apheresis platelets may result in a lower incidence of bacterial reactions (Ness, 2001). Pathogen reduction technology may, in the future, significantly reduce, if not eliminate, bacterial contamination (Lin, 1997; Zavizion, 2003).

Transfusion-Related Acute Lung Injury (TRALI)

TRALI usually presents during or within hours of transfusion. Its symptoms include dyspnea, hypoxemia, tachycardia, fever, hypotension, and cyanosis (Kleinman, 2004). Fever and hypotension, when present, are usually moderate and respond quickly to antipyretics and fluids. Characteristically, there is a lack of abnormal breath sounds. A chest X-ray usually shows pulmonary edema. By definition, there are no signs of cardiac failure. Patients with hematologic malignancies or cardiac disease appear to be at higher risk for TRALI (Silliman, 2003). This may reflect the fact that these patient groups receive the majority of platelet transfusions. The reported mortality is approximately 20%, depending on the severity of the lung injury and the underlying clinical status of the patient. There is a wide range of severity in this transfusion reaction; milder forms may not be readily recognized.

The differential diagnosis includes circulatory overload, bacterial contamination, allergic reactions, acute respiratory distress syndrome (ARDS), pulmonary embolism, and pulmonary hemorrhage. The diagnosis is established by findings of noncardiogenic pulmonary edema. Pulmonary artery wedge pressure is not elevated. Characteristically, TRALI resolves within 48–96 hours from outset (Popovsky, 1992). Failure of the patient to improve substantially after this time should call the diagnosis into question. Although chest X-ray findings may persist beyond 7 days, unlike ARDS, there appear to be no permanent pulmonary sequelae. A decrease in leukocyte or platelet count may be a useful clue in TRALI caused by transfusion of HLA class I antibodies (Cooling, 2002).

The treatment of TRALI is supportive. If a transfusion is in progress, it should be discontinued and blood bags from recently transfused units should be recovered. The blood bank should be consulted regarding the evaluation of TRALI. Usually, oxygen is indicated. Severely affected patients may require mechanical ventilation. Corticosteroids appear to be of little, if any, value. Diuresis is not indicated in the absence of signs of fluid overload.

TRALI has been attributed to the presence of antibodies in the plasma of the transfused unit that are directed against HLA or granulocyte antigens present on recipient leukocytes (Kopko, 2002). Plasma from multiparous female donors may carry a greater risk of TRALI (Palfi, 2001). It also has been attributed to the presence in the unit of lipid inflammatory mediators that activate already primed recipient neutrophils (from

Table 35–9 Indications for Irradiation of Blood Components for Prevention of TA-GVHD

Absolute indications

Congenital cellular immunodeficiency

Hematopoietic progenitor cell transplantation

Hodgkin disease

Granulocyte transfusions

Intrauterine transfusions (IUT)

Transfusion to neonates who have received IUT

Transfusions from biological relatives

Chemotherapy with purine analogs (fludarabine)

Probable indications

Low-birth-weight infants (< 1200 g)

Hematologic malignancies other than Hodgkin disease

HLA-matched platelet concentrates

High-dose chemotherapy, radiation therapy and/or aggressive immunotherapy

Controversial indications

Solid organ transplantation

Large-volume or exchange transfusion of infants who did not receive IUT

Aplastic anemia

Absolute lymphopenia (ALC < 500 μL)

Irradiation NOT indicated

HIV infection

Hemophilia

Small-volume transfusions of term infants who did not receive IUT

Elderly patients

Typical dose immunosuppressive therapy (other than purine analogs)

Immunocompetent surgical patients

Pregnancy

Red cell membrane, metabolic, or hemoglobin disorders (e.g., thalassemia, SCD)

Adapted from Gorlin, 2005.

surgery, trauma, or inflammation) to cause capillary injury and leakage (Silliman, 2003).

Graft-Versus-Host Disease

Transfusion-associated graft-vs.-host disease (TA-GVHD) can occur when viable donor T cells proliferate, are not recognized by the recipient's immune system as foreign, but recognize and reject the host as foreign. Patients with marked cellular immunodeficiencies are at risk of TA-GVHD (Table 35–9). These include congenital cellular immunodeficiencies (DiGeorge syndrome, SCIDS), immaturity of the immune system (intra-uterine transfusions, very low birth weight infants), disease-associated immunodeficiencies (Hodgkin disease), and therapy-associated cellular immunodeficiencies (hematopoietic progenitor cell transplantation, fludara-bine treatment). Humoral immunodeficiencies, such as common variable immunodeficiency (CVID), are not a risk factor for GVHD. HIV infection, although it may cause marked T cell dysfunction, does not increase the risk of TA-GVHD. Common immunosuppressive regimens for solid organ transplantation and typical chemotherapy regimen for solid tumors do not increase the risk of TA-GVHD. However, TA-GVHD has been reported with highly aggressive chemotherapy for neuroblastoma and some other tumors. Patients with normal immunity may be at risk of TA-GVHD if the recipient is homozygous for an HLA haplotype and the donor is heterozygous but shares one haplotype. In this case, recipient lymphocytes are unable to recognize transfused lymphocytes as foreign, but transfused cells see recipient cells as foreign (Fig. 35–1). This is most likely to occur with donations from close (first or second degree) relatives, but may also occur due to chance, particularly in populations that are relatively homogeneous (Aoun, 2003).

TA-GVHD typically manifests 2–50 days after transfusion. Characteristic findings include rash, diarrhea, fever, liver dysfunction, and pancytopenia. Mortality is greater than 90%, with most patients dying of infection. In contrast to the expected GVHD of allogeneic HPC transplantation, the bone marrow in TA-GVHD is of recipient type and is a target organ. Aggressive immunosuppressive treatments have been tried, but with rare

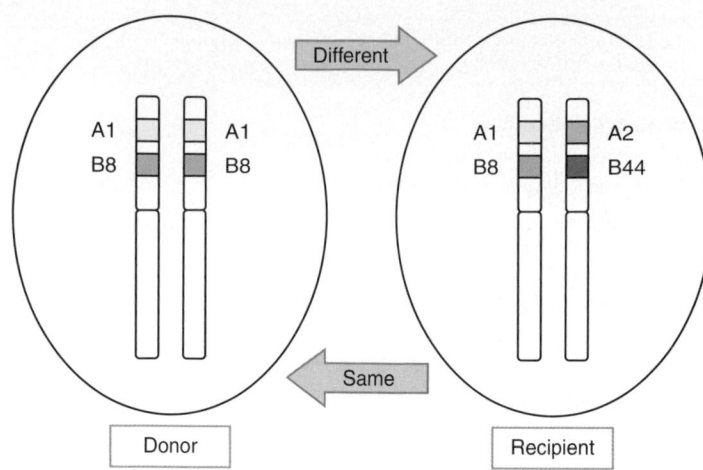

Figure 35–1 Mechanism of TA-GVHD in immunocompetent patients. The donor is homozygous at the HLA class I locus. The recipient is heterozygous, and shares one haplotype with the donor. Engrafted donor T cells recognize the recipient as foreign, but the recipient's T cells do not identify donor T cells as foreign.

exceptions have been unsuccessful. Thus, preventive measures are of paramount importance.

The minimum number of viable transfused T cells necessary to cause TA-GVHD has not been established, but it is clear that current leukocyte-reduction methods are not sufficient (Hayashi, 1993). Exposure to ionizing radiation (gamma rays or X-rays) can cause chromosomal damage and prevent replication of transfused leukocytes. Current FDA guidance suggests a midplane dose of 25 Gy, with a minimum dose of 15 Gy to any point of the blood container (see discussion of special components above). It is possible that pathogen-reduction technology based on nucleic acid modification may be effective in preventing TA-GVHD, but this remains to be established.

Hypotensive Reactions

Transfusion-associated hypotension is defined as hypotension occurring during transfusion in the absence of signs or symptoms of other transfusion reactions, such as fever, chills, dyspnea, urticaria, or flushing. The degree of hypotension required for the diagnosis is controversial but could be defined reasonably as a drop of at least 10 mmHg in systolic or diastolic arterial blood pressure from the pretransfusion baseline. However, if the immediate pretransfusion blood pressure is elevated from the patient's typical blood pressure and the arterial pressure does not fall below the patient's usual blood pressure, it should not be considered a hypotensive reaction. Hypotension begins during the transfusion and resolves quickly when the transfusion is discontinued. If hypotension persists beyond 30 minutes after discontinuation of the transfusion, another diagnosis should be strongly considered. Hypotensive reactions have been associated with red cell and platelet transfusions. Some reactions have been associated with the use of leukocyte-reduction filters (Fried, 1996; Abe, 1997).

If hypotension occurs, the transfusion should be discontinued and i.v. access maintained. The patient should be positioned with head down and feet elevated (Trendelenburg position), and isotonic fluids should be administered. Pressor support is indicated only if the hypotension is severe and refractory to i.v. fluids.

The cause of transfusion-associated hypotension has not been established definitively. However, the condition is most likely due to the release of bradykinin through activation of the contact pathway of coagulation. Some reactions have been associated with angiotensin-converting enzyme (ACE) inhibitor drugs in the recipient and/or the use of leukocyte-reduction filters. Angiotensin-converting enzyme is the major enzyme that breaks down bradykinin in the circulation. Some filters, particularly those with a net-negative surface charge, appear to cause activation of kallikrein and cleavage of high-molecular-weight kininogen that results in the release of bradykinin (Davenport, 1997; Shiba, 1997; Mair, 1998). However, there is variability because not all such filtered units show activation.

Nonimmune Hemolysis

Lysis of red cells can occur as a result of storage, handling, or transfusion conditions. Hyper- or hypo-osmotic fluids mixed with red cells can result in significant lysis. Patients who receive lysed red cells may tolerate them remarkably well. However, transient hemodynamic, pulmonary, and renal impairment may occur, and death due to transfusion of lysed red cells has been reported (Sazama, 1990). The transfusion of autologous blood from a patient with sickle hemoglobin can result in hemolysis and death

(DeChristopher, 1990). The clinical signs are usually hemoglobinemia and hemoglobinuria. Hyperkalemia may occur, particularly in patients with renal failure. Fever also may occur. Finding lysis of red cells in the transfused unit and excluding other causes, such as hemolytic transfusion reactions, establishes the diagnosis. All RBC units will show a slight degree of hemolysis with prolonged storage, but this will not result in clinical signs after transfusion. The principal reported complications of nonimmune hemolysis are renal failure and cardiac arrhythmia due to hyperkalemia. Hemolytic transfusion reactions can rarely occur when no red cell antibody is identifiable (Davey, 1980). Differentiation of this condition from nonimmune hemolysis may be impossible without careful investigation of the transfusion circumstances.

Should nonimmune hemolysis occur, the transfusion should be discontinued and i.v. access maintained. The blood bag, together with attached tubing and i.v. fluids, should be saved for further investigation. A hemolytic transfusion reaction needs to be ruled out. The serum potassium level should be checked and an electrocardiogram obtained to assess hyperkalemia. Care is supportive. Urine output should be maintained with hydration unless there is a contraindication such as renal failure.

Transfusion-Associated Circulatory Overload

Circulatory overload is an all-too-common and preventable transfusion reaction. It presents as congestive heart failure during or shortly after transfusion. Signs and symptoms can include dyspnea, orthopnea, cyanosis, tachycardia, elevated blood pressure, pulmonary edema, jugular venous distention, pedal edema, and headache. The differential diagnosis includes TRALI, allergic reactions, and causes of congestive failure not related to transfusion, such as valvular heart disease. Clearly, patients with pre-existing heart disease are at risk of circulatory overload with transfusion. The diagnosis of circulatory overload on clinical and radiologic examination may be difficult. Elevation of brain natriuretic peptide (BNP) can be helpful in making the diagnosis (Zhou, 2005).

Volume overload should be anticipated in at-risk patients and prevented readily. Blood should be transfused slowly. Although a transfusion usually should be completed within 4 hours, the duration may be extended if medically indicated. If more than 6 hours are required, however, alternative strategies should be considered. Small volumes can be transfused with adequate time between transfusions to allow for diuresis. To avoid additional donor exposures, a unit can be split sterilely and a portion retained in the blood bank for later transfusion. Units can also be concentrated by plasma removal. A diuretic can be administered before or during the transfusion.

Transfusion-Transmitted Disease

Improvements in donor screening and testing have resulted in dramatic reductions in transfusion-transmitted disease risks in the past two decades. For example, the risk of transmitting HIV by blood transfusion in the US has been reduced from approximately 1 in 100 in certain urban areas in the early 1980s to approximately 1 in 2 000 000 throughout the country at present. It is virtually impossible to accurately measure current risks of hepatitis and HIV transmission by epidemiological methods. Risk estimates for HIV, HBV, and HCV are now based on mathematical models that take into account probability of marker-negative window-phase donations, viral strains not reliably detected by current assays, persistent antibody-negative carriers, and testing errors (Dodd, 2002). Current (2004) risk estimates are summarized in Table 35–10.

Table 35–10 Approximate Current Per-Unit Risks of Infectious Disease Transmission

HIV	1 : 2 000 000
HBV	1 : 250 000–1 : 500 000
HCV	1 : 2 000 000
HTLV-I/II	1 : 3 000 000
West Nile virus	~ 1 : 7 000 000

Hepatitis

Historically, HCV has accounted for the majority of post-transfusion hepatitis (PTH). Approximately 10% of chronic HCV is attributable to blood transfusion (Alter, 1999). Post-transfusion hepatitis is asymptomatic in the majority of cases. Three patterns of transaminase elevation have been observed: monophasic, polyphasic, and plateau (Pastore, 1985). Approximately 75–85% of individuals have persistent HCV infection and about 50% of these have evidence of chronic hepatitis. As much as 10% of patients with HCV PTH eventually manifest clinical liver disease (Seeff, 1992). Acute PTH due to HBV is typically more severe with 25–30% of individuals having jaundice, with an incubation time of 40–60 days (Walsh, 1970; Seeff, 1975). Fewer than 10% of infected individuals progress to chronic hepatitis. If acquired before age 5 years, acute HBV infection is usually less severe, but the risk of chronic hepatitis is much greater. Hepatitis D virus (HDV) requires co-infection with HBV for replication. If acquired simultaneously with HBV, HDV can cause severe hepatitis and liver failure. If acquired during chronic HBV infections (superinfection), HDV significantly increases the risk of severe chronic liver disease. Transfusion-transmitted HDV is rare, and screening methods for HBV are also effective against HDV. Hepatitis A virus (HAV) and hepatitis E virus (HEV) have relatively short periods of viremia and do not progress to a chronic carrier state. Transmission of these viruses by transfusion is rare, but has occurred (Sherertz, 1984; Matsubayashi, 2004). Hepatitis G virus (HGV, GBV-C) has a prevalence rate of about 1% in asymptomatic blood donors (Roth, 1997). While it is clearly transmissible by transfusion, no causal relationship between GBV-C infection and hepatitis or chronic liver disease has been established (Alter, 1997).

Human Immunodeficiency Virus

The clinical manifestations of transfusion-transmitted HIV are similar to those of HIV infection acquired through other routes. An acute viral syndrome occurs in about 60% of cases. Untreated, asymptomatic infection persists for about 10 years before AIDS-defining illness occurs, although progression tends to be more rapid in older individuals (Blaxhult, 1990). The time to AIDS progression for transfusion recipients may be shorter than that for the implicated donor, but this may reflect the effect of age and other cofactors (Busch, 1994). Group O viral isolates are not reliably detected by current EIA tests. Currently, the prevalence of group O HIV in the US is low, but it is endemic in some parts of western Africa, and transfusion-transmission by emigrants from such areas has occurred (Pau, 1996).

Human T Cell Lymphotropic Viruses (HTLV)

HTLV-I is causally associated with adult T cell lymphoma/leukemia (ATL) and HTLV-associated myelopathy (HAM) (Manns, 1999; Hall, 1996). Most carriers are asymptomatic. ATL or HAM develops in a small minority of cases after a latent period of many years. HTLV-I is rare in the US. HTLV-II is prevalent in intravenous drug users in the US, and is also associated with HAM (Murphy, 1997). Blood donors who are HTLV-II-positive have a higher incidence of acute bronchitis, pneumonia, bladder or kidney infection, and arthritis; and HTLV-I-positive donors have a higher incidence of bladder or kidney infection and arthritis (Murphy, 2004).

Cytomegalovirus

CMV is common in the general population. In immunologically competent individuals it causes minor symptoms, but becomes latent in virtually all cases (Larsson, 1998). Approximately 50% of blood donors are CMV seropositive, although the estimated risk of transmission by a seropositive transfusion is about 1% (Preiksaitis, 1988). In patients with cellular immunodeficiency, CMV can cause pneumonitis, hepatitis, retinitis, and multisystem organ failure. CMV transmission can be minimized by the use of seronegative blood components, although many studies have shown a low rate of CMV infection developing in such patients. Whether this is due to failure to detect potentially infectious donors or whether viral transmission occurred by other routes in unclear. Several studies, including a prospective randomized trial, have shown that leukocyte-

reduced blood components are as effective as seronegative components in reducing the risk of CMV transmission (Bowden, 1995).

Parvovirus B-19

Parvovirus B-19 is also common in the general population. The incidence of viremia among blood donors is variable, with episodic peaks, but averages around 1 : 5000 (Hitzler, 2002). In most individuals, parvovirus B-19 causes a mild self-limited febrile illness. It is, however, trophic for erythrocyte precursors in the bone marrow, and can cause aplasia, particularly in the setting of accelerated erythropoiesis. Transfusion-transmitted parvovirus infection has been implicated in causing chronic anemia after bone marrow transplantation and in thalassemia (Cohen, 1997; Zanella, 1995).

West Nile Virus

West Nile virus (WNV) arrived in the US in 1999. From its initial outbreak in New York, it has spread across the country. Birds are the natural reservoir, with mosquitoes serving as the vector of transmission. Humans are an accidental host, with infection occurring during times of mosquito activity. Most acute WNV infections are asymptomatic, with a febrile illness occurring in about 1 in 5 infections and neuroinvasive disease in about 1 in 150 infections (Petersen, 2002). In 2002, 23 confirmed cases of transfusion-transmitted WNV were reported by the CDC (Pealer, 2003). In areas of peak WNV activity in 2002, the estimate rate of viremia among blood donors was 1.5 in 1000 (Biggerstaff, 2002). Donor screening for WNV by nucleic acid testing (NAT) was implemented in July 2003 in North America. Subsequently, rare cases of WNV transmission by blood transfusion have been reported, most likely due to low viral copy number that escaped detection (Macedo de Oliveira, 2004).

Malaria

About 1300 cases of malaria are reported annually in the US. Transfusion-transmission of malaria still occurs rarely (1–2 cases annually). The implicated donors usually have a history of travel to an endemic area (Mungai, 2001).

Babesiosis

Babesia species are endemic in North American mammals and are transmitted by ticks of the genus Ixodes. Many cases of babesiosis are asymptomatic or mild. However, it may be more severe in the asplenic or immunosuppressed patient. The parasite is capable of survival in refrigerated red cells. About 40 cases of transfusion-transmitted babesiosis have been reported in the US, although it is possible that the transmission in endemic areas may be as high as 1 in 1800 red cell units (Lux, 2003; Cable, 2001).

Trypanosoma cruzi

T. cruzi is the cause of Chagas' disease and is endemic in parts of Central and South America. There may be 50 000–100 000 chronic carriers of T. cruzi in the US, largely due to immigration (Kirchhoff, 1987). Rare cases of transfusion-transmitted Chagas' disease have been reported in the US (Nickerson, 1989). The risk is dependent on the demographics of the donor population. Seropositivity rates among blood donors have been estimated to be 1 : 7500 in Los Angeles, 1 : 9000 in Miami, and 1 : 25 000 nationally (Leiby, 2002). However, the rarity of confirmed transfusion-transmitted cases even in apparent high-risk areas suggests that seropositivity overestimates infectivity.

Transmissible Spongiform Encephalopathies

Transmissible spongiform encephalopathies (TSEs) are caused by a protein, called a prion, that is capable of assuming an abnormal configuration that is resistant to enzymatic degradation and serves as a template for further abnormal prion deposition. Variant Creutzfeldt–Jakob disease (vCJD) is a human TSE that emerged from an epidemic of bovine spongiform encephalopathy, probably as a result of the pathogenic prion entering the human food supply from affected cattle. The transmissibility of vCJD by blood in experimental models suggests that there is a possible risk of transmission by transfusion. The magnitude of such a risk is presently unknown. However, there have been two cases of prion acquisition (including one with vCJD) in individuals who received transfusions from donors who were themselves diagnosed with vCJD (Llewelyn, 2004; Peden, 2004).

Conclusion

The discovery of the A, B, and O blood groups by Carl Landsteiner in 1900 led to the widespread use of blood transfusion therapy early in the 20th century. This treatment directly afforded a remarkable evolution in surgical, trauma, and medical care. Although remarkable progress has been made in identifying and reducing transfusion-transmitted infections, the incidence of the principal noninfectious risks, TRALI and mistransfusion owing to clerical error, has remained stable for many years.

Increasing attention has been focused recently on these latter hazards, and it is hoped that this will lead to a substantial reduction in their occurrence. Despite the continuing risks of transfusion, it poses a much greater threat to withhold a blood component that is clinically indicated than to transfuse it.

References

Abe H, Ikebuchi K, Shimbo M, Sidiguchi S: Hypotensive reactions with a white cell-reduction filter: Activation of kallikrein-kinin cascade in a patient (abstract). Transfusion 37 1997; (Suppl):39S.

Adams RJ, McKie VC, Hsu L, et al: Prevention of a first stroke by transfusions in children with sickle cell anemia and abnormal results on transcranial Doppler ultrasonography. N Engl J Med 1998; 339:5–11.

This prospective randomized trial showed that chronic transfusion to maintain Hb S < 30% reduced the risk of stroke in children with sickle cell disease.

Adams RJ, Brambilla DJ, Granger S, et al: Stroke and conversion to high risk in children screened with transcranial Doppler ultrasound during the STOP study. Blood 2004; 103:3689–3694.

Alter HJ, Nakatsuji Y, Melpolder J, et al: The incidence of transfusion-associated hepatitis G virus infection and its relation to liver disease. N Engl J Med 1997; 336:747–754.

Alter MJ, Kruszon-Moran D, Nainan DV, et al : The prevalence of hepatitis C virus infection in the United States, 1988 through 1994. N Engl J Med 1999; 341:556–562.

Ambruso DR. Githens JH. Alcorn R. et al : Experience with donors matched for minor blood group antigens in patients with sickle cell anemia who are receiving chronic transfusion therapy. Transfusion 1987; 27:94–98.

Andreu G, Morel P, Forestier F, et al: Hemovigilance network in France: organization and analysis of immediate transfusion incident reports from 1994 to 1998. Transfusion 2002; 42:1356–1364.

Aoun E, Shamseddine A, Chehal A, et al: Transfusion-associated GVHD: 10 years' experience at the American University of Beirut-Medical Center. Transfusion 2003; 43:1672–1676.

AuBuchon JP, Cooper LK, Leach MF, et al: Experience with universal bacterial culturing to detect contamination of apheresis platelet units in a hospital transfusion service. Transfusion 2002; 42: 855–861.

Beard MJ, Cardigan R, Seghatchian J, et al: Variables determining blockage of WBC-depleting filters by Hb sickle cell trait donations. Transfusion 2004; 44:422–430.

Bhutani VK, Johnson L, Sivieri EM: Predictive ability of a predischarge hour-specific serum bilirubin for subsequent significant hyperbilirubinemia in healthy term and near-term newborns. Pediatrics 1999; 103:6–14.

Biggerstaff BJ, Petersen LR: Estimated risk of West Nile virus transmission through blood transfusion during an epidemic in Queens, New York City. Transfusion 2002; 42:1019–1026.

Blackall DP, Uhl L, Spitalnik SL: Transfusion Practices Committee. Cryoprecipitate-reduced plasma: rationale for use and efficacy in the treatment of thrombotic thrombocytopenic purpura. Transfusion 2001; 41:840–844.

Blaxhult A, Granath F, Lidman K, Giesecke J: The influence of age on the latency period to AIDS in people infected by HIV through blood transfusion. AIDS 1990; 4:125–129.

Boulis NM, Bobek MP, Schmaier A, Hoff JT: Use of factor IX complex in warfarin-related intracranial hemorrhage. Neurosurgery 1999; 45:1113–1118.

Bowden RA, Slichter SJ, Sayers M, et al: A comparison of filtered leukocyte-reduced and cytomegalovirus (CMV) seronegative blood products for the prevention of transfusion-associated CMV infection after marrow transplant. Blood 1995; 86:3598–3603.

This prospective randomized trial demonstrated that leukocyte reduction is equivalent to CMV seronegative blood components in preventing CMV transmission. However, CMV disease was more common in the group receiving leukocyte-reduced components, which is a point of controversy.

Boyan CP, Howland WS: Cardiac arrest and temperature of bank blood. JAMA 1963; 183:58–60.

British Committee for Standards in Haematology, Blood Transfusion Task Force: Guidelines for the use of platelet transfusions. Br J Haematol 2003; 122:10–23.

Busch MP, Operskalski EA, Mosley JW, et al: Epidemiologic background and long-term course of disease in human immunodeficiency virus type 1-infected blood donors identified before routine laboratory screening. Transfusion 1994; 34:858–864.

Butch SH, Oberman HA: The computer or electronic crossmatch. Transfusion Medicine Reviews 1997; 11:256–264.

Butch SH, Stoe M, Judd WJ: Solving the same-day admission identification problem. Transfusion 1994; 34(Suppl):93S.

Cable RG, Badon S, Trauem-Trend J, et al: Evidence for transmission of *Babesia microti* from Connecticut blood donors to recipients. Transfusion 2001; 41(Suppl)12S–13S.

Carson JL, Duff A, Poses RM, et al: Effect of anaemia and cardiovascular disease on surgical mortality and morbidity. Lancet 1996; 348:1055–1060.

This retrospective cohort study showed that low preoperative hemoglobin or a substantial operative blood loss increases the risk of death or serious morbidity more in patients with cardiovascular disease than in those without.

Carson JL, Poses RM, Spence RK, Bonavita G: Severity of anaemia and operative mortality and morbidity. Lancet 1988; 1(8588):727–729.

Castellino SM, Combs MR, Zimmerman SA, et al: Erythrocyte autoantibodies in paediatric patients with sickle cell disease receiving transfusion therapy: frequency, characteristics and significance. Br J Haematol 1999; 104:189–194.

Cohen BJ, Beard S, Knowles WA, et al: Chronic anemia due to parvovirus B19 infection in a bone marrow transplant patient after platelet transfusion. Transfusion 1997; 37:947–952.

Cooling L, Distenfeld A, Kopko PM, et al: Transfusion-related acute lung injury. JAMA 2002; 288:315–316.

Counts R, Haisch C, Simon T, et al: Hemostasis in massively transfused trauma patients. Ann Surg 1979; 190:91–96.

Dahlke MB, Weiss KL: Platelet transfusion from donors mismatched for crossreactive HLA antigens. Transfusion 1984; 24:299–302.

Davenport RD, Penezina OP: Cleavage of high molecular weight kininogen induced by filtration of platelet concentrates. Transfusion 1997; 37(Suppl):104S.

Davey RJ, Gustafson M, Holland PV: Accelerated immune red cell destruction in the absence of serologically detectable alloantibodies. Transfusion 1980; 20:348–353.

de la Roche MR, Gauthier L: Rapid transfusion of packed red blood cells: effects of dilution, pressure, and catheter size. Ann Emerg Med 1993; 22:1551–1555.

DeChristopher PJ, Orlina AR: Sudden death associated with autologous transfusion in a surgical patient with hemoglobin SC disease. ISBT & AABB 1990 Joint Congress: Book of Abstracts. Bethesda, MD: American Association of Blood Banks, 1990, p 119.

Dodd RY, Notari EP, IV, Stramer SL: Current prevalence and incidence of infectious disease markers and estimated window-period risk in the American Red Cross blood donor population. Transfusion 2002; 42:975–979.

Domen RE, Hoeltge GA: Allergic transfusion reactions. An evaluation of 273 consecutive reactions. Arch Pathol Lab Med 2003; 127:316–320.

Downes KA, Wilson E, Yomtovian R, Sarode R: Serial measurement of clotting factors in thawed plasma stored for 5 days. Transfusion 2001; 41:570.

Doyle S, O'Brien P, Murphy K, Fleming C, O'Donnell J: Coagulation factor content of solvent/detergent plasma compared with fresh frozen plasma. Blood Coagul Fibrinolysis 2003; 14:283–287.

Dzik WH, Anderson JK, O'Neill EM, et al: A prospective, randomized clinical trial of universal WBC reduction. Transfusion 2002; 42:1114–1122.

This prospective randomized trial showed that universal leukocyte reduction was associated with fewer febrile transfusion reactions, but not with in-hospital mortality, length of stay, or hospital costs. These latter points are controversial.

Federowicz I, Barrett B, Andersen J, et al: Characterization of reactions after transfusion of prestorage leukoreduced cellular blood components. Blood 1995; 86(Suppl):608a.

Fernandez F, Goudable C, Sie P, et al: Low haematocrit and prolonged bleeding time in uraemic patients: effect of red cell transfusions. Br J Haematol 1985; 59:139–148.

Fridey JL: Standards for Blood Banks and Transfusion Services, 22nd ed. Bethesda, MD: American Association of Blood Banks, 2003.

Fried MR, Eastlund T, Christie B, et al: Hypotensive reactions to white cell-reduced plasma in a patient undergoing angiotensin-converting enzyme inhibitor therapy. Transfusion 1996; 36:900–903.

Frohn C, Dumbgen L, Brand JM, et al: Probability of anti-D development in D– patients receiving D+ RBCs. Transfusion 2003; 43:893–898.

Gilleece MH, Dazzi F: Donor lymphocyte infusions for patients who relapse after allogeneic stem cell transplantation for chronic myeloid leukaemia. Leuk Lymph 2003; 44:23–28.

Gordon LI, Kwaan HC, Rossi EC: Deleterious effects of platelet transfusions and recovery thrombocytosis in patients with thrombotic microangiopathy. Sem Hematol 1987; 24:194–201.

Gorlin JB, Cable R: What is a unit? Transfusion 2000; 40:263–265.

Gorlin JB, Mintz PD: Transfusion-associated graft-vs-host disease. *In* Mintz PD (ed): Transfusion Therapy: Clinical Principles and Practice, 2nd ed. Bethesda, MD: AABB Press, 2005, p 585.

Hall WW, Ishak R, Zhu SW, et al: Human T lymphotropic virus type II (HTLV-II): epidemiology, molecular properties, and clinical features of infection. J Acquir Immune Defic Syndr Hum Retrovirol 1996; 13(Suppl 1):S204–S214.

Harkness DR, Byrnes JJ, Lian EC, et al: Hazard of platelet transfusion in thrombotic thrombocytopenic purpura. JAMA 1981; 246:1931–1933.

Hayashi H, Nishiuchi T, Tamura H, et al : Transfusion-associated graft-versus-host disease caused by leukocyte-filtered stored blood. Anesthesiology 1993; 79:1419–1421.

Hebert PC, Wells G, Blajchman MA, et al: A multicenter, randomized, controlled clinical trial of transfusion requirements in critical care. N Engl J Med 1999; 340:409–417.

This prospective randomized trial showed that a restrictive strategy of red-cell transfusion is at least as effective as, and possibly superior to, a liberal transfusion strategy in critically ill patients, with the possible exception of patients with acute myocardial infarction and unstable angina.

Heddle NM, Klama L, Singer J, et al: The role of the plasma from platelet concentrates in transfusion reactions. N Engl J Med 1994; 331:670–671.

This prospective randomized trial showed that most febrile reactions to platelet transfusion are due to a constituent in the plasma supernatant, most likely pyrogenic cytokines released during storage.

Heddle NM, Klama L, Meyer R, et al: A randomized controlled trial comparing plasma removal with white cell reduction to prevent reactions to platelets. Transfusion 1999; 39:231–238.

Heddle NM, Blajchman MA, Meyer RM, et al: A randomized controlled trial comparing the frequency of acute reactions to plasma-removed platelets and prestorage WBC-reduced platelets. Transfusion 2002; 42:556–566.

Heuft HG, Goudeva L, Sel S, Blaszczyk R: Equivalent mobilization and collection of granulocytes for transfusion after administration of glycosylated G-CSF (3 µg/kg) plus dexamethasone versus glycosylated G CSF (12 µg/kg) alone. Transfusion 2002; 42:928–934.

Hitzler WE, Runkel S: Prevalence of human parvovirus B19 in blood donors as determined by a haemagglutination assay and verified by the polymerase chain reaction. Vox Sang 2002; 82:18–23.

Horowitz B, Bonomo R, Prince AM, et al: Solvent/detergent-treated plasma: a virus-inactivated substitute for fresh frozen plasma. Blood 1992; 79:826–831.

Ibojie J, Greiss MA, Urbaniak SJ: Limited efficacy of universal leucodepletion in reducing the incidence of febrile nonhaemolytic reactions in red cell transfusions. Transfusion Med 2002; 12:181–185.

Kelley DL, Mangini J, Lopez-Plaza I, Triulzi DJ: The utility of ≤ 3-day-old whole-blood platelets in reducing the incidence of febrile nonhemolytic transfusion reactions. Transfusion 2000; 40:439–442.

Kirchhoff LV, Gam AA, Gilliam FC: American trypanosomiasis (Chagas' disease) in Central American immigrants. Am J Med 1987; 82:915–920.

Kleinman S, Caulfield T, Chan P, et al: Towards an understanding of transfusion related acute lung injury: Statement of a Consensus Panel. Transfusion 2004; 44:1774–1789.

This consensus panel statement summarizes the current understanding of the causes, incidence, outcomes, and strategies for reducing transfusion-related acute lung injury.

Kohan AI, Niborski RC, Rey JA, et al: High-dose intravenous immunoglobulin in non-ABO transfusion incompatibility. Vox Sang 1994; 67:195–198.

Kopko PM, Marshall CS, MacKenzie MR, et al: Transfusion-related acute lung injury: report of a clinical look-back investigation. JAMA 2002; 287:1968–1971.

Krumholz A, Ness PM, Hauser WA, et al: Adverse reactions in blood donors with a history of seizures or epilepsy. Transfusion 1995; 35:470–474.

Kuehnert MJ, Roth VR, Haley NR, et al: Transfusion-transmitted bacterial infection in the United States, 1998 through 2000. Transfusion 2001; 41:1493–1499.

Larsson LG, Welsh VJ, Ladd DJ: Acute intravascular hemolysis secondary to out-of-group platelet transfusion. Transfusion 2000; 40:902–906.

Larsson S, Soderberg-Naucler C, Wang FZ, Moller E: Cytomegalovirus DNA can be detected in peripheral blood mononuclear cells from all seropositive and most seronegative healthy blood donors over time. Transfusion 1998; 38:271–278.

Lazo A, Tassello J, Jayarama V, et al: Broad-spectrum virus reduction in red cell concentrates using INACTINE PEN110 chemistry. Vox Sang 2002; 83:313–323.

Leiby DA, Herron RM Jr, Read EJ, et al: *Trypanosoma cruzi* in Los Angeles and Miami blood donors: impact of evolving donor demographics on seroprevalence and implications for transfusion transmission. Transfusion 2002; 42:549–555.

Lin L, Cook DN, Wiesehahn GP, et al: Photochemical inactivation of viruses and bacteria in platelet concentrates by use of a novel psoralen and long-wavelength ultraviolet light. Transfusion 1997; 37:423–435.

Lin L, Dikeman R, Molini B, et al : Photochemical treatment of platelet concentrates with amotosalen and long-wavelength ultraviolet light inactivates a broad spectrum of pathogenic bacteria. Transfusion 2004; 44:1496–1504.

Linden JV, Wagner K, Voytovich AE, Sheehan J: Transfusion errors in New York State: an analysis of 10 years' experience. Transfusion 2000; 40:1207–1213.

This analysis of transfusion errors reported to the New York State Department of Health showed that transfusion errors are a significant risk. Most errors result from human actions and thus may be preventable. The majority of events occur outside the blood bank.

Llewelyn CA, Hewitt PE, Knight RS, et al: Possible transmission of variant Creutzfeldt–Jakob disease by blood transfusion. Lancet 2004; 363:417–421.

Lux JZ, Weiss D, Linden JV, et al: Transfusion-associated babesiosis after heart transplant. Emerg Infect Dis 2003; 9:116–119.

McCullough J, Weiblen BJ, Fine D: Effects of storage of granulocytes on their fate in vivo. Transfusion 1983; 23:20–24.

McCullough J, Vesole DH, Benjamin RJ, et al: Therapeutic efficacy and safety of platelets treated with a photochemical process for pathogen inactivation: the SPRINT Trial. Blood 2004; 104:1534–1541.

This prospective randomized trial showed that photochemically treated platelets are substantially equivalent to conventional platelets, although post-transfusion platelet count increments and days to next transfusion were decreased compared with conventional platelets.

Macedo de Oliveira A, Beecham BD, et al: West Nile virus blood transfusion related infection despite nucleic acid testing. Transfusion 2004; 44:1695–1699.

Mair B, Leparc GF: Hypotensive reactions associated with platelet transfusions and angiotensin-converting enzyme inhibitors. Vox Sang 1998; 74:17–30.

Mallouh AA, Asha M: Beneficial effect of blood transfusion in children with sickle cell chest syndrome. Am J Dis Child 1988; 142:178–182.

Manns A, Hisada M, La Grenade L: Human T-lymphotropic virus type I infection. Lancet 1999; 353:1951–1958.

Matsubayashi K, Nagaoka Y, Sakata H, et al: Transfusion-transmitted hepatitis E caused by apparently indigenous hepatitis E virus strain in Hokkaido, Japan. Transfusion 2004; 44:934–940.

Meryman HT, Hornblower M: Freezing and deglycerolizing sickle-trait red blood cells. Transfusion 1976; 16:627–632.

Mintz PD, Williams ME: Cerebrovascular accident during a delayed hemolytic transfusion reaction in a patient with sickle cell anemia. Ann Clin Lab Sci 1986; 16:214–218.

Moake J, Chintagumpala M, Turner N, et al: Solvent/detergent-treated plasma suppresses shear-induced platelet aggregation and prevents episodes of thrombotic thrombocytopenic purpura. 1994; Blood 84:490–497.

Moroff G, Holme S, AuBuchon JP, et al. Viability and in vitro properties of AS-1 red cells after gamma irradiation. Transfusion 1999; 39:128–134.

Mungai M, Tegtmeier G, Chamberland M, Parise M: Transfusion-transmitted malaria in the United States from 1963 through 1999. N Engl J Med 2001; 344:1973–1978.

Murphy EL, Fridey J, Smith JW, et al: HTLV-associated myelopathy in a cohort of HTLV-I and HTLV-II-infected blood donors. Neurology 1997; 48:315–320.

Murphy EL, Wang B, Sacher RA, et al: Respiratory and urinary tract infections, arthritis, and asthma associated with HTLV-I and HTLV-II infection. Emerg Infect Dis 2004; 10:109–116.

Murray DH, Pennell BJ, Weinstein SL, Olsen JD: Packed red cells in acute blood loss: Dilutional coagulopathy as a cause of surgical bleeding. Anesth Analg 1995; 80:336–342.

Muylle L, Joos M, Wouters E, et al. Increased tumor necrosis factor α (TNF α), interleukin 1, and interleukin 6 (IL-6) levels in the plasma of stored platelet concentrates: Relationship between TNF α and IL-6 levels and febrile transfusion reactions. Transfusion 1993; 33:195–199.

Ness P, Braine H, King K, et al: Single-donor platelets reduce the risk of septic platelet transfusion reactions. Transfusion 2001; 41:857–861.

Newman BH: Arterial puncture phlebotomy in whole-blood donors. Transfusion 2001; 41:1390–1392.

Newman BH, Waxman DA: Blood donation-related neurologic needle injury: evaluation of 2 years' worth of data from a large blood center. Transfusion 1996; 36:213–215.

Newman BH, Pichette S, Pichette D, Dzaka E: Adverse effects in blood donors after whole-blood donation: a study of 1000 blood donors interviewed 3 weeks after whole-blood donation. Transfusion 2003; 43:598–603.

Nickerson P, Orr P, Schroeder ML, et al: Transfusion-associated *Trypanosoma cruzi* infection in a non-endemic area. Ann Int Med 1989; 111:851–853.

Nussbaumer W, Schwaighofer H, Gratwohl A, et al: Transfusion of donor-type red cells as a single preparative treatment for bone marrow transplants with major ABO incompatibility. Transfusion 1995; 35:592–595.

Oberman HA: Controversies in transfusion medicine: Should a febrile transfusion response occasion the return of the blood component to the blood bank? Con. Transfusion 1994; 34:353–355.

O'Connell BA, Schiffer CA: Donor selection for alloimmunized patients by platelet crossmatching of random-donor platelet concentrates. Transfusion 1990; 30:314–317.

Ortolano GA, Freundlich LF, Holme S, et al: Detection of bacteria in WBC-reduced PLT concentrates using percent oxygen as a marker for bacteria growth. Transfusion 2003; 43:1276–1285.

Palfi M, Berg S, Ernerudh J, Berlin G: A randomized controlled trial of transfusion-related acute lung injury: Is plasma from multiparous blood donors dangerous? Transfusion 2001; 41:317–322.

Pastore G, Monno L, Santantonio T, et al: Monophasic and polyphasic pattern of alanine aminotransferase in acute non-A, non-B hepatitis. Clinical and prognostic implications. Hepato-Gastroenterology 1985; 32:155–158.

Pau CP, Hu DJ, Spruill C, et al: Surveillance for human immunodeficiency virus type 1 group O infections in the United States. Transfusion 1996; 36:398–400.

Pealer LN, Marfin AA, Petersen LR, et al: Transmission of West Nile virus through blood transfusion in the United States in 2002. N Engl J Med 2003; 349:1236–1245.

Peden AH, Head MW, Ritchie DL, et al: Preclinical vCJD after blood transfusion in a PRNP codon 129 heterozygous patient. Lancet 2004; 364:527–529.

Pennington J, Garner SF, Sutherland J, Williamson LM: Residual subset population analysis in WBC-reduced blood components using real-time PCR quantitation of specific mRNA. Transfusion 2001; 41:1591–600.

Perez P, Salmi LR, Folléa G, et al: Determinants of transfusion-associated bacterial contamination: results of the French Bacthem Case-Control Study. Transfusion 2001; 41: 862–872.

Petersen LR, Marfin AA: West Nile virus: a primer for the clinician. Ann Int Med 2002; 137:173–179.

Petz LD: 'Least incompatible' units for transfusion in autoimmune hemolytic anemia: should we eliminate this meaningless term? A commentary for clinicians and transfusion medicine professionals. Transfusion 2003; 43:1503–1507.

Petz LD, Garratty G, Calhoun L, et al: Selecting donors of platelets for refractory patients on the basis of

HLA antibody specificity. Transfusion 2000; 40:1446–1456.

This retrospective study showed that a strategy of selecting platelet donors based on the recipient's HLA antibody specificities was as effective as HLA matching or crossmatching and allowed for a much larger pool of potential donors.

Pineda AA, Zylstra VW, Clare DE, et al: Viability and functional integrity of washed platelets. Transfusion 1989; 29:524–527.

Popovsky MA, Chaplin HC Jr, Moore SB: Transfusion-related acute lung injury: A neglected, serious complication of hemotherapy. Transfusion 1992; 32:589–592.

Powell RW, Levine GL, Yang YM, Mankad VN: Acute splenic sequestration crisis in sickle cell disease: early detection and treatment. J Ped Surg 1992; 27:215–218.

Preiksaitis JK, Brown L, McKenzie M: The risk of cytomegalovirus infection in seronegative transfusion recipients not receiving exogenous immunosuppression. J Infect Dis 1988; 157:523–529.

Rao SV, Jollis JG, Harrington RA, et al: Relationship of blood transfusion and clinical outcomes in patients with acute coronary syndromes. JAMA 2004; 292:1555–1562.

Rebulla P, Finazzi G, Marangoni F, et al: The threshold for prophylactic platelet transfusions in adults with acute myeloid leukemia. N Engl J Med 1997; 337:1870–1875.

This prospective randomized trial demonstrated that prophylactic platelet transfusion at < 10 000/μL is as safe and effective as transfusion at < 10 000/μL in acute leukemia and substantially reduces the number of transfusions.

Roseff SD, Lugan NLC, Manno CS: Guidelines for assessing appropriateness of pediatric transfusion. Transfusion 2002; 42:1398–1413.

Roth WK, Waschk D, Marx S, et al: Prevalence of hepatitis G virus and its strain variant, the GB agent, in blood donations and their transmission to recipients. Transfusion 1997; 37:651–656.

Salama A, Berghofer H, Mueller-Eckhardt C: Red blood cell transfusion in warm-type autoimmune haemolytic anaemia. Lancet 1992; 340:1515–1517.

Sauer LA, France CR: Caffeine attenuates vasovagal reactions in female first-time blood donors. Health Psychol 1999; 18:403–409.

Sazama K: Reports of 355 transfusion-associated deaths: 1976 through 1985. Transfusion 1990; 30:583–590.

Schlossberg HR, Herman JH: Platelet dosing. Transfus Apheresis Sci 2003; 28:221–226.

Schmalzer EA, Lee JO, Brown AK, et al: Viscosity of mixtures of sickle and normal red cells at varying hematocrit levels. Implications for transfusion. Transfusion 1987; 27:228–233.

Seeff LB, Wright EC, Zimmerman HJ, McCollum RW: VA cooperative study of post-transfusion hepatitis, 1969–1974: incidence and characteristics of hepatitis and responsible risk factors. Am J Med Sci 1975; 270:355–362.

Seeff LB, Buskell-Bales Z, Wright EC, et al: Long-term mortality after transfusion-associated non-A, non-B hepatitis. N Engl J Med 1992; 327:1906–1911.

Seoud MA, Cantwell C, Nobles G, Levy DL: Outcome of pregnancies complicated by sickle cell and sickle-C hemoglobinopathies. Am J Perinatol 1994; 11:187–191.

Sherertz RJ, Russell BA, Reuman PD: Transmission of hepatitis A by transfusion of blood products. Arch Int Med 1984; 144:1579–1580.

Shiba M, Tadokoro K, Sawanobori M, et al: Activation of the contact system by filtration of platelet concentrates with a negatively charged white cell-removal filter and measurement of venous blood bradykinin level in patients who received filtered platelets. Transfusion 1997; 37:457–462.

Shimada E, Tadokoro K, Watanabe Y, et al: Anaphylactic transfusion reactions in haptoglobin-deficient patients with IgE and IgG haptoglobin antibodies. Transfusion 2002; 42:766–773.

Silliman CC, Boshkov LK, Mehdizadehkashi Z, et al: Transfusion-related acute lung injury: Epidemiology and a prospective analysis of etiologic factors. Blood 2003; 101:454–462.

Slavc I, Urban CH, Schwinger W, et al: ABO-incompatible bone marrow transplantation: Prevention of hemolysis by alkaline hydration with mannitol diuresis in conjunction with red cell reduced buffy coat bone marrow. Wien Klin Wochenschr 1992; 104:93–96.

Snyder EL, Mechanic S, Baril E, Davenport RD: Removal of soluble biologic response modifiers (complement and chemokines) by a bedside leukoreduction filter. Transfusion 1996; 36:707–713.

Spence RK, Carson JA, Poses R, et al: Elective surgery without transfusion: influence of preoperative hemoglobin level and blood loss on mortality. Am J Surg 1990; 159:320–324.

Strauss RG: Clinical perspectives of platelet transfusions: defining the optimal dose. J Clin Apheresis 1995; 10:124–127.

Strauss RG, Burmeister LF, Johnson K, et al: AS-1 red cells for neonatal transfusions: A randomized trial assessing donor exposure and safety. Transfusion 1996; 36:873–878.

Sweeney JD, Holme S, Moroff G: Storage of apheresis platelets after gamma radiation. Transfusion 1994; 34:779–783.

Trial to Reduce Alloimmunization to Platelets Study Group: Leukocyte reduction and ultraviolet B irradiation of platelets to prevent alloimmunization and refractoriness to platelet transfusions. N Engl J Med 1997; 337:1861–1869.

This prospective randomized trial demonstrated that reduction of leukocytes by filtration and ultraviolet B irradiation of platelets are equally effective in preventing alloantibody-mediated refractoriness to platelets during chemotherapy for acute myeloid leukemia. Platelets obtained by apheresis from single random donors provided no additional benefit as compared with pooled platelet concentrates from random donors.

Triulzi DJ, Blumberg N: Variability in response to cryoprecipitate treatment for hemostatic defects in uremia. Yale J Biol Med 1990; 63:1–7.

Uhlmann EJ, Isgriggs E, Wallhermfechtel M, Goodnough LT: Prestorage universal WBC reduction of RBC units does not affect the incidence of transfusion reactions. Transfusion 2001; 41:997–1000.

Vichinsky EP, Earles A, Johnson RA, et al: Alloimmunization in sickle cell anemia and transfusion of racially unmatched blood. N Engl J Med 1990; 322:1617–1621.

Vichinsky EP, Haberkern CM, Neumayr L, et al: A comparison of conservative and aggressive transfusion regimens in the perioperative management of sickle cell disease. N Engl J Med 1995; 333:206–213.

This prospective randomized trial showed that a conservative transfusion strategy (increase hemoglobin level to 10 g/dL) is as effective as an aggressive transfusion regimen (decrease the hemoglobin S level to < 30%) in preventing perioperative complications in patients with sickle cell anemia, and results in substantially fewer transfusions.

Vretzakis F, Papaziogas B, Matsaridou E, et al: Continuous monitoring of arterial blood gasses and pH during intraoperative rapid blood administration using a Paratrend sensor. Vox Sang 2000; 78:158–163.

Vyas GN, Holmadahl L, Perkins HA, Fudenberg HH: Serologic specificity of human anti-IgA and its significance in transfusion. Blood 1969; 34:573–581.

Wagner SJ, Robinette D: Evaluation of swirling, pH, and glucose tests for the detection of bacterial contamination in platelet concentrates. Transfusion 1996; 36:989–993.

Walsh JH, Purcell RH, Morrow AG, et al: Posttransfusion hepatitis after open-heart operations. Incidence after the administration of blood from commercial and volunteer donor populations. JAMA 1970; 211:261–265.

Wang SE, Lara PN Jr, Lee-Ow A, et al: Acetaminophen and diphenhydramine as premedication for platelet transfusions: A prospective randomized double-blind placebo-controlled trial. Am J Hematol 2002; 70:191–194.

Widmann FK: Controversies in transfusion medicine: Should a febrile transfusion response occasion the return of the blood component to the blood bank? Pro Transfusion 1994; 34:356–358.

Wu WC, Rathore SS, Wang Y, et al: Blood transfusion in elderly patients with acute myocardial infarction. N Engl J Med 2001; 345:1230 Controversies in transfusion medicine 1236.

Zanella A, Rossi F, Cesana C, et al: Transfusion-transmitted human parvovirus B19 infection in a thalassemic patient. Transfusion 1995; 35:769 Controversies in transfusion medicine 772.

Zavizion B, Serebryanik D, Serebryanik I, et al: Prevention of *Yersinia enterocolitica*, *Pseudomonas fluorescens*, and *Pseudomonas putida* outgrowth in deliberately inoculated blood by a novel pathogen-reduction process. Transfusion 2003; 43:135 Controversies in transfusion medicine 142.

Zhou L, Giacherio D, Cooling L, Davenport RD: Use of B-natriuretic peptide (BNP) as a diagnostic marker in the differential diagnosis of transfusion-associated circulatory overload (TACO). Transfusion 2005; 45:1056–1063.

CHAPTER 36

Hemapheresis

Jeffrey L. Winters MD, Alvaro A. Pineda MD

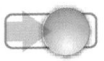

KEY POINTS

- Hemapheresis is the process of removing normal or abnormal components from circulating blood.

- Cytapheresis involves the removal of cellular components, while plasmapheresis involves the removal of plasma, the liquid component.

- Separation of the blood components is based upon either size (filtration instruments), density (centrifugation instruments), or a combination of both.

- Donor apheresis maximizes the collection of a scarce resource by allowing donors to donate only what is needed, returning the remaining components back to the donor.

- Donor apheresis is highly regulated. The donor eligibility requirements, frequency of donation, and amount of product allowed to be collected vary according to the components being collected, instruments being used for the collection, and the frequency of the apheresis donations.

- Peripheral blood hematopoietic progenitor cell collection has advantages over progenitor cells collected by bone marrow harvest, including faster time to engraftment, avoidance of general anesthesia for the donor, quicker donor recovery, and decreased expense.

- There is a dearth of randomized placebo-controlled clinical trials involving apheresis. To address this, the American Association of Blood Banks (AABB) and the American Society for Apheresis (ASFA) categorize diseases treated with apheresis according to the strength of the evidence supporting their use.

- Therapeutic cytoreduction for leukocytosis or thrombocytosis is indicated for primary disorders where symptoms of hyperviscosity or risk factors for complications are present.

- A 1–1.5 plasma volume plasma exchange will remove 70% of a substance located within the plasma. The treatment of additional plasma volumes results in the removal of a fixed percentage of the remaining substance leading to diminishing returns in treating more than 1.5 plasma volumes.

- Plasma exchange is nonselective, removing pathologic substances as well as beneficial substances such as coagulation factors and protein-bound drugs.

- Complications of donor apheresis are less common than complications seen with whole blood donation though the rate of reactions requiring hospitalization has been reported to be greater.

- The most common reactions to donor apheresis, in decreasing frequency, are: hematoma/pain; hypocalcemia due to the citrate anticoagulant; vasovagal reactions with syncope; and vasovagal reactions without syncope.

- Complications have been reported to occur in approximately 5% of patients undergoing therapeutic apheresis treatments. If complications due to central venous access placement are included, the complication rate has been reported to be 17%.

- The most common reactions due to therapeutic apheresis procedures, in decreasing frequency, are: transfusion reactions from replacement fluids; hypocalcemia due to citrate anticoagulant; hypotension; vasovagal reactions; tachycardia; respiratory distress; tetany/seizure; and rigors/chills.

Introduction

Definitions

The word apheresis is derived from the Greek word *aphairesis* which means 'to separate,' 'to take away by force,' or 'to remove.' Hemapheresis is the process of removing normal or abnormal blood constituents from circulating blood. It can be divided into cytapheresis, the removal of the cellular component of blood, and plasmapheresis, removal of the plasma fraction. Cytapheresis can be selective with removal of the red blood cells (erythropheresis), platelets (plateletpheresis), or leukocytes (leukapheresis). Plasmapheresis is, by its very nature, nonselective with the removal of all plasma constituents and replacement of the removed volume with an equal volume of plasma or, more commonly, a plasma substitute such as 5% albumin; when one or greater plasma volumes are removed and replaced with a similar volume of colloid or crystalloid a better phrase is plasma exchange or therapeutic plasmapheresis. Selective removal of specific components can be achieved through plasma perfusion. Here, plasma collected by plasmapheresis is then treated by perfusion through columns which selectively remove the substance of interest, either pathologic or not. The modified plasma is then returned to the patient.

Basic Principles

All of the early apheresis instruments separated whole blood into its components by centrifugation. Centrifugal force is applied to whole blood such that the various components separate according to their specific

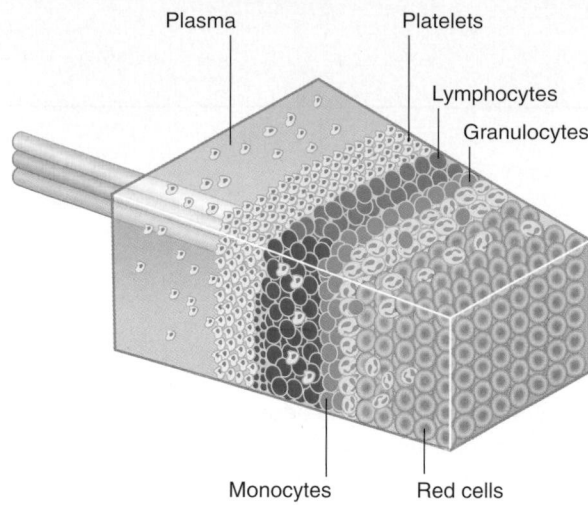

Figure 36–1 Separation of blood components within a centrifugal separation chamber. Blood components placed in a centrifuge are separated based upon their density. The densest elements (red blood cells) are furthest from the axis of rotation while the least dense (plasma) is closest. Image courtesy of Sergio Torloni, MD, Director of Transfusion Medicine, Mayo Clinic Scottsdale AZ.

gravity (density) with the most dense component layering the farthest from the axis of rotation and the least dense layering closest. Those components with intermediate densities would layer in between in order of increasing density. The order of density of blood components from least to most dense is shown in Figure 36–1 and is in the following order: plasma, platelets, lymphocytes, granulocytes, and red blood cells (Burgstaler, 2003). Some mixing does occur at the interfaces of the various layers resulting in some contamination with the components of the adjacent layers. For example, red cells are present within the granulocyte layer.

Centrifugation separators can be divided into two classes, intermittent flow and continuous flow centrifuges. In intermittent flow centrifuges, the bowl is filled with the whole blood to be separated and centrifugal force is applied. After the components are separated, the component of interest is removed. The centrifuge is then stopped and the bowl is emptied with contents returned to the patient/donor. The cycle is then repeated with whole blood being processed in discrete batches. In continuous flow centrifuges, each of the individual component layers are removed with the layer of interest being retained while the others are mixed together outside of the separation chamber and returned. This means that as volume is removed from the separation chamber, it can be continually replaced by whole blood, resulting in continuous separation. The chamber is not emptied until the entire procedure has been completed (Burgstaler, 2003).

In addition to centrifugation, apheresis can also be accomplished by filtration. In this method, components of whole blood are separated based not upon density but upon size. The whole blood flows over a membrane containing pores that are of a size such that only the component of interest can pass through. The remaining elements are then returned. These separators may be either hollow fiber or flat plate systems. The former consists of bundles of tubes containing pores within their walls. The blood enters into the tubes with the plasma exiting through the pores, where it is then collected, while the cellular elements exit from the opposite end of the tubes. The flat plate separators consist of two porous membranes. Whole blood flows between the membranes with the cellular elements being retained and collected at the opposite end of the plates while the plasma passes through the membranes and is collected from the exterior surface of the plate (Burgstaler, 2003).

Centrifugation and filtration can be combined. In these instruments, blood enters a stationary chamber containing a central rotating filter. As the filter rotates, the blood begins to move and separate into layers. The result is that the more dense elements move away from the filter with the plasma being located directly adjacent to the filter. The plasma can then pass through the filter and be drawn off while the cellular elements are collected from the periphery of the stationary chamber. The advantage of the combination of centrifugation and filtration in this arrangement is that the cellular elements cannot clog the pores of the filter. This means that filters with smaller surface areas, in comparison to filtration instruments, and lower g forces, in comparison to centrifugation instruments, can be used (Burgstaler, 2003).

Another basic aspect of apheresis is determining the blood volume of the donor/patient. This is necessary because of the need to limit the

amount of blood within the instrument and tubing connected to the donor/patient, the extracorporeal circuit, to avoid hypotension and complications. Previously, Standards for Blood Banks and Transfusion Services limited the extracorporeal blood volume for donors to 15% of the total blood volume (Standards Committee of the American Association of Blood Banks, 1997). It was therefore necessary to determine the donor's blood volume. This is most often accomplished through nomograms or as a calculation performed by the instrument used for the procedure. This requires the input of donor/patient-specific data by the instrument operator, typically height, weight, gender, and hematocrit. A number of equations and rules are available for this determination (Gilcher, 1996; Nadler, 1962). For example, Equations 36–1 and 36–2 can be used to determine blood volume in males and females respectively (Nadler, 1962):

$$\text{Males: } BV = (0.3669 \times H^3) + (0.03719 \times W) + 0.6041 \qquad (36\text{–}1)$$
$$\text{Females: } BV = (0.3561 \times H^3) + (0.03308 \times W) + 0.1833 \qquad (36\text{–}2)$$

where: BV = blood volume in liters, H = height in meters, W = weight in kilograms.

As the blood volume of tissues varies according to the ratio of adipose tissue present, such calculations may overestimate the blood volume in obese patients and underestimate it in muscular patients. These biases are partially corrected by formulas which cube the height of the patient (Mollison, 1998). The regulatory necessity to calculate blood volume has been simplified beginning with the 19th edition of Standards for Blood Banks and Transfusion Services. Instead of limiting the extracorporeal volume to 15%, the maximum amount allowed to be within the extracorporeal circuit is 10.5 mL/kg of the donor's weight (Standards Committee of the American Association of Blood Banks, 2004). Calculations of blood volume, however, are still necessary to 'prescribe' appropriate processing volumes during therapeutic cytapheresis. Additionally, for plasma exchanges the blood volume can be used to further calculate the plasma volume as given by Equation 36–3 (Buffaloe, 1983):

$$PV = BV\ [1 - (0.91)(0.96)VCH/100] \qquad (36\text{–}3)$$

where: PV = plasma volume in liters, VCH = venous centrifuge hematocrit.

Finally, the plasma volume can be used to calculate the exchange volume, the volume processed in a plasma exchange procedure as given by Equation 36–4 (Buffaloe, 1983):

$$EV = PV \times PVE \qquad (36\text{–}4)$$

where: EV = exchange volume in liters, PVE = desired number of plasma volumes to exchange.

These equations allow for the determination of the appropriate volumes to be processed in the various therapeutic procedures described in this chapter.

The final basic aspect of hemapheresis that is applicable to all procedures, therapeutic and donor, is venous access. In donor hemapheresis, peripheral venous access is used, usually the veins of the antecubital fossa. The use of central venous access in this setting, with the potential for serious complications, would be too risky for the donor. If a donor's peripheral venous access is such that it cannot be used, then another donor should be located. The possible exception to this would be the setting of allogeneic peripheral hematopoietic progenitor cell harvest where an alternative donor may not be available. Obviously, the risks to the donor and benefits to the recipient must be carefully considered and the donor must give informed consent before central venous access can be used.

In the setting of therapeutic hemapheresis procedures, it is often assumed that central access is essential due to damage to peripheral veins from previous medical treatment (e.g. chemotherapy) as well as the need for long-term therapy for some diseases. The Canadian Cooperative Multiple Sclerosis Study Group (Noseworthy, 1989) found that for 294 multiple sclerosis patients undergoing weekly plasma exchange procedures for 20 weeks, only 4.4% of patients could not be treated because of poor peripheral venous access. Of those who started the course of therapy, only 5.4% lost peripheral venous access such that the course could not be completed (Noseworthy, 1989). In a similar study, Grishaber et al. (Grishaber, 1992), looking at 46 patients with neurologic diseases requiring hemapheresis, found that 50% of patients could complete their course of therapy using peripheral access alone. Factors associated with the requirement of central venous access were Guillain–Barré syndrome or hospitalization within a medical intensive care unit (Grishaber, 1992). Contrary to popular belief, these authors also found no difference between peripheral venous access and central venous access with regard to the time required to perform the therapeutic procedures (Grishaber, 1992). These studies indicate that peripheral venous access, with its lower rate of complications, should be tried initially in therapeutic hemapheresis. Central venous access should be reserved for occasions in which peripheral access fails.

Table 36–1 Reported Benefits of Apheresis Platelet Products

Decreased donor exposure with decreased risk of transfusion-transmitted disease

Decreased donor exposure with delay in alloimmunization to HLA (Sintnicolaas, 1981)

Decreased risk of septic platelet transfusion reactions (Ness, 2001)

Pre storage leukocyte reduction with delay in alloimmunization to HLA (Trial to Reduce Alloimmunization to Platelets Study Group, 1997), decreased febrile transfusion reactions (Heddle, 1995), and decreased cytomegalovirus infection (Bowden, 1995)

When peripheral venous access is not possible, then both the hemapheresis service and the physician placing the catheter must determine the type of central catheter placed. Many routinely used central venous catheters are inadequate for hemapheresis because their walls are too soft and collapse, their length is too long or their diameter is too small. These will result in pressure alarms from the instruments. The ideal catheters should have relatively rigid walls to prevent collapse and large diameter with relatively short length to allow for maximum flow. Appropriate catheters include the Mahurkar dual-lumen catheter (Kendall, Mansfield, MA), PermCath (Kendall, Mansfield, MA), Hickman Hemodialysis and Plasmapheresis Catheters (C.R. Bard, Inc., Cranston, RI), and Neostar Pheres-Flow catheter (Horizon Medical Products, Inc., Manchester, GA). The Neostar catheter is specifically designed for long-term use in bone marrow or hematopoietic progenitor cell transplantation. Other catheters may be used, such as the Hickman dual-lumen vascular access catheter (C.R. Bard, Inc., Cranston, RI) or triple lumen catheters, but these can often only be used as return lines and not as draw lines, requiring peripheral access as well. Grishaber et al. (Grishaber, 1992) found unacceptable failure rates with these catheters and could not recommend their insertion solely for apheresis procedures. A rule of thumb is that if a catheter can be used for dialysis where flow rates are greater than those seen in apheresis, it can be used for apheresis.

Donor Cytapheresis

Donor Plateletpheresis

Benefits of Apheresis Platelets

The use of apheresis platelets has increased from 25% of platelets transfused in 1987 (Wallace, 1993) to 66% in 1999 (National Blood Data Resource Center, 2001). In part, this is due to the inability to increase platelets derived from whole blood donations. In addition, there is a perception that apheresis platelets offer advantages over those produced from whole blood. The reported benefits of apheresis platelet products are given in Table 36–1.

An additional advantage of apheresis platelets over pooled nonapheresis products is simplification of inventory management. Pooled products, because they are prepared in an open system, have a 4-hour shelf life after pooling. Apheresis products do not need to be pooled and as a result retain their 5-day shelf life. In situations where platelet products are initially requested but then not transfused, the use of apheresis products could avoid wastage. Of course, the disadvantages of apheresis platelets are the additional expense to obtain them, as well as limited availability in some areas.

Platelet Product Requirements

Standards for Blood Banks and Transfusion Services require that the minimum number of platelets in an apheresis product be 3.0×10^{11} in 90% of units tested (Standards Committee of the American Association of Blood Banks, 2004) while the Food and Drug Administration (FDA) requires a minimum of 3.0×10^{11} in 75% of units tested (CFR, 2003). These conflicting requirements will hopefully be synchronized in the future. The result of these requirements, however, is that an apheresis platelet product contains at least as many platelets as a pool of platelets from six whole blood donations.

Plateletpheresis Donor Selection

The donor requirements for plateletpheresis are the same as those for whole blood donation including a proscription on the use of a donor who has ingested an aspirin-containing medication within 36 hours as the sole source of platelets for a recipient (Standards Committee of the American Association of Blood Banks, 2004). Standards for Blood Banks and

Transfusion Services also require that the use of platelets from a donor taking 'medications known to irreversibly inhibit platelet function shall be evaluated' (Standards Committee of the American Association of Blood Banks, 2004). In addition to these requirements, hemapheresis and plateletpheresis specific requirements also exist. First, donors can donate as often as twice per week but cannot donate more than 24 times per year (Standards Committee of the American Association of Blood Banks, 2004). This limit on the number of donations is based upon the fact that early instruments produced platelet products containing significant numbers of lymphocytes (Strauss, 1994). This resulted in concerns that long-term platelet donation could result in lymphocyte depletion with subsequent disturbance in immune function. This will be discussed further in the section dealing with plateletpheresis donor concerns.

Individuals donating after whole blood donation, or after an instrument failure resulting in the inability to return the extracorporeal blood volume, must wait 8 weeks before donating by apheresis. Exceptions are if the extracorporeal volume of the instrument is less than 100 mL or if the loss of red cells is less than 200 mL. In these cases, the donor is eligible to donate by apheresis after the normal deferral period (Standards Committee of the American Association of Blood Banks, 2004).

Donors must also fulfill minimum platelet count requirements. At the initial donation, platelet counts for the donor are not required nor are they necessary as long as donation is not performed more frequently than every 4 weeks (Standards Committee of the American Association of Blood Banks, 2004). If the donor donates more frequently than every 4 weeks, the minimum acceptable platelet count is 150 000/µL (Standards Committee of the American Association of Blood Banks, 2003). This count may be determined either as a post-apheresis count, which is a count after one procedure determines eligibility for the next procedure, or as a pre-apheresis count (Standards Committee of the American Association of Blood Banks, 2004).

Donor selection for plateletpheresis may be influenced by a number of other factors in addition to regulatory considerations. The yield of a plateletpheresis procedure is determined, to a large extent, by the platelet count of the donor, with higher counts being associated with a higher yield (Glowitz, 1980; Goodnough, 1999). Female donors, on average, have higher platelet counts than males (Glowitz, 1980; Goodnough, 1999; Lasky, 1981). Some authors have found higher platelet yields in female donors compared to males (Glowitz, 1980; Lasky, 1981). This has not been seen in all studies, however (Dettke, 1998; Goodnough, 1999). In addition, the presence of a higher plasma volume in females enhances the separation and collection of platelets by some instruments and this could also contribute to the higher yield.

Additional donor considerations arise in the selection of platelet products for alloimmunized patients. These patients, through transfusion or previous pregnancies, develop antibodies to antigens expressed upon platelets, most frequently antibodies to HLA class I. The result is the development of an immune refractory state as defined by inadequate post-transfusion platelet increments as measured by platelet count collected between 10 minutes and 1 hour after the completion of a platelet transfusion. Antibodies toward platelet antigens are solely or partially responsible for a third of patients being refractory to platelet transfusion (Doughty, 1994). The presence of such a state requires the search for compatible platelet donors. Three general strategies have been employed to achieve this. First, if the specificities of the HLA alloantibodies and the HLA class I phenotype of the plateletpheresis donor are known, attempts can be made to obtain platelets from a donor lacking these antigens (Hussein, 1996; Schiffer, 1987). A second strategy that is used if the HLA class I type of the patient is known and the HLA antibody specificities are unknown or broad, is to attempt to match the HLA type of the patient and donor as closely as possible (Duquesnoy, 1978). Finally, if the HLA class I types of the recipient or potential donors are unknown or if poor increments continue despite HLA matching, platelet crossmatching can be performed. Such testing involves combining donor platelets with recipient serum in a solid-phase red blood cell adherence assay (Bock, 1989; Murphy, 1991; O'Connell, 1992; Schiffer, 1987).

Plateletpheresis Donor Concerns

The typical platelet donor experiences a drop in platelet count following donation of 20–29% (Heyns, 1985; Katz, 1981; Szymanski, 1973) with that among females typically being greater (Dettke, 1998; Rogers, 1995). The fall in platelet count does not correlate with the yield of the plateletpheresis procedure. That is, the fall is less than that predicted by the yield and represents mobilization of platelets from the spleen (Heyns, 1985). The time required for return to baseline following apheresis platelet donation is 4 days in males. A delay in increase of thrombopoietin levels causes delayed return to normal platelet counts in females (Dettke,

1998). In donors undergoing alternate day collections, platelet count and apheresis yields have been shown to return to baseline levels by day 10 of collection with stable counts and yields during subsequent collection procedures (Glowitz, 1980). A rebound elevation in platelet count with increased platelet yield following repeat procedures has also been seen (Szymanski, 1973). In donors with low platelet counts (150 000–180 000/mL), plateletpheresis using prolonged collection times to achieve the platelet yield required by regulations demonstrated no clinically significant problems in 291 procedures, despite post-procedure platelet counts as low as 69 000/mL (Rogers, 1995). The results of these studies indicate that even in donors undergoing repeated plateletpheresis, platelet counts return to normal levels promptly and bleeding complications are uncommon.

While studies have shown that platelet counts recover quickly following platelet donation, studies of the long-term effects of platelet donation on donor platelet counts are limited. Stohlawetz et al. examined levels of reticulated platelets, a measure of thrombopoiesis, following platelet donation in first-time donors and those who had undergone donation every other week for 18 months (Stohlawetz, 1998). Frequent donors demonstrated a significantly lower peak in reticulated platelet levels as well as a more prolonged rise (Stohlawetz, 1998). No difference in platelet counts was seen between the two groups but these findings led the authors to postulate that frequent apheresis platelet donation may lead to a 'relative exhaustion of thrombopoiesis' (Stohlawetz, 1998). Lazarus et al. retrospectively studied 939 donors who had donated 11 464 platelet donations over 4 years and found a significant and sustained decrease in platelet count that directly correlated with donation frequency (Lazarus, 2001). While regular donation resulted in lower platelet counts, clinically significant thrombocytopenia was not seen (Lazarus, 2001). These findings raise concerns that frequent apheresis platelet donations could produce thrombocytopenia.

Plateletpheresis using early hemapheresis instruments were associated with losses of donor lymphocytes as great as $5–10 \times 10^9$ per procedure (Strauss, 1994). Based upon studies involving therapeutic lymphocytapheresis and chronic thoracic duct drainage, it had been shown that abnormal cell-mediated immunity could be achieved by the loss of $1–1.5 \times 10^{11}$ lymphocytes within a few weeks (Strauss, 1994). As a result of this and studies showing decreased total lymphocytes, T lymphocytes, and IgG levels 8 months after donation, concerns about inducing immune suppression arose. This resulted in regulations limiting the number of plateletpheresis donations to 24 per year (Standards Committee of the American Association of Blood Banks, 2004), the warning of potential plateletpheresis donors about the possibility of lymphocyte depletion (Division of Blood and Blood Products, Center for Biologics Evaluation and Research, 1988), and some authors suggesting that donors should be deferred if their lymphocyte counts were below $1.2 \times 10^9/L$ (Strauss, 1994). More recent studies of donors donating with newer hemapheresis instruments have shown no differences in lymphocyte counts, lymphocyte subsets, or IgG levels in comparing nondonors, plateletpheresis donors, and whole blood donors (Lewis, 1999). In fact, the loss of lymphocytes over the course of 24 donations using modern hemapheresis equipment is equivalent to the loss of lymphocytes in a single whole blood donation (Strauss, 1994). Given the reports of decreased platelet counts with frequent apheresis, however, this restriction may still be warranted.

Donor Leukapheresis

Granulocyte Transfusions

Seven controlled trials comparing antibiotics versus antibiotics and granulocyte transfusions have appeared in the literature and were reviewed by Strauss (Strauss, 1993). In these studies, the granulocyte donors were stimulated with steroids. Granulocyte colony-stimulating factor (G-CSF) was not used. Five of seven trials reported at least partial success of granulocyte transfusion in treating infections in neutropenic patients whose infections were unresponsive to antibiotics. The data from these studies were subsequently analyzed by quantitative meta-analysis and demonstrated that dose of neutrophils transfused, as well as the survival rate of the controls, were primarily responsible for the differing success rates in the studies (Vamvakas, 1996). The authors stated that granulocyte transfusions should be considered in neutropenic patients with infections carrying a high mortality rate and that the highest possible granulocyte doses, $>4 \times 10^{10}$ neutrophils, should be used (Vamvakas, 1996). Since these early studies, only one randomized trial involving G-CSF stimulated donors has been published. This study demonstrated no difference between the study groups with regard to survival (Hubel, 2002). Most of the studies and reports describing granulocyte transfusions in adults have

dealt with neutropenic patients with unresponsive bacterial infections. Studies have looked at the utility of granulocyte transfusions in patients with fungal infections but the results of such trials have been mixed (van Burik, 2003).

Another group of patients frequently considered for granulocyte transfusions are septic neonates. Six controlled studies have been published evaluating granulocyte transfusions in this setting, four of which found benefit (Baley, 1987; Cairo, 1987, 1984; Christensen, 1982; Laurenti, 1981; Wheeler, 1987). Quantitative meta-analysis of these studies identified granulocyte dose as the primary reason for disagreement in the study outcomes. Those studies using buffy coat-derived granulocytes demonstrated no advantage, while those using leukapheresis-derived granulocytes demonstrated benefit (Vamvakas, 1996). Again, all of these trials were prior to the availability of G-CSF. No trials of transfusion of G-CSF stimulated granulocytes have been reported.

Granulocyte transfusions may benefit neutropenic patients, especially if large doses can be collected. Recommendations for whom to consider for granulocyte transfusions include adult patients who are profoundly neutropenic, are anticipated to remain neutropenic for at least 1 week, and whose infections have progressed despite appropriate antibiotic therapy (Schiffer, 1990). In addition, the patient should also have a possibility of recovery of granulocyte production. In neonates, indications for granulocyte transfusion are evidence of bacterial sepsis with an absolute neutrophil count below 3000/μL and decreased marrow store of neutrophils with less than 7% (of nucleated cells) metamyelocytes or more mature forms (Blanchette, 1991; Strauss, 1991).

Granulocyte Product Requirements

One of the critical factors in the success of granulocyte transfusions is the dose of granulocytes provided. Standards for Blood Banks and Transfusion Services require that 75% of granulocyte components collected have a minimum of 1.0×10^{10} granulocytes (Standards Committee of the American Association of Blood Banks, 2004). It must be realized that this dose represents a minimum, and that higher doses are desirable.

Granulocytes are stored at room temperature (20–24°C) without agitation and have an expiration date of 24 hours (Standards Committee of the American Association of Blood Banks, 2004). Neutrophils, however, undergo apoptosis throughout storage. Accumulation of transfused granulocytes at sites of inflammation decreases with increasing time of storage and they should therefore be transfused as soon as possible after collection (Price, 1979).

Granulocyte Donor Selection

As with plateletpheresis, leukapheresis donors must fulfill all of the requirements applicable to whole blood donation. In addition, platelets are also removed during the collection and the application of the 150 000/μL platelet count requirement to granulocyte donors may be prudent. Another consideration in selecting donors is ABO type of recipient and donor. Significant numbers of red blood cells are present within granulocyte products. Since the red cell content is greater than 2 mL, Standards for Blood Banks and Transfusion Services require than the product be crossmatch compatible (Standards Committee of the American Association of Blood Banks, 2004). If a granulocyte product could be generated with less than 2 mL of red cells, then ABO type could be ignored, as it does not influence transfused granulocyte survival or migration (McCullough, 1988).

Another consideration in donor selection is the cytomegalovirus status of the donor and recipient. Granulocyte transfusions have been linked to cases of CMV infection in CMV seronegative recipients (Buckner, 1983; Winston, 1980). Therefore, donors for CMV seronegative patients must also be CMV seronegative.

Finally, it is critical that HLA or crossmatch compatible donors be selected for alloimmunized patients. Studies of alloimmunized patients have demonstrated minimal to no recovery, survival, or localization to sites of infection using granulocytes from random donors (Dutcher, 1983; McCullough, 1986).

Granulocyte Donor Stimulation

Granulocyte dose is critical for the effectiveness of granulocyte therapy. The most commonly used method to increase granulocyte yield is to administer steroids to donors 10–12 hours prior to collection. The administration of oral prednisone (Jendiroba, 1998; MacPherson, 1976) or dexamethasone (Higby, 1977) increases granulocyte yield up to twice that of unstimulated donors. The effect of steroids appears to result from mobilization of granulocytes from marrow stores. Studies have shown no effect of steroid stimulation on the ability of neutrophils to phagocytose particles, phagocytose fungi, kill bacteria, or undergo chemotaxis when compared to granulocytes from nonstimulated donors (Glasser, 1977). In addition, steroid stimulation has been shown not to affect accumulation of transfused granulocytes at sites of injury (Price, 1979) and inhibits apoptosis during storage (Liles, 1995).

The availability of granulocyte colony-stimulating factor (G-CSF) has resulted in the ability to generate even larger granulocyte doses and has led to the resurgence of interest in granulocyte transfusions. Administration of 5 µg/kg of G-CSF either daily or every other day resulted in granulocyte collections four to five times those seen in unstimulated donors and greater than those seen with prednisone stimulation (Jendiroba, 1998). The use of G-CSF stimulated granulocyte transfusions has been shown to result in significant and sustained increments in neutrophil counts in patients (Adkins, 1997b). The optimum timing for granulocyte collection in G-CSF stimulated donors is 12 hours after administration of the G-CSF (Price, 1998).

As with steroids, concerns have arisen over the function of G-CSF stimulated granulocytes. Studies have demonstrated normal phagocytosis, chemotaxis, chemiluminescence, and superoxide anion production (Caspar, 1993) and normal accumulation at sites of injury (Adkins, 1997a). G-CSF has also been shown to enhance microbicidal activity (Lieschke, 1992) as well as inhibit neutrophil apoptosis during storage (Adachi, 1994). Concern has also been raised whether repeated doses of G-CSF will adversely affect granulocyte function. Again, enhanced phagocytosis and oxidative burst were seen with multiple G-CSF administrations (Joos, 2002).

Studies have been performed evaluating the effect of the combination of steroids and G-CSF (Dale, 1998; Liles, 1997). Eight milligrams of dexamethasone with either 300 or 600 µg of G-CSF resulted in higher granulocyte yields than either agent alone, resulting in a 10-fold increase in neutrophil count at 12 hours. The combination of dexamethasone and 600 µg resulted in a significantly greater yield than dexamethasone and 300 µg of G-CSF (Liles, 1997). Granulocyte function with this combined regimen demonstrated no defects (Dale, 1998). Subsequent studies comparing 450 µg versus 600 µg doses of G-CSF with 8 mg of dexamethasone found equivalency with regard to both the donor's absolute neutrophil count (ANC) at 12 hours and donor side effects (Liles, 2000). Finally, the route of administration of the G-CSF, when given with dexamethasone, also influences granulocyte kinetics. Subcutaneous administration gives a higher sustained ANC compared to i.v. administration (Stroncek, 2002).

Granulocyte Collection Procedure

Granulocyte yields can also be increased by enhancing the separation of the red blood cells and granulocytes during the centrifugation process. Red blood cells and granulocytes have similar densities and sedimentation rates, resulting in poor separation during centrifugation. The addition of sedimenting agents such as hydroxyethyl starch (HES) can improve this separation and thereby enhance granulocyte collection (Iacone, 1981). The mechanism of action of HES is the induction of rouleaux formation among the red blood cells. The resulting greater red cell sedimentation rate and a greater upward flow of plasma during centrifugation enhance separation (Lee, 1995b). Different types of HES include the high molecular weight hetastarch and the low molecular weight pentastarch. Both of these agents have been shown to have equivalent safety profiles (Strauss, 1986, 1987) though pentastarch has the benefit of being rapidly excreted. As a result, there is less danger of accumulation of the HES and possible complications (see discussion at end of chapter). While the safety profile of pentastarch may be superior, a controlled study has shown greater granulocyte yields with hetastarch (Lee, 1995b).

Granulocyte Donor Concerns

In addition to granulocytes, platelets and significant numbers of red blood cells are also present in the leukapheresis product. The donor's hematocrit typically drops by 7% following a granulocyte collection (Hester, 1995). This drop is due not only to loss of red blood cells but also due to dilutional effects of volume expansion caused by the HES used during the procedure. Platelet count typically drops by 22% after each procedure, an equivalent drop to that seen with plateletpheresis (Hester, 1995). Again, a degree of dilutional effect is present. An additional cause for a fall in platelet count is seen in donors stimulated with G-CSF (Bensinger, 1993). Healthy donors receiving G-CSF for 10 days typically have a decline in platelet count starting at day 8 with significant differences from baseline at days 10 and 11. The mechanism behind this effect is uncertain and may represent changed platelet distribution, decreased platelet production, or increased intravascular volume (Korbling, 1998). In addition, recovery of platelet count also appears to be prolonged, requiring 7–10 days among stem cell donors versus 4–6 days among platelet donors (Stroncek, 1996b).

Table 36–2 Short-Term Side Effects of Medications Used in Granulocyte Mobilization (Volk, 1999)

Medication	Side effects
Corticosteroids	Headache
	Flushing
	Insomnia
	Euphoria
	Palpitations
	Epigastric acidity
	Hyperglycemia
G-CSF	Bone pain
	Myalgias
	Arthralgias
	Headache
	Fever
	Chills
	Gastrointestinal discomfort
	Paresthesias
	Chest pain
	Edema
	Fatigue

Table 36–3 Diseases/Conditions that are Relative Contraindications to Medications Used for Granulocyte Mobilization (Korbling, 1998; Technical Manual Committee, 2002)

Medication	Condition
Corticosteroids	Hypertension
	Diabetes
	Peptic ulcer disease
G-CSF	Inflammatory conditions
	Gout
	Risk factors for thrombosis

G-CSF and corticosteroids can cause a number of other side effects (Table 36–2). These side effects are very common, occurring in 90% of allogeneic donors receiving G-CSF for hematopoietic progenitor cell (HPC) mobilization (Stroncek, 1996a), are usually mild and are treated symptomatically. For example, bone pain and headache, which tend to be dose related (Murata, 1999; Stroncek, 1996a), typically respond to mild analgesics. Nausea and vomiting are more common in women, and headache is more common in those under 35 (Murata, 1999). More significant side effects of G-CSF include splenic rupture, retinal hemorrhage, acute iritis, gouty arthritis, and thrombosis (Korbling, 1998; Volk, 1999). These are felt to represent exacerbation of underlying donor/patient illnesses. Donors, whether for granulocyte or allogeneic peripheral blood HPC collections, should be evaluated for these illnesses in determining suitability for donation (Table 36–3). A report has appeared in which an allogeneic peripheral blood HPC donor experienced a life-threatening capillary leak syndrome characterized by hypoxemia, ascites, pericardial effusion, pleural effusion, shock, and hepatocellular injury following G-CSF administration and HPC collection (Azevedo, 2001). This was felt to be due to apheresis activating the large number of neutrophils produced by the G-CSF administration (Azevedo, 2001).

While the short term effects of G-CSF are predominantly mild, the long-term effects are uncertain. Concerns have been expressed over the possibility of recipients developing hematologic diseases such as myelodysplasia or chronic myelogenous leukemia (Korbling, 1998; Volk, 1999). This is due in part to the occurrence of leukemic transformation after G-CSF therapy in 10–15% of patients with congenital neutropenia receiving long-term G-CSF therapy (Bonilla, 1994). In addition, studies of normal donors receiving G-CSF have demonstrated the induction of a small population of tetraploid myeloid cells (Kaplinsky, 2003) as well as temporary asynchronous allele replication and persistent aneuploidy, up to 265 days following G-CSF administration (Nagler, 2004). Studies with limited numbers of normal donors (3–281) and limited follow-up (12–60 months) have, however, reported no abnormalities in granulocyte and hematopoietic progenitor cell donors to date (Stroncek, 1997a; Volk, 1999). It has been estimated that in order to detect a 10-fold increase in the frequency of leukemia above the population background of 0.05%, a

Table 36–4 Advantages and Disadvantages of Double Red Blood Cell Collections

Advantages

Decreased incidence of donor reactions compared to whole blood donation (Wiltbank, 2002)

Decreased number of donors necessary to produce a given number of red blood cell units (Gilcher, 2003)

Standardized red blood cell dose (Gilcher, 2003)

Decreased amount of component processing (i.e., one set of laboratory tests for two units of red blood cells) (Beeler, 1997)

Decreased donor exposure if a patient receives both parts of a double red cell collection (Gilcher, 2003)

Disadvantages

Greater complexity of collection (Gilcher, 2003)

Greater time necessary for donation (Gilcher, 2003)

study following 2000 stimulated donors for a minimum of 10 years would be needed. Donors undergoing G-CSF stimulation should give informed consent prior to stimulation and appropriate institutional review should be obtained for use of G-CSF in this non-FDA-approved role. Recommendations have also been made that donor registries should be created to monitor for long-term consequences of G-CSF stimulation (Korbling, 1998).

Long-term steroid treatment is associated with a number of well-known side effects, including the development of posterior subcapsular cataracts (PSC). As these complications appear with chronic use, it would seem that short-term steroid stimulation of granulocyte donors should not be associated with such complications. This may not be the case, however. A double-blinded study compared the presence of cataracts in 9 apheresis platelet donors and 11 granulocyte donors matched for age, gender, and the number of respective donations (Ghodsi, 2001). The frequency of cataracts that are not associated with steroid administration was equivalent between the two groups but those associated with steroid administration, PSC, were statistically more frequent in the granulocyte donors when all eyes were considered (5 of 22 eyes versus 0 of 18, $p = 0.040$) (Ghodsi, 2001). The authors felt that steroid stimulation was the most likely explanation for this finding and recommended that additional studies be performed in an attempt to determine the risk of cataract formation with granulocyte stimulation (Ghodsi, 2001).

Donor Erythropheresis

Benefits of Erythropheresis

Either a single unit of red blood cells or the equivalent of two units of red blood cells can be collected by apheresis. With the current shortages of red blood cells in the US and the decreasing size of the donor pool, the collection of red blood cells, either with the concurrent collection of other blood products or as double red blood cells, can maximize collection of this scarce resource. Advantages and disadvantages of double red blood cell collections are given in Table 36–4.

Erythropheresis Product Requirements

The Standards for Blood Banks and Transfusion Services of the American Association of Blood Banks requires that red blood cells pheresis be collected and prepared by a method that is known to result in a mean hemoglobin of the unit of > 60 g or a packed red cell volume of 180 mL. In addition, at least 95% of the units sampled must have > 50 g of hemoglobin or 150 mL packed red cell volume (Standards Committee of the American Association of Blood Banks, 2004). If the red blood cell units are leukocyte reduced, then the mean hemoglobin must be > 51 g or 153 mL packed red cell volume. Here, at least 95% of tested units must have > 42.5 g of hemoglobin or 128 mL packed red blood cell volume (Standards Committee of the American Association of Blood Banks, 2004).

The FDA does not define product requirements for red blood cells, either single or double, collected by apheresis but instead states that 95% of the products collected must meet 'expected or target RBC volume' and 'any other target parameters specified in the device operator's manual' (Division of Blood and Blood Products, Center for Biologics Evaluation and Research, 2001). The FDA also defines how such validation and testing is to be performed, with the initial validation consisting of testing '100 consecutive RBC units' while subsequent testing must include at least

50 units per month, including both single and double red blood cell products. If a center collects less than 50 units, all units must be tested (Division of Blood and Blood Products, Center for Biologics Evaluation and Research, 2001).

Erythropheresis Donor Selection

Allogeneic apheresis red blood cell donors must meet the criteria defined by the FDA and AABB for whole blood donation. In addition, they are required to meet any other selection criteria defined by the device's operator manual (Division of Blood and Blood Products, Center for Biologics Evaluation and Research, 2001).

The FDA and the AABB do not define a minimum hemoglobin/hematocrit for double red cell donation. Instead, it is required that the collection center follow the instrument manufacturer's recommendations (Division of Blood and Blood Products, Center for Biologics Evaluation and Research, 2001; Standards Committee of the American Association of Blood Banks, 2004). The FDA does, however, require that the hemoglobin/hematocrit be determined by a quantitative method (Division of Blood and Blood Products, Center for Biologics Evaluation and Research, 2001). As a result, the copper sulfate method cannot be used to qualify a donor for double red cell donation.

The AABB limits the total volume of red blood cells removed such that the donor's hematocrit and hemoglobin are not < 30% and < 10 g/dL respectively, after volume replacement (Standards Committee of the American Association of Blood Banks, 2004). The FDA makes no specific limitations, requiring that manufacturer's recommendations be followed (Division of Blood and Blood Products, Center for Biologics Evaluation and Research, 2001).

The type of product collected determines the donation interval following hemapheresis red blood cell donations. Donors donating a single unit of red blood cells are deferred for 8 weeks. The exception to this would be that, as described in the section on donor plateletpheresis, they could donate platelets or platelets with concurrent plasma as long as the extracorporeal red blood cell volume of the collecting instrument is less than 100 mL (Division of Blood and Blood Products, Center for Biologics Evaluation and Research, 2001). Donors donating two units of red blood cells are deferred for 16 weeks and no automated or manual collections are allowed during this time (Division of Blood and Blood Products, Center for Biologics Evaluation and Research, 2001).

If a donor experiences an incomplete procedure, that is, the targeted collection is not reached, the FDA defines the length of deferral based upon the absolute loss of red blood cells during the initial collection as well as subsequent collections. If a donor has a red blood cell loss of > 300 mL, they are deferred for 16 weeks. If the loss is between 200–300 mL, they are deferred for 8 weeks. If the donor has a red cell loss of < 200 mL, they can donate within 8 weeks. If during the second donation the donor has a red blood cell loss of < 100 mL (total loss in 8 weeks < 300 mL), then they are deferred for 8 weeks from the second donation. If the 8-week loss is > 300 mL, they are deferred for 16 weeks from the second donation (Division of Blood and Blood Products, Center for Biologics Evaluation and Research, 2001).

Erythropheresis Donor Concerns

Due to the removal of two units of red blood cells, one of the most frequent concerns is whether reactions are more frequent with double red blood cell collections when compared to whole blood collections. Studies have demonstrated that there is not an increase in reactions with automated double red cell collections when compared to whole blood donation (Gorlin, 2003; Wiltbank, 2002). Wiltbank reported a lower rate of moderate and severe reactions with automated double red blood cell collection (6.8/10 000 and 1.2/10 000 collections respectively) compared to whole blood donations (14.5/10 000 and 1.2/10 000 collections respectively) (Wiltbank, 2002). The lower rate of reactions, despite the removal of a greater red blood cell mass, results from the fact that the donors are isovolemic at the end of the collection due to the infusion of saline.

Donors undergoing double red cell donation experience a transient fall in hematocrit of 9% (Taylor, 2002). This is due to red cell loss as well as the volume expansion from saline administration. Despite this fall, studies have shown minimal effects on donors following double red blood cell donations. Meyer et al. found in a study of 40 blood donors that double red blood cell donors took 1–2 days longer than whole blood donors to regain their baseline sense of well being (Meyer, 1993). Smith et al. found no significant differences in ambulatory monitored blood pressure and pulse among one unit red blood cell collections, two unit red blood cell collections, and sham collections (Smith, 1996). Quintana et al. found that double red blood cell donation did not have significant

Table 36–5 Combinations of Blood Products Available for Multicomponent Collections

Red blood cell and plasma
Red blood cell and platelet
Red blood cell, plasma, and platelet
Double red blood cell
Double or triple platelet
Platelet and single or double plasma
Double platelet and single plasma
Double or triple plasma

effects on exercise capacity as determined by examining maximal oxygen consumption decrease, anaerobic threshold, maximum heart rate, respiratory exchange ratio, and maximum power on days 0, 2, 7 and 14 following donation (Quintana, 1995).

A final concern with double red blood cell donations is whether donors making such donations are at a greater risk of developing iron deficiency than whole blood donors. Meyer et al. followed double red blood cell donors and whole blood donors for 1 year, measuring serum ferritin, serum iron, total iron-binding capacity, transferrin saturation, and zinc protoporphyrin/heme ratios. Half of the donors in each group received iron supplementation. No significant differences were found in iron balance between the double red cell donors and the whole blood donors (Meyer, 1993).

Multicomponent Apheresis Donation

With current instrumentation, different combinations of blood products can be collected from the same donor. This allows for the optimum utilization of each donor. For example, the maximum amount of plasma would be collected from an AB donor while their red blood cells, which frequently outdate before they are transfused, would not be collected. An O Rh negative or Rh positive donor would provide a double red blood cell collection, but plasma, which is usually in adequate supply, would not be collected. The various combinations of collections currently available are given in Table 36–5. It should be mentioned that all of the various regulations that apply to the individual apheresis collections with regard to donor criteria and donor frequency apply to multiple component collections. For example, a donor undergoing a double red cell collection with a concurrent plasma collection would have to meet the requirements for a double red cell collection as well as the requirements for frequent or infrequent plasma collection, as applicable.

Hematopoietic Progenitor Cell Collection

Benefits of Hematopoietic Progenitor Cell Collection

Hematopoietic progenitor cell (HPC) collection by hemapheresis provides a number of advantages, both to the donor and recipient, which have resulted in its replacement of bone marrow harvest in many patients. Donors tolerate hemapheresis better than bone marrow harvest as it does not require an operative procedure with the need for general anesthesia. As a result, the procedure is less expensive, more convenient as it can be undergone as an outpatient, and avoids the potential complications seen with general anesthesia and surgery. Also, the donor recovers more quickly from the procedure without the pain and temporary disability that often accompany bone marrow harvest (Lee, 1995a). The use of peripheral blood HPCs in transplantation restores hematopoietic and immune function more rapidly than bone marrow. This means fewer days of immune suppression and fewer exposures to allogeneic blood products in the recipient (Bensinger, 2001; Moog, 1998). Additionally, in autologous transplantation, collection of peripheral HPCs by hemapheresis can be performed when marrow involvement by malignancy or prior pelvic irradiation is present and would preclude bone marrow harvest (Lee, 1995a).

While HPC collection by hemapheresis provides a number of benefits over bone marrow harvest, it also has disadvantages when compared to bone marrow harvest. Disadvantages include possible adverse effects of mobilization regimens, a greater length of time required for collection, the possibility of a larger volume of component to be transfused at the time of transplantation, and the necessity of central venous access in many cases with the accompanying risks and complications (Lee, 1995a). In addition, there is conflicting evidence in allogeneic transplantation suggesting a greater frequency of chronic graft-versus-host disease (GVHD) (Brown, 1997; Duhrsen, 1988) or GVHD more refractory to standard therapy (Flowers, 2002). This may result from the larger number of T cells within peripheral blood stem cell products compared to bone marrow.

Autologous versus Allogeneic Hematopoietic Progenitor Cell Harvest

At first, peripheral HPC collections were limited to autologous transplantation. This was due to the use of chemotherapy as the method for mobilizing HPCs. Transplantation of HPCs collected in this way was limited to diseases such as solid malignancies, Hodgkin's disease and non-Hodgkin lymphomas, and multiple myeloma. The use of HPCs has subsequently expanded to include transplantation for leukemias, including chronic myelogenous leukemia (Gillespie, 1996; Lee, 1995a; Moog, 1998). As methods for mobilization that do not depend upon chemotherapy have become available, peripheral blood HPC collection has been applied to allogeneic donations as well. Initial use of peripheral HPC collection in this setting was limited to retransplant in recipients with recurrent disease or failure to engraft (Gillespie, 1996; Lee, 1995a; Moog, 1998). Currently, the use of allogeneic peripheral blood HPCs in initial transplants is becoming more widespread.

Hematopoietic Progenitor Cell Dose

An important factor in determining the success of HPC transplantation is the dose of HPCs infused. Unfortunately, a method for definitively enumerating HPCs is not available. It is known that HPCs are found within the mononuclear cell component of blood and as a result, the mononuclear cell count (MNC) has been used as an indicator of when to discontinue HPC collection. Studies have shown that a total dose of $6.0–6.5 \times 10^8$ MNC/kg is sufficient to produce rapid engraftment (Kessinger, 1989, 1995). While MNC does not correlate directly with HPC dose, it is convenient and easily measured.

A more exact way of measuring HPC dose is by determining colony-forming unit-granulocyte/macrophage (CFU-GM) colonies grown on soft agar. HPC collections that contain $0.5–2.0 \times 10^5$ CFU-GM/kg are associated with rapid engraftment (Bender, 1992). Unfortunately, CFU-GM assays are technically challenging and difficult to standardize. As a result, direct comparison of data between institutions and studies should be made with caution. In addition, the assay requires 2 weeks to complete.

A third method of determining HPC dose is the measurement of CD34+ cell count within the product. HPCs represent a subset of CD34+ cells. As a result, the measurement of CD34+ cells gives a better indication of HPC dose than MNC and also correlates with CFU-GM (Lee, 1995a). A minimum dose of CD34+ cells necessary for engraftment appears to be 2.5×10^6 CD34+ cells/kg (Bensinger, 1995; Korbling, 1995). This dose of CD34+ cells results in prompt engraftment of white blood cells. Bensinger, et al., however, found that the higher dose of 5.0×10^6 CD34+ cells/kg resulted in an equivalent engraftment of white blood cells as well as a more rapid engraftment of platelets (Bensinger, 1995). While CD34+ cell content is easier to measure than CFU-GM, it has also been plagued by difficulties in standardization due to variations in methodology (Lee, 1995a). Fortunately, the availability of kits and instruments from numerous manufacturers appears to be solving this problem.

It should be mentioned that in the setting of allogeneic HPC transplantation, as with many things in life, too much of a good thing may be bad. While minimal numbers of CD34+ cells/kg are needed for prompt engraftment, too many cells have been associated with an increased risk of chronic graft-versus-host disease in some studies (Heimfeld, 2003; Zaucha, 2001). Zaucha et al. found a higher incidence of extensive chronic graft-versus-host disease in allogeneic transplant patients receiving greater than 8.0×10^6 CD34+ cells/kg (Zaucha, 2001).

Some authors have suggested that the dose of CD34+ cells needed for engraftment may vary with the number of HPC collection procedures (Smolowicz, 1999). It is thought that a higher total dose is necessary when the CD34+ cells are collected over multiple procedures. This is felt to be due to changes in CD34+ cell subsets seen during the course of multiple collections (Smolowicz, 1999).

Hematopoietic Progenitor Cell Mobilization

Early attempts at harvesting hematopoietic progenitor cells from peripheral blood were successful but labor and resource intensive. The peripheral blood contains only 10% of the fraction of CD34+ cells found in the bone marrow (Lee, 1995a). This means that when HPCs are collected during steady state, i.e., without mobilization, the number of procedures necessary to achieve a sufficient dose may be large, for example 12 procedures in one study (Moog, 1998). This limits the utility of hemapheresis collection of HPCs during steady state.

IV

Table 36–6 Comparison of Different Mobilization Regimens (Gillespie, 1996)

Regimen	Approximate day when peak HPC concentrations are reached	Increase in HPCs above steady state
Chemotherapy	Day 14 after completion of chemotherapy	5–15×
Cytokines (G-CSF and GM-CSF)	Day 5 after initiation of cytokine therapy	60×
Chemotherapy and cytokines	Day 5 after initiation of cytokine therapy	1000×

Table 36–7 Factors that Negatively Influence Mobilization in Autologous Stem Cell Collections (Kessinger, 2003)

Age*
Presence of marrow involvement
Follicular NHL compared to diffuse NHL
Prior radiation therapy
Greater number of cycles of chemotherapy
Low platelet count
Low NK cell numbers
Prior rituximab therapy

* Not important if mobilized by chemotherapy. When G-CSF is given alone, younger donors/patients mobilize better than older ones (Bensinger, 1995; Moog, 1998).

The discovery that peripheral hematopoietic progenitor cells could be mobilized from the bone marrow meant that therapeutic doses of HPCs could be collected by hemapheresis in fewer procedures, making the method more attractive. Chemotherapy, cytokines, or a combination of chemotherapy and cytokines can mobilize HPCs from bone marrow (Gillespie, 1996; Lee, 1995a; Moog, 1998). Table 36–6 gives a general comparison of the effectiveness of these three mobilization regimens.

The regimen initially used for mobilization was chemotherapy. During the period of rebound hematopoiesis following chemotherapeutic treatment, the number of HPCs present within the peripheral blood increases dramatically (see Table 36–6). This allows for the effective collection of HPCs and also serves to decrease the tumor burden within the donor/recipient. The limitation of such a method of mobilization, however, is that it can only be applied to autologous transplants.

Cytokines, such as G-CSF and granulocyte/macrophage colony-stimulating factor (GM-CSF), also dramatically increase the presence of HPCs within the peripheral blood and have the additional benefit of having minimal short-term toxicity (see Table 36–2). This therefore allows for the mobilization of HPCs in normal donors and the use of hemapheresis in allogeneic transplantation. The mechanism of action of these cytokines is an indirect one with regard to their effects on HPCs. HPCs in the marrow are bound to stromal cells by adhesion molecules. These molecules include VLA-4 and CXCR4 on the HPCs and VCAM-1 and SDF-1 on the stromal cells. G-CSF increases the number of neutrophils in the marrow. This results in increases in proteolytic enzymes such as elastase and MMP-9, which are released by the neutrophils. These enzymes cleave VCAM-1 and SDF-1 resulting in release of the HPCs from the stromal cells, allowing them to enter the peripheral circulation (Lapidot, 2002).

Overall, the magnitude of increase in CD34+ cells with G-CSF and GM-CSF is the same, but differences in recipient recovery of hematopoiesis and donor side effects exist between the two agents. Recipients of GM-CSF-mobilized HPCs experience a longer period of time until recovery of platelet production than do recipients of G-CSF-mobilized HPCs (13 days versus 18 days) (Gillespie, 1996). Donors receiving GM-CSF, while experiencing the same symptoms as those receiving G-CSF, tend to have more severe side effects (Bolwell, 1994). The use of either G-CSF or GM-CSF in normal donors is associated with a peak in CD34+ cells at approximately 5 days following initiation of cytokine therapy (Bensinger, 1996). The use of G-CSF in normal donors for periods longer than 5 days has been associated with a decrease in the number of CD34+ cells collected after day 10 of stimulation (Stroncek, 1996a).

In addition to G-CSF and GM-CSF, a number of other cytokines and monoclonal antibodies against stem cell adhesion molecules are being evaluated for their effect of HPC mobilization. These include AMD-3100, stem cell factor, interleukin 3, c-kit ligand, and anti-VLA-4 (Filshie, 2002; Fruehauf, 2003; Gillespie, 1996; Lee, 1995a).

Finally, the effects of chemotherapy and cytokine mobilization are independent of one another. This means that by combining both mobilization regimens, even greater numbers of HPCs can be collected than when using either regimen alone.

In healthy allogeneic donors, the optimum mobilization regimen appears to be 10–16 µg/kg of G-CSF split into two doses and administered subcutaneously (Kroger, 2002). While G-CSF demonstrates a dose response, doses larger than 10–16 µg/kg result in more donor adverse effects without significant improvement in CD34+ cell yield. If a donor is a poor mobilizer, however, higher doses can be given (Kroger, 2002). Twice-daily dosing has been shown to be superior to single dosing in this setting. This is thought to be due to the relatively short half-life of G-CSF of 3–4 hours (Kroger, 2002).

In autologous donors, mobilization is complicated by the underlying disease as well as previous therapy. In autologous HPC collection, G-CSF

doses of > 16 µg/kg are needed. If poor mobilization occurs, the patient/donor may need to be remobilized with chemotherapy followed by growth factor or higher doses of growth factor (Kessinger, 2003).

In addition to these mobilization regimens, HPCs are also mobilized by the collection procedure itself. Studies of the kinetics of HPCs during hemapheresis procedures have shown that larger numbers of HPCs are recovered than would be expected based solely upon the number of cells present in the peripheral blood. This means that during the procedure, as HPCs are removed, additional HPCs are released from the marrow (Smolowicz, 1999).

Unfortunately, despite attempts to optimize mobilization regimens, not every patient collects a dose of peripheral blood HPCs sufficient for transplantation. Factors that have been found to adversely affect HPC harvest are given in Table 36–7. Some authors have found that the number of CD34+ cells within the bone marrow is a predictor of ability of a patient to mobilize and could be used to assist in deciding whether a patient should undergo hemapheresis or bone marrow harvest (Passos-Coelho, 1995a).

While mobilization increases the number of HPCs present in the peripheral blood, it can also have detrimental effects on the donor and on the HPC product. As discussed in the section on donor concerns in granulocyte collection, the use of G-CSF is associated with minimal short-term side effects as well as unknown long-term side effects. In the setting of autologous harvest, these effects and concerns are unimportant relative to the risks that the patient faces from their disease. In addition, the use of such agents in this setting accelerates white cell recovery following chemotherapy, a beneficial effect. In the setting of allogeneic donation, the uncertainty of long-term risks of cytokine mobilization must be explained to the donor during the consent process. Also, the delay in platelet recovery seen following G-CSF treatment and granulocyte collection is also seen with HPC harvest (Gillespie, 1996; Stroncek, 1996b). In autologous donors, this combined with marrow suppression from recent chemotherapy may result in the need for platelet transfusion. Mobilization is also associated with an increased risk of catheter thrombosis (Lee, 1995a). Finally, in addition to mobilizing HPCs, the regimens described previously have also been shown to mobilize tumor cells into the peripheral blood by some (Brugger, 1994; Gazitt, 1996) but not all authors (Passos-Coelho, 1995b). The study by Brugger, et al. demonstrated mobilization of tumor cells on days 1 through 7 following the start of chemotherapy in patients without bone marrow involvement and on days 9 through 16 in those with marrow involvement (Brugger, 1994). The mobilization of tumor cells in these later patients occurred within the time frame of HPC collection. Similarly, Gazitt, et al. found mobilization of plasma cells in multiple myeloma patients occurred later, days 5 and 6, than stem cells, days 1 through 3 (Gazitt, 1996). The differences in mobilization of tumor cells versus HPCs have led many to suggest that single collections early in the course of mobilization may be better than multiple collections. It should be realized that while tumor contamination does occur, the effect of this contamination on relapse is uncertain.

Hematopoietic Progenitor Cell Collection Procedure

One of the first things to consider in performing an HPC collection is when to initiate the collection. In allogeneic donors, initiating collection on the fifth day after the start of G-CSF administration appears to be the preferred practice. This is due to the relatively reproducible response of healthy allogeneic donors to G-CSF administration (Kroger, 2002). For autologous donors, a number of criteria can be used in determining whether to initiate therapy. Criteria that have been used include myelocytosis and rising monocyte levels (Lee, 1995a), total white blood cell count increase of twofold in 24 hours (Lee, 1995a), time of first platelet count increase (Gillespie, 1996), day 14 after initiation of chemotherapy (Gillespie, 1996), and a white blood cell (WBC) count of 10 000/µL (Dreger, 1993). With regard to this last indicator, Dreger et al. demonstrated a peak in CFU-GM 1–2 days after the WBC count reached 10 000/µL (Dreger, 1993). Starting collection at this time avoided missing the subsequent peak in CFU-GM. Another widely used method is serial CD34+ cell counts by flow cytometry. This can be used to detect a rise in CD34+ cells and trigger HPC harvest. Trigger levels described in the literature should be viewed with caution due to the current lack of standardization in CD34+ cell measurements (Lee, 1995a). Individual institutions must determine their own trigger criteria.

Once the decision to initiate collection has been made, a number of aspects of the procedure can be modified that will influence the quality of the product. First, the instrument used to collect the HPCs determines the characteristics of the product. A number of instruments are available with the two most commonly used being the CS3000 Plus (Baxter Healthcare Co, Round Lake, IL) and the COBE Spectra (Gambro BCT Inc., Lakewood CO). Direct comparison of these instruments has demonstrated no differences in their efficiency of collecting CD34+ cells (Stroncek, 1997b). It was found that the product produced by the COBE Spectra contained more neutrophils. This could be a significant finding if the HPC product is to be modified such as T cell depleted as these additional cells can interfere with the depletion process (Stroncek, 1997b).

Another variable to consider is the whole blood flow rate during the procedure. It would seem that higher flow rates would result in a higher volume processed and a concurrent larger number of HPCs collected. With the COBE Spectra, this does appear to be the case (Lin, 1995). With the CS3000, however, increased flow rates were associated with the detrimental effect of decreased mononuclear cell content of the product as well as the beneficial effect of decreased platelet count (Lin, 1995). This may have resulted from insufficient dwell time within the centrifugal field to allow for adequate centrifugation at the higher flow rate.

While the whole blood flow rate can adversely affect collection efficiency, the concept of increasing the amount of blood processed in order to increase the HPC yield is a valid one. Standard HPC collection involves the processing of approximately 1.5–3 blood volumes per procedure (Lee, 1995a). Alternatively, large-volume leukapheresis (LVL) involves processing greater than 5 blood volumes or greater than 15 liters (Reik, 1997). The benefits of such procedures include the collection of large numbers of HPC per procedure with the resulting need for fewer collection procedures as well as greater mobilization of HPCs during the procedure (Lee, 1995a; Moog, 1998). In addition to these, improved yield of HPCs in patients who mobilize poorly has also been seen (Smolowicz, 1997). Disadvantages of LVL include longer time required to complete the procedure as well as increased incidence of citrate reactions (see discussion at the end of the chapter) (Moog, 1998). In standard leukapheresis procedures, thrombosis of central catheters is the most common complication (Goldberg, 1995) but in LVL, citrate reactions predominate, occurring in 33% of donations (Lin, 1995). This is due to the greater amount of citrate anticoagulant that is infused. Some authors have attempted to minimize this by adding heparin to the anticoagulant for the procedure (Reik, 1997) and/or providing i.v. calcium supplementation during the procedure (Bolan, 2002; Buchta, 2003).

Hematopoietic Progenitor Cell Donor Concerns

In addition to the reactions associated with G-CSF as described under the section dealing with granulocyte collections and the concerns seen with large volume leukapheresis, thrombocytopenia is also a concern in both autologous and allogeneic HPC collections. Schlenke, et al. reported average platelet losses of 24.2 ± 12.5% during large-volume peripheral blood hematopoietic progenitor cell collections using the CS3000 (Schlenke, 2000). Smaller platelet loss has been reported using the Baxter Amicus (Burgstaler, 2004). In addition, patients undergoing autologous peripheral blood stem cell collections may also be thrombocytopenic from the chemotherapy routinely used as part of the mobilization regimen. Bleeding complications in these patients are uncommon (Goldberg, 1995). Patients may, however, require platelet transfusions prior to or after collections, depending upon their platelet count, in order to avoid bleeding complications.

Donor Plasmapheresis

Plasma Products

Two types of plasma products are collected by donor plasmapheresis, fresh frozen plasma and source plasma. Source plasma is plasma that is subsequently used to manufacture derivative products. These derivative products include albumin, immunoglobulins, coagulation factor

concentrates, and laboratory reagents. Fresh frozen plasma (FFP) is the liquid component of whole blood that has been frozen within 6–8 hours after collection. The benefit of collecting FFP by plasmapheresis is that 600–700 mL of plasma can be collected from a single donor. This can then be divided into multiple units of a volume equivalent to FFP derived from whole blood donations. Alternatively, the entire volume can be frozen as 'jumbo plasma.' These large units have the benefit of limiting donor exposure in patients requiring large volumes of FFP, such as in plasma exchange for thrombotic thrombocytopenic purpura. An additional benefit is that the large volume of collection can maximize the production of frequently used or rare products such as type AB FFP or IgA-deficient FFP.

Plasma Donor Selection

The donor criteria for plasmapheresis vary according to the frequency of donation. Donors donating plasma less frequently than every 4 weeks are classified as 'infrequent' donors and must fulfill whole blood donor requirements. If the donor donates more frequently than every 4 weeks, they are classified as a 'frequent' donor and must fulfill criteria outlined in the Code of Federal Regulations (CFR) (Standards Committee of the American Association of Blood Banks, 2004). These requirements are similar in many ways to those for whole blood donation with differences in the deferrals for malaria and transfusion-transmitted disease exposure (CFR, 2003). In addition, the CFR also requires that frequent plasma donors have a total serum protein of at least 6.0 g/dL and that this, as well as either a serum protein electrophoresis or quantitative immunodiffusion, be performed every 4 months (CFR, 2003). Finally, an annual examination by a physician is required. The CFR further limits the volume of plasma donated. Donors may not donate more than 1000 mL (1200 mL for donors weighing more than 175 lb) every 48 hours and no more than 2000 mL (2400 mL for donors weighing more than 175 lb) in a 7-day period (CFR, 2003).

Plasma Donor Concerns

The risks of donor plasmapheresis are those common to any hemapheresis procedure. In addition, concern arises over possible depletion of immunoglobulins or removal of coagulation factors faster than they can be replenished, especially in frequent donors. Studies of long-term donors (Wasi, 1991) as well as donors undergoing frequent donations (Ciszewski, 1993) have not supported these concerns.

Indications for Therapeutic Hemapheresis

Therapeutic apheresis procedures, both cytapheresis and plasmapheresis, have been used to treat a wide variety of illnesses, often without a clear scientific basis for expecting any benefit. There have been limited numbers of randomized controlled trials (Shehata, 2002). In this way, apheresis has been analogous to the blood letting of the early 18th century to which it has frequently been compared. As a result, it is difficult in some cases to determine for which diseases and disorders hemapheresis is truly indicated. To help in this determination, the American Society for Apheresis (ASFA) and the American Association for Blood Banks (AABB) have published lists, which are regularly updated, that provide recommendations for the use of apheresis (American Association of Blood Banks Hemapheresis Committee, 1995; American Society for Apheresis Clinical Applications Committee, 2000). Both lists place each disease/disorder into one of four categories. The categories and their definitions are given in Table 36–8. Table 36–9 lists the diseases that have been evaluated by the AABB and ASFA.

Table 36–8 ASFA/AABB Categorization of Apheresis Indications

Category	Description
I	Apheresis is standard and acceptable primary therapy. This is based upon well-designed randomized controlled trials or broad and noncontroversial published experience
II	Apheresis is generally accepted as a supportive or adjunct therapy. Randomized controlled trials are available for some disorders but others are supported only by small case series
III	There is a suggestion of benefit but insufficient evidence is present to establish the efficacy and/or clarify risk/benefit ratios
IV	Apheresis is not indicated. Controlled trials have shown no benefit

Introduction to the third special issue: Clinical applications of therapeutic apheresis, McLeod BC, Copyright © 2000 J Clin Apheresis 15:1–5. Reprinted with permission of Wiley-Liss, Inc., a subsidiary of John Wiley & Sons, Inc.

Table 36–9 Diseases Treated by Hemapheresis

Disorder	Hemapheresis procedure	ASFA category	AABB category
ABO-incompatible marrow transplants	Plasmapheresis	II	III
Acute central nervous system inflammatory demyelinating disease	Plasmapheresis	II	NC
Acute inflammatory demyelinating polyneuropathy (Guillain–Barré syndrome)	Plasmapheresis	I	I
AIDS	Plasmapheresis	NC	IV
Amyotrophic lateral sclerosis (ALS)	Plasmapheresis	NC	IV
Anti-basement membrane antibody disease (Goodpasture's syndrome)	Plasmapheresis	I	I
Aplastic anemia	Plasmapheresis	III	IV
Burns with shock	Plasmapheresis	NC	III
Chronic inflammatory demyelinating polyneuropathy (CIDP)	Plasmapheresis	I	I
Coagulation factor inhibitors	Plasmapheresis	II	III
Cold agglutinin disease	Plasmapheresis	NC	II
Cryoglobulinemia	Plasmapheresis	II	I
Cryoglobulinemia with polyneuropathy	Plasmapheresis	II	NC
Cutaneous T cell lymphoma	Photopheresis/leukapheresis	I/III	II/II
Demyelinating polyneuropathy with IgG/IgA	Plasmapheresis/immunoadsorption	I/III	NC
Drug overdose	Plasmapheresis	III	II
Eaton–Lambert syndrome	Plasmapheresis	II	II
Erythrocytosis/polycythemia vera	Erythropheresis/phlebotomy	II/I	NC
Familial hypercholesterolemia	Plasmapheresis/selective removal	II/I	I/NC
Recurrent focal segmental glomerulonephritis	Plasmapheresis	III	III
Heart transplant rejection	Plasmapheresis/photopheresis	III/III	NC
Hematopoietic progenitor cell collection	Leukapheresis	NC	I
Hemolytic disease of the newborn (maternal treatment)	Plasmapheresis	III	III
Hemolytic transfusion reaction	Erythropheresis	NC	III
Hemolytic uremic syndrome (HUS)	Plasmapheresis	III	II
Hepatic failure	Plasmapheresis	III	IV
Hypereosinophilia	Leukapheresis	NC	IV
Hyperviscosity	Plasmapheresis	II	I
Idiopathic thrombocytopenic purpura (ITP)	Plasmapheresis/staphylococcal A protein column	NC/II	IV/III
Inclusion-body myositis	Plasmapheresis/leukapheresis	III/IV	NC
Leukemia with hyperleukocytosis	Leukapheresis	I	I
Leukemia without hyperleukocytosis	Leukapheresis	NC	IV
Lupus nephritis	Plasmapheresis	NC	IV
Malaria (hyperparasitemia)	Erythropheresis	III	II
Multiple sclerosis (overall)	Plasmapheresis	NC	III
Relapsing	Plasmapheresis	III	NC
Progressive	Plasmapheresis/lymphapheresis	III/III	NC/NC
Myasthenia gravis	Plasmapheresis	I	I
Myeloma kidney	Plasmapheresis	II	NC
Multiple myeloma with polyneuropathy	Plasmapheresis	III	NC
Organ transplant rejection	Plasmapheresis/photopheresis/leukapheresis	NC/NC/NC	NC/III/III
Paraneoplastic syndromes	Plasmapheresis	III	NC
Pediatric autoimmune neuropsychiatric disorders associated with streptococcal infections (PANDAS)	Plasmapheresis	II	NC
Pemphigus vulgaris	Plasmapheresis/photopheresis	NC	II/NC
Phytanic acid storage disease (Refsum's disease)	Plasmapheresis	I	I
Platelet refractoriness due to alloantibodies	Plasmapheresis/staphylococcal A protein column	NC	III/NC
POEMS syndrome	Plasmapheresis	III	NC
Polymyositis/dermatomyositis	Plasmapheresis/leukapheresis	III/IV	IV/IV
Polyneuropathy with IgM	Plasmapheresis/immunoadsorption	II/III	NC
Post-transfusion purpura (PTP)	Plasmapheresis	I	I
Progressive systemic sclerosis (scleroderma)	Plasmapheresis/photopheresis/leukapheresis	III/NC/NC	III/III/NC
Psoriasis	Plasmapheresis	NC	IV
Quinine/quinidine-induced thrombocytopenia	Plasmapheresis	NC	II
Rapidly progressive glomerulonephritis	Plasmapheresis	II	II
Rasmussen's encephalitis	Plasmapheresis	III	III
Raynaud's disease	Plasmapheresis	III	NC

Table 36–9 Diseases Treated by Hemapheresis (*cont'd*)

Disorder	Hemapheresis procedure	ASFA category	AABB category
Red cell aplasia	Plasmapheresis	III	III
Renal transplant rejection	Plasmapheresis	IV	IV
Renal transplantation to remove HLA antibodies prior to transplant	Plasmapheresis	III	NC
Rheumatoid arthritis	Plasmapheresis/leukapheresis/immunoadsorption	NC/II/II	IV/III/NC
Schizophrenia	Plasmapheresis	NC	IV
Sickle cell anemia	Erythropheresis	I	I
Sickle cell anemia (maternal treatment in pregnancy)	Erythropheresis	NC	III
Stiff-man syndrome	Plasmapheresis	III	NC
Sydenham's chorea	Plasmapheresis	II	NC
Systemic amyloidosis	Plasmapheresis	IV	NC
Systemic lupus erythematosus (SLE)	Plasmapheresis	III	NC
Thrombocytosis (symptomatic)	Plateletpheresis	I	I
Thrombotic thrombocytopenic purpura (TTP)	Plasmapheresis	I	I
Thyroid storm	Plasmapheresis	NC	III
Vasculitis	Plasmapheresis	III	NC
Warm autoimmune hemolytic anemia	Plasmapheresis	III	III

See Table 36–8 for explanation of ASFA and AABB categories. NC = not categorized.

After Table 13–1, *Apheresis: Principles and Practice* (McLeod, 2003).

A discussion of all of the disorders listed in Table 36–9 is beyond the scope of this chapter. The interested reader is referred to three sources, the textbooks *Apheresis: Principles and Practice* (McLeod, 2003) and *Guidelines for Therapeutic Hemapheresis* (American Association of Blood Banks Hemapheresis Committee, 1995), both published by the AABB, and the special edition of the *Journal of Clinical Apheresis* entitled 'The Clinical Applications of Therapeutic Apheresis' published by the ASFA (American Society for Apheresis Clinical Applications Committee, 2000).

Therapeutic Cytapheresis

Therapeutic Plateletpheresis

Thrombocytosis

Thrombocytosis is defined as an increase in the number of platelets present in the blood. This can range from mild increases to increases resulting in platelet counts greater than 1 000 000/µL. It is in these later patients that concern arises. Thrombocytosis can result from a number of disease processes (Table 36–10). These processes can be primary or secondary (reactive) with the latter accounting for the majority (82%) in one study of patients with platelet counts greater than 1 000 000/µL (Buss, 1994).

The concern about patients with such high platelet counts is that complications could arise because of the extreme number of platelets present. Such complications include both thrombotic and hemorrhagic complications. Hemorrhagic complications consist predominantly of mucocutaneous bleeding (Schafer, 1996). Thrombotic complications include both microvascular thrombosis, such as erythromelalgia, and macrovascular thrombosis, such as myocardial infarction. Of cases of macrovascular thrombosis, arterial thrombosis predominates with the most frequent sites including the cerebrovascular, peripheral vascular, and coronary artery circulations (Schafer, 1996). These complications are rare in cases of secondary thrombocytosis (4%), but relatively common in primary causes (56%) (Buss, 1994). Risk factors found to be associated with these complications in primary thrombocytosis are given in Table 36–11.

Because of the concern over the occurrence of these complications, studies have focused on efforts to reduce these elevated platelet counts. Treatments include chemotherapeutic agents such as alkylating agents, radiophosphorus (^{32}P), and hydroxycarbamide (hydroxyurea) as well as other medications such as interferon alpha and Anagrelide (Schafer, 1996). All of these agents have been found to be effective in reducing platelet counts over a period of days to weeks but they also have significant side effects, including leukemogenesis with alkylating agents, ^{32}P, and hydroxycarbamide. As a result, and because of the low risk of complications in patients with secondary disorders, these interventions to reduce platelet count are not used in this setting and the underlying disorder is treated (Buss, 1994). In primary disorders, however, the decision is more difficult and controversial. Still, unless the patient is symptomatic from the elevated platelet count, many

Table 36–10 Diseases Associated with Thrombocytosis (Buss, 1994)

Primary	Essential thrombocythemia
	Agnogenic myeloid metaplasia
	Polycythemia vera
	Chronic myelogenous leukemia
Secondary (reactive)	Splenectomy
	Acute hemorrhage
	Iron deficiency
	Chronic inflammatory diseases
	Solid malignancies
	Rebound after myelosuppression

Reprinted from Am J Med Vol. 96, Buss DH, Cashell AW, O'Connor ML, et al: Occurrence, etiology, and clinical significance of extreme thrombocytosis: a study of 280 cases, pp. 247–253, Copyright 1994, with permission from Excerpta Medica, Inc.

Table 36–11 Factors Associated with Complications in Primary Thrombocytosis (Cortelazzo, 1990; Tefferi, 1994)

Thrombosis	Increasing age
	Previous thrombotic event
	Longer duration of thrombocythemia
Hemorrhage	Platelet count > 2 000 000/µL
	NSAID ingestion

authors recommend not treating. This is in part due to studies that have shown no convincing evidence that reducing the platelet count prevents complications (Schafer, 1984) as well as the fact that the platelet count does not correlate with the risk of thrombosis (Tefferi, 1994).

Therapeutic Plateletpheresis Indications

The role of hemapheresis in the treatment of thrombocytosis is to intervene when patients become symptomatic and to stabilize the patient's condition until medical management reduces the platelet count. As stated previously, platelet count does not correlate with the risk of thrombosis, even when the count is > 1 000 000/µL (Buss, 1994; Schafer, 1984, 1996; Tefferi, 1994). As a result, plateletpheresis should be used to treat those who are symptomatic from their elevated platelet counts. Additionally, plateletpheresis can also be used in the preoperative setting to reduce the platelet count and possibly prevent bleeding and in the treatment of pregnant women (Isbister, 1997). The benefit of plateletpheresis in this latter patient group is again uncertain, as there is a lack of correlation between platelet count and pregnancy outcome (Schafer, 1996). While hemapheresis is an adjunct to therapy and not a primary treatment modality, Baron, et al. did note that apheresis appeared to increase the sensitivity of the patients to busulfan therapy (Baron, 1993). This produced a greater platelet response, but also a greater danger of pancytopenia (Baron, 1993). It must be stressed that the effects of plateletpheresis in thrombocytosis are temporary, lasting hours to days, and medical management must be instituted at the same time.

Plateletpheresis procedures in this setting can be performed on any instrument that can collect platelets from donors. Typically, the goal of the procedure is to process 1–1.5 blood volumes (Baron, 1993) or to process for a defined length of time such as 3 hours (Burgstaler, 1994). In a study comparing apheresis systems' ability to reduce platelet counts, Burgstaler & Pineda found that processing for 3 hours resulted in a 43% reduction of platelet count using the COBE Spectra (Burgstaler, 1994). Just as there is no defined level at which thrombosis occurs, there is no defined target for platelet reduction. The patient's symptoms should be treated with their improvement/resolution being the desired end point.

Thrombocytosis is a category I indication for plateletpheresis according to the American Society for Apheresis (ASFA) (American Society for Apheresis Clinical Applications Committee, 2000).

Therapeutic Leukapheresis
Hyperleukocytosis

Hyperleukocytosis is an extreme elevation in white blood cell count. The causes of such elevations include malignant as well as nonmalignant disease with the former resulting in the highest counts. This can produce a number of syndromes including central nervous system leukostasis, characterized by neurologic deficits, and pulmonary leukostasis, characterized by poor oxygenation and chest pain (Isbister, 1997). Traditionally, the extremely elevated white blood cell counts have been felt to result in increased viscosity with changes in blood flow within the microvasculature. White blood cells, especially granulocytes, are more rigid than red blood cells (Isbister, 1997). It has been felt that, at these very high white blood cell counts, occlusion of the microvasculature can occur, resulting in leukostasis and ischemia. This, however, may not represent the entire picture. White blood cell count does not necessarily correlate with the onset of symptoms. More recent evidence suggests that the interactions of adhesion molecules expressed on the leukemic blasts and endothelial cells may also contribute to vascular occlusion and endothelial injury (Liesveld, 1997; Porcu, 2000; Stucki, 2001).

In addition to vascular occlusive symptoms of hyperleukocytosis, another potential problem resulting from markedly elevated white blood cell counts is the tumor lysis syndrome (Isbister, 1997). This occurs during the patient's initial chemotherapy and results from the release of tumor cell breakdown products producing damage to the kidneys and/or initiating disseminated intravascular coagulation.

Higher mortality rates occur during the first week of therapy among patients with white blood cell counts greater than 100 000/μL. These deaths were associated with a significantly greater number of CNS hemorrhages than in those with white cell counts < 50 000/μL (Dutcher, 1987). Similarly, the presence of pulmonary leukostasis is also associated with early mortality (Lester, 1985). In one study, average survival of patients with pulmonary leukostasis was 0.2 months versus 15.4 months in those with CNS leukostasis and 10.8 months in patients lacking leukostasis (Lester, 1985). As in thrombocytosis, the definitive treatment of these elevated white blood cell counts is to treat the underlying disease, in this case leukemia.

Therapeutic Leukapheresis Indications

As in therapeutic plateletpheresis, the role of leukapheresis in hyperleukocytosis is to decrease the white cell count in order to relieve symptoms and/or prevent tumor lysis syndrome. As with plateletpheresis, the indication for treating a patient is the presence of symptoms indicating leukostasis. Additionally, leukapheresis can be used to treat pregnant women in order to prolong pregnancy until the child can be delivered and the mother started on chemotherapy. Again, hemapheresis represents an adjunct to therapy and not a primary treatment modality. The definitive therapy is chemotherapy that should be begun at the same time or shortly after hemapheresis is initiated, as the reduction in white blood cell counts with leukapheresis is temporary. With this said, two things should be stated. While hemapheresis can reverse or lessen the leukostasis symptoms in some patients, no correlation has been found between the degree of leukoreduction, either as an absolute value or a percentage, and survival (Porcu, 1997). In addition, while leukapheresis may reduce 2-week mortality rates and increase complete remission rates, it does not appear to affect the long-term or overall survivals of these patients (Giles, 2001).

Leukapheresis procedures share similarities with granulocyte collections as previously described. Hydroxyethyl starch (HES) can be used to enhance the separation of the cellular components during centrifugation, resulting in more efficient white cell removal. This is especially important when the cells are more mature granulocytes, such as seen in chronic phase chronic myelogenous leukemia (CML). The total blood volume processed is usually 8–10 liters or two blood volumes (McLeod, 1993). With this strategy, reductions in white blood cell count of 50–85% have been reported (Burgstaler, 1994; Steeper, 1985). As in therapeutic plateletpheresis, there is no defined goal for the reduction of white blood cells, with improvement/resolution of the patient's symptoms being the end point.

Hyperleukocytosis is a category I indication for leukapheresis according to the ASFA (American Society for Apheresis Clinical Applications Committee, 2000).

Therapeutic Erythropheresis

Therapeutic erythropheresis, or red cell exchange (RCE), is a form of cytapheresis that removes the patient's red blood cells and replaces them with allogeneic red blood cells. This form of hemapheresis has occasionally been used to treat hyperparasitemia in malaria (Lercari, 1992; Rouvier, 1988) and other parasitic infections of red blood cells such as babesiosis (Evenson, 1998). It is most commonly used in the treatment of sickle cell anemia.

Sickle Cell Anemia

Sickle cell anemia is an autosomal recessive disorder present in 1 in 200–500 African-American newborns (Wayne, 1993) and is also seen in people from sub-Saharan and Western Africa, Arab countries, the Mediterranean basin, and India (Davies, 1997). It results from a mutation which substitutes a valine for a glutamic acid at position six of the β-globin chain of hemoglobin, producing hemoglobin S (Davies, 1997). This change decreases the solubility of hemoglobin when deoxygenated such that crystals form which alter the shape of the red blood cell and damage its membrane. Repeated episodes lead to irreversible sickling of the cell. Even in the absence of sickling, the red cells in sickle cell anemia are abnormally 'sticky.' The combination of this 'stickiness' and sickling leads to occlusion of small vessels, endothelial damage, and thrombosis (Davies, 1997; Wayne, 1993).

Sickle cell anemia is characterized by chronic hemolytic anemia and crises, episodes of acute illness. The crises are most often due to vascular occlusion and infarction and include crises of pain, aplasia, splenic sequestration, hemolysis, cerebrovascular accidents, acute chest pain syndrome, and priapism. They are treated by correcting factors that enhance sickling, namely dehydration, hypoxia and acidosis. This is done through hydration, alkalinization, and the administration of supplemental oxygen (Davies, 1997; Wayne, 1993). In addition, painful crises are also treated by the administration of analgesics. These crises can also be treated with red blood cell transfusion.

Red cell transfusion in sickle cell anemia can be divided into three categories: acute simple transfusion, chronic simple transfusion, and red cell exchange transfusion. Acute simple transfusion consists of the transfusion of red blood cells to increase oxygen-carrying capacity and is indicated for the treatment of symptomatic anemia, splenic sequestration crisis, aplastic crisis, blood loss, accelerated hemolysis, and preoperative preparation (Wayne, 1993). Chronic simple transfusion consists of regular transfusions of red blood cells in an attempt to suppress endogenous red cell production with the goal of keeping the percentage of red cells containing hemoglobin S below 30%. This form of therapy is indicated for cerebrovascular disease and debilitating vaso-occlusive symptoms. It can also be used to treat sickle cell disease complicated by pulmonary disease, cardiac disease, high-risk pregnancy, and preoperative preparation (Wayne, 1993).

RCE in sickle cell anemia is used to remove the hemoglobin S-containing red blood cells, replacing them with hemoglobin A-containing red cells. The goal of RCE is to leave the patient with a hematocrit of approximately 30% and a 'sicklecrit,' the percentage of cells containing hemoglobin S, less than 30% (Davies, 1997; Wayne, 1993). In order to do this, the fraction of red cells remaining (FCR) must be calculated based upon the patient's current hemoglobin S percentage and the desired hemoglobin S percentage. This can be calculated by Equation 36–5. If the patient's hematocrit is to be increased by the procedure, then the adjusted FCR must be calculated according to Equation 36–6 (COBE BCT, 1997). It should be noted that increasing the hematocrit too much can result in decreased oxygen delivery due to increased viscosity. This results from the fact that the sickle cells as well as the endothelium of these patients are 'stickier' than normal.

Table 36–12 Benefits of Red Blood Cell Exchange by Apheresis Compared to Simple or Chronic Transfusion (American Society for Apheresis Clinical Applications Committee, 2000)

Decreased amount of hemoglobin S without increasing hematocrit and, therefore, viscosity

Use of fewer units of red blood cells to achieve the same percentage of hemoglobin S

Decreased contribution to iron overload in chronically transfused patients

American Society for Apheresis Clinical Applications Committee: Clinical applications of therapeutic apheresis, McLeod BC, Copyright © 2000 J Clin Apheresis 15:1–5. Reprinted with permission of Wiley-Liss, Inc., a subsidiary of John Wiley & Sons, Inc.

$$\text{Desired FCR\%} = (\text{Desired hemoglobin S/Current hemoglobin S}) \times 100 \quad (36\text{–}5)$$

$$\text{Adjusted FCR\%} - \text{Desired FCR\%} \times (\text{Current hematocrit/Desired hematocrit}) \times 100 \quad (36.6)$$

These are then entered into the hemapheresis instrument along with other values to determine the volume of red blood cells necessary to perform the procedure. The benefits of RCE over the other strategies of transfusion are given in Table 36–12.

Acute chest syndrome is a crisis characterized by respiratory symptoms, chest and abdominal pain, infiltrates on chest radiograph, and an abnormal chest examination. It is thought that pain from rib splinting or fat embolism results in hypoventilation leading to atelectasis. This, in turn, causes hypoxia leading to occlusion of small vessels in the lung and possible thrombosis of the pulmonary arteries (Davies, 1997). It occurs in 20–50% of sickle cell patients and has a mortality rate of 2–14%. Repeated episodes may progress to chronic pulmonary disease (Wayne, 1993). RCE is used to remove the hemoglobin S-containing cells and has been associated with marked improvement in patients (Wayne, 1993).

Priapism is a painful, sustained erection and results from occlusion of vessels in the corpus cavernosum by sickled cells. It is associated with dehydration and acidosis. It is treated with supplemental oxygen, hydration, and analgesics (Wayne, 1993). If prolonged, over 6 hours, it is referred to as fulminant priapism and may require surgical intervention or RCE. A significant percentage of these patients will suffer from impotence if not treated (Davies, 1997). While RCE has been reported as effective in treating priapism, it is not without risks. A syndrome of neurologic events called ASPEN syndrome (association of sickle cell disease, priapism, exchange transfusion, and neurologic events) has been reported to occur in some patients treated with RCE. It consists of neurologic events ranging from headache and seizure activity to obtundation requiring ventilator support. The syndrome is thought to be due to decreased cerebral blood flow from the abrupt elevation in hematocrit as well as the release of vasoactive substances from the penile detumescence. Aggressive treatment has been associated with complete neurologic recovery (Siegel, 1993). Patients suffering from priapism undergoing RCE should be monitored for the symptoms of ASPEN syndrome.

Additional crises and disorders in sickle cell patients for which RCE is indicated include cerebrovascular accident, retinal artery vaso-occlusion, hepatic failure, and septic shock. RCE has also been used to decrease the percentage of hemoglobin S at the initiation of chronic simple transfusion therapy, to prevent sickling due to contrast dye during cerebral angiograms, and in preparation for surgery (Wayne, 1993). It should be noted that a study has shown no benefit of RCE versus a conservative transfusion regimen designed to increase the hemoglobin to 10 g/dL in preventing complications of surgery (Vichinsky, 1995).

Sickle cell anemia is a category I indication for erythropheresis according to the ASFA. Malaria and other parasitic diseases are category III indications (American Society for Apheresis Clinical Applications Committee, 2000).

Photopheresis

Photopheresis, also called extracorporeal photochemotherapy (ECP), is a form of leukapheresis. In this procedure, a small percentage of a patient's white blood cells are collected by intermittent flow hemapheresis. These cells are then treated by incubation with a psoralen compound and then exposed to ultraviolet A (UVA) irradiation within the instrument. Following this, the cells are reinfused into the patient (Zic, 1999). This then appears to result in an immunomodulatory effect. Depending upon the disease being treated, this may either stimulate or suppress an immune response. Currently, this therapy is approved by the FDA only for the treatment of cutaneous T cell lymphoma (CTCL).

Table 36–13 Characteristics Indicating Best Responders to Photopheresis among CTCL Patients (Zic, 2003)

Erythrodermic skin stage

WBC count < 15 000/mm^3

Disease of short duration

Normal percentage of CD8 cells

Immunocompetent patient

Absence of bulky lymph nodes or visceral disease

Presence of Sézary cells in the circulation

Photopheresis Indications

Cutaneous T cell Lymphoma. The first disease treated by photopheresis was cutaneous T cell lymphoma (CTCL). CTCL is a skin-based T cell lymphoma characterized by a long premalignant phase (4–10 years) of eczematous skin lesions. Following this, the disease progresses through a series of phases characterized by increasing skin involvement until the development of the tumor phase, characterized by cutaneous masses. CTCL may then progress to a leukemic phase known as Sézary syndrome where malignant T cells are found circulating in the blood. Median survivals depend upon the stage of the disease at diagnosis with 10-year survivals ranging from 20% for the tumor stage to 85% for the initial plaque phase (Zic, 1999).

In 1987, Edelson et al. reported responses in 64% of 37 CTCL patients treated with photopheresis. Subsequently, the use of photopheresis for the treatment of CTCL received FDA approval in 1988 (Zic, 2003). Combined analysis of over 400 patients reported in the literature has found an overall response rate of CTCL to photopheresis of 55.7% with 17.6% of patients having a complete response. Response rates vary from 64% for stage IB patients (generalized patches and plaques) to 27.3% for stage IVB (visceral involvement) (Zic, 2003). Factors predictive of response to photopheresis are given in Table 36–13. The median time until clearing of skin lesions in such patients is 11 months, with patients showing early response (clearing in 6–8 months) maintaining their response (Zic, 1999). Photopheresis has also been associated with longer survival from time of diagnosis (greater than 60 months among photopheresis-treated patients versus 31 months for patients receiving chemotherapy) (Christensen, 1991).

The mechanism of action of photopheresis in CTCL has not been completely elucidated. Photopheresis is known to induce a CD8+ T cell response toward expanded pathologic T cell clones within the patient (Zic, 2003). It is thought that this is due to the fact that upon exposure to UVA, 8-methoxypsoralen (8-MOP) reacts with cellular constituents, irreversibly binding to DNA, proteins, and lipids. This induces an increase in the number of HLA class I molecules present on the exposed cell as well as apoptosis. Interestingly, apoptosis occurs in exposed lymphocytes, including the malignant T cells, but not monocytes. The monocytes, due to their exposure to subphysiologic temperatures and contact with the walls of the tubing during collection and photoactivation, differentiate into immature dendritic cells (DC). These DC are then capable of phagocytosing the apoptotic malignant T cells and can then present the tumor antigens from these cells within their HLA class I molecules. Upon reinfusion of the UVA-exposed leukapheresis product, these antigen-presenting cells can then activate cytotoxic T cells, resulting in an immune response toward the abnormal T cell clones (Zic, 2003). This is associated with a shift in the patient's cytokine profile from that of a Th2 response to a Th1 response (Zic, 2003). The beneficial effects of the procedure do not result from the direct cytotoxicity of the 8-MOP and UVA on abnormal T cells or tumor cells as only 10–15% of the lymphocyte pool is harvested and less than 5% of cutaneous T cell lymphoma cells are treated (Christensen, 1991).

CTCL is a category I indication for photopheresis according to the ASFA (American Society for Apheresis Clinical Applications Committee, 2000).

Graft-Versus-Host Disease and Solid Organ Rejection. Chronic graft-versus-host disease (cGVHD) occurs in 27–50% of matched related sibling donor transplants and 42–72% of unrelated bone marrow or peripheral blood stem cell transplants (Foss, 2002). Factors associated with cGVHD are given in Table 36–14.

A number of studies have reported the use of photopheresis in cGVHD (Foss, 2002). In these studies, patients with cGVHD unresponsive to other therapies have shown improvement in skin, oral, and visceral (hepatic) lesions. These have been associated with normalization of CD4/CD8 ratios and decreased numbers of NK cells. Treatment allowed for tapering of steroid doses and maintenance of the response for a median of 12 months. There was no increase in infection rates or CMV activation in the patients studied (Foss, 2002). Those patients that were more likely to respond were those who started therapy within 10 months of transplant.

IV

Table 36–14 Factors Associated with the Development of Chronic Graft-Versus-Host Disease (Foss, 2002)

Increased donor age
Increased recipient age
HLA disparity
Unrelated donor
Prior acute GVHD
Alloimmunized female donor

Table 36–15 Diseases in which Photopheresis has been Reported as Effective (van Iperen, 1997; Zic, 1999)

Malignancy	Cutaneous T cell lymphoma (CTCL)
Graft-vs.-host disease	Mucocutaneous GVHD
	Hepatic GVHD
Organ rejection	Heart
	Kidney
	Lung
Autoimmune diseases	Systemic lupus erythematosus
	Rheumatoid arthritis
	Juvenile dermatomyositis
	Pemphigus vulgaris
	Epidermolysis bullosa acquisita
Infectious diseases	Chronic Lyme arthritis
	Aids-related complex (ARC)
Other diseases	Severe atopic dermatitis
	Psoriasis

As with CTCL, the mechanism behind photopheresis in cGVHD is unclear. It is remarkable that a therapy associated with immune activation in one disease is associated with immune suppression in another. In cGVHD patients, photopheresis is associated with a decrease in antigen recognition and processing by DC as well as decreased numbers of DC. This, in turn, decreases CD8 stimulation with a shift in Th1 response to a Th2 response through the inhibition of Th2 cytokine secretion (Foss, 2002). The result is decreased alloreactivity by T cells.

As with cGVHD, solid organ rejection is also a disorder of alloreactive T cells. Photopheresis has similarly been used to treat rejection in heart, lung, kidney, and liver transplant. In cardiac transplantation, the use of photopheresis has been reported to histologically reverse 89% of treated rejection episodes without side effects. Similar rates have been reported with other transplant types (Dall'Amico, 2002).

GVHD has not been categorized for photopheresis by ASFA (American Society for Apheresis Clinical Applications Committee, 2000). Solid organ rejection is a category III indication for photopheresis (American Society for Apheresis Clinical Applications Committee, 2000).

Other Diseases. Additional diseases that have been treated with photopheresis are listed in Table 36–15. These diseases have a common thread of T cell allo- or autoreactivity.

Photopheresis Procedure

The photopheresis procedure is performed using the UVAR XTS (Therakos, Inc., Exton PA). Following venipuncture, either 125 mL or 225 mL of whole blood is collected in a Latham centrifuge bowel where the components are separated. Heparin or acid-citrate-dextrose (ACD) can be used as the anticoagulant. The buffy coat is retained in a collection bag and the remaining blood components are returned to the patient. As this is an intermittent centrifuge, six cycles (125 mL bowl) or three cycles (225 mL bowl) of whole blood collection are performed in order to collect a 270 mL mononuclear cell (MNC) suspension. This consists of 80 mL of plasma, 90 mL of saline, and 100 mL of MNC. After completion of the collection, 8-MOP is added to the bag. The MNC suspension is then pumped through a photoactivation chamber. This consists of transparent acrylic plates between which is sandwiched a tortuous channel. Adjacent to the plate is a UVA light source that irradiates the 8-MOP-containing buffy coat. The MNC suspension is photoactivated for 30 minutes. Following the completion of photoactivation, the buffy coat is then reinfused. The total time necessary to perform a treatment is approximately 3 hours (Zic, 2003). A typical course of photopheresis consists of two treatments on consecutive days every 4 weeks (Christensen, 1991). Following improvement in disease

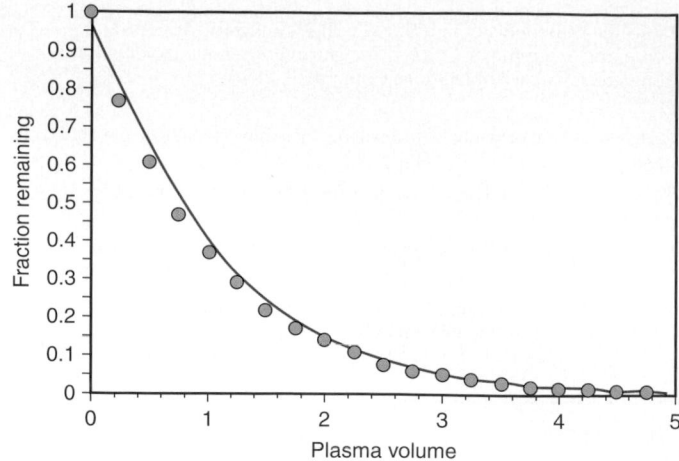

Figure 36–2 Removal of substances during plasma exchange. The removal of substances limited to the intravascular compartment, whether pathologic or normal can be predicted by an exponential equation (see Equation 36–7). A fixed percentage of the remaining substance is removed with each blood volume. This means that as the number of blood volumes processed increases, a progressively smaller amount of the substance is removed resulting in diminishing returns.

symptoms, the interval between procedures may be prolonged and the patient weaned from photopheresis.

An important aspect of this procedure is the clean separation of the whole blood into plasma and buffy coat. The product must allow the transmission of UVA light in order to photoactivate the 8-MOP. The presence of significant numbers of red blood cells within the leukapheresis product will reflect or absorb the UVA irradiation resulting in failure to photoactivate the product. As a result, it is critical that the hematocrit of the leukapheresis product be less than 7% (Zic, 1999). Similarly, it is important that excess plasma also not be present. Excess plasma will dilute the white blood cells, resulting in fewer passages of each cell through the photoactivation chamber (Zic, 1999).

Patients undergoing photopheresis are sensitive to sunlight (Knobler, 1993). They should avoid direct or indirect sunlight exposure for 24 hours following the completion of the procedure by covering exposed skin, using sunscreen, and wearing wrap-around UV protective eye wear. Another possible complication of photopheresis could be mutagenesis from DNA damage caused by the photoactivation of the 8-MOP. This theoretically could result in the reinfusion of cells with damaged DNA still capable of cell division. These cells could then give rise to hematologic malignancies. While evidence has not been found to support this concern, it is still a theoretical risk of the procedure (van Iperen, 1997).

Therapeutic Plasmapheresis

Efficacy of Removal

The goal of therapeutic plasmapheresis, better known as plasma exchange, is to remove a pathologic substance present within the plasma by removing the patient's plasma and replacing it with a substitution fluid. The removal is nonspecific in that all of the substances present in the plasma, including normal substances, are removed. The removal of a substance can be predicted by Equation 36–7 as shown in Figure 36–2 (Derksen, 1984b):

$$Y/Y_0 = e^{-x} \tag{36–7}$$

where Y = the final concentration of the substance, Y_0 = the initial concentration of the substance, and x is the total number of times the patient's volume is exchanged.

This model assumes that the intravascular compartment is closed and that exchange between the intra- and extravascular compartments does not occur. Based upon this equation, 30% of the initial quantity of a substance will remain within the patient's plasma after one plasma volume exchange and 10% will remain after the exchange of two plasma volumes. As more plasma volumes are exchanged, a fixed portion of the remaining substance is removed such that a smaller and smaller amount is removed. As can be seen in Figure 36–2, the marginal benefit of removing additional plasma volumes declines after 1.5–2 plasma volumes, so most therapeutic plasma exchange procedures are limited to 1–1.5 plasma volume exchanges.

The assumption that no exchange occurs between the intravascular and extravascular compartments during the procedure is not valid for all substances. As a result, the amount removed as well as the concentration in the plasma at the end of the procedure may not match that predicted.

For example, IgM is located predominantly within the intravascular space (76%) with influx from the extravascular space being negligible (Derksen, 1984b). As a result, during a plasmapheresis procedure the equation will accurately predict the removal of IgM. IgA, however, is evenly distributed between the intravascular space and the extravascular space and can move between the two compartments. During plasma exchange, as the concentration of IgA within the intravascular space falls, IgA within the extravascular space follows its concentration gradient and moves into the intravascular space. The result of this is that following the procedure, the plasma concentration of IgA is not as low as predicted and would lead one to believe that the procedure was not as efficient as expected (Derksen, 1984b). If one looks at the amount of substance removed by measuring the IgA within the collection bag, one would see that the total amount of IgA removed was greater than predicted and that the procedure was more efficient than expected. Not only was IgA being removed from the intravascular compartment but it was also being removed from the extravascular compartment (Derksen, 1984b).

Four patterns of removal in plasma exchange using 5% albumin as the replacement fluid have been identified. In the first pattern, seen with fibrinogen and C3, the concentration decreases greater than expected. This is probably due to the combination of removal and consumption of these factors during the hemapheresis procedure. In the second pattern, such as with IgM, cholesterol, and alkaline phosphatase; the change in concentration is what is predicted. These are substances confined to the intravascular space or with little exchange between compartments. In the third pattern, as seen with lactate dehydrogenase (LDH) and creatinine phosphokinase (CPK), the concentration is less than predicted due to movement of these substances between compartments. Finally, in the fourth pattern, concentrations are much greater than predicted or do not change at all and are due to rapid equilibration. This pattern is seen with small inorganic and organic molecules such as potassium, bicarbonate, and glucose (Orlin, 1980).

The pattern of removal of immunoglobulins during plasma exchange depends upon whether it is a normal immunoglobulin or a paraprotein. The removal of normal IgG has been reported to be predictable by Equation 36–7; it behaves as if it is entirely intravascular (Chopek, 1980; Orlin, 1980). Others, however, have reported behavior similar to a substance equilibrating between the two compartments (Derksen, 1984b). In the case of paraproteins, the removal of immunoglobulins may appear to be half of what is expected when looking at plasma concentrations (Chopek, 1980). This difference is attributed to expansion of the patient's plasma volume due to the presence of the paraprotein (Chopek, 1980). In other words, the plasma volume of the patient is greater than what is predicted by standard equations (e.g., Equation 36–3) such that if these are used to calculate a 1.5 plasma volume exchange, the real volume exchanged will be less.

In addition to the effect on the removal of the substance from the plasma, the distribution between the intravascular and extravascular compartments and the ability to move between these compartments will also influence the rise in plasma levels of the substance following plasma exchange. The concentration of substances that diffuse rapidly and have a large extravascular component will rise rapidly. The increase in the concentration of those substances that are predominantly intravascular will depend upon the rate of synthesis of the substance. Most substances return to normal levels within 48–72 hours. Exceptions to this include fibrinogen, complement, and immunoglobulins where mean recoveries at 48 hours were 65%, 65%, and 44% of initial values respectively. Cholesterol also shows a slow recovery with 67–72% of pre-apheresis values achieved 1 week after hemapheresis (Orlin, 1980).

For the majority of substances removed by plasma exchange, the rate of synthesis does not increase following the procedure (Derksen, 1984a). For some substances, especially the immunoglobulins, rebound may occur. Rebound is an increase in concentration following a procedure to a level greater than that seen initially (Dau, 1995; Derksen, 1984a). This may result from the removal of inhibitory substances by the procedure or removal of negative feedback on the responsible cell. As a result of this, concurrent treatment with cytotoxic agents during the procedure is suggested in order to prevent rebound (Dau, 1995). In addition, plasma exchange may enhance the efficacy of cytotoxic agents by increasing metabolic activity of autoreactive immune cells, making them more sensitive to such agents (Dau, 1995). Another point related to this is that plasma exchange will only temporarily decrease the level of a pathologic substance unless additional therapy is instituted to stop its production. This means that in most cases, plasma exchange should be viewed as an adjunct to other therapies.

Replacement Fluids

In therapeutic plasmapheresis, 1–1.5 plasma volumes are removed and therefore this volume must be replaced with another fluid. A number of replacement fluids are available, each of which has advantages and disadvantages. Replacement fluids used in plasma exchange include 5% albumin, fresh frozen plasma (FFP), cryo supernatant plasma (cryopoor plasma), saline, and hydroxyethyl starch (HES).

Albumin in a concentration of 5% is the most widely used replacement fluid. It is a hyperoncotic fluid for most patients and will therefore result in the net flow of fluid from the extravascular space. This can result in a mild dilutional anemia (Chopek, 1980). The main advantage of 5% albumin is that it does not transmit viral diseases. Disadvantages, however, are that it is expensive and has at times been in short supply because of FDA-mandated recalls. Hypotensive reactions due to prekallikrein activation (Alving, 1978) and febrile reactions due to pyrogens have been reported (Pool, 1995). Both of these reactions are rare. In addition, the albumin may not function comparably to the albumin present in the plasma before exchange. While exchange with 5% albumin provides physiologic concentrations of the protein, the drug and metabolite binding sites of this albumin are occupied by preservatives such as sodium caprylate and may not be available for normal physiologic functions (Koch-Weser, 1976). The standard practice is to use a 5% albumin solution for 60–70% of the replacement volume. The remaining volume is replaced by crystalloid (normal saline).

FFP is used as the primary replacement fluid in treating thrombotic thrombocytopenic purpura (TTP) (see discussion of this disease) and may also be used to prevent the dilutional coagulopathy seen with repeated plasma exchanges. FFP can also be used in the treatment of severe factor XI deficiency in a patient known to bleed from this defect who is to undergo a surgical procedure. As a concentrate for factor XI is not available and the quantity of FFP that would need to be infused to reach therapeutic levels would cause volume overload, exchange with FFP immediately prior to the surgical procedure can provide hemostasis. The advantages of FFP are that it is relatively inexpensive and provides physiologic concentrations of coagulation factors. The disadvantages are the danger of transmission of transfusion-transmitted viral diseases, transfusion reactions, the need to have an ABO compatible product, and an increase in the frequency of citrate reactions (see discussion at the end of the chapter). This last disadvantage results from the fact that the patient is infused not only with citrate anticoagulant but also the citrate within the FFP. When used to treat TTP, 60–70% of the replaced volume will be FFP with the remainder being normal saline. When used to prevent coagulopathy, two units of FFP can be given at the end of the procedure with the majority of the replacement volume being 5% albumin.

Cryopoor plasma is also used in the treatment of TTP, specifically in those unresponsive to plasma exchange with FFP. The advantages and disadvantages of cryopoor plasma are the same as those for FFP with the exception that cryopoor plasma does not provide physiologic concentrations of all coagulation factors, lacking fibrinogen and factor VIII.

Saline is used for a portion of most plasma exchange procedures (30–40%) as it is used to prime the instrument as well as to make the anticoagulant solution. The use of saline for greater volumes is problematic in that it is a crystalloid and not a colloid and can redistribute into the extravascular space resulting in hypotension and edema following the procedure. The advantages of saline are that it is inexpensive and does not carry the risks of transmitting disease.

The final option is the use of synthetic colloidal fluid such as hydroxyethyl starch (HES). HES is derived from plant starches and consists of large starch molecules that can be added to saline to generate a colloidal solution. Plasma exchanges using HES as the replacement fluid have been described (Burgstaler, 1990; Rock, 1997). The benefits of HES are that it is inexpensive and does not transmit disease. A disadvantage is that a small percentage of individuals will have allergic reaction to the HES (see discussion at end of chapter). Also, the high-molecular-weight HES hetastarch has a half-life of 25.5 hours, so significant amounts can persist after frequent plasma exchange procedures resulting in volume expansion and alterations in partial thromboplastin time, total protein, albumin, hematocrit, and fibrinogen (Rock, 1997). These changes are less frequent with pentastarch, a low-molecular-weight HES, because of its shorter half-life. HES has also been associated with changes in hemostasis (Rock, 1997), but is an alternative replacement solution for those who have reactions to albumin or FFP (Burgstaler, 1990). It can also be used in those who require plasma exchange but whose religious beliefs preclude the use of replacement fluids derived from blood.

Patient Concerns

Plasma exchange is a nonselective method of removing substances from plasma and as a result, many of the concerns about patients undergoing plasma exchange involve the removal of unintended substances such as therapeutic drugs and coagulation factors. Despite the fact that

IV

Table 36–16 Effect of Plasma Exchange on Medications as Reported in the Literature (Balogun, 2001; Hale, 2000; Hausfater, 2002; Kale-Pradhan, 1997; Mansur, 1995; McClellan, 1997; Przepiorka, 1994)

Medications that do not require dose supplementation because of insignificant removal, redistribution from tissue stores, or drug binding to red blood cells

Digoxin

Digitoxin

Prednisone

Prednisolone

Ciclosporin

Tacrolimus

Propranolol

Valproic acid

Phenobarbital

Ceftriaxone

Ceftazidime

Vancomycin

Medications that may require dose supplementation

Phenytoin*

Tobramycin

Interferon-α

* Monitoring of unbound phenytoin is necessary to determine the amount of supplementation, as total concentrations will lead to an overestimation (Kale-Pradhan, 1997). Mansur, et al. noted a rebound in plasma phenytoin levels 30 minutes after plasma exchange with a return to pre-apheresis levels at 120 minutes. As a result of this, signs of phenytoin toxicity could be seen despite a decrease in total body phenytoin levels (Mansur, 1995).

plasmapheresis has been a treatment modality for a variety of diseases for almost 30 years, little information is available with regard to its effects on therapeutic drugs. Theoretically, drugs which are highly protein or lipid bound should be efficiently removed by plasmapheresis. As in the discussion previously, the volume of distribution also influences the removal of a drug. For example, a highly protein bound drug which is predominantly limited to the intravascular compartment should be efficiently removed while a highly protein bound drug that is distributed throughout the body will not be efficiently removed. A poorly bound drug will also not be efficiently removed.

The effect of plasmapheresis on drug concentrations can be determined by calculating the drug half-life during plasma exchange (Sketris, 1986). These calculations could then be used to determine the necessary additional dosing that might be needed following plasma exchange. This has not been done with the majority of medications. The effect of plasma exchange on a variety of medications is given in Table 36–16. From a practical standpoint, since plasma exchange may remove a portion of a drug dose, drugs that are given once daily should be withheld until after the procedure, if possible. Drugs that are administered more often should also be scheduled so that they are not given directly prior to plasmapheresis.

Another possible way in which plasmapheresis and therapeutic drugs may interact is through the removal of enzymes necessary for metabolism and proteins necessary for transport. Plasma pseudocholinesterase is removed during plasmapheresis and as a result, neuromuscular blockade agents such as succinyl choline or mivacurium may have a prolonged effect in patients who have recently undergone plasma exchange (Naik, 2002; Wood, 1978). Such agents should be avoided immediately following plasma exchange.

Following plasma exchange using 5% albumin as a replacement fluid, decreases in the levels and activities of coagulation factors (Flaum, 1979; Orlin, 1980) as well as abnormal coagulation tests (Flaum, 1979) have been seen. Flaum et al. demonstrated significant decreases in the levels of factors V, VII, VIII, IX, X, and von Willebrand factor (vWF) activity following plasma exchange. These deficits returned to normal by 24 hours following plasma exchange with the exceptions of factors VIII, IX, and vWF activity, which had returned to normal at 4 hours (Flaum, 1979). Orlin & Berkman noted reductions in fibrinogen levels to 25% of pre-apheresis levels. Fibrinogen levels had reached 66% of pre-apheresis levels at 72 hours (Orlin, 1980). These studies indicate that a risk of bleeding exists in hemostatically challenged patients following plasmapheresis. This is especially true in patients undergoing serial procedures on consecutive days where sufficient time for recovery of hemostatic levels may not be possible. At-risk patients, such as those who have undergone or will undergo surgical procedures or biopsies in proximity to their plasma exchange, may require FFP as a portion of their replacement fluid. This should be given at the end of the procedure in order to prevent its removal.

In addition to an increased risk of bleeding, an increased risk of thrombosis is also possible. Because of the nonspecific nature of removal, inhibitors of coagulation, such as antithrombin, are also removed during plasma exchange (Chirnside, 1981; Volkin, 1982). This could theoretically lead to thrombosis.

Finally, platelets are also lost during therapeutic plasma exchange (Perdue, 2001). In a study of 71 patients undergoing therapeutic plasma exchange with the COBE Spectra, Fresenius AS104 (Fresenius HemoCare, Redmond WA), or the Haemonetics LN9000 (Haemonetics, Braintree, MA), platelet losses ranged from 0–71% (Perdue, 2001). Factors found to influence platelet losses included the instrument used, with the Fresenius AS104 having the greatest losses (18.6% vs. 2.6% and 1.6% for the Haemonetics LN9000 and the COBE Spectra respectively), as well as the disease for which patients are being treated. Of the patients treated in the study, those with hyperviscosity syndromes due to dysproteinemias had the greatest losses (Perdue, 2001). In this study, however, no bleeding complications occurred (Perdue, 2001). The greater losses with the Fresenius AS104 in comparison with the COBE Spectra were felt to be due to differences in g force and dwell time between the two instruments (Burgstaler, 2001).

Procedures for Selective Removal of Plasma Components

As previously discussed, plasmapheresis is nonselective. Each plasma exchange removes approximately 150 g of plasma proteins (110 g of albumin and 40 g of globulin) (Lysaght, 1985; Randerson, 1982) in order to eliminate 1–2 g of pathologic substance (Randerson, 1982). With repeated plasma exchanges, this can result in bleeding due to loss of coagulation factors, and immunodeficiency due to the loss of immunoglobulins. If other replacement fluids are used, additional risks may be present including disease transmission and allergic reactions. Because of these disadvantages, a number of procedures have been developed to selectively remove a plasma component, allowing the return of the patient's 'cleansed' plasma. The benefits of such procedures are that depletion of normal plasma components and the need for substitution fluids are avoided. The drawbacks to such procedures are that they are more expensive to perform than plasma exchange because of the costs of the selective removal columns.

Selective removal procedures most often involve an initial separation step where the cellular elements of whole blood are separated from the plasma. The plasma is then perfused through the selective removal device where the substance of interest is removed by chemical, physical, or immunological means. The treated plasma is then recombined with the cellular components and reinfused. The selective removal device may then be regenerated with the bound substance being removed and diverted to a waste collection bag. Following this, the selective removal device is used to treat additional plasma. If the device cannot be regenerated, then it is discarded. Examples of selective removal procedures are discussed in the following sections.

Staphylococcal A Protein Columns

Staphylococcal A protein is a bacterial cell wall component that can bind IgG molecules by their Fc receptor. In addition, it can also bind to an Fab domain encoded by the variable heavy chain (VH) clan III gene family (Matic, 2001). It strongly binds IgG1, IgG2, and IgG4 but variably binds IgG3, IgM, and IgA. Two types of staphylococcal A protein columns are available, the staphylococcal protein A-agarose (PAA) column (Immunosorba, Fresenius HemoCare, Redmond WA) and the staphylococcal protein A-silica (PAS) column (Prosorba, Fresenius HemoCare, Redmond WA). For both columns, patient's plasma is separated from the cellular elements using some other instrument, such as a centrifugal or filtration apheresis instrument. The plasma is then perfused through the columns.

The PAS column, once saturated, cannot be regenerated and is discarded, limiting the amount of plasma that can be treated to 2 L (Matic, 2001). The PAA column, however, can be perfused with an eluent buffer of pH 2.2 that removes the bound immunoglobulin. The eluent buffer is then flushed from the column with a buffer of pH 7.0 and the column is then available to treat additional plasma. The PAA column is used in a two-column system. The first column is perfused with plasma until it is saturated. Then the plasma flow is directed to the second column while the first is regenerated. This allows an unlimited volume of plasma to be

Table 36-17 Diseases Reported to Have Been Treated with Staphylococcal Protein A Columns (Levy, 2003; Matic, 2001)

Rheumatoid arthritis

Immune thrombocytopenic purpura (ITP)

HIV-related ITP

Alloimmune and autoimmune factor VIII and IX inhibitors

Anti-basement membrane disease (Goodpasture's syndrome)

Wegener's granulomatosis

Focal segmental glomerulosclerosis

Chemotherapy-induced thrombotic thrombocytopenic purpura (cTTP)

Refractory TTP

Systemic lupus erythematosus

Myasthenia gravis

Acute demyelinating polyneuropathy (Guillain–Barré syndrome)

Platelet alloimmunization

Solid malignancies

Table 36-18 Indications for Use of LDL Apheresis

Functional hypercholesterolemic homozygotes with an LDL cholesterol > 500 mg/dL

Functional hypercholesterolemic heterozygotes with an LDL cholesterol ≥ 300 mg/dL*

Functional hypercholesterolemic heterozygotes with an LDL cholesterol ≥ 200 mg/dL and documented coronary artery disease*

---

* A 6-month trial of maximal drug therapy and an American Heart Association Step II diet must be tried prior to the initiation of therapy.

---

treated but requires the use of a separate monitoring system (Citem 10, Fresenius HemoCare Redmond WA) to assure regeneration of the columns and to prevent the return of the eluent buffer to the patient. The PAA columns can be reused for up to 20 treatment sessions (Matic, 2001).

The mechanism of action of the PAA column is thought to be due to the binding of immunoglobulins with their removal (Matic, 2001). The mechanism of action of the PAS column is more complex. In addition to removing free immunoglobulin, the PAS column also removes circulating immune complexes. The total amount of immunoglobulins and complexes removed, however, may be very small and would not explain the efficacy of the procedure. It is felt that as opposed to simply removing substances, treatment with the PAS column produces immune modulation that allows the immune system to respond to the underlying disorder. This is thought to be mediated by a number of possible mechanisms. First, the presence of small immune complexes is thought to induce immune suppression, as these complexes cannot be removed by the reticuloendothelial system (RES) and result in an excess of antigen relative to antibody. By removing these, the antigen–antibody excess is reduced, removing the immune suppression. Second, when the IgG binds to staphylococcal protein A, complement is fixed. The generation of complement fragments in the column that are then infused into the patient may activate the immune system. Third, staphylococcal A protein is a T and B cell mitogen. Protein eluted from the column during the treatment may result in the proliferation of T and B cells. Finally, autoantibodies are thought to be controlled within the human body by anti-idiotypic antibodies. These are antibodies that bind to the Fab portion of the autoantibody. Treatment with the PAS column has been shown to result in an increase in anti-idiotypic antibodies. This could be due to changes in autoantibody conformation and immune complex size leading toward a greater immunogenicity of these antibodies (Levy, 2003).

The PAA column is FDA approved, under a humanitarian device exemption, for the treatment of factor VIII and IX inhibitors. The PAS column is FDA approved for the treatment of immune thrombocytopenic purpura (ITP) refractory to standard therapy, and rheumatoid arthritis (Matic, 2001). Additional diseases that have been treated with the PAA and PAS columns are given in Table 32-17. ITP and rheumatoid arthritis are category II indications for immunoadsorption according to the ASFA. Hemophilia with inhibitors has not been categorized by ASFA (American Society for Apheresis Clinical Applications Committee, 2000).

The use of staphylococcal A protein columns has been associated with a number of side effects. The types of side effects and the severity vary according to the column used. Side effects associated with the PAA column include musculoskeletal pain, nausea, vomiting, and hypotension. These effects have been seen with 26–30% of procedures (Huestis, 1996). Side effects with the PAS column include fever and chills, nausea, vomiting, pain, hypotension, dyspnea, allergic reactions, headache, hypertension and tachycardia. Reactions have been reported to occur in 34% of procedures (Huestis, 1996). It is thought that these reactions result from a number of mechanisms. As previously described, the binding of IgG to staphylococcal A protein fixes complement and many of these reactions could be explained by the infusion of activated complement fragments such as C5a. Other possible causes could be contamination of the column and subsequent infusion of endotoxin as well as leaching of staphylococcal A protein (Huestis, 1996). Most reactions are mild, starting up to 1 hour following treatment and lasting 1–2 hours. Severe reactions, including

death, have been reported more commonly with the PAS column than with the PAA column. The four patterns of severe reactions seen with the PAS column include anaphylaxis, vasculitis, large vessel thrombosis, and exacerbations of underlying disease (Huestis, 1996).

Selective Removal of Low-Density Lipoproteins

Plasma exchange or selective removal of low-density lipoproteins (LDL), also called LDL-apheresis, is indicated for the treatment of familial hypercholesterolemia in homozygotes as well as in heterozygotes unresponsive to drug therapy (Thompson, 1995). This disorder results in accelerated atherosclerosis due to the inability of the liver to clear LDL cholesterol from the blood. Criteria for the selection of patients to undergo either of these treatment options have been published (Gordon, 1994). Criteria for the treatment of patients with LDL apheresis are given in Table 36–18. Comparison of the life expectancy of patients treated with these techniques and their untreated siblings (Thompson, 1985) as well as series (Kamanabroo, 1988) and case reports (Leren, 1993) of treated patients have been reported. Significant reductions in cholesterol, improvements in xanthomas, disappearance of ECG abnormalities, regression of coronary artery lesions, improvement in exercise tolerance, and prolongation of life span have been seen (Kamanabroo, 1988; Leren, 1993; Matsuzaki, 2002; Thompson, 1985). A number of methods are available for the selective removal of LDL.

The first method is secondary or double filtration plasmapheresis. LDL is one of the largest plasma components and as such, filters can be constructed to allow its removal. In secondary filtration, plasma is separated from whole blood either by centrifugation, filtration or the combination of the two. The plasma is then passed through a second filter with pore size too small to allow the passage of the LDL. The resulting plasma filtrate contains 83% of the albumin, 68% of the IgG and 47% of the HDL cholesterol present in the original plasma. The filter, however, retains 94% of the LDL cholesterol, 92% of IgM, and 90% of fibrinogen. In comparison to plasma exchange, secondary filtration produced a similar decrease in LDL cholesterol but resulted in a smaller loss of HDL cholesterol (Leitman, 1989).

A second method of LDL-apheresis is heparin-induced extracorporeal low-density lipoprotein precipitation (HELP) (B Braun Medical Inc., Bethlehem PA). In this technique, plasma is separated from whole blood using a hollow fiber separator. A sodium acetate buffer of pH 4.84 containing heparin is added to the plasma to precipitate the LDL. This is then removed by filtration, with the heparin being adsorbed from the plasma by a diethylaminoethyl cellulose filter. The acetate and extra volume are then removed through bicarbonate dialysis/ultrafiltration. The treated plasma is then combined with the cellular elements and returned to the patient (Bambauer, 2003). Results of treatment in one trial demonstrated reductions in LDL cholesterol of greater than 30% with reductions in HDL and fibrinogen of 15 and 58% respectively (Lane, 1993).

A third method of removal is dextran sulfate absorption (Liposorber, Kaneka, Osaka, Japan). In this method two columns of dextran sulfate are used to continuously remove LDL cholesterol. Plasma is separated from whole blood using a hollow fiber separator and pumped through the dextran sulfate column. Treated plasma is then mixed with the cellular elements and returned to the patient. In the column, the negatively charged dextran sulfate interacts with the positively charged apolipoprotein B-100 of the LDL molecule, resulting in its removal. When the first column becomes saturated, flow is switched to the second column while the first is rinsed with 4.1% NaCl to remove the LDL cholesterol. Following this, the column is filled with heparin-containing normal saline and is ready to be used again (Bambauer, 2003). Studies using this system have demonstrated a 53% reduction of cholesterol with one plasma volume exchange (Thompson, 1995) as well as a 36% reduction in fibrinogen and a 5% loss of HDL (Schulzeck, 1992).

IV

Table 36-19 Conditions for which Plasmapheresis is Accepted

Neurologic disorders	Acute inflammatory demyelinating polyneuropathy (AIDP)
	Chronic inflammatory demyelinating polyneuropathy (CIDP)
	Myasthenia gravis
Hematologic disorders	Thrombotic thrombocytopenic purpura
	Hyperviscosity syndrome
Metabolic disorders	Familial hypercholesterolemia
Other disorders	Anti-basement membrane antibody disease (Goodpasture's syndrome)
	Cryoglobulinemia
	Glomerulonephritis
	Conditioning for renal transplant

The fourth method of LDL removal is immunoadsorption (Therasorb-LDL, Miltenyi Biotec, Cologne, Germany). In this system, two columns containing agarose beads covalently linked to sheep polyclonal anti-human apolipoprotein B-100 antibodies are used. Similarly to other methods, one column is perfused with plasma as the second one is regenerated. In this case, a glycine/HCl buffer is used to remove the bound ApoB-containing LDL (Bambauer, 2003). A study of the use of this form of LDL-apheresis demonstrated its ability to maintain cholesterol at levels of 165 mg% as well as to increase HDL (Richter, 1993).

The final available method is lipoprotein hemoperfusion (DALI, Fresenius, St. Wendel, Germany). This system consists of columns that contain polyacrylate-coated polyacrylamide beads. Like dextran sulfate, these beads are negatively charged resulting in the binding of the positively charged ApoB-containing LDL. For this column, plasma separation need not occur, as anticoagulated whole blood can be passed through the column. Unlike the systems previously described, the column is not regenerated but used only once. Different sizes of columns are available to treat different blood volumes (Bambauer, 2003; Bosch, 2001a).

Of the systems described previously, the dextran sulfate system and the HELP system are currently FDA approved for use in the US. Comparisons of these systems have shown similar reductions in LDL cholesterol, Lp(a), HDL, and other plasma components (Bambauer, 2003; Jovin, 1996; Matsuda, 1994; Parhofer, 2000) with the reductions in HDL, fibrinogen and other plasma components being less than that seen with plasma exchange. The systems have also demonstrated similar reaction rates but differ in cost and simplicity of operation (Matsuda, 1994).

Some systems, such as the HELP system and secondary filtration, remove additional plasma components such as fibrinogen. Because of the removal of large macromolecules other than LDL, these systems have been used to alter the blood flow characteristics in certain disease states. This form of apheresis has been referred to as rheophoresis. These devices have been used to treat age-related macular degeneration (Klingel, 2003), sudden sensorineural hearing loss (Suckfull, 1999, 2002), stroke (Jaeger, 1999), and myocardial ischemia (Jaeger, 1999).

Familial hypercholesterolemia is a category I indication for LDL apheresis according to the ASFA (American Society for Apheresis Clinical Applications Committee, 2000).

Therapeutic Plasmapheresis Indications

Table 36-19 lists selected disorders for which plasma exchange is indicated and which will be briefly discussed.

Neurologic Disorders

Acute Inflammatory Demyelinating Polyneuropathy. Guillain–Barré syndrome (GBS) is a neurologic disorder of immune origin. It is the most frequently encountered paralytic disorder (Ropper, 1992; Guillain–Barré Syndrome Study Group, 1985). It affects males more frequently than females and is more common with increasing age (Hughes, 1993). The disorder is characterized initially by leg weakness, which progresses proximally to involve the arm, face, and oropharyngeal muscles (Ropper, 1992). Sensory loss is mild but may include paresthesias of fingers and toes. Disease progression stops by the third week of the illness and then improves after a variable period of stability (Ropper, 1992).

The pathophysiology of GBS is thought to be one of antibody-mediated damage to peripheral nerve myelin followed by inflammatory response. Complement-fixing antibodies to peripheral myelin have been identified in patients (Koski, 1985). The titers of these antibodies correlate with the clinical course of the patients (Koski, 1986) as well as the response to plasmapheresis and relapse following plasmapheresis (Vriesendorp, 1991). Treatment of GBS consists of supportive care to provide adequate nutrition, ventilatory support, and avoidance of infection and pulmonary embolism (Ropper, 1992). IVIG is also beneficial to the treatment of GBS (Plasma Exchange/Sandoglobulin Guillain–Barré Syndrome Trial Group, 1997) but corticosteroids are not (Hughes, 1978) and may interfere with the response to hemapheresis (Mendell, 1985).

Plasma exchange is associated with improvement in disability, greater likelihood of recovering function, and a shortened course (Guillain–Barré Syndrome Study Group, 1985). Unfortunately, patients requiring ventilation support for several days before initiation of plasmapheresis are not likely to benefit immediately from the procedure. However, they have been found to have a shorter course of ventilator dependency (Guillain–Barré Syndrome Study Group, 1985). Plasmapheresis should be initiated within 14 days of the onset of symptoms (Plasma Exchange/Sandoglobulin Guillain–Barré Syndrome Trial Group, 1997; Guillain–Barré Syndrome Study Group, 1985) and should consist of five to six procedures over 8–13 days (Plasma Exchange/Sandoglobulin Guillain–Barré Syndrome Trial Group, 1997; Guillain–Barré Syndrome Study Group, 1985). Replacement fluid should be albumin. Treatments should continue for at least 10–14 days as cessation of plasmapheresis during the active phase of the disorder is characterized by relapse (Ropper, 1988). Ten percent of patients may relapse 16–21 days after therapy (Ropper, 1988).

A review of the Cochrane Neuromuscular Disease Group Register summarized the results of randomized and quasi-randomized trials of plasma exchange versus sham exchange or supportive therapy (Raphael, 2002). A total of six trials involving 649 patients were identified which fulfilled criteria for evaluation. According to the authors of the review, the results showed that TPE is the 'first and only treatment that has been proven to be superior to supportive treatment alone' (Raphael, 2002). In addition, the authors found that TPE was most effective if started within 7 days of disease onset; two sessions of TPE are superior to none in mild AIDP, four sessions are superior to two in moderate AIDP, and six sessions are no better than four in severe AIDP (Raphael, 2002).

AIDP is a category I indication for plasma exchange according to the ASFA (American Society for Apheresis Clinical Applications Committee, 2000).

Chronic Inflammatory Demyelinating Polyneuropathy. Chronic inflammatory demyelinating polyneuropathy (CIDP) is a neurologic disorder, probably of autoimmune origin, characterized by progressive or relapsing motor and/or sensory peripheral nerve dysfunction involving more than one limb and developing over 2 months (Cornblath, 1991). Hypo- or areflexia are also present, with nerve conduction studies indicating demyelination, and nerve biopsy showing demyelination and remyelination (Cornblath, 1991). Other causes of polyneuropathy, such as toxin exposure, must be excluded. Patients demonstrate a male predominance with the peak age of onset occurring in the 5th and 6th decades (Dyck, 1975). Patients typically present with burning dysesthesias, muscle pain, and shooting pains as well as distal muscle weakness (Dyck, 1975). The pathophysiology is thought to be immune-mediated damage to peripheral nerve myelin causing demyelination and subsequent nerve degeneration. Evidence in support of an immune mechanism includes the presence of demyelination in monkeys when given patient derived immune globulin (Heininger, 1984), deposition of immunoglobulin in nerve biopsies (Dalakas, 1980a), and monoclonal IgG in the CSF of some patients (Dalakas, 1980b). Some CIDP patients respond to corticosteroids but are prone to the complications of these medications because of the need for long-term treatment (Dyck, 1975). Intravenous immune globulin (IVIG) has also been found to be beneficial (van Doorn, 1990), especially in a select group of patients demonstrating specific findings (van Doorn, 1991).

The first double-blind, sham-controlled crossover study of plasma exchange in CIDP demonstrated an improvement in 5 of 15 patients undergoing two procedures per week for 3 weeks. The benefit of the therapy gradually disappeared 10–14 days following discontinuation (Dyck, 1986). A more recent study involving more frequent procedures (four the first week, three the second week, two the third week, and one the fourth week) demonstrated improvement in 80% of patients, usually becoming apparent on the 3rd to 6th days of treatment (Hahn, 1996). Unfortunately, 66% of responders relapsed after stopping therapy (Hahn, 1996). Comparison of plasmapheresis and IVIG has demonstrated similar rapid responses with both treatment modalities (Dyck, 1994). Therapy usually consists of an initial intensive course of four to six procedures over 2 weeks followed by one to two treatments per week or at longer intervals as tolerated. Improvement is usually seen within a week (Hahn, 1996) but only lasts 2 weeks (Dyck, 1986). Five-percent albumin is used as the replacement fluid.

CIDP is a category I indication for plasma exchange according to the ASFA (American Society for Apheresis Clinical Applications Committee, 2000).

Myasthenia Gravis. Myasthenia gravis (MG) is an autoimmune disorder characterized by weakness of voluntary muscle groups. It may involve only the extraocular muscles or be generalized, involving appendicular and trunk muscles. The presence of bulbar muscle weakness can lead to aspiration in the setting of a weakened diaphragm. This can result in severe respiratory compromise and was the major cause of death in these patients in the past. MG is caused by autoantibodies directed against the acetylcholine receptor on the motor endplate. These autoantibodies prevent the normal functioning of the receptor by increasing receptor turnover, blocking the binding of acetylcholine, and fixing complement with degradation of the receptor (Lindstrom, 1976; Maselli, 1994). The disorder can be associated with other autoimmune phenomena and is associated with thymic abnormalities including thymoma (Sanders, 1994). The treatment of myasthenia gravis is directed toward increasing the amount of acetylcholine at the motor endplate through the use of acetylcholine esterase inhibitors such as pyridostigmine and neostigmine, as well as decreasing the antibody production through immunosuppressive medications such as corticosteroids or azathioprine (Sanders, 1994). In addition, intravenous immune globulin (IVIG) has also been used to treat MG with beneficial effects and has been found to produce effects similar to plasma exchange (Gajdos, 1997).

Plasma exchange is performed to lower the level of anti-acetylcholine receptor antibody, though it has also been reported to be successful in the 10–15% patients with symptoms of MG who do not have detectable antibody. Intensive courses of plasma exchange are recommended for those patients with MG that have severe disease with impaired respiratory function, swallowing, and locomotion (Sanders, 1994) as well as to prepare patients for thymectomy or surgery (Iwasaki, 1993). This may consist of 1–1.5 plasma volume exchanges performed daily for 5–6 days (Dau, 1977). Patients with stable chronic disease who experience mild exacerbations can be treated with shorter courses, 2–3 plasma exchanges (Antozzi, 1991), and some patients can be treated with as few as 1–4 exchanges per month (Dau, 1980). The course of therapy should be individualized to the needs of the patient. Five-percent albumin is used as the replacement fluid. Concurrent immunosuppressive therapy is also performed to prevent rebound of the antibody (Dau, 1977).

Myasthenia gravis is a category I indication for plasmapheresis according to the ASFA (American Society for Apheresis Clinical Applications Committee, 2000).

Hematologic Disorders

Thrombotic Thrombocytopenic Purpura. Thrombotic thrombocytopenic purpura (TTP) is a disorder characterized by thrombocytopenia, microangiopathic hemolytic anemia, neurologic dysfunction, fever, and some degree of renal dysfunction. Laboratory abnormalities, in addition to thrombocytopenia, include schistocytes and nucleated red blood cells on peripheral smear as well as an elevated lactate dehydrogenase (LDH). While it has been assumed that the elevation in LDH is due to the hemolysis, a study of 10 patients has demonstrated that in the majority of patients, it is of hepatic origin (Cohen, 1998). TTP can also be divided into primary (idiopathic) and secondary TTP. Causes of secondary TTP include systemic lupus erythematosus (Nesher, 1994), bone marrow transplant (Pettitt, 1994), ciclosporin (Wiener, 1997), pregnancy (McCrae, 1997), ticlopidine (Bennett, 1998), HIV infection (Hymes, 1997), and a number of chemotherapeutic agents.

Primary TTP can be divided into several variants. Idiopathic initial episode TTP consists of a single episode not associated with any other cause. Intermittent TTP is characterized by relapses following the initial episode. Chronic relapsing TTP also consists of recurring episodes but these begin during childhood and recur at predictable intervals (Moake, 1995).

Histologic study of tissue from patients with TTP has demonstrated the presence of platelet thrombi within the microvasculature. Immunohistochemistry has demonstrated these to consist of platelets and von Willebrand factor (vWF) with little fibrin (Asada, 1985). In addition, studies have shown that early in the course of TTP, unusually large multimers of vWF (UL vWF) circulate in the patient's plasma (Moake, 1989). These multimers have an increased affinity for glycoprotein Ib-IX on platelets and are thought to induce platelet aggregation under high shear stress conditions. Normally, these UL vWF multimers are located within the endothelium and when released into the circulation are cleaved into smaller fragments by a metalloprotease called ADAMTS13 (Levy, 2001a). It has been demonstrated that in patients with idiopathic initial TTP, intermittent TTP, and ticlopidine-associated TTP, an autoantibody is present that decreases ADAMTS13 enzyme activity (Furlan, 1998a,b; Rice, 1998; Tsai, 1998). In chronic relapsing TTP, ADAMTS13 activity has been shown to be absent without the presence of an autoantibody representing a genetic deficiency in enzyme production (Furlan, 1997). This congenital syndrome of TTP is also known by the eponym of Schulman–Upshaw syndrome. Other than in patients with ticlopidine-induced TTP, and possibly HIV-induced TTP, neither autoantibodies nor a deficiency in ADAMTS13 enzyme activity appears to be involved in secondary TTP. A study of bone marrow transplant-associated TTP showed normal ADAMTS13 activity (van der Plas, 1999). It is postulated that endothelial damage in many of the secondary cases results in a release of UL vWF that may overwhelm protease activity. Similarly, studies of patients suffering from diarrhea-associated hemolytic uremic syndrome (HUS) also show normal ADAMTS13 activity (Tsai, 2001).

The primary treatment of TTP is plasmapheresis. Prior to the use of plasma exchange, the mortality rate of TTP was 95%. Following the widespread use of plasma exchange, the mortality rate has decreased to 15% (Rock, 1991). The mechanism of plasmapheresis is thought to be the combination of autoantibody removal, UL vWF removal, and ADAMTS13 infusion. An alternative therapy to plasma exchange is plasma infusion. In most cases, however, this is not as effective as plasma exchange (Rock, 1991). This is due to the fact that the volume of plasma that can be infused is limited by the ability of the patient's cardiovascular system to withstand the volume. Coppo et al. studied large-volume plasma infusion compared to plasma exchange. In their trial, they sought to infuse as much plasma as was given during a plasma exchange. They demonstrated no significant difference with regard to outcome between patients randomized to plasma exchange or plasma infusion. They did, however, see greater complications in the plasma infusion group due to volume overload, and 8 of the 19 patients in that arm had to be switched to plasma exchange because of this complication (Coppo, 2003). There are two settings in which plasma infusion is indicated in the treatment of TTP. First, patients with a genetic deficiency of ADAMTS13 as expressed as chronic relapsing TTP can be given regular fresh frozen plasma infusion to prevent exacerbation. In addition, plasma infusion can be used to treat a patient while arrangements are being made to perform plasma exchange. Additional therapies for TTP include antiplatelet medications (Amorosi, 1977), vincristine (Gutterman, 1982), splenectomy (Crowther, 1996), IVIG (Centurioni, 1995), ciclosporin (Hand, 1998), and corticosteroids (Bell, 1991).

The treatment of TTP consists of daily plasma exchange of 1–2 volumes using FFP as a replacement fluid until the platelet count is greater than 100 000–150 000/μL, the LDH is normalizing, and there is no evidence of neurologic dysfunction (Bell, 1991; Dawson, 1994). If the patient remains stable for 24–48 hours on plasma exchange, then tapering can be started by performing apheresis every other day (Dawson, 1994). It should be noted, however, that the benefits of tapering have not been proven (Bandarenko, 1998) and at some centers this is not done. Because patients may have an abrupt worsening of signs and symptoms with a longer course following early cessation of plasma exchange (Bell, 1991), many recommend tapering. Regardless, close monitoring of neurologic status, platelet count, and LDH should be performed during and after plasma exchange. In patients not responding to plasma exchange with FFP, switching to cryo supernatant-poor plasma as the replacement fluid may be beneficial and has been shown to induce remission in some patients (Rock, 1996). This is thought possibly to be due to the lack of vWF in cryo supernatant-poor plasma. Because of this finding, a frequent question is whether cryo supernatant-poor plasma should be routinely used as the replacement fluid in plasma exchange for TTP. The North American TTP Group performed a multi-institutional prospective randomized trial comparing FFP and cryo supernatant-poor plasma as replacement fluids in primary TTP during initial presentation. This trial showed the two replacement fluids to be equivalent in this population (Zeigler, 2001). In addition, cryo supernatant-poor plasma is not routinely available in many blood centers as it is discarded as a by-product of cryoprecipitate production.

While plasma exchange is effective in treating idiopathic TTP, its role in secondary cases lacking deficiency of ADAMTS13 is uncertain. Studies of plasmapheresis in the setting of bone marrow transplant-induced TTP have shown it to be ineffective (Sarode, 1995).

TTP is a category I indication for plasmapheresis according to the ASFA (American Society for Apheresis Clinical Applications Committee, 2000).

Hyperviscosity Syndrome. Hyperviscosity syndrome is characterized by mental status changes, a bleeding diathesis involving the mucosa and gastrointestinal tract, retinopathy with hemorrhage and papilledema, and hypervolemia with congestive heart failure (Foerster, 1993b). Hyperviscosity syndrome occurs in less than 5% of multiple myeloma patients but in as many as 70% of patients with Waldenström's macroglobulinemia (Foerster, 1993b). It may rarely be seen with polyclonal increases in immunoglobulin. The differences in frequencies in plasma cell disorders are due to the differences in the monoclonal proteins produced in these two diseases. In multiple myeloma, the immunoglobulins produced are usually either IgG or IgA, while in Waldenström's macroglobulinemia the protein is IgM. In hyperviscosity syndrome, the presence of large concentrations of paraprotein increases blood viscosity by causing sludging of the red blood cells and results in occlusion of the microcirculation with organ ischemia (McGrath, 1976). Symptoms usually occur when the viscosity increases to 4–6 Ostwald units (normal blood viscosity is 1.5–1.8 Ostwald units), but patients may be asymptomatic at very high protein concentrations and viscosities (Bloch, 1973). While the viscosity is dependent upon the concentration, demonstrating an exponential relationship (Bloch, 1973), it is also dependent upon the nature of the protein. The exponential nature of the relationship between concentration and viscosity means that after a critical concentration, small changes result in a large increase or decrease in viscosity.

The treatment of hyperviscosity syndrome is twofold. First, the long-term goal is to decrease paraprotein production with chemotherapy. The second goal is to decrease the protein concentration and improve blood flow. This second goal can be achieved with plasmapheresis by exchanging 1–1.5 plasma volumes with either 5% albumin or equal volumes of albumin and saline. In hyperviscosity syndrome due to an IgM monoclonal protein, one to two plasma exchanges may be sufficient to remove enough protein to improve viscosity, as IgM is located almost entirely within the intravascular space. With IgG or IgA paraproteins, the immunoglobulin is also present within the extravascular space and more procedures may be necessary to decrease the paraprotein levels. The goal of therapy should be relief of symptoms, with the subsequent frequency tailored to the needs of the patient. In instances of Waldenström's macroglobulinemia resistant to therapy, repeated plasmapheresis alone has been used to control hyperviscosity for extended periods of time, as long as 17 years (Salmon, 1997). It should be noted that because of the presence of extravascular immunoglobulin in multiple myeloma, patients might experience hypovolemia following procedures as oncotic pressure results in the movement of fluid from the intravascular space.

Hyperviscosity is a category II indication for plasmapheresis according to the ASFA (American Society for Apheresis Clinical Applications Committee, 2000).

Myeloma Kidney

Myeloma kidney occurs in multiple myeloma patients who excrete free light chains, Bence Jones proteins, in their urine. It is characterized by acute renal failure with the expected laboratory findings. It occurs in 3–9% of multiple myeloma patients (Bear, 1980; Johnson, 1980; Solling, 1988) and is associated with a poor prognosis. Myeloma kidney is caused by the filtration of monoclonal light chains with deposition in the renal tubules. This eventually leads to the dilation of the tubules as well as tubular atrophy and renal failure (Bernstein, 1982; Cohen, 1984; DeFronzo, 1978). Unlike hyperviscosity syndrome, the amount or characteristics of the light chain do not correlate with the disease. The diagnosis of myeloma kidney is made by renal biopsy. Prevention of the development of this complication is through treatment of the underlying disease. Additional treatment includes alkalization of the urine to enhance excretion of the protein.

Plasma exchange is used in the treatment of myeloma kidney to decrease the amount of light chains present. While this can also be accomplished with dialysis, plasmapheresis has been found to be more effective (Bear, 1980; Johnson, 1980; Solling, 1988). While renal failure in multiple myeloma is associated with poor prognosis, two controlled trials (Johnson, 1990; Zucchelli, 1984) have demonstrated recovery of renal function in some patients on dialysis by using the combination of chemotherapy and plasmapheresis. In myeloma kidney, the plasma exchange is performed daily to three times per week for 1–4 weeks until renal function improves. Subsequent therapy is performed as needed to maintain renal function (McGrath, 1976).

Myeloma kidney is a category II indication for plasmapheresis according to the ASFA (American Society for Apheresis Clinical Applications Committee, 2000).

Nephrologic Disorders

Anti-Basement Membrane Antibody Disease. Anti-basement membrane antibody disease (Goodpasture's syndrome) is a rare disorder characterized by the combination of pulmonary and renal hemorrhage. It affects men more commonly then women, and is most frequent between 18–35 years of age. The disorder is autoimmune with an antibody directed against type IV collagen within the glomerular and pulmonary basement membrane. The antibody is usually transient and may be triggered by damage to the respiratory system, as the syndrome is frequently preceded

by an infectious or chemical insult. Patients usually present with pulmonary symptoms of cough, hemoptysis, and dyspnea. Laboratory values show evidence of renal failure and renal inflammation. Mortality rate may be as high as 50%. The treatment of Goodpasture's syndrome focuses on suppressing the antibody production and inflammation as well as removing the antibody. The former goals are accomplished through the use of immunosuppressive agents such as cyclophosphamide and prednisone (Wiseman, 1993).

Plasmapheresis is used to remove the anti-basement membrane antibody. Treatment consists of 1–1.5 volume exchanges using 5% albumin for replacement. Therapy is usually performed daily for 7–14 days and, in the presence of concurrent immunosuppression, results in decreased antibody levels and clinical improvement (Erickson, 1979; Johnson, 1985; Pusey, 1983). As the antibody is only transiently present, treatment longer than 6 months is uncommon (Pusey, 1983). It should be noted that plasma exchange should be started early, as recovery of renal function is unlikely once scarring and atrophy of glomeruli and tubules occur (Johnson, 1978). Patients who present needing dialysis, who have a creatinine > 6.8 mg/dL, who are oliguric and who have 100% crescentic glomeruli on renal biopsy are unlikely to benefit from plasma exchange (Levy, 2001b). In this setting, plasma exchange may be reserved for the onset of pulmonary hemorrhage (Levy, 2001b). Patients with a creatinine of < 5.7 g/dL and who have less than 50% crescentic glomeruli on renal biopsy have overall and 'renal' survivals at 1 year of 100% and 95% respectively (Levy, 2001b).

Anti-basement membrane antibody disease is a category I indication for plasmapheresis according to the ASFA (American Society for Apheresis Clinical Applications Committee, 2000).

Cryoglobulinemia. Cryoglobulins are immunoglobulins that reversibly precipitate at cold temperature. Three categories of cryoglobulins exist. Type I cryoglobulin consists of a single monoclonal protein and is usually seen in multiple myeloma, Waldenström's macroglobulinemia or other lymphoproliferative disorders. Usually, the immunoglobulin is IgG or IgM (Foerster, 1993a). Type II cryoglobulin consists of a mixture of polyclonal immunoglobulins with a monoclonal protein, usually IgM, directed toward polyclonal IgG. Type II cryoglobulinemia is associated with chronic hepatitis C infection, autoimmune disorders, and IgM-producing malignancies (Foerster, 1993a). Finally, Type III cryoglobulin consists of polyclonal immunoglobulins, usually IgM, that have activity toward polyclonal IgG. They are associated with autoimmune conditions as well as infections (Foerster, 1993a). Cryoglobulins produce symptoms by precipitating in areas of low temperature, such as the skin or extremities, resulting in vascular occlusion. This produces a wide variety of symptoms including acrocyanosis, Raynaud's phenomenon, skin ulcers, skin purpura, and glomerulonephritis (Foerster, 1993a).

Cryoglobulin precipitation is dependent upon the concentration of the immunoglobulin. As the concentration of the immunoglobulin increases, the temperature at which the protein precipitates rises (Hillyer, 1996). As a result, some patients may experience symptoms with only small decreases in temperature such as those occurring in the distal extremities when patients are exposed to the outdoor environment.

The treatment of cryoglobulinemia is directed at the underlying disease (Berkman, 1980). In addition, plasma exchange can be used to reduce the protein concentration and thereby decrease the temperature at which precipitation occurs (Berkman, 1980; McLeod, 1980). Treatment usually consists of 1–1.5 volume exchange using 5% albumin. Again, the intensity, duration, and frequency of therapy are determined by patient symptoms. As these proteins precipitate at room temperature, blood warmers (both on the draw and return lines) may be necessary to prevent precipitation in the apheresis instrument. In some patients with high cryoglobulin concentrations and the resulting precipitation at higher temperatures, it may be necessary to perform the hemapheresis procedures at room temperatures of 37°C or higher to prevent precipitation (Hillyer, 1996).

Cryoglobulinemia, with or without polyneuropathy, is a category II indication for plasmapheresis according to the ASFA (American Society for Apheresis Clinical Applications Committee, 2000).

Glomerulonephritis. Many of the glomerulonephritides result from the deposition of antigen–antibody complexes within the glomeruli leading to glomerular damage. These complexes, as well as their constituent components, can be found circulating within the bloodstream. Because of this, it is theoretically possible for plasmapheresis to be used to remove these substances and thereby halt and possibly reverse further glomerular injury. A number of glomerulonephritides have been treated with plasmapheresis. As with many of the diseases treated by hemapheresis, investigations have been limited to case studies and small case series without randomized, controlled trials. The treatment of some selected glomerular kidney diseases is given in Table 36–20.

Table 36–20 Glomerulonephritides Treated with Plasma Exchange

Disease	ASFA/AABB category*	Putative substance removed	Reported efficacy
Primary focal segmental glomerulosclerosis (Bosch, 2001b)	NC/NC	50 kD permeability factor	Partial or complete remission of proteinuria in 44% of patients
Recurrent focal segmental glomerulosclerosis following renal transplant (Bosch, 2001b)	III/III	50 kD permeability factor	Long-term remission in 44% of adults and 74% of children
Lupus nephritis (Mistry-Burchardi, 2001)	NC/IV	Antinuclear antibodies, anti-DNA antibodies	No benefit over immunosuppression either alone or as adjunct therapy
Pauci-immune rapidly progressive glomerulonephritis (Gaskin, 2001)	NC/NC	Antineutrophil cytoplasmic antibodies (ANCA)	Possible benefit when renal function is impaired to the point where dialysis is required
IgA nephropathy (Chambers, 1999)	NC/NC	IgA	No conclusive evidence supporting the use in rapidly progressive glomerulonephritis due to IgA nephropathy

* See Table 36–8 for explanation of ASFA/AABB categories. NC = not classified.

Conditioning Therapy for Renal Transplantation

Kidney transplantation represents the current optimum therapy for chronic renal failure. Unfortunately, the supply of deceased donor kidneys is inadequate to meet the need for organs in the US with 50 000 people listed on the United Network for Organ Sharing (UNOS) deceased donor kidney waiting list (United Network for Organ Sharing, 2000). The waiting time for deceased donor kidney transplantation exceeds 4 years (United Network for Organ Sharing, 2001). If a patient is blood group O or blood group B, the average waiting time is even longer. In addition, 5000 of the 50 000 listed on the waiting list have panel reactive alloantibodies (PRA) > 80% (United Network for Organ Sharing, 2000). Fewer than 300 of these patients are transplanted each year, with many of the most highly sensitized patients requiring a perfect HLA-matched kidney. Because so few of these highly sensitized patients receive deceased donor kidneys, a waiting time cannot be calculated for this group (Stegall, 2002).

While these individuals await an ABO compatible or HLA compatible deceased donor kidney, their medical condition deteriorates. This wait is associated with a 5–8% mortality rate per year. Attempts to transplant ABO incompatible or crossmatch incompatible kidneys have, in the past, been associated with the development of hyperacute rejection. The preformed ABO isoagglutinins or anti-HLA antibodies bind to target antigens present upon the vascular endothelium of the incompatible organ at the time of reperfusion of the graft. The result is fixation of complement followed by endothelial injury, thrombosis, and occlusion of the microvasculature of the organ resulting in immediate loss of the organ. In order to circumvent hyperacute rejection and increase the availability of organs, a number of protocols have been developed which use plasmapheresis or immunoabsorption in combination with immunosuppression to reduce ABO isoagglutinin or anti-HLA antibody titers. These protocols have been reported to allow successful transplantation of incompatible kidneys from living donors.

Tanabe et al. used three to four immunoabsorption procedures and/or one to two double filtration plasmapheresis procedures in an attempt to reduce ABO isoagglutinin titers to less than 16 prior to transplantation of ABO incompatible living donor kidneys. This treatment, in conjunction with intensive immunosuppression and splenectomy at the time of transplantation, resulted in no instances of hyperacute rejection among 67 patients. Patient survival among ABO incompatible transplant recipients was equivalent to that of ABO compatible recipients. Graft survival was significantly less up to 3 years after transplant (79%) but showed equivalence at 4 years after transplant and beyond (Tanabe, 1998). Our group reported on the use of four plasma exchanges prior to transplant to reduce isoagglutinin titers to less than 4. This, and an intensive immunosuppression regimen with splenectomy, allowed for successful transplantation without hyperacute rejection among 26 ABO incompatible transplants (Winters, 2004). One-year graft and patient survivals were slightly lower than ABO compatible transplants performed during the same time period (89 vs. 96% and 94 vs. 99% respectively) (Gloor, 2003b).

Plasma exchange is associated with reductions in isoagglutinin scores and titers at the time of transplantation (Aikawa, 2001; Winters, 2004). Following transplant, however, titers will rise to levels greater than those seen at transplant but less than those seen initially (Aikawa, 2001; Winters, 2004). In addition, ABO antigen levels are maintained on the graft

(Aikawa, 2001). Despite these increases in antibody titers, rejection episodes are limited to the early transplant course and can be reversed with plasmapheresis and increased immunosuppression (Winters, 2004). Studies have suggested that 'accommodation' occurs in the setting of ABO incompatible kidney transplantation (Delikouras, 2003). This appears to be due to active self-protection of the graft through the alteration of gene expression (Park, 2003).

ABO incompatible organ transplantation is not categorized according to the ASFA (American Society for Apheresis Clinical Applications Committee, 2000).

A number of groups have reported success in transplanting crossmatch incompatible living donor kidneys using the combination of plasmapheresis, intravenous immunoglobulin (IVIG), immunosuppression, and splenectomy (Gloor, 2003a; Montgomery, 2000; Schweitzer, 2000). Four to six plasma exchanges with concurrent immunosuppressive therapy and IVIG were successful in converting patients with low-titer anti-HLA antibodies (< 16) to crossmatch compatibility on the day of transplantation. None of the patients treated developed hyperacute rejection. Acute humoral rejection episodes were seen in 43% of the patients treated by Gloor et al. but these episodes were reversed with additional plasmaphereses and steroids (Gloor, 2003a). Graft survivals of 100% (Schweitzer, 2000) and 79% (Gloor, 2003a) have been reported at 12 months following transplantation. Unlike ABO incompatible transplants, there have been reports of durable, sustained loss of donor-specific HLA antibodies following conditioning for and transplantation of crossmatch incompatible kidneys (Zachary, 2003). In addition, as in ABO incompatible accommodated transplants, crossmatch incompatible accommodated transplants demonstrate altered gene expression that results in the downregulation of apoptosis of the graft's endothelial cells (Salama, 2001).

Plasmapheresis for crossmatch incompatible renal transplantation has not been categorized by ASFA (American Society for Apheresis Clinical Applications Committee, 2000).

Donor/Patient Complications Common to all Hemapheresis Procedures

Hemapheresis procedures, both donor and therapeutic, are safe procedures with minimal risks of complications. The reaction rate among donors undergoing hemapheresis procedures has been found to be 2.18% (McLeod, 1998) and 0.81% (Despotis, 1999) by McLeod and Despotis et al. respectively. This is less than the 11–21% reaction rate reported for whole blood donation (Newman, 1997). However, the rate of serious reactions, those requiring hospitalization, has been found to be 0.01% (2 out of 19 736 donations) (Despotis, 1999) which is 20 times greater than that reported to occur with allogeneic whole blood donation (1 out of 198 119 donations, 0.0005%) (Popovsky, 1995). Therefore, while apheresis donation appears to have a lower reaction rate than whole blood donation, the risk of serious reactions is greater.

The most common of reactions seen by McLeod among apheresis donors were injuries due to venipuncture (McLeod, 1998). Table 36–21 lists the adverse effects to apheresis donation reported by McLeod, their frequency, and the comparable frequency among whole blood donors. As with whole blood donation, first time donors had reactions more frequently than repeat donors. Interestingly, reactions were found to be more frequent

IV

Table 36–21 Reaction Rates among Apheresis (McLeod, 1998) and Whole Blood (Newman, 1997) Donors

Reaction	Apheresis donations	Whole blood donations
Hematoma or pain	1.15%	9–16%
Citrate toxicity	0.4%	NA
Mild vasovagal	0.05%	2–5%
Vasovagal with syncope	0.08%	0.1–0.3%

Table 36–22 Reaction Rates among Patients undergoing Therapeutic Apheresis Procedures (McLeod, 1999)

Reaction	Frequency
Transfusion reactions	1.6%
Citrate toxicity	1.2%
Hypotension	1.0%
Vasovagal reactions	0.5%
Pallor and diaphoresis	0.5%
Tachycardia	0.4%
Respiratory distress	0.3%
Tetany and seizure	0.2%
Chills or rigors	0.2%

among platelet donors than either plasma or granulocyte donors (5.9 and 9.4% respectively versus 12%) and may have been due to a greater number of first time donors in this group (McLeod, 1998). Despotis et al. found associations of citrate and hypotensive reactions and donor weight, gender, and the type of collection instrument used. For venipuncture-related complications, only female gender was associated as a risk factor (Despotis, 1999). The instrument used for the collection also influenced reaction rates. McLeod found that the Fenwal CS3000 had fewer reactions than other instruments. This could possibly be due to lower citrate infusion rate with this instrument as well as the ability to perform single needle procedures with the other instruments. Such single needle procedures, which alternate between drawing and returning through the single intravenous line, result in larger extracorporeal volumes (McLeod, 1998). Despotis et al. noted that the relationship between donor weight and citrate reactions was different when comparing the COBE Spectra and the Fenwal CS3000. Donors with lower weights had a higher probability of citrate reactions on the Fenwal CS3000 while those with higher weights had a higher probability on the COBE Spectra. The authors of this study felt that this was due to the methods by which these instruments determine the anticoagulant infusion rate (Despotis, 1999).

Reactions among therapeutic hemapheresis procedures have been reported to occur in 4.75% of procedures (McLeod, 1999). The reactions identified and their overall frequencies are given in Table 36–22. The rate of reactions varied with regard to procedure, replacement fluid, and patient. For example, the reaction rates for plasma exchange using albumin was 3.35% as compared to 7.81% for plasmapheresis using plasma as the replacement fluid. Leukapheresis demonstrated a reaction rate of 5.71%, HPC collection had a rate of 1.66%, and no reactions occurred in the 18 patients who underwent therapeutic plateletpheresis. Patients with neurologic disorders were more likely to experience vasovagal reactions than other categories of patients (McLeod, 1999). It should be noted that the study by McLeod et al. did not include complications or reactions due to venous access. Other studies that have included these data have noted higher reaction rates with therapeutic hemapheresis. For example, Couriel & Weinstein noted adverse effects in 17% of therapeutic apheresis procedures (Couriel, 1994). These were predominantly mild, consisting of citrate reactions, but 6.15% of procedures were complicated by severe reactions, reactions that were life threatening or resulted in termination of the procedure. All of these reactions were due to central venous access and consisted of a pneumothorax, a hemopneumothorax, catheter-related bacteremia, and a sternocleidomastoid hematoma. The patient with the hemopneumothorax exsanguinated because of the complication (Couriel, 1994). While only one death due to therapy was reported by Couriel & Weinstein and no deaths attributable to therapeutic hemapheresis were reported in the study by McLeod et al., additional deaths have been reported by other authors. The majority of such deaths have been ascribed to cardiopulmonary arrest during hemapheresis with additional causes including anaphylaxis, pulmonary embolus, and vascular perforation due

to central venous access. Huestis et al. estimated a mortality rate for therapeutic hemapheresis of 3 per 10 000 procedures (0.03%) (Huestis, 1989) while Mokrzycki & Kaplan estimated the mortality rate, based on a review of the literature available to that time, to be 0.05% of procedures (Mokrzycki, 1994).

As discussed under the descriptions of each procedure, specific complications are associated with specific procedures, such as those seen due to G-CSF administration in granulocyte harvest. A discussion of complications and risks common to all hemapheresis procedures follows.

Electrolyte and Acid–Base Disturbances

Citrate is used as the primary anticoagulant in both donor and therapeutic apheresis procedures because it effectively prevents coagulation while being short acting and easily reversible, unlike heparin. Citrate ions chelate calcium ions producing a soluble complex. As a result, the chelated calcium ions are unavailable for biologic reactions such as the coagulation cascade. Within the apheresis instrument, plasma citrate concentrations reach 15–24 mmol/L, lowering the calcium ion concentration below 0.2–0.3 mmol/L, the level necessary for coagulation (Strauss, 1996). This ionized calcium level requires the infusion of approximately 500 mL of ACD-A solution and would be incompatible with life. Death does not occur, however because of compensatory mechanisms in the donor/patient. Upon return of the blood from the apheresis instrument to the donor/patient, the citrate is diluted throughout total extracellular fluid. In addition, the liver, kidneys, and muscles rapidly metabolize citrate, releasing the bound calcium (Strauss, 1996). Finally, the body also responds to the decrease in ionized calcium by increasing parathyroid hormone levels, resulting in mobilization of calcium from skeletal stores and increased absorption by the kidneys (Silberstein, 1986).

In therapeutic plasmapheresis procedures, the volume of plasma removed must be replaced by a similar volume of replacement fluid. In plasma exchange using either FFP or cryoprecipitate reduced plasma as replacement fluids, an additional source of citrate is infused in the form of the anticoagulant present in these solutions. It is therefore common for symptoms of citrate toxicity to be seen in these patients. In plasma exchange using albumin as a replacement fluid, it would be expected that citrate toxicity would be less of a problem. This, however, is not always the case. Normally, 40–55% of serum calcium is bound to albumin, with the unbound portion representing the physiologically active ionized calcium. Albumin preparations are depleted of this calcium and, as a result, bind calcium when infused during plasma exchange. This can lead to a drop in ionized calcium with the subsequent appearance of symptoms due to hypocalcemia. Goss & Weinstein demonstrated a higher incidence of citrate reactions as well as greater decreases in ionized calcium levels in neurology patients receiving plasma exchange with 5% albumin as the replacement fluid when compared to those receiving 10% pentastarch as the replacement fluid (Goss, 1999). A subsequent study demonstrated that the addition of calcium gluconate to the albumin preparation prior to administration more effectively reduced the incidence of citrate toxicity when compared to either i.v. calcium gluconate or oral calcium carbonate (Weinstein, 1996). The effect was due to the saturation of calcium binding sites on the albumin, thereby maintaining ionized calcium levels in the patient.

Despite compensatory mechanisms, citrate infusion can result in the decrease in ionized calcium levels to a point where symptoms develop in the donor/patient. These result from a decrease in ionized calcium to levels where excitability of nerve membranes increases to the point where spontaneous depolarization can occur (Strauss, 1996). The resulting signs and symptoms can include perioral paresthesias, acral paresthesias, shivering, light-headedness, twitching, and tremors. In addition, some patients also experience nausea and vomiting. As the ionized calcium levels fall further, these symptoms may progress to carpopedal spasm, tetany, and seizure (Strauss, 1996). It is therefore important to elicit the presence of the early symptoms from the donor/patient so that interventions can occur prior to the more severe symptoms. In addition to the symptoms described previously, prolongations of the QT interval on electrocardiogram, depressed myocardial contraction, and fatal arrhythmias have been reported (Strauss, 1996). Hypotension may also be seen with citrate reactions (Goodnough, 1999) and may be due to the depressed myocardial function mentioned and vascular smooth muscle relaxation (Bunker, 1962).

Factors which have been found to influence the rate of citrate reactions in donor and therapeutic apheresis include alkalosis due to hyperventilation (Strauss, 1996); the type of anticoagulant solution used, with ACD-A having more reactions than ACD-B (Szymanski, 1978); the rate of infusion of the anticoagulant solution (Strauss, 1996); the amount of citrate infused

(Strauss, 1996); and the donor's serum albumin level prior to the start of the collection procedure (Bolan, 2003a). It should be noted that intermittent flow hemapheresis procedures tend to have a greater frequency of citrate reactions, as there is a higher rate of citrate infusion when the separation chamber is emptied then during continuous apheresis procedures. Also, the method by which an instrument calculates the dose of anticoagulant may influence the rate of reactions among certain donor subgroups (Despotis, 1999).

The treatment of citrate reactions is relatively simple when the reactions are identified early. The treatment includes slowing the reinfusion rate to allow for dilution and metabolism of the citrate, increasing donor/patient blood to citrate ratio to decrease the amount of citrate infused, giving oral calcium in the form of calcium antacids, and giving intravenous calcium (Strauss, 1996).

The administration of oral calcium carbonate and its effects on citrate toxicity in apheresis platelet donors was studied by Bolan et al. (Bolan, 2003a,b). It was found that the administration of 2 g of calcium carbonate was associated with a statistically significant reduction in the severity of paresthesias (Bolan, 2003b). Physiologically, this dose was also associated with the greatest improvement in ionized and total calcium levels among the doses examined (Bolan, 2003a) but was not associated with a reduction in overall symptom development and did not affect the occurrence of more severe symptoms (Bolan, 2003b).

The administration of intravenous calcium, in the form of calcium gluconate or calcium chloride is usually not necessary in donor procedures but is common in the setting of therapeutic apheresis procedures. In hematopoietic progenitor cell (HPC) collections, the continuous infusion of either calcium gluconate or calcium chloride has been found to prevent hypocalcemic symptom development (Bolan, 2002; Buchta, 2003) with calcium chloride maintaining higher ionized calcium levels (Buchta, 2003). In a comparison of infusion of calcium gluconate continuously, prophylactically at the start of HPC collection, or at the time of symptom development, continuous infusion maintained higher calcium levels with insignificant changes in calcium levels with the other two modes of administration (Kishimoto, 2002). When given to treat symptoms, the usual dose is 10 mL of calcium gluconate i.v. infused over 10–15 minutes (Hester, 1983). In patients with low ionized calcium levels prior to the start of the procedure, calcium gluconate can be given prophylactically.

Magnesium is another physiologically important divalent cation. Similarly to calcium, magnesium is also bound by citrate. As a result, the infusion of citrate in the setting of plateletpheresis decreases ionized magnesium by 30% (Mercan, 1997). Mercan et al. also found that magnesium levels fall more rapidly than calcium during citrate infusion and recover more slowly (Mercan, 1997). Hypomagnesemia can induce signs and symptoms similar to hypocalcemia, including muscle spasms, muscle weakness, decreased vascular tone, and impaired cardiac contractility. In addition, hypomagnesemia can also impair calcium and potassium homeostasis, including the inhibition of the release of parathyroid hormone when markedly decreased (Mercan, 1997). As a result, patients with low magnesium levels prior to undergoing apheresis may exhibit signs and symptoms of citrate toxicity due to hypomagnesemia and not hypocalcemia. Patients who cannot rapidly metabolize citrate thereby releasing the bound cations may also be at risk (Kamochi, 2002). These symptoms may be unresponsive to the administration of calcium supplementation. To avoid hypomagnesemia, it is common at some institutions to measure magnesium levels prior to the initiation and supplement magnesium before performing procedures if indicated.

As described, citrate is rapidly metabolized. This process consumes hydrogen ions and as a result, the possibility of the development of metabolic alkalosis due to citrate infusion exists. The risk of this occurring is greatest in patients with renal disease who cannot adequately excrete bicarbonate (Kelleher, 1987) and in those receiving replacement fluids containing citrate (Dzik, 1988; Kelleher, 1987). A study comparing patients with TTP undergoing plasma exchange with FFP replacement to patients with myasthenia gravis undergoing plasma exchange with albumin demonstrated the increased frequency of metabolic alkalosis in the former group (Marques, 2001). The patients with TTP demonstrated a mean creatinine level of 1.3 mg/dL and a mean BUN of 24.8 mg/dL (Marques, 2001). While the metabolic alkalosis seen in these patients did not reach critical levels (> 35 mEq/L HCO_3^-) and resolved following the cessation of plasmapheresis, it was associated with critical drops in potassium (< 3.0 mEq/L) during the procedures (Mercan, 1997). The presence of alkalosis can worsen hypocalcemia (Edmondson, 1975) and slow citrate metabolism (Dzik, 1988). Unfortunately, the symptoms of metabolic alkalosis are nonspecific, usually presenting as worsening symptoms of hypocalcemia. The alkalosis resolves with time or dialysis and can be avoided by reducing the amount of citrate infused by adjusting the blood to citrate ratio and/or using replacement fluids lacking citrate (Pearl, 1985).

Metabolic alkalosis results in a shift in hydrogen ions from intracellular locations (in an attempt to compensate pH) with a concurrent flux of potassium into these cells to maintain electrical neutrality. The result is that significant drops in potassium can occur during large-volume hematopoietic progenitor cell collections in addition to those seen in the TTP patients described previously. Schlenke et al. found an average drop in potassium levels of $11.3 \pm 7\%$ in a study of 96 large-volume leukaphereses (Schlenke, 2000). Despite this decline, none of the patients in this study experienced symptoms attributable to hypokalemia. Symptoms of hypokalemia include weakness, hypotonia, or cardiac arrhythmia (Schlenke, 2000). Treatment of such complications would consist of replacement of the potassium, either orally or intravenously. A prudent option would be to prevent the reaction by determining the potassium level prior to the start of the procedure and supplementing if indicated.

Allergic, Anaphylactoid, and Anaphylactic Reactions

Allergic, anaphylactoid, and anaphylactic reactions result from the release of vasoactive substances such as histamine, leukotriene C_4, leukotriene D_4, prostaglandin D_2, and platelet-activating factor from mast cells and basophils. The release of these substances is mediated by the presence of IgE antibodies on the surface of these cells. When the target antigen binds to the IgE molecule, the substances listed previously are released. This in turn results in a variety of symptoms by causing contraction of smooth muscle, increased vascular permeability, and vasodilation. Mast cells and basophils can also be activated by complement-derived factors such as C3a and C5a which can be produce by antigen–IgG interactions and other mechanisms (Vamvakas, 2001). These types of reactions can range from mild urticarial reactions to life-threatening anaphylactic reactions. Signs and symptoms of these reactions include pruritus, urticaria, erythema, flushing, angioedema, upper airway obstruction, lower airway obstruction, hypotension, shock, nausea, vomiting, and diarrhea (Vamvakas, 2001).

Allergic reactions have been reported in both donors and patients undergoing hemapheresis procedures. Among donors, reactions have been reported among platelet, plasma, and granulocyte donors. In platelet and plasma donors, reactions to ethylene oxide gas used to sterilize the tubing sets used for the procedures have been described (Leitman, 1986; Muylle, 1986). These reactions have occurred predominantly in donors who had undergone numerous previous procedures. It is thought that during the procedures, ethylene oxide present within the plastic binds to proteins within the plasma. The proteins serve as carrier molecules and the ethylene oxide as a hapten with the result being an immune response with the generation of IgE antibodies toward ethylene oxide. In most of the donors who experienced allergic phenomenon, IgE antibodies to ethylene oxide were identified (Leitman, 1986). The reactions ranged from urticaria, flushing and periorbital edema (Leitman, 1986) to an anaphylactic reaction consisting of wheezing, flushing, swelling of the lips, and hypotension (Muylle, 1986). The overall rate of the reactions in one study was 1.0% of platelet donors. Interestingly, the reactions also showed an increased frequency with the Fenwal CS3000 than with the Haemonetics V-50 (Haemonetics, Braintree, MA). This was thought to be due to the fact that at the start of processing with the CS3000, a mixture of saline and anticoagulant that was used to prime the bag was infused into the patient. This was not the case with the V-50. It was postulated that this resulted in a bolus of ethylene oxide that produced the symptoms (Leitman, 1986).

Reactions have also been reported among granulocyte donors as well. Besides ethylene oxide reactions, another mechanism is possible. Granulocyte donors are exposed to hydroxyethyl starch (HES), either low molecular weight or high molecular weight, in order to enhance red cell sedimentation. While these substances are poor immunogens and have not been able to induce antibody formation, allergic reactions have occurred in the setting of HES use in hemapheresis (Dutcher, 1984) and as a volume expander (Ring, 1977). The mechanism behind the production of anaphylactoid reactions with HES is thought to be due to the ability of HES to activate the alternative complement cascade. This would result in the production of C3a and C5a, both of which can cause mast cell and basophil release (Dutcher, 1984). Reactions reported to occur with HES include mild urticarial reactions as well as severe reactions with respiratory and cardiac arrest. The rate of reactions in a study of patients receiving HES for volume expansion was 0.085% with severe (anaphylactic) reactions occurring in 0.006% (Ring, 1977). Reactions have occurred with both high molecular weight (hetastarch) (Ring, 1977) and low molecular weight (pentastarch) (Kannan, 1999) HES. Because of this risk, Dutcher et al.

recommended excluding people with a history of allergies as granulocyte donors (Dutcher, 1984).

Among therapeutic hemapheresis patients, either reactions to ethylene oxide or HES could occur. In addition, therapeutic plasmapheresis procedures frequently use plasma products, either FFP or cryosupernatant plasma, as replacement solutions. As a result, these patients are also at risk for allergic and anaphylactic reactions due to transfusion reactions. The most common allergic reaction within the setting of plasma product infusion is the urticarial reaction. This reaction occurs in 1–3% of plasma infusions and consists of hives scattered over the body. In 1 in 20 000–47 000 transfusions, anaphylaxis occurs (Vamvakas, 2001). The most common cause of this last reaction is the infusion of plasma containing IgA into an IgA-deficient individual who possesses anti-IgA antibodies (Vamvakas, 2001).

The treatment of allergic, anaphylactoid, and anaphylactic reactions depends upon their severity. In donor reactions, the procedure should be stopped. Simple reactions such as urticaria can then be treated with oral antihistamines, i.e., diphenhydramine. The same treatment can be done with therapeutic procedures though in this case, the procedure can be restarted following antihistamine administration. In addition, the patient can be premedicated with antihistamines before subsequent procedures.

Anaphylactic reactions are life threatening. The procedure, whether donor or therapeutic, must be immediately discontinued. The vascular access should be kept open using saline. For less severe reactions, epinephrine 0.3–0.5 mg can be given subcutaneously, with the dose being repeated every 20–30 minutes for up to three doses. In addition, aminophylline 6 mg/kg can be given for bronchospasm. This loading dose should be followed by an infusion of 0.5–1 mg/kg/hour. Volume expansion with normal saline or lactated Ringer's solution can be given for hypotension. Oxygen should be given for respiratory distress. For severe reactions, epinephrine 0.5 mg can be given intravenously, with repeated dosing every 5–10 minutes. Dopamine can also be given for hypotension unresponsive to volume. The airway must be protected and endotracheal intubation may be indicated (Vamvakas, 2001).

Obviously, the best course of action is to avoid such reactions. Donors who have experienced such reactions should be deferred from future donation. Patients with mild reactions should be premedicated with antihistamines. Those with severe reactions due to IgA should receive IgA-deficient replacement fluids. For most procedures, this could be albumin or saline. For procedures requiring plasma as a replacement fluid, as in plasma exchange for TTP, IgA-deficient plasma products must be used.

Angiotensin-Converting Enzyme Inhibitors

The use of angiotensin-converting enzyme (ACE) inhibitors by patients undergoing hemapheresis procedures is associated with reactions similar in many respects to the allergic reactions described previously. The reactions consist of flushing, hypotension, bradycardia, and dyspnea (Strauss, 1996). These have been seen in patients undergoing therapeutic plasma exchange (Owen, 1994), LDL-apheresis using dextran sulfate columns (Agishi, 1994), and treatment with staphylococcal A protein columns (Owen, 1994). These reactions result from activation of the kinin system and generation of bradykinin when patient plasma comes in contact with the negatively charged plastic of the apheresis set. Normally, bradykinin is rapidly inactivated by kininase I and II. ACE inhibitors, however, block the actions of these enzymes such that high levels accumulate producing the symptoms described previously (Strauss, 1996). During plasma exchange with albumin, prekallikrein-activating factor present in the albumin can also trigger the formation of bradykinin (Owen, 1994). Again, the presence of ACE inhibitors prevents degradation of this substance. These reactions can be avoided by withholding ACE inhibitors for 24–48 hours prior to hemapheresis procedures (Owen, 1994). Some newer ACE inhibitors have longer half-lives and withholding the drugs for longer periods or switching to ACE inhibitors with shorter half-lives may be necessary.

Hypovolemia and Vasovagal Reactions

Hypotension can be seen during both donor and therapeutic hemapheresis procedures. This can be the result of two different pathophysiologic mechanisms. In the first, hypotension results from intravascular volume depletion due to too much volume being present within the extracorporeal circuit. Such reactions are characterized by both increased vascular tone and an increased cardiac output as the sympathetic nervous system attempts to compensate for the hypovolemia (Strauss, 1996). Increasing both heart rate and contractility produces the increase in cardiac output. These reactions are not common among hemapheresis donors as Standards for Blood Banks and Transfusion Services limit the amount of volume that can be within the extracorporeal circuit to 10.5 mL/kg (Standards Committee of the American Association of Blood Banks, 2004) and the donors also fulfill health and weight requirements. In therapeutic procedures, the patient has an underlying disease that may make hypovolemia more likely. For example, the presence of hypotension has been found to be more common in patients with neurologic diseases (McLeod, 1999). Standards for Blood Banks and Transfusion Services do not prescribe limits on extracorporeal volume during therapeutic hemapheresis procedures, though the application of the limits used during donor hemapheresis procedures would seem prudent (Strauss, 1996).

The second mechanism causing hypotension during hemapheresis procedures is the vasovagal reaction. In this reaction, hypovolemia results in a decrease in blood pressure. As stated previously, the compensatory response is to increase cardiac output and vascular tone. During a vasovagal reaction, parasympathetic output, which normally counteracts sympathetic output, increases disproportionately, resulting in a slowing of heart rate and decreased vascular tone, leading to hypotension (Strauss, 1996). Factors that have been associated with such reactions in whole blood donors include younger age, low weight, first time donation, and inattentive staff (Newman, 1997). Tomita et al. examined the incidence of vasovagal reactions among apheresis donors and whole blood donors at the same collection center (Tomita, 2002). They noted that the incidence of these reactions among apheresis donors increased with age, unlike what has been reported with whole blood donors. The age-related increase in vasovagal reactions was even more common in women and thought to result from a lower circulating blood volume in these populations (elderly and women) leading to a greater percentage of the donor's blood being within the extracorporeal circuit during collection. The resulting greater drop in blood pressure during collection leads to more reactions. It was also noted that the incidence increased with increasing cycles during a collection and it was theorized that hypocalcemia was involved in the onset of vasovagal reactions (Tomita, 2002).

Hypovolemic and vasovagal reactions are treated similarly. The procedure should be temporarily interrupted and a fluid bolus should be infused. If the reaction is due to hypovolemia, the blood pressure should increase and the pulse rate should decrease in response to this intervention. If the reaction is due to a vasovagal reaction, this may not occur. Additional treatments for vasovagal reactions include placing the donor/patient in the Trendelenburg position (head down), applying cold compresses to the forehead and neck, and reassuring the donor/patient (Strauss, 1996).

Hydroxyethyl Starch and Coagulopathy

As discussed under the section dealing with plasmapheresis, the removal of plasma from a patient during a therapeutic hemapheresis procedure and the replacement of the volume with albumin or some other fluid that does not contain coagulation factors can result in mild, temporary abnormalities in coagulation. These changes are usually short lived, with return of most coagulation factors to normal levels within 24–48 hours. The use of HES, either as volume replacement or as a sedimenting agent, is also associated with changes in coagulation factor levels. Both high molecular weight HES, such as hetastarch, and low molecular weight HES, such as pentastarch, result in prolongation of the partial thromboplastin time (PTT) as well as decreases in fibrinogen levels. This is thought to result from the dilutional effects produced when these substances are infused. High molecular weight, but not low molecular weight HES, is also associated with decreases in factor VIII activity, factor VIII antigen, and von Willebrand factor (vWF) antigen as well as prolongation of bleeding time (Strauss, 1988). It is thought that this last effect is a result of the decrease in vWF antigen levels and may represent an acquired von Willebrand disease-like state. Because of these changes, a risk of coagulopathy exists with the use of these agents. This risk appears to be dose dependent. In the setting of volume expansion in critical care, the maximum dose of HES in order to avoid such complications has been suggested to be 20 mL/kg/24-hour period. Doses up to 3600 mL have been given in this setting without difficulty (Nearman, 1991). The danger in hemapheresis procedures is that multiple collections or therapeutic procedures may be necessary in a given donor/patient over consecutive days. Since HES, especially high molecular weight HES, has a long half-life, this may result in an accumulation of HES over the course of the hemapheresis procedures and the potential danger of coagulopathy.

Hydroxyethyl Starch and Other Side Effects

As has been mentioned, HES has a long half-life. This is dependent upon the metabolism of the HES by α-amylase and subsequent renal excretion of the breakdown products (Yacobi, 1982). Persistent pruritus due to deposition of HES in the skin has been reported as one of the most frequent complications of HES administration. Skin deposits have been detected for up to 4 years following administration (Sirtl, 1999; Stander, 2001).

In addition to skin deposition, a case report has appeared describing marrow and organ failure in a patient undergoing chronic plasma exchange (20 months) using HES as the replacement fluid. In this patient, foamy macrophages containing HES were found replacing bone marrow as well as infiltrating duodenal mucosa, liver, peritoneum, and dura mater. These cells were also present in ascitic fluid (Auwerda, 2002).

Air Embolus

Air embolus is a rare complication of hemapheresis procedures. It occurs when air enters the venous system through either a leak in the hemapheresis instrument or the venous access. Air entering the right ventricle and pulmonary artery results in obstruction to right ventricular output and pulmonary artery vasoconstriction (Montacer-Kuhssari, 1994). Symptoms of air embolism include dyspnea, tachypnea, cyanosis, tachycardia, and hypotension. The reason for the rarity of this complication is that all modern hemapheresis instruments possess sensors that can detect air within the extravascular circuit and stop the procedure. Should air embolism occur, however, the treatment consists of placing the donor/patient in the Trendelenburg position on their left side. This traps the air in the apex of the right ventricle, away from the pulmonary outflow tract, improving right ventricular outflow. With time, the air will dissolve.

Summary

In summary, hemapheresis represents a safe and effective technique for the production of needed blood components as well as for the treatment of a variety of diseases. While hemapheresis is often compared to the 18th century practice of bloodletting, it shares little with this practice. Hemapheresis is selective in what is removed from the donor/patient. In addition, hemapheresis is grounded in evidence-based medicine. While hemapheresis procedures are safe, they are not without risk and should only be applied to those diseases and disorders for which the possibility of benefit exists and for which evidence in support of this benefit has been shown.

References

Adachi S, Kubota M, Lin Y, et al: In vivo administration of granulocyte colony-stimulating factor promotes neutrophil survival in vitro. Eur J Haematol 1994; 53:129–134.

Adkins D, Goodgold H, Hendershott L, et al: Indium-labeled white blood cells apheresed from donors receiving G-CSF localize to sites of inflammation when infused into allogeneic bone marrow transplant recipients. Bone Marrow Transplant 1997a; 19:809–812.

Adkins D, Spitzer G, Johnston M, et al: Transfusions of granulocyte-colony-stimulating factor-mobilized granulocyte components to allogeneic transplant recipients: analysis of kinetics and factors determining posttransfusion neutrophil and platelet counts. Transfusion 1997b; 37:737–748.

Agishi T: Anion-blood contact reaction (ABC reaction) in patients treated by LDL apheresis with dextran sulfate-cellulose column while receiving ACE inhibitors. JAMA 1994; 271:195–196.

Aikawa A, Hadano T, Ohara T, et al: Donor specific antibody suppression in ABO incompatible kidney transplantation. Transplant Proc 2001; 33:395–397.

Alving BM, Hojima Y, Pisano JJ, et al: Hypotension associated with prekallikrein activator (Hageman-factor fragments) in plasma protein fraction. N Engl J Med 1978; 299:66–70.

American Association of Blood Banks Hemapheresis Committee: Guidelines for Therapeutic Hemapheresis. Bethesda, American Association of Blood Banks, 1995.

American Society for Apheresis Clinical Applications Committee: The clinical applications of therapeutic apheresis. J Clin Apheresis 2000; 15: 1–5.
A review of the state of the art of therapeutic apheresis. Includes classification of indications based upon the available scientific evidence, discussions of this evidence, and recommended treatment protocols.

Amorosi EL, Karpatkin S: Antiplatelet treatment of thrombotic thrombocytopenic purpura. Ann Intern Med 1977; 86:102–106.

Antozzi C, Gemma M, Regi B, et al: A short plasma exchange protocol is effective in severe myasthenia gravis. J Neurol 1991; 238:103–107.

Asada Y, Sumiyoshi A, Hayashi T, et al: Immunohistochemistry of vascular lesion in thrombotic thrombocytopenic purpura, with special reference to factor VIII related antigen. Thromb Res 1985; 38:469–479.

Auwerda JJ, Wilson JH, Sonneveld P: Foamy macrophage syndrome due to hydroxyethyl starch replacement: a severe side effect in plasmapheresis. Ann Intern Med 2002; 137:1013–1014.

Azevedo AM, Tabak DG: Life-threatening capillary leak syndrome after G-CSF mobilization and collection of peripheral blood progenitor cells for allogeneic transplantation. Bone Marrow Transplant 2001; 28:311–312.

Baley JE, Stork EK, Warkentin PI, et al: Buffy coat transfusions in neutropenic neonates with presumed sepsis: a prospective, randomized trial. Pediatrics 1987; 80:712–720.

Balogun RA, Sahadevan M, Sevigny J, et al: Impact of therapeutic plasma exchange on cyclosporine kinetics during membrane-based lipid apheresis. Am J Kidney Dis 2001; 37:1286–1289.

Bambauer R, Schiel R, Latza R: Low-density lipoprotein apheresis: An overview. Ther Apher Dial 2003; 7:382–390.

Bandarenko N, Brecher ME: United States Thrombotic Thrombocytopenic Purpura Apheresis Study Group (US TTP ASG): multicenter survey and retrospective analysis of current efficacy of therapeutic plasma exchange. J Clin Apheresis 1998; 13:133–141.

Baron BW, Mick R, Baron JM: Combined plateletpheresis and cytotoxic chemotherapy for symptomatic thrombocytosis in myeloproliferative disorders. Cancer 1993; 72:1209–1218.

Bear RA, Cole EH, Lang A, et al: Treatment of acute renal failure due to myeloma kidney. Can Med Assoc J 1980; 123:750–753.

Beeler SA, Giandelone JA, Axelrod FB: A blood center's motivation toward total apheresis collection. Transfusion 1997; 37(Suppl):113S.

Bell WR, Braine HG, Ness PM, et al: Improved survival in thrombotic thrombocytopenic purpura–hemolytic uremic syndrome. Clinical experience in 108 patients. N Engl J Med 1991; 325:398–403.

Bender JG, To LB, Williams S, et al: Defining a therapeutic dose of peripheral blood stem cells. J Hematother 1992; 1:329–341.

Bennett CL, Weinberg PD, Rozenberg-Ben-Dror K, et al: Thrombotic thrombocytopenic purpura associated with ticlopidine. A review of 60 cases. Ann Intern Med 1998; 128:541–544.

Bensinger W, Appelbaum F, Rowley S, et al: Factors that influence collection and engraftment of autologous peripheral-blood stem cells. J Clin Oncol 1995; 13:2547–2555.

Bensinger WI, Price TH, Dale DC, et al: The effects of daily recombinant human granulocyte colony-stimulating factor administration on normal granulocyte donors undergoing leukapheresis. Blood 1993; 81:1883–1888.

Bensinger WI, Buckner CD, Rowley S, et al: Treatment of normal donors with recombinant growth factors for transplantation of allogeneic blood stem cells. Bone Marrow Transplant 1996; 17:S19–S21.

Bensinger WI, Martin PJ, Storer B, et al: Transplantation of bone marrow as compared with peripheral-blood cells from HLA-identical relatives in patients with hematologic cancers. N Engl J Med 2001; 344:175–181.

Berkman EM, Orlin JB: Use of plasmapheresis and partial plasma exchange in the management of patients with cryoglobulinemia. Transfusion 1980; 20:171–178.

Bernstein SP, Humes HD: Reversible renal insufficiency in multiple myeloma. Arch Intern Med 1982; 142:2083–2086.

Blanchette VS, Hume HA, Levy GJ, et al: Guidelines for auditing pediatric blood transfusion practices. Am J Dis Child 1991; 145:787–796.

Bloch KJ, Maki DG: Hyperviscosity syndromes associated with immunoglobulin abnormalities. Semin Hematol 1973; 10:113–124.

Bock M, Heim MU, Schleich I, et al: Platelet crossmatching with Capture P: clinical relevance. Infusionstherapie 1989; 16:183–185.

Bolan CD, Cecco SA, Wesley RA, et al: Controlled study of citrate effects and response to i.v. calcium administration during allogeneic peripheral blood progenitor cell donation. Transfusion 2002; 42:935–946.

Bolan CD, Cecco SA, Yau YY, et al: Randomized placebo-controlled study of oral calcium carbonate supplementation in plateletpheresis: II. Metabolic effects. Transfusion 2003a; 43:1414–1422.

Bolan CD, Wesley RA, Yau YY, et al: Randomized placebo-controlled study of oral calcium carbonate administration in plateletpheresis: I. Associations with donor symptoms. Transfusion 2003b; 43:1403–1413.

Bolwell BJ, Goormastic M, Yanssens T, et al: Comparison of G-CSF with GM-CSF for mobilizing peripheral blood progenitor cells and for enhancing marrow recovery after autologous bone marrow transplant. Bone Marrow Transplant 1994; 14:913–918.

Bonilla MA, Dale D, Zeidler C, et al: Long-term safety of treatment with recombinant human granulocyte colony-stimulating factor (r-metHuG-CSF) in patients with severe congenital neutropenias. Br J Haematol 1994; 88:723–730.

Bosch T: Direct adsorption of lipoproteins from whole blood by DALI apheresis: technique and effects. Ther Apher 2001a; 5:239–243.

Bosch T, Wendler T: Extracorporeal plasma treatment in primary and recurrent focal segmental glomerular sclerosis: A review. Ther Apher 2001b; 5:155–160.

Bowden RA, Slichter SJ, Sayers M, et al: A comparison of filtered leukocyte-reduced and cytomegalovirus (CMV) seronegative blood products for the prevention of transfusion-associated CMV infection after marrow transplant. Blood 1995; 86:3598–3603.

Brown RA, Adkins D, DiPersio J, et al: Allogeneic peripheral blood stem cell transplantation is associated with an increased risk of chronic graft versus host disease. Blood 1997; 90:225a.

Brugger W, Bross KJ, Glatt M, et al: Mobilization of tumor cells and hematopoietic progenitor cells into peripheral blood of patients with solid tumors. Blood 1994; 83:636–640.

Buchta C, Macher M, Bieglmayer C, et al: Reduction of adverse citrate reactions during autologous large-

IV

volume PBPC apheresis by continuous infusion of calcium-gluconate. Transfusion 2003; 43:1615–1621.

Buckner CD, Clift RA, Thomas ED, et al: Early infectious complications in allogeneic marrow transplant recipients with acute leukemia: effects of prophylactic measures. Infection 1983; 11:243–250.

Buffaloe GW, Heineken FG: Plasma volume nomograms for use in therapeutic plasma exchange. Transfusion 1983; 23:355–357.

Bunker JP, Bendixen HH, Murphy AJ: Hemodynamic effects of intravenously administered sodium citrate. N Engl J Med 1962; 266:372–377.

Burgstaler EA: Current instrumentation for apheresis. In McLeod BC, Price TH, Weinstein R (eds): Apheresis: Principles and Practice, 2nd ed. Bethesda, AABB Press, 2003, pp 95–130.

Burgstaler EA, Pineda AA: Hydroxyethylstarch as replacement in therapeutic plasma exchange. Prog Clin Biol Res 1990; 337:395–397.

Burgstaler EA, Pineda AA: Therapeutic cytapheresis: continuous flow versus intermittent flow apheresis systems. J Clin Apheresis 1994; 9:205–209.

Burgstaler EA, Pineda A: Therapeutic plasma exchange: A paired comparison of Fresenius AS104 vs. COBE Spectra. J Clin Apheresis 2001; 16:61–66.

Burgstaler EA, Pineda AA, Winters JL: Hematopoietic progenitor cell large volume leukapheresis (LVL) on the Fenwall Amicus blood separator. J Clin Apheresis 2004; 19:103–111.

Buss DH, Cashell AW, O'Connor ML, et al: Occurrence, etiology, and clinical significance of extreme thrombocytosis: A study of 280 cases. Am J Med 1994; 96:247–253.

Cairo MS, Rucker R, Bennetts GA, et al: Improved survival of newborns receiving leukocyte transfusions for sepsis. Pediatrics 1984; 74:887–892.

Cairo MS, Worcester C, Rucker R, et al: Role of circulating complement and polymorphonuclear leukocyte transfusion in treatment and outcome in critically ill neonates with sepsis. J Pediatr 1987; 110:935–941.

Caspar CB, Seger RA, Burger J, et al: Effective stimulation of donors for granulocyte transfusions with recombinant methionyl granulocyte colony-stimulating factor. Blood 1993; 81:2866–2871.

Centurioni R, Bobbio-Pallavicini E, Porta C, et al: Treatment of thrombotic thrombocytopenic purpura with high-dose immunoglobulins. Results in 17 patients. Italian Cooperative Group for TTP. Haematologica 1995; 80:325–331.

Chambers ME, McDonald BR, Hall FW, et al: Plasmapheresis for crescentic IgA nephropathy: a report of two cases and review of the literature. J Clin Apheresis 1999; 14:185–187.

Chirnside A, Urbaniak SJ, Prowse CV, et al: Coagulation abnormalities following intensive plasma exchange on the cell separator. II. Effects on factors I, II, V, VII, VIII, IX, X and antithrombin III. Br J Haematol 1981; 48:627–634.

Chopek M, McCullough J: Protein and biochemical changes during plasma exchange. In Berkman EM and Umlas J (eds): Therapeutic Hemapheresis. Washington, American Association of Blood Banks, 1980, pp 13–52.

Christensen I, Heald P: Photopheresis in the 1990s. J Clin Apheresis 1991; 6:216–220.

Christensen RD, Rothstein G, Anstall HB, et al: Granulocyte transfusions in neonates with bacterial infection, neutropenia, and depletion of mature marrow neutrophils. Pediatrics 1982; 70:1–6.

Ciszewski TS, Ralston S, Acteson D, et al: Protein levels and plasmapheresis intensity. Transfus Med 1993; 3:59–65.

COBE BCT: COBE Spectra red blood cell exchange inservice student workbook. Lakewood, COBE BCT, 1997.

Code of Federal Regulations. 21 CFR 640, Washington, DC: Government Printing Office, 4-1-2003.

Cohen DJ, Sherman WH, Osserman EF, et al: Acute renal failure in patients with multiple myeloma. Am J Med 1984; 76:247–256.

Cohen JA, Brecher ME, Bandarenko N: Cellular source of serum lactate dehydrogenase elevation in patients with thrombotic thrombocytopenic purpura. J Clin Apheresis 1998; 13:16–19.

Coppo P, Bussel A, Charrier S, et al: High-dose plasma infusion versus plasma exchange as early treatment of thrombotic thrombocytopenic purpura/hemolytic-uremic syndrome. Medicine (Baltimore) 2003; 82:27–38.

Cornblath DR, Asbury AK, Albers JW, et al: Research criteria for diagnosis of chronic inflammatory demyelinating polyneuropathy (CIDP). Report from an ad hoc subcommittee of the American Academy of Neurology AIDS Task Force. Neurology 1991; 41:617–618.

Cortelazzo S, Viero P, Finazzi G, et al: Incidence and risk factors for thrombotic complications in a historical cohort of 100 patients with essential thrombocythemia. J Clin Oncol 1990; 8:556–562.

Couriel D, Weinstein R: Complications of therapeutic plasma exchange: a recent assessment. J Clin Apheresis 1994; 9:1–5.

Crowther MA, Heddle N, Hayward CP, et al: Splenectomy done during hematologic remission to prevent relapse in patients with thrombotic thrombocytopenic purpura. Ann Intern Med 1996; 125:294–296.

Dalakas MC, Engel WK: Immunoglobulin and complement deposits in nerves of patients with chronic relapsing polyneuropathy. Arch Neurol 1980a; 37:637–640.

Dalakas MC, Houff SA, Engel WK, et al: CSF 'monoclonal' bands in chronic relapsing polyneuropathy. Neurology 1980b; 30:864–867.

Dale DC, Liles WC, Llewellyn C, et al: Neutrophil transfusions: kinetics and functions of neutrophils mobilized with granulocyte-colony-stimulating factor and dexamethasone. Transfusion 1998; 38:713–721.

Dall'Amico R, Murer L: Extracorporeal photochemotherapy: a new therapeutic approach for allograft rejection. Transfus Apheresis Sci 2002; 26:197–204.

Dau PC: Plasmapheresis therapy in myasthenia gravis. Muscle Nerve 1980; 3:468–482.

Dau PC: Immunologic rebound. J Clin Apheresis 1995; 10:210–217.

Dau PC, Lindstrom JM, Cassel CK, et al: Plasmapheresis and immunosuppressive drug therapy in myasthenia gravis. N Engl J Med 1977; 297:1134–1140.

Davies SC, Roberts-Harewood M: Blood transfusion in sickle cell disease. Blood Rev 1997; 11:57–71.

Dawson RB, Brown JA, Mahalati K, et al: Durable remissions following prolonged plasma exchange in thrombotic thrombocytopenic purpura. J Clin Apheresis 1994; 9:112–115.

DeFronzo RA, Cooke CR, Wright JR, et al: Renal function in patients with multiple myeloma. Medicine (Baltimore) 1978; 57:151–166.

Delikouras A, Dorling A: Transplant accommodation. Am J Transplant 2003; 3:917–918.

Derksen RH, Schuurman HJ, Gmelig Meyling FH, et al: Rebound and overshoot after plasma exchange in humans. J Lab Clin Med 1984a; 104:35–43.

Derksen RH, Schuurman HJ, Meyling FH, et al: The efficacy of plasma exchange in the removal of plasma components. J Lab Clin Med 1984b; 104:346–354.

Despotis GJ, Goodnough LT, Dynis M, et al: Adverse events in platelet apheresis donors: A multivariate analysis in a hospital-based program. Vox Sang 1999; 77:24–32.

Dettke M, Hlousek M, Kurz M, et al: Increase in endogenous thrombopoietin in healthy donors after automated plateletpheresis. Transfusion 1998; 38:449–453.

Doughty HA, Murphy MF, Metcalfe P, et al: Relative importance of immune and non-immune causes of platelet refractoriness. Vox Sang 1994; 66:200–205.

Dreger P, Marquardt P, Haferlach T, et al: Effective mobilisation of peripheral blood progenitor cells with 'Dexa-BEAM' and G-CSF: Timing of harvesting and composition of the leukapheresis product. Br J Cancer 1993; 68:950–957.

Duhrsen U, Villeval JL, Boyd J, et al: Effects of recombinant human granulocyte colony-stimulating factor on hematopoietic progenitor cells in cancer patients. Blood 1988; 72:2074–2081.

Duquesnoy RJ: Donor selection in platelet transfusion therapy of alloimmunized thrombocytopenic patients. In Greenwalt TJ, Jamieson GA (eds): The blood platelet in transfusion therapy. New York, Alan R Liss, 1978, pp 229–243.

Dutcher JP, Schiffer CA, Johnston GS, et al: Alloimmunization prevents the migration of transfused indium-111-labeled granulocytes to sites of infection. Blood 1983; 62:354–360.

Dutcher JP, Aisner J, Hogge DE, et al: Donor reaction to hydroxyethyl starch during granulocytapheresis. Transfusion 1984; 24:66–67.

Dutcher JP, Schiffer CA, Wiernik PH: Hyperleukocytosis in adult acute nonlymphocytic leukemia: impact on remission rate and duration, and survival. J Clin Oncol 1987; 5:1364–1372.

Dyck PJ, Lais AC, Ohta M, et al: Chronic inflammatory polyradiculoneuropathy. Mayo Clin Proc 1975; 50:621–637.

Dyck PJ, Daube J, O'Brien P, et al: Plasma exchange in chronic inflammatory demyelinating polyradiculoneuropathy. N Engl J Med 1986; 314:461–465.

Dyck PJ, Litchy WJ, Kratz KM, et al: A plasma exchange versus immune globulin infusion trial in chronic inflammatory demyelinating polyradiculoneuropathy. Ann Neurol 1994; 36:838–845.

Dzik WH, Kirkley S: Citrate toxicity during massive blood transfusion. Transfus Med Rev 1988; 2:76–94.

Edmondson JW, Brashear RE, Li T: Tetany: Quantitative interrelationships between calcium and alkalosis. Am J Physiol 1975; 228:1082–1086.

Erickson SB, Kurtz SB, Donadio JV Jr, et al: Use of combined plasmapheresis and immunosuppression in the treatment of Goodpasture's syndrome. Mayo Clin Proc 1979; 54:714–720.

Evenson DA, Perry E, Kloster B, et al: Therapeutic apheresis for babesiosis. J Clin Apheresis 1998; 13:32–36.

Filshie RJ: Cytokines in haemopoietic progenitor mobilisation for peripheral blood stem cell transplantation. Curr Pharm Des 2002; 8:379–394.

Flaum MA, Cuneo RA, Appelbaum FR, et al: The hemostatic imbalance of plasma-exchange transfusion. Blood 1979; 54:694–702.

Flowers ME, Parker PM, Johnston LJ, et al: Comparison of chronic graft-versus-host disease after transplantation of peripheral blood stem cells versus bone marrow in allogeneic recipients: long-term follow-up of a randomized trial. Blood 2002; 100:415–419.

Foerster J: Cryoglobulins and cryoglobulinemia. In Lee GR, Bithell TC, Foerster J (eds): Wintrobe's Clinical Hematology. 9th ed. Philadelphia, Lea and Febiger, 1993a, pp 2284–2293.

Foerster J: Plasma cell dyscrasias: General considerations. In Lee GR, Bithell TC, Foerster J (eds): Wintrobe's Clinical Hematology. 9th ed. Philadelphia, Lea and Febiger, 1993b, pp 2202–2218.

Food and Drug Administration (Division of Blood and Blood Products, Center for Biologics Evaluation and Research): Guideline for the Collection of Platelets, Pheresis Prepared by Automated Methods. Bethesda, Maryland, 1988.

Food and Drug Administration (Division of Blood and Blood Products, Center for Biologics Evaluation and Research): Recommendations for Collecting Red Blood Cells by Automated Apheresis Methods. Bethesda, MD, Maryland, 2001.

Foss FM, Gorgun G, Miller KB: Extracorporeal photopheresis in chronic graft-versus-host-disease. Bone Marrow Transplant 2002; 29:719–725.

Fruehauf S, Seggewiss R: It's moving day: factors affecting peripheral blood stem cell mobilization and strategies for improvement. Br J Haematol 2003; 122:360–375.

Furlan M, Lammle B: Deficiency of von Willebrand factor-cleaving protease in familial and acquired thrombotic thrombocytopenic purpura. Baillières Clin Haematol 1998a; 11:509–514.

Furlan M, Robles R, Solenthaler M, et al: Deficient activity of von Willebrand factor-cleaving protease in chronic relapsing thrombotic thrombocytopenic purpura. Blood 1997; 89:3097–3103.

Furlan M, Robles R, Solenthaler M, Lammle B: Acquired deficiency of von Willebrand factor-cleaving protease in a patient with thrombotic thrombocytopenic purpura. Blood 1998b; 91:2839–2846.

Gajdos P, Chevret S, Clair B, et al: Clinical trial of plasma exchange and high-dose intravenous immunoglobulin in myasthenia gravis. Myasthenia Gravis Clinical Study Group. Ann Neurol 1997; 41:789–796.

Gaskin G, Pusey CD: Plasmapheresis in antineutrophil cytoplasmic antibody-associated systemic vasculitis. Ther Apher 2001; 5:176–181.

Gazitt Y, Tian E, Barlogie B, et al: Differential mobilization of myeloma cells and normal hematopoietic stem cells in multiple myeloma after treatment with cyclophosphamide and granulocyte-macrophage colony-stimulating factor. Blood 1996; 87:805–811.

Ghodsi Z, Strauss RG: Cataracts in neutrophil donors stimulated with adrenal corticosteroids. Transfusion 2001; 41:1464–1468.

Gilcher RO: Apheresis: principles and practice. In Rossi EC, Simon TL, Moss GS, Gould SA (eds): Principles of Transfusion Medicine. 2nd ed. Baltimore, Williams & Wilkins, 1996, pp 537–545.

Gilcher RO: It's time to end RBC shortages. Transfusion 2003; 43:1658–1660.

Giles FJ, Shen Y, Kantarjian HM, et al: Leukapheresis reduces early mortality in patients with acute myeloid leukemia with high white cell counts but does not improve long-term survival. Leuk Lymphoma 2001; 42:67–73.

Gillespie TW, Hillyer CD: Peripheral blood progenitor cells for marrow reconstitution: mobilization and collection strategies. Transfusion 1996; 36:611–624.

Glasser L, Huestis DW, Jones JF: Functional capabilities of steroid-recruited neutrophils harvested for clinical transfusion. N Engl J Med 1977; 297:1033–1036.

Gloor JM, DeGoey SR, Pineda AA, et al: Overcoming a positive crossmatch in living-donor kidney transplantation. Am J Transplant 2003a; 3:1017–1023.

Gloor JM, Lager DJ, Moore SB, et al: ABO-incompatible kidney transplantation using both A2 and non-A2 living donors. Transplantation 2003b; 75:971–977.

Glowitz RJ, Slichter SJ: Frequent multiunit plateletpheresis from single donors: Effects on donors' blood and the platelet yield. Transfusion 1980; 20:199–205.

Goldberg SL, Mangan KF, Klumpp TR, et al: Complications of peripheral blood stem cell harvesting: Review of 554 PBSC leukaphereses. J Hematother 1995; 4:85–90.

Goodnough LT, Ali S, Despotis G, et al: Economic impact of donor platelet count and platelet yield in apheresis products: Relevance for emerging issues in platelet transfusion therapy. Vox Sang 1999; 76:43–49.

Gordon BR, Stein E, Jones P, et al: Indications for low-density lipoprotein apheresis. Am J Cardiol 1994; 74:1109–1112.

Gorlin J, Stefan M: Evaluation of adverse events of donating two unit-red blood cells on a new automated component collection system. Transfusion 2003; 43(Suppl):43A.

Goss GA, Weinstein R: Pentastarch as partial replacement fluid for therapeutic plasma exchange: Effect on plasma proteins, adverse events during treatment, and serum ionized calcium. J Clin Apheresis 1999; 14:114–121.

Grishaber JE, Cunningham MC, Rohret PA, et al: Analysis of venous access for therapeutic plasma exchange in patients with neurological disease. J Clin Apheresis 1992; 7:119–123.

Guillain–Barré Syndrome Study Group: Plasmapheresis and acute Guillain–Barré syndrome. Neurology 1985; 35:1096–1104.

Gutterman LA, Stevenson TD: Treatment of thrombotic thrombocytopenic purpura with vincristine. JAMA 1982; 247:1433–1436.

Hahn AF, Bolton CF, Pillay N, et al: Plasma-exchange therapy in chronic inflammatory demyelinating polyneuropathy. A double-blind, sham-controlled, cross-over study. Brain 1996; 119:1055–1066.

Hale GA, Reece DE, Munn RK, et al: Blood tacrolimus concentrations in bone marrow transplant patients undergoing plasmapheresis. Bone Marrow Transplant 2000; 25:449–451.

Hand JP, Lawlor ER, Yong CK, et al: Successful use of cyclosporine A in the treatment of refractory thrombotic thrombocytopenic purpura. Br J Haematol 1998; 100:597–599.

Hausfater P, Cacoub P, Assogba U, et al: Plasma exchange and interferon-alpha pharmacokinetics in patients with hepatitis C virus-associated systemic vasculitis. Nephron 2002; 91:627–630.

Heddle NM: Febrile nonhemolytic transfusion reactions to platelets. Curr Opin Hematol 1995; 2:478–483.

Heimfeld S: Bone marrow transplantation: how important is CD34 cell dose in HLA-identical stem cell transplantation? Leukemia 2003; 17:856–858.

Heininger K, Liebert UG, Toyka KV, et al: Chronic inflammatory polyneuropathy. Reduction of nerve conduction velocities in monkeys by systemic passive transfer of immunoglobulin G. J Neurol Sci 1984; 66:1–14.

Hester JP, McCullough J, Mishler JM, et al: Dosage regimens for citrate anticoagulants. J Clin Apheresis 1983; 1:149–157.

Hester JP, Dignani MC, Anaissie EJ, et al: Collection and transfusion of granulocyte concentrates from donors primed with granulocyte stimulating factor and response of myelosuppressed patients with established infection. J Clin Apheresis 1995; 10:188–193.

Heyns AP, Badenhorst PN, Lotter MG, et al: Kinetics and mobilization from the spleen of Indium-111-labeled platelets during platelet apheresis. Transfusion 1985; 25:215–218.

Higby DJ, Henderson ES, Burnett D, et al: Filtration leukapheresis: effects of donor stimulation with dexamethasone. Blood 1977; 50:953–959.

Hillyer CD, Berkman EM: Plasma exchange in dysproteinemias. In Rossi EC, Simon TL, Moss GS, Gould SA (eds): Principles of Transfusion Medicine. 2nd ed. Baltimore, Williams & Wilkins, 1996, pp 569–575.

Hubel K, Carter RA, Liles WC, et al: Granulocyte transfusion therapy for infections in candidates and recipients of HPC transplantation: A comparative analysis of feasibility and outcome for community donors versus related donors. Transfusion 2002; 42:1414–1421.

Huestis DW: Risks and safety practices in hemapheresis procedures. Arch Pathol Lab Med 1989; 113:273–278.

Huestis DW, Morrison FS: Adverse effects of immune adsorption with staphylococcal protein A columns. Transfus Med Rev 1996; 10:62–70.

Hughes RA: Plasma exchange in Guillain–Barré syndrome and related disorders. Transfus Sci 1993; 14:3–8.

Hughes RA, Newsom-Davis JM, Perkin GD, et al: Controlled trial prednisolone in acute polyneuropathy. Lancet 1978; 2:750–753.

Hussein MA, Lee EJ, Fletcher R, et al: The effect of lymphocytotoxic antibody reactivity on the results of single antigen mismatched platelet transfusions to alloimmunized patients. Blood 1996; 87:3959–3962.

Hymes KB, Karpatkin S: Human immunodeficiency

virus infection and thrombotic microangiopathy. Semin Hematol 1997; 34:117–125.

Iacone A, Di Bartolomeo P, Di Girolamo G, et al: Hydroxyethyl starch and steroid improved collection of normal granulocytes with continuous flow centrifugation gravity leukapheresis. Haematologica 1981; 66:645–655.

Isbister JP: Cytapheresis: the first 25 years. Ther Apher 1997; 1:17–21.

Iwasaki Y, Kinoshita M, Ikeda K, et al: Neuropsychological function before and after plasma exchange in myasthenia gravis. J Neurol Sci 1993; 114:223–226.

Jaeger BR, Marx P, Pfefferkorn T, et al: Heparin-mediated extracorporeal LDL/fibrinogen precipitation – H.E.L.P. – in coronary and cerebral ischemia. Acta Neurochir Suppl (Wien.) 1999; 73:81–84.

Jendiroba DB, Lichtiger B, Anaissie E, et al: Evaluation and comparison of three mobilization methods for the collection of granulocytes. Transfusion 1998; 38:722–728.

Johnson JP, Whitman W, Briggs WA, et al: Plasmapheresis and immunosuppressive agents in antibasement membrane antibody-induced Goodpasture's syndrome. Am J Med 1978; 64:354–359.

Johnson WJ, Kyle RA, Dahlberg PJ: Dialysis in the treatment of multiple myeloma. Mayo Clin Proc 1980; 55:65–72.

Johnson JP, Moore J Jr, Austin HA III, et al: Therapy of anti-glomerular basement membrane antibody disease: analysis of prognostic significance of clinical, pathologic and treatment factors. Medicine (Baltimore) 1985; 64:219–227.

Johnson WJ, Kyle RA, Pineda AA, et al: Treatment of renal failure associated with multiple myeloma. Plasmapheresis, hemodialysis, and chemotherapy. Arch Intern Med 1990; 150:863–869.

Joos K, Herzog R, Einsele H, et al: Characterization and functional analysis of granulocyte concentrates collected from donors after repeated G-CSF stimulation. Transfusion 2002; 42:603–611.

Jovin IS, Taborski U, Muller-Berghaus G: Comparing low-density lipoprotein apheresis procedures: difficulties and remedies. J Clin Apheresis 1996; 11:186–170.

Kale-Pradhan PB, Woo MH: A review of the effects of plasmapheresis on drug clearance. Pharmacotherapy 1997; 17:684–695.

An extensive review of the literature concerning the effects of plasma exchange on drug clearance and metabolism. The article provides suggestions for therapy modification as well as future research.

Kamanabroo D, Ulrich K, Grobe H, et al: Plasma exchange in type II hypercholesterolemia. Prog Clin Biol Res 1988; 255:347–354.

Kamochi M, Aibara K, Nakata K, et al: Profound ionized hypomagnesemia induced by therapeutic plasma exchange in liver failure patients. Transfusion 2002; 42:1598–1602.

Kannan S, Milligan KR: Moderately severe anaphylactoid reaction to pentastarch (200/0.5) in a patient with acute severe asthma. Intensive Care Med 1999; 25:220–222.

Kaplinsky C, Trakhtenbrot L, Hardan I, et al: Tetraploid myeloid cells in donors of peripheral blood stem cells treated with rhG-CSF. Bone Marrow Transplant 2003; 32:31–34.

Katz AJ, Genco PV, Blumberg N, et al: Platelet collection and transfusion using the Fenwal CS-3000 cell separator. Transfusion 1981; 21:560–563.

Kelleher SP, Schulman G: Severe metabolic alkalosis complicating regional citrate hemodialysis. Am J Kidney Dis 1987; 9:235–236.

Kessinger A, Armitage JO, Smith DM, et al: High-dose therapy and autologous peripheral blood stem cell transplantation for patients with lymphoma. Blood 1989; 74:1260–1265.

Kessinger A, Bishop MR, Anderson JR, et al: Comparison of subcutaneous and intravenous administration of recombinant human granulocyte-macrophage colony-stimulating factor for

IV

peripheral blood stem cell mobilization. J Hematother 1995; 4:81–84.

Kessinger A, Sharp JG: The whys and hows of hematopoietic progenitor and stem cell mobilization. Bone Marrow Transplant 2003; 31:319–329.

Kishimoto M, Ohto H, Shikama Y, et al: Treatment for the decline of ionized calcium levels during peripheral blood progenitor cell harvesting. Transfusion 2002; 42:1340–1347.

Klingel R, Fassbender C, Fassbender T, et al: Clinical studies to implement rheopheresis for age-related macular degeneration guided by evidence-based-medicine. Transfus Apheresis Sci 2003; 29:71–84.

Knobler RM, Trautinger F, Graninger W, et al: Parenteral administration of 8-methoxypsoralen in photopheresis. J Am Acad Dermatol 1993; 28:580–584.

Koch-Weser J, Sellers EM: Binding of drugs to serum albumin (first of two parts). N Engl J Med 1976; 294:311–316.

Korbling M: Effects of granulocyte colony-stimulating factor in healthy subjects. Curr Opin Hematol 1998; 5:209–214.

Korbling M, Huh YO, Durett A, et al: Allogeneic blood stem cell transplantation: peripheralization and yield of donor-derived primitive hematopoietic progenitor cells (CD34+ Thy-1dim) and lymphoid subsets, and possible predictors of engraftment and graft-versus-host disease. Blood 1995; 86:2842–2848.

Koski CL, Humphrey R, Shin ML: Anti-peripheral myelin antibody in patients with demyelinating neuropathy: quantitative and kinetic determination of serum antibody by complement component 1 fixation. Proc Natl Acad Sci USA 1985; 82:905–909.

Koski CL, Gratz E, Sutherland J, et al: Clinical correlation with anti-peripheral-nerve myelin antibodies in Guillain–Barré syndrome. Ann Neurol 1986; 19:573–577.

Kroger N, Zander AR: Dose and schedule effect of G-GSF for stem cell mobilization in healthy donors for allogeneic transplantation. Leuk Lymphoma 2002; 43:1391–1394.

Lane DM, McConathy WJ, Laughlin LO, et al: Weekly treatment of diet/drug-resistant hypercholesterolemia with the heparin-induced extracorporeal low-density lipoprotein precipitation (HELP) system by selective plasma low-density lipoprotein removal. Am J Cardiol 1993; 71:816–822.

Lapidot T, Petit I: Current understanding of stem cell mobilization: the roles of chemokines, proteolytic enzymes, adhesion molecules, cytokines, and stromal cells. Exp Hematol 2002; 30:973–981.

Lasky LC, Lin A, Kahn RA, et al: Donor platelet response and product quality assurance in plateletpheresis. Transfusion 1981; 21:247–260.

Laurenti F, Ferro R, Isacchi G, et al: Polymorphonuclear leukocyte transfusion for the treatment of sepsis in the newborn infant. J Pediatr 1981; 98:118–123.

Lazarus EF, Browning J, Norman J, et al: Sustained decreases in platelet count associated with multiple, regular plateletpheresis donations. Transfusion 2001; 41:756–761.

Lee JH, Klein HG: Collection and use of circulating hematopoietic progenitor cells. Hematol Oncol Clin North Am 1995a; 9:1–22.

Lee JH, Leitman SF, Klein HG: A controlled comparison of the efficacy of hetastarch and pentastarch in granulocyte collections by centrifugal leukapheresis. Blood 1995b; 86:4662–4666.

Leitman SF, Boltansky H, Alter HJ, et al: Allergic reactions in healthy plateletpheresis donors caused by sensitization to ethylene oxide gas. N Engl J Med 1986; 315:1192–1196.

Leitman SF, Smith JW, Gregg RE: Homozygous familial hypercholesterolemia. Selective removal of low-density lipoproteins by secondary membrane filtration. Transfusion 1989; 29:341–346.

Lercari G, Paganini G, Malfanti L, et al: Apheresis for severe malaria complicated by cerebral malaria, acute respiratory distress syndrome, acute renal failure, and disseminated intravascular coagulation. J Clin Apheresis 1992; 7:93–96.

Leren TP, Fagerhol MK, Leren P: Sixteen years of plasma exchange in a homozygote for familial hypercholesterolemia. J Int Med 1993; 233:195–200.

Lester TJ, Johnson JW, Cuttner J: Pulmonary leukostasis as the single worst prognostic factor in patients with acute myelocytic leukemia and hyperleukocytosis. Am J Med 1985; 79:43–48.

Levy GG, Nichols WC, Lian EC, et al: Mutations in a member of the ADAMTS gene family cause thrombotic thrombocytopenic purpura. Nature 2001a; 413:488–494.

Levy J, Degani N: Correcting immune imbalance: The use of Prosorba column treatment for immune disorders. Ther Apher Dial 2003; 7:197–205.

Levy JB, Turner AN, Rees AJ, et al: Long-term outcome of anti-glomerular basement membrane antibody disease treated with plasma exchange and immunosuppression. Ann Intern Med 2001b; 134:1033–1042.

Lewis SL, Kutvirt SG, Bonner PN, et al: Effect of long-term platelet donation on lymphocyte subsets and plasma protein concentrations. Transfus Sci 1999; 18:205–213.

Lieschke GJ, Burgess AW: Granulocyte colony-stimulating factor and granulocyte-macrophage colony-stimulating factor (2). N Engl J Med 1992; 327:99–106.

Liesveld JL: Expression and function of adhesion receptors in acute myelogenous leukemia: parallels with normal erythroid and myeloid progenitors. Acta Haematol 1997; 97:53–62.

Liles WC, Dale DC, Klebanoff SJ: Glucocorticoids inhibit apoptosis of human neutrophils. Blood 1995; 86:3181–3188.

Liles WC, Huang JE, Llewellyn C, et al: A comparative trial of granulocyte-colony-stimulating factor and dexamethasone, separately and in combination, for the mobilization of neutrophils in the peripheral blood of normal volunteers. Transfusion 1997; 37:182–187.

Liles WC, Rodger E, Dale DC: Combined administration of G-CSF and dexamethasone for the mobilization of granulocytes in normal donors: optimization of dosing. Transfusion 2000; 40:642–644.

Lin JS, Burgstaler EA, Pineda AA, et al: Effects of whole blood flow rates on mononuclear cell yields during peripheral blood stem cell collection using Fenwal CS 3000 Plus. J Clin Apheresis 1995; 10:7–11.

Lindstrom JM, Seybold ME, Lennon VA, et al: Antibody to acetylcholine receptor in myasthenia gravis. Prevalence, clinical correlates, and diagnostic value. Neurology 1976; 26:1054–1059.

Lysaght MJ, Samtleben WS: Closed-loop plasmapheresis. In MacPherson JL, Kasprisin DO (eds): Therapeutic Hemapheresis. Boca Raton, CRC Press, 1985, pp 149–168.

McClellan SD, Whitaker CH, Friedberg RC: Removal of vancomycin during plasmapheresis. Ann Pharmacother 1997; 31:1132–1136.

McCrae KR, Cines DB: Thrombotic microangiopathy during pregnancy. Semin Hematol 1997; 34:148–158.

McCullough J, Clay M, Hurd D, et al: Effect of leukocyte antibodies and HLA matching on the intravascular recovery, survival, and tissue localization of 111-indium granulocytes. Blood 1986; 67:522–528.

McCullough J, Clay M, Loken M, et al: Effect of ABO incompatibility on the fate in vivo of 111indium granulocytes. Transfusion 1988; 28:358–361.

McGrath MA, Penny R: Paraproteinemia: Blood hyperviscosity and clinical manifestations. J Clin Invest 1976; 58:1155–1162.

McLeod BC: Introduction to the third special issue: Clinical applications of therapeutic apheresis. J Clin Apheresis 2000; 15:1–5.

McLeod BC, Sassetti RJ: Plasmapheresis with return of cryoglobulin-depleted autologous plasma (cryoglobulinpheresis) in cryoglobulinemia. Blood 1980; 55:866–870.

McLeod BC, Strauss RG, Ciavarella D, et al: Management of hematological disorders and cancer. J Clin Apheresis 1993; 8:211–230.

McLeod BC, Price TH, Owen H, et al: Frequency of immediate adverse effects associated with apheresis donation. Transfusion 1998; 38:938–943.

McLeod BC, Sniecinski I, Ciavarella D, et al: Frequency of immediate adverse effects associated with therapeutic apheresis. Transfusion 1999; 39:282–288.

McLeod BC, Price TH, Weinstein R (eds): Apheresis: Principles and Practice, 2nd ed. Bethesda, AABB Press, 2003.

A comprehensive textbook that addresses both donor and therapeutic apheresis including the history of apheresis, currently available instrumentation, and in-depth discussion of the mechanism of action and physiology of apheresis.

MacPherson JL, Nusbacher J, Bennett JM: The acquisition of granulocytes by leukapheresis: a comparison of continuous flow centrifugation and filtration leukapheresis in normal and corticosteroid-stimulated donors. Transfusion 1976; 16:221–228.

Mansur LI, Murrow RW, Garrelts JC, et al: Rebound of plasma free phenytoin concentration following plasmapheresis in a patient with thrombotic thrombocytopenic purpura. Ann Pharmacother 1995; 29:592–595.

Marques MB, Huang ST: Patients with thrombotic thrombocytopenic purpura commonly develop metabolic alkalosis during therapeutic plasma exchange. J Clin Apheresis 2001; 16:120–124.

Maselli RA: Pathophysiology of myasthenia gravis and Lambert–Eaton syndrome. Neurol Clin 1994; 12:285–303.

Matic G, Bosch T, Ramlow W: Background and indications for protein A-based extracorporeal immunoadsorption. Ther Apher 2001; 5:394–403.

Matsuda Y, Malchesky PS, Nose Y: Assessment of currently available low-density lipoprotein apheresis systems. Artif Organs 1994; 18:93–99.

Matsuzaki M., Hiramori K, Imaizumi T, et al: Intravascular ultrasound evaluation of coronary plaque regression by low density lipoprotein-apheresis in familial hypercholesterolemia: the Low Density Lipoprotein-Apheresis Coronary Morphology and Reserve Trial (LACMART). J Am Coll Cardiol 2002; 40:220–227.

Mendell JR, Kissel JT, Kennedy MS, et al: Plasma exchange and prednisone in Guillain–Barré syndrome: a controlled randomized trial. Neurology 1985; 35:1551–1555.

Mercan D, Bastin G, Lambermont M, et al: Importance of ionized magnesium measurement for monitoring of citrate-anticoagulated plateletpheresis. Transfusion 1997; 37:418–422.

Meyer D, Bolgiano DC, Sayers M, et al: Red cell collection by apheresis technology. Transfusion 1993; 33:819–824.

Mistry-Burchardi N, Schonermarck U, Samtleben W: Apheresis in lupus nephritis. Ther Apher 2001; 5:161–170.

Moake JL: Thrombotic thrombocytopenic purpura. Thromb Haemost 1995; 74:240–245.

Moake JL, McPherson PD: Abnormalities of von Willebrand factor multimers in thrombotic thrombocytopenic purpura and the hemolytic-uremic syndrome. Am J Med 1989; 87:9N–15N.

Mokrzycki MH, Kaplan AA: Therapeutic plasma exchange: Complications and management. Am J Kidney Dis 1994; 23:817–827.

Mollison PL, Engelfriet CP, Contreras M: Appendix 5. In: Blood Transfusion in Clinical Medicine, 10th ed. Malden, Blackwell Science, 1998, pp 561–561.

Montacer-Kuhssari J, Voller H, Keller F: Pulmonary air embolism. Intensive Care Med 1994; 20:166–167.

Montgomery RA, Zachary AA, Racusen LC, et al: Plasmapheresis and intravenous immune globulin provides effective rescue therapy for refractory humoral rejection and allows kidneys to be successfully transplanted into cross-match-positive recipients. Transplantation 2000; 70:887–895.

Moog R, Muller N: Technical aspects and performance in collecting peripheral blood progenitor cells. Ann Hematol 1998; 77:143–147.

Murata M, Harada M, Kato S, et al: Peripheral blood stem cell mobilization and apheresis: analysis of adverse events in 94 normal donors. Bone Marrow Transplant 1999; 24:1065–1071.

Murphy MF, Waters AH: Clinical aspects of platelet transfusions. Blood Coagul Fibrinolysis 1991; 2:389–396.

Muylle L, Baeten M, Avonts G, et al: Anaphylactoid reaction in platelet-pheresis donor with IgE antibodies to ethylene oxide. Lancet 1986; 2:1225.

Nadler SB, Hidalgo JU, Bloch T: Prediction of blood volume in normal human adults. Surgery 1962; 5:224.

Nagler A, Korenstein-Ilan A, Amiel A, et al: Granulocyte colony-stimulating factor generates epigenetic and genetic alterations in lymphocytes of normal volunteer donors of stem cells. Exp Hematol 2004; 32:122–130.

Naik B, Hirshhorn S, Dharnidharka VR: Prolonged neuromuscular block due to cholinesterase depletion by plasmapheresis. J Clin Anesth 2002; 14:381–384.

National Blood Data Resource Center (National Blood Data Resource Center): Comprehensive Report on Blood Collection and Transfusion in the United States in 1999. Bethesda, MD, Maryland, 2001.

Nearman HS, Herman ML: Toxic effects of colloids in the intensive care unit. Crit Care Clin 1991; 7:713–723.

Nesher G, Hanna VE, Moore TL, et al: Thrombotic microangiographic hemolytic anemia in systemic lupus erythematosus. Semin Arthritis Rheum 1994; 24:165–172.

Ness P, Braine H, King K, et al: Single-donor platelets reduce the risk of septic platelet transfusion reactions. Transfusion 2001; 41:857–861.

Newman BH: Donor reactions and injuries from whole blood donation. Transfus Med Rev 1997; 11:64–75.

Noseworthy JH, Shumak KH, Vandervoort MK: Long-term use of antecubital veins for plasma exchange. The Canadian Cooperative Multiple Sclerosis Study Group. Transfusion 1989; 29:610–613.

O'Connell BA, Lee EJ, Rothko K, et al: Selection of histocompatible apheresis platelet donors by cross-matching random donor platelet concentrates. Blood 1992; 79:527–531.

Orlin JB, Berkman EM: Partial plasma exchange using albumin replacement: Removal and recovery of normal plasma constituents. Blood 1980; 56:1055–1059.

Owen HG, Brecher ME: Atypical reactions associated with use of angiotensin-converting enzyme inhibitors and apheresis. Transfusion 1994; 34:891–894.

Parhofer KG, Geiss HC, Schwandt P: Efficacy of different low-density lipoprotein apheresis methods. Ther Apher 2000; 4:382–385.

Park WD, Grande JP, Ninova D, et al: Accommodation in ABO-incompatible kidney allografts, a novel mechanism of self-protection against antibody-mediated injury. Am J Transplant 2003; 3:952–960.

Passos-Coelho JL, Braine HG, Davis JM, et al: Predictive factors for peripheral-blood progenitor-cell collections using a single large-volume leukapheresis after cyclophosphamide and granulocyte-macrophage colony-stimulating factor mobilization. J Clin Oncol 1995a; 13:705–714.

Passos-Coelho JL, Ross AA, Moss TJ, et al: Absence of breast cancer cells in a single-day peripheral blood progenitor cell collection after priming with cyclophosphamide and granulocyte-macrophage colony-stimulating factor. Blood 1995b; 85:1138–1143.

Pearl DG, Rosenthal MH: Metabolic alkalosis due to plasmapheresis. Am J Med 1985; 79:391–393.

Perdue JJ, Chandler LK, Vesely SK, et al: Unintentional platelet removal by plasmapheresis. J Clin Apheresis 2001; 16:55–60.

Pettitt AR, Clark RE: Thrombotic microangiopathy following bone marrow transplantation. Bone Marrow Transplant 1994; 14:495–504.

Plasma Exchange/Sandoglobulin Guillain–Barré Syndrome Trial Group: Randomised trial of plasma exchange, intravenous immunoglobulin, and combined treatments in Guillain–Barré syndrome. Lancet 1997; 349:225–230.

Pool M, McLeod BC: Pyrogen reactions to human serum albumin during plasma exchange. J Clin Apheresis 1995; 10:81–84.

Popovsky MA, Whitaker B, Arnold NL: Severe outcomes of allogeneic and autologous blood donation: frequency and characterization. Transfusion 1995; 35:734–737.

Porcu P, Danielson CF, Orazi A, et al: Therapeutic leukapheresis in hyperleucocytic leukaemias: lack of correlation between degree of cytoreduction and early mortality rate. Br J Haematol 1997; 98:433–436.

Porcu P, Cripe LD, Ng EW, et al: Hyperleukocytic leukemias and leukostasis: A review of pathophysiology, clinical presentation and management. Leuk Lymphoma 2000; 39:1–18.

Price TH: Granulocyte colony-stimulating factor-mobilized granulocyte concentrate transfusions. Curr Opin Hematol 1998; 5:391–395.

Price TH, Dale DC: Blood kinetics and in vivo chemotaxis of transfused neutrophils: Effect of collection method, donor corticosteroid treatment, and short-term storage. Blood 1979; 54:977–986.

Przepiorka D, Suzuki J, Ippoliti C, et al: Blood tacrolimus concentration unchanged by plasmapheresis. Am J Hosp Pharm 1994; 51:1708.

Pusey CD, Lockwood CM, Peters DK: Plasma exchange and immunosuppressive drugs in the treatment of glomerulonephritis due to antibodies to the glomerular basement membrane. Int J Artif Organs 1983; 6(Suppl 1):15–18.

Quintana R, Smith KJ, James DS: Exercise performance in blood donors: a randomized, double blind comparison of sham, 1U, and 2U red cell donation. Transfusion 1995; 35(Suppl):14S.

Randerson DH, Blumenstein M, Habersetzer R, et al: Mass transfer in membrane plasma exchange. Artif Organs 1982; 6:43–49.

Raphael JC, Chevret S, Hughes RA, et al: Plasma exchange for Guillain–Barré syndrome. Cochrane Database Syst Rev 2:CD001798, 2002.
This is a comprehensive and critical review of all of the available literature concerning the effectiveness of plasma exchange in the treatment of AIDP.

Reik RA, Noto TA, Fernandez HF: Safety of large-volume leukapheresis for collection of peripheral blood progenitor cells. J Clin Apheresis 1997; 12:10–13.

Rice L, Tsai HM, Chow TW, et al: Increased von Willebrand factor (vWf)-platelet binding and decreased vWf-metalloproteinase in ticlopidine-induced thrombotic thrombocytopenic purpura (TTP). Blood 1998; 92(Suppl 2):706a.

Richter WO, Jacob BG, Ritter MM, et al: Three-year treatment of familial heterozygous hypercholesterolemia by extracorporeal low-density lipoprotein immunoadsorption with polyclonal apolipoprotein B antibodies. Metabolism 1993; 42:888–894.

Ring J, Messmer K: Incidence and severity of anaphylactoid reactions to colloid volume substitutes. Lancet 1977; 1:466–469.

Rock GA, Shumak KH, Buskard NA, et al: Comparison of plasma exchange with plasma infusion in the treatment of thrombotic thrombocytopenic purpura. N Engl J Med 1991; 325:393–397.

Rock G, Shumak KH, Sutton DM, et al: Cryosupernatant as replacement fluid for plasma exchange in thrombotic thrombocytopenic purpura. Members of the Canadian Apheresis Group. Br J Haematol 1996; 94:383–386.

Rock G, Sutton DM, Freedman J, et al: Pentastarch instead of albumin as replacement fluid for therapeutic plasma exchange. The Canadian Apheresis Group. J Clin Apheresis 1997; 12:165–169.

Rogers RL, Johnson H, Ludwig G, et al: Efficacy and safety of plateletpheresis by donors with low-normal platelet counts. J Clin Apheresis 1995; 10:194–197.

Ropper AE, Albert JW, Addison R: Limited relapse in Guillain–Barré syndrome after plasma exchange. Arch Neurol 1988; 45:314–315.

Ropper AH: The Guillain–Barré syndrome. N Engl J Med 1992; 326:1130–1136.

Rouvier B, Maudan P, Debue JF, et al: Traitement par erythropherese d'un acces pernicieux palustre. Ann Fr Anesth Reanim 1988; 7:257–260.

Salama AD, Delikouras A, Pusey CD, et al: Transplant accommodation in highly sensitized patients: a potential role for Bcl xL and alloantibody. Am J Transplant 2001; 1:260–269.

Salmon SE, Cassady RJ: Plasma cell neoplasms. *In* DeVita VT, Hellman S, Rosenberg SA (eds): Cancer: Principles and Practice of Oncology. 2nd ed. New York, Lippincott-Raven, 1997, pp 2344–2386.

Sanders DB, Scoppetta C: The treatment of patients with myasthenia gravis. Neurol Clin 1994; 12:343–368.

Sarode R, McFarland JG, Flomenberg N, et al: Therapeutic plasma exchange does not appear to be effective in the management of thrombotic thrombocytopenic purpura/hemolytic uremic syndrome following bone marrow transplantation. Bone Marrow Transplant 1995; 16:271–275.

Schafer AI: Bleeding and thrombosis in the myeloproliferative disorders. Blood 1984; 64:1–12.

Schafer AI: Management of thrombocythemia. Curr Opin Hematol 1996; 3:341–346.

Schiffer CA: Management of patients refractory to platelet transfusion – an evaluation of methods of donor selection. Prog Hematol 1987; 15:91–113.

Schiffer CA: Granulocyte transfusions: an overlooked therapeutic modality. Transfus Med Rev 1990; 4:2–7.

Schlenke P, Frohn C, Steinhardt MM, et al: Clinically relevant hypokalemia, hypocalcemia, and loss of hemoglobin and platelets during stem cell apheresis. J Clin Apheresis 2000; 15:230–235.

Schulzeck P, Olbricht CJ, Koch KM: Long-term experience with extracorporeal low-density lipoprotein cholesterol removal by dextran sulfate cellulose adsorption. Clin Investig 1992; 70:99–104.

Schweitzer EJ, Wilson JS, Fernandez-Vina M, et al: A high panel-reactive antibody rescue protocol for cross-match-positive live donor kidney transplants. Transplantation 2000; 70:1531–1536.

Shehata N, Kouroukis C, Kelton JG: A review of randomized controlled trials using therapeutic apheresis. Transfus Med Rev 2002; 16:200–229.
A summary of all of the randomized controlled trials involving therapeutic apheresis. Includes numerous tables summarizing the trials as well as recommendations concerning treatment protocols.

Siegel JF, Rich MA, Brock WA: Association of sickle cell disease, priapism, exchange transfusion and neurological events: ASPEN syndrome. J Urol 1993; 150:1480–1482.

Silberstein LE, Naryshkin S, Haddad JJ, et al: Calcium homeostasis during therapeutic plasma exchange. Transfusion 1986; 26:151–155.

Sintnicolaas K, Vriesendorp HM, Sizoo W, et al: Delayed alloimmunisation by random single donor platelet transfusions. A randomised study to compare single donor and multiple donor platelet transfusions in cancer patients with severe thrombocytopenia. Lancet 1981; 1:750–754.

Sirtl C, Laubenthal H, Zumtobel V, et al: Tissue deposits of hydroxyethyl starch (HES): dose-dependent and time related. Br J Anaesth 1999; 82:510–515.

Sketris IS, Parker WA, Jones JV: Effect of plasma exchange on drug removal. *In* Valbonesi M, Pineda

IV

AA, Biggs JC (eds): Therapeutic Hemapheresis. Milan, Wichtig Editore, 1986, pp 15–20.

Smith KJ, James DS, Hunt WC, et al: A randomized, double-blind comparison of donor tolerance of 400 mL, 200 mL, and sham red cell donation. Transfusion 1996; 36:674–680.

Smolowicz AG, Villman K, Tidefelt U: Large-volume apheresis for the harvest of peripheral blood progenitor cells for autologous transplantation. Transfusion 1997; 37:188–192.

Smolowicz AG, Villman K, Berlin G, et al: Kinetics of peripheral blood stem cell harvests during a single apheresis. Transfusion 1999; 39:403–409.

Solling K, Solling J: Clearances of Bence-Jones proteins during peritoneal dialysis or plasmapheresis in myelomatosis associated with renal failure. Contrib Nephrol 1988; 68:259–262.

Standards Committee of the American Association of Blood Banks, Menitove JE (ed): Standards for Blood Bank and Transfusion Services, 18th ed. Bethesda, American Association of Blood Banks, 1997.

Standards Committee of the American Association of Blood Banks, Silva MA (ed): Standards for Blood Banks and Transfusion Services, 23rd ed. Bethesda, American Association of Blood Banks, 2004.

Stander S, Szepfalusi Z, Bohle B, et al: Differential storage of hydroxyethyl starch (HES) in the skin: an immunoelectron-microscopical long-term study. Cell Tissue Res 2001; 304:261–269.

Steeper TA, Smith JA, McCullough J: Therapeutic cytapheresis using the Fenwal CS-3000 blood cell separator. Vox Sang 1985; 48:193–200.

Stegall MD, Dean PG, McBride MA, Wynn JJ: Survival of mandatorily shared cadaveric kidneys and their paybacks in the zero mismatch era. Transplantation 2002; 74:670–675.

Stohlawetz P, Stiegler G, Jilma B, et al: Measurement of the levels of reticulated platelets after plateletpheresis to monitor activity of thrombopoiesis. Transfusion 1998; 38:454–458.

Strauss RG: Transfusion therapy in neonates. Am J Dis Child 1991; 145:904–911.

Strauss RG: Therapeutic granulocyte transfusions in 1993. Blood 1993; 81:1675–1678.

Strauss RG: Effects on donors of repeated leukocyte losses during plateletpheresis. J Clin Apheresis 1994; 9:130–134.

Strauss RG: Mechanisms of adverse effects during hemapheresis. J Clin Apheresis 1996; 11:160–164.

Strauss RG, Hester JP, Vogler WR, et al: A multicenter trial to document the efficacy and safety of a rapidly excreted analog of hydroxyethyl starch for leukapheresis with a note on steroid stimulation of granulocyte donors. Transfusion 1986; 26:258–264.

Strauss RG, Villhauer PJ, Imig KM, et al: Selecting the optimal dose of low-molecular-weight hydroxyethyl starch (pentastarch) for granulocyte collection. Transfusion 1987; 27:350–352.

Strauss RG, Stansfield C, Henriksen RA, et al: Pentastarch may cause fewer effects on coagulation than hetastarch. Transfusion 1988; 28:257–260.

Stroncek DF, Clay ME, Petzoldt ML, et al: Treatment of normal individuals with granulocyte-colony-stimulating factor: donor experiences and the effects on peripheral blood CD34+ cell counts and on the collection of peripheral blood stem cells. Transfusion 1996a; 36:601–610.

Stroncek DF, Clay ME, Smith J, et al: Changes in blood counts after the administration of granulocyte-colony-stimulating factor and the collection of peripheral blood stem cells from healthy donors. Transfusion 1996b; 36:596–600.

Stroncek DF, Clay ME, Herr G, et al: Blood counts in healthy donors 1 year after the collection of granulocyte-colony-stimulating factor-mobilized progenitor cells and the results of a second mobilization and collection. Transfusion 1997a; 37:304–308.

Stroncek DF, Clay ME, Smith J, et al: Comparison of two blood cell separators in collecting peripheral blood stem cell components. Transfus Med 1997b; 7:95–99.

Stroncek DF, Matthews CL, Follmann D, et al: Kinetics of G-CSF-induced granulocyte mobilization in healthy subjects: effects of route of administration and addition of dexamethasone. Transfusion 2002; 42:597–602.

Stucki A, Rivier AS, Gikic M, et al: Endothelial cell activation by myeloblasts: Molecular mechanisms of leukostasis and leukemic cell dissemination. Blood 2001; 97:2121–2129.

Suckfull M: Fibrinogen and LDL apheresis in treatment of sudden hearing loss: a randomised multicentre trial. Lancet 2002; 360:1811–1817.

Suckfull M, Thiery J, Schorn K, et al: Clinical utility of LDL-apheresis in the treatment of sudden hearing loss: a prospective, randomized study. Acta Otolaryngol 1999; 119:763–766.

Szymanski IO: Ionized calcium during plateletpheresis. Transfusion 1978; 18:701–708.

Szymanski IO, Patti K, Kliman A: Efficacy of the Latham blood processor to perform plateletpheresis. Transfusion 1973; 13:405–411.

Tanabe K, Takahashi K, Sonda K, et al: Long-term results of ABO-incompatible living kidney transplantation: a single-center experience. Transplantation 1998; 65:224–228.

Taylor H, Sawyer S, Whitley P, et al: Donor safety and physiologic response to automated collection of double red cell collection on ALYX. J Clin Apheresis 2002; 17:143.

Technical manual committee, Brecher ME (ed): Technical Manual, 14th ed. Bethesda, American Association of Blood Banks, 2002.

Tefferi A, Hoagland HC: Issues in the diagnosis and management of essential thrombocythemia. Mayo Clin Proc 1994; 69:651–655.

Thompson GR, Miller JP, Breslow JL: Improved survival of patients with homozygous familial hypercholesterolemia treated by plasma exchange. Br Med J 1985; 291:1671–1673.

Thompson GR, Maher VM, Matthews S, et al: Familial Hypercholesterolaemia Regression Study: a randomised trial of low-density-lipoprotein apheresis. Lancet 1995; 345:811–816.

Tomita T, Takayanagi M, Kiwada K, et al: Vasovagal reactions in apheresis donors. Transfusion 2002; 42:1561–1566.

Trial to Reduce Alloimmunization to Platelets Study Group: Leukocyte reduction and ultraviolet B irradiation of platelets to prevent alloimmunization and refractoriness to platelet transfusions. N Engl J Med 1997; 337:1861–1869.

Tsai HM, Lian EC: Antibodies to von Willebrand factor-cleaving protease in acute thrombotic thrombocytopenic purpura. N Engl J Med 1998; 339:1585–1594.

Tsai HM, Chandler WL, Sarode R, et al: von Willebrand factor and von Willebrand factor-cleaving metalloprotease activity in Escherichia coli O157:H7-associated hemolytic uremic syndrome. Pediatr Res 2001; 49:653–659.

United Network for Organ Sharing, Department of Health and Human Services, Health Resources and Services Administration, Office of Special Programs, Division of Transplantation, United Network for Organ Sharing: US Scientific Registry for Transplant Recipients and the Organ Procurement and Transplantation Network: Annual report 2000. Transplant Data 1990–1999. Rockville MD, Richmond VA, Maryland, 2000.

United Network for Organ Sharing, Department of Health and Human Services, Health Resources and Services Administration. Office of Special Programs, Division of Transplantation: 2001 Annual Report of the US Organ Procurement and Transplantation Network and the Scientific Registry for Transplant Recipients: Transplant Data 1991–2000. Rockville MD, Richmond VA, Ann Arbor MI, Maryland, 2001.

Vamvakas EC, Pineda AA: Meta-analysis of clinical studies of the efficacy of granulocyte transfusions in the treatment of bacterial sepsis. J Clin Apheresis 1996; 11:1–9.

Vamvakas EC, Pineda A: Allergic and anaphylactic reactions. In Popovsky MA (ed): Transfusion Reactions, 2nd ed. Bethesda, AABB Press, 2001, pp 83–127.

van Burik JA: Granulocyte transfusions as treatment or prophylaxis for fungal infections? Curr Opin Investig Drugs 2003; 4:921–925.

van der Plas RM, Schiphorst ME, Huizinga EG, et al: von Willebrand factor proteolysis is deficient in classic, but not in bone marrow transplantation-associated, thrombotic thrombocytopenic purpura. Blood 1999; 93:3798–3802.

van Doorn PA, Brand A, Strengers PF, et al: High-dose intravenous immunoglobulin treatment in chronic inflammatory demyelinating polyneuropathy: a double-blind, placebo-controlled, crossover study. Neurology 1990; 40:209–212.

van Doorn PA, Vermeulen M, Brand A, et al: Intravenous immunoglobulin treatment in patients with chronic inflammatory demyelinating polyneuropathy. Clinical and laboratory characteristics associated with improvement. Arch Neurol 1991; 48:217–220.

van Iperen HP, Beijersbergen van Henegouwen GM: Clinical and mechanistic aspects of photopheresis. J Photochem Photobiol B 1997; 39:99–109.

Vichinsky EP, Haberkern CM, Neumayr L, et al: A comparison of conservative and aggressive transfusion regimens in the perioperative management of sickle cell disease. The Preoperative Transfusion in Sickle Cell Disease Study Group. N Engl J Med 1995; 333:206–213.

Volk EE, Domen RE, Smith ML: An examination of ethical issues raised in the pretreatment of normal volunteer granulocyte donors with granulocyte colony-stimulating factor. Arch Pathol Lab Med 1999; 123:508–513.

Volkin RL, Starz TW, Winkelstein A, et al: Changes in coagulation factors, complement, immunoglobulins, and immune complex concentrations with plasma exchange. Transfusion 1982; 22:54–58.

Vriesendorp FJ, Mayer RF, Koski CL: Kinetics of anti-peripheral nerve myelin antibody in patients with Guillain–Barré syndrome treated and not treated with plasmapheresis. Arch Neurol 1991; 48:858–861.

Wallace EL, Surgenor DM, Hao HS, et al: Collection and transfusion of blood and blood components in the United States, 1989. Transfusion 1993; 33:139–144.

Wasi S, Santowski T, Murray SA, et al: The Canadian Red Cross plasmapheresis donor safety program: changes in plasma proteins after long-term plasmapheresis. Vox Sang 1991; 60:82–87.

Wayne AS, Kevy SV, Nathan DG: Transfusion management of sickle cell disease. Blood 1993; 81:1109–1123.

Weinstein R: Prevention of citrate reactions during therapeutic plasma exchange by constant infusion of calcium gluconate with the return fluid. J Clin Apheresis 1996; 11:204–210.

Wheeler JG, Chauvenet AR, Johnson CA, et al: Buffy coat transfusions in neonates with sepsis and neutrophil storage pool depletion. Pediatrics 1987; 79:422–425.

Wiener Y, Nakhleh RE, Lee MW, et al: Prognostic factors and early resumption of cyclosporin A in renal allograft recipients with thrombotic microangiopathy and hemolytic uremic syndrome. Clin Transplant 1997; 11:157–162.

Wiltbank TB: Donor reaction rates: A preliminary comparison of automated vs. whole blood procedures. Transfusion 2002; 42(Suppl):67S.

Winston DJ, Ho WG, Young LS, et al: Prophylactic granulocyte transfusions during human bone marrow transplantation. Am J Med 1980; 68:893–897.

Winters JL, Gloor JM, Pineda AA, et al: Plasma exchange conditioning for ABO-incompatible renal transplantation. J Clin Apheresis 2004; 19:79–85.

Wiseman KC: New insights on Goodpasture's syndrome. ANNA J 1993; 20:17–26.

Wood GJ, Hall GM: Plasmapheresis and plasma cholinesterase. Br J Anaesth 1978; 50:945–949.

Yacobi A, Stoll RG, Sum CY, et al: Pharmacokinetics of hydroxyethyl starch in normal subjects. J Clin Pharmacol 1982; 22:206–212.

Zachary AA, Montgomery RA, Ratner LE, et al: Specific and durable elimination of antibody to donor HLA antigens in renal-transplant patients. Transplantation 2003; 76:1519–1525.

Zaucha JM, Gooley T, Bensinger WI, et al: CD34 cell dose in granulocyte colony-stimulating factor-mobilized peripheral blood mononuclear cell grafts affects engraftment kinetics and development of extensive chronic graft-versus-host disease after human leukocyte antigen-identical sibling transplantation. Blood 2001; 98:3221–3227.

Zeigler ZR, Shadduck RK, Gryn JF, et al: Cryoprecipitate poor plasma does not improve early response in primary adult thrombotic thrombocytopenic purpura (TTP). J Clin Apheresis 2001; 16:19–22.

Zic JA: The treatment of cutaneous T-cell lymphoma with photopheresis. Dermatol Ther 2003; 16:337–346.

Zic JA, Miller JL, Stricklin GP, et al: The North American experience with photopheresis. Ther Apher 1999; 3:50–62.

Zucchelli P, Pasquali S, Cagnoli L, et al: Plasma exchange therapy in acute renal failure due to light chain myeloma. Trans Am Soc Artif Intern Organs 1984; 30:36–39.

IV

CHAPTER 37

Tissue Banking and Progenitor Cells

Charlene A. Hubbell BS MT (ASCP) SBB, Lazaro Rosales MD

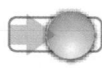

KEY POINTS

• A wide range of allogeneic tissues used for transplantation.

• Allograft tissue is screened, tested, and processed to improve its safety.

• Allograft tissue is stored by a variety of methods including cryopreservation.

• There are risks and complications associated with the use of allograft tissue.

• There is a wide range of assisted reproductive techniques available to infertile couples and individuals.

• Hematopoietic progenitor cells can be derived from multiple sources and transplanted in different ways depending on the needs of the recipient.

• Appreciate the balance between the graft-versus-host reaction and the graft-versus-leukemia effect.

Throughout the United States, tissue banks routinely provide hundreds of products that not only extend life, but also in many instances significantly improve the quality of life for the patients they serve. Over 400 000 bone allografts (American Association of Tissue Banks, 2004) and 46 000 corneas (Eye Bank Association of America, 2004) are transplanted annually in the US, a number that far exceeds the approximately 25 000 solid organ transplants per year (United Network for Organ Sharing, 2003). The clinical applications of allogeneic as well as autologous tissue and the types of tissue available have grown exponentially in the last two decades. Yet, aside from the patients and physicians served by these tissue banks, many people are unaware of the vast scope of activities in today's healthcare environment that are under the umbrella of tissue banking. In the last 20 years, tissue banking in the US has evolved from a system of incidental hospital bone or sperm banks to a system of regulated, accredited facilities, much like blood banks, providing an expanding variety of high-quality, carefully screened and tested products for use by physicians (Table 37–1).

Many tissue banks provide a wide range of products and services in skin, bone, and heart valve procurement; processing; and storage; while other tissue banks focus their services in specialized areas such as reproductive tissue or hematopoietic progenitor cells (HPCs). One bank may recruit donors, procure and process tissue such as skin for burn patients or bone for orthopedic repairs, while another may collect, process, and store HPCs for life-saving bone marrow transplants. Processing of musculoskeletal tissues and cardiac valves, which requires extensive equipment, personnel, and quality assurance, is primarily performed by a few large tissue banks, who subcontract with other tissues banks who in turn collect, store, and

issue these products. In addition, there has been an exponential growth in reproductive banks in the last two decades that provide assistance to infertile couples or individuals.

Sources of Tissue

Tissues used for transplantation come from two primary sources: living donors and deceased donors. Living donors may be individuals who donate for their own use (autologous HPCs or sperm), as directed donors for a given individual (allogeneic HPCs or sperm donation), or altruistically for unknown recipients (surgical discard bone, sperm donation, allogeneic HPCs through the National Marrow Donor Programs). The large majority of bone, skin, and cardiac valves used for transplantation, as well as eye tissue, come from deceased donors. Unlike solid organ donation where there is a need for the organs to be obtained while circulation is maintained, deceased donor tissue can be obtained for several hours after death and up to 24 hours later if the body is refrigerated. This substantially increases the number of available tissue donors. Because corneal tissue has relatively minimal contact with the circulatory system, some individuals who would otherwise be excluded as tissue donors may still be eye donors.

Deceased donor tissue is procured primarily from hospital operating rooms or morgues and medical examiners' offices. Harvesting of tissue is performed in a sterile or clean environment using aseptic techniques. Many tissues, such as bone, are then frozen for subsequent processing and refreezing or freeze-drying. Specialized tissues such as cornea are processed immediately and stored for only a short length of time (48–72 hours) before use. Tissue from living donors is procured either in the operating room (surgically salvaged bone or bone marrow) or in specialized clean environments that hemapheresis centers and sperm banks are equipped to provide. These tissues are collected sterilely, processed immediately, and either used in less than 24 hours or frozen for subsequent use.

Tissue Bank Activities

The major activities of tissue banks are outlined in Table 37–2. A major impetus for the movement to formal, accredited tissue banks in our nation was the concern about transfusion-transmitted disease. Like blood banks and transfusion services (see Chs 35 and 36), donor recruitment, screening, and testing are critical functions of the tissue bank. Since the early 1990s, cases involving disease transmission documented that careful screening by both medical record review and serologic testing as well as maintenance of detailed records was critical to safe tissue banking practices and thus acceptance of allograft tissue by both the public and healthcare providers. Concerns still remain that physicians who utilize these tissues recognize and report these adverse reactions, primarily infection, to the originating tissue bank. The Joint Commission on the

Table 37–1 Categories of Transplantable Tissue

Musculoskeletal
Bone
Cartilage
Meniscus
Tendon
Ligament
Fascia

Skin

Cardiovascular
Heart valves
Saphenous vein

Corneal (eye)

Reproductive
Sperm
Ova
Embryo

Hematopoietic
Bone marrow
Peripheral blood progenitor cells
Umbilical cord blood progenitor cells

Other
Ear ossicles
Dura mater
Parathyroids
Pancreatic islet cells

Table 37–2 Tissue Banking Activities

Donor recruitment and screening
Acquisition of tissues
Processing and storage of tissues
Provision of tissues for transplantation
Public and professional education
Quality assurance and record keeping
Recipient records

Table 37–3 Comprehensive Donor Testing

Donor screening
Review of medical history and medical records
Infectious diseases (including history of foreign travel)
Malignant disease
Collagen and immune complex diseases
History of genetic diseases
Trauma
Exposure to drugs, toxic substances or biological hazards
Physical examination of living donors
Review of autopsy records for deceased donors
Review of social history for risk behaviors

Donor serological testing
Antibody to human immunodeficiency virus
Antibody to human T cell lymphotropic virus
Antibody to hepatitis C virus
Hepatitis B surface antigen
Antibody to hepatitis B core antigen
Serological tests for syphilis
Bacteriologic testing of tissue product

Accreditation of Healthcare Organizations (JCAHO) has standards for tissue banking practices that are targeted primarily at the transplantation facility. These standards focus on the necessity for implantation facilities to keep clear, precise records regarding tissue receipt, storage, and use, so that all allogeneic tissues can be traced from donor to recipient. JCAHO standards also require institutions to establish a mechanism for physicians to report adverse reactions and the originating tissue bank to be notified. Accredited full service tissue banks, in the same manner as blood banks, investigate suspected reactions or complications extensively. 'Look-back' reviews should include review of the complications associated with other tissue from the same donor, current health of the donor if living, and quarantining of other tissue from the same donor. The American Association of Tissue Banks (AATB),* provides strict standards and accreditation for organizations involved in any area of tissue banking. Several states also require tissue banks to be licensed and the Food and Drug Administration (FDA) regulates the screening of donor tissue used for transplantation purposes (FDA, 2004). In addition, the FDA currently recommends that if specimens of cadaveric blood are used for infectious disease marker testing, a test specifically labeled by the manufacturer for such purpose be used. The FDA maintains a website (www.fda.gov/cber/tissue/prod/htm) which lists the manufacturers of tests which have been approved for this purpose.

Donor Screening

Tissue donors are carefully screened to prevent the transmission of bacterial, viral, and/or genetic disease as well as to ensure the quality of the

AATB, 1350 Beverly Rd. #220A, McLean, VA.

tissue obtained (Table 37–3). Unlike blood donors, with deceased tissue donors, information regarding the individual's medical and social history, not obtained from physicians' records, will come from the family or close friends. Reports in the early 1990s focused on the transmission of both human immunodeficiency virus (HIV) (Simonds, 1992) and hepatitis C (Conrad, 1995) from human tissue products. More recently, attention has focused on transmission of nonscreened viruses (Kainer, 2004) and other infectious agents such as Creutzfeldt–Jakob disease (Centers for Disease Control, 2003) by serologically negative tissue, emphasizing the need for careful screening of tissue and organ donors as well as laboratory testing. Asking the right questions in the correct manner is a critical function and needs to be performed by well-trained, experienced individuals who are able to identify possible risks in either the donor medical history, information about possible risk behaviors, or in available laboratory data. Other parts of the review process are targeted at ensuring the quality of the donated tissue. Musculoskeletal donors need to be carefully screened for any history of trauma that might result in a weakened structural bone graft. Sperm donations are reviewed not only for genetic disease but also to ensure viable sperm that will have a reasonable chance of resulting in successful fertilization. The use of umbilical cord blood for unrelated allogeneic bone marrow and peripheral blood transplantation requires screening and testing of the mother as well as the cord blood. When tissue is procured from living donors, with the exception of HPC, the tissue is frozen and quarantined for a minimum of 180 days; at the end of which, the donor serologic testing is repeated. This prevents the use of tissue from any donor who was in the 'window' period for HIV or hepatitis C; that is, they had been exposed to the virus but did not demonstrate antibody at the time of donation.

Cryopreservation

Tissues such as HPCs, sperm, skin, and some types of musculoskeletal tissue require the presence of viable cells and have a very short shelf life at refrigerator temperatures, and thus require cryopreservation. The goal of all cryopreservation techniques is to extend the usable storage period of the material being frozen by reducing the metabolic demand of the cells at lower temperatures without any loss of viability due to either the freezing or thawing procedures. Cryopreservation of animal sperm has been an established agricultural practice for decades and human researchers have been able to gain from their experiences. Generally, cryopreservation of human tissues makes use of cryoprotectant agents such as dimethyl sulfoxide (DMSO) or glycerol, balanced tissue culture medias, and some form of protein supplementation such as autologous plasma, albumin, or other colloidal suspensions. The actual freezing is often performed using a controlled-rate freezer, a mechanical device that controls the rate at which freezing of the tissue takes place, usually $-1°C/min$ down to temperatures of $-80°C$. DMSO is the cryoprotective agent of choice for tissues such as skin, HPCs, and other nucleated cell suspensions or tissues, while glycerol is generally used for the freezing of sperm. Cryoprotectant agents function by preventing formation of intracellular ice crystals during freezing, and balancing the osmotic pressure and concentration of intracellular versus extracellular water during the thawing process. The formation of extracellular ice crystals or too rapid an increase in extracellular osmotic pressure with resulting dehydration of the cell during thawing can result in damage to the cells and thus loss of viability. Cryoprotectant agents, such as DMSO, work by slowing the rate at which this change occurs (Gorin, 1986). Most tissue banks make use of liquid nitrogen and controlled-rate freezing processors that are programmed to compensate for the heat released, called the heat of fusion, at the change from the liquid state to the frozen state (Gorin, 1986). Uncompensated, the heat of fusion can result in decreased viability of the cells or tissue being frozen.

Once frozen, cryopreserved tissues are stored at a variety of temperatures from −80°C in a mechanical freezer to vapor (−100°C) or liquid (−196°C) phase liquid nitrogen. Expiration dates for cryopreserved tissues are generally 5 years, although these are arbitrary limits and the actual length of storage possible for many tissues has not been determined. Other tissues that do not require the presence of viable cells, such as structural bone, may be frozen or freeze-dried by a variety of other methods. Some freeze-dried tissues have expiration dates of 5 years, while others may be stored indefinitely.

Skin Banking

The most common use of allogeneic skin grafts is as a temporary cover for patients with extensive third-degree burns, until autologous or autogeneic skin can be recovered and grafted. Because of the concentration of histocompatibility antigens and antigen-presenting cells (APCs), all allogeneic skin grafts are eventually rejected (Medawar, 1946). When used to cover burns, the grafts are generally replaced periodically until autografting can be performed. Most deceased donor skin provided as an allograft is a split-thickness graft with a thin layer of epidermis without dermis, and therefore ABO matching is not required (Eastlund, 1998). As a temporary graft, however, split-thickness skin grafts provide vital, immediate cover, as a barrier against infection plus fluid, electrolyte, and heat loss from extensive burns, allowing for patient stabilization and for eventual autografting.

Generally, skin is harvested from deceased donors with uninfected, unblemished skin who have a body surface area less than 1.75 m². The skin is harvested with a dermatome from areas of the back, legs, and upper arms. The skin is generally disinfected before harvest and also soaked in antibiotic-containing tissue culture solution either until it is used or until it is frozen.

Skin can be stored at 2–8°C for several days (AATB, 2002) or cryopreserved and stored for several years. Because of today's needs for extensive review of the donor's history and laboratory records, skin grafts are more commonly frozen for subsequent use. The cryoprotectant of choice is 10–15% glycerol (AATB, 2002) and the graft is generally incubated for a period of time (20–30 minutes) in the freezing solution to allow the solution to permeate the graft. The skin is then frozen in strips supported by gauze mesh and frozen flat (Eastlund, 1996). Skin can be frozen with or without controlled-rate freezing and is easily stored at −50 to −80°C; however, lower temperatures are commonly used for longer storage by many tissue banks (Kearney, 1998). Frozen skin allografts are thawed rapidly at 37°C and either used immediately or washed with physiologic solutions to dilute the cryoprotectant.

The limited supply of human skin allografts has stimulated efforts targeted at xenogeneic substitutions, such as pigskin, artificial barriers and, more recently, attempts to culture and grow epithelial cells, thus expanding available autologous skin. Another homologous tissue product, which has gained widespread use, is Alloderm (Lifecell Corporation, The Woodlands, TX, USA), an acellular dermal matrix graft that is processed from human allograft skin. The tissue is enzymatically processed to remove the immunologically active cells, leaving behind an acellular collagen framework. It allows for fibroblast infiltration, collagen deposition, and neoepithelization. Because the immunologically active cells are removed, the graft is tolerated, not rejected, significantly longer than traditional human skin allografts. It not only has been employed as skin graft for burns, but also has applications in ophthalmic, plastic, ENT and dental surgeries (Shorr, 2000). It is a product made from allogeneic human tissue and must be used with the identical patient consents and tracking that are employed for other human tissue products.

Musculoskeletal Tissues

Bone banking had its beginnings several decades ago when physicians began to store surgical discard bone, mostly femoral heads from joint replacement surgery, for future use in other orthopedic procedures, usually spinal fusions. Generally, this involved simple storage of the bone in an unmonitored freezer somewhere in the hospital. Often there was no testing or processing of the surgical discard bone, no monitoring of storage conditions, no tracking of tissue sources or recipients and, in some situations, the original donor/patient was not even asked for consent. Today, these practices have been almost eliminated by the use of musculoskeletal tissue from registered, accredited tissue banks so that patients can confidently elect to have a bone allograft as part of a surgical procedure (Tomford, 1993). In addition to autogeneic bone grafts, living donor bone donation is still used as a source of some types of bone. Living donors are now screened and tested, and must provide informed consent. In addition, the bone tissue obtained is further processed to reduce the risk of infectious disease transmission, and detailed records of the source donor and recipient are kept for tracking and follow-up purposes.

Both surgical discard bone and deceased donor bone are processed in a similar fashion. Extraneous tissue, blood, and marrow elements are removed by high-pressure pulse washing and the tissue is soaked in antibiotic solutions. Bacteriologic culturing of the tissue is done at collection, during processing, and before freezing. Tissues that require the presence of viable cells, such as cartilage, femoral head, tibia, whole bone, or tendon, are usually washed, soaked, and frozen at temperatures between −60° and −150°C. With other tissues, where viability is not an issue, ethanol soaks may be used to remove lipid content, generally in the preparation of demineralized, lyophilized bone, which also decreases the infectivity of the tissue. Most bone tissue is further sterilized by the use of low-dose irradiation. In addition, lyophilization, which is possible with bone products such as cancellous and cortical bone chips, appears to also reduce the immunogenicity as well as infectivity of these products. The use of ethylene oxide to end-sterilize bone tissue has been generally eliminated, as adverse reactions were reported in multiple recipients (Jackson, 1990). The bone tissue is cut and shaped and then preserved either by freezing or freeze-drying.

Bone allografts serve mainly as a mechanical support and a framework for the host's bone-forming cells to replace lost tissue. The osteoinductive function of the allograft bone is dependent in part on the presence of certain growth factor glycoproteins (Mohan, 1991), but they do not appear to cause any significant allograft reaction on the part of the host. Because bone tissue is processed to remove blood, marrow, and other extraneous tissue, most studies have failed to demonstrate the presence of ABO antigens (Ezra-Cohen, 1961). The antigenicity of the resulting product is low and thus histocompatibility or blood type matching is not required. Because large osteoarticular grafts, such as whole bone–patellar-tendon grafts, are not extensively processed, they may contain residual red blood cells, and instances of immunization to Rh system antigens have been reported (Hill, 1974). Many surgeons using these larger grafts will attempt to provide Rh-compatible tissue to Rh-negative females of childbearing age.

In addition to autogeneic bone, allograft bone is used for spinal fusion surgery, replacement of failed prosthetic joints, packing of benign bone cysts, reconstruction of maxillofacial deficits, restoration of alveolar bone in periodontal pockets, and even replacement of resected bone for tumors such as osteosarcoma (Eastlund, 1996). Tendon and cartilage allografts are used primarily for knee repair surgery. Some patients will be confronted with the option of having autologous tissue recovered from their iliac crest for many elective orthopedic procedures, or receiving allograft tissue from a tissue bank. There are advantages and disadvantages to each (i.e., autograft vs. allograft). Autografts appear to incorporate quicker, are not immunogenic, and do not transmit disease; however, they are associated with longer anesthesia time, increased blood loss, and prolonged recovery from the donor site. Because of the wide supply of allografts, an exact fit can be made; there is no donor site recovery; and the surgical procedure is generally shorter. However, the risk of transmitted disease, although greatly reduced by today's procedures, is still present. For other purposes, use of autologous grafts is not possible.

Cardiac Valves

Human heart valves do not require the use of anticoagulants in patients subsequent to implantation, as do mechanical prosthetic or pig valves used for aortic valve replacement; hence, they provide a lower incidence of thromboembolism and infection. They are ideal for use in children, pregnant women, or patients with a history of bacterial endocarditis. They are utilized less often because procedures to place them are more technically difficult. Aortic and pulmonic valves are commonly procured from deceased organ donors when the whole heart is rendered unsuitable for transplantation due to events such as cardiac arrest, but that do not effect the integrity or function of the aortic or pulmonic valves. Procurement is performed in the operating room. The valves are carefully dissected with a cuff of myocardium, inspected for valve integrity, and frozen by controlled-rate freezing in liquid nitrogen using DMSO as the cryoprotective agent (O'Brien, 1988). While blood group antigens have been demonstrated on the endothelium of cryopreserved hearts, the major mechanical function of these is dependent only on the nonviable connective tissue. After transplantation, host cells eventually replace the donor endothelium. Several studies have documented that ABO compatibility is not necessary for long-term function of these allograft valves (Weipert, 1995). More recently, some cardiothoracic surgeons have attempted the use of saphenous vein allografts for coronary artery bypass procedures or for bypassing obstructed lower limb arteries when autografts are not available. Because the role of ABO matching in the long-term function of these tissues has been controversial, ABO-compatible tissue is generally used (Laub, 1992). Since the thawing of the allograft valves is generally performed by operating room personnel and not experienced tissue bank technologists, detailed instructions and protocols are necessary to prevent cracking of the valve. While the use of allograft valves has been a successful practice for several years, the results of most vein allograft studies to date are disappointing (Walker, 1993).

Cornea

Corneal transplantation has been regularly performed in the United States since 1961, although the first corneal transplant is recorded to have taken place in 1905. Currently, more than 46 000 corneal transplants are performed each year (Eye Bank Association of America, 1999). There are 108 accredited eye banks in the US involved in recruitment, screening, procurement, and transplantation of corneal tissue as well as public and professional education. Loss of vision due to corneal disease can result from infection, trauma, burns, or congenital diseases. Long-term (> 10 years) success rates for corneal allografts are well above 90%.

Corneal donation is possible from many donors where other tissues are not retrievable because of age, trauma, or disease. Corneal tissue is recovered from donors up to 80 years of age. Generally, eye enucleation is performed in the operating room or morgue from deceased donors within 6 hours of death. Subsequently, the cornea is then removed in a sterile environment in the eye bank and placed in supplemented, sterile tissue culture media. The corneas are stored at 4°C and are transplanted within 48–72 hours. This allows for appropriate serologic screening of the donor but ensures maximum viability of the graft.

The corneal graft has long been considered an 'immunologically privileged site' (Medawar, 1948). Because the cornea is almost entirely avascular, host APCs and effector lymphocytes do not circulate through the allograft cornea. Histocompatibility and blood group matching are therefore not required. In a small percentage of corneal grafts, vascularization occurs and some grafts are rejected. The use of human leukocyte antigen (HLA)-matched corneal transplants in an attempt to provide successful grafts for this group of patients has met with varying success rates (Volker-Dieben, 1987).

Reproductive Tissue

Due to the exponential growth in knowledge of fetal development as well as reproductive technologies, particularly in vitro fertilization (IVF), 1–3% of births in most western countries now occur with assisted reproductive technologies (Evers, 2202). Reproductive banks are currently able to assist more individuals and couples who wish to maintain or achieve fertility. Most reproductive banks in the US today function as for-profit corporations. Despite this and because of a number of factors including consumer demand, the need for consumer confidence and government regulation, sperm banks in the 21st century function with the highest medical and ethical standards and physicians and patients can make use of their services without concern. Guidelines and standards for anonymous-donation sperm banking have been established by the American Society for Reproductive Medicine and the American Association of Tissue Banks.

Reproductive banks serve two kinds of donors: client-directed donors and anonymous bank donors. Client-directed sperm donations are generally targeted to intimate partners of men who for a variety of reasons are concerned about future fertility. These include men who are about to undergo chemotherapy, radiation therapy, or surgery for malignant diseases that will affect their reproductive ability. Other men will predeposit their sperm prior to vasectomy as insurance against life changes when they may wish to father additional children. Individuals with low

sperm counts may bank their sperm to allow collection of sufficient gametes for fertilization of the intimate partner. Less frequently, males who have occupational exposure (such as nuclear power plant employees) that may lead to either infertility or the potential for genetic defects may elect to store their sperm. Sperm collected and stored for intimate partners is tested in the same manner that anonymous donor collections are screened. Semen from infected donors, which still may be usable by the intimate partner, must be quarantined and stored separately from other client deposits. Directed donations are also made to sperm banks for specific individuals who are not intimate partners.

Sperm banks also provide sperm from anonymous donors for infertile couples or individuals. Sperm banks maintain libraries of sperm donors so that individuals can select donors with similar physical characteristics such as hair and eye color, race, and the like. Anonymous sperm donors are rigorously screened not only to ensure safety for the recipient and potential offspring but also to provide the highest probability of successful fertilization. Sperm collected from anonymous donors is quarantined for 180 days prior to issue. During this 180 days, the donor is tested monthly, not only by the standard serologic assays employed for all tissue donors, but also for infections such as cytomegalovirus, *Neisseria gonorrhoeae*, and *Chlamydia*. Sperm donors are tested for genetic diseases such as Tay–Sachs disease, cystic fibrosis, sickle cell disease, and thalassemia. Generally, complete genetic karyotyping is performed on anonymous sperm donors (see Ch. 69). Collections are also examined for sperm number, function, and viability. Not until all of these criteria have been met and reviewed by the medical director of the sperm bank is tissue released for use.

In vitro fertilization and embryo banking are also offered by many reproductive banks as well as hospital-based fertility centers. Since the original success of IVF as a treatment for tubal obstruction in 1983 (Steptoe, 1983), significant advances have been made in this area which improve the success rate of IVF. They include technical innovations in culture media and embryo cryopreservation, as well as morphological criteria for the selection of the best embryo to transfer (Houghton, 2002). In addition to its use for women with fallopian disease, the success of intracytoplasmic sperm injection of the oocyte (Palermo, 1992) has made IVF the preferred technique for many infertile couples, utilizing either partner's sperm or donor sperm, as it results in higher fertilization rates as compared to artificial insemination (Boyle, 2004). In addition, IVF offers couples with certain genetic diseases such as hemophilia and cystic fibrosis, the opportunity for preimplantation genetic diagnosis with subsequent selection of embryos in an attempt to reduce the risk of disease transmission to their offspring.

Attempts at ova banking (egg banking) have not been as successful as embryo cryopreservation. Unfertilized ova have a very low rate of fertilization when subsequently thawed and attempts at IVF are made. In addition to freezing stimulated oocytes, attempts have also been made at cryopreserving ovarian tissue for future implantation. The latter has not resulted in a successful pregnancy in humans. Recent attempts to improve the success of oocyte banking have focused on modifications to both the culture medium and freeze–thaw temperature gradients (Boldt 2003). Female patients, confronted with loss of fertility due to age, disease, or chemotherapy and who have an intimate partner are still frequently guided to IVF with cryopreservation of the resulting embryos for later implantation. Donor sperm and IVF are often recommended for females without an intimate partner until oocyte cryopreservation demonstrates more promising results. Many reproductive banks also provide donor ova collection for infertile individuals. These donors are screened in the same manner that anonymous sperm donors are tested.

Collected semen is mixed with a glycerol–egg yolk solution that acts as a cryoprotectant, the egg yolk providing supplemental protein that assists in preserving the sperm during the thawing process. The semen–preservative mixture is aliquoted into straws or vials, precooled to a temperature of 5°C, frozen by controlled-rate freezing with liquid nitrogen, and stored in the liquid phase of liquid nitrogen at −196°C. Cryopreserved sperm can be used for either artificial insemination or in vitro fertilization. Client-directed donations are kept indefinitely, while anonymous sperm bank donor samples are usually stored for 5 years. For those individuals desiring artificial inseminations, these attempts are not always successful and individuals are counseled to deposit adequate sperm for several reproductive procedures.

The advent of all these technologies has raised many scientific as well as ethical issues. Disposition of unused embryos, preimplantation screening of embryos and multiple gestations, as well as unknown genetic risks to the health of children conceived through IVF (Lucifero, 2004), create the need for a multidisciplinary approach to this field to include members of public interest groups as well as scientific and medical professionals (Cetin, 2003).

IV

Table 37–4 Indications for Hematopoietic Transplantation

Acute myeloid leukemia

Acute lymphoblastic leukemia

Chronic myelogenous leukemia

Multiple myeloma

Non-Hodgkin lymphoma

Myelodysplastic syndromes

Hodgkin's disease

Neuroblastoma

Ewing's sarcoma

Rhabdomyosarcoma

Aplastic anemia

Sickle cell anemia

Thalassemia

Severe combined immunodeficiency

Hematopoietic Progenitor Cell Banking

Hematopoietic cell transplantation had its beginning about 40 years ago with bone marrow transplants performed between genetically identical individuals (identical twins) in the setting of high-dose, myeloablative chemotherapy and/or radiation therapy as an attempt to cure hematopoietic malignancies (Thomas, 1959). Earlier work had demonstrated the presence of colony-forming units (CFUs) or cells in the spleen or marrow of mice that were able to restore hematopoietic function to their lethally irradiated, genetically identical littermates (Lorenz, 1951). Restoration of hematopoiesis in the human recipient is dependent on the transplantation of sufficient numbers of the pluripotential hematopoietic progenitor cells that comprise about 1% of normal marrow cells and are capable of both replication and differentiation into all lineages of blood cells (see Ch. 30). The identification of the HLA system as the major histocompatibility system in man and the ability of tissue typing laboratories to identify individuals' HLA types at the allele level allowed for bone marrow transplantation to be performed between HLA-matched individuals, generally first-degree relatives, who were not genetically identical. Today, progenitor cell banks exist as highly specialized tissue banks that collect, process, store, and reinfuse HPC products obtained from bone marrow, peripheral blood, or even umbilical cord blood for patients with a wide variety of diseases (Table 37–4). Not only are HPC grafts performed in the traditional manner with the use of otherwise lethal doses of chemotherapy and/or radiation therapy (myeloablative transplants) in patients with malignant disease and to restore normal function in patients with defects of hematopoiesis (aplastic anemia, sickle cell anemia), hematopoietic transplants are also performed following minimal induction therapy in some patients (non-myeloablative transplants). Success of these transplants depends upon the 'graft-versus-disease' effect of donor T lymphocytes to eliminate residual disease in patients with malignant diseases. In the year 2000, approximately 18 000 patients worldwide were treated with some form of a hematopoietic graft (Storb, 2003). Terminology in transition is shown in Table 37–5.

Sources of Hematopoietic Grafts

Hematopoietic tissue for transplanting may come from one or more sources (Table 37–6). Individuals who have autologous or autogeneic grafts donate their own cells, which are frozen and thawed prior to high-dose chemotherapy and/or radiation therapy. Immediately following this myeloablative therapy, the patient's own cells are thawed and reinfused. The patient's own hematopoietic progenitor cells in the transplant will home and re-engraft in the marrow stroma and differentiate into mature blood cell-forming elements. Other patients who are not candidates for autologous transplantation, because of the presence of circulating tumor cells as in acute leukemias, will be candidates for an allogeneic transplant where the hematopoietic tissue comes from a closely HLA-matched individual. Hematopoietic tissue contains viable lymphocytes that are capable of recognizing the foreign HLA antigens of the host and creating a graft-versus-host (GVH) reaction. This immune response of the graft to the host can vary from mild (grade 1) to severe (grades 3 and 4). The GVH reaction, particularly grades 3 and 4, remains one of the most significant morbidity and mortality risks associated with allogeneic hematopoietic cell transplantation. For this reason, donors are selected who are the best

Table 37–5 Terminology in Transition

HPC	Hematopoietic progenitor cells, formerly hematopoietic stem cells
HPC, apheresis	Hematopoietic progenitor cells, apheresis, formerly peripheral blood progenitor cells or hematopoietic stem cells
HPC, marrow	Bone marrow-derived hematopoietic progenitor cells
HPC, umbilical cord blood	Cord blood-derived hematopoietic progenitor cells

Table 37–6 Comparison of Hematopoietic Progenitor Cell Sources and Products with Collection and Complications

	Cord blood (HPC, UCB)	Autologous (HPC, apheresis + marrow)	Allogeneic (HPC, apheresis + marrow)
Type of donor	Umbilical cord blood	Patient	Related or unrelated matched donor
Product	Cord blood progenitor/stem cells	Bone marrow or PB progenitor cells	Bone marrow or PB progenitor cells
Collection	Placenta umbilical cord at birth	Intraoperative marrow or hemapheresis	Intraoperative marrow or hemapheresis
Major complication	Insufficient progenitor cells	Recurrence of original disease	Graft-vs.-host disease

HPC, apheresis = PBPC = peripheral blood hematopoietic progenitor cells; HPC, marrow = BMPC = bone marrow hematopoietic progenitor cells; HPC, UCB = UCBPC = umbilical cord blood hematopoietic progenitor cells.

HLA match available. Donors may be HLA-matched siblings or other family members, or the patient may receive a graft from an unrelated HLA-matched individual identified through one of several worldwide donor registries. These registries, the largest in the US being the National Marrow Donor Program (NMDP), recruit healthy individuals who are willing to altruistically donate their bone marrow or peripheral blood progenitor cells (PBPCs) for an individual needing a transplant who does not have an HLA-matched related donor. Registry donors have their marrow or PBPCs obtained at a hospital or blood center close to their own home and the graft is then transported by courier to the transplant center. Anonymity is maintained for both donor and recipient. Because of the need for an almost perfect HLA match, registries must have millions of volunteers in order to have a reasonable chance of finding a match for a given patient. Because pluripotential hematopoietic progenitor cells do not express ABO antigens, they will engraft in the marrow stroma of ABO-incompatible individuals, thus abrogating the need for donors to be ABO compatible but requiring the removal of mature red cells from these grafts.

Bone Marrow

Bone marrow is harvested from the iliac crest of the donor in the operating room under sterile conditions. Donors will elect to have either general or spinal anesthesia. The amount of marrow to be collected is dependent on the recipient size. Generally, sufficient marrow is collected to provide 2×10^8 nucleated cells per kilogram of recipient body weight. For a 70-kg adult, this will generally require the collection of about 700 mL of marrow. The technique involves the collection of approximately 3–5 mL per aspiration into a heparinized syringe. Aspirating too large a volume from one site will result in the marrow being diluted with peripheral blood. Usually, two individuals will harvest marrow at the same time from each side of the donor iliac crest. As it is collected, the aspirated marrow is filtered through large-pore filters to remove bone spicules or clots, and supplemental anticoagulant is added. As the hematopoietic progenitor cells are contained within the nucleated cell fraction, the collected marrow is often further processed to reduce the volume by separating the buffy coat from a large proportion of the red cells and plasma volume. The buffy coat may be further processed to remove all red cells if the donor and recipient are ABO incompatible, or T cell-depleted if desired. Bone marrow from autogeneic donors is frozen and stored prior to use, while allogeneic marrow donations are generally not collected until the day of transplant and thus do not require storage.

While bone marrow harvested from the iliac crest was the original and longstanding source for HPCs for transplantation, the last decade has seen the development of technologies that allow the collection of these cells from the peripheral blood of both patients and normal donors and even from placental or cord blood.

Peripheral Blood Progenitor Cells

The stimulation for the development of technologies that would allow the collection of HPCs from peripheral blood was the potential for use in the autologous transplant setting where concern about marrow contamination with tumor cells is high. Because of the relative ease of hemapheresis collection over marrow harvest, progenitor cells obtained from the peripheral blood are increasingly being used in the allogeneic setting. One area where this may have a major impact is unrelated or volunteer donors, where more individuals may volunteer for the national marrow donor programs when hemapheresis is offered as an option over the traditional bone marrow harvest. The instrumentation and procedures used for peripheral blood progenitor cell harvest are described in Chapter 36.

Clearly, the greatest advantage of peripheral blood progenitor cells over marrow is the time to neutrophil and platelet engraftment, averaging 8–12 days for mobilized peripheral blood progenitor cells compared to 2–4 weeks for bone marrow (Gianni, 1989). This rapid recovery clearly reduces morbidity and mortality associated with profound neutropenia/thrombocytopenia as well as reducing costs associated with hospital stay, transfusion support, treatment of complications and so forth.

HPCs were known three decades ago to be present in the peripheral blood following chemotherapy recovery (Richman, 1976). It was later however, before hemapheresis systems were developed that would allow for the safe collection of adequate numbers of these cells to provide for engraftment of the recipient after chemotherapy (Kessinger, 1988). In the majority of patients undergoing autologous transplantation, large-volume apheresis collection (14–20 L/procedure) is now well established as an efficient means of collecting adequate numbers of HPCs in a reasonable number of procedures to provide for adequate hematopoietic recovery.

HPCs are morphologically undistinguishable from other mononuclear cells seen in the marrow or peripheral blood, yet collection of adequate numbers of cells is essential to enduring marrow engraftment in the recipient. Bone marrow collections have traditionally been targeted at collecting sufficient nucleated cells to ensure a minimum number of progenitor cells. Bone marrow grafts could be assayed for progenitor cell activity by the use of colony-forming assays (Iscove, 1971). In this technique, a sample of mononuclear cells from the graft is cultured in methylcellulose media supplemented with hematopoietic growth factors and essential amino acids for 10–14 days. At the end of this period, the plates are examined for the number and type of characteristic CFUs, including burst-forming unit-erythroid (BFU-E), granulocyte/macrophage (CFU-GM), and mixed colonies – granulocyte, erythrocyte, monocyte, megakaryocyte (CFU-GEMM). Clusters containing more than 50 cells are scored as a colony. Collections containing greater than 1×10^5 CFUs per kilogram of recipient weight are considered adequate.

As the collection of progenitor cell grafts moved to the use of peripheral blood hemapheresis procedures, it became necessary to develop an assay that could be completed on the same day and used to determine the number of hemapheresis collections required. Quantitation of the number of cells bearing the CD34 antigen by flow cytometry has become the widely accepted method for assessing the adequacy of peripheral blood progenitor cell collections. The CD34 antigen is restricted to primitive cells of all lineages (Civin, 1989). Collection of hemapheresis products using CD34+ cell enumeration as an index of graft efficacy has proven to result in enduring hematopoietic engraftment (Berenson, 1991). Standardization of the CD34 cell assay and availability of flow cytometric analysis have resulted in CD34+ cell measurements being used by most programs to determine the number and adequacy of peripheral blood progenitor cell collections (Sutherland, 1994). Generally, peripheral blood progenitor cells collections containing greater than 3×10^6 CD34+ cells per kilogram of recipient body weight are considered adequate to provide for neutrophil engraftment in 8–10 days.

Collection of HPCs in the nonmobilized patient or donor would require multiple apheresis procedures or collections, as the numbers of HPCs in the peripheral blood is about 1/10 to 1/100 of the numbers in the marrow. Thus, 'mobilization' therapies are required to increase the number of circulating HPCs and thus improve the efficiency of hemapheresis collection. Richman (1976) recognized that while there was a drop in the number of circulating CD34+ cells following chemotherapy, this was followed by a four- to fivefold increase in the percentage of circulating CD34+ cells just as the absolute neutrophil count began to recover, usually

around 14–21 days following therapy. This increase in circulating CD34+ cells is greatest with chemotherapeutic agents such as cytoxan and etoposide. If hemapheresis collection is performed in this window, large numbers of HPC can be recovered with a limited number of procedures even though the total white count may be less than 10 000/µL. As the period of increased numbers of circulating CD34+ cells is short (2–3 days), close monitoring of the patient's white count and peripheral blood CD34+ cell counts and timing of the hemapheresis collection are critical. In addition, some investigators have felt that collecting autologous HPCs in the recovery phase of chemotherapy decreases the likelihood of tumor cells contaminating the apheresis product. The use of hematopoietic growth factors such as granulocyte/macrophage colony-stimulating factor (GM-CSF) and granulocyte colony-stimulating factor (G-CSF) also result in a significant increase in the numbers of circulating CD34+ cells in the peripheral blood (Siena, 1989). Doses of 5–10 µg/kg of body weight for 4–5 days will result in a five- to tenfold increase in the number of HPCs in the peripheral blood. The use of G-CSF alone has proven to be more efficient than chemotherapy priming for the collection of CD34+ cells. The combination of chemotherapy priming and the use of growth factors (primarily G-CSF) results in the maximum mobilization of PBPCs and the need for the fewest number of hemapheresis procedures to collect a transplant dose of HPCs, a strategy employed by the majority of autogeneic transplant programs.

The use of G-CSF in the healthy allogeneic donor to mobilize HPCs has been investigated and, aside from mild effects such as bone pain and headache, is well tolerated (Anderlini, 1997). Increasingly, transplant programs are using peripheral blood instead of marrow as a source of HPCs for their allogeneic as well as autogeneic transplants. The higher risk of graft-versus-host disease (GVHD) in allogeneic recipients of peripheral blood HPCs versus marrow (Cutler, 2001) has stimulated trials of new technologies to modify these grafts (see below: T cell purging).

Umbilical Cord Blood

The fact that higher numbers of colony-forming unit cells or progenitor cells were present in umbilical cord blood was known for many years, but it was not until 1989 that the first attempts were made to use cells recovered from placenta umbilical cords for hematopoietic transplantation (Gluckman, 1989). The apparent success of many of these early cord blood transplants has led to the organization of several cord blood banks in the US and in Europe in an attempt to provide another source of progenitor cell tissue for patients requiring an allogeneic transplant. In addition, because the progenitor cells are obtained from cord blood, there appears to be a greater degree of tolerance for some degree of HLA incompatibility between the donor and recipient without the appearance of grades 3 or 4 GVH reaction; thus, hematopoietic transplantation might become available for some patients who otherwise have no HLA-matched donor (Laughlin, 2001). Umbilical cord progenitor cells are harvested by cannulation of the placental vessels either while the placenta is still in utero or, more commonly, following delivery, or by direct expression of the cord blood from the placenta following delivery. The number of HPCs recovered is directly proportional to the volume of cord blood collected, which varies with the size of the infant/placenta and also with the experience of the individual performing the collection (Wagner, 1992). Volumes ranging from 40–150 mL are common for experienced centers. This will result in approximately $4–11 \times 10^8$ nucleated cells being harvested. Collections that are not adequate in volume (< 40 mL) are usually discarded. Generally, umbilical cord blood collections are not further processed to reduce the volume and are frozen directly with DMSO and liquid nitrogen storage. Specially trained staff deployed to the delivery room are not distracted by the care of the mother and/or infant and also reduce the risk of bacterial contamination of the cord blood.

Careful medical history screening and testing of the mother are essential to ensure the safety of the cord blood product as well as the absence of genetic disease. In addition to the standard laboratory measurements for serologically transmittable disease, testing is also performed for viral and bacteriologic diseases.

While umbilical cord blood banking offers the exciting potential for a lesser degree of histocompatibility and thus availability for more patients, critical issues to be addressed are methods to expand the numbers of cells to provide adequate HPCs for larger recipients as well as the costs involved in establishing and maintaining cord blood banks (Grewal, 2003).

Non-Myeloablative Hematopoietic Grafts

Elimination of tumor cells may only be partially accomplished by the chemotherapy or radiation used in high-dose conditioning regimens. In addition, due to the increased morbidity and mortality associated with high-dose allogeneic HPC grafts, many patients, because of age or other comorbidities, are excluded as candidates for traditional HPC grafts. This and other data demonstrating a potential benefit from allogeneic versus autologous HPC grafts led to the investigation of non-myeloablative transplant protocols, also called reduced intensity allogeneic HPC grafts.

Early murine studies had shown that recipients of allogeneic grafts had better survival than recipients of syngeneic grafts (Barnes, 1957). Later studies in humans demonstrated this same 'graft-versus-leukemia effect' in patients transplanted for acute leukemias and it appeared to correlate with the development of chronic graft-versus-host disease in the recipient (Weiden, 1981). That this effect was dependent upon donor T lymphocytes was further demonstrated by the high relapse rate that occurred in patients receiving T cell-depleted HPC grafts (Marmont, 1989). Initial efforts focused on the infusion of donor T lymphocytes after the HPC graft in patients who had relapsed (Kolb, 1990). This technique became known as donor lymphocyte infusion (DLI). As these patients received no additional chemotherapy, the next approach was to attempt HPC peripheral blood grafts with no conditioning (Porter, 1999). It quickly became clear that some conditioning therapy, primarily immunosuppressive, was necessary to allow donor cells to engraft. Conditioning regimens in non-myeloablative HPC transplants are now focused on providing sufficient immunosuppression to allow engraftment of donor cells and not elimination of the tumor burden. The larger number of T lymphocytes in peripheral blood HPC grafts versus marrow appears to decrease the risk of graft rejection by overwhelming host T lymphocytes as well as favoring the development of a graft-versus-leukemia effect. DLI may also be given at a later date if there appears to be insufficient donor T cell engraftment or disease relapse.

In the non-myeloablative HPC grafts, disease control is mediated by recognition of host residual tumor cells by donor T cells and requires establishment of at least partial donor T lymphocyte chimerism if not full replacement by donor T cells. The kinetics of T cell engraftment in the non-myeloablative HPC transplants are such that up to a year may be required for the patient to achieve complete disease remission (Childs, 1999). This therapy is, therefore, not appropriate for patients with acute leukemia not in remission or other aggressive malignancies likely to relapse at an early date. While the morbidity and mortality associated with the conditioning regimen in non-myeloablative HPC grafts is lower, the risk of GVHD is the same as that seen following high-dose conditioning regimens. Because of the higher risk of GVHD as well as graft rejection in unrelated HPC grafts, particularly HLA mismatched ones, it remains to be seen if this group of patients will benefit from non-myeloablative HPC grafts (Niederwieser, 2003).

The reduced toxicity of the preparative regimen allows for its use in older patients and is also associated with less transfusion burden and shorter hospital stays (Weissinger, 2001). The reduced toxicity as well as improved outcomes seen with this therapy have contributed to its rapid growth in the hematopoietic transplant community. The European Group for Blood and Marrow Transplantation reported a 27% incidence of non-myeloablative HPC grafts in allogeneic transplant recipients in 2000 (Gratwohl, 2002).

Purging

Once hematopoietic progenitor cells are collected, either from the marrow or peripheral blood, it is often advantageous to further process the collected HPC product in an attempt to reduce possible tumor cell contamination or, in the allogeneic setting, to reduce the number of T lymphocytes. Two approaches, not mutually exclusive, have been taken. The first employs techniques targeted at eliminating tumor cells, so-called purging or negative-selection techniques. The second approach utilizes methods to separate and collect only the CD34+ hematopoietic progenitor cells, discarding the remaining cell fraction which presumably contains contaminating tumor cells. These methods are usually referred to as 'positive selection' techniques (Table 37–7).

Purging techniques originally employed a variety of both specific and nonspecific methods to remove the unwanted cell population. Original methods employed the use of cytotoxic drugs such as 4-hydroperoxycyclophosphamide (4-HC) and etoposide (VP-16) to remove contaminating tumor cells (Yeager, 1986). These methods are the in vitro equivalent of high-dose chemotherapy and thus the major negative effect is damage to HPCs. Other technologies included the use of lectins and/or rosetting to remove unwanted cell populations, particularly T cells. More recently, monoclonal antibodies targeted at a specific cell receptor have been used either with complement or coupled to immunotoxins such as ricin to actually lyse the contaminating tumor cell population. Also, with the advent of immunomagnetic bead technology, the monoclonal antibody can be coupled to an immunomagnetic bead. The antibody–bead–tumor cell complex is then removed by passing the cell suspension over a magnetic field

Table 37–7 Stem Cell Purging Methods

Positive selection

CD34+ cell selection
    Solid phase columns
    Magnetic beads

Negative selection

Pharmacologic
    4-Hydroperoxycyclophosphamide (4HC)
    Etoposide (VP-16)
Immunologic
    Tumor cell + MoAb + toxin
        Toxin = complement/ricin/other chemo
    Tumor cell + MoAb + solid phase
        Solid phase = bead column

where the unwanted cell populations will be retained and the HPCs are rinsed through and collected.

Positive selection techniques focus on the selective presence of the CD34 marker on hematopoietic progenitor cells and the availability of monoclonal antibodies targeted to this marker. While the original technology employed the use of a column to which the monoclonal antibody was bound, presently used methods utilize an immunomagnetic bead or sphere. The mononuclear cell fraction from either the bone marrow harvest or the progenitor cell hemapheresis collection is incubated with the monoclonal anti-CD34 or other monoclonal antibody of interest. A suspension of immunomagnetic beads labeled with a second antibody is then added. The second antibody binds to the monoclonal anti-CD34 antibody, creating a bead–target cell complex. When the cell suspension is subsequently passed over a magnetic field, the CD34+ cell–magnetic bead complex will be retained and the remaining mononuclear cell suspension containing either unwanted tumor cells or CD3+ T cells will be removed. The CD34+ progenitor cells are then freed from the magnetic beads by use of a releasing agent and the beads are removed by reapplication of the magnetic field, leaving a cell suspension that is approximately 90% CD34+ cells. The reduction in the total number of CD3+ T cells is about $3.5 \log_{10}$ depletion. The median recovery of CD34+ cells is approximately 50% of the starting numbers of CD34+ cells in the hemapheresis product. The benefit of both positive and negative selection purging of HPC grafts to reduce tumor cell contamination and reduce disease relapse rates has been controversial (de Lima, 2004). These techniques, with the exception of T cell depletion, have been widely investigated, but are still considered experimental.

T Cell Depletion

Techniques to reduce the number of T lymphocytes in allogeneic hematopoietic grafts, primarily marrow, have been targeted at reducing the incidence and severity of GVHD. Many of the techniques mentioned previously for purging of tumor cells, such as positive selection for CD34+ cells, have also been applied to the reduction of T cells in the graft (Table 37–8). Other techniques specifically targeting T cells have included soybean lectin agglutination, E-rosette formation, combinations of the two, counter-flow elutriation, and monoclonal antibodies.

Soybean lectin produces an agglutinin specific for the CD2 receptor on lymphocytes, thus agglutinating CD2+ T cells. The addition of a rosetting step with sheep erythrocytes removes the remaining T cells not agglutinated by the soybean lectin. This methodology results in a $2–3 \log_{10}$ depletion of T cells (Reisner, 1982). Current trials with monoclonal antibodies have focused on the use of anti-CD52 antibodies both in vitro for treatment of the HPC product as well as in vivo to reduce host T lymphocytes (Chakraverty, 2002).

Counter-flow elutriation is a method used for the depletion of T cells that utilizes the separation characteristic of cells in a centrifugal field, based on the size and density of various cell populations. One of the advantages of the system is that no chemotherapeutic agents or antibodies are added to the hematopoietic progenitor cell population; thus, there is no impairment of cell function. Buffy coat concentrates from harvested marrow are introduced into the centrifuge at different flow rates, allowing for the collection of cell fractions of different size and densities. The system is highly efficient at separating a CFU-GM-rich fraction from a CD3+ lymphocyte fraction. Since there are no changes made to the cells, the CD3+ fraction can be enumerated and partially added back to the CFU-GM fraction to provide a controlled dose of CD3+ cells, if clinically desired (Noga, 1990). Cell recovery is high, and since elutriation media

Table 37–8 T Lymphocyte Depletion Methods
Lectins
Soybean lectin with E-rosetting
Counterflow centrifugation
Immunologic
Antibody
Antibody + complement
Antibody + solid phase
Positive selection

are biocompatible, the product(s) can be reinfused without additional wash steps. The major disadvantage of the procedure is the cost of the required equipment and the need for experienced operators.

The introduction of immunomagnetic bead techniques for the positive selection of CD34+ cells has also led to the use of these techniques in the allogeneic setting for the resultant depletion of CD3+ T cells, particularly from peripheral blood progenitor cell collections. Immunomagnetic bead technology is easily applied to hemapheresis progenitor cell products as well as the larger-volume bone marrow harvest products. Many centers have reported success with these newer methods to reduce CD3+ T cells in allogeneic transplantation, particularly when the donor and recipient are not completely HLA matched (Henslee-Downey, 1997).

One additional advantage of either purging or positive selection techniques is that they result in a significantly reduced volume of progenitor cell product to be frozen, thawed, and reinfused into the patient. This greatly reduces tonicities associated with the reinfusion of DMSO-containing products as well as decreasing freezing and storage costs for the progenitor cell laboratory. Presently, licensed technologies for purging and/or positive selection to reduce tumor cell contamination are costly and additional data are needed to assess the clinical efficacy of these procedures for tumor cell reduction. Some centers have reported improved clinical outcomes by employing a combination of both purging and positive selection techniques (Clarke, 1998).

Both positive and negative selection techniques incur a concomitant loss of as much as 50% of the original number of CD34+ cells, from either agent toxicity (chemotherapeutics, complement), entrapment by magnetic beads complexes, or loss during required wash steps. The initial hemapheresis or bone marrow collection of CD34+ cells must be increased to allow for subsequent loss in processing. This may be difficult to accomplish in patients who are hard to mobilize.

The major disadvantage of T cell depletion is the resultant increase in the incidence of disease relapse. Patients who demonstrate mild GVHD appear to have a lower incidence of relapse of neoplastic disease than do those patients who have no GVHD. The presence of the donor T cell population is apparently critical to 'graft-versus-leukemia effect,' recognition of host antigens by the donor T cells generating an immune response that eliminates residual host tumor cells. More recent studies have also demonstrated a role for natural killer (NK) cells in the graft-versus-leukemia effect. Others have employed combinations of techniques such as CD34+ selection and counter-flow elutriation to create both a CD34+ cell-rich fraction, and an NK cell-rich/T cell-depleted fraction, taking advantage of the fact that the NK cells do appear to have antitumor effect but do not contribute to GVH effect (Skiera, 1999).

Cryopreservation of Hematopoietic Grafts

HPC grafts from all autogeneic and many allogeneic collections are cryopreserved and stored prior to use. The most common protocol

Table 37–9 Adverse Reactions Observed in Patients Transfused with Cryopreserved Progenitor Cell Products
Common
Chills
Nausea
Emesis
Fever
Headache
Dyspnea
Uncommon
Renal failure
Cardiac arrest
Hypotension
Sepsis
Contributing factors
Volume of product reinfused
Type and amount of cryoprotectant reinfused
Volume of incompatible red cells (allogeneic products)
Bacterial contamination

involves the use of 10% DMSO as a cryoprotective agent, controlled-rate freezing, and liquid nitrogen storage, either vapor or liquid phase. The use of DMSO provides significant improvement in post-thaw viability over agents such as glycerol. Because there are toxicities associated with the post-thaw infusion of progenitor cell products containing DMSO, other investigators have looked to the use of lower concentrations, addition of hetastarch, or other additives, but DMSO currently remains in use by the majority of programs. Attempts to wash products following thawing to reduce the amount of DMSO present resulted in significant loss of progenitor cells; strategies are now targeted at reducing the volume of the prefreezing product and thus lowering the amount of DMSO necessary.

Reinfusion of Progenitor Cell Products

Regardless of the source of the progenitor cell graft, HPCs are infused to the recipient in a manner very similar to any blood product transfusion. Pluripotential progenitor cells, with their unique membrane receptors, will home to the marrow space, engraft, and replicate. Products that have been cryopreserved with DMSO in most cases are thawed and immediately reinfused without washing. HPCs collected by hemapheresis that are not further processed may contain large numbers of red blood cells. Cryopreservation in DMSO does not maintain red blood cell membrane integrity and these products will contain a large amount of free hemoglobin when thawed. Recipient reactions will vary from mild, characterized by nausea, chills, or headache, to more severe reactions that can include hypotension, sepsis, renal failure, or even cardiac arrest (Stroncek, 1991). Such adverse reactions are shown in Table 37–9. Recipients of cryopreserved progenitor cell products are generally premedicated with antihistamines and/or antiemetics. Adequate hydration and the use of diuretics are also indicated to decrease renal toxicities associated with free hemoglobin and larger-volume infusions.

IV

References

American Association of Tissue Banks (AATB): Standards for Tissue Banking. McLean, VA, American Association of Tissue Banks, 2002.

American Association of Tissue Banks (AATB): Annual Statistical Report. McLean, VA, American Association of Tissue Banks, 2004.

Anderlini P, Korbling M, Dale D, et al: Allogenic blood stem cell transplantation: Consideration for donors. Blood 1997; 90:903–908.

Barnes DWH, Corp MJ, Loutit JF: Treatment of murine leukemia with X-rays and homologous bone marrow II. Br J Haematol 1957; 3:241–252.

Berenson RJ, Bensinger WI, Hill RS, et al: Engraftment after infusion of CD34+ marrow cells in patients with breast cancer or neuroblastoma. Blood 1991; 77:1717–1722.

Boldt J, Cline D, McLaughlin D: Human oocyte cryopreservation as an adjunct to IVF-embryo transfer cycles. Hum Reprod 2003; 18:1250–1255.

Boyle KE, Vlahos N, Jarow JP: Assisted reproductive technology in the new millennium: part II. Urology 2004; 63:217–224.

This, with part I, is an excellent review of current approaches to infertility.

Centers for Disease Control and Prevention (CDC): Update: Creutzfeldt–Jakob disease associated with cadaveric dura mater grafts – Japan, 1979–2003.

Morbidity & Mortality Weekly Report 2003; 52:1179.

Cetin I, Pardi G; A multidisciplinary approach to the future of reproduction. Placenta 2003; 24: s3–s4.

Chakraverty R, Peggs K, Chopra R, et al: Limiting transplantation-related mortality following unrelated donor stem cell transplantation by using a nonmyeloablative conditioning regimen. Blood 2002; 99:1071–1078.

Outlines the risks, benefits, and new methods in hematological transplants for patients without a matched related donor.

Childs R, Clave E, Contentin N, et al: Engraftment kinetics after nonmyeloablative allogenic peripheral blood stem cell transplantation: full donor T-cell chimerism precedes alloimmune responses. Blood 1999; 94:3234–3241.

Civin C, Trischman T, Fackler MJ, et al: Summary of CD34 cluster workshop section. *In* Knapp W, Dorken B, Gilks WR, et al: (eds): Leukocyte Typing IV. Oxford, Oxford University Press, 1989; pp 818–824.

Clarke E, Potter MN, Hale G, et al: Double T cell depletion of bone marrow using sequential positive and negative cell immunoaffinity or CD34+ cell selection followed by Campath-1M; effect on CD34+ cells and progenitor cell recoveries. Bone Marrow Transplant 1998; 22:117–24.

Conrad EU, Gretch D, Obermeyer KR, et al: The transmission of hepatitis C virus by tissue transplantation. J Bone Joint Surg 1995; 77-A:214–224.

Cutler C, Giri S, Jeyapalan S, et al: Acute and chronic graft-versus-host disease after allogenic peripheral blood stem-cell and bone marrow transplantation: a meta-analysis. J Clin Onc 2001; 19:3685–3691.

De Lima M, Shpall EJ: Ex-vivo purging of hematopoietic progenitor cells. Current Hematology Reports 2004; 3:257–264.
Good review of the methods and trials of ex-vivo purging.

Eastlund T: Tissue and organ preservation and transplantation. *In* Rossi EC, Simon TL, Moss GS, Gould SA (eds): Principles of Transfusion Medicine. Baltimore, Williams & Wilkins, 1996, pp 825–831.
An overview of current tissue transplantation practices including bone and skin allografts.

Eastlund T: The histo-blood group ABO system and tissue transplantation. Transfusion 1998; 38:975–988.

Evers JL: Female subfertility. Lancet 2002; 360:151–159.

Eye Bank Association of America: Annual Statistical Report. Washington, DC, Eye Bank Association of America, 1999.

Eye Bank Association of America: Annual Statistical Report. Washington, DC, Eye Bank Association of America, 2004.

Ezra-Cohen HE, Cook SF, et al: Blood typing compact human bone tissue. Nature 1961; 191:1267–1268.

Food and Drug Administration. Current good tissue practice for human cell, tissue and cellular and tissue-based product establishments, inspection and enforcement, final rule. 21 Code of Federal Regulations, parts 16, 1270 and 1271: November 24, 2004.

Gianni AM, Bregni M, Siena S, et al: Rapid and complete hematopoietic reconstitution following combined transplantation of autologous blood and bone marrow cells. A changing role for high-dose chemo-radiotherapy? Hematol, Oncol 1989; 7:139–148.

Gluckman E, Broxmeyer H, Auerbach A, et al: Hematopoietic reconstitution in a patient with Fanconi's anemia by means of umbilical-cord blood from an HLA-identical sibling. N Engl J Med 1989; 321:1174–1178.

Gorin NC: Collection, manipulation and freezing of haemopoietic stem cell. *In* Gladstone AH (ed): Clinics in Haematology. London, WB Saunders Company, 1986, pp 19–48.
A lengthy but comprehensive description of cell freezing physiology and practices.

Gratwohl A, Baldomero H, Passweg J, et al: Increasing use of reduced intensity conditioning transplants: report of the 2001 EBMT activity survey. Bone Marr Transp 2002; 30:813–831.

Grewal SS, Barker JN, Davies SM, Wagner JE: Unrelated donor hematopoietic cell transplantation: marrow or umbilical cord blood? Blood 2003; 101:4233–4244.

Henslee-Downey PJ, Abhyankar SH, Parrish RS, et al: Use of partially mismatched related donors extends access to allogeneic marrow transplant. Blood 1997; 89:3864–3872.

Hill Z, Vacl J, Kalasova E, et al: Haemolytic disease of the newborn due to anti-D antibodies in a Du positive mother. Vox Sang 1974; 27:92–94.

Houghton FD, Hawkhead JA, Humpherson PG, et al: Non-invasive amino acid turnover predicts human embryo developmental capacity. Hum Reprod 2002; 17:999–1005.

Iscove NN, Senn JS, Till JE, McCulloch EA: Colony formation by normal and leukemic human marrow cells in culture: Effect of conditioned medium from human leukocytes. Blood 1971; 37:1–5.

Jackson DW, Windler GE, Simon TM: Intraarticular reaction associated with the use of freeze-dried, ethylene oxide-sterilized bone-patella tendon-bone allografts in the reconstruction of the anterior cruciate ligament. Am J Sports Med 1990; 18:1–10.

Kainer MA, Linden JV, Whaley DN, et al: Clostridium infections associated with muscoskeletal-tissue allografts. N Engl J Med 2004; 350:2564–2571.

Kearney JN: Quality issues in skin banking: A review. Burns 1998; 24:299–305.

Kessinger A, Armitage JO, Landmark JD, et al: Autologous peripheral hematopoietic stem cell transplantation restores hematopoietic function following marrow ablative therapy. Blood 1988; 71:723–727.
Provides the earliest work and later refinements in autologous hematopoietic transplants by one of the first groups to describe this therapy.

Kolb HJ, Mittermulller J, Clemm CH, et al: Donor leukocyte transfusions for treatment of recurrent chronic myelogenous leukemia in marrow transplant patients. Blood 1990; 76:2462–2465.

Laub GW, Muralidharan S, Clancy R: Cryopreserved allograft veins as alternative coronary artery bypass conduits: Early phase results. Ann Thorac Surg 1992; 54:826–831.

Laughlin MJ, Barker J, Bambach B, et al: Hematopoietic engraftment and survival in adult recipients of umbilical-cord blood from unrelated donors. New Engl J Med 2001 344:1815–1822.
An excellent review of trials of umbilical cord blood transplants.

Lorenz E, Uphoff D, Reid TR, Shelton E: Modification of irradiation injury in mice and guinea pigs by bone marrow injections. Natl Cancer Inst 1951; 12:197–201.

Lucifero D, Chaillet JR, Trasler JM: Potential significance of genomic imprinting defects for reproduction and assisted reproductive technology. Hum Reprod 2004; 10:3–18.

Marmont AM, Gale RP, Butturini A, et al: T-cell depletion in allogenic bone marrow transplantation: progress and problems. Haematologica 1989; 74(3):235–248.

Medawar PB: Relationship between antigens of blood and skin. Nature 1946; 157:161–170.

Medawar PB: Immunity to homologous grafted skin. III. The fate of skin homografts transplanted to the brain, to subcutaneous tissue and to the anterior chamber of the eye. Br J Exp Pathol 1948; 29:58–62.

Mohan S, Baylink DJ: Bone growth factors. Clin Orthop 1991; 263:30–48.

Niederwieser D, Maris M, Shizuru JA, et al: Low-dose total body irradiation (TBI) and fludarabine followed by hematopoietic cell transplantation (HCT) from HLA-matched or mismatched unrelated donors and postgrafting immunosuppression with cyclosporine and mycophenolate mofetil (MMF) can induce durable complete chimerism and sustained remissions in patients with hematological diseases. Blood 2003; 101:1620–1629.

Noga SJ, Wagner JE, Rowley SD, et al: Using elutriation to engineer bone marrow allografts. Prog Clin Biol Res 1990; 333:345–359.

O'Brien MF, Stafford EG, Gardner MAH: Cryopreserved viable allograft aortic valves. *In*

Yankoh AC, Hetzer R, Miller DC, et al: (eds): Cardiac Valve Allografts 1972–1987. New York, Springer-Verlag, 1988, pp 311–318.

Palermo GD, Joris H, Devroey P: Pregnancies after intracytoplasmic injection of a single spermatozoan into an oocyte. Lancet 1992; 340:17–18.

Porter DL, Connors JM, Van Deerlin VM, et al: Graft-versus-tumor induction with donor leukocyte infusions as primary therapy for patients with malignancies. J Clin Oncol 1999; 17:1234.

Reisner Y, Kapoor N, Hodes MZ, et al: Enrichment for CFU-C from murine and human bone marrow using soybean agglutinin. Blood 1982; 59:360–363.

Richman CM, Weiner RS, Yankee RA: Increase in circulating stem cells following chemotherapy in man. Blood 1976; 47:1031–1039.

Shorr N, Perry J, Goldberg RA, et al: The safety and applications of acellular human dermal allograft in ophthalmic plastic and reconstructive surgery: a preliminary report. Ophthal Plast Reconstr Surg 2000; 16:223–230.

Siena S, Bregni M, Brando B, et al: Circulation of CD34+ hematopoietic stem cells in the peripheral blood of high-dose cyclophosphamide-treated patients: Enhancement by intravenous recombinant human granulocyte-macrophage colony stimulating factor. Blood 1989; 74:1905–1914.

Simonds RJ, Holmberg SD, Hurwitz RL, et al: Transmission of human immunodeficiency virus type 1 from a seronegative organ and tissue donor. N Engl J Med 1992; 326:726–732.

Skiera D, Zeller W, Zander AR: Graft engineering of G-CSF-mobilized allogenic leukapheresis products by counterflow centrifugal elutriation after CD34 column. J Hematol 1999; 8:299–304.

Steptoe P, Edwards R: Pregnancy in an infertile patient after transfer of an embryo fertilized in vitro. Brit Med J 1983; 286:1351–1352.

Storb R: Allogenic hematopoietic stem cell transplantation – yesterday, today, and tomorrow. Exp Hem 2003; 31:1–10.
Interesting, non-technical review by one of the leaders in hematopoietic transplantation.

Stroncek DF, Fautsch SK, Lasky LC, et al: Adverse reactions in patients transfused with cryopreserved marrow. Transfusion 1991; 31:521–526.

Sutherland DR, Keating A, Nayar R, et al: Sensitive detection and enumeration of CD34+ cells in peripheral blood and cord blood by flow cytometry. Exp Hematol 1994; 22:1003–1010.

Thomas ED, Lochte HL, Cannon JH, et al: Supralethal whole body irradiation and isologous marrow transplantation in man. J Clin Invest 1959; 38:1709–1716.

Tomford WW: Musculoskeletal Tissue Banking. New York, Raven Press, 1993.

United Network for Organ Sharing: 2002 Annual Report. United Network for Organ Sharing, Richmond, VA, 2003, p 1.

Volker-Dieben HJ, D'Amaro J, Kok-van Alphen CC: Hierarchy of prognostic factors for corneal allograft survival. Aust N Z J Ophthalmol 1987; 15:11–18.

Wagner WE, Broxmeyer HE, Cooper S: Umbilical cord and placental blood hematopoietic stem cells: Collection, cryopreservation and storage. J Hematother 1992; 1:167–175.

Walker PJ, Mitchell RS, McFadden PM: Early experience with cryopreserved saphenous vein allografts as a conduit for complex limb-salvage procedures. J Vasc Surg 1993; 18:561–568.

Weiden PL, Sullivan KM, Flourneoy N, et al: Antileukemic effects of chronic graft vs host disease. Contribution to improved survival after allogenic marrow transplantation. N Eng J Med 1981; 304:1529–1533.

Weipert J, Meisner H, Mendler N: Allograft implantation in pediatric cardiac surgery: Surgical experience from 1982–1994. Ann Thorac Surg 1995; 60(Suppl):S101–S104.

Weissinger F, Sandmaier BM, Maloney DG, et al: Decreased transfusion requirements for patients receiving nonmyeloablative allogenic hematopoietic stem cell transplants from HLA-identical siblings. Blood 2001; 98:3584–3588.

Yeager AM, Kaizer H, Santos GW, et al: Autologous bone marrow transplantation in patients with acute nonlymphocytic leukemia, using ex vivo marrow treatment with 4-hydroperoxycyclophosphamide. N Engl J Med 1986; 315:141–147.

IV

PART V

Hemostasis and Thrombosis

Edited by

Jonathan L. Miller MD PhD

CHAPTER 38

Coagulation and Fibrinolysis

Alvin H. Schmaier MD, Courtney D. Thornburg MD MS, Steven W. Pipe MD

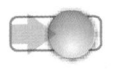

KEY POINTS

- Physiologic hemostasis consists of the plasma coagulation, fibrinolysis, and anticoagulation protein systems.

- Physiologic hemostasis is initiated by factor VIIa and tisssue factor.

- Physiologic hemostasis is not fully represented by current assays to detect coagulation abnormalities such as the activated partial thromboplastin time and prothrombin time.

- However, current assays to assess coagulation protein abnormalities have good diagnostic power to recognize specific defects in coagulation proteins.

- Acquired coagulation protein defects more commonly reflect general medical disorders than specific protein defects.

Overview of Coagulation and Fibrinolysis

Hemostasis, or the cessation of bleeding, occurs within the intravascular compartment lined with endothelium. Normal hemostasis and thrombosis involves a number of factors. These factors include platelets, granulocytes, and monocytes as well as the coagulation (clot forming), the fibrinolytic (clot lysing) and anticoagulant (regulating) protein systems. Each of the three protein systems balances the activities of the other. In addition, the integrity of the vessel wall endothelium is contributory. In recent years there has been a great evolution in our understanding of the physiologic hemostatic system (Fig. 38–1). For decades the hemostatic system has been referred to as the 'coagulation cascade' based upon the waterfall hypothesis of Ratnoff & Davies and MacFarland who published, almost simultaneously, a sequence of proteolytic reactions starting with factor XII (Hageman factor) activation and ending with formed thrombin proteolyzing fibrinogen to form a clot (Ratnoff, 1964; MacFarland, 1964). However, at the onset, this hypothesis for physiologic hemostasis was untenable. At the time of publication of these hypotheses, it was known that factor XII deficiency was not associated with bleeding (Ratnoff, 1955). Thus the physiologic basis for this system to be activated by factor XII was questioned. Further, by the mid-1970s the cofactors for factor XII activation, prekallikrein and high-molecular-weight kininogen, were identified, and deficiencies of these proteins were not associated with a bleeding state (Weuppers, 1972; Colman, 1975; Saito, 1975). Other mechanisms for physiologic hemostasis were sought. In 1977, Osterud and Rappaport recognized that factor VIIa is able to activate factor IX to factor IXa (Osterud, 1977). Later, Broze and colleagues recognized that the kinetics of tissue factor pathway inhibitor (TFPI) were such that under physiologic circumstances the factor VIIa–tissue factor complex cannot directly activate factor X but has to go through factor IX activation (Broze, 2003). These latter two studies indicate the important role of the factor VIIa–tissue factor pathway for physiologic hemostasis. A key remaining question was how does factor XI, whose deficiency is associated with bleeding, become activated under physiologic circumstances? In 1991, Gailiani and Broze found that formed thrombin can activate factor XI, resulting in amplification of the coagulation system under stress (Gailiani, 1991). Presently, physiologic hemostasis is believed to be an interacting system of activation and amplification of several zymogens that become serine proteases. The initiator of physiologic hemostasis is factor VIIa when bound to its cofactor tissue factor. Regulation of expression of tissue factor provides a major modulation of physiologic hemostasis. Thrombin in turn amplifies the process by activating factor XI, leading to additional factor IX activation. The fibrinolytic system's role is to lyse clot formed by thrombin. The anticoagulation system's role is to regulate all the enzymes of the coagulation and fibrinolytic systems so that there is no inappropriate excess of clotting or bleeding.

It is important for the pathologist to understand the physiologic basis of hemostasis. However, the clinical laboratory assays used to examine the coagulation system are based upon the original coagulation cascade hypothesis. Although these tests do not represent physiologic hemostasis, they are still very useful for diagnosis of potential bleeding disorders. Thus the pathologist needs to understand the distinction between physiologic coagulation, fibrinolysis, and anticoagulation and the tests that we use to measure these systems. This chapter endeavors to clarify this distinction for the reader. In the first part of this chapter, the details of physiologic coagulation, fibrinolysis, and the regulation of coagulation will be presented. In the second part of this chapter, a description of the assays performed to measure bleeding disorders will be presented, together with a discussion of the limitations of these assays for characterizing physiologic hemostasis. In the third part of this chapter, an overview of congenital bleeding disorders will be presented. Last, this chapter will present the acquired bleeding disorders, the most common forms of bleeding states one actually encounters.

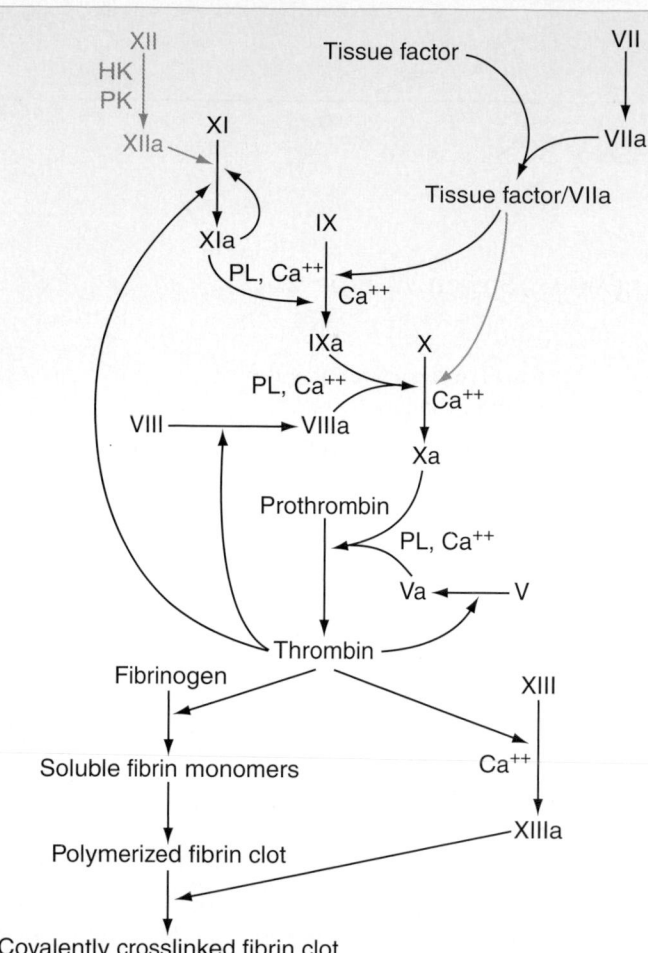

Figure 38–1 Schematic diagram of physiologic hemostasis. Note that the 'contact phase' factors comprising factor XII, HK (high molecular weight kininogen) and PK (prekallikrein) are shown grayed; although factor XI can be activated by this route under artificial *in vitro* conditions such as in the PTT test (see Fig. 38–8), this pathway is *not* believed to contribute to normal physiologic hemostasis. Similarly, whereas Tissue factor/VIIa can directly activate X to Xa in the *in vitro* PT test under conditions which supra-physiological concentrations of Tissue factor are employed, this reaction is shown as grayed because it does *not* contribute significantly to clot formation under normal *in vivo* physiological conditions. Normal clotting *in vivo* accordingly is initiated when sufficient Tissue factor/VIIa becomes available to activate factor IX to IXa. Subsequently, IXa in the presence of VIIIa activates X to Xa, which in turn activates prothrombin to thrombin in the presence of Va. Thrombin not only then proceeds to clot fibrinogen and to activate platelets (see Fig. 38–2), but additionally exerts critically important positive feedback by activating factors VIII and V. Thrombin has further been shown capable of activating factor XI, thereby providing an additional pathway for the activation of factor IX. PL (phospholipid present on the surface membranes of platelets *in vivo*) and Ca^{++} (calcium ions) contribute to reactions as indicated.

Physiologic Hemostasis

The physiologic hemostatic system, a tightly regulated balance between the formation and dissolution of hemostatic plugs modulated by a series of enzymes and scaffolding proteins, has two major parts. The first part of the physiologic hemostatic system is its cellular component, which consists mostly of platelets and endothelial cells but also includes neutrophils and monocytes. The second part is a large group of plasma proteins, which participate in clot formation (coagulation), dissolution of clots (fibrinolysis), and naturally occurring serine protease inhibitors that terminate activity of a number of enzymes of the coagulation and fibrinolytic systems.

Endothelium and Platelets

A number of factors are involved in coagulation and fibrinolysis reactions. Normal hemostasis involves interplay among the cellular components and proteins involved in clot formation and lysis. Normally, the endothelium that lines the vascular compartment contributes to its constitutive anticoagulant nature. Endothelial cells have glycosaminoglycans that bind antithrombin (Marcum, 1984). Thrombomodulin on endothelial cell membranes is a locus where protein C is activated by low levels of thrombin (Esmon, 1981). Intact

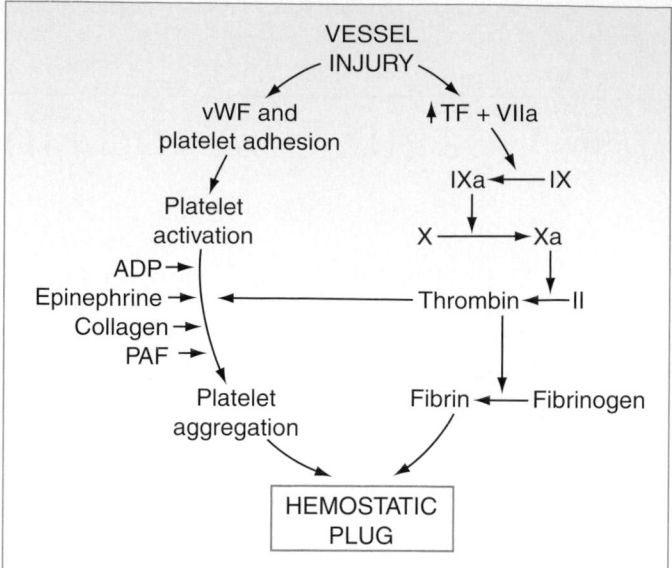

Figure 38–2 Schematic diagram of hemostasis. When a vessel is injured, platelets adhere to the injury site via von Willebrand factor (vWF). Upon adherence, the platelets are activated and release their granule contents. Released ADP and exposed collagen recruit more platelets to the injury site. Outward exposure of phosphatidylserine on the activated platelets further enhances phospholipid-dependent coagulation reactions (not shown). Simultaneously at the site of injury, tissue factor is up-regulated and with factor VIIa, activates factor IX to factor IXa and, sequentially, factor X to factor Xa, and prothrombin to thrombin. Thrombin stimulates more platelets, enhancing the platelet plug. Thrombin also proteolyses fibrinogen to form fibrin monomer that then polymerizes into a fibrin clot. These events occur on or about the activated platelet surface.

endothelial cells secrete an ectonucleotidase (ectoADPase), CD39, that degrades adenosine diphosphate (ADP) (Pinsky, 2002). Endothelial cells also secrete prostacyclin and nitric oxide, which prevent platelet activation (Hong, 1980; Palmer, 1987). Endothelial cells additionally bind plasminogen, tissue plasminogen activator, and single chain urokinase, all of which contribute to fibrinolysis and maintenance of an anticoagulant state (Barnathan, 1988; Cesarman, 1994). When a vessel wall is injured, collagen is exposed and platelets adhere to the site of injury. Von Willebrand factor helps platelets to adhere to the injured vessel wall by binding both to this exposed collagen and to the platelet receptor GP Ib–IX–V complex (He, 2003). This adhesion event activates platelets, initiating a signaling cascade within them (Zaffran, 2000). The stimulated platelets release the contents of their granules and help to generate thrombin on their surface. As a result of platelet activation and thrombin formation, the platelets aggregate and a hemostatic plug forms (Fig. 38–2).

Adjacent to the site of injury, tissue factor (TF) is upregulated in the subendothelium and forms a complex with factor VIIa (FVIIa). The complex of FVIIa–TF activates factor IX to factor IXa, which converts zymogen factor X to enzymatically active factor Xa (Fig. 38–1). In the presence of factor Va, factor Xa activates prothrombin (factor II) to thrombin (factor IIa), which is the major clotting enzyme. Under normal circumstances, the rate-limiting component of prothrombinase complex formation and the ultimate generation of thrombin activity is the concentration of factor Xa (Rand, 1996). Thrombin then proteolyzes fibrinogen to form fibrin. In static, *in vitro* systems, as little as 5–10 pM tissue factor is sufficient to induce clot formation leading to a 1000–2000-fold amplification of the process that brings the concentration of thrombin to 10–20 nM thrombin, which is sufficient to initiate clot formation (Mann, 2003). In a static model of blood coagulation, Mann and his colleagues have shown that the addition of 5 pM tissue factor results in an average clot time of 4.7 ± 0.2 min ($n = 35$ individual experiments). During the generation of thrombin in whole blood, there is a sequential activation of platelets, factors V and VIII, and liberation of fibrinopeptides A and B (see below) at an early stage of thrombin formation (Mann, 2003). Thrombin is additionally considered a major physiologic activator of platelets, together with other agonists such as collagen, ADP, platelet-activating factor (PAF), and epinephrine. Unactivated platelets probably circulate without promoting coagulation. When platelets are activated, their membrane becomes a site for more thrombin formation. Critical reactions to form factor Xa and thrombin are accelerated on the platelet surface. When perturbed or injured, endothelial cell membranes function similarly by expressing TF and factor V. Physiologically important coagulation and fibrinolytic reactions are likely to occur on the surface of cells

Table 38–1 Proteins of the Plasma Coagulation System

Surface-Bound Zymogens	Vitamin-K-Dependent Zymogens	Cofactors/Substrates
Factor XII	Factor VII	High M_r kininogen
Prekallikrein	Factor IX	Factor VIII
Factor XI	Factor X	Factor V
	Factor II	Fibrinogen
	Protein C	Protein S

in the intravascular compartment. Critical protein activation and inhibition reactions also occur on the membranes of activated neutrophils and monocytes.

Coagulation Protein System

Characterization of Coagulation Proteins

The proteins that comprise the coagulation system consist of zymogens and cofactors (Table 38–1). The zymogens of the coagulation system can be grouped into the phospholipid-bound proenzymes (zymogens) and the surface-dependent proenzymes. The phospholipid-bound zymogens make up the physiologically important hemostatic system. These proteins are vitamin-K-dependent. Vitamin K is required for an essential γ-carboxylation reaction that takes place on each of these proteins' glutamic acid residues located on their amino terminal ends (see Ch.41, Fig. 41–1). This carboxylation reaction allows these proteins to bind to phospholipid and cell membranes, where they are activated. Without this carboxylation reaction, these proteins do not function normally in the hemostatic system. These proenzymes include factor X, a 58 kDa protein; factor IX (Christmas factor), a 56 kDa protein; factor VII, a 50 kDa protein; and factor II (prothrombin), a 72 kDa protein.

The surface bound proenzymes are proteins of the plasma kallikrein/kinin system (Table 38–1). Surface-bound proenzymes include factor XII (Hageman factor), an 80 kDa protein; prekallikrein (Fletcher factor), an 85–88 kDa protein; and factor XI, a 160 kDa protein. These protein zymogens are also known as the 'contact system' because factor XII autoactivates when associated with a negatively charged surface such as a glass tube (Wiggins, 1979; Miller, 1980). The autoactivation of factor XII results in prekallikrein activation and in further amplification of factor XII, producing subsequent activation of factor XI. Formation of factor XIa then induces the series of proteolytic reactions (the coagulation 'cascade'), which *in vitro* results in thrombin formation and subsequent proteolysis by thrombin of fibrinogen to form a clot. However, deficiencies of factor XII and prekallikrein are not associated with bleeding. Therefore, this system cannot be a physiologic one for hemostasis. The autoactivation phenomenon of factor XII, however, allows for a common laboratory test, the activated partial thromboplastin time (PTT), which is used to assess the integrity of the coagulation system (see below). This assay is a useful one to assess many coagulation proteins but alone it does not describe physiologic hemostasis. Thus, it is important to be aware that assays to assess many coagulation proteins are based upon the non-physiologic event of factor XII autoactivation. Although absolutely essential for a normal PTT, the proteins of the plasma kallikrein/kinin system do not play a physiologic role in the activation of the coagulation system; rather, they participate in blood pressure regulation, fibrinolysis, and serve as a counterbalance to the renin/angiotensin system (Schmaier, 2002, 2003, 2004). Under physiologic circumstances *in vivo*, prekallikrein when assembled on endothelial cells is first activated by an endothelial enzyme, prolylcarboxypeptidase, and, secondly, factor XII is activated by the formed plasma kallikrein – events that are just the opposite of what takes place in a test tube (Shariat-Madar, 2002; Rojkjaer, 1998).

The hemostatic cofactors for the enzymatic reactions of the coagulation system may be considered to act as receptors for coagulation proteins. For example, high-molecular-weight kininogen serves as a receptor for prekallikrein binding to endothelial cells (Motta, 1998; Schmaier, 1988). Factors VIIIa and Va function as co-receptors of factors IXa and Xa, respectively (Miletich, 1978; Ahmad, 2000). All three of these proteins serve as cofactors that accelerate the reactions in which they participate. For example, high-molecular-weight kininogen accelerates the activation of prekallikrein and factor XI by factor XIIa. Factors VIIIa and Va accelerate factor X and prothrombin activation, respectively, by factors IXa and Xa. Each cofactor also functions as a substrate of one or more enzymes that participate in their formation and inactivation. High-molecular-weight kininogen is accordingly a substrate of factors XIIa, plasma kallikrein, and

factor XIa. Factors VIII and V are substrates of thrombin and of activated protein C. Fibrinogen is a substrate of thrombin.

Factor VIII (antihemophilic factor) is a 330 kDa protein. When activated to factor VIIIa, it is a cofactor for factor IXa in the activation of factor X. Its absence is associated with the most severe clinically recognized bleeding disorder, hemophilia A. Factor V is also a 330 kDa protein with homology to factor VIII. When activated to factor Va, it serves as a cofactor for factor Xa in the activation of factor II (prothrombin) to thrombin. Fibrinogen is a 330 kDa protein that is not only the main substrate of thrombin (factor IIa) but also the principal adhesive molecule subserving platelet aggregation. When it is proteolyzed by thrombin, a fibrin monomer is formed. This monomer associates end-to-end and side-to-side to form a fibrin clot. The clot is stabilized by activated factor XIII, a tissue transglutaminase that crosslinks the strands of associating fibrin. Tissue factor (TF) (47 kDa protein) is an essential cofactor for activated factor VIIa. It is found in most tissues and cells. Upregulation of TF results in the formation of complexes with factor VII that produce the initiation of hemostatic reactions. Last, high-molecular-weight kininogen (HK, also known as Fitzgerald factor or Williams factor) is a 120 kDa protein that acts as a cofactor for the activation of factor XII, prekallikrein, and factor XI on artificial surfaces and endothelial cell membranes. It is a substrate of kallikrein, activated factors XII and XI, and plasmin, and it is the parent compound for bradykinin, a biologically active peptide that regulates blood pressure and vascular biology. On endothelial cells, HK is a receptor for prekallikrein and factor XI, although there is significant factor XI binding to endothelial cells independent of HK (Mahdi, 2003).

Physiologic Protein Assemblies

There are certain critical protein assemblies in hemostatic reactions that accelerate these proteolytic reactions. The proteins of the coagulation system that are essential for hemostasis or control of bleeding were originally identified by observation of affected patients, and more recently through mouse knockout studies. Deficiencies in coagulation factors VIII and IX are the most severe bleeding disorders that occur in patients who survive gestation and birth. The rare patients who have apparent congenital deficiencies of coagulation factors VII, X, V, and II usually do not have severe bleeding states. In contrast, murine models have demonstrated that mouse embryos containing complete genetic knockouts of factors VII, X, V, or II die of massive hemorrhage during gestation or at birth. This information suggests that the human patient who has a deficiency of factors VII, X, V, or II may have some factor, albeit less than 1%, to allow for a more mild clinical phenotype than that seen in mouse models. Directly or indirectly, all of these proteins participate in two critically important assemblies that are essential for normal hemostasis: 'tenase' and 'prothrombinase.'

The *tenase* complex comprises the assembly of factor IXa and thrombin-activated factor VIIIa on phospholipid surfaces or cell membranes in an ordered structure with factor X to accelerate its activation to factor Xa. When all these components are present, the rate of factor X activation by factor IXa is increased 1.4×10^8-fold over the rate of factor X activation by factor IXa alone. The *prothrombinase* complex in analogous fashion comprises the assembly of factor Xa and thrombin-activated factor Va on phospholipid membranes or cell membranes in an ordered structure with factor II (prothrombin) to accelerate its activation to factor IIa (thrombin). When all these components are present, the rate of factor II activation by factor Xa is increased 1.7×10^8-fold over the rate of factor II activation by factor Xa alone. Since these coagulation reactions occupy critical regulatory points within the physiologic hemostatic system, they are also the target area of a number of anticoagulant agents that are currently in use or are being developed.

The Formation of Fibrin and the Fibrinolytic System

The six peptide chains of the fibrinogen molecule are organized into a structure described as having a central E domain and two terminal D domains. When thrombin is formed, it cleaves fibrinopeptide A from the Aα chain and fibrinopeptide B from the Bβ chain of fibrinogen in the E domain region (Doolittle, 1981). The remainder of this thrombin-proteolyzed fibrinogen is called soluble fibrin monomer. Soluble fibrin monomers then assemble with end-to-end and side-to-side association to form a non-covalent fibrin polymer (Fig. 38–3). Activated factor XIII, a transglutaminase, crosslinks fibrin monomeric subunits into an insoluble, cross-linked fibrin clot. When insoluble, cross-linked fibrin is made, a new linkage between the D domains of two adjacent fibrin monomers occurs, and in the process forms a neo-epitope of interaction (Fig. 38–3).

The fibrinolytic protein system consists of the zymogen plasminogen and its naturally occurring activators. Plasminogen is activated to the main clot-lysing enzyme, plasmin, by the endogenous tissue plasminogen

A

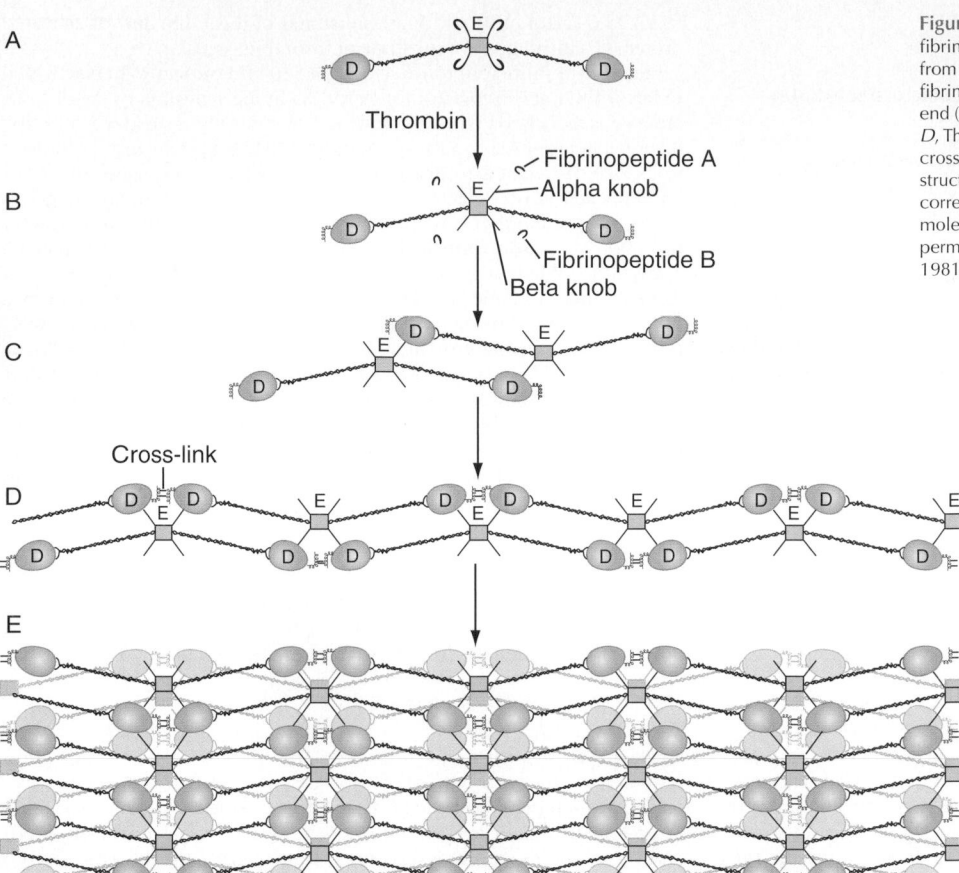

Thrombin

Fibrinopeptide A
Alpha knob

B

Fibrinopeptide B
Beta knob

C

Cross-link

D

E

Figure 38–3 Formation of a fibrin clot. *A,* Schematic of fibrinogen. *B,* Thrombin proteolyzes fibrinopeptides A and B from fibrinogen to leave soluble fibrin monomer. Soluble fibrin monomer then associates side-to-side (*C*) and end-to-end (not shown, for clarity) to form fibrin polymers. *D,* Thrombin-activated factor XIII (factor XIIIa) covalently crosslinks the fibrin polymers into an increasingly complex structure and ultimately insoluble clot (*E*). Note that 'E' corresponds to the central domain of the original fibrinogen molecule, and 'D' to the peripheral domains. (Modified with permission from Doolittle RF: Fibrinogen and fibrin. Sci Am 1981; 245:126–135.)

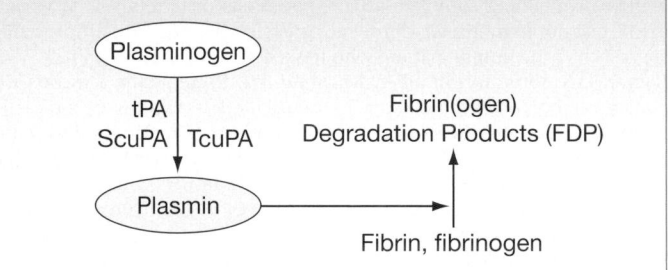

Figure 38–4 Fibrinolysis. Zymogen plasminogen is converted to plasmin by tissue plasminogen activator (tPA), single chain urokinase plasminogen activator (ScuPA), and two chain urokinase plasminogen activator (TcuPA). Formed plasmin degrades fibrinogen or fibrin to form fibrinogen or fibrin degradation products, respectively.

activator (tPA), single-chain urokinase plasminogen activator (ScuPA), and two-chain urokinase plasminogen activator (TcuPA). These activators are found in the endothelium as well as in granulocytes and monocytes. The natural plasminogen activators, tPA, ScuPA, and TcuPA, convert zymogen plasminogen to the active enzyme plasmin (Fig. 38–4). Plasminogen activator inhibitor-1 (PAI-1) is the major inhibitor of tPA and TcuPA. α_2-antiplasmin, a serine protease inhibitor (serpin), is the major inhibitor of formed plasmin. However, the plasma concentration of α_2-antiplasmin is only about half of the plasma concentration of plasminogen.

When plasmin is formed, it has multiple substrates. Plasmin will degrade soluble fibrinogen to produce fibrinogen degradation products (Fig. 38–5A). Plasmin cleaves fibrinogen into an X fragment of similar molecular mass by eliminating portions of the α chain (Marder, 1974). Plasmin then cleaves the X fragment asymmetrically between the D and E domains to produce fragment Y. Plasmin further degrades the Y fragment to produce soluble D and E domains that are called soluble fibrinogen degradation products or, in the case of fibrin digestion by plasmin, fibrin degradation products. Their presence indicates that plasmin has been formed. Plasmin will also degrade insoluble, crossed-linked fibrin (Fig. 38–5B). When it does so, it liberates a D–D dimer domain formed as result of the neo-epitope between these two domains (Fig. 38–5B) (Marder, 1976). The presence of soluble D-Dimer indicates that first thrombin has been

formed, then clotting has occurred, the clot has been cross-linked by factor XIIIa, and finally plasmin has been formed and has cleaved the insoluble, cross-linked fibrin clot. As will be discussed below, measuring D-Dimer is a confirmatory test for disseminated intravascular coagulation (DIC).

The Anticoagulation Protein Systems (Fig. 38–6)

Two major anticoagulant systems regulate the enzymes of the coagulation protein system to help to inhibit clot formation. These systems are the protein C/protein S system and the plasma serine protease inhibitor system. Antithrombin (antithrombin III) is the main serine protease inhibitor of coagulation enzymes of the plasma serine protease inhibitor system.

The protein C/protein S system is considered the major anticoagulant system *in vivo.* When activated, protein C, a 62 kDa vitamin-K-dependent protein, is an enzyme that functions as an inhibitor. Protein C is activated by thrombin that has bound to an endothelial cell protein called thrombomodulin. Activated protein C inactivates factors Va and VIIIa to decrease the rate of thrombin formation. Protein S, a 69 kDa vitamin-K-dependent protein, is not an enzyme. It is a cofactor, or receptor, for activated protein C on cell membranes. It allows activated protein C to bind to cell surfaces in such a manner as to orient itself to inactivate factors Va and VIIIa. The enzyme uses this cofactor as a receptor to localize its activity to perform its inhibitory function. Plasma protein S is in equilibrium between the free form and a bound form that is complexed to C4b-binding protein; only the free form functions as a cofactor for activated protein C. Activated protein C also binds to a protein on endothelial cells called endothelial cell protein C receptor (ECPR) and then activates protease activated receptor (PAR)1. Activation of PAR1 on endothelial cells may contribute to the anticoagulant function of activated protein C by liberating tissue plasminogen activator. Thus activated protein C both reduces thrombin formation and stimulates fibrinolysis to reduce thrombosis risk.

Antithrombin is a 58 kDa serine protease inhibitor that inhibits each of the following hemostatic enzymes: IIa, Xa, VIIa, IXa, XIa, kallikrein, and XIIa. It exerts its anticoagulant effect primarily by inhibiting factors IIa and Xa. The ability of antithrombin to function as an inhibitor of coagulation protein enzymes is potentiated by heparin. In fact, it is the presence of antithrombin that gives heparin its anticoagulant properties. In the presence of heparin, antithrombin is a 1000-fold more effective inhibitor of factor IIa.

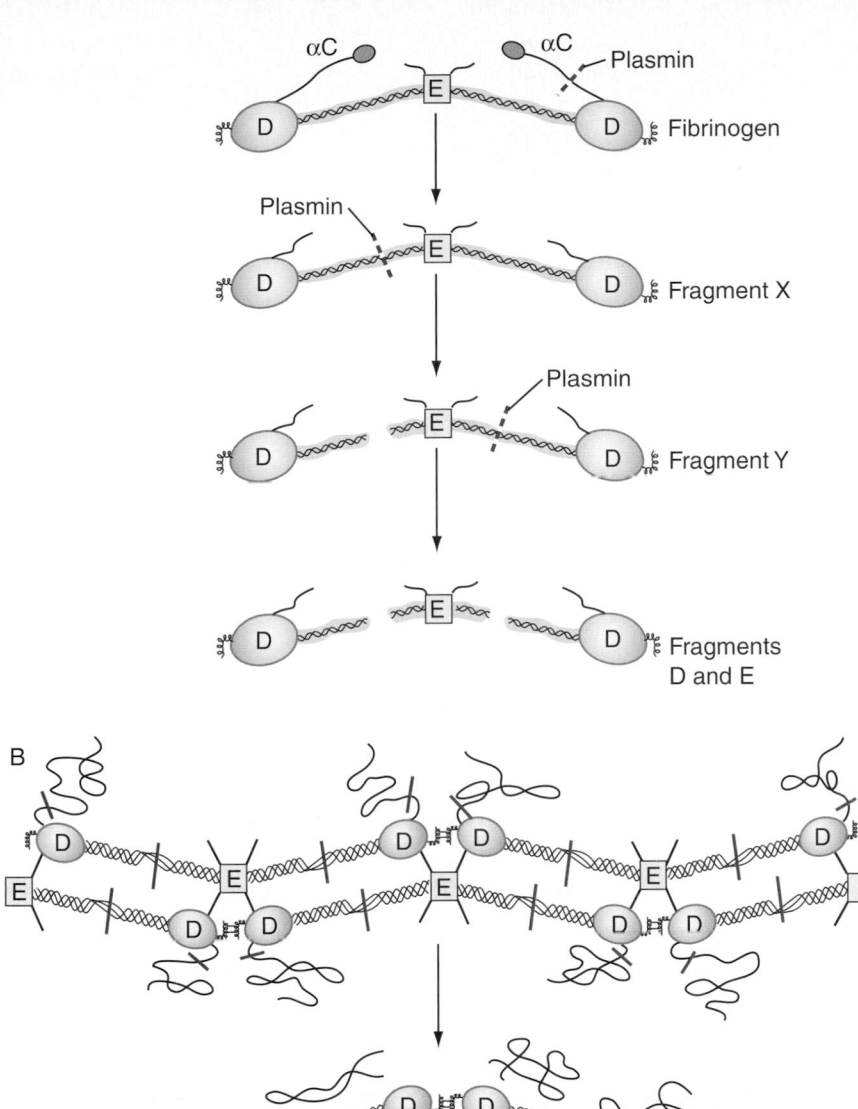

Figure 38–5 *Panel A*, Plasmin-cleaved soluble fibrinogen or fibrin. When plasmin cleaves fibrinogen, initially small portions from the α chain (αC) are removed to make Fragment X. Fragment X is then asymmetrically cleaved into Fragment D and Fragment Y. Fragment Y is further cleaved by plasmin into Fragments D and E. (Modified with permission from Greenberg CS, Lai T-S: Fibrin formation and stabilization. *In* Loscalzo J, Schafer AI (eds): Thrombosis and Hemorrhage, 3rd Edition. Philadelphia, PA, Lippincott, Williams & Wilkins, 2003, Fig. 5–3B, p 83.) *Panel B*, Plasmin-cleaved insoluble, cross-linked fibrin. When insoluble, cross-linked fibrin is proteolyzed by plasmin, the neo-epitope between the D-domains is preserved and the liberated fragment consists of the D-Dimer together with an E domain. (Modified with permission from Doolittle RF: Fibrinogen and fibrin. Sci Am 1981; 245:126–135.)

In addition to antithrombin, there are other serpins that regulate additional enzymes of the hemostatic and inflammatory systems. Heparin cofactor II is a serpin that specifically inhibits thrombin in the presence of dermatan sulfate. Protein Z inhibitor is a serpin that specifically inhibits factor Xa in the presence of its cofactor protein Z – a vitamin-K-dependent protein. C1 inhibitor (C1 esterase inhibitor) is the most potent inhibitor of factor XIIa, kallikrein, and factor XIa in plasma. Its main function is to regulate the amount of free bradykinin in the intravascular compartment (Han, 2002; Schmaier, 2002).

In addition to the serpins, there is another group of serine protease inhibitors – the Kunitz type. Tissue factor pathway inhibitor (TFPI), a Kunitz-type serine protease inhibitor, is the most potent inhibitor of the factor VIIa/tissue factor complex. Under physiologic conditions, TFPI prevents this complex from activating factor X directly. In order for TFPI to function, it forms a quaternary complex with factor VIIa/tissue factor and factor X. Another Kunitz-type serine protease inhibitor, the amyloid β-protein precursor, is present in platelets and brain and regulates factors XIa, IXa, Xa, VIIa/tissue factor, and plasmin (Van Nostrand, 1990; Schmaier, 1993, 1995; Mahdi, 1995, 2000). This inhibitor does not inhibit thrombin. The exact function of this inhibitor is not completely known but it is believed to be a cerebral anticoagulant.

Current Hypothesis for the Initiation of the Hemostatic System

Many proteins participate in coagulation reactions *in vitro*. However, fewer proteins are critical for hemostatic reactions *in vivo*. A more recent hypothesis to replace the original coagulation cascade hypothesis has been presented for hemostatic reactions (Gailiani, 1991). Coagulation protein

reactions are initiated by TF, which binds to factor VIIa. Tissue factor is ubiquitous throughout the body, although it is rich in brain, lung, and placenta. Its expression is upregulated after injury. Regulation of the expression of tissue factor is a major control mechanism for the initiation of hemostasis. Some investigators believe that there is circulating tissue factor, although this notion is currently not universally accepted. This complex then activates factor IX, leading in turn to factor X activation. It must be particularly noted that at the concentrations of factors ordinarily present in the body, TF-VIIa does *not* directly activate appreciable amounts of factor X because of the presence of TFPI– a point emphasized diagrammatically in Fig. 38–1 by the graying of this reaction – despite the ability of this reaction to predominate under the quite artificial conditions used for the *in vitro* 'PT' test (see below). Formation of factor Xa results in the activation of prothrombin to thrombin. Thrombin proteolyzes fibrinogen to form fibrin. Although TF-dependent coagulation reactions are rapidly inhibited by TFPI, if the stimulus for thrombin formation is sufficiently strong, coagulation is maintained through the activation of factor XI by thrombin (Meijers, 2000). Activation of factor XI to factor XIa results in increased activation of factor IX and eventually increased formation of thrombin. A further modulation of the hemostatic balance in the direction of clot formation is exerted by TAFI, the thrombin-activatable fibrinolysis inhibitor (also known as carboxypeptidase U). Among its actions, TAFI cleaves C-terminal lysine residues from fibrin, thereby decreasing binding of plasminogen to the clot and diminishing clot lysis (see review by Leurs and Hendriks, 2005).

Clinical Laboratory Hemostasis

When faced with a bleeding patient, the physician must use an analytic diagnostic approach to determine the cause of the problem. The

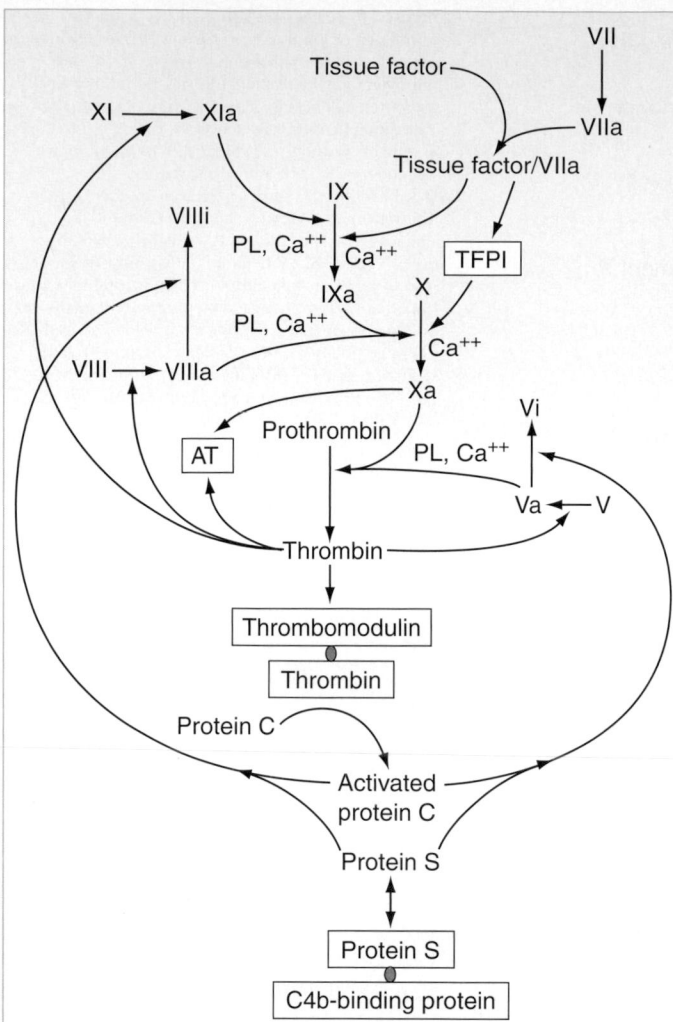

Figure 38–6 Natural inhibitors of coagulation: AT (antithrombin III, antithrombin); components of the protein C pathway (thrombomodulin, protein C, protein S); TFPI (tissue factor pathway inhibitor). For details of inhibitory mechanisms, see text.

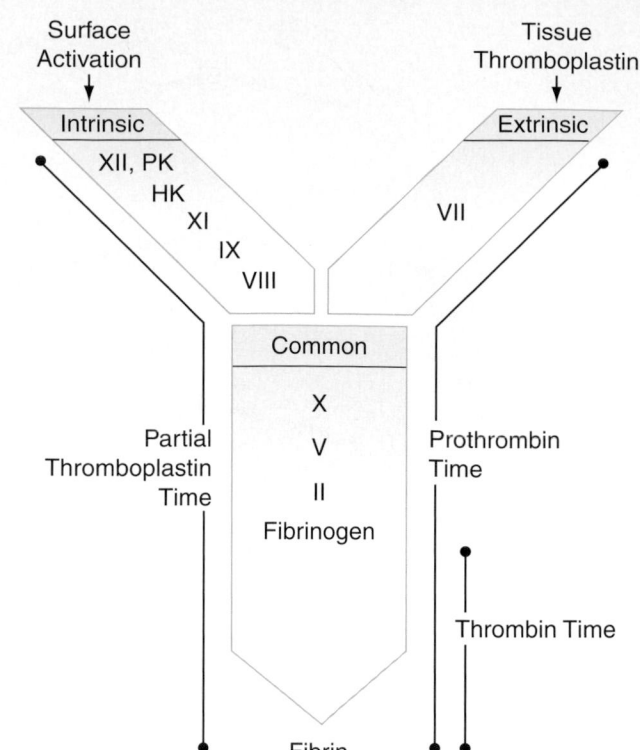

Figure 38–7 Organization of the coagulation system based upon current assays. The 'intrinsic' coagulation system consists of the proteins factors XII, XI, IX, and VIII and prekallikrein (PK) and high molecular weight kininogen (HK). The 'extrinsic' coagulation system consists of tissue factor (Tissue Thromboplastin) and factor VII. The 'common pathway' of the coagulation system consists of factors X, V, II, and fibrinogen (I).

Table 38–2 Patterns of Clinical Bleeding in Disorders of Hemostasis

Characteristics	Primary Hemostasis (Platelet/Vascular Problem)	Secondary Hemostasis (Coagulation Factor Problem)
Onset	Spontaneous, immediate after trauma	Delayed after trauma
Sites	Skin, mucous membranes	Deep tissues
Form	Petechiae, ecchymosis	Hematomas
Mucous membrane	Common (nasal, oral, gastrointestinal, genitourinary)	Less common
Other sites	Rare	Joint, muscle, central nervous system, retroperitoneal
Clinical examples	Thrombocytopenia, platelet defects, von Willebrand disease, scurvy	Factor deficiency, liver disease, acquired inhibitors

underlying etiology will in almost all cases derive from a defect or deficiency in a plasma protein, a defect in platelet number or function, or a defect in the adhesive interactions between platelets and the vessel wall.

Any coagulation protein defect can be a true protein deficiency, an inhibitor to the active site of the protein, an abnormal protein that cannot participate in its physiologic function(s), or arise as the result of enhanced clearance of the protein presenting with the appearance of a deficiency. In general, inhibitors to a coagulation protein are immunoglobulins, although hypergammaglobulinemic states or abnormal production of endogenous heparin, fibronectin, or cryoglobulins have also been reported as acquired inhibitors to coagulation proteins. Abnormal proteins that are present but do not function normally occur as a result of missense, deletion, and translocations of its DNA. Lastly, enhanced clearance of coagulation proteins usually occurs as a result of antigen–antibody complex formation. The resultant increased clearance of the protein gives the appearance of a deficiency, but the real mechanism is enhanced clearance.

Typical clinical presentations of bleeding disorders are shown in Table 38–2. In general, hemarthrosis and spontaneous soft tissue and intramuscular hemorrhage characterize plasma protein defects such as hemophilia A and B (factors VIII and IX deficiency). Soft tissue petechiae, purpura, or ecchymosis characterize von Willebrand disease or platelet number or function disorders. However, at times it is difficult to distinguish the potential mechanism for bleeding. Thus the clinical laboratory is essential for the definitive diagnosis of the bleeding disorder in the patient.

Physiologic Hemostasis Versus Clinical Assays

In the practice of clinical hemostasis, there is a dichotomy between physiologic hemostasis and the assays used in the clinical laboratory to

recognize coagulation protein defects. As indicated above in Figure 38–1, physiologic hemostasis is initiated by an increase in the formation of tissue factor/factor VIIa complexes. At present, there are no good assays in the clinical laboratory to assess this early event specifically. Instead, the relatively late event of actual clot formation is monitored. The two assays most commonly used to examine the coagulation system are (1) the activated partial thromboplastin time (PTT) induced by surface (contact) activation of the system; and (2) the prothrombin time (PT) induced by the addition of excess tissue factor. Contact activation of the coagulation system occurs in a test tube because factor XII associates with its glass surface or the presence of artificial, negatively charged particles in the reagent that results in factor XII autoactivation to factor XIIa, which in turn initiates the cascade of proteolytic reactions of the coagulation system. As

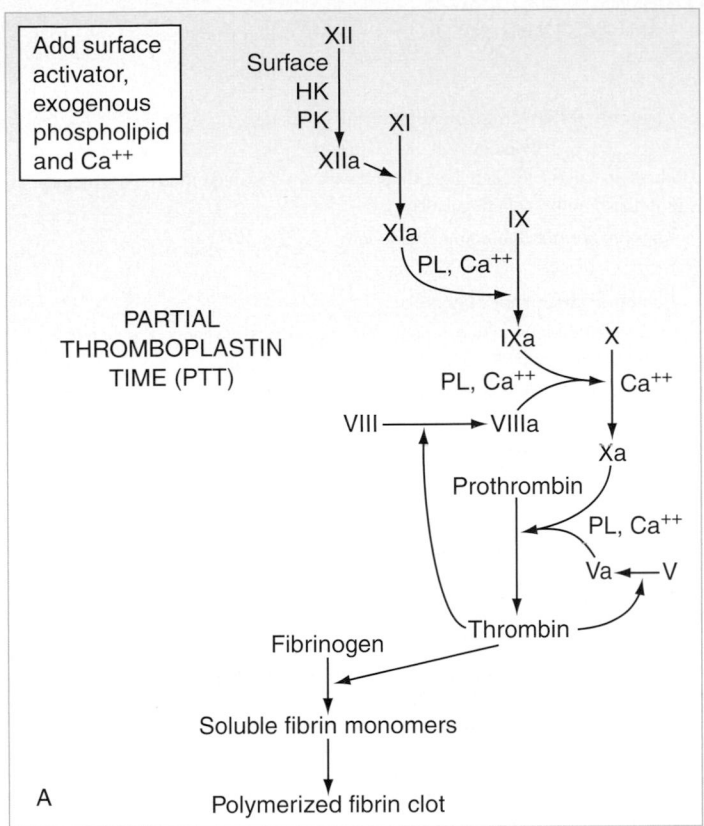

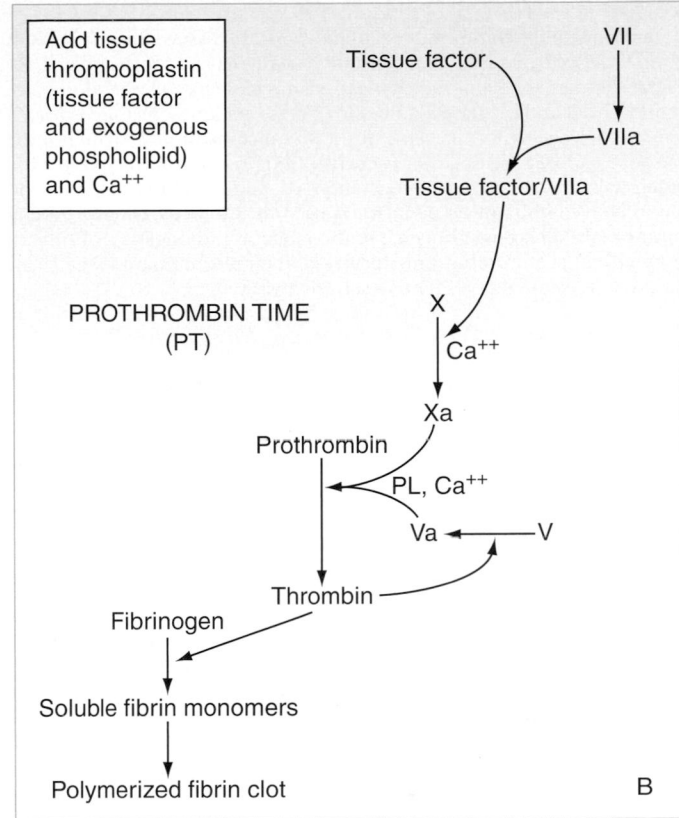

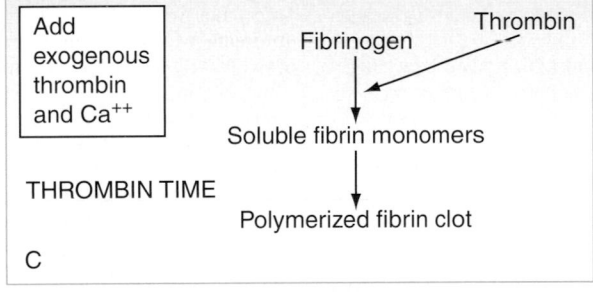

Figure 38–8 Coagulation Screening Tests. *Panel A*: The activated partial thromboplastin time (PTT) requires the presence of every protein except tissue factor and factor VII. *Panel B*: The prothrombin time (PT) requires tissue factor and factors VII, X, V, II, and fibrinogen. *Panel C*: In the Thrombin Time (or Thrombin Clotting Time) exogenous thrombin is added to plasma to proteolyze (clot) fibrinogen. The end point in each of these tests is the number of seconds until the detection of a clot, following addition of the indicated reagents to citrated platelet-free patient plasma. Since virtually all measuring systems employed detect formation of a polymerized fibrin clot whether or not there is any cross-linking of fibrin, none of the above tests will provide any information with respect to factor XIIIa activity.

will be seen below, this test measures more proteins than those necessary for physiologic hemostasis. In the PT test, the addition of excess tissue factor creates a very unphysiologic change in the normal stoichiometric relationship of factors, thereby allowing factor VIIa to overcome the inhibitory effect of tissue factor pathway inhibitor (TFPI) and favoring direct activation of factor X to factor Xa without the usual physiologic requirement to proceed by means of factor IX activation. Although neither test represents physiologic hemostasis, both assays are extremely useful for recognizing potential bleeding problems in a patient (see below).

Screening Tests for Coagulation Disorders

When approaching a patient with a bleeding problem in the clinical laboratory, several screening tests are used to classify and diagnose the basis of this disorder. 'Primary hemostasis' refers to platelet reactivity at the site of vessel injury and this material is covered in Chapter 39. The platelet count is an example of a screening assay for primary hemostasis. This section describes assays for 'secondary hemostasis' – i.e., the coagulation of plasma. When performed simultaneously on a sample of plasma, the results of these assays identify almost all of the diagnostic categories for a coagulopathy. Although it does not describe physiologic hemostasis, the 40 year old cascade hypothesis for hemostasis that underlies the clotting tests still has merit in explaining the mechanism(s) for clot formation seen

in the screening tests for coagulation reactions. In this hypothesis, coagulation proteins are classified as members of the 'intrinsic system', the 'extrinsic system', or the 'common pathway' (Fig. 38–7). This approach allows for a practical differential diagnosis of what protein(s) may be affected based upon the results of a series of screening tests. The specific coagulation factors involved in each test are shown schematically in Fig. 38–7. The methodological aspects of these tests (Fig. 38–8) are as follows:

Activated Partial Thromboplastin Time (PTT) (Fig. 38–8A)

To perform this common coagulation assay, a mixture of a negatively charged surface, phospholipid, and anticoagulated patient plasma is incubated for several minutes. The recommended anticoagulant is 3.2 g% sodium citrate since there is less variation in blood specimens from normal and patients on anticoagulants collected in this concentration of anticoagulant (Adcock, 1997, 1998). When whole blood is collected, the ratio of anticoagulant to whole blood is one part anticoagulant to nine parts whole blood. Calcium chloride is then added, and the time required for clot formation is measured. The PTT assesses the coagulation proteins of the so-called intrinsic system and the common pathways (see below). This assay is commonly referred to as the PTT, but it is really an 'activated' PTT, since its reagents contain a negatively charged surface that accelerates the rate of the reaction (Proctor, 1961).

To perform this common coagulation assay, tissue thromboplastin (animal-derived or recombinant) and patient plasma are incubated for several minutes, following which the plasma is recalcified by the addition of 30 mM CaCl$_2$, and the time required for clot formation is measured. The PT assesses the coagulation proteins of the so-called extrinsic system and the common pathway (see below) (Quick, 1935). Tissue thromboplastin has traditionally been a crude preparation of animal brain tissue factor. Presently, recombinant tissue factor is used in the preparation of several commercial PT reagents. In general, the range of prolongation of time of an abnormal prothrombin time increases when recombinant tissue factor is used. This fact makes for a more sensitive assay.

Thrombin Time (TT) or Thrombin Clotting Time (TCT) (Fig. 38–8C)

To perform this assay, purified exogenous thrombin is added to plasma to determine the time for clot formation. It is a direct measure of fibrinogen function and is used to ascertain if there is a defect in fibrinogen function. The thrombin time will be prolonged in hypofibrinogenemic states and if an abnormal protein fibrinogen (dysfibrinogenemia) is present.

Assays Used in Clinical Coagulation Testing

The basis of clinical coagulation testing is functional assays that examine the rate of clot formation. In these assays, a sequence of proteolytic reactions take place leading to thrombin formation and its proteolysis of fibrinogen (Mann, 2003). Proteolysis of fibrinogen results in clot formation, precipitation of soluble proteins, which is detected by either increased impedance or turbidity, or decreased optical clarity, etc., based upon the instrumentation used to measure the result. Any defect along the pathway to clot formation will give an abnormal result. Furthermore, since a series of reactions need to take place to get the final clot formation, any defect below a specific point will lead to an abnormal result above the defect. For example, an inhibitor of factor VIII will give an abnormal factor XI assay. Likewise, a deficient or abnormal fibrinogen will affect the results of all clotting tests.

All coagulation factors of the intrinsic system (XII, prekallikrein, high-molecular-weight kininogen, XI, IX, and VIII) are measured in assays using the PTT as its platform. These assays became readily available because of the recognition of patients with each factor deficient plasma that serves as substrate for them. For example, a factor VIII assay is a mixture of PTT reagent, factor-VIII-deficient plasma, and test (unknown) plasma. After incubation for a few minutes, the time to clot is initiated by the addition of calcium chloride. Factor VII, together with the coagulation factors of the common pathway (X, V, and II), is usually measured in assays using the PT as its platform. For example, a factor X assay is a mixture of PT reagent that contains tissue factor (thromboplastin), factor-X-deficient plasma, and test (unknown) plasma. After incubation for a few minutes, the time to clot is initiated by the addition of calcium chloride. The amount of factor present in a given patient sample is determined by comparing the patient sample against a standard curve made with plasma samples containing varying amounts of the specific factor mixed with the factor-deficient plasma and the appropriate PTT or PT reagent for the factor assay.

The coagulation-based assays are sensitive and specific. They are much simpler to perform than antigen assays for each of the coagulation proteins. Additional assays such as the thrombin time and reptilase time (see below) specifically examine the integrity of fibrinogen, since they add enzyme that proteolyzes fibrinogen to form a fibrin clot. When establishing a clinically useful thrombin time, it is important to reduce the thrombin concentration to about 4 U/mL so that the time of a normal assay is about 20 seconds. Such an assay will allow for sufficient sensitivity of the assay to detect subtle abnormalities in the protein. The coagulation-based assays examine the function of the protein; antigen assays establish the presence of these proteins; and, combined, both assays would be able to detect proteins with reduced function but with normal mass of the protein. Such a situation arises when examining fibrinogen. The most useful means to determine if there is an abnormal fibrinogen is to measure clottable fibrinogen and fibrinogen antigen. If fibrinogen clottability is less than 90% of the amount of fibrinogen antigen, this finding would suggest that the protein produced is abnormal in some way.

In addition to the clot-based assays, the modern coagulation laboratory performs antigen assays for various proteins. Further, chromogenic assays are used to measure certain enzymes (plasmin, activated protein C) and various plasma protease inhibitors (antithrombin, C1 inhibitor). The ability to neutralize the enzymatic activity of factor Xa or thrombin is a useful way to assay for the level of anticoagulants that inhibit factor Xa or thrombin. Further, a direct chromogenic assay for factor Xa has been

Table 38–3 Differential Diagnosis of Abnormal Coagulation Screening Tests

Abnormal partial thromboplastin time (PTT) alone
Associated with bleeding: VIII, IX, XI defects
Not-associated with bleeding: XII, prekallikrein (PK), high-molecular-weight kininogen, lupus anticoagulants

Abnormal prothrombin time (PT) alone
Factor VII defects

Combined abnormal PTT and PT
Medical conditions: anticoagulants, DIC, liver disease, vitamin K deficiency, massive transfusion
Rarely dysfibrinogenemias, factors X, V, and II defects

DIC = disseminated intravascular coagulation.

useful to assess the degree of anticoagulation of a patient on warfarin who also has lupus anticoagulants that interfere with the prothrombin time.

Interpretation of Screening Tests of the Coagulation System

Using the coagulation cascade hypothesis and its grouping of the proteins of the coagulation system, the screening tests for coagulation proteins can be used to identify various deficiencies or abnormalities in the coagulation proteins (Table 38–3, Fig. 38–7).

In the PTT, factor XII is activated by exposing this factor to an artificial negatively charged surface. As indicated above, this *in vitro* event initiates the sequence of reactions of the coagulation cascade. The PTT measures the proteins of the intrinsic coagulation system (factor XII, prekallikrein, high-molecular-weight kininogen, factor XI, factor IX, and factor VIII) and the proteins of the common pathway (factors X, V, II, and fibrinogen) (Fig. 38.8A). It is important to realize that there are different levels that a coagulation factor has to be decreased before the screening assays are sensitive, showing an abnormality. For example, most commercial PTT reagents will detect a decrease in factor VIII when the level of the protein is down to 35–45% normal (i.e. 0.35–0.45 U/mL). Alternatively, factor XII and high-molecular-weight kininogen need to be at a level of 10–15% normal before striking abnormalities are detected on the PTT. Similarly, factor VII levels below 35–40% will begin to be detected on the PT. When evaluating new lots of coagulation reagents, it is important to determine their level of sensitivity to detect coagulation protein deficiencies. Additionally, very high levels of factor VIII can mask a defect in other coagulation factors. High levels of factor VIII can also mask a low protein C level in a clot-based activated protein C assay.

The PT measures the extrinsic coagulation pathway of coagulation which consists of activated factor VII (factor VIIa) and tissue factor and the proteins of the common pathway (factors X, V, II, and fibrinogen) (Fig. 38.8B).

The thrombin time only measures the ability of exogenous thrombin to proteolyze (clot) fibrinogen (Fig. 38.8C). It is used to characterize fibrinogen function.

Knowing what each test measures, the following approach can be used to evaluate patients for bleeding risk who have one or more of these assays prolonged (Table 38–3, Fig. 38–7). For example, if a patient has an isolated prolonged PTT, determination of the patient's risk to bleed can begin with the addition of some historical information. If the isolated prolongation of the PTT in a male patient is associated with bleeding, then the differential diagnosis in decreasing likelihood of frequency is factor VIII, factor IX, or factor XI deficiency. These disorders will be discussed in the next section. If the PTT alone is prolonged and there is no history of bleeding, the most common cause is a lupus anticoagulant. The specific proteins of the so-called intrinsic coagulation system associated with a prolonged PTT but no bleeding history include, in decreasing frequency, factor XII, prekallikrein, and high-molecular-weight kininogen. Knowing about these latter three proteins is essential to evaluate a prolonged PTT even though the patient is not at bleeding risk, so that patients neither get unnecessary plasma replacement therapy nor experience unnecessary delays in scheduled surgical procedures.

Alternatively, if the patient has an isolated PT prolongation that is associated with bleeding, this finding usually indicates a partial factor VII deficiency. At times, defects in some common pathway proteins (fibrinogen, factors II, V, and X) may first appear as an isolated PT prolongation although, if severe, these latter protein defects will yield prolonged PT and PTT results. Usually, however, defects in the common pathway proteins (fibrinogen, factors II, V, X) result in a prolonged PT and PTT. However, when confronted with patient laboratory results of a prolonged PT and PTT, it is important not simply to consider the specific proteins mentioned above but also to address the differential diagnosis from general medical states such as anticoagulation therapy, disseminated intravascular coagulation, liver disease, vitamin K deficiency and massive transfusion. Each of these entities will be described below in the section on acquired bleeding disorders.

There are also a few rare bleeding disorders that will not be recognized on the routine blood coagulation and platelet screening tests. These entities include, in order of frequency, factor XIII defects, α_2-antiplasmin defects, plasminogen activator inhibitor-1 defects, and α_1-antitrypsin$_{PITTSBURGH}$. Factor XIII deficiency will be discussed below. α_2-Antiplasmin defects and plasminogen activator inhibitor-1 defects, both congenital and acquired, produce hyperfibrinolytic states as result of reduced inhibition of plasmin, tissue plasminogen activator, or urokinase, respectively. In addition to assaying specifically for these proteins, there are several screening tests that could be used for these rare disorders (see below). α_1-Antitrypsin$_{PITTSBURGH}$ is an exceedingly rare entity, which is a bleeding disorder resulting from a mutation in antitrypsin that results in potent thrombin inhibition, preventing any clot from forming.

Practical Approach to Patients with Coagulation Disorders

Patients with abnormal coagulation assays can be evaluated by the differential diagnosis of an isolated PTT abnormality, PT abnormality, or both. Specific coagulation protein defects will be discussed in more detail in the next section. When presented with a prolonged coagulation assay, the differential diagnosis is often between a true deficiency or an inhibitor to a specific coagulation protein. Two approaches can be performed to obtain a specific diagnosis. In the first approach, the specific defect of a prolonged coagulation assay can be obtained by performing all relevant coagulation factor assays. If any one test is decreased, then a specific coagulation factor inhibitor assay can be performed for that factor. One general approach to a specific inhibitor study can be performed by mixing various ratios of patient plasma to normal plasma (e.g. 1:1, 2:1, 4:1, 1:2, 1:4), incubating the samples for 2 h at 37°C, and then assaying the level of the specific factor in the mixture. Simultaneously, the patient plasma and the normal plasma used in the mixing study are also incubated under the same conditions. At the time of assay, the percentage activity of the specific factor under study in the normal plasma, patient plasma, and each of the mixtures are obtained. If the *observed value* at any given ratio of patient plasma to control plasma is less than the calculated *expected value* of mixing the two plasmas in the various ratios (e.g., 1:1, 2:1, 1:2, etc.), then one can conclude that an inhibitor is present in patient plasma that transfers to the normal plasma sample. For example, if there is 100% activity (1 U/mL) of the factor being studied in an undiluted sample, a 1:1 dilution of normal plasma with factor-deficient plasma should give a level of about 50% activity. If the same normal plasma was incubated with patient plasma 1:1 and the value came back 32% activity, one should conclude that there is something in patient plasma that transfers and inhibits the factor's activity in normal plasma, i.e., the definition of an inhibitor. This approach is a general, nonquantitative method for assessing a coagulation factor inhibitor. In the section on hereditary coagulation protein defects below, a specifically quantitative method for determining inhibitors to factor VIII will be presented and this approach is applicable to any factor that is measured by coagulant assay.

A second way to approach the problem of determining a specific coagulation factor defect is to begin with a mixing test of patient and normal plasma. Mixing studies based upon the PT or PTT are interpreted by the fact that a 50% level of any coagulation factor alone gives a normal PT and PTT value. The reason for this is that 50% of any coagulation factor will have a normal PT and PTT because both these screening assays have hyperbolic curves, i.e., a decrease in any one factor does not lead to a linear prolongation of either of these two assays. At 50% levels of any coagulation factor, the clotting time will fall in the normal range. Only with values well below 50% will the PT and PTT start to prolong. As indicated above, the sensitivity of the PT and PTT to prolongation with lowering of clotting factors varies as to the factor and the reagent made by the manufacturer. Thus, if patient plasma is mixed 1:1 with normal plasma, the PT or PTT should be normal if there were no inhibitory factor in the patient plasma. If, however, the mixture does not correct to within normal values, one can consider that there is something in patient plasma that interferes with function of the protein in normal plasma.

How one does screening assays for inhibitors has been somewhat subjective to individual laboratories. There are almost no studies that provide evidence-based laboratory medicine on how to proceed with inhibitor screening studies. Some of the approaches to the use of mixing studies have been developed for testing for lupus anticoagulants, which has its own peculiar aspects (Brandt, 1995a, b). Critical issues in performing mixing studies are the ratio of patient plasma to normal plasma (1:1 to 4:1), the time of incubation from mixing to assay (immediate to 2 h), and the assays to be used to measure the result (PT, PTT). One recent investigation aimed to examine the sensitivity and specificity of mixing studies to assess factor deficiencies and anticoagulants (Chang, 2002). In this study, patient and normal plasma were incubated for 37°C for 1 h before assay in ratios of 1:1 or 4:1 patient:normal. On a PTT mix of 1:1 with a percent correction of 70–75% calculated by a specific formula (see reference for formula), the sensitivity and specificity to recognize a factor deficiency or anticoagulant was 100%/33% or 33%/100%, respectively. When the percent correction was 50% calculated from ratio of 4:1 patient:normal in the plasma mix for the PTT, the sensitivity and specificity to recognize a factor deficiency or anticoagulant improved to 88%/100% or 100%/88%, respectively (Chang, 2002). Likewise, on a PT mix of 1:1 with a percentage correction of 70–75% calculated by a specific formula (see reference for formula), the sensitivity and specificity to recognize a factor deficiency or anticoagulant was 95%/50% or 50%/95% respectively (Chang, 2002). When the percentage correction was more than 40%, calculated from a ratio of 4:1 patient:normal in the plasma mix for the PT, the sensitivity and specificity for recognizing a factor deficiency or anticoagulant improved to 96%/100% or 100%/96% respectively (Chang, 2002). Further studies showed that assay after an immediate mix versus a 1 h incubation at 37°C had a lower sensitivity and specificity.

The above studies indicate one institution's approach towards screening mixing studies. Multiple factor deficiencies, such as when a patient is on warfarin, often do not correct since there are both deficiencies in plasma levels of proteins and the production of abnormal molecules as result of the carboxylation defect that function as inhibitors in coagulant-based assays. Once it is determined that an inhibitor is present, specific factor assays still need to be performed to isolate the specific protein that the inhibitor is directed toward. In general, our laboratory aims to find if a specific factor is affected when the screening tests are abnormal and then determine whether there is a specific inhibitor to the activity of that factor.

Hereditary Coagulation Protein Defects

As described above, protein or factor deficiencies can be quantitative or qualitative. In quantitative disorders, the factor level determined by routine clot-based methods (functional activity assays) is similar to the result obtained by immunologic (antigen) assays. In qualitative disorders, the functional assay result is decreased, but the antigen level is significantly higher or normal, indicating the presence of a dysfunctional protein or an inhibitor to the function of that protein.

Deficiency of Factor VIII (Hemophilia A) or Factor IX (Hemophilia B)

Hemophilia A (factor VIII deficiency) is the most common severe congenital bleeding disorder that allows for normal gestation and delivery, affecting 1 in 5000–10 000 males. Hemophilia B (factor IX deficiency) is also a severe congenital bleeding disorder, affecting 1 in 25 000–30 000 males. The factor VIII and IX genes are both located on the X chromosome such that hemophilia A and B are X-linked recessive disorders primarily affecting males. Females carrying a hemophilia mutation on one of their two X chromosomes are carriers. Hemophilia A can affect females when carriers have imbalanced Lyonization of the normal X chromosome, Turner's syndrome, or if they are daughters of an affected male and a carrier female.

Bleeding manifestations of hemophilia A and B, which are coagulation factor problems, include: hemarthrosis; soft tissue hematomas including bleeding into muscles; easy bruising; excessive bleeding with surgery, trauma, dental extraction, and circumcision; bleeding in the gastrointestinal or genitourinary tract; epistaxis; poor wound healing; and, uncommonly, umbilical stump bleeding (Table 38–2). Intracranial hemorrhages can occur, particularly following trauma. The severity of hemophilia is classified based on the plasma factor level (Table 38–4). Severe hemophilia presents with spontaneous bleeding two to four times per month and requires frequent treatment or prophylactic therapy with replacement factor products. At the other end of the spectrum, mild hemophilia presents with prolonged bleeding after trauma or major surgery and patients rarely need intravenous factor replacement.

Hemophilia is suspected based on bleeding symptoms or a family history of hemophilia. About one third of hemophilia A cases arise from

Table 38–4 Classification of Hemophilia A and B

	Classification		
	Severe	Moderate	Mild
Percentage of patients	50–70	10	30–40
Factor VIII or factor IX activity (%)	<1	1–5	6–30
Pattern of bleeding episodes	2–4 per month approx.	4–6 per year approx.	Uncommon
Etiology of bleeding	Spontaneous	Minor trauma	Major trauma Surgery

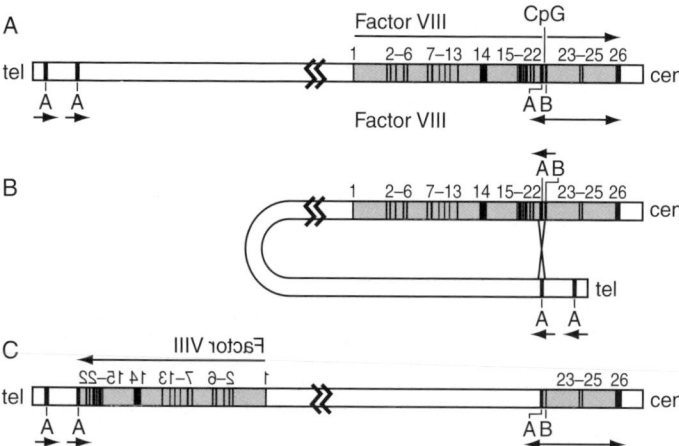

Figure 38–9 Factor VIII gene inversion in hemophilia A. The top panel illustrates a region of chromosome Xq28, with the factor VIII gene shaded. There are additionally two copies of a region having high homology to sequence within factor VIII, termed 'gene A', occurring upstream of factor VIII as well as a third copy of gene A present in inverse orientation within intron-22 of the factor VIII gene itself. The arrow on the top schematic indicates the direction of transcription. On line *B* a proposed homologous recombination is shown between the intron-22 copy of gene A and one of the two upstream copies. On line *C* crossover between these two identical regions, oriented as shown, results in an inversion of the sequence between the two recombined genes. Such a gene would block all factor VIII transcription. This figure represents one kind of recombination. A recombination can occur anywhere in the region of homology in the gene. (Redrawn with permission from Lakich D, Kazazian H, Antonarakis SE, Gitschier J. Inversion disrupting the factor VIII gene are a common cause of severe hemophilia A. Nat Gen 1993; 5:236–241.)

spontaneous mutations. The laboratory evaluation of hemophilia should include a PTT and PT. Diagnosis is confirmed by a factor VIII or factor IX assay. It is important to appreciate that two levels of the standard curve for factor VIII coagulant activity assays need to be prepared to fully characterize patients with severe factor VIII deficiency since the curve is not linear at lower values. In our institution, factor VIII levels above 10% are evaluated with a standard curve that spans 10–150% factor VIII activity. Low factor VIII levels are evaluated with a standard curve that ranges between 0.24% and 15% levels. The most common etiology of severe hemophilia A is a partial inversion of the factor VIII gene up to and including intron 22, which accounts for up to 40–45% of individuals with hemophilia (Naylor, 1992; Lakich, 1993) (Fig. 38–9). These inversions are due to homologous recombination between the region that includes the *F8A* gene in intron 22 and one of the two other homologous regions located more than 400 kb 5′ (telomeric) to the factor VIII gene (Lakich, 1993; Kaufman, 2001). Several types of these inversions have been described (Kaufman, 2001). If the intron 22 inversion is not detected, definition of the responsible mutation is difficult because of the large size of the factor VIII gene. In contrast, the factor IX gene is one third the size of the factor VIII complementary DNA and the mutations responsible for hemophilia B are easier to define by genetic analysis.

In addition to the above, more diagnostic testing may be required for patients with mild to moderate deficiency of factor VIII for whom there is no hemophilia A history (e.g. a female patient with low factor VIII and apparent autosomal inheritance). In patients with von Willebrand's disease, a secondary deficiency of factor VIII may occur (see Ch. 39), since factor VIII is normally bound to and stabilized by von Willebrand factor in the plasma (Weiss, 1977). Further, a unique von Willebrand factor

abnormality has been described in which a missense mutation in von Willebrand factor impairs the capacity of von Willebrand factor to bind to and promote factor VIII secretion into plasma. This abnormality, first described in a French patient from Normandy, has been named von Willebrand disease 'Normandy' or type 2N. It is recognized by having a patient with normal von Willebrand factor studies but reduced factor VIII levels whose inheritance is autosomal recessive rather than sex-linked (Schneppenheim, 1996).

Factor IX activity levels during childhood remain at about 75% of adult levels. There is a 25% increment in factor IX expression that begins at puberty in both sexes (Andrew, 1992). It has been assumed that this is a result of steroid hormone action. Interestingly, there is a rare form of factor IX deficiency, hemophilia B Leyden, which undergoes postpubertal phenotypic resolution. Patients with this condition present with hemophilia B in early childhood with factor IX activity ranging from less than 1% to 13% of normal. Plasma levels rise to as high as 70% of normal after the onset of puberty with resolution of bleeding complications (Reitsma, 2001). Mutations in hemophilia B Leyden have been identified in the promoter region of the factor IX gene, within which a consensus sequence for steroid receptor binding is located (Crossley, 1992).

Evaluation of Carriers

Detection of carriers is useful for prediction of symptoms and prenatal counseling. Carriers may have low enough factor VIII or IX levels to be symptomatic with easy bruising, menorrhagia, and hemorrhagic complications of surgery and trauma (Arun, 2001). In hemophilia A, if the mutation is known, the potential carrier may be tested for that mutation. Otherwise, the woman should be tested for the common intron 22 inversion. If available, detailed genetic analysis of the woman, affected male and intervening family members may define the mutation. These techniques provide an extremely high likelihood of detection of carriers when all family members are available for study. Otherwise, the woman's ratio of factor VIII activity to the level of von Willebrand factor antigen may be used to predict carrier status. Ratios less than 1 identify 91–99% of hemophilia A carriers (Fishman, 1982; Graham, 1986; Green, 1986). Prenatal diagnosis for the hemophilias can be performed at a number of high-risk obstetric centers either by chorionic villous sampling at 12 weeks gestation or by amniocentesis after the 16th week. If the genetic basis of the disease is known in a family, then mutational analysis or examination for the intron 22 inversion can be performed on the cell samples (Ljung, 1999; Arun, 2001). Fetoscopic blood sampling can be performed at 20 weeks gestation for coagulation factor analysis, although it carries a higher risk and is less precise. In hemophilia B, 30–40% of carriers will be missed by measurement of factor IX activity and mutation analysis is important for defining the carrier status (Graham, 1979; Ljung, 1999). Like hemophilia A, hemophilia B arises spontaneously in one third of patients.

Treatment of Hemophilia

Recombinant factor products are now the standard of care for treatment of hemophilia A and B in developed countries. Clotting factors are dosed based on weight and the desired plasma activity. Plasma with 100% clotting factor activity has 1 U/mL of that clotting factor. By convention, one unit of a coagulation factor is the amount of the factor present in 1 mL of normal pooled human plasma. Each unit of recombinant factor VIII/kg raises the plasma factor VIII activity by 2%, and each unit of recombinant factor IX/kg raises the plasma factor IX activity by about 1%. To raise the factor VIII plasma activity of a 70 kg man by 100%, the calculated dose will be as follows:

body weight (kg) × 0.5 international units/kg × factor VIII activity increase desired (%) = dose required, or

(70 kg) (0.5) (100) = 3500 units to be infused.

The plasma half life of factor VIII is about 12 h. To raise the factor IX plasma activity of a 70 kg man by 100%, the calculated dose will be:

body weight (kg) × desired factor IX increase (%) × 1 international unit/kg = dose required, or

(70 kg) (100) = 7000 units to be infused (Shapiro, 2005).

About one third of factor-IX-deficient patients have a lower recovery after recombinant factor IX infusion requiring a 20% higher dosing. The plasma half life of factor IX is about 24 h.

Complications of treatment

Inhibitor antibodies to factor VIII or IX are a significant complication of therapy. The incidence of inhibitors in patients with hemophilia A is approximately 15–35% and the incidence of inhibitors in patients with hemophilia B is approximately 1–4%. In hemophilia A, inhibitors are likely to develop if the individual is severely affected and if, in a previously untreated patient, there are 9–12 exposure days to therapy (Arun, 2001). Inhibitor testing in the hemophilia patient is warranted:

- if a patient's hemorrhage is not controlled with an appropriate dose of factor
- if the level of factor VIII plotted against time of factor infusion shows a too rapid fall-off curve
- if the level of factor in patient plasma seems to increase when the assay of the sample is performed at increased dilutions.

For example, in the latter case, one usually performs a factor level at several dilutions, e.g., 1:10, 1:20, 1:40. If the percentage activity of the factor at the greater dilution is significantly higher than the percentage activity seen at the lower dilution, one might conclude that something inhibiting the factor's activity is being diluted out. Recognizing such a phenomenon can be a first indication of an inhibitor developing in patient plasma.

The characterization of a specific inhibitor to factor VIII or factor IX or any other coagulation protein requires careful examination. A simple mixing test as described above for the PT and PTT can underestimate the presence of an inhibitor. Further, as indicated in the section above, there is no unanimity on how such mixing assays should be performed. It is recommended that when screening for a factor VIII or factor IX inhibitor a formal factor VIII or factor IX 'Bethesda' inhibitor assay be performed (Kasper, 1975). In general, this approach to assay for coagulation factor inhibitors is most reliable for all coagulation protein inhibitors. This assay standardizes the amount of plasma in the mixture, the time of incubation and normalizes the interpretation of the inhibitor so that it is universally interpretable. In this assay, 1 part patient plasma is mixed with 1 part normal plasma and incubated for 2 h at 37°C. The control is a 1:1 mix of pooled plasma with buffer. In a variation of the original Bethesda assay, the so-called Nijmegen modification, the control of pooled plasma is incubated with factor-VIII-deficient plasma and the normal pool used in the assay is buffered to prevent pH shifts during the 2 h incubation (Verbruggen, 1995). After incubation, the patient or control mixture is assayed for factor VIII activity and the percentage residual factor VIII activity is determined at each dilution by the ratio of patient mixture:control mixture. An arbitrary 'Bethesda unit' (BU) has been devised to quantify coagulation factor inhibitors. Thus, in the case of factor VIII, one BU is defined as the amount of patient plasma that destroys half the factor VIII activity in the control plasma (Fig. 38–10). Therefore, a patient's plasma producing a residual factor VIII activity of 50% is considered to contain one Bethesda unit of inhibitor per milliliter. If this same plasma had been diluted 10-fold before assaying for the inhibitor, then this result would indicate inhibitor values of 10 BU/mL. This assay is sensitive, but at times difficult to reproduce. It assumes that the normal plasma being used has 100% activity of factor VIII. The normal plasma used in this assay should be assayed and its level of factor VIII is that used in the calculation of the residual factor VIII after incubation with patient inhibitor plasma. Further, various dilutions of plasma may yield different estimates of the inhibitor titer. In deciding the level of Bethesda units, the dilution that comes closest to the 50% residual factor is chosen for calculation of the factor VIII inhibitor titer. This approach to determine the level of inhibitory units for any coagulation factor is readily adaptable to determine inhibitor levels for any other coagulation factor.

There are a number of therapeutic options for patients with inhibitors to factor VIII. Choosing which one to use has to be judicious since the expense of treating these patients can be a serious drain on the financial resources of an institution. The therapeutic options to treat factor VIII inhibitors include overwhelming the inhibitors with large doses of factor VIII; the use of 'bypassing agents' such as activated and non-activated prothrombin complex concentrates or recombinant factor VIIa (Abshire, 2004; Roberts, 2004; Zeitler, 2005); induction of immune tolerance through regular exposure to factor VIII with and without the use of immuno-suppressive drugs; and plasmapheresis that may include adsorption of antibody. The use of overwhelming inhibitors with massive doses of factor VIII or the use of recombinant factor VIIa are the most expensive forms of therapy by far. However, at times the use of recombinant factor VIIa can be life saving.

Hereditary Deficiencies of Other Coagulation Factors

The other hereditary deficiencies of coagulation factors have autosomal inheritance (Table 38–5). With the exception of factor XI deficiency, these disorders are very rare. However, they have a higher prevalence in areas where consanguineous marriage is practiced (Mannucci, 2004). In general, most patients with coagulation protein deficiencies of factors VII, X, V, and

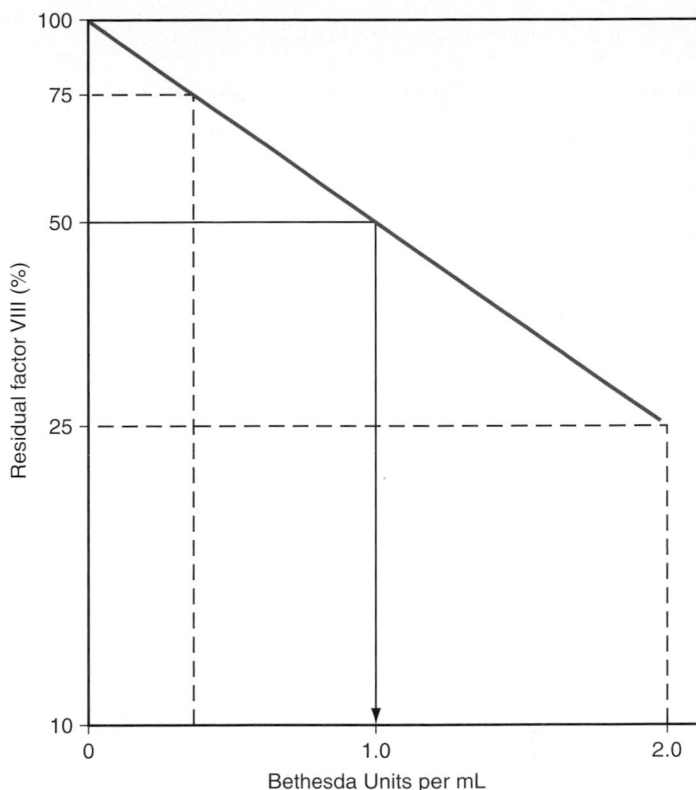

Figure 38–10 Expression of factor VIII inhibitor titer in Bethesda Units. In this assay for an inhibitor to factor VIII, the percent residual factor VIII activity in normal plasma is determined after incubation with patient plasma. By convention, one international Bethesda Unit of inhibitor is the amount of antibody that destroys 0.5 U factor VIII activity after 2 h incubation at 37°C. As shown in the figure, the percent residual factor VIII activity on a log scale is plotted against Bethesda Units/mL in a linear scale. In order for a sample to be evaluable in this assay, the level of factor VIII activity should fall between 25–75%. Patient samples that produce residual factor VIII activity below 25% need to be diluted further to find the 50% residual factor VIII activity point. (Redrawn with permission from Bockenstedt PL: Laboratory Methods in Hemostasis. In Loscalzo J, Schafer AI (eds): Thrombosis and Hemorrhage, 3rd ed. Lippincott Williams & Wilkins, Philadelphia, PA, 2003, Fig.21.7, p. 370.)

II probably have partial defects because they have relatively mild bleeding disorders. Most coagulation-based assays are insensitive to values below 5–10% factor levels. The presence of even this small level of coagulation factor can greatly influence bleeding risk. This assessment is based upon the findings with knockout mice that indicate that a true null of each of these proteins is associated with virtually 100% mortality from hemor-rhage before or at the time of birth. With hereditary factor deficiencies, heterozygous deficient individuals have approximately 50% (most commonly 30–60%) of the normal level of the affected factor. The symptoms of these disorders are quite variable (Table 38–6). Coagulation factor deficiencies may be suspected based on symptoms, family history, or abnormal screening tests and the laboratory confirms that diagnosis by specific factor assays. Once recognizing a specific protein deficiency, clinical grounds usually distinguish a congenital from an acquired defect (see below).

Differential Diagnosis of a Prolonged PTT and Normal PT

Factor XI

Factor XI deficiency is common in Ashkenazi Jews, in whom heterozygote frequency is 8% (Asakai, 1991). This ethnic population constitutes about 50% of the factor-XI-deficient patients seen in the United States. Most patients with factor XI deficiency rarely have spontaneous hemorrhages. Bleeding typically occurs following injury or surgery, particularly involving areas of the body with high fibrinolytic activity (mouth, nose, genitourinary tract) (Table 38–6). Women can experience menorrhagia and postpartum hemorrhage. Bleeding can occur in heterozygotes and does not necessarily correlate with the residual factor XI level (Leiba, 1965; Bolton-Maggs, 1988). However, the bleeding tendency may also be modified by additional defects such as hemophilia, von Willebrand's disease, and platelet function defects (Brenner, 1997). Diagnosis depends on the determination of factor XI activity below the reference range. Most

Table 38–5 Coagulation Factor Deficiencies

Factor	Gene Location	Normal Circulating Half-life	Incidence	Inheritance	Bleeding Severity
Fibrinogen	4q31.3–q32.1	2–4 days	1:1 million	Recessive	Mild–severe*
II	11p11.2	3–4 days	Very rare	Recessive	Mild–moderate
V	1q24.2	36 h	1:1 million	Recessive	Moderate
V and VIII combined	LMAN1:18q21.32 MCFD2:2p21	36 h for FV; 10–14 h for FVIII	1:2 million	Recessive	Mild–moderate
VII	13q34	3–6 h	1:500,000	Recessive	Mild–severe
VIII	Xq28	10–14 h	1:10,000	Sex-linked	Mild–severe
IX	Xq27	18–24 h	1:30,000	Sex-linked	Mild–severe
X	13q34	40–60 h	1:500,000	Recessive	Mild–severe
XI	4q35.2	40–70 h	Rare†	Recessive	Mild–moderate
XII	5q33-qter	50–70 days	Rare	Recessive	No bleeding
PK	4q33-q35	Not known	Very rare	Recessive	No bleeding
HK	3q27	9–10 h	Extremely rare	Recessive	No bleeding
XIII	A:6p25.1 B:1q31.3	11–14 days	<1:1 million	Recessive	Moderate–severe

* May be associated with thrombosis. † Rare except in those of Ashkenazi Jewish descent.

HK = high-molecular-weight kininogen; PK = prekallikrein.

Table 38–6 Clinical Manifestations of Coagulation Factor Deficiencies

Type of Bleeding	Coagulation Factor Deficiency
Easy bruising	FII, FVIII, FIX
Hematomas	FII, FVIII, FIX
Mucosal bleeding	FII, FVIII, FIX, FXI
Hemarthrosis	FVIII, FIX, FX
Postsurgical bleeding	Fibrinogen, FII, FV, FVII, FVIII, FIX, FX, FXI, FXIII
Intracranial bleeding	FVII, FVIII, FIX, FXIII
Delayed wound healing	Fibrinogen, FXIII
Umbilical cord bleeding	FX, FXIII
Miscarriage	Fibrinogen, FXIII
Thrombosis	Abnormal fibrinogens
Asymptomatic	FXII, prekallikrein, high M_r kininogen

widely used PTT reagents will have prolonged PTT results for patient samples with factor XI activity below 20–25% and mixed results when levels are 25–60%. The lower limit of the normal range is probably between 60% and 70% (Bolton-Maggs, 1995). Therefore, a normal PTT does not rule out a mild factor XI deficiency. In cases where there may be marked elevation of factor VIII, the PTT can be normalized even when other factors are reduced (Lawrie, 1998). In all patients with factor XI deficiency, preoperative management is critical to prevent bleeding complications. Patients with severe deficiency (factor XI <10–20%) should receive treatment with fresh frozen plasma to raise their factor XI levels. Usually, replacement therapy of 20 mL/kg loading dose with a maintenance dose of 5–10 mL/kg every 24 h is sufficient to cover patients with severe factor XI deficiency through elective surgery (Kessler, 1996). Patients with levels between 20–70% may bleed. A bleeding history and the nature of the proposed surgery will then guide the management. The development of inhibitors to factor XI in patients with factor XI deficiency has been described though these are rare (Salomon, 2003).

Factor XII, Prekallikrein and High-Molecular-Weight Kininogen

Factor XII deficiency, prekallikrein (PK), and high-molecular-weight kininogen (HK) deficiency are associated with a prolonged PTT, but are not associated with any bleeding risk. Factor XII deficiency is most common, occurring in all racial and ethnic backgrounds. It is associated with a very long PTT. Prekallikrein deficiency is less common, but seen in the United States in all ethnic groups. It is associated with a slightly prolonged PTT that corrects to normal when sitting on the bench for 1 h at 37°C. High-molecular-weight kininogen deficiency is a rare disorder. It too is associated with a very long PTT. These proteins are essential to have a normal PTT since in the PTT it is factor XII that autoactivates on the glass

tube surface or with the negatively charged particulate material in the PTT reagent that initiates the so-called cascade of proteolytic reactions that lead to *in vitro* thrombin formation as described above (Wiggins, 1979; Miller, 1980). Nevertheless, these protein deficiencies are *not* associated with bleeding – a point emphasized diagrammatically in Fig. 38–1 by the graying of this portion of the coagulation 'cascade'. Since no replacement therapy for hemostasis is necessary for factor XII, PK, or HK deficiencies, it is important to recognize these defects to prevent unnecessary transfusion. Furthermore, deficiencies of factor XII and HK have been associated with thrombosis risk. Although still experimental, data suggest that they contribute to the constitutive anticoagulant nature of the intravascular compartment (Ratnoff, 1968; Colman, 1992; Hasan, 2003; Zito, 2002). Factor XII and HK deficiencies give very long PTTs; prekallikrein deficiency gives a mildly prolonged PTT as indicated above. When a deficiency in the proteins of the kallikrein/kinin system is suspected, factor XII assays should be performed first since it is the most common.

Prolonged PTT and PT
Disorders of Fibrinogen

Fibrinogen (factor I) deficiencies may prolong the PT and PTT if the plasma concentration of the protein is sufficiently low, usually less than 100 mg/dL. Afibrinogenemia is autosomal recessive and represents the total absence of fibrinogen. It results in a bleeding disorder of variable severity (Fried, 1980; Lak, 1999). Umbilical stump and mucosal bleeding are most common, as well as an increased incidence of musculoskeletal and central nervous system bleeding. Patients also exhibit poor wound healing. Hypofibrinogenemia is a decreased level of normal fibrinogen and has a similar but milder pattern of bleeding. Both afibrinogenemia and hypofibrinogenemia are associated with recurrent miscarriage as well as antepartum and postpartum hemorrhage (Goodwin, 1989; Kobayashi, 2000). Paradoxically, there are reports of thrombotic events in patients with afibrinogenemia (Chafa, 1995; Lak, 1999; Dupuy, 2001).

Dysfibrinogenemia is a qualitative fibrinogen deficiency characterized by the production of a dysfunctional fibrinogen. Most patients with congenital dysfibrinogenemia are heterozygous, because of molecular defects in the produced protein, although rare homozygous cases have been reported. Dysfibrinogenemias are most commonly acquired in association with liver disease. The acquired dysfibrinogenemias are most commonly due to post-translational modifications of the fibrinogen protein as result of synthesis in an abnormal liver. In the clinical laboratory, both congenital and acquired homozygous cases have been reported. Dysfibrinogenemia patients are usually asymptomatic or have mild bleeding, but some cases have had thrombosis, with or without a bleeding history (Hanss, 2001). The thrombin time and reptilase time, which measure the clotting time during the conversion of fibrinogen into fibrin, are often prolonged in dysfibrinogenemia. When thrombin proteolyzes fibrinogen in the thrombin time, both fibrinopeptide A and B are released from the Aα and Bβ chains of fibrinogen. Reptilase clots fibrinogen by only liberating fibrinopeptide A (Funk, 1971). Proteolysis of fibrinopeptide A from fibrinogen is sufficient to induce clot formation. Fibrinopeptide B liberation increases the rate of association of the fibrin monomers but not the actual physiologic clot (Martinelli, 1980; Nawarawong, 1991). Bleeding risk is only associated with fibrinopeptide A release defects, not fibrinopeptide B release defects. Therefore, a patient can have a long PT and PTT from a fibrinopeptide B release defect and not have any bleeding risk. Hence the reason for using both the thrombin time and reptilase time to assess dysfibrinogenemias. Assays that measure clottable fibrinogen will show lower levels than assays that measure fibrinogen antigen. The ratio of clottable fibrinogen activity to fibrinogen antigen should be greater than 95%. Ratios less than that suggest a dysfibrinogenemia. Cryoprecipitate is a good source of fibrinogen when replacement is needed. Antifibrinolytic agents may reduce the bleeding associated with certain procedures such as dental extraction but should be avoided in those individuals at risk for or with a personal or family history of venous thrombosis.

Factor II Deficiency

Prothrombin deficiency may be the rarest inherited coagulation factor deficiency (1:2 000 000) (Bolton-Maggs, 2004). A true prothrombin deficiency in the mouse is incompatible with life after birth. Hypo-prothrombinemia (type I deficiency) manifests as a concomitant reduction in prothrombin activity and antigen levels. Bleeding symptoms include mucosal bleeding, hematomas and hemarthrosis. Dysprothrombinemia (type II deficiency) presents with reduced activity and normal antigen levels. The clinical presentation of dysprothrombinemia is less predictable and patients may be asymptomatic or have only mild bleeding manifestations (Bolton-Maggs, 2004). Depending on the sensitivity of the reagents, both the PT and PTT may be prolonged in prothrombin deficiency. However, a specific factor II assay is best if there is clinical suspicion or a positive family history in the presence of normal screening tests. A PT reagent-based prothrombin assay with factor-deficient plasma is most convenient. Prothrombin complex concentrates are the treatment of choice although fresh frozen plasma can serve as an alternative source of prothrombin.

Factor V Deficiency

Heterozygous factor V deficiency is asymptomatic. Homozygous factor V deficiency is rare (1:1 000 000), presenting in children with easy bruising and mucosal bleeding (Girolami, 1998; Lak, 1999). These individuals must have some functional factor V because 50% of true null mice die at the time of the development of the cardiovascular system (days 9–11) and the other half die at birth from hemorrhage (Cui, 1996). Hematomas and hemarthrosis may occur with injury but rarely spontaneously. It is associated with prolongation of both PTT and PT (but a normal thrombin time) and confirmed by a prothrombin time reagent-based, single-stage factor V assay. Patients with factor V deficiency should also have a factor VIII assay performed to evaluate for combined deficiency of factors V and VIII (Nichols, 1998; Zhang, 2004). The only suitable replacement product available is fresh frozen plasma. The replacement goal should be to elevate the factor V level to at least 15% (Peyvandi, 1999).

Factor X Deficiency

Heterozygous factor X deficiency is asymptomatic. Homozygous factor X deficiency is a severe bleeding disorder presenting in infancy. Symptoms include umbilical cord bleeding, mucosal bleeding, severe soft-tissue hematomas, and hemarthroses (Peyvandi, 1998a). One-stage PT-based factor X assays are sufficient for diagnosis, although additional assays are commercially available. Like all the vitamin-K-dependent clotting factors, it is important to exclude vitamin K deficiency or other acquired cause for the factor X deficiency before a diagnosis of an inherited deficiency is made. For example, factor X deficiency is the commonest factor deficiency associated with primary amyloidosis, occurring in 8.7% of patients (Uprichard, 2002) and probably due to adsorption of factor X on to amyloid fibrils. Current therapy for factor X deficiency includes prothrombin complex concentrates although recombinant VIIa has been used successfully to treat factor X deficiency associated with amyloidosis (Boggio, 2001).

Combined Deficiency of Factor V and Factor VIII

Combined factor V and factor VIII deficiency is a rare autosomal recessive disorder and results from a single gene defect rather than co-inheritance of defects in both factor V and factor VIII genes. Patients typically have factor V and factor VIII levels between 5% and 30%. In two thirds of patients this results from null expression of LMAN1 (previously known as ERGIC-53 (Nichols, 1998). LMAN1 shuttles between the endoplasmic reticulum and the Golgi and is believed to facilitate protein trafficking through the secretion pathway (Zhang, 2003). Others of the patients have a mutation of MCFD2, which directly interacts with LMAN1 (Zhang, 2003). Bleeding manifestations include epistaxis, easy bruising, menorrhagia and postpartum hemorrhage as well as bleeding following surgery, dental extractions, and trauma (Seligsohn, 1982; Peyvandi, 1998b) (Table 38–6). Testing usually demonstrates a disproportionate prolongation of the PTT compared to the PT. Replacement therapy includes both factor VIII concentrates and fresh frozen plasma (as a source of factor V).

Combined Deficiency of Vitamin-K-Dependent Clotting Factors

Combined deficiency of the vitamin-K-dependent clotting factors (factors II, VII, IX and X; VKCFD) occurs with vitamin K deficiency and hepatic dysfunction but it also results from heritable dysfunction of hepatic enzyme γ-glutamyl carboxylase (type I) or the vitamin K epoxide reductase enzyme complex (type II) (Brenner, 1998; Zhang, 2004; see also Ch. 41). Severely affected individuals may present as neonates with umbilical stump bleeding or spontaneous intracranial hemorrhage; in infancy or early childhood with hemarthroses, soft tissue hematomas or gastrointestinal hemorrhages; in adults with easy bruising, mucosal bleeding and bleeding following surgery (Table 38–6). Diagnosis is established by prolongation of both the PTT and PT and associated reductions in levels of the vitamin-K-dependent clotting factors. These patients may respond to vitamin K (oral or parenteral) with normalization of the PTT, PT and factor levels as well as resolution of bleeding symptoms. This fact makes the establishment of a diagnosis of an inherited abnormality difficult, since other acquired causes of vitamin K deficiency (hemorrhagic disease of the newborn, liver disease, and prolonged use of broad-spectrum antibiotics) or factitious warfarin administration could present similarly. For patients that do not respond fully to vitamin K administration, fresh frozen plasma can be used for acute bleeding or surgery.

Normal PTT and Prolonged PT

Factor VII Deficiency

Factor VII deficiency is common compared with the other rare hereditary coagulation factor deficiencies. The bleeding manifestations are quite variable, with epistaxis, mucosal bleeding and menorrhagia commonly reported (Peyvandi, 1997) (Table 38–6). Severe FVII deficiency is autosomal recessive, often presenting shortly after birth, and may have dramatic presentation with intracranial hemorrhage in 15–60% of cases (Ragni, 1981). The diagnosis is suspected with the finding of an isolated prolongation of the PT. However, factor VII, a vitamin-K-dependent clotting factor, is low in the newborn period and will also be low in the presence of vitamin K deficiency. Therefore, re-evaluation of infants with mild deficiencies is required after they reach a few months of age or after vitamin K replacement in older patients. Functional factor VII activity is measured by a PT-based, factor-VII-deficient plasma clotting assay. The use of recombinant human thromboplastin will yield results that are more likely to reflect *in vivo* factor VII levels. Samples for factor VII testing should also not be stored at 4°C as this can lead to cold activation of factor VII as result of C1 inhibitor inactivation and factor XIIa formation in the tube with factor VII activation (Kitchen, 1992). Cold activation of factor VII results in an overestimation of the actual plasma factor VII level. Therapeutic options include fresh frozen plasma, prothrombin complex concentrates and recombinant factor VIIa. For major surgery, plasma factor VII levels of at least 20% are sufficient (Bolton-Maggs, 2004).

Although factor VII deficiency is the classic example of an entity that will give a prolonged PT and a normal PTT, in certain instances, especially when recombinant human thromboplastin is used, mild defects in the common pathway proteins may present as only slight PT abnormalities. Mostly commonly, the defects will be dysfibrinogenemias, but mild deficiencies or inhibitors to factors X, V, and II may first present as slight PT-only defects.

Additionally, a prolonged PT but normal PTT may sometimes occur when there is a deficiency of a common pathway factor such as X, V, or II in conjunction with a marked elevation in the level of factor VIII. In this situation, the high factor VIII level may be capable of normalizing a PTT value that would otherwise have been increased due to the factor deficiency, but factor VIII of course would exert no comparable effect upon the PT.

Normal PTT and PT

Factor XIII deficiency

Factor XIII stabilizes the clot after a fibrin clot has formed. Therefore, the PT and PTT will be normal even with a severe factor XIII deficiency. Testing for factor XIII deficiency is suggested for individuals with a positive bleeding history, particularly with features such as delayed bleeding, umbilical stump bleeding or miscarriages, in which the PT and PTT are normal (Anwar, 1999) (Table 38–6). 30% of severely deficient factor-XIII-deficient patients die in middle age from spontaneous intracerebral hemorrhage unless they are receiving prophylactic therapy (Lorand, 1980). The diagnosis of severe factor XIII deficiency (<5% activity) can be confirmed with the 5 M urea clot stability test or a chromogenic assay. Clots formed with normal factor XIII activity remain stable in 5 M urea, while clots from factor-XIII-deficient patients dissolve in urea. The reason for this is that factor XIIIa initiates the formation of a new intermolecular γ-glutamyl-ε-lysine bridge between fibrin molecules (Lorand, 1980). This new interaction augments the mechanical rigidity of the clot structure and increases its resistance to lysis. Quantitative activity assays are available based on cross-linking of glycine-ethyl ester into a specific peptide (Fickenscher, 1991) or on incorporation of an amine substrate into fibrinogen (Kohler, 1998). Both assays employ thrombin activation of factor XIII. Acquired deficiency of factor XIII has been described in a variety of diseases, including Henoch–Schönlein purpura, isoniazid treatment for tuberculosis, various forms of colitis, erosive gastritis and some forms of leukemia (Board, 1993) although factor XIII level determination and therapeutic management is controversial. Since the half-life of factor XIII is very long, replacement with fresh frozen plasma is usually sufficient for most patients. Factor XIII concentrates and recombinant factor XIII are currently being evaluated in clinical trials.

Hereditary Hemorrhagic Disorders of Fibrinolysis

Hereditary bleeding disorders resulting from excessive fibrinolysis are rare. A deficiency of α_2-antiplasmin has been reported in a few families with a bleeding tendency (Fay, 1992; Aoki, 1980). While not recommended for routine use as a screening assay, the whole blood clot lysis time can be helpful as a first order test to detect deficiencies of α_2-antiplasmin. In brief, whole blood is allowed to clot, following which the time to clot lysis is recorded. In normal individuals, the presence of α_2-antiplasmin effectively prevents lysis from occurring in this *in vitro* setting even 24 h after initial clot formation. In contrast, in the presence of a severe deficiency of α_2-antiplasmin or in some fibrinolytic states, clot lysis can be observed after several hours. In such instances, follow-up testing specific for α_2-antiplasmin activity should be employed. Acquired α_2-antiplasmin deficiency commonly occurs in acute leukemia (Okajima, 1994; Schwartz, 1986). Plasma can also be admixed with dilute acid to precipitate a fraction relatively rich in plasminogen activator, plasminogen, and fibrinogen but relatively poor in antiplasmins. This 'euglobulin' fraction can subsequently be redissolved in buffer and clotted by recalcification, and the time for clot lysis then measured. Such *euglobulin clot lysis* is normally complete in 2–4 h but may be shortened with increased fibrinolysis, particularly in association with increased plasminogen activator activity. Plasminogen activator, plasminogen activator inhibitor, and plasminogen may of course also be quantitated individually.

Acquired Coagulation Protein Deficiencies

Acquired bleeding disorders are due to anticoagulation, disseminated intravascular coagulation, liver disease, vitamin K deficiency, massive transfusion, and unique inhibitors to coagulations proteins. The topic of anticoagulation has been examined in Chapter 41 and will not be discussed presently. In general, the appearance of a prolonged PT and PTT in a patient should first have the differential diagnosis, as discussed in the following section, of anticoagulants, DIC, liver disease, vitamin K deficiency, and massive transfusion. Only after these clinical states are excluded should the pathologist think of specific protein defects influencing the PT and PTT.

Disseminated Intravascular Coagulation

DIC is a clinicopathologic condition in which there is activation of the coagulation and fibrinolysis systems resulting in the simultaneous formation of thrombin and plasmin with consumption of coagulation factors and inhibitors of the system resulting in the clinical laboratory phenotype of a prolonged PT, PTT and thrombocytopenia. It arises in patients due to sepsis, malignancy, obstetrical complications, or massive tissue injury (Schmaier, 1991). DIC can arise during surgery as result of the release of thromboplastic material in the tissue. In circulatory arrest operations on the arch of the aorta or main pulmonary arteries, DIC is a frequent complication due to the chilling of the patient and tissue destruction. Abruptio placentae and placenta previa are associated with acute hemorrhagic DIC whereas retained dead fetus is associated with a

DIC that is not hemorrhagic but prothrombotic. DIC due to sepsis can also occur in the postoperative period. DIC with sepsis is most commonly seen with Gram-negative infections but can occur with Gram-positive infections and in the immunosuppressed patient with fungemia. The balance between thrombin and plasmin formation in the individual patient clinically translates into a prothrombotic versus hemorrhagic state, respectively.

The diagnosis of DIC depends on the appropriate clinical test results in the correct clinical setting. Finding a prolonged PT and PTT with a reduced fibrinogen and platelet count is usually DIC in the hospitalized patient until proven otherwise (Colman, 1972). This clinical laboratory phenotype of DIC most probably results from a hyperfibrinolytic state and is the form of DIC most commonly recognized. A prothrombotic state as the result of DIC is usually associated with a normal PT and PTT with a mildly reduced platelet count and normal or elevated fibrinogen. The diagnosis of DIC is made by the presence of a confirmatory test that shows the simultaneous presence of thrombin and plasmin formation. Currently, the D-Dimer assay is the confirmatory test that, if positive, shows that both thrombin and plasmin have been formed. The D-Dimer measures plasmin-cleaved, insoluble, cross-linked fibrin that originally arose from thrombin cleavage of fibrinogen (Figs 38–3 and 38–5B). D-Dimer assays are characteristic for DIC, but not pathognomonic. D-Dimer assays can be positive in individuals with resolving large vessel thrombosis and soft tissue hematomas. In the past, fibrin degradation (split) products (FDP) were used to recognize DIC (Fig. 38–5A). However, FDPs only indicate plasmin-cleaved fibrinogen, soluble fibrin, or insoluble fibrin. Their presence does not indicate plasmin-cleaved, insoluble, cross-linked fibrin. Fibrin monomer is the large molecular mass protein of fibrinogen that remains after fibrinopeptide A and B are liberated. It can be elevated in DIC but if the DIC is severe it can be absent. Thus, it is an unreliable assay to recognize DIC.

Liver Disease

It is important that liver disease is recognized in patients since, as discussed in Chapter 19, most coagulation factors are synthesized there. Thus, these patients have increased risk of bleeding. Patients with serious liver disease will have prolonged PT and PTT. Not only is the synthesis of these proteins reduced but those proteins made are at times abnormal, functioning as inhibitors of normal coagulation proteins. For example abnormal fibrinogens (dysfibrinogenemias) are very common in patients with liver disease. As already mentioned, if these proteins have defects in fibrinopeptide A or B release, the thrombin time will be abnormal; the reptilase time is abnormal in only fibrinopeptide A release defects. Overall, abnormal fibrinogens can be appreciated by an abnormal ratio of clottable fibrinogen (an activity measure) to fibrinogen antigen (measured by radial immunodiffusion or another immunoassay). Finding less activity in relation to the mass of the protein is characteristic of an abnormal molecule. Similarly, all the vitamin-K-dependent proteins (factors II, VII, IX, and X, proteins C, S, and Z) decrease in liver disease. These proteins may have abnormal γ-carboxylation reactions of the glutamic acid residues on the amino terminal portion of their protein, thus producing reduced factor activity, with relatively higher levels of that factor's antigen (see next section). In general, prekallikrein is one of the first proteins to be decreased in liver disease; fibrinogen is one of the last proteins to be decreased in liver disease. Factors VIII and V become absent in the anhepatic stage of liver transplantation but factor VIII is elevated in patients with inflammatory hepatocellular disease. Moreover, antithrombin and other serpin plasma protein inhibitors also decrease in liver disease. Thus these patients have reduced procoagulants and anticoagulants, adjusting the baseline for hemostasis at another level than that seen in normals.

Vitamin K Deficiency

Vitamin K, a lipid-soluble vitamin, is provided by dietary intake of leafy green vegetables and by synthesis of intestinal flora. In clinical medicine, vitamin K deficiency is mostly seen in the very ill patient on antibiotics who has subsisted on parenteral nutrition. Not infrequently, IV fluids are not supplemented with vitamin K. After 4–6 weeks of parenteral nutrition and antibiotic treatment, the patient becomes vitamin-K-deficient. Vitamin K deficiency can also be seen in patients who have anatomic bypass of the small intestine, malabsorption, biliary tract obstruction, and, rarely, reduced dietary intake. For example, alcoholics are often vitamin-K-deficient. Warfarin also inhibits the enzymatic pathway necessary for vitamin K utilization (see Fig. 41–1 in Ch. 41). Vitamin K has a critical role in the γ-carboxylation reaction of glutamic acid residues, γ-carboxyglutamic acid, of the so-called vitamin-K-dependent coagulation proteins, factors II, VII, IX, and X and proteins C, S, and Z. This reaction on certain amino acids on the amino terminus of these proteins is critical for these proteins to bind to cells and phospholipids so that they can participate in physiologic coagulation reactions. Thus these patients will have reduced clottable factor levels for the vitamin-K-dependent factors II, VII, IX, and X. If antigen levels of these patients are measured, they will be higher. In general, patients with a therapeutic level of warfarin (i.e., an INR between 2–3), have ~5–15% of clottable activity whereas their antigen levels measure 25–40%. As explained in Chapter 41, the international normalization ratio (INR) is a convention that the coagulation community has adopted to be able to interpret prothrombin times of patients on warfarin anticoagulation. Since there are many commercially available coagulation reagents and equipment to perform these assays, the INR was developed (Loeliger, 1985). The INR is the ratio of the (patient's PT/mean value of normal PT for the institution)^{ISI}. The ISI value for a reagent is a measure of the responsiveness of a given thromboplastin to reduction of the vitamin-K-dependent coagulation factors. It is provided by each manufacturer based upon the degree of variation of the thromboplastin from the World Health Organization (WHO) reference thromboplastin that has an assigned value of 1, as determined by the logarithm of a PT per second determined with the WHO standard (z) and x the logarithm of PT in seconds determined with the test preparation according to the equation $z = a_1 + b_1x$ (see Pollar, 1991 to determine the meaning of a_1 and b_1). If recombinant human thromboplastin is used, the ISI value is about 1. The higher the ISI value, the less sensitive the thromboplastin. Vitamin K usually is replaced by oral therapy. However, if necessary, parenteral replacement can be performed. IM versus IV is the preferred, safe route of administration.

Massive Transfusion

Massive transfusion has been defined as the replacement of more than 1.5 blood volume in 24 h. For example, in the 70 kg man, 7% of body weight or 4.9 kg or liters is the blood volume (~10 units). Hemostatic failure can result from dilution of clotting factors, DIC or acquired platelet dysfunction. Dilutional coagulopathy results from replacement with packed red blood cells and normal saline and a lack of clotting factors or platelets. Tests of hemostasis typically show prolongation of the PT and PTT, reduced fibrinogen and thrombocytopenia (Leslie, 1991).

In the past, attempts to avoid this problem by linking 1 unit of fresh frozen plasma to every 4–6 units of red blood cell transfusion were made. However, this strategy does not always correct all the hemostatic defects and may waste blood resources. It is important to remember that with 1.5 blood volume transfusion there is 10% anticoagulant that has been given to the patient. In a 70 kg person, the circulating amount of anticoagulant can be 735 mL. Some form of calcium infusion is useful to neutralize the circulating citrate anticoagulant. Current recommendations suggest that fresh frozen plasma and platelets should not be used prophylactically in massively transfused patients. However, bleeding associated with PT and PTT prolongation more than 1.5 times the laboratory mean should first prompt transfusion with cryoprecipitate to increase fibrinogen levels to more than 80–100 mg/dL. If bleeding persists, fresh frozen plasma transfusion is warranted, or platelet transfusion if there is significant thrombocytopenia.

Acquired Coagulation Protein Inhibitors

Acquired inhibitors to coagulation proteins occur and, in some cases, increase the risk of bleeding. The clinical laboratory phenotype of these patients depends upon the protein that the coagulation protein inhibitor is directed towards. The most common severe acquired coagulation protein inhibitor is that against factor VIII. These patients present with bleeding and a long PTT. Characteristically, one sees this inhibitor in elderly patients, patients with B-cell malignancies, patients with connective tissue disorders such as systemic lupus erythematosus, and post-partum. These patients are managed acutely with replacement therapy (high-dose factor VIII, activated vitamin-K-dependent coagulation factor concentrates, or rVIIa), but in the long term the management is immunosuppression with Cytoxan, prednisone, or rituximab (Lian, 1989; Aggarwal, 2005). Management decisions in these patients are influenced by the severity of bleeding and the height of the titer of the inhibitor to factor VIII as determined by the Bethesda assay.

Acquired deficiencies or inhibitors are also seen in a number of medical conditions. Systemic amyloidosis is associated with decreases in plasma factor X or IX as a result of adsorption of the coagulation proteins on to the amyloid protein (McPherson, 1977; Furie, 1981; Mumford, 2000). In the former the PT and PTT may be affected; in the latter, only the PTT. Hypergammaglobulinemic states seen with multiple myeloma or Waldenström's macroglobulinemia (immunoglobulin M) can be associated with pan-inhibitors to coagulation protein function (Glaspy, 1992). Dysfibrinogenemias are also common in these patients. These phenomena are recognized by performing specific factor assays against the one or more proteins affected at multiple dilutions of the patient plasma. In general, as the factor assay is performed at lower dilutions, e.g., 50%, 25%, and 10% of normal plasma, the degree of inhibition of the coagulation factor reduces, suggesting that, as one dilutes the plasma, the effect of the inhibitor is lost.

The last kind of inhibitor seen is the lupus anticoagulant or anti-phospholipid antibody that influences coagulation protein reactions. These inhibitors are dealt with in greater detail in Chapter 40. Briefly, these inhibitors are antibodies directed to epitopes of proteins bound to phospholipids. The antibodies are really to proteins and the influencing phospholipids can be acidic (phosphatidylserine, phosphatidylcholine) or neutral (phosphatidylethanolamine) (Lafer, 1981; Levine, 2002). Lupus anticoagulants variably interfere with the PTT and PT The degree of interference depends upon the nature of the commercial reagent. Characteristically, a lupus anticoagulant will have a greater effect on a coagulation assay, as the reagents in the assay are diluted out. For example, the degree of prolongation of a PT or PTT in a plasma sample will be greater at 1:50 dilution and 1:500 dilution of the assay reagent in a patient with a lupus anticoagulant than in a patient with a specific inhibitor to a coagulation protein. In the latter case, the inhibitor level will change only when one dilutes the patient plasma, not the reagent for the assay. Specific criteria have been developed to recognize lupus anticoagulants (Brandt, 1995a; Levine, 2002). In general assays that have some dilution of the coagulation reagent (dilute PT or tissue thromboplastin inhibition assay, dilute PTT, dilute Russell viper venom time (DRVVT), or kaolin clotting time) are useful but not specifically diagnostic assays for the condition (Levine, 2002). Paradoxically, these patients are not at a bleeding risk; rather they are at a thrombosis risk that at times can be a vicious prothrombotic state (Mueh, 1980, Rand, 2003). Antiphospholipid antibodies interfere with several anticoagulation mechanisms such as annexin V, thus enhancing prothrombinase on endothelial cells and prostacyclin production from endothelial cells. This topic is further discussed in Chapter 40.

V

References

Abshire T, Kenet G: Recombinant factor VIIa: review of efficacy, dosing regimens and safety in patients with congenital and acquired factor VIII or IX inhibitors. J Thromb Haemost 2004; 2:899–909.

Adcock DM, Kressin DC, Marlar RA: Effect of 3.2% vs 3.8% sodium citrate concentration on routine coagulation testing. Am J Clin Pathol 1997; 107:105–110.

Important paper that justifies the use of 3.2 g% sodium citrate as the anticoagulation standard for collection of samples for clinical coagulation testing

Adcock DM, Kressin DC, Marlar RA: Minimum specimen volume requirements for routine coagulation testing; dependence on citrate concentration. Am J Clin Pathol 1998; 109:595–599.

Aggarwal A, Grewal R, Green RJ, et al: Rituximab for autoimmune haemophilia: a proposed treatment algorithm. Haemophilia 2005; 11: 13–19.

Ahmad SS, Scandura JM, Walsh PN: Structural and functional characterization of platelet receptor-mediated factor VIII binding. J Biol Chem 2000; 275:13071–13081.

Andrew M, Vegh P, Johnston M, et al: Maturation of the hemostatic system during childhood. Blood 1992; 80:1998–2005.

Anwar R, Miloszewski KJ: Factor XIII deficiency. Br J Haematol 1999; 107:468–484.

Aoki N, Sakata Y, Matsuda M, Tateno K: Fibrinolytic states in a patient with congenital deficiency of alpha 2-plasmin inhibitor. Blood 1980; 55:483–488.

Arun B, Kessler CM: Clinical manifestations and therapy of the hemophilias. *In* Colman RW, Hirsh J, Marder VJ, et al (eds): Hemostasis and Thrombosis: Basic Principles and Clinical Practice,

4th edition. Philadelphia, PA, Lippincott-Raven, 2001.

Asakai R, Chung DW, Davie EW, Seligsohn U: Factor XI deficiency in Ashkenazi Jews in Israel. N Engl J Med 1991; 325:153–158.

Barnathan ES, Kuo A, van der Keyl H, et al: Binding of tissue type plasminogen activator to human endothelial cells: evidence for two distinct binding sites. J Biol Chem 1988; 263:7792–7799.

Board PG, Losowsky MS, Miloszewski KJ: Factor XIII: inherited and acquired deficiency. Blood Rev 1993; 7:229–242.

Boggio L, Green D: Recombinant human factor VIIa in the management of amyloid-associated factor X deficiency. Br J Haematol 2001; 112:1074–1075.

Bolton-Maggs PH, Young Wan-Yin B, McCraw AH, et al: Inheritance and bleeding in factor XI deficiency. Br J Haematol 1988; 69:521–528.

Bolton-Maggs PH, Patterson DA, Wensley RT, Tuddenham EG: Definition of the bleeding tendency in factor XI-deficient kindreds – a clinical and laboratory study. Thromb Haemost 1995; 73:194–202.

Bolton-Maggs PH, Perry DJ, Chalmers EA, et al: The rare coagulation disorders – review with guidelines for management from the United Kingdom Haemophilia Centre Doctors' Organisation. Haemophilia 2004; 10:593–628.

Brandt JT, Triplett DA, Alving B, Scharrer I: Criteria for the diagnosis of lupus anticoagulant: an update. Thromb Haemost 1995a; 74: 1185–1190.

Important paper that begins to define criteria for making a diagnosis of a lupus anticoagulant.

Brandt JT, Barna LK, Triplett DA. Laboratory identification of lupus anticoagulants: results of the secondary international workshop for identification of lupus anticoagulants. Thromb Haemost 1995b; 74:1597–1603.

Brenner B, Laor A, Lupo H, et al: Bleeding predictors in factor-XI-deficient patients. Blood Coagul Fibrinolysis 1997; 8:511–515.

Brenner B, Sanchez-Vega B, Wu SM, et al: A missense mutation in gamma-glutamyl carboxylase gene causes combined deficiency of all vitamin K-dependent blood coagulation factors. Blood 1998; 92:4554–4559.

Broze GJ Jr: The rediscovery and isolation of TFPI. J Thromb Haemost 2003; 1:1671–1675.

Cesarman GM, Guevara CA, Hajjar KA: An endothelial cell receptor for plasminogen/tissue plasminogen activator (t-PA). II. Annexin II-mediated enhancement of t-PA-dependent plasminogen activation. J Biol Chem 1994; 269:21198–21203.

Chafa O, Chellali T, Sternberg C, et al: Severe hypofibrinogenemia associated with bilateral ischemic necrosis of toes and fingers. Blood Coagul Fibrinolysis 1995; 6:549–552.

Chang SH, Tillema V, Scherr D: A percent correction formula for evaluation of mixing studies. Am J Clin Pathol 2002; 117:62–73.

An important paper that begins to provide some evidence-based laboratory medicine on how screening mixing studies should be performed.

Colman RW, Robboy SJ, Minna JD: Disseminated intravascular coagulation (DIC): an approach. Am J Med 1972; 52:679–689.

Colman RW, Bagdasarian A, Talarnos RC, et al: Williams trait. Human kininogen deficiency with diminished levels of plasminogen proactivator and prekallikrein associated with abnormalities of the Hageman factor-dependent pathways. J Clin Invest 1975; 56: 1650–1662.

Colman RW: Contributions of Mayme Williams to the elucidation of the multiple functions of plasma kininogens. Thromb Haemost 1992; 68:99–101.

Crossley M, Ludwi M, Stowell KM, et al: Recovery from hemophilia B Leyden: an androgen-responsive element in the factor IX promoter. Science 1992; 257:377–379.

Cui J, O'Shea KS, Purkayastha A, et al: Fatal haemorrhage and incomplete block to embryogenesis in mice lacking coagulation factor V. Nature 1996; 384:66–68.

Doolittle RF: Fibrinogen and fibrin. Sci Am 1981; 245:126–135.

Dupuy E, Soria C, Molho P, et al: Embolized ischemic lesions of toes in an afibrinogenemic patient: possible relevance to in vivo circulating thrombin. Thromb Res 2001; 102:211–219.

Esmon CT, Owen WG: Identification of an endothelial cell cofactor for thrombin-catalytic activation of protein C. Proc Natl Acad Sci USA 1981; 78:2249–2252.

Fay WP, Shapiro AD, Shih JL, et al: Brief report: complete deficiency of plasminogen-activator inhibitor type 1 due to a frame-shift mutation. N Engl J Med 1992; 327:1729–1733.

Fickenscher K, Aab A, Stuber W: A photometric assay for blood coagulation factor XIII. Thromb Haemost 1991; 65:535–540.

Fishman DJ, Jones PK, Menitove JE, et al: Detection of the carrier state for classic hemophilia using an enzyme-linked immunosorbent assay (ELISA). Blood 1982; 59:1163–1168.

Fried K, Kaufman S: Congenital afibrinogenemia in 10 offspring of uncle–niece marriages. Clin Genet 1980; 17:223–227.

Funk C, Gmür J, Herold R, Straub PW. Reptilase®-R – A new reagent in blood coagulation. Br J Haematol 1971; 21:43–52.

Furie B, Voo L, McAdam KP, *et al*. Mechanism of factor X deficiency in systemic amyloidosis. N Engl J Med 1981; 304:827–830.

Gailiani D, Broze G: Factor XI activation in a revised model of blood coagulation. Science 1991; 253:909–912.

Classic paper that presents for the first time the modern view of assembly and interaction of the proteins of the coagulation system.

Girolami A, Simioni P, Scarano L, et al: Hemorrhagic and thrombotic disorders due to factor V deficiencies and abnormalities: an updated classification. Blood Rev 1998; 12:5–51.

Glaspy JA: Hemostatic abnormalities in multiple myeloma and related disorders. Hematol Oncol Clin North Am 1992; 6:1301–1314.

Goodwin TM: Congenital hypofibrinogenemia in pregnancy. Obstet Gynecol Surv 1989; 44: 157–161.

Graham JB: Genotype assignment (carrier detection) in the haemophilias. Clin Haematol 1979; 8:115–145.

Graham JB, Rizza CR, Chediak J, *et al*: Carrier detection in hemophilia A: a cooperative international study. I. The carrier phenotype. Blood 1986; 67:1554–1559.

Green PP, Mannucci PM, Briet E, *et al*: Carrier detection in hemophilia A: a cooperative international study. II. The efficacy of a universal discriminant. Blood 1986; 67: 1560–1567.

Han ED, MacFarlane RC, Mulligan AN, *et al*: Increased vascular permeability in C1 inhibitor-deficient mice mediated by the bradykinin type 2 receptor. J Clin Invest 2002; 109:1057–1063.

Hanss M, Biot F: A database for human fibrinogen variants. Ann N Y Acad Sci 2001; 936:89–90.

Hasan AAK, Warnock M, Nieman M, et al: The mechanisms of Arg-Pro-Pro-Gly-Phe inhibition of thrombin. Am J Physiol Heart Circ Physiol 2003; 285:H183–H193.

He L, Pappan LK, Grenache DG, et al: The contributions of the alpha 2 beta 1 integrin to vascular thrombosis in vivo. Blood 2003; 102:3652–3657.

Hong SL: Effect of bradykinin and thrombin on prostacyclin synthesis in endothelial cells from calf and pig aorta and human umbilical cord vein. Thromb Res 1980; 18:787–795.

Kasper CK, Aledort L, Counts RB, et al: A more uniform measurement of factor VIII inhibitors. Thromb Diathes Haemorrh 1975; 34:869–872.

Kaufman RJ, Antonarakis SE, Fay PJ: Factor VIII and hemophilia A. In Colman RW, Hirsh J, Marder VJ, et al (eds): Hemostasis and Thrombosis, 4th Edition. Lippincott Williams & Wilkins, Philadelphia, PA, 2001, pp 135–156.

Kessler CM, Hoyer L, Feinstein DI: The hemophilias. In. McArthur JR, Schechter GP (eds): Hematology. The Educational Program of the American Society of Hematology. Washington, DC, American Society of Hematology, 1996, pp 95–105.

Kitchen S, Malia RG, Preston FE: A comparison of methods for the measurement of activated factor VII. Thromb Haemost 1992; 68: 301–305.

Kobayashi T, Kanayama N, Tokunaga N, et al: Prenatal and peripartum management of congenital afibrinogenaemia. Br J Haematol 2000; 109:364–366.

Kohler HP, Ariens RA, Whitaker P, Grant PJ: A common coding polymorphism in the FXIII A-subunit gene (FXIIIVal34Leu) affects cross-linking activity. Thromb Haemost 1998; 80:704.

Lafer EM, Rauch J, Andrzejewski C Jr, Mudd D, Furie B, Furie B, et al: Polyspecific monoclonal lupus autoantibodies reactive with both polynucleotides and phospholipids. J Exp Med 1981; 153:897–909.

Lak M, Keihani M, Elahi F, et al: Bleeding and thrombosis in 55 patients with inherited afibrinogenaemia. Br J Haematol 1999; 107:204–206.

Lakich D, Kazazian H, Antonarakis SE, Gitschier J. Inversion disrupting the factor VIII gene are a common cause of severe hemophilia A. Nat Gen 1993; 5:236–241.

Lawrie AS, Kitchen S, Purdy G, et al: Assessment of Actin FS and Actin FSL sensitivity to specific clotting factor deficiencies. Clin Lab Haematol 1998; 20:179–186.

Leiba H, Ramot B, Many A: Heredity and coagulation studies in ten families with Factor XI (plasma thromboplastin antecedent) deficiency. Br J Haematol 1965; 11:654–665.

Leslie SD, Toy PT. Laboratory hemostatic abnormalities in massively transfused patients given red blood cells and crystalloid. Am J Clin Pathol 1991; 96:770–773.

Levine JS, Branch W, Rauch J: The antiphospholipid syndrome. N Engl J Med 2002; 346:752–763.

Important paper that presents criteria for diagnosis of lupus anticoagulants and antiphospholipid antibody syndrome.

Lian EC, Larcada AF, Chiu A Y-Z : Combination immunosuppressive therapy after factor VIII infusion for acquired factor VIII inhibitor. Ann Intern Med 1989; 110:774–778.

Loeliger EA: ICSH/ICTH recommendation for reporting prothrombin time in oral anticoagulation control. Thromb Haemost 1985; 53:155–156.

Lorand L, Losowsky MS, Miloszewski KJM: Human factor XIII: fibrin-stabilizing factor. In: Spaet TH (ed): Progress in Hemostasis and Thrombosis, 1980; 5:245–29.

Ljung RCR: Prenatal diagnosis of haemophila. Haemophilia 1999; 5:84–87.

MacFarland, D: An enzyme cascade in the blood clotting mechanism, and its functions as a biochemical amplifier. Nature 1964; 202: 498–499.

McPherson RA, Onstad JW, Ugoretz RJ et al. Coagulopathy in amyloidosis: combined deficiency of factors IX and X. Am J Hematol 1977; 3:225–235.

Mahdi F, Van Nostrand, WE, Schmaier AH. Protease nexin-2/amyloid β-protein precursor inhibits factor Xa in the prothrombinase complex. J Biol Chem 1995; 270:23468–23474.

Mahdi F, Rehemtulla A, Van Nostrand WE, et al. Protease nexin-2/amyloid β-protein precursor regulates factor VIIa and the factor VIIa–tissue factor complex. Thrombosis Res 2000; 99: 267–276.

Mahdi F, Shariat-Madar Z, Schmaier AH: The relative priority of prekallikrein and factors XI/XIa assembly on cultured endothelial cells. J Biol Chem 2003; 278:43983–43990.

Mann KG. Thrombin formation. Chest 2003; 124:4S–10S.

Mannucci PM, Duga S, Peyvandi F: Recessively inherited coagulation disorders. Blood 2004; 104:1243–1252.

Marcum JA, McKenney JB, Rosenberg RD: Acceleration of thrombin-antithrombin complex formation in rat hindquarters via heparinlike molecules bound to endothelium. J Clin Invest 1984; 74:341–350.

Marder VJ, Budzynski AZ: Degradation products of fibrinogen and cross-linked fibrin-projected clinical applications. Thromb Diath Haemorrh 1974; 32:49–56.

Marder VJ, Budzynski AZ, Barlow GH: Comparison of the physio-chemical properties of fragment D derivatives of fibrinogen and fragment D-D of cross-linked fibrin. Biochim Biophys Acta 1976; 427:1–14.

Classic paper that described what a D-Dimer is.

Martinelli RA, Scheraga HA: Steady state kinetic study of the bovine thrombin-fribrinogen interaction. Biochemistry 1980; 19: 2343–2350.

Meijers JCM, Tekelenburg WL, Bouma BN, *et al*: High levels of coagulation factor XI as a risk factor for venous thrombosis. N Engl J Med 2000; 342:696–701.

Miletich JP, Majerus DW, Majerus PW: Patients with congenital factor V deficiency have decreased factor Xa binding sites on their platelets. J Clin Invest 1978, 62.824–831.

Miller G, Silberberg M, Kaplan AP: Autoactivability of human Hageman factor. Biochem Biophys Res Commun 1980; 92:803–810.

Motta G, Rojkjaer R, Hasan AAK *et al*: High molecular weight kininogen regulates prekallikrein assembly and activation on endothelial cells: A novel mechanism for contact activation. Blood 1998; 91:516–528.

Mueh JR, Herbst KD, Rapaport SI: Thrombosis in patients with the lupus anticoagulant. Ann Intern Med 1980; 92:156–159.

Mumford AD, O'Donnell J, Gillmore JD, et al: Bleeding symptoms and coagulation abnormalities in 337 patients with AL-amyloidosis. Br J Haematol 2000; 110:454–460.

Nawarawong W, Wyshock E, Meloni FJ, Weitz J, Schmaier AH: The rate of fibrinopeptide B release modulates the rate of clot formation: a study with an acquired inhibitor to fibrinopeptide B release. Br J Haematol 1991; 79:296–301.

Naylor JA, Green PM, Rizza CR, Giannelli F: Factor VIII gene explains all cases of haemophilia A. Lancet 1992; 340:1066–1067.

Nichols WC, Seligsohn U, Zivelin A, et al: Mutations in the ER-Golgi intermediate compartment protein ERGIC-53 cause combined deficiency of coagulation factors V and VIII. Cell 1998; 93:61–70.

Okajima K, Kohno I, Soe G, *et al*: Direct evidence for systemic fibrinogenolysis in patients with acquired alpha-2-plasmin inhibitor deficiency. Am J Hematol 1994; 45:16–24.

Osterud B, and Rappaport SI: Activation of factor IX by the reaction product of tissue factor and factor VII. Proc Natl Acad Sci USA 1977; 74: 5260–5264.

Palmer RMJ, Ferrige AG, Moncada S: Nitric oxide release accounts for the biologic activity of endothelium-derived relaxing factor. Nature 1987; 327:524–526.

Peyvandi F, Mannucci PM, Asti D, et al: Clinical manifestations in 28 Italian and Iranian patients with severe factor VII deficiency. Haemophilia 1997; 3:242–246.

Peyvandi F, Mannucci PM, Lak M, et al: Congenital factor X deficiency: spectrum of bleeding symptoms in 32 Iranian patients. Br J Haematol 1998a; 102:626–628.

Peyvandi F, Tuddenham EG, Akhtari AM, et al: Bleeding symptoms in 27 Iranian patients with the combined deficiency of factor V and factor VIII. Br J Haematol 1998b; 100:773–776.

Peyvandi F, and Mannucci PM: Rare coagulation disorders. Thromb Haemost 1999; 82: 1207–1214.

Pinsky DJ, Broekman MJ, Peschon JJ, et al: Elucidation of the thromboregulatory role of CD39/ectoapyrase in the ischemic brain. J Clin Invest 2002; 109:1031–1040.

Pollar L: Oral anticoagulation. *In* Kopke JA (ed): Practical Laboratory Hematology. New York, Churchill Livingstone, 1991.

An excellent description of what an INR is and how to calculate ISI values for thromboplastin reagents.

Proctor RR, Rapaport SI. The partial thromboplastin time with kaolin. A simple screening test for first stage plasma clotting factor deficiencies. Am J Clin Pathol 1961; 36:212–219.

The description of the APTT.

Quick AJ, Stanley-Brown M, Bancroft FW. A study of the coagulation defect in hemophilia and in jaundice. Am J Med Sci 1935; 190: 501–511.

The description of the prothrombin time

Ragni MV, Lewis JH, Spero JA, Hasiba U: Factor VII deficiency. Am J Hematol 1981; 10:79–88.

Rand MD, Lock JB, van't Veer C, et al: Blood clotting in minimally altered whole blood. Blood 1996; 88:3432–3445.

Rand JH: Antiphospholipid syndrome and lupus anticoagulants. *In* Loscalzo J, Schafer AI (eds): Thrombosis and Hemorrhage. Philadelphia, PA, Lippincott, Williams & Wilkins, 2003.

Ratnoff OD, Margolius Jr. A: Hageman trait: an asymptomatic disorder of blood coagulation. Trans Assoc Am Physicians 1955; 68:149–153.

Ratnoff OD, Davies E: Waterfall sequence for intrinsic blood coagulation. Science 1964; 145:1310–1312.

Ratnoff OD, Busse RJ, and Sheon RP: Medical intelligence: the demise of John Hageman. N Engl J Med 1968; 279:760–761.

Reitsma PH: Genetic principles underlying disorders of procoagulation and anticoagulation proteins. *In* Colman RW, Hirsh J, Marder VJ, et al (eds): Hemostasis and Thrombosis: Basic Principles and Clinical Practice, 4th edition. Philadelphia, PA, Lippincott-Raven, 2001.

Roberts HR, Monroe DM III, Hoffman M: Safety profile of recombinant factor VIIa. Semin Hematol 2004; 41:101–108.

Rojkjaer R, Hasan AAK, Motta G, et al: Factor XII does not initiate prekallikrein activation on endothelial cells. Thromb Haemost 1998; 80:74–81.

Saito H, Ratnoff OD, Waldmann R, Abraham JP: Fitzgerald trait: deficiency of a hitherto unrecognized agent, Fitzgerald factor, participating in surface mediated reactions of clotting, fibrinolysis, generation of kinins, and the property of diluted plasma enhancing vascular permeability. J Clin Invest 1975; 55:1082–1089.

Salomon O, Zivelin A, Livnat T, et al: Prevalence, causes, and characterization of factor XI inhibitors in patients with inherited factor XI deficiency. Blood 2003; 101:4783–4788.

Schmaier AH, Kuo A, Lundberg D, et al: Expression of high molecular weight kininogen on human umbilical vein endothelial cells. J Biol Chem 1988; 263:16327–16333.

Schmaier AH. Disseminated intravascular coagulation – pathogenesis and management. J Intens Care Med 1991; 6:209–228.

Schmaier AH, Dahl LD, Rozemuller AJM, et al: Protease nexin-2/amyloid β-protein precursor: A tight-binding inhibitor of coagulation factor IXa. J Clin Invest 1993; 92:2540–2545.

Schmaier AH, Dahl LD, Hasan AAK, et al: Factor IXa inhibition by protease nexin-2/amyloid β-protein precursor on phospholipid vesicles and cell membranes. Biochemistry 1995; 34: 1171–1178.

Schmaier AH: The plasma kallikrein/kinin system counterbalances the renin angiotensin system. J Clin Invest 2002; 109:1007–1009.

Schmaier AH: The kallikrein/kinin and the renin angiotensin systems have a multi-layered interaction. Am J Physiol – Reg Integr Comp Physiol 2003; 285:R1–R13.

Schmaier AH: The physiologic basis of assembly and activation of the plasma kallikrein/kinin system. Thromb Haemost 2004; 91:1–3.

Schneppenheim R, Budde U, Krey S, et al: Results of a screening for von Willebrand disease type 2N in patients with suspected haemophilia A or von Willebrand disease type 1. Thromb Haemost 1996; 76:598–602.

Schwartz BS, Williams EC, Conlan MG, Mosher DF: Epsilon-aminocaproic acid in the treatment of patients with acute promyelocytic leukemia and acquired alpha-2-plasmin inhibitor deficiency. Ann Intern Med 1986; 105: 873–877.

Seligsohn U, Zivelin A, Zwang E: Combined factor V and factor VIII deficiency among non-Ashkenazi Jews. N Engl J Med 1982; 307: 1191–1195.

Shapiro AD, Paola JD, Cohen A, et al: The safety and efficacy of recombinant human blood coagulation factor IX in previously untreated patients with severe or moderately severe hemophilia B. Blood 2005; 105: 518–525.

Shariat-Madar Z, Mahdi F, Schmaier AH. Identification and characterization of prolylcarboxypeptidase as an endothelial cell prekallikrein activator. J Biol Chem 2002; 277:17962–17969.

Paper that identifies a physiologic activator of the plasma kallikrein/kinin system, the so-called contact activation system.

Uprichard J, Perry DJ: Factor X deficiency. Blood Rev 2002; 16:97–110.

Van Nostrand WE, Schmaier AH, Farrow JS, Cunningham DD: Protease nexin-II (amyloid β-protein precursor): A platelet α-granule protein. Science 1990; 248:745–748.

Verbruggen B, Novakova I, Wessels H, et al: The Nijmegan modification of the Bethesda assay for FVIII:C inhibitors: improved specificity and reliability. Thromb Haemost 1995; 73: 247–251.

Paper that describes an improved way to perform specific inhibitor studies for factor VIII.

Weiss HJ, Sussman II, Hoyer LW: Stabilization of factor VIII in plasma by the von Willebrand factor. Studies on posttransfusion and dissociated factor VIII and in patients with von Willebrand's disease. J Clin Invest 1977; 60:390–404.

Weuppers KD, Cochrane CG: Plasma prekallikrein: isolation, characterization, and mechanism of action. J Exp Med 1972; 135: 1–20.

Wiggins RC, Cochrane CC: The autoactivability of human Hageman factor. J Exp Med 1979; 150:1122–1133.

Zaffran Y, Meyer SC, Negrescu E, et al: Signaling across the platelet adhesion receptor glycoprotein Ib-IX induces $\alpha_{IIb}\beta_3$ activation both in platelets and a transfected Chinese hamster ovary cell system. J Biol Chem 2000; 275:16779–16787.

Zeitler H, Ulrich-Merzenish G, Hess L *et al*: Treatment of acquired hemophilia by the Bonn-Malmö Protocol: documentation of an in vivo immunomodulating concept. Blood 2005; 105:2287–2293.

Zhang B, Cunningham MA, Nichols WC, et al: Bleeding due to disruption of a cargo-specific ER-to-

Golgi transport complex. Nat Genet 2003; 34:220–225.

Zhang B, Ginsburg D: Familial multiple coagulation factor deficiencies: new biologic insight from rare genetic bleeding disorders. J Thromb Haemost 2004; 2:1564–1572.

Zito F, Lowe GDO, Rumley A, et al: WOSCOPS Study Group. Association of the factor XII 46C>T polymorphism with risk of coronary heart disease (CHD) in the WOSCOPS study. Atherosclerosis 2002; 165:153–158.

CHAPTER 39

Blood Platelets and von Willebrand Disease

Jonathan L. Miller MD PhD, A. Koneti Rao MD

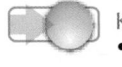 **KEY POINTS**
- Platelets are highly complex cells that participate in critical reactions central to hemostasis and thrombosis, including adhesion to subendothelium, secretion of granule contents, aggregation, and provision of membrane surface for activation of coagulation factors.

- Abnormalities of either platelet number or of platelet function can play an important role in the balance of hemostasis and thrombosis.

- Almost unique to laboratory medicine and pathology, assessment of platelet pathology may be determined in real time upon living cells obtained from the patient.

- Von Willebrand factor is a multimeric protein synthesized by endothelial cells and megakaryocytes that plays a central role in platelet adhesive interactions.

- Platelet counts and platelet function are affected by autoimmune processes, a wide variety of drugs, and a number of acquired disorders.

Normal Platelet Biology

Platelet Structure

Blood platelets are highly complex, anucleate cells that derive from bone marrow megakaryocytes. A well-prepared peripheral blood film offers the opportunity for evaluation of platelet numbers, size, distribution, and light microscopic structure. Although subtle abnormalities of platelet structure usually require electron microscopic analysis, gross absence or asymmetry of granulation and grossly aberrant platelet surfaces may be evident. In films from nonanticoagulated fingerstick specimens, some platelet clumping is an expected feature. In instances of observed abnormalities, artifacts resulting from improper specimen collection or handling should always be considered, and a repeat specimen should be obtained if a satisfactory explanation for the abnormality is not apparent.

In cases of suspected platelet structural abnormalities, electron microscopy allows much more precise characterization of the defect (White, 2004). It is essential that established protocols for the collection and processing of platelet specimens for ultrastructural study be followed meticulously, in order to avoid attributing changes occurring because of inadvertent in vitro activation to abnormalities truly characteristic of the platelets in vivo.

Normal features of the platelet that may be visualized ultrastructurally are shown in Figure 39–1. The outer surface of the platelet, the *glycocalyx*, is rich in glycoproteins. A submembranous band of *microtubules*, composed of the protein tubulin, provides structural support for the normally discoid cell. Contractile *microfilaments* may also be seen. These are composed principally of platelet actin and platelet myosin. An extensive *open canalicular system* within the platelet has been demonstrated by a variety of methods to be in direct communication with the extracellular environment. Often seen in close proximity to the open canalicular system is the *dense tubular system*. This system, apparently derived from the smooth endoplasmic reticulum, shows positive staining for platelet peroxidase activity (Breton-Gorius, 1972), in accord with its role as a site for arachidonic acid metabolism within the platelet. The dense tubular system also functions as a calcium-sequestering pump, providing low levels of cytoplasmic calcium in the resting platelet.

A variety of inclusions may be recognized within the platelet cytoplasm. Both *mitochondria* and *glycogen* may be identified. Lighter staining α *granules*, less frequent *dense core* (or 'bull's eye') *granules*, *lysosomes*, and *peroxisomes* may also be seen. The α granules contain a number of different proteins, including platelet fibrinogen, the platelet-derived growth factor (PDGF), von Willebrand factor (vWF), the factor V binding protein multimerin (Hayward, 1991; 1993), P-selectin (Stenberg, 1985; Berman 1986), β-thromboglobulin (βTG), and the heparin-neutralizing platelet factor (PF)4. The dense core granules are known to be the locus of stored, nonmetabolic pools of adenosine diphosphate (ADP), adenosine triphosphate (ATP), 5-hydroxytryptamine (5-HT), and calcium.

Platelet Membrane Glycoproteins

Detailed study of the platelet membrane glycoproteins has led to an improved understanding of platelet function. Through radioactive

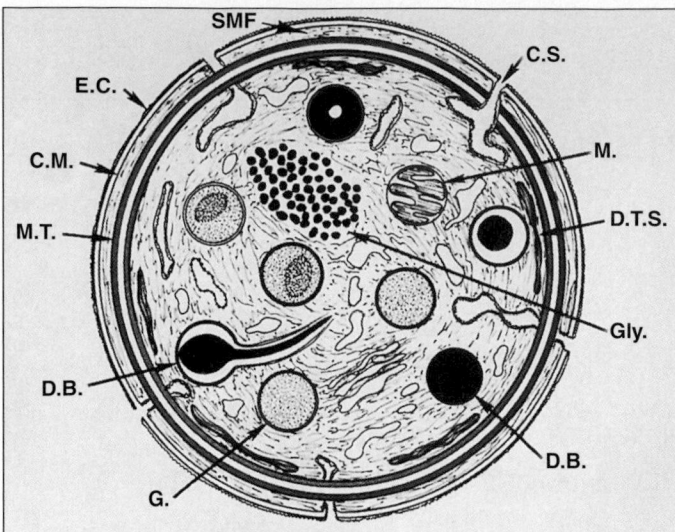

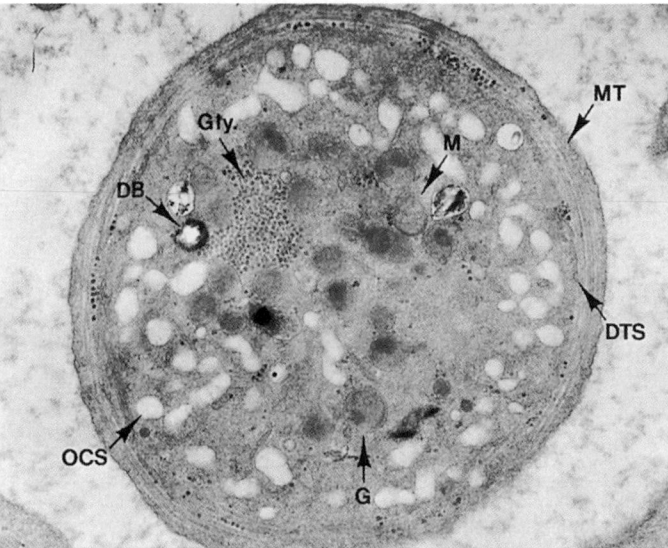

Figure 39–1 Discoid platelets. The diagram summarizes ultrastructural features observed in thin sections of discoid platelets cut in the equatorial plane. Components of the peripheral zone include the exterior coat (EC), trilaminar unit membrane (CM), and submembrane area containing specialized filaments (SMF) that form the wall of the platelet and line channels of the surface connected canalicular system (CS). The matrix of the platelet interior is the sol-gel zone containing actin microfilaments, structural filaments, the circumferential band of microtubules (MT), and glycogen (Gly). Formed elements embedded in the sol-gel zone include mitochondria (M), granules (G), and dense bodies (DB). Collectively they constitute the organelle zone. The membrane systems include the surface connected canalicular system (CS) and the dense tubular system (DTS), which serve as the platelet sarcoplasmic reticulum. The electron micrograph shows a platelet sectioned in the equatorial plane (×30 000) which reveals most of the structures indicated on the diagram. (With permission from White JG, Bloom AL, Forbes CD, Thomas DP, Tuddenham EGD (eds): Hemostasis and Thrombosis. New York, Churchill Livingstone, 1994.)

this receptor complex may alternatively be referred to as GP Ib/IX/V or GP Ib/V/IX, in recognition that GP V forms a tight, noncovalent association with GP Ib and GP IX.) Copy number for the remaining complexes is believed to be much lower. Analysis of a variety of polymorphisms within the major platelet membrane glycoproteins with respect to their possible association with increased thrombotic risk is currently under way in a number of laboratories (Kunicki, 2004; Yee, 2004). Such laboratory-based approaches, whether at the phenotypic or genotypic level, are likely to become increasingly important, particularly with respect to predicting individual patient responses to anti-thrombotic therapy (Michelson, 2000).

Although not readily visualized in electron micrographs of the platelet, platelet membrane phospholipids, and in particular phosphatidylserine, are additionally of significant functional importance. Due to phospholipid asymmetry, the negatively charged phosphatidylserine is not abundantly expressed in the outer membrane leaflet of the resting platelet (Fig. 39–3) (Zwaal, 2005); breakdown of this asymmetry upon platelet activation leads to the formation of a procoagulant platelet surface (Solum, 1999a). Monitoring of this activation-associated change in phospholipid exposure can be performed in the laboratory as increased binding of annexin V to the platelet surface using flow cytometry (Fig. 39–4).

Platelet Activities in Hemostasis and Their Laboratory Measurements

Platelet Activation

Through activation of the coagulation system, thrombin is produced, and serves as a very potent stimulus for platelet activation. Upon stimulation by thrombin, collagen, or various other agents, platelets change in shape from discoid to spherical, extend pseudopods, undergo internal contraction resulting in centralization of their α granules and dense core granules, and ultimately release from the cell the contents of these granules. Depending upon the strength of the stimulus, the contents of the α granules, dense core granules, or even lysosomal granules may be released. As a result of platelet activation, conformational changes in the glycoprotein IIb/IIIa complex occur (Frelinger, 1991; Phillips, 1991; Sims, 1991; Calvete, 1999), resulting in the formation of receptors capable of binding several plasma proteins, most notably fibrinogen (Bennett, 1979; Cox, 2004).

Following vascular injury, blood platelets rapidly adhere to the exposed subendothelium. Under lower shear conditions, such as those characteristic of the venous circulation, platelets may bind directly to exposed collagen by means of GP VI and GP Ia/IIa ($\alpha_2\beta_1$). Under the higher shear conditions present in the arterial circulation, adhesion is believed to be initiated by circulating vWF binding to exposed subendothelial collagen, and the surface-bound vWF then binding to the platelet via the platelet's GP Ib/IX receptor complex (Auger, 2005). In order for the formation of a stable platelet plug, however, GP IIb/IIIa must undergo a conformation change (Fig. 39–5), rendering it competent to bind fibrinogen. Fibrinogen serves as a major adhesive ligand for GP IIb/IIIa ($\alpha_{IIb}\beta_3$) (Auger, 2005), and in this capacity is an essential component underlying platelet aggregation. In the disease Glanzman thrombasthenia, described below, there is an absence of or defect in GP IIb/IIIa, resulting in defective platelet aggregation. Flow cytometry has proved useful not only for measuring the expression of the major glycoprotein receptors on the platelet surface but also for assessing t he ability of GP IIb/IIIa to undergo conformation change upon challenge of platelets with appropriate agonists (Fig. 39–6). In vivo, aggregates of platelets developing within vessels are termed thrombi.

In addition to the highly significant change in conformation of the platelet membrane GP IIb/IIIa complex that occurs as a result of platelet activation, there is also a remarkable translocation of P-selectin from its intracellular α-granule storage site to the platelet's outer membrane surface. Under conditions of platelet activation in which microparticles bud off from the platelet membrane, P-selectin is also exposed on the outer surface of the microparticles. Microparticle P-selectin, or P-selectin derived from other sources, is capable of binding to P-selectin glycoprotein ligand (PSGL)-1 expressed by monocytes, which in turn leads to the expression of circulating tissue factor (Cambien, 2004). Platelet P-selectin may also bind to PSGL expressed by neutrophils, injured endothelial cells, and a variety of other cells in particular disease states (Evangelista, 1999; Warkentin, 1999b; Andre, 2004; Cambien, 2004; Furie, 2004).

The initial laboratory evaluation of platelet disorders includes a platelet count. This measurement has now become a routine component of the complete blood count in an era of electronic particle counting instrumentation. Many instruments additionally provide a value for mean platelet volume (MPV), and may display a histogram of platelet volumes. In healthy individuals the MPV varies inversely with platelet count, so that interpretation of MPV values as abnormally low or high is best done with

labeling and, subsequently, chemical labeling with nonradioactive biotin (Fabris, 1992; Solum, 1995; Sachs, 2000) of surface glycoproteins, solubilization of the platelet membranes, electrophoretic separation of the solubilized proteins on polyacrylamide gels, and subsequent visualization of the gels, assessment of glycoproteins from patient platelets may be performed. In fact, the application of this methodology to the platelets of patients with a number of congenital bleeding disorders led to the discovery that these disorders were due to an absence of critical membrane glycoproteins. Moreover it was precisely the observation that multiple glycoprotein bands were absent in these patients, as illustrated in Figure 39–2, that led to the discovery that the major platelet glycoproteins existed in the form of multi-chain complexes. A summary of platelet membrane glycoproteins currently thought to function as receptors for adhesive ligands is presented in Table 39–1. Quantitatively, the GP IIb/IIIa receptor complex (also referred to as $\alpha_{IIb}\beta_3$) dominates, with approximately 50 000 copies per platelet, followed by the GP Ib/IX receptor complex at approximately 25 000 copies per platelet. (Note that

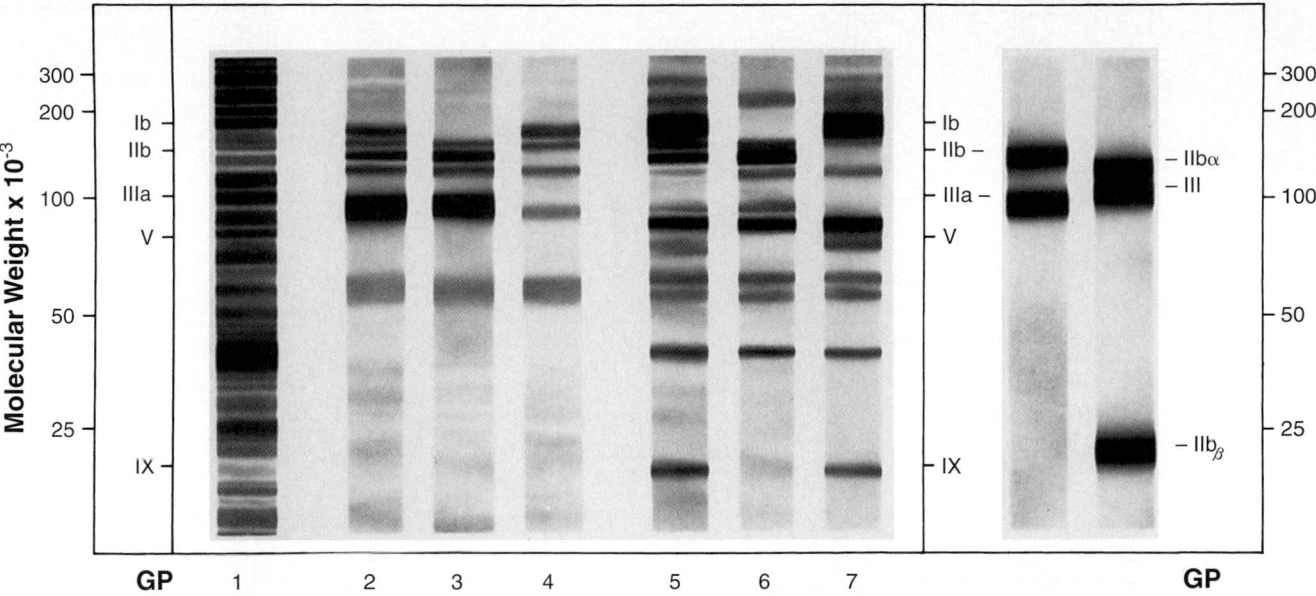

GP 1 2 3 4 5 6 7 **GP**

Figure 39–2 Analysis of platelet proteins and antiplatelet antibodies by SDS-polyacrylamide gel electrophoresis and immunoblotting. This figure is an artist's rendering of the original material to allow a clearer, more consistent presentation of typical analyses. Solubilized platelet proteins were separated by electrophoresis through a slab gel containing a 7–12% exponential gradient of polyacrylamide. All samples are unreduced, except for lane 9, in which the proteins are reduced with 5% β-mercaptoethanol. The ordinates mark the position of the major platelet membrane glycoproteins in the unreduced form; therefore, these notations are not applicable to lane 9. Lane 1 represents a Coomassie brilliant blue protein stain of normal whole platelets. Among the major membrane glycoproteins, only GP IIb is separated from other polypeptides and is present as a distinct band. Lanes 2–4 represent autoradiographs of platelet cell surface proteins labeled by lactoperoxidase-catalyzed radioiodination, and lanes 5–7 represent fluorographs of platelets labeled by sequential treatment with neuraminidase, galactose oxidase, and sodium [³H]borohydride (to label cell surface carbohydrate). Lanes 2 and 5 represent normal platelets. Lane 3 and 6 represent platelets from a patient with Bernard–Soulier syndrome. The lack of GP Ib can be seen with both techniques, whereas the apparent absence of GP V, GP IX, and a high-molecular-weight band that may contain complexes of GP Ib can only be seen in lane 6. Lanes 4 and 7 represent platelets from a patient with Glanzmann's thrombasthenia, demonstrating their deficiency of GP IIb and GP IIIa. Lanes 8 and 9 are Western blots of unreduced (lane 8) and reduced (lane 9) platelet proteins using a mixture of polyclonal rabbit anti-GP IIb and anti-GP IIIa antisera as the primary antibody. Disulfide bond reduction causes the dissociation of GP IIb into two subunits: GP IIb_α, with a slightly faster migration than GP IIb, and GP IIb_β, which can be seen at the position of $M_r = 22\,000$. GP IIIa is apparently rich in intramolecular disulfide bonds and assumes a larger size and slower electrophoretic migration after reduction. Lanes 8 and 9, left and right, respectively, occur in the smaller rectangular box on the far rigt. (With permission from Nurden AT, George JN, Phillips DR: Platelet membrane glycoproteins: their structure, function, and modification in disease. *In* Phillips DR, Shuman MA (eds): Biochemistry of Platelets. Orlando, Academic Press, 1986, pp 159–224.)

Table 39–1 Adhesive Platelet Membrane Glycoproteins

	Alternate Designation	Molecular Weight (Reduced)* α-Subunit	β-Subunit	Gene Family	Ligand	Function	Glycoprotein Expression†
GP IIb/IIIa	$\alpha_{IIb}\beta_3$	125 kDa, 23 kDa	110 kDa	Integrin	Fibr, vWF, FN, VN	Aggregation Adhesion	C, S
Vitronectin receptor	$\alpha_v\beta_3$	135 kDa, 25 kDa	110 kDa	Integrin	VN, ?vWF, fibr	Adhesion	C
GP Ic/IIa	VLA-5	135 kDa, 27 kDa	130 Da	Integrin	FN, laminin	Adhesion	C
α_6/IIa	VLA-6	125 kDa	130 kDa	Integrin	Laminin	Adhesion	C
GP Ia/IIa	VLA-2	167 kDa	130 kDa	Integrin	Collagen	Adhesion	C
GP Ib/IX		145 kDa, 24 kDa	17 kDa	Leucine-rich glycoprotein	vWF, THR	Adhesion	C
P-Selectin	GMP 140, PADGEM, CD-62	140 kDa		Selectin	PSGL-1, *O*-linked carbohydrate	Platelet–leukocyte interactions	S
PECAM-1	CD31	130 kDa		Immunoglobulin	?	Platelet–endothelial cell interactions	C
GP IV	GP IIIb, CD36	88 kDa		?	TSP, Collagen	Adhesion	C
GP VI		61 kDa		?	Collagen	Signaling	C
PETA-3		27 kDa		Tetraspan	?	?Aggregation	C

* Numbers separated by commas represent the molecular weight of disulfide-linked α- and β-chains of the respective receptor α- or β-subunit.

† C = constitutive expression; S = membrane expression requires platelet stimulation.

fibr = fibrinogen; FN = fibronectin; PETA-3 = platelet-endothelial cell tetraspan antigen-3; PSGL-1 = P-selectin-glycoprotein ligand-1; THR = thrombin; TSP = thrombospondin; VN = vitronectin; vWF = von Willebrand factor.

Source: modified with permission from Peerschke EIB, Lopez JA: Platelet membranes and receptors. *In* Loscalzo J, Schafer AI (eds): Thrombosis and Hemorrhage, 2nd ed. Baltimore, Williams & Wilkins, 1998, p 253.

reference to the patient's platelet count (Bessman, 1981, 1986). Some automated instruments additionally assess platelet maturity, as reflected by the RNA content of 'reticulated platelets' – analogous to reticulocyte measurements in the erythroid series, discussed below. Such measurements offer the opportunity to detect a thrombopoietic response from the bone marrow one or more days earlier than might be detected by more traditional approaches. Evaluation of the peripheral blood film should permit at least a rough corroboration of the measured count and platelet size distribution.

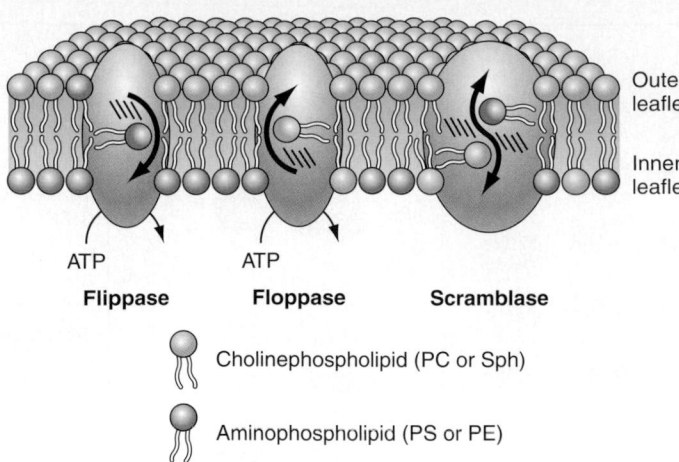

Figure 39–3 Transporter-controlled exchange of phospholipids between both lipid leaflets of the cell membrane. Unidirectional phospholipid transport by flippase is directed inward, whereas floppase promotes outward-directed transport. Both transporters are ATP-dependent and frequently move phospholipids against their respective concentration gradients. For example, aminophospholipid translocase (flippase) rapidly shuttles PS and PE from outer to inner leaflet, while ABCC1 (floppase) moves both choline- and aminophospholipids more slowly towards the outer leaflet. The concerted action of both transporters is thought to create a dynamic asymmetric steady state, in which the outer monolayer is rich in cholinephospholipids, whereas aminophospholipids predominantly occupy the inner leaflet. Bidirectional phospholipid transport is catalyzed by a scramblase, activation of which may occur following Ca^{2+} influx or when cells go into apoptosis. Since scramblase activity moves all major phospholipid classes back and forth between the two leaflets, it promotes collapse of membrane phospholipid asymmetry, with appearance of PS at the cells' outer surface. PC = phosphatidyl choline; SPH = sphingosine; PS = phosphatidyl-serine; PE = phosphatidylethanolamine. (Modified with permission from Zwaal RF, Comfurius P, Bevers EM: Surface exposure of phosphatidylserine in pathological cells. Cell Mol Life Sci 2005; 62:971–988.)

Because platelets may undergo variable degrees of activation and subsequent spreading in the preparation of the blood film, the apparent size distribution of platelets in the blood film may, in some cases, deviate significantly from actual volume distributions. In cases of severe thrombocytopenia below the established linearity of a given automated instrument, or whenever cellular fragments may be spuriously affecting the automated count, a manual phase contrast count with a hemocytometer chamber may be performed (Brecher, 1950). However, it must be kept in mind that such manual counts performed on a relatively small number of platelets have a much higher coefficient of variation than is obtained when the automated instruments are used within their linear ranges, and that, unless such counts are performed by an experienced individual, there is a significant opportunity for the introduction of error. The reference interval for the platelet count is approximately $150–400 \times 10^9/L$.

Screening Studies of Platelet Function

No currently available laboratory test faithfully reflects the platelets' ability to accomplish their enormously complex series of functions in a manner consistent with normal hemostasis. For many years the template bleeding time test has been used by many laboratories as a sort of 'global' test for the adequacy of primary hemostasis. In this procedure a disposable device is used that consists either of a spring-loaded blade that descends vertically into the epidermis (described in detail by Hoyer, 1982), or a blade that cuts the epidermis as it makes a rotary arc (Buchanan, 1989). In these tests a blood pressure cuff is placed around the upper arm and is inflated to maintain a constant pressure of 40 mmHg. A standardized cut is then made on the volar surface of the forearm, a timer is started, and at 30-second intervals the resulting drops of blood are blotted with filter paper (taking care that the paper does not directly touch the wound edge itself). When blood no longer stains the filter paper, the timer is stopped. Above platelet counts of $100 \times 10^9/L$, bleeding times should fall within the laboratory's established reference interval. Prolonged bleeding times in such cases are most frequently associated with the prior ingestion of drugs having an anti-platelet action (e.g., aspirin), von Willebrand disease, congenital platelet abnormalities, or acquired disorders of platelet function (e.g., uremia, as discussed below).

Whereas a carefully performed bleeding time test may provide useful information during the evaluation of a patient presenting with a history of increased bleeding, the usefulness of the bleeding time test is less clear in the frequently encountered context of preoperative hemostatic screening of asymptomatic patients. In an extensive review of published papers reporting the extent of clinical bleeding in a wide variety of settings, Rodgers and Levin (1990) concluded that the available data did not

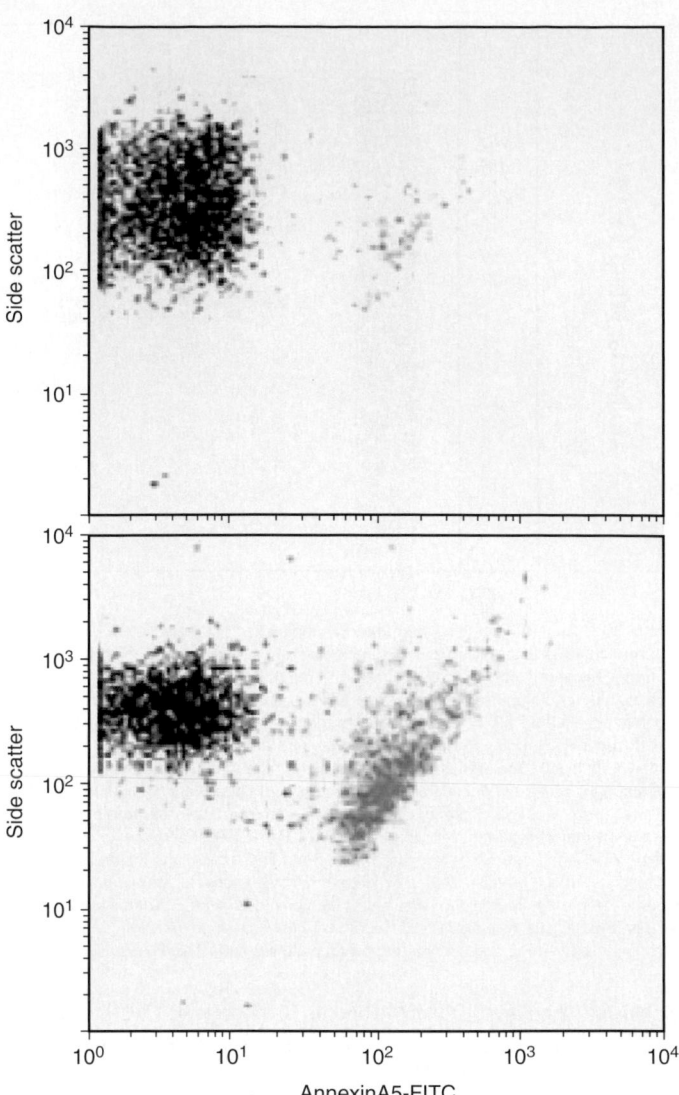

Figure 39–4 Flow cytometric analysis of the binding of fluorescently (FITC) labeled annexin A5 to activated platelets. Typical dot plots of fluorescence versus side scatter of (upper panel) control platelets and (lower panel) platelets activated by 10 μg/ml collagen plus 1 nM thrombin for min. Annexin A5 binding to PS-exposing platelet fraction is represented by the red dots. Scramblase is active in the annexin A5-positive platelets (red dots), whereas aminophospholipid translocase is active in the annexin A5-negative platelets (black dots). (Modified with permission from Zwaal RF, Comfurius P, Bevers EM: Surface exposure of phosphatidylserine in pathological cells. Cell Mol Life Sci 2005; 62:971–988.)

provide convincing evidence that the relationship between platelet count and bleeding time was predictively useful in the individual patient typically encountered in clinical practice. They additionally concluded that the degree of bleeding from a standardized template cut in the skin cannot be relied upon in an individual patient to predict the risk of bleeding elsewhere in the body, such as at operative sites. A prospective study of 40 patients with negative bleeding histories and no recent intake of nonsteroidal anti-inflammatory drugs who underwent coronary artery bypass surgery found no predictive relationship between the preoperative bleeding time test and either perioperative or postoperative bleeding (De Caterina, 1994). While most would agree that a dramatically prolonged bleeding time, in the absence of technical artifact, provides strong suspicion for an underlying disorder of primary hemostasis, the interpretation of only mildly or moderately prolonged bleeding times is decidedly less clear. Because of the limitation in predictive value, the risk of scarring, and the considerable technical expertise and performance time associated with performance of bleeding times, the use of this procedure has declined considerably in recent years. In parallel with this has been the increased popularity of in vitro measures of platelet reactivity, most notably the platelet function analyzer (PFA-100) instrument. In this instrument, anticoagulated whole blood is flowed under high shear force through a narrow hole punched out of a membrane coated with collagen and either epinephrine or ADP (Fig. 39–7A). The combination of biophysical shear and chemical stimulation initially promotes platelet adhesion to the outer

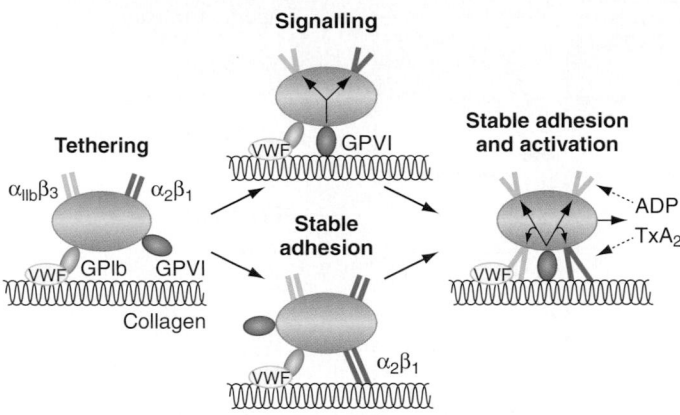

II Integrin in a low affinity, closed state

V Integrin in a high affinity, open state

Figure 39–5 Unifying model of platelet adhesion to collagen at arterial shear. Two different pathways by which human and mouse platelets firmly adhere to collagen at arterial shear are illustrated. In both, the majority of platelets are initially tethered to collagen via GP Ib/IX/V interacting with collagen-bound VWF (left), although a minority of platelets interact directly with collagen independently of VWF/GP Ib/IX/V. In the first pathway (upper), signaling from GP VI first leads to activation of integrins α2β1 (GP Ia/IIa) and αIIbβ3 (GP IIb/IIIa). Activated integrins then firmly attach the platelet to collagen, either directly (α2β1) or via collagen-bound VWF (αIIbβ3) (right). In the second pathway (lower), platelets first adhere to collagen via integrin α2β1, before GP VI engages collagen and induces activation. These two pathways are likely to reinforce each other and the events of thrombus formation. Release of secondary mediators (ADP and TxA2) would further potentiate these events (right). (Redrawn from Auger JM, Kuijpers MJ, Senis YA: Adhesion of human and mouse platelets to collagen under shear: a unifying model. FASEB J 2005;19:825–827.)

edges of the cut membrane, and subsequently platelet–platelet aggregation leads to full occlusion of the channel, which is recorded as 'closure time' (Fig. 39–7B). Whereas inhibition of the platelet cyclooxygenase pathway by aspirin (discussed more fully in Ch. 23) or other mild-moderate impairments of platelet function prolong closure times with the collagen/epinephrine membranes, only more profound impairment of platelet function or of vWF are typically capable of prolonging closure times in the collagen/ADP membranes. Thrombocytopenia or anemia also prolong closure times. Although abnormal in some platelet disorders, it is increasingly being recognized that the PFA-100 does not have sufficient sensitivity or specificity to be relied upon as a screening tool for platelet disorders (see Table 39–2; Hayward, 2006). Definitive identification of abnormalities on platelets of vWF requires more specialized studies.

Several additional ex vivo experimental systems have been developed in which shear forces play a major role. These include both variations of cone-and-plate viscometers and parallel plate flow chambers (Michelson, 2002). These devices offer the potential to detect inherited and acquired disorders relating to both platelets and vWF, depending, of course, on the level of severity of the particular disorder.

Platelet Aggregation and Secretion

Further evaluation of a suspected defect of platelet function can be obtained through laboratory study of platelet aggregation and secretion in response to a battery of platelet-stimulating agents. When citrated platelet-rich plasma is continuously stirred in a platelet aggregometer and a light beam passed through the suspension, platelet aggregation in response to an added chemical stimulus can be monitored by changes in light transmittance (Zucker, 1989). Discoid to spheroid shape change is seen as an initial decrease in transmittance, whereas the subsequent formation of platelet clumps allows more light to pass through the suspension to the photodetector and is recorded as an increase in light transmittance. In instruments equipped with a second channel for monitoring secretion, the release of ATP from platelet-dense granules is simultaneously measured (Fig. 39–8). This is accomplished by adding the firefly luminescence substrate

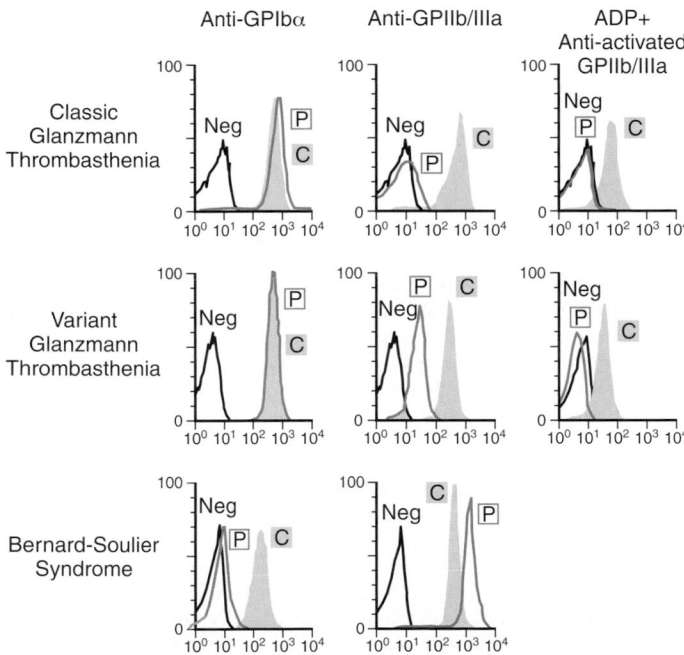

Figure 39–6 Flow cytometric evaluation of platelet membrane glycoprotein disorders. Platelets from normal controls (C) or from patients (P) were incubated with monoclonal antibodies against GP Ibα, GP IIb/IIIa, or a monoclonal antibody (Pac1) that recognizes only the conformationally altered 'active' form of GP IIb/IIIa that normally occurs following platelet stimulation with agonists (e.g., ADP). In the patient with classic Glanzmann thrombasthenia shown in the upper panel, there is a virtual absence of GP IIb/IIIa, although GP Ibα is present at normal levels. In the variant of Glanzmann thrombasthenia shown in the middle panel, while there appears to be an intermediate level of expression of GP IIb/IIIa, there is a more severe loss of ability to adopt the active conformation of this receptor upon stimulation of the platelets with ADP. In the patient with Bernard–Soulier syndrome shown in the lower panel, there is a severe deficiency of GP Ibα expression but no decrease of GP IIb/IIIa expression. (Modified with permission from Nurden AT, George JN: Inherited disorders of the platelet membrane: Glanzmann thrombasthenia, Bernard–Soulier syndrome, and other disorders. In Colman RW (ed.): Hemostasis and Thrombosis. Basic Principles and Clinical Practice, 4th ed. Philadelphia, Lippincott Williams & Wilkins, 2001.)

Table 39–2 PFA-100® closure times (CT) findings in congenital and acquired, non-drug-induced platelet disorders

	Total number of subjects reported	CADP CT	CEPI CT
Disorders with normal platelet counts			
Glanzmann thrombasthenia	23	P	P
Aspirin-like defect	6	N	P
P2Y$_{12}$ deficiency	4	N or P	N or P
Dense granule deficiency	30	N or P	N or P
Hermansky–Pudlak syndrome	44	N or P	N or P
Primary secretion defects	30	N	N or P
Platelet procoagulant defect	1	N	N
Disorders with reduced or normal platelet counts			
Bernard–Soulier syndrome	8	P	P
Platelet-type von Willebrand disease	3	P	P
Grey platelet syndrome	3	P	P
Wiskott–Aldrich syndrome	5	N or P	N or P
Hereditary macrothrombocytopenia associated with non-muscle Myosin Heavy Chain IIa syndromes	5	N	N or P
Macrothrombocytopenia of undefined cause	11	N or P	N or P
Undefined autosomal dominant thrombocytopenia	1	N	N
Primary bone marrow disorders			
Myelodysplastic or myeloproliferative syndromes, with or without thrombocytosis	69	N or P	N or P

Note, the data reported with CADP and CEPI cartridges, indicated as normal (N) or prolonged (P), are based on small numbers of reported
Source: modified with permission from Hayward CPM, Harrison P, Cattaneo M, et al: Platelet function analyzer (PFA)-100® closure time in the evaluation of platelet disorder and platelet function. J Thromb Haemost 2006; 4:312–319.

In vivo Haemostasis

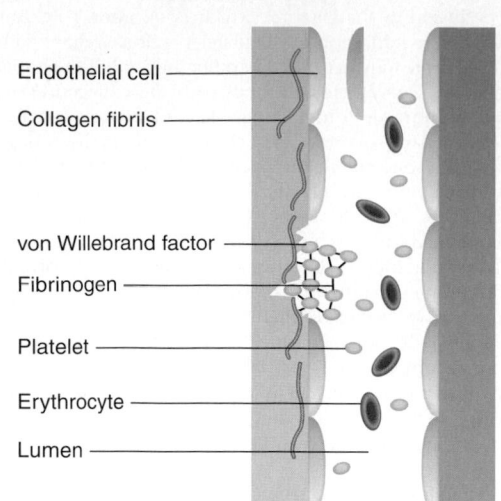

Endothelial cell
Collagen fibrils
von Willebrand factor
Fibrinogen
Platelet
Erythrocyte
Lumen

PFA-100

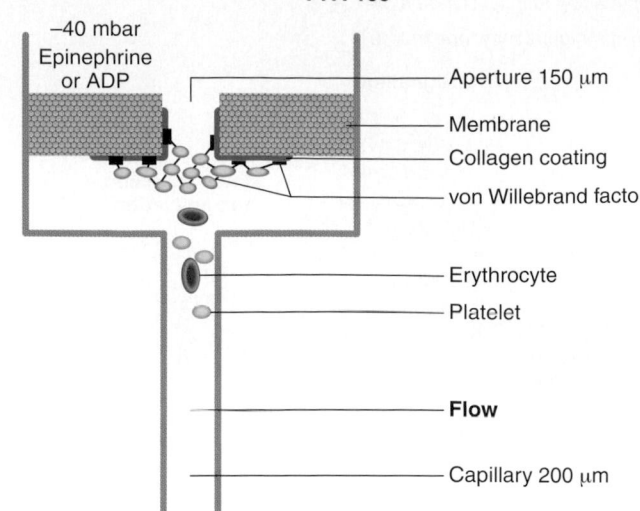

−40 mbar
Epinephrine
or ADP

Aperture 150 μm
Membrane
Collagen coating
von Willebrand factor

Erythrocyte
Platelet

Flow

Capillary 200 μm

Occlusion process
Collagen/epinephrine closure time: 110 sec.

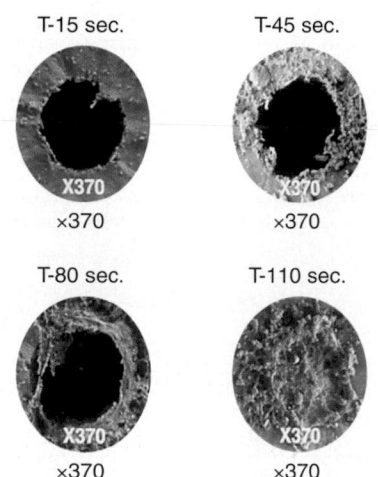

T-15 sec.   T-45 sec.

×370   ×370

T-80 sec.   T-110 sec.

×370   ×370

Figure 39–7 PFA-100. *A* (upper right), Diagrammatic representation of PFA-100 flow chamber. Following piercing of a membrane coated with collagen and either epinephrine or ADP, anticoagulated whole blood is exposed both to chemical stimuli and to the biophysical shear resulting from the forced flow through the narrow tubing used in the apparatus. While this in vitro environment shares some similar elements with in vivo hemostasis (shown diagrammatically at the left), it is important to remember that these environments are intrinsically quite different, and the PFA-100 may not always produce results identical to those observed in the far more complex *in vivo* environment. *B* (lower left), Illustration of progressive occlusion of the pierced aperture by platelet thrombi in a collagen/epinephrine membrane in the PFA-100 device. (Images provided by Dade Corporation.)

and enzyme, luciferin and luciferase, to the platelet-rich plasma; released ATP then functions as a cofactor in the light-producing luciferin–luciferase reaction, and light emission is recorded with a second photodetector. Because of separation of wavelengths, the aggregation and release channels can be monitored independently (Miller, 1984). The release of ATP may in most cases be assumed to reflect the release of the other constituents of dense granules, which are less easily measured (i.e., ADP, serotonin, calcium). Direct measurement of serotonin may also be performed (Holmsen, 1989). As an alternative to lumiaggregation studies, platelet secretion may be studied in parallel with aggregation by allowing the platelets to take up radioactive serotonin and then measuring the release of radioactivity from the platelets as they are challenged with aggregating agents (Lan, 2005).

As illustrated in Figure 39–9, there are multiple agonist receptors located on the platelet membrane. Following the binding of agonist to receptor, a complex series of internal signaling steps is initiated. A number of these natural agonists, together with several additional platelet stimuli, may be used in the diagnostic laboratory in an effort to determine if one or more of these agonist receptor/signaling pathways is not functioning normally. Frequently employed agonists include collagen, epinephrine, ADP, U46619 (a thromboxane A_2 [TxA_2] analog), ristocetin, arachidonic acid, and the calcium ionophore A23187. Although clearly of paramount importance as a platelet stimulus in vivo, thrombin is difficult to employ with platelet-rich plasma, because of interference from the formation of fibrin. The partially trypsinized γ-thrombin, however, retains platelet stimulating activity but largely lacks clotting activity and can be useful (Charo, 1977). Additionally, TRAP (thrombin receptor activating peptide, SFLLRN) sequences deriving from the extracellular 'tethered ligand' region of the platelet's G-protein-linked seven-transmembrane domain thrombin receptor (Furman, 1998) may be useful in platelet function testing.

By means of impedance measurement, the aggregation of platelets not only in PRP but also in whole blood may be evaluated (Cardinal, 1980).

Following the addition of a platelet agonist to the stirred sample, the conductance between two electrodes falls as platelets aggregate upon the electrode surfaces. The resulting curves of electrical impedance versus time share many similarities to those of light transmittance versus time, although characteristic differences between these two approaches are observed (Ingerman-Wojenski, 1984; Joseph, 1987). When impedance aggregometry is combined with ATP secretion measurement on whole blood samples (Ingerman-Wojenski, 1984), relatively rapid evaluation of platelet function, requiring only a small volume of blood, may be performed. Additionally, platelet aggregation in whole blood may be monitored optically by means of the coaggregation of fibrinogen-coated beads impregnated with a dye that absorbs light in the infrared region of the electromagnetic spectrum. This innovative approach has been introduced recently for assessing the effectiveness of treatment with a variety of platelet inhibitors (see Ch. 41).

The contractile abilities of activated platelets also result in contraction (or 'retraction') of formed clots. In the test tube, *clot retraction* may be quantitatively assessed (Taylor, 1970). In thrombocytopenia or Glanzmann thrombasthenia, clot retraction is delayed or incomplete. As demonstrated by monoclonal antibody inhibition studies (Coller, 1983), GP IIb/IIIa appears required for clot retraction. Although the tripeptide recognition sequence Arg–Gly–Asp (RGD) binding sites of fibrinogen play a major role in the binding of fibrinogen to GP IIb/IIIa, with subsequent fibrinogen-mediated platelet aggregation, recent studies have identified specific sites within the fibrinogen γ chain that appear to subserve clot retraction (Podolnikova, 2003). Since clot retraction markedly facilitates subsequent clot lysis (Carroll, 1981), through this process platelets may be playing an important role in facilitating the eventual lysis of the formed clot.

Role of Platelets in Coagulation

Not only do platelets serve as the key mediators of primary hemostasis, but they also play a vital role in coagulation. While the tissue factor

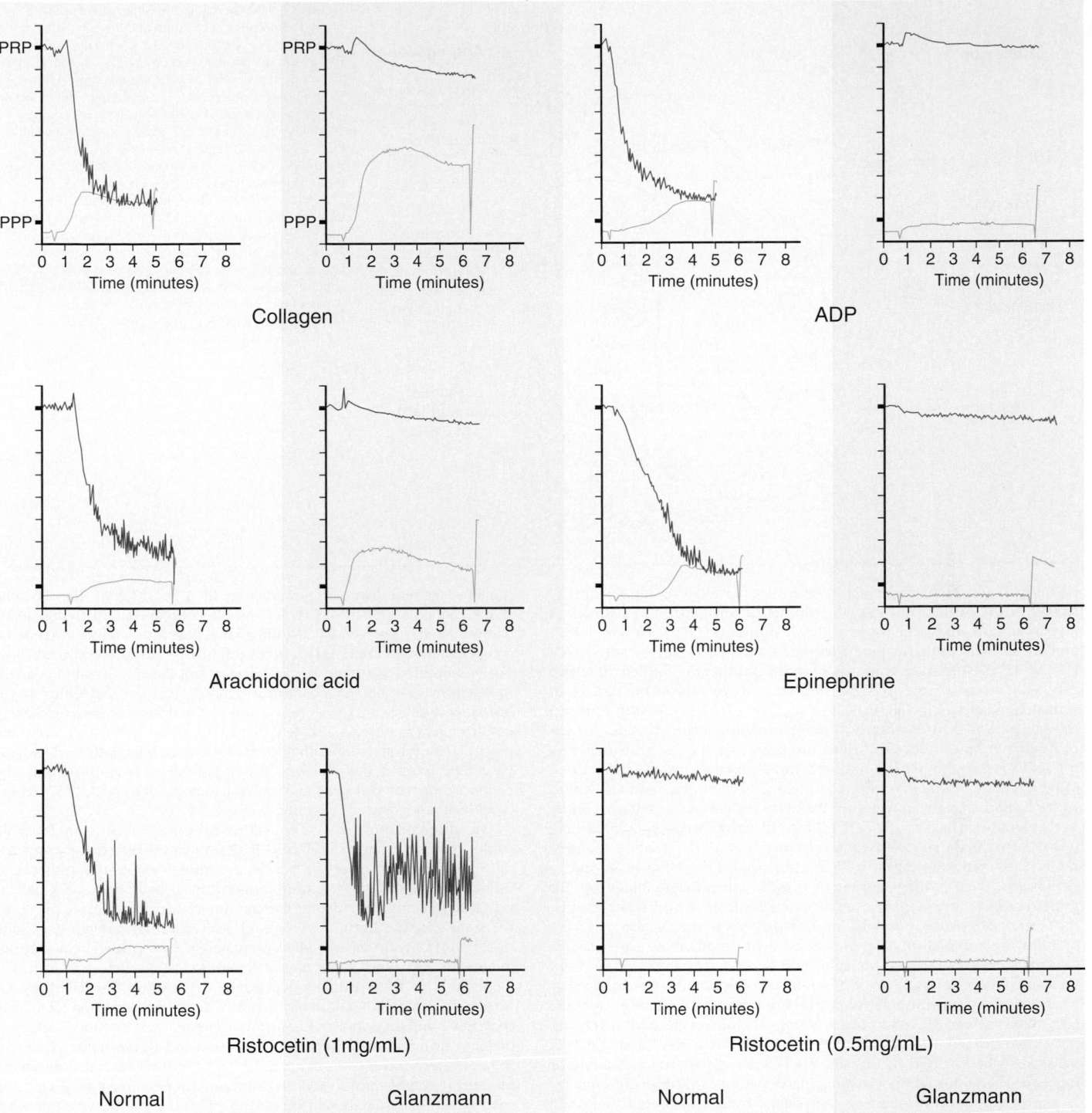

Collagen

ADP

Arachidonic acid

Epinephrine

Ristocetin (1mg/mL)

Ristocetin (0.5mg/mL)

| Normal | Glanzmann | Normal | Glanzmann |

Figure 39–8 Diagnostic platelet lumiaggregation studies in Glanzmann thrombasthenia. Simultaneously measured platelet aggregation and secretion of ATP (lumiaggregation). In each panel, the upper tracing displays platelet aggregation, with increasing aggregation shown as downward deflection. With platelet-rich plasma (PRP) initially set at 90% full vertical scale, and platelet-poor plasma (PPP) at 10%, the maximum possible downward deflection would be to the level of the PPP line. The lower tracing in each panel displays platelet secretion of ATP (monitored as luminescence when secreted ATP reacts with luciferin–luciferase reagent present in the cuvet) as an upward deflection. The abrupt deflection at the end of each secretion tracing represents the response to ATP added as an internal calibration standard. The simultaneous measurement of aggregation and a marker of dense granule secretion can potentially permit discrimination between a platelet disorder affecting the final step of platelet aggregation (as in this example of Glanzmann thrombasthenia), as opposed to an abnormality of a receptor for a specific platelet agonist or an abnormality of intracellular signaling that might impair secretory responses and even aggregation responses to the weaker platelet agonists (such as ADP or epinephrine), yet not markedly impair responses to the stronger platelet agonists (such as arachidonic acid or collagen). Note that the Glanzmann patient's platelets do aggregate uniquely to moderate or high concentrations of ristocetin: Even in the absence of GP IIb/IIIa to function as a receptor for platelet bridging by fibrinogen, ristocetin can facilitate the bridging together of platelets through the binding of plasma von Willebrand factor to the GP Ibα chains that are present in normal numbers in Glanzmann platelets (see Fig. 39–6). (Modified with permission from Miller JL, Schumackher H, Rock W, Stass S (eds): Handbook of Hematologic Pathology. New York, Marcel Dekker, 2000.)

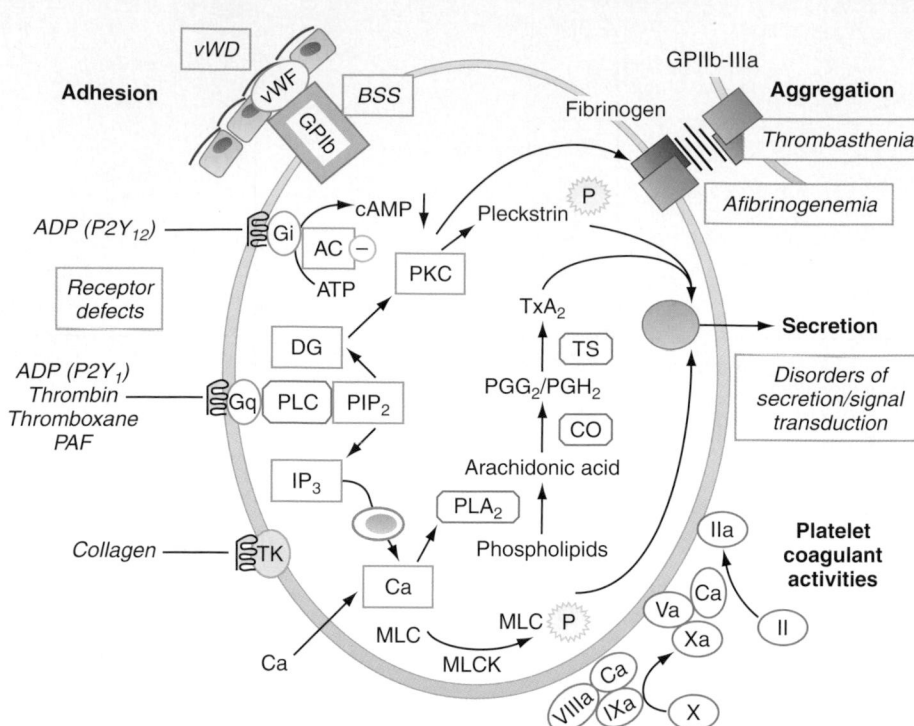

Figure 39–9 A schematic representation of selected platelet responses to activation and the congenital disorders of platelet function. AC = adenylyl cyclase; BSS = Bernard–Soulier syndrome; CO = cyclooxygenase; DG = diacylglycerol; G = GTP-binding protein; IP_3 = inositol trisphosphate; MLC = myosin light chain; MLCK = myosin light chain kinase; $P2Y_1$, $P2Y_{12}$ = G-protein-coupled ADP receptors; PAF = platelet activating factor; PGG_2/PGH_2 = prostaglandin arachidonic pathway intermediates; PIP_2 = phosphatidylinositol bisphosphate; PKC = protein kinase C; PLA_2 = phospholipase A_2; TK = tyrosine kinase; PLC = phospholipase C; TS = thromboxane synthase; $TxA2$ = thromboxane A_2; vWD = von Willebrand disease; vWF = von Willebrand factor. The Roman numerals in the circles represent coagulation factors and yellow Ps indicate phosphorylation. (Modified with permission from Rao AK: Congenital disorders of platelet function: disorders of signal transduction and secretion. Am J Med Sci 1998; 316:69–76.)

pathway involving the sequential formation of factors VIIa and Xa initially results in the formation of trace amounts of thrombin, this pathway is rapidly shut down by the tissue pathway inhibitor (TFPI) (Deykin, 1982) and by itself is probably not adequate to support normal hemostasis (Broze, 1990). The trace amounts of thrombin that are formed, however, may play a critical role in activating factor XI to XIa on the surface of activated platelets. Platelet activation (e.g., by ADP or collagen) results in the generation of high-affinity binding sites for factor XI. Either high-molecular-weight kininogen or prothrombin may then serve as cofactors for activation of the platelet-bound factor XI by thrombin (Baglia, 1998; Oliver, 1999). Moreover, specific interaction between residues within factor XI and a localized region of the platelet GP Ib α chain have recently been identified (Baglia, 2004a, b). Since it is now well appreciated that, unlike factor XI, the so-called 'contact factors' (factor XII, prekallikrein, high-molecular-weight kininogen, etc.) are not needed for effective secondary hemostasis, these findings appear to provide a reasonable framework for understanding how the platelet surface may facilitate the interplay between the tissue factor pathway and the intrinsic pathway of coagulation.

Following stimulation of platelets by agonists, there is a progressive loss of platelet membrane phospholipid asymmetry, which results from increased bilayer movement or 'flip-flop' of phosphatidylserine and other phospholipids from the internal to the external surface of the membrane (Fig. 39–3) (Hemker, 1983; Zwaal 2005). A proline-rich, transmembrane protein termed 'scramblase' (Fig. 39–3) (Comfurius, 1996; Zhou, 1997) is believed to be involved in this process (Zwaal, 2005). The availability of highly ordered phospholipoprotein surfaces permits activation of factors IX, X, and prothrombin to occur on the platelet surface. Platelets additionally contain endogenous factor V, which appears to play a key role in the formation of a receptor on the platelet surface for activated factor X (Miletich, 1978). Effector cell protease receptor (EPR)-1, a platelet-activation-dependent membrane protein (Bouchard, 1997), together with activated factor V, is required to mediate factor Xa binding to the surface of activated platelets in order to form a functional prothrombinase complex. The functional coagulation complexes are described further in the preceding chapter.

Intracellular Signaling Pathways

Considerable progress has been made in recent years in elucidating the signaling pathways underlying platelet function. These pathways characteristically involve receptor activation associated with initial outside-to-inside signaling, subsequent intracellular signaling, and finally inside-to-outside signaling that changes the conformation of GP IIb/IIIa so as to allow fibrogen binding. Following the primary event of an extracellular ligand binding to a specific platelet receptor (such as purinergic ADP receptors, adrenergic epinephrine receptors, thrombin receptors, etc.), receptor occupancy triggers a signal that is transduced by G proteins and other effectors (Fig. 39–9). A cascade of signaling events then ensues, including phosphorylation of specific proteins. As a result of these

processes, several discernible events may then be triggered. These include shape change, secretion of platelet granule contents, and a change in the conformational state of GP IIb/IIIa that makes this critical glycoprotein competent to bind fibrinogen or other adhesive proteins, as described above. The mobilization of arachidonic acid from membrane phospholipids, and its metabolism through the cyclooxygenase pathway to the potent proaggregatory agent TxA_2, is now a well defined intermediary mechanism occurring in response to a variety of platelet stimuli. However, even after potent cyclooxygenase-inhibiting agents such as acetylsalicylic acid (aspirin) have fully blocked this pathway, strong stimuli such as thrombin, high concentrations of collagen, and the calcium ionophore A23187 remain capable of producing full aggregatory responses.

Calcium plays a number of critical roles in platelet function. Since the conformational change in GP IIb/IIIa that makes this receptor competent to bind fibrinogen (see above) is dependent upon the presence of extracellular calcium, aggregation induced by virtually all platelet agonists is in turn calcium-dependent. An exception to this general principle occurs when the adhesive ligand vWF links platelets together through its binding to GP Ib/IX receptors on adjacent platelets (see below) – a calcium-independent process sometimes referred to as platelet *agglutination* to distinguish it from calcium-dependent aggregation mediated by GP IIb/IIIa. Calcium is additionally required for the promotion of platelet contractile and secretory mechanisms. Inherited and acquired defects in platelet calcium mobilization upon activation and agents that interfere with intra-platelet calcium fluxes (e.g., local anesthetics), calcium-binding proteins (e.g., phenothiazines), or extracellular free calcium (e.g., chelating agents) may accordingly be expected to produce inhibitory results when platelet function is tested.

Quantitative Platelet Disorders

Thrombocytopenia

Congenital thrombocytopenia

Congenital thrombocytopenias are being recognized with increasing frequency, and several distinct genetic abnormalities have been documented in such patients (Drachman, 2004). A diverse group of autosomal dominant syndromes including the May–Hegglin anomaly, Fechtner syndrome, Epstein syndrome, and Sebastian syndrome all share the feature of increased platelet size and have been shown to arise from mutations in the MYH9 gene encoding the nonmuscle myosin heavy chain II. Other congenital thrombocytopenias characterized by increased platelet size include Bernard–Soulier syndrome, velocardiofacial/DiGeorge syndrome, Paris–Trousseau thrombocytopenia, and mutations in transcription factor GATA1.

Table 39–3 Mechanisms of Platelet Destruction

Type of Thrombocytopenia	Specific Example(s)
Immune-Mediated	
Autoantibody-mediated platelet destruction by reticuloendothelial system (RES)	Primary immune thrombocytopenic purpura; 'secondary' immune thrombocytopenia associated with lymphoproliferative disease, collagen vascular disease, infections such as infectious mononucleosis, human immunodeficiency syndrome
Alloantibody-mediated platelet destruction by RES	Neonatal alloimmune thrombocytopenia; post-transfusion purpura; passive alloimmune thrombocytopenia; alloimmune platelet transfusion refractoriness
Drug-dependent, antibody-mediated platelet destruction by RES	Drug-induced immune thrombocytopenic purpura (e.g., quinine)
Platelet activation by binding of immunoglobulin G (IgG) Fc of drug-dependent IgG to platelet Fcγlla receptors	Heparin-induced thrombocytopenia
Non-Immune-Mediated	
Platelet activation by thrombin or proinflammatory cytokines	Disseminated intravascular coagulation; septicemia/systemic inflammatory response syndromes
Platelet destruction via ingestion by macrophages (hemophagocytosis)	Infections, certain malignant lymphoproliferative disorders
Platelet destruction through platelet interactions with altered von Willebrand factor	Thrombotic thrombocytopenic purpura; hemolytic uremic syndrome
Platelet losses on artificial surfaces	Cardiopulmonary bypass surgery; use of intravascular catheters
Decreased platelet survival associated with cardiovascular diseases	Congenital and acquired heart disease; cardiomyopathy; pulmonary embolism

Source: modified with permission from Warkentin TE, Kelton JG: Thrombocytopenia due to platelet transfusion and hypersplenism. *In* Hoffman R, Benz EJ Jr, Shattil SJ, et al (eds): Hematology: Basic Principles and Practice. Philadelphia, Elsevier Churchill Livingstone, 2005, pp 2305–2325.

Table 39–4 Clinical Features of Immunologic Thrombocytopenic Purpura

	Children	Adults
Occurrence		
Peak age (years)	2–4	15–40
Sex (F:M)	Equal	2.6:1
Presentation		
Onset	Acute (most with symptoms <1 week)	Insidious (most with symptoms >2 months)
Symptoms	Purpura (<10% with severe bleeding)	Purpura (typically bleeding not severe)
Platelet count	Most <20 000/μL	Most >20 000/μL
Course		
Spontaneous remission	83%	2%
Chronic disease	24%	43%
Response to splenectomy	71%	66%
Eventual complete recovery	89%	64%
Morbidity and mortality		
Cerebral hemorrhage	<1%	3%
Hemorrhagic death	<1%	4%
Mortality of chronic, refractory disease	2%	5%

See also George JN, Rizvi MA: Thrombocytopenia. *In* Beutler E, Lichtman MA, Coller BS, Kipps TJ, Seligsohn U (eds): Hematology. New York, McGraw-Hill, 2001, pp 1495–1539 for more detailed analysis of limitations pertaining to these distinctions.

Source: modified with permission from Diz-Kucukkaya R, Gushiken FC, Lopez JA: Thrombocytopenia. In. Lichtman MA, Beutler E, Kipps TJ, eds. Williams Hematology. 7th edn. New York: McGraw-Hill; 2006: 1758.

basophilic megakaryocytic forms should not be taken as evidence of a qualitative megakaryocytic disorder.

In contrast to estimations of megakaryocyte numbers, it is usually difficult to assess abnormalities in megakaryocyte size or lobulation pattern from biopsy or clot sections. This is because one section may sample only a small portion of the relatively large megakaryocyte cell. For such purposes a well prepared Wright–Giemsa stain on an aspirate smear or on a biopsy touch preparation is typically most helpful. Decreased numbers of circulating platelets may be seen with splenomegaly of any cause, because of the resulting increase in sequestration of platelets by the spleen. These considerations are discussed further in Chapters 29 and 30.

Immune thrombocytopenic purpura

As illustrated by a number of specific examples in Table 39–3, a wide variety of mechanisms may underlie thrombocytopenia resulting from increased platelet destruction. One of the most important and frequently encountered forms of enhanced consumption of platelets is the acquired disorder immune thrombocytopenic purpura (ITP). The clinical history will usually be most helpful in arriving at a tentative diagnosis, and in particular in distinguishing between the acute and chronic forms of ITP (Table 39–4). The study of platelet-associated immunoglobulins in patients suspected of having ITP has been widely employed in an effort to identify immune-mediated processes (Nowak, 1996). However, the predictive value of positive findings in such cases is in question, because immunoglobulin not influencing platelet survival or function may be associated with platelets in a wide variety of clinical settings (Kelton, 1982), and platelet-associated IgG may be nonspecifically elevated in disorders associated with elevated plasma IgG. Alternatively, a variety of enzyme-linked immunosorbent assay (ELISA) techniques are available, whereby either antibodies eluted from the patient's own platelets or patient serum is reacted against purified glycoprotein complexes typically immobilized in wells by murine monoclonal antibodies. Many pathologic antibodies may fail to recognize their epitopes within the glycoprotein targets provided in this artificial manner (especially in the case of GP Ib). Additionally, false-positive results may occur when using patient serum if human antimouse antibodies are present in sufficient titer.

A practice guideline published by the American Society of Hematology in 1996 (George, 1996) took a quite unenthusiastic view as to the value

Abnormalities in patients with the Wiskott–Aldrich syndrome and X-linked thrombocytopenia arise due to mutations in the *WAS* gene, with the patients characteristically having small platelets. In patients having the familial platelet disorder with predisposition to acute myeloid leukemia (FPD/AML), the autosomal dominant thrombocytopenia is secondary to mutations in the *CBFA2/AML1* gene, and the platelets are of normal size. Other causes of congenital thrombocytopenias include congenital amegakaryocytic thrombocytopenia, an autosomal recessive disorder associated with mutations in the thrombopoietin receptor *MPL*, the gray platelet syndrome, and thrombocytopenia with absent radii syndrome. Patients with congenital thrombocytopenias may have associated defects in platelet responses in addition to the decreased counts.

Establishing the etiology of a congenital thrombocytopenia in an individual case can be challenging, requiring specialized routine and molecular/cytogenetic techniques. Such techniques may include assay of plasma thrombopoietin, assay of the extracellular domain of platelet glycoprotein Ib α chain shed into the plasma ('glycocalicin'), and in vitro analysis of megakaryocytopoiesis (van den Oudenrijn, 2002).

Acquired aplastic anemias involving the erythroid and granulocytic lines as well as the megakaryocytic line are seen more commonly than are pure megakaryocytic aplasias. Toxic chemical exposures, viral illnesses, and, frequently, unexplained causes may underlie the aplasia.

Study of the bone marrow may be required in order to assess whether the thrombocytopenia is due at least in part to a failure of platelet production. Bone marrow aspirates are often less reliable than bone marrow biopsies for ascertaining the actual numbers of megakaryocytes present. In some instances abnormalities in megakaryocyte structure may be found, although the mere presence of an increased proportion of the more immature, actually provided by testing for platelet-associated immunoglobulins or antiplatelet antibodies in the evaluation of suspected ITP. Efforts to develop superior testing approaches have, however, continued. One highly innovative flow cytometric approach employs fluorescence resonance energy transfer between patient autoantibodies and known anti-GP IIb/IIIa or anti-GP Ib/IX monoclonal antibodies to increase the specificity of antibody detection (Koksch, 1995). However, this test has not been widely employed, because of difficulties in standardization. Some laboratories have also used the monoclonal antibody immobilization of platelet antigen (MAIPA) approach to detect autoantibody, either obtained directly from patient serum or eluted from patient platelets, which is directed at specific platelet glycoprotein complexes (Kiefel, 1987; Hewitt, 1994; Clofent-Sanchez, 1996; Cordiano, 1996). Because MAIPA assays preserve platelet target antigens in a more native form than most preceding techniques, MAIPA has generally achieved status as the 'gold standard' for the detection of specific antiplatelet antibodies. It is accordingly of interest that results closely matching those of the MAIPA assay have recently been reported employing an innovative, multicolor flow cytometric technique (Nguyen, 2004). Continuing evaluation of these and other techniques may be relevant, if laboratory methods are to occupy a central role in the evaluation of ITP (Beardsley, 1998).

Drug-induced thrombocytopenia

Drug-induced thrombocytopenia must always be considered as a cause for acute thrombocytopenia. This can be particularly difficult to identify in patients who are on multiple drugs. Certain drugs such as heparin, quinidine, gold, and sulfa antibiotics, however, have had a relatively higher frequency of causing thrombocytopenia than most other drugs. Particularly in the case of these drugs, the laboratory may play a helpful role in identifying the offending agent if an increase in patient antibody directed against a platelet target using one of the assays described above for ITP can be demonstrated by the in vitro inclusion of that drug in the assay. It is interesting that whereas virtually all normal platelets possess a binding site for antiplatelet antibodies arising in patients with a hypersensitivity to quinidine or to quinine, platelets from patients with Bernard–Soulier disease do not appear to have this receptor (Kunicki, 1978b). Berndt (1985) has provided evidence that such antibodies may be binding to glycoprotein IX, to the β subunit of glycoprotein Ib, or to a region defined by the association of glycoproteins Ib and IX. It has been suggested by Pfueller (1988), however, that quinine- and quinidine-induced thrombocytopenia may result from antibodies that are quite heterogeneous among patients, recognizing neoantigens composed either of various epitopes on the platelet surface and the drug, or of new conformations of platelet glycoproteins induced by the drug. Additionally, in some patients quinidine-dependent antibodies may also be directed against epitopes present within the GP IIb/IIIa complex (Pfueller, 1988; Chong, 1991; Visentin, 1991; Nieminen, 1992).

Platelet GP IIb/IIIa antagonist drugs such as abciximab, eptifibatide, tirofiban, and a number of other parenteral or oral agents have been developed to inhibit platelet responsiveness. A variety of techniques have been developed to monitor receptor occupancy of the GP IIb/IIIa in order to optimize dosage (Greilich, 1999; Quinn, 1999). In addition to the anticipated inhibition of platelet function, some patients may experience varying degrees of thrombocytopenia acutely following even a single exposure to GP IIb/IIIa antagonists (Madan, 1999). The acute thrombocytopenia results from drug-dependent, pre-existing antibodies that bind to the GP IIb/IIIa complex; additionally, drug-dependent antibodies may subsequently arise as an immune response to the drug administration (Aster, 2004).

Heparin-induced thrombocytopenia

Exposure by drug of an otherwise unexposed epitope of a naturally occurring platelet protein may also be the underlying etiology of heparin-induced thrombocytopenia (HIT). In this disorder, patients receiving heparin therapy develop antibodies that appear to bind by their Fab'_2 region to PF4 that has been released from their intracellular storage sites (Amiral, 1999). The HIT antibody specificity is thought to be directed against epitopes within PF4 that are exposed when heparin–PF4 complexes have formed (Rauova, 2005), as described in greater detail in Chapter 41. Assays have accordingly been developed that employ PF4 complexed to heparin or a similar partner molecule as a target for antibodies in the serum of patients suspected of having HIT (Amiral, 1992). In contrast to the antigen assays are a series of platelet activation assays, in which patient plasma or serum is incubated with washed test platelets and one or more of a variety of downstream events are then measured. Such events have included measurement of secretion of radioactive serotonin previously taken up by the platelets; chemiluminescent release of endogenous adenine nucleotide; platelet aggregation; and production of platelet microparticles (Warkentin, 1999a). Successful

performance of the platelet activation assays is technically demanding, and in particular is dependent upon the selection of platelet donors whose platelets are sensitive to activation by HIT sera. In general, the antigen assays tend to be more sensitive to the presence of HIT antibody formation than do the platelet activation assays, and can be useful for monitoring subclinical HIT antibody seroconversion (Zwicker, 2004). On the other hand, because of the greater sensitivity of the antigen assays for subclinical antibody detection, it has been suggested that the platelet activation assays may actually have greater positive predictive value for clinical HIT (Warkentin, 1999a). A recent study employing enzyme immunoassays has found, interestingly, that testing exclusively for IgG antibodies increases diagnostic specificity through avoidance of frequent nonpathogenic antibodies of the IgM and IgA classes (Warkentin, 2005a). Detailed guidelines for the integration of laboratory testing for HIT in patients receiving heparin have recently been published (Warkentin, 2004; Zwicker, 2004). Of particular note is the recent evidence-based guideline recommending against routine HIT antibody testing in the absence of thrombocytopenia, thrombosis, heparin-induced skin lesions, or other sequelae of HIT; routine platelet count monitoring of patients receiving heparin therapy, in contrast, can be of invaluable help in correctly identifying those patients requiring more specific HIT testing (Warkentin, 2004). In patients for whom a diagnosis of HIT is established, alternative forms of anticoagulant therapy need to be instituted, such as with the direct thrombin inhibitors lepirudin or argatroban. Laboratory monitoring of the direct thrombin inhibitors is discussed in Chapter 41.

In cases where the etiology of a patient's thrombocytopenia remains unclear despite thorough evaluation, assessment of platelet survival may be considered. This may be accomplished by labeling either the patient's own or heterologous platelets with a radioactive isotope and following the survival of the reinfused platelets. The chromium-51 and DF phosphorus-32 labels used in the past provide a number of methodologic problems, and have been largely supplanted by indium-111 (Heaton, 1979, 1989; Leissinger, 2001). While successful measurement of platelet life span using the nonradioactive label biotin has been reported in dogs (Heilmann, 1993) and in mice (Ault, 1995; Manning, 1996), this method has not been applied in humans. Assessment of platelet kinetics is not normally part of the evaluation of thrombocytopenic patients. In exceptional cases of chronic thrombocytopenias refractory to treatment, however, some groups have found measurement of platelet lifespan helpful in distinguishing between disorders of platelet production and platelet destruction, particularly in the context of a decision concerning possible splenectomy (Rossi, 2002; Bader-Meunier, 2003).

Thrombotic thrombocytopenic purpura

Until recently, the microangiopathic disorders referred to as thrombotic thrombocytopenic purpura (TTP) and the hemolytic–uremic syndrome (HUS) were widely considered to be close relatives better distinguished on the basis of clinical presentation than upon laboratory findings. This situation changed dramatically in 1998, with two independent groups (Furlan, 1998; Tsai, 1998) demonstrating that the pathogenesis of TTP was related to deficient activity of a plasma vWF-cleaving metalloproteinase, now known as ADAMTS-13. This results in unusually large vWF molecules (so-called 'UlvWF') that are capable of binding to platelets and producing platelet thrombi in the microcirculation (Moake, 1986; Tsai, 1998). In contrast, vWF-cleaving protease activity appears to be normal in HUS (Furlan, 1998). Both the sensitivity and the specificity of plasma ADAMTS-13 levels for the diagnosis of TTP have, however, been called into question in a number of studies. Thus neither the presence of a normal level of ADAMTS-13 (implying normal gene product) nor the absence of demonstrable neutralizing antibodies in the plasma of patients otherwise meeting clinical criteria for TTP is sufficient to exclude this diagnosis (George, 2004; Peyvandi, 2004). Patients with a variety of systemic connective tissue disorders (Mannucci, 2003), as well as those with ITP, disseminated intravascular coagulation, and a variety of other disorders have also been found to have decreased levels of ADAMTS-13 (Moore, 2001). The extent to which these findings reflect idiosyncrasies of the particular testing approaches employed to date, as opposed to reflecting shared or distinct pathophysiological mechanisms among these diverse disorders, is presently unresolved. Certainly the assays originally developed involved a great number of steps in the testing process, including reacting the patient's plasma with a protease-free vWF substrate previously denatured with guanidine or urea, performing gel electrophoresis on the degraded vWF, immunoblotting, and then demonstrating an abnormal persistence of higher-molecular-weight vWF multimers. There have been continual efforts to simplify and shorten the required time for ADAMTS-13 assays. One of the earliest modifications of this method was in the final step, where a technically less demanding ELISA assay of the residual ability of vWF to bind to a collagen-coated surface was substituted for vWF multimeric analysis (Gerritsen, 1999). More recently,

Table 39–5 Reactive Conditions in Which Elevated Platelet Counts May be Found

Transient processes
Acute blood loss
Recover ('rebound') from thrombocytopenia
Acute infection or inflammation
Response to exercise

Sustained processes
Iron deficiency
Hemolytic anemia
Asplenia (e.g., after splenectomy)
Cancer
Chronic inflammatory or infectious diseases
    Connective tissue disorders
    Temporal arteritis
    Inflammatory bowel disease
    Tuberculosis
    Chronic pneumonitis
    Drug reactions
    Vincristine
    All-*trans*-retinoic acid
    Cytokines
    Growth factors

Source: with permission from Schafer AI: Thrombocytosis. N Engl J Med 2004; 350:1211–1219.

Table 39–6 Clinical Findings That May Distinguish Between Clonal and Secondary (Reactive) Thrombocytosis

Finding	Clonal Thrombocytosis*	Secondary (Reactive) Thrombocytosis
Underlying systemic disease	No	Often clinically apparent
Digital or cerebrovascular ischemia	Characteristic	No
Large-vessel arterial or venous thrombosis	Increased risk	No
Bleeding complications	Increased risk	No
Splenomegaly	Yes, in about 40% of patients	No
Peripheral blood smear	Giant platelets	Normal platelets
Platelet function	May be abnormal	Normal
Bone marrow megakaryocytes:		
Number	Increased	Increased
Morphologic features	Giant, dysplastic forms with increased ploidy; associated with large masses of platelet debris	Normal

* Clonal thrombocytosis includes essential thrombocythemia and other myeloproliferative disorders

Source: with permission from Schafer AI: Thrombocytosis. N Engl J Med 2004; 350:1211–1219.

efforts have been directed towards the development of one-step, simplified assays of plasma proteolytic activity against molecules recapitulating the critical residues of vWF required for proteolysis by ADAMTS-13 (Kokame, 2004; Whitelock, 2004). While such assays offer the clear advantage of turn-around-times compatible with real-time diagnostic decision-making, their potential role in such decision-making is not yet clear.

Thrombocytosis

Increased platelet counts, or thrombocytosis, may be seen both as a benign, reactive process (Table 39–5) and as a manifestation of a myeloproliferative

Table 39–7 Classification of Inherited Disorders of Platelet Function

1. Defects in platelet–vessel wall interaction (disorders of adhesion)
  a. von Willebrand disease (deficiency or defect in plasma von Willebrand factor)
  b. Bernard–Soulier syndrome (deficiency or defect in GP Ib/IX)
2. Defects in platelet–platelet interaction (disorders of aggregation)
  a. Congenital afibrinogenemia (deficiency of plasma fibrinogen)
  b. Glanzmann's thrombasthenia (deficiency or defect in GP IIb/IIIa)
3. Disorders of platelet secretion and abnormalities of granules
  i. Storage pool deficiency
  ii. Quebec platelet disorder
4. Disorders of platelet secretion and signal transduction defects (primary secretion defects)
  i. Defects in platelet–agonist interaction (receptor defects)
    Receptor defects: thromboxane A_2, collagen, ADP, epinephrine
  ii. Defects in G-protein activation
    • $G\alpha_q$ deficiency
    • $G\alpha_s$ abnormalities
    • $G\alpha_{i1}$ deficiency
  iii. Defects in phosphatidylinositol metabolism
    Phospholipase C-β2 deficiency
  iv. Defects in calcium mobilization
  v. Defects in protein phosphorylation (pleckstrin)
    • PKC-θ deficiency
  vi. Abnormalities in arachidonic acid pathways and thromboxane A_2 synthesis
    • Impaired liberation of arachidonic acid
    • Cyclooxygenase deficiency
    • Thromboxane synthase deficiency
5. Defects in cytoskeletal regulation
  Wiskott–Aldrich syndrome
6. Disorders of platelet coagulant–protein interaction (membrane phospholipids defects)
  Scott syndrome
7. Miscellaneous

Source: modified with permission from Rao AK: Congenital disorders of platelet function: disorders of signal transduction and secretion. Am J Med Sci 1998; 316:69–76.

disorder (Griesshammer, 1999; Schafer, 2004). The blood film should confirm an electronic cell count, showing that the increased particles in fact correspond to platelets and not to cell fragments or other entities. The smear also affords an opportunity to assess deviations in platelet size, morphologic appearance, and clumping tendencies. Clues as to whether one is dealing with an autonomous clonal process or a reactive secondary process may be provided by a number of clinical and laboratory findings (Table 39–6).

It has been stated that reactive processes typically do not produce platelet counts over 1000×10^9/L but that myeloproliferative processes frequently do; nonetheless, this criterion is reliable neither for diagnosis nor for the decision as to whether to institute antiplatelet therapy. Particularly in the case of myeloproliferative syndromes, the individual patient may be asymptomatic, have a tendency to bleed, or have a tendency to develop thrombotic events; at present, the most appropriate clinical approach appears to be a response to such tendencies once they become evident. Unless additional risk factors are present, thrombotic events are less likely to occur in secondary than in primary thrombocytosis (Griesshammer, 1999). In documented cases of myeloproliferative syndromes there have been reports of abnormalities in platelet and megakaryocyte structure, platelet surface membrane receptors, platelet aggregation patterns, platelet coagulant activity, and arachidonic acid metabolism. Despite statistically significant abnormalities when populations of patients with myeloproliferative disorders or with reactive thrombocytosis are compared, in the individual patient platelet sizing parameters and platelet function studies are unlikely to be capable of differentiating these disorders (Sehayek, 1988).

Inherited Disorders of Platelet Function

Table 39–7 provides a classification based on the platelet functions or responses that are abnormal (Fig. 39–7). Although some of these disorders are rare, they shed enormous light on platelet physiology. In patients with defects in platelet–vessel-wall interactions (adhesion disorders), adhesion of platelets to subendothelium is abnormal. The two disorders in this group are von Willebrand disease (vWD), due to a deficiency or abnormality in plasma vWF, and the Bernard–Soulier syndrome (BSS), in which platelets are deficient in GP Ib (and GP V and GP IX); in both, platelet–vWF interaction is compromised. Disorders characterized by abnormal platelet–platelet interactions (aggregation disorders) arise because of a severe deficiency of plasma fibrinogen (congenital afibrinogenemia) or because of a quantitative or qualitative abnormality of the platelet membrane GP IIb–IIIa complex, which binds fibrinogen (Glanzmann thrombasthenia). Patients with defects in platelet secretion and signal transduction are a heterogeneous group lumped together for convenience of classification rather than on the basis of an understanding of the specific underlying abnormality. The major common characteristics in these patients, as currently perceived, are abnormal aggregation responses and an inability to release intracellular granule (dense) contents upon activation of platelet-rich plasma with agonists such as ADP, epinephrine, and collagen. In aggregation studies the second wave of aggregation is blunted or absent. A small proportion of these patients have a deficiency of dense granule stores (storage pool deficiency). In some of the other patients, the impaired secretion results from aberrations in the signal transduction events that govern end responses such as secretion and aggregation. Lastly, some patients have an abnormality in interactions of platelets with proteins of the coagulation system; the best described is the Scott syndrome. In addition to the above groups, there are patients who have abnormal platelet function associated with systemic disorders such as Down syndrome and the May–Hegglin anomaly, where the specific aberrant platelet mechanisms are still unclear.

Disorders of Platelet Adhesion

Bernard–Soulier syndrome

Bernard–Soulier syndrome is a rare autosomal recessive platelet function disorder resulting from an abnormality in platelet GP Ib–IX complex, which mediates the binding of vWF to platelets and thus plays a major role in platelet adhesion to the subendothelium, especially at the higher shear rates. GP Ib exists in platelets as a complex consisting of GP Ib, GP IX, and GP V. There are approximately 25 000 copies of GP Ib/IX on platelets, and these are reduced or abnormal in the BSS. Although GP V is also decreased in BSS platelets, it is not required for platelet surface GP Ib/IX expression. The bleeding time is markedly prolonged, the platelet counts are moderately decreased, and, on the peripheral smear, the platelets are increased in size. In platelet aggregation studies, the responses to the commonly used agonists ADP, epinephrine, thrombin, and collagen are normal. Characteristically, the aggregation in platelet-rich plasma in response to ristocetin is decreased or absent, a feature shared with patients with vWD. However, plasma vWF and factor VIII are normal in BSS. Secretion (dense granule) on activation with thrombin may be decreased.

The blood film from a patient with BSS may resemble that from some patients with ITP in that the platelets tend to be larger than normal and there is a mild to moderate thrombocytopenia. Findings in the aggregometer are almost the reciprocal of those in Glanzmann thrombasthenia: aggregation and release are normal with all agents *except* ristocetin. In addition, the release reaction induced by thrombin may be decreased.

Unlike vWD, in which there is also diminished platelet agglutination in response to ristocetin, in BSS the addition of exogenous vWF (present in plasma cryoprecipitate fractions) does not restore ristocetin-induced agglutination of platelets. This important difference is attributable to the finding that, whereas in vWD there is a deficiency in plasma vWF, in BSS the deficiency is in the platelet membrane receptor to which the vWF must bind for normal hemostasis.

When platelet surface membrane glycoproteins from patients with BSS are analyzed (Fig. 39–2), there is a striking decrease in glycoprotein Ib (Nurden, 1975). When very sensitive techniques for detection of this glycoprotein are employed, residual amounts of Ib may, however, be detected (Drouin, 1988; Finch, 1990). Molecular studies have identified a variety of specific point mutations or deletions in GP Ibα, GP Ibβ, and GP IX that, when present in homozygous or doubly heterozygous fashion, result in a classic BSS phenotype. A point mutation in the leucine-rich region of the GP Ibα chain may also produce a Bernard–Soulier phenotype even when expressed only by a single allele (Miller, 1992; Ware, 1993).

Abnormalities of Glycoprotein Ia/IIa and Glycoprotein VI

Nieuwenhuis (1985, 1986) reported the absence of the high-molecular-weight (168 kDa) glycoprotein Ia in a 33-year-old woman with a mild

bleeding disorder, whose platelets showed no response to collagen. Kehrel (1988) identified a second female patient with similar findings but whose platelets additionally had a lack of intact thrombospondin. Most interestingly, not only the bleeding tendency but also the structural and functional platelet abnormalities disappeared at the onset of menopause in this patient. Abnormalities of GP VI have been associated with increased bleeding tendencies; additionally, polymorphisms of GP VI are being studied as possible risk factors for thrombosis (Moroi, 1989; Arai, 1995; Nieswandt, 2001; Cabeza, 2004; Nurden, 2004; Yee, 2004).

Von Willebrand Disease

See section on 'von Willebrand factor and von Willebrand disease' below.

Disorders of Platelet Aggregation

Glanzmann Thrombasthenia

Glanzmann thrombasthenia is a rare autosomal recessive disorder characterized by markedly impaired platelet aggregation, a prolonged bleeding time, and relatively more severe mucocutaneous bleeding manifestations than most platelet function disorders (Nurden, 2001). It has been reported in clusters in populations where consanguinity is common. Normal resting platelets possess approximately 50 000–80 000 GP IIb/IIIa complexes on the surface. The primary abnormality in thrombasthenia is a quantitative or qualitative defect in the GP IIb/IIIa complex, a heterodimer consisting of GP IIb and GP IIIa whose synthesis is governed by distinct genes located on chromosome 17. Thus, thrombasthenia may arise due to a mutation in either gene, with decreased platelet expression of the complex. Because of this, fibrinogen binding to platelets on activation and aggregation are impaired. A variety of distinct mutations involving GP IIb and GP IIIa have been described in patients with thrombasthenia (French, 2000). Clot retraction, a function of the interaction of the GP IIb/IIIa with the platelet cytoskeleton, is also impaired.

In nonanticoagulated blood films prepared from patients with Glanzmann thrombasthenia, platelets are present in normal number and appearance but show a characteristic tendency to remain isolated, without the platelet–platelet clumping seen in normal blood films. The diagnostic hallmark of thrombasthenia is absence or marked decrease of platelet aggregation (Figure 39–8) in response to virtually all platelet agonists (except ristocetin), with absence of both the primary and secondary wave of aggregation; the shape change response is preserved. Platelet dense granule secretion may be decreased with weak agonists (e.g., ADP) but normal on activation with thrombin. Heterozygotes have approximately half the number of platelet GP IIb/IIIa complexes, but platelet aggregation responses are completely normal.

Because the platelet antigen Pl^{A1} is associated with glycoprotein IIIa, this antigen is typically decreased in patients with Glanzmann thrombasthenia (Kunicki, 1978a; von dem Borne, 1981). Relative estimation of platelet glycoprotein IIb/IIIa molecules through binding of specific monoclonal antibodies permits diagnosis of Glanzmann thrombasthenia by flow cytometry requiring only small volumes of blood for the assay (Montgomery, 1983; Kempfer, 1991). Although not ordinarily part of routine clinical diagnostic studies, platelet glycoprotein analyses such as are shown in Figure 39–2 were of considerable historical importance in demonstrating the structure–function relationships of such disorders. Definitive characterization of true homozygosity or compound heterozygosity for different mutations may be undertaken by molecular techniques (Bray, 1994; French, 1998; Rosenberg, 1998; Ruan, 1998; Gonzalez-Manchon, 1999). Although congenital afibrinogenemia is also characterized by a similar absence of platelet aggregation, in this disorder the PT, APTT, and thrombin time are markedly prolonged, whereas they are normal in thrombasthenia.

Disorders of Platelet Secretion and Signal Transduction

As a unifying theme, patients lumped in this heterogeneous group generally manifest impaired secretion of granule contents and absence of the second wave of aggregation upon stimulation of platelet-rich plasma with ADP or epinephrine; responses to collagen, thromboxane analog (U46619), arachidonic acid, and platelet-activating factor (PAF) may also be impaired. Conceptually, platelet function is abnormal in these patients either when the granule contents are diminished (storage pool deficiency, SPD) or when there is an aberration in the activation mechanisms governing aggregation and secretion (Table 39–6).

Deficiency of Granule Stores

The term SPD refers to patients with deficiencies in platelet content of dense granules (δ-SPD), α granules (α-SPD) or both types of granule (αδ-SPD) (Hayward, 1997; Rao, 2005b). The Quebec platelet disorder is an autosomal dominant bleeding disorder associated with abnormal proteolysis and deficiency of α-granule proteins (Kahr, 2001; McKay, 2004).

Patients with δ-storage pool deficiency (δ-SPD) have a mild to moderate bleeding diathesis associated with a prolonged bleeding time. In the platelet studies, the second wave of aggregation in response to ADP and epinephrine is absent or blunted, and the collagen response is markedly impaired. However, both impaired (Weiss, 1981) and normal (Ingerman, 1978) aggregation responses to arachidonic acid have been noted. The responses to epinephrine may also be variable; a second wave of aggregation is noted in some patients (Weiss, 1988). Interestingly, δ-SPD has been documented (Nieuwenhuis, 1987; Israels, 1990) in a number of patients with prolonged bleeding times and normal aggregation responses. Thrombin-induced secretion of acid hydrolases is also impaired in SPD platelets; this is corrected by addition of exogenous ADP.

Normal platelets possess three to eight dense granules (each 200–300 nm in diameter) (Israels, 1990). Under the electron microscope, dense granules are decreased in SPD platelets (White, 1971; Israels, 1990). Other methods to demonstrate a decrease in the dense granules include fluorescence microscopy after staining platelets with mepacrine (quinacrine), which localizes in the dense granules because of high affinity for ATP; and specific staining by uranyl ions (uranaffin reaction) of both the membrane and core of the dense granules. Flow cytometry can also be applied to assess the fluorescent staining of dense granules (Linden, 2004). By direct biochemical measurements, the total platelet and granule ATP and ADP contents are decreased (Holmsen, 1979) along with other dense granule constituents, calcium, pyrophosphate, and serotonin. Two-thirds of platelet ATP and ADP resides in the dense granules with a smaller amount in the metabolic pool, and there is proportionally more ADP than ATP in dense granules (Holmsen, 1979). Thus, in δ-SPD platelets the ratio of total ATP to ADP increases (>2.5) compared to normal platelets. Incubation of normal platelets with carbon-14-serotonin results in its incorporation into dense granules, and subsequent secretion upon activation. In SPD platelets the initial rate of uptake of carbon-14-serotonin is normal, but the saturation levels and its retention over 4–6 hours are decreased.

Other abnormalities reported in δ-SPD include decreased synthesis of prostaglandins, TxA$_2$ and malondialdehyde in platelets activated with collagen and epinephrine, but not arachidonate (Weiss, 1988), impaired liberation of arachidonic acid from membrane phospholipids (Rendu, 1978), and enhanced ADP- but not thrombin-induced rise in cytoplasmic Ca^{2+} levels (Lages, 1997). Platelet procoagulant activity (prothrombinase activity) induced upon activation has been reported to be impaired in association with an inability to maintain elevated intracellular Ca^{2+} levels (Weiss, 1997).

δ-SPD has been reported in association with other inherited disorders such as the Hermansky–Pudlak syndrome (HPS) (oculocutaneous albinism and increased reticuloendothelial ceroid), the Chediak–Higashi syndrome, the Wiskott–Aldrich syndrome, the thrombocytopenia–absent-radii syndrome and Griscelli syndrome (Menasche, 2000; Gunay-Aygun, 2004). The simultaneous occurrence of δ-SPD and defects in skin pigment granules, as in HPS, point to the interrelatedness of the two kinds of granules with respect to genetic control, a concept further advanced by animal models (Novak, 1984, 1985; Huizing, 2001; Gunay-Aygun, 2004).

Dense granule membranes possess the lysosomal proteins lysosomal-associated membrane protein (LAMP)2 and CD63 (granulophysin or LAMP3) (Nishibori, 1993; Israels, 1996) as well as P-selectin and GP IIb/IIIa. Granulophysin is deficient in HPS platelets (Gerrard, 1991). Studies with antigranulophysin antibody demonstrated the presence of the normal number of granules in platelets of two non-albino SPD patients (McNicol, 1994); these patients, therefore, have the granules but with reduced contents.

A substantial amount of our information in SPD has been obtained from patients with HPS, which is characterized by oculocutaneous albinism, platelet SPD, and lipofuscinosis (Gunay-Aygun, 2004). There is a large group of HPS patients in north-west Puerto Rico, where HPS occurs in 1 in every 1800 individuals (gene frequency 1 in 21) (Witkop, 1990). There are at least seven known HPS-causing genes leading to 7 subtypes of human HPS with most patients being in HPS-1 and from Puerto Rico (Gunay-Aygun, 2004). There are at least 14 mouse models of HPS reported to date; seven of these constitute models for the human subtypes (Gunay-Aygun, 2004). Together, the human and mouse models have been an invaluable source of information about vesicle formation and trafficking. The human

HPS subtypes are autosomal recessive, and the heterozygotes have no clinical findings. In addition to the albinism, which is variable between the HPS subtypes, most patients have congenital nystagmus and decreased visual acuity. There are two additional manifestations in HPS patients: granulomatous colitis and pulmonary fibrosis (Gunay-Aygun, 2004).

Chediak–Higashi syndrome is a rare autosomal recessive disorder characterized by SPD, oculocutaneous albinism, immune deficiency, neurological dysfunction, and the presence of giant cytoplasmic inclusions in different cells. (Huizing, 2001). Chediak–Higashi syndrome patients have defective cytotoxic T and natural killer (NK) cell function. It arises from mutations in the lysosomal trafficking regulator (LYST) gene on chromosome 1. The protein coded by this gene interacts with several proteins, including the SNARE complex protein HRS and signaling proteins, and participates in intracellular membrane fusion reactions and vesicle trafficking (Tchernev, 2002).

The rubric 'gray platelet syndrome' (GPS) has been derived from the initial observation by Raccuglia (1971) of a gray appearance of platelets with paucity of granules in peripheral blood smears from a patient with a lifelong bleeding disorder. Characterized by an isolated deficiency of α-granule contents, GPS patients have a lifelong bleeding diathesis of autosomal recessive inheritance, mild thrombocytopenia, and a prolonged bleeding time (Weiss, 1979; Gerrard, 1980). Under the electron microscope, platelets and megakaryocytes reveal absent or markedly decreased α granules (Levy-Toledano, 1981). The platelets are severely and selectively deficient in α-granule proteins: PF4, β-thromboglobulin, vWF, thrombospondin, fibronectin, factor V, high-molecular-weight kininogen, and PDGF(Gerrard, 1980; Nurden, 1982). Platelet aggregation responses have been variable. Responses to ADP and epinephrine were normal in most patients; in some patients aggregation responses to thrombin, collagen, and ADP have been impaired. Impaired thrombin-induced Ca^{2+} mobilization and an increase in Ca^{2+} transport has been reported in some patients.

Plasma levels of PF4 and βTG have been found to be raised (Gerrard, 1980), suggesting that the defect is not in their synthesis by megakaryocytes but in their packaging into granules. Studies on megakaryocytes cultured from peripheral blood of three GPS patients show that vWF is synthesized but is secreted into extracellular space instead of normal α-granule packaging (Drouin, 2001). The neutrophils from these patients also had decreased granules. There is increased reticulin in the bone marrow from GPS patients (Breton-Gorius, 1981; Levy-Toledano, 1981), attributed to elevated plasma PDGF levels. Using cDNA microarrays Hyman (2003) found upregulation of cytoskeletal proteins, including fibronectin 1, thrombospondins 1 and 2, and collagen VIα in fibroblasts from a GPS patient.

The Quebec platelet disorder is an autosomal dominant disorder associated with delayed bleeding and abnormal proteolysis of α-granule proteins due to increased amounts of platelet urokinase type plasminogen activator (Kahr, 2001; McKay, 2004). These patients are characterized by normal to reduced platelet counts, proteolytic degradation of soluble and membrane proteins of the α granules, deficiency of an α-granule factor V binding protein called multimerin, and defective aggregation selectively with epinephrine. Platelet factor V but not plasma factor V is degraded along with other α-granule proteins, fibrinogen, vWF, thrombospondin, osteonectin, fibronectin, and P-selectin. The platelets contain increased fibrinolytic activity. In contrast to the gray platelet syndrome, platelets appear morphologically normal under the light microscope. Patients with Quebec platelet disorder suffer from mucocutaneous bleeding, which is often delayed by 12–24 hours following injury and unresponsive to platelet transfusions but responsive to fibrinolytic inhibitors (McKay, 2004).

Defects in Platelet Signal Transduction

Signal transduction mechanisms encompass processes that are initiated by the interaction of agonists with specific platelet receptors and include responses such as G-protein activation and activation of effector enzymes such as phospholipase C and phospholipase A$_2$. If the key components in signal transduction are the surface receptors, the G-proteins, and the effectors, evidence now exists for specific platelet abnormalities at each of these levels.

Patients with defects in platelet–agonist interaction have impaired responses because of an abnormality in the platelet surface receptor for a specific agonist. Such receptor defects have been documented for epinephrine, collagen, ADP, and TxA$_2$ (Rao, 2004). Hirata (1994) described an Arg 60 to Leu mutation of the human TxA$_2$ receptor in a dominantly inherited bleeding disorder. Patients described by Cattaneo (1992; 1997) and Nurden (1995) have had a defect in the P2Y12 ADP receptor, which is coupled to inhibition of adenylyl cyclase. Because ADP and TxA$_2$ play a synergistic role in platelet responses to several agonists, these patients manifest abnormal responses to multiple agonists. More recently specific

V

deficiencies in the P2Y1(Oury, 1999) and P2X (Oury, 2000) ADP receptors have been documented. A few patients have been described in whom isolated blunting of platelet responses to collagen are associated with deficiencies in membrane glycoproteins GP Ia and GP VI (Kahn, 2004).

G-proteins are a heterogeneous group of proteins that link surface receptors and intracellular effector enzymes, and defects in G-protein activation can impair signal transduction. Patients with deficiencies at the level of $G\alpha_q$ (Gabbeta, 1997), and $G\alpha_{i1}$ (Patel, 2003) have been described. The patient with the $G\alpha_q$ deficiency had a mild bleeding disorder, abnormal aggregation and secretion responses to a number of agonists, and diminished GTPase activity (a reflection of G-protein α-subunit function) on activation. Essentially identical abnormal platelet findings have been reported in the $G\alpha_q$-deficient knockout mice (Offermanns, 1997).

Signal transduction is additionally impaired by defects in phospholipase C activation, calcium mobilization, and pleckstrin phosphorylation. Several patients have been identified who have a relatively mild bleeding diathesis and impaired dense granule secretion, although their platelets have normal granule stores and, in general, synthesize substantial amounts of TxA_2. On laboratory testing, these patients have abnormal aggregation and secretion particularly in response to weaker agonists (ADP, epinephrine, PAF); the response to relatively stronger agonists such as arachidonate and high concentrations of collagen may be normal. Such patients appear to be more common than those with SPD or defects in TxA_2 synthesis. Defects in early platelet activation events, including Ca^{2+} mobilization, phosphatidylinositol hydrolysis, and phosphorylation of pleckstrin (a protein phosphorylated by protein kinase C), have been described (Rao, 2004). Specific deficiencies at the level of phospholipase C-β_2 (Lee, 1996; Yang, 1996) and protein kinase C-θ (Sun, 2004) have been documented.

Activation of GP IIb/IIIa and platelet fibrinogen-binding is a prerequisite for aggregation and is a signal-transduction-dependent process. Defects in GP IIb/IIIa activation due to upstream signal transduction defects have been noted in some patients (Gabbeta, 1996).

A major platelet response to activation is liberation of arachidonic acid from phospholipids and its subsequent oxygenation to TxA_2, which plays a synergistic role in the response to several agonists. Patients have been described with impaired liberation of arachidonic acid from membrane phospholipids during platelet stimulation as well as with congenital deficiencies of cyclooxygenase and thromboxane synthase (Rao, 2004).

Defects in Cytoskeletal Assembly

Wiskott–Aldrich syndrome is an X-linked inherited disorder affecting T lymphocytes and platelets, characterized by thrombocytopenia, immunodeficiency, and eczema (Remold-O'Donnell, 1996). The bleeding manifestations are variable. Several platelet abnormalities, including dense granule deficiency and deficiencies of platelet GP Ib, GP IIb/IIIa, and GP Ia, have been reported. Wiskott–Aldrich syndrome arises from mutations in the gene coding for a novel protein of 502 amino acids that binds to several other signaling proteins including Cdc42 (a GTPase) and p47nck (a SH3-containing adapter protein) (Remold-O'Donnell, 1996; Zigmond, 2000). This protein constitutes a link between the cytoskeleton and signaling pathways, and is a key regulator of cytoskeletal assembly.

Disorders of Platelet Procoagulant Activities

Platelets play a major role in blood coagulation by providing the surface on which several specific key enzymatic reactions occur. As discussed previously, in resting platelets, there is an asymmetry in the distribution of some of the phospholipids such that phosphatidylserine (PS) and phosphatidylethanolamine are located predominantly on the inner leaflet while phosphatidylcholine has the opposite distribution. Platelet activation results in a redistribution with expression of PS on the outer surface, mediated by phospholipid scramblase (Fig. 39–3). The exposure of PS on the outer surface is an important event in the expression of platelet procoagulant activities. A few patients have been described in whom the platelet contribution to blood coagulation is impaired, and this is referred to as Scott syndrome (Weiss, 1994; Solum, 1999b). In these patients, who have a bleeding disorder, the bleeding time and platelet aggregation responses have been normal, along with a normal PT and PTT. In the patient described by Weiss (1994), platelet factor Xa binding sites as well as the binding of factors IXa and VIIIa were diminished, associated with a decreased surface expression of PS following platelet activation.

Relative Frequencies of Various Platelet Congenital Abnormalities

Thrombasthenia and BSS are rare disorders. Although there are no published data, patients currently classified in the heterogenous category

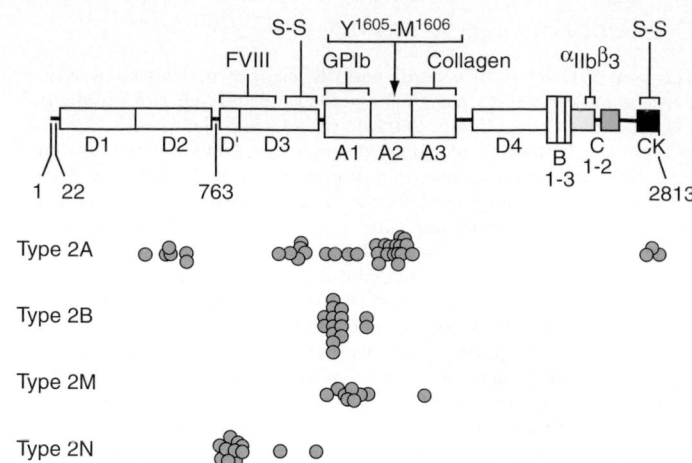

Figure 39–10 Structure of von Willebrand factor (vWF) and mutations in von Willebrand disease (vWD) type 2. The vWF precursor consists of a signal peptide (residues 1–22), a propeptide (residues 23–763), and the mature subunit (residues 764–2813). The locations are indicated for repeated domains (A, B, C, D, CK); binding sites for factor VIII (FVIII), platelet glycoprotein Ib (GP Ib), collagen, and integrin $\alpha_{IIb}\beta_3$; intersubunit disulfide bonds (S–S); and the Tyr–Met bond cleaved by ADAMTS13 (Y^{1605}–M^{1606}). Below the schematic structure of vWF are shown the locations of mutations that cause specific subtypes of vWD type 2. (Sadler JE: New concepts in von Willebrand disease. Annu Rev Med 2005; 56:175, fig. 1. Reprinted, with permission, from the *Annual Review of Medicine*, Volume 56 © 2005 by Annual Reviews www.annualreviews.org.)

of defects in platelet secretion and signal transduction probably constitute the more frequently encountered inherited platelet function abnormalities, excluding vWD. In our experience, the SPD is present in less than 10–15% of patients with congenital platelet defects. Abnormalities in thromboxane production occur in about 20% of these patients. A large proportion of the remaining patients with abnormal aggregation and secretion demonstrate adequate dense granule stores and produce substantial amounts of TxA_2. In some of these patients there is evidence for defects in the signaling mechanisms (Rao, 2004).

Von Willebrand Factor and von Willebrand Disease

Von Willebrand Factor Biology

Von Willebrand factor is a pivotal protein in hemostasis, playing key roles both in primary hemostasis and in secondary hemostasis. In the latter role, vWF serves as a carrier protein for factor VIII – in the absence of vWF, factor VIII is rapidly cleared from the plasma (see Ch. 39). With respect to primary hemostasis, vWF serves as an adhesive platelet ligand that tethers the platelet to exposed collagen at sites of vascular injury. vWF circulating in the blood plasma derives from secretion by endothelial cells. This secretion has a major constitutive component, but there is additionally a releasable pool of vWF that is stored in the endothelial Weibel–Palade bodies. Megakaryocytes also synthesize vWF, which is stored in the platelet α granules. This pool of vWF is released only upon platelet activation, as part of the more general platelet release reaction. Although such released vWF would generally not be capable of raising the overall level of vWF in the plasma appreciably, local increase of vWF at sites of injury may be significant.

The vWF gene is located on chromosome 12, and is 178 kB long, extending over 52 exons. The presence of a partial, but nonfunctional, duplication of the vWF gene on chromosome 22 (vWF pseudogene) is an important consideration in the design of primers for amplification of the vWF gene. Following cleavage of an N-terminal propolypeptide fragment, the mature 2050 amino acid vWF protein is composed of a series of functional domains, as shown in Figure 39–10. The individual vWF monomeric units are bound together by a series of disulfide bonds, occurring both near the N-termini and C-termini (Tsai, 2003). The resulting multimers may achieve molecular weights exceeding 20 MDa. Soon after their secretion into the blood, however, the vWF multimers undergo proteolytic trimming by the metalloproteinase ADAMTS13. Although there is a potential cleavage site between Tyr842 and Met843 within the A2 domain of each vWF multimer, following a certain degree of proteolysis, the ADAMTS13 proteolysis of potential sites within vWF comes to a halt – presumably due to steric hindrance of the ADAMTS13 penetrating deeper into the vWF multimeric structure. Deficiency of ADAMTS13, either due to a congenital abnormality or to the formation of autoantibodies against the enzyme, results in 'unusually large' vWF multimers circulating in the plasma. These forms are capable of spontaneously aggregating platelets, as well as forming large strands anchored to endothelial P-selectin (Padilla, 2004) that can result in RBC fragmentation – two characteristic attributes of the associated disorder termed thrombotic thrombocytopenic purpura (TTP).

At sites of vessel injury, vWF binds to exposed subendothelial collagen. Particularly under conditions of high shear, where there is relatively high blood flow through smaller-diameter vessels, the bound vWF and the GP Ibα on the surface of circulating blood platelets are able to bind together, effectively tethering the platelet to the injury site. This ligand–receptor interaction further produces an outside-to-inside signaling across the platelet membrane, leading to platelet activation. One component of this platelet activation consists of a subsequent inside-to-outside signaling event within GP IIb/IIIa that makes this receptor complex competent to bind the aggregatory ligand fibrinogen. In the clinical laboratory, vWF may be assayed antigenically, functionally, and even structurally. While vWF antigen was formerly quantified by a variety of gel electrophoretic approaches, it may now be measured with high precision by rapid methods such as ELISA or immunoturbometric procedures.

Von Willebrand Disease and its Subtypes

As shown in Table 39–8, there are a variety of clinical conditions associated with vWF abnormalities. In type 1 vWD, qualitatively normal vWF molecules are present in the plasma, but in quantitatively decreased amount. There is accordingly a normal distribution of vWF multimers across the entire size spectrum, albeit lower than normal amounts of each multimer (Fig. 39–11). In one sense, type 3 vWD represents an extreme extent of the quantitative abnormality, since there is a total absence of vWF gene product. However, whereas inherited type 1 vWD is typically expressed in autosomal dominant fashion, type 3 is autosomal recessive, with neither parent of an affected patient typically showing symptomatic disease. Since one of the key functions of vWF is to serve as a carrier molecule for factor VIII, type 3 patients not only suffer with respect to platelet function but also are at further hemostatic risk because of vanishingly low amounts of circulating factor VIII.

Patients with type 2 vWD have one or another of the many described qualitative abnormalities of this complex protein. For practical purposes, these abnormalities have been grouped into a small number of subtypes. In type 2A vWD, there is a lack of higher-molecular-weight multimers (Fig. 39–11), with corresponding loss of vWF functionality, due either to mutations that prevent proper multimerization or to mutations that increase the susceptibility of fully formed vWF to proteolysis by ADAMTS-13 or other proteolytic enzymes. Interestingly, in some instances vWF synthesized by megakaryocytes and stored in platelet α granules appears to have a fuller complement of vWF multimers than does the plasma vWF deriving from secretion by endothelial cells; this may reflect the protective effects from proteolysis due to sequestration within the α granules. In type 2B vWD, point mutations within the vWF molecule actually confer an increase-of-function capability with respect to its ability to bind the platelet GP Ib receptor. Binding of the abnormal type 2B vWF molecules to circulating platelets in the absence of appropriate hemostatic insult leads to an uncompensated depletion of the higher-molecular-weight multimers of plasma vWF (Fig. 39–11) and typically also to a mild–moderate thrombocytopenia. In the clinical laboratory this increase-of-function can be demonstrated by the ability of abnormally low concentrations (typically 0.3–0.5 mg/mL) of the modulator ristocetin to aggregate the platelet-rich plasma of such patients. In contrast, in the case of type 2A vWD or of type 1 vWD, the extent and/or rate of aggregation is decreased below normal at the standard ristocetin concentrations of 1.0–1.5 mg/mL. Patients with type 2M vWD share a similar decrease-of-function phenotype with type 2A vWD, but the mutations responsible for this vWD subtype do not result in a loss of the normal vWF multimeric structure. If, in contrast to testing the patient's own platelet-rich plasma, the patient's platelet-free plasma is tested for ristocetin cofactor activity, the observed level is decreased not only in type 1, type 2A, and type 2M, but also in type 2B, because of the acquired deficiency of high-molecular-weight multimers actually remaining in the patient's plasma. In type 1 vWD the level of vWF antigen and of ristocetin cofactor activity generally decline in parallel. In contrast, in the type 2 patients, there is typically a more dramatic decrease in ristocetin cofactor activity than in vWF antigen level, since it is precisely the missing higher-molecular-weight multimers that are critical to the vWF–platelet interaction that is measured by this functional assay. A similar discrepancy may be observed between WF collagen-binding activity and vWF antigen. Finally, patients with type 2N

Table 39–8 Classification of von Willebrand Disease

Type	Description
1	Partial quantitative deficiency of von Willebrand factor (vWF)
2	Qualitative deficiency of vWF
2A	Decreased platelet-dependent vWF function with selective deficiency of high-molecular-weight multimers
2B	Increased affinity for platelet glycoprotein Ib
2M	Decreased platelet-dependent vWF function with high-molecular-weight multimers present
2N	Markedly decreased binding of factor VIII to vWF
3	Complete deficiency of vWF

Source: adapted from Sadler JE: A revised classification of von Willebrand disease. Thromb Haemost 1994; 71:520 525.

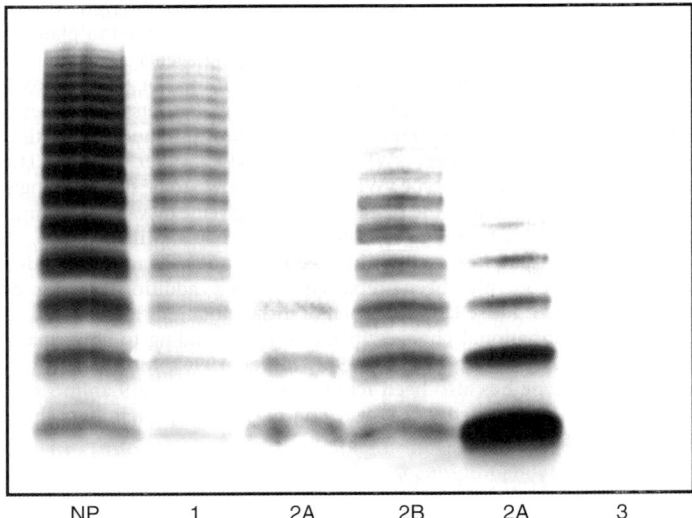

NP   1   2A   2B   2A   3

Figure 39–11 Multimer patterns in selected variants of vWD. Plasma samples were analyzed for vWF by SDS-agarose gel electrophoresis and Western blotting. Patterns are shown for pooled normal plasma (NP) and patients with the indicated types of vWD. Note that in both the 2A and 2B examples there is a relative loss of higher-molecular-weight multimers, although to varying extents. It is important to note that the actual extent of multimer loss is highly variable among patients of each subtype, and the differences in extent of multimer loss between the 2A and 2B subtypes illustrated in these particular examples should not be considered a basis for correctly distinguishing between these subtypes in diagnostic studies. Instead, functional studies are required to distinguish between the decrease-of-function 2A subtype and the increase-of-function 2B subtype (see text). (Adapted with permission from Sadler JE: New concepts in von Willebrand disease. Annu Rev Med 2005; 56:173–191 and Sadler JE: von Willebrand disease. In Bloom AL, Forbes CD, Thomas DP, Tuddenham EGD (eds): Hemostasis and Thrombosis. New York, Churchill Livingstone, 1994, pp 843–857.)

(Normandy) vWD have point mutations within the vWF molecule that specifically impair the ability of this molecule to bind factor VIII. Type 2N patients may accordingly show quite normal levels of vWF antigen and even ristocetin cofactor activity, but will prove to be responsible for abnormally low levels of circulating factor VIII. Since the vWF gene is transmitted autosomally, type 2N vWD should be suspected in cases where there appears to be an autosomal inheritance pattern of factor VIII deficiency. Definitive diagnosis is made by demonstrating impaired binding of normal factor VIII to the patient vWF, such as by ELISA assay, and by molecular diagnostic methods.

Whereas, at least conceptually, the basis for diagnosing type 2 and type 3 vWD seems clear, the same cannot be said for type 1 vWD (Sadler, 2003, 2005). The level of circulating vWF is a result of multigenic influences. Not only genes encoding vWF, but also genes encoding intracellular transporter proteins, ABO genes affecting post-translational modifications of the vWF molecule, genes affecting vWF proteolysis, and doubtlessly still other genetic factors influence the quantity and functionality of vWF. For example, individuals inheriting the same vWF genes may be anticipated to have 20% or lower circulating levels of vWF if they are of type O rather than type AB blood group type. In some instances this could make the difference between being considered normal or deficient in vWF level. Additionally, Sadler (2003) has argued that, because of the relatively high

ITP, disseminated intravascular coagulation, hemolytic–uremic syndrome, renal transplant rejection, multiple congenital cavernous hemangioma, MPD, acute and chronic leukemias, severe valvular disease, in patients undergoing CPB, and in platelet concentrates stored for transfusion.

Antiplatelet Antibodies and Platelet Function

Binding of an antibody to platelets may induce several effects, including accelerated destruction, platelet activation, cell lysis, aggregation, secretion of granule contents, and outward exposure of phosphatidylserine. Platelet–antibody interaction may lead to impaired function, both as a consequence of activation and due to antibody binding to specific glycoproteins. Patients with ITP have decreased platelet survival, and may have impaired platelet function and abnormally prolonged bleeding times even at adequate counts. Antibodies can induce platelet dysfunction by multiple mechanisms. In many patients the antibodies are directed against specific platelet surface membrane glycoproteins GP Ib (Woods, 1984a), GP IIb/IIIa (Woods, 1984b), GP Ia/IIa (Deckmyn, 1994), GP VI (Sugiyama, 1987; Boylan, 2004), and glycosphingolipids (van Vliet, 1987; Koerner, 1989). In one report the anti-GP VI antibody induced a clearance of the GP VI/FcRr complex from the platelet surface (Boylan, 2004). Some of these antibodies, in effect, induce acquired forms of BSS and thrombasthenia.

Drugs that Inhibit Platelet Function

Many drugs affect platelet function (Table 39–9). For several the effects on platelets have been studied in vitro, and the relevance of such findings to the drug levels achieved in clinical practice is not well established. Even among those shown to alter platelet responses ex vivo, the impact on hemostasis often remains unclear. Moreover, the impact of concomitant administration of multiple drugs, each with a mild effect on platelet function, is unknown, although this is clinically relevant. Because of their widespread use, aspirin and nonsteroidal anti-inflammatory agents are an important cause of platelet inhibition in clinical practice. Aspirin ingestion results in inhibition of platelet aggregation and secretion upon stimulation with ADP, epinephrine, and low concentrations of collagen. Aspirin irreversibly acetylates and inactivates the platelet cyclooxygenase, leading to the inhibition of synthesis of endoperoxides (PGG_2 and PGH_2) and TxA_2. Typically, 5–7 days are recommended after cessation of aspirin ingestion for studies intended to assess baseline platelet function. Several other nonsteroidal anti-inflammatory drugs also impair platelet function by inhibiting the cyclooxygenase enzyme and may prolong the bleeding time. Compared with aspirin, the inhibition of cyclooxygenase by these agents is generally short-lived and reversible. In the case of ibuprofen, for example, 24 hours after cessation of this medication is a sufficient interval for testing of baseline platelet function.

Ticlopidine and clopidogrel are orally administered thienopyridine derivatives that inhibit platelet function by inhibiting the binding of ADP to the platelet P2Y12 receptor. Both drugs prolong the bleeding time and inhibit platelet aggregation responses to several agonists, including ADP, collagen, epinephrine, and thrombin, to various extents depending on agonist concentrations. GP IIb/IIIa receptor antagonists are a class of compounds that inhibit fibrinogen binding and platelet aggregation. These include a monoclonal antibody against the GP IIb/IIIa receptor (abciximab), a synthetic peptide containing the KGD sequence (eptifibatide), and a peptidomimetic (tirofiban). They are potent inhibitors of aggregation (both primary and secondary) in response to all the usual agonists except ristocetin; they all prolong the bleeding time and are far more potent as platelet inhibitors than aspirin. Immune-mediated thrombocytopenia (secondary to drug-dependent antibodies) is a potential complication of the GP IIb/III antagonists (Aster, 2004; see also Ch. 42).

A host of other medications and agents, including food substances, inhibit platelet responses but the clinical significance for many is unclear. They have been reviewed elsewhere (Rao, 2005a). Given the increasing use of herbal medicines and food supplements, their role and interaction with pharmaceutical drugs needs to be considered in the evaluation of patients with unexplained bleeding.

Evaluation of Patients With Suspected Platelet Disorders

The evaluation of patients with a clinical history or symptoms suggesting a bleeding tendency involves consideration of the coagulation and

Table 39–9 Drugs That Affect Platelet Function

Cyclooxygenase inhibitors
  Aspirin
  Nonsteroidal anti-inflammatory agents
    Indomethacin, phenylbutazone, ibuprofen, sulfinpyrazone, sulindac, meclofenamic acid
ADP receptor antagonists
  Ticlopidine, clopidogrel
GP IIb/IIIa receptor antagonists
  c7E3 (abciximab), tirofiban, eptifibatride
Drugs that increase platelet cyclic AMP or cyclic GMP
Adenylate cyclase activators
  Prostaglandins I_2, D_2, E_1 and analogs
Phosphodiesterase inhibitors
  Dipyridamole
  Cilostazol
  Anagrelide
  Milrinone
  Methyl xanthines
    Caffeine, theophylline, aminophylline
Nitric oxide and nitric oxide donors
Antimicrobials
  Penicillins
  Cephalosporins
  Nitrofurantoin
  Hydroxychloroquine
  Miconazole
Cardiovascular drugs
  β-Adrenergic blockers (propranolol)
  Vasodilators (nitroprusside, nitroglycerin)
  Diuretics (furosemide)
  Calcium channel blockers
  Quinidine
  Angiotensin converting enzyme inhibitors
Anticoagulants
  Heparin
Thrombolytic agents
  Streptokinase, tissue plasminogen activator, urokinase
Psychotropics and anesthetics
  Tricyclic antidepressants
    Imipramine, amitriptyline, nortriptyline
  Phenothiazines
    Chlorpromazine, promethazine, trifluoperazine
  Local anesthetics
  General anesthesia (halothane)
Chemotherapeutic agents
  Mithramycin
  Carmustine
  Daunorubicin
Miscellaneous agents
  Dextrans and hydroxyethyl starch
  Lipid lowering agents (clofibrate, halofenate)
  ε-Aminocaproic acid
  Antihistaminics
  Ethanol
  Vitamin E
  Radiographic contrast agents
  Food items (omega-3 fatty acids, vitamin E, onions, garlic, ginger, cumin, turmeric, cloves, black tree fungus, Ginko)

Source: with permission from Rao AK: Acquired disorders of platelet function. *In* Colman RW (ed.): Hemostasis and Thrombosis: Basic Principles and Clinical Practice. Philadelphia, Lippincott Williams & Wilkins, 2006

fibrinolytic systems as well as of the blood platelets. A carefully conducted history can be the single most important factor leading to a diagnosis in many patients. Determination of whether the disorder is likely to be congenital or acquired is most important. A platelet count may help determine whether the bleeding tendency is explainable by decreased platelet numbers alone. A prolonged PFA-100 or bleeding time may help determine whether another abnormality is present. Because vWD is far more common than congenital disorders of platelet function, an evaluation of disordered primary hemostasis will frequently necessitate analysis of the factor VIII/vWF complex.

The bleeding manifestations in patients with inherited platelet function defects are highly variable. The usual reasons for referral for evaluation include mucocutaneous bleeding manifestations, excessive bleeding following a procedure or surgery, and a prolonged PFA-100 or bleeding time with a reasonable platelet count. In patients suspected to have a platelet function defect, the main widely available laboratory studies include a platelet count, PFA-100, and studies to assess platelet aggregation and secretion responses in vitro. The platelet studies are usually performed using platelet-rich plasma harvested from anticoagulated blood, and responses are monitored to various agonists including ADP, epinephrine, collagen, arachidonic acid, a TxA$_2$ analog (U46619), thrombin receptor peptides, and ristocetin. The patterns of responses observed may often provide clues to the nature of the underlying platelet defect, although specific techniques, largely available in research laboratories, are required to delineate the precise platelet mechanisms that are altered. Patients with classical thrombasthenia are characterized by the absence of both the primary and the secondary waves of aggregation in response to all the commonly used agonists except ristocetin with a normal shape change response. Impaired or absent response to ristocetin but with normal aggregation response to other agonists suggests vWD or BSS. In the latter disorder, the platelet counts are decreased and the platelet size is increased. Although these findings may occur in some variants of vWD (e.g., type 2B), plasma levels of vWF and factor VIII, as well as the multimeric pattern of vWF, are normal in BSS but abnormal in vWD. Patients with impaired granule secretion or diminished dense granule contents generally show a diminished or absent second wave of aggregation in response to ADP, epinephrine, and PAF, and blunted responses to other agonists (collagen, U46619), associated with markedly decreased release of granule contents.

Therapy of Congenital Platelet Function Defects

Platelet transfusions and 1-desamino-8D-arginine vasopressin (DDAVP) administration have been the mainstays of therapy of patients with inherited platelet defects. Because of the wide disparity in bleeding manifestations, therapeutic approaches need to be individualized. Platelet transfusions are effective in controlling the bleeding manifestations but come with potential risks associated with blood products including alloimmunization. Patients with thrombasthenia may develop antibodies against GP IIb/IIIa that compromise the efficacy of subsequent platelet transfusions. A viable alternative to platelet transfusions is intravenous administration of DDAVP, which was shown to shorten the bleeding time in a substantial number of patients with platelet function defects (Rao, 1995; Mannucci, 1998). The effect on the bleeding time lasted about 4–5 hours. This response appears to be dependent on the abnormalities leading to the platelet dysfunction. Most patients with Glanzmann thrombasthenia have not responded to DDAVP infusion with a shortening of the bleeding time. Responses in patients with disorders of platelet secretion, signal transduction, or storage pool deficiency have been variable with a shortening of the bleeding time in some patients. DDAVP administration induces a rise in plasma vWF, factor VIII, and tissue plasminogen activator. The abnormal in vitro platelet aggregation or secretion responses in patients with platelet defects are not corrected by DDAVP (Rao, 1995).

More recently, recombinant factor VIIa has developed into an important drug for the management of bleeding events in patients with Glanzmann thrombasthenia and some other inherited defects (Poon, 2000; Almeida, 2003). Additional approaches that have been utilized to improve hemostasis in patients with inherited platelet defects include a short (3–4 day) course of prednisone (20–50 mg) (Mielke, 1981) and the administration of antifibrinolytic agents such as ε-aminocaproic acid or tranexamic acid. Allogeneic bone marrow transplantation has now been successfully performed with complete correction in patients with thrombasthenia, although the development of antibodies directed against the GP IIb/IIIa complex remains a potential problem (Flood, 2005; Fujimoto, 2005).

References

Almeida AM, Khair K, Hann I: The use of recombinant factor VIIa in children with inherited platelet function disorders. Br J Haematol 2003; 121:477–481.

Amiral J: Antigens involved in heparin-induced thrombocytopenia. Semin Hematol 1999; 36:7–11.

Amiral J, Bridey F, Dreyfus M: Platelet factor 4 complexed to heparin is the target for antibodies generated in heparin-induced thrombocytopenia. Thromb Haemost 1992; 68:95–96.

Andre P: P-selectin in haemostasis. Br J Haematol 2004; 126:298–306.

Arai M, Yamamoto N, Moroi M: Platelets with 10% of the normal amount of glycoprotein VI have an impaired response to collagen that results in a mild bleeding tendency. Br J Haematol 1995; 89:124–130.

Aster RH, Curtis BR, Bougie DW: Thrombocytopenia resulting from sensitivity to GPIIb-IIIa inhibitors. Semin Thromb Hemost 2004; 30:569–577.

Auger JM, Kuijpers MJ, Senis YA: Adhesion of human and mouse platelets to collagen under shear: a unifying model. FASEB J 2005;

Ault KA, Knowles C: In vivo biotinylation demonstrates that reticulated platelets are the youngest platelets in circulation. Exp Hematol 1995; 23:996–1001.

Bader-Meunier B, Proulle V, Trichet C: Misdiagnosis of chronic thrombocytopenia in childhood. J Pediatr Hematol Oncol 2003; 25:548–552.

Baglia FA, Gailani D, Lopez JA: Identification of a binding site for glycoprotein Ibα in the Apple 3 domain of factor XI. J Biol Chem 2004a; 279:45470–45476.

Baglia FA, Shrimpton CN, Emsley J: Factor XI interacts with the leucine-rich repeats of glycoprotein Ibα on the activated platelet. J Biol Chem 2004b; 279:49323–49329.

Baglia FA, Walsh PN: Prothrombin is a cofactor for the binding of factor XI to the platelet surface and for platelet-mediated factor XI activation by thrombin. Biochemistry 1998; 37:2271–2281.

Beardsley DS, Ertem M: Platelet autoantibodies in immune thrombocytopenic purpura. Transfus Sci 1998; 19:237–244.

Bennett JS, Vilaire G: Exposure of platelet fibrinogen receptors by ADP and epinephrine. J Clin Invest 1979; 64:1393–1401.
Classic paper demonstrating that fibrinogen serves as the critical adhesive ligand for platelet aggregation.

Berman CL, Yeo EL, Wencel-Drake JD: A platelet alpha granule membrane protein that is associated with the plasma membrane after activation. Characterization and subcellular localization of platelet activation-dependent granule-external membrane protein. J Clin Invest 1986; 78:130–137.

Berndt MC, Chong BH, Bull HA: Molecular characterization of quinine/quinidine drug-dependent antibody platelet interaction using monoclonal antibodies. Blood 1985; 66:1292–1301.

Bessman JD: Automated blood counts and differentials. A practical guide. Baltimore, Johns Hopkins University Press, 1986.

Bessman JD, Williams LJ, Gilmer PR: Mean platelet volume. Am J Clin Pathol 1981; 76:289–293.

Boccardo P, Remuzzi G, Galbusera M: Platelet dysfunction in renal failure. Semin Thromb Hemost 2004; 30:579–589.

Bouchard BA, Catcher CS, Thrash BR: Effector cell protease receptor-1, a platelet activation-dependent membrane protein, regulates prothrombinase-catalyzed thrombin generation. J Biol Chem 1997; 272:9244–9251.

Boylan B, Chen H, Rathore V: Anti-GPVI-associated ITP: an acquired platelet disorder caused by autoantibody-mediated clearance of the GPVI/FcRgamma-chain complex from the human platelet surface. Blood 2004; 104:1350–1355.

Bray PF: Inherited diseases of platelet glycoproteins: considerations for rapid molecular characterization. Thromb Haemost 1994; 72:492–502.

Brecher G, Cronkite EP: Morphology and enumeration of human blood platelets. J Appl Physiol 1950; 3:365

Breton-Gorius J, Guichard J: Ultrastructural localization of peroxidase activity in human platelets and megakaryocytes. Am J Pathol 1972; 66:277–293.

Breton-Gorius J, Vainchenker W, Nurden A: Defective α-granule production in megakaryocytes from gray platelet syndrome: ultrastructural studies of bone marrow cells and megakaryocytes growing in culture from blood precursors. Am J Pathol 1981; 102:10

Broze GJJ, Girard TJ, Novotny WF: Regulation of coagulation by a multivalent Kunitz-type inhibitor. Biochemistry 1990; 29:7539–7546.

Buchanan GR, Holtkamp CA: A comparative study of variables affecting the bleeding time using two disposable devices. Am J Clin Pathol 1989; 91:45–51.

Budde U, van Genderen PJ: Acquired von Willebrand disease in patients with high platelet counts. Semin Thromb Hemost 1997; 23:425–431.

Cabeza N, Li Z, Schulz C: Surface expression of collagen receptor Fc receptor-gamma/glycoprotein VI is enhanced on platelets in type 2 diabetes and mediates release of CD40 ligand and activation of endothelial cells. Diabetes 2004; 53:2117–2121.

Calvete JJ: Platelet integrin GPIIb/IIIa: structure-function correlations. An update and lessons from other integrins. Proc Soc Exp Biol Med 1999; 222:29–38.

Cambien B, Wagner DD: A new role in hemostasis for the adhesion receptor P-selectin. Trends Mol Med 2004; 10:179–186.

Cardinal DC, Flower RJ: The electronic aggregometer: a novel device for assessing platelet behavior in blood. J Pharmacol Methods 1980; 3:135–158.

Carroll RC, Gerrard JM, Gilliam JM: Clot retraction facilitates clot lysis. Blood 1981; 57:44–48.

Castaman G, Lattuada A, Mannucci PM: Characterization of two cases of acquired transitory von Willebrand syndrome with ciprofloxacin: evidence for heightened proteolysis of von Willebrand factor. Am J Hematol 1995; 49:83–86.

Castillo R, Lozano T, Escolar G: Defective platelet adhesion on vessel subendothelium in uremic patients. Blood 1986; 68:337–342.

Cattaneo M, Lecchi A, Randi AM: Identification of a new congenital defect of platelet function characterized by severe impairment of platelet responses to adenosine diphosphate. Blood 1992; 80:2787–2796.

Cattaneo M, Lombardi R, Zighetti ML: Deficiency of (^{33}P)-2MeS-ADP binding sites on platelets with secretion defect, normal granule stores and normal thromboxane A_2 production. Thromb Haemost 1997; 77:986–990.

Charo IF, Feinman RD, Detwiler TC: Interrelations of platelet aggregation and secretion. J Clin Invest 1977; 60:866–873.

Classic paper characterizing monoclonal antibody inhibition of platelet GP IIb/IIIa.

Chong BH, Du X, Berndt MC: Characterization of the binding domains on platelet glycoproteins Ib-IX and IIb/IIIa complexes for the quinine/quinidine-dependent antibodies. Blood 1991; 77:2190–2199.

Clofent-Sanchez G, Lucas S, Laroche-Traineau J: Autoantibodies and anti-mouse antibodies in thrombocytopenic patients as assessed by different MAIPA assays. British Journal of Haematology 1996; 95:153–160.

Coller BS, Peerschke EI, Scudder LE: A murine monoclonal antibody that completely blocks the binding of fibrinogen to platelets produces a thrombasthenic-like state in normal platelets and binds to glycoproteins IIb and/or IIIa. J Clin Invest 1983; 72:325–338.

Classic paper characterizing monoclonal antibody inhibition of platelet GP IIb/IIIa.

Comfurius P, Williamson P, Smeets EF: Reconstitution of phospholipid scramblase activity from human blood platelets. Biochemistry 1996; 35:7631–7634.

Cooper B, Schafer AI, Puchalsky D: Platelet resistance to protaglandin D2 in patients with myeloproliferative disorders. Blood 1978; 52:618–626.

Cordiano I, Salvan F, Randi ML: Antiplatelet glycoprotein autoantibodies in patients with autoimmune diseases with and without thrombocytopenia. J Clin Immunol 1996; 16:340–347.

Cox D: Ligand-binding assays: fibrinogen. Methods Mol Biol 2004; 273:125–138.

De Caterina R, Lanza M, Manca G: Bleeding time and bleeding: An analysis of the relationship of the bleeding time test with parameters of surgical bleeding. Blood 1994; 84:3363–3370.

Deckmyn H, Zhang J, Van Houtte E: Production and nucleotide sequence of an inhibitory human IgM autoantibody directed against platelet glycoprotein Ia/IIa. Blood 1994; 84:1968–1974.

Deykin D, Janson P, McMahon L: Ethanol potentiation of aspirin-induced prolongation of the bleeding time. N Engl J Med 1982; 306:852–854.

Drachman JG: Inherited thrombocytopenia: when a low platelet count does not mean ITP. Blood 2004; 103:390–398.

Drouin A, Favier R, Masse JM: Newly recognized cellular abnormalities in the gray platelet syndrome. Blood 2001; 98:1382–1391.

Drouin J, McGregor JL, Parmentier S: Residual amounts of glycoprotein Ib concomitant with near-absence of glycoprotein IX in platelets of Bernard–Soulier patients. Blood 1988; 72:1086–1088.

Eigenthaler M, Ullrich H, Geiger J: Defective nitrovasodilator-stimulated protein phosphorylation and calcium regulation in cGMP-dependent protein kinase-deficient human platelets of chronic myelocytic leukemia. J Biol Chem 1993; 268:13526–13531.

Elliott MA, Tefferi A: Thrombosis and haemorrhage in polycythaemia vera and essential thrombocythaemia. Br J Haematol 2005; 128:275–290.

Evangelista V, Manarini S, Sıderı R: Platelet/polymorphonuclear leukocyte interaction: P-selectin triggers protein-tyrosine phosphorylation-dependent CD11β/CD18 adhesion: role of PSGL-1 as a signaling molecule. Blood 1999; 93:876–885.

Fabris F, Cordiano I, Mazzucato M: Labeling of platelet surface glycoproteins with biotin derivatives. Thromb Res 1992; 66:409–419.

Federici AB, Rand JH, Bucciarelli P: Acquired von Willebrand syndrome: data from an international registry. Thromb Haemost 2000; 84:345–349.

Finch CN, Miller JL, Lyle VA: Evidence that an abnormality in the glycoprotein Ib alpha gene is not the cause of abnormal platelet function in a family with classic Bernard–Soulier disease. Blood 1990; 75:2357–2362.

Flood VH, Johnson FL, Boshkov LK: Sustained engraftment post bone marrow transplant despite anti-platelet antibodies in Glanzmann thrombasthenia 1. Pediatr Blood Cancer 2005; 14 Mar (e-pub ahead of print).

Frelinger AL, Du X, Plow EF: Monoclonal antibodies to ligand-occupied conformers of integrin $\alpha_{IIb}\beta_3$ (glycoprotein IIb-IIIa) alter receptor affinity, specificity, and function. J Biol Chem 1991; 266:17106–17111.

French DL, Coller BS, Usher S: Prenatal diagnosis of Glanzmann thrombasthenia using the polymorphic markers BRCA1 and THRA1 on chromosome 17. Br J Haematol 1998; 102:582–587.

French DL, Seligsohn U: Platelet glycoprotein IIb/IIIa Receptors and Glanzmann's thrombasthenia. Arterioscler Thromb Vasc Biol 2000; 20:607–610.

Fujimoto T, Fujimura K, Kuramoto A: Abnormal Ca^{2+} homeostasis in platelets with myeloproliferative disorders: low levels of Ca^{2+} influx and efflux across the plasma membrane and increased Ca^{2+} accumulation into the dense tubular system. Thromb Res 1989; 53:99–108.

Fujimoto TT, Kishimoto M, Ide K: Glanzmann thrombasthenia with acute myeloid leukemia successfully treated by bone marrow transplantation 2. Int J Hematol 2005; 81:77–80.

Furie B, Furie BC: Role of platelet P-selectin and microparticle PSGL-1 in thrombus formation. Trends Mol Med 2004; 10:171–178.

Recent review of P-selectin and its roles in thrombosis and hemostasis.

Furlan M, Robles R, Galbusera M: von Willebrand factor-cleaving protease in thrombotic thrombocytopenic purpura and the hemolytic–uremic syndrome. N Engl J Med 1998; 339:1578–1584.

Landmark paper leading to the recognition of ADAMTS-13

Furman MI, Liu L, Benoit SE: The cleaved peptide of the thrombin receptor is a strong platelet agonist. Proc Natl Acad Sci USA 1998; 95:3082–3087.

Gabbeta J, Yang X, Kowalska MA: Platelet signal transduction defect with Gα subunit dysfunction and diminished Gαq in a patient with abnormal platelet responses. Proc Natl Acad Sci USA 1997; 94:8750–8755.

Gabbeta J, Yang X, Sun L: Abnormal inside-out signal transduction-dependent activation of glycoprotein IIb-IIIa in a patient with impaired pleckstrin phosphorylation. Blood 1996; 87:1368–1376.

George JN, Vesely SK, Terrell DR: The Oklahoma Thrombotic Thrombocytopenic Purpura-Hemolytic Uremic Syndrome (TTP-HUS) Registry: a community perspective of patients with clinically diagnosed TTP-HUS. Semin Hematol 2004; 41:60–67.

George JN, Woolf SH, Raskob GE: Idiopathic thrombocytopenic purpura: a practice guideline developed by explicit methods for the American Society of Hematology. Blood 1996; 88:3–40.

Gerrard JM, Lint D, Sims PJ: Identification of a platelet dense granule membrane protein that is deficient in a patient with the Hermansky–Pudlak syndrome. Blood 1991; 77:101–112.

Gerrard JM, Phillips DR, Rao GHR: Biochemical studies of two patients with the gray platelet syndrome: selective deficiency of platelet α granules. J Clin Invest 1980; 66:102

Gerritsen HE, Turecek PL, Schwarz HP: Assay of von Willebrand factor (vWF)-cleaving protease based on decreased collagen binding affinity of degraded vWF: a tool for the diagnosis of thrombotic thrombocytopenic purpura (TTP). Thromb Haemost 1999; 82:1386–1389.

Gill JC, Wilson AD, Endres-Brooks J: Loss of the largest von Willebrand factor multimers from plasma of patients with congenital cardiac defects. Blood 1986; 67:758–761.

Gonzalez-Manchon C, Fernandez-Pinel M, Arias-Salgado EG: Molecular genetic analysis of a compound heterozygote for the glycoprotein (GP) IIb gene associated with Glanzmann's thrombasthenia: disruption of the 674–687 disulfide bridge in GPIIb prevents surface exposure of GPIIb–IIIa complexes. Blood 1999; 93:866–875.

Gralnick HP, McKeown LP, Williams SB: Plasma and platelet von Willebrand's factor defects in uremia. Am J Med 1988; 85:806–810.

Greilich PE, Alving BM, Longnecker D: Near-site monitoring of the antiplatelet drug abciximab using the Hemodyne analyzer and modified thrombelastograph. J Cardiothorac Vasc Anesth 1999; 13:58–64.

Griesshammer M, Bangerter M, Sauer T: Aetiology and clinical significance of thrombocytosis: analysis of 732 patients with an elevated platelet count. J Intern Med 1999; 245:295–300.

Gunay-Aygun MHMGW: Molecular defects that affect platelet dense granules. Semin Thromb Hemost 2004; 30:537–547.

Hayward CPM: Inherited disorders of platelet α-granules. Platelets 1997; 8:197–209.

Hayward CP, Bainton DF, Smith JW: Multimerin is found in the alpha-granules of resting platelets and is synthesized by a megakaryocytic cell line. J Clin Invest 1993; 91:2630–2639.

Hayward CP, Warkentin TE, Horsewood P: Multimerin: a series of large disulfide-linked multimeric proteins within platelets. Blood 1991; 77:2556–2560.

Heaton WA, Davis HH, Melch MJ, et al: Indium-111: a new radionuclide label for studying human platelet kinetics. Br J Haematol 1979; 42:613

Heaton WA, Heyns ADP, Joist JH: Measurement of in vivo platelet turnover and organ distribution using ^{111}In-labeled platelets. Methods Enzymol 1989; 169:172–187.

Heilmann E, Friese P, Anderson S: Biotinylated platelets: a new approach to the measurement of platelet life span. Br J Haematol 1993; 85:729–735.

Hemker HC, van Rijn JL, Rosing J: Platelet membrane involvement in blood coagulation. Blood Cells 1983; 9:303–317.

Hewitt J, Burton IE: Incidence of autoantibodies to GPIIb/IIIa in chronic autoimmune thrombocytopenic purpura may be overestimated by the MAIPA. Br J Haematol 1994; 86:418–420.

Himmelfarb J, Holbrook D, McMonagle E: Increased reticulated platelets in dialysis patients. Kidney Int 1997; 51:834–839.

Hirata T, Kakizuka A, Ushikubi F: Arg60 to Leu mutation of the human thromboxane A_2 receptor in a dominantly inherited bleeding disorder. J Clin Invest 1994; 94:1662–1667.

Holmsen H: Secretable storage pools in platelets. Annu Rev Med 1979; 30:119–134.

Holmsen H, Dangelmaier CA: Measurement of secretion of serotonin. Methods Enzymol 1989; 169:205–211.

Hoyer L: The assessment of von Willebrand's disease. *In* Bloom AL (ed.): Methods of Hematology. New York, Churchill Livingstone, 1982, pp 106–121.

Huizing M, Anikster Y, Gahl WA: Hermansky–Pudlak syndrome and Chediak–Higashi syndrome: disorders of vesicle formation and trafficking. Thromb Haemost 2001; 86:233–245.

Hyman T, Huizing M, Blumberg PM: Use of a cDNA microarray to determine molecular mechanisms involved in grey platelet syndrome. Br J Haematol 2003; 122:142–149.

Ingerman CM, Smith JB, Shapiro S: Hereditary abnormality of platelet aggregation attributable to nucleotide storage pool deficiency. Blood 1978; 52:332–344.

Ingerman-Wojenski CM, Silver MJ: A quick method for screening platelet dysfunctions using the whole blood lumi-aggregometer. Thromb Haemost 1984; 51:154–156.

Israels SJ, McMillan EM, Robertson C: The lysosomal granule membrane protein, LAMP-2, is also present in platelet dense granule membranes. Thromb Haemost 1996; 75:623–629.

Israels SJ, McNicol A, Robertson C: Platelet storage pool deficiency: diagnosis in patients with prolonged bleeding times and normal platelet aggregation. Br J Haematol 1990; 75:118–121.

Joseph R, Welch KMA, D'Andrea G: Epinephrine does not induce platelet aggregation in citrated whole blood. Thromb Res 1987; 45:871–872.

Kahn ML: Platelet-collagen responses: Molecular basis and therapeutic promise. Semin Thromb Hemost 2004; 30:419–425.

Kahr WH, Zheng S, Sheth PM: Platelets from patients with the Quebec platelet disorder contain and secrete abnormal amounts of urokinase-type plasminogen activator. Blood 2001; 98:257–265.

Kaplan R, Gabbeta J, Sun L: Combined defect in membrane expression and activation of platelet GPIIb–IIIa complex without primary sequence abnormalities in myeloproliferative disease. Br J Haematol 2000; 111:954–964.

Kehrel B, Balleisen L, Kokott R: Deficiency of intact thrombospondin and membrane glycoprotein Ia in platelets with defective collagen-induced aggregation and spontaneous loss of disorder. Blood 1988; 71:1074–1078.

Kelton JG, Powers PJ, Carter CJ: A prospective study of the usefulness of the measurement of platelet-associated IgG for the diagnosis of idiopathic thrombocytopenic purpura. Blood 1982; 60:1050–1053.

Kempfer AC, Frontroth JP, Lazzari MA: Visualization of platelet glycoproteins Ib and IIIa by immunoenzymatic stain using avidin-biotin peroxidase complex. Thromb Res 1991; 64:395–404.

Kiefel V, Santoso S, Weisheit M: Monoclonal antibody-specific immunobilization of platelet antigens (MAIPA): a new tool for the identification of platelet-reactive antibodies. Blood 1987; 70:1722–1726.

Koerner TA, Weinfeld HM, Bullard LS: Antibodies against platelet glycosphingolipids: detection in serum by quantitative HPTLC-autoradiography and association with autoimmune and alloimmune processes. Blood 1989; 74:274–84.

Kokame K, Matsumoto M, Fujimura Y: VWF73, a region from D1596 to R1668 of von Willebrand factor, provides a minimal substrate for ADAMTS-13. Blood 2004; 103:607–612.

Koksch M, Rothe G, Kiefel V: Fluorescence resonance energy transfer as a new method for the epitope-specific characterization of anti-platelet antibodies. J Immunol Methods 1995; 187:53–67.

Kreuz W, Linde R, Funk M: Induction of von Willebrand disease type I by valproic acid. Lancet 1990; 335:1350–1351.

Kumar S, Pruthi RK, Nichols WL: Acquired von Willebrand disease. Mayo Clin Proc 2002; 77:181–187.

Kunicki TJ, Aster RH: Deletion of the platelet-specific alloantigen Pl^A1 from platelets in Glanzmann's thrombasthenia. J Clin Invest 1978a; 61:1225–1231.

Early paper demonstrating the relationship between a prominent platelet alloantigen and a major glycoprotein receptor.

Kunicki TJ, Head S, Salomon DR: Platelet receptor structures and polymorphisms. Methods Mol Biol 2004; 273:455–478.

Kunicki TJ, Johnson MM, Aster RH: Absence of the platelet receptor for drug-dependent antibodies in the Bernard–Soulier syndrome. J Clin Invest 1978b; 62:716–719.

Lages B, Weiss HJ: Enhanced increases in cytosolic Ca^{2+} in ADP-stimulated platelets from patients with δ-storage pool deficiency – a possible indicator of interactions between granule-bound ADP and the membrane ADP receptor. Thromb Haemost 1997; 77:376–382.

Lan Z, Schmaier AH: Platelet aggregation testing in platelet-rich plasma – description of procedures with the aim to develop standards in the field. Am J Clin Pathol 2005; 123:172–183.

Recent methodological review of platelet function testing.

Landolfi R, Marchioli R, Patrono C: Mechanisms of bleeding and thrombosis in myeloproliferative disorders. Thromb Haemost 1997; 78:617–621.

Lee SB, Rao AK, Lee K-H: Decreased expression of phospholipase C-β₂ isozyme in human platelets with impaired function. Blood 1996; 88:1684–1691.

Legrand C, Bellucci S, Disdier M: Platelet thrombospondin and glycoprotein IV abnormalities in patients with essential thrombocythemia: effect of α-interferon treatment. Am J Hematol 1991; 38:307–313.

Leissinger CA: Platelet kinetics in immune thrombocytopenic purpura and human immunodeficiency virus thrombocytopenia. Curr Opin Hematol 2001; 8:299–305.

Levesque H, Borg JY, Cailleux N: Acquired von Willebrand's syndrome associated with decrease of plasminogen activator and its inhibitor during hypothyroidism. Eur J Med 1993; 2:287–288.

Levy-Toledano S, Caen JP, Breton-Gorius J: Gray platelet syndrome: α-granule deficiency: its influence on platelet function. J Lab Clin Med 1981; 98:831.

Early paper characterizing the gray platelet syndrome.

Linden MD, Frelinger AL3, Barnard MR: Application of flow cytometry to platelet disorders. Semin Thromb Hemost 2004; 30:501–511.

Livio M, Gotti E, Marchesi D: Uraemic bleeding: role of anemia and beneficial effect of red cell transfusions. Lancet 1982; 2:1013–1015.

McKay H, Derome F, Haq MA, et al: Bleeding risks associated with inheritance of the Quebec platelet disorder. Blood 2004;104:159–165.

McNicol A, Israels SJ, Robertson C: The empty sack syndrome: a platelet storage pool deficiency associated with empty dense granules. Br J Haematol 1994; 86:574–582.

Madan M, Berkowitz SD: Understanding thrombocytopenia and antigenicity with glycoprotein IIb–IIIa inhibitors. Am Heart J 1999; 138:317–326.

Maldonado JE, Pintado T, Pierre RV: Dysplastic platelet and circulating megakaryocytes in chronic myeloproliferative diseases. I. The platelets: ultrastructure and peroxidase reaction. Blood 1974; 43:797–809.

Manning KL, Novinger S, Sullivan PS: Successful determination of platelet lifespan in C3H mice by in vivo biotinylation. Lab Anim Sci 1996; 46:545–548.

Mannucci PM: Hemostatic drugs. N Engl J Med 1998; 339:245–253.

Mannucci PM, Vanoli M, Forza I: Von Willebrand factor cleaving protease (ADAMTS-13) in 123 patients with connective tissue diseases (systemic lupus erythematosus and systemic sclerosis). Haematologica 2003; 88:914–918.

Menasche G, Pastural E, Feldmann J: Mutations in RAB27A cause Griscelli syndrome associated with haemophagocytic syndrome. Nat Genet 2000; 25:173–176.

Michelson AD (ed.): Platelets. Amsterdam: Academic Press; 2002.

Michelson AD, Furman MI, Goldschmidt-Clermont P: Platelet GP IIIa Pl(A) polymorphisms display different sensitivities to agonists. Circulation 2000; 101:1013–1018.

Mielke CH: Influence of aspirin on platelets and the bleeding time. Am J Med 1983; 74:72–78.

Mielke CH, Kaneshiro MM, Maher IA: The standardized normal Ivy bleeding time and its prolongation by aspirin. Blood 1969; 34:204–215.

Standardization of the bleeding time.

Mielke CH Jr, Levine PH, Zucker S: Preoperative prednisone therapy in platelet function disorders. Thromb Res 1981; 21:655–662.

Miletich JP, Jackson CM, Majerus PW: Properties of the factor Xa binding site on human platelets. J Biol Chem 1978; 253:6908–6916.

Miller JL: Platelet function testing: an improved approach utilizing lumi-aggregation and an interactive computer system. Am J Clin Pathol 1984; 81:471–476.

Miller JL: Platelet-type von Willebrand disease. Thromb Haemost 1996; 75:865–869.

Miller JL, Castella A: Platelet-type von Willebrand's disease: characterization of a new bleeding disorder. Blood 1982; 60:790–794.

Discovery of an increase-of-function mutation in the platelet receptor for vWF that mimics type 2B vWD.

Miller JL, Cunningham D, Lyle VA: Mutation in the gene encoding platelet glycoprotein Ibα in platelet-type von Willebrand disease. Proc Natl Acad Sci USA 1991; 88:4761–4765.

Miller JL, Kupinski JM, Castella A: Von Willebrand factor binds to platelets and induces aggregation in platelet-type but not type IIB von Willebrand disease. J Clin Invest 1983; 72:1532–1542.

Miller JL, Lyle VA, Cunningham D: Mutation of leucine-57 to phenylalanine in a platelet glycoprotein Ib alpha leucine tandem repeat occurring in patients with an autosomal dominant variant of Bernard–Soulier disease. Blood 1992; 79:439–446.

Miller JL, Ruggeri ZM, Lyle VA: Unique interactions of asialo von Willebrand factor with platelets in platelet-type von Willebrand disease. Blood 1987; 70:1804–1809.

Moake JL, Turner NA, Stathopoulos NA: Involvement of large plasma von Willebrand factor (vWF) multimers and unusually large vWF forms derived from endothelial cells in shear stress-induced platelet aggregation. J Clin Invest 1986; 78:1456–1461.

Moia M, Mannucci PM, Vizzotto L: Improvement in the haemostatic defect of uraemia after treatment with recombinant human erythropoietin. Lancet 1987; 8570:1227–1229.

Moliterno AR, Siebel KE, Sun AY: A novel thrombopoietin signaling defect in polycythemia vera platelets. Stem Cells 1998; 16:185–192.

Montgomery RR, Kunicki TJ, Taves C: Diagnosis of Bernard–Soulier syndrome and Glanzmann's thrombasthenia with a monoclonal assay on whole blood. J Clin Invest 1983; 71:385–389.

Development of immunological techniques for the diagnosis of inherited platelet disorders.

Moore A, Nachman RL: Platelet Fc receptor: increased expression in myeloproliferative disease. J Clin Invest 1981; 67:1064–1071.

Moore JC, Hayward CP, Warkentin TE: Decreased von Willebrand factor protease activity associated with thrombocytopenic disorders. Blood 2001; 98:1842–1846.

Moroi M, Jung SM, Okuma M: A patient with platelets deficient in glycoprotein VI that lack both collagen-induced aggregation and adhesion. J Clin Invest 1989; 84:1440–1445.

Nguyen XD, Dugrillon A, Beck C: A novel method for simultaneous analysis of specific platelet antibodies. SASPA. Br J Haematol 2004; 127:552–560.

Nieminen U, Kekomaki R: Quinidine-induced thrombocytopenic purpura: clinical presentation in relation to drug-dependent and drug-independent platelet antibodies. Br J Haematol 1992; 80:77–82.

Nieswandt B, Brakebusch C, Bergmeier W: Glycoprotein VI but not $\alpha_2\beta_1$ integrin is essential for platelet interaction with collagen. EMBO J 2001; 20:2120–2130.

Nieuwenhuis HK, Akkerman JW, Houdijk WP: Human blood platelets showing no response to collagen fail to express surface glycoprotein Ia. Nature 1985; 318:470–472.

Nieuwenhuis HK, Akkerman JWN, Sixma JJ: Patients with a prolonged bleeding time and normal aggregation tests may have storage pool deficiency: studies on one hundred six patients. Blood 1987; 70:620–623.

Nieuwenhuis HK, Sakariassen KS, Houdijk PM: Deficiency of platelet membrane glycoprotein Ia associated with a decreased platelet adhesion to subendothelium: a defect in platelet spreading. Blood 1986; 68:692–695.

Nishibori M, Cham B, McNicol A: The protein CD63 is in platelet dense granules, is deficient in a patient

V

with Hermansky–Pudlak syndrome, and appears identical to granulophysin. J Clin Invest 1993; 91:1775–1782.

Novak EK, McGarry MP, Swank RT: Correction of symptoms of platelet storage pool deficiency in animal models for Chediak–Higashi syndrome and Hermansky–Pudlak syndrome. Blood 1985; 66:1196

Novak EK, Swank RT, Hui SW: Platelet storage pool deficiency in mouse pigment mutations associated with seven distinct genetic loci. Blood 1984; 63:536–544.

Nowak G, Bucha E: Quantitative determination of hirudin in blood and body fluids. Semin Thromb Hemost 1996; 22:197–202.

Nurden AT, Caen JP: Specific roles for platelet surface glycoproteins in platelet function. Nature 1975; 255:720–722.

Classic paper beginning the field of platelet glycoprotein biology and pathophysiology.

Nurden AT, George JN: Inherited disorders of the platelet membrane: Glanzmann thrombasthenia, Bernard–Soulier syndrome, and other disorders. *In* Colman RW (ed.): Hemostasis and Thrombosis. Basic Principles and Clinical Practice, 4th ed. Philadelphia, Lippincott Williams & Wilkins, 2001, pp 921–943.

Nurden AT, Kunicki TJ, Dupuis D, et al: Specific protein and glycoprotein deficiencies in platelets isolated from two patients with the gray platelet syndrome. Blood 1982; 59:709–718.

Nurden P, Jandrot-Perrus M, Combrie R: Severe deficiency of glycoprotein VI in a patient with gray platelet syndrome. Blood 2004; 104:107–114.

Nurden P, Savi P, Heilmann E: An inherited bleeding disorder linked to a defective interaction between ADP and its receptor on platelets. Its influence on glycoprotein IIb–IIIa complex function. J Clin Invest 1995; 95:1612–1622.

Offermanns S, Toombs CF, Hu YH: Defective platelet activation in Gαq-deficient mice. Nature 1997; 389:183–186.

Oliver JA, Monroe DM, Roberts HR: Thrombin activates factor XI on activated platelets in the absence of factor XII. Arterioscler Thromb Vasc Biol 1999; 19:170–177.

Othman M, Notley C, Lavender FL, et al: Identification and functional characterisation of a novel 27-bp deletion in the macroglycopeptide-coding region of the GPIBA gene resulting in platelet-type von Willebrand disease. Blood 2005; 105:4330–4336.

Oury C, Lenaerts T, Peerlinck K: Congenital deficiency of the phospholipase C coupled platelet P2Y1 receptor leads to a mild bleeding disorder. Thromb Hemost 1999(Suppl): 20–21.

Oury C, Toth-Zsamboki E, Van Geet C: A natural dominant negative P2X1 receptor due to deletion of a single amino acid residue. J Biol Chem 2000; 275:22611–22614.

Padilla A, Moake JL, Bernardo A: P-selectin anchors newly released ultralarge von Willebrand factor multimers to the endothelial cell surface. Blood 2004; 103:2150–2156.

Patel YM, Patel K, Rahman S: Evidence for a role for Gαi1 in mediating weak agonist-induced platelet aggregation in human platelets: reduced Gαi1 expression and defective Gi signaling in the platelets of a patient with a chronic bleeding disorder. Blood 2003; 101:4828–4835.

Peyvandi F, Ferrari S, Lavoretano S: von Willebrand factor cleaving protease (ADAMTS-13) and ADAMTS-13 neutralizing autoantibodies in 100 patients with thrombotic thrombocytopenic purpura. Br J Haematol 2004; 127:433–439.

Pfueller SL, Bilston RA, Logan D: Heterogeneity of drug-dependent platelet antigens and their antibodies in quinine- and quinidine-induced thrombocytopenia: involvement of glycoproteins Ib, IIb, IIIa, and IX. Blood 1988; 72:1155–1162.

Phillips DR, Charo IF, Scarborough RM: GPIIb–IIIa: The responsive integrin. Cell 1991; 65:359–362.

Pincus MR, Dykes DC, Carty RP: Conformational energy analysis of the substitution of Val for Gly

233 in a functional region of platelet GPIbα in platelet-type von Willebrand disease. Biochim Biophys Acta 1991; 1097:133–139.

Podolnikova NP, Yakubenko VP, Volkov GL: Identification of a novel binding site for platelet integrins alpha IIb beta 3 (GPIIbIIIa) and alpha 5 beta 1 in the gamma C-domain of fibrinogen. J Biol Chem 2003; 278:32251–32258.

Poon MC, d'Oiron R: Recombinant activated factor VII (NovoSeven) treatment of platelet-related bleeding disorders. International Registry on Recombinant Factor VIIa and Congenital Platelet Disorders Group. Blood Coagul Fibrinolysis 2000; 11(Suppl 1):55–68.

Quinn M, Deering A, Stewart M: Quantifying GPIIb/IIIa receptor binding using 2 monoclonal antibodies: discriminating abciximab and small molecular weight antagonists. Circulation 1999; 99:2231–2238.

Raccuglia G: Gray platelet syndrome: a variety of qualitative platelet disorder. Am J Med 1971; 51:818

Rao AK: Acquired disorders of platelet function. *In* Clagett P (ed.): Hemostasis and Thrombosis: Basic Principles and Clinical Practice, 5th ed. Philadelphia, Lippincott, Williams & Wilkins 2005a, in press.

Rao AK: Inherited disorders of platelet secretion and signal transduction. *In* Clagett P (ed.): Hemostasis and Thrombosis: Basic Principles and Clinical Practice, 5th ed. Philadelphia, Lippincott, Williams & Wilkins, 2005b, in press.

Rao AK, Ghosh S, Sun L: Effect of mechanism of platelet dysfunction on response to DDAVP in patients with congenital platelet function defects. A double-blind placebo-controlled trial. Thromb Haemost 1995; 74:1071–1078.

Rao AK, Jalagadugula G, Sun L: Inherited defects in platelet signaling mechanisms. Semin Thromb Hemost 2004; 30:525–535.

Recent comprehensive review of platelet signaling biology and pathophysiology.

Rauova L, Poncz M, McKenzie SE: Ultralarge complexes of PF4 and heparin are central to the pathogenesis of heparin-induced thrombocytopenia. Blood 2005; 105:131–138.

Remold-O'Donnell E, Rosen FS, Kenney DM: Defects in Wiskott–Aldrich syndrome blood cells. Blood 1996; 87:2621–2631.

Remuzzi GD, Marchesi M, Livio AE: Altered platelet and vascular prostaglandin-generation in patients with chronic renal failure and prolonged bleeding times. Thromb Res 1978; 13:1007–1115.

Rendu F, Breton-Gorius J, Trugnan G: Studies on a new variant of the Hermansky–Pudlak syndrome: qualitative, ultrastructural, and functional abnormalities of the platelet-dense bodies associated with a phospholipase A defect. Amer J Hemat 1978; 4:387–399.

Rodgers RPC, Levin J: A critical reappraisal of the bleeding time. Semin Thromb Hemost 1990; 16:1–20.

Landmark article (and entire journal issue) demonstrating the poor predictive value of the bleeding time in a wide variety of clinical settings.

Rosenberg N, Dardik R, Rosenthal E: Mutations in the alphaIIb and beta3 genes that cause Glanzmann thrombasthenia can be distinguished by a simple procedure using transformed B-lymphocytes. Thromb Haemost 1998; 79:244–248.

Rossi G, Cattaneo C, Motta M: Platelet kinetic study in patients with idiopathic thrombocytopenic purpura (ITP) refractory or relapsing after corticosteroid treatment. Hematol J 2002; 3:148–152.

Ruan J, Peyruchaud O, Alberio L: Double heterozygosity of the GPIIb gene in a Swiss patient with Glanzmann's thrombasthenia. Br J Haematol 1998; 102:918–925.

Ruggeri ZM, Pareti FI, Mannucci PM: Heightened interaction between platelets and factor VIII/von Willebrand factor in a new subtype of von Willebrand's disease. N Engl J Med 1980; 302:1047–1051.

Classic article reporting discovery of the increase-of-function vWF mutation responsible for type 2B vWD.

Russell SD, Roth GJ: Pseudo-von Willebrand disease: A mutation in the platelet glycoprotein Ibα gene associated with a hyperactive surface receptor. Blood 1993; 81:1787–1791.

Sachs UJH, Kiefel V, Bohringer M: Single amino acid substitution in human platelet glycoprotein Ib beta is responsible for the formation of the platelet-specific alloantigen Iy(a). Blood 2000; 95:1849–1855.

Sadler JE: Von Willebrand disease type 1: a diagnosis in search of a disease. Blood 2003; 101:2089–2093.

Intriguing article questioning whether decreased levels of plasma vWF should simply be considered a risk factor for increased bleeding rather than an actual disease.

Sadler JE: New concepts in von Willebrand disease. Annu Rev Med 2005; 56:173–191.

Recent comprehensive review of von Willebrand factor biology and of von Willebrand disease.

Schafer AI: Deficiency of platelet lipoxygenase activity in myeloproliferative disorders. N Engl J Med 1982; 306:381–386.

Schafer AI: Bleeding and thrombosis in myeloproliferative disorders. Blood 1984; 64:1–12.

Classic paper exploring the relationship between platelets and myeloproliferative disorders.

Schafer AI: Thrombocytosis. N Engl J Med 2004; 350:1211–1219.

Sehayek E, Ben-Yosef N, Modan M: Platelet parameters and aggregation in essential and reactive thrombocytosis. Am J Clin Pathol 1988; 90:431–436.

Sims PJ, Ginsberg MH, Plow EF: Effect of platelet activation on the conformation of the plasma membrane glycoprotein IIb–IIIa complex. J Biol Chem 1991; 266:7345–7352.

Solum NO: Procoagulant expression in platelets and defects leading to clinical disorders. Arterioscler Thromb Vasc Biol 1999a; 19:2841–2846.

Solum NO, Holme PA, Pedersen TM: Detection of biotinylated proteins in crossed immunoelectrophoresis gels: Studies on platelet membrane receptors and microparticles. Electrophoresis 1995; 16:1408–1413.

Stenberg PE, McEver RP, Shuman MA: A platelet alpha-granule membrane protein (GMP-140) is expressed on the plasma membrane after activation. J Cell Biol 1985; 101:880–886.

Sugiyama T, Okuma M, Ushikubi F: A novel platelet aggregating factor found in a patient with defective collagen-induced platelet aggregation and autoimmune thrombocytopenia. Blood 1987; 69:1712–1720.

Sun L, Mao G, Rao AK: Association of CBFA2 mutation with decreased platelet PKC-θ and impaired receptor-mediated activation of GPIIb-IIIa and pleckstrin phosphorylation: proteins regulated by CBFA2 play a role in GPIIb-IIIa activation. Blood 2004; 103:948–954.

Takahashi H, Murata M, Moriki T: Substitution of Val for Met at residue 239 of platelet glycoprotein 16 alpha in Japanese patients with platelet-type von willebrand disease. Blood 1995; 85:727–733.

Taylor FB, Jr., Muller-Eberhard HJ: Qualitative description of factors involved in the retraction and lysis of dilute whole blood clots and in the aggregation and retraction of platelets. J Clin Invest 1970; 49:2068–2085.

Tchernev VT, Mansfield TA, Giot L: The Chediak–Higashi protein interacts with SNARE complex and signal transduction proteins. Mol Med 2002; 8:56–64.

Tsai HM: Shear stress and von Willebrand factor in health and disease. Semin Thromb Hemost 2003; 29:479–488.

Tsai HM, Lian EC: Antibodies to von Willebrand factor-cleaving protease in acute thrombotic thrombocytopenic purpura. N Engl J Med 1998; 339:1585–1594.

Landmark paper leading to the recognition of ADAMTS-13.

Ushikubi F, Ishibashi T, Narumiya S: Analysis of the defective signal transduction mechanism through the platelet thromboxane A$_2$ receptor in a patient with polycythemia vera. Thromb Hemost 1992; 67:144–146.

Van den Oudenrijn S, Bruin M, Folman CC, Bussel J, de Haas M, von dem Borne AE: Three parameters, plasma thrombopoietin levels, plasma glycocalicin levels and megakaryocyte culture, distinguish between different causes of congenital thrombocytopenia. Br J Haematol 2002; 117:390–398.

Vanhoorelbeke K, Cauwenberghs N, Vandecasteele G: A reliable von Willebrand factor: ristocetin cofactor enzyme-linked immunosorbent assay to differentiate between type 1 and type 2 von Willebrand disease. Semin Thromb Hemost 2002; 28:161–166.

Vanhoorelbeke K, Cauwenberghs N, Vauterin S: A reliable and reproducible ELISA method to measure ristocetin cofactor activity of von Willebrand factor. Thromb Haemost 2000; 83:107–113.

Van Vliet HH, Kappers-Klunne MC, van der Hel JW: Antibodies against glycosphingolipids in sera of patients with idiopathic thrombocytopenic purpura. Br J Haematol 1987; 67:103–108.

Vincentelli A, Susen S, Le Tourneau T: Acquired von Willebrand syndrome in aortic stenosis. N Engl J Med 2003; 349:343–349.

Visentin GP, Newman PJ, Aster RH: Characteristics of quinine- and quinidine-induced antibodies specific for platelet glycoproteins IIb and IIIa. Blood 1991; 77:2668–2676.

Von dem Borne AEG, van Leeuwen EF, von Reisz LE: Neonatal alloimmune thrombocytopenia: detection and characterization of the responsible antibodies by the platelet immunofluorescence test. Blood 1981; 57:649–656.

Ware J, Russell SR, Marchese P: Point mutation in a leucine-rich repeat of platelet glycoprotein Ib alpha resulting in the Bernard–Soulier syndrome. J Clin Invest 1993; 92:1213–1220.

Warkentin TE: Heparin-induced thrombocytopenia: a clinicopathologic syndrome. Thromb Haemost 1999a, 82:439–447.

Warkentin TE: Heparin-induced thrombocytopenia: a ten-year retrospective. Annu Rev Med 1999b; 50:129–147.

Warkentin TE, Greinacher A: Heparin-induced thrombocytopenia: recognition, treatment, and prevention: the Seventh ACCP Conference on Antithrombotic and Thrombolytic Therapy. Chest 2004; 126:311S–337S.
Recent comprehensive review of heparin-induced thrombocytopenia.

Warkentin TE, Kelton JG: Thrombocytopenia due to platelet destruction and hypersplenism. *In:* Hoffman R, Benz EJJr, Shattil SJ *et al*, editors: In: Hematology: Basic Principles and Practice. Philadelphia, Elsevier Churchill Livingstone, 2005a.2305–2325

Warkentin TE, Sheppard J-A I, Moore JC: Laboratory testing for the antibodies that cause heparin-induced thrombocytopenia: How much class do we need? J Lab Clin Med 2005b; 146:341–346.

Weiss HJ: Scott syndrome: a disorder of platelet coagulant activity. Semin Hematol 1994; 31:312–319.

Weiss HJ, Lages B: Platelet malondialdehyde production and aggregation responses induced by arachidonate, prostaglandin-G_2, collagen, and epinephrine in 12 patients with storage pool deficiency. Blood 1981; 58:27–33.

Weiss HJ, Lages B: The response of platelets to epinephrine in storage pool deficiency – evidence pertaining to the role of adenosine diphosphate in mediating primary and secondary aggregation. Blood 1988; 72:1717–1725.

Weiss HJ, Lages B: Platelet prothrombinase activity and intracellular calcium responses in patients with storage pool deficiency, glycoprotein IIb-IIIa deficiency, or impaired platelet coagulant activity – a comparison with Scott syndrome. Blood 1997; 89:1599–1611.

Weiss HJ, Meyer D, Rabinowitz R: Pseudo von Willebrand's disease: an intrinsic platelet defect with aggregation by unmodified human factor VIII/von Willebrand factor and enhanced adsorption of its high-molecular-weight multimers. N Engl J Med 1982; 306:326–362.
Discovery of an increase-of-function mutation in the platelet receptor for vWF that mimics type 2B vWD.

Weiss HJ, Witte LD, Kaplan KL: Heterogeneity in storage pool deficiency: Studies on granule-bound substances in 18 patients including variants deficient in -granules, platelet factor-4, β-thromboglobulin and platelet-derived growth factor. Blood 1979; 54:1296.

White JG: Electron microscopy methods for studying platelet structure and function. Methods Mol Biol 2004; 272:47–63.
Definitive methods of platelet electron microscopy.

White JG, Edson JR, Desnick SJ: Studies on platelets in a variant of the Hermansky–Pudlak syndrome. Am J Pathol 1971; 63:319

Whitelock JL, Nolasco L, Bernardo A: ADAMTS-13 activity in plasma is rapidly measured by a new ELISA method that uses recombinant VWF-A2 domain as substrate. J Thromb Haemost 2004; 2:485–491.

Witkop CJ, Babcock MN, Rao GHR: Albinism and Hermansky–Pudlak syndrome in Puerto Rico. Bol Asoc Puerto Rico 1990; 82:333–339.

Woods VL, Jr, Kurata Y, Montgomery RR, et al: Autoantibodies against platelet glycoprotein Ib in patients with chronic immune thrombocytopenic purpura. Blood 1984a; 64:1596–1560.

Woods, VL, Jr, Oh EH, Mason D, McMillan R: Autoantibodies against the platelet glycoprotein IIb/IIIa complex in patients with chronic ITP. Blood 1984b; 63:368–375.

Yang X, Sun L, Ghosh S: Human platelet signaling defect characterized by impaired production of 1,4,5 inositoltrisphosphate and phosphatic acid, and diminished pleckstrin phosphorylation. Evidence for defective phospholipase C activation. Blood 1996; 88:1676–1683.

Yee DL, Bray PF: Clinical and functional consequences of platelet membrane glycoprotein polymorphisms. Semin Thromb Hemost 2004; 30:591–600.

Zhou Q, Zhao J, Stout JG: Molecular cloning of human plasma membrane phospholipid scramblase. A protein mediating transbilayer movement of plasma membrane phospholipids. J Biol Chem 1997; 272:18240–18244.

Zigmond SH: How WASP regulates actin polymerization. J Cell Biol 2000; 150:117–120.

Zucker MB: Platelet aggregation measured by the photometric method. Methods Enzymol 1989; 169:117–133.

Zwaal RF, Comfurius P, Bevers EM: Surface exposure of phosphatidylserine in pathological cells. Cell Mol Life Sci 2005; 62:971–988.

Zwicker JI, Uhl L, Huang WY: Thrombosis and ELISA optical density values in hospitalized patients with heparin-induced thrombocytopenia. J Thromb Haemost 2004; 2:2133–2137.

CHAPTER 40

Laboratory Approach to Thrombotic Risk

Richard A. Marlar PhD, Louis M. Fink MD, Jonathan L. Miller MD PhD

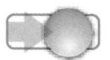

KEY POINTS

• The amount of clot formed is regulated by several important regulatory mechanisms. Under normal conditions these mechanisms control excess clot formation and halt venous thrombosis. The major systems are the antithrombin mechanism, the protein C–protein S system and the tissue factor pathway inhibitor mechanism

• Deficiencies, either genetic or acquired, of the main regulatory proteins (antithrombin, protein C and protein S) increase the risk for venous thrombosis

• Increased levels of the procoagulant factors or polymorphisms (causing functional change) also increase the risk for venous thrombosis. A very common polymorphism in factor V (factor V_Leiden) reduces the ability of activated factor V to be downregulated by activated protein C. Purported elevated levels of prothrombin (due to a specific polymorphism at base-pair 20210) and elevated levels of factor VIII also increase the risk for thrombosis development

• Other inherited or acquired defects in hemostasis (dysfibrinogenemia and fibrinolysis) and in nonhemostatic systems (homocysteine) also increase the risk of venous thrombosis

• Anti-phospholipid syndrome and lupus anticoagulant (LA) are autoimmune disorders that affect the coagulation system and increase the risk of venous and arterial thrombosis. The LA antibodies are heterogeneous and present with a variety of laboratory abnormalities that can only be detected with a battery of tests. An approach for the identification of antiphospholipid syndrome and lupus anticoagulant is presented

• When evaluating a patient for thrombotic risk, it is important to plan the timing of testing so as to avoid misinterpreting a decrease in natural anticoagulants secondary to consumption by thrombosis or to anticoagulation from inherited deficiencies

Hemostatic regulatory mechanisms limit the amount, location and duration of clot formation. Dysfunction in the major regulatory systems of blood coagulation may lead to the pathologic condition of excessive clot formation (thrombosis). Both genetic and acquired deficiencies or abnormalities of such regulatory factors are capable of increasing the risk for thromboembolism. This chapter will discuss a number of factors that influence the balance towards bleeding or towards thrombosis, and the role of the laboratory in identifying abnormalities associated with these factors.

Physiologic Anticoagulant Pathways

Antithrombin (formally termed antithrombin III) is a circulating plasma serine protease inhibitor that regulates thrombin and factor Xa, and to a lesser extent factors IXa, XIa, XIIa and VIIa (Stassen, 2004). The function of antithrombin is greatly enhanced on the endothelial cell surface by cell-bound glycosaminoglycans (heparan sulfate, dermatan sulfate, and the small amounts of heparin) (Fig. 40–1) and pharmacologically by heparin (see Ch. 41).

A second major antithrombotic regulatory system is the protein C pathway, with an apparent two-prong mechanism consisting of a major anticoagulant component (Fig. 40–2) and an indirect profibrinolytic component. The pathway is complex, with multiple factors that must interact to generate a multitiered mechanism (Esmon, 2003a, b). The central protein, protein C, is a vitamin-K-dependent plasma proenzyme. The system is initiated with the generation of excessive non-clot-bound thrombin that rapidly and tightly binds to an endothelial cell trans-membrane glycoprotein, thrombomodulin (TM in Fig. 40–2). Thrombin bound in this complex undergoes a dramatic change in substrate specificity. Whereas it formerly was the sine qua non procoagulant enzyme of the coagulation system and a potent activator of platelets, its new ability to activate protein C effectively renders thrombin a potent anticoagulant enzyme. Thrombomodulin-bound thrombin, together with the endothelial cell protein C receptor (EPCR), rapidly cleaves a small activation peptide from the protein C molecule (Stearns-Kurosawa, 1996; Esmon, 2004). This process generates an active serine protease enzyme, termed activated protein C (APC). A second vitamin-K-dependent inhibitory plasma protein, protein S (PS in Fig. 40–2), serves as a critical cofactor for APC. Protein S is a non-enzymatic cofactor molecule that binds in equilibrium to a large complement protein, C4b binding protein (Rigby, 2004). Only the unbound (or 'free') form of protein S possesses cofactor activity. The complex of APC and protein S at the phospholipid surface of platelets or other cells rapidly inactivates factor Va and factor VIIIa, thereby greatly diminishing thrombin generation in the procoagulant pathways (Esmon, 2003a, b). The protein C system also appears to exert significant, although indirect, profibrinolytic activity. This is believed to involve the thrombin-activated fibrinolytic inhibitor (TAFI) (van de Wouwer, 2004) and also the plasminogen activator inhibitor (PAI)-1. TAFI is a plasma carboxypeptidase that is rapidly activated by the thrombin–thrombomodulin complex (van de Wouwer, 2004). The active form of the carboxypeptidase cleaves C-terminal lysine residues from fibrin that has already undergone proteolytic cleavage by plasmin. Loss of these residues impairs the efficient binding of plasminogen-activating proteins to fibrin, thereby downregulating the fibrinolytic process. Activated protein C, via inactivation of factor Va, causes a decrease in thrombin generation, thus slowing TAFI activation. PAI-1 is inhibited by activated protein C, thereby increasing the overall fibrinolytic activity (Madden, 1991). Based on in vitro and animal experiments, the protein C system may also have other important defense properties, including anti-inflammatory activity and complement activity (Esmon, 2003a).

As shown in Figure 40–3, tissue factor pathway inhibitor (TFPI) is another regulatory system that controls the initiation of the tissue factor

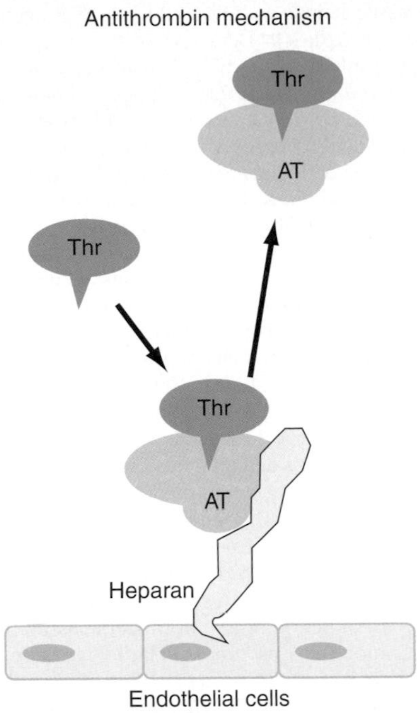

Antithrombin mechanism

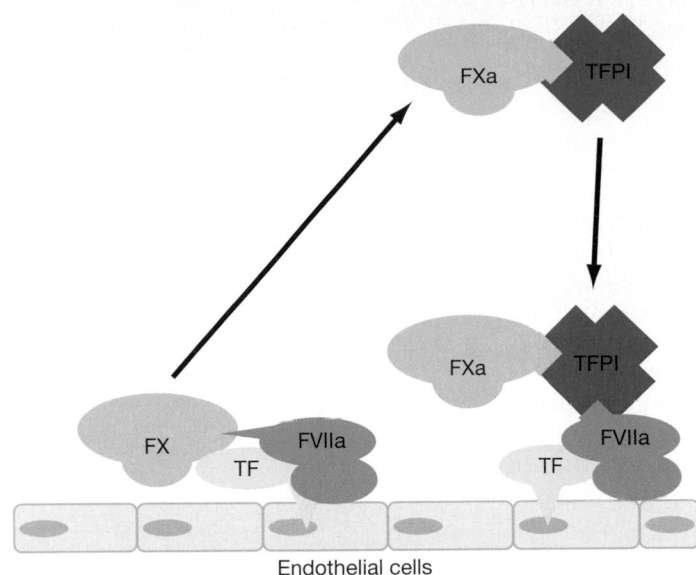

TFPI mechanism

Figure 40–3 Tissue factor pathway inhibitor mechanisms. FVIIa = factor VIIa; FXa = factor Xa; TF = tissue factor; TFPI = tissue factor pathway inhibitor.

Figure 40–1 Antithrombin inhibitor mechanisms. AT = antithrombin (formally termed antithrombin III); Heparan = heparan sulfate (a glycosaminoglycan); Thr = thrombin (or another coagulation enzyme such as factor X).

pathway (also referred to as the 'extrinsic pathway') of coagulation (Smithies, 2004). This inhibitor has two reactive binding sites: one for factor Xa that has previously been activated by tissue factor–factor VIIa, and a second for the tissue factor–factor VIIa complex itself (Esmon, 2003b). After some factor Xa is generated, then and only then can TFPI inhibit the tissue factor–factor VIIa complex. Binding of these proteins by TFPI removes their ability to contribute further to clot formation. TFPI accordingly provides a negative feedback mechanism for downregulating the coagulation process (Esmon, 2003b).

Thrombophilic Proteins or Factors

An imbalance between the procoagulant systems and the regulatory mechanisms can lead either to bleeding or thrombosis. An increase in the procoagulant factors or a decrease in the regulatory factors will tip the balance to excessive fibrin production, resulting in thrombus formation (Lane, 2000).

These imbalances can be caused either by genetic or acquired factors, or by a combination of both (Tables 40–1 and 40–2). However, the process leading to excessive fibrin formation is not as simple as a single factor being disproportionate to the other factors. Rather, it is a combination of mildly to moderately imbalanced factors that leads to excessive fibrin formation at the initial site of injury. This in turn leads to vessel occlusion and fibrin growth (Franco, 2001). This multifactorial paradigm in which these factors interact in a cooperative manner will lead to a significant risk for the development of thrombosis. Therefore a complete assessment of the recognized and established risk factors must be made to determine the overall risk potential for an individual. The following factors are the major known components involved in increased risk for thrombus development (see Table 40–1 for summary of prevalence and relative risk).

Antithrombin

Both hereditary and acquired deficiencies of antithrombin have been identified (Egeber, 1965; Bloemenkamp, 2003). Genetic deficiency of antithrombin is a rare disorder (1 in 10 000 individuals) in the general population and about 1% of patients diagnosed as having familial venous

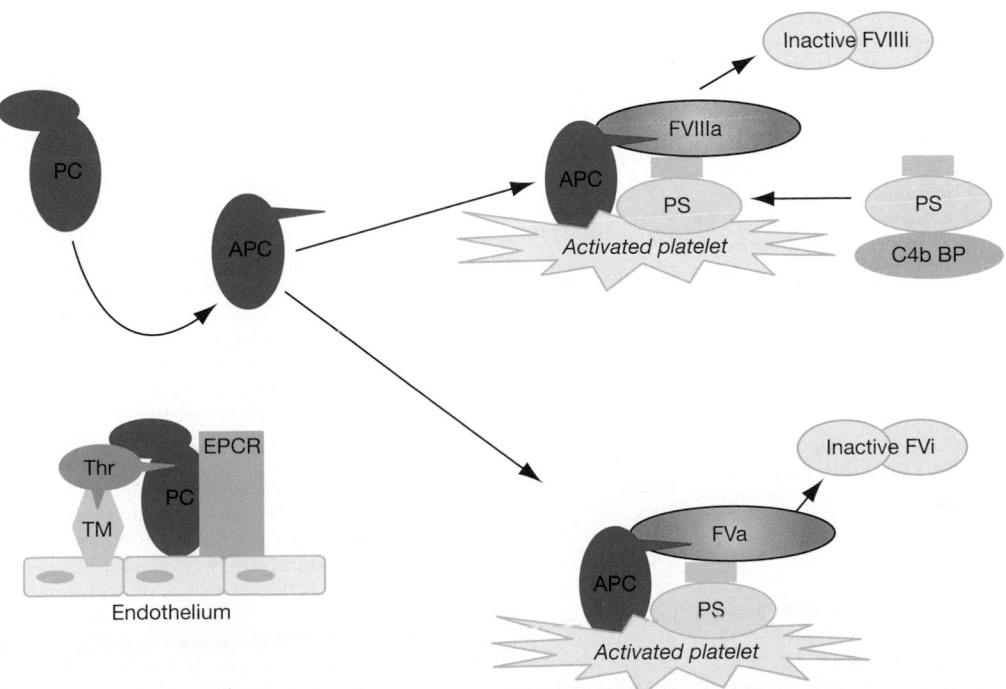

Figure 40–2 Protein C pathway. APC = activated protein C; C4b BP = complement factor 4b binding protein; EPCR = endothelial cell protein C receptor; FVa = factor Va; FVIIIa = factor VIIIa; PC = protein C; PS = protein S; Thr = thrombin; TM = thrombomodulin.

V

Table 40–1 Prevalence and Estimated Increased Thrombotic Risk of Thrombophilic Factors

Risk Factors for Thrombosis	Prevalence in General Population (%)	Prevalence in Thrombophilic Population (%)	Estimated Thrombotic Risk (-fold)
Decreased antithrombin	<0.01	<1	12–20
Decreased protein C	0.3	4–8	8–10
Decreased protein S	0.2	7–12	10–15
APC-R/factor V$_{Leiden}$	3–4*	10–40*	1.8–2.6
Prothrombin G20210A	2–3*	10–15*	1.5–2.2
Elevated factor VIII	10–15	20–35	2–4.5
Elevated fibrinogen	5–12	20–30	2–3
Dysfibrinogenemia	<0.01	0.3–0.8	1.5–3
Thrombomodulin mutations	<0.01	0.2–0.8	2–4
Elevated homocysteine	3–5	8–15	2–4.5
Lupus anticoagulant	<1.0	10–30	2–10
Oral contraceptives	N/A	N/A	2–3
Pregnancy	N/A	N/A	4–8

* Factor V$_{Leiden}$ and prothrombin-20210 prevalence in Caucasian population; however very low (<0.1%) in African and Asian populations

Table 40–2 Estimated Thrombotic Risk for Cooperativeness of Multiple Factors

Risk Factor 1	Risk Factor 2	Combined Risk (-fold)
Protein C	Factor V$_{Leiden}$	25–45
Protein S	Factor V$_{Leiden}$	25–50
Factor V$_{Leiden}$	Elevated Factor VIII	12–20
Factor V$_{Leiden}$	Oral contraceptives	8–20
Factor V$_{Leiden}$	Pregnancy	25–40

thrombosis (Adcock, 1997). Antithrombin is autosomal, having an apparent dominant expression and high penetrance, with a number of known mutants throughout the gene (Adcock, 1997; Lane, 1997). Heterozygous individuals have plasma antithrombin levels around 50% of normal and are usually symptomatic (in contrast to heterozygotes of factor deficiencies, who are usually asymptomatic). Both type I (decreased activity with concomitant decreased antigen) and type II (decreased activity with normal levels of antigen) mutations have been described in antithrombin-deficient individuals (Lane, 1997). Homozygous antithrombin deficiency is incompatible with life, except for unique type II mutations in the heparin binding region, where patients typically manifest venous thrombosis (Kuhle, 2001). The most common clinical presentation is deep venous thrombosis (DVT) in the lower extremities and pulmonary embolus (PE). Interestingly, thrombi may also occur in the retinal, mesenteric, and splenic veins (Bloemenkamp, 2003). Acquired deficiencies of antithrombin occur in disseminated intravascular coagulation (DIC) (Asakura, 2001), liver disease, the nephrotic syndrome, in the acute period following venous thrombosis, and during heparin therapy (Marlar, 1990b). In some cases acquired defects can have plasma levels down to 30–50% of normal and be mistaken for genetic deficiencies. In the newborn period antithrombin is also characteristically low, reaching adult levels by the age of 6 months (Streif, 1999)

Both antithrombin activity and antigen can be determined in plasma using commercial kits. Antithrombin activity is determined based on a chromogenic method utilizing factor Xa or thrombin as the inhibited enzyme. Antithrombin antigen is typically determined by enzyme-linked immunosorbent assay (ELISA) or by nephelometry. The normal ranges for both antithrombin activity and antigen are fairly narrow, usually around 80–120% of normal (Adcock, 1997; Kuhle, 2001).

Protein C

Protein C, the central protein in the protein C pathway, is a vitamin-K-dependent protein. Both genetic and acquired deficiencies of protein C increase the risk for thrombosis. Over 100 mutations have been described with both type I (decreased activity with concomitant decreased antigen)

and type II (decreased activity with normal levels of antigen) proteins (Lane, 1996). As shown in Table 40–1, surveys of the general population have found significant numbers of individuals with decreased levels of protein C. Interestingly, when plasma protein C levels, the types of mutation, and lifestyle are compared, no differences are noted between symptomatic and asymptomatic individuals. The difference between the asymptomatic and symptomatic protein C deficiencies is probably due to the further influence of additional thrombotic risk factors present within the symptomatic population (Marlar, 1990a). In homozygous protein C deficiency, severely deficient (<1% protein C activity) individuals manifest neurologic and ophthalmic complications during intrauterine development, and subsequently develop purpura fulminans and DIC during the newborn period (Peters, 1988; Marlar, 1990c). This disorder is incompatible with life unless treated with protein C replacement (fresh frozen plasma or protein C concentrate) and anticoagulant therapy. The plasma half-life of protein C is relatively short at 6–8 hours. The initiation of oral anticoagulant therapy (especially large loading doses) without overlap of prior heparin anticoagulation in individuals heterozygous for protein C deficiency can lead to an infrequent but devastating condition of thrombotic skin lesions known as warfarin-induced skin necrosis (Marlar, 1990b, Moll, 2004; Tai, 2004)

Testing for protein C is performed in plasma using either clotting- or chromogenic-based activity assays or one of several types of antigen assay. The activity assay measures the function of the molecule in plasma; however, there is the potential that chromogenic assays may erroneously report protein C molecules as functional that actually do not possess functionality with respect to their natural coagulant substrates. For this reason, a clotting-based assay is recommended to assess protein C functional activity (Rezende, 2004). In type I protein C deficiency, the functional activity and the antigen level are decreased to about 50% of normal, whereas in type II deficiency the functional level is decreased on average to 50% of normal but the antigen level is 100% of normal.

Protein S

Both genetic and acquired deficiencies of protein S are associated with an increased risk of thrombosis (Esmon, 2003a). As discussed previously, protein S, together with APC, binds to the phospholipid surface of a platelet or other cell, enhancing the enzymatic inactivation of factors Va and VIIIa (Hackeng, 1994; van Wijnen, 1996). About 40% of the protein S is free in plasma, whereas the remaining 60% is bound to the complement protein, C4b binding protein (C4b BP) (Nelson, 1992). Many pathological and physiological conditions can change the ratio of free and bound protein S, thereby effectively modulating the protein C inhibitory pathway (Mackie, 2001). The level of protein S characteristically decreases during pregnancy, with values averaging 60% of those of controls from the 10th week of pregnancy onwards (Cerneca, 1997).

The gene encoding protein S is autosomal and expressed with variable penetrance (Rezende, 2004). Over 50 mutations have been described with associated increase of thrombotic risk (Simmonds, 1998). The traditional quantitative type I deficiency (decreased protein S activity with concomitant decreased total antigen) and a qualitative type II deficiency (decreased protein S activity with normal levels of free and total antigen) have been reported. Because of the equilibrium between protein S and C4b BP, a third type of mutation has been identified (Simmonds, 1998): type III deficiency is similar to type I, but the decreased protein S activity is associated with normal free protein S yet decreased total protein S. Recent studies appear to show, however, that these rare type III individuals actually may not have increased risk for thrombosis (Brouwer, 2005; Libourel, 2005). Homozygous protein S deficiency with severely decreased protein S (<1% activity) has been reported with the same presentation and similar treatment as homozygous protein C deficiency (Brouwer, 2005). The symptoms are purpura fulminans and DIC during the newborn period, with ophthalmic and neurologic complications having developed in utero. This disorder is incompatible with life unless treated with replacement therapy (fresh frozen plasma) and anticoagulant therapy.

The determination of plasma protein S levels is performed by protein S clotting activity and antigenic assays for free protein S and total protein S antigen. The final diagnosis of protein S deficiency can be very difficult, because of the complexity of the protein S interaction with C4b BP (Nelson, 1992; Goodwin, 2002; Persson, 2003). The activity assay measures the functional fraction of protein S in the plasma sample, but falsely low protein S activity has been reported (Goodwin, 2002). Two types of antigen assay are available: Assays whose measurement includes both free protein S and the bound fraction are considered to be measuring the total amount of protein S in a plasma sample ('total protein S antigen'). Assays for free protein S measure only the unbound portion of protein S: This is achieved either by employing a monoclonal antibody specific for unbound protein

S or by including a precipitation step with polyethylene glycol in which the bound portion of the protein S molecules is removed (Comp, 1986; Goodwin, 2002; Persson, 2003). A clotting-based functional assay is recommended for the initial assessment of protein S. If the level is found to be decreased, reflex testing of both free and total protein S antigen should then be performed. Reaching a definitive diagnosis of congenital deficiency of protein S is challenging, given the complexity of the interaction of protein S with C4b BP, the acquired conditions that can change the equilibrium of the free and bound forms, and the presence of vitamin K antagonists (Simmonds, 1998; Mackie, 2001; Goodwin, 2002; Rezende, 2004).

Activated Protein C Resistance and Factor V$_{Leiden}$

Activated protein C resistance (APC-R) is said to be present when the addition of exogenous APC to plasma does not result in the anticipated prolongation of clotting time tests such as the partial thromboplastin time (PTT) (Dahlbäck, 1999). APC-R is considered one of the most common genetic risk factors for venous thrombosis; however, while the prevalence of this abnormality in the Caucasian population is on average 4%, prevalence is lower in the African and Asian populations (Ridker, 1995; Heijmans, 1998). APC normally enzymatically inactivates factors Va and VIIIa, prolonging the clotting time of plasma. In APC-R, the ability of APC to enzymatically degrade factor Va is significantly reduced. The polymorphism at one of the cleavage sites in factor Va is an arginine residue substituted by a glutamine residue (R506Q) that renders the site resistant to cleavage (Aparicio, 1996). The amino acid substitution is due to a single nucleotide change in the gene, termed factor V$_{Leiden}$ (Bertina, 1994). Factor V$_{Leiden}$ increases the relative risk of thrombosis by 2–3-fold in the heterozygous condition and by 8–12-fold in the homozygous individual (Svensson, 1997; De Stefano, 1999). There are numerous variations of the assay for APC-R, with some being fairly specific for factor V$_{Leiden}$. For APC-R assays, two clotting tests are performed: the first is in the presence of APC, and the second is in the absence of APC. If a ratio of the clotting time with added APC divided by the clotting time in the absence of APC is sufficiently high (usually >2.0), then there is an absence of APC-R or of factor V$_{Leiden}$. Lower ratios, in contrast, suggest that the sample is APC-resistant, and the patient may have factor V$_{Leiden}$. Depending on the method used, a number of acquired causes of APC resistance have been identified (Tripodi, 1997). Malignancy, antiphospholipid syndrome, pregnancy, and even hospitalization can cause an abnormal result (Cumming, 1995; Graf, 2003). The specific polymorphism of factor V$_{Leiden}$ is determined by molecular diagnostic methods (Aparicio, 1996; Tripodi, 1997).

Prothrombin-20210

A polymorphism in the prothrombin gene at base pair number 20 210 is a guanine to adenine substitution in the 3′-untranslated region of the gene (Colucci, 2004). It imparts a twofold increased risk for venous thrombosis (Eikelboom, 1999). Heterozygous individuals characteristically have levels of plasma prothrombin higher than in individuals lacking this polymorphism, although even these higher levels usually fall within the established reference interval for prothrombin activity of most laboratories. Accordingly, molecular diagnostic procedures are required for the diagnosis of prothrombin 20210 (Poort, 1996; Gruenewald, 2000). There is believed to be increased transcription of the gene into the gene product, probably resulting from an increase in time during which mRNA molecules are translated (De Stefano, 1999). Prothrombin 20210 is a common genetic risk factor for venous thrombosis in populations of European descent (about 3%), with lower prevalence in other, non-European populations (De Stefano, 1999).

Elevated Coagulation Factor Levels

In addition to an elevated level of prothrombin acting as a risk factor for thrombosis, elevation of several other coagulation factors has also been reported to impart an increased risk of thrombosis. As factors VII, VIII, IX, XI, or fibrinogen levels are elevated, the relative risks for developing thrombosis proportionately increase (1.5–6-fold) (Kannel, 1987; O'Donnell, 1997; Kyrle, 2000; Meijers, 2000; Weltermann, 2003). The most studied and most complex of these reported risk factors is factor VIII. Factor VIII is regulated by genetic mechanisms and additionally by physiologic mechanisms that increase factor VIII levels in times of stress and exercise. Some familial elevation of factor VIII has been reported but transiently high levels can be seen in patients with stress due to a variety of clinical conditions. Factor VIII levels of 120–150% have an increased risk of thrombosis of 1.5–2.0-fold; levels of 300–400% have an increased relative risk of 3–6-fold (O'Donnell, 1997).

Dysfibrinogenemia

Fibrinogen is the final protein in the formation of a clot and the major component in a venous thrombus. The published reports of abnormalities associated with increased risk of thrombosis due to dysfunctional fibrinogen molecules are rare (Haverkate, 1995). The incidence of recognized cases of dysfibrinogenemia in familial thrombosis is about 0.8%. Dysfibrinogenemias are thought to increase the risk of thrombosis about 2–6-fold. Presently, the only assays commonly employed to assess fibrinogen are functional assays of clottability and antigenic assays. As discussed in Chapter 39, an imbalance in the ratio of such assays provides an indication of a decrease-of-function dysfibrinogenemia. Unfortunately, subtleties in the ability of fibrinogen – and perhaps more importantly of the resulting fibrin – to bind proteins having an influence on the balance of hemostasis and thrombosis (e.g., tissue plasminogen activator) are not picked up by such assays. It is accordingly possible that the frequency by which dysfibrinogenemias underlie thrombotic events may be even higher than presently recognized

Hypofibrinolytic Mechanisms

Impaired function of the fibrinolytic system increases the risk of thrombosis, but there remains a lack of global clinical assays sufficiently robust to allow estimation of the degree of that risk (Collen, 1999). The euglobulin clot lysis time (ECLT or ELT) provides a measure of some aspects of the fibrinolytic system (Sartori, 2003). In brief, citrated plasma is diluted and acidified, resulting in the selective precipitation of many proteins, which include fibrinogen, plasminogen activator, and plasminogen, whereas other molecules including α_2-antiplasmin, remain in solution. This precipitated 'euglobulin fraction' is then redissolved in an appropriate buffer, clotted by thrombin, and the time to clot lysis measured. An abnormally prolonged euglobulin clot lysis time helps focus the subsequent laboratory evaluation on an underlying abnormality of a critical component of the fibrinolytic system. Such a result adds support to the decision to proceed to more detailed testing of the fibrinolytic system, such as specific assays for plasminogen activator, plasminogen, and other proteins upregulating or downregulating fibrinolysis.

Deficiencies of plasminogen, the major enzyme responsible for fibrin clot breakdown (see Ch. 38), have been reported, but the association with increased thrombotic risk is not well founded (Schulman, 1996). A polymorphism in the plasminogen activator inhibitor (PAI)-1 gene has had reports showing a slight increase in thrombotic risk, but is not well established and not recommended to be tested at this time (Iacoviello, 1998). Defects in plasminogen inhibitors (PAI-1 and PAI-2) and activators (tPA) regulated by the endothelial cell, white blood cells, and platelets are suspected, but not established, thrombotic risk factors (van der Bom, 1997). Assessment of the mechanical properties of clots throughout the period of their formation and subsequent lysis with the Thromboelastograph, Sonoclot®, or similar devices represents a quite different approach which, with sufficient standardization, may permit the detection of abnormal fibrinolysis (Vig, 2001; Salooja, 2001; Kamada, 2001). These types of instruments work by detecting the clot 'rigidity' or 'strength' during the clot formation and breakdown process. More details about the methodology can be reviewed in the following references: Vig, 2001; Salooja, 2001; Kamada, 2001.

Other Possible Defects

Abnormalities in several other coagulation regulatory proteins and platelet proteins have been reported. However, difficulty in assessment of these proteins and the lack of conclusive correlation with increased thrombotic risk has not yet established them as important risk factors for venous thrombosis.

Thrombomodulin (labeled as 'TM' in Fig. 40–2) defects have been reported by several groups to have good association with thrombosis (2–6-fold). Because there appear to be numerous defects spanning a large portion of the thrombomodulin gene, essentially detectable only through extensive sequencing, it is, however, still a challenge for clinical laboratories to detect these abnormalities (Ohlin, 1995; 1997).

Heparin cofactor II, a thrombin-specific inhibitor with homology to antithrombin, has not been demonstrated to be associated with increased risk of thrombosis (Tollefsen, 2002; Giri, 2005). The PLA-1/PLA-2 polymorphism of the platelet glycoprotein IIb/IIIa complex has been associated with an increased risk of arterial and venous thrombosis (Weiss, 1996). The effects of such polymorphisms are of increasing interest in the emerging study of antithrombotic pharmacogenetics. The PLA-1/PLA-2 polymorphism, as well as other platelet glycoprotein polymorphisms, is currently being critically assessed to determine its potential role as a clinical assay for thrombotic assessment (Lindoff, 1997; Heit, 2000; Robert 2000; Paganin, 2003). Additionally, the non-O types of the ABO blood groups have been reported as increased thrombotic risk factors compared with type O, possibly due to increased levels of von Willebrand factor and factor VIII (De Visser, 2003).

Acquired Hypercoagulable States

Numerous acquired conditions have been associated with an increased risk of venous thrombosis. The relative risk for many of these has been determined and appears to combine with the genetic causes to increase the overall risk for thrombosis. Common conditions having a strong association with venous thrombosis include: trauma, surgery and the postoperative state, pregnancy, immobility, obesity and diet, smoking, and previous thrombosis. Additionally, malignancy, chronic DIC, oral contraceptive use and hormone replacement use, heparin-induced thrombocytopenia, nephrotic syndrome, essential thrombocythemia, polycythemia vera, and inflammatory conditions have all been associated with an increased risk of venous thrombosis. Finally, as discussed in Chapter 39, abnormalities of the enzyme ADAMTS13 have been associated with the thrombotic disorder thrombotic thrombocytopenic purpura (TTP).

Antiphospholipid Syndrome and Lupus Anticoagulant

The antiphospholipid syndrome (APS) is one of the most commonly acquired risk factors of thrombosis and is a major cause of pregnancy loss. This syndrome appears to result from the formation of antibodies that are directed against β_2-glycoprotein I (β_2-GPI) or another phospholipid-binding protein (such as prothrombin, protein S, thrombomodulin, or others). These antibodies bind to various epitopes on the phospholipid-binding proteins. When this antibody–antigen interaction occurs in vivo, the result is prothrombotic. It is thus ironic that functional demonstration of the presence of APS-associated antibodies in the clinical laboratory is evidenced by the inhibition of procoagulant reactions. The term 'lupus anticoagulant' (LA) applied to such functionally demonstrable antibodies is accordingly misleading, since the corresponding in vivo effect is actually prothrombotic. It is further misleading, since most patients having LAs do not have lupus, despite this association having been noted in the original descriptions of this entity. Finally, despite the target for such antibodies being epitopes within phospholipid-binding proteins (see above), the original studies identifying these antibodies antigenically employed cardiolipin, phosphatidylserine, or other phospholipids within the binding assay, with the result that antibodies associated with the APS are still often referred to as 'anticardiolipin antibodies,' 'antiphosphatidylserine antibodies,' etc. Many of these 'antiphospholipid antibodies' (APAs) also generate false-positive results in biological tests for syphilis (VDRL) (Riboldi, 2003; McCrae, 2001; Galli, 2003).

The mechanisms by which APAs interfere with hemostatic processes appear to be multifactorial, likely reflecting the considerable diversity of phospholipid-associated target proteins playing critical roles in hemostasis and thrombosis. Reports of in vivo mechanisms include thrombomodulin or protein S inhibition, platelet activation, and endothelial cell activation. An important subset of such antibodies is against the prothrombin molecule. Such antibodies neutralize the prothrombin molecule and enhance the clearance of prothrombin from the blood. These antiprothrombin antibodies have been reported to be present in about 76% of patients with LA, even through the prothrombin levels are not decreased in plasma (Guerin, 1998).

In a number of studies, abnormal LA or anticardiolipin tests have been reported to occur in 2–15% of the apparently asymptomatic general population, with many of these antibodies being transitory (Galli 2003). Persistence of LAs, however, is associated with an approximately 30% risk of developing symptoms characteristic of APS. It is not unusual in the evolution of APS for there to be a demonstrable LA but not APA, or conversely a demonstrable APA but not LA. In ELISA-based assays of APA, separate determinations are made of IgG, IgM, and often also IgA classes of antibodies. There appears to be a relationship between level of APAs and thrombotic risk. Many laboratories interpret 'anticardiolipin' levels as mildly elevated, moderately elevated or highly elevated. However, the setting of precise upper cutoff limits to distinguish disease from normal in the different testing systems still remains to be standardized.

Recent studies by the de Groot laboratory have led to a proposed pathophysiological mechanism in which β_2-GPI first binds to platelet membranes and subsequently undergoes conformational change that exposes binding sites for anti-β_2-GPI antibody. Binding of the antibody in turn leads to platelet activation (de Groot, 2005). Laboratory testing to identify the subset of anti-β_2-GPI antibodies that may function by this pathophysiological mechanism will likely require an assay system that

replicates key features of the in vivo system, including the required conformational change of β_2-GPI (de Laat, 2006).

While there presently is no uniform approach for the diagnosis of LAs, it is clear that, because of the heterogeneity of these antibodies, the presence of a LA cannot be excluded simply by the failure to detect it in any single testing system. At a minimum, two distinct testing systems should be available to the laboratory (Brandt 1995a; Levine 2002) (Table 40–3). Most commonly, the PTT and the dilute Russell viper venom time (DRVVT) are employed for this purpose. The PTT and DRVVT are the main coagulation assays that are standardized and readily available on automated instruments. Since these assays recognize different aspects of the phospholipid-dependent coagulation reactions, they detect the majority of LA antibodies. LA-sensitive PTT reagents contain a mixture of phospholipids that interact with the LA antibodies at two critical points in the intrinsic system. The DRVVT uses a dilute concentration of phospholipids at a single phospholipid-dependent step within the coagulation pathway, which facilitates LA antibody detection.

As mentioned above, one commonly employed testing system for detection of LAs is the PTT. A LA typically will prolong the clotting time of the test performed on the patient's plasma. When patient plasma is then mixed in equal parts with normal control plasma, most LAs will also prolong the clotting time of the mixture by at least 5 seconds beyond the clotting time of the normal control plasma itself. Preincubation of the patient plasma with an appropriate source of phospholipid protein, however, can effectively 'neutralize' the LA, resulting in a significant shortening of the subsequently performed clotting time. Neutralizing substances range from purified 'hexagonal phase phospholipids' to the much more complex lysates of sequentially frozen and then thawed washed platelets (platelet neutralization procedure, PNP). As emphasized by Greaves and coworkers (Greaves, 2000; Jennings, 2002), attention to the many methodological details involved in LA testing can be critical to interpretation of the results. For example, employing a ratio of patient to control clotting times in each phase of testing in the DRVVT system (Fig. 40–4) and including a heparin neutralizing agent increases the robustness of this test system. Additionally, reagents employed in PTT testing for LAs should be carefully chosen with respect to having sufficient sensitivity to LAs.

Whereas specific factor inhibitors, such as those directed against factor VIII, are typically time- and temperature-dependent (see Ch. 38), LAs more commonly are immediate-acting even at room temperature. Of particular note, LAs are notorious for interfering with quantitative measurement of coagulation factors assayed in a PTT-based system. A telltale pattern that should itself arouse suspicion of a LA is a persisting

Table 40–3 Laboratory Approach to Lupus Anticoagulant Detection

Testing Stage	Method of Detection
Initial testing	The first step is prolongation of coagulation in at least one phospholipid-dependent in vitro coagulation assay with the use of platelet-poor plasma. These assays can be subdivided according to the portion of the coagulation cascade that they evaluate as follows: • The 'extrinsic' coagulation pathway (e.g., dilute PT) • The 'intrinsic' coagulation pathway (e.g., activated PTT) • The 'final common' coagulation pathway (e.g., DRVVT)
Mixing	The second step is a failure to correct the prolonged coagulation time by mixing the patient's plasma with normal plasma (Note that in some protocols a correction/neutralization step directly follows an abnormal initial testing step, with omission of a mixing step)
Correction/ Neutralization	The third step is confirmation of the presence of lupus anticoagulant antibodies by shortening or correction of the prolonged coagulation time after the addition of excess phospholipid or platelets that have been frozen and then thawed
Exclusion	The fourth step is ruling out other coagulopathies with the use of specific factor assays if the confirmatory test is negative or if a specific factor inhibitor is suspected

The use of two or more assays sensitive to lupus anticoagulant antibodies is recommended before the presence of lupus anticoagulant antibodies is excluded. At least one of these assays should be based on low phospholipid concentration (dilute PT, dilute activated PPT, colloidal silica clotting time, kaolin clotting time, or DRVVT). The two assays should evaluate distinct portions of the coagulation cascade (e.g., activated PTT and DRVVT). (Adapted from Levine 2002 and from Brandt 1995b.)

DRVVT = dilute Russell's viper venom time; PTT = partial thromboplastin time; PT = prothrombin time.

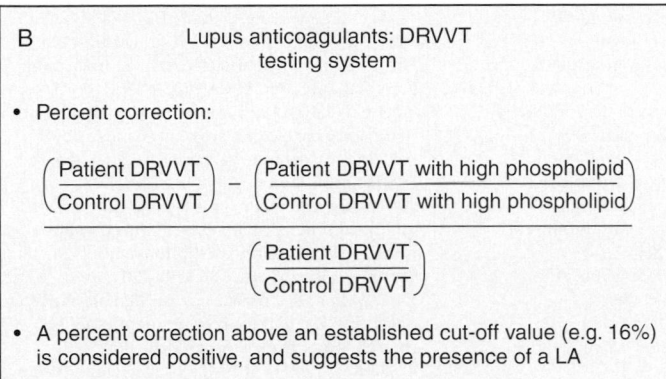

Figure 40–4 Example of dilute Russell viper venom test (DRVVT) in evaluation of a possible lupus anticoagulant (LA). *A* Description of the testing system. *B* Correction (neutralization) stage of DRVVT testing.

Table 40–4 Factors Affecting Measurements of Thrombophilic Factors

Physiological	Pathological	Pharmacological
Newborn	Disseminated intravascular coagulation (DIC)	Warfarin
Childhood	Thrombosis	Heparin
Pregnancy	Liver disease	Thrombin inhibitors
	Nephrotic syndrome	
	Diabetes	
	Hospitalization	

Table 40–5 Recommended Battery of Tests for Assessment of Thrombophilia

Test	Asymptomatic and no Anticoagulation	Symptomatic or Heparin or Oral Anticoagulation	Reflexive Testing
APC-R	APC-R		Factor V_{Leiden}
Factor V_{Leiden}		Factor V_{Leiden}	
Protein C	Protein C activity		Protein C antigen
Protein S	Protein S activity		Free PS antigen; total PS antigen
Antithrombin	Antithrombin activity		Antithrombin antigen
Prothrombin-20210	Prothrombin-20210	Prothrombin-20210	
Anti-phospholipid syndrome	Lupus anticoagulant; Anticardiolipin		Confirm in 6–8 weeks
Homocysteine	Homocysteine	Homocysteine	Homocysteine
Fibrinogen	Fibrinogen		Fibrinogen antigen
Factor VIII	Factor VIII		Confirm in 3–6 weeks

increase in apparent factor activity with increasing dilutions of patient plasma used in the assay: such apparent increases in factor activity result from corresponding dilutions of LA.

Hyperhomocysteinemia

Homocysteine is an amino acid that is an intermediate molecule for the production and regulation of the sulfur-containing amino acid methionine (Guba, 1996; Refsum, 1998; Cattaneo, 2001). Perturbations, either genetic or acquired, in the regulatory mechanism of this pathway can lead to elevated levels of homocysteine and to an associated increased risk of thrombosis. The most devastating of these is the cystathionine-β-synthetase (*CBS*) gene, which in the homozygous state leads to severe thrombosis and atherosclerosis (Mudd, 1985). Acquired causes, mostly associated with diet and vitamin intake, are also significant factors raising homocysteine levels in plasma. The associated risk for thrombosis by elevated homocysteine levels is a graded response, in which the higher the plasma level, the greater the risk. Of note, two common polymorphisms associated with the homocysteine metabolizing enzyme methylenetetrahydrofolate reductase (MTHFR) were initially thought to be associated with increased risk of thrombosis (Tosetto, 1997; Franco, 1999). However, major epidemiological studies have failed to confirm either an increased thrombotic risk for MTHFR polymorphisms or a corresponding increase in the plasma levels of homocysteine. Accordingly, evaluating MTHFR polymorphisms as a cause of venous thrombosis is not presently recommended (Franco, 1999; Legnani, 1997). Plasma levels of homocysteine, however, should be determined as part of such an investigation.

General Aspects of the Laboratory Evaluation for Thrombotic Risk

The laboratory evaluation of thrombophilia is complex and rapidly changing, including the appropriate tests to order, when to order them, and on whom to perform the testing. There is no global test to grade the thrombotic risk status of an individual, so that a series of individual tests must be ordered to obtain a good assessment of risk. Many physiological, pathological and pharmacological factors (Table 40–4) can influence some or all of the plasma-based tests, such as pregnancy, warfarin, DIC, liver disease, and age. Molecular diagnostic tests, in contrast, are not affected by such influences. From the laboratory perspective, the appropriate assays must be utilized. Whenever possible, activity assays should be used to determine the functionality of the molecule; simply determining the antigen level may miss the type II molecule and misidentify the patient as

normal (Rezende, 2004). A number of questions must be asked for every patient to be evaluated: Does the patient (and family) history actually justify an evaluation? Are the tests ordered appropriate to include the major accepted risk factors? Is the timing appropriate to provide the proper evaluation? Are there underlying therapeutic, pathologic, or physiologic conditions that interfere with the interpretations of the results?

Evaluations are ideally performed when the patient is asymptomatic and not on anticoagulation therapy. Unfortunately, the immediate post-thrombotic period before anticoagulation is a period when plasma factors are consumed, and erroneous diagnoses can be made. Heparin significantly decreases antithrombin levels, increases protein S levels, and may mask lupus anticoagulants (unless a heparin-neutralizing molecule such as protamine or polybrene is included in the assay). Warfarin decreases protein C and protein S levels. The only risk markers that can be evaluated at all times are the genetic markers assayed by molecular diagnostic techniques. Attempts have been made to circumvent the test abnormalities produced by oral anticoagulation by using ratios of protein C or protein S to one or another of the vitamin-K-dependent coagulation factors. However, the variability of such ratios can be considerable, inviting the opportunity for misdiagnosis, and this approach is not recommended. Underlying asymptomatic periods such as post-surgery and pregnancy also can decrease or change plasma factors, leading to erroneous diagnosis. Recommended tests and appropriate timing for their performance are detailed in Table 40–5.

Perhaps even more than in many other areas of clinical medicine, it is of critical importance to communicate the implications of these laboratory results to the patient in a manner that neither underestimates nor overestimates the role that thrombotic risk plays in that patient's life. Decisions such as whether or not to take oral contraceptives, management of pregnancies, and whether or not to undergo chronic anticoagulant therapy can be difficult for both patient and provider. In the case of inherited disorders, genetic counselors may play a critical role as well. In all such instances, knowledge not only of available testing but also of the limits in the interpretation of these tests can contribute greatly towards reaching the most appropriate clinical decisions.

Adcock DM, Fink L, Marlar RA: A laboratory approach to the evaluation of hereditary hypercoagulability. Am J Clin Pathol 1997; 108:434–449.

Aparicio C, Dahlbäck B: Molecular mechanisms of activated protein C resistance: properties of factor V isolated from an individual with homozygosity for the Arg506 to Gln mutation in the factor V gene. Biochem J 1996; 313:467–472.

Asakura H, Ontachi Y, Mizutani T, et al: Decreased plasma activity of antithrombin or protein C is not due to consumption coagulopathy in septic patients with disseminated intravascular coagulation. Eur J Haematol 2001; 67:170–175.

Bertina RM, Koeleman BP, Koster T, et al: Mutation in blood coagulation factor V associated with resistance to activated protein C. Nature 1994; 369:64–67.

Bloemenkamp KW, Helmerhorst FM, Rosendaal FR, et al: Thrombophilias and gynaecology. Best Pract Res Clin Obstet Gynaecol 2003; 17:509–528.

Brandt JT, Barna LK, Triplett DA: Laboratory identification of lupus anticoagulants: result of the Second International workshop for identification of lupus anticoagulants. Thromb Haemost 1995a; 74:1597–1603.

Brandt JT, Triplett DA, Alving B: Criteria for the diagnosis of lupus anticoagulants: an update. On behalf of the Subcommittee on Lupus Anticoagulant/Antiphospholipid Antibody of the Scientific and Standardisation Committee of the ISTH. Thromb Haemost 1995b; 74:1185–1190.

Brouwer JL, Veeger NJ, Schaaf W, et al: Difference in absolute risk of venous and arterial thrombosis between familial protein S deficiency type I and type III. Results from a family cohort study to assess the clinical impact of a laboratory test-based classification. Br J Haematol 2005; 128:703–710.

Cattaneo M Hyperhomocysteinemia and thrombosis. Lipids 2001; 36(Suppl):S13–S26.

Cerneca F, Ricci G, Simeone R, et al: Coagulation and fibrinolysis changes in normal pregnancy. Increased levels of procoagulants and reduced levels of inhibitors during pregnancy induce a hypercoagulable state, combined with a reactive fibrinolysis. Eur J Obstet Gynecol Reprod Biol 1997; 73:31–36.

Collen D: The plasminogen (fibrinolytic) system. Thromb Haemost 1999; 82:259.

Colucci M, Binetti BM, Tripodi A, et al: Hyperprothrombinemia associated with prothrombin G20210A mutation inhibits plasma fibrinolysis through a TAFI-mediated mechanism. Blood 2004; 103:2157–2161.

Comp PC, Thurnau GR, Welsh J, et al: Functional and immunologic protein S levels are decreased during pregnancy. Blood 1986; 68:881–885.

Conard J, Horellou MH, Van Dreden P, et al: Thrombosis and pregnancy in congenital deficiencies in AT III, protein C or protein S: study of 78 women. Thromb Haemost 1990; 63:319–320.

Cumming AM, Keeney S, Salden A, et al: The prothrombin gene G20210A variant: prevalence in a UK anticoagulant clinic population. Br J Haematol 1997; 98:353–55.

Cumming AM, Tait RC, Fildes S, et al Development of resistance to activated protein C during pregnancy. Br J Haematol 1995; 90: 725–727.

Dahlbäck B: Activated protein C resistance and thrombosis: molecular mechanisms of hypercoagulable state due to FVR506Q mutation. Semin Thromb Hemost 1999; 25:273–289.

De Groot PG, Derksen RH: Pathophysiology of the antiphospholipid syndrome. J Thromb Haemost 2005; 3:1854–1860.

De Laat B, Derksen RH, van Lummel M, et al: Pathogenic anti-β_2-GPI antibodies recognize domain I of β_2-GPI only after a conformational change. Blood 2006; 107.

De Stefano V, Martinelli I, Mannucci PM, et al: The risk of recurrent deep venous thrombosis among heterozygous carriers of both factor V Leiden and the G20210A prothrombin mutation. N Engl J Med 1999; 341:801–806.

De Visser MC, Sandkuijl LA, Lensen RP, et al: Linkage analysis of factor VIII and von Willebrand factor loci as quantitative trait loci. J Thromb Haemost 2003; 1:1771–1776.

Egeberg O: Inherited antithrombin III deficiency causing thrombophilia. Thromb Diath Haemorrh 1965; 13:516–520.

Eikelboom JW, Ivey L, Ivey J, et al: Familial thrombophilia and the prothrombin 20210A mutation: association with increased thrombin generation and unusual thrombosis. Blood Coagul Fibrinolysis 1999; 10:1–5.

Esmon CT: Inflammation and thrombosis. J Thromb Haemost 2003a; 1:1343–1348.

Good description of the regulatory mechanisms of hemostasis especially the protein C system.

Esmon CT: The protein C pathway. Chest 2003b; 124(Suppl):26S–32S.

Esmon CT: Structure and functions of the endothelial cell protein C receptor. Crit Care Med 2004; 32(Suppl):S298–S301.

Franco RF, Morelli B, Lourenco D, et al: A second mutation in the methylenetetrahydrofolate reductase gene and the risk of venous thrombotic disease. Br J Haematol 1999; 105:556–559.

Franco RF, Reitsma PH: Genetic risk factors of venous thrombosis. Hum Genet 2001; 109:369–384.

The authors review the common and important genetic risk markers for venous thrombosis.

Galli M, Luciani D, Bertolini G, et al: Lupus anticoagulants are stronger risk factors for thrombosis than anticardiolipin antibodies in the antiphospholipid syndrome: a systematic review of the literature. Blood 2003; 101:1827–1832.

Giri TK, Ahn CW, Wu KW, et al. Heparin cofactor II levels do not predict the development of coronary heart disease: the atherosclerosis risk in communities (ARIC) study [Letter to the editor]. Arterioscler Thromb Vasc Biol 2005; 25:2689–2690.

Goodwin AJ, Rosendaal FR, Kottke-Marchant K, et al: A review of the technical, diagnostic, and epidemiologic considerations for protein S assays. Arch Pathol Lab Med 2002; 126:1349–1366.

Graf LL, Welsh CH, Qamar Z, et al: Activated protein C resistance assay detects thrombotic risk factors other than factor V Leiden. Am J Clin Pathol 2003; 119:52–60.

Greaves M, Cohen H, Machin SJ, et al: Guidelines on the investigation and management of the antiphospholipid syndrome. Br J Haematol 2000; 109:704–715.

Gruenewald M, Germowitz A, Beneke H, et al: Coagulation factor II activity determination is not useful as a screening tool for the G20210A prothrombin gene allele [letter]. Thromb Haemost 2000; 84:141–142.

Guba SC, Fink LM, Fonseca V: Hyperhomocysteinemia: an emerging and important risk factor for thromboembolic and cardiovascular disease. Am J Clin Pathol 1996; 105:709–722.

Guerin J, Smith O, White B, Sweetman G, Feighery C, Jackson J: Antibodies to prothrombin in antiphospholipid syndrome and inflammatory disorders. Br J Haematol 1998; 102:896–902.

Hackeng TM, van't Veer C, Meijers JC, et al: Human protein S inhibits prothrombinase complex activity on endothelial cells and platelets via direct interactions with factors Va and Xa. J Biol Chem 1994; 269:21051–21058.

Haverkate F, Samama M: Familial dysfibrinogenemia and thrombophilia. Thromb Haemost 1995; 73:151–161.

Heijmans BT, Westendorp RG, Knook DL, et al: The risk of mortality and the factor V Leiden mutation in a population-based cohort. Thromb Haemost 1998; 80:607–609.

Heit JA, Mohr DN, Silverstein MD, et al: Predictors of recurrence after deep vein thrombosis and pulmonary embolism – A population-based cohort study. Arch Intern Med 2000; 160:761–768.

Iacoviello L, Burzotta F, Di Castelnuovo A, et al: The 4G/5G polymorphism of PAI-1 promoter gene and the risk of myocardial infarction: a meta-analysis. Thromb Haemost 1998.; 80:1029–1035

Jennings I, Greaves M, Mackie IJ, et al: Lupus anticoagulant testing: improvements in performance in a UK NEQAS proficiency testing exercise after dissemination of national guidelines on laboratory methods. Br J Haematol 2002; 119:364–369.

This is a current review of the most appropriate method for evaluating for the anti-phospholipid syndrome and lupus anticoagulation.

Kamada Y, Yamakage M, Niiya T, et al: Celite-activated viscometer Sonoclot can measure the suppressive effect of tranexamic acid on hyperfibrinolysis in cardiac surgery. J Anesth 2001; 15:17–21.

Kannel WB, Wolf PA, Castelli WP, D'Agostino RB: Fibrinogen and risk of cardiovascular disease: the Framingham Study. JAMA 1987; 258:1183–1186.

Koppelman SJ, Hackeng TM, Sixma JJ, et al: Inhibition of the intrinsic factor X activating complex by protein S: evidence for a specific binding of protein S to factor VIII. Blood 1995; 86:1062–1071.

Kuhle S, Lane DA, Jochmanns K, et al: Homozygous antithrombin deficiency type II (99 Leu to Phe mutation) and childhood thromboembolism. Thromb Haemost 2001; 86:1007–1011.

Kyrle PA, Minar E, Hirschl M, et al: High plasma levels of factor VIII and the risk of recurrent venous thromboembolism. N Engl J Med 2000; 343: 457–462.

Lane DA, Bayston T, Olds RJ, et al: Antithrombin mutation database: 2nd (1997) update. Thromb Haemost 1997; 77:197–211.

Lane DA, Gant PJ: Role of hemostatic gene polymorphisms in venous and arterial thrombotic disease. Blood 2000; 95:1517–1532.

A review paper on the important genetic thrombotic risk factors.

Lane DA, Mannucci PM, Bauer KA, et al: Inherited thrombophilia. Thromb Haemost 1996; 76:651–662.

Legnani C, Palareti G, Grauso F, et al: Hyperhomocyst(e)inemia and a common methylenetetrahydrofolate reductase mutation (Ala 223Val MTHFR) in patients with inherited thrombophillic coagulation defects. Arterioscler Thromb Vasc Biol 1997; 17:2924–1929.

Levine JS, Branch DW, Rauch J: The antiphospholipid syndrome. N Engl J Med 2002; 346:752–763. *Comprehensive review of antiphospholipid syndrome and lupus anticoagulants.*

Libourel EJ, Bank I, Veeger NJ: Protein S type III deficiency is no risk factor for venous and arterial thromboembolism in 168 thrombophilic families: a resprospective study. Blood Coagul Fibrinolysis 2005; 16-135-16-142.

Lindoff C, Ingemarsson I, Martinsson G, et al: Preeclampsia is associated with a reduced response to activated protein C. Am J Obstet Gynecol 1997; 176:457–460.

McCrae KR, Feinstein DI, Cines DB: Antiphospholipid antibodies and antiphospholipid syndrome. *In* Colman W, Hirsh J, Marder VJ, Clowes AW, George JN (eds): Haemostasis and thrombosis: basic principles and clinical practice. Philadelphia, Lippincott Williams & Wilkins, 2001, pp 1339–1356.

Meijers JC, Tekelenburg WL, Bouma BN, et al: High levels of coagulation factor XI as a risk factor for venous thrombosis. N Engl J Med 2000; 342:696–701.

Mackie IJ, Piegsa K, Furs SA, et al: Protein S levels are lower in women receiving desogestrel-containing combined oral contraceptives (COCs) than in women receiving levonorgestrel-containing COCs at steady state and on cross-over. Br J Haematol 2001; 113:898–904.

Madden RM, Levin EG, Marlar RA: Thrombin and the thrombin–thrombomodulin complex interaction with plasminogen activator inhibitor, type 1. Blood Coag Fibrinolysis 1991; 2:471–476.

Marlar RA, Adcock DM, Madden RM: Hereditary dysfunctional protein C molecules (type II): assay characterization and proposed classification. Thromb Haemost 1990a; 63:375–379.

Marlar RA, Mastovich S: Hereditary protein C deficiency: a review of the genetics, clinical presentation, diagnosis and treatment. Blood Coag Fibrinol 1990b; 1:319–330.

Marlar RA, Neumann A: Neonatal purpura fulminans due to homozygous protein C or protein S deficiencies. Semin Thromb Hemost 1990c; 16:299–309.

Moll S: Warfarin-induced skin necrosis. Br J Haematol 2004; 126:628.

Mudd SH, Skovby F, Levy HL, et al: The natural history of homocystinuria due to cystathionine β-synthase deficiency. Am J Hum Genet 1985; 37:1–31.

Nelson RM, Long GL: Binding of protein S to C4b-binding protein: mutagenesis of protein S. J Biol Chem 1992; 267:8140–8145.

O'Donnell J, Tuddenham EG, Manning R, et al: High prevalence of elevated factor VIII levels in patients referred for thrombophilia screening: role of increased synthesis and relationship to the acute phase reaction. Thromb Haemost 1997; 77:825–828.

Ohlin AK, Marlar RA: The first mutation identified in the thrombomodulin gene in a 45-year-old male presenting with thromboembolic disease. Blood 1995; 85:330–336.

Ohlin AK, Norlund L, Marlar RA: Thrombomodulin gene variations and thromboembolic disease. Thromb Haemost 1997; 78:396–400.

Paganin F, Bourde A, Yvin JL, et al: Venous thromboembolism in passengers following a 12-h flight: a case–control study. Aviat Space Environ Med 2003; 74:1277–1280.

Persson KE, Dahlbäck B, Hillarp A: Diagnosing protein S deficiency: analytical considerations. Clin Lab 2003; 49:103–110.

Peters C, Casella JF, Marlar RA, et al: Homozygous protein C deficiency: observations on the nature of the molecular abnormality and the effectiveness of warfarin therapy. Pediatrics 1988; 81:272–276.

Poort SR, Rosendaal FR, Reitsma PH, et al: A common genetic variation in the 3'-untranslated region of the prothrombin gene. Blood 1996; 88:3698–3703.

Refsum H, Ueland PM, Nygard O, et al: Homocysteine and cardiovascular disease. Annu Rev Med 1998; 49:31–62.

Rezende SM, Simmonds RE, Lane DA: Coagulation, inflammation, and apoptosis: different roles for protein S and the protein S-C4b binding protein complex. Blood 2004; 103:1192–1201.

Riboldi P, Gerosa M, Raschi E, et al: Endothelium as a target for antiphospholipid antibodies. Immunobiology 2003; 207:29–36.

Ridker PM, Miletich JP, Stampfer MJ, et al: Factor V Leiden and risks of recurrent idiopathic venous thromboembolism. Circulation 1995; 92:2800–2807.

Rigby AC, Grant MA: Protein S: a conduit between anticoagulation and inflammation. Crit Care Med 2004; 32(Suppl):S336–S341.

Robert A, Aillaud MF, Eschwege V, Randrianjohany et al: ABO blood group and risk of venous thrombosis in heterozygous carriers of factor V Leiden. Thromb Haemost 2000; 83:630–631.

Salooja N, Perry DJ: Thromboelastography. Blood Coag Fibrinolysis 2001; 12:327–337.

Sartori MT, Saggiorato G, Spiezia L, et al: Influence of the Alu-repeat I/D polymorphism in t-PA gene intron 8 on the stimulated t-PA release after venous occlusion. Clin Appl Thromb Hemostas 2003; 9:63–69.

Schulman S, Wiman B: The significance of hypofibrinolysis for the risk of recurrence of venous thromboembolism: Duration of Anticoagulation (DURAC) Trial Study Group. Thromb Haemost 1996; 75:607–611.

Simmonds RE, Ireland H, Lane DA, et al: Clarification of the risk for venous thrombosis associated with hereditary protein S deficiency by investigation of a large kindred with a characterized gene defect. Ann Intern Med 1998; 128:8–14.

Smithies MN, Weaver CB: Role of the tissue factor pathway in the pathogenesis and management of multiple organ failure. Blood Coagul Fibrinolysis 2004; 15(Suppl):S11–S20.

Stassen JM, Arnout J, Deckmyn H: The hemostatic system. Curr Med Chem 2004; 11:2245–2260.

Stearns-Kurosawa DJ, Kurosawa S, Mollica JS, et al: The endothelial cell protein C receptor augments protein C activation by the thrombin-thrombomodulin complex. Proc Natl Acad Sci USA 1996; 93:10212–10216.

Streif W, Mitchell LG, Andrew M: Antithrombotic therapy in children. Curr Opin Pediatr 1999; 11:56–64.

Svensson PJ, Zoller B, Dahlbäck B: Evaluation of original and modified APC-resistance tests in unselected outpatients with clinically suspected thrombosis and in healthy controls. Thromb Haemost 1997; 77:332–335.

Tai CY, Lerardi R, Alexander JB: A case of warfarin skin necrosis despite enoxaparin anticoagulation in a patient with protein S deficiency. Ann Vasc Surg 2004; 18:237–242.

Tollefsen DM: Heparin cofactor II deficiency. Arch Pathol Lab Med 2002; 126:1394–1400.

Tosetto A, Missiaglia E, Fressato M: The VITA project: C677T mutation in the methylenetetrahydrofolate reductase gene and the risk of venous thromboembolism. Br J Haematol 1997; 97:804–806.

Tripodi A, Negri B, Bertina RM, et al: Screening for the FV:Q506 mutation. Evaluation of thirteen plasma-based methods for their diagnostic efficacy in comparison with DNA analysis. Thromb Haemost 1997; 77:436–439.

Van de Wouwer M, Collen D, Conway EM: Thrombomodulin-protein C-EPCR system: integrated to regulate coagulation and inflammation. Arterioscler Thromb Vasc Biol 2004; 24:1374–1383.

Van der Bom JG, de Knijff P, Haverkate F, et al: Tissue plasminogen activator and the risk of myocardial infarction: the Rotterdam Study. Circulation 1997; 95:2623–2630.

Van Wijnen M, Stam JG, van't Veer C, et al: The interaction of protein S with the phospholipid surface is essential for the activated protein C-independent activity of protein S. Thromb Haemost 1996; 76:397–403.

Vig S, Chitolie A, Bevan DH, et al: Thromboelastography: a reliable test? Blood Coag Fibrinolysis 2001; 12:555–561.

Weiss EJ, Bray PF, Tayback M, et al: A polymorphism of a platelet glycoprotein receptor as an inherited risk factor for coronary thrombosis. N Engl J Med 1996; 334:1090–1094.

Weltermann A, Eichinger S, Bialonczyk C, et al: The risk of recurrent venous thromboembolism among patients with high factor IX levels. J Thromb Haemost 2003; 1:28–32.

V

Antithrombotic Therapy

Louis M. Fink MD, Richard A. Marlar PhD, Jonathan L. Miller MD PhD

KEY POINTS

• Warfarin is the most commonly used oral anticoagulant. It acts as a vitamin K antagonist and blocks γ-carboxylation of a series of glutamic residues during the synthesis of factors II, VII, IX, X, protein C and protein S. The resulting decreased functionality of the coagulation factors is monitored by prolongations of the prothrombin time/international normalized ratio.

• By binding to antithrombin and thereby increasing its ability to inhibit thrombin, factor Xa and, to a lesser extent other serine protease coagulation factors, heparin is considered to be an 'indirect' thrombin inhibitor. Heparin anticoagulant intensity is commonly monitored by prolongations of the partial thromboplastin time, with actual quantitation of heparin anticoagulant activity being assayed as anti-factor-Xa activity. In instances where it is necessary to monitor low-molecular-weight heparin therapy, this can only be done by measuring its anti-factor-Xa activity.

• Heparin-induced thrombocytopenia (HIT) is a complication of heparin therapy in which antibodies develop against complexes of platelet factor (PF)4 and heparin. In the most severe cases the resulting antibodies bind to platelets in such a manner as to activate them, leading to arterial and/or venous thrombosis. Both immunological and functional assays are employed in the evaluation of possible HIT.

• New anticoagulants are emerging that function as direct thrombin inhibitors or that directly inhibit factor Xa. Effectively monitoring the activity of these inhibitors, as well as identifying possible interference by these inhibitors upon the testing for other hemostatic abnormalities, presents new challenges to the diagnostic laboratory.

• Therapy directed towards the inhibition of platelet reactivity is increasingly being employed both in acute and chronic settings. The laboratory can monitor the resulting reactivity of platelets from treated patients and in some instances detect apparent resistance to aspirin or other therapeutic agents.

There is a wide array of agents that either alter the synthesis or action of coagulation factors, affect platelet function, or modify blood vessel responses. Prescribed and over-the-counter medicines having anticoagulant or antiplatelet activity are among the most common drugs dispensed. Such agents may behave as a 'double-edged sword' in that they may prevent the formation or extension of a thrombus but they can also produce or exacerbate bleeding. The clinical laboratory has a major role in the monitoring of antithrombotic therapy.

Pre-analytic Variables and Controls

All the standards for accuracy and precision for monitoring anticoagulant therapy are of little use if the blood sample is not obtained and processed in a defined manner. The Clinical and Laboratory Standards Institute (formerly the National Committee for Clinical Laboratory Standards) has provided useful guidelines for the collection, storage, and preparation of blood or plasma prior to coagulation testing that are presented as an Appendix at the end of this chapter (National Committee for Clinical Laboratory Standards, 1998).

For optimal reporting, the time and date of the sampling as well as the time of the last dose of the anticoagulant should be recorded. Laboratory results also need to be interpreted in conjunction with the clinical history for optimal regulation of anticoagulant therapy. Whenever there is a computed manipulation of the analytical output, such as the conversion of the prothrombin time (PT) from seconds to the international normalized ratio (INR; defined below), there must be a periodic check to see that the constants and the appropriate data manipulation are being performed as defined by the standard operating procedures for the laboratory.

Vitamin K Antagonists

Warfarin is the most commonly prescribed oral vitamin K antagonist. It is a racemic mixture of the stereoisomers (S)-warfarin and (R)-warfarin. The (S)-warfarin is more potent in producing an anticoagulant effect. Warfarin inhibits vitamin K reductase (vitamin K 2,3-epoxide reductase) and blocks the regeneration of the active form of vitamin K, which is necessary for the formation of γ-carboxyglutamic acid in a series of amino acid residues (termed the 'Gla domain') within factors II, VII, IX, X, protein C and protein S (Fig. 41–1). With decreasing extent of γ-carboxylation within the Gla domains, there is in turn a decreased ability of the affected proteins to be bound into the highly ordered protein-Ca^{2+}–phospholipid complexes that are critical components of the coagulation cascade (Ansell, 2004). Tests dependent upon proper functioning of these factors will become more abnormal with an increased intensity of oral anticoagulant therapy.

The degree of warfarin anticoagulation is typically measured in the PT testing system, although prolongations of the PTT are also typically observed. Since fibrinogen synthesis is not vitamin-K-dependent, the thrombin time (TT) remains normal. It must be stressed that the initial prolongation of the PT upon institution of warfarin therapy does not faithfully reflect the overall intensity of anticoagulation. The reason for this unintuitive observation is that while the relatively short half-life of factor VII (4–6 hours) underlies the contemporaneous prolongation of the PT, the half-lives of other vitamin-K-dependent factors actually extend to several days. Only when all these factors have reached a steady-state level of decreased γ-carboxylation should one anticipate that the overall diminution of the coagulation system (such as might be reflected by the actual production of thrombin) has been obtained. For this reason, a minimum of 4–6 days of oral anticoagulant therapy is generally recommended before assuming that laboratory monitoring actually reflects the steady-state level of anticoagulation. When a more rapid onset of effective anticoagulation is necessary, heparin is given prior to or along with the warfarin. After at least 4 days of combined therapy the heparin can be discontinued and the warfarin dose can be adjusted to the

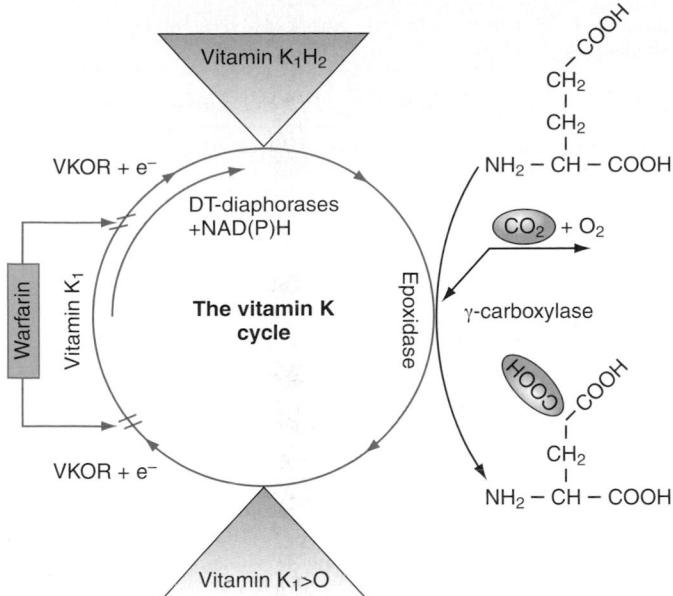

Figure 41–1 The vitamin-K-dependent γ-carboxylation system. The γ-carboxylase converts vitamin-K-dependent proteins to γ-carboxyglutamic-acid (Gla)-containing proteins by adding CO_2 to glutamic acid (Glu) residues in newly synthesized proteins. The γ-carboxylase requires reduced vitamin K_1 (vitamin K_1H_2) as a cofactor for this post-translational modification reaction. Concomitant with γ-carboxylation, vitamin K_1H_2 is converted to vitamin K_1 2,3-epoxide (vitamin K_1>O). The epoxide is reduced by the warfarin-sensitive enzyme vitamin K_1 2,3-epoxide reductase (VKOR) to the vitamin K_1H_2 cofactor. This cyclic interconversion of vitamin K metabolites constitutes the vitamin K cycle. At high tissue concentrations, vitamin K_1 quinone (vitamin K_1) can be reduced to vitamin K_1H_2 by the alternative pathway of the cycle. This pathway is catalyzed by NAD(P)H dehydrogenases (DT-diaphorases), which are not inhibited by warfarin (Wallin, 2004).

prescribed target INR. While warfarin therapy ordinarily produces a net anticoagulant effect, in certain settings (e.g., active heparin-induced thrombocytopenia), the resulting decrease in carboxylation and activity of protein C and/or protein S may dominate the hemostatic balance, resulting in purpura fulminans or other manifestations of venous thrombosis (Martin, 1998).

As discussed in Chapter 38, the PT is performed by first adding a source of tissue factor (thromboplastin) and phospholipid and then recalcifying the citrated platelet-free plasma. The time in seconds to subsequent clot formation is then determined by either mechanical or optical measurements. However, the actual degree of PT prolongation in response to warfarin therapy is highly dependent upon the particular thromboplastin reagent and instrument system employed. Cooperation among a number of laboratories in different countries resulted in the development of the international sensitivity index (ISI) and INR, which are now universally employed in an effort to improve standardization of PT reporting worldwide. In brief, the logarithms of PTs obtained on a prescribed series of normal and warfarinized patients, using the primary international reference thromboplastin or plasma calibrants, are plotted against the logarithms of PTs obtained using an individual thromboplastin reagent. The resulting slope of this plot is the ISI for that thromboplastin reagent and instrument combination (Adcock, 2002; Poller, 2004; van den Besselaar, 2004). The ratio of patient PT divided by mean normal PT for the local laboratory, raised to the power of the ISI defines the INR:

$$INR = \left| \frac{\text{Patient PT in seconds}}{\text{Mean of the normal PT in seconds}} \right|^{ISI}$$

Put in another way, the INR represents the PT ratio that would have been obtained if the international reference thromboplastin had actually been used for the patient testing.

As demonstrated by Ng (1993) and by Cunningham (1994), however, attainment of a fully assay-independent INR may be very difficult in practice.

Because of the importance of proper monitoring of oral anticoagulant therapy, it is important to emphasize several more points regarding the ISI and INR: The ISI must be correctly specified not only for each type but also for each new lot of thromboplastin, in conjunction with the specific instrument model being used in a given laboratory. The less sensitive thromboplastins (typically derived from brain or other tissues) have ISI values in the range of 2 or more, whereas the more sensitive tissue-derived

reagents have ISI values in the range of 1.0–1.7. Recombinant tissue factor is the most sensitive thromboplastin, with ISI values approaching 1.0. Most laboratories report results simply as an INR, but some additionally give the results as the PT in seconds, together with the mean PT value for that laboratory. During the initiation of anticoagulation, more frequent measurements of the PT may be required until the INR is stabilized. In plasma from patients treated with both heparin and warfarin, the anticoagulant contribution of the warfarin can be assessed if the heparin is first either removed or neutralized prior to performing the PT testing (see below). Unless a means becomes available for removal or neutralization of direct thrombin inhibitors (DTI), therapeutic intensities of such inhibitors can be sufficient to prolong the PT and accordingly influence the INR value (Tobu 2004; Walenga, 2004). While most lupus anticoagulants exert a more pronounced effect upon the PTT than the PT, the presence of a lupus anticoagulant may in some patients render the PT inaccurate as a means to monitor warfarin therapy. This may depend upon the reagents used (Moll, 1997). In such instances, a direct assay of factor X, using a chromogenic assay rather than a clotting assay, may aid in monitoring anticoagulant intensity (Rosborough, 2004).

The half-life of warfarin is between 20 and 60 hours with a mean plasma half-life of 40 hours. The maximum effect of a dose lasts for up to 48 hours after administration. The (S)-warfarin is metabolized by CYP2C9 and the (R)-warfarin is metabolized by the CYP1AZ and CYP3A4 enzymes. There are polymorphisms of the CYP2C9, and knowledge of the patient's allelic genes may have predictive value in determining which patients need higher or lower doses of warfarin (Higashi, 2002; Linder, 2002; Adcock, 2004). Genetic resistance to warfarin therapy is uncommon. In instances where there are marked and persistent inappropriate responses to warfarin, the metabolites can be measured using HPLC methodology (Lombardi, 2003) (see Ch. 4). These measurements can also be used to check compliance. Drugs affecting the (S)-warfarin metabolism may markedly alter the potency of the warfarin treatments. Some drugs or herbal medications induce the CYP450 and cause warfarin to be metabolized faster. They result in a decrease in the effects of warfarin. Other drugs inhibit the metabolism of warfarin and thus enhance its effect. There are several hundred compounds known to alter the metabolism of warfarin (Poller, 1996; Ansell, 2004). Antibiotics may either interfere with the metabolism of warfarin or suppress the gut flora, which supplies a significant amount of the vitamin K to humans. Foods, particularly green, leafy vegetables rich in vitamin K, may prevent adequate anticoagulation with warfarin. Warfarin products may have different potencies and any switching between types of coumadin may require more frequent monitoring and dosage adjustments (Bongiorno, 2004).

Warfarin is most commonly used for prevention of thromboembolic strokes in patients with atrial fibrillation. Additionally warfarin is used both prophylactically and therapeutically in a wide range of clinical settings, and may even be used on a lifelong basis in certain patients who have particularly high risk for recurrent thrombotic events. The American Association of Chest Physicians periodically reviews the guidelines for anticoagulant therapy and publishes its consensus report in the journal Chest (Hirsh, 2004a). The recommended treatment target is an INR of 2–3 for most patients with venous thromboembolic disease or atrial fibrillation (Ansell, 2004).

Because warfarin is influenced by liver function, diet, absorption from the gut, and cotreatment with other drugs or herbal medications, it is not uncommon for patients to present with INRs that are elevated or decreased. Mild elevations of INR can be treated by changing the dosage schedule. More significant elevations can be treated with 2 mg of vitamin K given orally. If there is a high risk of bleeding, higher doses of vitamin K can be administered. However, the patient may then become resistant to further warfarin therapy, and another anticoagulant may have to be substituted. If the patient is bleeding, fresh frozen plasma, activated prothrombin complexes or recombinant factor VIIa may be transfused to achieve hemostasis (Ansell, 2004).

Extreme care should be used in treating patients with warfarin. Warfarin should not be used in patients with any evidence of hemorrhage. Patients on warfarin should be checked for blood loss and anemia. Warfarin is teratogenic and should not be used in pregnant females (Bates, 2004). If there is suspicion of a deficiency state of protein C, heparin or another anticoagulant should be started before or concomitantly with warfarin therapy. In patients with heparin-induced thrombocytopenia, warfarin should not be used because it may lower the protein C and promote venous limb gangrene (Warkentin, 1997).

Monitoring of the INR is used to keep patients on warfarin therapy in a range that will prevent further thrombosis but not lead to bleeding. While an anticoagulant intensity goal INR of 2–3 defines the usual reference interval, still higher INRs may be sought in certain clinical settings.

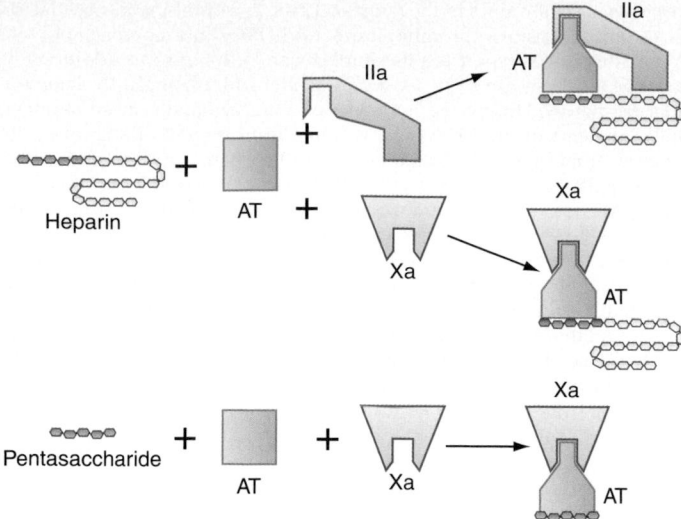

Figure 41–2 Hypothetical mechanisms for heparin/heparan sulfate regulation of protein–protein interactions. The interaction of antithrombin (AT) with thrombin (IIa) is catalyzed by a heparin-induced conformational change in ATIII and the nonspecific binding of thrombin to heparin (UFH) to bring the two proteins together (approximation model). Neither low molecular weight (LMWH) nor isolated pentasaccharide share this mechanism with UFH. The interaction of AT with the serine protease factor Xa (Xa) is catalyzed by a conformational change in ATIII by binding to a specific pentasaccharide sequence of heparin found in unfractionated heparain (UFH), LMWH, and the isolated pentasaccharide (fondaparinux). (Modified with permission from Nugent MA: Heparin sequencing brings structure to the function of complex oligosaccharides. Proc Natl Acad Sci USA 2000; 97:10301–10303.)

Patients, families and their caregivers should be educated about the therapy and should be informed about the importance of having their INR checked on a routine basis. Patients can be taught how to use point-of-care coagulometers to obtain an INR measurement (see below).

Heparin

Heparin is a polymer of sulfated glycosaminoglycans. Unfractionated heparin (UFH) is used either prophylactically or therapeutically for venous and arterial thrombosis. The molecular weight of UFH ranges from 20 000–50 000 daltons. UFH for systemic use is prepared from porcine intestine. For topical use UFH is prepared from bovine lung. Heparin is an 'indirect' thrombin inhibitor: rather than exerting its effects by binding directly to thrombin, it binds to antithrombin in such a manner as to increase the potency of antithrombin's inhibitory action of thrombin's serine esterase activity (Fig. 41–2). The anticoagulant effect is derived from inhibition of serine protease coagulation factors, with the most critical inhibition being that of factor IIa (thrombin) and factor Xa. However, there are additional effects of heparin. These include the release of tissue factor pathway inhibitor, increase in tissue plasminogen activator (t-PA) and fibrinolysis, and impairment of platelet function (Salzman, 1980). Unfractionated heparin can be given subcutaneously or intravenously. Its onset of action is rapid (Bussey, 2004; Hirsh, 2004b). It is important to achieve effective anticoagulation in patients with veno-occlusive disease, because sequestered thrombin may allow subsequent propagation of the thrombus (Hull, 1997).

A variety of methods can be used to measure unfractionated heparin. These include the PTT, the TT, protamine reversal, factor Xa inhibition and the activated clotting time (ACT) (see below). The PTT is the most commonly used assay, but the PTT reagents vary in their sensitivity to heparin, and changes in the lots of heparin or in the test reagents require a reassessment of the testing. The therapeutic range for the PTT should be determined by plotting the PTT against the direct heparin concentration measured by a factor Xa inhibition assay (Olson, 1998; 2004). The comparison between the PTT and the heparin levels of specimens should be done on patient samples and not on plasma spiked with heparin in vitro. This is because heparin induces changes in vivo that are not mimicked by adding exogenous heparins. There is not, however, uniform standardization at the present time with respect to PTT monitoring of heparin (Van der Velde, 1995; Francis, 2004a.). The PTT target range for UFH is defined by the anti-Xa heparin assay and should be provided to the treating physicians (van den Besselaar, 2002). The PTT is more sensitive to the effects of UFH than the PT, but high doses will also elevate the PT.

Table 41–1 Comparison of the Properties of LMWH, Fondaparinux and Idraparinux

Feature	LMWH	Fondaparinux	Idraparinux
Mode of administration	Subcutaneous	Subcutaneous	Subcutaneous
Bioavailability (%)	80–90	100	100
Half-life (h)	4	17	80
Target	Factor Xa and thrombin	Factor Xa	Factor Xa
Renal clearance	Yes	Yes	Yes
Neutralized by protamine sulfate	Partial	No	No

Source: from: Bates SM, Weitz JI: New anticoagulants: beyond heparin, low-molecular-weight heparin and warfarin. Br J Pharmacol 2005; 144:1017–1028.

Heparin contamination is a frequent cause for prolongation of the PTT and the TT, and in fact can complicate the performance of a number of clot-based tests. This is particularly true when samples are drawn from intravenous catheters. Some commercial test kits contain polybrene or other agents to neutralize heparin. The presence of heparin can be determined if a prolonged PTT shortens following treatment with heparinase (obtained from *Flavobacter heparinum*). In specimens with very prolonged PTTs a second treatment with heparinase may be necessary to remove all the heparin and produce a normal PTT. A similar approach can be employed in which heparin-binding cellulose (ECTEOLA) absorbs heparin from patient plasma. This absorption procedure has only minimal effects on the other coagulation factors, except for a slight reduction in factor IX (Hutt, 1972; Thompson, 1976; Cowan, 1981; Newman, 1995).

Heparin is used extensively to prevent thrombi from forming during cardiac bypass surgery. The activated clotting time is a whole-blood clotting assay where diatomaceous earth is often used as the activating agent. The ACT is most frequently used to monitor heparin in situations such as cardiopulmonary bypass surgery, and is most useful when the heparin levels are high (2–4 U/ml) and fluctuate widely. In these ranges the PTT is not useful. In instances where more precise monitoring is needed, factor Xa inhibition assays should be considered. Factor Xa inhibition assays are especially helpful when the patient is obese, in renal failure, pregnant, has a lupus anticoagulant, or manifests resistance to heparin. The factor Xa inhibition assays are less affected than the ACT by the presence of the protease inhibitor aprotinin, which is often used in cardiac surgery. When the patient is removed from cardiac bypass, heparin is usually reversed by treatment with protamine sulfate. The progress of protamine neutralization can be determined by titration of the ACT. Approximately 1 mg of protamine neutralizes 130 units of UFH. In rare cases where the patient is allergic to protamine, platelets can be administered to help neutralize the heparin (Hirsh, 2004b).

There are situations where patients appear to be resistant to heparin, although the definition of such resistance may be dependent upon the specific clinical setting:

In the context of venous thromboembolism, heparin resistance is defined as the need for more than 35 000 U/24 h to prolong the activated partial thromboplastin time into the therapeutic range. In contrast, during cardiac bypass procedures, the definition of heparin resistance is based on the ACT, with at least one ACT less than 400 s after heparinization and/or the need for exogenous antithrombin administration (Anderson, 2002).

Causes for heparin resistance include: massive thrombosis with release of heparin-binding proteins; elevated factor VIII levels (often evidenced by short baseline PTTs; treatment with aprotinin or nitroglycerine; severe obesity; antithrombin deficiency; heparin-induced thrombocytopenia; and cancer (Edson, 1967; Young, 1992; Bharadwaj, 2003; Francis, 2004a). In some instances of apparent heparin resistance as measured by the PTT, such as in the case of elevated factor VIII levels, simply changing to anti-factor Xa assays may be a more appropriate measure of the heparin level (Hirsh, 2004b).

Low-Molecular-Weight Heparins

Low-molecular-weight heparins (LMWH) are derived from unfractionated heparin. They have molecular masses in the range of 2000–10 000 daltons (Table 41–1). The LMWHs do not effectively allow the antithrombin to inactivate factor IIa because of their smaller size, but they can still inactivate factor Xa. Anti-Xa assays, rather than the PTT, are used when measurement of LMWH is needed (Boneu, 2001). The general therapeutic range for LMWH in patients being treated for venous thromboembolic disorders is different for each compound. Because of the decreased binding to plasma proteins, a predictable response to LMWH can be expected in most cases, and the LMWH can be given subcutaneously once or twice a day (Bounameaux, 2004; Harenberg, 2004). The plasma levels of LMWH are usually not monitored except when treating children, pregnant or markedly obese patients, or patients with renal failure. When monitoring is performed, blood is ordinarily drawn approximately 4 hours after the last dose, since this is when the peak level is anticipated to occur (Bounameaux, 2004; Harenberg, 2004).

The complications of osteopenia and heparin-induced thrombocytopenia (HIT) occur less frequently when LMWH are used rather than UFH (Pettila, 2002; Schulman, 2002). However, patients with established HIT should not be anticoagulated with LMWH: While LMWH are initially less immunogenic, once antibodies have actually been produced following UFH administration, pathological antigen–antibody interaction may also occur upon subsequent administration of LMWH (Warkentin, 1997; Schenk, 2003).

Heparin-induced Thrombocytopenia

Thrombocytopenias arising in the setting of heparin therapy occur in two forms. Nonimmune heparin-associated thrombocytopenia (HAT) is believed to result from platelet activation following the direct binding of heparin to platelets (Horne, 2001). The degree of thrombocytopenia is generally mild and transient. Of far greater concern are the immune-mediated processes, sometimes referred to as 'type II heparin-induced thrombocytopenia (HIT),' but more commonly simply as 'HIT.' Additionally, when venous and/or arterial thrombosis arise in the context of HIT, the entity is referred to as HITT – 'heparin-induced thrombocytopenia and thrombosis.' Recent studies (Rauova, 2005) suggest that UFH structures tetramers of platelet factor (PF)4 into ultralarge complexes (ULC) that are particularly antigenic. If multiple IgG molecules bind to the ULC, the Fc regions of these antibodies may then be oriented in a manner favoring their binding to the platelet's FcRIIA receptors, thereby causing signal transduction and subsequent platelet activation. Manifestations of such platelet activation include secretion of granular material and release of platelet microparticles whose outwardly facing phosphatidylserine may potentially promote thrombin generation and hence increased clotting. Antibodies to other chemokines that have shared sequence structures with PF4 (the CXC family of chemokines), including interleukin (IL)-8, interferon-8 inducible protein (IL-10), platelet basic protein and its proteolytic product β-thromboglobulin and neutrophil-activating protein-2, may also cause HIT (Greinacher, 1994; Amiral, 1996). HIT-associated antibodies may also cause endothelial cells and monocytes to activate tissue factor expression (Fig. 41–3). HIT occurs more frequently with exposure to bovine heparin than to porcine heparin. In the usual presentation, the platelet count drops at 5–10 days after the exposure to heparin. The platelets may drop to below 150 000/μL or decrease to levels of less than 50% of the peak platelet count or the count prior to initiation of heparin. When this occurs, all heparin treatment should be discontinued (including heparin flushes of catheters). In most cases, the platelet decrease is at 4–5 days from initiation of therapy, but in some cases the thrombocytopenia may occur as early as 2–3 days or persist after heparin is discontinued when the level of antibody is still high. Approximately one-third of patients with HIT-associated antibodies who are thrombocytopenic actually develop thromboses (Fig. 41–4). Venous thromboses are more common than arterial thromboses, and the lower limbs are more frequently involved. Formation of platelet microparticles with phosphatidylserine exposed on their outer surfaces probably promotes thrombin generation, and the subsequent venous thromboses (Warkentin, 2004). The patients may have areas of skin necrosis at the site of the heparin injections, acute systemic inflammatory reactions after a heparin bolus, and may show evidence of heparin resistance. Other causes of thrombocytopenia need to be ruled out. If the heparin is discontinued, the thrombocytopenia frequently abates in 9–10 days. However, the patient can be at risk for thrombosis for several weeks after discontinuing heparin.

A presumptive diagnosis of HIT is often made on clinical grounds, particularly in cases where the time course and extent of the drop in platelet count fit together convincingly with the patient's receipt of heparin therapy. In such cases, treatment decisions may be taken quite independently of whether or not the results of laboratory testing also point in this direction. In instances where a diagnosis of HIT appears more equivocal, laboratory testing for HIT may play a larger role in the subsequent clinical decision-making process. A test for HIT that had perfect sensitivity and specificity and that could be performed rapidly in a cost-effective fashion would of course be the ideal. Most laboratories presently employ a testing strategy in which the initial (or only) test is a readily performed PF4-ELISA immunoassay, with high sensitivity but somewhat less specificity. Functional tests are typically much more demanding to perform but can have the advantage of providing high specificity in addition to high sensitivity. A combination of the immunological and the functional tests have been reported to offer very high negative and positive predictive values (Francis, 2004b). A critical issue in the design of functional HIT tests is the choice of target upon which antibodies present in the patient's blood will act. Early tests employed platelet-rich plasma of normal donors. However, as has been analyzed in considerable detail (Warkentin, 2001), washing of these target platelets so as to remove the accompanying plasma can greatly improve test performance. In North America, the gold standard of functional testing for HIT has been the serotonin release assay (SRA), in which washed platelets that have taken up exogenous serotonin are challenged with patient plasma in the presence of optimal heparin concentrations, and the amount of released serotonin is taken as the endpoint. This test can be performed either by employing radiolabeled serotonin and measuring radioactivity in the platelet releasate, or by employing HPLC or other analytical methods to quantify the release of nonradioactive serotonin. Interestingly, in a number of European laboratories quite comparable results are obtained when aggregation in microtiter wells is employed as the functional end point using similarly washed platelets (Warkentin, 2001). An additional end point that has been explored is the formation of platelet microparticles, detectable by flow cytometric methods. A host of technical issues must be addressed in setting up any of these assays, including selection of platelet donors and whether or not to test these donors with respect to polymorphisms in FcRIIA. Blockade by monoclonal antibodies to the FcRIIA platelet receptor and/or inhibition of the functional responses by addition of quite high heparin concentrations have been employed by some groups in an effort to enhance specificity of the testing, although the utility of these measures remains a subject of discussion (Warkentin, 2001). Finally, it should be noted that, in those instances where the target epitope is atypical (i.e., not the anticipated epitopes within platelet PF4), while the highly specific immunoassays may then fail to detect the HIT-associated antibodies, this atypicality would not be expected to influence the functional assays.

A potential pitfall in the interpretation of HIT testing, particularly when immunoassays are performed, is the identification of immunoreactive antibodies in the absence of the clinical findings comprising true HIT. Presumably these antibodies represent a subclinical form of HIT at best, or a quite misleading biological false-positive result at worst (analogous to false-positive VDRL testing in the case of lupus anticoagulants). Appropriateness of the clinical setting (most typically falling platelet counts in reasonable temporal relationship to heparin administration) is accordingly of considerable importance when evaluating whether or not to perform such testing. The laboratory will sometimes be called upon, however, to perform HIT testing on asymptomatic individuals who have been positive for HIT at some time in the past. While it has been demonstrated that most HIT-associated antibodies do not show an anamnestic reappearance if the patient is rechallenged with heparin more than 6 months following loss of detectable antibody, close laboratory monitoring of such rechallenged patients is critical. In the event that an anamnestic response did develop, the re-emergence of antibody can be quite dramatic, requiring at least rapid detection of falling platelet counts, if not in fact more specific tests for HIT.

Point-of-Care Anticoagulant Monitoring

There are several types of point of care (POC) monitoring. The ACT is frequently used to guide heparin therapy during cardiac surgery and catheterizations. In the point of care instruments glass beads and kaolin are often used as activators. Basal levels must be greater than 300 s. to prevent microthrombi from forming during cardiac bypass surgery. The ACT may be influenced by the quantity and quality of platelets, temperature, lupus anticoagulants, levels of coagulation factors or hemodilution. Aprotinin, an antiprotease which helps prevent major blood loss with cardiac surgery, prolongs the ACT in kaolin-based assays, while leading to underestimates of heparin in celite-based assays.

There have been many new developments in the technology of POC monitors for oral anticoagulant therapy. Mechanical technologies using the magnetic motion of iron filings, motion flow detectors, thrombin cleavable fluorescent substrates, electrochemical detectors of impedance changes, and laser light dispersion technologies have been used to detect clot formation and transform the data into a reportable PT-INR. Each type

V

CHAPTER 41: Antithrombotic Therapy

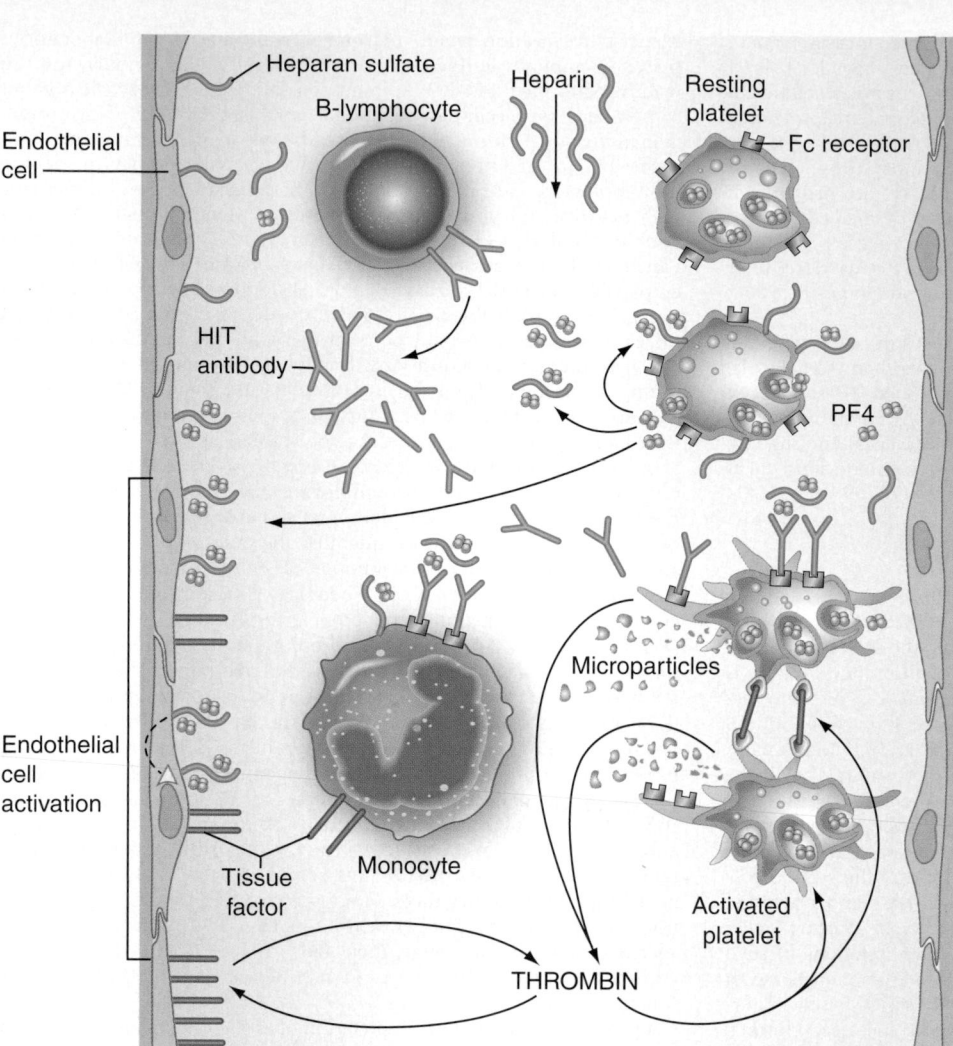

Figure 41–3 Pathogenesis of heparin-induced thrombocytopenia – a central role for thrombin generation. HIT-IgG antibodies bind to several identical epitopes on the same antigen complex, thus forming immune complexes that become localized to the platelet surface. The IgG immune complexes can cross-link the platelet FcγRIIa receptors, resulting in FcγRIIa-dependent platelet activation. The GP IIb/IIIa complex is not required for platelet activation. The activated platelets trigger a cascade of events that ultimately lead to activation of the coagulation pathways, resulting in thrombin generation. Activated platelets release their α-granule proteins, including PF4, leading to formation of more multimolecular PF4–heparin complexes, setting up a vicious cycle of platelet activation, triggering even more platelet activation. The activated platelets bind fibrinogen, recruit other platelets, and begin to form a primary clot. During shape change, procoagulant, platelet-derived microparticles are released, providing a phospholipid surface for amplifying thrombin generation. The released PF4 also binds to endothelial cell heparan sulfate, forming local antigen complexes to which HIT antibodies bind. Tissue factor expression on activated endothelial cells and monocytes further enhances thrombin generation. (Modified with permission from Warkentin TE, Greinacher A: Laboratory testing for heparin-induced thrombocytopenia. *In* Warkentin TE, Greinacher A (eds): Induced Thrombocytopenia, 2nd ed. New York, Marcel Dekker, 2001, pp 231–269.)

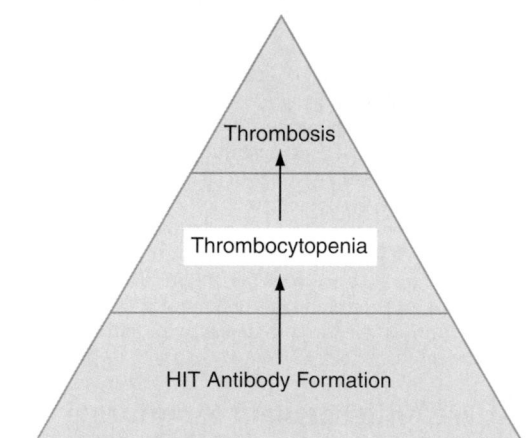

Figure 41–4 'Iceberg' model of heparin-induced thrombocytopenia. Development of actual thrombocytopenia develops in only a subset of those individuals who form HIT antibodies, and in turn only a subset of those with thrombocytopenia actually develop thrombosis. Note that thrombocytopenia is broadly defined, and includes patients with large relative falls in the platelet count, even if the platelet nadir is >150 × 10⁹/L. (Modified with permission from Warkentin TE, Greinacher A: Laboratory testing for heparin-induced thrombocytopenia. *In* Warkentin TE, Greinacher A (eds): Induced Thrombocytopenia, 2nd ed. New York, Marcel Dekker, 2001, pp 231–269.)

of POC-PT measurement must be characterized for use with specific patients (National Committee for Clinical Laboratory Standards, 2004). Comparisons of the results from different POC-PT instruments and laboratory-based instruments often are not comparable (Nutescu, 2004). Out-of-range POC INR should be retested in the clinical laboratory (Sunderji, 2005).

Direct Thrombin Inhibitors

Hirudin originally isolated from the salivary glands of leeches is available as a recombinant protein (Refludan®, lepirudin). It forms an essentially irreversible complex with thrombin. Lepirudin has been used in patients with HIT. The half-life of lepirudin is 90–120 minutes, and it is cleared by the kidneys. The anticoagulant activity has been monitored using the PTT, with a target range of 1.5–2.5× the baseline PTT (Call, 2004). However, in instances where a patient's baseline PTT is abnormal (e.g., in the presence of a lupus anticoagulant), monitoring by means of the PTT may be unreliable. One alternative to the PTT for monitoring DTIs is the ecarin clotting time (ECT), which employs the venom from *Echis carinatus*. The active enzyme of this venom is a metalloproteinase that converts prothrombin to meizothrombin – a reaction that is blocked by DTIs. A calibration curve for the ECT can be generated by directly spiking normal plasma with the DTIs in vitro (Nowak, 2001; Kolde, 2004). The DTI may inhibit the PT/INR, and anticoagulant monitoring during the bridging transition between DTI and vitamin K antagonist therapy is accomplished either by using a chromogenic assay for factor Xa or by discontinuing the DTI for several hours and then measuring the INR in patients after several days of vitamin K antagonist therapy (Hoppensteadt, 1997; Tobu, 2004; Walenga, 2004). A related DTI, bivalirudin, is a relatively short-acting molecule that has been approved for use in patients undergoing coronary angioplasty (Merry, 2004).

Argatroban, a synthetic DTI derived from L-arginine has also been approved for use in HIT. A rather wide window of 1.5–3.0× baseline PTT has been suggested for argatroban's target therapeutic range (Call, 2004). Alternative monitoring methodologies may help to narrow this range.

Argatroban is metabolized in the liver and can be used in patients with impaired renal function.

Ximelagatran is a dipeptide prodrug that can be taken orally. Following absorption from the small intestine, it is converted to the active DTI

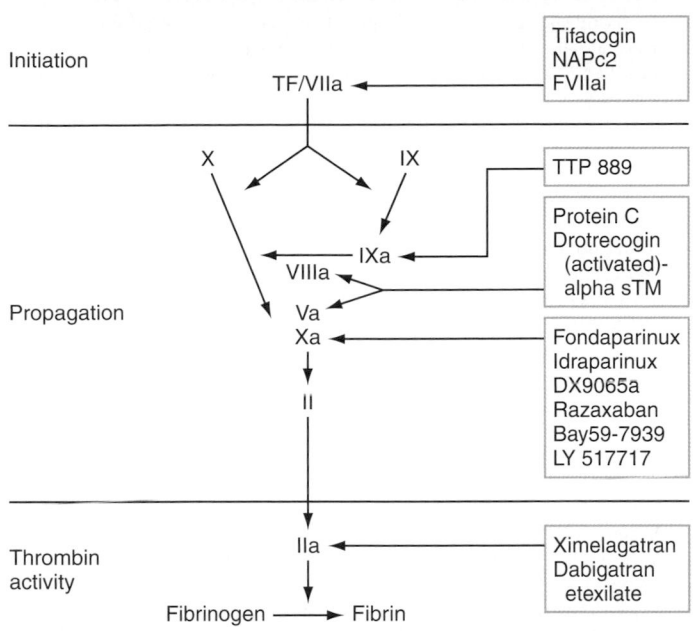

STEPS IN COAGULATION	COAGULATION CASCADE	DRUG
Initiation	TF/VIIa	Tifacogin NAPc2 FVIIai
	X IX	TTP 889
	IXa	Protein C Drotrecogin (activated)- alpha sTM
Propagation	VIIIa Va Xa	Fondaparinux Idraparinux DX9065a Razaxaban Bay59-7939 LY 517717
	II	
Thrombin activity	IIa	Ximelagatran Dabigatran etexilate
	Fibrinogen ⟶ Fibrin	

Figure 41–5 New anticoagulants and their targets in the coagulation pathway. (Redrawn from Br J Pharmacol. 2005 Feb 14; [Epub ahead of print] with permission.)

melagatran. Initial therapy may begin with intravenously administered melagatran, followed by oral ximelagatran. The efficacy to safety index of ximelagatran is comparable to warfarin. Few drugs interfere with the action of melagatran. While laboratory monitoring may not typically be required (Gustafsson, 2001; Francis, 2003; Kessler, 2004), laboratory monitoring may be performed in a similar manner to that of other DTIs (Fenyvesi, 2002). While not the ideal test to monitor melagatran activity, in emergency situations the PTT prolongation has been employed to monitor the effects of melagatran (Carlsson, 2005). Approximately 10% of patients treated with melagatran have elevations of their hepatic enzymes, leading to recommendations that alanine aminotransaminase be monitored in patients receiving this drug. Ximelagatran, however, is not presently approved for use in the USA.

Clearly DTIs are enjoying an increasing role in anticoagulation. At the present time they are used primarily in HIT patients. In the future, however, they may be anticipated to be used in a wider variety of clinical settings, and particularly for patients in whom it has proved difficult to stabilize anticoagulant intensity with more traditional agents.

New Anticoagulants

Until recently the choice of reagents for long-term anticoagulation was limited primarily to warfarin. A variety of new anticoagulants are being developed and tested to inhibit the various steps in the coagulation cascades (Mammen, 2004; Weitz, 2005; Hirsh, 2005). It is important for the laboratorian to keep abreast of the introduction of new agents, their requirements for laboratory monitoring, and the optimal methods for such monitoring. Drugs presently in development or approved are described in Table 41–1 and Figure 41–5. These include:

- Inhibitors of tissue factor/VII. A recombinant form of tissue factor pathway inhibitor is being tested: the polypeptide NAPc2 that binds factor Xa and inhibits FIIa.
- Indirect and direct factor Xa inhibitors. Indirect inhibitors require binding to antithrombin. Direct Xa inhibitors bind the active sites of factor Xa. Fondaparinux is an indirect Xa inhibitor that can be given subcutaneously daily. It does not form complexes with PF4 and is unlikely to cause HIT. Protamine does not reverse its effects. Idaparinux is an indirect factor Xa inhibitor that has a long half life and can be given subcutaneously on a weekly basis. Anti-factor-Xa agents (e.g. DPC906) that can be administered orally are being evaluated.
- Recombinant activated protein C, natural protein C, and recombinant thrombomodulin possess varying degrees of anticoagulant activity.

Activated protein C additionally may be employed to treat sepsis (Griffin, 2002; Liaw, 2004).

Antiplatelet Therapy

Several classes of compounds are currently employed to diminish platelet functionality. These include aspirin, other cyclooxygenase inhibitors, ADP receptor antagonists, and glycoprotein (GP) IIb/IIIa receptor antagonists. In contrast to treatment with the oral anticoagulants or with heparin, antiplatelet therapy has not traditionally been as closely monitored in the laboratory. Increasingly, however, the laboratory is coming to play a greater role. Questions that can potentially be answered by laboratory testing are: 1) whether or not a patient's platelets are resistant to inhibition by a particular agent; 2) what dose of agent is required to achieve a desired intensity of inhibition; 3) when, following termination of therapy, platelet function has returned to an adequate level to subserve significant hemostatic challenges such as surgery, and 4) whether thrombocytopenia observed following antiplatelet therapy may reasonably be attributed to that therapy itself.

Certainly, an agent that has enjoyed quite a long tenure in therapeutics is aspirin. As is widely known, aspirin irreversibly acetylates cyclooxygenase. In the case of the anucleate platelet, this effectively means that recovery from aspirin inhibition occurs only as platelets newly released from megakaryocytes enter the circulation. While human platelets circulate in the blood for an average of 10 days, there is already a substantial normalization of platelet functional responsiveness within 5–7 days following termination of aspirin therapy. This phenomenon may be due to the ability of thromboxane A_2, the active product from the platelet cyclooxygenase pathway of nonaspirinated platelets, to stimulate nearby platelets whose cyclooxygenase has been acetylated by aspirin. Attention has recently been given, however, to individual variations in the response of different patients to aspirin inhibition (Mason, 2004; Sanderson, 2005). Since relative resistance to the platelet inhibitory effects of aspirin may imply a need for additional or alternative antiplatelet treatment in some clinical settings, the laboratory can play a useful role in measuring such resistance. Presently there are two main approaches that have been employed to assess platelet resistance to aspirin. Because platelets are the principal cell type to produce thromboxane, assay of this substance provides a measure of the activity of platelet cyclooxygenase. Since thromboxane A_2 undergoes conversion to thromboxane B_2 and thence to the more stable 11-dehydro-thromboxane B_2, plasma assay of this metabolite has been developed as an indirect measure of platelet cyclooxygenase activity (Catella, 1986), and subsequently assay of urinary 11-dehydro-thromboxane B_2 assays has been employed for this purpose (Eikelboom, 2002). An alternative approach that more directly assesses actual platelet functionality is the measurement of platelet aggregation following stimulation of platelets in vitro by an agonist strongly dependent upon an intact cyclooxygenase pathway. Arachidonic acid or related compounds are frequently employed as agonists in such studies. Of great importance for validation of such functional assays, if they are to be capable of identifying aspirin resistance, is very tight standardization of testing procedure. While this may certainly be accomplished by carefully performed platelet aggregometry on platelet-rich plasma (see Ch. 39), newer methods are being developed to provide comparable information directly on anticoagulated whole blood. For example, optical platelet aggregation studies may be performed on a patient's whole blood to which has been added fibrinogen-coated plastic beads impregnated with an infrared dye (i.e., a dye that absorbs light in the infrared region of the electromagnetic spectrum). Following addition of arachidonic acid, the fibrinogen-coated beads coaggregate with the platelets, presumably by virtue of the fibrinogen binding to the conformationally active forms of GP IIb/IIIa on the stimulated platelets. Whereas absorbance by erythrocytes of light in the visible wavelength had previously precluded optical whole blood aggregometry, the introduction of infrared techniques has permitted rapid quantitation of platelet aggregation (as increasing infrared light transmittance) and of its inhibition by aspirin or other antiplatelet agents (Smith, 1999; Wang, 2003). Whole blood or platelet-rich plasma aggregation studies have also proved helpful in defined clinical settings such as percutaneous transluminal coronary angioplasty (PTCA) for assessing the degree of residual platelet reactivity following inhibition of platelets by abciximab, eptifibatide, and other antagonists of the platelet GP IIb/IIIa complex (see Ch. 39) (Hezard, 2000; Matzdorff, 2001). Detection of residual ADP purinergic receptors on the platelet surface following treatment by ticlopidine or clopidogrel may be assessed in a similar manner.

In addition to aggregometry, other methods may be employed to detect activation of the platelet by agonists, and consequently also the inhibition

V

of that activation by antiplatelet therapies. Flow cytometry may be employed for this purpose through the detection of markers of platelet activation. The translocation of P-selectin from the intracellular α granule of the resting platelet to the extracellular membrane following sufficient platelet stimulation provides one such marker, although the relatively small number of P-selectin molecules detectable even on the fully activated platelet limits the dynamic range of this marker. Antibodies sensitive to conformational change in the GP IIb/IIIa molecule associated with platelet activation potentially offer a greater dynamic range of signal, extending between fully nonactivated and fully activated platelets. Flow cytometric approaches have also been employed to monitor residual functionality of the GP IIb/IIIa complex following treatment of patients with the GP IIb/IIIa inhibitors (Hezard, 2000; Matzdorff, 2001), as well as to quantify platelet microparticles as an indicator of platelet activation (Craft, 2004).

In recent years there has been increasing interest in the possibility that molecular diagnostic testing of platelet polymorphisms may have a role in the individualization of antiplatelet therapy for individual patients. Most of the emphasis to date has been upon the major platelet membrane glycoproteins, although potentially other platelet molecules may prove to have important predictive value with respect to various therapeutic agents. Probably the polymorphism to date showing the greatest promise in this regard is the PLA^1/PLA^2 single amino acid polymorphism occurring within the GP IIb/IIIa receptor complex. Presence of the PLA^2 allele expressed not only in homozygous but even in heterozygous fashion appears capable of reducing the dose needed to achieve a comparable degree of platelet aggregation inhibition by various antiplatelet agents, including aspirin and the GP IIb/IIIa antagonist abciximab (Michelson, 2000).

With GP IIb/IIIa antagonists now being employed routinely in PTCA and other invasive procedures, there has been increasing recognition that thrombocytopenia can complicate this drug administration (Abrams, 2004). In some instances this fall in the platelet count appears to be due to an immediate interaction between drug and platelet, possibly due to preformed drug-dependent antibodies (Aster, 2004). In other instances the time course of the thrombocytopenia suggests development of antibodies either to the drug itself or to a neoepitope formed by binding of the drug to its platelet target (Curtis, 2002, 2004; Nurden, 2004). While definitively establishing such a drug-dependent etiology by laboratory methods is difficult, and at times may simply prove elusive, available methodologies currently employed for evaluation of such acquired thrombocytopenias include flow cytometry, monoclonal antibody-specific immobilization of platelet antigens (MAIPA), and related techniques (see Ch 39).

Appendix: Clinical and Laboratory Standards Institute Pre-analytic Guidelines

- The blood should be collected directly into the tube containing anticoagulant. Blood may be drawn through a vascular access device if it is flushed with saline and 6 dead space volumes of the vascular access device are discarded.
- In a direct draw the prothrombin time (PT) and partial thromboplastin time (PTT) are not affected if the first tube drawn is tested. Collection of blood through lines that have been flushed with heparin is to be avoided.
- The blood should be placed into an anticoagulated tube within 1 minute and mixed well, inverting at least four times. The tube should not be vigorously shaken.
- The anticoagulant should be 3.2% trisodium citrate. The ratio should be 9 parts blood and 1 part citrate.
- Inadequately filled or clotted specimens should be discarded.
- The specimen should be centrifuged and be platelet poor, which is defined as less than 10×10^9/L.
- Hemolyzed specimens are discarded.
- Icteric or lipemic specimens should be analyzed using a mechanical method to detect clotting.

Storage of Specimens

- PT determinations can be kept at 18–24°C either on separated plasma or spun cells, and tested within 24 hours. Cold activation of factor VII may occur at 2–4°C.
- Routine unheparinized specimens can be kept either centrifuged or uncentrifuged in an unopened tube on the cells at 18–24°C and tested within 24 hours. Specimens with unfractionated heparin (UFH) should be centrifuged within 1 hour of collection and the plasma tested within 4 hours.
- If testing is not done within 24 hours for the PT or 4 hours for the PTT, the plasma should be removed and frozen at –20°C and tested within 2 weeks or stored at –70°C and tested within 4 weeks. These frozen samples should be rapidly thawed with gentle mixing at 37°C and assayed immediately. These may be kept at 4°C and assayed within 4 hours.

Quality Control

- The quality control program should have a peer group for comparison. The laboratory should participate in a proficiency survey. The samples for this survey should be analyzed in the same manner as patient plasma samples.

References

Abrams CS, Cines DB: Thrombocytopenia after treatment with platelet glycoprotein IIb/IIIa inhibitors. Curr Hematol Rep 2004; 3:143–147.

Adcock DM, Johnston M: Evaluation of frozen plasma calibrants for enhanced standardization of the international normalized ratio (INR): a multi-center study. Thromb Haemost 2002; 87: 74–79.

Adcock DM, Koftan C, Crisan D, et al: Effect of plemorphisms of the cytochrome P450 CYP2C9 gene on warfarin anticoagulation. Arch Pathol Lab Med 2004; 128:1360–1363.

Amiral J, Marfaing-Koka A, Wolf M, et al: Presence of interleukin-8 or neutrophil-activating peptide-2 in patients with heparin-associated thrombocytopenia. Blood 1996; 88: 410–416.

Anderson JA, Saenko EL: Heparin resistance. Br J Anaesth 2002; 88:467–469.

Ansell J, Hirsh J, Poller L, et al: The pharmacology and management of the vitamin K antagonists. Chest 2004; 126: 204S–233S.
Excellent comprehensive review of oral anticoagulant therapy.

Aster RH, Curtis BR, Bougie DW: Thrombocytopenia resulting from sensitivity to GPIIb-IIIa inhibitors. Semin Thromb Hemost 2004; 30:569–577.
Important review of recently recognized thrombocytopenia secondary to anti-platelet therapy.

Bates SM, Greer IA, Hirsh J, et al: Use of antithrombotic agents during pregnancy. Chest 2004; 126: 627S–644S.

Bates SM, Weitz JI: New anticoagulants: beyond heparin, low-molecular-weight heparin and warfarin. Br J Pharmacol 2005; 144:1017–1028.

Current review of newer anti-thrombotic agents.

Bharadwaj J, Jayaraman C, Shrivastava R: Heparin resistance. Lab Hematol 2003; 9: 125–131.

Boneu B, de MP: How and when to monitor a patient treated with low molecular weight heparin. Semin Thromb Hemost 2001; 27:519–522.

Bongiorno RA, Nutescu EA: Generic warfarin: implications for clinical practice and perceptions of anticoagulation providers. Semin Thromb Hemost 2004; 30: 619–626.

Bounameaux H, de Moerloose P: Is laboratory monitoring of low-molecular-weight heparin therapy necessary? No. J Thromb Haemost 2004; 2:551–554.

Bussey H, Francis JH, Heparin Consensus Group: Heparin overview and issues. Pharmacotherapy 2004; 24:1035–1075.

Call JT, Deliargyris EN, Sane DC: Direct thrombin inhibitors in the treatment of immune-mediated heparin-induced thrombocytopenia. Semin Thromb Hemost 2004; 30: 297–304.

Carlsson SC, Mattsson C, Eriksson UG, et al: A review of the effects of the oral direct thrombin inhibitor ximelagatran on coagulation assays. Thromb Res 2005; 115: 9–18.

Catella F, Healy D, Lawson JA: 11-Dehydrothromboxane B2: a quantitative index of thromboxane A2 formation in the human circulation. Proc Natl Acad Sci USA 1986; 83:5861–5865.

Cowan JF, Khan MB, Vargo J, et al: An improved method for evaluation of blood coagulation in heparinized blood. Am J Clin Pathol 1981; 85: 60–64.

Craft JA, Masci PP, Roberts MS: Increased platelet-derived microparticles in the coronary circulation of

percutaneous transluminal coronary angioplasty patients. Blood Coagul Fibrinolysis 2004; 15:475–482.

Cunningham MT, Johnson GF, Pennell BJ, et al: The reliability of manufacturer-determined, instrument-specific international sensitivity index values for calculating the international normalized ratio. Am J Clin Pathol 1994; 102:128–133.

Curtis BR, Divgi A, Garritty M: Delayed thrombocytopenia after treatment with abciximab: a distinct clinical entity associated with the immune response to the drug. J Thromb Haemost 2004; 2:985–992.

Curtis BR, Swyers J, Divgi A: Thrombocytopenia after second exposure to abciximab is caused by antibodies that recognize abciximab-coated platelets. Blood 2002; 99:2054–2059.

Edson JR, Krivit W, White JG: Kaolin partial thromboplastin time: high levels of procoagulants producing short clotting times or masking deficiencies of other procoagulants or low concentrations of anticoagulants. J Lab Clin Med 1967; 70: 463–470.

Eikelboom JW, Hirsh J, Weitz JI: Aspirin-resistant thromboxane biosynthesis and the risk of myocardial infarction, stroke, or cardiovascular death in patients at high risk for cardiovascular events. Circulation 2002; 105:1650–1655.

Fenyvesi T, Jorg I, Harenberg J: Monitoring of anticoagulant effects of direct thrombin inhibitors. Semin Thromb Hemost 2002; 28:361–368.

Francis CW, Berkowitz SD, Comp PC, et al: Comparison of ximelagatran with warfarin for the prevention of venous thromboembolism after total knee replacement. N Engl J Med 2003; 349: 1703–1712.

Francis JL: A critical evaluation of assays for detecting antibodies to the heparin–PF4 complex. Semin Thromb Hemost 2004b; 30: 359–368.

Francis JL, Groce JB III: Challenges in variation and responsiveness of unfractionated heparin. Pharmacotherapy, 2004a; 24: 108S–119.

Greinacher A, Potzsch B, Amiral J, et al: Heparin-associated thrombocytopenia: isolation of the antibody and characterization of a multimolecular PF4–heparin complex as the major antigen. Thromb Haemost 1994; 71: 247–251.

Griffin JH, Zlokovic B, Fernandez JA: Activated protein C: potential therapy for severe sepsis, thrombosis, and stroke. Semin Hematol 2002; 39:197–205.

Gustafsson D, Nystrom J, Carlsson S, et al: The direct thrombin inhibitor melegatran and its oral prodrug H 376/95: intestinal absorption properties, biochemical and pharmacodynamic effects. Thromb Res 2001; 3:171–181.

Harenberg J: Is laboratory monitoring of low-molecular-weight heparin therapy necessary? Yes. J Thromb Haemostas 2004; 2: 547–550.

Hezard N, Metz D, Nazeyrollas P: Use of the PFA-100 apparatus to assess platelet function in patients undergoing PTCA during and after infusion of c7E3 Fab in the presence of other antiplatelet agents. Thromb Haemost 2000; 83:540–544.

Higashi MK, Veenstra DL, Kondo LM, et al: Association between CYP2C9 genetic variants and anticoagulation outcomes during warfarin therapy. JAMA 2002; 287: 1690–1698.

Hirsh J, Guyatt G, Albers GW, et al: The seventh ACCP conference on antithrombotic and thrombolytic therapy, evidence based guidelines. Chest 2004a; 126: 172S–178S.

Hirsh J, O'Donnell M, Weitz JI: New anticoagulants. Blood 2005; 105: 453–463.

Hirsh J, Raschke R: Heparin and low-molecular-weight heparin. Chest 2004b; 126: 188S–203S.

Hoppensteadt DA, Kahn S, Fareed J: Factor X values as a means to assess the extent of oral anticoagulation in patients receiving antithrombin drugs. Clin Chem 1997; 43: 1786–1788.

Horne MK III: Nonimmune heparin–platelet interactions: implications for the pathogenesis of heparin-induced thrombocytopenia. In Warkentin TE, Greinacher A (eds): Induced Thrombocytopenia, 2nd ed. New York, Marcel Dekker, 2001, pp 123–136.

Hull RD, Rasko GE, Brant RF, et al: Relation between the time to achieve the lower limit of the APTT therapeutic range and recurrent venous thromboembolism during heparin treatment for deep vein thrombosis. Arch Intern Med 1997; 157: 2562–2568.

Hutt ED, Kingdon HS: Use of heparinase to eliminate heparins inhibition in rowtime coagulation assays. J Lab Clin Med 1972; 79: 1027–1034.

Kessler CM: Current and future challenges of antithrombotic agents and anticoagulants: strategies for reversal of hemorrhagic complications. Semin Hematol 2004; 41: 44–50.

Kolde H: Haemostasis, 2nd ed. Basel, Pentapharm Ltd, 2004.

Lee DH, Warkentin TE: Frequency of heparin-induced thrombocytopenia. In Warkentin TE, Greinacher A (eds): Induced Thrombocytopenia, 2nd ed. New York, Marcel Dekker, 2001, pp 87–121.

Liaw PC, Esmon CT, Kahnamoui K: Patients with severe sepsis vary markedly in their ability to generate activated protein C. Blood 2004; 104:3958–3964.

Linder MW, Looney S, Adams, et al: Warfarin dose adjustments based upon CYP2C9 genetic polymorphisms. J Thromb Thrombolysis 2002; 14: 227–232.

Lombardi R, Chantarangkul V, Cattaneo M, et al: Measurement of warfarin in plasma by high

performance liquid chromatography (HPLC) and its correlation with the international normalized ratio. Thromb Res 2003; 111: 281–284.

Mammen EF: Current development in antithrombotic therapy. Semin Thromb Hemost 2004; 30: 605–607.

Martin DP, Schroeder TL, Levy ML: Vascular purpura and diseases of blood vessels. In Loscalzo J, Schafer AI (eds): Thrombosis and Hemorrhage, 2nd ed. Baltimore, Williams & Wilkins, 1998, pp 945–961.

Mason PJ, Freedman JE, Jacobs AK: Aspirin resistance: current concepts. Rev Cardiovasc Med 2004; 5:156–163.

Matzdorff AC, Kuhnel G, Kemkes-Matthes B: Comparison of GP IIB/IIIA inhibitors and their activity as measured by aggregometry, flow cytometry, single platelet counting, and the rapid platelet function analyzer. J Thromb Thrombolysis 2001; 12:129–139.

Merry AF: Bivalirudin, blood loss and graft patency in coronary artery bypass surgery. Semin Thromb Hemost 2004; 30:337–346.

Michelson AD, Furman MI, Goldschmidt-Clermont P: Platelet GP IIIa Pl(A) polymorphisms display different sensitivities to agonists. Circulation 2000; 101:1013–1018.

Moll S, Ortel TL: Monitoring warfarin therapy in patients with lupus anticoagulants. Ann Intern Med 1997; 127: 177–185.

National Committee for Clinical Laboratory Standards: Collection, transport, and processing of blood specimens for coagulation testing and general performance of coagulation assays; approved guideline H21-A3, 3rd ed. Wayne, PA, National Committee for Clinical Laboratory Standards, 1998, p. 18:20.

Excellent source of detailed information on guidelines for coagulation testing.

National Committee for Clinical Laboratory Standards: Point-of-care monitoring of anticoagulation therapy; approved guideline H49-A. Wayne, PA, National Committee for Clinical Laboratory Standards, 2004, p. 24:23.

Newman RS, Fagin AR: Heparin contamination in coagulation testing and a protocol to avoid it and the risk of inappropriate FFP transfusion. Am J Clin Pathol 1995; 104: 447–449.

Nowak G: Clinical monitoring of hirudin and direct thrombin inhibitors. Semin Thromb Hemost 2001; 27: 537–541.

Ng VL, Levin J, Corash L, et al: Failure of the International Normalized Ratio to generate consistent results within a local medical community. Am J Clin Path 1993; 99:689–694.

Nugent MA: Heparin sequencing brings structure to the function of complex oligosaccharides. Proc Natl Acad Sci USA 2000; 97:10301–10303.

Nurden P, Clofent-Sanchez G, Jais C: Delayed immunologic thrombocytopenia induced by abciximab. Thromb Haemost 2004; 92:820–828.

Nutescu EA: Point of care monitors for oral anticoagulant therapy. Semin Thromb Hemost 2004; 30: 697–702.

Olson JD: How to validate heparin sensitivity of the aPTT. CAP Today 2004; 18: 72–78.

Olson JD, Arkin CF, Brandt JT, et al: Laboratory monitoring of unfractionated heparin therapy. Arch Pathol Lab Med 1998; 122: 782–798.

Pettila V, Leinonem P, Markkola A, et al: Postpartum bone mineral density in women treated for thromboprophylaxis with unfractionated heparin or LMW heparin. Thromb Haemost 2002; 87: 182–186.

Poller L: International normalized ratios (INR): the first 20 years. J Thromb Haemost 2004; 2:849–860.

Poller L, Hirsh J: Oral anticoagualants. New York, Oxford University Press, 1996.

Rauova L, Poncz M, McKenzie SE, et al: Ultralarge complexes of PF4 and heparin are central to the

pathogenesis of heparin-induced thrombocytopenia. Blood 2005; 105: 131–138.

Provides insight into the mechanisms underlying HIT with respect to heparin and PF4 structures.

Rosborough TK, Shepherd MF: Unreliability of international normalized ratio for monitoring warfarin therapy in patients with lupus anticoagulant. Pharmacotherapy 2004; 24: 838–842.

Salzman EW, Rosenberg RD, Smith MH, et al: Effect of heparin and heparin fractions on platelet aggregation. J Clin Invest 1980; 65: 64–73.

Sanderson S, Emery J, Baglin T: Narrative review: aspirin resistance and its clinical implications. Ann Intern Med 2005; 142:370–380.

Schenk JF, Pindur G, Stephan B, et al: On the prophylactic and therapeutic use of danaparoid sodium (Orgaran) in patients with heparin-induced thrombocytopenia. Clin Appl Thromb Hemost 2003; 9: 25–32.

Schulman S, Hellgren-Wangdahl M: Pregnancy, heparin and osteoporosis. Thromb Haemost 2002; 87: 180–181.

Smith JW, Steinhubl SR, Lincoff AM: Rapid platelet-function assay: an automated and quantitative cartridge-based method. Circulation 1999; 99:620–625.

Sunderji R, Gin K, Shalansky K, et al: Clinical impact of point-of-care vs laboratory measurement of anticoagulation. Am J Clin Pathol 2005; 123: 184–188.

Thompson AR, Counts RB: Removal of heparin and protamine from plasma. J Lab Clin Med 1976; 88: 922–929.

Tobu M, Iqbal O, Hoppensteadt D, et al: Anti-Xa and anti-IIa drugs alter international normalized ratio measurements: Potential problems in the monitoring of oral anticoagulants. Clin Appl Thrombosis/Hemostasis 2004; 10: 301–309.

Van den Besselaar AMHP, Barrowcliffe TW, Houbouyan-Reveillard LL, et al: Guidelines on preparation, certification, and use of plasmas for ISI calibration and INR determination. J Thromb Haemost 2004; 2: 1946–1953.

Van den Besselaar AMHP, Sturk A, Reijnierse GLA: Monitoring of unfractionated heparin with the activated partial thromboplastin time: determination of therapeutic ranges. Thromb Res 2002; 107: 235–240.

Van der Velde EA, Poller L: The APTT monitoring of heparin – the ISTH/ICSH collaborative study. Thromb Haemost 1995; 73: 73–81.

Walenga JM, Hoppensteadt DA: Monitoring the new antithrombotic drugs. Semin Thromb Hemost 2004; 30: 683–695.

Wallin R, Hutson SM: Warfarin and the vitamin K-dependent gamma-carboxylation system. Trends Mol Med 2004; 10:299–302.

Wang JC, Aucoin-Barry D, Manuelian D: Incidence of aspirin nonresponsiveness using the Ultegra Rapid Platelet Function Assay – ASA. Am J Cardiol 2003; 92:1492–1494.

Warkentin TE: An overview of the heparin-induced thrombocytopenia syndrome. Semin Thromb Hemost 2004; 30: 273–283.

Warkentin TE, Elavathel LJ, Hayward CPM, et al: The pathogenesis of venous limb gangrene associated with heparin-induced thrombocytopenia. Ann Intern Med 1997; 127: 804–812.

Warkentin TE, Greinacher A: Laboratory testing for heparin-induced thrombocytopenia. In Warkentin TE, Greinacher A (eds): Induced Thrombocytopenia, 2nd ed. New York, Marcel Dekker, 2001, pp 231–269.

This chapter, as well as the entire book itself, provides an unusually comprehensive and helpful approach to the diagnosis of HIT.

Weitz JL, Bates SM: New anticoagulants. J Thromb Haemost 2005; 3:1843–1853.

V

PART VI

Immunology and Immunopathology

Edited by

H. Davis Massey MD PhD, Richard A. McPherson MD

Immunology and Immunologic Diseases

CHAPTER 42

Overview of the Immune System and Immunologic Disorders

Richard A. McPherson MD, Davis Massey MD PhD

KEY POINTS

- The immune system consists of cellular and humoral components that defend the body against invading microorganisms. Deficiency of individual factors of the immune system can leave an individual susceptible to different infections.

- The lymphoid cells of the immune system are composed of T cells, which act directly against foreign antigens, and B cells, which synthesize immunoglobulins that combine with foreign antigens. Antigen-presenting cells are crucial for cell-to-cell communication for the direction of an immune response.

- The mechanisms by which lymphocytes differentiate into T cells and B cells involve rearrangement of genes for the T cell antigen receptor and of genes for immunoglobulins respectively.

- Lymphocytes from patient specimens are characterized by detection of surface proteins, termed cluster of differentiation (CD) markers, that designate their subset and function.

- Additional cellular elements are natural killer lymphocytes plus neutrophils, eosinophils, and the effectors of IgE-mediated hypersensitivity – basophils and mast cells.

- In addition to immunoglobulins or antibodies, the other humoral elements include a cascading series of proteins in the complement system that results in enzymatic destruction of foreign cells and recruitment of cellular infiltrates by cytokine actions.

- Histocompatibility antigens play a major role in antigen presentation to T cells and also form the immunologic identity of an individual, which is important in rejection of organ transplants.

- Immunologic injuries can occur as a result of excessive response to specific antigenic exposures such as from allergies or from circulating immune complexes.

- Autoimmune diseases result when the mechanisms for maintaining immunologic tolerance to self-(auto)antigens fail resulting in formation of various autoantibodies plus activation of the cellular immune system against the patient's own tissues.

- Laboratory measurements of the immune system involve relatively simple techniques for counting lymphocytes and their subsets as well as for quantifying overall concentrations of immunoglobulins and complement proteins. More complex methods such as detection of gene rearrangements, autoantibody characterization, and allergen reactivity with IgE are useful for diagnosing various disorders of the immune system.

The immune system is structured to recognize, respond to, and destroy a wide variety of invading organisms such as bacteria, viruses, fungi, and parasites that would otherwise be capable of promoting infections harmful to the body. Discovery of the components of the immune system has very often followed investigations of serious infections and the specific reactions that the body uses to combat pathogenic organisms. In general, this immunologic function can be summarized as searching for foreign (or non-self) antigens that do not belong in the body and then destroying them. In this process, the immune system also maintains surveillance over the appearance of new or foreign antigens on tumor cells and also attempts to destroy them while leaving unharmed the normal (or self) antigens on healthy cells. Disease states may arise as a result of various aspects of immunologic function going awry. These include hypersensitivity reactions, autoimmune disease, various immunodeficiency disorders, and allogeneic organ/tissue transplantation, graft versus host disease and rejection; the quest for tolerance in transplantation continues. This overview highlights components of the immune system and their functions plus some of the significant clinical disorders of immunity.

Lymphoid cells

The lymphoid cells of the body consist of lymph nodes, spleen, cells at mucosal surfaces, and cells that circulate in the blood. They derive from multipotential hematopoietic stem cells, with their production moving progressively from the yolk sac in the embryo to the liver in the fetus and to the bone marrow in the infant through adult ages (Weissman, 1994). The various lymphoid cells are conveniently identified by the presence of unique protein markers on their surfaces that also endow those cells with particular functions.

T Lymphocytes

T lymphocytes undergo differentiation in the thymus. After originating in the bone marrow, they pass from the cortex to the medulla of the thymus, during which time they undergo maturation. This process involves selection such that self-reactive cells are eliminated while other cells are retained that can recognize antigens through interactions with molecules of the major histocompatibility complex (MHC) (Nossal, 1994; von Boehmer, 1994). T lymphocytes comprise about 60–70% of all lymphocytes in the blood, and they are also found in paracortical areas of lymph nodes and within periarteriolar sheaths in the spleen. During maturation, they undergo genetic programming in which the gene for the T-cell antigen receptor (TCR) is rearranged to produce protein receptors that are invariant in their antigen specificity for the lifespan of that T lymphocyte as well as for all its descendent cells.

The majority (>95%) of T lymphocytes have antigen receptors made of the α and β subunits linked with disulfide bonds to form a molecular

VI

heterodimer that resides on the outer membrane of the cell in association with the CD3 molecular complex (CD3 is a pan-T-cell marker). The α- and β-subunit TCR proteins have variable, joining, and constant regions (α also contains a diversity region), with corresponding encoding regions in the *TCR* gene that undergoes rearrangement, resulting in high specificity of binding for a particular antigen. The CD3 proteins assist transduction of the signal to the interior of the cell when an antigen binds to the TCR on the lymphocyte surface (Janeway, 1994; Weiss, 1994). A small percentage of T lymphocytes have a TCR composed of γ and δ subunits that similarly interact with CD3; these cells are generally found at mucosal surfaces of the gastrointestinal and respiratory tracts. T-cell proliferations may be characterized as neoplastic (clonal) versus benign (polyclonal) according to whether their DNA shows predominantly a single form of *TCR* gene rearrangement versus a complete spectrum of such rearrangements as normally occurs in a heterogeneous lymphocyte population.

Examination of T lymphocytes by flow cytometry uses a variety of surface markers. CD4 is found on about 60% of CD3+ cells; these are helper/inducer T cells that direct the function of other cells of the immune system by secreting cytokines that stimulate various functions. There are two distinct subpopulations of CD4+ helper cells: Th1, which secrete interleukin (IL)-2 and interferon (IFN)-γ; and Th2, which secrete IL-4 and IL-5. Th1 cells facilitate macrophage activities such as hypersensitivity and production of antibodies with opsonizing action; Th2 cells direct synthesis of other antibodies. The marker CD8 is found on about 30% of T cells (thus the normal ratio of CD4+ to CD8+ cells in the blood is typically 2:1). These CD8+ T cells exhibit cytotoxicity and suppressor activity in the immune response.

The mechanism of antigen recognition is different between the two subsets of T lymphocytes. CD4 molecules bind to the MHC class II molecules on antigen-presenting cells, whereas CD8 molecules interact with MHC class I molecules. Accordingly CD4+ cells recognize antigens only in the context of MHC class II antigens and CD8+ cells recognize them only through MHC class I antigens.

B Lymphocytes

B lymphocytes comprise roughly 10–20% of peripheral lymphocytes in the blood, and they also are found in bone marrow, lymph nodes, spleen, and other lymphatic tissues. In spleen and nodes they aggregate in lymphoid follicles. Differentiation of B lymphocytes occurs in the bone marrow, where both positive and negative selection take place, as well as at peripheral locations. Antigenic stimulation of B cells leads to formation of plasma cells that secrete immunoglobulins as the basis of specificity in humoral immunity. The B-cell–antigen-receptor complex uses immunoglobulin (Ig)M as the antigen-binding component. The

antigen specificity of immunoglobulins derives from a rearrangement process in which both heavy and light chain genes are realigned. The heavy chain has variable, diversity, joining, and constant regions, whereas the light chain gene has variable, joining, and constant regions. Maturation of an antibody response entails switching from IgM to another heavy chain type (usually IgG) due to further gene rearrangement, although the light chain type of a B cell remains fixed (Corcoran, 2005).

B cells also have on their surfaces receptors for complement (CD21, which is also the receptor for Epstein–Barr virus [EBV] and thus makes these cells susceptible to EBV infection) and for the Fc region of immunoglobulins; they also have CD19 and CD20, which are frequently used for immunologic identification of B cells.

Antigen-Presenting Cells

Macrophages function as mononuclear phagocytes in inflammation, and they also process ingested antigens and present them in association with MHC molecules on their membranes (Fig. 42–1). T cells are not activated by soluble antigens, and so presentation of antigens in this manner is necessary for T-cell stimulation and induction of cell-mediated immunity (Germain, 1994; Trombetta, 2005). Macrophages also secrete cytokines such as IL-1 for modulation of inflammatory processes, they can directly lyse tumor cells in their role of immunosurveillance, and they also are effector cells of some types of cell-mediated immunity (e.g., delayed hypersensitivity).

Dendritic cells (found in lymphoid tissues and in interstitial regions of other organs) and Langerhans cells (found in the epidermis) have extensive dendritic cytoplasmic processes that are rich in MHC class II molecules. Consequently they are very efficient at presenting antigens (although they are probably not phagocytic) and are considered to be extremely important at that task within the entire immune system (Park, 2005).

Natural Killer Cells

Natural killer (NK) cells constitute 10–15% of lymphocytes in the peripheral blood. They are neither T cells nor B cells and were formerly called 'null cells.' NK cells have the function of lysing other cells without prior sensitization. They can attack tumor cells, cells infected with viruses, and others as well; consequently, they form the initial defense against aberrant cells. NK cells are characterized by the surface markers CD16 and CD56, which are commonly used for their identification. CD16 is the Fc receptor for IgG and hence NK cells are able to lyse selectively those cells that are coated with antibodies (antibody-dependent cell-mediated cytotoxicity [ADCC], which is important in some hypersensitivity

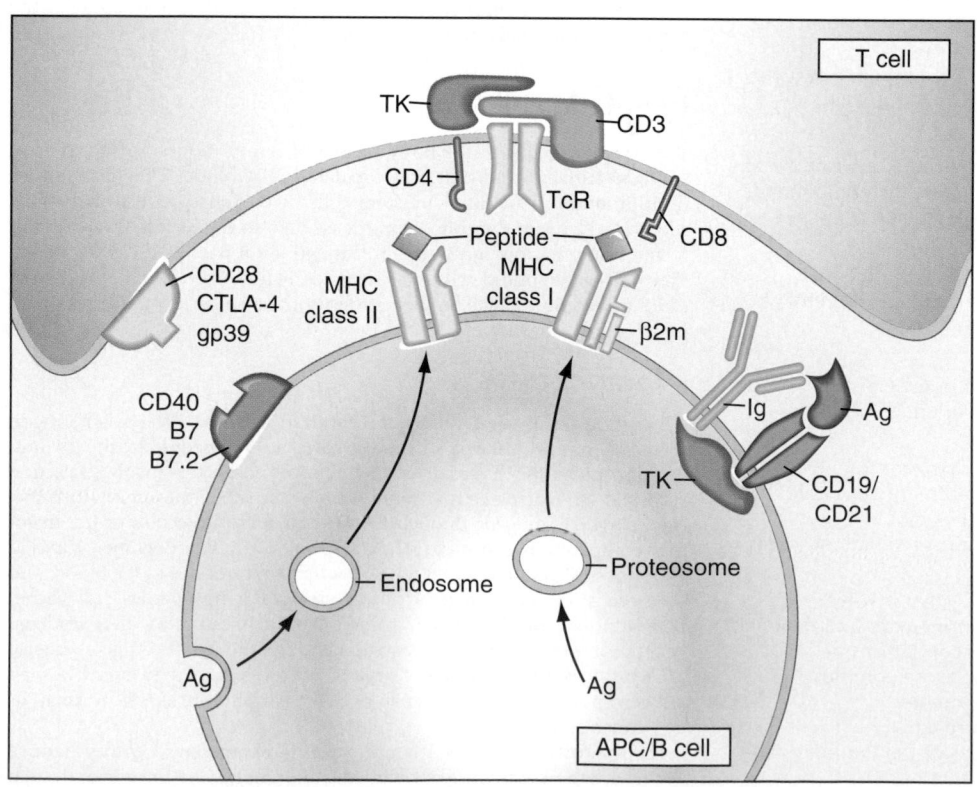

Figure 42–1 Cellular interactions in the immune system. Antigen-presenting cells (APC) process external or internal antigens (Ag) and present antigen peptide fragments, in association with an MHC molecule, to T cells. On the T cell, a specific antigen receptor (TCR), along with the co-receptor CD4 or CD8 molecule, recognizes the antigen–MHC complex. Cellular activation proceeds through the CD3 complex and activation of tyrosine kinases (TKs). The B-cell receptor is composed of membrane-bound Ig complexed to associated membrane proteins, and the CD19/21 co-receptor. On antigen recognition, cellular TKs are also activated. Co-stimulatory activation of T cells or B cells is provided by cellular receptors binding their ligands (the ligands B7 or B7.2 for T-cell co-stimulation through CD28 and CTLA-4 molecules, and the gp39 ligand for the B-cell CD40 molecule). (Redrawn with permission from Paul W, Seder R: Lymphocytic responses and cytokines. Cell 1994; 76:229 and Weiss A, Littman D: Signal transduction by lymphocyte antigen receptors. Cell 1994; 76:263.)

reactions). NK cells also secrete cytokines such as IFN-γ. Interestingly, NK cells are recognizable on examination of standard stained blood smears as large granular lymphocytes (Kronenberg, 2005).

Nonlymphoid cells

These cells are not genetically programmed to recognize specific antigens or to interact with lymphoid cells in the induction of an immune response. Instead, they are effectors of immune reactions that are triggered by various factors.

Neutrophils and Eosinophils

Neutrophils are drawn to regions of inflammation by chemoattractants; they then release from their granules toxic substances and enzymes that digest cellular structures indiscriminately; neutrophils also ingest cellular debris as do eosinophils and remove it from tissue sites.

Basophils and Mast Cells

Basophils (and their counterparts in tissues, the mast cells) have on their surfaces receptors that bind IgE. Uptake of IgE on to the membranes of basophils is apparently not specific by antigen that the IgE recognizes; instead, it is driven by mass action between the amount of total IgE and the available basophils. When the antigen (or allergen) comes into contact with IgE that recognizes it on the surface of basophils, those cells become activated and release substances such as histamines, which mediate some hypersensitivity. Thus, specificity of a basophil is directed by the particular IgE that is bound to its surface from the blood; theoretically, a basophil could have multiple different IgE molecules on its surface and so could react with many different allergens.

Humoral factors

Immunoglobulins

Antibody molecules can be bound to B-cell surfaces for stimulation of further immunoglobulin secretion; they also circulate in the blood and appear at mucosal surfaces of the respiratory and gastrointestinal tracts, where they are likely to come into contact with potentially pathogenic microorganisms. The major immunoglobulins in the blood are IgM, IgG, and IgA; these antibodies presumably arise following exposure to a multitude of foreign antigens and may remain for years with continued secretion to replace molecules that are lost through normal clearance of proteins from the circulation. At mucosal surfaces, the primary type of antibody is IgA in a special dimeric form that results from secretion at that site (Fagarasan, 2004) (see Ch. 46). The other immunoglobulins are IgD (which resides on B-cell surfaces, where it may be involved in immune signal transduction but does not achieve substantial concentrations as free molecules in the blood) and IgE (which functions through binding to surfaces of basophils and stimulates the release of vasoactive substances from those cells in the presence of specific allergens).

Immunoglobulins in the blood function by attaching to antigens on the surfaces of foreign cells, bacteria, viruses, and the like, and by facilitating their destruction through nonspecific effectors such as complement and NK cell activation. Disease monitoring by immunoglobulin testing includes qualitative analysis for clonal versus polyclonal detection (e.g., for diagnosis of multiple myeloma) and quantitative analyses both for overall concentrations of IgM, IgG, and IgA (to detect possible selective or combined deficiencies or overproduction of immunoglobulin classes) and for titers of specific antibodies against individual antigens (such as isohemagglutinins, pneumococcus, Haemophilus, tetanus, diphtheria, or other microorganisms).

Complement

This set of interacting proteins has the role of enzymatically destroying targets (e.g., cells, bacteria) to which they have been directed by antibodies or through other means (see Ch. 47). Measurements of complement components have two major utilities in clinical diagnosis: to detect congenital deficiencies (which are relatively rare) that may predispose to certain disorders such as infections or progression to autoimmune diseases) and to detect acquired reductions that reflect current activity of systemic autoimmune diseases such as systemic lupus erythematosus (Wen, 2004).

Cytokines

These soluble substances are the means by which cellular immune responses are regulated; they are short-acting mediators that are elaborated by some cells and diffuse to other cells where they act (Leonard, 2003). Many cytokines are pleiotropic, in that they can act on different cell types. They can act in an endocrine manner by stimulating cells at a distance; they can act on cells in their immediate vicinity (paracrine); they can also stimulate the same cells that secreted them (autocrine). The specific actions of cytokines include hematopoiesis through colony-stimulating factors (CSFs) that induce granulocyte and macrophage production, natural immune responses (through IL-1, tumor necrosis factor [TNF]-α, interferons, and IL-8), stimulation of lymphocyte growth and activation (through IL-2 and others), and activation of nonspecific inflammatory cells (see Ch. 47). Cytokines are still being discovered as more detail emerges concerning cell-to-cell communication.

Clinical use of cytokines includes both suppression of the immune response in allogeneic organ transplantation by drugs such as cyclosporine that blocks production of IL-2 and enhancement of the immune response in therapies against cancer or infections. These latter treatments are largely experimental, although it has been shown that pretreatment with antibodies against TNF-α can prevent deleterious Jarisch–Herxheimer reactions resulting from antibiotic treatment of Borrelia recurrentis infection in sheep (Fekade, 1996). This model very probably presages a host of new therapies by which immune responses will be selectively enhanced or suppressed according to particular clinical needs.

Histocompatibility antigens

The MHC (also called human leukocyte antigen complex, HLA) is encoded on human chromosome 6 and includes class I molecules (HLA A, B, and C), class II molecules (HLA DP, DQ, and DR), and the intervening class III molecules of some complement components and TNF-α and -β (see Ch. 48). The functions of class I and class II antigens have already been discussed briefly regarding how they participate in antigen presentation to T cells. These antigens were discovered and their highly polymorphic natures were described in studies of immune tolerance and rejection of transplanted allogeneic organs. Consequently, one of the most important clinical uses of HLA typing is in matching potential organ or tissue donors with recipients who are in need of a transplant. Another significant clinical application is in the typing of affected patients and their family members to establish their risk of developing some diseases that are associated with particular HLA types (e.g., ankylosing spondylitis with HLA B27) (see Ch. 49). Still another use of HLA typing is in providing matched platelets for patients who have become refractory to platelet transfusions due to HLA antibody formation after exposure to multiple donors (e.g., following transfusion support for chemotherapy or hematopoietic progenitor cell (HPC) transplantation (see Ch. 36)).

Mechanisms of Immunologic Injury

Immunologic responses can create injury to normal tissues as well as to invading organisms that may have triggered a response. These responses are conveniently classified into four types of hypersensitivity. Type I is anaphylactic or allergic in nature; it is mediated by IgE bound to the surface of basophils and mast cells. When specific antigens (or allergens) bind to surface IgE, the basophils are stimulated to release histamine and other vasoactive substances that are the immediate mediators of allergic reactions (Kemp, 2002). Clinical strategies for treatment of asthma and allergies have addressed different aspects of this sequence of events from counteracting the effects or release of histamine back to desensitization. Successful use of a recombinant humanized monoclonal antibody against IgE to treat such individuals has been demonstrated (Milgrom, 1999); this therapy could in the future be based in part on measurements of IgE concentrations in serum.

Type II occurs when antibodies bind to antigens on the surfaces of cells; damage may occur from binding and activation of complement (e.g., immune hemolysis), from antibody-dependent cell-mediated cytotoxicity (e.g., lysis of tumor cells or parasites), or antibody-mediated interference with cellular functions (e.g., autoantibodies against acetylcholine receptors in myasthenia gravis).

Type III results from immune complex formation, either between exogenous antigens such as bacteria or viruses and antibodies; or between endogenous autoantigens and autoantibodies. Typical tissue damage occurs in organs that contain numerous small blood vessels where

VI

circulating immune complexes deposit or in places where the endogenous antigens naturally occur.

Type IV is cell-mediated or delayed hypersensitivity, which depends on functioning CD4+ T cells or other cytotoxicity from CD8+ T cells. Type IV is the basis of immune reaction to viruses, fungi, protozoa, parasites, and also to intracellular microbes such as mycobacteria. Patients with acquired immunodeficiency syndrome (AIDS) are susceptible to infections with these and other opportunistic agents when they lose CD4+ T cells.

Laboratory Applications of Immunologic Assessment

The major areas in which immunologic testing has major clinical application are autoimmune diseases, organ/tissue transplantation and rejection, immunodeficiencies, and allergies.

The autoimmune disease may be systemic (see Ch. 51), restricted to specific organs (see Ch. 53), or involve vasculitis (see Ch. 52). Much of the testing is based on screening with techniques such as the antinuclear antibody followed by confirmatory testing with specific autoantigens such as double-stranded DNA. Other autoantibodies may be identified through indirect immunofluorescent assays that use organ sections to identify specific autoantibodies such as those directed against smooth muscle, mitochondria, parietal cells, and so forth. Technologic advancements have provided purified sources of many important autoantigens that will make future assays for autoantibodies more specific and certainly more easily automated.

Immunosuppressive therapy for rejection of allogeneic transplants and immunodeficiencies rely on testing for lymphocyte subsets with particular importance on T cells and CD4+ cells. In addition, congenital immunodeficiency states require more detailed analysis of the cellular and humoral elements of the immune system, usually beginning with a battery of more conventional tests for presence and function of lymphocytes, immunoglobulins, and complement, and proceeding when necessary to highly esoteric testing for rare disorders (see Chs 45 and 50).

Allergic disorders are typically evaluated through skin testing, measurement of total IgE concentrations in serum, and quantitation of specific IgE reactivities in serum with the common allergens of food, pollens, and other environmental factors (see Ch. 54).

As new discoveries of immunologic functions and new therapies appear, clinical diagnostic laboratories will probably have the opportunity to provide measurements of many more factors and activities to establish correct diagnoses and to monitor and adjust treatments.

References

Corcoran AE: Immunoglobulin locus silencing and allelic exclusion. Semin Immunol 2005; 17:141–154.

Fagarasan S: Regulation of IgA synthesis at mucosal surfaces. Curr Opin Immunol 2004; 16:277–283.

Fekade D, Knox K, Hussein K, et al: Prevention of Jarisch–Herxheimer reactions by treatment with antibodies against tumor necrosis factor α. N Engl J Med 1996; 335:311–315.

Germain R: MHC-dependent antigen processing and peptide presentation: providing ligands for T lymphocyte activation. Cell 1994; 76:287–299.

Janeway C, Bottomly K: Signals and signs for lymphocytic responses. Cell 1994; 76:275–285.

Kemp SF, Lockey RF: Anaphylaxis: a review of causes and mechanisms. J Allergy Clin Immunol 2002; 110:341–348.

An excellent review article covering the immunopathology, pathophysiology, and many causative agents of anaphylaxis, as well as its clinical management.

Kronenberg M: Toward an understanding of NKT cell biology: progress and paradoxes. Annu Rev Immunol 2005; 26:877–900.

This comprehensive review discusses the present state of knowledge of natural killer T cells.

Leonard WJ: Type 1 cytokines and interferons and their receptors. *In* Paul WE (ed.) Fundamental Immunology, 5th ed. Philadelphia, PA, Lippincott Williams & Wilkins, 2003, p 701.

Milgrom H, Fick RB, Su JQ, et al: Treatment of allergic asthma with monoclonal anti-IgE antibody. N Engl J Med 1999; 341:1966–1973.

Nossal G: Negative selection of lymphocytes. Cell 1994; 76:229–239.

Park C, Chio YS: How do follicular dendritic cells interact intimately with B cells in the germinal center? Immunol 2005; 114:2–10.

In this review, the function and interaction of follicular dendritic cells with B cells are nicely presented, with good illustrations.

Paul W, Seder R: Lymphocyte responses and cytokines. Cell 1994; 76:241–245.

Trombetta ES, Mellman I: Cell biology of antigen processing in vitro and in vivo. Annu Rev Immunol 2005; 23:975–1028.

This extensive review covers in detail the properties of antigen-presenting cells, and their regulation, processing, and transport of antigen.

Von Boehmer H: Positive selection of lymphocytes. Cell 1994; 76:219–228.

Wen L, Atkinson JP, Giclas PC: Clinical and laboratory evaluation of complement deficiency. J Allergy Clin Immunol 2004; 113:585–593.

This article presents a brief description of the three complement pathways, an organ system review of the effect of complement deficiencies, and a diagnostic screening approach for complement deficient states.

Weiss A, Littman D: Signal transduction by lymphocyte antigen receptors. Cell 1994; 76:263–274.

Weissman I: Developmental switches in the immune system. Cell 1994; 76:207–218.

CHAPTER 43

Immunoassay and Immunochemistry

Yoshihiro Ashihara PhD, Yasushi Kasahara PhD DMSc, Robert M. Nakamura MD

KEY POINTS

• Immunoassays are routinely employed in the clinical laboratory to identify and measure antigens and antibodies. Systems include particle agglutination assay, radioimmunoassay, enzyme immunoassay, fluorescent or chemiluminescent immunoassay and colorimetric immunoassay.

• The different classes of immunoassay will vary in sensitivity and precision, ease of use, resistance to interferences, shelf life, and hazardous exposures.

• Home testing and point-of-care testing has become more commonplace and sophisticated, as expertise in platform miniaturization has improved permitting the use of much smaller samples. However, issues of sensitivity and specificity remain to be fully investigated in these microsystems.

Immunoassays and Immunochemistry

General Characteristics of Antigen–Antibody Reaction

Biological ligands based on the affinity between molecules, such as enzyme and substrate, hormone and receptor, antigen and antibody, play an important role in living organisms. Specific recognition characteristics of immunoassays (antigen–antibody reactions) have become widely used as analytical tools, despite the wide range of methodologies available in clinical laboratory testing.

Immunoassays can be used for the detection of either antigens or antibodies. For antigen detection, the corresponding specific antibody should be prepared as one of the reagents. The reverse is true for antibody detection. The sensitivity of immunoassays has been enhanced through the development of new types of signal detection system and solid-phase technology. Immunoassays have been optimized to detect less than 0.1 pg/mL of antigen present in blood. They can be applied to the detection of haptens as small molecules; proteins and protein complexes as macromolecules; as well as of any antibody to allergens, infectious agents, and autologous antigens.

Characteristics of Antigens

Antigens can be defined as any substance that can represent antigenic sites (epitopes) to produce corresponding antibodies, from small molecules such as haptens and hormones, to macromolecules such as proteins, glycoproteins, glycolipids, and other natural products. Artificial chemical compounds can also be antigens acting as haptens. Antigens should have at least one epitope. Epitopes that can be recognized by antibodies include amino acid sequences of peptides in proteins and high-dimensional protein structures such as neoantigenic sites.

Characteristics of Antibodies

Immunoglobulin (Ig), an important plasma protein, refers to antibodies in the context of the biological functions of immunoglobulin specific to antigens. Antibodies, therefore, are produced in response to antigenic stimulation. Antibodies are formed of both functional and heterogeneous molecules that bind antigens via the antigen-binding site. There are five classes (isotypes) of immunoglobulin: IgG, IgM, IgA, IgD, and IgE. IgG is further divided into four subclasses, and both IgA and IgM have two subgroups. All known antibody molecules have a heavy chain with either a κ or a λ light chain. The molecular structure of antibodies is composed of variable regions and constant regions. The hypervariable domain (epitope-binding spot) can be assembled to interact with a wide variety of epitopes (antigen determinants). In laboratory medicine, two categories of antibodies can be distinguished: antibodies as reactants and antibodies as analytes. Antibodies as analytes are often classified by IgG, IgM, or IgA subtypes. Antibodies as reactants are prepared from antiserum obtained through animal immunization with purified antigen.

Polyclonal Antibodies

A polyclonal antibody can be obtained through immunization with an antigen, which presents various epitopes. In other words, antibody is generated that is specific against each epitope. The avidity of a polyclonal antibody to a complex antigen is usually stronger than a single monoclonal antibody. Carrier proteins may be needed for the immunization of rather small molecules, such as haptens or hormones.

Monoclonal Antibodies

Monoclonal antibodies (Koehler, 1975) have been developed using the following biotechnologies: somatic cell fusion, selection of the resulting hybridoma, and limiting dilution to obtain monoclonals. They are defined as uniform homogeneous antibodies directed to specific epitopes. An established cell line allows for the secretion of all reactive immunoglobulins specific to single epitopes. Monoclonal antibodies have made it possible to analyze molecules on an epitope-to-epitope basis because of their narrow specificity. Yet monoclonal antibodies do not have the ability to recognize the entire molecule, in contrast to polyclonal antibodies. For monoclonal antibodies, different antigens with a common epitope appear to be the same antigen. For instance CA 19-9 antibody (Magnani, 1983) as a tumor marker can detect different sizes and shapes of molecule that have common carbohydrate epitopes. Monoclonal antibodies enable the identification of isoenzymes, subtypes, isotypes of protein, and conformational changes of molecules, because they can discern the slightest differences in molecules.

Monoclonal antibodies may be cross-reactive with different antigens. This cross-reactivity can be explained by the probable existence of the same amino acid sequences, carbohydrates, or lipids on different molecules. Monoclonal antibody technology has allowed for the development of extremely useful and nearly ideal immunoassay systems for clinical laboratory testing.

The production methods and applications of monoclonal antibodies have been extensively reviewed (Nakamura, 1983; Zola, 1987). The advantages of monoclonal antibodies are as follows:

1. Monoclonal antibodies provide a well-defined reagent.
2. Monoclonal antibody production can yield an unlimited quantity of homogeneous reagent with highly consistent affinity and specificity.
3. Monoclonal antibodies can be prepared through immunization with a nonpurified antigen.

Monoclonal antibodies have certain limitations in their use, as follows:

1. Insufficient reactivity in precipitation or agglutination because network formation in the immunocomplex is weak or does not occur when single monoclonal antibodies are used.

2. Antigens with multiple heterogeneous epitopes are more difficult to characterize immunochemically with a single monoclonal antibody.

Antibody Production by Recombinant Technology

Skerra and Pluckthun (1988) have developed an expression system for the Fv fragment of variable domains of an antibody specific to phosphorylcholine using recombinant technology in *Escherichia coli*. This technology makes it possible to produce chimeric antibody fused to an enzyme.

A technology called phage display has emerged for the production of antibodies (Winter, 1994). In this method, antibody fragments of predetermined binding specificity are constructed from a repertoire of antibody variable region (V) genes, thereby eliminating the need for immunization and hybridoma technology. The V genes can be assembled in vitro. The phage selected from the repertoire by binding to antigen and antibody fragments is expressed in infected bacteria. Furthermore, the binding affinity of the antibodies is improved through the mutation. In the near future this technology will allow for the use of specific antibodies with high avidity.

Kinetics of Antigen–Antibody Reaction

Certain aspects of equilibrium or the law of mass action in chemistry can be applied to the antigen–antibody (Ag–Ab) reaction. The kinetics of the reversible Ag–Ab reaction is as follows (Steward, 1986):

$$Ag + Ab \underset{K_2}{\overset{K_1}{\rightleftharpoons}} AgAb,$$

where Ag represents free antigen, Ab represents free antibody sites, AgAb represents the antigen–antibody complex concentration, and K_1 and K_2 are the association and disassociation rate constants, respectively. The rate of formation of the antigen–antibody complex is represented as follows:

$$dt[AgAb]/dt = K_1 [Ag] [Ab] - K_2[AgAb],$$

and at equilibrium the net rate is zero. Therefore,

$$K_1/K_2 = [AgAb]/[Ag] [Ab] = K_a$$

(association equilibrium constant or affinity constant).

K_a is the parameter limited to site-to-site reactions, although antigens and antibodies often have multiple binding sites on the molecule. The apparent association constant for multiple antigen and antibody reactions may be referred to as *avidity* instead of affinity. The K_a value may be obtained from the following equations and experimental data:

$$[Ab] = [Ab]_t - [AgAb],$$

where [Ab] is the antibody concentration at equilibrium, and $[Ab]_t$ represents the total original antibody concentration.

$$K_a = B/([Ab]_t - B) F,$$

where *F* is free antigen or analyte, and *B* is bound antigen or analyte.

A Scatchard plot is produced when the amount of antigen bound (*B*) is plotted on the x-axis and the B/F ratio of analytes is plotted on the y-axis. Two parameters that can be determined from the Scatchard plot are the dissociation or affinity constant from the slope of the line and the concentration of antibody-binding sites from the x-intercept (Scatchard, 1949).

Overview of General Principles of Immunoassays

Classes of Immunoassay

A brief classification and list of features of various immunoassays appears in Table 43-1. Precipitation immunoassays provide the most simple method by which antigens and antibodies react with each other without involving the detection of any label. The resulting antigen–antibody complex in gel or liquid phase may be observed qualitatively as a precipitant by the naked eye and quantitatively with a detector.

The particle agglutination immunoassay (Kasahara, 1992b) uses inert particles as labels, as opposed to direct precipitation of the antigen–antibody complexes. Antigens or antibodies attached to particles such as erythrocytes, latex, or metal sol react with the analyte in the specimen. As a result of this immune reaction, the large particles show significant agglutination patterns that may be seen by the naked eye. Yalow (1959) reported on the development of a radioimmunoassay (RIA) using radioisotopes as labels. This breakthrough allowed for the quantitative detection of a trace level of analytes and contributed to the advancement of basic research and clinical medicine. Insulin, for example, was quantified by RIA, which subsequently replaced the insulin bioassay. RIA may be formatted in a solid-phase procedure for easy separation of bound and free labels. Since the

Table 43–1 Classification of Various Immunoassays and Their Characteristics

	Labels (Reporter Groups)	B/F Separation*	Signal Detection	Sensitivity
Precipitation immunoassays	Not required	Not required	Naked eye, turbidity, nephrometry	≈10 µg/mL[1]
Particle immunoassays	Blood cells, artificial particles (gelatin, particles, latex, etc.)	Not required	Naked eye, pattern analyzer, spectrophotometry, particle counting	≈5 ng/mL[2]
Radioimmunoassays	Radioisotopes (^{125}I, ^{3}H)	Required	Photon counting	≈5 pg/mL
Enzyme immunoassays	Enzymes	Required	Spectrophotometry, fluorometry, photon counting	≈5 pg/mL ≈0.1 pg/mL[3] (CL-EIA)
Fluorescent immunoassays	Fluorophores	Required	Photon counting	≈5 pg/mL[4]
Chemiluminescent immunoassays	Chemiluminescent compounds	Required	Photon counting	≈5 pg/mL[4]

* Washing step for separation of bound labels in immunocomplex from free labels. Homogeneous assays included are not required for B/F separation.

Data sources: (1) Ritchie, 1978; (2) Haux, 1988; (3) Isomura, 1994; (4) Sgoutas, 1989.

development of RIAs, the search for alternative labels to hazardous radioisotopes has intensified, with the aim of developing nonisotopic immunoassays using enzymes, fluorescent labels, and other reporter groups.

The enzyme immunoassay (EIA), using enzymes as labels, was developed in the early 1970s (Engvall, 1971; Van Weeman, 1971) and rapidly gained wide popularity. Enzymes can amplify signals depending on the turnover of enzyme catalytic activity. Efforts to improve substrates and to increase sensitivity have led to the introduction of chromophore, fluorophore, and later chemiluminescent compounds. Depending on the substrate chosen, the assay method can be defined as a fluorescent enzyme immunoassay or a chemiluminescent enzyme immunoassay (Thorpe, 1984).

Fluorescent immunoassays (FIAs) use fluorophores as labels. Fluorophores require optimal wavelength light energy for their excitation to produce detectable emission light. FIA sensitivity is likely to decrease because of the nonspecific background fluorescence present in biological specimens. Fluorophores that have a delayed fluorescence emission time of 100 ns (nanoseconds) are suitable for application on time-resolved FIA. The introduction of a new class of fluorescent compounds has resulted in improvements of FIA, such as the elimination of background noise. Sophisticated instrumentation has been introduced that can detect low concentrations (10–15 M) of analytes using FIAs.

Chemiluminescent immunoassays use chemiluminescent compounds as labels. Chemiluminescent compounds include chemically synthesized molecules as well as natural products such as aequorin. Unlike fluorophores, most chemiluminescent compounds require chemical rather than light energy to generate emission light. The reduction–oxidation reaction is a process common to all chemiluminescent assays. Signal amplification is not expected of chemiluminescent labels because chemiluminescent molecules generate just one photon through molecular decomposition. A series of new and innovative compounds for electrochemiluminescence have proved suitable for application on immunoassays. Metal chelate with tri-biphenyls emits light through a continuous reduction–oxidation reaction on the surface of electrodes (Blackburn, 1991).

In the various types of assay mentioned earlier, the main factors affecting assay sensitivity are the association constant (affinity or avidity) of the reactant, the signal intensity of the labels, and the signal:noise ratio of the detection signal reduced by either background from the signals themselves or by a nonspecific reaction.

Iodine-125 (^{125}I) isotopes require about 7 million molecules to generate 1 photon/s, based on half-life calculations of radioisotopes (Bounaud, 1987). Chemiluminescent substrates to enzymes can increase events by an order of magnitude six times greater than that of iodine-125. This is attributable to the catalytic amplification capacity of enzymes.

Conjugation Chemistry

Depending on the assay chosen, the method of conjugation that couples one molecule to others, such as enzymes (or cofactors) to antigens (or antibodies), or antigens (or antibodies) to solid phase, may vary. The coupling reaction applied should be performed under conditions that avoid the reduction of any of the biological activities of the protein. In the glutaraldehyde method (Avrameas, 1978), glutaraldehyde, with two (or possibly more) aldehyde groups as a coupling reagent, has been used for conjugation of protein amino groups. This method is based on mixed reactions, including aldol condensation at high pH (the pKa of the NH residue is 8.6–10.8). In this method, shown in Figure 43–1, the resulting conjugate has different forms because of the existence of multiple active

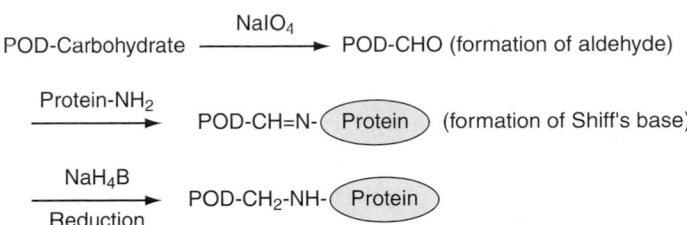

Figure 43–1 Coupling scheme for conjugation of protein with horseradish peroxidase (POD) based on the Nakane method.

sites for coupling. The periodate oxidation method (Nakane, 1966) for the conjugation of antibodies uses horseradish peroxidase, which contains carbohydrates in its molecules. The methods mentioned earlier are not suitable for regulation of site-specific reactions, such as when configurational stereospecificity of conjugates is required.

As shown in Figure 43–2, newer coupling methods (Kato, 1975; Kitagawa, 1978) have been developed using a sophisticated coupling reagent, m-maleimidobenzyl-N-hydroxysuccinimide ester (MBS). The MBS is a bivalent reagent consisting of an activated ester and maleimide, and can react with an NH_2 group and SH group, respectively. The carboxy group can also be used as specific site for conjugating with α- or ε-NH_2 residues of proteins using N-hydroxysuccinimide (NHS) as the coupling reagent. The NHS coupling reagent extends to conjugate protein or the carboxyl group introduced on the solid phase.

Characteristics of the Solid Phase

All heterogeneous immunoassays using conjugate with labels, including radioisotopes, require at least one separation step to distinguish the reacted immunocomplex (bound) from unreacted antigen (free). Immobilization of antigens or antibodies for solid phase is performed by covalent binding or physical adsorption through noncovalent interactions. Gel particles made of agarose, polyacrylamide, and plastic beads, or titer plates composed of polystyrene, have been used as the solid phase, as well as particles coated with iron oxide that can be separated by a magnetic field.

The inner wall of a tube or a microtiter well is commonly used as a solid phase. With these relatively large solid phases, shaking of the reaction mixture may be needed to shorten the time required for the immune reaction to take place. The prozone phenomenon or hook effect caused by high concentrations of the analyte is likely to be observed in one-step immunoassay when limited quantities of solid-phase antibody or labeled antibody are employed. Microtiter or strip-type plates may cause an 'edge effect.' This effect can be explained by the different kinetics of the immune reaction or enzyme activity with variations in temperature. A difference in temperature may be present between the wells located at the edge of the microtiter plate and the center of the plate. A difference of about 2°C may be observed with an infrared thermometer between the edge and center of wells at ambient temperature. The size and shape of the solid phase are critical factors affecting the immunoreaction kinetics and the capturing capacity of solid-phase antibody or antigen. Spherical small magnetic or latex particles with 3000 Å diameters provide a larger total surface area for immunoabsorbency than is usually obtained with other solid phases. The larger total surface area helps shorten the immunologic reaction time (Nishizono, 1991).

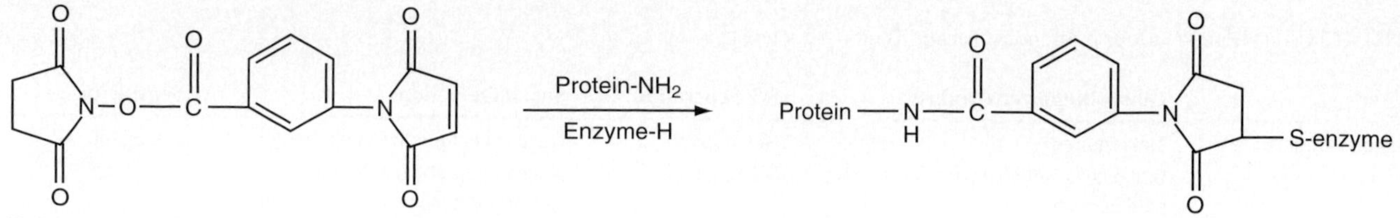

Figure 43–2 Preparation of enzyme–protein conjugate using heterobifunctional coupling reagent.

Table 43–2 Particles Used as Labels for Particle Agglutination Immunoassay

	Assay Method	Supply
Human erythrocyte	Direct hemagglutination (Landsteiner)	ABO blood type
	Erythrocyte antibody hemagglutination: titer plate/slide	Human immunodeficiency virus (HIV) antibody
Avian erythrocyte	Direct hemagglutination	Human influenza virus antibody
Fixed animal erythrocyte	Passive hemagglutination: titer plate	*T. pallidum* antibody
	Reverse passive hemagglutination: titer plate	Hepatitis B virus surface antigen
Latex	Reverse passive agglutination: slide	Chorionic gonadotropin
	Reverse passive agglutination: turbidimetry	Immunoglobulin E
	Reverse passive agglutination	Ferritin
Latex (color)	Immunochromatography	Human chorionic gonadotropin (hCG)
Microcapsule	Passive agglutination: titer plate	*Treponema pallidum* antibody
Gelatin particle	Passive agglutination: titer plate	HIV, *T. pallidum* antibody
	Reverse passive agglutination: CCD camera	Human hemoglobin (hHb)
Polypeptide particle	Passive and reverse agglutination	*T. pallidum* antibody, HBs antibody
Silicate particle	Passive agglutination: titer plate/CCD camera	*T. pallidum* antibody
Gold particle	Reverse agglutination enhancement photometry	Total estrogen
Metal sols	Reverse agglutination	hCG, hHb

Source: with permission from Kasahara Y: Principles and applications of particle immunoassay.*In* Nakamura RM, Kasahara Y, Rechnitz GA (eds): Immunochemical Assays and Biosensor Technology for the 1990s. Washington, DC, American Society for Microbiology, 1992, pp127–147.

The particles used for the particle agglutination assay are listed in Table 43–2. The phenomenon of particle agglutination (direct agglutination) caused by an immunoreaction was first observed in tests detecting antigen after incubation with infected patient serum. The agglutination of erythrocytes after incubation with serum led to the discovery of ABO blood types. Particle immunoassays are based on the agglutination principle and use the reactant of either an antibody or an antigen attached to the inert particle as a label, as opposed to direct precipitation of an antigen–antibody immunocomplex. As a label, the particle can significantly increase the immunoassay sensitivity regardless of whether the resulting agglutination is detected by the naked eye or with spectrophotometric instruments for quantification.

Erythrocytes, gelatin particles, liposomes, metal sols, and various kinds of latex particles, including latex modified with iron oxide or dyes, are all suitable solid phases. The diameter of particles used for agglutination reactions varies from 7–0.01 μm. No single theory can explain the kinetics of agglutination (Kasahara, 1992a) because of this wide variety of particle sizes used as labels. For particles larger than 3–5 μm in diameter, brownian motion of dispersed particles acting in accordance with the diffusion coefficient is not observed at room temperature. However, the theory of potential energy of interaction between particles, or the theory of colloidal coagulation reaction, can apply to small particles such as latex microparticles. The IgM antibody, being multivalent, is estimated to be 750 times more efficient than the bivalent IgG antibody in an agglutination reaction. The distance between particles in flocculation should be less than or equal to 120 Å because of the molecular length of the antibody. In summary, the important factors to consider in a solid-phase immunoreaction are the surface properties of particles, such as the charge and hydrophobicity, and the stability of dispersion.

Precipitin and Nephelometric Immunoassays

Background and Principles of Precipitin Reaction

The precipitate that forms when large complexes of antigen and antibody combine to form an insoluble lattice has been widely used to identify and quantify immunoprecipitin reactions. The modes of application of precipitin techniques have the advantages of sensitivity, specificity, and simplicity. The sensitivity limitation of these assays is a major consideration. Even under the best conditions of enhanced sensitivity afforded by the newer light-scattering techniques, the lower limit of sensitivity of immunoprecipitin assays remains in the range of 0.1–0.5 mg/dL. This lower limit of sensitivity appears to be quite sufficient for the quantification of many major serum proteins. The precipitin reaction forms the basis for many quantitative and qualitative immunochemical techniques now used in the clinical laboratory (Kabat, 1961).

Factors affecting the precipitin reaction were extensively investigated by Heidelberg in 1935, who found that the relative proportions of reactants; conditions of temperature, pH, and ionic strength of the medium; and the antibody characteristics of avidity and affinity were all equally important in the formation of the immune precipitate. On the pattern of precipitin formation it can be noted that there is a point at which precipitation is maximum or optimal, designated as the *point of equivalence*. Continued addition of antigen once the point of equivalence has been reached produces a solubilizing effect on the precipitate. The dynamic range suitable for the determination of analytes should be up to the zone of equivalence. Optimization of the antibody concentration as a reactant is necessary, in addition to optimization of buffer solutions. Typical precipitant reaction methods are as follows:

1. Qualitative Precipitant Assay Methods
   Single immunodiffusion (Williams, 1970)
   Double immunodiffusion (Garvey, 1977)
   Double immunodiffusion in two dimensions (Williams, 1970)
   Electroimmunodiffusion reaction (Ritzmann, 1975)
   Immunoelectrophoresis (Rose, 1973)
2. Semiquantitative Precipitant Assay Methods
   Single radial immunodiffusion (Fahey, 1965; Mancini, 1965)
   Single dimension electroimmunodiffusion (Axelsen, 1975) ('rocket' electrophoresis)
3. Nephelometric immunoassays
   A number of techniques for immunoprecipitin analysis have been developed that use light-scattering devices (Ritchie, 1978). The occurrence of immune complex formation has been related to the amount of such light scattering and has been used as a basis for antigen quantitation. Sophisticated instruments have been designed

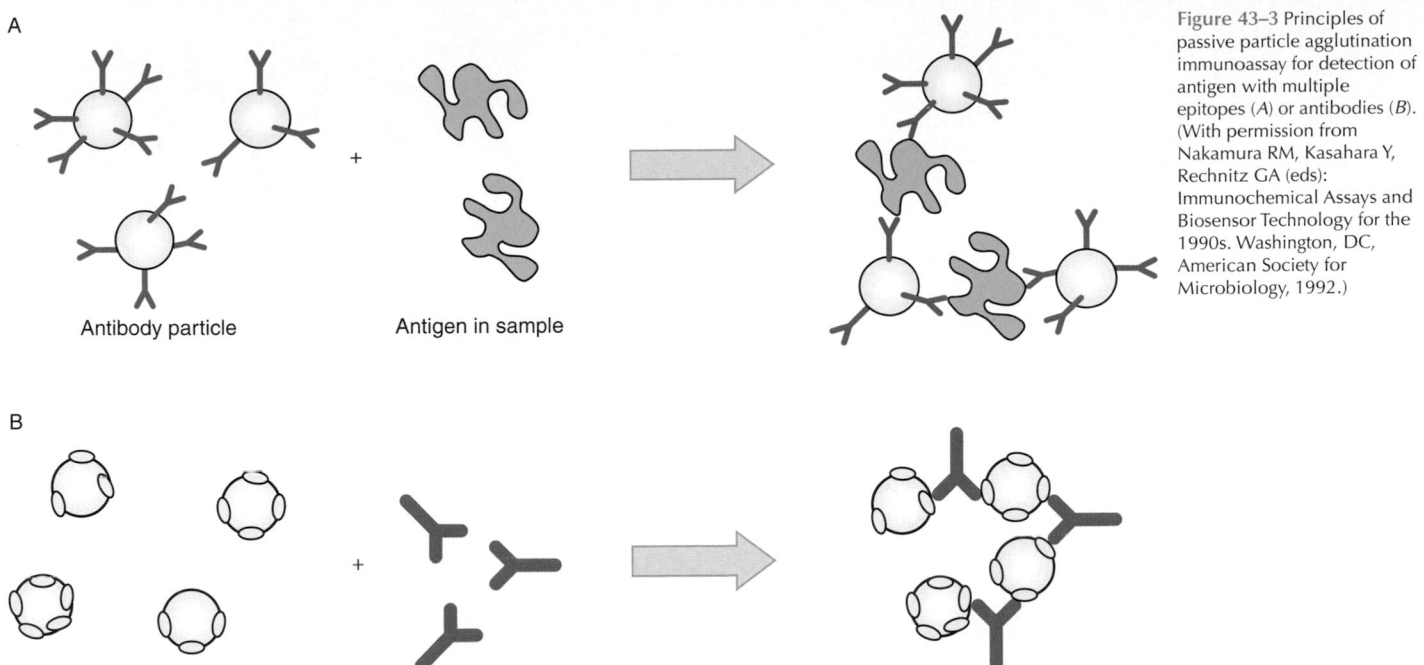

A

Antibody particle   Antigen in sample

B

Antigen or hapten   Antibody in sample
conjugate particle

Figure 43–3 Principles of passive particle agglutination immunoassay for detection of antigen with multiple epitopes (A) or antibodies (B). (With permission from Nakamura RM, Kasahara Y, Rechnitz GA (eds): Immunochemical Assays and Biosensor Technology for the 1990s. Washington, DC, American Society for Microbiology, 1992.)

to rapidly measure light scattering. Measurements of scattered light are generally referred to as *turbidimetry* or *nephelometry*.

Particle Immunoassay

Principles of Particle Agglutination

The agglutination reaction may be used to detect antibodies in specimens with specific antigens attached to a particle (passive or direct agglutination) (Fig. 43–3B). Reverse agglutination using a corresponding antibody attached to particles can be employed to detect soluble antigens in the specimen (Fig. 43–3A). A hapten unit single-binding site (for drugs, hormones, or small particles) does not form a cross-linking structure, and hence cannot become agglutinated unless it is immobilized on the solid phase. As shown in Figure 43–4A and B, when a particle or carrier immobilized with a hapten is used as a reactant, an agglutination inhibition reaction occurs that allows for the detection of the hapten. This assay is based on a competitive-type principle in which agglutination of hapten particles with a limited amount of antibody, whether free or attached to particles, is inhibited by the free hapten present in the specimen. Also, labeled particles can react with reactants fixed on the solid phase of the membrane. After immunoreaction, particles within the immunocomplex can be developed to show color on part of the membrane. This type of assay has been popular as a simple device for the qualitative detection of human chorionic gonadotropin (hCG) and other analytes.

Hemagglutination

Hemagglutination tests (Boyden, 1951) are simple to perform and do not require special equipment. For this reason, both advanced and developing countries have adopted a variety of hemagglutination tests. A popular worldwide hemagglutination test is used for the detection of antibody to *Treponema pallidum*, marketed as Serodia-TP, by Fujirebio, Inc. (Tokyo, Japan). In the United States, the hemagglutination test for *Treponema pallidum* was approved in 1981 by the Centers for Disease Control (CDC). It was also recommended by the World Health Organization (WHO) because of its superiority over other tests in terms of specificity and sensitivity (Kasahara, 1992b).

In the *Treponema pallidum* agglutination test, the reagent consists of sensitized and unsensitized sheep red cells and a serum diluent solution for the reconstitution of lyophilized sensitized cells as a positive control. Both qualitative and semiquantitative tests can be carried out using the following serum dilution protocol, using a titer plate as a reaction container as follows: Using a 25 µL pipette dropper, place four drops (100 µL) of serum diluent in well 1 (Fig. 43–5) and one drop in wells 2–4 for the qualitative assay (wells 2–8 are employed for the quantitative

assay). The resulting agglutination patterns are shown in Figure 43–6. Negative patterns, indicating that immunoreaction has not taken place, show condensed flocculation particles with a cross-packing structure at the bottom of the microtiter well. On the other hand, positive patterns, indicating that immunoreaction has occurred, show an expanded agglutination pattern of particles. Agglutinated particles cannot be sedimented any further to obtain condensation as negative patterns because their global shape is lost on account of the agglutination of particles. In the first and second rows, serum and unsensitized cells (negative control) were used, respectively. Specimens 1 and 2 show negative results. Specimens 3–8 show either negative or positive results, depending on the specimen dilution. Positive result is observed for both specimens 7 and 8 up to 1:2560 (rows 3–8).

Hemagglutination kits are now available for the detection of antibodies to hepatitis B virus (HBV), hepatitis type C (HCV), human immunodeficiency virus (HIV-l/2), thyroglobulin, thyroid microsome, and other substances. Reverse hemagglutination tests are used for the detection of HBV surface antigen, α-fetoprotein (AFP), human hemoglobin in stool specimens, and so forth. The sensitivity of hemagglutination tests is approximately 50 ng/mL for antigen (analyte) detection. Kemp (1988) developed a hemagglutination assay that uses a mouse monoclonal antibody specific to the surface antigen of human erythrocytes. The antibody can recognize an epitope common to different types of red cells or to abnormal cells, such as those found in sickle cell anemia. As shown schematically in Figure 43–7, blood cells in the specimens are used as the solid-phase particles, and the resulting agglutination can be observed by the naked eye. Bivalent antibodies are conjugated chemically so that one antibody specifically reacts with the surface epitopes of the blood cell, and the other is specific to the target antigen or analyte. The assay is applied for the detection of antibody to HIV as well as for the detection of various antigens. Unlike conventional agglutination formats, it does not require the separation of plasma or serum. This assay is simple and saves time and also has safety advantages, because it eliminates the need for serum separation for hazardous HIV- or HBV-positive specimens.

Gelatin Particle Agglutination

The development of a special gelatin particle with a highly hydrophilic surface that is able to prevent nonspecific binding of materials present in a specimen has provided an alternative to erythrocytes (Ikeda, 1984). The particle is made by phase separation and three-dimensional cross-linkage at 40°C and optimum pH. The resulting particle is fixed with formaldehyde or glutaraldehyde, and its diameter is about 3 µm. The physical properties of gelatin particles in comparison with those of erythrocytes are shown in Figure 43–8. A gelatin particle has no antigenicity and is therefore free from problems associated with heterophilic antibodies when erythrocytes are used as particles. This type of artificial particle requires much

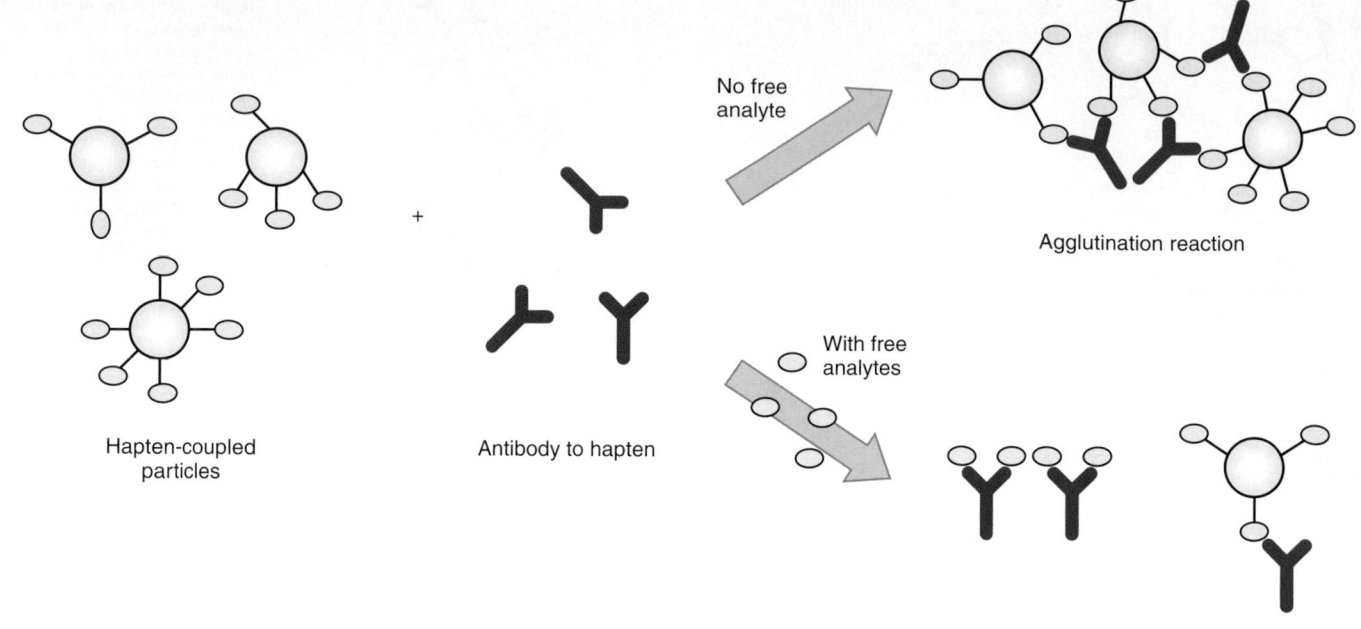

A

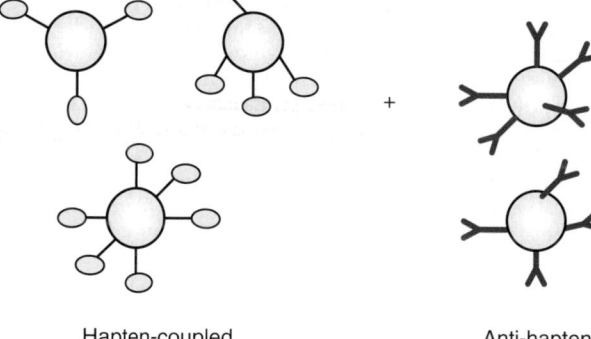

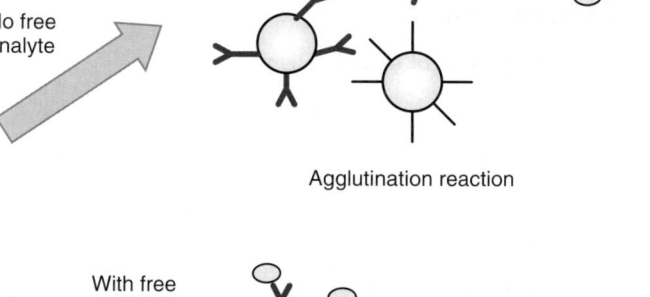

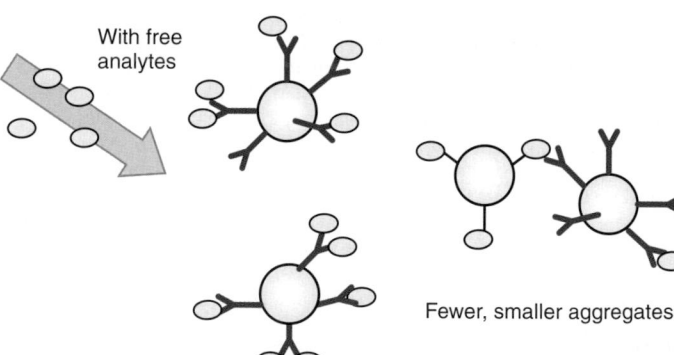

B

Figure 43–4 Principles of particle inhibition immunoassay for detection of antigen with single epitope (hapten), using antigen particle with free (*A*) or fixed (*B*) antibody. (With permission from Nakamura RM, Kasahara Y, Rechnitz GA (eds): Immunochemical Assays and Biosensor Technology for the 1990s. Washington, DC, American Society for Microbiology, 1992.)

less serum dilution to avoid nonspecific binding and guarantees more sensitive detection than with blood cells. Other synthetic particles (Hirayama, 1991) made from block copolymer composed of L-glutamic acid and derivatives have been developed by Hirayama (1991) as alternatives to gel particles. These synthetic particles can be stained with any color of dye because the particles themselves are colorless, as are gelatin particles. The gelatin particle agglutination test was initially applied to the detection of antibodies to human T-cell lymphotropic virus type I (HTLV-1), which was first discovered as a retrovirus in humans. This agglutination test (Ikeda, 1984) soon became particularly popular for blood screening for HIV, HBV, and HCV because of its high sensitivity and specificity and its simplicity, and the fact that strict temperature control is not required to perform the

tests. Gelatin particle agglutination can replace any assay based on hemagglutination, with the exception of assays using the red blood cells in specimens as particles.

Latex Agglutination

Latex agglutination (Galvin, 1984), using latex as particles, has been used for the detection of various analytes, such as hCG for qualitative pregnancy tests, and the quantitative detection of other plasma proteins with or without instrumentation. The format of this qualitative assay is simple. For example, one might only have to mix a couple of drops of latex labeled with reactant and specimen using a stick on a black slide. 2–3 minutes later, phase inversion agglutination resulting from the

TEST PROCEDURE OF SERODIA-TP^R (QUANTITATIVE ASSAY)

1. Drop absorbing diluent

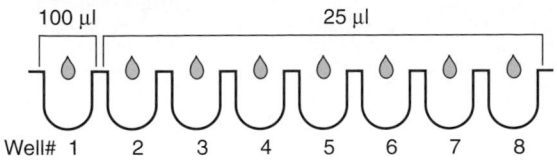

2. Add serum specimen

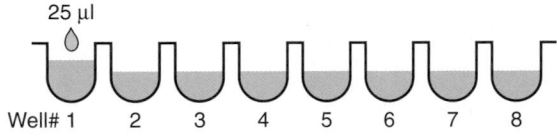

3. Make serum dilutions

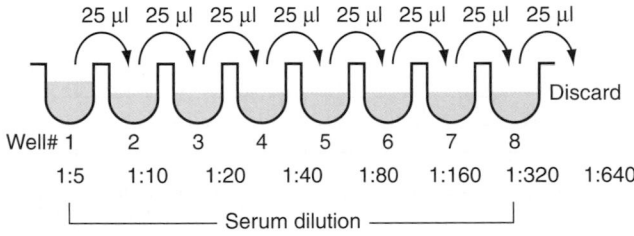

4. Drop cells

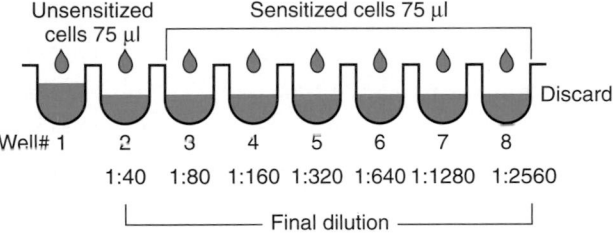

5. Mix on a tray mixer (automatic vibrator), cover plate, and incubate for two hours

6. Interpret

Figure 43–5 Hemagglutination assay for detection of *T. palladium* antigen (Serodia-TP, Fujirebio, Inc., Tokyo, Japan) based on semiquantitative test protocols. (With permission from Nakamura RM, Kasahara Y, Rechnitz GA (eds): Immunochemical Assays and Biosensor Technology for the 1990s. Washington, DC, American Society for Microbiology, 1992.)

---

immunoreaction can be observed by the naked eye. Latex agglutination was adapted for quantitative assays using light detection methods based on either turbidimetry (light absorption) or nephelometry (light scattering). With these techniques, latex agglutination achieves an enhanced sensitivity of subnanograms per milliliter, while the sensitivity of the assay measuring intact precipitation of the antigen antibody complex is less than 0.5 µg/mL.

Latex Turbidimetric Assay

Light adsorption (light loss by scattering on the surface of a particle) is proportional to the diameter of the particle and depends on the wavelength of light used. Most latex reagents commercially available use latex with a diameter of less than 1 µm and are applied in automated chemistry analyzers using photometric measuring principles. To further improve sensitivity, efforts were made to upgrade reagents and instrumentation, and to optimize the particle size, selection of appropriate wavelength, and improvement of computer software for integration of data. There are now automated systems that use latex particles and can perform about 200 tests per hour at a subnanogram-per-milliliter sensitivity.

Particle-Counting Immunoassay

The particle-counting immunoassay (Masson, 1986) uses optical cell counting to assess the decrease in the number of unagglutinated particles after an immunoreaction. In the particle-counting immunoassay format, either the rate assay, that is, the rate of decrease in the number of

---

unagglutinated particles, or the end point of the assay reaction can be measured. The end-point assay can be used to obtain a sensitivity at the nanogram-per-milliliter level; however, a longer incubation time is required for an end-point immunologic reaction.

Other Particle Immunoassays

Quasi-elastic scattering immunoassays were developed using a measurement of the change in response to particle size distribution (Yarmush, 1987). This technique uses a laser light beam to measure the reduction in the mean diffusion coefficient of particles as a result of immunoreaction. Other methods measure the change in angular anisotropy of scattered light with the increasing average size of the particle. Particles with diameters about equal to the size of a wavelength achieve a size-dependent angular variation of scattered light.

Summary

Indirect hemagglutination and gelatin particle agglutination tests using microtiter plates have been popular procedures for qualitative and semiquantitative determination of various analytes. These tests do not require additional instrumentation or strict temperature control. Most importantly, these tests guarantee a sensitivity equal to or higher than conventional enzyme immunoassays when applied to antibody detection of infectious agents. Latex as a solid phase provides great kinetic advantages, such as a shorter immunoreaction time. For this reason, it was possible to adapt latex for use in existing or sophisticated instruments by applying different principles, resulting in an assay sensitivity of about three orders of magnitude greater than standard immunoprecipitation assays. Latex is susceptible to interference from unknown factors present in specimens. To eliminate this problem, various absorbents have to be used in both the reagent and the incubation medium. The great advantage of particle immunoassay is its simplicity, because it does not require separation of bound and free reactants.

Radioimmunoassay

Background

Since RIA technology, using radioisotopes as labels, was first developed by Yalow and Berson (1959), it has been improved dramatically in sensitivity and precision. Numerous variations in the method have been introduced into the clinical laboratory. There are two main RIA techniques, competitive and noncompetitive heterogeneous formats, which require washing steps to separate bound and free labels (conjugates). The competitive assay follows the law of mass action, which specifies the reaction between analytes and binding proteins, receptors, and antibody. The key factor in assay optimization is the binding affinity of the antibody. The Scatchard plot of the ratio of bound to free antibody to analyte concentration is commonly used to evaluate antibody performance. Figure 43–9 shows the Scatchard plot for cyclosporine determination. As described in Kinetics of Antigen–Antibody Reaction, from the following equation:

$$B/F = K_a([Ab]_t - B),$$

the y-axis is the B/F ratio, which is proportional to free [Ab] from $[Ab]_t - B$, equal to free [Ag]. Therefore, K_a represents the slope of the plot. In this figure, the affinity constant K_a is 8.1×10^9 L/M for the antibody specific to cyclosporine. Radioactive emissions, such as gamma rays of iodine-125 labels, can be measured in terms of counts per minute (CPM) using a gamma scintillation counter. Typical radioisotopes used as labels and their properties are shown in Table 43–3. The choice of label affects the assay protocol considerably. For example, the most popular label, iodine-125, requires a rather short time for signal counting but has a limited shelf-life because of its short half-life. However, tritium (^{3}H) label requires a longer time for counting, thereby increasing the total assay time. Most RIAs now use iodine-125 as labels to expedite the conjugation process and to retain the biological activity of the reactants. A commonly used method for conjugation of iodine-125 with proteins is the chloramine-T method (Hunter, 1962). Tyrosine, in particular, has more reactivity with iodate because of its hydroxy group at the para-position on the aromatic ring. The signal can be measured in terms of CPM as gamma ray emissions. Unlike enzymes, isotopes as labels with a small Stokes radius are not likely to disrupt antigenic activity because of the lack of steric hindrance when isotopes are conjugated with small antigens (haptens).

Assay Principles and Methods

Various methods (antigen excess) based on the competitive binding reaction (Ekins, 1960) to antibodies between labeled antigens and

Agglutination patterns of Serodia-TP*

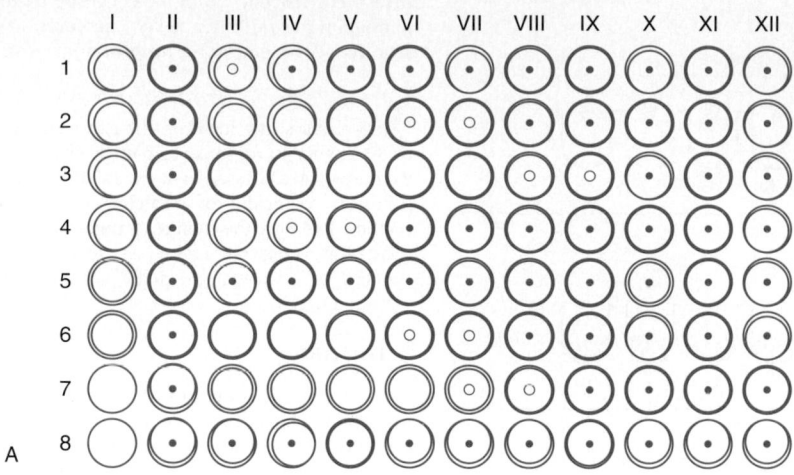

A

Row no.	I	II	III	IV	V	VI	VII	VIII	IX	X	XI	XII	
Type of cells added	Unsensitized cells		Sensitized cells										Result
Final dilution of serum specimen		1:40	1:80	1:160	1:320	1:640	1:1280	1:2560	1:5120	1:10240	1:20480	Medium control	Titer
Serum specimen													
No. 1	–	–		–		–		–	–	–	–	–	Inconclusive
No. 2	–	–	++	++	+	+	–	–	–	–	–	–	1:640
No. 3	–	–	++	++	++	++	++	+	–	–	–	–	1:2560
No. 4	–	–	+	+	–	–	–	–	–	–	–	–	1:160
No. 5	–	–	–	–	–	–	–	–	–	–	–	–	Negative
No. 6	–	–	++	++	++	+	–	–	–	–	–	–	1:640
No. 7	–	–	++	++	++	++	+	–	–	–	–	–	1:1280
No. 8	–	–	–	–	–	–	–	–	–	–	–	–	Negative

* Trade mark for agglutination test for *T. pallidum* antibody, Fujirebio, Inc., Tokyo, Japan

B

Figure 43–6 Hemagglutination patterns for detection of ant*i-T. pallidum* antibody (A) and interpretation as positive or negative at final serum dilution. (With permission from Nakamura RM, Kasahara Y, Rechnitz GA (eds): Immunochemical Assays and Biosensor Technology for the 1990s. Washington, DC, American Society for Microbiology, 1992.)

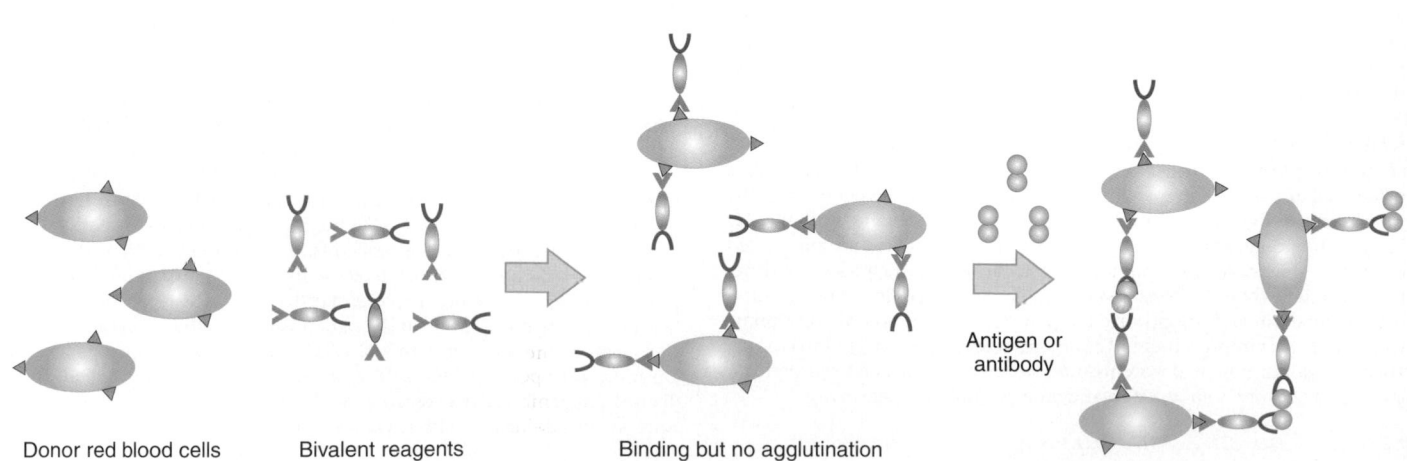

Donor red blood cells   Bivalent reagents   Binding but no agglutination

Antigen or antibody

Agglutination

Figure 43–7 Schematic presentation of an assay based on autologous erythrocyte agglutination, using erythrocytes in the specimen as particles. (With permission from Nakamura RM, Kasahara Y, Rechnitz GA (eds): Immunochemical Assays and Biosensor Technology for the 1990s. Washington, DC, American Society for Microbiology, 1992.)

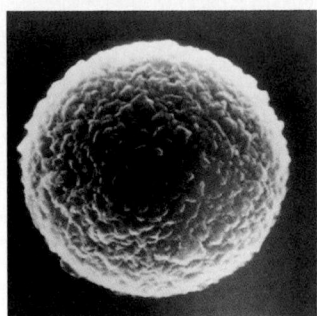

Physical properties	Carrier	
	Gelatin particles	Sheep erythrocytes
Diameter, μm	2 to 6	6
Specific gravity	1.05 to 1.10	1.10
Electrophoretic mobility; μm/s/V/cm	−0.75 to −1.85	−1.15

Figure 43–8 Electron micrograph (×25 000) and physical properties of gelatin particles in comparison with sheep erythrocytes. (With permission from Nakamura RM, Kasahara Y, Rechnitz GA (eds): Immunochemical Assays and Biosensor Technology for the 1990s. Washington, DC, American Society for Microbiology, 1992. pp 139)

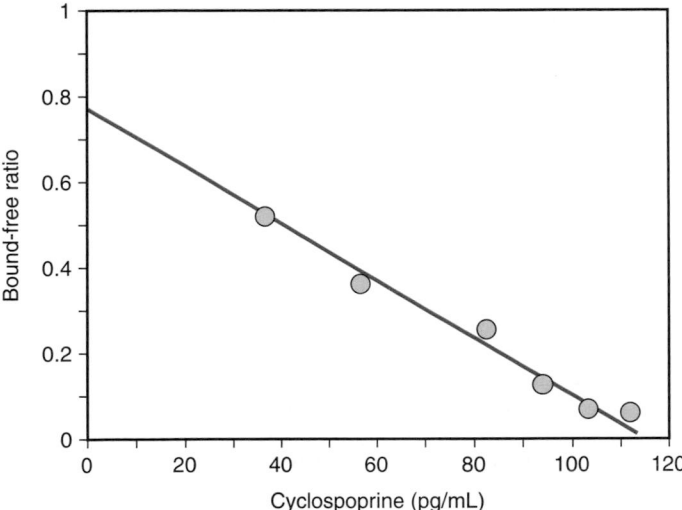

Figure 43–9 Scatchard plot of cyclosporine antibody binding characteristics ($K_a = 8.1 \times 10^9$ L/M)

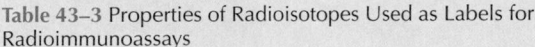

Table 43–3 Properties of Radioisotopes Used as Labels for Radioimmunoassays

Isotope	Half-Life	Type of Decay	Specific Activity (mCi/mmol)
Iodine-125	60 days	γ	2200
Iodine-131	8.1 days	β⁻, γ	16100
Hydrogen-3	12.3 years	β⁻	29
Carbon-14	5760 years	β⁻	6062
Phosphorus-32	14.3 days	β⁻	9120

nonlabeled antigens (analytes present in the specimen) have been developed for a wide variety of analytes. A conventional competitive method is shown in Figure 43–10. At first, a known amount of labeled antigen and antigen in the specimen are mixed and reacted competitively with a constant amount of antibody coated on a solid phase, such as sepharose beads or the inner wall of plastic tubes. After the immune reaction reaches its equilibrium, the mixture is washed for removing unreacted conjugates and antigens and the immune complex trapped on the solid phase is separated. The washing step is referred to as B/F (bound over free) separation. Applying the competitive principle, the plot of antigen-bound percentage against logarithmic concentration of analyte provides the standard curve shown in Figure 43–10. The CPM plot on the standard curve gives the concentration of analytes.

A second antibody method is shown in Figure 43–11. The first antibody specific to a particular antigen (analyte) reacts competitively with both the conjugate and the antigen. Then, the immune complex is captured by the second antibody specific to the first antibody, on the solid phase. When the second antibody is coated on a fine solid phase, the immune complex on the second reaction can be separated as a precipitant from the unreacted molecules. For antibody determination, labeled antibody and antibody in the specimen react competitively with the antigen (analyte) fixed on the solid phase. The steeper slope of the standard curve provides more precise data. Competitive methods require less amounts of antibody or antigen (analyte) than that for sandwich-type assays described below. Noncompetitive assays, originally demonstrated by Miles (1968), have recently become popular.

The immunoradiometric assays or sandwich assays (Fig. 43–12), have an alternative relationship between analyte and antibody. The classic competitive assay achieves an immunologic response with minimum amount of antibody, and the sandwich assay uses a large amount of antibody on the solid phase. Monoclonal antibody technology has made it possible to manufacture large amounts of specific antibodies at moderate costs, thereby allowing the sandwich assay to be exploited. The sandwich assay uses a stoichiometrically excess antibody and is more sensitive than the competitive assay. When background noise is completely omitted, the ultimate theoretical sensitivity of the sandwich

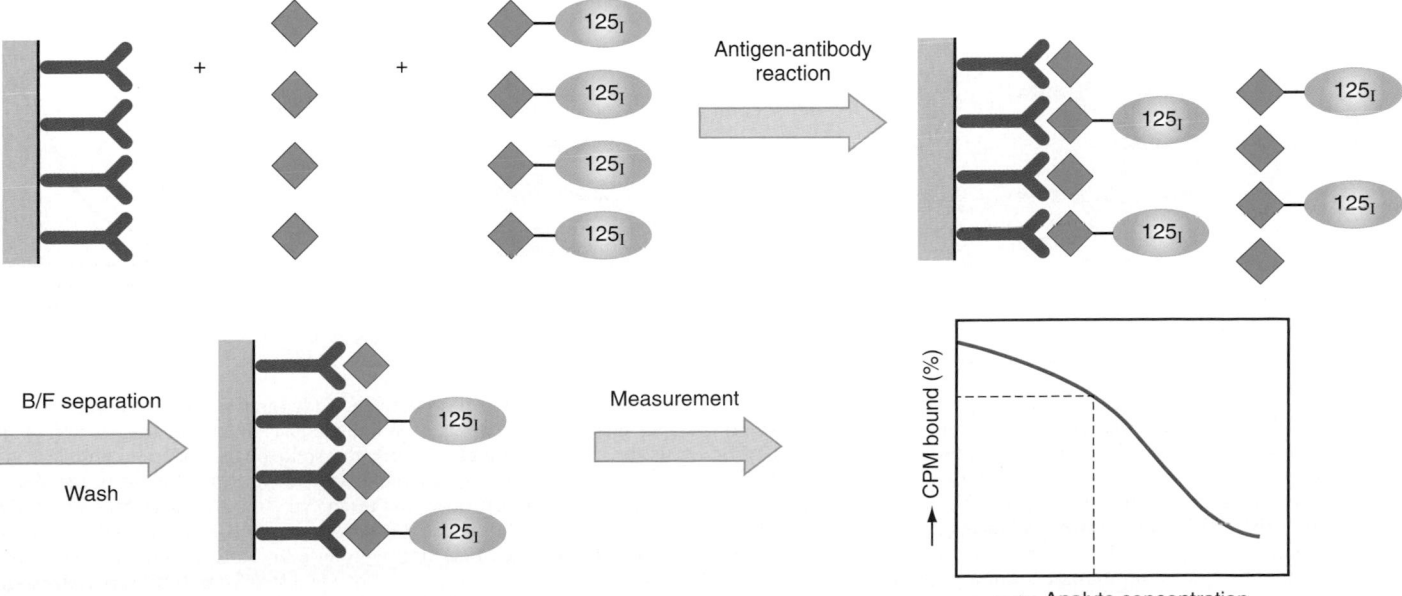

Figure 43–10 Assay principle of competitive RIA using first antibody as solid phase.

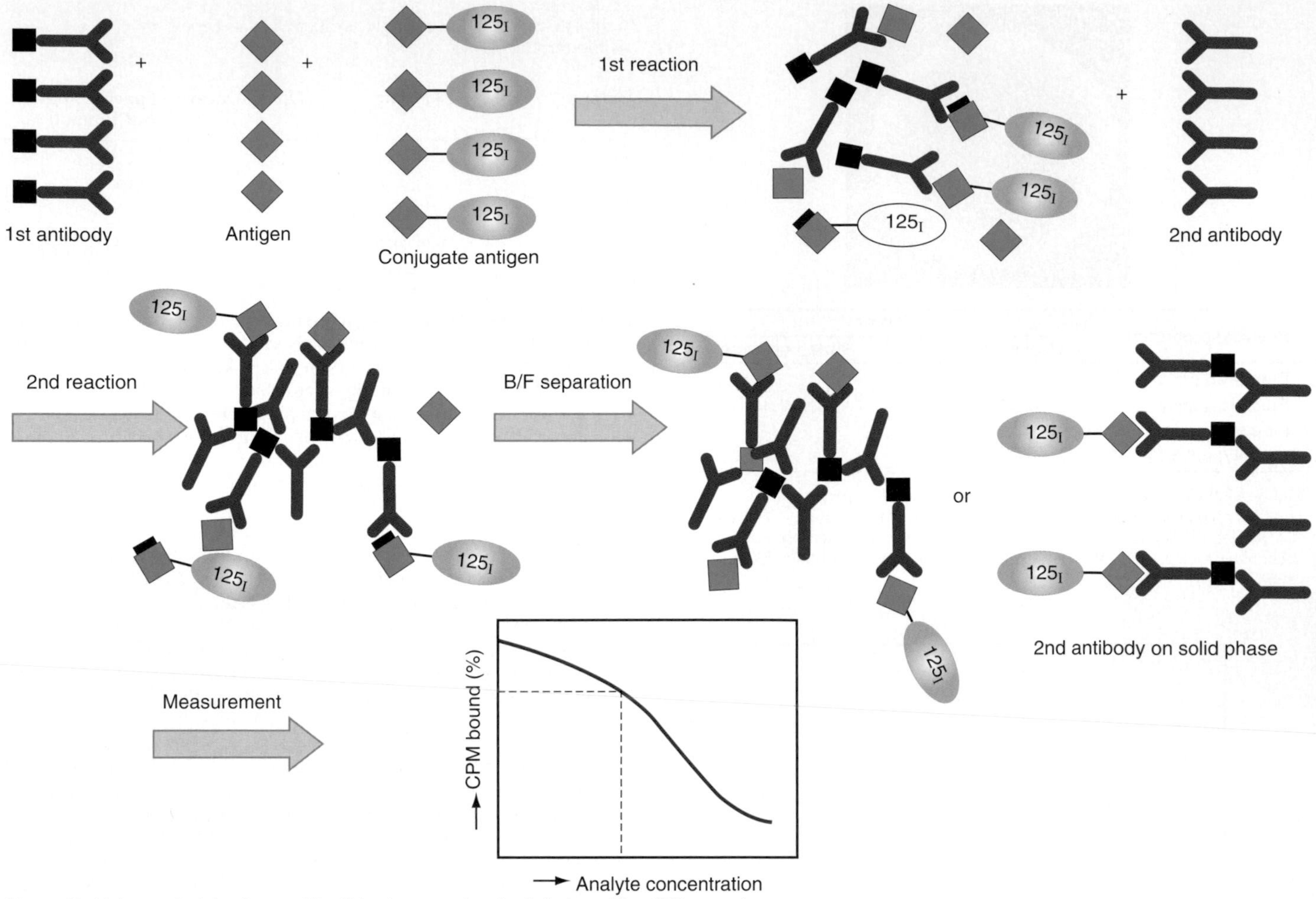

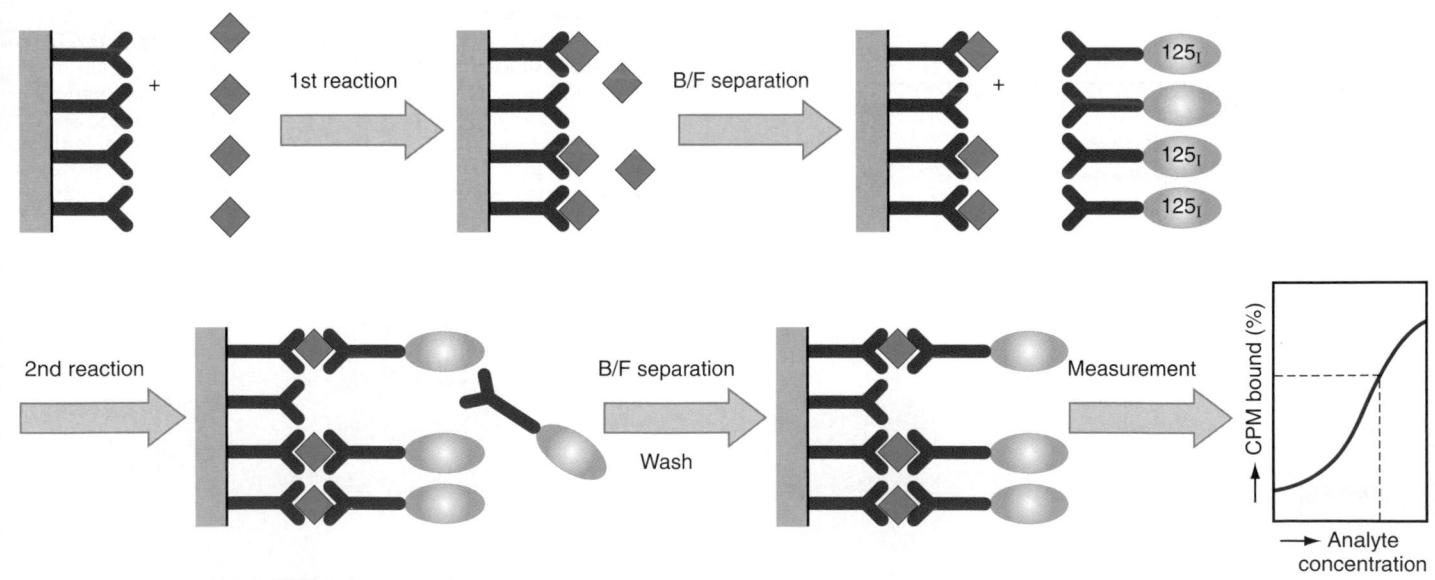

Figure 43–11 Assay principle of competitive RIA using second antibody for bound/free (B/F) separation.

Figure 43–12 Assay principle of sandwich RIA method using solid phase, also referred to as immunoradiometric assay. B/F = bound/free.

assay is one molecule of analyte, which is possible when the amount of antibody used in the assay system approaches infinity. As shown in Figure 43–12, the antibody on the solid phase first captures the antigen (analyte) in the specimen. Following B/F separation, the conjugate reacts with the antigen (analyte) fixed on the solid phase, and the signal can then be counted after the elimination of free conjugates through a washing step. This assay requires antigens with more than two antigenic sites. When two different antibodies (i.e., a solid-phase antibody specific to one antigenic site and a conjugate antibody specific to another antigenic site) are used, the assay protocol can be simplified by performing with a one-step

sandwich. Thus, the solid-phase antibody can mix with the antigen in the specimen and the conjugate simultaneously. Interference does not occur because the antibodies on both the solid phase and the conjugate are capable of recognizing different antigenic sites. In this assay the signal generated is proportional to the analyte concentration present in the specimen, as in the two-step sandwich assay. This assay method can be applied to antibody detection with an assay format using antigen as the solid phase and labeled antigen. For a two-step format, antigen as the solid phase and labeled antibody specific to the target antibody can be used. Using the sandwich format, assay sensitivity (Rodriguez-Espinosa, 1987) is

Table 43–4 Comparison of Radioimmunoassay, Heterogeneous Enzyme Immunoassay, and Homogeneous Enzyme Immunoassay

Assay	Immunological Reaction Steps	Enzyme Reaction Steps	Signal Detection Steps
Radioimmunoassay			
Sample + (Labeled analyte or Ab)-^{125}I	Immunoreaction with washing steps for separation	Not required	Radioactive decay (γ ray)
Heterogeneous Enzyme Immunoassay			
Sample + (Labeled analyte or Ab)- Enzyme	Immunoreaction with washing steps for separation	Enzyme reaction with additional reagent	Optical density: Fluorescence Luminescence
Homogeneous Enzyme Immunoassay			
Sample + (Labeled analyte or Ab)-Enzyme or cofactors	Immuno- and/or systemic reaction is carried out in one solution, which includes reagent for signal development of enzyme	Immuno- and/or systemic reaction is carried out in one solution, which includes reagent for signal development of enzyme	Optical density: Fluorescence Luminescence

high. An example is using immunoradiometric assay for the determination of the peptide hormone thyroid-stimulating hormone (TSH); the level of assay sensitivity is below 0.07 µU/mL of TSH, as compared with about 0.7 µU/mL with conventional competitive antigen-labeled assay.

Summary

Compared with other immunoassays, RIAs are advantageous for a number of reasons: (1) precision and high sensitivity, (2) ease of isotope conjugation, (3) signal detection without optimization, and (4) stability against interference from the assay environment, among others. Disadvantages of RIAs are the short shelf-life of the reagents and the need to protect against hazardous radioactivity. Furthermore, as discussed later, RIAs may not be applied to homogeneous immunoassays because signals from isotopes cannot modulate antigen–antibody reactions.

Enzyme Immunoassay

Background and Classification

Quantitative immunoassays using enzymes as labels were developed as an alternative to radioisotopes (Avrameas, 1971; Engvall, 1971; Van Weeman, 1971). The most widely used are the enzyme-linked immunoabsorbent assay (ELISA), the EIA, and the enzyme-multiplied immunoassay technique (EMIT), which is a registered trade name of SYVA Co. (Dade Behring Inc., Cupertino, CA) (Rubenstein, 1972). Essentially, heterogeneous EIAs are quite similar to RIAs, except that they use enzymes as labels. Enzymes make it possible to develop homogeneous EIAs, eliminating the otherwise necessary washing steps for B/F separation. Table 43–4 compares the features of heterogeneous and homogeneous EIAs with RIAs. Improvements in EIAs have provided many innovative formats with different degrees of speed, sensitivity, simplicity, and precision. The advantages and disadvantages of EIAs are listed in Table 43–5 (Nakamura, 1992a).

Heterogeneous Enzyme Immunoassays

The assay principle of heterogeneous EIAs is similar to that of RIAs, except that enzyme activity, not radioactivity, is measured. EIAs require a secondary process to obtain signals through the catalytic reaction of enzymes. As the solid phase for the separation of bound and free conjugates, microtiter plate wells, plastic beads, plastic tubes, magnetic particles, and latex with filters, among others, can be used. The use of small magnetic particles and latex allows shortening of the immunoreaction time, thereby reducing the total assay time. The development of substrates to be cleaved by enzymes was marked by the introduction of colorimetric and fluorometric substrates, and later chemiluminescent substrates, which increased the signal sensitivity. The enzymes commonly used in various heterogeneous EIAs are horseradish peroxidase, alkaline phosphatase, β-galactosidase, glucose oxidase, urease, and catalase. The most widely used enzymes as well as their characteristics are listed in Table 43–6. Assay sensitivity using enzymes may be determined by the turnover rate of each enzyme and selection of signal measurement in which chemiluminometry is the most sensitive method.

The assay format of heterogeneous EIAs, like RIAs, can be divided into competitive and noncompetitive assays (see Fig. 43–13). Competitive assays

Table 43–5 Advantages and Disadvantages of Enzyme Immunoassay

A. Advantages

1. Sensitive assays can be developed by the amplification effect of enzymes.
2. Reagents are relatively cheap and can have a long shelf-life.
3. Multiple simultaneous assays can be developed.
4. A wide variety of assay configurations can be developed.
5. Equipment can be inexpensive and is widely available.
6. No radiation hazards occur during labeling or disposal of wastes.

B. Disadvantages

1. Measurement of enzyme activity can be more complex than measurement of the activity of some types of radioisotopes.
2. Enzyme activity may be affected by plasma constituents.
3. Homogeneous assays at the present time have the sensitivity of 10^{-9} M and are not as sensitive as radioimmunoassays.
4. Homogeneous EIAs for large protein molecules have been developed but require complex immunochemical reagents.

EIA, enzyme immunoassay.

Source: with permission from Nakamura RM, Kasahara Y: Heterogeneous enzyme immunoassays. *In* Nakamura RM, Kasahara Y, Rechnitz GA (eds): Immunochemical Assays and Biosensor Technology for the 1990s. Washington, DC, American Society for Microbiology, 1992, pp 149–167.

Table 43–6 Characteristics of Typical Enzymes Used as Labels for Enzyme Immunoassay

Characteristics	Peroxidase (EC1.11.1.7)	Enzyme β-Galactosidase (EC3.2. 1.23)	Alkaline Phosphatase (EC3.1.3.1)
Source	Horseradish	*E. coli*	Bovine intestine
Molecular weight (daltons)	40 000	530 000	100 000
Specfic activity	250 U/mg	600 U/mg	25 000 U/mg
Turnover rate*	10 000	318 000	250 000
Measurement of enzyme	Colorimetry, fluorometry, luminometry	Colorimetry, fluorometry, luminometry	Colorimetry, fluorometry, luminometry
Highly sensitive measurement	Luminometry	Fluorometry	Luminometry
Method for enzyme labeling	Periodate oxidation (Nakane method)	Dimaleimide method, crosslinking reagent†	Glutaraldehyde method, crosslinking reagent

* Number of substrate molecules produced by a molecule of enzyme for one-minute reaction; molecule number/min.

† The reagent contains chemically reactive groups such as maleimide and succinimide.

COMPETITIVE ASSAY

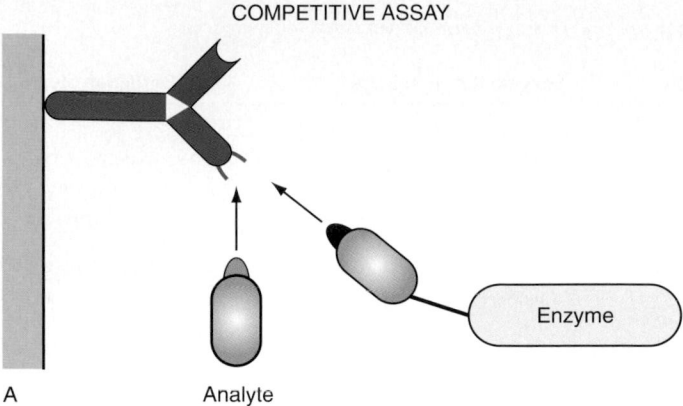

A   Analyte

NONCOMPETITIVE SANDWICH ASSAY

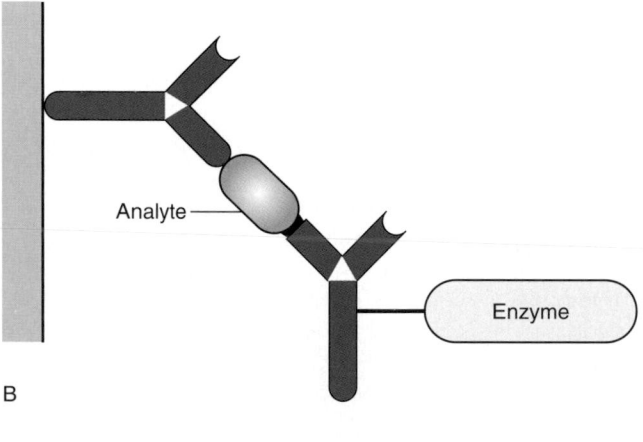

B

ANTIGEN ASSAY

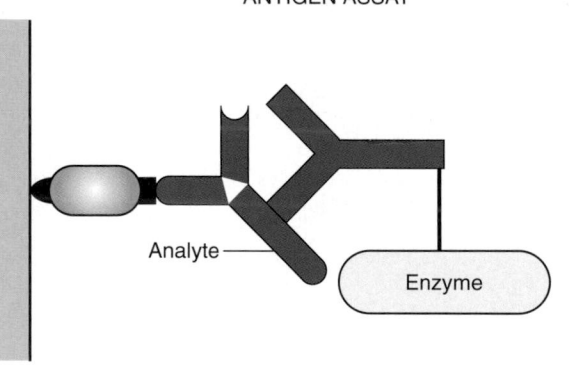

C

ANTIBODY ASSAY

Figure 43–13 Assay principles of heterogeneous enzyme immunoassay (EIA) using solid phase; (*A*) competitive assay and (*B and C*) non-competitive sandwich assay.

(analyte excess) use antigen-enzyme conjugates (Fig. 43–13*A*), while noncompetitive assays (reactant excess) include two-site immunometric sandwich assays and indirect assays to measure antibodies (Figs. 43–13*B* and *C*). Immunometric sandwich assays have now gained much popularity for the determination of antigen such as hormones, tumor markers, plasma proteins, and infectious agents. Indirect assays for antibody measurement (Fig. 43–13*C*) have been adopted for the detection of antibodies to infectious agents (e.g., HIV, HBV, HCV) and to autoantibodies.

Heterogeneous EIA (Fig. 43–13) consists of the following steps:

1. The solid-phase attached reactants are mixed with analyte, regardless of whether the assay is based on the competitive or the noncompetitive format.
2. Following the addition of conjugate and incubation, there are wash steps with a buffer solution containing a detergent, one or two steps

after the immunoreaction. The immunoreaction should reach certain yields to obtain a stable and precise assay.

3. The solid phase, with the immunocomplex containing either enzyme-labeled antigen or antibody, is incubated at constant temperature with the enzyme-substrate solution.
4. The enzyme reaction is stopped (not needed in rate assay), and the substrate reaction product is measured with various detectors depending on the substrate used.

Colorimetric Enzyme Immunoassay

In this assay, enzyme reaction is performed by using chromogenic substrates to develop a color by prime catalytic reaction. For example, horseradish peroxidase, catalyzing ABTS (diammonium salt of 2,2′-azino-di[3-ethyl-benzothiazoline-6-sulfonate])] with H_2O_2 to form a green color, and alkaline phosphatase, specific to the *p*-nitrophenyl phosphate, to form yellow color. Both enzymes are the most commonly used types of colorimetric enzyme immunoassay. A spectrophotometer is used to measure the optical density of the resulting chromogen. There are many instruments available allowing the measurement of optical density in tubes or microtiter plates, ranging from a fully automated system that performs sample pipetting and data printout to more simple manual devices. When the EIA reaction is performed on nitrocellulose membrane (Western blotting method) or other membranes, substrates that generate insoluble dyes are utilized. An hCG pregnancy test with an immunoassay format that is sold as an over-the-counter (OTC) test commonly uses either benzidine derivatives to react with peroxidase or indoxyl phosphate derivatives to react with alkaline phosphatase to generate insoluble dyes. The dye accumulating on the solid phase through enzyme reaction can be read by the naked eye. Theoretically, the measurement of optical density is limited to a range between 0 and 2.0. Therefore, the determination of optical density for analytes that require the determination of a wide dynamic range can be problematic, even when an excess amount of conjugate and solid phase with sufficient capturing capacity are used in a sandwich-type assay.

Efforts to improve EIAs, the milestone of nonisotopic immunoassays, have brought to light several disadvantages of RIAs, such as hazardous isotopic waste, radiolysis of labeled analytes, and the short half-life of iodine-125. Ishikawa (1989) developed an ultrasensitive EIA that is able to detect 3 fmol of specific IgG antibody. But to achieve this level of sensitivity, several tedious steps are required, such as immunocomplex transfer from a first solid phase to another solid phase to reduce background signals.

Fluorescent Enzyme Immunoassay

Fluorescent EIAs are identical to other EIAs except that they use fluorescent substrates. In the fluorescent EIA, a fluorophore is generated by an enzyme reaction. Following excitation of the fluorophore at its optimal light excitation wavelength, light at a characteristic wavelength is emitted. Instruments such as a fluorometer require both a supplier of the excitation light source and a photomultiplier tube as a detector of the emission fluorescence. There may be substances that emit fluorescent light present in the specimen. These substances may increase the background signal, which may interfere with the assay's sensitivity. Thus, close attention should be paid to the selection of substrates for EIAs to avoid these interfering factors. Compared with colorimetric EIAs, fluorescent assays generate a signal intensity that is at least one order of magnitude greater.

Chemiluminescent Enzyme Immunoassay

Chemiluminescent enzyme immunoassays (CL-EIA) use chemiluminescent substrates that react with various enzymes employed as labels. The chemiluminescent enzymatic reaction generates light, similar to bioluminescence, and involves the use of natural substrates such as luciferin-adenosine triphosphate (ATP). Over the past 20 years, much attention has been paid to the application of chemiluminescence in immunoassays, and a variety of systems consisting of substrates and enzymes have been developed. Current systems using either luminol derivatives to peroxidase with an enhancer or dioxetane derivatives to alkaline phosphatase achieve highly sensitive immunoassays. These assays are effective tools in practical diagnosis. The enzymatic oxidation reaction of luminol analogs has long been used for CL-EIA. Using peroxidase with H_2O_2 is a common method that is interchangeable with an alternative coupling enzyme producing H_2O_2, such as glucose oxidase or uricase. The discovery of enhancers by Thorpe (1985) for luminol-based chemiluminescence remarkably improved the assay's sensitivity. Enhancers include phenol derivatives and aromatic compounds. For example, luminol-peroxidase with *p*-iodophenol as an enhancer achieves a light emission increase of up to 2800-fold in the optimized reaction mixture. This assay is able to detect TSH at 0.04 µU/mL using serum as the specimen. However, oxidative reactions, such as those

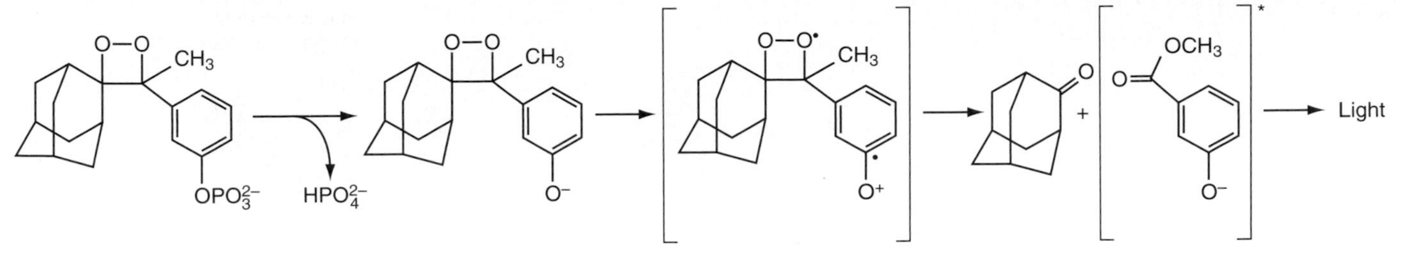

Figure 43–14 Adamantyl 1,2-dioxetane phenyl phosphate (AMPPD); a chemiluminescent substrate for alkaline phosphatase (ALP) detection. Hydrolytic phosphate cleavage by ALP triggers chemically initiated electron exchange luminescence (CIEEL) decomposition of AMPPD by releasing the electron-rich dioxetane phenolate (AMP-D). Charge transfer from the phenolate to the dioxetane ring takes place forming the charge transfer (CT) intermediate and subsequent breakdown of the cyclic peroxide. There is release of energy with light emission.

for luminol, are likely to be interfered with by multiple factors that cause increased nonspecific background signals (noise).

Bronstein (1989a) developed a chemiluminescent substrate for alkaline phosphatase that differs considerably from other compounds. This new substrate is known as AMPPD (disodium 3-(4-methylspiro-[1,2-dioxetane-3,2'-tricyclo-[3.3.1.1]decan]-4-yl) phenyl phosphate), an adamantyl dioxetane derivative. It requires no additional molecules for the emission of chemiluminescent light, unlike luminol, which needs oxidative compounds from outside the luminol molecules. AMPPD is a novel molecule that is a complete substrate because it is composed of the adamantyl group as a stabilizer of the entire molecule, the dioxetane bond as an energy source and phosphoryl ester as a cleavage site of the enzyme, and a phenyl group for chemiluminescence, all assembled within one molecule. The structure of the molecule and the reaction process for light generation are shown in Figure 43–14. Cleavage of phosphoester bond of AMPPD by alkaline phosphatase triggers chemically initiated electron exchange luminescence (CIEEL) by releasing electron-rich dioxetane. A chemiluminescent with a maximum wavelength of 477 nm can be detected within a couple of minutes to a few hours, depending on substrate concentration. The alkaline phosphatase with AMPPD assay system has a sensitivity of less than 10–21 mol (Bronstein, 1989b, 1991; Kricka, 1991).

CL-EIA uses AMPPD as a substrate to react with alkaline phosphatase, which is used as the enzyme label. CL-EIA can be performed on a fully automated instrument. This novel substrate made it possible to develop an extremely sensitive chemiluminescent enzyme immunoassay system. Ferrite particles 0.3 µm in diameter employed as the solid phase shorten the immunoreaction time to within 30 minutes and to provide a larger surface area for the immunoabsorbent. The relationship between the chemiluminescent signal and the concentration of analytes is linear up to about seven orders of dynamic range. The sensitivity of CL-EIA (Nishizono, 1991) was 10-fold greater than conventional RIAs when AFP was assayed; AFP was detected at a level of 30 pg/mL with an assay time of 30 minutes. Thus, the new chemiluminescent EIA systems are a definite improvement over RIAs in terms of sensitivity, time efficiency, and procedural simplicity and are gaining increasing popularity in the market.

Homogeneous Enzyme Immunoassays

Background

Two options are available to eliminate tedious assay procedures. One is to design fully automated instruments to access heterogeneous types of reagents, and the other is to develop innovative reagents that do not require the complicated washing steps, such as those needed for heterogeneous EIAs. Enzymes and their cofactors are advantageous labels in homogeneous EIAs because enzyme activity can be modulated easily by changing factors in the microenvironment of the Ag–Ab reaction. This is not the case when using radioisotope decay as the signal. At present, homogeneous EIAs are generally less sensitive than their heterogeneous counterparts. Conventional heterogeneous EIAs have sensitivity equal to that of RIAs in many applications, whereas homogeneous EIAs (Nakamura, 1988) remain one or two orders of magnitude less sensitive than RIAs. Homogeneous EIAs may require complex immunochemical reagents but the assay systems are rapid and simple, and are adaptable to conventional instruments. There are various types of homogeneous EIA. In each of these assays the antigen–antibody interaction modulates the activity of the enzyme or enzyme label in the presence of the substrate. Modulation of the enzyme activity reflects the degree of the immunochemical reaction. Table 43–7 lists the characteristics of typical homogeneous EIAs. Homogeneous EIAs can be classified as competitive or noncompetitive binding assays. Competitive assays usually

Table 43–7 Classification and Characteristics of Typical Homogeneous Enzyme Immunoassays

Name and Assay Type	Conjugate	Manner of Modulation
Competitive		
EMIT	Antigen with lysozyme,G6PD	Steric hindrance
SLFIA	Antigen with substrate	Steric hindrance
ARIS	Antigen with prosthetic group	Steric hindrance
Enzyme-channeling immunoassay	Antigen with G6PDH and hexokinase	Enhancement by proximity
Biotin-enzyme avidin immunoassay	Antigen with avidin	Steric hindrance
CEDIA	Antigen with fragments of	Steric hindrance
Noncompetitive		
Hybrid antibody immunoassay	Hybrid antibodies specific to antigen and to inhibitor	Steric hindrance
Proximal linkage immunoassay	Antibody with G6PDH and hexokinase	Substrate cascade by proximity
EIHIA	Antibody with amylase	Steric hindrance
Enzyme enhancement immunoassay	Antibody with β-galactosidase and succinyl antibody	Charge effect
AEST	Antibody with peroxidase	Stabilization

G6PD = glucose-6-phosphate dehydrogenase

Bold indicates that the enzyme name is spelled out and the enzyme is discussed in detail in the text.

Source: with permission from Kasahara Y: Homogeneous enzyme immunoassays. *In* Nakamura RM, Kasahara Y, Rechnitz GA (eds): Immunochemical Assays and Biosensor Technology for the 1990s. Washington, DC, American Society for Microbiology, 1992, pp 169–182.

consist of enzyme-labeled antigens. However, the antigen (analyte) may be conjugated to the substrate or a prosthetic group of the enzyme in other assay formats. In contrast, noncompetitive binding assays use a conjugate of antibody labeled with enzyme. Among the various methods reported, five homogeneous EIAs deserve our attention.

Enzyme-Multiplied Immunoassay Technique

EMIT, the first homogeneous EIA, was developed by Rubenstein (1972). The EMIT system is illustrated in Figure 43–15. In EMIT, the conjugation of enzymes to haptens does not disrupt enzyme activity; however, the binding of hapten-specific antibodies to haptens results in the inhibition of enzyme activity. Free haptens in the standard or sample relieve this inhibition by competing for antibodies. Thus, enzyme activity is proportional to the concentration of free haptens. As a general rule, the antibody inhibits the enzyme by inducing or preventing conformational changes necessary for enzyme activity (Rowley, 1975). The exception to the inhibition mechanism is the EMIT thyroxine assay, which uses malate dehydrogenase. In this assay, the thyroxine–malate-dehydrogenase conjugate is enzymatically inactive but it becomes activated when it is bound by thyroxine antibody (Ullman, 1979). It is believed that conjugated thyroxine inhibits the enzyme by binding to the active site, thus increasing the 'apparent' K_m of the substrate. The antibody reactivates the enzyme by 'pulling' the thyroxine out of the active site. In the EMIT assay system,

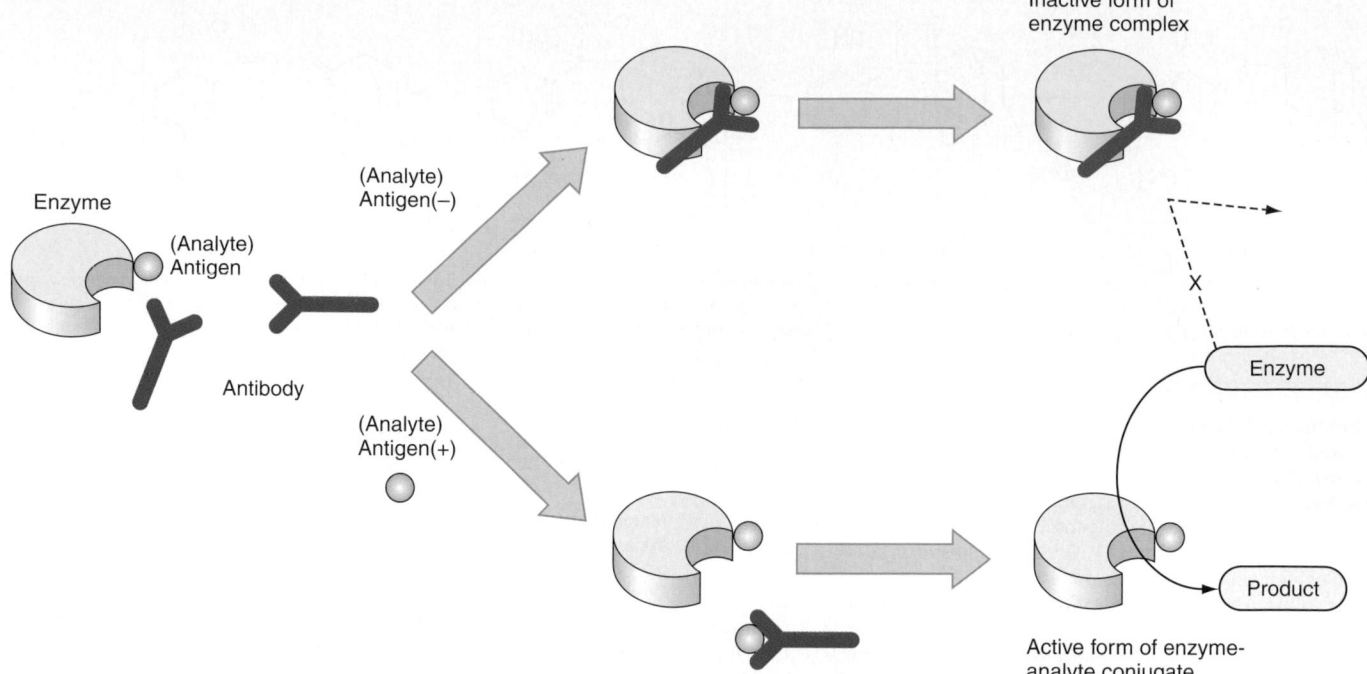

Figure 43–15 Enzyme-multiplied immunoassay technique (EMIT) system diagram: The activity of an enzyme as a label is inhibited by the binding of antibody to the antigen (analyte) conjugated with enzyme. The analyte is usually a hapten. Glucose-6-phosphate dehydrogenase (G6PD) and lysozyme are usually used as enzymes. In the assay, enzyme activity is proportional to concentration of analyte. (With permission from Nakamura RM, Kasahara Y, Rechnitz GA (eds): Immunochemical Assays and Biosensor Technology for the 1990s. Washington, DC, American Society for Microbiology, 1992.)

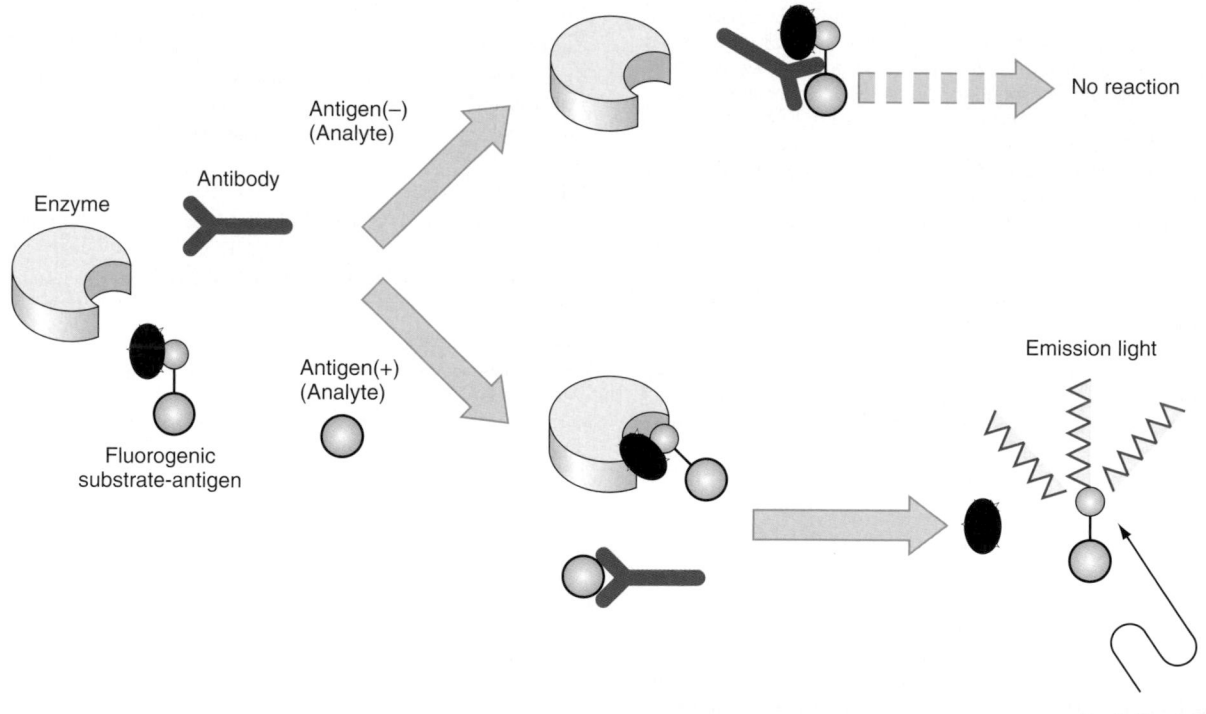

Figure 43–16 Substrate-labeled fluorescent immunoassay (SLFIA). The substrate β-galactosylumbeliferone is conjugated with the antigen (analyte) and forms a non-fluorescent substrate. The substrate can be cleaved by an enzyme β-galactosidase to form a fluorescent product. However, when the substrate–antigen conjugate is allowed to react with specific antibody to the antigen, there is no cleavage of the substrate complex with the β-galactosidase enzyme. In this assay, the concentration of the antigen (analyte) is directly proportional to the fluorescent intensity measured. (With permission from Nakamura RM, Kasahara Y, Rechnitz GA (eds): Immunochemical Assays and Biosensor Technology for the 1990s. Washington, DC, American Society for Microbiology, 1992.)

malate dehydrogenase and glucose-6-phosphate dehydrogenase (G6PD) have been found to be most useful because they are less likely to be affected by serum constituents. These assays generally measure drug at a concentration of milligrams per liter. However, the digoxin assay has a much lower limit of sensitivity, in the range of 0.8–2 μg/L.

Substrate-Labeled Fluorescent Immunoassay

The substrate-labeled fluorescent immunoassay (SLFIA) (Burd, 1977) uses a characteristic fluorogenic substrate, umbelliferyl β-galactoside, attached to the antigen (analyte) as a conjugate. Umbelliferone is the fluorescent product produced when the substrate is cleaved with β-galactosidase. The enzyme β-galactosidase cannot cleave the substrate–antigen complex when it reacts with the specific antibody. The free antigen (analyte) in the specimen solution competes with the antigen conjugated with the substrate to form the immunocomplex (Fig. 43–16). Antigen concentration in the sample is proportional to the fluorescent intensity of the cleaved fluorescent product. SLFIA can be used to assay drugs and haptens, as well as protein ligands such as IgG and IgM. A disadvantage of this method is

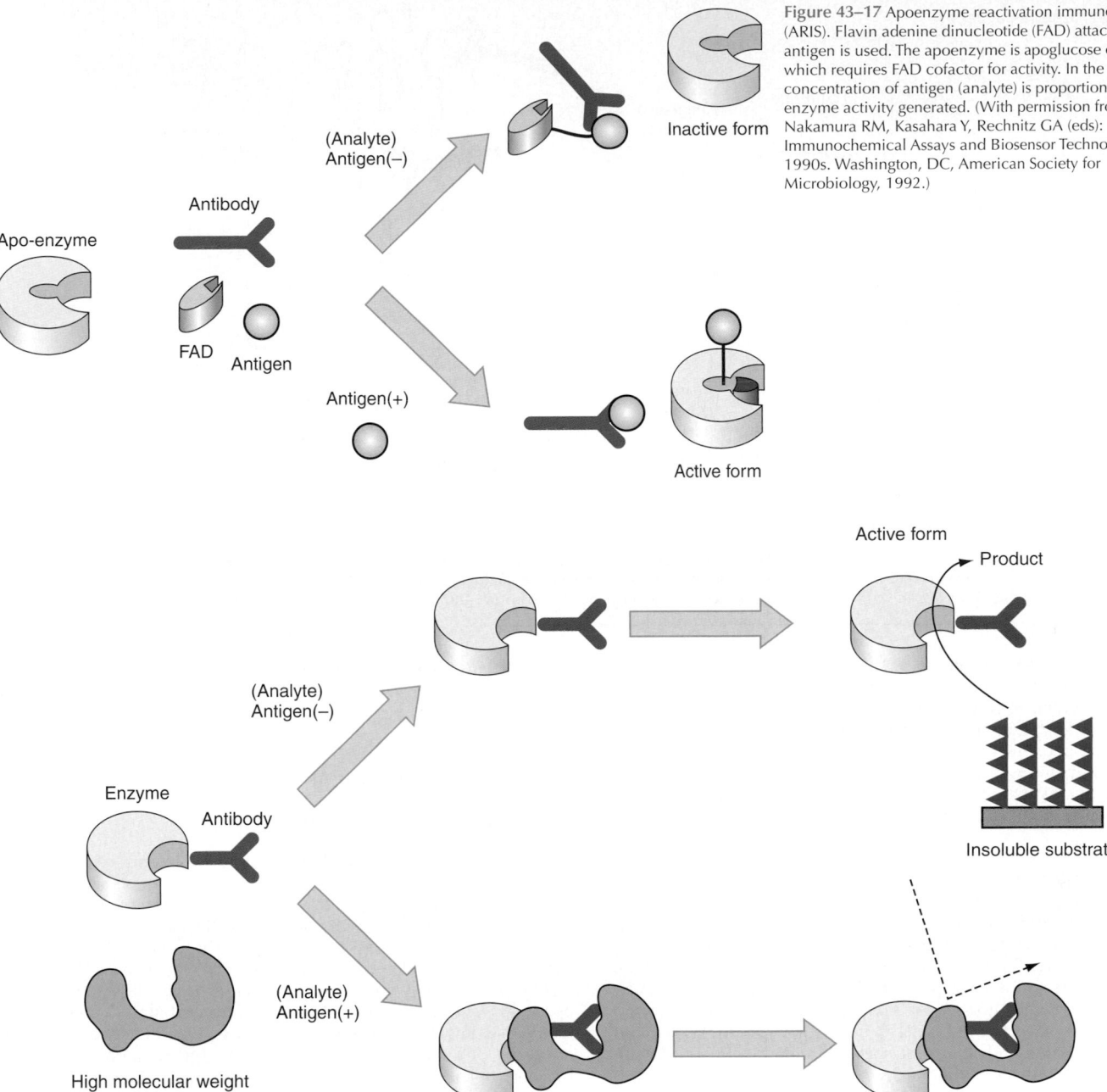

Figure 43–17 Apoenzyme reactivation immunoassay (ARIS). Flavin adenine dinucleotide (FAD) attached to the antigen is used. The apoenzyme is apoglucose oxidase which requires FAD cofactor for activity. In the assay concentration of antigen (analyte) is proportional to enzyme activity generated. (With permission from Nakamura RM, Kasahara Y, Rechnitz GA (eds): Immunochemical Assays and Biosensor Technology for the 1990s. Washington, DC, American Society for Microbiology, 1992.)

Figure 43–18 Enzyme inhibitory homogeneous immunoassay (EIHIA). The enzyme is α-amylase from *Bacillus subtilis* or dextranase from *Chaetomium gracile* is conjugated to the specific antibody to the high molecular weight antigen. The high-molecular-weight antigen can be ferritin or α-fetoprotein. The α-amylase enzyme is inactive when the enzyme antibody conjugate reacts with specific antibody. The active enzyme form can react with the starch insoluble substrate. The antigen concentration is directly proportional to the enzyme activity of assay reaction. (Redrawn from Nakamura RM, Kasahara Y, Rechnitz GA (eds): Immunochemical Assays and Biosensor Technology for the 1990s. Washington, DC, American Society for Microbiology, 1992s, pp 205–227.)

that the amplification properties of the enzyme are not utilized, and thus the assay system has limited sensitivity in the range of 10^{-9}–10^{-10} molar concentration of the analyte.

Apoenzyme Reactivation Immunoassay

The apoenzyme reactivation immunoassay (ARIS) is a homogeneous assay developed by Morris (1981) using the prosthetic group consisting of flavin adenine dinucleotide (FAD)-conjugated antigen (analyte) and glucose oxidase apoenzyme. As shown in Figure 43–17, the antigen (analyte) and a constant amount of analyte–FAD conjugate compete for a limited amount of specific antibody. At equilibrium, the level of free conjugate is proportional to the amount of antigen (analyte) in the specimen. The apoenzyme combines with the free but not the antibody-bound form of conjugate to reactivate glucose oxidase activity in proportion to the amount of free conjugate in the mixture. The active enzyme is generated in the procedure, and an amplification mechanism is also built into this assay. ARIS has been used to assay for theophylline and IgG (Morris, 1981, 1985). This FAD-labeled conjugate assay is readily adapted to the

measurement of high-molecular-weight proteins (e.g., thyroid binding globulin) (Schroeder, 1985) as well as other haptens like phenytoin and hormones.

Enzyme Inhibitory Homogeneous Immunoassay

The enzyme inhibitory homogeneous immunoassay (EIHIA), developed by Ashihara (1988), consists of antibody conjugated with enzyme and insoluble substrate. This assay is most suitable for the determination of large antigens (analytes). The EIHIA can be made to be homogeneous because the immunocomplex of conjugate with large antigen blocks the enzyme reaction with the solid substrate (Fig. 43–18). α-Amylase has been used as a labeled enzyme for the determination of ferritin and AFP. The immunoreaction of analyte with enzyme-labeled antibody can reach a plateau within 10 minutes; thus, EIHIA based on a noncompetitive binding assay requires less incubation time to achieve a sensitive detection level. Using this method, the measuring range of ferritin in serum is 10–800 ng/mL and for AFP it is 5–200 ng/mL. Dextranase has been used as an alternative enzyme (Nishizono, 1988). EIHIA has also been applied on a

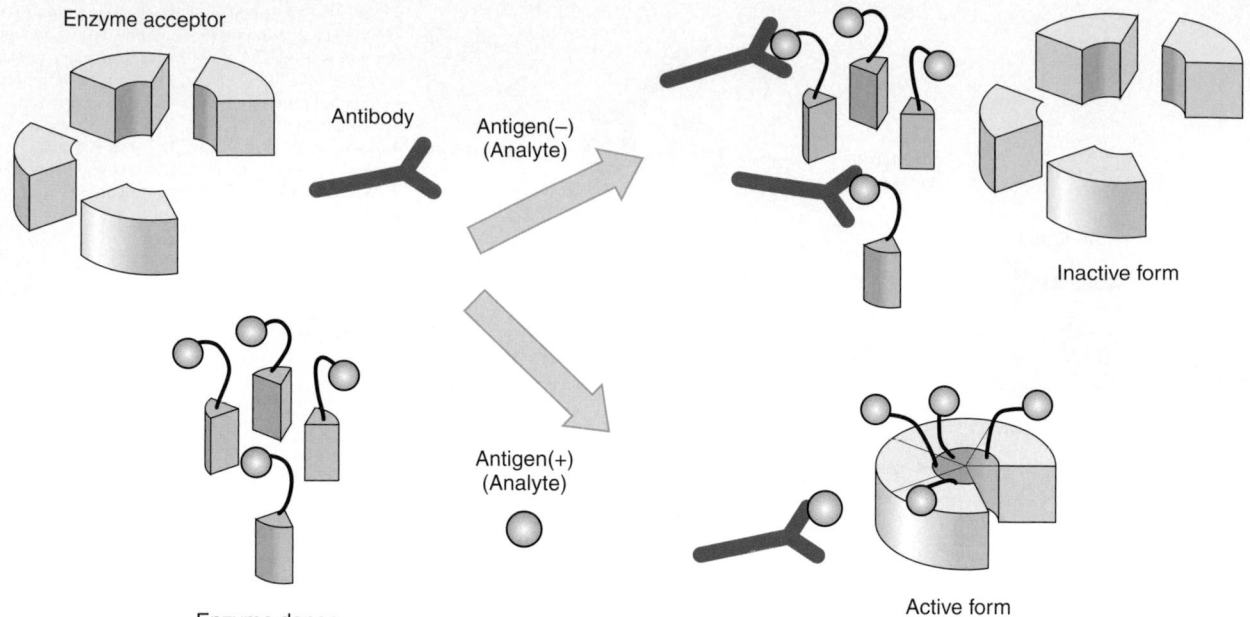

Enzyme acceptor

Antibody

Antigen(−)
(Analyte)

Inactive form

Enzyme donor

Antigen(+)
(Analyte)

Active form

Figure 43–19 Cloned enzyme donor immunoassay (CEDIA). Enzyme acceptors associate with enzyme donors to form an active β-galactosidase tetramer. The antibody inhibits the association of enzyme acceptor with enzyme donor–antigen conjugate. (Redrawn from Nakamura RM, Kasahara Y, Rechnitz GA (eds): Immunochemical Assays and Biosensor Technology for the 1990s. Washington, DC, American Society for Microbiology, 1992s, pp 205–227.)

simple dry-film format (Ashihara, 1991). The dry film consists of three major layers, each containing a developing zone for immunologic and enzymatic reaction, a barrier zone, and a color-developing zone. An inhibitor specific to human amylase present in serum is used to prevent serum background. The assay for serum C-reactive protein is completed in only six minutes by simply placing the specimen on the slide using dry chemistry instrumentation. Nevertheless, the sensitivity of the system remains inadequate for application to analytes such as tumor markers.

Cloned Enzyme Donor Immunoassay

The cloned enzyme donor immunoassay (CEDIA) was first achieved through the application of recombinant DNA technology to homogeneous immunoassays by Henderson (1986). Microgenics Corp. (Concord, CA) was able to engineer β-galactosidase protein into a large polypeptide (an enzyme acceptor) and a small polypeptide (an enzyme donor). Enzyme acceptors and enzyme donors assemble to form enzymatically active tetramers. In the assay (Fig. 43–19), a hapten antigen (analyte) is attached to an enzyme donor, and an analyte-specific antibody is used to inhibit the spontaneous assembly of the active enzyme. The antigens (analytes) in patient serum compete with the analytes in the analyte–enzyme-donor conjugate for antibody, modulating the amount of active β-galactosidase formed. The signal generated by enzyme substrates is directly proportional to the analyte concentration in the patient serum. The test for digoxin is a colorimetric assay that requires no serum pretreatment or predilutions. The assay system is suitable for use with automated chemistry analyzers.

Summary

EIAs can be applied to all antigen–antibody systems, including those involving serum protein, hormones, drugs, and other antigens and the antibodies directed against pathogens. Heterogeneous EIAs using chromogenic substrates can have a sensitivity comparable with that of RIAs, and they have gained wide acceptance for application in various immunoassays. Heterogeneous EIAs using sophisticated substrates that generate chemiluminescent light and small particles as the solid phase are sensitive enough to detect less than 1 pg/mL of analytes. Their sensitivity is thus much higher than that of RIAs. In addition, the assay manipulation is greatly simplified by fully automated instruments. Compared with heterogeneous EIAs, homogeneous EIAs have certain limitations in sensitivity, dynamic range, and large analyte application. Also, high background signals (noise) and relatively low assay signal are inevitable because of the elimination of washing steps for the separation of bound and free conjugates. The homogeneous EIAs are advantageous because they are based on a simple assay format and can be adapted to existing automatic instrumentation. At this time, heterogeneous EIA with fully automated instruments remains the best choice in terms of sensitivity and simplicity, as well as for safety reasons, because they do not require the use of radioisotopes.

Fluorescent Immunoassay

Background and Classification

Coons (1941) first introduced the use of fluorescent compounds as immunochemical labels to detect antigens in tissue sections. Immunofluorescence assays on tissue sections are currently very well established in the pathology laboratory. Over the past few years, many FIA procedures have been developed to detect the concentration of drugs, hormones, and a wide variety of proteins and polypeptides (Nakamura, 1992b). In the initial stages of development, analytic FIAs were hindered by a decrease in sensitivity because of background fluorescence of biological samples. Gradually, the sensitivity of fluorometric methods improved, and the detection of analytes at concentrations of 10–15 M became possible. Further advancements were achieved through improvements in instrumentation and the introduction of unique substrates with more optimal immunochemical and enzymatic reactions.

Selection of the fluorochrome label is important. The label should be stable and should demonstrate high molar extinction coefficient and quantum yield. It should also emit at appropriate wavelengths without interference with ligand–antibody reactions. When most fluorophores or fluorescent molecules are irradiated with light at appropriate wavelengths, an electron in the ground state is transited into the excited state of the molecule. As the electron returns to the ground state, physical energy is released in the form of a photon of lower energy (longer wavelength) than the exciting light. The fluorescence spectrum reveals a wavelength maximal emission, characteristic of a particular fluorescent compound. One of the typical labels, fluorescein isothiocyanate (FITC), has a less than 1 ns time interval between excitation and emission, whereas other compounds (i.e., europium) exhibit delayed fluorescence with an interval of several hundred nanoseconds. The various FIAs may be classified as follows: (1) heterogeneous and homogeneous, (2) ligand or antibody labeled, (3) competitive or noncompetitive, and (4) solid or nonsolid phase. The most common methods will be discussed.

Heterogeneous Fluorescent Immunoassay

Heterogeneous FIA procedures include a washing step to separate bound from free fluorescent labels. The assay procedure is similar to that of heterogeneous enzyme immunoassays and radioimmunoassays. Most of the commercially available assays use a solid-phase antigen or antibody

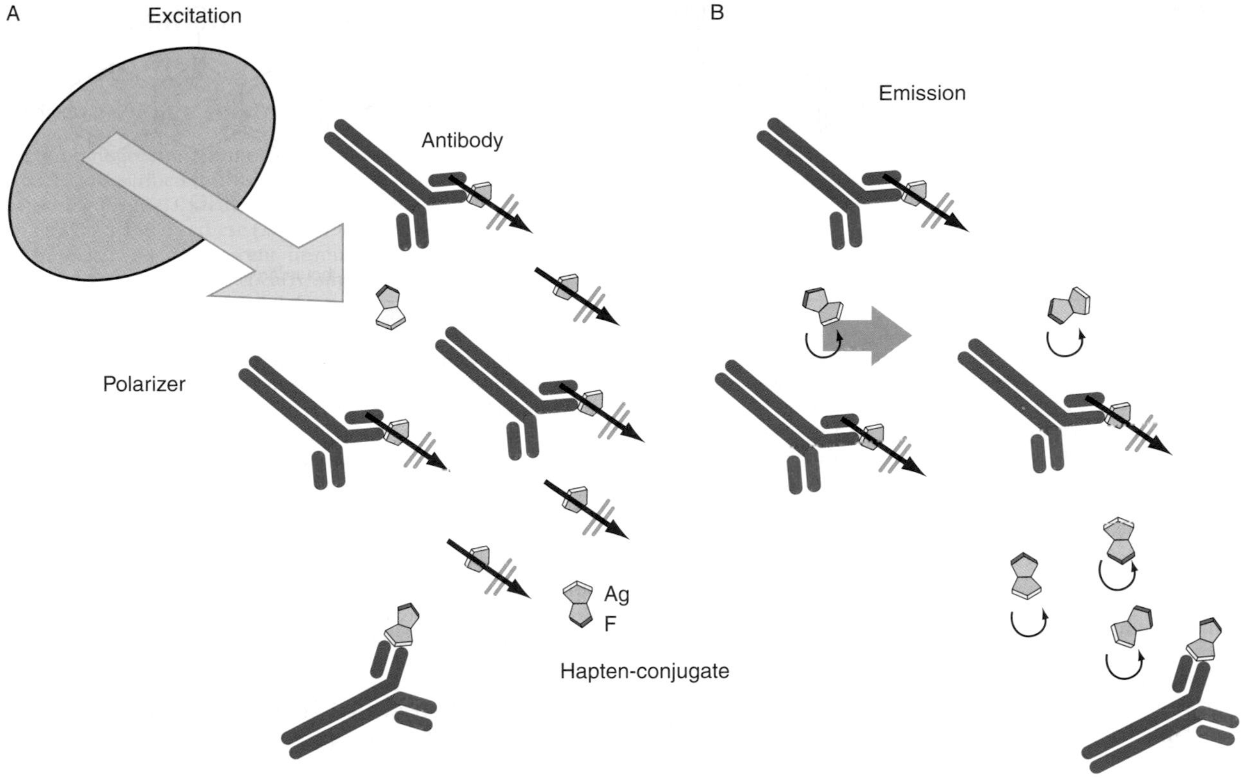

Figure 43–20 Assay principle of fluorescent polarization immunoassay (FPIA). *A* A polarized beam can excite both an unbound conjugate and the conjugate bound to antibody (Ab) exiting at the same angle as the irradiated beam. The conjugate consists of hapten (H) with a fluorescent molecule (F). *B* Orientation of the molecules at the time of fluorescence emission. Small hapten conjugates free from antibody can quickly change their orientation and fail to emit fluorescence. However, the conjugate bound to the antibody still remains at the same angle, because of its very slow movement, and it emits fluorescence.

system. The assay can be either competitive or noncompetitive, a property RIAs and EIAs also share.

Fluoroimmunometric Method

In the fluoroimmunometric method, analyte reacts with excess labeled antibodies in the solution. Residual labeled antibodies bind to excess solid-phase-bound antigens. The solid-phase matrix is washed and the fluorescence intensity is inversely related to the analyte concentration. This method is adaptable for the assay of haptens and complex proteins. Solid-phase FIA procedures were developed for the serologic assay of antibodies to rubella, toxoplasmosis, viral antigens, and antinuclear antibodies. Heterogeneous FIA methods for antigen determination were developed for serum proteins and hormones, including immunoglobulins, cortisol, progesterone, and thyroxine. The major advantage of heterogeneous FIAs is the significant reduction in interference by naturally fluorescent substances in patient samples, because of physical removal of interference factors during the separation step.

Radial Partition Immunofluorometric Assay

In radial partition immunoassays, radial chromatography is used and the assay is carried out on glass-fiber filter papers (Giegel, 1982). The procedure has been automated for the assay of hCG and several other analytes in serum (Rogers, 1986).

Time-Resolved Fluoroimmunoassay

This methodology makes use of special instrumentation and special fluorescent labels to increase assay sensitivity. It involves the use of fluorescent labels exhibiting delayed fluorescence with a time period of 100 ns or more between excitation and emission. Because most substances responsible for background fluorescence have a short decay period, the measurement of the delayed fluorescence signal will significantly reduce the effects of background fluorescence. This is accomplished with the time-resolved fluorometer, a special instrument that produces a fast light pulse that excites the fluorophore. Fluorescence is measured a little while after excitation. Thus, the effect of nonspecific background, which generally decays in less than 10 ns, can be removed (Halonen, 1973; Soini, 1983). The fluorophores exhibiting delayed fluorescence that have been used in these assays include (Soini, 1979) the following:

1. Pyrene derivatives with a decay time of almost 100 ns.
2. Rare earth metal chelate labels that have a very long decay time of almost 50–100 μs. These include europium (Eu^{3+}), samarium (Sm^{3+}), and terbium (Tb^{3+}).

Time-resolved fluoroimmunoassays have been developed to measure many analytes, including hCG, IgG, cortisol, insulin, and others.

Homogeneous Fluorescent Immunoassay

By definition, these immunoassays are performed on homogeneous specimen samples. They do not require the separation of bound from free conjugates and are usually not sensitive to background interference in the samples. Homogeneous FIAs also have the advantage of being quick to perform. However, when compared with heterogeneous assays, they show certain disadvantages. Homogeneous FIAs have a limited sensitivity near 10^{-10} mol with standard instrumentation. Labeled impurities in the sample may increase background interference. The assays require relatively pure labeled antigen or specific antibody, as well as special instrumentation to achieve a higher sensitivity.

Fluorescence Polarization Assay

A polarizing lens or prism can resolve light into rays in a single plane. When viewed at right angles to an excitation beam of vertically polarized light, fluorescent compounds in solutions emit partially polarized fluorescence. The fluorescence polarization principle was first applied to immunoassay procedures by Dandliker (1970, 1973). Polarized light transmitted through the sample can excite the fluorescent label regardless of binding to antibody. However, as shown in Figure 43–20, random thermal motion causes small molecules labeled with a hapten to tumble freely in solution, losing their polarized orientation. When the labeled antigen is bound to antibody with a molecular mass of over 160 kDa, the molecular motion is slowed enough to increase the polarized signal.

Studies using labeled antibody or antibody fragments showed no change in polarization upon mixing antigen and labeled antibody, even though immunoreaction had occurred. This method is most useful for the measurement of small antigens and haptens (Jolley, 1981). Abbott Laboratories has adapted this approach for the assay of many therapeutic and abused drugs on the TDx (Abbott Diagnostics, Abbott Park, IL). They developed a next generation analyzer the IMx, to measure molecules with

to capture the solid latex phase followed by B/F separation and the second immunoreaction of labeled antibody and the solid phase.

Sampling and Fluid Delivery Type

In general, fluid delivery is selected from two different types, either a disposable chip or a fixed-probe nozzle. Cross-contamination of samples should be avoided in all assay systems. The disposable chip can completely prevent cross-contamination. In the case of the fixed-probe system, even though the original sample is divided into several small aliquots, cross-contamination still occurs. Therefore, the disposable chip system is the best way to avoid cross-contamination and to also minimize biohazardous waste. On the other hand, the running cost of using chips for the assay is higher than that of the probe assay. The environmental effects of the disposable chip must also be considered.

Carryover

Carryover from an extremely high concentration of analyte in one sample to the next sample sometimes creates misjudgment in clinical diagnosis. A disposable plastic sample tube is the simplest way to prevent this problem. On the other hand, the fixed-probe nozzle has several cost advantages, as mentioned above. Thus, most of the technologies concerned with sample engineering have focused on minimizing sample carryover through washing and tip maintenance steps. Now, several fixed-probe tips have made it possible to limit carryover to less than the order of 10^{-7}. Even with such low carryover, some samples still create problems (e.g., a hepatitis B surface antigen [HBsAg] strong positive sample followed by a negative). In this case, a software system can be used to check the subsequent result by automatically retesting weekly positive values following strongly positive results.

Bound/Fixed Separation and Washing Systems

In a heterogeneous immunoassay, the bound conjugate has to be separated from free label. This B/F separation depends on the characteristics of the solid phase. The IMx and AxSYM systems use latex microparticles as the solid phase and employ a porous membrane to entrap the latex for separation of particles separating the solid phase from the liquid. The Diagnostics Product Corp., Los Angeles, CA has developed a unique cell for B/F separation systems, in which the reaction solution spins out from an inner cell to an outer waste cell while the bound phase stays in a solid-phase bead ($1/4''$ bead). An advantage of these formats is the avoidance of cross-contamination or carryover from one reaction mixture to the next, and no excess washing process is required. All other systems use magnetic particles and magnetic beads where easy and rapid separation can be achieved by applying a magnetic field.

New Systems for the Next Generation (Modular Systems)

Table 43–8 compares several of the commercial high-throughput immunoassay systems that have been introduced in the past few years. It shows the instrument specifications of each analyzer. By reducing the incubation and reaction times, a rapid result can be obtained in 10–25 minutes. Thus, a high-throughput machine performing 120–200 tests per hour is feasible. Furthermore, several manufacturers have demonstrated a new system concept that aligns the different analytical systems that are needed in a clinical laboratory. Many clinical laboratories have introduced an automated sample transporting line to which is connected different analytical instruments controlled independently. However, some analyzers are not amenable to this approach because the speed of the instrument or cycle time cannot easily be harmonized with the other software and hardware. To solve these problems, ARCHITECT (Abbott Laboratories) is an example of a new machine concept in which one system computer can control several immunoassay analyzers connected to one chemistry analyzer. Bayer Diagnostics (Tarrytown, NY) have also introduced the ADVIA IMS, based on a similar concept, which can perform clinical chemistry and immunoassay testing on a single platform. Several other combinations still under development are based on this concept, which will make it possible to simplify the clinical laboratory and to lower total cost.

Rapid and Simple Test Devices for Point-of-Care Testing

Background

A strong demand for a home test (e.g., hCG for pregnancy diagnosis) has simplified the immunoassay format: the test must be simple, rapid, and reproducible. With these goals in mind, many hCG tests have been developed and have resulted in the first-generation test format with a flow-through enzyme immunoassay.

Flow-Through Assay Devices (Immunofiltration Assay Devices)

Figure 43–23 illustrates schematically the typical device of flow-through type, the ICON hCG (Hybritech Incorporated, San Diego, CA), which consists of a porous membrane with immobilized anti-hCG antibody and

Table 43–8 New Generation of Heterogenous Immunoassay Systems

	AIA-21 Tosoh	ACS:Centaur Bayer Diagnostics	ARCHITECT Abbott	ADVIA IMS Bayer Diagnostics
Package of Reagent	Freeze-drying in portion package	Reagent pack (solution)	Solution in bottle	Dry bead in reaction cuvette
Reaction cuvette	Reagent cup	Disposable cuvette	Disposable cuvette	Reagent cup
Reaction principle	Fluorescent enzyme immunoassay	Chemiluminescent immunoassay	Chemiluminescent immunoassay	Chemiluminescent immunoassay
Labeled substance	Alkaline phosphatase	Acridinium ester	Acridinium ester	Alkaline phosphatase?
Enzyme substrate	4-methylumbelliferyl phosphate	None	None	Dioxetane phosphate?
Detector signal	Fluorescence	Chemiluminescence	Chemiluminescence	Chemiluminescence
Assay format	S-1, S-2, competitive	S-1, S-2, competitive	S-1, S-2, competitive	S-1, S-2, competitive
Pretreatment	Yes	Yes	Yes	?
Reaction Flow	Turntable	Turntable	Turntable	Turntable
Cycle time (s)	30	15	18	36
Reaction time (min)	10 or 40	7.5–36	29	20
Reaction temperature	37°C	37°C	37°C	37°C
Maximum analyte number	20	30	25	36
Throughput (test/h)	120	240	200	100
Solid phase	Magnetic bead	Magnetic particle	Magnetic particle	Magnetic particle
First result time (min)	50	8–40	30?	?
B/F separation	Magnetic field	Magnetic field	Magnetic field	Magnetic field
Sampling method	Pipetting probe	Disposable chip	Fixed probe	Pipetting probe (oil technology)
Sample autodilution	Yes	Yes	Yes	Yes

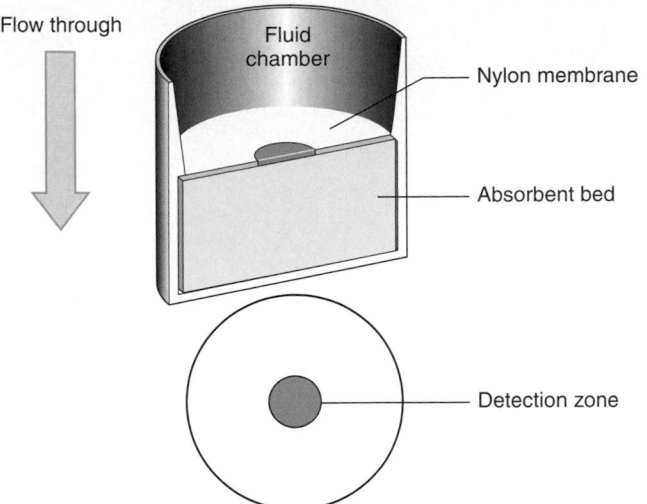

Figure 43–23 Flow-through immunoassay. Cross-section of Hybritech ICON and top view of the device. Capturing antibodies are immobilized at the center of a nylon membrane on which an absorbent bed is set to absorb unreacted sample fluid, labeled conjugate and washing buffer. The assay can be performed sequentially, similar to a two-step enzyme immunoassay.

an absorbent pad below the membrane (Valkirs, 1985). The assay principle and the procedure are as follows. Several drops of the urine sample are applied on the membrane. The urine is absorbed into the absorbent pad and then washing buffer is applied dropwise followed by a solution of alkaline-phosphatase-labeled anti-hCG antibody.

Dipping Strip

A dipping strip format has also been developed for reducing the materials cost, as compared to the flow-through format. In this format, the test strip contains a spotting area with antibody at the end of the strip. The assay can be performed as follows:

1. The strip is dipped in a sample cup containing the sample.
2. Then the strip is dipped in a washing cup.
3. Then the strip is dipped in labeling solution.
4. Finally the strip is dipped in color developer if needed.

Immunochromatographic Devices

To eliminate stepwise reagent additions for these two formats, further improvement has been accomplished by use of immunochromatographic techniques, which have led to a simple and rapid immunoassay. Immunochromatography consists of simultaneous B/F separation and signal generation followed by lateral flow on porous materials such as a

nitrocellulose membrane or glass fiber sheet. Through the capillary action of the membrane, the analyte in the sample can migrate from the proximal end to the distal end, where there is an absorbent pad set to maintain a constant capillary flow rate. The sample-loading zone, labeling zone, and detection zone are set between the two ends. The immunochromatographic method is classified into several formats. Figure 43–24 shows the typical immunochromatographic formats. The proximal end is employed as the sample loading port connected to a pad containing labeled antigen or antibody under which there is a nitrocellulose membrane in contact with the pad, serving as a fixed detection zone. The distal end of the membrane is attached to the absorbent pad as a source of capillary force. The sample, loaded by means of a dropper, reconstitutes the conjugate antibody or antigen labeled with colloidal gold or colored latex, which forms an immunocomplex with the analyte being detected, and the complex migrates to the detection zone. The antibody or antigen immobilized in the detection zone can capture the complex and form a positive red or blue line. Excess labeling substance migrates to the absorbent pad. The mobile phase for sample migration is the sample itself. Samples strongly colored because of the presence of a high concentration of bilirubin or hemoglobin, therefore, may interfere with the judgment in reading of the results by the naked eye. In this format, the signal to be read is produced directly in the detection zone as a concentrated zone of colored particles.

Yamauchi and colleagues (1997) have established a novel platform format in which EIA can be performed automatically, including a washing procedure. The device is depicted schematically in Figure 43–25. In this format, the positioning of each of the zones is completely different from that in the other immunochromatography formats mentioned previously. The proximal end has a developer solution, which makes it possible to carry out the washing process spontaneously with capillary force. The sample is applied to a pad in the center portion of the device that contains the labeled conjugate in dry form. The distal end connects to an absorbent pad. Two drops of sample are dropped on the sample pad to react with the conjugate following the reconstitution of the dried conjugate. The reaction mixture containing the immunocomplex formed between the analyte and the labeled antibody can spread to both ends. Once the reservoir of developing solution is ruptured, the dried substrate is reconstituted to become the soluble enzyme substrate in the detection zone. At this time, fluidic flow is directed towards the distal end. Serum components and the excess nonreacted conjugate can be washed away to the absorbent. If the sample contains analyte, then the immobilized antibody captures the complex in the detection zone to form a colored line. This method has some advantages, differing from other immunochromatographic devices developed by sample. In such devices, hemolytic serum or lipemic serum may interfere in the evaluation of the assay result by the naked eye because of high background color. However, the former type of device with a connected reservoir may not be interfered with by such colored components. This device has been useful to detect HBsAg, anti-HBs antibody (Yamauchi, 1997) and antibody to *T. pallidum* (Hasegawa, 1995). Most of the components such as the membrane, the absorbent pad, and the sample compartment have built-in housing as molded plastic.

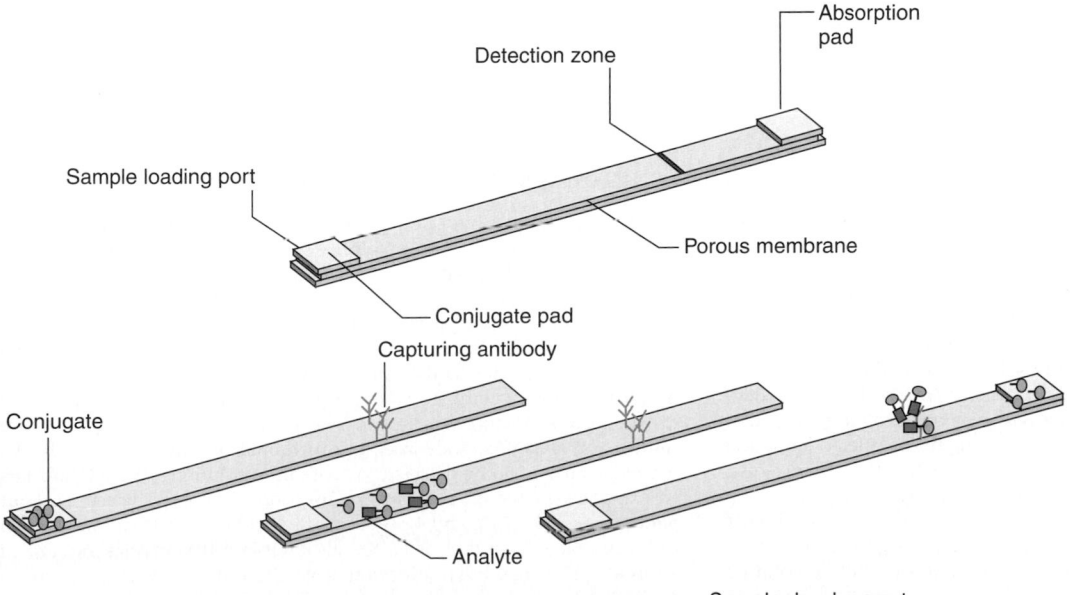

Figure 43–24 Typical immunochromatographic test strip by sample loading. Assay flows are illustrated in the lower part of the figure. In general form, proximal end of lateral flow serves as the sample loading portion consisting of a pad containing of antibody or antigen labeled with colored latex or colloidal gold. Analyte in the sample forms a complex with the conjugate and migrates to the detection zone thereby immobilizing the capturing antibody to form a positive colored line. Excess amounts of the conjugate and sample migrate to the distal end of the strip.

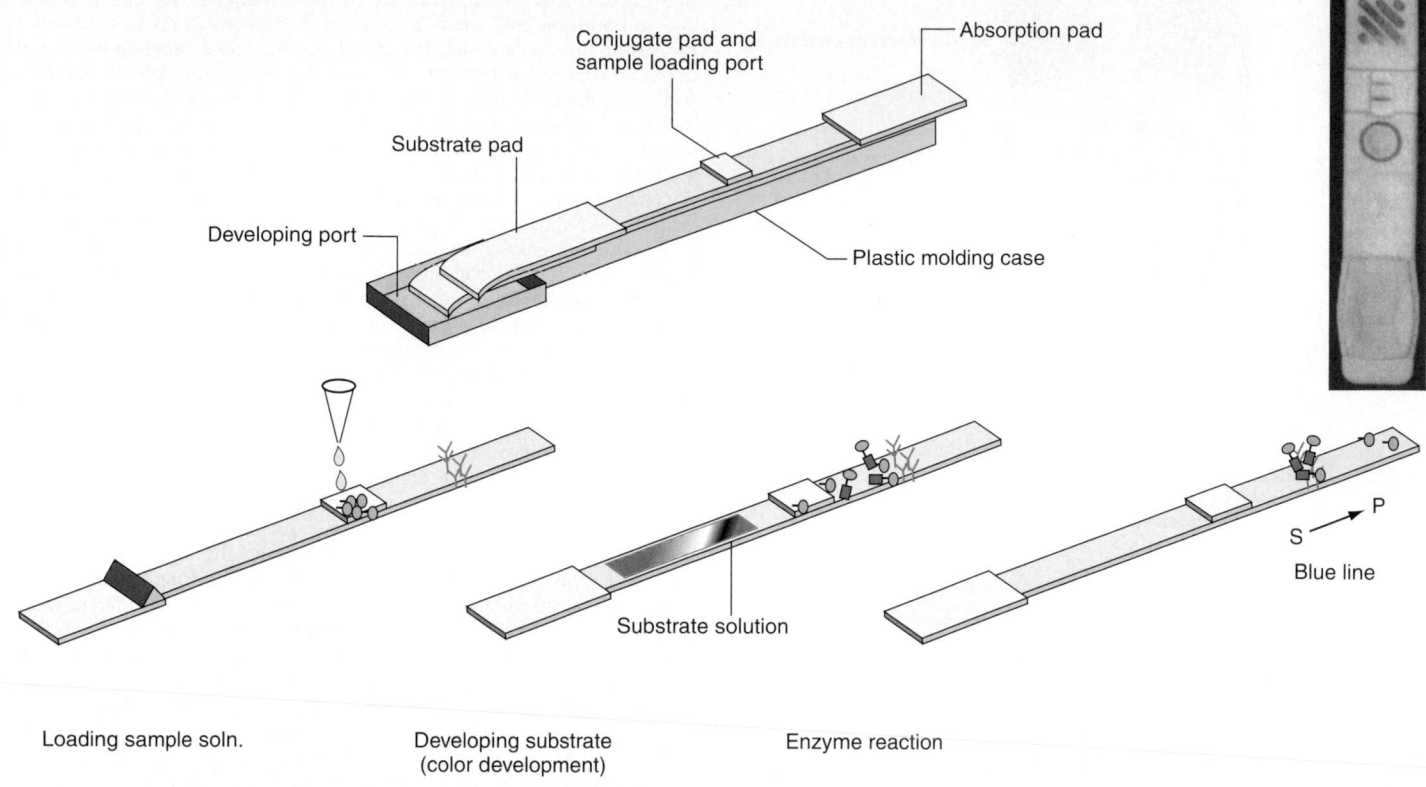

Figure 43–25 Immunochromatographic device using EIA. A sensitive amplification method is applied for immunochromatography using an enzyme. The sample is applied to the sample loading portion at the center of the strip. In this method, a developing solution is employed as the mobile phase which can serve as a washing buffer. The picture in the right part of the figure shows the plastic molded housing and assay results for TP antibody.

Summary

Rapid and simple immunoassay devices are summarized in Table 43–9. These devices can be classified into three major types – flow-through, dipping, and immunochromatography – and combination formats of these three types. Most of the immunochromatographic devices employ direct-labeled conjugate, colloidal metal, or colored latex. These types of format are actually well suited for direct migration of the immunocomplex, along with the migration of the sample solution. However, many of these devices require a large volume of sample, 100–200 μL. On the other hand, although developer is required, the EIA type device allows the assay to be carried out using a smaller amount of sample, 25 μL. The current stream of rapid tests for point-of-care testing is strongly oriented towards devices using immunochromatography because a skilled person, such as a home user or nurse, can perform the test correctly according to the manufacturer's directions, unlike other immunoassay devices (Kasahara, 1997).

Simultaneous multiple immunoassays

Background

Recent immunoassay advancements have led to the development of novel technology concepts that allow for simultaneous multiple detection as a way to reduce reagent cost. This means that anywhere from five to 100 analytes can be detected simultaneously in an individual sample. These technologies are classified into two broad categories in terms of the type of solid phase used. The first, microsectioning technology, is adapted to immunoassays using a microchip as the solid phase, and the second uses microparticles as the solid phase. In the second, two technologies have been applied to the recognition of individual assay analyte parameters. One is direct recognition of the solid phase using fluorolabeled latex, and the other involves the use of particles of different sizes. In the latter case, limited recognition is possible because the resolution is dependent on particle size. Miniaturized technologies such as these are considered highly advantageous to minimize the cost of reagents, save energy and protect the environment because of the small mass of reagent and sample volumes that they require.

MicroSpot Assay

The microchip solid surface is fractionated into small areas using microdotting technology. 100–200 reaction sites are produced in a 3 mm diameter area of a polystyrene flat plate (Ekins, 1998). In each site, a spotting area 80 μm in diameter receives a volume of less than 1 nL of solution ink-jetted automatically. In this method, ambient assay theory established by Ekins has been applied, and the sensitivity and the detection limit depend on the antibody occupancy but not on the surface area on the solid phase. The detection limit for TSH was found to be 0.01 mIU/L in an 18-hour assay using this ambient analyte assay method. Therefore, it is evident that a highly sensitive assay can be achieved even on the microspot area. Boehringer Mannheim, which later merged with Roche Diagnostics, applied an avidin-coated solid phase uniformly to the surface area and then ink-jetted biotin-binding antibody or antigen on the spot. Multiple parameters, including HIV antibody, HBsAg, anti-hepatitis-C antigens and rubella, could be detected simultaneously on a microchip made of polystyrene. The assay format is a three-step fluorescent immunoassay. Finally, a confocal laser scanner detects the fluorescent signal on the chip. This chip assay is also available for the application of DNA detection.

Multi-Analyte Microarray Immunoassay

Silzel and colleagues have developed an analyte mass assay that measures total analyte mass in a sample (Silzel, 1998). Therefore, the basic concept of this method is different from that of the ambient assay, which measures analyte concentration. A polystyrene film was employed as the solid phase. An 80 pL droplet was ink-jetted onto the film and DBCY5 was adopted as the labeling marker because of the long Stokes shift from the excitation wavelength at 670 nm to the emission wavelength at 710 nm, with near-infrared fluorescence emission. The detection apparatus used in this method consists of a microscope attached to a Pelitier-cooled charge-coupled device camera and a GaAlAs diode laser. In this format, 105 molecules of DBCY5 per 80 pL area could be detected in calibration solutions. The IgG subclass was applied to the present system for multiparameter detection. Four parameters, IgG1, 2, 3, and 4, were detected and the sensitivity was shown to be comparable to that of ELISA, although a much smaller amount of antibody (100 times less), sufficed to cover the surface area as compared to an ELISA plate.

Table 43–9 Simple and Rapid Immunoassay Device Specifications

Immunochromatographic Format

Assay Principle	Kit Name (Analyte)	Sample Specimens	Sample Volume (µL)	Mobile Phase	Reaction Time (min)	Sensitivity	Housing	Manufacturer
Immunochromatographic Format								
One step (all in one)	Helisal One Step (*Helicobacter pylori*)	Blood	50	Plasma	5	Equal to ELISA	MP	Cortics Diagnostics Ltd
	Biocard Troponin I test	Serum	150–200	Serum	15	0.1 ng/mL	MP	AniBiotech OY
	Clear View hCG II	Urine	?	Urine	5	25 mIU/mL	MP	Unipath Ltd
	Quick Vue one step hCG	Urine	3 drops (75?)	Urine	3	25 mIU/mL	MP	Quidel
	CARD-I-KIT Troponin I	Serum	4 drops (100?)	Serum	5–10	0.1 ng/mL	MP	AboaTech Ltd
	TROPT Troponin T	Blood	150	Plasma	5–15	0.1 ng/mL	MP	Roche Diagnostics*
	Determine HbsAg	Blood/serum	50	Plasma/serum	15	1 ng/mL?	TS	Abbott
	BioSign™ Tumor	Blood/serum	50	Developer	5–10	–	MP	Princeton BioMeditech Corporation
	HBs Insta Test	Blood/serum	200	Plasma/serum	15–20	0.5 ng/mL	MP	Morningstar Diagnostics
	EASY-SURE HbsAg Test	Serum	100–150	Serum	5–20	1 ng/mL	TC	West Wind Plus, Inc.
	PSA Rapid Screen Test	Blood	1 hanging drops	Developer	≈15	>4 ng/mL	MP	Craig Medical Distribution, Inc.
	Triage Cardiac (Myoglobin CK-MB Troponin-I)	Blood	?	Plasma	15	?	MP	Biosite Diagnostics†
	AMRAD ICT Hepatitis B	Blood/serum	?	Blood/serum	5–15	2 ng/mL	CC	Amrad Corporation Ltd
	Espline HbsAg	Plasma/serum	25	Developer	15	0.5 ng/mL	MP	Fujirebio, Inc.
	TestPack PLUS hCG	Serum/urine	25	Serum/urine	5	50 mIU/mL	MP	Abbott
Two steps	EASY-SURE HIV1/2 Test	Plasma/serum	40	Developer	10	–	CC	West Wind Plus, Inc.
Dip Strip Immunochromatographic methods								
	AimStickPBD	Urine	Dipping volume	Urine	3	200 mIU/mL		Orgenics
	Dainascreen HbsAg	Plasma/serum	25	Plasma/serum + conjugate solution	15	3.1 ng/mL	TS	Dainabot
Flow-through format								
	ICON-II hCG	Serum						
	NycoCard CRP	Whole blood/plasma	50	Buffer, etc.	2	10 µg/mL	TC	Nyco Diagnostics
	Chagas double spot test	Serum/plasma	1 drop	Buffer, etc.	10	?	MP	Morningstar Diagnostics
Immunochromatography and Flow Through Combination								
	DoubleCheck™ HbsAg	Serum/plasma	?	Buffer, etc.	15	2 ng/mL	MP	Orgenics

CC = card case; MP = molded plastic housing; TC = test card; TS = test strip.

* Towt, 1995. † Bruni, 1999.

Protein chips microfabricated with highly dense spotting sites having 1250 reaction sites per 1×2 cm have been developed by Zyomyx (Hayward, CA). The protein chip is composed of a silicon-based substrate as a solid phase and six lanes with a 5×50 array/lane (Peluso, 2003). Isomura *et al.* has employed the chip and applied a simultaneous fluorescent sandwich immunoassay for some target proteins, i.e., AFP, interleukin (IL)-6, Frk-2, c-Jun, Grb2, c-Src and H-Ras (Isomura, 2003). As shown in Figure 43–26, reaction sites are microfabricated to pillar structure and then coated with titanium oxide. The surface is coated with poly L-lysin polymer linking with polyethyleneglycol-biotin. After binding of streptavidin to the biotin, the solid streptavidin can bind to biotinylated antibodies. The assay can be performed in a flow device. The detection limit for IL-6 was found to be 5–50 000 ng/L in 3-hour assay, using this protein biochip assay method.

Flow Cytometric Immunoassay

Luminex (Austin, TX) has developed a simultaneous multiparameter fluorescent immunoassay using flow cytometric technology in which two types of fluorophore for recognition of the analyte serve to mark latex particles used as the solid phase (Fulton, 1997; Oliver, 1998). Two different types of fluorophore and fluorescence intensity mark the analyte mapping of each particle. More than 60 analytes can be detected

simultaneously in principle. The assay procedure is as follows. The sample is mixed with antibody labeled with R-phycoerythrin and a second antibody immobilized on latex as the solid phase. The mixture is incubated for 10–30 minutes and then injected into the flow system. 1000 particles are separated as in flow cytometry, and both an enhanced fluorescence signal from the excited R-phycoerythrin as a result of the labeling, and two fluorescence signals on the particle are detected simultaneously by laser scanner. Carson and colleagues have applied this approach to the simultaneous detection of 15 cytokines such as IL-1, IL-2, IL-4 and IL-6 (Carson, 1999). Simultaneous detection was less sensitive than the assay of individual cytokines. However, it is still a sensitive assay compared with conventional ELISA, and sensitivity was 100 pg/ml for IL-2, 10 pg/ml for IL-4, 100 pg/ml for granulocyte/macrophage colony-stimulating factor (GM-CSF) and 200 pg/ml for interferon-r.

Microchannel Assay Using Compact Disc

Gyros AB (Uppsala, Sweden) has developed a simultaneous microfluidic fluorescent immunoassay using a compact disc as microlaboratory technology in which the microfluidic flow can be obtained by centrifugal force (Poulsen, 2004). On the CD, 104 assays can be performed simultaneously by fluorescent column immunoassay. The solid phase

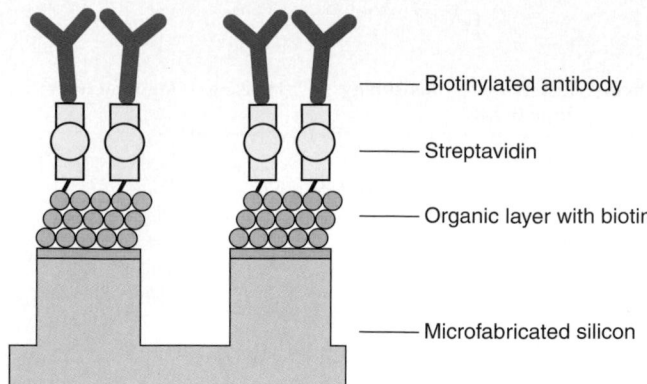

—— Biotinylated antibody

—— Streptavidin

—— Organic layer with biotin

—— Microfabricated silicon

Figure 43–26 Protein Biochip using FIA. Sandwich fluorescent immunoassay is applied for multiple detection using microfabricated silicon as a solid substrate. The surface of more than 1000 pillars is coated with organic polymer layer having biotin. Streptavidin bound to the biotin binds to biotinylated antibody specific to analyte can react with antigen in sample. The silicon device arraying different antibodies specific to different antigens is set in a molded plastic device.

consists of plastic microparticles binding with streptavidin. Specific antibody binding with biotin applies to the column. 100 nL of sample can be automatically metered by the separation of the hydrophobic breaking valve in which the wall has been coated with hydrophobic polymer. The valve can open by centrifugal force and several types of break settings in the channel of the CD makes it possible to perform a rapid and simple assay by changing the rpm to control reactions. This assay has been applied to the detection of human IgG. The sensitivity was 1 ng/ml.

Summary

Remarkable technological advancement in simultaneous assays has been achieved in the current decade. However, one of the tasks that remains to be achieved is the miniaturization of the assay in all of its aspects. For instance, mechanical or physicochemical difficulties in handling microvolumes of fluid, and sample evaporation during handling remain inevitable. Before it can be introduced successfully in routine clinical laboratories, both device technology and assay environment layout in the laboratory need to be improved.

From the point of view of clinical application, simultaneous multiple assays may not appear as attractive as might have been expected. In some cases, the sensitivity and specificity of this technique needs to be assessed more carefully. However, simultaneous multiple assays based on miniaturization technology should be the ultimate goal for laboratory diagnostics given the advantages they offer in terms of cost containment and reduction of burden on patients from phlebotomy, as well as clinical utility.

References

Actor JK, Kuffner T, Dezzutti CS, et al: A flash-type bioluminescent immunoassay that is more sensitive than radioimaging: quantitative detection of cytokine cDNA in activated and resting human cells. J Immunol Methods 1998; 211:65–77.

Alpha B, Lehn JM, Mathis G: Energy transfer luminescence of Eu(III) and Tb(III) cryptases of macrobicyclic polypyridine ligands. Angew Chem Int Ed Engl 1987; 26:266–267.

Ashihara Y, Hiraoka T, Makino Y, et al: Immunoassay for determining low- and high-Mr antigens with a dry multilayer film. Clin Chem 1991; 37:1525–1526.

Ashihara Y, Nishizono I, Miyagawa E, et al: Homogeneous enzyme immunoassay for high molecular weight antigen (I). J Clin Lab Anal 1988; 2:138–142.

Avrameas S, Guilbert B: Dosage enzymoimmunologique de proteines a l'aide d'immunoabsorbants et d'antigenes marques aux enzymes. CR Acad Sci 1971; 273:205–2707.

Avrameas S. Ternynck T, Guesdon JL: Coupling of enzymes to antibodies and antigens. Scand J Immunol 1978; 7 (Suppl):7–23.

Axelsen NH (ed.): Quantitative immunoelectrophoresis: new developments and applications. Scand J Immunol 1975; Suppl. 2: 1–230.

Babson AL, Olson DR, Palmieri T, et al: The IMMULITE assay tube: a new approach to heterogeneous ligand assay. Clin Chem 1991; 37: 1521–1522.

Blackburn GF, Shah HP, Kenten JH et al: Electrochemiluminescence detection for development of immunoassay and DNA probe assays for clinical diagnostics. Clin Chem 1991; 37:1534–1539.

Bounaud MP, Bounara JY, Bouin-Pineau MH, et al: Chemiluminescence immunoassay of thyrotropin with acridinium-ester-labeled antibody evaluated and compared with two other immunoassays. Clin Chem 1987; 33:2096–2100.

Boyd JC, Savory MG, Margrey M, et al: Adaptation of EMIT drug assays to a random-access automated clinical analyzer. Ann Clin Lab Sci 1985; 15: 39–44.

Boyden SV: The absorption of protein on erythrocytes treated with tannic acid and subsequent hemagglutination by antiprotein sera. J Exp Med 1951; 93:107–120.

Bronstein I, Edwards B, Voyta JC: 1,2-dioxetanes: novel chemiluminescent enzyme substrates.

Applications to immunoassays. J Biolumin Chemilumin 1989a 4:99–111.

Bronstein I, Juo RR, Voyta JC: Novel chemiluminescent adamantyl 1, 2 dioxetane enzyme substrate. *In* Stanley P, Kricka LJ (eds): Bioluminescence and Chemiluminescence. Chichester, UK, John Wiley & Sons, 1991, pp 74–82.

Bronstein I, Voyta J, Thorpe G, et al: Chemiluminescent assay of alkaline phosphatase applied in an ultra-sensitive enzyme immunoassay of thyrotropin. Clin Chem 1989b; 35:1441–1446.

Bruni J, McPherson P, Buechler K: A STAT cardiac marker system for detecting acute heart attacks. Am Clin Lab 1999; 18: 14–16.

Burd JF, Wong RC, Feeney JE, et al: Homogeneous reactant-labeled fluorescent immunoassay for therapeutic drugs exemplified by gentamicin determination in human serum. Clin Chem 1977; 23: 1402–1408.

Coons AH, Creech JH, Jones RN: Immunologic properties of an antibody containing a fluorescent group. Prop Soc Exp Biol Med 1941; 47:200.

Dandliker WB, de Saussure, VA: Fluorescence polarization in immunochemistry. Immunochemistry 1970;7:799–828.

Dandliker WB, Kelly RJ, Dandliker J, et al: Fluorescence polarization immunoassay. Theory and experimental method. Immunochemistry 1973; 10:219–227.

Ekins R: Ligand assays: from electrophoresis to miniaturized microarrays. Clin Chem 1998; 44: 2015–2030.

A new sensitive immunoassay in a miniaturized microarray format is described in this report. This method can be applied to immunoassays and to DNA/RNA analysis and may well revolutionize the diagnostic and pharmaceutical fields as the DNA chip and protein chip have.

Ekins RP: The estimation of thyroxine in human plasma by an electrophoretic technique. Clin Chem Acta 1960; 5:453.

Engvall E, Perlman P: Enzyme-linked immunosorbent assay (ELISA). Quantitative assay of immunoglobulin G. Immunochemistry 1971; 8:871–874.

Erler K: Elecsys immunoassay systems using electrochemiluminescence detection. Wien Klin Wochenschr Suppl 1998;3:5–10.

Fahey JL, McKelvey EM: Quantification determination of serum immunoglobulins in antibody-agar plates. J Immunol 1965; 94:84–90.

Fiore M, Mitchell J, Doan T, et al: The Abbott IMx automated benchtop immunochemistry analyzer system. Clin Chem 1988; 34:1726–1732.

Fulton RJ, McDade RL, Smith PL, et al: Advanced multiplexed analysis with the FlowMetrix system. Clin Chem 1997;43(9):1749–1756.

Galvin JP: Particle enhanced immunoassays – a review, diagnostic immunology. *In* Rippey JH, Nakamura RM (eds): Technology Assessment. Skokie, IL, College of American Pathologists, 1984, pp 18–30.

Garvey JS, Cremer NE, Sussdorf DH: Methods in Immunology, 3rd ed. Reading, MA, WA Benjamin, 1977, pp 273–327.

Giegel JL, Brotherton MM, Cronen P, et al: Radial partition immunoassay. Clin Chem 1982;28:1894–1898.

Halonen P, Meurman O, Lovgren T, et al: Detection of viral antigens by time resolved fluoroimmunoassay. *In* Bachman PA (ed): Current Topics in Microbiology and Immunology. New York, Springer-Verlag, 1973, pp 133–146.

Hasegawa A, Andoh A, Ashihara Y: Simple and rapid detection of antibodies to HIV-1/2 using immunochromatography (Abstract). IUVDT World STD/AIDS Cogress 1995, p 145.

Haux P, Dybois H, McGovern M, et al: Evaluation of the TIna-quant® ferritin assay on the Boehringer Mannheim/Hitachi 704 system. Clin Chem 1988; 34:1174 (Abstract).

Heidelberg M, Kendall FE: The precipitin reaction between type III pneumococcus polysaccharide and homologous antibody. J Exp Med 1935; 61: 563–591.

Henderson DR, Freidman SB, Harris JD, et al: CEDIA, a new homogeneous immunoassay system. Clin Chem 1986; 32: 1637–1641.

Hirayama C, Ihara H, Shibata M, et al: Polypeptide artificial carrier particles for use in passive agglutination immunoassay. Polymer J 1991; 23:161.

Hunter WH, Greenwood FC: Preparation of iodine-131-labeled human growth hormone of high specific activity. Nature 1962; 194:495–496.

Ikeda M: New agglutination test for serum antibodies to adult T-cell leukemia virus. Gann 1984; 75:845–848.

Ishikawa E, Kohono T: Development and application of sensitive enzyme immunoassay for antibodies. J Clin Lab Anal 1989; 3:252.

Isomura M, Honda N, Kawada A, et al: Development of a highly sensitive enzyme immunoassay for human calcitonin using solid phase coupled with multiple antibodies. Ann Clin Biochem 1999; 36: 629–635.

Isomura M, Okamura C, et al: Microfabricated protein biochip for multiple fluorescent sandwich immunoassay. Clin Chem 2003; 49(S6): A13

Isomura M, Ueno M, Shimada K, et al: Highly sensitive chemiluminescent enzyme immunoassay with gelatin-coated ferrite solid phase. Clin Chem 1994; 40:1830.

Jolley ME: Fluorescence polarization immunoassay for the determination of therapeutic drug levels in human plasma. J Anal Toxicol 1981; 5:236–240.

Kabat EA: Kabat and Meyer's Experimental Immunochemistry, 2nd ed. Springfield, IL, Charles C Thomas, 1961.

Kasahara Y: Homogeneous enzyme immunoassays. In Nakamura RM, Kasahara Y, Rechnitz GA (eds): Immunochemical Assays and Biosensor Technology for the 1990s. Washington, DC, American Society for Microbiology, 1992a, pp 169–182.

In this review, Kasahara describes the historical progression of immunoassay development, and reviews homogeneous enzyme immunoassays, addresses test sensitivity and procedure simplification, and their applicability to small haptens and large proteins.

Kasahara Y: Principles and applications of particle immunoassay. In Nakamura RM, Kasahara Y, Rechnitz GA (eds): Immunochemical Assays and Biosensor Technology for the 1990s. Washington, DC, American Society for Microbiology, 1992b, pp 127–147.

Kasahara Y, Ashihara Y: Simple devices and their possible application in clinical laboratory downsizing. Clin Chim Acta 1997; 267: 87–102

Immunochromatographic assays are powerful tools for point-of-care testing and near patient testing. This report describes immunochromatographic assays in a simplified immunoassay format for point-of-care testing and near patient testing, and discusses laboratory downsizing and laboratory automation with specific reference to the situation in Japan.

Kato K, Hamaguchi Y, Fukui H, et al: Enzyme-linked immunoassay, a simple method for synthesis of the rabbit antibody-β-D-galactosidase complex and its general applicability. J Biochem 1975; 78:423–425.

Kemp BE, Rylatt DB, Bundesen PG, et al: Autologous red cell agglutination assay for HIV-I antibodies: simplified test with whole blood. Science 1988;241:1352–1354.

Kitagawa T, Fujitake T, Taniyama H, et al: Enzyme immunoassay of viomycin, new cross-linking reagent for enzyme-labelling and a preparation method for antiserum of viomycin. J Biochem 1978; 83:1493–1501.

Koehler G, Milstein C: Continuous cultures of fused cells secreting antibody of predefined specificity. Nature 1975;256–495.

Kricka LJ: Chemiluminescent and bioluminescent techniques. Clin Chem 1991; 37:1472–1481.

In this review Kricka describes the characteristics and mechanisms of light emission from most of the chemiluminescent and bioluminescent molecules employed as detection signals in immunoassays and nucleic acid detection. This is an excellent review.

Magnani JL, Steplewski Z, Koprowski H: Identification of the gastrointestinal and pancreatic cancer-associated antigen detected by monoclonal antibody 19-9 in the sera of patients as a mucin. Cancer Res 1983; 43: 5489–5492.

Mancini G, Carbonara AO, Hereman JF: Immunochemical quantitation of antigens by single radial immunodiffusion. Immunochemistry 1965; 2:235.

Masson PL, Holy HW: Immunoassay by particle counting. In Rose NR, Friedman H, Fahey JL (eds): Manual of Clinical Laboratory Immunology, 3rd ed. Washington DC, American Society for Microbiology, 1986, 43–48.

Mathis G: Probing molecular interactions with homogeneous techniques based on rare earth cryptates and fluorescence energy transfer. Clin Chem 1995;41:1391–1397.

Mathis G: Rare earth cryptates and homogeneous fluoroimmunoassays with human sera. Clin Chem 1993;39:1953–1959.

Miles LEM, Hales CM: Labelled antibodies and immunological assay systems. Nature 1968; 219: 186–189.

Morris DL: Effect of antibodies to glucose oxidase in the apoenzyme reactivation immunoassay system. Anal Biochem 1985; 151: 235–41.

Morris DL, Ellis PB, Carrico FJ, et al: Flavin adenine dinucleotide as label in homogeneous colorimetric immunoassays. Anal Chem 1981; 53:658–665.

Nakane PK, Pierce GB:Enzyme-labeled antibodies: Preparation and application for localization of antigens. J Histochem Cytochem 1966;14:929–931

Nakamura RM, Monoclonal antibodies: Methods and clinical applications. Clin Physio Biochem 1983; 1: 160–72.

Nakamura RM: Fluorescence immunoassays. In Nakamura RM, Kasahara Y, Rechnitz GA (eds): Immunochemical Assays and Biosensor Technology for the 1990s. Washington, DC, American Society for Microbiology, 1992a, pp 205–227

Nakamura RM, Kasahara Y: Heterogeneous enzyme immunoassays. In Nakamura RM, Kasahara Y, Rechnitz GA (eds): Immunochemical Assays and Biosensor Technology for the 1990s. Washington, DC, American Society for Microbiology, 1992b, pp 149–167.

In this reference assay principles and assay performance are discussed, and practical application of heterogeneous enzyme immunoassays is described. This review will help the general reader gain an understanding of non-isotopic immunoassays, and will assist the researcher in developing enzyme immunoassays.

Nakamura RM, Robbins BA: Current status of homogeneous enzyme immunoassays. J Clin Lab Anal 1988; 2: 51.

Nargessi RD, Landon J, Smith DS: Use of antibodies against the label in non-separation non-isotopic immunoassay; 'indirect quenching' fluoroimmunoassay of protein. J Immunol Methods 1979; 26: 307–313.

Nishizono I, Ashihara Y, Tsuchiya H, et al: Homogeneous enzyme immunoassay for high molecular weight antigens (II). J Clin Lab Anal 1988; 2: 143–147.

Nishizono I, Iida S, Suzuki N, et al: Rapid and sensitive chemiluminescent enzyme immunoassay for measuring tumor markers. Clin Chem 1991; 37: 1639–1644.

Oliver KG, Kettman JR, Fulton RJ: Multiplexed analysis of human cytokines by use of the FlowMetrix system. Clin Chem 1998; 44: 2057–2060.

Patterson W, Werness P, Payne WJ, et al: Random and continuous-access immunoassays with chemiluminescent detection by Access automated analyzer. Clin Chem 1994; 40: 2042–2045.

Peluso P, Wilson D, Do D, et al: Optimizing antibody immobilization strategies for the construction of protein microarrays. Anal Biochem 2003; 312: 113–124.

Poulsen E, Sandegren F. CD microlaboratories – a fully automated solution for fast and flexible IgG quantification in biopharmaceutical process development. IBC Antibody Therapeutics, Nov 30–Dec 2, 2004. Available on line at: www.gyros.com/technology/tech_presentations.html.

Ritchie R: Automated immunoanalysis. New York, Marcel Decker, 1978.

Ritzmann SE, Daniels JC (eds): Serum protein abnormalities – diagnostic and clinical aspects. Boston, Little, Brown & Co., 1975.

Rodriguez-Espinosa J, Mora-Brugues J, Ordonez-Llanos J, et al: Technical and clinical performances of six sensitive immunoradiometric assays of thyrotropin in serum. Clin Chem 1987; 33:1439–1445.

Rogers LC, Kahn SE, Oeser TH, et al: The stratus immunofluorometric assay system evaluated for quantifying human chorionic gonadotropin in serum. Clin Chem 1986; 32: 1402.

Rose NR, Bigazzi PE (eds): Methods in Immunodiagnosis. New York, John Wiley & Sons, 1973, pp 1–30.

Rowley GL, Rubenstein JE, Huisjen J et al: Mechanism by which antibodies inhibit hapten-malate

dehydrogenase conjugates. J Biol Chem 1975; 250:3759–3766.

Rubenstein KE, Schneider RS, Ullman EF: Homogeneous enzyme immunoassay. A new immunological technique. Biochim Biophys Res Commun 1972; 47:846–851.

Scatchard G: The attractions of proteins for small molecules and ions. Ann NY Acad Sci 1949; 51:660–672.

Schroeder HR, Dean CL, Johnson PK, et al: Coupling aminohexyl-FAD to proteins with dimethyladipimidate. Clin Chem 1985; 31: 1432–1437.

Sgoutas DS, Barton EG, Hammarstrom M, et al: Four sensitive thyrotropin assays critically evaluated and compared. Clin Chem 1989; 25:1785–1789.

Silzel JW, Cercek B, Dodson C, et al: Mass-sensing, multianalyte microarray immunoassay with imaging detection. Clin Chem 1998; 44:2036–2203.

Skerra A, Pluckthun A: Assembly of a functional immunoglobulin Fv fragment in Escherichia coli. Science 1988; 240: 1038–1041.

Smith J, Osikowicz G: Abbott AxSYM random and continuous access immunoassay system for improved workflow in the clinical laboratory. Clin Chem 1993; 39: 2063–2069.

Soini E, Hemmila I: Fluoroimmunoassay: Present status and key problems. Clin Chem 1979; 25:353–361.

Soini E, Kojola H: Time resolved fluorometer for lanthanide chelates: a new generation of non isotopic immunoassays. Clin Chem 1983; 29:65–68.

Steward MW: Overview: introduction to methods used to study the affinity and kinetics of antibody–antigen reactions. In Weir M (ed): Handbook of Experimental Immunology, vol I; Immunochemistry, 4th ed. Oxford, Blackwell Scientific, 1986, p 25.

Thorpe GH, Haggart R, Kricka LJ, Whitehead TP: Enhanced luminescent enzyme immunoassays for rubella antibody, immunoglobulin E and digoxin. Biochem Biophys Res Commun 1984; 119: 481–487.

Thorpe GH, Kricka LJ, Moseley SB, Whitehead TP: Phenols as enhancers of the chemiluminescent horseradish peroxidase-luminol-hydrogen peroxide reaction: application in luminescence-monitored enzyme immunoassays. Clin Chem 1985; 31:1335–1341.

Towt J, Tsai SC, Hernandez MR, et al: ONTRAK TESTCUP: a novel, on-site, multi-analyte screen for the detection of abused drugs. J Anal Toxicol 1995; 19: 504–510.

Ullman EF, Schwartzberg M, Rubenstein KD: Fluorescent excitation transfer assay: A general method for determination of antigen. J Biol Chem 1976; 251: 4172–4178.

Ullman EF, Yoshida RA, Blakemore J, et al: Mechanism of inhibition of malate dehydrogenase by thyroxine derivatives and reactivation by antibodies: homogeneous enzyme immunoassay for thyroxine. Biochim Biophys Acta 1979 567:66–74.

Valkirs GE, Barton R. ImmunoConcentration™: a new format for solid-phase immunoassays. Clin Chem 1985; 31:1427–1431.

Van Weeman BD, Schuurs AHWM: Immunoassay using antigen enzyme conjugates. FEBS Lett 1971; 15:232..

Weeks I, Beheshti I, McCapra F, et al: Acridinium esters as high specific activity labels in an immunoassay. Clin Chem 1983; 29:1474–1479.

Williams CA, Chase MW (eds): Methods in Immunology and Immunochemistry, vol III. New York, Academic Press, 1970.

Winter G, Griffiths AD, Hawkins RE: Hoogenboom HR: Making antibodies by phage display technology. Annu Rev Immunol 1994; 12:433–455.

Wu AH, Wong SS, Waldron C, et al: Automated quantification of choriogonadotropin: analytical correlation between serum and urine with creatinine correction. Clin Chem 1987; 33:1424–1426.

Yalow RS, Berson SA: Assay of plasma insulin in human subjects by immunological methods. Nature 1959; 184:1648–1649.

Yamauchi S, Fujiwara Y, Hasegawa A, et al: Simple devices for sensitive and rapid detection of HBs-Ag and HBs-Ab by immunochromatography using enzyme (Abstract). Clin Chem, 1997; 43:S242.

Yarmush DM, Morel G, Yarmush ML: A new technique for mapping epitope specificities of monoclonal antibodies using quasi-elastic light scattering spectroscopy. J Biochem Biophys Methods 1987; 14:279–289.

Zola H: Monoclonal Antibodies: A Manual of Techniques. Boca Raton, Florida, CRC Press, 1987.

CHAPTER 44

Laboratory Evaluation of the Cellular Immune System

Roger S. Riley MD PhD, Jonathan Ben-Ezra MD

KEY POINTS

- Humoral immune tests assess production of specific antibody responses to past or recent infections, while cellular immune assays measure current immune responses.

- The immune system changes with age and nutritional status, so differences in test subject immune responses may be associated with immaturity, immunosenescence, or malnutrition and should be taken into account when evaluating the results of specific tests.

- Primary immunodeficiency may be associated with an increased incidence of malignancy; malignancy, chemotherapy, and radiotherapy can significantly suppress the immune response and alter cellular immune assay results.

- The evaluation of the cellular immune response is undertaken in a graduated sequence of stages that may include both in vitro and in vivo testing to identify areas of immune deficiency.

- Measurement of lymphocyte activation may be accomplished in vitro by flow cytometry using activation-specific fluorescent-labeled monoclonal antibodies and vital dyes. The usefulness of this approach has increased significantly with the development of fluorochromes with different excitation spectra.

Immune system understanding is greatly enhanced by detection of discrete abnormalities in patients with suspected immune deficiency. These advances have come from studies of normal immune cell differentiation and function, from experimental gene deletion, and from detailed analysis of human immunodeficiency syndromes. New experimental approaches have helped to elucidate the mechanisms and functional basis of immune dysregulation in patients with primary (congenital) genetic mutations of the immune system or secondary (acquired) congenital infections. Since immune deficiencies usually cannot be distinguished by clinical presentation of infections, genetic information is becoming an increasingly important component of diagnostic testing and interpretation. The mission of the clinical immunology laboratory is to translate new research leads into highly standardized and clinically relevant tests for the individual patient.

Studies of the human cellular immune system have focused mainly in three areas: (1) primary immune deficiency, which reveals the impact of congenital immune defects on host defense; (2) autoimmune diseases, where the effect of excessive or inappropriate immune activity is evident; and (3) acquired immune deficiency, in which infection damages the immune system directly, such as human immunodeficiency virus (HIV) infection. In addition, cellular immune defects of diseases with immune dysfunctional features, such as chronic infection, cancer, malnutrition, or traumatic injury, provide crucial insight into immune-mediated host defense.

The general concept of 'immunity' has been often equated with humoral immunity, the presence of potentially protective antibodies to an infectious agent introduced by natural infection or by immunization. Because immunology, as currently practiced in a clinical laboratory, is a relatively new science (Silverstein, 1979; Moulin, 1989; Good, 2002), it required the HIV epidemic to demonstrate the true impact of this powerful and mutable arm of the immune system. In contrast to humoral immunity, cellular immune function is both fundamentally complex and not easy to measure. Basic humoral immune tests measure the specific antibody product of a past response to a specific virus or microbe; by contrast, cellular immune assays measure current responses.

Since the majority of peripheral blood lymphocytes are resting cells, the cellular immune reaction must be recreated or generated freshly in the test system. The system must be capable of triggering the response, supporting the reaction by providing all needed elements available in vivo, as well as having a measurable end point. The field of cellular immunology changed dramatically during the 1980s, through the impact of major research efforts, including the use of monoclonal antibodies to identify immune cells, the development of analytic and sorting capabilities of the flow cytometer, the discovery of cytokine regulation of immune response, the birth of molecular immunology, and, above all, the tremendous need to understand and control the emerging HIV epidemic (Herzenberg, 2004). The appearance of HIV occurred virtually in parallel with the potential to identify CD4+ T cells. The first analyses of cellular immune functional deficiency in the acquired immunodeficiency syndrome (AIDS) were initially based on analysis of lymphocyte proliferative response (Masur, 1981; Siegal, 1981) and have since evolved into a range of functional approaches (Perfetto, 1997; Rosenberg, 1997; Zhou, 1998).

Table 44–1 Presentation of Possible Immunodeficiency

Frequent bacterial infection
Unusually severe systemic reaction to a virus
Development of infection with an unusual organism such as fungus or protozoan
Systemic reaction following live virus vaccination
Family history of recurrent infections
Exposure to the human immunodeficiency virus

This chapter presents current cellular immunologic tests in the light of future trends. Cellular immune assessment is moving away from single assays and single number fixed end points toward an integrated analysis of cell function at several levels that reflects cellular interactions as a dynamic process.

Clinical Criteria for Evaluation of Cellular Immunity: Implications for Interpretation

Decision to Test

Although in theory the interpretation of immune tests develops out of a careful differential approach towards screening, in practical terms, a patient's immune response is studied in the context of the current clinical presentation. However, immune tests may be expensive and time-consuming, so that choice of test is often dependent on clinical suspicion. Since there are few, if any, cellular immune tests that are totally and specifically diagnostic, interpretation should be approached with caution. The responsibility of the clinical immunology laboratory is to establish a sufficient range of tests to perform judicious testing for determination of nature and extent of the immune alteration, and to consider a range of potential causes when providing interpretation.

The decision to test immune response in a patient usually arises for one of the reasons described in Table 44–1. Increased or unexplained susceptibility to infection, increased severity of common infections, or unusual reaction to immunization are reasons for immune evaluation. Unusual infections, especially opportunistic agents or severe infections unresponsive to treatment, and certain allergic or atopic states may also prompt immune testing. In recent years, potential HIV infection has replaced possible primary immune deficiency as the leading presumptive diagnosis. However, as discussed subsequently, this may lead to underdiagnosis of primary immune deficiency disease.

Immune changes may accompany many clinical entities, including malignancies, hematologic diseases such as Fanconi anemia, hemophilia, immune thrombocytopenia, lymphoproliferative disorders such as histiocytosis, and the hemoglobinopathies such as sickle cell anemia and thalassemia, as well as a fairly wide range of chromosomal abnormalities such as DiGeorge syndrome, Down syndrome, Bloom syndrome, Williams congenital dyskeratosis, epidermolysis bullosa, and Duncan syndrome (X-linked lymphoproliferative disorder). Autoimmune diseases such as the rheumatic diseases, mixed connective tissue disease, type 1 diabetes, systemic lupus erythematosus, amyotrophic lateral sclerosis, multiple sclerosis, and myasthenia gravis may be associated with cellular immune changes and are further discussed elsewhere in this book.

Primary Versus Secondary Immune Deficiency

The principal features of primary immune deficiency, or suspected acquired immune deficiency due to HIV infection, must be distinguished from immune changes associated with other clinical conditions. Furthermore, traumatic injury such as burns or accidents resulting in major blood loss or organ damage often produce a period of vulnerability to infections. In addition, other conditions such as underlying premalignancy or undiagnosed infectious diseases may produce immune changes that could appear phenotypically identical to primary immunodeficiency.

While HIV infection can be readily diagnosed by direct testing, the clinical immunology laboratory is sometimes used as a proving ground before approaching the patient or guardian for informed consent for HIV testing. This is based on the observation that, at least among HIV-positive adults, an inverted CD4$^+$/CD8$^+$ ratio is virtually always found. Thus, as a result of the current AIDS epidemic, inverted CD4$^+$/CD8$^+$ ratio has become identified as a marker of HIV infection. However, there are a number of diseases involving the immune system other than HIV that can produce an inverted CD4$^+$/CD8$^+$ ratio or extremely low CD4$^+$ cell numbers. These include, but are not limited to, DiGeorge syndrome, benign thymoma, onset of hepatitis C virus (HCV) infection, Kawasaki disease, protein calorie malnutrition, and malignancy. Some examples of non-HIV-related inverted CD4$^+$/CD8$^+$ ratio and low CD4$^+$ numbers are shown in Table 44–2. The infant shown as Case 3 (Table 44–2) presented with multiple septic abscesses of the gastrointestinal tract and was thought to have a primary immune deficiency disorder. However, this evaluation occurred following a near-drowning episode in a bathtub later found to contain traces of drain cleaner. Caustic damage to the gastrointestinal tract produced the multiple unusual lesions and the peripheral T-lymphocyte subset imbalance. The T-lymphocyte subset imbalance, but not the gastrointestinal tract damage, resolved rapidly. This case also illustrates the need to conduct confirmatory testing as soon as possible when the patient is stable.

Primary immune deficiency disorders nearly always present in the context of infection or hematologic changes. Laboratory evaluation of these disorders requires a stepwise approach in order to minimize blood drawing and to choose logically among available tests for the purpose of differential diagnosis. Some presumptive diagnoses may appear to be too frequently suspected, for example, Wiskott–Aldrich syndrome, although this does need to be ruled out in cases of unexplained thrombocytopenia. However, Wiskott–Aldrich syndrome may be missed if response to mitogens alone is tested rather than response to antigens as well, and the immune defect may become more marked with time so that follow-up testing may be needed.

Table 44–2 Inverted CD4$^+$/CD8$^+$ Ratio, Low CD4$^+$ in Non-HIV Immunodeficiency

Case Study	Age	Lymphocyte Subsets % CD3$^+$	% CD4$^+$	% CD8$^+$	Abs No.	Diagnosis
1. Initial	3 years	56	26	29	209	Idiopathic CD4 deficiency
2. Initial	6 years	73	18	24	330	Dyskeratosis
3. Initial	3 months	29	15	10	762	Congenital R/O immunodeficiency
1 week	–	43	25	15	2846	Caustic gastrointestinal trauma
4. Initial	6 years	89	62	32	874	Red blood cell aplasia
3 years	–	93	36	57	272	–
5. Initial	3 months	83	51	31	2734	Noonan syndrome
5 months	–	76	18	48	96	–
6. Initial	4 months	36	25	7	304	Williams syndrome
1 year	–	51	42	12	2794	–
7. Initial	1 week	0	0	24	0	DiGeorge syndrome
8. Initial	12 years	64	20	33	ND	Thalassemia
9. Initial	8 years	65	26	47	ND	Immune neutropenia
10. Initial	50 years	74	18	51	ND	Uveal melanoma
1 day	–	72	45	35	ND	Post-hyperthermia

Abs No. = absolute number of CD4$^+$ T lymphocytes.

Clinical Significance of Tests of Immune Deficiency

An issue that often confronts the cellular immunology laboratory director is how to evaluate the potential clinical significance of impaired immune response in vitro. Studies of even relatively well defined disorders have shown that there may be very significant differences in clinical impact. However, the use of newer testing strategies can be helpful in subclassifying patients by level and extent of defect.

For example, the DiGeorge syndrome (DiGeorge, 1974) is classically a triad of thymic and parathyroid aplasia and conotruncal defects. Patients with the DiGeorge syndrome show marked differences in the severity of infections in spite of relatively similar findings of reduced numbers of mature T lymphocytes and a poor response to mitogens. Initially there was a very high degree of fatality associated with this syndrome. Improved surgical and anesthesia methods led to a significant decrease in the incidence of severe infections, although some infants still developed intractable and ultimately fatal infections (Bastian, 1989). Recently, it has been possible to use more exact lymphocyte phenotype analysis to determine the severity of the immune defect and to predict clinical outcome more accurately. Using longitudinal testing over several months and a multiple parametric approach, it now seems that severity may be predictable from consistently low CD4+ T-cell numbers, inverted CD4+/CD8+ ratio, and reduced lymphokine interleukin (IL)-2 production (Cunningham-Rundles, 1994). Investigation into the significance of monosomic deletions of chromosome 22q11.2, which are the leading cause of DiGeorge syndrome, velocardiofacial syndrome, and conotruncal anomaly face syndrome, illustrates the importance of new genetic information. Only DiGeorge syndrome was originally described as an immunodeficiency disorder. New studies looking at the frequency of immunodeficiency in the other clinical syndromes associated with the chromosome 22q11.2 microdeletion have shown that more than 75% of patients had evidence of immunocompromise (Sullivan, 1998). The severity of the immunodeficiency did not correlate with any particular phenotypic feature.

T-cell function may be as important or more important in HIV infection than loss of CD4+ T cells or rate of loss. In some virus-associated illnesses, there is considerable uncertainty as to how close the association is between immune deficit detected ex vivo and immune function in vivo (Landay, 1991; Lloyd, 1992). While current studies suggest that altered orthostatic response (Rowe, 1999) may explain some forms of chronic fatigue syndrome or that increased plasma levels of tumor necrosis factor (TNF)-α may be a disease marker (Moss, 1999), there is no clear understanding of cause and effect.

The Effect of Age on Immune Response

Current studies demonstrate that the immune system changes as part of the aging process (Burns, 2004). Although there is considerable variation in this and much is a consequence of altered nutritional status (Mazari, 1998; Lesourd, 2004), it is essential that the clinical laboratory provides relevant laboratory values for age-matched controls.

The study of pediatric patients presents particular issues for the laboratory diagnosis for immune deficiency. The development of the immune system in the child is not complete at birth and, in addition, children have not been exposed to a wide variety of abnormal environmental agents and may have vulnerability to infections (Zola, 1996). Congenital viral exposure or prematurity alone may be associated with immune abnormalities. Key differences in pediatric immune response include marked lymphocytosis at birth, elevation of B cells, increased CD4+/CD8+ T-cell ratio, few natural killer (NK) cells, and oligoclonal T-cell expansions (Yabuhara, 1990; Fletcher, 1992; Cunningham-Rundles, 1993; Wedderburn, 2001). These differences are reflected in marked differences in the normal range of lymphocyte subsets and must be taken into account in evaluation of results (Denny, 1992; Bonilla, 1997). Also, there are marked differences in response to various activators as compared to adults. The neonatal response of premature infants to certain microbial activators may be stronger than that of adults or full-term infants because of rapid changes in immune regulation (Veber, 1991; Cunningham-Rundles, 2000) or because of fundamental differences in perinatal programming (Prescott, 1998). The immune system of elderly individuals also shows changes in comparison to younger adults. In particular, cumulative alterations in critical B- and T-cell subpopulations, altered cell signaling and cytokine production, and other changes may contribute to the increased incidence of autoimmune disease and cancer in this group (Ginaldi, 2000; Fulop, 2003; Hakim, 2004). The deterioration of immune responses with increasing age has been designated 'immunosenescence' (Malaguarnera, 2001).

Malnutrition and Immune Response

Although it is generally believed that malnutrition is relatively rare in developed countries, growing evidence suggests that malnutrition is fairly common, especially in certain age groups (Pennington, 1996). Malnutrition is associated with immune deficiency and causes significant vulnerability to infections (Cunningham-Rundles, 1996; Keusch, 2003). For example, zinc deficiency can present as a profound immune deficiency, which may be related to the primary lack of zinc uptake at the gastrointestinal tract, to acrodermatitis enteropathica, or to lack of adequate zinc in the diet (Prasad, 1963; Moynahan, 1974). Persons with hypogammaglobulinemia and associated malabsorption affecting zinc levels may show poor proliferative response in vitro and infections that resolve with zinc repletion (Cunningham-Rundles, 1981). This is associated with the fact that zinc is required for the biological activity of thymic hormone, needed for the production of functionally mature T cells and for activation of T cells (Cunningham-Rundles, 1998). There is increasing evidence that micronutrient imbalance will alter immune response through specific effects on immune response (Amati, 2003). In many clinical settings, malnutrition may be a complicating factor. The interaction of infections with altered metabolism secondary to the acute phase response can cause temporal shifts in trace elements, leading to transient suppression of immune response. Physical stress may have a similar effect and lead to enhanced vulnerability to infections in the context of immune suppression (Cunningham-Rundles, 1999). This is a two-way process. Growth failure may be the first sign of HIV infection in an HIV+ child (Peters, 1998). For this as well as other reasons, immune evaluations should be an ongoing process in the context of continuing treatment or other testing.

Cancer

Primary immunodeficiency is associated with an increased incidence of cancer (Cunningham-Rundles, 1987) and it is increasingly clear that tumors develop in association with HIV infection (Krown, 1996; Aoki, 2004).

In the patient with cancer, generalized immune deficiency or reduction in response to antigenic challenge may appear in association with the development of primary malignancy, occur during metastasis, or be caused by the side effects of therapeutic intervention. Reduced immune response to nonspecific activators studied ex vivo in proliferation assays does correlate with stage of disease and has prognostic significance for survival (Heimdal, 1999). Inverted CD4+/CD8+ ratio and increased suppressor cell activity are often observed in untreated cancer patients and changes in cytokine production have been observed (Livingston, 1987; Smyth, 2004). Experimental studies have shown that tumors may be surprisingly immunogenic but drive the immune response towards a nonprotective response.

The development of new immunotherapeutic approaches is increasing, suggesting that response to tumor-specific antigens will be used more in the future (Schultes, 2004; Steinman, 2004; Waller, 2004). Immune response assays may also be used to track and evaluate response to treatments such as IL-2 (Lissoni, 1999) and cancer vaccines (Yannelli, 2004). In many patients, chemotherapy will produce transient suppression of immune response that resolves within a short period of time, while radiation may have longer-term effects (Katz, 1993). The assessment of immune response in the cancer patient requires highly selected and discriminating use of tests and activators, which reflect relevant processes, as well as specificity of response.

Methodologic Approach to Cellular Immune Testing

Human studies have been based on observation of peripheral blood immune cells because the peripheral compartment is most accessible and readily measured, but this approach may not reflect regional events. Knowledge of the differences between systemic and mucosal immune response may ultimately explain many current paradoxes arising when immune response measured in vitro or ex vivo is compared to host defense in vivo (Xu-Amano, 1993). Systemic cellular immune function appears to be regulated through functionally distinct T-helper-type cytokine patterns ('the cytokine network'), such that when T-helper type 1 (Th1) cytokines, IL-2, and interferon (IFN)-γ are produced, cellular immune host defense is favored. When T-helper type 2 (Th2) cytokines, IL-4, IL-5, IL-6, and II-10 are produced, B-lymphocyte response is induced (Balkwill, 1989; Yamamura, 1991).

In contrast to systemic immunity, the primary activity of the mucosal immune response is to protect the mucosa by blocking microbial, toxin, and antigen entry through secretion and transport of immunoglobulin

Table 44–3 Basic Scanning Immunology Studies

Complete blood count/differential

Lymphocyte subpopulation analysis (numbers and percentages of T and B cells) by flow cytometry

Lymphocyte activation in vitro to mitogens and microbial activators

Serum immunoglobulins, including immunoglobulin subclasses if evidence of clinical infections with encapsulated bacteria. In some cases, immunoglobulin levels are normal but heterogeneous nonbinding antibodies are produced; thus, additional studies are needed

Table 44–4 Confirming and First-Stage Analytical Studies

Radiograph for thymic shadow

Skin test

Natural killer cell activity (if child is 6 months or older)

Cytokine production in response to activation T-helper 1, T-helper 2 (IL-2, IFN-γ, IL-4, and so on)

Mixed lymphocyte culture reaction with patient as stimulator and patient as responder

Response to immunization

    Test for presence of age-appropriate specific antibodies

    Naturally occurring antibody response to isohemagglutinins (anti-A and -B blood group substances) if patient has A, B, or O blood type

Test for adenosine deaminase and purine nucleoside phosphorylase enzyme deficiency

(Ig)A to the lumen of the gut, a process mediated by a special type of memory T lymphocyte with reduced proliferative capacity capable of providing B-cell help (Tlaskalova-Hogenova, 2002; Cheroutre, 2004; Eckmann, 2004; Yuan, 2004). Both lamina propria T lymphocytes and intraepithelial T lymphocytes develop in relative independence of the thymus and function differently from peripheral blood T cells in using the CD2 signal transduction pathway rather than the T-cell receptor/CD3 pathway.

At present, tests of mucosal immunity are usually not performed in the clinical immunology laboratory and, with rare exceptions, the immune cells under study are from the peripheral blood compartment. For this reason, the use of in vivo skin testing and examination of humoral immune response to previously encountered vaccines is useful to the cellular immunologist, as these provide another means of assessment. In all cases, the use of a stepwise approach and repeated testing is highly informative.

Stages of Study: The Scanning Stage

The evaluation of immune function in a patient with possible immune deficiency is normally achieved in stages. The first stage is a scanning analysis of possible areas of deficiency and is outlined in Table 44–3. These scanning studies should be accompanied by appropriate flow cytometric analysis of lymphocyte subpopulations, and in children must include use of a B-cell marker to assess possible B-cell shifts, which may occur transiently in the neonate and be reflected in low T-cell populations. The use of an NK cell marker is also strongly recommended in young children over 3 months of age, since levels in this population may be reduced or absent at birth (Zola, 1983).

Since there is frequently a limitation on blood to be drawn for such studies it is essential that the first evaluation includes parallel studies, including a complete blood count (CBC), on the same specimen of blood. It is essential that a leukocyte differential be carried out.

The scanning stage will include a panel approach to assess mitogenic and antigenic proliferative response. The proliferative response of lymphocytes to a range of activators continues to be one of the most sensitive tools to assess normal function and, when this includes an appropriate T-cell and B-cell activator, it can be useful in defining the areas of defect. Although this is not always done, the use of multiple concentrations of each activator is strongly recommended.

In addition, the type of tube chosen to draw the blood is important. The use of lithium heparin or ethylenediaminetetraacetic acid (EDTA)-containing tubes is not recommended for any lymphocyte functional studies. Sodium heparin (preservative-free) or acid citrate dextrose (ACD) tubes must be used. Blood collected in heparinized tubes can also be used for flow cytometric analysis, although timing for specimen preparation and analysis is critical (Standards, 1992; Nicholson, 1993b).

The question of when the blood should be drawn is important. In general, most data have been obtained with blood drawn in the morning and there are circadian effects that may influence results. When this cannot be done, it is helpful to continue to maintain a uniformity of drawing time for an individual patient. This is most critical when measuring absolute numbers of T-lymphocyte subsets in the monitoring of HIV disease or as part of a clinical trial (Malone, 1990).

Functional studies need to be carried out on fresh anticoagulated blood whenever possible (or blood stored at room temperature in the dark for under 24 hours) before mononuclear cells are isolated. When blood is being sent by air or transport to a distant laboratory, it is extremely important to include a control specimen drawn in parallel from a healthy person to serve as an internal standard for the shipping process.

Stages of Study: The Confirming Stage

General Aspects

Once the screening of the individual has been achieved and evidence of potential gaps has been observed, these tests should be confirmed by repeat tests of aspects of the first series. Minimally, a positive and a negative (normal range and abnormal range) test should be carried out. Additional tests may sometimes be added to the panel, which may provide the beginning phase of analytical studies.

It is important to make appropriate arrangements to draw blood when a patient is in the most clinically stable state. Double baseline studies are recommended before intervention is undertaken, and these can encompass the confirming phase. In some cases of apparent immune deficiency there may be sequestration of immune cells, which is reflected in low percentages of T lymphocytes in the peripheral compartment, as illustrated in Table 44–2, Case 3. The confirmation stage should also include a careful re-evaluation of the patient's medical history and family history. Studies that may be used at this confirming stage are shown in Table 44–4.

Thymic Presence

The radiograph for thymic shadow may be inadequate, since the thymus is highly prone to stress depletion (Haynes, 1998). Although difficult to determine with accuracy, the actual size of the thymus assessed by magnetic resonance imaging (MRI) has been found to correlate with CD4$^+$ T-lymphocyte number in HIV infection (Vigano, 1999). Recent studies suggest that the human thymus can be thought of as a chimeric organ comprised of both central and peripheral lymphoid tissues. Haynes (1998) has postulated that thymic epithelial atrophy may in part derive from cytokines or other factors produced by peripheral immune cells within the thymic perivascular space. As described in the section on flow cytometry evaluation of T-lymphocyte subsets below, expression of normal maturation antigens acquired during thymic development will suffice to identify the presence of a working thymus.

The Skin Test

The use of a skin test panel can be important at this point. This approach to cellular immune assessment originally served as the departure point for the development of the cellular immune functional tests; it measures delayed-type hypersensitivity directly in vivo. Experience with the delayed type hypersensitivity skin test has shown good overall correlation between lack of reactivity, termed anergy, and immune deficiency (Deodhar, 1983; Maas, 1998) but has not been useful as an analytical tool to dissect out the reason for lack of response. The skin test is not very quantifiable. The use of the purified protein derivative (PPD) skin test to assess possible presence of Mycobacterium tuberculosis is an exception, although anergic individuals do not respond and, in addition, there are false positives in persons who have been vaccinated with bacille Calmette–Guérin (BCG) (Huebner, 1993).

Reasons for lack of skin test response are shown in Table 44–5. Some studies have been based on a de novo immunization skin test using dinitrofluorobenzene. While this was once used rather extensively, this approach is no longer considered useful because of ambiguities in the underlying mechanism of reaction. The introduction of the 'skin window' test may ultimately provide a more quantitative and informative measure of in vivo immune response because the reaction can be used to test autologous tumor response (Black, 1988). However, despite some reservations, the importance of the skin test as a convincing demonstration that immune defects noted in vitro may have prognostic significance in vivo should not be underestimated.

Stages of Study: Analytical Immune Studies

Analytical studies are outlined generally in Table 44–6. While complete description of these approaches is beyond the scope of this discussion, in

Table 44–5 Causes of Skin Test Anergy

Lack of appropriate antigenic history when panel does not include ubiquitous activators

Primary immunodeficiency

Viral infections

Malnutrition

Granulomatous diseases

Neoplasia

Table 44–6 Analytical and Immunoregulatory Studies

Development of activation antigens during response to stimulation, such as Tac antigen, transferrin receptor, upregulation for MHC class II on T cells, soluble receptors, and so on

Early activation response (e.g., calcium channels)

Immunoregulation

    Response to IL-1, IL-2, interferons

    Development of effector functions

    Immunoglobulin synthesis in vitro

    Cytotoxic T-cell activity

    Suppressor cell/factor analysis

Gene activation, cell cycle analysis

Response to immunization: de novo immunization

Table 44–7 Immunophenotyping Lymphocyte Subpopulations

Basic peripheral blood panel (whole blood, lysed red blood cells*)

    CD45/CD14

    Isotype mouse immunoglobulin controls

    CD3/CD19

    CD3/CD4

    CD3/CD8

    CD3-/CD56 and 16

Isolated mononuclear cells, activation panel[†]

    CD45/CD14

    Isotype mouse immunoglobulin controls

    CD3/CD25 (IL-2R)

    CD3/HLA-DR

* If low CD3, then repeat and add CD2. Further, monoclonals against T-cell receptor paired with CD3 may be added. Monocyte markers may also be evaluated. These may also be performed using three- or four-color reagents using CD45 gating.

[†] After 2 days of culture, remove cells and wash before staining with monoclonal antibodies listed; analyze control cells containing no activator, then analyze activated cells. Activators may include mitogen, IL-2, and/or interferon-γ.

general these studies are aimed at defining the underlying mechanism of immune defect and proceed through a series of steps. Although there are different possible ways of doing this, one good way is to assess the general level of defect by following the general plan of assessing presence of cell types and relative proportions of each in the light of areas of diminished general function and then to perform studies of effector function.

Differential Immune Function

There are two main immune cell types (Silverstein, 2003; Janeway, 2005): T lymphocytes (T cells) and B lymphocytes (B cells). T lymphocytes are defined by expression of the T-lymphocyte receptor, which binds to antigen and CD3, a surface determinant associated with the T-cell receptor that is essential for activation. T lymphocytes have different, clonally variable receptors for a large range of antigens, require thymic maturation for normal function, and mediate cellular immunity. B lymphocytes are identified by surface immunoglobulin (detected by monoclonal antibodies such as CD19 or CD20) and upon appropriate activation develop into plasma cells secreting specific antibody and thus mediate humoral immunity. Loss of the normal thymus will compromise T-lymphocyte function and affect T-dependent B-lymphocyte activation. Failure at the bone marrow level can affect both T-lymphocyte and B-lymphocyte immune response, although specific linkages may be involved. This is described in more detail later under 'Lymphocyte Proliferation as an In Vitro Method of Assessing Cellular Immunity'.

The distinction between specific and nonspecific immune response is a fundamental necessity in immune response, since the system must be able to distinguish between self and nonself (LeGuern, 2003; Smith, 2004). In general this is accomplished by the incorporation of the molecular complex major histocompatibility complex (MHC) self-antigen system into the antigen recognition phase. Antigen must be processed and presented in the context of self-MHC to be recognized and lead to response and the development of immune memory. The antigen processing function is carried out by antigen-presenting cells (APCs); the best studied is the monocyte. This response triggers lymphocyte activation and proliferation, and may include production of effector cells and triggering of B lymphocytes to produce antibody. This kind of immunity, often termed adaptive immunity, is retained as 'memory' and is typically elicited following immunization or natural infection (Owen, 1993; Sprent, 2002). Lack of expression of MHC class II antigen can be detected on lymphocytes by flow cytometry using monoclonal antibodies against HLA-DR or HLA-DQ and is a hallmark of MHC class II deficiency (Table 44–7).

A second fundamental type of immunity can be described as innate immunity, does not have memory, and is not improved by repeated contact (Janeway, 2002). This immunity is mediated by phagocytic cells, some of which, like the monocyte, can also process and present antigen, and NK cells. Unlike phagocytic cells, NK cells are not functionally

developed at birth, probably because the key cytokine, IFN-γ, which is needed for development and maturation of this system, is also downregulated at birth.

This third arm, represented by the NK cell, which is neither B-cell- nor exactly T-cell-like in having neither surface immunoglobulin nor a rearranged T-cell receptor (Yokoyama, 2004; Hamerman, 2005). This cell, once called the 'K' cell, 'null' cell, or 'third population,' has eluded conventional classification by cell lineage analysis. Currently, CD56 is considered the most definitive marker of the NK cell (Trinchieri, 1995). NK cells have been best known as cells that can kill nonspecifically (naturally) virally infected cells and bacteria and prevent tumor cell metastasis. However, NK cells also regulate T- and B-cell functions, and hematopoiesis. These functions of NK cells are probably dependent on their ability to produce lymphokines, particularly IFN-γ. NK cells are important for antigen-independent activation of phagocytic cells early in infection and for favoring the development of antigen-specific Th1 cells. The NK system is constitutively active and does not have to be primed by antigen to kill. When armed with specific antibody, however, these cells can kill specifically. Functional evaluation of this cell population can be readily achieved using a short-term chromium release assay (known as an NK cytotoxicity assay using K-562s as targets) or by flow cytometry (Hermans, 2004). Studies in the future will be performed to detect how NK cells bridge innate and adaptive immunity (Peritt, 1998).

Development of Immune Response

If cell populations have been determined to be essentially intact in the absence of activation, the issue of intrinsic failure may be studied by many different approaches, including the use of expanded lymphocyte surface marker analysis, including framework determinants to the T-cell antigen receptor (TCR), and activation antigens such as CD25, CD38, and HLA-DR (Table 44–7). Absence of MHC class II upregulation in response to IFN-γ is one example. Although cell populations may express a reference normal differentiation antigen, they may also coexpress others inappropriately, and this may be a key to functional abnormality. For example, CD8[+] T cells coexpressing CD38 are not functionally the same as CD8 cells that do not express this marker and are expanded in HIV disease (Giorgi, 1989). Absence of expression of certain molecules, such as CD28, is also an important indicator. In some primary immune deficiency syndromes, upregulation of the IL-2 receptor in response to IL-2 may be abnormal. Receptors may not be translocated normally or receptors may be shed prematurely (Cunningham-Rundles, 1990).

The development of the immune response may be kinetically abnormal, because of delayed secondary recruitment during the amplification phase. This should be tested by doing time course studies. In some cases, cytokines may not be made, or may be functionally altered. Effector functions may be missing or impaired. Evaluation of this may require a detailed approach. Attempts to restore response by cytokine addition may be useful, although this may circumvent the lesion through compensation rather than filling in the actual deficiency. New testing strategies may use whole blood rather than isolated mononuclear cells (Boccheri, 1995). This system provides an excellent ex vivo mirror of immune response, since the actual relationships among cells are not altered. Furthermore, this system can be used to measure cytokine production (Petrovsky, 1995; Suni, 1998).

VI

The cellular immunology laboratory is advised to choose basic analytical studies, which are normally done on a routine basis so that there is a basis of comparison. The establishment of laboratory normal ranges and maintenance of reagent quality control, especially for certain variable elements, is essential for accuracy and sensitivity of these tests.

Lymphocyte Proliferation as an In Vitro Method of Assessing Cellular Immunity

Cellular Immunology

Lymphocyte Activation and Proliferation

Although the immune system is classically divided into humoral and cellular components, this separation is in no way absolute, since there is considerable interdependence between B and T cells.

The most commonly measured functional cellular immune parameter is lymphocyte proliferation (Perfetto, 2002). Measurement of lymphocyte activation/proliferation has evolved substantially since the late 1950s and early 1960s, when cell division was determined by counting the number of lymphocytes that had transformed into blasts. The latter method was largely replaced by the quantification of incorporated radiolabeled nucleic acid precursors (tritiated thymidine) into newly synthesized DNA. Although this 'bulk assay' remains the most commonly used laboratory procedure to measure cellular proliferation, new reagents and new procedures have recently become available to assess lymphocyte activation and proliferation. These include the commercial availability of cell surface proliferation markers, the ability to measure the percentages of cells in specific phases of the cell cycle, the quantification of cell-associated and secreted cytokines/cytokine receptors, and the ability to assess the number of cell divisions in lymphocytes labeled with 'tracking dyes.' In this section we review the molecular events involved in T-lymphocyte activation and proliferation and review some of the new methods that have been developed to assess the functions of the cellular immune system.

Unraveling the Biochemical Pathways of Lymphocyte Activation

Following the specific interaction of mitogen or antigen/MHC with the appropriate lymphocyte receptors, several cellular processes occur, including changes in membrane transport, rearrangement of the cytoskeletal system (polarizing the lymphocyte toward APC), and activation of several signaling pathways (Harding, 2005). These changes ultimately lead to T-cell differentiation, cytokine secretion, proliferation, anergy, or apoptosis. Ongoing investigations are unraveling the complex molecular and biochemical pathways that drive the activated T cell down these pathways. Specific abnormalities in these pathways are constantly being discovered and underlie many of the primary immunodeficiency diseases. Unfortunately, abnormalities in a bulk proliferation assay indicate only that there is limited or no cell division and provide no information regarding the underlying abnormality in lymphocyte activation. More sophisticated assays are required to investigate the underlying T-cell abnormalities.

Antigen-Induced Activation of T Lymphocytes

Antigen/MHC-induced activation of T lymphocytes involves a series of complex and defined events that differ slightly between the activation of a naive T cell versus the activation of a memory T cell. Antigen is processed by B cells or monocytes, leading to the assembly of immunogenic peptides into the class I or class II products of the MHC genes (van der Merwe, 2003). The peptide/MHC complex is presented to T cells bearing the appropriate T-cell receptor. In addition, the APC expresses a series of adhesion and co-stimulatory molecules that interact with the appropriate ligand/counter receptors on the T-cell surface. Ligation of the T-cell receptor alone is not sufficient for the activation of the T cell, which has led to the development of the 'two signal model' for T cell activation (Bretscher, 1992, 2004). The first signal delivered via the TCR/CD4/CD8 modulates the transition of the T cell from the early stages of activation (i.e., G_0 to G_1). Signal two is delivered via the co-stimulatory pathways, most notably CD28 and to a lesser extent LFA-3, CD2, CD5, and CD7, and leads to the induction of IL-2 and other cytokine genes required for T-cell proliferation and differentiation to effector cells.

T-Cell Recognition, Activation, and Signal Transduction

The TCR complex is composed of a both a heterodimeric antigen recognition structure (i.e., the TCR) and a non-covalently bound transducing complex referred to as CD3 (Malissen, 2003). The TCR cannot be expressed on the cell surface without CD3 (Weiss, 1991) and has no inherent signaling capabilities of its own. The antigen recognition structure is composed of structurally divergent α and β chains (or less frequently the γ and δ chains) and the CD3-transducing complex is composed of five invariant polypeptide chains, α, β, ϵ, and a ζ-chain dimer. Each of the CD3 proteins contains a motif called the immune tyrosine activation motif (ITAM), which binds the SH2 domains of protein tyrosine kinases. The ζ chain (which exists as a ζ homodimer, a ζ with an η or a ζ with an Fc ϵ RI γ chain) contains 3 ITAMs and is the most significant component of the TCR complex involved in signal transduction from the TCR (Weiss, 1994; Alarcon, 2003). Originally described by Reth, these motifs play an essential role in the early events following T-cell activation (Reth, 1989; Irving, 1991). CD4 and CD8 molecules on the surface of T cells are also noncovalently attached to the TCR complex. They bind to HLA class II and class I molecules, respectively, on the APC and are also involved in transduction of activation signals. Processed antigen is presented to T cells in the context of the MHC antigens. In general, CD4+ T cells respond to exogenously processed antigens presented in the context of MHC Class II and CD8+ T cells respond to endogenously processed antigens presented in the context of MHC Class I. CD4 and CD8 are also associated with tyrosine kinases involved in the early events following T-cell activation. In addition to these interactions and the co-stimulatory molecule interactions, another group of molecules present (adhesion molecules) on both the APC and the responding T cell bind to each other and serve to increase the avidity of the binding.

Co-stimulatory molecules identified on APCs include B7 (CD80) (Linsley, 1991a), B7.2 (Azuma, 1993), heat stable antigen (HSA) (Liu, 1992), and others (Wingren, 1995; Foletta, 1998). On T cells, CD28 is the primary co-stimulatory molecule and binds B7; CTLA-4, on the other hand, binds both B7 and B7.2 and is involved in down-modulating T-cell activation (Linsley, 1991b). The receptor on T cells for HSA has not been identified. Antigen presentation in the presence of reagents that block the co-stimulatory molecules leads to anergic response (tolerance) on subsequent exposure to that specific antigen but does not affect the responses to other antigens (Tan, 1993). The ability to make nonimmunogenic transplantable tumors immunogenic by transfecting them with the *B7* gene (Chen, 1992; Baskar, 1993; Townsend, 1993; Janeway, 1994) suggests that co-stimulatory molecules play an important role in T-cell activation in vivo.

Signal Transduction Following Antigen-Specific Stimulation

The presentation of antigen to T cells leads to the aggregation of the TCR–CD3 complexes and the activation of protein tyrosine kinases (PTKs). The TCR itself has a small cytoplasmic tail with no known transducing activity. It is the associated ζ chains of the CD3 complex which contain the ITAM motifs and which have been shown to coprecipitate protein tyrosine kinase activity. Two well known classes of cytoplasmic PTK families are involved in the very early events following T-cell receptor aggregation, Src and Syk/ZAP-70. The signaling cascades downstream from the TCR–CD3 complex and the CD28 co-stimulatory pathway are fairly well understood (Foletta, 1998; Samelson, 2002). The activation of the TCR-associated tyrosine kinases ZAP70, p59^{fyn}, and p56^{lck} leads to activation of three pathways, p21^{ras}, calcium/calcineurin, and protein kinase C (PKC). Activation of p21^{ras} activates mitogen-activated protein kinases (MAPKs), which in turn phosphorylate several transcription factors, thereby regulating gene expression. The activation of the protein tyrosine kinases also activates phospholipase C, which hydrolyzes phosphatidyl inositol and leads to the generation of the second messengers diacyl glycerol (DAG) and inositol triphosphate (IP$_3$). DAG activates protein kinase C, and IP$_3$ leads to rapid and sustained increase in cytoplasmic calcium. The increase in free calcium activates the calmodulin-dependent phosphatase calcineurin. These events also lead to the induction of DNA-binding proteins and the transcription of numerous genes including *IL-2* and the IL-2 receptor required for T-cell proliferation.

Understanding the pathways leading to T-cell activation has led to the discovery of the molecular defects in several acquired immunodeficiency diseases and may ultimately help provide therapeutic strategies to correct the deficiencies (Rosen, 2000). For example, mutations in the protein tyrosine kinase ZAP70 have been reported and are associated with the autosomal form of severe combined immunodeficiency (SCID) syndrome in humans (Elder, 1998). Mutations in the common γ chain of the interleukin receptors IL-2, IL-4, IL-7, IL-9, and IL-15 lead to transduction abnormalities and are associated with the X-linked form of SCID (Noguchi, 1993). Interestingly, another form of autosomally inherited SCID is associated with mutations in the downstream Janus family protein tyrosine Jak3, the only signaling molecule associated with the common γ chain (Pesu, 2005). As more and more of the underlying abnormalities leading to T-cell immunodeficiency are being discovered, including at least 10 different molecular defects for SCID alone (Fischer, 2005), it has been proposed that the disorders should be classified using a comprehensive system that would identify the disorders according to abnormalities in differentiation, maturation, and function (Gelfand, 1993). These designations would begin to focus on the actual physiologic or biochemical defect and may ultimately provide new options for therapy, including gene therapy (Buckley, 2004; Conley, 2005).

T-Cell Responses

Recently, the designation of T-cell type I versus type II cytokine responses has been preferred for those T-cell responses that lead to cytokine secretion patterns known to be involved in cellular immunity versus cytokine secretion patterns observed in humoral immunity, respectively. Type I responses are characterized by the secretion of cytokines known to enhance inflammation (proinflammatory) and induce the activation and proliferation of T cells and monocytes, namely, IL-2, IFN-γ, and IL-12. Type II responses are characterized by the secretion of cytokines that suppress inflammation (anti-inflammatory) and stimulate B cells to divide and differentiate into immunoglobulin-secreting cells (i.e., IL-4, IL-5, IL-10, and IL-13). There is evidence suggesting that the secretion of type I cytokines regulates the secretion of type II cytokines and vice versa (Paul, 1993). For example, in the presence of IL-4 both in vivo (Chatelain, 1992) and in vitro (Seder, 1992, 1993), T cells will not develop into INF-γ-secreting cells (i.e., this environment favors the development of a humoral immune response). It has been suggested that the relative amounts of IL-4 and IL-12 that are present during the stimulation of naive T cells will shift the response one way or the other (Paul, 1994).

Several factors are involved in regulating the type of T-cell response that ensues after antigenic stimulation. In addition to the cytokine environment, there is evidence to suggest that the dose of antigen influences the type of response (Bretscher, 1992; Madrenas, 1995). The predominant response that develops following T-cell activation has significant clinical implications. It has been postulated that the development of a type I response to HIV infection may lead to protective immunity (Clerici, 1994). Clearly, a type II response is not protective, as most infected persons seroconvert and eventually succumb to a profound immunosuppression. Clerici and Shearer argue that repeated exposure to low-dose HIV-1 may lead to protective type I cellular immunity (Clerici, 1993, 1994). This group's results indicate that between 39% and 75% of HIV-1-seronegative and polymerase chain reaction (PCR)-negative high-risk individuals' peripheral blood mononuclear cells (PBMC) (homosexual men, intravenous drug users and infants born to HIV-1-positive mothers) secreted IL-2 in response to the *env* protein in vitro. These scientists propose that these seronegative high-risk individuals have developed protective cell-mediated immunity as a result of low-dose immunization or infection.

Methodology: Measurement of Lymphocyte Activation and Proliferation in the Evaluation of Cellular Immunodeficiency

Developmental defects, inherited genetic abnormalities, and acquired infections cause profound immunodeficiency states. Additionally, severe burns, trauma, and therapeutic intervention also lead to immuno-deficiency. Bulk assays can be used to ascertain whether or not an individual has a decreased T-cell proliferative response and have been available for some time but are limited both by poor reproducibility and by the limited information garnered from bulk assays. Recent technological developments have allowed for the production of a variety of reagents that can be used to assess multiple activities along the pathway of T-cell activation. These reagents include monoclonal antibodies specific for T-cell activation markers, reagents and systems for the detection of intracellular cytokines, and tracking dyes and nonradioactive DNA precursor developed to assess lymphocyte proliferation.

Procedures Used to Assess T-Cell Activation and Proliferation

The most common in vivo procedure used to assess cellular immunity is a simple skin test. A positive skin test for the detection of a delayed-type hypersensitivity response implies intact cellular immunity as well as intact monocyte chemotaxis (Borut, 1980; Ananworanich, 2002). Although skin testing is easily performed, negative results are difficult to interpret, especially in young children, and skin testing is not as sensitive as in vitro lymphocyte stimulation assays (Borut, 1980). Other in vivo correlates of cell-mediated immunity include contact sensitivity, granuloma formation, and allograft rejection.

Lymphocytes are unique in that they express surface receptors able to identify virtually any molecule or foreign substance (antigen). Structural diversity within these receptors is created by the differential rearrangement of the T-cell receptor genes. In general, there are only a limited number of circulating lymphocytes able to recognize any one antigen. In vivo, when a lymphocyte recognizes a foreign antigen, the cells proliferate rapidly in a clonal manner in order to generate a large number of both effector and memory cells.

The earliest methods used to assess lymphocyte proliferation involved manual counting of the actual number of cells before and after stimulation. Unfortunately, these procedures are time-consuming and replete with technical problems. Over the past several years new methods have been developed that measure different cellular events known to occur along the pathway of cell division. It must be emphasized that methods that measure early events in T-lymphocyte activation may or may not correlate with cell division.

Tritiated Thymidine Incorporation Assay ^{3}H (TdR Assay)

Most laboratories assess the proliferative capacity of lymphocytes by measuring the rate of incorporation of radiolabeled DNA nucleosides (tritiated thymidine) in a 4–24-hour pulse following prolonged incubation of peripheral blood mononuclear cell cultures with mitogens (3–4 days) or antigens (5–10 days)(Maluish, 1986). In general, only a limited number of T cells respond to any one antigen in vitro; therefore, cells must be cultured for 5–10 days in order to detect a response. Mitogens, on the other hand, will induce the rapid proliferation of up to 100% of the T cells. For this reason proliferation can be detected in 3–4 days and thus provides an effective screening tool. In vitro lymphocyte transformation in response to a mitogen was first reported by Nowell (Nowell, 1960). Mitogens in general are the most potent stimuli, as they activate the largest proportion of lymphocytes relative to alloantigens and then antigens.

Flow Cytometry in the Evaluation of Lymphocyte Activation and Proliferation

Bulk assays, in addition to their inherent technical problems, provide no information on the specific cell subsets that are responding. Flow cytometry with inherent multiparameter potential has become the instrument of choice for the analysis of cellular immunology. For a comprehensive review of flow cytometry and methods used to assess lymphocyte activation and proliferation, refer to Maluish or Perfetto (Maluish, 1986; Perfetto, 2002).

Another flow-cytometry-based method that has attained significant use in clinical laboratories is the measurement of lymphocytes in the various phases of the cell cycle. In general, cell cycle analyses are performed by measuring the level of fluorescence intensity emitted by DNA-staining dyes. The most common dye used is propidium iodide, which intercalates stoichiometrically into DNA (i.e., the amount or intensity of fluorescence is proportional to the amount of DNA in a cell). Using complex mathematical modeling, it is possible to measure the percentage of cells with a DNA content between 2c and 4c, which correlates with the percentage of cells in the 'S' phase of the cell cycle. Peripheral blood lymphocytes are in general in the resting phase of the cell cycle, with less than 5% of the cells in the 'S' phase.

Some laboratories have replaced the tritiated thymidine incorporation assays with a combination of cell surface marker induction assays and a measurement of the percentage of cells in various phases of the cell cycle following activation (Cost, 1993).

Recently, dyes have been developed that stably integrate into the membranes of live lymphocytes. After washing away excess dye, the lymphocytes are stimulated to divide. With each successive division the amount of dye per cell is halved. The fluorescence emitted from the cells after culture can be modeled and the number of cell divisions can be estimated. This methodology has recently been standardized into a kit that includes both the software required for analyses and the tracking dye (Sigma Immunochemicals, St. Louis, MO). An evaluation of 14 of the most commonly utilized tracking dyes reported that two of the dyes, PKH26 and carboxyfluorescein diacetate succinimidyl ester (CSFE), were the most suitable for their ability to quantify lymphocyte proliferation (Parish, 1999). This assay may provide the most accurate assessment of cell proliferative response in in vitro culture systems with the substantial advantage over standard bulk assays of allowing the measurement of specific lymphocyte subsets. CSFE indices appear to correlate more closely with TdR assays than the measurement of CD69+ cells (Angulo, 1998). The measurement of lymphocyte proliferation using the tracking dyes PKH26 and CSFE have been developed, optimized, and tested for their utility in clinical applications (Allsopp, 1998; Angulo, 1998).

The recently developed ability to measure the production of cell-associated cytokines at the single-cell level has significant potential as a clinical tool for the evaluation of the cellular immune response. Cells are stimulated for 4–6 hours in the presence of membrane-transport-blocking reagents (brefeldin A or monensin) to prevent the secretion of cytokines. Cells are then labeled with subset-specific monoclonal antibodies, fixed, permeabilized, and labeled with fluorescently tagged monoclonal antibodies specific for the cytokine of interest (Jung, 1993; Prussin, 1995). The assay has been developed with the presence of co-stimulatory antibodies for the sensitive detection of antigen responses in whole blood cultures after relatively short incubation periods (Suni, 1998). Special attention is being focused on the development of antibodies that recognize the nascent forms of the cytokines (within the Golgi) and the optimization of the timing of culture in order to detect maximal cytokine response (Mascher, 1999). Clinical studies have begun to demonstrate the potential utility of this technique. For example, patients suffering very severe burns and who show a shift to a Th2 cytokine response may be at increased risk for the development of multiple organ dysfunction syndrome (Zedler, 1999). This would be very advantageous, as there is currently no test to indicate which patients will go on to suffer this potentially fatal complication. Several studies are currently under way evaluating the clinical utility of this promising new technology. Expansion of this technique to incorporate the ability to simultaneously measure proliferation and specific cytokine synthesis at the single-cell level has been reported but has not yet been evaluated in a clinical setting (Mehta, 1997).

Clearly, new assays are being developed that measure different events involved in T-cell activation. There are methods and reagents available to measure the earliest phosphorylation/dephosphorylation events, through signal transduction, gene transcription, and cell division. As these methods are adapted for routine clinical use, we will have a veritable armamentarium of methods to assess many of the processes involved in lymphocyte activation and proliferation. Although many of these new technologies are still within the domain of research laboratories, the methods are constantly being simplified and adapted for use and evaluation in clinical laboratories.

Granulocyte Function in Cell-Mediated Immunity

Both monocytes and granulocytes are derived from a common parental precursor. Granulocytes are extremely important in the early inflammatory response, and abnormalities in their functions lead to profound deficiencies in cellular immunity. Abnormalities occur at any point in a series of processes required for granulocyte function, including difficulty in leaving the vasculature (diapedesis), movement toward the offending agent (chemotaxis, chemokinesis), engulfment of the offending agent (phagocytosis), and killing via the generation of toxic oxygen radicals.

Methodology: Flow and Image Cytometry

Since its development two decades ago, laser-based single-cell analysis (flow and image cytometry) has become an essential tool for the medical research laboratory and the standard of laboratory clinical practice in the study of the cellular immune response (Goetzman, 1993; Lamb, 2002; Herzenberg, 2004; Shapiro, 2004). The measures of immunocompetence and the immune modulation of specific surface markers and receptors, the lineage characterization by the immunophenotyping of lymphomas and leukemias, the definition of malignancy using specific chromosome probes, and the study of tumor heterogeneity by multiparameter DNA measures are commonly performed analyses in many laboratories, as detailed by many authors (Good, 2002; Goolsby, 2004; Herzenberg, 2004). The classification of cell types by these means enables the definition of biological and effector function on a molecular basis and allows the relationship of these measures to relate to disease process and definition. These are but a few of the applications that are possible using laser-based technologies.

Two major technologies are used. The first is characterized as flow-through, in which the particles being counted and their physical and chemical characteristics are measured by the particles passing in a fluid stream in a single-cell suspension (Keren, 1989; Givan, 2004; Stewart, 2004). In the second, known as static analysis, the particles are stationary and the stage or the laser moves as in image analysis (Martin-Reay, 1994). Image analysis technology is slowly making its mark in the laboratory in the evaluation of touch preparations or cytospins, chromosome preparations, and tissue sections for certain applications, such as DNA and fluorescence in situ hybridization (FISH). Advances in the availability of fluorescent probes for use in FISH and chromosome painting in recent years will make these analyses more relevant and useful tools in the clinical laboratory (Weinberg, 1993; Stewart, 2002). As in many techniques, including cell cycle analysis in DNA, each of the new markers and new techniques must be defined and evaluated and correlated with patient outcomes before deciding on absolute clinical utility or not. Instrumentation development combining the strengths of flow cytometry and the static advantages of image analysis has been introduced. These instruments, known as scanning laser cytometers, make the traditional flow cytometry measures of forward scatter, side scatter, and fluorescence on cells in suspension or fixed on to a glass slide. Experience with these systems will determine if this approach offers measurement advantages not available with the current flow cytometric and image system configurations (Martin-Reay, 1994).

The combined advances in electronic pulse processing, optics, and data storage with advances in computer technology and software have allowed the flow cytometry technology to become routine in the laboratory. Furthermore, the wide availability of workshop clustered monoclonal antibodies now numbering 339 (Zola, 2002) labeled in multicolor, directly conjugated, and in premixed formats has allowed the simultaneous detection of multiple surface antigens as well as cytoplasmic and nuclear constituents. The ability to perform multiparameter analysis is the greatest strength of flow cytometry. The measurement of both phenotypic and intracellular markers is now routine in many laboratories. The major manufacturers have made the art of flow cytometry into a routine laboratory measurement – a 'black box' science – much to the dismay of many (Chapman, 2000). As described, this black box approach phenomenon is largely the result of the use of flow cytometry in the phenotyping of T-cell subsets for the monitoring of patients with HIV (Shapiro, 1993; Mandy, 2004) (Fig. 44–1). Before the onset of the HIV epidemic, flow cytometry use in the laboratory was primarily for the characterization of leukemias and other hematologic malignancies and for DNA analysis of tumors for synthesis phase (S-phase) and DNA index (DI). Although flow cytometry technology may be more black box, the HIV epidemic brought the power of the flow cytometer to a much larger number of institutions and laboratories. This has allowed the technology to be an integral part of many diagnoses and an important adjunct in treatment of patients. Despite its simplification, many issues with regard to FDA regulation, proficiency testing, data management, and reproducibility of data remain. This is particularly true in the area of DNA analysis. It is not the purview of this chapter to describe all the nuances of a flow cytometer or image cytometer. Current flow cytometers all can adequately perform routine immunophenotyping and other assays. Most laboratory problems lie in the nonavailability of standard quality control reagents and calibrators and the lack of reliable, rapid methods for data transfer, and storage compatible with laboratory information systems. More important for clinicians is the understanding of the technology, the strengths, and the pitfalls in quality control and quality assurance, specimen preparation, and data interpretation.

The Hardware and Other Tools

The Light Source and Signal Processing

Today's clinical flow cytometer is rarely used for cell separation (i.e., cell sorting), and this property remains with research instruments in the highly specialized laboratory. Most multifaceted clinical flow cytometers use a single argon ion–air-cooled laser with a minimum of four photomultiplier tubes to perform three- or four-color immunophenotypic analysis (Shapiro, 1993; Chapman, 2000; Snow, 2004). Research laboratories interested in performing five or more colors of analysis with Hoescht's ultraviolet-stimulated probes use the larger water-cooled 5 W lasers in combination with the air-cooled lasers, although new instrument systems with new lasers are eliminating the need for water-cooled lasers. At present, commercial manufacturers of flow cytometers include Becton, Dickinson & Co. (San Jose, CA), Beckman Coulter, Inc. (Fullerton, CA), and Partec GmbH (Munster, Germany). Analytic software is provided by the instrument manufacturers, as well as by several independent software companies, including Tree Star, Inc. (Ashland, OR) and Verity Software (Topsham, ME).

The Flow Cell

Two common flow cells are in use in the clinical laboratory, but because most clinical instruments are used in the measurement of CD4+ cells in the monitoring of HIV disease, most clinical systems used a closed system

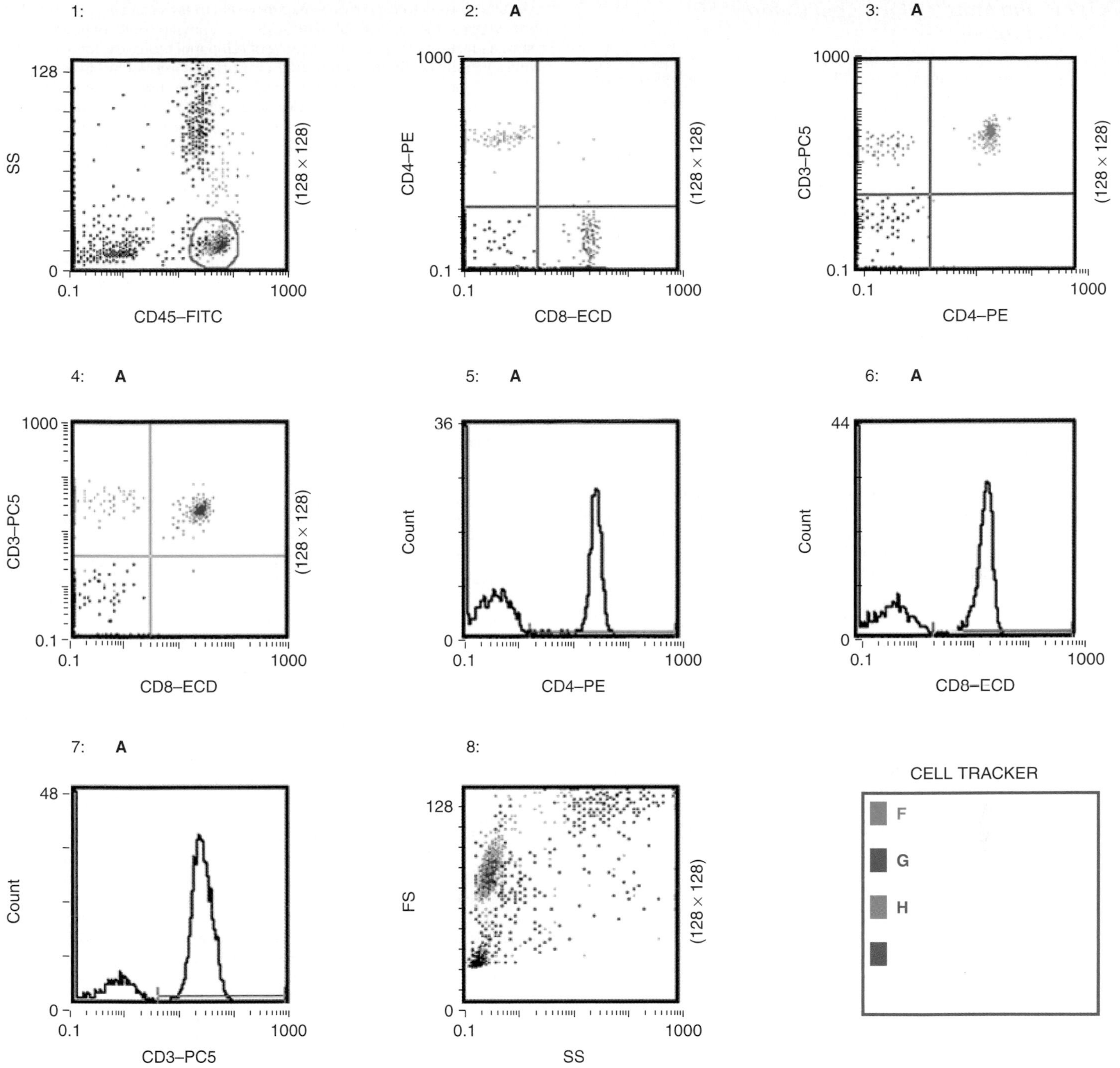

Figure 44–1 Use of four-color flow cytometry for the performance of peripheral blood lymphocyte subset enumeration. Histogram 1 demonstrates the use of CD45 fluorescence intensity (CD45-FITC) versus side scatter (SS) as a gating strategy to discriminate lymphocytes (gated area) from other peripheral blood cells. Histograms 2, 3, and 4 are dual parameter histograms of the gated lymphocyte population in which backgating was used to denote CD4+ lymphocytes by a green color and CD8+ lymphocytes by a red color. Histograms 5, 6, and 7 are single parameter histograms in which CD4+, CD8+ or CD3+ lymphocyte populations are differentiated from corresponding negative cells by a colored bar. Histogram 8 is a dual parameter display of SS vs. forward angle scatter (FS). In histograms 1 and 8, note the presence of scattered CD4+ or CD8+ cells outside of the lymphocyte gate. Directly conjugated monoclonal antibodies were conjugated with fluorescein isothiocyanate (FITC), phycoerythrin (PE), energy coupled dye (ECD), or a PE-Cy5 tandem (PC5).

as a biohazard precaution (Bogh, 1993; Chapman, 2000; McCoy, 2002). The first, known as a stream-in-air or flow-in-air flow cell, allows the optical measurement point to be directly on the sample stream. This type of flow cell minimizes the distance between the flow chamber and the sample injector tip and thus minimizes carryover between specimens and the sample wash time necessary between samples. This chamber allows greater sample flow rate variability than a closed system. Other advantages of the stream-in-air tips are important in cell sorting and are not considered here. In the closed system, often referred to as a quartz tip flow cell, the focal point is within the chamber. Disadvantages of these quartz systems are the thickness of the quartz and thus the diffraction of the laser beam or the scattering of the signal. Additionally, the relatively large cross-section $(200\,\mu m^2)$ makes the flow rate more difficult to control. The success of these quartz flow cells in the clinical system depends on the illumination and the collection optics. The major manufacturers have made many advances in these systems to provide both the safety and maximum sensitivity with the use of low-power, laser-based systems (Bogh, 1993).

Confounding are all the terms used in the definition of flow cytometry systems, which include the flow rate, the sheath pressure, the core size, the resulting particle velocity, the resulting coefficients of variation (CVs), and so forth. The most important factor for a laboratory worker to understand is that, in DNA analysis, the cells are analyzed at a slow flow rate to increase the time a particle spends in the beam, allowing greater sensitivity and better CVs. In immunophenotyping, sensitivity is typically not an issue, and the particle flow rate can be increased. Most clinical systems are compromises to accommodate the most common application of immunophenotypic analysis (Baumgarth, 2000). Research flow cytometers have much greater flexibility and operator control for controlling the sample flow rate, differential pressure, and time.

Colors and More Colors: Applications of Fluorochromes

Most laboratories are still using the most common fluorochromes, fluorescein isothiocyanate (FITC; 530 nm emission) and phycoerythrin (PE; 575 nm emission) for immunophenotyping and propidium iodide (PI) (625 nm emission) in the measurement of DNA (McCoy, 2002). FITC and PC are directly conjugated by the antibody of interest and simultaneously added to a patient's sample. The use of a secondary antibody such as a goat antimouse (GAM) IgG labeled with fluorescein is no longer necessary for extra sensitivity, and therefore the background fluorescence is minimized. Most clinically used antibodies in the study of HIV are premixed and prediluted for use in whole blood technologies. PI can be used simultaneously with cell surface made in multiparameter DNA analysis, although this requires preservation of the cell membrane (Clevenger, 1993).

New dyes that have become available to the clinical laboratory allow the simultaneous measurement of four colors with directly labeled monoclonal antibodies and excited with a single 488 nm laser. This availability is revolutionizing the current performance of flow cytometry in laboratory practice. These dyes with a red and far red emission include PE Texas Red tandems (625 nm emission), PE-Cy-5 tandems (675 nm emission), and allophycocyanin (675 nm emission), to name a few. The early tandems were problematic because of excess free PE in solution, leading to excess background fluorescence. New technologies for the synthesis of these dyes are exploding, solving most of the technical issues, and new dyes are constantly being added for use in the clinical laboratory (Clevenger, 1993a). With the availability of the red and far red dyes, an HIV subset analysis can be performed in a single tube with greater surety (Nicholson, 1993). A single tube with 1 µL of whole blood is simultaneously stained with CD45 PE-Cy-5, CD3 PE-Texas Red, CD8 FITC, and CD4 PE. With the new digitized signal processing, compensation (see below) is easily performed, and the analysis is performed using CD45 as a gating agent with side scatter (SSC) and the simultaneous analysis of CD3, CD4, and CD8.

Another interesting phenomenon is that these new dyes have allowed the use of fluorescence as a trigger in place of the usual forward light scatter parameter. This is possible because the far red dye spectra are not found in components of most cells or they do not have autofluorescence competition in nature as found with FITC. Furthermore, they can be excited at wavelengths that minimize the autofluorescence from cell constituents such as riboflavin. Therefore, when performing a rare event (cells present at <0.1% of total population) analysis using a fluorescent trigger, many cells can be analyzed very rapidly. This method is also used to label leukocytes in unloosed blood using fluorescence as a trigger. A dye is used that marks the leukocytes' nuclei or cytoplasm and not the erythrocytes.

The use of multicolor fluorescence has allowed the concept of multiparameter analysis to become a reality in most laboratories. The parameters can evaluate:

1. different functional subsets of a particular cell population using an intracellular fluorescent probes
2. use of several colors to identify small clusters of otherwise unidentifiable events (as in MRD)
3. activation status of cells in a particular disease stage (e.g., use of HLA-DR and CD38 on CD4 and CD8s in HIV staging using an anchor gate approach)
4. cell surface expression and the DI or S-phase of a particular cell population as in defining the CD19 S-phase in an acute leukemia.

Obviously, the possible combinations are nearly infinite and their sophistication enhanced by the specific dyes and DNA/RNA probes available. A discussion of some of these approaches and techniques follows.

Gating and Analysis

Immunophenotyping: Application to Routine and Leukemic Specimens

The analysis of cell populations with the flow cytometer uses a combination of parameters that, when applied, define a specific cell population. Flow cytometry uses parameters similar to those that have been used for many years in hematology, including size (forward light scatter), cytoplasmic granularity (side scatter), and affinities for specific dyes, and combine them with the immunologic tools already mentioned. These include multiple fluorescent dyes bound to antibodies or probes, DNA measurements as measured using either PI or 4'-6-diamidino-2-phenylindole (DAPI), and other nuclear markers. The key is the

simultaneous detection of these parameters in today's analytical systems. For many years, the clinical laboratory flow cytometer could only use three simultaneous measurements. Staining of cell populations was limited by the unavailability of directly conjugated monoclonal antibodies, necessitating the use of a secondary GAM reagent or the use of biotin-labeled antibodies. Definition of positive and negative populations in high-background cases made it necessary to use a subtraction channel-by-channel algorithm to define positive from negative (Bagwell, 1993). In cases in which the cell population had a defined boundary between negative and positive, a cursor was set so that no more than 2% of the events considered negative fell to the right of the cursor, defining the positive events when using a matched isotypic control. Although this approach seemed reasonable at the time (Lewis, 1993) and worked well with bright cell clusters, it has become quite cumbersome when identifying leukemic cells or performing analyses of cell activation markers. Leukemic cells were particularly problematic, because each leukemia has its own 'relative' fluorescent intensity and isotype controls may have little relevance. Applying hard and fast rules to cursor settings led to the underestimation of positive clusters. The failure of this approach is especially dramatic in the analysis of monoclonality by κ and λ light chain expression. Small but significant differences were often lost. Use of isotype controls in certain situations has been challenged on many fronts, both because of technical aberrations associated with their use and because of the added cost to the laboratory. New software algorithms have the capability of making intensity measurements and defining clusters based on population means intensities, including relative fluorescent intensities as well as actual MESF (Molecules of Equivalent Soluble Fluorophores) quantification (see below). Clearly, the need to remember what we are measuring and understanding the biology of the population of interest are important when designing an analysis protocol. Fortunately, some sophisticated software approaches and better reagents have allowed us to use multiparameter gating to define populations, rather than trying to make estimates of fluorescence expression using cursor values. Many investigators have used the multiparameter approach in defining cluster and other populations of interest (Loken, 1990; Baumgarth, 2000; Kraan, 2003; Stewart, 2004). These approaches take many forms, and a few are reviewed here.

With multicolor fluorescence came the need to analyze the number of cells expressing one or more colors at the same time on a particular cell population defined by forward angle light scatter (FALS) and SSC regions (Loken, 1977; Loken, 1976). When this method was first developed, scientists were basically thinking about the mathematics and the accounting of all cells and the number of these cells expressing one or more colors. A binary approach to this analysis was developed, known as Prism (Coulter, Hialeah, FL). These analysis regions were hard-gated and set into the instrument by the operator. They could not be redefined at a later time using list mode analysis, which caused a lot of frustration. This approach was later modified to allow some regating, and other manufacturers, as well as third-party software, made this prism binary approach on a post-analysis basis. Loken then defined bone marrow populations using CD45 versus SSC gating, a unique approach to defining the heterogeneous populations found in bone marrow (Loken, 1990; Stelzer, 1993). They and others (Borowitz, 1992) developed the concept of patterns defining specific leukemic states. Loken further promoted the use of CD45 and CD14 dual-parameter analysis gated on the lymphocyte region of FALS versus SSC for peripheral blood. Many agencies embraced and promoted this approach for most of the HIV flow cytometry panels in order to minimize the effect of contaminating monocytes in the lymphocyte population because they might interfere with a true CD4+ lymphocyte count, as monocytes have CD4 receptors on their surface (Passlick, 1989). Agencies promoting this type of analysis included the Centers for Disease Control and Prevention (Centers for Disease Control, 1992), the National Institute of Allergy and Infectious Disease, Division of AIDS (NIH, DAIDS; Calvelli, 1993), the National Committee for Clinical Laboratory Standards (NCCLS; Standards, 1992), and the College of American Pathologists. Unfortunately, even though this approach solved a lot of problems, it did not ensure that each tube in the panel had the same contents as the tube containing the CD45 and CD14, and the required purity correction might be overestimated, leading to incorrect values for CD4. These issues were reviewed during a conference held by the CDC, a year after the HIV guidelines for the performance of CD4 counts were published (Stelzer, 1993). Other analyses of this approach have been performed by the ACTG Flow Advisory Committee in the DAIDS Proficiency CD4/CD8 program (Kagan, 1993) and by the College of American Pathologists in their proficiency testing program (Homburger, 1993). A new approach to gating was evaluated in HIV panels that followed from Loken's original approach to bone marrow definition of clusters (Loken, 1990). Use of a CD45 as a gating parameter has simplified the analysis of bone marrow, leukemias, and HIV panels. In bone marrow and leukemia work-ups, the CD45 is usually set as the third or fourth color and is paired either with forward light scatter or side scatter; this allows the definition of a potential blast (malignant) population. The blast population is then defined using a panel of monoclonals using the three color parameters available. In the HIV, one-tube, four-color method, CD45 allows the definition of a large lymphocyte-gated region, which is secondarily gated for CD45. This can also be done without the use of the light scatter parameters, as previously described. (This can also be done using a two-tube, three-color panel.) Newer analytical reagents products (Becton-Dickinson and Beckman Coulter) include precounted beads in the tube containing monoclonal antibody, thus permitting an absolute lymphocyte count (known as a flow differential) to be performed at the same time as the lymphocyte subset enumeration. This removes the requirement of needing a hematology counter when performing T-cell enumerations and avoids the problems of white cell deterioration with shipping and the performance of an accurate differential to get accurate T-cell numbers. These methods are just becoming incorporated into ACTG HIV trial work and other laboratories.

Another gating strategy is the use of two- or three-color definition of a particular subset of interest. This approach, commonly now referred to as an anchor gate, uses the particular properties of some cells to investigate another set of parameters. When applied specifically to T lymphocytes, it is referred to as a T-gate (Mandy, 1992). Use of an anchor gate (Paxton, 1995) is especially useful when looking at activation markers, as in the HIV subsets of CD3/CD8 expressing CD38 and HLA-DR or looking at the expression of CD45Ra and CD45Ro against either CD3/CD4 or CD3/CD8. The advantage of this method is that it is intuitive and each color acts as a quality control check for the other subset. Furthermore, one has the choice to define the expression of biologically relevant markers in relation to functional or biologically relevant populations. This approach lends itself well to quantitative fluorescence (see histograms 2 and 3, respectively). Although the concept of quantitative fluorescence is not new, the techniques to measure fluorescence equivalents or fluorescence thresholds or other similar designations are. Quantitative fluorescent measurements will be described after DNA gating and analysis.

Another approach to anchor gating is in CD34 harvesting, which uses CD34 and CD45 staining with or without AAD as a viability assessment in the identification and enumeration of CD34 progenitor cells. These methods can also use beads to enumerate the number of cells recovered. The methods have great utility in bone marrow transplantation protocols in which progenitor cells are harvested from cord blood, bone marrow, or peripheral blood (e.g., the International Society for Hematotherapy and Graft Engineering) and reinfused. This approach has become the standard for most laboratories performing transplants. A commercial system called ProCount (Becton-Dickinson) uses a similar approach and reagents to automate the process. Complex immunophenotypic analysis with five or more monoclonal antibodies is becoming more common in clinical and research laboratories for the detection of minor lymphocyte subpopulations of clinical relevance in patients with autoimmune and immunodeficiency diseases, and for the detection of small, immunologically aberrant subpopulations for the detection of minimal residual disease in patients with hematologic malignancies. In this regard, multiparametric flow cytometric analysis using 17 fluorescent colors was recently reported (Perfetto, 2004).

DNA Analysis

General Aspects

Conceptually, the performance of DNA analysis should be less complex than immunophenotyping analysis but the review of published data and its prognostic capabilities as well as performance by laboratories on proficiency tests indicates otherwise (Nicholson, 1993b; Coon, 1994; Tirindelli, 1997). Since the publication of several thousand reports in the 1980s and early 1990s yielded conflicting findings regarding the diagnostic and prognostic significance of ploidy and S-phase activity in various human tumors, a DNA consensus conference was held and the proceedings were published in *Cytometry* (Shankey, 1993). This report was a historical review of major tumor types (in fresh, frozen, and paraffin samples) and the clinical value of the performance of ploidy by DI and the value of S-phase. These parameters were analyzed in terms of their effectiveness as prognostic markers. The 1994 College of American Pathologists Conference also looked at the previous markers and some additional potential tumor surrogates. In each case, the DI and S-phase were less predictable as prognostic markers than hoped. This was largely attributed to the variability in the technical performance and analysis of these assays (both instrument and samples preparation) and the inherent

risk of tumor heterogeneity and therefore the appropriate sampling of the tumor. Specific recommendations were made in each tumor type for the appropriate quality control measurements that should be performed and the proper deconvolution of the histograms. Since that time, the routine utilization of DNA analysis in the clinical laboratory has considerably declined. Because of the high degree of variability and lack of prognostic significance, it was suggested by some that clinical DNA measurements should be performed only by expert laboratories or completely eliminated (ASCO, 1996). The FDA to date has not cleared any methods and still considers this a research test. However, several groups have made significant inroads into solving some of the issues in analysis (Shankey, 2002). The future of this technique in clinical medicine are further discussed later in this chapter.

Sample Preparation

DNA preparative methods are reasonably simple and inexpensive to perform. Many references for the original methods exist, as well as many modifications. The most common methods are those used on fresh and frozen tissues developed by Krishan, Vindelov, Crissman, Steinkamp, and others (Rabinovitch, 1993; Vindelov, 1994) and those used on paraffin blocks with preparations of Hedley (Hedley, 1983). In each case, whether the cells are enucleated or the cell membrane is preserved, the DNA dye PI is the most commonly used in most clinical laboratories and has already been described. PI staining is straightforward as long as timing, saturation, and removal of RNA parameters are followed. Measures of the gross karyotypic abnormalities are made by comparing the peak (fluorescence intensity, PI uptake) of the tumor versus a diploid calibrator. Factors affecting this measurement include the CV of the peaks for both the calibrator and suspected tumor, the G_2/G_1 ratio, or the linearity of the instrument, linearity as measured by the deconvolution software package and percent of tumor present (sampling) in the sample (Shankey, 2002). It is common to find laboratories reporting out a diploid tumor result on a sample containing 'no' tumor. Tumors with near diploid values need stringent rules of interpretation, as does the definition of tetraploidy. Further problems occur in the definition of aggregates, doublets, debris, treatment of sliced and cut nuclei, and S-phase population. The descriptive and semiquantitative acronym BAD is used by the software analysis packages to model the effects of *b*ackground, *a*ggregates, and *d*oublets (Rabinovitch, 1993, 1994). The impact of this parameter on the analysis is controversial.

The resulting S-phase and DI measurements using a single-parameter mode of analysis (PI only) are subject to these deconvolution algorithms, leading to great interlaboratory variability (Coon, 1994). These deconvolution algorithms for DNA have been extensively studied (Wheeless, 1991; Shankey, 1993; Rabinovitch, 1993, 1994; Coon, 1994), but many models used for analysis need further study. The DNA consensus document makes specific recommendations applicable to certain tumor types and suggests that laboratories perform their analyses accordingly, but even with these guidelines there remains a level of ambiguity in the interpretation and performance for the clinical laboratory that contributes to the discordance of results in comparative studies as well as in proficiency tests (Coon, 1988, 1994; Wheeless, 1991). The difficulty in achieving consensus makes the interpretation of results more difficult for the novice laboratory as well as for clinicians who are trying to compare their laboratory results with the recent literature in the treatment of their patients. This is especially true in the classification of S-phase values. S-phase measures are subject to the effects of debris and aggregate modeling, as described by Rabinovitch and others (Coon, 1988; Bagwell, 1993; Rabinovitch, 1993, 1994; Shankey, 1993). Furthermore, it is critical that the decisions made with regard to which mathematical model is used for a particular tumor are kept constant and that the list mode data are retained without modeling in case further analysis is necessary.

Other approaches using DNA and RNA probes such as thymidine derivatives, bromodeoxyuridine (BrdU) and acridine orange (RNA) are used to improve the quality of the models in the estimation of proliferative and kinetic properties of a specific tumor. It is important to remember that proliferation measures are not the same as measures of S-phase quantification, which are a static model or a picture in time of all the cells being analyzed. The integration of the area for the number of cells between 2C and 4C in a DNA histogram is not capable of giving any information with regard to cells 'stuck' in S_0 (cells actually stop DNA synthesis) or measure the number of infiltrating normal cells that also might be proliferating. The S-phase value may often be higher than the actual proliferative capacity owing to artifacts of tumor heterogeneity. The single-parameter histogram yields reasonable results when dealing with an asynchronous, relatively homogeneous cell population. Pulse labeling is most commonly used in larger academic settings and is most often used to measure the effectiveness of radiation and chemotherapy by obtaining true measures of the G_0/G_1 cells as well as $G_2 + M$ compartments, which are not possible using single-parameter measures of S-phase.

Other approaches using nuclear and cytoplasmic probes as well as surface markers can be used to separate a population of interest from a mixture of cell types. This type of multiparameter analysis is especially useful in the measure of S-phase in hematologic malignancies. Specific blast populations can be identified by FITC fluorescence and FALS, and those events analyzed for DNA content and S-phase using PI. Staining methods are altered to preserve cell surface properties or nuclear properties (Clevenger, 1993; Ramaekers, 1993; Bauer, 1994; Carothers, 1994). These methods usually involve staining the surface marker of interest (e.g., KI-67, cyclin B1, cytokeratin, CD10) with the monoclonal antibody, fixing in an alcohol (or commercial fixation and permeabilization reagent), then treating with a detergent to allow penetration of PI or other nuclear dye. Staining methods are selectively modified to preserve specific membrane and nuclear properties specific to the probe of interest (Bauer, 1994).

DNA Studies of Interest

There has been an explosion of literature on the subject of apoptosis (i.e., programmed cell death) and its relevance to traditional DNA parameters and other phenotypic considerations. It is not within the scope of this chapter to handle this topic. Although many studies are ongoing, apoptotic measurements are still not part of the routine clinical laboratory procedures.

As mentioned earlier, laboratory DNA analysis has recently come under much scrutiny and, in some regions, these studies are no longer being reimbursed. Several investigators in the field have challenged the wholesale expulsion of this test from the laboratory, as it is quite useful in certain tumors. A set of retrospective breast cases is being re-examined by Bagwell and others to attempt to develop a unified prognostic model for node-negative breast cancer patients (Bagwell, 2004). It is hoped that these studies and others will resurrect what could be a useful prognostic and diagnostic tool the complexity of which was perhaps previously underestimated.

Quantitative Flow Cytometry: Fluorescence Intensity Measurements

The definition of cell types in immunologic terms such as effector cells implies the property of these cells to regulate, whether up or down, specific molecular functions through surface receptors. Known as immunologic phenotypes (Poncelet, 1993), these cells need other measurable properties to define their biological roles in maturation and in disease processes. One of the observed phenomena is the differential expression of cell surface antigens (CDs) in relative terms and in absolute quantitative terms. Before the availability of absolute measures, descriptive terms such as bright or dim, bimodal, and so forth, were used in the literature to describe a visual phenomenon of antigen density differences. Although descriptive, these terms are hard to define and to standardize between laboratories and between patients. They also lack precision in defining an event and cannot be objectively used to monitor patients' treatment or call definition (cell type) by measures of CD expression and their overlapping expression. Evidence suggests that quantitative differences in antigen expression in chronic lymphocytic leukemia and other leukemias may be important in determining the prognosis (Poncelet, 1985). These measures are also used in the definition of MRD and in the investigation of a viral effect or activation in HIV disease (Poncelet, 1991). The percent of a specific cell present often does not give the true clinical picture. This is particularly true in leukopenic cases and when the blast population is a relatively small percentage of total cells present.

Quantitative flow cytometry (QFCM) is defined as the quantification of fluorescence intensity (FI) as determined by the antibody-binding capacity of a given fluorochrome antibody conjugate, and is an indirect measure of the amount of cell surface antigen per individual cell (Stelzer, 1997; Marti, 2003) Investigators (Poncelet, 1985, 1986; Vogt, 1991, 1994) have described the use of polystyrene beads or cell lines coated with saturating amounts of antibody to determine the absolute number of receptors or antigenic sites per cell, also referred to as antigen density (Poncelet, 1993). ABC units are defined as a measure of relative antibody-binding capacity. This method does not need to match the fluorescein:protein (F/P) ratios, as both the cells and standards are being stained with the same antibody. The use of fluorescence intensity measurements should give the user a means to avoid this situation. More information can be obtained by referring to the 1997 US–Canadian consensus document reviewing the necessary parameters for standardization (Stelzer, 1997).

Although early in their development, quantitative phenotypes will help us define cluster analysis software programs for cell quantification and identification by establishing mean channel fluorescence intensity as a means of separating cells of different functional phenotypes.

Quality Control and Quality Assurance in the Cellular Laboratory

Throughout this chapter, we have tried to point out areas where the clinician as well as the laboratory must pay particular attention to the methods used and the interpretations made in the evaluation of the cellular response. Quality assurance and quality control parameters are not well defined in this area of the laboratory, and few absolute standards exist as compared with chemistry analytes or humoral antibody measures. The success of the cellular laboratory rests in its approach to the problem and the longitudinal assessment of the condition being diagnosed. It was clearly pointed out that baseline studies need to be repeated if the original evaluation is performed at a time of immunologic stress.

Basic parameters of diurnal variations in lymphocyte subsets are obvious but are often forgotten or overlooked. Malone pointed out that the variability in the CD4 measures of absolute counts is 50% due to biology and the other 50% due to other technical issues (Malone, 1990). Factors affecting the longitudinal evaluation of CD4 absolute counts in a clinical trial setting have been reviewed by Fei (1993). Furthermore, Fahey reviewed the prognostic value of both humoral and cellular assays in HIV (Fahey, 1990). In other clinical cellular assays, variability is inherent in the assay owing to lack of standard formats and methods as well as reagents. Furthermore, instrument calibration and sensitivity are not well monitored. Cytotoxic T-lymphocyte assays are particularly hard to standardize. Historic assays such as mitogen proliferation are also fraught with variability between laboratories. Therefore, laboratories offering these immunologic tests must have an extensive database by which they can interpret an individual patient's result. Cellular laboratories must establish normal ranges for their assays and be aware that adult normal ranges are not applicable to pediatric assays. This is particularly problematic because pediatric normal ranges are difficult to determine owing to lack of available subjects in the first year of life, and correct interpretation of laboratory results depends on these normal values. Comparisons of data between laboratories should be carefully undertaken.

When available, a cellular immunology laboratory must use the available standards in the performance of flow cytometry and DNA analysis and should be aware of the state and federal regulations with regard to the laboratory, including the Human Health and Services Clinical Laboratory Improvement Act of 1988. Furthermore, it should participate in proficiency testing, when available, and be involved in continuing education seminars, including competency evaluations for all personnel involved in testing. All assays performed in the laboratory must include a normal control and, when possible, in-process controls to establish the validity of the assay. Shipped samples must be carefully monitored for exposure to heat and cold and time since patient procurement. A clinical history should accompany the samples for particular studies being undertaken so that the laboratory director can take the correct approach to testing.

A consensus document with recommendations on the immuno-phenotypic analysis of hematologic neoplasia by flow cytometry has been published (Braylan, 1997). This document was painstakingly developed by concerned providers to the medical community to cover laboratory procedures, selection of antibodies for identification of neoplasms, data analysis and interpretation, medical reporting, and indications in the absence of standardized kits and other devices. The FDA has put into effect the Analyte Specific Regulation (Analyte Specific Regulation, November 21, 1997), which removes reagents such as monoclonals from research use status to ASRs. This rule does not allow manufacturers to tell laboratory users how to use their reagents. They cannot specify intended use. The ASR rule does provide for stable, well-defined reagents manufactured under good manufacturing practices. All laboratories using these reagents as a 'home brew test' must perform their own clinical trial and validation studies and must use a disclaimer in the final report. The consensus document allows a laboratory to perform their assays in a consistent manner and the definition of clinical significance across a large number of laboratories and institutions. The document is not a standard but is consistent with other published NCCLS standards already in use.

The cellular laboratory is faced with a more difficult job of interpretation because the data are not easily standardized. Furthermore, quality assurance of the sample and evaluation being performed depends on careful documentation of the biological and logical parameters that may influence the results. The future of tests used in the evaluation of the cellular component of the immune response resides in the development of new methods that may lend themselves to better standardization.

References

Alarcon B, Gil D, Delgado P, et al: Initiation of TCR signaling: regulation within CD3 dimers. Immunol Rev 2003; 191:38–46.

Allsopp CE, Nicholls SJ, Langhorne J: A flow cytometric method to assess antigen-specific proliferative responses of different subpopulations of fresh and cryopreserved human peripheral blood mononuclear cells. J Immunol Methods 1998; 214:175–186.

The authors of this paper describe a useful approach to analyzing lymphocyte proliferative responses to antigen that makes use of a stable membrane bound dye in combination with surface monoclonal antibody labels to identify subpopulations without the need for pre-sorting.

Amati L, Cirimele D, Pugliese V, et al: Nutrition and immunity: laboratory and clinical aspects. Curr Pharm Des 2003; 9:1924–1931.

Analyte Specific Regulation MD: Classification/reclassification; restricted devices; analyste specific reagents. Federal Regulation: 66243–62260, November 21, 1997.

Ananworanich J, Shearer WT: Delayed-type hypersensitivity skin testing. In Rose NR, Hamilton RG, Detrick B (eds): Manual of Clinical Laboratory Immunology, 6th ed. Washington, DC, ASM Press, 2002, pp 212–219.

Angulo R, Fulcher DA: Measurement of Candida-specific blastogenesis: comparison of carboxyfluorescein succinimidyl ester labelling of T cells, thymidine incorporation, and CD69 expression. Cytometry 1998; 34:143–151.

Aoki Y, Tosato G: Neoplastic conditions in the context of HIV-1 infection. Curr HIV Res 2004; 2:343–349.

ASCO: Clinical practice guidelines for the use of tumor markers in breast and colorectal cancer. Adopted May 17, 1996, by American Society of Clinical Oncology. J Clin Oncol 1996; 14:2843–2877.

Azuma M, Ito D, Yagita H, et al: B70 antigen is a second ligand for CTLA-4 and CD28. Nature 1993; 366:76–79.

Bagwell CB: Theoretical aspects of flow cytometry data analysis. In Bauer D, Duque RE, Shankey TV (eds): Clinical Flow Cytometry: Principles and Applications. Baltimore: Williams & Wilkins, 1993, pp 41–61.

Bagwell CB: DNA histogram analysis for node-negative breast cancer. Cytometry A 2004; 58:76–78.

Balkwill FR, Burke F: The cytokine network. Immunol Today 1989; 10:299–304.

Baskar S, Ostrand-Rosenberg S, Nabavi N, et al: Constitutive expression of B7 restores immunogenicity of tumor cells expressing truncated major histocompatibility complex class II molecules. Proc Natl Acad Sci USA 1993; 90:5687–5690.

Bastian J, Law S, Vogler L, et al: Prediction of persistent immunodeficiency in the DiGeorge anomaly. J Pediatr 1989; 115:391–396.

Bauer KD, Jacobberger JW: Analysis of intracellular proteins. Methods Cell Biol 1994; 41:351–376.

Baumgarth N, Roederer M: A practical approach to multicolor flow cytometry for immunophenotyping. J Immunol Methods 2000; 243:77–97.

This article describes basic multicolor flow cytometry, technical problems that may be expected, and artifacts frequently encountered, and offers suggestions for handling them.

Black MM, Zachrau RE, Hankey BF, et al: Skin window reactivity to autologous breast cancer. An index of prognostically significant cell-mediated immunity. Cancer 1988; 62:72–83.

Bocchieri MH, Talle MA, Maltese LM, et al: Whole blood culture for measuring mitogen induced T cell proliferation provides superior correlations with disease state and T cell phenotype in asymptomatic HIV-infected subjects. J Immunol Methods 1995; 181:233–243.

Bogh LD, Duling TA: Flow cytometry instrumentation in research and clinical laboratories. Clin Lab Sci 1993; 6:167–173.

Bonilla FA, Oettgen HC: Normal ranges for lymphocyte subsets in children. J Pediatr 1997; 130:347–349.

Borowitz MJ: Acute lymphoblastic leukemia. In Knowles DM (ed): Neoplastic Hematopathology. Baltimore, Williams & Wilkins, 1992, pp 1295–1314.

Borut TC, Ank BJ, Gard SE, et al: Tetanus toxoid skin test in children: correlation with in vitro lymphocyte stimulation and monocyte chemotaxis. J Pediatr 1980; 97:567–573.

Braylan RC, Atwater SK, Diamond L, et al: US–Canadian Consensus recommendations on the immunophenotypic analysis of hematologic neoplasia by flow cytometry: data reporting. Cytometry 1997; 30:245–248.

Bretscher P: The two-signal model of lymphocyte activation twenty-one years later. Immunol Today 1992; 13:74–76.

Bretscher P: Living with the ups and downs of the two signal model. Immunol Cell Biol 2004; 82:141–148.

Buckley RH: Molecular defects in human severe combined immunodeficiency and approaches to immune reconstitution. Annu Rev Immunol 2004; 22:625–655.

Burns EA: Effects of aging on immune function. J Nutr Health Aging 2004; 8:9–18.

Calvelli T, Denny TN, Paxton H, et al: Guideline for flow cytometric immunophenotyping: a report from the National Institute of Allergy and Infectious Diseases, Division of AIDS. Cytometry 1993; 14:702–715.

Carothers AD: Counting, measuring, and mapping in FISH-labelled cells: sample size considerations and implications for automation. Cytometry 1994; 16:298–304.

Centers for Disease Control C: Guidelines for the performance of CD4+ T-cell determinations in persons with human immunodeficiency virus infection. MMWR Morb Mortal Wkly Rep 1992; 41:1–17.

Chapman GV: Instrumentation for flow cytometry. J Immunol Methods 2000; 243:3–12.

Chatelain R, Varkila K, Coffman RL: IL-4 induces a Th2 response in Leishmania major-infected mice. J Immunol 1992; 148:1182–1187.

Chen L, Ashe S, Brady WA, et al: Costimulation of antitumor immunity by the B7 counterreceptor for the T lymphocyte molecules CD28 and CTLA-4. Cell 1992; 71:1093–1102.

Cheroutre H: Starting at the beginning: new perspectives on the biology of mucosal T cells. Annu Rev Immunol 2004; 22:217–246.

Clerici M, Shearer GM: A TH1→TH2 switch is a critical step in the etiology of HIV infection. Immunol Today 1993; 14:107–111.

Clerici M, Shearer GM: The Th1–Th2 hypothesis of HIV infection: new insights. Immunol Today 1994; 15:575–581.

Clevenger CV, Shankey TV: Cytochemistry II: Immunofluorescence measurement of intracellular antigens. In Bauer KD, Shankey TV (eds): Clinical Flow Cytometry: Principles and Applications. Baltimore, Williams & Wilkins, 1993, pp 157–175.

Conley ME: Molecular basis of immunodeficiency. Immunol Rev 2005; 203:5–9.

Coon JS, Deitch AD, de Vere White RW, et al: Interinstitutional variability in DNA flow cytometric analysis of tumors. The National Cancer Institute's Flow Cytometry Network Experience. Cancer 1988; 61:126–130.

Coon JS, Paxton H, Lucy L, et al: Interlaboratory variation in DNA flow cytometry. Results of the College of American Pathologists' Survey. Arch Pathol Lab Med 1994; 118:681–685.

Cost KM, Fineman D, Steger S: A flow cytometry-based screening assay for lymphocyte proliferation. Clin Immunol Newslett 1993; 13:82–85.

Cunningham-Rundles S: Issues in assessment of human immune function. In Military Strategies for Sustainment of Nutrition and Immune Function in the Field. Washington, DC, Institute of Medicine National Academy Press, 1999, pp 235–248.

Cunningham-Rundles S, Cervia JS: Malnutrition and host defense. In Walker WA, Watkins JB (eds): Pediatrics: Basic Science and Clinical Application, 2nd ed. New York, Marcel Dekker, 1996, pp 295–307.

Cunningham-Rundles S, Chen C, Bussel JB, et al: Human immune development: implications for congenital HIV infection. Ann NY Acad Sci 1993; 693:20–34.

Cunningham-Rundles C, Cunningham-Rundles S, Iwata T, et al: Zinc deficiency, depressed thymic hormones, and T lymphocyte dysfunction in patients with hypogammaglobulinemia. Clin Immunol Immunopathol 1981; 21:387–396.

Cunningham-Rundles S, Harbison M, Guirguis S, et al: New perspectives on use of thymic factors in immune deficiency. Ann NY Acad Sci 1994; 730:71–83.

Cunningham-Rundles S, Lin DH: Nutrition and the immune system of the gut. Nutrition 1998; 14:573–579.

Cunningham-Rundles S, Nessin M: Bacterial infections in the immunologically compromised host. In Nataro JP, Blaser MJ, Cunningham-Rundles S (eds): Persistent Bacterial Infections. Washington, DC, American Society of Microbiology Press, 2000, pp 145–164.

Cunningham-Rundles C, Siegal FP, Cunningham-Rundles S, et al: Incidence of cancer in 98 patients with common varied immunodeficiency. J Clin Immunol 1987; 7:294–299.

Cunningham-Rundles S, Yeger-Arbitman R, Nachman SA, et al: New variant of MHC class II deficiency with interleukin-2 abnormality. Clin Immunol Immunopathol 1990; 56:116–123.

Denny T, Yogev R, Gelman R, et al: Lymphocyte subsets in healthy children during the first 5 years of life. JAMA 1992; 267:1484–1488.

Deodhar SD: Basics in practical applications and standardization of techniques of cellular immunology. Lab Res Methods Biol Med 1983; 8:71–78.

DiGeorge AM: Congenital absence of the thymus and its immunologic consequences: Concurrence with congenital hypothyroidism. In Bergsma D (ed.): Birth Defects Immunologic Deficiency Disease in Man. White Plains, NY, The National Foundation–March of Dimes, 1974, vol 4(1), p 116.

Eckmann L: Innate immunity and mucosal bacterial interactions in the intestine. Curr Opin Gastroenterol 2004; 20:82–88.

Elder ME: ZAP-70 and defects of T-cell receptor signaling. Semin Hematol 1998; 35:310–320.

Fahey JL, Taylor JM, Detels R, et al: The prognostic value of cellular and serologic markers in infection with human immunodeficiency virus type 1. N Engl J Med 1990; 322:166–172.

Fei DT, Paxton H, Chen AB: Difficulties in precise quantitation of CD4+ T lymphocytes for clinical trials: a review. Biologicals 1993; 21:221–231.

Fischer A, Le Deist F, Hacein-Bey-Abina S, et al: Severe combined immunodeficiency. A model disease for molecular immunology and therapy. Immunol Rev 2005; 203:98–109.

Fletcher MA, Mosley JW, Hassett J, et al: Effect of age on human immunodeficiency virus type 1-induced changes in lymphocyte populations among persons with congenital clotting disorders. Transfusion Safety Study Group. Blood 1992; 80:831–840.

Foletta VC, Segal DH, Cohen DR: Transcriptional regulation in the immune system: all roads lead to AP-1. J Leukocyte Biol 1998; 63:139–152.

Fulop T, Jr, Larbi A, Dupuis G, et al: Ageing, autoimmunity and arthritis: perturbations of TCR signal transduction pathways with ageing – a biochemical paradigm for the ageing immune system. Arthritis Res Ther 2003; 5:290–302.

Gelfand EW: Abnormalities of signal transduction and T cell immunodeficiency. In Gupta S, Griscelli C (eds): New Concepts in Immunodeficiency Disease. New York, John Wiley & Sons, 1993, pp 231–248.

Ginaldi L, De Martinis M, Modesti M, et al: Immunophenotypical changes of T lymphocytes in the elderly. Gerontology 2000; 46:242–248.

Giorgi JV, Detels R: T-cell subset alterations in HIV-infected homosexual men: NIAID Multicenter AIDS cohort study. Clin Immunol Immunopathol 1989; 52:10–18.

Givan AL: Flow cytometry: an introduction. Methods Mol Biol 2004; 263:1–32.
This review article provides a thorough introduction to flow cytometry and is easy to read.

Goetzman EA: Flow cytometry: basic concepts and clinical applications in immunodiagnostics. Clin Lab Sci 1993; 6:177–182.

Good RA: Cellular immunology in a historical perspective. Immunol Rev 2002; 185:136–158.

Goolsby CL, Paniagua M, Marszalek L: Clinical flow cytometry: a transition in utilization. Cancer Treat Res 2004; 121:239–257.

Hakim FT, Flomerfelt FA, Boyiadzis M, et al: Aging, immunity and cancer. Curr Opin Immunol 2004; 16:151–156.

Hamerman JA, Ogasawara K, Lanier LL: NK cells in innate immunity. Curr Opin Immunol 2005; 17:29–35.

Harding CV, Neefjes J: Antigen processing and recognition. Curr Opin Immunol 2005; 17:55–57.

Haynes BF, Hale LP: The human thymus. A chimeric organ comprised of central and peripheral lymphoid components. Immunol Res 1998; 18:61–78.

Hedley DW, Friedlander ML, Taylor IW, et al: Method for analysis of cellular DNA content of paraffin-embedded pathological material using flow cytometry. J Histochem Cytochem 1983; 31:1333–1335.

Heimdal JH, Aarstad HJ, Klementsen B, et al: Peripheral blood mononuclear cell (PBMC) responsiveness in patients with head and neck cancer in relation to tumour stage and prognosis. Acta Otolaryngol 1999; 119:281–284.

Hermans IF, Silk JD, Yang J, et al: The VITAL assay: a versatile fluorometric technique for assessing CTL- and NKT-mediated cytotoxicity against multiple targets in vitro and in vivo. J Immunol Methods 2004; 285:25–40.

Herzenberg LA: Genetics, FACS, immunology, and redox: a tale of two lives intertwined. Annu Rev Immunol 2004; 22:1–31.

Homburger HA, Rosenstock W, Paxton H, et al: Assessment of interlaboratory variability of immunophenotyping. Results of the College of American Pathologists Flow Cytometry Survey. Ann NY Acad Sci 1993; 677:43–49.

Huebner RE, Schein MF, Bass JB, Jr: The tuberculin skin test. Clin Infect Dis 1993; 17:968–975.

Irving BA, Weiss A: The cytoplasmic domain of the T cell receptor zeta chain is sufficient to couple to receptor-associated signal transduction pathways. Cell 1991; 64:891–901.

Janeway CA, Jr, Bottomly K: Signals and signs for lymphocyte responses. Cell 1994; 76:275–285.

Janeway CA, Jr, Medzhitov R: Innate immune recognition. Annu Rev Immunol 2002; 20:197–216.

Janeway CA, Jr, Travers P, Walport M, et al: Immunobiology, 6th ed. New York, Garland Publishing, 2005.

Jung T, Schauer U, Heusser C, et al: Detection of intracellular cytokines by flow cytometry. J Immunol Methods 1993; 159:197–207.

Kagan J, Gelman R, Waxdal M, et al: NIAID Division of AIDS flow cytometry quality assessment program. Ann NY Acad Sci 1993; 677:50–52.

Katz P, Fauci AS: Immunosuppressives and immunoadjuvants. In Samter M, Talmage DW, Frank MM (eds): Immunological Diseases, 4th ed. Boston, Little, Brown & Co., 1993, pp 675–698.

Keren DF: Surface marker assays in immunodeficiency diseases. In Keren DF (ed.): Flow Cytometry in Clinical Diagnosis. Chicago, ASCP Press, 1989, pp 213–247.

Keusch GT: The history of nutrition: malnutrition, infection and immunity. J Nutr 2003; 133:336S–340S.

Kraan J, Gratama JW, Keeney M, et al: Setting up and calibration of a flow cytometer for multicolor immunophenotyping. J Biol Regul Homeost Agents 2003; 17:223–233.

Krown SE: AIDS-associated malignancies. Cancer Chemother Biol Response Modif 1996; 16:441–461.

Lamb LS, Jr: Hematopoietic cellular therapy: implications for the flow cytometry laboratory. Hematol Oncol Clin North Am 2002; 16:455–476.

Landay AL, Jessop C, Lennette ET, et al: Chronic fatigue syndrome: clinical condition associated with immune activation. Lancet 1991; 338:707–712.

LeGuern C: Regulation of T-cell functions by MHC class II self-presentation. TRENDS Immunol 2003; 24:633–638.

Lesourd B: Nutrition: a major factor influencing immunity in the elderly. J Nutr Health Aging 2004; 8:28–37.

Lewis DE: Cytochemistry I: Cell surface immunofluorescence. In Bauer KD, Duque RE, Shankey TV (eds): Clinical Flow Cytometry: Principles and Applications. Baltimore, Williams & Wilkins, 1993, pp 143–156.

Linsley PS, Brady W, Grosmaire L, et al: Binding of the B cell activation antigen B7 to CD28 costimulates T cell proliferation and interleukin 2 mRNA accumulation. J Exp Med 1991a; 173:721–730.

Linsley PS, Brady W, Urnes M, et al: CTLA-4 is a second receptor for the B cell activation antigen B7. J Exp Med 1991b; 174:561–569.

Lissoni P, Brivio F, Viviani S, et al: Which immunological parameters are clinically essential to monitor IL-2 cancer immunotherapy? J Biol Regul Homeost Agents 1999; 13:110–114.

Liu Y, Jones B, Aruffo A, et al: Heat-stable antigen is a costimulatory molecule for CD4 T cell growth. J Exp Med 1992; 175:437–445.

Livingston PO, Cunningham-Rundles S, Marfleet G, et al: Inhibition of suppressor-cell activity by cyclophosphamide in patients with malignant melanoma. J Biol Response Mod 1987; 6:392–403.

Lloyd A, Hickie I, Hickie C, et al: Cell-mediated immunity in patients with chronic fatigue syndrome, healthy control subjects and patients with major depression. Clin Exp Immunol 1992; 87:76–79.

Loken MR, Brosnan JM, Bach BA, et al: Establishing optimal lymphocyte gates for immunophenotyping by flow cytometry. Cytometry 1990; 11:453–459.

Loken MR, Parks DR, Herzenberg LA: Two-color immunofluorescence using a fluorescence-activated cell sorter. J Histochem Cytochem 1977; 25:899–907.

Loken MR, Sweet RG, Herzenberg LA: Cell discrimination by multiangle light scattering. J Histochem Cytochem 1976; 24:284–291.

Maas JJ, Roos MT, Keet IP, et al: In vivo delayed-type hypersensitivity skin test anergy in human immunodeficiency virus type 1 infection is associated with T cell nonresponsiveness in vitro. J Infect Dis 1998; 178:1024–1029.

McCoy JP, Jr: Basic principles of flow cytometry. Hematol Oncol Clin North Am 2002; 16:229–243.

Madrenas J, Wange RL, Wang JL, et al: Zeta phosphorylation without ZAP-70 activation induced by TCR antagonists or partial agonists. Science 1995; 267:515–518.

Malaguarnera L, Ferlito L, Imbesi RM, et al: Immunosenescence: a review. Arch Gerontol Geriatr 2001; 32:1–14.
This review provides a good summary of age-related changes that occur in both arms of the immune system.

Malissen B: An evolutionary and structural perspective on T cell antigen receptor function. Immunol Rev 2003; 191:7–27.

Malone JL, Simms TE, Gray GC, et al: Sources of variability in repeated T-helper lymphocyte counts from human immunodeficiency virus type 1-infected patients: total lymphocyte count fluctuations and diurnal cycle are important. J Acquir Immune Defic Syndr 1990; 3:144–151.

Maluish AE, Strong DM: Lymphocyte proliferation. In Rose NR, Friedman H, Fahey JL (eds): Manual of Clinical Laboratory Immunology. Washington, DC, American Society for Microbiology, 1986, pp 274–281.

Mandy FF: Twenty-five years of clinical flow cytometry: AIDS accelerated global instrument distribution. Cytometry A 2004; 58:55–56.

Mandy FF, Bergeron M, Recktenwald D, et al: A simultaneous three-color T cell subsets analysis with single laser flow cytometers using T cell gating protocol. Comparison with conventional two-color immunophenotyping method. J Immunol Methods 1992; 156:151–162.

Marti GE, Vogt RF, Jr, Stetler-Stevenson M: Clinical quantitative flow cytometry: 'Identifying the optimal methods for clinical quantitative flow cytometry'. Cytometry B Clin Cytom 2003; 55:59.

Martin-Reay DG, Kamentsky LA, Weinberg DS, et al: Evaluation of a new slide-based laser scanning cytometer for DNA analysis of tumors. Comparison with flow cytometry and image analysis. Am J Clin Pathol 1994; 102:432–438.

Mascher B, Schlenke P, Seyfarth M: Expression and kinetics of cytokines determined by intracellular staining using flow cytometry. J Immunol Methods 1999; 223:115–121.

Masur H, Michelis MA, Greene JB, et al: An outbreak of community-acquired *Pneumocystis carinii* pneumonia: initial manifestation of cellular immune dysfunction. N Engl J Med 1981; 305:1431–1438.

Mazari L, Lesourd BM: Nutritional influences on immune response in healthy aged persons. Mech Ageing Dev 1998; 104:25–40.

Mehta BA, Maino VC: Simultaneous detection of DNA synthesis and cytokine production in staphylococcal enterotoxin B activated CD4$^+$ T lymphocytes by flow cytometry. J Immunol Methods 1997; 208:49–59.

Moss RB, Mercandetti A, Vojdani A: TNF-alpha and chronic fatigue syndrome. J Clin Immunol 1999; 19:314–316.

Moulin AM: Immunology old and new: the beginning and the end. In Paulin MH (ed.): Essays on the History of Immunology. Toronto, Wall & Thompson, 1989, pp 292–298.

Moynahan EJ: Acrodermatitis enteropathica: a lethal inherited human zinc-deficiency disorder (Letter). Lancet 1974; 2:399–400.

Nicholson JK, Jones BM, Hubbard M: CD4 T-lymphocyte determinations on whole blood specimens using a single-tube three-color assay. Cytometry 1993a; 14:685–689.

Nicholson JKA, Green TA: Collaborating laboratories: selection of anticoagulants for lymphocyte immunophenotyping: effect of specimen age on results. J Immunol Methods 1993b; 165:31–35.

Noguchi M, Yi H, Rosenblatt HM, et al: Interleukin-2 receptor gamma chain mutation results in X-linked severe combined immunodeficiency in humans. Cell 1993; 73:147–157.

Nowell PC: Phytohemagglutinin: an initiator of mitosis in cultures of normal human leukocytes. Cancer Res 1960; 20:462–466.

Owen MJ, Jenkinson E: Ontogeny of the immune response. In Lachman PJ, Peters DK, Rosen FS (eds): Clinical Aspects of Immunology. Oxford, Blackwell Scientific, 1993, pp 3–12.

Parish CR: Fluorescent dyes for lymphocyte migration and proliferation studies. Immunol Cell Biol 1999; 77:499–508.

Passlick B, Flieger D, Ziegler-Heitbrock HW: Identification and characterization of a novel monocyte subpopulation in human peripheral blood. Blood 1989; 74:2527–2534.

Paul WE: Fundamental Immunology. New York, Bauer Press, 1993.

Paul WE, Seder RA: Lymphocyte responses and cytokines. Cell 1994; 76:241–251.

Paxton H, Pins M, Denton G, et al: Comparison of CD4 cell count by a simple enzyme-linked immunosorbent assay using the TRAx CD4 test kit and by flow cytometry and hematology. Clin Diagn Lab Immunol 1995; 2:104–114.

Pennington JA: Intakes of minerals from diets and foods: is there a need for concern? J Nutr 1996; 126:2304S–2308S.

Perfetto SP, Chattopadhyay PK, Roederer M: Seventeen-colour flow cytometry: unravelling the immune system. Nat Rev Immunol 2004; 4:648–655.

This paper describes a powerful form of flow cytometry capable of simultaneously examining several physical parameters and seventeen fluorescent colors.

Perfetto SP, Currier J, Birx DL: T-lymphocyte activation and cell signaling. In Rose NR, Hamilton RG, Detrick B (eds): Manual of Clinical Laboratory Immunology, 6th ed. Washington, DC: ASM Press, 2002, pp 224–237.

Perfetto SP, Hickey TE, Blair PJ, et al: Measurement of CD69 induction in the assessment of immune function in asymptomatic HIV-infected individuals. Cytometry 1997; 30:1–9.

Peritt D, Robertson S, Gri G, et al: Differentiation of human NK cells into NK1 and NK2 subsets. J Immunol 1998; 161:5821–5824.

Pesu M, Candotti F, Husa M, et al: Jak3, severe combined immunodeficiency, and a new class of immunosuppressive drugs. Immunol Rev 2005; 203:127–142.

Peters VB, Rosh JR, Mugrditchian L, et al: Growth failure as the first expression of malnutrition in children with human immunodeficiency virus infection. Mt Sinai J Med 1998; 65:1–4.

Petrovsky N, Harrison LC: Cytokine-based human whole blood assay for the detection of antigen-reactive T cells. J Immunol Methods 1995; 186:37–46.

Poncelet P, Carayon P: Cytofluorometric quantification of cell-surface antigens by indirect immunofluorescence using monoclonal antibodies. J Immunol Methods 1985; 85:65–74.

Poncelet P, George F, Lavabre-Bertrand T: Immunological detection of membrane bound antigens and receptors. Cells Tissues Methods Immunol Anal 1993; 3:389–417.

Poncelet P, Lavabre-Bertrand T, Carayon P: Quantitative phenotypes of B chronic lymphocytic leukemia B cells established with monoclonals antibodies from the B cell protocol. In Reinherz EL, Haynes BF, Nadler LM, et al (eds): Leukocyte Typing II. New York, Springer-Verlag, 1986, vol 2, pp 229–343.

Poncelet P, Poinas G, Corbeau P, et al: Surface CD4 density remains constant on lymphocytes of HIV-infected patients in the progression of disease. Res Immunol 1991; 142:291–298.

Prasad AS, Miale A, Jr, Farid Z, et al: Zinc metabolism in patients with the syndrome of iron deficiency anemia, hepatosplenomegaly, dwarfism, and hypogonadism. J Lab Clin Med 1963; 61:537–549.

Prescott SL, Macaubas C, Holt BJ, et al: Transplacental priming of the human immune system to environmental allergens: universal skewing of initial T cell responses toward the Th2 cytokine profile. J Immunol 1998; 160:4730–4737.

Prussin C, Metcalfe DD: Detection of intracytoplasmic cytokine using flow cytometry and directly conjugated anti-cytokine antibodies. J Immunol Methods 1995; 188:117–128.

Rabinovitch PS: Practical considerations for DNA content and cell cycle analysis. In Bauer KD, Duque RE, Shankey TV (eds): Clinical Flow Cytometry: Principles and Applications. Baltimore, Williams & Wilkins, 1993, pp 143–156.

Rabinovitch PS: DNA content histogram and cell-cycle analysis. Methods Cell Biol 1994; 41:263–296.

Ramaekers FC, Hopman AH: Detection of genetic aberrations in bladder cancer using in situ hybridization. Ann N Y Acad Sci 1993; 677:199–213.

Reth M: Antigen receptor tail clue. Nature 1989; 338:383–384.

Rosen FS: A brief history of immunodeficiency disease. Immunol Rev 2000; 178:8–12.

Rosenberg ES, Billingsley JM, Caliendo AM, et al: Vigorous HIV-1-specific CD4+ T cell responses associated with control of viremia. Science 1997; 278:1447–1450.

Rowe PC, Barron DF, Calkins H, et al: Orthostatic intolerance and chronic fatigue syndrome associated with Ehlers–Danlos syndrome. J Pediatr 1999; 135:494–499.

Samelson LE: Signal transduction mediated by the T cell antigen receptor: the role of adapter proteins. Annu Rev Immunol 2002; 20:371–394.

Schultes BC, Nicodemus CF: Using antibodies in tumour immunotherapy. Expert Opin Biol Ther 2004; 4:1265–1284.

Seder RA, Gazzinelli R, Sher A, et al: Interleukin 12 acts directly on CD4+ T cells to enhance priming for interferon gamma production and diminishes interleukin 4 inhibition of such priming. Proc Natl Acad Sci U S A 1993; 90:10188–10192.

Seder RA, Paul WE, Davis MM, et al: The presence of interleukin 4 during in vitro priming determines the lymphokine-producing potential of CD4+ T cells from T cell receptor transgenic mice. J Exp Med 1992; 176:1091–1098.

Shankey TV, Rabinovitch PS: DNA content flow cytometry. In Rose NR, Hamilton RG, Detrick B (eds): Manual of Clinical Laboratory Immunology, 6th ed. Washington, DC, ASM Press, 2002, pp 171–184.

Shankey TV, Rabinovitch PS, Bagwell B, et al: Guidelines for implementation of clinical DNA cytometry. International Society for Analytical Cytology. Cytometry 1993; 14:472–477.

Shapiro HM: Trends and developments in flow cytometry instrumentation. Ann NY Acad Sci 1993; 677:155–166.

Shapiro HM: The evolution of cytometers. Cytometry A 2004; 58:13–20.

Siegal FP, Lopez C, Hammer GS, et al: Severe acquired immunodeficiency in male homosexuals, manifested by chronic perianal ulcerative herpes simplex lesions. N Engl J Med 1981; 305:1439–1444.

Silverstein AM: History of immunology. Cellular versus humoral immunity: determinants and consequences of an epic 19th century battle. Cell Immunol 1979; 48:208–221.

Silverstein AM: Cellular versus humoral immunology: a century-long dispute. Nat Immunol 2003; 4:425–428.

Smith KA: The quantal theory of how the immune system discriminates between 'self and non-self'. Med Immunol 2004; 3:1–22.

Smyth MJ, Cretney E, Kershaw MH, et al: Cytokines in cancer immunity and immunotherapy. Immunol Rev 2004; 202:275–293.

Snow C: Flow cytometer electronics. Cytometry A 2004; 57:63–69.

Sprent J, Surh CD: T cell memory. Annu Rev Immunol 2002; 20:551–579.

Standards NCCL: Clinical applications of flow cytometry: Quality assurance and immunophenotyping of peripheral blood lymphocytes. NCCLS Document H42-T. Villanova, PA, National Committee for Clinical Laboratory Standards, 1992.

Steinman RM, Mellman I: Immunotherapy: bewitched, bothered, and bewildered no more. Science 2004; 305:197–200.

Stelzer GT, Marti G, Hurley A, et al: US–Canadian Consensus recommendations on the immunophenotypic analysis of hematologic neoplasia by flow cytometry: standardization and validation of laboratory procedures. Cytometry 1997; 30:214–230.

Stelzer GT, Shults KE, Loken MR: CD45 gating for routine flow cytometric analysis of human bone marrow specimens. Ann NY Acad Sci 1993; 677:265–280.

Stewart CC, Goolsby C, Shackney SE: Emerging technology and future developments in flow cytometry. Hematol Oncol Clin North Am 2002; 16:477–495, vii–viii.

Stewart CC, Stewart SJ: Multiparameter data acquisition and analysis of leukocytes. Methods Mol Biol 2004; 263.45–66.

Sullivan KE, Jawad AF, Randall P, et al: Lack of correlation between impaired T cell production, immunodeficiency, and other phenotypic features in chromosome 22q11.2 deletion syndromes. Clin Immunol Immunopathol 1998; 86:141–146.

Suni MA, Picker LJ, Maino VC: Detection of antigen-specific T cell cytokine expression in whole blood by flow cytometry. J Immunol Methods 1998; 212:89–98.

Tan P, Anasetti C, Hansen JA, et al: Induction of alloantigen-specific hyporesponsiveness in human T lymphocytes by blocking interaction of CD28 with its natural ligand B7/BB1. J Exp Med 1993; 177:165–173.

Tirindelli Danesi D, Spano M, Altavista P, et al: Quality control study of the Italian Group of Cytometry on flow cytometry DNA content measurements: II. Factors affecting inter- and intralaboratory variability. Cytometry 1997; 30:85–97.

Tlaskalova-Hogenova H, Tuckova L, Lodinova-Zadnikova R, et al: Mucosal immunity: its role in defense and allergy. Int Arch Allergy Immunol 2002; 128:77–89.

Townsend SE, Allison JP: Tumor rejection after direct costimulation of CD8+ T cells by B7-transfected melanoma cells. Science 1993; 259:368–370.

Trinchieri G: Natural killer cells wear different hats: effector cells of innate resistance and regulatory cells of adaptive immunity and of hematopoiesis. Semin Immunol 1995; 7:83–88.

Van der Merwe PA, Davis SJ: Molecular interactions mediating T cell antigen recognition. Annu Rev Immunol 2003; 21:659–684.

Veber MB, Cunningham-Rundles S, Schulman M, et al: Acute shift in immune response to microbial activators in very-low-birth-weight infants. Clin Exp Immunol 1991; 83:391–395.

Vigano A, Vella S, Principi N, et al: Thymus volume correlates with the progression of vertical HIV infection. AIDS 1999; 13:F29–34.

Vindelov LL, Christensen IJ: Detergent and proteolytic enzyme-based techniques for nuclear isolation and DNA content analysis. Methods Cell Biol 1994; 41:219–229.

Vogt RF, Jr, Cross GD, Phillips DL, et al: Interlaboratory study of cellular fluorescence intensity measurements with fluorescein-labeled microbead standards. Cytometry 1991; 12:525–536.

Vogt RF, Marti G, Schwartz A: Quantitative calibration of fluorescence intensity for clinical and research applications of immunophenotyping by flow cytometry. In Tyler H (ed.): Reviews in Biotechnology and Bioengineering. Norwood, N,: Ablex, 1994, vol 1.

Waller EK: Cellular immunotherapy and cancer. Semin Oncol 2004; 31:87–90.

Wedderburn LR, Patel A, Varsani H, et al: The developing human immune system: T-cell receptor repertoire of children and young adults shows a wide discrepancy in the frequency of persistent oligoclonal T-cell expansions. Immunology 2001; 102:301–309.

Weinberg DS: Relative applicability of image analysis and flow cytometry in clinical medicine. In Bauer KD, Duque RE, Shankey TV (eds): Clinical Flow Cytometry: Principles and Applications. Baltimore, Williams & Wilkins, 1993, pp 359–371.

Weiss A: Molecular and genetic insights into T cell antigen receptor structure and function. Annu Rev Genet 1991; 25:487–510.

Weiss A, Littman DR: Signal transduction by lymphocyte antigen receptors. Cell 1994; 76:263–274.

Wheeless LL, Coon JS, Cox C, et al: Precision of DNA flow cytometry in inter-institutional analyses. Cytometry 1991; 12:405–412.

Wingren AG, Parra E, Varga M, et al: T cell activation pathways: B7, LFA-3, and ICAM-1 shape unique T cell profiles. Crit Rev Immunol 1995; 15:235–253.

Xu-Amano J, Kiyono H, Jackson RJ, et al: Helper T cell subsets for immunoglobulin A responses: oral immunization with tetanus toxoid and cholera toxin as adjuvant selectively induces Th2 cells in mucosa associated tissues. J Exp Med 1993; 178:1309–1320.

Yabuhara A, Kawai H, Komiyama A: Development of natural killer cytotoxicity during childhood: marked increases in number of natural killer cells with adequate cytotoxic abilities during infancy to early childhood. Pediatr Res 1990; 28:316–322.

Yamamura M, Uyemura K, Deans RJ, et al: Defining protective responses to pathogens: cytokine profiles in leprosy lesions. Science 1991; 254:277–279.

Yannelli JR, Wroblewski JM: On the road to a tumor cell vaccine: 20 years of cellular immunotherapy. Vaccine 2004; 23:97–113.

Yokoyama WM, Kim S, French AR: The dynamic life of natural killer cells. Annu Rev Immunol 2004; 22:405–429.

Yuan Q, Walker WA: Innate immunity of the gut: mucosal defense in health and disease. J Pediatr Gastroenterol Nutr 2004; 38:463–473.

Zedler S, Bone RC, Baue AE, et al: T-cell reactivity and its predictive role in immunosuppression after burns. Crit Care Med 1999; 27:66–72.

Zhou Y, Kurihara T, Ryseck RP, et al: Impaired macrophage function and enhanced T cell-dependent immune response in mice lacking CCR5, the mouse homologue of the major HIV-1 coreceptor. J Immunol 1998; 160:4018–4025.

Zola H: The 8th Human Leucocyte Differentiation Antigens Workshop: potential new CD molecules. J Biol Regul Homeost Agents 2002; 16:119–124.

Zola H, Fusco M, Weedon H, et al: Reduced expression of the interleukin-2-receptor gamma chain on cord blood lymphocytes: relationship to functional immaturity of the neonatal immune response. Immunology 1996; 87:86–91.

Zola H, Moore HA, Bradley J, et al: Lymphocyte sub-populations in human cord blood: analysis with monoclonal antibodies. J Reprod Immunol 1983; 5:311–317.

CHAPTER 45

Laboratory Evaluation of Immunoglobulin Function and Humoral Immunity

Richard A. McPherson MD, H. Davis Massey MD PhD

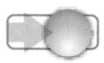

KEY POINTS

- There are five different classes of antibody: IgM, IgG, IgA, IgD, and IgE, each with a distinct heavy chain.

- There are two different light chain types: κ and λ.

- Antigens react with antibodies at the Fab region that contains variable regions of both heavy and light chains.

- The Fc region on the heavy chains determines what other proteins will bind to the antibody (e.g., complement).

- IgG is prevalent in blood and tissue fluids; IgM is found mainly in the blood; secretory IgA is found primarily on epithelial surfaces; IgD is bound mostly to B cells; IgE is bound largely to basophils and mast cells.

- Polyclonal increases in immunoglobulins occur as part of the immune response and may be found in chronic diseases.

- Monoclonal increases in immunoglobulins suggest a plasma cell dyscrasia.

- Diagnosis of disorders of immunoglobulins is aided by their quantitative measurement in addition to qualitative measures of their clonality by immunoelectrophoresis or immunofixation electrophoresis.

- Cryoglobulins can arise as excess monoclonal immunoglobulin (type I), which causes hyperviscosity, or as an IgM autoantibody against IgG (types II and III), which forms circulating immune complexes and causes vasculitis.

- Oligoclonal bands of immunoglobulin in cerebrospinal fluid suggest autoimmune disorder such as demyelinating disease or infection.

Antibodies are the effector molecules of humoral (B-cell-mediated) immunity. They are immunoglobulins that react specifically and bind with the antigens that stimulated their production. By mass, immunoglobulins comprise about 20% of plasma proteins in healthy individuals. Antibody activity is associated with the slowest migrating proteins on electrophoresis, the gamma-globulins. The focus of this chapter is to discuss the general structural and functional properties of immunoglobulins, their laboratory evaluation, and their clinical significance.

Structural Properties of Antibodies

Antibody Molecules

The molecular structure of antibodies has been well elucidated (Padlan, 1991; Poljak, 1991; Tedford, 1991). An immunoglobulin molecule is a Y-shaped glycoprotein. It has two identical antigen-binding sites at the tips of the Y (Fab region) and binding sites for complement components and/or various cell surface receptors on the tail of the Y (Fc region). Each immunoglobulin molecule is composed of two identical heavy (H) chains and two identical light (L) chains. These polypeptide chains are held together by noncovalent interactions that are stabilized by disulfide bonds. Parts of both the H and L chains form the antigen-binding sites. Each immunoglobulin L and H chain consists of a variable region of about 110 amino-acid residues at its amino-terminal end (the tips of the Y), which forms the antigen-binding site, linked to a constant region. The H constant region is three or four times larger than that of the L chain. Each chain is composed of repeating, similarly folded domains: an L chain has one variable region (V_L) and one constant region (C_L) domain, whereas the H chain has one variable region (V_H) and three or four constant region (C_H) domains (Fig. 45–1). The amino acid sequence variation in the variable regions of both L and H chains is for the most part confined to three small hypervariable regions that come together at the amino-terminal end of the molecule to form the antigen-binding site. Each antigen-binding site is only large enough to bind an antigenic determinant the size of five or six sugar residues.

There are five different heavy chain isotypes (γ, α, μ, δ, ϵ) and two light chain isotypes (κ and λ), with some of the isotypes having further subtypes. For example, γ has subtypes γ_1, γ_2, γ_3, and γ_4. The isotypes are formed as a result of variations in the constant regions of the heavy and light chains. These isotypic designations are the basis for the nomenclature of antibodies. Because the heavy chain alone determines effector functions, immunoglobulins are conveniently referred to by their heavy chain isotype (class) using an English letter terminology (IgG, IgA, IgM, IgD, and IgE).

Antibodies have two identical antigen-binding sites. An antigen-binding site is made up of amino acids from one H chain class and one L chain class. Thus, the four-chain Y monomer molecules (see Fig. 45–1) possess two identical antigen-combining sites and are said to be *bivalent*. Such antibody molecules can crosslink antigen molecules into a large lattice if the antigen molecules each have three or more antigenic determinants. Once the lattice reaches a certain size, it precipitates out of solution (Davies, 1983). This crosslinking is physiologically important because it enhances the engulfment of antigen, such as that expressed by bacteria, and by phagocytic leukocytes. It is also involved in activation of the complement system. In addition, crosslinking may be required for the triggering of antibody-producing cells (B lymphocytes) by antigen. The efficiency of antigen-binding and crosslinking reactions by antibodies is greatly increased by a flexible hinge region where the arms of the Y join the tail, allowing the distance between the two antigen-binding sites to vary.

Multivalence affects the avidity with which an antibody can bind certain types of antigens. A particulate antigen (such as a bacterium or virus) has

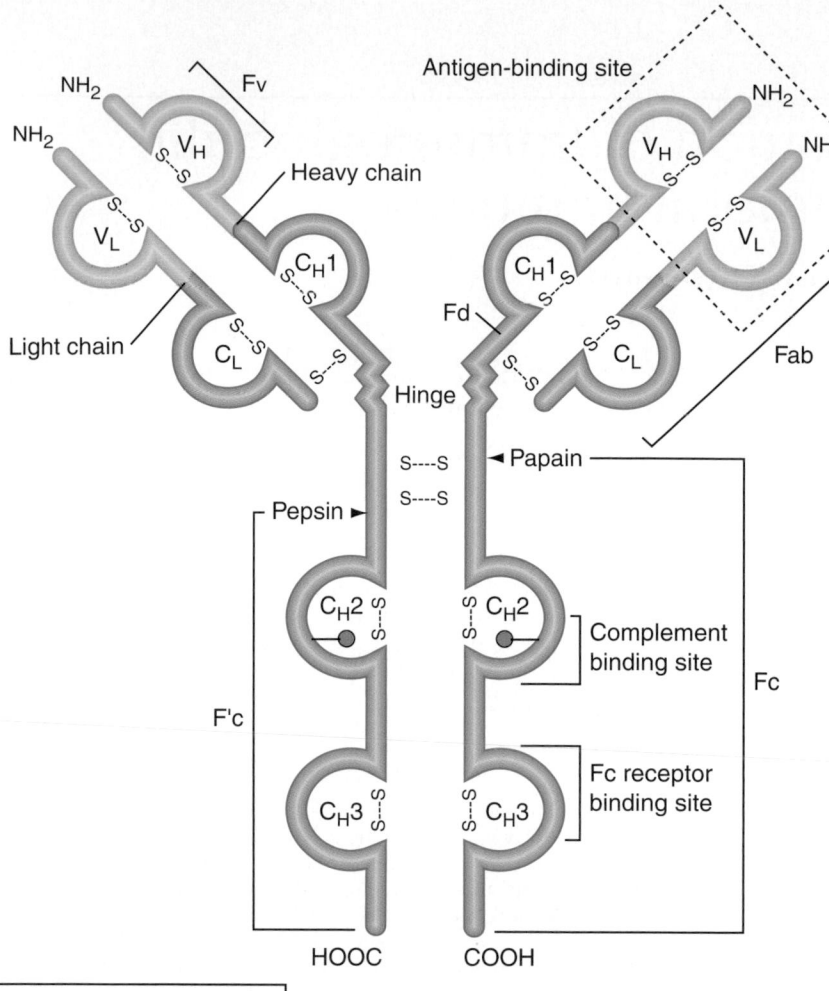

Figure 45–1 Schematic representation of immunoglobulin G molecule. The relative positions of the *interchain* disulfide bonds and the *intrachain* disulfide bonds that form the loop regions are shown. Each of the loops delineates the domain of the light and heavy chain labeled accordingly. The probable sties of enzymatic cleavage in the 'hinge' region by papain or pepsin are indicated,. The papain fragments are designated Fab and Fc. The pepsin fragments are Fc′ and Fab′2 (2 Fab fragments disulfide-linked). Digestion of Fab with pepsin under the proper conditions yields the fragment Fv (V_H and V_L noncovalently associated). The part of the heavy chain that contributes to the Fab fragment is designated Fd.

— ● Carbohydrate group
S---S Disulfide bond

repeating antigenic determinants on its surface. An antibody molecule may interact with a single particle in such a manner that both of its antigen-combining sites are bound to antigenic determinants on that particle rather than to antigenic determinants on two adjacent particles. When this type of binding occurs, the effective energy of interaction or avidity is greatly increased compared with that associated with monovalent attachments to two particles. This mechanism has been shown to be physiologically important in the neutralization of viruses by antibodies of relatively low binding affinity.

The protective effect of immunoglobulins is not due simply to their ability to bind antigen. They engage in a variety of biological activities mediated by the tail of the Y, the Fc region of the molecule. This part of the antibody molecule determines what will happen to the antigen once it is bound. Immunoglobulins with the same antigen-binding capacity can have a variety of different Fc regions and therefore different functional properties, such as activating the complement system and attaching to Fc receptors on macrophages, thereby aiding phagocytosis of antigens.

Because of its exposed location and loosely folded structure, the *hinge region* is readily attacked by various proteolytic enzymes. As the name suggests, the hinge region confers a certain amount of flexibility on the molecule, allowing it to assume the Y-shaped structure. This permits an antibody to become attached to a single particle (e.g., a bacterium) through both of its antigen-combining sites or, alternatively, to stretch out to its full length to join two particles. The unique properties conferred by the hinge region on Ig molecules are related to its rich content of proline and hydrophilic amino acid residues. The inter-H-chain disulfide bonds of IgG, IgA, and IgD molecules are located in the hinge region (Fig. 45–1).

The proteolytic enzymes papain and pepsin cleave antibody molecules into different characteristic fragments that lead to an understanding of the structure–function relationship of the protein. Papain cleavage produces two separate and identical Fab (fragment antigen-binding) fragments, each with one antigen-binding site, and one Fc fragment (so called because in nonhuman primates it readily crystallizes). On the other hand,

pepsin cleavage produces one F(ab′)₂ fragment, so-called because it consists of two covalently linked F(ab′) fragments (each slightly larger than a Fab fragment); the rest of the molecule is broken down into smaller fragments of various sizes (Fig. 45–1). Because F(ab′)₂ fragments are bivalent, they can still crosslink antigens and form precipitates. This is not true of the univalent Fab fragments. Neither of these fragments (subunits of antibodies) has the other biological properties of intact antibody molecules because they lack the tail (the Fc region) that mediates these properties. However, monovalent Fab is the form of post-immunization monospecific, affinity-purified ovine antibody that is used therapeutically in patients for such applications as removing toxic levels of digoxin (Digibind) or neutralizing crotalid snake venoms (CroFab).

Each B-cell clone makes antibody molecules with a unique antigen-binding site. Initially, the molecules are inserted into the plasma membrane, where they serve as cell surface receptors for antigen. When antigen binds to the membrane-bound antibodies, B cells are activated to multiply, differentiate to a plasma cell, and synthesize a large amount of soluble antibody with the same antigen-binding site, which is secreted into the blood. Humoral antibodies defend humans and animals against infection by inactivating viruses and bacterial toxins via its V_H/V_L domains and by recruiting complement and various cells to kill and ingest invading microorganisms via its C_L domains in the Fc region of the molecule. The biological properties of the various immunoglobulin domains are summarized in Table 45–1.

Antibody–Antigen Interaction

The binding of an antigen to antibody is reversible. The affinity and the number of binding sites contribute to the strength of an antibody–antigen interaction. This reversible binding is a result of many relatively weak noncovalent forces, including hydrophobic and hydrogen bonds, van der Waals forces, and ionic interactions. These weak forces are effective only when the antigen molecule is close enough to allow some of its atoms to

Table 45-1 Biological Properties of Immunoglobulin Domains

Domain	Known or Probable Function

C_H3	1. Cytotrophic reactions involving:
	  (a) Macrophages and monocytes
	  (b) Heterologous mast cells
	  (c) Cytotoxic killer (K) cells
	  (d) B cells
	2. Noncovalent assembly of heavy and light chains

C_H2	1. Binding of complement (C1q) 2. Control of catabolic rate
C_H1/C_L	1. Noncovalent assembly of heavy and light chains 2. Covalent assembly of heavy and light chains 3. Spacers between interdomain interactions involving antigen binding and effector functions
V_H/V_L	1. Antigen binding 2. Noncovalent bonding of heavy and light chains

Source: with permission from Dorrington KJ, Painter RH: Biological activities of the constant region of immunoglobulin G. *In* Mandel TE, et al (eds): Progress in Immunology III. Canberra, Australian Academy of Science, 1977.

fit into complementary recesses (regions) on the antibody surface. The complementary regions of a four-chain antibody unit are its two identical antigen-binding sites, whereas the corresponding region on the antigen is an antigenic determinant. Most antigenic macromolecules have many different antigenic determinants; if two or more of them are identical, the antigen is said to be multivalent.

The *affinity* of an antibody molecule reflects the tightness of the fit of an antigenic determinant to a single antigen-binding site, and it is independent of the number of antigenic sites. However, the total *avidity* of an antibody for a multivalent antigen, such as a polymer with repeating subunits, is defined as the total binding strength of all of its binding sites together. A typical IgG molecule binds at least 10,000 times more strongly to a multivalent antigen if both antigen-binding sites are engaged than if only one site is involved.

For the same reason, if the affinity of the antigen-binding sites in an IgG and an IgM molecule is the same, the IgM molecule (because it is a pentamer and thus has 10 binding sites) will have much greater avidity for a multivalent antigen than an IgG molecule (which has two binding sites). This difference in avidity is important in view of the fact that antibodies produced early in an immune response usually have much lower affinities than those produced later. The increase in the average affinity of antibodies produced as time passes after immunization is called *affinity maturation*. This occurs because the antibody response to an antigen is heterogeneous – that is, antibodies with different antigen-combining sites are elicited against the antigen by the responding clones of B lymphocytes. Because of its high total avidity, IgM (the major Ig class produced early in immune responses) can function even when each of its binding sites has only a low affinity.

The size of the antigen–antibody complex is determined by the valence of the antigen and the relative concentrations of the antigen and the antibody. The antigen–antibody precipitation reaction is based on the crosslinking of multivalent antigens by bivalent antibodies. If only one species of antibody (a monoclonal response) is present, molecules with only one antigenic determinant cannot be crosslinked. If an antigen is bivalent, it can form small cyclic complexes or linear chains with antibody, whereas an antigen with three or more antigenic determinants can form large three-dimensional lattices that readily precipitate. However, the majority of antisera elicited against an antigen contain a variety of different antibodies (a polyclonal response) that react with different determinants on the antigen and can cooperate in crosslinking the antigen. By contrast, homogeneous (monoclonal) antibodies can precipitate molecules only with repeating identical antigenic determinants.

Given valence conditions that allow the formation of large aggregates, the size of the antigen–antibody complexes that form depends critically on the relative molar concentrations of the two reactants. If there is an excess of either antigen or antibody, large complexes are unlikely to form (Fig. 45-2). This property is crucial to understanding seemingly paradoxical reactions in some immunoassays that depend on antigen–antibody complex formation. For example, a vast excess of antigen can completely saturate all antibody binding sites, leading to a negative signal (i.e., no agglutination, etc.). This phenomenon is sometimes referred to as the

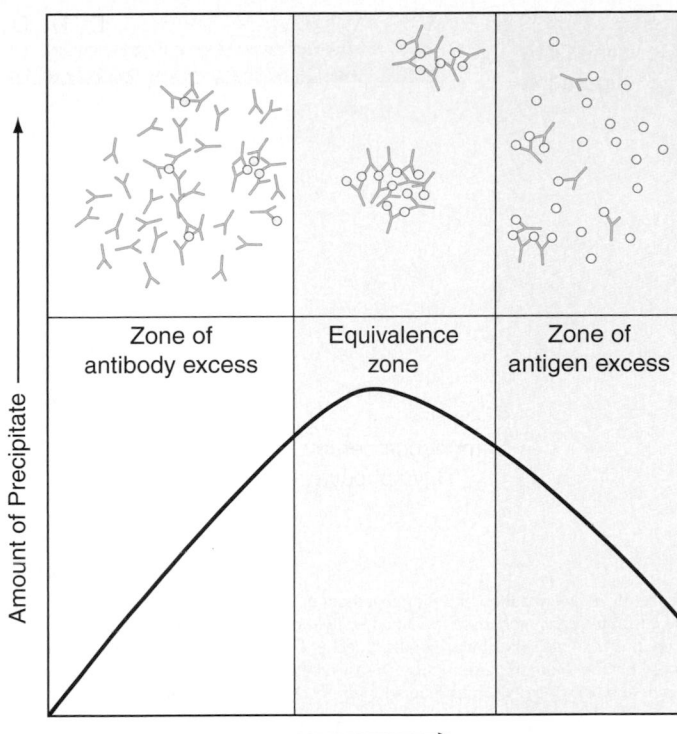

Amount of antigen (o) added to a fixed amount of antibody (Y)

Figure 45-2 Antibody and antigen concentrations influence the size of antigen–antibody complexes formed. The largest complexes form when both molecules are present at approximately the same molar concentration (zone of equivalence), whereas the smallest complexes form when the antigen is present in great excess, Note that the small complexes formed in antigen excess have only a few antibody molecules per complex; for this reason, they are inefficiently cleared from the extracellular fluids by macrophages.

'prozone effect.' The prozone effect remains a potential problem for modern assay systems, including syphilis testing in which extremely high titer antibodies can be missed unless the specimen is tested at dilutions (Smith, 2004) and even in immunofixation electrophoresis (see below, Fig. 45-6E).

The size and composition of antibody–antigen complexes are not only important in influencing precipitation reactions *in vitro*, they are crucial in determining the fate of the complexes in the body. Complexes formed at equivalence or in antibody excess have multiple protruding Fc regions and therefore bind strongly to Fc receptors in macrophages, which ingest and degrade them. Small complexes, formed in antigen excess, have only one Fc region per complex. Therefore, they bind poorly to Fc receptors on macrophages and are less efficiently destroyed. Instead, they may be deposited in small blood vessels in the skin, kidneys, joints, and brain, where they may activate the complement system, causing inflammation and the destruction of tissue.

Although it appears that antigen–antibody complexes have a rigid 'lock-and-key' appearance, antibodies are dynamic entities and undergo structural fluctuations (Karplus, 1983; Wilson, 1991). Conformational changes may even be required for the binding. These adjustments include side chain shifts of up to 20–30 nm, aromatic ring rotations, conformational changes, and even small rotations between V_H and V_L domains (Bhat, 1990; Standfield, 1990; Herron, 1991).

The Genetic Basis of Antibody Diversity

It is estimated that a human is able to make at least 10^6–10^9 different antibody molecules. Special genetic mechanisms have evolved to produce the very large number of immunoglobulin molecules that develop in response to antigen stimulation without the need for an excessive number of genes (Max, 2003).

Immunoglobulin molecules are produced by three separate gene pools encoding the κ, λ, and H chains, respectively. The gene pools for light and heavy chains reside on different chromosomes. In each pool, separate gene segments that encode for different parts of the variable regions of light and heavy chains can be brought together by site-specific recombination events during B-cell differentiation. The light chain gene pools contain one or more constant (C) genes and sets of variable (V) and joining (J) gene segments. The H-chain gene pool contains a set of C genes and sets of V,

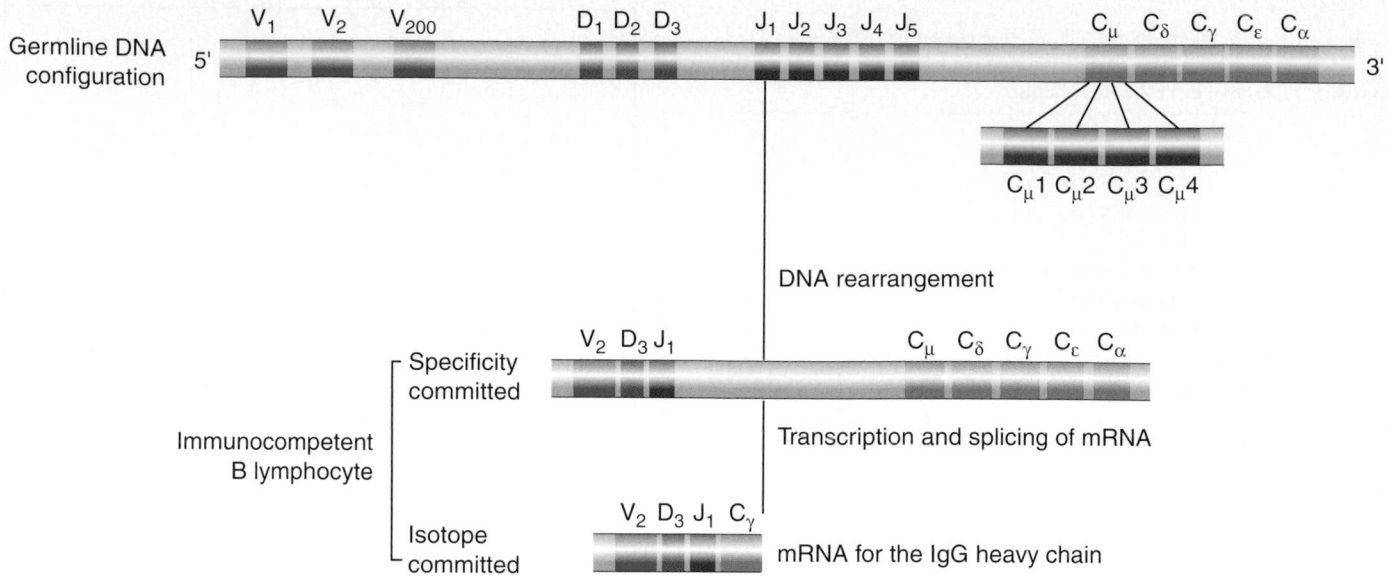

Figure 45–3 Organization and rearrangement of the heavy chain Ig genes (exons) on the mouse 12 chromosome. Each V_H gene also has a leader sequence, which is not shown. The constant region genes are identified by the heavy chain isotype, and more than one gene exists for the C_γ and C_α isotypes. Unlike C_γ and C_α genes, C_H genes are composed of multiple exons, as illustrated for the C_μ gene ($C_{\mu 1}$–$C_{\mu 4}$ domains.) The switch sites are located at the 5′ end of each of the C_H genes and are also not shown. The solid line represents the intervening sequences (introns) between the genes or gene segments. Each heavy chain is encoded by four distinct gene segments, V, D, J, and C. (Redrawn with permission from Marcu KB: Immunoglobulin heavy-chain constant region genes. Cell 1982; 29:719. Copyright © by Cell Press.)

diversity (D), and J gene segments. To make an antibody molecule, a V_L gene segment is recombined with a J_L gene segment to produce a V gene for the light chain; and a V_H gene segment is recombined with a D and J_H segment to produce a V gene for the heavy chain (Fig. 45–3). Each of the assembled gene segments is then cotranscribed with the appropriate constant region sequence to produce a messenger RNA molecule that encodes for the complete polypeptide chain. By variously combining inherited gene segments encoding for V_L and V_H regions, vertebrates can make thousands of different light chains and thousands of different H chains that can associate to form millions of different antibody molecules.

The baseline repertoire of antibody molecules can be expanded still further by somatic hypermutation, which seems to be activated by exposure to antigen. Thus, the selective role of antigen in the presence of somatic mutation appears to lead to a fine tuning of the immune response and to a virtually unlimited diversity of antibody molecules. Somatic point mutations in immunoglobulin genes occur in B cells (not germ cells) during the lifetime of the animal or of humans (Tonegawa, 1983). The somatic hypermutations are largely confined to the H-chain and L-chain variable region genes and the introns immediately surrounding them. It is estimated that close to one mutation will occur in either the H- or L-chain V region of an individual cell with each cell division. This not only increases antibody diversity but may also cause a change in the affinity with which the antibody binds its ligand. Those emerging B cells that can bind the antigen more avidly have an advantage over other B cells that do not bind the antigen as avidly. As the concentration of antigen falls, those B cells that have more avid receptors dominate the population of responding cells. This results in a greater affinity of the antibodies being produced on rechallenge than in the initial response. Thus, this process of somatic hypermutation can result in the presence in immunized individuals of high-affinity antibodies that are much more effective on a weight basis.

All B cells initially make IgM antibodies. Some later switch to make antibodies of other classes (isotypes: IgG, IgA, etc.) that have the same antigen-binding site (idiotype) as the original IgM antibodies (*allelic exclusion*) (Table 45–2). Such class switching in combination with allelic exclusion allows the same antigen-binding sites (same V_H and light chain) to be distributed among antibodies with many different biological properties (secondary effector functions) (Corcoran, 2005).

Thus, the gene organization mechanism permits the assembly of immunoglobulin molecules with a variety of specificities. Antibody diversity depends on the presence of multiple gene segments, their rearrangement into different sequences, the combination of different light and heavy chains in the assembly of immunoglobulin molecules, and somatic mutations.

General Properties of Immunoglobulins

The various classes of human immunoglobulins and their properties (Spiegelberg, 1974; Kolar, 2003) are summarized in Tables 45–3 and 45–4.

Table 45–2 Summary of Immunoglobulin Variants

Type of Variation	Distribution	Variant	Location	Examples
Isotypic	All variants present in serum of a normal individual	Classes	C_H	IgM, IgE
		Subclasses	C_H	IgA1, IgA2
		Types	C_L	κ, λ
		Subtypes	C_L	λOz$^+$, λOz$^-$
		Subgroups	V_L, V_H	$V_{\kappa I}$, $V_{\kappa II}$, V_{HI}, V_{HII}
Allotypic	Allelic forms not present in all individuals	Allotypes	Mainly C_H/C_L Occasionally V_H/V_L	Gm group (human γ chain; e.g., IgG1, G1m3, G1m17) b$_4$, b$_5$, b$_6$, b$_9$ (rabbit light chain)
Idiotypic	Antigenic individuality specific to each Ig molecule	Idiotypes	V_H/V_L	Determinant identified by antibody specific to an individual immunoglobulin

Source: modified with permission from Sell S: Immunology, Immunopathology, and Immunity, 4th ed. New York, Elsevier, 1987.

Immunoglobulin M

This glycoprotein is the major class of antibody secreted into the blood in the early stages of a *primary* antibody response. Normally, the secreted form of IgM is a pentamer composed of five four-chain units, a macroglobulin with a 19S sedimentation rate, and a molecular weight of 900 kDa. However, in human autoimmune disorders, such as systemic lupus erythematosus (SLE), the monomeric 7S form may be detected in appreciable amounts in serum. Selective IgM deficiency is a rare disorder associated with the absence of IgM and normal levels of other immunoglobulin classes. The cause of this disorder is unknown.

Because pentameric IgM has a total of 10 antigen-binding sites, it is more efficient than 7S monomeric IgM or IgG molecules in crosslinking antigen and in activating the complement system when bound to antigen. Thus, this high efficiency in binding and activating complement, coupled with its early appearance during the course of infection, makes IgM a particularly potent agent in combating microbial invasions.

Each IgM pentamer contains one copy of another polypeptide chain, called a J (*joining*) chain, which has a molecular weight of 15 kDa. This

Table 45–3 Physical Properties of Human Immunoglobulins

WHO Designation	IgM	IgG	IgA	IgD	IgE
Heavy chains	μ	γ	α	δ	ε
Heavy chain subclasses	μ_1, μ_2	$\gamma_1, \gamma_2, \gamma_3, \gamma_4$	α_1, α_2	–	–
Light chains	κ or λ	κ or λ	κ or λ	κ or λ	κ or λ
Molecular formula	IgM(κ) $(2\mu2\kappa)_5$ IgM(λ) $(2\mu2\lambda)_5$	IgG(κ) 2γ2κ IgG(λ) 2γ2λ	IgA(κ) $(2\alpha2\kappa)_{1-3}$ IgA(λ) $(1\alpha2\lambda_{1-3}$ IgA(κ) $(2\alpha2\kappa)_2 S^†$ IgA(λ) $(2\alpha2\lambda)_2 S$	IgD(κ) 2δ2κ IgD(λ) 2δ2λ	IgE(κ) 2ε3κ IgE(λ) 2ε2λ
Number of four-chain units per molecule	5	1	1–3	1	1
Heavy chain molecular weight, kDa	70	50–60	55	62	70
Light chain molecular weight, kDa	23	23	23	23	23
Sedimentation coefficient, S_{20W}	18.0–19.0	6.7–7.0	6.6–14.0	6.9–7.0	7.9–8.0
Molecular weight, kDa	900	143–160	159–447	177–185	187–200
Electrophoretic mobility	$\gamma^1–\beta^1$	$\gamma^2–\alpha^1$	$\gamma^2–\beta^2$	γ^1	γ^1
Carbohydrate content, %	7–14	2.2–3.5	7.5–9.0	12–13	11–12
Heavy chain allotypes	–	Gm	Am	–	–
Light chain allotypes	Km(κ)*	Km(κ)*	Km(κ)*	Km(κ)*	Km(κ)
Valency for antigen binding	5(10)	2	2.4 (? polymeric forms)	2	2
Number of domains on the heavy chains	5	4	4	4	5

* Formerly designated Inv marker.

† Dimer in external secretions carries secretory component -S.

Table 45–4 Properties of Human Immunoglobulins

	IgM	IgG	IgA	IgD	IgE
A. Physiologic					
Normal adult serum concentration, mg/mL	1.2–4.0	8.0–16.0	0.4–2.2	0.03	17–450 ng/mL
International units/mL	69–322	92–207	54–268	–	<100
Percentage total immunoglobulin	13	80	6	1	0.002
Intravascular distribution, %	41	48	76	75	51
Synthetic rate, mg/kg/day	2.2	35	24	0.4	0.003
Catabolic rate in serum, % per day (or half-life, days)	10.6 (5–6)	6 (18–23)	24 (5–6.5)	37 (2.8)	90
B. Biological					
Agglutinating capacity	+4	±	+2	–	–
Complement-fixing capacity via classical pathway	+4	+	–	–	–
Homologous anaphylactic hypersensitivity	–	–	–	–	+4
Heterologous guinea pig anaphylaxis	–	+	–	–	–
Fixation to homologous mast cells and basophils	–	±	–	–	+4
Cytophilic binding to macrophages	–	+	±	–	–
Placental transport to fetus	–	+	–	–	–
Rheumatoid factor-binding activity	–	+	–	–	–
Present in external secretions	±	+	+4	–	+2

Other characteristic properties:

IgM – Produced early in immune response, first effective defense against bacteremia

IgG – Combats microorganisms and their toxins in extravascular fluids

IgA – Defends external body surfaces

IgD – Present on lymphocyte surface of immunocompetent cells, important for B-cell activation and/or immunoregulation

accessory polypeptide is produced by IgM-secreting cells. It is an acidic glycoprotein with a high content of cysteine residues and thus is disulfide linked between two adjacent IgM monomeric Fc regions at the carboxy-terminal end. Presumably, oligomerization is initiated at this site.

IgM is also the first class of antibody to be produced by developing B cells. The immediate precursors of B cells, called pre-B cells, make μ chains but not light chains, which accumulate in the cells. Pre-B cells then begin to synthesize light chains, which combine with μ chains to form four-chain monomer IgM molecules. The two μ-chain and two light-chain component is inserted into the plasma membrane, where it functions as a receptor for antigen. At this point, the cells have become B lymphocytes and can respond to antigen.

Perhaps because of its large size, secreted pentamer IgM is not found to any significant extent in tissue spaces; it is confined to the blood circulation and does not cross the placenta. IgM is a minor component of secretory immunoglobulins at mucosal surfaces and in breast milk.

IgM is phylogenetically the most primitive of the immunoglobulins, and most variants of the genes from the μ chain appear to have evolved into heavy-chain genes for the other immunoglobulin classes. Additional physical and biological properties of IgM as well as the other classes of immunoglobulin are given in Tables 45–3 and 45–4.

Immunoglobulin G

IgG is the best studied isotype at both the structural and functional levels (Burton, 1985). Antibodies of this class constitute the major immunoglobulin in the blood. They are copiously produced during *secondary* immune response. The Fc region of IgG molecules binds to specific receptors on phagocytic cells, such as macrophages and polymorphonuclear leukocytes, thereby increasing the efficiency with which the phagocytic cells can ingest and destroy infecting microorganisms that have become coated with IgG antibodies in response to the infection. These receptors on antibodies attached to target cells also guide natural killer (NK) lymphocytes to destroy them through the process of antibody-dependent cell-mediated cytotoxicity (ADCC). The best known function of IgG is complement activation via the classical cascade. The Fc region of IgG can bind to and thereby activate the first component of the complement system, which unleashes a biochemical attack that kills the microorganisms. At least two molecules of IgG are required for complement activation compared to one molecule of IgM, which has five Fc regions.

IgG molecules are the only antibodies that can pass from mother to fetus. Cells of the placenta that are in contact with maternal blood have receptors that bind the Fc region of IgG molecules and mediate their passage to the fetus. The antibodies are first ingested by receptor-mediated endocytosis and then transported across the cell and released by exocytosis into the fetal blood. Other classes of antibodies do not bind to these receptors and therefore cannot pass across the placenta. The ability of IgG to cross the placenta provides a major line of defense against infection for the first weeks of an infant's life. Normally, the human fetus begins to receive significant quantities of maternal IgG transplacentally at around 12 weeks' gestation. The quantity increases steadily until, at birth, cord serum contains a concentration of IgG comparable to that of maternal serum. Barring any immunologic disorders, adult levels of IgG are reached by the seventh year of life and remain relatively constant thereafter.

IgG antibodies have a high diffusion coefficient, which enables them to diffuse into the extravascular body spaces more readily than other Ig classes. IgG, being the predominant immunoglobulin in these spaces, carries the major burden of neutralizing bacterial toxins and of binding microorganisms to enhance their phagocytosis. Furthermore, only IgG antibodies coating target cells, such as tumor cells, can sensitize them for extracellular killing by ADCC; the NK cells responsible for ADCC also possess Fc receptors for IgG.

There are four subclasses of human IgG, 1–4. The four subclasses reflect the existence of four antigenetically distinct H chains (γ1–γ4), which are similar but not identical in amino acid sequence and general properties. For example, IgG1 is the dominant subclass in adult humans. IgG3 is the most effective binder of complement, followed by IgG1 and IgG2. IgG4 in most cases fails completely to bind complement by the classical pathway. All the subclasses except IgG2 have been demonstrated to cross the placenta. A summary of the physical and biological properties of IgG is given in Tables 45–3 and 45–4 and for the subclasses in Table 45–5.

Immunoglobulin A

Antibodies of this class comprise the major class of antibody in secretions (milk, saliva, tears, and respiratory and intestinal secretions). It exists as a four-chain monomer (like IgG) or as a dimer of two such monomer units. IgA molecules in secretions are dimers that carry a single J chain, similar to the one associated with pentameric IgM, and an additional glycopolypeptide chain called *secretory component* (SC) of 70 kDa. IgA dimers pick up SC from the surface of the epithelial cells lining the intestine, bronchi, or the milk, salivary, or tear ducts. Secretory component is synthesized by the epithelial cells and is initially exposed on the nonluminal (external) surface of these cells, where it serves as a receptor for binding dimer IgA. The resulting dimer IgA–receptor complexes are ingested by receptor-mediated endocytosis, and transferred across the epithelial cell cytoplasm in the form of a membrane vesicle, which fuses with the plasma membrane on the luminal side of the epithelial cell. The extramembrane portion of the IgA receptor is then enzymatically cleaved and released as part of the secretory IgA molecule ($[\alpha_2, L_2,]_2$-Jα) into the lumen. The amino-terminus of the dimer IgA receptor remaining attached to dimer IgA is the SC (Fig. 45–4). Thus, the fully assembled dimeric secretory IgA molecule is the synthetic product of two distinct types of cells, plasma cells and epithelial cells. In addition to this transport role, SC may also protect the dimer IgA molecules from being digested by proteolytic enzymes in secretions.

In humans it has been possible to classify IgA antibodies into two subclasses, IgA1 and IgA2, based on differences in antigenic structure and variation in the arrangement of interchain disulfide bridges. Whereas IgA2

Table 45–5 Properties of Human Immunoglobulins G Subclasses

	IgG1	IgG2	IgG3	IgG4
A. Physiologic				
Percentage distribution of total normal serum IgG	66 ± 8	23 ± 8	7.3 ± 3.8	4.2 ± 2.6
Synthetic rate, mg/kg/day in serum	25	?	3.4	?
Fraction catabolic rate, % per day (half-life, day)	8 (23)	6.9 (23)	16.8 (7)	6.9 (23)
Ratio of κ/λ	1.4–2.4	1.0–1.1	1.1–1.3	5.0–7.0
Allotypic markers (Gm types)	a, z, f, x	n	bo, bi, bz g, st, etc.	?
B. Biological				
Complement-fixing capacity via classical, pathway	+2	±	+3	–
Heterologous skin-binding capacity	+	–	+	+
Placental transport to fetus	+	±	+	+
Macrophage receptor	+	–	+	–
Reaction with protein A	+	+	–	+
Dominant antibody activities:				
Antitetanus toxoid	+2	+	+	±
Antidiphtheria toxoid	+2	+	+	±
Antithyroglobulin	+2	+	+	±
Anti-DNA	+2	+2	±	±
Anti-Rh	+2	–	–	±
Anti-factor VIII	–	–	–	+
Antidextran	–	+	–	–
Antilevan	–	+	–	–
Antiteichoic acid	–	+	–	–
Number of interheavy chain disulfide bonds in hinge region	2	4	5	2
Position of light-heavy chain disulfide bond on the heavy chain	N214	N131	N131	N131

is a minor component of serum IgA, this subclass is the dominant form in secretions. Furthermore, secretory IgA reaches adult levels sooner than serum IgA. The IgA system in the intestinal tract of humans, for example, may be fully developed by two years of age, whereas serum IgA levels do not normally reach adult concentrations until 12 years of age.

Because of its presence near external membranes, secretory IgA constitutes a first line of defense against microorganisms in the external environment. It has been postulated that IgA inhibits the adherence of microorganisms to the surface of mucosal cells, thereby preventing their entry into body tissues. One property of secretory IgA that is important in this respect is its multivalence, which is associated with high avidity of binding to antigens; this may be especially relevant in the neutralization of viruses. Antiviral activity by IgA antibodies has been demonstrated in individuals given either of the polio vaccines. Secretory IgA may also combine with certain antigens in food, preventing their absorption into the bloodstream and thus reducing the incidence of allergic reactions. For example, IgA immunodeficiencies can lead to increased levels and incidence of humoral antibodies directed against antigens derived from food and intestinal organisms.

IgA possesses the following effective properties: it fixes complement through the alternative pathway; through a specific Fc receptor on macrophages it can serve as an opsonin for phagocytosis; and it can induce eosinophil degranulation through a specific receptor, which has implicated IgA in antiparasitic responses. The physical and biological properties of IgA are listed in Tables 45–3 and 45–4

Immunoglobulin D

Although only a minor component of the serum, IgD is a major membrane immunoglobulin found on the surface of a high proportion of B lymphocytes, especially in newborns. During the course of B-cell differentiation, these cells synthesize and display IgD molecules as well as IgM molecules. Whereas this appears to contradict the 'one-cell-one-immunoglobulin' rule, the antigen-binding sites (idiotype) of the two types of molecules and their light chains are identical. Only their C_H

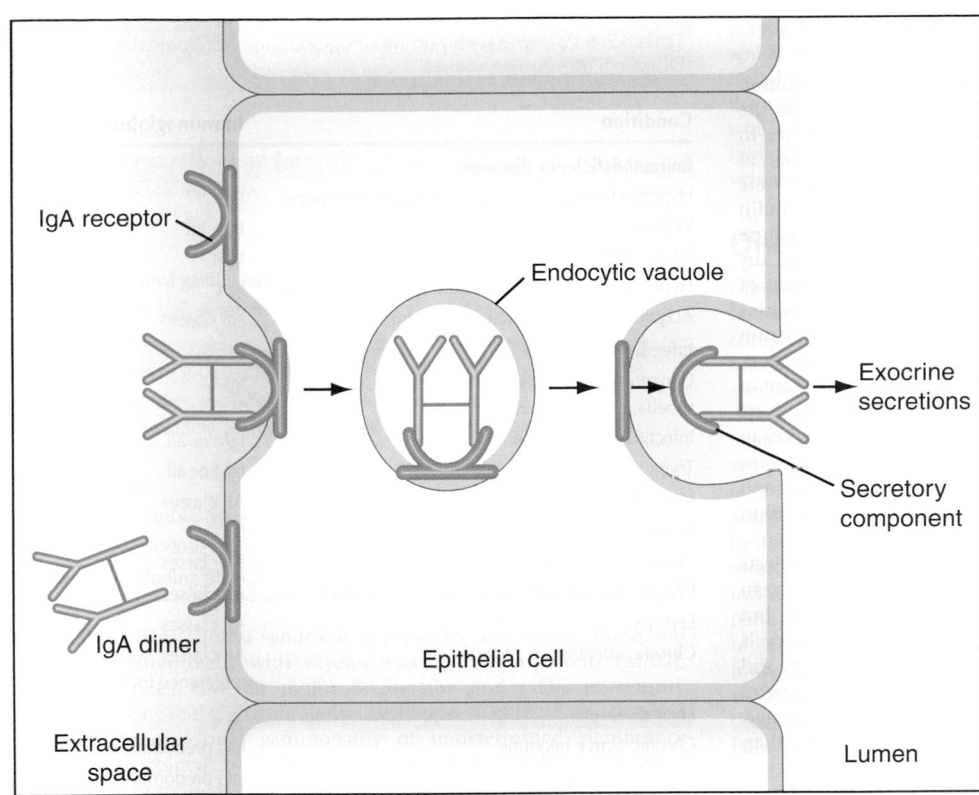

Figure 45–4 The mechanism by which the secretory component mediates the transport of a dimeric IgA molecule across an epithelial cell. The entire complex is transported from the extracellular fluid into the lumen of the epithelial tube. The secretory component is synthesized by the epithelial cell as a transmembrane glycoprotein and serves as a receptor on its basolateral surface for binding the IgA dimer. The receptor–IgA complex enters the cell in an endocytotic vesicle, which crosses the cell and is exocytosed at the apical surface. Cleavage of the receptor frees the dimer IgA for discharge at the exterior surface (lumen side). The portion of the receptor that remains attached to the IgA dimer is called the secretory component. This transport mechanism is responsible for depositing IgA in the various exocrine secretions (e.g., saliva, milk, bile, tears, and sweat), as well as in the mucous layer that protects the inner lining of the nasopharyngeal passages, intestine, and genitourinary tract.

regions differ. The membrane-bound IgD may serve as one of the receptors with which B cells bind antigen and are stimulated to undergo clonal proliferation. There is some evidence to suggest that IgM-bearing B cells can respond to certain T-independent antigens and that the acquisition of IgD is needed for B cells (IgM- and IgD-bearing) to respond to T-cell help required for T-dependent antigen responsiveness.

Furthermore, if IgD molecules are selectively removed from IgM- and IgD-bearing B cells by taking advantage of the much greater sensitivity of δ chain to papain, the cells are rendered susceptible to becoming tolerant. The precise role played by surface IgD in an immune response remains unknown, but the generally held view is that it turns on, turns off, or modulates (controls) B-cell division or differentiation.

IgD usually is detected in serum at about 6 months of age, and its concentration throughout life is always very low. In disease states, however, IgD concentration can vary greatly. In chronic infections, IgD serum levels increase, as do those of the other immunoglobulins. To date, no specific increase of IgD has been associated with a particular disease. Patients with allergies and autoimmune diseases do not show an abnormal IgD concentration. IgD is usually absent in hypogammaglobulinemic individuals.

To date, IgD has not been assigned a specific biological role as a humoral antibody. IgD activity against a number of antigens have been reported on occasion. Surface IgD, which has proteins like those of surface IgM, is a marker for mature B cells, and its role as a receptor is generally accepted even though the nature and purpose of the signal it transmits remains controversial (Carsetti, 1993; Roes, 1993). IgD does not bind complement, does not cross the placenta, and does not bind to cells through its Fc region. The secreted form of IgD as well as that of the other immunoglobulins lacks the carboxy-terminal transmembrane peptide that anchors it to the surface of B cells. Tables 45–3 and 45–4 list additional properties of IgD.

Immunoglobulin E

Of the various classes of immunoglobulin, IgE is present at the lowest serum concentration (Table 45–4). It has the ability to attach to human skin (homocytotropic antibody) and to initiate aspects of the allergic reaction (reaginic antibody). The biological activity of IgE is accounted for by its property of binding through the Fc region to basophils and to their tissue equivalent, mast cells. IgE may also be important in the humoral immune response to parasitic disease because it is often found at high levels in the serum of patients with helminthic infection. IgE may play a part in allowing white blood cells (WBCs), antibodies, and complement components to enter sites of inflammation leading to an immediate hypersensitivity reaction. IgE antibodies provide a striking example of

the *bifunctional* nature of antibody molecules. The Fc portion of the molecule binds to the target cells, whereas the Fab portion binds the allergen (see Ch. 54 for the role of IgE in allergic diseases and related assays).

Like IgA, IgE is produced mainly in the linings of the respiratory and intestinal tracts and is part of the external secretory system of antibody. A deficiency of IgE has been inconsistently associated with deficiency of IgA in individuals with impaired immunity who present with undue susceptibility to infection. IgE does not cross the placenta, and IgE-antigen complexes do not bind complement by the classical pathway (Table 45–4).

Summary

There are five different classes of antibody (IgM, IgG, IgA, IgD, and IgE), four subclasses of IgG antibody (IgG1, IgG2, IgG3, and IgG4), and two subclasses of IgA antibody (IgA1 and IgA2) in humans. Each of these antibody isotypes possesses a distinct H chain (μ, γ, α, δ, ε, γ_1, γ_2, γ_3, γ_4; and α_1, α_2, respectively). The H chains contain the Fc region of the antibody, which determines what other proteins will bind to the antibody and therefore the biological properties of the class and subclass. Either type of L chain (κ or λ) can be associated with any class of H chain.

The structural differences among the five classes of immunoglobulins correspond to functional differences in their sites of production and action, their relative levels of production in primary and secondary immune responses, and their roles as physiologic effectors. For example, IgG is prevalent in both blood and tissue fluids, whereas IgM is chiefly confined to the blood, and secretory IgA is found primarily on epithelial surfaces. IgD and IgE are principally bound to cells, IgD to B cells, and IgE to basophils and mast cells.

Clinical Significance of Immunoglobulins

Immunoglobulins play important roles in disease pathogenesis, diagnosis, prevention, and therapy.

Disease Pathogenesis

Monoclonal hyperimmunoglobulinemia is a prominent feature of multiple myeloma and Waldenström's macroglobulinemia. Antibodies against native antigens may result in autoimmune diseases, as discussed in Chapters 50 and 52. Hypo- or agammaglobulinemia is often the prime characteristic of some immunodeficiency disorders (see Ch. 49). Polyclonal hypergammaglobulinemia can result from chronic inflammation or other disorders such as cirrhosis of the liver due to excess pan-B cell stimulation.

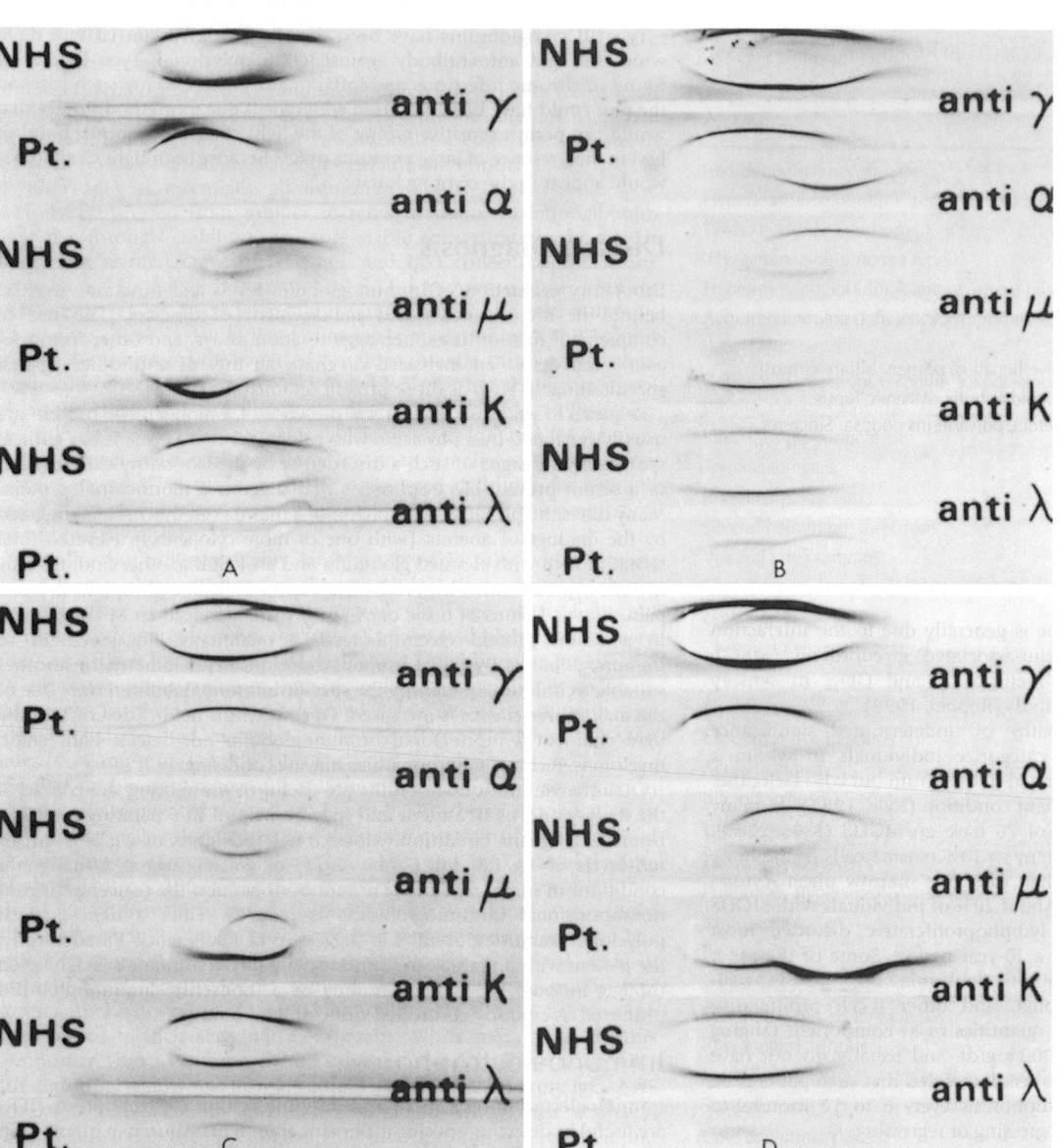

Figure 45–5 Monoclonal immunoglobulins demonstrated by serum immunoelectrophoresis. Aliquots of patient serum and a pool of normal human serum were subjected to electrophoresis on polyacrylamide at pH 8.6 (Poly-E-Film, Pfizer). The separated proteins were reacted overnight with antisera to (1) whole human serum; (2) a combination of IgG, IgA, and IgM; (3) γ, (4) α; (5) μ; (6) κ, and (7) λ chains, respectively. The membranes were washed and stained with Amido Black B. *A*, IgGκ M component. *B*, IgAλ M component. *C*, IgMGκ M component. *D*, κ-Light chain M component. *E*, λ-Heavy chain M component.

one is searching for a disruption of a normally smooth line – that is, by bowing, thickening, or changed mobility. Examples of IEP are shown in Figure 45–5. IEP is a useful technique but has limitations. It may identify the presence of heavy and light chains but does not ensure that one does indeed have an entire immunoglobulin molecule composed of two heavy chains and two light chains.

It is also possible, but unusual, for monoclonal immunoglobulins to be present in amounts below the level of detection of the system used. The lower level of detection can be estimated by diluting a known monoclonal immunoglobulin and testing it by IEP. Because monoclonal proteins of IgM, IgA, IgD, and IgE may be present in relatively small quantities compared with IgG, the light chain portion of the whole non-IgG immunoglobulin may not be detected by IEP. The inability to detect light chains of immunoglobulins in lesser concentrations in the presence of IgG of greater concentration is referred to as an umbrella effect. Therefore, other procedures may be required to rule out heavy-chain or Franklin's disease. It is possible that the serum being tested and the antibody being used are not in the proper concentrations and that the M component may be missed. Finally, it is possible that the antisera being used will not detect the available determinants on a particular M component. If one has a high index of suspicion, it may be useful to use a second antiserum from another source.

Immunofixation

IFE has virtually replaced IEP in the clinical laboratory because of its speed, sensitivity, and ease of interpretation; the two procedures are of comparable sensitivity. IFE also has the advantage of a more rapid readout because diffusion through gel is not required. Replicate samples of patient serum are subjected to electrophoresis through high-resolution gel before monospecific antisera are applied directly to the separated serum proteins. The gel is washed, and the protein–antibody conjugates are stained and read directly (Fig. 45–6). One lane is treated with a precipitating reagent that fixes all proteins in the same pattern as the serum protein electrophoresis. Maintaining all serum proteins in register with the immunofixed immunoglobulins adds to the ease of confirming and identifying monoclonal paraproteins.

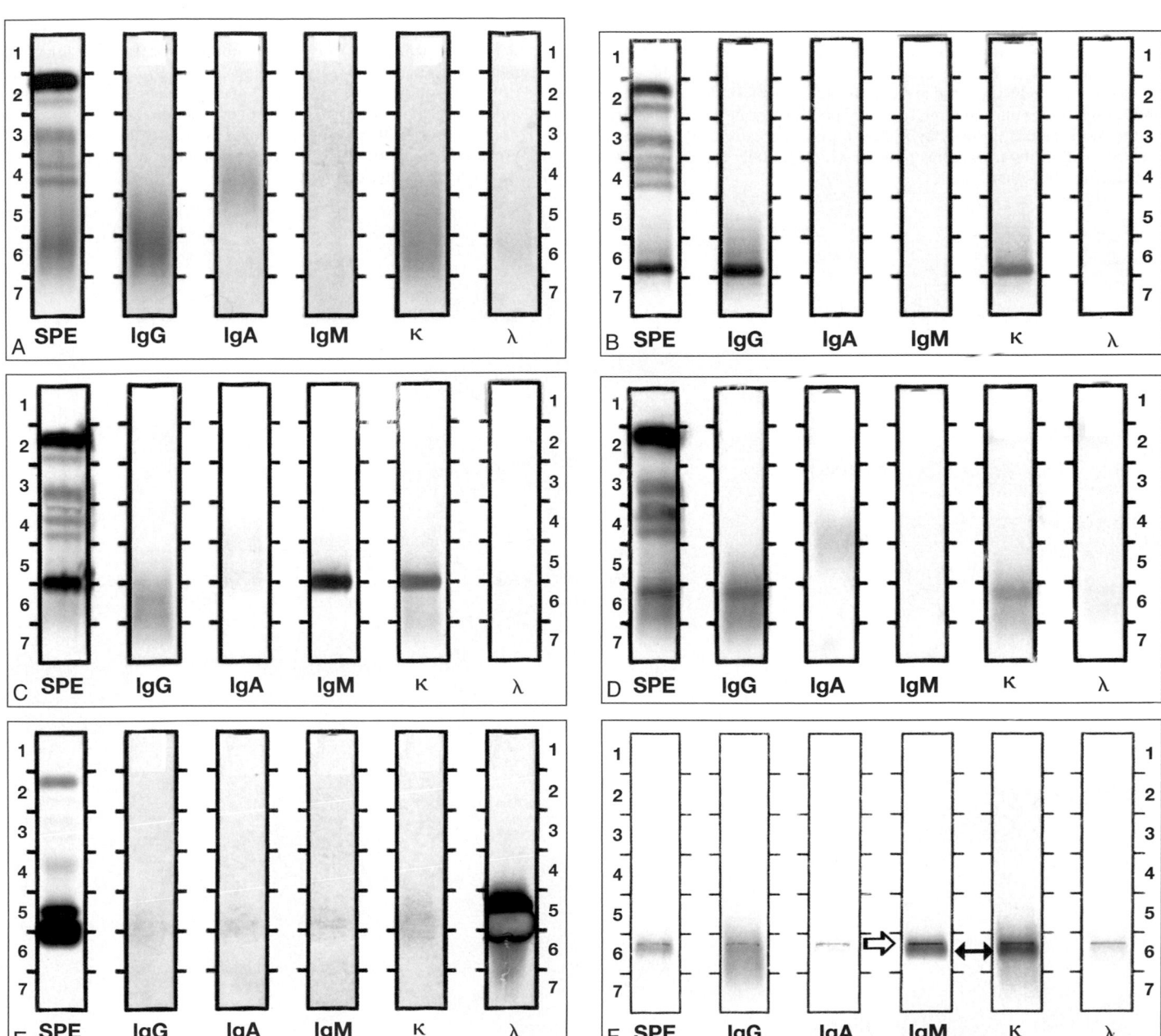

Figure 45–6 Monoclonal immunoglobulins demonstrated by serum immunofixation. Replicate samples of patient serum were subjected to electrophoresis through agarose at pH 8.6. The separated proteins were allowed to react with monospecific antisera and the gels were washed, fixed, and stained. *A*, Normal polyclonal pattern of immunoglobulins. *B*, Monoclonal IgGκ immunoglobulin (M-protein) in serum with loss of most normal polyclonal immunoglobulins. *C*, Monoclonal IgMκ immunoglobulin in serum. *D*, Minor band of IgGκ immunoglobulin in serum along with normal appearing immunoglobulins, possible MGUS. *E*, Two bands of λ light chains in urine. The lower band demonstrates antigen excess with artifactual clearing in its central region surrounded by a ring of immunofixed protein. The upper smaller band sometimes results from dimerization of free light chains through disulfide bonds. *F*, Type II mixed cryoglobulin precipitated from serum containing monoclonal IgMκ (solid arrow) and polyclonal IgG. Some undissolved cryoglobulin (open arrow) remained at the application point of each lane. A or anti-IgA = sample reacted with anti-IgA; G or IgG = sample reacted with anti-IgG; K or anti-κ = sample reacted with anti-κ; λ or anti-λ = sample reacted with anti-λ; M or anti-IgM = sample reacted with anti-IM; SP or SPE = sample not washed nor reacted with antisera (serum electrophoresis).

Occasionally, the concentration of the monoclonal protein in a patient's serum is so high that it exceeds the capacity of the reagent antibodies to form precipitating complexes by IFE. This phenomenon corresponds to the zone of antigen excess depicted in Figure 45–2. The result is a halo of precipitated complexes (where the concentrations are nearer to equivalence) with a clear central zone of antigen excess (Figure 45–6E). Although this result appears atypical, it is straightforward to interpret and to confirm by repeating the IFE with a greater dilution of patient serum (Keren, 1999).

Either technique may be applied to other body fluids, most commonly urine. Monoclonal light chains in the urine (Bence Jones protein) may be detected in more than half of patients with multiple myeloma (Isobe, 1971; Wells, 1974). Polyclonal light chains may be detected in patients with other disorders, usually as part of complete immunoglobulin molecules. Detection of Bence Jones protein by heat is reviewed in Chapter 27. IEP/IFE of urine is more specific and more sensitive than the older Bence Jones assay. IEP/IFE may be performed on urine samples with sufficient protein or subsequent to concentration by lyophilization or by selective membranes (Minicon, Amicon).

Immunoglobulins at very high concentrations can significantly increase the viscosity of blood leading to problems with organ perfusion. Measurements of the viscosity of serum have been done to assess this effect, but they are rarely used today because other methods for quantifying immunoglobulin concentrations such as nephelometry are widely practiced. Furthermore, serum viscosity by itself is a poor indicator of whole blood viscosity with cellular elements present, which is really the crucial factor clinically in the patient.

Cryoglobulin Testing

Testing for cryoglobulins in serum begins with a period of incubation in the cold (4°C) to detect turbidity or precipitate after 24 or 72 hours compared to an aliquot of the patient's serum kept at 37°C as a control for other precipitating substances not related to cold phenomena. Any cryoprecipitate is sedimented by centrifugation, washed briefly with cold saline to remove other serum proteins, and then redissolved (and dissociated) in warm saline for electrophoresis and immunofixation to identify immunoglobulin components (i.e., heavy and light chains).

Type I cryoglobulins typically form a relatively large volume of cryoprecipitate (e.g., up to 10 or even 20% of the serum volume – sometimes referred to as the 'cryocrit'). Upon immunofixation electrophoresis, type I cryoglobulins exhibit a single heavy chain and a single light chain type, often monoclonal IgM. The whole serum usually not treated with cryoprecipitation usually demonstrates a large amount of the same monoclonal band. The concentration of the band should fall after successful plasma exchange.

Type II cryoglobulins typically show only a small amount of cryoprecipitate that is less than 1% of the serum volume, and so quantitating the percentage of cryocrit is not analytically valid for serial measurements to monitor a patient's progress. IFE shows a monoclonal band of IgM plus polyclonal IgG (Figure 45–6F) This pattern is observed frequently due to its association with chronic hepatitis C.

IFE findings in type III cryoglobulin would be similar to those in type II with a relatively small amount of cryoprecipitate that demonstrates both polyclonal IgM and polyclonal IgG.

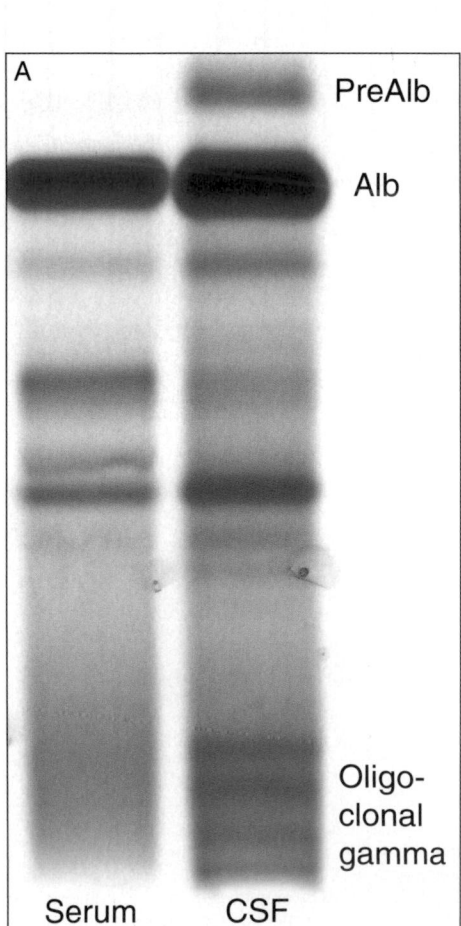

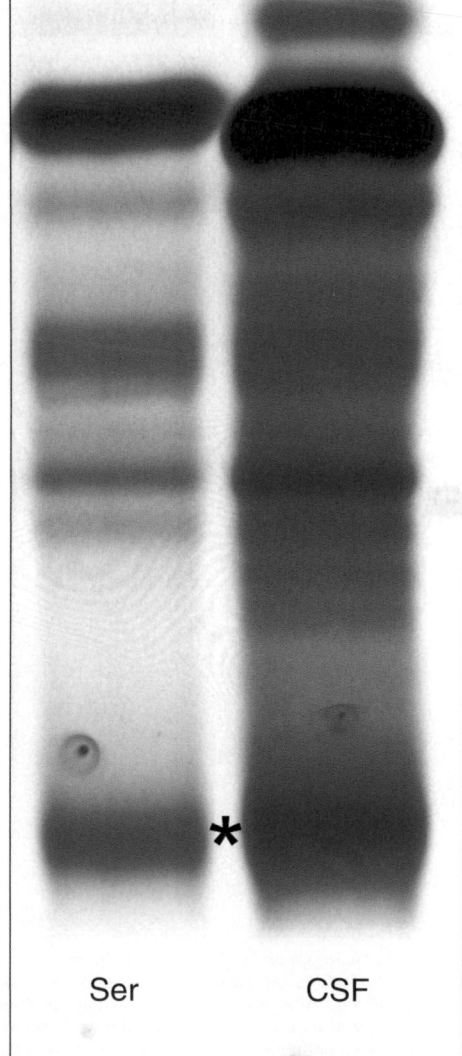

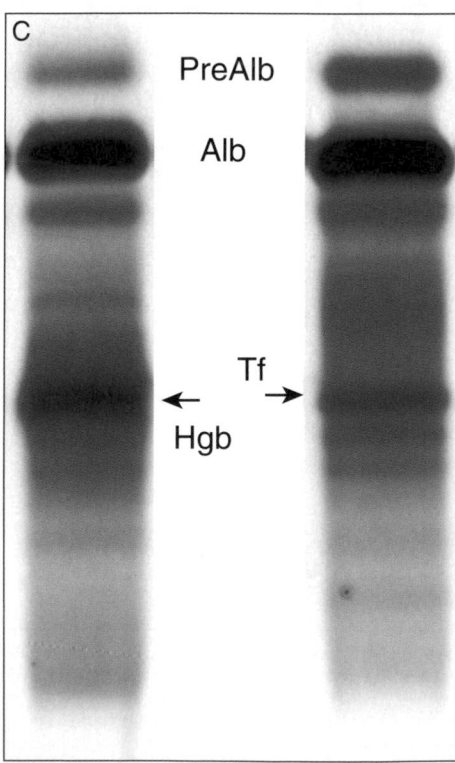

Figure 45–7 Protein electrophoretic patterns in serum and cerebrospinal fluid (CSF). A, Serum and CSF from the same patient showing positive oligoclonal bands in the γ region of the CSF but not in the patient's serum. B, Monoclonal band of immunoglobulin in both serum and CSF interpreted as negative for oligoclonal bands in CSF. C, Artifact of hemoglobin (Hgb) in CSF (left lane) adjacent to the position of transferrin (Tf) (right lane).

Oligoclonal Immunoglobulin Bands in Cerebrospinal Fluid

The evaluation of intrathecal synthesis of immunoglobulin is aided by high-resolution electrophoresis of cerebrospinal fluid protein that spreads out the γ region to display individual bands of different immunoglobulin clones. The interpretation of cerebrospinal fluid (CSF) protein electrophoresis requires simultaneous electrophoresis of the patient's serum to ensure that findings in the CSF are unique and not just the passive transfer of clonal immunoglobulins from the blood. Oligoclonal bands as a marker of synthesis of immunoglobulins in the central nervous system suggests the possibility of an autoimmune process such as a demyelinating disease. Another possibility is an immunologic response to CNS infection, so the interpretation of oligoclonal bands in CSF must be made in the context of other diagnostic findings such as cell counts, viral serologies, bacterial cultures, syphilis testing, nucleic acid amplification tests for viruses, etc.

The protein electrophoretic pattern of CSF and serum from a patient with multiple sclerosis is shown in Figure 45–7A. The CSF was concentrated and the serum was diluted to achieve comparable amounts of stainable protein in each application. CSF has a relatively higher concentration of prealbumin than does serum. Albumin is the predominant band in both fluids. The other significant band in CSF is transferrin, because of its small molecular size that permits ultrafiltration from blood into CSF. The higher-molecular-weight proteins in serum (α_2 plus β-lipoprotein) are absent from CSF. C3 is also identifiable in CSF plus a band of asialotransferrin in the β-2 region. After recognizing all these landmark proteins of CSF, oligoclonal bands should be evaluated in the γ region, which normally has only a small amount of polyclonal immunoglobulins. The oligoclonal bands in Figure 45–7A are discrete and clearly separate from one another.

Examination of serum and CSF sometimes shows a clonal band of immunoglobulin present in both (Figure 45–7B); however, this finding is not indicative of intrathecal synthesis and so is not a positive result for oligoclonal bands. Presumably it represents a clonal proliferation of plasma cells in the body with passive movement of the monoclonal antibody from blood into CSF.

Another distortion of the electrophoretic pattern occurs with release of hemoglobin into the CSF resulting in a major band in the β region close to transferrin (Figure 45–7C). This band of hemoglobin should not be confused with clonal immunoglobulin in CSF. Confirmation that this band is hemoglobin depends on visual examination of the CSF for blood or hemolysis (red color). A band of red hemoglobin can also be seen in the β region before staining the electrophoretic gel.

Disease Prevention and Therapy

Passive immunization is the administration of preformed antibodies obtained from another individual of the same species (homologous gammaglobulins) or a different species (heterologous gammaglobulins); it results in immediate protection against infection. The immunity is short-lived and decays as the antibodies are used and catabolized. Passive protection in neonatal life is based on transfer of maternal antibodies across the placenta or through colostrum (Pennington, 1991).

Pooled human γ-globulin is useful for temporary protection against several viral and bacterial infections (Berkman, 1990; Hammarström, 1990; Desai, 1991). Depending on the dose used and the time of administration, the disease may be modified to a mild form or entirely prevented. The effect is more complete and more predictable if one uses hyperimmune preparations made from the plasma of individuals who are either convalescing from the disease in question or have recently been immunized against it. Such preparations contain a higher concentration of specific antibodies. Antibodies may also be produced in animals, such as horses, and in the past these found widespread use. However, prior sensitization to foreign proteins may lead to clinical reactions such as anaphylaxis, serum sickness, pyrexia, and local Arthus reactions.

Monoclonal antibodies have revolutionized many areas of medicine, including research, diagnostics, and therapy. Murine, human, and humanized monoclonal antibodies have all been developed (Lefrano, 1990; Morrison, 1992; Mountain, 1992; Ward, 1992; Shin, 1993). Many monoclonal antibodies, often replacing polyclonal antisera, are used for diagnostic purposes (see Ch. 43). Perhaps the most important therapeutic applications of monoclonal antibodies are in the fields of transplantation and oncology (Stevenson, 1990; Vitetta, 1993; Neame, 1994). OKT3, a murine monoclonal antibody against the CD3 receptor on lymphocytes, is often used as an antirejection therapy to block the activity of cytotoxic T lymphocytes in renal transplant recipients (Ortho Multicenter Transplant Study Group, 1985). Many potential clinical applications of monoclonal antibodies are being evaluated. A recent example is the use of a monoclonal antibody against tumor necrosis factor-α to prevent Jarisch–Herxheimer reactions resulting from antibiotic treatment of Borrelia infection in sheep (Fekade, 1996). Anticytokine and antineutrophil adhesion molecule monoclonal antibodies may be effective in conditions associated with acute inflammation and cytokine release, for example, acid aspiration, ischemia, or reperfusion injury (myocardial infarction, hemorrhagic shock, aortic aneurysm repair); and antibodies inhibiting neutrophil adhesion may be effective in asthma, pulmonary fibrosis, meningitis, and cerebral malaria. It now seems reasonable to expect that a multitude of therapeutic applications will become available in the future, in which monoclonal antibodies will be designed to modulate the actions of one or more naturally occurring mediators of inflammation, infection, or malignant proliferations.

References

Atkinson JP, Waldmann TA, Stein SF, et al: Systemic capillary leak syndrome and monoclonal IgG gammopathy. Medicine 1977; 56:225.

Axelsson N, Hellen J: Frequency of M components in 6995 sera from an adult population. Br J Haematol 1968; 15:417.

Bachman R: The diagnostic significance of the serum concentration of pathological proteins. Acta Med Scand 1965; 178:801.

Benbassat J, Fluman N, Zlotnick A: Monoclonal immunoglobulin disorders: a report of 154 cases. Am J Med Sci 1976; 27:325.

Berkman SA, Lee ML, Gale RP: Clinical uses of intravenous immunoglobulins. Ann Intern Med 1990; 112:278.

Bhat TN, Bentley GA, Fischmann TO, et al: Small rearrangements in structures of Fv and Fab fragments of antibody D1.3 upon antigen binding. Nature 1990; 347:483.

Buckley RH: In Altman PL, Katz DD (eds): Human Health and Disease. Bethesda, MD, FASEB, 1977.

Burton DR: Immunoglobulin G: functional sites. Mol Immunol 1985; 22:161.

Cacoub P, Costedoat-Chalumeau N, Lidove O, Alric L: Cryoglobulinemia vasculitis. Curr Opin Rheumatol 2002;14:29–35.
This review presents an update on clinical findings in cryoglobulins with emphasis on patients with hepatitis C.

Carsetti R, Kohler G, Lamers MC: A role for immunoglobulin D: Interference with tolerance induction. Eur J Immunol 1993; 23:168.

Cassidy JT, Nordby GL, Dodge HJ: Biologic variation of human serum immunoglobulin concentrations: sex-age specific effects. J Chronic Dis 1974; 27:507.

Cohen HJ: Multiple myeloma in the elderly. Clin Geriatr Med 1985; 1:827.

Colls BM: Monoclonal gammopathy of undetermined significance (MGUS) – 31 year follow up of a community study. Aust NZ J Med 1999;29:500–504.
This clinical series demonstrated the long-term significance of MGUS.

Corcoran AE: Immunoglobulin locus silencing and allelic exclusion. Semin Immunol 2005; 17:141–154.

Cushman P, Grieco MH: Hyperimmunoglobulinemia associated with narcotic addiction. Am J Med 1973; 54:320.

Davies DR, Metzer H: Structural basis of antibody function. Ann Rev Immunol 1983; 1:87.

Desai RG: Recent advances in intravenous immunoglobulin therapy. Concluding remarks. Current trends and future directions. Cancer 1991; 68:1460.

Drouet E, Chapuis-Cellier C, Bosshard S, et al: Oligomonoclonal immunoglobulins frequently develop during concurrent cytomegalovirus (CMV) and Epstein–Barr virus (EBV) infections in patients after renal transplantation. Clin Exp Immunol 1999; 118:465.

Fekade D, Knox K, Hussein K, et al: Prevention of Jarisch–Herxheimer reactions by treatment with antibodies against tumor necrosis factor α. N Engl J Med 1996; 335:311.
This is an early clinical trial that showed how inflammatory reactions can be modulated by therapeutic antibodies.

Hammarström L, Smith CI: New and old aspects of immunoglobulin application. The use of intravenous IgG as prophylaxis and for treatment of infections. Infection 1990; 18:314.

Herron JN, He XM, Ballard DW: An antibody to single-stranded DNA: Comparison of the three-dimensional structures of the unliganded Fab and a deoxynucleotide–Fab complex. Proteins 1991; 11:159.

Isobe T, Osserman EF: Pathologic conditions associated with plasma cell dyscrasias: a study of 806 cases. Ann NY Acad Sci 1971; 190:507.

Karplus M, McCammon JA: Dynamics of proteins: elements and function. Annu Rev Biochem 1983; 53:263.

Kelly RH, Tardy TJ, Shah PM: Benign monoclonal gammopathy: a reassessment of the problem. Immunol Invest 1985; 14:193.

Keren DF: Procedures for the evaluation of monoclonal immunoglobulins. Arch Pathol Lab Med 1999; 123:126.
This review of laboratory procedures provides insight to modern measurements of monoclonal gammopathies.

Keren DF, Warren JS, Lowe JB: Strategy to diagnose monoclonal gammopathies in serum: High-resolution electrophoresis, immunofixation and kappa/lambda quantification. Clin Chem 1988; 34:2196.

Kolar G, Capra JD: Immunoglobulins: structure and function. In Paul WE (ed): Fundamental Immunology. Philadelphia, Lippincott, Williams & Wilkins, 2003, p 47.

Kyle RA: Monoclonal gammopathy of undetermined significance (MGUS): a review. Clin Haematol 1982; 11:123.

Kyle RA, Rajkumar SV: Monoclonal gammopathies of undetermined significance: a review. Immunol Rev 2003;194:112–139.
This is an updated and comprehensive assessment of patients with MGUS.

Lefrano G, Lefrano MP: Antibody engineering and perspectives in therapy. Biochemie 1990; 72:639.

Lichtman MA, Vaughan JH, Hames CG: The distribution of serum immunoglobulins, anti-γ-G globulins and antinuclear antibodies in White and Negro subjects in Evans County, Georgia. Arthritis Rheum 1967; 10:204.

Max EE: Immunoglobulins: Molecular genetics. In Paul WE (ed): Fundamental Immunology. Philadelphia, Lippincott, Williams & Wilkins, 2003, p 107.

Morrison SL: In vitro antibodies: strategies for production and application. Annu Rev Immunol 1992; 10:239.

Mountain A, Adair JR: Engineering antibodies for therapy. Biotechnol Genet Eng Rev 1992; 10:1.

Neame PB, Soamboonsrup P, Quigley JG, et al: The use of monoclonal antibodies and immune markers in the diagnosis, prognosis, and therapy of acute leukemia. Transfusion Med Rev 1994; 8:59.

Nickerson PW, Rush DN, Jeffery JR, et al: High serum levels of interleukin-6 in renal transplant recipients with monoclonal gammopathies. Transplantation 1994; 58:382.

Ortho Multicenter Transplant Study Group: A randomized clinical trial of OKT3 monoclonal antibody for acute rejection of cadaveric renal transplants. N Engl J Med 1985; 313:337.

Padlan EA: Anatomy of the antibody molecule. Mol Immunol 1991; 31:169.

Pennington JE: Immunoglobulin therapy in infectious disease. Cleveland J Med 1991; 58:309.

Poljak RJ: Structure of antibodies and their complexes with antigens. Mol Immunol 1991; 28:1341.

Radl J, Valentijn RM, Haaijman JJ, Paul LC: Monoclonal gammopathies in patients undergoing immunosuppressive treatment after renal transplantation. Clin Immunol Immunopathol 1985; 37:98.

Ritchie RF, Palomaki GE, Neveux LM, et al: Reference distributions for immunoglobulins A, G, and M: a practical, simple, and clinically relevant approach in a large cohort. J Clin Lab Anal 1998;12:363–370.
This manuscript presents reference ranges for immunoglobulins in a very large population by age and gender.

Roes J, Rajewski K: Immunoglobulin D (IgD)-deficient mice reveal an auxiliary receptor function for IgD in antigen-mediated recruitment of B-cells. J Exp Med 1993; 177:45.

Ropper AH, Gorson KC: Neuropathies associated with paraproteinemia. N Engl J Med 1998; 338:1601.

Schaefer AI, Miller JB, Lester EP, et al: Monoclonal gammopathy in hereditary spherocytosis: a possible pathogenetic relation. Ann Intern Med 1978; 88:45.

Shin SU, Wright A, Morrison SL: Hybrid antibodies. Int Rev Immunol 1993; 10:177.

Smith GS, Holman RP: The prozone phenomenon with syphilis and HIV-1 co-infection. South Med J 2004;97:379–382.
This recent case report reinforces the continuing need for vigilance in antigen–antibody based testing so as to avoid missing extremely high values of immune antibody due to the prozone effect.

Spielgelberg HL: Biological activities of immunoglobulins of different classes and subclasses. Adv Immunol 1974; 19:259.

Standfield RL, Fieser TM, Lerner RA, et al: Crystal structures of an antibody to a peptide and its complex with peptide antigen at 2.8 Å. Science 1990; 248:712.

Stanko CK, Jeffery JR, Rush DN: Monoclonal and multiclonal gammopathies after renal transplantation. Transplant Proc 1989; 21:3330.

Stevenson FK, George AJ, Glennie MJ: Anti-idiotypic therapy of leukemias and lymphomas. Chem Immunol 1990; 48:126.

Tedford MC, Stimson WH: Molecular recognition in antibodies and its application. Experientia 1991; 47:1129.

Tollerud DJ, Brown LM, Blattner WA, et al: Racial differences in serum immunoglobulin levels: Relationship to cigarette smoking, T-cell subsets, and soluble interleukin-2 receptors. J Clin Lab Anal 1995; 9:37.

Tonegawa S: Somatic generation of antibody-diversity. Nature 1983; 302:575.

Vitetta ES, Thorpe PE, Uhr JW: Immunotoxins: magic bullets or misguided missiles? Trends Pharmacol Sci 1993; 14:148.

Ward ES: Antibody engineering: The use of Escherichia coli as an expression host. FASEB J 1992; 6:2122.

Wells JV, Fudenberg HH: Paraproteinemias. DM 1:45, 1974.

Wilson IA, Stanfield RL, Rini JM, et al: Structural aspects of antibodies and antibody–antigen complexes. Ciba Foundation Symposium 1991; 159:13.

CHAPTER 46

Mediators of Inflammation: Complement, Cytokines, and Adhesion Molecules

H. Davis Massey MD PhD, Richard A. McPherson MD

VI

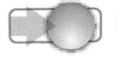

KEY POINTS

• The complement system is a group of circulating proteins that promote inflammation and host defense.

• Unregulated tissue damage is a possible complication of complement activation, and a large variety of circulating proteins exists, as well as tissue membrane-bound proteins that function to regulate complement activity.

• Complement component C3 is the central convergence point for all complement activation pathways.

• To track disease activity it is frequently necessary to measure serum complement levels, but it is important to recognize that serum complement measurements are snapshots of a dynamic process involving variable rates of complement consumption and production.

• Methods are available that allow accurate determination of serum levels of complement components.

• Functional complement assays are sensitive and precise tools for providing information about the activity of a complement component.

- The simplest functional assay of the classical pathway (CH_{50}) measures total hemolytic complement activity.

- Cytokines are soluble proteins released by cells over short distances to facilitate communication between cells, to assist in the upregulation or downregulation of the immune response, and to orchestrate associated inflammatory and reparative activities.

- Adhesion molecules are complex glycoproteins that bind living tissues together and mediate cell migration during embryogenesis, wound healing, and the inflammation response.

Structure and Function of the Complement System

The term 'complement' refers to a group of circulating glycoproteins that function to promote inflammation and serve an important role in host defense. Unregulated tissue damage is a possible complication of complement activation, and there exists a large variety of circulating glycoproteins as well as tissue membrane-bound proteins that function to regulate complement activity and down-regulate complement attack. The existence of this system of proteins was inferred late in the 19th century when it became clear that fresh serum had the ability to lyse gram-negative bacteria and cholera vibrios in the presence of specific antibody. As techniques for protein purification and identification became more sophisticated over the years, it was recognized that complement is a very complex system with many interacting proteins.

In general, the system functions to identify foreign cells and microorganisms and destroy them. This occurs either by direct lysis, by opsonization (the process of coating them with specific complement peptides recognized by specific receptors on phagocytes to aid ingestion), or by causing inflammation with the attraction of phagocytic cells. It also has become clear that complement plays a role in facilitating the immune response.

The complement system of proteins is older phylogenetically than that of acquired immunity (antibody) and is present in more primitive organisms. Presumably, it provides a level of natural immunity and host defense even in the absence of antibody. It does so via the mannan-binding lectin (MBL) pathway and the alternative complement pathway, both discussed below. Antibody provides a level of increased specificity and increased efficiency in mediating host defense. A detailed history of the discovery of complement and of the various complement pathways is provided elsewhere (Frank, 1998).

Nomenclature

There are three major pathways of complement activation in human serum: the classical pathway, the alternative pathway, and the MBL pathway (or MBLectin pathway). Figure 46–1 illustrates the reaction sequence of each pathway. Table 46–1 provides specific information on each plasma complement protein. The nomenclature for proteins of the complement system generally follows two conventions (World Health Organization, 1968; IUIS-WHO, 1981). For historical reasons, the nine proteins of the classical pathway are designated by the upper case letter C, which is then followed by the number that relates to their order of

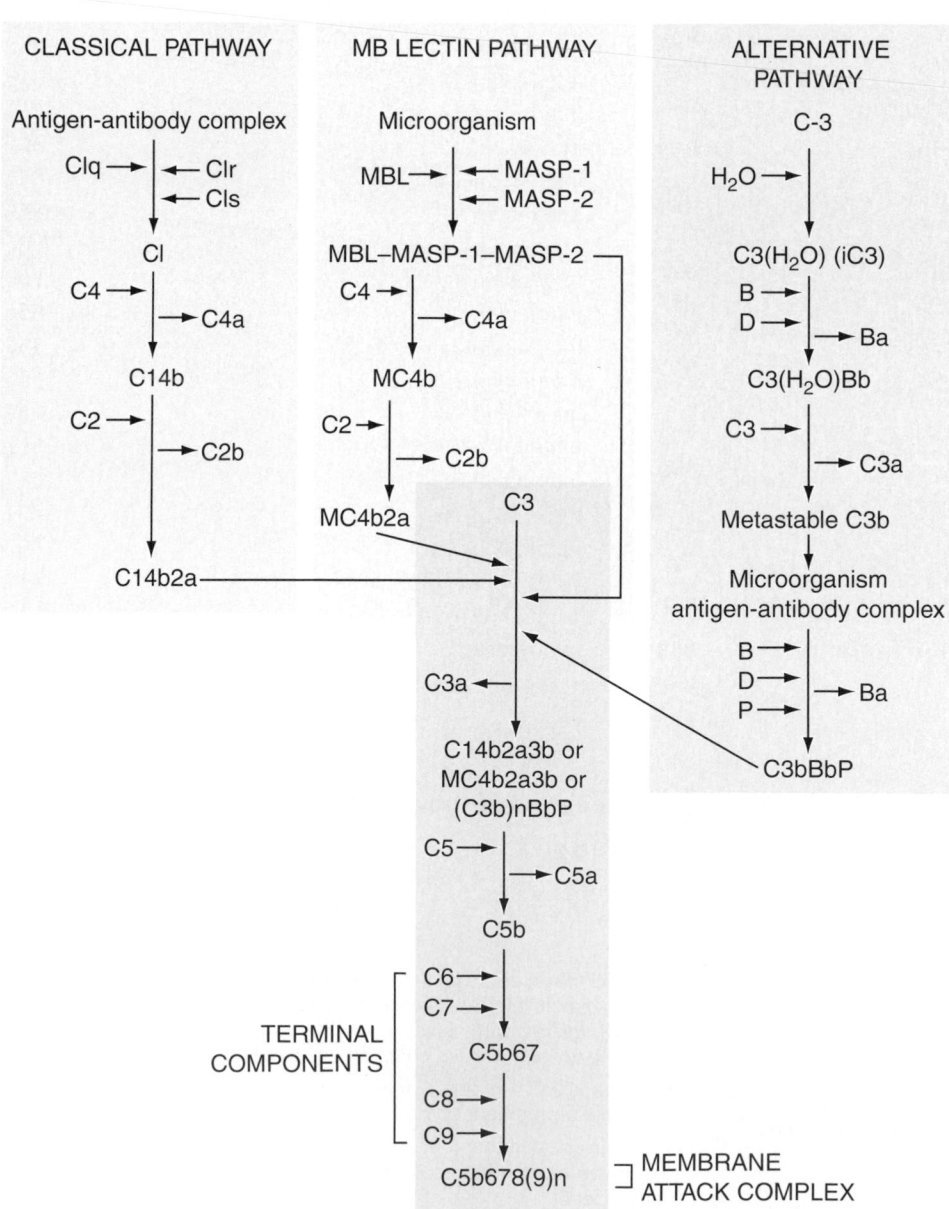

Figure 46–1 The components of the classical, MBLectin, and alternative pathways converge to form a convertase that cleaves C3. In the classical pathway, antigen–antibody complexes sequentially bind and activate C1, C4, and C2. In the MBLectin pathway, interaction of MBL with a carbohydrate on the surface of a microorganism leads to the formation of an enzymatic complex (MBL–MASP-1–MASP-2, termed M in the figure) that binds and activates C4 and C2. In the alternative pathway, C3 undergoes hydrolysis of its thioester bond, which induces a change in conformation, It then binds factor B (B), which is cleaved by factor D (D) to form a convertase that is stabilized by properdin (P). C3b, the cleavage product of C3, also has a cleaved thiolester bond and is capable of activating the alternative pathway, The C3b-containing convertase of all pathways continues sequentially by binding the late-acting component until the sequence of activation is complete.

Table 46–1 Complement Proteins in Human Plasma

Protein	Molecular Weight (kDa)	Chromosomal Location	Concentration (μg/mL)
Common to all pathways			
C3	185	19p13.3–p13.2	1200–1300
Classical pathway			
C1q	460	1p34.1–36.3	150
C1r	85	12p13	50
C1s	85	12p13	50
C4	205	6p21.3	300–600
C2	102	6p21.3	20
Alternative pathway			
Factor B	93	6p21.3	200
Factor D	24	Unknown	2
Properdin	55 (monomer)	Xp11.4–p11.2	25
MBLectin pathway			
MBL	200–400	10q11.2–q21	0.002–10
MASP-1	93	3q27–28	1.5–13
MASP-2	76	1p36.3–36.2	Unknown
Membrane attack complex			
C5	190	9q33	80
C6	110	5p13	45
C7	100	5p13	90
C8	150	1p32 (α, β chains), 9q22.3–q32 (γ chain)	55
C9	70	5p13	60
Control proteins			
C1inh	105	11q11–q13.1	240
C4bp	550	1q32	250
Factor I	88	4q25	35
Factor H	150	1q32	300–450
S protein	84	17q11	500
Clusterin	70	Unknown	50
Factor J	20	Unknown	≈5.4

appearance in the reaction sequence. A notable exception is C4, which acts before C2. Molecules that are part of the C1 complex are termed C1q, C1r, and C1s. Proteins reacting solely in the alternative pathway are called factors and are referred to by an upper case letter (e.g., factor B, factor D). In addition, fragments of complement proteins resulting from proteolytic cleavage are designated by a lower case letter (e.g., C4a, C4b) where 'a' represents the smaller fragment and 'b' represents the larger fragment. The exception to this rule is C2, where C2a is the larger fragment and C2b is the smaller fragment. Further degradation fragments of the large complement fragment of one component are designated by lower case letters (e.g., C3c, C3d). Components that have lost activity (i.e., are inactive) are usually designated by a prefixed lower case i (e.g., iC3b, iC4b). Polypeptide chains of a native complement protein are designated by Greek lower case letters (α, β, γ) except for C1q, the chains of which are termed A, B, and C. Single components or multicomponent complexes that have enzymatic activity are designated by a bar over the component(s). Proteins of the MBLectin pathway are designated by abbreviations of the proteins' names (e.g., MBL for mannan-binding lectin, MASP for MBL-associated serine protease). Regulatory proteins are designated by a descriptive title or letter (e.g., C4-binding protein, factor H). Membrane-bound regulatory proteins have been assigned CD numbers and descriptive titles (e.g., CD46 for membrane cofactor protein), and complement receptors are designated by numbers following the prefix CR (for complement receptors 1 to 4). The other complement receptors are designated by the component's symbol followed by the upper case letter R.

C3: Central Molecule of Complement Activation Pathways

The protein known as C3 is the central convergence point for the three complement activation pathways (the MBLectin pathway, the alternative pathway, and the classical pathway), which all proceed to lysis, phagocytosis, or regulation of the inflammatory response further down the cascade.

C3 is a two-chain molecule synthesized in many cells, particularly hepatocytes, formed from a single-chain molecule, pro-C3, and released into the circulation where it binds to foreign target surfaces. The α and β chains are stabilized by intrachain disulfide bonds; an interchain disulfide bond stabilizes α and β chain interaction (Fig. 46–2). The α chain contains a thiolester that imparts an unstable structure to the molecule. Although it is in the hydrophobic center of C3, the thiolester can be cleaved by gradual hydrolysis as water penetrates the molecule, activating the alternative complement pathway. C3 may also be cleaved rapidly by the action of C3 convertase releasing the 9 kDa C3a fragment from the α chain amino-terminus, from the larger C3b. C3b will go on to coat target proteins, thereby marking them for destruction, while C3a in the role of anaphylatoxin activates nearby cells to release mediators of inflammation (Wen, 2004). Either avenue results in marked conformational alteration of C3 (now termed C3b) that permits it to interact with cells expressing C3b receptors, in particular CR1 (C3b/C4b receptor, CD35). (Native C3 will not interact with C3b receptors.)

C3 activation and conversion to C3b (with thiolester cleavage) leads to covalent binding of C3b to the surface of a target such as a microorganism. The target becomes coated with C3b capable of interacting with cells expressing C3b receptors, including all phagocytes, B lymphocytes, and a subset of T lymphocytes. It is C3b that continues the complement cascade leading to lysis.

The Classical Pathway

The classical pathway of complement activation, described around the year 1900, was the first to be studied, and for this reason is called 'classical.'

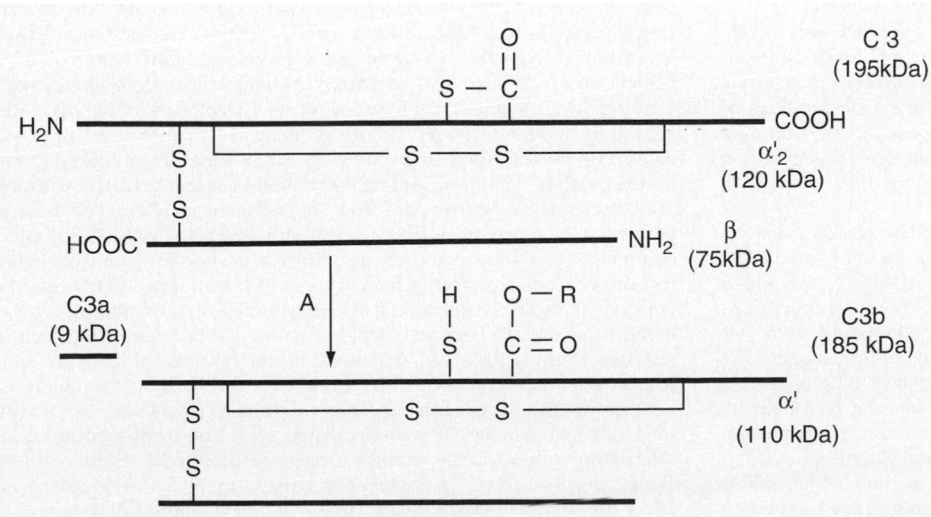

Figure 46–2 C3 cleavage by C3 convertase: The approximate molecular weight of each chain or fragment is given in kilodaltons (C3 convertase is represented by A).

It is evolutionarily the most recent of the three pathways described. The classical pathway is responsible for complement activation on most antibody-sensitized cells. Details of this pathway are published elsewhere (Fries, 1987; Volanakis, 1998). Nine numbered proteins comprise the classical pathway. Activation of the classical pathway usually requires interaction between an antigen and a C1-binding 'complementing' antibody. In humans, only immunoglobulin (Ig)M and IgG are effective at activating the classical pathway, except IgG4, which is unable to activate complement. Interestingly, a number of molecules, other than immunoglobulins, have the ability to activate the classical pathway via direct interaction with C1q. These include C-reactive protein, serum amyloid P component, β-amyloid, some Gram-negative bacteria, certain viruses, mycoplasmas, protozoa, and intracellular components such as DNA, mitochondrial membranes, and cytoskeletal filaments (Gewurz, 1993). Interestingly, apoptotic cells bind C1q (Korb, 1997) and have the ability to activate the classical pathway. This might be of critical importance in the elimination of apoptotic cells from the circulation. Prion diseases such as transmissible spongiform encephalopathy may be able to make use of complement system components such as C3 and C1q to facilitate localization within target cells (Mabbott, 2004).

Upon binding of immunoglobulin to a target, C1 binds to the immunoglobulin and becomes activated. C1 is a macromolecule of 740 kDa that comprises a single molecule of C1q complexed with two C1r and two C1s chains held together in the presence of calcium ions. Once bound to immunoglobulin, C1q adopts a conformational change that leads to autoactivation of the two C1r chains. Activated $C1s_2$ cleaves the next component in the cascade, C4. The larger fragment, C4b, becomes attached to the activator surface, whereas the smaller fragment, C4a, is released in the fluid phase. C4a is an anaphylatoxin and is described in a subsequent section of this chapter. Most of the generated C4b is hydrolyzed and remains in the fluid phase. Nevertheless, some of the generated C4b molecules bind to the activator surface as a cluster around the antigen–antibody-C1 site. A single antibody–antigen-C1 site can thus lead to the deposition of many C4b molecules.

In the presence of magnesium ions, C4b acts as a site for the binding and subsequent cleavage of C2. $C1s_2$, in association with C4b, cleaves C2 into two fragments. The larger fragment, C2a, remains bound to C4b, whereas the smaller one, C2b, is released in the fluid phase. This molecular complex, C4b2a, is unstable and has a relatively short half-life because of decay that results from the tendency of C2a to break away from the complex in an inactive form. The C4b2a complex is the classical pathway C3 convertase required for C3 binding and cleavage (Fig. 46–2). It is C2a as part of the C4b2a complex that enzymatically cleaves C3 in the next step of the activation cascade, and cleaves C5 in a later step. C2a cleaves C3 into a large fragment, C3b that binds to the activator surface and a smaller fragment, C3a that is released into the fluid phase where it serves as an anaphylatoxin. The newly generated C4b2a3b complex is the C5 convertase of the classical pathway that triggers deposition of terminal complement components on the target surface.

IgM and IgG differ in their ability to activate the classical pathway of complement. It appears that a single molecule of most IgM antibodies bound by multiple antibody sites to an antigen can bind one molecule of C1 and trigger a complete complement activation sequence. IgM, with its five antigen-binding sites, adopts a functionally active conformation on an antigenic surface that allows multiple interactions with antigens.

In contrast, C1 binding to IgG requires two molecules of IgG side by side in most experimental studies (Borsos, 1965). Because IgG antibodies bind to a target surface in a random fashion and, because antigens may not be evenly distributed on a target organism, the attachment of hundreds or thousands of IgG antibodies may be required to generate a C1-binding site. Classical pathway activation by IgG–antigen complexes is also shown to facilitate the alternative pathway (see next section) on the activator surface (Moore, 1981).

The ability of aggregated immunoglobulin to bind C1q has provided the basis for a number of tests designed to detect the presence of soluble immune complexes in patient blood samples. Radiolabeled C1q is added to the serum or plasma sample, and one of a number of techniques (e.g., polyethylene glycol precipitation) is used to separate free C1q from that bound to protein components of serum. The binding of C1q suggests the presence of immunoglobulin complexes in the serum or plasma sample (Zubler, 1976). Soluble immune complexes may also be measured by identification of C1q- or C3-bound immune complexes using enzyme-linked immunosorbent assay (ELISA) techniques (Stanilova, 2001). Detecting the presence of C1q in tissue specimens by direct visualization with immunofluorescently labeled anti-C1q antibodies may be used to identify immune complexes in biopsy specimens.

The Alternative Pathway

The presence of a second pathway of complement activation was first proposed by Pillemer (1954) but was accepted by the scientific community almost two decades later. This complement activation pathway appears to be important in early defense against pathogenic microorganisms (Pangburn, 1984). Though antibodies can activate this system, neither antibody nor lectin is required for activation. Initiation of the alternative pathway on an acceptor surface begins with deposition of active C3 on a surface that has no regulators of complement present on it, generating C3b fragments and allowing the process to continue as an unimpeded amplification loop (Wen, 2004). This depends on the ability of the carbonyl group of the exposed thiolester group of C3b to interact with either an amide or a hydroxyl group of a protein or a carbohydrate present on the surface of a target (Law, 1979). In serum, C3 is hydrolyzed at a rate of 0.2–0.4% of plasma pool per hour (Pangburn, 1981). C3 with a hydrolyzed thiolester undergoes a conformational change that allows it to interact with proteins that do not interact with native C3, and is termed $C3(H_2O)$ (also termed iC3). $C3(H_2O)$ then has the ability to interact with factor B in the presence of magnesium ions. Factor B, upon binding to $C3(H_2O)$, can interact with factor D and is cleaved to generate the so-called initiation C3 convertase $C3(H_2O)Bb$ and liberate a small fragment, Ba. This cleavage is mediated by factor D, a serine protease that adopts an active conformation upon recognition of its substrate and returns to an inactive conformation once proteolytic cleavage is accomplished (Volanakis, 1996).

The initiation C3 convertase cleaves C3 to generate metastable C3b at a continuously slow rate in the circulation. Metastable C3b can bind covalently to the activator surface and then, like $C3(H_2O)$, bind factor B. As in the initiation C3 convertase, factor D then cleaves factor B to generate the cell-bound C3 convertase C3bBb. This complex decays rapidly but is stabilized upon binding of properdin, which prolongs the half-life of the C3 convertase from 1 to 18 minutes (Fearon, 1975). This stabilized C3 convertase rapidly cleaves yet more C3, which can bind to the activator surface and is therefore referred to as the amplification C3 convertase of the alternative pathway. Amplification of C3b deposition to the activator surface leads to the formation of a C5 convertase ($C3b_2BbP$) (Kinoshita, 1988) that has the ability to trigger the activation of the terminal components of the complement system.

The Mannan-Binding Lectin Pathway

A third pathway of complement activation has been described recently that utilizes the serum protein MBL (also called mannose-binding lectin or mannose-binding protein), which is present in serum at about 1.5 µg/mL. MBL is formed in the liver and is found in all mammals and birds, and belongs to a family of molecules termed collectins (Epstein, 1996; Turner, 1996). The collectin family includes, in addition to MBL, lung surfactant proteins A and D (SP-A, SP-D), bovine conglutinin, and bovine CL-43 (Epstein, 1996). MBL is structurally related to C1q. MBL recognizes certain 'pathogenic' carbohydrates expressed on the surface of microorganisms, but does not recognize carbohydrates such as galactose and sialic acid, which are the terminal sugars expressed on mammalian glycoproteins (Epstein, 1996). This allows MBL to discriminate between self and non-self. MBL was reported to react with a wide range of acapsular Gram-positive and Gram-negative bacteria, viruses, yeasts, mycobacteria, parasites, and protozoa (Epstein, 1996). Upon recognition of its carbohydrate ligand, MBL adopts a conformational change that leads to activation of two MBL-associated serine proteases, MASP-1 and MASP-2 (Thiel, 1997). Both MASP-1 and MASP-2 share structural homology with C1r and C1s, suggesting similarity with the C1 complex ($C1qr_2s_2$). After activation, MASP-2 cleaves C4 to generate the classical pathway C3 convertase C4b2a (Vorup-Jensen, 1998). MASP-1 has the ability to cleave C3 (Matsushita, 1998), suggesting that it might trigger alternative pathway activation directly (Schweinle, 1989). Following the generation of classical pathway C3 convertase C4b2a by the MBL–MASP-1–MASP-2 complex, complement activation proceeds as in the classical pathway, with possible recruitment of the alternative pathway as well (Suankratay, 1998). Specific antibody–antigen complexes can also trigger the MBLectin pathway. It was demonstrated that a fraction of IgG molecules that lack terminal galactose residues (termed IgG-G0), as found in the plasma of patients with pathologic conditions such as rheumatoid arthritis, have the ability to interact with MBL and activate the classical pathway (Malhotra, 1995). MBL might play a role in the elimination of target organisms by phagocytes via an interaction with a specific receptor present on these cells (Hansen, 1998; Tenner, 1995), as well as modulate inflammatory and allergic responses, affect apoptotic cell clearance, and modulate the adaptive immune system (van de Wetering, 2004). Regulation of the MBLectin pathway appears to be mediated by C1 inhibitor (Matsushita, 1996) and α_2-macroglobulin (Terai, 1995).

Terminal Complement Components

All three main pathways of complement activation converge at the activation of C3 and the assembly of the membrane attack complex (MAC), which is formed by components C5 to C9. Upon formation of the classical, MBLectin (C4b2a3b), and alternative (C3b2Bb) pathway C5 convertases, C5 is cleaved. The larger fragment (C5b) can associate with the cell membrane and interact with C6. The next step involves the interaction of the C5b–6 complex with fluid-phase C7, forming a trimeric complex with amphiphilic properties (high affinity for the lipid constituents of the cell membrane) (Podack, 1979). C5b–7 inserts in the lipid bilayer of the cell membrane but is not sufficient for cell lysis to occur. C8 associates with this trimolecular complex via an interaction with exposed C5b. The C5b–8 complex penetrates the lipid bilayer further to form a small transmembrane pore to cause slow lysis of erythrocytes (Ramm, 1982). However, the insertion of multiple copies of C9 through the lipid bilayer via an initial interaction with the α chain of C8 is needed to produce the full cytolytic activity of the MAC (Plumb, 1998). It is believed that the C5b–8 complex serves as an initiator of C9 polymerization within the cell membrane. The MAC, by electron microscopy, has a hollow, cylinder-like structure formed by the assembly of its components in the presence of excess C9 (Podack, 1984). The mechanism by which the MAC disrupts the cell membrane is still controversial and may include the distortion of the lipid bilayer to form 'leaky patches' (Esser, 1991) or, more likely, the formation of a transmembrane pore with a hydrophilic center through which ions can pass freely (Bhakdi, 1991). The formation of the MAC induces lysis of certain bacteria and viruses, and of heterologous erythrocytes. Most nucleated cells resist MAC-induced cytotoxicity. This protection, especially from attack by one's own complement proteins, is mediated by membrane-associated regulatory molecules that prevent MAC formation (see below under Regulation of Complement Activation) as well as by shedding of the activated complement proteins by blebbing of the cell surface. Lysis of nucleated cells mediated by the MAC may occur but requires multiple MAC lesions to take effect (Koski, 1983). It has been proposed that the deposition of sublytic amounts of the MAC might protect the cell from subsequent complement attack (Reiter, 1992). Nucleated cells are protected from the effects of the MAC in part because of its active elimination from the cell surface by membrane repair linked to lipid turnover (Mold, 1998). MAC formation has a stimulating effect on several nucleated cell types. Among others, these effects include production of reactive oxygen radicals from neutrophils and macrophages, release of eicosanoids from phagocytic cells, induction of procoagulant activity in platelets and endothelial cells, proinflammatory activity in endothelial cells and smooth muscle cells, proliferation of smooth muscle cells and endothelial cells, and triggering of signal transduction pathways (Niculescu, 1993, 1999; Benzaquen, 1994; Sims, 1995; Kilgore, 1996; Tedesco, 1997; Mold, 1998).

Anaphylatoxins

Activation of complement via the classical, alternative, or MBLectin pathways leads to the generation of complement protein fragments that have important roles in various biological functions, including opsonization, phagocytosis, immunomodulation, and generation of inflammatory reactions.

Complement activation leads to proteolytic cleavage of many complement proteins with subsequent release of small fragments into the fluid phase that may have biological effects. Three of these released fragments are called anaphylatoxins. They are C4a, C3a, and C5a. Structural and functional characteristics of these molecules are described in an excellent review on the subject (Ember, 1998). C3a is a 9 kDa, peptide fragment released during selective proteolytic cleavage of the C3α chain by C2a (as a component of C3 convertase) in the classical and MBLectin activation pathway. It is also released by proteolytic cleavage of C3 by the enzymatically active peptide Bb, a component of the alternative pathway C3 convertase. C4a is a 8.7 kDa peptide released from C4 upon cleavage by C1s$_2$. C5a is an 11 kDa peptide released from the α chain of C5 by cleavage induced by either C2a in the classical and MBLectin pathway C5 convertase, or Bb in the alternative (and perhaps MBLectin) pathway C5 convertase. In general, anaphylatoxins are defined by their biological effects on smooth muscle cells, mast cells, small blood vessels, and peripheral blood leukocytes. The specific effects mediated by these peptides include degranulation of mast cells and basophils, with subsequent release of various mediators such as histamine and serotonin. Furthermore, they induce human neutrophil aggregation, smooth muscle contraction,

enhanced vascular permeability, and induction of thromboxane release from guinea pig macrophages, and stimulate mucus release from goblet cells (Marom, 1985). An especially important effect of the anaphylatoxins on basophils is to cause vasodilation via histamine release, leading to increased blood flow to sites of inflammation.

The function of C4a is generally similar to that of C3a. However, C4a is far less effective in its biological effects on a molar basis. C5a is by far the most potent of the human anaphylatoxins. The effect of C5a is 200-fold greater than C3a and 3000-fold greater than C4a in causing smooth muscle contraction of guinea pig ileum. It should be noted, however, that the relative effectiveness of these peptides is both tissue- and species-specific. It has been suggested that C3a is effective selectively in eosinophil localization to allergic sites, whereas C5a has an effect on many other cell types (DiScipio, 1999).

In addition to its role as an anaphylatoxin, C5a has many other important biological properties. The binding of C5a to neutrophils produces an increase in adhesion, aggregation, and induction of an oxidative response, and the release of lysosomal enzymes. Moreover, C5a is strongly chemotactic for monocytes and neutrophils, inducing the migration of the cells toward the source of complement activation. Thus, a local complement-activating inflammatory reaction can thereby induce increased blood flow to tissue and the adherence of neutrophils to local activated endothelium, and direct the migration of phagocytes to inflammatory sites along a chemotactic gradient. Neutrophils aggregated by C5a can embolize to the lung, causing changes in pulmonary gas exchange and even death. It is believed that C5a mediates much of the inflammation in the lungs caused by immune-complex formation (Ward, 1997). In a rat experimental sepsis model, it has been demonstrated that C5a may block the bactericidal functions of neutrophils if produced in excessive amounts, suggesting a role for complement activation in the high mortality rates observed in sepsis (Czermak, 1999).

The biological effects of anaphylatoxins are mediated via specific cell surface receptors described in the section on complement receptors.

Regulation of Complement Activation

Complement activation, although crucial to host defense, may produce profound tissue damage. Therefore, organisms have internal control mechanisms to: (1) limit overly widespread inflammation, (2) avoid excessive activation, and (3) protect host cells from inadvertent injury. A potent regulatory system consisting of fluid-phase and membrane-associated proteins has evolved to control complement activation at almost every step of the activation cascade (Table 46–2).

Fluid-Phase Regulators

Control of the first component of the classical pathway (C1) is mediated by C1-inhibitor (C1-Inh). C1-Inh blocks C1 autoactivation, C1 activation in the fluid phase, and C1 activation on weak activators of the classical pathway, but not on most immune complexes (Doekes, 1983). It is thought that C1-Inh has the ability to dislodge the entire C1qr$_2$s$_2$ complex from immunoglobulins with low binding affinity for C1q (Chen, 1998) and from targets sensitized with low doses of human IgG (Chen, 1998). In vitro, C1-Inh inactivates the mannan-binding lectin-associated serine proteases (MASP) (Matsushita, 1996). The activity of C4b is regulated by factor I (formerly referred to as the C3b/C4b inactivator) (Fries, 1987). Factor I cleaves the C4b α chain to generate two fragments, C4c and C4d; the latter fragment remains cell-bound. For proteolysis, a cofactor, C4-binding protein (C4BP), is required. C4BP is a 570 kDa protein that can also bind particle-bound and fluid-phase C4b and displace C2a from the classical pathway C3 convertase C4b2a (Gigli, 1979). Because of its crucial role in the three complement activation pathways, C3 is under rigid control. Fluid-phase C3b and C3(H$_2$O) are rapidly inactivated by factor I, which cleaves three peptide bonds on the α chain of C3b (Davis, 1982), thus generating an inactive form of the molecule, iC3b, which is incapable of engaging C5 or factor B. This factor I-mediated cleavage requires factor H as a cofactor. Factor H is a 150 kDa protein that binds C3b and has decay-accelerating activity toward the alternative pathway C3 convertase in addition to its cofactor activity for factor I-mediated cleavage of C3b. In addition to regulating C3b in the fluid phase, factor H binds to cell-bound C3b and triggers cleavage by factor I, thus limiting classical pathway activation (Ollert, 1995). Once C3b is cleaved into iC3b, which remains bound to the target surface, it can interact with complement receptor type 3 (CR3) present on phagocytic cells and promote phagocytosis.

There are a number of fluid-phase inhibitors of the terminal complement components that prevent the insertion of the membrane attack complex into cell membranes. S protein (different from protein S), also called vitronectin, binds the C5b–7 complex, thereby preventing its insertion in

CHAPTER 46: Mediators of Inflammation: Complement, Cytokines, and Adhesion Molecules

Table 46–2 Complement Regulatory Proteins

Protein	Molecular Weight (kDa)	Target	Mechanism of Action
Fluid phases			
C1 inhibitor	105	C1	Dissociates the C1 complex by binding to C1r and C1s
Factor H	150	C3b	Cofactor for C3b inactivation by factor I
C4-binding protein	550	C4	Cofactor for C4b inactivation by factor I
S-protein (vitronectin)	84	C5b-7	Inhibits the insertion of the MAC into cell membranes
Clusterin	70	C5b-7	Inhibits the insertion of the MAC into cell membranes
Factor J	20	C1, C3, B	Inhibits C1 complex formation, inhibits cleavage of C3 by Bb
Cell associated			
CR1	190*	C3b, C4b	Dissociation of C3/C5 convertases, cofactor for C3b and C4b inactivation by factor I
DAF (CD55)	70	C3bBb, C4b2a	Dissociation of C3/C5 convertases
MCP (CD46)	45–70	C3b (C4b)	Cofactor for C3b inactivation by factor I
CD59 (protectin)	18–20	C8, C9	Inhibition of formation of the MAC
HRF	65	C8, C9	Inhibition of formation of the MAC

* Most common isoform of CR1.

CR1 = complement receptor type 1; DAF = decay-accelerating factor; HRF = homologous restriction factor; MCP = membrane cofactor protein.

Table 46–3 Cell Receptors for Complement Protein Fragments

Receptor	Molecular Weight (kDa)	Ligand	Physiologic Role
CR1	190 (most common isoform)	C3b, C4b, iC3b	Phagocytosis, immune complex clearance
CR2	140	C3d, C3dg, iC3b	B-cell activation
CR3	165 (α chain) 95 (β chain)	iC3b, C3d, C3b	Phagocytosis, cellular adhesion
CR4	150 (α chain) 95 (β chain)	iC3b, C3b	Cellular adhesion
C1qRp*	126	C1q, MBL, SP-A	Phagocytosis
C3aR	48	C3a	Chemotaxis, degranulation of serosal-type mast cells, increase in vascular permeability
C5aR	43	C5a, C5a desArg	Chemotaxis, degranulation of serosal-type mast cells, cellular adhesion, increase in vascular permeability

* Other C1q receptors have also been described.

CR1 = complement receptor type 1; C1qRp = receptor for the collagenous region of C1q; CR2 = complement receptor type 2; CR3 = complement receptor type 3; C3aR = C3a receptor; CR4 = complement receptor type 4; C5a desArg = C5a lacking the terminal arginine residue following inactivation by carboxypeptidase-N; C5aR = C5a receptor; MBL = mannan-binding lectin; SP-A = surfactant protein A.

Regulatory control of terminal complement components of the membrane attack complex is achieved by homologous restriction factor (HRF) or C8-binding protein, and CD59 (also referred to as protectin, HRF-20, membrane inhibitor of reactive lysis, and P-18). HRF is expressed on erythrocytes, platelets, T-lymphocytes, B-lymphocytes, neutrophils, and monocytes (Morgan, 1994b), where it binds C8, and inhibits C9 polymerization (Morgan, 1994b). The second regulatory protein, CD59, is found on all circulating cells, endothelial cells, epithelial cells, spermatozoa, glomerular podocytes (Morgan, 1994b), and some cells of the central nervous system (Morgan, 1996). CD59 binds both the β chain of C8 and the b domain of C9 (Chang, 1994), inhibiting MAC formation on host cells. Because of their glycosyl phosphatidylinositol linkage to cell membranes, DAF, HRF, and CD59 are absent from the cells of patients with paroxysmal nocturnal hemoglobinuria (PNH) (Volanakis, 1988).

Complement Receptors

Receptors that bind activated complement components have been described in various cell types. These receptors control the biological effects of complement activation peptides and are linked to several other cellular functions as well (Table 46–3). The complement receptors that have been best studied are those that bind the degradation fragments of C3.

Complement receptor type 1 (CR1, CD35, C3b/C4b receptor) is a single-chain glycoprotein expressed on erythrocytes, mononuclear phagocytes, eosinophils, B lymphocytes, a subset of T lymphocytes, glomerular podocytes, follicular dendritic cells (Ahearn, 1998), and astrocytes (Morgan, 1996). It binds both C3b and C4b, to a lesser extent iC3b, and C1q as well (Klickstein, 1997). CR1 serves as a cofactor for factor-I-mediated cleavage of C3b, iC3b, and C4b and has decay-accelerating activity for both the classical and alternative pathway C3 and C5 convertases. A major physiologic role of CR1 is related to phagocytosis of complement-coated particles (opsonized particles). It is believed that erythrocyte CR1 has a major role in sequestering C3b- and iC3b-bearing immune complexes, removing them from the plasma and facilitating their transfer to degradation sites in the liver and the spleen (Birmingham, 1995). Decreased expression of erythrocyte CR1 may be associated with increased susceptibility to chronic forms of infection (Teixeira, 2001).

A receptor for the C3d fragment of C3 is found on human B cells, B-cell lines, follicular dendritic cells, some peripheral T cells, some T-cell lines, thymocytes (Ahearn, 1998), and astrocytes (Morgan, 1996), and is termed CR2 (CD21). CR2 has the ability to serve as a cofactor for factor-I-mediated cleavage of iC3b bound to targets (Mitomo, 1987), and is the receptor for

the cell membrane (Podack, 1977) and inhibiting C9 polymerization (Johnson, 1994). S protein binds C5b and C8 within the sC5b–9 complex (Su, 1996) and binds to the receptor C1q (Lim, 1996). Although the exact role of S-protein in regulating complement activation in vivo is uncertain, Peake et al. showed that S protein forms a complex with sC5b-9 when complement is activated in rabbits and that this complex still has the ability to block C9-mediated lysis of sensitized sheep erythrocytes bearing complement components 1–7 (Peake, 1996). Clusterin (also called Sp-40 or apolipoprotein J) is another fluid-phase inhibitor of the terminal complement components. Like vitronectin, clusterin prevents the insertion of the C5b–7 complex into the cell membrane (Choi, 1989) and regulates the membrane attack complex at both the C5b-7 and C9 levels (Berge, 1997).

Cell-Associated Regulatory Proteins

The regulation of complement activation must occur on host cell surfaces to limit inadvertent injury to those cells. Many of these regulatory proteins also act as complement receptors. One such protein is complement receptor type 1 (CR1), which binds activated C4b and C3b and serves as a cofactor their factor-I mediated cleavages (see next section for more). Control of cell-membrane-deposited C4b and C3b is also achieved by membrane cofactor protein (MCP, CD46). This protein is expressed by almost every cell, with the notable exception of erythrocytes, and serves as a cofactor for factor-I-mediated cleavage of C4b and C3b into C4c and C4d, and iC3b, respectively (Seya, 1986, 1989).

Another cell membrane-associated protein that controls complement activation at the level of the C3 and C5 convertases is decay-accelerating factor (DAF, CD55). DAF is expressed by all circulating cells, endothelial cells, and a number of epithelial cells (Morgan, 1994b), and accelerates the decay of C3 and C5 convertases of both the classical and alternative pathways.

Epstein–Barr virus on B cells causing infectious mononucleosis (Fingeroth, 1984). The major function of CR2 is thought to be the regulation of B-cell immune responses to antigen (Carroll, 1998b).

A third complement receptor, CR3 (also referred to as Mac-1, CD11b/CD18) is a member of the β_2 leukocyte integrin family of adhesion molecules. CR3 is expressed on mononuclear phagocytes, granulocytes, natural killer (NK) cells (Ahearn, 1998), and microglial cells (Morgan, 1996), and binds iC3b, and C3b and C3d (Brown, 1991). On phagocytes, CR3 triggers the phagocytic process in a fashion that parallels that of CR1. Another important role for CR3 is in the adhesion of monocytes and neutrophils to endothelial cells via an interaction with its ligand, intracellular adhesion molecule type 1 (ICAM-1). This allows accumulation of phagocytes at sites of tissue injury where endothelial cells become activated. CR3 may serve as a receptor for both human immunodeficiency virus (HIV)-1 and *Neisseria gonorrhoeae* infection of follicular dendritic cells and cervical epithelial cells, respectively (Edwards, 2001; Batjay, 2004).

Complement receptor type 4 (CR4, CD11c/CD18) is a glycoprotein that shares characteristics with CR3. It is also a member of the integrin family of adhesion molecules and is expressed on myeloid cells, dendritic cells, NK cells, activated B cells, some activated T cells, platelets (Ahearn, 1998), and microglial cells (Morgan, 1996). CR4 binds iC3b, and C3b to a lesser extent (Brown, 1991). The exact role of CR4 in terms of complement activation is unknown, but as this glycoprotein is an adhesion molecule it may serve to 'assist' neutrophil adhesion to the endothelium during inflammatory processes (Sengeløv, 1995).

A receptor for the anaphylatoxin C5a (C5aR) is expressed on neutrophils, monocytes, basophils, eosinophils, platelets, mast cells, liver parenchymal cells, lung vascular smooth muscle cells, lung and umbilical vascular endothelial cells, bronchial and alveolar epithelial cells, astrocytes, microglial cells (Ember, 1998), and human T cells (Nataf, 1999). C5a binding to the C5aR induces a wide variety of including chemotaxis of inflammatory cells; degranulation of mast cells; production of oxygen radicals; promotion of cell adhesion; production of leukotrienes and prostaglandins in neutrophils and eosinophils; and induction of acute phase proteins, cytokines, and antibodies (Ember, 1998).

Complement Biosynthesis

It is estimated that about 90% of plasma complement components are synthesized in the liver and are acute-phase proteins (i.e., their synthesis by the liver increases during inflammatory reactions to increase plasma levels). The hepatocyte produces the vast majority of complement components, with the exception of C1q, factor D, properdin, and C7 (Morgan, 1997a). C1q appears to be synthesized by epithelial cells, monocytes/macrophages, and fibroblasts. The main source of factor D is the adipocyte. Properdin is synthesized mainly by monocytes and macrophages with some synthesis occurring in lymphocytes and granulocytes. The majority of plasma C7 also appears to originate from monocytes and macrophages, although neutrophils were shown to store C7. Monocytes, macrophages, cells of the synovial tissues, and astrocytes have the ability to synthesize all the components of the classical and the alternative pathways. This may have important implications in tissue-specific inflammation, where a localized mechanism of host defense must be present to eliminate foreign particles efficiently. Production of complement components usually synthesized by hepatocytes or by extrahepatic cells often requires stimuli generated in inflammatory reactions such as interleukin-1α, interleukin-6, or interferon-γ. A good description of the regulation of complement protein synthesis by various cells is provided elsewhere (Colten, 1998).

Complement Genetics

Most of the complement components are inherited in an autosomal co-dominant fashion. The genes that encode complement proteins, receptors, and regulatory molecules have been cloned and assigned a chromosome location (Table 46–1). Interestingly, a linkage exists for a number of genes that code for complement-related molecules. These linkage groups include major histocompatibility complex (MHC) class III genes (C2, factor B, and C4), genes for the regulators of complement activation (C4-binding protein, CR1, CR2, DAF, MCP, and factor H), and genes for proteins of the membrane attack complex (C6, C7, and C9) (Schneider, 1999). Molecules within each of these three groups share structural homology, suggesting that complement proteins may have arisen from gene duplication of a limited number of ancestral genes. Almost all the complement-related proteins show polymorphism (i.e., multiple alleles exist with variable frequencies in humans). The most polymorphic complement component is C4, with more than 35 identified alleles (Schneider, 1997). Point mutations, insertions, or deletions of nucleic acids are usually linked to deficiencies in complement proteins (Schneider, 1997). Complement protein

polymorphism is assessed by both phenotypic and genotypic analysis. The details of these methods will not be discussed in this chapter and the reader is referred to Chapter 48 and others on the subject (Schneider, 1997; Mauff, 1996).

Complement and Acquired Immunity

It is becoming clear that the complement system has an important role to play in the establishment of acquired immune responses (Carroll, 2004). Depressed antibody responses to antigen stimulation were noted in animals transiently depleted in C3 (Pepys, 1974), animals with genetic deficiencies in C2, C4, or C3 (Ochs, 1983; Böttger, 1985; O'Neil, 1988), and in patients genetically deficient in either C2, C4, C3, or CR3 (Ochs, 1986). The recent development of 'knockout' mice lacking C4, C3, or complement receptors types 1 and 2 has allowed a better understanding of the role of complement in antibody responses to antigen. This effect has been reviewed recently (Carroll, 1998a, 1998b; Fearon, 1998).

Complement may influence the antibody response to an antigen in several ways. CR2 is present on the surface of B cells in association with CD19 and TAPA-1. Upon co-ligation of the B-cell receptor for antigen and CR2 (as would occur when antigen is complexed with C3d), the threshold for B-cell activation is dramatically lowered. Also, complement helps in the trapping of immune complexes by follicular dendritic cells in the spleen. This facilitates the formation of germinal centers where B cells acquire memory phenotype. A lack of one of the early components of the classical pathway of complement activation or lack of CR1 and/or CR2 may lead to markedly impaired immune responses to antigen and, in some cases, may lead to inability to mount a secondary antibody response. Complement may play a role in the generation of CD5-positive B cells, which give rise to 'natural' antibodies (Carroll, 1998a). Proper B-cell activation in response to an antigenic challenge also appears to depend, in some cases, on 'natural' antibody and complement activation (Boes, 1998; Lutz, 1999). Interestingly, complement seems important in the maintenance of B-cell tolerance to self-antigens. This appears to be dependent on complement component C4, and CR1 and CR2 (Prodeus, 1998). Finally, complement (especially C3) helps in the generation of an acquired immune response to antigen via antigen-presenting cells (APCs). The presence of C3 cleavage products on antigen enhances the uptake of antigen by APCs (B cells and other professional APCs expressing CR1 and/or CR2), thereby increasing the efficiency of antigen presentation to T cells with subsequent T-cell-mediated responses (Boackle, 1998; Kerekes, 1998).

Genetic Complement Deficiencies

Genetically controlled complement deficiencies are very rare, but they are of interest because they allow us to determine the role of complement components in various biological phenomena and in various disease states. In general, the absence of a complement component follows simple mendelian genetic principles and is usually inherited as an autosomal recessive trait. Heterozygous patients tend to have half the normal complement levels or less, and homozygous (deficient) patients have little or no detectable complement component activity. Deficiencies are known for every protein linked to complement activation (Table 46–4). The incidence of complete complement deficiency is estimated to be 0.03% of the general population (Wen, 2004), but with the discovery of the MBL pathway of complement activation came the surprising finding that deficiency in serum MBL is fairly common. It is estimated that approximately 5% of the population has one of the three recognized gene mutations that lead to MBL deficiency (Sumiya, 1997). There is a reported correlation between MBL deficiency and upper respiratory tract infections, especially between the ages of 6 and 18 months, demonstrating the importance of the MBLectin pathway in early childhood (Turner, 1996). A recent study suggested that variant MBL genes might be associated with as many as one third of all meningococcal infections in children (Hibberd, 1999). Purified MBL infusions are reported to correct the defect and susceptibility to infections in children with MBL deficiencies (Valdimarsson, 1998). Furthermore, there is a suggestion that MBL deficiency leads to autoimmune diseases such as systemic lupus erythematosus (SLE) (Turner, 1996) and is a risk factor for recurrent miscarriage (Christiansen, 1999).

Another feature of complement deficiency, especially in early classical pathway components (C1, C4, C2), is an association with autoimmune diseases such as SLE. Since complement is important in the clearance of immune complexes from the circulation, it may be that early complement component deficiency leads to improper handling of immune complexes, with their accumulation in tissues such as the kidney. Deficiency in C1 inhibitor leads to hereditary angioedema, a disease characterized by

Table 46–4 Inherited Deficiencies in Complement and Complement Related Proteins

Protein	Pattern of Inheritance	Major Clinical Correlates*
Common to all pathways		
C3	Autosomal recessive	Recurrent pyogenic infections, glomerulonephritis
Classical pathway		
C1q	Autosomal recessive	Glomerulonephritis, SLE
C1r	Autosomal recessive	Glomerulonephritis, SLE
C1s	Autosomal recessive	Glomerulonephritis, SLE
C4[†]	Autosomal recessive	SLE
C2[†]	Autosomal recessive	SLE, DLE, juvenile rheumatoid arthritic, glomerulonephritis
Alternative pathway		
Factor B	Autosomal recessive	*Neisseria meningitidis* infection
Factor D	Autosomal recessive	Recurrent pyogenic infections
Properdin	X-linked	Recurrent pyogenic infections, fulminant meningococcemia
MBLectin pathway		
MBL	Autosomal dominant	Recurrent infections
Membrane attack complex		
C5	Autosomal recessive	Recurrent disseminated neisserial infections, SLE
C6	Autosomal recessive	Recurrent disseminated neisserial infections
C7	Autosomal recessive	Recurrent disseminated neisserial infections, Raynaud disease
C8 (β or α–γ chains)	Autosomal recessive	Recurrent disseminated neisserial infections
C9	Autosomal recessive	None
Fluid-phase control proteins		
C1inh	Autosomal dominant or acquired	Hereditary angioedema, autoimmune diseases[‡]
C4bp	Autosomal recessive	Angioedema, Behçet's-like syndrome
Factor I	Autosomal recessive	Recurrent pyogenic infections
Factor H	Autosomal recessive	Recurrent pyogenic infections, glomerulonephritis
Cell-bound proteins		
CR1	Autosomal recessive[§]	Association between low erythrocyte expression and SLE
CR3	Autosomal recessive	Recurrent pyogenic infections, leukocytosis
DAF/CD59/HRF	Acquired	Paroxysmal nocturnal hemoglobinuria

* Note that some people with complement deficiencies, especially C2 and components of the membrane attack complex, are clinically well. A substantial number of patients with defects in C5–C9 have had autoimmune disease. Deficiencies of C1–C9 are associated with a CH_{50} of 0. Deficiencies of C1, C4 and C2 are associated with SLE and patients often have negative LE preps. Deficiencies of C3–C9 are associated with absent or low bactericidal activity in serum. Deficiency of C3 or C5 is associated with absent or diminished chemotactic activity of serum and may be associated with absent leukocyte response to infection.

† Deficiency in either C4 genes (*C4A* and *C4B*) is referred to as 'q0,' for quantity zero. Such deficiency is designated C4Aq0 or C4Bq0. Patients with such deficiencies have a higher than normal incidence of autoimmune diseases. Heterozygous C2-deficient individuals also have an increased incidence of autoimmune diseases.

‡ Approximately 85% of cases involve silent alleles, and 15% involve alleles encoding for acquired dysfunctional variant C1 inhibitor protein. In hereditary angioedema, the C1 level is normal or depressed, the C3 level is always normal, and the C4 level is depressed. In the acquired disease, C1 and C4 levels are depressed, the antigenic C1 inhibitor level usually is normal or high, and the functional C1 inhibitor level is very low.

§ Homozygosity for a low (not absent) numerical expression of CR1 on erythrocytes is detectable in vitro and may be associated with SLE. An acquired defect in the number of CR1 may also be operative.

Low, but not absent, levels of leukocyte CR3 are detectable in both parents of most CR3-deficient children.

DLE = disseminated lupus erythematosus; MBL = mannan-binding lectin; SLE = systemic lupus erythematosus.

recurrent episodes of subcutaneous and submucosal edema. This deficiency can be inherited or acquired following the development of autoantibodies to C1 inhibitor. And recently, a deficiency of factor H due to a novel homozygous factor H gene mutation has been described in an 8-month-old child that was associated with thrombotic microangiopathy and ultimately renal failure (atypical hemolytic uremic syndrome) (Licht, 2005).

Assessment of Complement Activity in Disease

Complement promotes inflammation or tissue damage during the immune response, and plays an important role in the pathogenesis of some diseases. In the latter situation, complement is often activated by an abnormal antibody (autoantibody), an immune complex, or by foreign material. To track disease activity in these cases, it is frequently necessary to measure serum complement levels, as with SLE, in which depressed serum C3 or C4 correlates with disease activity. In such instances nephelometric techniques are frequently employed (see Assays of Complement, below).

It is important to recognize that serum complement measurements are only snapshots of a dynamic process involving variable rates of complement consumption and production. Many of the complement proteins behave as acute-phase reactants, their serum levels rising dramatically in some inflammatory states while they may fall dramatically through catabolism in other inflammatory conditions such as autoimmune states. Depending on the rate of complement production and consumption, a normal serum complement level may be associated with tissue damage just as a decreased serum complement level may be. For example, patients with biliary cirrhosis have an increased catabolic rate of C3, and it has been suggested that C3 may play a role in the development of this disease. Nevertheless, the level of C3 in the serum of patients with biliary cirrhosis is almost always elevated. In this case, increased synthesis obscures the increased catabolism. It should also be recognized that complement function in various body compartments may differ. Serum complement levels in patients with seropositive rheumatoid arthritis may be normal or elevated, but in the joint compartment where tissue damage is greatest, joint fluid complement levels may be severely depressed.

Several investigators have attempted to identify which complement activation pathway predominates in mediating tissue damage or depressed complement levels in one illness or another by establishing the 'complement profile.' The simplest approach to this problem examines the levels of various components and assumes that decreased levels of a given component of one of the pathways of complement activation is more likely to occur when that pathway is activated. Therefore, if a patient has depressed levels of C3 and C4 and normal levels of factor B, the classical pathway is likely to be involved. If a patient has decreased levels of C3, factor B, and properdin, and normal levels of C4, alternative pathway activation is most likely. In this way, determining the levels of a limited number of components can provide a great deal of information.

An important advance in this area is the use of ELISA to detect stable complexes formed in serum during complement activation. These assays are highly sensitive and can readily demonstrate which pathway of complement is activated in various disease states (Morgan, 1994a).

On activation, many complement proteins express new antigens (neoantigens) that are not revealed on the native plasma protein. The neoantigen present on the MAC but not present on native terminal components is perhaps the most interesting. Antibody to this neoantigen exists and has been used to study the level of neoantigen by immunofluorescence as well as by ELISA (Falk, 1983; Sanders, 1985). The neoantigen level is elevated in blood and spinal fluid in many patients with ongoing complement activation (Sanders, 1986). Moreover, it is present in tissues at sites of terminal complex deposition. For example, it is present in lesional tissue in the glomeruli of patients with glomerulonephritis (Falk, 1983) and in lesional skin at sites of active SLE (Biesecker, 1982). Unlike C3 deposited in normal skin of patients with SLE and a positive lupus band test, the MAC neoantigen is found only in lesions.

Complement in Disease States

Rheumatologic Diseases

Deficiency of an early complement component (C1, C4, or C2) is often associated with autoimmune disease (Wen, 2004). The rheumatologic disease that has been evaluated most extensively in terms of the contribution of complement to disease activity is SLE (Agnello, 1986; Atkinson, 1986; Liu, 2004). The incidence of a deficiency of complement components C1q, C4, and C2 is 90%, 75%, and 15%, respectively in those with SLE (Pickering, 2000); the incidence of SLE is also increased in those with MBL deficiencies (Kilpatrick, 2002). Large amounts of immune complexes are formed in this disease, both circulating and tissue-bound. These immune complexes activate complement, and complement activation products contribute to ongoing inflammation. C3 and C4 levels are often reduced in SLE and, in general, low levels are found in patients with active disease. Some suggest that a low C4 level is the best indicator of ongoing active disease. However, there are patients with active disease who show normal C4 levels. According to others, the level of circulating sC5b–9 or neoantigen of the MAC might serve as a better indicator of active disease (Gawryl, 1988). As discussed earlier, complement appears to play an essential role in the clearance of immune complexes from the circulation, particularly those that contain IgM or IgG complement-activating isotypes. C3b deposition on the immune complex results from complement activation, which allows interaction with cells that possess a C3b receptor (CR1). Upon binding to erythrocytes via CR1, immune complexes are prevented from diffusing from the plasma to tissues where they could cause damage. Erythrocytes that bear immune complexes circulate to the liver where immune complexes are removed by a process that does not shorten the life span of the red cell (Cornacoff, 1983; Birmingham, 1995). In diseases in which complement is activated and these immunologically active products are formed in the circulation, the number of CR1 per red cell is decreased. This may result from removal of some of the CR1 upon removal of the immune complex from the erythrocyte in the liver (Ross, 1985). In addition to SLE, erythrocytes from patients with chronic cold agglutinin disease, PNH, autoimmune hemolytic anemia, Sjögren's syndrome, and mycoplasmal pneumonia are reported to have reduced erythrocyte CR1, suggesting that immune deposits have been removed from erythrocytes in these diseases (Ross, 1985; Atkinson, 1986).

The complement proteins act as acute-phase reactants and levels may not be depressed even in situations in which complement activation occurs. Normal or elevated serum complement levels are found in juvenile rheumatoid arthritis, palindromic arthritis, pseudogout, gout, Reiter syndrome, and gonococcal arthritis. At the same time, depressed levels of complement in joint fluid have been shown to exist in a number of other rheumatologic conditions, including rheumatoid arthritis. Depressed total hemolytic complement activity (CH_{50}; see below under Assays of Complement) and the presence of cleavage products of C3 and factor B are thought to represent intra-articular activation in the synovial fluid of most patients with seronegative rheumatoid arthritis, SLE, pseudogout, gout, Reiter syndrome, and gonococcal arthritis. This is not true of fluids obtained from patients with degenerative arthritis.

Hereditary Angioedema

Hereditary angioedema is a potentially life-threatening condition marked by submucosal and subcutaneous, nonpruritic and non-erythematous swelling. It usually resolves within 48–72 hours but may instead be fatal when it involves the laryngeal mucosa. The cause of hereditary angioedema is a heterozygous deficiency of C1-Inh. Because C1-Inh is regulator of various components of the clotting, complement, and kinin-generating pathways, the actual pathway involved in the genesis of episodes of hereditary angioedema is difficult to pinpoint. Several types of hereditary angioedema have been identified, including type I in which patients have a reduced (30% or less) level of functional or antigenic C1-Inh, and a type II in which, although present at normal levels, the C1-Inh protein has reduced or absent activity (Wen, 2004).

Infectious Diseases

As mentioned earlier and as evidenced by clinical findings in patients with genetically controlled complement deficiencies, the complement system plays a crucial role in defense against microorganisms. Patients with Gram-negative septicemia and pyogenic infections often have deficiency of C3, the primary opsonin, or components of the alternative pathway. Complement might be involved in tissue damage associated with chronic infection. It is known that patients with HBsAg-positive infectious hepatitis have an early fall in serum C3, which later returns to normal. This may be associated with signs of immune complex disease (i.e., arthralgia). In a similar fashion, complement appears to play an important role in many parasitic infections, including leishmaniasis, trypanosomiasis, giardiasis, and malaria. In those with recurrent infections by *N. gonorrhoeae* or *Neisseria meningitidis*, a deficiency of MAC or properdin may be suspected. A thorough discussion of the interactions between the complement system and parasites, bacteria, and viruses may be found in several excellent reviews (Frank, 1988; Fishelson, 1994; Moffitt, 1994; Kozel, 1996; Cooper 1998). However, it is important to recognize that serum complement levels are in general not a reliable index of disease activity in these conditions.

The role of complement in the adult respiratory distress syndrome (ARDS), a common occurrence in patients with severe trauma or overwhelming sepsis, has been studied. There is evidence of massive activation of complement in these patients, suggesting that bacteria and bacterial products activate complement (Hammerschmidt, 1980). Both the classical and alternative pathways appear to be activated (Langlois, 1988). Inflammatory factors such as neutrophil-activating factor and C5a are formed. There is evidence that neutrophils infiltrate the lung, and neutrophil oxidative products and proteases are thought to be responsible for much of the pulmonary damage that occurs. Recent evidence has identified a possible role for complement, through complement receptors, in the infection of follicular dendritic cells by the HIV virus (Doepper, 2002; Stoiber, 2005). A similar role for the MAC has been postulated in prion diseases, (see Neurologic Diseases, below).

Renal diseases

Complement appears to be of key importance in glomerular damage in many of the glomerulonephritides (West, 1998). This is usually demonstrated by the deposition of C3 or other components, within or near the glomerular basement membrane. Moreover, the MAC has been recognized in the damaged glomeruli in patients with glomerulonephritis and SLE. Patients with serum sickness due to immune complexes in the circulation have been shown to have glomerular injury. On serum analysis, these patients show activation of the classical or alternative pathways, or both. Traditionally, it has been believed that complexes are deposited in glomeruli as they filter the plasma that contains immune complexes. Once deposited, these complexes activate complement. An alternative view is that antibodies to glomerular structures form immune complexes in the kidney that then activate complement to cause local damage (Daha, 1979). Although antibodies to glomerular basement membrane structures are clearly of importance in Goodpasture syndrome, their overall role in glomerulonephritis is more questionable. The role of complement in interstitial and tubular disease is less clear; however, there are those who believe that complement functions in these disorders as well. Interestingly, especially in some patients with a rare form of glomerulonephritis (membranoproliferative glomerulonephritis, type II) with very low C3 levels, a protein termed C3 nephritic factor (C3NeF or NF_a) stabilizes the alternative pathway C3 convertase. This factor is an autoantibody directed against Bb that extends the half-life of the alternative pathway C3 convertase by more than 10 times (Daha, 1979, 1976). C3NeF appears to protect the alternative pathway C3 convertase from decay dissociation by factor H (Fearon, 1980). C3NeF is believed to be responsible for the very low C3 levels present in these patients but is not thought to play a central role in the development of nephritis. Complement components C4, C3, and C1q are routinely searched for in the glomeruli of renal biopsies using immunofluorescence microscopy as part of the evaluation of glomerular disease.

Dermatologic Diseases

Complement is thought to play a part in ongoing tissue damage in a variety of dermatologic illnesses. These include bullous pemphigoid, pemphigoid gestationis, cicatricial pemphigoid, epidermolysis bullosa acquisita, dermatitis herpetiformis, and pemphigus vulgaris (Yancey, 1998). It should be noted that serum complement levels are usually normal or elevated in these inflammatory states, and the importance of complement in these conditions is suggested by immunofluorescence analysis of tissue biopsies and by studies of blister fluid. Gammon et al. (1984) developed an in vitro model useful for the study of anti-basement-membrane-zone antibody-mediated skin disorders. These authors have shown conclusively that C5a is a key element in the pathogenesis of bullous pemphigoid and epidermolysis bullosa acquisita. C5a acts as the chemoattractant necessary for the influx of neutrophils into the sites of subsequent tissue damage in these diseases.

Hematologic Diseases

In many types of autoimmune hemolytic anemia, complement plays an important role in the opsonization of erythrocytes, leading to their clearance by cells of the reticuloendothelial system. However, even in those cases in which complement is clearly involved, serum complement levels are usually normal. Complement is particularly important in the clearance of cells coated with IgM cold-reactive autoantibodies with anti-I specificity. These autoantibodies (cold agglutinins) are associated with lymphoproliferative disorders following infections, or they may be isolated findings, especially in the elderly. Cold agglutinins generally bind erythrocytes optimally at the sub-physiologic temperatures found in some areas of the body like the tip of the nose, fingers, and ears. They usually mediate cell lysis when the circulating erythrocytes return to core body temperatures. Not all cold agglutinins are IgM antibodies. The syndrome of paroxysmal cold hemoglobinuria (PCH), for example, results from the cold-reactive Donath–Landsteiner IgG antibodies, which bind to cells at temperatures below 37°C but mediate lysis upon warming. Although the antibody is different, the pathophysiologic effects are similar.

Other autoantibodies that activate complement bind more efficiently at warm temperatures. In general, these warm-reactive antibodies are of the IgG isotype. In some cases, these antibodies may be associated with lymphoproliferative malignancies and viral infections. Most IgG warm-reactive antibodies found in autoimmune hemolytic anemia have Rh specificity and are poor complement activators as opposed to cold agglutinins and anti-A and anti-B blood group antibodies. However, some antibodies, like Tja, activate complement well and cause lysis.

In a rare acquired hemolytic anemia, termed paroxysmal nocturnal hemoglobinuria (PNH), patients experience recurrent episodes of intravascular hemolysis. Lysis of erythrocytes in these patients is believed to proceed via the alternative pathway (Rosse, 1998; Jarva, 1999), although serum complement levels are always normal and the direct antiglobulin test is always negative. The defect in PNH is a lack of glycosyl phosphatidylinositol-linked proteins on the surface of the patient's cells resulting from mutations in the phosphatidylinositol glycan A (pig-A) gene. Among other proteins linked via this cell membrane anchor are DAF and CD59, two molecules that control complement activation at the level of the C3 convertase, and C8 and C9, respectively (see above under Regulation of Complement Activation). It is believed that the lysis of erythrocytes in PNH patients is due to uncontrolled complement activation on the surface of these cells. Recently, it was reported that, although lack of both DAF and CD59 from the surface of erythrocytes of PNH patients is responsible for the increased sensitivity to complement-mediated lysis, CD59 deficiency leads to greater sensitivity to cell lysis than DAF deficiency (Shichishima, 1999).

Recently, the ability to modulate complement activity and take advantage of classic pathway activation has been accomplished with the use of a designed antibody specific for the B-cell marker CD20. The monoclonal antibody, C2B8, is marketed as rituximab and is a chimeric (mouse/human) antibody that activates complement-mediated destruction of cells bearing CD20 through binding C1q. Therapies of this sort may hold promise in the treatment of lymphoid neoplasia and systemic autoimmune processes (Reff, 1994).

Neurologic Diseases

The role of the complement system in diseases of the nervous system has become evident in recent years. This is somewhat surprising, since the blood–brain barrier effectively blocks complement penetration into spinal fluid. Complement activation was demonstrated in diseases like myasthenia gravis, multiple sclerosis, cerebral lupus, Guillain–Barré syndrome, and Alzheimer's disease (Morgan, 1994a, 1997b; Shin, 1998). Deposition of complement proteins was demonstrated in diseased tissue and complement activation was shown in the cerebrospinal fluid (CSF) of patients of most of these diseases. Presumably, inflammation causes a breakdown in the blood–brain barrier with local penetration of complement proteins. Moreover, some cells synthesize complement proteins. There is evidence that complement activation might be involved in myelin damage, thus leading to both central and peripheral nervous system illnesses. Complement was also shown to be involved in Alzheimer disease and Pick disease. In Alzheimer disease, a peptide derived from amyloid and termed β-A4 binds C1q and activates complement in senile plaques of the diseased brain. Interestingly, the most abundant glial cell type, the astrocyte, was shown in vitro to synthesize all of the complement proteins under inflammatory conditions (Morgan, 1996). Furthermore, astrocytes and microglial cells express complement receptors in vitro (Morgan, 1997a). Therefore, despite the blood–brain barrier, the brain has the ability to mount a potent complement-dependent inflammatory reaction as a defense mechanism. Complement components may play a facilitating role in the neuropathology of prion diseases. The neuronal loss associated with transmissible spongiform encephalitis may be related to MAC formation on neuronal surfaces, and the presence of extracellular C3b and C1q in disease-associated prion protein deposits (Kovacs, 2004).

Cardiovascular Diseases

The involvement of the complement system in myocardial ischemia/reperfusion injury is well accepted. This has been reviewed recently (Lucchesi, 1997a). The mechanism by which complement contributes to acute myocardial infarction in patients is still unclear. Nevertheless, deposition of components of the classical and alternative pathways has been demonstrated in the affected myocardium along with C5b–9. The production of anaphylatoxins that accompany complement activation appears to be responsible for the local inflammatory reaction. The most dramatic demonstration of an effect of complement, especially the terminal complement components (C5b–9), has come from an animal model of coronary artery occlusion (Kilgore, 1998). Rabbits with genetically controlled C6 deficiency showed significantly reduced infarct size as compared to normal rabbits. In addition, neutrophil infiltration was significantly reduced in C6-deficient rabbits, suggesting the crucial role of terminal complement components in the generation of local inflammation.

Complement also appears to play a role in the development of atherosclerotic lesions (Torzewski, 1997). Again, the exact mechanism by which complement contributes to the development of atherosclerotic lesions is not clear. However, deposition of the terminal complement components (C5b–9) has been demonstrated in intimal thickenings and fibrous plaques. Activation of the complement system is associated with pre-lesional stages and progression of atherosclerotic lesions (Niculescu, 1987; Seifert, 1989). C6-deficient rabbits were shown to be less susceptible than normal rabbits to cholesterol-induced atherosclerotic lesions (Schmiedt, 1998).

Biocompatibility

Many of the biomaterials that are implanted in the body activate complement, particularly the alternative complement pathway (Mollnes, 1997). On contact with blood or tissue fluids, these materials may activate complement and produce local inflammation or tissue damage. Materials must be tested for their complement-activating activity before they are widely used.

Organ Transplantation

The success of organ transplantation has created a major problem, a shortage of human organs to meet the demands for an ever-growing number of patients awaiting such a surgical procedure. Therefore, the use of animal donors such as the pig is proposed by many in the field as a logical alternative to human organs. However, vascularized porcine organs are susceptible to an intense rejection reaction, termed hyperacute rejection, when implanted in nonhuman primates or humans (Dalmasso, 1992; Platt, 1998). This reaction is mediated by antibody binding to

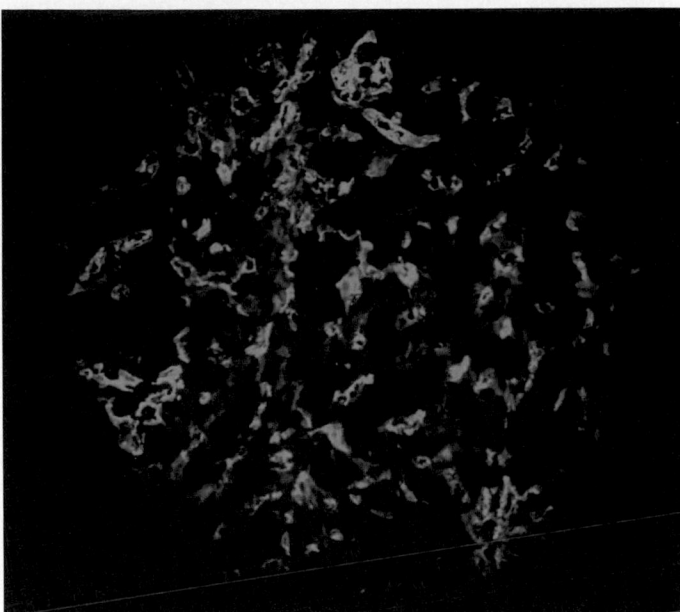

Figure 46–3 Fluorescence-labeled antibody to complement fragment C4d stains peritubular capillaries in a transplant kidney biopsy. In the early post-transplant setting this staining pattern is a marker of humoral rejection. (40×, fluorescein isothiocyanate).

vascular endothelial cells and complement activation. Complement activation was shown to be crucial in tissue damage in hyperacute rejection of xenografts. Complement activation on xenogeneic endothelial cells leads to their activation (i.e., endothelial cells adopt a procoagulant phenotype), which leads to intravascular and interstitial thrombosis and hemorrhage. Such an intense reaction is due to the inability of porcine cell-associated complement-regulatory molecules such as DAF, MCP, and CD59 to control human complement activation. Therefore, the success of this promising therapeutic intervention relies on proper control of complement activation. The role of complement in the rejection of human organs (allografts) is less well accepted but it is likely that complement activation contributes to some extent to acute and chronic rejection episodes (Baldwin, 1995). Along these lines, identification of C4d in the peritubular capillaries of renal transplant biopsies by immunofluorescence microscopy has proved useful in the recognition of humoral rejection (Fig. 46–3) (Onitsuka, 1999).

Clinically Useful Complement Inhibitors

Complement activation undoubtedly contributes to tissue damage observed in a variety of human diseases. Therefore, the use of agents that block complement activation should prove useful to limit tissue damage. Unfortunately, there are no such agents available for widespread clinical use. Research is underway to develop complement inhibitors that will prove efficient and safe. Since complement is crucial in the control of infection, a suitable complement inhibitor should not interfere with this complement function. Also, C3a and C5a are known to be potent inducers of inflammatory reactions. Therefore, a desirable inhibitor should act at the level of the classical and alternative C3 convertases to avoid production of these anaphylatoxins. Many inhibitors have been produced recently and are currently being developed. For a more complete description of the inhibitors of the complement system, the reader is referred to reviews on the subject (Makrides, 1998; Wagner, 1998).

As discussed earlier, CR1 is a potent regulator of both the classical and alternative pathways of complement. It accelerates the decay of the C3 and C5 convertases of both pathways and serves as a cofactor for factor-I-mediated cleavage of C4b, C3b, and iC3b. This molecule therefore represents an excellent candidate for therapeutic inhibition of the complement system in disease states. A soluble, recombinant form of CR1, termed sCR1, was produced and shown to retain all of the membrane-bound native protein properties. In a variety of animal models of human disease where complement activation is known to play a role, the use of sCR1 significantly ameliorated the disease process. These include, among others: pig heart xenotransplantation in *Cynomolgus* monkeys (Pruitt, 1994), alveolitis in a pulmonary Arthus reaction model (Mulligan, 1992), ischemia/reperfusion myocardial tissue injury (Weisman, 1990),

demyelination in an experimental allergic encephalomyelitis model in rats (Piddlesden, 1994), and glomerulonephritis (Couser, 1995). sCR1 has now entered phase I clinical trials in patients with myocardial infarcts and patients with burn-induced ARDS.

Another complement inhibitor is a humanized single-chain antibody to human C5. The advantage of such an antibody is that it allows the blocking of complement activation without release of C5a and deposition of C5b-9, which are known to promote potent tissue damage due to inflammation and cellular activation. Monoclonal antibody to C5 was shown in animal models to interfere with hyperacute rejection of porcine organs in in vitro perfusion systems (Kroshus, 1995), to prevent the onset of arthritis in a mouse model of collagen-induced arthritis (Wang, 1995), to reduce glomerulonephritis in a mouse model of SLE (Wang, 1996), and to reduce the infarct size in a rat model of myocardial ischemia/reperfusion injury model (Vakeva, 1999). The humanized anti-C5 antibody was shown to be a potent inhibitor of the complement system in vitro (Evans, 1995). Results from clinical trials suggest that this antibody can significantly reduce damage to the myocardium in patients undergoing cardiopulmonary bypass surgery (Rollins, 1998).

Preparations of pooled human IgG for intravenous use (IVIG) are being used in a number of autoimmune and inflammatory diseases such as idiopathic thrombocytopenic purpura, Kawasaki disease, Guillain–Barré syndrome, and myasthenia gravis (Dwyer, 1992). However, the exact mechanism by which IVIG exerts its beneficial action is unclear and may include blockade of antibodies via idiotype–anti-idiotype interactions, blockade of IgG Fc receptors on phagocytic cells, modulation of T- and B-cell functions, and selection of immune repertoires. However, IVIG clearly has an effect on the complement system (Frank, 1992). IVIG was shown to interfere with the classical pathway-dependent Forssman shock reaction in guinea pigs (Basta, 1989) and to prolong porcine cardiac xenograft survival in nonhuman primates (Magee, 1995). Furthermore, treatment of patients with dermatomyositis with high-dose IVIG inhibited the deposition of C3b and C5b-9 on endomysial capillaries normally seen in these patients (Basta, 1994). IVIG inhibits complement activation via its Fc portion. The exact mechanism by which IVIG blocks complement activation on target surfaces is still incompletely understood. Reports have shown that IVIG might prevent complement-mediated tissue damage by interacting directly with C1 or by preventing C4 from binding to the target cell (Mollnes, 1995; Miletic, 1996).

As mentioned above, C1-Inh is absent or reduced in the serum of those with hereditary angioedema, and has been administered as a therapeutic concentrate during acute attacks. Because C1-inhibitor is also often reduced in severe inflammatory states generally, concentrates of C1-Inh have been shown to have promising clinical utility in conditions including septic shock, reperfusion injury, hyperacute transplant rejection, and PNH (Kirschfink, 2001; Davis, 2004).

Assays of Complement

General Principles

Methods that allow accurate determination of levels of each of the components of the classical, alternative, and MBLectin pathways as well as several enzymes and regulators of the complement system are available. However, many of these assays are not available in routine clinical laboratories and are restricted to research laboratories. We will focus our attention on techniques that do not require a laboratory skilled in complement research for their performance. The reader is referred to other publications for details relative to methods that require more specialized techniques (Whaley, 1985; Harrison, 1986; Dodds, 1997; Giclas, 1997; Würzner, 1997). Complement assays can be divided into two types: those that measure complement proteins as antigens in biological fluids and those that measure the functional activity of a given component. Both types of technique have advantages and disadvantages. Methods for antigenic (immunochemical) analysis are generally simpler to perform. These antigenic assays are highly specific, require fewer specialized reagents, are cheaper, and are considerably less time-consuming. Antibodies to human complement proteins and purified human complement proteins are commercially available. The *Linscott's Directory of Immunological and Biological Reagents* (2004) is a useful guide to commercially available complement reagents. In these assays, either serum or plasma can be used, and the commonly available methods of freezer storage (−20°C) are sufficient. For these reasons, antigenic assays are easily adaptable to a clinical laboratory. On the other hand, antigenic assays do not provide information about the activity of a component because they may detect degradation products as well as functionally active components. The presence in serum of small fragments of a protein with antigenic activity may confuse the results. Some antigenic assays use radial immunodiffusion. In these assays, a protein fragment may diffuse more rapidly than the parent molecule, which may result in falsely high levels. As an example, the most commonly employed antigenic assays for C3 measures its major degradation product, C3c, by radial immunodiffusion. For accurate measurements of C3c, the specimen should be thawed at 37°C for a number of days to allow for complete conversion of C3 to C3c. In fact, this is not usually done and thus can represent a source of error, although the error is small and not usually of clinical consequence. In general, antigenic assays are not as sensitive as functional assays and may not detect low levels of a component present in certain body fluids. The sensitivity of antigenic assays depends to some degree on the strength of the antibody employed, and with the usual assays, as little as $10\,\mu g/mL$ of protein antigen can be measured.

Kits are available that use inhibition of binding of radiolabeled substrate to detect various complement peptides. Such kits are available for measurement of C3a, C4a, and C5a. The usefulness of these measurements is still debated. A detailed report on procedures for measuring the functional lytic activity and the antigenic levels of each of the components of the alternative pathway is available (Minta, 1983). Assays designed to measure the functional activity of the control proteins factors H and I in human serum have also been reported but require specialized reagents that may not be commercially available (Gaither, 1979). ELISA assays have been developed for the measurement of split products of complement proteins or complexes formed following complement activation. Kits are commercially available (Quidel, San Diego, CA). These kits measure breakdown products of complement proteins as they are generated after complement activation using specific monoclonal antibodies. Complement activation via the classical pathway can be measured by following the levels of C4d in serum versus those of C4. Also, the measurement by ELISA of C1r–C1s–C1inh complexes provides a measure of complement activation via the classical pathway. Activation of the alternative pathway can be measured by ELISA by assessing levels of Bb, or C3bBbP, or C3bP complexes in circulation (Mayes, 1984). Measurement of as little as 10–20 ng/mL of C3bP in serum has been reported. This assay may also be used to measure surface-bound activation complexes. Activation via either pathway can be monitored by measuring levels of iC3b, or sC5b-9, the soluble form of the membrane attack complex. Recently, an ELISA test for the measurement of serum or plasma MBL complex activity has been developed that eliminates interference by components of the classical pathway (Petersen, 2001; Kuipers, 2002). In addition, ELISA kits are available that measure the generation of anaphylatoxins in serum/plasma. Since C3a and C5a are rapidly converted to their inactive desArg fragments by carboxypeptidase-N in serum, these assays utilize monoclonal antibodies specific for C3a-desArg and C5a-desArg. Because of their high sensitivity, these ELISA assays provide an excellent tool to assess complement activation in biological fluids via either the classical pathway or the alternative pathway. Nevertheless, these kits are generally expensive and require that the user establish a standard dilution curve. Therefore, limited numbers of specimens can be run in a single kit.

Functional Evaluation of the Classical Pathway

Functional complement assays are sensitive and precise tools for providing information about the activity of a complement component. Some of these methods may be used to quantify activity at the molecular level, and others to express complement function in arbitrary units. Commercial reagents are available for titrating each component of the classical or alternative pathways. Assays that measure the total hemolytic activity in a specimen (CH_{50}) or the functional activity of isolated complement components in general use sheep erythrocytes as targets of complement-mediated lysis. Sheep erythrocytes are more sensitive to antibody- and complement-mediated lysis than erythrocytes from other species. The alternative pathway of complement activation (AH_{50}) is easily measured using rabbit erythrocytes. These cells are particularly sensitive to antibody-independent lysis mediated by human serum. In addition, a functional hemolytic assay using chicken erythrocytes to assess functional mannose-binding levels in serum has been developed, which the authors claim is useful for large-scale testing of patient samples (Petersen, 2001; Kuipers, 2002). A useful summary of the clinical significance of CH_{50} and AH_{50} testing is provided in Table 46–5.

The simplest functional assay of the classical pathway measures total hemolytic complement. The absence of any one of the nine components, as occurs in homozygous genetically deficient patients, generally results in a total hemolytic complement titer (CH_{50}) of zero. However, a normal value does not exclude the possibility of reduced levels of individual

Table 46–5 CH_{50} and AH_{50} Interpretation

1 Test Result	2 Interpretation
CH_{50} very low or 0 (AH_{50} normal)	Missing C1q, C1r, C1s, C2, or C4
AH_{50} very low or 0 (CH_{50} normal)	Missing properdin, or (very rarely) factor B or factor D
CH_{50} and AH_{50} very low or 0	Missing C3, C5, C6, C7, C8, or C9
Late components low (especially C3) CH_{50} and AH_{50} low	Missing factor H or factor I

Source: Adapted from Wen BS, Atkinson J, Giclas PC: Clinical and laboratory evaluation of complement deficiency. J Allergy Clin Immunol 2004;113:585–593.

components in test subjects. When a patient's history and symptoms suggest a possible deficiency, hemolytic or antigenic titrations of individual components may be required. Often, a CH_{50} titer will be an adequate functional measure of complement activity. In the CH_{50} assay, commercially available antibodies added to sheep red blood cells react with antigen on red cell surfaces, forming immune complexes. Patient test serum is then added to the mixture as the source of classic pathway complement. Complement in the test serum will bind the immune complex previously formed on the sheep red cells, leading to activation of the classical complement pathway and to red cell lysis. By titrating the addition of patient test serum it is possible to calculate the complement activity present in the patient sample, and to express that activity as the reciprocal of the dilution that causes lysis of 50% of red cells in the assay (the CH_{50}). The complement titer is expressed in CH_{50} units (the reciprocal of the dilution of the complement source that lyses 50% of sensitized sheep erythrocytes).

Serial dilutions of the specimen are prepared and added to EA. In this case, the 50% end point is determined by the Von Krogh transformation of the data. This empirically derived formula converts the S-shaped dose-response curve into a linear function. Values of $Y/1-Y$ are calculated in which Y is the fraction of red cells lysed in a test dilution. A graph is constructed in which the log of the relative volume of complement is plotted against the log of $Y/1-Y$ values. Usually, a straight line is obtained, and the titer is calculated by determining the relative volume of complement at which $Y/1-Y = 1.0$ (or 50% lysis). That value is divided into the reciprocal of original serum dilution (1:60 for human serum) to calculate the concentration of serum complement that lyses 50% of the cells. The complement titer represents the number of 50% hemolytic units that are present in 1.0 mL of undiluted serum (Mayer, 1961; Rapp, 1970).

Clinical laboratories may use one of two commercially available variations on this classic test to perform the CH_{50} assay. One is based on the lysis of liposomes, releasing a marker enzyme, and the other an ELISA that detects the final C9 neoantigen formed with complete activation of the classic pathway.

Functional Evaluation of the Alternative Pathway

In this assay, human serum (usually first diluted 1:5) is serially diluted and added to rabbit erythrocytes that are not sensitized with specific antibody, in a buffer that contains magnesium ions and ethylene glycol tetraacetic acid (EGTA) to chelate calcium ions (calcium ions are required for classical pathway activation, not for alternative pathway activation) (Pangburn, 1988). The alternative pathway titer is designated AH_{50} and represents the final dilution of human serum in the assay that lyses 50% of the rabbit erythrocytes. A graph similar to that described for total hemolytic complement titration is produced to determine the AH_{50}. Human serum may at times possess 'natural' antibody to a carbohydrate widely expressed on cells of species other than humans and nonhuman primates. A high concentration of serum mixed with rabbit erythrocytes may induce agglutination, which can be misleading in interpreting an AH_{50} titer (Tomlinson, 1997). Therefore, it may be useful to absorb the serum with washed, packed rabbit erythrocytes on ice for 15–30 minutes to remove a certain proportion of natural antibodies, hence reducing cell agglutination in the assay.

Functional Assay of C1-inhibitor

Assays for the assessment of C1-Inh function have been developed. One in common use is an ELISA-based assay that measures formation of a complex between biotinylated C1s and C1-Inh on an avidin-coated solid phase. A second test makes use of steric hindrance created by the binding of inhibitor to C1r, preventing the subsequent binding of antibody to C1r. During radial immunodiffusion of C1r, unbound and therefore active C1r quantities will increase as the amount of C1-Inh present decreases.

Complement Levels by Antigenic Assays

For use in antigenic assays, the specimen (either serum or plasma) is stored frozen (−20°C or lower). Bacterial contamination may cause protein denaturation or fragmentation, whereas freezing and thawing do not usually have a major adverse effect on antigenic levels. For certain complement assays, the specimen is diluted in saline to achieve the correct concentration range for accurate measurement.

Antigenic analyses of complement proteins make use of one of several immune precipitin techniques. Single radial immunodiffusion using the method of either Fahey or Mancini is a commonly used method for calculating specific protein quantities. In both methods, antigen is added to wells in a gel that contains antibody, and rings of precipitation are formed. The Fahey method employs antibody that is not in excess. The diffusion time at which results are read is thus critical. Diffusion end points are not reached and can lead to inaccurate measurements of antigenic complement levels. The Mancini method uses excess antibody in the gel and is more sensitive and accurate. Most commercial firms preparing immunodiffusion plates use the Mancini method. Radial immunodiffusion kits are available for all components of the classical and alternative pathways. These kits consist of plates coated with a thin layer of 2% agarose containing monospecific antibody. Protein standard serum (a stabilized pool of normal human serum) is supplied, usually in pre-diluted solutions. Each standard solution contains a specific amount of the particular protein being measured for use in construction of the reference curve.

Nephelometric methods are also used to measure complement component levels and in some instances may be comparable to those obtained with radial immunodiffusion (Bossuyt, 2002); they are commonly used in hospital laboratories to measure serum C3 and C4.

Kinins and the Kinin-Generating System

The kinin-generating system is another inflammatory response pathway present in plasma that controls the generation of peptides important in the inflammatory response. It will be described briefly here. For more details, the reader is referred to recent reviews on the subject (Sharma, 1990; Kozin, 1992; Margolius, 1995; Vio, 1998). The most important biologically active peptide generated by the system appears to be bradykinin, a nonapeptide with potent activity in many biological systems. It is active in increasing vascular permeability, vasodilation, hypotension, induction of pain, contraction of many types of smooth muscle cells, and activation of the phospholipase A_2 system with activation of cellular arachidonic acid metabolism. Although in many respects similar to the complement system, the plasma kinin-generating system is simpler because it is composed of only four plasma proteins. The major proteins of the kinin-generating system as currently understood are Hageman factor, clotting factor XI, prekallikrein, and high-molecular-weight kininogen.

On interacting with negatively charged surfaces, such as those experimentally supplied by glass or naturally by many biologically active materials such as lipid A of Gram-negative bacterial endotoxin, Hageman factor is cleaved and activated. Proteolytic enzymes including kallikrein can cleave and activate Hageman factor as well. The cleaved Hageman factor (αHFa) has proteolytic activity and further activates and cleaves additional Hageman factor molecules to generate more αHFa.

αHFa activates factor XI to factor XIa, resulting in activation of the intrinsic coagulation cascade. αHFa also cleaves the single-chain prekallikrein into a two-chain molecule, kallikrein, with the chains linked by disulfide bonds. The cleaved prekallikrein has proteolytic enzymatic activity located on the lower-molecular-weight chain. The activated kallikrein cleaves high-molecular-weight kininogen at several sites, releasing bradykinin.

Bradykinin has a short half-life because it is rapidly cleaved by kininase and by angiotensin-converting enzyme in the lung to form low-molecular-weight peptides that lack biological activity.

Bradykinin has been postulated to play a role in a variety of diseases. Free bradykinin and lysyl-bradykinin have been found in the nasal fluid in rhinitis. A pathogenic role for bradykinin has also been suggested in diseases ranging from asthma to hereditary angioedema, as well as other kinds of swelling disorder, including inflammation. Clearly, the exact role of the kinin-generating system in disease is not fully understood. However, bradykinin and its derivatives are undoubtedly important in the swelling and pain associated with inflammation.

Table 46–6 Functional Classes of Cytokines

Area of Activity	Cytokine	Action
Innate immunity	IL-1, TNF, IL-6, IL-12, IFNγ	Protect against viral infection, recruit leukocytes, stimulate acute inflammatory response
Lymphocyte growth, differentiation, and activation	IL-2, IL-4, IL-12, IL-15, TGFβ	NK, B cell, and T cell growth factors, down-regulate immune response
Inflammatory cell activation	IFNγ, IL-5, TNF, TNFβ	Induce acute inflammation, activate macrophages, eosinophils, neutrophils, and endothelial cells
Chemokinesis	IL-8 superfamily members	Released from T cells and other cells as 'homing' signals for B and T cells
Hematopoiesis	Colony-stimulating factors (CSF-GM, CSF-G), stem cell factor	Stimulate progenitor and stem cells

When grouped according to major activity, many cytokines share similar and apparently overlapping activities.

Cytokines

Cytokines are soluble proteins released by capable cells to permit usually short-distance communication between cells. These mediators are released to assist in the upregulation or downregulation of the immune response, and to orchestrate associated inflammatory and reparative activities. Secretion and binding of cytokines is the cellular equivalent of connecting to the internet. The prevailing milieu of cytokines within a region of an organism creates a web of communication between cells. Cytokine signals are received at the cell surface not only as single messages but also in complex, subtle synergistic and antagonistic combinations that coordinate processes including the stimulation of hematopoiesis, the orchestration of directed leukocyte migration (chemokinesis), activation of various inflammatory cells, stimulation of lymphocyte development and maturation, and processes related to the immune response. In order to respond to specific cytokine messages, cells display thousands of surface cytokine receptors, arrayed as so many antennae. Using these receptors, cells sample, process, and respond to combinations of soluble and substrate-bound cytokines in a manner dependent on surface receptor density and state of activation.

The term 'cytokine' refers to the soluble products of 'cells' in the generic sense. Many cell types are capable of producing cytokines, but for the most part it is the T cell and the macrophage that are virtual cytokine factories, and for this reason many familiar cytokines are known as interleukins (ILs). The biologic actions of a given cytokine may overlap with that of other cytokines (Table 46–6) and are often dependent upon both the circumstance in which it is secreted and the responding cell type. In addition, a given cytokine may be produced and released by several different cell types, including lymphoid cells, stromal cells (such as fibroblasts, osteocytes and endothelial cells), and epithelial cells. The range of influence of these soluble proteins may extend over the long range (systemically) when released into the circulation (endocrine effect), as with the pyrogen IL-1, or its action may be local only, producing an effect on the cell releasing it (autocrine effect), or its neighboring cells. IL-2 released by T cells has an autocrine proliferative effect through the IL-2 receptor (CD_{25}). In the thymus, cytokines such as IL-7 released from thymic epithelial cells affect thymocyte maturation in a paracrine fashion. The majority of cytokines bind to high affinity receptors that transducer signal to the cell nucleus through JAK/STAT signaling pathways, although other pathways including MAPK, cAMP, and PI3-kinase are used as well. Because of the profound biologic effects of these powerful proteins, attempts at mass-producing and therapeutically administering cytokines are ongoing. Clinical laboratory detection and measurement of them may become commonplace.

Bioassays are sometimes the 'gold standard' for detecting cytokine activity, but they are usually time-consuming and unmanageable in the hospital laboratory. ELISA kits are widely available for many of the cytokines described in the text. Molecular techniques (polymerase chain reaction, in situ hybridization) are employed in more sophisticated laboratories to identify the presence of cytokines with great sensitivity and to localize a cytokine more precisely to particular cell type.

VI

Interleukin-1

The IL-1 cytokine family contains three proteins: IL-1α and IL-1β (the two agonist components), and IL-1 receptor antagonist (IL-1RA), a naturally occurring receptor-specific antagonist (Dinarello, 1998). Two IL-1 receptors have been described: a widely expressed 80 kDa type I receptor (IL-1RI) that transduces signal when bound to either IL-1α or IL-1β, and a more restricted (to neutrophils, monocytes, and B cells) 67 kDa type II receptor (IL-1RII). IL-1RII does not transduce an intracellular signal, even when bound to its preferred ligand, IL-1β, and it therefore has been described as a 'decoy' receptor that acts as a 'sink' for IL-1β molecules. Once bound to ligand, IL-1RI associates with an accessory protein (IL-1RAcP). Together they signal the nucleus through several macrotubule-associated protein (MAP) kinase pathways that activate nuclear transcription factors including NF-κB, among others (O'Neill, 1996). The antagonist molecule IL-1RA is capable of binding IL-1RI and IL-1RII, but does not trigger intracellular signal transduction.

As a primary regulator of immune and inflammatory responses, IL-1 exhibits myriad biological effects (Rosenwasser, 1998). It optimizes major histocompatibility antigen/T-cell receptor complex (MHC/TCR)-mediated T helper (Th) cell activation and enhances the activity of T-cell-derived cytokines such as IL-2 through up-regulation of the IL-2 receptor. IL-1 stimulates hematopoietic progenitor cell (HPC) proliferation in synergy with hematopoietic colony-stimulating factors, and when administered alone it mobilizes a bone marrow-derived neutrophilia. Evidence indicates a role for IL-1 in promoting the growth and proliferation of some leukemic cell lines but it is directly cytotoxic to some virally infected and to some tumor cells.

IL-1's ability to stimulate arachidonic acid metabolism and its ability to induce production and release of other cytokines accounts for much of its proinflammatory activity. At sites of inflammation, IL-1 causes up-regulation of adhesion molecule receptors on the vascular endothelium and stimulates chemokine production, leading to local accumulation of leukocytes. IL-1 is responsible for the production of acute phase reactants by the liver (e.g., complement, C-reactive peptide) at the expense of housekeeping proteins such as albumin. To pay the amino acid cost of this massive new peptide synthesis, IL-1 promotes the breakdown of muscle, thereby accounting for the myalgia that accompanies some illnesses. IL-1 contributes to vascular dilation and hypotension in septic shock through the induction of nitric oxide (NO) within endothelial cells, and may be a significant mediator of cardiogenic shock as well.

In the central nervous system (CNS), IL-1 promotes fever, anorexia, slow-wave sleep and lethargy, as well as the release of corticosteroids from the hypothalamus. Within the joint spaces, IL-1 promotes synovial cell proliferation, deposition of collagen, and resorption of cartilage and bone; actions that have implications for inflammatory conditions such as rheumatoid arthritis.

When administered to humans in low doses, IL-1 causes profound febrile and hypotensive reactions similar to those induced by low doses of endotoxin. There is an accompanying mild increase in hematopoiesis, which can decrease the nadir and shorten the period of marrow suppression in those receiving marrow-suppressive chemotherapy (Iizumi, 1991). However, the beneficial effect of IL-1 administration is limited by its profound toxicity.

Monitoring IL-1or IL-1RA levels in serum and other body fluids may be useful in the diagnosis and monitoring of disease activity. Along these lines, urinary levels of IL-1β are elevated in patients with immune-complex glomerulonephritis, and may serve as a useful non-invasive means of following disease activity (Hrvacevic, 2001). When measured in the appropriate clinical setting that includes chest pain, significant elevation of IL-1RA has been noted to occur before elevation of markers of myocardial necrosis such as troponin I, and may be an early marker of impending myocardial infarction (Patti, 2004). Children with Langerhans cell histiocytosis have elevated IL-1RA serum levels that decrease following successful chemotherapy, providing a potentially sensitive means of tracking disease activity after treatment (Rosso, 2003).

Interleukin-2

IL-2 is a 15.5 kDa, 133-amino-acid glycoprotein member of the four α-helical bundle family of cytokines (Bazan, 1990). The receptor for IL-2 (IL-2R) is a tripartite membrane complex that exists in three cellular forms: a high-affinity complex of α, β, and γ subunits, an intermediate affinity complex of β and γ subunits, and a lower affinity receptor made of IL-2Ra alone. Only IL-2Raβγ and IL-2Rβγ are capable of transducing signal after ligand binding. In T cells and natural killer (NK) cells, IL-2 activates intracellular pathways, including JAK/STAT. Gene targets of IL-2-activated

signaling pathways include bcl-2, c-myc, c-jun, and c-fos (Gomez, 1998). Because they share β and γ chain receptor subunits, IL-2 and IL-15 have overlapping biological activities. Both cytokines stimulate in vitro proliferation of activated CD4/CD8+ T cells, γ/δ T-cell subsets, and NK cells (Burton, 1994), while promoting the cytolytic function of cytotoxic T lymphocytes and lymphokine-activated killer (LAK) cells (Burton, 1994; Grabstein, 1994). In addition, both cytokines can induce proliferation of stimulated B cells, and synthesis of IgM. IL-2 is chemotactic for T cells as well (Armitage, 1995; Wilkinson, 1995). In vivo, IL-2 may play an indispensable role in maintenance of self-tolerance, since animals deficient in IL-2 develop immune deficiency and autoimmune conditions such as hemolytic anemia and inflammatory bowel disease (Willerford, 1995). Mice lacking IL-2Rβ spontaneously develop T-cell activation and plasma cell differentiation from B cells, with increased serum levels of IgG and IgE (Suzuki, 1995; Wang, 1996). This suggests that IL-2 may provide for induction of anergy or apoptosis in activation-induced T-cell death.

Measuring IL-2 levels in patients with malignant disease may provide useful prognostic information. The level of IL-2 secretion in whole blood cultures of patients with small-cell carcinoma of the lung at the time of diagnosis is lower in those patients with reduced survival following chemotherapy (Fischer, 2000). Anti-cytokine therapy using monoclonal antibody directed against IL-2R (daclizumab and basiliximab) has been used with some success in preventing rejection in renal transplantation (Jacobsohn, 2002, 2004).

Interleukin-3

IL-3 activity was first detected in cultures of splenic lymphocytes from nude mice, where it induced the enzyme 20-α-hydroxysteroid dehydrogenase (Ihle, 1981). It is a 26 kDa protein expressed on a restricted population of cells, including activated T cells, NK cells, mast cells, and some megakaryocytes (Blalock, 1999). Optimal synthesis of IL-3 requires T-cell activation via the TCR/CD3 complex. This initiates the intracellular pathways leading to activation of NF-κB, which enters the nucleus to transactivate IL-3 gene expression (Link, 1992; Park, 1993). The IL-3 receptor (IL-3R) is a member of the cytokine receptor gene family and has a ligand-specific α chain noncovalently associated with a signal-transducing β chain. IL-3 target cells include T- and B-cell precursors in vitro. In vivo administration of IL-3 in pharmacologic doses produces increased red cell, leukocyte, and platelet production in mice (Metcalf, 1986). A role for IL-3 in development of contact hypersensitivity is suggested, since IL-3-deficient mice exhibit poorly developed hapten-specific delayed-type hypersensitivity (Mach, 1998). In addition, evidence points to a role for IL-3 in the normal development of the CNS (Chiang, 1996).

Interleukin-4

IL-4 performs important functions in regulating antibody production, hematopoiesis, inflammation, and the development of effector T-cell responses. It is a complex protein with many intramolecular disulfide bonds and glycosylation sites whose gene has been mapped to chromosome 5. Production of IL-4 is highly regulated and is restricted to a subset of activated T cells, mast cells, basophils, and eosinophils (Paul, 1991). The biological effects of IL-4 are mediated through high-affinity IL-4 receptors (IL-4R) composed of a ligand-specific α chain and a signal-transducing γ chain shared by several other cytokines including interleukins 2, 7, 9, 13, 15, and 21. IL-4 activates B cells and promotes their differentiation, reflecting the fact that IL-4 was first described in supernatants of activated T-cell cultures and dubbed B-cell growth factor. In addition to inducing expression of CD23 and MHC molecules on B cells, it regulates B-cell apoptosis and isotype switching, particularly IgG1 and IgE (Brown, 1997). In the realm of hematopoiesis, IL-4 stimulates colony formation by erythroid, megakaryocyte, mast cell, and granulocyte/monocyte precursors, while promoting development of CD8+ and CD4+ Th subsets (Sillaber, 1991; Erard, 1993).

In the inflammatory response, IL-4 induces proliferation of endothelial cells, and causes up-regulation of endothelial cell adhesion molecules permitting increased leukocyte adhesion to vessel surfaces before they migrate into sites of local inflammation. In addition, IL-4 is chemotactic for eosinophils and promotes monocyte and T-cell cytotoxicity (Tepper, 1989; Crawford, 1993). Increased levels of IL-4 are found in allergic diseases such as atopic dermatitis and hay fever (Tepper, 1989). Elevated IL-4 levels in the tears and blood of atopic patients as determined by ELISA suggests a role for IL-4 in allergic disease and may serve as a marker for disease severity (Paranos, 1998; Fujishima, 1995). IL-4 also confers a degree of protection from some extracellular parasites, and decreases harmful autoimmune responses by inhibiting prolonged T cell responses

(Finkelman, 1986; Rapoport, 1993). IL-4 plays a part in tumor immunity as well through promoting NK effector cell and macrophage tumoricidal activity (Bosco, 1990). At the same time, IL-4 is implicated in the growth of human T-cell leukemias in vitro. Because it is associated with a switch of effector CD8[+] cells to non-cytotoxic cells, IL-4 may play a role in the progression of the acquired immunodeficiency syndrome (AIDS) (Erard, 1993).

Interleukin-5

IL-5 is a 45 kDa, 134-amino-acid, disulfide-linked homodimer, which plays a pivotal role in the maturation, activation and survival of eosinophils, and in the development of atopic disease and eosinophilia. The IL-5 gene resides on chromosome 5 in a cluster of genes encoding IL-3, IL-4, and granulocyte–macrophage colony-stimulating factor (GM-CSF). The receptor for IL-5 (IL-5R) consists of a ligand-specific α chain, and a signal-transducing β chain common to the receptors for IL-3 and GM-CSF (Tavernier, 1991). The intracytoplasmic domains of the α- and β-subunits contain regions involved in binding JAK-2 and JAK-1, respectively, which are necessary for signal transduction. IL-5 is produced by Th2 cells, mast cells, NK cells, B cells, eosinophils, malignant cells, and some virally transformed cells. It promotes the differentiation, migration, activation, degranulation, and survival of eosinophils. IL-5 is responsible for inducing accumulation, activation, and degranulation of eosinophils after antigenic challenge, possibly through its mild chemotactic activity, its ability to bring about upregulation of certain adhesion molecules present on eosinophils such as CD11b, and through promoting IgG-induced granule release (Wang, 1989; Fujisawa, 1990; Walsh, 1991).

The role of IL-5 in human disease may include promoting the basement membrane damage seen in bullous pemphigoid, promoting eosinophil infiltration at sites of parasite infestation, and promoting the production of antithyrotropin receptor antibodies in Graves disease. In addition, the local eosinophilia of Hodgkin disease may be associated with the Reed–Sternberg cell's ability to release IL-5. In allergic responses, IL-5 release from tissue mast cells may serve to promote eosinophil accumulation in the tissues (Lalani, 1999). Among infectious diseases, decreased serum IL-5 levels appear to correlate well with HIV-1 disease progression as a predictor of immunodeficiency in infected children born to HIV-1 infected mothers (Resino, 2001).

Currently, ELISA is employed for in vitro IL-5 measurement, and immunofluorescence techniques allow localization of IL-5 to specific cells, while in situ hybridization permits precise localization of IL-5 within individual cells.

Interleukin-6

IL-6 was initially identified in the supernatants of helper T-cell cultures as an agent capable of inducing proliferation of and immunoglobulin secretion by B-cells. However, its actions extend to many target cells and it is now recognized as an important immune, hematopoietic, and proinflammatory cytokine (Hirano, 1998). IL-6 is secreted as a 184-amino-acid peptide of about 21 kDa, depending on extent of glycosylation. The gene encoding IL-6 has been mapped to chromosome 7 (Hirano, 1986). The IL-6 receptor (IL-6R) complex (Hirano, 1998) is a member of the cytokine receptor superfamily and is composed of an 80 kDa ligand-specific α-binding chain (IL-6Rα) and a noncovalently associated β-signaling chain, gp130. The β-subunit is shared by other receptors, including those for IL-11 and GM-CSF. This may account for the observed functional redundancy of these cytokines' activities. The combined IL-6R complex forms a high-affinity receptor for IL-6, permitting signal transduction through JAK/STAT pathways.

A variety of cells produce IL-6, including T and B cells, monocytes and macrophages, fibroblasts, keratinocytes, synoviocytes, chondrocytes, and endothelial cells. IL-6 acts upon T cells, hepatocytes, hematopoietic progenitors, and neuronal cells. It is a powerful growth factor for human myeloma and plasmacytoma cell lines, and has an autocrine or paracrine action among human myelomas transplanted to mice. Among hepatocytes, IL-6 stimulates production of various acute-phase reactants and, in IL-6 knockout mice, acute-phase reactant and Ig release are greatly reduced. Among hematopoietic cells, IL-6 causes proliferation and differentiation of T cells, enhances multipotential hematopoietic progenitor colony formation, and induces megakaryocyte maturation. It stimulates osteoclast formation and the proliferation of vascular smooth muscle cells, and induces platelet-derived growth factor production. In the CNS, IL-6 supports survival of cholinergic neurons, while in the reproductive system it induces secretion of human chorionic gonadotropin from trophoblasts.

Abnormalities of IL-6 production have been observed among patients with rheumatoid arthritis, and a significant correlation has been noted between synovial fluid concentrations of IL-6 and IgG in rheumatoid arthritis patients (Hirano, 1988; Hermann, 1989). In animal models, administration of IL-6 appears to play a part in the development of severe and accelerated membranoproliferative glomerulonephritis, resembling similar changes found in patients with SLE (Ryffel, 1994). Transgenic mouse studies suggest a role for IL-6 in the development of type 1 diabetes and in the generation of malignant monoclonal plasmacytomas (Suematsu, 1989; Hirano, 1991).

Clinical evidence suggests that determination of serum IL-6 levels in neonates (Kuster, 1998) and in cancer chemotherapy patients (de Bont, 1999) may help to identify those neonates at imminent risk of sepsis and those cancer patients whose febrile episodes are due to chemotherapy rather than sepsis. Levels of IL-6 in the breath condensate of patients with non-small-cell carcinoma of the lung as measured by ELISA are increased over those of controls. Early detection of increased IL-6 by this noninvasive means in at-risk populations may advance the date of disease detection and permit post-therapy monitoring for recurrent disease (Carpagnano, 2002).

Interleukin-7

IL-7 was first identified as a 25 kDa murine glycoprotein that showed proliferative in vitro effects on pre-B cells (Namen, 1988). Though initially described as a B-cell growth factor, IL-7 subsequently was found to be critical to T- and B-cell lymphopoiesis, as well as a mobilizer of myeloid progenitor cells (Grzegorzewski, 1994). The active cytokine is produced by epidermal keratinocytes, intestinal epithelial cells, and stromal cells of the bone marrow and thymus. The IL-7 receptor (IL-7R) is a member of the hematopoietin receptor superfamily, sharing a γ chain in common with receptors for interleukins 2, 4, 7, 9, 13, and 21, which partly explains the overlapping and redundant effects these cytokines have on T-cell populations.

Mice transgenic for IL-7 develop increased numbers of B and T cells and their progenitors. Neutralizing antibodies to IL-7R administered to mice resulted in greatly reduced numbers of thymocytes and marrow B-lineage cells, with reduced numbers of B and T cells in spleen and lymph nodes (Peschon, 1994). Knockout mice for IL-7 and IL-7R show still greater reductions of the same cell populations. Because of its important lymphopoietic function, IL-7 accelerates T- and B-cell reconstitution in lethally irradiated mice, with minimal effect on the myeloid compartment. IL-7 stimulates growth and increases cytotoxic activity among mature T cells and cytotoxic T cells, respectively. In vitro, T cells isolated from the intestinal lamina propria proliferate in response to exogenous IL-7 and show increased ability to respond to anti-CD3 antibody and IL-2, suggesting a role for this cytokine in enhancing cell-mediated immune responses (Watanabe, 1995). Clinical roles for IL-7 have been suggested that range from increasing the T-cell compartments of those suffering from AIDS to treating cancers via its LAK-enhancing activity.

Interleukin-8 and the Chemokines

IL-8, a member of the chemokine superfamily, is responsible for the accumulation of neutrophils at sites of inflammation (Hoch, 1996), and induces calcium translocation, chemotaxis, shape change, actin polymerization, and possibly respiratory burst activity within these cells as well. It is also chemotactic for basophils and a subset of CD4/CD8[+] T cells. Several cell types produce the small IL-8 peptide, including endothelial cells, epithelial cells, fibroblasts, neutrophils, monocytes, macrophages, and T cells.

IL-8 is released in response to various stimuli such as lipopolysaccharide and leukotrienes, and though it can exist as a non-covalently-bound homodimer, it has its greatest chemotactic activity as a monomer (Paolini, 1994). Two receptors, both members of the seven-transmembrane domain receptor superfamily, mediate the biological effect of IL-8: IL-8 receptor A (IL-8RA) and IL-8 receptor B (IL-8RB). IL-8RA apparently has higher ligand affinity and specificity, while IL-8RB demonstrates lower ligand affinity and specificity and is able to bind other IL-8-related chemoattractant proteins. Intradermal injection of IL-8 causes intense and immediate infiltration of neutrophils around venules with a local plasma exudate. To reach areas of inflammation, however, leukocytes must first traverse the local endothelium. This is in part facilitated by IL-8, which alters neutrophil integrin expression by activating CD11b/CD18 to its high-affinity conformation, and triggers shedding of L-selectin. IL-8 forms part of the cell-surface-bound chemoattractant gradient upregulated on endothelial cells in the vicinity of inflammation that activated leukocytes follow. As a soluble protein, IL-8 forms a chemotactic gradient within tissues, guiding extravasated leukocytes to sites of inflammation. IL-8 also may be stored in Weibel–Palade bodies, where it is available for immediate synthesis-

VI

independent release (Rot, 1996). Interestingly, though it acts predominantly as a chemoattractant, increased IL-8 levels within the circulatory system are associated with decreased neutrophil accumulation at sites of inflammation, though a systemic neutrophilia is observed (Hechtman, 1991). This suggests an anti-inflammatory function for IL-8 as well.

Since the identification of IL-8 as the first chemokine in 1987, the chemokine superfamily has been growing. Chemokines act as chemoattractants by activating leukocyte integrins, particularly LFA-1, MAC-1, and VLA-4, to bind endothelial cell ICAM-1 and VCAM-1. Chemokines also are critical to hematopoiesis, angiogenesis, activation of T cells and NK cells, to the pathogenesis of HIV, and in the development of the CNS. The superfamily is presently divided into four families based on the positions of the first and second of four cysteines in the amino-acid sequence. The CXC family (α family) has one amino acid separating the first two cysteines; the CC family (β family) has no intervening amino acid; in the C family (γ family), members have lost cysteines one and three; and the CX3C chemokine family (δ family) has three intervening amino acids. The CXC family is further divided into members having a glutamate–leucine–arginine (E–L–R) motif in their amino-terminal sequence, and possessing angiogenic activity and neutrophil chemotactic activity. Those members lacking the E–L–R motif are generally lymphocyte chemoattractants and lack angiogenic activity. The CC chemokine family is the largest family and contains members chemotactic for monocytes, lymphocytes, eosinophils, basophils, mast cells, and NK cells. Its members may also regulate hematopoiesis within the marrow cavity, and induce mast cell and eosinophil degranulation. Lymphotactin is the only member of the C family of chemokines. It has highest expression in the thymus, where it may serve to recruit immature T-cell precursors from the bone marrow. Other functions of this chemokine are not yet defined. The CX3C chemokine family also has but one member at present, fractalkine (neurotactin). Anchored to cell surfaces by a mucin-like stalk, the extracellular portion may be released from cell surfaces to act as a chemoattractant for monocytes, T cells, and NK cells in vitro. A role for fractalkine in the inflammatory process is suggested by its upregulation on endothelium in the CNS of mice with experimental autoimmune encephalomyelitis (EAE), in the presence of tumor necrosis factor (TNF). Because fractalkine is also expressed within the normal brain, it may also play a nonpathologic role there.

Chemokines may promote disease progression. Studies have highlighted the role of IL-8 in various inflammatory states from the chronic arthritides to sepsis. Some have suggested measuring IL-8 levels in urine as a means of monitoring the severity of glomerular disease (Wada, 1994). In sepsis, IL-8 is central to neutrophil accumulation in various organs, and to progression to endstage disease development. Other chemokines including RANTES (regulated on activation, normal T cell expressed and secreted), GROα, and MIP-1α are active in septic shock, and may provide targets for therapeutic intervention. In granulomatous responses, the presence of MIP-1α correlates with granuloma formation. Similarly, in EAE, the animal model for multiple sclerosis, disease progression and relapse is positively affected by the administration of neutralizing antibodies to MIP-1α and MCP-1. Measurement of IL-8 along with C reactive protein in neonates has permitted sensitive detection and identification of cases of true early neonatal sepsis, and reduced unnecessary antibiotic administration (Franz, 2001, 2004).

Interleukin-9

The human IL-9 protein contains 144 amino acids and its gene has been mapped to chromosome 5, where genes for other growth factors and growth factor receptors (IL-3, IL-4, IL-5, GM-CSF, and CSF-1R) cluster. cDNA for the IL-9 receptor (IL-9R) encodes a 522-amino-acid ligand-specific α chain member of the hematopoietic receptor superfamily, which associates with a signal-transducing γ chain that is shared with interleukins 2, 4, 7, 13, 15, and 21. The fact that a common receptor subunit is employed by these cytokines may explain some of the observed redundancies of activity among them. Upon IL-9 binding, the γ chain transmits signal through JAK/STAT pathways (Yin, 1995).

IL-9 functions during the immune response, and has growth factor and anti-apoptotic activity in transformed cell lines. In humans, IL-9 expression is apparently limited to CD4+ CD45 RO-positive T-cell subsets (memory T cells), and to CD45-RA+ T cells in the presence of IL-4 and IL-10 (Houssiau, 1995). Freshly isolated T cells in long-term culture eventually respond to a growth-promoting activity of IL-9, and in murine cultures T cells eventually undergo tumor transformation (Uyttenhove, 1988). Interestingly, 5–10% of transgenic mice that overproduce IL-9 spontaneously develop lymphoblastic lymphomas (Renauld, 1994), and IL-9 is produced in the tumor cells of Hodgkin's lymphoma and anaplastic lymphoma (Merz, 1991). The latter raises the possibility of an IL-9 autocrine loop (Demoulin, 1998). Recently, serum IL-9 levels as measured by a novel ELISA technique were shown to be elevated especially in nodular sclerosis Hodgkin's lymphoma (Fischer, 2003). Within the hematopoietic system, IL-9 and erythropoietin appear to support the maturation of erythroid progenitors in vitro, and may promote colony-forming-unit–granulocyte–macrophage (CFU-GM) growth from CD34+ progenitors. IL-9 exerts growth-promoting activity on mast cell lines, and may regulate mast cell differentiation as well (Eklund, 1993). It is suggested that IL-9 induces mast cell-dependent resistance to parasites in vivo, and with IL-4 may facilitate IgE and IgG production (Louahed, 1995). A role for IL-9 within the CNS is suggested by its ability to support increased neurite extension and promote excitability among cultures of immortalized mouse progenitor hippocampal cell lines (Mehler, 1993).

Animal studies suggest a role for IL-9 in the development of asthma and bronchial hyper-reactivity (Soussi-Gounni, 2001), and may stimulate respiratory epithelial goblet cell hyperplasia during repair thereby promoting excessive mucus production (Vermeer, 2003). Therapies aimed at IL-9 blockade may ultimately prove valuable in controlling the undesirable remodeling associated with reactive airway disease.

Interleukin-10

IL-10 is a potent anti-inflammatory cytokine that has been mapped to chromosome 1 (Fiorentino, 1989). It is a 160-amino-acid protein with a molecular mass of 18.5 kDa (Kim, 1992). The IL-10 receptor (IL-10R) is mainly expressed on hematopoietic cells, and binds dimerized IL-10 molecules (Tan, 1995). IL-10 signal transduction is mediated through the JAK/STAT pathway (Lalani, 1997). Though many cell types including Th2 cells, CD4+ and CD8+ T cells, monocytes and macrophages, mast cells, keratinocytes, eosinophils, epithelial cells, and several tumor cells are capable of producing IL-10, it is the monocyte that produces the bulk of IL-10 in most inflammatory conditions (Lalani, 1997). Because it may be produced in an autocrine fashion and regulates its own production through a negative-feedback loop, IL-10 regulates the inflammatory response from within the inflammatory focus as needed (Tan, 1995). IL-10 acts to inhibit the production of proinflammatory cytokines such as IL-1α, IL-1β, IL-3, IL-6, IL-8, TNF, G-CSF, GM-CSF, and chemokines including IL-8 and MIP-1α, by suppressing transcription of their corresponding genes (Goldman, 1997). IL-10 also suppresses release of free oxygen radicals and inhibits nitric-oxide dependent microbicidal activity within macrophages (Fleming, 1996).

In allergic conditions such as asthma, IL-5 production is a crucial initiating event. In vitro, IL-10 prevents IL-5 production in Th0, Th2, and resting T cells and downregulates MHC class II expression among APCs. It also inhibits MIP-1α expression in human neutrophils, monocytes, and macrophages; inhibits production of chemoattractants active at sites of chronic inflammation; and may directly inactivate eosinophil function and hasten eosinophil death. These findings suggest the potential for IL-10 to limit chronic airway inflammation (Pretolani, 1999).

IL-10 may participate in the induction and perpetuation of SLE, and disease activity correlates with IL-10 titers (Houssiau, 1995). It is implicated in other autoimmune diseases including myasthenia gravis, Graves disease, Sjögren syndrome, polymyositis, psoriasis, systemic sclerosis, pemphigus vulgaris, bullous pemphigoid, and Kawasaki disease (Lalani, 1997). In addition, detection of elevated serum IL-10 as determined by ELISA in patients with small-cell carcinomas of the lung and adenocarcinomas of the colon may be a useful predictor of clinically undetectable disease progression (De Vita, 1999, 2000), and in febrile patients with cancer its detection may be useful in identifying those cases due to infection rather than to neoplasm-related fever, allowing earlier appropriate therapy to be initiated (Kallio, 2001).

Interleukin-11

IL-11 is a 23 kDa cytokine with numerous effects on many tissues, including bone marrow, brain, gut, and testis. The gene encoding it is mapped to chromosome 19, and its three-dimensional structure probably contains four α-helical motifs (Czupryn, 1995). The IL-11 receptor (IL-11R) is formed from the noncovalent association of a ligand-specific α chain and a signal-transducing β chain, gp130. The IL-6R complex also uses the gp130 subunit as its signaling chain, accounting for some of the overlap in the action of these cytokines (Cherel, 1996). When associated with IL-11Rβ (gp130), binding affinity for IL-11 is high and a biological signal is generated through the formation of gp130 homodimers. These are thought to activate transduction pathways including JAK kinases, MAPK kinases, ribosomal S6 protein kinases, and Src family kinases (Fuhrer, 1996). IL-11 mRNA has been detected in many stimulated tissues, including fibroblasts, epithelial cells, chondrocytes, synoviocytes, osteoblasts, and glioblastoma cells.

Evidence indicates that IL-11 is a potent anti-inflammatory cytokine (Redlich, 1996; Trepicchio, 1998). Its hematopoietic effects (Du, 1995) include a role in megakaryocytopoiesis and the stimulation of erythropoiesis, macrophage proliferation and differentiation, and B-cell immunoglobulin production. In addition, it regulates the differentiation and maturation of progenitor myeloid cells in combination with stem cell factor, and may play a role in lymphopoiesis. In chemotherapy patients, IL-11 therapy improves recovery of hematopoiesis and immune function, and reduces morbidity of bone-marrow-suppressive chemotherapy.

IL-11 has extensive nonhematopoietic effects as well (Du, 1995). IL-11 may function in pulmonary inflammation and is produced by stimulated alveolar and pulmonary epithelial cells in large quantities. Respiratory viruses are strong stimulators of IL-11 synthesis in the lung, and IL-11 is detected in the nasal secretions of children with upper respiratory tract infections (Einarsson, 1996). IL-11 also may be involved in the growth control of gastrointestinal epithelial cells, since it is shown to reversibly inhibit proliferation of intestinal crypt stem cell lines in vitro. IL-11 may also be able to confer mucosal protection to the gastrointestinal epithelium after radiation and chemotherapy (Keith, 1994).

Other activities of IL-11 include osteoclast development in vitro, a role in the survival of both sensory and motor neurons, stimulation of acute-phase reactant release in vitro and in vivo, and regulation of extracellular matrix (ECM) metabolism. In tumor biology, IL-11 acts synergistically with other cytokines to promote the growth of human leukemia cell lines and stimulates leukemic blast colony formation (Hu, 1993; Lemoli, 1995). A beneficial thrombocytopoietic effect has been detected in patients with Crohn's disease receiving recombinant IL-11 (Sands, 1999).

Interleukin-12

IL-12 is a 70 kDa, heterodimeric cytokine encoded by two separate genes (Trinchieri, 1994). The IL-12 receptor (IL-12R) is a member of the hematopoietin receptor superfamily and has significant homology with gp130 and the G-CSF and leukemia inhibitory factor receptors. IL-12 promotes differentiation of human Th1-like cells, readies them for increased production of interferon-γ (IFN-γ), and increases the cytolytic abilities of NK and T cells (Heufler, 1996). It is produced mainly by monocytes and macrophages, dendritic cells (professional APCs) and, to a smaller extent, by neutrophils and keratinocytes. Its production is down regulated by IL-10 and TGF-β, and its synthesis is increased by IFN-γ. IL-12 synthesis is rapidly induced in phagocytic cells by certain bacterial strains and by intracellular pathogens including protozoa and fungi, and to a lesser extent, viruses.

IL-12 plays a vital role as a proinflammatory cytokine. In models of septic shock involving intraperitoneal injections of endotoxin in mice, IL-12 is found to promote the overproduction of IFN-γ, which by a positive-feedback loop induces the release of still more IL-12. Ultimately, overproduction of IFN-γ causes death of the animal. The important role of IL-12 in this series of events is highlighted by the observation that injection of neutralizing anti-IL-12 antibodies into subject mice rescues about 90% of them from death (Trinchieri, 1994). Evidence suggests that IL-10 inhibits IL-12 production by phagocytes, and that IL-12 itself may stimulate IL-10 production, thereby serving as a negative regulator of its own production (Meyaard, 1996). Experimental animal evidence suggests an exacerbating role for IL-12 in certain autoimmune diseases, including autoimmune diabetes, arthritis, the animal model for multiple sclerosis (EAE), and colitis (Trinchieri, 1997). But in allergic conditions, IL-12 plays an ameliorative role through its capacity to downregulate production of IL-4, IL-5, and IgE. The effect is striking in antigen-induced airway hyper-responsiveness in mouse models (Gavett, 1995).

IL-12 has significant antitumor and antimetastatic effects in mouse models in vivo (Zitvogel, 1995). However, gastrointestinal, liver, and hematologic toxicity has been noted in clinical trials with rIL-12 among patients with renal cell carcinoma. Because of its role in promoting Th1 memory responses to vaccines, IL-12 may be important as a vaccine adjuvant. When expressed as a ratio with serum IL-10, serum IL-12 measurement may help to identify cancer patients with infection-related fevers, permitting prompt and appropriate antibiotic therapy (Kallio, 2001).

Interleukin-13

IL-13 is a 12 kDa, 132-amino-acid protein whose gene has been mapped to chromosome 5 in the gene cluster containing IL 3, IL-4, IL-5, IL-9, and GM-CSF. It is thought to possess an α-helical structure, with four α-helices and two β-pleated sheets. The IL-13 receptor (IL-13R) is expressed on B cells, monocytes, basophils, eosinophils, mast cells, endothelial cells, fibroblasts, keratinocytes, and certain tumor cells. Apparently, it is not expressed on human T lymphocytes. IL-13 and IL-4 share a common receptor component, gp140, that serves as the low-affinity receptor (IL-13Ra) for IL-13 and as the type II receptor (IL-4Ra) for IL-4. Not surprisingly, then, IL-13 elicits many of the biological actions of IL-4. When bound to ligand, IL-13R and IL-4R transducer signal via the JAK/STAT pathways (Burd, 1995; Keegan, 1996). IL-13 is released from Th0, Th1, and Th2 subsets of CD4/CD8⁺ T-cell clones in response to antigen-specific stimulation or polyclonal activation, and from mast cells, basophils, and eosinophils after stimulation through their high-affinity IgE receptors (CD23) (Keegan, 1996). It is for the most part an anti-inflammatory cytokine that is capable of inhibiting the production of proinflammatory cytokines such as IL-1α and IL-1β, IL-12, and IFN-γ by lipopolysaccharide-activated monocytes. IL-13 is able to induce secretion of IgE from cultured human B cells and to increase expression of the proinflammatory adhesion molecule VCAM-1 on endothelial cells. This fact, and the observation that IL-13 synthesis is increased in atopic conditions in the lungs of asthmatics and in patients with chronic sinusitis while it is decreased in response to corticosteroid administration, highlight the importance of IL-13 to allergic conditions (de Vries, 1998). At the same time, IL-13 appears to attenuate the allergic response by downregulating the ability of endothelial cells and airway smooth muscle cells to release the T lymphocyte and inflammatory cell chemoattractant RANTES (Tony, 1994). It is chemotactic to monocytes, and promotes proliferation of activated B cells, and in vitro appears to promote megakaryocyte colony formation and enhance proliferation of murine bone marrow progenitor cells. Its downregulation of tissue factor production and upregulation of thrombomodulin production further highlight its anti-inflammatory nature.

Interleukin-14

IL-14 may have been named prematurely, but refers to high-molecular-weight- B-cell growth factor, a protein that causes B-cell proliferation and inhibition of immunoglobulin secretion (Ambrus, 1993).

Interleukin-15

IL-15 is a 14–15 kDa protein first identified as a cell growth factor in the supernatants of a monkey kidney epithelial cell line (Grabstein, 1994). Although its primary amino acid sequence is unique, its three-dimensional structure closely resembles that of other members of the four α-helix bundle family of cytokines, which includes IL-2, a cytokine with similar functional activities. The gene encoding IL-15 has been mapped to chromosome 4, close to the gene for IL-2 (Anderson, 1995). The IL-15 receptor (IL-15R) is composed of three protein subunits: a ligand-specific IL-15Rα chain, and a β and γ chain that are identical with the β and γ chains of IL-2R. This arrangement accounts for similar activities of IL-15 and IL-2. IL-15R utilizes JAK/STAT pathways during signal transduction (Johnston, 1995).

Macrophages, fibroblasts, keratinocytes, epithelial cells, and other tissues secrete IL-15 but, unlike IL-2, it is not secreted by lymphocytes. Nonetheless, the tissue distribution of IL-15 is broad, with mRNA transcripts also identified in monocytes and macrophages, Langerhans cells, dendritic cells, and endothelial cells. IL-15 mRNA appears to be stored in translationally inactive pools that are available for translation early in the innate response to infection. IL-15 production by macrophages in the initial phase of microbial infection may serve to activate NK cells as part of the response to infection (Cosman, 1995).

As with IL-2, IL-15 is shown to participate in co stimulation of T-cell proliferation, induction of cytokine activity in T cells, proliferation of NK cells, and activation of B-cell proliferation and immunoglobulin release (Kirman, 1998). Unlike IL-2, IL-15 may anabolically increase skeletal muscle mass and has been shown to stimulate mast cell proliferation in vitro and in vivo. IL-15 is chemotactic for T cells, recruiting them to sites of inflammation, and such a role has been suggested in the synovium of patients with rheumatoid arthritis (McInnes, 1996). Other evidence points to a role for IL-15 production in inflammatory conditions such as ulcerative colitis, hepatitis C, and sarcoidosis. In these conditions, IL-15 may serve to recruit activated lymphocytes into areas of inflammation where they would be able to release additional proinflammatory cytokines and exert cytotoxic effects (Kirman, 1998). In patients with postoperative methicillin-resistant Staphylococcus aureus (MRSA) enterocolitis, serum IL-15 was found to rise prior to the onset of diarrhea. But serum IL-15 levels remained unchanged in MRSA-related infections at sites other than the colon, suggesting a role for IL-15 in the pathogenesis of MRSA enterocolitis, and providing a serum marker disease severity (Mayumi, 1999).

Interleukin-16

Initially recognized as a chemoattractant factor in cultures of mitogen-stimulated human peripheral blood mononuclear cells (Center, 1982), IL-16 is now recognized as a proinflammatory T-cell chemoattractant. Mitogen-stimulated lymphocytes produce IL-16 as a precursor molecule that is cleaved and secreted. Only after aggregating into homotetramers does IL-16 appear to possess biological activity (Bazan, 1996). The gene encoding IL-16 has been mapped to chromosome 15. Surface CD4 appears to serve as the surface receptor for soluble IL-16 and is absolutely required for biological signaling (Cruikshank, 1994). IL-16 is released from T cells following stimulation with mitogens, antigen, histamine, and serotonin. Cultured eosinophils and mast cells also release IL-16 in the presence of GM-CSF, and either PMA or calcium ionophore, respectively.

IL-16 serves as a chemoattractant for CD4[+] T cells and other peripheral immune cells expressing CD4, including monocytes and eosinophils. It is a competence growth factor for and stimulates cell cycle progression in human CD4[+] T cells (Cruikshank, 1994). In addition, IL-16 promotes increased adhesion to the ECM by eosinophils, and upregulates HLA-DR expression among monocytes (Wan, 1995). The in vivo result may be increased accumulation of primed, cytokine-responsive CD4[+] T cells at sites of inflammation, which are protected from TCR-mediated activation-induced T-cell death (Cruikshank, 1994).

Interleukin-17

IL-17 is a 32 kDa proinflammatory cytokine secreted as covalently bound homodimers from a restricted set of activated human memory T cells (Yao, 1995; Fossiez, 1996). The gene encoding this cytokine has been mapped to chromosome 2. IL-17 is expressed predominantly by CD4[+] CD45-RO memory T cells in response to a variety of activation (Fossiez, 1996). Studies in mice suggest that in contrast to the restricted expression of IL-17, the IL-17 receptor (IL-17R) is a widely distributed novel protein especially abundant in spleen and kidney. Recent evidence implicates the JAK/STAT signaling pathway in transducing signals from the IL-17R (Subramaniam, 1999).

An in vivo role for IL-17 in protection from bacterial infection has been suggested and, because of its ability to induce production of high levels of cytokines, including IL-6, IL-18, and MCP-1, it may serve to regulate inflammatory processes (Dalrymple, 1996). Unlike its presumed protective role in infectious states, IL-17 is believed to cause joint inflammation and promote bone and cartilage destruction in autoimmune inflammation, and has been identified in the synovial fluids of patients with rheumatoid arthritis (Leonaviciene, 2004).

Interleukin-18

IL-18 is an approximately 18 kDa protein produced by activated macrophages, Kupffer cells, osteoblasts, and keratinocytes (Torigoe, 1997). Formation of biologically active IL-18 requires processing of a 24 kDa precursor by caspase-1 (ICE) in Kupffer cells. The IL-18 receptor (IL-18R) is identical to the IL-1R-related protein (IL-1Rrp) (Torigoe, 1997) and, when bound to ligand, IL-18R induces NF-κB DNA binding. High- and low-affinity IL-18Rs are identified but their roles in signal transduction are unclear. The primary function of IL-18 appears to be induction of IFN-γ in activated Th1 cells and anti-CD40-activated B cells (in the presence of IL-12). IL-18 also induces T-cell synthesis of GM-CSF and IL-6, and promotes cytotoxicity among NK cells by permitting exocytosis of perforins and granzyme A (Ushio, 1996). Physiologic roles for IL-18 may include defense against infection and a role in tumor rejection. Through suppression of IgE production, IL-18 may dampen the allergic response (Yoshimoto, 1997) but unregulated IL-18 production is associated with liver parenchyma damage in animal models. IL-18 may play a part in the pathogenesis of hemophagocytic lymphohistiocytosis through induction of Th1 cells. Measuring IL-18 levels in the peripheral blood of affected patients may provide a means of monitoring smoldering disease activity in hemophagocytic lymphohistiocytosis (Takada, 1999).

Serial laboratory measurements of IL-18 gene expression by polymerase chain reaction may be useful in predicting impending renal allograft rejection (Simon, 2004), while high serum IL-18 levels may help to identify those patients likely to succumb to postoperative shock (Emmanuilidis, 2002).

Interleukin-19

IL-19 is a member of the IL-10 family-related molecules that include IL-20, IL-22, IL-24, IL-26, and IL-10. It was initially identified in monocytes stimulated with lipopolysaccharide (Gallagher, 2000) and, because its expression could be upregulated by IL-4 and downregulated by IFN-γ, a role for it in regulating the Th1/Th2 system was proposed by its discoverers, who later showed that IL-19 may be able to influence T-cell maturation (Gallagher, 2004). As with most of the recently described cytokines, the physiologic role of IL-19 is not defined. Recent investigation of the physiologic role of IL-19, however, suggests that it may function within the skin and that single-nucleotide polymorphisms in the IL-19 (and IL-20) gene may influence susceptibility to psoriasis (Koks, 2004). Others have suggested a role for IL-19 in the pathogenesis of asthma through its upregulation of Th2 cytokine in animal studies (Liao, 2004). Although a specific receptor for it has not yet been identified, IL-19 does appear capable of binding to the IL-20 receptor complex and by so doing is able to initiate STAT3 phosphorylation (Dumoutier, 2001).

Interleukin-20

As mentioned above, IL-20 is a member of the IL-10 family of related molecules. The molecule was initially identified through the use of a bioinformatics algorithm that also led to the identification of the IL-10 cytokine family gene cluster (Blumberg, 2001). Further investigation with transgenic mice overexpressing IL-20 suggests a role for IL-20 in the pathogenesis of skin diseases, since the pups of these mice develop significant epidermal abnormalities. Keratinocytes express the receptor for IL-20 on their surfaces and, upon receptor binding (possibly in autocrine fashion), IL-20 induces keratinocyte proliferation and upregulation of inflammatory cytokines including TNF (Rich, 2003) through the STAT3 signaling pathway (Blumberg, 2001). As with IL-19, single-nucleotide polymorphisms in the IL-20 gene may influence susceptibility to some forms of psoriasis (Kingo, 2004). Others have demonstrated IL-20 expression in cultured glial cells after lipopolysaccharide stimulation, indicating a possible role for IL-20 in infection (Hosoi, 2004), and in hematopoiesis through its effect as a stimulator of colony formation by CD34[+] multipotential progenitors (Liu, 2003).

Interleukin-21

IL-21 is a member of the IL-2 cytokine family that includes IL-4, IL-7, IL-9, IL-13, IL-15, and IL-2. Members of this family compose the type I superfamily of cytokines, which share a common γ chain structure. Produced by activated T-cells, IL-21 both upregulates and downregulates the immune response, depending upon the signaling context (Strengell, 2002; Mehta, 2004), by modulating T- and B-cell proliferation and the cytolytic activity and maturation of NK cells (Parrish-Novak, 2002; Sivori, 2003). Studies with rIL-21 in human B-cells also point to a role for IL-21 in IgG1 and IgG3 isotype switching (Pene, 2004). A disease specific role for IL-21 comes indirectly through animal studies in which mice with highly elevated IL-21 levels appear to develop an autoimmune condition resembling SLE (Ozaki, 2004). There may be therapeutic potential to IL-21 administration, since IL-21-treated mice seem to maintain tumor immunity against thymoma in a syngeneic tumor model (Moroz, 2004).

Interleukin-22

IL-22 is a primarily Th1-cell-derived cytokine with homology to IL-10 and the other molecules of the IL-10 family: IL-19, IL-20, IL-24, and IL-26. Unlike its homolog IL-10, IL-22 does not appear to regulate the immune activities of B-cells but probably functions as an inducer of acute-phase reactants (Xu, 2001; Nagem, 2002). Because the IL-22 receptor mRNA expression is highest in pancreas, liver, small intestine, colon, and kidney, pulmonary alveolar macrophages, and pneumocytes, IL-22 may serve to regulate the immune response in those tissues. Along these lines, Western blotting for IL-22 in the bronchial lavage fluids of patients with acute respiratory distress syndrome and sarcoidosis has demonstrated lower IL-22 levels than in normal controls, suggesting a role for IL-22 in pulmonary inflammation (Whittington, 2004).

Interleukin-23

IL-23 is composite cytokine produced by activated macrophage and dendritic cells, composed of the IL-12-specific subunit p19 and the IL-12 subunit p40, together forming a unique functional cytokine capable of inducing long-lasting Th1 and cytotoxic T lymphocyte immune responses, and may play an important role in autocrine stimulation of antigen-presenting cells at the time of initial immune response to antigen (Puccetti, 2002). As a consequence, IL-23 may become useful as a strong adjuvant for creating lasting Ag-specific T cell vaccines directed against poorly antigenic substances such as viral DNA (Ha, 2004). It is argued that IL-23 assists in the recruitment and activation of inflammatory cells that induce chronic inflammation and granuloma formation as a response to infection (Langrish, 2004), and provides antitumor activity through its modulation of specific T-cell subsets (Lo, 2003). Mouse studies suggest that IL-23 may exacerbate the inflammation associated with autoimmune arthritis (Murphy, 2003).

Interleukin-24

IL-24 is a potent immunosuppressive cytokine discovered in human melanoma cells, and is a homolog of the IL-10-family molecules. It is produced by activated peripheral blood mononuclear cells and macrophages, induces Th1 type cytokine secretion from peripheral blood mononuclear cells (Caudell, 2002), and binds to its receptor located on keratinocytes. First identified as a melanocyte differentiation factor (MDA-7), when delivered by an adenoviral vector, IL-24 is capable of inducing apoptosis of malignant cells, including melanoma cells, without damaging supporting stromal cells (Sarkar, 2002) and, in concert with free-radical-generating agents such as arsenic trioxide, may potentially be a useful therapy for renal cell carcinoma (Yacoub, 2003). IL-24 may also have antiangiogenic effects, since in vivo it inhibits angioneogenesis around implanted human lung tumors in mice (Ramesh, 2003). Yet IL-24 may also be tumor-supportive in the early stages of some epithelial neoplasms that induce IL-24 production and take advantage of its autocrine growth effects (Shinohara, 2004).

Interleukin-25

IL-25 is a member of the IL-17 cytokine family and is an important mediator of IL-4, IL-5, IL-13, and eotaxin production. It is produced by activated Th2 cells and mast cells, and may be an important link in the development and amplification of allergic responses and disease (Fort, 2001). Mice administered IL-25-expressing adenovirus intranasally developed epithelial cell hyperplasia, increased mucus secretion, and airway hyper-reactivity, and production of IL-4, IL-5, IL-13, and eotaxin mRNA in the lung, with eosinophilia of bronchoalveolar lavage specimens and lung tissues. In addition, following fungal infection of the gut and lung, IL-25 mRNA expression was increased in this model (Hurst, 2002).

Interleukin-26

IL-26 is the most recent member of the IL-10 family of molecules and is produced mainly by T memory cells. IL-26 was first identified as a secretion of T-cells transformed by herpesvirus saimiri, and appears to be capable of inducing IL-8 and IL-10 secretion, and CD54 surface expression by keratinocytes and colon carcinoma cells. By affecting epithelial and mucosal surfaces, IL-26 may modulate mucosal and cutaneous immune responses (Hor, 2004).

Interleukin-27

The heterodimeric product of activated antigen-presenting cells, IL-27 functions early in the immune response by fueling the rapid proliferation of naive Th1 CD4+ T-cells, both through its own action and synergistically with IL-12 by stimulating the production of IFN-γ (Pflanz, 2002). In this way it may help provide resistance to intracellular infections such as *Leishmania* or *Toxoplasma* spp. (Hunter, 2004). In B cells, IL-27 may induce IgG2a-class switching, and may eventually be therapeutically useful in treating allergic diseases through induction of class IgG2a switching as well as by regulating Th1 differentiation (Yoshimoto, 2004).

Transforming Growth Factor-β

TGF-β is a 25 kDa cytokine with three isoforms: TGF-β1, TGF-β2, and TGF-β3 (McCartney-Francis, 1998). Bioactive peptide associates with ECM components or carriers such as α_2-macroglobulin, albumin, or IgG, which facilitate TGF-β uptake and catabolism. TGF-β is important to the development, growth, and differentiation of epithelial cells. It also plays a role in carcinogenesis, inflammation, repair, and angiogenesis. Its biological signal is transduced to the nucleus via Smad proteins (members of the MAD-related family) (Lopez-Casillas, 1993; Derynck, 1996). TGF-β is produced by every leukocyte lineage from lymphocytes to macrophages and dendritic cells, and it acts in both an autocrine and paracrine fashion. In TGF-β knockout mice, 50–60% of embryos demonstrate failure of angiogenesis and hematopoiesis, and spontaneously abort, while in transgenic mice overexpressing TGF-β, the consequence is pulmonary hypoplasia and lack of respiratory epithelial differentiation, causing perinatal death. TGF-β serves as both a proliferation factor and an inhibitor of growth. It inhibits the growth of most epithelial cell types and leukocytes. In mice, over- or underexpression of TGF-β causes hypo or

hyperproliferation (carcinoma) of epithelial cells (Norgaard, 1995). In humans, aggressiveness of melanoma and colon carcinoma cell lines increases with increasing loss of responsiveness to TGF-β. TGF-β may also serve as a tumor suppresser, since antibodies to TGF-β increase tumor-forming ability of colon carcinoma cells in vitro. TGF-β suppresses the inflammatory response and promotes healing through inhibiting T- and B-cell proliferation, inhibiting NK cell function, inducing cytokine antagonists, downregulating integrin expression, and inhibiting IgG release. During wound healing TGF-β promotes fibroblast proliferation and the synthesis of collagen. However, overproduction of TGF-β not only quells the inflammatory response but pushes healing too far, producing exuberant fibrosis and excessive scarring (Wahl, 1994). Therapy aimed at blocking the fibrogenic effect of TGF-β has been studied in recipients of organ transplants in whom immunosuppressant agents have induced ischemia and associated fibrosis, and in those with the connective tissue disease scleroderma. In these conditions, anti-TGF-β antibody has been used with some success to ameliorate progressive interstitial fibrosis (Sule, 2003; Khanna, 2004).

Tumor Necrosis Factor

TNF (previously TNF-α) is a 17 kDa proinflammatory cytokine (Beutler, 1985). Its name derives from its ability to kill tumor cells and to induce hemorrhagic necrosis in tumors transplanted to mice. The majority of TNF effects are mediated through two high-affinity cell surface receptors: TNFR-I (CD120a, 55 kDa) and TNFR-II (CD120b, 75 kDa) (Hohmann, 1989). These receptors mediate signals for cell proliferation and programmed cell death (apoptosis). TNFR-I has within its intracellular domain a motif referred to as the 'death domain' that is required for transduction of the apoptotic signal. Mainly macrophages and monocytes produce TNF but other cells, including lymphocytes, mast cells, neutrophils, keratinocytes, astrocytes, microglial cells, smooth muscle cells, and tumor cells, produce it as well. TNF may act locally in a paracrine fashion but also acts at distant sites in the manner of endocrine hormones. The biological effects of TNF are numerous (Kollias, 1999) and include a direct cytotoxic effect, modulation of cell growth and differentiation, and a role in chronic inflammatory conditions and infection. In addition, TNF is responsible for the wasting syndrome of malignancy and of major parasitic infections. Through the stimulation of neutrophils, TNF increases phagocytosis, degranulation, and respiratory burst activity. Additional proinflammatory effects include inducing increased formation of platelet-activating factor in neutrophils, stimulating the secretion of arachidonic acid, enhancing antibody-dependent cell-mediated cytotoxicity, and increasing neutrophil adherence to TNF-activated endothelium via upregulation of E-selectin. Animal models implicate TNF in rheumatoid arthritis and inflammatory bowel disease in which TNF exercises a proinflammatory effect through activation of endothelial cells and induction of neutrophil chemotactic chemokines. In addition, a role for TNF in inflammatory demyelinating diseases of the CNS has been proposed on the basis of several multiple sclerosis studies in humans (Kollias, 1999). Therapeutic administration of anti-TNF monoclonal antibody (infliximab) or antibody-receptor fusion proteins (etanercept) for the treatment of rheumatoid arthritis and Crohn's disease, and potentially for graft-versus-host disease, is currently under investigation and appears promising (Furst, 2003).

Interferon-γ

IFN-γ (Samuel, 1991) is a 40–70 kDa homodimeric, 143-amino-acid protein mapped to chromosome 12. T cells and NK cells are the only known sources of IFN. T cells produce it in response to antigen or mitogen stimulation, and NK cells produce it in response to IL-2 or anti-CD16 antibodies, or in the presence of activated macrophages (Carson, 1995). In vitro, IFN-γ is a strong stimulator of macrophages and strongly enhances their tumoricidal activity. It causes upregulation of MHC molecules on many cell types, including APCs. In addition, it regulates antibody production by B cells (Snapper, 1987), and stimulates Th1 cells. In response to infection, IFN-γ induces macrophages to kill intracellular microorganisms through the production of oxidative metabolites and proteases. Clinically, IFN-γ has been used to improve the bactericidal ability of phagocytes in those with chronic granulomatous diseases (Bolinger, 1992).

Cell Adhesion Molecules

The glue that binds living tissues into complex multicellular organisms is comprised in part of the adhesion molecules described subsequently. These complex glycoproteins permit cell migration during embryogenesis

Table 46–7 Major Integrins and their Ligands

Integrin	Name	Ligands
$\alpha_1\beta_1$	VLA-1, CD49a/CD29	Collagen, LMN
$\alpha_2\beta_1$	VLA-2, CD49b/CD29	Collagen, LMN
$\alpha_3\beta_1$	VLA-3, CD49b/CD29	Collagen, LMN, FBN
$\alpha_4\beta_1$	VLA-4, CD49d/CD29	VCAM-1, FBN
$\alpha_5\beta_1$	VLA-5, CD49e/CD29	FBN
$\alpha_6\beta_1$	VLA-6, CD49f/CD29	LMN
$\alpha_7\beta_1$	CD49g/CD29	LMN
$\alpha_8\beta_1$	CD49h/CD29	FBN
$\alpha_L\beta_2$	LFA-1, CD11a/CD18	ICAM-1, -2, -3
$\alpha_M\beta_2$	Mac-1, CD11b/CD18	ICAM-1, iC3b
$\alpha_X\beta_2$	p150, 95, CD11cCD18	FBGN, iC3b
$\alpha_D\beta_2$	–	ICAM-3, VCAM-1
$\alpha_{IIb}\beta_3$	GP IIb/IIIa, CD41/CD61	FBGN, vWF, FBN, VN
$\alpha_V\beta_3$	CD51/CD61	VN, FBGN
$\alpha_4\beta_3$	CD49d/-	MadCAM-1, FBN, ICAM-1
$\alpha_E\beta_7$	–	E-cadherin

FBGN = fibrinogen; FBN = fibronectin; ICAM = intercellular adhesion molecule; LFA = lymphocyte functional antigen; LMN = laminin; VCAM = vascular cell adhesion molecule; VN = vitronectin; vWF = von Willebrand factor.

and wound healing, and govern the leukocyte trafficking and homing critical to lymphopoiesis and the immune response. Adhesion molecules are conventionally divided into five groups based on structural homology: cadherins, mucins, integrins, selectins, and immunoglobulin superfamily molecules. Cadherins are mostly expressed on epithelial cells and interact with each other in a calcium-dependent manner. Mucins are heavily glycosylated proteins that mainly interact with selectins. Immunoglobulin superfamily members have immunoglobulin-like domains and interact with integrins, selectins, and each other. Integrins and selectins are discussed.

Integrins

The integrin family (Gonzalez-Amaro, 1999) of adhesion molecules provides a critical physical link between those things external to the cell (other cells and the ECM) and those things within the cell (the cytoskeleton, intracytosolic molecules, and nucleus). Each integrin family member is composed of a heterodimer of noncovalently linked α and β subunits (Table 46–7). The major integrins are divided into four subfamilies, differing in patterns of expression and ligand specificity. The α_1 integrins, also known as the very late activation antigens (VLAs) are created from the association of a β_2-chain subunit (CD29) with any one of the α chain subunits (CD49a–CD49h). They are expressed on all cells requiring firm anchoring to the ECM, and on circulating leukocytes, platelets, and some tumor cells. The β_2 integrins, which tend to be expressed mainly by leukocytes and myeloid cells, result from the association of the β_2 chain subunit (CD18) with any of several α subunits. When combined with the α_L (CD11a) subunit, the β_2 integrin LFA-1 (CD11a/CD18) is formed. LFA-1 plays a crucial role in leukocyte adhesion to vascular endothelium during transendothelial migration. The β_2-chain subunit, in association with the α_M subunit (CD11b), forms Mac-1 (CD11b/CD18), an integrin expressed on myeloid cells and mononuclear phagocytes. The α integrin subunits are 120- to 180 kDa membrane proteins with short intracytoplasmic domains, a long extracellular fragment with seven homologous domains, and several metal ion-binding motifs (metal ion-dependent adhesion sites, MIDAS) thought to function in converting an integrin from an inactive to an active conformation. Both α and β subunits bind to ligand, but the α subunit is generally thought to provide ligand specificity.

The intracytoplasmic tails of α and β integrin subunits associate with cytoskeletal components to transduce intracytoplasmic signals. In the process of signal transduction, integrins associate and interact with other cell membrane-associated proteins, cytoskeletal components, and noncytoskeletal cytoplasmic components. The integrin-associated protein (IAP or IAP 50) designated CD47, a member of the immunoglobulin superfamily, is one such membrane-associated protein that, mainly through association with β_3 integrins, may function as a signal transducer. Other membrane-associated proteins involved in integrin signaling

include caveolin-1 and CD9, which are involved in cell membrane caveola formation and platelet aggregation, respectively. Cytosolic molecules including integrin cytoplasmic domain-associated protein (ICAP-1) help orchestrate the complex activity of β_1-integrin-mediated cell migration.

Perhaps the best-studied intracytoplasmic associations of integrin molecules are those with the cytoskeleton-associated proteins α-actinin, talin, filamin, vinculin, tensin, and paxillin. These cytoskeleton proteins, through their association with β_1, β_2, and β_3 integrin subunits, bridge integrin and cytoskeleton and direct cell migration, phagocytosis, stress fiber formation at focal contact sites, and intracellular signal transduction, as well as linking separate cytoskeletal proteins.

The pattern of integrin distribution is wide, especially among those integrins (mostly β_1) involved in anchoring cells to components of the general ECM such as collagen and laminin. For those integrins mediating attachment to less widely distributed components, tissue distribution is more restricted.

Selectins

The selectin family (Gonzalez-Amaro, 1999) contains three homologous proteins. L-selectin (CD62L) is expressed by most leukocytes, especially lymphocytes, and is thought to play an important role in naive and memory lymphocyte homing or trafficking to lymph nodes through high endothelial venules (HEV). L-selectin also tethers neutrophils to activated endothelial cells in regions of inflammation. Its ligands include Glycam (glycan-bearing cell adhesion molecule)-1, MadCAM (mucosal addressin cell adhesion molecule)-1 and CD34. P-selectin (CD62P) is stored in the α granules and Weibel–Palade bodies of platelets and endothelial cells, respectively, and is expressed on the cell surface after cell activation. Once on the cell surface, P-selectin binds neutrophils, lymphocytes, and monocytes via its ligands, Lewis-X-, and Lewis-A-family-type complex carbohydrate groups. E-selectin (CD62E) is found on the surface of activated endothelial cells only and recognizes ligands similar to those recognized by P-selectin. It plays a recognition role for homing effector and memory T cells as they localize to sites of inflammation. Selectins interact with carbohydrate moieties such as sialyl–Lewis X and sialyl–Lewis A, and possibly other ligands including integrins and glycolipids. The full extent of physiologic selectin ligands has not been determined but it is expected that the list will include molecules expressed on leukocytes and endothelium, since selectins are important to leukocyte–leukocyte and leukocyte–endothelium interactions.

The role of selectins is twofold: to mediate cell–cell interaction and to contribute to cell activation by intracytoplasmic signaling. As with integrins, selectins are critical to the initial tethering and rolling of leukocytes along activated endothelium prior to extravasation. After binding a soluble form of the mucin-like glycoprotein GlyCAM-1 (a high endothelial venule product), L-selectin is able to mediate the activation of β_1 integrins and their adhesion to fibronectin. P- and E-selectin may also serve as signal-transducing receptor molecules, since a rise in intracellular free Ca^{2+} within leukocytes adhering to endothelial cells is linked to these selectin molecules (Huang, 1993).

Leukocyte Extravasation

Expression of integrin molecules is dependent on cell activation and may be upregulated or downregulated in response to specific cues from the external environment, including local cytokine stimulation or immune interaction. Leukocyte integrin interaction with endothelial cells is critical to the evolution of the inflammatory and immune responses. In addition, homing of lymphoid cells to their sites of residence and the intravascular spread of metastases all involve similar endothelial interactions mediated through surface integrins and another set of cell adhesion molecules, the selectins and their ligands.

The extravasation of leukocytes occurs during cell homing as with the trafficking of γ/δ T cells to Peyer's patches, and as a part of the inflammatory response. Both processes involve similar steps, using different adhesion molecules. In inflammation the process begins with local release of proinflammatory cytokines such as TNF, IL-1, and IFN-γ, which activate the local endothelium to increase surface expression of adhesion molecules including members of the immunoglobulin superfamily, VCAM-1 and ICAM-1. In addition, endothelial cells release chemotactic agents including IL-8, forming a surface-bound and a soluble chemotactic gradient recognizable by transmigrating inflammatory cells, which localize them to the inflammatory focus.

This process for white cells (Fig. 46–4) involves: (1) tethering of the passing leukocyte to the endothelial surface mainly by endothelial selectins (E- and P-selectin) and their leukocyte ligand Sialyl-Lewis X-

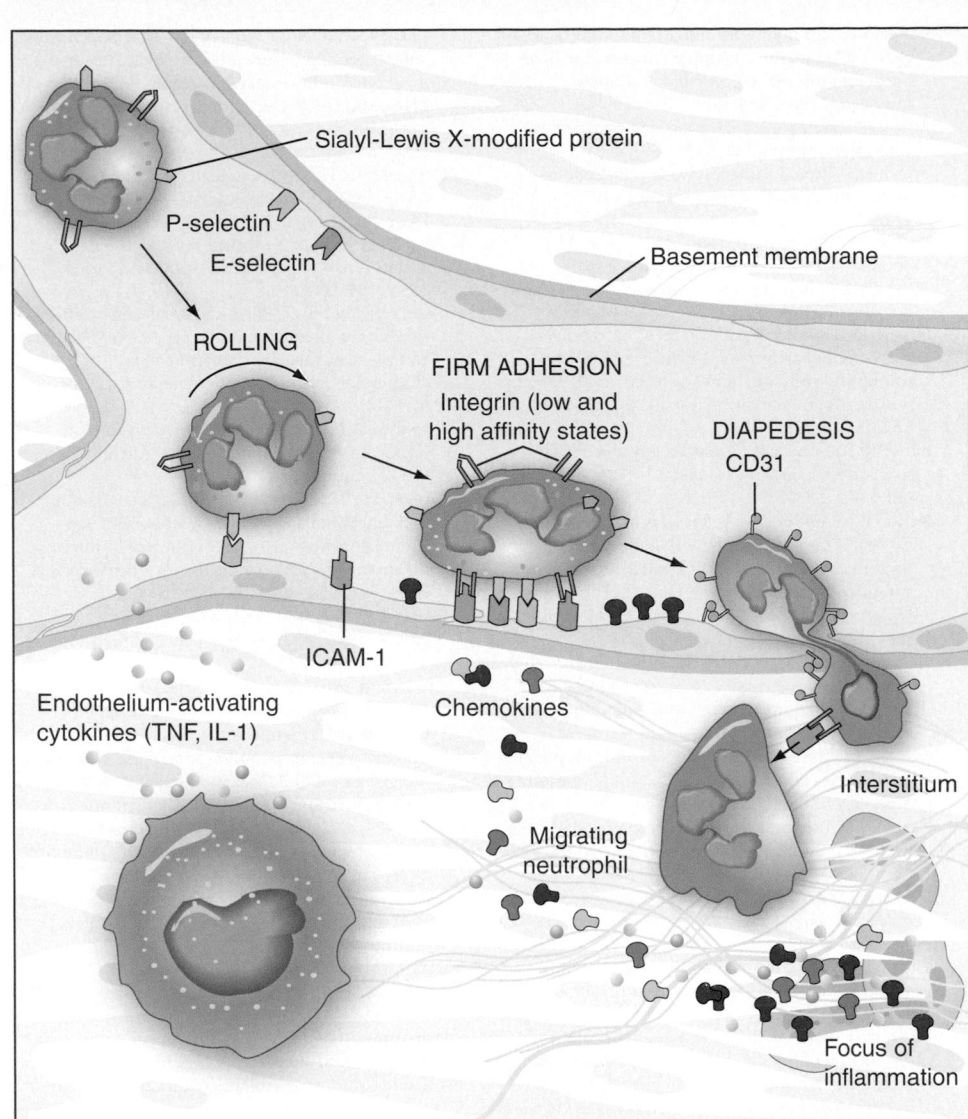

Figure 46–4 Adhesion molecules on the surfaces of leukocytes and activated endothelial cells guide the movement of white blood cells from the bloodstream to foci of tissue inflammation. Direction is provided by a chemotactic gradient. ICAM = intracellular adhesion molecule; IL = interleukin; TNF, tumor necrosis factor.

modified glycoprotein; and (2) leukocyte rolling, in which through rapid sequential surface expression of mainly leukocyte VLA-4 and $\alpha_4\beta_7$ integrin, the shear force provided by the bloodstream rolls leukocytes along the endothelial surface, thereby bringing these integrins into contact with their endothelial ligands, VCAM-1 and MAdCAM-1, respectively. In the case of neutrophils, rolling is mediated by selectins alone. As they roll, leukocyte cell adhesion molecules trigger biochemical events leading to (3) leukocyte activation, and conversion of its integrins to an activated state of increased avidity. This leads to increased leukocyte–endothelial cell adhesion, and eventually (4) to arrest of leukocyte rolling, and (5) leukocyte transmigration of the endothelium with the assistance of the homotypic adhesion molecule CD31 expressed on both white cells and the endothelium, while following a chemotactic gradient. It is still a matter of debate whether leukocytes pass directly through individual endothelial cells or merely pass between adjacent endothelial cells. Endothelial cell retraction early in the inflammatory response would seem to make movement between endothelial cells easier. Once through the endothelium, integrin-mediated cell migration through the extracellular matrix along a chemotactic gradient completes the leukocyte journey to a focus of inflammation.

Deficiency states for β_2 integrins (leukocyte adhesion deficiency type I) and congenital defects in the expression of selectins and their ligands demonstrate the indispensable role these receptors play in producing the inflammatory response and in lymphocyte trafficking. In these patients, neutrophils are unable to exit the bloodstream and migrate to sites of inflammation or infection, creating in effect a state of immune suppression with increased susceptibility to bacterial infection and a paradoxical peripheral neutrophilia (Bullard, 1996). The events surrounding septic shock, thrombosis, reperfusion injury, and metastases also require integrin and selectin activity. This knowledge has led to the therapeutic use of monoclonal antibodies, soluble adhesion molecule ligands, and other interventions including antisense oligonucleotides to overcome adhesion-molecule-mediated disease (Buckley, 1996; Gonzalez-Amaro, 1998).

Perspectives

Complement, cytokines, and adhesion molecules all play a role in disease states. In recognition of this, therapies have been designed to directly trigger or block various cytokines and complement components as part of the treatment of disease. The recent introduction of chimeric monoclonal antibodies designed to block or advantageously trigger these components (i.e., rituximab, daclizumab, infliximab, etanercept, and others) marks the beginning of what may become a routine means of treating or ameliorating disease. The clinical laboratory detection and measurement of the native proteins and the clinically administered therapeutic agent will become increasingly commonplace.

References

Agnello V: Lupus diseases associated with hereditary and acquired deficiencies of complement. Springer Semin Immunopathol 1986; 9:161.

Ahearn JM, Rosengard AM: Complement receptors. *In* Volanakis JE, Frank MM (eds): The Human Complement System in Health and Disease, New York, Marcel Dekker, 1998, p 167.

Ambrus JL, Jr, Pippin J, Joseph A, et al: Identification of a cDNA for a human high-molecular-weight B-cell growth factor. Proc Natl Acad Sci USA 1993; 90: 6330–6334.

Anderson DM, Johnson L, Glaccum MB, et al: Chromosomal assignment and genomic structure of Il15. Genomics 1995; 25:701–706.

Armitage RJ, Macduff BM, Eisenman J, et al: IL-15 has stimulatory activity for the induction of B cell proliferation and differentiation. J Immunol 1995; 154:483–490.

Atkinson JP: Complement activation and complement receptors in systemic lupus erythematosus. Springer Semin Immunopathol 1986; 9:179.

Baldwin WM, Pruitt SK, Brauer RB, et al: Complement in organ transplantation. Transplantation 1995; 59:797.

Basta M, Dalakas MC: High-dose intravenous immunoglobulin exerts its beneficial effect in patients with dermatomyositis by blocking endomysial deposition of activated complement fragments. J Clin Invest 1994; 94:1729.

Basta M, Kirshbom P, Frank MM, et al: Mechanism of therapeutic effect of high-dose intravenous immunoglobulin. Attenuation of acute, complement-dependent immune damage in a guinea pig model. J Clin Invest 1989; 84:1974.

Batjay Z, Speth C, Erdei A, Dierich MP: Cutting edge: productive HIV-1 infection of dendritic cells via complement receptor type 3 (CR3, CD11b/CD18). J Immunol 2004; 173:4775–4778.

Benzaquen LR, Nicholson-Weller A, Halperin JA: Terminal complement proteins C5b-9 release basic fibroblast growth factor and platelet-derived growth factor from endothelial cells. J Exp Med 1994; 179:985.

Berge V, Johnson E, Hogasen K: Clusterin and the terminal complement pathway synthesised by human umbilical vein endothelial cells are closely linked when on co-cultured agarose beads. APMIS 1997; 105:17.

Beutler B, Greenwald D, Hulmes JD, et al: Identity of tumour necrosis factor and the macrophage-secreted factor cachectin. Nature 1985; 316:552–554.

Bhakdi S, Tranum Jensen J: Complement lysis: a hole is a hole. Immunol Today 1991; 12:318.

Biesecker G, Lavin L, Ziskind M, et al: Cutaneous localization of the membrane attack complex in discoid and systemic lupus erythematosus. N Engl J Med 1982; 306:264.

Birmingham DJ: Erythrocyte complement receptors: Crit Rev Immunol 1995; 15:133.

Blalock WL, Weinstein-Oppenheimer C, Chang F, et al: Signal transduction, cell cycle regulatory, and anti-apoptotic pathways regulated by IL-3 in hematopoietic cells: possible sites for intervention with anti-neoplastic drugs. Leukemia 1999; 13:1109–1166.

Blumberg H, Conklin D, Xu WF, et al: Interleukin 20: discovery, receptor identification, and role in epidermal function. Cell 2001; 104:9–19.

Boackle SA, Morris MA, Holers VM, et al: Complement opsonization is required for presentation of immune complexes by resting peripheral blood B cells. J Immunol 1998; 161:6537.

Boes M, Prodeus AP, Schmidt T, et al: A critical role of natural immunoglobulin M in immediate defense against systemic bacterial infection. J Exp Med 1998; 188:2381.

Bolinger AM, Taeubel MA: Recombinant interferon gamma for treatment of chronic granulomatous disease and other disorders. Clin Pharmacol 1992; 11:834–850.

Borsos T, Rapp HJ: Complement fixation on cell surfaces by 19S and 7S antibodies. Science 1965; 150:505.

Bosco M, Giovarelli M, Forni M, et al: Low doses of IL-4 injected perilymphatically in tumor-bearing mice inhibit the growth of poorly and apparently nonimmunogenic tumors and induce a tumor-specific immune memory. J Immunol 1990; 145:3136–3143.

Bossuyt X, Sneyers L, Marien G, Vranken G: Novel nephelometric assay for measurement of complement 3d. Ann Clin Biochem 2002; 39:34–38.

Böttger EC, Hoffman T, Hadding U, et al: Influence of genetically inherited complement deficiencies on humoral immune response in guinea pigs. J Immunol 1985; 135:4100.

Brown EJ: Complement receptors and phagocytosis. Curr Opin Immunol 1991; 3:76.

Brown MA, Hural J: Functions of IL-4 and control of its expression. Crit Rev Immunol 1997; 17:1–32.

Buckley TL, Bloemen PG, Henricks PA, et al: LFA-1 and ICAM-1 are crucial for the induction of hyperreactivity in the mouse airways. Ann NY Acad Sci 1996; 796:149–161.

Bullard DC, Kunkel EJ, Kubo H, et al: Infectious susceptibility and severe deficiency of leukocyte rolling and recruitment in E-selectin and P-selectin double mutant mice. J Exp Med 1996; 183:2329–2336.

Burd PR, Thompson WC, Max EE, Mills FC: Activated mast cells produce interleukin 13. J Exp Med 1995; 181:1373–1380.

Burton JD, Bamford RN, Peters C, et al: A lymphokine, provisionally designated interleukin T and produced by a human adult T-cell leukemia line, stimulates T-cell proliferation and the induction of lymphokine-activated killer cells. Proc Natl Acad Sci USA 1994; 91:4935–4939.

Carpagnano GE, Resta O, Foschino-Barbaro MP, et al: Interleukin-6 is increased in breath condensate of patients with non-small cell lung cancer. Int J Biol Markers 2002; 17:141–145.

Carroll MC: The role of complement and complement receptors in induction and regulation of immunity. Annu Rev Immunol 1998a; 16:545.

Carroll MC: The complement system in regulation of adaptive immunity. Nat Immunol 2004; 5:981–986.
This article describes the intricate interaction that exists between complement activation products and T and B cell responses, and the nature of the link that exists between the innate and adaptive immune responses.

Carroll MC, Prodeus AP: Linkages of innate and adaptive immunity. Curr Opin Immunol 1998b; 10:36.

Carson WE, Ross ME, Baiocchi RA, et al: Endogenous production of interleukin 15 by activated human monocytes is critical for optimal production of interferon-gamma by natural killer cells in vitro. J Clin Invest 1995; 96:2578–2582.

Caudell EG, Mumm JB, Poindexter N, et al: The protein product of the tumor suppressor gene, melanoma differentiation-associated gene 7, exhibits immunostimulatory activity and is designated IL-24. J Immunol 2002; 168:6041–6046.

Center DM, Cruikshank W: Modulation of lymphocyte migration by human lymphokines. I. Identification and characterization of chemoattractant activity for lymphocytes from mitogen-stimulated mononuclear cells. Immunol 1982; 128:2563–2568.

Chen C-H, Lam CK, Boackle RJ: C1 inhibitor removes the entire $C1qr_2s_2$ complex from anti-C1Q monoclonal antibodies with low binding affinities. Immunology 1998; 95:648.

Cherel M, Sorel M, Apiou F, et al: The human interleukin-11 receptor alpha gene (IL11RA): genomic organization and chromosome mapping. Genomics 1996; 32:49–53.

Chiang CS, Powell HC, Gold LH, et al: Macrophage/microglial-mediated primary demyelination and motor disease induced by the central nervous system production of interleukin-3 in transgenic mice. J Clin Invest 1996; 97:1512–1524.

Choi N-H, Mazda T, Tomita M: A serum protein, SP-40,40, modulates the formation of the membrane attack complex of complement on erythrocytes. Mol Immunol 1989; 26:835.

Christiansen OB, Kilpatrick DC, Souter V, et al: Mannan-binding lectin deficiency is associated with unexplained recurrent miscarriage. Scand J Immunol 1999; 49:193.

Colten HR, Garnier G: Regulation of complement protein gene expression. In Volanakis JE, Frank MM

(eds): The Human Complement System in Health and Disease, New York, Marcel Dekker, 1998, p 217.

Cooper NR: Complement and viruses. In Volanakis JE, Frank MM (eds): The Human Complement System in Health and Disease. New York, Marcel Dekker, 1998, p 393.

Cornacoff JB, Hebert LA, Smead WL, et al: Primate erythrocyte-immune complex-clearing mechanism. J Clin Invest 1983; 71:236.

Cosman D, Kumaki S, Ahdieh M, et al: Interleukin-15 and its receptor. Ciba Foundation Symposium 1995; 195:221–229.

Couser WG, Johnson RJ, Young BA, et al: The effects of soluble complement receptor type 1 on complement-mediated experimental glomerulonephritis. J Am Soc Nephrol 1995; 5:1888.

Crawford DH, Catovsky D: In vitro activation of leukaemic B cells by interleukin-4 and antibodies to CD40. Immunology 1993; 80:40–44.

Cruikshank WW, Center DM, Nisar N, et al: Molecular and functional analysis of a lymphocyte chemoattractant factor: association of biologic function with CD4 expression. Proc Natl Acad Sci USA 1994; 91:5109–5113.

Czermak BJ, Sarma V, Pierson CL, et al: Protective effects of C5a blockade in sepsis. Nat Med 1999; 5:788.

Czupryn MJ, McCoy JM, Scoble HA: Structure–function relationships in human interleukin-11. Identification of regions involved in activity by chemical modification and site-directed mutagenesis. J Biol Chem 1995; 270:978–985.

Daha MR, Fearon DT, Austen KF: C3 nephritic factor (C3NeF): stabilization of fluid phase and cell-bound alternative pathway convertase. J Immunol 1976; 116:1.

Daha MR, van Es LA: Further evidence for the antibody nature of C3 nephritic factor (C3NeF). J Immunol 1979; 123:755.

Dalmasso AP: The complement system in xenotransplantation. Immunopharmacology 1992; 24:149.

Dalrymple SA, Slattery R, Aud DM, et al: Interleukin-6 is required for a protective immune response to systemic Escherichia coli infection. Infect Immun 1996; 64:3231–3235.

Davis AE, III: Biological effects of C1 inhibitor. Drug News Perspect 2004; 17:439–446.

Davis AE III, Harrison RA: Structural characterization of factor I mediated cleavage of the third component of complement. Biochemistry 1982; 21:5745.

De Bont ES, Vellenga E, Swaanenburg JC, et al: Plasma IL-8 and IL-6 levels can be used to define a group with low risk of septicaemia among cancer patients with fever and neutropenia. Br J Haematol 1999; 107:375–380.

De Vita F, Orditura M, Galizia G, et al: Serum interleukin-10 levels in patients with advanced gastrointestinal malignancies. Cancer 1999; 86:1936–1943.

De Vita F, Orditura M, Galizia G, et al: Serum interleukin-10 levels as a prognostic factor in advanced non-small cell lung cancer patients. Chest 2000; 117:365–373.

De Vries JE: The role of IL-13 and its receptor in allergy and inflammatory responses. J Allergy Clin Immunol 1998; 102:165–169.

Demoulin JB, Renauld JC: Interleukin-9 and its receptor: an overview of structure and function. Int Rev Immunol 1998; 16:245–364.

Derynck R, Zhang Y: Intracellular signaling: the mad way to do it. Curr Biol 1996; 63:1226–1229.

DiScipio RG, Daffern PN, Jagels MA, et al: A comparison of C3a and C5a-mediated stable adhesion and rolling eosinophils in postcapillary venules and transendothelial migration in vitro and in vivo. J Immunol 1999; 162:1127.

Dodds AW, Sim RB (eds): Complement. A practical approach. Oxford, IRL Press, 1997.

Doekes G, Es LA, Daha MR: C1 inactivator: its efficiency as a regulator of classical complement pathway activation on soluble IgG aggregates. Immunology 1983; 49:215.

Doepper S, Kacani L, Falkensammer B, et al: Complement receptors in HIV infection. Curr Mol Med 2002; 2:703–711.

Du X, Williams DA: Update on development of interleukin-11. Curr Opin Hematol 1995; 2:182–188.

Dumoutier L, Leemans C, Lejeune D, et al: Cutting edge: STAT activation by IL-19, IL-20 and mda-7 through IL-20 receptor complexes of two types. J Immunol 2001; 167:3545–3549.

Dwyer JM: Manipulating the immune system with immune globulin. N Engl J Med 1992; 326:107.

Edwards JL, Brown EJ, Ault KA, Apicella MA: The role of complement receptor 3 (CR3) in *Neisseria gonorrhoeae* infection of human cervical epithelia. Cell Microbiol 2001; 3:611–622.

Einarsson O, Geba GP, Zhu Z, et al: Interleukin-11: stimulation in vivo and in vitro by respiratory viruses and induction of airways hyperresponsiveness. J Clin Invest 1996; 97:915–924.

Eklund KK, Ghildyal N, Austen KF, Stevens RL: Induction by IL-9 and suppression by IL-3 and IL-4 of the levels of chromosome 14-derived transcripts that encode late-expressed mouse mast cell proteases. J Immunol 1993; 151:4266–4273.

Ember JA, Engels MA, Hugli TE: Characterization of complement anaphylatoxins and their biological responses. *In* Volanakis JE, Frank MM (eds): The Human Complement System in Health and Disease. New York, Marcel Dekker, 1998, p 241.

Emmanuilidis K, Weighardt H, Matevossian E, et al: Differential regulation of systemic IL-18 and IL-12 release during postoperative sepsis: high serum IL-18 as an early predictive indicator of lethal outcome. Shock 2002; 18:301–305.

Epstein J, Eichbaum Q, Sheriff S, et al: The collectins in innate immunity. Curr Opin Immunol 1996; 8:29.

Erard F, Wild MT, Garcia-Sanz JA, Le Gros G: Switch of CD8 T cells to noncytolytic CD8–CD4 cells that make TH2 cytokines and help B cells. Science 1993; 260:1802–1805.

Esser AF: Big Mac attack: complement proteins cause leaky patches. Immunol Today 1991; 12:316.

Evans MJ, Rollins SA, Wolff DW, et al: In vitro and in vivo inhibition of complement activity by a single-chain Fv fragment recognizing human C5. Mol Immunol 1995; 32:1183.

Falk RJ, Dalmasso AP, Kim Y, et al: Neoantigen of the polymerized ninth component of complement: characterization of a monoclonal antibody and immunohistochemical localization in renal disease. J Clin Invest 1983; 72:560.

Fearon DT: The alternative pathway of complement: a system for host resistance to microbial infection. N Engl J Med 1980; 303:259.

Fearon DT: The complement system and adaptive immunity. Semin Immunol 1998; 10:355.

Fearon DT, Austen KF: Properdin: binding to C3b and stabilization of the C3b-dependent C3 convertase. J Exp Med 1975; 142:856.

Fingeroth JD, Weiss JJ, Tedder TF, et al: Epstein Barr virus receptor of human B lymphocytes is the C3d receptor CR2. Proc Natl Acad Sci USA 1984; 81:4510.

Finkelman FD, Katona IM, Urban JF Jr, et al: Suppression of in vivo polyclonal IgE responses by monoclonal antibody to the lymphokine B-cell stimulatory factor 1. Proc Natl Acad Sci USA 1986; 83:9675–9678.

Fiorentino DF, Bond MW, Mosmann TR. Two types of mouse T helper cell. IV. Th2 clones secrete a factor that inhibits cytokine production by Th1 clones. J Exp Med 1989; 170:2081–2095.

Fischer JR, Schindel M, Bulzebruck H, et al: Long-term survival in small cell lung cancer patients is correlated with high interleukin-2 secretion at diagnosis. J Cancer Res Clin Oncol 2000; 126:730–733.

Fischer M, Bijman M, Molin D, et al: Increased serum levels of interleukin-9 correlate to negative prognostic factors in Hodgkin's lymphoma. Leukemia 2003; 17:2513–2516.

Fishelson Z: Complement-related proteins in pathogenic organisms. Springer Semin Immunopathol 1994; 15:345.

Fleming SD, Campbell PA: Macrophages have cell surface IL-10 that regulates macrophage bactericidal activity. J Immunol 1996; 156:1143–1150.

Fort MM, Cheung J, Yen D, et al: IL-25 induces IL-4, IL-5, and IL-13 and Th2-associated pathologies in vivo. Immunity 2001; 15:985–995.

Fossiez F, Djossou O, Chomarat P, et al: T cell interleukin-17 induces stromal cells to produce proinflammatory and hematopoietic cytokines. J Exp Med 1996; 183:2593–2603.

Frank MM: Introduction and historical notes. *In* Volanakis JE, Frank MM (eds): The Human Complement System in Health and Disease. New York, Marcel Dekker, 1998, p 1.

Frank MM, Basta M, Fries LF: The effects of intravenous immune globulin on complement-dependent immune damage of cells and tissues. Clin Immunol Immunopathol 1992; 62:S82.

Frank MM, Fries LF: The role of complement in defence against bacterial disease. Baillière's Clin Immunol Allergy 1988; 2:335.

Franz AR, Bauer K, Schalk A, et al: Measurement of interleukin 8 in combination with C-reactive protein reduced unnecessary antibiotic therapy in newborn infants: a multicenter, randomized, controlled trial. Pediatrics 2004; 114:1–8.

Franz AR, Steinbach G, Kron M, Pohlandt F: Interleukin-8: a valuable tool to restrict antibiotic therapy in newborn infants. Acta Paediatr 2001; 90:1025–1032.

Fries LF, Frank MM: Molecular mechanisms of complement action. *In* Stamatoyannopoulos G, Nienhuis AW, Leder P, Majerus PW (eds): The Molecular Basis of Blood Diseases. Philadelphia, WB Saunders, 1987, p 450.

Fuhrer DK, Yang YC: Activation of Src-family protein tyrosine kinases and phosphatidylinositol 3-kinase in 3T3-L1 mouse preadipocytes by interleukin-11. Exp Hematol 1996; 24:195–203.

Fujisawa T, Abu-Ghazaleh R, Kita H, et al: Regulatory effect of cytokines on eosinophil degranulation. J Immunol 1990; 144:642–646.

Fujishima H, Takeuchi T, Shinozaki N, et al: Measurement of IL-4 in tears of patients with seasonal allergic conjunctivitis and vernal keratoconjunctivitis. Clin Exp Immunol 1995; 102:395–398.

Furst DE, Schiff MH, Fleischmann RM, et al: Adalimumab, a fully human anti tumor necrosis factor-alpha monoclonal antibody, and concomitant standard antirheumatic therapy for the treatment of rheumatoid arthritis: results of STAR (Safety Trial of Adalimumab in Rheumatoid Arthritis). J Rheumatol 2003; 30:2563–2571.

Gaither TA, Hammer CH, Frank MM: Studies of the molecular mechanisms of C3b inactivation and a simplified assay of 1H and the C3b inactivator (C3bINA). J Immunol 1979; 123:1195.

Gallagher G, Dickensheets H, Eskdale J, et al: Cloning, expression and initial characterization of interleukin-19 (IL-19), a novel homologue of human interleukin-10 (IL-10). Genes Immun 2000; 1:442–450.

Gallagher G, Eskdale J, Jordan W, et al: Human interleukin-19 and its receptor: a potential role in the induction of Th2 responses. Int Immunopharmacol 2004; 4:615–626.

Gammon WR, Inman AO, Wheeler CE Jr: Differences in complement-dependent chemotactic activity generated by bullous pemphigoid and epidermolysis bullosa acquisita immune complexes: demonstration by leukocytic attachment and organ culture methods. J Invest Dermatol 1984; 83:57.

Gavett SH, O'Hearn DJ, Li X, et al: Interleukin 12 inhibits antigen-induced airway hyperresponsiveness, inflammation, and Th2 cytokine expression in mice. J Exp Med 1995; 182:1527–1536.

Gawryl MS, Chudwin DS, Langlois PF, Lint TF: The terminal complement complex, C5b-9, a marker of disease activity in patients with systemic lupus erythematosus. Arthritis Rheum 1988; 31:188.

Gewurz H, Jiang H, Ying S-C, et al: Nonimmune activation of the classical complement pathway. Behring Inst Mitt 1993; 93:138.

Giclas PC (ed.): Complement, immune complexes, and cryoglobulin. *In* Rose NR, Conway de Macario E, Folds JD, et al (eds): Manual of Clinical Laboratory Immunology, 5th ed. Washington, DC, ASM Press, 1997, p 179.

Gigli I, Fujita T, Nussenzweig V: Modulation of the classical pathway C3 convertase by plasma proteins C4b-binding protein and C3b inactivator. Proc Natl Acad Sci USA 1979; 76:6596.

Goldman M, Velu T, Petrolani M: Interleukin-10. Actions and therapeutic potentials. Biodrugs 1997; 7:6–14.

Gomez J, Gonzalez A, Martinez A: Rebollo A: IL-2-induced cellular events. Crit Rev Immunol 1998; 18:185–220.

Gonzalez-Amaro R, Diaz-Gonzalez F, Sanchez-Madrid F: Adhesion molecules in inflammatory diseases. Drugs 1998; 56:977–988.

This article provides an excellent and in-depth review of the process of leukocyte diapedesis. Pharmacologic therapeutic blocking of this process is discussed.

Gonzalez-Amaro R, Sanchez-Madrid F: Cell adhesion molecules: selectins and integrins. Crit Rev Immunol 1999; 19:389–429.

Grabstein KH, Eisenman J, Shanebeck K, et al: Cloning of a T cell growth factor that interacts with the beta chain of the interleukin-2 receptor. Science 1994; 264:965–968.

Grzegorzewski K, Komschlies KL, Mori M, et al: Administration of recombinant human interleukin-7 to mice induces the exportation of myeloid progenitor cells from the bone marrow to peripheral sites. Blood 1994; 83:377–385.

Ha SJ, Kim DJ, Baek KH, et al: IL-23 induces stronger sustained CTL and Th1 immune responses than IL-12 in hepatitis C virus envelope protein 2 DNA immunization. J Immunol 2004; 172:525–531.

Hammerschmidt D, Weaver L, Hudson L, et al: Association of complement activation and elevated plasma-C5a with adult respiratory distress syndrome. Lancet 1980; 1:947.

Hansen S, Holmskov U: Structural aspects of collectins and receptors for collectins. Immunobiology 1998; 199:165.

Harrison RA, Lachman PJ: Complement technology. *In* Weir DM, Herzenberg LA, Blackwell C (eds): Handbook of Experimental Immunology, 4th ed. Oxford, Blackwell Scientific, 1986, p 39.1.

Hechtman DH, Cybulsky MI, Fuchs HJ, et al: Intravascular IL-8. Inhibitor of polymorphonuclear leukocyte accumulation at sites of acute inflammation. J Immunol 1991; 147:883–892.

Hermann E, Fleischer B, Mayet WJ, et al: Correlation of synovial fluid interleukin 6 (IL-6) activities with IgG concentrations in patients with inflammatory joint disease and osteoarthritis. Clin Exp Rheumatol 1989; 7:411–414.

Heufler C, Koch F, Stanzl U, et al: Interleukin-12 is produced by dendritic cells and mediates T helper 1 development as well as interferon-gamma production by T helper 1 cells. Eur J Immunol 1996; 26:659–668.

Hibberd ML, Sumiya M, Summerfield JA, et al: Association of variants of the gene for mannose-binding lectin with susceptibility to meningococcal disease. Lancet 1999; 353:1049.

Hirano T: Interleukin 6 (IL-6) and its receptor: their role in plasma cell neoplasias. Int J Cell Cloning 1991; 9:166–184.

Hirano T: Interleukin 6 and its receptor: ten years later. Int Rev Immunol 1998; 16:249–284.

Hirano T, Matsuda T, Turner M, et al: Excessive production of interleukin 6/B cell stimulatory factor-2 in rheumatoid arthritis. Eur J Immunol 1988; 18:1797–1801.

Hirano T, Yasukawa K, Harada H, et al: Complementary DNA for a novel human interleukin (BSF-2) that induces B lymphocytes to produce immunoglobulin. Nature 1986; 324:73–76.

Hoch RC, Schraufstatter IU, Cochrane CG: In vivo, in vitro and molecular aspects of IL-8 and the IL-8 receptors. Lab Clin Med 1996; 128:134–145.

Hohmann HP, Remy R, Brockhaus M, van Loon AP: Two different cell types have different major receptors for human tumor necrosis factor (TNF alpha). J Biol Chem 1989; 264:14927–14934.

Hor S, Pirzer H, Dumoutier L, et al: The T-cell lymphokine interleukin-26 targets epithelial cells through the interleukin-20 receptor 1 and interleukin-10 receptor 2 chains. J Biol Chem 2004; 279:33343–33351.

Hosoi T, Wada S, Suzuki S, et al: Bacterial endotoxin induces IL-20 expression in the glial cells. Brain Res Mol Brain Res 2004; 130:23–29.

Houssiau FA, Schandene L, Stevens M, et al: A cascade of cytokines is responsible for IL-9 expression in human T cells. Involvement of IL-2, IL-4, and IL-10. J Immunol 1995; 154:2624–2630.

Hrvacevic R, Dimitrijevic D, Spasic P, et al: [Interleukin-1 beta in patients with primary immunocomplex glomerulonephritis]. Vojnosanit Pregl 2001; 58:33–38.

Hu JP, Cesano A, Santoli D, et al: Effects of interleukin-11 on the proliferation and cell cycle status of myeloid leukemic cells. Blood 1993; 81:1586–1592.

Huang AJ, Manning JE, Bandak TM, et al: Endothelial cell cytosolic free calcium regulates neutrophil migration across monolayers of endothelial cells. J Cell Biol 1993; 120:1371–1380.

Hunter CA, Villarino A, Artis D, Scott P: The role of IL-27 in the development of T-cell responses during parasitic infections. Immunol Rev 2004; 202:106–114.

Hurst SD, Muchamuel T, Gorman DM, et al: New IL-17 family members promote Th1 or Th2 responses in the lung: in vivo function of the novel cytokine IL-25. J Immunol 2002; 169:443–453.

Ihle JN, Lee JC, Rebar L: T cell recognition of Moloney leukemia virus proteins. III. T cell proliferative responses against gp70 are associated with the production of a lymphokine inducing 20 alpha-hydroxysteroid dehydrogenase in splenic lymphocytes. J Immunol 1981; 127:2565–2570.

Iizumi T, Sato S, Iiyama T, et al: Recombinant human interleukin-1 beta analogue as a regulator of hematopoiesis in patients receiving chemotherapy for urogenital cancers. Cancer 1991; 68:1520–1523.

IUIS-WHO Nomenclature Committee: nomenclature of the alternative activating pathway of complement. J Immunol 1981; 127:1261.

Jacobsohn DA, Vogelsang GB: Novel pharmacotherapeutic approaches to prevention and treatment of GVHD. Drugs 2002; 62:879–889.

Although specifically addressing GVHD, this article provides insight into the pharmacologic blocking and regulating of the cytokine response.

Jacobsohn DA, Vogelsang GB: Anti-cytokine therapy for the treatment of graft-versus-host disease. Curr Pharm Des 2004; 10:1195–1205.

Jarva H, Meri S: Paroxysmal nocturnal haemoglobimuria: the disease and a hypothesis for a new treatment. Scand J Immunol 1999; 49:119.

Johnson E, Berge V, Hogasen K: Formation of the terminal complex on agarose beads: further evidence that vitronectin (complement S-protein) inhibits C9 polymerization. Scand J Immunol 1994; 39:281.

Johnston JA, Bacon CM, Finbloom DS, et al: Tyrosine phosphorylation and activation of STAT5, STAT3, and Janus kinases by interleukins 2 and 15. Proc Natl Acad Sci USA 1995; 92:8705–8709.

Kallio R, Surcel HM, Bloigu A, Syrjala H: Balance between interleukin-10 and interleukin-12 in adult cancer patients with or without infections. Eur J Cancer 2001; 37:857–861.

Keegan AD, Ryan JJ, Paul WE: IL-4 regulates growth and differentiation by distinct mechanisms. Immunologist 1996; 4:194–198.

Keith JCJ, Albert L, Sonis ST, et al: IL-11, a pleiotropic cytokine: exciting new effects of IL-11 on gastrointestinal mucosal biology. Stem Cells 1994; 12:79–84.

Kerekes K, Prechl J, Bajtay Z, et al: A further link between innate and adaptive immunity: C3 deposition on antigen-presenting cells enhances the proliferation of antigen-specific T cells. Int Immunol 1998; 10:1923.

Khanna AK, Plummer MS, Hilton G, et al: Anti-transforming growth factor antibody at low but not high doses limits cyclosporine-mediated nephrotoxicity without altering rat cardiac allograft survival: potential of therapeutic applications. Circulation 2004; 110:3822–3829.

Kilgore KS, Flory CM, Miller BF, et al: The membrane attack complex of complement induces interleukin-8 and monocyte chemoattractant protein-1 secretion from human umbilical vein endothelial cells. Am J Pathol 1996; 149:953.

Kilgore KS, Park JL, Tanhehco EJ, et al: Attenuation of interleukin-8 expression in C6-deficient rabbits after myocardial ischemia/reperfusion. J Mol Cell Cardiol 1998; 30:75.

Kilpatrick DC: Mannan-binding lectin: clinical significance and applications. Biochim Biophys Acta 2002; 1572:401–413.

Kim JM, Brannan CI, Copeland NG, et al: Structure of the mouse IL-10 gene and chromosomal localization of the mouse and human genes. J Immunol 1992; 148:3618–3623.

Kingo K, Koks S, Nikopensius T, et al: Polymorphisms in the interleukin-20 gene: relationships to plaque-type psoriasis. Genes Immun 2004; 5:117–121.

Kinoshita T, Takata Y, Kozono H, et al: C5 convertase of the alternative complement pathway: Covalent linkage between two C3b molecules within the trimolecular complex enzyme. J Immunol 1988; 141:3895.

Kirman I, Vainer B, Nielsen OH: Interleukin-15 and its role in chronic inflammatory diseases. Inflamm Res 1998; 47:285–289.

Kirschfink M, Mollnes TE: C1-inhibitor: an anti-inflammatory reagent with therapeutic potential. Expert Opin Pharmacother 2001; 2:1073–1083.

Klickstein LB, Barbashov SF, Liu T, et al: Complement receptor type 1 (CR1, CD35) is a receptor for C1q. Immunity 1997; 7:345.

Koks S, Kingo K, Ratsep R, et al: Combined haplotype analysis of the interleukin-19 and -20 genes: relationship to plaque-type psoriasis. Genes Immun 2004; 5:662–667.

Kollias G, Douni E, Kassiotis G, Kontoyiannis D: The function of tumour necrosis factor and receptors in models of multi-organ inflammation, rheumatoid arthritis, multiple sclerosis and inflammatory bowel disease. Ann Rheum Dis 1999; 58(Suppl 1):132–139.

Korb LC, Ahearn JM: C1q binds directly and specifically to surface blebs of apoptotic human keratinocytes. J Immunol 1997; 158:4525.

Koski CL, Ramm LE, Hammer CH, et al: Cytolysis of nucleated cells by complement: cell death displays multi-hit characteristics. Proc Natl Acad Sci USA 1983; 80:3816.

Kovacs GG, Gasque P, Strobel T, et al: Complement activation in human prion disease. Neurobiol Dis 2004; 15:21–28.

Kozel TR: Activation of the complement system by pathogenic fungi. Clin Microbiol Rev 1996; 9:34.

Kozin F, Cochrane CH: The contact activation system of plasma: biochemistry and pathophysiology. *In* Gallin JI, Goldstein IM, Snyderman R (eds): Inflammation: Basic Principles and Clinical Correlates, 2nd ed. New York, Raven Press, 1992, p 103.

Kroshus TJ, Rollins SA, Dalmasso AP, et al: Inhibition with an anti-C5 monoclonal antibody prevents acute cardiac tissue injury in an ex vivo model of pig-to-human xenotransplantation. Transplantation 1995; 60:1194.

Kuipers S, Aerts PC, Sjoholm AG, et al: A hemolytic assay for the estimation of functional mannose-binding lectin levels in human serum. J Immunol Methods 2002; 268:149–157.

Kuster H, Weiss M, Willeitner AE, et al: Interleukin-1 receptor antagonist and interleukin-6 for early diagnosis of neonatal sepsis 2 days before clinical manifestation. Lancet 1998; 352:1271–1277.

Lalani I, Bhol K, Ahmed AR: Interleukin-10: biology, role in inflammation and autoimmunity. Ann Allergy Asthma Immunol 1997; 79:469–483.

Lalani T, Simmons RK, Ahmed AR: Biology of IL-5 in health and disease. Ann Allergy Asthma Immunol 1999; 82:317–332.

Langlois PF, Gawryl MS: Complement activation occurs through both classical and alternative pathways prior to onset and resolution of adult respiratory distress syndrome. Clin Immunol Immunopathol 1988; 47:152.

Langrish CL, McKenzie BS, Wilson NJ, et al: IL-12 and IL-23: master regulators of innate and adaptive immunity. Immunol Rev 2004; 202:96–105.

Law SK, Lichtenberg NA, Levine RP: Evidence for an ester linkage between the labile binding site of C3b and receptive surfaces. J Immunol 1979; 123:1388.

Lemoli RM, Fogli M, Fortuna A, et al: Interleukin-11 (IL-11) acts as a synergistic factor for the proliferation of human myeloid leukaemic cells. Br J Haematol 1995; 91:319–326.

Leonaviciene L, Bradunaite R, Astrauskas V: [Proinflammatory cytokine interleukin-17 and its role in pathogenesis of rheumatoid arthritis]. Medicina (Kaunas) 2004; 40:419–422.

Liao SC, Cheng YC, Wang YC, et al: IL-19 induced Th2 cytokines and was up-regulated in asthma patients. J Immunol 2004; 173:6712–6718.

Licht C, Weyersberg A, Heinen S, et al: Successful plasma therapy for atypical hemolytic uremic syndrome caused by factor H deficiency owing to a novel mutation in the complement cofactor protein domain 15. Am J Kidney Dis 2005; 45:415–421.

Lim BL, Reid KBM, Ghebrehiwet B, et al: The binding protein for globular heads of complement C1q, gC1qR. Functional expression and characterization as a novel vitronectin binding factor. J Biol Chem 1996; 271:26739.

Link E, Kerr LD, Schreck R, et al: Purified I kappa B-beta is inactivated upon dephosphorylation. J Biol Chem 1992; 267:239–246.

Liu L, Ding C, Zeng W, et al: Selective enhancement of multipotential hematopoietic progenitors in vitro and in vivo by IL-20. Blood 2003; 102:3206–3209.

Liu CC, Manzi S, Danchenko N, Ahearn JM: New advances in measurement of complement activation: lessons of systemic lupus erythematosus. Curr Rheumatol Rep 2004; 6:375–381.

Lo CH, Lee SC, Wu PY, et al: Antitumor and antimetastatic activity of IL-23. J Immunol 2003; 171:600–607.

Lopez-Casillas F, Wrana JL, Massague J: Betaglycan presents ligand to the TGF beta signaling receptor. Cell 1993; 73:1435–1444.

Louahed J, Kermouni A, Van Snick J, Renauld JC: IL-9 induces expression of granzymes and high-affinity IgE receptor in murine T helper clones. J Immunol 1995; 154:5061–5070.

Lucchesi BR, Kilgore KS: Complement inhibitors in myocardial ischemia/reperfusion injury. Immunopharmacology 1997; 38:27.

Lutz HU: How pre-existing, germline-derived antibodies and complement may help induce a primary immune response to nonself. Scand J Immunol 1999; 49:224.

Mabbott NA: The complement system in prion diseases. Curr Opin Immunol 2004; 16:587–593.

McCartney-Francis NL, Frazier-Jessen M, Wahl SM: TGF-beta: aA balancing act. Int Rev Immunol 1998; 16:553–580.

Mach N, Lantz CS, Galli SJ, et al: Involvement of interleukin-3 in delayed-type hypersensitivity. Blood 1998; 91:778–783.

McInnes IB, al Mughales J, Field M, et al: The role of interleukin-15 in T-cell migration and activation in rheumatoid arthritis. Nat Med 1996; 2:175–182.

Magee JC, Collins BH, Harland RC, et al: Immunoglobulin prevents complement-mediated hyperacute rejection in swine-to-primate xenotransplantation. J Clin Invest 1995; 96:2404.

Makrides SC: Therapeutic inhibition of the complement system. Pharmacol Rev 1998; 50:59.

Malhotra R, Wormald MR, Rudd PM, et al: Glycosylation changes of IgG associated with rheumatoid arthritis can activate complement via tha mannose-binding protein. Nat Med 1995; 1:237.

Margolius HS: Kallikreins and kinins. Some unanswered questions about system characteristics and roles in human disease. Hypertension 1995; 26:221.

Marom Z, Shelhammer J, Berger M, et al: Anaphylatoxin C3a enhances mucous glycoprotein release from human airways in vitro. J Exp Med 1985; 161:657.

Matsushita M, Endo Y, Fujita T: MASP (MBL-associated serine protease 1). Immunobiology 1998; 199:340.

Matsushita M, Fujita T: Inhibition of mannose-binding protein-associated serine protease (MASP) by C1 inhibitor (C1 INH). Mol Immunol 1996; 33:44.

Mauff G, Würzner R: Complement genetics. In Herzenberg LA, Weir DM, Blackwell C (eds): Weir's Handbook of Experimental Immunology, 5th ed, vol 2. Malden, MA, Blackwell Science, 1996, p 77.1.

Mayer MM: Complement and complement fixation. In Kabat EA, Mayer MM (eds): Experimental Immunochemistry, 2nd ed. Springfield, IL, Charles C Thomas, 1961, p 133.

Mayes JT, Schreiber RD, Cooper NR: Development and application of an enzyme-linked immunoabsorbent assay for the quantification of alternative complement pathway activation in human serum. J Clin Invest 1984; 73:160.

Mayumi T, Takezawa J, Takahashi H, et al: IL-15 is elevated in the patients of postoperative enterocolitis. Cytokine 1999; 11:888–893.

Mehler MF, Rozental R, Dougherty M, et al: Cytokine regulation of neuronal differentiation of hippocampal progenitor cells. Nature 1993; 362:62–65.

Mehta DS, Wurster AL, Grusby MJ: Biology of IL-21 and the IL-21 receptor. Immunol Rev 2004; 202:84–95.

Merz H, Houssiau FA, Orscheschek K, et al: Interleukin-9 expression in human malignant lymphomas: unique association with Hodgkin's disease and large cell anaplastic lymphoma. Blood 1991; 78:1311–1317.

Metcalf D, Begley CG, Johnson GR, et al: Effects of purified bacterially synthesized murine multi-CSF (IL-3) on hematopoiesis in normal adult mice. Blood 1986; 68:46–57.

Meyaard L, Hovenkamp E, Otto SA, Miedema F: IL-12-induced IL-10 production by human T cells as a negative feedback for IL-12-induced immune responses. J Immunol 1996; 156:2776–2782.

Miletic VD, Hester CG, Frank MM: Regulation of complement activity by immunoglobulin. I. Effect of immunoglobulin isotype on C4 uptake on antibody-sensitized sheep erythrocytes and solid phase immune complexes. J Immunol 1996; 156:749.

Minta JO, Gee AP: Purification and quantitation of the components of the alternative pathway. Methods Enzymol 1983; 93:375–408.

Mitomo K, Fujita T, Iida K: Functional and antigenic properties of complement receptor type 2, CR2. J Exp Med 1987; 165:1424.

Moffitt MC, Frank MM: Complement resistance in microbes. Springer Semin Immunopathol 1994; 15:327.

Mold C: Cellular responses to the membrane attack complex. In Volanakis JE, Frank MM (eds): The Human Complement System in Health and Disease. New York, Marcel Dekker, 1998, p 309.

Mollnes TE: Biocompatibility: complement as mediator of tissue damage and as indicator of incompatibility. Exp Clin Immunogenet 1997; 14:24.

Mollnes TE, Høgasen K, Hoass BF, et al: Inhibition of complement-mediated red cell lysis by immunoglobulins is dependent on the Ig isotype and its C1 binding properties. Scand J Immunol 1995; 41:449.

Moore FD, Fearon DT, Austen KF: IgG on mouse erythrocytes augments activation of the human alternative complement pathway by enhancing deposition of C3b. J Immunol 1981; 126:1805.

Morgan BP: Clinical complementology: recent progress and future trends. Eur J Clin Invest 1994a; 24:219.

Morgan BP, Gasque P: Expression of complement in the brain: role in health and disease. Immunol Today 1996; 17:461.

Morgan BP, Gasque P: Extrahepatic complement biosynthesis: where, when and why? Clin Exp Immunol 1997a; 107:1.

Morgan BP, Gasque P, Singhrao S, et al: The role of complement in disorders of the nervous system. Immunopharmacology 1997b; 38:43.

Morgan BP, Meri S: Membrane proteins that protect against complement lysis. Springer Semin Immunopathol 1994b; 15:369.

Moroz A, Eppolito C, Li Q, et al: IL-21 enhances and sustains CD8+ T cell responses to achieve durable tumor immunity: comparative evaluation of IL-2, IL-15, and IL-21. J Immunol 2004; 173:900–909.

Mulligan MS, Yeh CG, Rudolph AR, et al: Protective effects of soluble CR1 in complement- and neutrophil-mediated tissue injury. J Immunol 1992; 148:1479.

Murphy CA, Langrish CL, Chen Y, et al: Divergent pro- and antiinflammatory roles for IL-23 and IL-12 in joint autoimmune inflammation. J Exp Med 2003; 198:1951–1957.

Nagem RA, Colau D, Dumoutier L, et al: Crystal structure of recombinant human interleukin-22. Structure (Camb) 2002; 10:1051–1062.

Namen AE, Schmierer AE, March CJ, et al: B cell precursor growth-promoting activity. Purification and characterization of a growth factor active on lymphocyte precursors. J Exp Med 1988; 167:988–1002.

Nataf S, Davoust N, Ames RS, et al: Human T cells express the C5a receptor and are chemoattracted to C5a. J Immunol 1999; 162:4018.

Niculescu F, Badea T, Rus H: Sublytic C5b-9 induces proliferation of human aortic smooth muscle cells. Role of mitogen activated protein kinase and phosphatidylinositol 3-kinase. Atherosclerosis 1999; 142:47.

Niculescu F, Rus H, Shin S, et al: Generation of diacylglycerol and ceramide during homologous complement activation. J Immunol 1993; 150:214.

Niculescu F, Rus HG, Vlaicu R: Immunohistochemical localization of C5b-9, S-protein, C3d and apolipoprotein B in human arterial tissues with atherosclerosis. Atherosclerosis 1987; 65:1.

Norgaard P, Hougaard S, Poulson HS, Spang-Thomsen M: Transforming growth factor beta and cancer. Cancer Treat Rev 1995; 21:367–403.

Ochs HD, Wedgwood RJ, Frank MM, et al: The role of complement in the induction of antibody responses. Clin Exp Immunol 1983; 53:208.

Ochs HD, Wedgwood RJ, Heller SR, et al: Complement, membrane glycoproteins, and complement receptors: their role in regulation of the immune response. Clin Immunol Immunopathol 1986; 40:94.

Ollert MW, Davis K, Bredehorst R, et al: Classical complement pathway activation on nucleated cells. Role of factor H in the control of deposited C3b. J Immunol 1995; 155:4955.

O'Neil KM, Ochs HD, Heller SR, et al: Role of C3 in humoral immunity. Defective antibody production in C3-deficient dogs. J Immunol 1988; 140:1939.

Onitsuka S, Yamaguchi Y, Tanabe K, et al: Peritubular capillary deposition of C4d complement fragment in ABO-incompatible renal transplantation with humoral rejection. Clin Transplant 1999; 13 Suppl 1:33–37.

Ozaki K, Spolski R, Ettinger R, et al: Regulation of B cell differentiation and plasma cell generation by IL-21, a novel inducer of Blimp-1 and Bcl-6. J Immunol 2004; 173:5361–5371.

Pangburn MK: Alternative pathway of complement. Methods Enzymol 1988; 162:639.

Pangburn MK, Müller-Eberhard HJ: The alternative pathway of complement. Springer Semin Immunopathol 1984; 7:163.

Pangburn MK, Schreiber RD, Müller-Eberhard HJ: Formation of the initial C3-convertase of the alternative pathway. Acquisition of C3b-like activities by spontaneous hydrolysis of the putative thioester in native C3. J Exp Med 1981; 154:856:4458.

Paolini JF, Willard D, Consler T, et al: The chemokines IL-8, monocyte chemoattractant protein-1, and I-309 are monomers at physiologically relevant concentrations. J Immunol 1994; 153:2704–2717.

Paranos S, Pravica V, Bonaci B, Stojkovic-Mostarica M: [Interleukin 4, total and allergen-specific immunoglobulin E antibodies in the blood of individuals with an atopic constitution]. Srp Arh Celok Lek 1998; 126:92–96.

Park JH, Kaushansky K, Levitt L: Transcriptional regulation of interleukin 3 (IL3) in primary human T lymphocytes. Role of AP-1- and octamer-binding proteins in control of IL3 gene expression. J Biol Chem 1993; 268:6299–6308.

Parrish-Novak J, Foster DC, Holly RD, Clegg CH: Interleukin-21 and the IL-21 receptor: novel effectors of NK and T cell responses. J Leukoc Biol 2002; 72:856–863.

Patti G, D'Ambrosio A, Mega S, et al: Early interleukin-1 receptor antagonist elevation in patients with acute myocardial infarction. J Am Coll Cardiol 2004; 43:35–38.

Paul WE: Interleukin-4: A prototypic immunoregulatory lymphokine. Blood 1991; 77:1859–1870.

Peake PW, Sreenstein JD, Pussell BA, et al: The behaviour of human vitronectin in vivo: effects of complement activation, conformation and phosphorylation. Clin Exp Immunol 1996; 106:416.

Pene J, Gauchat JF, Lecart S, et al: Cutting edge: IL-21 is a switch factor for the production of IgG1 and IgG3 by human B cells. J Immunol 2004; 172:5154–5157.

Pepys MB: Role of complement in the induction of antibody production in vivo. J Exp Med 1974; 140:126.

Peschon JJ, Morrissey PJ, Grabstein KH, et al: Early lymphocyte expansion is severely impaired in interleukin 7 receptor-deficient mice. J Exp Med 1994; 180:1955–1960.

Petersen SV, Thiel S, Jensen L, et al: An assay for the mannan-binding lectin pathway of complement activation. J Immunol Methods 2001; 257:107–116.

Pflanz S, Timans JC, Cheung J, et al: IL-27, a heterodimeric cytokine composed of EBI3 and p28 protein, induces proliferation of naive CD4+ T cells. Immunity 2002; 16:779–790.

Pickering MC, Botto M, Taylor PR, et al: Systemic lupus erythematosus, complement deficiency, and apoptosis. Adv Immunol 2000; 76:227–324.

Piddlesden SJ, Storch MK, Hibbs M, et al: Soluble recombinant complement receptor type 1 inhibits inflammation and demyelination in antibody-mediated demyelinating experimental allergic encephalomyelitis. J Immunol 1994; 152:5477.

Pillemer L, Blum L, Lepow IH, et al: The properdin system and immunity. I. Demonstration and isolation of a new serum protein, properdin, and its role in immune phenomena. Science 1954; 120:279.

Platt JL: New directions for organ transplantation. Nature 1998; 392:11.

Plumb ME, Sodetz JM: Proteins of the membrane attack complex. In Volanakis JE, Frank MM (eds):

VI

CHAPTER 46: Mediators of Inflammation: Complement, Cytokines, and Adhesion Molecules

The Human Complement System in Health and Disease. New York, Marcel Dekker, 1998, p 119.

Podack ER, Biesecker G, Müller-Eberhard HJ: Membrane attack complex of complement: generation of high affinity phospholipid binding sites by fusion of five hydrophilic plasma proteins. Proc Natl Acad Sci USA 1979; 76:897.

Podack ER, Kolb WP, Müller-Eberhard HJ: The sC5b-7 complex: formation, isolation, properties and subunit composition. J Immunol 1977; 119:2024.

Podack ER, Tschopp J: Membrane attack by complement. Mol Immunol 1984; 21:589.

Pretolani M: Interleukin-10: an anti-inflammatory cytokine with therapeutic potential. Clin Exp Allergy 1999; 29:1164–1171.

Prodeus AP, Goerg S, Shen L-M, et al: A critical role for complement in maintenance of self-tolerance. Immunity 1998; 9:721.

Pruitt SK, Kirk AD, Bollinger RR, et al: The effect of soluble complement receptor type 1 on hyperacute rejection of porcine xenografts. Transplantation 1994; 52:868.

Puccetti P, Belladonna ML, Grohmann U: Effects of IL-12 and IL-23 on antigen-presenting cells at the interface between innate and adaptive immunity. Crit Rev Immunol 2002; 22:373–390.

Ramesh R, Mhashilkar AM, Tanaka F, et al: Melanoma differentiation-associated gene 7/interleukin (IL)-24 is a novel ligand that regulates angiogenesis via the IL-22 receptor. Cancer Res 2003; 63:5105–5113.

Ramm LE, Whitlow MB, Mayer MM: Size of the transmembrane channels produced by complement proteins C5b-8. J Immunol 1982; 129:1143.

Rapoport MJ, Jaramillo A, Zipris D, et al: Interleukin 4 reverses T cell proliferative unresponsiveness and prevents the onset of diabetes in nonobese diabetic mice. J Exp Med 1993; 178:87–99.

Rapp HJ, Borsos T (eds): Molecular Basis of Complement Action. New York, Appleton-Century-Crofts, 1970.

Redlich CA, Gao X, Rockwell S, et al: IL-11 enhances survival and decreases TNF production after radiation-induced thoracic injury. J Immunol 1996; 157:1705–1710.

Reff ME, Carner K, Chambers KS, et al: Depletion of B cells in vivo by a chimeric mouse human monoclonal antibody to CD20. Blood 1994; 83:435–445.

Reiter Y, Ciobotariu A, Fischelson Z: Sub-lytic complement attack protects tumor cells from lytic doses of antibody and complement. Eur J Immunol 1992; 22:1207.

Renauld JC, van der Lugt N, Vink A, et al: Thymic lymphomas in interleukin-9 transgenic mice. Oncogene 1994; 9:1327–1332.

Resino S, Sanchez-Ramon S, Bellon JM, et al: Impaired interleukin-5 (IL-5) production by T cells as a prognostic marker of disease progression in human immunodeficiency virus type 1 (HIV-1)-infected children. Eur Cytokine Netw 2001; 12:253–259.

Rich BE: IL-20: a new target for the treatment of inflammatory skin disease. Expert Opin Ther Targets 2003; 7:165–174.

Rollins SA, Fitch JCK, Sherman S, et al: Anti-C5 single chain antibody therapy blocks complement and leukocyte activation and reduces tissue damage in CPB patients. Mol Immunol 1998; 35:397.

Rosenwasser LJ: Biologic activities of IL-1 and its role in human disease. Allergy Clin Immunol 1998; 102:344–350.

Ross GD, Yount WJ, Walport MJ, et al: Disease-associated loss of erythrocyte complement receptors (CR1, C3b receptors) in patients with systemic lupus erythematosus and other diseases involving autoantibodies and/or complement activation. J Immunol 1985; 135:2005.

Rosse WF: Paroxysmal nocturnal hemoglobinuria and complement. In Volanakis JE, Frank MM (eds): The Human Complement System in Health and Disease. New York, Marcel Dekker, 1998, p 481.

Rosso DA, Ripoli MF, Roy A, et al: Serum levels of interleukin-1 receptor antagonist and tumor necrosis factor-alpha are elevated in children with

Langerhans cell histiocytosis. J Pediatr Hematol Oncol 2003; 25:480–483.

Rot A, Hub E, Middleton J, et al: Some aspects of IL-8 pathophysiology. III: chemokine interaction with endothelial cells. J Leukoc Biol 1996; 59:39–44.

Ryffel B, Car BD, Gunn H, et al: Interleukin-6 exacerbates glomerulonephritis in (NZB × NZW)F1 mice. Am J Pathol 1994; 144:927–937.

Samuel CE: Antiviral actions of interferon. Interferon-regulated cellular proteins and their surprisingly selective antiviral activities. Virology 1991; 183:1–11.

Sanders ME, Koski CL, Robbins D, et al: Activated terminal complement in cerebrospinal fluid in Guillain–Barré syndrome and multiple sclerosis. J Immunol 1986; 136:4456.

Sanders ME, Schmetz MA, Hammer CH, et al: Quantitation of activation of the human terminal complement pathway by ELISA. J Immunol Methods 1985; 85:245.

Sands BE, Bank S, Sninsky CA, et al: Preliminary evaluation of safety and activity of recombinant human interleukin 11 in patients with active Crohn's disease. Gastroenterology 1999; 117:58–64.

Sarkar D, Su ZZ, Lebedeva IV, et al: mda-7 (IL-24) Mediates selective apoptosis in human melanoma cells by inducing the coordinated overexpression of the GADD family of genes by means of p38 MAPK. Proc Natl Acad Sci USA 2002; 99:10054–10059.

Schmiedt W, Kinscherf R, Deigner H-P, et al: Complement C6 deficiency protects against diet-induced atherosclerosis in rabbits. Arterioscler Thromb Vasc Biol 1998; 18:1790.

Schneider PM, Rittner C: Complement genetics. In Dodds AW, Sim RB (eds): Complement. A Practical Approach. New York, Oxford University Press, 1997, p 165.

Schneider PM, Würzner R: Complement genetics: biological implications of polymorphism and deficiencies. Immunol Today 1999; 20:2.

Schweinle JE, Ezekowitz RAB, Tenner AJ, et al: Human mannose-binding protein activates the alternative complement pathway and enhances serum bactericidal activity on a mannose-rich isolate of Salmonella. J Clin Invest 1989; 84:1821.

Seifert, Hugo F, Hansson GK, et al: Prelesional complement activation in experimental atherosclerosis. Terminal C5b-9 complement deposition coincides with cholesterol accumulation in the aortic intima of hypercholesterolemic rabbits. Lab Invest 1989; 60:747.

Sengeløv H: Complement receptors in neutrophils. Crit Rev Immunol 1995; 15:107.

Seya T, Atkinson JP: Functional properties of membrane cofactor protein of complement. Biochem J 1989; 264:581.

Seya T, Turner JR, Atkinson JP: Purification and characterization of a membrane protein (gp45–70) that is a cofactor for cleavage of C3b and C4b. J Exp Med 1986; 163:837.

Sharma JN, Moshin SS: The role of chemical mediators in the pathogenesis of inflammation with emphasis on the kinin system. Exp Pathol 1990; 38:73.

Shichishima T, Saitoh Y, Terasawa T, et al: Complement sensitivity of erythrocytes in a patient with inherited complete deficiency of CD59 or with the Inab phenotype. Br J Haematol 1999; 104:303.

Shin ML, Rus H, Niculescu F: Complement system in central nervous system disorders. In Volanakis JE, Frank MM (eds): The Human Complement System in Health and Disease. New York, Marcel Dekker, 1998, p 499.

Shinohara S, Rothstein JL: Interleukin 24 is induced by the RET/PTC3 oncoprotein and is an autocrine growth factor for epithelial cells. Oncogene 2004; 23:7571–7579.

Sillaber C, Strobl H, Bevec D, et al: IL-4 regulates c-kit proto-oncogene product expression in human mast and myeloid progenitor cells. J Immunol 1991; 147:4224–4228.

Simon T, Opelz G, Wiesel M, et al: Serial peripheral blood interleukin-18 and perforin gene expression

measurements for prediction of acute kidney graft rejection. Transplantation 2004; 77:1589–1595.

Sims PJ, Wiedmer T: Induction of cellular procoagulant activity by the membrane attack complex of complement. Semin Cell Biol, 1995; 6:275.

Sivori S, Cantoni C, Parolini S, et al: IL-21 induces both rapid maturation of human CD34+ cell precursors towards NK cells and acquisition of surface killer Ig-like receptors. Eur J Immunol 2003; 33:3439–3447.

Snapper CM, Paul WE: Interferon-gamma and B cell stimulatory factor-1 reciprocally regulate Ig isotype production. Science 1987; 236:944–947.

Soussi-Gounni A, Kontolemos M, Hamid Q: Role of IL-9 in the pathophysiology of allergic diseases. J Allergy Clin Immunol 2001; 107:575–582.

Stanilova SA, Slavov ES: Comparative study of circulating immune complexes quantity detection by three assays – CIF-ELISA, C1q-ELISA and anti-C3 ELISA. J Immunol Methods 2001; 253:13–21.

Stoiber H, Pruenster M, Ammann CG, Dierich MP: Complement-opsonized HIV: the free rider on its way to infection. Mol Immunol 2005; 42:153–160.

Strengell M, Sareneva T, Foster D, et al: IL-21 up-regulates the expression of genes associated with innate immunity and Th1 response. J Immunol 2002; 169:3600–3605.

Su HR: S-protein/vitronectin interaction with the C5b and the C8 of the complement membrane attack complex. Int Arch Allergy Immunol 1996; 110:314.

Suankratay C, Zhang X-H, Zhang Y, et al: Requirement for the alternative pathway as well as C4 and C2 in complement-dependent hemolysis via the lectin pathway. J Immunol 1998; 160:3006.

Subramaniam SV, Cooper RS, Adunyah SE: Evidence for the involvement of JAK/STAT pathway in the signaling mechanism of interleukin-17. Biochem Biophys Res Commun 1999; 262:14–19.

Sule SD, Wigley FM: Treatment of scleroderma: an update. Expert Opin Investig Drugs 2003; 12:471–482.

Sumiya M, Summerfield JA: The role of collectins in host defense. Semin Liver Dis 1997; 17:311.

Suzuki H, Kundig TM, Furlonger C, et al: Deregulated T cell activation and autoimmunity in mice lacking interleukin-2 receptor beta. Science 1995; 268:1472–1476.

Takada H, Ohga S, Mizuno Y, et al: Oversecretion of IL-18 in haemophagocytic lymphohistiocytosis: a novel marker of disease activity. Br J Haematol 1999; 106:182–189.

Tan JC, Braun S, Rong H, et al: Characterization of recombinant extracellular domain of human interleukin-10 receptor. J Biol Chem 1995; 270:12906–12911.

Tavernier J, Devos R, Cornelis S, et al: A human high affinity interleukin-5 receptor (IL5R) is composed of an IL5-specific alpha chain and a beta chain shared with the receptor for GM-CSF. Cell 1991; 66:1175–1184.

Tenner AJ, Robinson SL, Ezekowitz RAB: Mannose binding protein (MBP) enhances mononuclear phagocyte function via a receptor that contains the 126,000Mr component of the C1q receptor. Immunity 1995; 3:485.

Tepper RI, Pattengale PK, Leder P: Murine interleukin-4 displays potent anti-tumor activity in vivo. Cell 1989; 57:503–512.

Teixeira JE, Martinez R, Camara LM, Barbosa JE: Expression of complement receptor type 1 (CR1) on erythrocytes of paracoccidiodomycosis patients. Mycopathology 2001; 152:125–133.

Thiel S, Vorup-Jensen T, Stover CM, et al: A second serine protease associated with mannan-binding lectin that activates complement. Nature 1997; 386:506.

Tomlinson S, Nussenzweig V: Human alternative complement pathway-mediated lysis of rabbit erythrocytes is enhanced by natural anti-gal α 1–3gal antibodies. J Immunol 1997; 159:5606.

Tony HP, Shen BJ, Reusch P, Sebald W: Design of human interleukin-4 antagonists inhibiting interleukin-4-dependent and interleukin-13-dependent responses in T-cells and B-cells with high efficiency. Eur J Biochem 1994; 225:659–665.

Torigoe K, Ushio S, Okura T, et al: Purification and characterization of the human interleukin-18 receptor. J Biol Chem 1997; 272:25737–25742.

Torzewski J, Bowyer DE, Waltenberger J, et al: Processes in atherogenesis: complement activation. Atherosclerosis 1997; 132:131.

Trepicchio WL, Dorner AJ. Interleukin-11. A gp130 cytokine. Ann N Y Acad Sci 1998; 856:12–21.

Trinchieri G: Function and clinical use of interleukin-12. Curr Opin Hematol 1997; 4:59–66.

Trinchieri G: Interleukin-12: a cytokine produced by antigen-presenting cells with immunoregulatory functions in the generation of T-helper cells type 1 and cytotoxic lymphocytes. Blood 1994; 84:4008–4027.

Turner MW: Mannose-binding lectin: the pluripotent molecule of the innate immune system. Immunol Today 1996; 17:532.

Ushio S, Namba M, Okura T, et al: Cloning of the cDNA for human IFN-gamma-inducing factor, expression in *Escherichia coli*, and studies on the biologic activities of the protein. J Immunol 1996; 156:4274–4279.

Uyttenhove C, Simpson RJ, Van Snick J: Functional and structural characterization of P40, a mouse glycoprotein with T-cell growth factor activity. Proc Natl Acad Sci USA 1988; 85:6934–6938.

Vakeva AP, Agah A, Rollins SA, et al: Myocardial infarction and apoptosis after myocardial ischemia and reperfusion. Role of the terminal complement components and inhibition by anti-C5 therapy. Circulation 1998; 97:2259.

Valdimarsson H, Stefansson M, Vikingsdottir T, et al: Reconstitution of opsonizing activity by infusion of mannan-binding lectin (MBL) to MBL-deficient humans. Scand J Immunol 1998; 48:116.

Van de Wetering JK, van Golde LM, Batenburg JJ: Collectins: players of the innate immune system. Eur J Biochem 2004; 271:1229–1249.

Vermeer PD, Harson R, Einwalter LA, et al: Interleukin-9 induces goblet cell hyperplasia during repair of human airway epithelia. Am J Respir Cell Mol Biol 2003; 28:286–295.

Vio CP, Olavarria V, Gonzalez C, et al: Cellular and functional aspects of the renal kallikrein system in health and disease. Biol Res 1998; 31:305.

Volanakis JE: Structure, molecular genetics, and function of complement control proteins: An update. Year Immunol 1988; 3:275.

Volanakis JE: Overview of the complement system. *In* Volanakis JE, Frank MM (eds): The Human Complement System in Health and Disease. New York, Marcel Dekker, 1998, p 9.

Volanakis JE, Narayana SV: Complement factor D, a novel serine protease. Protein Sci 1996; 5:553.

Vorup-Jensen T, Jensenius JC, Thiel S: MASP-2, the C3 convertase generating protease of the MBLectin complement activating pathway. Immunobiology 1998; 199:348.

Wada T, Yokoyama H, Tomosugi N, et al: Detection of urinary interleukin-8 in glomerular diseases. Kidney Int 1994; 46:455–460.

Wagner E, Frank MM: Development of clinically useful agents to control complement-mediated tissue damage. *In* Volanakis JE, Frank MM (eds): The Human Complement System in Health and Disease. New York, Marcel Dekker, 1998, p 527.

Wahl SM: Transforming growth factor beta: The good, the bad, and the ugly. J Exp Med 1994; 180:1587–1590.

Walsh GM, Wardlaw AJ, Hartnell A, et al: Interleukin-5 enhances the in vitro adhesion of human eosinophils, but not neutrophils, in a leucocyte integrin (CD11/18)-dependent manner. Int Arch Allergy Appl Immunol 1991; 94:174–178.

Wan HC, Lazarovits AI, Cruikshank WW, et al: Expression of alpha 4 beta 7 integrin on eosinophils and modulation of alpha 4-integrin-mediated eosinophil adhesion via CD4. Int Arch Allergy Immunol 1995; 107:343–344.

Wang JM, Rambaldi A, Biondi A, et al: Recombinant human interleukin 5 is a selective eosinophil chemoattractant. Eur J Immunol 1989; 19:701–705.

Wang R, Rogers AM, Rush BJ, Russell JH: Induction of sensitivity to activation-induced death in primary CD4+ cells: A role for interleukin-2 in the negative regulation of responses by mature CD4+ T cells. Eur J Immunol 1996; 26:2263–2270.

Wang Y, Rollins SA, Madri JA, et al: Anti-C5 monoclonal antibody therapy prevents collagen-induced arthritis and ameliorates established disease. Proc Natl Acad Sci U S A 1995; 92:8955.

Ward PA: Recruitment of inflammatory cells into lung: roles of cytokines, adhesion molecules and complement. J Lab Clin Med 1997; 129:400.

Watanabe M, Ueno Y, Yajima T, et al: Interleukin 7 is produced by human intestinal epithelial cells and regulates the proliferation of intestinal mucosal lymphocytes. J Clin Invest 1995; 95:2945–2953.

Weisman HF, Bartow T, Leppo MK, et al: Soluble human complement receptor type 1: in vivo inhibitor of complement suppressing post-ischemic myocardial inflammation and necrosis. Science 1990; 249:146.

Wen L, Atkinson JP, Giclas PC: Clinical and laboratory evaluation of complement deficiency. J Allergy Clin Immunol 2004; 113:585–593.
This article provides a practical clinical approach to complement deficiency testing as well as an overview of the complement system.

West C: Complement and glomerular disease. *In* Volanakis JE, Frank MM (eds): The Human Complement System in Health and Disease. New York, Marcel Dekker, 1998, p 571.

Whaley K (ed): Methods in Complement for Clinical Immunologists. Edinburgh, Churchill Livingstone, 1985.

Whittington HA, Armstrong L, Uppington KM, Millar AB: Interleukin-22: a potential immunomodulatory molecule in the lung. Am J Respir Cell Mol Biol 2004; 31:220–226.

Wilkinson PC, Liew FY: Chemoattraction of human blood T lymphocytes by interleukin-15. J Exp Med 1995; 181:1255–1259.

Willerford DM, Chen J, Ferry JA, et al: Interleukin-2 receptor alpha chain regulates the size and content of the peripheral lymphoid compartment. Immunity 1995; 3:521–530.

World Health Organization: Nomenclature of complement. Bull WHO 1968; 39:934.

Würzner R, Mollnes TE, Morgan BP: Immunochemical assays for complement components. *In* Johnstone AP, Turner MW (eds): Immunochemistry 2. A Practical Approach. Oxford, Oxford University Press, 1997, p 197.

Xu W, Presnell SR, Parrish-Novak J, et al: A soluble class II cytokine receptor, IL-22RA2, is a naturally occurring IL-22 antagonist. Proc Natl Acad Sci USA 2001; 98:9511–9516.

Yacoub A, Mitchell C, Brannon J, et al: MDA-7 (interleukin-24) inhibits the proliferation of renal carcinoma cells and interacts with free radicals to promote cell death and loss of reproductive capacity. Mol Cancer Ther 2003; 2:623–632.

Yancey KB, Lawley TJ: Role of complement in diseased and normal skin. *In* Volanakis JE, Frank MM (eds): The Human Complement System in Health and Disease. New York, Marcel Dekker, 1998, p 597.

Yao Z, Fanslow WC, Seldin MF, et al: Herpesvirus Saimiri encodes a new cytokine, IL-17, which binds to a novel cytokine receptor. Immunity 1995a; 3:811–821.

Yin T, Keller SR, Quelle FW, et al: IL-9 induces tyrosine phosphorylation insulin receptor substrate-1 via JAK tyrosine kinases. J Biol Chem 1995; 270:20497–20502.

Yoshimoto T, Okada K, Morishima N, et al: Induction of IgG2a class switching in B cells by IL-27. J Immunol 2004; 173:2479–2485.

Yoshimoto T, Okamura H, Tagawa YI, et al: Interleukin 18 together with interleukin 12 inhibits IgE production by induction of interferon-gamma production from activated B cells. Proc Natl Acad Sci USA 1997; 94:3948–3953.

Zitvogel L, Tahara H, Robbins PD, et al: Cancer immunotherapy of established tumors with IL-12. Effective delivery by genetically engineered fibroblasts. J Immunol 1995; 155:1393–1403.

Zubler RH, Lambert PH: The 125I-C1q binding test for the detection of soluble immune complexes. *In* Bloom BR, David JR (eds): In Vitro Methods in Cell-Mediated and Tumor Immunity. New York, Academic Press, 1976, p 565.

CHAPTER 47

Human Leukocyte Antigen: The Major Histocompatibility Complex of Man

H. Davis Massey MD PhD, Richard A. McPherson MD

KEY POINTS

- MHC class I molecules include HLA-A, HLA-B, and HLA-C, while MHC class II molecules include HLA-DR, HLA-DQ, and HLA-DP; these are the classic 'transplantation' antigens.

- MHC genes are closely linked and segregate en bloc to offspring.

- Characterization of *HLA* alleles and molecules has been combined with clinical protocols to maximize donor and recipient compatibility, and to minimize the impact of the immune response on the transplanted organ. Advances in this area have contributed to the development of transplantation as a successful treatment modality for the replacement of diseased tissue.

- HLA matching usually includes evaluation of at least three loci, *HLA-A, HLA-B,* and *HLA-DR.* Individuals matched, at whatever resolution, for all three loci are termed 6/6 matches or 0 mismatches.

- Patients can be sensitized to specific foreign HLA molecules through transfusion, pregnancy, or prior transplantations. Assessment of compatibility between the recipient and the possible donor includes the testing for this sensitization.

- Several methods are available for HLA typing, including serologic and cellular typing approaches, and DNA-based typing. DNA-based typing has significant advantages over the other methods.

Survival depends on the ability of the immune system to recognize and to respond to a multitude of foreign substances (antigens). Although this defense mechanism is basic to survival in a hostile world of microorganisms, this same defense system has a negative impact when transplanting tissue from one individual to another or when malfunctioning triggers autoaggressive reactions. The major histocompatibility complex (MHC) genes encode proteins that are essential to immune recognition: the class I and class II molecules (Fig. 47–1). In the human, the class I molecules include human leukocyte antigen (HLA) HLA-A, HLA-B, and HLA-C, and the class II molecules include HLA-DR, HLA-DQ, and HLA-DP. These molecules are the classical transplantation antigens. Other molecules encoded within the MHC are the class III molecules (see Ch. 48). These include the MHC-linked complement components (C2, C4, and Bf), 21-hydroxylase (CYP21), heat shock protein (Hsp)70, and tumor necrosis factor (TNF).

During an infection, the invading microorganism may either infect or be engulfed by cells and may then be degraded into peptide fragments. Inside the cell, MHC class I or class II molecules bind antigenic fragments derived from the microorganism. Once antigenic fragments have bound to the MHC molecules and have translocated to the cell surface, receptors on T lymphocytes interact with the complex of antigen fragment–MHC molecule, triggering both humoral and cellular immune responses (Fig. 47–2). T-cell-specific cell-surface molecules, CD4 and CD8, act to strengthen this cellular interaction and to transmit activation signals. Other cell-surface molecules act to increase the affinity of cellular interactions (e.g., CD2 and its ligand, CD58 [LFA-3] or CD11a/CD18 [LFA-1] and its ligand, CD54 [ICAM-1]) and to transmit co-stimulatory signals (e.g., CD28 and its ligands,

HLA Class II Region

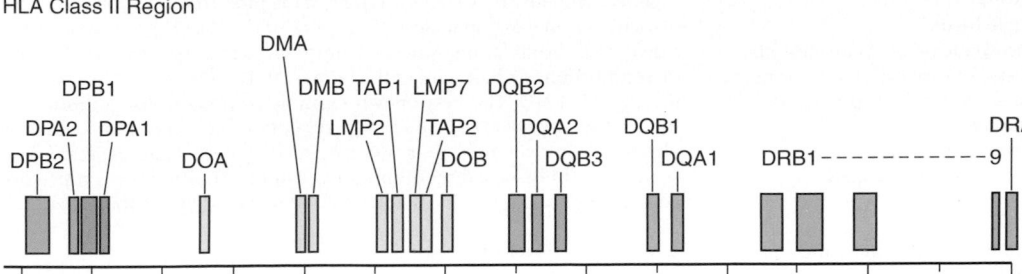

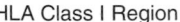

Figure 47–1 Map of the *MHC* gene complex on chromosome 6. *HLA-DPB2* in the HLA class II region is located closest to the centromere. *HLA-F* is the most telomeric. The region between *HLA-DRA* and *HLA-B* is not shown. (With permission from the Anthony Nolan Bone Marrow Trust, www.anthonynolan.org.uk/HIG.)

HLA Class I Region

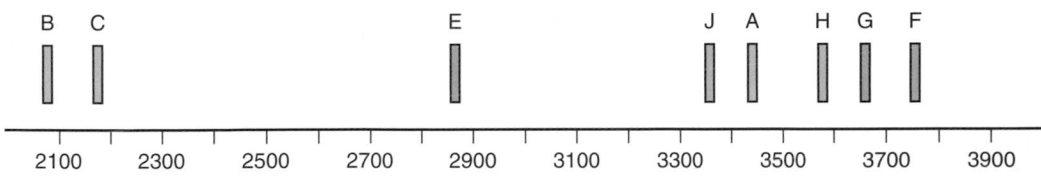

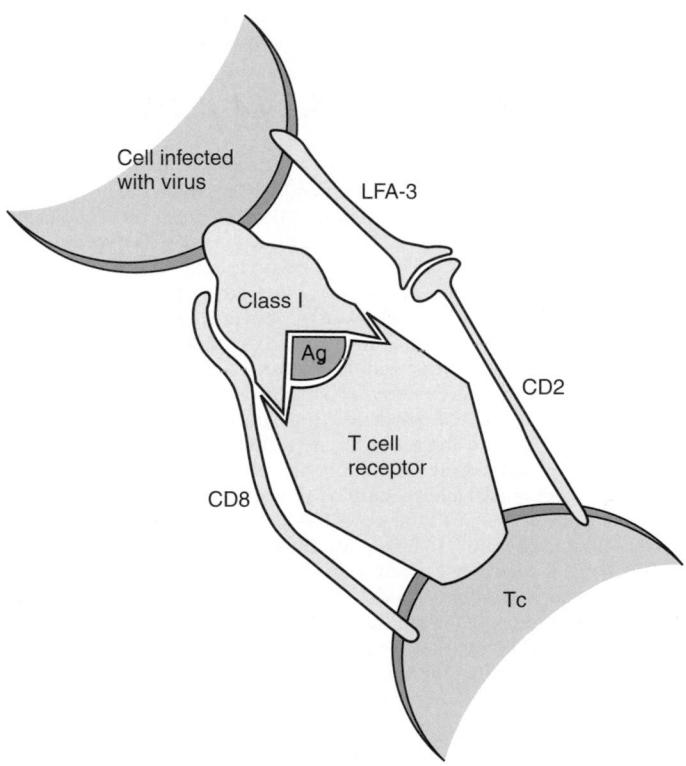

Figure 47–2 Model of the molecular interactions involved in antigen recognition.

CD80/CD86 [B7] and CD40 and its ligand, CD154). Polymorphism in the genes that specify the MHC class I and class II molecules affects the antigen-binding specificity of the molecules, resulting in differences in immune responses among members of the species. The same pattern of interactions between a cell bearing an MHC class I or class II antigen fragment complex and a T lymphocyte occur not only in the recognition of invading pathogens but also in the recognition of foreign class I and class II molecules (alloantigens) (see Ch. 48) and in the recognition of self-antigens (autoantigens) (see Ch. 48).

Because donor MHC class I and class II molecules are recognized by the recipient's immune system as foreign antigens, it is beneficial to ensure that donor and recipient are histo- (i.e., tissue) compatible (i.e., HLA-matched). Class I and class II molecules have great allelic diversity in a population, so ensuring compatibility between donor and recipient is often a difficult task requiring collaboration among the medical staff, the clinical HLA typing personnel, and the donor tissue coordinators (e.g., large organ-sharing networks and registries or banks of hematopoietic progenitor cell donors).

The genetics, structure, function, nomenclature, and techniques of detection of the human MHC gene products, HLA-A, -B, and -C (class I)

Table 47–1 Websites on HLA Transplantation

Address	Information
www.ashi-hla.org	American Society for Histocompatibility and Immunogenetics, HLA typing standards
www.ebi.ac.uk/imgt/hla	HLA sequence database, tools for allele submission and sequence manipulation
www.anthonynolan.org.uk/hig	World Health Organization nomenclature information
www.ihwc.org or www.ihwg.org	International Histocompatibility Workshop
www.marrow.org	National Marrow Donor Program
www.bmdw.org	Bone Marrow Donors Worldwide
www.worldmarrow.org	World Marrow Donor Association
www.ibmtr.org	International Bone Marrow Transplant Registry
www.ctstransplant.org	Collaborative Transplant Study
www.unos.org	United Network for Organ Sharing
www.nhgri.nih.gov	National Human Genome Research Institute

and HLA-DR, -DQ, and -DP (class II) are discussed in this chapter. Also discussed is the importance of HLA matching for transplantation. In addition to references listed at the end of the chapter, Table 47–1 lists helpful web page addresses that provide both reference material and updates of clinical outcome.

Genetics of the Major Histocompatibility Complex

Basic Genetics

Mendel's first law, the law of segregation, is based on the principle that hereditary traits are determined by factors that are distributed to progeny. In any one individual, these factors, or genes as they are now called, are present on chromosomes (see Ch. 69). Each gene may have multiple forms (i.e., alleles). Because humans are diploid, there are two genes per pair of homologous chromosomes. In meiosis, the chromosomes segregate randomly during formation of the gametes (ova or sperm) so that only one of each pair of chromosomes (i.e., a haploid number) is transmitted by any given gamete. The double, or diploid number of chromosomes, is restored when the male and female gamete fuse to form the zygote. Thus, for a trait determined by one gene, there will always be four possible genetic combinations in the offspring, each with equal probability of occurrence. These laws of segregation and random assortment apply to the genes of the MHC system. Definitions are given below for genetic terms that will be used in this chapter (Crow, 1976; www.nhgri.nih.gov) as listed in Table 47–1.

Gene The unit factor of inheritance.

Chromosome Carriers of the unit factors of inheritance.

VI

Locus The position of a gene on a chromosome.

Allele An alternative form of a gene at a single locus.

Homozygous Having identical alleles at a locus, one on each chromosome.

Heterozygous Having different alleles at a locus, one on each chromosome.

Codominance The state in which the allele at each locus expresses its characteristic effect equally in the heterozygote.

Genotype The genetic composition of an organism or individual.

Phenotype The observable characteristics produced by the genes.

Polymorphic Having two or more common distinct genotypes maintained in a population.

Homologous chromosomes The two members of a chromosome pair that have corresponding gene loci, one derived from each parent.

Crossing over The exchange of segments between homologous chromosomes. This process may also be termed recombination.

Allo-(antigen, graft) Refers to antigenic differences between individuals of a single species.

Auto-(antigen, graft) Refers to tissue or antigens of the same individual (i.e., self).

Composition of the MHC

The major histocompatibility gene complex in humans is located on the short arm of chromosome 6 (i.e., 6p21). It spans 3600 kb (kilobases) and includes 224 identified gene loci, of which 128 are predicted to be expressed. Approximately 40% of the expressed genes are estimated to have an immune system function (Aguado, 1999). The HLA genes of the MHC are located in six subregions: *HLA-A, HLA-C, HLA-B, HLA-DR, HLA-DQ,* and *HLA-DP* (Fig. 47–1). Each subregion encodes a minimum of one cell surface glycoprotein. With only one exception, the HLA genes are highly polymorphic – that is, each of the HLA genes has multiple alleles in the human population. Indeed, the HLA genes are the most polymorphic loci known in man (Parham, 1995; Table 47–1, www.anthonynolan.org/uk/hig). Because the HLA genes specify molecules that play an important role in the immune response, the polymorphism is believed to be essential to the survival of the species and to be maintained in the population by selection.

Localization of MHC Genes

The genes of the MHC were assigned to the short arm of chromosome 6 (6p) on the basis of cytogenetic studies of aberrant chromosomes (i.e., chromosomes that have undergone a translocation). The map order and positioning of the MHC genes was determined by meiotic linkage analyses (i.e., studies of crossing over in families) and molecular biology techniques including gene cloning, DNA sequencing, and pulsed field gel electrophoresis. The latter technique detects the presence of genes on single long fragments of DNA. The map order of genes within the MHC is *HLA-A, -C, -B, -DR, -DQ, -DP,* with *HLA-A* being distal to the centromere (Fig. 47–1).

Inheritance

The MHC genes are closely linked – that is, they segregate en bloc to the offspring. The complex of linked genes that resides on one of the pair of homologous chromosomes and that segregates en bloc to the offspring is termed a *haplotype*. Each individual inherits two MHC haplotypes – one from each parent – and thus has two alleles for each of the genes. These alleles are codominantly expressed. The inheritance of the MHC genes follows the rules of segregation set down by Mendel. Within a family, each child inherits one MHC haplotype from the mother and one from the father. By convention, the paternal haplotypes are designated *a* and *b* and the maternal haplotypes *c* and *d*. Thus, there are four possible MHC genotypes in the offspring: *ac, ad, bc,* and *bd*. Since the chance of inheriting a given haplotype is random, the probability of occurrence of any one of the four genotypes is one in four for each mating. In a family with five children, at least two of the children will be HLA-identical (assuming no crossing over). Although the MHC genes are closely linked, families have been reported in which a crossover has occurred. The frequency of crossing over between two linked genes was thought to be a measure of the distance separating the genes; however, molecular data have suggested the existence of recombination 'hot' spots in the intervening DNA that can increase or decrease the likelihood of recombination during meiosis (Uematsu, 1988).

Linkage Disequilibrium

The observation that alleles at different genetic loci occur in the population on the same haplotype significantly more frequently than would be expected on the basis of chance alone is called *linkage disequilibrium*. The expected frequency of two alleles (f1, f2) is the product of the gene frequency of each allele in that population ($[f_{expected} = f1 \times f2]$). The observed frequency is determined from family studies within the same population. Linkage disequilibrium is a hallmark of the human MHC and extends from *HLA-A* through *HLA-DQ*. The best known example of linkage disequilibrium is the A1,Cw7,B8,DR17(3),DR52,DQ2 haplotype in Caucasians, which is observed approximately four times more frequently than expected. The significance of linkage disequilibrium as it applies to immune competence and disease is discussed in Chapter 48 under Extended Haplotypes.

Ethnic Variation

The accumulated data from the study of the world population groups (Dausset, 1973; Imanishi, 1992; Cadavid, 1997; Bugawan, 1999) demonstrate that the frequencies of HLA alleles differ significantly among ethnic population groups. MHC haplotypes and linkage disequilibrium of alleles also differ. These observations must be taken into account when developing unrelated allograft hematopoietic progenitor cell donor registries and banks such as the United States National Marrow Donor Program (NMDP) (Perkins, 1994). Both the allele and haplotype frequencies dictate the number of volunteers required to find an HLA-matched unrelated donor for any patient. Some patients (i.e., those with rare or unusual types) cannot find closely matched unrelated donors from among the more than 6 million volunteers listed in all donor registries worldwide (Beatty, 1995; Mori, 1997). Improvement in methods for engraftment of progenitor cells from partially HLA-mismatched donors may allow transplantation in patients for whom close matches cannot be found (see Ch. 37).

Class I Molecules – *HLA-A, HLA-B, HLA-C* Subregions

The HLA-A and -B molecules were the first MHC molecules to be described in humans (Dausset, 1981; van Rood, 1993). Because these molecules were defined by antibody responses to white blood cells (WBCs), they were called human leukocyte 'antigens.' Leukocyte antibodies were observed in humans as early as the 1920s, but it was not until the 1950s that a systematic study began. In 1952, Dausset convincingly demonstrated the existence of leukocyte antibodies (leukoagglutinins). Because these leukoagglutinins did not react with leukocytes from the antibody producer but did react with a percentage of leukocytes from red cell group O unrelated individuals, he suggested that these leukoagglutinins were alloantibodies. Shortly thereafter, Payne (1964) reported that sera from patients who had febrile nonhemolytic blood transfusion reactions frequently contained leukoagglutinins that demonstrated allospecificity. In 1958, Dausset described the first HLA alloantigen 'MAC' (now HLA-A2 + HLA-28) and showed it to be genetically determined.

Originally, the leukocyte specificities were thought to be the products of a single locus. A two-locus model, each locus with multiple alleles, was established through HLA studies in families by the identification of recombinational events that separated the two allelic series. These two allelic series were called the first or LA (now HLA-A) and the second, or four series (now HLA-B). These names derived from the description of the LA 1, 2, 3 allelic series by Payne in 1967 and of the 4a, 4b allelic series by van Rood in 1969. A third locus was first proposed in 1970; however, it was not confirmed until 1975 when a family with a recombination between HLA-B and the new locus was identified. This third locus was designated HLA-C following the 1975 International Histocompatibility Workshop. Dausset (1981) was awarded the Nobel Prize for Medicine in 1980 for his original work on the human HLA system.

Structure of Class I Molecules

The classical class I molecules, termed HLA-A, HLA-B, and HLA-C in the human, are heterodimers consisting of a transmembrane glycosylated polypeptide (heavy chain, 44 kDa) noncovalently associated with β_2-microglobulin (12 kDa) (Fig. 47–3) (Bjorkman, 1990). The heavy chain of the class I molecule spans the cell membrane and is oriented with its amino-terminus on the outside of the cell. β_2-Microglobulin is associated with the extracellular region of the heavy chain and is necessary for cell surface expression. The extracellular region of the class I heavy chain is divided into three domains designated α_1, α_2, and α_3, each consisting of about 90 amino acid residues. The amino-terminal α_1 domain contains a glycosylation site at the asparagine residue in position 86. The transmembrane segment of approximately 24 amino acids is mostly hydrophobic, whereas the intracellular carboxy-terminal segment of the molecule consists mainly of hydrophilic residues with a cluster of basic residues adjacent to the cytoplasmic surface of the cell membrane.

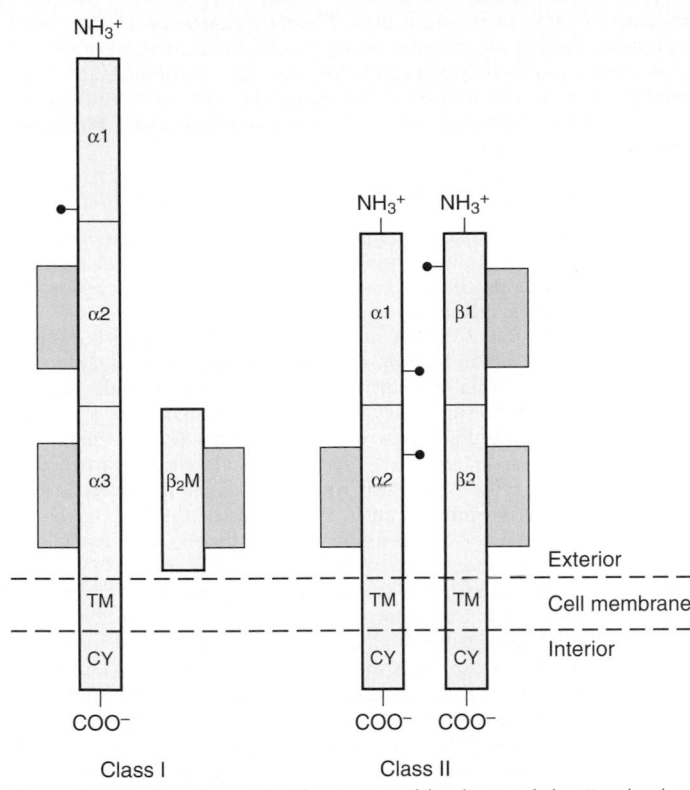

Figure 47–3 A schematic model of the structure of the class I and class II molecules.

Polymorphism of class I molecules (Table 47–2) (Bodmer, 1997, 1999) is defined by the use of (1) class I specific antibodies (alloantisera and monoclonal antibodies) that bind to the HLA molecules; (2) cytotoxic T lymphocytes (CTLs) that recognize and kill in response to stimulation by foreign or allogeneic class I molecules in vitro; (3) isoelectric focusing of isolated class I molecules; (4) polymerase chain reaction (PCR)-based DNA typing of class I alleles; and (5) nucleotide sequencing of class I alleles. Most of the class I polymorphism arises from amino acid sequence differences clustered in the α_1 and α_2 domains of the heavy chain. The α_3 domain is highly conserved among HLA class I molecules.

Fresh insights into the structure of the HLA molecule came when the three-dimensional structure of the class I molecule was defined using X-ray crystallography (Bjorkman, 1987). The structure of the extracellular portion is shown in Figure 47–4. The molecule consists of two pairs of structurally similar domains: α_1 has the same tertiary conformation as α_2, while α_3- and β_2-microglobulin have similar tertiary conformations. The α_3- and β_2-microglobulin domains are each composed of two antiparallel β-pleated sheets, one with four strands and one with three strands, connected by a disulfide bond. The α_3 and α_2 domains interact with one another through these β-pleated sheets and their structure closely resembles that described for an immunoglobulin constant region domain. The α_1 and α_2 domains are paired to form an eight-strand β-pleated sheet. This sheet is topped by two α-helices forming a groove at the top of the molecule. This groove is the site for the binding of antigenic peptide fragments by the class I molecule (Fig. 47–4). The sides and bottom of the groove are formed by side chains of the amino acids that comprise the helices and β-pleated sheets. Many of the amino acids that line this groove are polymorphic, creating allele-specific differences in antigen binding specificity among the different class I allelic products (Stern, 1994). Other residues in the helical regions of the groove interact with the T-cell receptor during recognition of the class I-antigenic fragment complex by a T lymphocyte (see Fig. 47–2).

Table 47–2 Examples of WHO Recognized HLA Antigens (Specificities) Defined by Serologic Typing and HLA Alleles Defined by DNA Sequencing

HLA-A Antigens	HLA-DQ Antigens	HLA-A Alleles[†]	HLA-DQA1 Alleles[‡]	HLA-DBQ1 Alleles[‡]
A1	DQ1	A*0101–0104N	DQA1*0101-*0105	DQB1*0501-*0504
A2	DQ2	A*02011-*0230	DQA1*0201	DQB1*06011-*0615
A203	DQ3	A*03011-*0304	DQA1*03011–0303	DQB1*0201-*0203
A210	DQ4	A*1101-*1105	DQA1*0401	DQB1*03011-*0309
A3	DQ5(1)	A*2301	DQA1*05011-*0505	DQB1*0401-*0402
A9	DQ6(1)	A*2402101-*2420	DQA1*06011-*06012	
A10	DQ7(3)	A*2501-*2502		
A11	DQ8(3)	A*2601-*2612		
A19	DQ9(3)	A*2901-*2904		
A23(9)		A*3001-*3007		
A24(9)		A*31012-*3104		
A2403		A*3201-*3203		
A25(10)		A*3301-*3304		
A26(10)		A*3401-*3402		
A28		A*3601		
A29(19)		A*4301		
A30(19)		A*6601-*6603		
A31(19)		A*68011-*6809		
A32(19)		A*6901		
A33(19)		A*7401-*7403		
A34(10)		A*8001		
A36				
A43				
A66(10)				
A68(28)				
A69(28)				
A74(19)				
A80				

Each column of the table is independent. Numbers in parentheses indicate the broad serologic specificity. The serologic type may be listed without the broad specificity. For example, both A23(9) and A23 are correct designations.

[†] HLA-A alleles specify HLA-A antigens. The antigen A1 is specified by either A*0101 or A*0102 or A*0103 alleles. A*0104N is a null or nonexpressed allele.

[‡] HLA-DQA1 and HLA-DQB1 alleles specify HLA-DQ antigens. The antigen DQ5 (1) is specified by several different DQA1 and DQB1 combinations including (1) DQA1*0101 and DQB1*0501 and (2) DQA1*0101 and DQB1*0502 alleles. In the past, serologic split designations were given to specificities that appeared to identify the antigen specified by a single HLA allele (e.g., A2 splits A203, A210; B7 split B703; B39 splits B3901 and B3902). It is now recognized that other alleles may also encode antigens that carry these serologic specificities and the WHO Nomenclature Committee has recommended that these splits be discontinued.

Source: adopted from www.anthonynolan.org.uk/HIG, with permission of SGE Marsh.

VI

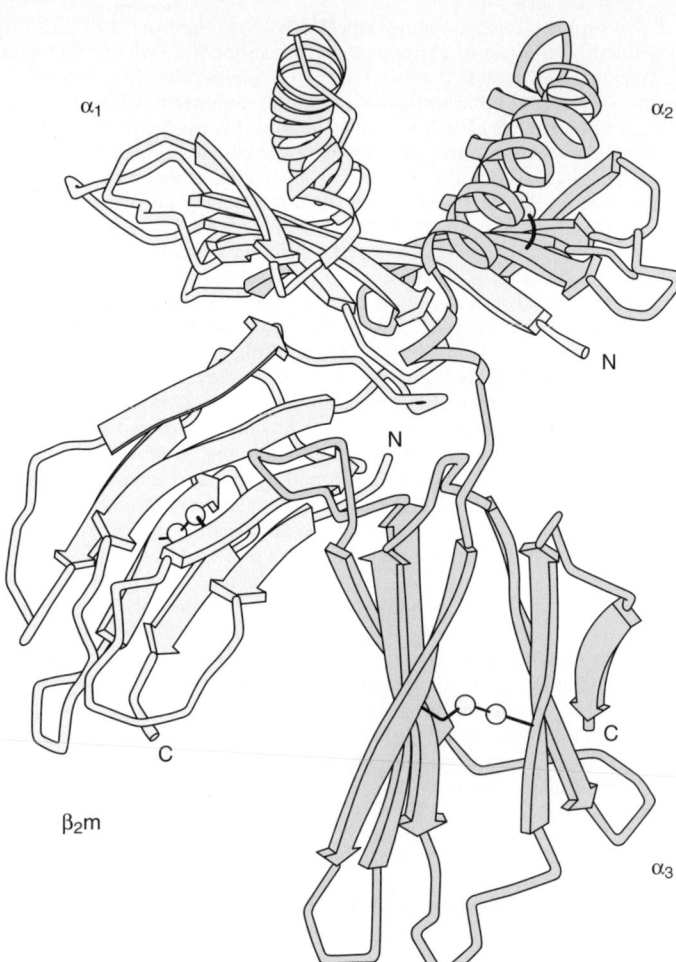

Figure 47–4 Three-dimensional model of the extracellular portion of a class I molecule. (With permission from Bjorkman PJ, Saper MA, Samraoui B, et al: Structure of the human class I histocompatibility antigen, HLA-A2. Nature 1987; 329:506.)

Organization of Class I Genes

The HLA heavy chains are encoded within the MHC on chromosome 6 (Fig. 47–1) (Shiina, 1999) and are highly polymorphic, whereas β_2-microglobulin is encoded on chromosome 15 and is not known to be polymorphic in humans. The typical class I gene is encoded by eight exons. The first exon encodes the 5' untranslated region and a hydrophobic leader peptide. Exons 2–4 encode the three extracellular domains; exon 5 encodes the transmembrane region. The sixth and seventh exons encode the cytoplasmic region and the eighth exon encodes the 3' untranslated region including the poly(A) addition site. The intervening sequences (termed introns) between the exons are transcribed into RNA but are removed during messenger RNA (mRNA) splicing.

Regulation of Class I Gene Expression

HLA class I molecules are expressed as transmembrane glycoproteins on the surface of many cell types. However, the level of the surface expression can vary extensively (Singer, 1990). The resting level of class I molecules is highest on lymphoid cells; class I molecules are undetectable on the membrane of certain other cell types such as brain cells, muscle cells, and sperm cells. Sequence elements located upstream of class I genes bind

regulatory factors that control the cell surface expression of the class I molecules. During an immune response, the cell surface expression of class I genes can be upregulated by cytokine (e.g., interferon-γ and TNF) binding to upstream regulatory elements. Tumors and certain viruses (e.g., human immunodeficiency virus [HIV]) can suppress class I expression (Brodsky, 1999).

Function of Class I Molecules

The HLA-A, -B, and -C molecules play key roles in an immune response. First, in the *adaptive* immune response, class I molecules bind peptides derived from proteins either degraded or synthesized in the cytosol and display them on the cell surface for perusal by the antigen receptors on T lymphocytes (see Ch. 44). Presentation of antigen by class I molecules allows T cells to detect and mount a cytotoxic response to foreign material (e.g., a virus or abnormal proteins from a malignant cell). In the cytosol, intracellular antigens (including self-proteins and viral or abnormal proteins) are broken down into peptide fragments (Rock, 1999). The peptide fragments are transported to the endoplasmic reticulum where they bind to the groove at the top of newly synthesized class I molecules and then are carried to the cell surface (Pamer, 1998; Hansen, 1997b) (Fig. 47–2). Four genes, located in the class II region of the MHC (Figs 47–1 and 47–5), are involved in this process. Two of these genes (*LMP2* and *LMP7*) encode components of the proteosome complex, a macromolecular structure that degrades proteins within the cytosol (Tanaka, 1997). The other two genes (*TAP1* and *TAP2*) encode components of peptide transporters that move peptides from the cytosol into the endoplasmic reticulum (Momburg, 1998). CD8+ CTLs recognize the processed peptide in conjunction with the class I molecule (Jorgensen, 1992). In the experimental system used to dissect this mechanism, CTLs were generated by in vitro stimulation with virally infected autologous cells. The recognition and lysis of the target cell was specific for the priming virus strain. The recognition also was affected by allelic polymorphism of class I molecules, as only virally infected target cells sharing the appropriate class I allelic product(s) with the responder were lysed (Zinkernagel, 1997a, 1997b). The latter requirement is termed 'MHC restriction.' Zinkernagel and his collaborator Doherty were awarded the Nobel Prize for Medicine in 1996 in recognition of the importance of the concept of MHC restriction to immunology.

Second, the surface expression of class I molecules has a protective function in the *innate* immune response by preventing target cell lysis effected by natural killer (NK) cells. Unlike CTLs, NK cells do not require activation through the recognition of peptide bound to the class I molecule but can lyse and destroy target cells lacking classical HLA class I molecule expression on the cell surface. Through this innate mechanism, NK cells play an important role in surveillance against viruses and tumor cells that down-regulate expression of the class I molecule to avoid recognition by CTLs (Lanier, 1998; Long, 1999).

There are two groups of NK receptors: (1) the C-type lectin receptor CD94/NKG2 whose genes reside on chromosome 12, and (2) the killer cell immunoglobulin-like receptors (KIRs) encoded by genes on chromosome 19. NK cell function appears to be regulated by a balance between positive signaling receptors that initiate and inhibitory receptors that suppress cell activation. Both groups of receptors recognize HLA class I ligands. For example, the KIR2D receptors differentiate between HLA-C ligands based on the presence of specific amino acid residues at codons 77 and 80 (i.e., asn77lys80 vs. ser77asn80). Another NK receptor, KIR3D, recognizes the HLA-Bw4/Bw6 polymorphism. A third NK receptor, CD94/NKG2, recognizes the HLA-E molecule complexed with the HLA leader peptide from some of the allelic products of HLA-A, -B, -C, and -G molecules (Brooks, 1999).

NK cells can specifically recognize and lyse allogeneic cells that do not express the specific class I molecules expressed by the effector cell (i.e., 'missing self') (Valiante, 1997). This could potentially occur even in apparently HLA-matched transplant pairs where one member of the pair is homozygous and the other is heterozygous (e.g., donor: Bw4,Bw6; recipient: Bw6). Thus Bw4-specific NK cells from the donor might lyse

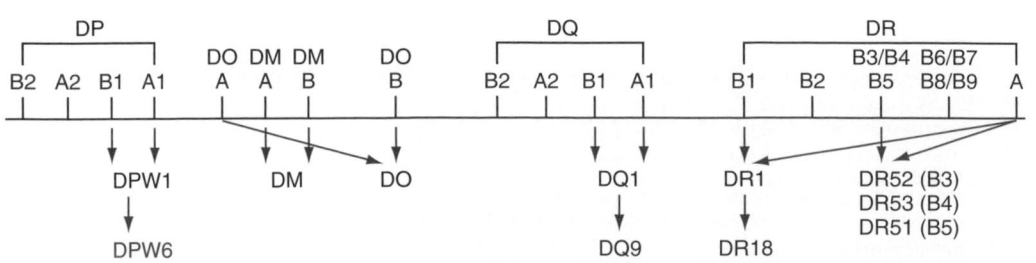

Figure 47–5 Map of the class II region of the human MHC. Gene products encoded by each subregion are listed. Not all genes are included.

cells without Bw4 from the recipient in a hematopoietic progenitor cell graft. This response may be unidirectional in some settings. In the example, the donor does not lack any HLA molecule present in the recipient; thus, the recipient NK cells will not detect any missing self. Since NK cells are relatively radioresistant and comprise a subpopulation of about 10–15% of peripheral blood lymphocytes, the NK response could be substantial; however, the extent of the role of NK activity in affecting transplant outcome is not known at present (Ruggeri, 1999).

Other Class I Genes

As many as 20 additional nonclassical or class Ib genes have been identified within the class I region of chromosome 6p by gene cloning (Aguado, 1999). Many of these are pseudogenes; however, several encode and express class I-like mRNA and/or molecules, HLA-E, HLA-F, and HLA-G. These molecules may be key mediators of both adaptive and innate immune responses (O'Callaghan, 1998). Their genes are homologous to classical class I genes in structure and the polypeptides encoded by these loci also associate with β_2-microglobulin. However, just as a high level of allelic polymorphism is a hallmark of the *HLA-A*, *HLA-B*, and *HLA-C* loci, a low level of polymorphism of the *HLA-E*, *HLA-F*, and *HLA-G* loci is a defining feature of these genes. In addition, by comparison with classical class I molecules, the cell surface expression of nonclassical class I molecules is low and the distribution of these class Ib molecules on specific cell types varies.

HLA-G

HLA-G is expressed principally on extravillous cytotrophoblast cells at the fetal–maternal interface, where it is thought to play a role in materno-fetal tolerance (Le Bouteiller, 1999). HLA-G, as a ligand for at least three NK and other cell inhibitory receptors, protects the invading placental tissue from the cytolytic action of NK cells. Although HLA-G has the capability to bind and present processed antigen (i.e., peptides) to T cells, the diversity of peptides bound by HLA-G appears to be lower than the diversity of peptides bound by classical class I molecules. Regulation of the expression of HLA-G also differs from the classical class I genes, as the gene contains no interferon response signal; thus, it is not interferon-inducible. It has been hypothesized that the soluble forms may act as specific immunosuppressors during pregnancy (Le Bouteiller, 1999). Recent evidence supports this hypothesis. *HLA-G* transcripts are present in great number in placental extravillous membranes in the first trimester, while at term, transcript numbers decline sharply, in keeping with the theory that HLA-G provides protection for the allogeneic embryo from maternal NK cell surveillance (Agrawal, 2003). This putative role raises the possibility that HLA-G may play a role in tolerance for transplanted tissues. Along these lines, it is interesting to note that liver–kidney transplant recipients with high concentrations of HLA-G in their sera had low numbers of acute rejection episodes and may therefore require less immunosuppressive therapy (Creput, 2003).

HLA-E

HLA-E may play a role in protecting a target cell from NK-cell-mediated lysis. HLA-E molecules bind a set of almost identical hydrophobic peptides derived from the leader sequences of the classical class I and HLA-G heavy chains. HLA-E displays these bound peptides at the cell surface for recognition by NK cells, providing a check for the integrity of the antigen-presenting pathway (Lee, 1998a, 1998b; O'Callaghan, 1998). Skin grafting in a transgenic mouse model suggests that HLA-E may be recognized as a transplantation antigen (Pacasova, 1999). Recent studies suggest that host NK cells may be able to recognize HLA-E on allogeneic cells, and possibly tolerate it, even when it is bound to donor peptides. With this finding comes the potential for exploiting this tolerance in pursuit of preventing NK-cell-mediated graft rejection and graft-versus-host disease (GVHD) (Matsunami, 2002).

HLA-F

The role of HLA-F is unknown. Computer modeling predicts that certain amino acid residues of HLA-F could contribute to a putative peptide-binding groove, consistent with a role in antigen presentation by HLA-F (O'Callaghan, 1998). To date, HLA-F appears to be normally expressed only on the surface of extravillous trophoblasts that have invaded the maternal decidua, and has also been found on the surfaces of lymphoblastoid cell lines infected with Epstein–Barr virus (Ishitani, 2003)

Class II Molecules – *HLA-DR, HLA-DQ, HLA-DP* Subregions

The class II molecules in humans were first recognized by their ability to stimulate allogeneic T cells in the mixed leukocyte culture (MLC). During the 1975 International Histocompatibility Workshop, the MLC was used to define the HLA-D allelic series (Thorsby, 1975). Because MLCs required 7 days before results could be obtained, a rapid serologic detection of HLA-D was sought. In 1975, it was determined that alloantisera contained antibodies reactive with molecules closely associated with the specificities previously identified as HLA-D by cellular techniques (Dausset, 1981). Following the 1977 International Histocompatibility Workshop, these serologic specificities were termed DR, for D-related specificities, since HLA-D and HLA-DR were observed to be associated but not identical to each other. Serologic testing coupled with genetic and immunochemical studies identified additional class II molecules, DR52, DR53, DR51, and DQ. Cellular techniques identified still another class II molecule in the late 1970s (Shaw, 1981). This molecule (now termed HLA-DP) was initially described as a secondary B-cell antigen (SB) because it was usually weak or undetectable in a primary MLC and required a secondary phase stimulation in culture for detection. Subsequently, the DNA coding sequences and locations of these genes within the MHC were further characterized using molecular biology techniques (Beck, 1999).

Structure of Class II Molecules

The class II HLA-DR, -DQ, and -DP molecules are heterodimers consisting of two noncovalently associated transmembrane glycoproteins, an α chain (33–35 kDa) and a β chain (26–28 kDa) (Fig. 47–3) (Gorga, 1992). Both polypeptide chains span the cell membrane and are oriented with their amino termini on the outside of the cell. The extracellular regions of the α- and β-polypeptides are each divided into two domains, designated α_1 and α_2 and β_1 and β_2, and each domain consists of approximately 90 amino acid residues. The α chain has two carbohydrate moieties, one high-mannose and one complex-type glycan, at amino acids 78 and 118, respectively. β Chains have one complex-type oligosaccharide at amino acid 19. The amino-terminal α_1 and β_1 domains of α and β chains contain the polymorphic residues, while the membrane proximal α_2 and β_2 domains are highly conserved and are homologous to immunoglobulin constant region domains. A region of approximately 12 amino acids in length connects the second extracellular domain to the hydrophobic transmembrane region (23 amino acids) and a small intracytoplasmic domain (8–15 amino acids).

Based on crystallography, the class II molecule is similar in structure to the class I molecule (Brown, 1993) (Fig. 47–4). In the class II molecule, the α_1 and β_1 domains of the α and β chains form an eight-stranded β-pleated sheet topped by two α-helices to form the antigen-binding groove at the top of the molecule. The α_2 and β_2 domains each form two antiparallel β-pleated sheets that support the groove at the top. As with class I, many of the amino acids that line the antigenic peptide-binding groove are polymorphic, creating differences in peptide-binding specificities for the different class II allelic products.

Like the class I molecules, the class II molecules are highly polymorphic (Table 47–2) (Bodmer, 1997, 1999; Marsh, 2002). Class II polymorphism is defined by (1) class II specific antibodies (alloantisera and monoclonal antibodies), which bind to class II molecules; (2) alloproliferative T cells that recognize and proliferate in response to foreign class II molecules in vitro; (3) two-dimensional gel electrophoresis of isolated class II molecules; (4) hybridization of restriction endonuclease digests of DNA encoding class II genes using locus-specific probes (a technique that detects restriction fragment length polymorphism [RFLP]); (5) PCR-based DNA typing of class II alleles; and (6) nucleotide sequencing of class II genes. Most of the class II polymorphism arises from amino acid sequence differences localized in the α_1 and β_1 domains of the two polypeptide chains.

Organization of Class II Genes

In contrast to the class I molecules, both the α and β chains of the class II molecules are encoded within a 1100 kb section of the MHC region (Figs 47–1 and 47–5) (Beck, 1999). The class II region includes three subregions – DR, DQ, and DP – each of which encodes at least one expressed *A* (encoding an α chain) and *B* (encoding a β chain) gene. Sequence comparisons suggest that both class I and class II genes arose through a successive series of gene duplications during the evolution of this gene complex. The original duplication in the class II region most likely gave rise to primordial *A* and *B* genes. More recent gene duplications generated the *DR*, *DQ*, and *DP* subregions containing multiple genes.

A typical *A* gene contains five exons encoding: (1) the 5' untranslated region and leader sequence; (2) α_1 domain; (3) α_2 domain; (4) connecting peptide, transmembrane region, cytoplasmic tail, and a portion of the 3' untranslated region; and (5) the remainder of the 3' untranslated region including the poly(A) addition signal. A typical β-chain gene is similar to the α-chain gene but has an extra exon for the cytoplasmic tail.

DR Subregion

The DR subregion encodes either one or two DR molecules depending on the haplotype (Bodmer, 1997, 1999). The subregion contains a single expressed DRA gene that is similar in different haplotypes, differing only in a single conservative amino acid substitution found in the cytoplasmic domain.

The most centromeric DRB gene, DRB1 (Fig. 47–5), encodes a highly polymorphic β chain that, when associated with the α chain, exhibits serologic specificities DR1–DR18. This molecule is the predominant class II molecule on the cell surface, accounting for well over half of the total cell surface class II molecules. There are multiple nucleic acid and, hence, amino acid sequence differences among DRB1 alleles.

The second expressed DRB gene, present only in some class II haplotypes, is located between the DRB1 locus and the DRA locus (Fig. 47–5). In cells expressing DR alleles, DRB1*03, *11, *12, *13, *14, the second DRB gene is termed DRB3. (HLA nomenclature is described subsequently.) The DRB3 gene is polymorphic, although at present the number of identified alleles is approximately 10 times less than the number of DRB1 alleles. The DRB3 product combined with the DRA product forms the DR molecule, which carries the DR52 serologic specificity. In cells expressing DRB1*04, *07, and *09 alleles, the second DRB gene is termed DRB4. The DRB4 product combined with the DRA product forms the molecule that carries the serological specificity DR53. Lastly, in cells expressing DRB1*15 and *16 alleles, the second DRB gene is termed DRB5. This DRB5 product combined with the DRA product carries the DR51 serological specificity. Haplotypes expressing DRB1*01, *08, or *10 alleles do not usually carry a second expressed DRB locus. There are exceptions to these associations. For example, a haplotype carrying DRB1*15 without a DRB5 locus has been described (Wade, 1993).

DQ Subregion

One set of A and B genes, DQA1 and DQB1, encode the DQ heterodimer that carries the DQ1–9 serologic specificities (Table 47–2 and Fig. 47–5) (Bodmer, 1997, 1999). DQ molecules represent approximately 15–20% of the total class II molecules expressed on the cell surface. As both DQA1 and DQB1 loci are polymorphic and because the protein products can associate in trans as well as in cis, heterozygotes may potentially express four different DQ molecules on their cell surfaces (Fig. 47–6). Other DQ-like A and B genes in the DQ subregion such as DQA2 and DQB2 are very similar to the DQA1 and DQB1 genes; however, no functional protein products are expressed.

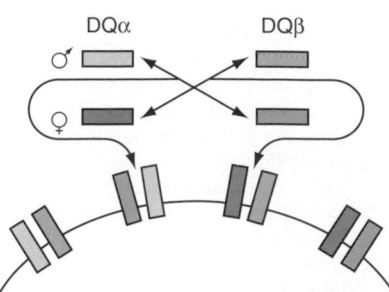

Cis association

DQα   DQβ

Cell surface

Trans association

DQα   DQβ

Figure 47–6 Model of the *cis* and *trans* associations of DQα and DGβ chains.

DP Subregion

The DP subregion contains two sets of A and B genes (Fig. 47–5). One set, DPA1 and DPB1, encodes the DP protein product; the other set is made up of pseudogenes. Both DPA1 and DPB1 genes are highly polymorphic (Bodmer, 1997, 1999). The level of DP expression on the cell surface is very low.

Linkage Disequilibrium of Genes in the Class II Region

Specific combinations of DRB1/DRB3, DRB1/DRB4, DRB1/DRB5, and DQA1/DQB1 alleles are common. The DQA1/DQB1 combinations found may be controlled in part by the ability of α and β chains to pair (Kwok, 1993). In addition, certain DR and DQ alleles are inherited together more frequently than expected, resulting in linkage disequilibrium in a population. The frequency of these combinations differs strikingly among different ethnic population groups. For example, both the DRB1*1101, DQB1*0501 (DR11[5]), DQ5[1] and the DRB1*0901, DQB1*0303(DR9, DQ9[3]) haplotypes frequently are found in populations of direct African heritage; whereas these DR–DQ combinations are rarely found in populations of Caucasoid heritage. Crossing over between the DP loci and the DR/DQ loci is common. Thus, there is minimal linkage disequilibrium between the DR/DQ and the DP alleles. Lists of the common DRB1/DQA1/DQB1 haplotypes have been published (Begovich, 1992; Imanishi, 1992).

Regulation of Class II Gene Expression

Class II molecules, HLA-DR, -DQ and -DP, are constitutively expressed on antigen-presenting cells (APCs) of the immune system, including monocytes, macrophages, dendritic cells, and B lymphocytes. DNA sequences found upstream of the coding sequences in class II genes are critical to expression. Binding of proteins to these regions regulates the expression of class II genes. Alterations in the ability of DNA-binding proteins to interact with the 5′ regulatory DNA sequences eliminating the expression of class II genes leads to an immunodeficiency called the 'bare lymphocyte syndrome' (Kovats, 1994; Mach, 1996). Class II genes are inducible by interferon (IFN)-γ in many cell types (Glimcher, 1992; Mach, 1996) and expression may be affected by other cytokines (Guardiola, 1993). Expression of class II molecules in APCs may be modulated, particularly in dendritic cells, following antigen deposition and inflammation. The level of antigenic peptide-class II complex expression as well as the presence of a co-stimulatory signal on the mature APC may play an important role in transplantation and in autoimmune diseases (Nepom, 1991; Banchereau, 1998) (see Ch. 48).

Function of Class II Molecules

Class II molecules act as antigen receptors in the immune response (Fig. 47–2), binding antigenic peptide fragments processed from exogenous antigens such as bacteria. The exogenous antigens enter the cell through the endocytic pathway and are degraded into peptide fragments in late endosomes where they encounter and bind to the newly assembled class II molecules (Watts, 1997). Binding of processed protein peptide fragments to the class II molecule is facilitated by two proteins encoded within the class II region of the MHC, DM and DO (Fig. 47–5). Peptide binding is affected by polymorphic residues located in the groove of the class II molecule. The complex of antigenic fragment bound to the class II molecule is then transported to the cell surface for display to and recognition by circulating T cells.

Antigen receptors on CD4⁺ T lymphocytes interact with the class II-antigenic fragment complex triggering activation of the cell (Jorgensen, 1992). In the experimental system used to dissect this mechanism, effector T lymphocytes were stimulated in vitro with autologous APCs previously incubated with antigen. As observed for class I, the recognition of the antigenic fragment by the effector T cell is influenced by MHC allelic polymorphism. The effector T cell is specific for the priming antigenic peptide in conjunction with the particular class II allelic product that originally presented the antigen (MHC restriction) (Rosenthal, 1973).

Each T cell activated by recognition of the complex of antigen fragment bound to class II molecule can perform one or several functions (Paul, 1994). The CD4⁺ T cell can help B lymphocytes to differentiate to antibody-producing plasma cells, or it can help other T lymphocytes to differentiate to either cytotoxic cells or cells with suppressor function. In addition, the T cell itself can function either as a cytotoxic cell, directly killing cells with the appropriate target (i.e., cells expressing class II MHC molecules complexed with the specific antigen), or as a cell with suppressor function causing a dampening of the immune response. T cells also produce a number of biologically important molecules (such as IFN-γ) that augment the immune response and increase the expression of MHC molecules on target cells. In addition, T cells produce growth factors such as interleukin (IL)-2. These growth factors affect a wide range of cells from hematopoietic progenitor cells to mature lymphocytes.

Other Class II Genes

At least four other class II genes, *DOA*, *DOB*, *DMA*, and *DMB*, have been described that express protein products (Fig. 47–5). The proteins encoded by the *DMA* and *DMB* genes form the DM heterodimer. The proteins encoded by the *DOA* and *DOB* genes form the DO heterodimer. These gene products are not detected on the cell surface but rather are expressed inside the cell, localized to specialized intracellular compartments where newly synthesized class II (DR, DQ, DP) molecules bind their antigenic peptides. The DM molecule regulates peptide binding to HLA-DR, -DQ, -DP, serving both a chaperone-like and an editor-like function (Morris, 1994) that favors the presentation of stably bound peptides. The DO molecule negatively regulates the function of DM (van Ham, 1997).

Characteristics of Antigenic Fragments Bound by MHC Class I and Class II Molecules

The function of class I and class II molecules as antigen-binding receptors is similar; however, the peptides they bind have different characteristics (Cresswell, 1994; Engelhard, 1994). Peptides derived from proteins synthesized de novo in the cell (endogenous antigens such as viral antigens), associate with class I molecules in the endoplasmic reticulum. In contrast, peptides from soluble and particulate antigens taken up by the cell into the endocytic pathway (exogenous antigens) bind with class II molecules in an endosomal compartment. Both class I and class II molecules can alternatively bind self-peptides found in these compartments. Self-peptides result from the normal degradation of cellular proteins. Some of these self-peptides are fragments of histocompatibility molecules themselves. Usually, the self-peptides bound to MHC molecules do not trigger T lymphocytes, as they are molecules to which the immune system of the individual is tolerant. These self-peptides may, however, trigger immune responses initiating a self-destructive process leading to autoimmunity (Nepom, 1991) (see Chs 50–52).

Peptide binding to MHC molecules occurs only when the peptide fragment is of a suitable length and contains a particular amino acid sequence or motif that allows it to bind to one or more of the MHC molecules expressed in that individual. An example of a motif for a peptide that binds to the HLA molecule encoded by *A*0201* is leucine (or methionine or isoleucine) at residue 2 of the peptide, a hydrophilic amino acid at residue 3, and a valine (or leucine or isoleucine or alanine) at residue 9. The amino acids that make up the motif are referred to as 'anchor' residues of the peptide. Different HLA molecules, either molecules encoded by different alleles at the same locus (*HLA-A*0203, *0211*, or **0301*) or molecules encoded by different loci (*B*4001* or *DRB1*0406*) bind peptides with different motifs. The amino acids forming the peptide motif bind to the MHC molecule in pockets found within the antigen-binding groove (Stern, 1994). The polymorphic amino acids of the MHC molecules line this groove and thus create differences in peptide-binding specificities for the different MHC molecules.

The peptides bound to class I molecules are 9–10 amino acids in length. Both the carboxy- and amino-terminal ends of the peptide are buried in the class-I-binding groove forming a 'closed' peptide–MHC complex. The peptides bound to class II molecules vary in length from 12 to 30 amino acids. While maintaining the requirement for specific motif residues nested in the central portion of the peptide, both the carboxy- and amino-terminal ends of the peptide extend outside the class-II-binding groove forming an 'open' peptide–MHC complex (Stern, 1994).

Recognition of Foreign MHC Molecules

Allorecognition involves the recognition by a T lymphocyte of a foreign MHC molecule on a cell from a second (allogeneic) individual. Upon recognition, the interaction triggers a series of events resulting in activation of the T cell and the initiation of an immune response not unlike the recognition of pathogens. Based on data from models of vascularized organ transplantation (Sayegh, 1996). The *direct* pathway for allorecognition involves the stimulation of recipient T cells by the donor MHC–peptide complex (i.e., direct recognition of intact foreign MHC molecules). The second route of allorecognition, the *indirect* pathway, involves the stimulation of recipient T cells by self-MHC molecules presenting peptide fragments from donor cells. Indirect presentation occurs when antigen-processing cells of the recipient ingest cellular material from the grafted tissue, degrade the material intracellularly, and display the allogenic peptide(s) complexed with self-MHC molecules. Peptides derived from polymorphic regions of donor MHC molecules are the major candidates for stimulation of the indirect immune response (Suciu-Foca, 1998; Gould, 1999; Harris, 1999).

Tandem Repeats and Single Nucleotide Polymorphisms in the MHC

Over 300 short tandem repeats (STRs) have been identified within the human MHC region (Foissac, 1997). Multiple single nucleotide polymorphisms (SNPs) are also present. A study by Abbal (1997) examined six STR loci within the MHC in a population of unrelated individuals and found strong linkage disequilibrium between specific HLA haplotypes and the STR markers. Since these markers cover a larger region of the MHC than the classical HLA markers now used, they may provide a more comprehensive approach to identifying MHC-identical individuals. These markers might, for example, be used to identify a recombinant MHC haplotype within a family (Carrington, 1996) and to enhance the probability that any unidentified histocompatibility genes in the MHC are matched. Molecular methods have been developed to identify both STRs and SNPs that are accurate and reproducible (Carrington, 1998).

Minor Histocompatibility Molecules

Minor histocompatibility antigens (mHags) are immunogenetic peptides that bind to MHC molecules and can be recognized by T cells to undesirable GVHD, but in the setting of leukemic recipients, can produce the beneficial condition graft-versus-leukemia. Achieving the proper balance of acceptable GVHD and sufficient graft-versus-leukemia is problematic. In MHC-identical progenitor cell grafts, GVHD may be induced by mHag differences between the recipient and donor (Mutis, 1999). The mHags can be any polymorphic gene product encoded outside the MHC that differs between donor and recipient and which stimulates a T-cell response (Goulmy, 1997; Simpson, 1998). Like other protein antigens, the polymorphic protein must be processed into antigenic fragments and the polymorphic peptide fragment(s) must bind within the groove of MHC molecules. Because of the requirement for antigen presentation by MHC molecules, any polymorphic peptide must carry a motif suitable for MHC-specific binding. Thus, not all individuals can present and respond to all mHags even if there is a difference between donor and recipient. Most mHags are presented to CD8+ T cells by MHC class I molecules. T-cell responses are initiated when the T-cell receptor recognizes complexes formed by the polymorphic peptides of the mHags bound to the MHC molecules expressed on APCs.

The mHags were originally defined by skin graft rejection and by cytotoxic assays with T-cell clones. These polymorphic peptides have restricted binding to class I MHC molecules, so biochemical definition of the minor histocompatibility antigenic peptide components was accomplished by the elution, purification, and sequencing of the mHag peptide bound to a specific MHC molecule (den Haan, 1995). Recent studies have demonstrated the potential significance of mHags in clinical transplantation (Goulmy, 1997, 1996; Martin, 1997; Dupont, 1998). mHag-specific cytotoxic T lymphocytes have been demonstrated in patients with GVHD (Mutis, 1999). Recipient disparity for one mHag (HA-1) was associated with an increased risk of acute GVHD after marrow transplantation using genotypically HLA-identical sibling donors, though this may not always be the case. Recently, HA-1 disparity has been shown to be associated with ongoing graft-versus-leukemia and suppression of progenitor leukemia cells in some patients (Kircher, 2004; Kloosterboer, 2004). The importance of matching for other mHags (HA-2, HA-3, HA-4, HA-5, H-Y) is less clear. DNA-based techniques to detect differences in mHags have been developed (Tseng, 1998; Wilke, 1998) and are being used in studies to measure the impact of these disparities on the outcome of transplantation.

HLA Nomenclature

Serologic and Cellular Specificities

HLA terminology is designated by a World Health Organization (WHO) Committee for HLA Nomenclature (Table 47–2) (Bodmer 1999, 1997).

VI

Historically, serologic and cellular defined specificities localized on the HLA protein molecules were assigned based on results of international workshops during which typing reagents were exchanged among participating laboratories (13th International Histocompatibility Workshop Web site, Table 47–1). (The 14th HLA and Immunogenetics workshop will be convened during November 2005 in Melbourne, Australia.) The assignments include the name of the HLA molecule and a numerical designation based on the order in which the serologically defined specificity was defined. For example, HLA-A1 (or just A1) was the first HLA-A specificity to be assigned and HLA-A80 was the most recent. Over time, older serologically defined specificities were 'split' as the definition became more discriminating. The narrowest definition of the specificity is called the subtypic or private specificity. The broader, shared specificities are called supertypic specificities. For example, B44 and B45 are subtypic specificities of the supertypic specificity B12. Thus, a cell that is either B44$^+$ or B45$^+$ must also be positive for B12.

In serologic testing, some alloantisera bind to more than one HLA allelic product, a phenomenon termed *cross-reactivity*. This serologic cross-reactivity among allelic products of the *HLA-A* and *HLA-B* loci has been extensively studied and has been used to cluster molecules within cross-reactive antigen groups (CREGs) (Rodey, 1987). Class I molecules within a CREG share one or more determinants that are not shared by molecules in another CREG. An antigenic determinant (epitope) shared among members of a CREG is called a *public specificity*. Some of the CREG reactivity can be explained by the sharing of amino acid sequences among the HLA molecules in a CREG (Terasaki, 1992). The inclusion of HLA specificities within a CREG is not standard, as different sets of antibodies produce unique reaction patterns and two different investigators with different sets of reagents may identify slightly different CREG groups. However, the various CREG groupings overlap considerably (Ellison, 1994).

The HLA-Bw4 and Bw6 specificities are broad, public epitopes that reside on the same molecule as the *HLA-B* locus subtypic specificities, but at a different site. Thus Bw4 and Bw6 are a diallelic system, and all *B* locus (and some *A* locus) molecules carry either Bw4 or Bw6 specificities. The region of the HLA molecule carrying the Bw4/Bw6 specificities has been identified in the α_1 helix between amino acid residues 77 and 83 (Parham, 1991).

The WHO designated serologic specificities localized to the class II molecules, HLA-DR and -DQ, have been assigned as described for the class I molecules (Bodmer, 1999, 1997) (Table 47–2). Six HLA-DP types were originally defined by cellular techniques. Class II HLA-DP molecules are not adequately defined serologically.

There are 26 HLA-D specificities that were identified by MLC. All the HLA-D specificities retain the 'w' designation, as these specificities are defined functionally by the measurement of stimulation of a responder cell. The stimulation is generated by differences in the DR molecules expressed on a stimulator cell and, to a lesser extent, additional stimulation by the DQ and DP molecules.

DNA-Based Allele Designations

Nucleotide sequencing has been used to identify the many different alleles encoding the HLA molecules. Currently, a single serologically defined specificity may reside on two to more than 25 different allelic products (Table 47–2). Each HLA allele is designated by the name of the gene locus followed by an asterisk and a four- to seven-digit number indicating the allele. For example, A*0201 is an allele of the *HLA-A* gene; B*1510 is an allele of the *HLA-B* gene; DPB1*0101 is an allele of the *HLA-DPB1* gene; and DQA1*0601 is an allele of the *HLA-DQA1* gene.

The first two numbers in the numerical designation of each allele are frequently based on the serologic type of the resultant molecule and/or the nucleotide sequence similarity to other alleles in the group. For example, the HLA-A molecule expressed by the A*0201 allele bears the A2 serologic specificity defining the HLA-A2 antigen. However, the HLA-B molecule expressed by the B*1510 allele does not bear the B15-associated serologic specificity but rather the B71 serologic specificity defining the B71 antigen. It was designated B*1510 because of its predicted amino acid sequence similarity to B15 antigens. Cells expressing DRB1*0103 were serologically typed as DR-blank, DR1, or even DR13. Nucleotide sequencing identified an allele with a similar DNA structure to alleles bearing the DR1 serologic specificity (e.g., DRB1*0101 and *0102) and the name of this allele was based on that structural similarity. When a unique serologic specificity was later identified, the DR antigen determined by DRB1*0103 was given the DR103 serologic designation. The third and fourth numbers in the allele designation refer to the order in which the allele was described. For example, A*0201 was the first A2 allele to be sequenced and A*0203 was the third.

Some alleles may differ in the DNA sequence of their coding regions but their predicted amino acid sequence does not differ (often termed a silent or synonymous substitution). These combinations of alleles are identified by a five-digit designation. The first four numbers are shared, while the fifth digit is used to distinguish the unique nucleic acid sequences of the alleles (e.g., B*27051 and B*27052). In addition, two or more alleles may have a seven-digit name in which the first four digits are shared (e.g., DRB4*0103101 and DRB4*0103102). Digits five through seven indicate that the two alleles differ only outside the protein coding region. In the example listed here, the difference affects the RNA splice site of DRB4*0103102 resulting in loss of expression of the allele (Sutton, 1989). Finally, alleles that are not expressed as proteins at the cell surface may have an N added to their names (e.g., A*0215N, DRB4*0103102N) to indicate 'null.' Since each allele has a unique numerical designation, the N designation is not always written (i.e., A*0215 and A*0215N are the same allele).

New alleles are described in regular reports of the WHO HLA Nomenclature Committee (Table 47–1, www.anthonynolan.com/HIG/nomenc.html; Bodmer, 1999), and the nucleotide sequences of all alleles are deposited in a computerized databank (GenBank, EMBL, IMGT/HLA databases). Currently, there are, for example, over 349 *HLA-A* alleles assigned. New alleles are continually being identified and can be accessed through the web site.

Techniques for Identifying HLA Polymorphism

Histocompatibility testing or HLA typing or tissue typing is performed in a limited number of laboratories because it uses specialized procedures and reagents. Commercially available kits can be obtained for both DNA-based and serologic testing; however, interpretation of the test results requires considerable experience and knowledge. Histocompatibility laboratories usually are found in medical centers that have organ and/or hematopoietic progenitor cell transplantation programs. HLA testing techniques are discussed in general in this section. For detailed procedures, the reader should refer to the most recent American Society for Histocompatibility and Immunogenetics (ASHI) *Laboratory Manual*, 4th edition (2001) (see Table 47–1 for the ASHI web site). HLA testing laboratories are accredited through ASHI, the European Foundation for Immunogenetics, and other organizations.

DNA-Based Typing of Class I and Class II Alleles

Although serologic and cellular typing of HLA antigens has been extremely useful, there are a number of technical drawbacks to these techniques. With the advent of rapid and reliable methods for the isolation and characterization of class I and II genes and the determination of the nucleotide sequences of class I and II alleles, it has become possible to use DNA-based methods for HLA typing. DNA-based typing of HLA alleles is now a commonly used technique in HLA typing laboratories (Hurley, 1997a; Middleton, 1999).

In contrast to other forms of testing, DNA-based typing has five significant advantages.

1. It is *specific*. The specificity of each DNA typing reagent (i.e., synthetic oligonucleotide primers and probes) is clearly defined and is based on a specific, known nucleotide sequence. Since the oligonucleotides used as DNA typing reagents are synthetic, reagents are not limited and there should be no lot-to-lot variation in specificity.
2. It is *flexible*. New reagents can be designed as new alleles are discovered and unique nucleotide sequences identified. The testing can be carried out at several levels of resolution depending on the typing requirements and the time available for the testing.
3. It is more *robust* than other techniques. DNA typing does not require viable lymphocytes and is not influenced by the health of the patient. Furthermore, DNA-based testing is highly reproducible when standard methodologies such as sequence specific oligonucleotide probe (SSOP) testing is used in conjunction with a standard test protocol (Ng, 1996; Hurley, 2000a).
4. It can be used for *large-scale* typing. The batching of samples facilitated by automated and computerized methodologies reduces cost and errors. DNA-based methods are particularly applicable for the HLA typing of large numbers of volunteers for donor registries.
5. It can *discriminate* by detecting the full extent of HLA diversity. HLA alleles can specify HLA proteins that are indistinguishable using serologic typing. For example, an individual carrying the DRB1*0401 allele would have the same serologic type (DR4) as an individual carrying the DRB1*0412 allele (DR4). Thus, DRB1*0401 and DRB1*0412 are splits of the broad specificity DR4. These splits are identified by DNA typing. Serologic reagents specific enough to define

this split are not available. Currently, over 30 subdivisions of DR4 have been defined. There are many other examples of splits defined using DNA typing that cannot be identified using serologic typing; some are listed in Table 47–2.

The problems with serologic typing are particularly acute when typing some population groups. For example, populations of direct African origin can express class I and class II antigens that are difficult to identify with the currently available serologic reagents (Bozon, 1997; Yu, 1997; Mytilineos, 1998). DNA-based HLA typing has greatly improved the ability to define HLA types in these populations.

Preparation and Amplification of DNA

Any cell with a nucleus can be used as a source of DNA. While red blood cells do not contain nuclei, other cells in the blood, such as lymphocytes, are a good source of DNA. Cell lines such as Epstein–Barr-virus-transformed B lymphocytes are also a good source of DNA. As transformed cells can be grown in culture in the laboratory, they provide a replenishable supply of DNA and are used to provide reference DNA for quality control of typing procedures.

DNA is usually prepared from a small quantity (0.2–1 mL) of whole blood. Many different protocols can be used to isolate DNA from cells, and commercial kits are also available for the preparation of DNA. The sensitivity of detection of HLA types is enhanced greatly by the amplification of DNA encoding HLA genes using the PCR technique (Saiki, 1988). A pair of synthetic oligonucleotides (primers) should be complementary to sequences flanking a specific HLA gene are utilized to generate millions of copies of that gene for use in the HLA typing reaction. Some typing reactions utilize primer sequences that are shared by all alleles at an HLA locus; other typing procedures utilize primer sets that are shared by only a subset of alleles at a locus. Annealing of the primers to sample DNA during the PCR reaction uses reaction conditions that guarantee that the primers will bind to perfectly matched sequences (target sequences) and not to sequences of other loci or other alleles that are not matched. By adjusting the temperature of the annealing component of the PCR reaction, the typing laboratory can control the specificity of the amplification.

Sequence-Specific Priming

One method of identification of HLA alleles uses sequence-specific primers (SSPs) in the PCR reaction (Olerup, 1992; Bunce, 1995). These primers anneal to denatured DNA containing the HLA alleles from which the primer sequences were derived. In the subsequent PCR reaction, only these selected alleles are amplified. DNA amplified by the primers is identified by gel electrophoresis or, if the DNA is labeled with a dye during amplification, by fluorescence. This procedure is useful in typing a small number of samples within a short time period. Commercial kits are available.

Sequence-Specific Oligonucleotide Hybridization.

It has been possible to use hybridization of SSOPs to amplified DNA to identify alleles (Gao, 1991; Williams, 1997; Cao, 1999). The use of several different oligonucleotide probes to define a specific HLA allele or the use of sequence-specific priming coupled with hybridization with panels of probes is usually required. A set of oligonucleotides capable of identifying each allele is hybridized to denatured PCR-amplified DNA attached to a solid support. Hybridization conditions are adjusted so that the probes will anneal to denatured DNA containing the HLA alleles from which the oligonucleotide sequence was derived. The oligonucleotides are labeled with a tag for detection of hybridization. For example, the oligonucleotide might be coupled to an enzyme such as alkaline phosphatase. Following addition of a substrate, alkaline phosphatase cleaves the substrate to yield a colored compound or to produce light (chemiluminescence). After visualization, the pattern of hybridization can be read to determine the alleles present. Figure 47-7 illustrates the approach using an oligonucleotide probe for the DQB1 allele, DQB1*0302, to identify patients with insulin-dependent diabetes who carry this allele (Todd, 1987). The SSOP method is highly accurate, specific, and reliable (Ng, 1996; Hurley, 2000a). It is often used in situations where many samples are typed in large batches. Commercial kits using this method are available.

In a related procedure, called the reverse format, the oligonucleotide probes are bound to a solid support (Bugawan, 1994). DNA from the samples to be tested is amplified using primers labeled with, for example, biotin. The amplified DNA is then hybridized to the immobilized probes, which contain sequences found in the alleles present in the DNA. After visualization (using an avidin-linked detection system), the pattern of hybridization can be read to determine the alleles present. This procedure is useful for typing both small and large numbers of samples. Commercial kits utilizing this method are available.

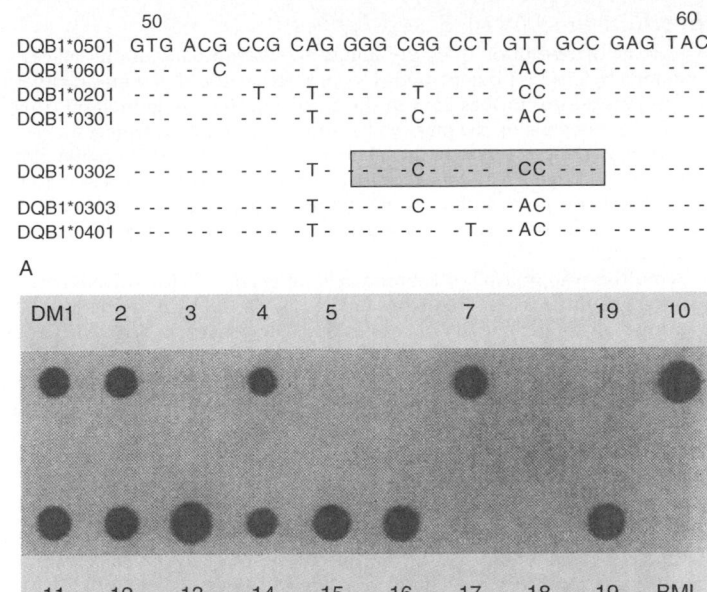

	50								60		
DQB1*0501	GTG	ACG	CCG	CAG	GGG	CGG	CCT	GTT	GCC	GAG	TAC
DQB1*0601	- - -	- - C	- - -	- - -	- - -	- - -	- - -	- AC	- - -	- - -	- - -
DQB1*0201	- - -	- - -	- T -	- T -	- - -	- T -	- - -	- CC	- - -	- - -	- - -
DQB1*0301	- - -	- - -	- T -	- - -	- C -	- - -	- AC	- - -	- - -	- - -	- - -
DQB1*0302	- - -	- - -	- T -	- - -	- C -	- - -	- CC	- - -	- - -	- - -
DQB1*0303	- - -	- - -	- T -	- - -	- C -	- - -	- AC	- - -	- - -	- - -
DQB1*0401	- - -	- - -	- T -	- - -	- - -	- T -	- AC	- - -	- - -	- - -

A

B

Figure 47–7 A, Nucleotide sequences of several DQB1 alleles. The sequences presented cover the codons for amino acids 50–60. A dash indicates that the nucleotide is identical to the top sequence. An oligonucleotide that is specific for the DQB1*0302 sequence is boxed. B, Oligonucleotide dot blot analysis of 17 insulin-dependent diabetes mellitus patients (DM1–19) and one control, BML. Amplified DNA containing class II DQB1 sequences for the patients was attached to a membrane and hybridized to the labeled oligonucleotide specific for the DQB1*0302 sequence (described previously). Positive hybridization signals indicate the patients who carry this DBQ1 gene sequence (patients DM1, 2, 4, 7, 10–16, 19). (With permission from Todd JA, Bell J, McDevitt HO: HLA-DQ β gene contributes to susceptibility and resistance to insulin-dependent diabetes mellitus, Nature 1987; 329:599.)

Sequence-Specific Conformational Polymorphism or Heteroduplex Analysis

Another, although little used, method of identification of HLA alleles analyzes the mobility of amplified DNA, either denatured (sequence-specific conformational polymorphism [SSCP]) or as a renatured DNA duplex (heteroduplex analysis), following electrophoresis (Arguello, 1996). The mobility of the DNA is compared to the mobility of amplified DNA from known HLA alleles to define an HLA allele. This procedure is useful in typing a small number of samples and particularly in comparisons between individuals, for example, within a family.

Nucleic Acid Sequencing

A final method of identification of HLA alleles involves the direct determination of the DNA sequences of the HLA alleles carried by an individual (sequence-based typing [SBT]). Alleles are identified either following PCR amplification to separate the alleles based on SSPs or as a mixture of two alleles. Sequencing is labor-intensive and highly complex but will be used frequently to determine the HLA match at an allele level between hematopoietic progenitor cell transplant patients and their prospective donors (Petersdorf, 1995a; Rozemuller, 1996; Scheltinga, 1997). Efforts to develop automated SBT methodologies have yielded several potentially promising high-throughput approaches. These include the use of denaturing high-performance liquid chromatography (HPLC), which is reported to provide greater typing resolution than can be achieved by PCR-based sequencing approaches (Etokebe, 2003), and the so-called pyrosequencing technique. Pyrosequencing is a real-time, non-electrophoretic DNA sequencing method that uses luciferase–luciferin light emission as a detection signal as nucleotides are incorporated into target DNA. A unique signal is created for each allelic variant, which is distinguished by recognition software (Nordstrom, 2000). Pyrosequencing by means of high-throughput systems permits processing of hundreds of individual specimens daily. In addition, reference-strand-mediated conformation analysis (RSCA) has been employed in high-throughput systems to achieve discrimination between HLA alleles differing by as little as one nucleotide. The technology detects differences between alleles by measuring their conformation-dependent mobility in polyacrylamide gels after they have been labeled with locus-specific fluorescent tags (Arguello, 1998).

Resolution of DNA-Based Typing

The level of resolution (i.e., the ability to discriminate among alleles) obtained by DNA typing methods is controlled by the choice and number of primers and/or probes used in the assay and the typing method. This choice may depend on the time available for performing the typing, the cost of the typing, the expertise of the laboratory personnel, and the purpose of the typing. Large-scale donor registry typing is usually carried out at low–intermediate resolution, while typing of a potential hematopoietic progenitor cell donor for a specific patient will be carried out at allele-level resolution.

A multistep approach is often used to identify *HLA* alleles by DNA-based typing. For this reason, HLA types defined by DNA-based typing may be reported at different levels of resolution. Low-resolution (or generic or serologic)-level DNA-based typing produces a result that is similar in appearance and detail to a serologic type. For example, a DNA-defined type, *DRB1*11* or *DRB1*11XX*, is the approximate equivalent of the serologic type DR11. The 'XX' indicates that the allele was not further defined. At this level of resolution, it is not possible to determine which of the more than 30 *DRB1*11* alleles is carried by the individual being tested. Although serologic typing can be as informative as low-resolution typing, results are more reliable with DNA-based testing. Intermediate-resolution-level DNA-based typing may narrow the choices by listing several different possibilities for the type of an individual, (e.g., *DRB1*1101* or *DRB1*1104*). Finally, high-resolution-level (or allele-level) DNA-based typing identifies the specific allele carried by an individual (e.g., *DRB1*1104*). Since identification of *HLA* alleles may be based on partial sequence information, it is possible that the interpretation of the results will miss alleles that were unknown at the time of the typing (Hurley, 1997b). For this reason, laboratories are cautioned to maintain their raw typing data (i.e., which primers and probes were positive and negative and the nucleotide sequences of the reagents) so that the results can be reinterpreted as new alleles are described.

Serologic Detection of Class I and Class II Molecules

Lymphocyte microcytotoxicity testing, which was originally used in the mouse system by Gorer and Amos and later modified by Terasaki and McClelland for use in the human system, has been used for HLA typing since the 1960s. Serologic testing for HLA-A, -B can be reproducible under controlled, standardized conditions; however, in large-scale testing (e.g., for registries), error rates may increase (Bozon, 1997; Yu, 1997). The reproducibility for serologically determined HLA-C and class II specificities is much lower. HLA-DP is not usually defined by serology. The microcytotoxicity serologic assay is still used fairly widely for class I specificities (HLA-A, -B) but has been supplanted by DNA-based testing for HLA-C and for class II specificities (HLA-DR, -DQ, -DP) in most typing laboratories. DNA-based testing with its greater resolution is used to determine the HLA type of unrelated individuals and of family members especially if the segregation of HLA cannot be accurately discriminated by serology (e.g., families where parents are not available or families where parents share an HLA antigen). For example, an offspring inherits DR4 from each parent and so is DR4 *antigen* homozygous (DR4,DR4). However, high-resolution DNA typing might identify two distinct alleles of the DR4 antigen, *DRB1*0401* and *DRB1*0403* (*DRB1*04 allele* heterozygote), providing informative data for haplotype segregation analysis.

Lymphocyte Preparation

Lymphocytes used routinely in HLA serologic typing assays are readily obtained from peripheral whole blood by layering on to a Ficoll–Hypaque gradient to separate the blood cells by density centrifugation. The separated peripheral blood lymphocytes (PBLs) can be used for HLA-A, -B, -C typing. To test for HLA-DR, -DQ serologic specificities, it is necessary either to enrich for B lymphocytes or to use a special two-color fluorescent technique to simultaneously differentiate between the unseparated B cells and T cells.

Lymphocyte Microcytotoxicity Assay

The HLA phenotype is determined by testing the unseparated lymphocyte preparation (PBL) or T lymphocytes (for HLA-A, -B, -C) or the enriched B lymphocytes (for HLA-DR, -DQ) against a panel of well-characterized HLA alloantisera. The assay is a two-stage test. During the sensitization stage, the lymphocytes are incubated with the antisera. Prescreened and standardized rabbit serum as a source of complement is added in excess and the mixture is incubated for an additional period. If the lymphocytes carry a cell-surface molecule recognized by complement-fixing antibodies

in the alloantiserum, the antibodies bind to the cells and the cells are subsequently lysed following the addition of complement. The assay is terminated with the addition of fluorescein diacetate and ethidium bromide for fluorescent detection procedures, or with either eosin and formalin or trypan blue and ethylenediaminetetraacetic acid (EDTA) for dye visualization methods. Reactions are read for percentage lysis and numerically graded.

HLA Typing Sera Trays

HLA typing reagents are derived from the sera of alloimmunized individuals (multiparous women, transplant recipients, multitransfused patients, and planned immunization of humans). Multi-well plates of human alloantisera (i.e., HLA typing trays) are commercially available. Because of the antigenic complexity of HLA antigens, several antisera should be used to define each specificity. Most laboratories use trays from at least two different vendors or may use locally derived alloantisera. Since many alloantisera are not truly monospecific and many exhibit some cross-reactivity, the reactivity of each antiserum must be thoroughly tested and known to the individual interpreting the results. This requires stringent quality control of each new lot of typing trays with well characterized reference cells. Since the titer and the specificity of antibody formed by a sensitized individual may not remain constant over time, supplies of antisera are limited. In an attempt to create a consistent and unlimited supply of reagents, some companies have produced monoclonal antibodies. These monoclonal reagents are not available for all HLA specificities.

Cross-Reactivity

HLA alloantisera may react with more than one HLA allelic product. This phenomenon can result from polyspecificity of the antisera and/or from cross-reactivity and is responsible for the complex reactivity patterns of some alloantisera. Polyspecific sera contain two or more HLA-specific antibodies that can be adsorbed to remove one antibody with little effect on the reactivity of the other(s). Cross-reactive antisera contain, most frequently, a single antibody that reacts with an antigenic determinant shared among several different HLA allelic products (i.e., CREG or broad determinants, as previously discussed) (Rodey, 1994). Cross-reactions occur most frequently among allelic products encoded by the same locus but can occur between allelic products encoded by different loci (e.g., A2 + B17).

Cellular Detection of Class II Molecules

The response of one cell in tissue culture to the alloantigens on the surface of a second cell is called the mixed leukocyte culture or mixed lymphocyte reaction (Hartzman, 1971). The MLC is considered an in vitro measure of class II disparity between individuals recognizing determinants found on class II molecules, which are known collectively as HLA-D. The T-cell response is made unidirectional by preventing cells from one of the two individuals from replicating by treating those cells with radiation or mitomycin-C prior to addition to the culture. The MLC represents a summation response of a responder cell to differences in the multiple determinants on HLA class II molecules (DR, DQ, and DP) encoded by the irradiated stimulator cell haplotypes. The response to DR molecules appears to predominate.

Use of the MLC in clinical laboratories to determine histocompatibility has declined because of limitations inherent in the technique. The MLC can be influenced by the health of the patient, the type of disease, and history of prior transfusion (Mickelson, 1996). For these reasons the MLC assay has been replaced by the more precise DNA-based typing methods. Currently, in some transplantation centers, the MLC is used to identify renal allograft recipients with specific hyporeactivity to donor HLA molecules following transplantation as a guideline for tapering of immunosuppression (Reinsmoen, 1993).

Limiting dilution analysis to define the frequency of donor cytotoxic (CTL_p) or helper (HTL_p) T lymphocytes has been used to predict the extent of allorecognition in hematopoietic progenitor cell transplantation (Madrigal, 1997). The correlations of these frequencies with subsequent events such as the extent of GVHD is still controversial.

Tissue/Organ Transplantation

Long-term survival of solid organ and hematopoietic progenitor cell grafts represents one of the most challenging goals in medical science. Renal transplantation is the therapy of choice for most patients with end-stage renal disease. Hematopoietic progenitor cell, heart, lung, liver, and pancreas transplantation are gaining wide acceptance as therapeutic procedures with successful outcome. The primary obstacle to solid organ and to hematopoietic progenitor cell transplantation is immunologically

Table 47–3 Therapeutic Drugs, Mechanism of Action and Monitoring Methods

Drug	Mechanism(s) of Action	Monitoring Methods*
Azathioprine	Purine antagonist; blocks cell proliferation	Routine labs, pharmacokinetic studies, pharmacodynamic studies
Glucocorticoids	Blocks cytokine gene transcription; inhibits T-cell proliferation and T-cell-dependent immunity	Routine labs, pharmacokinetic studies
Cyclosporine	Inhibits expression of nuclear regulatory proteins and T-cell activation genes	Routine labs, pharmacokinetic studies, pharmacodynamic studies
FK506	Inhibits expression of nuclear regulatory proteins and T-cell activation genes	Routine labs, pharmacokinetic studies
Mycophenolate mofetil	Inhibits purine biosynthesis, thereby suppressing T- and B-cell proliferation	Routine labs, pharmacokinetic studies, pharmacodynamic studies
Rapamycin	Inhibits DNA and protein synthesis, blocking T-cell proliferation; inhibits antigen-driven B-cell proliferation	Routine labs, pharmacokinetic studies, pharmacodynamic studies

* Routine labs include serum creatinine, BUN, CBC, liver enzymes, etc. Pharmacokinetic studies include measurement of trough levels and calculation of area under the curve (AUC). Pharmacodynamic study refers to measuring the biological effect of the drug at its target site.

Source: adapted from: Massey D, King A, Riley R: Renal Allograft Dysfunction in Kidney Transplant. American Society for Clinical Pathology, Clinical Chemistry Check Sample 2003; 43:19–38.

mediated rejection of the foreign tissue. Therefore, the success of allografting is dependent on the ability to deter the immune reaction, which may be accomplished by: (1) histocompatibility matching between the donor and the recipient; (2) immunosuppressive therapy of the recipient (see Table 47–3 for a list of common immunosuppression drugs and laboratory approaches used to monitor them) (Suthanthiran, 1996); and (3) ultimately achieving specific unresponsiveness to donor alloantigen(s) (i.e., tolerance) (Remuzzi, 1995).

Genetic Basis of Transplantation

The genetic basis of transplantation was first determined in 1916 as a result of tumor transplantation experiments in mice and was subsequently extended to transplants of normal tissue (Snell, 1981) It was demonstrated that skin grafts within inbred strains that were homozygous at histocompatibility loci (i.e., syngeneic grafts) were successful but grafts between two different inbred strains (allografts) were rejected. Furthermore, allografts from either parent inbred strain (two copies of the same MHC genes; homozygous) to first generation (F1) hybrids (one copy of each of the two different sets of MHC genes from two homozygous parents) survived in all animals; whereas, grafts from F1 hybrid offspring to either parent (one haplotype mismatch) did not survive. These observations established the laws of transplantation. In 1948, the factors or genes determining the fate of allografts were named histocompatibility or H genes. Also in 1948, the major histocompatibility locus in the mouse, H-2, was defined by Gorer (Snell, 1981). There are other histocompatibility or H antigens, which are termed mHags. Although called minor, mismatching for these antigens can have major effects (Goulmy, 1997; Dupont, 1998).

As convincing evidence already existed in experimental animal models that molecules encoded by the MHC represent the major genetic barrier to successful allografting, HLA typing was used in humans to determine and to optimize compatibility between graft donor and recipient. Initially, the influence of HLA antigens on graft survival was investigated by grafting of nonvascularized skin between family members. As in studies with inbred mice, skin grafts between HLA-identical siblings survived significantly longer than grafts between one-haplotype-matched siblings, parents, or unrelated donors. These observations were extended to renal transplantation during the late 1960s and early 1970s. The most recent data from the international Collaborative Transplant Study (CTS) in Heidelberg and from the United Network for Organ Sharing (UNOS) Registry in the United States (analyzed at UCLA), confirm the MHC as the major genetic barrier to transplantation for renal grafts (Cecka, 1999; Opelz, 1999) (Fig. 47–8); for current updates see the web sites listed in Table 47–1. The data for hematopoietic progenitor cell transplantation also reaffirms the role of the MHC in transplant outcome as measured by both patient survival and GVHD (Hansen, 1999) (Fig. 47–9).

Histocompatibility Matching

HLA Matching

Although the level of HLA match is an important element in transplant outcome, histocompatibility matching means different things in different settings and strategies for matching vary. Criteria differ with variables that

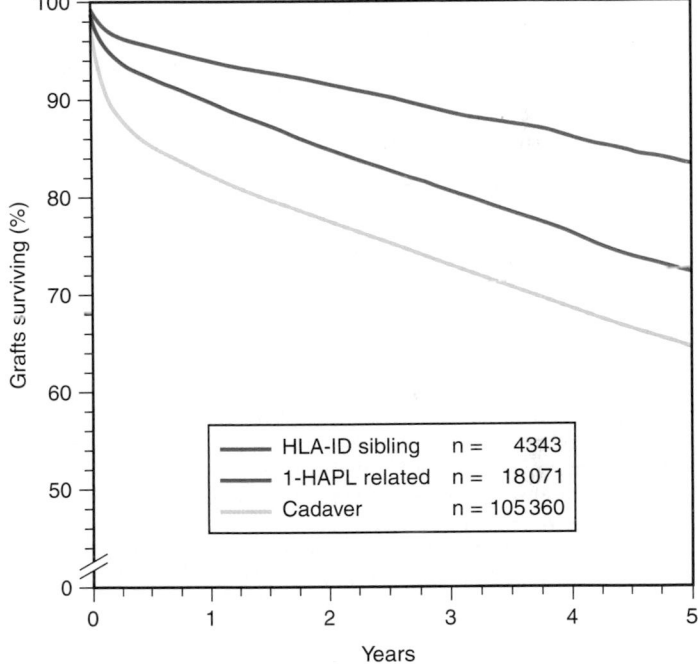

Figure 47–8 Five-year renal allograft (first transplant) survival of three categories of histocompatibility: HLA-identical siblings; one-haplotype living related; cadaver donor. Grafts from HLA-identical sibling donors (both HLA chromosomes matched) have the best outcome. Numbers of transplants studied are indicated (regression p <0.0001). (With permission from Opelz G, Wujcak T, Dohler B, et al: HLA compatibility and organ transplant survival. Rev Immunogenet 1999; 1:334.)

include the type of graft (e.g., solid vascularized organ versus hematopoietic progenitor cell), the disease (e.g., chronic myelogenous leukemia versus aplastic anemia), the age of the patient, and the clinical protocol (e.g., marrow versus umbilical cord blood; T cell depletion of marrow versus non-T-cell depletion) (see Ch. 37).

Matching usually includes evaluation of at least three loci, HLA-A, HLA-B, and HLA-DR. Individuals matched, at whatever resolution, for all three loci are termed 6/6 matches or 0 mismatches. Zero mismatches (a term used in solid organ transplantation) may also refer to donor/recipient pairs, where the donor has no detectable HLA differences from the recipient – that is, where the donor is homozygous for the alleles at one or more of the loci (e.g., homozygous donor: A*0101; B*0801; DRB1*0301; heterozygous recipient: A*0101, A*0301; B*0801, B*0702; DRB1*0301, DRB1*1501). Individuals matched for four of six alleles or antigens are termed 4/6 matches. Apparent differences in the level of match can arise because of the typing methodology used to assign HLA types (e.g., serologic versus DNA-based typing). The serologic and DNA nomenclatures, although they are related, can differ. The definition of a match can also vary depending on the typing resolution. A patient and donor may appear to be

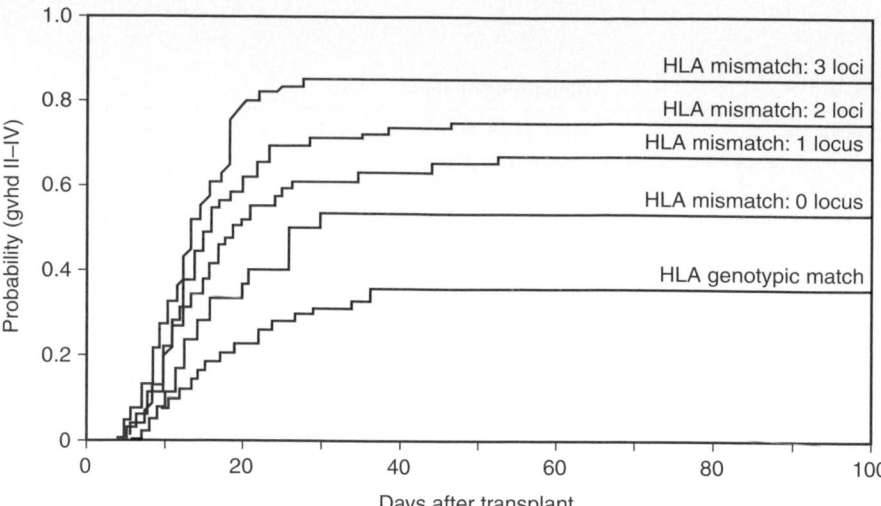

Figure 47–9 Probability of grades II–IV acute graft-versus-host disease (GVHD) in HLA-identical sibling (HLA genotypic match) and haploidentical related marrow donor transplants variably matched for HLA-A, -B, or DR/Dw (HLA mismatch: 3 loci, 2 loci, 1 locus or 0 loci). Matching for HLA-A, -B, and -DR was defined by serology, and matching for HLA-Dw was defined by MLC or by typing for *HLA-DRB1* alleles with sequence specific oligonucleotide probe (SSOP). All patients received unmodified marrow (without T-cell depletion) following a conditioning regimen that included total body irradiation,. Cyclosporine and methotrexate were given for GVHD prophylaxis. (With permission from Hansen JA, Yamamoto K, Petersdorf E, et al: The role of HLA matching in hematopoietic cell transplantation. Rev Immunogenet 1999; 1:359, copyright © 1999 Munksgaard International Publishers Ltd, Copenhagen, Denmark.)

matched at the serologic level (e.g., recipient: A2, A26; donor: A2, A26); however, the pair may be mismatched at the level of HLA alleles (e.g., recipient: *A*0201, A*2601*; Donor *A*0205, A*6601*).

Matching for classical HLA molecules at the allele level could optimize outcome for all grafts (both vascular organs and hematopoietic progenitor cells) (Petersdorf, 1998; Opelz, 1999). However, because of the extremely large number of HLA alleles, allelic-level matching is difficult. Therefore, the level of matching that ensures a good outcome for the largest number of patients of all ethnic populations must be considered.

Following hematopoietic progenitor cell transplantation, subtypic determinants or allelic differences initiate important cytotoxic T-cell responses leading to graft rejection and GVHD. Indeed, studies have shown that high-resolution matching for class I and class II alleles of the donor and recipient can improve outcome after unrelated marrow transplantation. Recent data suggest that multiple mismatches are detrimental to outcome; however, the impact neither of single mismatches nor of specific loci has yet been well defined (Petersdorf, 1998; Sasazuki, 1998; Hansen, 1999). Only a minority of patients awaiting transplantation will receive grafts from fully allele-matched donors (Hurley, 2000b). To enable all patients to benefit from life-saving transplantations, identifying allele mismatches that are well tolerated would allow the selection of mismatched donors to be prioritized according to the biologic risk of specific HLA mismatches.

Optimal matching for solid organ grafts may differ from matching requirements for hematopoietic progenitor cell transplantation. Recent data suggest that both the HLA loci matched and the level of resolution of HLA testing contribute to renal graft outcome (Opelz, 1999). Currently, UNOS facilitates sharing of cadaveric kidneys based on subtypic specificities. As subtypic matches are infrequently identified, it has been proposed that the HLA class I molecules be matched for the broader CREG determinants. CREG may define immunodominant determinants recognized in the humoral immune response. Rodey (1994) showed that 80–90% of the HLA alloantibodies formed by kidney recipients following transplantation are directed to CREG determinants. CREG determinants are shared among different class I HLA molecules and, in contrast to subtypic specificities, have a similar distribution among ethnic population groups. Rare subtypic specificities are included within the CREG. As the number of CREGs is less than the number of subtypic specificities, the probability of a CREG-level match is greater than for a subtypic or allele-level HLA class I match. Therefore, allocation of organs based on CREG matching should result in a higher probability of matched grafts being distributed equitably to recipients of all ethnic populations. CREG matching for the allocation of kidneys has been characterized as immunologically flawed and its observed positive effect in prolonging graft survival and reducing immunosuppressant requirements has been attributed entirely to the effect of HLA matching (Egfjord, 2003). Others cite a positive role for CREG matching in reducing HLA sensitization among minority recipients of renal transplants (Crowe, 2003).

Other strategies focus on matching for biologically relevant fragments of MHC molecules (e.g., epitope matching) (Suciu-Foca, 1998; Harris, 1999). Until recently, direct recognition of alloantigens was thought to be the main pathway for graft rejection responses. However, studies suggest that the indirect response plays a significant role in graft rejection, at least of solid organ grafts (Sayegh, 1996). If the indirect pathway is activated, then the peptide epitopes generated by proteolytic breakdown of the HLA molecule and not the HLA molecule itself would be the immunogenic stimulus. New innovative strategies can then be designed for defining allowable mismatches based on recognition of the peptide fragments. For example, a strategy could consider whether the mismatched donor HLA molecules would be perceived as immunogenic in the recipient (i.e., whether the recipient HLA molecules would bind and present these epitopes). Theoretically, one could identify foreign HLA peptide sequences not presented by specific recipient HLA molecules and thus define allowable mismatches for given HLA molecules.

The inherent complexity in the interpretation of HLA typing results and in the selection of a donor makes it critical to include an expert in histocompatibility testing. Experts in HLA typing will know the strengths and weaknesses of each method of typing as well as the frequency of alleles and haplotypes in the population, information important in both the search for and the selection of a suitable donor.

HLA-Specific Antibody Detection in Recipient Serum

Patients can be sensitized to specific foreign HLA molecules through transfusion, pregnancy, or prior transplantations. Assessment of compatibility between the recipient and the possible donor includes the testing for this sensitization. Recipient serum is tested prior to transplantation on a panel (lymphocytes or immobilized soluble HLA molecules) of known HLA profile to measure panel reactive antibody (PRA). At the time of transplantation, the recipient serum is tested with the prospective donor lymphocytes to identify specific reactivity to the potential donor in the donor-specific crossmatch. While the techniques used to detect antibody binding may differ among laboratories, the purpose remains to obtain a profile of the immunologic risk factors of a recipient on the waiting list, which will aid the medical team in both pretransplantation and post-transplantation decisions. The binding of antibody in the *current* serum of the recipient to the T lymphocytes of the donor is a contraindication to renal transplantation.

Serum Screening (PRA)

Thorough characterization of the antibody profile in patients awaiting transplantation aids in the interpretation of the pretransplantation donor-specific crossmatch. The goals of a PRA screen are:

1. To identify the level of presensitization of the patient to HLA antigens. A patient with PRA in excess of 60% (i.e., serum from the patient reacts to specificities found in at least 60% of the panel) has a decreased likelihood of a negative donor-specific crossmatch and, thus, of receiving a transplant from an unrelated transplant.
2. To identify the HLA specificity of the antibodies to predict the HLA antigen(s) to be avoided when donors are selected.
3. To identify patients with irrelevant antibodies (e.g., IgM autoantibodies) so that appropriate techniques may be selected to avoid false-positive readings at the time of the donor specific crossmatch.

Characterization of HLA-specific antibody present in the recipient serum requires testing on a selected panel of well-defined HLA specificities. Lymphocytes or soluble antigen from a sufficient number of individuals must be included in the screening panel to ensure that all but the rarest HLA-directed antibody will be detected. As far as possible, the screening panel should remain the same so that results are comparable over time. Renal transplantation recipients frequently form antibodies to CREGs rather than to subtypic specificities (Rodey, 1994, 1997) so the analyses of panel reactivity should consider identification of CREG as well as of subtypic specificities. Identification of antibody specificities in patients awaiting transplantation aids in preselecting a potential donor for whom the recipient will have a negative final crossmatch. Computer programs assist in this selection (Claas, 1999; Duquesnoy, 1999).

The frequency of the screening and the selection of the assays used for the screening procedure are decisions based on the immunologic profile of the individual recipient. The decreased use of blood transfusions has negated the requirement for screening monthly serum samples on all patients (ASHI web site; Table 47–1). The presence of both HLA class-I- and class-II-specific antibodies is detected by serum testing on a panel of lymphocytes (e.g., by direct complement-dependent cytotoxicity or antiglobulin-augmented cytotoxicity assays) or on a panel of soluble HLA molecules immobilized either on plates (i.e., enzyme linked immunosorbent assay [ELISA]) or on beads (i.e., flow cytometry). (The assays are described in detail in the ASHI manual [2001].) An advantage of the solid phase soluble antigen assay is that it can be designed to detect only IgG, HLA class-I-specific antibodies.

Serum samples from potential recipients should be stored at –70°C and protected from carbon dioxide and from evaporation. The stored characterized serum samples will be used in the donor-specific crossmatch to assess compatibility with a prospective donor.

Donor-Specific Crossmatch

The lymphocyte crossmatch tests for the presence of antibodies, if any, in the serum of the potential recipient that react with lymphocytes of the specific donor. In the crossmatch test, the lymphocyte is the target cell of choice, since it expresses high levels of HLA molecules and is easy to isolate. This test is probably the most important contribution of the HLA tissue typing laboratory to clinical renal transplantation. The purpose of the crossmatch is to prevent hyperacute rejection and to detect antibodies that identify immunologic risk factors in patients awaiting transplantation. The occurrence of hyperacute rejection is significantly correlated with a positive direct complement-dependent cytotoxicity (CDC) crossmatch between donor T lymphocytes and recipient serum at the time of transplantation. Reactivity of the current valid serum of the recipient to the T lymphocytes of the donor is a contraindication to renal graft transplantation. Detection of donor-reactive antibodies in noncurrent recipient serum samples is not a contraindication but may represent risk for graft loss other than immediate hyperacute rejection (Cardella, 1982; Geddes, 1999). A donor-specific crossmatch also is used to predict hematopoietic progenitor cell graft failure in some centers (Hansen, 1997a).

Requirements and methods for the donor-specific crossmatch are stated in the standards of the American Society for Histocompatibility and Immunogenetics (Table 47–1) and in the ASHI procedure manual (2001). Acceptable techniques at the present include the Amos modified CDC, extended incubation time CDC, the antiglobulin-augmented CDC, and flow cytometry.

Antibody Detection Techniques

Different laboratories may use different combinations of assays to detect antibody. The level of sensitization detected will vary with the assay. The antibody specificity detected will vary with the target cell.

Direct Complement-Dependent Cytotoxicity

Direct CDC includes all assays that use the addition of complement to detect the direct binding of antibody to lymphocytes. Fixation of complement by the antibody–antigen complexes on the cell surface results in cell death or cytotoxicity. CDC methods include the basic technique (no wash step before addition of complement), the Amos-modified technique (wash step added before addition of complement), and extended-time incubation techniques. The wash step removes serum, which may contain substances that hinder complement activation. The advantages of direct CDC techniques are that they are reproducible and the correlation with the incidence of hyperacute rejection is excellent.

Indirect Crossmatch Techniques

Indirect techniques include the antiglobulin-augmented cytotoxicity (AHG) technique and flow cytometry. Both use a reagent specific for human immunoglobulin to augment detection of HLA-directed antibody. Indirect techniques detect the presence of antibodies specific for CREGs that frequently go undetected in direct CDC assays. The advantages of the flow cytometry assay include the discrimination of the subclass of the cell-bound immunoglobulin (IgG versus IgM) and the characterization of the target cell binding the alloantibody (T lymphocyte versus B lymphocyte versus monocyte).

Autoantibodies

The presence of circulating autoantibodies in the recipient is not known to be deleterious. Thus, an autocrossmatch should be performed, preferably when the patient is put on the transplantation waiting list. If autoantibodies are present, the sera used for donor crossmatching should have the autoreactivity removed. Autoantibodies are primarily IgM and HLA-specific antibodies are primarily IgG (Barger, 1989). Either heat inactivation at 63±1°C or reduction with the chemical agents dithioerythritol (DTE) or dithiothreitol (DTT) of any potential IgM antibodies are used to differentiate between IgM and IgG antibodies in the serum samples. If the heat-inactivated or DTT-treated serum sample is negative, even though the untreated sample is positive, most centers will proceed with transplantation. However, DTT or heat inactivation should be used with caution, since not all HLA-specific antibodies are IgG and since, if not properly controlled, both procedures can remove IgG activity as well as IgM.

B-Cell Antibodies

A crossmatch using donor B lymphocytes (B-cell crossmatch) may be performed in sensitized patients in some centers. A positive donor-specific B-cell crossmatch is not a contraindication to transplantation. The clinical significance has not been resolved, but a positive test may be a risk factor, particularly in patients who had previously been transplanted. Antibodies detected in a B-cell crossmatch can be (1) class II, HLA-DR, -DQ-specific, (2) weak HLA-A, -B, -C-specific antibodies (B cells have a higher density of class I molecules and are more sensitive to complement-dependent assays than are T cells), and/or (3) non-HLA-specific antibodies (e.g., autoantibodies). To interpret a positive B-cell crossmatch, it may be necessary to adsorb recipient sera with platelets before performing the donor crossmatch. (Platelets express class I but not class II molecules.) The two most commonly used B-cell crossmatch techniques are the CDC and the flow cytometry assays.

Selection of Recipient Serum Samples for Donor Crossmatch

For patients with no detectable sensitization (i.e., 0% PRA), the most recent serum sample available can be used for the donor-specific crossmatch. If the patient has pre-existing antibodies or has had a recent sensitizing event, a current serum sample (i.e., within 48 hours of transplantation) should be collected. For sensitized recipients, representative samples, including the most reactive or 'peak' serum sample, are tested in most centers, as a donor-positive noncurrent sample may be considered to be a risk factor, particularly in the patient who rejected a primary graft early in the post-transplantation period (Mahoney, 1996).

Renal Transplantation

Current practice is to select donors for recipients who are ABO-compatible, T-cell donor-specific crossmatch-negative with appropriate recipient sera, and the best available HLA match. The original finding that kidney grafts between HLA-identical siblings survive significantly longer than grafts transplanted between HLA-mismatched siblings or parent–sibling combinations has been consistently confirmed. Figure 47–8 shows a recent analysis of the five-year survival of renal allografts from the international CTS registry among three categories of donors: (1) HLA-identical sibling, 84% survival; (2) one-haplotype living-related, 73% survival; (3) all cadaver, 66% survival. The impact of the matching for MHC in living-related transplantation is clearly observed by comparing categories 1 and 2. Similar results are observed in the UNOS database (Cecka, 1999).

Although outcome analyses of living-related grafts confirm the role of the MHC as the major genetic barrier to successful graft outcome, the demonstration and acceptance of a positive influence of HLA matching in graft outcome for unrelated cadaveric transplantation has been more controversial. However, the long-term survival data from collaborative, multicenter studies are consistent in showing a highly significant effect of HLA matching on graft survival in cadaveric renal transplantation (Cecka, 1999; Opelz, 1999). Moreover, two recent single-center studies, one from Europe (Oslo) and one from North America (Toronto) have reported significant improvement in graft survival as a function of HLA match (Geddes, 1999; Leivestad, 1999). A single center may require prioritization based on HLA match to transplant sufficient recipients with well-matched grafts to achieve statistical significance in outcome analysis. Although the numbers are smaller, a highly significant influence of HLA matching has been observed on the outcome of kidney grafts from living unrelated donors (Opelz, 1999).

Zero mismatched (0 MM) grafts from cadaver donors survive significantly better and approximately as well as grafts from HLA-identical siblings (Figs 47–8); thus, UNOS mandates the sharing of 0 MM kidneys. Graft survival in patients following first kidney transplantations decreases stepwise as the number of mismatches increases from 0 MM to 6 MM (Cecka, 1999; Opelz, 1999). However, to ensure equitable sharing of organs for all recipients, including those with rare HLA haplotypes, new algorithms for prioritizing recipients on the waiting list have been adopted by organ-sharing programs (Opelz, 1999). The most recent outcome data for both graft and patient survival can be accessed through the CTS web site (www.ctstransplant.org).

Matching of the initial graft not only increases survival time for that graft, but it decreases the probability of recipient sensitization and facilitates retransplantation. The accumulation of highly sensitized patients on the waiting list is a significant problem in many centers, as the patients wait for long periods of time and may present difficult clinical management problems (Sanfilippo, 1992).

Nonrenal Organ Transplantation

Survival of heart, liver, lung, and pancreas grafts is good, with between 58% and 67% of first grafts surviving at 5 years. Donors are not usually matched for HLA type, and a pretransplant donor crossmatch is not routinely performed. Serum antibody screens are recommended to identify the state of sensitization as an immunologic risk factor for the recipient. If feasible, the graft recipients and cadaveric donors of nonrenal vascularized grafts should be typed for HLA to allow for retrospective analyses. Recent international CTS data show no effect of HLA matching on the outcome of liver transplantation; however, the CTS data do show a significant impact of matching for HLA-A, -B, and -DR on the outcome of first heart transplants (Opelz, 1999). The acceptable period for cold ischemia preservation may limit the extent of HLA matching possible for heart transplantation.

Allogeneic Hematopoietic Progenitor Cell Transplantation

Allogeneic hematopoietic progenitor cell transplantation is performed for hematologic malignancies and disorders, bone marrow failure, certain inherited metabolic disorders such as lipid storage diseases, and congenital immunodeficiency syndrome. From a histocompatibility standpoint, the best donor is either self (autogeneic transplant) if the malignancy is not one that involves the bone marrow or the disease is not genetic, or an identical twin (syngeneic transplant). Progenitor cells from an HLA-identical sibling donor are a frequent source. These donor cells usually will be genetically identical to the patient across the entire MHC region. The use of a sibling donor also increases the probability that non-HLA genes that might affect transplantation success and which are not well defined (i.e., minor histocompatibility genes) are more likely to be matched (Goulmy, 1997). Haploidentical family members may also be chosen as donors (Aversa, 1998), although there is a greater risk of severe GVHD from mismatched HLA donors. Based on data from the International Bone Marrow Transplant Registry (IBMTR) (Table 47–1; www.ibmtr.org), over 16 000 allogeneic bone marrow transplants were performed from 1996 to 1997; 75% used related donors.

Most patients (≈70%) do not have an HLA-matched sibling and may be considered for transplantation with cells from an HLA-matched, unrelated donor. To facilitate the search for a matched donor, national registries of unrelated donors have been developed around the world (Hansen, 1996). The NMDP in the United States is such a registry and contains over 3.9 million HLA-typed donors, making it the largest unrelated donor registry in the world (Perkins, 1994; see Table 47–1; www.marrow.org).

Hematopoietic progenitor cell grafts are among the most difficult of all clinical procedures for several reasons (Madrigal, 1997; Hansen, 1997a). First, at the time of transplantation, the recipients are nearly totally immunodeficient, either because of inherited deficiency (severe combined immunodeficiency [SCID]) or because of the pretransplantation conditioning (cytotoxic chemotherapy and irradiation). Conditioning is required to eliminate malignant cells and to prevent the immune system of the recipient from rejecting the donor progenitor cells, which are infused several days after conditioning. The amount of cytotoxic pretreatment is high enough to eliminate circulating leukocytes, nearly eliminate platelets, and abrogate production of new erythrocytes. Thus, the recipient is profoundly susceptible to all types of infection and would certainly die if not rescued by extraordinary medical care and the transfused progenitor cells.

The second risk is the potential of immunologic attack of the recipient by the transplanted allogeneic progenitor cells resulting in GVHD. GVHD has several forms and can be fatal. In spite of the difficulties, a number of transplant centers have achieved exceptional success. Recent reports from single institutions and the IBMTR suggest leukemia-free survival of 40–60% at 5 years after unrelated hematopoietic progenitor cell transplantation of patients with chronic myelogenous leukemia in chronic phase (Table 47–1, www.ibmtr.org) (Hansen, 1998). Survival for patients with severe aplastic anemia transplanted with cells from unrelated donors varies from 30% to 50% at 5 years depending on patient age (see Table 47–1, NMDP at www.marrow.org and www.ibmtr.org) and survival rates of nearly 90% have been reported in some centers (Deeg, 1998).

In addition to marrow as a source of hematopoietic progenitor cells, the collection of hematopoietic progenitor cells from growth-factor-mobilized peripheral blood (Anderlini, 1997) or umbilical cord blood progenitor cells (Cairo, 1997) increases the availability of unrelated donors. New approaches to immunosuppression, including less aggressive conditioning protocols (e.g., 'minitransplants') (Storb, 1999), may extend the availability of progenitor cell transplantation as a therapeutic procedure to patients presently excluded either by age or by organ dysfunction. Hematopoietic progenitor cell transplantation can also be used to generate immune responses directed at malignant cells. Relapse of disease following transplantation is greater for patients receiving an HLA-matched graft, suggesting that some degree of mismatching may be beneficial in stimulating an immune response against tumor cells (Beatty, 1993). As problems surrounding this most difficult procedure are overcome, hematopoietic progenitor cell transplantation may become one of the most widely used methods for the treatment of a variety of diseases (see Ch. 38).

HLA Typing for Progenitor Cell Transplantation

Many factors, including histocompatibility, influence the outcome of hematopoietic progenitor cell transplantation (Madrigal, 1997). The pretransplantation work-up includes HLA-A, -B, and -DR typing of all available members of the immediate family to identify a matched related donor and to establish inheritance of haplotypes. DNA-based typing for class II genes has become standard and DNA-based typing for class I genes has been implemented in many centers. Typing of the extended family, allele-level (i.e., high-resolution) typing of specific HLA class I and class II loci, typing of other loci within the MHC (short tandem repeats or complement loci), or use of other tests (e.g., crossmatching; cytotoxic T-cell precursor measurements) to measure compatibility may also be appropriate (Hurley, 1999).

The level of HLA typing resolution required differs for hematopoietic progenitor cell and renal transplantation. It is likely that higher-resolution HLA typing is required to match donor and recipient for progenitor cell transplantation than is required for renal transplantation because progenitor cell transplantation involves the transfer of an entire immune system to the patient. Current research is focused on defining the loci that must be considered in donor selection, the level of resolution that must be used for matching, and the additive effect of multiple mismatches. The level of matching required may vary for each disease or protocol. Evidence suggests that matching unrelated donor and recipient for HLA-A, -B, -DRB1 alleles is related to an improved outcome. The impact of matching at other HLA loci (e.g., HLA-C and HLA-DQ) is under evaluation. Single mismatches may be tolerated; however, multiple mismatches appear to have a negative impact on outcome (Petersdorf, 1995b, 1998; Hansen, 1997a; Madrigal, 1997; Sasazuki, 1998). Furthermore, the positive effect of histocompatibility matching on outcome must be balanced by the positive impact of transplantation early in the course of the disease. Data from the IBMTR and the NMDP show that survival following transplantation is reduced as the disease phase advances (data on web sites listed in Table 47–1).

Summary

The HLA class I and class II molecules encoded within the major histocompatibility complex have a significant role in the specificity and character of immune responses. The extensive polymorphism of these molecules provides the diversity needed to ensure survival in an environment of hostile and adaptive pathogens. Unfortunately, this ability of the immune system to distinguish self from non-self extends to the recognition of foreign HLA molecules following tissue transplantation. Definition and characterization of HLA alleles and molecules have been combined with clinical protocols to maximize compatibility and to minimize the impact of the immune response on foreign tissue. These advances have contributed to the development of transplantation as a successful treatment modality for the replacement of diseased tissue.

References

Abbal M, Cambon-Thomsen A, Foissac A, et al: Microsatellites in the HLA region: potential applications in bone marrow transplantation. Transplant Proc 1997; 29:2374.

Agrawal S, Pandey MK: The potential role of HLA-G polymorphism in maternal tolerance to the developing fetus. J Hematother Stem Cell Res 2003; 12:749–756.

Aguado B, Bahram S, Beck S, et al: Complete sequence and gene map of a human major histocompatibility complex. Nature 1999; 401:921.
Contains the first complete sequence and gene map of an MHC region and represents the collaborative effort of an international group of researchers.

American Society for Histocompatibility and Immunogenetics: Laboratory Manual, 4th ed. Lenexa, KS, ASHI, 2000.

Anderlini P, Korbling M, Dale D, et al: Allogeneic blood stem cell transplantation: considerations for donors. Blood 1997; 90:903.

Arguello JR, Little AM, Bohan E, et al: High resolution HLA class I typing by reference strand mediated conformation analysis (RSCA). Tissue Antigens 1998; 52:57–66.
Describes the use of RSCA in separating polymorphic HLA alleles using an automated technology that may provide rapid high-throughput HLA analysis with the additional advantage of time and cost saving.

Arguello R, Avakian H, Goldman JM, et al: A novel method for simultaneous high resolution identification of HLA-A, HLA-B, and HLA-Cw alleles. Proc Natl Acad Sci USA 1996; 93:10961.

Aversa F, Tabilio A, Velardi A, et al: Treatment of high-risk acute leukemia with T-cell-depleted stem cells from related donors with one fully mismatched HLA haplotype. N Engl J Med 1998; 339:1186.

Banchereau J, Steinman RM: Dendritic cells and the control of immunity. Nature 1998; 392:245.

Barger BO, Shroyer TW, Hudson SL, et al: Successful renal allografts in recipients with a positive standard, DTE negative crossmatch. Transplant Proc 1989; 21: 746.

Beatty PG, Anasetti C, Hansen JA, et al: Marrow transplantation from unrelated donors for treatment of hematologic malignancies: effect of mismatching for one HLA locus. Blood 1993; 81:249.

Beatty PG, Mori M, Milford E: Impact of racial genetic polymorphism on the probability of finding an HLA-matched donor. Transplant 1995; 60:778.

Beck S, Trowsdale J: Sequence organization of the Class II region of the human MHC. Immunol Rev 1999; 167:201.

Begovich AB, McClure GR, Suraj VC, et al: Polymorphism, recombination and linkage disequilibrium within the HLA Class II region. J Immunol 1992; 148:249.

Björkman PJ, Parham P: Structure, function and diversity of Class I major histocompatibility complex molecules. Annu Rev Biochem 1990; 59:253.

Bjorkman PJ, Saper MA, Samraoui B, et al: Structure of the human Class I histocompatibility antigen, HLA-A2. Nature 1987; 329:506.

Bodmer JG, Marsh SGE, Albert ED, et al: Nomenclature for factors of the HLA system, 1996. Tissue Antigens 1997; 49:297.

Bodmer JG, Marsh SGE, Albert ED, et al: Nomenclature for factors of the HLA system, 1998. Tissue Antigens 1999; 53:407.

Bozon MV, Delgado JC, Selvakumar A, et al: Error rate for HLA-B antigen assignment by serology: Implications for proficiency testing and utilization of DNA-based typing methods. Tissue Antigens 1997; 50:387.

Brodsky FM, Lem L, Solache A, et al: Human pathogen subversion of antigen presentation. Immunol Rev 1999; 168:199.

Brooks AG, Borrego F, Posch PE, et al: Specific recognition of HLA-E, but not classical, HLA Class I molecules by soluble CD94/NKG2A and NK cells. J Immunol 1999; 162:305.

Brown JH, Jardetzky TS, Gorga JC, et al: Three-dimensional structure of the human Class II histocompatibility antigen HLA-DR1. Nature 1993; 364:33.

Bugawan TL, Apple R, Erlich HA: A method for typing polymorphism at the HLA-A locus using PCR amplification and immobilized oligonucleotide probes. Tissue Antigens 1994; 44:137.

Bugawan TL, Mack SJ, Stoneking M, et al: HLA Class I allele distributions in six Pacific/Asian populations: Evidence of selection of the HLA-A locus. Tissue Antigens 1999; 53:311.

Bunce M, O'Neill CM, Barnardo MC, et al: Phototyping: comprehensive DNA typing for HLA-A, B, C, DRB1, DRB3, DRB4, DRB5 & DQB1 by PCR with 144 primer mixes utilizing sequence-specific primers (PCR-SSP). Tissue Antigens 1995; 46:355.

Cadavid LF, Watkins DI: Heirs of the jaguar and the anaconda: HLA, conquest and disease in the indigenous populations of the Americas. Tissue Antigens 1997; 50:209.

Cairo MS, Wagner JE: Placental and/or umbilical cord blood: an alternative source of hematopoietic stem cells for transplantation. Blood 1997; 90:4665.

Cao K, Chopek M, Fernandez-Vina MA: High and intermediate resolution DNA typing systems for Class I HLA-A, -B, -C genes by hybridization with sequence specific oligonucleotide probes (SSOP). Immunogenetics 1999; 1:53.

Cardella CJ, Falk JA, Nicholson MJ, et al: Successful renal transplantation in patients with T-cell reactivity to donor. Lancet 1982; 2:1240.

Carrington M, Chadwick R, Cullen M, et al: Characterization of 12 microsatellite loci of the human MHC in a panel of reference cell lines. Immunogenetics 1998; 47:131.

Carrington M, Wade J: Selection of transplant donors based on MHC microsatellite data. Hum Immunol 1996; 50:151.

Cecka M: The UNOS scientific renal transplant registry. In Cecka M, Terasaki P (eds): Clinical Transplants 1998. Los Angeles, CA, UCLA Tissue Typing Laboratory, 1999, p 1.

Claas FHJ, De Meester J, Witvliet MD, et al: Acceptable HLA mismatches for highly immunized patients. Rev Immunogenet 1999; 1:73.

Creput C, Le Friec G, Bahri R and et al: Detection of HLA-G in serum and graft biopsy associated with fewer acute rejections following combined liver-kidney transplantation: possible implications for monitoring patients. Hum Immunol 2003; 64:1033–1038.

Cresswell P: Assembly, transport, and function of MHC Class II molecules. Annu Rev Immunol 1994; 12:259.

Crow JF: Genetics Notes, 7th ed. Minneapolis, MN, Burgess Publishing, 1976.

Crowe DO: The effect of cross-reactive epitope group matching on allocation and sensitization. Clin Transplant 2003; 17(Suppl 9):13–16.

Dausset J: The Nobel Lectures in Immunology. Lecture for the Nobel Prize for Physiology or Medicine, 1980: The major histocompatibility complex in man. Science 1981; 213:1469.

Dausset J, Colombani J (eds): Histocompatibility Testing 1972. Copenhagen, Munksgaard, 1973.

Deeg HJ, Leisenring W, Storb R, et al: Long-term outcome after marrow transplantation for severe aplastic anemia. Blood 1998; 91:3637.

Den Haan JMM, Sherman NE, Blokland E, et al: Identification of a graft versus host disease-associated human minor histocompatibility antigen. Science 1995; 268:1476.

Dupont B: Induction of a MINOR into the MAJOR league? Genomic identification of a human minor histocompatibility antigen. Tissue Antigens 1998; 52:303.

Duquesnoy RJ, Marrari M: HLAMATCHMAKER: a molecularly based donor selection strategy for highly allosensitized patients. Hum Immunol 1999; 60:S10.

Egfjord M, Jakobsen BK, Ladefoged J: No impact of cross-reactive group human leucocyte antigen class I

matching on long-term kidney graft survival. Scand J Immunol 2003; 57:362–365.

Ellison MD, Bennett LE, Edwards EB, et al: Multivariate analysis of verified national data to assess the impact of HLA mismatch level on kidney graft survival. J Am Soc Nephrol 1994; 5:1003.

Engelhard VH: Structure of peptides associated with Class I and Class II molecules. Annu Rev Immunol 1994; 12:181.

Etokebe GE, Opsahl M, Tveter AK and et al: Physical separation of HLA-A alleles by denaturing high-performance liquid chromatography. Tissue Antigens 2003; 61:443–450.
Describes the application of HPLC to the task of identifying polymorphic HLA-A alleles in an automated high throughput setting.

Foissac A, Crouau-Roy B, Faure S, et al: Microsatellites in the HLA region: an overview. Tissue Antigens 1997; 49:197.

Gao X, Moraes JR, Miller S, et al: DNA typing for Class II HLA antigens with allele-specific or group-specific amplification. V. Typing for subsets of HLA-DR1 and DR'Br'. Hum Immunol 1991; 30:147.

Geddes C, Cole E, Wade J, et al: Factors influencing long-term primary cadaveric kidney transplantation – importance of functional renal mass versus avoidance of acute rejections – the Toronto Hospital experience 1985–1997. In Cecka M, Terasaki P (eds): Clinical Transplants 1998. Los Angeles, CA, UCLA Tissue Typing Laboratory, 1999, p 195.

Glimcher LH, Kara CJ: Sequences and factors: a guide to MHC Class-II transcription. Annu Rev Immunol 1992; 10:13.

Gorga JC: Structural analysis of Class II major histocompatibility complex proteins. Crit Rev Immunol 1992; 11:305.

Gould DS, Auchincloss H: Direct and indirect recognition: the role of MHC antigens in graft rejection. Immunol Today 1999; 20:77.

Goulmy E: Human minor histocompatibility antigens: new concepts for marrow transplantation and adoptive immunotherapy. Immunol Rev 1997; 157:125.

Goulmy E, Schipper R, Pool J, et al: Mismatches of minor histocompatibility antigens between HLA-identical donors and recipients and the development of graft-versus-host disease after bone marrow transplantation. N Engl J Med 1996; 334:281.

Guardiola J, Maffei A: Control of MHC Class II gene expression in autoimmune, infectious, and neoplastic diseases. Crit Rev Immunol 1993; 13:247–268.

Hansen JA: Development of registries of HLA-typed volunteer marrow donors. Tissue Antigens 1996; 47:460.

Hansen JA, Gooley TA, Martin PJ, et al: Bone marrow transplants from unrelated donors for patients with chronic myeloid leukemia. N Engl J Med 1998; 338:962.

Hansen JA, Petersdorf E, Martin PJ, et al: Hematopoietic stem cell transplants from unrelated donors. Immunol Rev 1997a; 157:141.

Hansen JA, Yamamoto K, Petersdorf E, et al: The role of HLA matching in hematopoietic cell transplantation. Rev Immunogenet 1999; 1:81.

Hansen TH, Lee DR: Mechanism of Class I assembly with β-2 microglobulin and loading with peptide. Adv Immunol 1997b; 64:105.

Harris PE, Cortesini R, Suciu-Foca N: Indirect allorecognition in solid organ transplantation. Rev Immunogenet 1999; 1:19.

Hartzman RJ, Segall M, Bach ML, et al: Histocompatibility matching. VI. Miniaturization of the mixed leukocyte culture test: a preliminary report. Transplantation 1971; 11:268.

Hurley CK: Acquisition and use of DNA-based HLA typing data in bone marrow registries. Tissue Antigens 1997b; 49:323.

Hurley CK, Baxter-Lowe LA, Begovich AB, et al: The extent of HLA Class II allele level disparity in unrelated bone marrow transplantation: analysis of 1,259 National Marrow Donor Program donor-recipient pairs. Bone Marrow Transplant 2000b; 25:385.

Hurley CK, Maiers M, Ng J, et al: Large-scale DNA-based typing of HLA-A and HLA-B at low resolution is highly accurate, specific, and reliable. Tissue Antigens 2000a; 55:352.

Hurley CK, Tang T, Ng J, et al: HLA typing by molecular methods. In Rose NR, Conway de Macario E, Folds JD, et al (eds): Manual of Clinical Laboratory Immunology, 5th ed. Washington, DC, ASM Press, 1997a, p 1098.

Hurley CK, Wade JA, Oudshoorn M, et al: A special report: histocompatibility testing guidelines for hematopoietic stem cell transplantation using volunteer donors. Hum Immunol 1999; 60:347.

Imanishi T, Akaza T, Kimura A, et al: Allele and haplotype frequencies for HLA and complement loci in various ethnic groups. In Tsuji K, Aizawa M, Sasazuki T (eds): HLA 1991. New York, Oxford University Press, 1992, vol 1, p 1065.

Ishitani A, Sageshima N, Lee N, et al: Protein expression and peptide binding suggest unique and interacting functional roles for HLA-E, F, and G in maternal-placental immune recognition. J Immunol 2003; 171:1376–1384.

Jorgensen JL, Reay PA, Ehrich EW, et al: Molecular components of T-cell recognition. Annu Rev Immunol 1992; 10:835.

Kircher B, Wolf M, Stevanovic S, et al: Hematopoietic lineage-restricted minor histocompatibility antigen HA-1 in graft-versus-leukemia activity after donor lymphocyte infusion. J Immunother 2004; 27:156–160.

Kloosterboer FM, Luxemburg-Heijs SA, van Soest RA, et al: Direct cloning of leukemia-reactive T cells from patients treated with donor lymphocyte infusion shows a relative dominance of hematopoiesis-restricted minor histocompatibility antigen HA-1 and HA-2 specific T cells. Leukemia 2004; 18:798–808.

Kovats S, Drover S, Marshall WH, et al: Coordinate defects in human histocompatibility leukocyte antigen Class II expression and antigen presentation in bare lymphocyte syndrome. J Exp Med 1994; 179:2017.

Kwok WW, Kovats S, Thurtle P, et al: HLA-DQ allelic polymorphisms constrain patterns of Class II heterodimer formation. J Immunol 1993; 150:2263.

Lanier LL: NK cell receptors. Annu Rev Immunol 1998; 16:359.

Le Bouteiller P, Blaschitz A: The functionality of HLA-G is emerging. Immunol Rev 1999; 167:233.

Lee N, Goodlett DR, Ishitani A, et al: HLA-E surface expression depends on binding of TAP-dependent peptides derived from certain HLA Class I signal sequences. J Immunol 1998a; 160:4951.

Lee N, Llano M, Carretero M, et al: HLA-E is a major ligand for the natural killer inhibitory receptor CD94/NKG2A. Proc Natl Acad Sci USA 1998b; 95:5199.

Leivestad T, Reisaeter AV, Brekke IB, et al: The role of HLA matching in renal transplantation: experience from one center. Rev Immunogenet 1999; 1:343.

Long EO: Regulation of immune responses through inhibitory receptors. Annu Rev Immunol 1999; 17:875.

Mach B, Steimle B, Martinez-Soria E, et al: Regulation of MHC Class II genes: lessons from a disease. Annu Rev Immunol 1996; 14:301.

Madrigal JA, Scott I, Argello R, et al: Factors influencing the outcome of bone marrow transplants using unrelated donors. Immunol Rev 1997; 157:153.

Mahoney RJ, Norman DJ, Colombe BW, et al: Identification of high- and low-risk second kidney grafts. Transplantation 1996; 61:1349.

Marsh SG, Albert ED, Bodmer WF, Bontrop RE, et al: Nomenclature for factors of the HLA system, 2002. Tissue Antigens 2002; 60:407–64.

Martin PJ: How much benefit can be expected from matching for minor antigens in allogenic marrow transplantation? Bone Marrow Transplant 1997; 20:97.

Matsunami K, Miyagawa S, Nakai R, et al: Modulation of the leader peptide sequence of the HLA-E gene up-regulates its expression and down-regulates natural killer cell-mediated swine endothelial cell lysis. Transplantation 2002; 73:1582–1589.

Mickelson EM, Longton G, Anasetti C, et al: Evaluation of the mixed lymphocyte culture (MLC) assay as a method for selecting unrelated donors for marrow transplantation. Tissue Antigens 1996; 47:27.

Middleton D: History of DNA typing for human MHC. Rev Immunogenet 1999; 1:11.

Momburg F, Hammerling GJ: Generation and TAP-mediated transport of peptides for major histocompatibility complex Class I molecules. Adv Immunol 1998; 68:191.

Mori M, Beatty PG, Graves M, et al: HLA gene and haplotype frequencies in the North American population. Transplant 1997; 64:1017.

Morris P, Shaman J, Attaya M, et al: An essential role for HLA-DM in antigen presentation by Class II major histocompatibility molecules. Nature 1994; 368:551.

Mutis T, Gillespie G, Schrama E, et al: Tetrameric HLA Class I-minor histocompatibility antigen peptide complexes demonstrate minor histocompatibility antigen-specific cytotoxic T lymphocytes in patients with graft-versus-host disease. Nat Med 1999; 5:839.

Mytilineos J, Lempert M, Scherer S, et al: Comparison of serological and DNA PCR-SSP typing results for HLA-A and HLA-B in 421 black individuals – a collaborative transplant study report. Hum Immunol 1998; 59:512.

Nepom GT, Erlich H: MHC Class-II molecules and autoimmunity. Annu Rev Immunol 1991; 9:493.

Ng J, Hurley CK, Carter C, et al: Large-scale DRB and DQB1 oligonucleotide typing for the NMDP registry: progress report from year 2. Tissue Antigens 1996; 47:21.

Nordstrom T, Ronaghi M, Forsberg L, et al: Direct analysis of single-nucleotide polymorphism on double-stranded DNA by pyrosequencing. Biotechnol Appl Biochem 2000; 31 (Pt 2):107–112. *Describes the technology behind pyrosequencing, and its specific application to the task of sequencing and verifying the presence of single nucleotide polymorphisms in double-stranded DNA.*

O'Callaghan CA, Bell JI: Structure and function of the human MHC Class Ib molecules HLA-E, HLA-F and HLA-G. Immunol Rev 1998; 163:129.

Olerup O, Zetterquist H. HLA-DR typing by PCR amplification with sequence specific primers (PCR-SSP) in 2 hours: an alternative to serological DR typing in clinical practice including donor-recipient matching in cadaveric transplantations. Tissue Antigens 1992; 39:225.

Opelz G, Wujciak T, Dohler B, et al: HLA compatibility and organ transplant survival. Rev Immunogenet 1999; 1:56.

Pacasova R, Martinozzi S, Bouloues HJ, et al: Cell surface expression and allogenic function of a human non-classical Class I molecule (HLA-E) in transgenic mice. J Immunol 1999; 162:5190.

Pamer E, Cresswell P: Mechanisms of MHC Class I-restricted antigen processing. Annu Rev Immunol 1998; 16:323.

Parham P, Adams EJ, Arnett KL: The origins of HLA-A, B, C polymorphism. Immunol Rev 1995; 143:141.

Parham P, Lawlor DA: Evolution of Class I major histocompatibility complex genes and molecules in humans and apes. Hum Immunol 1991; 30:119.

Paul WE, Seder RA: Lymphocyte responses and cytokines. Cell 1994; 76:241.

Payne R, Tripp M, Weigle J, et al: A new leukocyte isoantigen system in man. Cold Spring Harbor Symp Quant Biol 1964; 29:285.

Perkins HA, Hansen JA: The US National Marrow Donor Program. Am J Pediatr Hemotol Oncol 1994; 16:30.

Petersdorf EW, Gooley TA, Anasetti C, et al: Optimizing outcome after unrelated marrow transplantation by comprehensive matching of HLA Class I and II alleles in the donor and recipient. Blood 1998; 92:3515.

Petersdorf EW, Hansen JA: A comprehensive approach for typing the alleles of the HLA-B locus by automated sequencing. Tissue Antigens 1995a; 46:73.

Petersdorf EW, Longton GM, Anasetti C, et al: The significance of HLA-DRB1 matching on clinical outcome after HLA-A, B, DR identical unrelated donor marrow transplantation. Blood 1995b; 86:1606.

Reinsmoen NL, Matas AJ: Evidence that improved late transplant outcome correlates with the development of in vitro donor antigen-specific hyporeactivity. Transplant 1993; 55:1017.

Remuzzi G, Perico N, Carpenter CB, Sayegh MH: The thymic way to transplantation tolerance. J Am Soc Nephrol 1995, 5:1639.

Rock KL, Goldberg AL: Degradation of cell proteins and the generation of MHC Class I-presented peptides. Annu Rev Immunol 1999; 17:739.

Rodey GE, Fuller TC: Public epitopes and the antigenic structure of the HLA molecules. CRC Crit Rev Immunol 1987; 7:229.

Rodey GE, Neylan JF, Whelchel JD, et al: Epitope specificity of HLA Class I alloantibodies. I. Frequency analysis of antibodies to private versus public specificities in potential transplant recipients. Hum Immunol 1994; 39:272.

Rodey GE, Revels K, Fuller TC: Epitope specificity of HLA Class I alloantibodies. II. Stability of cross-reactive group antibody patterns over extended time periods. Transplantation 1997; 63:885.

Rosenthal AS, Shevach EM: Function of macrophages in antigen recognition by guinea pig T lymphocytes. I. Requirement for histocompatible macrophages and lymphocytes. J Exp Med 1973; 138:1194.

Rozemuller EH, Tilanus MGJ: A computerized method to predict the discriminatory properties for Class II sequencing based typing. Hum Immunol 1996; 46:27.

Ruggeri L, Capanni M, Casucci M, et al: Role of natural killer cell alloreactivity in HLA-mismatched hematopoietic stem cell transplantation. Blood 1999; 94:333.

Saiki RK, Gelfand DH, Stoffel S, et al: Primer-directed enzymatic amplification of DNA with a thermostable DNA polymerase. Science 1988; 239:487.

Sanfilippo FP, Vaughn WK, Pilers TH, et al: Factors affecting the waiting time of cadaveric kidney transplant candidates in the United States. JAMA 1992; 267:247.

Sasazuki T, Juji T, Morishima Y, et al: Effect of matching of Class I HLA alleles on clinical outcome after transplantation of hematopoietic stem cells from an unrelated donor. N Engl J Med 1998; 339:1177.

Sayegh MH, Carpenter CB: Role of indirect allorecognition in allograft rejection. Int Rev Immunol 1996; 13:221.

Scheltinga SA, Johnston-Dow LA, White CB, et al: A generic sequencing based typing approach for the identification of HLA-A diversity. Hum Immunol 1997; 57:120.

Shaw S, Kavathas P, Pollack MS, et al: Family studies define a new histocompatibility locus, SB, between HLA-DR and GLO. Nature 1981; 293:745.

Shiina T, Tamiya G, Oka A, et al: Genome sequencing analysis of the 1.8 Mb entire human MHC Class I region. Immunol Rev 1999; 167:193.

Simpson E, Roopenian D, Goulmy E: Much ado about minor histocompatibility antigens. Immunol Today 1998; 19:108.

Singer DS, Maguire J: Regulation of the expression of Class I MHC genes. CRC Crit Rev Immunol 1990; 10:235.

Snell GD: Studies in histocompatibility. Science 1981; 213:172.

Stern LJ, Wiley DC: Antigenic peptide binding by Class I and Class II histocompatibility proteins. Structure 1994; 2:245.

Storb R, Yu C, McSweeney P: Mixed chimerism after transplantation of allogeneic hematopoietic cells. *In* Thomas D, Blume KG, Forman SJ (eds): Hematopoietic Cell Transplantation, 2nd ed. Oxford, Blackwell Science, 1999, p 287.

Suciu-Foca N, Harris PE, Cortesini R: Intramolecular and intermolecular spreading during the course of organ allograft rejection. Immunol Rev 1998; 164:241.

Suthanthiran M, Morris RE, Strom TB: Immunosuppressants: cellular and molecular mechanisms of action. Am J Kidney Dis 1996; 28:159.

Sutton VR, Kienzle BK, Knowles RW: An altered splice site is found in the *DRB4* gene that is not expressed in HLA-DR7, Dw11 individuals. Immunogenetics 1989; 29:317.

Tanaka K, Tanahashi N, Tsurumni C, et al: Proteosomes and antigen processing. Adv Immunol 1997; 64:1.

Terasaki PI, Takemoto S, Park MS, et al: HLA epitope matching. Transfusion 1992; 32:775.

Thorsby E, Piazza A: Joint Report II. Typing for HLA-D determinants (LD-1 or MLC). *In* Kissmeyer-Nielsen F (ed): Histocompatibility Testing. Copenhagen, Munksgaard, 1975, p 414.

Todd JA, Bell JI, McDevitt HO: HLA-DQβ gene contributes to susceptibility and resistance to insulin-dependent diabetes mellitus. Nature 1987; 329:599.

Tseng L-H, Lin M-T, Martin PJ, et al: Definition of the gene encoding the minor histocompatibility antigen HA-1 and typing for HA-1 from genomic DNA. Tissue Antigens 1998; 52:305.

Uematsu Y, Fischer-Lindahl K, Steinmetz M, et al: The same recombinational hot spots are active in crossing-over between wild/wild and wild/inbred mouse chromosomes. Immunogenetics 1988; 27:96.

Valiante NM, Uhrber M, Shilling HG, et al: Functionally and structurally distinct NK cell receptor repertoires in the peripheral blood of two human donors. Immunity 1997; 7:739.

Van Ham SM, Tjin EPM, Lillemier BF, et al: HLA-DO is a negative modulator of HLA-DM mediated MHC Class II peptide loading. Curr Biol 1997; 7:950.

Van Rood JJ: HLA and I. Annu Rev Immunol 1993; 11:1.

Wade JA, Hurley CK, Hastings A, et al: Combinational diversity in DR2 haplotypes. Tissue Antigens 1993; 41:113.

Watts C: Capture and processing of exogenous antigens for presentation of MHC molecules. Annu Rev Immunol 1997; 15:821.

Wilke M, Pool J, den Haan JMM, et al: Genomic identification of the minor histocompatibility antigen HA-1 locus by allele-specific PCR. Tissue Antigens 1998; 52:312.

Williams F, Mallon E, Middleton D: Development of PCR-SSOP for HLA-A typing of bone marrow registry donors. Tissue Antigens 1997; 49:61.

Yu N, Ohashi M, Alosco S, et al: Accurate typing of HLA-A antigens and analysis of serological deficiencies. Tissue Antigens 1997; 50:380.

Zinkernagel RM: Cellular immune recognition and the biological role of major transplantation antigens. Biosci Rep 1997a; 17:91.

Zinkernagel RM: The Nobel Lectures in Immunology. The Nobel Prize for Physiology or Medicine, 1996. Cellular immune recognition and the biological role of major transplantation antigens. Scand J Immunol 1997b; 46:421.

CHAPTER 48

The Major Histocompatibility Complex and Disease

Julio C. Delgado, M.D., Edmond J. Yunis, M.D.

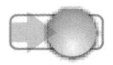

KEY POINTS

• The major histocompatibility complex (MHC) genomic region contains several genes with immune-related functions.

• The recent identification of several genes within the MHC has increased the possibility of defining the genetic basis of immunity.

• The clustering of immune-related genes in the MHC region may not be coincidental and may be the result of evolutionary forces joining genes with similar functions.

• The MHC is associated with more diseases than any other region on the human genome.

• Non-random associations of fixed stretches of MHC DNA complicate the study of susceptibility genes but also provide the means for their identification.

• There are methods for detecting associations or linkage between polymorphisms found with the MHC and disease.

• Although class I and class II encoded proteins are distinguished by structural and functional similarities shared by the members of each class, class III molecules can only be defined as non-I and non-II, because their genes and their products have no common features and are not recognized by T cells.

• Despite convincing genetic association studies showing the importance of the class III region in health and disease, neither the genes responsible for disease nor the underlying mechanism of pathology is known for many of the associated conditions.

• Almost half the genes within the MHC class III region play roles in the innate immune system, including members of the complement fixation cascade (C4, C2, BF) and tumor necrosis factor family.

• Deficiency of the second component of the complement system has been reported only in Caucasians, and it is the most common complement protein deficiency state in that population.

• Complete C4 deficiency is extremely rare. The level of C4 in the serum of patients with C4 null alleles is extremely variable and cannot be used reliably to detect heterozygotes for complete deficiency because there is no correlation between the level of C4 and the number of expressed C4 genes.

• Extended haplotypes are highly characteristic of an ethnic subgroup and have lower frequencies or do not occur at all in other ethnic groups.

• It is critical to know the ethnic distribution of a disease-associated MHC allele in order to evaluate whether the allele in patients is increased compared with ethnically matched control populations and is in fact truly a marker for the ethnic distribution of the disease.

• A major problem with MHC gene associations is their incomplete penetrance, making ordinary formal segregation and linkage studies very difficult, if not impossible to carry out.

Introduction

Understanding the role of the major histocompatibility complex (MHC) in immune responses and in the pathogenesis of disease requires defining polymorphisms in the class I and class II regions, as well as genes in the central region of the MHC, sometimes called the non-HLA region or class III region. It should be mentioned from the outset that there are DNA regions where recombinations occur more frequently than expected, i.e. in the interval from HLA-DR to HLA-DP. Of particular importance is the fact that there are constellations of DNA, or fixed DNA, wherein recombinations are rarely observed. The two major constellations are the complement region in the central region, and HLA-DR, DQ in the class II region. Furthermore, analysis of MHC haplotypes in many populations has led us to recognize that a sizable proportion of individuals have ethnic-group-specific haplotypes that appear to be identical in the interval from HLA-B to HLA-DR, DQ. These haplotypes, known as extended haplotypes, should be considered fixed genetic units that, together with MHC variants that are

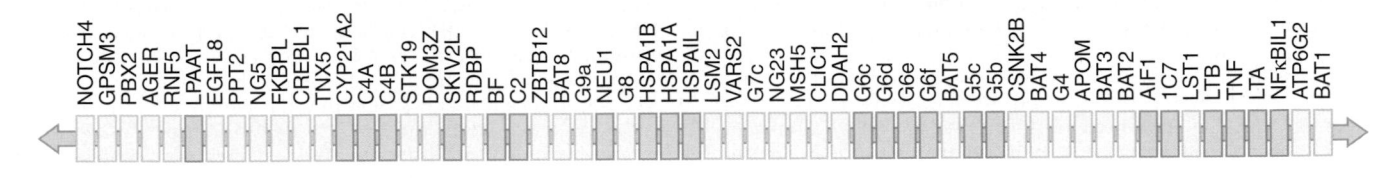

Figure 48.1 Gene map of the class III region of the major histocompatibility complex. Shown in order but not to scale are 58 genes from centromere to telomere. Genes representing 'immune loci' are marked by green boxes.

not part of these haplotypes, serve to help us understand immune responses and disease association. The variants of class I and class II genes have been described in detail in Chapter 47. In this chapter, we will discuss the non-HLA region genes, extended haplotypes, disease associations and methods for detecting the association of diseases with genetic markers.

Overview of The Human Major Histocompatibility Complex DNA Sequence

It is not surprising that the completion of the MHC DNA sequence preceded the completion of the total human genome sequence by almost four years (MHC Sequencing Consortium, 1999). The rush to complete the entire MHC sequence followed the need to understand the biology and genetics of the mouse MHC (H-2) and human leukocyte antigen (HLA) regions, which were initially provided by murine inbred experiments and serological typing (reviewed in Klein, 1986). Although the MHC was discovered over 50 years ago, its nature has only been resolved in the last two decades, with the advent of DNA cloning and the discovery of the structure of class I and class II molecules (Bjorkman, 1987; Brown, 1993).

The MHC located in the short arm of chromosome 6 spans approximately 4 Mb and contains over 200 identified loci, by far the most gene-dense region of the human genome sequenced to date (reviewed in Beck, 2000). It also encodes the most polymorphic human proteins, the class I and class II molecules, some of which have over 500 allelic variants to date (Marsh, 2004). More than 40% of the total expressed loci in the MHC have been associated with immune-related functions. This clustering of immune-related genes in the MHC region may not be coincidental and may be the result of evolutionary forces joining genes with similar functions.

Traditionally, the MHC region has been classified into three regions from telomere to centromere: HLA class I, non-HLA class III and HLA class II. HLA class I and class II gene functions have been reviewed in detail in the preceding chapter. We will concentrate our review on the MHC class III region and will later return to HLA class I and class II genes when we discuss disease associations.

Genes in the Non-HLA or Class III Region

The human MHC class III, or central MHC region, located between the class I and class II regions, is the most gene-dense region of the human genome. Specifically, the MHC class III region contains approximately 60 genes in ≈700 kb sequence, with an average gene size of ≈8.5 kb (Xie, 2003), compared to the entire human genome which contains, on average, fewer than 11 genes per megabase and an average gene size between 27 and 45 Mb (Lander, 2001; Heilig, 2003). Although class I and class II encoded proteins are distinguished by structural and functional similarities shared by the members of each class, class III molecules can only be defined as non-I and non-II, because their genes and their products have no common features and are not recognized by T cells. The entire class III region has been analyzed using pulse field gel electrophoresis and by cloning in artificial yeast chromosome and cosmid vectors (Dunham, 1987; Sargent, 1989; Spies, 1989; Kendall, 1990; Ragoussis, 1991; Xie, 2003). Figure 48–1 shows a genetic map of the MHC class III region.

Despite convincing genetic association studies showing the importance of the class III region in health and disease, neither the genes responsible for disease nor the underlying mechanism of pathology is known for many of the associated conditions. One reason for this is the fact that the functions of nearly half the genes in the MHC class III region are not completely known. Recently, a high-throughput yeast two-hybrid system has been used to look into the function of 27 intracellular proteins encoded within the MHC class III region (Lehner, 2004). The yeast two-hybrid system is a method by which a protein–protein interaction is identified in vivo through reconstitution of the activity of a transcriptional activator (Fields, 1989). The method is based on the properties of the GAL4 protein, which consists of separable domains responsible for DNA-binding and transcriptional activation (Fields, 1989). Plasmids encoding two hybrid proteins, one consisting of the GAL4 DNA binding domain fused to protein X and the other consisting of the GAL4 activation domain fused to protein Y, are constructed and introduced into yeast. Thus, a putative interaction between protein X and Y would lead to the transcriptional activation of a reporter gene containing a binding site for GAL4 (Chien, 1991). Notably, this study has revealed that approximately one third of the analyzed proteins encoded within the MHC class III region may have a role in mRNA processing, which again suggests clustering of functionally related genes within this region of the human genome. Specifically, four of the proteins in the MHC class III region (LSM2, UAP56, DOM3z, and SKIV2L) are orthologs of yeast proteins involved in mRNA processing, while another five proteins (BAT2, STK19, CLIC1, PBX2, and BAT5) were found to interact with proteins previously implicated in RNA processing. Three proteins (STK19, PBX2, and NELF-E or RDBP) were found to interact with proteins implicated in transcriptional regulation.

The region closer to class II genes contains several genes, including NOTCH-4, a member of the NOTCH signaling protein family that has been tentatively linked to schizophrenia (Skol, 2003; Wassink, 2003) and alopecia areata (Tazi-Ahnini, 2003). TNXB encodes tenascin-X, a large extracellular matrix protein expressed in connective tissues. Mutations of TNXB are a cause of the Ehlers–Danlos syndrome (Burch, 1997). Polymorphisms of TNXB have also been recently linked to schizophrenia (Wei, 2004). Close to NOTCH-4 is RAGE (receptor for advanced glycosylation end products), a member of the immunoglobulin superfamily (IgSF). Mutations of both RAGE genes in mice have been important for research into septic shock (Liliensiek, 2004).

As previously mentioned, almost half the genes within the MHC class III region play roles in the innate immune system, including members of the complement fixation cascade (C4, C2, BF) and tumor necrosis factor family, which will be discussed in greater detail later in this chapter. Three other members of the IgSF are also located within the MHC class III regions: 1C7 and the less characterized G6f and G6b genes. The 1C7 gene, located between LST1 and LTB, encodes the NKp30 protein responsible for triggering NK cells (Pende, 1999), and it is specifically involved in the killing of dendritic cells (Ferlazzo, 2002). The NFKBIL1 (NF-κB-inhibitor-like) gene is also located in this region (Albertella, 1994). Much interest has recently been focused on the NFKBIL1 protein, after a single nucleotide polymorphism (SNP) in the promoter of its gene was linked to rheumatoid arthritis (Okamoto, 2003). Other immune-related genes (e.g. LY6 family members, LST1 and AIF1) are likely to function as part of immune/inflammatory control (Holzinger, 1995; Utans, 1995; Ribas, 1999). Finally, the genes for the microsomal enzyme steroid P450 21-hydroxylase (CYP21) and three members of the major heat-shock protein 70 family are also contained in the MHC class III region and will be discussed later.

Tumor Necrosis Factor and Lymphotoxin α and β Genes

Tumor necrosis factor (TNF) and lymphotoxin α (LTα) and β (LTβ) are potent immunomodulatory cytokines produced in response to inflammatory stimuli. TNF and LTα proteins are each encoded by separate genes (*TNF* and *LTA*) and share approximately 34% amino acid identity (Carroll, 1987). TNF and LTα are either maintained as cell surface molecules or released from cells. LTα is retained on the cell surface via a *trans* membrane region. Surface TNF does not result from the presence of a *trans* membrane region but rather from an association with LTβ (Browning, 1993). LTβ encoded by *LTB* has 21% and 24% amino acid identity with TNF and LTα, respectively.

To date, several TNF promoter polymorphisms, located at −1030, −862, −856, −574, −375, −307, −243, −237 and +70 nucleotides relative to the transcription start site, have been identified (Wilson, 1992; Brinkman, 1994; D'Alfonso, 1994; Hamann, 1995; Zimmerman, 1996; Higuchi, 1998; Uglialoro, 1998). The endonucleases, EcoRI and NcoI, have revealed polymorphic patterns within the *LTA* gene (Partanen, 1988; Messer, 1991). The polymorphic site for the EcoRI enzyme is located in exon 4, whereas the site for NcoI has been mapped to the first intron of the *LTA* gene. DNA sequences consisting of varying lengths of TC/GA or AC/GT repeats or microsatellites within the *TNF* gene region have been identified using polyacrylamide gel sequencing (Nedospasov, 1991). There are five microsatellites: *TNFa* and *TNFb* microsatellites are located 3.5 kb telomeric to the *LTA* gene and 7 and 13 alleles have been identified respectively for *TNFa* and *TNFb*, respectively. The *TNFc* microsatellite is located in intron 1 of the *LTA* gene and has two alleles. *TNFd* and *TNFe* microsatellites, also located in intron 1, have seven and three alleles, (Jongeneel, 1991).

Throughout the past decade, the *TNF* loci have been the center of intense attention concerning the relevance of its promoter polymorphisms to susceptibility to various autoimmune and infectious diseases. This work remains controversial both at the genetic level and more importantly with regards to functional relevance. As recently demonstrated for some of the *TNF* promoter SNPs, these gene variations may be ethnic-specific markers for other linked and unidentified factors that may impact host immune response in the development of autoimmune diseases and susceptibility or resistance to infectious diseases in a given population (Delgado, 2002). Polymorphisms in the *TNF* promoter region have been correlated in large-scale population studies with cerebral malaria (McGuire, 1994), rheumatoid arthritis (Criswell, 2004), coronary heart disease (Nicaud, 2002), type 2 diabetes (Heijmans, 2002; Kubaszek, 2003), Alzheimer's disease (McCusker, 2001), ankylosing spondylitis (McGarry, 1999) mortality to septic shock (Mira, 1999) and mucocutaneous leishmaniasis (Cabrera, 1995). The TNF microsatellites *d3* and *b4* were found in higher frequencies in two distinct populations with clozapine-induced agranulocytosis (Turbay, 1997). Other TNF microsatellites have been associated with rheumatoid arthritis (Mu, 1999) and systemic lupus erythematosus (Sturfelt, 1996). In relation to *LTA* polymorphisms, large-scale analysis has linked both promoter and coding SNPs within the *LTA* gene to myocardial infarction (Ozaki, 2002, 2004).

Heat-Shock Protein 70 Genes

Stress proteins, or heat-shock proteins, are expressed in response to a variety of stress stimuli on cells. This response has been observed in all species examined to date. The family of stress proteins 70 kDa in size has a high amino acid sequence identity from primitive eukaryotes to humans. Several studies have identified loci for heat-shock protein 70 (HSP70) on chromosomes 6, 14, 21 and at least one other autosomal chromosome (Hunt, 1985; Sargent, 1989). Three genes encoding members of the HSP70 family are located telomeric to the *C2* locus (*HSPA1L*, *HSPA1A*, and *HSPA1B*, formerly known as *HSP70-Hom*, *HSP70–1*, and *HSP70–2*, respectively).

Sequence analysis of *HSPA1A* and *HSPA1B* genes has shown that they are intronless genes that encode an identical protein product of 641 amino acids. *HSPA1L* is also an intronless gene that encodes a protein of 641 amino acids and has 90% sequence identity with *HSPA1A* (Milner, 1990). Because of the high degree of sequence similarity between the coding regions of the various different *HSP70* genes, DNA probes corresponding to coding regions tend to cross-hybridize. There are however, sufficient sequence differences between the 5′ and 3′ untranslated regions to design oligonucleotide primers and probes to allow the specific amplification and hybridization of the three genes (Milner, 1992).

Three nucleotide substitutions have been detected in the 5′ flanking and untranslated regions of *HSPA1A*: an A to C transversion at position −110, a T to C transition at position +120, and a G to C transversion at position +190. Variations at position −110 and +120 have been shown to influence its mobility in polyacrylamide gel electrophoresis. Three allelic forms have been recognized: *HSPA1A A* (slow), *B* (fast) and *C* (intermediate). Oligonucleotide probes containing sequence variations at position −110

and +120 can also detect the three alleles after specific PCR amplification of the *HSPA1A* gene.

In *HSPA1B*, a G to A transition at position 1267 results in the loss of a *Pst* I restriction site. Hybridization of *Pst* I-digested genomic DNA with an *HSP70* probe results in a polymorphic fragment of DNA either 8.5 kb or 9 kb in length. Recently, a C to T transition has been identified at position −179 of *HSPA1B* (Temple, 2004). In the *HSPA1L* gene, there is a T to C transition at position 2437 that lies within an *Nco* I restriction site and yields two allelic fragments of 1.5 kb and 0.5 kb.

The *HSP70* gene cluster has lately drawn attention due to a recent study that linked both *HSPA1L* and *HLA-B*5701* loci to hypersensitivity to the antiretroviral drug abacavir (Martin, 2004). Other polymorphisms in the *HSP70* genes have been correlated to cytokine response in trauma (Schroder, 2003), Parkinson disease (Wu, 2004) and risk of clozapine-induced agranulocytosis in Ashkenazi Jews (Corzo, 1995).

C2, C4 and BF Genes

The *C2* and *C4* and *BF* genes encode proteins that play a major role in the activation of the complement system and are therefore, critical components of both innate and adaptive immunity. C2, C4 and factor B proteins are encoded in a 120 kb region of genomic DNA about 300 kb from *HLA-DR* and 600 kb from *HLA-B* (Carroll, 1984). C2 and factor B show considerable amino-acid sequence identity and share a number of physicochemical and functional characteristics, suggesting that the two genes arose by tandem duplication of a factor-B-like ancestral gene. Both are serine proteases (of the SERPIN family of plasma proteins) and mediate cleavage of C3 during activation of their respective complement pathways. C4, on the other hand, is related structurally and functionally to C3 and C5, and, by virtue of containing a highly reactive internal thiolester, is related to C3 and the protease inhibitor α_2 macroglobulin.

C2, C4 and BF Typing

The C2, C4 and factor B proteins encoded within the MHC class III demonstrate inherited structural variants that can be studied by using techniques that detect differences in net surface charge due to amino acid differences. Two methods are used to separate these proteins: (1) high-voltage agarose gel electrophoresis, which detects variations in mobility due to charge differences between proteins at a given pH and (2) isoelectric focusing in thin-layer polyacrylamide gels, which shows differences in isoelectric points. Proteins can be visualized either by immunofixation electrophoresis using insolubility of antigen–antibody complexes or by detection of functional hemolytic activity with overlay gels in which antibody-sensitized sheep erythrocytes are combined with complement-deficient serum (Alper, 1983).

At the protein level, C2 shows minor polymorphism by isoelectric focusing. The alleles for C2 are *C* (common), a less common *B* (basic) allele with three rare basic variants, and four rare *A* (acidic) variants (Jahn, 1990). The polymorphic site for the *C2*B* allele is carried by the C2a fragment. The C2 protein is genetically polymorphic in a wide variety of ethnic groups, although *C2*C* accounts for over 90% of *C2* genes in most populations (Alper, 1976; Meo, 1977). In Caucasian and Asian populations, *C2*B* accounts for 5–10% of *C2* genes. There is a non-expressed allele (*C2*QO*), which is found in 2% of the Caucasian European population (Truedsson, 1993a). For C2 typing, proteins are separated by isoelectric focusing in polyacrylamide gels and visualized by C2-induced hemolysis in overlay gels. Diluted normal human serum can replace C2-deficient serum as a reagent because C2 is the limiting factor in the classical pathway.

There are two distinct but closely related loci for the C4 protein (*C4A* and *C4B*), presumably the result of tandem gene duplication, that encode for two forms of C4. The genetics of *C4* is extraordinarily complex, not only at the genetic level but also at the protein level. It has been shown that the number of *C4* genes in humans varies from two to six and in exceptional cases, eight (Chung, 2002). Three quarters of *C4* genes carry endogenous retrovirus sequences that might confer intrinsic protection against exogenous retroviral infections (Schneider, 2001). Recent data suggest a negative correlation between the presence of endogenous retrovirus sequences and the level of C4 proteins, as well as a direct relationship between the number of genes and C4 protein levels (Yang, 2003).

At the protein level, C4A and C4B differ only by four amino acid residues in the α chain between positions 1101 and 1106. C4B is several times more hemolytically active than C4A, but C4A is more active at inhibiting the formation and dissolution of immune complexes than C4B. C4A variants usually carry Rodgers antigenic determinants (a

Val–Asp–Leu–Leu epitope of the C4A chain), and C4B variants carry Chido determinants (an Ala–Asp–Leu–Arg epitope of the α chain of C4B). There is extensive genetic polymorphism detectable in C4A and C4B proteins among populations, over 35 variants having been observed by agarose gel electrophoresis and DNA-based typing methods (Awdeh, 1980; Sim, 1986; Schneider, 1996; Hui, 2004). Among the C4A and C4B allotypes, the most common alleles are C4A*3 and C4B*1. C4A*4, C4A*2, C4B*2 and C4B*5 show a worldwide general distribution. C4A*6 is also observed in many populations, with the exception of some Mongoloid groups. C4B*3 is identified mainly in African and Caucasian groups.

C4 typing requires a combination of several techniques: (1) Immunofixation electrophoresis after treatment with neuraminidase. The patterns produced show three bands for each variant with some overlap occurring between certain variants. Additional treatment of the sample with carboxypeptidase reduces each variant to a single band. (2) Detection of C4A versus C4B by functional hemolytic assay. This method distinguishes C4A or C4B overlapping patterns because C4B variants have 5–10 times the hemolytic activity of C4A variants. (3) Rodgers (C4A) or Chido (C4B) serologic reactivity. The serum is incubated with either human anti-Rodgers or human anti-Chido to test for inhibition of agglutination with appropriate positive erythrocytes. Alternatively, C4 variants can be typed for Chido or Rodgers reactivity by immunoblotting. There are two ways to detect null alleles of C4 heterozygotes. Electrophoresis of C4 null (C4A QO and C4B QO) samples demonstrates an absence of bands in homozygotes but in heterozygotes requires quantification by visual inspection, crossed immunoelectrophoresis, or densitometric scanning of the immunofixation patterns. An alternative method is to determine the presence and ratios of the C4A and C4B α chains after sodium dodecyl sulfate polyacrylamide gel electrophoresis of immunoprecipitates. More recently, DNA-based typing methods including sequence-specific primer (SSP) amplification, restriction fragment length polymorphisms (RFLP) analysis and direct DNA sequencing have been used to complement inconclusive C4A and C4B protein allotyping (reviewed in Schneider, 2003).

Factor B is synthesized by the BF gene. Human factor B is highly polymorphic with more than 20 variants identified to date, including several dysfunctional proteins, those present in low concentration and null alleles. Factor B typing is normally performed by combination of agarose electrophoresis and/or isoelectric focusing at the protein level combined with PCR analysis at the DNA level (Geserick, 1998). Using these methods it is possible to identify two very common alleles, BF*F and BF*S, two less common alleles, BF*F1 and BF*S1, and a host of rare alleles. Variants are named for their decimal fraction migration in gel electrophoresis: BF F to BF F1 for fast variants and BF S to BF S1 for slow variants. In European Caucasian populations, BF*F has a frequency of 0.2, BF*S of 0.77, BF*F1 of 0.01, BF*S1 of 0.01, and rare alleles account only for 0.002. BF*S is most common in Caucasian, Mongoloid, and Australoid populations, while BF*F is most common in Negroid populations. BF*F1 is observed in African groups as well as in some Caucasian populations.

Disease Associations with C2, C4 and BF Genes

Deficiency of the second component of the complement system has been reported only in Caucasians, and it is the most common complement protein deficiency state in that population (Silverstein, 1960; Klemperer, 1966). People with complete C2 deficiency are homozygous for null C2 alleles (C2*Q0 for quantity zero). C2*Q0 results from a 28 bp gene deletion that generates a frame shift and a stop codon 14-bp distal to the end of exon 6 (Johnson, 1992). Remarkably, C2*QO has a gene frequency of approximately 0.01 among Caucasians. Rarely, C2 deficiency is the result of missense mutations resulting in impaired C2 secretions that have been termed C2 deficiency type II (Wetsel, 1996). Although C2 deficiency can lead to disease, the majority of patients remain asymptomatic. Up to 25% of homozygotes for C2 deficiency have increased susceptibility to bacterial infections due to alleged abnormal antibody response (Densen, 1991; Alper, 2003). Between 20% and 40% of reported C2 deficiency cases have a systemic-lupus-like disease (Truedsson, 1993b; Sullivan, 1994).

There is a high incidence of C4 null alleles in the general population. C4A*Q0 and C4B*Q0 result from gene deletions, premature stop codons, and other mutations that result in transcription failure (Braun, 1990; Lokki, 1999). 35% of individuals of all races do not express one C4A or C4B gene (i.e. carry C4A*Q0 or C4B*Q0), 8–10% carry two null alleles, and fewer than 1% do not express three alleles. Complete C4 deficiency (trans C4A*Q0, C4B*Q0) haplotypes are extremely rare (Hauptmann, 1986). The C4A*Q0 allele, particularly in homozygous individuals or those with complete C4 deficiency, has been associated with systemic and discoid lupus erythematosus (Dunckley, 1987; Nousari, 1999). This susceptibility probably relates to defective handling of immune complexes (Fielder, 1983). Children homozygous for C4B*Q0 have a 3.5-fold greater incidence of bacterial meningitis (Colten, 1992). The level of C4 in the serum of patients with C4 null alleles is extremely variable and cannot be used reliably to detect heterozygotes for complete deficiency because there is no correlation between the level of C4 and the number of expressed C4 genes (Truedsson, 1989).

The absence of any identified homozygous factor B deficiency in humans has led to the notion that the condition might be lethal during embryonic development. Based on inheritance patterns and serum levels, some heterozygotes from BF*Q0 have been identified as having reduced protein products (Siemens, 1992). The BF F variant has been associated with higher protein concentration but lower hemolytic activity than BF S (Lokki, 1991).

Complotypes

The four genes of the complement region occupy approximately 120 kb of genomic DNA (Carroll, 1984). The C2 and BF genes are located in very close proximity, separated by less than 2 kb, but BF and C4A are separated by about 30 kb. C4A and C4B are about 10 kb apart. Alleles of the complement genes occur as a unit at the population level and show striking linkage disequilibrium in haplotypes determined by family studies. That is to say, they occur together as sets on the same chromosome more frequently than expected from the frequencies of their individual alleles and with no well documented recombinations. For these reasons, haplotypes of the four complement loci have been called complotypes, as an abbreviation for 'complement haplotypes' (Alper, 1983). Although their order from telomere to centromere is C2, BF, C4A, C4B (Fig. 48–1), for clarity in using variant alleles to designate complotypes, the positions of BF and C2 are transposed. Thus, BF*S, C2*C, C4A*QO, C4B*1 is a complotype that in abbreviated form is SC01. There are more than a dozen complotypes in Caucasians that have frequencies of about 0.01 or higher (Table 48–1). In the majority of populations, the SC31 complotype is most common. In Negroid populations, FC31 is common, as is SC42 in Asian Mongoloids.

Extended Haplotypes

Based on the study of the distribution of complotypes in relation to HLA-B and HLA-DR specificities on normal Caucasian haplotypes determined in family studies, it became evident that there was striking linkage disequilibrium involving the whole region. One could easily recognize HLA-B, complotype, DR allele sets that showed statistically significant three-point linkage disequilibrium (Fig. 48–2) and defined what are regarded as extended haplotypes (Awdeh, 1983). A shorthand nomenclature for extended haplotypes has been designed by enclosing HLA-B, complotype, and HLA-DR variants in brackets. Thus, the most common extended haplotype in Caucasians is [HLA-B8, SC01, DR3]. Extended haplotypes are highly characteristic of an ethnic subgroup and have lower frequencies or do not occur at all in other ethnic groups (Alper, 1992; Fraser, 1990).

Initial studies defined extended haplotypes as the genomic interval between HLA-B and DR. It was then evident that other uncharacterized MHC alleles in the interval were likely to be included. Despite the fact that HLA-A alleles have shown limited variation for extended haplotypes, only half such haplotypes show unique and significant HLA-A allele associations (Alper, 1982). The HLA-Cw locus was by far the last to be characterized. Based on genetic distance and previously incomplete typing data of HLA-B/Cw pairs, it was evident that conserved haplotypes would also include the HLA-Cw genetic region. Thus, different HLA-Cw alleles have been recently associated with different extended haplotypes (Table 48–2) (Clavijo, 1998). Furthermore, several TNF and HSP allele systems and microsatellites have also been studied in relation to extended haplotypes (Table 48–3). More recently, models have been created to describe the variable sizes of stretches of conserved DNA in the MHC using the known frequencies of four different kinds of small blocks (<0.2 Mb) of relatively conserved DNA sequence: HLA-Cw/B; TNF; complotype; and HLA-DR/DQ (Yunis, 2003). Using HLA allele identification and TNF microsatellites, Yunis and colleagues have shown that some extended haplotypes extend to the HLA-A and HLA-DPB1 loci, which form fixed genetic units of at least 3.2 Mb of DNA. Intermediate fragments of extended haplotypes also exist, which are, nevertheless, larger than any of the four small blocks. This complexity of genetic fixity at various levels should be taken into account in studies of genetic disease association, immune response control, and human diversity.

Extended haplotypes, which account for at least 30% of normal Caucasian haplotypes, have relatively fixed gross structure and DNA sequence and carry very similar, if not identical alleles, even when they are

CHAPTER 48: The Major Histocompatibility Complex and Disease

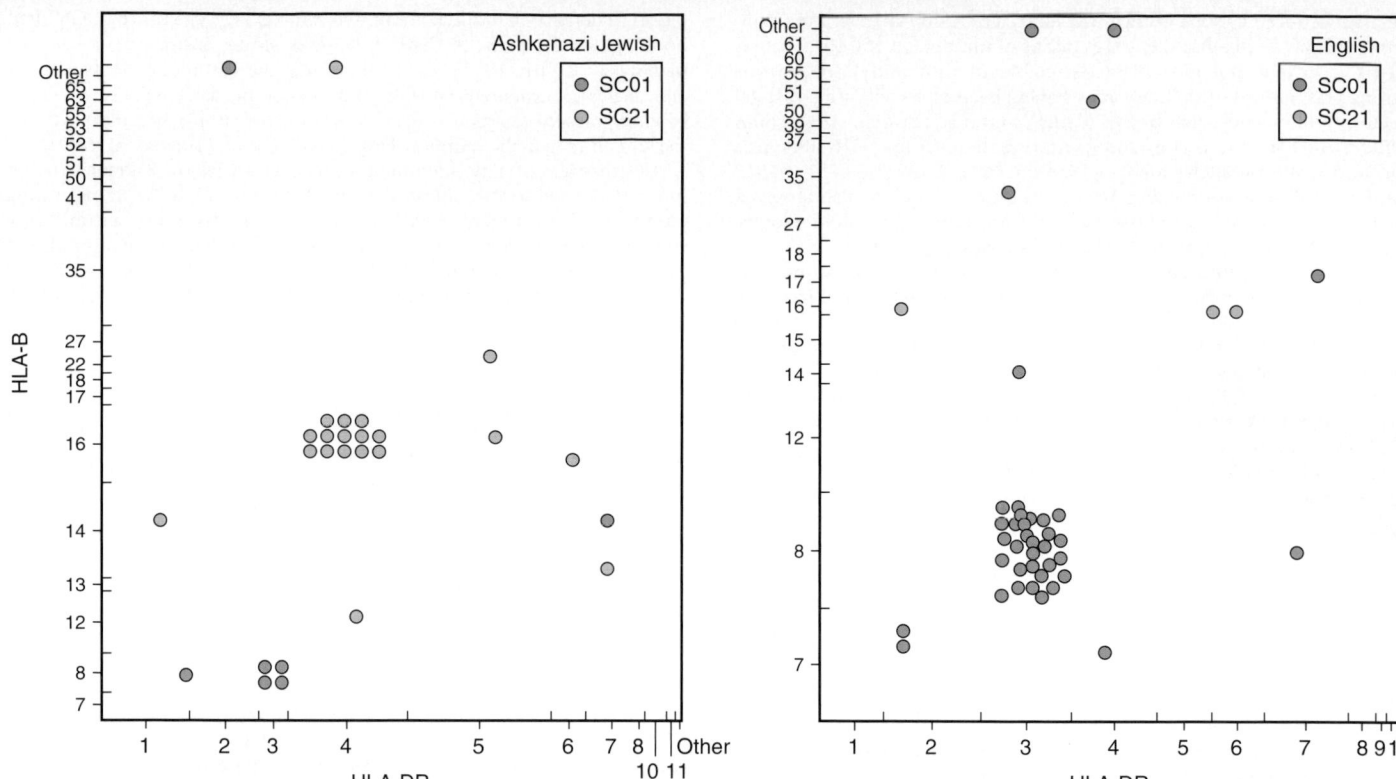

Figure 48–2 The haplotype distribution of the complotypes (haplotypes of complement alleles) *SC01* (*BF*S, C2*C, C4A*QO, C4B*1*) and *SC21* (*BF*S, C2*C, C4A*2, C4B*1*) in relation to *HLA-B* alleles on the ordinate and *HLA-DR* alleles on the abscissa. The heights and widths representing each HLA specificity are proportional to allele frequencies for the respective populations. Clustering represents linkage disequilibrium and flags the extended haplotypes (*HLA-B16(38), SC21, DR4*) in the Ashkenazi Jews and (*HLA-B8, SC01, DR3*) in the English and, to a much lesser extent, the Jews. (From Alper CA, Awdeh Z, Yunis EJ: Conserved, extended MHC haplotypes. Exp Clin Immunogenet 1992; 9:5, fig. 4. Copyright S. Karger AG, Basel.)

found in apparently unrelated individuals. The frequency of extended haplotypes is more likely to be underestimated than overestimated since haplotypes must be determined from family studies involving thousands of unrelated index cases. Recently, the MHC reference sequence (MHC Sequencing Consortium, 1999) has been used as the starting point for numerous studies trying to ascertain multiple common and rarer extended haplotypes (Walsh, 2003; John, 2004; Stewart, 2004). These studies will help to facilitate the identification of precise disease loci and may help to better understand events such as recombination and polymorphism. Studies using high-resolution sperm typing techniques suggest the

presence of regions of low recombination within the MHC (Jeffreys, 2001). One such region was described near the *LTA* gene, where a lower than expected recombination rate was seen between *HLA-A* and *HLA-B* (Cullen, 2002). The effect of these regions of low recombination on disease association remains unknown. Furthermore, recent reports (based on linkage disequilibrium (LD) analysis applied to SNPs data without pedigree analysis), describing the existence of blocks of conserved DNA sequences within the human genome separated by sites of high recombination activity, have been questioned (Jeffreys, 2001; Gabriel, 2002). These reports identifying blocks of conserved DNA within the MHC differ from studies using haplotype LD analysis defined by family studies (Dawkins, 1999; Yunis, 2003). It appears that LD analysis using SNP data

Table 48–1 Common Complotypes in Normal Chromosomes of Caucasoid Populations

Complotype	Frequency (%)
SC31	0.430
SC01	0.127
FC31	0.096
SC30	0.053
SC42	0.040
SC61	0.034
FC30	0.031
FC01	0.029
SC02	0.029
SC21	0.022
SB42	0.019
SC33	0.014
SC2(1,2)*	0.013
SC32	0.011

Complotypes are given as abbreviated letters and numbers, with four alleles in arbitrary order: *BF, C2, C4A,* and *C4B*.

* *C4B* locus is heteroduplicated.

Table 48–2 Common Extended MHC Haplotypes

Extended Haplotype	HLA-Cw allele	Ethnicity
[HLA-B8, SC01, DR3, DQ2]	0701	Northern Europe
[HLA-B7, SC31, DR2, DQ6]	0702	Northern Europe
[HLA-B44, FC31, DR7, DQ2]	1601	Europe
[HLA-B44, SC30, DR4, DQ7/8]	0501	Europe
[HLA-B57, SC61, DR7, DQ2/3]	0602	Northern Europe
[HLA-B14, SC22, DR1, DQ1]	0802	Northern Europe
[HLA-B35, SC31, DR5, DQ3]	0401	Southern Europe
[HLA-B38, SC21, DR4, DQ8]	1203	Ashkenazi Jews
[HLA-B15, SC33, DR4, DQ8]	0304	Northern Europe
[HLA-B18, F1C30, DR3, DQ2]	0501	Basques, Sardinia, Spain
[HLA-B18, S042, DR2]*	1203	Northern Europe
[HLA-B42, FC(1,90)0, DR3]†	1/01	African

Data from normal Caucasoid population chromosomes from Boston.

* Data from patients with C2 deficiency (Clavijo, 1998).

† Data from chromosomes of normal black population living in Boston (Clavijo, 1999).

Table 48–3 *TNF* and *HSP* Gene Polymorphisms in Relation to Common Extended Haplotypes

| | Complotype | | | | HSP | | | | TNF markers | | | | | | |
HLA-DR	C4B	C4A	BF	C2	1B	1A	e	d	-307	-856	-862	a	b	HLA-B	HLA-Cw
3	1	0	S	C	8.5	C	3	1	2	1	1	2	3	8	0701
2	1	3	S	C	9	A	3	3	1	1	1	11	4	7	0702
7	1	3	F	C	9	A	3	3	1	1	1	7,8	4	44	1601
4	0	3	S	C	9	A	3	3	1	1	1	6,7	5	44	0501
7	1	6	S	C	9	A	3	4	1	1	1	2	5	57	0602
5	1	3	S	C	9	A	3	3	1	1	1	5	5	35	0401
1	1,2	2	S	C	9	A	1	4	1	1	2	2	1	14	0802
4	1	2	S	C	9	A	3	3	1	2	1	10	4	38	1203
4	3	3	S	C	9	A	1	4	1	1	2	2	1	62	0304
2	2	4	S	0	9	A	3	3	1	2	1	10	4	18	1203
3	0	3	F1	C	8.5	C	3	4	1	1	1	1	5	18	0501

The number or letters under each column refers to a particular allele variant of the complement, heat-shock protein (*HSP*), tumor necrosis factor (*TNF*) microsatellite or *TNF* promoter polymorphisms that are associated with the HLA specificities as noted. See text for explanation. In the case of *TNF-307*, 1 and 2 represent the *-307/G* and *-307/A* variants, respectively. *TNF-856/C* allele is noted as 1 and the *TNF-856/T* allele is 2. The *TNF-862/C* TNF allele is noted as 1 and the *-862/A* as 2.

Source: data extracted and modified from Clavijo, 1998.

alone lacks the power to distinguish individual variations between sizes of DNA blocks and their frequency distribution among populations. Thus, SNPs studies should be performed in individuals whose blocks have already been determined by family studies in order to elucidate the relationship between the presence of small or larger sizes of blocks.

MHC Disease Associations

The MHC is associated with more diseases than any other region on the human genome. We have reviewed the concepts about complotypes and extended haplotypes in order to be able to understand the relevance of a rather extensive literature on MHC markers of disease. Most of the MHC markers of disease reported to date are contained within extended haplotypes. It is probably because of this simple fact that so many MHC-allele associated diseases have been reported, since it is not a single base pair but over 3 million base pairs of conserved DNA that comprise the marker. For example, complement alleles such as *BF*F1* and *C4B*3* have been linked to type 1 diabetes because the extended haplotypes that carry them, [*HLA-B18, F1C30, DR3*] and [*HLA-B62, SC01, DR3*], are more common in these patients than in the general population. This association means that haplotypes comprised of 3 million bases or more in length of conserved genomic DNA carry susceptibility alleles for type 1 diabetes. It is also critical to know the ethnic distribution of an associated MHC allele in order to evaluate whether the allele in patients is increased compared with ethnically matched control populations or is in fact truly a marker for the ethnic distribution of the disease. Furthermore, it is more difficult to map the genes responsible for disease in Caucasian Americans than in African Americans or Asian Americans because the level of genetic diversity is lower in Caucasians. When results of the MHC project become available, in which consanguineous MHC haplotypes from populations of different ethnicity were chosen for sequencing analysis (Allcock, 2002), investigators will have the opportunity to identify genes responsible for disease within smaller fragments of DNA.

There are a remarkable number of diseases that show an association with MHC genes. Most MHC disease associations are autoimmune and do not show clear-cut mendelian inheritance. There are many problems that confound attempts to understand the inheritance mechanisms by which these diseases occur, and an analysis of MHC markers in patients and their families has only clarified the picture marginally. A major problem with MHC gene associations is their incomplete penetrance, making ordinary formal segregation and linkage studies very difficult, if not impossible, to carry out. This is seen most clearly in monozygotic twins who presumably have identical genes. If one such twin has one of these diseases (e.g., type 1 diabetes mellitus), the other twin does not necessarily have the disease. For type 1 diabetes, the concordance rate appears to be no higher than 50% (Rubinstein, 1977; Barnett, 1981). This suggests that penetrance of a disease in a completely susceptible host is incomplete. Although there is excellent reason to consider genes in the MHC as determinants of type 1 diabetes susceptibility, only 15% of MHC-identical siblings of diabetic patients have insulin-dependent diabetes. This difference between 50%

and 15% is evidence for the influence of genes at a second, non-MHC-linked locus (or loci), and also suggests the influence of other factors, such as environmental factors, in determining susceptibility.

Incomplete penetrance makes the assignment of a specific mode of inheritance difficult and makes the likelihood of finding families with more than one affected member within one or more generations low. Families are frequently used to determine modes of inheritance. Another complicating factor is the inability to determine whether or not we are studying a group of patients homogeneous in terms of genetic determination. About 5–6% of random families with a type 1 diabetic proband will have a second affected child. Of these sibling pairs, approximately 60% will be MHC-identical, 35% will be haploidentical, and a few percent will share no MHC haplotypes. This pattern suggests recessive inheritance of an MHC-linked susceptibility gene for the disease. At the very least, however, family studies provide highly useful haplotype data and usually allow the assignment of homozygosity for an HLA marker in probands. They have also established that MHC association in most of the diseases of interest is based on linkage between a susceptibility gene and the MHC.

Yet another unknown is the number of different susceptibility alleles for a disease in any specific population. In this regard, extended haplotypes can be helpful because, if increased in patients, they probably represent a single susceptibility allele that could be anywhere in the region of fixity. However, some patients have only portions of these haplotypes, and this provides little information about the location of specific allele involvement. Furthermore, it appears likely that many MHC-associated diseases are polygenic. Because of these problems, we will begin our discussion of MHC disease association with disorders that show mendelian inheritance and 100% penetrance, at least for the primary biochemical defect. We have already reviewed two of these disorders earlier in the chapter: C2 and C4 protein deficiencies.

Hereditary Hemochromatosis and the *HFE* gene

Hemochromatosis is an autosomal recessive disease and is the most common hereditary metabolic disease in Caucasians. Hemochromatosis consists of an inherited metabolic defect in iron metabolism resulting in failure to control iron absorption in the setting of increasing iron stores, leading to tissue iron overload and eventually to organ damage (reviewed in Adams, 2000). The most common manifestations of hemochromatosis are cirrhosis of the liver, hepatocellular carcinoma and cardiomyopathy. The discovery of the hereditary hemochromatosis (*HH*) gene in the MHC was based on the early finding of an increased frequency of the *HLA-A3* allele in HH patients (Simon, 1976). After years of effort in the vicinity of the *HLA-A* locus, the *HFE* gene was found several megabase pairs away (Feder, 1996). *HFE* encodes a 343 amino-acid protein that belongs to a group named MHC class-I-related molecules because of their similarities to HLA class I molecules.

The *HFE* gene has two common missense mutations: the C282Y mutation, resulting in the substitution of a tyrosine for a cysteine, and the H63D mutation, resulting in the substitution of an aspartate for a histidine. Unlike the H63D mutation, the C282Y mutation interferes with

Table 48–4 Examples of Association Between HLA and Disease

Disease	Ethnicity	HLA Antigen	Reference
Ankylosing spondylitis	Caucasian, Asian, African	B27	Khan, 1992; Rubin, 1994
Gluten-sensitive enteropathy	Caucasian	DRB1*0301, DQB1*0201, DQA1*0501	Marsh, 1992; Goggins, 1994
		DRB1*0701, DQB1*0201, DQA1*0501	
Pemphigus vulgaris	Jews	B38, DR4, DQ8; B35, DR4, DQ8	Ahmed, 1990
	Non-Jews	B55, DR6, DQ5	Ahmed, 1991
Cicatricial pemphigoid	Caucasian	DR4, DQB1*0301	Yunis, 1994; Delgado, 1996
Multiple sclerosis	Caucasian	DRB1*1501, DQB1*0602, DQA1*0102	Marrosu, 1992
Narcolepsy	Caucasian, Jews	DRB1*1501, DQB1*0602, DQA1*0102	Kwon, 1995; Rogers, 1997
Type 1 diabetes (susceptibility)	Caucasian	DR3 or DR4, DQB1*0302, DQA1*0301	Thomson, 1984; Kockum, 1993; Noble, 1996
Type 1 diabetes (resistance)	Caucasian	DRB1*1501, DQB1*0602	Noble, 1996
Rheumatoid arthritis	Caucasian	DR4 (DRB1*0401; DRB1*0404)	MacGregor, 1995
HIV infection			
Rapid progression to AIDS	Caucasian	B35, Cw4	Kaslow, 1996; Carrington, 1999
Slow progression to AIDS	Caucasian	B27, B57	Kaslow, 1996; Keet, 1999
HIV viremia control	Caucasian	Bw4	Flores-Villanueva, 2001
Tuberculosis	Asian (Cambodia)	DQB1*0503	Goldfeld, 1998
	Asian (India, Indonesia)	DR2	Bothamley, 1989; Rajalingam, 1996

the protein interaction with β_2-microglobulin, abolishing the cell-surface expression of HFE (Feder, 1997; Waheed, 1997). A homozygous C282Y mutation is present in the majority of HH Caucasian patients. The C282Y mutation has a remarkably high allelic frequency in northern European populations (0.05–0.1%) and is rare in non-Caucasian populations. The H63D mutation is present at high frequency in control Caucasians (>0.1%) and was also found in non-Caucasian populations; however, its role in HH remains unclear.

Congenital Adrenal Hyperplasia due to 21-Hydroxylase Deficiency

Immediately 3′ to each C4 locus are two loci for the adrenal steroid enzyme 21 hydroxylase (CYP21A and CYP21B) (Carroll, 1985; Higashi, 1986; White, 1986). The two genes are highly homologous but three mutations cause premature termination of the transcription of the CYP21A gene, rendering it a pseudogene (White, 1988). Congenital adrenal hyperplasia is clinically heterogeneous, with a severe salt-wasting form, a milder late onset form manifested largely by masculinization in girls, and a mild cryptic form. The MHC linkage of this disorder was discovered before any MHC associations were detected and before it was known that the CYP21 loci were located within the MHC. Subsequently, studies found that 20% or more European Caucasian patients with the salt-wasting form carried the rare extended haplotype [HLA-A1, Cw6, B47, FC(91)0, DRB1*07, DRB4*0101, DQA1*0201, DQB1*0201] (Fleischnick, 1983). It has been shown that this haplotype has a deletion of both C4B and CYP21B, thus explaining the severity of symptoms and complete deficiency of the enzyme in homozygotes for this haplotype. Among patients with milder and cryptic disease, a different extended haplotype is common: [HLA-B65, SC2(1,2), DR1] (Sinnott, 1991). This haplotype is common, particularly in southern Europe, and has a frequency of over 0.01% in Caucasians living in Boston. In all forms of 21-hydroxylase deficiency, the bulk of MHC haplotypes are not extended, and there is a great variety of complotypes, suggesting that many independent mutations have led to either deletion or derangement of the CYP21B gene.

Specific Diseases Without Evidence of Mendelian Inheritance and with MHC Associations

Table 48–4 lists some MHC-associated diseases and their markers. This list is not exhaustive, and we shall discuss only a few of the diseases in greater detail.

Type 1 Diabetes

The most studied of all MHC-linked diseases is type 1 diabetes mellitus (Nepom, 1991; Thorsby, 1992; Winter, 1993; Lernmark, 1999). Alleles of the HLA class II genes DQB1, DQA1, and DRB1 in the MHC region are major determinants of genetic predisposition to type 1 diabetes. Several alleles of each of these three loci are associated with either susceptibility or protection from disease. There are striking increases in the frequency of HLA-DR3 and HLA-DR4 among Caucasian patients (Thomson, 1984; Jenkins, 1991). Using molecular-based HLA typing analysis, the increase in DR4 is found primarily in the subset of DR4 in linkage disequilibrium with DQB1*0302 (Kockum, 1993). Although the latter gene is now considered a major marker and perhaps a primary determinant of type 1 diabetes susceptibility, it is present in only 70% of Caucasian patients. Even among those who carry it, there is variability in the relative risk for diabetes: DRB1*0401, DQB1*0302 and DRB1*0402, DQB1*0302 are highly associated with the disease, while DRB1*0404, DQB1*0302 is less so. In many Caucasian patient populations with type 1 diabetes there is an excess of DR3/DR4 heterozygotes over the number of DR3 or DR4 homozygotes predicted by the Hardy–Weinberg equilibrium (Kockum, 1999). In addition, the relative risks for some DR-DQ genotypes are not simply the sum or product of the relative risks for the single haplotype. For example, the risk of the DRB1*03–DQB1*02/DRB1*0401–DQB1*0302 genotype is often found to be higher than for the individual DRB1*03–DQB1*02 and DRB1*0401–DQB1*0302 homozygous genotypes. It has been hypothesized that this synergy occurs through the formation of highly susceptible trans-encoded HLA-DQB1 and HLA-DQA1 heterodimers (Koeleman, 2004). DQA1*0301 is present on all DR4-positive haplotypes, whether or not they carry DQB1*0302, and it is possible that DQA1*0301 may contribute to risk itself. On the other hand, DRB1*1501, DQB1*0602 is negatively associated with type 1 diabetes. Individuals heterozygous for DRB1*1501, DQB1*0602 who also carry a susceptibility gene for type 1 diabetes on the other haplotype are nonetheless not at risk for the disease (dominant protection), as expected with a recessive disorder (Noble, 1996). A recently proposed model for type 1 diabetes, which assumes that DQB1 is a direct determinant of susceptibility, suggests a hierarchy of affinities among different class II molecules that compete for binding to the same type 1 diabetes-peptide (Nepom, 1990). Susceptibility occurs if a gene product (for example, DQB1*0302) binds and presents the type 1 diabetes peptide. In the presence of a high-affinity (DRB1*1501) competitor this event does not occur. Another model proposes that codon 57 of the DQB-encoded chain plays a critical role in the pathogenesis of type 1 diabetes. The presence of a nonaspartic acid at position 57 of DQB1 has been suggested as an important determinant of susceptibility to type 1 diabetes mediated by the DQB1 genes (Lee, 2001; Siebold, 2004). The excess presence of valine or serine at this position in diabetic patients carrying the HLA-DR3 or DR4 haplotypes supports this concept.

Rheumatoid Arthritis

The association between MHC markers and rheumatoid arthritis (RA) is well documented (Nepom, 1992; Ollier, 1992; Auger, 1998). For most of the populations studied, the primary associated marker is HLA-DR4 (MacGregor, 1995). In Caucasians, for example, the most common RA-associated DR4 alleles are DRB1*0401 and DRB1*0404, and in Japanese, Israeli, and Chinese patients it is DRB1*0405. Other HLA-DR specificities are also associated with RA: DR1 has been reported in association with RA in Caucasian, Japanese, Spanish, Greek, and Israeli patients; *DR3* in Kuwaitis; *DR6* in Yakima American Indians; *DR9* in Chileans; and *DR10* in Spanish, Greek, and Israeli patients (reviewed in Zanelli, 2000). To explain this broad spectrum of different *HLA-DR* associations with RA, it has been proposed that a shared DRB1 peptide sequence is involved in conferring RA susceptibility (Penzotti, 1996; Garavito, 2004). The alleles associated with RA share a highly conserved sequence of amino acids in their third hypervariable region (amino acids 67–74). These residues could affect the binding of peptides and their presentation to T cells (Hammer, 1995). Thus, if an arthritogenic peptide exists, it may preferentially bind to molecules with the RA DRB1 sequence. As yet, no such arthritogenic peptide has been identified. An alternative explanation may involve molecular mimicry between the shared RA DRB1 and antigenic sequences of a pathogen that can induce RA (reviewed in Albani, 1992). Sequence homology has been found between the shared RA sequence and a HSP from *Escherichia coli* (Auger, 1998). RA differs clinically from juvenile rheumatoid arthritis (JRA) and the HLA associations with JRA are quite different. Furthermore, other *HLA-DR* associations vary among JRA clinical subsets (Stastny, 1993). For example, it has been reported that the frequency of haplotype *HLA-DRB1*0801, DQA1*0401, DQB1*0402* is increased in the whole pauciarticular group and in patients with the persistent pauciarticular form. The haplotype *HLA-DRB1*1301, DRB3*0101, DQA1*0103, DQB1*0603* was also associated with patients with persistent pauciarticular JRA (Fernandez-Vina, 1994). In keeping with the view that the polyarticular form of JRA is RA occurrence in the young, *DRB1*0401* shows a strong association.

HIV-1 Infection and AIDS Progression

Over 70 publications on HLA association with human immunodeficiency virus (HIV) progression have been published to date, covering few ethnic groups. Most of these studies have limited power because of scarce patient and control samples or use overlapping risk groups, which makes comparisons between studies difficult. Furthermore, at least half of the studies have been performed using serologic typing of HLA specificities, increasing the degree of inconsistency between them. Despite these limitations and thanks to the development of more precise PCR-based methods for HLA typing in the last decade (reviewed in the previous chapter), some relatively clear and consistent associations have emerged in relation to HIV infection and acquired immunodeficiency syndrome (AIDS) progression, primarily in Caucasian patients. *HLA-B35*, an antigen predominantly found in Caucasians, is the most consistently described HLA antigen associated with rapid progression to AIDS (Kaslow, 1996; Carrington, 1999), while *HLA-B*27* and *HLA-B*57*, which are rare alleles in most populations, have been consistently associated with slower progression to AIDS in Caucasians (Kaslow, 1996; Hendel, 1999; Keet, 1999). HLA-B molecules can be categorized by the presence of a *Bw4* or *Bw6* epitope, which is defined by two different amino acid sequences at residues 79–83 at the carboxyl end of the α_1 helix of the HLA class I binding groove (Salter, 1989). Flores-Villanueva and colleagues have recently demonstrated that profound suppression of HIV-1 viremia is significantly associated with homozygosity for *HLA-B* alleles that share the HLA-Bw4 epitope (Flores-Villanueva, 2001). Further analysis of large population-based studies, especially those including cohorts from different ethnicities, such as African and Asian populations, are urgently needed to confirm previous results and to discover potentially new associations in different ethnicities infected with various HIV-1 subtypes. Such studies will also be valuable for the development of HIV vaccination strategies involving the induction of ethnicity-specific HLA-restricted CD8[+] T-cell responses in populations at greater risk for HIV infection.

Tuberculosis

Several alleles of the HLA class II DR2 serotype have been associated with susceptibility to progressive clinical tuberculosis (Bothamley, 1989; Khomenko, 1990; Rajalingam, 1996; Teran-Escandon, 1999). More recently, *HLA-DQB1*0503* has been associated with progressive clinical tuberculosis in Cambodia (Goldfeld, 1998). This association is particularly intriguing as the *DQB1*0503* allele encodes a change at amino-acid position 57 of the β chain (β57) that influences the charge in the putative peptide binding pocket, P9, of the DQ molecule. As reviewed in greater detail in the previous chapter, peptides bind in an extended conformation to a groove in the HLA class II molecule that contains antigen-specific pockets formed by polymorphic side chains (Brown, 1993; Stern, 1994). HLA-DQ molecules, encoded by polymorphic HLA-DQ α and β chain genes, bind peptides with certain amino acids that are anchored at specific positions within peptide-binding pockets, termed P1, P4 and P9 pockets, in the

HLA-DQ molecular groove (Lee, 2001; Siebold, 2004). The amino acid at codon 57 of the HLA-DQ β chain is critical for the peptide binding specificity of the P9 pocket and is dependent upon whether there is an aspartic acid or a nonaspartic acid at the position (Kwok, 1996; Nepom, 1996; Quarsten, 1998). The *DQB1*0503* allele encodes the negatively charged aspartic acid at position 57 in place of the more common, uncharged and hydrophobic amino acid alanine. Thus, it is possible that the MHC-restricted presentation of peptides by tuberculosis-infected macrophages is affected in the group of patients that express this particular pocket, leading to a diminished immunogenic response. HLA association studies investigating whether or not sets of HLA alleles have shared binding specificities associated with susceptibility to tuberculosis, combined with functional experiments testing the ability of these alleles to bind *Mycobacterium tuberculosis* peptides and stimulate effector T-cell responses, are currently under way.

Methods of Detecting Association or Linkage of Diseases with Genetic Markers

Genetic Polymorphism

Genetic polymorphism is defined as the occurrence of two or more alleles at one gene, each with appreciable frequency in the same population. The frequency has been arbitrarily defined to be higher than 1%. There are two groups of genetic polymorphisms: balanced or stable and transient. A balanced or stable polymorphism occurs when two or more alleles are maintained in a population by selection. The heterozygous advantage is the classic example of balanced polymorphism. A transient polymorphism represents a phase of allelic changes driven by genetic drift or by selection. Polymorphism of a gene can be stable in one population and transient in another depending on the effect of selection.

Gene and Phenotype Frequencies

To determine genetic polymorphism, it is necessary to find a representative sample of the population, assess the individuals, count the genes and estimate the number of genes contained in the entire population. For example, assuming that a population of 100 individuals has been studied for a particular genetic trait or allele at a given gene, we can define the phenotype frequency as the number of individuals carrying the trait or the genetic variant. To calculate the frequency (f) of an allele, the frequency of each allele is added and then divided by the total number of analyzed alleles:

$$f(x) = \frac{f(x)}{f(x) + f(y) + f(z)}.$$

It is possible to calculate the gene frequency (g) without knowing the mode of inheritance by using the formula:

$$g = 1 - \sqrt{f}.$$

Strength of Association

Several methods have been devised for detecting the degree of association of genetic markers with hypothesized genes for disease susceptibility. One method is to compute the risk of disease among individuals carrying a specific allele of a polymorphic system. In this computation, the relative risk (RR), or odds ratio, calculates the risk of carrying a marker in a population of diseased individuals compared with a control population. This strength of association is the delta of Bergston and Thomson (Svejgaard, 1983), which is the same as the etiologic fraction (EF) (Miettinen, 1976). If, in a patient population, 'a' individuals carry the specific character but 'b' individuals do not, and in the control (normal) population, 'c' individuals carry the character, we may then write the information conveniently in the 2×2 table:

	Character-Positive	Character-Negative
Patient	a	b
Control	c	d

The frequency of the character in this patient population (h_p) is:

$$h_p = \frac{a}{a+b}.$$

The relative risk (RR), or odds ratio, is defined as:

$$RR = \frac{a \times d}{b \times c}.$$

Etiologic fraction (EF) is defined as:

$$EF = \frac{RR-1}{RR} \times \frac{a}{a+b}$$

$$= \frac{RR-1}{RR} \times h_p.$$

Similarly, in decreased risk, for which the RR is less than 1, the preventive factor (PF) can be used:

$$PF = \frac{(1-RR)\, h_p}{RR(1-h_p)+h_p}.$$

The EF and PF fractions can vary between 0 (no association) and 1.0 (maximal association). Apart from providing estimates of having a marker if one already has a disease, these calculations ignore the mode of genetic determination of the disease in question. This is particularly problematic for recessive or more complicated modes, in which both haplotypes are important for determining disease but heterozygotes and homozygotes for a given marker are given the same weight, i.e., both are positive for the marker.

Analysis of Mode of Inheritance Based on Sibling Pairs

The analysis of mode of inheritance based on sibling pairs was introduced to help overcome the problems of incomplete penetrance of disease genes and variations in the age of onset (Penrose, 1935). The analysis is based on the assumption that if HLA and/or genes closely linked to HLA have no influence on the development of a disease, then the affected sibling pairs will share HLA haplotypes with a normal frequency: 25% will share both haplotypes, 50% will share one, and 25% will share no haplotypes. Thus, observed and expected distributions of haplotype sharing are compared. If susceptibility genes or their closely linked markers are rare and fully penetrant in a purely recessively determined disease, the distribution of two-, one- and no-haplotype-sharing sibs would be 100, 0, and 0. For dominant determination, the ratio would be 33, 66, and 0. What is observed in diabetes, for example (Rubinstein, 1977), is 60, 35, and 5, closer to recessive than dominant predictions. Once the mode of inheritance has been established, the disease gene frequency and penetrance can be determined (Thomson, 1977).

Analysis of Mode of Inheritance Based on Population Studies

Thomson and Bodmer (1977) have devised a method for analyzing population data for markers closely linked to susceptibility loci for diseases with incomplete penetrance. In essence, this method predicts the proportion of homozygotes, heterozygotes, and noncarriers for the linked marker that is expected in cases of dominant or recessive inheritance. The greatest difference between the two modes of inheritance is observed by the proportion of individuals who are homozygous for the marker. Application of this method to HLA-B27 and ankylosing spondylitis led, on statistical grounds, to the rejection of a recessive mechanism. Thus, it was concluded that susceptibility to ankylosing spondylitis is inherited as a dominant trait.

Similarly, the same method of analysis was applied to the distribution of BF*F1 among 1107 patients with type 1 diabetes mellitus (Raum, 1981). For dominant inheritance 1.89 homozygotes were predicted, and for recessive inheritance 6.2 homozygotes were predicted. Seven BF*F1 homozygotes were found, a result that is consistent only with recessive

inheritance. Other modes of inheritance that could be rejected by these observations include simple dominant, epistatic (disease resulting from the presence of non-allelic genes), and overdominant (disease with greater penetrance when two specific alleles are present than when other combinations, including homozygosity for each specific allele, occur). Although a mixed model with different penetrance for homozygotes and heterozygotes could not be completely ruled out, other considerations make such a model unsatisfactory.

Lod Score Method

The lod score is a statistical measure of linkage between a marker locus, such as in the MHC and a disease susceptibility gene (Sutton, 1980). In the equation for calculating the lod score: (1) the Z value is the ratio of the maximum likelihood of finding linkage ($P(F_1/\theta)$) to that of no linkage at a particular recombination value of θ and (2) the $\theta(q)$ value, or recombination frequency, is a measure of distance from a given locus corresponding to maximum Z value. The lod score expresses the probability that alleles at two loci will segregate together, in terms of the ratio between the observed and the predicted recombination frequency if they assort independently. Various values of (q) from 0 to 0.5 are substituted into the following equation:

$$P(F_1/\theta) = 1/2\,[\theta^r(1-\theta)^{n-r} + \theta^{n-r}(1-\theta)^r],$$

where n = the number of children in a given family and r = the number of recombinants. The probability of obtaining a pedigree for a given value of θ (recombination frequency from 0 to 0.5), which is expressed as the ratio of $P(F_1/\theta)$ in a family at a given recombination fraction θ (from 0 to 0.5) to $P(F_1/0.5)$ in the same family assuming no recombination, can be expressed as the lod score (Z). The lod score is the sum of all z values where Z is:

$$z = \log_{10} \frac{P(F_1/\theta)}{P(F_1/0.5)}.$$

Values of Z greater than zero favor linkage, and those less than or equal to zero are against linkage. In general, a Z value greater than 3 (for some values of 0<0.5) means that the odds in favor of linkage are 1000 to 1 (p value = 0.05), as opposed to no linkage or independence. It is easier to calculate linkage for codominant traits, i.e. HLA, than for recessive traits. In studies that examine the linkage of HLA and disease, the parents may have recessive or dominant impenetrant susceptibility genes. There are basic problems in using the lod score method in detecting linkage of partially penetrant genes, apart from impenetrant susceptible siblings. If susceptibility genes are common, as appears to be the case in type 1 diabetes, for example, apparent crossovers or nonidentical sibs could suggest additional susceptibility genes in a parent.

Summary

The MHC comprises many alleles at many loci. The high resolution typing of class I and class II MHC genes, and the identification of genes between and near them has increased the possibility of defining the genetic basis of immune responses and diseases of unknown etiology, such as autoimmune diseases in man. The nonrandom association of markers to immune responses or associations with autoimmune diseases, due to the presence of fixed stretches of MHC DNA and extended haplotypes and their fragments in the population, complicates the study of susceptibility genes but also provides the means for their identification. Even though the human MHC is the most intensively investigated region of the genome, not all the expressed genes within the MHC have been identified. It is probable that some unidentified MHC genes, rather than one already identified, are susceptibility genes for some human MHC-associated diseases.

References

Adams P, Brissot P, Powell LW: EASL International Consensus Conference on Haemochromatosis. J Hepatol 2000; 33:485–504.

Ahmed AR, Wagner R, Khatri K, et al: Major histocompatibility complex haplotypes and class II genes in non-Jewish patients with pemphigus vulgaris. Proc Natl Acad Sci USA 1991; 88:5056–5060.

Ahmed AR, Yunis EJ, Khatri K, et al: Major histocompatibility complex haplotype studies in Ashkenazi Jewish patients with pemphigus vulgaris. Proc Natl Acad Sci USA 1990; 87:7658–7662.

Albani S, Tuckwell JE, Esparza L, et al: The susceptibility sequence to rheumatoid arthritis is a cross-reactive B cell epitope shared by the Escherichia coli heat shock protein dnaJ and the

histocompatibility leukocyte antigen DRB10401 molecule. J Clin Invest 1992; 89:327–331.

Albertella MR, Campbell RD: Characterization of a novel gene in the human major histocompatibility complex that encodes a potential new member of the I kappa B family of proteins. Hum Mol Genet 1994; 3:793–799.

Allcock RJ, Atrazhev AM, Beck S, et al: The MHC haplotype project: a resource for HLA-linked association studies. Tissue Antigens 2002; 59:520–521.

Alper CA: Inherited structural polymorphism in human C2: evidence for genetic linkage between C2 and Bf. J Exp Med 144:1111–1115, 1976.

Alper CA, Awdeh ZL, Raum DD, et al: Extended major histocompatibility complex haplotypes in man: role of alleles analogous to murine t mutants. Clin Immunol Immunopathol 1982; 24:276–285.

Alper CA, Awdeh Z, Yunis EJ: Conserved, extended MHC haplotypes. Exp Clin Immunogenet 1992; 9:58–71.

Alper CA, Raum D, Karp S, et al: Serum complement 'supergenes' of the major histocompatibility complex in man (complotypes). Vox Sang 1983; 45:62–67.

Alper CA, Xu J, Cosmopoulos K, et al: Immunoglobulin deficiencies and susceptibility to infection among homozygotes and heterozygotes for C2 deficiency. J Clin Immunol 2003; 23:297–305.

Auger I, Toussirot E, Roudier J: HLA-DRB1 motifs and heat shock proteins in rheumatoid arthritis. Int Rev Immunol 1998; 17:263–271.

Awdeh ZL, Alper CA: Inherited structural polymorphism of the fourth component of human complement. Proc Natl Acad Sci USA 1980; 77:3576–3580.

Awdeh ZL, Raum D, Yunis EJ, et al: Extended HLA/complement allele haplotypes: evidence for T/t-like complex in man. Proc Natl Acad Sci USA 1983; 80:259–263.

Barnett AH, Eff C, Leslie RD, et al: Diabetes in identical twins. A study of 200 pairs. Diabetologia 1981; 20:87–93.

Beck S, Trowsdale J: The human major histocompatability complex: lessons from the DNA sequence. Annu Rev Genomics Hum Genet 2000; 1:117–137.

Bjorkman PJ, Saper MA, Samraoui B, et al: Structure of the human class I histocompatibility antigen, HLA-A2. Nature 1987; 329:506–512.
This landmark paper shows the first crystal structure of an HLA class I molecule associated to a peptide.

Bothamley GH, Beck JS, Schreuder GM, et al: Association of tuberculosis and M. tuberculosis-specific antibody levels with HLA. J Infect Dis 1989; 159:549–555.

Braun L, Schneider PM, Giles CM, et al: Null alleles of human complement C4. Evidence for pseudogenes at the C4A locus and for gene conversion at the C4B locus. J Exp Med 1990; 171:129–140.

Brinkman BM, Giphart MJ, Verhoef A, et al: Tumor necrosis factor alpha-308 gene variants in relation to major histocompatibility complex alleles and Felty's syndrome. Hum Immunol 1994; 41:259–266.

Brown JH, Jardetzky TS, Gorga JC, et al: Three-dimensional structure of the human class II histocompatibility antigen HLA-DR1 [see comments]. Nature 1993; 364:33–39.
This landmark paper shows the first crystal structure of an HLA class II molecule associated to a peptide.

Browning JL, Ngam-ek A, Lawton P, et al: Lymphotoxin beta, a novel member of the TNF family that forms a heteromeric complex with lymphotoxin on the cell surface. Cell 1993; 72:847–856.

Burch GH, Gong Y, Liu W, et al: Tenascin-X deficiency is associated with Ehlers–Danlos syndrome. Nat Genet 1997; 17:104–108.

Cabrera M, Shaw MA, Sharples C, et al: Polymorphism in tumor necrosis factor genes associated with mucocutaneous leishmaniasis. J Exp Med 1995; 182:1259–1264.

Carrington M, Nelson GW, Martin MP, et al: HLA and HIV-1: heterozygote advantage and B*35-Cw*04 disadvantage [see comments]. Science 1999; 283:1748–1752.

Carroll MC, Campbell RD, Bentley DR, et al: A molecular map of the human major histocompatibility complex class III region linking complement genes C4, C2 and factor B. Nature 1984; 307:237–241.

Carroll MC, Campbell RD, Porter RR: Mapping of steroid 21-hydroxylase genes adjacent to complement component C4 genes in HLA, the major histocompatibility complex in man. Proc Natl Acad Sci USA 1985; 82:521–525.

Carroll MC, Katzman P, Alicot EM, et al: Linkage map of the human major histocompatibility complex including the tumor necrosis factor genes. Proc Natl Acad Sci USA 1987; 84:8535–8539.

Chien CT, Bartel PL, Sternglanz R, et al: The two-hybrid system: a method to identify and clone genes for proteins that interact with a protein of interest. Proc Natl Acad Sci USA 1991; 88:9578–9582.

Chung EK, Yang Y, Rennebohm RM, et al: Genetic sophistication of human complement components C4A and C4B and RP-C4-CYP21-TNX (RCCX) modules in the major histocompatibility complex. Am J Hum Genet 2002; 71:823–837.

Clavijo OP, Delgado JC, Awdeh ZL, et al: HLA-Cw alleles associated with HLA extended haplotypes and C2 deficiency. Tissue Antigens 1998; 52:282–285.

Clavijo OP, Delgado JC, Yu N, et al: HLA-Cw*1701 is associated with two sub-Saharan African-derived HLA haplotypes: HLA-B*4201, DRB1*03 and HLA-B*4202 without DRB1*03. Tissue Antigens 1999; 54:303–306.

Colten HR, Rosen FS: Complement deficiencies. Annu Rev Immunol 10:809–834, 1992.

Corzo D, Yunis JJ, Salazar M, et al: The major histocompatibility complex region marked by HSP70-1 and HSP70-2 variants is associated with clozapine-induced agranulocytosis in two different ethnic groups. Blood 1995; 86:3835–3840.

Criswell LA, Lum RF, Turner KN, et al: The influence of genetic variation in the HLA-DRB1 and LTA-TNF regions on the response to treatment of early rheumatoid arthritis with methotrexate or etanercept. Arthritis Rheum 2004; 50:2750–2756.

Cullen M, Perfetto SP, Klitz W, et al: High-resolution patterns of meiotic recombination across the human major histocompatibility complex. Am J Hum Genet 2002; 71:759–776.

D'Alfonso S, Richiardi PM: A polymorphic variation in a putative regulation box of the TNFA promoter region. Immunogenetics 39:150–154, 1994.

Dawkins R, Leelayuwat C, Gaudieri S, et al: Genomics of the major histocompatibility complex: haplotypes, duplication, retroviruses and disease. Immunol Rev 1999; 167:275–304.

Delgado JC, Baena A, Thim S, et al: Ethnic-specific genetic associations with pulmonary tuberculosis. J Infect Dis 2002; 186:1463–1468.

Delgado JC, Turbay D, Yunis EJ, et al: A common major histocompatibility complex class II allele HLA-DQB1* 0301 is present in clinical variants of pemphigoid. Proc Natl Acad Sci USA 1996; 93:8569–8571.

Densen P: Complement deficiencies and meningococcal disease. Clin Exp Immunol 1991; 86(Suppl 1):57–62.

Dunckley H, Gatenby PA, Hawkins B, et al: Deficiency of C4A is a genetic determinant of systemic lupus erythematosus in three ethnic groups. J Immunogenet 1987; 14:209–218.

Dunham I, Sargent CA, Trowsdale J, et al: Molecular mapping of the human major histocompatibility complex by pulsed-field gel electrophoresis. Proc Natl Acad Sci USA 1987; 84:7237–7241.

Feder JN, Gnirke A, Thomas W, et al: A novel MHC class I-like gene is mutated in patients with hereditary haemochromatosis. Nat Genet 1996; 13:399–408.

Feder JN, Tsuchihashi Z, Irrinki A, et al: The hemochromatosis founder mutation in HLA-H disrupts beta2-microglobulin interaction and cell surface expression. J Biol Chem 1997; 272:14025–14028.

Ferlazzo G, Tsang ML, Moretta L, et al: Human dendritic cells activate resting natural killer (NK) cells and are recognized via the NKp30 receptor by activated NK cells. J Exp Med 2002; 195:343–351.

Fernandez-Vina M, Fink CW, Stastny P: HLA associations in juvenile arthritis. Clin Exp Rheumatol 1994; 12:205–214.

Fielder AH, Walport MJ, Batchelor JR, et al: Family study of the major histocompatibility complex in patients with systemic lupus erythematosus: importance of null alleles of C4A and C4B in determining disease susceptibility. Br Med J (Clin Res Ed) 1983; 286:425–442.

Fields S, Song O: A novel genetic system to detect protein–protein interactions. Nature 1989; 340:245–246.

Fleischnick E, Awdeh ZL, Raum D, et al: Extended MHC haplotypes in 21-hydroxylase-deficiency congenital adrenal hyperplasia: shared genotypes in unrelated patients. Lancet 1983; 1:152–156.

Flores-Villanueva PO, Yunis EJ, Delgado JC, et al: Control of HIV-1 viremia and protection from AIDS are associated with HLA-Bw4 homozygosity. Proc Natl Acad Sci USA 2001; 98:5140–5145.

Fraser PA, Moore B, Stein R, et al: Complotypes in individuals of African origin: frequencies and possible extended MHC haplotypes. Immunogenetics 1990; 31:89–93.

Gabriel SB, Schaffner SF, Nguyen H, et al: The structure of haplotype blocks in the human genome. Science 2002; 296:2225–2229.

Garavito G, Yunis EJ, Egea E, et al: HLA-DRB1 alleles and HLA-DRB1 shared epitopes are markers for juvenile rheumatoid arthritis subgroups in Colombian mestizos. Hum Immunol 2004; 65:359–365.

Geserick G, Otremba P, Schroder H, et al: Reference typing report for complement factor B. Exp Clin Immunogenet 1998; 15:261–263.

Goggins M, Kelleher D: Celiac disease and other nutrient related injuries to the gastrointestinal tract. Am J Gastroenterol 1994; 89:S2–S17.

Goldfeld AE, Delgado JC, Thim S, et al: Association of an HLA-DQ allele with clinical tuberculosis. JAMA 1998; 279:226–228.
The first report of an MHC gene associated with susceptibility to pulmonary tuberculosis.

Hamann A, Mantzoros C, Vidal-Puig A, et al: Genetic variability in the TNF-alpha promoter is not associated with type II diabetes mellitus (NIDDM). Biochem Biophys Res Commun 1995; 211:833–883.

Hammer J, Gallazzi F, Bono E, et al: Peptide binding specificity of HLA-DR4 molecules: correlation with rheumatoid arthritis association. J Exp Med 1995; 181:1847–1855.

Hauptmann G, Goetz J, Uring-Lambert B, et al: Component deficiencies. 2. The fourth component. Prog Allergy 1986; 39:232–249.

Heijmans BT, Westendorp RG, Droog S, et al: Association of the tumour necrosis factor alpha-308G/A polymorphism with the risk of diabetes in an elderly population-based cohort. Genes Immun 2002; 3:225–228.

Heilig R, Eckenberg R, Petit JL, et al: The DNA sequence and analysis of human chromosome 14. Nature 2003; 421:601–607.

Hendel H, Caillat-Zucman S, Lebuanec H, et al: New class I and II HLA alleles strongly associated with opposite patterns of progression to AIDS. J Immunol 1999; 162:6942–6946.

Higashi Y, Yoshioka H, Yamane M, et al: Complete nucleotide sequence of two steroid 21-hydroxylase genes tandemly arranged in human chromosome: a pseudogene and a genuine gene. Proc Natl Acad Sci USA 1986; 83:2841–2845.

Higuchi T, Seki N, Kamizono S, et al: Polymorphism of the 5′-flanking region of the human tumor necrosis factor (TNF)-alpha gene in Japanese. Tissue Antigens 1998; 51:605–612.

Holzinger I, de Baey A, Messer G, et al: Cloning and genomic characterization of LST1: a new gene in the human TNF region. Immunogenetics 1995; 42:315–322.

Hui J, Oka A, Tomizawa M, et al: Identification of two new C4 alleles by DNA sequencing and evidence for a historical recombination of serologically defined C4A and C4B alleles. Tissue Antigens 2004; 63:263–269.

Hunt C, Morimoto RI: Conserved features of eukaryotic hsp70 genes revealed by comparison with the nucleotide sequence of human hsp70. Proc Natl Acad Sci USA 1985; 82:6455–6459.

Jahn I, Uring-Lambert B, Arnold D, et al: C2 reference typing report. Complement Inflamm 1990; 7:175–182.

Jeffreys AJ, Kauppi L, Neumann R: Intensely punctate meiotic recombination in the class II region of the major histocompatibility complex. Nat Genet 2001; 29:217–222.

Jenkins D, Fletcher J, Penny MA, et al: DRB genotyping supports recessive inheritance of DR3-associated susceptibility to insulin-dependent diabetes mellitus. Am J Hum Genet 1991; 49:49–53.

John S, Shephard N, Liu G, et al: Whole-genome scan, in a complex disease, using 11,245 single-nucleotide polymorphisms: comparison with microsatellites. Am J Hum Genet 2004; 75:54–64.

Johnson CA, Densen P, Hurford RK, Jr., et al: Type I human complement C2 deficiency. A 28-base pair gene deletion causes skipping of exon 6 during RNA splicing. J Biol Chem 1992; 267:9347–9353.

Jongeneel CV, Briant L, Udalova IA, et al: Extensive genetic polymorphism in the human tumor necrosis factor region and relation to extended HLA

VI

haplotypes. Proc Natl Acad Sci USA 1991; 88:9717–9721.

Kaslow RA, Carrington M, Apple R, et al: Influence of combinations of human major histocompatibility complex genes on the course of HIV-1 infection. Nat Med 1996; 2:405–411.

Keet IP, Tang J, Klein MR, et al: Consistent associations of HLA class I and II and transporter gene products with progression of human immunodeficiency virus type 1 infection in homosexual men. J Infect Dis 1999; 180:299–309.

Kendall E, Sargent CA, Campbell RD: Human major histocompatibility complex contains a new cluster of genes between the HLA-D and complement C4 loci. Nucleic Acids Res 1990; 18:7251–7257.

Khan MA, Kellner H: Immunogenetics of spondyloarthropathies. Rheum Dis Clin North Am 1992; 18:837–864.

Khomenko AG, Litvinov VI, Chukanova VP, et al: Tuberculosis in patients with various HLA phenotypes. Tubercle 1990; 71:187–192.

Klein J: Natural History of Major Histocompatibility Complex. New York, John Wiley & Sons, 1986.

Klemperer MR, Woodworth HC, Rosen FS, et al: Hereditary deficiency of the second component of complement (C'2) in man. J Clin Invest 1966; 45:880–890.

Kockum I, Sanjeevi CB, Eastman S, et al: Complex interaction between HLA DR and DQ in conferring risk for childhood type 1 diabetes. Eur J Immunogenet 1999; 26:361–372.

Kockum I, Wassmuth R, Holmberg E, et al: HLA-DQ primarily confers protection and HLA-DR susceptibility in type I (insulin-dependent) diabetes studied in population-based affected families and controls. Am J Hum Genet 1993; 53:150–167.

Koeleman BP, Lie BA, Undlien DE, et al: Genotype effects and epistasis in type 1 diabetes and HLA-DQ trans dimer associations with disease. Genes Immun 2004; 5:381–388.

Kubaszek A, Pihlajamaki J, Komarovski V, et al: Promoter polymorphisms of the TNF-alpha (G-308A) and IL-6 (C-174G) genes predict the conversion from impaired glucose tolerance to type 2 diabetes: the Finnish Diabetes Prevention Study. Diabetes 2003; 52:1872–1876.

Kwok WW, Domeier ME, Johnson ML, et al: HLA-DQB1 codon 57 is critical for peptide binding and recognition. J Exp Med 1996; 183:1253–1258.

Kwon OJ, Peled N, Miller K, et al: HLA class II analysis in Jewish Israeli narcoleptic patients. Hum Immunol 1995; 44:199–202.

Lander ES, Linton LM, Birren B, et al: Initial sequencing and analysis of the human genome. Nature 2001; 409:860–921.

Lee KH, Wucherpfennig KW, Wiley DC: Structure of a human insulin peptide-HLA-DQ8 complex and susceptibility to type 1 diabetes. Nat Immunol 2001; 2:501–507.

Lehner B, Semple JI, Brown SE, et al: Analysis of a high-throughput yeast two-hybrid system and its use to predict the function of intracellular proteins encoded within the human MHC class III region. Genomics 2004; 83:153–167.

Lernmark A: Type 1 diabetes. Clin Chem 1999; 45:1331–1338.

Liliensiek B, Weigand MA, Bierhaus A, et al: Receptor for advanced glycation end products (RAGE) regulates sepsis but not the adaptive immune response. J Clin Invest 2004; 113:1641–1650.

Lokki ML, Circolo A, Ahokas P, et al: Deficiency of human complement protein C4 due to identical frameshift mutations in the C4A and C4B genes. J Immunol 1999; 162:3687–3693.

Lokki ML, Koskimies SA: Allelic differences in hemolytic activity and protein concentration of BF molecules are found in association with particular HLA haplotypes. Immunogenetics 1991; 34:242–246.

McCusker SM, Curran MD, Dynan KB, et al: Association between polymorphism in regulatory region of gene encoding tumour necrosis factor alpha and risk of Alzheimer's disease and vascular dementia: a case–control study. Lancet 2001; 357:436–439.

McGarry F, Walker R, Sturrock R, et al: The -308.1 polymorphism in the promoter region of the tumor necrosis factor gene is associated with ankylosing spondylitis independent of HLA-B27. J Rheumatol 1999; 26:1110–1116.

MacGregor A, Ollier W, Thomson W, et al: HLA-DRB1*0401/0404 genotype and rheumatoid arthritis: increased association in men, young age at onset, and disease severity. J Rheumatol 1995; 22:1032–1036.

McGuire W, Hill AV, Allsopp CE, et al: Variation in the TNF-alpha promoter region associated with susceptibility to cerebral malaria. Nature 1994; 371:508–510.

Marrosu MG, Muntoni F, Murru MR, et al: HLA-DQB1 genotype in Sardinian multiple sclerosis: evidence for a key role of DQB1 *0201 and *0302 alleles. Neurology 1992; 42:883–886.

Marsh MN: Gluten, major histocompatibility complex, and the small intestine. A molecular and immunobiologic approach to the spectrum of gluten sensitivity ('celiac sprue'). Gastroenterology 1992; 102:330–354.

Marsh SG: Nomenclature for factors of the HLA system, update July 2004. Eur J Immunogenet 2004; 31:215–216.

Martin AM, Nolan D, Gaudieri S, et al: Predisposition to abacavir hypersensitivity mediated by HLA-B*5701 and a haplotypic Hsp70-Hom variant. Proc Natl Acad Sci USA 2004; 101:4180–4185.

Meo T, Atkinson JP, Bernoco M, et al: Structural heterogeneity of C2 Complement protein and its genetic variants in man: a new polymorphism of the HLA region. Proc Natl Acad Sci USA 1977; 74:1672–1675.

Messer G, Spengler U, Jung MC, et al: Polymorphic structure of the tumor necrosis factor (TNF) locus: an NcoI polymorphism in the first intron of the human TNF-beta gene correlates with a variant amino acid in position 26 and a reduced level of TNF-beta production. J Exp Med 1991; 173:209–219.

MHC Sequencing Consortium: Complete sequence and gene map of a human major histocompatibility complex. The MHC sequencing consortium. Nature 1999; 401:921–923.

Miettinen O: Estimability and estimation in case-referent studies. Am J Epidemiol 1976; 103:226–235.

Milner CM, Campbell RD: Structure and expression of the three MHC-linked HSP70 genes. Immunogenetics 1990; 32:242–251.

Milner CM, Campbell RD: Polymorphic analysis of the three MHC-linked HSP70 genes. Immunogenetics 1992; 36:357–362.

Mira JP, Cariou A, Grall F, et al: Association of TNF2, a TNF-alpha promoter polymorphism, with septic shock susceptibility and mortality: a multicenter study. Journal of the American Medical Association 1999; 282:561–568.

Mu H, Chen JJ, Jiang Y, et al: Tumor necrosis factor a microsatellite polymorphism is associated with rheumatoid arthritis severity through an interaction with the HLA-DRB1 shared epitope. Arthritis Rheum 1999; 42:438–442.

Nedospasov SA, Udalova IA, Kuprash DV, et al: DNA sequence polymorphism at the human tumor necrosis factor (TNF) locus. Numerous TNF/lymphotoxin alleles tagged by two closely linked microsatellites in the upstream region of the lymphotoxin (TNF-beta) gene. J Immunol 1991; 147:1053–1059.

Nepom BS, Nepom GT, Coleman M, et al: Critical contribution of beta chain residue 57 in peptide binding ability of both HLA-DR and -DQ molecules. Proc Natl Acad Sci USA 1996; 93:7202–7206.

Nepom GT: A unified hypothesis for the complex genetics of HLA associations with IDDM. Diabetes 1990; 39:1153–1157.

Nepom GT, Erlich H: MHC class-II molecules and autoimmunity. Annu Rev Immunol 1991; 9:493–525.

Nepom GT, Nepom BS: Prediction of susceptibility to rheumatoid arthritis by human leukocyte antigen genotyping. Rheum Dis Clin North Am 1992; 18:785–792.

Nicaud V, Raoux S, Poirier O, et al: The TNF alpha/G-308A polymorphism influences insulin sensitivity in offspring of patients with coronary heart disease: the European Atherosclerosis Research Study II. Atherosclerosis 2002; 161:317–325.

Noble JA, Valdes AM, Cook M, et al: The role of HLA class II genes in insulin-dependent diabetes mellitus: molecular analysis of 180 Caucasian, multiplex families. Am J Hum Genet 1996; 59:1134–1148.

Nousari HC, Kimyai-Asadi A, Provost TT: Generalized lupus erythematosus profundus in a patient with genetic partial deficiency of C4. J Am Acad Dermatol 1999; 41:362–364.

Okamoto K, Makino S, Yoshikawa Y, et al: Identification of I kappa BL as the second major histocompatibility complex-linked susceptibility locus for rheumatoid arthritis. Am J Hum Genet 2003; 72:303–312.

Ollier W, Thomson W: Population genetics of rheumatoid arthritis. Rheum Dis Clin North Am 1992; 18:741–759.

Ozaki K, Inoue K, Sato H, et al: Functional variation in LGALS2 confers risk of myocardial infarction and regulates lymphotoxin-alpha secretion in vitro. Nature 2004; 429:72–75.

Ozaki K, Ohnishi Y, Iida A, et al: Functional SNPs in the lymphotoxin-alpha gene that are associated with susceptibility to myocardial infarction. Nat Genet 2002; 32:650–654.

Partanen J, Koskimies S: Low degree of DNA polymorphism in the HLA-linked lymphotoxin (tumour necrosis factor beta) gene. Scand J Immunol 1988; 28:313–316.

Pende D, Parolini S, Pessino A, et al: Identification and molecular characterization of NKp30, a novel triggering receptor involved in natural cytotoxicity mediated by human natural killer cells. J Exp Med 1999; 190:1505–1516.

Penrose LS: The detection of autosomal linkage in pairs of brothers and sisters of unspecified parentage. Ann Eugen 1935; 6:133.

Penzotti JE, Doherty D, Lybrand TP, et al: A structural model for TCR recognition of the HLA class II shared epitope sequence implicated in susceptibility to rheumatoid arthritis. J Autoimmun 1996; 9:287–293.

Quarsten H, Paulsen G, Johansen BH, et al: The P9 pocket of HLA-DQ2 (non-Aspbeta57) has no particular preference for negatively charged anchor residues found in other type 1 diabetes-predisposing non-Aspbeta57 MHC class II molecules. Int Immunol 1998; 10:1229–1236.

Ragoussis J, Monaco A, Mockridge I, et al: Cloning of the HLA class II region in yeast artificial chromosomes. Proc Natl Acad Sci USA 1991; 88:3753–3757.

Rajalingam R, Mehra NK, Jain RC, et al: Polymerase chain reaction-based sequence-specific oligonucleotide hybridization analysis of HLA class II antigens in pulmonary tuberculosis: relevance to chemotherapy and disease severity. J Infect Dis 1996; 173:669–676.

Raum D, Awdeh Z, Alper CA: BF types and the mode of inheritance of insulin-dependent diabetes mellitus (IDDM). Immunogenetics 1981; 12:59–74.

Ribas G, Neville M, Wixon JL, et al: Genes encoding three new members of the leukocyte antigen 6 superfamily and a novel member of Ig superfamily, together with genes encoding the regulatory nuclear chloride ion channel protein (hRNCC) and an N ω-N ω-dimethylarginine dimethylaminohydrolase homologue, are found in a 30-kb segment of the MHC class III region. J Immunol 1999; 163:278–287.

Rogers AE, Meehan J, Guilleminault C, et al: HLA DR15 (DR2) and DQB1*0602 typing studies in 188 narcoleptic patients with cataplexy. Neurology 1997; 48:1550–1556.

Rubin LA, Amos CI, Wade JA, et al: Investigating the genetic basis for ankylosing spondylitis. Linkage studies with the major histocompatibility complex region. Arthritis Rheum 1994; 37:1212–1220.

Rubinstein P, Suciu-Foca N, Nicholson JF: Genetics of juvenile diabetes mellitus. A recessive gene closely linked to HLA D and with 50 per cent penetrance. N Engl J Med 1977; 297:1036–1040.

Salter RD, Parham P: Mutually exclusive public epitopes of HLA-A, B, C molecules. Human Immunology 1989; 26:85–89.

Sargent CA, Dunham I, Trowsdale J, et al: Human major histocompatibility complex contains genes for the major heat shock protein HSP70. Proc Natl Acad Sci USA 1989; 86:1968–1972.

Schneider PM, Mauff G: Complement C4 protein and DNA typing methods. Methods Mol Biol 2003; 210:269–295.

Schneider PM, Stradmann-Bellinghausen B, Rittner C: Genetic polymorphism of the fourth component of human complement: population study and proposal for a revised nomenclature based on genomic PCR typing of Rodgers and Chido determinants. Eur J Immunogenet 1996; 23:335–344.

Schneider PM, Witzel-Schlomp K, Rittner C, et al: The endogenous retroviral insertion in the human complement C4 gene modulates the expression of homologous genes by antisense inhibition. Immunogenetics 2001; 53:1–9.

Schroder O, Schulte KM, Ostermann P, et al: Heat shock protein 70 genotypes HSPA1B and HSPA1L influence cytokine concentrations and interfere with outcome after major injury. Crit Care Med 2003; 31:73–79.

Siebold C, Hansen BE, Wyer JR, et al: Crystal structure of HLA-DQ0602 that protects against type 1 diabetes and confers strong susceptibility to narcolepsy. Proc Natl Acad Sci USA 2004; 101:1999–2004.

Siemens I, Brenden M, Mauff G, et al: Apparently non-expressed alleles of factor B (BF) code for hypomorphic proteins. Immunogenetics 1992; 37:24–28.

Silverstein AM: Essential hypocomplementemia: report of a case. Blood 1960; 16:1338–1341.

Sim E, Cross SJ: Phenotyping of human complement component C4, a class-III HLA antigen. Biochem J 1986; 239:763–767.

Simon M, Bourel M, Fauchet R, et al: Association of HLA-A3 and HLA-B14 antigens with idiopathic haemochromatosis. Gut 1976; 17:332–334.

Sinnott PJ, Costigan C, Dyer PA, et al: Extended MHC haplotypes and CYP21/C4 gene organisation in Irish 21-hydroxylase deficiency families. Hum Genet 1991; 87:361–366.

Skol AD, Young KA, Tsuang DW, et al: Modest evidence for linkage and possible confirmation of association between NOTCH4 and schizophrenia in a large Veterans Affairs Cooperative Study sample. Am J Med Genet 2003; 118B:8–15.

Spies T, Bresnahan M, Strominger JL: Human major histocompatibility complex contains a minimum of 19 genes between the complement cluster and HLA-B. Proc Natl Acad Sci USA 1989; 86:8955–8958.

Stastny P, Fernandez-Vina M, Cerna M, et al: Sequences of HLA alleles associated with arthritis in adults and children. J Rheumatol Suppl, 1993; 37:5–.

Stern LJ, Brown JH, Jardetzky TS, et al: Crystal structure of the human class II MHC protein HLA-DR1 complexed with an influenza virus peptide. Nature 1994; 368:215–221.

Stewart CA, Horton R, Allcock RJN, et al: Complete MHC haplotype sequencing for common disease gene mapping. Genome Res 2004; 14:1176–1187.

This landmark report is the first of what will undoubtedly be many reports of the fine structure of MHC haplotypes to map the genetic variants that confer disease susceptibility.

Sturfelt G, Hellmer G, Truedsson L: TNF microsatellites in systemic lupus erythematosus – a high frequency of the TNFabc 2-3-1 haplotype in multicase SLE families. Lupus 1996; 5:618–622.

Sullivan KE, Petri MA, Schmeckpeper BJ, et al: Prevalence of a mutation causing C2 deficiency in systemic lupus erythematosus. J Rheumatol 1994; 21:1128–1133.

Sutton HE: An Introduction to Human Genetics, 3rd ed. Philadelphia, PA, WB Saunders, 1980.

Svejgaard A, Platz P, Ryder LP: HLA and disease 1982 – a survey. Immunol Rev 1983; 70:193–218.

Tazi-Ahnini R, Cork MJ, Wengraf D, et al: *Notch4*, a non-HLA gene in the MHC is strongly associated with the most severe form of alopecia areata. Hum Genet 2003; 112:400–403.

Temple SE, Cheong KY, Ardlie KG, et al: The septic shock associated HSPA1B1267 polymorphism influences production of HSPA1A and HSPA1B. Intensive Care Med 2004; 30:1761–1767.

Teran-Escandon D, Teran-Ortiz L, Camarena-Olvera A, et al: Human leukocyte antigen-associated susceptibility to pulmonary tuberculosis: molecular analysis of class II alleles by DNA amplification and oligonucleotide hybridization in Mexican patients. Chest 1999; 115:428–433.

Describes the first sequence-based gene map of a human MHC

Thomson G: HLA DR antigens and susceptibility to insulin-dependent diabetes mellitus. Am J Hum Genet 1984; 36:1309–1317.

Thomson G, Bodmer W (1977). The genetic analysis of HLA and disease association. *In* Dausset J, Svejgaard A (eds) HLA and Disease. Copenhagen, Munksgaard.

Thorsby E, Ronningen KS: Role of HLA genes in predisposition to develop insulin-dependent diabetes mellitus. Ann Med 1992; 24:523–531.

Truedsson L, Alper CA, Awdeh ZL, et al: Characterization of type I complement C2 deficiency MHC haplotypes. Strong conservation of the complotype/HLA-B-region and absence of disease association due to linked class II genes. J Immunol 1993; 151:5856–5863.

Truedsson L, Awdeh Z, Yunis EJ, et al: Quantitative variation of C4 variant proteins associated with many MHC haplotypes. Immunogenetics 1989; 30:414–421.

Truedsson L, Sturfelt G, Nived O: Prevalence of the type I complement C2 deficiency gene in Swedish systemic lupus erythematosus patients. Lupus 1993b; 2:325–327.

Turbay D, Lieberman J, Alper CA, et al: Tumor necrosis factor constellation polymorphism and clozapine-induced agranulocytosis in two different ethnic groups. Blood 1997; 89:4167–4174.

Uglialoro AM, Turbay D, Pesavento PA, et al: Identification of three new single nucleotide polymorphisms in the human tumor necrosis factor-alpha gene promoter. Tissue Antigens 1998; 52:359–367.

Utans U, Arceci RJ, Yamashita Y, et al: Cloning and characterization of allograft inflammatory factor-1: a novel macrophage factor identified in rat cardiac allografts with chronic rejection. J Clin Invest 1995; 95:2954–2962.

Waheed A, Parkkila S, Zhou XY, et al: Hereditary hemochromatosis: effects of C282Y and H63D mutations on association with beta2-microglobulin, intracellular processing, and cell surface expression of the HFE protein in COS-7 cells. Proc Natl Acad Sci USA 1997; 94:12384–12389.

Walsh EC, Mather KA, Schaffner SF, et al: An integrated haplotype map of the human major histocompatibility complex. Am J Hum Genet 2003; 73:580–590.

Wassink TH, Nopoulos P, Pietila J, et al: NOTCH4 and the frontal lobe in schizophrenia. Am J Med Genet 2003; 118B:1–7.

Wei J, Hemmings GP: TNXB locus may be a candidate gene predisposing to schizophrenia. Am J Med Genet 2004; 125B:43–49.

Wetsel RA, Kulics J, Lokki ML, et al: Type II human complement C2 deficiency. Allele-specific amino acid substitutions (Ser189 → Phe; Gly444 → Arg) cause impaired C2 secretion. J Biol Chem 1996; 271:5824–5831.

White PC, New MI, Dupont B: Structure of human steroid 21-hydroxylase genes. Proc Natl Acad Sci USA 1986; 83:5111–5115.

White PC, Vitek A, Dupont B, et al: Characterization of frequent deletions causing steroid 21-hydroxylase deficiency. Proc Natl Acad Sci USA 1988; 85:4436–4440.

Wilson AG, di Giovine FS, Blakemore AI, et al: Single base polymorphism in the human tumour necrosis factor alpha (TNF alpha) gene detectable by NcoI restriction of PCR product. Hum Mol Genet 1992; 1:353.

Winter WE, Chihara T, Schatz D: The genetics of autoimmune diabetes. Approaching a solution to the problem. Am J Dis Child 1993; 147:1282–1290.

Wu YR, Wang CK, Chen CM, et al: Analysis of heat-shock protein 70 gene polymorphisms and the risk of Parkinson's disease. Hum Genet 2004; 114:236–241.

Xie T, Rowen L, Aguado B, et al: Analysis of the gene-dense major histocompatibility complex class III region and its comparison to mouse. Genome Res 2003; 13:2621–2636.

Yang Y, Chung EK, Zhou B, et al: Diversity in intrinsic strengths of the human complement system: serum C4 protein concentrations correlate with C4 gene size and polygenic variations, hemolytic activities, and body mass index. J Immunol 2003; 171:2734–2745.

Yunis EJ, Larsen CE, Fernandez-Vina M, et al: Inheritable variable sizes of DNA stretches in the human MHC: conserved extended haplotypes and their fragments or blocks. Tissue Antigens 2003; 62:1–20.

A recent review of MHC extended haplotypes and smaller haplotype blocks, and an update of their allele compositions in the world's populations.

Yunis JJ, Mobini N, Yunis EJ, et al: Common major histocompatibility complex class II markers in clinical variants of cicatricial pemphigoid. Proc Natl Acad Sci USA 1994; 91:7747–7751.

Zanelli E, Breedveld FC, de Vries RR: HLA class II association with rheumatoid arthritis: facts and interpretations. Hum Immunol 2000; 61:1254–1261.

Zimmerman PA, Guderian RH, Nutman TB: A new TNFA promoter allele identified in South American Blacks. Immunogenetics 1996; 44:485–486.

CHAPTER 49

Immunodeficiency Disorders

Kimberly W. Sanford MD MT(ASCP), Susan D. Roseff MD

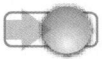

KEY POINTS

• Primary immunodeficiencies are a group of single gene disorders.

• Because of the complexity of diagnosing a primary immunodeficiency, the cooperation of the clinician, research scientist, and clinical pathologist is required.

• A logical approach to the diagnosis of primary immunodeficiency disorders based on staged diagnostic testing is necessary because of the complex nature of the immune system.

• Preparation for specimen collection, handling, and delivery to a specialty laboratory is required for performing complex immunologic assays.

• As a result of technologic advances, molecular genetic testing is increasingly employed in diagnosing primary immunodeficiency disorders.

Primary immunodeficiencies are a group of single-gene disorders that result in defects in the immune system. The manifestations can vary in the degree of severity, the types of symptom exhibited, or both. These conditions, when unrecognized and left untreated, can result in death. A genetic defect may result in loss of a critical enzyme, cause developmental arrest in one aspect of the immune system, cause loss of a structural component, or create a nonfunctional protein. Most of these disorders are X-linked, causing a disproportionate number of affected males, approximately 70% of patients with primary immunodeficiency disorders (Puck, 1997a). The majority of primary immunodeficiencies are detected before 20 years of age, but diagnosis can be delayed because recognition requires a high degree of clinical suspicion. Over 100 primary immunodeficiency disorders are described; however, more than 90% of such patients are affected by fewer than 20 primary immuno-deficiency disorders (Puck, 1997a). Whereas primary immunodeficiency disorders are due to single gene mutations, secondary immuno-deficiencies may be due to malnutrition, viral infections, hematologic and other types of malignancy, chemotherapeutic treatments for malignancies, and immunosuppressive medications for treatment of a variety of disorders.

The natural physical barriers of the body are the first line of defense against invading microbes, and include skin, mucus at exposed mucosal surfaces, and ciliated cells of the respiratory, intestinal, and genital tracts. In addition to physical barriers, immunologic functions of the body exert continual surveillance through acquired and innate modes of action. The acquired immunologic response is specific, requiring previous antigen exposure for sensitization, and improves with each subsequent challenge from a given antigen. These responses are the result of a proliferation of antigen-specific B and T cells, which are stimulated after cellular receptors bind to antigens. B cells produce antigen-specific antibodies to eliminate extracellular antigens. T cells assist B cells to produce antigen-specific antibodies and also kill cells that are virally infected. Innate responses do not require prior antigen exposure and are comprised of phagocytic cells (macrophages, neutrophils and monocytes), complement, cytokines, and acute phase reactants (Delves, 2000).

The immune system is an interlocking group of immune cells and immune functions, in which any defect may result in an immunodeficiency. The incidence of primary immunodeficiency diseases in the United States is estimated at about 1 in 200 000 liveborn infants, excluding selective immunoglobulin A (IgA) deficiency (Winkelstein, 2000). The most common immunodeficiency, selective IgA deficiency, has an incidence of 1 in every 328 healthy blood donors (Clark, 1983). As a whole, the estimated incidence of diagnosed primary immunodeficiency diseases is 1/10 000 (Smith, 1999; Immune Deficiency Foundation, 1992; Shearer, 1994). Data from Australia and Norway estimate the incidence of primary immunodeficiencies at 2.1 per 100 000 (Baumgart, 1997) and 6.8 per 100 000, respectively (Ryser, 1988; Stray-Pedersen, 1997; Matamoros, 2000).

For unknown reasons, approximately half the reported immune defects involve defective antibody production due to low numbers of B cells or B cells with decreased production of antigen-specific antibody. Decreased antigen-specific antibody production most frequently manifests as recurrent pulmonary or sinus infections, as well as bacterial septicemia (Noroski, 1998). These infections are typically caused by encapsulated bacteria such as *Streptococcus pneumoniae* or *Haemophilus influenzae*. Defective T-cell immunity is characteristically associated with opportunistic, viral, and fungal infections, such as *Candida albicans*, *Mycobacterium avium intracellulare* (MAI), and *Pneumocystis carinii* (Buckley, 2000). The type of infection a patient acquires may point towards the type of cellular immune defect (Fig. 49–1). There is also an association of primary immunodeficiency disorders with autoimmune diseases, as well as malignant neoplasms and especially lymphomas (Smith, 1999).

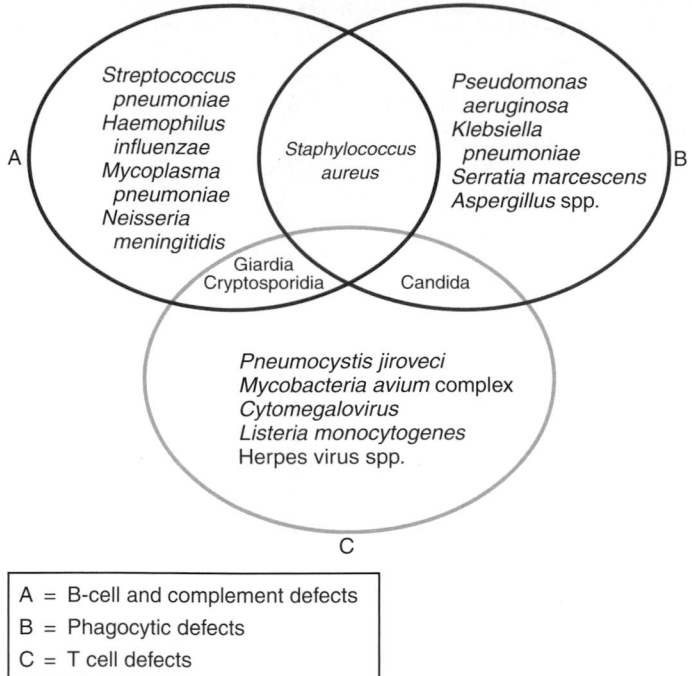

A = B-cell and complement defects
B = Phagocytic defects
C = T cell defects

Figure 49–1 Infections associated with cellular immune defects.

clinical assessment and laboratory investigation, even without a history of severe or unusual infections. In one study of 70 patients with primary immunodeficiency disorders, approximately 18.6% had a family history of an immunodeficiency (Kobrynski, 2002).

Awareness of common clinical presentations can aid physicians in identifying individuals who are more likely to have a primary immune defect. The clinical signs and symptoms of primary immunodeficiency are presented in Figure 49–2. In addition to these warning signs, the physician should be alerted by elements in the history that are unusual, such as a history of autoimmune disease, significant lymphadenopathy, the need for an adult to have a myringotomy, severe herpes zoster or herpes zoster appearing in a young child, or intractable diarrhea or ulcerative colitis diagnosed in a child less than 1 year old. These additional signs and symptoms should prompt an evaluation for a possible immune defect.

It is not practical to investigate all immunologic systems in all patients, so the clinical picture and age of the patient will point the investigator to the portion of the immune system that is most likely to be affected. Taking a careful history and performing a thorough physical examination can narrow the possibilities to defects involving T cells, B cells, granulocytes, or the complement system. The role of these host defenses and their correlation with different immunodeficiency disorders is presented in Figure 49–3.

It is also important to pay attention to the clinical circumstances and not to dwell exclusively on the number or severity of infectious episodes (Atkinson, 2000). For example, when an infectious process involves the same anatomic site repeatedly, the etiology is more likely to be structural and not a failure of one of the host defenses. Examples of this include chronic osteomyelitis in one location, recurrent episodes of pneumonia that affect only one lobe of the lung, or recurrent infections of a surgical wound. Additionally, some primary immunodeficiency disorders, such as chronic granulomatous disease, may present later in life than expected; however, it is still important to keep these disorders in the differential diagnosis (Lukela, 2005)

Clinical Signs and Symptoms of Immune Deficiency

Most frequently, an increased susceptibility to recurrent infection is the first clinical indication of an immune defect. The type of recurrent infection provides insight into the immune defect and helps guide the clinician evaluating the patient. Therefore the most critical part of the medical evaluation is obtaining a complete medical history. Identifying children with immune deficiency presents a significant challenge to pediatricians, since infections are a common occurrence in normal childhood but can also be the principal manifestation of a primary immune deficiency. Therefore, frequent and prolonged infections, coupled with failure to thrive, or opportunistic infections require a thorough immunologic work-up (Puck, 1999). A confirmed report of an immunodeficiency disease occurring in a sibling or first-degree relative should also prompt careful

Evaluation of the Immune System

Based on the above considerations, when an immune defect is suspected, the evaluation of the immune system is best approached in stages, performing basic screening tests first and turning to more complex testing as indicated. For example, if a patient presents with strong clinical symptoms suggestive of a B- or T-cell disorder but a normal lymphocyte count, further investigation by a lymphocyte enumeration panel is warranted. An overview of this staged approach is given in Figure 49–4 and a basic testing algorithm for immunodeficiencies is provided in Figure 49–5.

VI

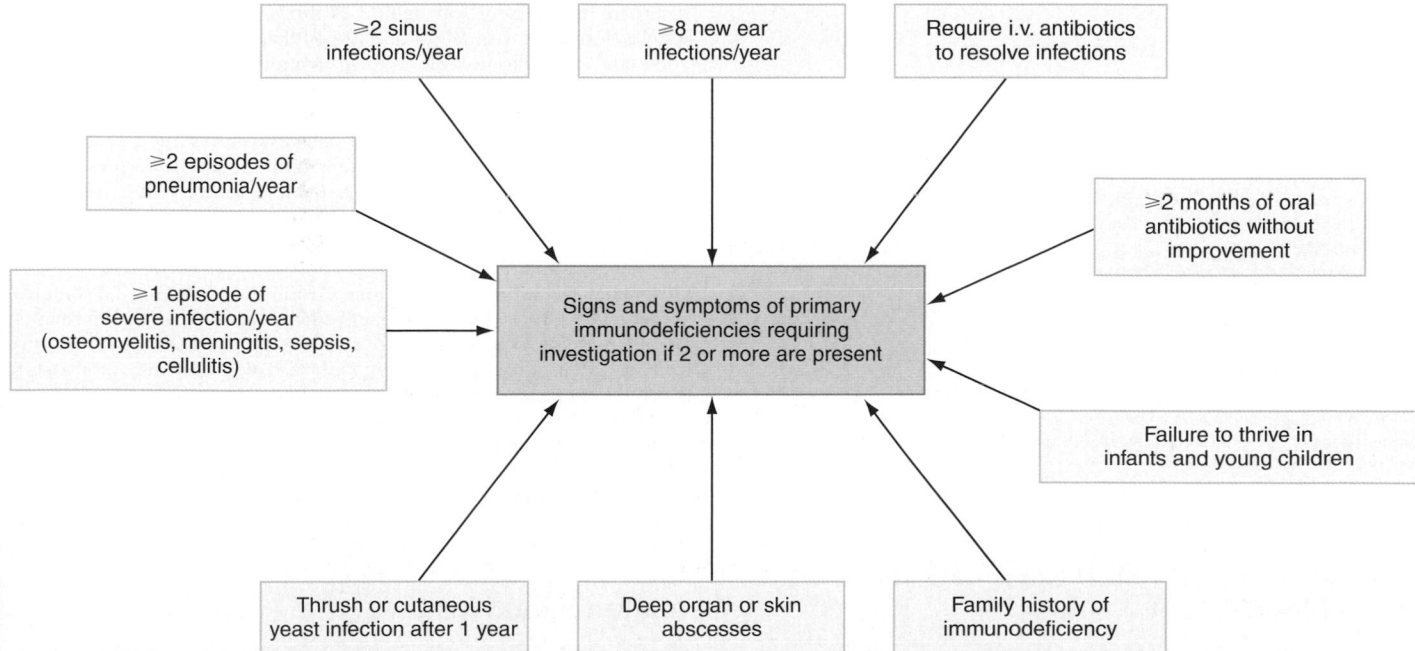

Figure 49–2 Clinical signs and symptoms of primary immunodeficiencies.

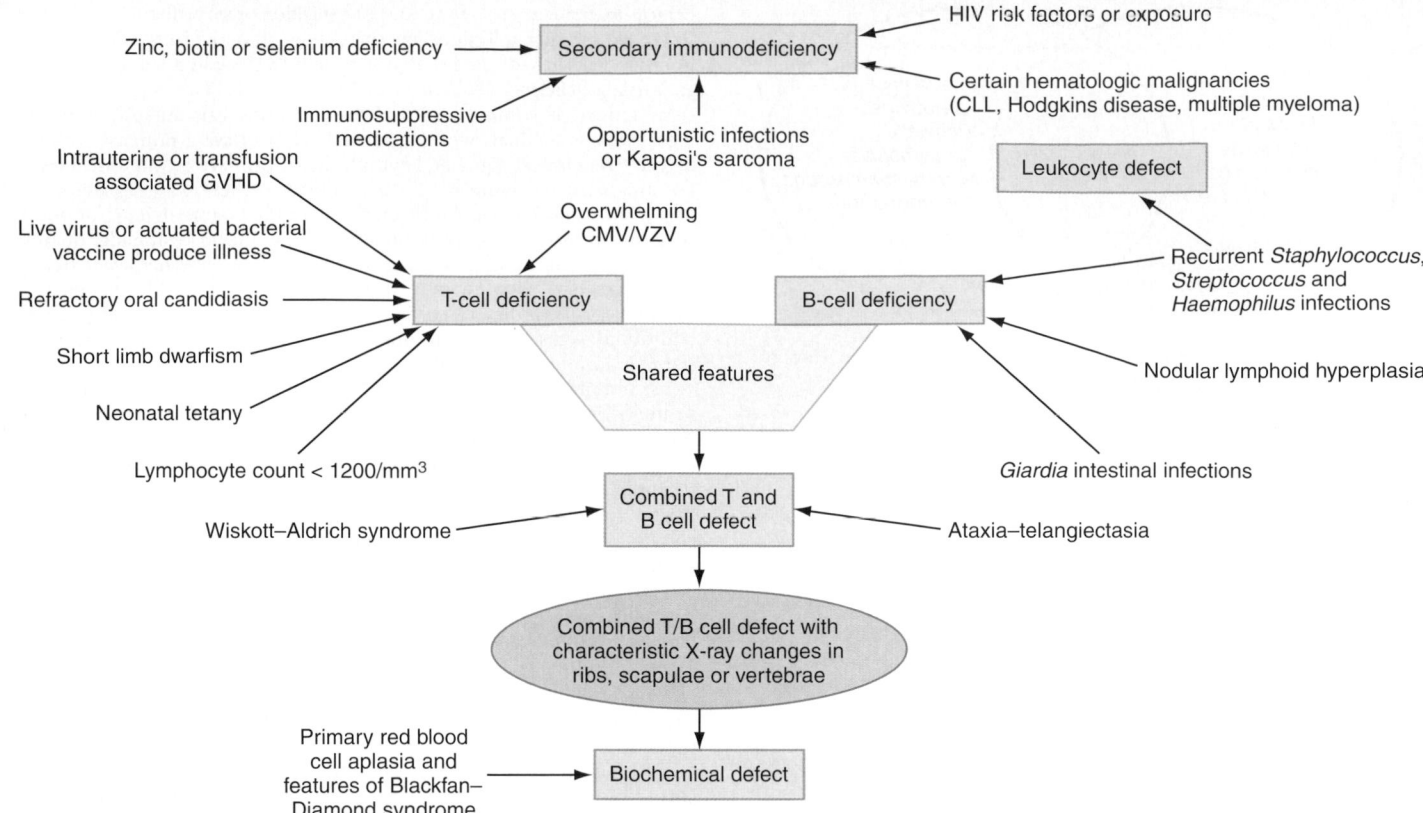

Figure 49–3 Patterns of immunodeficiency disorders. CLL = chronic lymphoid leukemia; CMV = cytomegalovirus; GVHD = graft-versus-host disease; HIV = human immunodeficiency virus; VZV = varicella zoster virus.

Primary investigation

- History and physical examination
- CBC/differential
- X-rays
- Quantitative immunoglobulins (IgG, IgM, IgA)
- Review previous culture results
- Pulmonary function testing

Secondary investigation

- Titers for vaccines administered (tetanus, diphtheria, pneumococcus)
- IgG subclass analysis
- Lymphocyte enumeration panel (CD3, CD4, CD8, CD19, CD16, CD56)
- Complement levels (CH50, C3, C4)
- Skin testing
- Mononuclear cell proliferation studies
- NBT

Tertiary investigation

- Enzyme studies
  (Adenosine deaminase, purine nucleotide phosphorylase)
- NK cell cytotoxic studies
- Phagocyte studies
- Histology and immunohistochemistry analysis (or flow cytometry)
  of lymph nodes or lymphoid organs
- Cytokine production
- Advanced complement studies
- Molecular biology

Figure 49–4 Staged approach for laboratory investigation of primary immunodeficiencies. CBC = complete blood count; NBT = nitroblue tetrazolium slide test; NK cell = natural killer cell.

First-Level Investigations

Clinical History, Physical Examination and Initial Blood Count

A thorough clinical history provides the primary clues in diagnosing a primary immunodeficiency disorder. The typical history includes recurrent, persistent infections or infections caused by unusual microbes. The clinician will be guided by the types of infection the patient has acquired. Patients with immunoglobulin deficiencies typically report an increased number of bacterial infections. Repeated viral, fungal, or other opportunistic infections are associated with T-cell immunodeficiencies. Patients with phagocytic defects will usually report a history of infections with catalase-positive bacteria, such as *Staphylococcus* spp. Complement deficiencies are most frequently associated with *Streptococcus pneumoniae* or *Neisseria* spp. infections (Fig. 49–1) (Lindegren, 2004).

The physical examination may reveal findings that are characteristic for particular primary immunodeficiency disorders. Patients with primary immunodeficiency diseases are pale, lethargic, and appear chronically ill. Infants or young children affected with primary immunodeficiency disorders may present with failure to thrive, so monitoring height and weight is important. Small or absent peripheral lymph nodes, tonsils, or adenoids are indicative of X-linked agammaglobulinemia (Lindegren, 2004). In addition to respiratory infections, the infant may also experience rhinitis, conjunctivitis, hematologic, gastrointestinal, and autoimmune disorders (Fleisher, 2003). In contrast, patients with chronic granulomatous disease (CGD) and common variable immunodeficiency present with normal or enlarged peripheral lymph nodes (Buckley, 2000). The genetic defect in Wiskott–Aldrich syndrome causes immune deficiencies and thrombocytopenia, which result in increased bruisability, petechiae, and eczematous skin rashes (Zhu, 1997).

The first test performed to examine the immune system is the complete blood count. A white blood count and differential will provide information on the morphology and number of small lymphocytes (diameter <10 μm). The normal parameters vary, based on the age of the patient, and therefore must be interpreted using age appropriate normal ranges. At a minimum, regardless of age, one expects more than 1200 small lymphocytes per cubic millimeter. Since few (≈10%) of the lymphocytes are B lymphocytes, an absolute lymphocyte deficiency primarily reflects T-cell deficiency. Part of the first visit should also include obtaining all previous medical records, including pathology reports or slides, and results of previous cultures and X-rays.

Immunoglobulins

Since antibody deficiency diseases are more common than other immune defects, the first emphasis should be placed on investigation of

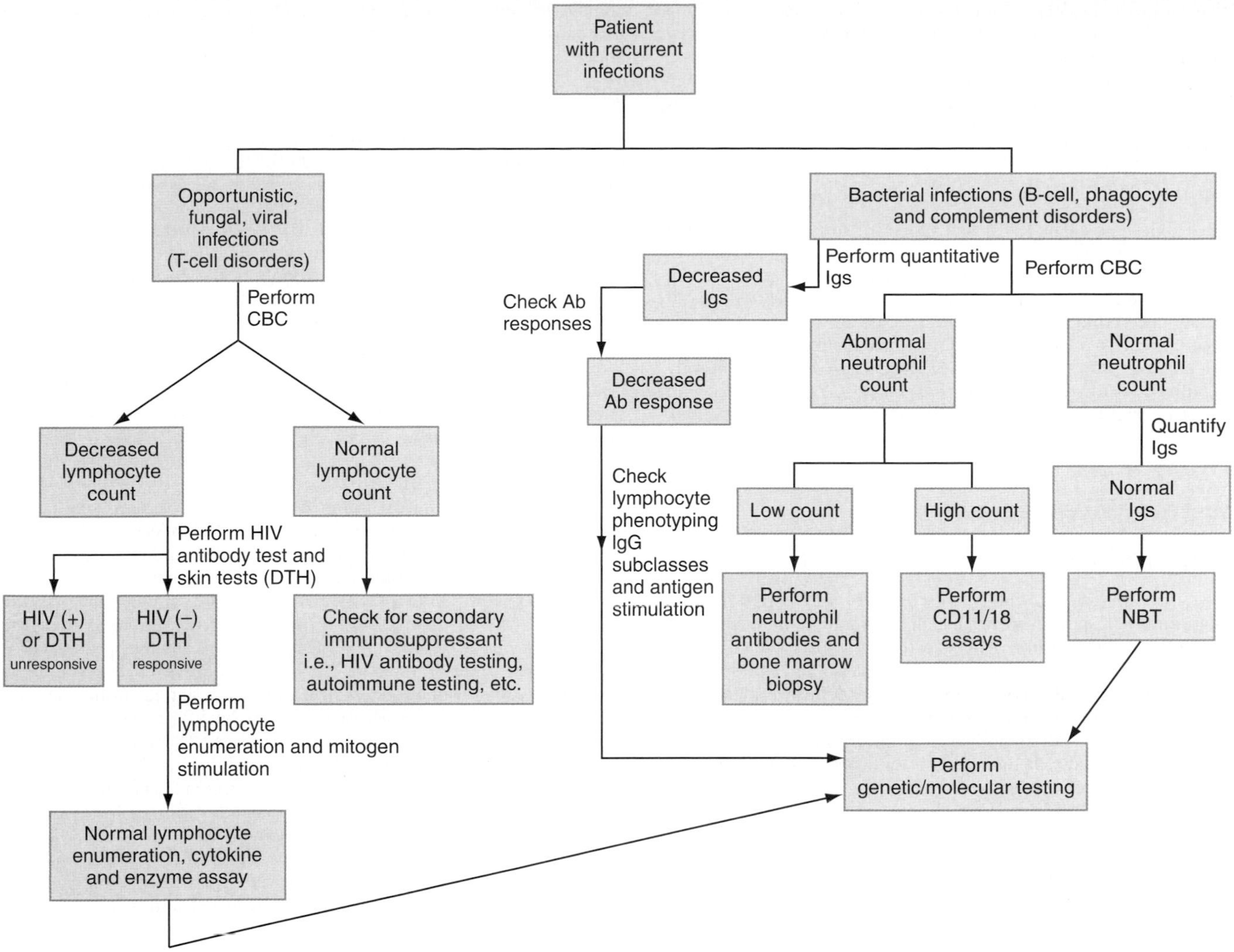

Patient
with recurrent
infections

Opportunistic,
fungal, viral
infections
(T-cell disorders)

Perform
CBC

Decreased
lymphocyte
count

Normal
lymphocyte
count

Perform HIV
antibody test and
skin tests (DTH)

HIV (+)
or DTH
unresponsive

HIV (−)
DTH
responsive

Check for secondary
immunosuppressant
i.e., HIV antibody testing,
autoimmune testing, etc.

Perform
lymphocyte
enumeration and mitogen
stimulation

Normal lymphocyte
enumeration, cytokine
and enzyme assay

Bacterial infections (B-cell, phagocyte
and complement disorders)

Perform quantitative
Igs

Perform CBC

Check Ab
responses

Decreased
Igs

Decreased
Ab response

Check
lymphocyte
phenotyping
IgG
subclasses
and antigen
stimulation

Abnormal
neutrophil
count

Normal
neutrophil
count

Quantify
Igs

Low count

High count

Normal
Igs

Perform
neutrophil
antibodies and
bone marrow
biopsy

Perform
CD11/18
assays

Perform
NBT

Perform
genetic/molecular testing

Figure 49–5 Testing algorithm for immunodeficiencies. Ab = antibody; CBC = complete blood count; DTH = delayed-type hypersensitivity skin test (PPD); HIV = human immunodeficiency virus; Igs = immunoglobulins; NBT = nitroblue tetrazolium slide test.

immunoglobulins and their production (Stiehm, 1996). Approximately half of primary immunodeficiency disorders are related to either inadequate antibody production or nonfunctional antibodies (Noroski, 1998). Quantitative immunoglobulin assays are readily available in all commercial and larger hospital laboratories and only require small volumes of serum to perform (see Chs 19 and 45). Since immunoglobulin values increase with age, comparison to age-matched normal ranges is necessary for correct interpretation.

For the first few months of life, IgG is the major immunoglobulin found in infant serum and is maternal in origin. At approximately 3 months of age, dissipation of maternal IgG concentration, combined with a lag in production by the infant, creates a nadir in IgG levels. However, primarily IgM and secondarily IgA are synthesized by the infant; thus, the presence of these two immunoglobulins is convincing evidence that X-linked agammaglobulinemia, characterized by pan-hypogammaglobulinemia, is not present. Therefore, IgA, IgM, and IgG should be quantified simultaneously.

IgA is often not present in significant amounts until 6 months of age; however, after 1 year of age, IgA levels that remain decreased indicate that this is a permanent defect (Plebani, 1986). Some IgA-deficient patients may be asymptomatic or have mild symptoms such as increased respiratory or gastrointestinal infections; however some patients may experience severe or fatal anaphylactic reactions to plasma in blood products that contain IgA (Lindegren, 2004).

Hyper-IgM syndrome, an X-linked T-cell inherited disorder, is characterized by normal to elevated levels of IgM with markedly low levels of IgA, IgG, and IgE (Levy 1997; Ramesh, 1998; Buckley, 2000). However, marked elevations of IgE are almost always part of the hyper-IgE syndrome (Buckley, 1978) and are common in Wiskott–Aldrich syndrome, some isolated T-cell deficiencies, and CGD. Wiskott–Aldrich syndrome also characteristically shows marked elevation of serum IgA combined with low IgM concentrations (Ochs, 1998).

A simple way to assess functional antibody levels in children is to check for isohemagglutinins directed against ABO antigens the patient lacks, since their presence will indicate active functional antibody production (Fleisher, 2003). Isohemagglutinins are naturally occurring antibodies that form some time after 2–3 months of age, however testing for these antibodies is not valid for children 4–6 months of age because of the persistence of maternal immunoglobulin. Additionally, because of relative immaturity, or perhaps inadequate exposure, children with normal immunity may have low concentrations of isohemagglutinins until 5–10 years of age (Brecher, 2002).

Radiological Imaging

X-rays, computed tomography (CT), and magnetic resonance imaging (MRI) studies can be helpful in assessing immune deficiencies. Chronic interstitial pneumonia is common in infants, children, or adults with T-cell deficiencies, and should be confirmed on chest X-ray. With time, many patients with primary B-cell deficiency (agammaglobulinemia, common variable immunodeficiency) may develop chronic pulmonary fibrosis or bronchiectasis (Sweinberg, 1991; Cunningham-Rundles, 1999). Chest CT in a patient who has recurrent respiratory tract infections is the best means of investigating for bronchiectasis; if these changes have developed, further investigation is clearly warranted.

In the past, lateral views of the neck were used to assess pharyngeal lymphoid tissue in children. However, X-rays are not recommended for evaluation of cervical lymphoid tissue, because the information they provide is more easily obtained by alternative methods. Frontal views of the chest may reveal an absence of the thymic shadow in infants but, since the thymus can easily shrink because of stress, evaluation of thymic size by this method is not reliable. Bony abnormalities, however, can alert the radiologist to an immunologic problem presenting in childhood. A subset of patients with immune deficiencies involving abnormalities of T cells, or both T and B cells, have short-limbed dwarfism. These patients show

VI

characteristic lesions, usually in the metaphyseal regions of the long bones. Patients with infant-onset adenosine deaminase deficiency show readily identifiable skeletal abnormalities of ribs and hips (Lindegren, 2004). Bony abnormalities may be present in patients with the hyper-IgE syndrome; these abnormalities include diffuse osteoporosis, fractures that occur with little trauma, craniosynostosis, and midline bony defects (Grimbacher, 1999).

Pulmonary Functions

Immune deficiency, especially if it has persisted for some time, will often affect the pulmonary system and its function, as previously mentioned. Therefore complete lung volumes, with forced expiratory volumes, should be tested even if the chest X-ray is normal. Patients with both T- and B-cell defects are subject to pulmonary infections, resulting in bronchospasm, restrictive or obstructive disease, or combinations of these abnormalities. Those patients who are both IgA and IgG2-deficient have significantly abnormal pulmonary function tests and there may be a causal relationship between these deficiencies and deterioration of lung function (Bjorkander, 1985).

Second-Level Investigations

Antibody Production

Investigation of specific antibody production may only require monitoring immune responses to vaccine antigens and is the most direct method to assess B-cell function. This is a useful approach for patients with a history of recurrent bacterial infections and low-normal quantitative immunoglobulin concentrations. The definitive method to assess decreased quantitative immunoglobulins is to measure antigen specific preimmunization levels and postimmunization antibody levels approximately 4 weeks later. If the child or adult has received the usual immunizations in the past, antibody titers for these vaccine antigens can be measured. The most useful vaccine responses to assess are those for tetanus, diphtheria, Haemophilus, and pneumococcus; many commercial laboratories have developed sensitive tests, such as enzyme-linked immuno-sorbent assays (ELISA), that can be used to assess antibody production. Evaluation of immune responses to vaccine must include pre-immunization serum antibody concentrations and the patient's age, since these factors affect antibody response. The testing laboratory provides guidelines for appropriate antibody responses. In general, a fourfold increase in protein antigens and a twofold increase in polysaccharide antigens are expected.

Antibody responses to tetanus toxoid and diphtheria toxoid are useful to evaluate responses to T-cell-dependent protein antigens. Assessment of B-cell function requires evaluation of responses to carbohydrate antigens, which activate B cells directly. It is important to use carbohydrate antigens that are not conjugated to proteins, such as meningococcal and pneumococcal polysaccharide antigens (Balmer, 2003). Children less than 2 years old will not respond to unconjugated carbohydrate antigens (Barrett, 1984) and no live virus vaccines should be administered to the child, or any family member, until an immune deficiency is ruled out (Go, 1996).

IgG Subclasses

IgG consists of four subclasses, IgG1 through IgG4, distinguished by both structural and biological differences (Normansell, 1987; Schur, 1987). Although individual roles for each of the IgG subclasses have not been established, antibodies to carbohydrate antigens are concentrated in the IgG2 subclass, and many bacterial cell wall antigens are composed of carbohydrates (Scott, 1988). Thus, absence of an IgG2 response could result in a failure to develop protection against bacterial infection. This relationship is most convincing in the occasional patient with IgA deficiency who also has a deficiency of IgG2 subclass and lacks an antibody response to vaccines for pneumococcus. IgG subclass deficiency has also been implicated as the cause of recurrent infections in patients with normal or near normal IgG levels (Oxelius, 1979; Wedgwood, 1986; Shackelford, 1990; Gross, 1992; Popa, 1994).

The biological significance of IgG subclass deficiency is not always clear and some individuals who completely lack genes for IgG2, IgA, and IgE are healthy (Lefranc, 1982; Migone, 1984). IgG1 is the first type of subclass response to carbohydrate antigens, and conversion to an IgG2 response occurs as the individual matures (Scott, 1988). There is no evidence that those who are restricted to only IgG1 responses are at any disadvantage. To determine the biological significance of IgG subclass deficiency, testing of specific antibody production, usually by administering vaccines such as

tetanus, diphtheria, Haemophilus, and a pneumococcal vaccine is mandatory. Only patients with a clear antibody deficiency for multiple antigens would be considered to have a significant immune defect.

T-Cell Immunity

Migration of stem cells from the bone marrow to the thymus results in development of T cells (Kruisbeek, 1999). During development of T cells in the thymus, many surface molecules are turned on and off in a regulated manner. These surface molecules are identified by their cluster of differentiation (CD). The CD markers help distinguish the stage of maturation and function of lymphocytes (Buckley, 2000). Despite the regression of the thymus over time, T-cell development persists throughout life (Jamieson, 1999). Unlike antibodies produced by B cells, which recognize antigens in their natural state, T cells recognize peptides along with MHC molecules after processing by antigen presenting cells through CD3, the T cell receptor (Buckley, 2000).

Monoclonal antibodies are useful for detection of CD markers on lymphocytes and enable rapid enumeration of T cells and T-cell subsets. This can be done using small volumes of whole blood. The CD designation subdivides T cells (as a group, CD3+) into two major subsets, CD4+ and CD8+ T cells. CD4+ T cells are referred to as 'helper' cells, which are involved in initiation of immune reactions, cytokine secretion, and augmentation of B-cell responses. CD8+ T cells also release cytokines and are associated with cytolytic (killer) functions. CD4+ and CD8+ markers on T cells serve as signaling molecules and work in conjunction with major histocompatibility class (MHC) I and II antigens to amplify and stabilize engagement of T-cell receptors (TCR) with antigens. CD4+ cells recognize antigens that are presented in the context of MHC class II antigens, and CD8+ cells recognize antigens presented in context with MHC class I antigens (Buckley, 2000). Immunodeficiency diseases resulting from defective generation of T cells may result in a total loss or low numbers of CD3+ T cells, thereby creating similar effects on the T-cell subsets, CD4+ and CD8+ cells. For example, DiGeorge syndrome results in low numbers of CD3+ cells (Hong, 1998). MHC class II deficiency results in a low number of CD4+ cells (Klein, 1993) and an abnormality of Zap-70, a signaling molecule integral to the activity of the T-cell receptor, leads to reduced numbers of CD8+ T cells (Elder, 1998). If an immune defect is suspected, a panel of T-cell markers is examined by flow cytometry and the percentage and absolute count of cells in each set are compared with age appropriate normal ranges (Illoh, 2004).

T-Cell Functional Assessment

A clinical history of opportunistic infections and a decreased absolute lymphocyte count in a complete blood count should prompt further investigation of a patient's T-cell function (Fleisher, 2003). Mucocutaneous candidiasis is another indication of defective T-cell function and is characterized by extension of infection from the mucous membranes on to contiguous skin and may involve the fingernails with granulomatous inflammation (Atkinson, 2000; Lilic 2001). Delayed-type hypersensitivity (DTH) skin tests are commonly used as measures of T-cell function, because they measure the ability to recall, recognize and present antigen, mobilize T cells, and generate a specific inflammatory response. Despite a normal absolute lymphocyte count, DTH skin tests should be performed when there is a suspicion of a T-cell defect. However, these tests are hard to interpret in infants since they may not have had sufficient exposure to respond to antigens to mount an immunogenic response and a reduced or absent response may be normal. Hypersensitivity skin testing should incorporate more than one antigen (Kniker, 1985). In order to ensure proper administration and appropriate interpretation of test results, the personnel must be well trained (Fleisher, 2003).

Insight into the capability of T cells can be gained by performing functional assessments of in vitro proliferative responses to different stimuli. Mitogens, antigens, and alloantigens are stimuli that will cause proliferation of T cells. Mitogens are usually plant extracts that lack specificity and stimulate both CD4+ and CD8+ T lymphocytes. Alloantigens on unrelated donor cells also stimulate CD4+ and CD8+ cells in a relatively nonspecific way. Patients with significant T-cell deficiency may still show proliferative responses to these stimulators, indicating the presence of T cells but not their ability to clear infectious agents from the host. Nonetheless, the proliferative responses to specific antigens is a good indicator of the host's ability to resist infection (Lane, 1985). In the case of specific antigens, tetanus, diphtheria, and Candida are commonly used, although sufficient exposure to these antigens is required. Therefore, these are not reliable antigens for testing infants during the first year of life. A measure of specific T-cell responses that is useful in infants is to culture peripheral blood mononuclear cells with mitogenic concentrations of anti-CD3 monoclonal antibody. This stimulator normally causes proliferation of all CD3+ T cells, while absence of proliferation demonstrates a severe T-cell defect (Hong, 1996).

Polymorphonuclear Killing Assays

Testing neutrophil function requires careful planning, since specimens may be transported over long distances to large reference laboratories for testing. Blood collected from a patient should be submitted to the investigating laboratory as soon as possible, since neutrophils undergo apoptosis rapidly after collection. If the blood must be stored or transported it should be collected in a preservative such as ethylenediaminetetraacetic acid (EDTA) or citrate in a polypropylene tube and maintained at room temperature (20–25°C). This will decrease metabolic activity and minimize adhesion of cells to the wall of the tube. Even under optimal conditions cells can only be maintained for approximately 24–36 hours (Kuijpers, 1999).

Neutropenia or neutrophil dysfunction results in recurrent bacterial or fungal infections in the skin, lymph nodes, liver, lungs, or bones. This most commonly occurs with myelosuppressive therapies to treat malignant neoplasms. These disorders must be distinguished from CGD, in which there is normal phagocytosis but defective intracellular killing of infectious organisms, resulting in abscess or granuloma formation in the liver, bones, and lungs (Lekstrom-Himes, 2000). CGD inheritance is most commonly X-linked or autosomal recessive, due to mutations involving chromosome locations 16p24, 7q11.23, or 1q25. These changes result in defects in one of the four subunits of NADPH oxidase, the enzyme that catalyzes the formation of hydrogen peroxide. This error causes failure of the metabolic burst in granulocytes following phagocytic ingestion of bacteria (Meischl, 1998). As a result, molecular oxygen is not reduced to superoxide and other free radicals, such as hydroxyl radical and hydrogen peroxide, which are all important components of the intracellular mechanism of bacterial death (Babior, 1978). CGD is therefore characterized by recurrent infections with catalase-producing organisms, such as *Staphylococcus aureus*, which are capable of destroying the hydrogen peroxide produced by granulocytes. Therefore, catalase-positive organisms survive intracellular ingestion, multiply, and cause a granulomatous tissue response that, when excessive, can obstruct the gastrointestinal and genitourinary tracts. Chronic infections with *Serratia* spp., *Klebsiella* spp., *Burkholderia cepacia*, and *Aspergillus* spp. are particularly problematic (Gallin, 1983, 1990). However, patients with CGD do not experience this problem with catalase-negative organisms.

The fundamental biological characteristic of CGD leukocytes is that they will phagocytose bacteria normally but will not kill them. This provides the basis of a bacterial killing assay for CGD. Historically, the nitroblue tetrazolium (NBT) slide test has been the laboratory assay to screen for CGD and is performed by reference laboratories (Park, 1968). In this assay the patient's neutrophils are incubated with nitroblue tetrazolium, a pale yellow dye, which is then activated by phorbol-myristate acetate (PMA), a strong, receptor-independent activation stimulus. Functional neutrophils phagocytose, reduce and precipitate the NBT dye, forming intracellular deposits of black formazan. These deposits are indicative of a rapid activation of NADPH-oxidase enzyme, causing reduction of oxygen by NADPH to superoxide that is subsequently catalyzed to hydrogen peroxide by superoxide dismutase (SOD). A technician then microscopically scores neutrophils that contain intracellular black formazan deposits (Kuijpers, 1999). However, the NBT slide test has been replaced in many laboratories by a flow cytometry test that detects intracellular oxidation of dichlorofluorescein di-acetate dihydrorhodamine 123 (O'Gorman, 1995). These nonfluorescent dyes, once oxidized, will produce intracellular fluorescent products that are detected by flow cytometry. Flow cytometry is a more objective and reliable method of identifying intracellular products.

The hyper-IgE syndrome (Buckley, 1978) is phenotypically similar to CGD, with recurrent skin and pulmonary abscesses; however, defective polymorphonuclear leukocyte function is not a predominant finding of this disease (Buckley, 1978). In addition, this syndrome also includes bone abnormalities, unusual facies, and cutaneous candidiasis. The immune defect in the hyper-IgE syndrome is still poorly defined, and although it has been mapped to chromosome 4, the host defect or specific gene has still not been classified. Demonstration of IgE levels over 2000 IU/mL (but as high as 20 000–60 000 IU/ml) with the appropriate clinical manifestations points towards the diagnosis (Grimbacher, 1999). There are no diagnostic or confirmatory tests currently available for hyper-IgE and it is primarily recognized by clinical presentation (Grimbacher, 1999).

Complement Evaluation

A number of congenital defects of the complement system have been described, although this is not a frequent cause of primary immuno-deficiency disorders. The defects are typically associated with absence of one of the complement molecules or a nonfunctional complement protein, thereby reducing the ability of complement to bind to the surface of invading microorganisms. Individual defects lead to distinct clinical syndromes such as hereditary angioedema or paroxysmal nocturnal hemoglobinuria, a propensity for recurrent bacterial infections, or autoimmune disease (Schneider, 1999). Many of the genetically based deficiencies of the classical activating pathway (C1, C2, C3, C4) and of the terminal components (C5, C6, C7, C8, and C9) can be detected by using antibody-sensitized sheep erythrocytes in a total hemolytic complement assay (CH_{50}). This assay tests for the functional integrity of C1–C9. Many commercial laboratories perform this assay but, in order to get accurate results, freshly drawn serum or plasma that is then frozen must be used. Therefore, logistics must be carefully coordinated if specimens must be sent to a distant location. Deficiencies of alternative pathway component factors D, H, and I and properdin are uncommon but can be detected by a hemolytic assay using unsensitized rabbit erythrocytes as potent activators of the alternative pathway. If one of these assays is abnormal, the identification of individual deficient components rests on specialized functional and immunochemical tests that are specific for each component (see Ch. 46).

Third-Level Investigations

Enzyme Measurements for Metabolic Defects

Deficiencies of the enzymes adenosine deaminase and purine nucleoside phosphorylase are related to purine metabolism and result in an immune deficiency. Patients with adenosine deaminase deficiency have findings similar to those of severe combined immunodeficiency syndrome (SCID), a collection of genetic disorders in which there is a severe defect in the function or development of B and T cells. In contrast to SCID, patients deficient in adenosine deaminase have chondro-osseous dysplasia, resulting in skeletal abnormalities, and more severe lymphopenia. Deficient adenosine deaminase is caused by mutation of the gene located on chromosome 20q13.2–q13.11, resulting in toxic accumulation of metabolites that inhibit cell replication and cause apoptosis of lymphocytic cell lines (Buckley, 2000). Lack of adenosine deaminase initially causes loss of T cells (CD4+ T cells in particular) and subsequently B cells, leading to the common form of severe combined T- and B-cell deficiency (SCID) (Hirschhorn, 1995). As with many primary immune defects first recognized in the severe homozygous form, adenosine deaminase deficiency has also been diagnosed in adults with CD4 lymphopenia and significant T-cell defects as a heterozygous partial deficiency (Shovlin, 1994).

Purine nucleoside phosphorylase deficiency is characterized by recurrent infections, lymphopenia, neurological abnormalities, and autoimmune disorders (Myers, 2004). This enzyme deficiency causes a decrease of T cells with minimal or no effect on the B cells. Purine nucleoside phosphorylase enzymes are usually measured in erythrocyte lysates (Kizaki, 1977) but, if blood products have been administered within the previous 3 months, the assay may be unreliable. More recently, capillary electrophoresis has been proposed as an alternative inexpensive assay that offers high separation flexibility in diagnosis of errors in metabolism and is capable of determining purine nucleoside phosphorylase or adenosine deaminase enzyme activity and the presence of toxic metabolites (Carlucci, 2003).

Natural Killer Cell Assays

Natural killer (NK) cells are a subset of lymphocytes that often function with T cells to eradicate intracellular organisms. Complete deficiency of NK cells is rare and is characterized by recurrent herpes infections (Fleisher, 2003). NK cells have the morphology of a large granular lymphocyte and express a unique group of cellular surface markers: CD16, CD56, and CD57 (Trinchieri, 1989). NK cells can easily be quantified by detecting these surface markers using flow cytometry. However, to assess functional activity of NK cell function, chromium release assays, which use chromium-51-loaded K-562 cell lines, have traditionally been performed (Biron, 1989). This older assay has limitations, since it is more labor-intensive, incorporates radioactive materials, and cannot identify the cellular mechanisms for cell death of the target cells. These disadvantages have driven the development of newer, non-radioactivity-based methods, including fluorescent labeling techniques in combination with flow cytometry, to assess NK cell function. Another technique uses a colorimetric substrate to detect granzyme B, the serine protease found in the granules of cytotoxic T lymphocytes and NK cells, and has a key role in granule mediated apoptosis by cleaving cellular substrates (Hoppner, 2002; Ewen, 2003).

VI

Additional Phagocyte Analyses

There are genetic defects of the innate immune system related to the formation or function of granules within neutrophils. Myeloperoxidase is the predominant enzyme detected in the primary granules of granulocytes and catalyzes the formation of hypochlorous acid (HOCL), which is capable of killing microorganisms (Kuijpers, 1999). However its absence is not usually associated with clinical symptoms, with the notable exception of patients with diabetes mellitus, who experience an increased susceptibility to disseminated candidiasis (Lanza, 1998). Myeloperoxidase deficiency, inherited as an autosomal recessive defect, is one of the most commonly inherited disorders of neutrophils but its clinical significance is unknown (Lehrer, 1969; Klebanoff, 1999). Approximately half of affected patients have a deficiency of myeloperoxidase while the remainder have normal concentrations but possess a structural defect in the enzyme (Nauseef, 1998).

Chédiak–Higashi syndrome and specific granule deficiency are congenital defects resulting in phagocyte granular disorders. Chédiak–Higashi syndrome is an autosomal recessive disorder in which all lysosome-containing cells have giant abnormal granules. In neutrophils, there is fusion of the primary and secondary granules, causing a delay of fusion with the phagosomes and resulting in recurrent bacterial infections. Patients with Chédiak–Higashi syndrome have a mild neutropenia, normal immunoglobulin levels, peripheral nerve defects, mild cutaneous and ocular albinism, mild platelet dysfunction, and periodontal disease (Introne, 1999).

Neutrophil-specific granule deficiency is a rare disorder characterized by recurrent bacterial infections of the skin and lungs. Patients lack the secondary or specific granules of the neutrophils, which play an important role in acute inflammation and do not allow for proper migration of neutrophils. Morphologic examination of stained neutrophils shows the characteristic abnormalities in specific granule deficiency (Ganz, 1988).

Patients with leukocyte adhesion deficiency (LAD) type 1; a defect in the integrin CD18, the common β-chain of LFA-1, Mac-1, and p150,95 molecules) (Anderson, 1987) are susceptible to all infections seen in CGD patients, along with otitis media and poor wound healing. Normally, as pathogens cause tissue damage and inflammation, adhesion molecules on vascular endothelium are upregulated and recognized by passing neutrophils bearing the appropriate counterligands, ultimately leading to accumulation of neutrophils at sites of inflammation (see Ch. 46). Patients with LAD lack the adhesion molecules necessary for diapedesis, resulting in tissue neutropenia and therefore more infections (Arnaout, 1993). This abnormality starts after birth and is marked by delayed cord separation, chronic skin ulcers, periodontitis, impaired wound healing, and leukocytosis. Deficient leukocytes demonstrate defects of adherence and adhesion-dependent functions such as spreading, phagocytosis, and chemotactic orientation (Anderson, 1987).

LAD type 2 predominantly affects neutrophils and macrophages, with faulty expression of the selectin ligand sialyl-Lewis[x] and failure to convert GDP mannose to fucose, and results in a clinical syndrome similar to type 1. It is also responsible for expression of the rare Bombay blood group (LAD-2) on red blood cells (Etzioni, 1993).

Leukocyte mobility is usually evaluated by directed migration through membrane filters or under agarose (Nelson, 1975; Cates, 1981). Counting the number of cells at a particular end point or 'stop filter' microscopically, or by radioactive labeling, has the disadvantage of measuring only the fastest cells. This may give an inaccurate assessment of the majority of the patient's neutrophils and it is actually better to count the number of cells at different points along the filter (Kuijpers, 1999). Injections of epinephrine and steroids, which cause polymorphonuclear leukocytes to demarginate and leave the marrow reserves, are used to further assess polymorphonuclear leukocyte mobility. A disorder of actin, important in polymorphonuclear leukocyte migration, has been described (Southwick, 1988).

Adhesion proteins on the surface of neutrophils can be functionally tested with different immobilized ligands bound to a monolayer of endothelial cells attached to a glass slide and can be measured after pretreatment with chemoattractants. The rolling, attachment, and migration of neutrophils can be monitored over periods of time by a video camera. Phagocytosis can now be assessed by flow cytometry in which the neutrophils are incubated with fluorescence-labeled microorganisms, the sample is washed to remove labeled undigested microorganisms, and the cells with ingested labeled microorganism are counted (Kuijpers, 1999). Much in the same fashion, flow cytometry may be used to assess killing of microbes, by employing vital dyes that distinguish live from dead organisms after incubation with neutrophils (Martin, 1992). Degranulation may be assessed by measuring expression of granule membrane proteins on the neutrophil cell surface by means of flow cytometry (Kuijpers, 1999).

Cytokines and Cytokine Receptors

Immune responses are regulated by soluble mediators called cytokines that produce a multiplicity of immune events through interactions with appropriate cytokine receptors on tissue and inflammatory cells. Cytokines serve an important role as messengers within the immune system and in conjunction with the rest of the body to regulate immune responses (Mire-Sluis, 1998). By studying immune deficient patients and gene-knockout mice our understanding of the role cytokines play in our host defenses has expanded. Deficiencies in interleukin (IL)-12 and interferon (IFN)-γ increase susceptibilities to salmonella and mycobacterial infections (de Jong 1998). Impaired secretions or responses to IL-12 impair granuloma formation and therefore allow for unregulated growth of mycobacterial organisms (Jouanguy, 1999). Recent studies show that the pathophysiology of many of these disorders may be the result of defective cytokine signaling which causes dysfunction or arrested development of B, T, and NK cells (Kelly, 2003). Most notably, human X-linked SCID is associated with defects in the interleukin receptor gene (IL2RG), which codes for a common gamma chain (γc) a shared component of several cytokine receptors such as IL-4F, IL-7R, IL-9R, IL-15R. The impaired production of γc leads to cytokine dysfunction and lack of development of the affected lymphoid cells (Malek, 1999). Additionally, the JAK3 gene encodes for a tyrosine kinase used for signal transduction through γc-containing cytokine receptors. Defects in this gene have been identified in patients with autosomal recessive SCID. IL-7 is a cytokine with a key role in T-cell development and a genetic defect in the α subunit of the IL-7 receptor has been identified in patients with a rare disorder of B+ SCID (Notarangelo, 2000).

Additional Cell Surface Markers

MHC Class I and II Molecules

Congenital mutations affecting the expression of MHC class I and class II expression have been described. Class II molecules are found primarily on the antigen-presenting cells, which initiate the acquired immune response. As one might predict, genetic defects of MHC class II (from mutations involving MHC class II gene transcriptional activation) result in a profound immune deficiency state (Klein, 1993), known as MHC class II deficiency, using World Health Organization nomenclature. This is referred to as bare lymphocyte syndrome type II and is characterized by lack of expression of MHC II molecules on cellular surfaces. Thymic education and selection of immature T cells is compromised because of loss of antigen processing by MHC class II molecules. The quantity of B and T cells is normal in patients with bare lymphocyte syndrome; however, they have decreased CD4+ counts as a result of loss of proper antigen processing. As a result, these patients are unable to respond to foreign antigens and present with recurrent bacterial, fungal, viral, and protozoal infections. They do not respond to skin testing (type IV delayed type hypersensitivity), have a decreased ability to respond to mixed lymphocyte reactions, and have panhypogammaglobulinemia (Nekrep, 2003). An interesting facet of this syndrome is that there is no genetic defect of the MHC class II genes. Instead, a defect occurs in one of the four genes that encode the four regulatory factors that are essential for the surface expression of MHC class II antigens (Reith, 2001).

The elimination of foreign antigen can be accomplished by CD8+ T-cell binding to MHC class I antigens that are expressed on nearly all nucleated cells. Strangely, the immune defects that result from MHC class I deficiency, a mutation involving either of the MHC class I cytoplasmic peptide transporters TAP-1 or TAP-2, produce an immune defect characterized by severe lung disease that becomes apparent in later childhood (Donato, 1995; de la Salle, 1999). This immune deficiency was previously named type I bare lymphocyte syndrome or HLA class I deficiency and is characterized by a decrease in CD8+ cells and NK cell activity (Yabe, 2002). The diagnosis of both defects involves examining the expression of these MHC antigens on peripheral blood lymphoid cells by flow cytometry (Illoh, 2004).

Treatment by targeting cell surface receptors

Recent case reports describe therapies that target cell surface receptors to treat complications associated with primary immunodeficiency disorders. An example is anti-CD20 (rituximab) a monoclonal antibody directed against the CD20 antigen, found on B lymphocytes, used to deplete peripheral benign and malignant B lymphocytes. Successful treatment using these monoclonal antibodies has been reported for IgM autoantibody (reactive at 37°C)-mediated autoimmune hemolytic anemia in a child with common variable immunodeficiency and a lymphoproliferative disorder in a child with Wiskott–Aldrich syndrome by depleting peripheral B cells in patients (Sebire, 2003; Wakim, 2004).

Using Novel Immunogens to Assess Antibody Production

Another valuable tool to evaluate specific antibody responses is vaccination with neoantigens such as the bacteriophage Φ X174 and keyhole limpet hemocyanin. These neoantigens may also be used to evaluate patients receiving immunoglobulin replacement therapy, since monitoring antibody responses to standard vaccines while receiving passive infusion of pooled immunoglobulins is not possible. Primary and secondary responses may be monitored since the neoantigens provoke a primary IgM response, and then, upon re-exposure, cause a secondary IgG response (Curtis, 1970; Ochs, 1971). Using Φ X174 clearance patterns and isotypes, a patient's response can be measured, thereby further defining various degrees and subsets of B-cell deficiency (Ochs, 1971). Currently, this evaluation is only available in some academic institutions using research protocols (Fleisher, 2004).

Molecular Genetics and Prenatal Diagnosis

A number of the genes involved in the primary immune deficiency syndromes have now been identified, cloned, and sequenced (Conley, 1992; Puck, 1993; Derry, 1994; Ramesh, 1998; Vihinen, 1999). In many cases, mouse knockout models have been produced to further study the effects of genes on immune function. In the past, more traditional methods of screening for genetic mutations responsible for immunodeficiencies were used, such as dideoxy fingerprinting and single-strand conformational polymorphism (Sarkar, 1992; Sheffield, 1993; Puck, 1997b). More recent advances using fluorescence-based sequencing, which uses fluorescently labeled dideoxynucleotide terminators, allows for a simple and sensitive identification of DNA sequence variations in individuals. Automated multichannel capillary sequences is an automated method of rapidly detecting fluorescence-based sequences for multiple patients within hours, and makes direct sequencing for genetic mutations responsible for immune deficiencies practical (Niemela, 2000). Identification of mutated genes facilitates genetic counseling for prenatal diagnosis and aids in the detection of carrier status for defective genes. It also assists in the evaluation of previously undefined immune disorders. An excellent example of how these advanced techniques are enhancing our understanding of primary immunodeficiency disorders is exhibited by hyper-IgM syndrome. Previously, this was categorized as a single disorder, but genetic sequencing has revealed five distinct genetic defects affecting B or T cells with variable phenotypes (Durandy, 2004).

Analysis of immune deficiencies with known genetic defects involves testing specific sites on DNA to detect specific mutations. Different methods such as polymerase chain reaction (PCR) may be used to detect the presence or absence of a particular gene and immunoblotting or flow cytometry can be used to detect protein products and confirm a diagnosis of primary immunodeficiency when the gene product is absent. An example when determining the etiology of an immunodeficiency is important in SCID, a heterogenous group of immunodeficiencies characterized by a number of different molecular defects. Distinguishing between various molecular defects in SCID has implications for treatment, antenatal diagnosis, and carrier testing. It is important to determine if a patient has X-linked SCID since this may be treated using gene therapy. JAK3-deficient SCID is clinically indistinguishable from X-linked SCID, but gene therapy is not effective (Cavazzana-Calvo, 2000). Previously, testing to distinguish between these molecular defects took several weeks to complete since the JAK3-deficient SCID is encoded by 23 exons. This required DNA analysis using single-stranded conformational polymorphism analysis and sequencing of all affected exons. More rapid screening methods can now be used to get an expeditious diagnosis, with time-consuming genetic analysis being performed for subsequent confirmation. These protein based assays employ flow cytometric analysis of γc, immunoblotting for JAK3 and γc, and detection of IL-2 induced tyrosine phosphorylation of JAK3 (Gilmour, 2001). However, in defects characterized by nonfunctional protein products, these assays are not useful.

With advances in technology, the ability to detect a wider range of immune defects prenatally is possible. If the specific mutation is known, or if the inheritance pattern is known to be X-linked, analysis of linked polymorphic markers or specific mutation detection can be performed. Chorionic villus samples, amniocyte DNA prepared directly from fetal cells, or cultured and expanded cell lines can be analyzed (Durandy, 1985).

Many of the primary immunodeficiencies are rare disorders that can be difficult to diagnose and in these cases genetic mutation detection is the most reliable method. These specialized tests are not readily available and physicians may have difficulty locating laboratories to perform the necessary genetic analysis. There are mutation registries and databases available to provide information about tests for clinical data, immune status, antibody response, cellular function, and enzyme assays. Additionally, some online registries contain information about laboratories that perform these assays that increases awareness of testing availability and the ability to obtain an exact and prompt diagnosis (Samarghitean, 2004).

Summary

Assessment of host defenses is an extraordinarily complex process entailing the cooperation of the clinician, research scientist, and clinical pathologist. A logical approach, based on appreciation of the multiple systems involved in host defense and various diagnostic options, can help lead to the identification of the underlying disorder. The impressive success of modern therapy, incorporating new antimicrobials, recombinant DNA technology, bone marrow transplantation, and gene therapy, allows more precise delineation and characterization of immunologic deficiency state. This in turn improves the recognition and ultimately the treatment of these patients.

References

Anderson DC, Springer TA: Leukocyte adhesion deficiency: an inherited defect in the MAC-1, LFA-1, and p150,95 glycoproteins. Annu Rev Med 1987; 38:175.

Arnaout MA, Michishita M: Genetic abnormalities in leukocyte adhesion molecule deficiency. In: Gupta S, Griscelli C, eds. New concepts in immunodeficiency diseases. Chichester, West Sussex: John Wiley 1993:191–202.

Atkinson JC, O'Connell A, Aframian D: Oral manifestations of primary immunological diseases. J Am Dent Assoc 2000; 131:345–356

Babior BM: Oxygen-dependent microbial killing by phagocytes first of two parts. N Engl J Med 1978; 298:721–725.

Balmer P, North J, Baxter D, et al: Measurement and interpretation of pneumococcal IgG levels for clinical management. Clin Exp Immunol 2003; 133:364–369.

Barrett DJ, Lee CG, Ammann AJ, Ayoub EM: IgG and IgM pneumococcal polysaccharide antibody responses in infants. Pediatr Res 1984;18:1067–1071.

Baumgart KW, Britton WJ, Kemp A, et al: The spectrum of primary immunodeficiency disorders in Australia. J Allergy Clin Immunol 1997;100:415–423.

Biron CA, Byron KS, Sullivan JL: Severe herpes virus infections in an adolescent without natural killer cells. N Engl J Med 1989; 320:1731–1735.

Bjorkander J, Bake B, Oxelius VA, Hanson LA: Impaired lung function in patients with IgA deficiency and low levels of IgG2 or IgG3. N Engl J Med 1985; 313:720–724.

Brecher M, ed: Technical Manual. Bethesda, MD, American Association of Blood Banks, 2002.

Buckley RH, Becker WG: Abnormalities in the regulation of human IgE synthesis. Immunol Rev 1978; 41:288–314.

Buckley RH: Primary immunodeficiency diseases due to defects in lymphocytes. N Engl J Med 2000; 343:1313–1324.

Carlucci F, Tabucchi A, Aiuti A, et al: Capillary electrophoresis in diagnosis and monitoring of adenosine deaminase deficiency. Clin Chem 2003; 49:1830–1838.

Cates KL: Defects in neutrophil chemotaxis. Clin Immunol Allergy 1981; 1:603.

Cavazzana-Calvo M, Haein-Bey S, de Saint BG, et al: Gene therapy of human severe combined immunodeficiency (SCID) -X1 disease. Science 2000; 288:66–72.

Clark JA, Callicoat PA, Brenner NA, et al : Selective IgA deficiency in blood donors. Am J Clin Pathol 1983; 80:210–213.

Conley ME: Molecular approaches to analysis of X-linked immunodeficiencies: Annu Rev Immunol 1992; 10:215–238.

Curtis JE, Hersh EM, Harris JE, et al: The human primary immune response to keyhole limpet haemocyanin: interrelationships of delayed hypersensitivity, antibody response and in vitro blast transformation. Clin Exp Immunol 1970; 6:473–491.

Cunningham-Rundles C: Common variable immunodeficiency: clinical and immunological features of 248 patients. J Appl Biomaterials 1999; 92:34–48.

De Jong R, Altare F, Haagen IA, et al: Severe mycobacterial and salmonella infections in interleukin-12 receptor-deficient patients. Science 1998; 280:1435–1438.

De la Salle H, Zimmer J, Fricker D, et al: HLA class I deficiencies due to mutations in subunit 1 of the peptide transporter TAP-1. J Clin Invest 1999; 103:R9–R13.

Delves PJ, Roitt IM. The immune system, first of two parts. N Engl J Med 2000; 343;1:37–49.

A general overview of the immune system and the function of the innate and acquired responses as well as the role of B and T cells. This article also provides a glossary of commonly used immunologic terms that clinicians may find useful.

Derry JM, Ochs HD, Francke U: Isolation of a novel gene mutated in Wiskott–Aldrich syndrome. Cell 1994; 78:635–644.

VI

Donato L, de la Salle H, Hanau D, et al: Association of HLA class I antigen deficiency related to a *TAP2* gene mutation with familial bronchiectasis. J Pediatr 1995; 127:895–900.

Durandy A, Dumez Y, Griscelli C: Prenatal diagnosis of severe hereditary immunologic deficiencies. Arch Fr Pediatr 1985; 42:163–167.

Durandy A, Revy P, Fischer A: Human models of inherited immunoglobulin class switch recombination and somatic hypermutation defects (hyper-IgM syndromes). Adv Immunol 2004; 82:295–330.

Elder ME: ZAP-70 and defects of T cell receptor signaling. Semin Hematol 1998; 35:310–320.

Etzioni A, Harlan JM, Pollack S, et al: Leukocyte adhesion deficiency (LAD) II: A new adhesion defect due to absence of sialyl Lewis X, the ligand for selectins. Immunodeficiency 1993; 4:307–308.

Ewen C, Kane KP, Shostak I, et al: A novel cytotoxicity assay to evaluate antigen-specific CTL responses using a colorimetric substrate for granzyme B. J Immunol Methods 2003; 279:89–101.

Fleisher RA, Oliveira JB: Functional and molecular evaluation of lymphocytes. J Allergy Clin Immunol 2004;114:227–234.

Fleisher TA: Evaluation of suspected immunodeficiency. Medical Laboratory Observer 2003; February:10–21.
An overview of the application of laboratory methods to evaluate immune defects and includes a continuing education test.

Gallin JI: Recent advances in chronic granulomatous disease. Ann Intern Med 1983; 99:657–674.

Gallin JI, Malech HL: Update on chronic granulomatous diseases of childhood. JAMA 1990; 263:1533–1537.

Ganz T, Metcalf JA, Gallin JI, et al: Microbicidal/cytotoxic proteins of neutrophils are deficient in two disorders: Chediak–Higashi syndrome and 'specific' granule deficiency. J Clin Invest 1988; 82:552–556.

Gilmour KC, Cranston T, Loughlin S, et al: Rapid protein-based assays for the diagnosis of T-B+ severe combined immunodeficiency. Br J Haematol 2001; 112:671–676.

Go E and Ballas Z: Anti-pneumococcal antibody response in normal subjects. J Allergy Clin Immunol 1996; 98:205–215.

Grimbacher B, Schaffer AA, Holland SM, et al: Genetic linkage of hyper-IgE syndrome to chromosome 4. Am J Hum Genet 1999; 65:735–744.

Gross S, Blaiss MS, Herrod HG: Role of immunoglobulin subclasses and specific antibody determinations in the evaluation of recurrent infection in children. J Pediatr 1992; 121:516–522.

Hirschhorn R: Adenosine deaminase deficiency: molecular basis and recent developments. Clin Immunol Immunopathol 1995; 76:S219–S226.

Hong R: Disorders of the T-cell system. *In* Stiehm ER (ed.): Immunologic Disorders of Infants and Children, 4th ed. Philadelphia, PA, WB Saunders, 1996, pp 339–408.

Hong R: The DiGeorge anomaly (CATCH 22, DiGeorge/velocardiofacial syndrome). Semin Hematol 1998; 35:282–290.

Hoppner M, Luhm J, Schlenke P, et al: A flow-cytometry based cytotoxicity assay using stained effector cells in combination with native target cells. J Immunol Methods 2002; 267:157–163.

Illoh O.Current applications of flow cytometry in the diagnosis of primary immunodeficiency diseases. Arch Pathol Lab Med 2004; 128:23–31.

Immune Deficiency Foundation: The clinical presentation of the primary immunodeficiency diseases (physician's primer). Towson, MD, Immune Deficiency Foundation, 1992. Available on line at: www.primaryimmune.org/pubs/book_phys/book_phys.htm.

Introne W, Boissy RR, Gahl WA: Clinical, molecular and cell biological aspects of Chediak–Higashi syndrome. Mol Genet Metab 1999; 68:283–303.

Jamieson BD, Douek DC, Killian S, et al: Generation of functional thymocytes in the human adult. Immunity 1999; 10:569–575.

Jouanguy F, Doffinger R, Dupuis S, et al: IL-12 and IFN-gamma in host defense against mycobacteria and salmonella in mice and men. Curr Opin Immunol 1999; 11:3416–3451.

Kelly J, Leonard WJ: Immune deficiencies due to defects in cytokine signaling. Curr Allergy Asthma Rep 2003; 5:396–401.

Kizaki H, Sakurada T: Simple micro-assay methods for enzymes of purine metabolism. J Lab Clin Med 1977; 89:1135.

Klebanoff SJ: Myeloperoxidase. Proc Assoc Am Physicians 1999; 111:383–389.

Klein C, Lisowska-Grospierre B, LeDeist F, et al: Major histocompatibility complex class II deficiency: clinical manifestations, immunologic features, and outcome. J Pediatr 1993; 123:921–928.

Kniker WT, Lesourd BM, McBryde JL, Corriel RN: Cell-mediated immunity assessed by multitest CMT skin testing in infants and preschool children. Am J Dis Child 1985; 139:840–845.

Kobrynski L: Evaluation of a clinical scoring system for the identification of patients with a possible primary immunodeficiency (Abstract 379). Presented at the Federation of Clinical Immunology Society Meeting, 2002.

Kuijpers TW, Weening RS, Roos D: Clinical and laboratory work-up of patients with neutrophil shortage or dysfunction. J Immunol Methods 1999; 232:211–229.
This article provides a succinct overview of clinical signs and symptoms exhibited by patients, the physiology of the antimicrobial system of neutrophils, the mechanisms of assays to diagnose these aberrations, and potential treatments for affected patients.

Kruisbeek AM: Regulation of T cell development by the thymic microenvironment. Semin Immunol 1999; 11:1–70.

Lane HC, Depper JM, Greene WC, et al: Qualitative analysis of immune function in patients with the acquired immunodeficiency syndrome: evidence for a selective defect in soluble antigen recognition. N Engl J Med 1985; 313:79–84.

Lanza F. Clinical manifestation of myeloperoxidase deficiency. J Mol Med 1998; 76:676–681.

Lefranc M-P, Lefranc G, Rabbitts TH: Inherited deletion of immunoglobulin heavy chain constant region genes in normal human individuals. Nature 1982; 300:760.

Lehrer RI, Cline MJ: Leukocyte myeloperoxidase deficiency and disseminated candidiasis: the role of myeloperoxidase in resistance to infection. J Clin Invest 1969; 48:1478.

Lekstrom-Himes JA, Gallin JI: Primary immunodeficiency diseases due to defects in phagocytes. N Engl J Med 2000; 343:1703–1714.
This review article provides an overview of the immunodeficiencies due to phagocytic defects. Also features tables summarizing the syndromes with the corresponding genetic defect as well as clinical and microscopic photographs to demonstrate the manifestations of the immunodeficiencies.

Levy J, Espanol-Boren T, Thomas C: Clinical spectrum of X-linked hyper IgM syndrome. J Pediatr 1997; 131:47–54.

Lilic D, Gravenor I: Immunology of chronic mucocutaneous candidiasis. J Clin Pathol 2001; 54:81–3.

Lindegren ML, Kobrynski L, Rasmussen SA : Applying public health strategies to primary immunodeficiency diseases: A potential approach to genetic disorders. MMWR 2004; 53(RR01):1–29.
Summary of a workshop convened by CDC to discuss strategies to improve clinical outcomes of patients with primary immunodeficiencies. This summary discusses incidence and birth prevalence of primary immunodeficiency, newborn screening methods, morbidity and mortality data, and information for primary immunodeficiency registries.

Lukela M, DeGuzman D, Weinberger S, et al: Unfashionably late. N Engl J Med 2005; 352:64–69.

Malek T, Porter B, He Y. Multiple γc-dependent cytokines regulate T-cell development. Immunol Today 1999; 20:71–76.

Martin E, Bhakdi S. Flowcytometric assay for quantifying opsonophagocytosis and killing of Staphylococcus aureus by peripheral blood leukocytes. J Clin Microbiol 1992; 30:2246–2255.

Matamoros Flori N, Mila Llambi J, Espanol Boren T, et al : Primary immunodeficiency syndrome in Spain: first report of the National Registry in Children and Adult. Clin Immunol 2000; 20:477–485.

Meischl C, Roos D: The molecular basis of chronic granulomatous disease. Springer Semin Immunopathol 1998; 19:417–434.

Migone N, Oliviero S, De Lange G, et al: Multiple gene deletions within the human immunoglobulin heavy-chain cluster. Proc Natl Acad Sci USA 1984; 81:5811.

Mire-Sluis AR, Thorpe R (eds): Cytokines. San Diego, CA, Academic Press, 1998.

Myers LA, Hershfield MS, Neale WT, et al: Purine nucleoside phosphorylase deficiency (PNP-def) presenting with lymphopenia and developmental delay: successful correction with umbilical cord blood transplantation. J Pediatr 2004; 145:710–712.

Nauseef WM: Insights into myeloperoxidase biosynthesis from its inherited deficiency. J Mol Med 1998; 76:661–668.

Nekrep N, Fontes JD, Geyer M, Peterlin BM: when the lymphocyte loses its clothes. Immunity 2003; 18:453–457.

Nelson RD, Quie PG, Simmons RL: Chemotaxis under agarose: a new and simple method for measuring chemotaxis and spontaneous migration of human polymorphonuclear leukocytes and monocytes. J Imunol 1975; 115:1650.

Niemela JE, Puck JM, Fisher RE, et al: Efficient detection of thirty-seven new IL-2RG mutations in human X-linked severe combined immunodeficiency. Clin Immunol 2000; 95:33–38.

Normansell DE: Human immunoglobulin subclasses. Diagn Clin Immunol 1987; 5:115–128.

Noroski LM, Shearer WT: Screening for primary immunodeficiencies in the clinical immunology laboratory. Clin Immunol Immunopathol 1998; 86:237–245.

Notarangelo LD, Giliani S, Mella P, et al: Combined immunodeficiencies due to defects in signal transduction: defects of the gamma-JAK3 signaling pathway as a model. Immunobiology 2000; 202:106–119.

Ochs HD: The Wiskott–Aldrich syndrome. Semin Hematol 1998; 35:332–345.

Ochs HD, Davis SD, Wedgwood RJ: Immunologic responses to bacteriophage ΦX174 in immunodeficiency diseases. J Clin Invest 1971; 50:2559–2568.

O'Gorman MR, Corrochano V: Rapid whole-blood flow cytometry assay for diagnosis of chronic granulomatous disease. Clin Diagn Lab Immunol 1995; 2:227–232.

Oxelius VA: Quantitative and qualitative investigations of serum IgG subclasses in immunodeficiency diseases. Clin Exp Immunol 1979; 36:112–116.

Park BH, Fikrig SM, Smithwick EM: Infection and nitro-blue-tetrazolium reduction by neutrophils. A diagnostic aid. Lancet 1968; 2:532.

Plebani A, Ugazio AG, Monafo V, Burgio GR: Clinical heterogeneity and reversibility of selective immunoglobulin A deficiency in 80 children. Lancet 1986; 12:829–831.

Popa V: Airway obstruction in adults with recurrent respiratory infections and IgG deficiency. Chest 1994; 105:1066–1072.

Puck JM: Primary immunodeficiency diseases. JAMA 1997a;278:1835–41.

Puck JM: Genetic aspects of primary immunodeficiencies. In Ochs HD, Smith Die, Puck JM, eds. Primary Immunodeficiency Diseases: A Molecular and Genetic Approach. New York, Oxford University Press, 1999.

Puck JM, Deschenes SM, Porter JC, et al: The interleukin-2 receptor γ chain maps to Xq13.1 and is mutated in X-linked severe combined immunodeficiency. Hum Mol Genet 1993; 2:1099.

Puck JM, Middleton L, Pepper AE: Carrier and prenatal diagnosis of X-linked severe combined immunodeficiency: mutation detection methods and utilization. Hum Genet 1997b; 99:628–633.

Ramesh N, Seki M, Notarangelo LD, Geha RS: The hyper IgM (HIM) syndrome. Springer Semin Immunopathol 1998; 19:383–399.

Reith W, Mach B: The bare lymphocyte syndrome and the regulation of MHC expression. Annu Rev Immunol 2001; 19:331–373.

Ryser O, Morrell A, Hizid WE: Primary immunodeficiencies in Switzerland: first report of the nation registry in adults and children. J Clin Immunol 1988; 8:479–485.

Samarghitean C, Valiaho J, Vihinen M: Online registry of genetic and clinical immunodeficiency diagnostic laboratories, IDdiagnostics. J Clin Immunol 2004; 24:53–61.

Sarkar G, Yoon Hs, Sommer SS. Dideoxy fingerprinting (ddE): a rapid and efficient screen for the presence of mutations. Genomics 1992; 13:441–443.

Schneider PM, Wurzner R: Complement genetics: biological implications of polymorphisms and deficiencies. Immunol Today 1999; 20:2–5.

Schur PH: IgG subclasses – a review. Ann Allergy 1987; 58:89–96.

Scott MG, Schackelford PG, Briles ED, Nahm MH: Human IgG subclasses and their relation to carbohydrate antigen immunocompetence. Diagn Clin Immunol 1988; 5:241–248.

Sebire NJ, Haselden S, Malone M, et al: Isolated EBV lymphoproliferative disease in a child with Wiskott–Aldrich syndrome manifesting as cutaneous lymphomatoid granulomatosis and responsive to anti-CD20 immunotherapy. J Clin Pathol 2003; 56:555–557.

Shackelford PG, Granoff DM, Madassery JV, et al: Clinical and immunologic characteristics of healthy children with subnormal serum concentrations of IgG2. Pediatr Res 1990; 27:16.

Shearer WT, Paul ME, Smith CW, Huston DP: Laboratory assessment of immune deficiency disorders. Immunol Allergy Clin North Am 1994:14:265–299.

Sheffield VC, Beck JS, Kwitek AE, et al: The sensitivity of single stand conformation polymorphism analysis for the detection of single base substitutions. Genomics 1993; 16:325–332.

Shovlin CL, Simmon HA, Fairbanks LD, et al: Adult onset immunodeficiency caused by inherited adenosine deaminase deficiency. J Immunol 1994; 153:2331–2339.

Smith CIE, Ochs HD, Puck JM: Genetically determined immunodeficiency diseases: a perspective. In: Ochs HD, Smith CIE, Puck JM, eds. Primary Immunodeficiency Diseases: A Molecular and Genetic Approach. New York, Oxford University Press, 1999.

Southwick FS, Dabiri GA, Stossel TP: Neutrophil actin dysfunction is a genetic disorder associated with partial impairment of neutrophil actin assembly in three family members. J Clin Invest 1988; 82:1525–1531.

Stiehm ER, Conley ME: Immunodeficiency disorders: general considerations. In Stiehm ER (ed.): Immunologic Disorders of Infants and Children, 4th ed. Philadelphia, PA, WB Saunders, 1996, pp 201–252.

Stray-Pedersen A, Abrahamsen TG, Froland SS: Primary immunodeficiency diseases in Norway. Clin Immunol 1997; 17:333–339.

Sweinberg SK, Wodell RA, Grodofsky MP, et al: Retrospective analysis of the incidence of pulmonary disease in hypogammaglobulinemia. J Allergy Clin Immunol 1991; 88:96–104.

Trinchieri G: Biology of natural killer cells. Adv Immunol 1989; 47:187–376.

Vihinen M, Kwan SP, Lester T, et al: Mutations of the human BTK gene coding for bruton tyrosine kinase in X-linked agammaglobulinemia. Hum Mutat 1999; 13:280–285.

Wakim M, Shah A, Arndt PA, et al: Successful anti-CD20 monoclonal antibody treatment of severe autoimmune hemolytic anemia due to warm reactive IgM autoantibody in a child with common variable immunodeficiency. Am J Hematol 2004; 76:152–155.

Wedgwood RJ, Ochs HD, Oxelius VA: IgG subclass levels in the serum of patients with primary immunodeficiency. Monogr Allergy 1986; 20:80.

Winkelstein JA, Marino MC, Johnston RB Jr, et al: Chronic granulomatous disease. Report on a national registry of 368 patients. Medicine (Baltimore) 2000; 79:155–169.

Yabe T, Kawamura S, Masako S, et al: A subject with a novel type I bare lymphocyte syndrome has tapasin deficiency due to deletion of 4 exons by Alu-mediated recombination. Blood 2002; 100:1496–1498.

Zhu Q, Watanabe C, Liu T, et al : Wiskott–Alrich syndrome/X-linked thrombocytopenia: WASP gene mutations, protein expression, and phenotype. Blood 1997; 90:2680–2689.

VI

CHAPTER 50

Clinical and Laboratory Evaluation of Systemic Rheumatic Diseases

Carlos Alberto von Mühlen MD PhD, Robert M. Nakamura MD

KEY POINTS

- There are many types of autoantibody to intracellular and nuclear antigens in the various systemic rheumatic diseases. Currently, it is considered important not only to detect the presence and quantity of the intracellular and nuclear autoantibody in the patient, but also to identify its immunological specificity.

- Past studies have shown that distinct diagnostic profiles of autoantibodies are observed in many of the rheumatic diseases. Some of the diseases are characterized by the presence or absence of a specific antibody, or by differences in the quantitative level or titer of the autoantibody.

- Much progress has been made in improvement of the sensitivity, specificity, and quality control of the many laboratory tests for the detection of autoantibodies to intracellular and nuclear antigens.

- Immunofluorescence microscopy using human cellular extracts, such as HEp-2 cells, allows for the sensitive detection of serum antibodies that react very specifically with various cellular proteins and nucleic acids.

- Widely used tests for screening of intracellular autoantibodies are immunofluorescence microscopy and the immunoenzyme tests. The secondary definitive tests for specific identification of autoantibodies to nuclear antigens are immunodiffusion, immunoprecipitation, particle agglutination, enzyme-linked immunosorbent assay (ELISA), and immunoblotting methods.

- Molecular biologists have used many of the autoantibodies as biological probes and have elucidated the biological functions of several of the autoantigens.

Introduction and Classification of Systemic Rheumatic Diseases

The rheumatic diseases are characterized by the presence of one or more autoantibodies that may be directed against components of the surface, cytoplasm, nuclear envelope, or nucleus of the cell. The last group, autoantibodies to nuclear antigens (ANAs), is a hallmark of the systemic rheumatic diseases (Tan, 1982, 1989; Nakamura, 1985, 1986, 1992; von Mühlen & Tan, 1994). Many of the rheumatic diseases have a distinctive

Table 50–1 Systemic Rheumatic Diseases and Related Disorders

1. Systemic lupus erythematosus (SLE)
2. Discoid lupus erythematosus (DLE)
3. Lupus-like syndromes
4. Drug-induced lupus erythematosus
5. Sjögren's syndrome
6. Scleroderma/CREST syndrome (calcinosis cutis, Raynaud's phenomenon, esophageal dysmotility, sclerodactyly, and telangiectasia)
7. Rheumatoid arthritis (RA)
8. Dermatomyositis and polymyositis
9. Overlap syndromes
   a. Mixed Connective Tissue Disease (MCTD)
   b. RA and SLE (Rupus)
   c. SLE and scleroderma (Lupoderma)
   d. Scleroderma and dermatomyositis (Sclerodermatomyositis)
   e. Other
10. Systemic vasculitis
    a. Takayasu's arteritis
    b. Giant cell arteritis and polymyalgia rheumatica
    c. Wegener's granulomatosis
    d. Polyarteritis nodosa and Churg–Strauss syndrome
    e. Leukocytoclastic vasculitis
    f. Other
11. Poorly defined connective tissue disease syndromes

Table 50–2 1997 Update of the 1982 Revised Criteria for Classification of Systemic Lupus Erythematosus

1. Malar rash
2. Discoid rash
3. Photosensitivity
4. Oral ulcers
5. Nonerosive arthritis
6. Serositis (pleuritis or pericarditis)
7. Renal disorder (persistent proteinuria, cellular casts)
8. Neurologic disorder
9. Hematological disorder
   a. hemolytic anemia with reticulocytosis, OR
   b. leukopenia <4000/mm^3 on ≥2 occasions, OR
   c. lymphopenia <1500/mm^3 on ≥2 occasions, OR
   d. thrombocytopenia <100 000/mm^3 in the absence of offending drug
10. Immunologic disorder
    a. anti-DNA: antibody to native DNA in abnormal titer, OR
    b. anti-Sm: presence of antibody to Sm nuclear antigen, OR
    c. positive finding of antiphospholipid antibodies based on: 1) an abnormal serum level of IgG or IgM anticardiolipin antibodies, 2) a positive test result for lupus anticoagulant using a standard method, or 3) a false-positive test result for syphilis known to be positive for at least 6 months and confirmed by *Treponema pallidum* immobilization or fluorescent treponemal antibody absorption test
11. Positive antinuclear antibody
    An abnormal titer of antinuclear antibody by immunofluorescence or an equivalent assay at any point in time and in the absence of drugs known to be associated with 'drug-induced lupus' syndrome

The proposed classification is based on 11 criteria. For the purpose of identifying patients in clinical studies, a person shall be said to have SLE if any four or more of the 11 criteria are present, serially or simultaneously, during any interval of observation (Hochberg, 1997).

profile of autoantibodies with diagnostic specificities. Moreover, the biochemical and biological functions of many of the antigens involved in deoxyribonucleic acid (DNA) replication, splicing of ribonucleic acid (RNA) precursor, and RNA processing were elucidated (Tan, 1989). Classification of the various rheumatic diseases has been difficult because of a lack of a firm etiologic basis for most of the diseases. A comprehensive classification was developed by Decker and the glossary subcommittee of the American College of Rheumatology (Decker, 1986), still in use. Our abridged classification of the systemic rheumatic diseases and related disorders is shown in Table 50–1.

Systemic Lupus Erythematosus and Related Lupus-Like Disorders

Systemic lupus erythematosus (SLE) is the prototype systemic rheumatic disease and has the following significant features (Nakamura, 1994a):
1. SLE is a non-organ-specific autoimmune disease in which the tissue injury is mediated primarily by DNA–anti-DNA immune complexes.
2. It is a multisystem disease that affects persons of all ages and both sexes, although it is most prevalent in women during childbearing years.
3. The disease demonstrates a hyperactive immune system with multiple abnormalities.
4. Patients with SLE demonstrate a heterogeneous and polyclonal antibody response, with autoantibody formation reaction involving similar mechanisms to those seen in a typical immune response to foreign immunogens (Fatenejad, 1998)
5. The typical case of SLE has an average of three different circulating antibodies present simultaneously. The prevalence of antibodies varies over a wide range, and more than 110 different types of autoantibodies have been identified in SLE (Sherer, 2004).

Etiologic Factors in Systemic Lupus Erythematosus

The etiology is still poorly known. Some of the important etiologic factors in SLE are (1) endocrine–metabolic, (2) environmental, and (3) genetic (Chan, 1989). The strongest risk factor for the development of SLE is female gender (Hochberg, 1990). SLE has been considered to have a possible viral etiology (Pincus, 1982). The presence of antinuclear antibodies was determined in female laboratory workers with varying degrees of exposure to blood from patients with SLE. The presence of anti-native-DNA antibodies was higher in laboratory workers than in an unexposed nonlaboratory group of women (p <0.001) (Zarmbinski, 1992). These results help support a hypothesis that a transmissible agent that can cause autoantibody formation may exist in the blood of patients with SLE.

Certain chemicals have been implicated in SLE (Hochberg, 1990). The syndrome of drug-induced lupus with hydralazine, procainamide, and isoniazid has been studied for clues to the pathogenesis of SLE. There have been varying reports that show the acetylation mechanism as a risk factor in SLE. Studies have demonstrated a greater concordance rate of SLE among monozygotic and dizygotic twins (Block, 1975). The concordance of SLE was present in 11 (58%) of 19 monozygotic twins. The end result of the interaction of multiple etiologic factors is polyclonal activation of B cells in SLE patients with production of a wide spectrum of antibodies (Nakamura,1994a; Sherer, 2004).

What Are the Diagnostic Criteria for Systemic Lupus Erythematosus?

In 1971, the American College of Rheumatology (ACR; previously the American Rheumatism Association [ARA]), published preliminary criteria for the classification of SLE (Cohen, 1971). Patients were considered to have SLE if four of the criteria were met sequentially or simultaneously during any interval of observation. In 1982, the Subcommittee for SLE Criteria of the ARA published revised criteria that incorporated new immunologic knowledge and improved the disease classification of SLE (Tan, 1982b). The 1982 revised criteria for classification of SLE included 11 categories, adding (1) abnormal titer of antinuclear antibody by immunofluorescence or an equivalent assay, and (2) antibody to native DNA and/or Sm antigen. In contrast to the 1971 criteria, the 1982 criteria removed Raynaud's phenomenon and alopecia because of their lack of sensitivity and specificity.

When the 1982 ARA Criteria for Classification of SLE were compared with the 1971 criteria, there was definite improvement in sensitivity and specificity. The 1982 criteria showed a 96.7% sensitivity and 96% specificity when evaluated with known SLE and control patients (Tan, 1982). In 1997, an update of the criteria was published, in which the LE cell test was dropped and anticardiolipin antibodies were added (Table 50–2). These changes were emphasized in the 'Guidelines for referral and management of SLE in adults' by the ACR Ad Hoc Committee on SLE Guidelines (Gladman, 1999).

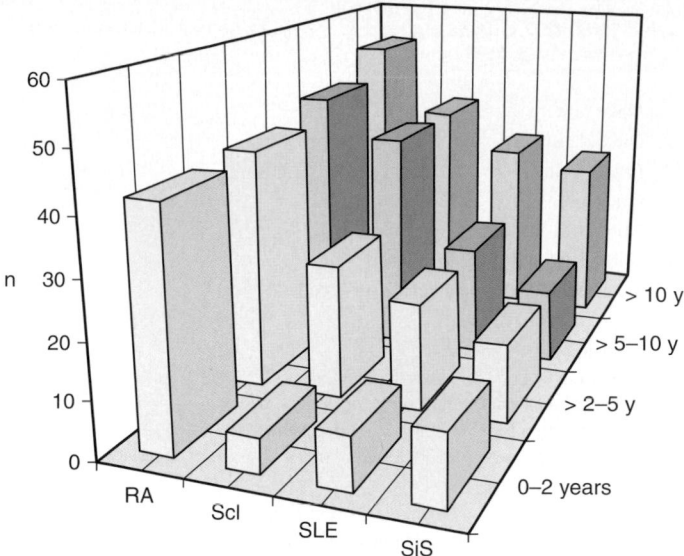

Figure 50–1 Classification criteria fulfilled by 99 patients with anti-U1nRNP antibodies during more than 10 years of observation. Many patients in this cohort were classified as undifferentiated connective tissue disease in the first 2 years of clinical symptoms, while 43 individuals could be classified as having rheumatoid arthritis (RA). The number of RA-classified patients did not grow significantly towards the end of the study, but diagnoses of systemic lupus erythematosus (SLE) and scleroderma (Scl) were fulfilled more often ($p = 0.02$ and 0.0008 respectively, Chi-square for trend). Patients developing SLE had low titers of anti-U1nRNP antibodies and were HLA-DR2/3. Those developing Scl had high anti-U1nRNP titers and were HLA-DR4. SjS = Sjögren syndrome. Source: von Mühlen CA, Genth E, Mierau R, unpublished data.

What Are 'Lupus-Like' Syndromes and Diseases?

There are many diseases and syndromes that may share certain clinical features with SLE but are not SLE and have differing etiologies and pathogeneses. Diseases that have been listed in this category include vasculitis, cryoglobulinemia, relapsing polychondritis, lymphoproliferative diseases, rheumatic fever, glomerulonephritis, syphilis, lupoid hepatitis, drug-induced lupus, and occult malignancy (Panush, 1993). There is a very broad category of patients who demonstrate fewer than four of the 1982 ARA classification criteria for SLE (Lazaro, 1989; Lom-Orta, 1980; Schur, 1993) but are considered to have 'lupus like' illnesses. These patients have been classified as follows: (1) undifferentiated rheumatic disease, (2) nonrheumatic disease, (3) overlap syndrome, and (4) incomplete, latent or incipient lupus. Schur recommended, similarly to the early ARA criteria for the diagnosis of rheumatoid arthritis (RA), that patients be labeled as having classic SLE (many criteria), definite SLE (four or more criteria), probable SLE (three criteria), or possible SLE (two criteria). The patients with two or three criteria may be considered as incomplete, incipient, or latent, as well as possible and probable lupus (Schur, 1993).

If these patients are followed, some stay with mild symptoms – and as such remain labeled as 'undifferentiated connective tissue disease' (UCTD), a few may develop definite SLE, but many evolve into other diseases with a better prognosis. Actually, up to 75% of patients with UCTD never fulfill diagnostic criteria for specific systemic rheumatic diseases (Mosca, 2004). In our hands, 99 patients with anti-U1nRNP antibodies followed for 10 years, many diagnosed as UCTD when entering the cohort, developed characteristic signs and symptoms of rheumatoid arthritis, Sjögren syndrome, systemic lupus or scleroderma (Fig. 50–1), according to their human leukocyte antigen (HLA) profile and antibody titers.

Autoantibody Profile in Systemic Lupus Erythematosus

Characteristic of SLE is the presence of a broad spectrum of autoantibodies, including antibody to native DNA (dsDNA), chromatin, Sm antigen, U1nRNP, SS-A/Ro, SS-B/La, and several other nonhistone protein or nonhistone protein–RNA complexes (Nakamura, 1994a; Sherer, 2004). Polyclonality of antibodies is seen in SLE and scleroderma, and is rarely seen in the other systemic rheumatic diseases. Anti-native-DNA, anti-Sm, anti-ribosomal-RNP, and antibody to proliferating cell nuclear antigen (anti-PCNA) are generally specific for SLE. SLE is characterized by a heterogeneous and polyclonal antibody response, and the usual case of SLE has an average of three different circulating antibodies present

Table 50–3 Antigens and Autoantibodies in Systemic Lupus Erythematosus

Antigen	Molecular Structure	Autoantibody Frequency (%)
Native DNA	Double-strand DNA	40–90
Denatured DNA	Single-strand DNA	70
Histones	H1, H2A, H2B, H3, H4	50–70
Chromatin (nucleosome)	DNA-histones complex	50–90
Sm	Proteins 29 (B'), 28 (B), 16 (D), and 13(E) kDa, complexed with U1, U2, and U4-U6 snRNAs; spliceosome component	15–30
Nuclear RNP (U1nRNP)	Proteins 70, 33(A), and 22 (C) kDa, complexed with U1 snRNA; spliceosome component	30–40
SS-A/Ro	Proteins 60 and 52 kDa, complexed with Y1-Y5 RNAs	24–60
SS-B/La	Phosphoproteins 48 kDa, complexed with Y1 nascent RNA Pol transcripts	9–35
Ku	Proteins 86 and 66 kDa, DNA-binding proteins	1–19
hnRNP protein A1	Nuclear protein 34 kDa	31–37
PCNA	Protein 36 kDa; auxiliary protein of DNA polymerase	3
Ribosomal RNP	Phosphoproteins 38, 16, and 15 kDa associated with ribosomes	10–20
Hsp-90	Heat-shock protein 90 kDa	5–50
Golgi complex	Golgins, giantin	Unknown
HMG-17	DNA-associated proteins, 9 to 17 kDa	34–70
β_2-glycoprotein I	Anionic phospholipids, cardiolipin	25

Frequencies are mostly related to patients with active disease.

PCNA = proliferating cell nuclear antigen; RNP = ribonucleoproteins.

Source: modified from Nakamura, 1994a; Krapf, 1996; Sherer, 2004.

simultaneously. The prevalence of autoantibodies varies over a wide range. Antibodies to native DNA and chromatin are detectable in up to 90% of patients, and antibodies to PCNA and cyclin or Alu-RNA protein are seen in 3% or fewer (von Mühlen, 1995) (Table 50–3).

Antibodies to Native DNA or Double-Stranded DNA

Anti-double-stranded-DNA (ds-DNA) antibodies are rather specific for SLE and are observed at a frequency of 40–90% in SLE patients with active disease (Buskila, 1992; Rekvig, 2003). There have been many earlier reports of antibodies to ds-DNA in diseases other than SLE. However, current thinking is that the reactive antibodies to DNA in the other diseases were actually anti-single-stranded-DNA antibodies. The ds-DNA antibody tests often used ds-DNA preparations contaminated with denatured or single-stranded DNA. One possible exception could appear in primary Sjögren's syndrome, a disease sometimes difficult to differentiate from SLE in older people. Antibody to DNA plays a definite role in the pathogenesis of SLE. In studies of SLE patients, antibody to DNA is followed by the appearance of circulating DNA antigen, a sequence of events that results in the formation of immune complexes. Such DNA–anti-DNA immune complexes, mostly containing complement-activating IgG3, have a special tropism for basement membranes and are readily deposited in the kidney glomeruli. This initiates kidney damage through inflammatory mechanisms that end up with complement activation and cell lysis (Okamura, 1993). Earlier methods for detection of DNA antibodies were the insensitive precipitation method, complement fixation, and passive hemagglutination. Current methods used are radioimmunoassay (RIA), indirect immunofluorescence (IFA) on *Crithidia luciliae*, and enzyme-linked immunosorbent assay (ELISA) (Buskila, 1992; Kavanaugh, 2002). These can detect anti-DNA in 75–90% of active untreated SLE patients. Transient increases in anti-DNA antibodies were recently described in RA patients treated with anti-TNF therapy (Allanore, 2004; Bobbio-Pallavicini, 2004). Occasional clinical lupus-like cases may occur in this situation (Swale, 2003; Eriksson, 2005).

Antibodies to Sm and Nuclear Ribonucleoprotein

Precipitating antibodies to Sm antigen have been considered highly specific markers for SLE (Tan, 1989). Antibodies to both Sm and nuclear ribonucleoproteins (nRNP) are found in patients with SLE. The Sm and nRNP antigens were clearly associated, because the nRNP could not be biochemically isolated from the Sm antigen. Lerner and Steitz (1979) used the tools of molecular biology to show that Sm and nRNP antigens were subcellular particles comprised of small nuclear RNAs complexed with proteins. The particle bound by anti-nRNP is composed of an RNA component designated U1 (U for uridine-rich), complexed to at least seven proteins varying in molecular mass from 12 to 68 kDa (Tan, 1989), found at a frequency of 30–40% in active SLE (Ter Borg, 1990).

The antigens of Sm consist of several proteins, conventionally called B1 (29 kDa), D (16 kDa), and E (13 kDa) (Tan, 1989). Purified anti-B1/B antibodies cross-react with the D protein and vice versa, but no cross-reaction is observed in a smaller percentage of SLE sera. Thus, there are at least two epitopes on the B1/B protein recognized by anti-Sm sera. Antigens reactive with anti-Sm and antinuclear RNA are therefore in assemblies of interactive proteins and RNAs engaged in precursor nRNA splicing (Tan,1989). No characteristic clinical features are apparent in SLE patients with anti-Sm antibodies (Barada, 1981), although some authors claim these autoantibodies to be associated with renal disease or to disorders of the central nervous system. Patients who have antibodies to only nRNP have a low frequency of antibodies to DNA and a low frequency of clinically apparent renal disease (Ter Borg, 1990). Anti-Sm and anti-nRNP antibodies may be detected by immunodiffusion, passive hemagglutination, or counterimmunoelectrophoresis. However, the above-mentioned methods do not accurately distinguish between antibodies against different small nuclear-RNA-associated polypeptides. The reactivities with individual RNAs and polypeptides can be best demonstrated by RNA immuno-precipitation and immunoblotting techniques, respectively. Immunoblotting has been found to be more sensitive than conventional methods for the detection of anti-Sm and anti-nRNP (Nakamura, 1994b). Currently, the most widely used laboratory tests for the detection of anti-Sm and anti-nRNP antibodies are immunodiffusion and ELISA. These tests can differentiate between Sm and nRNP antibodies but cannot define the specific antibody epitopes present in patients' sera. The antibody specificity and epitopes are best determined by Western and Northern blotting methods.

Antibodies to SS-A/Ro and SS-B/La

Patients with SLE can have antibodies to SS-A/Ro alone or may have both anti-SS-A/Ro and anti-SS-B/La. Having anti-SS-A/Ro alone is strongly associated with HLA DR2 and with being young (<22 years of age at onset). The presence of both anti-SS-A/Ro and anti-SS-B/La in SLE is associated with HLA-DR3 and is seen in older patients (>50 years of age at disease onset) (Hochberg, 1985). A study of 55 patients with SLE showed that patients with anti-SS-A/Ro alone had much more serious renal disease (Hochberg, 1985). The SLE patients with only anti-SS-A/Ro also had a higher incidence of concomitant anti-DNA antibodies than those SLE patients with both the anti-SS-A/Ro and anti- SS-B/La antibodies (Chan, 1989). Anti-SS-A/Ro autoantibodies have been closely associated with the appearance of nephritis, vasculitis, lymphadenopathy, photosensitivity and leukopenia in SLE patients. Anti-SS-B/La antibodies, like anti-SS-A/Ro antibodies, are antibodies noteworthy for their strong association with Sjögren's syndrome, occurring in more than two thirds of patients with this disorder. The SS-B/La antigen is a cellular protein bound to a small RNA species, forming a small RNP that may function in processing of RNA polymerase III transcripts (Chan, 1989).

Clinical Subsets of Systemic Lupus Erythematosus Associated with Antibodies to SS-A/Ro

Elevated levels of SS-A/Ro antibodies are related to several clinical autoimmune disorders, including: (1) subacute cutaneous lupus erythe-matosus, (2) neonatal lupus erythematosus syndrome with congenital heart block and cutaneous lesions, (3) homozygous C2 and C4 deficiency with SLE-like disease, (4) primary Sjögren's syndrome vasculitis, rheumatoid factor positivity and severe systemic symptoms, (5) ANA-negative SLE

patients, and (6) SLE with interstitial pneumonitis (Bylund, 1991). Precipitating antibodies to SS-A/Ro are seen in 65–95% of patients with anti-SS-A/Ro associated subsets, and more than 90% of the patients have anti-SS-A/Ro levels when detected by ELISA methods (Bylund,1991).

Anti-Ku and Anti-Ki Antibodies

The Ku-antigen system consists of a pair of proteins called p70/p80 (Francoeur, 1986; Reeves, 1992). These proteins have a high affinity for DNA and are known to be DNA-binding proteins, interacting covalently with the ends of native DNA. With the use of both immunoprecipitation and immunoblot assays, the Ku autoantibody was found in 10% of SLE sera and was not detected in 100 scleroderma sera examined. In studies with an enzyme immunoassay, Reeves showed that 39% of SLE, 55% of mixed connective tissue disease (MCTD), and 40% of scleroderma patients had low levels of antibody to Ku protein (Reeves, 1992). Anti-Ki antibody was first reported in Japan (Tojo, 1981) and was observed in approximately 10% of SLE patients. A relationship was observed between anti-Ki and the clinical features of arthritis, pericarditis, and pulmonary hypertension in SLE patients. The Ki antigen was purified from rabbit thymus and had a molecular weight of 32 kDa. Sakamoto (1989) developed an ELISA and observed anti-Ki antibodies in 21% (30/140) of SLE patients, while 11 of 140 were positive for anti-Ki by double-immunodiffusion tests.

Antibodies to P Ribosomal Proteins

Some 10–20% of SLE sera show autoantibodies targeting three ribosomal phosphoproteins of 15, 18, and 38 kDa in Western blot assays. Association of anti-rRNPs with major central nervous system disorders in SLE, mainly psychotic symptoms, was reported in a retrospective study (Bonfa, 1987). No association was shown with cognitive impairment or depression in lupus patients. Significant differences in the prevalence of anti-rRNP are found among races. These antibodies occur in a higher frequency together with anti-Sm and anti-U1nRNP antibodies in SLE (Yalaoui, 2002). The etiopathogenic role of anti-rRNP in central nervous system symptoms of lupus patients is not conclusive so far (Nakamura, 1997; Isshi, 1998). Recent observations in bigger samples of SLE patients showed association of anti-rRNP antibodies with hemolytic anemia, leukopenia, alopecia, malar rash, proteinuria, and neurologic complications (Hoffman, 2004; Mahler 2006). There was no correlation with disease activity.

Proliferating Cell Nuclear Antigen Multiprotein Complex

Antibodies to PCNA proteins are detected in 3% of patients with active SLE and show no distinctive clinical associations (Miyachi, 1978; Kaneda, 2004). A possible association with central nervous system features, such as transverse myelitis, has been seen in our own patients (von Mühlen & Nakamura, unpublished results). The PCNA complex has been characterized as cell-cycle-related, and PCNA antibodies have been useful probes in the study of agents regulating DNA replication, cell proliferation, and blast transformation.

Antiphospholipid Antibodies in Systemic Lupus Erythematosus

The lupus anticoagulant/antiphospholipid antibody syndrome is characterized by the presence of circulating antibodies to phospholipids and clinical features of arterial and venous thrombosis, thrombocytopenia, hemolytic anemia, miscarriages, and several systemic symptoms. Anti-phospholipid antibodies have been found frequently in patients with SLE, and also in other disorders such as infectious diseases (McNeil, 1991; Alarcón-Segovia, 1992). Antiphospholipid antibodies are found in up to 60% of patients with SLE. This is a very heterogeneous family of antibodies, functionally and immunochemically (McNeil, 1991). Cardiolipin (anionic phospholipid) has been widely used for the detection of antiphospholipid antibodies. The majority of anticardiolipin antibodies cross-react with zwitterionic phospholipids (McNeil, 1991). Antibodies to anionic phospholipids may be IgG or IgM, whereas antibodies to zwitterionic phospholipids are more frequently IgM.

Antibodies to phospholipids are identified in SLE patients in three ways (Alarcón-Segovia, 1992): (1) serologically false-positive test for syphilis by a positive Venereal Disease Research Laboratory (VDRL) test, which is a flocculation assay using carbon particles coated with cholesterol, lecithin (phosphatidylcholine), and cardiolipin; (2) the lupus anticoagulant assay, which is a prolongation of the kaolin partial thromboplastin time that is not corrected by normal plasma; and (3) cardiolipin immunoassay with the use of cardiolipin or other negatively charged phospholipids as antigens and β_2-glycoprotein I as co-factor. Patients with SLE will usually react with a negatively charged phosphate group present in cardiolipin, phosphatidic acid, phosphatidylserine, or phosphatidylinositol.

Harris (1987, 1990) convened international workshops to improve the precision and accuracy of antiphospholipid antibody immunoassays. Reference sera were prepared and standard units (GPL and MPL) were defined. One GPL (MPL) unit is equivalent to 1 mg/mL of an affinity-purified standard IgG (IgM) sample. However, Lopez (1992) suggested that an IgA-specific assay for antiphospholipid antibody is important in assessing the antiphospholipid syndrome in patients with SLE. A higher prevalence of the IgA isotype seems to be found in black persons.

Newly developed assays for β_2-glycoprotein I autoantibodies seem to bring specificity to the findings, since it was described that the β_2-glycoprotein is the specific epitope for anti-phospholipid autoantibodies (Obermoser, 2004). Furthermore, IgA antibodies targeting β_2-glycoprotein I, or antibodies recognizing a complex of β_2-GP I/oxLDL (oxidized low-density lipoprotein) seem to be pathogenic in atherosclerotic vascular disease (Staub, 2003; Matsuura, 2004; Ranzolin, 2004).

Chronic Discoid Lupus and Other Cutaneous Variants

A benign form of lupus may present as 'discoid' (coin- or disc-shaped) cutaneous lesions without symptoms of systemic disease. This disorder is called chronic discoid lupus erythematosus (CDLE) (Sontheimer, 1992; Wallace, 1992). The clinical and laboratory characteristics of CDLE have not been clearly delineated since adoption of the revised 1982 American College of Rheumatology Criteria for The Classification of SLE. The skin lesions of CDLE are as follows: (1) persistent localized erythema, (2) adherent scales, (3) follicular plugging, (4) telangiectasis, and (5) atrophy (Wallace, 1992). Subacute cutaneous lupus erythematosus (SCLE), another similar skin condition, consists of papulosquamous or nonscarring lesions with a major association to SS-A/Ro autoantibodies. Also, additional variants of CDLE, such as lupus panniculitis (also called lupus profundus) and urticarial lupus, have been described (Sontheimer, 1992).

Wallace (1992) has defined CDLE as the fulfillment of the description of CDLE or SCLE, or one of the variants of SLE, in which the 1982 ACR/Criteria for SLE are not met. Unfortunately, CDLE is a cutaneous autoimmune disorder that lacks any unifying diagnostic serological abnormality. It is a mild form of lupus erythematosus that uncommonly disseminates to SLE. Otherwise, there is considerable overlap between CDLE and SLE, since up to 15% of patients with SLE have cutaneous discoid lesions. About 6–12% of patients with SLE had discoid lupus for a varying number of years before the onset of systemic disease (Wallace, 1992). Antinuclear antibodies are commonly found, with estimates of prevalence in discoid lupus from 6–50%. The sex ratio of discoid lupus (2 females:1 male) is much less biased toward females than the systemic form.

Drug-induced Lupus Erythematosus, Antihistone, and Antichromatin Antibodies

Characteristic of drug-induced lupus is the presence of histone autoantibodies. Histones are basic molecular proteins containing high molar ratios of the positively charged amino acids lysine and arginine. Histones are found in eukaryotic cells closely associated with genomic DNA. The subunit of this histone–DNA complex is called a nucleosome, which has two molecules of each of the 'core' histones (H2A, H2B, H3, and H4) and one molecule of H1, along with DNA of about 200 base pairs in length (Rubin, 1985, 1987).

In studies of drug-induced lupus, the liver enzyme acetyltransferase appears to play an important role (Woosley, 1987). Acetyltransferase is an enzyme that can acetylate drugs such as hydralazine and procainamide, playing an important role in detoxification and excretion of the drug. Patients with low levels of acetyltransferase were more prone to develop ANA and clinical symptoms than patients who were treated with hydralazine and had phenotypically high levels of acetyltransferase. Patients with high levels of enzyme and who were rapid acetylators were not immune to the development of ANA. These patients, however, took a longer and larger cumulative dose of hydralazine before developing disease. These findings concerning acetyltransferase phenotypes have been confirmed in patients treated with procainamide (Rubin, 1988). Procainamide is the most common drug involved in drug-induced autoimmunity. Hydralazine, quinidine, and other drugs have also been implicated as causing drug-induced autoimmunity.

In drug-induced lupus, antibodies to single-stranded DNA and histones are present. In SLE, on the other hand, antibodies to double-stranded native DNA, Sm, and U1nRNP antigens are often present, in addition to

the antibodies to histones. Procainamide is used to treat patients with cardiac arrhythmias, and most patients eventually develop antihistone antibodies. However, only 10–20% of procainamide-treated patients develop symptomatic autoimmune disease (Rubin, 1988). In the asymptomatic patients, the antihistone antibody is predominantly IgM and displays broad reactivity with all of the individual histones. Patients with symptomatic disease develop a unique type of IgG antihistone antibody, which, rather than reacting with individual histones, shows specific reactivity with the histone H2A–H2B dimer complex (Rubin, 1988). Thus, the IgG anti-(H2A–H2B) is a useful diagnostic marker, with high sensitivity and specificity for symptomatic disease, in contrast to the benign form of procainamide-induced autoimmunity, with IgM antibodies to the individual histone. In both types of drug-induced lupus erythematosus (hydralazine and procainamide), IgM antibodies were present in higher concentrations than IgG antibodies.

Some 50% of all patients treated with procainamide developed ANAs after 1 year of treatment (Tan, 1989). The slow acetylators developed ANAs more rapidly than the rapid acetylators (Woosley, 1987). All patients on prolonged procainamide treatment developed a positive ANA response irrespective of acetylator phenotype.

Since antihistone antibodies are found in many other conditions, more specific antibodies such as antichromatin are replacing assays for antihistones. Synonyms for antichromatin antibodies are LE cell factor, antinucleosome, antideoxyribonucleoprotein (DNP), and anti-(H2A–H2B-DNA). They are found in 75% of all patients with SLE, in up to 100% of drug-induced lupus patients, and in 20–50% of patients with autoimmune hepatitis type I (lupoid hepatitis). In SLE patients, antichromatin antibodies correlate better with kidney disease than anti-dsDNA (Burlingame, 2002, 2004; Cervera, 2003).

Sjögren's Syndrome

Sjögren's syndrome is a chronic progressive inflammatory autoimmune disease marked by dryness of the eyes, mouth, and other mucous membranes (Schumacher, 1993; Ramos-Casals, 2005). The disease may evolve from exocrine glands to a systemic disorder, as well as to B-cell lymphoproliferative transformation. It is much more frequently found in women than men, with an increasing prevalence throughout adult life. Often associated with Sjögren's syndrome is another rheumatic disease, such as RA, SLE, primary biliary cirrhosis, or systemic sclerosis (Table 50–4). The affected salivary or lacrimal glands are infiltrated with aggregates of lymphocytes. Extraglandular manifestations include lymphadenopathy, cutaneous vasculitis, and interstitial pneumonitis.

The disease has been classified into (1) primary Sjögren syndrome, which is not associated with another connective tissue disease, and (2) secondary Sjögren's syndrome, in which RA or some other autoimmune disorder is present. Sjögren's syndrome is known to occur in a primary form, with the sicca complex (keratoconjunctivitis sicca and xerostomia) as its hallmark feature. Autoantibodies in Sjögren's syndrome are normally restricted to SS-A/Ro and SS-B/La antigens (Tan, 1989) but we have seen patients with other specificities alone, like anti-Golgi complex or anti-NuMA. The anti-SS-A/Ro and anti-SS-B/La are present in SLE but in lower prevalences than in Sjögren's syndrome. Anti-SS-B/La is seen in 60% of Sjögren's syndrome patients and in 35% of SLE patients, and anti-SS-A/La is seen in 40% and 15%, respectively (von Mühlen, 1995). The presence of anti-SS-A/Ro, when associated with anti-SS-B/La, is indicative of primary Sjögren's syndrome, at times coexisting with SLE. The presence of anti-SS-B antibodies is less than 1% in RA (Tan, 1988). There is a striking association between anti-SS-A/Ro and the presence of both systemic and

---

Table 50–4 Frequent clinical associations with Sjögren's syndrome.

1. Rheumatoid arthritis
2. Systemic lupus erythematosus
3. Polydermatomyositis
4. Mixed connective tissue disease
5. Primary biliary cirrhosis
6. Necrotizing systemic vasculitis
7. Autoimmune thyroiditis
8. Chronic active hepatitis
9. Mixed cryoglobulinemia
10. Hypergammaglobulinemic purpura

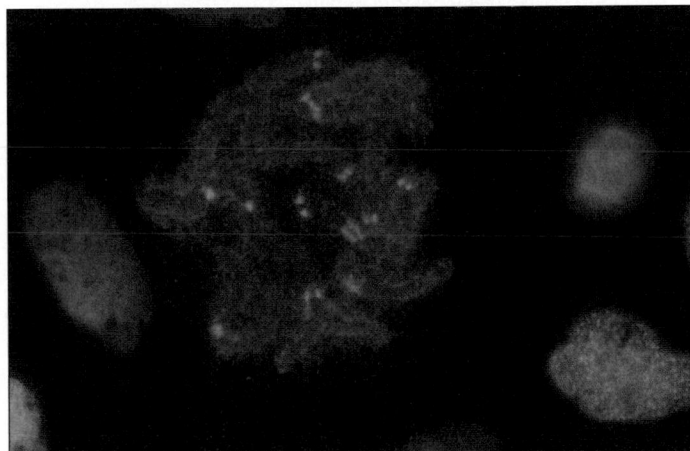

Figure 50–2 Antinuclear antibody in Sjögren's syndrome. Fine speckled nuclear pattern by indirect immunofluorescence assay on HEp-2 cells, characteristic for the presence of anti-SSA/Ro autoantibodies.

cutaneous vasculitis (Bylund, 1991). The association of SS-A/Ro antibody and vasculitis has been observed in patients with unclassified connective tissue disease. Determination of anti-α-fodrin autoantibodies, which are also found in RA sera, does not add much to the diagnosis of Sjögren's syndrome (Ruffatti, 2004; Zandbelt, 2004). The antinuclear antibody pattern of fine speckled staining is characteristic of Sjögren's syndrome (Fig. 50–2).

Scleroderma

Systemic sclerosis (scleroderma) is a multisystem connective tissue disorder of unknown etiology in which vascular lesions and tissue fibrosis are prominent features. The etiology of systemic sclerosis remains obscure. Patients with systemic sclerosis spontaneously produce autoantibodies against nuclear, nucleolar, and mitochondrial antigens (Reimer, 1990; Rothfield, 1992; Ho, 2003; Cepeda, 2004), which are of diagnostic and prognostic significance (Harris, 2003). A scleroderma patient usually has a restricted heterogeneity of autoantibody types, so an individual patient rarely has more than one autoantibody detected. Table 50–5 lists the various types of autoantibodies described in scleroderma.

Patients with rapidly progressive and diffuse cutaneous involvement affecting the distal and often proximal extremities and trunk are at greater risk of developing early visceral involvement. Included in the classification of scleroderma is a large subset of patients who have a form of the CREST (calcinosis cutis, Raynaud's phenomenon, esophageal dysmotility, sclerodactyly, and telangiectasia) syndrome. The subset of CREST patients may make up 20–30% of all scleroderma patients (Fritzler, 1980). Patients with the CREST variant have a limited cutaneous involvement confined to the distal extremities of the fingers and face, and usually a better prognosis and clinical course than patients with diffuse cutaneous involvement (Fig. 50–3).

Antibodies to Centromere Antigens

The autoantibodies to centromere antigens were detected initially by immunofluorescence microscopy. The centromere antigen was localized to the region of the condensing metaphase chromosomes. In immunoblotting studies, the centromere antigens consist of three proteins: 16 kDa, 80 kDa, and 120 kDa. Autoantibodies to centromere proteins are present in 50–80% of patients with the CREST subset. 25% of patients with idiopathic Raynaud's phenomenon with other signs or symptoms of CREST have anticentromere antibodies (Rothfield, 1992). Anticentromere antibodies are most often associated with a lower frequency of pulmonary fibrosis and mortality, although an increased risk for pulmonary hypertension has been described (Cepeda, 2004).

Antibodies to Scl-70 (DNA Topoisomerase I)

A major autoantigen is Scl-70, which was initially detected as a 70 kDa protein. This was later recognized as a degradation product of a 95 kDa protein, DNA topoisomerase I (Tan, 1989). The antigen was localized in punctate distribution in the nucleoplasm and nucleolus. In early studies, autoantibodies to Scl-70 were detected in 20% of unselected scleroderma patients by immunodiffusion studies (Tan, 1982a). In later studies, Scl 70

Table 50–5 Autoantigens and Autoantibodies in Scleroderma

Autoantigen	Molecular Structure	Autoantibody Frequency
Scl-70	100 kDa native and 70 kDa degradation product; DNA topoisomerase I	70% in diffuse scleroderma; 20–59% in all patients; 13% in CREST
Centromere	Proteins 17, 80, and 140 kDa, localized at inner and outer kinetochore plates	57–82% in CREST; 8% in diffuse form
RNA Pol I	RNA Pol I complex of subunit proteins, 210–211 kDa	4–20% in scleroderma; 13% in diffuse form
RNA Pol II	Transcripts mRNA	4%
RNA Pol III	Transcripts 5S rRNA, tRNA	23% in scleroderma; 45% in diffuse form; 6% in CREST
Fibrillarin	Protein 34 kDa, component of U3 RNP particle	6–8%; 5% in diffuse form; 10% in CREST
U1nRNP	Spliceosome complex	2–5% in all patients; 24% in polymyositis/scleroderma overlap
PM-Scl	Complex of 11 proteins, 110–120 kDa	2–5%; 24% in polymyositis/scleroderma overlap
Ku	DNA-binding protein	1–14% in scleroderma; 26–55% in polymyositis/scleroderma overlap
Th/To	Protein 40 kDa, complexes with 7S and 8S RNAs	4–10% in scleroderma; 1–11% in diffuse form; 8–19% in CREST; up to 3% in polymyositis/scleroderma overlap
NOR-90	Protein 90 kDa, human upstream binding factor, localized in nucleolus organizer region	Rare

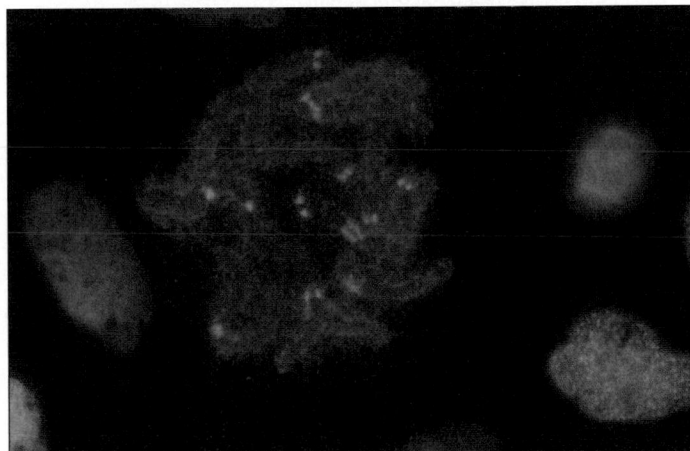

Figure 50–3 Systemic sclerosis (scleroderma): special study. Centromere decoration in rat Indian muntjac preparation with anticentromere antibody.

autoantibodies were found in 75% of patients with the diffuse, severe form of scleroderma by immunodiffusion tests (Jarzabek-Chorzelska, 1986). This latter finding was probably caused by better preservation of topoisomerase I antigen in the tests, as well as the demonstration of higher prevalence of Scl-70 autoantibody in patients with the diffuse severe form of scleroderma (Nakamura, 1992). In summary, in many literature series anti-Scl70 autoantibodies are associated with diffuse cutaneous involvement, increased frequency of pulmonary fibrosis, and higher mortality.

Antibodies to RNA Polymerases

Three RNA polymerases catalyze the transcription of genes into RNA (von Mühlen, 1994). Autoantibodies targeting RNA polymerases tend to occur together in the same patients, appear to be specific for scleroderma, and are mostly detected in individuals with diffuse scleroderma. There is an association with diffuse cutaneous disease, interstitial lung fibrosis, renal crisis, and higher mortality (Harris, 2003; Cepeda, 2004; Ioannidis, 2005).

Autoantibodies to the Nucleolar Antigen Fibrillarin (U3-snRNP)

The name fibrillarin comes from the antigen localization in the dense fibrillar component of nucleoli. Antifibrillarin antibodies are seen most often in young men with scleroderma, minimal joint involvement, and pulmonary hypertension (von Mühlen, 1994; Harris, 2003).

Antibodies Targeting the Nucleolar Organizing Region

Nucleolar organizing region (NOR)-90 antibodies recognize the RNA polymerase I transcription factor hUBF (human upstream binding factor) in the fibrillar center of the nucleolus. NORs are regions where the nucleolus reforms after mitosis, with clusters of ribosomal RNA genes, and sites where Scl-70, U3-RNA/fibrillarin, NOR-90, and RNA polymerase I antigens can be detected (von Mühlen, 1994; Fritzler, 1995; Dagher, 2002).

Rheumatoid Arthritis

Rheumatoid arthritis is a systemic autoimmune disorder characterized by chronic, symmetric, and erosive arthritis of the peripheral joints. A large percentage of the patients have elevated titers of serum rheumatoid factors. There may be associated nonarticular manifestations, such as subcutaneous nodules, vasculitis, interstitial fibrosis, and anemia. Sjögren's and Felty's syndromes commonly occur in RA. The primary cause of the disease is unknown. Most patients with RA have the class II MHC alleles DR4, DR1, or both (Schumacher, 1993). RA is associated with several autoantibodies, which can serve as diagnostic and prognostic markers (Aho, 1994; Viander, 1997; Firestein, 2003). These include:

1. Rheumatoid factor (RF)
2. Antifillagrin antibodies (also known as anti-citrullinated-protein antibodies [ACPA]; Table 50-6):
   a) Antikeratin antibodies (AKA)
   b) Antiperinuclear factor (APF) (Fig. 50-4)
   c) Antibodies to citrullinated peptides (often referred to as anti-CCP [anti-cyclic-citrullinated-peptide])
   d) Anti-Sa antibodies, targeting citrullinated vimentin
3. Anti-RA33.

They all may possibly precede the onset of clinical RA (Klareskog, 2004).

Rheumatoid Factor

Rheumatoid factor (RF) is an antibody directed against the Fc portion of the IgG molecule. Studies of monoclonal and polyclonal RF have shown polyreactive RF with binding specificity for substances other than IgG, such as nuclear components (Schumacher, 1993). The polyreactive RF is usually of the IgM class with low affinity. RF is not specific for RA and is often seen in cases of chronic infection and other systemic inflammatory conditions. RF in rheumatic diseases has considerable immunochemical heterogeneity. In addition to the common IgM RF, both IgA RF and IgG RF have been detected. IgA RF has been related to more severe disease with erosions. The group of RFs are among the only autoantibodies clearly shown to be involved in disease pathogenesis (Smolen, 1998).

Antikeratin Antibody

Antikeratin antibody reacts against the stratum corneum of rat esophagus (Young, 1979). AKA is a fairly specific but not very sensitive marker for RA.

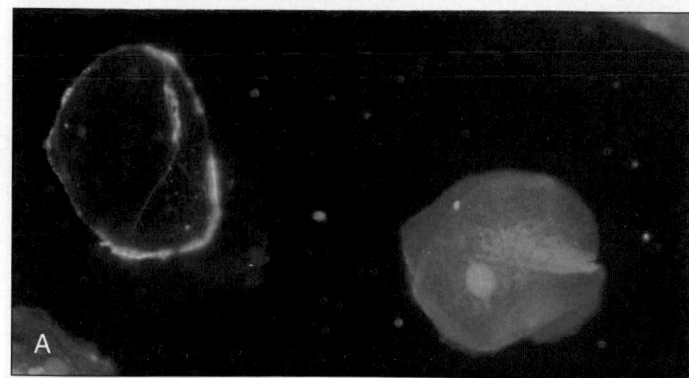
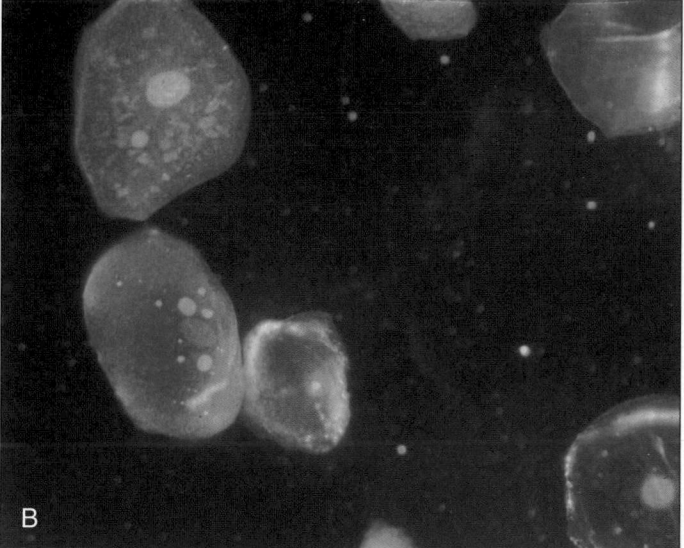

Figure 50–4 Antiperinuclear factor (APF) in rheumatoid arthritis. *A*, Negative preparation for APF using oral mucosa cells as substrate in indirect immunofluorescence. *B*, positive preparation for APF – note dense homogeneous granules around nuclei counterstained with ethidium bromide (orange color).

The occurrence of positive reactions in RA sera is 36–59% while it is 0–3% in normal healthy individuals (Aho, 1994). Most antikeratin-positive sera are also reactive with antiperinuclear factor, suggesting that both antigens share some similarities. It was demonstrated that AKA reacts with water-soluble acidic–neutral isoforms of fillagrin in the epidermis and molecular forms of (pro)fillagrin in the rat esophagus epithelium, instead of cytokeratin (Simon, 1993; Sebbag, 2004).

Antiperinuclear Factor (APF)

This antibody is reactive with perinuclear keratohyalin granules of buccal mucosa cells (Nienhuis, 1964). The nonstandard amino acid citrulline seems to be an essential component in epitopes recognized by these autoantibodies (Schellekens, 1998). This immunofluorescence test is sensitive but less specific than AKA in RA patients. APF-positive tests in RA patients have been reported to range from 49–87% (Janssens, 1988; Aho, 1994), and up to 5% in other connective tissue diseases or in normal controls. Both AKA and APF have been described in early seronegative RA, bringing clear improvement to the diagnosis of the disease.

Anti-Citrullinated-Peptides

Antibodies to citrullinated peptides (CCP) detected by ELISA constitute early, specific markers for RA (van Venrooij, 2004; Vossenaar, 2004; Hoffman, 2005). The antigen used in most assays is citrullinated fillagrin. The unusual amino acid citrulline is generated by action of the enzyme peptidyl arginine deiminase (PAD), which generates a post-translational modification of peptides containing arginine. A second generation ELISA is claimed to reach 98% specificity for the diagnosis of RA, with 70% sensitivity, which is a major improvement over the RF test (Lee, 2003; Sebbag, 2004). Furthermore, anti-CCP antibodies can be detected in 50% of patients with early RA, at a time when RF is negative, allowing for improved diagnosis and early specific treatment. Many series in the

Table 50–6 Autoantibodies in common use in rheumatoid arthritis

	IgM RF 1940	APF IIF 1964	Anti-CCP1 ELISA 1998	Anti-CCP2 ELISA 2002	Anti-CCP3 ELISA 2005
Sensitivity (%)	66–85	60 (39–87)	60	69	74
Specificity (%)	72	95 (73–99)	92	95–98	96

APF = antiperinuclear factor; CCP = cyclic citrullinated peptide (1, 2, and 3 refers to first, second, and third generation assays respectively); RF = rheumatoid factor. See text for references.

Table 50–7 Autoantigens and Autoantibodies in Polymyositis and Dermatomyositis

Autoantigen	Molecular Structure	Antibody Frequency (%)
Jo-1	Histidyl tRNA synthetase protein, 52 kDa	23–36
PL-7	Threonyl tRNA synthetase protein, 80 kDa	4 in polymyositis
PL –12	Alanyl tRNA synthetase protein, 110 kDa	3
Mi-2	Nuclear protein complex, proteins 53 and 61 kDa	15–35 in polymyositis; 5–9 in dermatomyositis
Signal recognition particle (SRP)	Protein 54 kDa complexed with 7 SL RNA	4–5 in polymyositis; does not occur in dermatomyositis
PM-Scl	Complex of 11 proteins, 110–20 kDa	8–12 in polymyositis; 25 in polymyositis/scleroderma overlap
U1nRNP	Spliceosome complex	4–17 in polymyositis/dermatomyositis
56 kDa	56 kDa, RNP component	80
5 EJ	Glycyl-tRNA synthetase	<3 in polymyositis
OJ	Isoleucyl-tRNA synthetase	<3 in polymyositis

Source: data from Tan (1988), Nakamura (1992) and von Mühlen (1994).

literature point to associations with erosive, more severe and progressive disease (Forslind, 2004; Kastbom, 2004; Sebbag, 2004).

Anti-CCP antibodies are rarely found in other clinical conditions, such as viral infections (mainly hepatitis C), Lyme disease, Graves disease, SLE, and Sjögren's syndrome (both with associated erosive articular disease). Children with juvenile RA generally do not benefit from this laboratory test, as its sensitivity is only 0.2–3%. Positive results are seen in the polyarticular, RF-positive subset of children that commonly evolves to the erosive, adult form of RA (Low, 2004).

On the other hand, anti-CCP autoantibodies may better discriminate between patients with rheumatoid arthritis and patients with polyarticular manifestations associated with hepatitis C virus infection (Bombardieri, 2004). Many authors now suggest that the anti-CCP test should greatly improve accuracy for RA disease classification if added to the modified 1987 criteria of the American College of Rheumatology.

Anti-RA33

Hassfeld (1989) has reported an antinuclear antibody (anti-RA33) that may be specific for RA. From extracts of HeLa cells, an antigen of approximately 33 kDa was found to react with 36% of 95 sera from RA patients and with only one of 170 control patients. The antigen was termed RA33, and the autoantibody has no discernible relationship to other nuclear antibodies. Anti-RA33 was not related to antihistone. Immunoblot analyses with soluble extracts from HeLa cells showed an autoantibody targeting a 33 kDa antigen (anti-RA33) in 30% of Austrian RA patients but in no patients with ankylosing spondylitis or psoriatic arthritis (Aho, 1994). However, the prevalence of anti-RA33 in Finnish RA was found to be a low 6% (Aho, 1994). Anti-RA33 autoantibodies may also be found in mixed connective tissue disease and in SLE (Steiner, 1996).

Polymyositis and Dermatomyositis

Polymyositis is an inflammatory disease of striated muscle of unknown etiology. It is characterized by the presence of inflammatory infiltrates in the skeletal muscle, with associated muscle fiber necrosis and degeneration (Targoff, 1992). When the disease is accompanied by typical skin changes, it is called dermatomyositis. Polymyositis is characterized serologically by the presence of a number of autoantibodies of various specifications directed against different transfer RNA (tRNA) synthetases (von Mühlen, 1994; Targoff, 2002) (Table 50–7). These autoantibodies define a subgroup of patients with polymyositis, arthralgia, interstitial lung disease, and poorer prognosis than patients without the autoantibodies.

Antibodies to Jo-1 (histidyl tRNA synthetase) occur in 23–36% of polymyositis patients, most with interstitial lung disease (Targoff, 1992).

Autoantibodies to threonyl and alanyl tRNA-synthetase occur at a lower prevalence in autoimmune myositis. In patients with a clinical syndrome showing overlapping features of polymyositis and scleroderma, an antibody called anti-PM-Scl has been reported (Tan, 1988). The anti-PM-Scl antibody reacts with a complex of 11 polypeptides ranging from 110–120 kDa. Anti-PM-Scl shows staining of nucleolus and nucleoplasm in substrate cells by indirect immunofluorescence microscopy. Antibodies directed to Mi-2, a DNA-dependent, nucleosome-stimulated ATPase remodeling factor (Wang, 2001), are considered specific for dermatomyositis (von Mühlen, 1995). Attention is being called to the presence of antibodies to the 52 kDa component of SSA/Ro in a certain proportion of patients with polymyositis/dermatomyositis (Peene, 2002).

Concept of Overlap Syndromes

Overlap syndrome is a term used when patients exhibit symptoms of more than one disease (Pope, 2002). For example, patients who meet the diagnostic criteria for SLE and also have typical manifestations suggestive of a second diagnosis, such as RA, have been described (Lazaro, 1989). It is uncertain whether overlap syndromes may represent the coexistence of two or more different diseases, or whether the syndrome is a distinct entity.

Mixed Connective Tissue Disease

The concept of MCTD was initially proposed by Sharp and colleagues in 1972. The 20 patients described in the initial report had a combination of features usually associated with SLE, systemic sclerosis, and polymyositis. Characteristically, a high titer of autoantibody to a nuclear ribonucleoprotein was found in all the patients by hemagglutination (Sharp, 1972). The lack of renal and neurologic abnormalities and the excellent response of these patients to small doses of oral corticosteroids initially justified the classification as a separate group from SLE and systemic sclerosis. However, the concept of MCTD as a separate group has changed with time. Many feel that MCTD represents an overlap of systemic sclerosis, SLE, and polymyositis (Nimelstein, 1980). A group of patients originally diagnosed as MCTD was restudied 8 years later and showed a general evolution out of the overlap pattern to one of single disease, and scleroderma was the most prevalent diagnosis (Nimelstein, 1980). There appears to be a large overlap that becomes apparent when the above-mentioned criteria are applied to a certain population of patients, and the studies do not completely support the existence of MCTD as an individual clinical entity. Recently, it was shown that antibodies to a subunit of nRNP appearing in apoptotic blebs, named U1–70K, is a superior marker for early MCTD than autoantibodies to U1nRNP (Hof, 2005).

Molecular Biology and Functions of Certain Nuclear and Intracellular Autoantigens

Many of the intracellular autoantibodies, including the autoantibodies to nuclear antigens (ANAs), have been identified as diagnostic markers for the rheumatic diseases, such as SLE, scleroderma, Sjögren's syndrome, MCTD, drug-induced lupus and polymyositis/dermatomyositis (Tan, 1989). The autoantibodies in human diseases have been used as tools to study various molecular biological functions and mechanisms. ANAs have been used to screen cDNA expression libraries, with later identification of autoantigens. Biological functions that the autoantibodies have been demonstrated to inhibit include pre-mRNA splicing, DNA replication, DNA repair, transcription, transcription of rRNA, microtubule-based chromosome movement during mitosis, and aminoacetylation of tRNAs (Tan, 1988, 1989, 1997a; Casiano, 1996).

Profiles of Autoantibodies in Various Systemic Rheumatic Diseases

It has been observed that distinct profiles of ANA are seen in different systemic rheumatic diseases, characteristics of which include the presence or absence of certain antibodies and differences in the mean titers of these antibodies (Nakamura, 1986; Tan, 1988; Bizzaro, 2004). Nonetheless, one should be aware of the low positive predictive value of the ANA test in settings with low prevalence of systemic rheumatic diseases and in aging populations (Slater, 1996). The following features are noteworthy:

1. Multiple ANAs are frequently seen in SLE, often with high levels of anti-dsDNA antibodies in active disease.
2. Distinctiveness of anti-Sm, anti-rRNP, and anti-PCNA for SLE.

VI

Table 50–8 Decision Chart for the Identification of Selected Autoantibodies Using HEp-2 Cells and Their Disease Association

1. Nuclear pattern

Envelope (rim)

Punctate, mitotic-figure-negative	→ Primary biliary cirrhosis
Continuous, mitotic-figure-negative	→ Chronic liver diseases
Homogeneous, mitotic-figure-positive	→ SLE, drug-induced SLE

Speckled

Large	→ hnRNP in SLE
Coarse	→ Sm, RNP in SLE, MCTD
Fine	→ SS-A/Ro, SS-B/La in SLE, Sjögren's syndrome
Pleomorphic	→ PCNA in SLE
Discrete	
Mitotic-figure-positive	→ Centromere in scleroderma
Mitotic-figure-negative	→ p95 (Sp100) in primary biliary cirrhosis

2. Nucleolar pattern

Homogeneous	→ PM-Scl in scleroderma
Clumpy	→ Fibrillarin in scleroderma
Speckled	
Mitotic figure punctate	→ RNA pol I, NOR-90 in scleroderma
Mitotic figure homogeneous	→ Scl-70 in scleroderma

3. Cytoplasmic pattern

Dense, fine speckles	→ Jo-1, PL-7, PL-12 in polymyositis/dermatomyositis
Homogeneous	→ rRNP in SLE and juvenile SLE
Fibrillar	→ Actin, myosin in MCTD, primary biliary cirrhosis, chronic autoimmune hepatitis
Segmental	→ α-actinin, vinculin in myasthenia gravis, Crohn's disease, ulcerative colitis
Reticular	→ Mitochondria in primary biliary cirrhosis
Polar	→ Golgi in Sjögren's syndrome, SLE, viral infections
Spindle apparatus	→ NuMA in Sjögren's syndrome, SLE; midbody, p330^d in cancer

MCTD = mixed connective tissue disease; NuMA, nuclear mitotic-associated antigen; PCNA, proliferating cell nuclear antigen; SLE = systemic lupus erythematosus.

Source: modified from Krapf AR, von Mühlen CA, Krapf FE, et al: Atlas of Immunofluorescent Autoantibodies. Munich, Urban & Schwarzenberg, 1996.

3. Restriction of ANA in drug-induced lupus to antihistone and/or antichromatin (antinucleosome) antibodies.
4. Antibodies to U1nRNP or nuclear antibodies to RNP present in several rheumatic diseases with different frequencies.
5. The restriction of ANA in MCTD to U1nRNP (by disease definition), or nuclear RNP antibodies.
6. Sjögren's syndrome sera are characterized primarily by the presence of antibodies to SS-A/Ro and SS-B/La.
7. Patients with scleroderma showing a profile consisting of antibodies to Scl-70, the centromere/kinetochore antigens, and other nucleolar antigens such as fibrillarin and Th/To.
8. The frequent presence of RF, anti-citrullinated-proteins (AKA, APF, anti-CCP), and anti-RA33 in RA.
9. The presence of Jo-1, Mi-2, and PM-Scl autoantibodies in polymyositis/dermatomyositis.
10. Autoantibodies such as anti-centromere, anti-CCP, and anti-dsDNA, may antedate overt clinical disease by many years.

Decision Chart for the Diagnostic Work-Up of Autoimmune Diseases

Immunofluorescence microscopy using human cellular substrates, such as HEp-2 cells, allows for the sensitive detection of serum antibodies that react very specifically with various cellular proteins and nucleic acids. This technique is nowadays essential in immunology laboratories committed to the routine diagnosis of human autoimmune diseases. From a positive immunofluorescence test result, one is able to associate the specific pattern to the presence of a distinct autoantibody in that particular patient's serum. Since distinct autoantibody patterns occur in each disease, as discussed above, the laboratorian offers the clinician the real possibility of narrowing down the diagnostic chase. A decision chart developed with those issues in mind is found in Table 50–8, and the cytoplasmic pattern classification for use in the routine laboratory is found in Table 50–9. Figures 50–5, 50–6, and 50–7 depict some examples of immunofluorescence patterns as seen in our laboratories.

Diagnostic Methods in Autoantibody Detection

The commonly used methods for autoantibody detection are listed in Table 50–10. Widely used tests for screening of intracellular autoantibodies are immunofluorescence microscopy (IFM) and the immunoenzyme tests with many distinct antigens combined (Nakamura, 1994b), sometimes called 'anti-ENA.' The secondary definitive tests for specific identification of ANA are immunodiffusion, immunoprecipitation, particle agglutination, immunoenzyme, and immunoblotting methods (Teodorescu, 1992). A search for the presence of ANAs by immunofluorescence in HEp-2 cells will be positive 98% of the time, when screening SLE patients with active disease. In other words, a negative test will usually rule out an SLE diagnosis.

Standardization of the indirect immunofluorescence (IF)-ANA has been difficult (Nakamura, 1992; Feltkamp, 1996; Smolen, 1997). Many factors are involved in the performance of IF-ANA tests. They include (1) substrate and fixative variations, (2) microscopic optics, (3) method and quantitation of results, (4) establishment of reference ranges, (5) interpretation of results, (6) reference sera, and (7) specificity and avidity of the ANA. The ANA Standardization Committee of the World Health Organization recommends that laboratories should (1) report IF-ANA results at both 1:40 and 1:160 dilutions, and (2) supply information on percentage of normal individuals who are positive at these dilutions in their own experience (Tan, 1997b).

Bylund and Nakamura (Bylund, 1991) have shown the importance of SS-A/Ro autoantibody determination in screening tests for autoantibodies to nuclear antigens. The detection of anti-SS-A/Ro requires implementation and adherence to several technical and quality assurance recommendations. With use of the appropriate substrate cells containing the SS-A/Ro antigen, many of the so-called ANA-negative lupus erythematosus patients will show a positive test by the indirect immunofluorescence test. Immunoprecipitin and double immunodiffusion analyses have been used to determine the specificity of several ANAs. Assay specificity in double immunodiffusion is generally dependent on the quality of other control sera used in the procedure, as well as the nature of the antigen preparation. Immunodiffusion tests are not very sensitive but positive tests have a high degree of specificity. Immunodiffusion commercial kits are available for the detection of antibodies to RNP, Sm, SS-A/Ro, SS-B/La, and Scl-70, as well as other less prevalent markers (Nakamura, 1994b).

An increasing number of enzyme immunoassays have been developed with the use of standard purified and recombinant antigens (Saitta, 1992). Many of these enzyme immunoassays have proved to be more sensitive than comparable immunodiffusion methods. Thus, because of the high sensitivity of enzyme immunoassays, one needs to determine carefully the reference range of normal patients and the proper cut-off values. Compared with immunodiffusion tests, ELISA tests showed much greater sensitivity but had lower specificity (Nakamura, 1992). Further, ELISA tests were frequently positive at low titers in sera of patients with rheumatic diseases other than SLE. For example, the presence of antibodies to Sm as assayed by immunodiffusion is considered to be highly specific for SLE. However, in ELISA tests the Sm antibody was positive in 23% of 54 RA patients, 25% of 24 systemic sclerosis patients, 9% of 11 polymyositis patients, and 2% of 59 normal patients (Maddison, 1985). Increasing sensitivity and decreasing specificity might result in false-positive test results. Furthermore, clinical associations with distinct autoantibodies were mainly determined using immunodiffusion techniques.

New commercial ELISA kits developed for screening purposes claim to detect a variety of autoantibodies in one single assay, but having 'total' fractions of cellular antigens in one ELISA well is not technically feasible nowadays. Those assays are not 100% sensitive for the screening of antinuclear antibodies, as they cannot detect autoantibodies such as antinucleolar-specific, PCNA or distinct NuMA types. Reported results using those kits, for the moment, should correctly specify to physicians which

Table 50–9 Classification of Cytoplasmic Patterns in Indirect Immunofluorescence

Cytoplasmic Patterns in IIF (Cell Substrate)	Representative Antigens	Disease and Clinical Associations
1. Fibrous		
Stress fibers – linear cytoskeletal fibers, sometimes with small, discontinuous granular deposits (HEp-2, fibroblasts)	Actin Nonmuscle myosin	Both in chronic active hepatitis, liver cirrhosis, and myasthenia gravis; actin in autoimmune hepatitis, Crohn's disease, PBC, long term hemodialysis, NHS, but rare in DCTD
Filamentous – filaments and fibrils spreading out from the nuclear rim (HEp-2, PtK2 epithelial cells)	Vimentin Keratin	Antivimentin often caused by cross-reaction with anti-α helix antibodies, detected in many kinds of infectious or inflammatory conditions, and in long-term hemodialysis; rare in DCTD; both seen in NHS; keratin is major system in ALD (69%), also common in DCTD and psoriasis
Segmental – small segments of fibers (periodic dense bodies) are decorated (HEp-2, fibroblasts)	α-Actinin, vinculin Tropomyosin	Myasthenia gravis, Crohn's disease, ulcerative colitis
2. Speckled		
Fine speckled – scattered small speckles, mostly with homogeneous or dense fine speckled background (HEp-2)	Many of the aminoacyl-tRNA-synthetases, mainly Jo-1	Polymyositis; 'Jo-1 syndrome' (myositis and interstitial lung disease)
Dense fine speckled – cloudy, almost homogeneous throughout the cytoplasm (HEp-2)	rRNP, ribosomal phosphoproteins	Neuropsychiatric SLE
Granular pole – perinuclear, arrow-shaped, coarse granular, corresponding to the lamellar stacks of the Golgi complex (HEp-2)	Golgi apparatus	Rare in SLE, SjS, RA, MCTD, Wegener's granulomatosis, and other systemic rheumatic diseases; reported in idiopathic cerebellar ataxia, paraneoplastic cerebellar degeneration, and viral infections, including EBV and HIV
Coarse reticular – coarse diffuse reticular and granular (HEp-2)	Proteins in the inner mitochondrial membrane (mainly M2)	PBC; systemic sclerosis (43%); rare in other DCTD; centromere antibodies are frequently associated
Scattered small speckled – countable cytoplasmic speckles irregularly distributed (HEp-2)	Lysosomes/ endosomes/ peroxisomes/ proteasomes	Limited scleroderma, glioblastoma and other neurologic diseases, idiopathic pleural effusion
Fine reticular – fine diffuse reticular and granular (HEp-2)	Endoplasmic reticulum (?); other unknown proteins	CLD; detected in all types of (chronic) inflammatory conditions
ANCA – pANCA – irregular perinuclear staining; cANCA – dense, fine or coarse speckles (peripheral blood granulocytes, HL-60 leukemia cell line)	pANCA targets myeloperoxidase; cANCA targets PR3 (proteinase 3)	First reported in systemic vasculitis with necrotizing glomerulonephritis and inflammatory pulmonary disease; Wegener's granulomatosis (cANCA) and other necrotizing vasculitis (pANCA); cathepsin-G is the main antigen in ulcerative colitis, Crohn's disease, and primary sclerosing cholangitis; autoimmune hepatitis; vasculitis in PTU therapy; recently reported in RA (32%); IgM ANCA in tuberculosis and malaria

ANCA = antineutrophil cytoplasmic antibodies; ALD = alcoholic liver disease; CLD = chronic liver diseases; DCTD = diffuse connective tissue diseases; EBV = Epstein–Barr virus; HIV = human immunodeficiency virus; IIF = indirect immunofluorescence test; MCTD = mixed connective tissue disease; NHS = normal human serum; PBC = primary biliary cirrhosis; PM = polymyositis; PTU = propylthiouracil; RNP = ribonucleoprotein; SjS = Sjögren's syndrome; SLE = systemic lupus erythematosus.

Source: modified from Humbel, 1993; used with permission from von Mühlen, 1994; Stinton, 2004.

types of autoantibody were tested, so as not to imply that a particular sample is 'negative for all nuclear antibodies.' Each ELISA test kit in such a situation should be validated for the antibody specificities that it can actually detect (von Mühlen, 2002).

More recently, multiplexed assays are being incorporated into the routine work of bigger laboratories. The so called multiplexed fluorescent microsphere immunoassay uses spectral addresses, allowing for the simultaneous determination of several autoantibodies all in one incubation with no wash steps. We recently demonstrated that results for a proprietary multiplexed assay compared very favorably with results from established ELISAs (Martins, 2004): agreement, sensitivity, and specificity, respectively, for five nuclear antigens evaluated were as follows: SSA, 99.1%, 100.0%, and 98.8%; SSB, 98.6%, 88.9%, and 99.5%; Sm, 97.6%, 95.8%, and 97.9%; RNP, 97.2%, 92.7, and 98.8%; Scl-70, 93.6%, 50.0%, and 99.0%. The multiplexed microsphere-based immunoassay seems to be a sensitive and specific method for the detection and semiquantification of common antibodies in human sera. Clusters of clinically important autoantibodies, such as those in SLE or in systemic vasculitis, may be rapidly tested in a single batch.

Variations in Methodologies Used for Detection of Autoantibodies to Nuclear and Intracellular Antigens

Probably the best studies regarding different methods for detection of autoantibodies to intracellular antigens were reported by a European Consensus Study Group. The European Consensus Study Group for the Detection of Autoantibodies to Intracellular Antigens in Rheumatic Diseases was formed in 1988 and has conducted four annual workshops

from 1989–1992 (van Venrooij, 1991; Charles, 1992). In 1988 and 1989, consensus workshops were conducted to define interlaboratory concordance in the detection of autoantibody specificities in rheumatic diseases. A total of 28 laboratories participated in the study and used various methodologies. The objectives of the consensus study initiated in 1989 were (1) to define the interlaboratory consensus in detecting autoantibodies and specificities, (2) to test whether discrepancies were due to the methodology used, and (3) to make recommendations for improved quality of results with improved sensitivity and specificity.

Enzyme-Linked Immunosorbent Assays

In the 1988 and 1989 studies, many false-positive reactions were noted. False-positive reactions were caused by poor blocking reagents in the procedure; also, impure antigen preparations were used. In the 1990 and 1991 cooperative study, laboratories using ELISA performed very well, with few false-positive or extraneous negative results. The ELISA assays also performed well in sorting out sera with multiple specificities.

The percentage of clinical laboratories using ELISA increased from 25% to 47% over the 4-year period from 1989–1992. Homburger and colleagues reported a comparison between a commercial ELISA and IF-ANA on HEp-2 cells, concluding that both methods were substantially equivalent for detecting clinically relevant ANA in patients with systemic rheumatic diseases (Homburger, 1998). Reaching an opposite conclusion, Emlen and O'Neill tested six commercial ELISA kits and concluded for the existence of significant differences in the detection of ANA by immunofluorescence and ELISA (Emlen, 1997). A group of international scientists joined by the World Health Organization reported on the performance of many commercial ELISAs, showing that (1) no single manufacturer was clearly superior to others in terms of their products' overall sensitivity, specificity, and precision, and (2) areas that needed

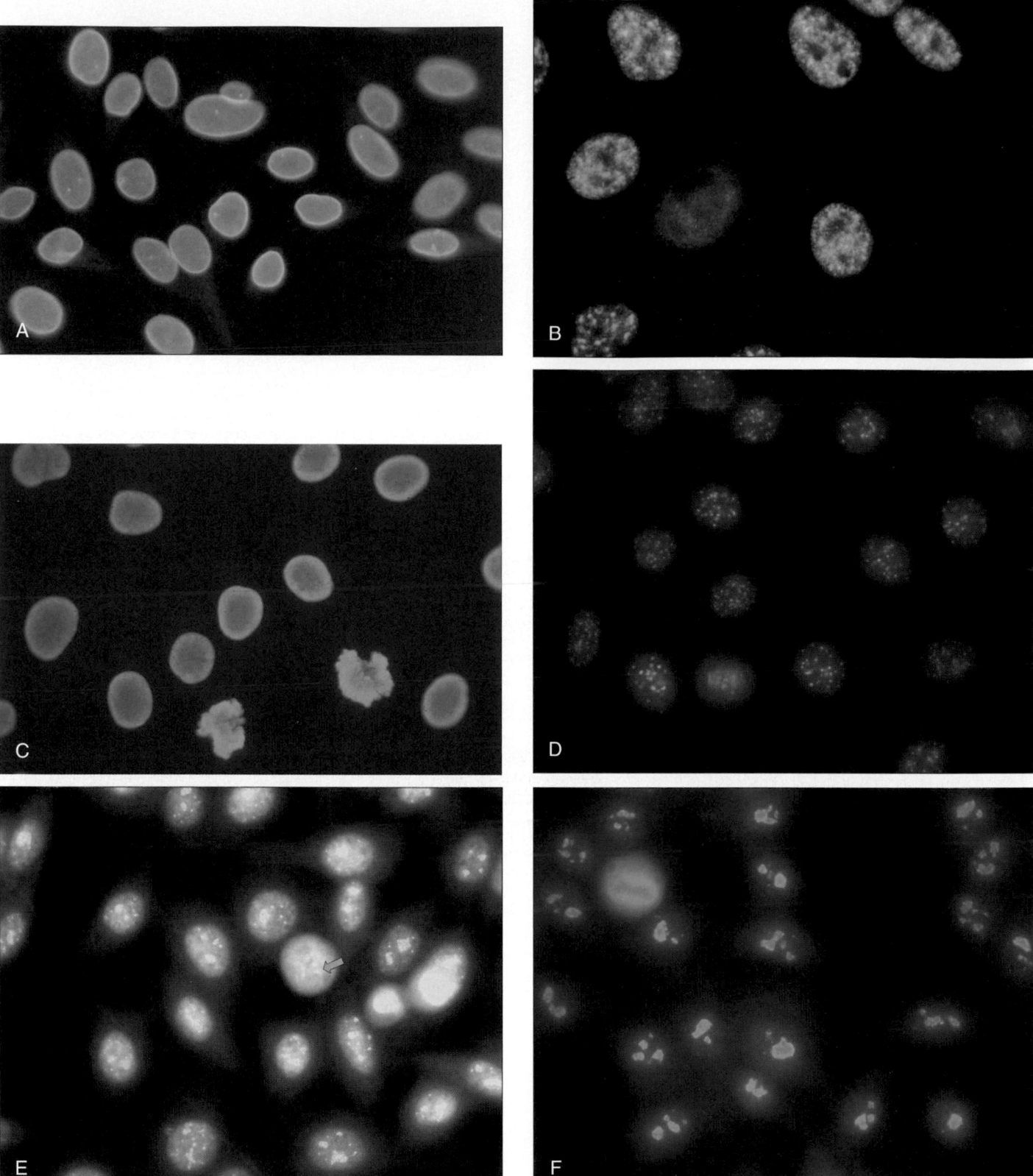

Figure 50–5 Indirect immunofluorescence with autoantibodies to nuclear and nucleolar antigens in HEp-2 cells, 400×, fluorescein isothiocyanate (FITC) stain.
A, Autoantibodies to lamin proteins A, B and C of the nuclear envelope give a homogeneous nuclear pattern in HEp-2 cells, associated with a continuous nucleoplasmic rim. No rim is seen when the antibodies are specifically directed to histones or dsDNA. Previous reports of a peripheral pattern elicited by anti-dsDNA antibodies were probably due to fixation artifacts. *B*, The speckled nucleoplasmic pattern is characteristic of autoantibodies directed to the so-called 'extractable nuclear antigens,' as the anti-U1nRNP shown here. The nucleoli and metaphase cells are negative. *C*, Anti-dsDNA autoantibodies, with homogeneous pattern in interphase as well as in metaphase cells. *D*, Anticentromere autoantibodies, typically found in patients with the limited form of scleroderma (CREST syndrome) but also in primary biliary cirrhosis. Distinct speckles are seen in the interphase nuclei, one for each chromosome pair, which aggregate in the metaphase plates during cell division. *E*, Autoantibodies to NOR-90 and RNA-polymerase I elicit the same pattern in HEp-2 cells, with nucleolar speckles and dots along some spindles of metaphase cells (arrow). They can be differentiated by other assays, such as immunoblot or immunoprecipitation. *F*, Autoantibodies targeting fibrillarin (U3-nRNP) give a clumpy staining of all nucleoli.

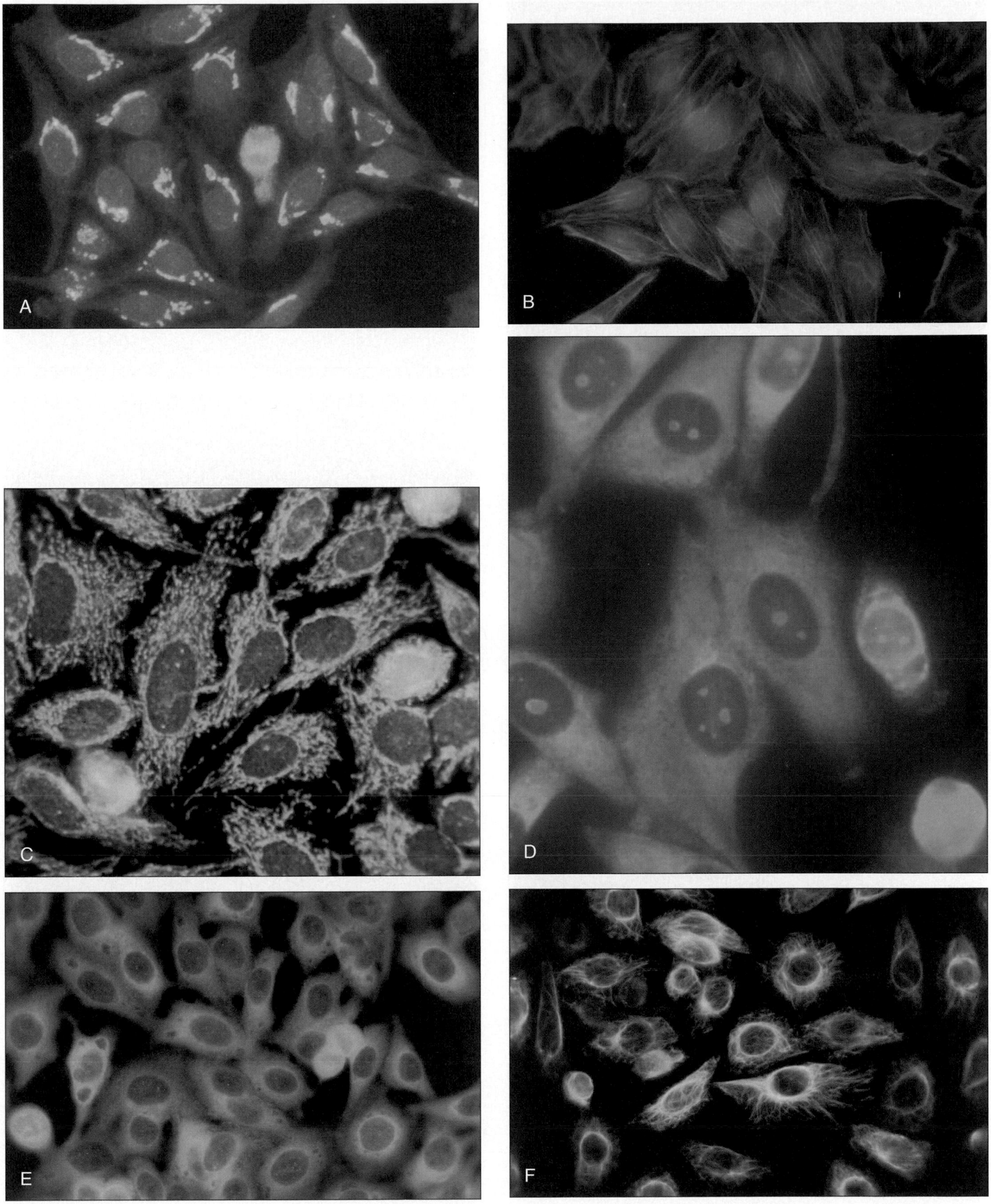

Figure 50–6 Indirect immunofluorescence of HEp-2 cells with autoantibodies to distinct cytoplasmic antigens, 400×, FITC stain. *A*, The characteristic pattern of autoantibodies to the Golgi organelle is seen, with granules arranged in clusters at one pole of the cell and sparing the nuclei. *B*, Autoantibodies to nonmuscle myosin decorate the stress fibers of the cytoskeleton (nuclei staining in blue with DAPI). These antibodies are found in patients with myasthenia gravis and chronic liver diseases. *C*, Anti-mitochondrial autoantibodies display a coarse granular pattern involving the whole cytoplasm, mostly seen in primary biliary cirrhosis. *D*, Dense granular, almost homogeneous, cytoplasmic pattern obtained with anti-rRNP antibodies. They target ribosomal phosphoproteins, and are clinically associated with central nervous system manifestations in patients with systemic lupus erythematosus. As can be noticed in the picture, not uncommonly such antibodies also stain the nucleoli in a homogeneous pattern, although weakly. *E*, Homogeneous decoration of the cytoplasm conferred by autoantibodies to PL-7 in polymyositis. *F*, Antikeratin antibodies are seen as filamentary staining of cytoskeletal stress fibers and constitute the major specificity found in alcoholic liver disease (69%); they are also common in rheumatoid arthritis (36–59%), psoriasis, and healthy individuals.

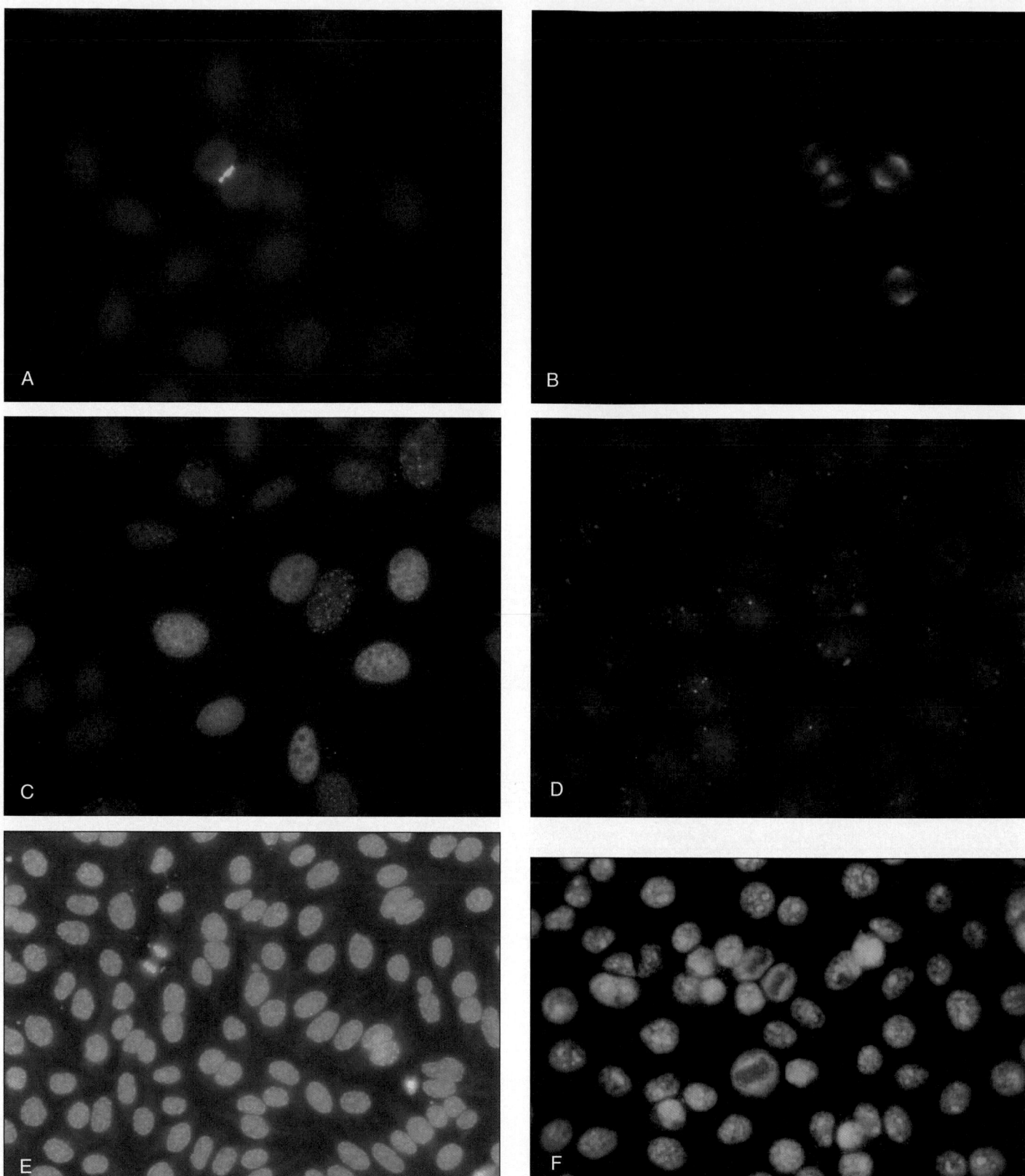

Figure 50–7 Some other distinct patterns in indirect immunofluorescence of HEp-2 cells, 400×, FITC stain. *A,* Cells at the end of metaphase show antigens condensing in the midbody, also called the intercellular bridge region. *B,* The spindle poles of dividing cells can be decorated with antibodies targeting the mitotic apparatus, such as NuMA. *C,* PCNA-autoantibodies give a mosaic of nucleoplasmic patterns, ranging from homogeneous to distinct speckled, according to the phases of cellular division (details in the text). *D,* The pattern obtained with anti-p80-coilin autoantibodies, where one can see between one and eight nucleoplasmic dots. *E,* One of the most common patterns seen in the routine laboratory, dense fine speckled nuclear in interphase as well as in mitotic cells. This is a nonspecific autoantibody, found in systemic connective tissue diseases but also in interstitial cystitis, breast cancer, and allergic reactions. *F,* Nuclear and nucleolar stainings are seen with anti-Ku autoantibodies. Chromosomes in mitotic cells are negative (see clinical associations in text).

Table 50–10 Methods for Detection of Autoantibodies to Nuclear and Intracellular Antigens

Method	Antigen Source	Sensitivity and Use
Immunofluorescence microscopy	Tissue sections; cell lines	Sensitive assay, often used for screening
Double immunodiffusion (Ouchterlony)	Tissue and cell extracts	Requires precipitin reaction; high specificity but not very sensitive
Counterimmuno-electrophoresis	Tissue and cell extracts	Increased sensitivity and speed as compared with immunodiffusion procedure
Immunoblotting, Western blot	Cell extracts	Very sensitive; permits detection of antibodies against soluble and insoluble antigens
Dot blot, linear blot (line immunoassays)	Purified native or recombinant antigens	Qualitative assay, average sensitivity
ELISA	Purified native or recombinant antigens	Very sensitive; quantitative; high throughput; can determine antibody class; low cost
Microsphere multiplexed assay	Purified native or recombinant antigens	Very sensitive (compares to ELISA); semiquantitative; rapid; expensive proprietary technology

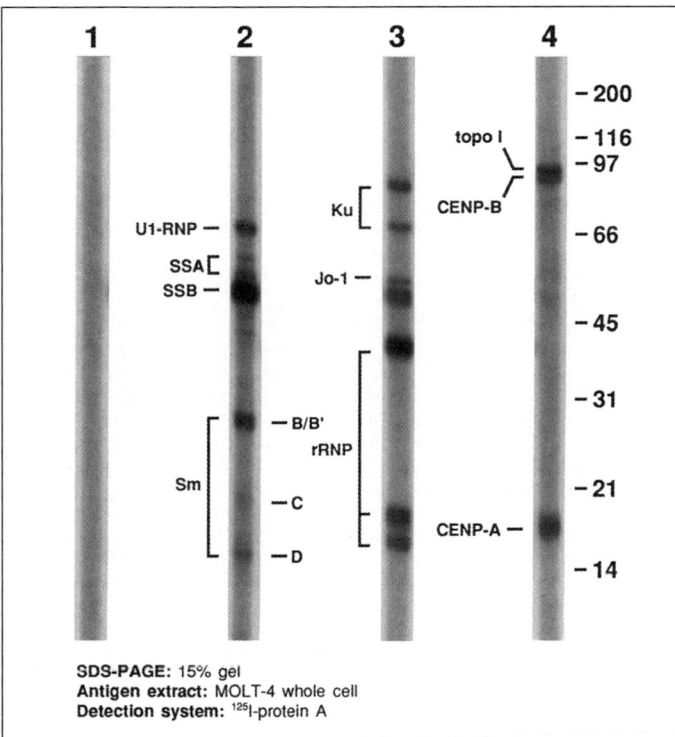

SDS-PAGE: 15% gel
Antigen extract: MOLT-4 whole cell
Detection system: ¹²⁵I-protein A

Figure 50–8 Immunoblotting analysis of common autoantibodies seen in rheumatic diseases. In *lane 1* the nitrocellulose strip was probed with a normal human serum (negative control), and no reactivity is seen as expected. The next three lanes show distinct bands obtained by mixing positive control sera containing known specificities. *Lane 2* depicts reactivities to the ribonucleoproteins (RNP) SSA (52 and 60 kDa), SSB (48 kDa), Sm (B/B', 28 kDa, and D, 14 kDa) and U1nRNP (the 70 kDa protein and a faint band around 19 kDa, the C antigen. The A protein, with 32 kDa and also characteristically recognized by U1nRNP antibodies, is not seen in this experiment). *Lane 3* shows the bands obtained by using the human prototype antisera to Jo-1 (52 kDa), Ku (2 bands around the 70 and 80 kDa regions), and ribosomal RNP (15, 18 and 37 kDa). The small band above the 52 kDa antigen is not identified. *Lane 4* displays the bands most commonly seen using sera from scleroderma patients, e.g., anti-DNA topoisomerase I (Scl-70, 95 kDa), and anti-centromere antibodies (16 kDa, CENP-A, and 80 kDa, CENP-B). On the right, positions in kilodaltons of the broad-range molecular weight standards can be seen. (With permission from von Mühlen CA, Tan EM: Autoantibody specificities in autoimmune rheumatic diseases. Rev Bras Reumatol 1994; 34:173.

improvement were in kits for the detection of antibodies to dsDNA and to Sm antigens (Tan, 1999). Great care should be exercised when selecting ELISA reagents and commercial kits. A good source of quality control data for the best commercial reagents is the periodic review of the College of American Pathologists in Immunology.

Immunoblotting

This technique is very sensitive and is an important method for characterization of the specific nature of many autoantibodies. One important advantage is that a specific antibody can be identified with the use of crude cell extract antigen preparations (Fig. 50–8). The European Consensus Study observed the following with the immunoblotting test (Nakamura, 1994b):

1. The antigen preparation is very important in the immunoblotting procedure.

2. The detection of antibodies to nRNP, Sm, and Scl-70 was acceptable. This sensitive method is helpful in the detection of multiple specificities of antibodies in the same specimen.
3. The method requires careful controls to monitor molecular-weight bands. For example, histone bands can be confused with a centromeric antigen (CENP-A, 19 kDa), and Scl-70 (topoisomerase I) can be confused with other 100 kDa bands.
4. Protein degradation can occur in the antigen cell extract used for immunoblotting, especially Scl-70 and centromere antigens.
5. The anti-Sm is distinguished by the presence of anti-D (the D antigen is a 16 kDa protein contained in all major nRNP particles).
6. Anti-SS-B/La is readily detected by immunoblotting. Anti-SS-A/Ro is poorly detected by immunoblotting and is insensitive, because SS-A/Ro may not demonstrate the proper structure for recognition.

VI

References

Aho K, Paluso T, Kurki P: Marker antibodies of rheumatoid arthritis: diagnostic and pathogenic implications. Semin Arthritis Rheum 1994; 23:379.

Alarcón-Segovia D, Perez-Vasquez ME, Villa AR, et al: Preliminary classification criteria for the antiphospholipid syndrome within systemic lupus erythematosus. Semin Arthritis Rheum 1992; 21:275.

Allanore Y, Sellam J, Batteux F, Job Deslandre C, Weill B, Kahan A: Induction of autoantibodies in refractory rheumatoid arthritis treated by infliximab. Clin Exp Rheumatol 2004; 22:756.

Barada FA, Andrews BS, Davis JS, Taylor RP: Antibodies to Sm in patients with systemic lupus erythematosus. Correlation of Sm antibody titers with disease activity and other laboratory parameters. Arthritis Rheum 1981; 24:1236.

Bizzaro N, Wiik A: Appropriateness in anti-nuclear antibody testing: from clinical request to strategic laboratory practice. Clin Exp Rheumatol 2004; 22:349.

Block SR, Winfield JB, Lockshin MC, et al: Studies of twins with systemic lupus erythematosus: A review of the literature and presentation of 12 additional sets. Am J Med 1975; 59: 533.

Bobbio-Pallavicini F, Alpini C, Caporali R, Avalle S, Bugatti S, Montecucco C: Autoantibody profile in rheumatoid arthritis during long-term infliximab treatment. Arthritis Res Ther 2004;6:R264.

Bombardieri M, Alessandri C, Labbadia G, Iannuccelli C, Carlucci F, Riccieri V, Paoletti V, Valesini G: Role of anti-cyclic citrullinated peptide antibodies in discriminating patients with rheumatoid arthritis from patients with chronic hepatitis C infection-associated polyarticular involvement. Arthritis Res Ther 2004; 6:R137.

Bonfa E, Golombek SJ, Kaufman LD et al: Association between lupus psychosis and anti-ribosomal P protein antibodies. N Engl J Med 1987; 317:265.

Burlingame RW, Cervera R: Anti-chromatin (anti-nucleosome) autoantibodies. Autoimmun Rev 2002;1:321.

Burlingame RW: Recent advances in understanding the clinical utility and underlying cause of antinucleosome (antichromatin) autoantibodies. Clin Appl Immunol Rev 2004; 4:351.
Antichromatin antibodies are a hallmark of lupus disease, and this review brings all important data that justify the assertion.

Buskila D, Shoenfeld Y: Anti-DNA antibodies. In Lahita RG (Ed): Systemic Lupus Erythematosus, 2nd ed. New York, Churchill Livingstone, 1992, p 205.

Bylund DJ, Nakamura RM: Importance of detection of SS-A/Ro autoantibody in screening immunofluorescence tests for autoantibodies to nuclear antigens. J Clin Lab Anal 1991; 5:212.

Casiano CA, Tan EM: Recent developments in the understanding of antinuclear antibodies. Int Arch Allergy Immunol 1996; 111:308.

Cepeda EJ, Reveille JD: Autoantibodies in systemic sclerosis and fibrosing syndromes: clinical indications and relevance. Curr Opin Rheumatol 2004;16:723.

Cervera R, Vinas O, Ramos-Casals M, et al: Anti-chromatin antibodies in systemic lupus erythematosus: a useful marker for lupus nephropathy. Ann Rheum Dis 2003; 62:431.

Chan EK, Tan EM: Epitopic targets for autoantibodies in systemic lupus erythematosus and Sjögren's syndrome. Curr Opin Rheumatol 1989; 1: 376.

Charles PJ, van Venrooij WJ, Maini RN: The consensus workshops for the detection of autoantibodies to intracellular antigens in rheumatic diseases, 1989–1992. Clin Exp Rheumatol 1992; 10:507.

Cohen AS, Reynolds WE, Franklin EC, et al: Preliminary criteria for the classification of systemic lupus erythematosus. Bull Rheum Dis 1971; 21:643.

Dagher JH, Scheer U, Voit R, et al: Autoantibodies to NOR 90/hUBF: longterm clinical and serological followup in a patient with limited systemic sclerosis suggests an antigen driven immune response. J Rheumatol 2002;29:1543.

Decker JL: Glossary Subcommittee of ARA Committee on Rheumatologic Practice. Arthritis Rheum 1986; 26:1029.

Emlen W, O'Neill L: Clinical significance of antinuclear antibodies: comparison of detection with immunofluorescence and enzyme-linked immunosorbent assays. Arthritis Rheum 1997; 40:1612.

Eriksson C, Engstrand S, Sundqvist KG, Rantapää-Dahlqvist S: Autoantibody formation in patients with rheumatoid arthritis treated with anti-TNF. Ann Rheum Dis 2005; 64:403.

Fatenejad S, Bennett M, Moslehi J, Craft J: Influence of antigen organization on the development of lupus autoantibodies. Arthritis Rheum 1998; 41:603.

Feltkamp TEW: Antinuclear antibody determination in a routine laboratory. Ann Rheum Dis 1996; 55:723.

Firestein GS: Evolving concepts of rheumatoid arthritis. Nature 2003; 423:356.

Forslind K, Ahlmén M, Eberhardt K, Hafström I, Svensson B: Prediction of radiological outcome in early rheumatoid arthritis in clinical practice: role of antibodies to citrullinated peptides (anti-CCP). Ann Rheum Dis 2004; 63:1090.

Francoeur AM, Peebles CL, Gomper PT, Tan EM: Identification of Ki (Ku, p70/p80) autoantigens and analysis of anti-Ki autoantibody reactivity. J Immunol 1986; 136:1648.

Fritzler MJ, Kinsella TD, Garbutt E: The CREST syndrome: a distinct serologic entity with anticentromere antibodies. Am J Med 1980; 69:520.

Fritzler MJ, von Muhlen CA, Toffoli SM, et al: Autoantibodies to the nucleolar organizer antigen NOR-90 in children with systemic rheumatic diseases. J Rheumatol 1995; 22:521.

Gladman DD, Urowitz MB, Esdaile JM, et al: Guidelines for referral and management of systemic lupus erythematosus in adults. Arthritis Rheum 1999; 42:1785.

Harris EN: The second International Anticardiolipin Standardization Workshop: the Kingston Antiphospholipid Antibody Study (KAPS) groups. Am J Clin Pathol 1990; 94: 476.

Harris EN, Gharavi AE, Patel SP, Hughes ERV: Evaluation of the anticardiolipin test: report of an international workshop held 4 April 1986. Clin Exp Immunol 1987; 68:215.

Harris ML, Rosen A: Autoimmunity in scleroderma: the origin, pathogenetic role, and clinical significance of autoantibodies. Curr Opin Rheumatol 2003; 15:778.

Hassfeld W, Steiner G, Hartmuth K, et al: Demonstration of a new antinuclear antibody (anti RA-33) that is highly specific for rheumatoid arthritis. Arthritis Rheum 1989; 32:1515.

Ho KT, Reveille JD: The clinical relevance of autoantibodies in scleroderma. Arthritis Res Ther 2003; 5:80.

Hochberg MC: Systemic lupus erythematosus. Rheum Dis Clin North Am 1990; 16:617.

Hochberg MC: Updating the American College of Rheumatology revised criteria for the classification of systemic lupus erythematosus (letter). Arthritis Rheum 1997; 40:1725.

Hochberg MC, Boyd RE, Ahearn JM, et al: Systemic lupus erythematosus: a review of clinical laboratory features and immunogenetic markers in 150 patients with emphasis on demographic subsets. Medicine 1985; 64:285.

Hof D, Cheung K, de Rooij DJRAM, et al: Autoantibodies specific for apoptotic U1–70K are superior serological markers for mixed connective tissue disease. Arthritis Res Ther 2005; 7:R302.

Hoffman IE, Peene I, Meheus L, et al: Specific antinuclear antibodies are associated with clinical features in systemic lupus erythematosus. Ann Rheum Dis 2004; 63:1155.

Hoffman IE, Peene I, Pottel H, et al: Diagnostic performance and predictive value of rheumatoid factor, anti-citrullinated peptide antibodies, and the HLA shared epitope for diagnosis of rheumatoid arthritis. Clin Chem 2005; 51:261.

Homburger HA, Cahen YD, Griffiths J, Jacob GL: Detection of antinuclear antibodies: comparative evaluation of enzyme immunoassay and indirect immunofluorescence methods. Arch Pathol Lab Med 1998; 122:993.

Humbel RL: Detection of antinuclear antibodies by immunofluorescence. In Van Venrooij WJ, Maini RN (eds): Manual of Biological Markers of Disease. Dordrecht, Kluwer Academic, 1993, pp 1–16.

Ioannidis JP, Vlachoyiannopoulos PG, Haidich AB, et al: Mortality in systemic sclerosis: an international meta-analysis of individual patient data. Am J Med 2005;118:2.

Isshi K & Hirohata S: Differential roles of the anti-ribosomal P antibody and antineuronal antibody in the pathogenesis of central nervous system involvement in systemic lupus erythematosus. Arthritis Rheum 1998; 41:1819.

Janssens X, Veys EM, Verbruggen G, Declecq L: The diagnostic significance of the antiperinuclear factor for rheumatoid arthritis. J Rheumatol 1988; 15:1346.

Jarzabek-Chorzelska M, Balszczyk M, Jablonska S, et al: Scl-70 antibody, a specific marker of systemic sclerosis. Br J Dermatol 1986; 115:393.

Kaneda K, Takasaki Y, Takeuchi K, et al: Autoimmune response to proteins of proliferating cell nuclear antigen multiprotein complexes in patients with connective tissue diseases. J Rheumatol 2004;31:2142.

Kastbom A, Strandberg G, Lindroos A, Skogh T: Anti-CCP antibody test predicts the disease course during 3 years in early rheumatoid arthritis (the Swedish TIRA project). Ann Rheum Dis 2004; 63:1085.

Kavanaugh AF, Solomon DH: Guidelines for immunologic laboratory testing in the rheumatic diseases: anti-DNA antibody tests. Arthritis Rheum 2002; 47:546.

Klareskog L, Alfredsson L, Rantapaa-Dahlqvist S, et al: What precedes development of rheumatoid arthritis? Ann Rheum Dis 2004; 63(Suppl 2): ii28.

Krapf AR, von Mühlen CA, Krapf FE, et al: Atlas of Immunofluorescent Autoantibodies. Munich, Urban & Schwarzenberg, 1996.

Lazaro MA, Maldonado-Cocco JA, Catoggio LJ, et al: Clinical and serological characteristics of patients with overlap syndrome: Is mixed connective tissue disease a distinct clinical entity? Medicine 1989; 68:58.

Lee DM, Schur PH: Clinical utility of the anti-CCP assay in patients with rheumatic diseases. Ann Rheum Dis 2003; 62:870.

Lerner MR, Steitz JA: Antibodies to small nuclear RNAs complexed with proteins are produced by patients with systemic lupus erythematosus. Proc Natl Acad Sci USA 1979; 76:5495.

Lom-Orta H, Alarcón-Segovia D, Diaz-Jouanen E: Systemic lupus erythematosus. Differences between patients who do and who do not fulfill classification criteria at the time of diagnosis. J Rheumatol 1980; 7:831.

Lopez LR, Santos ME, Espinoza LR, La Rosa FG: Clinical significance of immunoglobulin A versus immunoglobulins E and M anticardiolipin antibodies in patients with systemic lupus erythematosus: correlation with thrombosis, thrombocytopenia, and recurrent abortion. Is J Clin Pathol 1992; 98:447.

Low J, Chauhan A, Kietz D, et al: Determination of anti-cyclic citrullinated peptide antibodies in the sera of patients with juvenile idiopathic arthritis. J Rheumatol 2004; 31:1829.

McNeil HP, Chesterman CH, Krilis SA: Immunology and clinical importance of antiphospholipid antibodies. Adv Immunol 1991; 49:193.

Maddison PF, Skinner RP, Vlachoviannopoulos P, et al: Antibodies to nRNP, Sm, Ro (SSA) and La (SSB) detected by ELISA: their specificity and inter-relations in connective tissue disease sera. Clin Exp Immunol 1985; 62:337.

Mahler M, Kessenbrock K, Szmyrka M, et al: International multicenter evaluation of autoantibodies to ribosomal P proteins. Clin Vaccine Immunol 2006; 13:77–83.

Martins TB, Burlingame R, von Muhlen CA, et al: Evaluation of multiplexed fluorescent microsphere immunoassay for detection of autoantibodies to nuclear antigens. Clin Diagn Lab Immunol 2004;11:1054.

Matsuura E, Lopez LR: Are oxidized LDL/beta2-glycoprotein I complexes pathogenic antigens in autoimmune-mediated atherosclerosis? Clin Dev Immunol 2004;11:103.

Miyachi K, Fritzler MJ, Tan EM: Autoantibody to nuclear antigen in proliferating cells. J Immunol 1978; 121:2228.

Mosca M, Baldini C, Bombardieri S: Undifferentiated connective tissue diseases in 2004. Clin Exp Rheumatol 2004; 22:S14.

Nakamura RM: Role of autoantibody tests in the diagnostic evaluation of neuropsychiatric systemic lupus erythematosus (NPSLE). Clin Lab Med 1997; 17:379.

Nakamura RM, Bylund DJ: Contemporary concepts for clinical and laboratory evaluation of systemic lupus erythematosus and 'lupus-like' syndromes. J Clin Anal 1994a; 8:347.

Nakamura RM, Bylund DJ, Tan EM: Current status of available standards for quality improvement of assays for the detection of autoantibodies to nuclear and intracellular antigens. J Clin Lab Anal 1994b; 8:360.

Nakamura RM, Peebles CL, Rubin RL, et al: Autoantibodies to nuclear antigens. In Advances in Laboratory Tests and Significance in Systemic Rheumatic Diseases, 2nd ed. Chicago, IL, American Society of Clinical Pathology, 1985, p 1.

Nakamura RM, Tan EM: Recent advances in laboratory tests and the significance of autoantibodies to nuclear antigens in systemic rheumatic diseases. Clin Lab Med 1986; 6:41.

Nakamura RM, Tan EM: Update on autoantibodies to intracellular antigens in systemic rheumatic diseases. Clin Lab Med 1992; 12:1.

Nienhuis RLF, Mandema E: A new serum factor in patients with rheumatoid arthritis: the perinuclear factor. Ann Rheum Dis 1964; 23:302.

Nimelstein SH, Brody S, McShane D, and Holman HR: Mixed connective tissue disease: a subsequent evaluation of the original 25 patients. Medicine 1980; 59:239.

Obermoser G, Bitterlich W, Kunz F, Sepp NT: Clinical significance of anticardiolipin and anti-beta2-glycoprotein I antibodies. Int Arch Allergy Immunol 2004;135:148.

Okamura M, Kanayama Y, Amastu K, et al: Significance of enzyme-linked immunosorbent assay (ELISA) for antibodies to double-stranded and single-stranded DNA in patients with lupus nephritis: correlation with severity of renal histology. Ann Rheum Dis 1993; 52:14.

Panush RS, Greer JM, Morshedian KK: What is lupus? What is not lupus? Rheum Dis Clin North Am 1993; 19:223.

Peene I, Meheus L, Veys EM, De Keyser F: Diagnostic associations in a large and consecutively identified population positive for anti-SSA and/or anti-SSB: the range of associated diseases differs according to the detailed serotype. Ann Rheum Dis 2002; 61:1090.

Pincus T: Studies regarding a possible function for viruses in the pathogenesis of systemic lupus erythematosus. Arthritis Rheum 1982; 25:847.

Pope JE: Scleroderma overlap syndromes. Curr Opin Rheumatol 2002;14:704.

Ramos-Casals M, Tzioufas AG, Font J: Primary Sjögren's syndrome: new clinical and therapeutic concepts. Ann Rheum Dis 2005; 64:347.

Ranzolin A, Bohn JM, Norman GL, et al: Anti-beta2-glycoprotein I antibodies as risk factors for acute myocardial infarction. Arq Bras Cardiol 2004; 83:141.

Rekvig OP, Nossent JC: Anti-double-stranded DNA antibodies, nucleosomes, and systemic lupus erythematosus: a time for new paradigms? Arthritis Rheum 2003; 48:300.

Reeves WH: Antibodies of the p70/p80 (Ku) antigens in systemic lupus erythematosus. Rheum Dis Clin North Am 1992; 18:391.

Reimer G: Autoantibodies against nuclear, nucleolar, and mitochondrial antigens in systemic sclerosis (scleroderma). Rheum Dis Clin North Am 1990; 16:169.

Rothfield NF: Autoantibodies in scleroderma. Rheum Dis Clin North Am 1992; 18:483.

Rubin RL: Autoimmune reactions induced by procainamide and hydralazine. *In* Kammuller M, Bloksma M, Siemen W (eds): Autoimmunity and Toxicology: Immune Dysregulation Induced by Drugs and Chemicals. Amsterdam, Elsevier, 1988, p 119.

Rubin RL, McNally EM, Nusinow SR, et al: IgG antibodies to the histone complex H2A–H2B characterize procainamide-induced lupus. Clin Immunol Immunopathol 1985; 36:49.

Rubin RL, Waga S: Antihistone antibodies in systemic lupus erythematosus. J Rheumatol 1987; 14(Suppl 13):118.

Ruffatti A, Ostuni P, Grypiotis P, et al: Sensitivity and specificity for primary Sjögren's syndrome of IgA and IgG anti-alpha-fodrin antibodies detected by ELISA. J Rheumatol 2004; 31:504.

Saitta MR, Keene JD: Molecular biology of nuclear autoantigens. Rheum Dis Clin North Am 1992; 18:283.

Sakamoto M, Takasaki Y, Yamanaka K, et al: Purification and characterization of Ki antigen and detection of anti-Ki antibody by enzyme-linked immunosorbent assay in patients with systemic lupus erythematosus. Arthritis Rheum 1989; 32:1554.

Schellekens GA, de Jong BAW, van den Hoogen FHJ, et al: Citrulline is an essential constituent of antigenic determinants recognized by rheumatoid arthritis-specific autoantibodies. J Clin Invest 1998; 101:273.

Schumacher HR, Klippel JH, Koopman WJ: Primer on the Rheumatic Diseases, 10th ed. Atlanta, GA, Arthritis Foundation, 1993.

Schur PH: Clinical features of SLE. *In* Kelly WN, Harris ED, Ruddy S, Sledge CB (eds): Textbook of Rheumatology, vol 2, 4th ed. Philadelphia, PA, WB Saunders, 1993, p 1017.

Sebbag M, Chapuy-Regaud S, Auger I, et al: Clinical and pathophysiological significance of the autoimmune response to citrullinated proteins in rheumatoid arthritis. Joint Bone Spine 2004; 71:493.

Very informative account, with historic highlights, for these important group of autoantibodies specifically seen in rheumatoid arthritis.

Sharp GC, Irwin WS, Tan EM, et al: Mixed connective tissue disease: an apparently distinct rheumatic disease syndrome associated with a specific antibody to an extractable antigen (ENA). Am J Med 1972; 52:148.

Sherer Y, Gorstein A, Fritzler MJ, Shoenfeld Y: Autoantibody explosion in systemic lupus erythematosus: more than 100 different antibodies found in SLE patients. Semin Arthritis Rheum 2004; 34:501.

Most complete account of autoantibodies prevalence and specificities in systemic lupus erythematosus, comprising antibodies that target nuclear, cytoplasmic, phospholipid, cell membrane and other antigens.

Simon M, Girbal E, Sebbag M, et al: The cytokeratin filament-aggregating protein fillagrin is the target of the so-called 'antikeratin antibodies,' autoantibodies specific for rheumatoid arthritis. J Clin Invest 1993; 92:1387.

Slater CA, Davis RB, Shmerling RH: Antinuclear antibody testing: a study of clinical utility. Arch Intern Med 1996; 156:1421.

Smolen JS, Steiner G: Are autoantibodies active players or epiphenomena? Curr Opin Rheumatol 1998; 10:201.

Smolen JS, Steiner G, Tan EM: Standards of care: the value and importance of standardization. Arthritis Rheum 1997; 40:410.

Sontheimer RD, Gilliam JN: Systemic lupus erythematosus and the skin. *In* Lahita RG (ed.): Systemic Lupus Erythematosus, 2nd Ed. New York, Churchill Livingstone, 1992, p 657.

Staub HL, Norman GL, Crowther T, et al: Antibodies to the atherosclerotic plaque components beta2-glycoprotein I and heat-shock proteins as risk factors for acute cerebral ischemia. Arq Neuropsiquiatr 2003; 61:757.

Steiner G, Skriner K, Hassfeld W, Smolen JS: Clinical and immunological aspects of autoantibodies to RA33/hnRNP-A/B proteins – a link between RA, SLE and MCTD. Mol Biol Rep 1996; 23:167.

Stinton LM, Eystathioy T, Selak S, et al: Autoantibodies to protein transport and messenger RNA processing pathways: endosomes, lysosomes, Golgi complex, proteasomes, assemblyosomes, exosomes, and GW bodies. Clin Immunology 2004; 110:30.

Swale VJ, Perrett CM, Denton CP, et al: Etanercept-induced systemic lupus erythematosus. Clin Exp Dermatol 2003; 28:604.

Tan EM: Autoantibodies to nuclear antigens (ANA): their immunobiology and medicine. Adv Immunol 1982; 33:167.

Tan EM, Chan EKL, Sullivan KF, Rubin RL: Antinuclear antibodies (ANAs): diagnostically specific immune markers and clues toward the understanding of systemic autoimmunity. Clin Immunol Immunopathol 1988; 47:121.

Tan EM: Antinuclear antibodies: diagnostic markers for autoimmune diseases and probes for cell biology. Adv Immunol 1989; 44:93.

This is a classic review paper in the field of autoantibodies, their clinical associations and molecular nature of autoantigens, written by a scientist that discovered many of the most important autoantibody markers in Rheumatology.

Tan EM: Autoantibodies and autoimmunity: a three-decade perspective. A tribute to Henry G Kunkel. Ann NY Acad Sci 1997a; 815:1.

Tan EM, Cohen AS, Fries JF, et al: The 1982 revised criteria for the classification of systemic lupus erythematosus. Arthritis Rheum 1993; 25:1271.

Tan EM, Feltkamp TEW, Smolen JS, et al: Range of antinuclear antibodies in 'healthy' individuals. Arthritis Rheum 1997b; 40:1601.

Tan EM, Smolen JS, McDougal JS et al: A critical evaluation of enzyme immunoassays for detection of antinuclear antibodies of defined specificities. I. Precision, sensitivity, and specificity. Arthritis Rheum 1999; 42:455.

This paper is a first in trying to shed light into the difficult task of standardization of laboratory practices. Many useful recommendations for researchers, technicians, and clinicians help understand ELISA results.

Targoff IN: Autoantibodies in polymyositis. Rheum Dis Clin North Am 1992; 18:455.

Targoff IN: Laboratory testing in the diagnosis and management of idiopathic inflammatory myopathies. Rheum Dis Clin North Am 2002; 28:859.

Teodorescu M, Froelich CJ: Laboratory evaluation of systemic lupus erythematosus. *In* Lahita RG (ed.): Systemic Lupus Erythematosus, 2nd ed. New York, Churchill Livingstone, 1992, p 345.

Ter Borg EJ, Groen H, Horst G, et al: Clinical association of antiribonucleoprotein antibodies in patients with systemic lupus erythematosus. Sem Arthritis Rheum 1990; 20:164.

Tojo T, Kaburaki J, Hayakawa M, et al: Precipitating antibody to a soluble nuclear antigen 'Ki' with specificity for systemic lupus erythematosus. Ryumachi 1981; 21(Suppl): 129.

Van Venrooij WJ, Charles P, Maini RN: The consensus workshops for the detection of autoantibodies to intracellular antigens in rheumatic diseases. J Immunol Methods 1991; 140:507.

Van Venrooij WJ, Vossenaar ER, Zendman AJ: Anti-CCP antibodies: the new rheumatoid factor in the serology of rheumatoid arthritis. Autoimmun Rev 2004; 3 Suppl 1:S17.

Viander M: Clinically useful antibody assays – systemic rheumatic diseases. *In* Lefkovits I (ed.): Immunology Methods Manual. San Diego, CA, Academic Press, 1997, pp 1610–1624.

Von Mühlen CA, Tan EM: Autoantibody specificities in autoimmune rheumatic diseases. Rev Bras Rheumatol 1994; 34:173.

Von Mühlen CA, Tan EM: Autoantibodies in the diagnosis of systemic rheumatic diseases. Sem Arthritis Rheum 1995; 24:323.

Very thorough description of major autoantibodies in systemic rheumatic diseases, with clinical associations and molecular data for autoantigens.

Von Mühlen CA, Nakamura RM: Guidelines for selecting and using laboratory tests for autoantibodies to nuclear, nucleolar and other related cytoplasmic antigens. *In* Nakamura RM, Keren DF, Bylund DJ (eds): Clinical and Laboratory Evaluation of Human Autoimmune Diseases. Chicago, IL, ASCP Press, 2002, pp 183–198.

Vossenaar ER, van Venrooij WJ: Anti-CCP antibodies, a highly specific marker for (early) rheumatoid arthritis. Clin Applied Immunol Rev 2004: 4:239.

Historic and clinical discussion of anti-CCP autoantibodies, presenting some evidence for a possible etiologic role of the autoantibodies in rheumatoid arthritis.

Wallace DJ, Pistiner M, Nessim S, et al: Cutaneous lupus erythematosus without systemic lupus erythematosus: Clinical and laboratory features. Semin Arthritis Rheum 1992; 21:221.

Wang HB, Zhang Y: Mi2, an auto-antigen for dermatomyositis, is an ATP-dependent nucleosome remodeling factor. Nucleic Acids Res 2001; 29:2517.

Woosley RL, Drager DE, Reidenber MM, et al: Effect of acetylator phenotype on the rate at which procainamide induces antinuclear antibodies and the lupus syndrome. N Engl J Med 1987; 298:1157.

VI

Yalaoui S, Gorgi Y, Hajri R, et al: Autoantibodies to ribosomal P proteins in systemic lupus erythematosus. Joint Bone Spine 2002; 69:173.

Young BJJ, Mallya RK, Leslie RDG, et al: Anti-keratin antibodies in rheumatoid arthritis. Br Med J 1979; ii: 97.

Zandbelt MM, Vogelzangs J, Van De Putte LB, et al: Anti-alpha-fodrin antibodies do not add much to the diagnosis of Sjögren's syndrome. Arthritis Res Ther 2004; 6:R33-R38.

Zarmbinski MN, Messner RP, Mandel JS: Anti-dsDNA antibodies in laboratory workers handling blood from patients with systemic lupus erythematosus. J Rheumatol 1992; 19:1380.

CHAPTER 51

Vasculitis

Rex M. McCallum MD, David J. Bylund MD

KEY POINTS

- The etiology and pathogenesis of vasculitides remain obscure and poorly understood, and may vary between different forms of vasculitis.

- There is no widely accepted standard classification system for idiopathic vasculitides.

- The diagnosis of idiopathic systemic necrotizing vasculitides requires a high degree of suspicion.

- There are no pathognomonic clinical laboratory tests in patients with systemic necrotizing vasculitides.

- Antineutrophil cytoplasmic autoantibody (ANCA) tests are most valuable when selectively ordered in clinical situations where some form of ANCA-associated vasculitis is a serious consideration, and should not be used as a screening test.

- Detection of ANCA, particularly the association of c-ANCA with Wegener's granulomatosis, has become an important adjunct in diagnosis of systemic necrotizing vasculitis.

- c-ANCA immunofluorescence pattern should be confirmed using PR-3 ELISA.

- p-ANCA pattern on indirect fluorescence microscopy is diagnostically nonspecific so p-ANCA-positive sera should be tested in ELISA for MPO-ANCA

- Tissue biopsy with histologic confirmation of vasculitis remains the most important laboratory test for diagnosis of systemic necrotizing vasculitis.

The clinical, laboratory, and pathological expressions of systemic necrotizing vasculitis are protean. Clinicians face a patient who presents with a wide array of confusing and conflicting symptoms and/or signs. Diagnosis of a systemic necrotizing vasculitic syndrome requires thorough evaluation that correlates an individual patient's history and physical examination with laboratory, imaging, and pathologic data. Although vasculitis can occur anywhere in the body, distinctive patterns of disease have been defined and their identification point to particular disorders with specific treatment and prognosis (Langford 1995, 2003).

Systemic necrotizing vasculitis is characterized pathologically by inflammation causing vascular lesions. These lesions may include the proliferation of intimal cells inside the lumen of vessels and narrowing or even closing that space, causing ischemia and possible infarction of anatomic structures distal to the site of vascular injury. Also, the vessel wall may thin and weaken until an aneurysm forms or the vessel ruptures.

Idiopathic (primary) vasculitis occurs when vascular inflammatory damage is the principal clinicopathologic finding and there is no other underlying illness. Secondary vasculitis occurs when vasculitic lesions accompany an underlying disorder (Table 51–1). This chapter focuses on idiopathic vasculitis and those clinical laboratory tests useful for its diagnosis and management. Since methods of diagnosis and management in secondary vasculitides concentrate on the underlying disorders, they are discussed in the appropriate chapters of this book. However, comments related to laboratory evaluation of end-organ damage in idiopathic vasculitis are relevant to secondary vasculitis.

Classification

There is no widely accepted standard classification system for idiopathic vasculitides. Historically, their classification has been based on various combinations of clinical and pathologic findings (Jennette, 1997, 1998b), although working classifications have improved in recent years as a result of efforts at standard nomenclature (Hunder, 1990; Jennette, 1994b; Hoffman, 1998a; Langford 2003). The classification scheme provided in Table 51–2 is modified from the one used at the National Institutes of Health (Langford, 1995). Table 51–3 contains the names and definitions of vasculitides adopted by the Chapel Hill Consensus Conference on the nomenclature of systemic vasculitis (Jennette, 1994b). The close association of antineutrophil cytoplasmic autoantibodies (ANCA) with the small-vessel necrotizing vasculitides has contributed to new thoughts in classification (Falk, 2004). These schemes were not intended for use in diagnosing the individual patient (Langford, 2003).

Pathogenesis of Vasculitis

The etiology and pathogenesis of vasculitides remains obscure and poorly understood, and may vary between different forms of vasculitis (Langford, 2003). Most idiopathic vasculitides are attributed to immune-mediated vascular injury induced by any of several mechanisms, including: (1) immune-complex deposits; (2) direct autoantibody binding, either to vessel wall structures (e.g., endothelium or basement membrane antigens) or to neutrophils when vasculitis is associated with ANCA; and, (3) T-cell-

VI

Table 51.1 Secondary Systemic Necrotizing Vasculitides

Drug-related vasculitis
Foreign-protein-related vasculitis
Vasculitis associated with infection
Vasculitis in malignancies
Lymphomatoid granulomatosis
Hypocomplementemic urticarial vasculitis
Hypergammaglobulinemic purpura
Cryoglobulinemic vasculitis
Radiation vasculitis
Transplant vasculitis (vascular rejection)
Connective-tissue-disease-associated vasculitis
Rheumatoid arthritis
Systemic lupus erythematosus
Sjögren syndrome
Scleroderma
Dermatomyositis/polymyositis
Sarcoidosis
Relapsing polychondritis
Antiphospholipid antibody syndrome
Behçet disease

Source: adapted from Langford CA, McCallum RM: Idiopathic vasculitis. *In* Belch JJF, Zurier RB (eds): Connective Tissue Diseases. London, Chapman & Hall, 1995, p 179, with permission.

Table 51.2 Idiopathic (Primary) Systemic Necrotizing Vasculitides

Small-vessel vasculitis
Wegener's granulomatosis
Henoch–Schönlein purpura
Primary angiitis of the central nervous system

Medium-vessel vasculitis
Churg–Strauss syndrome
Polyarteritis nodosa
Kawasaki disease

Large-vessel vasculitis
Giant cell (temporal) arteritis
Takayasu's arteritis

Table 51.3 Names and Definitions of Vasculitides from the Chapel Hill Consensus

	Conference
Large-vessel vasculitis	
Giant cell (temporal) arteritis	Granulomatous arteritis of the aorta and its major branches, with a predilection for the extracranial branches of the carotid artery. Often involves the temporal artery. Usually occurs in patients older than 50 and often associated with polymyalgia rheumatica.
Takayasu's arteritis	Granulomatous inflammation of the aorta and its major branches. Usually occurs in patients younger than 50.
Medium-sized-vessel vasculitis	
Polyarteritis nodosa (classic)	Necrotizing inflammation of medium-sized or small arteries without glomerulonephritis or vasculitis of the arterioles, capillaries, or venules.
Kawasaki disease	Arteritis involving the large, medium-sized, and small arteries, and associated with mucocutaneous lymph node syndrome. Coronary arteries are often involved. Aorta and veins may be involved. Usually occurs in children.
Small-vessel vasculitis	
Wegener's granulomatosis	Granulomatous inflammation involving the respiratory tract, and necrotizing vasculitis affecting small to medium-sized vessels (capillaries, venules, arterioles, and arteries). Necrotizing glomerulonephritis is common.
Churg–Strauss	Eosinophil-rich and granulomatous inflammation involving the respiratory tract, and necrotizing vasculitis affecting small to medium-sized vessels, and associated with asthma and eosinophilia.
Microscopic polyangiitis	Necrotizing vasculitis, with few or no immune deposits, affecting small vessels (capillaries, venules, or arterioles).
Henoch–Schönlein purpura	Vasculitis with IgA dominant immune deposits, affecting small vessels (capillaries, venules, or arterioles).
Essential cryoglobulinemic vasculitis	Vasculitis with cryoglobulin immune deposits, affecting small vessels, (capillaries, venules, or arterioles). Typically involves skin, gut, and glomeruli, and is associated with arthralgias, and arthritis.
Cutaneous leukocytoclastic vasculitis	Isolated cutaneous leukocytoclastic angiitis without systemic vasculitis or glomerulonephritis

mediated inflammation (Jennette, 1994a) (Table 51–4). The pathogenic effects of these different mechanisms all unite in a final common pathway of vascular injury that activates humoral and cellular mediators of inflammation. Adhesion molecules that are involved in the normal immune response appear to mediate the pathologic immune responses noted in vasculitis. Quantitative and qualitative abnormalities of cytokine production are noted in systemic vasculitis. Increased levels of interleukin (IL)-1, IL-2, IL-6, tumor necrosis factor (TNF)-α, and TNF-β (Grau, 1989; Arimura, 1993), as well as increased production of TNF-α by circulating mononuclear cells (Deguchi, 1990), have been reported. These mediators initiate the infiltration of inflammatory cells, activation of complement and coagulation cascades, and up-regulation of other inflammatory molecules (Conn, 1993; Niles, 1995; Sneller, 1997, Langford 2003). Substantial evidence of direct ANCA involvement in vasculitis tissue damage exists, including recombinant-activating-gene-deficient mice that develop vasculitis when infused with antimyeloperoxidase antibodies and propylthiouracil, which accumulates in neutrophil granules and is associated with an ANCA-associated vasculitis (Seo, 2004b). Finally, an association between the Birmingham Vasculitis Activity Score and extent of disease and the number of activated B cells has been described (Seo, 2004b).

Perspective on Use of Clinical Laboratory Tests

When evaluating patients with complicated multisystem disease, the clinician's goal is accurate diagnosis to the level that defines proper treatment. Since there are no pathognomonic clinical or laboratory features of vasculitis, the physician must use combinations of clinical, laboratory, imaging, and pathologic findings to recognize patterns of disease. This may allow specific diagnosis or classification of the patient's disease as one in a group of vasculitic disorders with similar treatment, even when no specific entity is identifiable.

Deciding that a patient has vasculitis strictly on the basis of clinical symptoms is fraught with risks because of the large number of differential diagnostic possibilities and the lack of pathognomonic findings. Consequently, histologic or angiographic confirmation of vasculitis should be obtained from tissue biopsy or angiography for definitive diagnosis prior to therapy (Mandell, 1994; Langford, 2003).

Clinical laboratory tests are of limited value in establishing a specific diagnosis of vasculitis (Mandell, 1994; Langford, 2003), although clinicians use these tests to assist in identifying patterns of organ involvement characteristic of vasculitis, evaluating the extent and severity of end-organ damage, distinguishing idiopathic vasculitis from alternative secondary forms, and establishing baseline values for management. The association of ANCA with certain idiopathic vasculitides is an important aid in diagnosis and management. ANCA are discussed in detail subsequently.

Table 51.4 Potential Mechanisms of Vessel Damage in Selected Primary Vasculitis Syndromes

Immune complex formation
Hepatitis-B-associated polyarteritis nodosa
Henoch–Schönlein purpura
Essential mixed cryoglobulinemia

Production of antineutrophil cytoplasmic antibodies
Wegener's granulomatosis
Microscopic polyangiitis
Churg–Strauss syndrome

Pathogenic T-lymphocyte responses and granuloma formation
Giant cell (temporal) arteritis
Takayasu's arteritis
Wegener's granulomatosis
Churg–Strauss syndrome

Table 51.5 Antibodies Associated with Vasculitis

Antibody	Disease Association	Principal Test Method(s)
ANCA, usually c-ANCA	Wegener's granulomatosis	IFM, ELISA
ANCA, c-ANCA or p-ANCA	Microscopic polyangiitis	IFM, ELISA
Anti-C1q antibodies	Hypocomplementemic urticarial vasculitis	C1q binding
Hepatitis B antibodies	Hepatitis-B-associated polyarteritis nodosa	ELISA
ANA	Systemic lupus erythematosus	IFM, ELISA
Mixed cryoglobulins	Cryoglobulinemic vasculitis	Cryoprecipitation, IEP, IF
SSA (Ro), SSB (La)	Sjögren syndrome	IFM, ELISA, ID
Rheumatoid factor	Rheumatoid arthritis	LA, ELISA
Hepatitis C antibodies	Hepatitis-C-associated polyarteritis nodosa	EIA
Anti-DNA	Systemic lupus erythematosus	IFM, ELISA

ANA = antinuclear antibodies; ANCA = antineutrophil cytoplasmic autoantibodies; c-ANCA = cytoplasmic ANCA; EIA = enzyme immunoassay; ELISA = enzyme-linked immunosorbent assay; ID = immunodiffusion; IEP = immunoelectrophoresis; IF = immunofixation; IFM = indirect immunofluorescence microscopy; LA = latex agglutination; p-ANCA = perinuclear ANCA.

When evaluating a patient whose differential diagnoses includes vasculitis, use the following principles regarding the use and interpretation of clinical laboratory tests.

Routine Tests

Patients whose history and physical examination suggest idiopathic vasculitis often have a confusing array of multisystem complaints that have been occurring for some time. First-order tests include the following: cultures for infectious agents (particularly if the patient has fever), complete blood count with differential count, erythrocyte sedimentation rate (ESR), urinalysis, blood chemistry panel, and tests for specific organ function, such as the liver.

Special Tests

Special tests help to differentiate idiopathic vasculitis from alternatives in the working differential diagnosis. Relevant laboratory tests would include those to identify the circulating autoantibodies listed in Table 51-5 and immune complexes. Directed tissue biopsy for histologic confirmation of vasculitis, with or without angiography, is considered the definitive test for idiopathic vasculitis.

Some Test Patterns in Vasculitis

Certain patterns of clinical laboratory test results are useful:
- Finding leukopenia and/or thrombocytopenia in idiopathic vasculitides is rare and suggest alternative diagnoses such as systemic lupus erythematosus, neoplasm, bone marrow disorders, lymphomatoid granulomatosis, or hypersplenism (Mandell, 1994).
- ESR, although a nonspecific finding, is typically elevated in idiopathic vasculitides. If the ESR before therapy is not elevated, the diagnosis is probably not giant cell (temporal) arteritis or Wegener's granulomatosis.
- Vasculitis with histologic features of polyarteritis nodosa associated with pancytopenia can be seen in patients with hairy cell leukemia (Mandell, 1994).
- Anemia with hemoglobin less than 9 g/dL results from conditions other than anemia of chronic disease, such as hemolysis, occult bleeding, or renal disease (Mandell, 1994).
- When polyarteritis nodosa is suspected, serologic tests for liver function, hepatitis B virus (HBV), hepatitis C virus (HCV), and cytomegalovirus (CMV) should be obtained (Golden, 1994; Mandell, 1994; Langford 2003). Similarly, serologic tests for hepatitis B and C viruses are appropriate when a patient has cryoglobulins, leukocytoclastic vasculitis on cutaneous biopsy, and/or renal disease.
- Elevated serum creatine kinase or aldolase may indicate myositis or muscle ischemia (Mandell, 1994).
- Testing for antinuclear antibodies (ANA) and rheumatoid factor (RF) is useful only when connective tissue disease or arthritis is suspected.
- Patients with rheumatoid vasculitis have high-titer RF.
- Peripheral blood eosinophilia occurs in a wide variety of inflammatory disorders. About 15–20% of patients with polyarteritis nodosa or Wegener's granulomatosis may have eosinophilia but not at the high levels seen in Churg–Strauss syndrome.
- Identification of cytoplasmic-ANCA (c-ANCA) supports the diagnosis of Wegener's granulomatosis in patients with clinical findings of Wegener's granulomatosis.

- Untreated patients with Wegener's granulomatosis do not have leukopenia.
- First morning urine, both before and after centrifugation, should be carefully examined for protein, hematuria, cells, and casts, which accompany the glomerulonephritis that may occur in vasculitides. If renal amyloidosis is in the differential diagnosis, proteinuria is typically seen without cells.

Antineutrophil Cytoplasmic Antibody

ANCA reacts with neutrophil cytoplasmic antigens (Tervaert, 1991; Jennette, 1993a) that were previously shielded (Seo, 2004b). Identification of ANCA has become an important adjunct in diagnosis of systemic necrotizing vasculitis (Niles, 1993; Seo, 2004b).

Detection Methods

Several laboratory methods, including indirect fluorescence microscopy (IFM), enzyme-linked immunosorbent assay (ELISA), radioimmunoassay, Western blotting, dot blotting, flow cytometry, immunoprecipitation, and capture enzyme immunoassay techniques have been used to detect ANCA (Wieslander, 1991; Roberts, 1992; Seo, 2004b). IFM and ELISA are the most common test methods used for this purpose. IFM is the most sensitive widely used method for ANCA detection.

IFM is done using isolated normal human neutrophils as substrate. These neutrophils are cytocentrifuged against multiwell glass slides, fixed with 99% ethanol, and then incubated with dilutions of patients' sera. Neutrophils may also be attached to slides by adherence, smear, or drop techniques (Roberts, 1990, 1992). Slides are stained with a fluorescein-labeled polyspecific antihuman immunoglobulin (Ig) conjugate; polyspecific conjugate is recommended because IgM and IgA c-ANCA occur (Roberts, 1992). Slides are read on a fluorescence microscope. Using IFM, there are three patterns of neutrophil staining: c-ANCA, perinuclear ANCA (p-ANCA), and 'atypical patterns' (Seo, 2004b).

C-ANCAs are characterized by finely granular staining of neutrophil cytoplasm with central accentuation between the nuclear lobes; the nucleus itself does not stain (Fig. 51–1). Criteria useful for differentiating c-ANCA from nonspecific cytoplasmic staining due to other autoantibodies include: (1) lack of central accentuation, (2) less than 95% of neutrophils demonstrate cytoplasmic staining, (3) non-neutrophil specificity (e.g., lymphocytes on the slide should not stain when true ANCA is present), and (4) heterogeneous cytoplasmic granularity (Roberts, 1992; Savige, 1998).

P-ANCAs are characterized by staining of the perinuclear area (Fig. 51–2), although nuclear staining mimicking ANA may occur when this autoantibody is present in high titers (Niles, 1993). The perinuclear staining pattern that defines p-ANCA is caused by redistribution of target antigens from the neutrophil cytoplasm to the nuclear region when ethanol is used to prepare human neutrophils as substrate (Jennette, 1993a) (Fig. 51–3). When

VI

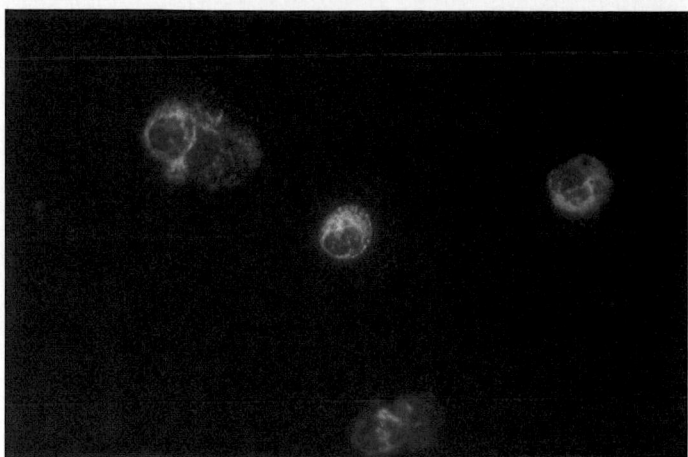

Figure 51–1 Antineutrophil cytoplasmic antibody-cytoplasmic pattern (c-ANCA). Most ethanol-fixed neutrophils show finely granular, cytoplasmic fluorescence with central accentuation. There is no nuclear staining. (×400)

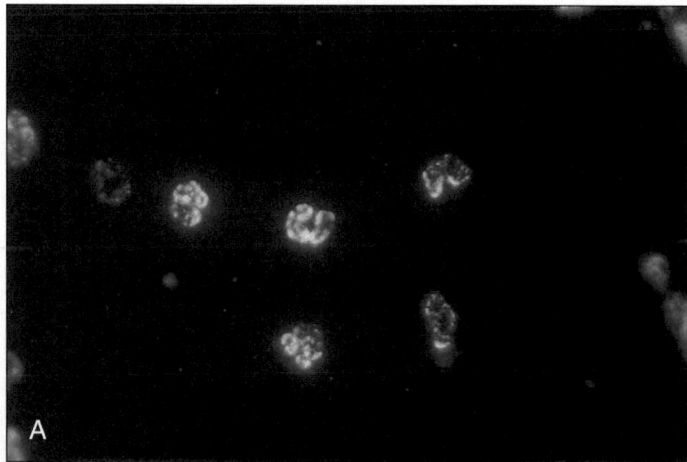

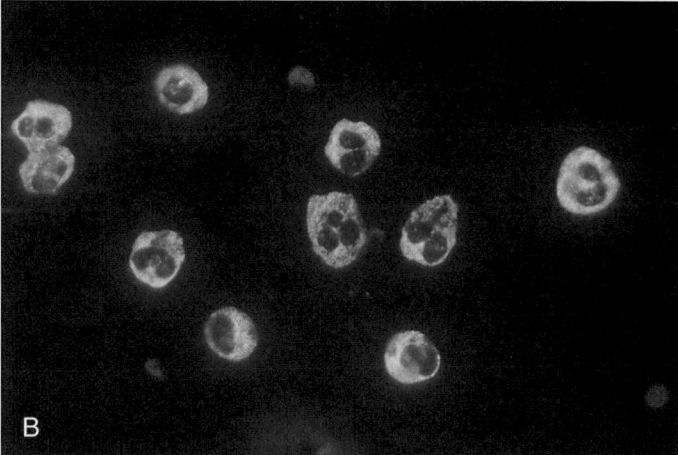

Figure 51–2 Antineutrophil cytoplasmic antibody-perinuclear pattern (p-ANCA). Most ethanol-fixed neutrophils show perinuclear and nuclear fluorescence without cytoplasmic staining. (A, ×400) that is cytoplasmic when formalin rather than alcohol is used to fix neutrophils (B, ×400)

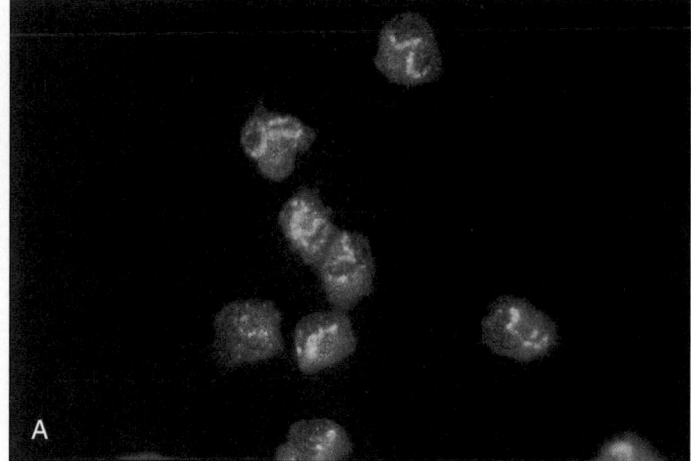

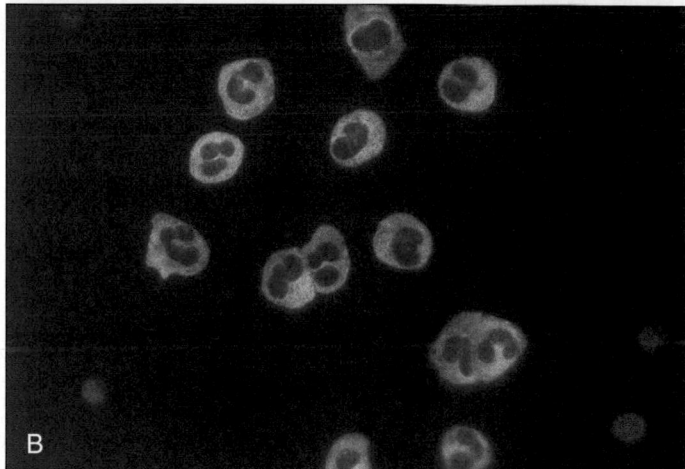

Figure 51–3 Atypical perinuclear-antineutrophil cytoplasmic antibody pattern on ethanol-fixed neutrophils shows perinuclear fluorescence (A, ×500) but no fluorescence when formalin rather than alcohol is used to fix neutrophils (B, ×500)

formalin rather than alcohol is used to fix neutrophils, target antigen is immobilized, and the immunofluorescent staining pattern is then cytoplasmic (Jennette, 1993a). The role of using formalin-fixed neutrophils to detect ANCA in routine diagnostic work remains controversial (Chowdhury, 1999). Distinguishing p-ANCA from 'atypical patterns' is difficult (Seo, 2004b).

Antigenic Specificity

The antigenic specificity of c-ANCA has been identified as a 29 kDa neutral serine protease, proteinase 3 (PR-3), located within azurophilic granules

of neutrophils and peroxidase-positive lysosomes of monocytes (Roberts, 1992; Niles, 1993; Seo 2004b). Proteinase-3 is also found on the plasma membrane of resting neutrophils and monocytes in many patients (Seo, 2004b). P-ANCA in vasculitis is usually due to autoantibodies against myeloperoxidase (MPO-ANCA) (Falk, 1988). Interestingly, many p-ANCAs are not directed at MPO but rather are directed at other neutrophil cytoplasmic enzymes, including elastase, lactoferrin, lactoperoxidase, lysozyme, azurocidin, or cathepsin G (Jennette, 1993a; Niles, 1993; Hoffman, 1998b). ANCA patterns should be confirmed with more specific tests for PR-3 and MPO, the antibodies most often associated with vasculitis (Savige, 2000; Langford 2003; Seo, 2004b).

ELISAs for detecting autoantibodies to PR-3 (PR-3-ANCA) show good correlation with the presence of c-ANCA when experienced observers perform IFM (Niles, 1993; Roberts, 1992). An ELISA for detecting PR-3-ANCA must be carefully validated, with particular attention to using proven techniques for solid-phase antigen preparation and to using either background subtraction or a specific absorption step to control for nonspecific binding of immunoglobulin to the solid-phase (Roberts, 1992; Niles, 1993; Wang, 1997). Efforts to standardize solid phase ELISAs are being made in Europe (Hagen, 1996, 1998).

Licensed commercial ELISAs for both PR-3 and MPO are available. Most use standard direct antigen coating of polystyrene microwell plates so that antigen purity is of critical importance in defining analytic sensitivity and specificity (Niles, 1993; Roberts, 1992). Attempts to preserve native antigen conformation are important, since ANCAs to PR-3 are directed against conformational epitopes (Hoffman, 1998b).

The correlation between p-ANCA and detection of MPO on ELISA, however, is not good (Roberts, 1992). Several autoantibodies, including ANA, antineutrophil elastase, and granulocyte-specific ANA (GS-ANA) can produce p-ANCA pattern on IFM. Therefore, sera that produce nuclear fluorescence on IFM require additional testing to confirm MPO-ANCA. MPO-ELISA is recommended to confirm anti-MPO specificity because true ANA or GS-ANA and MPO-ANCA are known to occur concurrently. IFM using Hep-2 cells does not adequately make this distinction because ANA and MPO-ANCA can occur together, and GS-ANA may be negative on Hep-2 cells (Roberts, 1992; Specks, 1994).

ELISA has limitations and, ultimately, each laboratory must carefully verify a manufacturer's claims so that the clinician can receive information on performance characteristics. This proves especially important in confusing clinical situations where there may be discrepancies between clinical presentation and laboratory results and/or discordant results between IFM and ELISA tests.

In summary, it is recommended that a combination of IFM and ELISA be used to detect ANCA specific for PR-3-MPO. There must be careful attention given to quality control, reporting, and situations when ANCA is detected in nonvasculitic autoimmune diseases (Savige, 2003).

Disease Associations

Vasculitis

Both PR-3-ANCA (c-ANCA) and MPO-ANCA (p-ANCA) are associated with Wegener's granulomatosis, polyarteritis nodosa, microscopic polyangiitis, Churg–Strauss syndrome, idiopathic pauci-immune necrotizing vasculitis and crescentic glomerulonephritis, and polyangiitis overlap syndromes (Niles, 1993; Langford, 2003; Seo, 2004b). PR-3-ANCA is identified in about 70–80% of patients with active Wegener's granulomatosis, whereas MPO-ANCA is identified in less than 10% of such patients (Wiik, 2002; Seo, 2004b). Some 80–90% of patients with active microscopic polyarteritis have either PR-3-ANCA (30%) or MPO-ANCA (60%) (Wiik, 2002). MPO-ANCA is identified in patients with Churg–Strauss syndrome or pauci-immune glomerulonephritis in 50–80% of patients with active disease; rarely, this latter group of diseases may be associated with PR-3-ANCA rather than MPO-ANCA (Langford, 2003; Seo, 2004b).

Coexistence of ANCA and antiglomerular basement membrane (anti-GBM) antibodies has been reported (Bonsib, 1993; Niles, 1993).

Inflammatory Disease of Gastrointestinal and Hepatobiliary Tracts

A variety of serologic tests including p-ANCA are emerging that are relevant to the diagnosis and treatment of ulcerative colitis, Crohn's disease (Sandborn, 2004), and disorders of the hepatobiliary system (Jennette, 1993b). P-ANCAs have been reported in about 75–80% of patients with active ulcerative colitis or primary sclerosing cholangitis (Klein, 1991; Lo, 1993; Ellerbroek, 1994), about 75% of patients with chronic active hepatitis, about 30% of patients with primary biliary cirrhosis (Kallenberg, 1992; Mulder, 1993), and 20% of patients with Crohn's disease (Roberts, 1992; Jennette, 1993b). Target antigen specificities in inflammatory bowel disease have not been fully defined, although autoantibodies against lactoperoxidase, bactericidal permeability-increasing protein (Hoffman, 1998b), lactoferrin (Peen, 1993), and cathepsin G have been reported (Jennette, 1993b). The majority of adult patients with ulcerative colitis have detectable p-ANCA that is sensitive to DNAase, which helps to differentiate p-ANCA in inflammatory bowel disease from p-ANCA in other disorders such as autoimmune hepatitis and primary sclerosing cholangitis (Nakamura, 2003). A subgroup of patients with Crohn's disease with p-ANCA may have colon involvement that mimics the clinical presentation of ulcerative colitis.

Other Diseases

ANCAs have also been reported in other diseases, including drug-induced lupus erythematosus, systemic lupus erythematosus, Felty syndrome and rheumatoid arthritis, Sjögren syndrome, polymyositis and dermatomyositis, juvenile rheumatoid arthritis, reactive arthritis, relapsing polychondritis, antiphospholipid antibody syndrome, myelodysplastic syndromes, human immunodeficiency virus (HIV) infection, chromomycosis, invasive amoebiasis, subacute bacterial endocarditis, cystic fibrosis, and certain neoplasms (Jennette, 1993b; Peter, 1993; Hoffman, 1998b; Choi, 2000). In the connective tissue disorders, ANAs that mimic p-ANCAs must be excluded. Many patients treated with hydralazine appear to develop MPO-ANCA (Roberts, 1992). Propylthiouracil-associated vasculitis has been associated with positive ANCA (Hoffman, 1998b; Langford, 2003).

Test Interpretation

Interpretation of ANCA tests must consider several factors (Hagen, 1998; Hoffman, 1998a; Vassilopoulos, 1999; Seo, 2004a):

- ANCA tests should not be used as a screening test in nonselected patient groups where the prevalence of vasculitis is low (Langford, 1998a).

- ANCA tests are most valuable when selectively ordered in clinical situations where some form of ANCA-associated vasculitis is a serious consideration.
- c-ANCA immunofluorescence pattern should be confirmed using PR-3 ELISA (Savige, 1999; Langford, 2003; Seo, 2004b).
- Anti-PR3 reactivity is most often seen in active Wegener's granulomatosis or polyarteritis nodosa but may be seen in idiopathic crescentic glomerulonephritis or Churg–Strauss syndrome.
- c-ANCA in Wegener's granulomatosis is considered highly sensitive in signaling active systemic disease (Vassilopoulos, 1999).
- Predictive value of an increased c-ANCA titer as a harbinger of Wegener's granulomatosis relapse is controversial, since not all increases in c-ANCA titer are followed by worsening Wegener's granulomatosis (Specks, 1994; Langford, 2003).
- Rise in ANCA titer is a risk factor for a flare but is insufficient to adjust immunosuppressant medications on this basis alone (Langford, 2003; Seo, 2004b)
- p-ANCA pattern on IFM is diagnostically nonspecific.
- p-ANCA-positive sera should be tested in ELISA for MPO-ANCA (Savige, 1999; Seo, 2004b).
- MPO-ANCA is most often seen in polyarteritis nodosa, idiopathic crescentic glomerulonephritis, or Churg–Strauss syndrome; however, it may be seen in Wegener's granulomatosis.
- Neither a diagnosis of systemic necrotizing vasculitis nor a decision to treat should be based solely on a positive ANCA test result.
- A negative ANCA should not be used to exclude disease.

Ultimately, the interpretation of a test for ANCA depends on the experience of individual clinicians that treat vasculitis and the pattern of disease manifested by the patient at hand (Jennette, 1998a, Langford, 2003; Seo, 2004b).

Synopses of Major Idiopathic Vasculitic Syndromes

Polyarteritis Nodosa

Epidemiology

Polyarteritis nodosa, like all idiopathic vasculitides, is an uncommon disease. Estimates of the prevalence of polyarteritis nodosa have varied from 4.6 per 1 000 000 in England and 9.0 per 1 000 000 in Olmstead County, Minnesota, to 77 per 100 000 in an Alaskan Eskimo population hyperendemic for hepatitis B (Conn, 1993; Langford, 1995). Polyarteritis nodosa may occur in either gender and at any age but is more common in men (male:female ratio = 2:1) between 40 and 60 years old (Langford, 1995). There is no observed racial predilection (Conn, 1993). Older series of patients with polyarteritis nodosa contain patients who would now be thought to have microscopic polyangiitis (Langford, 2003).

Clinical Features

The clinical manifestations of classic polyarteritis nodosa are highly variable. Patients often present with such nonspecific symptoms as fever, weight loss, and malaise. Hypertension is common and can be an important diagnostic clue. Although polyarteritis nodosa can occur in virtually any organ system, symptomatic involvement of skin, joints, peripheral nerves, gastrointestinal tract, and nonglomerular renal vessels dominate the clinical picture (Conn, 1993; Savage, 2000; Langford, 2003). Tests indicating abnormal liver function suggest the possibility of concurrent hepatitis B infection (Langford, 1995, 2003; Savage, 2000). Pulmonary involvement in classic polyarteritis nodosa is rare and even controversial. Although some investigators think pulmonary polyarteritis nodosa occurs (Lie, 1989), others believe that such patients have Churg–Strauss syndrome or Wegener's granulomatosis, in which pulmonary involvement is common (Langford, 1995; Fauci, 1998). The course of polyarteritis nodosa is characterized by remissions, relapses and, if untreated, high mortality (Fauci, 1998). 5-year survival rate with treatment is estimated to be 80% and fewer than 10% of patients relapse (Langford, 2003).

Clinical Laboratory Findings

Results of clinical laboratory tests, although diagnostically nonspecific, reflect the systemic inflammatory nature of polyarteritis nodosa. Typically, one finds normochromic anemia, neutrophilic leukocytosis, hypoalbuminemia, hypergammaglobulinemia, and a markedly elevated ESR. Measurement of serum creatinine and blood urea nitrogen (BUN),

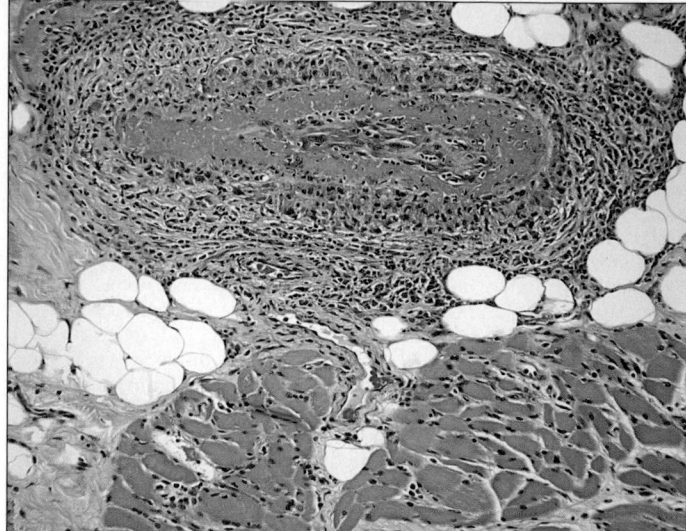

Figure 51–4 Polyarteritis nodosa. Skeletal muscle biopsy reveals circumferential panmural necrotizing arteritis of a small muscular artery with mixed cell inflammation, fibrinoid necrosis, and proliferative endarteritis. Eosinophils are a prominent component of the inflammation in this case but there are no granulomas (Hematoxylin and eosin [H&E], ×200).

together with urinalysis to check for proteinuria, hematuria, and abnormal sediment, are important for evaluating renal function. The positive ANA or RF found in 10–40% of these patients may be associated with decreased levels of complement components C3 and C4. Serologic tests for hepatitis B, hepatitis C, and HIV should be obtained in all patients with polyarteritis nodosa (Conn, 1993; Langford, 1995, 2003). Eosinophilia is seen only rarely and, when present in high levels, should lead to consideration of Churg–Strauss syndrome (Fauci, 1998).

Diagnosis

Polyarteritis nodosa can be difficult to diagnose given its nonspecific presentation, potential for diverse and diffuse organ involvement, and low prevalence. However, once suspected, a diagnosis is based on angiography and/or the histologic demonstration of polyarteritis nodosa on biopsy of tissue from symptomatic site(s), such as muscle, nerve, kidney, and testes. Pathologically, polyarteritis nodosa is a focal but panmural necrotizing arteritis of small and medium-sized muscular arteries (Fig. 51–4), preferentially occurring at vessel branch points. Necrotizing mixed cell inflammation with fibrinoid necrosis, either circumferential or segmental, in the vessel wall is the hallmark lesion of active polyarteritis nodosa. Microaneurysm or aneurysmal dilatation are also characteristic of acute phase polyarteritis nodosa. The inflammatory process heals with fibrosis that may lead to proliferative endarteritis. An admixture of active and/or healing lesions adjacent to normal segments of blood vessel is a characteristic feature (Langford, 1995).

Angiography may be especially valuable in identifying gastrointestinal abnormalities or when a potential biopsy site is unavailable. In particular, angiography should be considered before attempting a closed needle biopsy of the liver or kidney in patients suspected to have polyarteritis nodosa, since the predilection for aneurysms at these sites increases the risk of severe bleeding (Langford, 1995).

Treatment and Prognosis

Patients are treated with glucocorticoids. The goal of glucocorticoid therapy is control of the disease without significant complications from the drug itself. Cyclophosphamide may be used for patients with severe polyarteritis nodosa (gastrointestinal, cardiac, and central nervous system [CNS] involvement), those failing corticosteroids alone, and to spare steroid in patients having significant corticosteroid adverse effects (Langford, 1995, 2003; Jayne, 2000; Watts, 2000). The prognosis has greatly improved with the use of glucocorticoids, extending the 5-year survival rate from 13% to 50–60%. The majority of deaths are within the first year but, whether before or after 1 year of disease, mortality most often results either from infection as a complication of treatment or from sequelae of vessel obliteration, such as myocardial infarction or stroke (Langford, 1995). Polyarteritis nodosa associated with hepatitis infection and HIV should be accompanied by antiviral or antiretroviral therapy respectively (Langford, 2003).

Churg–Strauss Syndrome

Epidemiology

Churg–Strauss syndrome is thought to be a rare clinical condition and a prevalence of 3 per 1 000 000 people has been estimated (Conn, 1993; Langford, 2003). Churg–Strauss syndrome typically begins between ages 15 and 69 years, with 38 years as the median age for onset of vasculitis (Langford, 1995).

Clinical Features

Churg–Strauss syndrome, also called allergic angiitis and granulomatosis, is a systemic necrotizing vasculitis characterized by vascular and extravascular granulomatous inflammation, multiple organ involvement, and associations with allergic rhinitis, severe asthma, fever, and hypereosinophilia (Fauci, 1998; Langford, 1995, 2003). Clinical manifestations of Churg–Strauss syndrome may resemble those of polyarteritis nodosa in many respects but differ in that lung disease is typical and renal disease is uncommon, usually less severe in Churg–Strauss syndrome than in polyarteritis nodosa (Fauci, 1998).

The clinical course of Churg–Strauss syndrome is often divided into three distinct phases, although in reality these three phases are not always identifiable or may overlap (Langford, 1995, 2003): (1) a prodromal phase characterized by allergic respiratory disease, (2) an eosinophilic phase characterized by peripheral blood and tissue hypereosinophilia, and (3) a vasculitic phase. Cardiac involvement, either transmural eosinophilic carditis or coronary vasculitis, occurs in 25–62% of patients and is the major cause of death (Langford, 1995, 2003). Involvement with sites such as the heart, CNS, gastrointestinal tract, and kidney are associated with a poor prognosis (Langford, 2003).

Clinical Laboratory Findings

A hallmark of Churg–Strauss syndrome is striking peripheral blood eosinophilia, which may be seen at any phase of the disease. The peripheral blood eosinophil count reaches 1000 eosinophils per μL in 80% or more of patients (Conn, 1993); however, eosinophilia may not be found in all patients because of prior steroid treatments for asthma or the wide and rapid fluctuation in the eosinophil count that can occur in this disorder. Normalization of the eosinophil count in response to steroid treatment is a feature of Churg–Strauss syndrome, distinguishing it from the hypereosinophilic syndrome, in which eosinophilia may be steroid-resistant. The degree of eosinophilia may correlate with the activity of the vasculitic disease in some patients.

Other laboratory findings are nonspecific. Anemia, leukocytosis, and increased ESR frequently accompany the vasculitic phase. Serum IgE levels may be elevated. Serum RF may be identified but the titer is usually low. Serum complement is reported as normal (Conn, 1993). Unlike polyarteritis nodosa, no association between Churg–Strauss syndrome and hepatitis B has been described (Langford, 1995).

Diagnosis

Historically, the diagnosis of Churg–Strauss syndrome has been made solely on histologic demonstration of necrotizing eosinophilic vasculitis, eosinophilic tissue infiltration, and extravascular granuloma. In practice, however, few biopsy specimens contain all these findings. To increase the likelihood of identifying and diagnosing Churg–Strauss syndrome, the emphasis can be shifted from these diagnostic indicators to include clinical features. One study has recommended the following criteria:

1. Asthma (Katzenstein 2000).
2. Peripheral blood eosinophilia in excess of 1.5×10^3 cells/μL.
3. Systemic vasculitis involving two or more extrapulmonary organs (Conn, 1993).

Definitive diagnosis still requires demonstration of biopsy-proven vasculitis. Open-lung biopsy frequently does not confirm all histologic features of Churg–Strauss syndrome and must be considered before the institution of therapy if there is concern over possible infection. When clinical symptoms so indicate, useful biopsy specimens are most often obtained from muscle, sural nerve, prostate, and kidney. The differential diagnosis of Churg–Strauss syndrome includes polyarteritis nodosa, Wegener's granulomatosis, and the hypereosinophilic syndrome (Langford, 1995, 2003).

Treatment and Prognosis

Corticosteroids are the basis for treatment. The utility of immunosuppressive therapy with azathioprine or cyclophosphamide is not well studied (Langford, 1995). Early diagnosis of Churg–Strauss syndrome and corticosteroid treatment has led to these patients having a 5-year survival rate of 62%. Congestive heart failure and myocardial infarction cause 48% of all deaths in Churg–Strauss syndrome. Cerebral hemorrhage, renal failure, gastrointestinal perforation or hemorrhage, status asthmaticus, and respiratory failure also cause the demise of Churg–Strauss patients. All these features should lead to strong consideration of cytotoxic agent (cyclophosphamide) therapy in conjunction with corticosteroids (Langford, 1997). Shortness of the interval between the onset of asthma and the onset of vasculitis is considered an unfavorable prognostic sign.

Microscopic Polyangiitis

Epidemiology

Microscopic polyangiitis was recently distinguished from polyarteritis nodosa and little is known about its epidemiology.

Clinical Features

Microscopic polyangiitis occurs in a heterogeneous group of patients who, by definition, have a systemic necrotizing vasculitis of small vessels with few or no immune deposits (Langford, 2003). The sentinel features of microscopic polyangiitis are glomerulonephritis, pulmonary hemorrhage, mononeuritis multiplex, and fever, similar to Wegener's granulomatosis (Langford, 2003; Seo, 2004b). Presentation is often acute and severe. Neurologic disease (peripheral or central) manifests in 60–70%, arthralgias/arthritis in 40–60%, and cutaneous disease in 50–65% of patients (Langford, 2003).

Clinical Laboratory Findings

Chest radiographs reveal nodules, infiltrates, or alveolar hemorrhage in up to 70% of patients. Proteinuria and hematuria compatible with glomerulonephritis occur in 75–90% of patients. Electromyography/nerve conduction velocity reveals evidence of peripheral neurologic disease in up to two thirds of patients. CNS imaging may show evidence of central neurologic disease in 10% of people with microscopic polyangiitis (Langford, 2003).

Diagnosis

Microscopic polyangiitis is diagnosed when tissue biopsy reveals small-to-medium-vessel nongranulomatous necrotizing vasculitis. In the lung, capillaritis is seen in the face of alveolar hemorrhage and the absence of the linear immunofluorescence that would be seen in Goodpasture's syndrome). Renal biopsy reveals focal segmental necrotizing glomerulonephritis with few to no immune complexes (Langford, 2003).

Treatment and Prognosis

Patients with life threatening disease in the lungs, kidneys, or nerves should be treated with cyclophosphamide (2 mg/kg/day) and prednisone (1 mg/kg/day) in a manner similar to the treatment of Wegener's granulomatosis (see below) (Langford, 2003). Less severe disease may be treated with corticosteroids alone. 5-year survival is estimated to be 74% and relapses occur in one third of patients (Langford, 2003).

Wegener's Granulomatosis

Epidemiology

Detailed annual incidence and prevalence data for Wegener's granulomatosis are not available, but Wegener's granulomatosis is estimated to be less common than polyarteritis nodosa. Wegener's granulomatosis occurs in persons of any age, race, or sex, although it affects predominantly Caucasians and has a slight male predominance (Conn, 1993). The mean age at onset is 41 years (Langford, 1995). Males and females are equally affected (Langford, 2003).

Clinical Features

Wegener's granulomatosis is a clinicopathologic syndrome of unknown etiology characterized pathologically by necrotizing granulomatous inflammation of the upper and lower respiratory tracts, focal segmental glomerulonephritis, and necrotizing vasculitis, predominantly involving medium and small arteries. Wegener's granulomatosis presents in the ear/nose/throat regions with sinusitis, nasal obstruction or ulceration, otitis media, or hearing loss (Lie, 1989; Fauci, 1998). 45% of patients have lung involvement at presentation, and 85% manifest lung disease sometime during the course of their disease. Common lung manifestations include pulmonary infiltrates, pulmonary nodules, hemoptysis, or pleuritis (Fauci,

1998). Although renal disease initially afflicts only about 18% of these patients, 80% demonstrate glomerulonephritis at some time in the course of the syndrome (Fauci, 1998). Other common signs of systemic illness include skin rash, arthralgias, fever, eye manifestations, and weight loss (Lie, 1989; Fauci, 1998). Although patients with Wegener's granulomatosis limited to the respiratory tract without renal involvement have been described ('limited Wegener's granulomatosis'), more than 50% of patients with such limited disease at presentation eventually develop more generalized disease (Langford, 1995).

Clinical Laboratory Findings

Clinical laboratory findings typical of Wegener's granulomatosis include moderate leukocytosis without striking eosinophilia, mild normochromic anemia, and thrombocytosis (Conn, 1993; Langford, 1995). Leukopenia is not seen in the untreated patient and thus helps to distinguish Wegener's granulomatosis from other disorders. The presence of c-ANCA supports the diagnosis. Circulating immune complexes, measurable by C1q binding, may be found together with normal complement levels and hypergammaglobulinemia; immunoglobulins of the IgA subclass are often elevated (Conn, 1993; Langford, 1995). Indicators of glomerular involvement include microscopic or gross hematuria, proteinuria, red blood cell casts, and/or elevated serum creatinine and BUN. More than 50% of patients are RF-positive, but ANA are usually absent (Langford, 1995; Fauci, 1998). Serologic tests for anti-GBM autoantibody are negative. Prior to treatment, 80% of these patients have an elevated ESR.

Diagnosis

Although clinical and laboratory findings may be suggestive, a diagnosis of Wegener's granulomatosis should be made only when there is biopsy-proven, histologic confirmation or when c-ANCA is established in the patient with sinusitis, pulmonary infiltrate or nodule, and glomerulonephritis (Langford, 1998b, 2003). Pulmonary tissue obtained via open-lung biopsy offers the best opportunity to make an accurate diagnosis (Langford, 1995). Transbronchial biopsy does not yield adequate tissue for diagnosis more than 90% of the time. Although head and neck tissue is more directly accessible, characteristic pathologic features are found in fewer than 23% of such biopsy specimens. Diagnostically useful tissue from the head and neck region is best obtained from, in decreasing order of frequency, paranasal sinuses, nasal tissue, and subglottic region. Glomerular changes in renal biopsy tissue, although suggestive of Wegener's granulomatosis, are rarely diagnostic (Langford, 1995).

Although the morphologic spectrum of Wegener's granulomatosis is broad, the hallmark pathologic lesion in Wegener's granulomatosis is necrotizing granulomatous vasculitis. Affected vessels undergo fibrinoid necrosis with early infiltration by polymorphonuclear leukocytes followed by mononuclear cells. Pulmonary tissue may reveal any combination of necrosis, vasculitis, and granulomatous inflammation; microabscesses and scattered multinucleated giant cells in a highly inflammatory background may also occur (Yi, 2001) (Fig. 51–5). However, biopsy specimens often do not include all of these characteristic features. The most common finding found on renal biopsy is segmental necrotizing glomerulonephritis, which is present to varying degrees in 80% of specimens. Renal vasculitis not related to glomeruli is unusual and present in only 8% of biopsies.

Many disorders can mimic Wegener's granulomatosis, including infectious or noninfectious granulomatous diseases, Churg–Strauss syndrome, Goodpasture's syndrome, idiopathic midline granuloma, lymphomatoid granulomatosis, and neoplasms of the upper airway or lungs (Fauci, 1998). Of these, infection is an important consideration, since misdiagnosis can have fatal consequences when mistakenly treated with immunosuppressive therapy (Langford, 1995).

Treatment and Prognosis

A regimen of daily oral cyclophosphamide and corticosteroids is the therapy of choice for Wegener's granulomatosis. Using this regimen, the National Institutes of Health reported that marked improvement or partial remission was achieved in 91% of patients, with complete remission in 75%. An overall mortality rate of 20% was noted, 13% of which could be completely or partially attributed to Wegener's granulomatosis. Despite this marked improvement in survival and remission compared to 100% mortality in untreated patients, relapse and morbidity from both disease and treatment were noted. One half of the complete remissions were followed by one or more relapses, which occurred 3 months to 16 years after achieving remission (Langford, 1995; de Groot, 2001). Methotrexate is an alternative to cyclophosphamide in patients who do not have immediately life-threatening diseases (Langford, 1997). Also, methotrexate (20–25 mg/week) or azathioprine (2 mg/kg/day) can be given

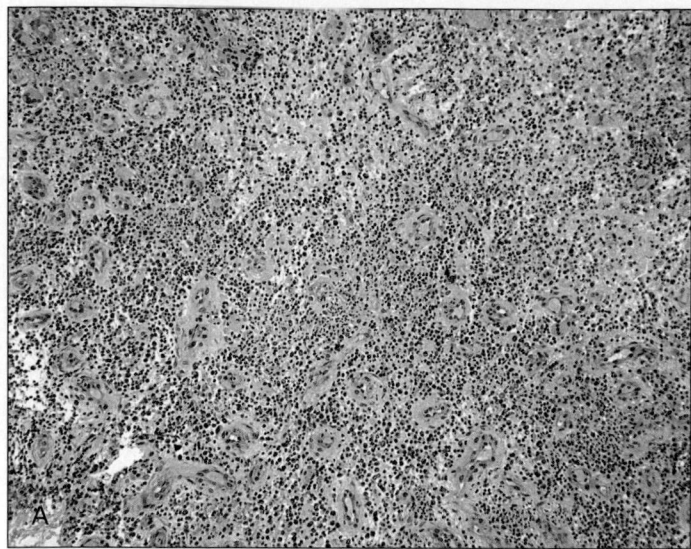

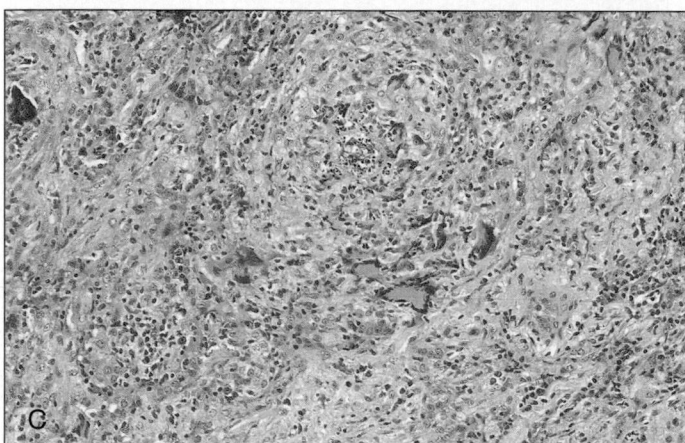

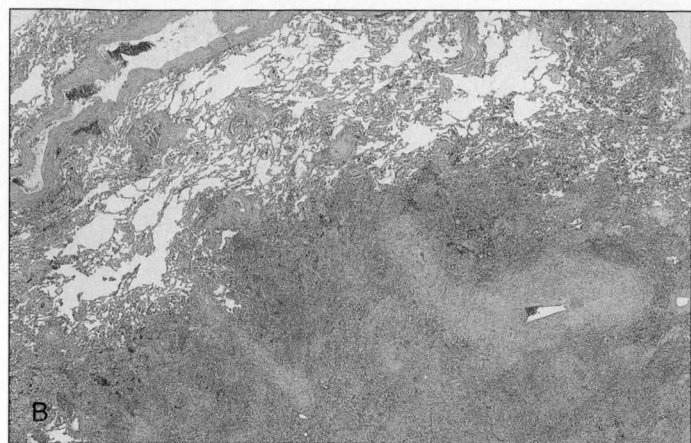

Figure 51–5 Wegener's granulomatosis. Paranasal sinus tissue reveals a florid mixed inflammatory cell infiltrate in a granulation tissue-type background. Inflammatory cells include multinucleated giant cells and neutrophil microabscesses (A, H&E, ×200). Lung biopsy reveals nodular inflammation with necrosis (B, H&E, ×20) and granulomatous vasculitis (C, H&E, ×200).

to maintain remission after 3–6 months of cyclophosphamide to induce remission. This therapy is given for an additional 1–2 years (Langford, 2003). During the first year of Wegener's granulomatosis, the extent of renal disease is the factor most closely related to prognosis (Koldingsnes, 2002). Thereafter, lung involvement becomes the most important prognostic indicator, and glomerulonephritis does not appear to significantly affect prognosis.

Lymphomatoid Granulomatosis

Lymphomatoid granulomatosis is considered to be an unusual lymphoproliferative disorder that may evolve into malignant lymphoma in approximately 50% of patients. Lymphomatoid granulomatosis mainly affects the lungs, where it clinically mimics Wegener's granulomatosis. However, characteristic histologic findings include prominent blood vessel infiltration ('angiocentric') and destruction mimicking vasculitis (Fig. 51–6), but cellular morphology is more suggestive of lymphoma or lymphoproliferative disorder (Langford, 1995). There are no specific clinical laboratory tests.

Henoch–Schönlein Purpura

Epidemiology

Henoch–Schönlein purpura occurs primarily in children between the ages of 4 and 11 years (Conn, 1993) but also afflicts some adults. It presents most commonly in the spring and classically follows an upper respiratory infection (Conn, 1993; Langford, 2003). Henoch–Schönlein purpura has a 3:2 male predominance (Langford, 1995).

Clinical Features

Henoch–Schönlein purpura, sometimes referred to as anaphylactoid purpura, is a systemic small vessel vasculitis classified as a subgroup of hypersensitivity vasculitis. The etiology is not known. Typical clinical findings include nonthrombocytopenic palpable purpura, arthralgias, renal disease, and gastrointestinal tract abnormalities (Langford, 1995,

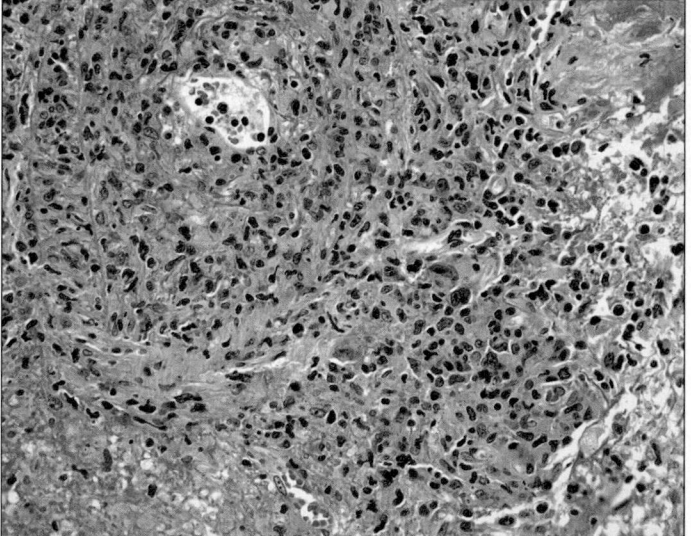

Figure 51–6 Lymphomatoid granulomatosis. Lung biopsy reveals admixtures of large atypical lymphoid cells and histiocytes with prominent blood vessel infiltration ('angiocentric') and destruction mimicking vasculitis. The atypical lymphoid cells are malignant B-cells. (H&E, ×400; case courtesy of Dr Robert W. Sharpe).

2003). Some 70% of Henoch–Schönlein purpura patients manifest gastrointestinal signs and symptoms, which include colicky abdominal pain associated with nausea and vomiting, blood or mucus in the stool, life-threatening gastrointestinal hemorrhage, and intussusception (Langford, 1995). The associated renal disease is characterized by focal proliferative glomerulonephritis that has variable clinical expression from isolated hematuria with red blood cell casts, to acute renal failure, to rare chronic renal failure (Lie, 1989; Langford, 1995; Fauci, 1998).

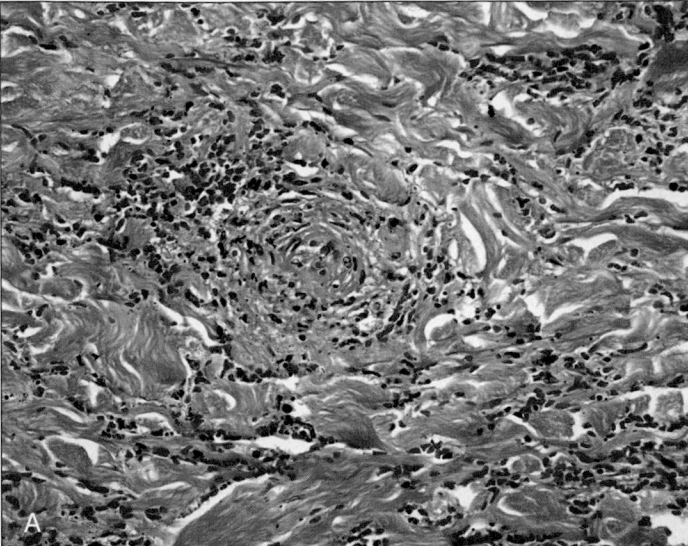

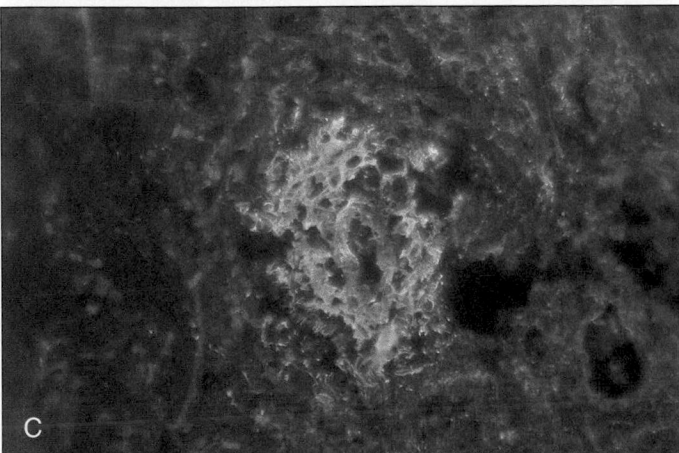

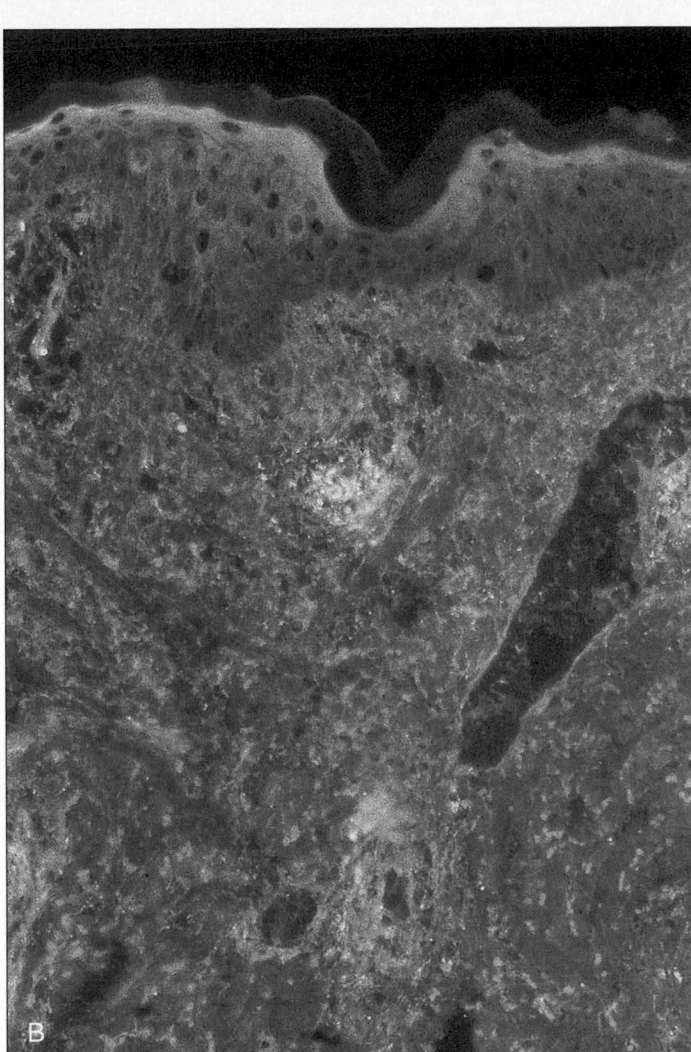

Figure 51–7 Henoch–Schönlein purpura. Skin biopsy reveals leukocytoclastic vasculitis with fibrinoid necrosis of small blood vessels in the superficial dermis associated with abundant perivascular nuclear leukocytoclastic debris (A, H&E, ×400). Direct immunofluorescence of the skin biopsy reveals granular vascular IgA immunofluorescence (B, ×200) and corresponding vascular and perivascular fibrinogen immunofluorescence (C, ×500).

Clinical Laboratory Findings

Clinical laboratory studies in Henoch–Schönlein purpura are nonspecific and are primarily useful in excluding other disorders and seeking evidence of renal involvement. Leukocytosis and elevated ESR may be seen. Tests of complete blood count with platelet count and of coagulation are important in the evaluation of cutaneous purpura; in Henoch–Schönlein purpura, purpura are not from thrombocytopenia. Stool guaiacs should be performed intermittently to look for evidence of occult blood loss. Serum complement levels are usually normal, although an association between Henoch–Schönlein purpura and the congenital absence of complement component C2 has been reported (Conn, 1993). Urinalysis and serum creatinine measurements should be performed at the onset of illness and twice weekly until systemic signs have ceased (Langford, 1995). Skin biopsy of the purpura reveals leukocytoclastic vasculitis with IgA deposition (Langford, 2003) (Fig. 51–7).

Diagnosis

Difficulty in diagnosing Henoch–Schönlein purpura is rare, except when the involvement of other major sites precedes appearance of palpable purpura. Unlike other systemic necrotizing vasculitides, diagnosis is clinical, with laboratory studies being used to rule out other disorders. Renal biopsy, which demonstrates proliferative glomerulonephritis, is typically not necessary for diagnosis, although it is used to assess disease severity and estimate prognosis. Disorders to be considered in the differential diagnosis include any that cause acute abdomen, nephritis, or purpura (Langford, 1995).

Treatment and Prognosis

Treatment is supportive and there is no specific treatment of proven benefit for nephritis in Henoch–Schönlein purpura. Although glucocorticoids may be useful for decreasing edema, joint pain, and abdominal discomfort, sustained glucocorticoid therapy is not helpful, since it does not decrease the risk of recurrent disease or improve renal prognosis (Langford, 1995). Nonsalicylate pain relievers for analgesia may soothe joint and soft-tissue discomfort. Therapy for adults is similar to that for children, although hypertension in adults must be carefully controlled (Langford, 1995).

Prognosis for this generally self-limited disease, lasting 6–16 weeks, is good (Conn, 1993). The mortality rate is about 1–3% (Langford, 1995) and renal disease is the major cause of death (Langford, 1995). Those who have an acute nephritic presentation, particularly with nephrotic syndrome, have the worst outcome, with fewer than 50% returning to normal renal function and urinalysis in 2 years. The percentage of glomeruli with crescents may also be a useful prognostic indicator; however, it is important to realize that the course of Henoch–Schönlein purpura can be extremely variable. Patients having severe clinical or histologic abnormalities may recover fully, and those with mild changes can progress to renal insufficiency. The disease recurs in 25–40% of patients and largely consists of skin manifestations. Deterioration or improvement may be most notable during the first 2–3 years after resolution of the acute episode, although significant changes in outcome have also been seen later than that. Regular follow-up with measurements of blood pressure and urinalysis is extremely important for at least the first 5 years following an episode of Henoch–Schönlein purpura (Langford, 1995, Langford, 2003).

Giant Cell (Temporal) Arteritis

Epidemiology

Giant cell arteritis is a relatively common vasculitic disorder. Epidemiologic studies have shown increased incidence with age; one study that included biopsy-proven giant cell arteritis demonstrated an annual incidence rate of

VI

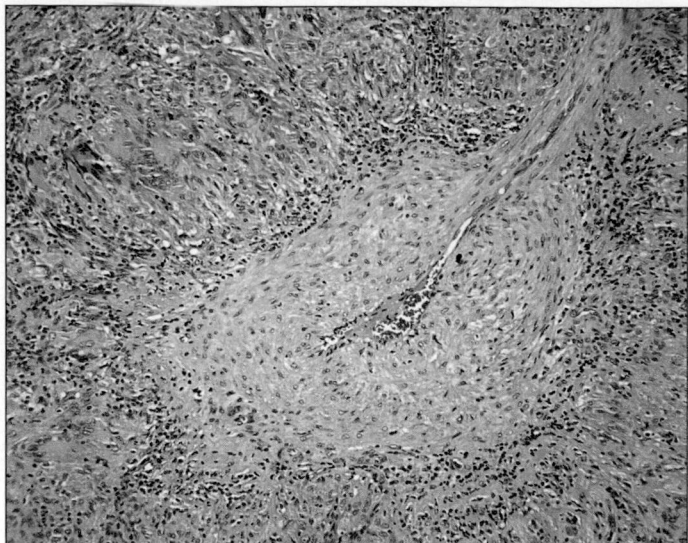

Figure 51–8 Giant cell (temporal) arteritis. Temporal artery biopsy reveals panmural mononuclear cell infiltration with prominent giant cells associated with disruption of the internal elastic lamina (H&E, ×200)

23.3 per 100 000 persons older than 50 years (Conn, 1993). Nearly all cases of giant cell arteritis begin after age 50 and involve women twice as often as men (Langford, 2003).

Clinical Features

Giant cell arteritis is a systemic disease characterized by granulomatous vascular inflammation involving medium to large arteries. Although arteries in multiple sites can be affected, giant cell arteritis classically involves the temporal artery and/or other branches of the carotid artery (Fauci, 1998). Clinical manifestations include fever, headache, diplopia, and jaw claudication in patients over 50 years of age. Ischemic optic neuritis can lead to sudden blindness, particularly in untreated patients (Fauci, 1998). Giant cell arteritis is closely associated with polymyalgia rheumatica, which is characterized by stiffness and pain of the neck, shoulders, lower back, hips, and thighs that is worse in the morning and better with activity of the day (Fauci, 1998; Langford, 2003). Findings on physical examination can include temporal artery tenderness, nodularity, and absent pulsations (Langford, 2003).

Clinical Laboratory Findings

Characteristic laboratory findings include an elevated ESR and a normochromic anemia. Serum alkaline phosphatase is commonly elevated. Hypergammaglobulinemia and increased levels of complement and immune complexes have been reported (Fauci, 1998).

Diagnosis

Diagnosis is based on identifying typical clinical manifestations and a high ESR in an elderly patient who may or may not also have symptoms of polymyalgia rheumatica (Fauci, 1998). Diagnosis is confirmed by biopsy of the temporal artery showing panmural mononuclear cell infiltration, which can be granulomatous with giant cells and typically reveals disruption of the internal elastic lamina (Langford, 2003) (Fig. 51–8).

Treatment and Prognosis

Giant cell arteritis is treated with glucocorticoids, and the clinical response to this therapy is usually dramatic. The prognosis is good, since most patients achieve and maintain complete remission after glucocorticoid therapy (Fauci, 1998). Unfortunately, recovery of eyesight following blindness secondary to giant cell arteritis is rare, even with rapid and high-dose corticosteroid therapy (Hayreh, 2002). Treatment is begun with 60 mg of prednisone daily with taper starting in 2–4 weeks and patients often requiring 2 years of corticosteroid therapy (Langford, 2003).

Takayasu's Arteritis

Epidemiology

Like many of the idiopathic vasculitides, Takayasu's arteritis is uncommon, and the epidemiology of the disease is not accurately known. This disorder is most prevalent in adolescent and young females between the ages of 10

and 30 years; in fact, 80–90% of cases occur in females. Although more common in Japan, this disease has no proven racial or geographic restrictions (Conn, 1993; Fauci, 1998).

Clinical Features

Takayasu's arteritis is a granulomatous vasculitis of medium to large elastic arteries that causes vascular stenosis or occlusion or aneurysm; there is strong predilection for the aortic arch and its large branches, including pulmonary arteries (Langford, 1995, 2003; Fauci, 1998; Johnston, 2002). This disorder is sometimes called the aortic arch syndrome or pulseless disease. Patients present with acute systemic symptoms including fever, malaise, night sweats, and weight loss. Ischemia in organs receiving their blood supply through the affected vessel(s) causes organ-specific symptoms and signs (Smetana 2002). In the chronic obliterative phase, arterial pulses are decreased or absent in involved arteries (Langford, 1995), most commonly in the subclavian artery (Fauci, 1998). Vascular bruits and hypertension are common (Langford, 1995). Other findings include aortic regurgitation, cardiomegaly secondary to aortic or pulmonary hypertension, and stroke (Fauci, 1998). Takayasu's arteritis may progress slowly, may stabilize, or may rapidly cause death (Fauci, 1998).

Clinical Laboratory Findings

Laboratory studies of Takayasu's arteritis define a systemic inflammatory disorder (Langford, 1995). The ESR is elevated in 7–100% of patients with active disease, which tends to return to normal over time. ESR is believed to be a reliable index of inflammatory activity and has been used as a tool to monitor the effectiveness of therapy. Resolution of the disease, both symptomatically and angiographically, has been found to correlate with decline of the ESR, although one surgical series observed that 44% of patients felt to be quiet clinically were not upon arterial biopsy (Langford, 2003).

Hematologic studies often show mild to moderate normochromic anemia and/or mild leukocytosis. RF and ANA are usually negative. There may be hypergammaglobulinemia, hyperfibrinogenemia, and hypo-albuminemia (Conn, 1993). Circulating immune complexes may be present in up to 50% of these patients but do not appear to correlate with disease activity.

Diagnosis

Takayasu's arteritis is diagnosed by correlating data from history, physical examination, and angiography. The disease should be considered as a diagnostic possibility in any young female who lacks or has a markedly decreased peripheral pulse rate or who has blood pressure discrepancies and/or arterial bruits (Fauci, 1998). Characteristic angiographic findings help confirm the clinical diagnosis. Biopsy for tissue confirmation of diagnosis is seldom required or done (Fauci, 1998; Langford, 2003). The predilection of this syndrome for young females is an important feature that often separates it from other possible diagnoses, particularly giant cell arteritis (Langford, 1995).

Treatment and Prognosis

In patients with active disease, corticosteroid therapy is the initial treatment of choice. If active disease persists despite corticosteroids, cyclophosphamide or methotrexate may be administered. Vasodilators, anticoagulants, and nonsteroidal anti-inflammatory agents are used for symptomatic relief. Surgical intervention may be necessary for symptomatic vascular stenosis or occlusion (Langford, 1995; Hoffman, 2003).

The clinical course of Takayasu's arteritis is variable. Although spontaneous remissions occur, most patients require treatment. Prognosis appears to be related to the presence and severity of complications. Major complications include Takayasu's retinopathy, secondary hypertension, aortic valve insufficiency, and aortic/arterial aneurysm (Langford, 1995). Overall survival declines from 72–97% at 5 years to 59% at 10 years, as the number and/or severity of these complications increases (Langford, 1995; Nordborg, 2003). Disease-related deaths usually occur from vascular complications, such as congestive heart failure, stroke, myocardial infarction, and aneurysm rupture (Langford, 1995).

Primary Angiitis of the Central Nervous System

Epidemiology

Primary angiitis of the central nervous system (PACNS) is a rare condition where difficulty in making a definitive diagnosis hinders epidemiologic studies. PACNS is slightly more common in males than females (4:3) and begins at a mean age of 43 years (Langford, 1995).

Clinical Features

Patients with PACNS present with headaches; focal neurologic deficits, and altered mental status, paraparesis, quadriparesis, cranial neuropathies, seizures, and ataxia (Calabrese, 1997; Fauci, 1998). Initial symptoms are more generalized and focal symptoms and signs generally develop later in the course of the disease (Langford, 1995). 15% of cases have spinal cord involvement (Calabrese, 1997). The course may be rapidly progressive or wax and wane over a long time period. Systemic symptoms are rare.

Clinical Laboratory Findings

Laboratory studies are not useful in making a diagnosis of PACNS but they do play an important role in excluding other disease processes. The ESR is elevated in most, but not all, patients. Anemia has been seen in only 17% of them, and other hematologic parameters are usually normal. RF, ANA, and ANCA are typically absent. However, the cerebrospinal fluid (CSF) is usually abnormal, with findings that include increased opening pressure, elevated protein, and lymphocytic pleocytosis. Since the CSF can also be completely normal, such testing does not always rule out the possibility of vasculitis (Langford, 1995).

Diagnosis

The diagnosis of PACNS remains one of exclusion. Proposed diagnostic criteria have included CNS dysfunction that is not explained by clinical, laboratory, or neurologic investigation; documentation by angiogram and/or biopsy of an arteritis within the CNS; and no evidence of a systemic vasculitis or other condition to which the angiographic or pathologic features could be secondary.

Given the difficulty with certainty regarding the last criterion and the poor discriminatory power of angiography regarding inflammatory versus noninflammatory vascular disease (Calabrese, 1997), CNS biopsies are underused. The role of brain biopsy in the diagnosis of PACNS remains controversial, although some advocate that such biopsy is essential to make a definitive diagnosis (Calabrese, 1997). Precluding the widespread application of brain biopsy has been not only its invasive nature but also the inconsistency of demonstrating histologic vasculitis given the patchy nature of the process. Biopsy yield may be increased by obtaining samples of both parenchyma and leptomeningeal vessels. Given the difficulty in obtaining diagnostic certainty for this disease, biopsy is equally important to rule out other possible etiologies. Histologically, there is segmental mixed inflammation with necrosis involving predominantly small and medium-sized cranial arteries. Granulomatous inflammation may be present. Thrombosis is often noted; extracranial arteries are rarely involved (Langford, 1995; Rhodes, 1995). Therefore, differential diagnoses must be carefully considered in all cases and used in deciding appropriate tests both to support a diagnosis of PACNS and to exclude other processes. The combination of normal magnetic resonance imaging and CSF has strong negative predictive value and excludes consideration of PACNS in most clinical situations (Calabrese, 1997).

Treatment and Prognosis

Aggressive treatment is indicated for patients in whom other disorders are ruled out, the diagnosis of PACNS is supported, and there is evidence of progressive neurologic difficulties (Calabrese, 1997). Combination therapy using corticosteroids and daily cyclophosphamide is advocated; however, the prognosis of PACNS is poor, with 60–70% of patients dying from their disease within 1 year of diagnosis (Langford, 1995).

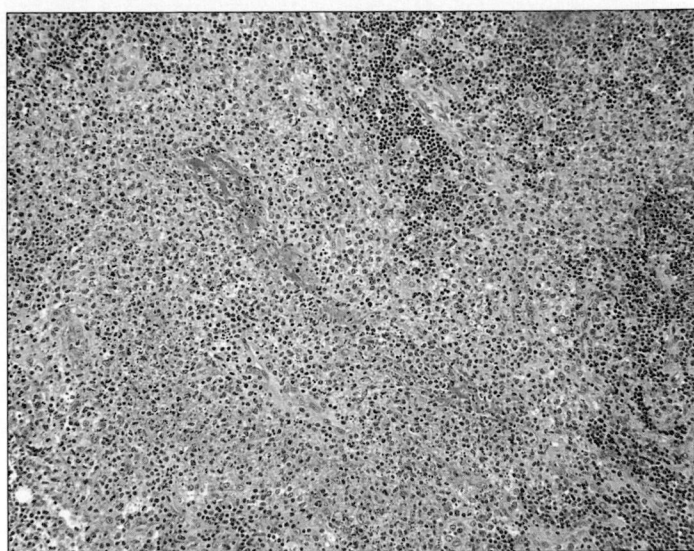

Figure 51–9 Kawasaki disease. Lymph node biopsy reveals necrotizing vasculitis with fibrin thrombi and mixed inflammation including neutrophils (H&E, ×200; case courtesy of Dr Robert W. Sharpe).

Kawasaki Disease

Kawasaki disease, or mucocutaneous lymph node syndrome, is a form of vasculitis involving small and medium arteries (Fig. 51–9). This disease typically occurs in children who present with cervical lymphadenitis and alterations in skin and mucous membranes. Kawasaki disease is usually self-limited, but arteritis causes coronary aneurysms in 25% of patients. Death occurs in up to 3% of patients, usually from coronary vasculitis. Antiendothelial cell autoantibodies have been demonstrated in patients with Kawasaki disease (Fauci, 1998).

Summary

The diagnosis of idiopathic systemic necrotizing vasculitides requires a high degree of suspicion and can be difficult because of the large number of differential diagnostic considerations. There are no pathognomonic clinical laboratory tests in patients with systemic necrotizing vasculitides, but such tests are useful for defining the extent and patterns of organ involvement. ANCA and its associations with systemic necrotizing vasculitis, particularly the association of c-ANCA with Wegener's granulomatosis, has become an important serologic test used in the evaluation these patients. However, clinicians and laboratorians using this test must thoroughly understand the operating characteristics, including limitations, of the test as performed in their laboratory. Tissue biopsy of symptomatic site(s) with histologic confirmation of necrotizing vasculitis remains the most important laboratory procedure for diagnosis of systemic necrotizing vasculitides.

References

Arimura Y, Minoshima S, Kamiya Y: Serum myeloperoxidase and serum cytokines in anti-myeloperoxidase antibody-associated glomerulonephritis. Clin Nephrol 1993; 40:256–264.

Bonsib SM, Goeken JA, Kemp JD: Coexistent anti-neutrophil cytoplasmic antibody and antiglomerular basement membrane antibody associated disease = report of six cases. Mod Pathol 1993; 6(5):526–530.

Calabrese L, Duna GF, Lie JT: Vasculitis in the central nervous system. Arthritis Rheum 1997; 40:1189–1201.

Choi HK, Lamprecht P, Niles JL: Subacute bacterial endocarditis with positive cytoplasmic antineutrophil cytoplasmic antibodies and anti-proteinase 3 antibodies. Arthritis Rheum 2000; 43:226–231.

Chowdhury SM, Broomhead V, Spickett GP: Pitfalls of formalin fixation for determination of antineutrophil cytoplasmic antibodies. J Clin Pathol 1999; 52:475–477.

Conn DL, Hunder GG, O'Duffy JD: Vasculitis and related disorders. In Kelley WN, Harris ED, Jr, Ruddy S, et al. (eds): Textbook of Rheumatology. 4th ed. Philadelphia, PA, WB Saunders, 1993, p 1077.

De Groot K, Adu D, Savage CO, EUVAS (European Vasculitis Study Group): The value of pulse cyclophosphamide in ANCA-associated vasculitis: meta-analysis and critical review. Nephrol Dial Transplant 2001; 16:2018–2027.

Deguchi Y, Shibata N, Kishimoto S: Enhanced expression of the tumour necrosis factor/cachectin gene in peripheral blood mononuclear cells from patients with systemic vasculitis. Clin Exp Immunol 1990; 81:311–314.

Ellerbroek PM, Oudkerk Pool M, Ridwan BU, et al: Neutrophil cytoplasmic antibodies (p-ANCA) in ulcerative colitis. J Clin Pathol 1994; 47:257–262.

Falk RJ, Jennette JC: Anti-neutrophil cytoplasmic autoantibodies with specificity for myeloperoxidase in patients with systemic vasculitis and idiopathic necrotizing and crescentic glomerulonephritis. N Engl J Med 1988; 318:1651–1657.

Falk RJ, Jennette JC: Thoughts about the classification of small vessel vasculitis. J. Nephrol 2004; 17(Suppl 8):S3–S9.

Fauci AS: The vasculitis syndromes. In Fauci AS, Braunwald E, Isselbacher KJ, et al. (eds): Harrison's Principles of Internal Medicine, 14th ed. New York, McGraw-Hill, 1998, pp 1910–1922.

Golden MP, Hammer SM, Wanke CA, Albrecht MA: Cytomegalovirus vasculitis. Case reports and review of the literature. Medicine 1994; 73:246–255

Grau GE, Roux-Lombard P, Gysler C, et al: Serum cytokine changes in systemic vasculitis. Immunology 1989; 68:196–198.

Hagen EC, Andrassy K, Csernok E, et al: Development and standardization of solid phase assays for the detection of anti-neutrophil cytoplasmic antibodies (ANCA): a report on the second phase of an international cooperative study on the standardization of ANCA assays. J Immunol Methods 1996; 196:1–15.

Hagen EC, Daha MR, Hermans J, et al: Diagnostic value of standardized assays for anti-neutrophil cytoplasmic antibodies in idiopathic systemic vasculitis. EC/BCR project for ANCA assay standardization. Kidney Int 1998; 53:743–753.

Hayreh SS, Zimmerman B, Kardon RH: Visual improvement with corticosteroid therapy in giant cell arteritis. Report of a large study and review of literature. Acta Ophthalmol Scand 2002; 80:353–367.

Hoffman GS: Classification of the systemic vasculitides: antineutrophil cytoplasmic antibodies, consensus and controversy. Clin Exp Rheumatol 1998a; 16:111–115.

Hoffman GS, Specks U: Antineutrophil cytoplasmic antibodies. Arthritis Rheum 1998b; 41:1521–1537.

Hoffman GS: Large-vessel vasculitis: unresolved issues. Arthritis Rheum 2003; 48:2406–2414.

Hunder GG, Arend WP, Bloch DA, et al: The American College of Rheumatology 1990 criteria for the classification of vasculitis. Introduction. Arthritis Rheum 1990; 33:1065–1067.

Jayne D: Evidence-based treatment of systemic vasculitis. Rheumatology 2000; 39:585–595.

Jennette JC: Pathogenic potential of anti-neutrophil cytoplasmic autoantibodies. Lab Invest 1994a; 70:135.

Jennette JC, Ewert BH, Falk RJ: Do antineutrophil cytoplasmic autoantibodies cause Wegener's granulomatosis and other forms of necrotizing vasculitis? Rheum Dis Clin North Am 1993a; 19:1–14.

Jennette JC, Falk RJ: Antineutrophil cytoplasmic autoantibodies in inflammatory bowel disease. Am J Clin Pathol 1993b; 99:221–223.

Jennette JC, Falk RJ: Small-vessel vasculitis. N Engl J Med 1997; 337:1512–1523.

Jennette JC, Falk RJ: Vasculitis. In Rose NR, Mackay IR (eds): The Autoimmune Diseases, 3rd ed. San Diego, CA, Academic Press, 1998a, pp 705–724.

Jennette JC, Falk RJ, Andrassy K, et al: Nomenclature of systemic vasculitides. Proposal of an international consensus conference. Arthritis Rheum 1994b; 37:187–192.

Outlines important conclusions and proposals made at the Chapel Hill Consensus Conference on the Nomenclature of Systemic Vasculitis.

Jennette JC, Wilkman AS, Falk RJ: Diagnostic predictive value of ANCA serology. Kidney Int 1998b; 53:796–798.

Johnston SL, Lock RJ, Gompels MM: Takayasu arteritis: a review. J Clin Pathol 2002; 55:481–486.

Excellent review of the history, clinical features, differential diagnoses, classification, immunology and treatments of this rare but well-known disorder.

Kallenberg CG, Mulder AH, Tervaert JW: Antineutrophil cytoplasmic antibodies: a still-growing class of autoantibodies in inflammatory disorders. Am J Med 1992; 93:675–682.

Klein R, Eisenburg J, Weber P, et al: Significance and specificity of antibodies to neutrophils detected by western blotting for the serological diagnosis of primary sclerosing cholangitis. Hepatology 1991; 14:1147–1152

Koldingsnes W, Nossent H: Predictors of survival and organ damage in Wegner's granulomatosis. Rheumatology 2002; 41:572–581.

Langford CA: New developments in the treatment of Wegener's granulomatosis, polyarteritis nodosa, microscopic polyangiitis, and Churg–Strauss syndrome. Curr Opin Rheumatol 1997; 9:26–30.

Langford CA: The diagnostic utility of c-ANCA in Wegener's granulomatosis. Cleve Clin J Med 1998a; 65:135–140.

Langford CA: Treatment of polyarteritis nodosa, microscopic polyangiitis, and Churg–Strauss syndrome: where do we stand? Arthritis Rheum 2001; 44:508–512.

Langford CA: Vasculitis. J Allergy Clin Immunol 2003; 111:S602–S612.

Excellent current review of vasculitis.

Langford CA, Klippel JH, Balow JE, et al: Use of cytotoxic agents and cyclosporine in the treatment of autoimmune disease, Part 2: Inflammatory bowel disease, systemic vasculitis, and therapeutic toxicity. Ann Intern Med 1998b; 129:49–58.

Langford CA, McCallum RM: Idiopathic vasculitis. In Belch JJF, Zurier RB (eds): Connective Tissue Diseases. London, Chapman & Hall, 1995, p 179.

Lie JT: Systemic and isolated vasculitis: a rational approach to classification and pathologic diagnosis. Pathol Annu 1989; 24:25–114.

Lo SK, Chapman RWG, Cheeseman P, et al: Antineutrophil antibody: a test for autoimmune primary sclerosing cholangitis in childhood? Gut 1993; 34:199–202.

Mandell BF, Hoffman GS: Differentiating the vasculitides. Rheum Dis Clin North Am 1994; 20:409–442.

Mulder AH, Horst G, Haagsma EB, et al: Prevalence and characterization of neutrophil cytoplasmic antibodies in autoimmune liver diseases. Hepatology 1993; 17:411–417.

Nakamura RM, Matsutani M, Barry M: Advances in clinical laboratory tests for inflammatory bowel disease. Clin Chim Acta 2003; 335:9–20.

Niles JL: Value of tests for antineutrophil cytoplasmic autoantibodies in the diagnosis and treatment of vasculitis. Curr Opin Rheumatol 1993; 5:18–24.

Niles JL, McCluskey RT: Vasculitis. In Colvin RB, Bhan AK, McCluskey RT (eds): Diagnostic Immunopathology, 2nd ed. New York, Raven Press, 1995, p 95.

Nordborg E, Nordborg C: Giant cell arteritis: epidemiological clues to its pathogenesis and an update on its treatment. Rheumatology 2003; 43:413–421.

Peen E, Almer S, Bodemar G, et al: Anti-lactoferrin antibodies and other types of ANCA in ulcerative colitis, primary sclerosing cholangitis, and Crohn's disease. Gut 1993; 34:56–62.

Peter HH, Metzger D, Rump A, et al: ANCA in diseases other than systemic vasculitis. In Anonymous. Proceedings of the 5th International ANCA Workshop, August 31–September. Cambridge, UK, St John's College, 1993, p 12.

Rhodes RH, Madelaire C, Petrelli M, et al: Primary angiitis and angiopathy of the central nervous system and their relationship to systemic giant cell arteritis. Arch Pathol Lab Med 1995; 119:334–349.

Roberts DE: Antineutrophil cytoplasmic autoantibodies. Clin Lab Med 1992; 12:85–98.

Roberts DE, Peebles C, Daggett R: A simplified method of preparing neutrophil slides in the examination for antibodies to cytoplasmic antigens. J Clin Pathol 1990; 43:83–84.

Sandborn WJ. Serologic markers in inflammatory bowel disease: state of the art. Rev Gastroenterol Disord 2004; 4:167–174.

State of the art review of emerging serologic tests relevant to ulcerative colitis and Crohn's disease.

Savage CO, Harper L, Cockwell P, et al: ABC of arterial and vascular disease: Vasculitis. Br Med J 2000; 320:1320–1328.

Savage J, Davies D, Falk RJ, Jennette JC, Wiik A. Antineutrophil cytoplasmic antibodies and associated diseases: a review of the clinical and laboratory features. Kidney Int 2000; 57:846–862.

Discusses a number of advances related to ANCA testing, diagnostic criteria for the ANCA-associated vasculitides, and the complications associated with treatment.

Savige J, Dimech W, Fritzler M, et.al: Addendum to the International Consensus Statement on testing and reporting of antineutrophil cytoplasmic antibodies. Quality control guidelines, comments, and recommendations for testing in other autoimmune diseases. Am J Clin Pathol 2003 120:312–318.

Savige J, Gillis D, Benson E, et al: International Consensus Statement on Testing and Reporting of Antineutrophil Cytoplasmic Antibodies (ANCA). Am J Clin Pathol 1999; 111:507–513.

Savige JA, Paspaliaris B, Silvestrini R: A review of immunofluorescent patterns associated with antineutrophil cytoplasmic antibodies (ANCA) and their differentiation from other antibodies. J Clin Pathol 1998; 51:568–575.

Seo P, Stone JH: Large-vessel vasculitis. Arthritis Rheum 2004a; 1:128–139.

Seo P, Stone JH: The antineutrophil cytoplasmic antibody-associated vasculitides. Am J Med 2004b; 117:39–50.

Current review of the ANCA-associated vasculitides that discusses the role of ANCA assays in diagnosis and treatment, and outlines an approach to the evaluation and management of these diseases.

Smetana GW, Shmerling RH: Does this patient have temporal arteritis? JAMA 2002; 287:92–101.

Sneller MC, Fauci AS: Pathogenesis of vasculitis syndromes. Med Clin North Am 1997; 81:221–242.

Specks U, Homburger HA: Laboratory medicine and pathology: anti-neutrophil cytoplasmic antibodies. Mayo Clin Proc 1994; 69:1197–1198.

Tervaert JW, Limburg PC, Elema JD, et al: Detection of autoantibodies against myeloid lysosomal enzymes: a useful adjunct to classification of patients with biopsy-proven necrotizing arteritis. Am J Med 1991; 91:59–66.

Vassilopoulos D, Hoffman GS: Clinical utility of testing for antineutrophil cytoplasmic antibodies. Clin Diagn Lab Immunol 1999; 6:645–651.

Wang G, Csernok E, deGroot K: Comparison of eight commercial kits for quantitation of antineutrophil cytoplasmic antibodies (ANCA). J Immunol Methods 1997; 208:203–211.

Watts RA, Scott DGI, Pusey CD, Lockwood CM: Vasculitis – aims of therapy. An overview. Rheumatology 2000; 39:229–237.

Wieslander J: How are antineutrophil cytoplasmic autoantibodies detected? Am J Kidney Dis 1991; 18:154–158.

Wiik A: Rational use of ANCA in the diagnosis of vasculitis. Rheumatology 2002; 41:481–483.

Yi ES, Colby TV: Wegener's granulomatosis. Semin Diagn Pathol 2001; 18:34–46.

CHAPTER 52

Organ-Specific Autoimmune Diseases

David J. Bylund MD, Robert M. Nakamura MD

KEY POINTS

• The dominant clinical feature of organ-specific autoimmune diseases is chronic inflammation, generally localized in a single organ specific for each individual disease.

• The etiology of virtually all the organ-specific autoimmune diseases remains elusive.

• Direct immunofluorescence is essential for resolving the microscopic differential diagnosis of acantholytic and subepidermal bullous disorders.

• The presence of circulating autoantibodies at significant titers is often useful in establishing the etiology of autoimmune liver disorders.

• Antimitochondrial antibodies are the most specific and sensitive diagnostic markers for primary biliary cirrhosis (PBC). As a general guideline, an AMA titer greater than or equal to 1:160 is highly predictive of PBC.

• The prevalence of gluten-sensitive enteropathy/celiac sprue in the US population is considered to be much greater than previous estimates.

• In gluten-sensitive enteropathy/celiac sprue, IgA antiendomysial autoantibodies detect tissue transglutaminase (tTG), the primary autoantigen in gluten-sensitive enteropathy (GSE). Enzyme-linked immunosorbent assays are now available for the detection of anti-tTG. Their identification is considered diagnostically sensitive and specific for GSE alone or GSE associated with dermatitis herpetiformis.

• For specificity reasons, the use of assays to detect DNAase-sensitive p-ANCA and antibodies to *Saccharomyces cerevisiae* should be limited to patients with colitis and should not be applied to the general population.

• Technical advances in enzyme-linked immunosorbent assays have made this technology available in most clinical laboratories so that many assays for organ-specific autoantibodies (e.g.; thyroid, kidney, pancreatic islet cells, peripheral and central nervous system) are more widely available where indirect immunofluorescence microscopy is not feasible.

Autoimmune disorders can be categorized broadly into either systemic or organ-directed diseases (Nakamura, 2002). In this chapter, we discuss most of the organ-directed autoimmune diseases listed in Table 52–1.

The dominant clinical feature of these autoimmune disorders is chronic inflammation, generally localized in a single organ specific for each individual disease. Within this group of autoimmune disorders, familial clustering of diseases occurs with remarkable frequency. The relevant autoantibodies may or may not be species-specific but they do exhibit specificity for an antigen present in the diseased organ or tissue.

Included in this chapter are some diseases with autoantibodies and inflammatory lesions restricted to one, or a few, organ(s) that combine clinicopathologic features of both organ-specific and systemic autoimmune diseases. Autoimmune liver disorders, such as primary biliary cirrhosis (PBC) or autoimmune hepatitis, are examples of diseases in this group. Except for autoantibodies to thyroid receptors, the pathogenesis of autoantibodies in organ-specific diseases remains largely unproven.

Detection Methods

Direct immunofluorescence microscopy (DIFM) is the laboratory method used to detect immune deposits in a patient's tissue. Indirect immunofluorescence microscopy (IIFM), briefly described below, is the method most commonly used to detect circulating autoantibodies to specific target organs or tissues. Clinical laboratories are using enzyme-linked

Table 52–1 Organ-Specific Autoimmune Diseases

Organ Disease	Autoantibody	Detection Method(s)
Thyroid Gland		
Autoimmune thyroiditis	Thyroid peroxidase	ELISA; IIFM using unfixed monkey thyroid
	Thyroglobulin	IIFM using methanol-fixed monkey thyroid; passive hemagglutination; latex agglutination
Graves disease	TSH receptor	Radioreceptor binding assay; cAMP bioassay
Adrenal Gland		
Addison's disease	Adrenocortical	IIFM on unfixed monkey or human adrenal cortex
Parathyroid Gland		
Parathyroid	Parathyroid endothelial proteins	IIFM on unfixed bovine parathyroid gland
Pancreas		
Type 1A diabetes mellitus	Islet cells	IIFM on unfixed human pancreas, blood group O
	Insulin-associated	Radioimmunoprecipitation
	Antiglutamic acid decarboxylase	ELISA, RIA, immunoblotting
Muscle		
Dermatomyositis/polymyositis	PM-1, Jo-1	ELISA; immunodiffusion
Gastrointestinal Tract		
Atrophic gastritis	Gastric parietal cell	IIFM – mouse stomach/kidney
Pernicious anemia	Intrinsic factor	Radioactive vitamin B_{12} binding assay
	Salivary duct cells	IIFM – unfixed human salivary gland
	Gastric parietal cell	IIFM – human, monkey, mouse, or rat gastric mucosa substrate
Ulcerative colitis	Colon; lipopolysaccharide	IIFM – human or rat colon; hemagglutination
	DNAase sensitive p-ANCA associated	IIFM – ethanol-fixed neutrophils
Crohn's disease	ASCA	ELISA
Celiac disease	Tissue transglutaminase	ELISA
	IgA endomysial	IIFM – monkey esophagus
	Gliadin	ELISA
Liver		
Autoimmune hepatitis	Smooth muscle	IIFM – mouse stomach/kidney
	Liver–kidney microsomal	IIFM – mouse stomach/kidney; ELISA
	ANA	Hep-2 cells
Primary biliary cirrhosis	Mitochondrial (M2)	IIFM – mouse stomach/kidney; ELISA
Primary sclerosing cholangitis	p-ANCA	IIFM – ethanol-fixed neutrophils
Neurologic		
Myasthenia gravis	AChR	Immunoprecipitation of iodine-125 α-bungarotoxin-conjugated AChR (human skeletal muscle); ELISA
Demyelinating diseases (i.e., multiple sclerosis)	Myelin; tubulin; myelin basic protein; myelin-associated glycoprotein	IIFM – mammalian spinal cord; ELISA; immunoblotting
Kidneys		
Anti-GBM disease	Glomerular and lung basement membrane	ELISA
Skin		
Pemphigus	ICS (desmogleins)	DIFM on skin biopsy specimen; IIFM on monkey or guinea pig esophagus
Pemphigoid	BMZ (hemidesmosomal proteins)	DIFM on skin biopsy; IIFM on monkey esophagus
Dermatitis herpetiformis	Tissue transglutaminase	ELISA
	IgA endomysial	Monkey esophagus
Paraneoplastic pemphigus	ICS and BMZ	DIFM on skin biopsy; IIFM on rat bladder urothelium
Linear IgA dermatosis	IgA BMZ	DIFM on human skin biopsy; IIFM on monkey esophagus
IgA Pemphigus	IgA ICS	DIFM on human skin biopsy; IIFM on monkey esophagus

AChR = acetylcholine receptor; ASCA = antibodies to *Saccharomyces cerevisiae*; BMZ = basement membrane zone; cAMP = cyclic adenosine monophosphate; DIFM = direct immunofluorescence microscopy; ELISA = enzyme-linked immunosorbent assay; ICS = intercellular spaces; IIFM = indirect immunofluorescence microscopy; p-ANCA = perinuclear antineutrophil cytoplasmic antibody; RIA = radioimmunoassay; TSH = thyroid-stimulating hormone.

immunosorbent assays (ELISA) more frequently as technical aspects of this method have improved.

Indirect Immunofluorescence Microscopy

This test procedure is essentially the same except for the substrate used to bind target autoantibodies. The general procedure follows:

1. Prepare screening dilution of patient sera, or serial dilutions, and appropriate controls in phosphate buffered saline (PBS).
2. Use a moisture chamber to incubate for 20–30 minutes diluted sera and controls layered over cryostat tissue sections of the substrate on multiwell glass slides. Do not allow the slides to dry.
3. Remove slides from the moisture chamber. Briefly but carefully wash each entire slide two to three times using PBS at room temperature. Then wash slides in PBS for 15 minutes, changing the wash once during this period.
4. Remove one slide at a time from the PBS wash, blot each slide dry, and place each in a moisture chamber. Dispense diluted fluorescein-labeled conjugate over each well. Incubate slides at room temperature for 20 minutes. Do not allow slides to dry.
5. Wash slides for 10 minutes in PBS that contains Evan's blue counterstain.
6. Mount coverslips.
7. View slides under a fluorescence microscope.
8. Store slides in the dark at 4°C.

Table 52–2 Autoimmune Skin Diseases

Immunologic Findings Essential for Diagnosis

Epidermal intercellular spaces

Pemphigus

Paraneoplastic pemphigus

Basement membrane zone

Pemphigoid

Gestational pemphigoid

Epidermolysis bullosa acquisita

Linear IgA dermatosis

Chronic bullous dermatosis of childhood

Dermal papillae ± basement membrane zone

Dermatitis herpetiformis

Immunologic Findings Useful for Diagnosis

Cutaneous Manifestations in Systemic Rheumatic Diseases

Dermatomyositis/polymyositis

Lupus erythematosus

Mixed connective tissue disease

Relapsing polychondritis

Sjögren syndrome

Systemic sclerosis

Vasculitis

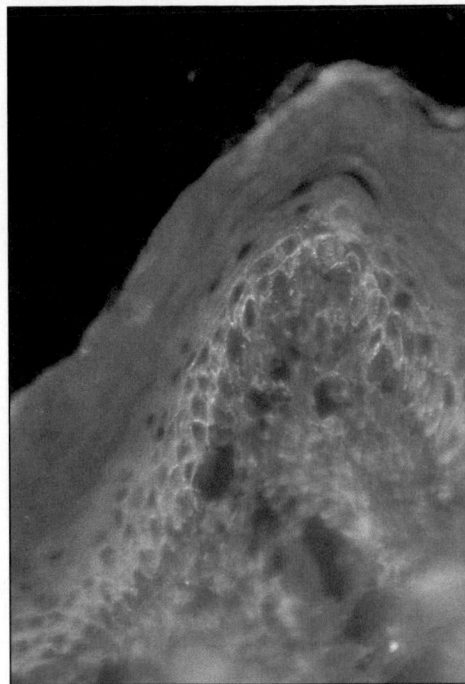

Figure 52–1 Direct immunofluorescence microscopy of skin lesion in pemphigus shows linear/granular C3 deposition on the cell surfaces (intercellular spaces) of mainly basal keratinocytes without basement membrane zone immunofluorescence (×400).

Skin

Detection of autoantibodies is highly useful in the work-up for cutaneous bullous disease. In patients with autoimmune skin diseases, autoantibodies include those to basement membrane zone (BMZ), epidermal intercellular spaces (ICS), or dermal blood vessels, as summarized in Table 52–2. Several excellent technical reviews are available that detail the use of immunofluorescence for examining skin (Crosby 1993; Flotte, 1995).

Pemphigus

Pemphigus refers to a group of disorders that are characterized clinically by blisters and histologically by acantholysis. There are three major subtypes of pemphigus: pemphigus vulgaris, pemphigus foliaceus, and paraneoplastic pemphigus (Nousari, 1999a). Each of these subtypes is characterized by autoantibodies to desmosomal adhesion molecules. Both IIFM to detect circulating autoantibodies and the more informative DIFM to identify tissue-bound autoantibodies are used for initial evaluations to maximize diagnostic sensitivity.

Pemphigus Vulgaris

Pemphigus vulgaris is a rare disorder that occurs in all racial and ethnic groups, although the incidence is slightly increased in the Jewish population. The disease affects either sex and most commonly occurs in individuals between 40 and 60 years old (Becker, 1993). Desmoglein 3 is the major antigen in pemphigus vulgaris (Naparstek, 1993; Lin, 1998). ELISAs to detect anti-desmoglein-3 are available.

Direct immunofluorescence microscopy

DIFM of perilesional skin shows linear/granular immunoglobulin G (IgG) and C3 ICS immunofluorescence without BMZ staining (Fig. 52–1). This pattern is often described as 'chicken wire' and preferentially stains the lower one half of the epidermis. IgG, especially IgG4, is present in nearly 100% of patients whereas C3 is present in 50–100% of patients, usually in acantholytic areas (Becker, 1993; Flotte, 1995; Lin, 1998). In 30–50% of patients, IgA or IgM immunoreactants are seen (Izuno, 1986). C3 immunofluorescence only, without IgG, is described in drug-induced pemphigus and in impetigo (Nousari, 1997).

Indirect immunofluorescence microscopy

IIFM should detect circulating IgG autoantibodies to the surfaces of squamous epithelial cells in 100% of patients with active disease (Nousari, 1997). Monkey esophagus is considered the best tissue substrate (Fig. 52–2).

The presence of pemphigus vulgaris autoantibodies is abnormal at any titer. The titer generally correlates with disease activity, and increasing titers may be predictive of relapse (Becker, 1993; Crosby, 1993). Exceptions to this correlation do occur, however, so serial testing of IgG titers to monitor these

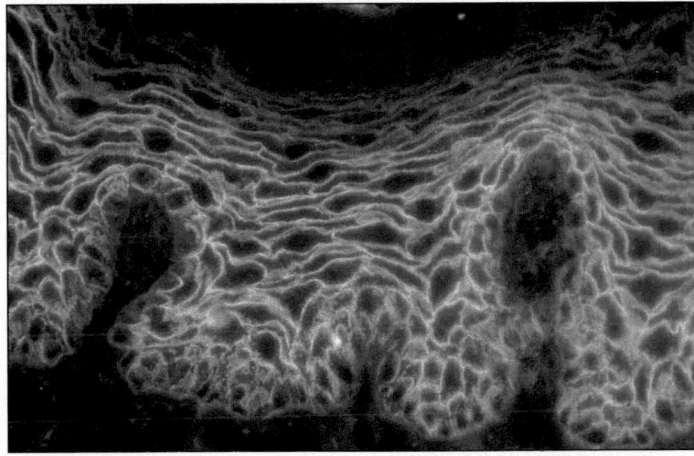

Figure 52–2 Indirect immunofluorescence microscopy in pemphigus shows linear IgG immunofluorescence on the cell surfaces of epithelial cells (intercellular spaces) using mouse esophagus as tissue substrate (×250).

patients must be carefully correlated with the clinical findings. Patients who have only oral mucosal lesions may not have detectable circulating pemphigus vulgaris autoantibodies. In these patients, diagnosis is made using DIFM (Izuno, 1986).

Low titers of ICS-like autoantibodies may be infrequently detected in diverse conditions such as skin burns, penicillin or other drug allergy, toxic epidermal necrolysis, systemic lupus erythematosus (SLE), myasthenia gravis, pemphigoid, and lichen planus. Rarely, they are seen in healthy individuals (<1%) (Becker, 1993; Mutasim, 1993b; Nousari, 1997).

Pemphigus Foliaceus

The subsets of pemphigus foliaceus include idiopathic pemphigus foliaceus, endemic pemphigus foliaceus (fogo selvagem), drug-induced pemphigus foliaceus, and pemphigus erythematosus (PE). Desmoglein 1 is the major antigen in pemphigus foliaceus (Lin, 1998; Naparstek, 1993). ELISAs to detect anti-desmoglein -1 are available.

Direct immunofluorescence microscopy

For all forms of pemphigus foliaceus except pemphigus erythematosus, the DIFM pattern is similar to pemphigus vulgaris. In some cases, the staining predominates in the superficial epidermis at the level of the

VI

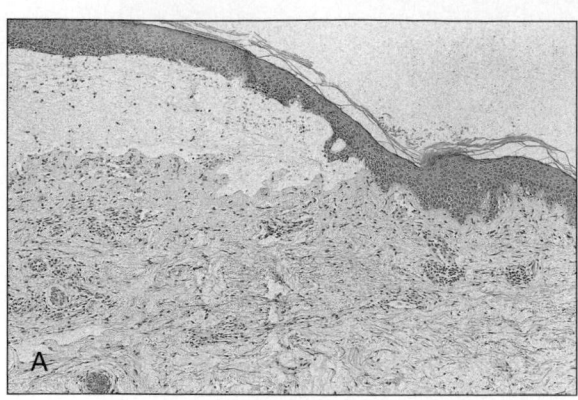

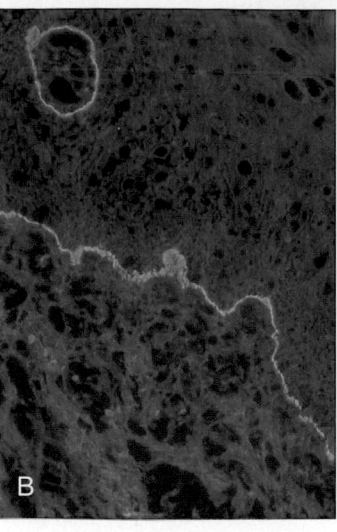

Figure 52–3 Skin biopsy of pemphigoid reveals a subepidermal split, non-necrotic epidermis, and variable inflammation often with prominent eosinophils (A, hematoxylin and eosin [H&E], ×100). Direct immunofluorescence microscopy reveals intense linear C3 deposition along the basement membrane zone (B, ×400).

stratum granulosum. In pemphigus erythematosus, there is linear IgG staining of epidermal ICS combined with granular immunoreactants along the BMZ.

Indirect immunofluorescence microscopy

IIFM should detect circulating IgG ICS autoantibodies in virtually 100% of pemphigus foliaceus patients with active disease (Nousari, 1997). About 90% of these pemphigus foliaceus patients have detectable autoantibodies when monkey esophagus is used for indirect studies. Guinea pig esophagus is somewhat more sensitive in that it detects the remaining 10% of patients and the indirect titers tend to run higher than those obtained when using monkey esophagus (Jiao, 1997).

Paraneoplastic Pemphigus

Paraneoplastic pemphigus, an uncommon disorder characterized by painful blisters or erosions of mucous membranes and skin, is a condition of patients with neoplasms. These blisters or erosions usually erupt in the mouth, but other mucosal sites have been reported. Malignant neoplasms that have been associated with paraneoplastic pemphigus include malignant lymphoma, chronic lymphocytic leukemia, thymoma, bronchogenic squamous cell carcinoma, and sarcomas. Rarely, paraneoplastic pemphigus is associated with benign neoplasms (Camisa, 1993; Mutasim, 1993c; Flotte, 1995).

The following criteria to define paraneoplastic pemphigus have been proposed by Mutasim (1993c):

- Painful mucosal erosions and a polymorphous skin eruption, with papular lesions progressing to blisters and erosive lesions affecting trunk, extremities, and palms and soles, associated with an occult or clinically known neoplasm.
- Suprabasilar acantholysis, keratinocyte necrosis, and vacuolar interface changes on light microscopic tissue sections.
- IgG ICS combined with linear/granular complement and IgG along the BMZ.
- Circulating ICS autoantibodies that bind to rodent bladder urothelium and monkey/guinea pig esophagus.
- Immunoprecipitation of a complex of four keratinocytic proteins bound by the autoantibodies; this is mainly a research tool but may provide helpful clinical information in difficult cases.

Paraneoplastic pemphigus associated with malignant neoplasms signals an extremely poor prognosis. Although clinical improvement or remission of mucocutaneous lesions after tumor resection has been reported, treatment for malignancy-associated paraneoplastic pemphigus is supportive. Paraneoplastic pemphigus associated with a benign neoplasm remitted after tumor resection (Mutasim, 1993c).

Direct immunofluorescence microscopy

DIFM of perilesional skin and/or mucosa from patients with paraneoplastic pemphigus detects IgG ICS immunoreactant with or without complement components. Granular or, less commonly, linear BMZ deposits of complement components (C3, C1q) are also present in addition to IgG ICS immunofluorescence (Mutasim, 1993c).

Indirect immunofluorescence microscopy

IIFM using monkey esophagus and rodent bladder urothelium demonstrates IgG immunoreactant both in ICS and along the BMZ. The binding to rodent (rat or mouse) bladder epithelium is an important differential finding that distinguishes paraneoplastic pemphigus from other types of pemphigus (Liu, 1993; Mutasim, 1993c).

IgA Pemphigus (Intercellular IgA Dermatosis)

Direct immunofluorescence microscopy

Intercellular IgA dermatosis is a rare intraepidermal vesiculobullous disorder. Direct studies show linear ICS immunofluorescence for IgA that is suprabasilar, and particularly accentuated in the upper epidermis.

Indirect immunofluorescence microscopy

IIFM detects circulating IgA anti-ICS autoantibodies (Teraki, 1991; Flotte, 1995).

Pemphigoid

Bullous Pemphigoid

Bullous pemphigoid is a subepidermal bullous disease of unknown cause that can occur in patients of any age but mainly affects adults older than 60 years (Fig. 52–3A). This disorder typically involves flexor surfaces of the arms, legs, groin, axilla, and lower abdomen. The oral mucous membranes may be affected but such lesions are rarely the presenting or predominant sign, a point that differentiates pemphigoid from pemphigus vulgaris.

The major antigens in bullous pemphigoid are two keratinocytic hemidesmosomal proteins, an intracellular 230 kDa protein (bullous pemphigoid antigen 1) and a transmembrane 180 kDa protein (bullous pemphigoid antigen 2) (Nousari, 1997; Lin, 1998).

Direct immunofluorescence microscopy

DIFM of unblistered, perilesional skin from the edge of a fresh blister is diagnostically sensitive and typically demonstrates linear BMZ immunofluorescence in nearly 100% of patients (Fig. 52–3B). C3 and IgG, or C3 alone, are the predominant immunoreactants. Also, IgA and/or IgM may be present in up to 25% of patients, usually in weaker intensity and in combination with IgG (Izuno, 1986; Crosby, 1993; Korman, 1993).

A linear epidermal BMZ pattern can be identified in several disparate clinical disorders, including benign mucous membrane pemphigoid, epidermolysis bullosa acquisita, gestational pemphigoid (herpes gestationis), and bullous lupus erythematosus.

To help separate these disorders, salt-split direct skin biopsies are useful (Domloge-Hultsch, 1991). In bullous pemphigoid and gestational pemphigoid, linear IgG is localized to the epidermal side, or roof, of the split. Linear C3 immunofluorescence, however, may be seen along epidermal and dermal locations. In epidermolysis bullosa acquisita and bullous lupus erythematosus, immunoreactants are seen along the dermal side of the split (Nousari, 1997). Clinical correlation then becomes important in resolving diagnostic alternatives.

Indirect immunofluorescence microscopy

Bullous pemphigoid is serologically characterized by the presence of circulating autoantibodies to the BMZ, either cutaneous or oral mucosa. IIFM detects circulating IgG anti-BMZ autoantibodies in about 50% of patients with pemphigoid but sensitivity increases to 70–80% if normal human salt-split skin is used as substrate (Izuno, 1986; Domloge-Hultsch,

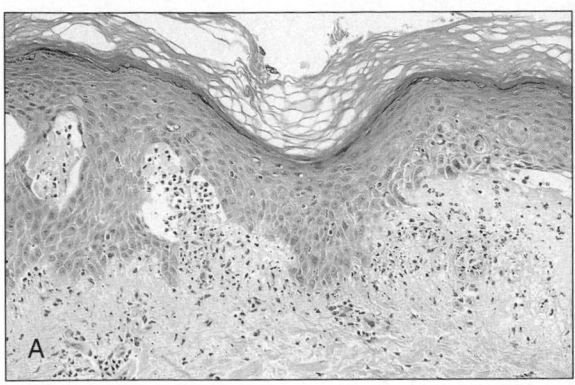
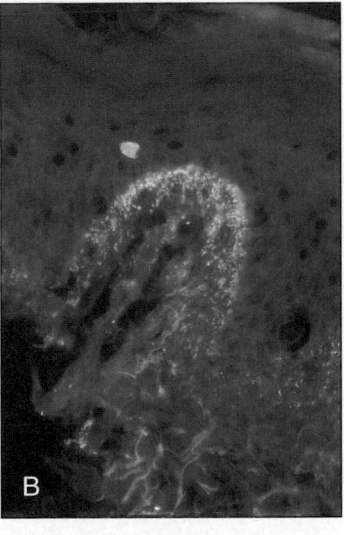

Figure 52–4 Skin biopsy of dermatitis herpetiformis reveals a subepidermal split, non-necrotic epidermis, and neutrophilic microabscesses in the tips of dermal papillae (*A*, H&E, ×200). Direct immunofluorescence microscopy reveals granular IgA immunofluorescence in the tips of dermal papillae and, to a lesser extent, along the basement membrane region (*B*, ×400).

1991; Nousari, 1997). In bullous pemphigoid, autoantibodies bind only to the roof of salt-split skin in 80% of patients. In epidermolysis bullosa acquisita and bullous lupus erythematosus, autoantibodies bind to the dermal base, or floor, of the split in 50% of patients (Domloge-Hultsch, 1991; Crosby, 1993; Korman, 1993).

Benign Mucous Membrane Pemphigoid

Benign mucous membrane pemphigoid, or cicatricial pemphigoid, consistently affects oral and ocular mucosa. Other mucosal sites of these lesions can be the nasopharynx, larynx, genitalia, rectum, and esophagus (Mutasim, 1993a). Scarring follows the healing of lesions, and blindness is the most feared complication.

Direct immunofluorescence microscopy

The DIFM pattern is similar to that seen in bullous pemphigoid. Sensitivity is 90% but increases if additional biopsies are taken. Chronic localized scarring pemphigoid, also known as cicatricial pemphigoid of Brunsting-Perry, is a variant of benign mucous membrane pemphigoid that is localized to the head and neck region (Sarret, 1991). In this variant, DIFM demonstrates IgG only along the BMZ without IgA or IgM; circulating anti-BMZ autoantibodies are also rare (Izuno, 1986).

Indirect immunofluorescence microscopy

IIFM detects circulating IgG autoantibodies in fewer than 33% of benign mucous membrane pemphigoid patients when oral mucosal substrate is used but only in 5–15% of patients using standard substrates (Sarret, 1991; Crosby, 1993; Nousari, 1997). Salt-split human skin studies may reveal deposits of IgA, IgG, or both in about 80% of these patients (Sarret, 1991).

There is no correlation between the presence and titer of autoantibodies and disease activity.

Gestational Pemphigoid

Infrequently, the subepidermal bullous disease gestational pemphigoid (herpes gestationis) develops during or soon after pregnancy (Izuno, 1986). Lesions are typically pruritic and located predominantly on the abdomen and/or extremities.

Direct immunofluorescence microscopy

With DIFM, one typically finds linear C3 BMZ deposits. Associated IgG deposits are detected in 30–40% of cases but IgA and IgM are rare (Izuno, 1986).

Indirect immunofluorescence microscopy

Linear C3 deposits only may be visualized along the BMZ, but often autoantibody titers are too low to be seen using standard IIFM substrates. Complement may be detected, however, if complement immunofixation using normal human salt-split skin is used as substrate (Izuno, 1986; Nousari, 1997).

Epidermolysis Bullosa Acquisita and Bullous Lupus Erythematosus

Epidermolysis bullosa acquisita and bullous lupus erythematosus are acquired subepidermal blistering diseases characterized by the presence of autoantibodies to type VII collagen in BMZ protein (Gammon, 1993). Epidermolysis bullosa acquisita can occur at any age but most commonly

presents in adults who are 40–50 years old. There is neither an ethnic nor a sex predilection. All such patients are afflicted with a combination of blisters, erosions, scars, milia, and dyspigmentation of skin, most often located on trauma-susceptible extensor skin surfaces such as knees, elbows, and dorsa of hands and feet (Gammon, 1993). Bullous lupus erythematosus occurs in patients with lupus erythematosus.

Direct immunofluorescence microscopy

Using DIFM, patients with epidermolysis bullosa acquisita and bullous lupus erythematosus have linear BMZ immunoreactants that most commonly consist of IgG and C3. Using direct salt-split skin biopsy tissue, the linear immunoreactants are localized at the dermal, or floor, aspect of the induced blister.

Indirect immunofluorescence microscopy

Only about 40% of epidermolysis bullosa acquisita patients have demonstrable autoantibodies when human skin without salt treatment is used as substrate. Using indirect salt split skin technique, circulating autoantibodies can be identified in about 50–85% of patients (Fine, 1994; Nousari, 1997).

Dermatitis Herpetiformis

Dermatitis herpetiformis is a severely pruritic subepidermal bullous disease associated with gluten-sensitive enteropathy (Fig. 52–4A). Dermatitis herpetiformis is also associated with HLA-B8, DR3 histocompatibility types (Crosby, 1993).

Direct immunofluorescence microscopy

The direct biopsy should be from perilesional skin because a lesional skin biopsy may be negative. DIFM detects granular IgA in the tips of dermal papillae in approximately 80–100% of dermatitis herpetiformis patients (Flotte, 1995) (Fig. 52–4B). There may be concomitant IgA deposits along the BMZ. C3 deposits are often found with IgA, but IgG and/or IgM are detected infrequently (Izuno, 1986).

Indirect immunofluorescence microscopy

Patients with dermatitis herpetiformis do not have detectable anti-BMZ autoantibodies. However, antiendomysial IgA autoantibodies are detected in 80% of dermatitis herpetiformis patients. These autoantibodies are identified by their characteristic immunofluorescence pattern in the subepithelial muscularis mucosa of monkey esophagus (Peters, 1989).

Linear IgA Dermatosis

Linear IgA dermatosis is an uncommon acquired subepidermal blistering disorder that is now considered a distinct clinical entity rather than being a variant of dermatitis herpetiformis as was once thought (Izuno, 1986; Crosby, 1993). Many cases are thought to be idiopathic but drug-induced and systemic-disorder-related forms are described (Kuechle, 1994; Nousari, 1995, 1999; Bouldin, 2000). Chronic bullous dermatosis of childhood is similar to linear IgA dermatosis, both clinically and immunopathologically (Elenitsas, 1995).

Direct immunofluorescence microscopy

In nearly 100% of cases, DIFM demonstrates intense linear IgA deposits along the BMZ but none in dermal papillae (Izuno, 1986). Although

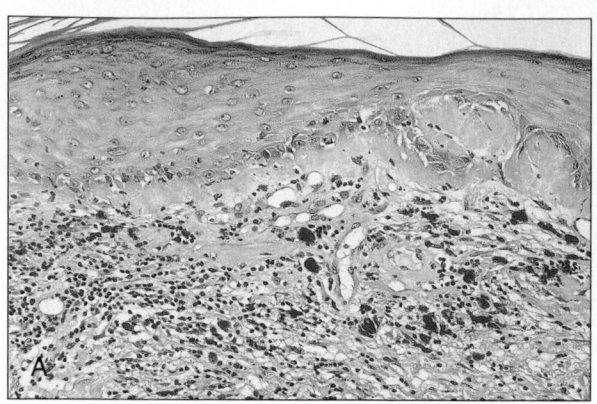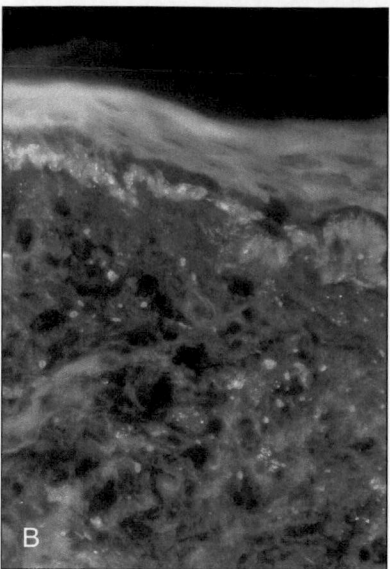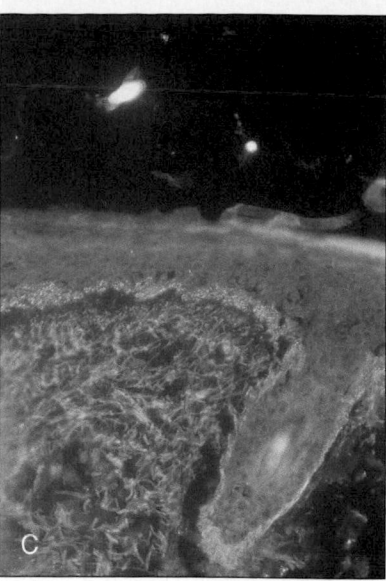

Figure 52–5 Skin biopsy of lupus erythematosus reveals epidermal atrophy, vacuolar alteration of basal keratinocytes, marked thickening of the basement membrane zone, perivascular and interstitial mainly lymphocytic inflammation, and melanin incontinence (*A*, H&E, ×500). Direct immunofluorescence microscopy reveals continuous granular C3 (*B*, ×500) and C1q (*C*, ×200) immunofluorescence along the basement membrane zone.

occasional cases may show concomitant weak C3 BMZ staining, immunoreactants other than IgA are not usually present.

Indirect immunofluorescence microscopy

Circulating IgA anti-BMZ autoantibodies can be detected with IIFM in about 10–30% of cases (Crosby, 1993; Flotte, 1995).

Lupus Erythematosus

Lupus erythematosus (Fig. 52–5A) is a disorder characterized serologically by the presence of multiple autoantibodies, including antinuclear antibodies, anti-native-DNA, antihistones, and anti-Sm.

Direct immunofluorescence microscopy

With DIFM, one sees characteristic coarse, granular, continuous deposits of immunoglobulins and complement along the epidermal BMZ in 50–95% of SLE patients (Izuno, 1986). BMZ deposits of the complement membrane attack complex C5b–9 in lesional skin may be a marker for SLE (Helm, 1993).

Whereas these patients commonly have deposits of IgG, IgM and complement component (C3 and/or C1q) (Fig. 52–5B and C), immunoglobulins of all classes may be identified (Izuno, 1986). When nonlesional skin concurrently contains immunoglobulins IgG, IgA, and/or IgM in the typical pattern, the diagnosis is more likely than not SLE (Izuno, 1986).

Although characteristic, this reaction pattern can be seen in other disorders, such as mixed connective tissue disease, dermatomyositis, graft-versus-host reaction, drug eruptions, and vasculitis (Izuno, 1986). Therefore, it is mandatory to correlate direct results with both the clinical presentation and the results of light microscopic study of a skin biopsy. This information is then interpreted in the context of an individual's direct findings to categorize the clinical type of lupus erythematosus. Many publications cite the utility of DIFM for the purpose of diagnosing SLE from biopsied skin, with or without lesions, and from sun-exposed or sun-protected sites. In patients diagnosed with SLE, normal sun-exposed skin proves positive about 70% of the time, whereas normal sun-protected skin is positive in about 40% of patients (Izuno, 1986). However, the potential for predicting disease activity or renal involvement in this way remains controversial (Izuno, 1986). Perhaps the most practical clinical application of laboratory testing comes in the differential diagnosis of SLE from discoid lupus erythematosus. Up to 95% of individuals with discoid lupus erythematosus have coarse, granular, continuous BMZ deposits similar to those of SLE (Izuno, 1986). However, positive DIFM findings in discoid lupus erythematosus are confined to lesional skin, whereas skin with or without lesions can give positive DIFM findings in SLE (Izuno, 1986).

Subacute cutaneous lupus erythematosus is characterized clinically by arthritis, mild systemic manifestations, and anti-SS-A/Ro autoantibodies. DIFM of skin biopsies from these patients detects BMZ immunoglobulin and/or complement deposits in only 50% of lesional skin biopsies and 30% of uninvolved skin biopsies (Izuno, 1986). IIFM is positive in 50–70% of patients with subacute cutaneous lupus erythematosus.

Other major systemic autoimmune diseases do not offer diagnostically specific findings by either DIFM or IIFM. Although some patients have granular IgM deposits along the BMZ, this immunopathologic finding is considered to be a completely nonspecific marker that may be detected not only in autoimmune disease but also in a large number of inflammatory dermatitides or in sun-exposed skin of clinically normal individuals (Izuno, 1986).

Vasculitis

Vasculitis (see Ch. 51) in the skin has a number of synonyms, including leukocytoclastic vasculitis, allergic vasculitis, and hypersensitivity angiitis/vasculitis. Histologically, small blood vessels of the dermis show endothelial cell swelling, neutrophilic exocytosis, nuclear debris ('leukocytoclasis'), and necrosis in conjunction with extravasated red blood cells.

Direct immunofluorescence microscopy

Biopsy of such a lesion within 24 hours of onset may display vascular deposits of IgM, C3, fibrinogen, and sometimes IgG. A negative result does not exclude vasculitis. Biopsy of a lesion older than 24 hours may not be helpful, since nonspecific fibrinogen staining may be the only finding. Histologic confirmation of the diagnosis is therefore essential. Henoch–Schönlein purpura is diagnosed when granular IgA, with or without C3, vascular immunofluorescence is seen in the appropriate clinical setting.

Liver

Autoantibodies

Antinuclear Autoantibodies

Antinuclear antibodies (ANAs) are most commonly detected by IIFM, although ELISAs for identification of specific autoantibodies are becoming popular in clinical laboratories. ANAs are a very heterogeneous group, and almost all subtypes that occur in rheumatologic disorders are found in persons with autoimmune hepatitis. Either homogeneous or speckled ANA patterns on Hep-2 cells are more commonly identified in patients with autoimmune hepatitis. Also reported in liver disease are specific autoantibodies to double-stranded DNA (Manns, 1992). ANAs in titers greater than 1:80 are detected in about 80% of patients with autoimmune hepatitis (Nakamura, 1991). However, ANAs may also be found in about 60% of patients with PBC, 50% of patients with alcohol-related liver disease, 40% of patients with viral hepatitis type B, and 25% of autoimmune hepatitis patients who also have anti-liver–kidney microsomal autoantibodies (LKMs) (Nakamura, 1991). Anticentromere autoantibodies can be identified in 10–15% of PBC patients.

Antimitochondrial Autoantibodies

Nine separate mitochondrial antigens have been identified that react with antimitochondrial antibodies (AMAs). AMAs directed at M2 and M9 antigens are considered the most important diagnostic markers of PBC (Bylund, 1992).

Table 52–3 Autoimmune Liver Diseases

	ANA	LKM	SLA	SMA	AMA	Anti-HCV	p-ANCA	ACA	Therapy
Autoimmune hepatitis									
Type 1	+	–	–	+	–	–	±	–	Immunosuppression
Type 2a	–	+	–	–	–	–	–	–	Immunosuppression
Type 2b	–	+	–	–	–	+	–	?	
Type 3	–	–	+	±	±	–	–	–	Immunosuppression
Type 4	–	–	–	+	–	–	–	–	Immunosuppression
PBC	–	–	–	–	+	–	–	–	Supportive; transplant
PSC	–	–	–	–	–	–	+	–	Supportive; transplant
AiC	+	–	–	–	–	–	–	+	Immunosuppression

ACA = anti-carbonic-anhydrase; AiC = autoimmune cholangitis; AMA = antimitochondrial antibodies; ANA = antinuclear antibodies; HCV = hepatitis C virus; LKM = liver–kidney microsomal antibodies; p-ANCA, perinuclear antineutrophil cytoplasmic antibodies; PBC = primary biliary cirrhosis; PSC = primary sclerosing cholangitis; SLA = antibodies against soluble liver antigens; SMA = smooth muscle antibodies.

Source: modified from Manns MP: Autoimmune diseases of the liver. Clin Lab Med 1992; 12:25–40.

AMAs detected using IIFM on a substrate of rodent stomach/kidney tissue block show a typical pattern of fluorescence that reflects homogeneous cytoplasmic staining of kidney tubules and stomach parietal cell regions; distal tubules are also positive. This distal tubular staining is an important point in differentiating the reactivity of AMAs from that of LKMs, which do not stain distal renal tubules.

The M2 autoantigen is a heterogeneous mix containing several components of the mitochondrial 2-oxo-acid dehydrogenase complex. The dominant M2 autoantigen in patients with PBC is the 70 kDa E2 subunit of pyruvate dehydrogenase (PDH-E2) (Manns, 1992). The second most common mitochondrial autoantigen is the 50 kDa E2 subunit of branched-chain oxo-keto-acid-dehydrogenase (BCOADH-E2) (Manns, 1992). A group of serum autoantibodies called naturally occurring mitochondrial autoantibodies (NOMAs) have been found in persons having close contact with PBC patients and even in laboratory technicians processing PBC sera (Bylund, 1992). NOMAs are rarely produced in PBC patients but are observed in sera from patients with Epstein–Barr virus infection, cytomegalovirus infection, and other infectious disorders. NOMAs are directed at epitopes on the M2 and M9 antigens in PBC but not to the same antigens as AMAs (Bylund, 1992). Although the significance of NOMAs is uncertain, their presence in persons associated with PBC patients has raised questions about possible contagious agents in the serum of these patients (Bylund, 1992).

Smooth Muscle Autoantibodies

Smooth muscle autoantibodies (SMAs) are found in approximately 50% of patients with classic autoimmune hepatitis and often they occur with ANAs (Nakamura, 1991). When accompanying liver disease, SMAs are directed against F-actin, which is part of the liver cell cytoskeleton in close association with the liver cell plasma membrane (Nakamura, 1991). The SMA titer is typically greater than or equal to 1:80 in serum from a patient with autoimmune hepatitis. However, low titers of SMA can be detected in patients with other diseases, and in apparently healthy individuals (Nakamura, 1991).

IIFM on a tissue substrate of rodent stomach is commonly used to detect SMA, which stain the muscularis propria of stomach in a uniform and consistent pattern. Specific staining of muscularis mucosae and walls of blood vessels is characteristic. If a rodent stomach/kidney tissue block is used as substrate, there may be faint staining in glomerular mesangial zones due to the presence of F-actin in this region. If Hep-2 cells are used instead of other substrates, IIFM reveals 'cable-like' cytoplasmic staining when SMA is present.

Liver–Kidney Microsomal Autoantibodies

LKMs stain the microsomes of hepatocytes and proximal renal tubules when detected using a rodent stomach/kidney tissue block as the substrate for IIFM. The distal renal tubules are characteristically negative for immunofluorescence. The simultaneous occurrence of AMA and LKM, although possible, is extremely unlikely.

ELISAs that detect LKM are becoming available for use in clinical laboratories. The presence of LKM can also be confirmed by using Western blotting, although this assay is not generally available outside research laboratories.

Using the Western blotting procedure, LKMs have been grouped into three subtypes on the basis of their target antigens (Manns, 1992). A 50 kDa component of cytochrome P-450 IID6 has been identified as the major antigen for LKM-1 (Manns, 1992). LKM-2, directed at cytochrome P-450 IIC9, was found in patients taking ticrynafen (Manns, 1992), a drug that is no longer on the American market. LKM-3 has been identified in sera from patients with chronic viral hepatitis type D (Manns, 1992).

Other Liver Autoantibodies

The remaining groups of hepatic autoantibodies include anticytoskeleton, anticytosol, antiliver membrane, antinuclear lamins, liver-specific, and asialoglycoprotein receptor autoantibodies. All these have been identified in patients with autoimmune liver diseases, but their use as diagnostic markers is not currently widespread (Nakamura, 1991).

Liver Diseases

Table 52–3 lists typical serologic profiles in autoimmune hepatitis, PBC, and primary sclerosing cholangitis. These are typically chronic disorders defined by elevated concentrations of serum transaminases for at least 6 months.

Common clinical differential diagnoses include alcohol-related liver disease, drug-induced liver injury, viral hepatitides, and fatty liver of diabetes mellitus or obesity. Less common differential diagnoses include idiopathic hemochromatosis, Wilson's disease, α_1-antitrypsin deficiency, and hepatic involvement in systemic diseases.

Autoimmune Hepatitis

Autoimmune hepatitis classically occurs in females around 35 years old, who present with high concentrations of serum aminotransferases, hypergammaglobulinemia, amenorrhea, arthralgias, and circulating autoantibodies such as ANA, SMA, and LKM. By definition, these patients have no serologic evidence of viral hepatitis, Wilson's disease, or other diseases in the differential diagnosis. Histologically, liver biopsy typically shows chronic hepatitis with interface activity (Fig. 52–6A). The patient's response to corticosteroids is dramatic, and failure to respond sheds doubt on the diagnosis of autoimmune hepatitis.

Autoimmune hepatitis is a heterogeneous group of disorders of uncertain etiology. There are no pathognomonic features. The International Autoimmune Hepatitis Group (IAHG) has integrated clinical and laboratory features at patient presentation into a scoring system for definite or probable diagnosis of autoimmune hepatitis. Table 52–4 lists clinical laboratory parameters used as criteria to diagnose autoimmune hepatitis; other criteria and scoring interpretations are in the references (Johnson, 1993; Manns, 1998). Importantly, the absence of ANA, SMA, or LKM does not exclude this diagnosis.

Although autoimmune hepatitis subtypes based on autoantibody patterns are presented in the medical literature, the clinical utility of such subtyping is uncertain, and the IAHG did not recommend subdivision of autoimmune hepatitis on the basis of autoantibody profiles. From a clinical perspective, autoimmune hepatitis can be viewed as a chronic liver disease characterized by the presence of a variety of autoantibodies. Most experts seem to agree that autoimmune hepatitis types 1 and 2 are the major forms of this disease, whereas additional subtypes are still at issue.

Since the various subtypes are widely quoted, subclassification of autoimmune hepatitis according to its serologic profile is briefly discussed here.

VI

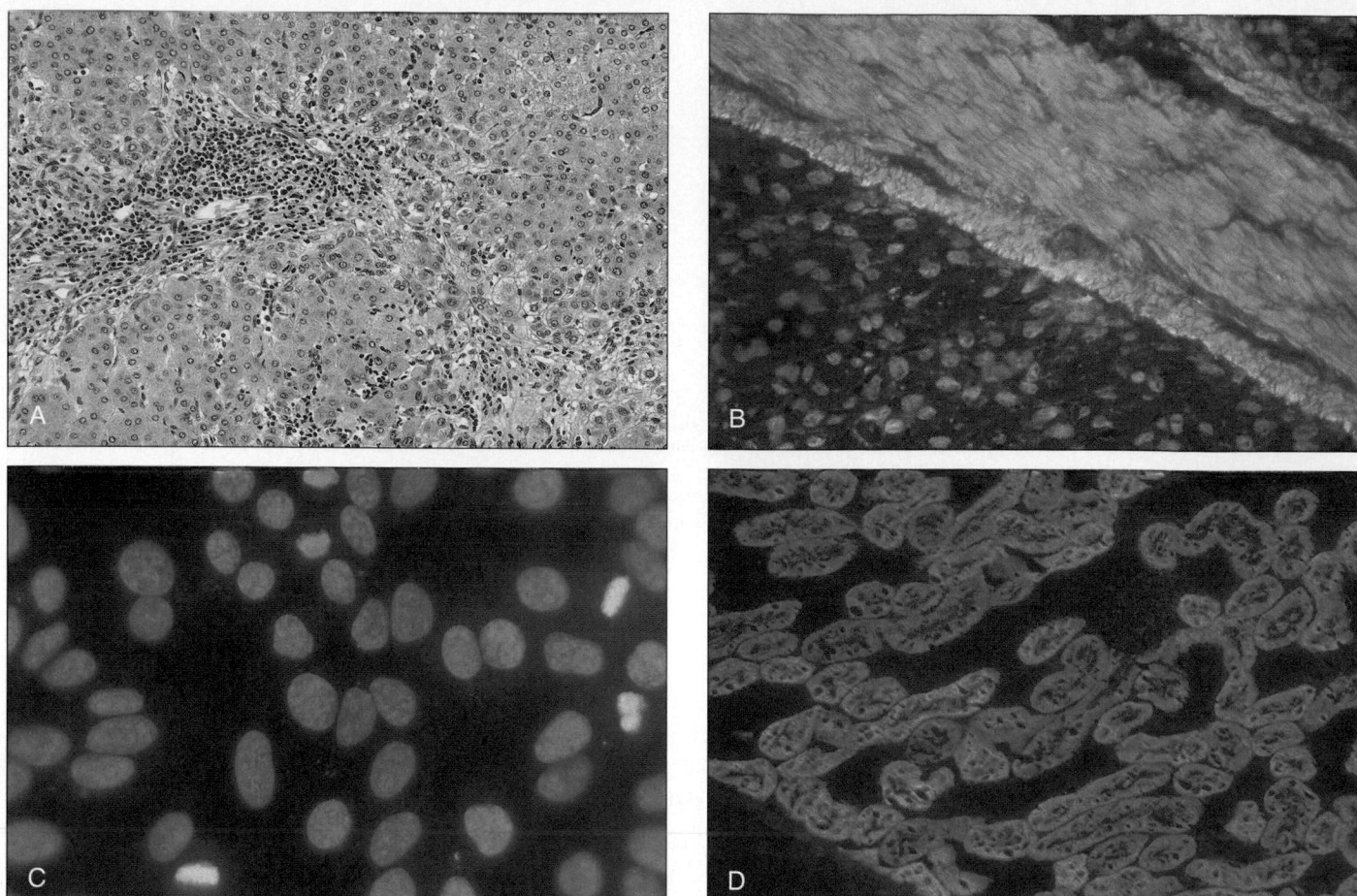

Figure 52–6 Liver biopsy in untreated autoimmune hepatitis shows prominent portal and lobular inflammation with interface activity and often numerous plasma cells at the leading edge of inflammation (A, H&E, ×500). IIFM in this instance reveals combined smooth muscle antibodies and antinuclear antibodies using mouse stomach/kidney as substrate (B, ×200). The ANA pattern in liver disease is often homogeneous (C, ×400). IIFM of liver–kidney microsomal autoantibodies using mouse stomach/kidney as substrate. There is finely granular cytoplasmic immunofluorescence of proximal renal tubules, not distal tubules (D, ×200).

ANAs characterize classical, type 1, autoimmune-type hepatitis. SMAs are also frequently detected (Fig. 52–6B and C). Although AMAs are specific and sensitive diagnostic markers for PBC, as described below, AMAs can also be detected in about 15% of patients with both clinical and histologic features of autoimmune hepatitis, including clinical improvement in response to immunosuppressive therapy. Such patients are regarded as having a syndrome with features that 'overlap' both autoimmune hepatitis and PBC. The AMA titer in this autoimmune hepatitis subgroup is rarely greater than 1:40 (Bylund, 1992). Additionally, the antigen specificity of these AMAs is similar to that seen in classical PBC (Manns, 1992). Liver disease in which LKMs are detected (Fig. 52–6D), so-called type 2 autoimmune hepatitis, has been subdivided into two subgroups, types 2a and 2b. Usually, patients with this variant are negative for ANA and SMA. However, thyroid microsomal, thyroglobulin, and parietal cell autoantibodies are frequently detected. Type 2 autoimmune hepatitis is characterized by low IgA levels, and hypergammaglobulinemia is less prominent than in type 1 (Manns, 1992). Type 2a occurs in young females, who have high titers of LKM-1, negative serology for hepatitis C virus, and active but steroid-responsive disease.

The type 2b variant occurs in older patients, and there is less of a female preponderance. These patients have low titers of LKM-1, manifest milder liver disease, and are often serologically positive for hepatitis C virus. Their disease tends to be less responsive to immunosuppression than the 2a type.

A third subgroup of autoimmune hepatitis, separated from other subgroups on the basis of identifying serum anti-soluble-liver autoantibody (SLA), has been proposed by some investigators (Manns, 1992). Although this may become an important autoantibody to identify because it has been reported as the only serologic marker in about 25% of patients with autoimmune hepatitis, reliable tests to detect SLA are technically difficult and, as yet, are not routinely available in clinical laboratories (Manns, 1992).

It may be that high titers of SMA directed against F-actin characterize a fourth subgroup of autoimmune hepatitis that is frequently observed in young children (Manns, 1992).

Primary Biliary Cirrhosis

PBC is a chronic, progressive, cholestatic disorder typically occurring in young or middle-aged females. Patients may be asymptomatic or have symptoms of cholestasis (itch). Laboratory studies demonstrate an elevation in alkaline phosphatase with or without hyperbilirubinemia, as well as increased IgM and AMA. Associated extrahepatic immunologic phenomena such as Raynaud's phenomenon, sicca complex, rheumatoid arthritis, thyroiditis, scleroderma, or celiac disease may occur (Bylund, 1992; Manns, 1992). Histologically, the liver shows various stages of nonsuppurative destructive cholangitis (Fig. 52–7A).

AMAs are the most specific and sensitive diagnostic markers for PBC (Fig. 52–7B and C). As a general guideline, an AMA titer greater than or equal to 1:160 is highly predictive of PBC, although about 10% of PBC patients have AMA titers of 1:16 or less (Bylund, 1992). About 95% of patients with typical features of PBC have been shown to have anti-M2 and/or anti-M9 AMA, whereas the remaining 5% of patients are AMA negative.

The cause of PBC is unknown and several pathogenetic mechanisms are proposed regarding the immune-related bile duct injury characteristic of this disorder (Gershwin, 2000). Although this disease is classically associated with serum AMA, T-cell-mediated immune injury to intrahepatic interlobular bile ducts dominates tissue lesions (Batts, 1991; Manns, 1991, 1988; Poupon, 1996). The discovery of retroviral antibody in PBC patients has been ascribed to either an autoimmune response or immune reactivity to viral proteins that share antigenic determinants with retroviruses (Mason, 1998).

The diagnosis of AMA negative PBC derives from the clinical presentation, liver biopsy findings, and cholangiogram to exclude primary sclerosing cholangitis.

Primary Sclerosing Cholangitis

Primary sclerosing cholangitis typically occurs in males with a history of inflammatory bowel disease and/or diarrhea. In 50% of these patients,

Clinical Laboratory Parameters	Score
Table 52–4 Laboratory Parameters and Score for Autoimmune Hepatitis Diagnosis	

Clinical Laboratory Parameters	Score
Biochemistry	
Ratio of Increased Alkaline Phosphatase to Aminotransferase	
>3.0	−2
<3.0	+2
Total Serum Globulin, γ-Globulin, or IgG (× Upper Normal Limit)	
>2.0	+3
1.5–2.0	+2
1.0–1.5	+1
<1.0	0
Autoantibodies (IIFM)	
Adults	
ANA, SMA, LKM	
>1:80	+3
1:80	+2
1:40	+1
<1:40	0
Children	
ANA, LKM	
>1:20	+3
1:10 or 1:20	+2
<1:10	0
SMA	
>1:20	+3
1:20	+2
<1:20	0
AMA	
Detected	−2
Not detected	0
Adults and Children (if ANA, SMA, LKM not detected)	
Other Liver Autoantibodies (SLA, ASGP-R, LC-1)	
Detected	+2
Not detected	0
Viral Markers	
Acute HAV or HBV	−3
HCV by ELISA and/or RIBA	−2
HCV RNA by PCR	−3
Other active viral infection	−3
Seronegative for known viruses	+3
Genetic Factors	
HLA B8-DR3 or DR4 allotype	+1

Source: adapted from Johnson PJ, McFarlane IG: Convenors on behalf of the panel. Meeting report: International autoimmune hepatitis group. Hepatology 1993; 18:998–1008.

ulcerative colitis is the inflammatory bowel disease linked with primary sclerosing cholangitis. A diagnosis of primary sclerosing cholangitis is typically based on cholangiography, which reveals a characteristic beading pattern of bile ducts due to multifocal strictures at those sites (Fig. 52–8A). The hallmark histologic lesion is fibrous cholangitis of large and/or small bile ducts, although in practice a wide spectrum of chronic inflammatory lesions is seen on liver biopsy (Fig. 52–8B).

Routine biochemical studies demonstrate an elevation in alkaline phosphatase and an increase of aminotransferases with or without hyperbilirubinemia. Although ANA may be present, AMA are not.

Furthermore, a high prevalence of atypical perinuclear antineutrophil cytoplasmic antibodies (p-ANCA) detected with IIFM on ethanol- and formalin-fixed neutrophils displays has been reported (Manns, 1992; Lo, 1994; Gur, 1995; Bansi, 1996).

Autoimmune Cholangitis/Cholangiopathy

Autoimmune cholangitis/cholangiopathy is a chronic cholestatic liver disease that does not appear to be a variant of primary sclerosing cholangitis (Goodman, 1995; Tsui, 1997). The clinical presentation and histologic appearance of the liver resemble PBC, but serologic findings mimic autoimmune hepatitis type 1. AMAs are not detected. Additionally, an autoantibody to carbonic anhydrase has been detected in some autoimmune cholangitis patients (Gordon, 1995).

Although the connection between autoimmune cholangitis and PBC is not resolved, autoimmune cholangitis may be the same as AMA-negative PBC. Generally, autoimmune cholangitis patients respond to immunosuppression.

Thyroid Gland

Thyroid Diseases

Autoimmune thyroid diseases include Graves disease and Hashimoto's thyroiditis (Burek, 1995).

Graves Disease

The patient who has Graves disease presents with symptoms of hyperthyroidism and diffuse goiter. The peak incidence is in the third to fourth decades of life, and the female/male ratio is 4–8:1; 60–70% of these patients additionally manifest ocular disturbances (Patrick, 1993). Laboratory data show an increase in levels of triiodothyronine (T_3) and thyroxine (T_4) and in the uptake of T_3. Therapy is directed at reducing the thyroid's ability to respond to stimulation by autoantibodies. This can be achieved by subtotal thyroidectomy, by administration of radioactive iodine, or by use of antithyroid drugs such as propylthiouracil or methimazole (Patrick, 1993).

Hashimoto's Thyroiditis

Hashimoto's thyroiditis is the most common form of thyroiditis, and is functionally characterized by a slow progression to hypothyroidism. In patients with hypothyroidism, T_3 and T_4 levels and T_3 uptake are low and amounts of thyroid-stimulating hormone (TSH) increase abnormally (Patrick, 1993). The incidence of Hashimoto's thyroiditis peaks during the third to fifth decades, with a female/male ratio of 10:1. Autoantibodies directed against thyroglobulin (anti-Tg) and thyroid peroxidase (anti-TPO) antigens are clinically the most important for diagnosis (Patrick, 1993), but up to 20% of the adult female population with no clinical disease have detectable anti-Tg and/or anti-TPO, raising questions about their pathogenic significance (Patrick, 1993). Thyroid hormone replacement is reserved for patients with proven hypothyroidism.

There are similarities between Graves disease and Hashimoto's thyroiditis (Utiger, 1991). Both are associated with HLA-B8; both share fundamentally similar pathogenesis, and it is believed that Graves disease may progress to Hashimoto's thyroiditis (Utiger, 1991; Patrick, 1993).

Autoantibodies

Three major autoantibodies are important in autoimmune thyroid diseases, including anti-TPO, anti-Tg, and autoantibody to thyroid stimulating hormone receptor (anti-TSHR) (Naparstek, 1993). Although anti-TPO and anti-Tg are considered to be markers of autoimmune thyroid disease, their etiologic role has not been proved. They may occur as well in other organ-directed autoimmune diseases. Anti-TSHR, however, clearly plays a causal role in autoimmune thyroid disease (Naparstek, 1993).

Anti-Thyroid Peroxidase Autoantibodies

Anti-TPO is directed to a 105 kDa antigen that is contained within the microsomal fraction of thyroid epithelial cell cytoplasm (Burek, 1995). ELISA is becoming a common available method for detecting anti-TPO.

Historically, IIFM has been a popular and sensitive method for detecting anti-TPO ('antimicrosomal antibodies'). The IIFM test uses unfixed and air-dried human or monkey cryostat tissue sections as substrate. Positive sera stain the cytoplasm of thyroid follicular epithelial cells but do not stain their nuclei (Fig. 52–9A). Anti-TPO must be differentiated from AMA when coarse granular cytoplasmic staining is noted; testing sera on mouse stomach/kidney tissue block can do this.

Anti-TPO can be detected in sera from patients with either Graves disease or Hashimoto's thyroiditis, and its presence and titer correlate strongly with active clinical disease (Burek, 1995). There is some controversy among investigators about whether determination of anti-TPO alone is sufficient to reliably detect autoimmune thyroid disease (Nordyke, 1993;

VI

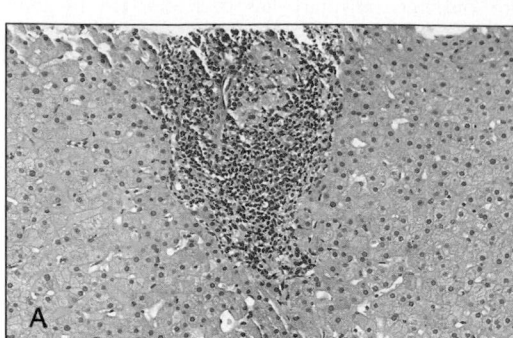
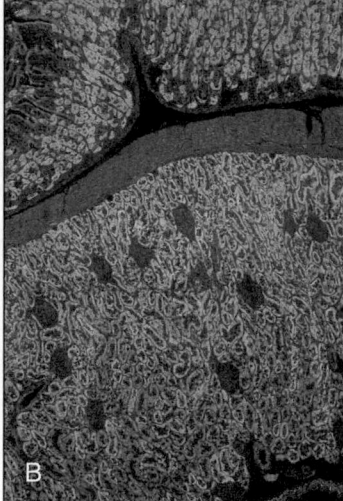
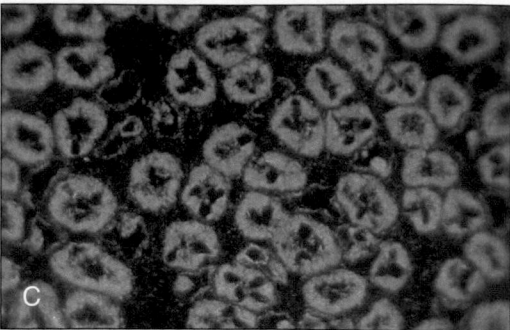

Figure 52–7 Liver biopsy in primary biliary cirrhosis shows variable portal inflammation with nonsuppurative lymphocytic cholangitis and in this example a florid duct lesion with granulomatous inflammation centered on an interlobular bile duct (A, H&E, ×200). IIFM reveals diffuse immunofluorescence of renal tubules, including distal tubules (B, ×200) that has a homogeneous cytoplasmic appearance at higher power (C, ×500).

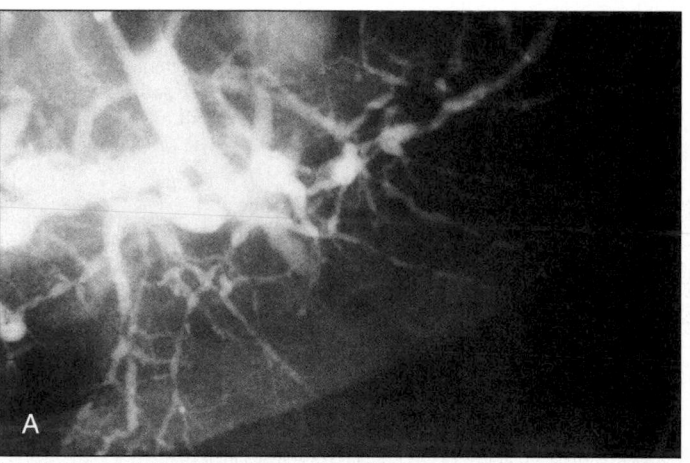
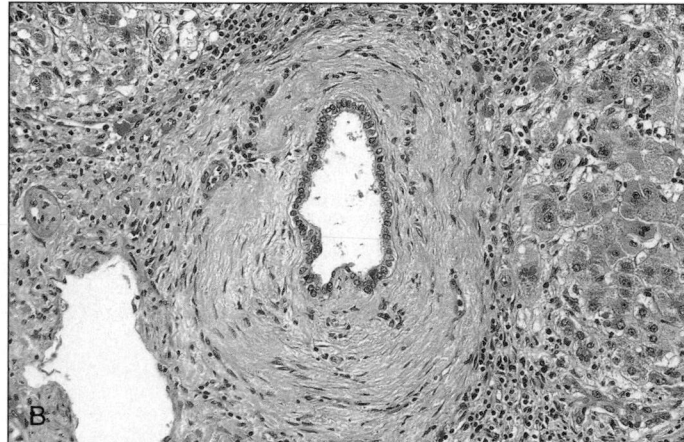

Figure 52–8 Cholangiogram in primary sclerosing cholangitis reveals the characteristic beading pattern of bile ducts due to multifocal strictures at those sites (A). Liver biopsy reveals prominent periduct fibrosis in the characteristic 'onion-skin' pattern (B, H&E, ×500).

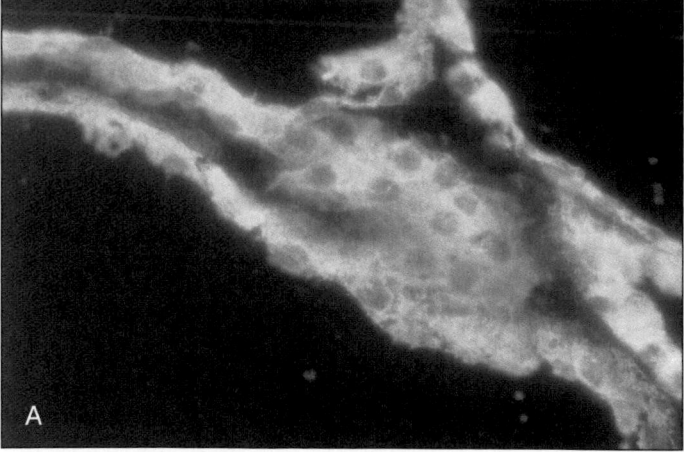
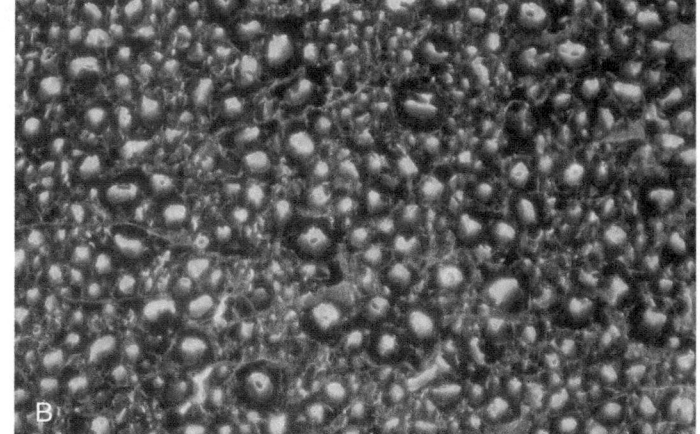

Figure 52–9 Indirect immunofluorescence microscopy of thyroid microsomal autoantibodies using unfixed monkey thyroid tissue as substrate (A, ×400) and of thyroglobulin autoantibodies using methanol-fixed cryostat tissue sections of monkey thyroid gland (B, ×200).

Kaplan, 1999). The pathogenic role of anti-TPO remains unclear (Naparstek, 1993).

Anti-Thyroglobulin Autoantibodies

Anti-Tg is targeted against thyroglobulin, which is the storage form of thyroid hormones within thyroid gland follicles (Burek, 1995). Several methods are available for measuring anti-Tg, including quantitative passive hemagglutination, IIFM, and ELISA.

Quantitative passive hemagglutination with either chromic chloride hemagglutination or tanned red blood cells is the most widely used and sensitive method for detecting anti-Tg (Burek, 1995). Anti-Tg detected by hemagglutination is identified in titers greater than 1:1000 in about 80% of patients with Hashimoto's thyroiditis (Burek, 1995). Patients with Graves disease (60%) or thyroid carcinoma (30%), or other autoimmune disorders such as pernicious anemia or Sjögren syndrome, and 3–18% of apparently normal individuals, may also have anti-Tg, but their hemagglutination titers are usually (>90%) less than 1:1000 (Burek, 1995).

To locate anti-Tg, IIFM is done using methanol-fixed cryostat tissue sections of monkey thyroid gland (Fig. 52–9B). Fixation is required to prevent loss of thyroglobulin during washing steps. Three patterns of immunofluorescence are described when anti-Tg is present (Burek, 1995): (1) floccular pattern, (2) dull colloid spaces but bright peripheral fluorescence, and (3) diffuse, bright, uniformly staining colloid in a 'ground-glass' pattern attributed to the anti-Tg reaction with CA2. (Burek, 1995). CA2, or so-called second colloid antigen, is detected as the only serologic marker of autoimmune thyroiditis in the 5–8% of patients who are positive by IIFM but negative for anti-Tg and anti-TPO using other methods (Bigazzi, 1992).

Anti-Thyroid-Stimulating Hormone Receptor Autoantibodies

Anti-TSHR autoantibodies consist of two groups of autoantibodies that can either stimulate or block TSHRs causing, respectively, hyperthyroidism or hypothyroidism. Anti-TSHR autoantibodies that bind to these receptors and stimulate thyroid hormone production are referred to as thyroid-stimulating immunoglobulins (TSIs), whereas anti-TSHR autoantibodies that bind to receptors and block the binding and function of TSH are referred to as thyroid-binding inhibitory immunoglobulins (TBIIs) (Mooij, 1993; Brunt, 1995). TSIs probably cause the hyperthyroidism in Graves disease (Wilkin, 1990; Bigazzi, 1992; Brunt, 1995). Their prevalence varies from 55% to 95%, depending on the method of detection (Bigazzi, 1992; Brunt, 1995). TSIs, which are usually of the IgG class, stimulate production of thyroid hormones by activating the adenylate cyclase system after binding to TSHRs (Patrick, 1993).

Detection of anti-TSHR is complex and is not part of routine clinical testing. The test may be useful for confirming Graves disease in hyperthyroid patients with equivocal results in routine laboratory studies (Bigazzi, 1992). Additionally, one of the anti-TSHR assays may be used to monitor patients' hormone replacement therapy or to diagnose neonatal thyrotoxicosis (Bigazzi, 1992).

There are two main classes of assays for anti-TSHRs, namely, bioassays and binding assays; their methodologic aspects are reviewed elsewhere (Bigazzi, 1992; Patrick, 1993; Gupta, 1988). Newer assays of a patient's serum based on stimulation of cyclic adenosine monophosphate (cAMP) in rat thyroid cells, maintained in tissue culture, may prove to be an improvement over the technically difficult bioassays (Burek, 1995).

TSIs are measured in bioassays that determine increased TSHR-mediated activity either by measuring the release of cAMP or by measuring the uptake of iodide by thyroid cells maintained in culture (Brunt, 1995). TBIIs are measured either by determining binding inhibition of radiolabeled TSH to its receptor or by using cAMP bioassays (Brunt, 1995).

Kidney

Glomerulonephritis

Glomerulonephritis is a major cause of primary renal disease. Immune-mediated mechanisms are thought to have an important role in the pathogenesis of glomerulonephritis, although experimental confirmation of such putative autoimmune mechanisms is still lacking.

DIFM has an important role in the study and diagnosis of glomerulonephritis (Fig. 52–10). The patterns of immune reactants can be divided broadly into those that cause either granular or linear deposits within glomeruli or other kidney structures examined with DIFM. Granular deposits have been attributed to immune complexes (ICs) that settle out of circulating blood or form in situ (McCluskey, 1995). DIFM patterns of immune deposits associated with major glomerular diseases are summarized in Table 52–5. Thorough reviews of these disorders are available in several texts (Heptinstall, 1992; McCluskey, 1995). However, for this discussion, only antiglomerular basement membrane (anti-GBM) autoantibodies are presented in some additional detail.

Antiglomerular Basement Membrane Disease

Patients with anti-GBM disease vary in clinical presentation in that about 50% have renal-limited disease and the other 50% have both renal and pulmonary symptoms. This latter presentation is often called Goodpasture syndrome. Rarely, patients with anti-GBM disease may have pulmonary-limited disease (Wilson, 1987).

Diagnosis of anti-GBM disease requires detection of anti-GBM auto-antibodies to the NC1 domain of type IV collagen (McCluskey, 1995), the

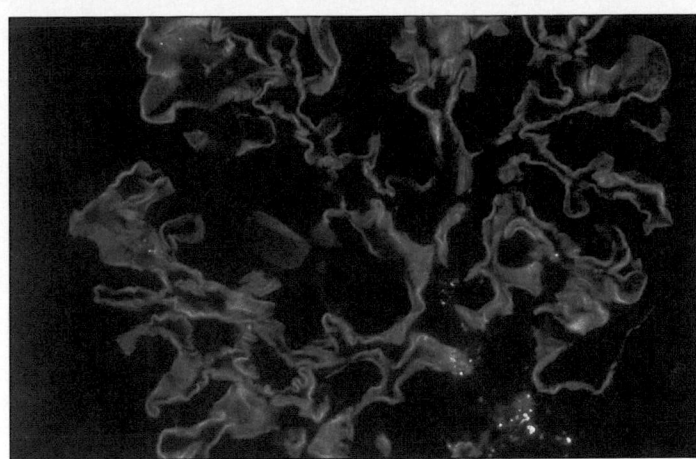

Figure 52–10 Direct immunofluorescence microscopy reveals global and linear glomerular basement membrane immunofluorescence in antiglomerular basement membrane disease (×400).

Table 52–5 Major Glomerular Diseases with Direct Immunofluorescent Findings

Immunofluorescent Pattern and Disease	Immune Reactant(s)
Granular, Mesangial and GBM Deposits	
Acute poststreptococcal glomerulonephritis	Scattered C3 ± IgG, IgM
Diffuse proliferative lupus nephritis	IgG, IgA, IgM, C3
Membranoproliferative glomerulonephritis (MPGN, type I)	C3, IgG, IgM
Idiopathic immune complex crescentic glomerulonephritis	IgG, C3 ± IgM
Dense deposit disease (MPGN, type II)	C3 (globular) ± IgM
Chronic infections (e.g., bacterial endocarditis)	IgG, IgM, C3
Granular, Mesangial Predominant	
Lupus nephritis	
Mesangial	IgG, C3; usually IgM and IgA
Focal proliferative	IgG, C3, IgA; focal capillary loop deposits
Henoch–Schönlein purpura	IgA predominant; IgG, IgM, C3
IgA Nephropathy	IgA predominant; often IgG, IgM, C3
Granular, GBM Predominant	
Membranous lupus nephritis	IgG, C3, IgA, IgM
Mixed cryoglobulinemia	IgM, IgG, C3; intravascular masses
Linear GBM	
Anti-GBM nephritis	IgG, C3; IgA and IgM infrequent
Light chain nephropathy	Usually κ light chain, may be in TBM, blood vessels, interstitium

GBM = glomerular basement membrane; TBM = tubular basement membrane.

Modified from McCluskey RT, Collins AB, Niles JL: Kidney. In Colvin RB, Bhan AK, McCluskey RT (eds): Diagnostic Immunopathology, 2nd ed. New York, Raven Press, 1995, p 109.

VI

so-called Goodpasture's antigen. Methods for detecting circulating anti-GBM have included IIFM, ELISA, and radioimmunoassay (RIA) (Wilson, 1987; McCluskey, 1995); some investigators have additionally developed a sensitive Western blot test (McCluskey, 1995). Because IIFM is difficult to standardize and requires experience to perform, methods for detection have focused instead on validation of quantitative RIA or ELISA. Currently, a licensed commercial ELISA kit is available for the measurement of anti-GBM. This assay determines patient values from a standard curve and reports negative, borderline, or positive ranges. Most patients with active anti-GBM disease appear to have values greater than 100 units. Although borderline values can be seen in both active and quiescent anti-GBM disease, we have also seen such values in patients with renal disorders that are not anti-GBM disease.

The coexistence of antineutrophil cytoplasmic antibodies (ANCA) has been documented in some patients with rapidly progressive glomerulonephritis (McCluskey, 1995). The coexistence of these two autoantibodies has varied from 0–40% of patients with rapidly progressive glomerulonephritis, accompanied by some evidence that the presence of ANCA in patients with anti-GBM disease affords a better renal prognosis (McCluskey, 1995).

Adrenal Gland

Addison's Disease

Nontuberculous chronic adrenocortical insufficiency, or Addison's disease, has an estimated prevalence of 3–6 cases per 100 000 people (Muir, 1993). 65–70% of such patients have circulating autoantibodies to adrenal cortex cells, demonstrable using IIFM on frozen sections of human adrenal cortex (Muir, 1993; Patrick, 1993; Burek, 1995). 21-Hydroxylase and 17α-hydroxylase are two autoantigens that have been identified as reactive with adrenocortical autoantibodies (Song, 1994; Devendra, 2004). Adrenocortical autoantibodies are not found in Addison's disease caused by tuberculosis or other exogenous agents (Patrick, 1993). Importantly, about 45% of asymptomatic individuals with serum adrenocortical autoantibodies develop impaired adrenocortical function within 2.5 years after the autoantibody is identified (Muir, 1991).

Addison's disease associated with autoantibodies is most commonly diagnosed in persons between the ages of 20 and 50 years and is two to three times more frequent in females when diagnosed after the age of 30 (Muir, 1993; Patrick, 1993).

Laboratory tests show metabolic acidosis, hyperkalemia, hyponatremia, and low levels of serum chloride and bicarbonate. Plasma cortisol levels are also low and adrenocorticotropic hormone levels are elevated (VanArsdel, 1993). Consequently, therapy consists of replacing glucocorticoids and mineralocorticoids (Patrick, 1993).

Addison's disease associated with autoantibodies can occur by itself but is more commonly accompanied by other autoimmune disorders as part of an autoimmune polyglandular syndrome (Muir, 1993). These companion diseases may include autoimmune thyroiditis, pernicious anemia, or insulin-dependent diabetes mellitus (Patrick, 1993).

In addition to adrenocortical autoantibodies, other adrenal autoantibodies have been detected in patients with Addison's disease, including steroid cell autoantibodies and autoantibodies that bind adrenocorticotropic hormone receptors (Muir, 1993).

Pancreas

Diabetes Mellitus

Diabetes mellitus (see Ch. 16) is the diagnostic term applied to a group of metabolic disorders that share hyperglycemia as their common link (Eisenbarth, 1995). That it is a serious diagnosis is documented by the fact that acute and chronic multiorgan diabetic complications account for about 15% of total US health care expenditures. However, significant progress has been made in the care of diabetic patients with the knowledge that aggressive blood glucose control reduces the risk for development of and progression to vascular complications.

Clinical Subtypes

The major clinical subgroups of diabetes mellitus are: type 1A for immune-mediated diabetes; type 1B for non-immune-mediated diabetes with severe insulin deficiency; and, a subgroup of adults with type 2 diabetes with anti-islet autoantibodies that is termed latent autoimmune diabetes mellitus (American Diabetes Association, 1997; Devendra, 2004). Type 2 diabetes mellitus was formerly termed non-insulin-dependent diabetes and most commonly occurs in obese individuals older than 30 years.

The major types of circulating autoantibody in type 1A diabetes mellitus are the following: islet cell autoantibodies (ICAs); glutamic acid decarboxylase autoantibodies (anti-GAD); insulin autoantibodies (IAAs); and insulinoma associated-2 and -2-β autoantibodies (Lan, 1996; Schmidli, 1998; Devendra, 2004).

Islet Cell Autoantibodies

IIFM is the classical method used for detection of ICAs (Atkinson, 1993b). Frozen sections of human pancreas are used as the tissue substrate to

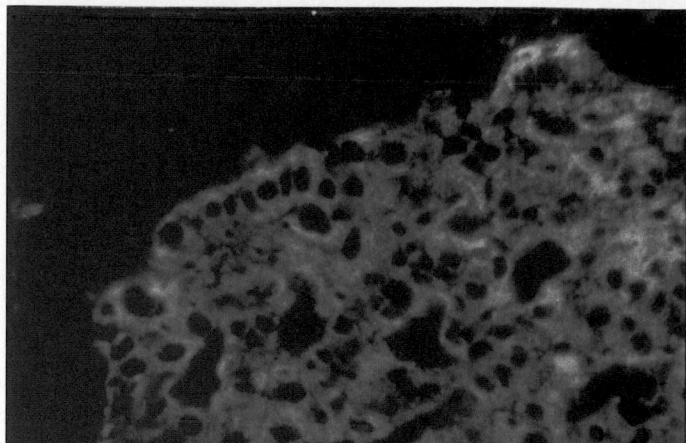

Figure 52–11 Indirect immunofluorescence microscopy of islet cell autoantibodies using human blood group O pancreas as substrate (×400).

detect specific, finely granular, cytoplasmic fluorescence in all cells of pancreatic islets (Fig. 52–11). Human blood group O is recommended as substrate to reduce nonspecific background interference due to ABO isohemagglutinins. Using IIFM, ICAs are detectable in about 80% of patients with newly diagnosed type 1A diabetes, 3–4% of nondiabetic relatives of patients with type 1A diabetes, and only 0.5% of clinically normal subjects (Atkinson, 1994). ICAs include autoantibodies specifically reactive with anti-GAD as well as non-GAD-reactive ICAs (Kaufman, 1992; Atkinson, 1993).

ICA should be titered in Juvenile Diabetes Foundation (JDF) units in reference to an 80 unit standard serum from the Immunology of Diabetes Workshop; titers greater than 20 JDF units seem to have prognostic significance (Maclaren, 1992). Commercial ICA assays using primate substrate are available.

Insulin Autoantibodies

Insulin autoantibodies (IAAs) are identified in about 50% of patients with type 1A diabetes at the time of diagnosis and before insulin therapy begins (Atkinson, 1994). IAAs are usually measured using a technically demanding competitive radioimmunoprecipitation assay. This assay cannot distinguish between IAAs occurring spontaneously and those that occur as a result of insulin therapy. Therefore, IAAs need to be measured before insulin is administered.

Glutamic Acid Decarboxylase Autoantibodies

Anti-GAD are detected in most newly diagnosed type 1A diabetes patients and in about 80% of prediabetic, first-degree relatives of patients (Hagopian, 1993; Schatz, 1995). The two GAD autoantigens, classified by molecular mass, are designated GAD65 and GAD67 (Atkinson, 1993a). Anti-GAD are directed primarily at the GAD65 isoform, which is found mainly in pancreatic islets and in the central nervous system (CNS), where it functions as an enzyme responsible for formation of the inhibiting neurotransmitter γ-aminobutyric acid (Maclaren, 1988; Barmeier, 1992; Kaufman, 1992; Luhder, 1994). The GAD67 form predominates in peripheral nerves (Atkinson, 1993; Falorni, 1994).

GADAs are also associated with the rare stiff man syndrome (Eisenbarth, 1995). Interestingly, a high percentage of these patients have type 1A diabetes.

Interpretation and Clinical Utility of Autoantibodies in Type 1A Diabetes

ICA, anti-GAD, IAA, and IA-2 autoantibodies are used currently as predictive markers for diabetes. ICA is a specific marker associated with an elevated risk of developing type 1A diabetes, but ICAs do not persist. Anti-GAD is usually detected before the diagnosis of diabetes and usually declines in titer after the onset of clinical diabetes (Schatz, 1994). Initial screening for autoantibodies associated with type 1A diabetes has been limited to ICA and IAA (Devendra, 2004).

Identification of islet autoantibodies can be used to confirm autoimmunity in patients with acute diabetes, which differentiates type 1A from type 1B diabetes. The use of these markers to identify individuals at risk for type 1A is being evaluated to determine the need for metabolic studies that would assess subclinical glucose intolerance and call for immunotherapy in the preclinical phase of diabetes (Maclaren, 1992). Measurement of anti-GAD using ELISA may eventually improve the feasibility of widespread screening for this autoantibody.

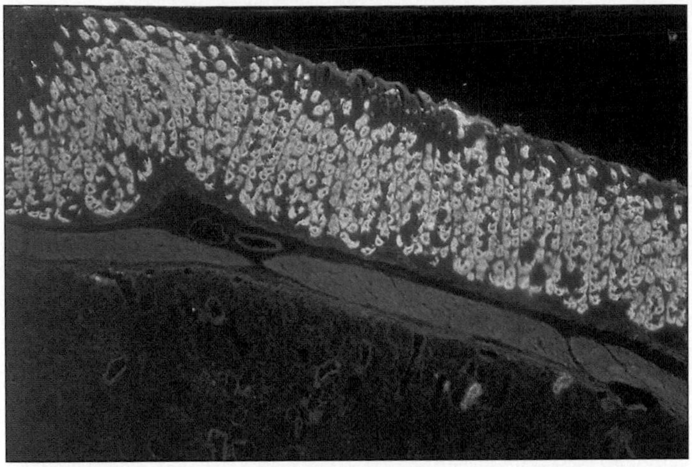

Figure 52–12 Indirect immunofluorescence microscopy of gastric antiparietal cell autoantibodies using mouse stomach/kidney as substrate (×400).

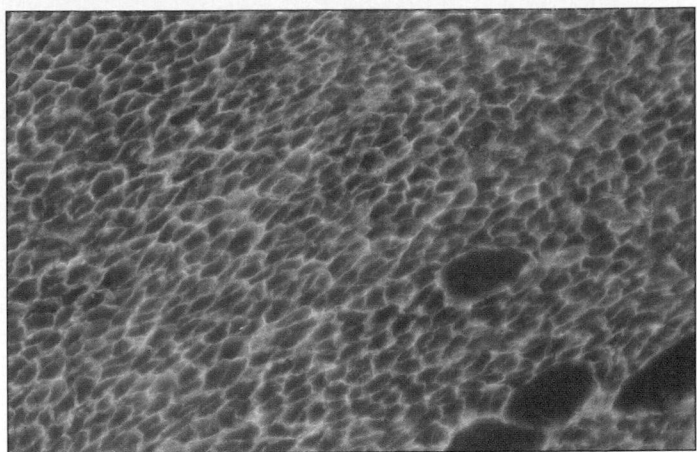

Figure 52–13 Indirect immunofluorescence microscopy of IgA endomysial autoantibodies using monkey esophagus as substrate (×400).

In addition to the autoantibodies discussed above, patients with diabetes also may have anti-TPO, antiparietal cell, and antiadrenocortical autoantibodies, so diabetes patients should be screened for these autoantibodies at least once (Maclaren, 1992).

Gastrointestinal Tract

Pernicious Anemia

Pernicious anemia is characterized by histamine-fast achlorhydria, hypergastrinemia, and vitamin B_{12} deficiency (Brown, 1995). The insidious onset of neurologic symptoms and development of megaloblastic anemia are typical features of the clinical course (Patrick, 1993). Morphologically, biopsy of the stomach body mucosa contains evidence of chronic atrophic gastritis.

Pernicious anemia is associated with circulating antiparietal cell (APC) autoantibodies in 90% of patients and to intrinsic factor (anti-IF) in 60–75% of patients, although anti-IF may be more specific for pernicious anemia (Brown, 1995; Burek, 1995). APCs are detected by IIFM performed on mouse stomach/kidney tissue blocks. This combined tissue block allows identification of specific parietal cell staining when there is no concomitant staining of renal tubules as would be seen in the presence of AMAs (Fig. 52–12).

Anti-IF is most commonly detected by RIA. Of the two known types of anti-IF, type 1 anti-IF, or blocking autoantibody, prevents the binding of IF to vitamin B_{12}, and type 2, or binding autoantibody, reacts with free or complexed vitamin B_{12} to inhibit the action of IF (Patrick, 1993; Karen, 1994). Type 1 anti-IF is considered more diagnostically sensitive and specific for pernicious anemia (Karen, 1994). However, identification of either APCs or anti-IF is not required for diagnosis of pernicious anemia. Pernicious anemia can occur in association with other autoimmune diseases, such as autoimmune thyroiditis or Addison's disease, and may be a part of either autoimmune polyglandular syndrome 1 or autoimmune polyglandular syndrome 2 (Patrick, 1993).

Gluten-Sensitive Enteropathy

Gluten-sensitive enteropathy (GSE), or celiac sprue, is a small-bowel disease characterized by malabsorption of gastrointestinal fat. Until recently, GSE was considered to be a rare disease in the United States but now the prevalence is considered much greater than previously estimated, affecting about 1% of the US population (Ferguson, 1997; NIH Consensus, 2004; Rostom, 2004). Patients may have nongastrointestinal manifestations that dominate the clinical presentation, such as anemia, neurological symptoms, and autoimmune diseases (Green, 2003). Hypersensitivity to gluten, or gluten derivatives, is the cause of GSE (Brown, 1995). Small-bowel biopsy from a patient with GSE is variably abnormal but characteristic changes include villous atrophy, crypt elongation, intraepithelial lymphocytes, and crypt mitoses.

Patients with GSE manifest several humoral immune alterations. Interestingly, serum IgA levels are usually elevated in GSE patients except those with an IgA deficiency, which does occur in GSE patients more commonly than in normal individuals (Brown, 1995). Patients with GSE may have circulating IgA antiendomysial, antireticulin, and/or antigliadin autoantibodies. IgA antiendomysial autoantibodies are detectable by IIFM using monkey esophagus as tissue substrate (Fig. 52–13). IgA antiendomysial autoantibodies detect tissue transglutaminase (tTG), the primary autoantigen in GSE (Dieterich, 1997). ELISA is now available for the detection of anti-tissue transglutaminase (anti-tTG). Their identification is considered diagnostically sensitive and specific for GSE alone or GSE associated with dermatitis herpetiformis (GSE-DH) (Talal, 1997). Measuring the titer of IgA antiendomysial autoantibody may be used to monitor a patient's compliance with a gluten-free diet (Karen, 1994).

Antireticulin autoantibodies are detected by IIFM on a mouse stomach/kidney combined tissue block. These autoantibodies are detectable in adults (40%) as well as children (60%) with GSE and also in adults with GSE-DH (20%). However, antireticulin autoantibodies are diagnostically nonspecific and are generally no longer considered to be useful in the diagnosis of GSE, being present also in patients with Crohn's disease, myasthenia gravis, Sjögren syndrome, and other connective tissue disorders.

Antigliadin autoantibodies are detected by ELISA in almost all patients with GSE or GSE-DH (Brown, 1995). The target antigen, gliadin, is purified from gluten and used in a solid-phase ELISA to detect these autoantibodies. Like IgA endomysial autoantibodies, antigliadin autoantibodies can be used to monitor a patient's adherence to a gluten-free diet. Antigliadin antibodies are less specific than anti-tTG and anti-endomysial antibodies.

A patient suspected of having GSE should be tested while on a normal gluten-containing diet. In suspected patients without chronic liver disease, the presence of anti-tTG and/or IgA anti-endomysial antibodies in the appropriate clinical setting is supportive of GSE. However, most clinicians consider histologic confirmation on small-bowel biopsy to be necessary to establish the diagnosis. Negative serology does not exclude a diagnosis of GSE and IgA deficiency should be considered in patients with a suggestive clinical presentation. If IgA deficiency is identified, an IgG-tTg or IgG anti-endomysial antibody test should be performed (NIH Consensus, 2004).

Compliance with a gluten-restricted diet can be monitored by anti-tTG, IgA anti-endomysial, or gliadin levels.

Ulcerative Colitis and Crohn's Disease

A wide variety of inflammatory conditions affect the gastrointestinal tract. Ulcerative colitis and Crohn's disease are the two most common disorders within the group of idiopathic inflammatory bowel diseases. In recent years, several serologic markers have become useful in the evaluation of patients with inflammatory bowel disease. These markers include p-ANCA, antibodies to Saccharomyces cerevisiae (ASCA), antipancreatic antibody, OmpC antibody, I-2 antibody, and antibodies to anaerobic coccoid rods (Nakamura, 2003).

The majority of adult patients with ulcerative colitis (60–80%) have detectable p-ANCA that is sensitive to DNase, which helps differentiate p-ANCA in inflammatory bowel disease from p-ANCA in other disorders such as autoimmune hepatitis and primary sclerosing cholangitis (Nakamura, 2003). 10–30% of patients with Crohn's disease may also have p-ANCA and this subgroup may have colon involvement that mimics the clinical presentation of ulcerative colitis.

ASCA is expressed in up to 70% of patients with Crohn's disease and appears to be highly specific (Vasiliauskas, 2000). The antibodies are directed against oligomannosidic epitopes on Saccharomyces cerevisiae (Nakamura, 2003). ELISA is available for detection of ASCA.

VI

For specificity reasons, the use of these tests should be limited to patients with colitis and should not be applied to the general population.

Nervous System

Myasthenia Gravis

Myasthenia gravis is a neuromuscular disorder characterized by use-associated muscular weakness, fatigue, and the presence of antiacetylcholine receptor (anti-AChR) autoantibodies. AChRs, located in postsynaptic membranes of skeletal muscle fibers, bind acetylcholine (ACh) from nerve endings, which causes a muscle contraction when enough ACh has been released (Naparstek, 1993; Rose, 1995). Anti-AChR autoantibodies interfere with this neuromuscular function, resulting in muscle weakness and fatigue.

Anti-AChR autoantibodies are detected in about 90% of myasthenia gravis patients (Rose, 1995). Radiolabeled α-bungarotoxin (α-BTx) is used in competitive RIAs to measure different forms of anti-AchR (Barna, 1995). α-BTx is a protein from snake venom that essentially irreversibly binds AChR, but it binds to ACh receptors at a site different from binding sites for anti-AchR (Rose, 1995). AChRs are obtained from extracts of denervated human skeletal muscle, such as from diabetic amputations, or from tissue cell culture. For testing, the AChRs are labeled with α-BTx then incubated with patients' serum to allow any anti-AChR autoantibodies present to bind to AChRs at sites near the α-BTx binding site. After incubation, the radiolabeled complexes are precipitated by polyvalent antihuman immunoglobulin, and the washed precipitate is counted for radioactivity, after correction for nonspecific binding. The degree of radioactivity in the precipitate is directly proportional to the amount of anti-AChR in the patient's serum.

Modifications of this binding assay can be used to identify anti-AChR blocking and modulating autoantibodies. In a blocking assay, patients' sera containing anti-AChR is allowed to incubate with AChRs before addition of α-BTx. The basis for this technique is the premise that anti-AChR capable of blocking α-BTx binding also blocks ACh binding to AChRs (Rose, 1995). The amount of radioactivity in the precipitate is, therefore, inversely proportional to the amount of anti-AChR in patient's sera.

Modulating anti-AChR autoantibodies are thought to accelerate AChR degradation, but their measurement in the clinical laboratory is technically difficult and not widely performed.

Multiple Sclerosis

Multiple sclerosis is a relatively common demyelinating disease involving the white matter of the brain and spinal cord. It occurs more frequently in females than males (2:1 ratio) and is usually evident during young adulthood, with a wide variety of possible clinical manifestations. About 50% of these patients undergo alternating periods of active disease and remissions, whereas the remainder follow a chronic progressive course (Steinman, 1993; McFarland, 1995). The diagnosis of multiple sclerosis derives from clinical findings and exclusion of all other disorders.

Although the cause of multiple sclerosis is unknown, autoimmune mechanisms are considered important in the pathogenesis of this disease (McFarland, 1995). There are not, however, any characteristic circulating autoantibodies in multiple sclerosis that are accepted as diagnostic enough for routine measurement in clinical laboratories.

However, laboratory examination of cerebrospinal fluid (CSF) does provide important information that supports a diagnosis of multiple sclerosis in an appropriate clinical setting (Barna, 1987). Synthesis of IgG increases abnormally within the CNS of multiple sclerosis patients, so that measurement of the IgG index and IgG synthetic rate provides useful, but not specific, test results (Valenzuela, 1987; Zweiman, 1991; Karen, 1994; McFarland, 1995). Evaluation of CSF for oligoclonal bands is also useful in the appropriate clinical setting, since they are identified in greater than 90% of multiple sclerosis patients; however, their presence is not diagnostically specific, since they can be detected in patients with such diverse disorders as neurosyphilis, CNS vasculitis, Lyme disease, subacute sclerosing panencephalitis, Creutzfeldt–Jakob disease, stroke, Guillain–Barré syndrome, and neoplasms (Karen, 1994). Serum protein electrophoresis must also be performed to ensure that CSF oligoclonal bands are not from serum leakage into the CSF. CSF oligoclonal bands are usually measured by high-resolution agarose electrophoresis of concentrated CSF (Karen, 1994).

Neuropathies

The focus of much recent attention is a group of neurologic syndromes affecting either the CNS or peripheral nervous system and associated with autoantibodies (Naparstek, 1993). These autoantibodies are detected either by ELISA, IIFM, or immunohistochemistry. The importance of identifying such autoantibodies will undoubtedly increase as/if clinical studies correlate their presence with either a particular disease or a therapeutic benefit. However, to date, these autoantibodies are not disease-specific and can even occur after trauma to the nervous system. Autoantibodies to primary neural components include those to neuronal proteins or to neuronal gangliosides (Zeballos, 1992; Darnell, 2003).

Neuronal Protein Autoantibodies

A subgroup of patients with paraneoplastic cerebellar degeneration has anti-Yo autoantibodies that are usually detected about the time a malignant neoplasm is discovered. Anti-Yo are detectable as cytoplasmic Purkinje cell fluorescence by using IIFM on human cerebellar tissue. Identification of anti-Yo in a patient with no known malignancy should initiate careful evaluation for a malignant neoplasm (Zeballos, 1992).

Anti-Ri are neuron-specific autoantibodies whose identification appears limited to patients with breast carcinoma and paraneoplastic opsoclonus (Zeballos, 1992). Anti-Ri are characterized by fluorescence of neuronal nuclei on IIFM.

Anti-Hu are also neuron-specific autoantibodies visible as neuronal nuclear fluorescence on IIFM. These autoantibodies may be identified in patients with small cell lung carcinoma and paraneoplastic encephalomyelitis (Zeballos, 1992).

Neuronal Ganglioside Autoantibodies

Gangliosides are glycolipid components found in the outer membranes of peripheral nerve cells (Naparstek, 1993). Peripheral motor neuropathies may occur in patients with IgM monoclonal gammopathies whose IgM paraprotein reacts with the gangliosides GM_1 or GD_{1b} (Zeballos, 1992). Although anti-GM_1 or anti-GD_{1b} can be identified in a wide variety of neurologic syndromes, their presence in high titers is more characteristic of motor neuron disease than other alternatives (Zeballos, 1992).

Other Organs

Heart

Myocardial Autoantibodies

Autoantibodies to the myocardium have been reported as a part of several conditions that damage cardiac striated muscle, including myocardial infarction, following cardiac surgery, and cardiomyopathies, although their identification may help differentiate immune-mediated cardiomyopathy from other causes of myocarditis (Naparstek, 1993; Burek, 1995). IIFM on frozen sections of monkey heart is used to detect myocardial autoantibodies. Specific myocardial staining can also be determined by excluding reactivity on noncardiac skeletal muscle. Unfortunately, AMA and/or heterophile autoantibodies can cause fluorescent staining that may be confused with that caused by myocardial autoantibodies.

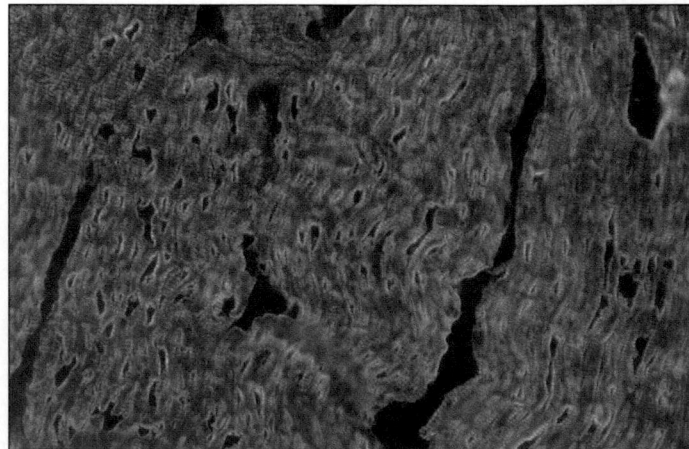

Figure 52–14 Indirect immunofluorescence microscopy of skeletal muscle autoantibodies on frozen sections of monkey thigh skeletal muscle (×400).

Muscle

Skeletal Muscle Autoantibodies

Skeletal muscle autoantibodies have limited clinical applicability. Low titers (<1:30) may be seen in apparently healthy individuals, whereas some patients with myopathic disorders may have titers up to 1:60. Although high titers (>1:60) of skeletal muscle autoantibodies have been found in patients with myasthenia gravis, anti-AChR assays have greater clinical utility in diagnosing or monitoring myasthenia gravis. Skeletal muscle autoantibodies are detected by IIFM on frozen sections of monkey thigh skeletal muscle (Fig. 52–14).

Summary

Autoantibodies have an important role in the study of patients with organ-specific autoimmune disease. Detection of these autoantibodies may be important in diagnosis of some organ-specific autoimmune diseases, such as Graves disease, but more often they are supportive rather than essential for diagnosis. Similarly, although some of these autoantibodies are directly involved in pathogenesis of a disease – pemphigus, for example – their presence is often a marker of underlying immunologic injury attributable to another disease mechanism, as is the case in type 1A diabetes mellitus. Newer techniques in molecular biology have disclosed, and will continue to disclose, the specific nature of many antigens targeted by these autoantibodies. It is hoped that this work will elucidate underlying disease mechanisms, allowing improved diagnostic tests and perhaps new directions in therapy. Technical advances in ELISA have made this technology available in most clinical laboratories so that many assays for organ-specific autoantibodies are more widely available where IIFM is not feasible.

References

American Diabetes Association: Report of the Expert Committee on the Diagnosis and Classification of Diabetes Mellitus. Diabetes Care 1997; 20:1183–1197.

Atkinson MA, Kaufman D, Newman D, et al: Islet cell cytoplasmic autoantibody reactivity to glutamate decarboxylase in insulin-dependent diabetes. J Clin Invest 1993a; 91:350–356.

Atkinson MA, Maclaren NK: Islet cell autoantigens in insulin-dependent diabetes. J Clin Invest 1993b; 92:1608–1616.

Atkinson MA, Maclaren NK: The pathogenesis of insulin-dependent diabetes mellitus. N Engl J Med 1994; 331:1428–436.

Bansi DS, Fleming KA, Chapman RW: Importance of antineutrophil cytoplasmic antibodies in primary sclerosing cholangitis and ulcerative colitis: prevalence, titre, and IgG subclass. Gut 1996; 38:384–389.

Barmeier H, Ahlmeen J, Landin-Olsson M, et al: Quantitative analysis of islet glutamic acid decarboxylase p64 autoantibodies in insulin-dependent diabetes mellitus. Autoimmunity 1992; 13:187–196.

Barna BP, Gupta MK: Laboratory analyses of blood. In Barna BP (ed.): Laboratory Handbook of Neuroimmunologic Disease. Chicago, IL, ASCP Press, 1995, p 106.

Barna BP, Valenzuela R, Gupta MK: Laboratory analyses of cerebrospinal fluid. In Barna BP (ed.): Laboratory Handbook of Neuroimmunologic Disease. Chicago, IL, ASCP Press, 1995, p 65.

Batts KP, Ludwig J: Histopathology of autoimmune chronic active hepatitis, primary biliary cirrhosis, and primary sclerosing cholangitis. In Krawitt EL, Wiesner RH (eds): Autoimmune Liver Disease. New York, Raven Press, 1991, pp 75–92.

Becker BA, Gaspari AA: Pemphigus vulgaris and vegetans. In Dermatologic Clinics, Vol II. Philadelphia, PA, WB Saunders, 1993, pp 429–452.

Bigazzi PE, Burek CL, Rose NR: Antibodies to tissue-specific endocrine, gastrointestinal, and surface receptor antigens. In Rose NR, de Macario EC, Fahey JL, et al (eds): Manual of Clinical Laboratory Immunology, 4th ed. Washington, DC, American Society for Microbiology, 1992, p 765.

Bouldin MB, Clowers-Webb HE, Davis JL, et al: Naproxen-associated linear IgA bullous dermatosis: case report and review. Mayo Clin Proc 2000; 75:967–970.

Brown WR, Claman HN, Strober W: Immunologic diseases of the gastrointestinal tract. In Frank MM, Austen KF, Claman HN, et al (eds): Samter's Immunologic Diseases, 5th ed. Boston, MA, Little, Brown & Co, 1995, vol II, p 1151.

Brunt LM: Immunologic disorders of the thyroid gland and autoimmune polyendocrinopathies. In Frank MM, Austen KF, Claman HN, et al (eds): Samter's Immunologic Diseases, 5th ed. Boston, MA, Little, Brown & Co, 1995, vol II, p 975.

Burek CL, Rose NR: Autoantibodies. In Colvin RB, Bhan AK, McCluskey RT (eds): Diagnostic Immunopathology, 2nd ed. New York, Raven Press, 1995, pp 207–230.

Bylund DJ, McHutchison J, Nakamura RM: Antimitochondrial antibodies in primary biliary cirrhosis. Clin Immunol Newsletter 1992; 12:1–5.

Camisa C, Helm TN: Paraneoplastic pemphigus is a distinct neoplasia-induced autoimmune disease. Arch Dermatol 1993; 129:883–886.

Crosby DL, Diaz LA: Autoimmune diseases of the skin. In Altman LC (ed): Immunology and Allergy Clinics of North America: Autoimmune Diseases. Philadelphia, PA, WB Saunders, 1993, p 395.

Darnell RB, Posner JB: Paraneoplastic syndromes involving the nervous system. N Engl J Med 2003; 349:1543–1554.
An up-to-date and comprehensive review of paraneoplastic antibodies.

Devendra D, Yu L, Eisenbarth GS: Endocrine autoantibodies. Clin Lab Med 2004; 24:275–303.
State-of-the-art review of endocrine organ autoimmunity.

Dieterich W, Ehnis T, Bauer M, et al: Identification of tissue transglutaminase as the autoantigen of celiac disease. Nat Med 1997; 3:797–780.

Domloge-Hultsch N, Bisalbutra P, Gammon WR, et al: Direct immunofluorescence microscopy of 1 mol/L sodium chloride-treated patient skin. J Am Acad Dermatol 1991; 24:946–951.

Eisenbarth GS, Castano L: Diabetes mellitus. In Frank MM, Austen KF, Claman HN, et al (eds): Samter's Immunologic Diseases, 5th ed. Boston, MA, Little, Brown & Co, 1995, vol II, p 1007.

Elenitsas R, Jaworksy C, Murphy GF: Diagnostic methodology: immunofluorescence. In Murphy GF (ed.): Dermatopathology. A Practical Guide to Common Disorders. Philadelphia, PA, WB Saunders, 1995, pp 29–45.

Falorni A, Grubin CE, Takei I, et al: Radioimmunoassay detects the frequent occurrence of autoantibodies to the Mr 65,000 isoform of glutamic acid decarboxylase in Japanese insulin-dependent diabetes. Autoimmunity 1994; 19:113–125.

Ferguson A: Celiac disease, an eminently treatable condition, may be underdiagnosed in the United States. Am J Gastroenterol 1997; 92:1252–1254.

Fine J-D: Laboratory tests for epidermolysis bullosa. Dermatol Clin 1994; 12:123–132.

Flotte TJ, Margolis RJ, Mihm MC Jr: Skin. In Colvin RB, Bhan AK, McCluskey RT (eds): Diagnostic Immunopathology, 2nd ed. New York, Raven Press, 1995, p 123.

Gammon WR, Briggaman RA: Epidermolysis bullosa acquisita and bullous systemic lupus erythematosus. Diseases of autoimmunity to Type VII collagen. Dermatol Clin 1993; 11:535–547.

Gershwin ME, Ansari AA, Mackay IR, et al: Primary biliary cirrhosis: an orchestrated immune response against epithelial cells. Immunol Rev 2000; 172:210–225.

Goodman ZD, McNally PR, Davis DR, et al: Autoimmune cholangitis: a variant of primary biliary cirrhosis. Clinicopathologic and serologic correlations in 200 cases. Dig Dis Sci 1995; 40:1232–1242.

Gordon SC, Quattrociocchi-Longe TM, Khan BA, et al: Antibodies to carbonic anhydrase in patients with immune cholangiopathies. Gastroenterology 1995; 108:1802–1809.

Green PHR, Jabri B: Coeliac disease. Lancet 2003; 362:383–391.
Excellent review of celiac disease.

Gupta MK: Recent advances in laboratory tests for autoantibodies to thyrotropin receptor protein in Graves' disease. Clin Lab Med 1988; 8:303–323.

Gur H, Shen G, Sutjita M, et al: Autoantibody profile of primary sclerosing cholangitis. Pathobiology 1995; 63:76–82.

Hagopian WA, Karlsen AE, Gottsater A, et al: Quantitative assay using recombinant human islet glutamic acid decarboxylase (GAD65) shows that 64K autoantibody positivity at onset predicts diabetes type. J Clin Invest 1993; 91:368–374.

Helm KF, Peters MS: Deposition of membrane attack complex in cutaneous lesions of lupus erythematosus. J Am Acad Dermatol 1993; 28:687–691.

Heptinstall RH: Pathology of the Kidney, 4th ed. Boston, MA, Little, Brown & Co, 1992.

Izuno GT: Cutaneous immunofluorescence. Clin Lab Med 1986; 6:85–102.

Jiao D, Bystryn J-C: Sensitivity of indirect immunofluorescence, substrate specificity, and immunoblotting in the diagnosis of pemphigus. J Am Acad Dermatol 1997; 37:211–216.

Johnson PJ, McFarlane IG: Convenors on behalf of the panel. Meeting report: International autoimmune hepatitis group. Hepatology 1993; 18:998–1008.
Excellent summary of clinical laboratory parameters including serology useful in the diagnosis and classification of autoimmune hepatitis.

Kaplan MM: Clinical perspectives in the diagnosis of thyroid disease. Clin Chem 1999; 45:1377–1383.

Karen DF: Immunology and serology. In Jacobs DS, DeMott WR, Finley PR, et al (eds): Laboratory Test Handbook, 3rd ed. Hudson, OH, Lexi-Comp, 1994, p 627.

Kaufman DL, Erlander MG, Clare-Salzer M, et al: Autoimmunity to two forms of glutamate decarboxylase in insulin-dependent diabetes mellitus. J Clin Invest 1992; 89:283–292.

Korman NJ: Bullous pemphigoid. Dermatol Clin 1993; 11:483–498.

Kuechle MK, Stegemeir E, Maynard B, et al: Drug-induced linear IgA bullous dermatosis: report of six cases and review of the literature. J Am Acad Dermatol 1994; 30:187–192.

Lan MS, Wasserfall C, Maclaren NK, et al: IA-2, a transmembrane protein of the protein tyrosine phosphatase family, is a major autoantigen in insulin-dependent diabetes mellitus. Proc Natl Acad Sci USA 1996; 93:6367–6370.

Lin M-S, Liu Z, Drolet BA, et al: Cutaneous autoimmune diseases. In Rose NR, Mackay IR (eds): The Autoimmune Diseases, 3rd ed. San Diego, Academic Press, 1998, pp 545–570.

Liu AY, Valenzuela R, Helm TN, et al: Indirect immunofluorescence on rat bladder transitional epithelium: a test with high specificity for paraneoplastic pemphigus. J Am Acad Dermatol 1993; 28:696–699.

Lo SK, Fleming KA, Chapman RW: A 2-year follow-up study of anti-neutrophil antibody in primary sclerosing cholangitis: relationship to clinical activity, liver biochemistry and ursodeoxycholic acid treatment. J Hepatol 1994; 21:974–978.

Luhder F, Schlosser M, Mauch L, et al: Autoantibodies against GAD65 rather than GAD67 precede the onset of type 1 diabetes. Autoimmunity 1994; 19:71–80.

McCluskey RT, Collins AB, Niles JL: Kidney. In Colvin RB, Bhan AK, McCluskey RT (eds): Diagnostic Immunopathology, 2nd ed. New York, Raven Press, 1995, p 109.

McFarland HF, McFarlin DE: Immunologically mediated demyelinating diseases of the central and peripheral nervous system. In Frank MM, Austen KF, Claman HN, et al (eds): Samter's Immunologic Diseases, 5th ed. Boston, MA, Little, Brown & Co, 1995, vol II, p 1081.

Maclaren N: Immunology of diabetes mellitus. Ann Allergy 1992; 68:5–9.

Maclaren NK: Prespectives in diabetes: How, when, and why to predict IDDM. Diabetes 1988; 37:1591–1594.

Manns MP: Cytoplasmic autoantigens in autoimmune hepatitis: Molecular analysis and clinical relevance. Semin Liver Dis 1991; 11:205–214.

Manns MP: Autoimmune diseases of the liver. Clin Lab Med 1992; 12:25–40.

Manns MP, Lüttig B, Obermayer-Straub P: Autoimmune diseases: The liver. In Rose NR, Mackay IR (eds): The Autoimmune Diseases, 3rd ed. San Diego, CA, Academic Press, 1998, pp 511–544.

Manns MP, Nakamura RM: Autoimmune liver diseases. In Deodhar S (ed): Clinics in Laboratory Medicine. Philadelphia, PA, WB Saunders, 1988, pp 281–301.

Mason AL, et al: Retroviral antibodies in primary biliary cirrhosis. Lancet 1998; 351:1620–1624.

Mooij P, Drexhage HA: Autoimmune thyroid disease. Clin Lab Med 1993; 13:683–697.

Muir A, Maclaren NK: Autoimmune diseases of the adrenal glands, parathyroid glands, gonads, and hypothalamic-pituitary axis. Endocrinol Metab Clin North Am 1991; 20:619–644.

Muir A, Schatz DA, Maclaren NK: Autoimmune Addison's disease. Springer Semin Immunopathol 1993; 14:275–284.

Mutasim DF, Pelc NJ, Anhalt GJ: Cicatricial pemphigoid. In Dermatologic Clinics. Bullous Diseases, vol II. Philadelphia, PA, WB Saunders, 1993a, pp 499–510.

Mutasim DF, Pelc NJ, Anhalt GJ: Drug-induced pemphigus. In Dermatologic Clinics. Bullous Diseases, vol II. Philadelphia, PA, WB Saunders, 1993b, pp 463–471.

Mutasim DF, Pelc NJ, Anhalt GJ: Paraneoplastic pemphigus. In Dermatologic Clinics. Bullous Diseases, vol II. Philadelphia, PA, WB Saunders, 1993c, pp 473–481.

Nakamura RM. Concepts of autoimmunity and autoimmune diseases. In: Nakamura RM, Bylund DJ, Keren DF (eds): Clinical and Laboratory Evaluation of Human Autoimmune Diseases. Chicago, IL, ASCP Press, 2002, pp 13–35.
Succinct overview of the immune system, tolerance, principal factors associated with development of autoimmune disease, and classification of autoimmune disease.

Nakamura RM, Bylund DJ: Diagnostic significance of autoantibodies in autoimmune chronic active hepatitis. Clin Immunol Newsletter 1991; 11:161–167.

Nakamura RM, Matsutani M, Barry M: Advances in clinical laboratory tests for inflammatory bowel disease. Clin Chim Acta 2003; 335:9–20.

Naparstek Y, Plotz PH: The role of autoantibodies in autoimmune disease. Annu Rev Immunol 1993; 11:79–104.

NIH Consensus: National Institutes of Health Consensus Development Conference Statement Celiac Disease June 28–30, 2004. Available on line at: http://consensus.nih.gov/cibs/118/118celiacPDF.pdf.
Consensus and state-of-the-science statements on celiac disease with summary statements of key elements for management and future research.

Nordyke RA, Gilbert FI, Miyamoto LA, et al: The superiority of antimicrosomal over antithyroglobulin antibodies for detecting Hashimoto's thyroiditis. Arch Intern Med 1993; 12;153:862–865.

Nousari HC, Anhalt GJ: Bullous skin diseases. Curr Opin Immunol 1995; 7:844–852.

Nousari HC, Anhalt GJ: Skin diseases. In Rose NR, Conway de Macario E, Folds JD, et al (eds): Manual of Clinical Laboratory Immunology, 5th ed. Washington, DC, ASM Press, 1997, pp 997–1004.
Possibly the best synopsis of autoimmune skin diseases.

Nousari HC, Anhalt GJ: Pemphigus and bullous pemphigoid. Lancet 1999a; 354:667–672.

Nousari HC, Kimyai-Asadi A, Caeiro JP, et al: Clinical, demographic, and immunohistologic features of vancomycin-induced linear IgA bullous disease of the skin. Medicine 1999b; 78:1–8.

Patrick C: Organ-specific autoimmune diseases. Immunol Ser 1993; 58:423–436.

Peters MS, McEvoy MT: IgA antiendomysial antibodies in dermatitis herpetiformis. J Am Acad Dermatol 1989; 21:1225–1231.

Poupon R, Poupon RE: Primary biliary cirrhosis. In Zakim D, Boyer TD (eds): Hepatology – A Textbook of Liver Disease, 3rd ed. Philadelphia, PA, WB Saunders, 1996, pp 1329–1365.

Rose JW, McFarlin DE: Myasthenia gravis. In Frank MM, Austen KF, Claman HN, et al (eds): Samter's Immunologic Diseases, 5th ed. Boston, MA, Little, Brown & Co, 1995, vol II, p 1061.

Rostom A, Dube C, Cranney A, et al. Celiac Disease. Summary, Evidence Report/Technology Assessment No. 104. (Prepared by the University of Ottawa Evidence-based Practice Center, under Contract No. 290–02–0021.) AHRQ Publication No. 04-E029–1. Rockville, MD: Agency for Healthcare Research and Quality, 2004.

Sarret Y, Hall R, Cobo LM, et al: Salt-split human skin substrate for the immunofluorescent screening of serum from patients with cicatricial pemphigoid and a new method of immunoprecipitation with IgA antibodies. J Am Acad Dermatol 1991; 24:952–958.

Schatz D, Krischer J, Horne G, et al: Islet cell antibodies predict insulin-dependent diabetes in United States school age children as powerfully as in unaffected relatives. J Clin Invest 1994; 93:2403–2407.

Schatz D, Winter W: Recent advances in the immunopathogenesis of insulin-dependent diabetes mellitus. Curr Opin Pediatr 1995; 7:459–465.

Schmidli RS, Colman PG, Cui L, et al: Antibodies to the protein tyrosine phosphatases IAR and IA-2 are associated with progression to insulin-dependent diabetes (IDDM) in first-degree relatives at-risk for IDDM. Autoimmunity 1998; 28:15–23.

Song YH, Connor EL, Muir A, et al: Autoantibody epitope mapping of the 21-hydroxylase antigen in autoimmune Addison's disease. J Clin Endocrinol Metab 1994; 78:1108–1112.

Steinman L: Misguided assaults on the self produce multiple sclerosis, juvenile diabetes and other chronic illnesses. Promising therapies are emerging. Sci Am 1993; 269:106–114.

Talal AH, Murray JA, Goeken JA, et al: Celiac disease in an adult population with insulin-dependent diabetes mellitus: use of endomysial antibody testing. Am J Gastroenterol 1997; 92:1280–1283.

Teraki Y, Amagai N, Hashimoto T, et al: Intercellular IgA dermatosis of childhood. Selective deposition of monomer IgA1 in the intercellular space of the epidermis. Arch Dermatol 1991; 127(2):221–224.

Tsui WMS, Lam TW: The mystery of autoimmune cholangitis: a new entity or variant? Adv Anat Pathol 1997; 4:64–69.

Utiger RD: The pathogenesis of autoimmune thyroid disease. N Engl J Med 1991; 325:278–279.

Van Arsdel PP: Autoimmune endocrinopathies. In: Altman LC, ed. Immunology and allergy clinics of North America: autoimmune diseases. Philadelphia: Saunders; 1993:371.

Valenzuela R, Barna BP: Calculation of CNS IgG synthesis. In Barna BP (ed.): Laboratory Handbook of Neuroimmunologic Disease. Chicago, IL, ASCP Press, 1995, p 97.

Vasiliauskas EA, Kam LY, Karp LC, et al. Marker antibody expression stratifies Crohn's disease into immunologically homogeneous subgroups with distinct clinical characteristics. Gut 2000; 47:487–496.

Wilkin TJ: Receptor autoimmunity in endocrine disorders. N Engl J Med 1990; 323:1318–1324.

Wilson CB: Immune aspects of renal diseases. JAMA 1987; 258:2957–2961.

Zeballos RS, McPherson RA: Update of autoantibodies in neurologic disease. Clin Lab Med 1992; 12:61–83.

Zweiman B, Lisak RP: Autoantibodies: autoimmunity and immune complexes. In Henry JB (ed): Clinical Diagnosis and Management by Laboratory Methods, 18th ed. Philadelphia, PA, WB Saunders, 1991, p 885.

CHAPTER 53

Allergic Diseases

Henry A. Homburger MD

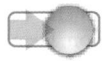

KEY POINTS

• Immunoglobulin E (IgE) is the most important trigger molecule for allergic inflammation.

• Laboratory tests that establish a high likelihood of allergic disease have assumed increased importance since the results justify referrals to allergy specialists and enable primary care physicians to decide whether or not to manage patients within their own practices.

• New drug treatments for allergic diseases such as monoclonal anti-IgE antibodies require demonstration of an elevated IgE level or the presence of IgE antibodies in serum as justification for their use.

• Clinical investigations of the natural history of allergic diseases in children have shown a reproducible sequence of sensitization to allergens that makes it increasingly important to establish the diagnosis of allergy at an early age in order to ameliorate the progression to serious diseases like asthma.

• Tests for IgE and IgE antibodies are ordered principally for diagnosis.

• Measurement of IgE in children and adults is of limited value in the diagnosis of allergic disease. The highest serum IgE levels typically occur in patients with hypersensitivity to several allergens and combinations of asthma, atopic dermatitis, and rhinitis. An elevated level carries a high predictive value for allergic disease.

• The measurement of IgE antibodies is useful and can be recommended in the following clinical situations:

  – the evaluation of children with a strong family history of allergic disease and early clinical signs of disease

  – the evaluation of children and adults suspected of having allergic respiratory disease to establish the diagnosis and to define the specificity of allergen sensitivity to pollens, dusts, fungal antigens, and foods

  – to confirm the clinical expression of sensitivity to foods in patients with anaphylactic sensitivity or with asthma, angioedema or cutaneous disease

  – to evaluate sensitivity to insect venom allergens, particularly as an aid in defining venom specificity in those cases in which skin tests are equivocal

  – to confirm the diagnosis of penicillin hypersensitivity in patients with anaphylactic sensitivity

  – to confirm the presence of IgE antibodies to certain occupational allergens, for example, natural rubber latex.

• Testing for IgE antibodies is not useful for evaluating the effects of immunotherapy or in excluding the diagnosis of anaphylactic sensitivity to insect venoms in treated patients. Tests for IgE antibodies are indicated only in patients who have had a thorough medical history and physical examination.

Allergic diseases are common in both children and adults. Estimates of the cumulative prevalence of allergic diseases in the United States range as high as 30% (Sly, 1999; Downs, 2001). According to recent data, more than 31 million individuals suffer from asthma, of which more than 9 million are children (Weiss, 2001). Recent epidemiologic studies point to an alarming increase in the incidence of asthma. Like many large categories of disease, estimates of the total yearly cost of allergic diseases run to the tens of billions of dollars. Taken collectively, allergic diseases are a major public health problem.

It is well documented that the clinical signs and symptoms of allergic diseases are difficult to distinguish from other etiologies (Host, 2003). The clinical manifestations may be relatively mild and self limited, as in seasonal allergic rhinitis, or severe with marked morbidity, as in asthma. Laboratory tests are useful in the evaluation of patients with allergic disease, but knowledge of the basic mechanisms of immediate hypersensitivity and awareness of the empirical relationships between test results and their diagnostic predictive values are needed to optimize testing. This chapter addresses these subjects, beginning with a review of the biology of immediate hypersensitivity and the 'allergic phenotype,' and proceeding to a detailed discussion of laboratory tests applied to the diagnostic evaluation of children and adults with allergic diseases. Emphasis is placed on identifying the minimum numbers of tests needed to achieve high positive and negative predictive values in different clinical situations. Specific mention is also made of clinical applications in which laboratory testing is not cost effective or may lead to erroneous clinical conclusions

Mechanisms of Immediate Hypersensitivity

Immunoglobulin E (IgE) is the most important trigger molecule for allergic inflammation. In the late 1960s, investigators working independently in two laboratories described a new class of human immunoglobulin that was responsible for the skin-sensitizing activity of serum from patients with allergic diseases (Bennich, 1969; Ishizaka, 1966). This immunoglobulin, originally called IgND, was later named IgE (Ishizaka, 1967). In the years that followed, investigators have focused on discovering the basic biologic mechanisms of immediate hypersensitivity, including mechanisms that control IgE production by immunocompetent B lymphocytes, and that promote the recruitment of inflammatory cells and release of vasoactive

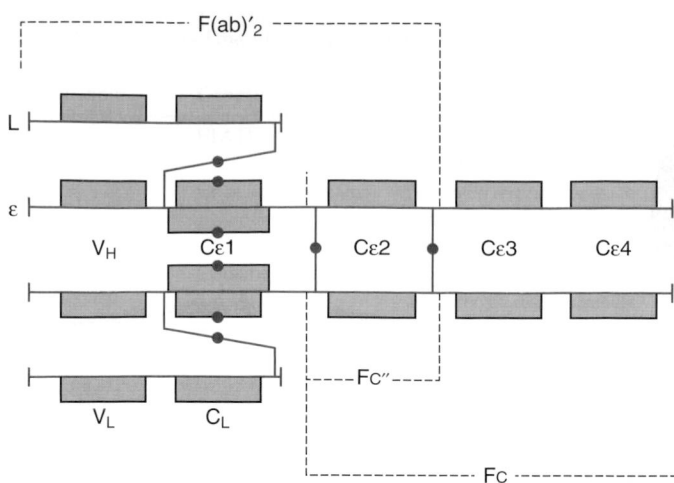

Figure 53–2 IgE structure.

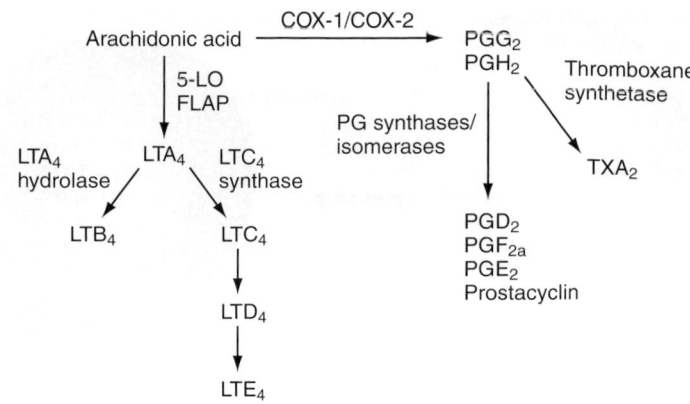

Figure 53–3 Metabolism of arachidonic acid. COX = cyclooxygenase; PG = prostaglandin; TX = thromboxane; LT = leukotriene; 5-LO = 5-lipoxygenase; FLAP = 5-lipoxygenase activating protein.

for IgE (Fcε RI) located diffusely on the plasma membranes of effector cells. Binding of IgE antibodies to Fcε RI is reversible but of very high affinity (Ka = $10^{10}\,M^{-1}$) (Wank, 1983). While IgE antibodies in blood have a half-life of only 2–3 days, the half-life of IgE antibodies bound to Fcε RI on mast cells is estimated to be more than 10 days. The number of receptors per cell ranges from 40 000 to 500 000. Higher numbers of receptors are found on cells cultured in the presence of IgE, possibly reflecting upregulation of Fcε RI expression by IgE. Fcε RI is a multimetric receptor, composed of α, β, and γ subunits as follows: α_1, β_1, and γ_2. IgE antibodies are bound by the α subunit; the β and γ subunits contain transmembrane regions that function in transmembrane signaling (Ravetech, 1991).

Fcε RI molecules are mobile within the plasma membranes of sensitized cells, as indicated by capping studies performed with fluorescein-conjugated anti-IgE antibodies. This mobility over short distances is believed to be important for the release of mediators from mast cells and basophils. Extensive studies with basophils and mast cells sensitized in vitro with IgE myeloma proteins or with specific IgE antibodies have shown that crosslinking (or bridging) of occupied IgE receptors by multivalent antigens or by intact anti-IgE antibodies or their F(ab')$_2$ fragments triggers release of histamine, but univalent haptens or Fab fragments of anti-IgE antibodies do not.

The initial signal for release of pre-formed mediators and for the synthesis and release of prostaglandins and leukotrienes from IgE-sensitized mast cells is crosslinking of Fcε RI by multivalent allergen. Degranulation is accomplished by a process of exocytosis. Receptor aggregation by allergen leads to methylation of membrane phospholipids, activation of adenylate cyclase, a transient increase in intracellular cyclic adenosine monophosphate (cAMP) and influx of Ca^{2+} ions which promotes fusion of granule and cell membranes during exocytosis. Increased intracellular Ca^{2+} also activates cytosolic phospholipase A_2, which promotes synthesis of arachidonic acid derived from membrane lipids. Free arachidonic acid is metabolized in mast cells to PGD$_2$ by enzymes of the cyclooxygenase (COX) pathway (COX-2, PG synthase, and isomerase), and to the cysteinyl leukotrienes LTB$_4$, LTC$_4$, LTD$_4$, and LTE$_4$ by enzymes of the 5-lipoxygenase pathway (Church, 2003) (Fig. 53–3).

Histamine is the best known mediator of allergic inflammation. Injected intradermally, histamine produces a characteristic weal and flare reaction that results from simultaneous vasoconstriction of postcapillary venules and neurogenic erythema (Petersen, 1997). Histamine in mast cells is contained in preformed granules with approximately 3–8 pg of histamine per cell. After release from mast cells, histamine interacts with specific, G-protein-coupled receptors termed H1–H4 (Wess, 1997; Gether, 2000; Church, 2003). Engagement of the H1 histamine receptor leads to activation of phospholipase C with subsequent protein kinase C activation and Ca^{2+} mobilization that causes the cellular responses associated with allergic inflammation. The effects of histamine are mediated by different receptors in different tissues. H1 receptors in the airway promote contraction of bronchial smooth muscle and mucus production, while H2 receptors in the stomach promote acid secretion. H3 and H4 receptors are found on histaminergic nerves and bone marrow cells, respectively. Histamine is degraded by two enzymatic pathways, with the major metabolite, N-methyl imidazole acetic acid (MIAA) resulting from the sequential methylation and deamination of histamine by the enzymes histamine N-methyl transferase and monoamine oxidase. Most secreted histamine is excreted in the urine as MIAA, with small amounts appearing undegraded.

The most abundant proteins in mast cell granules are neutral proteases, of which tryptase and chymase are the most familiar. As noted above, mast cells are categorized by their content of these two proteases. MCt cells predominate in the mucosa of the gut and in the airway while MCtc cells are found in connective tissues of the skin and gut submucosa. Human mast cell tryptase is a tetramer comprised of 31–38 kDa subunits with a molecular mass of approximately 130 kDa (Schwartz, 1981). Two cDNA subunits of tryptase termed α and β have been cloned from human mast cells that bear approximately 90% sequence homology with one another (Miller, 1990). Most tryptase in human serum is in the α form and is believed to be released constitutively from mast cells. β Tryptase is stored in secretory granules as a noncovalent complex with the proteoglycan heparin and is released upon cellular activation. Consequently, α tryptase provides an estimate of mast cell mass and β tryptase is a marker of mast cell activation and release of mediators (Schwartz, 1987). The half life of tryptase in circulation is approximately 90 minutes (Schwartz, 1989). In addition to having enzymatic activity, tryptase promotes growth of fibroblasts and smooth muscle cells, activates mast cells, and promotes release of the chemoattractant IL-8 from epithelial cells (Cairns, 1996).

Newly synthesized prostaglandins and leukotrienes are important proinflammatory allergic mediators. The principal prostaglandin mediator of mast cells is PGD$_2$ (Fig. 53–3). PGD$_2$ is much more potent than histamine on a molar basis but is released in smaller quantities than histamine by activated mast cells (Church, 2003). PGD$_2$ and its metabolite, $9\alpha,11\beta$ PGF$_2$ promote constriction of airway smooth muscle, peripheral vasodilatation and inhibition of platelet aggregation. IgE-mediated mast cell activation also results in synthesis and release of the cysteinyl leukotrienes LTC$_4$, LTD$_4$ and LTE$_4$ (Fig. 53–3). These molecules are extremely potent bronchoconstrictors, up to 1000 times more potent than histamine, and they promote increased vascular permeability and mucus production. In the early allergy literature, the leukotrienes were referred to as slow-reacting substance of anaphylaxis (SRS-A). Their role in the asthmatic response is demonstrated by clinical trials that show effective elimination of much of the early asthmatic response to allergen by administration of leukotriene antagonists (Findlay, 1992). Allergic inflammation often proceeds in two stages, an immediate response to allergen contact that occurs within minutes followed by a late reaction that occurs up to 24 hours following allergen exposure. This biphasic response occurs commonly in asthma. Both stages of the allergic response depend upon the presence and engagement of cell-bound IgE antibodies. The initial response reflects the effects of histamine, prostaglandin, and leukotriene mediators. The late response is caused by the recruitment of inflammatory cells, including eosinophils and neutrophils, at sites of allergic inflammation, followed by release of mediators from these activated cells. This late response is facilitated by the release of cytokines and chemoattractants from activated mast cells that promote the infiltration and degranulation of inflammatory leukocytes.

Laboratory Testing in the Evaluation of Allergic Diseases

The Rationale for Testing

Laboratory tests for allergic diseases have been available for more than 30 years (Wide, 1967). Immunoassays for total IgE protein (IgE) and allergen-specific IgE antibodies (IgE antibodies) in serum have been the mainstays.

During most of this time, there has been only modest interest in performing a full repertoire of tests on site in hospital clinical laboratories and many institutions have elected to send specimens to reference laboratories for testing. More recently, the use of laboratory tests in the evaluation of patients with allergic diseases has been driven by the shift to managed care health plans, development of new therapeutic drugs for the treatment of allergic diseases, improvements in the analytical methods for measuring IgE antibodies, and improved knowledge about the natural history of development of allergic diseases especially in children. Prior to the era of managed care, it was usually possible for a child or adult with symptoms and signs of allergy to be seen by an allergy specialist without prior medical evaluation. This is no longer the case for many patients whose health plans require that they be evaluated initially by primary care physicians. In this paradigm, laboratory tests that establish a high likelihood of allergic disease assume increased importance since the results justify referrals to allergy specialists and enable primary-care physicians to decide whether or not to manage patients within their own practices. In addition, new drug treatments for allergic diseases such as monoclonal anti-IgE antibodies require demonstration of an elevated IgE level or the presence of IgE antibodies in serum as justification for their use (Soler, 2001; Lanier, 2003). There have also been significant improvements in the analytic methods for measuring IgE antibodies. As detailed below, the current generation of test methods bears little resemblance to the original tests introduced shortly after the discovery of IgE. Finally, and perhaps most importantly, clinical investigations of the natural history of allergic diseases in children have shown a reproducible sequence of sensitization to allergens that makes it increasingly important to establish the diagnosis of allergy at an early age in order to ameliorate the progression to serious diseases like asthma (Wahn, 2000).

In the field of clinical allergy, tests for IgE and IgE antibodies are ordered principally for diagnosis. Results may have prognostic significance or serve as a guide to specific therapies such as allergen avoidance or immunotherapy, but laboratory data have little role in evaluating the response to such therapies or in monitoring the course of disease. Furthermore, the usefulness of diagnostic test results is determined empirically by whether or not it is difficult to establish an accurate diagnosis on clinical grounds and by studies of clinical outcomes that may justify trials of drug therapy without a specific etiologic diagnosis (so called empiric therapy) (Gendo, 2004). Nevertheless, in many clinical situations definitive management requires that the offending allergens be identified unequivocally. For example, it is necessary to define allergen specificity in cases of anaphylactic sensitivity to foods, drugs and insect venom allergens, in patients in whom allergen immunotherapy is indicated as treatment, and in patients with occupational allergies or sensitivity to allergens such as natural rubber latex.

In Vivo Test Techniques: Skin Tests and End Organ Challenge Tests

It is not possible to discuss the use of laboratory tests in the diagnosis and management of allergic diseases without mentioning in vivo tests of immediate hypersensitivity, particularly the skin test and end-organ challenge tests. In vivo tests are considered the standards of diagnostic accuracy and reliability. The ability to reproduce a specific allergic reaction by in vivo challenge is regarded by most allergy specialists as the most sensitive technique for demonstrating the presence of immediate hypersensitivity and for defining its allergen specificity.

Skins tests are performed by intradermal injection and by skin prick methods (Demoly, 1998). The response to intradermal injection of an allergen extract is graded by measuring the diameter of the weal and erythema reaction immediately following the injection. A 1+ reaction corresponds to a 5–10 mm weal. A response of this magnitude is usually regarded as evidence for specific sensitivity to an allergen. Highly sensitive individuals often develop weal diameters greater than 15 mm with pseudopods. Skin tests performed by the prick method make use of more concentrated allergen exacts, up to 1000-fold greater concentrations than are used for intradermal testing, and grading is often omitted. Mean weal diameters in millimeters are recorded as an indication of the degree of sensitivity. A more quantitative estimate of sensitivity to a given allergen can be obtained by the technique of end-point titration. This technique is a modification of the intradermal and skin prick methods. Serial, tenfold dilutions of a standardized allergen extract are used, beginning with the most dilute solution. The endpoint of sensitivity is defined as the greatest dilution that produces a 1+ reaction.

End-organ challenge tests are useful clinically and for investigative purposes. Adaptations of this technique include the bronchial provocation test in the diagnosis of asthma; the rhinoconjunctive challenge test in the diagnosis of allergic rhinitis; the food elimination and challenge test in the

Age	Mean (kU/L)	+ 1SD (kU/L)
6 weeks	0.6	2.3
3 months	1.0	4.1
6 months	1.8	7.3
9 months	2.6	10
12 months	3.2	13
2 years	5.7	23
3 years	8.0	32
4 years	10	40
5 years	12	48
6 years	14	56
7 years	16	63
8 years	18	71
9 years	20	78
10 years	22	85
*Adults	13.2	41

Table 53–3 Serum IgE Reference Ranges in Children and Adults

* In adults the mean +2 SD cut-off is 127 kU/L. See text for explanation.

diagnosis of food-induced asthma, and the sting challenge in the diagnosis of anaphylactic sensitivity to insect venom. The application of challenge tests in routine clinical situations is limited by the requirement for well standardized allergen extracts of defined potency and by the limited number of allergens that can be tested in an individual on a single occasion. As an example, food elimination and challenge procedures require periods of abstinence of several days, during which time inadvertent consumption of a particular food may invalidate the test.

Measurement of IgE: Analytic Methods and Reference Ranges

A variety of immunochemical methods have been used to measure IgE including competitive displacement immunoassays, immunometric (sandwich) assays with radiolabeled and enzyme-labeled second stage antibodies and enhanced sensitivity nephelometry (Homburger, 1998). Nonisotopic immunometric assays are the most widely used methods. The most popular commercial method uses anti-IgE antibody bound to a high-capacity cellulose solid phase to capture IgE in a test sample, after which bound IgE is detected with an enzyme-labeled second-stage antibody that generates a fluorescent product. The amount of product is proportional to the amount of IgE captured in the first stage of the assay. This assay is capable of measuring concentrations of IgE in the range of 2–5000 kU/L (1 kU equals approximately 2.4 μg of IgE). Assay calibrators used in commercial products are traceable to an international standard (WHO preparation 75/502 for human IgE).

There have been a number of studies of the serum concentrations of IgE in healthy, nonallergic children and adults. Synthesis of IgE occurs in the human fetus as early as the 11th week of gestation, but cord serum typically contains less than 1 kU/L of IgE (Homburger, 1998). Serum concentrations of IgE in children increase slowly with age and reach adult levels at approximately 10 years of age (Table 53–3). In both children and adults, studies of healthy subjects have yielded frequency histograms of IgE measurements that are positively skewed with 95% confidence intervals that are seemingly high compared to the mean levels of IgE. Consequently, many laboratories report reference ranges that are logarithmically transformed, and the upper limit of 'normal' is portrayed as +1 SD of an age related, geometric distribution (Table 53–3). This convention is confusing to many clinicians, and it has become common practice to regard 100 kU/L as the upper limit of normal in non allergic adults.

Measurement of IgE: Clinical Applications

The measurement of IgE protein in serum has been thoroughly evaluated for its clinical usefulness as a screening test in the diagnosis of various allergic diseases, for its predictive value as an indicator of the likelihood of the development of allergic disease in asymptomatic infants and children, and as a prognostic indicator in adults with certain types of chronic allergic disease. Measurement of IgE may also be useful in the evaluation of patients suspected of having immunodeficiency diseases, parasitic diseases, or the rare hyper-IgE syndrome.

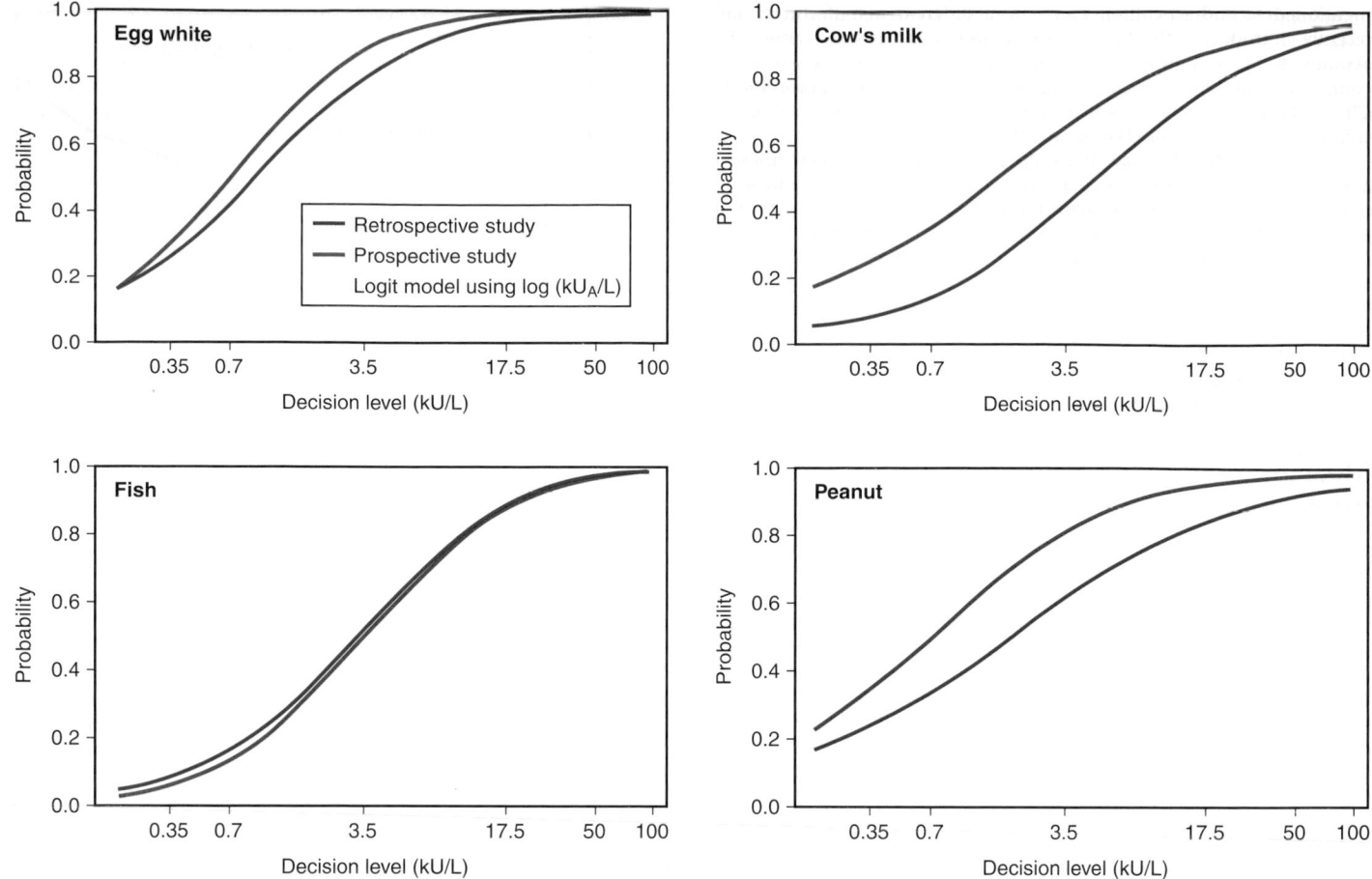

Figure 53–5 Probability of reacting to food allergens at increasing levels of IgE antibodies. (With permission from Sampson HA: Utility of food-specific IgE concentrations in predicting symptomatic food allergy. J Allergy Clin Immunol 2001; 107:891–896.)

testing, it is important to be selective in the initial testing of children with respiratory signs and symptoms in order to avoid unnecessary testing. Data from clinical investigations support complementary approaches: the use of small panels of individual inhalant allergens and use of the multiallergen IgE antibody test to test for several antibodies simultaneously.

The allergens chosen for testing in children with respiratory diseases depend upon the age of the child and the scope of clinical manifestations (Table 53–4). After age 3 or 4, it is common in atopic children to develop IgE antibodies to indoor aeroallergens including house dust mites, animal epithelia (cat and dog), and cockroach. The last antibody specificities to develop in children are to common outdoor aeroallergens, including molds and pollen inhalants of trees, grasses, and weeds. There is no agreement on the minimum number of inhalant allergens that should be tested when evaluating children with respiratory symptoms, but there is consensus that testing should include house dust mites, cat or dog epithelium, a ubiquitous mold species (e.g., *Alternaria tenuis*), and appropriate pollen allergens (Host, 2003). Testing for IgE antibodies to pollen allergens is indicated in older children especially if symptoms are seasonal and tests can be performed at the time that symptoms are manifest. It is well known that the levels of IgE antibodies to seasonal inhalants vary with the seasons, and there is little utility in performing tests for IgE antibodies to pollen inhalants when the allergens are not present in the environment, since the results may be falsely negative. The multiallergen IgE antibody test is an efficient way to screen for the presence of IgE antibodies to pollen allergens. A positive result indicates the presence of IgE antibodies to at least one of the allergens on the immunosorbent, but is not specific for a particular allergen. As such, a positive result is useful to identify patients who might benefit from further testing with individual allergen reagents.

In adults with respiratory allergic rhinitis or allergic (extrinsic) asthma, tests for IgE antibodies are reliable for identifying sensitivity to all classes of allergen. The most common sensitivities are to common aeroallergens, including house dust mite, cockroach, animal epithelia, mold spores, pollen allergens, and organic dust allergens (Hamilton, 2004). Testing is indicated in cases in which the results are likely to influence the choice of treatment modality (Gendo, 2004). In adults suspected of having allergic rhinitis, IgE antibody tests are most useful in making the diagnosis when

Table 53–4 Selected IgE Antibody Tests for Evaluating Children with Clinical Signs of Allergy

Age (years)	Signs of Disease	Allergens
Younger than 3	Eczema with or without wheezing and otitis	Common foods: egg white, milk, wheat, soy; house dust mites (*Dermatophagoides farinae* and *Dermatophagoides pteronyssinus*)
Older than 3 or 4	Rhinitis, wheezing, asthma	Common perennial inhalants: house dust mites, cat or dog, cockroach, *Alternaria tenuis*
Older than 3 or 4	Rhinitis, wheezing, asthma with seasonal exacerbations	Common perennial inhalants, as above, plus pollen inhalants (tree, grass, or weed pollens)

the pretest probability of disease is relatively low (less than 30%). Such patients typically do not have clinical findings that strongly suggest an allergic etiology. In this situation, positive test results greatly increase the post-test probability of disease for most common aeroallergens, including animal epithelia, molds, and pollens. Among patients with a strong clinical history (prominent nasal symptoms and allergen triggers), testing is less likely to be useful and empirical treatment is often indicated. The results of several studies indicate that skin tests and second-generation IgE antibody tests have essentially equivalent diagnostic utility in adults with allergic rhinitis, and either test modality can be used to identify allergens for inclusion in immunotherapy regimens (Gendo, 2004). The use of allergen immunotherapy in adults with asthma is more controversial, with only some studies showing clear efficacy. The decision to test for IgE antibodies in adults with asthma must be made on a case-by-case basis, with testing more likely to be useful in patients with clear-cut allergen triggers or occupational exposure to unique allergens.

New drug treatments for allergic diseases have become available in recent years. In particular, the treatment of severe persistent allergic asthma has been influenced by the introduction of anti-IgE pharmacotherapy

(Busse, 2001; Soler, 2001; Lanier, 2003). Anti-IgE drugs are humanized mouse monoclonal antibodies to IgE that bind to the ε heavy chain and inhibit binding of IgE antibodies to receptors on mast cells. By interfering with binding of IgE antibodies to effector cells, anti-IgE antibody effectively blocks the release of inflammatory mediators that results from exposure to allergen. The results of clinical studies of anti-IgE pharmacotherapy of asthma have shown reduced rates of disease exacerbation and reduced requirements for corticosteroid drugs in treated patients (Soler, 2001; Lanier, 2003).

In order for a physician to treat a patient with anti-IgE, it is necessary to document that the patient has IgE antibodies to perennial aeroallergens and an elevated baseline level of serum IgE (30–700 kU/L). Anti-IgE has also been tested successfully in patients with peanut allergy and in patients with severe allergic rhinitis.

As noted earlier, the availability of quantitative assays for IgE antibodies has extended the usefulness of testing for several clinical applications (Yunginger, 2000). One such area is in the evaluation of hypersensitivity to food allergens. Measurement of IgE antibodies is indicated to evaluate patients with food-induced symptoms that affect several end organs, including the skin, gastrointestinal tract, airways, and even systemic reactivity. The gold standard for determining hypersensitivity to a food allergen is the double-blind, placebo-controlled food challenge. Recent data indicate that the levels of IgE antibodies can be used to predict the responses to food challenge for several common foods (Fig. 53–5). These results define the levels of IgE antibodies below which the probabilities of obtaining a negative result exceed 95% and above which a challenge is not necessary. Similar attempts to define cut-offs for IgE antibody levels that predict reactivity to inhalant aeroallergens have failed to define levels that can be used across different practice situations (Soderstrom, 2003).

IgE antibody testing is useful in the diagnosis of suspected sensitivity to Hymenoptera venom(s). Individuals sensitive to the venoms of honey bees, yellow jackets, hornets, or wasps may manifest signs of anaphylaxis following a sting; urticaria, angioedema, bronchospasm, or cardiovascular collapse may ensue. The reported death rate from sting-induced systemic reactions is 30–40 cases annually, but this figure probably underestimates the true incidence. The natural history of untreated venom sensitivity is not completely known. In many patients with documented anaphylactic sensitivity, it is possible to elicit a clinical history of progressively more severe reactions to successive sting episodes. On the other hand, venom sensitivity apparently ameliorates spontaneously in some individuals. The decision to treat a patient with venom immunotherapy is based upon clinical assessment of the risk of anaphylaxis to possible future stings.

The most reliable indicator of venom sensitivity is the response to a deliberate sting challenge; but, this test is not widely performed and is rarely required in previously untreated patients to establish the diagnosis of venom sensitivity. Venom skin tests and IgE antibody tests are useful to confirm the clinical impression of venom sensitivity and to define its specificity. Comparative studies indicate that skin testing is a more sensitive diagnostic modality, with only approximately 80% of skin-test-positive patients having elevated venom specific IgE antibodies (Golden, 2003). Venom IgE antibody tests are useful primarily to confirm the results of skin tests, to define the allergen specificity of venom hypersensitivity, and in selected patients to identify venom sensitivity when a positive clinical history is not confirmed by intradermal venom skin testing (Golden, 2003).

With the exception of the sting challenge, there is no in vitro or in vivo test that reliably predicts the clinical response to an insect sting in a treated patient following venom immunotherapy. Although the levels of IgG antibodies in serum increase markedly with venom immunotherapy, no cut-off level has been defined that can be used to identify those patients who are no longer at risk. Semiquantitative estimates of IgG antibodies are not useful clinically, and the levels of IgE antibodies following treatment bear no consistent relationship to the clinical status. The decision to discontinue venom immunotherapy is based on clinical studies that show high protection rates after approximately 3 years of treatment (Yunginger 1998).

Measurements of IgE antibodies have also been applied to the diagnosis of drug allergy. Although many drugs and their metabolites are capable of eliciting synthesis of antibodies, clinical data and the results of IgE antibody measurements are available only for the penicillins and their metabolites and for certain polypeptide drugs including insulin. Penicillin and its isomer, penicillanic acid, combine with serum proteins through amide linkages to create allergenic moieties: penicilloyl-protein and penicillenic acid-protein are so called major and minor antigenic determinants, respectively (Fig. 53–6). Measurable levels of IgM and IgG antibodies specific for the penicilloyl determinant occur commonly in

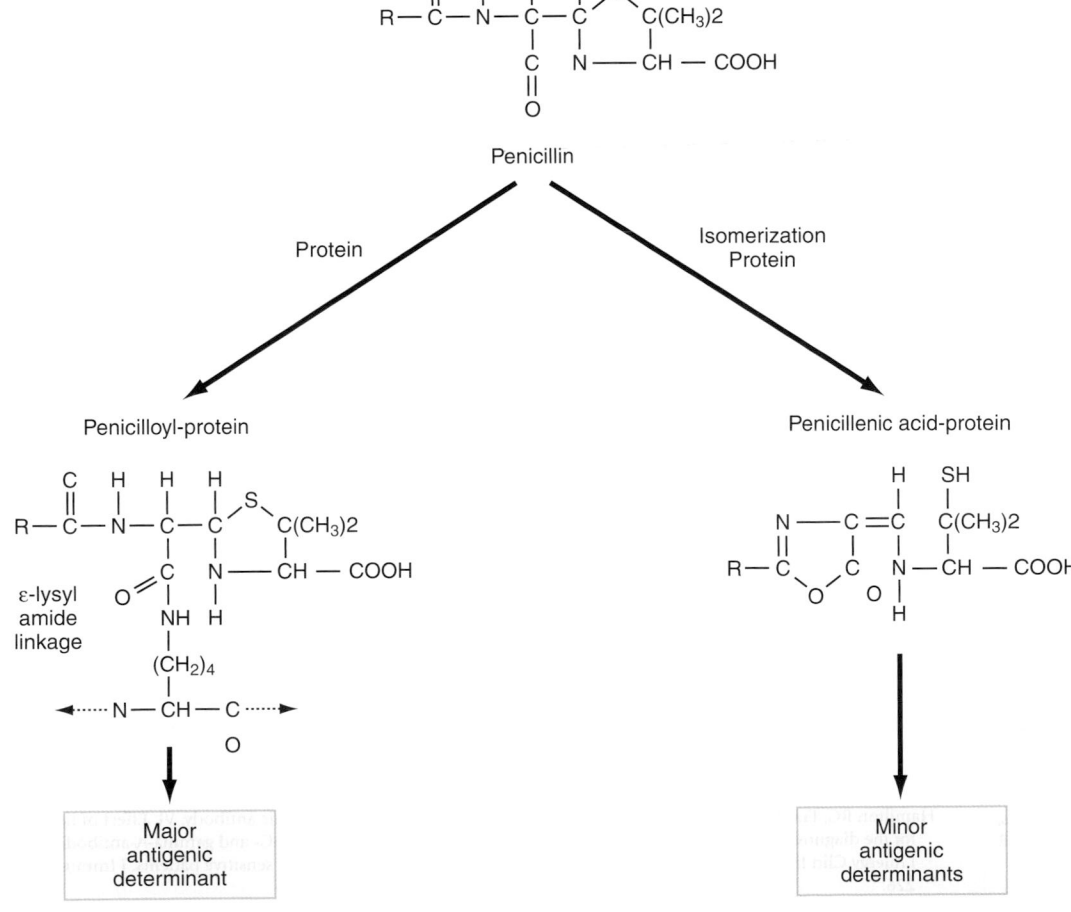

Figure 53–6 Allergens derived from penicillin.

PART VII

Medical Microbiology

Edited by

Gail L. Woods MD, Richard A. McPherson MD

Introduction

Viruses are the most frequent cause of human infectious diseases and are responsible for a spectrum of illness ranging from the trivial colds to fatal immunoimpairment caused by human immunodeficiency virus (HIV) destruction of CD4+ T lymphocytes. Virology evolved rapidly from electron microscopy characterization of viral morphology to the development of cell culture methods for vaccine development to the detailed delineation of the viral biochemistry needed to engineer antiviral therapy.

There are now straightforward cell culture procedures for isolation of many viruses and sophisticated molecular techniques for viral identification and for quantitative assessment of response to therapy; both community and university hospitals can offer testing for respiratory, central nervous system, gastrointestinal, and disseminated viral infections. Accurate and timely diagnosis is fundamental for optimal patient management, promotion of appropriate use of antiviral drugs, reduction of unnecessary tests and superfluous antibiotics, and efficient implementation of nursing precautions to limit nosocomial spread (Aitken, 2001). Additional benefits of accurate diagnosis include focused public health control and prevention initiatives for influenza, HIV, arbovirus, and enterovirus infections. Interestingly, the failure to identify traditional viruses in apparent outbreaks led to prompt characterization by the Centers for Disease Control and Prevention of the west Nile virus (WNV) meningoencephalitis epidemic and variant coronavirus responsible for severe acute respiratory syndrome (SARS).

Several excellent references provide detailed information about taxonomy and pathogenicity of human viruses (Fields, 2001; Murray, 2003). This chapter reviews the common viral syndromes that generate the majority of testing in a typical hospital laboratory. Organization and staffing, equipment and supplies, specimen collection and test selection are discussed, along with isolation and identification methods. Most hospitals have a case mix of common viral infections in healthy and immunocompromised children and adults to support a virology service. Table 54–1 summarizes test volumes and recovery rates for Lutheran General Hospital, a community hospital with adult and pediatric primary care and high risk obstetrics, neonatology, hematology–oncology, and HIV services. Hospitals with different medical specialty profiles recover the same viruses, with variations in the relative isolation percentages. Average detection time for most viruses is often 2 days or less (on the same time scale as routine bacterial cultures) and reflects the use of rapid antigen assays, shell vial cultures with short incubation schedules, and nucleic acid amplified tests. Overall recovery rates for viruses are high – 16–23% – several times greater than for routine bacterial blood or stool cultures, mycobacterial cultures, or ova and parasite exams (Costello, 1996). Many common viruses exhibit seasonal variations (Fig. 54–1). Influenza, respiratory syncytial virus, and parainfluenza virus 1 and 2 circulate every winter. Adenovirus, parainfluenza virus 3, cytomegalovirus, and herpes simplex infections occur year-round. Enterovirus disease clusters in late summer and early autumn. These temporal patterns influence laboratory staffing needs, which are most taxing in pediatric hospitals.

There are three principal viral diagnostic laboratory methods, and each has advantages and limitations (Fig. 54–2). Culture and antigen detection require either viable virus or relatively intact viral fragments; specimens

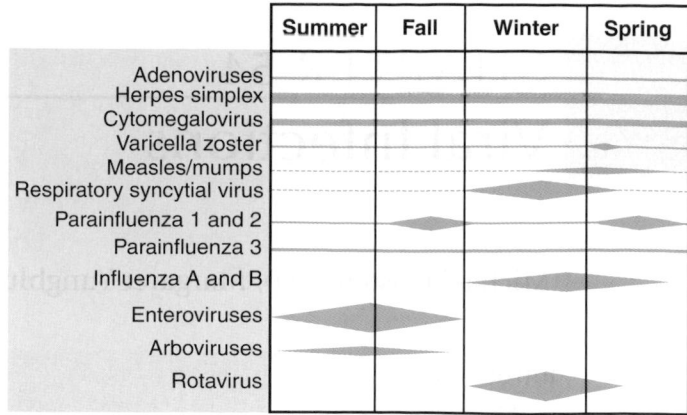

Figure 54–1 Seasonal variation of viral infections.

must be collected during active viral replication. Amplified nucleic acid tests (NAAT) have the highest sensitivity and, because of the relative stability of DNA and RNA, allow more latitude for collection; however, interpretation may be more difficult because positivity may persist into the recovery phase. Molecular assays can separate active infection from latent infection by targeting an actively replicating component of the viral genome; reverse-transcriptase polymerase chain reaction (RT-PCR) assay for cytomegalovirus (CMV)-specific RNA identifies active viral replication while DNA-specific PCR is also positive with latency. Traditional serologic diagnosis requires paired sera from both the acute and convalescent stages of infection to demonstrate a significant rise in specific viral antibody titer. Detection of virus-specific IgM antibody can diagnose acute illness from a single serum obtained during the acute or early convalescent period. Virus-specific IgG antibody tests are typically used to document immune status.

All necessary materials and reagents for virus isolation, antigen assays, and serologic procedures are available from commercial suppliers. The number of viruses that can be detected or quantified by NAATs continues to grow, and several are commercially produced. Home-configured procedures require considerable technical expertise, and all molecular methods demand stringent quality control to guarantee accuracy and to minimize contamination. Despite these constraints, NAATs are particularly helpful for identifying viruses that propagate slowly or not at all in cell culture, and their sensitivity and quantitative accuracy is superior to conventional procedures.

Viral Culture

Virus propagation in tissue culture was developed over 50 years ago and is still a versatile and comprehensive diagnostic approach. Many clinically significant viruses replicate in vitro, and virus recovery correlates well with acute disease. However, culture is labor-intensive, requires technical proficiency, and means at least one-day turnaround for positive results. Replication in newborn mice or embryonated eggs may be essential for some fastidious viruses but is rarely performed outside research facilities (Nalonen, 1998). Tissue culture cells are divided into three categories: primary cell cultures, diploid cell lines, and heteroploid cell lines. Primary cell cultures are prepared directly from the parent organ (e.g., monkey or rabbit kidney) by mincing and trypsinization and the mixture is transferred to a tube or shell vial where the cells attach and form a confluent monolayer on the glass surface. Overlay medium with buffered isotonic inorganic salts, glucose, amino acids, vitamins, and cofactors at a physiologic pH sustains cell viability. Eagle minimum essential medium in Earl or Hanks balanced salt solution is a versatile nutrient system, and is usually supplemented with a low concentration of protein-rich/immunoglobulin-poor fetal bovine serum to maintain a healthy monolayer but not promote cell proliferation. Diploid cell lines are usually human diploid fibroblasts (HDF) derived from lung or newborn foreskin, and the majority of cells have a normal diploid chromosome number. Cells are propagated in serum-rich growth medium and can be serially subcultured 20–50 times; examples include MRC-5, WI-38, and foreskin fibroblasts. Heteroploid cell lines are derived from malignant tumors and can be passaged indefinitely, they are aneuploid and divide rapidly. Heteroploid lines include HEp-2 (laryngeal carcinoma), HeLa (cervical carcinoma), and A549 (laryngeal carcinoma).

Primary cultures must be checked for contamination with endogenous virus. Diploid and heteroploid cell lines should be tested periodically for

CHAPTER: 54 Viral Infections

Table 54–1 Viral Detection for Community Hospital Laboratory – percentage of and typical detection times (Lutheran General Hospital, Park Ridge, IL)

Virus	% Positive Specimens 1995	% Positive Specimens 1998	% Positive Specimens 2004	Typical Detection Times
Herpes simplex virus	34	25	22	1–2 days
Cytomegalovirus	3	4	4	3 days
Adenoviruses	5	6	8	3 days
Influenza A virus	6	11	9	2 days
Enterovirus	8	7	10	4 days
Varicella zoster virus	2	1	<1	3–5 days
Influenza B virus	1	<1	4	2 days
Parainfluenza virus	6	4	10	2 days
Respiratory syncytial virus	27	41	31	8–48 hours
Measles and mumps	<1	0	0	5 days
Total specimens processed	3323	3040	2750	
Recovery of viruses	21%	23%	16%	

Standard tube cell monolayer

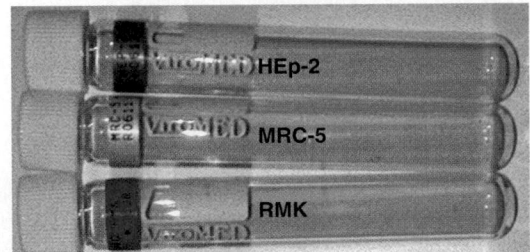

Centrifugation-enhanced
Shell vial monolayer

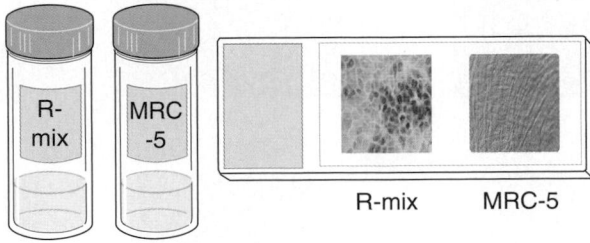

R-mix   MRC-5

Detection of viral antigen-nucleic acid in direct specimen

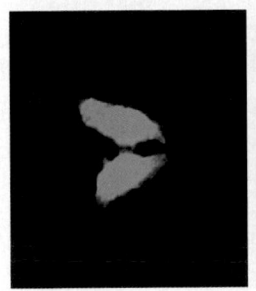

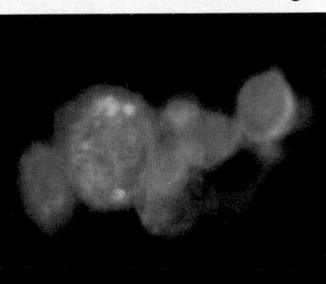

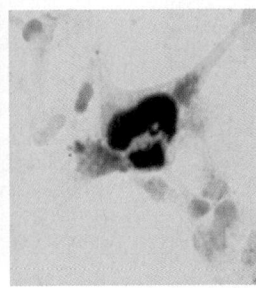

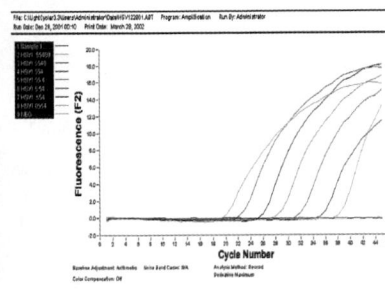

Influenza
DFA/NP aspirate

VZV DFA
Vesicular lesion

CMV *in situ*
Hybridization
Lung biopsy

HSV PCR amplification - CSF

Serological detection of virus-specific antibodies

Demonstration of immunity
IgG: HAV, HBsAg, rubella, measles,
    mumps, VZV

Diagnosis of acute infection
IgM: HAV, HBc, EBV-VCA, measles,
    mumps, rubella, parvovirus B19,
    MNV (other arboviruses)

Diagnosis of chronic infection
IgG: HIV, HCV, HLTV

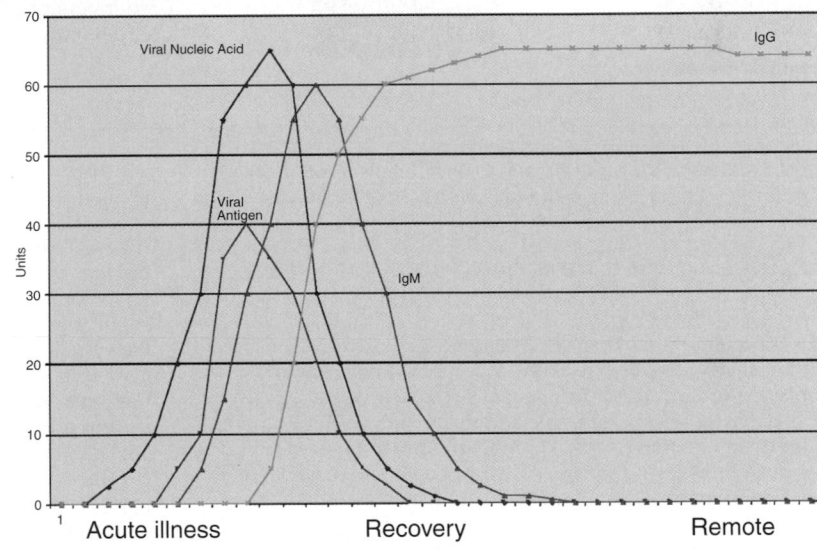

Figure 54–2 Laboratory methods for diagnosis of viral infections.

Mycoplasma contamination and continued sensitivity to viral infection. The suppliers of purchased cells should perform these quality control responsibilities. 'Hybrid' cells are a new concept; the monolayer is a mixture of two cell types that together support growth of a wide range of viruses. R-Mix contains A549 and mink lung cells with added trypsin and will recover the respiratory agents – influenzas, parainfluenzas, respiratory syncytial virus (RSV), and adenovirus. E-Mix contains Buffalo green monkey kidney and A549 cells to maximize recovery of enteroviruses. Viruses differ somewhat in their ability to replicate in culture, so critical specimens should be inoculated to a variety of cell lines to maximize recovery. Figure 54–3 shows the viral preferences for some common cell lines; all are available commercially and can be supplied in tubes, shell vials, or bulk flasks. Each laboratory should select sufficient lines to cover the usual viral pathogens in its patient population, and can vary the number and type to meet seasonal demands (Chapin, 2003; Clarke, 2004).

Viral replication in tube monolayers is identified by inspecting the cell sheet with an inverted phase-contrast microscope for cytopathic changes caused by virus proliferation. Tube monolayers are versatile: a single cell line may support growth of several viruses, each producing distinctive cytopathic effect (CPE) or other identifying features (hemagglutination, hemadsorption, interference). CPE may develop in 1–3 days (herpes simplex virus [HSV]) or may not be recognized for 5–20 days (RSV, varicella zoster virus [VZV], CMV); therefore, cultures may need extended incubation for 2 weeks or more. With the shell vial technique, the cell sheet rests on a round coverslip, monolayer side up, in a shell vial. The specimen is inoculated into the vial, which is then centrifuged to enhance viral attachment to the cell surface. After 1–3 days' incubation, the monolayer is tested for specific viral antigen, usually with a fluorescent antibody stain (Gleaves, 1985; Clarke, 2004). Shell vials are ideal for identification of a single virus (HSV) or limited number of viruses (RSV and influenza), and for faster detection of slow-growing agents such as CMV and VZV. HSV vesicular genital lesions are excellent candidates for shell vial culture; sensitivity is almost 100% compared with traditional tube culture and turnaround for negative specimens is decreased from 1 week to 1 day. Shell vials are comparable or superior to tube methods for

VII

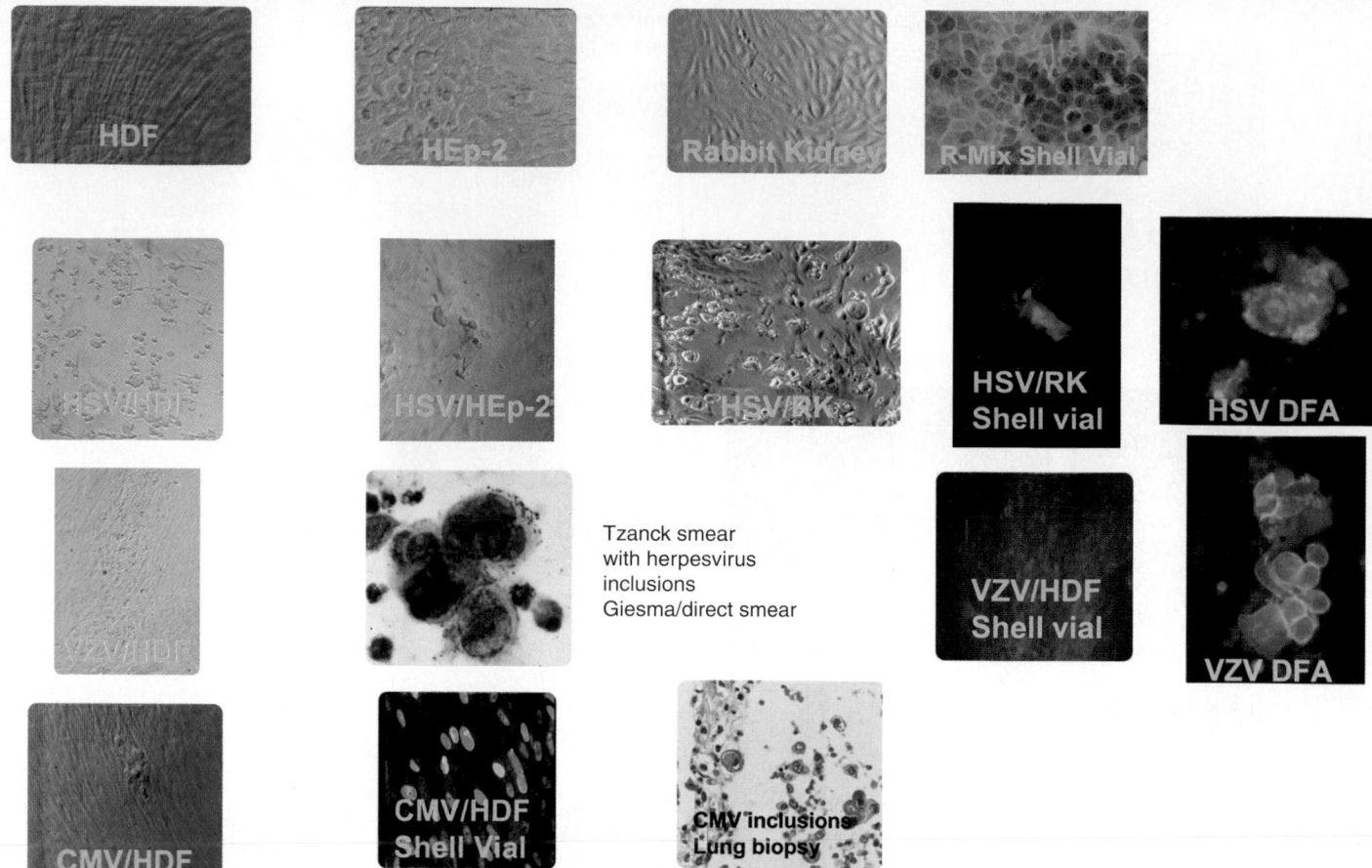

Figure 54–3 Viral growth in cell culture lines and viral detection in patient samples.

recovery of CMV from urine, but backup tube culture is recommended to maximize CMV recovery from peripheral blood, body fluids and tissue biopsies.

Viral Antigen Detection and Molecular Detection

Rapid identification by direct methods is especially useful when specific antiviral therapy is available (for HSV, VZV, CMV, influenza) and when nosocomial control is a factor (influenza, RSV, rotavirus and VZV). Viral antigen is detected with comparable sensitivity and specificity by both direct fluorescent antibody (DFA) and enzyme immunoassay (EIA) methods. DFA has the advantage of microscopic visualization of the specimen's cell content, so sample adequacy can be easily verified (Rossier, 1989); but DFA procedures are labor-intensive and may be unfeasible during seasonal respiratory viral outbreaks with high specimen demand. EIA methods require less subjective interpretive judgment than DFA, but the automatic assessment of sample quality is lost. DFA is best performed with an epifluorescence microscope, and positive and negative controls must be run routinely. Many EIA procedures are engineered for individual specimen testing with positive and negative control verification incorporated into a single-use cassette. Automated EIA procedures for batch testing combine washing, spectrophotometric, and data processing components into a self-contained system; positive and negative controls are standard with each run and the reading for the patient sample is interpreted using an established cut-off value.

Nucleic acid hybridization and molecular amplification tests detect viruses by recognizing specific segments of the viral DNA or RNA genome. In situ hybridization (ISH) is a direct probe technique used in surgical pathology to identify human papillomavirus (HPV), CMV, HSV and parvovirus B19; specificity is excellent but suboptimal sensitivity limits the clinical value. NAATs raise the sensitivity of molecular diagnosis beyond that of antigen assay and culture by sequential exponential duplication of the viral oligonucleotide target (PCR, strand displacement amplification [SDA] and nucleic acid sequence-based amplification [NASBA]), or by amplification of an attached chemiluminescent signal label (hybrid capture and branched DNA [bDNA] methods). PCR and bDNA amplification have become standard for quantitative monitoring of HIV

and hepatitis C virus (HCV) (Nolte, 2003). PCR is the most sensitive method for diagnosis of enterovirus meningitis and HSV encephalitis (Tang, 1998; Read, 1999; Romero, 2003); PCR detection of Epstein–Barr virus (EBV) in spinal fluid is diagnostic of central nervous system lymphoma in patients with acquired immunodeficiency syndrome (AIDS). The clinical utility of PCR was greatly expanded with introduction of 'real-time' amplification. Amplification steps and detection of amplicon take place in the same closed tube; multiple specimens can be run simultaneously and detection cycle number is proportional to viral copy number. Quantitative CMV PCR in bronchoalveolar fluid is predictive of viral pneumonia in bone marrow transplant patients and sentinel surveillance of CMV PCR of blood predicts infection in solid organ transplant recipients. Automation of NAATs, particularly with incorporation of internal standards and procedural steps configured to avoid amplicon crosscontamination, has accelerated throughput time and reduced false-negative and false-positive errors. Commercial products are limited at present, but several kits for identification of common viral pathogens are in development. Strict adherence to specimen collection and processing requirements must be maintained to preserve viral nucleic acid and maximize detection.

Direct electron microscopy visualization of viral particles using phosphotungstic acid negative staining has been helpful in evaluation of viral gastroenteritis, since rotavirus, enteric adenovirus, norovirus, astrovirus, and calicivirus replicate poorly or not at all in standard cell monolayers but have distinctive ultrastructural features.

Viral Serology

Serologic diagnosis of viral infection is attractive because serum specimens are easy to obtain, transport, and store. Viral serology has two major applications: diagnosis of recent infection and determination of immunity. Evidence of current/recent infection requires demonstration of virus-specific IgM during the acute stage of illness or demonstration of a fourfold or greater rise in virus-specific IgG titer between acute and convalescent sera. Specific IgM is usually found in blood during the first week of primary infection and typically becomes undetectable within 1–3 months; EIA methods are more sensitive and may identify persistent IgM for approximately twice as long as immunofluorescent assays. Specificity and sensitivity of IgM assays are improved by removal of rheumatoid factor

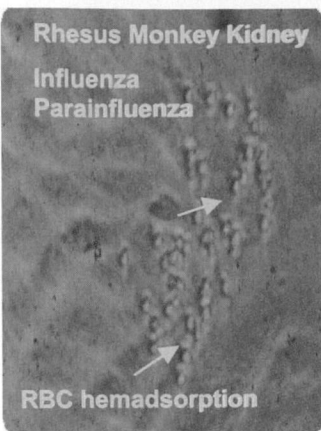

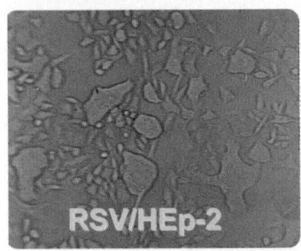

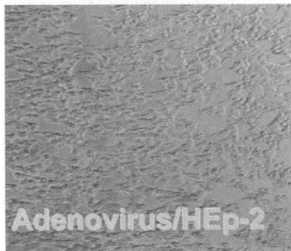

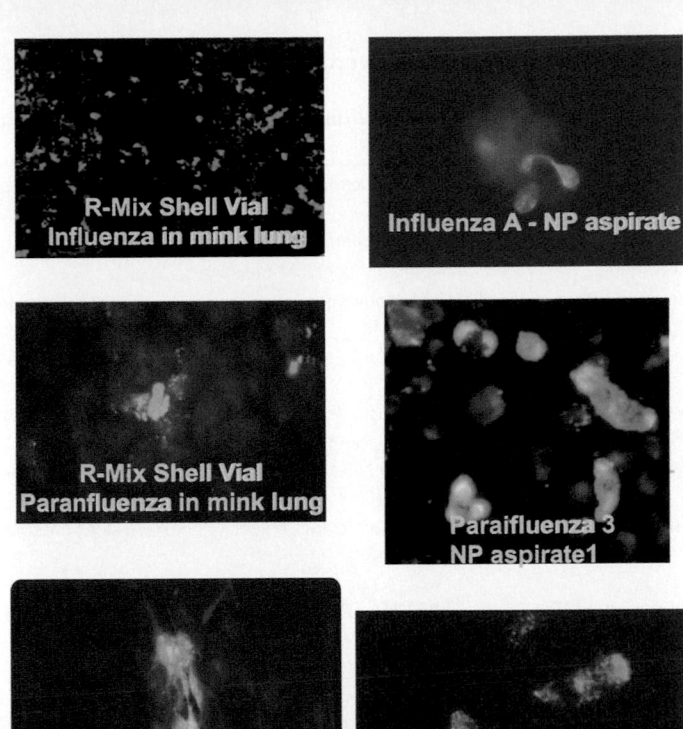

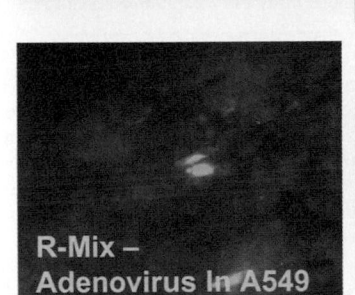

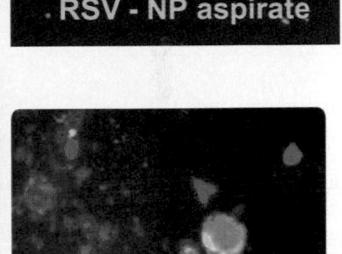

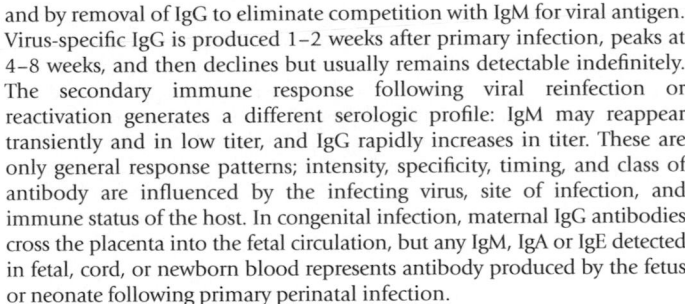

Figure 54–3 (cont'd)

and by removal of IgG to eliminate competition with IgM for viral antigen. Virus-specific IgG is produced 1–2 weeks after primary infection, peaks at 4–8 weeks, and then declines but usually remains detectable indefinitely. The secondary immune response following viral reinfection or reactivation generates a different serologic profile: IgM may reappear transiently and in low titer, and IgG rapidly increases in titer. These are only general response patterns; intensity, specificity, timing, and class of antibody are influenced by the infecting virus, site of infection, and immune status of the host. In congenital infection, maternal IgG antibodies cross the placenta into the fetal circulation, but any IgM, IgA or IgE detected in fetal, cord, or newborn blood represents antibody produced by the fetus or neonate following primary perinatal infection.

Serology is particularly helpful if specimen quality or transportation conditions have been suboptimal for culture or direct antigen testing. If viral disease was not suspected at initial evaluation, then serology may be the only diagnostic tool available once the opportunity for culture or antigen assays has passed. Serology is a logical diagnostic choice for viruses that require complex isolation procedures (EBV, human herpesvirus 6) or animal inoculation (arboviruses, some Coxsackie A viruses) or are a biohazardous risk (HIV, arboviruses, hemorrhagic fever viruses). For some infections, serology is fast and cheap; both measles and mumps can be diagnosed by culture but IgM-specific antibody is detectable within 3 days of the onset of illness. Rubella virus grows in cell culture but IgM serology is much simpler. Virus may no longer be present when symptomatic infection develops; WNV and other arboviruses are often cleared from spinal fluid by the time the patient develops encephalitis, making serology the preferred diagnostic method. Infections with a prolonged prodrome often have detectable antibody when the patient becomes symptomatic (EBV and CMV mononucleosis). Specific situations for serologic diagnosis are listed in Figure 54–2.

Specimen Collection and Transportation

Success with any diagnostic test is contingent upon proper specimen collection and transportation. The laboratory must have realistic guidelines for optimal specimen handling and a specimen ejection policy, and then circulate this information to the clinical staff and nursing units (Table 54–2). Specimens for culture, antigen and NAATs should be obtained during acute illness when viral shedding is highest; virus recovery is unreliable during convalescence.

Viral transport medium (VTM) contains a buffered salt solution, protein stabilizer, pH indicator, and antibiotics to inhibit bacterial and fungal contaminants. Multipurpose viral, chlamydial, and mycoplasmal transport media have been developed (M4, FlexTrans); most formulations can stabilize viruses for 24 hours or less (Johnson, 1990). All specimens except blood samples should be transported and stored until setup at 4°C. Room temperature transport of specimens may be unavoidable in some circumstances but physicians should appreciate the negative effect on recovery. Blood samples for virus isolation should be held at room temperature at all times and processed for culture the day of collection. Viral cultures are best set up the day specimens arrive in the laboratory, preferably within 36 hours of collection; at least one culture inoculation session should be scheduled during weekend shifts. Specimens should only be frozen (–20°C) as a last resort; blood and urine for CMV isolation or respiratory specimens for RSV should not be frozen.

Equipment and Supplies

Most virology equipment is relatively inexpensive and already in use in the microbiology and immunology laboratory sections. A class II biosafety laminar flow cabinet must be used for culture setup and whenever cultures

Table 54–2 Specimen collection for common viral syndromes

Syndrome	Common Viruses	Preferred Specimen and Transport Conditions	Specimen Quality Validation	Most Useful Tests
Bronchiolitis/bronchitis	RSV, PIV, adenovirus, influenza A and B	Nasopharyngeal aspirate, swab BAL; transport on ice	Ciliated columnar cells or alveolar macrophages	DFA, EIA, culture; nucleic acid test
Influenza	Influenza A and B			
Pneumonia	RSV, PIV, influenza A, adenovirus			
Conjunctivitis	HSV, adenoviruses, enteroviruses, VZV	Conjunctival scrapings swab in VTM; transport on ice	Epithelial cells	DFA, culture, nucleic acid test
Vesicular rash	HSV, VZV	Vesicular fluid/cells in VTM or slide smear for DFA; transport on ice	Epithelial cells	Nucleic acid test, culture, DFA
Meningitis	Enteroviruses, HSV, west Nile/arboviruses	CSF; transport on ice		Nucleic acid test, culture, IgM serology
Encephalitis	HSV, west Nile/arboviruses, rabies	CSF, fresh brain tissue; transport on ice		Nucleic acid test, culture, IgM serology
Enteritis	Rotavirus, norovirus, enteric adenoviruses	Fresh stool; transport promptly	Swab must be covered with stool	Rotavirus and adenovirus – EIA; norovirus – RNA amplification
Disseminated viral infection	CMV, HSV, VZV, adenovirus	Blood, tissue biopsy, BAL, CSF; transport immediately		Nucleic acid amplification (quantitative for CMV), culture
	HIV	Blood		Serology, HIV viral load
Prenatal/neonatal viral infection	HSV 1 and 2, CMV, enterovirus, parvovirus B19, Rubella	CSF, vesicular fluid, tissue biopsy, amniotic fluid, urine; transport immediately		Nucleic acid amplification, culture, serology

BAL = bronchoalveolar lavage; CMV = cytomegalovirus; CSF = cerebrospinal fluid; DFA = direct fluorescent antibody; EIA = enzyme immunoassay; HIV = human immunodeficiency virus; HSV = herpes simplex virus; PIV = parainfluenza virus; RSV = respiratory syncytial virus; VTM = viral transport medium; VZV = varicella zoster virus.

are manipulated, to protect the technologist from infectious aerosol and to reduce tissue culture contamination. A centrifuge with covered carriers to accommodate shell vials should be available. Incubators to maintain uninoculated cells and to incubate inoculated cultures are needed, preferably with an internal outlet for hook-up of a roller drum. Also needed are an inverted phase-contrast microscope to identify CPE in cell culture monolayers, and an epifluorescence microscope for DFA and indirect immunofluorescence assay (IFA) procedures, and freezer space at –20°C (–70°C, if available, is also desirable) for specimen and reagent storage. Liquid nitrogen is expensive and not essential for laboratories that purchase cell lines.

All essential supplies and reagents for identifying the common viruses are commercially available. Cell cultures are nourished by a balanced salt solution (Hanks or Earle) with added buffers, serum, and a nutrient mixture such as Eagle minimum essential medium (MEM). Eagle MEM is a precisely defined formulation of amino acids, sugars, vitamins, cofactors, and other metabolic requirements for the cell monolayer. Fetal bovine or calf serum (FBS) is a popular nutritional and hormonal supplement added to MEM; 5–10% FBS is used for cell culture growth medium and 2% for maintenance medium. Trypsin (0.25% solution), phosphate-buffered saline (PBS), glutamine and sodium bicarbonate solutions, VTM and antibiotic mixtures for specimen decontamination should also be stocked in the laboratory as needed (Clarke, 2004).

Laboratories undertaking viral diagnostic services for the first time should consider beginning with straightforward testing such as HSV culture. Influenza, RSV, and rotavirus assays and cultures can be added during the winter months. CMV identification is a priority for a hospital with immunocompromised patients. Enterovirus isolation could be offered initially for the summer and autumn. VZV, adenovirus, and parainfluenza virus cultures and antigen assays would be reasonable additions as staff time and expertise increases. The laboratory should be familiar with specimen collection and transport requirements of public health laboratories and reference laboratories that provide supplementary serology, antigen assay, and NAATs so that send-out specimens are processed efficiently.

Clinical Viral Infectious Syndromes

One approach to laboratory diagnosis separates viral infections into specific clinical syndromes; this encourages the physician to associate a reasonable but limited group of viruses with the patient's illness. The requisition/order screen should be designed to require specific patient demographic data, clinical diagnosis and suspected virus(es) so that the laboratory effort can be streamlined and focused on rapid, high-yield, and efficient testing. In this chapter the following viral diseases are discussed:

Herpetic mucocutaneous infections
Pediatric and adult respiratory syndromes
Infectious mononucleosis
Congenital and neonatal infections
Viral central nervous system infections
Viral exanthems and cutaneous infections
Viral enteric infections
Viral hepatitis and HIV and retrovirus infection
Viral infections in the immunocompromised host

Herpetic Mucocutaneous Infections

The Herpesviridae family contains two viruses that characteristically produce infections in the skin and squamous mucous membrane surfaces of the body: HSV and VZV. Both are commonplace and, while usually not life threatening, the effectiveness of acyclovir therapy has produced demand for prompt laboratory diagnosis, particularly for HSV (Corey, 2005). Acyclovir resistance has now been documented, as high as 10% in bone marrow transplant patients (Szatanek, 2004). VZV is discussed in the viral exanthem section of this chapter.

HSV is ubiquitous and infects all racial groups worldwide. The two strains of HSV (serotype 1 and serotype 2) share many molecular and biological features and both preferentially infect squamous epithelium; however, each has a unique antigenic profile and a somewhat distinctive epidemiology. HSV1 is transmitted via saliva to infect oropharyngeal and labiofacial surfaces. Lesions may develop on the exposed skin of wrestlers (herpes gladiatorum) or the hands of medical personnel after direct salivary contact (herpetic whitlow). Initial HSV1 infection usually occurs before puberty; primary infection is often asymptomatic, though a substantial minority develop fever and painful gingivostomatitis. HSV1 cases of genital ulcer disease have been reported (Ribes, 2001).

HSV1 directly infects ectodermal cells; as the virus replicates itself, squamous cells lose their cytoplasmic integrity, leak fluid, and separate from one another to create a vesicle. Surface bacteria convert the vesicle to a pustule, which then ulcerates when damaged epithelial cells completely lyse. Herpetic lesions heal without scarring as the epidermal layers regenerate. The immediate immune response involves natural killer cells, cytotoxic T lymphocytes, and production of neutralizing antibody. Despite cellular and humoral factors, however, HSV1 is able to migrate through sensory nerve fibers to the trigeminal ganglion and persist indefinitely in a dormant state in the neuronal nucleus (Corey, 2005). HSV episodically reactivates and travels back down neurosensory axons to the mouth and lips, where it again replicates in squamous cells. Most recurrent herpes infections are asymptomatic or produce transient vesicles with only cosmetic significance. With severe impairment of cell-mediated immunity (in AIDS and transplant patients), reactivation infection may be severe or even fatal. Encephalitis is another rare but devastating HSV1 infection. Both these complications are discussed in later sections of this chapter.

HSV2 infection is found principally in genital squamous surfaces and is transmitted through intimate sexual contact. About 40 million Americans are probably infected, with estimates of 1 million new cases annually. HSV2 recovery from children is most unusual and raises concern about sexual abuse; beginning with adolescence, however, seroprevalence rises steadily through middle age and is proportional to the number of sexual partners (Fleming, 1997). In the United States, HSV2 seroprevalence is 22%; in persons 13 years of age or older, the age-adjusted seropositivity has risen 30% since 1980. HSV2 produces the same pattern of primary and recurrent mucocutaneous lesions seen with oral HSV1. Latency is established in sacral neural ganglia, but reactivation rates are at least twice as high as with HSV1 and transient meningitis may occur. Primary and recurrent HSV2 lesions heal completely in people with normal cellular immune function. The principal concern is exposure of infants during vaginal delivery; neonatal herpes is discussed later in this chapter.

Specimen Collection and Handling Guidelines

HSV is probably the easiest and fastest human virus to cultivate in cell culture; antigen assays are also relatively straightforward procedures. Specimen collection is simple, and HSV is sufficiently durable that stat transport and laboratory handling are not essential.

Cell Culture Isolation of Herpes Simplex Virus

Swab specimens in VTM with antibiotics can tolerate room temperature (22°C) transportation delay of 12 hours with only modest viral loss. Specimens should be inoculated to cell culture the day of receipt, but overnight refrigeration is acceptable. HSV isolation is still the practical gold standard diagnostic test and is more sensitive than any antigen assay. HSV grows exceptionally well in a variety of cell lines; human fibroblasts (WI-38, MRC-5, foreskin) are popular choices but rabbit kidney, mink lung, HeLa, rhabdomyosarcoma (RD), Vero, and HEp-2 cell lines are also useful. Primary monkey kidney (PMK) is not reliable. Two tissue culture tubes (e.g., one rabbit kidney [RK] and one MRC-5) are usually inoculated; the procedure is summarized in Figure 54–4.

HSV replicates rapidly; CPE usually develops by the second or third day of incubation. Cultures from genital lesions that fail to show HSV CPE after 5–7 days of incubation are reported as negative; because other viruses (VZV, adenovirus, enterovirus, etc.) may be recovered from central nervous system (CNS), corneal, oral, and other nongenital sites, these cultures should be incubated for 2 weeks. Individual HSV-infected cells first become swollen and rounded (ballooning change), with cellular damage spreading rapidly across the monolayer. HSV2 frequently causes syncytium formation as the cytoplasmic membranes of infected cells coalesce (Fig. 54–4). This CPE is characteristic of but not unique for HSV; changes caused by other viruses, toxins, or even trichomonads may be confused with HSV CPE, so confirmation with a DFA stain is recommended. Monolayer cells are scraped off, transferred to a glass slide, fixed in acetone, and then stained with either monoclonal or polyclonal HSV antibodies (Lipson, 1991). Type-specific monoclonal DFA stains can distinguish HSV1 from HSV2; this information often adds little to the clinical impression, and serotyping may be reserved for cases with medicolegal concerns or clinical ambiguity.

The demand for HSV cultures led to the use of shell vial centrifugation-enhanced culture, in which viral antigen can be identified in the monolayer by DFA staining after only 1 day of incubation (Gleaves, 1985) (Fig. 54–4).

Direct Detection of Herpes Simplex Virus

A direct smear from a herpetic vesicle that is stained with Giemsa reagent may demonstrate viral multinucleated syncytial epithelial giant cells and intranuclear inclusions. The Tzanck smear is not specific for HSV infection (identical changes are seen in VZV chickenpox and shingles) and it is positive in only 67% of herpetic lesions at the vesicle stage. Immunostaining of direct smears (Fig. 54–3) with fluorescein- or immunoperoxidase-labeled HSV antibodies eliminates confusion with VZV, and viral antigen can be identified in cells that do not yet have nuclear inclusions or syncytium formation. However, when compared with culture, DFA staining has at

least a 20–30% false-negative error (Moseley, 1981; Lafferty, 1987). All negative direct specimen test results must be considered as potential false negatives that should be validated by parallel culture. On the other hand, PCR diagnosis of mucocutaneous genital herpes infection is 20–30% more sensitive than culture and can result in a marked decrease in turn around time compared with culture (Espy, 2000). PCR is superior for identification of asymptomatic mucocutaneous viral shedding, eight times more sensitive than culture (Cone, 1994). In evaluation of genital ulcer disease, multiplex NAAT showed 100% sensitivity for HSV detection along with substantially improved diagnosis of chancroid and primary syphilis (Orle, 1996).

Serologic Diagnosis

There is broad antigenic homology between HSV1 and HSV2, so accurate serologic testing requires antigens that are serotype-specific. EIA and Western blot methods that use unique HSV1 and HSV2 glycoprotein G (gG) envelope antigens do not detect crossreacting antibodies (Ashley, 1988; Morrow, 2003). The most valuable application of HSV2 specific antibody testing is serological assessment of pregnant women to predict neonatal transmission risk (Ashley, 1999; Cherpes, 2003).

Viral Respiratory Tract Infections

Every year there are several million outpatient visits and hospitalizations in the United States for respiratory tract infections, the majority of which are viral in origin. Infections range from trivial colds to serious laryngotracheobronchitis (croup), bronchiolitis, and pneumonia. Colds and pharyngitis are usually managed clinically with no laboratory testing; however, the number of antigen assay and culture requests for lower respiratory viral infection diagnosis can account for a sizable part of work load, particularly in winter (Table 54–1). Influenza viruses and RSV are the most important respiratory pathogens in adults; RSV, parainfluenza virus, influenza virus, and adenovirus are most significant in young children.

Influenza

Influenza A and B viruses cause annual cold weather outbreaks of acute febrile upper and lower respiratory tract illness with characteristic accompanying systemic features. Influenza A is usually more common than B, and produces more serious disease (Fig. 54–5). Influenza antigens change through point mutations in the genome (antigenic drift, influenza A and B) and through recombination of human and animal viral RNA segments (antigenic shift, influenza A), so antibodies from prior infections may not be protective in subsequent outbreaks. Influenza is easily spread person to person in aerosol droplets or on contaminated hands (Troanor, 2005).

Influenza virus replicates rapidly in the ciliated columnar cells of the pharynx and tracheobronchial tree. Onset of fever is usually abrupt; viral respiratory epithelial necrosis causes sore throat and cough, but associated myalgias, headache, and generalized weakness are typically more severe than respiratory symptoms. Uncomplicated influenza usually resolves after 4–5 days. Every year there are approximately 100 000 hospitalizations and 20 000 deaths in the United States linked to influenza. In a minority of patients, acute viral necrosis extends into the alveolar lining cells, producing severe potentially fatal pneumonia (Yeldandi, 1994). Most deaths are caused by secondary bacterial bronchopneumonia as the virus-damaged respiratory tract becomes infected with *Staphylococcus aureus*, *Streptococcus pneumoniae*, *Haemophilus influenzae*, or other bacteria from the pharynx. Secondary staphylococcal infection is particularly worrisome due to the now widespread distribution of community acquired methicillin-resistant *S. aureus*. Bacterial superinfection is more common in patients with pre-existing chronic lung disease or congestive heart failure. Myocarditis, meningoencephalitis, Reye syndrome, and Guillain–Barré syndrome are rare complications.

Influenza is diagnosed best during the first 2–3 days of illness when viral shedding is maximal. RT-PCR is the most sensitive method for diagnosis but is not widely available (Erdman, 2003; Templeton, 2004). Culture is the next most sensitive diagnostic test; nasopharyngeal secretions/nasopharyngeal aspirate (NPA) samples are ideal and expectorated sputum is acceptable if bronchial columnar cells, alveolar macrophages, or neutrophils are present; nasopharyngeal swabs and throat swabs may be satisfactory but often are suboptimal samples that cannot be assessed for adequacy. Shell vial culture with 1–2 days' incubation has excellent sensitivity (Dunn, 2004), and can affect management of the index patient or prophylaxis of contacts. Culture with traditional cell monolayers and red cell hemadsorption (Fig. 54–3) may not yield a positive result for 2–7 days.

VII

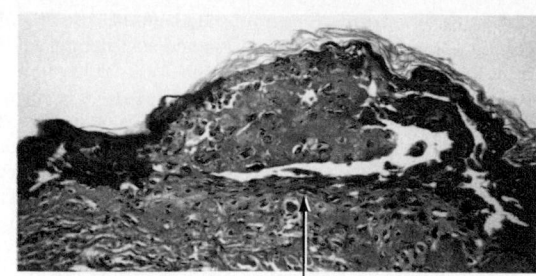

Sample fluid and cells

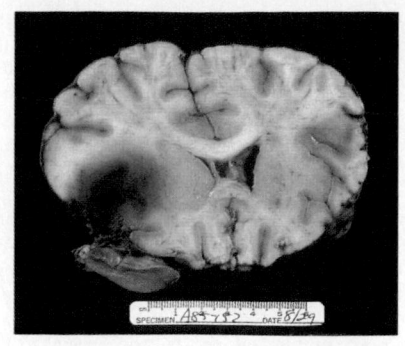
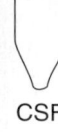

CSF, minimum 1ml.
Tissue biopsy or vesicle swab
in VTM; vortex, wring out swab.

CSF/body fluid
Min. 1 ml.

CSF

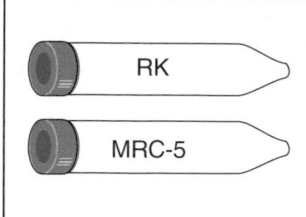

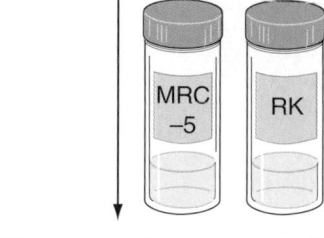

Purify viral DNA/remove inhibitors

Discard maintenance media from cell culture tubes. Inoculate 0.2–0.4 ml. VTM supernatant/tube. Hold tubes at 35C for 60 min. for viral adsorption. Discard inoculum fluid; add 2 ml. fresh maintenance medium. Incubate at 35 C for 5–7 days.

Check daily for CPE

Discard maintenance media from shell vials. Centrifuge shell vials at 700 x G for 60 min. Discard inoculum fluid; add 1 ml. fresh maintenance medium. Incubate at 35C for 16–36 hours.

Add sample to master mix and run amplified assay. Ideal assay amplifies and detects amplicons simultaneously (real time).

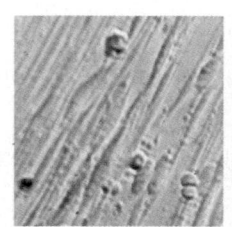
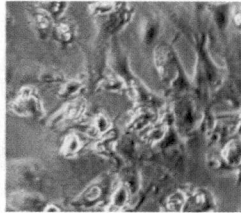

MRC-5   Rabbit kidney

Remove maintenance medium, wash monolayer 2x with PBS, fix with acetone for 10 min. Air-dry. DFA stain monolayer for HSV antigen. Report positive and negative results.

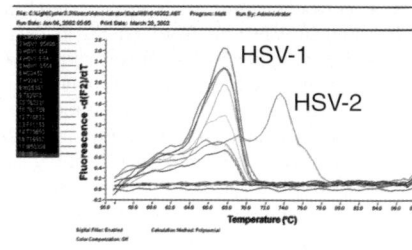

Real time HSV PCR

HSV-1

HSV-2

Confirm positive CPE with DFA stain to HSV antigen. Report all negative cultures at 5–7 days.

Melt temperature differentiation of HSV-1 and HSV-2

Figure 54–4 Traditional tube and shell vial cultures for herpes simplex virus (HSV) and HSV DNA amplification. CPE = cytopathic effect; CSF = cerebrospinal fluid; DFA = direct fluorescent antibody; PBS = phosphate-buffered saline; PCR = polymerase chain reaction; VTM = viral transport medium.

DFA stain of influenza antigen is useful for rapid diagnosis; NPA samples contain abundant virus-infected columnar epithelial cells and are the preferred specimen. Sensitivity ranges from 77–93% for detection of influenza A and from 70–80% for influenza B (higher in pediatric patients); specificity is greater than 95%, and is heavily influenced by the experience of the microscopist and specimen quality. Throat and nasopharyngeal swabs generally lack sufficient columnar cells for DFA staining. Commercial immunochromatographic EIA methods are rapid, easy to perform, and have good sensitivity for influenza antigen detection if performed with NPA; sensitivity with throat swabs is lower and throat swabs are considered suboptimal. Optical immunoassay of influenza A and B neuraminidase antigen also has good diagnostic sensitivity for NPS (80%) and for expectorated sputum (83%) (Mulford, 1999). Sensitivity is dependent on specimen quality; the best overall sample is NPA in both adult and pediatric groups; NPA collection is reviewed in Figure 54–6. EIA methods should be backed up with culture during non-epidemic periods since positive predictive value is poor in low prevalence settings.

Respiratory Syncytial Virus Bronchiolitis

RSV is the most important cause of serious lower respiratory viral disease in infants and young children (Anderson, 1990; Hall, 1998, 2001). RSV is transmitted by droplet aerosol and outbreaks recur every winter (Fig. 54–5). There is no vaccine for RSV. Immunity to RSV is incomplete and of short duration; multiple infections of decreasing intensity occur throughout life, although RSV may cause severe pulmonary disease in the elderly and in the immunocompromised host (Pohl, 1992; Falsey, 2005). RSV, like influenza, infects ciliated columnar epithelial cells from the nasopharynx to the distal bronchioles. The most serious RSV presentation is bronchiolitis; this occurs in babies under 1 year of age whose small terminal airways are easily occluded by necrotic epithelial cells and inflammatory debris. Bronchiolar obstruction leads to air trapping and hypoxia, which may be severe. Most critical RSV infections occur in premature infants, in children with underlying cardio-pulmonary disease or immunodeficiencies, and in transplant recipients;

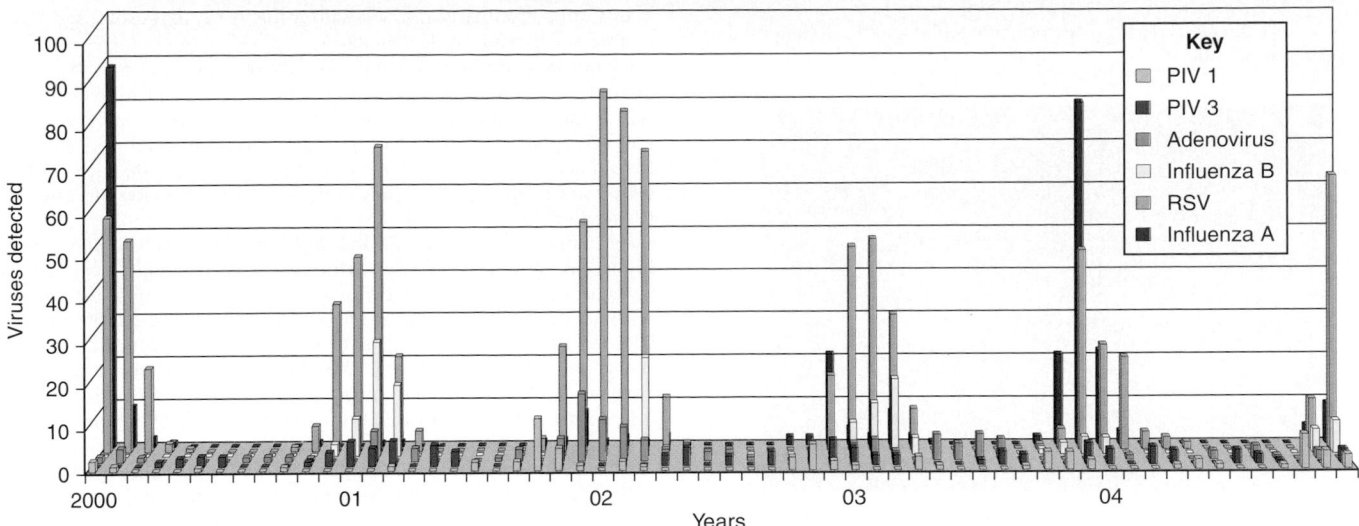

Figure 54–5 Seasonal variation of respiratory viral infections.

prophylaxis with RSV immunoglobulin is useful for premature infants (Meissner, 2003).

Rapid RSV diagnosis in the hospitalized patient is important for implementing infection control measures to prevent nosocomial spread (Hall, 1998). RSV is a particularly fragile and labile virus and may not remain viable if specimen transport is delayed. Once inoculated into cell culture, it replicates slowly with late development of CPE (Fig. 54–3); isolation times range from 3–10 days (Arens, 1986; Tristram, 2003). Shell vial culture improves RSV recovery somewhat and shortens isolation time to 2 days (Dunn, 2004). Detection of RSV antigen in respiratory secretions by DFA staining or by EIA is as sensitive as or superior to culture and result availability is clinically relevant, and rapid tests have become the definitive practical methods for RSV diagnosis in children (Ohm-Smith, 2004). EIA is easy and rapid to perform; however, stat kit reagents are somewhat expensive and methods do not include an automatic mechanism to verify specimen adequacy. DFA requires more time and interpretive expertise but it can easily be expanded to assay multiple viruses and confirmation of specimen quality is simple. RT-PCR has superior sensitivity over all other methods and is more reliable for geriatric specimens but is not yet readily available (Falsey, 2002; Perkins, 2005).

Croup

Croup is most commonly caused by parainfluenza virus (PIV) (Henrickson, 2003). PIV1 and PIV2 peak during cold weather; PIV3 causes disease year-round. PIVs (particularly PIV3) are the second most frequent viral lower respiratory tract infections in young children (Fig. 54–5). Viral epithelial necrosis and mucosal edema in the larynx, trachea, and large bronchi narrow the airway, producing hoarseness, barking cough, and the stridorous obstructed breathing pattern characteristic of croup. Immunity is transient and repeat infections are common; however, in older children and adults, symptoms are less severe and are centered in the upper respiratory tract. Culture of NPA is the most sensitive current method of diagnosis, but DFA demonstration of PIV antigen in NPA has good sensitivity, ranging from 69–85% (Costello, 1993). DFA-negative specimens should be cultured to maximize recovery.

Metapneumovirus

Human metapneumovirus (hMPV) is a recently recognized RNA virus, genus *Metapneumovirus*. Like RSV, hMPV causes a range of respiratory infections including upper airway disease, lower airway bronchitis and bronchiolitis, influenza-like syndrome, and pneumonia; hMPV has been implicated in 4–21% of infants with acute bronchiolitis (Maggi, 2003; Xepapadaki, 2004). Very young children, the elderly and the immuno-compromised account for most symptomatic infections, similar to RSV (Stockton, 2002; van den Hoogen, 2001, 2004). Seasonality somewhat similar to RSV, and infections recur throughout life. hMPV respiratory disease tends to be less harsh than RSV; coinfections with the two viruses are often more severe than infections with either alone (Konig, 2004).

Diagnosis of hMPV is currently limited to detection by RT-PCR; this is the 'gold standard' but is not realistic for most community hospitals. hMPV may grow in LLC-MK2 cells or Vero cells, but growth takes up to 14 days with no detectable CPE (Deffrasnes, 2005). Culture of NPA and bronchial specimens using a shell vial culture format and anti-hMPV monoclonal antibody DFA staining of the monolayer has been developed, and more widespread use of culture may lead to a better understanding of the true incidence of hMPV infection (Ebihara, 2005; Landry, 2005).

Specimen Collection

The respiratory myxoviruses and adenovirus all can infect ciliated columnar epithelial cells from the nasopharynx to the alveoli, so when lower airway disease (croup, bronchiolitis, pneumonia, or influenza) is suspected, the upper respiratory mucosa is still the easier and more accessible site to sample for culture or antigen assay. Specimens should be collected during the first few days of illness when viral replication is greatest. A throat swab placed in VTM with antibiotics may be accepted for influenza culture but yield is 10–20% less; expectorated sputum is also adequate for culture (Kimball, 1983; Yungbluth, 1998), particularly in adults who are coughing productively.

NPA can be collected by inserting a catheter attached to a syringe through the nares to the nasopharynx and instilling 1–3 mL of saline, and then aspirating mucosal secretions directly back into the syringe. All specimens should be transported on ice promptly to minimize RSV loss. Specimen quality should be verified before performing culture or antigen assay. NPA with at least two ciliated columnar epithelial cells per 250× field yields a fourfold greater recovery of respiratory viral pathogens (Table 54–3).

Virus Antigen Assay

Figure 54–6 outlines a culture and antigen assay procedure for respiratory virus diagnosis. Reproducible and accurate viral antigen detection by DFA requires interpretive expertise, so if possible, both viral culture and antigen assay should be done to maximize recovery. Hospitals with a large pediatric service routinely test respiratory specimens for a panel of viruses (RSV, influenza A and B, PIVs, and adenovirus) during winter months if budgets permit. Adults should be tested for influenza virus; RSV should also be considered for elderly patients. The NPA sample is used for EIA testing, and then is washed in PBS and centrifuged; the supernatant is used for virus culture; if DFA stains for viral antigens are ordered, the cell button is resuspended in PBS and spread on Teflon and poly-L-lysine-coated slides. Air-dried smears are fixed with 100% acetone and stained for viral antigen(s) using specific fluorescein conjugated antibodies with Evans blue counterstain. NPA cytospin preparations may increase cell recovery (Landry, 2000). Note the number of ciliated columnar epithelial cells and the degree of nonspecific staining caused by residual background mucus or neutrophils. Figure 54–3 shows NPA DFA stains positive for influenza A, parainfluenza 3, RSV, and adenovirus. Fluorescein-conjugated antisera are tested for specificity with a panel of known positive tissue culture control cells; reagent lots should show consistent cellular stain distribution and intensity. Overall,

Table 54–3 Virus recovery from Nasopharyngeal Aspirates: Relationship to Specimen Adequacy

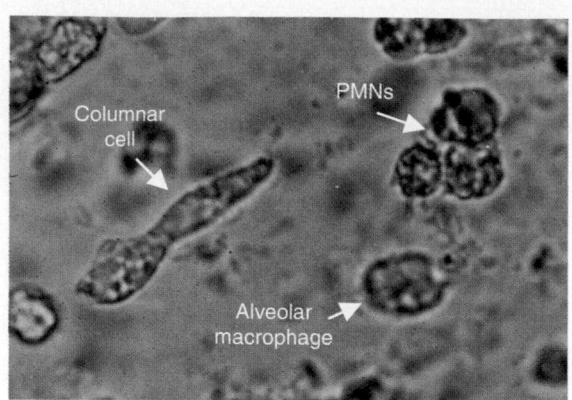

Sample (n = 2173)	Number of Specimens	% with Positive Virus Recovery
Nasopharyngeal secretions with <1 columnar cells per 250× field	243	6
Nasopharyngeal secretions with >2 columnar cells per 250× field	1930	27

11% of specimens had insufficient cells and required recollection.

DFA methods have excellent specificity and sensitivity (Hughes, 1988; Landry, 2000).

Several EIAs are commercially available for RSV and influenza A. The specificity and sensitivity of these products is quite good, comparable to DFA staining (Hughes, 1988; Thomas, 1991; Miller, 1993; Ohm-Smith, 2004; Weinberg, 2005). NPA should be checked for the presence of ciliated columnar epithelial cells; a wet mount slide prepared by mixing one drop of specimen with one drop of saline is scanned at 250× to verify that sufficient nasopharyngeal columnar cells are present (Table 54–3). Swab specimens from the throat or nasopharynx contain too little cellular material for cytologic prescreening.

Virus Isolation

The same specimen requirements and restrictions for antigen assays also apply to virus culture. NPA cultures in nonimmunocompromised adults and children can be modified to accommodate seasonal epidemics of influenza, RSV and PIV (Fig. 54–6). At a minimum, virology laboratories should attempt to isolate RSV and influenza during the winter; if staffing permits, PIV and adenovirus can be included for pediatric patients. Culture improves overall diagnostic yield beyond antigen assay by approximately 10–20% for all agents but RSV. Culture setup also can be expanded to recover viruses that are not included in the antigen assay panel. At present, hMPV culture is not offered in most hospitals.

Throat swabs for influenza culture only should be placed in VTM with antibiotics at collection and transported promptly, preferably on ice. Sputum that contains lower respiratory tract cells and/or acute inflammation is also acceptable for influenza culture and should be placed in VTM with antibiotics. The VTM vial should be vortexed vigorously; culture inoculation should not be delayed past 24 hours, and the day of collection is obviously preferable. For prompt recovery, the supernatant is inoculated into duplicate shell vials (either two trypsinized Madin–Darby canine kidney (MDCK) or two Rhesus monkey kidney (RMK)), which are refed after centrifugation with FBS-free MEM (bovine serum may contain antibodies to influenza virus). After 1–2 days' incubation at 35°C, shell vial monolayers are DFA-stained for influenza antigen. If staffing permits, a single back-up tube of RMK or MDCK also can be inoculated, incubated on a roller drum, and then checked for viral growth by adding fresh guinea pig red blood cells. Influenza virus, like PIV and measles, does not consistently produce CPE; however, these viruses make hemagglutinin antigens at the tissue culture surface, and guinea pig red cell adherence to the monolayer indicates hemadsorbing virus is present. A daily testing schedule for hemadsorption is preferable (Minnich, 1987). When hemadsorption is observed, the monolayer cells must be tested with a set of antisera to determine which virus is present. Figure 54–3 shows a RMK shell vial monolayer positive for influenza A after 2 days of incubation and

a RMK tube monolayer infected with influenza A that exhibits guinea pig erythrocyte hemadsorption on day 3.

Figure 54–6 outlines a shell vial culture procedure for NPA using a 'hybrid' cell monolayer that contains both A549 and mink lung (MvL) cells, which together support growth of RSV, influenza A and B, adenovirus and the parainfluenzas. Compared with traditional cell lines, this hybrid cell mix has overall recovery rates of 96–100%, with shortened turnaround time and overall reduced cost of materials and labor (Schindler, 1999).

Laboratories that culture for RSV only should consider using shell vials in place of traditional tubes to reduce recovery time. HEp-2 or A-549 cells in Eagle MEM supplemented with 2–5% fetal bovine serum support RSV replication. Cell culture tube monolayers should be checked daily for CPE for 10 days. Figure 54–3 shows typical RSV multinucleated cellular syncytium CPE, a pattern that is influenced by the cation content and freshness of the maintenance medium (Shahrabadi, 1988; Tristram, 2003). Adenovirus also replicates in HEp-2 and A-549 cell lines, and produces a grape-like rounding and swelling of monolayer cells, usually by 5–7 days; shell vial culture shorten adenovirus detection to 3 days (Fig. 54–3).

There are a number of serologic methods for detecting specific antiviral antibodies but none is practical for rapid diagnosis and clinical management. Serologic diagnosis is most useful for public health epidemiology studies.

Infectious Mononucleosis and Related Infections

Infectious mononucleosis is a common systemic lymphoproliferative disease usually caused by primary EBV infection. EBV is part of the Herpesviridae family, and like HSV, eventually infects the majority of the population worldwide. EBV is spread by saliva; primary infection in early childhood is usually asymptomatic but if delayed until the teen or young adult years often produces classic infectious mononucleosis. There are approximately 150 000 mononucleosis cases annually in the United States (Cohen, 2000; Schooley, 2005). EBV first infects the pharyngeal epithelium, so sore throat and fever typically mark the onset of infectious mononucleosis. EBV is strikingly lymphotrophic; it attaches to the C3d receptor (CD21) on the surface of B lymphocytes and initiates a polyclonal B-cell blastic proliferation that generates a polyclonal array of nonspecific IgM antibodies. The cell-mediated immune system responds with natural killer cells and CD8+ cytotoxic T lymphocytes to eradicate infected B cells. EBV-infected B lymphocytes accumulate in lymph nodes throughout the body, and defensive cytotoxic T lymphocytes infiltrate nodal interfollicular areas, spleen, and liver and circulate as atypical lymphocytes in the peripheral blood (Strickler, 1993). As cell-mediated factors control EBV replication, infectious mononucleosis symptoms diminish, and lymphadenopathy, splenomegaly and hepatitis subside.

Like other herpesviruses, EBV persists in a latent state. A small percentage of B lymphocyte nuclei contain Epstein–Barr-encoded RNA (EBER) and the Epstein–Barr nuclear antigen (EBNA) and latent membrane protein antigens that maintain the dormant EBV genome in the immortalized B cells. CD8+ T lymphocytes restrain EBV proliferation in these chronically infected B cells but asymptomatic EBV reactivation is common and up to 20% of healthy adults sporadically shed infectious virus in saliva. With impaired cell-mediated immunity (AIDS, organ transplantation, X-linked lymphoproliferative disease), EBV cannot be held in check, and overt diseases such as oral hairy leukoplakia and B cell lymphoproliferative disease and lymphoma may develop. EBV DNA and EBER are identified by NAAT in the spinal fluid of patients with primary CNS lymphoma and by ISH in transplant recipients who develop B cell lymphoproliferative disease during immunosuppressive therapy. EBV is also linked to nasopharyngeal carcinoma in Asians and to African Burkitt's lymphoma; EBV apparently functions as an initiator and then proliferative factors such as coinfection or immune dysregulation lead to malignancy.

Serologic Diagnosis

Cytotoxic T lymphocytes and apoptotic lymphocytes circulate in the blood in infectious mononucleosis (Fisher, 1996); atypical lymphocytosis (>10% total lymphocytes) is relatively insensitive for diagnosing EBV mononucleosis but has overall specificity of at least 95%. EBV can be cultivated in lymphoblastoid cell lines but positivity does not differentiate primary infection from reactivation. Serologic testing is the principal laboratory method for infectious mononucleosis diagnosis (Schooley, 2005). The polyclonal B lymphocyte proliferation of acute EBV infection generates a variety of transitory but generally harmless autoantibodies such as IgM anti-i (cold agglutinin), rheumatoid factor, and antinuclear antibody. Perhaps the most unusual immunoglobulins produced in infectious

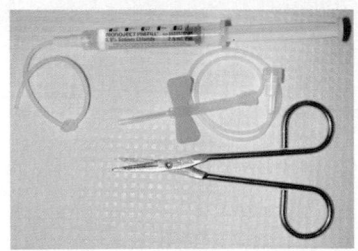

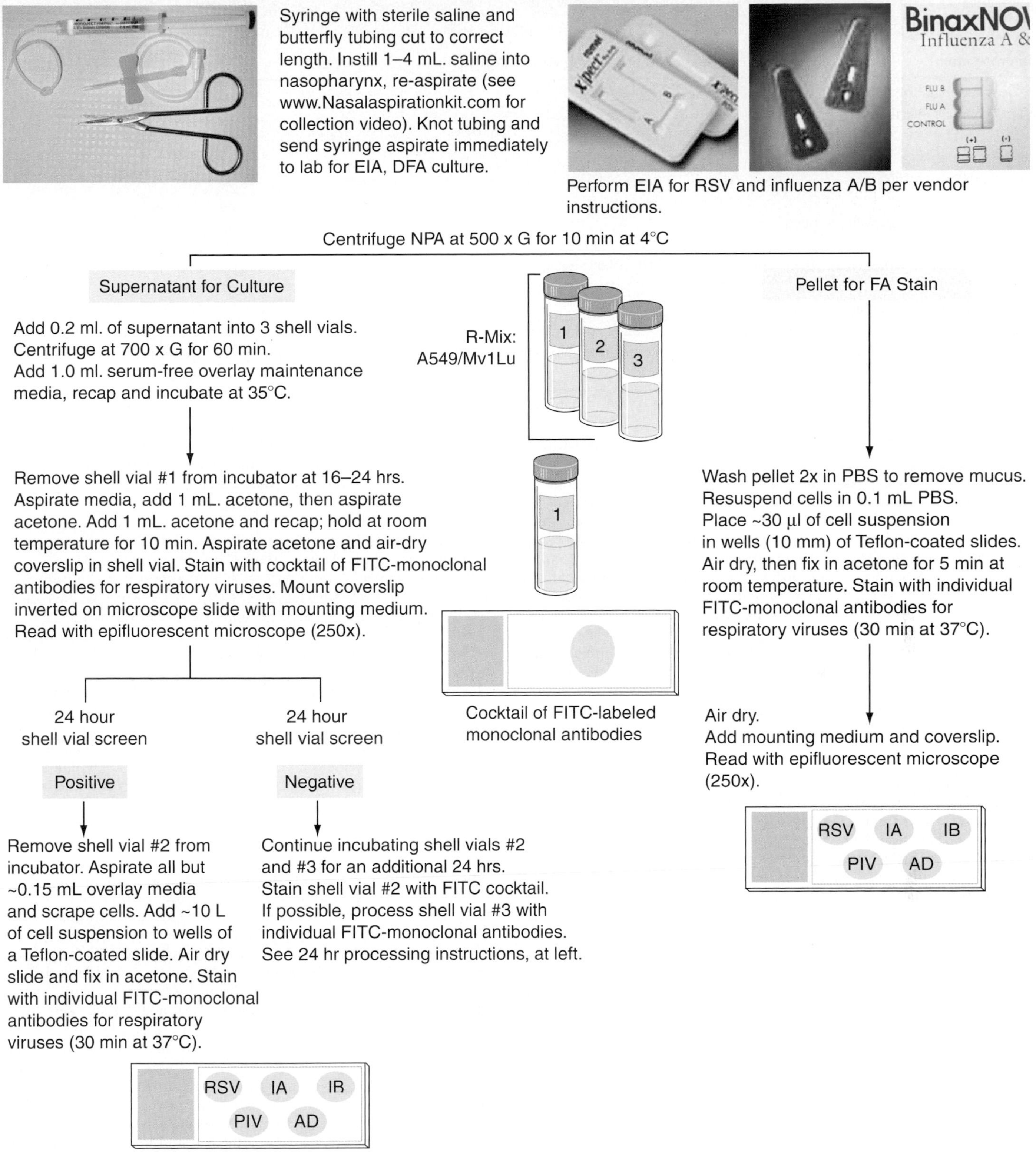

Syringe with sterile saline and butterfly tubing cut to correct length. Instill 1–4 mL. saline into nasopharynx, re-aspirate (see www.Nasalaspirationkit.com for collection video). Knot tubing and send syringe aspirate immediately to lab for EIA, DFA culture.

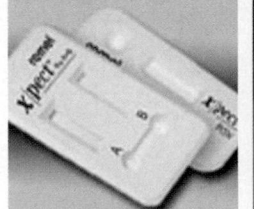
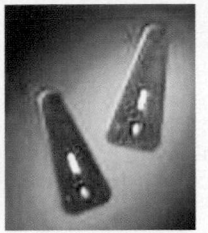
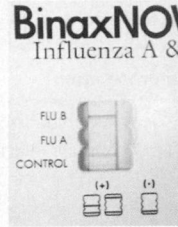

Perform EIA for RSV and influenza A/B per vendor instructions.

Centrifuge NPA at 500 x G for 10 min at 4°C

Supernatant for Culture

Add 0.2 ml. of supernatant into 3 shell vials.
Centrifuge at 700 x G for 60 min.
Add 1.0 ml. serum-free overlay maintenance media, recap and incubate at 35°C.

R-Mix: A549/Mv1Lu

Pellet for FA Stain

Remove shell vial #1 from incubator at 16–24 hrs. Aspirate media, add 1 mL. acetone, then aspirate acetone. Add 1 mL. acetone and recap; hold at room temperature for 10 min. Aspirate acetone and air-dry coverslip in shell vial. Stain with cocktail of FITC-monoclonal antibodies for respiratory viruses. Mount coverslip inverted on microscope slide with mounting medium. Read with epifluorescent microscope (250x).

Wash pellet 2x in PBS to remove mucus. Resuspend cells in 0.1 mL PBS. Place ~30 μl of cell suspension in wells (10 mm) of Teflon-coated slides. Air dry, then fix in acetone for 5 min at room temperature. Stain with individual FITC-monoclonal antibodies for respiratory viruses (30 min at 37°C).

24 hour shell vial screen

24 hour shell vial screen

Cocktail of FITC-labeled monoclonal antibodies

Air dry.
Add mounting medium and coverslip.
Read with epifluorescent microscope (250x).

Positive

Negative

Remove shell vial #2 from incubator. Aspirate all but ~0.15 mL overlay media and scrape cells. Add ~10 L of cell suspension to wells of a Teflon-coated slide. Air dry slide and fix in acetone. Stain with individual FITC-monoclonal antibodies for respiratory viruses (30 min at 37°C).

Continue incubating shell vials #2 and #3 for an additional 24 hrs. Stain shell vial #2 with FITC cocktail. If possible, process shell vial #3 with individual FITC-monoclonal antibodies. See 24 hr processing instructions, at left.

| RSV | IA | IB |
| PIV | AD | |

| RSV | IA | IR |
| PIV | AD | |

Figure 54–6 Laboratory diagnosis of respiratory viral infections with direct antigen assays enzyme immunoassay (EIA) and direct fluorescent antibody (DFA) and shell vial culture. FITC = fluorescein isothiocyanate; PBS = phosphate-buffered saline; RSV = respiratory syncytial virus.

mononucleosis are the Paul–Bunnell heterophile antibodies. These IgM-class antibodies have affinity for sheep, horse, and bovine erythrocytes, and are not directed against any EBV antigens. They are apparently random antibodies produced during EBV-induced B lymphocyte polyclonal proliferation; they emerge during the first week of infectious mononucleosis, decline during convalescence, and are usually undetectable by 3–6 months. Various heterophile antibodies develop during serum sickness and occasionally in other viral infections; however, heterophile antibody with strong affinity for beef erythrocyte antigens unchanged by adsorption with guinea pig kidney antigen (the differential absorption

test) is specific for acute EBV infectious mononucleosis. Several commercial assays directly mix patient serum on a slide with a suspension of guinea pig kidney antigen followed by addition of preserved equine or bovine erythrocyte antigen, often bound to latex particles; agglutination occurs almost immediately if infectious mononucleosis heterophile antibody is present. Rapid agglutination tests and solid phase modifications are approximately 80–90% sensitive, with a false-positive rate of less than 2% and a positive predictive value of 95% or greater, and are excellent point of care assays (Farhat, 1993; Linderholm, 1994; Gerber, 1996; Rogers, 1999). Their chief limitation is sensitivity: heterophile antibody is present in over

Table 54–4 Serologic profiles in Epstein–Barr virus infection

Interpretation	Heterophile Antibodies (IgM)	VCA (IgM)	VCA (IgG)	EA (IgG)	EBNA-1 (IgG)
Never infected (susceptible)	–	–	–	–	–
Current primary infection	+/– (50–85%)*	+ (70–100%)	+ (98–100%)	+ (60–80%)	– (0%)
Infectious mononucleosis	++	++	++	++	–
Recent primary infection	–/+	–/+	++	+	–
Remote past infection	–	–	++	+	+
Immunodeficient patient with persistent activation	+/–	–/+	++	++	+/–

Atypical serological profiles may require further testing (VCA-IgG avidity testing, Western blot, or polymerase chain reaction) for evaluation

* Positive results are lower in younger patients.

EA = early antigen; EBNA = Epstein–Barr nuclear antigen; VCA = viral capsid antigen.

Source: adapted from Hess RD: Minireview. Routine Epstein–Barr virus diagnostics from the laboratory perspective: still challenging after 35 years. J Clin Microbiol 2004; 42:3381–3387

90% of teens and adults but in fewer than 40% of younger children with EBV infectious mononucleosis.

As EBV evolves from primary infection into latency, various EBV antigens are sequentially expressed, and the specific antibodies generated are valuable markers of the stage of infection. The structural nucleocapsid protein viral capsid antigen (VCA) is produced during acute lytic infection; VCA IgM is a specific and sensitive marker of acute primary EBV infection; VCA IgG is usually present with onset of symptoms and persists for life. The early antigens (EAs) (DNA polymerase and thymidine kinase) are produced during acute infection and active EBV replication; antibody to EA-D is present in recent infection, but EA-R antibody is a persistent late marker. As acute mononucleosis subsides, a small percentage of Epstein–Barr-immortalized B lymphocytes escape immune destruction and latently retain EBV DNA as a circularized episome; EBNA is responsible for duplication and survival of this episome. Therefore, EBNA IgG typically develops after acute EBV infection has resolved.

The serologic patterns encountered in the various stages of EBV infection are summarized in Table 54–4. IFA serologic assays use lymphoblastoid cell lines with EBV production arrested at specific stages for expression of specific antigens; IFA methods are sensitive and specific, but have some interpretive subjectivity. EIA methods using purified or recombinant VCA show better than 95% sensitivity and almost 100% specificity, and have the advantage of objective interpretation and automated processing (Gerber, 1996; Chan, 1998; Tranchard-Bunel, 1999; Hess, 2004). Most physicians rely upon demonstration of atypical lymphocytes in peripheral blood, rapid heterophile screens, and IgM and IgG VCA for diagnosis of infectious mononucleosis. Quantitative tube heterophile reference methods, IgG-EBNA, and IgG-EA are procedurally more complex and have less practical applicability.

Heterophile-Negative Infectious Mononucleosis

Of the many patients who present with typical clinical features of infectious mononucleosis, 70% or more have a positive heterophile test, identifying EBV as the cause. Of the 30% who lack heterophile antibody, up to half are IgM-VCA positive, which also verifies acute EBV infection. In approximately 15% of patients with a febrile lymphoproliferative mononucleosis syndrome, primary infection with *Toxoplasma gondii*, CMV, human herpesvirus 6 (HHV6), or HIV is demonstrated; in the remaining 5–10%, no etiology is established.

Toxoplasmosis is discussed in Chapter 61; accurate diagnosis is most critical in pregnancy, in immunocompromised hosts and in chorioretinitis (Remington, 2004). Primary CMV infection acquired in childhood is usually asymptomatic, whereas teens and adults may have a systemic febrile lymphoproliferative illness (Wreghitt, 2003). Isolation of CMV from saliva or urine is not helpful, because asymptomatic reactivation and shedding is so common. Recovery of CMV from circulating leukocytes is valid and sensitive but is expensive and time-consuming compared with serodiagnosis. CMV IgM IFA serology is complicated by the fact that CMV-infected substrate cells express receptors for immunoglobulin Fc; the anticomplement IFA method (ACIF) is procedurally more complex but reduces this false-positive error. IgM-specific EIAs have overall accuracy that is comparable to ACIF-IFA IgM assay and have less interpretive subjective variation (Smith, 1987; VanEnk, 1991; Roseff, 1993).

HHV6 is another ubiquitous lymphotrophic virus with affinity for T cells. HHV6 causes roseola infantum (exanthem subitum), a common febrile exanthem in young children (Braun, 1997; Zerr, 2005). Delay of primary infection past childhood is associated with mononucleosis (Akashi, 1993). Both IFA- and EIA-specific IgM assays can diagnose acute infection; virus can be identified in saliva and blood with PCR but this is impractical for routine diagnosis (Steeper, 1990; Chiu, 1998; Zerr, 2005).

Infection with HIV1 can produce an acute illness that clinically mimics EBV mononucleosis (Kessler, 1987). Up to 50% of patients develop fever, lymphadenopathy, atypical lymphocytosis and occasionally mild hepatocellular damage or meningoencephalitis. Standard anti-HIV EIA usually fails to detect specific IgG antibody during this early phase of infection, but quantification of plasma HIV by RT-PCR is typically high (10^5 copies/mL) (Henrard, 1994). EIA, Western blot, and IFA serologic tests all become positive for HIV antibodies within 1–3 months, as features of acute infection resolve (Schupbach, 2003).

Figure 54–7 shows an algorithmic approach for the serologic evaluation of a patient with symptoms of acute mononucleosis. Despite extensive laboratory testing for these acknowledged causes of mononucleosis, no etiologic agent is identified in 5–10% of cases.

Chronic Fatigue Syndrome

Both the medical and lay press have discussed at length a clinical entity characterized by persistent disabling fatigue accompanied by fever, pharyngitis, tender lymphadenopathy, arthralgias, and myalgias (Holmes, 1987, 1988; Klonoff, 1992). While the clinical features of this syndrome suggest an infectious cause, none has yet been clearly identified. Initial reports implied that EBV, either as chronically persistent primary or reactivated infection, was responsible because many patients had high titers to EBV VCA and EA. However, serologic tests were neither standardized nor reproducible, and EBV culture and ISH performed on saliva and circulating leukocytes showed no difference between chronic fatigue patients and normal controls. Some studies have suggested a role for CMV, *T. gondii*, HHV6 and HHV7, and human T-cell leukemia virus (HTLV), but other reports have failed to verify a causative role (Gold, 1990; Reeves, 2000). Immunologic and serologic testing is not helpful for diagnosis or prognosis. Chronic fatigue syndrome remains defined by clinical signs and symptoms rather than laboratory test results (Lloyd, 1998; Gantz, 2001).

Congenital and Perinatal Viral Infections

The pregnant uterus is a sterile secluded environment that shelters the fetus from external microbial injury. Maternal vaginal bacteria that ascend through a flawed cervical barrier cause many infections in pregnancy, but maternal infection also can spread hematogenously to the fetus across the placenta or can directly involve the baby at the time of vaginal delivery. These perinatal infections are collectively named TORCH infections, for *toxoplasma* (see Ch. 61), *rubella*, *cytomegalovirus*, *herpes* simplex virus, and *other* organisms such as HIV, parvovirus, enterovirus, and *Treponema pallidum* (see Ch. 58). Infections with these agents may be silent or cause only minor symptoms in the mother; however, the immature fetal

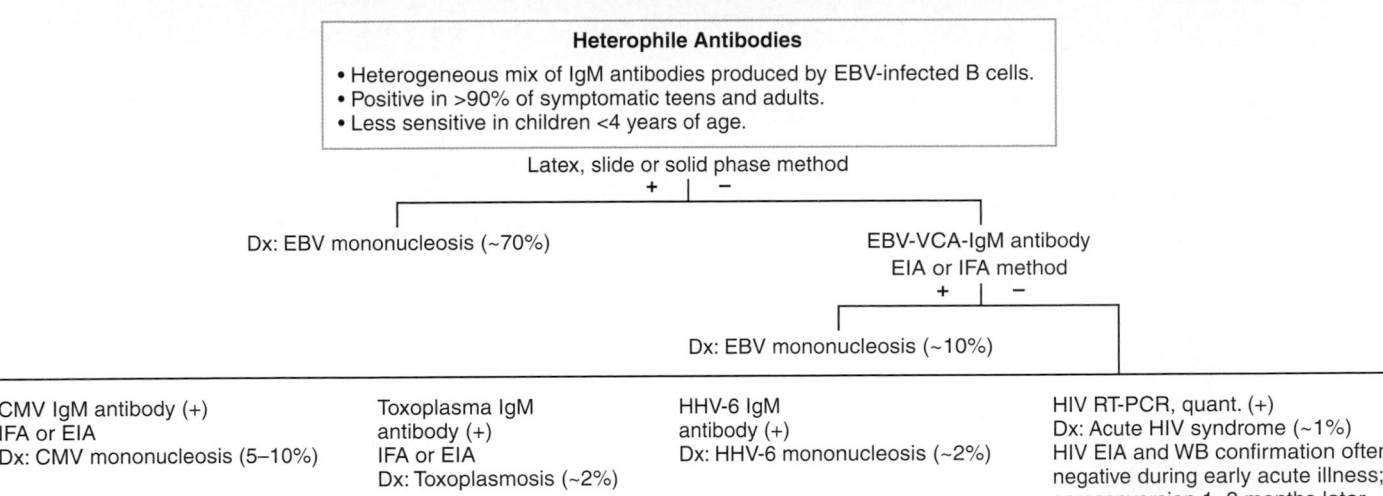

Figure 54–7 Serologic evaluation of patients with clinical symptoms of acute infectious mononucleosis and atypical lymphocytosis. No diagnosis is established in 5–10% of cases. CMV = cytomegalovirus; Dx = diagnosis; EBV = Epstein–Barr virus; EIA = enzyme immunoassay; HHV = human herpes virus; HIV = human immunodeficiency virus; IFA = indirect fluorescent antibody; Ig = immunoglobulin; RT-PCR = reverse-transcriptase polymerase chain reaction; VCA = viral capsid antigen; WB = Western blot.

immune system does not generate an effective cellular or humoral response, and tissue necrosis may be severe or even fatal.

Diagnosis of perinatal infections centers on two issues: identification of acute maternal infection (particularly primary infection) and verification of involvement of the fetus or newborn. Maternal infection is best established by recovery of the suspected organism but for many organisms this is impractical and serologic demonstration of specific IgM antibody, while imperfect, is the first-line diagnostic test. Maternal infection crosses the placenta in 30–60% of cases. Ultrasound may detect fetal organ damage (microcalcifications, microcephaly, hydrocephalus, organomegaly, hydrops, etc.), but recovery of the organism by culture, demonstration of its antigen or genome in fetal blood or tissues, or detection of specific antibody, is required to prove fetal infection. Test selection for diagnosis of common perinatal and congenital infection is summarized in Table 54–5. Routine screening of all pregnant women for immunity to rubella is standard care but testing for toxoplasma, HSV, and CMV antibodies is not advised. IgM serologic methods in particular may show inter- and intra-laboratory variation, with false-negative and false-positive errors; IgG assays do not differentiate primary from recurrent or latent maternal infection and cannot predict fetal involvement. Testing should be reserved for mothers with suspected infection.

Cytomegalovirus

CMV is the most common intrauterine infection and affects 1% of liveborn babies in the US. About 90% of these infants are asymptomatic at birth; isolation of CMV from urine or saliva or detection of IgM CMV may be the only marker of congenital infection. The symptomatic 10% may present with jaundice, hepatosplenomegaly, and pancytopenias; approximately 10% of these will die and the remainder will suffer permanent neurologic sequelae. Primary CMV infection in the mother is often viremic, with risk of hematogenous transplacental fetal infection and prenatal tissue injury (Stagno, 1982; Revello, 2002). Reactivation CMV infection in the mother can also cross the placenta but maternal IgG CMV antibody also traverses the placenta and is somewhat protective; these infants are usually asymptomatic but 5–15% have sensory neural hearing loss or neurodevelopmental difficulties (Istas, 1995). Maternal reinfection with a new CMV strain has a greater risk of causing a symptomatic congenital infection (Boppana, 2001).

IgM-specific assays have shifted from complement fixation, IFA, and anticomplement IFA methods to EIA tests that use refined recombinant CMV antigens and IgM capture to improve specificity and sensitivity. IgM may persist for more than 3 months in at least one third of adult women, obscuring somewhat the interpretive value of a positive result during pregnancy. CMV IgG avidity testing may be useful in dating recent vs. remote infection, similar to assessment of toxoplasma serology in pregnancy (Revello, 2002; Remington, 2004). Identification of CMV viremia in a nonimmunocompromised pregnant woman through shell vial culture of peripheral blood leukocytes or detection of CMV pp65 antigenemia or CMV DNA by PCR in blood is conclusive evidence of primary maternal infection. However, risk of fetal involvement is

estimated at about 40% and no test performed on the mother can predict fetal infection accurately.

The most reliable prenatal tests to verify fetal infection are viral culture and PCR detection of CMV in amniotic fluid, which have a combined sensitivity of 75–92% (Revello, 2002). Virus in amniotic fluid indicates overflow shedding from an infected fetus and a positive result has 100% specificity for disease. Detection of CMV-IgM in fetal cord blood is less sensitive(55–60%), because of delay in fetal immune response following exposure; cordocentesis CMV DNA PCR has sensitivity of 84%. High CMV viral load in amniotic fluid has been proposed as an indicator of severity of fetal tissue damage.

IgM CMV in cord blood collected at delivery is also diagnostic but is false-negative in 30% (Fowler, 1992). Recovery of CMV by culture or PCR from newborn urine, saliva, cerebrospinal fluid (CSF), or blood is also very sensitive; PCR DNA detection is almost 100% sensitive. Specimens must be collected during the first 2 weeks after birth to avoid confusion with postnatally acquired infection (Nelson, 1995; Revello, 2002). There is no defined predictive value of monitoring viral load. Typical CMV nuclear inclusions in urine cytology preparations are specific but very insensitive; even autopsy material may have few remaining diagnostic cells if tissue necrosis is advanced.

Rubella

Rubella (German measles) is highly communicable and produces mild fever and a transient rash in children and adults. All infections are viremic, and transplacental spread during the first trimester produces devastating teratogenic cardiac, ocular, and brain malformations (Schluter, 1998). Rubella is no longer endemic in the US because of widespread vaccination; genome analysis demonstrates that most recent rubella cases are imported from Latin America. Routine prenatal screening is standard practice. Only four cases of congenital infection have been identified since 2001, three of which occurred in immigrant mothers (MMWR, 2005). When acute rubella is suspected in a pregnant woman, the most straightforward diagnostic method is assay of maternal serum for antirubella IgM by EIA or IFA. Culture of rubella is technically complex and not routinely available. RT-PCR for rubella virus RNA performed on amniotic fluid is 100% sensitive and specific and can also be performed on placenta and autopsy tissues (Revello, 1997; Mace, 2004). The congenitally infected newborn is IgM-positive and also excretes rubella in urine for months to years.

Herpes Simplex Virus

Primary acquisition of genital HSV during pregnancy carries a high risk of ascending herpetic chorioamnionitis with spontaneous abortion, preterm labor, and mucocutaneous exposure of the baby during vaginal delivery (Brown, 1987). Primary genital HSV infection rather than recurrences put the baby at great risk for two reasons: the total number of lesions is often higher with primary infection, and maternal serum contains IgM but little or no IgG for transplacental passive protection of the baby (Prober, 1987).

Most babies have a vertex presentation during labor, so the scalp and face are the first to encounter HSV in the maternal tract; viral exposure on

Table 54–5 Laboratory testing for congenital and perinatal infections

Pathogen	Maternal Serology	Culture, Antigen Assay, Amplified Nucleic Acid Tests	Fetal or Newborn Serology
Cytomegalovirus	IgM EIA IgG avidity	CMV culture: maternal blood CMV culture: newborn urine, saliva, blood, tissues (first 2 weeks) CMV nuclear inclusions: tissues CMV PCR: amniotic fluid, in utero cord blood CMV PCR: newborn blood, tissues	IgM EIA
Herpes simplex virus	IgM EIA for HSV1 and HSV2 (glycoprotein G)	HSV PCR or culture: newborn conjunctiva, oral mucosa, skin, CSF HSV nuclear inclusions: newborn tissues, skin lesions	IgM EIA or IFA
Enterovirus		Amplified probe: newborn CSF, blood, tissues, throat Enterovirus culture: newborn blood, CSF, tissues, stool, throat Request enterovirus typing from Public Health Laboratory	
Parvovirus B19	IgM EIA or IFA PB19 PCR: blood	PB19 PCR: maternal blood Ground glass viral nuclear inclusions in erythroblasts PB19 ISH in erythroblasts PB19 PCR: placenta, fetal tissues, blood	IgM EIA
Hepatitis B virus	HBsAg, HBc-IgM, Anti-HBsAg	Quantitative PCR, newborn vaccination and immune globulin	
Human immunodeficiency virus	HIV EIA and Western blot HIV RNA quantification	Newborn HIV DNA PCR HIV RNA RT-PCR after 3 months age	Monitor HIV EIA for possible seroreversion (6–18 months)
Rubella	IgM EIA or IFA	Rubella culture: newborn urine Rubella RT-PCR: amniotic fluid, placenta, fetal or newborn tissue	IgM EIA or IFA

HBc = hepatitis B core antigen; HBsAg = hepatitis B surface antigen; CMV = cytomegalovirus; CSF = cerebrospinal fluid; EIA = enzyme immunoassay; HIV = human immunodeficiency virus; HSV = herpes simplex virus; IFA = indirect immunofluorescence assay; Ig = immunoglobulin; ISH = in situ hybridization; PCR = polymerase chain reaction.

the chest wall and buttocks occurs in breech delivery. Vesicles develop where skin and mucous membranes are directly inoculated with virus. Since the newborn immune response is still immature, a baby's chief resource for modifying infection is maternal IgG-HSV; when this passive protection is lacking, viral replication and visceral dissemination can proceed unchecked (Whitley, 1988). Conjunctival and oral mucosa and skin lesions are usually rich in virus; if dissemination occurs, any visceral organ can be infected.

Obstetrical management is based on several findings. Routine HSV culture of all mothers or infants at the time of delivery has a 0.2% yield and is not recommended (Prober, 1988). Prenatal HSV surveillance cultures of women with known recurrent genital herpes fails to predict which mothers will shed virus at the time of delivery (Arvin, 1986).

Studies of women who experienced their first recognized episode of genital herpes during pregnancy demonstrated that half had true primary genital herpes, and they had a high rate of complications (herpetic amnionitis, preterm labor, severe neonatal infections); almost half of mothers who acquired their primary infection shortly before labor had severely affected babies (Brown, 1997). Mothers with recurrent genital herpes had a much lower rate of neonatal infection, with involvement confined to mucocutaneous sites and no visceral dissemination (Brown, 1987, 1991).

It is accepted practice that women in labor who have genital lesions suspicious for herpes are managed with cesarean section to prevent possible exposure of the baby. Women with a history of recurrent genital herpes can deliver vaginally if active lesions are not present but careful

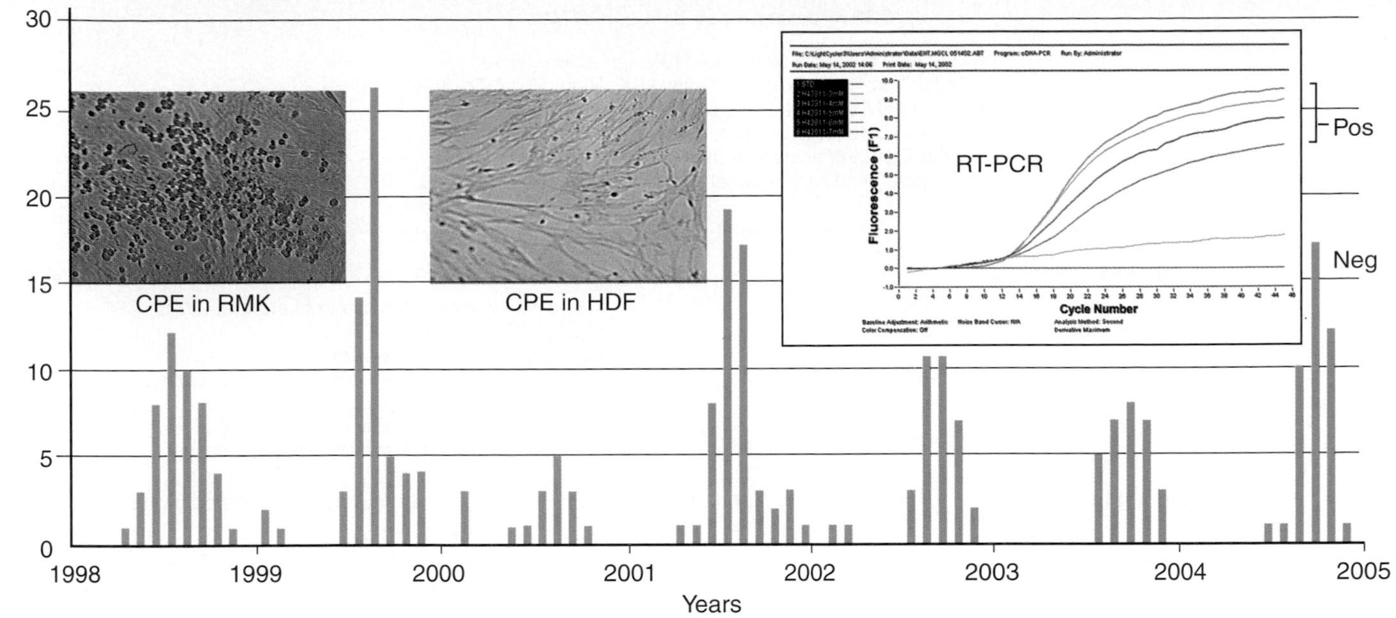

CPE in RMK

CPE in HDF

RT-PCR

Pos

Neg

Figure 54–8 Enterovirus detection by cytopathic effect (CPE) in cell cultures and by reverse transcriptase-polymerase chain reaction (RT-PCR). Seasonal variation with warm weather peaks of activity. HDF = human diploid fibroblasts; RMK = Rhesus monkey kidney. (Advocate Lutheran General Hospital, Park Ridge, IL.)

clinical monitoring of their newborns (including HSV culture of conjunctiva, oral mucosa, and any suspicious cutaneous lesions) is warranted. Neonatal herpes infection may be silent for up to several days before disease becomes apparent. Despite antiviral therapy, disseminated infection is often fatal; infants with infection confined to the central nervous system who survive are always severely retarded.

Laboratory diagnosis of HSV infection was discussed above. Type-specific HSV serology is now available and can identify seronegative women with seropositive partners, highlighting risk for acquiring infection during pregnancy (Ashley 1999; Cherpes, 2003). Tzanck smears and rapid antigen assays are often positive for vesicle lesions but cannot replace culture (which yields a positive result in 24 hours, especially when shell vials are used). Identification of HSV DNA by PCR in neonatal serum, spinal fluid, or mucocutaneous lesions has greater sensitivity than culture and is particularly valuable for detection of virus in CSF and for following therapy in babies with known CNS involvement (Kimberlin, 1996, 2004).

Human Immunodeficiency Virus, Parvovirus, Enterovirus and Hepatitis B Virus

HIV can spread hematogenously to the fetus, with placental trophoblast and Hofbauer macrophages acting as a cellular reservoir. However, approximately 75% of perinatal infections are acquired at delivery when the baby is exposed to maternal blood. Perinatal risk of HIV acquisition varies from 13–45%, depending on maternal HIV-1 viral load, but transmission rates are reduced to less than 2% by administration of antiviral drugs to the mother during pregnancy and labor and to the newborn (Watts, 2002). HIV is also transmissible postpartum in leukocytes in breast milk.

Diagnosis of maternal HIV infection is straightforward (positive EIA for HIV antibody with Western blot confirmation). Routine screening is strongly recommended in the first trimester and seropositive mothers should be offered antiviral prophylaxis. Maternal IgG crosses the placenta and persists in infant blood for up to 15 months, so standard EIA HIV serologic tests cannot be used to diagnose neonatal infection. Variations of both EIA and Western blot tests for detection of IgM and IgA antibodies (neither IgA nor IgM are passively transferred to the fetus and represent antibody made by the baby) can accurately identify an infected baby; sensitivity is age-dependent, and testing is not reliable in the first 3 months after birth. HIV p24 antigen assay also has suboptimal sensitivity during the immediate postnatal period (Quinn, 1991; Sison, 1992). If infection occurred in utero, newborn blood is positive for HIV DNA that has been transcribed and integrated into his circulating lymphoid cells. HIV-DNA PCR has a diagnostic sensitivity of over 95% at 1 month of age (Rogers, 1989; Bremer, 1996). HIV RNA RT-PCR assay is positive at birth if the baby was infected transplacentally, and becomes positive within

several weeks when the baby was infected during delivery. HIV RNA RT-PCR is also used for quantitative monitoring to assess the baby's response to antiretroviral therapy.

Parvovirus B19 (PB19) causes the benign, self-limited childhood exanthem erythema infectiosum (fifth disease) (Heegaard, 2002; Young, 2004). Approximately 50% of young women are seronegative and infection in pregnancy has a 25% risk of fetal infection; fetal death estimates vary from 2–38% (Alder, 1993). PB19 targets erythroid progenitor cells; virolytic cytotoxicity causes fetal anemia, hydrops, and intrauterine demise (Anand, 1987; Tolfvenstam, 2001). Infected erythroblasts have characteristic ground-glass nuclear inclusions. Parvovirus can only be cultivated in human bone marrow containing erythrocytic precursor cells. Acute infection is diagnosed serologically by detecting specific IgM in maternal or fetal blood, or by ISH or PCR detection of viral DNA in amniotic fluid or cord blood (Bruu, 1995; Zerbini, 1996).

Enterovirus infection is very common, with 10 million or more cases each year in the US. Many enteroviral infections are viremic; maternal infection just prior to delivery spreads virus across the placenta to the fetus and the baby is born with disseminated virus but with no passively acquired maternal IgG antibody to modify infection. Nosocomial outbreaks with nursery personnel as the source of virus have also been reported. Echovirus 11 is particularly virulent, causing hepatocellular necrosis and meningoencephalitis that is often fatal. Coxsackie B viruses can produce neonatal myocardial injury (Bryant, 2004). Perinatal infection with other enteroviruses usually is benign. RT-PCR and NASBA NAATs that detect a common sequence present in all enteroviruses have excellent sensitivity, superior to standard culture (Abzug, 1995; Landry, 2003). Echovirus grows well in shell vial and standard tube cultures (PMK, HDF, and RD cell lines); suitable specimens for viral culture include neonatal blood, CSF, throat, and rectal swab samples, or tissues from fatal cases. Typing of enterovirus can usually be obtained through regional or national public health laboratories (Modin, 1986).

Maternal infection with hepatitis B virus is often transmitted vertically; the baby may be infected transplacentally or during delivery with exposure to maternal blood. Screening for hepatitis B surface antigen (HbsAg) is standard prenatal care; if the maternal screen is positive, then immediately after birth the newborn is given hepatitis B virus (HBV) immune globulin along with the first dose of the HBV vaccination series (Poland, 2004).

Viral Meningitis and Encephalitis

Several thousand viral infections of the central nervous system occur each year in the US and morbidity and mortality varies considerably. Accurate and prompt laboratory diagnosis aids patient management and is important for public health interventions to control arbovirus insect vectors and investigate waterborne sources. Viral proliferation in the

CSF or brain biopsy tissue in VTM*

- Amplified nucleic acid test for HSV and enteroviruses
- Cell culture: inoculation of E-mix, HDF, PMK, RK, HEp-2, RD, etc.
- Additional CSF/tissue, freeze at −20°C
- Collect acute phase serum; freeze portion at −20°C
- Refer CSF and acute serum to public health laboratory for
  seasonal West Nile/regional arbovirus IgM antibody testing

Diagnosis established

(+) Amplified nucleic acid test for HSV or enterovirus
(+) Virus isolation in cell culture
(+) WNV/regional arbovirus IgM

No viral infection identified – further testing as clinically indicated

- Amplified nucleic acid testing of stored (−20°C) CSF
- VZV, EBV, HIV, CMV, JC virus, etc.
- Collect convalescent serum
- Consult with public health/reference laboratory;
  provide clinical history and travel history.
  Send paired acute and convalescent sera
  and frozen CSF/tissue for additional testing.

Aseptic meningitis	Meningoencephalitis/encephalitis	Immunocompromised patient
• Enteroviruses • WNV, other regional arboviruses • HIV • HSV2 • EBV • Travel-associated arboviruses • VZV measles, mumps, adenovirus	• WNV, other regional arboviruses • HSV • Enteroviruses • EBV • Travel-associated arboviruses • VZV, measles, RSV, influenza, adenovirus • Rabies	• CMV, HSV, VZV • HIV • EBV • JC virus • Enteroviruses • HHV6

* Consult with Public Health/Reference laboratory for volume of CSF needed for all amplified nucleic acid tests and serology ordered.
0.5 cm³ tissue biopsy usually sufficient for imprints, surgical pathology, comprehensive microbiology, and amplified nucleic acid tests.

Figure 54–9 Laboratory diagnosis of viral meningitis and encephalitis. CMV = cytomegalovirus; CSF = cerebrospinal fluid; EBV = Epstein–Barr virus; HDF = human diploid fibroblasts; HHV = human herpes virus; HIV = human immunodeficiency virus; HSV = herpes simplex virus; PMK = primary monkey kidney; RD = rhabdomyosarcoma; RK = rabbit kidney; RSV = respiratory syncytial virus; VTM = viral transport medium; VZV = varicella-zoster virus; WNV = West Nile virus.

meningeal layers covering the brain induces acute inflammation with fever, headache, nuchal rigidity, and CSF pleocytosis. In encephalitis, virus replicates within the brain parenchyma; inflammation and tissue necrosis may be diffuse or may produce a space-occupying lesion with mass effect. Many viruses are associated with either meningitis or encephalitis but overlap injury with involvement of both anatomic sites (meningoencephalitis) is common, particularly with arbovirus infection (Fig. 54–9).

Viral encephalitis is not infrequent in the US; annual reported cases average about 2000. Accurate diagnosis is limited by the fact that some neurotropic viruses are fastidious and require molecular methods for detection. Arboviruses and HSV cause most acute encephalitis in the US. HSV encephalitis usually is a reactivation of latent HSV1 that tracks (via the olfactory or trigeminal cranial nerves) into the cerebral cortex, producing a large necrotic mass. There are about 700 cases of herpes encephalitis each year; the pattern is sporadic and nonseasonal. Progression is rapid and mortality is high but early diagnosis and acyclovir treatment reduce both mortality and the level of permanent disability (Whitley, 1995; Mitchell, 1997).

Mosquitoes are vectors for hundreds of neurotropic viruses worldwide, but only five arboviruses (arthropod borne) are encountered regularly in the US: west Nile, the eastern and western equines, St Louis, and California–LaCrosse encephalitis viruses. Arboviruses are a heterogeneous group and mosquito transmission is their common denominator; the most frequent in North America are in the flavivirus, togavirus, and bunyavirus families. Prior to the WNV outbreak, total annual US arboviral cases varied between 100 and 2000; disease peaked when mosquito populations were greatest. Severity and mortality is highest with the eastern equine virus, the least frequent of the group (Calisher, 1994). The WNV outbreak originated in 1999 in New York and then traveled in infected birds from the east coast across America and involved all states by 2004. The estimated total number of human WNV infections is currently about 1 million; approximately 200 000 patients have become clinically ill with disease ranging from simple fever to meningitis, encephalitis, and flaccid poliomyelitic paralysis; both long-term encephalitic and paralytic disabilities have been reported, along with many fatalities (Nash, 2001; Petersen, 2004). Mosquito bites are the typical route of acquisition, but blood transfusion and organ transplantation also accounted for several cases (Iwamoto, 2003; Pealer, 2003; Kleinman, 2005). Blood donations are now screened for WNV by NAAT, effectively interrupting this mechanism of spread (Busch, 2005). At the time of presentation with CNS disease, WNV and many other arboviruses often cannot be cultured

from blood or spinal fluid; therefore, diagnosis hinges on EIA for specific IgM antibody in CSF and serum. NAAT can also be performed on CSF along with direct sequencing of virus if needed. State health departments and reference laboratories offer a range of tests for common regional arboviruses but hundreds of arboviruses are endemic outside the US in Asia, Africa, Latin America, and parts of eastern Europe. Testing for arbovirus infection in travelers is available through public health laboratories; provide a detailed travel history and clinical information along with blood, CSF, or tissue specimens submitted for culture, nucleic acid detection, or serological diagnosis (Fig. 54–9). Current information about global arbovirus activity and risk to tourists is available at www.cdc.gov/travel.

There are more than 60 enteroviruses, some of which produce encephalitis (Coxsackie virus and echovirus); paralytic polio caused by poliovirus necrosis of spinal cord or brainstem motor neurons has been eliminated in most of the world, with residual disease in Africa and Asia. Rabies virus travels via nerve fibers directly to the CNS and produces necrotizing brain damage; bat rather than canine strains account for most disease in the US; a recent outbreak was traced to transplanted organs from a donor who had died with undiagnosed rabies (Plotkin, 2000; Smith, 2003; MMWR, 2004). Measles, mumps, EBV mononucleosis, and chickenpox rarely are complicated by acute encephalitis (Cherry, 1998); HHV6 has also produced focal cerebral injury (Isaacson, 2005). HIV replication in CNS glial cells can cause progressive dementia in advanced AIDS (Atwood, 1993). Opportunistic necrotizing brain infections with HSV, CMV, and VZV as well as JC polyomavirus destruction of oligodendroglia may also develop in the immunocompromised host, discussed below.

Enteroviruses cause 75% of viral meningitis in the United States, usually relatively benign and transient disease. Enteroviruses spread easily from person to person via fecal–oral means, and there is distinct seasonality, with annual summer–fall outbreaks (Fig. 54–6); most clinically recognized infections are in children. Chronic severe meningoencephalitis can develop in patients with hypogammaglobulinemia; any enteroviral CNS infection with an encephalitis component is more virulent and may leave permanent sequelae (McKinney, 1987). Acute HIV infection occasionally produces acute meningeal inflammation (Schupbach, 2003). About 1% of primary HSV2 genital herpes infections are accompanied by transient meningitis; HSV2 is the major cause of Mollaret's benign recurrent lymphocytic meningitis. Mumps, measles, and adenovirus infections rarely produce acute meningitis.

Table 54-6 Laboratory Diagnosis of Common Viral Exanthems

Exanthem	Virus	Culture/Antigen and Nucleic Acid Assays	Serology
Chicken pox/shingles	Varicella zoster	Tzanck smear DFA smear Cuture (shell vial most sensitive), PCR*	IgM-EIA (chickenpox) IgG-EIA for immunity following chicken pox Commercial VZV-IgG tests are not reliable for documenting immunity post-vaccination
Enteroviral rash (hand, foot, and mouth disease)	Enteroviruses	Culture, RT-PCR	
Measles	Measles	Culture*	IgM-EIA or IFA*
Rubella	Rubella	Culture*	IgM-EIA*
Erythema infectiosum	Parvovirus B19		IgM-EIA or IFA*
Exanthem subitum	HHV6	Co-culture in lymphoblasts*	IgM-EIA*
Anogenital condyloma	Papillomaviruses	Hybrid capture amplified assay; low/high risk types	
HSV	HSV1 and HSV2	Amplified probe, culture, DFA smear	HSVgG1 and gG2G glycoprotein specific antibody IgM*

If smallpox is considered for a patient with vesicular lesions, contact local health authorities for specific instructions.

* Test available at research and reference laboratories.

DFA = direct fluorescent antibody; EIA = enzyme immunoassay; HSV = herpes simplex virus; HHV = human herpes virus; IFA = indirect fluorescent antibody; RT-PCR = reverse transcriptase polymerase chain reaction; VZV = varicella zoster virus.

Laboratory Diagnosis

Comprehensive laboratory evaluation of viral CNS disease is beyond the scope of most hospitals. A streamlined plan for stepwise testing based on the clinical scenario can coordinate in house testing with efficient use of reference laboratory and public health laboratory services (Fig. 54–9). For immunocompetent patients, initial testing of spinal fluid/brain biopsy tissue using NAATs for HSV and enterovirus plus virus culture can be paired with serum and CSF assays for IgM antibodies to the prevalent regional seasonal arboviruses. If clinically indicated, CSF reserved at −20°C and paired acute and convalescent sera can be referred for more extensive arbovirus testing in public health laboratories and for culture and additional NAATs for the less common causes of viral meningitis or encephalitis. The 1999 WNV outbreak was quickly identified because of cooperative and coordinated efforts between hospital and government laboratories (MMWR, 1999). Despite extensive evaluation, an infectious cause for encephalitis is often not identified (Glaser, 2003).

Immunocompromised patients may develop CNS disease with the same viruses that afflict the healthy host; in addition, several opportunistic viral infections may also produce CNS involvement. JC polyomavirus, CMV, VZV, and HSV can cause CNS disease; CNS B-lymphocytic lymphoma is almost always related to EBV infection; PCR for EBV in CSF is diagnostic of CNS lymphoma. NAATs are available that are more sensitive than culture or electron microscopy and can be performed on CSF as well as brain biopsy tissue (Koralnik, 2005).

The most practical approach for diagnosis of viral encephalitis is NAAT performed on CSF. RT-PCR identification of enterovirus and PCR of HSV, VZV, EBV, CMV, and HHV6 are more sensitive than virus recovery by cell culture from either CSF or brain tissue; several home-brew assays and commercial systems have been developed (Abzug, 1995; Domingues, 1998; Tang, 1999a; Landry, 2003; Romero, 2003; DeBiasi, 2004). Preliminary screening of CSF for elevated protein and pleocytosis is advisable since herpesviruses are rarely, if ever, identified when protein and cell count are normal (Tang, 1999a). Brain biopsy is still performed on occasion, usually when tumor or nonviral infection is also a clinical consideration (Whitley, 1989). A 0.5 cm³ biopsy is sufficient for surgical pathology examination, imprint smears for direct examination, NAATs, and comprehensive culture for all infectious organisms. HSV isolation in cell culture is discussed above; recovery of other viruses should also be attempted, so the specimen should be inoculated to all cell lines that the laboratory carries. Imprints stained with DFA reagents can demonstrate HSV-infected cells. Some arboviruses and enteroviruses require animal inoculation for replication; if needed, tissue should be frozen at −20°C and the specimen forwarded to a public health or reference laboratory.

Enteroviruses are the most common agents of acute aseptic meningitis; NAATs (RT-PCR and NASBA) are the gold standard for enterovirus identification in CSF, with yields of 128–142% compared with cell culture recovery (Rotbart, 1994, 1997; Kessler, 1997; Romero, 1999; Landry, 2003). 10–100 µL of CSF is needed for RT-PCR; simplified microtiter test formats have reduced turnaround time to 6 hours. Several tissue lines

(PMK, HDF, HEp-2, RD, and Buffalo green monkey) support growth of many enteroviruses and also HSV, VZV, measles, mumps, and adenovirus; E-mix hybrid shell vial culture is also an excellent choice for culture of enteroviruses and related agents (Huang, 2002). From 0.1–0.2 mL of CSF should be inoculated directly into each tube or shell vial without delay. Enterovirus CPE begins as focal pyknotic change with individual cell rounding which then rapidly progresses across the cell monolayer (Fig. 54–8). CPE is identified within 4 days in up to 69% of positive cultures. Shell vials and tube monolayers can be stained with panenterovirus DFA reagents (Lipson, 2001). Enterovirus specific typing is available in public health laboratories.

Viral Exanthems and Common Cutaneous Infections

Several viruses primarily target the skin; some infect the squamous epidermis through direct inoculation (oral and genital herpes, warts caused by human papillomavirus or molluscum poxvirus) but exanthems are caused by viruses that spread hematogenously to skin and mucous membranes (VZV, measles, rubella, enteroviruses, parvovirus, HHV6) (Cherry, 1993). Many of these benign childhood exanthems are diagnosed clinically with no laboratory testing; several are preventable with vaccination. However, viral culture, antigen identification, or serologic confirmation may be helpful to define the extent of disease in severe cases, to apply infection control precautions efficiently in hospitalized patients, or to select appropriate antiviral therapy. Laboratory diagnostic procedures are summarized in Table 54-6.

VZV causes both varicella (chickenpox) and zoster (shingles). In chickenpox, VZV is spread through infected respiratory aerosol droplets, multiplies in the nasopharynx, and then enters the bloodstream and travels to the skin (Arvin, 1996). Replication in the squamous epithelium produces pruritic vesicles that rapidly progress to ulcers, which eventually crust over and heal without scarring – similar to HSV skin lesions. In healthy children, systemic symptoms are mild and sequelae are rare. In adults, pregnant women, neonates, and immunocompromised patients, disease is often more severe; pneumonia and visceral involvement may develop in addition to typical skin lesions (Gershon, 1976). After chickenpox resolves, latent VZV infection is established in sensory neural ganglia (Arvin, 1996); with reactivation, VZV spreads from trigeminal or dorsal root ganglia back to the skin, and produces painful cutaneous vesicles with dermatome distribution (shingles, zoster). Zoster is most common in the elderly and the immunocompromised; when it occurs in teens and young adults, HIV infection should be suspected. Any vesicular rash that raises the possibility of smallpox should be immediately reported to local public health officials.

Vesicle fluid is rich with virus and is the ideal specimen for culture and DFA staining (Fig. 54–3). VZV replicates in HDF cell lines. Traditional tube culture is slow and insensitive; shell vial culture has better yield (up to 75%) and allows more rapid detection (Brinker, 1993). Specimen

VII

collection is identical to that for HSV vesicles (Fig. 54–4). Culture setup is also similar to herpes culture; however, tubes are held for 2 weeks and shell vial monolayers are stained at 3 and 5 days with VZV DFA reagent. VZV CPE develops in HDF as small patches of rounded, swollen, refractile cells. Because the behavior of VZV in tissue culture may be somewhat fastidious, DFA stain of vesicle cells for viral antigen is the most sensitive, rapid and practical diagnostic test (Schrim, 1989). RT-PCR assays have also been developed (Tang, 1999b; Weidmann, 2003).

Of the approximately 70 enterovirus serotypes, several produce vesicular or maculopapular eruptions (Coxsackie B1 and A9, and echoviruses 2, 4, 9, 11, 19, and 33), usually during summer months. Hand–foot–mouth disease (Coxsackie A16) in young children presents with vesicles on the tongue and palmar and plantar skin. Adult family members of infected children occasionally also develop symptomatic disease. Laboratory diagnosis is limited to cell culture and RT-PCR; vesicles from the soles and palms should be completely unroofed and the exposed squamous cells vigorously swabbed. Cell culture identification of enterovirus was described earlier. DFA stains and serology are impractical for diagnosis of enteroviral exanthems (Cherry, 1963; DeChamps, 1988).

Measles is highly contagious and presents with both systemic and respiratory features (fever, conjunctivitis, coryza, oral lesions, cough, and a generalized maculopapular erythematous rash). Vaccination has dramatically curtailed measles but it persists in impoverished countries; morbidity and mortality are high because of accompanying pneumonia and malnutrition. Virus can be isolated from the nasopharynx but acute infection is most easily diagnosed serologically by detecting measles-specific IgM. Immunity following natural infection presumably is lifelong, verified by the presence of specific IgG; however, immunity following vaccination may fade during the late teen years. Reinfection occurring in this setting may be atypical and serologic diagnosis is particularly helpful.

Parvovirus B19 causes erythema infectiosum (fifth disease), a common childhood febrile illness with a distinctive maculopapular rash that gives the face a 'slapped cheek' appearance (Young, 2004). PB19 infection in adults often produces arthralgias. Parvovirus infects erythroblastic precursor cells in the bone marrow and may provoke aplastic crisis in patients with hemoglobinopathy or HIV infection. Primary infection during pregnancy can cause fetal red cell aplasia with hydrops fetalis. Laboratory diagnosis was discussed earlier in this chapter.

Rubella virus produces German measles, a mild febrile illness with a transient maculopapular rash (Cherry, 1993). Infection in children is inconsequential, although adult rubella may be associated with arthralgias. The only serious complication of rubella is transplacental spread to the fetus, with risk of congenital malformation. Acute infection is diagnosed by detection of virus-specific IgM. Verification of immune status is determined with specific IgG screening.

HHV6, a lymphotrophic virus that infects lymphocytes, is the cause of exanthem subitum (roseola infantum), a common illness of early childhood with high fever and development of a fleeting maculopapular rash as fever abruptly subsides (Salahuddin, 1986; Prober, 2005; Zerr, 2005). Primary HHV6 infection in older children and adults produces a systemic, febrile lymphoproliferative illness resembling acute mononucleosis (discussed earlier); it may cause pneumonitis in immunosuppressed patients (Cone, 1993). Laboratory diagnosis was reviewed earlier.

Human papillomaviruses are ubiquitous and found in all societies; there are hundreds of HPV types defined by unique DNA sequences, and various HPV types target different skin or mucosal sites in the body. Most HPV warty cutaneous infections of the hands and feet are transient and of no medical consequence. Sexual encounters transmit HPV types that are associated with anogenital condylomatous disease. Low-risk HPV types generally lead to low-grade squamous intraepithelial proliferative lesions that frequently resolve. Infection with high risk HPV types carries a much greater likelihood of persistent viral infection in the squamous epithelium of the cervix, vagina, vulva or perineum, which can evolve from a low- to high-grade dysplastic intraepithelial lesion and progress over time to invasive squamous carcinoma. The histopathological and cytopathological characteristics of HPV lesions are well described in standard pathology texts. However, HPV detection has been enhanced by the use of NAATs; the hybrid capture signal amplification method is most widely used and can identify both high-risk and low-risk HPV types in liquid-based cervical cytology specimens (Burd, 2003). Several strategies have been suggested for efficient use of adjuvant or reflex HPV testing to maximize detection and follow-up management (Kim, 2002; Kulasingham, 2002; Wright, 2002).

Viral Gastroenteritis

Viral gastroenteritis causes major morbidity and mortality worldwide, most significantly in young children in developing nations; in the US, viral enteritis is rarely fatal but causes at least 3 million episodes annually and approximately 200 000 pediatric hospitalizations (Parashar, 1998). The viruses responsible are a diverse group, and all are ubiquitous. Severe debilitating diarrhea with rotavirus, enteric adenoviruses, caliciviruses, astrovirus, and coronavirus is largely confined to infants and young children. All treatment is supportive (Thielman, 2004).

Rotaviruses cause most cases of watery diarrhea in infants and young children in the US (Musher, 2004); symptomatic infections occasionally develop in elderly adults in nursing homes. Transmission is fecal–oral; epidemics occur during cold weather in temperate climates and year-round in tropical regions. Dehydration with electrolyte imbalance is the most serious complication. Rotavirus can survive transiently on inanimate surfaces; enteric isolation precautions must be followed to prevent nosocomial or daycare spread.

Adenovirus serotypes 40 and 41 are associated with gastroenteritis and account for 10–20% of pediatric cases. Adenovirus enteritis is clinically similar to rotavirus disease but has no seasonality. Coronavirus and astrovirus have caused nosocomial and daycare center outbreaks (Mitchell, 1993), mild gastroenteritis in adults, and diarrhea in HIV patients (Grohmann, 1993).

Norovirus and morphologically related caliciviruses (Sapporo, Hawaii, Snow Mountain, etc.) cause epidemic acute gastroenteritis, characterized by nausea and vomiting that are more intense than the accompanying diarrhea. Norovirus is nonenveloped and can survive on inanimate surfaces as well as in contaminated water, shellfish, and prepared foods; it has been identified in several community and national epidemics and cruise ship and daycare outbreaks. All age groups are vulnerable but older children and adults are the usual victims (Hedberg, 1993; MMWR, 2001; Griffin, 2003).

Laboratory Diagnosis

Gastroenteritis viruses grow poorly or not at all in standard cell lines. Diagnosis had been based on the distinctive morphology of each virus when stool samples are negatively stained with phosphotungstic acid and examined by electron microscopy. Viruses can be accurately identified by EM (Petric, 2003), but the service is not available in most laboratories. Rotavirus diagnosis has the most significant clinical relevance; rapid detection of rotavirus antigen in stool is easily and accurately accomplished with latex agglutination and immunoassays. All methods have excellent specificity and EIA is slightly more sensitive (Thomas, 1994; Dennehy, 1999). Rapid diagnosis is useful for patient cohorting and infection control measures to contain nosocomial spread. An accurate and sensitive commercial EIA for enteric adenovirus antigen detection is available, if needed. EIA and RT-PCR assays and genotype-relatedness studies have been developed for norovirus and other gastroenteric viruses (Atmar, 2001; Burton-MacLeod, 2004; Pang, 2004); testing is performed in public health laboratories, and has been quite helpful in evaluating food-related outbreaks.

Viral Hepatitis and Retroviral Infection

Many viruses are hepatotoxic. Yellow fever virus and other hepatotropic arboviruses cause massive hepatocellular necrosis. Atypical T lymphocytes aggregate in the liver and cause transient hepatic injury during EBV, CMV, HHV6, and HIV acute mononucleosis syndrome. Adenovirus, HSV, VZV, CMV, and echoviruses occasionally produce aggressive hepatitis in the immunocompromised (Hierholzer, 1992). However, hepatitis A, B, C, D, and E virus infections characteristically lead to lytic hepatocyte injury and account for most clinical cases of infectious hepatitis (Iwarson, 1992).

Hepatitis A virus (HAV) and hepatitis E virus (HEV) are nonenveloped agents with fecal-oral transmission; inadequate sewage treatment and crowded living conditions are linked to waterborne outbreaks and HAV has been spread in contaminated foods. HAV is a picornavirus, distinct from but related to the enteroviruses. Children in daycare and crowded institutions and their caregivers are at increased risk for HAV hepatitis (Cuthbert, 2001; Iwarson, 1992; Emerson, 2004). Acute disease in children is mild and often asymptomatic; adults occasionally develop severe infection, but fulminant hepatitis and death are rare; IgM antibody is the most practical marker of acute infection. Recovery is complete with no chronic infectious state. HAV vaccines are now available (Craig, 2004). HEV is related to caliciviruses; outbreaks occur in developing countries and in refugee camps with suboptimal food and water sanitation but are unusual in industrialized nations. Teens and young adults are most commonly affected; mortality is rare, except in pregnant women where death rates may reach 20% (Duff, 1998). HEV does not cause chronic infection. IgG antibody develops promptly and persists at low titers indefinitely; specific-IgM is a reliable test of acute infection (Schlauder, 2003).

HBV is easily transmitted through blood and classically acquired through transfusions, needle sharing, or occupational injury with contaminated sharps. Infection may be acquired transplacentally during pregnancy, and sexual contact and household exposure to virus in body fluids are also important routes of spread. Acute infection is frequently symptomatic, with much of the liver damage inflicted by CD8+ cytotoxic T lymphocytes; 1% develop fulminant fatal massive hepatocellular necrosis. HBV can also persist as a chronic infection. Up to 90% of infants born with HBV vertically acquired in utero become chronic carriers, compared with 25% of infected children and 10% of adults. Even in apparently resolved infections, HBV DNA persists despite host production of antibodies to core and e antigens. Hepatocellular T-cell damage is ongoing in chronic infection. Unrelenting inflammation progresses to cirrhotic scarring in at least 2% of chronic infections (Lok, 2002; Ganem, 2004); HBV-induced cirrhosis is a risk factor for hepatocellular carcinoma. HBV infection and sequelae are largely preventable; vaccination of neonates and children has significantly decreased the incidence of pediatric chronic infection and hepatocellular carcinoma (Chang, 1997; Poland, 2004). Response to antiviral therapy in chronically infected patients can be monitored with quantitative assay of HBV DNA viral load (Shyamala, 2004).

HBV coinfection or superinfection with δ hepatitis virus (HDV) accelerates hepatocyte damage and mortality (rates as high as 30%) (Polish, 1993). HDV is an incomplete virus that requires HBV surface antigen for full expression and replication. HDV may be transmitted from person to person in household situations in endemic areas (South America, Africa, Italy) but transfusion and intravenous drug abuse are the principal risk factors in the US (Hadziyannis, 1997).

HCV is estimated to infect 4 million Americans and is the leading cause of non-A non-B hepatitis; since the advent of serologic testing and NAAT, transfusion-associated HCV has dropped dramatically (Cuthbert, 1994; Lauer, 2001; National Institutes of Health, 2002; Stramer, 2004). Parenteral drug abuse and inadvertent puncture wounds in healthcare workers are known means of transmission but no source is identified in many cases. Transmission of HCV during pregnancy or through sexual and household contact is much less efficient than transmission of HBV and HIV. Fulminant and fatal acute hepatitis is rare; however, HCV clearance by cytotoxic T lymphocytes is inadequate in most patients. About 80% of infections become chronic, with hepatocellular fibrosis that may progress to cirrhosis (20%) and hepatocellular carcinoma (1–4% per year in cirrhotic patients). Coinfection with HIV or HBV, as well as ethanol use, accelerates the natural course; superinfection with HAV can provoke fulminant hepatitis. Treatment with pegylated α-interferon and ribavirin produces sustained remission in chronic HCV disease and may significantly modify or prevent serious long-term sequelae (McHutchison, 1998). However, response rates are lower for genotype 1, which represents 75% of infections in the US (Zein, 2000).

Third-generation screening HCV antibody chemiluminescence and enzyme immunoassays (CIA and EIA) use an expanded number of refined viral antigens; sensitivity and specificity are between 95% and 98% (Richter, 2002; Ismail, 2004). Because of the high rate of chronic HCV disease and favorable outcome with antiviral therapy, an algorithm for efficient testing that begins with a CIA or EIA HCV antibody screen has been recommended by the CDC. A screening HCV antibody result with a high signal-to-cutoff ratio has a high probability of being a true positive with chronic infection; quantitative HCV PCR is then appropriate to verify viremia and begin antiviral treatment. A low signal-to-cutoff HCV antibody screen result has a high likelihood of being a false positive, so confirmation with a third-generation recombinant immunoblot assay (RIBA) is useful before proceeding with viral load testing (MMWR, 2003). The CDC algorithmic strategy outlines a logical testing sequence that minimizes unnecessary, costly testing and provides helpful information in a timely fashion for treatment. Hepatitis GB virus-C, a flavivirus related to HCV, has been identified in post-transfusion hepatitis. However, since the clinical significance of GBV-C is not well characterized, routine GBV-C antibody and RNA testing are not recommended in patients with chronic hepatic disease (Hadziyannis, 1998). Interestingly, coinfection with GBV-C and HIV appears to induce host antiviral activity against HIV and prolong survival (Xiang, 2001).

None of the hepatitis viruses replicates in standard culture cell lines. Detection of specific IgM and IgG antibodies and specific viral antigens designates the stage of infection with each virus; quantitative viral load NAATs are used to monitor response to treatment of chronic infection.

Table 54–7 summarizes virological and serological markers with viral hepatitis.

Human Immunodeficiency Virus and Retrovirus Infections

HIV-1 is a retrovirus in the Lentiviridae family that now has worldwide distribution. HIV infects and destroys CD4+ T lymphocytes and eventually leads to debilitating opportunistic infections and malignancies (Stein, 1992; Schupbach, 2003). HIV is also neurotropic and can cause acute meningitis and slow destructive encephalopathy (Atwood, 1993). The HIV-2 strain present in west Africa is somewhat less pathogenic with reduced risk of transmission and progression to AIDS.

Half of individuals acutely infected with HIV experience mononucleosis-like symptoms before entering an asymptomatic latent stage. During acute infection, circulating HIV RNA levels are high but antibody may not yet be detectable. Median time for CD4+ cell destruction sufficient to develop full features of AIDS is 10–11 years; 5–10% of individuals develop AIDS in 3 years and 5–10% of individuals maintain stable CD4+ counts and remain asymptomatic indefinitely (Munoz, 1995). Children vertically infected at birth often show accelerated progression.

There are several commercial EIA screening tests for HIV antibody made with an array of recombinant and purified HIV antigens; third-generation kits have overall excellent specificity and sensitivity and may detect HIV antibody as early as 2–4 weeks post-infection. Fourth-generation EIA tests that combine screening for HIV antibody with detection of HIV antigens have even greater sensitivity in recognizing early infection. Nevertheless, blood banks in industrialized countries routinely test donor blood for HIV RNA by NAAT to identify donors in the false-negative window (Busch, 2000; Ly, 2001; Candotti, 2003; Schupbach, 2003; Stramer, 2004). US blood banks test for HIV-2 antibody, and it is standard screening in Africa and Europe. A positive EIA HIV antibody screen should be repeated and then confirmed with an additional test, such as immunofluorescence assay or Western blot assay (Carlson, 1987). Western blot is the more popular verification method and demonstrates antibodies that react with specific HIV antigens; Western blot is less sensitive than EIA but a classic positive band pattern provides convincing serologic evidence of HIV infection (MMWR, 1991). Laboratory reporting of all HIV serology test results should be concise and avoid use of ambiguous or confusing comments (Hewitt, 1992).

HIV is propagated in tissue culture by co-cultivating infected patient lymphocytes or tissues with normal donor lymphocytes that have been stimulated with phytohemagglutinin, interleukin-2, and interferon. Culture is complex, expensive, and dangerous and should not be attempted in hospital laboratories. HIV culture has been largely supplanted by NAATs; RT-PCR, NASBA, transcription mediated amplification (TMA), and bDNA methods are commercially available. In addition to routine testing of donor blood, NAAT has also been proposed as a component of routine HIV screening (Pilcher, 2005). Antiretroviral treatment has dramatically improved survival and quality of life for HIV patients (Freedberg, 2001; Aberg, 2004). HIV RNA quantitative assays to measure viral load in plasma has revolutionized monitoring of anti-retroviral therapy; treatment-related reductions of HIV RNA more than 0.5–1.0 log copies/mL correlate with slower clinical progression. Noncompliance has led to the emergence of drug-resistant HIV mutants, which can be identified with genotypic and phenotypic assays. Genotypic methods sequence HIV genes to identify mutant oligonucleotides that are linked to drug resistance, and have the most clinical utility. Phenotypic testing is complex and involves amplification of protease and reverse-transcriptase genes in the suspect patient virus, insertion of these genes into a test virus, and then in vitro susceptibility testing of this laboratory-constructed virus against specific antiviral drugs. A 'virtual phenotype' can be approximated from the genotypic mutation data to ascertain the likelihood of in vitro phenotypic actual susceptibility, with the two methods often showing excellent correlation (Shafer, 2002; Hirsch, 2003; Clavel, 2004).

In utero or perinatal transmission from HIV-infected mothers can be dramatically reduced with treatment. Proviral HIV DNA PCR assay is primarily used to diagnose vertically transmitted HIV infection during the first few months of life (see Congenital and Perinatal Infections, above). HTLV infects CD4+ T lymphocytes and causes adult T-cell leukemia; adult T-cell leukemia occurs in 2–4% of individuals infected with HTLV-1 in endemic areas of Japan (Folks, 1998). HTLV-1 also causes myelopathy/tropical spastic paraparesis, a chronic degenerative neurological disease characterized by progressive lower extremity weakness, spasticity, and loss of sensory function and bladder control (Manns, 1999). HTLV-II has been isolated from patients with T-cell hairy cell leukemia but the association is unclear. EIA antibody assays are available and are used by blood banks to screen donated blood.

VII

CHAPTER: **54** Viral Infections

Table 54–7 Serologic and Virologic Tests for Hepatitis Viruses

	IgM anti-HAV	Anti-HAV (IgG + IgM)	HBsAg	Anti-HBs	IgM anti-HBc	Anti-HBc (IgG + IgM)	HBeAg	Anti-HBe	HBV-DNA	Anti-HCV screen	HCV RIBA	HCV-RNA Quant.	Anti-HDV	Anti-HEV
HAV – acute	+	+												
HAV – remote	–	+												
HBV – early			+	–	+	+	+	–	+					
HBV – window			–	–	+	+	–	–	+					
HBV – resolving			–/+	+	–	+	–/+	+	–/+					
HBV – chronic			+	–/+	–	+	+/–	+/–	+					
HBV – remote			–	+	–	+/–	–	+/–	–/+					
HCV – Screen*										+ low S/C	Confirm with RIBA			
HCV – acute										+ high S/C				
HCV – chronic										+/–	+/–	Perform RNA quant. +		
HCV – remote										+	+	–		
HDV – superinfection			+	–	–	+	–	+/–	–				+	
HEV														+

+ = positive; – = negative

* See MMWR 2003; 52: RR-03 for detailed algorithm for testing and reporting.

HAV = hepatitis A virus; HBc = hepatitis B core antigen; HBeAg = hepatitis B e antigen; HBsAg = hepatitis B surface antigen; HBV = hepatitis B virus; HCV = hepatitis C virus; HDV = δ hepatitis virus; HEV = hepatitis E virus; quant. = quantification; RIBA = recombinant immunoblot assay; S/C = signal-to-cutoff ratio.

Viral Infections in Immunocompromised Hosts

The immune response to viral infection is a complex interaction of both humoral and cellular factors. The cell-mediated immune system responds to acute infection with natural killer large granular lymphocytes that circulate through blood and tissues, identify host cells with viral ('non-self') antigens, and destroy them by proteolytic lysis. Viral antigens are processed by macrophages and presented to B and T lymphocytes. CD4+ cells produce cytokines that promote clonal expansion of sensitized cytotoxic CD8+ cells, which then eliminate host cells harboring viral antigen. Any impairment of the normal interactions among macrophages, CD4+, CD8+, and natural killer cells reduces host ability to control viral disease. Cell-mediated immunity is also critical in suppressing viruses that have established latency (such as HSV, CMV, and EBV). In healthy individuals, most reactivation infections with these viruses are asymptomatic or produce limited disease confined to a discrete anatomic area (genital or oral herpes, for example). With impaired cellular immune function, recurrent infections may be locally aggressive or may disseminate and produce severe multiorgan damage.

The number of immunocompromised patients continues to increase. Corticosteroids, chemotherapy and radiation, immunosuppressive drugs to prevent transplant rejection, and HIV obliteration of CD4+ lymphocytes all damage cellular immune regulation and increase vulnerability to viral infections. Primary infections, such as EBV mononucleosis, influenza, and chickenpox, are often more severe. HPV anogenital condylomas show accelerated progression to squamous dysplasia and carcinoma. The most serious viral diseases often are reactivation of endogenous dormant organisms (CMV, HSV, and VZV). Necrotizing oral and perianal HSV lesions, and zoster with multidermatome involvement may occur. Reactivated EBV is linked to CNS lymphoma in AIDS patients and to post-transplant lymphoproliferative disorders, as described above.

The most common opportunistic viral infections in HIV and transplant patients are caused by CMV (Drew, 1992a; Sia, 2000). Adult AIDS patients with CD4 cell counts below 100/mm³ are at risk for reactivation of latent CMV. Retinitis is a frequent complication; CMV pneumonia and gastrointestinal and CNS involvement are also common, and widely disseminated multiorgan disease at autopsy is not unusual (Drew, 1992b). CMV disease may also develop from primary infection in pediatric HIV patients and also in seronegative transplant recipients. Primary CMV infection carries an increased risk of disease relapse in solid organ transplant recipients. Serology has little practical value for diagnosing acute primary CMV infection in this setting. IgM production may be impaired in marrow and stem cell recipients, and IgG seroconversion requires acute and convalescent specimens. Serology is very useful for screening blood donors to limit transfusion of CMV-positive blood products to naive patients, and in assessing donor and recipient serostatus. EIA screens for CMV-IgG are most sensitive, have objective endpoints, and avoid the interpretive problems of complement binding in IFA procedures.

Typical cytomegalic inclusions are specific for identifying CMV infection in biopsy samples and bronchoalveolar lavage, but hematoxylin and eosin staining is insensitive. Sensitivity improves somewhat with immuno-peroxidase or in situ hybridization stains, but isolation of virus has higher diagnostic accuracy. CMV replicates almost exclusively in HDF cell lines; growth is slow, with incubation times of 7 days or more before CPE develops. The infected fibroblast initially retains its fusiform shape as the nucleus becomes swollen and refractile; the entire cell eventually becomes rounded and distorted, and virus spreads into adjacent fibroblasts, producing an enlarging patch of damaged cells (Fig. 54-3).

CMV recovery is shortened to 1–2 days with shell vial culture (Gleaves, 1984, 1987). HDF monolayers are inoculated by centrifugation with peripheral blood leukocytes (harvested by density gradient separation), bronchoalveolar lavage (BAL) fluid, or homogenized tissue; after a 16–40 hour incubation, the monolayer is stained with fluorescein-conjugated antibody to CMV early antigen. Infected fibroblasts show homogeneous fluorescence of the entire nucleus (see Fig. 54-3). CMV burden is usually high in infected endstage HIV patients, and culture has excellent diagnostic sensitivity with tissue and BAL specimens (95–100%). Shell vial culture of peripheral blood leukocytes has turnaround advantages, but sensitivity is only 75% compared with tube monolayer inoculation, so back-up tube culture is recommended. Recovery of CMV in both standard tube and shell vial cultures is optimized when specimens are inoculated immediately to fresh cell monolayers; yield is reduced if inoculation is delayed (Brumback, 1997; Roberts, 1997). Another advantage of shell vial culture is that results are semiquantitative (Buller, 1992; Slavin, 1992); a standard inoculum of cells (leukocytes or BAL cells) and a count of fluorescent CMV nuclei in the shell vial monolayer can generate a figure that has clinical value in estimating severity of infection, for monitoring response to therapy, and for predicting prognosis. CMV is the most common cause of viremia in compromised patients; however VZV, HSV, adenovirus, and occasionally enterovirus may be recovered. HDF and A549 traditional tube cultures held for 14 days will recover these agents as well as CMV (Stanberry, 1994). When immunosuppression is severe, AIDS patients and transplant recipients are at risk for other viral infections with specific organ or site involvement. Central nervous system infections are described above. Adenovirus, HSV, and VZV may present with pneumonitis; herpetic infection (HSV and VZV) may develop initially in esophageal and mucocutaneous sites and then disseminate. For this reason, mucosal, cutaneous or tissue biopsy specimens should be inoculated to a comprehensive series of cell lines to maximize recovery.

CMV infection in solid organ and allogeneic marrow transplant recipients has serious implications. Virus can directly damage transplanted organs, and toxicity from antiviral drugs or reduction/modulation of immunosuppressive therapy may threaten graft survival. CMV viremia is a sensitive marker of active viral replication with potential graft endangerment and risk of opportunistic pneumonia. Early detection allows preemptive use of antiviral agents with improved transplant conservation and decreased morbidity. Surveillance CMV blood culture using traditional tubes is a poor predictor for development of CMV disease and has not been helpful in making treatment adjustments (Falagas, 1997). Shell vial surveillance cultures have better prognostic value, but sequential quantitative assays of CMV pp65 antigen in peripheral blood and PCR detection of CMV DNA in blood are more sensitive and identify viremia earlier (Boeckh, 1998; Mendez, 1998; Sia, 2000; Razonable, 2002). CMV antigen assay is performed by IFA or immunoperoxidase staining of peripheral blood neutrophils for CMV antigen (Gerna, 1992; Storch, 1994; Erice, 1995; Landry, 1996); neutropenia is the principal practical limitation. Quantitative CMV PCR measurements are useful predictors of CMV disease in liver and renal transplant patients (Drouet, 1995). A sustained elevated CMV DNA copy number is a good predictor of retinitis risk in HIV patients with low CD4 levels (Rasmussen, 1997). NAAT for CMV mRNA has the potential advantage of specificity for active viral replication. The appearance of CMV in the blood has the ability to forecast systemic CMV disease; quantitative DNA methods can also be used to assess response to antiviral agents. Antiviral susceptibility testing method using plaque reduction assay or genotypic assay of mutations associated with resistance may be indicated in patients who do not respond to therapy (Erice, 1999; Sia, 2000; Razonable, 2002).

References

Aberg JA, Gallant JE, Anderson J, et al: Primary care guidelines for management of persons infected with HIV: recommendations of the HIV Medicine Association of the Infectious Diseases Society of America. Clin Infect Dis 2004; 39:609–629.

Abzug MJ, Loeffelholz M, Rotbart H: Diagnosis of neonatal enterovirus infection by polymerase chain reaction. J Pediatr 1995; 126:447–450.

Aitken C and Jeffries DJ: Nosocomial spread of viral disease. Clin Microbiol Rev 2001; 14:528–546.

Akashi K, Eizuru Y, Sumiyoshi Y, et al: Brief report: severe infectious mononucleosis-like syndrome and primary HH6 infection in an adult. N Engl J Med 1993; 329:168–171.

Alder SP, Manganello AM, Koch WL, et al: Risk of human parvovirus B19 infections among school and hospital employees during endemic periods. J Infect Dis 1993; 168:361.

Anand A, Grayes B, Brown T, et al: Human parvovirus infection in pregnancy and hydrops fetalis. N Engl J Med 1987; 316:183, 1987.

Anderson LJ, Parker RA, Stikas RL, et al: Association between respiratory syncytial virus outbreaks and lower respiratory tract deaths of infants and young children. J Infect Dis 1990; 161:640.

Arens MQ, Swierkosz EM, Schmidt RR, et al: Enhanced isolation of respiratory syncytial virus in cell culture. J Clin Microbiol 1986; 23:800.

Arvin AM: Varicella zoster virus. Clin Microbiol Rev 1996; 9:361–381.

Arvin AM, Hensleigh PA, Prober CG, et al: Failure of antepartum maternal cultures to predict the infant's risk of exposure to herpes simplex virus at delivery. N Engl J Med 1986; 315:796.

Ashley RL, Milton J, Lee F, et al: Comparison of Western blot (immunoblot) and glycoprotein G-specific immunodot assay for detecting antibodies to herpes simplex virus types 1 and 2 in human sera. J Clin Microbiol 1988; 26:662.

Ashley RL, Wald A: Genital herpes: review of the epidemic and potential use of type-specific serology. Clin Microbiol Rev 1999; 12:1–8.

Atmar RL, Estes MK: Diagnosis of noncultivatable gastroenteritis viruses, the human caliciviruses. Clin Microbiol Rev 2001; 14:15–37.

Atwood WJ, Berger JR: Human immunodeficiency virus type 1 infection of the brain. Clin Microbiol Rev 1993; 6:339.

Boeckh M, Boivin G: Quantitation of cytomegalovirus: methodologic aspects and clinical applications. Clin Microbiol Rev 1998; 11:533.

Boppana SB, Rivera LB, Fowler KB, et al: Intrauterine transmission of cytomegalovirus to infants of women with preconceptional immunity. N Engl J Med 2001; 344:1366–1371.

Braun DK, Dominguez G, Pellet PE: Human herpesvirus 6. Clin Microbiol Rev 1997; 10:521.

Bremer JW, Lew JF, Cooper GV, et al: Diagnosis of infection with HIV-1 by a DNA polymerase chain reaction among infants enrolled in the Women and Infants' Transmission Study. J Pediatr 1996; 129:198–207.

Brinker JP, Doern GV: Comparison of MRC-5 and A-549 cells in conventional cultures and shell vial assays for the detection of varicella-zoster virus. Diagn Microbiol Infect Dis 1993; 17:75.

Brown ZA, Benedetti J, Ashley R, et al: Neonatal herpes simplex virus infection in relation to asymptomatic maternal infection at the time of labor. N Engl J Med 1991; 325:1247.

Brown ZA, Selke S, Xeh J, et al: The acquisition of herpes simplex virus during pregnancy. N Engl J Med 1997; 337:509–515.

Brown ZA, Vontver LA, Benedetti J, et al: Effects on infants of a first episode of genital herpes during pregnancy. N Engl J Med 1987; 317:1246.

Brumback BG, Solejack SN, Morris MV, et al: Comparison of culture and the antigenemia assay for detection of cytomegalovirus in blood specimens submitted to a reference laboratory. J Clin Microbiol 1997; 35:1819.

Bruu AL, Nordbo SA: Evaluation of five commercial tests for detection of immunoglobulin M antibodies to human parvovirus B19. J Clin Microbiol 1995; 33:1363–1365.

Bryant PA, Tingay D, Dargaville PA, et al: Neonatal coxsackie B virus infection – a treatable disease? Eur J Pediatr 2004; 163:223–228.

Buller RS, Bailey TC, Ettinger NA, et al: Use of a modified shell vial technique to quantitate cytomegalovirus viremia in a population of solid organ transplant recipients. J Clin Microbiol 1992; 30:2620.

Burd EM: Human papillomavirus and cervical cancer. J Clin Microbiol 2003; 16:1–17.

Burton-MacLeod JA, Kane EM, Beard RS, et al: Evaluation and comparison of two commercial enzyme-linked immunosorbent assay kits for detection of antigenically diverse human noroviruses in stool samples. J Clin Microbiol 2004; 42:2587–2595.

Busch MP: Closing the windows on viral transmission by blood transfusion. In Stramer SL (ed.): Blood Safety in the New Millennium. Bethesda, MD, American Association of Blood Banks, 2000.

Busch MP, Tobler LH, Saldanha J, et al: Analytical and clinical sensitivity of West Nile Virus RNA screening and supplemental assays available in 2003. Transfusion 2005; 45:492–499.

Calisher CH: Medically important arboviruses of the United States and Canada. Clin Microbiol Rev 1994; 7:89.

Candotti D, Richetin A, Cant B, et al: Evaluation of a transcription-mediated amplification-based HCV and HIV-RNA duplex assay for screening individual blood donations; a comparison with a minipool testing system. Transfusion 2003; 43:215–225.

Carlson JR, Lee J, Henrichs SH, et al: Comparison of indirect immunofluorescence and Western blot for detection of anti-human immunodeficiency virus antibodies. J Clin Microbiol 1987; 28:494.

Chan KH, Luo RX, Chen HL, et al: Development and evaluation of an EBV immunoglobulin M ELISA based on the 18-kilodalton matrix protein for diagnosis of primary EBV infection. J Clin Microbiol 1998; 26:3359.

Chang MH, Chen CJ, Lai MS, et al: Universal hepatitis B vaccination in Taiwan and the incidence of hepatocellular carcinoma in children. Taiwan childhood hepatoma study group. N Engl J Med 1997; 336:1855–1859.

Chapin KC, Westenfeld FW: Reagents, stains, media and cell lines: virology. In Murray PR (ed.): Manual of Clinical Microbiology, 8th ed. Washington, DC, ASM Press, 2003.

Cherpes TL, Ashley RL, Meyn LA, et al: Longitudinal reliability of Focus glycoprotein G-based type-specific enzyme immunoassays for detection of herpes simplex virus types 1 and 2 in women. J Clin Microbiol 2003; 41:671–674.

Cherry JD: Contemporary infectious exanthems. Clin Infect Dis 1993; 16:199.

Cherry JD, Shields WD: Enecphalitis and meningoencephalitis. In Cherry JD, Feigin RD (eds): Textbook of Pediatric Infectious Diseases, 4th ed. Philadelphia, PA, WB Saunders, 1998.

Cherry JD, Lerner AM, Klein JO, et al: Coxsackie A9 infections with exanthems with particular reference to urticaria. Pediatrics 1963; 31:819.

Chiu SS, Cheung CY, Tse CY, et al: Early diagnosis of primary human herpesvirus 6 infection in childhood: serology, polymerase chain reaction, and viral load. J Infect Dis 1998; 178:1250.

Clarke L: Selection, maintenance and observation of uninoculated monolayer cell cultures. Viral culture: isolation of viruses in cell cultures. In Eisenberg HD (ed.): Clinical Microbiology Procedures Handbook, 2nd ed. Washington, DC, ASM Press, 2004.

Clavel F, Hance AJ: HIV drug resistance. N Engl J Med 2004; 350:1023–1035.

Cohen JI: Epstein–Barr virus infection. N Engl J Med 2000; 343:481–492.

Cone RW, Hackman RC, Haung M, et al: Human herpesvirus 6 in lung tissue from bone marrow transplant patients with pneumonia. N Engl J Med 1993; 329:156.

Cone RW, Hobson AC, Brown Z, et al: Frequent detection of genital herpes simplex virus DNA by polymerase chain reaction among pregnant women. JAMA 1994; 272:792.

Corey L: Herpes simplex virus. In Mandell GL, Bennett JE, Dolin R (eds): Principles and Practice of Infectious Diseases, 6th ed. Philadelphia, PA, Elsievier Churchill Livingstone, 2005.

Costello M, Smernoff NT, Yungbluth M, et al: Laboratory diagnosis of viral respiratory infections. Lab Med 1993; 24:152.

Craig AS, Schaffner W: Prevention of hepatitis A with the hepatitis A vaccine. N Engl J Med 2004; 350:476–481.

Cuthbert JA: Hepatitis C: Progress and problems. Clin Microbiol Rev 1994; 7:505.

Cuthbert JA: Hepatitis A: old and new. Clin Microbiol Rev 2001; 14:38–58.

DeBiasi RL, Tyler KL: Molecular methods for diagnosis of viral encephalitis. Clin Microbiol Rev 2004; 17:903–925.

DeChamps C, Peigue-Lafeuille HH, Laveran H, et al: Four cases of vesicular lesions in adults caused by enterovirus infections. J Clin Microbiol 1988; 26:2182.

Deffrasnes C, Cote S, Boivin G: Analysis of replication kinetics of the human metapneumovirus in different cell lines by real-time PCR. J Clin Microbiol 2005; 43:488–490.

Dennehy PH, Harhn M, Nelson SM, et al: Evaluation of the ImmunoCardSTAT! rotavirus assay for detection of group A rotavirus in fecal specimens. J Clin Microbiol 1999; 37:1977.

Domingues RB, Lakeman FD, Mayo MS, Whitley FJ: Application of competitive PCR to cerebrospinal fluid samples from patients with herpes simplex encephalitis. J Clin Microbiol 1998; 36:2229–2234.

Drew WL: Cytomegalovirus infection in patients with AIDS. Clin Infect Dis 1992a; 14:608.

Drew WL: Nonpulmonary manifestations of cytomegalovirus infection in immunocompromised patients. Clin Microbiol Rev 1992b; 5:204.

Drouet E, Colimon R, Michelson S, et al: Monitoring levels of human cytomegalovirus DNA in blood after liver transplantation. J Clin Microbiol 1995; 33:389.

Duff P: Hepatitis in pregnancy. Semin Perinatol 1998; 22:277–283.

Dunn JJ, Woolstenhulme RD, Langer J, et al: Sensitivity of respiratory virus culture when screening with R-mix fresh cells. J Clin Microbiol 2004; 42:79–82.

Ebihara T, Endo R, Ma X, et al: Detection of human metapneumovirus antigens in nasopharyngeal secretions by an immunofluorescent antibody test. J Clin Microbiol 2005; 43:1138–1141.

Emerson SU, Purcell RH: Running like water – the omnipresence of hepatitis E. N Engl J Med 2004; 351:2367–2368.

Erdman DD, Weinberg GA, Edwards KM, et al: GeneScan reverse transcription–PCR for detection of six common respiratory viruses in young children hospitalized with acute respiratory illness. J Clin Microbiol 2003; 41:4298–4303.

Erice A: Resistance of human cytomegalovirus to antiviral drugs. Clin Microbiol Rev 1999; 12:286–297.

Erice A, Holm MA, Sanjuan MV, et al: Evaluation of CMV-vue antigenemia assay for rapid detection of cytomegalovirus in mixed-leukocyte blood fractions. J Clin Microbiol 1995; 33:1014.

Espy MJ, Ross TK, Teo R, et al: Evaluation of LightCycler PCR for implementation of laboratory diagnosis of herpes simplex virus infections. J Clin Microbiol 2000; 38:3116–3118.

Falagas ME, Snydman DR, Ruthazer R, et al: Surveillance cultures of blood, urine, and throat specimens are not valuable for predicting cytomegalovirus disease in liver transplant recipients. Clin Infect Dis 1997; 24:824.

Falsey AR, Formica MA, Walsh EE: Diagnosis of respiratory syncytial virus infection: comparison of reverse transcription-PCR to viral culture and serology in adults with respiratory illness. J Clin Microbiol 2002; 40:817–820.

Falsey AR, Hennessey PA, Formica MA, et al: Respiratory syncytial virus in elderly and high-risk adults. N Engl J Med 2005; 352:1749–1759.

Farhat SE, Finn S, Chua R, et al: Rapid detection of infectious mononucleosis-associated heterophile antibodies by a novel immunochromatographic assay and a latex agglutination test. J Clin Microbiol 1993; 31:1597.

Fields BN: Fields Virology, 4th ed. Philadelphia, PA, Lippincott-Raven, 2001.

Fisher MS, Guerra CG, Hickman JR, et al: Peripheral blood lymphocyte apoptosis. A clue to the diagnosis of acute infectious mononucleosis. Arch Pathol Lab Med 1996; 120:951.

Fleming DT, McQuillan GM, Johnson RE, et al: Herpes simplex virus type 2 in the United States, 1976 to 1994. N Engl J Med 1997; 337:1105.

Folks TM, Khabbaz RF: Retroviruses and associated diseases in humans. In Mahy BWJ, Collier L (eds): Microbiology and Microbial Infections. Virology. New York, Oxford University Press, 1998.

Fowler KB, Stagno S, Pass RF, et al: The outcome of congenital cytomegalovirus infection in relation to maternal antibody status. N Engl J Med 1992; 326:663.

Freedberg KA, Losina E, Weinstein MC, et al: Cost effectiveness of combination antiretroviral therapy for HIV disease. N Engl J Med 2001; 344:824–831.

Ganem D, Prince AM: Hepatitis B virus infection – natural history and clinical consequences. N Engl J Med 2004; 350:1118–1129.

Gantz NM, Coldsmith EE: Chronic fatigue syndrome and fibromyalgia resources on the world wide web: a descriptive journey. Clin Infect Dis 2001; 32:938–948.

Gerber MA, Shapiro DE, Ryan RW, et al: Evaluation of enzyme-linked immunosorbent assay procedure for determining specific Epstein–Barr virus serology and of rapid test kits for diagnosis of infectious mononucleosis. J Clin Microbiol 1996; 34:3240–3241.

Gerna G, Revello MG, Percivalle E, et al: Comparison of different immunostaining techniques and monoclonal antibodies to the lower matrix phosphoprotein (pp65) for optimal quantitation cytomegalovirus antigenemia. J Clin Microbiol 1992; 30:1232–1237.

Gershon AA, Raker R, Steinberg S, et al: Antibody to varicella-zoster virus in parturient women and their offspring during the first year of life. Pediatrics 1976; 58:692.

Glaser CA, Gilliam S, Schnurr D, et al: In search of encephalitis etiologies: diagnostic challenges in the California Encephalitis Project, 1998–2000. Clin Infect Dis 2003; 36:731–742.

Gleaves CA, Lee CF, Kirsch L, et al: Evaluation of a direct fluorescein-conjugated monoclonal antibody for detection of cytomegalovirus in centrifugation culture. J Clin Microbiol 1987; 25:1548.

Gleaves CA, Smith TF, Shuster EA, et al: Rapid detection of cytomegalovirus in MRC-5 cells inoculated with urine specimens by using low speed centrifugation and monoclonal antibody to an early antigen. J Clin Microbiol 1984; 19:917.

Gleaves CA, Wilson DJ, Wold AD, et al: Detection and serotyping of herpes simplex virus in MRC-5 cells by use of centrifugation and monoclonal antibodies 16h postinoculation. J Clin Microbiol 1985; 21:29.

Gold D, Bowden R, Sixbey J, et al: Chronic fatigue: a prospective clinical and virologic study. JAMA 1990; 264:48.

Griffin DA, Donaldson KA, Paul JH, et al: Pathogenic human viruses in coastal waters. Clin Microbiol Rev 2003; 16:129–143.

Grohmann GS, Glass RI, Pereira HG, et al: Enteric viruses and diarrhea in HIV infected patients. Enteric Opportunistic Infections Working Group. N Engl J Med 1993; 329:14.

Hadziyannis, SJ: Review: hepatitis delta. J Gastroenterol Hepatol 1997; 12:289–298.

Hadziyannis, SJ: Fulminant hepatitis and the new G/GBV-C flavivirus. J Viral Hepat 1998; 5:15–19.

Hall CB: Respiratory syncytial virus. In Cherry JD, Feigin RD (eds): Textbook of Pediatric Infectious Diseases, 4th ed. Philadelphia, PA, WB Saunders, 1998.

Hall CB: Medical progress: RSV and parainfluenza. N Engl J Med 2001; 344:1917–1928.

Hedberg CW, Osterholm MT: Outbreaks of food-borne and water borne gastroenteritis. Clin Microbiol Rev 1993; 6:199.

Heegaard ED, Brown KE: Human Parvovirus B19. Clin Microbiol Rev 2002; 15:485–505.

Henrard Dr, Phillips J, Windsor I, et al: Detection of human immunodeficiency virus type 1 p24 antigen and plasma RNA. Relevance to indeterminate serology tests. Transfusion 1994; 34:376.

Henrickson KJ: Parainfluenza viruses. Clin Microbiol Rev 2003; 16:242–264.

Hess RD: Minireview. Routine Epstein–Barr virus diagnostics from the laboratory perspective: still challenging after 35 years. J Clin Microbiol 2004; 42:3381–3387.

Hewitt DJ, Peddecord KM, Francis DP, et al: Content and design of laboratory report forms for human immunodeficiency virus type 1 antibody testing. Am J Clin Pathol 1992; 98:1992.

Hierholzer JC: Adenoviruses in the immunocompromised host. Clin Microbiol Rev 1992; 5:262.

Hirsch MS, Brun-Vezinet F, Clotet B, et al: Antiretroviral drug resistance testing in adults infected with HIV1: 2003 recommendations of an International AIDS Society-USA panel. Clin Infect Dis 2003; 37:113–128.

Holmes GP, Kaplan JE, Gantz NM, et al: Chronic fatigue syndrome: a working case definition. Ann Intern Med 1988; 108:387.

Holmes GP, Kaplan JE, Stewart JA, et al: A cluster of patients with a chronic mononucleosis-like syndrome. Is Epstein–Barr virus the cause? JAMA 1987; 257:2297.

Huang YT, Yam P, Huimin Y, et al: Engineered BGMK cells for sensitive and rapid detection of enteroviruses. J Clin Microbiol 2002; 40:366–371.

Hughes JH, Mann DR, Hamparian VV, et al: Detection of respiratory syncytial virus in clinical specimens by viral culture, direct and indirect immunofluorescence, and enzyme immunoassay. J Clin Microbiol 1988; 26:588.

Isaacson E, Glaser CA, Gorghani B, et al: Evidence of human herpesvirus 6 in 4 immunocompetent patients with encephalitis. Clin Infect Dis 2005; 40:890–893.

Ismail N, Fish GE, Smith MB: Laboratory evaluation of a fully automated chemiluminescence immunoassay for rapid detection of HbsAg, antibodies to HbsAg and antibodies to hepatitis C virus. J Clin Microbiol 2004; 42:610–617.

Istas AS, Dermmier GJ, Dubbins JC, et al: Surveillance for congenital CMV disease. Report from the National Congenital CMV Disease Registry. Clin Infect Dis 1995; 20:665.

Iwamoto M, Jernigan DB, Gausch A, et al: Transmission of West Nile Virus from an organ donor to four transplant recipients. N Engl J Med 2003; 348:2196–2203.

Iwarson I: The five main types of hepatitis: an alphabetical update. Scand J Infect Dis 1992; 24:129.

Johnson EB: Transport of viral specimens. Clin Microbiol Rev 1990; 3:120.

Kessler HA, Blaau W, Spear J, et al: Diagnosis of human immunodeficiency virus infection in seronegative homosexuals presenting with an acute viral syndrome. JAMA 1987; 258:1196–1199.

Kessler HH, Sanker B, Rabenau H, et al: Rapid diagnosis of enterovirus infection by a new one-step reverse transcription-PCR assay. J Clin Microbiol 1997; 35:976–977.

Kim JJ, Wright TC, Goldie SJ: Cost effectiveness of alternative triage strategies for atypical squamous cells of undetermined significance. JAMA 2002; 287:2382–2390.

Kimball AM, Foy HM, Cooney MK, et al: Isolation of respiratory syncytial and influenza viruses from the sputum of patients hospitalized with pneumonia. J Infect Dis 1983; 147:181.

Kimberlin DW: Neonatal herpes simplex infection. Clin Microbiol Rev 2004; 17:1–13.

Kimberlin DW, Lakeman FD, Arvin AM, et al: Application of the polymerase chain reaction to the diagnosis and management of neonatal herpes simplex virus disease. J Infect Dis 1996, 174:1162.

Kleinman S, Glynn SA, Busch M, et al: The 2003 West Nile Virus United States epidemic: the America's Blood Centers experience. Transfusion 2005; 45:469–479.

Klonoff DC: Chronic fatigue syndrome. Clin Infect Dis 1992; 15:812.

Konig B, Konig W, Arnold R, et al: Prospective study of human metapneumovirus infection in children less than 3 years of age. J Clin Microbiol 2004; 42:4632–4635.

Koralnik IJ: Neurologic diseases caused by HIV-1 and opportunistic infections. In Mandell GL, Bennett JE, Dolin R (eds): Principles and Practice of Infectious Diseases, 6th ed. Philadelphia, PA, Elsievier Churchill Livingstone, 2005.

Kulasingham SL, Hughes JP, Kiviat NB, et al: Evaluation of human papillomavirus testing in primary screening for cervical abnormalities. JAMA 2002; 288:1749–1757.

Lafferty WE, Krofft S, Remmington M, et al: Diagnosis of herpes simplex virus by direct immunofluorescence and viral isolation from samples of external genital lesions in a high prevalence population. J Clin Microbiol 1987; 25:323.

Landry ML, Ferguson D: SimulFluor respiratory screen for rapid detection of multiple respiratory viruses in clinical specimens by immunofluorescence staining. J Clin Microbiol 2000; 38:708–711.

Landry ML, Ferguson D, Cohen S, et al: Detection of human metapneumovirus in clinical samples by immunofluorescence staining of shell vial centrifugation cultures prepared from three different cell lines. J Clin Microbiol 2005; 43:1950–1952.

Landry ML, Ferguson D, Stevens-Ayers T, et al: Evaluation of CMV Brite Kit for detection of cytomegalovirus pp65 antigenemia in peripheral blood leukocytes by immunofluorescence. J Clin Microbiol 1996; 34:1337.

Landry ML, Garner R, Ferguson D: Comparison of the NucliSens Basic Kit (nucleic acid sequence-based amplification) and the Argene Biosoft Enterovirus Consensus Reverse Transcription-PCR Assays for rapid detection of enterovirus RNA in clinical specimens. J Clin Microbiol 2003; 41:5006–5010.

Lauer GM, Walker BD: Hepatitis C virus infection. N Engl J Med 2001; 345:41–52.

Linderholm M, Bowman J, Juto P, et al: Comparative evaluation of nine kits for rapid diagnosis of infectious mononucleosis and Epstein–Barr virus-specific serology. J Clin Microbiol 1994; 32:259.

Lipson SM, David K, Shaikh F, et al: Detection of precytopathic effect of enteroviruses in clinical specimens by centrifugation-enhanced antigen detection. J Clin Microbiol 2001; 39:2755–2759.

Lipson SM, Salo RJ, Leonardi GP: Evaluation of five monoclonal antibody-based kits or reagents for the identification and culture confirmation of herpes simplex virus. J Clin Microbiol 1991; 29:466.

Lloyd AR: Chronic fatigue and chronic fatigue syndrome: shifting boundaries and attributions. Am J Med 1998; 105:7S.

Lok A: Chronic hepatitis B. N Engl J Med 2002; 346:1682–1683.

Ly TD, Martin L, Daghfal D, et al: Seven Human Immunodeficiency Virus (HIV) antigen-antibody combination assays: evaluation of HIV seroconversion sensitivity and subtype detection. J Clin Microbiol 2001; 39:3122–3128.

Mace M, Cointe D, Six C, et al: Diagnostic value of RT-PCR of amniotic fluid for prenatal diagnosis of congenital rubella infection in pregnant women with confirmed primary rubella infection. J Clin Microbiol 2004; 42:4818–4820.

McHutchison JG, Gordon SC, Schiff ER, et al: Interferon alfa-2b alone or in combination with ribavirin as initial treatment for chronic hepatitis C. N Engl J Med 1998; 352:1426–1432.

McKinney RE, Katz SL, Wilfert CM: Chronic enteroviral meningoencephalitis in agammaglobulinemic patients. Rev Infect Dis 1987; 9:334–356.

Maggi F, Pifferi M, Vatteroni M, et al: Human metapneumovirus associated with respiratory tract infections in a 3-year study of nasal swabs from infants in Italy. J Clin Microbiol 2003; 41:2987–2991.

Manns A, Hisada M, LaGrenade K: Human T-lymphotrophic virus type 1 infection. Lancet 1999; 353:1951.

Meissner HC, Long SS: Revised indications for the use of palivizumab and respiratory syncytial virus immune globulin intravenous for prevention of RSV infections. Pediatrics 2003; 112:1447–1452.

Mendez JC, Espy MJ, Smith TF, et al: Evaluation of PCR primers for early diagnosis of cytomegalovirus infection following liver transplantation. J Clin Microbiol 1998; 36:526.

Miller H, Milk R, Diaz-Mitoma K, et al: Comparison of the VIDAS RSV assay and the Abbott Testpack RSV with direct immunofluorescence for detection of respiratory syncytial virus in nasopharyngeal aspirates. J Clin Microbiol 1993; 31:1336.

Minnich II, Ray CG: Early testing of cultures for detection of hemadsorbing viruses. J Clin Microbiol 1987; 25:421.

Mitchell DK, Vaan R, Morrow AL, et al: Outbreaks of astrovirus gastroenteritis in day care centers. J Pediatr 1993; 123:725.

Mitchell PS, Espy MJ, Smith TF, et al: Laboratory diagnosis of central nervous system infections with herpes simplex virus by PCR performed with cerebrospinal fluid specimens. J Clin Microbiol 1997; 35:2873.

MMWR: Interpretive criteria used to report Western blot results for HIV-1-antibody testing – United States. Morbid Mortal Weekly Rep 1991; 40:692.

MMWR: Outbreak of West Nile-like viral encephalitis – New York, 1999. Morbid Mortal Weekly Rep 1999; 48:845.

VII

MMWR: Norwalk-like viruses. Public health consequences and outbreak management. Morbid Mortal Weekly Rep 2001; 50(RR09); 1–18.

MMWR: Alter MJ, Kuhnet WL, Finelli L: Guidelines for laboratory testing and result reporting of antibody to hepatitis C virus. Morbid Mortal Weekly Rep 2003; 52:RR-3.

MMWR: Investigation of rabies infections in organ donor and transplant recipients – Alabama, Arkansas, Oklahoma and Texas, 2004. Morbid Mortal Weekly Rep 2004; 53:586–589.

MMWR: Achievements in Public Health: elimination of rubella and congenital rubella syndrome – United States, 1969–2004. Morbid Mortal Weekly Rep 2005; 54:279–282.

Modin JF: Perinatal echovirus infection: Insights from a literature review of 61 cases of serious infection and 16 outbreaks in nurseries. Rev Infect Dis 1986; 8:918.

Morrow RA, Friedrich D, Krantz E: Performance of the Focus and Kalon enzyme-linked-immunosorbent assays for antibodies to herpes simplex virus type 2 glycoprotein G in culture-documented cases of genital herpes. J Clin Microbiol 2003; 41:5212–5214.

Moseley RC, Corey L, Benjamin D, et al: Comparison of viral isolation, direct immunofluorescence, and indirect immunoperoxidase techniques for detection of genital herpes simplex virus infection. J Clin Microbiol 1981; 13:913.

Mulford WS, Buller RS, Lewis L, et al: Evaluation of the Biostar Flu Optical Immunoassay (OIA) for rapid detection of influenza virus in pediatric and adult patients. Clinical Virology Symposium, 1999, Abstract S9.

Munoz A, Kirby AJ, He YD, et al: Long-term survivors with HIV-1 infection: incubation period and longitudinal patterns of CD4+ lymphocytes. J Acquir Immun Defic Syndr Hum Retrovirol 1995; 8:496–505.

Murray PR (ed.): Manual of Clinical Microbiology, 8th ed. Washington, DC, ASM Press, 2003.

Musher DM, Musher BL: Contagious acute gastrointestinal infections. N Engl J Med 2004; 351:2417–2427.

Nalonen PE, Madeley CR: The laboratory diagnosis of viral infection. In Collier L, Balows A, Sussman M (eds): Microbiology and Microbial Infections, 9th ed. New York, Oxford University Press, 1998.

Nash D, Mostashari F, Fine A, et al: The outbreak of West Nile Virus infection in the New York City area in 1999. N Engl J Med 2001; 344:1807–1814.

National Institutes of Health: Consensus Statement of Management of Hepatitis C. National Institutes of Health 2002; 19:10–12.

Nelson CT, Istas AS, Wilkerson MK, et al: PCR detection of cytomegalovirus DNA in serum as a diagnostic tool for congenital CMV infection. J Clin Microbiol 1995; 33:314.

Nolte FS, Caliendo AM: Molecular detection and identification of microorganisms. In Murray PR (ed.): Manual of Clinical Microbiology, 8th ed. Washington, DC, ASM Press, 2003.

Ohm-Smith MJ, Nassos Ps, Haller BL: Evaluation of the Binax NOW, BD Directigen and BD Directigen EZ assays for detection of respiratory syncytial virus. J Clin Microbiol 2004; 42:2996–2999.

Orle KA, Gates CA, Martin DH, et al: Simultaneous PCR detection of Haemophilus ducreyi, Treponema pallidum, and herpes simplex virus types 1 and 2 from genital ulcers. J Clin Microbiol 1996; 34:49.

Pang X, Lee B, Chiu L, et al: Evaluation and validation of real-time reverse-transcriptase PCR assay using the LightCycler system for detection and quantitation of norovirus. J Clin Microbiol 2004; 42:4679–4685.

Parashar UD, Holman RC, Clarke MJ, et al: Hospitalizations associated with rotavirus diarrhea in the United States: 1993 through 1995: surveillance based on new ICD-9-CM rotavirus-specific diagnostic code. J Infect Dis 1998; 177:13.

Pealer LN, Marfin AA, Petersen LR, et al: Transmission of West Nile Virus through blood transfusion in the United States in 2002. N Engl J Med 2003; 349:1236–1245.

Perkins SM, Webb DL, Torrance SA, et al: Comparison of a real-time reverse transcription PCR assay and a culture technique for quantitative assessment of viral load in children naturally infected with respiratory syncytial virus. J Clin Microbiol 2005; 43:2356–2362.

Petersen LR, Hayes EB: Westward ho? – the spread of West Nile Virus. N Engl J Med 2004; 351:2257–2259.

Petric M, Tellier R: Rotaviruses, caliciviruses, astroviruses and other diarrheic viruses. In Murray PR (ed.): Manual of Clinical Microbiology, 8th ed. Washington, DC, ASM Press, 2003.

Pilcher CD, Fiscus SA, Nguyen TQ, et al: Detection of acute infections during HIV testing in North Carolina. N Engl J Med 2005; 352:1873–1883.

Plotkin SA: Rabies. Clin Infect Dis 2000; 30:4–12.

Pohl C, Green M, Wald ER, et al: Respiratory syncytial virus infections in pediatric liver transplant recipients. J Infect Dis 1992; 165:166.

Poland GA, Jacobson RM: Prevention of Hepatitis B with the Hepatitis B vaccine. N Engl J Med 2004; 351:2832–2838.

Polish LB, Gallagher M, Fields H, et al: Delta hepatitis: molecular biology and clinical epidemiological features. Clin Microbiol Rev 1993; 6:211.

Prober C: Sixth disease and the ubiquity of human herpesviruses. N Engl J Med 2005; 352:753–755.

Prober CG, Hensleigh PA, Boucher F, et al: Use of routine viral cultures at delivery to identify neonates exposed to herpes simplex virus. N Engl J Med 1988; 318:887.

Prober CG, Sullender WM, Yasukawa II, et al: Low risk of herpes simplex virus infections in neonates exposed to the virus at the time of vaginal delivery to mothers with recurrent genital herpes simplex virus infections. N Engl J Med 1987; 316:240.

Quinn TC, Klein RL, Halsey N, et al: Early diagnosis of perinatal HIV infection by detection of viral-specific IgA antibodies. JAMA 1991; 266:3439.

Rasmussen L, Zipeto D, Wolitz RA, et al: Risk for retinitis in patients with AIDS can be assessed by quantitation of threshold levels of cytomegalovirus DNA burden in blood. J Infect Dis 1997; 176:1146.

Razonable RR, Paya CV, Smith TF: Role of the laboratory in diagnosis and management of cytomegalovirus infection in hematopoietic stem cell and solid organ transplant recipients. J Clin Microbiol 2002; 40:746–752.

Read SJ, Kurtz JB: Laboratory diagnosis of common viral infections of the central nervous system by using a single multiplex PCR screening assay. J Clin Microbiol 1999; 37:1352.

Reeves WC, Stamey FR, Black JB, et al: Human herpesviruses 6 and 7 in chronic fatigue syndrome: a case-control study. Clin Infect Dis 2000; 31:48–52.

Remington JS, Thulliez P, Montoya JG: Minireview: recent developments in the diagnosis of toxoplasmosis. J Clin Microbiol 2004; 42:941–945.

Revello MG, Baldanti F, Sarasini A, et al: Prenatal diagnosis of rubella virus infection by direct detection and semiquantitation of viral RNA in clinical samples by RT-PCR. J Clin Microbiol 1997; 35:708.

Revello MG, Gerna G: Diagnosis and management of human cytomegalovirus infection in the mother, fetus and newborn infant. Clin Microbiol Rev 2002; 15:680–715.

Ribes JA, Steele AD, Seabolt JP, et al: Six year study of the incidence of herpes in genital and nongenital cultures in a central Kentucky Medical Center patient population. J Clin Microbiol 2001; 39:3321–3325.

Richter SS: MiniReview: Laboratory assays for diagnosis and management of hepatitis C virus infection. J Clin Microbiol 2002; 40:4407–4412.

Roberts TC, Buller RS, Gaudreault M, et al: Effects of storage temperature and time on qualitative and quantitative detection of cytomegalovirus in blood specimens by shell vial culture and PCR. J Clin Microbiol 1997; 35:2224.

Rogers MF, Ou C, Rayfield M, et al: Use of the polymerase chain reaction for early detection of the proviral sequences of HIV in infants born to seropositive mothers. N Engl J Med 1989; 320:1649.

Rogers R, Windust A, Gregory J: Evaluation of a novel dry latex preparation for demonstration of infectious mononucleosis heterophile antibody in comparison with three established tests. J Clin Microbiol 1999; 37:95.

Romero JR: Reverse-transcription polymerase chain reaction detection of the enteroviruses. Arch Pathol Lab Med 1999; 123:1161–1169.

Romero JR, Kimberlin DW: Molecular diagnosis of viral infections of the central nervous system. Clin Lab Med 2003; 23:843–865.

Roseff SD, Campos JM: Detection of cytomegalovirus antibodies in serum using the TransSTAT-CMV and CMV Scan assays. Am J Clin Pathol 1993; 99:539.

Rossier JE, Miller HR, Phipps PH: Rapid viral diagnosis by immunofluorescence. Ottawa, University of Ottawa Press, 1989.

Rotbart HA, Ahmed A, Hickey S, et al: Diagnosis of enterovirus infection by polymerase chain reaction of multiple specimen types. Pediatr Infect Dis J 1997; 16:409.

Rotbart HA, Sawyer MH, Fast S, et al: Diagnosis of enteroviral meningitis by using PCR with a colorimetric microbial detection assay. J Clin Microbiol 1994; 32:2590.

Salahuddin SZ, Ablashi DV, Markham PD, et al: Isolation of a new virus HBLV, in patients with lymphoproliferative disorders. Science 1986; 234:596.

Schindler S, Sholtis W, Hadziyannis E, et al: Rapid detection of respiratory viruses using a mink lung/A549 mixed cell line. Clinical Virology Symposium, 1999, Abstract S16.

Schlauder GG, Dawson GJ: Hepatitis E virus. In Murray PR (ed.): Manual of Clinical Microbiology, 8th ed. Washington, DC, ASM Press, 2003.

Schluter WW, Reef SE, Redd SC, et al: Changing epidemiology of congenital rubella syndrome in the United States. J Infect Dis 1998; 178:636.

Schooley RT: Epstein-Barr virus (infectious mononucleosis). In Bennett JE, Dolin R (eds): Principles and Practice of Infectious Diseases, 6th ed. Philadelphia, Elsevier Churchill Livingstone, 2005.

Schrim J, Meulenberg G, Pastoorm P, et al: Rapid detection of varicella zoster virus in clinical specimens using monoclonal antibodies on shell vials and smears. J Med Virol 1989; 28:1.

Schupbach J: Human immunodeficiency viruses. In Murray PR (ed.): Manual of Clinical Microbiology, 8th ed. Washington, DC, ASM Press, 2003.

Shafer RW: Genotypic testing for HIV-1 drug resistance. Clin Microbiol Rev 2002; 15:247–277.

Shahrabadi MS, Lee PW: Calcium requirement for syncytium formation in HEp-2 cells by respiratory syncytial virus. J Clin Microbiol 1988; 26:139.

Shyamala V, Arcangel P, Cottrell J, et al: Assessment of the Target-Capture PCR Hepatitis B Virus DNA Quantitative Assay and comparison with commercial HBV DNA quantiative assays. J Clin Microbiol 2004; 42:5199–5204.

Sia IG, Patel R: New strategies for prevention and therapy of cytomegalovirus infection and disease in solid organ transplants. Clin Microbiol Rev 2000; 13, 83.

Sison A, Campos JM: Laboratory methods for early detection of HIV type 1 in newborns and infants. Clin Microbiol Rev 1992; 5:238.

Slavin MA, Gleaves CA, Schoch HG, et al: Quantification of cytomegalovirus in bronchoalveolar fluid after allogeneic marrow transplantation by centrifugation culture. J Clin Microbiol 1992; 30:2776.

Smith, J: Rabies virus. In Murray PR (ed.): Manual of Clinical Microbiology, 8th ed. Washington, DC, ASM Press, 2003.

Smith RF, Elder BL: Evaluation of Cytomegelisa immunoglobulin M assay and comparison with indirect fluorescent antibody testing of QAE-Sephadex A50-treated sera. Am J Clin Pathol 1987; 87:230.

Stagno S, Pass RF, Dworsky ME, et al: Congenital cytomegalovirus infection: the relative importance of primary and recurrent maternal infection. N Engl J Med 1982; 306:945–949.

Stanberry LR, Floyd-Reising A, Connelly BL, et al: Herpes simplex viremia: report of eight pediatric cases and review of the literature. Clin Infect Dis 1994; 18:401.

Steeper TA, Horwitz CA, Ablashi DV, et al: The spectrum of clinical and laboratory findings resulting from human herpesvirus-6 in patients with mononucleosis-like illnesses not resulting from Epstein–Barr virus or cytomegalovirus. Am J Clin Pathol 1990; 93:776.

Stein DS, Korvick JA, Vermund SH, et al: CD4 lymphocyte cell enumeration for prediction of clinical course of human immunodeficiency virus disease: a review. J Infect Dis 1992; 165:352.

Stockton J, Stephenson I, Fleming D, et al: Human metapneumovirus as a cause of community acquired respiratory illness. Emerg Infect Dis 2002; 8:897–901.

Storch GA, Buller RS, Bailey TC, et al: Comparison of PCR and pp65 antigenemia assay with quantitative shell vial culture for detection of cytomegalovirus in blood leukocytes from solid organ transplant recipients. J Clin Microbiol 1994; 32:997.

Stramer SL, Glynn SA, Kleinman SH, et al: Detection of HIV-1 and HCV infections among antibody-negative blood donors by nucleic acid-amplification testing. N Engl J Med 2004; 351:760–768.

Strickler JG, Fedeli F, Horwitz CA, et al: Infectious mononucleosis in lymphoid tissue. Histopathology, in situ hybridization and differential diagnosis. Arch Pathol Lab Med 1993; 117:269.

Szatanek CD, Aymard M, Thouvenot D, et al: Surveillance Network for herpes simplex virus resistance to antiviral drugs: 3-year followup. J Clin Microbiol 2004; 42:242–249.

Tang YW, Hibbs JR, Tau KR, et al: Effective use of polymerase chain reaction for diagnosis of central nervous system infection. Clin Infect Dis 1999a; 29:803.

Tang YW, Mitchell, PS, Espy MJ, et al: Molecular diagnosis of herpes simplex virus infections in the central nervous system. J Clin Microbiol 1999b; 37:2127.

Tang YW, Rys PN, Rutledge BJ, et al: Comparative evaluation of colorimetric microtiter plate systems for detection of herpes simplex virus in cerebrospinal fluid. J Clin Microbiol 1998; 36:2714.

Templeton KE, Scheltinga SA, Beersma MF, et al: Rapid and sensitive method using multiplex real-time PCR for diagnosis of infections by influenza A and B viruses, respiratory syncytial virus and parainfluenza viruses. J Clin Microbiol 2004; 42:1564–1569.

Thielman NM, Guerrant RL: Acute infectious diarrhea. N Engl J Med 2004; 350:38–47.

Thomas EE, Book LE: Comparison of two rapid methods for detection of RSV (TestPack RSV and Ortho RSV ELISA) with direct immunofluorescence and virus isolation for the diagnosis of pediatric RSV infection. J Clin Microbiol 1991; 29:632.

Thomas EE, Roscoe DL, Brook L, et al: The utility of latex agglutination assays in the diagnosis of pediatric viral gastroenteritis. Am J Clin Pathol 1994; 101:742.

Tolfvenstam T, Papadogiannakis N, Norbeck O, et al: Frequency of human parvovirus B19 infection in intrauterine fetal death. Lancet 2001; 357:1494–1497.

Tranchard-Bunel D, Gras-Masse H, Bourez B, et al: Evaluation of an Epstein–Barr Immunoglobulin M ELISA using a synthetic convergent peptide library, or mixotope, for diagnosis of primary EBV infection. J Clin Microbiol 1999; 37:2366.

Tristram DA: Respiratory syncytial virus. In Murray PR (ed.): Manual of Clinical Microbiology, 8th ed. Washington, DC, ASM Press, 2003.

Troanor JJ: Influenza virus. In GL, Bennett JE, Dolin R (eds): Principles and Practice of Infectious Diseases, 6th ed. Philadelphia, Elsievier Churchill Livingstone, 2005.

Van den Hoogen BG, de Jong JC, Goren J, et al: A newly discovered human pneumovirus isolated from young children with respiratory tract disease. Nat Med 2001; 7:719–724.

Van den Hoogen BG, Osterhaus DM, Fouchier RA: Clinical impact and diagnosis of human metapneumovirus infection. Pediatr Infect Dis J 2004; 23(1 Suppl):S25–S32.

VanEnk RA, James KK, Thompson KD: Evaluation of three commercial enzyme-linked immunosorbent assays for detection of herpes simplex virus antigen. Am J Clin Pathol 1991; 95:428.

Watts DH: Management of HIV infection in pregnancy. N Engl J Med 2002; 346:1879–1891.

Weidmann M, Meyer-Konig U, Hufert FT: Rapid detection of herpes simplex virus and varicella zoster virus by real-time PCR. J Clin Microbiol 2003; 41:1565–1568.

Weinberg A, Walker ML: Evaluation of three immunoassay kits for rapid detection of influenza virus A and B. Clin Diagn Lab Immunol 2005; 12:367–370.

Whitley RJ, Cobbs CG, Alford CA: Disease that mimics herpes simplex virus encephalitis. JAMA 1989; 262:234.

Whitley RJ, Corey L, Arvin A, et al: Changing presentation of herpes simplex virus infections in neonates. J Infect Dis 1988; 158:109.

Whitley RJ, Lakeman F: Herpes simplex virus infection of the central nervous system: therapeutic and diagnostic considerations. Clin Infect Dis 1995; 20:414–420.

Wreghitt RG, Teare EL, Sule O, et al: Cytomegalovirus infection in immunocomptetent patients. Clin Infect Dis 2003; 37:1603–1606.

Wright TC, Cox JT, Massad LS, et al: 2001 consensus guidelines for the management of women with cervical cytological abnormalities. JAMA 2002; 287:2120–2129.

Xepapadaki P, Psarras S, Bossios A, et al: Human metapneumovirus as a causative agent of acute bronchiolitis in infants. J Clin Virol 2004; 30:267–270.

Xiang J, Wunschmann S, Diekema DJ, et al: Effect of coinfection with GB Virus C on survival among patients with HIV infection. N Engl J Med 2001; 345:707–714.

Yeldandi AV, Colby TV: Pathologic features of lung biopsy specimens from influenza pneumonia cases. Hum Pathol 1994; 25:47.

Young NS, Brown KE: Parvovirus B19. N Engl J Med 2004; 350:586–597.

Yungbluth M, Costello M, Cutler C, Levin M: Rapid shell vial culture of sputum for influenza A virus: implications for infection control. Abstract #1689, Interscience Conference on Antimicrobial Agents and Chemotherapy, September 1998, San Francisco.

Zein NN: Clinical significance of hepatitis C virus genotypes. Clin Microbiol Rev 2000; 13:223–235.

Zerbini M, Musiani M, Gentilomi G, et al: Comparative evaluation of virological and serological methods in prenatal diagnosis of parvovirus B19 fetal hydrops. J Clin Microbiol 1996; 34:603–608.

Zerr DM, Amalia SM, Selke SS, et al: A population-based study of primary human herpesvirus 6 infection. N Engl J Med 2005:352:768–776.

Websites and E-mail Addresses

Centers for Disease Control and Prevention: http://www.cdc.gov/
Many journals, articles, materials free

Infectious Diseases Society of America: http://www.idsociety.org
Care and treatment guidelines free

World Health Organization: http://www.who.int/

Association for Professionals in Infection Control and Epidemiology: http://www.apic.org/

Medscape: http://www.medscape.com

American Society for Microbiology: http://www.asmusa.org
Many articles and materials free

European Society for Clinical Virology: http://www.eur.nl/FGG/VIRO/ESCV/

National Centers for Infectious Diseases: http://www.cdc.gov/ncidod/

National Institutes of Health: http://www.nih.gov

New England Journal of Medicine: http://www.nejm.org

Pan American Society for Clinical Virology: http://www.virology.org/

All the Virology on the WWW: http://www.virology.net

Johns Hopkins Infectious Disease: http://www.hopkins-id.edu/

Mike.Costello@advocatehealth.com

myungbluth@reshealthcare.org

VII

CHAPTER 55

Chlamydial, Rickettsial, and Mycoplasmal Infections

Gail L. Woods MD, David H. Walker MD

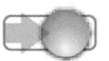 **KEY POINTS**

• *Chlamydia trachomatis* is the most common bacterial cause of sexually transmitted disease in the United States.

• The most sensitive method for detecting *C. trachomatis* is nucleic acid amplification.

• *Chlamydophila pneumoniae* (formerly *Chlamydia pneumoniae*) is responsible for at least 10% of community-acquired pneumonias. Infection is most often diagnosed serologically.

• Treatable rickettsial infections, including life-threatening Rocky Mountain spotted fever, epidemic typhus, scrub typhus, human monocytotropic ehrlichiosis, and human granulocytotropic anaplasmosis, are seldom diagnosed serologically during the acute stage of illness, owing to absence of an early antibody response.

• Immunohistochemistry and molecular diagnostics are effective in diagnosing rickettsioses and ehrlichioses, respectively, but are not generally available.

• Q fever endocarditis is a chronic infection that is usually diagnosed by detecting a high titer (= 1:800 by immunofluorescent antibody assay) of antibodies against *Coxiella burnetii* phase I antigen.

• The clinicoepidemiologic diagnosis of cat scratch disease can be confirmed serologically by antibodies to *Bartonella henselae* or by polymerase chain reaction testing of lymph node aspirates.

• Pneumonia due to *Mycoplasma pneumoniae* is often diagnosed on the basis of clinical manifestations alone. Definitive diagnosis requires detection of specific IgM, a fourfold change in IgG antibody titer between acute and convalescent serum specimens, or detection of nucleic acid in sputum or other respiratory specimen by nucleic acid amplification.

Human infections caused by chlamydias, rickettsiae, and mycoplasmas are discussed separately because the responsible pathogens differ from most other bacteria in several ways: the organisms are smaller, the structure of their cell walls is different, and chlamydias and many rickettsias are obligately intracellular parasites.

Chlamydial Infections

The chlamydias have a tropism for columnar epithelial cells. They have a cell wall similar to that of Gram-negative bacteria; they contain both deoxyribonucleic acid (DNA) and ribonucleic acid (RNA), have prokaryotic ribosomes, and synthesize their own proteins, nucleic acids, and lipids; they divide by binary fission; and they are susceptible to particular antibiotics. Unlike most bacteria, the chlamydias are 'energy parasites;' they lack cytochromes and so cannot synthesize high-energy adenosine triphosphate (ATP) metabolites. For this reason, they are obligate intracellular bacteria and cannot replicate outside cells.

The chlamydias are classified in the order Chlamydiales, family Chlamydiaceae, the only family that contains human pathogens (Everett, 1999). There are two genera and three species pathogenic for humans: *Chlamydia trachomatis*, *Chlamydophila* (formerly *Chlamydia*) *psittaci*, and *Chlamydophila* (formerly *Chlamydia*) *pneumoniae*. Features useful for differentiating the three species are shown in Table 55–1. These genera also contain six other species that have not been associated with infections in humans. There are three biovars of *C. trachomatis*: mouse pneumonitis, lymphogranuloma venereum (LGV), and trachoma, the latter two of which preferentially infect humans. The LGV biovar contains four serovars (L1, L2, L2a, L3), and there are 15 serovars included in the trachoma biovar: A, B, Ba, and C are associated with trachoma, whereas D–K, Da, Ia, and Ja are associated with genital infections.

Structure

Two morphologically distinct forms of chlamydia are recognized. The elementary body is a dense, spherical form, 0.2–0.4 μm in diameter, that contains prokaryotic ribosomal RNA and has a rigid cell wall due to extensive disulfide crosslinking of cell wall proteins. It is the infectious form of the organism, capable of limited extracellular survival. The reticulate body, 0.6–1.0 μm in diameter, is the intracellular, metabolically active form, incapable of surviving outside cells. The closed circular DNA of both forms is compactly organized in a central nucleoid and has a genome of 1.0–1.2 million nucleotide base pairs.

Two components of the outer membrane of the chlamydial elementary body have diagnostic importance. The most prominent is the major outer membrane protein (MOMP), a transmembrane protein with serovar-, species-, genus-, and family-reactive epitopes defined by monoclonal antibodies. Infection with chlamydias induces MOMP-specific antibodies but their role in protective immunity is unclear. The chlamydial outer membrane also contains a lipopolysaccharide (LPS) antigen, which is the major antigen detected in genus-specific serologic tests for chlamydial infection.

Table 55–1 Features Useful for Differentiating Species of *Chlamydia* and *Chlamydophila* Pathogenic for Humans

Parameter	*Chlamydia trachomatis*	Species *Chlamydophila psittaci*	*Chlamydophila pneumoniae*
Sulfa susceptibility	Susceptible	Resistant	Resistant
Glycogen staining of inclusion	Positive	Negative	Negative
Elementary body shape	Round	Round	Pear-shaped or round

Monoclonal antibodies and monospecific polyvalent antisera to the LPS or MOMP are used in direct fluorescent antibody (DFA) tests and enzyme immunoassays (EIAs) to detect chlamydial antigen in clinical specimens.

Replication

Chlamydias replicate in the cytoplasm of infected host cells. The developmental cycle begins with attachment of the elementary body to a microvillus on a susceptible columnar cell via heparin bridges. The elementary body travels down the microvillus and localizes in indentations of the host cell plasma membrane. There the chlamydia enters the host cell in an endosome, where *C. psittaci*, *C. pneumoniae*, and *C. trachomatis* remain during their intracellular development. Endosomes containing elementary bodies of *C. psittaci* do not become acidified or fuse with cellular lysosomes; those containing *C. trachomatis* elementary bodies fuse with one another and perhaps with lysosomes. Within 6–8 hours after the elementary body enters the host cell, changes in its cell wall result in a transition to the reticulate body and subsequent initiation of DNA, RNA, and protein synthesis and its division by binary fission. Host cell mitochondria migrate to and are positioned against the enlarging endosome, allowing the reticulate body to utilize host cell ATP. Reticulate bodies begin to reorganize 18–24 hours after infection and, presumably when nutrients are depleted, they mature into elementary bodies, which are released from the host cell. Cells infected with *C. psittaci* usually are severely damaged and the organisms are released by cell lysis within 48 hours. In contrast, the inclusion of *C. trachomatis* appears to be extruded by fusion of the inclusion membrane with the plasma membrane 72–96 hours after infection, leaving a lesion in the surviving host cell membrane.

Chlamydia trachomatis

C. trachomatis is the most common cause of sexually transmitted disease in the United States, and in trachoma-endemic regions of the Middle East, North Africa, and northern India it is an important cause of blindness.

Epidemiology, Pathology, and Clinical Manifestations

Humans are the only known natural host for all strains of *C. trachomatis*. The clinical manifestations and organ specificity of human infections with *C. trachomatis* are determined by both the mechanism of transmission and the properties of the infecting strain. Epidemiologically, *C. trachomatis* infections are divided into three categories: classic trachoma, sexually transmitted infections of adults, and perinatal ocular and respiratory tract infections.

Classic trachoma is an important cause of blindness in areas where public sanitation is inadequate and personal hygiene poor, and it is the most common cause of preventable blindness worldwide (Solomon, 2004). Typically, the infection is transmitted among children via fingers, fomites, and probably flies. In endemic areas, acute chlamydial conjunctivitis of adults or infants is uncommon but most children become chronically infected within a few years of birth. Repeated exposure to *C. trachomatis* eventually results in chronic follicular keratoconjunctivitis, conjunctival scarring, and pannus formation (invasion of vessels into the cornea).

C.-trachomatis-induced sexually transmitted infections of adults include LGV and urethritis/cervicitis and the associated complications. LGV is endemic in Asia, Africa, and South America. In the United States, approximately 500 cases are reported each year; the disease affects males more frequently than females and is most common in persons of low socioeconomic status living in the southeastern states, in homosexual men, and in persons who have visited LGV-endemic countries outside the United States. LGV is transmitted sexually, although transmission by fomites and by aerosols produced during laboratory accidents has caused pneumonitis, pleural effusions, and mediastinal or hilar lymphadenopathy (Jones, 2000). The reservoirs of infection probably are persons with asymptomatic or ignored symptomatic urethral, cervical, or anorectal infection.

LGV is the only infection caused by *C. trachomatis* that produces multisystem involvement and constitutional manifestations. During the primary phase, a small, painless vesicle or a nonindurated papule or ulcer develops, often on the external genitalia, 3 days to 3 weeks after exposure, and heals quickly without scarring. The secondary stage, characterized by suppurative regional lymphadenopathy, fever, chills, anorexia, headache, myalgias, and arthralgias, begins 2–6 weeks after exposure. Histologic examination of affected lymph nodes shows granulomas surrounding stellate abscesses. Involved lymph nodes become matted and eventually suppurate, producing draining fistulas that heal with scarring over several months. The fibrosis and resultant abnormal lymphatic drainage are responsible for the urethral or rectal strictures or induration and lymphedema of the genitalia that develop during the third stage.

Each year in the United States an estimated 3 million non-LGV *C. trachomatis* infections occur in sexually active adolescents and young adults, and the annual costs associated with untreated chlamydial infections and their complications are estimated to exceed $2 billion (Peipert, 2003). The clinical spectrum of sexually transmitted infections due to non-LGV strains of *C. trachomatis* is similar to disease caused by *Neisseria gonorrhoeae* (see Ch. 56). In men, *C. trachomatis* is responsible for 30–50% of cases of nongonococcal urethritis, but as many as 85–90% of men who harbor *C. trachomatis* in the urethra are asymptomatic (Peipert, 2003). Rarely, urethritis caused by *C. trachomatis* progresses to epididymitis. Among homosexual males, non-LGV strains of *C. trachomatis* have been associated with proctitis. The organism also has been recovered from the urethra of as many as 70% of men with untreated Reiter syndrome associated with urethritis (Keat, 1983). Genital infection with *C. trachomatis* is probably more prevalent in women than in men. Risk factors for chlamydial infection in sexually active women are young age (<25 years), intercourse at an early age, inconsistent use of barrier contraceptives, multiple sexual partners, and being single or divorced, black, or of low socioeconomic status. Infection of the endocervix with *C. trachomatis* is often asymptomatic but at least one third of women have signs of infection on physical examination. The most common sign is mucopurulent cervicitis, which can spread to the urethra and urinary bladder, resulting in the 'acute urethral syndrome' of abacteriuric pyuria, or to the endometrium and fallopian tubes, producing endometritis or salpingitis. Untreated infections of the upper reproductive tract may progress to pelvic inflammatory disease or cause scarring and dysfunction of the oviduct transport system, which could result in infertility, ectopic pregnancy, or chronic pelvic pain. Intraperitoneal spread of the infection may cause acute peritonitis, perihepatitis (Fitz-Hugh–Curtis syndrome), periappendicitis, or perisplenitis. Chlamydial infection in pregnancy has been associated with preterm labor, premature rupture of membranes, low birth weight, neonatal death, and postpartum endometritis. A small percentage of adults with chlamydial genital infections develop inclusion conjunctivitis.

In developed countries where sexually transmitted infection with *C. trachomatis* is epidemic, the organism may be transmitted from infected mother to infant during passage through the birth canal. Data from studies in North America indicate that 60–70% of infants exposed to *C. trachomatis* during vaginal delivery become infected with the organism, whereas infection after cesarean section is uncommon (Jones, 2000). *C. trachomatis* is recovered from the conjunctiva of infected infants after 1–2 weeks and from the nasopharynx soon thereafter. The rate of isolation from the conjunctiva falls by 5–6 weeks, but *C. trachomatis* can be recovered from the nasopharynx, conjunctiva, rectum, and vagina (usually without producing symptoms) for several months.

Inclusion conjunctivitis, the most common manifestation of infection with *C. trachomatis* in infants, develops in nearly 80% of infants whose conjunctival culture or cytologic examination demonstrates the organism (Jones, 2000). A mucopurulent discharge appears 2–25 days after birth, and the conjunctiva becomes inflamed and edematous. Symptoms usually resolve without therapy in several months with no sequelae, although scarring can occur.

Approximately 20–30% of infants who acquire infection with *C. trachomatis* at birth develop interstitial pneumonitis. The illness begins between 2 weeks and 3 months of age (peak, 3–6 weeks) with nasal congestion, followed by a distinctive staccato cough with tachypnea and rales but no fever. About one half have or have had conjunctivitis. Symptoms last several weeks, but inspiratory rales and chest roentgenographic changes may persist for months.

Chlamydophila (Formerly Chlamydia) psittaci

Pneumonia associated with exposure to birds was described in Switzerland in 1879. The disease was rare in the United States and Europe

VII

until the late 1920s, when pet tropical birds became fashionable. The pathogen was isolated by Bedson from human and avian tissue in 1930 during an investigation of an outbreak at the London Zoo.

Epidemiology

Infection caused by *Chlamydophila* (formerly *Chlamydia*) *psittaci* (called psittacosis) occurs worldwide. Psittacine birds are considered the major reservoir but most species of birds can be infected with the organism. Infected birds may be obviously ill and die of the disease, but frequently they have mild signs such as anorexia, diarrhea, lethargy, and ruffled feathers. Human illness is sporadic and has been associated with exposure to parrots, canaries, pigeons, sparrows, ducks, cockatiels, fowl (especially turkeys), and occasionally mammals. Owners of pet birds account for about half of the 40–60 cases reported in the United States each year. Pet shop employees, pigeon fanciers, zoo workers, veterinarians, and others who work with birds are at increased risk of infection. Outbreaks have occurred in turkey processing plants, principally among workers who killed the birds and plucked their feathers and those who eviscerated carcasses (Centers for Disease Control, 1990). Over the past two decades the prevalence of psittacosis in the United States has declined dramatically as a result of adding tetracycline to poultry feed, requiring medication of commercially imported psittacine birds before entering the country, and breeding parakeets domestically.

C. psittaci is present in the blood, tissues, excreta, and feathers of infected birds and may be shed for months after acute infection. Infection usually is transmitted to humans via inhalation of infectious aerosols derived from feces, fecal dust, and secretions of *C. psittaci*-infected birds, but may result from handling contaminated plumage or tissues, from bird bites, or from mouth-to-beak contact. Contact with birds does not have to be close or prolonged. Person-to-person spread of *C. psittaci* is rare.

Pathogenesis and Pathology

C. psittaci enters the body via the respiratory tract and is transported to the macrophages of the liver and spleen, where the organisms replicate. They then enter the blood and travel to the lungs, the primary target of infection, and other organs. Histologic examination of lung tissue shows lymphocytes in the alveolar and interstitial spaces and mucus plugging of the bronchioles. Small hemorrhages and macrophages with intracytoplasmic inclusions may be seen. The hilar lymph nodes, liver, and spleen may be enlarged and contain foci of necrosis, and in fatal cases the myocardium, pericardium, meninges, brain, and adrenals may be involved.

Clinical Manifestations

After an incubation period of 1–2 weeks, psittacosis begins either abruptly with chills and fever or more gradually with increasing fever and malaise. Persistent dry, hacking cough, occasionally productive of blood-streaked mucoid sputum, is prominent. The heart rate is often slow relative to body temperature and a diffuse, severe headache is usual. Malaise, anorexia, painful myalgias, and arthralgias are common, and a macular rash (Horder spots) resembling the rose spots of typhoid fever may occur. Decreased mentation may develop at the end of the first week of illness and a few persons have gastrointestinal complaints. *Chlamydophila psittaci* is a rare cause of destructive endocarditis; most affected persons have a history of rheumatic heart disease or congenital valvular abnormalities (Jones, 1982).

Chlamydophila (Formerly Chlamydia) pneumoniae

In 1986, a unique chlamydial organism, initially considered to be a strain of *C. psittaci*, was associated with acute respiratory tract disease in humans. The organism was named TWAR for the laboratory identifying letters of the first two isolates: TW-183, isolated in 1965 from the eye of a control child in a trachoma vaccine trial in Taiwan, and AR-39, recovered the same year from the throat of a student with pharyngitis at the University of Washington. Soon after its recognition, data from DNA homology and electron microscopic studies showed that this unique organism was a separate species, designated as *Chlamydia pneumoniae*, which has been reclassified as *Chlamydophila pneumoniae* (Campbell, 1987; Chi, 1987; Cox, 1988; Everett, 1999). Strains of *C. pneumoniae* and *C. psittaci* have 10% or less DNA sequence homology, and under some conditions the elementary body of *C. pneumoniae* is pear-shaped, whereas under other conditions it is round, like the elementary bodies of *Chlamydophila psittaci* and *Chlamydia trachomatis*.

Epidemiology

The epidemiology of infection with *Chlamydophila pneumoniae* is based on data from retrospective studies of sera collected during respiratory tract illnesses. About 50% of adults have antibodies to *C. pneumoniae*. Antibody prevalence rates are low in children, increase sharply in teenagers, continue to increase until middle age, and remain high into old age; and rates are 10–25% higher for males. Data from retrospective and prospective serologic studies indicate that disease caused by *C. pneumoniae* is endemic in the United States and epidemic in Scandinavia and Finland but does not occur with any consistent seasonal periodicity (Grayston, 1990, 1989). *C. pneumoniae* appears to be a primary human pathogen, transmitted from person to person without an avian or animal reservoir. The mechanism and place of transmission, incubation period, and infectiousness of the organism have not yet been determined.

Pathogenesis

The pathogenesis of infection with *C. pneumoniae* is unknown. Because the illness is generally mild and self-limited, autopsy studies are unavailable.

Clinical Manifestations

It is estimated that *C. pneumoniae* is responsible for at least 10% of community-acquired pneumonias (Grayston, 1990). The pneumonia usually is mild with a single subsegmental infiltrate but it may be severe, especially in elderly persons and in those with chronic disease. It often begins with pharyngitis and hoarseness, followed by persistent cough. Although pneumonia is the most common syndrome associated with *C. pneumoniae* infection, serologic studies during epidemics among military trainees have shown that only about 10% of infections with *C. pneumoniae* result in pneumonia, suggesting that infection is frequently mild or asymptomatic and unrecognized. Other manifestations of *C. pneumoniae* infection are bronchitis, pharyngitis, fever of undetermined origin, otitis, influenza-like illness, myocarditis, endocarditis, and possibly atherosclerosis, although the latter is controversial (Campbell, 1998; Maraha, 2004).

Laboratory Diagnosis

Chlamydia trachomatis

Specimens for detection of *C. trachomatis* are determined by the type of disease suspected (Table 55–2). Screening women at risk for genital *C. trachomatis* infection (described earlier) has been shown to decrease the rate of pelvic inflammatory disease, thus preventing subsequent reproductive sequelae (Nelson, 2001). The transport system selected must be approved for the test method that is used. Specific collection techniques are discussed in Chapter 63. Most infections involve mucous membranes, and specimens should be collected directly from the involved surface and must contain an adequate sample of infected epithelial cells. Purulent discharge is not an appropriate specimen and should be removed before a sample is collected with a swab or brush. Of the types of swabs available, Dacron- or rayon-tipped swabs are preferred. Swabs with wooden shafts should be avoided because wood is toxic to the organism. Calcium alginate swabs may be toxic to the chlamydias or to the cells that support their growth. Cotton-tipped swabs are acceptable but are occasionally toxic to the chlamydias. Collection of urine for nucleic acid amplification testing should follow the recommendations of the manufacturer.

Cell Culture
Cell culture is the reference method for diagnosis of chlamydial infections and should be performed when the diagnosis is disputed and in cases of

Table 55–2 Specimens for Detection of *Chlamydia trachomatis*

Disease	Specimen
Mucopurulent cervicitis	Endocervical swab, urine
Acute urethral syndrome (women)	Urethral swab, urine
Acute endometritis	Endometrial aspirate
Acute salpingitis	Fallopian tube biopsy
Nongonococcal urethritis (men)	Urethral swab, urine
Inclusion conjunctivitis	Conjunctival scrapings/swab
Trachoma	Conjunctival scrapings/swab
Lymphogranuloma venereum	Lymph node aspirate, biopsy of ulcerated lesion, serum
Pneumonitis (infants)	Serum, tracheobronchial aspirate, nasopharyngeal swab

Urine is acceptable for some enzyme-linked immunoassays and for the commercial nucleic acid amplification tests.

suspected sexual assault or abuse. Cell lines most commonly used are McCoy or Buffalo green monkey cells. Both have equivalent sensitivity but the latter cells are easier to maintain and more resistant to cytotoxic substances, and they have been associated with more inclusions and larger inclusions (Krech, 1989). Adding cycloheximide (0.5–1.5 μL/mL) to the growth medium enhances sensitivity. Cell monolayers are grown on glass coverslips in shell vials or 24-well plates or on the surface of polystyrene 96-well or 48-well culture dishes. To enhance recovery of *C. trachomatis*, specimens are sonicated or agitated on a vortex mixer before inoculation to release elementary bodies from host cells, and inoculated shell vials or culture dishes are centrifuged. After incubation for 48–72 hours, monolayers are fixed and stained with fluorescein-conjugated monoclonal antibodies. If a 96-well culture system is used, passaging specimens that are negative for *C. trachomatis* at 48 hours may enhance detection; however, passaging does not significantly increase detection in shell vials or 24-well plates.

Nonculture Direct Detection Methods

Direct Fluorescent Antibody Tests. The DFA test allows direct visualization of *C. trachomatis* elementary bodies in smears of clinical specimens. Total processing time is 30–60 minutes. It is the only test that permits direct assessment of specimen adequacy. Specimens with columnar or metaplastic squamous cells are acceptable, whereas those with few columnar cells, excessive amounts of mucus, or predominance of squamous cells are not. However, interpretation of the smear is subjective, and operator fatigue can be a problem in high-volume situations.

Monoclonal antibodies are available from several manufacturers. Antibodies directed against the species-specific MOMP of *C. trachomatis* appear to be more specific, and produce more intense fluorescence than those directed against the chlamydial LPS (Cles, 1988). Occasionally, even the species-specific antibodies stain bacteria other than *C. trachomatis*, perhaps because of nonspecific immunoglobulin binding or crossreactivity. Staining organisms other than *C. trachomatis* is especially frequent with rectal specimens; therefore, for this site, culture is preferred, although some DFA reagents are approved for evaluation of rectal samples. Monoclonal antibody cross reactivity between Chlamydiaceae and *Bartonella* has also been reported.

The sensitivity of the DFA test has varied from 50% to almost 100% compared with culture as the standard, and specificity is ≥95%. Sensitivity depends on the prevalence of infection in the population being evaluated and the number of elementary bodies required for a positive result (Barnes, 1989), and in general, is greater with lower cutoff values for elementary bodies and in populations with high prevalence of disease.

Enzyme Immunoassays. EIAs detect chlamydial LPS with monoclonal or polyclonal antibodies labeled with an enzyme that converts a colorless substrate into a colored product. Both solid-phase systems, which use plastic or beads coated with the antibody, and membrane systems are commercially available. Total processing time ranges from 15–30 minutes for membrane systems to 3–4 hours for solid-phase systems. Advantages of EIA are the objective interpretation of results and ease of use for batching large numbers of specimens.

As with DFA, the sensitivities of EIAs vary (from about 70–100%) compared with culture as the standard and tend to be higher in populations with a high prevalence of disease, such as persons attending a sexually transmitted disease clinic (Barnes, 1989; Mills, 1992; Clarke, 1993; Ehret, 1993; Kluytmans, 1993; Warren, 1993). The specificity of EIA is 95% or higher. Causes of false-positive results are the presence of a bacterial urinary tract infection (Demaio, 1991) or contamination of the specimen with cervical mucus or vaginal secretions. The latter problem can be reduced by improving the specimen collection technique (removing cervical mucus and obtaining a true endocervical sample) and by using blocking antibodies (Mills, 1992).

Nucleic Acid Hybridization Tests. A commercially available acridinium-ester-labeled DNA probe complementary to *C. trachomatis* ribosomal RNA allows direct detection of *C. trachomatis* in urogenital and conjunctival specimens. The test requires a water-bath and a luminometer. Total processing time is 2–3 hours. The sensitivity of the probe test compared with culture as the reference method varies for both endocervical samples and urethral swab specimens in men (76–97%) (Iwen, 1991; Kluytmans, 1991, 1994; Blanding, 1993; Clarke, 1993; Warren, 1993; Centers for Disease Control, 2002b). The specificity of the probe test is 97% or greater, and it can be improved with a probe competition assay (Woods, 1996).

Nucleic Acid Amplification. Several nucleic acid amplification tests for direct detection of *C. trachomatis* in endocervical swab specimens, male urethral swab specimens, and male and female urine samples are commercially available. Total time to a result is 2–5 hours, depending on the test used and the number of samples being processed. Data from several studies comparing nucleic acid amplification and cell culture indicate that the amplification tests are highly specific and more sensitive than culture (Goessens, 1997; Carroll, 1998; Ferrero, 1998; Mahony, 1998; Puolakkainen, 1998; Toye, 1998; Wylie, 1998; Vincelette, 1999; van der Pol, 2001; Koumans, 2003; Boyadzhyan, 2004; Gaydos, 2004).

Verification of Nonculture Tests

Experts at the Centers for Disease Control and Prevention (CDC) recommend that positive nonculture test (DFA, EIA, probe, nucleic acid amplification) results are verified with a supplemental test if a false-positive result is likely to have adverse medical, social, or psychological consequences (Centers for Disease Control, 1993, 2002b). In low-prevalence populations, verification should probably be routine but might be selective in high-prevalence populations. Culture confirmation is optimal but requires a second specimen collected either during the first visit or during a return visit. EIA-blocking assays, a probe competition assay, evaluation of the transport medium with a DFA test, or repeating samples positive by nucleic acid amplification using a different target are alternative verification methods.

Serologic Tests

Serologic tests have little value for diagnosis of chlamydial genital infections for two reasons. First, antibodies to *C. trachomatis* persist after the infection resolves, so a positive serologic test does not necessarily correlate with active disease. Second, many serologic tests are not specific for *C. trachomatis* because they detect genus-specific antibodies. Exceptions are diagnosis of LGV and *C. trachomatis* pneumonitis in infants. Because LGV has a long latent period and clinical diagnosis often is delayed, antibodies are generally present when the acute phase serum is collected, and a fourfold rise in titer between acute and convalescent phase serum samples often cannot be documented. Thus, a single or stable complement fixation titer of 1:64 or greater supports a presumptive diagnosis of LGV. For diagnosis of *C. trachomatis* pneumonitis in infants, detection of immunoglobulin M (IgM) antibodies by microimmunofluorescence may be the method of choice (a titer of 1:32 or greater is diagnostic).

Chlamydophila psittaci

C. psittaci can be grown in cell culture but this is recommended only for specially equipped laboratories with experienced personnel because the organism is especially virulent and has been associated with laboratory-acquired infections. Infection with *C. psittaci* is usually diagnosed serologically, preferably by testing acute and convalescent phase sera. A fourfold or greater rise in complement-fixing antibody titers between specimens in a patient with symptoms of psittacosis supports the diagnosis. A single titer of 1:32 or greater in an individual with a compatible illness is presumptive evidence of psittacosis. Antibodies usually are detected by the end of the second week of illness, but early antibiotic therapy can delay their appearance for several weeks. False-positive rises in antibody titer occur uncommonly in individuals with legionnaires' disease.

Chlamydophila pneumoniae

Diagnosis of *C. pneumoniae* infection is based predominantly on serologic tests (Grayston, 1990). The microimmunofluorescence test with the TWAR antigen is specific for *C. pneumoniae*. IgM antibodies appear about 3 weeks after the onset of primary illness, usually decline over the next 2–6 months to a level that cannot be detected, and may not reappear with reinfection. IgG antibodies are detected 6–8 weeks after the onset of the primary illness, persist for life, and may rise 1–2 weeks following reinfection. Serologic test results consistent with acute infection include a fourfold or greater rise in IgG titer between acute and convalescent phase serum samples, a single IgG titer of 1:512 or greater, or an IgM titer of 1:16 or greater. *C. pneumoniae* can be isolated in cell culture but it is more difficult to grow than *C. trachomatis* (Roblin, 1992).

Treatment

Tetracyclines are the treatment of choice for infections with chlamydias. For genital infections due to *C. trachomatis*, recommended regimens are azithromycin (1 g orally, 1 dose) or doxycycline (100 mg orally twice a day for 7 days); other effective agents include erythromycin, ofloxacin, or levofloxacin (Centers for Disease Control, 2002a). Ocular infections with *C. trachomatis* require systemic treatment with a tetracycline (for adults) or erythromycin or sulfisoxazole (for neonates); topical therapy suppresses symptoms but does not eradicate the organism. Macrolides are acceptable alternative agents for infections caused by *C. pneumoniae*. Sulfonamides are ineffective against both *C. psittaci* and *C. pneumoniae*.

Rickettsial Infections

Rickettsia is a concept that developed historically as the molecular and physical nature of viruses were defined (Weiss, 1988). In contrast with human viral agents, which also require eukaryotic host cells for their intracellular replication, rickettsias have a Gram-negative bacterial cell wall and their growth is inhibited by particular antibiotics. Rickettsias are further differentiated from other obligately intracellular bacteria by their ecology and frequent transmission by arthropod vectors. The traditional taxonomic scheme of rickettsias based on such phenotypic characteristics as intracellular growth and arthropod vector transmission requires substantial modification in light of contemporary gene sequence analyses. Genera that contain rickettsias pathogenic for humans are *Rickettsia*, *Orientia*, *Ehrlichia*, *Anaplasma*, *Neorickettsia*, *Coxiella*, and *Bartonella* (formerly *Rochalimaea*) (Dumler, 2001; Yu, 2003). Despite their historical association with rickettsiology and arthropod transmission, *Bartonella* are cultivable in cell-free medium and do not belong in the order Rickettsiales (Brenner, 1993), which includes the genera *Rickettsia*, *Orientia*, *Ehrlichia*, *Anaplasma*, and *Neorickettsia*, which are more closely related to one another than to *Coxiella*. Grouped by genus, the following diseases are presented in this chapter: *Rickettsia* – Rocky Mountain spotted fever, boutonneuse fever, African tick bite fever, rickettsialpox, and murine typhus; *Orientia* – scrub typhus; *Ehrlichia* – human monocytotropic ehrlichiosis caused by *Ehrlichia chaffeensis* and human infection with *Ehrlichia ewingii*; *Anaplasma*, human granulocytotropic anaplasmosis; *Coxiella* – Q fever; and *Bartonella* – cat scratch disease, bacillary angiomatosis and peliosis, trench fever, and South American bartonellosis. The diseases of each genus comprise cohesive clinical and pathologic groupings, and overall the rickettsial diseases pose a similar set of diagnostic challenges with similar technical approaches to their solution.

Infections Caused by Organisms of the Genus Rickettsia

Structure and Function

Spotted fever group and typhus group rickettsias are genetically closely related bacteria that have a thin ($0.3–0.5 \times 1–2\,\mu m$) bacillary morphology and a Gram-negative cell wall containing lipopolysaccharide with antigenic components that distinguish the two groups. All *Rickettsia* species reside free in the cytosol of the host cell and divide by binary fission. Rickettsias attach to the host cell via a protein adhesin, enter by induced phagocytosis, and escape from the phagosome (Walker, 1984; Li, 1992, 1998; Uchiyama, 1999). These functions can occur within minutes and are associated with phospholipase activity apparently of rickettsial origin (Silverman, 1992). Spotted fever group rickettsias are propelled within cells and during release from the cell by stimulating polymerization of host cell F-actin at one pole (Heinzen, 1993; Gouin, 2004). Rickettsias that manifest this activity (e.g., *Rickettsia rickettsii*) escape earlier from host cells and spread more quickly to other cells than those lacking this activity (e.g., *Rickettsia prowazekii*), which divide intracellularly to massive numbers before the host cell bursts and the organisms are released. According to the molecular phylogeny, *Rickettsia* species that are pathogenic for humans have evolved into three genogroups (Table 55–3) (Roux, 1995, 1997; Stothard, 1995). The typhus group includes *R. prowazekii* and *Rickettsia typhi*. The core spotted fever group contains *R. rickettsii*, *Rickettsia conorii*, *Rickettsia japonica*, *Rickettsia africae*, *Rickettsia parkeri*, *Rickettsia honei*, *Rickettsia sibirica*, *Rickettsia aeschlimannii*, and *Rickettsia slovaca*. A newly recognized clade contains *Rickettsia akari*, *Rickettsia australis*, and *Rickettsia felis*. *R. akari* and *R. australis* were traditionally considered to be relatively distant members of the spotted fever group, with which they share lipopolysaccharide antigens.

Rocky Mountain Spotted Fever

The most severe of all the rickettsioses, Rocky Mountain spotted fever, has a substantial case-fatality rate, currently 5%, even among previously healthy, immunocompetent children and young adults (Dalton, 1995a; Paddock, 1999). *R. rickettsii* normally resides in nature in ticks: *Dermacentor variabilis*, the American dog tick, in the eastern two thirds of the United States and California; *Dermacentor andersoni*, the Rocky Mountain wood tick, in the western United States; *Rhipicephalus sanguineus*, the brown dog tick, in Mexico; and *Amblyomma cajennense* in South America. These ticks maintain *R. rickettsii* as they moult from stage to stage (larva, nymph, and adult) and transovarially from generation to generation. Fewer than 1 per 1000 ticks carries virulent *R. rickettsii*, which seems to be mildly pathogenic for ticks (Niebylski, 1999). New lines of ticks become infected by feeding on

rickettssemic rodents, replenishing the population of organisms transovarially maintained in ticks (Gage, 1990).

Infections occur when and where humans encounter *R. rickettsii*-infected ticks (Helmick, 1984). Although Rocky Mountain spotted fever has been documented in recent years in nearly every state except Hawaii, Alaska, and Vermont, the highest incidence is in the south Atlantic states from Maryland to Georgia and the south central states of Oklahoma, Missouri, Arkansas, and Tennessee. Most cases occur in late spring and summer but, particularly in the southern latitudes, a few cases may occur even in winter. The highest incidence is in children and others who are exposed to ticks during outdoor activities. Fatality/case ratios are higher for persons older than 30 years. Fulminant Rocky Mountain spotted fever (death by the fifth day of illness) occurs in association with moderate hemolysis, for example, in African American males with glucose-6-phosphate dehydrogenase (G6PD) deficiency (Walker, 1983).

Rickettsias are injected via the infected tick's salivary gland secretions into the patient's dermis after 6–10 hours of tick feeding and spread hematogenously throughout the body. The vascular endothelium is the target of intracellular infection, with some invasion into adjacent vascular smooth muscle cells. Infected endothelium is injured by reactive-oxygen-species-induced damage to cell membranes and possibly by phospholipase activity (Silverman, 1992, 1997). Damage to the endothelium results in increased vascular permeability, edema, hypovolemia, and hypotension. The life-threatening consequences of vascular injury in the central nervous system (CNS) and lung are rickettsial meningoencephalitis and noncardiogenic pulmonary edema. Early in the course, lesions show endothelial rickettsias without thrombi or a cellular response. Late in the course, the characteristic lymphohistiocytic perivascular infiltrate appears as interstitial pneumonia, interstitial myocarditis, perivascular glial nodules of the brain, and similar vascular lesions in the dermis, gastrointestinal tract, liver, skeletal muscles, and kidneys. Severe injury may be accompanied by focal hemorrhages but seldom by microinfarcts, except in the white matter of the brain.

The clinical illness usually begins with fever, headache, and myalgia 2–14 days after a tick bite (Kaplowitz, 1981). Nausea, vomiting, abdominal pain and tenderness, and diarrhea occur more frequently in the first 3 days of illness. The rash, which usually appears between days 3 and 5, typically begins as macules around the wrists and ankles and, later, on the arms, legs, and trunk. The lesions become maculopapular and in half of cases a central petechia appears in many of the maculopapules. Characteristic involvement of the palms and soles occurs in half of cases as a late manifestation. Renal failure is a feature of severe illness. CNS involvement is ominous; seizures and coma occur in 8–10% of cases overall, often preceding a fatal outcome. Thrombocytopenia occurs in half of cases, but disseminated intravascular coagulation is rare (Elghetany, 1999).

African Tick Bite Fever, Boutonneuse Fever and Other Spotted Fevers

R. conorii has been isolated in southern Europe; northern, eastern, and southern Africa; Israel; Turkey; India; Pakistan; Russia; Georgia; and the Ukraine. The ecology of *R. conorii* and the epidemiology of boutonneuse fever are closely tied to ticks, especially *R. sanguineus*, which maintain the rickettsias transovarially and transmit the infection to humans while feeding (Walker, 1991). Imported cases are diagnosed in travelers returning to the United States and northern Europe from the Mediterranean basin. The fatality rate among hospitalized patients is 1.4–5.6%, particularly in patients with underlying diseases. A milder disease caused by *R. africae* occurs with a probably higher frequency in travelers returning from southern Africa (McQuiston, 2004). The clinical illness resembles that recently associated in the Americas with *R. parkeri*, which is essentially conspecific with *R. africae* (Paddock, 2004). Tick bite eschars are often multiple, regional lymphadenopathy is observed frequently, and rash is typically sparse, sometimes vesicular, and often absent. *R. sibirica* has been isolated in Russia, China, Mongolia, and Pakistan. *R. japonica* has been documented in Japan infection, and *R. japonica* (strain *heilongjiangiensis*) occurs also in China and Russia. Human infections with *R. australis* occur only in Australia, and infection with *R. honei* has been documented in Australia and Thailand. After an average incubation period of 7 days, these illnesses begin with fever, headache, and myalgias. Frequently, an eschar can be discovered by careful examination of the skin at this time. The pathology of these spotted fevers is well described in the tache noire or eschar at the site of tick bite inoculation of rickettsias (Walker, 1988a). Endothelial infection and injury by *R. conorii* in the eschar result in dermal and epidermal necrosis and perivascular edema. The host defenses that effect killing of intracellular rickettsias include cytokines secreted by T lymphocytes and macrophages, which infiltrate around the infected

Table 55–3 *Rickettsia, Orientia, Ehrlichia, Anaplasma, Neorickettsia, Coxiella,* and *Bartonella* Infections

Etiologic Agent	Disease	Geographic Distribution	Transmission
Spotted Fevers			
R. rickettsii	Rocky Mountain spotted fever	North, Central, and South America	Tick bite
R. conorii	Boutonneuse fever	Southern Europe, Africa, Russia, Georgia, Middle East, Indian subcontinent	Tick bite
R. africae	African tick bite fever	Southern and eastern Africa, Caribbean	Tick bite
R. parkeri	American tick bite fever	North and South America	Tick bite
R. sibirica	North Asian tick typhus	Russia, China, Mongolia, Pakistan, Europe, Africa	Tick bite
R. japonica	Japanese spotted fever	Japan, China	Tick bite
R. honei	Flinders Island spotted fever	Australia, southeastern Asia	Tick bite
R. slovaca	Tick-borne lymphadenopathy	Europe	Tick bite
Typhus Fevers			
R. prowazekii	Epidemic typhus	Potentially worldwide; in recent decades in Africa, South America, Central America, Mexico, Asia	Feces of human body louse
R. prowazekii	Brill–Zinsser disease	Worldwide; wherever persons with past epidemic typhus now reside	Recrudescence of latent infection
R. prowazekii	Flying squirrel typhus	United States	Presumably feces of flea or louse of flying squirrel
R. typhi	Murine typhus	Worldwide in tropics and subtropics	Flea feces
Other Rickettsial Fevers			
R. akari	Rickettsialpox	United States, Ukraine, Croatia, Korea	Mite bite
R. australis	Queensland tick typhus	Eastern Australia	Tick bite
R. felis	Flea-borne spotted fever	Worldwide	Presumably flea bite or feces
Scrub Typhus			
Orientia tsutsugamushi	Scrub typhus	SE Asia, Japan, China, Sri Lanka, India, Asiatic Russia, Tadzhikistan, Indonesia, Western Pacific, Northern Australia	Chigger bite
Ehrlichioses			
E. chaffeensis	Human monocytotropic ehrlichiosis	United States, Africa, Asia	Tick bite
E. ewingii	Ehrlichiosis ewingii	United States	Tick bite
Anaplasma phagocytophila	Human granulocytotropic anaplasmosis	United States, Eurasia	Tick bite
Neorickettsia sennetsu	Sennetsu rickettsiosis	Asia	Not known
Coxiellosis			
C. burnetii	Q fever	Worldwide	Inhalation of aerosols from infected animals, possibly ingestion of animal products
Bartonelloses			
B. bacilliformis	Oroya fever, verruga peruana	Western South America	Sandfly bite
B. henselae	Cat scratch disease, bacillary angiomatosis and peliosis, endocarditis	Worldwide	Kitten scratch or bite
B. clarridgeiae	Cat-scratch-like disease	Probably worldwide	Presumed cat scratch or bite
B. quintana	Trench fever, endocarditis	Worldwide	Feces of *Pediculus* louse

dermal blood vessels and cytotoxic CD8⁺ T lymphocytes (Herrero-Herrero, 1987; Valbuena, 2002). Activation of endothelial cells by cytokines, including γ-interferon and tumor necrosis factor-α, results in intracellular rickettsicidal activity, and ultimate clearance is mediated by cytotoxic T lymphocytes. Disseminated endothelial infection results in maculopapular rash, meningoencephalitis, and vascular lesions in the lungs, kidneys, gastrointestinal tract, and heart (Walker, 1985). Multifocal hepatocellular necrosis and granuloma-like lesions correlate with moderately increased concentrations of hepatic transaminases (Walker, 1986).

Rickettsialpox

R. akari is maintained in nature by transovarial transmission in the gamasid mite, *Liponyssoides sanguineus,* an ectoparasite of the domestic mouse, *Mus musculus. R. akari* has been isolated only in the United States, Croatia, the Ukraine, and Korea, perhaps more an indication of the paucity of rickettsial investigations than the actual distribution of this rickettsial species.

A papule develops during the approximately 10-day incubation period at the site of mite bite and progresses to become a 1–2.5 cm eschar. Illness begins with chills, fever, malaise, severe headache, and myalgia. Rash, which appears 2–6 days later, is initially maculopapular, later papular, and in classic cases pustular, then vesicular. Some patients also suffer nausea, vomiting, pharyngitis, photophobia, splenomegaly, and nuchal rigidity.

Histopathologic examination of the eschar reveals coagulative necrosis of the epidermis, underlying vascular injury, and a perivascular lympho-histiocytic infiltrate in which macrophages appear to be the main target cell of infection (Brettman, 1981; Kass, 1994; Walker, 1999b). Regional lymphadenopathy and cutaneous rash presumably reflect lymphogenous and hematogenous spread, respectively.

Flea-borne Spotted Fever

A widely dispersed organism, *R. felis* is maintained transovarially in cat fleas (*Ctenocephalides felis*) with apparent involvement of opossums in a zoonotic cycle. Human infections have been documented in North America, Europe, and Asia (Schriefer, 1994a; Zavala-Velazquez, 2000; Raoult, 2001; Parola, 2003).

Murine Typhus and Louse-borne Typhus

Endemic flea-borne *R. typhi* infection, murine typhus, is presently the most important typhus group infection in the United States and causes extensive morbidity throughout the warm regions of the world (Azad, 1990). Historically, epidemic louse-borne *R. prowazekii* infections have

VII

had a major impact on the outcome of military campaigns as well as scourging general populations disrupted by war, famine and natural disasters (Zinsser, 1935; Patterson, 1993). *R. prowazekii* continues to cause disease in some poverty-stricken areas of the world and reappears in situations such as the civil war in Burundi, the extreme poverty of indigenous populations of the Andes, and the unsettled social and economic conditions of Russia. Recrudescence of latent *R. prowazekii* infections can occur years after the primary infection in immigrants from typhus-afflicted areas. Endemic transmission of *R. prowazekii* from a natural infectious cycle of flying squirrels and their ectoparasites occurs in the United States (McDade, 1980; Reynolds, 2003).

Murine typhus occurs particularly in tropical and subtropical coastal areas where *Rattus rattus*, *Rattus norvegicus*, and the Oriental rat flea abound (Azad, 1990). The fleas imbibe rickettsias in the blood of infected rats and maintain the infection for their normal life span. Transovarian transmission occurs only at low levels; thus, horizontal transmission to other rats is a key factor in maintenance of *R. typhi* in nature. Other mammal-arthropod cycles maintain the rickettsias and result in transmission of infections to humans (e.g., the cat flea, *C. felis*, and the opossum in Texas and California) (Schriefer, 1994b).

Humans are believed to become infected by intradermal inoculation of infected flea feces into skin excoriated by scratching. However, inhalation of a rickettsial aerosol from dried infected flea feces or inoculation by flea bite may account for transmission in some cases. After an incubation period of 1–2 weeks, illness begins with fever accompanied in some cases by severe headache, chills, myalgias, and nausea. A macular or maculopapular rash, most prominent on the trunk, appears on day 5 or 6 in 80% of patients with fair skin and in 20% with darkly pigmented skin. A small proportion of patients have cough and pulmonary infiltrates. Severely ill patients may also suffer coma, seizures, and other neurologic signs. Approximately 10% of hospitalized patients require admission to the intensive care unit, and 1–2% of murine typhus patients die (Dumler, 1991).

The pathologic lesions of murine typhus include endothelial swelling and perivascular lymphohistiocytic infiltrates involving the blood vessels in the dermis, CNS, lungs, heart, gastrointestinal tract, and kidneys (Walker, 1989). The most serious consequences are meningoencephalomyelitis and diffuse alveolar injury.

Rickettsias as Agents of Bioterrorism

R. prowazekii and *R. rickettsii* are select agents, the possession of which is restricted by law to registered scientists in approved institutions where rigorous security and safety regulations are applied to the laboratories. These organisms exist in nature, can be recovered and propagated, and are infectious via a stable aerosol with infectivity of as little as a single bacterium.

Case-fatality rates of 15–25% in previously healthy persons would occur without prompt diagnosis and treatment. The potential for genetically engineered resistance to the only effective antibiotics, tetracycline and chloramphenicol, would render these cases of typhus and Rocky Mountain spotted fever untreatable. Although the case-fatality rates would be lower, bioterrorist dispersed *R. typhi* or *R. conorii* could also create terror and overwhelm the medical and public health systems.

Laboratory Diagnosis

Unlike most infectious diseases for which precise diagnosis is sought during the acute phase of illness, when critical therapeutic decisions are made, rickettsial diseases are usually diagnosed acutely purely on clinicoepidemiologic suspicion and are treated empirically on a presumptive basis (Kaplowitz, 1981). Serologic diagnosis, which is often mistakenly sought early in the course of illness, provides the majority of laboratory confirmed diagnoses by demonstration of a fourfold or greater rise in titer only during convalescence. Even with the most sensitive serologic methods, fewer than 20% of patients have detectable specific antibodies to rickettsias when presenting to the physician for medical attention. Other approaches to diagnosis at the time of presentation include immuno-histologic demonstration of rickettsias in cutaneous lesions, immuno-cytologic identification of rickettsias in circulating detached endothelial cells, detection of rickettsial DNA in blood and tissue specimens by polymerase chain reaction (PCR) (Furuya, 1995; Schriefer, 1994a; Sexton, 1994; Williams, 1994), and cultivation of rickettsias from blood or tissue specimens; but these tests are not available in most clinical laboratories.

Rickettsias were originally demonstrated in tissues of patients with Rocky Mountain spotted fever and epidemic louse-borne typhus by Wolbach using Giemsa stain during and shortly after World War I. This method, essentially a lost art, requires careful attention to details of fixation and staining of rickettsias, and is not performed successfully in this manner in contemporary histology laboratories. A modified Brown–Hopps method

stains a small fraction of organisms, which appear as thin bacilli within endothelial cells. A more sensitive and specific approach to visualization of rickettsias in tissue section is immunohistology, either immunofluorescence or immunoenzyme staining, using antibodies specific for the spotted fever or typhus group (Kaplowitz, 1983; Walker, 1989, 1997b, 1999b; Dumler, 1990). Staining of skin biopsies from patients with Rocky Mountain spotted fever by histochemistry has a sensitivity of 70% and a specificity of 100%. Patients with boutonneuse fever, African tick bite fever, murine typhus, and rickettsialpox have also been diagnosed by immunohistologic detection of rickettsias in rash and eschar lesions. A monoclonal antibody to a spotted-fever-group-specific epitope on the cell wall lipopolysaccharide demonstrates *R. rickettsii*, *R. conorii*, *R. akari*, *R. japonica*, *R. australis*, *R. africae*, *R. honei*, and *R. sibirica* in formalin-fixed, paraffin-embedded tissues, and a typhus group lipopolysaccharide-specific monoclonal antibody is similarly useful for detecting *R. typhi* and *R. prowazekii* (Walker, 1997b). Currently, reagents for diagnostic immunohistology of rickettsioses are not commercially available, but it is feasible that kits could be developed for rickettsial-group-specific diagnosis using antibodies produced in research laboratories.

A unique diagnostic approach is the immunocytologic demonstration of *R. conorii* in detached, circulating endothelial cells captured from patient blood samples by immunomagnetic beads coated with a monoclonal antibody to a surface antigen of human endothelial cells (Drancourt, 1992; La Scola, 1996a). In boutonneuse fever patients, this method has a sensitivity of 58% for examination of a single blood sample and may be used in patients prior to the onset of rash, which must be present for selection of the site of skin biopsy for immunohistologic diagnosis.

PCR has been applied successfully to the diagnostic detection of *R. rickettsii*, *R. conorii*, *R. japonica*, *R. africae*, *R. parkeri*, *R. felis*, *R. sibirica*, *R. slovaca*, *R. aeschlimannii*, *R. typhi*, and *R. prowazekii* from clinical samples including biopsy of eschar or rash, peripheral blood, buffy coat, plasma, necropsy tissue, and arthropod vectors removed from patients. This approach may fail to detect rickettsial nucleic acids early in the course of or after development of immunity or effective antimicrobial treatment (Tzianabos, 1989; Schriefer, 1994a; Sexton, 1994; Furuya, 1995; Roux, 1999; Walker, 2003; Fournier, 2004).

Isolation of rickettsias is achieved frequently in antibiotic-free, centrifugation-enhanced shell vial cell culture in reference and research laboratories with biosafety level-3 containment and specialized expertise.

The 'gold standard' serologic test for rickettsioses is the indirect immunofluorescent antibody (IFA) assay (Kaplan, 1986). The indirect immunoperoxidase antibody test yields similar results. For spotted fever and typhus-group rickettsial infections in the United States, IFA titers of 1:64 or greater are considered to be diagnostic in a compatible clinicoepidemiologic situation. In countries where there is a high prevalence of persons with antibodies to these rickettsias, due hypothetically to stimulation by nonpathogenic rickettsias or subclinical or undiagnosed infection, higher titers are required to establish the diagnosis. In any event, a fourfold rise in IFA antibody titer to at least a titer of 1:64 is diagnostic. The sensitivity of the IFA for Rocky Mountain spotted fever is 94–100%, and the specificity is 100%. With a cutoff titer for IgG of 1:128 and for IgM of 1:32, the indirect immunoperoxidase test yields similar results and has the advantage of requiring only a light microscope instead of an ultraviolet microscope.

Commercially available serologic tests include indirect immuno-fluorescence, latex agglutination, and standard solid-phase enzyme immunoassay (Kelly, 1995). Latex agglutination and solid-phase enzyme immunoassay provide diagnostically useful information, require less expensive equipment to perform, but generally are not considered as reliable as the IFA. The Weil–Felix tests, which measure agglutination of *Proteus vulgaris* strains OX-19 and OX-2 (Kaplan, 1986), are insensitive and nonspecific and should not be used except in developing countries in which no other method can be performed.

Treatment

Spotted fever and typhus group rickettsioses are treated effectively with doxycycline, tetracycline, or chloramphenicol (Raoult, 1991). Fluoro-quinolones, azithromycin, and clarithromycin are active against some rickettsias in vitro. Ciprofloxacin, ofloxacin, and perfloxacin have been used successfully to treat boutonneuse fever, and azithromycin and clarithromycin have been used to treat mild boutonneuse fever in children, but these agents have not been evaluated and are not recommended for treatment of Rocky Mountain spotted fever.

Scrub Typhus Caused by *Orientia tsutsugamushi*

The Gram-negative cell wall of *Orientia* (formerly *Rickettsia*) *tsutsugamushi* differs from that of spotted fever and typhus group rickettsias; it has an ultrastructurally thicker outer leaflet and thinner inner leaflet of the outer envelope, different major proteins, and lacks lipopolysaccharide and peptidoglycan (Tamura, 1995). Scrub typhus rickettsias grow in the cytoplasm of the host cell and are released via a process involving pinching off a host cell membrane-bound rickettsia. *O. tsutsugamushi* is transovarially maintained in mites of the genus *Leptotrombidium* (Traub, 1978). Infected ova hatch into larvae, the only stage that feeds on an animal host. Rats become infected after rickettsia-containing larvae (chiggers) feed on the rats' tissue fluids, but feeding mite larvae that acquire rickettsias do not pass the infection to their offspring. Thus, humans and rats are only accidental, nonessential, dead-end hosts of scrub typhus rickettsias. Scrub typhus occurs in countries within the triangle formed by Japan, Pakistan, and northern Australia. Infection is acquired in areas of dense vegetation where abundant rat populations harbor large populations of chiggers.

O. tsutsugamushi infects endothelial cells more extensively than macrophages (Moron, 2001). The basic pathologic lesion is vascular injury with perivascular lymphohistiocytic inflammation, which is present in the cutaneous chigger-inoculation site of rickettsias, the brain, lung, heart, gastrointestinal tract, and kidney.

After incubation for 6–21 days, illness begins with fever, headache and, in some patients, myalgia, cough, and gastrointestinal symptoms (Watt, 1999). An eschar develops in half of westerners, usually prior to the onset of fever, but seldom in indigenous patients. Likewise, a macular or maculopapular rash occurs in half of westerners with primary infection, 2–9 days after the onset of illness. Severely ill patients may develop hypotension, meningoencephalitis, acute renal failure, and hemorrhagic phenomena. Unless treated with appropriate antimicrobial medications, 7% of cases are fatal. Scrub typhus may occur in trekkers and other travelers exposed to chiggers in endemic areas. For the diagnosis of scrub typhus in an endemic region, a titer of 1:400 or greater by IFA is 96% specific and 48% sensitive. The criterion of a fourfold increase in titer to 1:200 or greater yields a specificity of 98% and sensitivity of 54%. Indirect immunoperoxidase is a similar method that does not require a fluorescent microscope. *Proteus mirabilis* strain OX-K agglutination is more readily available, but insensitive. Serologic assays using a recombinant 56 kDa antigen representing the major immunodominant surface protein, including a dipstick test on a rapid lateral flow assay and a IgM capture enzyme immunoassay, have given highly promising results that await commercialization. (Jang, 2003; Jiang, 2003).

PCR has been applied to the diagnosis of scrub typhus for more than a decade (Murai, 1992; Furuya, 1993; Kawamori, 1993; Sugita, 1993) and has been demonstrated to be effective in practice (Manosroi, 2003). Real-time PCR offers the opportunity for a highly sensitive, specific diagnosis with prompt turnaround time (Jiang 2004).

Treatment with a tetracycline drug such as doxycycline or with chloramphenicol is effective except among some cases in northern Thailand, where rifamycin and azithromycin may be alternatives (Watt, 1996, 2000).

Infections Caused by Organisms of the Genera *Ehrlichia* and *Anaplasma*

Structure and Function

The family Anaplasmataceae consists of four genera, *Ehrlichia*, *Anaplasma*, *Neorickettsia*, and *Wolbachia*. Ehrlichias and anaplasmas are small (0.5 µm), tick-borne, obligately intracellular, Gram-negative coccobacilli that reside in a cytoplasmic vacuole of white blood cells (Yu, 2003). This intravacuolar microcolony of bacteria stained by Wright–Giemsa method resembles a mulberry and thus is called a morula (Latin for mulberry). *Neorickettsia*, similar small obligately intracellular bacteria, reside in trematode parasites in aquatic snails, insects, and fish and are transmitted by ingestion of this parasitized host, e.g., *Neorickettsia helminthoeca* in trematode-parasitized salmon eaten by dogs in the Pacific northwest. *Wolbachia* reside in arthropods and filarial worms, e.g., *Onchocerca volvulus*, in which they play a role in the pathogenesis of the human illness.

Long known and studied as agents of veterinary diseases, *Ehrlichia* and *Anaplasma* have recently emerged as human pathogens. The reasons are primarily their recent discovery in humans, their rapid characterization with contemporary molecular tools, and increasing populations and geographic distribution of particular ticks that depend on deer as a host. The well documented human pathogens in the United States are *E. chaffeensis*, *E. ewingii*, and *Anaplasma phagocytophila*. *Neorickettsia sennetsu* is the agent of the disease in Asia resembling infectious mononucleosis.

Human Monocytotropic Ehrlichiosis

E. chaffeensis is transmitted by ticks, primarily *Amblyomma americanum*, the Lone Star tick, but also *D. variabilis* and *Ixodes pacificus* (Anderson, 1992a;

Ewing, 1995; Kramer, 1999). Cases are predominantly rural and seasonal (68% occur from May to July) (Fishbein, 1994; Olano, 2003a). Deer are a documented reservoir, and infected dogs are also a potential reservoir host. Ticks become infected when feeding as larvae or nymphs, carry the ehrlichias as they moult from stage to stage, and transmit the infection during a subsequent blood meal. Human monocytotropic ehrlichiosis has been reported in 47 states; most cases have occurred within the range of *A. americanum* in the third of the United States south of a line from New Jersey to Kansas. The number of reported cases is particularly high in Oklahoma, Missouri, Arkansas, Tennessee, and Maryland.

Since the first case of human ehrlichiosis was reported in the United States in 1987, more than 1000 patients with laboratory-confirmed *E. chaffeensis* infection have been documented at the CDC and more than 2000 cases at one commercial laboratory (Fishbein, 1994). Fatalities have occurred in approximately 3% of cases, a rate that would be much higher without effective antibiotic treatment in many patients (Fichtenbaum, 1993; Fishbein, 1994). The severity is reflected in the admission of 41–62% of patients to a hospital (Fishbein, 1994; Olano, 2003a, 2003b). Although severe cases often affect older persons, children are also susceptible to the illness (Schultz, 1997). The median duration of illness in a large CDC series, including treated cases, was 23 days. Signs and symptoms depict a systemic disease that has no clinically diagnostic features: fever (97%), headache (81%), myalgia (68%), anorexia (66%), nausea (48%), vomiting (37%), rash (6% at onset, 25% during the first week, and 36% overall), regional lymphadenopathy (29%), cough (26%), pharyngitis (26%), diarrhea (25%), abdominal pain or tenderness (22%), photophobia (27%), and confusion (20%) (Fishbein, 1994; Olano, 2003b). Severe complications include adult respiratory distress syndrome, disseminated intravascular coagulation, and renal insufficiency. Clinical laboratory findings include leukopenia (60%), thrombocytopenia (68%), and elevated hepatic transaminases (86%). CNS involvement manifested by seizures and coma has been documented by cerebrospinal fluid (CSF) pleocytosis, increased protein concentration and *E. chaffeensis* in CSF, and the presence of cerebral lesions at autopsy (Dunn, 1992; Ratnasamy, 1996; Walker, 1997a). Severity is age-dependent (Olano, 2003a). In immuno-compromised patients, including those with the acquired immunodeficiency syndrome (AIDS), human monocytotropic ehrlichiosis can be an overwhelming infection with massive growth of ehrlichias and a fatal outcome (Paddock, 1993; Walker, 1997a). Mild infections have also been documented. *E. chaffeensis* establishes persistent infection in its natural hosts and in one reported human case (Dumler, 1993b).

After entry via tick bite, *E. chaffeensis* spreads by the lymphatic and/or hematogenous routes. Ehrlichial morulas have been identified in monocytes and macrophages in the bone marrow, peripheral blood (rarely), hepatic sinusoids, spleen, lymph nodes, meninges, kidney, gastrointestinal tract, and epicardium (Dumler, 1993a; Walker, 1997a; Sehdev, 2003). Bone marrow examination frequently reveals granulomas, myeloid hyperplasia, and megakaryocytosis. Other reported lesions include perivascular lymphohistiocytic infiltrates in the kidney, meninges, brain, and heart; interstitial mononuclear pneumonitis; foci of apoptosis-like cell death in the liver, lymph node, and spleen; diffuse reticulo-endothelial hyperplasia; erythrophagocytosis; and cholestasis.

Human Infection with Ehrlichia ewingii

Recognized first as a canine pathogen in 1971, *E. ewingii* is also transmitted by *A. americanum* ticks (Ewing, 1971; Anziani, 1990). It shares antigens with *E. chaffeensis* but infects mainly neutrophils. A high proportion of infected patients are immunocompromised, suggesting that immunocompetent patients may be relatively resistant to the illness (Buller, 1999, Paddock, 2001).

Human Granulocytotropic Anaplasmosis

More than 1000 cases of human granulocytic ehrlichiosis have been documented, with most of the cases in the upper midwest (Wisconsin and Minnesota) and northeastern states (New York, Connecticut, Rhode Island, and New Jersey) of the United States but with confirmed autochthonous infections southward along the eastern seaboard and in California and Europe (Bakken, 1994; Aguero-Rosenfeld, 1996; Petrovec, 1997; Horowitz, 1998). Infection is transmitted by *Ixodes scapularis*, *I. pacificus*, and *Ixodes ricinus* ticks. The white-footed mouse (*Peromyscus leucopus*) and other small mammals are likely reservoir hosts in the United States, and red deer, sheep, goats, and cattle in Europe (Hodzic, 1998). The pathology is poorly defined, with the observation of morula-containing neutrophils in peripheral blood and various organs, infiltrates of reticuloendothelial organs with foamy macrophages, multiorgan perivascular lymphohistiocytic infiltrates, and focal hepatocellular apoptosis (Walker, 1997a). Fatality is frequently associated with secondary opportunistic fungal and viral infections (Hardalo, 1995).

Human granulocytotropic anaplasmosis varies from asymptomatic to severe, with many diagnosed patients requiring hospitalization (Bakken, 1994). Infection is fatal in fewer than 1% of cases. The illness begins with chills, fever, headache, and myalgia. Thrombocytopenia occurs in most cases and leukopenia in nearly half. Hepatocellular injury is manifested as elevated hepatic enzymes, and severely ill patients may have septic shock-like illness with multiorgan involvement.

Laboratory Diagnosis

Isolation of ehrlichias and anaplasmas from human blood in antibiotic-free cell culture has been accomplished more often for A. phagocytophila (in HL-60 cells) than E. chaffeensis (in DH-82 cells), only once for E. canis (in an asymptomatic person), and has yet to be reported for E. ewingii (Dawson, 1991; Edelman, 1996; Goodman, 1996; Perez, 1996; Childs, 1999). Amplification of ehrlichial DNA by PCR using species-specific primers is an efficient diagnostic tool for all the human ehrlichioses (Anderson, 1992b; Chen, 1994; Everett, 1994; Buller, 1999; Comer, 1999). For human monocytotropic ehrlichiosis, the sensitivity of PCR is reported as 79–100% and for granulocytotropic anaplasmosis caused by A. phagocytophila, 48–86% (Anderson, 1992b; Everett, 1994). Lateness in the course, a lower level of ehrlichiemia and tetracycline treatment reduce the sensitivity of detection of ehrlichias by PCR. Target genes that have been validated clinically include 16S rRNA (rrs), 120 kDa glycoprotein, groESL, nadA, and VLPT for E. chaffeensis, rrs for E. ewingii, and rrs, ank-1, msp2, and ftsZ for A. phagocytophila (Dumler, 2004). Although in many cases a laborious task, identification of morulas in peripheral blood neutrophils provides a diagnosis of human anaplasmosis or ehrlichiosis and can be performed in any clinical laboratory. It is a more sensitive approach for A. phagocytophila infection (30–80%) than for E. chaffeensis (7–17% in immunocompetent patients and a very high proportion of immunocompromised patients (Hamilton, 2004)). It is important to avoid false-positive interpretation caused by toxic granulations, Döhle bodies, superimposed platelets, apoptotic bodies, or contaminant particles. Immunohistochemical identification of E. chaffeensis can be performed in tissue specimens (Dumler, 1993a; Yu, 1993).

Serologic diagnosis is the usual approach to the diagnosis of human ehrlichiosis, using cell-culture-propagated E. chaffeensis and A. phagocytophila antigens in IFA assays (Nicholson, 1997; Walls, 1999; Olano, 2003b). This method is very sensitive for the demonstration of seroconversion to a titer of 1:64 or greater 2–4 weeks after disease onset. The expected serologic result on acute serum is absence of detected antibodies. Thus, treatment should be initiated empirically on the basis of clinical and epidemiologic factors and not withheld pending laboratory confirmation. Opinion as to a diagnostic single serum titer for E. chaffeensis ranges from 1:64 to 1:256. Cross-reactivity of A. phagocytophila and E. chaffeensis is observed in approximately 20% of patients with human monocytotropic ehrlichiosis and human granulocytic ehrlichiosis. Thus, particularly in geographic regions where these infections overlap; indeed, if there is a possibility of travel-associated exposure, it is essential to determine antibody titers against both organisms. A fourfold difference in titer determines the infecting agent. Cases with twofold or less difference are classified as ehrlichiosis of indeterminate etiology.

Distinguishing E. chaffeensis from E. ewingii serologically is more problematic because the latter has yet to be cultivated. Western immuno-blotting is a useful research tool at present for distinguishing infection with E. chaffeensis with its distinctive 120 kDa protein and 28 kDa protein family from infection with A. phagocytophila with its major 42–49 kDa protein patterns (Asanovich, 1997; Chen, 1997a, 1997b; Zhi, 1997). Serologic assays using these and other recombinant proteins show promise for future development (Yu, 1999; Knowles, 2003).

Treatment

Doxycycline is the drug of choice for the treatment of these human ehrlichioses (Bakken, 1994; Fishbein, 1994). The use of chloramphenicol is controversial as it has been reported to shorten the course of human monocytotropic ehrlichiosis (Fishbein, 1994) and to be associated with a fatal outcome. Cell culture studies show E. chaffeensis and A. phagocytophila to be resistant to it and the commonly prescribed β-lactams, macrolides, aminoglycosides, and sulfonamide drugs (Branger, 2004; Brouqui, 1992; Klein, 1997). Anaplasma phagocytophila is susceptible to rifampin and rifabutin in cell culture, and rifampin has been used to treat a limited number of pregnant women and children successfully (Krause, 2003).

Infections Caused by Coxiella burnetii

Structure and Function

C. burnetii is quite distant phylogenetically from other pathogenic rickettsias and is the only one classified in the γ group of the Proteobacteria. These Gram-negative bacteria vary morphologically from rods to cocci, and by electron microscopic examination there are two distinct forms: large cells (0.5–1.2 μm) and small dense cells (0.5 μm), which have been proposed to represent a developmental cycle that includes a spore-like form.

Much emphasis has been placed on a laboratory phenomenon associated with cultivation of C. burnetii by prolonged passage in cell culture or eggs, namely, loss of the organisms' ability to synthesize the entire lipopolysaccharide. This change from synthesis of the full to a truncated lipopolysaccharide, analogous to the conversion from smooth to rough phenotype by Enterobacteriaceae, has been designated phase variation from phase I to phase II. Phase I is found in nature and in infected persons and animals; phase II occurs in the laboratory owing to deletions of genes without selective advantage under conditions of passage outside of its hosts.

Coxiella burnetii enters its target cell, the macrophage, by phagocytosis after interaction with $\alpha_v\beta_3$ integrin and is highly adapted (e.g., synthesis of superoxide dismutase and acid phosphatase) to the acidic conditions in the phagolysosome, where replication by transverse binary fission occurs.

Q Fever

The name Q fever was derived from the unknown status of its etiology when the clinicoepidemiologic syndrome was first described as query fever. The ecology of C. burnetii includes silent infections in animals: many species of ticks, ungulates (particularly sheep, cattle, and goats), other mammals (including cats and wild rabbits), fish, birds, and marsupials (Marrie, 1988, 1997). Humans usually are infected by inhalation, especially of aerosols that originate in infected birth products of domestic livestock and pets and possibly also by ingestion of unpasteurized contaminated milk (Fishbein, 1992). Many human infections occur as an occupational disease among abattoir workers, farmers, and veterinarians. However, urban nonoccupational cases are by no means rare in some populations in which they have been evaluated, such as among immunocompromised patients in France (Brouqui, 1993).

The majority of human infections are asymptomatic (Marrie, 1990). Acute illness is often a self-limited, undifferentiated febrile illness, pneumonia, hepatitis, or meningoencephalitis (Drancourt, 1991; Tissot Dupont, 1992). Individual patients with myalgias, anorexia, and headache are unlikely to be investigated diagnostically for Q fever, even though this syndrome is the most likely clinical presentation of this infection and accounts for a substantial proportion of patients with these symptoms in some populations. Manifestations of Q fever pneumonia vary: cough may be nonproductive or absent, and the pneumonia may be severe and progress rapidly or be detected as multiple rounded or segmental radiographic infiltrates without pulmonary symptoms. Q fever hepatitis may have a clinical presentation similar to acute viral hepatitis or the pathologic presentation of granulomatous hepatitis.

Chronic Q fever is considered synonymous with C. burnetii endocarditis but also occurs less frequently as infection of an aneurysm or vascular prosthesis or osteomyelitis (Marrie, 1990; Brouqui, 1993). Chronic Q fever endocarditis usually involves previously damaged aortic or mitral valves as an afebrile illness that may manifest with heart failure, hepatosplenomegaly, changing cardiac murmurs, and weight loss. Disease associated with circulating immune complexes includes vasculitis-based purpuric rash or glomerulonephritis.

The pathology of acute Q fever includes mixed interstitial–alveolar–bronchiolar pneumonia with mononuclear inflammatory cells and granulomatous inflammation of the liver and bone marrow (Walker, 1988b). Q fever granulomas often contain a clear central vacuole and a surrounding ring of fibrin as well as epithelioid macrophages. These doughnut granulomas are neither pathognomonic lesions nor the only form of granuloma that occurs in the liver and bone marrow of Q fever patients. The involved cardiac valves in Q fever endocarditis have a small vegetation and show a mixed subacute and chronic inflammation with many foamy macrophages having the cytoplasm filled with C. burnetii (Lepidi, 2003).

Laboratory Diagnosis

The laboratory diagnosis of Q fever is most often accomplished by demonstration of antibodies to C. burnetii (Fournier, 1996, 1998). Serologic methods employ both phase I and phase II antigens and often evaluate class-specific antibody production. Enzyme immunoassay and indirect IFA tests are highly specific and are more sensitive than complement fixation. In acute Q fever, antibodies to phase II antigens appear earliest after infection, and antibodies to phase I may be detected as early as 2 weeks after the onset of illness. In general, acute Q fever is associated with high titers to phase II antigens and lower titers to phase I antigens. By IFA, an anti-phase II IgG titer of 1:200 or greater and anti-phase II IgM titer of 1:50 or greater have a sensitivity of 58% and specificity of 92% in acute Q fever. In chronic Q fever, antibodies to phase I are present at a higher titer (e.g., IgG-IFA anti-phase I titer of 1:800 or greater) and antibodies to phase II are generally equal to or lower than the phase I titer. An IgA response to phase I antigens is often observed in patients with chronic Q fever. A titer of 1:128 or greater against phase I antigen by the complement fixation test is also considered diagnostic of chronic Q fever, although some patients have lower titers. Because of cross-reactivity of *Bartonella henselae* and *Bartonella quintana* with *C. burnetii*, a serologic diagnosis of *Bartonella* endocarditis should not be made until anti-*C.-burnetii* titers have been determined (La Scola, 1996b). In Q fever endocarditis, the anti-*C. burnetii* titer is substantially higher than the anti-*Bartonella* titer. An IFA containing both *C. burnetii* and *B. henselae* effectively distinguishes the infecting bacterium (Rolain, 2003b).

PCR assays have been developed against diverse target genes, and during the first 2 weeks of acute Q fever real-time PCR of serum is more sensitive (24%) than IFA serology (14%) (Fournier, 2003). It is likely that PCR of blood or buffy coat would detect a greater proportion of cases with *Coxiella*.

Other methods for the diagnosis of chronic Q fever endocarditis include immunohistologic staining (sensitivity 32%), electron microscopy, culture (sensitivity 64%), and PCR (sensitivity 75%) detection of *C. burnetii* (Lepidi 2003). *Coxiella burnetii* can be recovered from the blood or infected cardiac valves by in vitro cultivation using a centrifugation-enhanced shell vial HEL cell culture system. This method can identify the presence of coxiellas within 7 days but should be attempted only within cell culture facilities approved for biohazard containment level 3.

Treatment

Doxycycline is effective in shortening the course of acute Q fever when administered during the first 3 days after the onset of illness (Levy, 1991). Fluoroquinolones or a combination of macrolide and rifampin are alternative medications for patients who cannot be treated with tetracycline. Treatment of chronic *C. burnetii* endocarditis requires prolonged administration of doxycycline and a quinolone, which often does not eradicate the infection (Marrie, 1997). Successful treatment is indicated by a slow fall in anti-phase I IgG titer below 1:200, when discontinuation of treatment can be considered. Cardiac valve replacement is often performed for hemodynamic reasons.

Infections Caused by Organisms of the Genus *Bartonella*

Structure and Function

The genus *Bartonella* has been removed from the order Rickettsiales (Brenner, 1993; Birtles, 1996). The human pathogens, *B. quintana* (the etiologic agent of trench fever, a major louse-borne disease in World Wars I and II and among homeless persons), *B. henselae* (the etiologic agent of cat scratch disease), *Bartonella elizabethae* and *Bartonella vinsonii* (associated with infective endocarditis), and *Bartonella bacilliformis* (a sandfly-transmitted bacterium that causes febrile acute hemolytic anemia and chronic verruga peruana cutaneous lesions in South America), have been cultivated in blood-enriched media in the presence of 5% CO_2. These facultative intracellular Gram-negative bacilli do not produce acid from carbohydrates and usually reside within erythrocytes in their natural mammalian hosts. Among numerous newly described species of *Bartonella*, *Bartonella clarridgeiae* is a suspected second agent of cat scratch disease (Kordick, 1997).

Cat Scratch Disease, Bacillary Angiomatosis, and Bacillary Peliosis

B. henselae is transmitted to humans by the scratch or bite of infected kittens, which are bacteremic for many months while appearing healthy (Tappero, 1993; Chomel, 1995; Bergmans, 1997; Heller, 1997). The bacteria are transmitted from cat to cat by the cat flea (Chomel, 1996; Higgins, 1996). The nature of the disease is largely host-determined. In immunocompetent hosts, 80% are younger than age 21 years and present with a cutaneous papule or pustule at the inoculation site and self-limited regional lymphadenopathy. Fewer than 2% of patients suffer complications such as hematogenously disseminated involvement of the liver, spleen, lung, bone, CNS, retina, conjunctiva, or skin (Liston, 1996; Wade, 2000; Verdon, 2002). The histopathology of cat scratch disease lesions is granulomas surrounding stellate microabscesses. In severely immunocompromised patients, *B. henselae* infection is manifested by fever and bacteremia or by cutaneous or visceral angioproliferative lesions.

The latter are characterized by lobular vascular proliferations of plump endothelial cells with clusters of small capillaries surrounding ectatic capillaries separated by edematous, mucinous, or fibrotic stroma containing clusters of neutrophils, neutrophil debris, and granular microcolonies of bartonellas. In the skin these lesions are designated *bacillary angiomatosis*; in the liver and spleen, *hepatic* and *splenic peliosis*. Dissemination to other sites may occur also. The angioproliferative lesions of *B. henselae* and *B. quintana* in immunocompromised patients are indistinguishable, and they are quite similar to the verruga peruana of *B. bacilliformis* (Koehler, 1997). *B. henselae*, *B. quintana*, *B. vinsonii* subsp. *berkhoffii* and *B. elizabethae* have been documented as agents of infective endocarditis. (Drancourt, 1995; Roux 2000).

Trench Fever and Bacillary Angiomatosis

B. quintana causes prolonged bacteremia in convalescent humans, the apparent reservoir. Infections were recognized to be transmitted from person to louse (*Pediculus humanus corporis*) to another person in front-line trenches during World War I (Bruce, 1921). Among French homeless persons, 14% are bacteremic, of whom 80% are afebrile (Brouqui, 1999).

Louse feces laden with *B. quintana* are scratched into the skin, and approximately 8 days later an illness of variable severity begins. Manifestations include fever, generally lasting less than a week, headache, myalgias, pretibial pain, and an evanescent macular rash. Relapses often occur at 4- or 5-day intervals. Bacteremia persists for weeks, months, or longer, serving as a source for infecting lice, even when the person feels relatively healthy. Cases occur at present in alcoholic and homeless populations in American and European cities (Spach, 1995; Foucault, 2002).

Oroya Fever and Verruga Peruana

South American bartonellosis, manifested as an acute illness called Oroya fever or as chronic cutaneous lesions called verruga peruana, is transmitted by the bite of a *Lutzomyia* sandfly. Asymptomatic long-term human carriers are the reservoirs of *B. bacilliformis*. After an incubation period of approximately 3 weeks, Oroya fever begins insidiously with anorexia, headache, malaise, and low-grade fever, or abruptly with chills, high fever, headache, and mental status changes. Bartonellas invade the red blood cells and cause erythrocytic changes that result in erythrophagocytosis and anemia. Verruga peruana, characterized by red to purple nontender nodules that appear in crops over 1–2 months and persist for months to years, follows Oroya fever or occurs without prior symptoms (Arias-Stella, 1986; Walker, 1999a).

Laboratory Diagnosis

Lysis release of intraerythrocytic bacteria followed by centrifugation and incubation at 35°C in humid CO_2 atmosphere on chocolate or Columbia blood agar for more than a month has been used to recover *B. henselae* and *B. quintana* from patients (Tierno, 1995). These *Bartonella* organisms are Gram-negative bacilli, 0.2–0.5 μm in diameter and 1–3 μm long. *B. henselae* are oxidase-, catalase-, and urease-negative and do not utilize carbohydrates. Identification is accomplished by twitching motility in wet mounts, immunofluorescent staining, analysis of fatty acid composition, DNA sequencing or hybridization (Scott, 1996). Polymerase chain reaction detects *B. henselae* DNA in 31% of lymph node biopsies and 55% of lymph node aspirates (Bergmans, 1996). *B. bacilliformis* may be cultivated from blood by inoculation of Columbia blood agar supplemented with 5% defibrinated blood or other blood- or hemin-supplemented media with detection of colonies after an average of 18 days.

Formerly the diagnosis of cat scratch disease required a combination of clinical, epidemiologic, and pathologic criteria. Histopathologic studies, including Warthin–Starry stain and immunohistochemistry, have been used to support the diagnosis of bacillary angiomatosis and cat scratch disease. Oroya fever may be diagnosed by visualization of intra-erythrocytic bartonellas, appearing as cocci or bacilli, occasionally with curved or ring forms, in peripheral blood carefully stained by the Giemsa method to avoid misinterpretation of artifacts. Diagnosis of *B. henselae* and *B. quintana* infections is usually accomplished by the serologic demonstration of antibodies by indirect immunofluorescence or enzyme immunoassay (Dalton, 1995b). Serologic diagnosis of *Bartonella* endocarditis should include measurement of antibody titers against *C. burnetii*, which may stimulate cross-reacting antibody titers against *Bartonella* (Maurin, 1997; Rolain, 2003a). The titers against *C. burnetii* phase I are much higher than the anti-*Bartonella* titers in chronic Q fever endocarditis, and Western immunoblotting after crossabsorption yields a definitive diagnosis if necessary (Houpikian, 2003). Real-time PCR can also be used to establish the diagnosis of *Bartonella* endocarditis (Zeaiter, 2003).

VII

Centers for Disease Control and Prevention: Screening Tests To Detect *Chlamydia trachomatis* and *Neisseria gonorrhoeae* Infections. MMWR 2002b; 51:RR-15 *Discusses nonculture tests, both amplified and nonamplified, for diagnosis of genital infection with C. trachomatis and N. gonorrhoeae.*

Chandler DKF, Grabowski MW, Barile MF: *Mycoplasma pneumoniae* attachment: Competitive inhibition by mycoplasmal binding component and by sialic acid containing glycoconjugates. Infect Immun 1982; 38:598.

Chanock RM, Hayflick L, Barile MF: Growth on artifical medium of an agent associated with atypical pneumonia and its identification as a PPLO. Proc Natl Acad Sci USA 1962; 48:41.

Chen SM, Cullman LC, Walker DH: Western immunoblotting analysis of the antibody responses of patients with human monocytotropic ehrlichiosis to different strains of *Ehrlichia chaffeensis* and *Ehrlichia canis*. Clin Diagn Lab Immunol 1997a; 4:731.

Chen SM, Dumler JS, Bakken JS, et al: Identification of a granulocytotropic *Ehrlichia* species as the etiologic agent of human disease. J Clin Microbiol 1994; 32:589.

Chen SM, Yu X-J, Popov VL, et al: Genetic and antigenic diversity of *Ehrlichia chaffeensis*: comparative analysis of a novel human strain from Oklahoma and previously isolated strains. J Infect Dis 1997b; 175:856.

Chi EY, Kuo CC, Grayston JT: Unique ultrastructure in the elementary body of *Chlamydia* sp. strain TWAR. J Bacteriol 1987; 169:3757.

Childs JE, Sumner JW, Nicholson WL, et al: Outcome of diagnostic tests using samples from patients with culture-proven human monocytic ehrlichiosis: Implication for surveillance. J Clin Microbiol 1999; 37:2997.

Chomel BB, Abbott RC, Kasten RW, et al: *Bartonella henselae* prevalence in domestic cats in California: risk factors and association between bacteremia and antibody titers. J Clin Microbiol 1995; 33:2445.

Chomel BB, Kasten RW, Floyd-Hawkins KA, et al: Experimental transmission of *Bartonella henselae* by the cat flea. J Clin Microbiol 1996; 34:1952.

Clarke LM, Sierra MF, Daidone BJ, et al: Comparison of the Syva Microtrak enzyme immunoassay and Gen-probe Pace 2 with cell culture for diagnosis of cervical *Chlamydia trachomatis* infection in a high-prevalence female population. J Clin Microbiol 1993; 31:968–971.

Cles LD, Bruch K, Stamm WE: Staining characteristics of six commercially available monoclonal immunofluorescence reagents for direct diagnosis of *Chlamydia trachomatis* infections. J Clin Microbiol 1988; 26:1735.

Clyde WA Jr, Kenny GE, Schachter J: Laboratory diagnosis of chlamydial and mycoplasmal infections. *In*: Drew WL (ed.): Cumitech 19. Washington, DC, American Society for Microbiology, 1984.

Comer JA, Nicholson WL, Sumner JW, et al: Diagnosis of human ehrlichiosis by PCR assay of acute-phase serum. J Clin Microbiol 1999; 37:31.

Cox RL, Kuo CC, Grayston JT, et al: Deoxyribonucleic acid relatedness of *Chlamydia* sp. strain TWAR to *Chlamydia trachomatis* and *Chlamydia psittaci*. Int J Syst Bacteriol 1988; 38:265.

Dalton MJ, Clarke MJ, Holman RC, et al: National surveillance for Rocky Mountain spotted fever, 1981–1992: Epidemiologic summary and evaluation of risk factors for fatal outcome. Am J Trop Med Hyg 1995a; 52:405.

Dalton MJ, Robinson LE, Cooper J, et al: Use of *Bartonella* antigens for serologic diagnosis of cat-scratch disease at a national referral center. Arch Intern Med 1995b; 155:1670.

Dawson JE, Anderson BE, Fishbein DB, et al: Isolation and characterization of an *Ehrlichia* sp. from a patient diagnosed with human ehrlichiosis. J Clin Microbiol 1991; 29:2741.

DeGirolami PC, Madoff S: *Mycoplasma hominis* septicemia. J Clin Microbiol 1982; 16:566.

Demaio J, Boyd RS, Rensi R, et al: False-positive Chlamydiazyme results during urine sediment analysis due to bacterial urinary tract infections. J Clin Microbiol 1991; 29:1436.

Drancourt M, George F, Brouqui P, et al: Diagnosis of Mediterranean spotted fever by indirect immunofluorescence of *Rickettsia conorii* in circulating endothelial cells isolated with monoclonal antibody-coated immunomagnetic beads. J Infect Dis 1992; 166:660.

Drancourt M, Mainardi JL, Brouqui P, et al: *Bartonella* (*Rochalimaea*) *quintana* endocarditis in three homeless men. N Engl J Med 1995; 332:419.

Drancourt M, Raoult D, Xeridat B, et al: Q fever meningoencephalitis in five patients. Eur J Epidemiol 1991; 7:134.

Dumler JS, Barbet AF, Bekker CP, et al: Reorganization of genera in the families *Rickettsiaceae* and *Anaplasmataceae* in the order *Rickettsiales*: unification of some species of *Ehrlichia* with *Anaplasma*, *Cowdria* with *Ehrlichia* and *Ehrlichia* with *Neorickettsia*, descriptions of six new species combinations and designations of *Ehrlichia equi* and 'HE agents' as subjective synonyms of *Ehrlichia phagocytophilia*. Int J Syst Evol Microbiol 2001; 6:2145.

Dumler JS, Brouqui P: Molecular diagnosis of human granulocytic anaplasmosis. Expert Rev Mol Diagn 2004; 4:559.

Dumler JS, Dawson JE, Walker DH: Human ehrlichiosis: hematopathology and immunohistologic detection of *Ehrlichia chaffeensis*. Hum Pathol 1993a; 24:391.

Dumler JS, Gage WR, Pettis GL, et al: Rapid immunoperoxidase demonstration of *Rickettsia rickettsii* in fixed cutaneous specimens from patients with Rocky Mountain spotted fever. Am J Clin Pathol 1990; 93:410.

Dumler JS, Sutker WL, Walker DH: Persistent infection with *Ehrlichia chaffeensis*. Clin Infect Dis 1993b; 17:903.

Dumler JS, Taylor JP, Walker DH: Clinical and laboratory features of murine typhus in south Texas, 1980–1987. JAMA 1991; 266:1365.

Dunn BE, Monson TP, Dumler JS, et al: Identification of *Ehrlichia chaffeensis* morulae in cerebrospinal fluid mononuclear cells. J Clin Microbiol 1992; 30:2207.

Edelman DC, Dumler JS: Evaluation of an improved PCR diagnostic assay for human granulocytic ehrlichiosis. Mol Diagn 1996; 1:41.

Ehret JM, Leszczynski JC, Douglas JM, et al: Evaluation of Chlamydiazyme enzyme immunoassay for detection of *Chlamydia trachomatis* in urine specimens from men. J Clin Microbiol 1993; 31:2702.

Elghetany TM, Walker D: Hemostatic changes in Rocky Mountain spotted fever and Mediterranean spotted fever. Am J Clin Pathol 1999; 112:159.

Everett ED, Evans KA, Henry RB, et al: Human ehrlichiosis in adults after tick exposure: Diagnosis using polymerase chain reaction. Ann Intern Med 1994; 120:730.

Everett KDE, Bush RM, Andersen AA: Emended description of the order Chlamydiales, proposal of Parachlamydiaceae fam. nov. and Simkaniaceae fam. nov., each containing one monotypic genus, revised taxonomy of the family Chlamydiaceae, including a new genus and five new species, and standards for the identification of organisms. Int J Syst Bacteriol 1999; 49:415.

Ewing SA, Dawson JE, Kocan AA, et al: Experimental transmission of *Ehrlichia chaffeensis* (Rickettsiales: Ehrlichieae) among white-tailed deer by *Amblyomma americanum* (Acari: Ixodidae). J Med Entomol 1995; 32:368.

Ewing SA, Roberson WR, Buckner RG, Hayat CS: A new strain of *Ehrlichia canis*. J Am Vet Med Assoc 1971; 159:1771.

Fernald GW, Collier AM, Clyde WA Jr: Respiratory infections due to *Mycoplasma pneumoniae* in infants and children. Pediatrics 1975; 55:327.

Ferrero DV, Meyers HN, Schultz DE, Willis SA: Performance of the Gen-Probe amplified *Chlamydia trachomatis* assay in detecting *Chlamydia trachomatis* in endocervical and urine specimens from women and urethral and urine specimens from men attending sexually transmitted disease and family planning clinics. J Clin Microbiol 1998; 36:3230.

Fichtenbaum CJ, Peterson LR, Weil GJ: Ehrlichiosis presenting as a life-threatening illness with features of the toxic shock syndrome. Am J Med 1993; 95:351.

Fishbein DB, Dawson JE, Robinson LE: Human ehrlichiosis in the United States, 1985 to 1990. Ann Intern Med 1994; 120:736.

Fishbein DB, Raoult D: A cluster of *Coxiella burnetii* infections associated with exposure to vaccinated goats and their unpasteurized dairy products. Am J Trop Med Hyg 1992; 47:35.

Fournier PE, Casalta JP, Habib G, et al: Modification of the diagnostic criteria proposed by the Duke endocarditis service to permit improved diagnosis of Q fever endocarditis. Am J Med 1996; 100:629.

Fournier PE, Marrie T-J, Raoult D: Diagnosis of Q fever. J Clin Microbiol 1998; 36:1823.

Fournier PE, Raoult D: Comparison of PCR and serology assays for early diagnosis of acute Q fever. J Clin Microbiol 2003; 41:5094.

Fournier PE, Raoult D: Suicide PCR on skin biopsy specimens for diagnosis of rickettsioses. J Clin Microbiol 2004; 42:3428.

Foucault C, Barrau K, Brouqui P, et al: *Bartonella quintana* bacteremia among homeless people. Clin Infect Dis 2002; 35:684.

Foucault C, Raoult D, Brouqui P: Randomized open trial of gentamicin and doxycycline for eradication of *Bartonella quintana* from blood in patients with chronic bacteremia. Antimicrob Agents Chemother 2003; 47:2204.

Furuya Y, Katayama T, Yoshida Y, et al: Specific amplification of *Rickettsia japonica* DNA from clinical specimens by PCR. J Clin Microbiol 1995; 33:487.

Furuya Y, Yoshida Y, Katayama T, et al: Serotype-specific amplification of *Rickettsia tsutsugamushi* DNA by nested polymerase chain reaction. J Clin Microbiol 1993; 31:1637.

Gage KL, Burgdorfer W, Hopla CE: Hispid cotton rats (*Sigmodon hispidus*) as a source for infecting immature *Dermacentor variabillis* (Acari: Ixodidae) with *Rickettsia rickettsii*. J Med Entomol 1990; 27:615.

Gaydos CA, Theodore M, Dalesio N, et al: Comparison of three nucleic acid amplification tests for detection of *Chlamydia trachomatis* in urine specimens. J Clin Microbiol 2004; 42: 3041.

Geary SJ, Gabridge MG: Characterization of a human lung fibroblast receptor site for *Mycoplasma pneumoniae*. Isr J Med Sci 1987; 23:462.

Goessens WHF, Mouton JW, vanDer Meijden WI, et al: Comparison of three commercially available amplification assays, AMP CT, LCx, and COBAS AMPLICOR, for detection of *Chlamydia trachomatis* in first-void urine. J Clin Microbiol 1997; 35:2628.

Goodman JL, Nelson C, Vitale B, et al: Direct cultivation of the causative agent of human granulocytic ehrlichiosis. N Engl J Med 1996; 334:209.

Gouin E, Egile C, Dehoux P, Villiers, V, et al: The RickA protein of *Rickettsia conorii* activates the Arp2/3 complex. Nature 2004; 427–457.

Grayston JT, Campbell LA, Kuo CC, et al: A new respiratory pathogen: *Chlamydia pneumoniae* strain TWAR. J Infect Dis 1990; 161:618.

Grayston JT, Wang SP, Kuo CC, et al: Current knowledge on *Chlamydia pneumoniae*, strain TWAR, an important cause of pneumonia and other acute respiratory diseases. Eur J Clin Microbiol Infect Dis 1989; 8:191.

Hamilton KS, Standaert SM, Kinney MC: Characteristic peripheral blood findings in human ehrlichiosis. Mod Pathol 2004; 17:512.

Hammerschlag MR, Alpert S, Rosner I, et al: Microbiology of the vagina in children: normal and potentially pathogenic organisms. Pediatrics 1978; 62:57.

Hardalo CJ, Quagliarello V, Dumler JS: Human granulocytic ehrlichiosis in Connecticut: report of a fatal case. Clin Infect Dis 1995; 21:910.

Heinzen RA, Hayes SF, Peacock MG, et al: Directional actin polymerization associated with spotted fever group rickettsia infection of vero cells. Infect Immun 1993; 61:1926.

Heller R, Artosis M, Xemar V, et al: Prevalence of *Bartonella henselae* and *Bartonella clarridgeiae* in stray cats. J Clin Microbiol 1997; 35:1327.

Helmick CG, Bernard KW, D'Angelo LJ: Rocky Mountain spotted fever: clinical, laboratory, and epidemiological features of 262 cases. J Infect Dis 1984; 150:480.

Herrero-Herrero JI, Walker DH, Ruiz-Beltran R: Immunohistochemical evaluation of the cellular immune response to *Rickettsia conorii* in 'taches noires.' J Infect Dis 1987; 155:802.

Higgins JA, Radulovic S, Jaworski DC, et al: Acquisition of the cat scratch disease agent *Bartonella henselae* by cat fleas (Siphonaptera: Pulicidae). J Med Entomol 1996; 33:490.

Hodzic E, Fish D, Maretzki CM, et al: Acquisition and transmission of the agent of human granulocytic ehrlichiosis by *Ixodes scapularis* ticks. J Clin Microbiol 1998; 36:3574.

Horowitz HW, Aguero-Rosenfeld ME, McKenna DF, et al: Clinical and laboratory spectrum of culture-proven human granulocytic ehrlichiosis: comparison with culture-negative cases. Clin Infect Dis 1998; 27:1314.

Houpikian P, Raoult D: Western immunoblotting for *Bartonella* endocarditis. Clin Diag Lab Immunol 2003; 10:95.

Iwen PC, Blair TMH, Woods GL: Comparison of the Gen-probe Pace 2™ system direct fluorescent-antibody, and cell culture for detecting *Chlamydia trachomatis* in cervical specimens. Am J Clin Pathol 1991; 95:578.

Jang W-J, Huh M-S, Park K-H, et al: Evaluation of an immunoglobulin M capture enzyme-linked immunosorbent assay for diagnosis of *Orientia tsutsugamushi* infection. Clin Diag Lab Immunol 2003; 10:394.

Jiang J, Chan T-C, Temenak JJ, et al. Development of a quantitative real-time polymerase chain reaction assay specific for *Orientia tsutsugamushi*. Am J Trop Med Hyg 2004; 70:351.

Jiang J, Marienau KJ, May LA, et al. Laboratory diagnosis of two scrub typhus outbreaks at Camp Fuji, Japan in 2000 and 2001 by enzyme-linked immunosorbent assay, rapid flow assay, and Western blot assay using outer membrane 56-kD recombinant proteins. Am J Trop Med Hyg 2003; 69:60.

Jones RB, Batteiger BE: *Chlamydia trachomatis* (trachoma, perinatal infections, lymphogranuloma venereum, and other genital infections). *In* Mandell GL, Bennett JE, Dolin R (eds): Principles and Practice of Infectious Diseases, 5th ed. New York, Churchill Livingstone, 2000, p 1989.

Jones RB, Priest JB, Kuo C. Subacute chlamydial endocarditis. JAMA 1982; 247:655.

Kaplan JE, Schonberger LB: The sensitivity of various serologic tests in the diagnosis of Rocky Mountain spotted fever. Am J Trop Med Hyg 1986; 35:840.

Kaplowitz LG, Fischer JJ, Sparling PF: Rocky Mountain spotted fever: a clinical dilemma. Curr Clin Top Infect Dis 1981; 2:89.

Kaplowitz LG, Lange JV, Fischer JJ, et al: Correlation of rickettsial titers, circulating endotoxin, and clinical features in Rocky Mountain spotted fever. Arch Intern Med 1983; 143:1149.

Kass EM, Szaniawski WK, Levy H, et al: Rickettsialpox in a New York City hospital, 1980 to 1989. N Engl J Med 1994; 331:1612.

Kawamori F, Akiyama M, Sugieda M, et al: Two-step polymerase chain reaction for diagnosis of scrub typhus and identification of antigenic variants of *Rickettsia tsutsugamushi*. J Vet Med Sci 1993; 55:749.

Keat A, Thomas BJ, Taylor-Robinson D: Chlamydial infection in the etiology of arthritis. Br Med Bull 1983; 39:168.

Kelly DJ, Chan CT, Paxton H, et al: Comparative evaluation of a commercial enzyme immunoassay for the detection of human antibody to *Rickettsia typhi*. Clin Diagn Lab Immunol 1995; 2:356.

Klein JO, Buckland D, Finland M: Colonization of newborn infants by mycoplasmas. N Engl J Med 1969; 280:1025.

Klein MB, Nelson CM, Goodman JL: Antibiotic susceptibility of the newly cultivated agent of human granulocytic ehrlichiosis: Promising activity of quinolones and rifamycins. Antimicrob Agents Chemother 1997; 41:76.

Kluytmans JAJW, Goessens WHF, Mouton JW, et al: Evaluation of Clearview and Magic Lite tests, polymerase chain reaction, and cell culture for detection of *Chlamydia trachomatis* in urogenital specimens. J Clin Microbiol 1993; 31:3204.

Kluytmans JAJW, Goessens WHF, vanRijsoort-Vos JH, et al: Improved performance of Pace 2 with modified collection system in combination with probe competition assay for detection of *Chlamydia trachomatis* in urethral specimens from males. J Clin Microbiol 1994; 32:568.

Kluytmans JAJW, Niesters HGM, Mouton JW, et al: Performance of nonisotopic DNA probe for detection of *Chlamydia trachomatis* in urogenital specimens. J Clin Microbiol 1991; 29:2685.

Knowles TT, Alleman AR, Sorenson HL, et al: Characterization of the major antigenic protein 2 of *Ehrlichia canis* and *Ehrlichia chaffeensis* and its application for serodiagnosis of ehrlichiosis. Clin Diag Lab Immunol 2003; 10:520.

Koehler JE, Sanchez MA, Garrido CS, et al: Molecular epidemiology of *Bartonella* infections in patients with bacillary angiomatosis-peliosis. N Engl J Med 1997; 337:1876.

Kordick DL, Hilyard EJ, Hadfield TL, et al: *Bartonella clarridgeiae*, a newly recognized zoonotic pathogen causing inoculation papules, fever, and lymphadenopathy (cat scratch disease). J Clin Microbiol 1997; 35:1813.

Koumans EH, Black CM, Markowitz LE, et al: Comparison of methods for detection of *Chlamydia trachomatis* and *Neisseria gonorrhoeae* using commercially available nucleic acid amplification tests and a liquid pap smear medium. J Clin Microbiol 2003; 41:1507.

Kramer VL, Randolph MP, Hui LT, et al: Detection of the agents of human ehrlichioses in ioxdid ticks from California. Am J Trop Med Hyg 1999; 60:62.

Krause PJ, Corrow CL, Bakken JA: Successful treatment of human granulocytic ehrlichiosis in children using rifampin. Pediatrics 2003; 112:e652.

Krech T, Bleckmann M, Paatz R: Comparison of buffalo green monkey cells and McCoy cells for isolation of *Chlamydia trachomatis* in a microtiter system. J Clin Microbiol 1989; 27:2364.

La Scola B, Raoult D: Diagnosis of Mediterranean spotted fever by cultivation of *Rickettsia conorii* from blood and skin samples using the centrifugation-shell vial technique and by detection of *R. conorii* in circulating endothelial cells: a 6-year follow-up. J Clin Microbiol 1996a; 34:2722.

La Scola B, Raoult D: Serological cross-reactions between *Bartonella quintana*, *Bartonella henselae*, and *Coxiella burnetii*. J Clin Microbiol 1996b; 34:2270.

Lepidi H, Houpikian P, Liang Z, et al: Cardiac valves in patients with Q fever endocarditis: microbiological, molecular, and histologic studies. J Infect Dis 2003; 187:1097.

Levy PY, Drancourt M, Etienne J, et al: Comparison of different antibiotic regimens for therapy of 32 cases of Q fever endocarditis. Antimicrob Agents Chemother 1991; 35:533.

Li H, Walker DH: Characterization of rickettsial attachment to host cells by flow cytometry. Infect Immun 1992; 60:2030.

Li H, Walker DH: rOmpA is a critical protein for the adhesion of *Rickettsia rickettsii* to host cells. Microb Pathog 1998; 24:289.

Liston TE, Koehler JE: Granulomatous hepatitis and necrotizing splenitis due to *Bartonella henselae* in a patient with cancer: case report and review of hepatosplenic manifestations of bartonella infection. Clin Infect Dis 1996; 22:951.

Loens K, Ursi D, Goossens H, Ieven M: Molecular diagnosis of *Mycoplasma pneumoniae* respiratory tract infections. J Clin Microbiol 2003; 41:4915.
Discusses various nucleic acid amplification methods that have been examined for direct detection of M. pneumoniae in respiratory specimens. Includes a discussion of specimen processing and quality control.

McDade JE, Shepard CC, Redus MA, et al: Evidence of *Rickettsia prowazekii* infections in the United States. Am J Trop Med Hyg 1980; 29:277.

McMahon DK, Dummer JS, Pasculle AR, et al: Extra-genital *Mycoplasma hominis* infections in adults. Am J Med 1990; 89:275.

McQuiston JH, Paddock CD, Singleton J, Jr, et al: Imported spotted fever rickettsioses in United States travelers returning from Africa: a summary of cases confirmed by laboratory testing at the Centers for Disease Control and Prevention, 1999–2000. Am J Trop Med Hyg 2004; 70:98.

Mahony J, Chong S, Jang D, et al: Urine specimens from pregnant and nonpregnant women inhibitory to amplification of *Chlamydia trachomatis* nucleic acid by PCR ligase chain reaction, and transcription-mediated amplification; identification of urinary substances associated with inhibition and removal of inhibitory activity. J Clin Microbiol 1998; 36:3122.

Manosroi J, Chutipongvivate S, Auwanit W, et al: Early diagnosis of scrub typhus in Thailand from clinical specimens by nested polymerase chain reaction. Southeast Asian J Trop Med Public Health 2003; 34:831.

Maraha B, Berg H, Kerver M, et al: Is the perceived association between *Chlamydia pneumoniae* and vascular diseases biased by methodology? J Clin Microbiol 2004; 42:3937.

Marrie TJ (ed.): Q fever. Vol. I: The Disease. Boca Raton, FL, CRC Press, 1990.

Marrie TJ, Durrant H, Williams C, et al: Exposure to parturient cats: a risk factor for acquisition of Q fever in maritime Canada. J Infect Dis 1988; 158:101.

Marrie TJ, Raoult D: Q fever – a review and issues for the next century. Int J Antimicrob Agents 1997; 8:145.

Maurin M, Eb F, Etienne J, et al: Serological cross-reactions between *Bartonella* and *Chlamydia* species: implications for diagnosis. J Clin Microbiol 1997; 35:2283.

Mills RD, Young A, Cain K, et al: Chlamydiazyme plus blocking assay to detect *Chlamydia trachomatis* in endocervical specimens. Am J Clin Pathol 1992; 97:209.

Moron CG, Popov VL, Feng H-M, et al: Identification of the target cells of *Orientia tsutsugamushi* in human cases of scrub typhus. Mod Pathol 2001; 14:752.

Murai K, Tachibana N, Okayama A, et al: Sensitivity of polymerase chain reaction assay for *Rickettsia tsutsugamushi* in patients' blood samples. Microbiol Immunol 1992; 36:1145.

Nelson HD, Helfand M: Screening for chlamydial infection. Am J Prev Med 2001; 20(3S):95–107.

Nicholson WL, Comer JA, Sumner JW, et al: An indirect immunofluorescence assay using a cell culture-derived antigen for detection of antibodies to the agent of human granulocytic ehrlichiosis. J Clin Microbiol 1997; 35:1510.

Niebylski ML, Peacock MG, Schwan TG: Lethal effect of *Rickettsia rickettsii* on its tick vector (*Dermacentor andersoni*). Appl Environ Microbiol 1999; 65:773.

Olano JP, Hogrefe W, Seaton, et al: Clinical manifestations, epidemiology, and laboratory diagnosis of human monocytotropic ehrlichiosis in a commercial laboratory setting. Clin Diag Lab Immunol 2003a; 10:891.

Olano JP, Masters E, Hogrefe W, et al: Human monocytotropic ehrlichiosis, Missouri. Emerg Infect Dis 2003b; 9:1579.

Paddock CD, Folk SM, Shore GM, et al: Infections with *Ehrlichia chaffeensis* and *Ehrlichia ewingii* in persons coinfected with human immunodeficiency virus. Clin Infect Dis 2001; 33:1586.

Paddock CD, Greer PW, Ferebee TL, et al: Hidden mortality attributable to Rocky Mountain spotted fever: immunohistochemical detection of fatal, serologically unconfirmed disease. J Infect Dis 1999; 179:1469.

Paddock CD, Suchard DP, Grumbach KL, et al: Brief report: Fatal seronegative ehrlichiosis in a patient with HIV infection. N Engl J Med 1993; 329:1164.

Paddock CD, Sumner JW, Comer JA, et al: *Rickettsia parkeri*: a newly recognized cause of spotted fever rickettsiosis in the United States. Clin Infect Dis 2004; 38:805.

Parola P, Miller RS, McDaniel, et al: Emerging rickettsioses of the Thai–Myanmar border. Emerg Infect Dis 2003; 9:592.

Patterson KD: Typhus and its control in Russia, 1870–1940. Med Hist 1993; 37:361.

Peipert JF: Genital chlamydial infections. N Engl J Med 2003; 349:2424.

Provides an excellent overview of genital infections with C. trachomatis, including epidemiology, screening strategies, and treatment.

Perez M, Rikihisa Y, Wen B: *Ehrlichia canis*-like agent isolated from a man in Venezuela: antigenic and genetic characterization. J Clin Microbiol 1996; 34:2133.

Petrovec M, Furlan SL, Zupanc TA, et al: Human disease in Europe caused by a granulocytic *Ehrlichia* species. J Clin Microbiol 1997; 35:1556.

Phillips LE, Goodrich KH, Turner RM, et al: Isolation of *Mycoplasma* species and *Ureaplasma urealyticum* from obstetrical and gynecological patients by using commercially available medium formulations. J Clin Microbiol 1986; 24:377.

Ponka A: The occurrence and clinical picture of serologically verified *Mycoplasma pneumoniae* infections with emphasis on central nervous system, cardiac, and joint manifestations. Ann Clin Res 1979; 11(Suppl 24):1.

Puolakkainen M, Hiltunen-Back E, Reunala T, et al: Comparison of performances of two commercially available tests, a PCR assay and a ligase chain reaction test, in detection of urogenital *Chlamydia trachomatis* infection. J Clin Microbiol 1998; 36:1489.

Raoult D, Drancourt M: Antimicrobial therapy of rickettsial diseases. Antimicrob Agents Chemother 1991; 35:2457.

Raoult D, Fournier PE, Vandenesch F, et al: Outcome and treatment of *Bartonella* endocarditis. Arch Intern Med 2003; 163:226.

Raoult D, La Scola B, Enea M, et al: A flea-associated rickettsia pathogenic for humans. Emerg Infect Dis 2001; 7:73.

Ratnasamy N, Everett ED, Roland WE, et al: Central nervous system manifestations of human ehrlichiosis. Clin Infect Dis 1996; 23:314.

Reynolds MG, Krebs JW, Comer JA, et al: Flying squirrel-associated typhus, United States. Emerg Infec Dis 2003; 9:1341.

Roblin PM, Dumornay W, Hammerschlag MR: Use of HEp-2 cells for improved isolation and passage of *Chlamydia pneumoniae*. J Clin Microbiol 1992; 30:1968.

Rolain JM, Fournier PE, Raoult D, et al: First isolation and detection by immunofluorescence assay of *Bartonella koehlerae* in erythrocytes from a French cat. J Clin Microbiol 2003a; 41:4460.

Rolain JM, Lecam C, Raoult D: Simplified serological diagnosis of endocarditis due to *Coxiella burnetii* and *Bartonella*. Clin Diag Lab Immunol 2003b; 10:1147.

Rolain JM, Maurin M, Bryskie A, et al: *In vitro* activities of telithromycin (HMR 3647) against *Rickettsia rickettsii*, *Rickettsia conorii*, *Rickettsia africae*, *Rickettsia typhi*, *Rickettsia prowazekii*, *Coxiella burnetii*, *Bartonella henselae*, *Bartonella quintana*, *Bartonella bacilliforis*, and *Ehrlichia chaffeensis*. Antimicrob Agents Chemother 2000; 44:1391.

Roux V, Fykrn S, Wyllie S, Raoult D: *Bartonella vinsonii* subsp. *berkhoffii* as an agent of afebrile blood culture-negative endocarditis in a human. J Clin Microbiol 2000; 38:1698.

Roux V, Raoult D: Phylogenetic analysis of the genus *Rickettsia* by 16S rDNA sequencing. Res Microbiol 1995; 146:385.

Roux V, Raoult D: Body lice as tools for diagnosis and surveillance of reemerging disease. J Clin Microbiol 1999; 37:596.

Roux V, Rydkina E, Eremeeva M, Raoult D: Citrate synthase gene comparison, a new tool for phylogenetic analysis, and its application for the rickettsiae. Int J Syst Bacteriol 1997; 47:252.

Schriefer ME, Sacci JB, Jr., Dumler JS, et al: Identification of a novel rickettsial infection in a patient diagnosed with murine typhus. J Clin Microbiol 1994a; 32:949.

Schriefer ME, Sacci JB, Higgins A, et al: Murine typhus: updated roles of multiple urban components and a second typhus like rickettsia. J Med Entomol 1994b; 31:681.

Schultze GE, Jacobs RF: Human moncytic ehrlichiosis in children. Pediatrics 1997; 100:E10.

Scott MA, McCurley TL, Vnenckjones CL, et al: Cat scratch disease – detection of *Bartonella henselae* DNA in archival biopsies from patient with clinically, serologically, and histologically defined disease. Am J Pathol 1996; 149:2161.

Sehdev AES, Dumler JS: Hepatic pathology in human monocytic ehrlichiosis. Am J Clin Pathol 2003; 119:859.

Sexton DJ, Kanj SS, Wilson K, et al: The use of a polymerase chain reaction as a diagnostic test for Rocky Mountain spotted fever. Am J Trop Med Hyg 1994; 50:59.

Silverman DJ: Oxidative cell injury and spotted fever group rickettsiae. *In* Anderson BE (ed.): Rickettsial Infection and Immunity. New York, Plenum Press, 1997, p 79.

Silverman DJ, Santucci LA, Meyers N, et al.: Penetration of host cells by *Rickettsia rickettsii* appears to be mediated by a phospholipase of rickettsial origin. Infect Immun 1992; 60:2733.

Solomon AW, Peeling RW, Foster A, Mabey DCW: Diagnosis and assessment of trachoma. Clin Microbiol Rev 2004; 17:982.

Provides an excellent review of trachoma, including an historical perspective, an overview of the developmental cycle, clinical presentation, and laboratory diagnosis.

Spach DH, Kanter AS, Dougherty MJ, et al: *Bartonella* (*Rochalimaea*) *quintana* bacteremia in inner-city patients with chronic alcoholism. N Engl J Med 1995; 332:424.

Stothard DR, Fuerst PA: Evolutionary analysis of the spotted fever and typhus groups of *Rickettsia* using 16S rRNA gene sequences. Syst Appl Microbiol 1995; 18:52.

Sugita Y, Yamakawa Y, Takahasi K, et al: A polymerase chain reaction system for rapid diagnosis of scrub typhus within six hours. Am J Trop Med Hyg 1993; 49:636.

Tamura A, Ohashi N, Urakami H, et al: Classification of *Rickettsia tsutsugamushi* in a new genus, *Orientia* gen. nov., as *Orientia tsutsugamushi* comb. nov. Int J Syst Bacteriol 1995; 45:589.

Tappero JW, Mohle-Boetani J, Koehler JE, et al: The epidemiology of bacillary angiomatosis and bacillary peliosis. JAMA 1993; 269:770.

Taylor-Robinson D, Furr PM, Webster ADB: *Ureaplasma urealyticum* causing persistent urethritis in a patient with hypogammaglobulinemia. Genitourin Med 1985; 61:404.

Taylor-Robinson D, McCormack WM: Medical progress: the genital mycoplasmas. N Engl J Med 1980; 302:1003.

Tierno PM, Jr, Inglima K, Parisi MT: Detection of *Bartonella* (*Rochalimaea*) *henselae* bacteremia using BacT/Alert blood culture system. Am J Clin Pathol 1995; 104:530.

Tissot Dupont HL, Raoult D, Brouqui P, et al: Epidemiologic features and clinical presentation of acute Q fever in hospitalized patients: 323 French cases. Am J Med 1992; 93:427.

Toye B, Woods W, Bobrowska M, Ramotar K: Inhibition of PCR in genital and urine specimens submitted for *Chlamydia trachomatis* testing. J Clin Microbiol 1998; 36:2356.

Traub R, Wisseman CL Jr, Farhang-Azad A: The ecology of murine typhus – a critical review. Trop Dis Bull 1978; 75:237.

Tzianabos TB, Anderson BE, McDade JE: Detection of *Rickettsia rickettsii* DNA in clinical specimens by using polymerase chain reaction technology. J Clin Microbiol 1989; 27:2866.

Uchiyama T: Role of major surface antigens of *Rickettsia japonica* in the attachment to host cells. *In* Raoult D, Brouqui P (eds): Rickettsiae and Rickettsial Diseases at the Turn of the Third Millenium. Paris, Elsevier, 1999, p 182.

Valbuena G, Feng H-M, Walker DH: Mechanisms of immunity against rickettsiae. New perspectives and opportunities offered by unusual intracellus parasites. Microbes Infect 2002; 4:625.

Van der Pol B, Ferrero DV, Buck-Barrington L, et al: Multicenter evaluation of the BDProbeTec ET system for detection of *Chlamydia trachomatis* and *Neisseria gonorrhoeae* in urine specimens, female endocervical swabs, and male urethral swabs. J Clin Microbiol 2001; 39:1008.

Verdon R, Geffray L, Collet T, et al: Vertebral osteomyelitis due to *Bartonella henselae* in adults: a report of 2 cases. Clin Infect Dis 2002; 35: e141.

Vincelette J, Schirm J, Bogard M, et al: Multicenter evaluation of the fully automated COBAS AMPLICOR PCR test for detection of *Chlamydia trachomatis* in urogenital specimens. J Clin Microbiol 1999; 37:74.

Wade N, Levi L, Jones M, et al: Optic disk edema associated with peripapillary serous retinal detachment: an early sign of systemic *Bartonella henselae* infection. Am J Ophthalmol 130:327, 2000.

Waites KB, Talkington DF: *Mycoplasma pneumoniae* and its role as a human pathogen. Clin Microbiol Rev 2004; 17:697.

Provides an in-depth review of M. pneumoniae, including taxonomy, pathogenesis, clinical syndromes, diagnosis, and treatment.

Walker DH: Pathology of Q fever. *In* Walker DH (ed.): Biology of Rickettsial Diseases, vol 1. Boca Raton, FL, CRC Press, 1988b, p 17.

Walker DH, Bouyer DH: Rickettsia. *In* Murray PR, Baron EJ, Jorgensen JH, et al (eds): Manual of Clinical Microbiology, 8th ed. Washington, DC, ASM Press, 2003, p 1005.

Walker DH, Dumler JS: Human monocytic and granulocytic ehrlichioses. Discovery and diagnosis of emerging tick-borne infections and the critical role of the pathologist. Arch Pathol Lab Med, 1997a; 121:78.

Walker DH, Feng HM, Ladner S, et al: Immunohistochemical diagnosis of typhus rickettsioses using an histochemical diagnosis of typhus rickettsioses using an anti-lipopolysaccharide monoclonal antibody. Mod Pathol 1997b; 10:1038.

Walker DH, Fishbein DB: Epidemiology of rickettsial diseases. Eur J Epidemiol 1991; 7:237.

Walker DH, Gear JHS: Correlation of the distribution of *Rickettsia conorii*, microscopic lesions, and clinical features in South African tick bite fever. Am J Trop Med Hyg 1985; 34:361.

Walker DH, Guerra H, Maguina C: *Bartonelloses*. *In* Guerrant RL, Walker DH, Weller PF (eds): Tropical Infectious Diseases: Principles, Pathogens, and Practice: Philadelphia, PA, Churchill Livingstone, 1999a, p 482.

Walker DH, Hawkins HK, Hudson P: Fulminant Rocky Mountain spotted fever: its pathologic characteristics associated with glucose-6-phosphate dehydrogenase deficiency. Arch Pathol Lab Med 1983; 107:121.

Walker DH, Hudnall SD, Szaniawski WK, Feng HM: Monoclonal antibody-based immunohistochemical diagnosis of rickettsialpox: the macrophage is the principal target. Mod Pathol 1999b; 12:529.

Walker DH, Occhino C, Tringali GR, et al: Pathogenesis of rickettsial eschars: the *tache noire* of boutonneuse fever. Hum Pathol 1988a; 19:1449.

Walker DH, Parks FM, Betz TG, et al: Histopathology and immunohistologic demonstration of the distribution of *Rickettsia typhi* in fatal murine typhus. Am J Clin Pathol 1989; 91:720.

Walker DH, Staiti A, Mansueto S, et al: Frequent occurrence of hepatic lesions in boutonneuse fever. Acta Trop 1986; 43:175.

Walker TS: Rickettsial interactions with human endothelial cells in vitro: adherence and entry. Infect Immun 1984; 44:205.

Walls JJ, Aguero-Rosenfeld M, Bakken JS, et al: Inter- and intralaboratory comparison of *Ehrlichia equi* and human granulocytic ehrlichiosis (HGE) agent strains for serodiagnosis of HGE by the immunofluorescent-antibody test. J Clin Microbiol 1999; 37:2968.

Warren R, Dwyer B, Plackett M, et al: Comparative evaluation of detection assays for *Chlamydia trachomatis*. J Clin Microbiol 1993; 31:1663.

Watt G, Chouriyagune C, Ruangweerayud R, et al: Scrub typhus infections poorly responsive to antibiotics in northern Thailand. Lancet 1996; 348:86.

Watt G, Kantipong P, Jongsakul K, et al: Doxycycline and rifampicin for mild scrub-typhus infections in northern Thailand: a randomized trial. Lancet 2000; 356:1057.

Watt G, Walker DH: Scrub typhus. *In* Guerrant RL, Walker DH, Weller PF (eds): Tropical Infectious Diseases, Principles, Pathogens, and Practice. Philadelphia, PA, Churchill Livingstone, 1999, p 592.

Weiss E: History of rickettsiology. *In* Walker DH (ed.): Biology of Rickettsial Diseases. Boca Raton, FL, CRC Press, 1988, vol I, p 15.

Williams WJ, Radulovic S, Dasch GA, et al: Identification of *Rickettsia conorii* infection by polymerase chain reaction in a soldier returning from Somalia. Clin Infect Dis 1994; 19:93.

Wood JC, Lu RM, Peterson EM, et al: Evaluation of Mycotrim-GU for isolation of *Mycoplasma* species and *Ureaplasma urealyticum*. J Clin Microbiol 1985; 22:789.

Woods GL, Garza DM: Use of Gen-Probe probe competition assay as a supplement to probes for direct detection of *Chlamydia trachomatis* and *Neisseria gonorrhoeae* in urogenital specimens. J Clin Microbiol 1996; 34:177.

Wylie JL, Moses S, Babcock R, et al: Comparative evaluation of Chlamydiazyme, PACE 2, and AMP-CT assays for detection of *Chlamydia trachomatis* in endocervical specimens. J Clin Microbiol 1998; 36:3488.

Yajko DM, Balston E, Wood D, et al: Evaluation of PPLO, A7B, E, and NYC agar media for the isolation of *Ureaplasma urealyticum* and *Mycoplasma* species from the genital tract. J Clin Microbiol 1984; 19:73.

Yu X-J, Brouqui P, Dumler JS, et al: Detection of *Ehrlichia chaffeensis* in human tissue by using a species specific monoclonal antibody. J Clin Microbiol 1993; 31:3284.

Yu X-J, Crocquent-Valdes PA, Cullman LC, et al: Comparison of *Ehrlichia chaffeensis* recombinant proteins for serologic diagnosis of human monocytotropic ehrlichiosis. J Clin Microbiol 1999; 37:2568.

Yu X-J, Walker DH: The order *Rickettsiales*. *In* Dworkin M, et al (eds): The Prokaryotes: An Evolving Electronic Resource for the Microbiological Community, 3rd ed. New York, Springer-Verlag, 2003. Available on line at: http://link.springer-ny.com/link/service/books/10125.

Zavala-Velazquez JE, Ruiz-Sosa JA, Sanchez-Elias RA, et al: *Rickettsia felis* rickettsiosis in Yucatán. Lancet 2000; 356:1079.

Zeaiter Z, Fournier PE, Greub G, et al: Diagnosis of *Bartonella* endocarditis by a real-time nested PCR assay using serum. J Clin Microbiol 2003; 41:919.

Zhi N, Rikihisa Y, Kim HY, et al: Comparison of major antigenic proteins of six strains of the human granulocytic ehrlichiosis agent by Western immunoblot analysis. J Clin Microbiol 1997; 35:2606.

Zinsser H (ed): Rats, Lice, and History. New York, Little, Brown, 1935.
Very readable historical account of the toll that disease takes, especially in times of conflict.

VII

CHAPTER 56

Medical Bacteriology

Gerri S. Hall PhD, Gail L. Woods MD

KEY POINTS

• Bacteria can be categorized based on the Gram stain reaction (Gram-positive or Gram-negative), shape (cocci, bacilli, coccobacilli, spirochete), preferred atmosphere (aerobic, microaerophilic, anaerobic), and presence or absence of spores; and they can be identified based on key biochemical tests, antigenic components (e.g., cell wall antigens, toxins), and/or molecular features.

• Among the Gram-positive cocci, the most important human pathogens (and the infections they commonly cause) are *Staphylococcus aureus* (skin and soft tissue infections, bacteremia, toxic shock syndrome), *Streptococcus pyogenes* (pharyngitis and its nonsuppurative complications, skin and soft tissue infections), *Streptococcus agalactiae* (neonatal bacteremia and meningitis), *Streptococcus pneumoniae* (community-acquired pneumonia, meningitis), and *Enterococcus faecalis* and *Enterococcus faecium* (nosocomial urinary tract infections and bacteremia).

• Among the Gram-positive bacilli, the most important human pathogens (and the infections they commonly cause) are *Listeria monocytogenes* (meningitis, bacteremia), *Nocardia* species (pneumonia, soft tissue infections, brain abscess), *Bacillus anthracis* (skin and soft tissue infections, pneumonia; a bioterrorism agent), and *Corynebacterium diphtheriae* (diphtheria), which is rarely encountered in the clinical laboratory in the United States.

• Among the Gram-negative cocci, the most important human pathogens (and the infections they commonly cause) are *Neisseria meningitidis* (meningitis) and *Neisseria gonorrhoeae* (gonorrhea).

• The Gram-negative bacilli include Enterobacteriaceae, many of which are normal flora in the gastrointestinal tract, nonfermentative Gram-negative bacilli (e.g., *Pseudomonas aeruginosa*), which are found in the environment and cause human infections when the host defenses are compromised, halophilic organisms (*Vibrio* species), microaerophilic bacteria (*Campylobacter, Helicobacter*), fastidious organisms (*Legionella* species, *Bordetella* species, *Francisella tularensis, Brucella* species, *Haemophilus* species), and miscellaneous infrequently encountered bacteria.

• Among the Enterobacteriaceae, the most important human pathogens (and the infections they commonly cause) are *Escherichia coli* (urinary tract infection, diarrhea, bacteremia), *Klebsiella pneumoniae* and *Klebsiella oxytoca* (urinary tract infection, pneumonia), *Proteus* species (urinary tract infection), *Salmonella* species (diarrhea, typhoid fever), *Shigella* species (diarrhea), *Enterobacter* species (nosocomial pneumonia, urinary tract infection, bacteremia) and *Serratia* species (nosocomial pneumonia).

• Among the anaerobes, the most important human pathogens (and the infections they commonly cause) are *Bacteroides fragilis* group (intra-abdominal infections, abscesses) and *Clostridium* species, especially *Clostridium perfringens* (soft tissue infections, food poisoning), *Clostridium tetani* (tetanus), and *Clostridium difficile* (antibiotic-associated diarrhea).

A wide variety of bacterial species may be recovered from clinical specimens. To appropriately assess the clinical significance of these organisms, an understanding of the normal bacterial flora present at different anatomic locations is essential. In some cases the number of organisms present can be extremely high; for example, 10^6 organisms/cm^2 of skin, 10^9 organisms/mL of oral secretions, and 10^{11} organisms/g of colon contents. It is important to obtain samples with minimal contamination from the normal flora. This may be difficult, but can be optimally achieved if proper procedures are followed. These procedures, along with processing techniques that serve to enhance recovery of pathogenic microorganisms, are discussed in Chapter 63. This chapter begins with a short discussion of laboratory procedures used to process a specimen for bacterial culture, followed by a more in-depth discussion of the bacterial species that are commonly considered to be human pathogens.

Specimen Processing

Gram's Stain

Few would argue that direct examination of a specimen with the Gram's stain is one of the most valuable procedures performed by the microbiology laboratory. The Gram's stain result provides rapid information that is used by the clinician for selecting appropriate antimicrobial therapy and it also helps the laboratory technologist assess the quality of the specimen and the extent to which certain organisms recovered in culture will be worked up. Organisms present in abundant quantity in specimens containing many white blood cells are given more attention than those that are present in few numbers in the absence of white blood cells.

To prepare a smear for staining, an aliquot of the most purulent or bloody portion of the specimen is placed on a clean microscopic slide in a manner that provides both thick and thin areas. For sterile body fluids, a cytocentrifuge may be used to concentrate the specimen by 10–100 times (Peterson, 1988). The material on the slide is allowed to air-dry, fixed with methanol or gentle heat, and then stained with the Gram's stain reagents (crystal violet, Gram's iodine, alcohol, and safranin). Organisms that have a Gram-positive cell wall will resist decolorization with methanol and retain the purple color of the crystal violet; organisms that have a Gram-negative cell wall will be decolorized and stain red with safranin.

Stained smears are initially examined using a low-power objective to look for large structures, such as nematode larvae, Curschmann's spirals, large granules, grains, bacterial microcolonies, or fungal forms. An oil

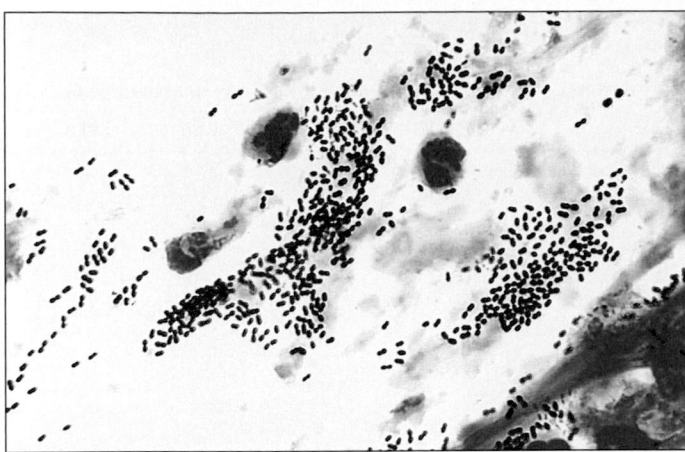

Figure 56–1 Gram's stain of a sputum smear shows neutrophils, debris, and Gram-positive diplococci, suggestive of pneumococcal infection (oil immersion).

immersion lens is then used to assess the type of bacteria present. Because 10^5 organisms/mL must be present in order to see one organism per oil immersion field (1000×), smears must be examined carefully to detect small numbers of organisms.

The organisms observed should be evaluated for size, shape, and Gram's reaction and reported with as much description as possible; reporting the presence of Gram-positive cocci in pairs that resemble *Streptococcus pneumoniae* (Fig. 56–1) is more helpful than simply reporting Gram-positive cocci in chains. The presence of white or red blood cells should be quantified and reported, along with any intracellular bacteria observed. Correlation of the Gram stain observations with culture results is a good way to check on the quality of the stains and culture. Demonstration of many bacteria on the Gram stain that do not grow out in culture may indicate unusual organisms that require more specialized media, inability of the laboratory personnel to recognize certain colonial types in culture, or could suggest a false-positive Gram stain result due to contamination of reagents or collection materials, such as swabs, or incorrect interpretation of the Gram stain results. Gram stain results could also indicate the need to inoculate additional media for a specific specimen. For example, finding many Gram-negative coccobacilli in a respiratory specimen could indicate the need for a chocolate plate to recover *Haemophilus* sp., which would not be recovered on a blood agar plate. Other stains, such as the acridine orange stain, can be utilized for staining blood culture bottles, cerebrospinal fluid (CSF) or buffy coat preparations. This is a type of fluorescent stain that provides a rapid and, at times, more sensitive stain for bacteria and fungi (Mirrett, 1982). Bacteria and fungi will produce an orange fluorescence, while mammalian cells will stain green. Some experience is required for accurate interpretation of the acridine orange stain, and correct preparation of the smears is necessary to avoid too much cellular material, which can result in 'too much' cellular DNA and mask the presence of any bacterial DNA.

Culture Techniques

Media for culture is selected to provide the optimal conditions for growth of pathogens commonly encountered at a particular site or in a particular type of specimen. Consideration is given to special growth requirements of bacteria associated with a given type of infection or to the necessity of selecting certain pathogenic bacteria from a mixed population of indigenous flora. Therefore, the media chosen may include selective and differential media in addition to standard enrichment agar.

Blood-supplemented agar is a good general growth medium and demonstrates the hemolytic action of the colonies on the red blood cells. Antibiotics or chemicals can be added to create a selective medium such as colistin–nalidixic acid (CNA) agar or phenylethyl alcohol (PEA) agar, which are used to inhibit the growth of Gram-negative bacilli while permitting Gram-positive bacteria to grow. Heating the blood to make chocolate agar and adding vitamin supplements creates an enriched medium with available hemin (X factor) and nicotinamide adenine dinucleotide (V factor) for the isolation of *Haemophilus* spp. and other fastidious bacteria. Gram-negative bacilli may be separated from Gram-positive bacilli by using a bile salt and dye in a medium such as MacConkey's agar, which additionally divides the colonies into lactose-positive and lactose-negative colonies, thus making it both selective and differential. Guidelines for the selection of media to be used with different types of specimens are shown in Table 56–1.

Bacterial cultures are generally incubated at 35°C and examined initially after 18–24 hours of incubation. Added CO_2 in concentrations of 5–10% CO_2 is either essential or stimulatory to the growth of *Neisseria gonorrhoeae*, *Haemophilus influenzae*, and *S. pneumoniae*, and should be used whenever feasible. Exceptions to this recommendation are those cultures on differential and selective media in which the pH alteration (which can be affected by added CO_2) is used to differentiate colony types (e.g., xylose–lysine–deoxycholate [XLD] agar, Hektoen enteric [HE] agar).

For recovery of anaerobes, inoculated media should be placed into an anaerobic environment as quickly as possible. There are several types of anaerobic culture systems available. One of these is the anaerobic jar, in which water is added to a CO_2 and H_2 generator package and O_2 is catalytically converted with H_2 to water with palladium-coated alumina pellets contained in a lid chamber. A modification of this system is a transparent plastic bag containing its own gas generator and palladium catalyst, and designed to hold an agar plate.

Another approach to anaerobic culture is the anaerobic glove box or chamber, which consists of a large, clear plastic, airtight chamber filled with an oxygen-free gas mixture of nitrogen, hydrogen, and carbon dioxide. Specimens, plates, and tubes are introduced into or removed from the chamber through a gas interchange lock. Anaerobiosis is maintained by palladium catalysts and the hydrogen gas in the chamber. All manipulations within the chamber are done with neoprene gloves sealed to the chamber wall or, for 'gloveless' systems, through a hole with sleeves that seal tightly around the forearms. The chambers contain internal incubators that maintain the incubation temperature. Each of the anaerobe systems has its advantages and disadvantages but they are all equally effective for isolating clinically significant anaerobic bacteria from specimens.

Bacterial cultures should be examined routinely after 18–24 hours of incubation. The exception to this is the anaerobe culture, which is generally examined at 48 hours to allow these slower-growing bacteria to produce visible colonies. In general, solid media are held for 48 hours, with liquid media held for an additional 24–48 hours. If this is different for specific organisms, it will be mentioned in the text.

A preliminary report is issued when the culture is first examined, and this report is updated as additional information becomes available. Certain results (e.g., positive blood or CSF Gram's stain, isolation of an organism requiring infection control measures) are reported to the health care provider as soon as the information becomes available. Final reports are issued when all work on a culture has been completed.

Medically Important Bacteria

Gram-Positive Cocci

Staphylococcus

Characteristics

Staphylococci are catalase-positive spherical cocci, often appearing in grape-like clusters in stained smears (Fig. 56–2). They grow well on any peptone-containing nutrient medium under aerobic and anaerobic conditions, and may produce hemolysis of various species of animal blood and yellow or orange pigment on certain types of agar. Growth of staphylococci is readily detected on blood agar plates or in various types of nutrient broth. A selective medium for the isolation of *Staphylococcus aureus* is one containing 7.5–10% NaCl with mannitol.

Tests useful for distinguishing staphylococci from micrococci (generally considered nonpathogenic) are listed in Table 56–2 (Kloos, 1999). *S. aureus* is differentiated from other species of staphylococci principally by its production of coagulases, which are capable of clotting plasma. Two antigenically distinct forms of coagulase have been recognized; one bound to the cell wall is called clumping factor and is detected with the slide coagulase test, and the other is free from the cell wall and is detected with the tube coagulase test (often considered the definitive test for the presence of coagulase enzyme). There are commercial latex agglutination products that detect clumping factor and protein A in *S. aureus* with good sensitivity and specificity. These assays may be appropriate in situations where reproducibility of the test is in question due to the inexperience of the technologists performing the assay. There is also a fluorescence in situ hybridization (FISH) product (*S. aureus* PNA FISH from AdvanDx, Woburn, MA) for the differentiation of *S. aureus* from coagulase negative staphylococci in a blood culture bottle found positive for Gram-positive cocci in clusters.

Clinical Manifestations and Pathogenesis

S. aureus may be present among the indigenous flora of the skin, eye, upper respiratory tract, gastrointestinal tract, urethra and, infrequently,

Table 56–1 Guidelines for Media Selection for Various Specimens

Specimen	Media for Recovery of Aerobic and Facultatively Anaerobic Bacteria					Media for Recovery of Anaerobic Bacteria		
	BAP	MAC or EMB	CBA	Broth[†]	Other	BAP[*]	BBE	PEA
Body cavities					Consider the use of BCB for large volumes of fluids			
Fluids								
Cerebrospinal	X		X	X (for shunt specimens)				
Peritoneal	X	X	X		BCB	X	X	X
Pleural; pericardial	X		X	X	BCB	X		
Synovial	X		X	X	BCB			
Wounds								
Aspirate	X	X	X			X	X	X
Swab[‡]	X	X						
Tissue[§]	X	X	X	X		X	X	X
Respiratory tract								
Sputum	X	X	X					
Throat	X							
Bronchiolar lavage	X	X	X		CYE[♯]			
Brush; washings	X	X	X			X[¶]	X[¶]	X[¶]
Nasal	X							
Genitourinary								
Vaginal/rectal for group B			LIM		Selective or chromogenic			
Streptococcus (GBS)					GBS media			
Other	X	X	X		GC media[‖]	X	X	X
Cervix					GC media			
Urethra/penis					GC media			
Urine								
Mid-void	X	X			Screen; chromagar			
Suprapubic aspirate	X	X						
Feces			X	EB	HE or XLD; Campy			
Eye	X	X	X**			X**		
Ear; internal aspirate	X	X				X		
Vascular catheters	X							

Specific guidelines for individual organisms will be included where they are described in text.

[*] Consider a CDC BAP or a *Brucella* blood agar, or other 'enriched' BAP for anaerobic recovery; a laked blood agar plate with antibiotics may also be appropriate.
[†] Supplemented thioglycollate the usual broth; however; for aerobes, a brain–heart infusion may be adequate. [‡] Not recommended for anaerobic cultures. [§] If specific organisms, or situations, other media may be added. [¶] If a protected bronchoscope is used for collection of the specimen. [‖] Thayer–Martin or Martin–Lewis or other media enriched for recovery of *N. gonorrhoeae*. ** If *Propionibacterium acnes* is suspected in cases of endophthalmitis, a thioglycollate broth and/or anaerobic BAP may be used.

BAP = blood agar plate; BCB = blood culture bottles; BBE = *Bacteroides* bile esculin agar; Campy = Campylobacter-selective medium; CBA = chocolate blood agar; CYE = charcoal yeast extract; for *Legionella* or *Nocardia* requests; EB = enrichment broth, such as GN or Selenite Broth; same for rectal swabs, minus the *Campylobacter*-selective culture; EMB = eosin methylene blue; HE = Hektoen enteric agar; LIM = enrichment broth for Group B Streptococcus; MAC = MacConkey agar; PEA = phenylethyl alcohol; XLD = xylose–lysine–deoxycholate agar.

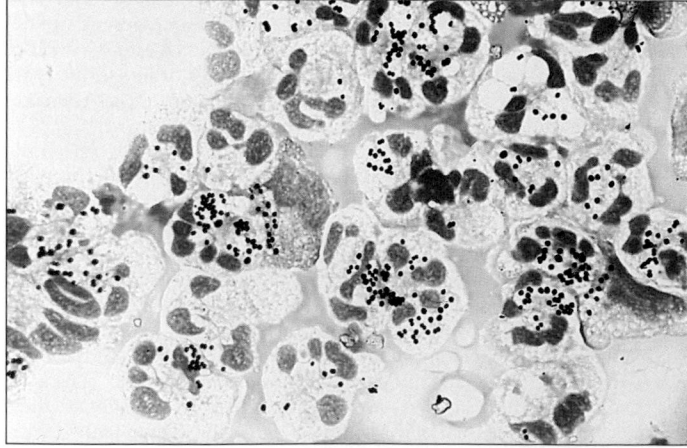

Figure 56–2 Cytocentrifuge preparation of cerebrospinal fluid stained with Gram's stain shows many neutrophils, smooth amorphous material, and Gram-positive cocci in pairs, short chains, and clusters, suggestive of staphylococcal infection (oil immersion).

Table 56–2 Tests Differentiating Staphylococci from Micrococci

	Staphylococci	Micrococci
Lysostaphin susceptibility	S	R
Aerobic acid production from glycerol	+	–
Anaerobic acid production from glucose	+	–
Lysozyme (50 µg disk)	R	S
Bacitracin susceptibility (0.04 U)	R	S
Modified oxidase	–	+

Adapted from: Mahon CR, Manuselis G: Textbook of Diagnostic Microbiology, 2nd ed. London, WB Saunders, 2000, p 332.

vagina. Infection may, therefore, arise from an endogenous or an exogenous source. Factors of importance in the development of infections due to *S. aureus* include breaks in the continuity and integrity of mucosal and cutaneous surfaces, the presence of foreign bodies or implants, prior viral diseases, antecedent antimicrobial therapy, and underlying diseases with defects in cellular or humoral immunity.

Infections caused by *S. aureus* may affect multiple organ systems. Among the most common are those involving the skin and its appendages, such as impetigo, folliculitis, mastitis, and infections of surgical wounds. *S. aureus* is among the leading causes of bacteremia in hospitalized patients, and it may cause endocarditis, particularly in persons with left-sided valvular heart disease and in intravenous drug users. *S. aureus* is the most common cause of spinal epidural abscess and suppurative intracranial phlebitis, and may be recovered from brain abscesses, typically following trauma. Meningitis caused by *S. aureus* is uncommon and generally follows head trauma or a neurosurgical procedure.

S. aureus is responsible for many cases of osteomyelitis, is the most common cause of septic arthritis in prepubertal children, and is occasionally responsible for septic arthritis in adults. In the tropics, it may cause spontaneous deep abscesses of muscles, predominantly affecting malnourished persons who have a concomitant parasitic infection (Chiedozi, 1979). *S. aureus* is an infrequent cause of community-acquired pneumonia but a common cause of nosocomial pneumonia, which usually follows aspiration of endogenous nasopharyngeal organisms. Predisposing factors include infection with measles or influenza A viruses, cystic fibrosis, and immune deficiency. Urinary tract infections caused by *S. aureus* are rare but pyelonephritis, intrarenal and perirenal abscesses can be found.

Several factors play a role in the virulence of *S. aureus*. The capsule, if present, has antiphagocytic properties. Cell-wall peptidoglycans have endotoxin-like activity, stimulating the release of cytokines by macrophages, activation of complement, and aggregation of platelets. Protein A, an immunologically active substance in the cell wall, has antiphagocytic properties that are based on its ability to bind the Fc fragment of immunoglobulin (Ig)G. Other surface proteins designated as microbial-surface components recognizing adhesive matrix molecules (MSCRAMM) may play an important role in the ability of staphylococci to colonize host tissues.

S. aureus produces numerous toxins. The exotoxin TSST-1 is responsible for toxic shock syndrome and enterotoxins A–E are responsible for staphylococcal food poisoning. The exfoliative toxins, epidermolytic toxins A and B, cause skin erythema and separation seen in scalded skin syndrome. Various enzymes are also produced including protease, lipase, and hyaluronidase, all of which destroy tissue and probably function to facilitate the spread of the infection.

Toxin-mediated diseases caused by *S. aureus* include scalded skin syndrome, food poisoning, and toxic shock syndrome. Scalded skin syndrome occurs in infants infected with a strain of *S. aureus* producing exfoliative toxin. The illness begins abruptly with erythema, followed in 2–3 days by the formation of flaccid bullae, which slough, leaving denuded areas that eventually resolve completely. Staphylococcal food poisoning, characterized by nausea, vomiting, abdominal cramps, and diarrhea, occurs 1–6 hours after ingestion of foods contaminated with preformed staphylococcal enterotoxin.

Toxic shock syndrome is a multisystem disease affecting individuals who have no antibodies to TSST-1 and are colonized or infected with strains of *S. aureus* producing TSST-1 or rarely enterotoxin B or C. The illness is most common in women 15–25 years of age who use tampons during menstruation, but also may occur in nonmenstruating individuals, including women in the postpartum period, persons with a surgical wound or other focal infections, and individuals who have had a surgical procedure in the nose or sinuses. Toxic shock syndrome begins abruptly with fever, myalgias, vomiting, and diarrhea followed by hypotension, hypovolemic shock, and an erythematous rash that frequently involves the palms and soles and desquamates in 1–2 weeks. The diagnosis is clinical; isolation of *S. aureus* from any site is not required. Full recovery is the rule, although repeated episodes may occur.

More recently, cases of community-acquired infection with *S. aureus* that are oxacillin-resistant have become more common. In these isolates, a toxin referred to as Panton–Valentine leucocidin toxin (PVL), which has rarely been associated with hospital-acquired strains of *S. aureus* (Vandenesch, 2003), has been found. PVL has been shown to be responsible for necrotizing skin and soft tissue infections and infrequently demonstrated to cause a necrotizing and occasionally fatal pneumonia. (Francis, 2005) The individuals at risk are predominantly children involved in contact sports and individuals who are living in institutions, such as prisons. (MMWR, 2003; Pan, 2003)

Infections caused by coagulase-negative species of *Staphylococcus* usually occur in association with foreign bodies, especially implanted prosthetic valves, joints, and shunts. *S. epidermidis* is the species most frequently involved in such infections. *S. saprophyticus* is an important cause of bacteriuria, particularly in sexually active young women. *S. hemolyticus*, although a relatively rare isolate in clinical specimens, can be resistant to vancomycin, an agent to which most coagulase-negative staphylococci are susceptible.

Laboratory Diagnosis

The observation microscopically of typical rounded, Gram-positive cocci in clusters in smears of material taken from previously unopened or undrained lesions or in smears of broth from a positive blood culture is indicative of staphylococcal infection.

S. aureus produces coagulase, an enzyme that binds plasma fibrinogen, causing the organisms to agglutinate or plasma to clot; almost all other staphylococci do not. Over 95% of isolates of *S. aureus* are identified by the slide coagulase test, which detects cell-bound enzyme (clumping factor); and almost all isolates are identified by the tube coagulase tests, which detects free coagulase.

The slide coagulase test is performed by mixing a dense emulsion of organism with plasma on a glass slide. The test is positive if clumping occurs within 30 seconds. *Staphylococcus lugdunensis* and *Staphylococcus schleiferi* are two other staphylococci that may give a positive result with this test. A control that consists of emulsifying the suspect colony in saline should be run with each slide test to be certain that autoagglutination does not occur. If autoagglutination is present, the slide test results should be considered insufficient for determination of the coagulase nature of the isolate.

For the tube coagulase test, several colonies are transferred into a tube containing plasma that is incubated at 35°C for 4 hours and then examined for clot formation. If no clot has formed, the tube is reincubated at room temperature and re-examined after a total of 20 hours of incubation. The test should be examined after 4 hours because most isolates of *S. aureus* produce a clot within this interval and because some strains produce a fibrinolysin that can lyse the clot and thus produce a false-negative reaction if the test is only observed after 20 hours. *Staphylococcus intermedius* and *Staphylococcus hyicus* will also be positive with the tube coagulase test, but are primarily pathogens of animals and are only rarely encountered in human specimens.

Several commercial latex agglutination assays are available for rapid identification of *S. aureus*. These assays detect protein A and clumping factor, and some also detect capsular polysaccharide, which improves the ability to detect methicillin (oxacillin)-resistant *S. aureus*. *S. saprophyticus* and *Staphylococcus sciuri* are two other staphylococcus species that may be latex-agglutination-positive.

Many species of coagulase-negative staphylococcus have been recognized; however, with the exception of *S. saprophyticus*, which is resistant to novobiocin, identification of these isolates to the species level is not practical or clinically indicated. If necessary, attempts to identify these isolates to the species level may be made using commercially available identification kits, which have been found to have an accuracy of between 70% and more than 90% (Bannerman, 2003). Alternatively, isolates may be sent to a reference laboratory capable of performing standard biochemical assays or molecular assays such as 16S rRNA analysis (Lee, 2001). Staphylococci may be classified into strains for epidemiologic purposes in attempting to identify common sources of infections on the basis of their susceptibility to different bacteriophages, plasmid profiles, cellular fatty acids, electrophoresis of multilocus enzymes, or chromosomal molecular typing (pulsed field gel electrophoresis and repetitive polymerase chain reaction [rep-PCR]). These tests are generally available only through reference laboratories.

Antimicrobial Susceptibility

More than 90% of staphylococci are resistant to penicillin. Because resistance is due to an inducible plasmid-encoded β-lactamase, sensitivity to penicillin should be confirmed after a period of induction (Clinical and Laboratory Standards Institute/NCCLS, 2003a) with a β-lactam agent.

Resistance to the penicillinase-resistant penicillins (methicillin, oxacillin, nafcillin) occurs in up to 80% of coagulase-negative staphylococci and up to 50% of *S. aureus*. Resistance to this group of antimicrobial agents is mediated by the *mecA* gene, which encodes an altered penicillin binding protein, PBP2a. Resistance typically is heterogeneous, meaning that only rare cells (1 in 10^4–10^8) express the resistance trait. Because of this, specific guidelines must be followed to ensure detection: a 1 µg oxacillin disk has been traditionally used for disk diffusion testing. More recently, the CLSI (formerly NCCLS) has suggested that, if disk diffusion is used as the method of detection of oxacillin-resistant *S. aureus* (MRSA), a 30 µg cefoxitin disk test is a better indicator than oxacillin. To predict the presence of *mecA*-mediated resistance in *S. aureus* (and *S. lugdunensis*), CLSI recommends that isolates with zone sizes of >20 mm can be reported as susceptible (S) and those with zone sizes <19 mm be reported as oxacillin resistant (R) (Velasco, 2005). For coagulase-negative staphylococci (except *S. lugdunensis*), >25 mm = S and <24 mm = R (Clinical and Laboratory Standards Institute/NCCLS 2005). Oxacillin in cation-supplemented Mueller–Hinton broth containing 2% NaCl should be used for microdilution testing, and agar plates and microtiter trays should be incubated a full 24 hours at 35°C. To screen isolates of *S. aureus* for oxacillin resistance, Mueller–Hinton agar supplemented with 4% NaCl and containing 6 μg/mL of oxacillin is spot inoculated with a cotton swab, and plates are incubated for 24 hours. Several assays have been developed for rapid detection of oxacillin resistance. These include nucleic acid amplification, nucleic acid probe assays for *mecA*, and latex agglutination assays for PBP2a (the MRSA Screen Test, Denka-Seiken Co., Tokyo, Japan), and the PBP 2′ (Oxoid Ltd., Basingstoke, UK) (Chediac-Tannoury, 2003; Chapin, 2004). For detection of MRSA in nasal swabs, two approaches can be used. There are newer chromogenic media specific for the detection of MRSA that require overnight incubation but allow for easy detection of specific-colored colonies that are MRSA (Perry, 2004). IDI (Infectio Diagnostics, Inc., Canada, recently Gene-Ohm) has a PCR-based assay, run on the Smart Cycler instrument (Cepheid, Sacramento, CA), that can detect MRSA directly in clinical specimens in less than 90 minutes (Warren, 2004). Although oxacillin-resistant staphylococci may appear to be susceptible to cephalosporins, they should be considered resistant to all β-lactam agents (penicillins and cephalosporins), including carbapenems. Hospital-acquired strains usually are resistant to many non-β-lactam antibiotics as well. The newly recognized CA-MRSA strains still remain susceptible to most non-β-lactam antibiotics (Daum, 2002).

Clindamycin may be used to treat staphylococcal infections. An inducible resistance, due to mechanisms involving a class of enzyme-inactivating genes referred to as *erm* genes, may not be detected in routine susceptibility testing. This *erm* gene also confers crossresistance to the macrolides (erythromycin, for example) and streptogramins (quinupristin–dalfopristin). An isolate of *S. aureus* that is resistant to erythromycin but susceptible to clindamycin in a minimum inhibitory concentration (MIC) test (broth or agar dilution or E-test) should be evaluated for inducible resistance to clindamycin by the 'D' test, as follows. A 15 μg erythromycin disk and a 2 μg clindamycin disk are placed 15 mm apart on the surface of a blood agar plate inoculated with the isolate in question. After overnight incubation, if there is inducible resistance to clindamycin, there will be a blunting of the clindamycin zone of inhibition on the side near the erythromycin disk, giving the appearance of a 'D zone' (Clinical and Laboratory Standards Institute/NCCLS, 2005)

Vancomycin resistance, although rarely seen in *S. aureus*, is a serious issue that laboratories need to be aware of and screen for. Isolates of VISA (vancomycin intermediately susceptible *S. aureus*) have MICs in the intermediate range (8–16 μg/mL) (Cosgrove, 2004). There have been three reported cases of vancomycin-resistant *S. aureus* with vancomycin MICs as high as 1024 μg/mL (Centers for Disease Control, 2004b). Because the latter have not been uniformly detected in automated systems for susceptibility testing, the Centers for Disease Control and Prevention (CDC) recommends that all *S. aureus* isolates tested on an automated instrument are also tested by a vancomycin screen assay to insure that the correct MIC is determined. This is usually done by inoculating 100 μl of a 0.5 McFarland suspension of the *S. aureus* to a blood agar plate containing 6 μg/mL of vancomycin and incubating overnight. Screen-positive isolates that have elevated vancomycin MIC values (4 μg/mL) should be sent to a reference lab for confirmation, and confirmed cases should be referred to the CDC.

Streptococcus and Enterococcus

Characteristics

Streptococci are catalase-negative, Gram-positive, spherical, ovoid, or lancet-shaped cocci, often seen in pairs or chains. They are facultatively anaerobic. Some strains require added CO_2 for their initial isolation but may lose this requirement in subcultures. Streptococci can be broadly classified according to the hemolytic reaction on blood agar (Table 56–3). Those strains that completely hemolyze the red cells about their colonies are called β-hemolytic and can be further categorized into the Lancefield groups based on serologically reactive carbohydrates. Important members of this group include *Streptococcus pyogenes* (group A) and *Streptococcus agalactiae* (group B). Figure 56–3 is a Gram stain of *S. pyogenes* (group A Streptococcus) in a specimen from abscess material on the arm of a patient with cellulitis. Those that produce partial hemolysis (cause 'greening' of the agar) are α-hemolytic. An important member of this group is *S. pneumoniae*. Streptococci that do not hemolyze blood are γ-hemolytic. An important member of this group is *Streptococcus bovis*. Some *S. agalactiae* may also be γ-hemolytic. Most of the remainder of the α- and γ-hemolytic streptococci are collectively called 'viridans' streptococci, including *Streptococcus mutans*, *Streptococcus sanguis*, *Streptococcus mitis*, *Streptococcus salivarius*, and *Streptococcus anginosus*. The group of organisms previously referred to as nutritionally variant (pyridoxal-, B_6-, or thiol-dependent, satelliting) streptococci have now been assigned to the genus *Abiotrophia* or *Granulicatella*.

Table 56–3 Classification of Streptococci and Enterococci

Hemolysis	Lancefield Group	Species
β	A	*Streptococcus pyogenes*
	B	*Streptococcus agalactiae*
	C	*Streptococcus dysgalactiae*
	D	*Enterococcus* sp.
α or γ	D	*Enterococcus* sp
	D	*Streptococcus bovis*
	None	Viridans group*
α	None	*Streptococcus pneumoniae*

* Small colony variants of Lancefield group A, C, F, or G, or nongroupable strains, can be any hemolysis

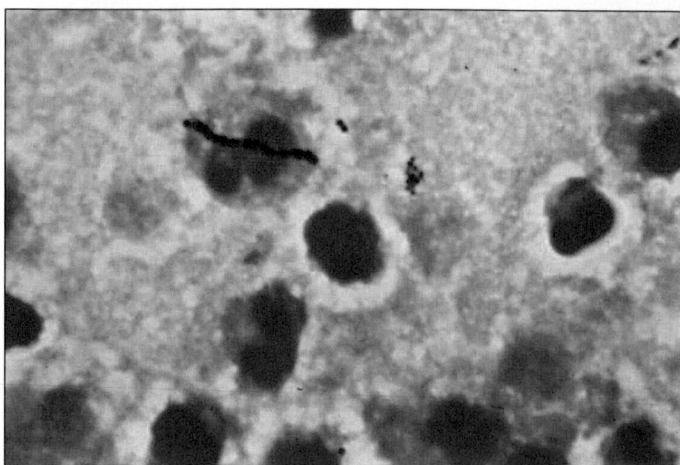

Figure 56–3 Gram stain of *Streptococcus pyogenes* (group A streptococcus) from a case of cellulitis.

Members of the genus *Enterococcus*, previously designated as group D streptococci because their cell-wall antigens reacted with the group D antisera, are sufficiently different from the other members of the genus *Streptococcus* to be considered a separate genus. These organisms are Gram-positive cocci that occur singly, in pairs, and in short chains. They are facultatively anaerobic. Most enterococci are α- or γ-hemolytic on blood agar but some may exhibit β-hemolysis. The most common species are *Enterococcus faecium* and *Enterococcus faecalis*; yellow motile strains of the enterococci, usually non-pathogenic, include *Enterococcus cassilflavus* and *Enterococcus gallinarum*. These latter two species are usually intrinsically vancomycin-resistant, and it is important to differentiate them from vancomycin-resistant *E. faecium* or *E. faecalis*.

Other genera of catalase negative Gram-positive cocci that may be isolated from clinical specimens include *Leuconostoc*, *Pediococcus*, *Stomatococcus*, *Gemella*, *Aerococcus*, and *Lactococcus* spp. These organisms are considered to have low virulence potential and are generally only pathogenic in the compromised host. Some of these isolates may, however, be confused with viridans streptococci, in particular, and their differentiation is important because of their lower virulence and their potential for vancomycin resistance. Further differentiation should be considered if a vancomycin-resistant viridans streptococci is being considered.

Clinical Manifestations and Pathogenesis

One of the most common clinical manifestations of the group A streptococci is pharyngitis. This may be accompanied by scarlet fever, a punctate exanthem overlying diffuse erythema that usually appears first on the neck or upper chest, becomes generalized, and then desquamates. Skin infections caused by group A *Streptococcus* include cellulitis, erysipelas, and pyoderma. Acute rheumatic fever, characterized by carditis, polyarthritis, erythema marginatum, chorea, and subcutaneous nodules, may occur 1–5 weeks after group A streptococcal pharyngitis. Acute glomerulonephritis may develop 10 days to 3 weeks after group A streptococcal pharyngitis or pyoderma.

Beginning in the late 1980s, serious group A streptococcal clinical syndromes including necrotizing fasciitis, myositis, malignant scarlet fever, bacteremia, and toxic shock syndrome began to be seen with increasing frequency. These have been associated with high morbidity rates and mortality rates of up to 30% or more. The reason for this increase is not completely understood but appears to be related to changes in the prevalence of organisms having an enhanced 'virulence potential' (Kaplan, 2005).

S. pyogenes produces numerous virulence factors. One of the most important is the antiphagocytic cell wall M protein. Antibodies against the specific M protein confer lifelong type-specific immunity; however, because over 60 M protein types exist, infection with a group A *Streptococcus* possessing a different M protein may occur. Another important cell-wall component is lipoteichoic acid, which permits bacterial adherence to the respiratory epithelium. *S. pyogenes* also elaborates about 20 extracellular products, including enzymes (streptolysins, hyaluronidase, streptokinase, deoxyribonucleases [DNases], and nicotinamide adenine dinucleotidase [NADase]) and erythrogenic toxins. Streptolysin O, an antigenic, oxygen-labile enzyme, produces subsurface hemolysis on blood agar plates; and streptolysin S, a nonantigenic, oxygen-stable enzyme, produces surface hemolysis. Neither streptolysin has a proven role in the pathogenesis of human disease. Streptokinase promotes fibrinolytic activity by converting plasminogen to plasmin, and hyaluronidase may enhance the spread of the organism through connective tissue. The pathogenic significance of the DNases and of NADase is unknown. Pyrogenic (erythrogenic) toxins (serotypes A, B, C) are produced by isolates of *S. pyogenes* infected with a specific temperate bacteriophage. Their pyrogenicity is caused by a direct action on the hypothalamus. Streptococcus group A has also been found to possess superantigens (SAGs) with high mitogenic capabilities; these have been associated with cases of more severe streptococcal infections, such as necrotizing fasciitis or toxic shock syndrome (Kotb, 2002).

The pathogenesis of acute rheumatic fever is not fully understood. Certain M protein types of *S. pyogenes* may be rheumatogenic. The presence of complexes of immunoglobulin and the C3 component of complement along the sarcolemmal sheaths of cardiac myofibers from individuals with rheumatic carditis suggests that myocardium results from the production of antibodies directed against a streptococcal cell wall M protein that crossreacts with myocardial tissue. Moreover, a heart- or tissue-crossreactive antigen of *S. pyogenes* that shares immunologic epitopes with, but is distinct from, the M protein has been identified (Barnett, 1990). The renal damage in acute glomerulonephritis is caused by deposits of circulating streptococcal–antistreptococcal immune complexes in the glomeruli and the subsequent activation of complement. Cell-mediated reactions to an altered glomerular basement membrane or activation of the alternate complement pathway also may be involved.

The most common infections caused by group B streptococci are neonatal sepsis, pneumonia, and meningitis. Colonization of the maternal genital tract is associated with colonization of infants and risk of neonatal disease, with early-onset infections occurring within the first few days after delivery and late-onset infections appearing after 1 week of age. To reduce the incidence of neonatal disease, the CDC published specific guidelines to allow for early identification and treatment of women colonized with group B *Streptococcus* as well as identification and treatment of neonates at risk for developing disease (Schuchat, 1996; Centers for Disease Control, 2004a). All pregnant women at 35–37 weeks gestation should have vaginal/rectal specimens collected and processed for detection of group B *Streptococcus*. Results of this test should be available during labor so appropriate prophylaxis can be given to the mother before delivery, to prevent infection to the newborn. Group B streptococcal infections in adults include postpartum endometritis, urinary tract infections, bacteremia, skin and soft-tissue infections, pneumonia, endocarditis, meningitis, arthritis, and osteomyelitis.

Group C and G streptococci are similar to *S. pyogenes* in that they cause a wide range of infections, including bacteremia, endocarditis, meningitis, arthritis, and respiratory and skin infections. The pharyngeal infection caused by these streptococci is similar to that of group A streptococci except that the nonsuppurative sequelae of rheumatic fever do not occur.

Infections caused by *S. pneumoniae* are pneumonia, meningitis (especially in infants and the elderly), spontaneous bacteremia (in persons who do not have a spleen), otitis, sinusitis, and spontaneous peritonitis. *S. pneumoniae* is normal flora of the upper respiratory tract of 25–50% of preschool children, 36% of primary-school-age children and nearly 20% of adults, termed carriers (Hendley, 1975; Lopez, 1999). Its spread is enhanced by upper respiratory tract infections and crowding. Pneumonia may develop when the host immune defenses are impaired. Most cases are endogenous, following aspiration of oral secretions containing normal flora that include *S. pneumoniae*. Person-to-person transmission during epidemics occurs by droplet aerosols. The major virulence factor of *S. pneumoniae* is its antiphagocytic polysaccharide capsule, and strains with a thick, mucoid

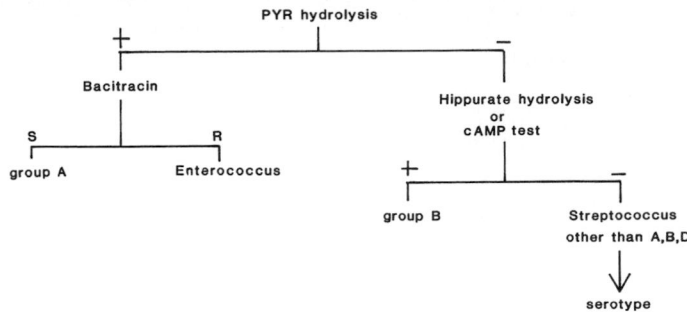

Figure 56–4 Decision tree of tests to presumptively name the β-hemolytic species of *Streptococcus*. (+ = positive result; − = negative result; S = susceptible; R = resistant.) (With permission from Woods GL, Gutierez Y: Diagnostic Pathology of Infectious Diseases. Philadelphia, Lea & Febiger, 1993.)

capsule are especially virulent. Vaccines designed to protect against infection by pneumococci of many of the predominant capsular polysaccharide types are available. A new vaccine is available for use in infants and children to prevent invasive pneumococcal disease.

Bacterial endocarditis is the most common infection caused by viridans streptococci; others include abscesses in the brain or liver, bacteremia, and dental caries. *S. bovis* bacteremia has been associated with malignancies of the gastrointestinal tract. Enterococci are not highly pathogenic; however, they are a common cause of urinary tract infections in hospitalized persons. They may also cause endocarditis, bacteremia, and wound infections. Vancomycin-resistant enterococci offer a greater potential for infection, especially in immunocompromised patients and patients with implanted foreign devices (Shay, 1995; Orloff, 1999).

Laboratory Diagnosis

Streptococci grow well on blood or chocolate agar. Blood agar is preferred because the hemolytic properties of the organism can be assessed. When culturing vaginal/rectal swabs from pregnant women specifically for group B streptococci, specimens should first be inoculated to a selective broth, such as LIM or Carrot broth, or on to selective agar, Granada agar, to enrich for this organism (Schuchat, 1996, Claeys, 2001; Gupta, 2004; Heelan, 2005). Tests that may be used in the clinical microbiology laboratory to presumptively name the β-hemolytic species of *Streptococcus* are shown in Figure 56–4. Over 99% of isolates of group A *Streptococcus* are susceptible to bacitracin, but a very small percentage of isolates of group B *Streptococcus* and 10–20% of isolates of groups C and G *Streptococcus* are also susceptible. Therefore, results of the bacitracin susceptibility test provide a presumptive identification. An isolate may be called group A *Streptococcus* presumptively, based on the hydrolysis of the L-pyrrolidonyl-β-naphthylamide (PYRase) test (Wellstood, 1987). All isolates of group A *Streptococcus* and over 99% of isolates of *Enterococcus* are PYRase-positive. Identification of group A *Streptococcus* is confirmed by serotyping, using latex agglutination, or a nucleic acid probe. A nucleic acid probe (Gen-Probe, San Diego, CA) for the direct detection of Group A *Streptococcus* in throat swabs is also available (Chapin, 2002).

Group A *Streptococcus* may be detected directly in throat swab specimens by using commercial kits designed to generate a rapid result. These tests are highly specific but, given their low sensitivity, varying in different studies from 31–95% (Wegner, 1992; Carroll, 1996), a negative direct test should be followed by culture or probe. Serologic tests to detect antibodies in acute and convalescent serum samples to streptolysin O and DNase B are used primarily to diagnose acute rheumatic fever and acute glomerulonephritis following infection with group A *Streptococcus*.

An isolate that is β-hemolytic and hydrolyzes hippurate or has a positive CAMP test reaction presumptively is called group B *Streptococcus*. Isolates of presumed group B *Streptococcus* from sterile body sites should be identified by serotyping (using latex agglutination or coagglutination tests) or by using a chemiluminescent DNA probe. The DNA probe can also be used to identify group B streptococci growing in LIM or other selective broth cultures. (Daly, 1991; Bourbeau, 1997) Isolates of β-hemolytic groups C, D, F, and G *Streptococcus* are identified by serotyping with latex agglutination reagents. The IDI-Smart Cycler assay mentioned above can be used to detect Group B *Streptococcus* directly in vaginal-rectal specimens or can be used to detect group B *Streptococcus* in culture, such as LIM broth (Picard, 2004).

Latex agglutination assays are available for direct detection of group B *Streptococcus* (as well as *S. pneumoniae*, some serotypes of *Neisseria meningitidis*, *Escherichia coli*, and *H. influenzae* type b) in CSF, serum, and urine. Because these assays have been shown to have sensitivities

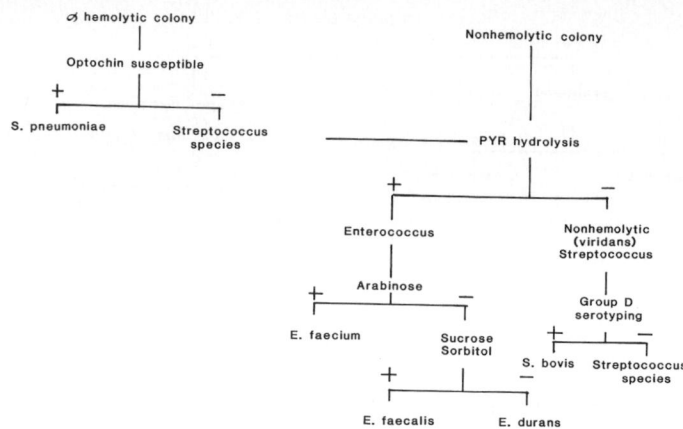

Figure 56–5 Decision tree of tests to presumptively name the α-hemolytic species of *Streptococcus* and *Enterococcus*. (+ = positive result; − = negative result; S = susceptible; R = resistant.) (With permission from Woods GL, Gutierez Y: Diagnostic Pathology of Infectious Diseases. Philadelphia, Lea & Febiger, 1993.)

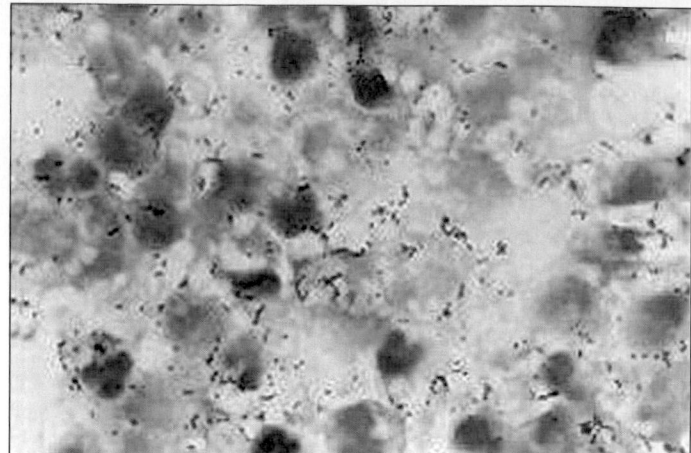

Figure 56–6 Gram stain of a viridans *Streptococcus*, specifically a member of the milleri group, from a brain abscess.

Table 56–4 Characteristics Differentiating Enterococcus, Leuconostoc, Pediococcus and Aerococcus

	Enterococcus	Aerococcus	Leuconostoc	Pediococcus
Gram stain	Pairs and short chains	Tetrads	Cocci, coccobacilli, and rods; pairs and chains	Tetrads and pairs; spherical cells
Hemolysis	β or α or γ	α or γ	α or γ	α or γ
Bile esculin	+	V	V	+
Growth in 6.5% NaCl	+	+	V	V
PYR	+	*	−	−
LAP	+	*	−	+
Vancomycin susceptibility	S/R	S	R	R

LAP = leucine aminopeptidase; PYR = L-pyrrolidonyl-β-naphthylamide; V = variable reactions.

* *Aerococcus urinae* is PYR- and LAP-positive; *Aerococcus viridans* is PYR-positive and LAP-negative.

equivalent to or lower than a Gram stain, may give false-positive results, do not in general provide additional useful information above that provided by the CSF Gram stain, and hence do not add clinical utility, and because the rapid bacterial antigen tests are much more expensive and labor-intensive than the Gram's stain, most laboratories no longer offer these tests or strictly limit their use (Thomas, 1994).

Tests used to presumptively identify α- and γ-hemolytic streptococci and enterococci are shown in Figure 56–5. α-Hemolytic colonies that are mucoid or flattened with a depressed center are suggestive of *S. pneumoniae* and should be tested for susceptibility to ethylhydroxycupreine hydrochloride, more commonly called optochin (P disk) and bile solubility. *S. pneumoniae* is susceptible to both; other α-hemolytic streptococci are resistant to optochin and variable in response to bile. A urinary antigen assay for detection of *S. pneumoniae* can be performed as well (Sopena, 2005).

α-Hemolytic colonies that are not *S. pneumoniae* and γ-hemolytic colonies are tested for PYRase hydrolysis; enterococci are PYRase-positive, viridans streptococci are negative. Moreover, all enterococci grow in the presence of 6.5% NaCl; viridans streptococci do not. Enterococci hydrolyze esculin in the presence of bile (causing visible growth and blackening of the agar), but up to 10% of the viridans streptococci also are bile–esculin-positive. Additional biochemical assays are required to identify enterococci to the species level (Facklam, 1989a). The majority of clinical isolates are *E. faecalis*.

α-Hemolytic streptococci that are optochin-resistant and PYRase-negative and γ-hemolytic streptococci that are PYRase-negative and do not grow in 6.5% NaCl are grouped as nonhemolytic (viridans) streptococci. Identification of the individual species of viridans streptococci requires conventional biochemical testing (Coykendall, 1989). Kit systems to identify these organisms are also commercially available. Full identification of species members of the viridans streptococci is usually not necessary. The members of viridans streptococci belonging to the milleri streptococci, since they are usually recognized by their characteristic 'caramel' odor, can be reported, if present, to alert clinicians about this group of viridans because of their propensity for abscess formation and their uniform susceptibility to penicillin. Figure 56–6 is an example of a Gram stain of a member of the milleri group of viridans streptococci from a brain abscess.

There are no vancomycin-resistant streptococci; however, occasionally a 'viridans'-like isolate is reported as vancomycin-resistant. Usually this is an enterococcus but it could also be a member of some more uncommon genera such as *Leuconostoc* or *Pediococcus*. If vancomycin resistance has been demonstrated, it would be important to differentiate the intrinsically vancomycin-resistant *Leuconostoc* and *Pediococcus* from enterococci that have acquired vancomycin-resistance. The characteristics that might be used to accomplish this are listed in Table 56–4 (reviewed by Facklam, 1989b). Included in this table is differentiation from *Aerococcus* sp. as well, because of their similarity to *Enterococcus* sp.

Members of the genus *Abiotrophia* will not grow in the absence of pyridoxal. Often they are first recognized as satellite colonies growing around a colony of *S. aureus*. Differential characteristics of *Abiotrophia defectiva* and *Abiotrophia adiacens* are reviewed elsewhere (Ruoff, 1990).

Antimicrobial Susceptibility

The antibiograms of groups A, B, C, and G *Streptococcus* are predictable (all are susceptible to penicillin); therefore, routine antimicrobial susceptibility testing of these organisms is unnecessary unless penicillin cannot be used, as in the case of a penicillin allergy. In the latter situations, testing for resistance to macrolides, clindamycin, and the tetracyclines may be warranted. Inducible resistance to clindamycin may occur with *Streptococcus* (i.e., group B *Streptococcus*) and a D zone test as described above for *S. aureus* may be warranted if the streptococcal isolate is found resistant to erythromycin. Specific guidelines for streptococcal D testing have not yet been published. Because *S. pneumoniae* with intermediate or high-level resistance to penicillin (MIC 0.12–1.0 μg/mL or ≥2 μg/mL, respectively) are found worldwide, isolates should be screened for susceptibility to penicillin using disk diffusion with a 1 μg oxacillin disk. Isolates that are not susceptible by this method must be further evaluated by macrodilution or microdilution testing, using Mueller–Hinton broth supplemented with lysed horse blood or the E test to determine the penicillin MIC. Resistance to the third-generation cephalosporins also occurs; therefore, isolates should be tested for susceptibility to these antimicrobial agents as well.

Susceptibility testing should be performed on isolates of nonhemolytic (viridans) streptococci from sterile body sites, because resistance to penicillin does occur. *Enterococcus* spp. should also be tested, primarily to identify high-level resistance to penicillin or ampicillin, high-level resistance to streptomycin and gentamicin, and resistance to vancomycin (Tenover, 1993). Enterococci are resistant to vancomycin (MIC >32 μg/mL) because of the presence of resistance genes, referred to as the *van* genes. Although many of these genes have been described, the most common are *vanA*, *vanB*, and *vanC*. The *vanA* and *vanB* genes, conferring high level resistance and predominantly found in *E. faecium* and *E. faecalis* (although most are *E. faecium*), are acquired, plasmid-borne genes and can create infection control problems involving transmission of this resistance. Differentiation of this vancomycin resistance from that of the intrinsic and lower level

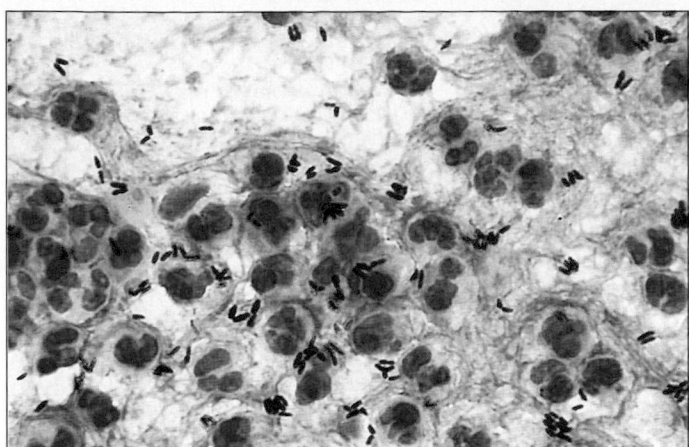

Figure 56–7 Sputum stained with Gram's stain shows many neutrophils, amorphous debris, and coryneform Gram-positive bacilli (oil immersion).

resistance (*vanC* genes) in the yellow, motile species of *Enterococcus* should be done in laboratories and reported as such to the infection control team.

Gemella and Aerococcus spp.

Other non-streptococcal Gram-positive, catalase negative cocci of increasing importance are those that belong to the genera *Gemella* and *Aerococcus*. *Gemella* sp. (*Gemella haemolysans* and *Gemella morbillorum*) resemble viridans streptococci, although they usually produce smaller colonies. *G. haemolysans* has been associated with endocarditis and meningitis. Gram stain usually demonstrates diplococci with adjacent sides flattened that can be confused with a *Neisseria* sp. because cells can easily become decolorized. *G. haemolysans* is aerobic and *G. morbillorum* anaerobic. The latter usually appears as cocci in pairs or short chains. Both are PYR-positive, 6% NaCl and esculin-hydrolysis-negative (to differentiate them from enterococci). *G. morbillorum* is leucine-aminopeptidase (LAP)-positive as well. Both are usually susceptible to penicillin. As with other Gram-positive cocci, if there is doubt about the morphology of the organism, i.e., whether it is a short rod or a coccus, performing the Gram stain from a broth culture will usually resolve the difficulty.

Two major species of *Aerococcus* may be clinically relevant and/or isolated from clinical specimens: *Aerococcus urinae* and *Aerococcus viridans*. Both resemble viridans streptococci or enterococci on agar plates; however, in Gram stains they usually appear in tetrads. *A. urinae* has recently been recognized as a pathogen in urinary tract infections; in addition, it has been isolated from the blood in cases of endocarditis. *A. urinae* is PYR-negative and LAP-positive, in contrast to *A. viridans*, which is PYR-positive and LAP-negative (Table 56–4). Both will grow in the presence of 6.5% NaCl. Neither are anaerobes, and *A. viridans* will usually not grow under anaerobic conditions.. *A. urinae* is usually susceptible to penicillin and nitrofurantoin but may be resistant to sulfonamides. There has been variability in its response to trimethoprim (Ruoff, 2003).

Gram-Positive Rods

Corynebacterium and Arcanobacterium

Characteristics

The corynebacteria, or 'diphtheroids,' as they are sometimes called, appear in the Gram's stained smear as slightly curved, Gram-positive rods with nonparallel sides and sometimes wider ends, giving a clubbed appearance (Fig. 56–7). These organisms are catalase-positive. There are more than 46 species of *Corynebacterium*. Most are rarely pathogenic in humans; notable exceptions are *Corynebacterium diphtheriae* and its closely related species or varieties *Corynebacterium ulcerans* and *Corynebacterium pseudotuberculosis*. The medically relevant *Arcanobacterium* spp. include *Arcanobacterium haemolyticum*, *Arcanobacterium pyogenes*, and *Arcanobacterium bernardiae*. *Arcanobacterium* species also appear as irregular Gram-positive rods in the Gram's stain but can be easily differentiated from the corynebacteria by the negative catalase reaction.

Clinical Manifestations and Pathogenesis

At the initial site of infection on the epithelial cells of the tonsils and oropharynx, *C. diphtheriae* elaborates an exotoxin that causes local cell necrosis and subsequent inflammation. The exotoxin produced by strains

of *C. diphtheriae* infected with a specific bacteriophage, is absorbed into the circulation. Distribution of exotoxin through the bloodstream can produce degenerative changes in the heart, nervous system, and kidneys. The toxin molecule consists of two fragments: A, containing the enzymatically active site, and B, comprising the receptor binding site. Once in the cell, protein synthesis is disrupted. The bacteria and exotoxin produce a serum exudate and cellular infiltrate of the mucous membrane in the pharynx. Exudative lesions coalesce, forming a grayish black adherent pseudo-membrane, which is characteristic of diphtheria. Although toxin production and pathogenicity are often considered to be synonymous, pseudomembranes may form in persons infected with nontoxigenic strains. Extension of the pseudomembrane superiorly into the nasopharynx or inferiorly into the larynx may be so marked as to produce respiratory obstruction. Although *C. diphtheriae* infections of other parts of the body do occur, the most frequent ones observed in the United States today are those of the skin. Transmission of *C. diphtheriae* is by droplet nuclei from the respiratory tract or by contact from cutaneous foci of infection.

Because they are part of the normal flora of the skin and mucous membranes, it is difficult to establish the etiologic role of the other corynebacteria. The clinical significance is generally increased if the organism is observed in the Gram's stained smear in association with leukocytes, is isolated from a sterile site, and is isolated from multiple samples. *Corynebacterium jeikeium* has been clearly associated with infections of implanted prosthetic materials (e.g., heart valves, CSF, and joints), has caused subacute bacterial endocarditis, and has been involved in a variety of opportunistic infections. *Corynebacterium ureolyticum* has been associated with urinary tract infection as well as bacteremia, endocarditis, and wound infections (Nebreda-Mayoral, 1994) When identified, *Corynebacterium striatum* and *Corynebacterium amycolatum* are the most common normal flora skin coryneforms. They may become pathogenic and of note, are often resistant to β-lactam antibiotics, a characteristic usually attributed only to *C. jeikeium*. (Crabtree, 2003)

A. haemolyticum has been associated with pharyngitis and wound and soft tissue infections. (Gaston, 1996) *A. pyogenes* and *A. bernardiae* are associated with abscess formation.

Laboratory Diagnosis

Because of the relative rarity of diphtheria in the United States today, the diagnosis may be overlooked clinically and the laboratory may easily fail to recognize it in cultures. A tentative diagnosis must always be provided to the laboratory so that the specimen can be handled appropriately. Specimens should be obtained with a cotton- or polyester-tipped swab from the inflamed regions of the nasopharynx, and if possible beneath the pseudomembrane. If skin lesions are suspected of being positive for *C. diphtheriae*, the most appropriate specimen would be an aspirate of the lesion. Corynebacteria will grow on routine blood-containing agar; however, cystine-tellurite (CT) blood agar or Tinsdale medium are preferred. On CT medium, colonies of *C. diphtheriae* are gray or black after 48 hours of incubation. Colonies may be large or small and flat or convex. Colonies of species other than *C. diphtheriae* may produce black colonies on CT or Tinsdale media, although these will usually be smaller. If a laboratory does not have CT or Tinsdale medium and a request for *C. diphtheriae* is made, colistin–nalidixic agar (CNA) can be used, although it will be more difficult to recognize possible *C. diphtheriae* strains.

The classification of the oral and skin corynebacteria or diphtheroids is difficult and confusing. The differential characteristics of some species are shown in Table 56–5. Commercial identification systems are available to identify many of the members of this group of organisms (Gavin, 1992; Hudspeth, 1998) Isolates of suspected *C. diphtheriae* must be tested for production of exotoxin. The elaboration of toxin may be detected in vitro with the Elek immunodiffusion test; however, this is generally not done in a routine clinical laboratory. Isolates should be sent to a state health laboratory or a reference lab where this can be performed. Alternatively, PCR-based tests have been described that may be used for detection of the toxin gene (Efstratiou, 2000). *C. jeikeium* often produces a characteristic metallic sheen on the surface of blood agar plates. *C. striatum* and *C. amycolatum* are common skin flora and can be responsible for infections; whether they need to be specifically identified is controversial and can be difficult. These latter strains are often resistant to many antibiotic agents, more typical of *C. jeikeium*.

Arcanobacterium spp. are β-hemolytic on sheep blood agar. Colonies on sheep blood agar are small after 48 hours of incubation and the hemolysis may go unnoticed. Growth and hemolysis is best in a CO$_2$-enhanced environment. *Arcanobacterium* spp. are catalase negative. Biochemical reactions that are used to determine the species of corynebacteria are also useful for the *Arcanobacterium* spp. (Funke, 1997). *A. haemolyticum* produces phospholipase D, which is responsible for the reverse CAMP

Table 56–5 Differential Characteristics of Some Species Within the Genus *Corynebacterium* and Related Organisms

Test	*C. diphtheriae*	*C. ulcerans*	*C. pseudotuberculosis*	*C. jeikeium*	*Arcanobacterium haemolyticum*	*Arcanobacterium pyogenes*
Catalase	+	+	+	+	−	−
Hemolysis	v	+	+		+	+
Gelatinase	−	+	−	−	−	+
Urease	−	+	+	−	−	−
Nitrate reduction	v	−	v	−	−	−
Sucrose fermentation	−	−	v	−	v	v

+ = positive; − = negative; v = variable.

reaction with the *S. aureus*. This organism inhibits the hemolysis around the *S. aureus* streak, producing an inverted triangle of no hemolysis.

Antimicrobial Susceptibility

Although antitoxin remains the only specific method of treatment of diphtheria, antibiotics are administered to patients with disease and to asymptomatic carriers of toxigenic strains. *C. diphtheriae* is usually inhibited by penicillins and the macrolides. The antimicrobial susceptibilities of other species of corynebacteria or diphtheroids are far less predictable. *C. jeikeium* is usually resistant to the penicillins and cephalosporins, variably susceptible to most other antibiotics, and almost uniformly susceptible to vancomycin. Other species of *Corynebacterium* sp., however, may be similarly resistant to β-lactam antibiotics. The therapy of infections caused by these organisms is often complicated by the presence of compromised host defenses and implanted prosthetic materials. Arcanobacteria are sensitive to penicillin and other β-lactams, rifampin, tetracycline, and the macrolides. There may be reduced activity by fluoroquinolones and the aminoglycosides (Funke, 2003).

Prevention

The methods of prevention of diphtheria are almost exclusively active and passive immunization programs with supplemental antibiotics to eliminate the carrier state of toxigenic strains during epidemics.

Listeria

Characteristics

Listeria spp. are nonbranching, non-spore-forming Gram-positive rods. Optimal growth of *Listeria monocytogenes* (Fig. 56–8), the only species of *Listeria* pathogenic for humans, is observed between 30°C and 37°C; however, growth may occur as low as 4°C. Colonies are small after 24 hours and will exhibit a narrow zone of β-hemolysis on blood agar. A characteristic tumbling motility of saline suspensions of the colonies occurs at room temperature but rarely at 35°C. This same temperature-dependent motility is also noted in semisolid media, where growth appears as an umbrella shape in the top of the medium.

Clinical Manifestations and Pathogenesis

L. monocytogenes is found in soil, dust, water, silage, sewage, and raw, unpasteurized milk. Transmission of the organism by foods such as coleslaw, pasteurized milk, and soft cheeses has resulted in several major epidemics in North America and Europe (Fleming, 1985; Linnan, 1988; MacDonald, 2005). According to data from microbiological surveys of food, *L. monocytogenes* has been detected in 2–3% of dairy products, 20% of soft cheeses and processed meats, 30% of certain vegetables (cabbages, radishes), and up to 50% of raw meat and poultry (Broome, 1993). A transient carrier state is found in 2–20% of animals and humans.

Defects in the immune system probably are involved in production of disease because many persons with listeriosis are immunosuppressed. Macrophages and T lymphocytes are the most important host defenses against *L. monocytogenes*. The virulence of *L. monocytogenes* is related to production of listeriolysin O, a 52-kDa protein with hemolytic and cytotoxic properties that is secreted under conditions of low pH and low iron concentration, as would exist in a phagolysosome. The protein is postulated to bind irreversibly to cholesterol in the lysosome membrane, causing its disruption and allowing unrestricted bacterial multiplication within the phagocyte cytoplasm.

Clinical manifestations of listeriosis differ in pregnant women, neonates, and immunocompromised individuals, which are the high-risk groups. Listeriosis during pregnancy, most common in the third trimester, presents as a flu-like illness. Bacteremia occurs concomitantly, during which time the uterine contents are infected. Progression to amnionitis

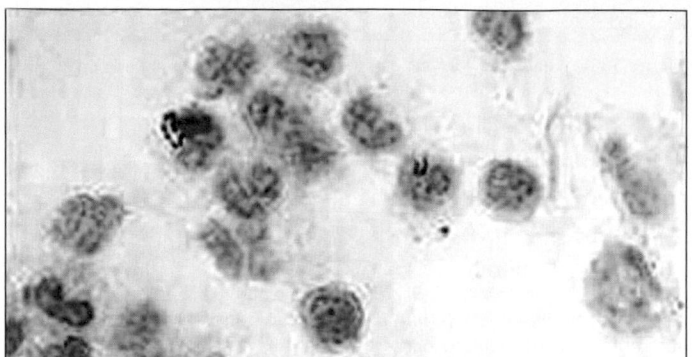

Figure 56–8 Gram stain of a cerebrospinal fluid sample that grew *Listeria monocytogenes*. The short bacilli are seen inside white blood cells.

may induce premature labor or septic abortion in 3–7 days. Infection in the mother is self-limited because the source of the infection is removed with delivery of the infected fetus and uterine contents. Neonatal listeriosis may have an early or late onset. Early-onset disease, manifested at birth or a few days thereafter, results from in utero infection. Infants present with temperature instability, hemodynamic compromise, and respiratory distress; widely disseminated granulomas, particularly involving the placenta, posterior pharynx, and skin, are characteristic of the illness but are not always present. Late-onset disease, affecting full-term infants of mothers with uncomplicated pregnancies, is assumed to be acquired postpartum, but in most cases the source is unknown. Clinical manifestations of meningitis become apparent several days to weeks after birth.

Nonperinatal listeriosis usually occurs in immunosuppressed individuals, but in about one third of the cases no risk factor is identified. Approximately half of these infections are manifested as meningitis; other forms of central nervous system (CNS) listeriosis include cerebritis and brain stem and spinal cord abscesses. Primary bacteremia or focal infections outside the CNS are uncommon. Food-associated disease with *L. monocytogenes* has become more common in recent years and immunocompromised patients, such as those with leukemias, bone marrow transplants and patients on immunosuppressive therapies, are cautioned against eating uncooked dairy meals for fear of infection with this organism.

Laboratory Diagnosis

Colonies are small, grayish blue and surrounded by a narrow zone of β-hemolysis on blood agar. A positive catalase reaction differentiates *L. monocytogenes* from the similarly appearing group B streptococci. Organisms are motile at room temperature and produce acid from glucose, trehalose, and salicin. Other biochemical characteristics of *L. monocytogenes* and differences between *Listeria* and *Erysipelothrix* are listed in Table 56–6.

Antimicrobial Susceptibility

L. monocytogenes is usually sensitive to penicillin, ampicillin, erythromycin, chloramphenicol, tetracycline, and gentamicin. Cephalosporins should not be tested against *Listeria* sp., since they are ineffective in vivo regardless of the in vitro result. Resistance to chloramphenicol, macrolides, and tetracyclines has been found in several clinical isolates (Bille, 2003). Ampicillin, alone or in combination with an aminoglycoside, has been used successfully in the treatment of infections caused by *L. monocytogenes*. Trimethoprim–sulfamethoxazole may be used as alternative therapy in penicillin-allergic patients.

Table 56–6 Differential Characteristics of *Listeria monocytogenes* and *Erysipelothrix rhusiopathiae*

Test	L. monocytogenes	E. rhusiopathiae
β-Hemolysis	+	–
Growth at 4°C	+	–
Catalase	+	–
Motility	+	–
Esculin hydrolysis	+	–
Gluconate utilization	+	–
Voges-Proskauer	+	–
H₂S in triple sugar iron agar	–	+

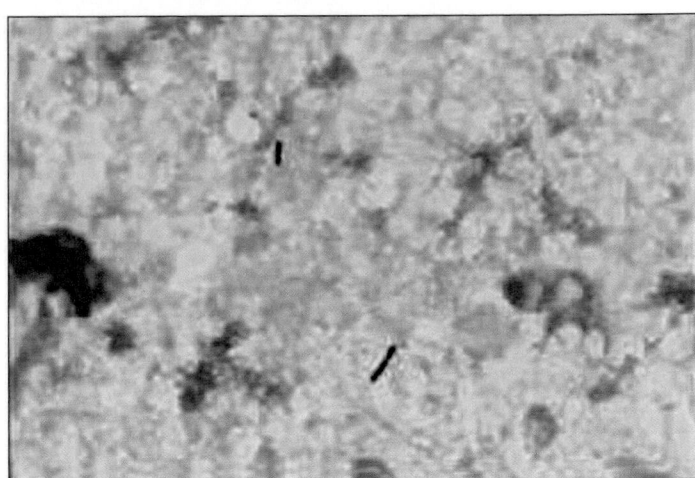

Figure 56–9 Gram stain of *Bacillus cereus* in pleural fluid.

Erysipelothrix

Characteristics

Erysipelothrix rhusiopathiae is a catalase-negative, non-spore-forming, nonmotile, facultatively anaerobic Gram-positive bacillus that has a worldwide distribution. Cells from smooth-phase colonies are small, straight, or slightly curved rods, while those from rough colonies are long and filamentous.

Clinical Manifestations and Pathogenesis

E. rhusiopathiae is usually transmitted to humans from animals by means of skin wounds produced with contaminated objects or in contact with blood, flesh, viscera, or feces of infected animals. *E. rhusiopathiae* is widespread in nature in wild and domestic animals, birds, fish, and decaying organic matter and causes infection in swine, sheep, rabbits, cattle, birds, and fowl. At risk of infection with this organism are butchers, abattoir workers, fishermen, fish handlers, poultry processors, and veterinarians. The most common form of erysipeloid is a local cutaneous infection manifested by pain, swelling, and a cutaneous eruption characterized by a slowly progressive, slightly elevated, violaceous zone around the site of inoculation. The swelling and erythema migrate peripherally and the lesion involutes without desquamation. Systemic disease is rare, but there are numerous case reports of septicemia and endocarditis. Also rarely reported have been cases of arthritis and brain abscess.

Laboratory Diagnosis

Biopsy or tissue aspirates from erysipeloid lesions are the best specimens for culture. The organisms are located deep in the subcutaneous layer of the leading edge of the lesion; therefore, swabs of the surface of the skin are not useful. The organism will grow on blood or chocolate blood agar, but may require up to 7 days for growth. Conventional blood culture media are suitable for its isolation from blood.

E. rhusiopathiae is oxidase- and catalase-negative. Characteristically, it produces H₂S in triple sugar iron agar (TSIA). It is nonmotile, does not reduce nitrates to nitrites, and ferments glucose and lactose. A trait highly characteristic of *E. rhusiopathiae* is the 'pipe cleaner' pattern of growth in gelatin stab cultures that are incubated at 22°C. This organism can be readily distinguished from *Listeria* spp. (see Table 56–6).

Antimicrobial Susceptibility

Erysipelothrix is susceptible to the penicillins, cephalosporins, imipenem, erythromycin, clindamycin, chloramphenicol, tetracyclines, and fluoroquinolones, but is resistant to sulfonamides, aminoglycosides, and vancomycin.

Bacillus

Characteristics

The members of this genus are strictly aerobic or facultatively anaerobic, rod-shaped, spore-forming, Gram-positive, and catalase-positive. Figure 56–9 is a Gram stain of *Bacillus* sp. seen in pleural fluid. With the notable exception of *Bacillus anthracis*, they are usually motile by means of lateral or peritrichous flagella. Some strains will stain Gram-negatively and, because of their variable oxidase reactions, are confused with Gram-negative bacilli. The most reliable diagnostic characteristic of the genus is spore formation, which occurs optimally and on a variety of media under aerobic conditions at 25–30°C. In Gram-stained smears, endospores are detectable by the presence of unstained defects or holes within the cell. The spores themselves can be stained by any one of several methods.

Clinical Manifestations and Pathogenesis

Of the numerous species of *Bacillus*, *B. anthracis* is the only one that is uniformly and highly pathogenic. Great care must be exercised when handling material suspected of harboring this species. Work should be performed in biological safety cabinets by gloved, gowned, masked, and immunized personnel; work surfaces must be disinfected with 5% hypochlorite or 5% phenol; and all supplies, materials, and equipment must be decontaminated. Because *B. anthracis* spores have been used as a means of bioterrorism, cultures containing suspect *B. anthracis* should be handled only by reference or public health laboratories.

Three forms of anthrax are recognized: cutaneous, inhalation, and intestinal. In its cutaneous form, anthrax produces a small, red, macular lesion that progresses to a vesicle and finally necrosis with formation of a characteristic black eschar. Regional lymphadenopathy and septicemia may occur. The mortality in untreated cases with this form of disease is approximately 20%. Inhalation of anthrax spores can lead to acute bronchopneumonia, mediastinitis, and septicemia ('woolsorter's disease'). The mortality in recognized cases of this form of disease is nearly 100%. Intestinal anthrax follows the ingestion of contaminated food and is manifested by nausea, vomiting, and diarrhea. In some cases there is gastrointestinal bleeding, followed by prostration, shock, and death. Septicemia can occur in all three forms of anthrax and may lead to a fatal, purulent meningitis.

A major factor in the organism's pathogenic capabilities is its glutamyl polypeptide capsule, which inhibits phagocytosis; anticapsular antibodies do not protect against the disease. A complex toxin with three components (edema factor, protective antigen, and lethal factor) is responsible for the signs and symptoms of anthrax.

Humans become infected with anthrax by contact with and inhalation or ingestion of infected animals, their carcasses, or their byproducts. Cattle, sheep, horses, and goats are the animals most frequently infected and provide a ready source of vegetative organisms that sporulate and perpetuate the environmental contamination.

Although usually saprophytic, other species of *Bacillus* can cause disease. *Bacillus cereus* has been associated with ear infection, pneumonia, post-traumatic ocular wound infection, septicemia, and endocarditis. Patients with pneumonia and septicemia are often immunosuppressed. Bacteremia is frequently associated with intravenous drug use and with contaminated intravascular devices.

Two forms of gastroenteritis are associated with *Bacillus* species. Food poisoning caused by *Bacillus* may occur within 1–6 hours following the ingestion of food that has been contaminated with *B. cereus* that has produced a preformed heat-stable toxin. The major manifestations of *Bacillus* food poisoning are nausea, vomiting, cramps, and occasionally diarrhea. Typically, this form of *Bacillus* gastroenteritis results from the bulk preparation of foods that are not reheated prior to being served. *B. cereus* type 1 grows particularly well in fried rice and is more heat-resistant than other types, so this form of gastroenteritis is frequently seen in association with consumption of cooked rice in Chinese restaurants. The second form of gastroenteritis caused by *Bacillus* spp. results from the contamination of meat and vegetable dishes and is characterized by the onset of cramps and diarrhea 8–16 hours following ingestion of the contaminated food. In this instance, the major manifestations of *B. cereus* infection are caused by the production of a heat-labile enterotoxin.

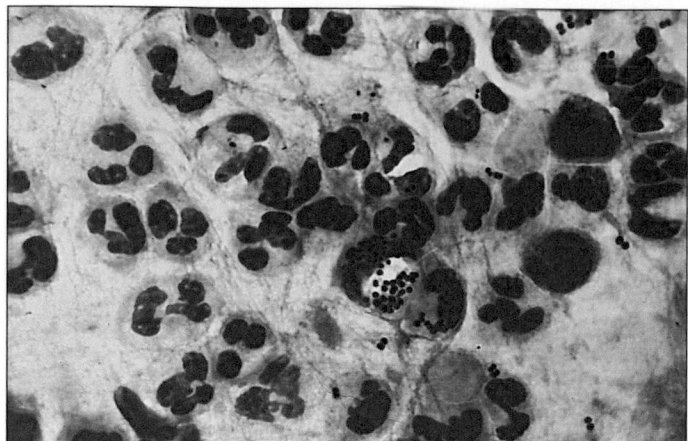

Figure 56–12 Sputum smear stained with Gram's stain shows many neutrophils and intracellular Gram-negative diplococci, suggestive of *Neisseria meningitidis* infection (oil immersion).

membranous white, yellow, pink, or red colonies. Colonies of *Streptomyces* are dry to chalky, heaped or folded, gray-white to yellow, and have the odor of a musty basement. A wide variety of pigments are produced that color the substrate and hyphae. Some species do not produce aerial hyphae. As with the *Nocardia* spp., complete identification of these members of the aerobic actinomycetes often requires molecular sequencing methods (Garter, 2004).

Gram-Negative Bacteria – Cocci

Neisseria

Characteristics

These genera are nonmotile, catalase- and oxidase-positive, aerobic, Gram-negative cocci that are often arranged in pairs with flattened adjacent surfaces, giving the appearance of kidney or coffee beans (Fig. 56–12). These organisms are somewhat fastidious, in some instances requiring the addition of blood, serum, cholesterol, or oleic acid to the medium to counteract growth inhibitors, such as fatty acids. *N. gonorrhoeae* and *N. meningitidis* generally require prompt incubation in CO_2 for growth; however, this is strain-dependent, varies with the phase of the organism's growth curve, and is often lost in subcultures. *N. meningitidis* and most *N. gonorrhoeae* are not inhibited by the presence of vancomycin or lincomycin, colistin, and nystatin, a characteristic that is particularly useful in their selective isolation from specimens contaminated with other bacteria. Rarely, isolates of *N. gonorrhoeae* (especially AUH strains, which require arginine, uracil, and hypoxanthine) are susceptible to vancomycin.

Clinical Manifestations and Pathogenesis

Although opportunistic infections caused by species of *Neisseria* other than *N. gonorrhoeae* and *N. meningitidis* have occasionally been reported in compromised hosts, these species are generally nonpathogenic. *N. meningitidis* may colonize the mucous membranes of the upper respiratory tract, an event that is usually followed in 7–10 days by the formation of bactericidal and hemagglutinating antibodies, which may not eliminate the carrier stage but conveys group-specific immunity. In a few cases, disease results shortly after colonization, most frequently in the form of meningococcemia and meningitis. The organism also has a tendency to invade serous membranes and joint tissues, with the development of pleuritis, pericarditis, and arthritis. Carriage of *N. meningitidis* in the nasopharynx occurs in 5–15% of healthy individuals, and may be higher in confined groups such as military recruits. A direct correlation between carrier rates and incidence of disease has not been established, with the possible exception of members of large households or households with an infant or childhood case during epidemics of disease. *N. meningitidis* has also been isolated from genital sources, where its clinical significance is uncertain. When cultured from these sources, bacteria may be misidentified as *N. gonorrhoeae* unless appropriate tests for distinguishing these species are performed.

The principal virulence factor of *N. meningitidis* is a lipopolysaccharide–endotoxin complex, which in experimental animals activates the clotting cascade, depositing fibrin in small vessels, producing hemorrhage in the adrenals and other organs, altering peripheral vascular resistance, and leading to shock and death.

The pathogenesis and clinical manifestations of *N. gonorrhoeae* infections differ somewhat from those of *N. meningitidis*. Pathogenic types (1 and 2) of *N. gonorrhoeae* adhere by means of pili, which are not produced by nonpathogenic types (3 and 4), to various human cells. These antigenically heterogeneous pili, which represent one of the principal virulence factors of *N. gonorrhoeae*, may inhibit phagocytosis and stimulate strain-specific antibody formation. Other possible virulence factors of *N. gonorrhoeae* are less clearly defined. Both *N. gonorrhoeae* and *N. meningitidis* produce an IgA protease, which may also be important in their pathogenesis, because IgA is the antibody class that predominates in secretions on mucous membranes.

Laboratory Diagnosis

The single most important element in the laboratory diagnosis of infections caused by *N. meningitidis* and *N. gonorrhoeae* is the specimen, including proper selection, collection, and transport to the laboratory (see Ch. 63). The pathogenic species are sensitive to drying and extremes of temperature, and material must be cultured promptly to enhance recovery. They are mesophilic and grow poorly, if at all, at room temperature. Many require prompt incubation in CO_2 (2–8%) for primary isolation. Media containing chocolatized blood are commonly used for cultures and should contain antibiotics (i.e., vancomycin or lincomycin, as well as colistin, nystatin or anisomycin, and trimethoprim) if the specimen is contaminated with indigenous flora. Vancomycin-susceptible gonococci will grow on media containing lincomycin; however, because of the synergistic interaction of lincomycin and trimethoprim, the latter must be omitted from media containing lincomycin. Direct inoculation of specimens 'at the bedside' followed by prompt incubation at 35°C in CO_2 is optimal. This can be accomplished in several ways: placing the medium into a candle jar; placing the medium in a sealed bag containing a citric acid bicarbonate tablet; or using a medium contained within a bottle having a CO_2 atmosphere. If any of these culture systems must be mailed to a reference laboratory for processing, they must first be incubated overnight to ensure growth of the organisms.

An isolate from a urogenital specimen showing the appropriate colony appearance on a selective medium presumptively may be called *N. gonorrhoeae* based on results of the Gram's stain and oxidase and catalase tests. Gram-stained smears prepared from colonies of *N. gonorrhoeae* should show typical Gram-negative diplococci, but organisms may occur in tetrads, especially from young cultures. All species of *Neisseria* are oxidase positive, and all species except *N. elongata* are catalase positive. Because *Neisseria* other than *N. gonorrhoeae* may be recovered from urogenital sites, confirmatory testing is strongly recommended and is required for all isolates from extragenital sites and when sexual abuse is suspected (preferably by more than one method).

Confirmation of *N. gonorrhoeae* and identification of the other *Neisseria* spp. are based on growth and biochemical characteristics (Table 56–8) (Knapp, 1988). The standard method of identification is detection of acid production from carbohydrates in a cystine trypticase acid (CTA) base medium and other conventional biochemical tests. However, given the drawbacks of the conventional methods, more rapid identification tests are used in most clinical laboratories. Tests for direct detection of *N. gonorrhoeae* and *N. meningitidis* in clinical specimens are also available. Typing of isolates of *N. gonorrhoeae* and *N. meningitidis* is done primarily for epidemiologic studies.

With the standard method of identification, acid production from glucose, maltose, lactose, sucrose, and fructose in a CTA base medium and a carbohydrate-free control are tested. Tubes are inoculated, incubated at 35–37°C in ambient air, and examined at 24-hour intervals until reactions are interpretable or for 72 hours. Expected results for the species of *Neisseria* are shown in Table 56–8. Occasionally, however, an isolate of *N. meningitidis* yields aberrant carbohydrate reactions: glucose-negative, maltose-negative, or asaccharolytic. If *N. meningitidis* is strongly suspected in these cases, the identification can be confirmed by slide agglutination, using pooled polyvalent grouping antisera or sera specific for individual serogroups. In addition to conventional carbohydrate degradation tests, reduction of nitrates and nitrites, and DNase production should be evaluated. The latter is especially useful for identification of *Moraxella catarrhalis*, which is DNase positive (*Neisseria* spp. are DNase negative). Drawbacks to conventional tests are the requirement for a heavy inoculum, the need to work with pure cultures, long turnaround time, and failure of some fastidious strains of *N. gonorrhoeae* to grow.

Several commercial systems detect acid production from carbohydrates, usually in 1–4 hours (Knapp, 1988). The inoculum must be prepared from a pure culture of the isolate, so identification is generally available 24 hours after isolation. Acid reactions of some of *N. gonorrhoeae* and, to a lesser extent, *N. meningitidis* may be difficult to interpret or are aberrant

Table 56–8 Differentiation of Species of *Neisseria* and *Moraxella catarrhalis*

	N. gonorrhoeae	*N. meningitidis*	*N. cinerea*	*N. lactamica*	*N. sicca*	*N. subflava*	*N. flavescens*	*N. mucosa*	*M. catarrhalis*
Growth									
Thayer–Martin medium	+*	+	–	+	–	–	+	–	†
Nutrient agar, 25°C	–	–	–	–	+	+	–	+	+
Oxidase	+	+	+	+	+	+	+	+	+
β-Galactosidase	–	–	–	+	–	–	–	–	–
Reduction of nitrate	–	–	–	–	–	–	–	+	+
DNase	–	–	–	–	–	–	–	–	+
Production of acid from									
Glucose	+	+	–‡	+	+	+	–	+	–
Maltose	–	+	–	+	+	+	–	+	–
Lactose	–	–	–	+	–	–	–	–	–
Sucrose	–	–	–	–	+	D§	–	+	–
Fructose	–	–	–	–	+	–	–	–	–

* Most vancomycin-susceptible strains will not grow on Thayer–Martin medium. † Some strains positive and others negative. ‡ Weak reaction may occur in rapid carbohydrate utilization tests. § Biovar. *perflava*, +; biovar. *flava*, –.

+ = ≥90% of strains positive; – = ≥90% of strains negative; D = variable.

with some kits, and strains of *N. gonorrhoeae* that are weak producers of acid from glucose may appear to be glucose-negative. Some strains of *Neisseria cinerea*, which does not produce acid from glucose, can appear glucose-positive in certain systems.

Enzyme substrate tests provide rapid identification (1–4 hours) only of isolates of oxidase-positive, Gram-negative diplococci recovered on a selective medium (Kellogg, 1995; Knapp, 1988). They are valuable for differentiating maltose-negative strains of *N. meningitidis* from *N. gonorrhoeae*, but color changes may be subtle and if misinterpreted could cause isolates of *N. meningitidis* and other *Neisseria* spp. to be incorrectly called *N. gonorrhoeae*. Moreover, strains of *N. cinerea* and *Kingella denitrificans* that grow on gonococcus-selective media could be misidentified as *N. gonorrhoeae* if not confirmed with other procedures. Commercial products that combine enzyme substrate tests with modified conventional tests provide accurate identification of species of *Neisseria* and *Haemophilus* (Janda, 1987, 2002).

Immunologic tests for *N. gonorrhoeae*, in particular coagglutination can be used to confirm the biochemical identification of *N. gonorrhoeae*. Three tests are available for this, the Phadebact Monoclonal GC Test (Boule Diagnostics AB, Huddinge, Sweden) the GonoGen I (New Horizons Diagnostics, Columbia, MD) and the GonoGen II (New Horizons Diagnostics). There have been both false positive and false negative results reported with these reagents. (Dillon, 1988; Kellogg, 1995, Janda, 1993). A chemiluminescent nucleic acid probe for detection of *N. gonorrhoeae* can be used for culture confirmation or direct detection of the organism in endocervical or urethral swab specimens (Limberger, 1992; Hale, 1993; Janda, 1993). Nucleic acid amplification assays for use on endocervical or urethral swab specimens and urine are also available and may increase sensitivity when compared to the nucleic acid probe and culture techniques, largely because the problem with organism viability is not an issue. (Carroll, 1998; Kehl, 1998).

Latex agglutination assays are available for direct detection of *N. meningitidis* antigens in CSF, serum, and urine. As discussed previously (see *Streptococcus*), the sensitivity of these assays has been found to be less than or equal to that of the Gram stain and the results of such testing appear to have little impact on patient care (Granoff, 1986; Maxson, 1994; Perkins, 1995; Bhisitkul, 1994); therefore, many laboratories have stopped offering this test.

Antimicrobial Susceptibility

Despite the occasional recovery of *N. meningitidis* strains with a decreased susceptibility to penicillin, penicillin G remains the drug of choice for treatment of meningococcal meningitis (Janda, 2003). Decreased susceptibility of *N. meningitidis* to penicillin is thought to be due to decreased binding of penicillin by altered meningococcal cell-wall penicillin-binding proteins, PBP2 and PBP3. Other species of *Neisseria* have also demonstrated this lowered affinity to penicillin (Saez-Nieto, 1992; Janda, 2003). Other agents that have good activity against *N. meningitides* include the extended-spectrum cephalosporins and chloramphenicol. Rifampin, minocycline, and the fluoroquinolones may be used for

prophylaxis among household contacts. Currently, there are no standardized methods of susceptibility testing or breakpoints in the CLSI documents; however, these will very probably be included in newer supplements in coming years. The CLSI does recommend that either a broth microdilution or an agar dilution MIC test with cation supplemented Mueller–Hinton Broth (with 2–5% laked horse blood) or Mueller–Hinton Agar (with 5% [vol/vol] sheep blood) be used if testing is done. Enrichments such as IsoVitaleX (1%) may also be needed. In laboratories where susceptibility testing of *N. meningitidis* is not available, β-lactamase testing can be performed by using the chromogenic cephalosporin test, the cefinase nitrocefin disk test if there is a suspicion of lowered susceptibilities or clinical failure on penicillin. If positive, isolates can then be shipped to a reference laboratory for further testing.

Because there is widespread resistance of *N. gonorrhoeae* to penicillin and tetracycline (Fox, 1997), the current recommendations for treatment include the extended-spectrum cephalosporins or the newer fluoroquinolones. Although there does not appear to be any resistance to the cephalosporins, resistance to the fluoroquinolones has been documented. Therefore, susceptibility testing should be performed if symptoms persist after treatment. β-Lactamase production can be detected using a chromogenic cephalosporin. Disk diffusion using GC agar with 1% growth supplement is recommended to determine the susceptibility of *N. gonorrhoeae* to the cephalosporins, quinolones, and spectinomycin. The CLSI document recommends the agar dilution method or a disk diffusion method for testing of *N. gonorrhoeae* (Clinical and Laboratory Standards Institute/NCCLS 2003b). In addition, an E-test can be performed. For some agents, only a susceptible breakpoint is available since there have been no documented resistant strains as yet. If one identifies a 'nonsusceptible' result with a third-generation cephalosporin, for example, confirmation tests and referral to a reference lab should be strongly considered (Clinical and Laboratory Standards Institute/NCCLS, 2005).

Prevention

A polysaccharide vaccine against *N. meningitidis* serogroups A, C, Y, and W135 is licensed in the United States and is recommended for military personnel, for persons living in epidemic areas of developing countries, for individuals with a nonfunctional or absent spleen and for college students. Antibiotic prophylaxis should be limited to household contacts and those who have had contact with patients' oral secretions. Rifampin is currently the drug of choice.

The use of pre-exposure antibiotics to prevent gonococcal diseases is discouraged because of the potential risks of sensitization and the emergence of resistant strains. The sole exception to this rule is the application of silver nitrate solution or erythromycin ointment to the eyes of newborns to prevent gonococcal (and chlamydial) ophthalmia.

Moraxella catarrhalis

M. catarrhalis may be carried in the oropharynx of healthy children and adults. It is an encapsulated organism, and extending from its outer membrane are pili that serve as adhesins. The most common infections it

VII

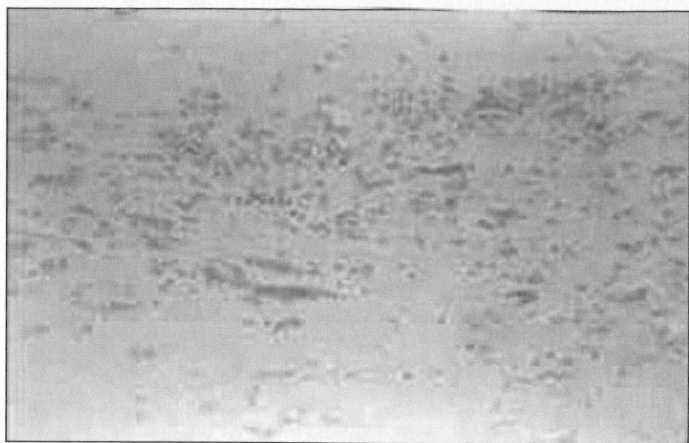

Figure 56–13 Gram stain of *Moraxella catarrhalis* in a sputum specimen. Note the intracellular Gram-negative diplococci that resemble *Neisseria* sp.

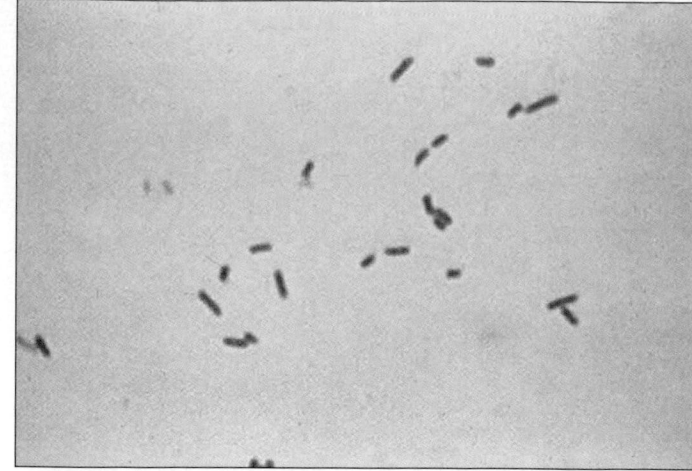

Figure 56–14 Gram stain of a urine positive for *E. coli*. The short, plump Gram-negative rods are typical of any member of the Enterobacteriaceae

causes are bronchitis, otitis, sinusitis, and pneumonia (especially in persons with underlying chronic lung disease) (Catlin, 1990). *M. catarrhalis* is an infrequent cause of bacteremia, endocarditis, meningitis, urogenital infections, and ophthalmia neonatorum. Figure 56–13 is the Gram stain of a sputum in which *M. catarrhalis* is seen in large quantities inside and outside of polymorphonuclear leukocytes. *Moraxella catarrhalis* used to be contained in the *Neisseria* genera and was then transferred to the *Branhamella* genus for a short period of time. *M. catarrhalis* is a coccus and morphologically resembles *Neisseria* sp., unlike other members of the genus *Moraxella* (for example, *Moraxella lacunata*, *Moraxella osloensis* and *Moraxella atlantae*), which appear as rods. *M. catarrhalis* bacteria are oxidase- and catalase-positive, but can be differentiated from *Neisseria* sp. in their ability to grow readily on blood and chocolate agar, their lack of oxidative metabolism (sugars will be negative), and their production of DNase. Nearly all isolates of *M. catarrhalis* produce β-lactamase, which can be detected using nitrocefin. Although they should be assumed to be resistant to penicillin because of this, these isolates generally remain susceptible to cephalosporins, trimethoprim–sulfamethoxazole, and β-lactamase inhibitor combinations.

Gram-Negative Bacteria – Bacilli

The Gram-negative bacilli are a complex group. They are broken down into the following: Enterobacteriaceae, those that are found normally in the gastrointestinal tract or colonize and cause infections there primarily; nonfermentative Gram-negative bacilli, which are not usually found as part of the normal flora of humans but rather are environmental bacteria; non-Enterobacteriaceae that can cause gastrointestinal infections, such as *Vibrio* and *Campylobacter*; agents of infections with specific epidemiological characteristics, such as *Legionella* and *Francisella*; other Gram-negative bacilli, including *Haemophilus* spp., and miscellaneous genera.

Enterobacteriaceae

Characteristics

The Enterobacteriaceae are aerobic and facultatively anaerobic, non-spore-forming, non-motile or peritrichously flagellated, oxidase-negative, Gram-negative bacilli that produce acid fermentatively from glucose and reduce nitrates to nitrites. Figure 56–14 is a Gram stain of *E. coli* but could represent any member of the Enterobacteriaceae. The genera included in this group are: *Budvicia*, *Buttiauxella*, *Cedecea*, *Citrobacter*, *Edwardsiella*, *Enterobacter*, *Escherichia*, *Ewingella*, *Hafnia*, *Klebsiella*, *Kluyvera*, *Leclercia*, *Leminorella*, *Moellerella*, *Morganella*, *Obesumbacterium*, *Pragia*, *Pantoea*, *Photorhabdus*, *Proteus*, *Providencia*, *Rahnella*, *Salmonella*, *Serratia*, *Shigella*, *Tatumella*, *Trabulsiella*, *Xenorhabdus*, *Yersinia*, and *Yokenella*. Only a few of these will be discussed here.

Clinical Manifestations and Pathogenesis

Enterobacteriaceae are found on plants, in soil, in water, and in the intestines of humans and animals. They have been associated with many clinical infections, including abscesses, pneumonia, meningitis, septicemia, and urinary tract infections. Those commonly associated with human infection include *E. coli*, *Klebsiella* spp., *Proteus* spp., *Enterobacter* spp., *Salmonella* spp., *Shigella* spp., *Serratia* spp., *Citrobacter* spp., and *Providencia* spp. Figure 56–15 is a Gram stain of CSF from a newborn child that was culture positive for *E. coli*. In the urinary tract, those frequently isolated are

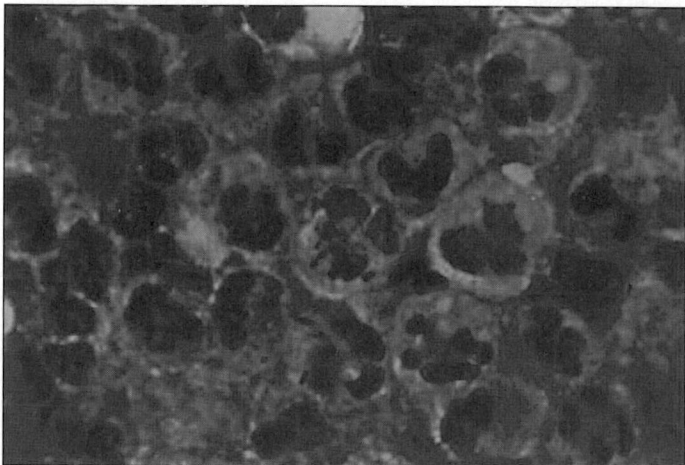

Figure 56–15 Gram stain of a cerebrospinal fluid specimen from a neonate containing Gram-negative bacilli that grew *Escherichia coli*.

E. coli, *Proteus mirabilis*, and *Klebsiella pneumoniae*. Gram-negative pneumonias associated with the Enterobacteriaceae are frequently caused by *K. pneumoniae*. Gram-negative bacteremias related to the Enterobacteriaceae are frequently caused by *E. coli*, *K. pneumoniae*, and *P. mirabilis*. Infections acquired in the hospital are likely to be caused by members of the antibiotic-resistant genera, such as *Citrobacter*, *Enterobacter*, and *Serratia*. Enterobacteriaceae associated with diarrhea include *Shigella* spp., *Salmonella* spp., *E. coli* (enterohemorrhagic (Shiga-toxin-producing), enterotoxigenic, enteroinvasive, enteropathogenic, enteroadherent), and *Yersinia* spp. Shigellas are rarely isolated from sources other than the gastrointestinal tract, while salmonellas are more frequently isolated from other sources, such as urine or blood.

Endotoxins that are present within the cell walls of the Enterobacteriaceae, as well as other Gram-negative bacilli, are responsible for much of the morbidity and mortality resulting from infections associated with these bacteria. Endotoxins consist of lipid and polysaccharide moieties with small amounts of amino acids, and are often referred to as lipopolysaccharides. Lipopolysaccharides may elicit fever, chills, hypotension, granulocytosis, thrombocytopenia, disseminated intravascular coagulation, and activation of both the classic and alternate complement pathways. Endotoxic shock is the result of Gram-negative septicemia with endotoxin reacting with macrophages, leukocytes, platelets, complement, and other serum proteins to increase the blood levels of proteolytic enzymes and vasoactive substances, and resulting in pooling of blood, increased peripheral vasoconstriction, and diminution in cardiac output. It has become clear that the lethal effects of endotoxin are dependent on macrophage activation and responsiveness, and that the production of cachectin from the activated macrophage plays a major role in causing profound shock and multiple organ injury (Tracey, 1988).

Other pathogenetic factors of the Enterobacteriaceae include the K1 antigen, which is associated with a high percentage of strains of *E. coli*

Table 56–9 Differentiation of Aerobic Gram-Negative Bacilli

Test	Escherichia coli	Klebsiella pneumoniae	Klebsiella oxytoca	Proteus mirabilis	Proteus vulgaris	Shigella spp.	Citrobacter freundii
Indole	+	−	+	−	+	D	−
Methyl red	+	− or +	D	+	+	+	+
Voges–Proskauer	−	+	+	− or +	−	−	−
Citrate (Simmons)	−	+	+	D	D	−	+
H₂S (triple sugar iron agar)	−	−	−	+	+	−	+
Urease	−	+	+	+	+	−	D
Phenylalanine deaminase	−	−	−	+	+	−	−
Lysine decarboxylase	+ or −n−	+	+	−	−	−	−
Arginine dihydrolase	− or +	−	−	−	−	−	D
Ornithine decarboxylase	D	−	−	+	−	D	− or +
Motility	+ or −	−	−	+*	+*	−	+
Acid produced from lactose	+	+	+	−	−	−	+ or (+)

* Swarm on blood and chocolate agar.

+ = ≥90% positive reactions within two days; − = ≥90% negative reactions; (+) = positive reactions in three to seven days; + or − = reactions of most strains positive; − or + = reactions of most strains negative; D = different reactions [+, (+), or −].

causing neonatal meningitis; the capsule of *K. pneumoniae*, which, like that of the pneumococcus, inhibits phagocytosis; the Vi antigen of *Salmonella* serotype *typhi*, which may interfere with intracellular killing of this organism; and various surface antigens, such as fimbriae, that mediate adherence of the organism to mucosal surfaces.

Plasmid-mediated factors appear to play an important role in the invasive properties of *Salmonella*, *Shigella*, and enteroinvasive strains of *E. coli*. Moreover, the heat-labile enterotoxins (LT) and heat-stable enterotoxins of *E. coli* are plasmid-mediated. LT stimulates adenylate cyclase in mucosal cells of the small intestine, which, in turn, activates cAMP, which causes secretion of fluid and electrolytes into the intestinal lumen and produces watery diarrhea. In contrast, heat-stable (ST) enterotoxins appear to activate guanylate cyclase.

Laboratory Diagnosis

The isolation of Gram-negative bacilli from contaminated specimens is greatly facilitated by the use of differential and selective media (Table 56–10). Eosin methylene blue (EMB) and MacConkey's agar can be used interchangeably as minimally selective and differential media to initially select for and differentiate lactose-fermenting from non-lactose-fermenting Gram-negative bacilli. XLD and HE agars are more selective differential media that are especially useful to select for *Salmonella* spp. and *Shigella* spp. in heavily contaminated specimens such as stool. Bismuth sulfite is a highly selective medium, especially useful for the detection of salmonellae in endemics or epidemics. *Salmonella* spp. produce H₂S and are easily recognized by the production of colonies with black centers on XLD, HE, and bismuth sulfite agars. An enrichment medium, such as selenite-F or Gram-negative (GN) broth, may be useful to detect low numbers of *Salmonella* spp. and *Shigella* spp. in stool. Cefsulodin–irgasan–novobiocin (CIN) agar incubated at room temperature is selective and differential for the recovery of *Yersinia enterocolitica*. Colonies will appear as bull's-eyes with red centers and transparent borders. MacConkey agar with sorbitol as the fermentable sugar is a differential medium that is capable of differentiating the sorbitol-fermentation-negative *E. coli* 0157:H7 associated with hemolytic uremic syndrome from most other *E. coli*.

For some of the Enterobacteriaceae, a few simple colonial characteristics or biochemical reactions can be used to presumptively identify an isolate. For example, *Proteus* spp. swarm on blood agar, *Klebsiella* spp. form mucoid colonies, *Serratia marcescens* may produce a red pigment, *Salmonella* spp. produce H₂S, and *E. coli* is indole-positive. Definitive identification of these and other species require additional biochemical testing. Innumerable schemes based on the use of conventional biochemical media have been described for the identification of the Enterobacteriaceae. Differential characteristics of the Enterobacteriaceae most commonly encountered in the clinical laboratory are shown in Table 56–10. Commercially prepared kits and automated devices are available and offer convenience and accuracy in the identification of the vast majority of isolates belonging to the Enterobacteriaceae. In some instances, the identification is accurately made in a few hours. Semiautomated systems may also combine the identification and antimicrobial susceptibility testing together in a single

disposable unit. In general, accuracy of identification among these systems is very high and comparable.

The classification of the Enterobacteriaceae has undergone considerable revision in recent years as the result of DNA hybridization and relatedness studies. Because phenotypic groupings on the basis of biochemical reactions are not always consistent with their DNA relatedness, the use of tribes (e.g., Klebsielleae, Proteeae) for grouping species within the Enterobacteriaceae has been discontinued.

Historically, the genus *Salmonella* has been divided into the following species: *S. typhi*, *Salmonella paratyphi* A and B, *Salmonella choleraesuis*, *Salmonella typhimurium*, and *Salmonella enteritidis*. Because all groups have been found to be genetically very closely related, current terminology now recognizes only two species, *S. enterica* and *S. bongori* (rarely isolated from humans), each of which contains multiple subspecies. There are six subspecies of *S. enterica*, with subspecies I (*S. enterica* subsp. *enterica*) the usual human isolate. There are more than 2000 serotypes of *Salmonella*, the majority being in the subspecies *enterica*. Serotyping is based on immunologic reactivity of the heat-stable somatic 'O' antigens, which are predominantly lipopolysaccharide in content, and heat-labile flagellar 'H' antigens. In the United States, *Salmonella* serotypes *typhimurium* and *enteritidis* are the most common. *Salmonella* serotype *typhi* also produces a heat-labile capsular polysaccharide Vi antigen. In practice, most clinical laboratories identify isolates as *Salmonella* spp. based on biochemical reactions and use group-specific immunologic reagents to assign isolates to a specific serogroup. Commercial slide agglutination tests to differentiate large serogroups, A, B, C, and D, are useful in differentiating the typhoidal salmonella from nontyphoidal strains. *S.* serotype *typhi* carries the D serogroup and Vi antigen. Further identification of the specific serotype is generally performed only by State Health Departments or other reference laboratories. Isolates biochemically resembling *Shigella* are also classified by the reactivity of the 'O' antigen, as are isolates of *E. coli* that are identified as potential causes of diarrhea, hemolytic uremic syndrome, or thrombotic thrombocytopenic purpura. Such *E. coli* are classified by the type of toxin produced as well. Commercial kits are available to identify *E. coli* 0157 and to detect some types of toxins in culture or stool specimens; however, this type of testing often is referred to the State Health Departments.

Antimicrobial Susceptibility

The susceptibility of the Enterobacteriaceae to various antimicrobial agents is highly variable. Susceptibility to ampicillin is expected among strains of *E. coli* and *P. mirabilis*, for example (although resistance is increasing in both), but not expected among most other clinically significant members of the Enterobacteriaceae. Resistance to first-generation cephalosporins (cefazolin, cephalothin) is expected for *Enterobacter* spp., *Serratia* spp., *Citrobacter* spp., *Proteus vulgaris*, *Providencia* spp., *Morganella* spp., and *Yersinia* spp.; susceptibility to the third-generation cephalosporins (ceftriaxone, cefotaxime, ceftazidime, for example) remains for many of the members of the Enterobacteriaceae. However, the presence of extended-spectrum β-lactamases and *Amp-C* genes, which are recognized by resistance to third-generation cephalosporins, are increasing in selected strains. Most

Table 56–9 Differentiation of Aerobic Gram-Negative Bacilli *Continued*

Yersinia enterocolitica	Enterobacter cloacae	Serratia marcescens	Morganella morganii	Providencia alcalifaciens	Salmonella Serotype choleraesuis	Salmonella Serotype typhi	Salmonella Serotype paratyphi A
D	−	−	+	+	−		−
+	−	+ or −	+	+	+	+	+
+ (25°C)/ −(37°C)	+	+	−	−	−	−	−
−(25°C)	+	+	−	+	(+)	−	−
−	−	−	−	−	D	+	− or +
+	D	− or +	+	−	−	−	−
−	−	−	+	−	−	−	−
−	−	−	−	−	+	+	−
−	+	−	−	−	(+)	− or (+)	− or +
+	+	+	−	+	−	+	−
+ + (25°C)/−(37°C)	+	+	+ or −	+	+	+	+
D	D	−	−	−	−	−	−

Table 56–10 Enteric Differential and Selective Media

Medium	Gram-Positive Bacteriostatic Agent	Fermentable Carbohydrate	Indicator	Colony Color Fermenter	Nonfermenter	Category
Eosin methylene blue (EMB)	Eosin Y Methylene blue	Lactose*	Eosin Y Methylene blue	Red or black with sheen	Colorless	S, D
MacConkey	Crystal violet Bile salts	Lactose	Neutral red	Red	Colorless	S, D
Xylose-lysine-deoxycholate (XLD)	Bile salts	Xylose Lactose Sucrose	Phenol red	Yellow	Red	S, D
Hektoen enteric (HE)	Bile salts	Salicin Lactose Sucrose	Bromthymol blue	Yellow-orange	Green, blue-green	S, D
Salmonella–shigella (SS)	Bile salts	Lactose	Neutral red	Red	Colorless	S
Bismuth sulfite (BS)	Brilliant green	Glucose	Bismuth sulfite	†	†	S
Thiosulfate citrate bile salts sucrose (TCBS)‡	Bile salts pH 8.6	Sucrose	Thymol blue Bromthymol blue	Yellow	Colorless	S, D

* Levine's formulation. † H$_2$S-producing salmonellae have black colonies. ‡ Used for isolation of vibrios.

D = differential; S = selective.

Enterobacteriaceae are susceptible to aminoglycosides and fluoro-quinolones. It is very unusual for a member of the Enterobacteriaceae to be resistant to carbapenems (e.g., imipenem, meropenem, or ertapenem), and, if resistance is found, this should be confirmed before carbapenem resistance is reported. Because the susceptibility pattern of the Enterobacteriaceae is unpredictable, as a general rule susceptibility testing should be performed if antimicrobial therapy is being considered. No susceptibility testing need be performed if antimicrobial therapy is not instituted, as for uncomplicated enteric infections due to salmonellas, where therapy may actually prolong the carrier state, or when there is a mixed flora infection and individual susceptibilities may not be appropriate.

Plesiomonas

Characteristics

Plesiomonas shigelloides, the only species in the genus *Plesiomonas*, is a facultatively anaerobic, oxidase- and catalase-positive, glucose-fermenting, Gram-negative rod. Recent molecular genetic evidence demonstrates that the genus *Plesiomonas* is most closely related to the genus *Proteus*. Therefore, it has been placed into the Enterobacteriaceae family (Farmer, 2003) as the only oxidase-positive member of this group of Gram-negative bacilli.

Clinical Manifestations and Pathogenesis.

P. shigelloides is found in aquatic environments that are limited geographically by its minimum growth temperature of 8°C. It may be found in fresh and estuarine water, usually in tropical countries. It has been implicated as a cause of gastroenteritis, especially following the ingestion of uncooked shellfish. The diarrheal stool specimen frequently contains polymorphonuclear leukocytes and red blood cells, although a cholera-like illness may also occur. Gastroenteritis may occur in sporadic cases, as well as in outbreaks. Extraintestinal manifestations of infection with *P. shigelloides* include meningitis, septicemia, cellulitis, arthritis, and endophthalmitis (Ampofo, 2001).

Relatively little is known about virulence factors of *P. shigelloides* as yet. The organism appears to have invasive properties, and there are some data suggesting enterotoxigenic activity (Brenden, 1988).

Laboratory Diagnosis

P. shigelloides can be isolated on a variety of nonselective and enteric-selective media, including HE agar. Acid production from lactose is variable but on enteric media the organism usually appears to be a non-lactose-fermenter. It is indole-positive; reduces nitrates to nitrites; produces catalase; is methyl-red-positive; and ferments glucose, maltose, and trehalose (Brenden, 1988).

Antimicrobial Susceptibility

P. shigelloides is susceptible to a variety of antimicrobial agents, including cephalosporins, trimethoprim–sulfamethoxazole, imipenem and the quinolones (Abbott, 2003b). Susceptibility to the penicillins is variable, because of the presence of a β-lactamase similar to that of *Aeromonas* spp.

Gram-Negative Bacteria – Nonfermentative Bacilli

A group of Gram-negative bacilli that do not ferment glucose and other sugars are often lumped together under the heading of 'non-fermenters.' They account for about 15% of the Gram-negative bacilli isolated from

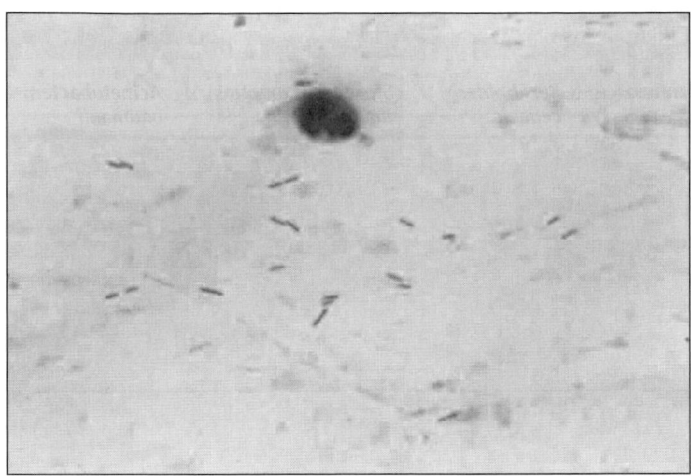

Figure 56–16 Gram stain of *Pseudomonas aeruginosa* in a sputum specimen. Note the longer, Gram-negative bacilli compared to Figure 56–13.

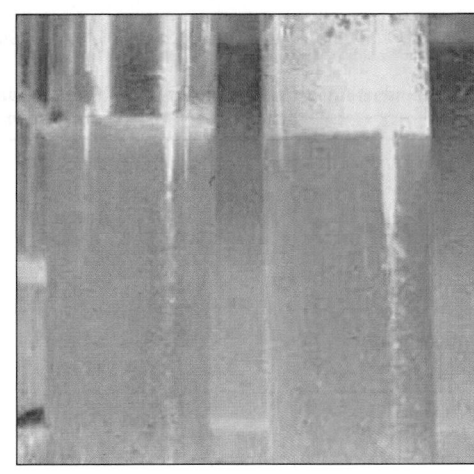

Figure 56–17 Extracted pyocyanin pigment from *Pseudomonas aeruginosa*.

hospitalized patients. Although there are many genera of non-fermenters, 75% of the clinically relevant ones are *Pseudomonas aeruginosa*; the majority of the other 25% are either *Acinetobacter* sp., *Stenotrophomonas maltophilia*, or *Burkholderia cepacia*. As a group, they are environmental bacteria, not usually found as part of the normal flora of the human body except as colonizers in hospitalized patients. They can be readily isolated from water, soil, vegetables, plants, and hospital surfaces. Although there are no uniform biochemical characteristics, they are often oxidase-positive, lactose-negative colonies on selective media such as MacConkey's agar (although some of the species do not grow on this media) and they are often resistant to many of the antibiotics that are effective against members of the Enterobacteriaceae. The four main species mentioned above, as well as a few others, will be discussed in this chapter.

Pseudomonas
Characteristics
The genus *Pseudomonas* has undergone extensive revision and now many of the species that were previously classified in this genus have been reclassified into the genera *Burkholderia*, *Stenotrophomonas*, *Comamonas*, *Shewanella*, *Ralstonia*, *Methylobacterium*, *Sphingomonas*, *Acidovorax*, and *Brevundimonas*. Of the species that remain, *P. aeruginosa* is the most significant human pathogen. Figure 56–16 is the Gram stain of *P. aeruginosa* in a sputum specimen.

Pseudomonads are strictly aerobic, catalase-positive, oxidase-positive, Gram-negative bacilli. Their metabolism is respiratory and never fermentative with oxygen as the terminal electron acceptor. Some pseudomonads are motile by means of polar flagella.

Clinical Manifestations and Pathogenesis
Pseudomonads are found in moist environments. Some of the more unusual habitats for these organisms include cosmetics, swimming pools, hot-tubs, and the inner soles of sneakers. The latter can lead to puncture wounds that are infected with *P. aeruginosa*. The species causing the greatest morbidity and mortality today is *P. aeruginosa*. Other species of *Pseudomonas*, although often isolated from clinical specimens, are only occasionally involved in disease.

P. aeruginosa is ubiquitous in the hospital environment, existing almost anywhere there is moisture, including medical equipment and disinfectant solutions and soaps. It is only rarely found as part of the normal flora of healthy people but in hospitalized patients the rates of colonization increase with the length of hospitalization. *P. aeruginosa* may produce serious infection in patients with burns, traumatic, and operative wounds; following urinary tract manipulation; in patients with diseases of the hematopoietic, reticuloendothelial, and lymphoid systems; and in those with impaired cellular or humoral defenses. Pulmonary infection occurs commonly in patients with cystic fibrosis. The mortality rate is highest in severely leukopenic (<1000 polymorphonuclear neutrophils/mm³) patients.

P. aeruginosa produces a slime polysaccharide, an endotoxin, and proteases that inactivate components of complement, thereby inhibiting to some degree opsonization and the inflammatory response and perhaps contributing to its invasiveness. Exotoxin A promotes cellular damage and tissue invasion and is toxic for macrophages.

Laboratory Diagnosis
The presence of *P. aeruginosa* in cultures can often be suspected because of its musty grape-like (or corn tortilla) odor, the rough or ground-glass appearance of its colonies on sheep blood agar, and the presence of one or both of two pigments: a 'blue-green' fluorescent pigment (Figure 56–17) and/or a metallic sheen due to pyoverdin pigment. Its identification can be made easily with a positive oxidase reaction, an alkaline slant/neutral butt reaction in TSIA, growth at 42°C, and the formation of sheen and/or pigment on the slants of TSIA and *Pseudomonas* P agar. Additional tests that can be performed are shown in Table 56–11. Tests of carbohydrate utilization should be carried out in O-F basal medium, which contains a minimal quantity of peptone and a relatively large quantity of carbohydrate and so can provide detection of the very small quantities of acid formed by this group of bacteria. Reactions are usually complete within 48 hours but may require as long as seven days.

Antimicrobial Susceptibility
As a general rule, susceptibility testing should be performed for all clinically significant isolates of *P. aeruginosa*. Hospital strains of *P. aeruginosa* may be resistant to many classes of antibiotic. Isolates are often susceptible to the aminoglycosides, the carboxy- and ureidopenicillins, ceftazidime or cefepime, carbapenems, and the quinolones. However, multiple resistance is increasing, especially in intensive care units and in patients who have longstanding *Pseudomonas* infections, such as patients with cystic fibrosis and other chronic syndromes (Friedland, 2004; Hauser, 2005). Laboratories are being asked to test additional antibiotics, especially colistin or polymyxin B, when these resistant isolates are encountered. The CLSI has recently provided breakpoints for testing of polymyxin B that can be interpreted for polymyxin B or colistin (Clinical and Laboratory Standards Institute/NCCLS 2005).

Acinetobacter
Characteristics
Organisms in this genus are short, rod-shaped to spherical, non-motile, oxidase-negative, strictly aerobic, and Gram-negative. In a Gram-stained smear they often appear in pairs and may be difficult to decolorize.

Clinical Manifestations and Pathogenesis
Acinetobacter spp. are commonly found in soil and water and uncommonly found on the skin and mucous membranes of healthy people. Little is known about virulence factors in this group of organisms, but they do appear to form small amounts of endotoxin. Although usually nonpathogenic, they have been increasingly associated with nosocomial septicemia, pneumonia, bacteriuria, and wound infection.

Laboratory Diagnosis
Acinetobacter spp. can be distinguished readily from the pseudomonads on the basis of their lack of motility, inability to reduce nitrates, and negative oxidase reaction. They may produce characteristic purplish colonies on MacConkey's agar. There are over 25 species but their differentiation biochemically is difficult and they are often lumped together in the *Acinetobacter calcoaceticus*–*Acinetobacter baumanii* complex. The glucose oxidizing (saccharolytic strains), nonhemolytic clinical strains are usually referred to as *A. baumanii*; the nonsaccharolytic strains (non-glucose-oxidizers) are either *Acinetobacter lwoffi*, if non-hemolytic, or *Acinetobacter haemolyticus* if hemolytic (Gerner-Smidt, 1991). The more clinically relevant species is *A. baumanii*.

VII

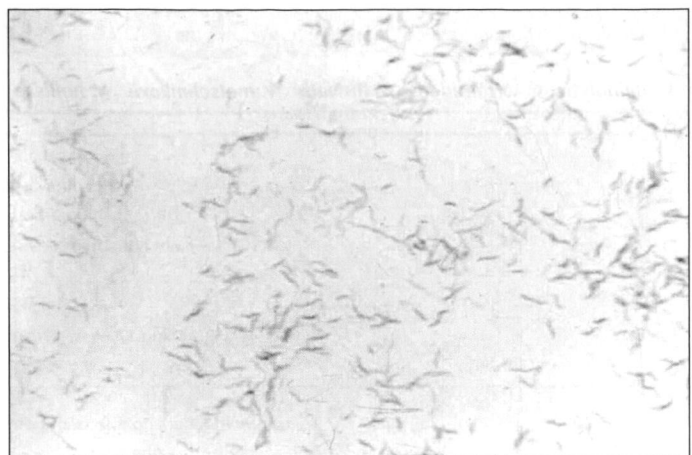

Figure 56–18 *Campylobacter jejuni* Gram stain: note the 'comma-shaped' appearance of the bacilli.

difficult to detect in conventional susceptibility testing methods, including automated systems (Rossolini, 1996). *Aeromonas* spp. have been found to maintain resistance plasmids of both the Enterobacteriaceae and *Pseudomonas* spp.

Campylobacter

Characteristics

Campylobacter spp. are small (0.5–8 μm long × 0.2–0.5 μm wide), motile, non-spore-forming, curved (comma-shaped) or S-shaped Gram-negative bacilli that grow optimally in an atmosphere containing 5–10% oxygen and, therefore, are considered to be microaerophilic. Figure 56–18 is the Gram stain of a *Campylobacter jejuni* from culture. *C. jejuni* is the most common cause of bacterial enteritis in the United States. Other *Campylobacter* spp. associated with enteritis are *Campylobacter coli*, *Campylobacter lari*, and *Campylobacter upsaliensis*. *Campylobacter fetus* subsp. *fetus* is a cause of septic thrombophlebitis, arthritis, peritonitis, abscesses, and pericarditis (Penner, 1988), especially in persons with an underlying chronic disease.

Clinical Manifestations and Pathogenesis

C. jejuni is found worldwide as a commensal of the gastrointestinal tract of wild or domesticated cattle, sheep, swine, goats, dogs, cats, and fowl, especially turkeys and chickens. It is the most common cause of bacterial enteritis in the United States, with an estimated occurrence of 1000 cases per 100 000 individuals. The incidence of infection in the UK and other developed nations is similar to the United States, and the incidence in underdeveloped countries is probably even higher. Infections generally occur in the summer and fall and are commonly the result of ingestion of improperly cooked foods, usually poultry. In addition, several outbreaks of *C. jejuni* enteritis have been linked to unpasteurized milk and to defects in municipal water systems. The spectrum of illness ranges from asymptomatic to severely ill. The diarrhea produced may be with or without blood or fecal leukocytes. Symptoms can last up to one week and are generally self-limited. Extraintestinal infections may also occur, including bacteremia, reactive arthritis, urinary tract infections, and meningitis. *C. jejuni* is the most recognized antecedent cause of Guillain–Barré syndrome. The pathogenesis of this organism is not completely understood; it appears to first colonize the intestinal mucous layer and then is able to translocate through the epithelial surface to the underlying tissue.

The major habitat of *C. fetus* subsp. *fetus* is the intestine of sheep and cattle; it also may be found in the genital tract of these animals, their placentas, the gastric contents of their aborted fetuses, and, less frequently, in other animals and birds. The mechanisms of transmission of infection to humans are not understood completely. Direct contact with an infected animal is possible, but fewer than one third of infected individuals have a history of environmental or occupational exposure. Contaminated food or water may be a vehicle for infection, or infection may originate from an endogenous source.

Laboratory Diagnosis

A single stool specimen is generally adequate to detect enteric pathogens, including *Campylobacter* spp. Examination for fecal leukocytes is not recommended because they may be present in as few as 25% of the cases. An enzyme immunoassay (EIA) is available for direct detection of *Campylobacter jejuni* and *Campylobacter coli* antigens in stool specimens. (Tolcin, 2000; Dediste, 2003)

Several media can be used for the selective isolation of *Campylobacter* spp., including charcoal–cefoperazone–deoxycholate agar, charcoal-based selective medium, semisolid blood-free motility medium, Skirrow's medium, and *Campylobacter* agar with 5% sheep blood and five antimicrobials (cephalothin, trimethoprim, vancomycin, polymyxin B, and amphotericin B). Most *Campylobacter* spp. require a microaerobic environment (5% O_2, 10% CO_2, and 85% N_2), which can be produced using commercially available gas generator packs. The amount of oxygen in a candle jar is too low to support the growth of *Campylobacter* spp. and should not be used. Incubation of the plates at 42°C increases the selectivity for *C. jejuni*.

If *Campylobacter* spp. are suspected in a blood culture based on clinical history or appearance of an organism in the Gram's stain, the broth should be subcultured to a nonselective blood agar plate and incubated at 37°C in a microaerobic environment.

In general, *Campylobacter* spp. produce gray, flat, irregular, spready colonies, which may become round, convex, and glistening as the moisture content in the media is reduced. A typical Gram stain appearance and a positive oxidase reaction from a colony growing on selective media at 42°C can be reported as *Campylobacter* spp. *C. jejuni* is able to hydrolyze hippurate and is susceptible to nalidixic acid and resistant to cephalothin. *C. coli* is hippuricase-negative.

Strains of *C. fetus* subsp. *fetus* are resistant to nalidixic acid, fail to hydrolyze hippurate, and do not ordinarily grow at 42°C.

Antimicrobial Susceptibility

C. jejuni is variably susceptible to antimicrobial agents. Most are not susceptible to penicillins or cephalosporins. For intestinal infection, erythromycin is the drug of choice, with quinolones used as alternative therapy. Treatment is often not warranted, however, for simple gastroenteritis with *Camplyobacter* sp. in an otherwise healthy individual. Resistance to both agents has been encountered. There are currently no standardized methods for susceptibility testing of this group of organisms; however, a CLSI document giving guidelines for testing is available now in a proposed format (CLSI, M-4SP).

Helicobacter

Characteristics

Helicobacter spp. are spiral-shaped or curved Gram-negative non-spore-forming bacilli, measuring 0.3–1.0 μm wide and 1.5–10 μm in length. They are motile by multiple bipolar or monopolar flagella, are microaerobic, and have a respiratory metabolism.

Clinical Manifestations and Pathogenesis

Helicobacter spp. are found in the gastrointestinal tracts of mammals and birds. Transmission from one host to another occurs through both oral–oral and fecal–oral routes. *Helicobacter pylori* is considered to be one of the 'gastric' helicobacters. In the stomach it lives within or beneath the mucous layer adjacent to the epithelium. It is also found transiently in the duodenum, saliva, and feces.

Infection with *H. pylori* may result in acute gastritis symptoms. Most infected patients develop chronic active gastritis, which may lead to nonulcer dyspepsia or duodenal ulcers. *H. pylori* has been associated with 90% of duodenal ulcers and nearly all gastric ulcers. Infection with *H. pylori* has also been associated with gastric carcinoma and gastric lymphoma (Parsonnet, 1991, 1994; Murray, 1993). The prevalence of gastritis associated with *H. pylori* increases with age, suggesting that the organism is acquired as people become older.

The 'enteric' helicobacters, such as *Helicobacter* (formerly *Campylobacter*) *cinaedi*, and *Helicobacter fennelliae*, have been implicated in cases of gastroenteritis. Rarely, these organisms may invade the bloodstream and be isolated from cultures of blood.

Laboratory Diagnosis

Typically, nonculture methods have been utilized to diagnose *H. pylori* infection. One such test is the urea breath test. This is a noninvasive test that detects urease activity of *H. pylori* by measuring ^{14}C and ^{13}C-labeled CO_2 in the patient's expelled air after ingestion of labeled urea. Serologic assays are also widely used in symptomatic patients to detect antibodies against *H. pylori*, however since the majority of adults will have been exposed to *H. pylori*, this can be a nonspecific test, except as an epidemiologic or surveillance tool. In some cases, biopsies of the affected tissues are obtained and examined histologically using the hematoxylin and eosin or Giemsa stain for the presence of organisms with the morphology typical of *H. pylori*. Because the organism hydrolyzes urea very rapidly, a portion of the gastric biopsy may be placed directly into urea broth or onto urea-containing agar to detect urea hydrolysis in 1–24 hours (CLO

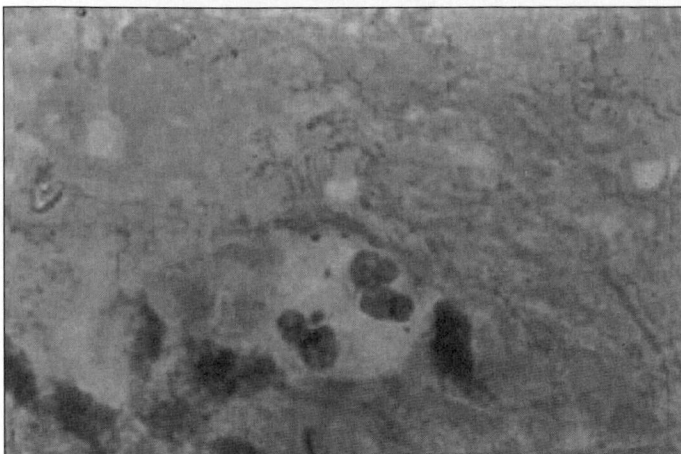

Figure 56–19 Gram stain of a *Haemophilus influenzae* cocco-bacillus in a brain abscess.

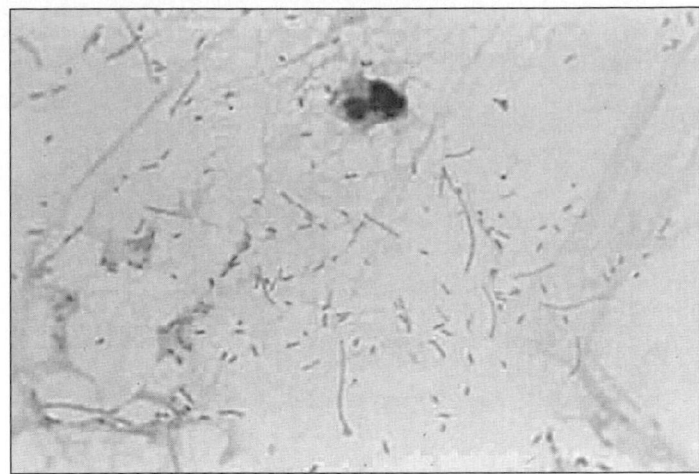

Figure 56–20 Note the pleomorphic nature of the *Haemophilus influenzae* seen in this Gram stain of cerebrospinal fluid.

test). A commercially available EIA for detection of *H. pylori* antigen in stool is a noninvasive alternative for diagnosis of *H. pylori* infection (Premier Platinum HpSA, Meridian Bioscience, Cincinnati, OH). Sensitivity of this assay is as high as 89% with specificities up to 95% (Montiero, 2001). PCR has also been reported as a sensitive method for detection of *H. pylori* (Makristathis, 1998).

For culture, tissue specimens should be maintained at 4°C and processed within 2 hours of collection. Transport media include *Brucella* broth with 20% glycerol, cysteine Albemi broth with 20% glycerol, isotonic saline with 4% glucose, and Stuart's transport media. Processed specimens may be inoculated to one of several media, including brain–heart infusion (BHIA), *Brucella*, Columbia, or Skirrow's supplemented with horse blood, horse serum, or sheep blood. The addition of vancomycin, amphotericin, and cefsulodin are recommended as selective agents. Inoculated media should be incubated in a microaerobic atmosphere (5–10% CO_2, 80–90% N_2, and 5–10% O_2) under high humidity at 35°C for 5–7 days. Addition of 5–8% H_2 in the atmosphere enhances growth of *H. pylori*. *H. pylori* generally produces small, gray, translucent colonies on these media, has the characteristic Gram-negative spiral appearance in stained smears, and is oxidase-, catalase-, and urease-positive. Feces are generally not cultured for the enteric helicobacters. *Helicobacter* spp. will grow and be detected by the automated blood culture systems in use in many laboratories, but may require incubation for longer than the standard 5 days.

Antimicrobial Susceptibility

Multidrug regimens are used to treat *H. pylori* infection. These usually include two antibiotics (metronidazole, clarithromycin, tetracycline, or amoxicillin) and an 'antiacid' drug. Strains resistant to metronidazole and clarithromycin have been reported. For susceptibility testing, the CLSI recommends agar dilution using Mueller–Hinton agar plus 5% sheep blood (Clinical and Laboratory Standards Institute/NCCLS, 2005). Interpretive breakpoints are only given for clarithromycin.

Haemophilus

Characteristics

Members of the genus are oxidase-positive, facultatively anaerobic, small, Gram-negative, pleomorphic rods or coccobacilli with a potential requirement for X (hemin) and/or V (NAD) factor. Figure 56–19 shows a *H. influenzae* bacterium in a brain abscess specimen.

Clinical Manifestations and Pathogenesis

Most *Haemophilus* spp. are normal inhabitants of the upper respiratory tract. Some may reside in the gastrointestinal or urogenital tract. Person-to-person spread occurs by respiratory droplets. Infections caused by *Haemophilus* spp. range from conjunctivitis and otitis media to meningitis and endocarditis. Those that are generally considered human pathogens are *H. influenzae*, *Haemophilus parainfluenzae*, *Haemophilus ducreyi*, and *Haemophilus aphrophilus*.

The major virulence factor of *H. influenzae* is the polysaccharide capsule, of which there are six serotypes (a–f). Strains that do not possess a capsule are referred to as nontypeable. Endotoxin is not produced by *H. influenzae*, and this species is rapidly killed once ingested by macrophages unless antibody, complement, or the phagocytes are deficient. The role of antibodies in immunity is also poorly understood. Antibodies develop with age, presumably following natural infection

with *H. influenzae* or with crossreacting antigenic organisms, so that most persons older than 15 years have antibodies. Which antibodies and the level of those antibodies that is protective remain unknown.

Since the introduction of a vaccine for *H. influenzae* type b in the mid 1980s there has been a sharp drop in the incidence of invasive infection such as meningitis and epiglottitis due to this organism (Centers for Disease Control, 1994). Figure 56–20 demonstrates the pleomorphic nature of the *H. influenzae* that was seen in this CSF specimen. Nontypeable strains of *H. influenzae* are most frequently associated with acute otitis media and acute exacerbations of chronic bronchitis. *H. parainfluenzae* is usually a commensal in the upper respiratory tract but may also cause serious illness, such as endocarditis. *H. aphrophilus*, another upper respiratory tract commensal, can cause endocarditis, brain abscess, pneumonia, meningitis, and bacteruria. *H. ducreyi* is responsible for the sexually transmitted disease chancroid.

Laboratory Diagnosis

The isolation of *Haemophilus* spp. usually requires the presence of X and/or V factor in the culture medium. The former is most frequently supplied by the incorporation of heat-lysed ('chocolatized') blood cells in agar, although it may also be provided by whole human, horse, or rabbit blood cells. The V factor (NAD) is commonly supplied either by the incorporation of yeast extract or other appropriate supplements in the medium or by a suspension of staphylococci, which is streaked across the agar surface and about which satellite colonies of dependent strains of *Haemophilus* spp. grow. The differential characteristics of members of this genus are listed in Table 56–13.

The requirements for X and V factors are determined by absence or presence of growth on media containing these factors. An alternative method to test for X factor dependence is the porphyrin test described by Kilian (1974), which determines the ability of dependent species to use δ-aminolevulinic acid in the biosynthesis of porphobilinogen and porphyrins. The formation of porphobilinogen can be detected by adding Kovac's reagent to the reaction mixture and observing the development of a red color in the aqueous phase. Alternatively, the formation of porphyrins in the reaction mixture can be demonstrated by red fluorescence under a Wood's lamp. Hemolytic properties of *Haemophilus* spp. can be determined on rabbit or horse blood agar.

H. aphrophilus must often be distinguished from species such as *Actinobacillus actinomycetemcomitans*, *Cardiobacterium hominis*, and *Eikenella corrodens* (Table 56–14), all of which have been associated with subacute bacterial endocarditis.

The cultivation of *H. ducreyi* from chancroid lesions is problematic. A Gram-stained smear of material from the lesion may be helpful if Gram-negative bacilli in pairs or in rows ('schools of fish') are seen. Figure 56–21 shows a 'typical' Gram stain of *H. ducreyi* from clinical material. Material may be inoculated onto GC medium base plus 1% hemoglobin, 5–10% fetal calf serum, 1% IsoVitaleX (BBL Microbiology Systems), and 3 µg/mL of vancomycin or Mueller–Hinton agar plus 5% horse blood, 1% cofactor–vitamin–amino acid enrichment and 3 µg/mL vancomycin.

Antimicrobial Susceptibility

Currently, the CLSI recommends testing *H. influenzae* isolated from blood or CSF against ampicillin, chloramphenicol, a third-generation cephalosporin, and meropenem (Clinical and Laboratory Standards Institute/NCCLS,

Table 56–13 Differential Characteristics of Medically Important *Haemophilus* Species

	Porphyrin	X-Factor-Dependent	V-Factor-Dependent	CO$_2$ Enhancement	Hemolysis*	Catalase
Haemophilus influenzae	–	+	+	+	–	+
Haemophilus haemolyticus	–	+	+	–	+	+
Haemophilus parahaemolyticus	+	–	+	–	+	V
Haemophilus ducreyi	–	+	–	V	–	–
Haemophilus parainfluenzae	+	–	+	V	–	V
Haemophilus aphrophilus	+	–	–	+	–	–
Haemophilus paraprophilus	+	–	–	+	–	–

* On horse and rabbit blood.

Source: adapted from: Mahon CR, Manuselis G: Textbook of Diagnostic Microbiology, 2nd edn. London, WB Saunders, 2000, p 435.

Table 56–14 Differential Characteristics of *Haemophilus aphrophilus, Actinobacillus actinomycetemcomitans, Cardiobacterium hominis, Eikenella corrodens*, and *Kingella kingae*

Test	H. aphrophilus	A. actinomycetemcomitans	C. hominis	E. corrodens	K. kingae
Oxidase	+/–	–/W	+	+	+
Catalase	–	+	–	–	–
δ-ALA utilization	+	+	+	+	+
V-requirement	–	–	–	–	–
Indole	–	–	+	–	–
Urease	–	–	–	–	–
Lysine decarboxylase	–	–	–	+	–
Acid from glucose	+	+	+	–	(+)
Sucrose	+	–	+	–	–
Lactose	+	–	–	–	–
Mannitol	–	+	D	–	–
Xylose	–	D	–	–	–

δ-ALA = δ-aminolevulinic acid; W = weak.

For key to symbols, see Table 56–9.

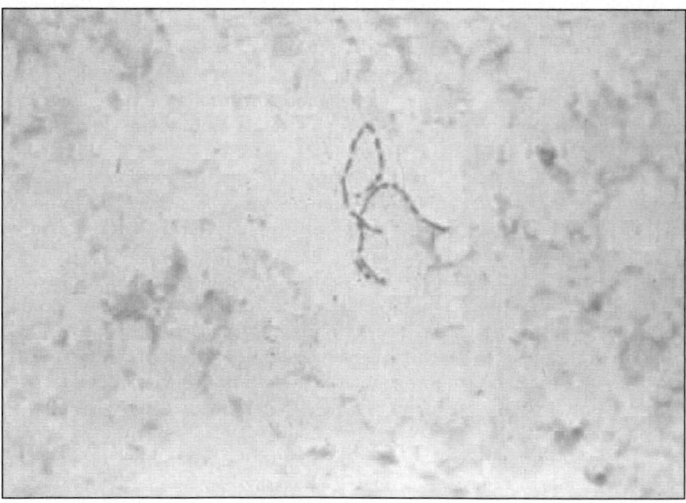

Figure 56–21 *Haemophilus ducreyi* bacilli from a genital lesion.

2003a). Resistance to ampicillin may be as high as 40–60% in the United States, varying geographically. Resistance to ampicillin is usually mediated by the production of β-lactamase; however, rare isolates are resistant on the basis of alterations in outer membrane permeability or affinity to penicillin-binding proteins. Resistance to second- or third-generation cephalosporins has not been documented in the United States. Susceptibility testing of *H. influenzae* requires the use of *Haemophilus* test medium (HTM). The recommended treatment for *H. ducreyi* infection is erythromycin; alternative agents include azithromycin, ciprofloxacin, ceftriaxone, amoxicillin–clavulanate, and trimethoprim–sulfamethoxazole. Although there are not many data on the susceptibility of other *Haemophilus* spp to antibiotics, resistance is assumed higher than among *H. influenzae* strains. (Kilian, 2003)

Gram-Negative Bacteria – The HACEK Bacteria

There are five small Gram-negative coccobacilli that are part of the normal oral flora and are occasionally associated with bacterial endocarditis and rarely other infections. They are opportunists that enter the blood stream, settle on damaged heart valves, and cause a relatively slowly progressive, indolent form of endocarditis. They typically require an additional 1–2 days before they are isolated in blood cultures, and are uniformly susceptible to many antimicrobial agents. The word HACEK stands for: *Haemophilus* sp. (*influenzae, parainfluenzae*, and *aphrophilus* most commonly), *Actinobacillus actinomycetemcomitans, Cardiobacterium hominis, Eikenella corrodens*, and *Kingella* sp. Differential characteristics of the members of this group are listed in Table 56–14.

Haemophilus sp.

H. influenzae was discussed above in this chapter. *H. aphrophilus* is also part of the HACEK group. It does not require X or V factor, hence can easily grow on blood and chocolate agars. It does not require CO$_2$ for growth. It is usually susceptible to β-lactam agents; treatment often entails combination therapy with a β-lactam and aminoglycoside.

Actinobacillus

Characteristics

A. actinomycetemcomitans is a Gram-negative, non-spore-forming coccobacillus or short rod. It grows both aerobically and anaerobically. The addition of 5–10% CO$_2$ enhances growth. Colonies on blood agar appear slowly and remain small.

Clinical Manifestations and Pathogenesis

The actinobacilli are found in the mucous membranes of the respiratory and genitourinary tract of humans and animals. They generally cause disease only in immunocompromised individuals or when they are accidentally introduced into healthy surrounding tissue, for example, by trauma. *A. actinomycetemcomitans* has a low level of pathogenicity. It derives its name from its frequent association with actinomycotic lesions. In recent years, however, it has most frequently been reported as a cause of subacute bacterial endocarditis, periodontitis, and brain abscess. Two virulence factors are known: a leukotoxin and a collagenase.

Laboratory Diagnosis
A. actinomycetemcomitans grows on blood and chocolate agar. After 24–72 hours, colonies are 1–3 mm in diameter with a central wrinkling. The organism is catalase positive, oxidase negative or weakly positive, and urease negative. Additional biochemical assays must be used to differentiate it from other slowly growing, somewhat fastidious Gram-negative bacilli (Table 56–14).

Antimicrobial Susceptibility
This organism is resistant to penicillin but is usually susceptible to many other antibiotics including the cephalosporins, β-lactam–β-lactamase inhibitor combinations, fluoroquinolones, and tetracycline.

Cardiobacterium hominis
Characteristics
C. hominis is a Gram-negative, non-spore-forming bacillus that is part of the normal oral flora. It is a facultative anaerobe that does not require CO_2, although growth is enhanced in microaerophilic conditions. Growth occurs on blood and chocolate agar but not on MacConkey's agar and is better at longer than 48 hours.

Clinical manifestations and pathogenesis
Cardiobacterium hominis can cause subacute bacterial endocarditis, similar to other HACEK members; it may also be responsible for cases of periodontitis.

Laboratory Diagnosis
Colonies at 48 hours incubation are small and may have a yellow pigment, although most are white. The organism is generally oxidase- and indole-positive but negative for catalase, urease, esculin, and nitrate reduction. Acid may be produced from glucose, maltose and sucrose.

Antimicrobial susceptibility
Isolates are usually susceptible to penicillins and cephalosporins, aminoglycosides, and tetracyclines. Resistance to clindamycin is common. No β-lactamases have been reported as yet.

Eikenella
Characteristics
Formerly classified as *Bacteroides corrodens*, the 'corroding bacilli' that are facultatively anaerobic have been assigned to the species *Eikenella corrodens*. *E. corrodens* organisms are oxidase-positive, catalase-negative, nonfermentative, Gram-negative bacilli, colonies of which may corrode or pit agar. Growth is enhanced by 5–10% CO_2 and usually requires the presence of X factor in the medium.

Clinical Manifestations and Pathogenesis
Little is known about factors contributing to the organism's virulence and it has a low level of pathogenicity for animals. *E. corrodens* resides predominantly in the oral cavity and is isolated frequently from the upper respiratory tract. Like other HACEK bacteria, it is responsible for subacute bacterial endocarditis. It has been recovered from abscesses, cellulitis, and wound infections, often following human bites. Infections are usually mixed with other organisms.

Laboratory Diagnosis
Growth is observed on blood or chocolate agar but not MacConkey agar. The most striking features of *E. corrodens* in culture are the distinctive odor of bleach and characteristic pitting of the agar; however, pitting does not occur with all strains. The colonies appear slowly (2–4 days) and are generally small (0.5–1.0 mm in diameter). *E. corrodens* must usually be distinguished from other fastidious, slowly growing Gram-negative bacilli (Table 56–14).

Antimicrobial Susceptibility
E. corrodens is susceptible to the penicillins, quinolones, and tetracycline, variably susceptible to aminoglycosides, and resistant to clindamycin and metronidazole.

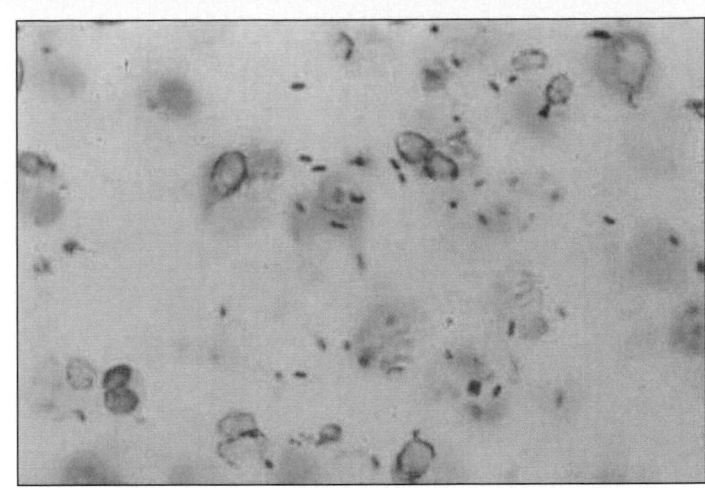

Figure 56–22 *Legionella pneumophila* in a clinical specimen stained with a Dieterle silver stain.

Kingella sp.
Characteristics
Kingella has three recognized species: *K. kingae* (the HACEK species), *Kingella oralis*, and *Kingella denitrificans*. They are Gram-negative rods to coccobacilli, requiring increased CO_2 for optimum growth. Colonies will grow on blood (β-hemolytic) and chocolate, but not MacConkey agar after 2 days.

Clinical Manifestations and Pathogenesis
K. kingae is the most pathogenic of the three species. It is a member of the HACEK group, causing a indolent, slowly progressive endocarditis. In addition, it is associated with septic arthritis/osteomyelitis, usually in children, and septicemia.

Laboratory Diagnosis
K. kingae is oxidase-positive and produces acid from glucose, although in delayed fashion. Indole and catalase are negative.

Antimicrobial susceptibility
K. kingae is susceptible to penicillin and most other antibiotics to which other members of the HACEK group are susceptible.

Miscellaneous Gram-Negative Bacilli

Legionella
Characteristics
Legionella spp. are non-spore-forming, faintly staining, thin, Gram-negative bacilli. *Legionella* spp. were first recognized to cause human disease during an epidemic of pneumonia that occurred among members of the Pennsylvania American Legion who had gathered in Philadelphia to celebrate the 1976 bicentennial. There are now over 20 named species and a number of unnamed species. The majority of clinical cases have been due to *Legionella pneumophila*, serogroup 1. Figure 56–22 demonstrates the excellent staining of *Legionella* spp with a Dieterle silver stain.

Clinical Manifestations and Pathogenesis
Legionella spp. are found in the environment in association with water. Growth within environmental protozoa is thought to be an important factor for survival of the organism in the environment. Transmission to humans occurs through exposure to contaminated water (e.g., through faucets, shower heads, or public fountains). Human-to-human infection or laboratory-acquired infections are not known to occur.

Infections can be subclinical, pulmonary, or extrapulmonary. Infection is usually manifested as an acute, fibrinopurulent pneumonia with lobular distribution. Histologically, there is an alveolar infiltrate of neutrophils and macrophages, accompanied by fibrin and red blood cell extravasation. *Legionella* spp. may be found within alveolar macrophages. Figure 56–23 is the Gram stain of sputum of a patient with *L. pneumophila* pneumonia. *L. pneumophila* has also been isolated from cultures of blood.

Laboratory Diagnosis
Legionella spp. may be isolated on BCYE agar supplemented with growth factors, including L-cystine, ferric salt, and α-ketoglutarate. This medium may be made selective for culture of nonsterile body sites by the addition

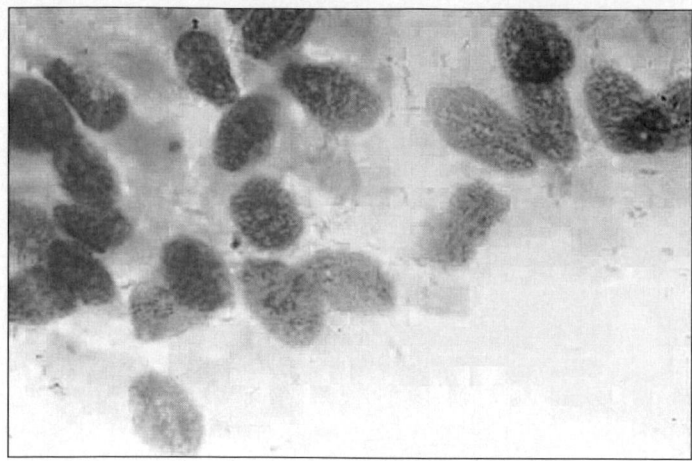

Figure 56–23 *Legionella pneumophila* faintly staining negative with Gram stain of pulmonary infiltrate.

Figure 56–24 Gram stain of culture of *Legionella pneumophila*.

of cefamandole, polymyxin B, and anisomycin or polymyxin B, anisomycin, and vancomycin (Edelstein, 1987). Chocolate agar may also support the growth of legionellae. Treatment of sputum with a weak acid (0.2 M HCl/KCl pH 2.2) for 4 minutes or heat (60°C) for 2 minutes may help to reduce contamination from other organisms but will reduce the number of legionellas as well.

Inoculated media should be incubated for 5 days in a humid atmosphere containing no more than 2–5% CO_2. Colonies will often appear iridescent and have a sticky consistency. Isolates with the typical Gram's stain morphology should be subcultured to blood agar, where no growth will be observed. These organisms may be weakly oxidase- and catalase-positive, will be gelatinase-positive, and often motile. The identification of this organism is most accurately achieved using type-specific antibody assays. Figure 56–24 is a Gram stain of *L. pneumophila* from culture.

Legionella spp. may be detected or identified by direct fluorescent antibody (DFA) staining of specimens or colonies in cultures. The sensitivity of the DFA examination of respiratory specimens has ranged from 25–75% but is considerably higher in open lung biopsies. However, use of this test has decreased due to the availability of more sensitive tests, e.g., the urine antigen assay and/or direct PCR methods. Cross-reactions in the DFA assays have been reported between *L. pneumophila* and other *Legionella* spp., as well as with some strains of *Bordetella pertussis*, *Pseudomonas fluorescens*, and *Bacteroides fragilis*. Sensitivity of DFA for detection of other species in sputum is not known (Edelstein, 1987).

The urine antigen test for *L. pneumophila* serogroup 1 has a reported sensitivity of 80–90%, although it should be noted that antigenuria may persist for many months following infection. Use of the urinary antigen test in and out of the ICU has been shown to have a positive impact on patient case. (Edelstein, 1987; Garbino, 2004; Sopena, 2005).

The diagnosis of legionellosis can also be established serologically by detecting a fourfold or greater rise in antibody titer to at least 1:128. A single antibody titer of 1:256 is presumptive evidence of past infection. The sensitivity of serologic diagnosis for disease caused by species other

than *L. pneumophila* serogroup 1 is not known, and specificity of antibody tests for disease caused by other species is less than that of *L. pneumophila* serogroup 1 (Edelstein, 1987). PCR assays for direct detection of *Legionella* sp. in clinical specimens and for sequencing identification of cultured isolates have been developed. Sensitivities of 64–100%, and specificities of 88–100% have been reported (Stout, 2003). Use of these assays can provide more rapid results especially when used in direct specimen testing; in addition, identification of species other than *L. pneumophila*, which is the problem with DFA and serology, could increase the demand for such assays.

Antimicrobial Susceptibility

Because of the intracellular nature of *Legionella* sp. in clinical infections, in vitro susceptibility test results do not predict the clinical response of antibiotics. Susceptibility testing should not be performed. Therapy generally consists of erythromycin and rifampin. Other agents that have been used include trimethoprim–sulfamethoxazole, quinolones, clarithromycin, and azithromycin.

Bordetella

Characteristics

Bordetellas are strictly aerobic, nonfermentative, minute coccobacilli requiring nicotinic acid, cysteine, and usually methionine but not X or V factor for growth. Phase variation from smooth virulent strains to rough avirulent strains occurs after cultivation on artificial media.

Clinical Manifestations and Pathogenesis

Bordetella spp. are found in the respiratory tracts of warm-blooded animals. *Bordetella bronchiseptica* primarily causes kennel cough in dogs, although it may rarely cause pertussis-like symptoms in immuno-compromised human hosts. *Bordetella parapertussis*, which infects both humans and lambs, is an uncommon human pathogen. Infection may be asymptomatic or may cause a pertussis-like illness, or most frequently bronchitis. *B. pertussis*, the etiologic agent of whooping cough, only causes disease in humans.

B. pertussis, *B. parapertussis*, and *B. bronchiseptica* produce a number of virulence factors. Adenylate cyclase toxin inhibits immune effector and other cell functions by creating a high intracellular level of cyclic adenosine 3',5'-phosphate. Tracheal cytotoxin causes cell ciliostasis and cell death. Filamentous hemagglutinin, pertactin, and fimbras are involved in adhesion. *B. pertussis* also uniquely produces pertussis toxin, which inhibits intracellular signal transduction factors by transferring adenosine diphosphate ribose to G proteins of cells.

It is thought that, in a pertussis infection, the organism first attaches to the ciliated epithelium of the respiratory tract and immune effector cells by means of the fimbras, filamentous hemagglutinin, pertussis toxin, and pertactin. Pertussis toxin and adenylate cyclase toxin work together to inhibit the host's immune system and the tracheal cytotoxin damages the respiratory epithelium. As a result, there is inflammation and epithelial necrosis; leukocytosis and lymphocytosis; accumulation of secretions; cough; and ultimately bronchopneumonia, hypoxic episodes, and encephalopathy.

B. pertussis contains a protective antigen that when combined with antibody abolishes its infectivity. It appears, however, that both cellular and humoral immunity are needed to eradicate the organism.

Laboratory Diagnosis

The rate of isolation of *B. pertussis* from patients declines with the duration of illness. The most commonly recommended specimen is the nasopharyngeal swab; however, nasopharyngeal aspirates collected with a soft rubber catheter have provided higher rates of isolation in some people's hands. A more invasive specimen such as fluid collected by bronchoalveolar lavage may also be cultured. In general, swabs or aspirates should be inoculated on to suitable media, such as Regan–Lowe agar, at the patient's bedside. For shipment to reference laboratories, the inoculated medium should be incubated for at least 24 hours prior to transport to allow some initial growth of the organism.

Direct examination of smears stained with fluorescein-conjugated *B. pertussis* monoclonal or polyclonal antiserum may provide a rapid diagnosis. Because the sensitivity of the DFA is low, culture also must be performed to rule out a false-negative DFA result. False-positive DFA reactions can occur, especially when a polyclonal antibody is used. Direct detection of *B. pertussis* in clinical specimens by means of PCR is quickly replacing the DFA in many laboratories and is rapidly becoming the primary method for detection of *B. pertussis*. Commercial products are available; these should enhance the reproducibility of results between laboratories (Khanna, 2005). PCR test results, however, may remain positive longer than results with culture or DFA, even with appropriate antimicrobial therapy. PCR methods for the direct detection of *B. parapertussis* in clinical specimens are also available (Dragsted, 2004).

Cultures, when done, should be incubated in a humid environment at 35°C without addition of CO_2. *B. pertussis* grows slowly and colonies may not be visible for 3–4 days. Cultures should be held for 7–12 days before being discarded as negative. Colonies of *B. pertussis* are small, smooth, round, and shiny and may have the appearance of a drop of mercury. Organisms with the typical colony morphology and Gram's stain appearance should be subcultured to blood agar to verify the absence of growth on this medium. Positive catalase and oxidase reactions and negative urease can be used for presumptive identification of an organism as *B. pertussis*. *B. parapertussis* grows more rapidly and will grow on blood agar and occasionally on MacConkey agar. Colonies are oxidase-negative and catalase- and urease-positive. *B. bronchiseptica* grows well on both blood and MacConkey agars and is the most biochemically active of the three. It is catalase-, oxidase-, urease-, and nitrate-reduction-positive.

Antimicrobial Susceptibility
Antimicrobial agents probably play no role in the therapy of pertussis but nasopharyngeal cultures become negative after 1–2 days of treatment, which may prevent bacterial complications in patients with the disease and may be effective in preventing spread of the disease to nonimmune contacts. Susceptibility testing is not indicated for *B. pertussis*. Erythromycin is the drug of choice for treatment and prophylaxis; trimethoprim–sulfamethoxazole is an acceptable alternative.

Brucella spp.
Characteristics
Brucellas are small, Gram-negative coccobacillary organisms (0.5–0.7 µm × 0.6–1.5 µm). In smears, they occur singly, in pairs, or in short chains and have been described as having the appearance of sand. They are nonmotile, strictly aerobic, and catalase- and usually oxidase-positive organisms. Growth in the laboratory is often enhanced by the presence of 5–10% CO_2 and requires complex media, which is improved by the addition of blood or serum. Of the recognized species, *Brucella melitensis*, *Brucella abortus*, *Brucella suis*, and *Brucella canis* are human pathogens.

Clinical Manifestations and Pathogenesis
Brucella spp. are intracellular parasites that infect a wide range of animal species (including humans) and have also been found in some insects and ticks. They are important veterinary and human pathogens. The preferential hosts are sheep and goats for *B. melitensis*, cattle for *B. abortus*, swine for *B. suis*, and dogs for *B. canis*; however, each species may occasionally infect other animals. Humans become infected by inhaling the organism; by direct contact with infected material, including animal carcasses, fetal membranes, vaginal discharge, fetuses, skin, or mucous membranes; or by ingestion of unpasteurized milk or milk products from infected animals. There are approximately 100 cases of human brucellosis reported per year in the United States. A common risk factor is consumption of imported cheese made from unpasteurized goat's milk.

Local lymphadenopathy often occurs with dissemination and secondary localization in the reticuloendothelial system and formation of granulomas in the liver, spleen, bone, genitourinary tract, lungs, and soft tissues. Organisms may be seen within phagocytes. Signs and symptoms are often variable and nonspecific, with chills, fever, sweats, and anorexia occurring frequently. The fever is characteristically diurnal ('undulant').

Laboratory Diagnosis
Brucella spp. are most often recovered from blood and bone marrow and less often from material obtained from spleen and liver abscesses. The organism grows on standard laboratory media including *Brucella*, blood, chocolate, and trypticase soy agar. Some strains will grow on MacConkey agar. *Brucella* spp. will grow in media used for culturing blood specimens. Many references recommend incubating blood cultures for at least 21 days with blind subculture performed early and late in the incubation period; however, these recommendations may not be necessary with newer automated blood culture systems, some of which have been shown to reliably recover *Brucella* spp. in 5 days or less without blind subculture (Bannatyne, 1997; Yagupsky, 1997). *Brucella* spp. are recognized as Class A bioterrorism organisms and as such should only be handled in public health laboratories and/or the CDC. The identification and testing of this organism are described here for completeness but should not be performed in sentinel labs, which includes most hospital laboratories.

Solid media should be incubated in an atmosphere containing 5–10% CO_2. These organisms grow slowly and even after 48 hours of incubation colonies may be difficult to see. Organisms can be presumptively identified as *Brucella* spp. based on a characteristic Gram-stain appearance and positive catalase, oxidase, and urease results. Urease activity is manifested rapidly (about 15 minutes) by *B. suis* and more slowly (2–24 hours) by *B. melitensis* and *B. abortus*. Because brucellosis can be laboratory acquired, the laboratory personnel should be notified if this organism is suspected, and all manipulations of possible *Brucella* spp. should be conducted in a biological safety cabinet.

Identification of *Brucella* spp. to the species level requires tests for CO_2 requirement, H_2S production, urea hydrolysis, dye sensitivity, and phage sensitivity. Most hospital laboratories refer this testing to the State Health Departments or other reference laboratories. Use of molecular tools, such as PCR will probably become more effective means of detecting cases of brucellosis in the future (Queipo-Ortuno, 2005).

The diagnosis of brucellosis can be made serologically. A minimum titer of 1:160 in a standard tube agglutination test is suggestive of the diagnosis; however, evidence of recent brucellosis can be accepted only when a fourfold or greater rise in titer occurs during the first month or two of illness. Prozone effect can occur in patients with titers as high as 1:640 so that all sera from patients with suspected disease should be diluted to at least 1:1280. Crossreactivity with *Francisella tularensis* and with *V. cholerae*, including cholera vaccination, occurs.

Antimicrobial Susceptibility
Treatment consists of combinations of tetracycline, aminoglycosides, rifampin, and trimethoprim–sulfamethoxazole for prolonged periods of time. Although treatment failures do occur, they are not due to antimicrobial resistance and susceptibility testing is not recommended.

Pasteurella
Characteristics
The pasteurellas are facultatively anaerobic, oxidase- and catalase-positive, nonmotile, Gram-negative bacteria that range morphologically from coccobacilli to long filamentous rods. Of the eight species known to infect humans (*Pasteurella multocida*, *Pasteurella bettyae*, *Pasteurella canis*, *Pasteurella dagmatis*, *Pasteurella stomatis*, *Pasteurella pneumotropica*, *Pasteurella haemolytica*, *Pasteurella aerogenes*), *P. multocida* is the most important human pathogen. *Pasteurella* spp. are phenotypically similar to the *Actinobacillus* spp. and DNA–DNA hybridization studies and comparisons of the 16S rRNA have shown that *P. pneumotropica*, *P. haemolytica*, and *P. aerogenes* are more closely related to the genus *Actinobacillus* than to the genus *Pasteurella*.

Clinical Manifestations and Pathogenesis
Pasteurella spp., especially *P. multocida*, are found as commensals in the upper respiratory tract of fowl and mammals and are frequently isolated from animal bite or scratch wounds. Cat bites more often become infected than dog bites. Local infections can become systemic, and there have been a number of reports of septicemia, osteomyelitis, and meningitis. Pasteurellae have been associated with respiratory tract infections, including sinusitis, peritonsillar abscess, mastoiditis, pulmonary abscess, pneumonia, empyema, bronchitis, and bronchiectasis, usually in patients with chronic pulmonary disease.

Laboratory Diagnosis
Pasteurellae grow well on blood agar and are only rarely able to grow on Gram-negative differential media, such as EMB or MacConkey agar. The finding of a Gram-negative bacillus that grows on blood agar only and is oxidase- and indole-positive and ONPG-negative provides strong presumptive evidence for the isolation of *P. multocida*, the most frequently encountered species. In addition, susceptibility to penicillin, as evidenced by a wide zone of inhibition around a penicillin disk on a blood agar plate is good evidence that the isolate is *P. multocida*.

Antimicrobial Susceptibility
Resistance to antimicrobial agents is rarely seen in human isolates. Pasteurellas are usually susceptible to penicillin and tetracycline and many other antibiotics. Penicillin is the therapeutic drug of choice.

Francisella
Characteristics
F. tularensis is a very small, strictly aerobic, coccoid to pleomorphic rod-shaped, Gram-negative bacillus that requires cystine or cysteine for growth. Faint bipolar staining occurs with aniline dyes.

Clinical Manifestations and Pathogenesis
F. tularensis is found in both wild and domesticated animals, birds, arthropods, water, mud, and animal feces. The primary reservoir for this organism is the cottontail rabbit. Transmission to humans occurs through

VII

tick bite, direct cutaneous inoculation from an infected animal, conjunctival inoculation, inhalation, or ingestion of undercoocked infected animal meat or contaminated water. Several forms of the disease occur, including ulceroglandular, glandular, oculoglandular, oropharyngeal, intestinal, pneumonic, and typhoidal. Approximately 100–200 cases of tularemia are reported each year in the United States. *F. tularensis* is considered to be one of the class A agents of bioterrorism, and because of this, work-up of suspected cases is limited to approved laboratories. Most clinical laboratories are considered sentinel laboratories and, if *F. tularensis* is suspected, isolates should be sent to state health departments or other selected laboratories.

Tularemia manifests after an incubation period of 1–10 days in various forms. Headache, fever, chills, vomiting, and myalgias characteristically occur at the onset. In ulceroglandular disease, lymphadenitis and lymphadenopathy occur in the region draining the primary lesion. The lesion is initially papular and later ulcerative. Oculoglandular disease is characterized by inflammation of the conjunctiva and usually a papule of the lower lid with lymphadenitis of the preauricular, parotid, submaxillary, and anterior cervical nodes. The intestinal form of tularemia is characterized by ulcerative lesions of the mouth, throat, and upper gastrointestinal tract.

Virulence appears to be related to a smooth colonial morphology. Repeated subcultures result in an alteration from smooth to rough colonies, with a concomitant loss of virulence. Highly virulent strains for humans have citrulline ureidase activity and ferment glycerol, and are most often associated with tick-borne disease in rabbits. Toxins have not been recognized.

Tularemia should be suspected in anyone who has been in an endemic area, has had contact with wild animals or livestock, has a history of tick bite, has been engaged in farming operations, has drunk impure water, or has been exposed to cultures or infected animals in the laboratory. Trappers, hunters, fur and meat industry workers, agricultural workers, and laboratory personnel are at greatest risk. Because of its protean manifestations, tularemia is readily confused with many other diseases, such as brucellosis, anthrax, sporotrichosis, typhoid fever, tuberculosis, histoplasmosis, and syphilis.

Laboratory Diagnosis

Material suitable for examination includes fluid or curettings from the primary lesion, aspirates of enlarged regional nodes, sputum, pharyngeal washes, and gastric aspirates. Bacterial isolation is difficult because the organism has special growth requirements and grows slowly, allowing for overgrowth by other organisms present in the specimen. The organism grows on glucose–cysteine agar supplemented with 5% defibrinated rabbit blood, chocolate agar with IsoVitalX, or BCYE agar. Some isolates may even grow on blood agar or trypticase soy agar. If the clinical material is contaminated with other organisms, penicillin, polymyxin B, and cycloheximide can be added to inhibit their growth. Special care must be exercised in handling infected material to prevent aerosolization or direct contact with the skin. Clinicians should always notify laboratory personnel if *F. tularensis* is suspected so that the proper precautions can be taken to prevent exposure to this organism.

Cultures are incubated at 35°C with or without added CO_2. Colonies usually appear within 2–4 days, and are blue-gray to white, round, smooth, and slightly mucoid. On blood-containing agar, a small zone of α-hemolysis may be seen. Because working with the organism in the laboratory is dangerous, suspected isolates should be sent to a reference laboratory such as the CDC for confirmation with a slide agglutination or direct fluorescent antibody test.

The diagnosis of *F. tularensis* can be established serologically. Agglutination titers as low as 1:40 in the absence of previous disease are diagnostic and may rise within the first 3 weeks to levels of 1:640 or greater. *Brucella* agglutinins may also rise nonspecifically, but usually to a considerably lower level (Johansson, 2004).

Antimicrobial Susceptibility

Streptomycin is bactericidal, while the tetracyclines and chloramphenicol are bacteriostatic to *F. tularensis*. Because relapses may occur after treatment with bacteriostatic agents, streptomycin is the agent of choice.

Gardnerella
Characteristics

Gardnerella vaginalis is a thin, Gram-variable rod or coccobacillus. Over the years this organism, in its association with bacterial vaginosis, has been called *Haemophilus vaginalis* and *Corynebacterium vaginale*, further demonstrating its Gram variable appearance. Catalase is not produced and cells are nonmotile. Growth is best observed after 48 hours of incubation

in a 5% CO_2-enriched atmosphere. Colonies are small and exhibit β-hemolysis on media containing rabbit or human blood.

Clinical Manifestations and Pathogenesis

This organism is associated with bacterial vaginosis but is not the cause. It has been found in the blood of patients with postpartum fever and can also cause infections in newborns. *G. vaginalis* is a part of the anorectal flora of healthy adults of both sexes, as well as of children. It is part of the endogenous vaginal flora of women of reproductive age.

Laboratory Diagnosis

Diagnosis of bacterial vaginosis does not require culture. The diagnosis is made by direct examination of vaginal secretions for the presence of clue cells (epithelial cells covered with bacteria on the cell margins), small Gram-negative rods and coccobacilli, the absence of lactobacilli (Gram-positive thin rods), a pH greater than 4.5, and a fishy amine odor after addition of 10% potassium hydroxide (KOH) to the secretions. A scored Gram stain is the laboratory test that should be performed when vaginal discharge is submitted for the diagnosis of bacterial vaginosis (Nugent, 1991). Alternatively, there is a nucleic acid probe (Affirm, Becton Dickinson Microbiology Systems, Sparks, MD) that tests for a high concentration of *G. vaginalis* as a marker for bacterial vaginosis (Briselden, 1994)When observed in culture the organism is presumptively identified based on hemolysis on human blood bilayer Tween agar after 48 hours of incubation.

Antimicrobial Susceptibility.

Susceptibility testing of *G. vaginalis* is not recommended, and no guidelines exist for performing this testing. Metronidazole is the drug of choice for bacterial vaginosis. Systemic infections due to *G. vaginalis* may be treated with ampicillin because this organism has not been found to produce β-lactamase.

Capnocytophaga

Capnocytophaga is a genus of Gram-negative, facultatively anaerobic, Gram-negative rods to filamentous bacteria. Species include *Capnocytophaga ochraceus*, *Capnocytophaga canimorsus* (formerly DF-2), *Capnocytophaga gingivalis*, and *Capnocytophaga sputigena* among others. *C. canimorsus* is part of the oral flora of dogs and cats; the others can be found as part of the normal human oral flora.

Clinical manifestations and pathogenesis

C. ochraceus can cause transient bacteremia or endocarditis in immuno-compromised and immunocompetent patients (Parenti, 1985). It also has been associated with periodontitis. *C. canimorsus* is a cause of a fatal septicemia following wound infections subsequent to the bite of dogs or cats. Patients with this fatal septicemia have predisposing factors of a prior splenectomy or alcoholism (Lion, 1996). Meningitis, endocarditis, arthritis and eye infections have also been documented with *C. canimorsus*. Figure 56–25 is a Wright' s stain of *C. canimorsus* seen in a blood film of patient with *C. canimorsus* septicemia. Note the intracellular nature of the bacilli.

Isolation of *Capnocytophaga* spp. requires inoculation of blood or chocolate agar and incubation in a 5–10% CO_2 environment, generally for more than 24 hours. Colonies are usually slightly pigmented yellow or orange and may spread because of a 'sliding' motility. Gram stains often show long, thin, spindle shaped cells, almost fusiform in appearance. Figure 56–26

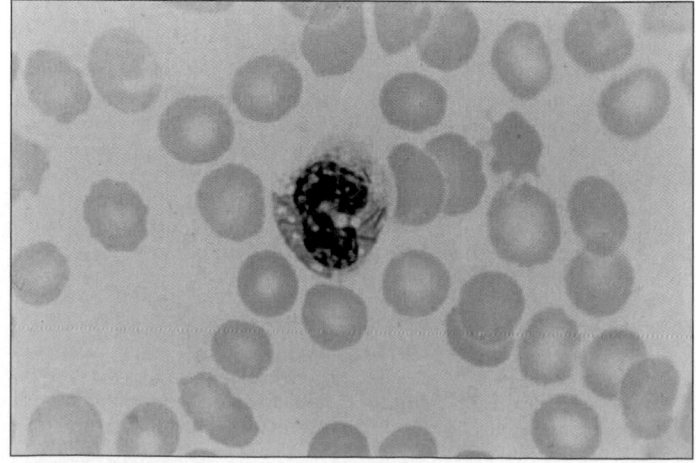

Figure 56–25 Blood smear positive for *Capnocytophaga canimorsus* in patient with septicemia (Wright's stain).

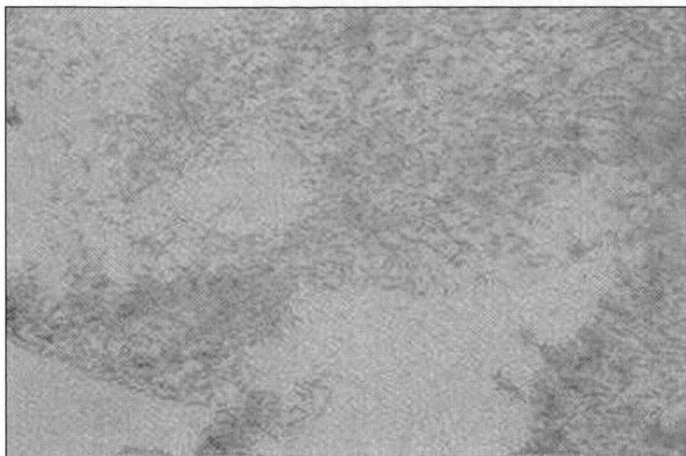

Figure 56–26 Gram stain of *Capnocytophaga ochraceus.* Note the fusiform bacilli.

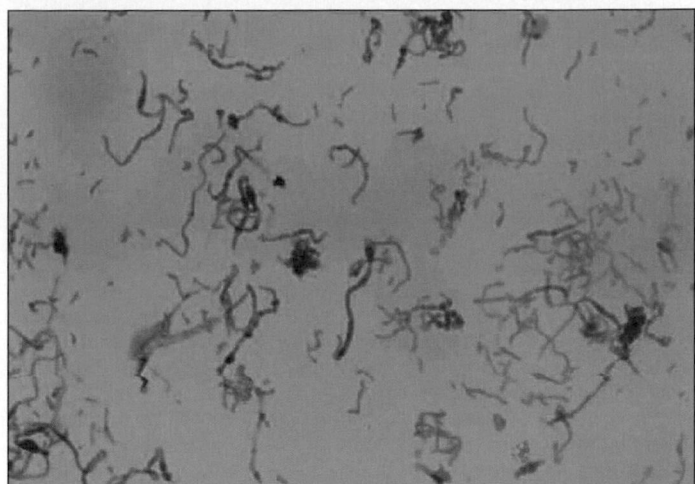

Figure 56–27 Gram stain of *Streptobacillus moniliforme* from culture. (Courtesy of Dr Nancy Cornish.)

shows the Gram stain of *C. ochraceus,* demonstrating the fusiform bacilli. *C. ochraceus* is oxidase- and catalase-negative; *C. canimorsus* is oxidase- and catalase-positive. *Capnocytophaga* spp. are usually susceptible to many antibiotics, including β-lactams, macrolides, tetracycline, clindamycin, and quinolones. They are resistant to the aminoglycosides. There have been occasional β-lactamases described in this genus, although response to the β-lactam/β-lactamase inhibitor combinations has been good (Jolivet-Gougeon, 2000).

Calymmatobacterium
Characteristics
Calymmatobacterium granulomatis is a Gram-negative, nonmotile, encapsulated, pleomorphic rod that may be cultured in yolk sacs or on fresh egg yolk medium. The organism possesses antigenic determinants similar to those of *Klebsiella* spp., leading some experts to classify it among the Enterobacteriaceae.

Clinical Manifestations and Pathogenesis
The organism does not produce disease in animals. In humans, it causes granuloma inguinale (donovanosis), characterized by ulcerogranulomatous lesions of the skin and mucosa of the genital and inguinal areas.

Laboratory Diagnosis
A fragment of tissue removed from the margin of an ulcer is pressed and rubbed against a glass slide and stained with Wright's or Giemsa stain. The finding of small, straight or curved, pleomorphic rods with rounded ends and characteristic polar granules, giving a 'safety pin' appearance within mononuclear cells, is the most effective way of establishing the diagnosis.

Antimicrobial Susceptibility
The tetracyclines, erythromycin, ampicillin, and chloramphenicol are active against *C. granulomatis.* Resistance may develop to streptomycin.

Streptobacillus
Characteristics
Streptobacillus is a facultatively anaerobic, fermentative, nonencapsulated, and nonmotile Gram-negative rod, frequently occurring in chains or long filaments, and often with a series of oval to elongated bulbous swellings, giving a string-of-beads appearance. The microscopic morphology varies with time, being more homogeneously filamentous in young cultures and becoming fragmented into irregular coccobacilli with age. L-phase organisms having a 'fried egg' appearance may occur spontaneously on agar and become stabilized if penicillin is incorporated in the medium. Figure 56–27 is a smear of *Streptobacillus moniliformis* from culture of patient with rat-bite fever.

Clinical Manifestations and Pathogenesis
S. moniliformis occurs as indigenous flora in the upper respiratory tract of wild and laboratory rodents. Infection (rat bite fever or Haverhill disease) in humans follows rodent bites, ingestion of contaminated food, or traumatic injury. Local lymphangitis and lymphadenitis may develop up to 3 weeks later, followed by fever, chills, malaise, and later a general morbilliform maculopapular or petechial rash. Some patients develop a migratory polyarthritis. Endocarditis has been reported. The histopathology is nonspecific chronic inflammation.

Laboratory Diagnosis
The organism grows on heart infusion agar supplemented with heat-inactivated horse serum and yeast extract. Inoculated media should be incubated at 35°C in a humid environment containing an atmosphere of 10% CO_2.

Colonies in broth form as fluff balls, while those on agar are small and slightly translucent to opaque with a slightly irregular edge. L-phase variants may form on agar. Because this organism is relatively inert, identification of *S. moniliformis* is complex. Biochemical tests must be performed in heart infusion agar or broth supplemented with yeast extract and horse serum.

Antimicrobial Susceptibility
S. moniliformis is susceptible to penicillin; however, aminoglycosides or tetracycline must also be used to treat L-forms.

Prevention and Control
Because 10–65% of rats are infected with the organism, their control and precautions against bites represent the only effective methods of control of the disease.

Anaerobic Bacteria

It is important to re-emphasize that anaerobes represent a major component of the indigenous flora of the skin and mucous membranes; therefore, their isolation and identification is contingent on the proper selection and collection of specimens, as well as on their proper transport to the laboratory. Anaerobic infections are frequently mixed, consisting of several species of anaerobes or of anaerobes with facultatively anaerobic bacteria; therefore, the first task in examining an anaerobic culture is to separate facultatively anaerobic from obligate anaerobic bacteria. With experience, the more commonly isolated anaerobes can often be recognized on the basis of their colonial and microscopic morphologies and presumptively identified on the basis of a few additional tests. Definitive identification is based on biochemical reactions, physiologic and genetic characteristics, and pathogenicity and toxin neutralization tests.

The extent to which anaerobes are identified varies according to the facilities and expertise available, the interest of the laboratory personnel and clinical staff, and the clinical utility of the information available from the laboratory.

Definitions and Characteristics
An anaerobe requires an atmosphere with reduced oxygen tension for its growth and fails to grow on the surface of solid media in an atmosphere of room air with 10% CO_2. A facultatively anaerobic bacterium will grow in either the presence or absence of room air. The term *microaerophile* has not been strictly defined but is commonly applied to bacteria, usually campylobacters and streptococci, that grow only or preferentially in an atmosphere with reduced O_2 and with increased CO_2.

Pathogenesis and Virulence Factors
Little is known about the factors responsible for the pathogenic and virulence properties of most anaerobes other than the clostridia. Endotoxic, proteolytic, and heparinase activities have been identified among the Bacteroidaceae. The polysaccharide capsule of *B. fragilis* promotes abscess

VII

formation. The clostridia, on the other hand, elaborate potent exotoxins, including lethal and necrotizing toxins, hemolysins, lecithinases, gelatinases, and hyaluronidases.

While clostridial infection may be either exogenous or endogenous in origin, disease caused by other anaerobes usually originates endogenously from the normal indigenous anaerobic flora of a contiguous mucous membrane, the integrity of which has been disrupted by surgery, instrumentation, trauma, or malignancy. Essential to the establishment of anaerobes in the infectious process is a decrease in the oxidation-reduction potential (E_h) of the area, which may result from a failure of its blood supply or from the multiplication of other bacteria at the site.

Although clostridial infections and intoxications are unquestionably of major medical importance, the role of other anaerobes in causing cellulitis and myonecrosis has been recognized only relatively recently. Most isolates of Clostridium perfringens are the result of simple contamination of a wound. In such instances, the clostridia may multiply in cellular debris, a hematoma, or necrotic tissue without observable clinical symptomatology. Anaerobic cellulitis is a necrotizing process of the soft tissues. Its onset is gradual but it can progress rapidly and extensively. Gas is produced; however, the process typically does not involve muscle. In addition to or instead of clostridia, the bacteriology of anaerobic cellulitis may involve anaerobic cocci and anaerobic Gram-negative bacilli.

In contrast to anaerobic cellulitis, gas gangrene or clostridial myonecrosis is an acute and rapidly progressive invasive process producing marked changes in muscles. Distinguishing between anaerobic cellulitis and gas gangrene is critical in order to avoid performing unnecessarily aggressive and mutilating surgery in the former condition.

The histotoxic clostridia associated with gas gangrene include C. perfringens, Clostridium novyi, Clostridium septicum, Clostridium histolyticum, Clostridium sporogenes, and Clostridium bifermentans. While C. perfringens has been the species most frequently involved in gas gangrene, the prevalence of the other species in this process has varied widely.

Tetanus and botulism are described as intoxications rather than infections because their manifestations are related to the elaboration of potent neurotoxins. Botulism is most frequently due to the ingestion of home-processed foods that have been improperly preserved or canned; however, sporadic outbreaks of the disease have been associated with commercially processed food and with wounds infected with the organism. The incubation period for botulism is short: signs and symptoms usually occur between 18 and 36 hours following ingestion of contaminated food. Of the seven antigenic types of botulinum toxin known, type A is the most common in cases of food poisoning in North America, followed by types B, E, and F. The toxin is absorbed from the intestinal tract and, rarely, from an infected wound and ultimately attaches to motor nerve terminals, thereby preventing acetylcholine release at the nerve endings.

Tetanus typically occurs in nonimmunized persons within the first 2 weeks following a traumatically acquired puncture, laceration, or abrasion. Cases have been reported to occur postoperatively; following dental work, childbirth, and abortion; or in association with stasis and decubitus ulcers. The toxin, tetanospasmin, is transported to gangliosides in the CNS via the lymphatics and bloodstream, and by migration through the perineural spaces of peripheral nerves.

Clostridium difficile is the major cause of nosocomial diarrhea and the primary pathogen responsible for pseudomembranous colitis. It is a rare cause of abscesses, wound infections, osteomyelitis, pleuritis, peritonitis, septicemia, and urogenital tract infections. Carriage rates of C. difficile and its toxins are high (50% or more) in neonates, but disease is rare (Bartlett, 1997). Colonization, with or without toxin production, may be maintained for several months; but when the adult flora becomes established at 6–12 months of age, colonization rates fall and only about 3% of normal healthy adults are colonized with the organism. C. difficile almost always is acquired in the hospital by persons receiving antimicrobial agents via direct or indirect exposure to human or inanimate reservoirs. Although the penicillins and cephalosporins are implicated most frequently, any antimicrobial agent may trigger C. difficile-associated disease. Disease rarely occurs without antibiotic exposure but cases have been reported following therapy with antineoplastic agents that have antibacterial activity. Pseudomembranous colitis is a toxin-mediated illness in which microbial invasion of the mucosa is not known to occur. C. difficile produces two toxins. Toxin A, a weakly cytopathic toxin, is predominantly responsible for the enterotoxic activity of the organism. Toxin B, a potent cytotoxin, appears to play a minor role in human disease, although toxin-A-negative, B-positive strains have been isolated from symptomatic patients (Johnson, 1998). Use of a PCR assay in the laboratory for detection of both toxin A and toxin B may increase the sensitivity (Lemee, 2004).

As previously mentioned, other anaerobic bacteria, particularly the anaerobic cocci and Gram-negative bacilli, have been associated with

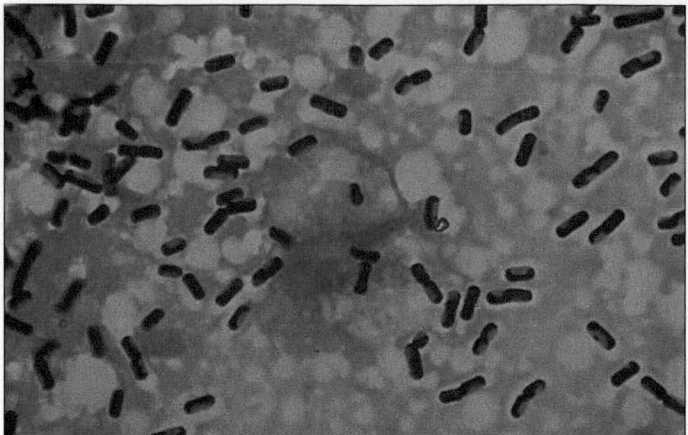

Figure 56–28 Gram stain of a smear of exudate from a wound that had gas bubbles shows large, boxcar-shaped, Gram-positive bacilli, suggestive of clostridial disease (oil immersion).

anaerobic cellulitis in addition to or instead of the histotoxic clostridial species. These organisms are part of the indigenous flora of the mucous membranes of the oral cavity and of the gastrointestinal and genitourinary tracts. As such, they are encountered in aspiration pneumonias, lung abscesses, empyemas, intra-abdominal infections and abscesses, pelvic abscesses, brain abscesses, and bacteremias. Anaerobic intra-abdominal infections commonly follow abdominal and especially colon surgery, and are most frequently associated with the B. fragilis group. Clinically significant anaerobic bacteremias are also most frequently caused by this species.

Laboratory Diagnosis

Identifying anaerobic bacteria to the species level can be quite complex; however, the extent to which isolates of anaerobic bacteria are identified varies widely and may be limited to basic information that is of clinical utility. For example, the mixed anaerobic flora from a site such as a decubitus ulcer, perirectal fistula, or intra-abdominal abscess may simply be reported as mixed fecal flora without specific identification of its components. Determining the species of an isolate may be limited to those present in pure culture from a normally sterile body fluid or site and can be readily accomplished by any one of several commercially available biochemical assay-containing kits or using gas–liquid chromatography. One should understand that the clinical value of any report of the presence of anaerobic bacteria is directly related to the speed of reporting such results from the laboratory. Identification procedures that require 1–2 weeks to complete are generally of academic interest only.

Because of their rapid progression and considerable morbidity and mortality, the initial diagnosis and management of diseases caused by the clostridia must be based on their clinical presentation and manifestations. In some patients with tetanus, no primary wound is evident. When a wound is present, organisms typical of C. tetani are seldom seen in stained smears, even though they may be recovered from cultures. Moreover, because of this organism's widespread distribution in nature, its isolation from a wound is not necessarily indicative of the diagnosis of tetanus. Laboratory confirmation of botulism requires detection of the toxin in serum, wounds, gastric contents, feces, or the food suspected of causing the disease. Procedures for extracting the toxin and for performing mouse neutralization tests are complex; therefore, it is suggested that the appropriate materials be referred to the CDC for examination. Telephone consultation should be made in such instances to ensure that the requisite specimens are properly collected and transported and that the appropriate authorities are alerted.

In cases of suspected anaerobic cellulitis or gas gangrene, the laboratory can be helpful by examining exudate or tissue microscopically. The finding of numerous, large, 'boxcar'-shaped, Gram-positive bacilli (Fig. 56–28) provides presumptive confirmation of the diagnosis. Stained smears may also be diagnostic of anaerobic streptococcal myositis. Cultures of exudate, tissue, and blood should also be performed. Once again, the level or extent of identification varies considerably among laboratories; however, C. perfringens may be easily identified by its Gram's-stained morphology, the production of double zones of hemolysis on blood agar, and a positive Nagler's reaction on egg yolk agar. Laboratory diagnosis of C. difficile diarrhea is most rapidly accomplished by detecting the toxin directly in stool using an EIA or cell culture assay. Alternatively, C. difficile recovered

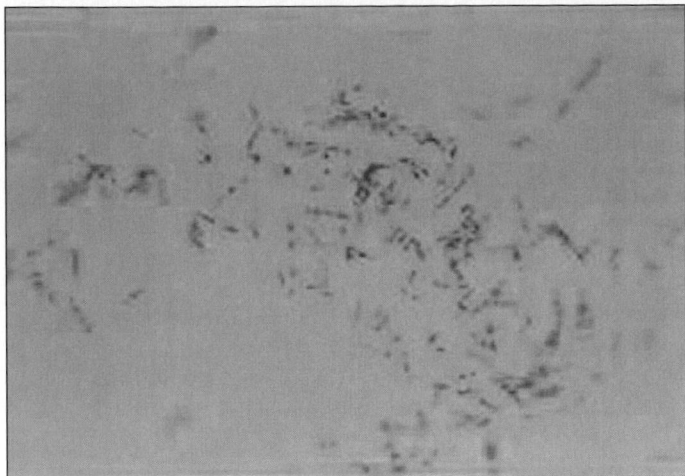

Figure 56–29 Gram stain of *Bacteroides fragilis* from broth culture.

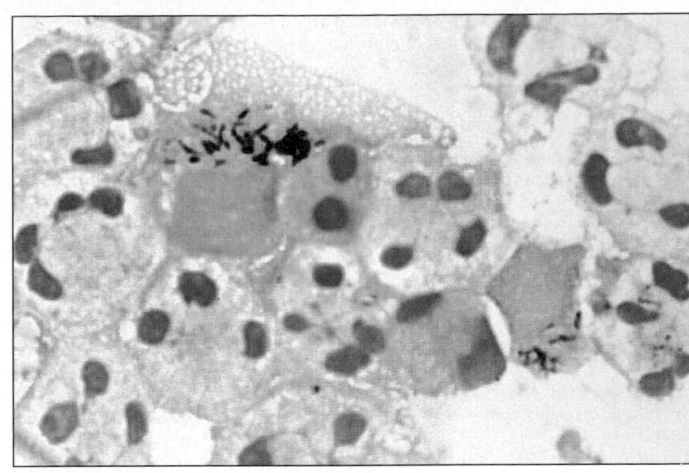

Figure 56–30 Gram stain *of Propionibacterium acnes* from vitreous fluid.

from stool may be tested for toxin production. PCR methods for detection of the toxins of *C. difficile* have been reported (Lemee, 2004).

One of the most common group of anaerobic bacteria of clinical importance is the *B. fragilis* complex. Isolates from this complex will grow selectively on *Bacteroides* bile esculin medium, and have characteristic Gram stain morphology as seen in Figure 56–29. These Gram-negative bacilli are found as normal flora throughout much of the gastrointestinal and genitourinary tract. Infections caused by the complex include abdominal abscess, pelvic abscess, bacteremia, and brain abscess. Rarely they may be involved in pulmonary disease. Although most anaerobic infections are polymicrobial, *B. fragilis* alone may be responsible for the above infections.

An anaerobic Gram-positive bacillus, *Propionibacterium acnes*, has been associated with cases of endophthalmitis that occur after cataract surgery. In addition, *P. acnes* may be associated with ventricular shunt infections in patients with hydrocephalus; rarely *P. acnes* can cause endocarditis, septic arthritis, or other infections. Isolation of this organism may require extended incubation, often up to 10 days. Figure 56–30 is a Gram stain of *P. acnes* in vitreous fluid from a patient months after cataract surgery.

Antimicrobial Susceptibility

Susceptibility testing of anaerobic bacteria is generally unnecessary. The major indications for testing are clinical settings in which decisions regarding the selection of agents are critical because of (1) the failure of usual therapeutic regimens and persistence of infection, (2) the key role of antimicrobial agents in determining the outcome of infection, or (3) the difficulty in making empiric therapeutic decisions based on precedent. Infections from which isolates should be tested are brain abscess, endocarditis, osteomyelitis, joint infections, infections of prosthetic devices or vascular grafts, and refractory or recurrent bacteremia (Clinical and Laboratory Standards Institute/NCCLS, 2004). Testing under these circumstances should include some members of the *B. fragilis* group, other *Bacteroides* species, certain fusobacteria, *C. perfringens*, and *Clostridium ramosum*. Some agents, such as metronidazole, chloramphenicol, imipenem, ampicillin–sulbactam, and ticarcillin–clavulanate, are almost always active against anaerobic bacteria and need not be tested for clinical purposes. Thus, testing should be limited to alternative agents with unpredictable activity, such as penicillin, clindamycin, cefoxitin, cefotetan, and third-generation cephalosporins. Although an agar dilution method has been recommended for reference purposes, testing in the clinical laboratory is generally performed by the microdilution or Etest method. Batch testing of saved isolates on a yearly basis is recommended to develop antibiograms for empiric use by clinicians and to monitor for possible resistance development.

References

Abbott SL: *Aeromonas. In* Murray PR, Baron EJ, Jorgensen JH, et al (eds): Manual of Clinical Microbiology, 8th ed. Washington, DC, American Society for Microbiology, 2003a, pp 701–705.

Abbott SL: *Klebsiella, Enterobacter, Citrobacter, Serratia, Plesiomonas, and Other Enterobacteriaceae. In* Murray PR, Baron EJ, Jorgensen JH, et al (eds): Manual of Clinical Microbiology, 8th ed. Washington, DC, American Society for Microbiology, 2003b, pp 684–700.

Provides an excellent discussion of the biochemical tests useful for identification of Enterobacteriaceae.

Ampofo K, Graham P, Ratner A, et al: Plesiomonas shigelloides sepsis and splenic abscess in an adolescent with sickle-cell disease. Pediatr Inf Dis J 2001; 20:1178–1179.

Bannatyne RM, Jackson MC, Memish S: Rapid diagnosis of *Brucella* bacteremia by using the BACTEC 9240 system. J Clin Microbiol 1997; 35:2673.

Bannerman T: *Staphylococcus, Micrococcus,* and other catalase positive cocci that grow aerobically. *In* Murray PR, Baron EJ, Jorgensen JH, et al (eds): Manual of Clinical Microbiology, 8th ed. Washington, DC, American Society for Microbiology, 2003, pp 384–404.

Provides an excellent overview of the biochemical tests useful for identification of aerobic catalase-positive Gram-positive cocci. Additionally, it includes a discussion of the important resistance mechanisms and tests that allow detection of resistant isolates.

Barnett LA, Cunningham MW: A new heart-cross-reactive antigen in *Streptococcus pyogenes* is not M protein. J Infect Dis 1990; 162:875.

Bartlett JG: *Clostridium difficile* infection: pathophysiology and diagnosis. Semin Gastrointest Dis 1997; 8:12.

Bhisitkul DM, Hogan AE, Tanz RR: The role of bacterial antigen detection tests in the diagnosis of bacterial meningitis. Pediatr Emerg Care 1994; 10:67.

Bille J, Rocourt J, Swaminathan B: *Listeria* and *Erysipelothrix. In* Murray PR, Baron EJ, Jorgensen JH, et al (eds): Manual of Clinical Microbiology, 8th ed. Washington, DC, American Society for Microbiology, 2003, pp 461–471.

Bourbeau PP, Heiter BJ, Figdore M: Use of GenProbe AccuProbe Group B Streptococcus test to detect group B streptococci in broth cultures of vaginal-anorectal specimens from pregnant women: comparison with traditional culture method. J Clin Microbiol 1997; 35:144–7.

Brenden RA, Miller MA, Janda JM: Clinical disease spectrum and pathogenic factors associated with *Plesiomonas shigelloides* infection in humans. Rev Infect Dis 1988; 10:303.

Briselden AM, Hillier SL: Evaluation of Affirm VPmicrobial identification test for *Gardnerella vaginalis* and *Trichomonas vaginalis.* J Clin Microbiol 1994; 32:148–152.

Broome CV: Listeriosis: can we prevent it? New monitoring techniques are helping to prevent this relatively rare but frequently fatal food-borne disease. ASM News 1993; 59:444.

Carroll K, Reimer L: Microbiology and laboratory diagnosis of upper respiratory tract infections. Clin Infec Dis 1996; 23.4442.

Carroll KC, Aldeen WE, Morrison M, et al: Evaluation of the Abbott LCx ligase chain reaction assay for detection of *Chlamydia trachomatis* and *Neisseria gonorrhoeae* in urine and genital swab specimens from a sexually transmitted disease clinic population. J Clin Microbiol 1998; 36:1630.

Catlin BW: *Branhamella catarrhalis*: an organism gaining respect as a pathogen. Clin Microbiol Rev 1990; 3:293.

Centers for Disease Control: Progress toward elimination of *Haemophilius influenzae* type b disease among infants and children United States, 1987–1993. Morbid Mortal Wkly Rep 1994; 43:144.

Centers for Disease Control: Laboratory Practice for prenatal Group B Streptococcus screening – seven states, 2003. Morbid Mortal Wkly Rep 2004a; 53:506–509.

Centers for Disease Control: Vancomycin resistant *S. aureus* – New York, 2004. Morbid Mortal Wkly Rep 2004b; 53:322–323.

Chapin KC, Blake P, Wilson CD: Performance characteristics and utilization of rapid antigen test, DNA probe, and culture for the detection of Group A Streptococcus in an acute care clinic. J Clin Microbiol 2002; 40:4207–4210.

Chapin KC, Musgnug MC: Evaluation of the PBP2a Latex agglutination assay for identification of methicillin resistant *Staphylococcus aureus* directly from blood cultures. J Clin Microbiol 2004;42:1283 1284.

VII

Chediac-Tannoury R, Araj GF: Rapid MRSA detection by Latex Kit. Clin Lab Sci 2003;16:198–202.

Chiedozi LC: Pyomyositis: review of 205 cases in 112 patients. Am J Surg 1979; 137:255.

Claeys G, Verschraegen G, Temmerman M: Modified Granada Agar Medium for detection of Group B Streptococcus carriage in pregnant women. Clin Microbiol Infect 2001; 7:22–24.

Clinical and Laboratory Standards Institute/NCCLS: Methods for Antimicrobial Susceptibility Testing of Anaerobic Bacteria; Approved Standard, 6th ed. CLSI/NCCLS Publication M11-A6. Wayne, PA, NCCLS, 2004.

Clinical and Laboratory Standards Institute/NCCLS: Methods for Antimicrobial Dilution and Disk Susceptibility Testing of Infrequently Isolated Fastidious Bacteria — Proposed Guideline. CLSI/NCCLS publication M45-P. Wayne, PA, CLSI 2005.

Clinical and Laboratory Standards Institute/NCCLS: Methods for Dilution Antimicrobial Susceptibility Tests for Bacteria that Grow Aerobically; Approved Standard, 7th ed. CLSI/NCCLS Document M7-A5. Wayne, PA, CLSI, 2006a.
Essential for laboratories that perform antimicrobial susceptibility testing by broth dilution.

Clinical and Laboratory Standards Institute/NCCLS: Performance Standards for Antimicrobial Disk Susceptibility Tests: Approved Standard, 9th ed. CLSI, NCCLS Document M2-A9. Wayne, PA, CLSI, 2006b.
Essential for laboratories that perform antimicrobial susceptibility testing by disk diffusion.

Clinical and Laboratory Standards Institute/NCCLS: Performance Standards for Antimicrobial Susceptibility Testing; 16th Informational Supplement. M100-S16. Vol 26(1). Wayne, PA, CLSI, 2006c.
Essential for appropriate interpretation and reporting of antibacterial susceptibility test results.

Cloud JL, Woods GL: Nocardia species in the era of sequencing technology. Abstract of Paper read at ASM General Meeting, May 2004.

Cosgrove SE, Carroll KC, Perl TM: S. aureus with reduced susceptibility to vancomycin. Clin Infect Dis 2004; 39:539–545.
Provides an excellent discussion of the mechanism of reduced susceptibility to vancomycin in S. aureus and tests that allow its detection.

Coykendall AL: Classification and identification of the viridans streptococci. Clin Microbiol Rev 1989; 2:315.

Crabtree JH, Garcia NA: Corynebacterium striatum peritoneal dialysis catheter exit site infections. Clin Nephrol 2003; 60:270–274.

Daly JA, Clifton NA, Seskin KC, et al: Use of rapid, nonradioactive DNA probes in culture confirmation tests to detect Streptococcus agalactiae, Haemophilus influenzae, and Enterococcus spp. from pediatric patients with significant infections. J Clin Microbiol 1991; 29:80–82.

Daum RS, Ito T, Hiramatsu K: A novel methicillin resistant cassette in community-acquired MRSA isolates of diverse genetic backgrounds. J Infect Dis 2002; 186:1344–1347.

Dediste A, Vandenberg O, Vlaes L, et al: Evaluation of the ProSpecT Microplate Assay for detection of Campylobacter: a routine laboratory perspective. Clin Microbiol Infect 2003; 9:1085–1089.

Dillon JR, Carballo M, Pauze M: Evaluation of eight methods for identification of pathogenic Neisseria species: Neisseria-Kwik, RIM-N, Gonobio-Test, Minitek, Gonochek II, GonoGen, Phadebact monoclonal GC OMNI test, and Syva Microtrak Test. J Clin Microbiol 1988; 26:493.

Dragsted DM, Dohn B, Madsen J, et al: Comparison of culture and PCR for detection of Bordetella pertussis and Bordetella parapertussis under routine laboratory conditions. J Med Microbiol 2004; 53:745–754.

Edelstein PH: Laboratory diagnosis of Legionnaires' disease. Semin Respir Infect 1987; 2:235.

Efstratiou A, Engler KH, Mazurova IK, et al: Current approaches to the laboratory diagnosis of diphtheria. J Infect Dis 2000; 181 :S138–S145.

Facklam RR, Collins MD: Identification of Enterococcus species isolated from human infections by a conventional test scheme. J Clin Microbiol 1989a; 27:731.

Facklam RR, Hollis D, Collins MD: Identification of gram-positive coccal and coccobacillary vancomycin-resistant bacteria. J Clin Microbiol 1989b; 27:724.

Farmer JJ: Enterobacteriaceae:Introduction and Identification. *In* Murray PR, Baron EJ, Jorgensen JH, et al (eds): Manual of Clinical Microbiology, 8th ed. Washington, DC, American Society for Microbiology, 2003, pp 643.

Fleming DW, Cochi SL, MacDonald KL, et al: Pasteurized milk as a vehicle of infection in an outbreak of listeriosis. N Engl J Med 1985; 312:404.

Fox KK, Knapp JS, Holmes KK, et al: Antimicrobial resistance in Neisseria gonorrhoeae in the United States 1988–1994: the emergence of decreased susceptibility to the fluoroquinolones. J Infect Dis 1997; 175:1396.

Francis JS, Doherty MC, Lopatin U, et al: Severe community onset pneumonia in healthy adults caused by methicillin resistant Staphylococcus aureus carrying the Panton Valentine Leucocidin gene. Clin Infect Dis 2005; 40:100–107.

Friedland I, Gallagher G, King T, et al: Antimicrobial susceptibility patterns in P. aeruginosa: data from a multicenter intensive care unit surveillance study (ISS) in the United States. J Chemother 2004; 16:437–441.

Funke G, Bernard KA: Coryneform Gram-positive rods. *In* Murray PR, Baron EJ, Jorgensen JH, et al (eds): Manual of Clinical Microbiology, 8th ed. Washington, DC, American Society for Microbiology, 2003, pp 472–501.

Funke G, Renaud FNR, Freney J, Riegel P. Multicenter evaluation of the updated and extended API (RAPID) Coryne database 2.0. J Clin Microbiol 1997; 35:3122–3126.

Gales AC, Jones RN, Forward KR, et al: Emerging importance of multidrug-resistant Acinetobacter species and Stenotrophomonas maltophilia as pathogens in seriously ill patients: geographic patterns, epidemiological features, and trends in the SENTRY antimicrobial surveillance program (1997–1999). Clin Infect Dis 2001; 32:104–113.

Garbino J, Bornand JE, Uckay I, et al: Impact of the Legionella urinary antigen test on the management and improvement of antibiotic use. J Clin Pathol 2004; 57:1302–1305.

Gaston DA, Zurowski SM. Arcanobacterium haemolyticum pharyngitis and exanthem. Three case reports and a literature review. Arch Dermatol 1996; 132:61–64.

Gavin SE, Leonard RB, Briselden AM, Coyle MB. Evaluation of the rapid CORYNE identification system for Corynebacterium sp. and other coryneforms. J Clin Microbiol 1992; 30:1692–1695.

Gerner-Smidt P, Tjernberg I, Ursing J: Reliability of phenotypic tests for identification of Acinetobacter species. J Clin Microbiol 1991; 29:277–282.

Granoff DM, Murphy TV, Ingram DL, et al: Use of rapidly generated results in patient management. Diagn Microbiol Infect Dis 1986; 4(Suppl):157S.

Gupta C, Briski LE: Comparison of 2 culture media and 3 sampling techniques for sensitive and rapid screening of vaginal colonization by group B Streptococcus in pregnant women. J Clin Microbiol 2004; 42:3975–3977.

Gurtler V, Mayall BC, Seviour R: Can whole genome analysis refine the taxonomy of the genus Rhodococcus. FEMS Microbiol Rev 2004; 28:377–405.

Hale YM, Melton ME, Lewis JS, et al: Evaluation of the Pace 2 Neisseria gonorrhoeae assay by three public health laboratories. J Clin Microbiol 1993; 31:451.

Hauser AR, Siriam P: Severe P. aeruginosa infections: tracking the conundrum of drug resistance. Postgrad Med 2005; 117:41–48.

Heelan JS, Struminsky J, Lauro P, Sung CJ: Evaluation of a new selective enrichment broth for detection of Group B Streptococcus in pregnant women. J Clin Microbiol 2005; 43:896–897.

Hendley JO, Sande MA, Stewart PM, et al: Spread of Streptococcus pneumoniae in families. Carriage rates and distribution of types. J Infect Dis 1975; 132:55.

Hudspeth MK, Hunt S, Citron DM, Goldstein EJ: Evaluation of the RAPID ID CB Plus system for identification of Corynebacterium sp. and other gram positive rods. J Clin Microbiol 1998; 36:543–547.

Janda JM: Recent advances in the study of the taxonomy, pathogenicity, and infectious syndromes associated with the genus Aeromonas. Clin Microbiol Rev 1991; 4:397.

Janda WM, Guthertz LS, Kokka RP, et al: Aeromonas species in septicemia: laboratory characteristics and clinical observations. Clin Infect Dis 1994; 19:77.

Janda WM, Knapp JS: Neisseria and Moraxella catarrhalis. *In* Murray PR, Baron EJ, Jorgensen JH, et al (eds): Manual of Clinical Microbiology, 8th ed. Washington, DC, American Society for Microbiology, 2003, pp 585–608.

Janda JM, Malloy PJ, Schreckenberger PC: Clinical evaluation of the Vitek Neisseria–Haemophilus identification card. J Clin Microbiol 1987; 25:37.
Provides an excellent review of methods useful for identification of the aerobic Gram-negative diplococci.

Janda WM, Montero MC, Wilcoski LM: Evaluation of the Bacti Card Neisseria for identification of pathogenic Neisseria and Moraxella catarrhalis. Eur J Clin Microbiol Infect Dis 2002; 21:875–879.

Janda WM, Wilcoski KL, Mandel P, et al: Comparison of monoclonal-based methods and a ribosomal ribonucleic acid probe test for Neisseria gonorrhoeae culture confirmation. Eur J Clin Microbiol Infect Dis 1993; 12:177–184.

Johansson A, Forsman M, Sjostedt A: The development of tools for diagnosis of tularemia and typing of Francisella tularensis. Acta Pathol Microbiol Immunol Scand 2004; 112:898–907.

Johnson S, Gerding DN: Clostridium difficile-associated diarrhea. Clin Infect Dis 1998; 26:1027.

Jolivet-Gougeon A, Buffet A, Dupuy C, et al: In vitro susceptibilities of Capnocytophaga isolates to β-lactam antibiotics and β-lactamase inhibitors. Antimicrob Agents Chemother 2000; 44:3186–3188.

Kaper JB, Morris JG Jr, Levine MM: Cholera. Clin Microbiol Rev 1995; 8:48.

Kaplan EL: Pathogenesis of acute rheumatic fever and rheumatic heart disease: evasive after half a century of clinical, epidemiological, and laboratory investigations. Heart 2005; 91:3–4.

Kehl SC, Georgakas K, Swain GR, et al: Evaluation of the Abbott LCx assay for detection of Neisseria gonorrhoeae in endocervical swab specimens from females. J Clin Microbiol 1998; 36:3549.

Kellogg JA, Orwig LK: Comparison of GonoGen, GonoGen II, and MicroTrak direct fluorescent antibody test with carbohydrate fermentation for confirmation of culture isolates of Neisseria gonorrhoeae. J Clin Microbiol 1995; 33:474.

Khanna M, Fan J, Pehler-Harrington K, et al: The pneumoplex assays, a multiplex PCR enzyme-hybridization assay that allows the simultaneous detection of 5 organisms, Mycoplasma pneumoniae, Chlamydophila pneumoniae, Legionella pneumophila, Legionella micdadei, Bordetella pertussis and its real-time counterpart. J Clin Microbiol 2005; 43:565–571.

Kilian M: A rapid method for the differentiation of Haemophilus strains. Acta Pathol Microbiol Scand 1974; 82:835.

Kilian M: Haemophilus. *In* Murray PR, Baron EJ, Jorgensen JH, et al (eds): Manual of Clinical Microbiology, 8th ed. Washington, DC, American Society for Microbiology, 2003, pp 623–635.

Kiska DL, Kerr A, Jones MC, et al: Accuracy of four commercial systems for identification of Burkholderia cepacia and other gram-negative nonfermenting bacilli recovered from patients with cystic fibrosis. J Clin Microbiol 1996;34:886–891.

Kloos WE, Bannerman TL: Staphylococcus and Micrococcus. *In* Murray PR, Baron EJ, Pfaller MA, et al (eds): Manual of Clinical Microbiology, 7th ed. Washington, DC, American Society for Microbiology, 1999, pp 264–282.

Knapp JS: Historical perspective and identification of *Neisseria* and related species. Clin Microbiol Rev 1988; 1:415.

Kotb M, Norrby-Teglund A, McGeer A, et al: An immunogenetic and molecular basis for differences in the outcome of invasive Group A streptococcal infections. Nat Med 2002; 8:1398–1404.

Lee MK and Park AJ: Rapid species identification of coagulase negative staphylococci by rRNA spacer length polymorphisms. J Infect 2001; 42; 189–194.

Lemee L, Dhalluin A, Testelin S, et al: Multiplex PCR targeting tpi (triose phosphate isomerase), tcdA (Toxin A), and tcdB (Toxin B) genes for toxigenic culture *of Clostridium difficile*. J Clin Microbiol 2004;42:5710–5714.

Limberger RJ, Biega R, Evancoe A, et al: Evaluation of culture and the Gen-Probe Pace 2 assay for detection of *Neisseria gonorrhoeae* and *Chlamydia trachomatis* in endocervical specimens transported to a state health laboratory. J Clin Microbiol 1992; 30:1162.

Linnan MJ, Mascola L, Lou XD, et al: Epidemic listeriosis associated with Mexican-style cheese. N Engl J Med 1988; 319:823.

Lion C, Escande F, Burdin JC: *Capnocytophaga camimorsus* infections in humans: review of the literature and a case report. Eur J Epidemiol 1996; 12:521–533.

Logan NA, Turnbull PCB: *Bacillus* and recently derived genera. *In* Murray PR, Baron EJ, Pfaller MA, et al (eds): Manual of Clinical Microbiology, 7th ed. Washington, DC, American Society for Microbiology, 1999, pp 357–369.

Lopez R, Cima MD, Vazquez F, et al: Epidemiologic studies of *S. pneumoniae* carriage in healthy primary school aged children. Eur J Clin Microbiol Infect Dis 1999; 18:771–776.

MacDonald PD, Whitwam RE, Boggs JD, et al: Outbreaks of listeriosis among Mexican immigrants as a result of consumption of illicitly produced Mexican-style cheese. Clin Infect Dis 2005; 40:677–682.

Makristathis A, Pasching E, Schutze K, et al: Detection of *H. pylori* in stool specimens by PCR and antigen enzyme immunoassay. J Clin Microbiol 1998; 36:2772–2774.

Maxson S, Lewno MJ, Schutze GE: Clinical usefulness of cerebrospinal fluid bacterial antigen studies. J Pediatr 1994; 125:235.

Mirrett S, Lauer BA, Miller GA, Reller LB: Comparison of acridine orange, methylene blue, and gram stain for blood cultures. J Clin Microbiol 1982; 14:562–566.

MMWR: Methicillin resistant *S. aureus* infections among competitive sports participants-2000–2003. Morbid Mortal Wkly Rep 2003; 52:793–798.

Montiero L, de Mascarel A, Sarrasqueta AM, et al: Diagnosis of *Helicobacter pylori* infection: noninvasive methods compared to invasive methods and evaluation of two new tests. Am J Gastroenterol 2001; 96:353–358.

Murray DM: Clinical relevance of infection by *Helicobacter pylori*. Clin Microbiol Newslett 1993; 15:33.

Nebreda-Mayoral T, Munoz-Bellido JL, Garcia-Rodriguez JA: Incidence and characteristics of urinary tract infections caused by *Corynebacterium urealyticum* (*Corynebacterium* group D2). Eur J Clin Microbiol Infect Dis 1994; 13:600–604.

Nugent RP, Krohn MA, Hillier SL: Reliability of diagnosing bacterial vaginosis is improved by a standardized method of Gram stain interpretation. J Clin Microbiol 1991; 29:297–301.

Orloff SL, Bush AM, Olyaei AJ, et al: Vancomycin resistant enterococcus in liver transplant patients. Am J Surg 1999; 177:418–422.

Pan ES, Diep BA, Carlton HA, et al: Increasing prevalence of MRSA infections in California jails. Clin Infect Dis 2003; 37:1384–1388.

Parenti DM, Snydman DR: *Capnocytophaga* species: infections in nonimmunocompromised and immunocompromised hosts. J Infect Dis 1985; 151:140–147.

Parsonnet J, Friedman GD, Vandersteen DP, et al: *Helicobacter pylori* infection and the risk of gastric carcinoma. N Engl J Med 1991; 325:1127.

Parsonnet J, Hansen S, Rodriquez L, et al: *Helicobacter pylori* infection and gastric lymphoma. N Engl J Med 1994; 330:1267.

Patel JB, Wallace RJ, Brown-Elliott BA, et al: Sequence-based identification of aerobic actinomycetes. J Clin Microbiol 2004; 42:2530–2540.

Penner JL: The genus *Campylobacter*: a decade of progress. Clin Microbiol Rev 1988; 1:157.

Perkins MD, Mirrett S, Reller LB: Rapid bacterial antigen detection is not clinically useful. J Clin Microbiol 1995; 33:1486.

Perry JD, Davies A, Butterworth LA, et al: Development and evaluation of a chromagar media for methicillin resistant *S. aureus*. J Clin Microbiol 2004; 42:4519–4523.

Peterson LR, Shanholtzer CJ: Using the microbiology laboratory in the diagnosis of pneumonia. Semin Respir Infect 1988; 3:106.

Picard FJ, Bergeron MG: Laboratory detection of Group B streptococci for prevention of perinatal disease. Eur J Clin Microbiol Infect Dis 2004; 23:665–671.

Queipo-Ortuno MI, Colmenero JD, Baeza G, Morata P: Comparison between LightCycler Real-Time Polymerase Chain Reaction (PCR) assay with serum and PCR-enzyme-linked immunosorbent assay with whole blood samples for the diagnosis of human brucellosis. Clin Infect Dis 2005; 40:260–264.

Rossolini GM, Walsh T, Amicosante G: The *Aeromonas* metallo-β-lactamases: genetics, enzymology, and contribution to drug resistance. Microb Drug Resist 1996; 2:245–251.

Ruoff KL: Update on nutritionally variant streptococci (*Streptococcus defectivus* and *Streptococcus adjacens*). Clin Microbiol Newslett 1990; 12:97.

Ruoff KL: *Aerococcus, Abiotrophia*, and other infrequently isolated aerobic catalase-negative, Gram-positive cocci. *In* Murray PR, Baron EJ, Jorgensen JH, et al (eds): Manual of Clinical Microbiology, 8th ed. Washington, DC, American Society for Microbiology, 2003, pp 434–444.

Saez-Nieto JA, Lujan R, Berron S, et al: Epidemiology and molecular basis of penicillin-resistant *Neisseria meningitis* in Spain: A 5-year history (1985–1989). Clin Infect Dis 1992; 14:394.

Schuchat A, Whitney C, Zangwill K: Prevention of perinatal group B streptococcal disease: a public health perspective. Morbid Mortal Wkly Rep 1996; 45:RR-7:1.

Shay DK, Maloney SA, Montecalvo M, et al: Epidemiology and mortality risk of vancomycin resistant enterococcal blood stream infections. J Infect Dis 1995; 172:993–1000.

Sopena N, Sabia M, Neunos 2000 Study Group: Multicenter study of hospital-acquired pneumonia in the non-ICU patient. Chest 2005; 127:213–219.

Stout JE, Rihs JD, Yu VL: *Legionella. In* Murray PR, Baron EJ, Jorgensen JH, et al (eds): Manual of Clinical Microbiology, 8th ed. Washington, DC, American Society for Microbiology, 2003, pp 809–823.

Discusses the tests useful for diagnosis of Legionnaire's disease and methods for identification of Legionella species.

Tenover FC, Tokars J, Swenson J, et al: Ability of clinical laboratories to detect antimicrobial agent-resistant enterococci. J Clin Microbiol 1993; 31:1695.

Thomas JG: Routine CSF antigen detection for agents associated with bacterial meningitis: another point of view. Clin Microbiol Newsl 1994; 16:89–95.

Tolcin R, LaSalvia MM, Kirkley BA: Evaluation of the Alexin ProSpecT Campylobacter Microplate Assay. J Clin Microbiol 2000; 38:3853–5.

Tracey KJ, Lowry SF, Cerami A: Cachectin: a hormone that triggers acute shock and chronic cachexia. J Infect Dis 1988; 157:413.

Vandenesch F, Naimi T, Enright MC, et al: Community-acquired methicillin resistant *S. aureus* carrying the Panton Valentine Leucocidin gene: worldwide emergence. Emerg Infec Dis 2003; 9:978–984.

Velasco D, DelMar Tomas M, Cartelle M, et al: Evaluation of different methods for detection of methicillin (oxacillin) resistance in *Staphylococcus aureus*. J Antimicrob Chemother 2005; 55:379–382.

An excellent review of methods for detection oxacillin-resistant S. aureus.

Warren DK, Liao RS, Merz LR, et al: Detection of methicillin resistant *S. aureus* directly from nasal swab specimens by a real-time PCR assay. J Clin Microbiol 2004; 42:5578–5581.

Wegner D, Witte D, Schrantz R: Insensitivity of rapid antigen detection methods and single blood agar plate culture for diagnosing streptococcal pharyngitis. JAMA 1992; 267:695.

Welch DF, Muszynski MJ, Pai CH, et al: Selective and differential medium for recovery of *Pseudomonas cepacia* from the respiratory tracts of patients with cystic fibrosis. J Clin Microbiol. 1987; 25:1730–1734.

Wellstood SA: Rapid, cost-effective identification of group A streptococci and enterococci by pyrrolidonyl-β-naphthylamide hydrolysis. J Clin Microbiol 1987; 25:1805.

Wilson JP, Turner AP, Kirchner KA, et al: Nocardial infections in renal transplant recipients. Medicine 1989; 68:38.

Woods GL, Gutierez Y: Diagnostic Pathology of Infectious Diseases. Philadelphia, PA, Lea & Febiger, 1993.

Yagupsky P, Peled N, Press J, et al: Comparison of BACTEC 9240 peds plus medium and Isolator 1.5 microbial tube for detection of *Brucella melitensis* from blood cultures. J Clin Microbiol 1997; 35:1382.

Further Reading

Finegold SM: Anaerobic Bacteria in Human Disease. New York, Academic Press, 1977.

Forbes B, Sahm D, Weissfeld A (eds): Bailey and Scott's Diagnostic Microbiology, 11th ed. St Louis, MO, CV Mosby, 2002.

Koneman EW, Allen SD, Janda W, et al: Color Atlas and Textbook of Diagnostic Microbiology, 5th ed. Philadelphia, PA, JB Lippincott, 1997.

Krieg NR, Holt JC (eds): Bergey's Manual of Systematic Bacteriology, Vol 1. Baltimore, MD, Williams & Wilkins, 1984.

Mandell GL, Bennett JE, Dolin R (eds): Principles and Practice of Infectious Diseases, 5th ed. New York, Churchill Livingstone, 2000.

Murray PR, Baron EJ, Jorgensen JH, et al (eds): Manual of Clinical Microbiology, 8th ed. Washington, DC, American Society for Microbiology, 2003.

Washington JA II (ed): Laboratory Procedures in Clinical Microbiology, 2nd ed. New York, Springer-Verlag, 1985.

VII

CHAPTER 57

In Vitro Testing of Antimicrobial Agents

Michael B. Smith MD, Gail L. Woods MD

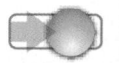

KEY POINTS

• The minimum inhibitory concentration (MIC), or the lowest concentration of antibiotic that inhibits the visible growth of an organism in vitro, is distinguished from the breakpoint, or the concentration of antibiotic (expressed as an MIC), that determines whether an isolate is categorized as susceptible, intermediate, or resistant.

• MIC values are determined by inhibitory testing methods, which include macrobroth dilution, microbroth dilution, and Epsilometer (E-test). Disk diffusion testing, which is a qualitative rather than a quantitative test, does not directly result in an MIC value but is based on direct correlation of inhibitory zone sizes with MIC values.

• Whatever method of susceptibility testing is used, standardized conditions of media, inoculum concentration, and incubation time and temperature are required to produce accurate and reproducible results. These conditions are published by the Clinical and Laboratory Standards Institute (CLSI) and represent standard of practice for laboratories.

• Commercial automated instrument systems are available for rapid, high-volume susceptibility testing; however, despite the advantage of speed and efficiency these systems allow, it must be remembered that all these systems have specific weaknesses. In addition to expense associated with them, some systems are associated with problems in detecting specific resistance phenotypes.

• Both the indications for susceptibility testing of individual isolates and the selection of what antibiotics to test and report should be determined by individual laboratories on the basis of recommendations published by the CLSI in close consultation with the medical and infectious disease staff of the facility.

• Cumulative antimicrobial susceptibility reports (antibiograms) are to be published by laboratories, based on CLSI guidelines, on at least an annual basis. These compilations are crucial for use by physicians in initiating empirical treatment and by pharmacists in monitoring the need for new antibiotics and in attempting to control drug costs by highlighting the use of less expensive antibiotics.

• The use of bactericidal susceptibility tests (minimum bactericidal concentration, killing rate studies, and serum bactericidal test) are purported to have utility in certain specific circumstances related to either evaluation of a new antibiotic's characteristics, therapy of specific types of infections, the use of several antibiotics together, or assessment of the efficacy of an antibiotic under simulated in vivo conditions. These tests are technically demanding, their use controversial, and most laboratories either refer these tests to reference laboratories and/or limit their use to infectious disease physicians.

The selection of a particular antibiotic agent depends on a number of factors, including the site of infection; host factors such as the patient's immune status, hepatic and renal function, or history of allergies; the absorption characteristics, pharmokinetic properties, and dosage requirements of the drug; local susceptibility and resistance patterns; personal experience with individual antibiotics; cost of individual antibiotics; and susceptibility of the isolate to the antibiotic, if known. Although, in many cases, the selection of initial treatment is made on an empiric basis, susceptibility testing is important to aid in modifying therapy, if indicated. Modification may be necessary if 1) the infecting organism is resistant to the antibiotic given, 2) the dose of the antibiotic is not appropriate, or 3) an equally effective but less expensive drug can be used.

Definitions

As more is learned of the mechanisms of antimicrobial resistance, molecular methods for determining resistance have become available. These methods are currently in the minority relative to the conventional or phenotypic methods, and are mostly limited to specific applications for specific species. In contrast, at least one, and in many cases, several methods of the phenotypic type are used in most microbiology laboratories that perform antimicrobial susceptibility testing. These methods can detect the phenotypic expression of a resistance mechanism in a given isolate. Examples include broth dilution, agar dilution, disk diffusion, and gradient diffusion (E-test). Additionally, commercial systems based on phenotypic methods are used in many laboratories that have a need for systems amenable to high volume throughput.

Interpretive categories have been established for specific antibiotic-pathogen combinations by the Clinical and Laboratory Standards Institute (CLSI, formerly the National Committee for Clinical Laboratory Standards [NCCLS]). These categories include 'susceptible,' 'intermediate,' and 'resistant,' and definitions of the categories are provided in CLSI publications delineating performance standards for dilution testing (National Committee for Clinical Laboratory Standards, 2003a) and diffusion disk testing (National Committee for Clinical Laboratory Standards, 2003b). While these particular publications are not revised every year, the CLSI publishes a yearly informational supplement (National Committee for Clinical Laboratory Standards, 2005) that contains updates and changes to the performance standards. Susceptible implies that an infection due to a specific isolate can be appropriately treated with the recommended dosage of antibiotic. Resistant implies that the isolate will not or is unlikely to respond to achievable concentrations of the antibiotic using normal doses. Between these two categories is the intermediate category, which was created to act as a 'buffer' to prevent technical factors involved in performing susceptibility testing from resulting in major discrepancies in interpretation. The intermediate category also implies that an infection caused by the specific isolate can be treated with an antibiotic if treated with high doses or if the infection is in an anatomic site where the antibiotic is concentrated, for example, β-lactam antibiotics in the urine. It is important to remember, however, that these tests and interpretations are in vitro estimates of antimicrobial activity. Antimicrobial activity in vivo depends on many factors, including dosage, route of administration, immune status, distribution space of the antibiotic, pharmokinetic characteristics of the antibiotic, and the hepatic and/or renal functional status of the patient. These factors will play into the patient's response to therapy, and must be considered in the physician's assessment and treatment plan. Susceptibility testing is thus an adjunct to the patient's treatment and does not in of itself completely predict a patient's response to therapy.

Antimicrobial susceptibility tests may be categorized according to the end point being used, inhibition or killing. Most tests used in the clinical microbiology laboratory use inhibition. There are limited uses for determining lethal activity of an antibiotic in vitro.

The inhibitory parameter that forms the basis for the majority of susceptibility tests is the minimum inhibitory concentration (MIC). The MIC is the lowest concentration of antibiotic that inhibits the visible growth of an organism in an in vitro system. MIC results are dependent not only on the relationship between the organism and the antibiotic but on a host of environmental factors that affect the interaction between the organisms and the antibiotic in the system. These factors include the pH of and ion concentrations in the culture medium used, the temperature at which the system is incubated, the incubation atmosphere, the amount of organism inoculated, and the length of time the system incubates. In order to have intra- and interlaboratory reproducibility, and have different laboratories obtain the same results, these variables must be standardized. In the United States, the CLSI is responsible for standardizing methods and quality control, and periodically publishes detailed updates of standards, to which laboratorians can refer.

The MIC must be distinguished from the interpretive breakpoint. The breakpoint is the level of antibiotic, quantitatively expressed as the MIC, that determines whether the isolate is categorized as susceptible, intermediate, or resistant. Breakpoints allow the MIC to be used as an instrument to help predict the infected patient's response to therapy (Mouton, 2002). In this context, the microbiological breakpoint must be distinguished from the clinical breakpoint. While the microbiological breakpoint will separate different isolates on the basis of their susceptibility to an antibiotic along a bimodal distribution, the clinical breakpoint will allow an assessment of the probability of a patient's response to therapy (Mouton, 2002). If the isolate is susceptible, if the MIC for that species–drug combination is below the clinical breakpoint that allows categorization as susceptible, the likelihood of therapeutic success is good and, if the isolate is resistant, the likelihood of therapeutic failure is more likely. It should be evident that determining a clinical breakpoint is complex and depends not only on the relationship between the antibiotic and the microorganism and any resistance mechanisms the pathogen may possess, but also on the relationship between the drug and the patient. The concentration of the drug that can be obtained in the various compartments of a patient's body (blood, cerebrospinal fluid [CSF], urine, etc.), and hence the amount of antibiotic available to combat infection, is dependent on the pharmokinetic/pharmacodynamic properties of the drug, which, in turn, are modified by the state of function of various systems in a patient, such as the hepatic or renal systems. Numerous trials examining all these factors must be undertaken, and the data collated and analyzed, with breakpoints determined after extensive study. The CLSI publishes breakpoints for use by clinical laboratories in the United States, and evaluates and updates them on a yearly basis (National Committee for Clinical Laboratory Standards, 2005).

Inhibitory Methods for Susceptibility Testing

Dilution Testing

In dilution testing, a standardized amount of microorganism is inoculated into a series of tubes, wells, or dishes that contain a range of concentrations of the antibiotic in a vehicle, such as broth or agar, usually starting with an integral power of 2 (e.g., 128 μg/mL) and decreasing on a log_2 basis (e.g., 64, 32, 16, 8, 4) to the lowest concentration to be tested. For the purposes of convenience and economy, it has become common to limit the range of concentrations of each antimicrobial tested to those concentrations that encompass the breakpoints that distinguish between susceptible and resistant. Indeed, some commercial systems contain only a single concentration of an antimicrobial agent.

The broth macrodilution method is performed using standard test tubes, and the tubes are viewed by the unaided eye to determine whether growth

is present. The broth macrodilution system is no longer used by most clinical microbiology laboratories because of its labor-intensive nature, but this methodology is the foundation of most modern susceptibility testing systems. Similarly, the agar dilution method, where the antibiotic being tested is incorporated into solid agar in Petri dishes, is an older, labor-intensive method that is little used by modern microbiology laboratories for routine testing. However, since the isolate being tested is placed on the agar as a single spot, the agar dilution method can allow the testing of multiple isolates on a single plate. Additionally, some more fastidious species that do not grow as well in broth media can be tested with this method. With the exception of the *Bacteroides fragilis* group, agar dilution is the only standardized method that is CLSI-approved for susceptibility testing of anaerobe species (National Committee for Clinical Laboratory Standards, 2004).

Broth microdilution is the most common dilution method used in the modern microbiology laboratory, and this method is the basis for most commercial systems. Commercially prepared and disposable microtiter trays containing antibiotics exist as standalone devices, which are manually inoculated and read by visualization, or as components of automated systems that are read by spectrophotometric methods. Currently, although there are a number of systems that are Food and Drug Administration (FDA)-approved for automated susceptibility testing in the United States, the two systems used in greatest numbers are the Vitek system (bioMerieux Vitek, Hazelwood, MO) and the Microscan system (Baxter Diagnostics, Inc., Sacramento, CA). These systems have been in existence for a number of years, have extensive databases, and have the advantage of computerized software that allows collection of antibiogram data and expert interpretation systems that assist in interpretations. Because of the labor associated with preparing microtiter trays in-house, and the extensive quality assurance testing necessary when preparing the trays, commercially prepared trays and systems are very popular. They are, however, somewhat expensive, and the antibiotics available on a given tray may not conform exactly to what is on the formulary of the institution.

Epsilometer

The Epsilometer, or E-test (AB Biodisk, Solna, Sweden), is a plastic strip with an increasing gradient of antibiotic on one side of the strip and a continuous MIC scale on the opposite side. The strip is placed on the surface of an agar plate that has been inoculated with the isolate, and antibiotic will diffuse into the surrounding agar in a gradient that corresponds to the gradient on the strip. If the isolate is susceptible, an ellipse of inhibition of growth will occur in the bacterial growth on the plate, and the point on the MIC scale on the strip where the ellipse of inhibition intersects is the MIC (Fig. 57–1). The MIC obtained by the E-test has been shown to correlate well with that obtained by either agar or broth dilution for many bacterial species–antibiotic combinations (Baker, 1991). The method is useful because it allows testing of single antibiotics against specific isolates, which has particular utility when testing those fastidious bacteria that grow better on special agar media (e.g., *Haemophilus influenzae*). There are limitations, however, and the method is too expensive to use as a laboratory's routine method for most susceptibility testing. Some pH-susceptible antibiotics may give MIC values that do not correlate exactly with broth dilution methods (Gerrado, 1996).

Disk Diffusion

In the disk diffusion test (Kirby-Bauer), which is largely limited to rapidly growing aerobic and facultatively anaerobic bacteria, a paper disk containing a specified amount (not concentration) of antimicrobial is applied to an agar surface that has been inoculated with a standardized inoculum of the isolate. Testing is done on a 150 mm diameter agar plate that allows testing up to 12 antibiotics at once. The antibiotic diffuses into the agar medium from the disk, resulting in a zone of growth inhibition at the point at which a critical concentration of the antimicrobial in the medium inhibits growth of the bacteria at a standardized point in time (16–18 hours) (Fig. 57–2). The diameter of the zone of inhibition has been shown to be inversely related to the MIC. The relationship between the two can be expressed as a linear regression line, and zone diameter equivalents of susceptible, intermediate, and resistant interpretations can be extrapolated from their intercepts on the regression line with the corresponding MIC values.

Disk diffusion is a simple method that provides a qualitative susceptibility result. It allows easy modification of the battery of antibiotics that are being tested and is inexpensive relative to other methods. For laboratories with a high volume, however, the lack of automation may be prohibitive. Further, although there are modifications that can allow testing of some more fastidious species (e.g., *Streptococcus pneumoniae* and other *Streptococcus*

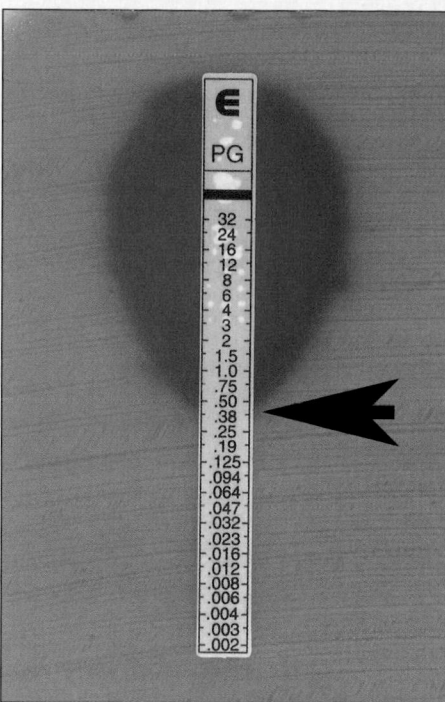

Figure 57–1 Epsilometer or E-test. A gradient of antibiotic (penicillin in this example) is incorporated into the plastic strip, which is placed on the agar surface on which an organism has been streaked (*Streptococcus pneumoniae*). The intersection of the zone of inhibition with the numerical scale on the strip is read as the MIC (arrow).

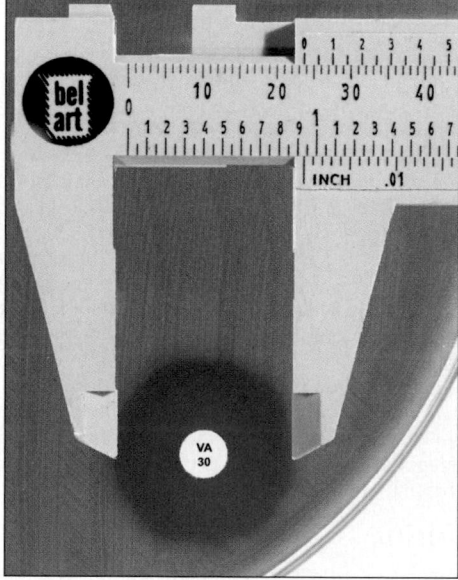

Figure 57–2 Disk diffusion. The zone of inhibition around the antibiotic disk (vancomycin in this case) on the agar surface on which the organism (*Streptococcus pneumoniae*) has been streaked is measured. The result is either susceptible, intermediate, or resistant, based on the zone size.

species, *Haemophilus influenzae*, *Neisseria gonorrhoeae*), many other fastidious species and anaerobes cannot be tested by this methodology (National Committee for Clinical Laboratory Standards, 2003b).

Direct Tests for β-lactamase

The direct β-lactamase tests are not inhibitory tests but phenotypic tests that detect the presence of β-lactamase production by an organism. They are discussed with the inhibitory tests because they, like the inhibitory tests, are commonly used in clinical laboratories. There are three basic types of direct test: the acidometric, the iodometric, and chromogenic. The chromogenic method is the most susceptible and specific, has replaced the other types in usual laboratory use, and is the only type discussed here. The chromogenic test consists of a paper disk impregnated with a chromogenic cephalosporin (nitrocefin). A loopful of the bacteria to be

tested is simply smeared on to the disk and, if the organism is producing β-lactamase, hydrolysis of the chromogenic cephalosporin will occur and the disk color will change from yellow to red, usually within a minute but the disks should be observed for up to 15 minutes for a final reading. A positive test indicates that the bacteria will not respond to penicillinase-susceptible penicillins. The test is useful in testing susceptibility of a number of species, including *H. influenzae*, *Moraxella catarrhalis*, *Staphylococcus* spp., *Enterococcus* spp., and Gram-negative anaerobes (excluding the *B. fragilis* group). It should be noted that for some species (e.g., *Staphylococcus*), a positive test is indicative of penicillinase production, however, a negative test is inconclusive. Staphylococcal β-lactamases are inducible rather than constitutive like the other species listed. If a staphylococcal isolate tests negative with the nitrocefin test, it must be exposed to sub-lethal levels of a β-lactam (growth from around the edge of the inhibitory zone around a β-lactam containing disk, such as oxacillin, on a disk diffusion plate is a simple source) and the test repeated.

Technical Considerations in Testing

Whatever method of dilution or disk diffusion testing a laboratory selects, utilization of a standardized procedure is of the utmost importance in producing accurate and reproducible results. In the United States, professional organizations (e.g., the American Society for Microbiology, Infectious Diseases Society of America), governmental agencies, and private industry work together on a consensus basis under the guidance of the Area Committee on Microbiology of the CLSI. These groups have worked together within the Subcommittee on Antimicrobial Susceptibility Testing under the Area Committee on Microbiology to produce a series of documents that describe standardized procedures for susceptibility testing of aerobic and facultatively anaerobic bacteria (National Committee for Clinical Laboratory Standards, 2003a, 2003b), anaerobic bacteria (National Committee for Clinical Laboratory Standards, 2004), mycobacteria, nocardiae and other aerobic actinomycetes (National Committee for Clinical Laboratory Standards, 2003c), filamentous fungi (National Committee for Clinical Laboratory Standards, 2000b), and yeasts (National Committee for Clinical Laboratory Standards, 2002c, 2004). The Subcommittee on Antimicrobial Susceptibility Testing revises the texts of each document on a 3-year cycle, and reviews and revises the tables detailing MIC breakpoints or zone diameter breakpoints on a yearly basis. The standardized procedures published by the CLSI represent standard of laboratory practice, and laboratories should ensure that the most current tables and texts are on hand, and the revisions in the tables and texts are incorporated into the methods and policies of the laboratory.

Medium

One important variable in susceptibility testing is composition of the medium. Currently, for testing aerobic and facultative bacteria, the CLSI recommends Mueller–Hinton agar or broth, because it demonstrates good batch-to-batch reproducibility; is low in sulfonamide, trimethoprim, and tetracycline inhibitors; and supports the growth of most nonfastidious bacterial pathogens. Some bacteria, such as streptococci, do not grow well on or in unsupplemented Mueller–Hinton agar or broth, a problem overcome by adding defibrinated sheep blood or lysed horse blood to the medium at a final concentration of 2–5% (v/v).

Various components of or supplements to Mueller–Hinton media may affect susceptibility test results. For broth dilution and disk diffusion tests, variation in the concentration of calcium, magnesium, and zinc will affect the results of testing (National Committee for Clinical Laboratory Standards, 2003a, 2003b). Excess calcium and magnesium will cause *Pseudomonas aeruginosa* isolates to appear more resistant when tested against aminoglycosides and all bacteria when tested against tetracyclines; decreased levels of these cations will result in false susceptibility. The level of calcium ions also affects testing results for daptomycin, and zinc ion content will influence results with the carbapenems. The pH of the media will also influence the results of testing, and it must be between 7.2 and 7.4 for accurate results. A pH below this range may cause drugs such as aminoglycosides, quinolones, and macrolides to lose potency, and others (e.g., penicillins) to appear to have excessive activity. A pH higher than 7.4 can result in the opposite affect.

For agar or broth dilution testing, supplementation of Mueller–Hinton agar or broth, respectively, with 2% NaCl (w/v) is recommended to improve detection of oxacillin (methicillin)-resistant staphylococci (National Committee for Clinical Laboratory Standards, 2003a). An alternative approach to detecting oxacillin-resistant *Staphylococcus aureus* or coagulase-negative staphylococci is the oxacillin screening-plate procedure (National Committee for Clinical Laboratory Standards, 2003a). By adding 4% NaCl (w/v) and 6 μg oxacillin/mL to Mueller–Hinton agar and inoculating the agar with an aliquot of a 0.5 McFarland suspension of the isolate, oxacillin-resistant staphylococci can be detected (National Committee for Clinical Laboratory Standards, 2003a). Enterococci that are resistant to vancomycin can be detected by a similar agar screening procedure, using 6 μg/mL vancomycin-supplemented BHI agar (National Committee for Clinical Laboratory Standards, 2003a).

Other medium-related issues of note are related to susceptibility testing of fastidious organisms. For *Haemophilus* species, *Haemophilus* test medium (HTM) is recommended for the MIC broth dilution (agar dilution is not validated for the genus) or disk diffusion testing; and for *N. gonorrhoeae*, GC agar is indicated (National Committee for Clinical Laboratory Standards, 2003a, 2003b). Mueller–Hinton medium that is as thymidine-free as possible is important to the accurate determination of the susceptibility of an isolate to trimethoprim–sulfamethoxazole. Some species can utilize thymine or thymidine in the media to bypass the mechanism of action of trimethoprim and sulfonamides, resulting in false resistance. Thymidine phosphorylase may be incorporated into the media to improve the reliability of testing with trimethoprim–sulfamethoxazole.

For susceptibility testing of anaerobes, agar dilution using *Brucella* agar supplemented with laked sheep blood, hemin, and vitamin K$_1$ (Wadsworth method) is the reference method, and the only CLSI-approved method by which susceptibility testing on most anaerobe species can be carried out (National Committee for Clinical Laboratory Standards, 2004). The disk diffusion method and the broth dilution method currently are not recommended for anaerobes because of poor correlation with the agar dilution method. The exception to this is with the *B. fragilis* group, where broth microdilution using *Brucella* broth with hemin, vitamin K, and 5% lysed horse blood is an approved option. The number of antibiotics that can be tested using microbroth dilution is more limited than with agar dilution.

Other medium related issues affect disk diffusion. For example, the agar depth in plates must be 4 mm, otherwise the diffusion gradient of the antibiotic will be affected. False resistance will occur if the agar is too deep, and false susceptibility results if the agar is not deep enough. When Mueller–Hinton is supplemented with blood, the zones of growth inhibition may be 2–3 mm smaller than those obtained with unsupplemented agar. Sheep blood supplementation may also result in indistinct zone margins around trimethoprim–sulfamethoxazole disks or a film of growth with the zone of inhibition.

Inoculum

Variations in inoculum size are responsible for a significant amount of the day-to-day variation in susceptibility test results. Use of the proper inoculum is particularly important in the accurate detection of resistance to oxacillin in staphylococci and to extended-spectrum penicillins and cephalosporins by Gram-negative isolates with class I β-lactamases (e.g., *Enterobacter*, *Citrobacter*, *Pseudomonas*). The CLSI recommends an inoculum suspension with a density equal to a 0.5 McFarland (compared to a turbidity standard of BaSO$_4$ suspension) for testing in disk diffusion (which gives a final bacterial concentration of $1–2 \times 10^8$ CFU/mL) (National Committee for Clinical Laboratory Standards, 2003b). For broth dilution, the 0.5 McFarland suspension is diluted such that the final concentration of bacteria is 5×10^5 CFU/mL (National Committee for Clinical Laboratory Standards, 2003a). The importance of accurate inoculum density is well illustrated by the frequent occurrence of a high rate of susceptibility of *Enterobacter cloacae* to ampicillin in laboratories using microbroth dilution systems. While the susceptibility rate should not exceed 5% with this species, laboratories reporting a rate greater than this are not infrequent (sometimes up to 40%). This is directly attributable to too low a density of inoculum. Users of broth microdilution methods must assess quantitation of their inoculum density on a regular basis.

A second factor related to inoculum is the method of preparation. There are two preparation methods. The first is the growth method, where three to five colonies of bacteria are inoculated into broth and incubated until growth results in a turbidity equivalent to a 0.5 McFarland standard. The other is the direct colony suspension method, where colonies from an 18–24 hour old plate are used to create a suspension equivalent to a 0.5 McFarland standard. For most species, either of these two methods are equivalent. For more fastidious species, such as *H. influenzae*, *S. pneumoniae*, other streptococci, or *N. gonorrhoeae*, or to detect oxacillin resistance in staphylococci, the direct colony suspension method is recommended (National Committee for Clinical Laboratory Standards, 2003a, 2003b).

Incubation

Incubation conditions will also affect testing results. General recommendations are overnight incubation (16–20 hours) in ambient air at 35°C; however, exceptions exist. Isolates of *S. pneumoniae*, *H. influenzae*, and *N.*

gonorrhoeae require incubation in an atmosphere of 5% CO$_2$, and *S. pneumoniae* and *N. gonorrhoeae* should be incubated for 20–24 hours rather than 16–20 hours. Staphylococci and enterococci also must be incubated for a full 24 hours to ensure detection of resistance to oxacillin and vancomycin, respectively. For anaerobes, agar dilution plates are to be incubated for 42–48 hours, and broth microdilution plates for 46–48 hours. *Candida* species are incubated 46–50 hours when tested by broth dilution, while *Cryptococcus neoformans* requires incubation for 70–74 hours. For further details, the appropriate CLSI standards should be consulted.

Commercial Automated Instrument Systems

According to results from a recent survey of method preferences and testing accuracy by the College of American Pathologists, most clinical microbiology laboratories in the United States now use microdilution-based systems, and most use automated commercial systems (Jones, 2001). One reason for this shift from the disk diffusion test to automated dilution technology is the efficiency gained from replicate inoculation of combined systems for identification and susceptibility testing, and from data management software that are features of many of these systems. Another reason relates to the misconception that MIC values are more accurate and what physicians prefer. However, many physicians other than those specializing in infectious diseases have difficulty in interpreting and utilizing MIC values, requiring laboratories to report interpretive categories along with an MIC. Further, as there are no studies demonstrating definitive clinical superiority of MIC values over reporting just interpretive categories in routine practice (not surprising since the two are highly correlated statistically), the choice of whether to utilize dilution testing or diffusion testing can be made on convenience and economic grounds.

There are many commercially available systems from which to choose. Before purchasing such a system, the laboratory director should consider whether the advantages of replicate inoculation and the data management systems outweigh the added cost of these systems as compared with the simplicity and economy offered by the disk diffusion test. There is a tendency to consider the disk diffusion test archaic and too unsophisticated for modern laboratory practice; however, this test provides accurate results that are easily understood by health care providers and suffice in nearly all clinical situations, and it is economical and flexible. The lack of automation of the test may, however, be an impediment for a high-volume laboratory.

The selection of a particular automated system must be based on a number of considerations. These include test volume, the technical expertise required, the need for data management, the need for a common system for bacterial identification, compatibility with laboratory information systems, cost of equipment (purchase or lease), cost of disposable supplies, reagents, and service contracts, and availability of space. With the VITEK system (bioMerieux, Hazelwood, MO) antimicrobial agents are contained in wells within a plastic card, with 35 or 40 well formats. The system consists of a filler–sealer module, a reader incubator, a computer module, a data terminal, and a printer. The Vitek 2 system has now replaced the original iteration of the system. While the original system monitored turbidity within the wells, the Vitek 2 combines both a multichannel fluorometer and a photometer to record fluorescence, turbidity, and colorimetric data at 15 minute intervals, allowing identification and susceptibility results within 4–15 hours.

There are a number of microdilution systems in which antimicrobial reagents are provided in either a frozen or lyophilized state. Selection of these systems is based not only on the availability of storage space (freezers) for the trays but also on the hands-on time required for each system. The Microscan Walkaway (Dade Microscan, Sacramento, CA) incubates and scans anywhere from 40–96 microdilution trays that have been rehydrated and inoculated manually. The system can read conventional panels after overnight incubation by turbidimetry, or rapid panels that use fluorometric methodology.

The Sensititre Automated Reading and Incubation System (ARIS, TREK Diagnostic Systems, Inc., Cleveland, OH) also detects fluorescence in the Sensititre trays, and the system is fully automated. Sensititre offers two tray setups, one which comes with fluorogenic substrate in the wells and is used with either the automated ARIS or a semi-automated Autoreader, and one which requires addition of the fluorogenic substrate, which can be read manually (without the substrate) or with the Autoreader or ARIS. Of the currently FDA approved systems, the Vitek 2, Microscan, and ARIS offer walkaway capability, freeing technologists for other duties in the laboratory.

Speed of susceptibility testing is heavily promoted by manufacturers of these systems, however, only a few studies have examined whether faster reporting of susceptibility results has actual clinical or financial importance. In a nonrandomized study, Matsen (1985) reported the results of both a 2–5 hour susceptibility system and the disk diffusion test, and then questioned physicians as to whether receiving a faster result influenced their choice of antimicrobial therapy. In 31.7% of instances, physicians indicated that, based on the rapid results, they started a different antibiotic from the one they would have otherwise; another 17% of physicians indicated that they 'probably' would have. In a prospective, randomized study of 794 general surgical patients, Vincent (1985) provided rapid results for half of the patients and conventional results for the other half. They found that antimicrobial therapy was modified in 14.5% of instances in the group of patients for which rapid results were provided and in 8.8% of instances in the group of patients for which conventional results were provided (p <0.001); however, there was no statistically significant difference between the two groups with respect to length of stay in the hospital.

Doern and colleagues (1994) evaluated the clinical impact of rapid bacterial identification and antimicrobial susceptibility testing in hospitalized patients in a tertiary-care medical center. The mean times to reporting identification and susceptibility results, respectively, were 9.6 hours and 11.3 hours for the rapid test group, and 19.6 hours and 25.9 hours in the overnight test group (p <0.0005). There were no significant differences between the two groups with respect to demographic descriptors, other than the length of time to reporting results. The mean lengths of hospitalization were the same for both groups, but mortality rates were lower in the rapid test group (8.8% vs 15.3%). Moreover, for patients in the rapid test group there were significantly fewer laboratory tests, imaging procedures, days of intubation, and days in the intensive care unit; the length of time elapsed prior to alterations in antimicrobial therapy was shorter; and overall patients' cost of hospitalization were significantly lower. In a similar study, Barenfanger (1999) found no difference in mortality between groups for whom rapid susceptibility test results were available when compared to patients for whom routine reporting of results was carried out (mean difference 5.2 hours). They did, however, note significant decreases in length of stay (mean difference, 2.0 days; p = 0.0006) and in total cost of hospital stay (mean difference, $2395; p = 0.04) for those patients for whom rapid susceptibility test results were available.

While there appears to be a valid case for the benefits of the automated susceptibility systems, it must be remembered that they, like all systems, have weaknesses. In addition to the expense associated with the purchase of these systems and their supplies, automated systems, particularly when used in the 3–5-hour 'rapid' mode, have been associated with some problems in detecting specific resistance phenotypes. For example, the Microscan Rapid Pos MIC panels have been associated with difficulty in detecting vancomycin resistance in enterococci (Tenover, 1995). Additionally, Jorgensen and colleagues (2004) recently described inability of automated broth systems (Vitek 2 in this study) to detect inducible clindamycin resistance in staphylococci. Despite shortcomings, these systems can have an important role in susceptibility testing in high-volume laboratories, as long as the occasional weaknesses in the systems are compensated for by additional testing methodology.

Indications for Susceptibility Testing

The necessity of performing susceptibility testing varies with the infecting species. For bacteria, rapidly growing aerobic or facultatively anaerobic bacteria require testing if susceptibility to the antimicrobial agent of choice is unpredictable. If the susceptibility profile is predictable, it is not necessary in most cases to do testing on an isolate. For example, resistance to penicillin in Streptococcus pyogenes has not been reported in the United States, so it is appropriate to treat a patient with S. pyogenes pharyngitis with penicillin without susceptibility testing. However, if the patient is allergic to the primary choice of antibiotic used to treat an infection, and susceptibility to the alternative choice antibiotic is unpredictable, testing is warranted. If the patient in the previous example were allergic to penicillin and the physician wished to treat with erythromycin, then testing would be appropriate, since only approximately 60% of isolates of S. pyogenes are susceptible to erythromycin in the United States (Jacobs, 2003). It is important to remember that testing of isolates should be limited to those isolates that are clinically significant, as testing of isolates that are 'contaminants' or 'normal flora' is expensive, time consuming, and may cause unnecessary administration of antibiotics (Bates, 1991); therefore, it should be avoided. In some patients, however, species normally considered normal flora or contaminants may be clinically significant. These patients are frequently immunocompromised and susceptibility testing may be warranted in these circumstances.

In the past, antibiotic therapy for infections caused by anaerobes was often empirical, as the susceptibility profiles of anaerobic species were thought to be relatively predictable, susceptibility testing had not been standardized, and there was limited proof that susceptibility testing correlated with clinical outcome. Recent literature has demonstrated, however, that susceptibility patterns of many anaerobes are changing, and that, at least for some species, in vitro susceptibility correlates with clinical outcome (Nguyen, 2000; Snydman, 2002). The CLSI currently recommends testing of individual isolates from specific infections, including brain abscess, endocarditis, osteomyelitis, joint infection, infection of prosthetic devices or vascular devices, and bacteremia (National Committee for Clinical Laboratory Standards, 2004). Additionally, species that are commonly resistant or particularly virulent, such as some species of Bacteroides, Prevotella, Fusobacterium, Clostridium, Bilophila, and Sutterella warrant testing. Currently, the only CLSI-approved susceptibility testing method for all species of clinically relevant anaerobes is the agar dilution method (National Committee for Clinical Laboratory Standards, 2004). The only exception is the B. fragilis group, for which broth microdilution has been approved (National Committee for Clinical Laboratory Standards, 2004). Laboratories that do not have the capability to perform agar dilution may wish to perform broth microdilution on those isolates of B. fragilis group that warrant testing and refer other species that require testing to a reference laboratory. For other isolates not described above, susceptibility testing of archived isolates of anaerobes can be performed on a periodic basis (recommended annually by the CLSI) in a surveillance protocol to detect changes in resistance patterns, either by the laboratory or a reference laboratory.

Unlike the situation with anaerobes, all initial isolates of Mycobacterium tuberculosis complex (MTBC) should be tested for susceptibility to primary antituberculous drugs and, if there is clinical evidence of therapeutic failure or failure of cultures to convert to negative after 3 months, testing should be repeated (National Committee for Clinical Laboratory Standards, 2003c). Guidelines exist for testing of some slowly growing nontuberculous mycobacteria (Mycobacterium avium complex, Mycobacterium kansasii, Mycobacterium marinum) and the rapidly growing mycobacteria (Mycobacterium fortuitum group, Mycobacterium chelonae, Mycobacterium abscessus, Mycobacterium mucogenicum, Mycobacterium smegmatis group). Similarly, recommendations exist for susceptibility testing for the aerobic actinomycetes (Nocardia species, Actinomadura spp., Rhodococcus spp., Gordona spp., Tsukamurella spp., Streptomyces spp.). In general, testing of the nontuberculous mycobacteria and aerobic actinomycetes involves variations of the broth dilution method, and commercial systems can be used for a few of the species. Since the drugs tested vary with the species and there are method variations, CLSI document M24-A (National Committee for Clinical Laboratory Standards, 2003c) should be consulted for details. It should be emphasized that some of these species can exist as transient colonizers of the respiratory tract or may be recovered as contaminants, so adherence to criteria to assess clinical significance prior to susceptibility testing, as outlined in CLSI document M24-A, is strongly recommended.

Although a similar situation exists with fungi, that is, both yeasts and moulds may exist as transient colonizers or contaminants, with the increase in immunocompromised patients in the last several decades the prevalence of systemic fungal infections has increased. Additionally, many new antifungal agents have been developed, and resistance to some antifungal agents has begun to appear, particularly among the yeasts (especially some Candida species), both to older agents and the newer agents such as the azole derivatives. Both broth dilution and disk diffusion procedures have been standardized for some yeasts (primarily Candida species and Cryptococcus neoformans) and antifungals (National Committee for Clinical Laboratory Standards, 2002c, 2004). Currently, the testing standards have not been validated for the dimorphic fungi, such as Histoplasma capsulatum or Blastomyces dermatitidis. In fact, for yeasts, interpretive guidelines exist only for Candida species and the drugs fluconazole, itraconazole, and flucytosine; the clinical relevance of any other drug–species combination is not known (National Committee for Clinical Laboratory Standards, 2002c). Broth dilution procedures utilizing conidia or sporangiospores of some moulds such as Aspergillus spp., Fusarium spp., Rhizopus arrhizus, Pseudoallescheria boydii, and Sporothrix schenckii (National Committee for Clinical Laboratory Standards, 2002b) have been standardized, however, interpretive breakpoints are not available as yet, and the clinical relevance of the association between a mould species and its MIC to a particular drug has not been established. Currently, the CLSI recommends determining MIC values on mould species to use as an aid in managing invasive infections with a filamentous fungus when the utility of azole drugs is uncertain, or to establish antibiograms for these fungi at particular institution (National Committee for Clinical Laboratory Standards, 2002c).

Selection of Antibiotics for Testing

The selection of antimicrobial agents for testing is complicated by the expanding spectrum and number of antibiotics available and the growing list of resistance phenotypes that are being identified in pathogenic bacteria. Testing of all available agents is neither practical nor warranted. Selection of what agents should be tested begins with the institution's Pharmacy and Therapeutics Committee, with the objective of coordinating the antibiotics to be tested and reported with those in the formulary. This coordination is important for a number of reasons. First, most laboratories use commercially prepared microdilution panels for susceptibility testing. Manufacturers offer a variety of panel configurations that are designed to correspond as closely as possible with those agents in hospital formularies, but disparities between the agents on the panels and those in the hospital formulary often exist. The laboratory may be faced with either testing more than one panel for a particular pathogen, or paying a premium price for a customized panel. In many cases, more agents are tested than are available in the formulary, so the laboratory must suppress the reporting of some agents. Second, it is not usually necessary to report susceptibility testing results for multiple representatives of the same spectrum class (e.g., cefotaxime, ceftizoxime, and ceftriaxone), as results of a representative agent can usually be generalized to the class. This applies even when more than one is available in the formulary. Third, because manufacturers of commercial antimicrobial susceptibility testing systems must submit data to the FDA validating the accuracy of their systems relative to any newly approved antibiotic, there is often a lag between approval of the agent for clinical use and its incorporation in the susceptibility testing product. Thus a new antimicrobial agent may be approved for an institution's formulary before the laboratory has the capability of testing its activity in vitro.

Both the CLSI standards for dilution and disk diffusion (National Committee for Clinical Laboratory Standards, 2003a, 2003b), and the yearly informational supplement (National Committee for Clinical Laboratory Standards, 2005), list antimicrobial agents that should be considered for testing for Enterobacteriaceae, *P. aeruginosa*, *Staphylococcus* spp., *Enterococcus* spp., *Haemophilus* spp., *N. gonorrhoeae*, *S. pneumoniae*, and other *Streptococcus* spp. In the most recent informational supplement (National Committee for Clinical Laboratory Standards, 2005), separate recommendations are made for *Acinetobacter* spp., *Burkholderia cepacia*, and *Stenotrophomonas maltophilia*. The drugs are listed in four groups, with group A containing drugs that are recommended for testing and reporting against all isolates, and group B containing agents that are suggested for testing against all isolates but may be reported only in certain circumstances (e.g., when the isolate is resistant to drugs in group A). Group C contains supplemental or alternative agents that can be tested and reported in institutions that harbor resistant strains, for treating unusual organisms, or for use by infection control practitioners as epidemiologic tools. Finally, group D contains agents that should be tested and reported only on isolates from urine.

Within each of these groupings of antibiotics, more drugs are listed than need be tested (National Committee for Clinical Laboratory Standards, 2003a, 2003b; 2005). Within the boxes of the tables, antibiotics that usually have similar interpretive results and clinical efficacy are grouped together, implying that testing results for one can often be generalized to other drugs in the group (although not always), and if an agent is listed with another agent separated by an 'or,' this implies there is identical crossresistance or susceptibility between the agents. For example, mezlocillin, ticarcillin, and piperacillin are listed together for primary testing for *P. aeruginosa*. Because it is generally recommended that *Pseudomonas*-active penicillins not be used alone (Gribble, 1983) and because it has not been demonstrated that seriously ill patients have significant differences in outcome between regimens consisting of different penicillins plus an aminoglycoside, it is felt that differences in degrees of activity of the *Pseudomonas*-active penicillins in vitro are not clinically important, and selection of a *Pseudomonas*-active penicillin for the institution's formulary (and therefore in vitro testing) may be based on the list of approved indications for use and its ease of acquisition and administration relative to the other drugs in the class. In contrast, while the two first-generation cephalosporins cephalothin and cefazolin are listed together in group A for Enterobacteriaceae, resistance and susceptibility to one agent is not predictive for all other first-generation cephalosporins. While resistance to cephalothin is predictive of resistance to the other first-generation cephalosporins cefadroxil, cephalexin, and cephalin, it is not predictive of resistance to cefazolin (National Committee for Clinical Laboratory Standards, 2005).

With respect to β-lactams, it is important to test penicillin against staphylococci and streptococci, ampicillin against enterococci and Enterobacteriaceae, and oxacillin against staphylococci. Testing of the cephalosporins is more problematic. In addition to the issue of first-generation cephalosporins mentioned above, there is debate over which second-generation (if any) should be tested against Enterobacteriaceae. The CLSI lists the second-generation cephalosporins cefamandole, cefonicid, cefuroxime, and the cephamycins (also considered second-generation) cefmetazole, cefotetan, and cefoxitin in group B (test and report selectively) to be considered when an isolate is resistant to the first-generation cephalosporins. Selection depends on which one, if any, an institution's Pharmacy and Therapeutics Committee has chosen for the formulary and for what indications. If one or more of the second-generation cephalosporins are available in the institution for perioperative prophylaxis only, there may be no need for routine testing of these agents. On the other hand, if cefoxitin or cefotetan is used in the institution for anaerobic infections, then testing them against any Enterobacteriaceae that may be present in a mixed aerobic-anaerobic infection may be useful.

Testing of the cephamycins may have additional utility in a situation where the broad-spectrum or third-generation cephalosporins are not useful, when an isolate of Enterobacteriaceae possesses an extended-spectrum β-lactamase (ESBL). These enzymes, mutants of the common TEM and SHV β-lactamases, result in resistance to the cephalosporins and monobactams (aztreonam) but not to the cephamycins (cefmetazole, cefoxitin, cefotetan) or carbapenems (imipenem, meropenem, ertapenem). They are found in Enterobacteriaceae, primarily *Klebsiella* spp. and *Escherichia coli*, in the United States currently, but have been reported in several other species in Europe, including *Enterobacter* spp., *Citrobacter* spp., and *Proteus mirabilis*, and in *Salmonella* spp. in Europe, Latin America, and the Western Pacific (Sturenburg, 2003b). Detection of these ESBLs can be problematic, as the isolate may appear susceptible to cephalosporins by routine testing. Screening, using specific MIC breakpoints for third-generation cephalosporins or aztreonam, or disk diffusion zone sizes for these same antimicrobials (National Committee for Clinical Laboratory Standards, 2005), along with the confirmatory tests using combinations of third-generation cephalosporins with and without β-lactamase inhibitors, is necessary to identify these isolates. Testing for ESBLs in *Klebsiella pneumoniae*, *K. oxytoca*, *E. coli*, and *P. mirabilis* is considered on an institutional basis, based on prevalence, therapeutic considerations, and infection control issues in the particular institution (National Committee for Clinical Laboratory Standards, 2005). Many automated susceptibility systems have tests to detect ESBLs, although difficulties in identifying certain ESBL phenotypes (e.g., cefotaximase or ceftazidimase phenotypes) have been reported and a high proportion of 'indeterminate' results requiring additional testing are limiting factors for some systems (Sanders, 2000; Leverstein-van Hall, 2002; Livermore, 2002; Sturenburg, 2003a).

Aside from the issue of ESBLs, there are only slight variations in activity against Enterobacteriaceae among cefoperazone, cefotaxime, ceftizoxime, ceftriaxone, and ceftazidime. Thus, even though more than one of these compounds may be in the formulary, consideration may be given to testing only one of these agents against isolates. Cefoperazone and ceftazidime are third-generation cephalosporins that have good activity against *Pseudomonas aeruginosa*. Since ESBLs having preferential activity against ceftazidime have been reported, and β-lactamases with preferential activity against cefoperazone are known, limiting testing of these agents to isolates of *P. aeruginosa* to avoid selecting for the emergence of strains of Enterobacteriacea with these β-lactamase phenotypes may be a useful policy for some institutions.

For enterococci, testing isolates for vancomycin resistance has become a necessity for many institutions, as the number of enterococcal isolates that are resistant continues to grow. In 2002, 27.5% of isolates involved in ICU infections from hospitals in the National Nosocomial Infections Surveillance (NNIS) were vancomycin-resistant enterococci (VRE) (NNIS, 2003). Some automated systems have had difficulties in the past with detecting all phenotypes of vancomycin resistance, and many laboratories have used alternate methods (disk diffusion, agar screen, or E-test) to screen for VRE (Kohner, 1997; Endtz, 1998). Although improvements have been made, and detection for many resistant phenotypes is very good, some systems still have difficulty detecting some phenotypes such as the *vanC* strains (d'Azevedo, 2001; Garcia-Garrote, 2000; van Den Braak, 2001; Fahr, 2003). Fortunately, the clinical significance of this intrinsic low-level vancomycin resistance, found in *Enterococcus gallinarum* and *Enterococcus casseliflavus*, is unknown so this may have minimal importance. Further, screens for high-level resistance to gentamicin and streptomycin should be performed on all enterococcal isolates from sterile body sites, and clinicians should be informed that combination therapy with penicillin or ampicillin plus an aminoglycoside is indicated for serious enterococcal infections. As with vancomycin, improvements in systems have made detection of high-level resistance fairly accurate; however, some are better than others and each system has peculiarities, such as better accuracy with one drug than with the other (Garcia-Garrote, 2000; d'Azevedo, 2001; Fahr, 2003; Murdoch, 2003). If a laboratory is going to use an automated system, familiarity with weaknesses in the system is important, so that alternate methods can be instituted to insure accuracy. For blood or CSF isolates, the CLSI recommends testing enterococci for β-lactamase production, as described earlier. Additionally, susceptibility results for aminoglycosides (except high-level concentrations), cephalosporins, clindamycin, and trimethoprim–sulfamethoxazole should not be reported, as the isolates may appear susceptible in vitro but the agents are not effective clinically. Similar reporting prohibitions exist for *Salmonella* and *Shigella* spp. (aminoglycosides, first- and second-generation cephalosporins) and oxacillin-resistant *Staphylococcus* spp. (all β-lactams and β-lactam–β-lactamase inhibitor combinations).

Oxacillin resistance in *Staphylococcus* spp. has become a significant problem in the United States, with 57.1% of *S. aureus* (MRSA – methicillin-resistant *Staphylococcus aureus*) and 89.1% of coagulase-negative *Staphylococcus* (CNS) isolates involved in nosocomial ICU infections reported to the NNIS in 2002 being resistant (NNIS, 2003). The CLSI lists oxacillin (as a surrogate for methicillin) in group A, as a test and report drug for all *Staphylococcus* spp. isolates (National Committee for Clinical Laboratory Standards, 2005). Most commonly, oxacillin resistance in *Staphylococcus* spp. is due to altered penicillin binding protein production (PBP 2a) mediated by the *mecA* gene, although less commonly the phenotype is due to either hyperproduction of β-lactamase or the production of altered intrinsic PBP. Isolates that possess the *mecA* gene can express it either heterogeneously or homogenously. While those isolates that express the gene homogenously will be easily detected by most available testing methods, those that express the gene heterogeneously are more problematic. These isolates may appear susceptible by dilution testing, including the commercial automated systems, giving MIC values in the susceptible or borderline range, and may be misclassified (Sakoulas, 2001; Swenson, 2001; Felten, 2002). CLSI document M100-S15 (National Committee for Clinical Laboratory Standards, 2005) describes an oxacillin-salt agar screening test for S. *aureus* and a cefoxitin disk diffusion test for use with either *S. aureus* or CNS. Tests that detect the *mecA* gene or PBP 2a are considered the most accurate of available tests (National Committee for Clinical Laboratory Standards, 2005). There are two FDA approved latex tests that detect PBP 2a, the MRSA-Screen (Denka-Seiken Co., Ltd., Tokyo, Japan) and the PBP 2′ latex agglutination test (Oxoid Ltd., Basingstoke, United Kingdom), and an FDA-approved DNA probe, the Velogene Rapid MRSA Identification Assay (Remel, Lenexa, KS). For CNS, which have different oxacillin MIC breakpoints and disk diffusion diameters from *S. aureus*, the cefoxitin disk diffusion test has been shown to have approximately the same sensitivity as broth dilution but a greater specificity (National Committee for Clinical Laboratory Standards, 2005). The commercial dilution systems also show a reduced specificity and a reduced sensitivity relative to detection of methicillin resistant CNS in some studies (Horstkotte, 2002, 2004; Ligozzi, 2002). There are fewer options for testing CNS relative to *S. aureus*, as the oxacillin–salt agar screen cannot be used for CNS, and the MRSA-Screen (Denka-Seiken Co., Tokyo, Japan) is not FDA approved for CNS. While the PBP 2′ latex agglutination test (Oxoid, Basingstoke, UK) is approved by the FDA for use with CNS, no literature is available to assess its performance.

The isolation of *S. aureus* with reduced susceptibility to vancomycin (VISA), and then most recently the identification of several isolates in the United States that were resistant to vancomycin (VRSA) has heightened the importance of susceptibility of testing *S. aureus* against vancomycin (Tenover, 2004). While the broth microdilution method described in CLSI document M7-A6 (National Committee for Clinical Laboratory Standards, 2003a) will correctly detect vancomycin resistance in a VRSA isolate, Tenover and associates (2004) note that the second VRSA was not identified as resistant to vancomycin by the automated susceptibility systems on which it was tested. Consequently, the CLSI recommends that, when using either an automated susceptibility test system or agar dilution, a BHI vancomycin agar screen plate containing 6 µg/ml of vancomycin should also be inoculated with the *S. aureus* isolate in question to ensure detection of either VISA or VRSA (National Committee for Clinical Laboratory Standards, 2005). Similarly, the vancomycin disk diffusion method will not detect VISA, and VRSA may be difficult to detect by this method, so the vancomycin agar screen plates are also recommended when a laboratory has used the disk diffusion methodology for susceptibility testing (National Committee for Clinical Laboratory Standards, 2005). Finally, it is recommended that any *S. aureus* isolate with an MIC above the susceptible breakpoint (e.g., >4 µg/ml) for vancomycin is sent to a reference laboratory for confirmatory testing.

With high rates of penicillin resistance in S. *pneumoniae* seen worldwide (approximately 20% [Jacobs, 2003]), and increasing rates of resistance to

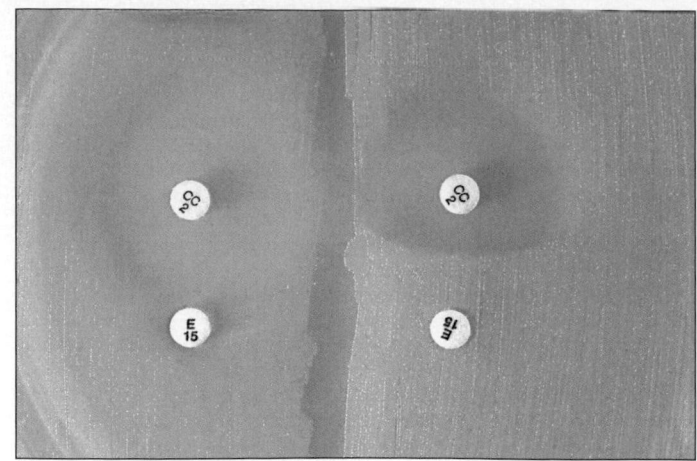

Figure 57–3 Disk induction or 'D' test. The *Staphylococcus aureus* isolate on the left demonstrates erythromycin (E) resistance but susceptibility to clindamycin (CC). The *S. aureus* isolate demonstrates inducible clindamycin resistance with blunting of the zone of inhibition around the clindamycin disk adjacent to the erythromycin disk.

other drugs as well, susceptibility testing of this pathogen is required whenever isolated from sterile body sites. The oxacillin screen disk diffusion method can be used. The test is accurate in categorizing an isolate as susceptible if the zone size is more than 20 mm. However, zone sizes less than this can be seen with susceptible, intermediate, or resistant isolates, so MIC testing is necessary when the zone size is less than 19 mm. Other agents to consider testing depend on the body site from which it is isolated. For example, for isolates from CSF, the CLSI recommends testing penicillin, cefotaxime or ceftriaxone, meropenem, and vancomycin by broth dilution, since disk diffusion interpretive standards for cephalosporins or the carbapenems for *S. pneumoniae* do not exist (National Committee for Clinical Laboratory Standards, 2005). It should also be noted that the interpretive standards for the cephalosporins are different depending on the body site from which the *S. pneumoniae* was isolated (meningitis vs non-meningitis), and interpretations and reporting will therefore vary depending on the source. The CLSI recommends reporting only meningitis interpretations for isolates from the central nervous system and reporting both meningitis and non-meningitis interpretations for all other isolates. For non-life-threatening infections, agents to consider testing and reporting are penicillin, erythromycin (which will predict susceptibility to other macrolides), and trimethoprim–sulfamethoxazole by broth dilution or disk diffusion; since disk diffusion interpretive standards exist for these drugs, disk diffusion testing can be utilized.

For streptococci other than *S. pneumoniae*, the drugs to be tested and the method required depend on the species/complex. For *S. pyogenes* (Lancefield group A) or *Streptococcus agalactiae* (group B), susceptibility testing for the primary drug of choice for treatment, penicillin, is not necessary because resistant strains have not been reported. The same is true if vancomycin is used to treat infections with these species. If the patient is penicillin-allergic, and another drug such as a macrolide is considered for therapy, erythromycin may be tested, and will predict susceptibility to other macrolides. The CLSI recommends testing erythromycin and clindamycin for pregnant women who are colonized with Group B streptococci and allergic to penicillin (National Committee for Clinical Laboratory Standards, 2005). Isolates that are resistant to erythromycin but susceptible to clindamycin should be tested for 'inducible' resistance to clindamycin mediated by the *erm* gene (macrolide, lincosamide, streptogramin B resistance) using the 'D-zone approximation test,' with closely approximated erythromycin and clindamycin disks (National Committee for Clinical Laboratory Standards, 2005) (Fig. 57–3). This type of inducible resistance has been described in various Gram-positive cocci, including staphylococci. Some institutions have begun testing staphylococcal isolates for this type of resistance in certain situations or routinely (Fiebelkorn, 2003; Jorgensen, 2004). The prevalence of this type of resistance in various Gram-positive species may vary from institution to institution. Surveying for the prevalence of inducible clindamycin resistance in Gram-positive cocci in an institution to determine and implement the most cost-effective testing policy is a reasonable and logical strategy for (Schreckenberger, 2004).

For viridans streptococci, any isolate from a sterile body site and implicated in a serious infection, such as endocarditis, should be tested for penicillin susceptibility (Quinn, 1988). As interpretive standards for the disk diffusion method for this organism–agent combination do not exist, testing must be accomplished by an MIC method (National Committee for Clinical Laboratory Standards, 2005). Testing for susceptibility to cephalosporins is also warranted, as some viridans streptococci may exhibit relative resistance to third-generation cephalosporins (Wilcox, 1993). Vancomycin is the recommended alternative to β-lactam drugs for viridans streptococcal therapy but, because no resistant strains have been reported, testing against vancomycin is not necessary. For identification purposes, however, evaluating susceptibility to vancomycin would be reasonable, as resistance in the isolate would indicate that the isolate is not a viridans streptococcus but most probably a member of the intrinsically vancomycin-resistant genera such as *Leuconostoc* or *Pediococcus*.

For some species, the β-lactamase test may be sufficient for many purposes. For example, in non-life-threatening infections, a β-lactamase test will predict the susceptibility of *H. influenzae* to ampicillin or amoxicillin, and it is reasonable to test for β-lactamase alone. The prevalence of β-lactamase-positive *H. influenzae* is approximately 30% in the United States, and the β-lactamase-negative, ampicillin-resistant (BLNAR) strains, which will not be detected by β-lactamase testing, are rare (Jacobs, 2003). Given that susceptibility testing for *H. influenzae* requires specialized media (HTM), this simplifies testing and may save time and money. If the incidence of BLNAR is high in a given area, disk diffusion or dilution testing of ampicillin using HTM can be done. Such testing may be necessary for isolates from serious infections, such as meningitis, where the CLSI recommends that only susceptibility results for penicillin, a third-generation cephalosporin, chloramphenicol, and meropenem be reported (National Committee for Clinical Laboratory Standards, 2005).

β-Lactamase testing used to be recommended for isolates of *N. gonorrhoeae*. However, since neither penicillin or ampicillin is used to treat gonorrhea, it is no longer necessary but may be useful for epidemiologic purposes only. MIC interpretive standards for *N. meningitides* have been included in CLSI document M100-S15 (National Committee for Clinical Laboratory Standards, 2005) for the first time. A survey of US isolates from cases of meningococcal disease in 1997 by the Centers for Disease Control did not demonstrate any isolates resistant to penicillin (*n* = 121), although three were intermediate and three isolates were resistant to rifampin, a drug commonly used in chemoprophylaxis of exposures (Rosenstein, 2000). The authors of this report suggest that, while the low prevalence of antibiotic resistance in this pathogen does not warrant routine susceptibility testing in the United States, it should be considered for isolates from patients who do not respond appropriately to therapy.

In contrast, resistance to antimicrobial agents among anaerobic bacteria has been increasing in recent years. For example, the *B. fragilis* group, *Prevotella* spp., *Porphyromonas* spp., and *Clostridium* spp. are showing increasing resistance to the β-lactams and to clindamycin (Falagas, 2000; National Committee for Clinical Laboratory Standards, 2004). However, such trends are not limited to these species or these agents. The CLSI has suggested groupings (primary and supplemental) of antibiotics for testing that depend both on species, and on the presence or absence of β-lactamase in the isolate (for non-*B. fragilis*-group Gram-negative anaerobes). For *B. fragilis* group and other β-lactamase-positive Gram-negative anaerobes, the primary group includes a β-lactam–β-lactamase combination, cefoxitin or cefotetan, a carbapenem, and metronidazole (National Committee for Clinical Laboratory Standards, 2004). For β-lactamase-negative isolates, ampicillin or penicillin, clindamycin, and metronidazole comprise the primary group to be tested. *Clostridium* spp. (other than *Clostridium perfringens*) have the same groupings as β-lactamase-positive Gram-negative species, except that clindamycin can also be tested. *C. perfringens*, anaerobic Gram-positive cocci, and other anaerobic Gram-positive bacilli have the same groupings as β-lactamase-negative Gram-negative isolates. Testing in a given institution may be limited by the demanding nature of agar dilution testing, necessary for all species except the *B. fragilis* group, and referral of isolates to a reference laboratory may be necessary.

For MTBC, all initial isolates should be tested for susceptibility to primary anti-tuberculous drugs (National Committee for Clinical Laboratory Standards, 2003c). Additionally, if the patient fails to respond to therapy, or cultures fail to become negative by 3 months after initiation of therapy, testing should be repeated. Testing results should be available as quickly as possible, and it is recommended that laboratories provide results to clinicians within 28 days of receiving the initial specimen (Bird, 1996). Several commercial rapid broth-based methods that correlate with the slower agar proportion reference method are available for use and FDA-approved (although not for all drugs), including a nonradiometric automated method, the BACTEC MGIT 960 (Scarpano, 2004). The full panel of primary drugs includes isoniazid at two concentrations (critical and high concentration), rifampin, ethambutol, and pyrazinamide. Some laboratories test only the critical concentration of isoniazid, rifampin, and ethambutol, based on: (1) the population served; (2) the prevalence of drug resistance; (3) drugs used in the community; and (4) the availability

of testing for the secondary drugs required when resistance to rifampin or any two primary drugs is detected (National Committee for Clinical Laboratory Standards, 2003c).

Selecting Antibiotics to be Reported

Selecting antibiotics to report for a given isolate should take into account not only the results of the testing itself but also a number of other factors. For example, drugs that are not effective in treating infections of the central nervous system, such as clindamycin, macrolides, tetracyclines, fluoroquinolones, or most first- and second-generation cephalosporins, must not be reported for isolates from CSF (National Committee for Clinical Laboratory Standards, 2005). Drugs that are only indicated for urinary tract infections (e.g., nitrofurantoin) should not be reported for isolates from sputum. These prohibitions are relatively simple and self-evident. Other considerations in reporting may be more complicated. Many laboratories use 'cascade' reporting to encourage physicians to use equally effective but less expensive antibiotics first, rather than the 'newest' or most heavily commercially promoted, in order to lower institutional pharmacy expenses. For example, second or third-generation cephalosporins will be reported only if the isolate is resistant to first-generation cephalosporins. Similarly, some institutions require the approval of infectious disease physicians (or other 'gate-keeper' providers) prior to the use of some antibiotics. This may be on grounds of expense or, even more importantly, the control of resistance phenotypes within the institution. It has been demonstrated in prospective studies (Project ICARE: Intensive Care Antimicrobial Resistance Epidemiology) that the frequent use of vancomycin and third-generation cephalosporins is associated with the increased prevalence of vancomycin-resistant enterococcus (VRE) in intensive care units and that, by limiting the use of vancomycin, the prevalence can be decreased (Fridkin, 2001, 2002). Finally, institutions may attempt to influence antibiotic usage not by limiting the antimicrobials that are reported but by publishing cost data for individual agents, either along with a susceptibility report or in a separate format to which physicians can refer (discussed in the following section). Any of these reporting strategies may involve some resistance from providers, so careful consultation and cooperation on the part of the laboratory with the medical staff, infectious disease physicians, and the institution's Pharmacy and Therapeutics Committee are important in establishing local reporting policy.

Cumulative Antimicrobial Susceptibility Reports

Since susceptibilities can vary considerably depending on the geographic locale, patient demographics, and antibiotic usage patterns in an institution, it is the responsibility of the microbiology laboratory to compile and publish a cumulative antimicrobial susceptibility report (antibiogram) of the pathogens isolated at the institution on at least an annual basis. The reports, usually published as tables on a small pocket card, should list the most significant pathogens isolated in the institution and the percentage susceptible to the antimicrobials on the institution's formulary. These reports are used by physicians to guide empiric therapy until specific susceptibility data are available. Additionally, the data can be used by infection control personnel to detect emerging resistance patterns and design measures to contain outbreaks of resistant species, and by the pharmacy to identify the need for new antimicrobials for the formulary, determine when some antibiotics are no longer effective, and monitor prescribing patterns (Critchley, 2004). Additionally, by including cost data on the antibiogram, institutions may attempt to encourage physicians to use less expensive but still effective agents, and thus decrease pharmaceutical costs.

The National Committee for Clinical Laboratory Standards (2002a) provides guidance to laboratories on the preparation of antibiograms and includes suggestions on data selection, validation, and presentation along with important considerations relating to limitations of the data and an example of an antibiogram. By using the CLSI guidelines and providing timely, up-to-date data, laboratories can both assist in proper patient management and infection control and help the pharmacy in the difficult task of controlling resistance and managing antibiotic usage in the institution. To accomplish this, CLSI standards relating to compilation of an antibiogram, annual updating, and distribution to appropriate infection control and medical staff yearly should be met. To assess how well microbiology laboratories at US medical facilities were faring in meeting these standards, Ernst and colleagues surveyed 494 medical facilities and found that while most (95%) were compiling antibiograms, only 60% fully met all three standards (Ernst, 2004). Approximately three quarters of laboratories updated the antibiogram on an annual basis, and slightly fewer published and distributed the antibiogram to the medical staff and infection control. Those that were able to accomplish all three standards were more likely to be larger laboratories that provided on-site services, had a referral laboratory function, and had more personnel working in the laboratory.

Bactericidal Tests

There are three major categories of bactericidal test: (1) determination of the minimum concentration of an antimicrobial required to kill a microorganism, otherwise known as the minimum bactericidal or lethal concentration (MBC or MLC); (2) determination of the killing rate (time-kill rate or killing curve); and (3) determination of the highest dilution of a patient's serum required to kill a microorganism, otherwise known as the serum bactericidal or lethal titer (SBT or SLT). The use of any of these tests is influenced by the indications, methodology, and interpretation of results.

Minimum Bactericidal or Lethal Concentration

There is general agreement that determining the MBC or MLC should be part of the initial investigation of a new antimicrobial agent. There is, however, less agreement over whether the test is indicated for clinical use with isolates of streptococci from patients with endocarditis, staphylococci from patients with endocarditis or osteomyelitis, and Enterobacteriaceae or *Pseudomonas* from patients with meningitis. In part, some of the controversy stems from biological and technical variables affecting the results of MBC determinations (National Committee for Clinical Laboratory Standards, 1999b). To determine the MBC or MLC, serially diluted (on a $\log_2$ basis) antimicrobial in broth is inoculated with a standardized suspension of the test organism, as described for determination of the MIC. After incubation at 35°C for 24 hours, those tubes exhibiting no visible growth are subcultured on to an antibiotic-free agar medium. The MBC or MLC is defined as the lowest concentration of antimicrobial agent that is bactericidal or lethal to at least 99.9% of the original inoculum. Among the biological variables of the test are (1) the persistence phenomenon in which a small number (usually <0.1%) of the bacterial inoculum, 'persisters,' survive antibiotic exposure but remain susceptible if retested against the antibiotic, usually a cell wall active agent; (2) the paradoxical effect in which the proportion of surviving cells increases with the concentration of antibiotic, again most frequently observed with the cell-wall-active antibiotics; and (3) tolerance, a much misunderstood phenomenon. Both 'persisters' and the paradoxical effect are thought to be related to the slowing of the rate of growth of the bacteria by the antibiotic, which results in decreased killing effect (National Committee for Clinical Laboratory Standards, 1999b). Tolerant organisms, strictly defined, are those in which viability is lost slowly and those in which the bacteriostatic–bacteriolytic response to antibiotics is changed in the direction of bacteriostasis (Handwerger, 1985). However, tolerance has also been defined as an MBC:MIC ratio of 32 or more, despite the many technical problems that influence MBC results and procedural variations in determining MBCs (Sherris, 1986). As pointed out by Sherris (1986), the MBC is defined by the lowest concentration of antibiotic yielding l0.1% survivors or less at the least accurate portion of the killing curve (i.e., 18–24 hours). The number of survivors after overnight incubation with a cell-wall-active antibiotic is invariably greater if the inoculum is in the stationary rather than the logarithmic phase (Handwerger, 1985; Sherris, 1986). The most frequent technical problems that result in a greater proportion of bacteria in the stationary phase is use of cultures that have been growing more than 8 hours (National Committee for Clinical Laboratory Standards, 1999b). Additional technical artifacts include the survival of bacteria in the condensate above the meniscus of antibiotic-containing broth, subculture volume, antibiotic carryover in subcultures, and lack of test reproducibility. Assuming that these technical problems can be controlled, determination of an end point (MBC) can be based on rejection criteria published by Pearson (1980). However, because tolerance is defined by a delayed rate of killing, the most reliable method for its detection is a simplified time-kill study of the organism, comparing the quantity of bacteria that remain viable after 5–6 hours of incubation in the presence of an antibiotic concentration 4–8 times its MIC with the quantity present at 2-hour or zero-time readings (Handwerger, 1985; Sherris, 1986).

Considering all the biological and technical problems associated with bactericidal testing and defining tolerance, it is not surprising that the interpretation of published clinical studies of infections caused by purportedly 'tolerant' organisms is fraught with difficulty, especially infection with staphylococci, for which technical variables have major consequences (Handwerger, 1985). For these reasons, most laboratories do not determine MBCs of cell-wall-active antibiotics against staphylococci.

There are data from studies of experimental viridans streptococcal endocarditis in animals suggesting that penicillin may be less effective against infection due to tolerant strains than against nontolerant strains (Handwerger, 1985; Wilson, 1985); however, there is little information regarding the clinical significance of such strains (Wilson, 1985). Handwerger and Tomasz (Handwerger, 1985) have speculated that nontolerant bacteria may manifest a phenotypically tolerant response in an endocardial lesion because of their high density, diminished metabolic activity, and slow growth rate in vegetations. Because some strains of viridans streptococci are resistant (MIC ≥4 μg/mL) to penicillin, it certainly is necessary to determine the MIC of viridans streptococci isolated from patients with endocarditis or other life-threatening infections. Because patients with endocarditis caused by tolerant viridans streptococci may be at greater risk of relapse and may require 4–6 weeks of therapy with penicillin and an aminoglycoside (Wilson, 1985), it may be reasonable to determine the MBC of such strains.

Killing Rate Studies

Determination of the rate of killing by an antibiotic is the method by which not only tolerance but also synergy or antagonism of two or more antibiotics is best determined. Furthermore, bactericidal, rather than bacteriostatic, activity appears to be a requirement for therapy of bacterial meningitis (Sande, 1981). In the case of Gram-negative bacillary (other than *H. influenzae*) meningitis, MBCs of cephalosporins may correlate poorly with outcome in contrast with the results of 6-hour time-kill rate studies (Eng, 1987). Time-kill studies of antimicrobials, singly or in combination, may therefore be more predictive of outcome than MBCs in those instances in which bactericidal therapy is necessary for cure (Bayer, 1985; Drake, 1985; Eng, 1987). Results of combination studies by the time-kill method also correlate better with the results of combination studies in experimental animal models of infection than do results of such studies obtained by the checkerboard method (Bayer, 1985), perhaps once again because the end point of the checkerboard method is determined at 18–24 hours, which is the least accurate end of the killing curve (Sherris, 1986). In killing rate studies, quantitative cultures are made at varying intervals (e.g., 0, 4, 8, 12, and 24 hours) following the inoculation of the antibiotic-containing medium. Bactericidal activity is defined as 99.9% killing of the final inoculum, determined by noting a decrease in CFUs/mL on the plotted time-kill curve of 3 $\log_{10}$ or more (National Committee for Clinical Laboratory Standards, 1999b). When antimicrobials are tested in combination, synergy is usually defined by a reduction in CFUs/mL between the combination and its most active constituent of 2 $\log_{10}$ or more, assuming that at least one of the constituents does not affect the growth curve of the test organism when used alone. In the case of enterococci, this requirement poses no difficulties because clinically attainable concentrations of penicillins or aminoglycosides are not bactericidal; however, the requirement may pose problems in tests of other microorganisms, which may be susceptible to each of the antimicrobials used in the combination. In the latter instance, synergy may be defined only when there is a reduction in CFUs/mL of 2 $\log_{10}$ or more between the combination of each of two antimicrobials present in concentrations representing one fourth of their respective MBCs, compared with the more active constituent alone at a concentration of one half its MBC (Hallander, 1982).

As with MBC determinations, carryover of antimicrobial agents in quantitative subcultures is problematic and requires that any antimicrobial present be inactivated or that samples removed for subculture be sufficiently diluted that drug carryover effects are eliminated, if possible. Whether carryover occurs, particularly at test concentrations of 16 times the MIC or greater, can be ascertained by streaking a 10–100 μL aliquot of a subculture dilution across an agar surface, allowing a 20-minute absorption time, and then streaking the entire agar surface with the test organism and observing for inhibition of growth at the site of the initial streak after incubation for 24 hours (National Committee for Clinical Laboratory Standards, 1999b). Another problem that may complicate interpretation of kill-kinetic studies is regrowth occurring between 6–8 hours and 24 hours of incubation of the test. In such instances, it is appropriate to determine whether antimicrobial inactivation has occurred or whether prolonged incubation has selected out a resistant subpopulation. By determining the MIC at 0 and 24 hours against an American Type Culture Collection (ATCC) reference strain, antibiotic inactivation can be inferred if the MIC is markedly higher at 0 hours than at 24 (National Committee for Clinical Laboratory Standards, 1999b).

Serum Bactericidal Test

The principal objective of the serum bactericidal test is to determine the activity of one or more antimicrobial agents that are present in serum against an organism that has been isolated from the patient. By using different modifications, bactericidal activity can be determined relative to the MBC (serum bactericidal titer), the rate over time (serum bactericidal rate), or the magnitude of bactericidal activity and its duration (National Committee for Clinical Laboratory Standards, 1999a). Practically, the peak and trough serum bactericidal titers are the most easily determined. This is done by obtaining a serum sample from the patient at the anticipated peak and/or trough levels of the antimicrobial agents that the patient is receiving. The serum sample is then diluted in broth, pooled human serum, or a mixture of broth and pooled human serum that has been supplemented with cations (when testing aminoglycosides or fluoroquinolones against *P.*

aeruginosa). A standardized suspension of the organism is then added to the serially diluted serum, and the tubes are incubated overnight at 35°C. The serum inhibitory titer is the highest dilution of serum that visibly inhibits the growth of the organism. Subcultures may be made of each tube containing the serum dilutions that do not have visible growth to determine the highest dilution of serum that was bactericidal to the test organism.

Although there is much controversy over the clinical value of the serum bactericidal test, it should be apparent that all the technical issues involved in bactericidal testing are also involved in this test. Moreover, the serum bactericidal test involves two additional variables: (1) the timing of blood collection, and (2) the type of diluent (i.e., broth, serum, or a combination thereof) used in the test. Once again, because of variations in methodology and technical variables affecting such tests, correlation between specific bactericidal titers and outcome of antimicrobial therapy has been difficult to establish.

References

Baker CN, Stocker SA, Culver DM, Thornsberry C: Comparison of the E-test to agar dilution, broth microdilution, and agar diffusion susceptibility testing techniques by using a special challenge set of bacteria. J Clin Microbiol 1991; 29:533.

Barenfanger J, Drake C, Kacich G: Clinical and financial benefits of rapid bacterial identification and antimicrobial susceptibility testing. J Clin Microbiol 1999; 37:1415.

This interesting study demonstrates the potential benefits of rapid identification of and susceptibility testing against bacterial isolates using commercial susceptibility systems. Potential benefits in patient outcome, length of stay, and hospital costs are discussed.

Bates DW, Goldman L, Lee TH: Contaminant blood cultures and resource utilization. The true consequences of false-positive results. JAMA 1991; 265:365.

Bayer AS, Lam K: Efficacy of vancomycin plus rifampin in experimental aortic valve endocarditis due to methicillin-resistant *Staphylococcus aureus*: in vitro–in vivo correlations. J Infect Dis 1985; 151:157.

Bird BR, Denniston MM, Huebner RE, Good RC: Changing practices in mycobacteriology: a follow-up survey of state and territorial public health laboratories. J Clin Microbiol 1996; 34:554.

Critchley IA, Karlowsky JA: Optimal use of antibiotic resistance surveillance systems. Clin Micrbiol Infec 2004; 10:502–511.

D'Azevedo PA, Dias CA, Goncalves ALS, et al: Evaluation of an automated system for the identification and antimicrobial susceptibility testing of enterococci. Diag Microbiol Infect Dis 2001; 40:157.

Doern GV, Vautour R, Gaudet M, et al: Clinical impact of rapid in vitro susceptibility testing and bacterial identification. J Clin Microbiol 1994; 32:1757.

This interesting study demonstrates the potential benefits of rapid identification of and susceptibility testing against bacterial isolates using commercial susceptibility systems. Potential benefits in patient outcome, length of stay, and hospital costs are discussed.

Drake TA, Sande MA: Studies of the chemotherapy of endocarditis: correlation of in vitro, animal model, and clinical studies. Rev Infect Dis 1985; 5(Suppl 2):S345.

Endtz HP, van Den Braak N, van Blekum A, et al: Comparison of eight methods to detect vancomycin resistance in enterococci. J Clin Microbiol 1998; 36:592.

Eng RHK, Chjerubin CE, Pechere J-C, Beam TR: Treatment failures of cefotaxime and latamoxef in meningitis caused by *Enterobacter* and *Serratia* spp. J Antimicrob Chemother 1987; 20:903.

Ernst EJ, Diekema DJ, Bootsmiller BJ, et al: Are United States hospitals following national guidelines for the analysis and presentation of cumulative antimicrobial susceptibility data? Diag Microbiol Infec Dis 2004; 49:141.

Fahr AM, Eigner U, Armbrust M, et al: Two-center collaborative evaluation of the performance of the BD Phoenix Automated Microbiology System for identification and antimicrobial susceptibility

testing of *Enterococcus* spp. and *Staphylococcus* spp. J Clin Microbiol 2003; 41:1135.

Falagas ME, Siakavellas E: *Bacteroides, Prevotella,* and *Porphyromonas* species: a review of antibiotic resistance and therapeutic options. Int J Antimicrob Agents 2000; 15:1.

Felten A, Grandry B, Lagrange PH, Casin I: Evaluation of three techniques for detection of low-level methicillin-resistant *Staphylococcus aureus* (MRSA): a disk diffusion method with cefoxitin and moxalactam, the Vitek 2 system, and the MRSA-Screen latex agglutination test. J Clin Microbiol 2002; 40:2766.

Fiebelkorn KR, Crawford SA, McElmeel ML, Jorgensen JH: Practical disk diffusion method for detection inducible clindamycin resistance in *Staphylococcus aureus* and coagulase-negative staphylococci. J Clin Microbiol 2003; 41:4740.

Fridkin SK, Edwards JR, Courval JM, et al: The effect of vancomycin and third-generation cephalosporins on the prevalence of vancomycin-resistant enterococci in 126 US adult intensive care units. Ann Intern Med 2001; 135:175.

Fridkin SK, Lawton R, Edwards JR, et al: Monitoring antimicrobial use and resistance: comparison with a national benchmark on reducing vancomycin use and vancomycin-resistant enterococci. Emerg Infect Dis 2002; 8:702.

These two references demonstrate the utility of antibiotic susceptibility testing and cumulative antibiotic susceptibility monitoring in changing practice patterns and the effect that changing antibiotic use patterns can have on reducing the prevalence of a virulent pathogen.

Garcia-Garrote F, Cercenado E, Bouza E: Evaluation of a new system, VITEK 2, for identification and antimicrobial susceptiblity testing of enterococci. J Clin Microbiol 2000; 38:2108.

Gerrado SH, Citron DM, Claros MC, Goldstein EJC: Comparison of E-test to broth microdilution method for testing *Streptococcus pneumoniae* susceptibility to levofloxacin and three macrolides. J Clin Microbiol 1996; 40; 2413.

Gribble MJ, Chow AW, Naiman SL, et al: Prospective randomized trial of piperacillin monotherapy versus carboxypenicillin-aminoglycoside combination regimens in the empirical treatment of serious bacterial infections. Antimicrob Agents Chemother 1983; 24:388.

Hallander HO, Dornbusch K, Gezelius L, et al: Synergism between amingoglycosides and cephalosporins with antipseudomonal activity: interaction index and killing curve method. Antimicrob Agents Chemother 1982; 22:743.

Handwerger S, Tomasz A: Antibiotic tolerance among clinical isolates of bacteria. Rev Infect Dis 1985; 7:368.

Horstkotte MA, Knobloch JKM, Rohde H, et al: Rapid detection of methicillin resistance in coagulase-negative staphylococci with the VITEK 2 System. J Clin Microbiol 2002; 40:3291.

Horstkotte MA, Knobloch JKM, Rohde H, et al: Evaluation of the BD PHOENIX automated microbiology system for detection of methicillin resistance in coagulase-negative staphylococci. J Clin Microbiol 2004; 42:5041.

Jacobs MR, Felmingham D, Appelbaum PC, et al: The Alexander project 1998–2000: susceptibility of

pathogens from community-acquired respiratory tract infection to commonly used antimicrobial agents. J Antimicrob Chemother 2003; 52:229.

Jones RN: Method preferences and test accuracy of antimicrobial susceptibility testing: updates from the College of American Pathologists microbiology surveys. Arch Pathol Lab Med 2001; 125:1285.

A description of the types of susceptibility testing performed by participating laboratories, systems used, and their respective accuracies against specific proficiency test isolates. Potential reporting errors by laboratories are also highlighted.

Jorgensen JH, Crawford SSA, McElmeel ML, Fiebelkorn KR: Detection of inducible clindamycin resistance of staphylococci in conjunction with performance of automated broth susceptibility testing. J Clin Microbiol 2004; 42:1800.

Kohner PC, Patel R, Uhl JR, et al: Comparison of agar dilution, broth microdilution, E-test, disk diffusion, and automated vitek methods for testing susceptibilities of *Enterococcus* spp. to vancomycin. J Clin Microbiol 1997; 35:3258.

Leverstein-van Hall M, Fluit AC, Paauw A, et al: Evaluation of the Etest ESBL and the BD Phoenix, VITEK 1, and VITEK 2 automated instruments for detection of extended spectrum beta-lactamases in multiresistant *Esherichia coli* and *Klebsiella* spp. J Clin Microbiol 2002; 40:3703.

Ligozzi M, Bernini C, Bonora MG, et al: Evaluation of the VITEK 2 System for identification and antimicrobial susceptibility testing of medically relevant Gram-positive cocci. J Clin Microbiol 2002; 40:1681.

Livermore DM, Struelens M, Amorim J, et al: Multicentre evaluation of the VITEK 2 Advanced Expert System for interpretive reading of antimicrobial resistance tests. J Antimicrob Chemother 2002; 49:289.

Matsen JM: Means to facilitate physician acceptance and use of rapid test results. Diagn Microbiol Infect Dis 1985; 3:S73.

Mouton JW: Breakpoints: current practice and future perspectives. Int J Antimicrob Agents 2002; 19:323.

Interesting discussion of the concept and rationale behind the antibiotic breakpoint. The distinction between the microbiologic and clinical breakpoint is discussed. Recommendations for improving the accuracy and utility of the breakpoint are made.

Murdoch DR, Mirrett S, Harrell LJ, et al: Comparison of Microscan broth dilution, Synergy Quad plate agar dilution, and disk diffusion screening methods for detection of high-level aminoglycoside resistance in *Enterococcus* species. J Clin Microbiol 2003; 41: 2703.

National Committee for Clinical Laboratory Standards: Methodology for the Serum Batericidal Test; Approved Guideline. CLSI Document M21-A. Wayne, PA, CLSI, 1999a.

National Committee for Clinical Laboratory Standards: Methods for Determining Bactericidal Activity of Anitmicrobial Agents. Approved Guidelines. CLSI Document M26-A. Wayne, PA, CLSI, 1999b.

National Committee for Clinical Laboratory Standards: Analysis and Presentation of Cumulative Antimicrobial Susceptiblity Test Data; Approved Guideline. CLSI Document M39-A. Wayne, PA, CLSI, 2002a.

VII

National Committee for Clinical Laboratory Standards: Reference Method for Broth Dilution Antifungal Testing of Filamentous Fungi; Approved Standard. CLSI Document M38-A. Wayne, PA, CLSI, 2002b.

National Committee for Clinical Laboratory Standards: Reference Method for Broth Dilution Antifungal Susceptibility Testing of Yeasts; Approved Standard, 2nd ed. CLSI Document M27-A2. Wayne, PA, 2002c.

National Committee for Clinical Laboratory Standards: Methods for Dilution Antimicrobial Susceptibility Tests for Bacteria That Grow Aerobically; Approved Standard, 6th ed. CLSI Document M7-A6. Wayne, PA, CLSI, 2003a.

National Committee for Clinical Laboratory Standards: Performance Standards for Antimicrobial Disk Susceptibility Tests; Approved Standard, 8th ed. CLSI Document M2-A8, Wayne, PA, CLSI, 2003b.

National Committee for Clinical Laboratory Standards: Susceptiblity Testing of Mycobacteria, Nocardiae, and Other Aerobic Actinomycetes; Approved Standard. CLSI Document M24-A. Wayne, PA, CLSI, 2003c.

National Committee for Clinical Laboratory Standards: Methods for Antimicrobial Susceptibility Testing of Anaerobic Bacteria; Approved Standard, 6th ed. CLSI Document M11-A6. Wayne, PA, CLSI, 2004.

National Committee for Clinical Laboratory Standards: Performance Standards for Antimicrobial Susceptibility Testing; 15th Informational Supplement. CLSI Document M100-S15. Wayne, PA, CLSI, 2005.

Nguyen MH, Yu VL, Morris AJ, et al: Antimicrobial resistance and clinical outcome of *Bacteroides* bacteremia: findings of a multicenter prospective observational trial. Clin Infect Dis 2000; 30:870.

Important study that demonstrates the changing susceptibility patterns of a genus of anaerobic bacteria over time, the correlation of appropriate antibiotic treatment with patient outcome, and the importance of susceptibility testing in guiding treatment.

NNIS: National Nosocomial Infections Surveillance (NNIS) System Report, Data Summary from January 1992 through June 2003. Am J Infect Control 2003; 31:481.

Pearson RD, Steigbigel RT, Davis HY, Chapman SW: Method for reliable determination of minimum lethal antibiotic concentrations. Antimicrob Agents Chemother 1980; 18:699.

Quinn JP, Divincenzo CA, Lucks DA, et al: Serious infections due to penicillin-resistant strains of viridans streptococci with altered penicillin-binding proteins. J Infect Dis 1988; 157:764.

Rosenstein NE, Stocker SA, Popvic T, et al: Antimicrobial reistance of *Neisseria meningitidis* in the United States, 1997. The Active Bacterial Core Surveillance (ABCs) Team. Clin Infect Dis 2000; 30: 212.

Sakoulas G, Gold HS, Venkataraman L, et al: Methicillin-resistant *Staphylococcus aureus*: comparison of susceptibility testing methods and analysis of *mecA*-positive susceptible strains. J Clin Microbiol 2001; 39:3946.

Sande MA: Antibiotic therapy of bacterial meningitis: lessons we've learned. Am J Med 1981; 71:507.

Sanders CC, Peyret M, Smith Moland E, et al: Ability of the VITEK 2 Advanced Expert System to identify β-lactam phenotypes in isolates of *Enterobacteriaceae* and *Pseudomonas aeruginosa*. J Clin Microbiol 2000; 38:570.

Scarpano C, Ricordi P, Ruggiero G, Piccoli P: Evaluation of the fully automated BACTEC MGIT 960 System for testing susceptibility for *Mycobacterium tuberculosis* to pyrazinamide, streptomycin, isoniazid, rifampin, and ethambutol and comparison with the radiometric BACTEC 460TM method. J Clin Microbiol 2004; 42:1109.

Schreckenberger PC, Ilendo E, Ristow KL: Incidence of constitutive and inducible clindamycin resistance in *Staphylococcus aureus* and coagulase-negative staphylococci in a community and a tertiary care hospital. J Clin Microbiol 2004; 42:2777.

Sherris JC: Problems in in vitro determination of antibiotic tolerance. Antimicrob Agents Chemother 1986; 30:633.

Snydman DR, Jacobus NV, McDermott LA, et al: National survey on the susceptibility of *Bacteroides* *fragilis* group: report and analysis of trends for 1997–2000. Clin Infect Dis 2002; 35:S126.

Sturenburg E, Mack D: Extended-spectrum β-lactamases: implications for the clinical microbiology laboratory, therapy, and infection control. J Infect 2003a; 47:273.

Sturenburg E, Sobottka I, Feucht HH, et al: Comparison of BDPhoenix and VITEK2 automated antimicrobial susceptibility test systems for extended-spectrum beta-lactamase detection in *Escherichia coli* and *Klebsiella* species clinical isolates. Diagn Microbiol Infect Dis 2003b; 45:29.

Swenson JM, Williams PP, Killgore G, et al: Performance of eight methods, including two new rapid methods for detection of oxacillin resistance in a challenge set of *Staphylococcus aureus* organisms. J Clin Microbiol 2001; 39:3785.

Tenover FC, Swenson JM, O'Hara CM, Stocker SA: Ability of commercial and reference antimicrobial susceptibility testing methods to detect vancomycin resistance in enterococci, J Clin Microbiol 1995; 33:1524.

Tenover FC, Weigel LM, Appelbaum PC, et al: Vancomycin-resistant *Staphylococcus aureus* isolate from a patient in Pennsylvania. Antimicrob Agents Chemother 2004; 48: 275.

Van Den Braak N, Goessens W, van Belkum A, et al: Accuracy of the VITEK 2 system to detect glycopeptide resistance in enterococcci. J Clin Microbiol 2001; 39:351.

Vincent P, Izard D, Lebrun T, et al: Intaret cliniques des resultats rapides de bacteriologie ou de l'infection nosocomiales: comparaison avec les methodes traditionelles. Presse Med 1985; 14:1697.

Wilcox MH, Winstanely TG, Douglas CWI, et al: Susceptibility of alpha-hemolytic streptococci causing endocarditis to benzylpenicillin and ten cephalosporins. J Antimicrob Chemother 1993; 32:63.

Wilson WR, Geraci JE: Treatment of streptococcal infective endocarditis. Am J Med 1985; 75(Suppl 6B):128.

CHAPTER 58

Spirochete Infections

P. Rocco LaSala MD, Michael B. Smith MD

KEY POINTS

- While some exceptions and variations exist, human diseases caused by spirochetes typically have a natural history with sequential clinical manifestations that reflect three general phenomena: (a) early, local proliferation of the organisms at the site of inoculation, (b) spirochetemia with systemic dissemination, and (c) persistence of small numbers of microbes at various sites.

- Although direct detection of spirochetes causing human disease is sometimes possible (microbiologic culture, microscopy, genomic amplification, etc.), a diagnosis more often relies upon the demonstration of a patient's serologic response to the offending agent.

- Venereal syphilis is a historic sexually transmitted disease caused by *Treponema pallidum* subspecies *pallidum*.

- In the early stages of disease, venereal syphilis may be diagnosed using direct microscopic visualization.

- Serologic detection of syphilis, by far the most common mode of diagnosis, comprises methods that semi-quantitatively measure antibody to various lipoproteins and methods that qualitatively measure antibody to treponeme-specific antigens.

- Yaws, endemic syphilis (bejel) and pinta are not sexually transmitted, are endemic to various tropical and Middle Eastern regions, and are caused by *T. pallidum* subsp. *pertenue*, *T. pallidum* subsp. *endemicum*, and *T. carateum*, respectively.

- Presumptive diagnosis of the endemic trepanematoses can often be made based on clinical and epidemiologic data; however, like venereal syphilis, serologic and direct microscopic techniques may also prove useful.

- The most common tick-borne disease in North America and Europe, Lyme disease is caused by *Borrelia burgdorferi* sensu stricto, *Borrelia garinii* and *Borrelia afzelii*.

- Typical clinical manifestations if Lyme disease include erythema migrans (early localized disease), neuroborreliosis (early disseminated or late-stage disease) and/or Lyme arthritis (late-stage disease).

- As no single laboratory test performs sufficiently in all clinical scenarios, a diagnosis of Lyme disease must be based upon a combination of (a) clinico-epidemiologic characteristics, (b) host serologic response (as measured by ELISA/IFA and immunoblot), (c) molecular evidence, and/or (d) culture results.

- Epidemic, louse-borne relapsing fever has a worldwide distribution and is caused by *Borrelia recurrentis*.

- Endemic, tick-borne relapsing fever has a limited geographic distribution and is caused by several *Borrelia* species, including *Borrelia hermsi* and *Borrelia turicata*.

- Acute-onset of high fever and constitutional symptoms followed by cycles of evanescence and recrudescence are frequently recognized in both forms of relapsing fever.

- Diagnosis of relapsing fever is most often established through the demonstration of spirochetes in peripheral blood smears stained by a Giemsa technique.

- One of the most common zoonotic diseases throughout the world, leptospirosis is caused by various serovars of different species within the genus *Leptospira*.

- Although leptospirosis is usually subclinical or mild and flu-like, a small proportion of patients develop severe constitutional symptoms in addition to gastrointestinal/hepatic disease, meningitis, renal failure and/or myocarditis (also referred to as Weil's disease).

- While *Leptospira spp.* can be cultivated in vitro, diagnosis is usually made by demonstrating seroconversion.

- *Brachyspira aalborgi* and *Brachyspira pilosicoli* have each been demonstrated in and isolated from the colons of humans with diarrheal disease, but pathogenic etiology has not been firmly established. Demonstration of spirochetes along the colonic epithelial cell borders using routine, immunohistochemical or in situ hybridization microscopy from biopsy material is more commonly performed than cultivation or genomic amplification assays.

Spirochetes are slender bacteria occurring in the form of spirals with one or more complete rotations in the helix. They are Gram-negative but can only be visualized by darkfield or phase microscopy, silver impregnation and immunohistochemical stains in tissue sections. Flagella-like organelles, termed periplasmic fibrils or axial filaments, that are attached near the poles of the bacteria permit a corkscrew-like motility. While many commensal and nonpathogenic species of spirochetes exist, human disease is limited to infections by members of three genera: *Treponema*, *Borrelia*, and *Leptospira*. Widely diverse from an epidemiological standpoint, spirochetes within these genera demonstrate a number of pathogenic, and hence clinical, similarities upon acquisition by humans (Schmid, 1989). Additionally, spirochete-like bacteria such as *Spirillum minor* and *Anaerobiospirillum succiniciproducens* have been implicated in human diseases. Although *Brachyspira* species have been associated with gastrointestinal syndromes, definitive causation by these bacteria for disease has not been universally accepted.

Treponema

The genus *Treponema* contains two species that cause disease in humans. *Treponema pallidum* is divided into three subspecies, each of which is the etiologic agent of a distinct clinical entity: subspecies *pallidum*, *pertenue*, and *endemicum*, are the etiologic agents of venereal syphilis, yaws, and endemic syphilis (bejel), respectively. Pinta is caused by the second pathogenic species, *Treponema carateum*.

Classic Treponemal Diseases

Syphilis

Description

T. pallidum subsp. pallidum, the etiologic agent of venereal syphilis, is a thin (0.2 µm) spirochete, 6–20 µm in length with 10–13 coils. The spirochete has corkscrew motility with an undulating central flexion. It is readily killed by heat, cold, desiccation, disinfectants, and osmotic changes.

Epidemiology

Man is the only natural reservoir for T. pallidum subsp. pallidum. Transmission is by direct contact with active lesions, primarily through sexual contact. The probability that an infected individual will transmit the disease to his or her partner is approximately 30–50% (Larsen, 1995). Alternatively, vertical transmission across the placenta, the second most common mode of infection, may result when either a latently infected female becomes pregnant or when a pregnant woman becomes infected (Wicher, 2001). Although much less frequent, the infection can be transmitted by nonsexual contact with an active lesion, the transfusion of fresh blood products from an infected person (organisms cannot survive more than 24–48 hours under conditions of blood bank storage), by accidental needle stick, or when handling laboratory specimens.

The incidence of venereal syphilis in the United States declined dramatically with the advent of penicillin after World War II and remained stable until the 1980s, when the prevalence of syphilis increased, probably because of the association of increased drug use and sexual promiscuity in certain populations. While the global prevalence of syphilis remains strikingly variable (Gerbase, 1998; Peeling, 2004), the United States experienced a continuous decline in infection rates among women of childbearing age throughout the 1990s, which was paralleled by a comparable decrease in congenital syphilis incidence (Centers for Disease Control and Prevention, 2003, 2004a). Despite the establishment of a National Plan to Eliminate Syphilis from the United States (Centers for Disease Control and Prevention, 1999), however, disease incidence among homosexual men continues to increase (Centers for Disease Control and Prevention, 2003).

Pathogenesis and Pathology

T. pallidum subsp. pallidum penetrates an intact mucous membrane or gains access to tissue through abraded skin, multiplies at the inoculation site, and then enters the lymphatic and circulatory system and spreads throughout the body. In laboratory animals, infections have been produced with as few as four spirochetes (Cumberland, 1949). Clinical lesions appear when a critical mass of organisms is reached locally ($\approx 10^7$ spirochetes); therefore, the incubation period is directly related to the size of the initial inoculum and varies from 3 days to 3 months (Magnuson, 1956).

The host immunologic response to T. pallidum subsp. pallidum is influenced by the structure of the bacterium. The outer membrane is a phospholipid bilayer with few demonstrable protein antigens. The most important antigens for the host immune response appear to be lipoproteins within the periplasmic space (Chamberlain, 1989; Cox, 1992; Salazar, 2002). Additionally, the bacterium appears to be able to coat itself with host proteins. The net effect is to delay the humoral response, reducing its effectiveness because the spirochetes are in extravascular locations by the time antibodies are produced. Furthermore, it has been demonstrated in animal models that the cellular immune response is down-regulated in syphilis, despite the ineffective humoral response (Fitzgerald, 1992).

This delayed and attenuated immune response allows T. pallidum subsp. pallidum to disseminate and to produce a chronic infection. The course of syphilis can be divided into predictable stages. The primary stage, the development of a chancre, occurs at a median of 3 weeks, although a primary lesion does not develop in all patients. In some cases, because of its painless nature, the lesion passes without notice. Healing in anywhere from 2–8 weeks, the chancre gives way to the secondary stage. Seen a mean of six weeks after inoculation (range, 2–12 weeks), this stage is characterized by widespread dissemination via the bloodstream and the development of mucocutaneous and organ involvement with the presence of constitutional symptoms. The secondary stage resolves, and the infection enters a period of latency, during which the patient shows no manifestations of the infection. The first 4 years of this period are termed the early latent period, and it is during this period that relapses can occur, with the majority of relapses occurring within the first year. This is followed by the late latent period, during which time relapses do not occur. Anywhere from 10–25 years after the primary stage, one third of untreated patients develop tertiary syphilis, with the most serious manifestations in the cardiovascular system or the central nervous system (CNS).

Whatever organ involved or whatever stage of the disease, the histologic hallmark of syphilis is an obliterative endarteritis showing a concentric endothelial and fibroblastic proliferation with an associated mononuclear cell infiltrate rich in plasma cells. Endarteritis results from the binding of spirochetes to endothelial cells via fibronectin molecules that have attached to the surface of the bacteria (Thomas, 1986). Treponemes are demonstrable in the tissues with silver-impregnation and immunohistochemical stains. With progression of the disease, both the plasma cell infiltrate and the concentration of treponemes lessen in intensity.

The recent elucidation of the complete genomic sequence of T. pallidum subsp. pallidum may provide insights into the pathogenesis of this organism (Fraser, 1998). For example, researchers have been able to verify the absence of many particular enzymatic pathways typically found in other cultivable bacterial pathogens. One particularly interesting finding was a series of duplicated genes, termed T. pallidum repeats (tprA–tprL), which encode homologous membrane proteins that may impart the means of antigenic variability and immunologic escape (Centurion-Lara, 1999). Their roles in such, as well as their putative cellular location, however, remain vague (Hazlett, 2001). Nonetheless, as functions have thus far been ascribed or extrapolated to only about two thirds of the proteins encoded by the 1041 open reading frames (Singh, 1999), much work yet remains.

Clinical Manifestations

Syphilis is a chronic infection with a multiplicity of expressions, primarily related to the stage at which it presents. The primary chancre is characteristically ulcerated with raised, firm edges, a smooth base and notable for an absence of an exudate or pain. Usually single, multiple chancres can occur in up to one third of patients. Patients with previous infection can present with atypical lesions, such as a small papule, or may not develop a lesion at all. Regional lymphadenopathy, with moderately enlarged, rubbery, nonsuppurative lymph nodes, is seen in some patients.

Dissemination results in the secondary stage, and patients present with signs and symptoms of a systemic illness. More than 90% develop a rash that begins on the trunk and extremities (although any body surface can be involved) as small macules that progress to papules, and in some patients to pustules over a period of weeks. The appearance of the rash on the palms and soles is characteristic, and enlargement and coalescence of papules produces the pale plaques of condyloma lata. Approximately the same number (90%) have generalized lymphadenopathy, and three quarters can suffer from fever, malaise, anorexia, arthralgia, pharyngitis, and weight loss. Mucous patches are seen in up to one third of cases. About 40% develop CNS symptoms, although only 1–2% develop acute aseptic meningitis (Lukehart, 1988). The remainder show headache and meningismus, uveitis, sensorineural hearing loss, and cranial nerve involvement.

The tissue destruction of tertiary syphilis becomes evident 10–25 years after the primary infection. Cardiovascular syphilis occurs as a result of weakening of the tunica media and results in an aneurysm of the ascending aorta with aortic valve insufficiency and narrowing of the coronary artery ostia. Syphilitic gummas (i.e., areas of gummatous necrosis), ranging in size from microscopic to large tumors, most commonly involve the skin, skeletal system, and mucocutaneous tissues but may affect any organ. Both cardiovascular syphilis and gummas became much less frequent after the advent of antibiotic treatment. By contrast, because antibiotics are often administered in doses insufficient to cross the blood–brain barrier in bactericidal concentrations, neurosyphilis still occurs with some frequency (Mohr, 1976; Greene, 1980). This manifestation of syphilis is classified as either meningovascular or parenchymatous, although overlap is common.

Meningovascular syphilis occurs 5–10 years after initial infection and clinically presents as seizures, stroke, and aphasia. Multiple small infarcts due to the characteristic endarteritis in the CNS are the etiology of this form. Parenchymatous neurosyphilis, which presents 15–30 years after initial infection, is a degenerative process with loss of neurons and myelinated tracts resulting in a complex of neurologic and psychiatric manifestations, including general paresis, tabes dorsalis, and pupillary abnormalities. Some patients lack any clinical signs or symptoms, but demonstrate cerebrospinal fluid (CSF) abnormalities such as pleocytosis, increased protein, a reactive Venereal Disease Research Laboratory (VDRL) test, or antibody against T. pallidum, indicating CNS infection. Such patients have been described as having 'asymptomatic neurosyphilis' (Tramont, 2000).

Congenital syphilis also occurs clinically in two forms: an early or infantile form and a late form occurring after a latent period of 5–30 years. Although the traditional view that infection of the fetus occurs only in the second trimester is no longer accepted, congenital syphilis is more often a cause of early than of late abortion (Harter, 1976; Blanc, 1981). Necrotizing funisitis, or inflammation of the umbilical cord, is characteristic of congenital syphilis, although typically present in only the most severe cases. In the infantile form, a diffuse rash with sloughing of the skin and osteochondritis and periostitis are characteristic; however, affected newborns may be asymptomatic (Dorfman, 1990; Ikeda, 1990). Diffuse fibrosis of the liver (hepar lobatum) and lung (pneumonia alba) are also seen. After a latent period, the late form presents in childhood or adulthood with a wide variety of signs and symptoms; however, the triad of interstitial keratitis, Hutchinson's teeth, and eighth nerve deafness is classic. Periostitis, saber shins, and saddle deformity of the nose are also seen frequently.

Syphilis and human immunodeficiency virus (HIV) infection are frequently seen in the same patient, as both diseases share common risk factors. Studies that have examined the association have demonstrated no difference in stage at clinical presentation between patients with concomitant syphilis and acquired immunodeficiency syndrome (AIDS) and those without AIDS (Hutchinson, 1991; Gourevitch, 1993). Whether AIDS has an effect on the clinical course of primary and secondary syphilis is currently controversial. Some experts cite a predilection for the infection to present with an atypical and more severe rash, greater constitutional symptoms, and a more malignant course in AIDS patients (Tramont, 2000; Collis, 2001). Others, including one prospective study, indicate little difference in disease manifestations between AIDS and non-AIDS patients (Hutchinson, 1991; Musher, 1990; Rolfs, 1997). Furthermore, although it has been proposed that AIDS patients with syphilis show an increased propensity to develop neurosyphilis, and to develop it more rapidly, than non-AIDS patients (Johns, 1987; Musher, 1990), this remains a contested issue given (a) the shortcomings of current neurosyphilis diagnostic criteria (Collis, 2001) and (b) an apparent lack of correlation between early CNS treponemal invasion and HIV status (Lukehart, 1988). A recent multicenter prospective study showed that CSF nontreponemal tests were more likely to remain positive following therapy in HIV-infected individuals than in HIV-uninfected patients (Marra, 2004). However, it remains to be seen if such laboratory evidence of treatment failure is a true reflection of potential clinical relapse or simply an immunologic peculiarity unique to this population. Nevertheless, AIDS patients do show a high incidence of eye involvement, with anterior uveitis being the most common manifestation of *T. pallidum* infection (Tramont, 2000).

Yaws

Yaws (also called frambesia tropica, pian, parangi, paru, buba, or bouba) is a chronic disease caused by *T. pallidum* subsp. *pertenue*. This disease, which has afflicted residents of the tropics since antiquity, is prevalent in rural areas of tropical countries with heavy rainfall. After a decline in the 1950s due to large campaigns to control the treponematoses, the incidence of yaws has increased in some areas (Engelkens, 1991a; Antal, 2002).

Yaws is contracted during childhood prior to age 15 years by direct contact, with breaks in the skin allowing entry of the treponemes. Early lesions generally appear an average of 3 weeks later but may not develop for months. One or several papules appear, most frequently on the lower extremities, and then ulcerate or progress to papillomatous lesions. Numerous treponemes are found in these lesions. Spontaneous resolution is usual; however, relapses preceded by malaise, fever, and generalized lymphadenopathy followed by disseminated skin lesions are common. Most patients enter a period of latency during which no clinical signs or symptoms are evident. For most, the disease shows no further manifestations; however, approximately 10% develop late yaws, which shows irreversible, destructive lesions of bone, cartilage, soft tissue, and the skin (Engelkens, 1991a; Antal, 2002). Cardiovascular and CNS lesions similar to those seen in syphilis have been reported to occur (Roman, 1986).

Endemic Syphilis

Endemic syphilis (bejel) is a nonvenereal chronic infection caused by infection with *T. pallidum* subsp. *endemicum*. The disease is ancient and, while it is no longer as widespread as it once was, still occurs in the Middle East and Africa in hot, dry climates. In Sahelian Africa, the disease has been increasing in prevalence (Engelkens, 1991b).

The disease is transmitted by direct contact with active lesions, contaminated fingers, and eating or drinking utensils. Crowded living conditions and poor hygiene are common. Children aged 2–15 years are primarily infected, although the disease can be found in adults in the same family, and those adults who did not suffer from the disease in childhood can be infected by their children.

The inoculum is small and the primary lesions of early endemic syphilis, most frequent on the oropharyngeal mucosa, are often not apparent. Often, the initial clinical manifestations of the disease are in a secondary stage, with mucous patches, condyloma lata, angular stomatitis, generalized

lymphadenopathy, and painful osteoperiostitis. This is followed by a latent period of variable length. The late stage is characterized by tissue destruction of the skin, bones, and cartilage, with a predilection for the nose and palate (so-called gangosa), and sometimes laryngeal involvement.

Pinta

Pinta (carate, mal de pinto, azul) is caused by infection with *T. carateum*. The disease is endemic in rural tropical Central and South America and recently has reappeared in Mexico and Colombia, two countries from which it was eradicated in the 1950s (Englekens, 1991). Children under the age of five years are primarily affected. Inoculation is thought to occur via nonvenereal skin or mucous membrane contact. Characterization of the pathogenesis of the disease is difficult because, unlike other treponematoses that are pathogenic in humans, an animal model is unavailable and the treponeme cannot be cultured continuously.

While similar to other treponemal infections that have early and late stages, there is frequent overlap of stages in pinta. A primary papule or plaque develops at the site of inoculation after weeks to months, with or without localized lymphadenopathy. The primary lesion resolves and several months to years later disseminated secondary lesions, or pintids, which resemble scaly psoriasiform plaques, appear and remain for long periods or resolve and recur. In late pinta, lesions demonstrate hypopigmentation and skin atrophy or hyperkeratosis, which can persist for life. The skin appears to be the only organ affected in this disease (Antal, 2002).

Laboratory Diagnosis of Treponematoses

Because the etiologic agents of the human treponematoses cannot be isolated by routine culture methods, detection is either by direct visualization of the organisms in material from lesions or indirectly by immunologic methods. Each stage of the treponematoses requires a particular testing modality. In the early stages when lesions are present, direct microscopy is used. In later stages, serologic tests are employed. Nonspecific nontreponemal tests are used for screening, and the specific treponemal tests are used for confirmation. It is important to realize that none of these commonly used laboratory tests is capable of distinguishing between the closely related species and subspecies of pathogenic treponemes, and differentiation must be made on clinical and epidemiologic grounds.

Darkfield Microscopy

When direct sampling of lesions is possible, such as in primary, secondary, or early congenital syphilis (chancres, mucous patches, or condyloma lata), the lesion should be cleansed with sterile water (no soap or antiseptic) then gently abraded. Pressure is applied, causing serous exudate to collect in the lesion. A drop of the fluid is placed on a slide and a coverslip placed over the fluid. The specimen must be examined immediately, as visualization of motility is necessary for definitive identification. Because of their narrow width, treponemes cannot be visualized by conventional light microscopy. Darkfield microscopy, which uses a condenser that allows light rays to hit the treponemes at an oblique angle, causing the light to reflect off the treponemes, which then appear as bright objects on a dark background, is necessary. The darkfield examination can be positive several weeks before a positive serologic test and has a sensitivity of 80% in diagnosing syphilis (Larsen, 1995). Because of possible confusion with commensal treponemes in the mouth, it is not recommended that this technique be utilized for oral lesions. Additionally, there are three species of *Treponema* that are normal inhabitants of the genital region (*Treponema phagedensis*, *Treponema refringens*, and *Treponema minutum*) that potentially could be confused with *T. pallidum* on darkfield examination. Careful cleaning of the area is important in reducing the likelihood of this happening.

Fluorescence Microscopy

Fluorescein isothiocyanate (FITC)-labeled antibodies specific for *T. pallidum* can be used for direct detection of treponemes in lesions, obviating the need to observe motility of the bacteria. The test can be applied to tissue fluid that has been dried and fixed to the slide (direct fluorescent antibody [DFA-TP]) or paraffin-embedded tissue sections (direct fluorescent antibody tissue test [DFAT-TP]). Monoclonal antibodies are commercially available, and can be used in these tests instead of the previously used, less specific Reiter treponeme adsorbed polyclonal antibodies obtained from syphilitic rabbits and humans. When used to examine fluid from fresh lesions, both the DFA-TP and DFAT-TP have a sensitivity of approximately 100%, compared to the Stiener silver impregnation stain in congenital syphilis (Larsen, 1995). Since these tests are specific for the pathogenic treponemes, they are preferred for examination of oral lesions.

Immunohistochemical Microscopy

In a manner similar in principle to fluorescence microscopy, monoclonal and polyclonal antibodies with specificities for spirochetes, treponemes, or *T. pallidum* have been used by pathologists for the detection of these organisms in paraffin-embedded tissues (Guarner, 2000; Hoang, 2004). In contrast to immunofluorescence, however, immunohistochemistry does not require the use of rather expensive fluorescent microscopes. With this technique anti-treponemal antibodies bound to spirochetes in tissue sections are detected after a series of immunologic reactions, which typically consist of a species-specific biotinylated antiglobulin conjugate followed by an enzyme-conjugated streptavidin complex. After development of the enzyme with an appropriate chromogenic substrate, organisms, when present, are highlighted against a pale counterstained background. This allows easy detection of rare bacteria and affords the capability for histologic localization. The procedure reportedly offers an improvement in sensitivity and specificity over the silver impregnation stains for the detection of treponemes, but this is largely dependent upon the source of primary antibody.

Nontreponemal Serologic Tests

The nontreponemal assays detect the presence of antibodies to lipoprotein material from damaged cells and cardiolipin from treponemes and as a consequence are not specific for *Treponema*. These tests are used to screen for disease and to monitor the course of the disease after treatment. Standard tests include the VDRL reagin slide, rapid plasma reagin (RPR) circle card, unheated serum reagin (USR), and toluidine red unheated serum (TRUST) tests. A nontreponemal enzyme-linked immunosorbent assay (ELISA) has also been approved by the United States Food and Drug Administration (FDA), although it is not yet considered a standard test (Larsen, 1998). All the tests use a phospholipid (cardiolipin) antigen fortified with lecithin and cholesterol in a colloidal particle. Flocculation is the end point for the standard tests, whereas absorbance values are calculated spectrophotometrically in the ELISA. Serum, rather than plasma, is the preferred specimen for all tests, and heating of the serum to eliminate nonspecific reactions is required in the VDRL. Addition of choline chloride to the RPR and USR eliminates the need for heating the specimen. The antibody–antigen reactions in the VDRL and USR are assessed using a microscope at 100×, while the addition of charcoal to the RPR and dye to the TRUST make the reactions macroscopically visible.

The antibodies detected by these tests generally develop 1–4 weeks after the appearance of the primary chancre. The time at which the specimen is taken during the primary stage, therefore, could affect the sensitivity. The titer rises, remains high during the first year and then gradually declines. The test spontaneously reverts to negative in 25% of patients. Both false-negative and false-positive tests occur. False-negative tests are associated with high titers of antibody (prozone phenomenon), which can be seen especially in secondary syphilis. This situation can be resolved by diluting the specimen prior to testing. False-positive results occur temporarily with acute illnesses such as hepatitis, other viral infections, and pregnancy; or chronically with the connective tissue diseases (Larsen, 1995).

Positive standard tests are titered by repeating the tests with twofold dilutions of specimen. This is a major drawback to the provisional ELISA format, however. Although it affords the ability for high sample throughput, semiquantitative analysis via serial dilutions have not been adequately evaluated in the ELISA. Titers from standard tests are used to determine the efficacy of treatment. A fourfold decrease in titer at 12 months in early syphilis and a fourfold decrease at 6 months and an eightfold decrease at 12 months in late syphilis is evidence of adequate treatment (Romanowski, 1991). Patients treated in early syphilis are more likely to revert to negative than those treated in late syphilis (Fiumara, 1980; Brown, 1985).

The screening of certain populations for syphilis requires the use of particular specimens or tests. For example, when screening for congenital syphilis, the mother's serum is a better specimen than cord blood or neonatal blood, which have been used in the past (United States Public Health Service, 1968). Neonatal serum may occasionally be tested semiquantitatively, however, in order to compare titers with maternal serum. When the former is significantly higher than the latter, one may reason that the neonatal antibody source is not likely to be the sole result of transplacental diffusion. Another example is in the diagnosis of neurosyphilis, which requires a positive serum treponemal test in addition to either a positive VDRL on CSF or some CSF abnormality (e.g., elevated white blood cell count or protein level) (Centers for Disease Control and Prevention, 2002). The VDRL is very specific, albeit insensitive, for the diagnosis of neurosyphilis. It can be negative in 22–69% of patients with active neurosyphilis, and its sensitivity in inactive neurosyphilis may be as low as 10% (MacLean, 1996). Despite this, none of the other non-treponemal tests are useful in detecting this late complication of syphilis, and treponemal tests suffer from lack of specificity, with false positives due to transudation of antibody across the blood–brain barrier.

There have been reports of various aberrant nontreponemal test results with patients coinfected with HIV and syphilis, including delayed seroconversion; however, seronegative syphilis does not appear to be prevalent in AIDS patients (Flores, 1995). The false-positive rate is slightly increased in AIDS patients (4% vs 1% in non-AIDS); however, at least one study associated the increased rate of positivity with intravenous drug abuse rather than HIV infection itself (Flores, 1995; Larsen, 1995; Hernandez-Aguado, 1998). False-negative results also occur in AIDS patients with syphilis because of an exaggerated nontreponemal antibody response that occurs in some patients, with the resultant prozone effect (Gourevitch, 1993). Furthermore, as mentioned previously, nontreponemal antibody titers do not decline (so-called 'seroreversion') in some AIDS patients with syphilis despite therapy, although some believe this is more related to the stage at which treatment was initiated, rather than HIV infection, as this has also been reported in non-AIDS patients (Larsen, 1995).

Treponemal Serologic Tests

These tests detect the presence of antibodies to treponemal antigens and are used to confirm a positive nontreponemal screening test, or confirm infection in the face of a negative nontreponemal test in late or latent disease, which can occur in 30% of patients with tertiary syphilis (Larsen, 1995). The fluorescent treponemal antibody absorption test (FTA-ABS), one of the two standard treponemal tests, is an indirect fluorescent antibody test. It involves the addition of heated patient serum, which has been adsorbed with antigen of the nonpathogenic Reiter treponeme to remove cross-reacting antibodies, to a slide on which *T. pallidum* subsp. *pallidum* (Nichols strain) has been fixed, followed by the addition of FITC-labeled anti-human globulin. Visible treponemes on fluorescent microscopy indicate the presence of antibody to the pathogenic treponemal species in the patient's serum. The second test, which is preferred by many laboratories because of its relative simplicity, is the microhemagglutination-*T. pallidum* test (MHA-TP). Absorbed serum is added to sheep red blood cells sensitized with *T. pallidum* (Nichols strain) sonicate in a microtiter tray. Agglutination of the red cells will be produced by antibody containing serum. Generally, the MHA-TP and FTA-ABS are equivalent, except in the primary stage of syphilis, where the FTA-ABS shows greater sensitivity (Hart, 1980; Augenbraun, 1998). Sensitivities and specificities of the various nontreponemal and treponemal serologic tests are summarized in Table 58–1 (Larsen, 1995).

Treponemal-specific antibody develops in primary syphilis and can be detected for the patient's lifetime irrespective of therapy, although there are exceptions. AIDS patients have shown a greater tendency to revert to seronegativity after treatment (Haas, 1990). The FTA-ABS usually is the first test to become positive, followed by the MHA-TP, and then the nontreponemal tests shortly thereafter. Treponemal tests are not used for screening in the clinical setting, as approximately 1% of the population can show false-positive results. False-positive FTA-ABS results occurred in the elderly, in persons with connective tissue diseases, and in persons infected with related organisms, such as *Borrelia* (Larsen, 1995). The frequency of false-positive results with the MHA-TP is reportedly lower than with the FTA-ABS (Larsen, 1995).

As with the nontreponemal serologic tests, ELISAs that use *Treponema*-specific antigens have also become available for use in clinical laboratories.

Table 58–1 Sensitivities of Serologic Tests for Syphilis in Different Stages of Disease

Test	Stage of Syphilis (% Sensitivity)			
	Primary	Secondary	Latent	Late
VDRL	78 (74–87)	100	95 (88–100)	71 (37–94)
RPR	86 (77–100)	100	98 (95–100)	73
FTA-ABS	84 (70–100)	100	100	96
MHA-TP	76 (69–90)	100	97 (97–100)	94

Numbers in parentheses represent ranges of sensitivities in studies at the Centers for Disease Control and Prevention.

FTA-ABS = fluorescent treponemal antibody absorption; MHA-TP = microhemagglutination assay for antibodies to *Treponema pallidum*; RPR = rapid plasma reagin; VDRL = Venereal Disease Research Laboratory.

Source: data are from Larsen SA, Steiner BM, Rudolph AH: Laboratory diagnosis and interpretation of tests for syphilis. Clin Microbiol Rev 1995; 8:1.

Again, these offer the advantages of a format amenable to high-volume testing and objective interpretation. Sensitivity and specificity of the various products commercially available are comparable to the FTA-ABS and MHA-TP (Lefevre, 1990; Norgard, 1993). These tests have been used as screening tests in specific environments such as the screening of blood donors and, in conjunction with a nontreponemal test, in a high-volume laboratory that serves a high-prevalence population (Reisner, 1997; Aberle-Grasse, 1999). Enzyme immunoassay (EIA) tests using nontreponemal antigens and IgM-specific formats are also available and have been used for screening and diagnosis of congenital syphilis, respectively (Stoll, 1993; Hooper, 1994; Larsen, 1998).

Molecular tests, such as the Western blot and the polymerase chain reaction (PCR), are available in some reference laboratories. The Western blot has been recommended in the diagnosis of congenital syphilis (Larsen, 1995). PCR has been advocated for the diagnosis of neurosyphilis, particularly in AIDS patients, although studies have not demonstrated advantages over currently used methods (Marra, 1996). Because of the present lack of standardization in primer design, DNA extraction techniques and method of amplicon detection, PCR will probably remain outside the diagnostic armamentarium for at least the immediate future (Wicher, 1999).

Treatment of Treponematoses

T. pallidum subspecies and *T. carateum* are uniformly susceptible to penicillin and other β-lactam antibiotics. Treatment of primary, secondary, and early latent syphilis is a single intramuscular injection of benzathine penicillin G. Yaws, pinta, and endemic syphilis are treated with the same antibiotic, although at a lower dose (Engelkens, 1991a, 1991b). Household contacts of patients with the latter three diseases are also treated. For patients who are allergic to penicillin, doxycycline or tetracycline are used. Macrolide antibiotics are no longer recommended, as efficacy has been shown to be less than 90% (Schroeter, 1972). A pronounced worsening in clinical course, termed the Jarisch–Herxheimer reaction, may be seen upon treatment of venereal syphilis patients, although symptoms are frequently not as severe as in treatment of relapsing fever spirochetes (Griffin, 1998). For late latent syphilis or syphilis of unknown duration, benzathine penicillin G in multiple doses is given. Stage of disease does not affect treatment for yaws, pinta, or endemic syphilis (Engelkens, 1991a, 1991b). High-dose intravenous aqueous penicillin G is given for neurosyphilis and congenital syphilis. For patients coinfected with HIV and *T. pallidum*, current Centers for Disease Control and Prevention (CDC) guidelines do not recommend any change in therapy (Centers for Disease Control and Prevention, 2002). Indeed, prospective studies have failed to show any benefit of 'enhanced' or alternative therapies for early syphilis and neurosyphilis, respectively, among HIV-infected persons (Rolfs, 1997; Marra, 2000). On the other hand, some authorities suggest that, given a propensity to develop neurosyphilis even in the face of treatment for primary syphilis, AIDS patients should be treated with higher doses of penicillin (Musher, 1991; Tramont, 2000).

Other Treponemal Diseases

Description

A number of spirochetes belonging to the treponeme molecular group (TRE)-1, previously referred to as pathogen-related oral spirochetes (PROS) and various species of *Treponema* (e.g., *Treponema denticola* and *Treponema socranski*), have been recovered with increased frequency and in higher numbers from the gingiva of patients with ulcerative gingivitis and chronic periodontitis compared to patients with healthy gingiva (Riviere, 1995, 1996; Loesche, 2001). Although originally thought to resemble *T. pallidum*, on the basis of immuno-crossreactivity and in vitro invasive properties, these putative pathogens are rather genetically heterogeneous – only distantly related to *T. pallidum* – and can be induced to express crossreactive surface antigens (Choi, 1996; Riviere, 1999)

Pathogenesis

A definitive causal relationship between the spirochetes and these diseases has not been firmly established; however, their presence in significant numbers, more commonly in diseased than healthy tissue, suggests at least an association with gingivitis/periodontitis. Because of the fact that a number of other nontreponemal bacteria (e.g., genera *Prevotella*, *Actinobacillus*, *Porphyromonas*, etc.) have also been associated with these clinical manifestations, the current debate seems primarily to involve determining whether culpability belongs to specific virulent organisms among them or rather to the overall diversity of organisms contained within the plaque biofilm (Loesche, 2001).

Diagnosis

Like the commensal species of *Treponema* found in the genital area, some oral *Treponema* species can be cultured under strict anaerobic conditions using a variety of nonroutine, enriched broth media (Choi, 1996; Riviere, 1999). Other species, including the majority associated with periodontal disease, have not been cultured in vitro (Loesche, 2001). Detection of these organisms has been with monoclonal antibodies against *T. pallidum*, with which they crossreact. More recently, other investigators have employed a variety of genetic amplification tools in an effort to identify and characterize them (Paster, 2001; Hutter, 2003). These 'molecular expeditions' are conducted by using primers that target conserved bacterial sequences and either PCR to amplify rRNA genes or reverse-transcriptase PCR (RT-PCR) to amplify the rRNA itself. The resultant products can then be cloned in *Escherichia coli* and sequenced in order to determine phylogenic relationships.

Treatment

For years, treatment has been aimed primarily at reducing the overall bacterial burden by removing the plaque biofilm, both above and below the gumline, through physical manipulation (e.g., surgical debridement). Recently, the addition of various antimicrobial regimens, including systemic antibiotics and locally applied agents, has been shown to be a potentially beneficial adjunct (Loesche, 2001).

Leptospira

Description

The genus *Leptospira* is composed of 18 genomic species, many containing both pathogenic and nonpathogenic strains, and over 260 serovars (Perolat, 1998; Brenner, 1999). Previously, *Leptospira* was divided into three species: *L. interrogans* (pathogenic), *Leptospira biflexa* (nonpathogenic); and *Leptospira parva* (nonpathogenic), based on biochemical properties. However, it has become evident that such properties, in addition to pathogenicity and antigenicity, are not consistently predictive of genetic relatedness (Levett, 2001). Leptospires are tightly coiled with hooked ends, 0.1 μm in width by 6–20 μm in length, and demonstrate a spinning motility. They survive in alkaline fresh water but are killed by acid pH, salt-water, and drying.

Epidemiology

Leptospirosis is perhaps the most widespread global zoonosis and, although identified nearly 100 years ago, is still considered an important emerging disease. Individual serovars show geographic preferences as well as particular ecological niches. The organism is carried by many rodents, and feral and domestic animals; however, the rat is one of the most frequent reservoirs and an important source of infection in man. Contact with urine-contaminated water and entry of the bacteria through cuts or mucosal surfaces is a frequent mode of infection. Those with occupational exposure (miners, farmers and field workers, veterinarians, fish farmers, and sewage workers) or recreational exposure (camping near or swimming in infected waterways) are at greater risk. The incidence in the United States is 40–120 cases per year; however, the disease is thought to be underreported (Farr, 1995).

Pathology and Pathogenesis

After entry into the circulation, the organisms disseminate widely, including into the CNS and eye. Damage to endothelium in infected tissues results in local ischemia and hemorrhage. Hepatocellular damage and renal tubular damage also occur. The liver may have a characteristic yellow-green color, but histologic changes are nonspecific and include ballooning degeneration, acidophilic bodies, regeneration, and cholestasis; and leptospires can be found in around 25% of cases (Dooley, 1976). The kidney shows a chronic interstitial nephritis, necrosis of proximal tubules, and granular or hyaline casts, with intratubular leptospires in around 65% (Arean, 1962). Pulmonary manifestations include congestion and edema, alveolar hemorrhage, pleural effusion and occasional hyaline membrane formation (Arean, 1962; Ramachandran, 1977). Myocarditis, meningitis/encephalitis, and myositis may also be seen (Arean, 1962). The mechanisms for endothelial, hepatic, and renal damage are unknown but may be immune-mediated.

Clinical

Typically, infection with leptospires presents as a mild, influenza-like illness (anicteric form) or is subclinical and never recognized; a minority suffer from a more severe form, characterized by jaundice, that has a 5–10% fatality rate (icteric form or Weil's disease). Leptospirosis is biphasic, beginning after an incubation period of 2–20 days, with the abrupt appearance of chills, fever, headache, myalgia, back pain, abdominal pain,

VII

anorexia, and nausea and vomiting. During this phase, termed the bacteremic phase, wide dissemination of bacteria occurs. The bacteremic phase lasts 4–7 days and is followed by a short remission of several days, after which the immune phase, characterized by the appearance of antibodies to the organism, meningitis, uveitis, rash, and hepatic and renal damage, occurs. A pretibial rash has been associated with infection by serovar *autumnalis* (Fort Bragg fever). In many, the immune phase is mild and lasts only 1–3 days. About half of patients have clinical signs of meningitis and a CSF pleocytosis during the second week of illness. In the small percentage of patients who suffer from Weil's disease, the two phases merge with persistent high fever, jaundice, and bleeding, followed by oliguric renal failure, shock, and myocarditis. Mortality has been reported to be 5–10% in Weil's disease (Edwards, 1960; Arean, 1962; Levett, 2001).

Laboratory Diagnosis

Leptospires can be isolated from the CSF, blood, and tissues early in the bacteremic phase (first 10 days), and from urine during the immune phase (second week to up to 30 days). Culture requires a semisolid medium (Fletcher's or Ellinghausen–McCullough–Johnson–Harris [EMJH]), which is incubated in the dark for 4–6 weeks at 25°–30°C. Urine requires alkalinization unless cultured immediately. Leptospires grow 1–3 cm below the surface of the medium and may form a linear disk of growth. Material from this location should be examined by darkfield microscopy weekly for the characteristic spinning leptospires with hooked ends. Leptospiral antigens, detected either directly in clinical specimens (e.g., ELISA, radioimmunoassay, immunomagnetic capture) or in processed tissue samples (e.g., immunofluorescence, immunohistochemistry), have also been used with variable success in the diagnosis of leptospirosis.

The majority of cases, however, are diagnosed serologically. Agglutinating antibodies appear during the first week of illness, peak around 3–4 weeks, and may persist for years. Antibodies can be detected serologically, using bacterial antigens either by a macroscopic or microscopic agglutination test, a hemagglutination test, or EIA testing. The microscopic agglutination test, which employs antigen from live bacteria, is the established serological reference method but is used primarily in a research setting. Recently, a modified EIA dipstick test that detects *Leptospira*-specific antibodies has been used with success in settings with minimal laboratory facilities (Gussenhoven, 1997; Yersin, 1999). Molecular methods, including hybridization techniques and PCR, have also been used to detect leptospiral DNA in infected patients (Vinetz, 1996; Levett, 2001).

Treatment

Severe disease requires aqueous penicillin G or ampicillin intravenously, while less severe disease can be treated with oral ampicillin, amoxicillin, or doxycycline. Prophylaxis with doxycycline provides protection for individuals in high-exposure environments (Farr, 1995). Immunization of domestic livestock and pets has reduced danger of infection from these animals to high-risk populations such as veterinarians and farmers. Risk is not completely eliminated, as infection has been shown to occur in immunized animals, with transmission of the disease to humans (Feigin, 1973).

Borrelia

The genus *Borrelia* contains several pathogenic and nonpathogenic species from two clades, the Lyme borreliosis group (also termed *Borrelia burgdorferi* sensu lato [s.l.]) and the relapsing fever group. The former has been divided into several genospecies by molecular analyses, three of which have been implicated in human disease: *B. burgdorferi* sensu stricto (s.s.), *Borrelia garinii*, and *Borrelia afzelii*. The relapsing fever group contains a variety of species that can be isolated from argasid (soft) ticks (e.g., *Borrelia hermsii* and *Borrelia turicatae*), ixodid (hard) ticks (e.g., *Borrelia lonestari* and *Borrelia miyamotoi*) and the human body louse (*Borrelia recurrentis*). Morphologically similar to the treponemes, members of the *Borrelia* genus are helical bacteria ranging in size from 5–30 μm long by 0.2–0.5 μm wide. They are actively motile, contain 7–22 periplasmic flagella (axial filaments), and multiply by binary fission. Unlike *Treponema* spp. however, *Borrelia* exhibit a multitude of immunogenic proteins on their outer membrane surfaces, and many species can be cultivated in/on artificial media. Moreover, the intricacies of the *Borrelia* genome, with its 910 kB linear chromosome and 21 linear and circular plasmids, render it a considerably more complex genus than *Treponema* (Porcella, 2001).

What follows is a description of the two major clinical disease forms of human borreliosis, each of which is vector-borne. As such, these entities must often be considered, both from an epidemiologic and from a clinical standpoint, in conjunction with other infectious agents transmitted by identical tick vectors. Examples include the flaviviral agents of tick-borne

encephalitis, various bacteria of the Rickettsiaceae, Ehrlichiaceae and Francisellaceae families as well as the protist *Babesia microti*, all of which can be transmitted by ixodid ticks. Clinical and diagnostic information relating to these and other vector-borne diseases may be found elsewhere in this book.

Lyme Disease

The most common tick-borne illness in North America and Europe today (Wang, 1999), Lyme disease (Lyme borreliosis) was so named during the 1970s following an epidemic of oligoarticular arthritis encompassing several communities in eastern Connecticut, chief among them the town of Old Lyme (Steere, 1977a, 1977b). Epidemiologic inquiry soon established an association between Lyme disease (then referred to as Lyme arthritis) and the hard tick *Ixodes scapularis* (previously *Ixodes dammini*) (Steere, 1978). Within 4 years, Burgdorfer and colleagues had (1) isolated a novel spirochete species from an ixodid tick collected in New York, (2) reproduced the characteristic primary dermal lesions of Lyme disease in tick-fed rabbit models and (3) demonstrated seroreactivity to antigens of this novel spirochete both in the rabbit model and in convalescent sera from human cases (Burgdorfer, 1982). The contemporary 'immunologic' variations on Koch's postulates were thereby fulfilled (Fredricks, 1996). The implicated organism was subsequently recognized as a member of the genus *Borrelia* and named *B. burgdorferi* in honor of its discoverer. In retrospect, different aspects of the multisystem inflammatory ailment now commonly known as Lyme disease had been recognized and described both in Europe (Afzelius, 1910; Bannwarth, 1941) and in the United States (Scrimenti, 1970) prior to the epidemic in Connecticut. Yet the present body of knowledge pertaining to Lyme borreliosis can be attributed in large part to the establishment and identification of its infectious etiology spawned by the New England outbreak.

Epidemiology and Pathogenesis

A total of 11 different genospecies of *Borrelia* from the Lyme borreliosis group have been phylogenetically characterized, three of which are well-established human pathogens. *B. burgdorferi* s.s. causes Lyme disease in North America, Europe and Asia, whereas *B. garinii* and *B. afzelii* cause similar, but subtly different illnesses in Europe and Asia (van Dam, 2002). Although other *Borrelia* species have been isolated from patients with Lyme-disease-like illnesses on occasion, their relative impact on overall disease burden remains undetermined.

Geographic distributions of *B. burgdorferi* s.l. and consequent regional prevalence of Lyme disease are the result of complex enzootic cycles involving one or several tick vectors of the *Ixodes ricinus* complex, various animal reservoirs and incidental hosts. Seasonal variability in disease onset often parallels the life cycle and questing periods of ixodid ticks (Falco, 1999). In the United States, *B. burgdorferi* s.s. is endemic in the north-east, upper mid-west and north-west regions, where the annual incidence of Lyme disease focally exceeds 100 cases/100 000 population. The overall number of reported cases, however, is considerably lower in the north-west than in the other two endemic foci (Centers for Disease Control and Prevention, 2004b). This discrepancy is partly attributable to the distinct enzootic cycles of the regions. In the north-west, perpetuation of *B. burgdorferi* s.s. in nature involves *Ixodes spinipalpis* ticks, which feed on the spirochete's principal animal reservoir, the dusky-footed woodrat, but not on humans. The ticks acquire and transmit infection between susceptible and infected reservoir hosts. However, the western black-legged tick (*Ixodes pacificus*), which feeds primarily on reptiles and humans, occasionally becomes infected after conceding its preferences and feeding on the woodrat. A potential consequence of this event is human infection. Yet because of the infrequency of such a concession on the part of *I. pacificus*, the overall incidence of Lyme disease remains fairly low in the region. By contrast, the chief vector in the mid-west and north-east, *I. scapularis* (black-legged or deer tick), promiscuously feeds on humans as well as on the spirochete's principal animal reservoir, the white-foot mouse. This results in proficient transmission to humans and an extremely high disease incidence, exceeding 1000 cases/100 000 population in certain communities (Shapiro, 2000; Steere, 2001). The most important tick vectors in Europe and Asia include *I. ricinus* (sheep tick) and *Ixodes persulcatus*, respectively, whereas primary animal reservoirs for *B. afzelii* and *B. garinii* are small rodents, voles and/or various avian species (Fukunaga, 1995; Wang, 1999; Parola, 2001).

Many other epidemiologic factors contribute to the transmission dynamics of *B. burgdorferi* s.l.. High vector densities and infection rates, abundance and infectivity of reservoir hosts and increased likelihood of human exposure all enhance the risk of Lyme disease (Parola, 2001). Furthermore, amplification of *Borrelia* in nonreservoir, dead-end hosts may also influence regional disease incidence. Such has been postulated the case in the north-eastern United States, where high population densities of white-tailed deer are thought to contribute to extremely high human infection rates (Steere, 2000). Another important transmission variable relates to the nature and duration of vector attachment during feeding. Hard-tick life cycles consist of three developmental stages, each of which secures only one blood meal before transition to the next stage (or oviposition, in the case of an adult). Because *B. burgdorferi* s.l. is not efficiently transmitted vertically in *Ixodes* spp., larvae acquire the spirochete while feeding upon an infected host (Shapiro, 2000; Scoles, 2001). The larval form, consequently, is usually not a direct vector for human infection (Patterson, 2003). Upon taking a blood meal, the larvae soon molt to become nymphs. Both nymphal and adult forms are capable of feeding on and transmitting infection to humans but the former are considerably smaller and much more likely to go unrecognized while attached. Given that the transmission of *Borrelia* to a susceptible host appears to be enhanced by longer feeding durations (Piesman, 1987; Sood, 1997), the nymph is almost certainly the primary vector for human transmission (Falco, 1999; Nadelman, 2001).

As with *T. pallidum*, the genomic sequence of *B. burgdorferi* s.s. has been completely characterized (Fraser, 1997), revealing a number of biosynthetic 'gaps' in addition to a few seemingly important lipoproteins. The latter include a group of outer surface proteins (Osp), A–F, which are encoded by plasmids, differentially expressed in vector and mammal environments, and highly immunostimulatory (de Silva, 1997; Porcella, 2001). Also, a lipoprotein, VlsE, which has the capability to undergo extensive antigenic variation, has also been recently recognized in *B. burgdorferi* (Zhang, 1998; Porcella, 2001). The diversity of symptoms observed in Lyme borreliosis is probably due to the direct effects of spirochete dissemination as well as to the extent of the host immune response (Sigal, 1997; Whooten, 2001). Many animal models of Lyme borreliosis have been developed, some of which have been useful for investigating the dynamics of *Borrelia* dissemination (e.g., tissue localization within heart, skin, and joints) in addition to specific cellular interactions (e.g., with host glycosaminoglycans and plasminogen) (Steere, 2000; Sigal, 1997). The mouse model has been particularly valuable in uncovering details of immunologic responses in Lyme disease (Whooten, 2001). A paucity of cultivable organisms or detectable genomic material within lesions of longstanding, treatment-resistant disease, such as occur in Lyme arthritis, suggests a pathogenic mechanism other than direct spirochete injury, however. Autoimmune events have been postulated, since an association between Lyme arthritis and HLA-DR4 has been established, and a recent report of an autoantigen candidate, leukocyte function antigen-1, further substantiates this hypothesis (Gross, 1998; Steere, 2004).

Clinical Manifestations

Rather analogous to syphilis, the clinical progression of Lyme borreliosis has been divided into three general stages: (1) an early localized phase, in which a primary lesion develops in the vicinity of the inoculation site, (2) an early disseminated phase when the spirochetes spread systemically and cause a variety of cardiac, neurologic, and/or dermatologic manifestations, and (3) a late phase, which may be heralded by other neurologic and/or dermatologic phenomena in addition to rheumatologic disease. Yet, because symptom overlap occurs during early disseminated and late persistent infection, some investigators have abstained from using this clinical staging system, preferring instead simply to incorporate duration of illness into both diagnostic and therapeutic considerations (Kaiser, 1998; Nadelman, 1998). Asymptomatic seroconversion or subclinical disease has also been reported to occur in as many as 7% of persons within endemic areas (Steere, 2003). Given the wide diversity of symptoms, Lyme borreliosis, like syphilis, has been aptly labeled 'the great imitator.'

The earliest stage begins roughly 1 week following the bite of an infected tick, at which time a characteristic rash, descriptively termed erythema migrans, develops near the inoculation site in a majority of patients (the exact proportion depends upon case definition or study inclusion criteria). The lesion begins as a painless red macule or papule and subsequently expands to become an erythematous patch measuring up to 70 cm (Nadelman, 1996). Erythema migrans is typically painless, occasionally demonstrates central pallor, imparting a 'target-like' or 'bullseye' appearance, and may be accompanied by nonspecific symptoms such as fever, fatigue, headache, and myalgia, as well as regional lymphadenopathy (Nadelman, 1996; Smith, 2002). Histologic analysis reveals superficial, perivascular dermatitis comprised of lymphocytes, macrophages, and abundant plasma cells, and the organisms can sometimes be visualized in tissue sections treated with silver impregnation stains or by immunohistochemical techniques (Duray, 1997). Unlike the lesions of syphilis, vasculitis is not a typical histologic feature of erythema migrans

Dissemination of *Borrelia* portends the second stage of clinical illness, in which many organ systems may be affected. Smaller, secondary erythema migrans lesions arising in multiple sites are one of the more common signs of early dissemination (Shapiro, 2000). Neurologic manifestations (neuroborreliosis) affect up to 15% of US patients, with symptoms including cranial nerve palsy (commonly the facial nerve), lymphocytic meningitis, and a variety of peripheral neuropathies (e.g., painful radiculitis) (Steere, 2001; Halperin, 2002). These manifestations are collectively referred to as 'Bannwarth syndrome' in some European countries (Kaiser, 1998). Somewhat rarer, cardiac involvement in the form of transient atrioventricular block or myocarditis has also been reported in approximately 5% of patients with Lyme disease (Steere, 2001). Other sites potentially affected include the musculoskeletal system (e.g., fatigue, malaise), liver (e.g., mild, transient hepatitis) and eyes (e.g., conjunctivitis, neuroretinitis) (Lesser, 1995; Steere, 2000).

In the United States, the most common manifestation of untreated, late-stage Lyme disease is arthritis, which develops in well over one half of untreated patients (Steere, 2000). Typically mono- or oligoarticular in extent, large joints such as the knee are frequently involved (Steere, 1977a, 2001). Symptoms of pain and swelling begin acutely several weeks to months following spirochete inoculation and last for several days to months (median 1 week) (Steere, 1977b). Whether the result of autoimmunity or persistent infection, many patients continue to experience intermittent recurrences of migratory arthritis followed by prolonged disease-free periods (Nadelman, 1998). Conversely, late-stage manifestations of persistent Lyme borreliosis in European patients often involve neurologic or cutaneous organs. The former may overlap clinically with early disseminated neuroborreliosis and include chronic lymphocytic meningitis and peripheral neuropathies (e.g., sensory polyneuritis, pareses, etc.). In addition, CNS manifestations such as myelitis and spastic–ataxic gait disturbances, as well as short-term cognitive dysfunction, have been noted (Kaiser, 1998; Halperin, 2002). A chronic dermatologic phenomenon known as acrodermatitis chronica atrophica has also been associated with late Lyme borreliosis in Europe. As the name implies, the lesions are present on hands, wrists, elbows, and feet. They are often symmetrical and are characterized histologically by a lymphomononuclear and, to a lesser extent, granulocytic infiltrate with progressive epidermal thinning, hyperkeratosis and dermal atrophy (Aberer, 1991; Duray, 1997). Other well-established or controversial long-term dermatologic manifestations include *Borrelia* lymphocytoma, cutaneous B-cell lymphoma, morphea, and lichen sclerosis et atrophica (Duray, 1997; McGinley-Smith, 2003).

Variations in clinical manifestations, particularly during the late stages of Lyme disease, have been partly ascribed to inherent traits of the organisms themselves, whether genospecies or strain specific. For instance, *B. afzelii* (previously group VS461) has been disproportionately isolated from lesions of erythema migrans and acrodermatitis chronica atrophica in Europe as compared to other genospecies of *Borrelia* (van Dam, 1993; Balmelli, 1995; Wang, 1999). By contrast, *B. garinii* is more frequently implicated in European cases of neuroborreliosis (Balmelli, 1995; Wang, 1999). Furthermore, recent study from the United States demonstrated that particular molecular subtypes of *B. burgdorferi* s.s. may be associated with invasive properties that more frequently lead to spirochetemia (Wormser, 1999). Additional observations that corroborate the notion that certain *Borrelia* strains may cause distinctive clinical diseases include: (1) serologic responses among patients with particular clinical symptoms may be preferential toward antigens from specific *Borrelia* sources; and (2) certain genospecies appear to have different properties in vitro (Dressler, 1994; Norman, 1996; Wang, 1999).

In the vast majority of patients, clinical manifestations of Lyme disease respond to appropriate antibiotic therapy (Shadick, 1999; Seltzer, 2000; Wormser, 2000). Yet, a small subset may continue to experience persistent, subjective symptoms such as musculoskeletal pain, fatigue, neurocognitive deficits, etc. despite treatment – a condition that has variably been termed 'post-Lyme-disease syndrome', 'chronic Lyme disease' or 'treatment-resistant borreliosis' (Klempner, 2002). To date, prospective studies have shown little to no benefit of antibiotic therapy over placebo in reducing the symptoms of this syndrome, and isolation of *Borrelia* or amplification of *Borrelia* genes have been almost uniformly unsuccessful (Klempner, 2002). Moreover, retrospective case-controlled studies illustrate that frequency of objective signs among 'chronic Lyme disease' patients is similar to age-matched controls without a history of Lyme disease (Shadick, 1999; Seltzer, 2000). As with the similarly nebulous diagnoses of fibromyalgia and chronic fatigue syndrome to which it has been compared (Steere, 2002), much remains to be learned about the pathogenesis, diagnosis, and management of 'chronic Lyme disease.'

During recent years several reports have documented erythema-migrans-like lesions in patients residing in the southern United States. Occasionally

VII

referred to as southern tick-associated rash illness (STARI), the lesions are preceded by the bite of the Lonestar tick, *Amblyomma americanum*, and have not yielded any *B. burgdorferi* s.s. isolates to date (Kirkland, 1997; James, 2001). Instead, a novel agent, *B. lonestari* sp. nov., of the relapsing-fever group, has been tentatively implicated (Varela, 2004). Because *B. burgdorferi* s.s. does occur naturally within this geographic area (Oliver, 2003), future epidemiologic work should determine the details and extent of disease caused by each of these organisms in the region.

Laboratory Diagnosis

Issued for surveillance purposes, the most recent CDC case definition of Lyme disease emphasizes clinical findings and physical examination – the development of physician-diagnosed erythema migrans in a patient with a possible tick exposure is considered diagnostic (Centers for Disease Control and Prevention, 1997). Laboratory confirmation is required only for less specific, objective signs that would be expected to develop later in the disease course (e.g., arthritis, cranial neuritis, cardiac conduction defects, etc.). Other experts agree that laboratory testing, particularly indirect methodologies such as serologic tests, should not be performed as stand-alone diagnostic modalities, but rather should serve as tools to assist in confirming or refuting clinical suspicions (Luger, 1990; Tugwell, 1997; Brown, 1999). Reports highlighting the concepts of pretest probability based on epidemiologic and clinical factors, as well as likelihood ratios and test predictive values, thoroughly demonstrate the futility and high cost of such a stand-alone approach (Seltzer, 1996; Tugwell, 1997; Nichol, 1998). In fact, Lyme disease testing for patients with only nonspecific symptoms like fatigue, headache, or myalgia (i.e., when pretest probability is = 0.2), even in endemic areas using accurate laboratory assays, can lead to more false-positive than true-positive results (Tugwell, 1997). Exacerbated by widespread anxiety on the part of the public and a general misunderstanding by many health-care providers, the current diagnostic confusion surrounding Lyme borreliosis can perhaps be best dealt with by taking a thorough look at the indications for and limitations of laboratory testing.

Culture

Culture usually offers the 'gold-standard' in diagnostic tests for infectious diseases in which the causative agent does not also colonize the human body. Yet, despite the fact that cultivation of *Borrelia* spp. is readily achievable and often not as time-consuming as for other pathogenic microorganisms (Reed, 2002), most clinical and commercial diagnostic laboratories do not offer this testing alternative. Several modifications of the broth-based Barber–Stoenner–Kelly medium have been shown not only to support the growth of *Borrelia* spp. but also to be useful in their recovery from biopsy tissue of erythema migrans lesions and large-volume plasma collections during the early, acute phase of disease (Nadelman, 1996; Steere, 1998; Wormser, 2001) Given the specificity of organism isolation and the absence of measurable antibody in most patients with *B. burgdorferi* s.l. infection during the early phase of clinical illness, culture would seem to be a very practical diagnostic modality. However, reliance on darkfield microscopy or fluorescent antibodies for the detection and identification of positive cultures, high media and reagent costs, wide reported sensitivity ranges (doubtless the result of variability in quantity of tissue/blood cultured and timing of specimen collection) and the requirement that invasive procedures be performed on the patient (e.g., tissue biopsy) have probably all contributed to the test's general unpopularity outside the research arena. Importantly, recovery of *Borrelia* from CSF, synovial fluid or other samples collected beyond the early phases of disease is so frequently unsuccessful as to be of little diagnostic utility. For this reason, additional laboratory testing for Lyme borreliosis is an important adjunct.

Serologic Tests

Detection of *Borrelia*-specific antibody production during Lyme disease may be accomplished using a variety of methodologies that express results in terms of total immunoglobulin (Ig) or class-specific IgG or IgM. Immunofluorescent antibody (IFA) assays, which typically contain antigen in the form of whole-cell *B. burgdorferi* s.s. fixed to glass slides, were popular in the 1980s but have been largely superseded by the more automated and less subjective ELISA. This assay uses antigens that are recombinantly produced or derived from partially purified extracts of *Borrelia* organisms.

As with all serologic responses to infectious etiologies, a multitude of variables potentially affect the performance of assays developed to detect them. False-negative and false-positive results may consequently serve only to confound clinical impressions. Early in the course of Lyme disease, absence of antibody (or levels below the limit of detection) can lead to false-negative serologic results. It would seem that this might be partly circumvented with assays that detect IgM specifically, because IgM production precedes the development of an IgG response (Shapiro, 2000; Reed, 2002). Yet reported sensitivities of both IgM and IgG ELISAs during the acute phase of disease have generally been quite low, although variable. With time, as the disease progresses and patients seroconvert, test sensitivity increases (Engstrom, 1995; Brown, 1999; Liang, 1999). Specificity of the IFA and ELISA may also be adversely affected by crossreacting antibodies to a variety of microorganism- and host-derived proteins. Some of these include pathogenic spirochetes (e.g., relapsing fever group of *Borrelia* and treponemes), other bacteria (e.g., *Helicobacter pylori*) and viruses (e.g., Epstein–Barr) as well as antinuclear antigens present in autoimmune disorders such as systemic lupus erythematosus (Brown, 1999; Reed, 2002). Previous immunization with the OspA subunit Lyme disease vaccine may lead to false-positive ELISA and IFA results as well, given that this lipoprotein is typically an integral antigenic component of these tests (Steere, 1998).

Additional factors that may also contribute to test limitations include the composition of antigen contained in the particular assay (which is poorly standardized at present), the level of quality control within the testing facility, the interpretive levels at which positive and negative (and indeterminate) optical density, or index values are set, the particular bacterial strain responsible for infection, the patient's individual immune response and or the method of comparison (i.e., whether the patient truly has Lyme disease).

In an effort to increase the accuracy of serologic testing as a whole, the CDC has proposed the use of a two-tiered algorithm in which all positive and indeterminate results by ELISA or IFA are subsequently tested by another methodology, the Western blot (Centers for Disease Control and Prevention, 1995). In this assay, proteins extracted from low-passaged *B. burgdorferi* s.s. are quantitatively standardized and then separated by electrophoresis on the basis of size and charge. Following transfer to a membrane substrate, control and test sera (in addition to a panel of monoclonal antibodies for reference and calibration) are then incubated with the *Borrelia* proteins. Nonspecific immunoglobulin is removed by washing, whereas antibody with *Borrelia* specificity is bound and subsequently detected with an enzyme-linked conjugate. This technique provides the capability to detect and analyze antibodies against particular proteins. Interpretation is somewhat subjective, and criteria defining positive results vary somewhat. The CDC recommendations are as follows: IgM blot positivity if two of the following bands are present: 24 (OspC), 39 (BmpA), and 41 (flagellin) kDa; IgG blot positivity if five of the following bands are present: 18, 21 (OspC), 28, 30, 39 (BmpA), 41 (flagellin), 45, 58, 66, and 93 kDa (Centers for Disease Control and Prevention, 1995). In theory, this approach provides a highly sensitive first-round test that should detect most cases of Lyme disease, followed by a highly specific assay that should exclude false-positive results from the preceding round (Dressler, 1993; Ledue, 1996). In reality, however, the high degree of inter- and intralaboratory variability and less than ideal sensitivity observed in ELISA and IFA studies, in addition to the wide ranges of reported performance for the Western blot, suggest that such may not be the case (Engstrom, 1995; Aguero-Rosenfeld, 1996; Ledue, 1996; Bakken, 1997). Nonetheless, improvement in overall testing performance using the algorithm has been described, again with the caveat that immunoblot results may also be significantly influenced by the stage of disease during which testing is performed (Engstrom, 1995; Johnson, 1996). A slight departure from this algorithm – Western blot testing only on sera with indeterminate results from the first round – has been advocated by the American College of Physicians (1997) and may be slightly more sensitive than the CDC recommendation in detecting Lyme disease patients (identified by surveillance case definition) in endemic areas (Trevejo, 1999). Also, newer ELISA formats utilizing recombinant antigens may ultimately serve to increase accuracy even further (Gomes-Solecki, 2000; Bacon, 2003).

Peak antibody titers generally plateau between 7 and 30 days following the development of erythema migrans, with the degree of reactivity (i.e., number of bands by Western blot or optical density reading by ELISA) often being higher in patients with early dissemination (Aguero-Rosenfeld, 1996). Beyond 30 days, most patients with Lyme disease will have developed an IgG response and should not be tested with IgM assays alone (Centers for Disease Control and Prevention, 1995). Several reports have suggested that therapeutic intervention early in the course of disease may abrogate the antibody response and lead to 'seronegative' Lyme disease (Aguero-Rosenfeld, 1996; Ledue, 1996; Dattwyler, 1988). Although one retrospective European study demonstrated that treatment had no statistically significant effect on ultimate seroreactivity, the authors did note a trend toward higher seropositivity incidence and titer among patients who did not receive antibiotics (Plorer, 1993). Finally, because the duration of both IgG and IgM detection may last many years after successful eradication of the spirochete, there appears to be no role in monitoring antibody levels during convalescence for determination of disease activity and response to therapy or in assessing IgM positivity as a means of establishing the timing of infection (Hilton, 1997; Kalish, 2001).

A number of other laboratory-based immunologic techniques have been evaluated for potential use in the diagnosis of Lyme disease. Several reports have indicated that *Borrelia*-specific antibodies detected by IFA, ELISA, and/or Western blot in CSF and synovial fluid samples may be useful in confirming neuroborreliosis and Lyme arthritis, respectively, particularly when compared to serum levels (Cruz, 1991; Hansen, 1991). As of 1999, however, no commercially available kits had been cleared for such use by the US FDA (Brown, 1999). Another methodology that showed promise in the identification of 'seronegative' Lyme disease cases, the T-cell proliferative assay, was probably too complex and insensitive to gain widespread appeal among diagnostic laboratories (Dressler, 1991). A recent strategy employing precipitation and disassociation of *Borrelia*-specific IgM from circulating immune complexes prior to capture on solid phase and quantitation shows promise (Brunner, 2001). Lastly, an antigen capture assays used on CSF or urine has been reported (Coyle, 1995; Klempner, 2001) but is not presently recommended for diagnostic purposes without further validation studies (Tugwell, 1997).

Molecular tests

Alternative testing methodologies for Lyme borreliosis have been strongly sought after, given the overall low sensitivity of culture and serologic assays. In the early 1990s, researchers set their sights on genomic amplification techniques, which were relatively new to the diagnostic armamentarium at that time. Since then, several modifications of the PCR using various genetic targets and amplicon detection methods have been applied to a variety of specimen types in search of *Borrelia* nucleic acids.

Samples from which *B. burgdorferi* s.l. could not be readily isolated were the primary focus of initial investigations on PCR utility. Studies of PCR analyses on joint aspirate samples from patients with Lyme arthritis demonstrated excellent sensitivity and specificity rates when several primer sets were used (Nocton, 1994; Dumler, 2001). After the results were compared with clinical information, it became apparent (1) that detection of *Borrelia* nucleic acids was more frequently associated with a history of absent or inadequate antimicrobial therapy and (2) that PCR positivity disappeared following appropriate treatment (Nocton, 1994). Further inquiry into a performance discrepancy of primer sets targeting genomic (e.g., rRNA genes) versus plasmid-derived (e.g., *OspA* and *OspB*) DNA revealed that the latter is present in higher quantities within joint spaces in Lyme arthritis (Persing, 1994). This phenomenon, termed 'target imbalance,' seems to be unique to the inflammatory-spirochete milieu of synovial fluid in Lyme arthritis and probably accounts for the higher sensitivity observed in tests that target the *OspA* gene (Lebech, 2002). By contrast, studies of amplification assays on CSF from patients with acute or chronic neuroborreliosis have demonstrated only a minimal to moderate improvement in sensitivity over culture (Nocton, 1996; Dumler, 2001). Partly the result of study inclusion criteria, the extremely wide reported sensitivity ranges are also probably due to the extremely low numbers of *Borrelia* genomic copies (i.e., levels near lower detection limits) in the CSF of affected patients (Schmidt, 1997). As a general rule, successful amplification occurs more frequently during the early stages of neurologic disease (Lebech, 2002).

The PCR has likewise been applied to specimens collected during the primary and early disseminated stages of Lyme borreliosis. Nucleic acid detection in tissue from erythema migrans lesions has been successful, and such an approach may offer improvement in both sensitivity and turnaround time over culture (Dumler, 2001). Testing of blood and plasma has also been attempted but is limited by the frequent presence of inhibiting substances as well as by the timing of sample collection (Schmidt, 1997). Initial reports of urine testing by PCR were encouraging because of the ease of specimen collection and high sensitivity, but these findings have not been consistently reproduced (Brettschneider, 1998; Lebech, 2002). Additionally, detection of *Borrelia* genetic material extracted directly from ixodid tick vectors may be useful from an epidemiologic standpoint but should not be relied upon for diagnosis or management of patients from whom the ticks were removed (Sood, 1997; Dumler, 2001).

In time, developments in technology and improvements in understanding will continue to lend themselves to new, creative uses for the PCR beyond simply diagnosis. For instance, the technique has been readily used alongside restriction fragment length polymorphism (RFLP) and DNA sequencing for subcategorization of *Borrelia* isolates for taxonomic purposes (Wang, 1999). The use of labeled, internal hybridization probes within the reaction vessel has afforded the ability to detect and quantify amplification

products in real time. Although not yet typically performed in diagnostic laboratories, these quantitative assays have provided clues about *Borrelia* transmission dynamics and pathogenesis (Pahl, 1999; Wang, 2002). In contrast to cases of human immunodeficiency virus or hepatitis C virus, monitoring therapeutic responses by PCR has not been firmly established as beneficial in Lyme disease (Schmidt, 1997). However, the relationships between *Borrelia* genetic material in joints affected by Lyme arthritis, antibiotic therapy, and symptomatic outcome suggest that it may in the future (Nocton, 1994; Steere, 2004).

As with most amplification techniques, use of the PCR for diagnosis of Lyme disease is limited by many factors, including polymerase inhibitors, low target levels, potential for contamination, primer choices, and method of amplicon detection. Whatever the application, sensitivity and specificity of molecular tests are imperfect. Accordingly, negative results alone should never be used to exclude a diagnosis while positive results out of context should not confirm a diagnosis. Misinterpretations such as these may lead to dismal consequences if not resolved early (Patel, 2000; Molloy, 2001). Importantly, because most patients with late manifestations of Lyme disease will have evidence of seroreactivity by the time of presentation (thereby fulfilling the CDC case definition), PCR studies are probably best used during early Lyme disease prior to a serologic response. Of utmost importance is correlation of laboratory data with clinical impression, irrespective of whether such data is derived through serological or molecular means.

Treatment and Prevention

The Infectious Disease Society of America (IDSA) has recently published a set of guidelines for the management of patients with suspected or proven Lyme borreliosis (Wormser, 2000). To summarize, a large body of evidence in the form of randomized, prospective, double-blind studies has consistently demonstrated that a 2–3-week course of oral doxycycline or ampicillin is highly efficacious in the treatment of early, uncomplicated Lyme disease. Cefuroxime is also effective but not recommended as first-line therapy because of cost. In patients unable to tolerate any of these regimens or for whom such regimens would be contraindicated, macrolide therapy may be an acceptable alternative. Extended treatment courses of this standard oral regimen are also considered to be effective in the majority of patients with Lyme arthritis in the absence of neurologic manifestations. However, parenteral therapy with ceftriaxone (or penicillin as an alternative) may be used in cases of arthritis relapse. This same intravenous regimen is also recommended for patients with third-degree heart block and/or neuroborreliosis. Of note, the majority of prospective therapeutic trials, upon which these IDSA recommendations are based, have end points defined in terms of clinical responses (i.e., disappearance of symptoms) rather than on the eradication of *Borrelia*.

A somewhat more hotly contested issue surrounds the use of prophylactic antibiotic therapy following recognition and removal of a feeding tick. Early prospective studies employing 10-day oral regimens of antimicrobial prophylaxis failed to establish any benefit over placebo (Warshafsky, 1996). Factors that further confound the matter include: (1) the extremely low success rate of *Borrelia* transmission to humans (1–3%), even in hyperendemic areas where tick infection rates may exceed 50% (Shapiro, 1992; Nadelman, 2001); (2) the frequency with which tick bites are not recognized among patients with Lyme disease (up to 75% of patients) (Nadelman, 1996); (3) the inaccuracy of tick species identification and estimates of feeding duration by non-entomologists (Falco, 1998); and (4) the potential costs of widespread antibiotic use (e.g., financial, unanticipated side effects, bacterial resistance). A more recent investigation demonstrated that a single 200 mg dose of doxycycline administered after removal of an *I. scapularis* tick significantly reduced the incidence of subsequent development of erythema migrans (Nadelman, 2001). Once again, interpretations of the study were mixed (Bellovin, 2001; Leenders, 2001; Shapiro, 2001).

Primary Lyme disease prevention strategies that are generally agreed upon include interventions that decrease both the likelihood and duration of vector attachment and feeding. Use of insect repellants, acaricides, and barrier clothing such as long pants and long-sleeved shirts, as well as the performance of daily 'tick checks', each have a theoretical if not proven value in reducing human cases of ixodid-tick-borne diseases (Poland, 2001; Hayes, 2003). The one most widely accepted and thoroughly tested prevention strategy, human vaccination, is no longer commercially available however (Hitt, 2002). This subunit vaccine containing a lipidized, recombinant Osp-A antigen was shown to significantly reduce the incidence of Lyme borreliosis following a three-step immunization schedule (Steere, 1998). Because of low sales, and perhaps an unfounded fear of complications, the product was withdrawn from the market in 2002.

Relapsing fever can be divided into two distinctive entities based on microbiologic and epidemiologic features. Epidemic, louse-borne relapsing fever (LBRF) occurs worldwide, reflecting the ubiquitous distribution of its transmission vector, *Pediculus humanus* (Johnson, 2000). While the disease has been largely eradicated from most developed nations, documented occurrences persist in parts of east Africa and South America (Sundnes, 1993; Raoult, 1999). Humans are the only known reservoir for the causative agent, *B. recurrentis*. Successful transmission between them does not require that the vector feeds upon an uninfected person. Rather, when an infected louse is crushed, susceptible hosts are exposed and infected via contaminated hemolymph (Johnson, 2000).

Endemic, tick-borne relapsing fever (TBRF) has a slightly narrower geographic distribution, which parallels that of its primary transmission vectors, argasid ticks of the genus *Ornithodoros*. North American areas of disease endemicity include the Pacific north-west, the northern and central Rocky Mountains and parts of the Sierra range of California (*Ornithodoros hermsi* habitats) as well as the arid flatlands of Mexico, Texas and New Mexico (*Ornithodoros turicata* habitats) (Dworkin, 2002). The disease is also well-documented in parts of Africa and Europe (Parola, 2001). In the past, *Borrelia* spp. causing TBRF were considered to have a high degree of tick-vector specificity and were named after the *Ornithodoros* species from which they were isolated (Davis, 1942). Thus, *B. hermsi* and *B. turicatae* are associated with *O. hermsi* and *O. turicata*, respectively. However, recent reports demonstrating the presence of relapsing-fever-group *Borrelia* nucleic acids in several *Ixodes* tick species, many captured in regions of Lyme endemicity, may challenge this assumption (Fukungaga, 1995; Scoles, 2001; Fraenkel, 2002). Furthermore, because (1) serologic cross-reactivity between organisms from the two borreliosis clades is highly likely (Schwan, 1996), and (2) relapsing-fever-like spirochetes have been shown to produce disease in localities heretofore considered non-endemic for TBRF (Breitschwerdt, 1994), the clinical and diagnostic implications of these reports will undoubtedly spark renewed research in the relapsing fever agents.

Transmission dynamics and, therefore, epidemiologic factors associated with TBRF are considerably different from those of Lyme disease. Argasid ticks feed nocturnally and for much shorter durations than ixodid ticks (Parola, 2001). Yet, because they harbor *Borrelia* in their salivary secretions, soft ticks can successfully inoculate spirochetes within minutes of feeding (Dworkin, 2002). Although *Ornithodoros* ticks can transmit *Borrelia* vertically (transovarial) and maintain the bacteria in nature for extended periods, several mammalian hosts also contribute to spirochete persistence (Dworkin, 2002). Human cases often occur in small clusters following exposure to the vector while sleeping in rustic cabins or seldom-occupied rural dwellings (*O. hermsi*) or in caves (*O. turicata*) (Rawlings, 1995; Dworkin, 1998).

Clinical features of LBRF and TBRF are somewhat similar. Following an approximately 7-day incubation period, infected patients experience the acute onset of high fever (38.9–40.0°C) accompanied by nonspecific symptoms such as headache, malaise, arthralgia, and fatigue (Southern, 1969; Dworkin, 1998). Minor hemorrhagic manifestations are not uncommon and may be related to transient thrombocytopenia. Hepato-splenomegaly is identified more frequently in patients with LBRF (Southern, 1969). Neurologic involvement in the form of meningitis, seventh nerve palsy, myelitis, and encephalitis, have all been reported (Cadavid, 1998). Almost as suddenly as they begin, symptoms subside after 3–6 days in most patients, only to relapse roughly 1 week later (Johnson, 2000). Similar episodes of symptomatic recurrence may continue up to as many as 13 times, but more typically resolve after two or three relapses (Southern, 1969). These waves of recrudescence are believed to be due to the organism's extraordinary ability to vary its surface-protein antigenic makeup under immune selective pressures, thus expanding and contracting in number as new antibodies are produced (Rich, 2001; Dworkin, 2002). Left untreated, LBRF appears to have a higher mortality rate than its tick-borne counterpart, but the contributive effects of other factors (e.g., famine, war) often accompanying LBRF may obscure direct comparisons (Dworkin, 2002). Nevertheless, self-limited cases of probable TBRF have been reported (Rawlings, 1995; Dworkin, 1998).

Microscopic examination of peripheral blood samples obtained during febrile episodes has been the traditional laboratory approach to diagnosis of relapsing fever. *Borrelia* organisms may be visualized in wet mounts using a darkfield technique or in fixed smears stained with Wright–Giemsa, acridine orange or specific fluorescent antibodies. Drawbacks to microscopy include: (1) the requirement of a fairly high spirochetemic burden, although this may be obviated by collection of samples during febrile periods; (2)

observer inexperience or unfamiliarity with clinical differential; and (3) the inability to identify the causative *Borrelia* to the species level. Cultivation of the spirochetes is possible, although difficult, and is rarely performed in clinical settings. Demonstration of serologic response using techniques such as IFA, ELISA, and Western blot has been used with variable success. The degree of *Borrelia* antigenic variability may limit serologic assay sensitivity, whereas crossreactivity with other spirochetes, in particular those of the Lyme borreliosis group, may affect specificity. Newer tests utilizing a 34 kDa recombinant protein, GlpQ, appear to be more specific for the relapsing fever spirochetes (Porcella, 2000; Schwan, 1996). At present, molecular methods such as PCR play little, if any, role in the routine diagnosis of relapsing fever. However, given their extreme power of strain and/or species discrimination (Wormser, 1999; Bunikis, 2004), these techniques may one day play a vital part in the elucidation of borreliosis etiology in regions where both relapsing fever and Lyme disease spirochetes are found.

Successful treatment of LBRF may be accomplished using a single oral dose of tetracycline or erythromycin, whereas 5–10 days of therapy with either of these agents is recommended for TBRF (Johnson, 2000). Parenteral administration of a β-lactam may be considered in the case of meningitis or encephalitis (Cadavid, 1998). Whatever the antibiotic, symptoms of the Jarisch–Herxheimer reaction are not uncommon and may be particularly severe in the louse-borne form of disease. This reaction usually occurs within a few hours of antibiotic initiation and is typified by an increase in temperature (0.5–1°C) with rigors, systemic hypotension and leukopenia. As with other shock-like syndromes, the proposed mechanism of Jarisch–Herxheimer reaction involves a cytokine 'storm,' with tumor necrosis factor-α, interleukin-6 and interleukin-8 as major orchestrating components (Griffin, 1998).

Prevention strategies for TBRF include rodent-proofing rural cottages or cabins to avoid immigration and colonization by soft ticks, use of insecticides around such dwellings, use of topical repellents while sleeping and altogether avoiding overnight excursions into known *Ornithodoros* habitats. Prevention of LBRF may be effected through good personal hygiene and delousing procedures (Johnson, 2000). No vaccine is currently available.

Rat-bite fever

Description

Spirillum minus is a Gram-negative, tightly coiled bacterium 2–5 μm in length by 0.5 μm in width, with bipolar tufts of flagella, more closely related to *Neisseria* species than members of the family Spirochaetaceae.

Epidemiology

Infection with *S. minus* in humans results in a relapsing fever called sodoku, most cases of which have been described in Japan, although cases have occurred worldwide. This bacterium is part of the respiratory flora of rats and is transmitted by a bite. Oral ingestion is not reported to be a source of infection for humans. The disease is very rare in the United States. Research laboratory workers and world travelers are the groups at risk for infection (Anderson, 1983; Signorini, 2002).

Pathogenesis and Pathology

The pathogenesis of *S. minus* is poorly understood. Dissemination from the original bite occurs soon after inoculation. In the few postmortem descriptions of fatal cases, epithelial necrosis and a mononuclear infiltrate in the dermis at the original bite site; a perivascular mononuclear infiltrate in the dermis from the site of the rash; hyperplasia of lymph nodes; and hemorrhage and necrosis in the liver, spleen, kidney, myocardium, and meninges have been described (Washburn, 1995).

Clinical

The bite wound initially heals but, 1–4 weeks later, an indurated lesion, which may ulcerate, appears at the bite site. Febrile periods recur, separated by afebrile periods of 3–7 days. Fever can be accompanied by myalgia, headache, and vomiting. Half of patients have a macular rash that may form large plaques (Taber, 1979). Resolution in 3–8 weeks usually occurs, but relapses and complications such as endocarditis, meningitis, myocarditis, and nephritis can occur (Washburn, 1995). The mortality for untreated cases in the preantibiotic era was 6–10% (Washburn, 1995).

Laboratory Diagnosis

S. minus can be propagated only in mice or guinea pigs by intraperitoneal inoculation. Demonstration of the organisms can be accomplished by staining exudate from the lesion or lymph nodes by a Wright–Giemsa stain or visualization by darkfield microscopy. Serologic tests are not available; however, up to 50% of patients can have a false-positive nontreponemal test for syphilis (Taber, 1979).

Treatment

Intravenous aqueous penicillin G is the therapy of choice, with tetracycline used in penicillin-allergic patients.

Anaerobiospirillum succiniciproducens

Description

Anaerobiospirillum succiniciproducens is a Gram-negative, spiral-shaped bacterium measuring 0.6–0.8 μm in width by 4–8 μm in length. It shows a corkscrew-like motility and possesses bipolar multitrichous flagella. Like *Spirillum* spp., members of the genus *Anaerobiospirillum* are not true spirochetes. Rather, they are more closely related to the genus *Aeromonas* than to either the *Treponema* or *Borrelia* genus.

Epidemiology

This anaerobic bacterium can be part of the normal flora of healthy cats and dogs but has also recently been demonstrated in association with severe feline ileocolitis (De Cock, 2004). An association of similar illness in humans with exposure to these pets has been suggested but not definitively established (Malnick, 1990; Goddard, 1998). *A. succiniciproducens* has been associated with diarrheal illness in normal patients and with septicemia in patients with predisposing illnesses. The gastrointestinal tract in these patients has been postulated as the source for entry into the circulatory system (McNeil, 1987; Tee, 1998). The incidence of infection is low but has been increasing, thought to be primarily due to better detection by improved culture technique (Goddard, 1998).

Clinical

Patients with gastroenteritis suffer from abdominal pain, vomiting, and diarrhea for 3–7 days; those without underlying illnesses recover uneventfully (Malnick, 1990). Septicemia has occurred in patients with underlying illnesses, including alcoholism, atherosclerosis, malignancy, diabetes mellitus, and gingivitis (Goddard, 1998; Pienaar, 2003). Fatalities have occurred in about one third of the cases of septicemia.

Laboratory Diagnosis

A. succiniciproducens grows well in automated blood culture systems (Tee, 1998). After subculture on chocolate or blood agar, moist and spreading colonies 1–2 mm in diameter appear after 2–3 days. Useful identifying biochemical reactions include a negative catalase, indole, and oxidase; production of succinic acid and acetic acid from glucose as demonstrated by gas-liquid chromatography; and no growth at 25°C or 42°C. A selective medium has been developed by Malnick et al. (Malnick, 1990).

Treatment

Because of the uncommon nature of this infection, optimal therapy for septicemia has not been established. In vitro, most isolates tested have been susceptible to carbenicillin, cefoxitin, chloramphenicol, and metronidazole and resistant to vancomycin and clindamycin; however, testing has been limited and is not standardized (Shlaes, 1982; McNeil, 1987).

Agents of Intestinal Spirochetosis

Description

Two species of spirochete, *Brachyspira aalborgi* and *Brachyspira pilosicoli* (formerly designated as a member of the genus *Serpulina*), have been found in the colon of humans. These organisms are Gram-negative, 0.2–0.4 μm in diameter, and 4–8 μm in length. Four to six flagella are present subterminally at each end near the pointed ends of the bacteria.

Epidemiology and Clinical

B. pilosicoli, along with *Brachyspira hyodysenteriae*, causes porcine intestinal spirochetosis, a diarrheal disease in young pigs. Although strains related to these species have been recovered from dogs, birds, and other animals (Korner, 2003). It is unknown whether animals act as reservoirs for human infection. In contrast, *B. aalborgi* was named after its isolation from the colon of a human patient (Hovind-Hougen, 1982) but is less well-characterized overall. The association of intestinal spirochetes with disease is not firmly established, as the bacteria have been identified in both symptomatic and asymptomatic individuals. Homosexual men have shown a higher prevalence than other populations (Teglbjaerg, 1990). Diarrhea, abdominal pain, rectal bleeding, and discharge have been attributed to intestinal spirochetosis (Teglbjaerg, 1990). Additionally, *B. pilosicoli* has been isolated from the blood of critically ill and immunocompromised patients, the clinical significance of which is uncertain (Trott, 1997; Kanavaki, 2002).

Pathology and Pathogenesis

The spirochetes are easily seen on biopsy specimens as a dark blue 'fringe' on the surface of colonic epithelial cells with sparing of the goblet cells. Silver impregnation stains demonstrate the organisms well. The epithelial cells appear normal and there is no increased inflammation in the lamina propria. Electron microscopy demonstrates that the bacteria attach to the surface of colonic epithelial cells end-on and are oriented perpendicular to the lumen (Teglbjaerg, 1990). Invasion into epithelial and mucosal macrophages has been demonstrated in both symptomatic and asymptomatic patients (Teglbjaerg, 1990). Pathogenesis has not been established.

Laboratory Diagnosis

Spirochetes can be detected in stool by darkfield microscopy and cultured from stool or biopsy specimens on trypticase soy agar with 5–10% horse or calf blood. The addition of spectinomycin and polymyxin B makes the media selective (Teglbjaerg, 1990). On media incubated anaerobically, pinpoint, weakly β-hemolytic colonies develop in 3 days to 4 weeks, depending on the strain. Fluorescent in situ hybridization assays and amplification techniques followed by RFLP analysis have both been used for the detection and/or identification of spirochetes from tissue biopsy samples (Calderaro, 2003; Jensen, 2004). Moreover, amplification of *Brachyspira* genes from DNA extracted directly from feces of infected animals has also been successful (Atyeo, 1998).

Treatment

Although antimicrobial susceptibilities of *Brachyspira* spp. have been published, standardized testing of a large number of isolates has not been described (Karlsson, 2003). Patients suffering from symptoms and intestinal spirochetosis have reportedly responded to metronidazole (Teglbjaerg, 1990).

References

Aberer E, Klade H, Hobisch G. A clinical, histological, and immunohistochemical comparison of acrodermatitis chronica atrophicans and morphea. Am J Dermatopathol 1991; 13:334.

Aberle-Grasse J, Olton SL, Notari E, et al: Predictive value of past and current screening tests for syphilis in blood donors: changing from a rapid plasma reagin test to an automated specific treponemal test for screening. Transfusion 1999; 39:206.

Afzelius A: Verhanlungen der dermatologischen Gesellschaft zu Stockholm. Arch Dermatol Syphilis 1910; 101:405.

Aguero-Rosenfeld ME, Shoop E, Johnson RC: Immunoblot interpretation criteria for serodiagnosis of early Lyme disease. J Clin Microbiol 1996; 33:419.

American College of Physicians: Guidelines for laboratory evaluation in the diagnosis of Lyme disease. Ann Intern Med 1997; 127:1106.

Anderson LC, Leary SL, Manning PJ: Rat-bite fever in animal research laboratory personnel. Lab Anim Sci 1983; 33:292.

Antal GM, Lukehart SA, Meheus AZ: The endemic treponematoses. Microbes Infect 2002; 4:83.
This extensive review provides descriptions of the causative agents and their principal pathogenic mechanisms as well as diagnostic and treatment options. Its depiction of each of the clinical diseases and their individual impact on various human populations, however, is extraordinary.

Arean VM: The pathologic anatomy and pathogenesis of fatal human leptospirosis (Weil's disease). Am J Pathol 1962; 40:393.

Atyeo RF, Oxberry SL, Combs BG, Hampson DJ: Development and evaluation of polymerase chain reaction tests as an aid to diagnosis of swine dysentery and intestinal spirochetosis. Lett Appl Microbiol 1998; 26:126.

Augenbraun M, Roits R, Johnson R, et al: Treponemal specific tests for the serodiagnosis of syphilis. Sex Transm Dis 1998; 25:549.

Bacon RM, Biggerstaff BJ, Schriefer ME, et al: Serodiagnosis of Lyme disease by kinetic enzyme-linked immunosorben assay using recombinant VlsE1 peptide antigens of *Borrelia burgorferi* compared with 2-tiered testing using whole cell lysates. J Infect Dis 2003; 187:1187.

Bakken LL, Callister SM, Wand PJ, et al: Interlaboratory comparison of test results for detection of Lyme disease by 516 participants in the Wisconsin State Laboratory of Hygiene/ College of American Pathologists Proficiency Testing Program. J Clin Microbiol 1997; 35:537.

Balmelli T, Piffaretti JC: Association between different clinical manifestations of Lyme disease and different species of *Borrelia burgdorferi sensu lato*. Res Microbiol 1995; 146:329.

VII

Bannwarth A: Chronische lymphocytäre Meningitis, entzundliche polyneuritis und 'rheumatismus.' Arch Psychiatr Nervenkr 1941; 113:284.

Bellovin SM: Correspondence. N Engl J Med 2001; 345:1349.

Blanc WA: Pathology of the placenta, membranes, and umbilical cord in bacterial, fungal, and viral infections in man. *In* Naeye RL, Kissane JM, Kaufman N (eds): International Academy of Pathology Monograph. Baltimore, MD, Williams & Wilkins, 1981, p 67.

Breitschwerdt EB, Nicholson WL, Kiehl AR, et al: Natural infections with *Borrelia* spirochetes in two dogs from Florida. J Clin Microbiol 1994; 32:352.

Brenner DJ, Kaufmann AF, Sulzer KR, et al: Further determination of DNA relatedness between serogroups and serovars in the family Leptospiraceae with a proposal for *Leptospira alexanderi* sp. nov. and four new *Leptospira* genomospecies. Int J Syst Bacteriol 1999; 49:839.

Brettschneider S, Bruckbauer H, Klugbauer N, et al: Diagnostic value of PCR for detection of *Borrelia burgdorferi* in skin biopsy and urine samples from patients with skin borreliosis. J Clin Microbiol 1998; 36:2658.

Brown SL, Hansen SLH, Langone JJ: Role of serology in the diagnosis of Lyme disease. JAMA 1999; 281:62.
Explores the performance characteristics of serologic techniques in the diagnosis of Lyme disease and demonstrates the role that corroborating clinical and epidemiologic factors should play.

Brown ST, Zaidi A, Larsen SA, et al: Serological response to syphilis treatment. JAMA 1985; 253:1296.

Brunner M, Sigal LH: Use of serum immune complexes in a new test that accurately confirms early Lyme disease and active infection with *Borrelia burgdorferi*. J Clin Microbiol 2001; 39:3213.

Bunikis J, Tsao J, Farmpo U, et al: Typing of *Borrelia* relapsing fever group strains. Emerg Infect Dis 2004; 10:1661.

Burgdorfer W, Barbour AG, Hayes SF, et al: Lyme disease – a tick-borne spirochetosis? Science 1982; 216:1317.

Cadavid D, Barbour AG: Neuroborreliosis during relapsing fever: review of the clinical manifestations, pathology, and treatment of infections in human and experimental animals. Clin Infect Dis 1998; 26:151.

Calderaro A, Villanacci V, Conter M, et al: Rapid detection and identification of *Brachyspira aalborgi* from rectal biopsies and faeces of a patient. Res Microbiol 2003; 154:145.

Centers for Disease Control and Prevention: Recommendations for test performance and interpretation from the Second National Conference on Serologic Diagnosis of Lyme Disease. JAMA 1995; 274:937.

Centers for Disease Control and Prevention: Case definitions for public health surveillance. MMWR 1997; 46(RR-10):20.

Centers for Disease Control and Prevention: The National plan to eliminate syphilis from the United States. 1999. Available on line at http://www.cdc.gov/stopsyphilis/Plan.pdf

Centers for Disease Control and Prevention: Sexually transmitted diseases treatment guidelines. MMWR Recomm Rep 2002; 51(RR-6):1.
Developed as a tool to guide therapy of many sexually transmitted diseases, these recommendations also include many valuable diagnostic considerations for a variety of presentations

Centers for Disease Control and Prevention: Primary and secondary syphilis – United States, 2002. MMWR 2003; 52:1117.

Centers for Disease Control and Prevention: Congenital syphilis – United States, 2002. MMWR 2004a; 53:716.

Centers for Disease Control and Prevention: Lyme disease – United States, 2001–2002. MMWR 2004b; 53:365.

Centurion-Lara A, Castro C, Barret L, et al: *Treponema pallidum* major sheath protein homolog Tpr K is a target of opsonic antibody and the protective immune response. J Exp Med 1999; 189:647.

Chamberlain NR, Brandt ME, Erwin AL, et al: Major integral membrane protein immunogens of *Treponema pallidum* are proteolipids. Infect Immun 1989; 57:2872.

Choi BK, Wyss C, Gobel UB: Phylogenetic analysis of pathogen-related oral spirochetes. J Clin Microbiol 1996; 34:1922.

Collis TK, Celum CL: The clinical manifestations and treatment of sexually transmitted diseases in human immunodeficiency virus-positive men. Clin Infect Dis 2001; 32:611.

Coyle PK, Schutzer SE, Deng Z, et al: Detection of *Borrelia burgdorferi*-specific antigen in antibody-negative cerebrospinal fluid in neurologic Lyme disease. Neurology 1995; 45:2010.

Cox DL, Chang P, McDowall AW, et al: The outer-membrane, not a coat of host proteins, limits antigenicity of virulent *Treponema pallidum*. Infect Immun 1992; 60:1076.

Cruz M, Hansen K, Ernerudh J, et al: Lyme arthritis: oligoclonal anti-*Borrelia burgdorferi* IgG antibodies occur in joint fluid and serum. Scand J Immunol 1991;33:61.

Cumberland MC, Turner TB: Rate of multiplication of *Treponema pallidum* in normal and immune rabbits. Am J Syphilis 1949; 33:201.

Dattwyler RJ, Volkman DJ, Luft BJ, et al: Seronegative Lyme disease: dissociation of specific T- and B-lymphocyte responses to *Borrelia burgdorferi*. N Engl J Med 1988; 319:1441.

Davis GE: Species unity or plurality of the relapsing fever spirochetes. *In* Moulton FR (ed.): A Symposium on Relapsing Fever in the Americas. Washington, DC, American Association for the Advancement of Science, 1942.

De Cock HE, Marks SL, Stacy BA, et al: Ileocolitis associated with *Anaerobiospirillum* in cats. J Clin Microbiol 2004; 42:2752.

De Silva AM, Fikrig E: Arthropod- and host-specific gene expression by *Borrelia burgdorferi*. J Clin Invest 1997; 99:377.

Dooley JR, Ishak KG: Leptospirosis. *In* Binford CC, Conner DH (eds): Pathology of Tropical and Extraordinary Diseases, vol I. Washington, DC, Armed Forces Institute of Pathology, 1976, p 101.

Dorfman DH, Glaser JH: Congenital syphilis presenting in infants after the newborn period. N Engl J Med 1990; 323:1299.

Dressler F, Ackerman R, Steere AC: Antibody responses to the three genomic groups of *Borrelia burgdorferi* in European Lyme borreliosis. J Infect Dis 1994; 169:313.

Dressler F, Whalen JA, Reinhart BN, et al: Western blotting in the serodiagnosis of Lyme disease. J Infect Dis 1993; 167:392.

Dressler F, Yoshinari NH, Steere AC: The T-cell proliferation assay in the diagnosis of Lyme disease. Ann Intern Med 1991; 115:533.

Dumler JS: Molecular diagnosis of Lyme disease: review and meta-analysis. Mol Diagn 2001; 6:1.
Successfully accomplishes the feat of assembling a multitude of diverse molecular data in order to illustrate the overall performance characteristics and utility of amplification assays on different clinical specimens.

Duray PH, Chandler FW: Lyme disease. *In* Conner DH, Chandler FW, Schwartz DA, et al (eds): Pathology of Infectious Diseases. Stamford, CT, Appleton & Lange, 1997, p 635.

Dworkin MS, Anderson DE Jr, Schwan TG, et al: Tick-borne relapsing fever in the northwestern United States and southwestern Canada. Clin Infect Dis 1998; 26:122.

Dworkin MS, Schwan TG, Anderson DE: Tick-borne relapsing fever in North America. Med Clin North Am 2002; 86:417.
Instructive review of endemic relapsing fever that provides a description of the causative spirochetes, epidemiologic, tick-vector ecologic and pathogenic factors that lead to human disease, and clinical manifestations of relapsing fever. Laboratory diagnostic techniques, treatment and prevention issues are also highlighted.

Edwards GA, Olmm BM: Human leptospirosis. Medicine 1960; 39:117.

Engelkens HJ, Judanarson J, Orange AP, et al: Endemic treponematoses. Part I: Yaws. Int J Dermatol 1991a; 30:77.

Engelkens HJ, Niemel PL, van der Sluis JJ, et al: Endemic treponematoses. Part II: Pinta and endemic syphilis. Int J Dermatol 1991b; 30:231.

Engstrom SM, Shoop E, Johnson RC: Immunoblot interpretation criteria for serodiagnosis of early Lyme disease. J Clin Microbiol 1995; 33:419.

Falco RC, Fish D, D'Amico V: Accuracy of tick identification in a Lyme disease endemic area. JAMA 1998; 280:602.

Falco RC, McKenna DF, Daniels TJ, et al: Temporal relation between *Ixodes scapularis* abundance and risk for Lyme disease associated with erythema migrans. Am J Epidemiol 1999; 149:771.

Farr RW: Leptospirosis. Clin Infect Dis 1995; 21:1.

Feigin RD, et al: Human leptospirosis from immunized dogs. Ann Intern Med 1973; 79:777.

Fitzgerald TJ: The TH_1/TH_2 switch in syphilitic infection: is it detrimental? Infect Immun 1992; 60:3475.

Fiumara NJ: Treatment of primary and secondary syphilis. Serological response. JAMA 1980; 243:2500.

Flores JL: Syphilis: A tale of twisted treponemes. West J Med 1995; 163:552.

Fraenkel CJ, Garpmo U, Berglund J: Determination of novel *Borrelia* genospecies in Swedish *Ixodes ricinus* ticks. J Clin Microbiol 2002; 40:3308.

Fraser CM, Casjens S, Huang WM, et al: Genomic sequence of a Lyme disease spirochete, *Borrelia burgdorferi*. Nature 1997; 390:580.

Fraser CM, Norris SJ, Weinstock GM, et al: Complete genome sequence of *Treponema pallidum*, the syphilis spirochete. Science 1998; 281:375.

Fredricks DN, Relman DA: Sequence-based identifications of microbial pathogens: a reconsideration of Koch's postulates. Clin Microbiol Rev 1996; 9:18.

Fukunaga M, Takahashi Y, Tsuruta Y, et al: Genetic and phenotypic analysis of *Borrelia miyamotoi* sp. nov., isolated from the ixodid tick *Ixodes persulcatus*, the vector for Lyme disease in Japan. Int J Syst Bacteriol 1995; 45:804.

Gerbase AC, Rowley TR, Heymann DHL, Berkley SFB, Plot P: Global prevalence and incidences estimates of selected curable STD. Sex Transm Infect 1998;11(Suppl 1):S12.

Goddard WW, Bennett SA, Parkinson C: *Anaerobiospirillum succiniciproducens* septicaemia: important aspects of diagnosis and mangement. J Infect 1998; 37:68.

Gomes-Solecki MJC, Dunn JJ, Luft BJ et al: Recombinant chimeric *Borrelia* proteins for diagnosis of Lyme disease. J Clin Microbiol 2000; 38:2530.

Gourevitch MN, Selwyn PA, Devanay K, et al: Effects of HIV infection on the serologic manifestations and response to treatment of syphilis in intravenous drug users. Ann Intern Med 1993; 118:350.

Greene BM, Miller NR, Bynum TE: Failure of penicillin G benzathine in the treatment of neurosyphilis. Arch Intern Med 1980; 140:1117.

Gross DM, Forsthumber T, Tary-Lehmann M, et al: Identification of LFA-1 as a candidate autoantigen in treatment-resistant Lyme arthritis. Science 1998; 281:703.

Guarner J, Southwick K, Greer P, et al: Testing umbilical cords for funisitis due to *Treponema pallidum* infection, Bolivia. Emerg Infect Dis 2000; 6:487.

Gussenhoven GC, van der Hoorn MAWG, Goris MGA, et al: Leptodipstick, a dipstick assay for detection of leptospira-specific immunoglobulin M antibodies in human sera. J Clin Microbiol 1997; 35:92.

Haas JS, Bolan G, Larsen SA, et al: Sensitivity of treponemal tests for detecting prior treated syphilis during human immunodeficiency virus infection. J Infect Dis 1990; 162:862.

Halperin JJ: Nervous system Lyme disease. Vector Borne Zoonotic Dis 2002; 2:241.

Hansen K, Lebech AM: Lyme neuroborreliosis: a new sensitive diagnostic assay for intrathecal synthesis of *Borrelia burgdorferi*-specific immunoglobulin. Ann Neurol 1991;30:197.

Hart G: Screening to control infectious diseases: evaluation of control programs for gonorrhea and syphilis. Rev Infect Dis 1980; 2:701.

Harter C, Bernischke K: Fetal syphilis in the first trimester. Am J Obstet Gynecol 1976; 124:705.

Hayes EB, Piesman J: How can we prevent Lyme disease? N Engl J Med 2003; 348:2424.

Hazlett KRO, Sellati TJ, Nguyen TT, et al: The TprK protein of *Treponema pallidum* is periplasmic and is not a target of opsonic antibody or protective immunity. J Exp Med 2001; 193:1015.

Hernandez-Aguado I, Bolumar F, Moreno R, et al: False positive tests for syphilis associated with human immunodeficiency virus and hepatitis B virus infection among intravenous drug abusers. Eur J Clin Microbiol Infect Dis 1998; 17:784.

Hilton E, Tramontanno A, DeVoti J, Sood SK: Temporal study of immunoglobulin M seroreactivity to *Borrelia burgdorferi* in patients treated for Lyme borreliosis. J Clin Microbiol 1997; 35:774.

Hitt E: Poor sales trigger vaccine withdrawal. Nat Med 2002; 8:311.

Hoang MP, High WA, Molberg KH: Secondary syphilis: a histologic and immunohistochemical evaluation. J Cutan Pathol 2004; 31:595.

Hooper NE, Malloy DC, Passen S: Evaluation of a *Treponema pallidum* enzyme immunoassay as a screening test for syphilis. Clin Diagn Lab Immunol 1994; 1:477.

Hovind-Hougen K, Birch-Andersen A, Henrik-Neilsen R, et al: Intestinal spirochetosis: morphological characterization and cultivation of the spirochete *Brachyspira aalborgi* gen. nov., sp. nov. J Clin Microbiol 1982; 16:1127.

Hutchinson CM, Rompalo AM, Reochart CA, et al: Characteristics of syphilis in patients attending Baltimore STD clinics – multiple high risk subgroups and interchange with human immunodeficiency virus infection. Arch Intern Med 1991; 151:511.

Hutter G, Schlagenhauf U, Valenza G, et al: Molecular analysis of bacteria in periodontitis: evaluation of clone libraries, novel phylotypes and putative pathogens. Microbiology 2003; 149:67.

Ikeda MK, Jenson HB: Evaluation and treatment of congenital syphilis. J Pediatr 1990; 117:843.

James AM, Liveris D, Wormser GP, et al: *Borrelia lonestari* infection after a bite by an *Amblyomma americanum* tick. J Infect Dis 2001; 183:1810.

Jensen TK, Teglbjaerg PS, Lindboe CF, Boye M: Demonstration of *Brachyspira aalborgi* lineages 2 and 3 in human colonic biopsies with intestinal spirochaetosis by specific fluorescent in situ hybridization. J Med Microbiol 2004; 53:341.

Johns DR, Tierney M, Felsenstein D: Alteration in the natural history of neurosyphilis by concurrent infection with the human immunodeficiency virus. N Engl J Med 1987; 316:1569.

Johnson BJ, Robbins KE, Bailey RE, et al: Serodiagnosis of Lyme disease: accuracy of a two-step approach using flagella-based ELISA and immunoblotting. J Infect Dis 1996; 174:346.

Johnson WD, Golightly LM: *Borrelia* species (relapsing fever). *In* Mandell J, Bennett J, Dolin R (eds): Principles and Practice of Infectious Diseases. 5th ed. New York, Churchill Livingstone, 2000, p 2502.

Kaiser R: Neuroborreliosis. J Neurol 1998; 245:247.

Kalish RA, McHugh G, Granquist J, et al: Persistence of immunoglobulin M or immunoglobulin G antibody responses to *Borrelia burgdorferi* 10–20 years after active Lyme disease. Clin Infect Dis 2001; 33:780.

Kanavaki S, Mantadakis E, Thomakos N, et al: *Brachyspira* (*Serpulina*) *pilosicoli* spirochetemia in an immunocompromised patient. Infection 2002; 30:175.

Karlsson M, Fellstrom C, Gunnarsson A, et al: Antimicrobial susceptibility testing of porcine *Brachyspira* (*Serpulina*) species isolates. J Clin Microbiol 2003; 41:2596.

Klempner MS: Controlled trials of antibiotic treatment in patients with post-treatment chronic Lyme disease. Vector Borne Zoonotic Dis 2002; 2:255.

Klempner MS, Schmid CH, Hu L et al: Intralaboratory reliability of serologic and urine testing for Lyme disease. Am J Med 2001; 110:217.

Kirkland KB, Klimko TB, Meriwether RA, et al: Erythema migrans-like rash illness at a camp in North Carolina. Arch Intern Med 1997; 157:2635.

Korner M, Gebbers JO: Clinical significance of human intestinal spirochetosis – a morphologic approach. Infection 2003; 5:341.

Focuses on a compilation of evidence that ascribes pathogenic traits to the organisms heretofore only associated with intestinal spirochetosis.

Larsen SA, Johnson RE: Diagnostic tests. *In*: Larson SA, Pope V, Johnson RE, Kennedy EJ (eds): A Manual of Tests for Syphilis, 9th ed. Washington DC, American Public Health Association, 1998, p 1.

Larsen SA, Steiner BM, Rudolph AH: Laboratory diagnosis and interpretation of tests for syphilis. Clin Microbiol Rev 1995; 8:1.

Lebech AM: Polymerase chain reaction in diagnosis of *Borrelia burgdorferi* infections and studies on taxonomic classification. Acta Pathol Microl Immunol Scand Suppl 2002; 105:1.

Ledue TB, Collins MF, Craig WY: New laboratory guidelines for serologic diagnosis of Lyme disease: evaluation of the two-test protocol. J Clin Microbiol 1996; 34:2343.

Leenders ACAP: Correspondence. N Engl J Med 2001; 345:1349.

Lefevre J, Bertrand CMA, Bauriaud R: Evaluation of the Captia enzyme immunoassays for detection of immunoglobulins G and M to *Treponema pallidum* in syphilis. J Clin Microbiol 1990; 28:1704.

Lesser RL: Ocular manifestations of Lyme disease. Am J Med 1995; 24:60S.

Levett PN: Leptospirosis. Clin Microbiol Rev 2001; 14:296.

A comprehensive, yet concise review of historic, epidemiologic, clinical and diagnostic features of leptospirosis.

Liang FT, Steere AC, Marques AR, et al: Sensitive and specific serodiagnosis of Lyme disease by enzyme-linked immunosorbent assay with a peptide based on an immunodominant conserved region of *Borrelia burgdorferi* VlsE. J Clin Microbiol 1999; 37:3990.

Loesche WJ, Grossman NS: Periodontal disease as a specific, albeit chronic, infection: diagnosis and treatment. Clin Microbiol Rev 2001; 14:727.

Luger SW, Krauss E: Serologic tests for Lyme disease. Interlaboratory variability. Arch Intern Med 1990; 150:761.

Lukehart S, Hook EW, Baker-Zander SH, et al: Invasion of the central nervous system by *Treponema pallidum*. Implications for diagnosis and therapy. Ann Intern Med 1988; 109:855.

McGinley-Smith DE, Tsao SS: Dermatoses from ticks. J Am Acad Dermatol 2003; 49:363.

MacLean S, Luger A: Finding neurosyphilis without the Venereal Disease Research Laboratory Test. Sex Transm Dis 1996; 23:392.

McNeil MM, Martone WJ, Dowell VR Jr: Bacteremia with *Anaerobiospirillum succiniciproducens*. Rev Infect Dis 1987; 9:737.

Magnuson HJ, Thomas SW, Olansky S, et al: Inoculation syphilis in human volunteers. Medicine (Baltimore) 1956; 35:33.

Malnick H, Williams K, Phil-Eboise J, et al: Description of a medium for isolating *Anaerobiospirillum* sp., a possible cause of zoonotic disease from diarrheal feces and blood of humans and use of the medium in a survey of human canine and feline feces. J Clin Microbiol 1990; 28:1380.

Marra CM, Boutin P, McArthur JC, et al: A pilot study evaluating ceftriaxone and penicillin G as treatment agents for neurosyphilis in human

immunodeficiency virus-infected individuals. Clin Infect Dis 2000; 30:540.

Marra CM, Gary DW, Kuypers J, et al: Diagnosis of neurosyphilis in patients infected with human immunodeficiency virus type I. J Infect Dis 1996; 174:219.

Marra CM, Maxwell CL, Tantalo L, et al: Normalization of cerebrospinal fluid abnormalities after neurosyphilis therapy: does HIV status matter? Clin Infect Dis 2004; 38:1001.

Mohr JA, Griffits W, Jackson R, et al: Neurosyphilis and penicillin levels in cerebrospinal fluid. JAMA 1976; 236:2208.

Molloy PJ, Persing DH, Berardi VP: False positive results of PCR testing for Lyme disease. Clin Infect Dis 2001; 33:412.

Musher DM: Syphilis, neurosyphilis, penicillin, and AIDS. J Infect Dis 1991; 163:1201.

Musher DM, Hamill RJ, Baughn RE: Effect of human immunodeficiency virus (HIV) on the course of syphilis and on the response to treatment. Ann Intern Med 1990; 113:872.

Nadelman RB, Nowakowski J, Fish D et al: Prophylaxis with single-dose doxycycline for the prevention of Lyme disease after *Ixodes scapularis* tick bite. N Engl J Med 2001; 345:79.

Nadelman RB, Nowakowski J, Forseter G, et al: The clinical spectrum of early Lyme borreliosis in patients with culture-confirmed erythema migrans. Am J Med 1996; 100:502.

Nadelman RB, Wormser GP: Lyme borreliosis. Lancet 1998; 352:557.

Nichol G, Dennis DT, Steere AC et al: Test-treatment strategies for patients suspected of having Lyme disease: a cost effective analysis. Ann Intern Med 1998; 128:37

Nocton JJ, Bloom BJ, Rutledge BJ, et al: Detection of *Borrelia burgdorferi* DNA by polymerase chain reaction in cerebrospinal fluid in Lyme neuroborreliosis. J Infect Dis 1996; 174:623.

Nocton JJ, Dressler F, Rutledge BJ, et al: Detection of *Borrelia burgdorferi* DNA by polymerase chain reaction in synovial fluid from patients with Lyme arthritis. N Engl J Med 1994; 330:229.

Norgard MV: Clinical and diagnostic issues of acquired and congenital syphilis encompassed in the current syphilis epidemic. Curr Opin Infect Dis 1993; 6:9.

Norman GL, Antig JM, Bigaignon G, Hogrefe WR: Serodiagnosis of Lyme borreliosis by *Borrelia burgdorferi* sensu stricto, *B. garinii*, and *B. afzelii* Western blots (immunoblots). J Clin Microbiol 1996; 34:1732.

Oliver JH, Lin T, Gao L, et al: An enzootic transmission cycle of Lyme borreliosis spirochetes in the southeastern United States. Proc Natl Acad Sci USA 2003; 100:11642.

Pahl A, Kuhlbrandt U, Brune K, et al: Quantitative detection of *Borrelia burgdorferi* by real-time PCR. J Clin Microbiol 1999; 37:1958.

Parola P, Raoult D: Ticks and tickborne bacterial diseases in humans: an emerging infectious threat. Clin Infect Dis 2001; 32:897.

Paster BJ, Boshces SK, Galvin JL, et al: Bacterial diversity in human subgingival plaque. J Bacteriol 2001; 183:3770.

Patel R, Grogg KL, Edwards WD, et al: Death from inappropriate therapy for Lyme disease. Clin Infect Dis 2000; 31:1107.

Patterson FC, Winn WC: Practical identification of hard ticks in the parasitology laboratory. Pathol Case Rev 2003; 8:187.

Peeling RW, Mabey DCW: Syphilis. Nat Rev Microbiol 2004;2:448.

Perolat P, Chappel RJ, Adler B, et al: *Leptospira fainei* sp. nov. isolated from pigs in Australia. Int J Syst Bacteriol 1998; 48:851.

Persing DH, Rutledge BJ, Rys PN, et al: Target imbalance: disparity of *Borrelia burgdorferi* genetic material in synovial fluid from Lyme arthritis patients. J Infect Dis 1994; 169:668.

Pienaar C, Kruger AJ, Venter EC, Pitout JD: *Anaerobiospirillum succiniciproducens* bacteraemia. J Clin Pathol 2003; 56:316.

VII

Piesman J, Mather TN, Sinsky RJ, et al: Duration of tick attachment and *Borrelia burgdorferi* transmission. J Clin Microbiol 1987; 25:557.

Plorer A, Sepp N, Schmutzhard E, et al: Effects of adequate versus inadequate treatment of cutaneous manifestations of Lyme borreliosis on the incidence of late complications and late serological status. J Invest Dermatol 1993; 100:103.

Poland GA: Prevention of Lyme disease: a concise review of the evidence. Mayo Clin Proc 2001; 76:713.

Porcella SP, Raffel SJ, Schrumpf ME, et al: Serodiagnosis of louse-borne relapsing fever with glycerophosphodiester phosphodiesterase (GlpQ) from *Borrelia recurrentis*. J Clin Microbiol 2000; 38:3561.

Porcella SF, Schwan TG: *Borrelia burgdorferi* and *Treponema pallidum*: a comparison of functional genomics, environmental adaptations, and pathogenic mechanisms. J Clin Invest 2001; 107:651.

Ramachandran S, Perera MVF: Cardiac and pulmonary involvement in leptospirosis. Trans R Soc Trop Med Hyg 1977; 71:56.

Raoult D, Birtles RJ, Montoya M, et al : Survey of three bacterial louse-associated diseases among rural Andean communities in Peru: prevalence of epidemic typhus, trench fever, and relapsing fever. Clin Infect Dis 1999 29:434.

Rawlings JA: An overview of tick-borne relapsing fever with emphasis on outbreaks in Texas. Tex Med 1995; 91:56.

Reed KD: Laboratory testing for Lyme disease: possibilities and practicalities. J Clin Microbiol 2002; 40:319.

Reisner BS, Mann L, Tholcken C, et al: Use of the *Treponema pallidum* specific Captia Syphilis IgG assay in conjunction with the rapid plasma reagin test to test for syphilis. J Clin Microbiol 1997; 35:1141.

Rich SM, Sawyer SA, Barbour AG: Antigen polymorphism in *Borrelia hermsii*, a clonal pathogenic bacterium. Proc Natl Acad Sci USA 2001; 98:15038.

Riviere GR, Smith KS, Carranza N, et al: Subgingival distribution of *Treponema denticola*, *Treponema socranskii*, and pathogen-related oral spirochetes: prevalence and relationship to periodontal status of sampled sites. J Periodontol 1995; 66:829.

Riviere GR, Smith KS, Tzagaroulaki E, et al: Periodontal status and detection frequency of bacteria at sites of periodontal health and gingivitis. J Periodontol 1996; 67:109.

Riviere GR, Smith KS, Willis SG, Riviere KH: Phenotypic and genotypic heterogeneity among cultivable pathogen-related oral spirochetes and *Treponema vincentii*. J Clin Microbiol 1999;37:3676.

Rolfs RT, Joesoef MR, Hendershot EF, et al: A randomized trial of enhanced therapy for early syphilis in patients with and without human immunodeficiency virus infection. The syphilis and HIV study group. N Engl J Med 1997; 337:307.

Roman GC, Roman LN: Occurrence of congenital, cardiovascular, visceral, neurologic, and neuro-opthalmologic complications in late yaws: a theme for future research. Rev Infect Dis 1986; 8:760.

Romanowski M, Sutherland R, Fick GH, et al: Serologic response to treatment of infectious syphilis. Ann Intern Med 1991; 114:1005.

Salazar JC, Hazlett KRO, Radolf JD: The immune response to infection with *Treponema pallidum*, the stealth pathogen. Microbes Infect 2002; 4:1133.

Schmid GP: Epidemiology and clinical similarities of human spirochetal diseases. Rev Infect Dis 1989;11(Suppl 6):S1460.

Short review offering interesting pathogenetic and clinical correlations between the major spirochete diseases.

Schmidt BL: PCR in laboratory diagnosis of human *Borrelia burgdorferi* infections. Clin Microbiol Rev 1997; 10:185.

Schroeter AL, Lucas JA, Price EV, et al: Treatment for early syphilis and reactivity of serologic tests. JAMA 1972; 221:471.

Schwan TG, Schrumpf ME, Hinnebusch BJ, et al: GlpQ: an antigen for serological discrimination between relapsing fever and Lyme borreliosis. J Clin Microbiol 1996; 34:2483.

Scoles GA, Papero M, Beati L, Fish D: A relapsing fever group spirochete transmitted by *Ixodes scapularis* ticks. Vector Borne Zoonotic Dis 2001; 1:21.

Scrimenti RJ: Erythema chronicum migrans. Arch Dermatol 1970;102:104.

Seltzer EG, Gerber MA, Cartter ML, et al: Long-term outcomes of persons with Lyme disease. JAMA 2000; 283:609.

Seltzer EG, Shapiro ED: Misdiagnosis of Lyme disease: when not to order serologic tests. Pediatr Infect Dis J 1996; 15:762.

Shadick NA, Phillips CB, Sangha O, et al: Musculoskeletal and neurologic outcomes in patients with previously treated Lyme disease. Ann Intern Med 1999; 133:919.

Shapiro ED: Doxycycline for tick bites – not for everyone. N Engl J Med 2001; 345:133.

Shapiro ED, Gerber MA: Lyme disease. Clin Infect Dis 2000; 31:533.

Shapiro ED, Gerber MA, Holabird NB, et al: A controlled trial of antimicrobial prophylaxis for Lyme disease after deer-tick bites. N Engl J Med 1992; 327:1769.

Shlaes DM, Dul MJ, Lerner PI: *Anaerobiospirillum* bacteremia. Ann Intern Med 1982; 97:63.

Sigal LH: Lyme disease: a review of aspects of its immunology and immunopathogenesis. Annu Rev Immunol 1997; 15:63.

Signorini L, Colombini P, Cristini F, et al: Inappropriate footwear and rat-bite fever in an international traveler. J Trav Med 2002; 9:275.

Singh AE, Romanowski B: Syphilis: review with emphasis on clinical, epidemiologic, and some biologic features. Clin Microbiol Rev 1999; 12:187.

Smith RP, Schoen RT, Rahn DW, et al: Clinical characteristics and treatment outcome of early Lyme disease patients with microbiologically confirmed erythema migrans. Ann Intern Med 2002; 136:421.

Sood SK, Salzman MB, Johnson BJB, et al: Duration of tick attachment as a predictor of the risk of Lyme disease in an area in which Lyme disease is endemic. J Infect Dis 1997; 175:996.

Southern PMJ, Sanford JP: Relapsing fever: a clinical and microbiological review. Medicine 1969; 48:129.

Steere AC: *Borrelia burgdorferi* (Lyme disease, Lyme borreliosis). *In* Mandell J, Bennett J, Dolin R (eds): Principles and Practice of Infectious Diseases, 5th ed. New York, Churchill Livingstone, 2000, p 2504.

Steere AC: A 58-year old man with a diagnosis of chronic Lyme disease. JAMA 2002; 288:1002.

Steere AC: Lyme disease. N Engl J Med 2001; 345:115.

Steere AC, Broderick TF, Malawista SE: Erythema chronicum migrans Lyme arthritis. Epidemiologic evidence for a tick vector. Am J Epidemiol 1978; 108:312.

Steere AC, Glickstein L: Elucidation of Lyme arthritis. Nat Rev Immunol 2004; 4:143.

Steere AC, Malawista SE, Hardin JA, et al: Erythema chronicum migrans and Lyme arthritis. The enlarging clinical spectrum. Ann Intern Med 1977a; 86:685.

Steere AC, Malawista SE, Syndman DR, et al: Lyme arthritis: an epidemic of oligoarticular arthritis in children and adults in three Connecticut communities. Arthritis Rheum 1977b; 20:7.

Steere AC, Sikand VK, Meurice F, et al: Vaccination against Lyme disease with recombinant *Borrelia burgdorferi* outer-surface lipoprotein A with adjuvant. Lyme Disease Vaccine Study Group. N Engl J Med 1998; 339:209.

Steere AC, Sikand VK, Schoen RT, Nowakowski J: Asymptomatic infection with *Borrelia burgdorferi*. Clin Infect Dis 2003; 37:528.

Stoll BJ, Lee FK, Larsen S, et al: Clinical and serologic evaluation of neonates for congenital syphilis: a continuing diagnostic dilemma. J Infect Dis 1993; 167:1093.

Sundnes KO, Haimanot AT: Epidemic of louse-borne relapsing fever in Ethiopia. Lancet 1993; 342:1213.

Taber LH, Feigin RD: Spirochetal infections. Pediatr Clin North Am 1979; 26:377.

Tee W, Korman TM, Waters MJ, et al: Three cases of *Anaerobiospirillum succiniciproducens* bacteremia confirmed by 16s rRNA gene sequencing. J Clin Microbiol 1998; 36:1209.

Teglbjaerg PS: Intestinal spirochetosis. Curr Top Pathol 1990; 81:247.

Thomas DD, Baseman JB, Alderete JF, et al: Enhanced levels of attachment of fibronectin-primed *Treponema pallidum* to extracellular matrix. Infect Immun 1986; 52:736–741.

Tramont EC: *Treponema pallidum* (syphilis). *In* Mandell J, Bennett J, Dolin R (eds): Principles and Practice of Infectious Diseases, 5th ed. New York, Churchill Livingstone, 2000, p 2474.

Trevejo RT, Krause PJ, Sikand VK, et al: Evaluation of two-test serodiagnostic method for early Lyme disease in clinical practice. J Infect Dis 1999; 179:931.

Trott DJ, Jensen NS, Saint Girons I, et al: Identification and characterization of *Serpulina pilosicoli* isolates recovered from the blood of critically ill patients. J Clin Microbiol 1997; 35:482.

Tugwell P, Dennis DT, Weinstein A, et al: Laboratory evaluation in the diagnosis of Lyme disease. Ann Intern Med 1997; 127:1109.

Explores the performance characteristics of serologic techniques in the diagnosis of Lyme disease and demonstrates the role that corroborating clinical and epidemiologic factors should play.

United States Public Health Service: Syphilis, a synopsis. Publication No. 1660. Washington, DC, US Government Printing Office, 1968.

Varela AS, Luttrell MP, Howerth EW, et al: First culture isolation of *Borrelia lonestari*, putative agent of southern-tick associated rash illness. J Clin Microbiol 2004; 42:1163.

Van Dam AP: Diversity of *Ixodes*-borne *Borrelia* species – clinical, pathogenetic, and diagnostic implications and impact on vaccine development. Vector Borne Zoonotic Dis 2002; 2:249.

Van Dam AP, Kuiper H, Vos K, et al: Different genospecies of *Borrelia burgdorferi* are associated with distinct clinical manifestations of Lyme borreliosis. Clin Infect Dis 1993; 17:708.

Vinetz JM, Glass GE, Flexner CE, et al: Sporadic urban leptospirosis. Ann Intern Med 1996; 125:794.

Wang G: Direct detection methods for Lyme *Borrelia*, including the use of quantitative assays. Vector Borne Zoonotic Dis 2002; 2:223.

Wang G, van Dam AP, Dankert J: Molecular typing of *Borrelia burgdorferi* sensu lato: taxonomic, epidemiological and clinical implications. Clin Microbiol Rev 1999; 12:633.

Warshafsky S, Nowakowski J, Nadelman RB, et al: Efficacy of antibiotic prophylaxis for prevention of Lyme disease. J Gen Intern Med 1996; 11:329.

Washburn RG: *Spirillum minus* (rat bite fever). *In* Mandell GL, Bennett JE, Dolin R (eds): Principles and Practice of Infectious Disease, 4th ed. New York, Churchill Livingstone, 1995, p 2155.

Whooten RM, Weis JJ: Host–pathogen interactions promoting inflammatory Lyme arthritis: use of mouse models for dissection of disease purposes. Curr Opin Microbiol 2001; 4:274.

Wicher K, Horowitz HW, Wicher V: Laboratory methods of diagnosis of syphilis for the beginning of the third millennium. Microbes Infect 1999; 1:1035.

Wicher V, Wicher K: Pathogenesis of maternal–fetal syphilis revisited. Clin Infect Dis 2001; 33:354.

Wormser GP, Bittker S, Cooper D, et al: Yield of large-volume blood cultures in patients with early Lyme disease. J Infect Dis 2001; 184:1070.

Wormser GP, Liveris D, Nowakowski J, et al: Association of species subtypes of *Borrelia burgdorferi* with hematogenous dissemination in early Lyme disease. J Infect Dis 1999; 180:720.

Wormser GP, Nadelman RB, Dattwyler RJ, et al: Practice guidelines for the treatment of Lyme Disease. Clin Infect Dis 2000; 31(Suppl 1):S1.

Yersin C, Bovet P, Smits H, et al: Field evaluation of a one-step dipstick assay for the diagnosis of human leptospirosis in the Seychelles. Trop Med Int Health 1999; 4:38.

Zhang JR, Norris SJ: Genetic variation of the *Borrelia burgdorferi* gene *vlsE* involves cassette-specific, segmental gene conversion. Infect Immunol 1998; 66:3698.

CHAPTER 59

Mycobacteria

Gail L. Woods MD

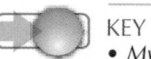

KEY POINTS

- *Mycobacterium tuberculosis* complex is the only mycobacterium that is transmitted from person-to-person and, therefore, is of public health importance.

- The Mantoux skin test is useful for identifying persons with latent tuberculosis infection.

- For optimal detection of mycobacteria in clinical specimens, laboratories should use a fluorochrome stain and both a liquid and a solid medium for culture.

- Nucleic acid amplification tests provide direct detection of *M. tuberculosis* complex in respiratory specimens.

- Susceptibility testing to the primary antituberculous agents (isoniazid, rifampin, ethambutol, and pyrazinamide) should be performed on all initial isolates of *M. tuberculosis* complex.

- Infections caused by nontuberculous mycobacteria are acquired from the environment (e.g., water).

- The nontuberculous mycobacteria most commonly encountered in the clinical laboratory are: *Mycobacterium avium* complex, which causes pulmonary disease and, in immune compromised patients, disseminated disease; the rapidly growing mycobacteria *Mycobacterium abscessus*, *Mycobacterium chelonae*, and *Mycobacterium fortuitum* group, which most often cause skin and soft tissue infections; *Mycobacterium kansasii*, which causes pulmonary infection; and *Mycobacterium marinum*, which causes skin and soft tissue infections.

Mycobacteria are aerobic, nonmotile, acid–alcohol fast, slightly curved or straight bacilli. The organisms contain high-molecular-weight (60–90 carbons) mycolic acids in their cell wall that on pyrolysis release C_{22} to C_{26} straight-chain saturated long chain acids. Their guanine plus cytosine DNA-base content ratios are in the range of 62–70 mol%.

Mycobacterium tuberculosis, *Mycobacterium bovis*, *Mycobacterium africanum*, and '*Mycobacterium canettii*' are the human pathogens that comprise the *M. tuberculosis* complex (MTBC). These organisms, the 'tubercle bacilli,' are the etiologic agents of human tuberculosis. Mycobacteria other than the MTBC have been called 'atypical' because they differ from the tubercle bacilli. The terms 'nontuberculous mycobacteria' and 'mycobacteria other than tubercle bacilli,' however, are preferred, because these organisms are not atypical but simply have characteristics distinct from those of *M. tuberculosis*.

In 1957, Runyon proposed that the nontuberculous mycobacteria (NTM) be divided into four groups based on colony pigmentation and growth rate on a solid medium (Table 59-1) (Runyon, 1959). This classification system, however, has limits. For example, *Mycobacterium kansasii* is usually a photochromogen but rarely is nonchromogenic or scotochromogenic. Members of the *Mycobacterium avium* complex (MAC) are nonchromogenic in Runyon's scheme, but some isolates produce slightly pigmented colonies, potentially causing incorrect classification as a scotochromogen. *Mycobacterium szulgai* is a scotochromogen at 37°C and a photochromogen at 25°C. Moreover, when a liquid medium is used for mycobacterial culture as is currently recommended (see below), growth rates used by Runyon for classification do not apply. *Mycobacterium leprae*, which is unique among mycobacteria by virtue of the fact that it has not yet been cultivated in vitro, is discussed separately.

Mycobacterium tuberculosis Complex

Mycobacterium tuberculosis

Today tuberculosis is a global problem. Worldwide, an estimated 8–10 million new cases of tuberculosis and 2–3 million deaths due to tuberculosis occur each year. In much of the world, tuberculosis is the leading cause of death from any one infectious agent, directly responsible for an estimated 7% of all deaths and 26% of all preventable deaths worldwide (Murray, 1990; Snider, 1994).

In the United States, tuberculosis was the leading cause of death at the turn of the 20th century. Mortality then decreased, initially because of public health efforts to house tuberculosis patients in sanatoria to improve their nutrition and ventilation, and later because of antituberculous drugs. Between 1953, when tuberculosis became notifiable on a national basis, and 1984 the incidence steadily decreased, by about 5–6% each year (Rieder, 1989). The rate of decline slowed dramatically from 1984–1985, and then the downward trend reversed. From 1985–1992, the number of tuberculosis cases reported to the Centers for Disease Control and Prevention (CDC) increased by about 20%, that is, over 51 000 more cases were reported than would have been expected had the decline continued (Centers for Disease Control and Prevention, 1993). Of the metropolitan areas, the most marked rise was reported in New York City. Factors

Table 59–1 Runyon's Classification of the Nontuberculosis Mycobacteria

Classification	Description of Colonies
Photochromogen	Not pigmented unless exposed to light (optimally during their early growth and with good aeration of the surface)
Scotochromogen	Pigmented when grown in the dark and in light
Nonphotochromogen	Not pigmented when grown in the dark or in light
Rapid grower	Growth on solid media in ≤7 days

contributing to the excessive number of cases were the epidemic spread of human immunodeficiency virus (HIV); a deterioration in the health-care infrastructure; and increases in the numbers of cases among the homeless, migrant workers, immigrants, and residents of long-term care facilities such as correctional facilities and nursing homes (Ellner, 1993). In addition to the resurgence of tuberculosis in the United States, another concern was multidrug-resistant tuberculosis (MDR-TB), defined as disease caused by *M. tuberculosis* that is resistant to two or more primary antimycobacterial agents used in the United States to treat tuberculosis (see below under Treatment). Since 1992, the incidence of tuberculosis has declined each year and MDR-TB has become uncommon (Centers for Disease Control and Prevention, 1998, 2004). However, despite the overall decline, high rates continue to be reported in foreign-born persons (predominantly those born in Mexico, the Philippines, Vietnam, India, and China), who accounted for 53% of the total tuberculosis cases reported in 2003, and in racial/ethnic minorities, especially the non-Hispanic black population.

M. tuberculosis is transmitted primarily via inhalation of dried residues of small infected droplets (1–10 μm in diameter) but also by direct inoculation of abraded skin, an event most likely to occur when pathologists or other laboratory personnel handle infected tissues. The most important source of infection is an undiagnosed person with cavitary (and sputum-smear-positive) pulmonary disease. The risk of active pulmonary disease is low after one exposure to the organism but increases under conditions of stress or in a confined environment where repeated exposures to the organism occur. Most persons who become infected with *M. tuberculosis* do not develop active disease. The lifetime risk of active disease is 5–10% for immune competent persons. For persons infected with both *M. tuberculosis* and HIV, in contrast, the risk of developing tuberculosis is 7–10% per year.

The specific structures, antigens, and mechanisms responsible for the virulence of *M. tuberculosis* are unknown, but cord factor and sulfatides have been associated with the ability of virulent strains to produce disease. In vitro, cord factor is responsible for the morphologic appearance of cells of *M. tuberculosis* – serpentine cords of bacilli in close parallel arrangements. This growth pattern correlates with the presence in the bacillus of trehalose 6,6'-dimycolate. When this glycolipid is injected into mice, it inhibits neutrophil migration, elicits granuloma formation, and stimulates protection against virulent infection; its specific role in the pathogenesis of human tuberculosis, however, remains unknown. Sulfatides are peripherally located glycolipids that inhibit fusion of secondary lysosomes with bacilli-containing phagosomes within a macrophage, possibly promoting intracellular survival of the organism.

The usual host response to infection with *M. tuberculosis* is activation of the cell-mediated immune system. During primary (initial) infection, inhaled bacilli travel to the alveolar spaces, where they are ingested by resident macrophages. These macrophages are unable to kill the mycobacteria, which multiply intracellularly during the first several days after infection. Macrophages infected with mycobacteria migrate to regional tracheobronchial lymph nodes and present the sensitizing antigen(s) to immunocompetent T cells, or they enter the lymphatics and blood and travel back to the lungs (primarily the apices) and to distant organs such as lymph nodes, kidneys, epiphyseal areas of the long bones, vertebral bodies, and meninges where bacilli continue to multiply until the cellular immune response is activated.

Immunocompetent T cells migrate from regional lymph nodes to the site of infection in the lung. There they release chemotactic, migration-inhibitory, and mitogenic cytokines, which stimulate recruitment of blood-derived monocytes and lymphocytes, macrophage and lymphocyte division, and macrophage activation. The activated macrophages have enhanced microbicidal activity, and they produce cytokines such as interleukin-1, interferon-γ, and tumor necrosis factor that stimulate or regulate other components of the immune system, properties that help control infection. The cytokines and lytic enzymes released by the macrophages also contribute to the concomitant local tissue destruction. With time, the activated T-cell population declines and is replaced by long-lived memory immune T cells, which protect against reinfection with *M. tuberculosis* and provide some crossprotection against infection with other mycobacteria. Despite the limitation of further mycobacterial multiplication in primary and metastatic foci by the activated macrophages and memory T cells, a residual nidus of infection remains indefinitely in the lung (most frequently in the apex, where the oxygen tension is high) and less often in distant sites. Therefore, the potential for reactivation of disease in these quiescent foci exists during periods of immunosuppression.

The primary focus of pulmonary infection, called the Gohn lesion, is usually subjacent to the pleura in the lower part of the upper lobes or the upper part of the lower lobes of one lung, corresponding to areas of the lung that receive the greatest volume flow of inspired air. Lesions (tubercles) are well-circumscribed, 1–2 cm diameter areas of grayish white consolidation with soft to necrotic centers. Similar appearing tubercles typically are found in the regional tracheobronchial lymph nodes, and these plus the primary lung lesion are termed the Gohn complex. Microscopically, tubercles are composed of well circumscribed caseating or noncaseating granulomas; organisms may be seen in sections stained with an acid-fast stain. With time these lesions are replaced by hyalinized fibrous tissue and eventually calcify. The lesions of miliary tuberculosis are small (one to several millimeters in diameter), distinct, yellow-white areas of consolidation without gross caseation that histologically resemble tubercles. The ability to form granulomas depends on the immunocompetence of the host. Individuals infected with HIV, for example, may have extensive necrosis without granuloma formation, many neutrophils, microabscesses, and numerous acid-fast bacilli (AFB).

In the United States, pulmonary tuberculosis accounts for about 85% of cases of active disease. Manifestations of pulmonary disease vary. The clinical presentation may be insidious, with gradual onset of constitutional symptoms over months; catarrhal, with productive cough often attributed to a bad cold or lingering bronchitis; pneumonia or 'flu-like,' with high fever, aches and pains, and cough; hemoptoic with acute onset of blood-streaked sputum; or pleuritic. Extrapulmonary tuberculosis may be localized but more commonly involves multiple organs with or without concurrent lung infection. Multiorgan tuberculosis, historically a disease of infants and young children, currently predominates among the elderly and immunocompromised individuals, especially those infected with both HIV and *M. tuberculosis* (Chaisson, 1987; Kim, 1990).

Mycobacterium bovis

M. bovis may be transmitted from cattle to humans by drinking contaminated raw milk or by respiratory exposure to live infected cattle or their carcasses, from person to person via respiratory exposure, from humans to cattle via exposure to urine from persons with urinary tract infections due to *M. bovis*, and from cattle to cattle probably by respiratory secretions. *M. bovis* also may be transmitted to cattle from wild animal reservoirs such as the bush-tailed possum in New Zealand and possibly the badger in Switzerland and Great Britain (Grange, 1987).

Between 1900 and 1930, *M. bovis* was responsible for 6–30% of cases of tuberculosis in the United States and the UK (Karlson, 1970; Grange, 1987). Declining rates of human tuberculosis caused by *M. bovis* are due to milk pasteurization and cattle inspection programs. Since 1950, *M. bovis* has accounted for fewer than 1% of cases of human tuberculosis in North America. Most infections are extrapulmonary, involving cervical and mesenteric lymph nodes, the intestines, bones, and kidneys. Uncommonly, infection follows intravesical instillation of bacille Calmette–Guérin (BCG) for treatment of superficial bladder carcinoma (Centers for Disease Control and Prevention, 1985; Kristjansson, 1993).

Mycobacterium africanum

M. africanum, the 'African' tubercle bacillus, was first recovered from persons in west Africa (Castets, 1968). The modes of transmission, pathogenesis, and clinical manifestations of disease caused by *M. africanum* are the same as those associated with *M. tuberculosis*. Although it has been isolated primarily from individuals in Africa, the prevalence of infection with *M. africanum* worldwide is difficult to assess because it may not be correctly identified in many laboratories. Identification requires sophisticated molecular typing methods, such as spoligotyping (spacer oligotyping), that generally are available only in research or reference laboratories (Mostowy, 2004). Recently, five isolates of MTBC in California were identified as *M. africanum*, two of which were from patients who had neither lived in Africa nor had known connection with a source case from Africa (Desmond, 2004).

VII

Table 59–2 Mycobacteria infrequently recovered or infrequently causing human disease

Mycobacterium species	Associated infections
Slowly growing mycobacteria	
M. asiaticum	Pulmonary disease
M. celatum	Pulmonary disease, disseminated disease in immunocompromised persons
M. conspicuum	Disseminated disease in immunocompromised persons
M. flavescens	Pulmonary disease
M. genavense	Disseminated disease in immunocompromised persons
M. interjectum	Lymphadenitis
M. lentiflavum	Pulmonary disease, lymphadenitis
M. malmoense	Pulmonary disease
M. scrofulaceum	Pulmonary disease, disseminated disease, lymphadenitis, and rarely conjunctivitis, osteomyelitis, granulomatous hepatitis
M. shimoidei	Pulmonary disease
M. terrae complex*	Tenosynovitis, pulmonary disease
M. thermoresistabile	Pulmonary disease, cutaneous infection
M. triplex	Pulmonary disease, lymphadenitis
Rapidly growing mycobacteria	
M. goodii	Traumatic osteomyelitis, pulmonary disease
M. mageritense	Surgical wounds, pulmonary disease, catheter-related sepsis
M. neoaurum	Catheter-related infections
M. peregrinum	Post-traumatic wounds and/or osteomyelitis
M. smegmatis	Soft tissue infections following trauma or surgery
M. wolinskyii	Surgical and traumatic wounds, osteomyelitis

* Includes *M. terrae, M. nonchromogenicum, M. triviale*

'Mycobacterium canettii'

M. canettii is the smooth strain of *M. tuberculosis*. Like *M. tuberculosis*, *M. canettii* is niacin- and nitrate-positive but it grows more rapidly than *M. tuberculosis*, as colonies are typically visible on solid media in about 6 days. The first human isolate was from a cervical lymph node of a Somali child in 1993 (van Soolingen, 1997). *M. canettii* has also been isolated from an AIDS patient with mesenteric tuberculosis who was living in Switzerland at the time of diagnosis but had previously worked for many years in Africa (Pfyffer, 1998).

Nontuberculous Mycobacteria

In general, little is known about the antigens associated with the virulence of the NTM; however, such antigens presumably are responsible for persistence of the organisms within the monocyte–macrophage system of the host. The immune response to infection with these mycobacteria also is poorly understood. With current molecular techniques, over 100 species of mycobacteria have been identified. Select potential pathogens are reviewed in the following sections. Some of the infrequently encountered mycobacteria and the infections with which they have been associated are listed in Table 59–2 (DeChairo, 1973; Cianciulli, 1974; Schroder, 1977; Edwards, 1978; Weitzman, 1981; Casimir, 1982; Blacklock, 1983; Tsukamura, 1983; Davison, 1988; Wallace, 1988; Neeley, 1989; Coyle, 1992; Wald, 1992; Henriques, 1993; Butler, 1994; Maschek, 1994; Smith, 2000; Piersimoni, 2004). A more extensive description of the more recently described and infrequently isolated mycobacteria is found in the excellent review by Tortoli (2003). *Mycobacterium gordonae*, the 'tap water bacillus,' is a common laboratory contaminant and rarely causes disease in humans (Weinberger, 1992).

Mycobacterium avium Complex

M. avium and *Mycobacterium intracellulare* have such similar growth characteristics and biochemical reactions that they often are not distinguished in the clinical microbiology laboratory; isolates of both species are reported as MAC. MAC bacilli are ubiquitous in the environment. They have been isolated from water, soil, food, house dust, and several animals, but the specific environmental sources responsible for human infection are not known (Inderlied, 1993; Falkinham, 1996). The most likely portal of entry is the gastrointestinal tract but transmission via the respiratory tract is also possible. From sites of colonization, organisms enter the blood and infect many organs, especially those of the monocyte–macrophage system. Prior to the epidemic of the acquired immunodeficiency syndrome (AIDS), MAC was the second most frequently isolated mycobacteria in the United States, following *M. tuberculosis*. The percentage of isolates of MAC then increased, equaling or even surpassing the number of isolates of *M. tuberculosis* in some parts of the country.

For many years, pulmonary disease caused by MAC occurred most frequently in elderly white men who had underlying chronic lung disease or who had undergone gastrectomy; but since the mid- to late 1980s, it has become more common in persons without predisposing factors, especially older women (Prince, 1989; Dhillon, 2000). Disseminated MAC occurs almost exclusively in immunosuppressed individuals, especially persons with advanced AIDS. In the United States, MAC was the most common cause of systemic bacterial infection in patients with AIDS in the late 1980s and early 1990s (Horsburg, 1991a). The numbers of such cases, however, decreased since the widespread availability of highly active antiretroviral therapy (Centers for Disease Control and Prevention, 1999). The major risk factor for disseminated MAC in AIDS patients is the degree of immune dysfunction, indicated by the CD4+ lymphocyte count, as the disease is rare in individuals whose CD4+ lymphocyte count is over 50/μL.

Manifestations of disease caused by MAC depend on the site and the extent of infection. Pulmonary infection may be asymptomatic or it may present as bronchiectasis or mimic tuberculosis. Disseminated disease in persons without AIDS is manifested by fever, weight loss, bone pain, lymphadenopathy, hepatosplenomegaly, and skin lesions. In those with AIDS, persistent fever, weight loss, and diarrhea are most common; anorexia, weakness, lymphadenopathy, or hepatomegaly also may occur (Inderlied, 1993). Significant laboratory abnormalities are anemia and elevated alkaline phosphatase. Cervical lymphadenitis caused by MAC most often affects children but also occurs in adults. Other manifestations of infection with MAC are synovitis, genitourinary tract disease, cutaneous lesions, deep infection of the hand, osteomyelitis, meningitis, ulcers of the colon, and pericarditis (Wolinsky, 1979; Woods, 1987; Inderlied, 1993).

The histologic findings of lesions caused by MAC vary. Caseating granulomas with AFB, indistinguishable from tuberculosis; pulmonary interstitial fibrosis with organizing pneumonia; necrotizing granulomatous vasculitis resembling Wegener's granulomatosis; and, especially in persons with AIDS, aggregates of foamy macrophages containing many intracellular AFB may be seen.

Mycobacterium kansasii

M. kansasii, first described as the 'yellow bacillus,' accounted for 3% of mycobacterial isolates in the United States in 1979 and 1980; the highest numbers were reported from California, Texas, Louisiana, Illinois, and Florida (Buhler, 1953; Good, 1982). The natural reservoir of *M. kansasii* is unknown; however, it has been recovered from water samples (Falkinham, 1996). Pulmonary disease is most common in males 50–60 years of age living in urban areas, among certain occupational groups (miners, welders, sandblasters, and painters), and among individuals with pneumoconioses and chronic obstructive pulmonary disease. Disseminated disease generally affects persons with impaired cellular immunity.

The most common manifestation of disease caused by *M. kansasii* is chronic cavitary pulmonary lesions, usually involving the upper lobes. Extrapulmonary manifestations include cervical lymphadenitis in children, cutaneous disease, musculoskeletal involvement (carpal tunnel syndrome, synovitis, arthritis, tendinitis and fasciitis, or osteomyelitis), disseminated disease, isolated genitourinary tract disease, and pericarditis.

The histologic findings of lesions caused by *M. kansasii* vary and include caseating or noncaseating granulomas and, especially in skin lesions, necrosis or foci of acute and chronic inflammation without well-formed granulomas. AFB are common in lung and lymph node tissue but are seen less frequently in tissue from other sites.

Mycobacterium xenopi

M. xenopi was first isolated from a toad in 1957 and was recognized as a human pathogen in 1965 (Costrini, 1981). It has been cultured from hot- and cold-water taps, hospital hot-water generators and storage tanks, and other environmental sources. In Great Britain, *M. xenopi* is found more often in coastal than inland areas, and birds are a possible natural reservoir. Most pulmonary infections caused by *M. xenopi* have been reported from Europe and Great Britain; it is an uncommon cause of mycobacterial disease in the United States. Disease has occurred only in adults, more frequently in males than females. Most persons have pre-existing lung damage or another predisposing condition, such as an extrapulmonary malignancy, alcoholism, diabetes mellitus, or immuno-suppressive therapy. Pulmonary disease may be chronic, subacute, or acute; symptoms are indistinguishable from those associated with disease caused by *M. kansasii*. Focal extrapulmonary infections (osteomyelitis, arthritis, lymphadenitis) and disseminated disease are uncommon, but the latter has been reported in persons with AIDS (Tecson-Tumang, 1984).

Mycobacterium simiae

M. simiae was first isolated from monkeys from India in 1965 (Karassova, 1965). The organism is found in monkeys and has been recovered from tap water in hospitals. An infrequent human pathogen, *M. simiae* has been associated with chronic pulmonary disease, osteomyelitis, and disseminated disease.

Mycobacterium marinum

M. marinum was recognized as a human pathogen in 1951 (Norden, 1951). Human infection is typically acquired via trauma to the skin during contact with contaminated nonchlorinated fresh or salt water, but it may be acquired via trauma unassociated with water contact or contact with water in the absence of preceding trauma. A single papulonodular lesion usually appears 2–3 weeks after inoculation, most commonly on the elbow, knee, foot, toe, or finger, and often becomes verrucous or ulcerated. Occasionally, an abscess forms at the site of inoculation, and several secondary nodules develop and progress centrally along the lymphatics, resembling sporotrichosis (see Ch. 60). In immunocompromised persons, cutaneous lesions may become disseminated. Extracutaneous mani-festations are uncommon: synovitis, osteomyelitis, and ocular and laryngeal lesions have been reported (Woods, 1987).

The histology of skin lesions varies with the stage of infection. Early on, neutrophil aggregates are surrounded by histiocytes. Later, lymphocytes, epithelioid histiocytes, occasional Langhans giant cells, and foci of fibrinoid necrosis are seen. In lesions present for over 6 months, aggregates of lymphocytes are found in the dermis. Stains for AFB are usually negative but organisms may be seen within histiocytes.

Mycobacterium haemophilum

M. haemophilum first was described in 1978, but very probably was the nonculturable AFB recognized in skin ulcers in 1972 and 1974 (Lomwardias, 1972; Feldman, 1974; Sompolinsky, 1978). The organism is unique among the mycobacteria in its growth requirement for hemoglobin or hemin. Human infections caused by *M. haemophilum* are uncommon, usually seen in persons who have an underlying immunodeficiency such as lymphoma, exogenous immunosuppression after organ transplantation, or AIDS, but a few cases of lymphadenitis in otherwise healthy children have been reported (Centers for Disease Control and Prevention, 1991). Disease most commonly is manifested by multiple cutaneous nodules, ulcers, or painful swellings, typically involving the extremities, that occasionally become abscesses and open fistulas draining purulent material. Micro-scopically, lesions show foci of necrosis without caseation surrounded by a polymorphous inflammatory infiltrate with occasional Langhans giant cells in the lower dermis. AFB are seen singly or in small clusters, often within cells.

Mycobacterium ulcerans

M. ulcerans is endemic in areas of Zaire, Uganda, Nigeria, Ghana, Cameroon, Malaysia, New Guinea, Guyana, Mexico, and Australia located between latitudes 25° N and 38° S. In all endemic areas disease is slightly more common in males. The natural reservoir of *M. ulcerans* and the usual route of its transmission to humans are unknown.

Eponyms for disease caused by *M. ulcerans* are Bairnsdale ulcer, for the area in Australia where it was first recognized, and Buruli ulcer or Buruli disease after the area of Uganda reporting the most cases. The disease begins as one or, rarely, multiple painless boils or subcutaneous lumps on an exposed area, most often the leg, that possibly was a site of previous trauma. After several weeks the lump ulcerates, and satellite nodules and ulcers may appear. Lymph nodes typically are not enlarged, and affected individuals are afebrile and without systemic symptoms unless lesions become secondarily infected with bacteria.

Table 59–3 Infections caused by the more commonly encountered rapidly growing mycobacteria

Infection	*Mycobacterium* species	Risk factors
Skin/soft tissue	M. fortuitum, M. chelonae, M. abscessus, M. mucogenicum, M. immunogenum	Trauma, surgery, use of whirlpool footbaths in nail salons (M. fortuitum)
Osteomyelitis	M. fortuitum	Trauma, surgery
Pneumonia	M. abscessus, M. fortuitum (rare)	Cystic fibrosis, bronchiectasis, chronic vomiting
Hypersensitivity pneumonitis	M. immunogenum, M. chelonae	Employment in metal-working industries and exposure to aerosolized oil
Disseminated disease	M. chelonae, M. abscessus	Steroids, organ transplant, collagen vascular disease, chronic renal failure, impaired cell-mediated immunity, leukemia, lymphoma
Prosthetic valve endocarditis	M. chelonae	Contaminated valve
Corneal infections	M. chelonae, M. fortuitum, M. immunogenum	Trauma
Catheter-related infections	All 5 species	Indwelling catheter, immunosuppression

Rapidly Growing Mycobacteria

The most commonly encountered rapidly growing mycobacteria are *Mycobacterium abscessus*, *Mycobacterium chelonae*, and the *Mycobacterium fortuitum* group; *Mycobacterium mucogenicum* and *Mycobacterium immunogenum* are recovered from clinical specimens less often. Infections caused by these rapidly growing mycobacteria are shown in Table 59–3. Infrequently isolated rapidly growing mycobacteria and the infections with which they have been associated are listed in Table 59–2. Rapidly growing mycobacteria have been cultured from soil, freshwater lakes and rivers, seawater, waste water from hospitals, drinking water, raw milk, and dust. Skin and soft tissue infections due to rapidly growing mycobacteria typically follow a penetrating injury (trauma or surgical procedure) with possible soil or water contamination. Outbreaks have been associated with administration of diphtheria–pertussis–tetanus–polio vaccines, histamine injections, lidocaine administration using a jet injector, contaminated hemodialyzers, placement of contaminated porcine heterograft valves, use of foot baths in nail salons, and liposuction (Wallace, 1983; Brown-Elliott, 2002).

Primary cutaneous disease caused by rapidly growing mycobacteria is manifested by localized cellulitis, draining abscesses, or minimally tender nodules. Lesions typically develop 3 weeks to 12 months (most often 4–6 weeks) after a penetrating injury in persons with an intact immune system. Osteomyelitis is an occasional complication, especially following puncture wounds to the feet. Postoperative infections are characterized by a nonhealing wound or breakdown of a healed wound with serous drainage in a person with minimal systemic symptoms. They generally develop 3 weeks to 3 months after the procedure, especially median sternotomy, augmentation mammaplasty, or insertion of a percutaneous catheter. Disseminated disease, which typically occurs in immunocompromised (especially due to corticosteroid therapy) adults, is manifested by multiple, recurrent skin and soft tissue abscesses; no primary source of infection is evident. Chronic pulmonary disease is most often seen in patients with underlying cystic fibrosis or bronchiectasis, is usually caused by *M. abscessus*, and typically resembles disease due to *M. kansasii* or MAC, except that cavitation is uncommon. Endocarditis involving a prosthetic valve usually becomes manifest 4–12 weeks after surgery. Rarely, rapidly growing mycobacteria cause keratitis and corneal ulceration after trauma, or cervical lymphadenitis. A more thorough description of disease caused by rapidly growing mycobacteria is found in the excellent review by Brown-Elliott and Wallace (Brown-Elliott, 2002).

Lesions caused by rapidly growing mycobacteria are characterized histologically by necrosis with minimal caseation and a mixed inflam-matory infiltrate composed of neutrophils and granulomas with foreign body or Langhans giant cells; lipid-laden macrophages are seen occasionally. Clumps of extracellular AFB are found within aggregates of neutrophils in less than a third of cases. In lung tissue, foamy macrophages are frequent, a pattern resembling lipoid pneumonia.

VII

Mycobacterium leprae

Mycobacterium leprae is the etiologic agent of leprosy (also called Hansen's disease). Although it does not belong to the MTBC and, therefore, could be considered a 'nontuberculous mycobacteria,' it is discussed separately because it is unique among the mycobacteria by virtue of the fact that it has not been cultivated. Useful animal models of infection are the mouse foot pad model and the nine-banded armadillo.

M. leprae has been recognized in nearly every part of the world at some time. An estimated 10–15 million persons in the world have leprosy; approximately 62% are in Asia and 34% are in Africa (Binford, 1982). About 6000 persons in the United States have leprosy; most are immigrants, but some cases develop in persons indigenous to the Gulf Coast states, California, and Hawaii (Neill, 1985).

Leprosy predominantly affects humans but is also a natural infection of wild armadillos in Louisiana and Texas, and spontaneous cases have been described in mangabey monkeys (Hastings, 1988). The mechanism of transmission of *M. leprae* is unknown, but person-to-person spread via aerosolization of organisms from the nose of a person with active lepromatous disease (see below), which then contacts the nasal mucosa of another individual, is the favored theory. Transmission also may occur through intact skin or via penetrating wounds, such as thorns or the bite of an arthropod. Breast milk from lactating women with lepromatous disease contains bacilli that may be transmitted to infants, and transplacental transmission of *M. leprae* is possible. Cases of human leprosy following contact with armadillos have been reported (Lumpkin, 1983). Moreover, the discovery of a naturally occurring leprosy-like disease among armadillos and the fact that sporadic cases of leprosy occur in persons who have no known contact with human leprosy suggest that nonhuman sources of *M. leprae* may exist (Blake, 1987).

Most persons effectively resist infection with *M. leprae*. Resistance depends on an effective cell-mediated immune response to *M. leprae* antigens, as occurs in tuberculoid leprosy. In persons who lack specific cell-mediated immunity to these antigens, bacilli multiply within macrophages, eventually resulting in widely disseminated lepromatous leprosy. The defect in cellular immunity, which may involve T-lymphocyte function or their interaction with macrophages, is apparently specific for antigens to *M. leprae* rather than a generalized defect.

The lesions of leprosy develop after a 2–5-year incubation period, varying in appearance depending on the host's immune response. Leprosy always involves peripheral nerves, almost always involves the skin, and frequently involves mucous membranes. The three cardinal signs of the disease are skin lesions, areas of cutaneous anesthesia, and enlarged peripheral nerves.

The system outlined by Ridley and Jopling (presented below) is used most commonly to classify the spectrum of clinical and histopathologic forms of leprosy (Ridley, 1964). Indeterminate leprosy, the earliest sign of disease, is characterized by one or a few hypopigmented skin macules with minimal local sensory loss. In about 75% of cases the disease heals spontaneously; in the rest it progresses, often after a prolonged period.

The polar types of leprosy – lepromatous leprosy, the widespread anergic form of the disease, and tuberculoid leprosy, the localized form – are stable clinically. Lepromatous leprosy is characterized by cutaneous lesions ranging from diffuse generalized skin involvement to widespread, symmetrically distributed nodules (called lepromas) filled with organisms. Lesions generally involve the cooler parts of the body surface – the anterior third of the eye, the nasal mucosa, and the superficial peripheral nerve trunks. In advanced disease, lesions are accompanied by sensory loss from involvement of dermal nerve fibers. Microscopically, lesions show foamy histiocytes containing many AFB; few or no lymphocytes; minimal intraneural inflammation; and many AFB in nerves, the perineurium, blood vessel walls, and arrector muscles. In tuberculoid leprosy, one or a few well circumscribed anesthetic macules or plaques develop, often accompanied by an enlarged peripheral nerve near the skin lesions. Histologically, lesions demonstrate noncaseating granulomas in the nerves and dermis, extending to involve the basal layer of the epidermis; there are few, if any, AFB. Borderline leprosy, a clinically unstable condition, encompasses the types of disease between the polar forms. It may develop features more closely resembling tuberculoid disease, a process termed upgrading; or features more like lepromatous disease, called downgrading.

Skin Testing

The tuberculin skin test is useful for identifying persons infected with MTBC but it does not differentiate active disease from infection. Persons infected with MTBC develop a hypersensitivity reaction to proteins of the bacilli, which comprise the skin test reagent – purified protein derivative (PPD). The preferred method of skin testing is the Mantoux test, performed by intracutaneous injection of 0.1 mL of intermediate-strength (5 tuberculin units) PPD-S. The reaction is interpreted after 48–72 hours by measuring the diameter of induration in millimeters (Huebner, 1993). Induration of 5 mm or more is a positive result in persons infected with HIV, those who have had recent close contact with someone who has infectious tuberculosis, and those who have chest X-ray findings consistent with old healed tuberculosis. A reaction of 10 mm or more is positive in persons who do not meet the above criteria but who have other risk factors for tuberculosis. Included in this group are foreign-born persons from countries where the prevalence of tuberculosis is high (such as Asia, Africa, or Latin America); injection drug users; medically underserved, low-income populations, especially racial or ethnic minorities; residents of long-term care facilities; and persons who have a medical condition associated with an increased risk of tuberculosis (e.g., silicosis, gastrectomy, jejunoileal bypass, 10% or more below ideal body weight, chronic renal failure, diabetes mellitus, treatment with high-dose corticosteroids or with other immunosuppressive drugs, and malignancies). A reaction of 15 mm or more is positive in all other persons. Interpretation is difficult in person immunized with BCG.

False-positive PPD reactions result from infection with nontuberculous mycobacteria. False-negative reactions may be due to poor technique or improper storage of the reagent. If the test is administered appropriately, false-negative reactions are uncommon in relatively healthy people but occur in up to 20% of individuals with known tuberculosis when they are first tested. Most of these false-negative reactions are attributed to the general illness and revert to positive after 2–3 weeks of therapy when health is restored. Factors causing a state of general anergy, such as protein malnutrition, concurrent viral infection, sarcoidosis, malignancy (especially lymphoma), immunosuppressive or corticosteroid therapy, and infection with HIV, also may cause a false-negative tuberculin reaction.

The Mantoux test generally remains positive as long as viable bacilli persist in quiescent foci. However, the reaction may wane below positive with increasing age, a phenomenon that occurs most frequently in those over age 55 years. In these individuals the reaction will be boosted (or become positive) if retesting is performed as early as 1 week after the first test, a reaction termed the booster effect.

Skin test reagents prepared from nontuberculous mycobacteria include PPD-A (*M. avium*), PPD-B (*M. intracellulare*), PPD-F (*M. fortuitum*), PPD-G (*Mycobacterium scrofulaceum*), and PPD-Y (*M. kansasii*). In the United States, these reagents were once available from the CDC; however, this service was discontinued because antigens were not standardized and the skin reactions were difficult to interpret.

Laboratory Diagnosis

Specimens

Specimens recommended for diagnosis of mycobacterial infections are listed in Table 59–4. Samples from contaminated sites such as sputum and other respiratory secretions, gastric secretions, urine, and feces must be decontaminated prior to inoculation of media to prevent the normal flora from overgrowing and thus masking the presence of mycobacteria, which grow more slowly. Concentrating the specimen after decontamination increases the sensitivity of smear and culture. Specimens from normally sterile body sites such as blood, cerebrospinal fluid (CSF), pleural and peritoneal fluid, and tissues may be inoculated directly without decontamination.

Processing and inoculation of specimens for mycobacterial culture should be performed in a biological safety cabinet. The *N*-acetyl-l-cysteine (NALC)-sodium hydroxide procedure (Fig. 59–1) is the most common method used in the clinical laboratory to liquify, decontaminate, and concentrate specimens for detection of mycobacteria. Potentially contaminated specimens should be refrigerated if they cannot be processed immediately. Before proceeding to the steps outlined in Figure 59–1, additional handling is necessary for some specimens. Gastric lavage specimens should be processed immediately but, if a delay cannot be avoided, 10% sodium hydroxide should be added until the pH of the sample (measured with pH paper) is neutral. If more than 10 mL of gastric secretions is collected, the sample is centrifuged at 3000 to 3600 *g* for 20 to 30 minutes, the supernatant is decanted, and the sediment is processed as shown in Figure 59–1. For feces, 1 to 2 g of a formed sample or 5 mL of a liquid specimen is placed in a 50-mL centrifuge tube, and sterile filtered distilled water is added to give a volume of 10 mL. The suspension is agitated on a vortex mixer, filtered through gauze, and then processed as

Table 59–4 Mycobacterial diseases and specimens for diagnosis

Disease	Common Mycobacterium Species	Specimens
Pneumonia	*M. tuberculosis, M. kansasii, M. avium* complex, *M. abscessus*	Sputum (early morning, deep cough, on 3 consecutive days), BAL fluid, lung tissue, pleural fluid, gastric contents
Disseminated	*M. tuberculosis, M. avium* complex	Blood, bone marrow, involved tissue
Lymphadenitis	*M. tuberculosis, M. avium* complex	Lymph node aspirate or biopsy
Skin, soft tissue	*M. fortuitum, M. abscessus, M. chelonae, M. marinum, M. haemophilum M. leprae*	Aspirate or biopsy of lesion Smears of nasal secretions and skin slits, biopsy of lesion
Musculoskeletal	*M. tuberculosis, M. fortuitum, M. marinum, M. kansasii*	Joint fluid, synovium, bone
Meningitis	*M. tuberculosis*	Cerebrospinal fluid
Brain abscess	*M. tuberculosis*	Abscess material
Genitourinary	*M. tuberculosis, M. bovis* BCG	Urine (early morning), involved tissue – kidney, bladder (*M. bovis* BCG), endometrium, fallopian tube, prostate, seminal vesicles, epididymis
Gastrointestinal	*M. tuberculosis, M. bovis, M. avium* complex	Tissue, feces
Peritonitis	*M. tuberculosis*	Peritoneal biopsy, peritoneal fluid
Hepatitis	*M. tuberculosis, M. avium* complex,	Liver tissue
Pericarditis	*M. tuberculosis*	Pericardium, pericardial tissue
Catheter-related infections	Rapidly growing mycobacteria	Blood

BAL = bronchoalveolar lavage; BCG = bacille Calmette–Guérin.

Source: modified with permission from Woods GL: Mycobacteria. In Woods GL, Gutierrez Y (eds): Diagnostic Pathology of Infectious Diseases. Philadelphia, PA, Lea & Febiger, 1993, p 378.

Transfer 10 mL (maximum) of sputum, urine, or other fluid specimen to sterile, disposable plastic 50-mL conical centrifuge tube

↓

Add equal volume of NALC–2% NaOH (prepared fresh each day of use) and tighten cap

↓

Mix on vortex mixer, 15 to 30 seconds

↓

Let mixture stand at room temperature for 15 minutes (45 minutes for stool specimens)

↓

Add 30 mL of phosphate buffer (pH 6.8); cap tubes and invert to mix

↓

Centrifuge at 3000 to 3600 x *g* for 15 minutes (or 2500 x *g* for 20 minutes)

↓

Decant supernatant; resuspend sediment in 1.5 to 2 mL of sterile water of buffer

↓   ↓

Prepare smear for staining   Inoculate media

Figure 59–1 Protocol for decontamination, using 2% sodium hydroxide *N*-acetyl-L-cysteine, and concentration of specimens for detection of mycobacteria by smear and culture.

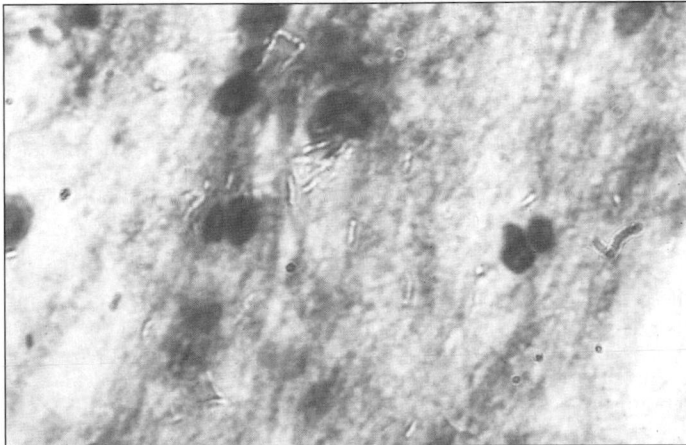

Figure 59–2 Smear of a sputum specimen stained with Gram's stain shows 'ghost cells' (mycobacterial culture grew *Mycobacterium tuberculosis*: Gram's stain, ×400).

Microbial Stains

In smears stained with the Gram stain, most mycobacteria appear as slender, poorly stained, beaded Gram-positive bacilli, but sometimes the bacilli do not take up the crystal violet or safranin and appear 'Gram-neutral' or as 'Gram-ghosts' (Fig. 59–2). Similar ghost images of bacilli may be found in macrophages in smears stained with the Wright or Papanicolaou stain. In general, specimens (except blood) collected from persons with suspected mycobacterial infection should be examined microscopically for organisms. However, to improve cost efficiency, many laboratories do not prepare smears of specimens in which AFB rarely are seen, such as CSF, urine, and bone marrow. To prepare a smear, two to three drops of the concentrated sediment are spread uniformly on a microscope slide, which then is fixed at 80°C for 15 minutes or for 1–2 hours at 65° to 70°C on an electric hot plate.

Two types of stain detect AFB: carbol fuchsin (the classic Ziehl–Neelsen stain, which requires heating, and the cold Kinyoun stain) and the preferred fluorochrome stains (auramine–rhodamine and auramine-O), which are more sensitive. Smears stained with a carbol fuchsin stain are examined at 800–1000× magnification (oil immersion). Smears stained with a fluorochrome stain are examined at lower magnifications (250× and 400×), which allows visualization of more fields in less time. Cells of some rapidly growing mycobacteria stain poorly with fluorochromic stains and may not be detected; therefore, when the latter organisms are suspected pathogens (e.g., in postsurgical wound infections), restaining

outlined. Urine specimens are divided into two to four 50-mL centrifuge tubes and centrifuged at 3000 to 3600 *g* for 30 minutes. The supernatant is decanted, leaving about 2 mL of sediment in each tube. Tubes are mixed on a vortex mixer, sediments are combined and, if necessary, distilled water is added to give a volume of 10 mL, which then is decontaminated as shown in Figure 59–1.

Table 59–5 Guidelines for Reporting Smears for Acid-Fast Bacilli

No. of AFB with Carbol Fuchsin Stain (1000×)	No. of AFB with Fluorochrome Stain (450×)	Report
0	0	No AFB seen
1–2/300 F (3 sweeps)	1–2/70 F (1½ sweeps)	Doubtful; repeat
1–9/100 F	2–18/50 F (1 sweep)	1+
1–9/10 F	4–36/10 F	2+
1–9/F	4–36/F	3+
>9/F	>36/F	4+

AFB = acid-fast bacilli; F = field; sweep = scanning full length of a smear.

Source: modified with permission from Kent PT, Kubica GP: Public Health Mycobacteriology: A Guide for the Level III Laboratory. Atlanta, GA, Department of Health and Human Services, 1985.

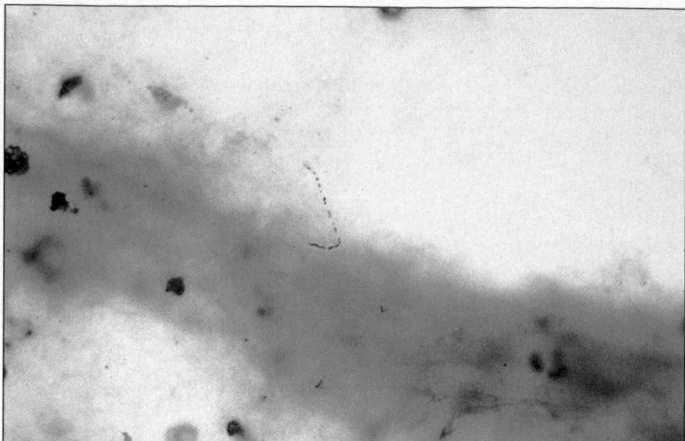

Figure 59–4 Smear of an aspirate from an enlarged cervical lymph node shows a large, crossbarred acid-fast bacillus (*Mycobacterium kansasii*; Kinyoun, ×400). (Courtesy of Vick J. Schnadig, M.D., Department of Pathology, University of Texas Medical Branch, Galveston, TX.)

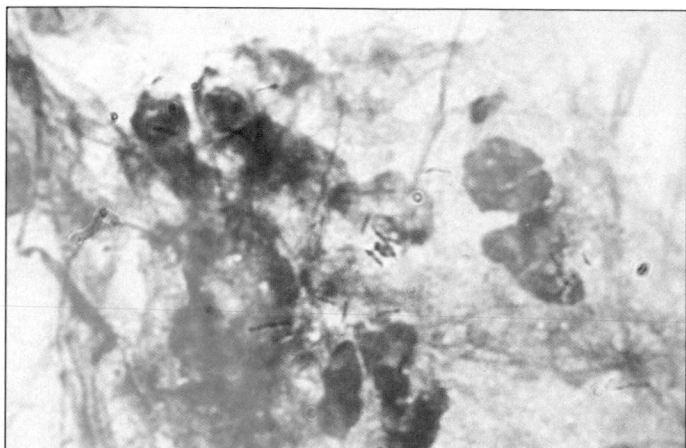

Figure 59–3 Smear of a sputum specimen shows acid-fast bacilli (*Mycobacterium tuberculosis*; Kinyoun, ×400).

negative fluorescent smears with a carbol fuchsin stain is reasonable. Results are reported after viewing 100 fields and should include a statement indicating whether the smear was prepared directly from the specimen or after decontamination and concentration. Guidelines for reporting results of smears stained for AFB are shown in Table 59–5 (Kent, 1985).

In smears stained with carbol fuchsin, AFB typically appear as purple to red, slightly curved rods (1–10 μm long and 0.2–0.6 μm wide), which often are beaded or banded (Fig. 59–3) but may also appear coccoid or filamentous. In general, the appearance of AFB does not provide a species identification; however, cells of certain species have features that may be useful diagnostically. The formation of 'cords' in smears of broth cultures is typical (but not diagnostic) of *M. tuberculosis*. Cells of *M. kansasii* often appear as crossbarred bacilli (Fig. 59–4), larger than *M. tuberculosis* and resembling a 'shepherd's crook.' Cells of MAC are typically pleomorphic, occasionally coccobacillary, and stain positively with the periodic-acid–Schiff (PAS) stain. Cells of *M. marinum* are typically longer and broader than those of *M. tuberculosis* and often show cross-banding. Cells of *M. leprae* stain weaker than most other mycobacteria.

The specificity of stains for AFB typically is 99% or more, and the sensitivity about 25% to about 75% (Strumpf, 1979; Murray, 1980; Rickman, 1980). False-positive results (positive stain, negative culture) may be caused by nonviable organisms, such as might occur in patients receiving antituberculosis therapy; prolonged decontamination, killing mycobacteria as well as contaminating bacteria; or crosscontamination during the staining procedure. Factors that influence the sensitivity of smear results include: (1) patient population (persons with cavitary lesions are more likely than those without cavities to have a smear-positive sputum), (2) specimen type (respiratory specimens are more likely than other specimen types to be positive), (3) the number of specimens examined, (4) number of AFB present in the sample (5000–10 000 organisms/mL of specimen are needed for a positive result), (5) the species present (specimens containing *M. tuberculosis* or *M. kansasii* are more likely to be positive than are those that contain other mycobacteria), (6) observer experience, and (7) stain used. Fluorochromic stains are more

sensitive and easier to read than carbol fuchsin stains and are recommended by experts at the CDC (Tenover, 1993). The CDC also suggests that for respiratory specimens, results of stained smears be reported within 24 hours of specimen receipt, which means processing seven days a week.

Culture Methods

For optimal recovery of mycobacteria from clinical specimens, experts at the CDC recommend that both a broth and a solid medium should be inoculated and that the culture system used should detect mycobacterial growth within a mean of 14 days (Tenover, 1993). In general, broth is more sensitive than solid media and provides more rapid detection of mycobacterial growth (Stager, 1991; Anargyros, 1990; Abe, 1992). Broth systems currently available are the BACTEC 460TB radiometric system (BD Biosciences), SEPTI-CHEK AFB (BD Biosciences), BBL Mycobacteria Growth Indicator Tubes (MGIT; BD Biosciences), the ESP Culture System II (Trek Diagnostic Systems), and BacT/Alert MB (Organon Teknika).

Two types of solid medium are used for mycobacterial culture: egg-based (Löwenstein–Jensen) and agar-based (Middlebrook 7H10, 7H11, and selective 7H11). These media are available in screw-cap tubes and flasks; agar-based media also are available in Petri dishes. Flasks are preferred to screw-cap tubes for safety reasons and because they provide a larger surface area for mycobacterial growth. Specimens from cutaneous lesions should be inoculated to one egg- or agar-based medium, and to ensure recovery of *M. haemophilum* (see below) they also should be plated on chocolate agar, 5% sheep blood Columbia agar, Mueller–Hinton agar with Fildes supplement, or Löwenstein–Jensen containing 2% ferric ammonium citrate. To recover *Mycobacterium genavense* (from specimens or subcultures of liquid to solid media), solid media must be supplemented with mycobactin J. All cultures should be incubated at 37°C in an atmosphere of 5–10% CO_2, and tubed media should be incubated in a slanted position with caps loose for at least 1 week to ensure even distribution of the inoculum over the surface. For specimens from cutaneous sites, a second set of cultures should be inoculated and incubated at 30°C, because some mycobacteria that cause skin lesions – *M. marinum*, *M. haemophilum*, *M. chelonae*, and *M. ulcerans* – grow optimally at the lower temperature. All cultures should be examined weekly for at least 6 weeks.

The major advantage of culture on solid media is that it allows visualization of colony morphology and pigmentation, which is useful diagnostically, especially for distinguishing colonies of *M. tuberculosis* from those of some NTM. The colony appearance and growth characteristics of the commonly encountered mycobacteria are outlined in Table 59–6. Disadvantages of conventional solid media are prolonged time to growth of mycobacteria (colonies often are not visible on tubed solid media for 3–4 weeks or more) and low sensitivity. Inoculation of Middlebrook agar plates, which then are examined under the microscope, allows more rapid detection of colonies (Welch, 1993), but this procedure is labor-intensive, thus prohibiting its use in many clinical laboratories.

The semiautomated radiometric BACTEC TB460 system uses broth media (one for blood [13A] and another for all other specimen types [12B]) that contain ^{14}C-labeled palmitic acid substrate. Each specimen is inoculated into one vial, and an antibiotic mixture is added to specimens other than blood. Vials are incubated in ambient air at 37°C for 5–6 weeks. To ensure recovery of *M. genavense*, blood cultures (especially those

Table 59–6 Colony Morphology and Growth Characteristics of Mycobacteria Commonly Isolated in the Clinical Laboratory

Mycobacterium Species	Colony Morphology	Pigment	Growth Rate (weeks)	Comments
Slowly growing mycobacteria				
M. tuberculosis	Rough	N (buff)	3–6	Generally niacin and nitrate positive
M. bovis	Rough; thin or transparent on LJ	N (colorless to buff)	4–6	Generally niacin & nitrate negative; resistant to PZA
M. avium complex	Smooth; small, thin, transparent or large, opaque, domed; ± rough	N	3–6	Colonies of some isolates become lightly pigmented with prolonged incubation; grows at 42°C
M. kansasii	Rough, ± smooth, β-carotene crystals	P	3–6	Rare strains are N or S
M. gordonae	Smooth	S	3–6	Common laboratory contaminant; rare strains are N
M. marinum	Wrinkled, shiny; smooth, hemispherical; (rarely) rough, dry	P	2	Optimal growth, 30–33°C
M. xenopi	Smooth, filamentous extensions ('bird's nest')	S	3–6	Growth at 42°C
M. simiae	Smooth	P (±N)	3–6	Pigment production often requires prolonged exposure to light
M. haemophilum	Rough, ± smooth	N	3–6	Optimal growth, 20–32°C; requires hemin for growth
M. malmoense	Smooth, dysgonic	Colorless	2–3	
M. terrae complex	Smooth (M. terrae), rough (M. triviale), intermediate (M. nonchromogenicum)	N	3–6	
M. scrofulaceum	Smooth, globoid	S	2–3	
M. szulgai	Smooth or rough	S, 37°C; P, 25°C	3–6	
Rapidly growing mycobacteria				
M. abscessus	Smooth; ± rough, wrinkled	N	<1	
M. fortuitum group	Wrinkled	N	<1	Branching filaments often are present on periphery of colonies
M. chelonae	Smooth	N	<1	
M. mucogenicum	Smooth, usually mucoid	N	<1	

N = nonchromogenic, P = photochromogenic, S = scotochromogenic, PZA = pyrazinamide.

collected from patients with AIDS) should be incubated for 8–10 weeks. Bacilli multiply in the broth and utilize the labeled substrate, releasing $^{14}CO_2$ into the head space above the broth. Bottles are manually loaded onto the BACTEC TB460, which measures the amount of $^{14}CO_2$ and calculates a growth index (GI). A GI greater than 10 suggests that mycobacteria are present, and when the GI reaches 50–100, a smear of the broth is stained for AFB. Vials containing AFB are subcultured to a solid medium, and direct tests for identification (discussed in the following section) may be performed. For positive mycobacterial blood cultures from patients with AIDS, subculture to Middlebrook 7H11 agar containing mycobactin J should be done to allow recovery of *M. genavense* if initial subcultures from the broth show no growth, or the positive broth should be sent to a reference laboratory prepared to do the appropriate tests.

SEPTI-CHEK AFB is a biphasic mycobacterial culture system that consists of a broth medium and agar media on an enclosed paddle, similar to the biphasic blood culture system described in Chapter 63. The broth is inoculated with the specimen, the paddle is attached to the top of the bottle, and the system is inverted to allow the broth to flow over the agar media. The system is incubated 6–8 weeks at 35–37°C in 5–7% CO_2, and at regular intervals the broth is subcultured to the solid medium on the paddle by inverting the system. The sensitivity of this system is similar to that of the BACTEC TB460 (D'Amato, 1991; Isenberg, 1991; Abe, 1992). Time to detection of growth, however, is longer than with the BACTEC TB460, although more rapid than conventional solid media.

The MGIT consists of 4 mL of modified 7H9 broth and a fluorescent indicator embedded in silicone in the bottom of a 16×100 mm glass tube. Tubes are inoculated with the specimen, an antibiotic mixture to inhibit growth of contaminating bacteria and a mycobacterial growth enrichment are added, and the tubes are capped and incubated at 37°C for up to 8 weeks. To detect mycobacterial growth, tubes are manually placed on top of a 365 nm UV transilluminator or in front of a Wood's lamp. The appearance of strong fluorescence in the sensor (a bright orange color on the bottom of the tube and meniscus) indicates growth. Alternatively, tubes may be incubated in the totally automated BACTEC 960 instrument, which continuously monitors tubes for fluorescence and signals those that are positive. MGIT is as sensitive as the BACTEC TB460 for recovery of

mycobacteria but the mean time to detection of growth is a few days longer with MGIT (Cornfield, 1997; Pfyffer, 1997b; Hanna, 1999).

In addition to the BACTEC MGIT 960, three other fully automated continuously monitoring systems for growth and detection of mycobacteria are commercially available: the BACTEC 9000MB system (BD Biosciences) (Pfyffer, 1997a; Zanetti, 1997), the MB/BacT system (Organon Teknika) (Rohner, 1997; Brunello, 1999), and the ESP Culture System II (Trek Diagnostic Systems) (Tholcken, 1997; Woods, 1997). With each system, bottles are incubated in the respective instrument, where they are monitored for changes in production or production and consumption of various gases, indicating growth of mycobacteria or other organisms. In general, these systems perform comparably to the BACTEC TB460 and have the advantages of being fully automated, and thus less labor-intensive, and nonradiometric.

Tests for Identification of Mycobacteria

Identification of mycobacteria has traditionally been based on rate of growth on solid media, colony morphology, colony pigmentation with and without exposure to light, and results of biochemical tests (described in detail elsewhere [Kent, 1985]). Biochemical test results, however, are not usually available for several weeks to months after colonies appear on solid media, and for identification of MTBC especially, more rapid methods are recommended (Tenover, 1993). Additionally, biochemical testing not infrequently does not provide an unequivocal identification at the species level.

Currently, the most rapid method for diagnosis of pulmonary tuberculosis is the use of a nucleic acid amplification test for direct detection of MTBC in clinical specimens (Piersimoni, 2003). These tests, however, do not differentiate the species in the MTBC. Two nucleic acid amplification tests are available worldwide for testing respiratory specimens: Amplified Mycobacterium Tuberculosis Direct Test (Gen-Probe, Inc.) and AMPLICOR *Mycobacterium tuberculosis* Test (Roche Diagnostic Systems, Inc.). The BDProbeTec ET System (BD Biosciences) is available outside the United States only. The AMPLICOR assay is cleared by the Food and Drug Administration (FDA) for testing AFB smear positive respiratory specimens only. The Gen-Probe test is approved for

VII

testing both smear-positive and smear-negative respiratory specimens. Data suggest that nucleic acid amplification tests may be useful in AFB smear-negative patients at high risk for tuberculosis (e.g., persons infected with HIV and incarcerated persons in correctional facilities), allowing more rapid diagnosis and earlier initiation of treatment (Gamboa, 1998; Bergmann, 1999). The sensitivity of nucleic acid amplification tests is generally slightly lower for nonrespiratory specimens but they may be useful for diagnosis of some cases of extrapulmonary tuberculosis, especially when the AFB smear is positive.

The BACTEC TB NAP (para-nitro-α-acetyl-amino-β-hydroxypropio-phenone) test differentiates members of the MTBC from NTM within 4–5 days after AFB are detected in a BACTEC 12B vial (Gross, 1985). A volume of broth from the positive 12B vial is injected into two fresh bottles of 12B medium, one with and one without NAP. An increase in the GI in the bottle without NAP and no increase in the GI in the bottle containing NAP indicates that the isolate is a member of MTBC, because only those species are susceptible to, and thus inhibited by, NAP. This test, however, does not differentiate between species of the MTBC.

Chemiluminescent DNA probes allow identification of a few species or species complex of mycobacteria within 1–2 hours after sufficient growth is present (on solid or in a liquid medium) (Evans, 1992; Goto, 1992; Lebrun, 1992; Reisner, 1994). Commercial probes specific for MTBC, MAC, *M. avium*, *M. intracellulare*, *M. gordonae*, and *M. kansasii* are currently available. Testing requires minimal equipment (i.e., luminometer, sonicator, and heating block). Disadvantages of the probes include failure to identify some isolates of MAC, especially when testing growth from a liquid medium, false-positive results with the MAC probe when testing aliquots of broth cultures, and rare false-positive results with the MTBC probe (Bull, 1992; Lebrun, 1992; Butler, 1994).

High-performance liquid chromatography allows identification of mycobacterial colonies on a solid medium or growth in a liquid medium in 2–4 hours. The most sophisticated identification method is sequencing hypervariable regions of the 16S ribosomal RNA gene (Patel, 2000; Cloud, 2002; Hall, 2003). Both techniques, which are technically more complex and require expensive equipment, are performed predominantly in research and large reference laboratories.

Susceptibility Testing

Standardized guidelines for susceptibility testing of mycobacteria now exist (Clinical and Laboratory Standards Institute, formerly National Committee for Clinical Laboratory Standards, 2003). For MTBC, testing may be performed on isolated colonies or a positive broth culture (indirect test) or on sputum specimens that are AFB smear-positive (direct test). Agar proportion is the standard method of testing susceptibility of MTBC to antituberculosis agents. With this method, isolates showing greater than 1% resistance to a single concentration of drug are considered resistant to that drug. However, because the turnaround time for results is a minimum of 21 days after plates are inoculated, use of an FDA-approved liquid-based system that provides results equivalent to those of agar proportion is recommended (Tenover, 1993; Clinical and Laboratory Standards Institute, 2003). With the currently available liquid-based systems, results generally available are 5–7 days after bottles are inoculated (Bergmann 1998, 2000; Scarparo, 2004).

Susceptibility testing may be performed on clinically significant isolates of the NTM (Wallace, 1997; Clinical and Laboratory Standards, 2003); however, for some species, there may be little correlation between susceptibility test results and clinical response to drug therapy. For isolates of rapidly growing mycobacteria, broth microdilution testing of amikacin, cefoxitin, ciprofloxacin, clarithromycin, doxycycline (or minocycline), imipenem (*M. fortuitum* only), sulfamethoxazole (or trimethoprim–sulfamethoxazole), and tobramycin (*M. chelonae* only) is recommended (Woods, 1999; Clinical and Laboratory Standards, 2003). Broth dilution (either macrodilution or microdilution) should be used to test susceptibility of isolates of MAC to clarithromycin only (clarithromycin results predict azithromycin) (Inderlied, 1997; Wallace, 1997; Clinical Laboratory and Standards Institute, 2003). Isolates of *M. kansasii* initially should be tested for susceptibility to rifampin only. Rifampin-resistant *M. kansasii* should be tested against rifabutin, ethambutol, streptomycin, clarithromycin, amikacin, ciprofloxacin, and sulfamethoxazole (or trimethoprim–sulfamethoxazole).

Treatment

Initial isolates of MTBC from all patients with tuberculosis should be tested for susceptibility to the primary antituberculosis agents isoniazid, rifampin, pyrazinamide, and ethambutol. Susceptibility testing should be repeated if the patient continues to produce culture-positive sputum after

Table 59–7 Treatment of infections with commonly encountered pathogenic mycobacteria

Mycobacterium Species	Surgery	Antimicrobial Therapy Agents	Duration (months)
*M. tuberculosis**	–	INH, RIF, EMB, and PZA	6
M. avium complex Pulmonary	±	CLARI (or AZITHRO), RIF (or RBT), and EMB	Until culture-negative 12
Disseminated	–	CLARI (or AZITHRO) and EMB, ± RBT	Lifelong
Lymphadenitis	+	–	
M. kansasii	–	INH, RIF, and EMB	18
M. marinum	±	CLARI, DOX, SXT, or RIF and EMB	1–2 after clinical resolution (3 minimum)
M. fortuitum group[†]	±	AMK, CFX, IMI, SXT, QUIN[‡], LNZ	1–2 after clinical resolution
M. chelonae[†]	±	CLARI, TOBRA, IMI, GATI (or MOXI)	1–2 after clinical resolution
M. abscessus[†]	±	CLARI, AMK, IMI, CFX, GATI (or MOXI)	1–2 after clinical resolution

– = not indicated; ± = may be indicated; + = definitely indicated; AZITHRO = azithromycin; CLARI = clarithromycin; DOX = doxycycline; EMB = ethambutol; GATI = gatifloxacin; IMI = imipenem; INH = isoniazid; LNZ = linezolid; MOXI = moxifloxacin; PZA = pyrazinamide; QUIN = quinolone; RBT = rifabutin; RIF = rifampin; SXT = trimethoprim–sulfamethoxazole.

* Pyrazinamide is given only for the first 2 months; ethambutol may be discontinued if the isolate is susceptible to isoniazid and rifampin. This regimen is for drug-susceptible isolates only. [†] Regimen is based on results of susceptibility testing. Serious disease is treated with 2- or 3-drug combination therapy. [‡] Most isolates are susceptible to ciprofloxacin, levofloxacin, gatifloxacin, and moxifloxacin

3 months of therapy (Tenover, 1993). If the isolate is resistant to rifampin only or to two or more primary agents, susceptibility to secondary drugs (streptomycin, ethionamide, kanamycin, capreomycin, ofloxacin, and rifabutin) also should be evaluated. The chemotherapeutic regimen currently recommended for treatment of tuberculosis (Table 59–7) should be initiated before susceptibility test results are available, but treatment should be altered based on those results if an isolate is found to be resistant. Medications should be administered by directly observed therapy. Regimens commonly used to treat infections caused by the most frequently encountered NTM also are listed in Table 59–7 (Wolinsky, 1979; Wallace, 1983, 1994, 1997; Inderlied, 1993; Brown-Elliott, 2002). For many NTM, the optimal duration of therapy is not known, but the intervals indicated in Table 59–6 have been successful in some cases.

Prevention

Mycobacterium tuberculosis

Four general strategies for controlling tuberculosis are described (Centers for Disease Control and Prevention, 1988). The most important is early identification and adequate treatment of persons with infectious tuberculosis. This measure renders the infected person noncontagious within a few weeks and eventually results in cure. The second strategy entails identification and treatment of individuals with noncontagious tuberculosis: extrapulmonary disease, primary pulmonary disease in children, bacteriologically unconfirmed pulmonary disease, and infection with *M. tuberculosis* not yet causing disease (i.e., positive skin test or Quantiferon Gold, normal chest X-ray, no symptoms).

The third strategy involves creation of a safe environment in situations where the risk of transmitting infection is high: autopsy suites, sputum induction cubicles, chest clinic waiting areas, correctional facilities, some shelters for the homeless, and mycobacteriology laboratories. To accomplish this, several issues must be addressed (Segal-Maurer, 1994). Rooms housing infectious patients or in which potentially infectious specimens are handled should be under negative pressure, and air likely to be contaminated with infectious droplet nuclei should be exhausted to the outside. A single-pass ventilation system (best accomplished by locating air supply outlets at the ceiling level and exhaust inlets near the floor) and a minimum of six air changes per hour (12 exchanges per hour for autopsy suites) are recommended. Universal precautions must be followed when handling all specimens, and both specimens and cultures must be handled in a certified, class II biological safety cabinet. Moreover, a particulate respirator that filters out particles 1–5 μm in diameter should be worn, and personnel should be trained in a respiratory program; the standard surgical mask is not adequate.

The fourth strategy is vaccination with the BCG vaccine, an attenuated vaccine derived from a strain of *M. bovis* by Calmette and Guérin in France. The efficacy of the BCG vaccine in prevention of tuberculosis is controversial, but a meta-analysis of the literature has suggested that the vaccine reduces the risk of tuberculosis by 50% (Colditz, 1994). In the United States, the BCG vaccine is recommended only for infants and children who have negative tuberculin skin tests and who belong to selected population groups (Centers for Disease Control and Prevention, 1988): (1) those at high risk of intimate and prolonged exposure to persistently untreated or ineffectively treated persons with infectious pulmonary tuberculosis, who cannot be removed from the source of exposure, and for whom long-term preventive therapy is not possible; (2) those exposed continuously to persons with tuberculosis due to strains resistant to isoniazid and rifampin; and (3) those in groups in which the rate of new infections is greater than 1% per year and for whom the usual surveillance and treatment programs have been attempted but are not feasible. The BCG vaccine is not recommended for health-care workers in the United States. The current recommendation for protection of health-care workers is adequate surveillance, which includes periodic tuberculin skin or Quantiferon Gold testing (at least yearly and more frequently for persons in high-risk groups) and isoniazid preventive therapy for persons who have recently converted from tuberculin-skin-test-negative to -positive and for persons who are tuberculin-skin-test-positive and are close contacts

of individuals with tuberculosis or who have medical conditions such as diabetes, renal failure, or immunosuppression associated with therapy or disease (Centers for Disease Control and Prevention, 1988).

The BCG vaccine should not be given to immunocompromised persons and should be given with caution to those at risk of infection with HIV. Disseminated *M. bovis* in patients with AIDS and *M. bovis* lymphadenitis in symptomatic HIV-infected infants have occurred following BCG vaccination (Centers for Disease Control and Prevention, 1985; Blanche, 1986). However, disseminated *M. bovis* has not been reported in asymptomatic persons infected with HIV. In populations where the risk of tuberculosis is high, the World Health Organization recommends that the BCG vaccine be given to HIV-infected children at birth or soon thereafter. It should not be given to children with symptomatic HIV infection or, in populations where the risk of tuberculosis is low, to persons known or suspected to be infected with HIV (World Health Organization, 1987).

Mycobacterium avium Complex

Disseminated MAC in patients with AIDS is associated with considerable morbidity and a shortened duration of survival (Horsburgh, 1991b; Nightingale, 1992); therefore, prevention of the disease is desirable. Because MAC is ubiquitous in the environment, the most reasonable approach to prevention is chemoprophylaxis. Currently, the United States Public Health Service and the Infectious Diseases Society of America recommend clarithromycin or azithromycin prophylaxis in AIDS patients with CD4+ cell counts under 50/μL (Centers for Disease Control and Prevention, 1997). If neither of these drugs can be tolerated, rifabutin is an alternative prophylactic agent for MAC disease.

References

Abe C, Hosojima S, Fukasawa Y, et al: Comparison of MB-Check, BACTEC, and egg-based media for recovery of mycobacteria. J Clin Microbiol 1992; 30:878–881.

Anargyros P, Astill DSJ, Lim ISL: Comparison of improved BACTEC and Lowenstein–Jensen media for culture of mycobacteria from clinical specimens. J Clin Microbiol 1990; 28:1288–1291.

Bergmann, JS, Fish G, Woods GL: Evaluation of the BBL MGIT (Mycobacterial Growth Indicator Tube) AST SIRE system for antimycobacterial susceptibility testing of *Mycobacterium tuberculosis* to 4 primary antituberculous drugs. Arch Pathol Lab Med 2000; 124:82–86.

Bergmann, JS, Woods GL: Evaluation of the ESP culture system II for testing susceptibilities of *Mycobacterium tuberculosis* isolates to four primary antituberculous drugs. J Clin Microbiol 1998; 36:2940–2943.

Bergmann JS, Yuoh G, Fish G, Woods GL: Clinical evaluation of the enhanced Gen-Probe amplified mycobacterium direct test for rapid diagnosis of tuberculosis in prison inmates. J Clin Microbiol 1999; 37:1419–1425.

Binford CH, Meyers WM, Walsh GP: Leprosy. JAMA 1982; 247:2283–2292.

Blacklock ZM, Dawson DJ, Kane DW, McEvoy D: *Mycobacterium asiaticum* as a potential pulmonary pathogen for humans: a clinical and bacteriologic review of five cases. Am Rev Respir Dis 1983; 127:241–244.

Blake LA, West BC, Lary CH, et al: Environmental nonhuman sources of leprosy. Rev Infect Dis, 1987; 9:562–567.

Blanche S, LeDeist F, Fischer A: Longitudinal study of 18 children with perinatal LAV/HTLV III infection: attempt at prognostic evaluation. J Pediatr 1986; 109:965–970.

Brown-Elliott AB, Wallace RJ Jr: Clinical and taxonomic status of pathogenic nonpigmented or late-pigmenting rapidly growing mycobacteria. Clin Microbiol Rev 2002; 15:716–746.
Excellent review of the taxonomy of the rapidly growing mycobacteria. Also includes a discussion of the laboratory tests for identification and the usual antimicrobial susceptibility patterns.

Brunello F, Favari F, Fontana R: Comparison of the MB/BacT and BACTEC 460 TB systems for recovery

of mycobacteria from various clinical specimens. J Clin Microbiol 1999; 37:1206–1209.

Buhler VB, Pollak A: Human infection with atypical acid-fast organisms. Am J Clin Pathol 1953; 23:363–374.

Bull TJ, Shanson DC: Rapid misdiagnosis by *Mycobacterium avium-intracellulare* masquerading as tuberculosis in PCR/DNA probe tests. Lancet 1992; 340:1360.

Butler WR, O'Connor SP, Yakrus MA, et al: Cross-reactivity of genetic probe for detection of *Mycobacterium tuberculosis* with newly described species *Mycobacterium celatum*. J Clin Microbiol 1994; 32:536.

Casimir MT, Fainstein V, Papadopolous N: Cavitary lung infection caused by *Mycobacterium flavescens*. South Med J 1982; 75:253.

Castets M, Boisvert H, Grumback F, et al: Les bacilles tuberculeux de type africaine. Rev Tuberc Pneumol 1968; 32:179.

Centers for Disease Control and Prevention: Disseminated *Mycobacterium bovis* infection from BCG vaccination of a patient with acquired immunodeficiency syndrome. Morbid Mortal Wkly Rev 1985; 34:227.

Centers for Disease Control and Prevention: Use of BCG vaccines in the control of tuberculosis: a joint statement by the ACIP and the Advisory Committee for the Elimination of Tuberculosis. Morbid Mortal Wkly Rev 1988; 37:663.

Centers for Disease Control and Prevention: *Mycobacterium haemophilum* infection – New York City Metropolitan Area, 1990–1991. Morbid Mortal Wkly Rev 1991; 40:636.

Centers for Disease Control and Prevention: Summary of notifiable diseases, United States, 1992. Morbid Mortal Wkly Rev 1993; 41:59.

Centers for Disease Control and Prevention: USPHS/IDSA guidelines for prevention of opportunistic infections in persons infected with human immunodeficiency virus. Morbid Mortal Wkly Rev 1997; 46(RR-12):1.

Centers for Disease Control and Prevention: Tuberculosis morbidity – United States, 1997. Morbid Mortal Wkly Rev 1998; 47:253.

Centers for Disease Control and Prevention: Surveillance for AIDS-defining opportunistic illnesses, 1992–1997. Morbid Mortal Wkly Rev 1999; 48(SS-2):1.

Centers for Disease Control and Prevention: Trends in Tuberculosis – United States, 1998–2003. Morbid Mortal Wkly Rev 2004; 53:209–14.

Chaisson RE, Schecter GF, Theuer CP, et al: Tuberculosis in patients with the acquired immunodeficiency syndrome: clinical features, response to therapy, and survival. Am Rev Respir Dis 1987; 136:570.

Cianciulli FD: The radish bacillus (*Mycobacterium terrae*): saprophyte or pathogen? Am Rev Respir Dis 1974; 109:138.

Clinical and Laboratory Standards. Susceptibility testing of Mycobacteria, Nocardia, and other aerobic actinomycetes. Approved Standard M24-A. Wayne, PA, National Committee for Clinical Laboratory Standards, 2003.

Cloud JL, Neal H, Rosenberry R, et al: Identification of *Mycobacterium* spp. by using a commercial 16S ribosomal DNA sequencing kit and additional sequencing libraries. J Clin Microbiol 2002; 40:400–406.

Colditz GA, Brewer TF, Berkey CS, et al: Efficacy of BCG vaccine in prevention of tuberculosis: meta-analysis of the published literature. JAMA 1994; 271:698.

Cornfield DB, Beavis KG, Greene JA, et al: Mycobacterial growth and bacterial contamination in the Mycobacteria Growth Indicator Tube and BACTEC 460 culture system. J Clin Microbiol 1997; 35:2068.

Costrini AM, Mahler DA, Gross WM, et al: Clinical and roentgenographic features of nosocomial pulmonary disease due to *Mycobacterium xenopi*. Am Rev Respir Dis 1981; 123:104.

Coyle MB, Carlson LC, Wallis CK, et al: Laboratory aspects of '*Mycobacterium genavense*,' proposed species isolated from AIDS patients. J Clin Microbiol 1992; 30:3206.

D'Amato RF, Isenberg HD, Hochstein L, et al: Evaluation of the Roche Septi-Chek AFB system for recovery of mycobacteria. J Clin Microbiol 1991; 29:2906.

Davison MB, McCormack JG, Blacklock ZM, et al: Bacteremia caused by *Mycobacterium neoaurum*. J Clin Microbiol 1988; 26:762.

DeChairo DC, Kittredge D, Meyers A, et al: Septic arthritis due to *Mycobacterium triviale*. Am Rev Respir Dis 1973; 108:1224.

Desmond E, Ahmed AT, Probert WS, et al: *Mycobacterium africanum* cases, California. Emerg Infect Dis 2004; 10:921–923.

Dhillon SS, Watanakunakorn C: Lady Windermere syndrome: middle lobe bronchiectasis and *Mycobacterium avium* complex infection due to

VII

voluntary cough suppression. Clin Infect Dis 2000; 30:572.

Edwards MS, Huber TW, Baker CJ: *Mycobacterium terrae* synovitis and osteomyelitis. Am Rev Respir Dis 1978; 117:161.

Ellner JJ, Hinman AR, Dooley SW, et al: Tuberculosis symposium: emerging problems and promise. J Infect Dis 1993; 168:537.

Evans KD, Nakasone AS, Sutherland PA, et al: Identification of *Mycobacterium tuberculosis* and *Mycobacterium avium-Mycobacterium intracellulare* directly from primary BACTEC cultures by using acridinium-ester-labeled DNA probes. J Clin Microbiol 1992; 30:2427.

Falkinham JO, III: Epidemiology of infection by nontuberculous mycobacteria. Clin Microbiol Rev 1996; 9:177.

In-depth review of the epidemiology of the more commonly encountered nontuberculous mycobacteria, including M. avium complex, M. kansasii, and M. marinum, as well as M. simiae and M. xenopi.

Feldman RA, Hershfield E: Mycobacterial skin infection by an unidentified species. A report of 29 patients. Ann Intern Med 1974; 80:445.

Gamboa F, Fernandez G, Padilla E, et al: Comparative evaluation of initial and new versions of the Gen-Probe Amplified Mycobacterium Tuberculosis Direct Test for direct detection of *Mycobacterium tuberculosis* in respiratory and nonrespiratory specimens. J Clin Microbiol 1998; 36:684.

Good RC, Snider DE Jr: Isolation of nontuberculous mycobacteria in the United States. J Infect Dis 1982; 146:829.

Goto M, Oka S, Okuzumi K, et al: Evaluation of acridinium-ester-labeled DNA probes for identification of *Mycobacterium tuberculosis* and *Mycobacterium avium-Mycobacterium-intracellulare* complex in culture. J Clin Microbiol 1992; 30:2473.

Grange JM, Collins CH: Bovine tubercle bacilli and disease in animals and man. Epidemiol Infect 1987; 92:221.

Gross WM, Hawkins JE: Radiometric selective inhibition tests for differentiation of *Mycobacterium tuberculosis*, *Mycobacterium bovis*, and other mycobacteria. J Clin Microbiol 1985; 21:565.

Hall L, Doerr KA, Wohlfiel SL, et al: Evaluation of the MicroSeq System for identification of mycobacteria by 16S ribosomal DNA sequencing and its integration into a routine clinical mycobacteriology laboratory. J Clin Microbiol 2003; 41:1447–1453.

Hanna BA, Ebrahimzadeh A, Elliott LB, et al: Multicenter evaluation of the BACTEC MGIT 960 System for recovery of mycobacteria. J Clin Microbiol 1999; 37:748.

Hastings RC, Gillis TP, Krahenbuhl JL, et al: Leprosy. Clin Microbiol Rev 1988; 1:330.

Henriques B, Hoffner SE, Petrini B, et al: Infection with *Mycobacterium malmoense* in Sweden: report of 221 cases. Clin Infect Dis 1993; 18:596.

Horsburgh CR Jr: *Mycobacterium avium* complex infection in the acquired immunodeficiency syndrome. N Engl J Med 1991a; 324:1332.

Horsburgh CR Jr, Havlik JA, Illis DA, et al: Survival of patients with acquired immune deficiency syndrome and disseminated *Mycobacterium avium* complex infection with and without antimycobacterial chemotherapy. Am Rev Respir Dis 1991b; 144:557.

Huebner RE, Schein MF, Bass JB Jr: The tuberculin skin test. Clin Infect Dis 1993; 17:968.

Inderlied CB: Microbiology and minimum inhibitory concentration testing for *Mycobacterium avium* complex prophylaxis. Am J Med 1997; 102:2.

Inderlied CB, Kemper CA, Bermudez LEM. The *Mycobacterium avium* complex. Clin Microbiol Rev 1993; 6:266.

Isenberg HD, D'Amato RF, Heifets L, et al: Collaborative feasibility study of a biphasic system (Roche Septi-Chek AFB) for rapid detection and isolation of mycobacteria. J Clin Microbiol 1991; 29:1719.

Karassova V, Weiszfeiler J, Krasznay E: Occurrence of atypical mycobacteria in macacus rhesus. Acta Microbiol Acad Sci Hung 1965; 12:275.

Karlson AG, Carr DT: Tuberculosis caused by *Mycobacterium bovis*. Ann Intern Med 1970; 73:979.

Kent PT, Kubica GP: Public health mycobacteriology: a guide for the level III laboratory. Atlanta, GA, Department of Health and Human Services, 1985.

Kim JH, Langston AA, Gallis HA: Miliary tuberculosis: epidemiology, clinical manifestations, diagnosis, and outcome. Rev Infect Dis 1990; 12:583.

Kristjansson M, Green P, Manning HL, et al: Molecular confirmation of bacillus Calmette–Guérin as the cause of pulmonary infection following urinary tract instillation. Clin Infect Dis 1993; 17:228.

Lebrun L, Espinasse R, Poveda JD, et al: Evaluation of nonradioactive DNA probes for identification of mycobacteria. J Clin Microbiol 1992; 30:2476.

Lomwardias S, Madge GE: Chaetoconidium and atypical acid-fast bacilli in skin ulcers. Arch Dermatol 1972; 106:875.

Lumpkin LR III, Cox GF, Wolf JE: Leprosy in five armadillo handlers. J Am Acad Dermatol 1983; 9:899.

Maschek H, Georgii A, Schmidt RE, et al: *Mycobacterium genavense* autopsy findings in three patients. Am J Clin Pathol 1994; 101:95.

Mostowy S, Onipede A, Gagneux S, et al: Genomic analysis distinguishes *Mycobacterium africanum*. J Clin Microbiol 2004; 42:3594–3599.

Murray CJ, Styblo K, Rouillon A: Tuberculosis in developing countries: burden, intervention, and cost. Bull Int Union Tuberc Lung 1990; 65:6.

Murray PR, Elmore C, Krogstad D: The acid-fast stain: a specific and predictive test for mycobacterial disease. Ann Intern Med 1980; 92:512.

Guidelines for testing susceptibility of M. tuberculosis complex, rapidly growing mycobacteria, and select slowly growing mycobacteria, including M. avium complex, M. kansasii, and M. marinum.

Neeley SP, Denning DW: Cutaneous *Mycobacterium thermoresistible* infection in a heart transplant recipient. Rev Infect Dis 1989; 11:608.

Neill MA, Hightower AW, Broome CV: Leprosy in the United States, 1971–1981. J Infect Dis 1985; 152:1064.

Nightingale SD, Byrd LT, Southern PM, et al: Incidence of *Mycobacterium avium–intracellulare* complex bacteremia in human immunodeficiency virus-positive patients. J Infect Dis 1992; 165:1082.

Norden A, Linell F: A new type of pathogenic *Mycobacterium*. Nature 1951; 168:826.

Patel JB, Leonard DGB, Pan X, et al: Sequence-based identification of *Mycobacterium* species using the MicroSeq 500 16S rDNA bacterial identification system. J Clin Microbiol 2000; 38:246–251.

Pfyffer GE, Auchenthaler ER, van Embden JD, *et al*: *Mycobacterium canettii*, the smooth variant of *M. tuberculosis*, isolated from a Swiss patient exposed in Africa. Emerg Infect Dis 1998; 4:631.

Pfyffer GE, Cieslak C, Welscher HM, et al: Rapid detection of mycobacteria in clinical specimens by using the automated BACTEC 9000 MB system and comparison with radiometric and solid culture systems. J Clin Microbiol 1997a; 35:2229.

Pfyffer GE, Welscher HM, Kissling P, et al: Comparison of the Mycobacteria Growth Indicator Tube (MGIT) with radiometric and solid culture for recovery of acid-fast bacilli. J Clin Microbiol 1997b; 35:364.

Piersimoni C, Goteri G, Nista D, et al: *Mycobacterium lentiflavum* as an emerging causative agent of cervical lymphdenitis. J Clin Microbiol 2004; 42:3894–3897.

Piersimoni C, Scarparo C: Relevance of commercial amplification methods for direct detection of *Mycobacterium tuberculosis* complex in clinical samples. J Clin Microbiol 2003; 41:5355–5365.

Excellent review of the commercial nucleic acid amplification tests for direct detection of M. tuberculosis complex in clinical specimens.

Prince DS: Infection with *Mycobacterium avium* complex in patients without predisposing conditions. N Engl J Med 1989; 321:863.

Reisner BS, Gatson AM, Woods GL: Use of Gen-Probe AccuProbes to identify *Mycobacterium avium* complex, *Mycobacterium tuberculosis* complex, *Mycobacterium kansasii*, and *Mycobacterium gordonae* directly from BACTEC TB broth cultures. J Clin Microbiol 1994; 32:2995.

Rickman TW, Moyer NP: Increased sensitivity of acid-fast smears. J Clin Microbiol 1980; 11:618.

Ridley DS, Jopling WH: Classification of leprosy according to immunity: a five group system. Int J Lepr 1964; 34:255.

Rieder HL, Cauthen GM, Kelly GD, et al: Tuberculosis in the United States. JAMA 1989; 262:385.

Rohner P, Ninet B, Metral C, et al: Evaluation of the MB/BacT system and comparison to the BACTEC 460 system and solid media for isolation of mycobacteria from clinical specimens. J Clin Microbiol 1997; 35:3127.

Runyon EH: Anonymous mycobacteria in pulmonary disease. Med Clin North Am 1959; 43:273.

Classic description of the different groups of nontuberculous mycobacteria.

Scarparo C, Ricordi P, Ruggiero G, Piccoli P: Evaluation of the fully automated BACTEC MGIT 960 for testing susceptibility of *Mycobacterium tuberculosis* to pyrazinamide, streptomycin, isoniazid, rifampin, and ethambutol and comparison with the radiometric BACTEC 460TB method. J Clin Microbiol 2004; 42:1109–14.

Schroder KH, Juhlin I: *Mycobacterium malmoense* sp. nov. Int J Syst Bacteriol 1977; 27:241.

Segal-Maurer S, Kalkut GE: Environmental control of tuberculosis: continuing controversy. Clin Infect Dis 1994; 19:299.

Smith DS, Lindholm-Levy P, Huitt GA, et al: *Mycobacterium terrae*: Case reports, literature review, and in vitro antibiotic susceptibility testing. Clin Infect Dis 2000; 30:444.

Snider DE Jr, La Montagne JR: The neglected global tuberculosis problem: a report of the 1992 World Congress on Tuberculosis. J Infect Dis 1994; 169:1189.

Sompolinsky D, Lagziel A, Naveh D, et al: *Mycobacterium haemophilium* sp. nov., a new pathogen of humans. Int J Sys Bacteriol 1978; 28:67.

Stager CE, Libonati JP, Siddiqi SH, et al: Role of solid media when used in conjunction with the BACTEC system for mycobacterial isolation and identification. J Clin Microbiol 1991; 29:154.

Strumpf IJ, Tsang AY, Sayre JW: Re-evaluation of sputum staining for the diagnosis of pulmonary tuberculosis. Am Rev Respir Dis 1979; 119:599.

Tecson-Tumang FT, Bright JL: *Mycobacterium xenopi* and the acquired immunodeficiency syndrome. Ann Intern Med, 1984; 100:461–46.

Tenover FC, Crawford JT, Huebner RE, et al: The resurgence of tuberculosis: is your laboratory ready? J Clin Microbiol 1993; 31:767.

Tholcken CA, Huang S, Woods GL: Evaluation of the ESP culture system II for recovery of mycobacteria from blood specimens collected in isolation tubes. J Clin Microbiol 1997; 35:2681.

Tortoli E: Impact of genotypic studies on mycobacterial taxonomy: the new mycobacteria of the 1990s. Clin Microbiol Rev 2003; 16:319–354.

Excellent discussion of the more recently described species of slowly growing and rapidly growing mycobacteria. Includes information regarding epidemiology, clinical manifestations, phenotypic characteristics, and antimicrobial susceptibility.

Tsukamura M, Kita N, Otsuka W, et al: A study of the taxonomy of the *Mycobacterium nonchromogenicum* complex and report of six cases of lung infection due to *Mycobacterium nonchromogenicum*. Microbiol Immunol 1983; 27:219.

Van Soolingen D, Hoogenboezem T, de Haas PEW, et al: A novel pathogenic taxon of M. *tuberculosis* complex, Canetti: characterization of an exceptional isolate from Africa. Int J Syst Bacteriol 1997; 47:1236.

Wald A, Coyle MB, Carlson LC, et al: Infection with a fastidious mycobacterium resembling

Mycobacterium simiae in seven patients with AIDS. Ann Intern Med 1992; 117:586.

Wallace RJ Jr, Dunbar D, Brown BA, et al: Rifampin-resistant *Mycobacterium kansasii*. Clin Infect Dis 1994; 18:736.

Wallace RJ Jr, Glassroth J, Griffith DE, et al: Diagnosis and treatment of disease caused by nontuberculous mycobacteria. Am J Respir Crit Care Med 1997; 156:S1.

Excellent review of the laboratory diagnosis and treatment of the commonly encountered nontuberculous mycobacteria, including M. avium complex, M. kansasii, M. marinum, and the rapidly growing mycobacteria.

Wallace RJ Jr, Nash DR, Tsukamura M, et al: Human disease due to *Mycobacterium smegmatis*. J Infect Dis 1988; 158:52.

Wallace RJ Jr, Swenson JM, Silcox VA, et al: Spectrum of disease due to rapidly growing mycobacteria. Rev Infect Dis 1983; 5:657.

Weinberger M, Berg SL, Feuerstein IM, et al: Disseminated infection with *Mycobacterium gordonae*: report of a case and critical review of the literature. Clin Infect Dis 1992; 14:1229.

Weitzman I, Osadczyi D, Corrado ML, et al: *Mycobacterium thermoresistible*: a new pathogen for humans. J Clin Microbiol 1981; 14:593.

Welch DF, Guruswamy AP, Sides SJ, et al: Timely culture for mycobacteria which utilizes a microcolony method. J Clin Microbiol 1993; 31:2178.

Wolinsky E: Nontuberculous mycobacteria and associated diseases. Am Rev Respir Dis 1979; 119:107.

Woods GL: Mycobacteria. *In* Woods GL, Gutierrez Y (eds): Diagnostic Pathology of Infectious Diseases. Philadelphia, PA, Lea & Febiger, 1993, p 378.

Woods GL, Bergmann JS, Witebsky FG, *et al*: Multisite reproducibility of results obtained by the broth microdilution method for susceptibility testing of *Mycobacterium abscessus*, *Mycobacterium chelonae*, and *Mycobacterium fortuitum*. J Clin Microbiol 1999; 37:1676–1682.

Woods GL, Fish G, Plaunt M, Murphy T: Clinical evaluation of Difco ESP culture system II for growth and detection of mycobacteria. J Clin Microbiol 1997; 35:121.

Woods GL, Washington JA II: Mycobacteria other than *Mycobacterium tuberculosis*: review of microbiologic and clinical aspects. Rev Infect Dis 1987; 9:275.

World Health Organization: Special Programme on AIDS and Expanded Programme on Immunization – joint statement: consultation on human immunodeficiency virus (HIV) and routine childhood immunization. Wkly Epidemiol Rep 1987; 62:297.

Zanetti S, Ardito F, Sechi L, et al: Evaluation of a nonradiometric system (BACTEC 9000 MB) for detection of mycobacteria in human clinical samples. J Clin Microbiol 1997; 35:2072.

VII

CHAPTER 60

Mycotic Diseases

Peter C. Iwen, Ph.D.

KEY POINTS

- Opportunistic fungal pathogens have emerged as common causes of invasive disease in the compromised host.

- Histopathologic examination of deep tissue is the gold standard for the rapid detection and recognition of fungal pathogens causing invasive infection.

- Micromorphologic and phenotypic methods continue to be the main mechanisms for the identification of fungal pathogens in culture, although molecular techniques have begun to show promise in this area.

- *Candida albicans* continues to be the most common fungal species causing human disease, however, non-*albicans Candida* species are rapidly becoming more widespread in causing invasive disease and tend to develop resistance to standard antifungal treatments more readily.

- True pathogenic dimorphic fungal pathogens are frequent causes of mild infection in people living in endemic areas; however, invasive disease, whether recurrent or primary, is becoming more common in immunocompromised hosts.

- Recent introduction of new antifungal agents and the progression of resistance among moulds and yeast have added importance to the development and standardization of antifungal susceptibility testing.

Medical mycology is the science devoted to the study of fungi and their relationship to human disease. It encompasses single-celled yeast and filamentous moulds, agents of superficial skin infections (cutaneous mycoses) and disseminated deep-seated visceral disease (systemic mycoses), and established historical pathogenic fungi (true pathogens) and saprophytic fungi elevated to the status of pathogen by modern therapies and diseases (opportunistic pathogens). Modern therapies such as high-dose chemotherapy to treat cancer, solid organ transplantation, and immunosuppressive infections such as acquired immunodeficiency syndrome have allowed the fungi to emerge as major causes of human disease (Wingard, 1995; Ponton, 2000; Blumberg, 2001; Fleming, 2002; Stevens, 2002; Clark, 2004). Although medical mycology education has been lacking in general for the medical profession, pathologists, who have been nurtured in the surgical pathology suite, have received a general understanding in the recognition of fungal pathogens (Steinbach, 2003a). Overall, the general lack of education in this area is troublesome, since the identification of most fungi is accomplished by skilled human observation rather than by machines. The macroscopic counterpart of the surgical specimen is the colonial morphology of the isolated fungus on agar media; as in anatomic pathology, definitive analysis of the problem must await microscopic observation.

The goal of this chapter is to present the fundamentals of medical mycology with an emphasis on practical issues and those fungal pathogens encountered regularly in the laboratory. For a review on the many emerging fungal pathogens that have been reported in the literature, the reader is referred to the several reference texts available for information on the unusual saprophytic fungi that, increasingly, are implicated as etiologic agents in severely immunosuppressed patients (De Hoog, 2000; Ponton, 2000). For a comprehensive atlas of the histopathology of fungal infections refer to the publication by Chandler and Kaplan (Chandler, 1987a). Finally, while not included in the fungal kingdom, the infections caused by the achlorophyllous algae are discussed in this chapter because the characteristics of the algae and the diseases they produce resemble those of fungi more than those of other infectious agents.

Since this chapter reports specifically on fungal mycoses, other types of fungal disease are not discussed. Excellent reviews are available for reference to these other diseases including noninvasive allergic responses to fungi (Schubert, 2004; Thakar, 2004), poisoning by the ingestion of poisonous fungi (mushroom poisoning or mycetismus) (McPartland, 1997; Broussard, 2001), and intoxication by ingesting of fungal toxins (mycotoxicosis) (Bennett, 2003).

Nomenclature, Taxonomy, and Fungal Morphology

Overview

The first hurdle for the beginning mycologist is nomenclature and its handmaiden, taxonomy. The members of the fungal kingdom (Eumycota) are eukaryotic cells that have the capability to reproduce by both sexual and asexual methods. They are classified into phyla by the nature of their sexual reproductive structures or lack thereof (Guarro, 1999). Fungi that have recognized sexual reproductive structures (perfect fungi) are classified into the Zygomycetes, Ascomycetes, or Basidiomycetes on the basis of the type of sexual reproductive structure produced. Fungi that lack recognized sexual reproductive structures are classified in the phylum Deuteromycetes, also called the fungi imperfecti, on the basis of their asexual reproductive structures. Once the sexual phase (called the teleomorph) of a deuteromycete becomes recognized, the organism is reclassified into one of the other phyla. In practice, however, the old familiar name of the imperfect asexual phase, the anamorph, is usually retained. For example, few people know *Histoplasma capsulatum*, *Blastomyces dermatitidis*, and *Cryptococcus neoformans* by their respective teleomorphic names, *Ajellomyces capsulatus*, *Ajellomyces dermatitidis*, and *Filobasidiella neoformans*, respectively. In contrast, the sexual phase *Pseudallescheria boydii* and its asexual phase *Scedosporium apiospermum* are both recognized terms used in common practice. Generally, the anamorphic (asexual) name is used to describe a fungal species in the laboratory, although many exceptions to this rule exist.

Much of fungal taxonomy is related to structural details since both classification and laboratory identification are heavily dependent on morphology. A glossary of important terms used in medical mycology is displayed in Table 60–1. In this chapter, a simplified conceptual approach is used to recognize the pathogens that are most commonly encountered in the clinical laboratory. For practical purposes, a few general characteristics shown in Table 60–2 serve as the basis for identification of fungi in the laboratory.

As mycologists learn more about fungi, reclassification of organisms occurs on a regular basis. The influence of molecular techniques in the taxonomic characterization of fungi has had a profound impact not only on the reclassification of fungal pathogens but also on the recognition of pathogens not previously reported as causes of human disease (De Hoog, 2000; Bastola, 2004).

The Fungal Colony

Two morphologic forms of fungus are recognized: yeasts and moulds. Yeasts are unicellular organisms that usually reproduce asexually by budding to produce a daughter cell. The colonial mass of yeast is a collection of distinct individual organisms that macroscopically resembles bacterial colonies on the surface of agar. Yeast colonies are usually smooth with a regular edge. When the colonies become heaped and dull, as *Candida albicans* often is, they may resemble those of staphylococci. Yeast produce catalase, so the incautious microbiologist who does not perform Gram's stain or a wet prep may mistake a yeast colony for a bacterium and provide an entirely misleading report. The presence of pseudohyphae is a characteristic of yeast belonging to the genus *Candida*. The pseudohyphae of yeast are often visible macroscopically as filamentous extensions from the edges of the colony, known colloquially as 'feet' (Fig. 60–1).

In contrast to yeast, moulds are filamentous fungi which are multicellular. The term 'mould' is becoming more common in use by mycologists although the term 'mold' has also been historically recognized and is used

Table 60–1 Glossary of Commonly Used Terms in Medical Mycology

Term	Definition
Aerial mycelium	Hyphae produced above the surface of the agar media
Anamorph	Asexual form of fungal sporulation (imperfect state)
Arthroconidium	Conidium derived from the fragmentation of specialized hypha
Ascocarp (ascoma)	Fruiting structure that contains asci (several types exist)
Ascospore	Sexual spore contained within an ascus
Ascus (pl., asci)	Sac-like structure that contains ascospores
Basidiospore	Sexual spore formed on an outgrowth of a basidium
Basidium	Structure that contains basidiospores, e.g., mushroom
Blastoconidium	Asexual spore formed by budding of the yeast cell
Chlamydospore	Thick-walled resting or survival structure (also called chlamydoconidium)
Cleistothecium	Enclosed ascocarp, composed of layers of hyphae (ascospores released by rupture)
Collarette	Funnel-shaped structure at the apex of a phialide
Columella	An extension of the sporangiophore into the base of the sporangium
Conidiogenous cell	Cell that produces conidia
Conidiophore	Specialized hyphal structure that carries the conidia
Conidium (pl. conidia)	Asexual reproductive structure formed in any manner that does not involve cleavage
Dematiaceous	Pigmented in dark color
Glabrous	Smooth, referring to colonial morphology
Hypha (pl. hyphae)	Vegetative unit of a mould
Intercalary	Borne within a hypha
Macroconidium	Larger of two types of conidium produced by a mould
Microconidium	Smaller of two types of conidium produced by a mould
Mould	Filamentous fungus that reproduces by sexual or asexual means (also called mold)
Mycelium	Mass of hyphae that make up the thallus of a mould
Perithecium	Enclosed ascocarp with a pore at the top through which the ascospores are discharged
Phialide (sterigmata)	Cell with opening through which conidia are produced
Pseudohypha	Connected yeast cells (blastoconidia) that resemble a hypha but contain areas of constriction between adjacent cells
Septum (pl. septa)	Crosswall in a hypha
Sporangiophore	Stalk bearing the sporangium
Sporangiospore	Asexual spore produced within a sporangium
Sporangium	Sac-like structure in which the asexual sporangiospores develop
Teleomorph	Sexual form of a fungal sporulation (perfect state)
Terminal	Borne at the end of a hypha
Vegetative mycelium	Hyphae produced on the surface or extending into the agar media
Vesicle	Enlarged or swollen cell, often at the end of a conidiophore or sporangiophore which may also be within hyphae
Yeast	Single-cell fungus that reproduces by budding or by fission

VII

routinely to describe these fungi. The filamentous nature of the mould gives the colonies a wooly, fluffy, or velvety appearance, sometimes punctuated with a granular or powdery aspect that is produced by the formation of asexual reproductive structures (Fig. 60–2). At other times, the colony may have a glabrous (smooth) appearance.

The distinction between moulds and yeasts is not firmly established. Some yeast also develops a visually macroscopic filamentous component. *Trichosporon* species are yeast that develops such filamentous extensions, whereas *Exophiala jeanselmei* is a dematiaceous yeast that develops a mycelium as it matures. The ultimate in fence-sitting is exemplified by the dimorphic fungi, which exhibit a mould form under some conditions and a nonmould form in other circumstances. The most important dimorphic fungi are systemic pathogens that behave as moulds in the environment

Table 60–2 Characteristics Useful for the Identification of Fungi

Characteristic	Examples
Type of macroscopic growth	Colonies of unicellular organisms (yeast)
	Colonies of filamentous organisms (moulds)
Morphology of yeast	Budding
	Budding with pseudohyphae
	Round yeast with capsules
	Budding yeast with collarettes
Morphology of filamentous structures	True septate hyphae
	True nonseptate hyphae (or sparsely septate)
Pigment of hyphae	Hyaline (lightly or nonpigmented)
	Dematiaceous (darkly pigmented)
Morphology of asexual reproductive structures	Conidia
	Spores
Morphology of sexual reproductive structures (rarely demonstrated)	Ascospores
	Cleistothecium
	Perithecium
Growth rate	Slow (>10 days)
	Medium (4–10 days)
	Fast (<4 days)
Inhibition by cycloheximide	Many saprobic fungi
Optimal growth temperature (occasional value)	25–30°C
	35–37°C
	40–42°C
	50–58°C
Biochemical tests	Assimilation
	Fermentation
	Enzymatic degradation (e.g., urease)
	Growth enhancement
Conversion from mould to yeast phase	Supplanted by DNA probe tests in most laboratories
Immunologic detection of antigens or antibodies	*Cryptococcus, Histoplasma, Coccidioides, Blastomyces, Aspergillus*
Molecular characteristic of DNA	*Histoplasma, Coccidioides, Blastomyces*

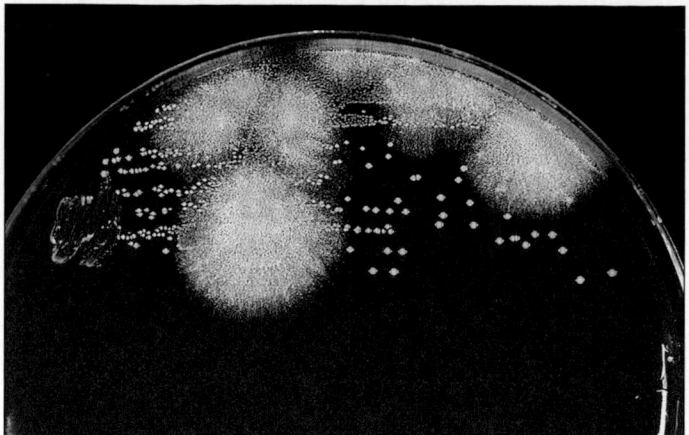

Figure 60–2 Green, powdery surface of the colonies of *Aspergillus fumigatus* overlies white masses of mycelium. Adjacent bacterial colonies contrast with the filamentous fungus. (Sheep blood agar)

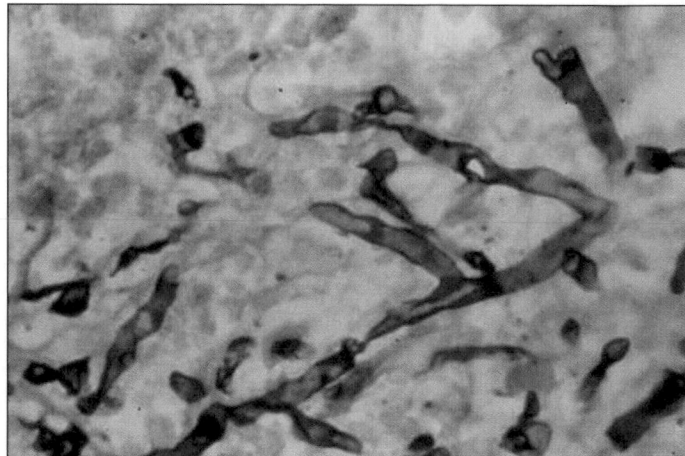

Figure 60–3 Characteristic wide, nonseptate hypha of a zygomycete in lung tissue. (Gomori's methenamine silver stain; ×400)

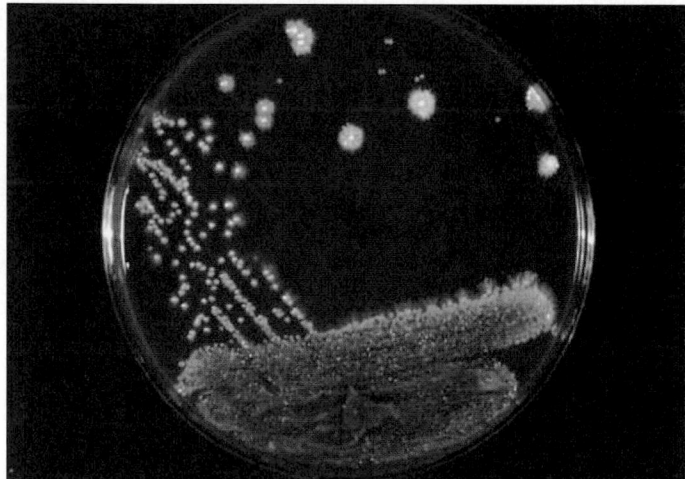

Figure 60–1 Filamentous extensions from the periphery of colonies of *Candida albicans* are known colloquially as feet.

and on agar media at 25–30°C. In contrast, the tissue form is either a yeast (such as *B. dermatitidis, H. capsulatum,* and *Sporothrix schenckii*) or, in the case of *Coccidioides immitis,* a yeast-like structure called a spherule. When cultivated in vitro at 37°C, the tissue form is reproduced by these fungi. Other less common or publicized agents also exhibit dimorphism. For instance, *Penicillium marneffei,* a distinctive member of that widely dispersed genus, grows as a mould on laboratory media at 25–30°C, but a yeast-like form is found in human tissues. The sclerotic bodies found in tissues of patients with chromoblastomycosis are a vegetative form arrested between a mould and yeast form of the dematiaceous fungi, which appear as moulds when grown on solid media at room temperature. Reverse dimorphism is exemplified by *Malassezia furfur,* which produces both yeast cells and hyphae in the cutaneous lesions of pityriasis versicolor. In the laboratory, the hyphal form is rarely seen unless special culture conditions are provided (Marcon, 1992).

Structure of Yeast and Hyphae

The morphology of the fungus is an important characteristic for the identification of both yeasts and moulds. The filamentous structure of a mould is referred to as hyphae (singular, hypha), with a mass of hyphae known as a mycelium. The mycelium growing on the surface of or within the agar is known as the vegetative mycelium, whereas filamentous extensions above the colony are called aerial mycelium. True hyphae may have crosswalls that contain pores for communication through the hyphae or crosswalls that are complete, dividing the hyphae into multiple cells. Hyphae that have crosswalls are called septate, whereas those without crosswalls are referred to as aseptate. Some fungi that have septate hyphae also have either aseptate or septate specialized hyphae (conidiophores) that bear asexual reproductive structures. Conversely, some so-called nonseptate fungi have occasional crosswalls and should perhaps be better designated as sparsely septate. It is important, therefore, to evaluate the mycelium as a whole.

The width of the hyphae and the angle of branching are important clues to the fungal identity. The Zygomycetes, such as *Rhizopus* spp., have broad, ribbon-like hyphae and branch predominantly at right angles (Fig. 60–3), whereas hyaline moulds such as *Aspergillus* spp. have narrow hyphae and branch at acute angles (dichotomous branching) (Fig. 60–4). The designation of a fungus as *Aspergillus* on the basis of hyphal morphology in a smear or tissue section is, in truth, only a statement of the a priori odds for this pathogen group. It is better simply to describe the characteristics of the hyphae.

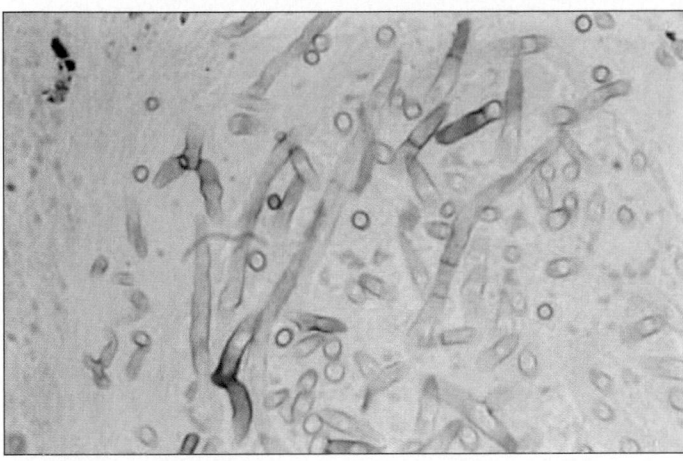

Figure 60–4 Characteristic narrow branching, septate hyphae of a hyaline mould in tissue, (Gomori's methenamine silver stain, ×400)

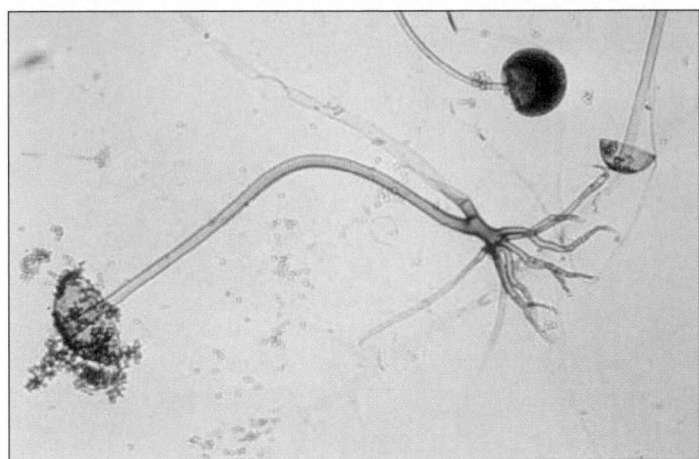

Figure 60–6 Sporangiophores of *Rhizopus* spp. supporting sporangia which contain sporangiospores. Rhizoids arise from the hyphae near the origin of the sporangiophores. (Lactophenol cotton blue stain; ×100)

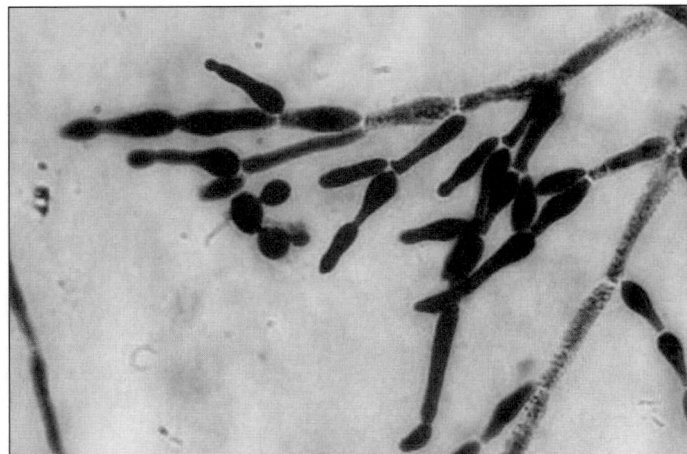

Figure 60–5 Chains of elongated budding yeasts of *Candida albicans* producing pseudohyphae observed in sputum. (Gram's stain; ×1000)

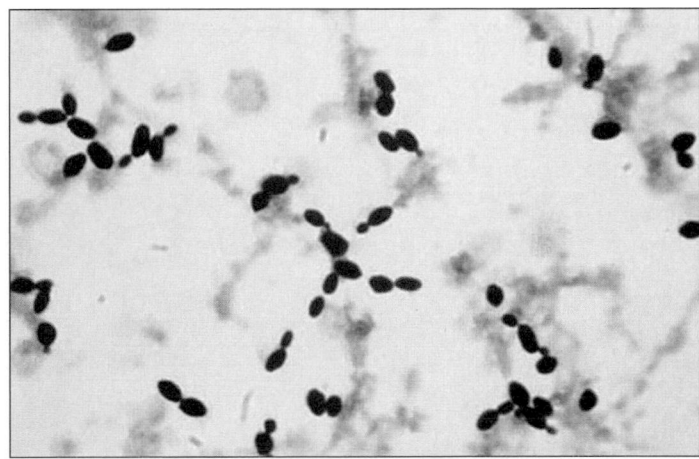

Figure 60–7 Budding and nonbudding yeast cells detected in a blood culture bottle sample. (Gram's stain; ×1000)

Yeasts reproduce asexually by the formation of blastoconidia where the daughter cell usually appears at one end of a yeast cell and eventually enlarges to form a new yeast cell. This process is also referred to in a more generic sense as budding. If a series of daughter cells do not detach fully from the originating cells, a pseudohypha (plural, pseudohyphae) is produced. Pseudohyphae are distinguished from true hyphae by the presence of a constriction at the junction of adjacent cells and the restriction in size of the daughter cell to that of the parent (Fig. 60–5). In contrast, the walls of true hyphae are parallel without constrictions. *C. albicans* and some strains of *Candida tropicalis* may produce pseudohyphae that have the appearance of true hyphae, depending on growth conditions, and differentiation of *Candida* from hyaline moulds such as *Aspergillus* in tissue sections on occasion may be problematic. In contradistinction, *Cryptococcus* spp. produces only budding yeast and rarely rudimentary or primitive pseudohyphae, but true hyphae are not formed.

Hyphal Pigment

Some mould hyphae can be characterized by the production of a dark pigment. The hyphae of dematiaceous fungi contain a melanin pigment that imparts a brown coloration to the hyphae in microscopic preparations and causes colonies of the fungi to appear dark green, brown, or black. Superimposed dyes in stained smears, wet preps, or histologic sections may partially obscure the color, which can be more obvious in unstained preparations. Those fungi that lack dark hyphal pigmentation are referred to as hyaline (clear or colorless). This term may not fully reflect the fungal species appearance, since in some cases a light pigmentation may produce colored colonies and asexual reproductive structures of some hyaline moulds may have green, brown, or black pigments that impart a color to the surface of the colony once the reproductive structures have formed. The true appearance of these moulds can usually be discerned by observing the back of the colony, which maintains a light coloration. In contrast, both the front (obverse) and back (reverse) of dematiaceous colonies usually demonstrate the dark pigment.

Reproductive Structures

The primary means for identification of mould fungi is by characterization of asexual reproductive structures. For yeast, phenotypic studies are the mainstay in identification with asexual reproductive structures serving as ancillary clues in the identification process. The two principal asexual structures are spores (which may also be present as sexual structures) and conidia. Asexual spores (called sporangiospores) are produced by cleavage within an encompassing structure called a sporangium (Fig. 60–6). Conidia (singular, conidium) are much more diverse and form by differentiation from the tip or side of a fertile hypha, such as a conidiophore, or by hyphal differentiation. Unfortunately, the interchangeable use of the terms conidium and spore in the literature has led to confusion. Sporulation and spores are often used as general terms for asexual reproduction, and the term spore is sometimes used when conidium would have been more accurate.

The principal means of asexual reproduction in yeast is by the formation of blastoconidia, i.e., budding. A bud starts as a softening of the cell wall of the mother cell, followed by expansion of the cell wall (blown out) and migration of nucleus and cytoplasm to the swollen area. A septum seals the boundary between the daughter and parent cell (Fig. 60–7). If separation does not occur, a pseudohypha results, as discussed earlier.

The portions of the vegetative mycelium that differentiate into conidia are referred to as conidiogenous cells. Specialized hyphae that support the conidia are termed conidiophores, which may be either the conidiogenous cell itself arising from the vegetative mycelium or may be a supporting hypha. In *Aspergillus* spp., the conidiophore, which is aseptate, enlarges at the tip to form a swollen vesicle (Fig. 60–8). Conidiogenous cells, now termed phialides (formerly sterigmata), arise from the vesicle to support

VII

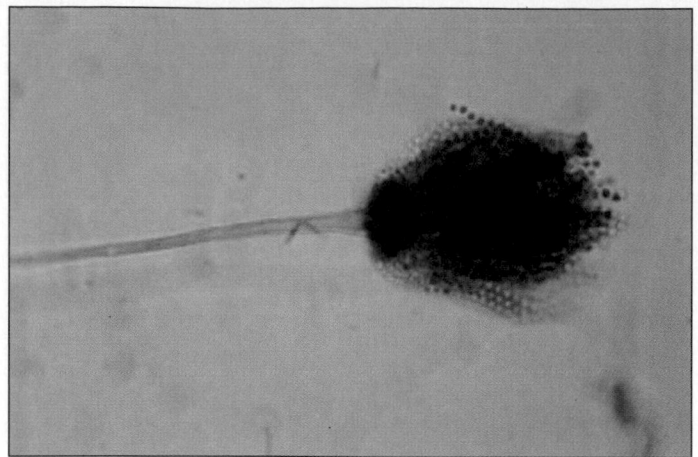

Figure 60–8 Fruiting head of *Aspergillus fumigatus*. The conidiophore is swollen at the tip to form a vesicle and phialides arise from the upper half of the vesicle with chains of conidia present that align parallel to the long axis of the conidiophore. (Lactophenol cotton blue stain; ×400)

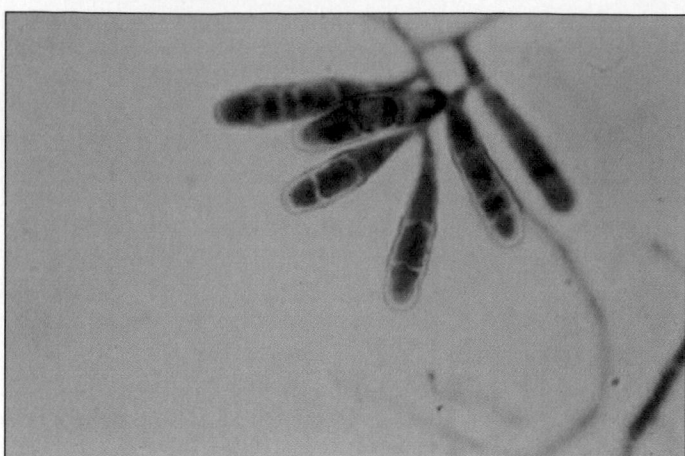

Figure 60–10 Macroconidia of *Epidermophyton floccosum*. The typical blunt-ended macroconidia occur in aggregates along the hyphae with the absence of microconidia. (Lactophenol cotton blue stain; ×400)

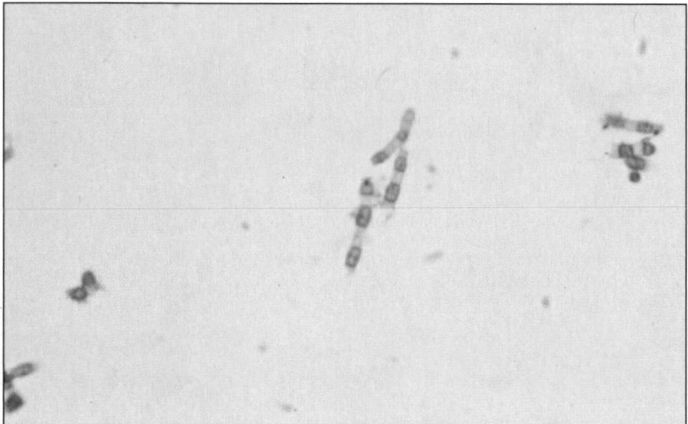

Figure 60–9 Arthroconidia of *Coccidioides immitis*. Alternating barrel-shaped arthroconidia are separated by thin-walled, empty disjunctor cells within portions of the hyphae. (Lactophenol cotton blue stain; ×400)

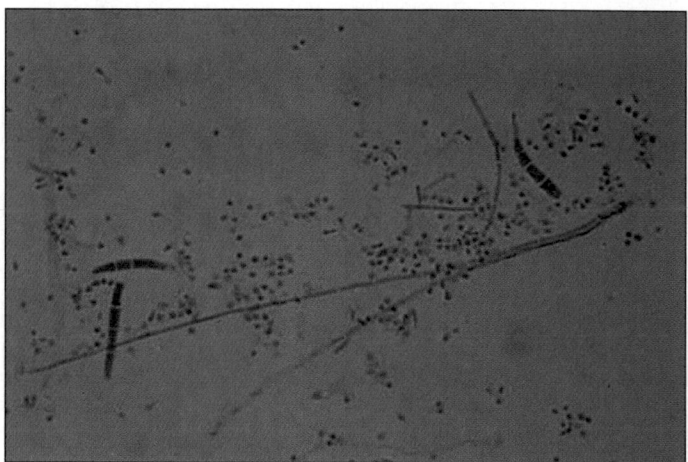

Figure 60–11 Elongated microconidia of *Trichophyton mentagrophytes* are lined up along the surface of the hypha. (Lactophenol aniline blue stain; ×400)

chains of conidia. Some species of *Aspergillus* produce a row of phialides, which occur on a row of sterile cells called metulae, with the conidia arising from the distal phialides. The Zygomycetes produce structures called sporangiophores that support the sporangium and its enclosed sporangiospores (Fig. 60–6). An extension of the apex of the sporangiophore into the sporangium is termed the columella.

Thallic conidiogenesis is a process in which the conidium does not develop until a septum is formed between the conidium and the parent cell. The conidium originates from the whole of the parent cell. The most important human pathogens that exhibit thallic conidiogenesis are the dermatophytes and the dimorphic fungus *C. immitis*. As conidiogenesis progresses in *Coccidioides*, barrel-shaped conidia called arthroconidia are produced that fragment easily and are disseminated with little difficulty, resulting in the high degree of infectivity demonstrated by this important human pathogen (Fig. 60–9). The thallic conidia of the dermatophytes are separated by size into two types, large septated macroconidia (Fig. 60–10) and small, one-celled microconidia that are simpler structures (Fig. 60–11).

The other type of conidiogenesis is called blastic conidiogenesis, where the protoplasm of the conidiogenous cell is blown out or blasted to form the conidium. The simplest form of blastic conidiogenesis is the budding process by which many yeast, including *Candida* spp., develop. As with thallic conidia, blastoconidia are divided into two types, dependent on whether the entire cell wall is or is not involved in the process. A further division of blastic conidiogenesis is made among those species in which the outer cell wall does not participate in the process (called enteroblastic conidiogenesis). In enteroblastic fungi, phialidic and annellidic conidiogenous cells have been recognized. Phialides are conidiogenous cells that often have a collarette at the apices, produced when the tip releases the first conidium. The collarette may be a conspicuous, flask-shaped structure, as observed in *Phialophora* spp., or an inconspicuous structure, as seen in *Aspergillus* spp. In contrast, annellides are conidiogenous cells that rupture to

leave a distinct ring of cellular material at the base of the conidium when it separates from the annellide. Formation of sequential conidia at the base pushes the oldest cell to the tip of the chain and leaves a series of rings or annellations at the apex of the annellide, providing a record of past events, like rings on a tree. Although important for the microscopic identification of some mould fungi, the fine details of these structures may be difficult to visualize using the light microscope.

The differentiation of the various conidial structures is the key to correct identification of many fungal isolates. In some cases, the pertinent morphologic features are easily discerned; however, as in surgical pathology, pattern recognition is an essential tool for identification of the most common pathogens and saprobes. It is also important to appreciate the salient features of the entire morphologic preparation without primarily focusing on outliers or aberrant structures, just as it is important for the surgical pathologist to appreciate the tissue pattern without being distracted by an occasional atypical cell. Developing conidial structures of *Aspergillus* or *Paecilomyces*, for instance, may resemble the structures of *Penicillium*, and the observer must not be misled into thinking that two moulds are present. At the same time, the possibility of a mixed culture must be remembered. Mycologists must use a low-powered objective for initial observation, however: the detail of cellular subsets in that low-powered picture must be appreciated for study at a higher magnification.

The fine art of mycologic diagnosis rests in the appreciation and differentiation of the cellular details, and in some instances the task requires great subtlety and considerable experience. Sometimes, the isolate must be coaxed to produce the necessary diagnostic structures by selection of the appropriate media (Table 60–3). In general, enriched media favor the propagation of vegetative mycelium, whereas asexual reproductive structures are encouraged by basal (starving) media. Subculture on to water agar or potato flake agar is a general technique for encouraging the development of conidial structures. The colors of *Aspergillus* colonies are best studied on

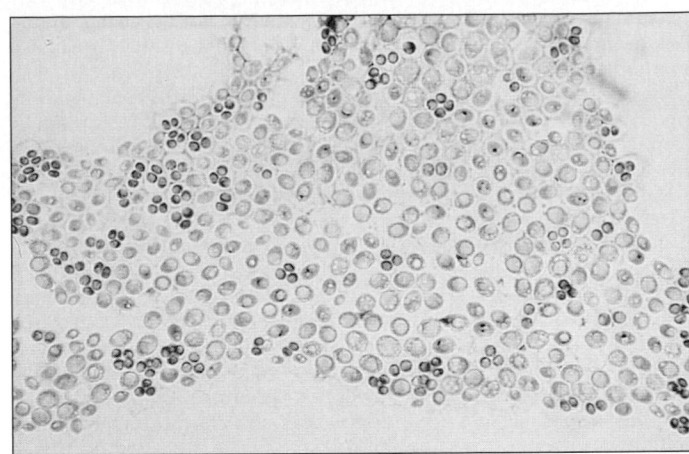

Table 60–3 Media for the Identification and Isolation of Fungi

Medium	Main function
Ascospore medium, V-8 agar	Ascospore development
Bird (niger) seed agar	Demonstration of melanin in *Cryptococcus neoformans*
Brain–heart infusion agar with blood	To enhance recovery of dimorphic fungi
Christensen urea agar	Differentiation of *Trichophyton rubrum* and *T. mentagrophytes*
CHROMagar	Chromagenic mixture to identify yeast species
Cornmeal agar with Tween 80	Visualize yeast morphology
Czapek-Dox agar	Identification of *Aspergillus* species
Potato dextrose agar with 1% glucose	Pigment development of *T. rubrum* and mould morphology
Potato flake agar	Pigment development of *T. rubrum* and mould morphology
Sabouraud dextrose (SAB) agar	General purpose fungal growth medium (traditional formulation or Emmon's modification)
SAB agar with cycloheximide	Selective medium to inhibit saprophytic fungi (antibacterials such as chloramphenicol or gentamicin also included)
Slide culture (various agars)	Study of microscopic structure and its origin
Trichophyton agars	Differentiation of *Trichophyton* species

Figure 60–12 Ascospores of *Saccharomyces cerevisiae* are contained in naked asci. The ascospores are colored red by the acid-fast stain. (Ziehl–Neelsen stain, ×1000)

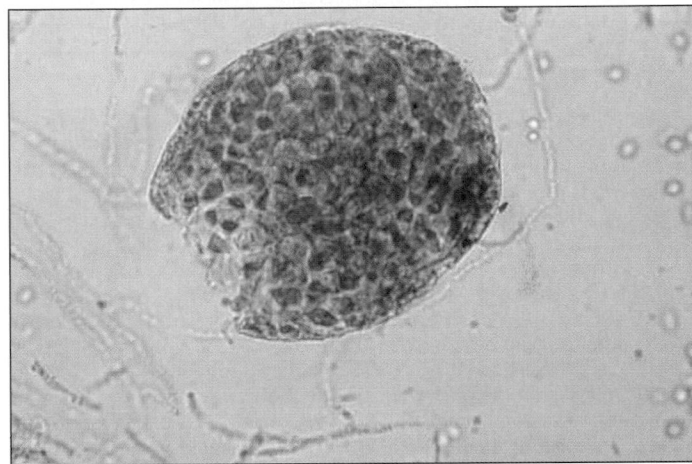

Figure 60–13 Cleistothecium of *Pseudallescheria boydii*. This sexual reproductive structure is specifically referred to as an ascus containing ascospores. (Lactophenol cotton blue stain; ×400)

Czapek–Dox agar, whereas *Trichophyton rubrum* is encouraged to produce red pigment on potato flake agar or cornmeal agar with 1% glucose.

Experience also is important to determine whether a subculture has been incubated sufficiently long for the diagnostic structures to form. Root-like structures (rhizoids) that develop from the hyphae of some zygomycetes are important differentiating features, but they may not be detected if observation is terminated prematurely. It must be admitted that some of the techniques necessary for complete differentiation are difficult or even beyond the reach of most clinical laboratories. For instance, the dematiaceous pathogen *Exophiala (Wangiella) dermatitidis* produces blastic conidia with phialides and annellides. The presence of annellides was not recognized when the mould was studied with the light microscope, however, and this organism was once classified as *Phialophora dermatitidis*. Recognition that annellides were formed by the isolate led to its assignment to a new genus, *Exophiala*, which contained both phialides and annellides. However, the genus *Wangiella* continues to be suggested, since the phialides do not reproduce obvious collarettes, which is the predominate feature of this genus. Subsequently, there continues to remain a disagreement as to whether this species belongs in the genus *Exophiala* or in the genus *Wangiella* (McGinnis, 1999).

Sexual reproductive structures are of occasional value in the general mycology laboratory for the identification of common pathogens and saprophytes. A variety of sexual structures may be produced, although they are infrequently encountered in vitro. The two structures most likely to be demonstrated in the laboratory are the naked asci of *Saccharomyces cerevisiae* and the cleistothecium of *P. boydii* (the sexual phase of *S. apiospermum*), *Aspergillus nidulans*, or the *Aspergillus glaucus* group. The naked asci of *Saccharomyces* resemble oval yeast cells in which one to four individual haploid ascospores are enclosed (Fig 60–12). Ascospore formation in *Saccharomyces* spp. can be encouraged by incubation on certain agar media, such as V-8 juice agar, but this effort usually is not necessary, since commercial yeast identification systems can readily identify the isolate. The ascospores may be visualized in wet preparations but are detected more reliably using an acid-fast stain. A cleistothecium is a sexual fruiting body (ascocarp) in which the ascospores are entirely enclosed and can only be released by rupture of the cleistothecial wall (Fig. 60–13). The wall is composed of single or multiple layers of specialized hyphae. A perithecium is similar to a cleistothecium but contains an opening at the apex of the pear-shaped structure.

Although asexual and rarely sexual reproductive structures are necessary for the identification of fungi, especially moulds, some isolates refuse to produce either of these structures for diagnosis. The colonies consist only of vegetative and aerial hyphae morphologically and are subsequently described as sterile hyphae or mycelia sterilia. The identification under this circumstance requires specialized molecular methods which are not available in most routine diagnostic laboratories (Yeo, 2002; Iwen, 2003).

Dimorphism

Demonstration of dimorphism is the traditional approach to definitive identification of an important group of systemic pathogens. In most laboratories, the initial isolate is the mould phase because the culture plates usually are incubated at 25–30°C. Conversion to the tissue phase is accomplished by incubating a subculture at 37°C. The transition from mould to yeast morphology may occur grudgingly, and hyphal forms are often intermixed with the yeast cells. Some isolates may never be successfully converted. A rich medium, such as brain–heart infusion agar with a blood supplement, should be included, particularly when working with *H. capsulatum*. Brain-heart infusion agar or cysteine hemoglobin agar has been recommended for optimal conversion of *B. dermatitidis*. Media for conversion of *C. immitis* have been described but are not often used. Similarly, inoculation of animals is infrequently employed in clinical laboratories. Introduction of molecular probes has considerably simplified the task of definitive identification for these fungi and eliminated the need to demonstrate both phases of the dimorphic fungi (Reiss, 2000). Nucleic acid hybridization tests for these three dimorphic pathogens are marketed by GEN-PROBE, Inc. (San Diego, CA). Demonstration of the characteristic yeast or yeast-like phase in tissue strongly supports the diagnosis of a dimorphic fungus; however, culture of the pathogen with identification is still necessary for disease confirmation.

Diagnostic Techniques

Laboratory Safety

Inoculation of specimens and manipulations of mould colonies should be performed in a biological safety cabinet to prevent dissemination of the highly mobile fungal conidia and spores. Scrupulous attention to cleaning

VII

the surfaces of both the biological safety cabinet and incubator should also be maintained. Separate safety cabinets for the study of isolated moulds may minimize contamination of other clinical samples.

The greatest hazard to laboratory personnel comes from handling mould cultures of the dimorphic pathogens *C. immitis* and *H. capsulatum*. Both of these isolates are classified as risk group 3 pathogens, requiring biosafety level 3 practices and facilities for propagating and manipulating of cultures, as well as for the processing of soil or other environmental materials known or likely to contain infectious conidia (Department of Health and Human Services, 1999). Kwon-Chung and Bennett (Kwon-Chung, 1992) recommend inoculating screw-capped tubes if these pathogens are suspected. Unfortunately, in most areas of the United States, the diagnosis may not be appreciated before the pathogen is isolated. The plate can be flooded with 4% formaldehyde solution (10% formalin) and left at room temperature for several hours or overnight to sterilize the culture before microscopic examination is performed. Obviously, such a course is irreversible, so it is best to have colonies growing on other plates or tubes as a reserve.

It is worth noting that the tissue phase of dimorphic pathogens is not infectious by the airborne route, so there is little or no biohazard in handling tissue specimens from patients with histoplasmosis or coccidioidomycosis. A possible exception to this rule might occur if *C. immitis* grew in its mould phase within a lung cavity that connected with the bronchial tree.

Specimen Collection and Transport

The correct specimen for submission to the mycology laboratory depends on the clinical presentation and the organ system affected. A summary of the major categories of disease produced by fungi, along with suggested specimens, is presented in Table 60–4.

Yeast, particularly *Candida* spp., may be recovered on occasion from swab specimens, especially from purulent lesions. Swabs may be used for sampling oral or vaginal lesions suggestive of candidiasis and may be adequate for collecting specimens from patients with chronic external otitis, in which large numbers of *Aspergillus* conidia are usually present. Swabs are, however, decidedly inferior tools for collecting specimens in most areas of infectious disease. Particularly troubling is that swab fibers may be mistaken for hyphal elements upon direct examination of clinical specimens. A firm but politically flexible policy of rejecting swabs under most cases for fungal culture should be accompanied by assiduous and persistent educational efforts.

The best specimens for mycologic diagnosis are scrapings, curettings, aspirates, and lesion biopsies. Hairs infected with dermatophytic fungi (e.g., *Microsporum canis*) fluoresce under a long-wavelength ultraviolet light (Wood's lamp) and can be specifically selected for examination. The cutaneous lesions of dermatophytosis (ringworm) are characterized by an active advancing edge with central healing, so that scrapings can be collected from the edge of the process. Hair, nails, and skin scrapings should be sent to the laboratory in a clean, dry container. Biopsy samples should be sent in a sterile container with sterile saline or a transport medium to prevent drying of the sample. Most samples can be handled as one would any other samples submitted for bacterial observation and culture.

Direct Examination

Most clinical specimens can be examined directly for the presence of a fungal pathogen, although negative results are not sensitive enough to rule out the presence of a fungus. Multiple techniques are employed for the direct examination of clinical material. It is important to remember that the manipulation of specimen material may render the material not acceptable for culture, so, in those cases where culture is warranted, specimens must be separated before performing this type of examination.

Wet Preparation
The simplest method for direct examination of a specimen is the observation of a suspension placed on a slide and cover slip under reduced light. For those specimens that are dry or viscous, the addition of a wetting agent such as saline is necessary prior to observation. For specimens that contain distracting tissue debris and cells, such as vaginal secretions, nails, and skin scrapings, a solution of potassium hydroxide (KOH) may be used as a means to dissolve the tissue material so the fungal elements may be more visible (Table 60–5).

Gram Stain
This commonly used microbiologic stain is particularly useful for the detection of yeast. Most yeast stain partially or completely gram-positive and are generally differentiated from the bacteria due to their larger size and by the presence of budding cells (Fig. 60–5). The hyphae of moulds appear either gram-positive or gram-negative by this stain but stain less reliably than yeast cells and are easily missed in clinical specimens using this method.

Giemsa or Wright stains
In cases where histoplasmosis is suspected, these hematologic stains are useful for demonstrating the yeast cells within macrophages.

India Ink Preparation
The polysaccharide capsule of *C. neoformans* can be demonstrated by negative staining using India ink particles; especially evident when examining infected cerebrospinal fluid (Table 60–6). When examined with the light microscope, the capsule stands out as a clear space around the fungal cell, with ink particles bouncing off the edge as brownian motion occurs (Fig. 60–14). When budding yeast cells are demonstrated along with the capsule in the cerebrospinal fluid of infected patients, the specificity of the diagnosis of cryptococcal meningitis is ensured. Other potentially encapsulated fungi, such as *Rhodotorula* spp. or other cryptococcal species, are infrequent pathogens and can be eliminated from practical consideration under this circumstance. Although the capsules are usually large in direct examination of specimens, isolation of the pathogen on agar media is usually characterized with the production of a much diminished capsule that is not so obvious. Unfortunately, some *C. neoformans* strains are poorly encapsulated and therefore the sensitivity of the India ink test is generally less than 50% in patients who are not infected with human immunodeficiency virus (HIV). The direct detection of antigen in cerebrospinal fluid or serum, however, using a latex agglutination or enzyme immunoassay technique has increased the sensitivity to close to 100%. These techniques have basically replaced the use of India ink as a direct diagnostic technique, although the India ink technique is still useful when the antigen test is not immediately available and for examination of capsules in cells from isolated colonies that suggest *C. neoformans*. The India ink test appears to have greater sensitivity in patients who are infected with HIV, perhaps because of the greater number of yeast cells present (Chuck, 1989).

Histochemical Stains
Surgical pathologic examination of biopsy material is a common practice for the identification of suspect fungal infections. A number of stains have proved to be useful to recognize fungal elements in tissue and to show the immunologic response to infection. The periodic-acid–Schiff (PAS) method is useful for demonstrating internal details. The Gomori's methenamine silver (GMS) technique is considered one of the better stains for demonstrating fungi because it provides high contrast with minimal background staining, thus allowing for the demonstration of sparsely present fungal elements in the sample. The hematoxylin and eosin (H&E) stain is best used for studying the host reaction and for determining whether a fungus is hyaline (colorless) or dematiaceous (naturally pigmented). When the GMS stain is combined with H&E as a counterstain, the detailed morphology of both tissue and fungus can be studied (Swisher, 1982). Other more specialized stains include Mayer's mucicarmine stain for the demonstration of the mucoid capsule of *C. neoformans* and the Fontana–Masson stain for the demonstration of melanin or melanin-like substances in the lightly pigmented agents of phaeohyphomycosis. A book by Chandler and Kaplan (Chandler, 1987a) gives more details of the use of stains to detect fungi in tissue.

Calcofluor White Stain
This fluorochrome compound, a whitener used in the textile and paper industries, binds to the chitin in the walls of fungal cells and fluoresces white (Fig. 60–15) or apple green (depending on the filter combination used) when exposed to short-wavelength ultraviolet light from a fluorescence microscope (Table 60–7) (Hageage, 1984). Calcofluor white can also be mixed with potassium hydroxide to clear the specimen for easier observation of fungi. As is true with all fluorescent staining, care must be used in interpreting the results, since nonspecific staining of substances that resemble fungal elements may also occur.

Isolation in Culture

Selection of *Media*
All specimens should be inoculated on to a general purpose fungal growth medium (Table 60–3). The traditional medium used is Sabouraud dextrose agar, which has a pH of 5.5–5.6 and was designed for the isolation of dermatophytic fungi. Emmons's modification of Sabouraud dextrose agar, which contains less glucose, with a pH of 6.8–7.0, is more widely used in the clinical mycology lab as a general growth medium because of its wide application for the culture of fungi. Inhibitory mould agar and potato dextrose agar are also used as general isolation medium in

Table 60–4 Major Clinical Syndromes and Commonly Associated Pathogens

Clinical Presentation/ Organ System	Patient Group	Likely Pathogen(s)	Specimen(s)
Skin, hair, or nail infection	All	Dermatophytes *Candida* *Malassezia*	Skin scraping Hair Nail clipping
Subcutaneous tissues	All	*Coccidioides immitis* *Blastomyces dermatitidis* *Sporothrix schenckii*	Lesion biopsy
	Patient with mycetoma	*Scedosporium apiospermum* *Madurella* *Nocardia** *Streptomyces** *Actinomadura**	
Primary pneumonia	All	*Histoplasma capsulatum* *Blastomyces dermatitidis* *Cryptococcus neoformans*	Sputum Bronchoalveolar lavage Transbronchial biopsy Surgical lung biopsy
	Immunodeficient	*Aspergillus* *Fusarium* Zygomycetes *Scedosporium apiospermum* *Pneumocystis jiroveci*	
Gastrointestinal infection	Immunodeficient	*Candida* *Aspergillus* Zygomycetes	Scrapings Curettings Lesion, biopsy
Urinary tract infection	All	*Candida*	Urine
Endocarditis	All	*Candida* *Fusarium*	Blood
Meningitis	Immunodeficient	*Cryptococcus neoformans* *Candida*	Cerebrospinal fluid
Encephalitis and brain abscess	Immunodeficient	Zygomycetes *Aspergillus* *Nocardia asteroides** *Cladophialophora bantiana*	Brain biopsy
Osteomyelitis	All	*Coccidioides immitis* *Blastomyces dermatitidis* *Cryptococcus neoformans*	Bone biopsy
Keratitis	All	*Aspergillus* *Fusarium*	Scraping
External otitis	All	*Aspergillus*	Scraping Swab
Sinusitis	All	*Aspergillus* *Fusarium* Dematiaceous moulds	Biopsy Curettings
Burn wounds		*Aspergillus* Zygomycetes *Fusarium* *Scedosporium apiospermum*	Skin biopsy
Vaginitis	All	*Candida*	Vaginal secretions
Intravenous catheter infection	Indwelling catheter	*Candida* *Malassezia furfur* (newborns)	Catheter tip Blood
Disseminated infection	All	*Histoplasma capsulatum* *Blastomyces dermatitidis* *Coccidioides immitis*	Blood Tissue biopsy
	Immunodeficient	*Candida* Zygomycetes *Aspergillus* *Fusarium* *Scedosporium apiospermum* *Cryptococcus neoformans* Potentially any fungus	Blood Tissue biopsy

* Bacterial pathogens

the laboratory. Rinaldi (1982) described a simplified modification of potato dextrose agar that uses a preparation of potato flakes available in grocery stores. It is easier to prepare than the traditional potato-based medium and functions equivalently. Potato flake agar is advantageous for moulds, because the diagnostically useful asexual reproductive structures develop more readily on this agar than on Sabouraud dextrose medium.

For specimens from nonsterile sites or sites that are likely to be contaminated, inoculation of a nonselective agar and a selective agar in

VII

Table 60–5 KOH Preparation

1. Place one drop of 10% KOH (potassium hydroxide) on a clean glass slide.
2. Immerse an aliquot of the specimen in the drop of KOH on the slide.
3. Gently heat the mixture by passing the slide through a Bunsen burner flame several times. Do not allow the mixture to boil.
4. Cover slip the slide and examine at 100× and 400× magnification using reduced light. Excessively tenacious specimens may require additional heating.
5. KOH may also be used as a simple mounting medium without heating.

(The addition of lactophenol aniline blue or Calcofluor white stain with the KOH will enhance the visibility of fungal elements.)

Table 60–6 India Ink Preparation for Presumptive Identification of *Cryptococcus neoformans*.

1. Centrifuge the cerebrospinal fluid for a minimum of 10 minutes.
2. Place one drop of India ink on a clean glass slide.
3. Mix with a drop of sediment obtained from the spun fluid and cover slip.
4. Search for encapsulated yeast using the 400× magnification.

(Colonies growing on agar may also be mixed directly with India ink on a slide to confirm the presence of capsules.)

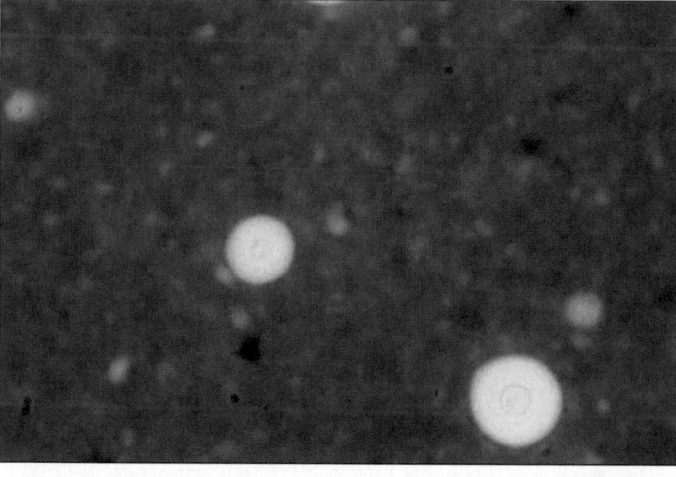

Figure 60–14 India ink preparation of cerebrospinal fluid containing *Cryptococcus neoformans*. This yeast produces a characteristic polysaccharide capsule around the budding yeast cells (×400)

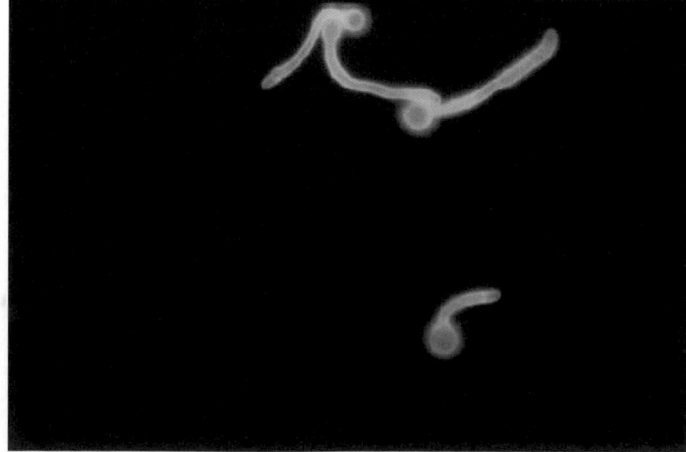

Figure 60–15 Calcofluor white stain of *Candida albicans* in culture. When viewed with a fluorescence microscope the chitinous walls of the fungus will fluoresce. Germ tubes are shown, which are produced following incubation of the yeast in serum. (Courtesy of Dr Brian Harrington, CDC Public Health Image Library)

Table 60–7 Calcofluor White Stain

1. Place specimen on a clean glass slide.
2. Mix with Calcofluor white reagent.
3. Using a fluorescent microscope, examine the preparation for fungal elements at 100–400× magnification (will typically appear bluish white against a dark background).

(Calcofluor white may be substituted for lactophenol aniline blue stain when studying microscopic morphology of culture isolates.)

tandem is recommended. The most commonly employed selective agars employ cycloheximide to inhibit saprophytic fungi and an antibacterial agent (usually chloramphenicol or gentamicin) to inhibit bacteria. For tissue specimens, especially when a dimorphic fungus might be the etiologic agent, an enriched agar, such as brain–heart infusion agar with blood and supplemented with antibiotics may be added.

A recent addition for the cultivation of yeast from clinical specimens is the selective and differential medium called CHROMagar *Candida*. This medium uses a chromagenic mixture that allows selective isolation of yeasts and simultaneously identifies colonies of *C. albicans*, *C. tropicalis*, *C. glabrata*, and *Candida krusei*. This medium has proven to be useful to detect mixed cultures of *Candida* spp. within a single specimen (Pfaller, 1996).

Inoculation and Incubation

The processing of clinical specimens for fungal detection requires careful handing since some processes commonly used to prepare specimens for bacterial culture, e.g., grinding in a homogenizer, may be too disruptive for the fungal organism. Inoculation of scrapings or curettings on to and into the agar at multiple points of the agar surface is a reliable technique for culture. Tissue should be teased or minced, after which the fragments are similarly inoculated.

Plates or tubes should be incubated in ambient air at 25–30°C. A controlled temperature incubator is essential. It is not necessary to incubate parallel plates or tubes at 37°C for recovery of the yeast phase of dimorphic fungi, because little additional yield results. Most fungi grow within a 2-week incubation period and, among commonly isolated fungi, only the dimorphic fungi such as *H. capsulatum* and *B. dermatitidis* are frequently detected after 14 days of incubation. General recommendations for incubation time are 7 days to detect for the presence of yeast in mouth, throat, or vagina; 21 days to detect for fungal pathogens in tissues and sterile body fluids other than blood; and up to 28 days for respiratory, bone marrow, blood specimens, and specimens in which a dimorphic fungus is suspect. In general, all other specimens should be incubated for up to 14 days. Plates should be examined at least twice during the first week, when rapidly growing isolates may appear, and at least weekly thereafter.

Blood cultures

Recovery of fungi from blood requires special attention and can be accomplished by inoculating broth media, by using a biphasic broth-agar system, or by the lysis centrifugation technique (Isolator, Wampole, Cranbury, NJ). The Isolator system consists of a tube containing a solution that lyses erythrocytes and leukocytes (Cockerill, 1996, Reimer, 1997). After the blood is drawn into the tube by vacuum, the lysed contents, including any microbes, are centrifuged into a pellet, which is removed and plated on to the surface of agar plates. The Isolator system has been proven to be especially valuable for the detection of *H. capsulatum* in blood. Although the Isolator system is considered the most sensitive method for detection of fungemia, this system is also somewhat more susceptible to contamination, either through handling of the system during processing or by airborne spores that settle on to the agar plates (Reimer, 1997). Since a high percentage of fungemias are caused by yeast, development of continuous-read automated culture methods have become the mainstay for detection including the BACTEC system (Becton Dickinson, Sparks, MD) or the BacT-Alert system (Organon Teknika, Durham, NC). Since yeasts are aerobic organisms, aerobic culture bottles are employed for detection. Bottles with specific lysis medium are available, but many laboratories have had success using the standard blood culture bottles for fungal detection. Molecular methods had proved to be useful for the identification of fungal species directly from blood culture bottles (Iwen, 2004). These methods show applicability as potential rapid and reliable techniques for the identification of fungi.

Growth Rate

The rate of growth of fungal isolates provides a useful clue to diagnostic possibilities. In general, the pathogenic dimorphic and dematiaceous

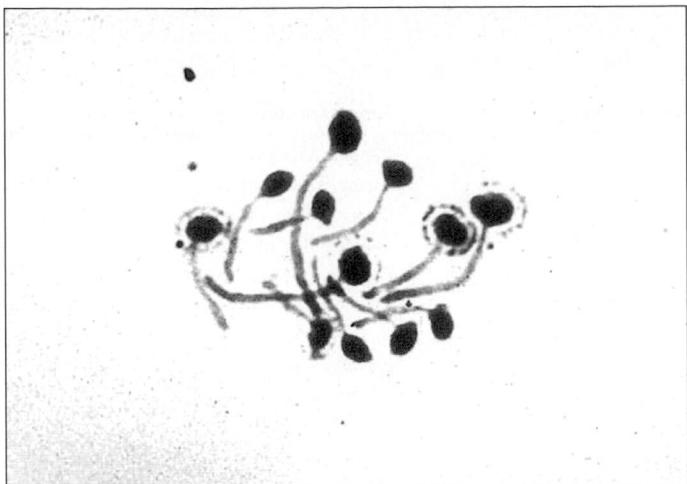

Figure 60–16 Germ tubes have extended from the yeast cells of *Candida albicans*. There is no constriction at the junction of yeast cell and germ tube. The walls of the germ tube are parallel. Human serum was incubated for two hours at 37°C. (Gram stain×400)

fungi grow slower, requiring a week or more for colonies to appear. The significance of rapid growing mould colonies that appear after prolonged incubation on mycologic media should be questioned as possible contaminants. However, there are many exceptions to this generalization and laboratory staff need to be aware that fungi such as *C. immitis*, a classic pathogen, may grow quickly on nonfungal medium. Protocols on how to handle fungal growth on bacterial cultures are needed to prevent unnecessary exposure of laboratory personnel to highly infectious fungal pathogens that may be encountered.

Growth Temperature

Growth at an elevated temperature is occasionally a useful differential tool in the identification of fungi. Most moulds grow best at 25–30°C. Most yeasts however, grow well at 35–37°C and are often recovered first on enriched blood agar plates in the bacteriology laboratory. In some cases, growth of a fungus at elevated temperatures is useful for the differentiation of species.

Morphologic Identification

Some of the morphologic studies necessary for the identification of fungal isolates can be accomplished with colonies from the original isolation plates but it is often necessary to transfer portions of colonies to new or different media (subculture) in order to demonstrate diagnostic structures. Table 60–3 describes some of the common media used for the identification of fungal species. One of the more common medium used is cornmeal agar supplemented with Tween 80 (CM-T80) for the visualization of yeast morphology. The recognition of pseudohyphae with chlamydoconidia on this medium is confirmatory for *C. albicans*. Other morphologic features can help to categorize the yeast into groups to assist in the separation into species. Although biochemical tests are important for identifying yeast isolates, morphologic examination provides an important check on the biochemical information, especially if a commercial identification system has been used.

Yeast Morphology

The germ tube test is an important initial step in the identification of yeast isolates. Germ tubes, which are elongated, finger-like extensions from a yeast cell, are the beginnings of a true hypha (Fig. 60–16). This structure can be differentiated from pseudohyphae by the lack of a constriction at the junction of germ tube and yeast cell and by the parallel cell walls in the germ tube. True germ tubes are formed by both *C. albicans* and *Candida dubliniensis* after growth in serum at 37°C for no longer than 4 hours. In many laboratories with well trained staff, the germ tube in combination with results of morphology on CM-T80 agar is considered confirmatory for the identification of *C. albicans/C. dubliniensis*.

The traditional germ tube test involves inoculation of a tube of serum (Table 60-8). After observation of the isolate for germ tubes at 37°C, incubation is continued for subsequent study of hyphal morphology and chlamydoconidia formation at 25–30°C. Thus, all the information necessary can be collected with one procedure. Cornmeal agar may be substituted but, regardless of the medium used, incubation conditions must be carefully controlled and the test monitored with controls in order to

Table 60–8 Serum Germ Tube Test

1. Aseptically transfer several colonies of yeast to a 12 × 75 mm test tube containing approximately 0.5 mL of serum (human, fetal calf, bovine or rabbit).
2. Incubate the tube at 37°C for 2–4 hours.
3. Place one drop of the mixture on a clean glass slide and cover slip.
4. Examine for germ tubes using 400× magnification and reduced light.

Table 60–9 Yeast Morphology Test

1. Streak a light inoculum of yeast onto a section of a cornmeal agar containing Tween 80.
2. Cover slip the area inoculated.
3. Incubate at 25–30°C for 24–72 hours.
4. Observe under 100× and 400× magnification using reduced light for morphologic structures.

Table 60–10 Rapid Testing for Presumptive Identification of Yeast Following Formation of Colonies

Characteristic	Likely organism
Urease production	*Cryptococcus neoformans*
Germ tube production	*Candida albicans*
Pseudohyphae present	*Candida* species
Chlamydospores present	*Candida albicans*
Lipid growth requirement	*Malassezia furfur*
Red colonial pigmentation	*Rhodotorula* species
Ascospore formation	*Saccharomyces cerevisiae*
Trehalose assimilation	*Candida glabrata*

achieve good results. The traditional Dalmau technique for demonstration of chlamydoconidia on cornmeal agar is detailed in Table 60–9 (McGinnis, 1980).

Mould Morphology

The simplest method for examination of moulds is the Cellophane tape mount, using clear tape and staining with lactophenol aniline (cotton) blue (LPAB) stain. If diagnostic structures are not observed, incubation can be continued and the process repeated. The traditional method for observing mould morphology is to tease the mycelium apart with inoculating needles and examine the teased hyphae with LPAB stain.

Occasionally, it may be necessary to perform a slide culture to preserve easily disrupted conidial structures in their original relationships. The classic approach involves cutting squares of an appropriate agar medium (usually Sabouraud dextrose or potato dextrose agar) which are suspended on a slide supported by glass rods in a Petri dish to which sterile water is added for maintenance of humidity.

If a mould isolate is suspected of being a dimorphic fungus (e.g., growth on cycloheximide-containing medium), a slide culture should not be performed and a Cellophane tape test or teased preparation should be examined only after the preparation has been sealed in a biosafety cabinet certified for use. Lactophenol aniline blue is fungicidal, but sealing the cover slip with nail polish before observation provides additional protection. Alternatively, the culture may be flooded with 10% formalin (4% formaldehyde solution) and incubated at room temperature overnight before manipulating the mould.

Biochemical Identification

Biochemical tests are at the heart of identification schemes for yeast and are occasionally useful for the identification of moulds. A number of rapid tests for the presumptive identification of yeast are given in Table 60–10.

Biochemical characterization of yeast may be accomplished by study of fermentation or assimilation patterns. Assimilation testing, which is used more extensively in the laboratory, assesses the ability of an isolate to use a carbohydrate as the sole source of carbon needed for growth or of nitrate as the sole source of nitrogen. The Wickerham auxanographic method uses a basal medium in which a particular carbohydrate or nitrate serves as the nutrient. Growth of the yeast is the end point of a positive test. This rather cumbersome reference method is not detailed because it has been replaced in most laboratories by one of five commercial identifications systems: API 20C (BioMérieux, Hazelwood, MO), Vitek Systems (BioMérieux, Hazelwood, MO), MicroScan (Dade Behring MicroScan, Sacramento, CA), the UniYeastTek System (Remel Laboratories, Lenexa, KS), and the RapID Yeast Plus System (Innovative Diagnostics Systems, Norcross, GA). All five systems perform well, as judged by reports in the literature and by proficiency testing surveys of the College of American Pathologists (Dooley, 1994; Fenn, 1994; Riddle, 1994; Crist, 1996; Bernal, 1998; Espinel-Ingroff, 1998; Ramani, 1998). Since no one system is known to be 100% accurate for the identification of yeast species, a combination of methods is usually considered.

In addition to fermentation and assimilation studies, stimulation of growth by biochemical compounds is a secondary test in the differentiation of certain *Trichophyton* spp. (Weitzman, 1983). Inclusion of inositol and thiamine in various combinations into agar media (*Trichophyton* agars) allows assessment of growth-stimulating properties. The end point of the test, relative growth in comparison to a basal medium, is subjective and both positive and negative controls should be included.

The test for urease production in cryptococci is of general utility in the clinical laboratory to differentiate cryptococci from *Candida* spp., particularly in respiratory specimens (Canteros, 1996). *C. neoformans* is a pulmonary and systemic pathogen, whereas *Candida* spp. are frequent inhabitants of the upper airways but uncommon causes of primary pneumonia. Urease may be produced by other nonpathogenic species of *Cryptococcus*, by *Rhodotorula* species, and by some isolates of *Trichosporon beigelii* and *C. krusei*. Urease production can be tested by inoculation of the yeast isolate on to a slant of Christensen urea agar or into urea broth. Alkalinization of the medium after production of NH_3 by urea-splitting organisms is detected by inclusion of a pH indicator in the system. Colonies that have macroscopically visible pseudohyphae (feet) or that grow on cycloheximide-containing agar need not be tested, because *Cryptococcus* does not produce pseudohyphae in vitro and does not grow in the presence of cycloheximide.

Biochemical tests also play an ancillary role in the identification of dermatophytic moulds. Production of urease within 4 days helps differentiate *Trichophyton mentagrophytes* (urease-positive) from *T. rubrum* (urease-negative). The isolate should be subcultured to a slant of Christensen urea agar and incubated at 25–30°C for at least 3 days. A positive reaction is strong production of urease, evidenced by alkalinization of the medium.

If biochemical tests are the heart of yeast identification systems, confirmation of the identification by examination of yeast morphology on agar media is the soul. Using morphologic observation as a check can save embarrassing mistakes that would be made if automated or packaged systems were trusted implicitly.

Serologic Identification

Immunologic tests are available both for detection of antigen and antibodies to selected fungal pathogens (Hamilton, 1998, McLintock, 2004). Tests for antibodies have proven useful for the diagnosis and management of immunocompetent patients with histoplasmosis and coccidioidomycosis. With the availability of well standardized commercial reagents, both complement fixation and immunodiffusion testing have been used. Serodiagnostic antibody testing for other fungal pathogens has not been widely accepted because of low sensitivity and specificity. Additionally, the inability of immunocompromised patients to mount a humoral response makes antibody testing less useful in this type of patient.

Tests to detect fungal antigens or metabolic byproducts in serum or other body fluids, on the other hand, have seen shown to be more useful for the diagnosis and management of fungal disease. One of the most widely used antigen detection tests is the cryptococcal antigen test for the diagnosis of cryptococcal infection (de Repentigny, 1992). The polysaccharide capsule of *C. neoformans* becomes dissolved in the serum and cerebrospinal fluid which can be detected using either latex-based agglutination testing commercially available from a number of companies or the enzyme immunoassay. The titer of *Cryptococcus* polysaccharide in cerebrospinal fluid is also helpful to monitor therapy over time.

Antigen detection for the diagnosis of histoplasmosis has proven to be useful when testing either serum, urine, or bronchoalveolar lavage fluid is used (Wheat, 2002, 2003a) Antigen testing plays a special role in the diagnosis of disseminated and diffuse acute pulmonary histoplasmosis. As a screening test, *H.-capsulatum*-specific antigen has been detected in urine

Table 60–11 Genomic Targets Utilized for the Detection and Identification of Fungal Pathogens

Gene target	Fungal species
Actin	*Candida albicans*
Alkaline proteinase	*Aspergillus fumigatus*
Chitin synthetase	Dermatophyte species
Cytochrome b	*Candida albicans*
Dihydrofolate reductase	*Pneumocystis jiroveci (carinii)*
Heat-shock protein	*Candida albicans*
IgE binding protein	*Aspergillus* species
Mitochondrial rRNA	*Pneumocystis jiroveci*
Secretory aspartate proteinase	*Candida albicans*
Thymidylate synthase	*Pneumocystis jiroveci*
rDNA complex (5S gene)	*Candida albicans, Pneumocystis jiroveci*
rDNA complex (18S gene)	Multiple
rDNA complex (28S gene)	*Aspergillus fumigatus, Candida albicans*
rDNA complex (IGS regions)	*Aspergillus fumigatus*
rDNA complex (ITS regions)	Multiple

IGS = intergenic spacer region; ITS = internal transcribed spacer region.

Source: modified with permission from Iwen PC: Molecular detection and typing of fungal pathogens. Clin Lab Med, 2003; 23: 781–799.

of 90% of patients with disseminated infection and 80% of patients with acute pulmonary histoplasmosis (Wheat, 2003b).

Recently a commercial Food and Drug Administration (FDA)-approved enzyme-linked immunosorbent assay (ELISA; Platelia *Aspergillus* ELISA; Bio-Rad, Marnes-la-Coquette, France) for the detection of galactomannan antigenemia became available for the rapid diagnosis of invasive aspergillosis (Herbrecht, 2002). This test has been shown to be useful when testing multiple serum samples from high-risk patients; however, several variables have now been reported to affect the reliability of the result of testing (Walsh, 2004b). Treatment with piperacillin–tazobactam or amoxicillin–clavulanate may cause false-positive galactomannan results. Additionally, false-positive results are more common in children than in adults.

Skin tests have been used for epidemiologic study of some infections but have limited utility for diagnostic purposes.

Molecular Identification

Molecular techniques for the evaluation of fungi have shown rapid advances since the mid 1990s (Reiss, 2000; Chen, 2002). In mycology, nucleic acid assays have been used in studies involving phylogenetics, epidemiologic typing, gene expression regulation, identification from culture, and direct detection/identification from clinical material (Iwen, 2003). One of the greatest needs for clinical medicine is to develop rapid detection and identification methods that can be applied directly to clinical specimens. This need stems not only from the inability of current laboratory tests to provide a timely result but also from the fact that fungal infections in immunocompromised patients usually appear suddenly, progress rapidly, and are often fatal unless treatment is started early in the course of infection.

An initial goal for any molecular assay is to define the genetic loci within the genome to be used as the molecular target. Numerous areas within the fungal genome have been evaluated, with most of the current work using sequence areas within the ribosomal DNA (rDNA) gene complex as the target region (Table 60–11) (Iwen, 2003). This section of the genome includes the relatively conserved areas of the 18S, 5.8S, and 28S genes and the variable DNA sequence areas of the intervening internal transcribed spacer (ITS) regions called ITS1 and ITS2. All three genes within the rDNA complex and the ITS1 and ITS2 regions have been used in studies on the molecular evaluation of fungi. Sequence homology within the rDNA genes and differences within the spacer regions are the genetic basis for the organization of the fungi into taxonomic groups (Bastola, 2004). Most of the molecular assays being developed currently use either a variable domain region of the 18S gene or one or both of the ITS regions as molecular targets (Iwen, 2002).

The commercially available molecular assays for testing fungi and a majority of the 'home brew' amplification methods are used for culture confirmation only. The licensed nonamplified probe tests developed by

GenProbe (Accuprobe, San Diego, CA) have been successful for the identification of *H. capsulatum*, *B. dermatitidis*, and *C. immitis* from culture. More recently, amplification assays using a variety of identification methods have been developed to identify fungal pathogens from culture (Iwen, 2003). These methods include direct sequence analysis of amplified DNA, genus/species-specific primers, genus/species-specific probing of the amplicon, rDNA restriction fragment length polymorphism analysis, automated capillary electrophoresis, hybridization enzyme immunoassays, and microchip electrophoresis resolution.

The molecular amplification approach has also been successfully applied to the detection of fungal DNA directly from clinical samples (Iwen, 2003). Much of the current research in this area centers on the detection of *Pneumocystis* (*carinii*) *jiroveci* in respiratory samples and the detection/identification of *Candida* species and *Aspergillus* species from blood and respiratory specimens (Chen, 2002). Additional clinical specimens such as deep tissue, dermatologic samples, and ocular fluids have also shown some success when tested directly for the presence of fungal DNA.

Although most molecular testing has centered on the use of conventional polymerase chain reaction (PCR) methodology, many modified approaches to this procedure have also been applied. Some of these approaches include assays such as multiplex PCR and nested PCR to increase the sensitivity of testing (Shin, 1999). In multiplex PCR, more than one target sequence is amplified by including multiple pairs of primers in the reaction. With nested PCR, a second set of primers that are internal to the original set are used to re-amplify the target DNA using the amplicon from the first PCR as the template.

The latest revolution in molecular testing involves using rapid-cycle real-time PCR. The platform of testing in this methodology involves thermal cycling combined with fluorescence monitoring of the amplified product during. The capacity not only to detect and identify a fungal pathogen rapidly but also to quantify fungal DNA in a sample adds to the applicability of this technology. Two commercially available instruments, the GeneAmp 5700 (along with its updated version the Prism 7700) from Applied Biosystems, which uses the fluorescent-labeled TaqMan probes, and the LightCycler from Roche Applied Science, which uses the fluorescence resonance energy transfer (FRET) probe technique, have both been used to evaluate fungi with encouraging results (Loeffler, 2000; Guiver, 2001).

Susceptibility Testing

For many years, few antifungal chemotherapeutic agents were available, with amphotericin B virtually the only agent effective against most systemic pathogens. Although this potent antifungal agent was frequently toxic, resistance to therapy was rare. The recent introduction of new antifungal agents and the subsequent development of resistance among mould and yeast pathogens has added new impetus to the development and standardization of tests for laboratory guidance of antifungal chemotherapy (Ellis, 2002; Pfaller, 2002, 2004; Hajjeh, 2004). The Clinical and Laboratory Standards Institute (CLSI, formerly the National Committee for Clinical Laboratory Standards) has developed reference macrodilution and microdilution broth methods for antifungal susceptibility testing of yeasts (Clinical and Laboratory Standards Institute, 2002b) and moulds (Clinical and Laboratory Standards Institute, 2002a) (Espinel-Ingroff, 2002, CLSI, 2002a, CLSI, 2002b). The CLSI M27-A2 document (Clinical and Laboratory Standards Institute, 2002b) has been approved for the testing of *Candida* species and *C. neoformans*. It describes interpretive breakpoints for fluconazole, flucytosine, and itraconazole. The CLSI M38-A method (Clinical and Laboratory Standards Institute, 2002a) has been developed for in vitro susceptibility testing of the more common rapid growing filamentous fungi that can cause invasive disease such as *Aspergillus* species, *Fusarium* species, *Rhizopus* species, *Pseudallescheria boydii*, and the mycelial form of *Sporothrix schenckii*. No interpretive breakpoints have been established to evaluate in vitro testing of mould fungi.

Since both reference methods are time consuming to perform, simplified alternatives to these methods have been assessed to include the E-test agar-gradient minimum inhibitory concentration (MIC) method (AB Biodisk, Piscataway, NJ) and the Sensititre Yeast One method (TREK Diagnostics Systems, Cleveland, Ohio). Both methods have been shown to be reliable for the testing of moulds and yeast to the standard antifungal agents (Espinel-Ingroff, 2002, 2003, 2004; Maxwell, 2003; Pfaller, 2003a, 2003b; Castro, 2004). The Yeast One plate has been cleared by the FDA for the testing of *Candida* species with fluconazole, itraconazole, and flucytosine in the clinical laboratory. Both methods have also been shown to be reliable for the testing of caspofungin, posaconaozle, ravuconazole, and voriconazole (Espinel-Ingroff, 2002; Maxwell, 2003; Pfaller, 2003c; Castro, 2004).

While susceptibility testing of all fungal isolates is not recommended, testing may be warranted in the following situations: (1) as part of periodic surveys that establish antibiograms for isolates in an institution; (2) to help in the management of refractory oropharyngeal candidiasis in patients with apparent therapeutic failure; and (3) to aid in the management of invasive candidiasis when the use of azole antifungal agents is uncertain. Future studies are needed to determine the relationship between the MIC and patient response to therapy before routine antifungal susceptibility testing becomes clinically useful (Rex, 2001; Patterson, 2002).

Candidiasis, Cryptococcosis, and Other Infections Caused by Yeast

The Genus *Candida*

Candida spp. are the most important of the yeast pathogens (Pfaller, 1998). With the increased use of immunosuppressive therapies, the use of broad-spectrum antibiotics, and the aging of the population, yeasts have assumed a large place among nosocomial pathogens (Pfaller, 2004). *Candida* species are now the fourth most common cause of hospital-acquired blood stream infections in the United States, with *C. albicans* accounting for more than 50% of infections followed by *Candida glabrata* and the less common species *C. tropicalis*, *Candida parapsilosis*, *C. krusei*, and *Candida lusitaniae* (Pfaller, 2002).

Risk Factors

Candida infections are limited in extent and severity if the host is normal. Since *Candida* species are a part of the normal flora in the gastrointestinal tract, on mucous membranes, and on the skin, infections occur as an opportunity. For instance, the use of broad-spectrum antibacterial therapy upsets the balance of colonizing flora on the mucous membranes of the oral cavity and the gastrointestinal tract by eliminating the predominant competing bacterial flora. In some locations, such as the female genital system, the cause of a disruption in the normal flora balance may not be obvious. In cutaneous sites, such as the groin, excessive moisture predisposes an individual to *Candida* infection.

Severe and invasive disease develops when host defenses are compromised. Diabetes, immunosuppressive diseases or therapies, and neutropenia as a result of disease (e.g., acquired immunodeficiency syndrome) or treatment with high-dose chemotherapy are common risk factors. Bloodstream infections, including fungal endocarditis, are fostered by use of indwelling vascular lines as is common practice in the management of hospitalized patients (Kojic, 2004).

Clinical Diseases

Although *C. albicans* is by far the most common pathogen within the genus *Candida*, the frequency of the non-*albicans* species has increased (Wingard, 1995; Pfaller, 2004). Numerous reports describe invasive infections caused by *C. tropicalis*, *C. parapsilosis*, *C. glabrata*, *C. krusei*, and *C. lusitaniae* (Weems, 1992; Minari, 2001; Redding, 2002; Hawkins, 2003).

Resistance to imidazole antibiotics (e.g., ketoconazole, fluconazole, or itraconazole) is unfortunately developing in isolates of *Candida* species. *C. glabrata* and *C. krusei*, in particular, are intrinsically more resistant to this class of antifungal agent than is *C. albicans* (Pfaller, 2002, 2003b). *C. lusitaniae*, an infrequently isolated pathogen, is prone to develop resistance to amphotericin in vivo (Hawkins, 2003).

Cutaneous disease

Cutaneous disease is the most frequent infection caused by the *Candida* species, typically presenting as erythematous lesions of the skin, sometimes accompanied by a creamy, white exudate or scaling (Vazquez, 2002). Moist conditions predispose to infection, such as diaper rash in infants or infection of skin folds (intertrigo) in adults. Common sites are in the groin (a form of jock itch), between fingers and toes, under the female breast, and in the axilla. Workers who must immerse their hands in water for long periods of time are particularly at risk for infections of the skin of the hands, nails (onychomycosis), or the nail bed (paronychia). A chronic cutaneous disease is an uncommon manifestation of *Candida* infection in patients with defective cellular immunity (Kirkpatrick, 2001).

Oral candidiasis

Oral candidiasis is usually manifest as creamy white patches overlying erythematous buccal mucosa (thrush) (Akpan, 2002). Symptoms are usually minimal but dysphagia may result from heavy infections. Fissuring at the corners of the mouth is common and may be the primary complaint. Oral candidiasis is a common initial infection in patients

VII

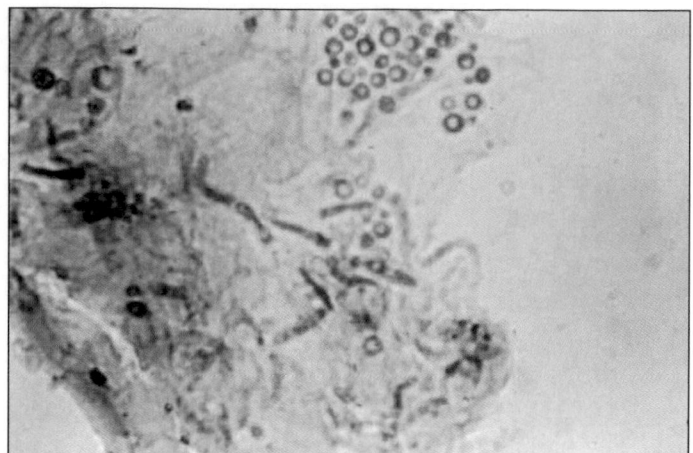

Figure 60–19 Skin scrapings from a lesion of pityriasis versicolor. The yeast and short hyphal forms (spaghetti and meatball appearance) are characteristic of *Malassezia furfur*. (Lactophenol cotton blue stain; ×400)

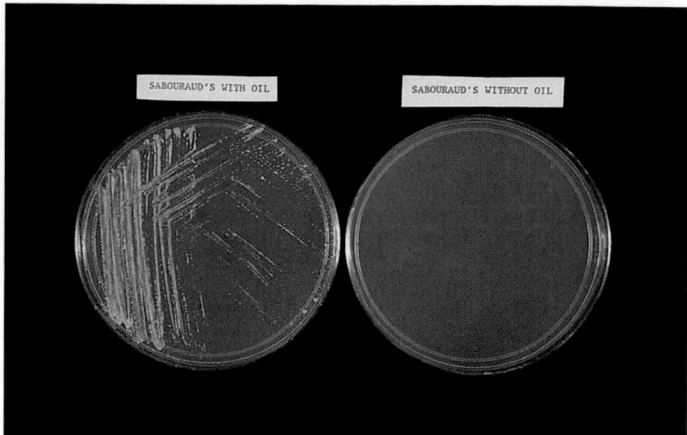

Figure 60–20 Abundant growth of *Malassezia furfur* is evident on a plate that was overlaid with oil before the inoculum was applied. There is no growth on a companion plate without oil. (Sabouraud dextrose agar)

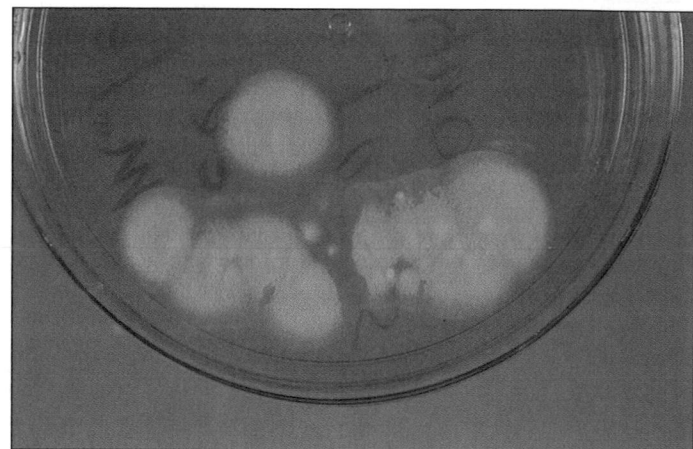

Figure 60–21 An aerial mycelium arises from the yeast-like colony of *Geotrichum candidum*. (Sabouraud dextrose agar)

are the most common presentation, but depigmenting lesions are more obvious in dark-skinned persons and may be accentuated by suntans in light-skinned individuals. The ill effects are purely cosmetic but may be considerably troublesome. Hypopigmented lesions must be differentiated from vitiligo. Therapy consists of topical application of fungicidal creams or rinses.

Systemic infection

Systemic infection occurs almost invariably in infants who have received intravascular infusions of lipid. Diluted lipid solution supports the growth of *M. furfur* by supplying long-chain fatty acids that are also found on the skin and must be supplied in the laboratory for isolation of the yeast. Infected infants are often asymptomatic but fever, leukocytosis, and thrombocytopenia may be present. Pneumonia is the most common systemic manifestation of disease, probably resulting from emboli from infected intravenous catheters. Removing the infected catheter is therapeutic.

Pathology of Malassezia Infection

The diagnosis of pityriasis versicolor usually is made clinically or by demonstrating yeast and short hyphal forms (similar in appearance to spaghetti and meatballs) in KOH preparations of skin scrapings (Fig. 60–19). The addition of Calcofluor white or other fungal stain enhances detection, because the fungal cells are small and difficult to visualize when unstained. When biopsied, hyperkeratosis, acanthosis, and dermal mononuclear infiltrates may be seen. Little is known of the pathology of systemic infection with *M. furfur*, because biopsies are infrequently performed and lethal infection is uncommon. In rare fatal cases, vasculitis, septic infarcts, and granulomatous inflammation have been described in many organs, including the lung, liver, and kidney.

Laboratory Diagnosis

Culture for *M. furfur* is rarely requested in cutaneous disease, and direct observation of yeast in KOH preparations is usually done in the physician's office. This yeast should be sought in cultures of blood and intravenous catheter tips from neonates. Before inoculation, a drop of sterile olive oil is added to the surface of a suitable agar medium, such as Sabouraud dextrose agar or sheep blood agar. Within 2–3 days, light brown colonies, often with a dry appearance, appear in the oil overlay. An initial clue to this pathogen is lack of growth in the absence of oil or stimulation of growth by the presence of an oil overlay (Fig. 60–20). *M. pachydermatis* is not dependent on long-chain fatty acids for growth.

The identification of the isolate can be confirmed by microscopic examination of the yeast cells, which measure 3–7 μm in size. The budding process in *Malassezia* is unusual, because it occurs as an enteroblastic process with the formation of phialides. The bud is broad-based and the collarettes of the phialides may be observed with the light microscope as a distinct dark ring separating the mother and daughter cells.

Other Yeast and Yeast-like Pathogens

Blastoschizomyces capitatus (formerly *Trichosporon capitatum*) is a rare cause of disseminated infection that resembles candidiasis (Martino, 2004). A morphologically similar fungus, *Geotrichum candidum*, is also a rare cause

of pulmonary or disseminated disease (Schiemann, 1998). *Geotrichum* and *Trichosporon* produce smooth, yeast-like colonies that later develop aerial mycelium, like new hair growth on a bald head (Fig 60–21). Both species produce arthroconidia, which lack the disjunctor cells seen in *C. immitis*. *Saccharomyces cerevisiae* (Ponton, 2000), *Rhodotorula* species (Anatoliotaki, 2003), and *Hansenula* species (Ma, 2000) are saprophytic yeast but rarely cause disease. Demonstration of the yeast in tissues or isolation from multiple specimens, even from sterile sites, is required to document the role of the unusual yeast in an infectious process. *S. cerevisiae* is baker's yeast and is perhaps best known to students of mycology for its salutary effects on malt and hops.

Mycoses Caused by Dimorphic Fungi

The thermally dimorphic fungi are the most pathogenic organisms encountered in a clinical mycology laboratory. In the United States, the most important dimorphic pathogens are *Histoplasma capsulatum* var. *capsulatum*, *Blastomyces dermatitidis*, *Coccidioides immitis*, and *Sporothrix schenckii*. *Sporothrix* is widely distributed throughout the world while the other organisms are predominantly found in North America, where they have distinct geographic distributions (Fig. 60–22). Epidemic disease is most common with *Histoplasma* and *Coccidioides* and less common with *Sporothrix* and *Blastomyces*. The tissue phase of *Coccidioides* is a unique structure called the spherule while the other genera produce a yeast phase in vivo that may also grow as yeast if incubated at 37°C in vitro.

The Genus *Histoplasma*

H. capsulatum is subdivided into two varieties, *H. capsulatum* var. *capsulatum* (hereafter referred to *H. capsulatum*) and *H. capsulatum* var. *duboisii*. Both of these fungal pathogens are geographically restricted and acquisition of infection does not overlap in most cases. *H. capsulatum* var. *capsulatum* is found primarily along the Ohio, Mississippi, and St Lawrence rivers but

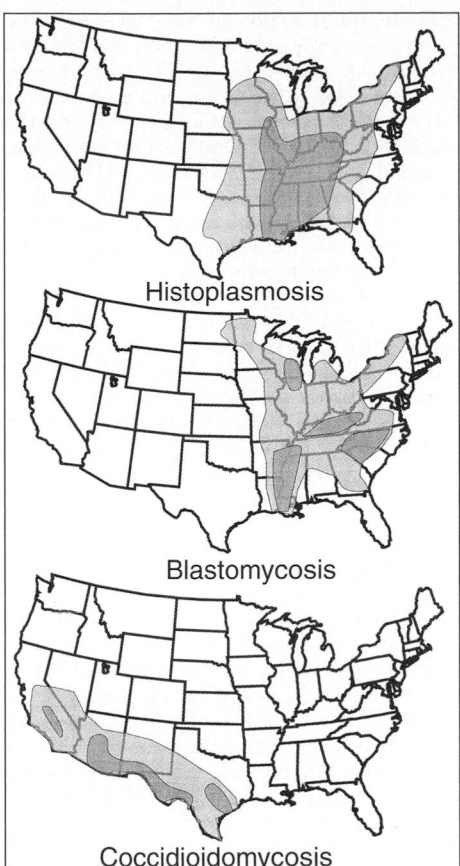

Figure 60–22 Geographic distribution of dimorphic fungal infections in the United States. The areas of greatest endemicity (dark shading) and lesser endemicity (light shading) are illustrated. Sporadic cases may also occur in other areas outside the endemic zones.

may have worldwide distribution. *H. capsulatum* var. *duboisii*, on the other hand, is limited to equatorial Africa and is associated with a disease referred to as African histoplasmosis. Distinguishing characteristics of the tissue phase can be observed to distinguish these two pathogens; however, lack of travel to the endemic area in Africa can generally rule out infection with the var. *duboisii*.

Risk Factors

The primary risk factor for acquiring infection is living in one of the endemic regions of the United States. In some areas, more than 90% of the population reacts positively to histoplasmin skin testing. Growth of *H. capsulatum* in the soil is stimulated by bird guano, although the fungus does not infect the bird. Once growing in the soil, the fungus sporulates and produces conidia, which, during activities that generate aerosols, can be inhaled into the lungs. A classic history for a patient with acute pulmonary histoplasmosis is recent cleaning of a chicken coop. Occupationally acquired histoplasmosis has been reported, leading the US Department of Health and Human Services to issue a document outlining measures for protecting workers at risk (Department of Health and Human Services, 1997). Epidemic acute disease has occurred in individuals vacationing in areas where this fungus in endemic. For example, there were 221 cases among students from 37 colleges in 18 states who had vacationed in Acapulco, Mexico in March of 2001 (Centers for Disease Control and Prevention, 2001a). Most of these patients had visited a common source point, thus leading to spore exposure. Chronic pulmonary histoplasmosis occurs primarily in patients with chronic obstructive pulmonary disease, whereas disseminated infection occurs in patients with immunologic deficits, especially of the cellular immune system. Infection with HIV has become an important risk factor for fatal disseminated infection.

Clinical Diseases

The magnitude of the exposure and the immune status of the host influence the clinical manifestations of disease. Exposure to low concentrations of spores from the environment in a normal host is typically asymptomatic. A majority of adults living in an endemic area are seropositive but have no clinical evidence of infection.

Acute pulmonary infection

Individuals who are exposed to large numbers of conidia may develop a flu-like syndrome with high fever, chills, fatigue, cough, and pleuritic or retrosternal chest pain. More severely affected individuals may be ill for several weeks but resolution usually is complete without antifungal therapy in the normal host. If focal granulomatous inflammation has occurred, calcification of the focus typically leaves a well circumscribed coin lesion, which may be seen on the chest radiograph.

Granulomatous and fibrosing mediastinitis

These types of manifestations involve the lymph nodes in the mediastinum. Granulomatous disease is characterized by enlarged lymph nodes, which may obstruct the airways, superior vena cava pulmonary vessels, or the esophagus. Fistulae can form within the lymph nodes and adjacent mediastinal structures. Fibrosing disease is a reaction that occurs in the mediastinum in individuals predisposed to an excessive response to *Histoplasma* antigens. Both granulomatous and fibrosing diseases are thought to progress independently.

Chronic pulmonary histoplasmosis

This debilitating disease occurs primarily in patients with chronic obstructive pulmonary disease, most of whom are middle-aged men. Calcification and cavitations occur, which may mimic chronic pulmonary tuberculosis and pulmonary neoplasia.

Disseminated Histoplasmosis

Dissemination of yeast through the reticuloendothelial system may occur as a part of acute pulmonary histoplasmosis, resulting in healed granulomas, which often calcify, especially in the spleen. Clinically, disseminated infection occurs in two classes of patient. The first group consists of individuals at the extremes of age who do not have a recognized immunosuppressive condition but may have an immune system that is incompletely developed or diminished by age in ways that are incompletely understood. The second group is patients with recognized immuno-suppressive diseases or therapies. Before the 1980s, the diseases were predominantly hematologic neoplasms; more recently HIV infection has become the most common risk factor (McKinsey, 1998). Progression of disease may be rapid or insidious.

Infection of the reticuloendothelial system may result in lymphadenopathy, hepatosplenomegaly, or thrombocytopenia (Wheat, 2003b). Destruction of the adrenal cortex by the granulomatous process may be sufficiently extensive to cause hormonal insufficiency. Central nervous system infection may be manifested as chronic meningitis, intracerebral granulomas, or both. Endovascular infection includes endocarditis with large, bulky vegetations. Any part of the gastrointestinal tract may be affected, and the ulcerating lesions may suggest a neoplasm macroscopically. The hallmark of disease is an oropharyngeal ulcer, which may cause hoarseness, dysphagia, or a painful lesion on the tongue or gingiva. In patients with HIV infection, the symptoms of disseminated histoplasmosis may resemble those produced by the virus, including fever, lymphadenopathy, anemia, leukopenia, thrombocytopenia, weight loss, and fatigue (McKinsey, 1998).

Solitary cutaneous lesions are rare but may follow direct introduction of the fungus into the dermis.

Pathology of Histoplasmosis

As a facultative intracellular pathogen, *H. capsulatum* is found predominantly in macrophages. The pathologic lesions consist of collections of infected macrophages, noncaseating granulomas, or caseating granulomas. The histopathologic lesions are similar to those produced by *Mycobacterium tuberculosis*. The intracellular yeast are often well demonstrated by H&E staining (Fig. 60–23). The periodic-acid–Schiff and methenamine silver techniques are more sensitive, and the silver stain is essential for demonstration of old yeast cells in healed granulomas. This yeast, presumably no longer viable, may be enlarged and distorted in morphology. The differential diagnosis of the yeast forms includes small forms of *B. dermatitidis*, *Penicillium marneffei*, *Leishmania* species, or *Candida* spp., especially *C. glabrata*. The larger size of *Candida* yeast cells (other than *C. glabrata*) or the clinical presentation, usually suggests the proper diagnosis. The yeast of *H. capsulatum* in caseating granulomas are sufficiently distinctive to provide a presumptive diagnosis, but unusual granulomatous presentations of *P. (carinii) jiroveci* must be differentiated.

Laboratory Diagnosis

The yeast form in tissue may be demonstrated histologically or in preparations of respiratory secretions, fluids, peripheral blood, bone marrow, or tissue imprints. Wet preparations and Calcofluor white may be

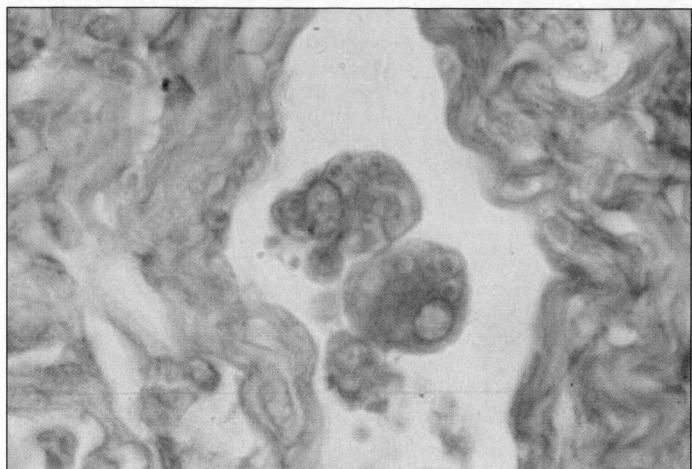

Figure 60–23 Yeast cells of *Histoplasma capsulatum* in macrophages. The presence of intracellular small, round to oval yeast-like cells in tissue is a characteristic pathologic finding in histoplasmosis (Hematoxylin and eosin stain; ×1000)

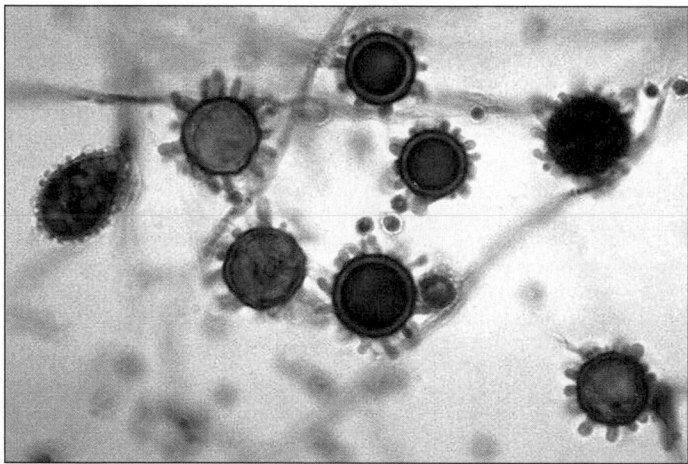

Figure 60–24 Tuberculate macroconidia with microconidia of *Histoplasma capsulatum* in culture. These structures are characteristic of the environmental mould form of this dimorphic fungus. (Lactophenol cotton blue stain; ×400; CDC Public Health Image Library)

used but the morphology of tissue and yeast cells is best seen with Giemsa staining, because the details of nuclear morphology can be assessed. The yeast cells measure 3–5 μm in diameter, have a single nucleus, and bud with a narrow neck.

If disseminated infection is suspected, blood cultures for *Histoplasma* should be performed. The Isolator technique appears to be the most sensitive technique for recovering the yeast phase from blood. Other clinical specimens should be inoculated to an enriched agar, such as brain–heart infusion agar supplemented with sheep blood, which is incubated at 25–30°C.

Colonies of *H. capsulatum* usually appear after incubation for 10–14 days but occasionally require incubation for up to 4 weeks. On primary isolation medium at 25–30°C, they are fluffy and vary from white to buff-brown in color. The diagnostic asexual forms include microconidia and macroconidia. The microconidia, which are produced first, resemble the structures produced by *B. dermatitidis*. The more characteristic macroconidia have roughened projections from the periphery of the conidia, a configuration referred to as tuberculate (Fig. 60–24). The macroconidia of the saprophyte *Sepedonium* may be confused with *Histoplasma*, so differentiation of these two fungi is important. The macroscopic appearance of the colonies, rate of growth, growth of *H. capsulatum* on media containing cycloheximide, the presence of yeast forms in tissue, and the clinical history are usually sufficient to distinguish these fungi. Final identification most often is provided by nucleic acid hybridization probe testing. Conversion of the mould to the yeast phase also confirms the identification, but this is often exceedingly difficult and has been supplanted in most clinical laboratories by molecular techniques (Accuprobe, GenProbe, San Diego, CA). Exoantigen testing is another possible identification method but it too is rarely, if ever, used.

Serologic tests for the detection of anti-*Histoplasma* antibodies (i.e., immunodiffusion and complement fixation) have several limitations (Wheat, 2003a). A 2–6 week delay after exposure is required for the production of antibodies, reducing the value of this testing for the diagnosis of acute histoplasmosis. Once patients are infected with *H. capsulatum*, antibody levels remain detectable for many years. Antibodies to *H. capsulatum* and *B. dermatitidis* crossreact. Additionally, patients with immune dysfunction may not produce detectable levels of antibodies. Antigen detection, on the other hand, has been shown to be useful for the diagnosis of histoplasmosis. The sensitivity of urine antigen detection for diagnosis is greatest in patients with disseminated disease (up to 92%) or acute pulmonary histoplasmosis (75–80%) (Wheat, 2002, 2003a, 2003b). Antigen detection also is useful for following the effect of therapy on fungal burden; failure of antigen concentrations in urine or serum to fall during therapy suggests treatment failure. Moreover, an increase in antigen levels in a previously treated individual suggests a relapse of disease.

The histoplasmin skin test antigen has been useful for epidemiologic studies but should never be used for diagnosis. Not only does the high frequency of positive tests in endemic areas cloud the interpretation, but the skin test can cause an individual to become seropositive, further confusing the issue.

The Genus *Blastomyces*

B. dermatitidis is the sole species within the genus *Blastomyces*, although the difference in yeast conversion rates between American and African isolates suggest that different taxa may be involved (Gueho, 1997). Endemic areas for this pathogen are the soil in the Eastern part of the United States, mainly in areas adjacent to the Mississippi and Ohio river basins; areas northwest of the Great Lakes in Canada; and areas within Africa. Recent reports suggest, however, that the endemic area for blastomycosis may be larger than originally described with reports of disease in patients from previously non-endemic areas in Colorado and Nebraska (Centers for Disease Control and Prevention, 1999a; DeGroote, 2000; Veligandla, 2002).

Risk Factors

Most cases of blastomycosis (also referred to as North American blastomycosis) are sporadic with an environmental source not often found. Small outbreaks do occur, and the fungus has been isolated from soil at the outbreak sites (Klein, 1986). There are no recognized specific risk factors for blastomycosis, although severe, disseminated infection has been described in immunocompromised patients. HIV infected patients who reside in endemic areas are particularly at risk for infection (Pappas, 2002).

Clinical Diseases

As with most other endemic dimorphic fungi, the portal of entry is through the respiratory tract, where the infection may be asymptomatic, transient or insidiously progressive (Bradsher, 2003). Chronic pulmonary blastomycosis with low-grade fever, weight loss, and localized pulmonary infiltrates may suggest neoplastic disease, for which diagnostic studies, including bronchoalveolar lavage, fine-needle aspiration of the lung, or surgical lung biopsy may be undertaken (Lemos, 2002). Dissemination of yeast from the lung most commonly results in cutaneous or skeletal infection. The central nervous system and genitourinary systems are involved less frequently. The cutaneous lesions often are hypertrophic or ulcerative, and may be locally destructive. The lesions may be mistaken for squamous cell carcinoma of the skin (Bradsher, 1997). Secondary involvement of the skin over bony lesions also occurs. A delay in diagnosis is not uncommon, especially when patients have no history of exposure to an endemic area (Veligandla, 2002).

Pathology of Blastomycosis

The characteristic histologic response to *B. dermatitidis* is a mixture of acute inflammation with microabscess formation and granulomatous inflammation. In cutaneous lesions, pseudoepitheliomatous hyperplasia of the epidermis overlying the inflammation is characteristic. The yeast cells are most often found in the microabscesses or within multinucleated giant cells. They can frequently be demonstrated in tissue sections stained with H&E, but organisms may be more readily visible when stained with periodic-acid–Schiff or methenamine silver stains. The thick-walled yeast cells measure 8–15 μm in diameter and maintain a broad-base during the budding process. An artifactual separation of the cytoplasm from the cell wall in formalin-fixed preparations may give the appearance of a double wall. Although nonbudding yeast cells must be differentiated from the yeast cells of *C. neoformans* and from the developing spherules of *C.*

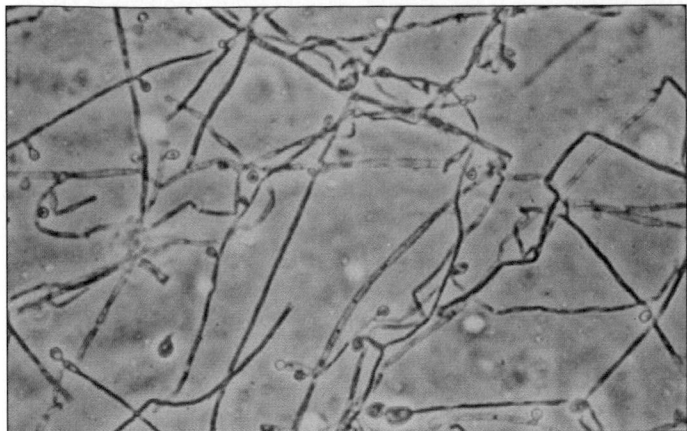

Figure 60–25 Mould form of *Blastomyces dermatitidis* in culture. The lollipop appearance of the conidium on a conidiophore is characteristic of the environmental mould form for this dimorphic fungus. (Lactophenol cotton blue stain; ×400)

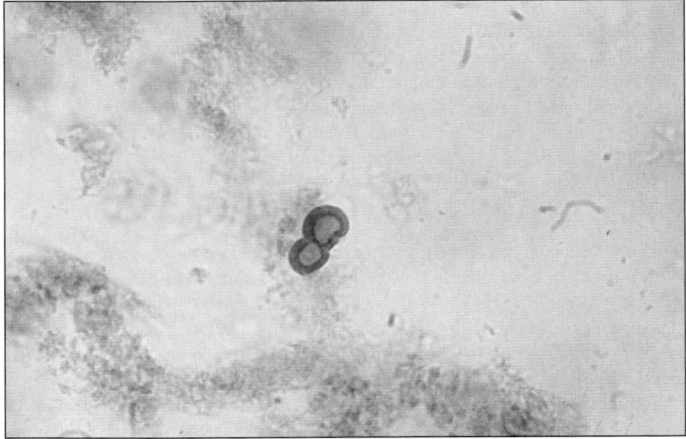

Figure 60–26 Budding yeast cells of *Blastomyces dermatitidis* in culture. When cultures are incubated at 37°C, large, broad-based budding yeast with a double-contoured all are detected which are characteristic for the yeast phase of this dimorphic fungus. (Lactophenol cotton blue stain; ×400)

immitis, the diagnosis of blastomycosis can generally be made by observation of the characteristic yeast forms in tissues by an experienced pathologist (Bradsher, 2003).

Laboratory Identification

Direct demonstration of the yeast cells may be accomplished in tissue sections or in wet preparations of aspirated fluids and imprints of tissues. Calcofluor white staining may enhance the detection of the yeast. Growth is somewhat more rapid than that of *Histoplasma*; fluffy white to buff colonies, which often cannot be distinguished from *H. capsulatum*, usually appear within 1–2 weeks. The microconidia resemble those of *H. capsulatum* (Fig. 60–25), but macroconidia are not formed. A saprophytic mould, *Chrysosporium* resembles *Blastomyces*, but does not develop a yeast phase and does not grow on media that contain cycloheximide. Conversion to the yeast phase may occur on routine media incubated at 37°C with hemoglobin and cysteine containing agar used specifically for this purpose (Fig. 60–26). Once again, demonstration of the yeast form in tissue serves as a reasonable substitute for demonstration of dimorphism in the laboratory. The nucleic acid probe testing colony material is the preferred method for confirming the identification in most laboratories (Accuprobe, GenProbe, San Diego, CA). Recently, an in situ hybridization protocol for the identification of yeast-like organisms in tissue sections using specific and pan fungal oligonucleotides complementary to the 18S and 28S rDNA was published showing a sensitivity of 90% and specificity of 97% for the detection of *B. dermatitidis* DNA (Hayden, 2001).

Although the complement fixation test has been used as a serologic test for the diagnosis of blastomycosis, this test has considerable limitations and should be used only as an adjunct to culture of the fungus. A *Blastomyces* antigen test, similar to the *Histoplasma* antigen test, also is available in a reference laboratory; however, data regarding its utility and reliability are lacking.

The Genus *Coccidioides*

C. immitis was considered until recently to be the sole etiologic agent of coccidioidomycosis. Phylogenetic studies by Fisher et al. showed the existence of two genetically distinct *C. immitis* clades, one called the California clade (*C. immitis*) and the other called the non-California clade (*Coccidioides posadasii*) (Fisher, 2002). Although there is a strong difference in genotype between these two species, the phenotypic differences are minimal, arguing against separation of the species (Cox, 2004). The coccidioidal organisms are soil-dwelling fungi found in the southern portions of California and in other areas of the southwestern United States (especially southern Arizona, southern New Mexico, and west Texas), northern Mexico, and Central and South America (especially Venezuela) (Kirkland, 1996). Arizona has seen a dramatic increase in cases over the years, with a disproportionate rate of infection occurring in people over the age of 65 years and in those with HIV infection (Centers for Disease Control and Prevention, 1996, 2003; Leake, 2000).

Another interesting 'twist' to these agents is the recent classification by the US Department of Health and Human Services of *C. immitis* and *C. posadasii* as select agents of bioterrorism (Centers for Disease Control and Prevention, 2002; Department of Health and Human Services, 2002a). This designation suggests that these pathogens could be used as potential bioweapons and establishes strict federal regulations to be followed for individuals who possess and transport these agents and for the reporting of confirmed infections (Deresinski, 2003). Individuals have questioned the rationale and justification for classifying the *Coccidioides* as select agents due to the burden placed on diagnostic laboratories (Fierer, 2002).

Risk Factors

Residence in an endemic area is the primary risk factor for the development of infection, since the arthroconidia of the mould phase are in the soil and easily disseminated through the air (Chiller, 2003; Crum, 2004). A classic example of epidemic coccidioidomycosis occurred in a group of archeology workers in a dig at the Dinosaur National Monument in northeastern Utah in 2001. Ten workers within this group developed pulmonary coccidioidomycosis during an excavation, and eight of these individuals required hospitalization (Petersen, 2004). Another outbreak of disease occurred in individuals attending the World Championship of Model Airplane Flying in Kern County, California in October 2001. This outbreak illustrated the importance of cooperation within the international community for epidemiologic evaluation, since competing teams from over 30 countries were potentially involved in the outbreak (Centers for Disease Control and Prevention, 2001b)

Suggestions have been made that genetic factors influence the frequency of severe and disseminated infection, but the nature of this association is incompletely understood (Cox, 2004). Disseminated infection is more common in black people and Filipino people than in white people. Asians, Native Americans, and Mexicans also appear to be at increased risk. Adult women develop erythema nodosum more commonly than men in response to primary *Coccidioides* infection, but disseminated infection occurs more common in adult men than in women. Immunosuppressive infection or disease is an important risk factor for disseminated infection with HIV infected patients at particular risk for disseminated disease (Woods, 2000).

Clinical Diseases

Primary coccidioidomycosis is most frequently asymptomatic, as indicated by the high prevalence of positive results of skin tests for the coccidioidal antigens in endemic areas. Symptomatic disease usually is manifested as fever with cough or chest pain, or both, and may mimic bacterial pneumonia clinically (Chiller, 2003). Erythema nodosum and erythema multiform, which may accompany the primary infection, are good prognostic signs. Solitary pulmonary nodules may persist as consequences of the primary pulmonary infection.

Disseminated infection most commonly affects the skin, skeletal system, and meninges. Skin lesions include papules, ulcers, draining sinuses, and subcutaneous abscesses. Arthritis most often results from involvement of adjacent bones. The meningitis may be acute but is more commonly indolent and chronic.

Pathology of Coccidioidomycosis

The tissue response to *C. immitis* is granulomatous, with or without caseation. Developing spherules are typically found in macrophages and multinucleated giant cells (Fig. 60–27). Endospores within the spherules measure 2–5 µm in size (Fig 60–28). Spherules measure up to 200 µm in diameter, and developing spherules have a large range of sizes. The differential diagnosis of developing spherules primarily includes nonbudding forms of *B. dermatitidis* or *C. neoformans*. The spherules must

VII

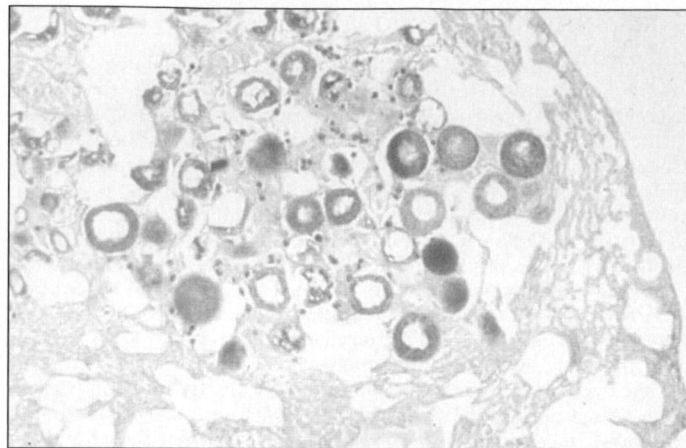

Figure 60–27 Spherules of *Coccidioides immitis* in tissue. The observation of these large structures in tissue is diagnostic for coccidioidomycosis. (Hematoxylin and eosin stain, ×100)

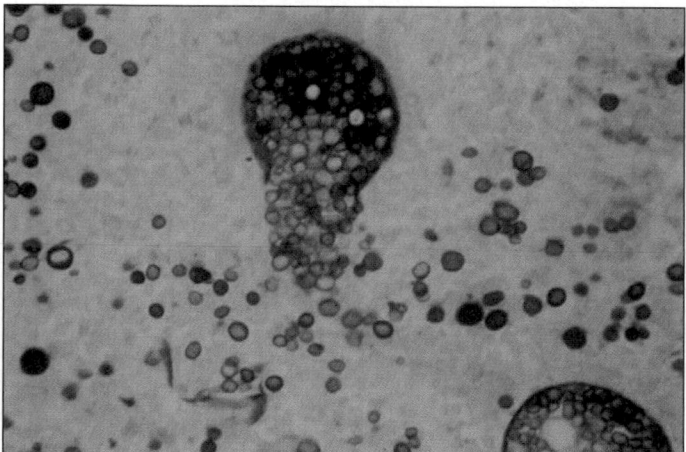

Figure 60–28 Spherules of *Coccidioides immitis* in tissue showing endospore release. At maturity, the spherule ruptures and releases endospores which in turn mature to become spherules. When seen in tissue, these immature endospores may be confused with other smaller yeast. (Gomori's methenamine silver stain; ×1000)

be differentiated from the fungal forms in adiaspiromycosis and rhinosporidiosis, both of which are uncommon infections in the United States.

Laboratory Diagnosis

As with other dimorphic fungi, the possibility of infection should be pursued fully. Spherules may be demonstrated in sputum or bronchoalveolar lavage fluid, but the sensitivity of direct exam for these structures is generally low. Calcofluor white staining following digestion of the specimen with KOH may increase the sensitivity. If cavitary disease is present, hyphae may be present in clinical specimens, although this is rare. In contrast to the other dimorphic pathogens, the possibility of communicability of arthroconidia directly from the specimen exists under this circumstance.

C. *immitis* grows rapidly (less than 1 week) on media with or without cycloheximide and may even appear on blood agar plates in the bacteriology laboratory. The arthroconidia of the *Coccidioides* are highly infectious and easily transmitted by aerosolization. Infection of laboratory workers is a major concern, so inoculated cultures should be handled with great care in a biosafety cabinet. The National Institutes of Health has classified *Coccidioides immitis* (along with *H. capsulatum*) as a risk group 3 biological agent: agents that are associated with serious or lethal human disease for which preventive or therapeutic interventions may not be available (Department of Health and Human Services, 1999). Biosafety level 3 containment is suggested when handling specimens known or very likely to contain this organism (Department of Health and Human Services, 2002a, 2002b). If Petri dishes have been inoculated, they must be carefully taped to prevent accidental dislodging of the lid. The colonies of the *Coccidioides* are extremely variable in appearance, ranging from velvety or cottony to granular or powdery. The colonial morphology may change

as the colony and arthroconidia develop. Most isolates are white, but a variety of colors may be observed and a diffusible pigment may be produced by some strains. Cultures often become gray with age. If *C. immitis* is suspected, some mycologists prefer to sterilize the culture before examination of the colonies by flooding the container with 10% formalin, followed by overnight incubation. In cases where specimens are suspect of containing *Coccidioides*, screw-capped slants should be used instead of plates. Conversion of the mould form to the tissue form is not routinely performed since specialized synthetic broth is generally required for this to occur. Differentiation between *C. immitis* and *C. posadasii* is not generally available in clinical laboratories; therefore, laboratories report the result as *C. immitis*.

The alternating barrel-shaped arthroconidia with empty disjuncture cells are distinctive of *C. immitis* (Fig. 60–9) but must be differentiated from other organisms that produce arthroconidia, such as *Trichosporon*, *Geotrichum*, and some members of the family Gymnoascaceae. Confirmation of the identification is most commonly accomplished by the nucleic acid hybridization probe test.

In contrast to histoplasmosis and blastomycosis, serologic analysis with the complement fixation test is useful for assessing the extent and prognosis of coccidioidomycosis (Pappagianis, 1990). Of the serologic techniques available, complement fixation has been studied most extensively. Antibodies are detected approximately 2–6 weeks after infection. The height of the titer is an indication of the likelihood of disseminated disease and a rising titer bodes a poor outcome. Skin testing does not confound the diagnosis by producing a seroconversion, as in histoplasmosis, but the high prevalence of skin test positivity decreases the usefulness of the test. Patients with disseminated infection may demonstrate anergy to the skin test antigen.

The Genus *Sporothrix*

The only known pathogen within the genus is *Sporothrix schenckii*, of which there are two varieties: *S. schenckii* var. *schenckii* and *S. schenckii* var. *luriei*. The var. *luriei* differs from var. *schenckii* only by morphology in host tissue by producing large and often septated budding cells. Only three cases of *S. schenckii* var. *luriei* have been reported in the literature, none from the United States (Padhye, 1992). *S. schenckii* var. *schenckii* (hereafter called *S. schenckii*) is a dimorphic fungus present worldwide in soil, plants, and decaying vegetation (Bustamante, 2001). It has been associated with numerous outbreaks, with one major outbreak occurring among florists and nursery and forestry workers who handled contaminated sphagnum moss grown in Wisconsin (Centers for Disease Control and Prevention, 1988). Although considered an endemic dimorphic fungus, *S. schenckii* exhibits epidemiologic differences that separate it from the other classic endemic dimorphic fungi (De Araujo, 2001). The mode of entry for the fungus is usually through traumatic implantation (vs. inhalation), the disease produced is usually a localized subcutaneous infection (vs. pulmonary), and the incidence of systemic infection is rare.

Risk Factors

Although *S. schenckii* is common in vegetation throughout the world, it does not appear to be a plant pathogen. Epidemics have been caused by exposure to plant products, such as sphagnum moss used in gardening (Coles, 1992). An unusual epidemic occurred among members of a college fraternity in Florida, who were building a wall with bricks packed in contaminated straw while consuming copious amounts of beer (Sanders, 1971). The only predisposing factor that has been identified with any frequency is consumption of alcohol. It is interesting that the stereotype of the patient at risk for sporotrichosis is the 'alcoholic rose gardener.'

Clinical Diseases

The overwhelming predominant clinical form of sporotrichosis is involvement of the cutaneous and subcutaneous tissues. A papule at the portal of entry may ulcerate and spread the pathogen through regional lymphatics, resulting in a series of lesions progressing up the affected limb (referred to lymphocutaneous sporotrichosis). Dissemination to osteo-articular structures and viscera is uncommon and appears to occur more often in patients who have a history of alcohol abuse or immuno-suppression, especially patients with AIDS (Kauffman, 2000)

Pathology of Sporotrichosis

The histologic responses to *Sporothrix* and *Blastomyces* are similar. Granulomatous inflammation may be accompanied by small collections of polymorphonuclear neutrophils. In the skin, pseudoepitheliomatous hyperplasia of the epidermis is common. The yeast cells of *S. schenckii* are pleomorphic, round or elongated, resembling cigars, but they are rarely

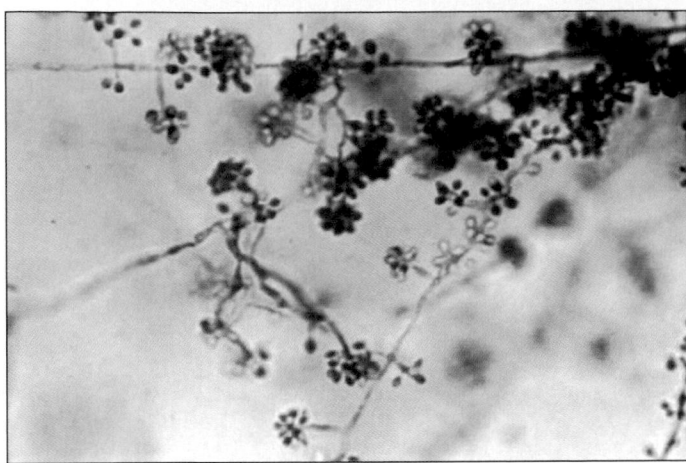

Figure 60–29 Sympodial conidia of *Sporothrix schenckii* are borne in clusters at the tips of lateral conidiophores. (Lactophenol cotton blue stain; ×400)

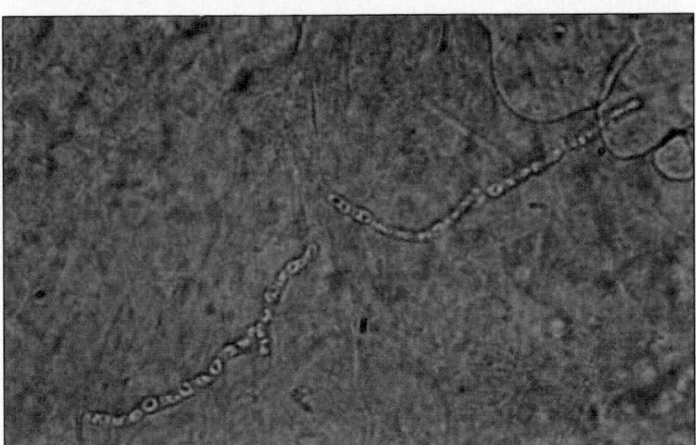

Figure 60–30 Hyphae of a dermatophyte are demonstrated in a scraping from the edge of a tinea lesion. The presence of thin-segmented hyphae in this clinical setting establishes the diagnosis of dermatophytosis but does not define the specific etiology. (KOH preparation; ×400)

seen in tissue. A tissue reaction to the fungus may result in radiating eosinophilic material up to 10 μm in thickness around the yeast cell, known as the Splendore–Hoeppli phenomenon. This distinctive tissue reaction is uncommon and not specific for sporotrichosis. The differential diagnosis of the skin lesions includes mycobacterial infections, especially *Mycobacterium marinum* (swimming pool granuloma) in the United States and cutaneous leishmaniasis in the tropics.

Laboratory Diagnosis

The preferred specimen is an aspirate, curetting, or biopsy of the skin lesion. *S. schenckii* grows well on primary isolation media with cycloheximide incubated at 25–30°C. The colonies, which may be moist or smooth (glabrous), are often light colored initially, and turn darker with increasing age. *S. schenckii* produces two types of conidium; thin-walled hyaline conidia arranged as a rosette around the apex of a conidiophore and thick-walled, dark, sessile conidia attached directly to the hyphae. The thin-walled microconidia are borne on conidiophores that arise at right angles from the hyphae. They may be arranged sympodically around an expanded vesicle at the tip of the conidiophore, producing an arrangement that has been described as a floret (Fig. 60–29). Similar structures are produced by *Acremonium* species, which have rarely been reported as a cause of human disease, and by an uncommon isolated saprophyte, *Ophiostoma stenoceras*. These moulds are differentiated from *Sporothrix* by the inability to grow on media with cycloheximide and the absence of a yeast phase. Conversion of the mould phase to yeast is accomplished by incubation of the isolate at 37°C in an atmosphere of 5% CO_2 on an enriched medium, such as brain–heart infusion agar supplemented with sheep blood, or chocolate agar.

Skin tests and serologic assays for the diagnosis of sporotrichosis have been described but are not readily available.

Other Dimorphic Fungi

H. capsulatum var. *duboisii* causes cutaneous and systemic diseases in Africa. The yeast are larger than those of *H. capsulatum* var. *capsulatum*, and the walls are thicker, resembling the cells of *B. dermatitidis*, but without the broad-based buds. *Paracoccidioides brasiliensis*, which is restricted to the soil in Central and South America, produces cutaneous, pulmonary, and disseminated infections collectively called paracoccidioidomycosis (Mann, 1996). The characteristic tissue phase yeast cells of *Paracoccidioides* have multiple peripheral buds, producing an appearance that has been compared to a mariner's wheel. *Penicillium marneffei* is the fourth most common cause of disseminated opportunistic infection in patients with AIDS in Thailand, southern China, and other parts of south-east Asia where it is endemic (Duong, 1996). The environmental source for this fungus is still unknown but recent reports suggest that bamboo rats may play some role in the epidemiology of the infection caused by this fungus (Chariyalertsak, 1996). This species is unique among the penicillia in being dimorphic, producing in tissue yeast-like cells that are oval or cylindrical and may have crosswalls (Cooper, 2000).

Dermatophytoses

Dermatophytic fungi are common and important causes of human morbidity (Howard, 1999; Hainer, 2003). Generally, the infections are mild and rarely do the fungi associated with these infections cause invasive disease (Chastain, 2001). Three genera are recognized as causes of dermatophytosis: *Microsporum*, *Trichophyton*, and *Epidermophyton*. Other moulds, such as *Acremonium* species, *Fusarium* species, and *Scopulariopsis* species, have caused infections of the nails (onychomycosis) (Gupta, 2004). As a group, the dermatophytic fungi are distributed worldwide, but individual species may have a more restricted geographic distribution. Dermatophytes may also be found in strict association with humans (anthropophilic), with animals (zoophilic), or with soil (geophilic).

Risk factors

Dermatophyte infections (tinea) result from contact with the relevant source of the fungus, which may also provide a clue to the diagnosis. For instance, infection of the face in farmers who lean against their cows as they milk the animals is characteristically caused by *Trichophyton verrucosum*, a zoophilic dermatophyte that is found in cattle. The importance of geographic variation in dermatophytic pathogens is illustrated by a study of an epidemic of cutaneous fungal infection among American troops during the Vietnam War (Allen, 1973). The majority of the infections were caused by a heavily sporulating variant of *T. mentagrophytes* that had not been recognized in the United States. Skin disorders caused by the dermatophytic fungi have also become more frequently recognized in sports where there is direct contact between the athletes, such as wrestling (Kohl, 2000; Adams, 2002; Nenoff, 2002).

Clinical Diseases

Dermatophytes produce infection of the epidermis, hair, and nails (Rinaldi, 2000). Infection is often referred to as ringworm (or tinea), a name derived from the advancing, serpiginous nature of the lesions (especially evident on the skin). The clinical terminology uses the Latin name tinea followed by the body part involved, such as tinea capitis (scalp), tinea barbae (beard), tinea corporis (trunk and limbs), tinea pedis (foot), tinea cruris (groin), and tinea unguium (nail, which is also called onychomycosis). With occasional exceptions, *Epidermophyton floccosum* infects the skin only, *Microsporum* spp. infect the scalp and skin, while the *Trichophyton* spp. infect the skin, scalp, and nails. *Trichophyton tonsurans* is the most common cause of tinea capitis in the United States. *M. canis* is a common cause of scalp infection, particularly in children (Aly, 2000; Gupta, 2000). When deep infection of the hair follicles occurs, a boggy inflammatory process called a kerion results; *T. mentagrophytes* and *T. verrucosum* are particularly associated with kerion formation. *T. mentagrophytes*, *T. rubrum*, and *M. canis* are commonly found in tinea corporis and tinea pedis. The lesions produced by *T. rubrum* are often chronic and intractable, whereas *E. floccosum* is a common cause of tinea cruris.

Laboratory Diagnosis

Treatment of dermatophyte infections is not directed by the specific identification of the isolate, so that demonstration of hyphae in skin scrapings (using a KOH preparation) is frequently the only diagnostic technique performed before the initiation of therapy (Fig. 60–30). The size and morphology of hyphae suggest the involvement of dermatophytes in the infection. Confirmation of the species is useful for confirming that

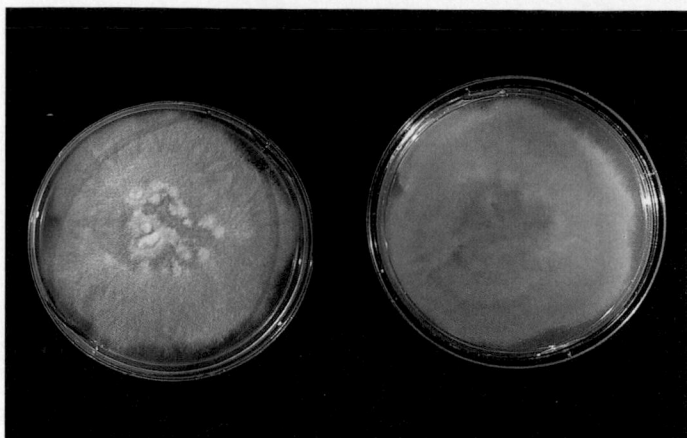

Figure 60–31 A fluffy white *Microsporum canis* colony (left) has the characteristic lemon yellow pigment, which may also be seen on the reverse of the colony (right). (Sabouraud dextrose agar with cycloheximide)

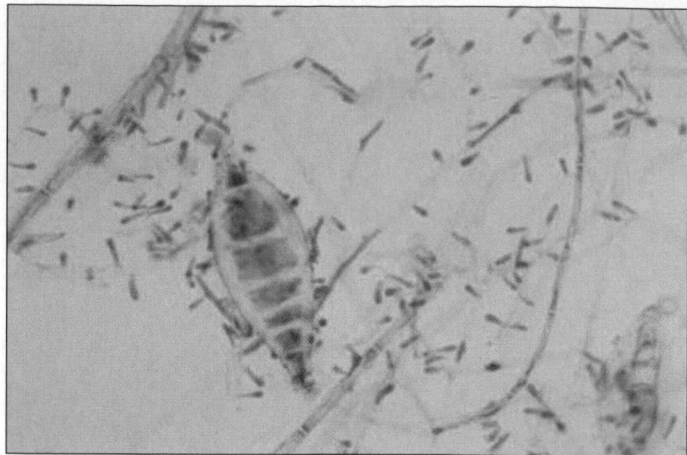

Figure 60–32 Thick-walled, roughened, tapered, spindle-shaped macroconidia of *Microsporum canis* with thin, septate hyphae. (Lactophenol cotton blue stain; ×400)

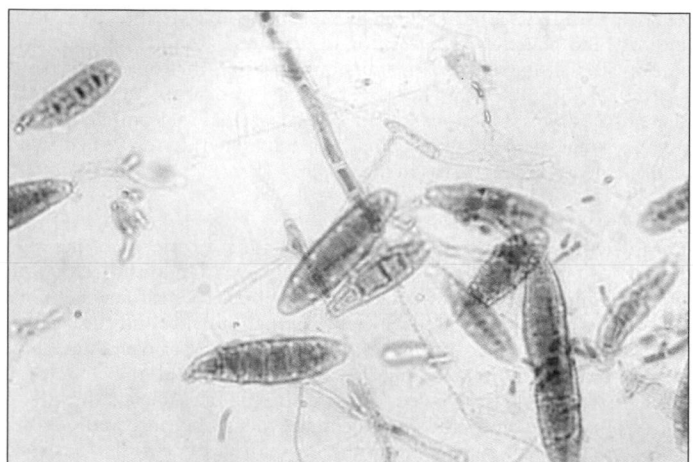

Figure 60–33 Thick-walled, smooth macroconidia of *Microsporum gypseum*. (Lactophenol cotton blue stain; ×400)

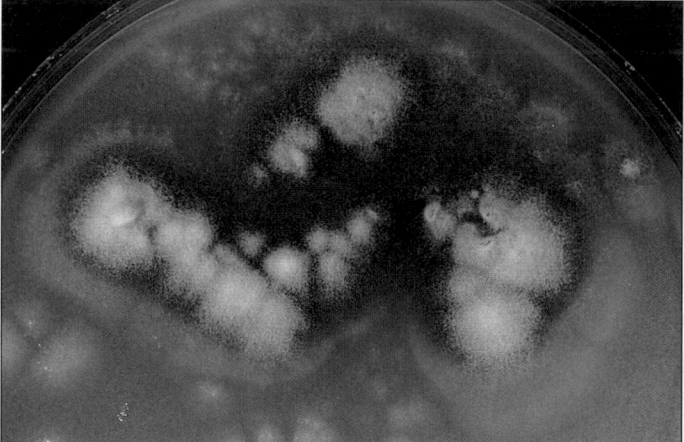

Figure 60–34 Fluffy white colonies of *Trichophyton rubrum* with diffusible red pigment, which may also be seen on the reverse of the colony. (Potato dextrose agar)

the hyphae did, in fact, belong to a dermatophytic fungus, for assessing the probable source of the infection, and for assessing the increased likelihood for chronic, relapsing infections (especially when *T. rubrum* is identified). Skin scrapings, nail, and hair can be examined in KOH preparations, which may incorporate Calcofluor white to facilitate the detection of hyphae. Care must be taken when reading this type of preparation, since tissue fragments, fibers, and cholesterol crystals may be mistaken for hyphae by the inexperienced observer.

When a hair infection is suspected, the infected hairs should be removed for analysis. Fungi such as *Microsporum audouinii*, *M. canis*, or *Microsporum ferrugineum* cause the hairs to fluoresce with a long-wavelength ultraviolet light (Wood's lamp). In the United States, tinea capitis due to a fluorescing fungus is most probably caused by *M. canis*, because the other two species are uncommon. Microscopic examination of the infected hair by an experienced observer may suggest the etiologic agent, based on the appearance and location of the arthroconidia. In ectothrix colonization, as occurs with *M. canis* and *M. audouinii* infection, arthroconidia are external to the hair shaft. Endothrix invasion, as seen in infection with *T. tonsurans*, is characterized by arthroconidia within the hair shaft. In favic infection, hyphae, air bubbles, or tunnels and fat droplets are present in the intrapilar area.

Infected hairs, nail scraping, or scrapings of the edges of skin lesions should be submitted to the laboratory in a clean, dry container or placed on the surface of primary isolation medium supplied by the laboratory. Sabouraud dextrose agar was designed for recovery of dermatophytic fungi and is also effective for isolating *Candida* spp., especially *C. albicans*, which may produce similar infections of the skin and nails. Dermatophytes are not inhibited by cycloheximide, which will inhibit many saprophytic fungi. All dermatophytic fungi have septate, hyaline hyphae and produce macroconidia and/or microconidia in various combinations. Arthroconidia and chlamydoconidia may also be produced but the morphology of the macroconidia, and especially the microconidia, are more important for identification. The sexual stages of many of the dermatophytes have been identified but they are not encountered in the clinical laboratory. A combination of both micromorphologic features and some phenotypic testing is used to differentiate the dermatophytes (Caddell, 2002).

Microsporum species produce characteristic macroconidia, which are the key diagnostic structures. In some cases, microconidia, which are not as useful diagnostically, also are produced. *M. audouinii*, a classic anthropophilic agent of ringworm, often does not produce diagnostic structures, which makes identification difficult. *M. canis*, the most frequently isolated zoonotic species of this genus, produces a characteristic lemon yellow pigment in culture (Fig. 60–31), which is intensified by growth on potato flake agar. The macroconidia of this species are illustrated in Figure 60–32. The macroconidia of *Microsporum gypseum*, the most common isolated geophilic species, are illustrated in Figure 60–33.

The genus *Trichophyton* includes the most commonly isolated dermatophytic fungi: *T. rubrum* (Fig. 60–34), *T. verrucosum*, *T. mentagrophytes* (Figs 60–11 and 60–35), and *T. tonsurans* (Fig. 60–36). The colonies may have a fluffy, granular or, less commonly, glabrous appearance. Macroconidia, which are useful for identification, may be produced, especially in strains that produce powdery colonies, but unfortunately

they are usually absent. Microconidia are formed more commonly. When present, the macroconidia are thin-walled, smooth, and contain variable numbers of septa. Interpretation of the microscopic morphology in some isolates can be difficult, because overlap occurs frequently. To help in this matter, additional tests are useful. In particular, the *Trichophyton* agars are helpful in the characterization of nutritional requirements among members of the genus. Seven media have been described; however, the first four are the most useful for identification purposes. In combination, these media allow for the assessment of dependency on inositol, thiamine, or both compounds together.

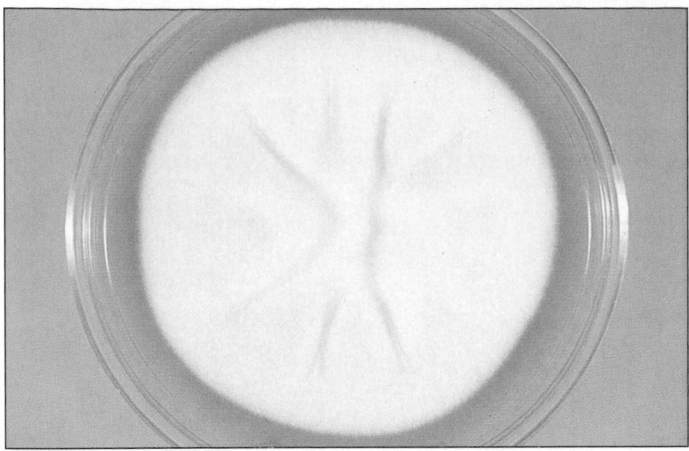

Figure 60–35 Fluffy white colony with radial folds of *Trichophyton mentagrophytes*. (Sabouraud dextrose agar with cycloheximide)

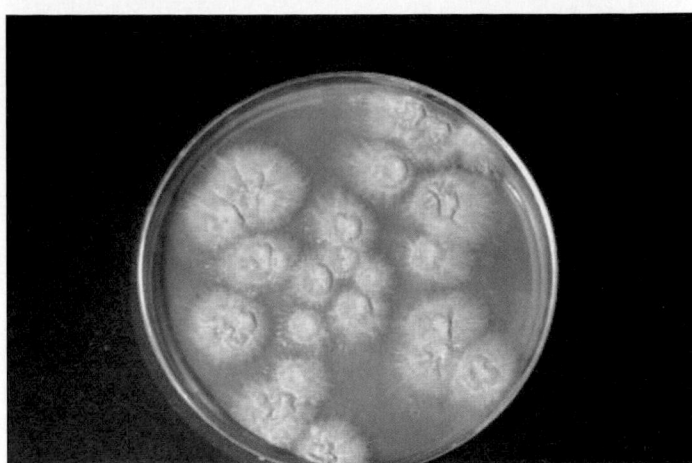

Figure 60–37 The suede-like texture and yellowish green color are characteristic of *Epidermophyton floccosum*. (Sabouraud dextrose agar with cycloheximide)

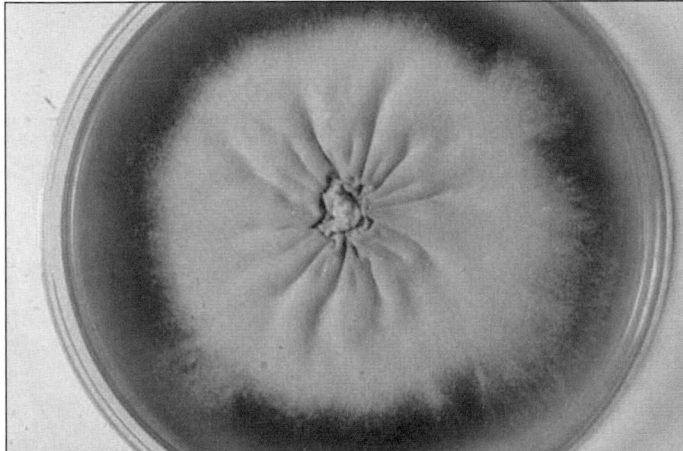

Figure 60–36 A flat colony showing pale yellow coloration with a reddish-brown pigmentation at the periphery characteristic of *Trichophyton tonsurans*. Radial furrowing of the thallus as seen is also common. (Sabouraud dextrose agar with cycloheximide)

Medium	Constituents	Interpretation of Stimulated Growth
T1	Basal medium agar	To compare with other formulations
T2	Inositol	Stimulated by inositol alone
T3	Inositol + thiamine	Stimulated only when both compounds present
T4	Thiamine	Stimulated by thiamine alone

Differentiation of *T. mentagrophytes* and *T. rubrum* is facilitated by several nonmorphologic tests as well. A diffusible pigment may be produced by both species, but the intensely red pigment of *T. rubrum* is enhanced by culture on potato flake agar or cornmeal agar with 1% dextrose. Production of urease within 3–5 days by *T. mentagrophytes* but not by *T. rubrum* also helps differentiate these two species. Finally, the hair penetration test can be used as a differential test. *T. mentagrophytes* produces wedge-shaped defects in hairs in vitro whereas *T. rubrum* grows on the outside of the hair without penetration. Use of both morphologic and nonmorphologic approaches provides the most accurate identification of isolates.

The only pathogen within the genus *Epidermophyton* is *E. floccosum*, an anthropophilic fungus that is an important cause of tinea cruris and, less commonly, tinea pedis. Colonies, which are initially brownish yellow, gray, or khaki brown, become velvety and folded as they mature (Fig. 60–37). *E. floccosum* produces no microconidia, but distinctive macroconidia provide the clues to the identification (Fig. 60–10). These structures have smooth external walls, with up to four crosswalls and a club shape and they tend to 'flocculate,' hence the species name.

Although the examination of micromorphologic structures and the comparison of results to phenotypic testing is generally reliable for the identification of dermatophyte species, molecular approaches have also recently been initiated to study the dermatophytes (Iwen, 2002; Kac, 2000). These studies have not only been conducted for diagnostic applications (Makimura, 2001), but also for phylogenetic (Graser, 2000a, 2000b) and epidemiologic evaluations (Kac, 2000).

Mycoses Caused by Dematiaceous Moulds

The dematiaceous moulds (also called the black moulds) are a fascinating and complex group of fungi characterized by the formation of a dark pigment due to the production of melanin in the cell walls of hyphae or conidia or both (Brandt, 2003). These fungi are soil and plant saprophytes and historically considered rare causes of disease in humans; however, they are now considered emerging fungal pathogens (Silveira, 2001).

Clinical Diseases

The clinical spectrum of diseases caused by these fungi includes eumycotic mycetoma (pl. mycetomata) and chromoblastomycosis, predominantly in hosts with normal immune systems, and phaeohyphomycosis, which is most common among immunocompromised patients (Rinaldi, 1996; McGinnis, 2003; Sanche, 2003). These diseases are frequently diagnosed on the basis of a unique histologic picture of the fungus in tissue followed by isolation of the fungus in culture and morphologic evaluation of the reproductive structures. The classification of black moulds has undergone numerous changes over the years, which increases the difficulty in identifying the etiologic agent (McGinnis, 1999; 2003). For a comprehensive morphologic description of the dematiaceous fungi, the reader is referred to a reference book by Sigler (2003). Although, a detailed description of the clinical and mycologic aspects of the diseases caused by the dematiaceous fungi is beyond the scope of this chapter, a brief description of the major types of disease entities is presented.

Dematiaceous moulds, such as *Stachybotrys chartarum*, although not generally associated with invasive disease, have been associated with a condition known as 'sick building syndrome,' although this association has been questioned (Miller, 2003). For a review on this subject, refer to a manuscript by Kuhn and Ghannoum (Kuhn, 2003).

Mycetoma

Mycetoma is a localized, chronic granulomatous infection of the cutaneous and subcutaneous tissues with the formation of a sinus tract and frequent involvement of the contiguous bones. In most cases, the disease is confined to the hands or feet (also called 'Madura foot') of individuals such as farmers, field hands, and others who are in contact with contaminated soil-laden materials. Both bacteria classified as aerobic actinomycetes (actinomycotic mycetoma) and filamentous fungi (eumycotic mycetoma) may cause mycetoma. Additionally, hyaline fungal pathogens (nonpigmented) can also cause this disease. For a review on actinomycotic mycetoma, refer to an article written by McNeil and Brown (McNeil, 1994). Mycetoma occurs after a traumatic injury with a contaminated object such as a splinter, thorn, or any other penetrating item. The clinical disease is characterized by the formation of a necrotic lesion at the site of inoculation. Although over 25 mould species have been known to cause this disease, the most common causative agents of eumycotic mycetoma are *Madurella mycetomatis*, *Scedosporium apiospermum*, *Leptosphaeria senegalensis*, and *Madurella grisea* (Bustamante, 2003; Ahmed, 2004). *S. apiospermum* (teleomorph, *Pseudallescheria boydii*, discussed in more detail later with the hyalohyphomycoses) is considered the most

VII

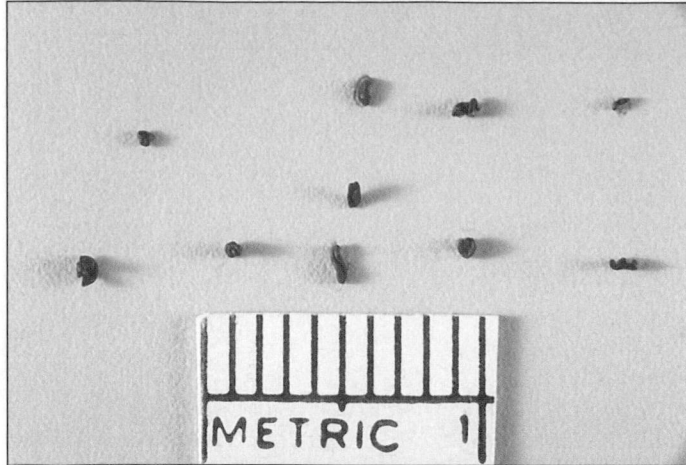

Figure 60–38 Image showing various sized granules of the fungus *Madurella grisea* composed of black masses of hyphae. (CDC Public Health Image Library)

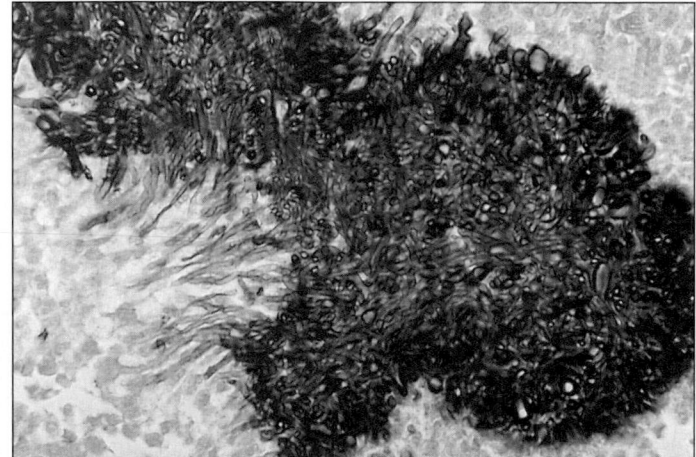

Figure 60–39 Histologic appearance of 'black grain mycetoma' due to *Madurella mycetomatis*. (Gridley stain, ×1000) (Courtesy of Dr Libero Ajello, CDC Public Health Image Library.)

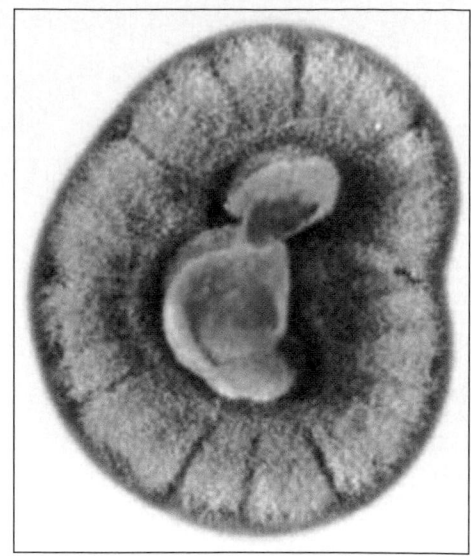

Figure 60–40 Close-up of a dematiaceous fungus growing on Sabouraud dextrose agar.

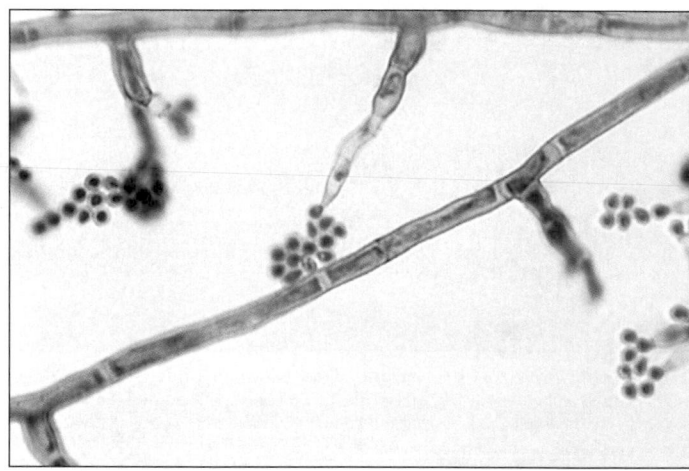

Figure 60–41 Image showing phialides with terminal conidia of *Madurella mycetomatis*. (Lactophenol cotton blue stain) (Courtesy of Dr Lucille K. George, CDC Public Health Image Library)

common cause of this disease in the United States; however, this fungal species does not produce dark pigmentation within tissue and so is not considered a dematiaceous fungus.

A definitive diagnosis of a mycetoma can be achieved by the demonstration of sclerotia (also referred to as grains or granules) in a tissue biopsy, in draining exudates from a sinus tract, or in material aspirated from an unopened sinus (Fig. 60–38). These grains are microscopically composed of broad, interwoven, septate hyphae 2–5 μm in diameter (Fig. 60–39). For dematiaceous fungi, these grains are associated with a dark pigment and generally called black grains, while sclerotia of nondematiaceous fungi consist of nonpigmented hyphae called white grains. Identification of the etiologic agent requires culture on standard fungal media such as Sabouraud dextrose agar, which may take 4 weeks or longer to grow because of the slow growth of these species (Fig. 60–40). Once isolated, the fungal species is identified, using the gross colony morphology and pigmentation along with close observation of the micromorphologic characteristics of the reproductive structures following sporulation (Fig. 60–41). In cases where sporulation does not occur, physiologic tests such as carbohydrate and nitrate utilization may aid in identification. A number of molecular techniques using a variety of targets have also been developed to help in the identification of the etiologic agent (Iwen, 2002).

Chromoblastomycosis

Chromoblastomycosis (chromomycosis) is a chronic infection of the skin and soft tissue characterized by the presence of muriform fungal structures called sclerotic bodies within the infected tissues. The disease is distinguished by the formation of a painless verrucous plaque or nodule at the site of inoculation with healing areas of the lesion evident and the formation of scar materials. The most common etiologic agents are the black moulds *Fonsecaea pedrosi*, *Phialophora verrucosa*, and *Cladophialophora carrionii*, although numerous other species may also be involved (Baddley,

2003a). The distinguishing feature is the presence of round, nonhyphal, brown cells (sclerotic bodies) in tissues. These structures, which divide by producing a septal plane, are diagnostic of the entity but do not provide a clue as to the species identification of the mould. Culture and recognition of the morphologic features of the isolate are again needed to identify the infecting species.

Pheohyphomycosis

Pheohyphomycosis (from the Greek word *phaeo*, meaning 'dark') was a term originally proposed by Ajello et al in 1974 as a histopathologic entity to cover all infections 'caused by fungi that develop in tissue in the form of dark-walled dematiaceous septate mycelial elements'(Ajello, 1974). Over the years, pheohyphomycosis has become more recognized as a cause of subcutaneous and systemic diseases characterized by the formation of pigmented septate hyphae in tissue. Although both chromoblastomycosis and eumycotic mycetoma are caused by dematiaceous fungi, they are distinguished from pheohyphomycosis by the appearance in tissue of sclerotic bodies and mycotic granules, respectively.

Phaeohyphomycosis ranges from an indolent subcutaneous lesion, probably resulting from direct inoculation of fungi at the site, to a devastating, destructive infection that is almost always fatal. The subcutaneous form of the disease is characterized by the formation of a solitary asymptomatic subcutaneous nodule or cyst usually in an immuno-competent individual, but this also may occur in transplant recipients (Clancy, 2000). The most common dematiaceous fungi associated with this condition are *Exophiala jeanselmei*, *Wangilla dermatitidis*, and *Phialophora* species (Perfect, 2003). This disease may become chronic with little observable clinical change for years. Systemic pheohyphomycosis, on the other hand, has emerged as a more common infection, especially in individuals with chemotherapy induced neutropenia. In a review of 101 cases of primary central nervous system pheohyphomycosis from 1966–2002, *Cladophialophora bantiana* accounted for 48% of the cases, by far the most common species responsible for cerebral disease (Revankar, 2004). The next most common species was *Ramichloridium mackenzei* (13% of cases). Interestingly, over half of these cases occurred in individuals with no known underlying immunodeficiency. In another review of 72 cases of disseminated pheohyphomycosis, leukemia was reported as the most common underlying condition, and the most common pathogen was *Scedosporium prolificans* (42%), followed by *Bipolaris spicifera* (8.3%) and *Wangiella dermatitidis* (*Exophiala dermatitidis*) (7%) (Revankar, 2002). Overall, the mortality was 79%. In most cases of pheohyphomycosis, the diagnosis may be difficult, since many of the etiologic agents are often considered to be contaminants when isolated from culture. In tissue, the presence of irregularly swollen, septate hyphal forms with yeast-like structures that stain with a melanin-specific Masson–Fontana stain is presumptive for the diagnosis of pheohyphomycosis.

Zygomycosis

The zygomycetes are important causes of invasive fungal infection in compromised hosts (Eucker, 2001; Freifeld, 2004; Pagano, 2004). *Rhizopus* spp. are the most common organisms isolated from patients with zygomycosis with *Rhizopus (oryzae) arrhizus* and *Rhizopus microsporus* var. *rhizopodiformis* the species causing a majority of cases (Ribes, 2000). Other less common species include *Absidia corymbifera*, *Apophysomyces elegans*, *Cunninghamella bertholletiae*, and *Rhizomucor pusillus* (Iwen, 2005). The invasive diseases caused by these fungi have historically been called mucormycosis and phycomycosis, but zygomycosis is the more frequent term, used as a more precise term relating diseases to the taxonomic classification (Freifeld, 2004).

Risk Factors

Diabetes, steroid use, neutropenia, infant prematurity, stem cell or solid organ transplantation, and the use of deferoxamine are well-described risk factors for the development of zygomycosis (Freifeld, 2004). In general, most of these conditions are associated with impairment of normal leukocyte immune function. Diabetic ketoacidosis has long been recognized as a major risk factor for the development of zygomycosis in humans. Ketoacidotic serum has been shown to stimulate the growth of *Rhizopus* (Artis, 1982).

Clinical Diseases

One of the two most common clinical presentations of zygomycosis is rhinocerebral disease (also called sinus–orbital or craniofacial zygomycosis). The infection begins as an undifferentiated sinusitis but the hyphae rapidly break through the thin walls of the sinus and extend up into the orbit, forward into the skin of the face, and back up into the cranial cavity. The typical risk factor for this type of infection is diabetes mellitus, and most patients are in ketoacidosis at the time the infection develops. Rhinocerebral disease may progress rapidly, and death often results. Thrombosis of the carotid artery or cavernous sinus may occur.

The second major presentation of zygomycosis is pulmonary disease, which may be followed by hematogenous dissemination. The infection begins as an undifferentiated pneumonia, which may be complicated by hemoptysis and cavitation. Disseminated infection is common and the outcome is almost uniformly fatal. The risk factors for pulmonary infection are neutropenia and immunosuppression, particularly by hematologic malignancy (Pagano, 2004).

A less common presentation of zygomycosis is infection of skin and soft tissues (Alsuwaida, 2002; Oh, 2002). The hyphae may reach the skin by the hematogenous route, by direct extension from a deep focus, or by introduction from the outside. Contaminated adhesive tape has been reported as a source of primary cutaneous disease in the compromised patient (Alsuwaida, 2002). Other rare cases of zygomycosis include primary involvement of the gastrointestinal tract, the heart, the brain, or the kidneys (Freifeld, 2004).

Pathology of Zygomycosis

The histopathology is dominated by necrosis of tissue, regardless of the site of infection. The propensity for these moulds to invade through the walls of arteries and veins, producing thrombosis, leads to extensive coagulative necrosis (Chandler, 1987b). The hyphae appear as ribbons of broad hyphae that are often twisted and collapsed with a variable width from 5–20 μm (Fig. 60-3). Septa are sparse and are usually not observed

Table 60–12 Histopathologic Features of the Zygomycetes in Comparison to Other Fungi that Occur as Nonpigmented Hyphae in Tissue

Characteristic	Zygomycetes*	Aspergillus†	Fusarium
Hyphal characteristics			
Width (μm)	Variable (5–10)	Consistent (3–6)	Consistent (3–8)
Branching pattern	Haphazard	Dichotomous	Right angle
Septation frequency	Rare	High	High
Reproductive structures in tissue	Absent	May be present where infected area communicates with air	Chlamydoconidia sometimes present
Angioinvasive	Yes	Yes	Yes

In all cases, a definitive diagnosis of the species requires isolation and identification of the fungus on synthetic media.

* Entomophthorales are included in this group with the hyphal fragments in tissue generally coated by amorphous eosinophilic Splendore–Hoeppli material and a lack of angioinvasiveness noted.

† Due to hyphal degeneration or host immune response or both, the hyphae of the *Aspergillus* species may exhibit atypical morphologic forms that may cause problems in the differential diagnosis.

Source: modified with permission from Freifeld AG, Iwen PC: Zygomycosis. Semin Respir Crit Care Med 2004; 25: 221–231.

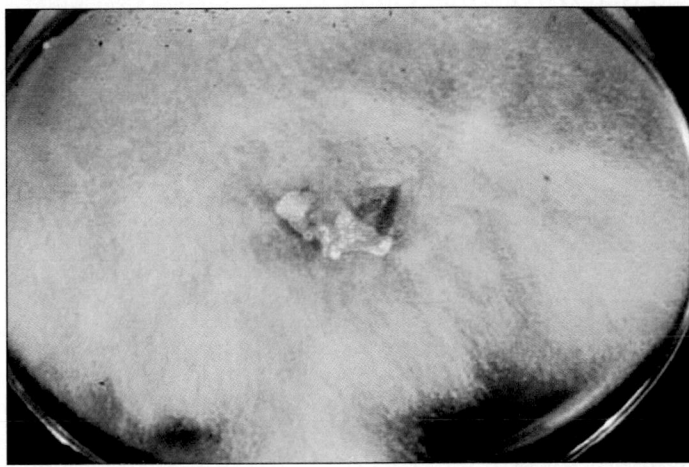

Figure 60–42 A fluffy gray colony of *Rhizopus* species fills the space within the Petri dish (lid lifter). (Sabouraud dextrose agar)

in tissue, but an overlay of the exterior walls of collapsed hyphae may be mistaken for septa. Swollen segments of hyphae and hyphae cut in cross-section may be incorrectly interpreted as yeast cells. Branching tends to occur at right angles in a haphazard pattern. These hyphal characteristics along with the angioinvasive property of these fungi are highly suggestive of a zygomycosis. A comparison of the histologic features of the zygomycetes with other nonpigmented hyphae in tissue is given in Table 60–12. The hyphae of these moulds often stain better with H&E than with the methenamine silver method.

Laboratory Diagnosis

Zygomycetes often are considered common contaminants within the mycology laboratory, but the potential clinical implications of isolates should be carefully investigated before they are dismissed as saprophytes. Collaboration between the pathologist and laboratory personnel is important because demonstration of hyphae in tissue demonstrates that an isolated mould was present in vivo and is not an environmental contaminant. The broad, sparsely septate hyphae may be demonstrated in tissue sections or in imprint smears of tissue, using the Calcofluor white stain. Tissue should be minced or teased, rather than homogenized, after which it is inoculated on to the surface of a primary isolation agar. Zygomycetes are inhibited by cycloheximide so nonselective fungal medium should be included when performing fungal cultures.

Zygomycetes grow rapidly (within 48–72 hours) and produce abundant aerial hyphae that quickly reach the lid of the Petri dish, colloquially referred to as 'lid lifters.' The colonies are characterized as wooly, initially white, turning gray to black as the spores are developed (Fig 60–42).

Rhizopus spp. produce unbranched sporangiophores that support sporangia (60–350 µm) with an ellipsoidal columella and containing sporangiospores. The sporangiospores are oval and frequently have a brown pigment (Fig 60–6). An important diagnostic feature for *Rhizopus* is the presence of hyaline to brown root-like structures called rhizoids, which develop at the point where the sporangiophores arise. In contrast to *Rhizopus*, the rhizoids of *Absidia* species arise from the stolons between conidiophores. The sporangiophores are pear-shaped rather than round, and a collarette is visible around the columella when the sporangium disintegrates. *Mucor* species do not produce rhizoids, the conidiophores are usually more branched than those of other zygomycetes, and growth does not occur above 37°C. *Rhizomucor*, which is morphologically intermediate between *Rhizopus* and *Mucor*, has rudimentary rhizoids and branched conidiophores, and grows at temperatures as high as 58°C. *Mucor* spp. were once believed to be the second most recognized cause of zygomycosis. This is no longer the case since *Mucor corymbifera* has been reassigned to the genus *Absidia* as *Absidia corymbifera*, and *Mucor pusillus* has been reclassified in the genus *Rhizomucor* as *Rh. pusillus*. *Mucor* spp. are now considered a distant third as causes of zygomycosis, well behind the *Rhizopus* species and *A. corymbifera* in occurrence (Ribes, 2000). Although the genera of the zygomycetes can be readily recognized, few mycology labs have the ability to identify species, which requires mating studies (for the production of zygospores) or molecular analysis using sequence comparison mechanisms (Weitzman, 1995; Yeo, 2002).

Aspergillosis, Fusariosis, and Other Mycoses Caused by Hyaline Fungi

This large group of saprophytic fungi, frequently encountered in the clinical laboratory, contains some of the most important pathogenic moulds. These moulds are collectively classified as hyaline because they produce non-pigmented hyphae, and the disease is called hyalohyphomycosis. The number of species within this group capable of causing human disease is large and continues to expand as immunosuppressive therapies become more common. Since it is beyond the scope of this chapter to discuss the full range of organisms involved, the reader is referred to an atlas of clinical fungi for more detail on the variety of species causing hyalohyphomycosis (De Hoog, 2000). By far, the most recognized hyaline moulds causing human disease are classified in the Eurotiales (*Aspergillus*, *Paecilomyces*, and *Penicillium*), the Microascales (*Scedosporium* and *Scopulariopsis*), and the Hypocreales (*Cylindrocarpon*, *Fusarium*, and *Trichoderma*). In this section, detailed consideration will be given to *Aspergillus* spp. and *Fusarium* spp., the hyaline moulds most commonly associated with invasive human disease.

The Genus *Aspergillus*

Aspergillosis is a term used to describe infection caused by species of the genus *Aspergillus*. This group of organisms has the ability to produce a wide spectrum of infections, including mycotoxicosis, allergic manifestations, and superficial infection in the normal host; localized noninvasive infection in hosts with tissue damage or foreign body obstruction; and invasive infection in the compromised host (Bodey, 1989). Reviews by Etzel (2002) and Judson (2004) are recommended for more information on intoxication by ingestion of *Aspergillus* toxin and allergic manifestations associated with *Aspergillus* spore exposure, respectively.

Aspergillus fumigatus is considered the most common species associated with human diseases, followed by *Aspergillus flavus*, although in some institutions *A. flavus* has emerged as the most common species detected (Bodey, 1989; Iwen, 1993). The third most common species is either *Aspergillus niger* or *Aspergillus terreus* (Iwen, 1998a, Perfect, 2001; Marr, 2002a). Resistance of *A. terreus* to amphotericin B makes invasive disease caused by this species particularly challenging to treat (Iwen, 1998a; Sutton, 1999; Baddley, 2003b; Steinbach, 2004). Other rare species of *Aspergillus* have also been associated with invasive disease (Iwen, 1998b; Marr, 2002a).

Risk Factors

The Hyphomycetes are ubiquitous fungi to which all of us are exposed on a regular basis. They are resident in vegetation of all types and ubiquitous in the environment. Nosocomial infections are not uncommon, and hospital construction has been linked to numerous cases in the literature (Iwen, 1994; Warnock, 2001). Engineering infection control through facility design to protect high risk patients from spore exposure have been done to provide a safer environment for patients (Noskin, 2001).

The most important risk factors for invasive aspergillosis are immunosuppressive disease, high-dose chemotherapy with or without transplantation, and solid organ transplantation (Denning, 1998a, 1998b; Fishman, 2002; Marr, 2002b; Ergin, 2003). Neutropenia is a prominent predisposing factor for disease; however, serious invasive disease may also occur in individuals who are not immunosuppressed by chemotherapy or malignancy (Denning, 2004). Invasive disease in entirely normal individuals is rare, however. Wound infection has been a problem in patients with extensive burn wounds and in individuals who are exposed to materials contaminated with conidia, a situation reminiscent of the zygomycetes (Holzheimer, 2002). Fungus balls may occur in the lung of patients with chronic obstructive lung disease, bronchiectasis, or old cavities caused by tuberculosis (Judson, 2004).

Clinical Diseases

The spectrum of invasive disease caused by *Aspergillus* species is broad. These fungi have a low pathogenicity in humans, and rarely cause disease in the immunologically competent individual. However, immunocompromised patients are at risk for invasive disease, especially those patients with prolonged granulocytopenia or graft-versus-host disease, and those undergoing immunosuppressive therapy or receiving corticosteroid treatment (Kontoyiannis, 2002). Since *Aspergillus* spores are normal in the environment, the most common primary site of infection is the lower respiratory tract and to a lesser extent, the paranasal sinuses.

Ocular infections

Keratomycosis usually follows trauma to the eye, especially in patients who have been treated with topical steroids. Pain and blurring of vision follow the traumatic episode and, if it is not treated, the infection may extend into the anterior chamber. Enucleation of the eye may be necessary if the process is not halted. A review by Thomas on the current perspectives on ophthalmic mycoses describes in more detail the clinical features associated with diseases involving the orbit and eye (Thomas, 2003).

Otic infections

Otomycosis is an infection of the external ear, usually caused by *A. niger* or *A. fumigatus*. Pain, decreased hearing, and a discharge are accompanied by a fluffy green or black growth in the ear canal. Extension beyond the external ear is rare, but may occur in immunosuppressed patients (Vennewald, 2003).

Sinus infection

Fungal sinusitis can be classified into four primary categories: acute fulminate invasive disease, chronic indolent invasive disease, fungus ball, and allergic disease (Morpeth, 1996). Spread of the fungus from the sinus into adjacent tissues (acute or chronic invasive disease) is frequently dependent on the host immunologic responses and the presence of metabolic ketoacidosis, although invasive infection has also been reported in apparently healthy individuals (Parikh, 2004; Sivak-Callcott, 2004). Many different *Aspergillus* species have been involved in invasive disease, with *A. flavus* as the most common species in some reports (Iwen, 1997).

Cutaneous infection

Aspergillus species may infect the skin after dissemination from another site, usually pulmonary, in either HIV-infected or immunocompromised patients, or the infection may be a primary case after direct exposure to a cutaneous source (Arikan, 1998; van Burik, 1998). Recognized risk factors include immunosuppression, but local factors that abrogate defense mechanisms of the skin are also important, such as may occur with burn wounds and surgical wounds, especially if occlusive dressings are present. Dissemination to the skin from another primary source is difficult to treat and frequently results in death.

Primary pulmonary infection

Primary pulmonary aspergillosis is the most common mould infection in immunocompromised patients, especially those with hematologic malignancies treated with intensive chemotherapy (Herbrecht, 2004). Acute invasive pulmonary disease is usually associated with severely immunocompromised persons; however. less invasive and noninvasive diseases that affect the lungs, such as aspergillomas (fungus ball), chronic necrotizing pulmonary aspergillosis, semi-invasive aspergillosis, chronic invasive pulmonary aspergillosis, symptomatic pulmonary aspergillosis, and *Aspergillus* pseudotuberculosis, have also been described. The predilection of *Aspergillus* to invade blood vessels leads to infarction and hemorrhage in the lungs and may cause hematogenous spread to other organs (Saubani, 2002)

Dissemination infection

Dissemination from the lung or other sites may involve any organ system. The propensity of hyphae to invade vascular structures and cause thrombosis leads to infarcts and abscesses in multiple organs. Single or

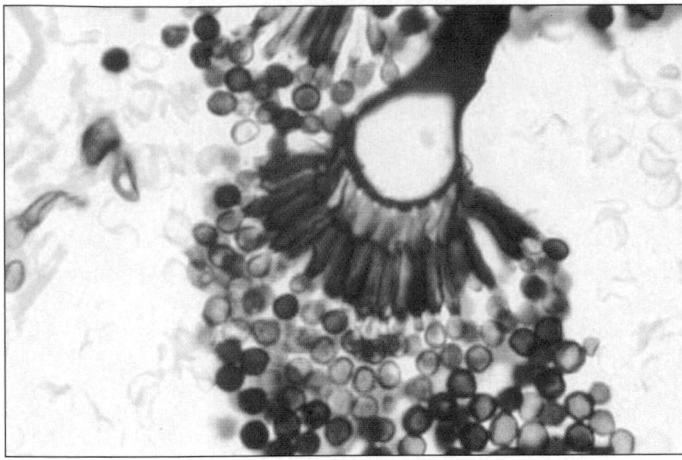

Figure 60–43 A fruiting head of *Aspergillus* is demonstrated within a pulmonary mycetoma (fungus ball). The phialides and conidia are well demonstrated. Although the hyphae of *Aspergillus* are not etiologically diagnostic, demonstration of the fruiting head documents the presence of this genus. (Hematoxylin and eosin stain, ×400)

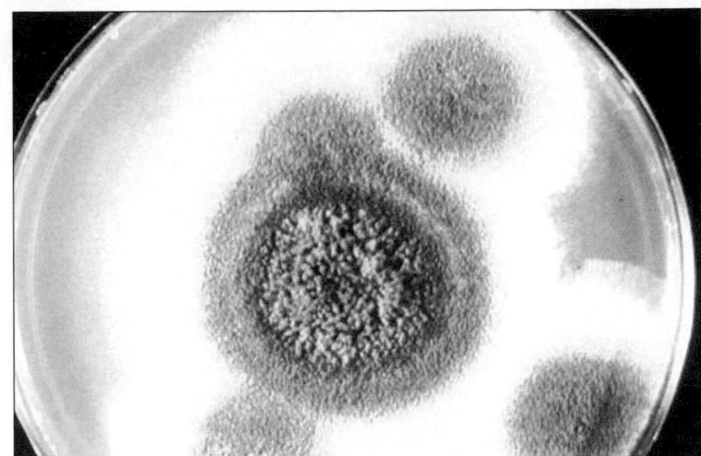

Figure 60–44 Fluffy colonies with granular areas produced by fruiting heads of *Aspergillus flavus*. The development of yellow or green coloration within the white colonies is characteristic. (Sabouraud dextrose agar)

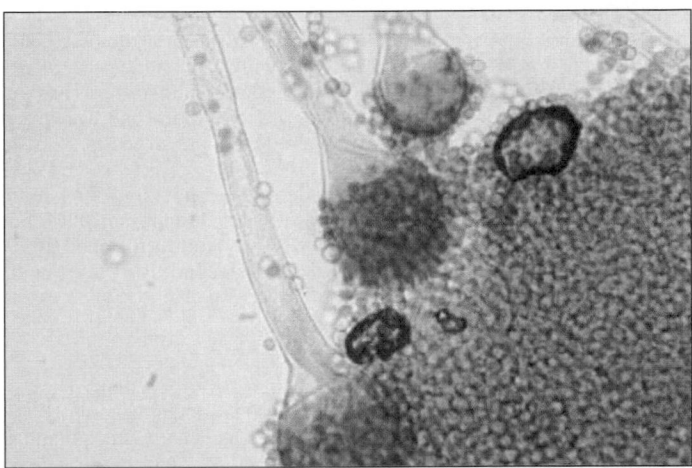

Figure 60–45 The fruiting head of *Aspergillus flavus* is uniseriate and biseriate. The phialides extend around much of the vesicle with a roughened (spiny) appearance of the conidiophore present. (Lactophenol cotton blue stain; ×400)

multiple organs, including the brain, skin, kidneys, pleura, heart, esophagus, liver, or any other site may be involved (Denning, 1998a).

Pathology of Aspergillosis

The histologic appearance of *Aspergillus* infection is similar to that observed with the other hyaline mould infections, and differentiation among genera and species is usually not possible except in unusual cases where sporulation within the tissue cavity has occurred. The tissue reaction may be granulomatous but is more commonly dominated by polymorphonuclear neutrophils, unless the patient is severely neutropenic. Vascular invasion, thrombosis, and infarction often are prominent features. The hyphae are thin (2–5 μm), septate, and branch at acute angles (dichotomous) (Fig. 60–4). H&E stain often color the hyphae well, but the morphology may be demonstrated to advantage with the periodic-acid–Schiff or methenamine silver techniques. The histologic appearance of aspergilli and zygomycetes can be differentiated on the basis of on size, hyphal characteristics, and the presence of septations (Table 60–12).

When the pathologic process is a fungus ball, the hyphae may stain poorly using histopathologic stains. Hyphae in a cavity that is in contact with air, as in the lung or sinuses, may develop fruiting heads, an event that permits identification as *Aspergillus* (Fig. 60–43). The conidiophores, which are not septate and may be wider than the vegetative hyphae, should not be confused with zygomycetes. Thick-walled Hülle cells and cleistothecia have been described in vivo. When the patient is immunocompetent and the histologic response is granulomatous, the hyphae may be fragmented and confined to the cytoplasm of macrophages and multinucleated giant cells. The granulomatous response to *Aspergillus* in the lung may be mistaken for bronchocentric granulomatosis, usually in patients who have allergic disease (Nagata, 1990).

Laboratory Diagnosis

Aspergilli are saprophytic fungi but should never be dismissed as contaminants without consultation with the attending physician. Isolation from a sterile site or repeated isolation from respiratory specimens suggests clinical significance. Hyphae may be demonstrated directly in clinical specimens in imprint preparations or wet preparations. Calcofluor white is useful for demonstrating the mould in specimens. It is important to obtain tissue, fluid, scrapings, or curettings for examination. Tissue should be teased or minced and inoculated directly on to the surface of the isolation medium. These moulds grow rapidly but most are or partially completely inhibited by cycloheximide. The colonies of many of these moulds teem with conidia. To prevent contamination of the worker and other cultures, the colonies should be manipulated carefully in a biological safety cabinet, after which the surfaces of the safety cabinet should be thoroughly wiped with a fungicidal solution. Maintenance of isolated moulds in plastic bags while continuing incubation also reduces the probability of contaminating other cultures.

The identification of *Aspergillus* species is made by study of the reproductive structures and the macroscopic appearance of the culture. Careful attention to details of the conidial head is needed for species identification (Klich, 2002). *A. fumigatus* is a common mould isolated in mycology laboratories. The fungus grows rapidly, producing colonies with a fluffy appearance. The development of fruiting heads imparts a blue-green appearance to the colony (Fig. 60–2). Examination of the colony with a dissecting microscope reveals the conidiophores with their expanded vesicles as small globes projecting above the vegetative mycelium. The conidiophore is smooth, relatively short (300–500 μm), and expanded into a flask-shaped vesicle. The phialides develop in a single row (uniseriate), and most commonly develop only on the upper two-thirds of the vesicle parallel to the axis of the conidiophore (Fig. 60–8). The conidia are roughened (echinulate) and round to oval in shape.

The second most important pathogen in the genus *Aspergillus* is *A. flavus*. The colonies grow rapidly and have a velvety yellow to green appearance once fruiting heads develop (Fig. 60–44). The conidiophore is long (400–700 μm), ending in a vesicle that may be elliptical or round. The conidiophore is rough and stubbly. A single or double (biseriate) row of phialides occurs over the whole vesicle or the upper three quarters (Fig. 60–45). Round to oval conidia appear yellow-green *en masse* and measure 3–4.5 μm.

Aspergillus terreus can be differentiated from the other species by the production of a cinnamon brown colony with microscopic characteristics that include short conidiophores (<250 μm) and biseriate phialides.

Although the gold standard for diagnosing invasive aspergillosis is a positive culture from sterile tissue with histologic evidence of mycelial invasion, the need for invasive techniques to obtain the specimen, the delayed time required for culture, and the rapidity with which the aspergilli can spread make diagnosis problematic. Non-culture-based methods for the diagnosis of aspergillosis have been developed (Wheat, 2003c). Recently, a commercial serologic assay (Platelia Aspergillus ELISA; Bio-Rad, Marnes-la-Coquette, France) using the double-sandwich enzyme-linked immunosorbent assay for the detection of galactomannan antigenemia was cleared by the US Food and Drug Administration for the rapid diagnosis of invasive aspergillosis. The sensitivity of the test has

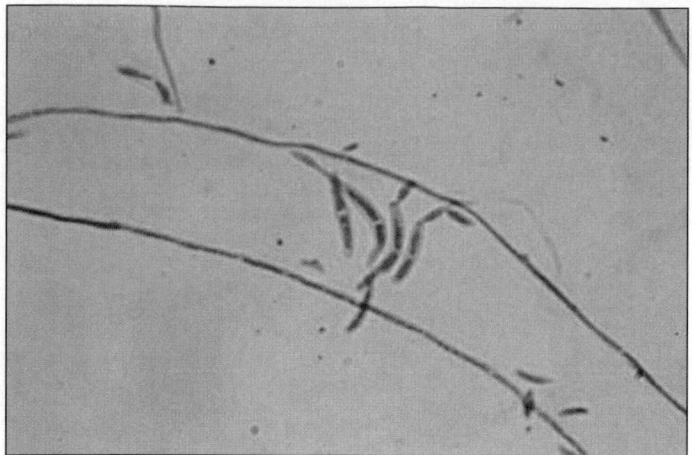

Figure 60–46 Canoe-shaped conidia of *Fusarium* species. The conidia are often septate. (Lactophenol cotton blue stain; ×400)

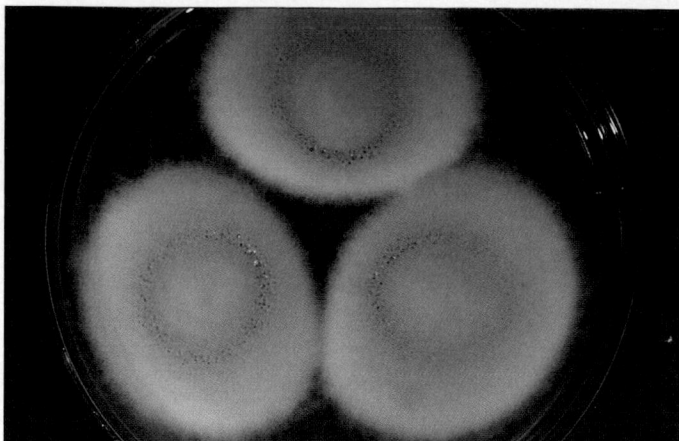

Figure 60–47 A developing colony of *Scedosporium apiospermum* with the characteristic mousy gray coloration. (Sabouraud dextrose agar)

ranged from less than 50% to 95% and the specificity from less than 70% to 100%, suggesting that it will not replace careful microbiologic and clinical evaluation (Herbrecht, 2002). Variables that affect the performance of this assay include antimicrobial therapy (piperacillin–tazobactam and amoxicillin–clavulanate can cause a false-positive result) and age (false-positive results are more common in children than in adults) (Walsh, 2004a).

Molecular methods have also been developed, not only for culture confirmation of *Aspergillus* species (Henry, 2000; de Aguirre, 2004), but also for the direct detection of fungal DNA in clinical material (Iwen, 2002). The results have shown promise, but considerable work needs to be done before these assays become commercially available.

The Genus *Fusarium*

Fusarium species have been implicated in a number of infectious diseases, including keratomycosis (Thomas, 2003), burn wounds (Latenser, 2003), and invasive disease in immunocompromised patients (Sampathkumar, 2001; Jensen, 2004; Lionakis, 2004; Nucci, 2004). They are now considered the second most common pathogenic moulds causing invasive disease (Dignani, 2004). The histopathologic picture is essentially identical to that observed with invasive aspergillosis (angioinvasive and acute branching-septate hyphae). However, fungemia with positive blood cultures are common in disseminated fusariosis but rarely occur with aspergillosis (Lionakis, 2004).

Colonies of *Fusarium* develop rapidly, producing a fluffy aerial mycelium, which often has a pink, lavender, or salmon color. Diffusible pigments may be seen in the surrounding agar. Simple or branched phialides develop directly from the hypha without a separate conidiophore. Short oval microconidia may be produced, but the distinctive structure is a canoe-shaped or crescent-shaped macroconidium, which may have one or more septa (Fig. 60–46). The species frequently implicated in human infection include *Fusarium solani*, *Fusarium oxysporum*, and *Fusarium moniliforme*, however, the recognition of species although important for epidemiologic purposes, does not impact therapeutic decisions. The ability to identify species in the mycology laboratory is difficult, usually requiring a reference laboratory with experience in recognition of the subtle details concerning the reproductive structures. Additionally, molecular technology using sequence areas within the ribosomal DNA gene complex have shown promise for the rapid and accurate identification of *Fusarium* species (Hennequin, 1999; Iwen, 2002).

The Genus *Scedosporium*

The two members of this genus associated with systemic infection are *S. apiospermum* (teleomorph *Pseudallescheria boydii*, previously known as *Allescheria boydii* and *Petriellidium boydii*) and *Scedosporium (inflatum) prolificans* (Steinbach, 2003b). These fungi are ubiquitous saprophytic moulds found in the soil and decaying vegetation. *S. prolificans* is an uncommon cause of disseminated infection (Grosbell, 1999); whereas *S. apiospermum*, although most often associated with a subcutaneous infection (mycetoma), is a more common cause of invasive disease in the immunocompromised patient (Nesky, 2000; Castiglioni, 2002; Nonaka, 2002; Nucci, 2003). *P. boydii* is the sexual phase of this pathogen, whereas *S. apiospermum* is the imperfect, asexual phase. The mould grows rapidly

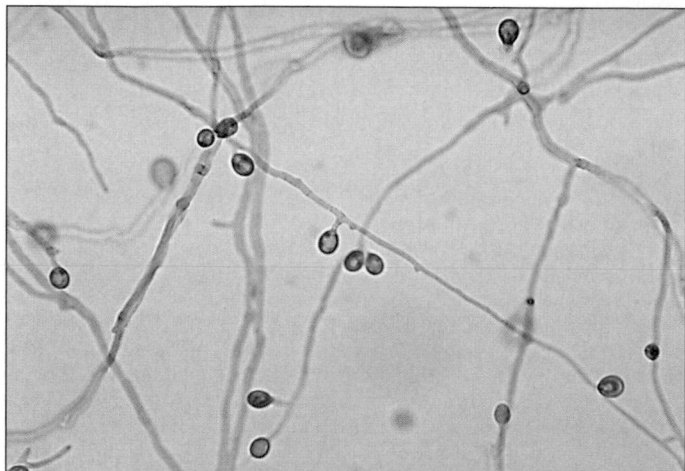

Figure 60–48 The tadpole- or sperm-shaped microconidia of *Scedosporium apiospermum* gave this organism its name. (Lactophenol cotton blue stain; ×400)

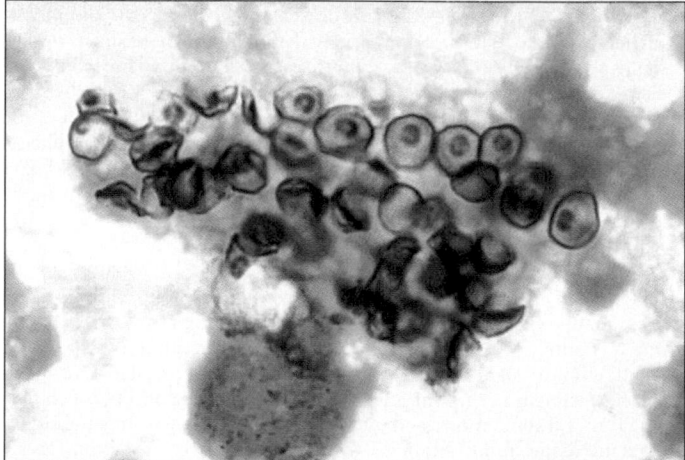

Figure 60–49 Cysts of *Pneumocystis jiroveci* in a smear from bronchoalveolar lavage. (Methenamine silver stain; ×400) (Courtesy of Dr Russell K. Brynes, CDC Public Health Image Library)

on isolation medium, producing a fluffy colony, which develops a brownish gray to dark gray ('mousy') color after incubation for several days. The culture darkens still more with continued incubation (Fig. 60–47). This mould may grow on media that contain up to 8 mg/mL of cycloheximide. The asexual phase is characterized by single or small clusters of annelloconidia on a straight or branched conidiophore that may develop terminally or laterally from the vegetative hyphae. The conidia are light brown and have an oval, sperm-like morphology (Fig. 60–48). In the sexual phase, brown cleistothecia (ascus) contain ascospores (Fig. 60–13).

The cleistothecia, which are found most readily at the edges of the colony, develop best on nutritionally deficient media, such as cornmeal agar, V-8 juice agar, or potato dextrose (potato flake) agar. Strictly speaking, the isolate should be reported as *P. boydii* if the cleistothecia are demonstrated and as *S. apiospermum* if the asexual conidia are the only diagnostic structures observed.

Other Septate Hyaline Moulds

There is a long list of hyaline moulds that are environmental saprophytes of low virulence and usually not associated with clinical disease when isolated in the mycology laboratory (Walsh, 2004b). As mentioned earlier, any mould may be pathogenic under the right conditions. In most cases, the host defenses of the patient are compromised in some way or the fungus is introduced into the body by trauma or medical manipulations. Increasing numbers of case reports document saprophytic fungi producing infections of deep tissue and systemic organs (Hilmarsdottir, 2000; Rodriguez-Villalobos, 2003; Schinabeck, 2003; Hall, 2004). Demonstration of hyphae in tissue is extremely important for documenting the pathogenicity of these saprophytic isolates, with culture necessary for species recognition. Molecular methods are becoming more useful for the identification of these unusual pathogens (Iwen, 2000)

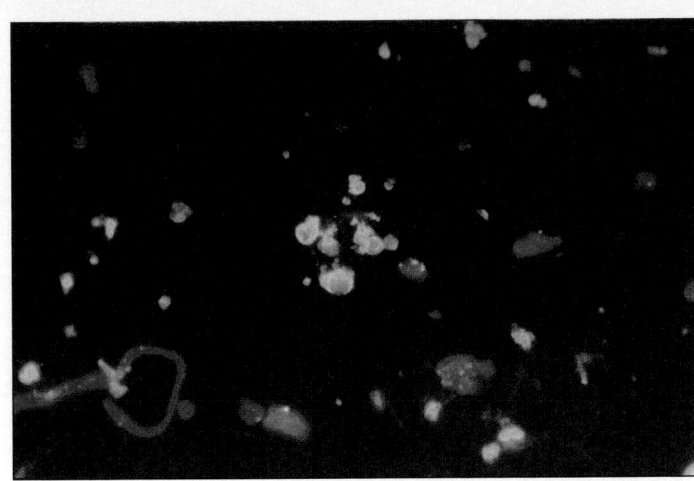

Figure 60–50 Immunofluorescence microscopy showing the presence of *Pneumocystis jiroveci*. (×560) (Courtesy of Lois Norman, CDC Public Health Image Library)

Pneumocystis Pneumonia

The taxonomic position of *P. (carinii) jiroveci* has undergone changes over the years. Originally, it was described as a protozoan with the morphologic forms identified as trophozoites, cysts, and sporozoites. This protozoan hypothesis remained predominant until Edman and colleagues., through DNA analysis, reported on the similarity of this organism to the fungi (Edman, 1988). More recently, information has shown that the organism has very different DNA sequences when identified from different mammal hosts. As a means to address this issue, the *Pneumocystis Working Group* in 1994 proposed the name *P. carinii* f. sp. *hominis* as a special form (formae specialis) of the organism causing *P. carinii* pneumonia (PCP) in humans (Pneumocystis Working Group, 1994). Subsequently, those attending the International Workshop on Opportunistic Protists in 2001 began the process to rename the species to *P. jiroveci* (pronounced 'yee row vet zee') (Frenkel, 1999; Stringer, 2002). Although controversial (Hughes, 2003), the name has now become widely accepted as the 'microbe that causes PCP in humans.' The acronym PCP now stands for *Pneumocystis* pneumonia.

Risk Factors

Pneumocystis jiroveci (human-derived *Pneumocystis*) is a pathogen capable of causing a broad spectrum of clinical presentation. It was first recognized in outbreaks of pulmonary disease among malnourished infants in Eastern Europe during and after World War II (called 'interstitial plasma cell pneumonia') (Cushion, 2003). More recently, it became a major cause of life-threatening pneumonia in 60–80% of HIV-infected adults in America and western Europe and subsequently became one of the AIDS-defining illnesses (Centers for Disease Control and Prevention, 1999b). Although still considered a serious problem within this patient population, the incidence of disease in people with AIDS has decreased to less than 10% of patients because of the availability of highly active antiretroviral therapy, the increasing use of anti-PCP prophylaxis, and improved awareness of the infection (Wolff, 2003). The disease should also be considered in any immunosuppressed patient who presents with fever, respiratory symptoms, or infiltrate on chest radiograph (Dei-Cas, 2000). Initially, clinical disease was thought to be due to reactivation of latent childhood infection in immunosuppressed cases, but studies now show that the organism can be transmitted between humans by the airborne route (Nevez, 2003; Totet, 2003). In individuals with compromised immune systems (e.g., HIV infection, chemotherapeutic regimens, organ transplantation), a potentially severe and fatal pneumonia can occur. Disseminated disease may also be present via spread through the lymphatic and blood routes, but this is uncommon. Although rare, infection has been documented in patients without a predisposing illness (Al Soub, 2004).

Clinical Diseases

Pneumonia is the most common manifestation of *P. jiroveci* infection (Wilkin, 1999). The onset may be acute or insidious. Symptomatic adults frequently present with dyspnea, a nonproductive cough, an inability to breathe deeply, chest tightness, and night sweats. The classic radiologic feature of PCP is fine, bilateral, perihilar interstitial shadowing; however other radiographic pictures may be present (Barry, 2001). Often, radiographic infiltrates are much more extensive than would be suggested by the degree of symptoms. Concurrent infection with other agents, particularly cytomegalovirus or *C. neoformans*, is common. The infection is often fatal if untreated. The most common extrapulmonary sites of infection are the thyroid, liver, bone marrow, lymph nodes, and spleen (Wazir, 2004).

Pathology of Pneumocystis Pneumonia

The definitive diagnosis of PCP requires the demonstration of cysts or trophozoites within clinical specimens (Fig. 60–49). Historically, this required an open-thorax lung biopsy because of the low number of organisms present in other respiratory specimens and the lack of sensitive diagnostic tests. Although open lung biopsy is still considered one of the most sensitive tests for the detection of this disease, other specimens such as induced sputum and bronchoalveolar lavage have proved to be reliable specimens for diagnosis (Rodriguez, 2004). The classic histopathologic findings of PCP in sections of lung stained with H&E are widening of the alveolar septa with an infiltrate of mononuclear cells and a foamy exudate within the alveolar spaces (sometime referred to as honeycombed exudates) (Woods, 2003). This exudate consists of aggregated cysts and trophozoites. The cyst form of *P. jiroveci* can be illustrated in tissue using the methenamine silver stain. The cysts, which are 5–6 μm in diameter, stain brown to black and have the characteristic cup-shaped or crescent-shaped morphology. *Pneumocystis* cysts do not bud, a feature that can be used to distinguish this organism from other fungi found in tissue.

Laboratory Diagnosis

P. jiroveci has been cultivated in cell cultures but serial maintenance of subcultures has not been accomplished. The standard for diagnosis is staining bronchoalveolar lavage fluid with an immunofluorescent monoclonal antibody directed against surface epitopes for *Pneumocystis* cysts and trophozoites (Cushion, 2003). The life cycle of *P. jiroveci* involves development of sporozoites within a cyst, after which the sporozoites are released. In patients with HIV infection, sufficient numbers of organisms are produced that sputum induced with saline by a skilled respiratory therapist may provide the diagnosis. The experience with sputum has varied in different centers, however, and the yield is very low in patients who have underlying diseases other than HIV. The advent of fluorescein-conjugated monoclonal antibodies to detect *P. jiroveci* in clinical specimens has proven to be a specific and sensitive method for identification (Fig. 60–50) (Kovacs, 2001). The immunofluorescence technique has been more sensitive in histochemical stains in some reports but the skill and care of the observers undoubtedly play a role in the comparative sensitivity of the techniques (Cushion, 2003). It should be noted that the cysts of *P. jiroveci* may occasionally be encountered in Gram-stained preparations, although this technique is not a sensitive method for detecting them.

Polymerase chain reaction assays have recently been evaluated but these have remained predominately research tools (Cushion, 2003). They are especially useful for testing samples with low organism burden, such as induced sputum, especially as an alternative for patients in whom bronchoscopy is contraindicated. A variety of genetic targets such as the internal transcribed spacers of the rRNA complex, microchondrial rRNA, and the major surface glycoprotein genes, have proved to be useful (Iwen, 2002).

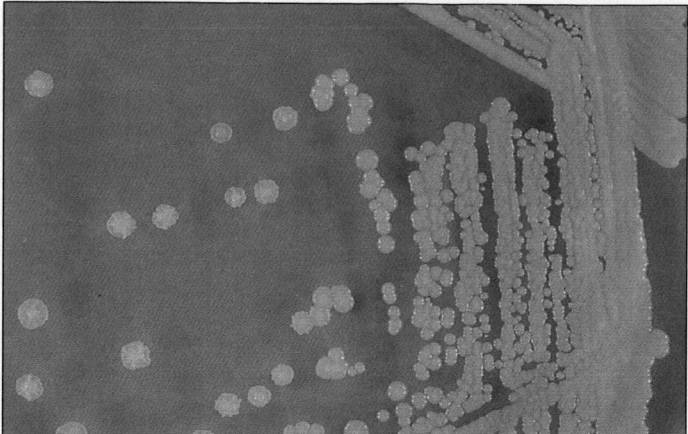

Figure 60–51 Colonies of *Prototheca wickerhamii* are yeast-like. (Sabouraud dextrose agar)

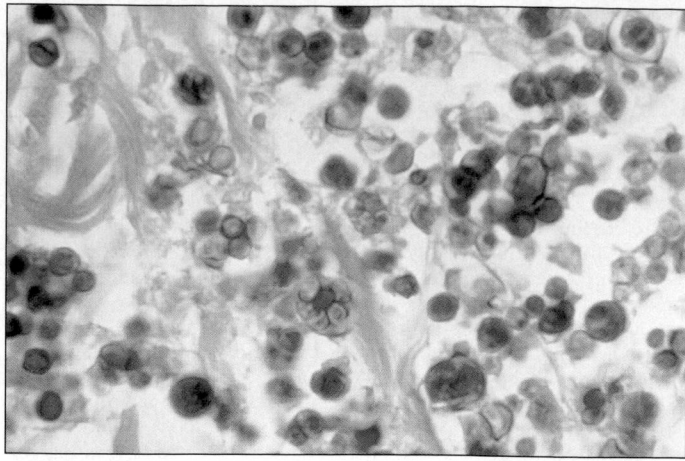

Figure 60–52 Histopathologic changes in protothecosis of the skin and mucous membrane of the nose due to *Prototheca wickerhamii*. Septation of the algal cells leads to multiple intracellular bodies and structures known as morula. (Courtesy of Dr William Kaplan, CDC Public Health Image Library)

Protothecosis

Protothecosis is an infection caused by achlorophyllic algae of the genus *Prototheca* (Thiele, 2002; Kantrow, 2003; Leimann, 2004). Most human infections are caused by *Prototheca wickerhamii*; however, rare cases have also been caused by *Prototheca zopfii* (Lass-Florl, 2004). Although these species are classified as algae, they are included in this chapter because of the resemblance of the infections to fungal disease. *Prototheca* are found in fresh and marine waters and probably gain entrance to the body through superficial wounds. Some patients are immunocompetent, but serious underlying diseases, such as diabetes mellitus, or immunosuppressive therapies often predispose patients to infection with these pathogens. Other patients have received injections of corticosteroids at the site of infection or have had musculoskeletal infection, particularly involving the tendons. The infections commonly involve the skin and subcutaneous tissue, with subsequent involvement of underlying tendons.

The algae grow readily on fungal isolation media that do not contain cycloheximide, and the colonies resemble those of *Candida* species (Fig. 60–51). The algal cells have a characteristic appearance, in which multiple daughter cells (sporangiospores) develop within the mother cell (sporangium), resembling a spherule (Chandler, 1978). These structures can also be demonstrated in histologic sections, where they must be differentiated from dimorphic fungi (Fig. 60–52). They may be seen in H&E preparations and stain well with the periodic-acid–Schiff or methenamine silver methods. *Prototheca* species are included in the databases of commercial yeast identification systems, such as API 20C (BioMérieux, Hazelwood, MO) and Vitek systems (BioMérieux, Hazelwood, MO).

References

Adams BB: Dermatologic disorders of the athlete. Sports Med 2002; 32:309–321.

Ahmed AO, van Leeuwen W, Fahal A, et al: Mycetoma caused by *Madurella mycetomatis*: a neglected infectious burden. Lancet Infect Dis 2004; 4:566–574.

Ajello L, George L, Steigbigel R: A case of phaeohyphomycosis caused by a new species of *Phialophora*. Mycologia 1974; 66:190–198.

Akpan A, Morgan R: Oral candidiasis. Postgrad Med J 2002; 78:455–459.

Allen AM, Taplin D: Epidemic *Trichophyton mentagrophytes* infections in servicemen. Source of infection, role of environment, host factors, and susceptibility. JAMA 1973; 226:864.

Al Soub H, Taha RY, El Deeb Y, et al: *Pneumocystis carinii* pneumonia in a patient without a predisposing illness: case report and review. Scand J Infect Dis 2004; 36:618–621.

Alsuwaida K: Primary cutaneous mucormycosis complicating the use of adhesive tape to secure the endotracheal tube. Can J Anaesth 2002; 49:880–882.

Aly R, Hay RJ, Del Palacio A, Galimberti R: Epidemiology of tinea capitis. Med Mycol 2000; 38 (Suppl 1):183–188.

Anatoliotaki M, Mantadakis E, Galanakis E, Samonis G: *Rhodotorula* species fungemia: a threat to the immunocompromised host. Clin Lab 2003; 49:49–55.

Arikan S, Uzun O, Cetinkaya Y, et al: Primary cutaneous aspergillosis in human immunodeficiency virus-infected patients: two cases and review. Clin Infect Dis 1998; 27:641–643.

Artis WM, Fountain JA, Delcher HK, Jones HE: A mechanism of susceptibility to mucormycosis in diabetic ketoacidosis: transferrin and iron availability. Diabetes 1982; 31:1109–1114.

Baddley JW, Dismukes WE: Chromoblastomycosis. *In* Dismukes WE, Pappas PG, Sobel JD (eds): Clinical Mycology. New York, Oxford University Press, 2003a, pp 399–404.

Baddley JW, Pappas PG, Smith AC, Moser SA: Epidemiology of *Aspergillus terreus* at a university hospital. J Clin Microbiol 2003b; 41:5525–5529.

Barry SM, Johnson MA: *Pneumocystis carinii* pneumonia: a review of current issues in diagnosis and management. HIV Med 2001; 2:123–132.

Bastola DR, Otu HH, Doukas SE, et al: Utilization of the relative complexity measure to construct a phylogenetic tree for fungi. Mycol Res 2004; 108:117–125.

Bennett JW, Klich M: Mycotoxins. Clin Microbiol Rev 2003; 16:497–516.

Bernal S, Martin Mazuelos E, Chavez M, et al: Evaluation of the new API *Candida* system for identification of the most clinically important yeast species. Diagn Microbiol Infect Dis 1998; 32:217–221.

Blumberg HM, Jarvis WR, Soucie JM, et al: Risk factors for candidal bloodstream infections in surgical intensive care unit patients: the NEMIS prospective multicenter study. The National Epidemiology of Mycosis Survey. Clin Infect Dis 2001; 33:177–186.

Bodey GP, Vartivarian: Aspergillosis. Eur J Clin Microbiol Infect Dis 1989; 8:413–437.

Bonacini M: Medical management of benign esophageal disease in patients with human immunodeficiency virus infection. Dig Liver Dis 2001; 33:294–300.

Borst A, Theelen B, Reinders E, et al: Use of amplified fragment length polymorphism analysis to identify medically important *Candida* spp., including *C. dubliniensis*. J Clin Microbiol 2003; 41:1357–1362.

Bradsher RW: Clinical features of blastomycosis. Semin Respir Infect 1997; 12:229–234.

Bradsher RW, Chapman SW, Pappas PG: Blastomycosis. Infect Dis Clin North Am 2003; 17:21–40.

Brandt ME, Warnock DW: Epidemiology, clinical manifestations, and therapy of infections caused by dematiaceous fungi. J Chemother 2003; 15 Suppl 2:36–47.

Broussard BN, Aggarwal A, Lacey SR, et al: Mushroom poisoning: from diarrhea to liver transplantation. Am J Gastroenterol 2001; 96:3195–3198.

Bustamante B, Campos PE: Endemic sporotrichosis. Curr Opin Infect Dis 2001; 14:145–149.

Bustamante B, Campos PE: Eumycetoma. *In* Dismukes WE, Pappas P, Sobel JD (eds): Clinical Mycology. New York, Oxford University Press, 2003, pp 390–398.

Caddell JR: Differentiating the dermatophytes. Clin Lab Sci 2002;15:13–15.

Canteros CE, Rodero L, Rivas MC, Davel G: A rapid urease test for presumptive identification of *Cryptococcus neoformans*. Mycopathologia 1996; 136:21–23.

Castiglioni B, Sutton DA, Rinaldi MG, et al: *Pseudallescheria boydii* (Anamorph *Scedosporium apiospermum*). Infection in solid organ transplant recipients in a tertiary medical center and review of the literature. Medicine (Baltimore) 2002; 81:333–348.

Castro C, Serrano MC, Flores B, et al: Comparison of the Sensititre YeastOne colorimetric antifungal panel with a modified CLSI M38-A method to determine the activity of voriconazole against clinical isolates of *Aspergillus* spp. J Clin Microbiol 2004; 42:4358–4360.

Centers for Disease Control and Prevention: Epidemiologic notes and reports multistate outbreak of sporotrichosis in seedling handlers, 1988. Morb Mortal Wkly Rep 1988; 37:652–653.

Centers for Disease Control and Prevention: Coccidioidomycosis: Arizona, 1990–1995. Morb Mortal Wkly Rep 1996; 45:1069–1073.

Centers for Disease Control and Prevention: Blastomycosis acquired occupationally during prairie dog relocation – Colorado, 1998. Morb Mortal Wkly Rep 1999a; 48:98–100.

Centers for Disease Control and Prevention: CDC surveillance summaries, surveillance for AIDS-defining opportunistic illnesses, 1992–1997. Morb Mortal Wkly Rep 1999b; 48:1–22.

Centers for Disease Control and Prevention: Outbreak of acute respiratory febrile illness among college students – Acapulco, Mexico, March 2001. Morb Mortal Wkly Rep 2001a; 50:261.

Centers for Disease Control and Prevention: Coccidioidomycosis among persons attending the world championship of model airplane flying: Kern County, California, October 2001. Morb Mortal Wkly Rep 2001b; 50:1106–1107.

Centers for Disease Control and Prevention: Laboratory security and emergency response guide for laboratories working with select agents. Morb Mortal Wkly Rep 2002; 51:1–6.

Centers for Disease Control and Prevention: Increase in coccidioidomycosis – Arizona, 1998–2001. Morb Mortal Wkly Rep 2003; 52:109–112.

Chandler FW, Kaplan W: Pathologic Diagnosis of Fungal Infections. Chicago, IL, ASCP Press, 1987a.
This atlas provides a practical foundation for the pathologic diagnosis of diseases caused by the fungi, actinomycetes, and algae.

Chandler FW, Kaplan W, Callaway CS: Differentiation between *Prototheca* and morphologically similar green algae in tissue. Arch Pathol Lab Med 1978; 102:353–356.

Chandler FW, Watts JC: Zygomycosis. *In* Chandler FW, Watts JC (eds): Pathologic Diagnosis of Fungal Infections, vol 1. Chicago, IL, American Society of Clinical Pathologists, 1987b, pp 85–96.

Chariyalertsak S, Vanittanakom P, Nelson KE, et al: *Rhizomys sumatrensis* and *Cannomys badius*, new natural animal hosts of *Penicillium marneffei*. J Med Vet Mycol 1996; 34:105–110.

Chastain MA, Reed RJ, Pankey GA: Deep dermatophytosis: report of 2 cases and review of the literature. Cutis 2001; 67:457–462.

Chen SC, Halliday CL, Meyer W: A review of nucleic acid-based diagnostic tests for systemic mycoses with an emphasis on polymerase chain reaction-based assays. Med Mycol 2002; 40:333–357.

Chiller TM, Galgiani JN, Stevens DA: Coccidioidomycosis. Infect Dis Clin North Am 2003; 17:41–57.

Chuck SL, Sande MA: Infections with *Cryptococcus neoformans* in the acquired immunodeficiency syndrome. N Engl J Med 1989; 321:794.

Clancy CJ, Wingard JR, Hong Nguyen M: Subcutaneous phaeohyphomycosis in transplant recipients: review of the literature and demonstration of in vitro synergy between antifungal agents. Med Mycol 2000; 38:169–175.

Clark R, Powers R, White R, et al: Nosocomial infection in the NICU: a medical complication or unavoidable problem? J Perinatol 2004; 24:382–388.

Clinical and Laboratory Standards Institute: Reference Method for Broth Dilution Antifungal Susceptibility Testing of Filamentous Fungi; Approved Standard (M38-A). Wayne, PA, CLSI, 2002a.

Clinical and Laboratory Standards Institute: Reference method for broth dilution antifungal susceptibility testing of yeasts; approved standard (M27-A2) (ed 2nd). Wayne, PA, CLSI, 2002b.

Clinical and Laboratory Standards Institute: Abbreviated Identification of Bacteria and Yeast; Approved Guideline (M35-A). Wayne, PA, CLSI, 2002c.

Cockerill FRI, Torgerson CA, Reed GS, et al: Clinical comparison of Difco ESP, Wampole Isolator, and Becton Dickinson Septi-Chek aerobic blood culturing systems. J Clin Microbiol 1996; 34:20–24.

Coles FB, Schuchat A, Hibbs JR, et al: A multistate outbreak of sporotrichosis associated with sphagnum moss. Am J Epidemiol 1992; 136:475–487.

Collazos J: Opportunistic infections of the CNS in patients with AIDS: diagnosis and management. CNS Drugs 2003; 17:869–887.

Cooper CR, Jr., Haycocks NG: *Penicillium marneffei*: an insurgent species among the penicillia. J Eukaryot Microbiol 2000; 47:24–28.

Cox RA, Magee DM: Coccidioidomycosis: host response and vaccine development. Clin Microbiol Rev 2004; 17:804–839.

Crist AE, Jr., Johnson LM, Burke PJ: Evaluation of the Microbial Identification System for identification of clinically isolated yeasts. J Clin Microbiol 1996; 34:2408–2410.

Crum NF, Lederman ER, Stafford CM, et al: Coccidioidomycosis: a descriptive survey of a reemerging disease. Clinical characteristics and current controversies. Medicine (Baltimore) 2004; 83:149–175.

Cushion MT: Pneumocystis. *In* Murray PR, Baron EJ, Jorganesen JH, et al. (eds): Manual of Clinical Microbiology, 8th ed. Washington, DC, ASM Press, 2003, vol 2, pp 1712–1725.

De Aguirre L, Hurst SF, Choi JS, et al: Rapid differentiation of *Aspergillus* species from other medically important opportunistic molds and yeasts by PCR-enzyme immunoassay. J Clin Microbiol, 2004; 42:3495–350.

De Araujo T, Marques AC, Kerdel F: Sporotrichosis. Int J Dermatol 2001; 40:737–742.

DeGroote MA, Bjerke R, Smith H, Rhodes III LC: Expanding epidemiology of blastomycosis: clinical features and investigation of 2 cases in Colorado. Clin Infect Dis 2000; 30:582–584.

De Hoog GS, Guarro J, Gene J, Figueras MJ: Atlas of Clinical Fungi. Utrecht, Netherlands, Centraalbureau voor Schimmelcultures, 2000.

Dei-Cas E: *Pneumocystis* infections: the iceberg? Med Mycol 2000; 38 (Suppl 1):23–32.

Denning DW: Invasive aspergillosis. Clin Infect Dis 1998a; 26:781–803.

Denning DW: Aspergillosis in 'nonimmunocompromised' critically ill patients. Am J Respir Crit Care Med 2004; 170:580–581.

Denning DW, Marinus A, Cohen J, et al: An EORTC multicentre prospective survey of invasive aspergillosis in haematological patients: diagnosis and therapeutic outcome. EORTC Invasive Fungal Infections Cooperative Group. J Infect 1998b; 37:173–180.

Denning DW, Riniotis K, Dobrashian R, Sambatakou H: Chronic cavitary and fibrosing pulmonary and pleural aspergillosis: case series, proposed nomenclature change, and review. Clin Infect Dis 2003; 37 (Suppl):S265–S280.

Department of Health and Human Services: Histoplasmosis: protecting workers at risk. Washington, DC, CDC, 1997.

Department of Health and Human Services: Biosafety in Microbiological and Biomedical Laboratories (ed 4th). Washington, DC, US Government Printing Office, 1999.

Department of Health and Human Services: Possession, use, and transfer of select agents and toxins. 42 CFR, Part 73. Washington, DC, Federal Register, 240:76886–76905, 2002a.

Department of Health and Human Services: NIH Guidelines for research involving recombinant DNA Molecules. Washington, DC, Federal Register, 66FR 57970:Appendix B, 2002b.

De Repentigny L: Serodiagnosis of candidiasis, aspergillosis, and cryptococcosis. Clin Infect Dis 1992; 14 (Suppl 1):S11–S22.

Deresinski S: *Coccidioides immitis* as a potential bioweapon. Semin Respir Infect 2003; 18:216–219.

Dignani MC, Anaissie E: Human fusariosis. Clin Microbiol Infect 2004; 10 (Suppl 1):67–75.

Dooley DP, Beckius ML, Jeffrey BS: Misidentification of clinical yeast isolates by using the updated Vitek yeast biochemical card. J Clin Microbiol 1994; 32:2889–2892.

Duong TA: Infection due to *Penicillium marneffei*, an emerging pathogen: review of 155 reported cases. Clin Infect Dis 1996; 23:125–130.

Edman JC, Kovacs JA, Masur H, et al: Ribosomal RNA sequence shows *Pneumocystis carinii* to be a member of the fungi. Nature 1988; 334:519–522.

Ellepola AN, Hurst SF, Elie CM, Morrison CJ: Rapid and unequivocal differentiation of *Candida dubliniensis* from other *Candida* species using species-specific DNA probes: comparison with phenotypic identification methods. Oral Microbiol Immunol 2003; 18:379–388.

Ellis M: Invasive fungal infections: evolving challenges for diagnosis and therapeutics. Mol Immunol 2002; 38:947–957.

Ergin F, Arslan H, Azap A, et al: Invasive aspergillosis in solid-organ transplantation: report of eight cases and review of the literature. Transpl Int 2003; 16:280–286.

Espinel-Ingroff A: Evaluation of broth microdilution testing parameters and agar diffusion Etest procedure for testing susceptibilities of *Aspergillus* spp. to caspofungin acetate (MK-0991). J Clin Microbiol 2003; 41:403–409.

Espinel-Ingroff A, Pfaller M, Messer SA, et al: Multicenter comparison of the Sensititre YeastOne colorimetric antifungal panel with the CLSI M27-A2 reference method for testing new antifungal agents against clinical isolates of *Candida* spp. J Clin Microbiol 2004; 42:718–721.

Espinel-Ingroff A, Rezusta A: E-test method for testing susceptibilities of *Aspergillus* spp. to the new triazoles voriconazole and posaconazole and to established antifungal agents: comparison with CLSI broth microdilution method. J Clin Microbiol 2002; 40:2101–2107.

Espinel-Ingroff A, Stockman L, Roberts G, et al: Comparison of RapID yeast plus system with API 20C system for identification of common, new, and emerging yeast pathogens. J Clin Microbiol 1998; 36:883–886.

Etzel RA: Mycotoxins. JAMA 2002; 287:425–427.

Eucker J, Sezer O, Graf B, Possinger K: Mucormycoses. Mycoses 2001; 44:253–260.

Fenn JP, Segal H, Barland B, et al: Comparison of updated Vitek yeast biochemical card and API 20C yeast identification systems. J Clin Microbiol 1994; 32:1184–1187.

Fierer J, Kirkland T: Questioning CDC's 'Select Agent' criteria. Science 2002; 295:43.

Filler SG, Kullberg BJ: Deep-seated candidal infections. *In* Calderone RA (ed): *Candida* and Candidiasis. Washington, DC, ASM Press, 2002, pp 341–348.

Fisher MC, Koenig G, White TJ, Taylor JW: Molecular and phenotypic description of *Coccidioides posadasii* sp. nov., previously recognized as the non-California population of *Coccidioides immitis*. Mycologia 2002; 94:73–84.

Fishman JA: Overview: fungal infections in the transplant patient. Transpl Infect Dis 2002; 4 (Suppl 3):3–11.

Fleming RV, Walsh TJ, Anaissie EJ: Emerging and less common fungal pathogens. Infect Dis Clin North Am 2002; 16:915–933.

Freifeld AG, Iwen PC: Zygomycosis. Sem Resp Care Med 2004; 25:221–231.

Frenkel JK: *Pneumocystis* pneumonia, an immunodeficiency-dependent disease: a critical historical overview (with a Latin redescription of *Pneumocystis jiroveci* of humans in conformance with the International Code of Botanical Nomenclature). J. Eucaryot Microbiol 1999; 46:89S–92S.

Graser Y, Kuijpers AF, El Fari M, et al: Molecular and conventional taxonomy of the *Microsporum canis* complex. Med Mycol 2000a; 38:143–153.

Graser Y, Kuijpers AF, Presber W, deHoog GS: Molecular taxonomy of the *Trichophyton rubrum* complex. J Clin Microbiol 2000b; 38:3329–3336.

Grosbell IB, Morris ML, Gallo JH, et al: Clinical, pathologic and epidemiologic features of infection with *Scedosporium prolificans*: four cases and review. Clin Microbiol Infect 1999; 5:672–686.

Guarro J, GeneJ, Stchigel AM: Developments in fungal taxonomy. Clin Microbiol Rev 1999; 12:454–500.
A review to update our present understanding of the systematics of pathogens and opportunistic fungi.

Gueho E, Leclerc MC, de Hoog GS, Dupont B: Molecular taxonomy and epidemiology of *Blastomyces* and *Histoplasma* species. Mycoses 1997; 40:69–81.

Guiver M, Levi K, Oppenheim BA: Rapid identification of *Candida* species by TaqMan PCR. J Clin Pathol 2001; 54:362–366.

Gupta AK, Ryder JE, Summerbell RC: Onychomycosis: classification and diagnosis. J Drugs Dermatol 2004; 3:51–56.

Gupta AK, Summerbell RC: Tinea capitis. Med Mycol 2000; 38:255–287.

Hageage GJ, Harrington B: Use of calcofluor white in clinical mycology. Laboratory Medicine 1984; 15:109.

Hainer BL: Dermatophyte infections. Am Fam Physician 2003; 67:101–108.

Hajjeh RA, Sofair AN, Harrison LH, et al: Incidence of bloodstream infections due to Candida species and in vitro susceptibilities of isolates collected from 1998 to 2000 in a population-based active surveillance program. J Clin Microbiol 2004; 42:1519–1527.

Hall VC, Goyal S, Davis MD, Walsh JS: Cutaneous hyalohyphomycosis caused by Paecilomyces lilacinus: report of three cases and review of the literature. Int J Dermatol 2004; 43:648–653.

Hamilton AJ: Serodiagnosis of histoplasmosis, paracoccidioidomycosis and penicilliosis marneffei: current status and future trends. Med Mycol 1998; 36:351–664.

Hawkins JL, Baddour LM: Candida lusitaniae infections in the era of fluconazole availability. Clin Infect Dis 2003; 36:14–18.

Hayden RT, Qian X, Roberts GD, Lloyd RV: In situ hybridization for the identification of yeastlike organisms in tissue section. Diagn Mol Pathol 2001; 10:15–23.

Hennequin C, Abachin E, Symoens F, et al: Identification of Fusarium species involved in human infection by 28S rRNA gene sequencing. J Clin Microbiol 1999; 37:3586–3589.

Henry T, Iwen PC, Hinrichs SH: Identification of Aspergillus species using internal transcribed spacer regions 1 and 2. J Clin Microbiol 2000; 38:1510–1515.

Herbrecht R, Letscher-Bru V, Oprea C, et al: Aspergillus galactomannan detection in the diagnosis of invasive aspergillosis in cancer patients. J Clin Oncol 2002; 20:1898–1906.

Herbrecht R, Natarajan-Ame S, Letscher-Bru V, Canuet M: Invasive pulmonary aspergillosis. Pulmon Fungal Infect 2004; 25:191–202.

Hilmarsdottir I, Thorsteinsson SB, Asmundsson P, et al: Cutaneous infection caused by Paecilomyces lilacinus in a renal transplant patient: treatment with voriconazole. Scand J Infect Dis 2000; 32:331–332.

Holzheimer RG, Dralle H: Management of mycoses in surgical patients – review of the literature. Eur J Med Res 2002; 7:200–226.

Howard RM, Frieden IJ: Dermatophyte infections in children. Adv Pediatr Infect Dis 1999; 14:73–107.

Hughes WT: Pneumocystis carinii vs. Pneumocystis jiroveci: another misnomer (response to Stringer et al.). Emerg Infect Dis 2003; 9:276–277.

Iwen PC: Molecular detection and typing of fungal pathogens. Clin Lab Med 2003; 23:781–799.
This article provides an overview on some of the basic molecular mycology assays used in clinical mycology research for diagnostic and epidemiologic typing purposes.

Iwen PC, Davis JC, Reed EC, et al: Airborne fungal spore monitoring in a protective environment during hospital construction, and correlation with an outbreak of invasive aspergillosis. Infect Control Hosp Epidemiol 1994; 15:303–306.

Iwen PC, Freifeld AG, Bruening TA, Hinrichs SH: Use of a panfungal PCR assay for detection of fungal pathogens in a commercial blood culture system. J Clin Microbiol 2004; 42:2292–2293.

Iwen PC, Freifeld AG, Sigler L, et al: Molecular identification of Rhizomucor pusillus as a cause of sinus-orbital zygomycosis in a patient with acute myelogenous leukemia. J Clin Microbiol 2005; 43:5819–5821.

Iwen PC, Hinrichs SH, Rupp ME: Utilization of the internal transcribed spacer regions as molecular targets to detect and identify human fungal pathogens. Med Mycol 2002; 40:87–109.

Iwen PC, Reed EC, Armitage JO, et al: Nosocomial invasive aspergillosis in lymphoma patients treated with bone marrow or peripheral stem cell transplants. J Clin Microbiol 1993; 14:131–139.

Iwen PC, Rupp ME, Bishop MR, et al: Disseminated aspergillosis caused by Aspergillus ustus in a patient following allogeneic peripheral stem cell transplantation. J Clin Microbiol 1998b; 36:3713–3717.

Iwen PC, Rupp ME, Hinrichs SH: Invasive mold sinusitis: 17 cases in immunocompromised patients and review of the literature. Clin Infect Dis 1997; 24:1178–1184.

Iwen PC, Rupp ME, Langnas AN, et al: Invasive pulmonary aspergillosis due to Aspergillus terreus: 12-year experience and review of the literature. Clin Infect Dis 1998a; 26:1092–1097.

Iwen PC, Sigler L, Tarantolo S, et al: Pulmonary infection caused by Gymnascella hyalinospora in a patient with acute myelogenous leukemia. J Clin Microbiol 2000; 38:375–381.

Jensen TG, Gahrn-Hansen B, Arendrup M, Bruun B: Fusarium fungaemia in immunocompromised patients. Clin Microbiol Infect 2004; 10:499–501.

Judson MA: Noninvasive Aspergillus pulmonary disease. Semin Respir Critical Care Med 2004; 25:203–219.

Kac G: Molecular approaches to the study of dermatophytes. Med Mycol 2000; 38:329–336.

Kantrow SM, Boyd AS: Protothecosis. Dermatol Clin 2003; 21:249–255.

Kauffman CA, Hajjeh R, Chapman SW, Group MS: Practice guidelines for the management of patients with sporotrichosis. Clin Infect Dis 2000; 30:684–687.

Kirkland T, Fierer J: Coccidioidomycosis: a reemerging infectious disease. Emerg Infect Dis 1996; 2:192–199.

Kirkpatrick CH: Chronic mucocutaneous candidiasis. Pediatr Infect Dis J 2001; 20:197–206.

Klein BS, Vergeront JM, Weeks RJ, et al: Isolation of Blastomyces dermatitidis in soil associated with a large outbreak of blastomycosis in Wisconsin. N Engl J Med 1986; 314:529–534.

Klich MA: Identification of Common Aspergillus species. Utrecht, Netherlands, Centraalbureau voor Schimmelcultures, 2002.

Kohl TD, Lisney M: Tinea gladiatorum: wrestling's emerging foe. Sports Med 2000; 29:439–447.

Kojic EM, Darouiche RO: Candida infections of medical devices. Clin Microbiol Rev 2004; 17:255–267.

Kontoyiannis DP, Bodey GP: Invasive aspergillosis in 2002: an update. Eur J Clin Microbiol Infect Dis 2002; 21:161–172.

Kovacs JA, Gill VG, Meshnick S, Masur H: New insights into transmission, diagnosis and drug treatment of Pneumocystis carinii pneumonia. JAMA 2001; 286:2450–2460.

Kuhn DM, Ghannoum MA: Indoor mold, toxigenic fungi, and Stachybotrys chartarum: infectious disease perspective. Clin Microbiol Rev 2003; 16:144–172.

Kwon-Chung KJ, Bennett JE: Medical Mycology. Philadelphia, PA, Lea & Febiger, 1992.

Kwon-Chung KJ, Sorrell TC, Dromer F, et al: Cryptococcosis: clinical and biological aspects. Med Mycol 2000; 38 (Suppl 1):205–213.

Lass-Florl C, Fille M, Gunsilius E, et al: Disseminated infection with Prototheca zopfii after unrelated stem cell transplantation for leukemia. J Clin Microbiol 2004; 42:4907–4908.

Latenser BA: Fusarium infections in burn patients: a case report and review of the literature. J Burn Care Rehabil 2003; 24:285–288.

Lazcano O, Speights VO, Jr, Strickler JG, et al: Combined histochemical stains in the differential diagnosis of Cryptococcus neoformans. Mod Pathol 1993; 6:80–84.

Leake JA, Mosley DG, England B, et al: Risk factors for acute symptomatic coccidioidomycosis among elderly persons in Arizona, 1996–1997. J Infect Dis 2000; 181:1435–1440.

Leimann BC, Monteiro PC, Lazera M, et al: Protothecosis. Med Mycol 2004; 42:95–106.

Lemos LB, Baliga M, Guo M: Blastomycosis: the great pretender can also be an opportunist. Initial clinical diagnosis and underlying diseases in 123 patients. Ann Diagn Pathol 2002; 6:194–203.

Lionakis MS, Kontoyiannis DP: Fusarium infections in critically ill patients. Pulmon Fungal Infect 2004; 25:159–170.

Liu PY: Cryptococcal osteomyelitis: case report and review. Diagn Microbiol Infect Dis 1998; 30:33–35.

Loeffler J, Henke N, Hebart H, et al: Quantification of fungal DNA by using fluorescence resonance energy transfer and the light cycler system. J Clin Microbiol 2000; 38:586–590.

Ma JS, Chen PY, Chen CH, Chi CS: Neonatal fungemia caused by Hansenula anomala: a case report. J Microbiol Immunol Infect, 2000; 33:267–27.

McGinnis MR: Laboratory Handbook of Medical Mycology. New York, Academic Press, 1980.

McGinnis MR, Padhye AA: Fungi causing eumycotic mycetoma. In Murray PR, Baron EJ, Jorganesen JH, et al (eds): Manual of Clinical Microbiology. Washington, DC, ASM Press, 2003, pp 1148–1856.

McGinnis MR, Sigler L: Some medically important fungi and their common synonyms and names of uncertain application. Clin Infect Dis 1999; 29:728–730.

McKinsey DS: Histoplasmosis in AIDS: advances in management. AIDS Patient Care STDs 1998; 12:775–781.

McLintock LA, Jones BL: Advances in the molecular and serological diagnosis of invasive fungal infection in haemato-oncology patients. Br J Haematol 2004; 126:289–297.

McNeil MM, Brown JM: The medically important aerobic actinomycetes: epidemiology and microbiology. Clin Microbiol Rev 1994; 7:357–417.

McPartland JM, Vilgalys RJ, Cubeta MA: Mushroom poisoning. Am Fam Physician 1997; 55:1797–1812.

Makimura K: Species identification system for dermatophytes based on the DNA sequences of nuclear ribosomal internal transcribed spacer 1. Nippon Ishinkin Gakkai Zasshi 2001; 42:61–67.

Mann BJ, Baylis BW, Urbanski SJ, et al: Paracoccidioidomycosis: case report and review. Clin Infect Dis 1996; 23:1026–1032.

Marcon MJ, Powell DA: Human infections due to Malassezia spp. Clin Microbiol Rev 1992; 5:101–119.

Marr KA, Carter RA, Crippa F, et al: Epidemiology and outcome of mould infections in hematopoietic stem cell transplant recipients. Clin Infect Dis 2002b; 34:909–917.
An assessment of the incidence and risks for mold infections in a large database of hemotopoietic stem cell transplant recipients with an emphasis on the emerging fungal pathogens.

Marr KA, Patterson T, Denning D: Aspergillosis. Pathogenesis, clinical manifestations, and therapy. Infect Dis Clin North Am 2002a; 16:875–894.

Martino R, Salavert M, Parody R, et al: Blastoschizomyces capitatus infection in patients with leukemia: report of 26 cases. Clin Infect Dis 2004; 38:335–341.

Maxwell MJ, Messer SA, Hollis RJ, et al: Evaluation of Etest method for determining fluconazole and voriconazole MICs for 279 clinical isolates of Candida species infrequently isolated from blood. J Clin Microbiol 2003; 41:1087–1090.

Miller JD, Rand TG, Jarvis BB: Stachybotrys chartarum: cause of human disease or media darling? Med Mycol 2003; 41:271–291.

Minari A, Hachem R, Raad I: Candida lusitaniae: a cause of breakthrough fungemia in cancer patients. Clin Infect Dis 2001; 32:186–190.

Morpeth JE, Rupp NT, Dolen WK, et al: Fungal sinusitis; an update. Ann Allergy Asthma Immun 1996; 76:128–13.

Nagata N, Sueishi K, Tanaka K, Iwata Y: Pulmonary aspergillosis with bronchocentric granulomas. Am J Surg Pathol 1990; 14:485–488.

Narani N, Epstein JB: Classifications of oral lesions in HIV infection. J Clin Periodontol 2001; 28:137–145.

Nenoff P, Handrick W, Haustein UF: Sports-induced infections – an overview. Wien Med Wochenschr 2002; 152:574–577.

Nesky MA, McDougal EC, Peacock Jr JE: *Pseudallescheria boydii* brain abscess successfully treated with voriconazole and surgical drainage: case report and literature review of central nervous system pseudallescheriasis. Clin Infect Dis 2000; 31:673–677.

Nevez G, Totet A, Jounieaux V, et al: *Pneumocystis jiroveci* internal transcribed spacer types in patients colonized by the fungus and in patients with pneumocystosis from the same French geographic region. J Clin Microbiol 2003; 41:181–186.

Nonaka D, Yfantis H, Southall P, Sun CC: Pseudallescheriasis as an aggressive opportunistic infection in a bone marrow transplant recipient. Arch Pathol Lab Med 2002; 126:207–209.

Noskin GA, Peterson LR: Engineering infection control through facility design. Emerg Infect Dis 2001; 7:354–357.

Nucci M: Emerging moulds: *Fusarium, Scedosporium* and Zygomycetes in transplant recipients. Curr Opin Infect Dis 2003; 16:607–612.

Nucci M, Marr KA, Queiroz-Telles F, et al: *Fusarium* infection in hematopoietic stem cell transplant recipients. Clin Infect Dis 2004; 38:1237–1242.

Oh D, Notrica D: Primary cutaneous mucormycosis in infants and neonates: case report and review of the literature. J Pediatri Surg 2002; 37:1607–1611.

Padhye AA, Kaufman L, Durry E, et al: Fatal pulmonary sporotrichosis caused by *Sporothrix schenckii* var. *luriei* in India. J Clin Microbiol 1992; 30:2492–2494.

Pagano L, Offidani M, Fianchi L, et al: Mucormycosis in hematologic patients. Haematologica 2004; 89:207–214.

Pappagianis D, Zimmer BL: Serology of coccidioidomycosis. Clin Microbiol Rev 1990; 3:247–268.

Pappas PG, Dismukes WE: Blastomycosis: Gilchrist's disease revisited. Curr Clin Top Infect Dis 2002; 22:61–77.

Parikh SL, Venkatraman G, DelGaudio JM: Invasive fungal sinusitis: a 15-year review from a single institution. Am J Rhinol 2004; 18:75–81.

Patterson TF: Fungal susceptibility testing: where are we now? Transpl Infect Dis 2002; 4 Suppl 3:38–45.

Perfect JR, Casadevall A: Cryptococcosis. Infect Dis Clin North Am 2002; 16:837–874.

Perfect JR, Cox GM, Lee JY, et al: The impact of culture isolation of *Aspergillus* species: a hospital-based survey of aspergillosis. Clin Infect Dis 2001; 33:1824–1833.

Perfect JR, Schell WA, Cox GM: Phaeohyphomycoses. *In* Dismukes WE, Pappas P, Sobel JD (eds): Clinical Mycology. New York, Oxford University Press, 2003, pp 271–282.

Petersen LR, Marshall SL, Barton-Dickson C, et al: Coccidioidomycosis among workers at an archeological site, northeastern Utah. Emerg Infect Dis 2004; 10:637–642.

Pfaller JB, Messer SA, Hollis RJ, et al: In vitro susceptibility testing of *Aspergillus* spp.: comparison of Etest and reference microdilution methods for determining voriconazole and itraconazole MICs. J Clin Microbiol 2003a; 41:1126–1129.

Pfaller MA, Diekema DJ: Rare and emerging opportunistic fungal pathogens: concern for resistance beyond *Candida albicans* and *Aspergillus fumigatus*. J Clin Microbio 2004; 142:4419–4431.
A minireview of selected emerging fungal agents and less common agents of opportunistic mycoses with an emphasis on what is known of their susceptibility and resistance to both new and established antifungal agents.

Pfaller MA, Diekema DJ, Boyken L, et al: Evaluation of the Etest and disk diffusion methods for determining susceptibilities of 235 bloodstream isolates of *Candida glabrata* to fluconazole and voriconazole. J Clin Microbiol 2003b; 41:1875–1880.

Pfaller MA, Diekema DJ, Jones RN, et al: Trends in antifungal susceptibility of *Candida* spp. isolated from pediatric and adult patients with bloodstream infections: SENTRY Antimicrobial Surveillance Program, 1997 to 2000. J Clin Microbiol 2002; 40:852–856.

Pfaller MA, Diekema DJ, Messer SA, et al: In vitro activities of voriconazole, posaconazole, and four licensed systemic antifungal agents against *Candida* species infrequently isolated from blood. J Clin Microbiol 2003c; 41:78–83.

Pfaller MA, Houston A, Coffmann S: Application of CHROMagar *Candida* for rapid screening of clinical specimens for *Candida albicans, Candida tropicalis, Candida krusei*, and *Candida (Torulopsis) glabrata*. J Clin Microbiol 1996; 34:58–61.

Pfaller MA, Jones RN, Doern GV, et al: International surveillance of bloodstream infections due to *Candida* species: frequency of occurrence and antifungal susceptibilities of isolates collected in 1997 in the United States, Canada, and South America for the SENTRY Program. The SENTRY Participant Group. J Clin Microbiol 1998; 36:1886–1889.

Pneumocystis Working Group: Nomenclature of *Pneumocystis*. Eukaryot Microbiol 1994; 41:1215–1225.

Ponton J, Ruchel R, Clemons KV, et al: Emerging pathogens. Med Mycol 2000; 38 (Suppl 1):225–236.

Ramani R, Gromadzki S, Pincus DH, et al: Efficacy of API 20C and ID 32C systems for identification of common and rare clinical yeast isolates. J Clin Microbiol 1998; 36:3396–3398.

Redding SW, Kirkpatrick WR, Coco BJ, et al: *Candida glabrata* oropharyngeal candidiasis in patients receiving radiation treatment for head and neck cancer. J Clin Microbiol 2002; 40:1879–1881.

Reimer LG, Wilson ML, Weinstein MP: Update on detection of bacteremia and fungemia. Clin Microbiol Rev 1997; 10:444–465.

Reiss E, Obayashi T, Orle K, et al: Non-culture based diagnostic tests for mycotic infections. Med Mycol 2000; 38 (Suppl 1):147–159.

Revankar SG, Patterson JE, Sutton DA, et al: Disseminated phaeohyphomycosis: review of an emerging mycosis. Clin Infect Dis 2002; 34:467–476.

Revankar SG, Sutton DA, Rinaldi MG: Primary central nervous system phaeohyphomycosis: a review of 101 cases. Clin Infect Dis 2004; 38:206–216.

Revenga F, Paricio JF, Merino FJ, et al: Primary cutaneous cryptococcosis in an immunocompetent host: case report and review of the literature. Dermatology 2002; 204:145–149.

Rex JH, Pfaller MA, Walsh TJ, et al: Antifungal susceptibility testing: practical aspects and current challenges. Clin Microbiol Rev 2001; 14:643–658.

Ribes JA, Vanover-Sams CL, Baker DJ: Zygomycetes in human disease. Clin Microbiol Rev 2000; 13:236–301.
A review exploring the diversity of the zygomycetes and their disease manifestations and the taxonomy and the relationship of the zygomycete to other fungal pathogens.

Riddle DL, Giger O, Miller L, et al: Clinical comparison of the Baxter MicroScan Yeast Identification Panel and the Vitek Yeast Biochemical Card. Am J Clin Pathol 1994; 101:438–442.

Rinaldi MG: Use of potato flakes agar in clinical mycology. J Clin Microbiol 1982; 15:1159.

Rinaldi MG: Phaeohyphomycosis. Dermatol Clin 1996; 14:17–53.

Rinaldi MG: Dermatophytosis: epidemiological and microbiological update. J Am Acad Dermatol 2000; 43:S120–S124.

Rodriguez M, Fishman JA: Prevention of infection due to *Pneumocystis* spp. in human immunodeficiency virus-negative immunocompromised patients. Clin Microbiol Rev 2004; 17:770–782.

Rodriguez-Villalobos H, Georgala A, Beguin H, et al: Disseminated infection due to *Cylindrocarpon (Fusarium) lichenicola* in a neutropenic patient with acute leukaemia: report of a case and review of the literature. Eur J Clin Microbiol Infect Dis 2003; 22:62–65.

Sampathkumar P, Paya CV: *Fusarium* infection after solid-organ transplantation. Clin Infect Dis 2001; 32:1237–1240.

Samuel R, Bettiker RL, Suh B: AIDS related opportunistic infections, going but not gone. Arch Pharm Res 2002; 25:215–228.

Sancak B, Rex JH, Paetznick V, et al: Evaluation of a method for identification of *Candida dubliniensis* bloodstream isolates. J Clin Microbiol 2003; 41:489–491.

Sanche SE, Sutton DA, Rinaldi MG: Dematiaceous fungi. *In* Anaissie EJ, McGinnis MR, Pfaller MS (eds): Clinical Mycology. New York, Churchill Livingstone, 2003, pp 325–351.

Sanders E: Cutaneous sporotrichosis. Beer, bricks, and bumps. Arch Intern Med 1971; 127:482–483.

Saubani AO, Chandrasekar PH: The clinical spectrum of pulmonary aspergillosis. Chest 2002; 121:1988–1999.

Schiemann R, Glasmacher A, Bailly E, et al: *Geotrichum capitatum* septicaemia in neutropenic patients: case report and review of the literature. Mycoses 1998; 41:113–116.

Schinabeck MK, Ghannoum MA: Human hyalohyphomycoses: a review of human infections due to *Acremonium* spp., *Paecilomyces* spp., *Penicillium* spp., and *Scopulariopsis* spp. J Chemother 2003; 15 (Suppl 2):5–15.

Schubert MS: Allergic fungal sinusitis. Otolaryngol Clin North Am 2004; 37:301–326.

Shin JH, Nolte FS, Holloway BP, Morrison CJ: Rapid identification of up to three *Candida* species in a single reaction tube by a 5' exonuclease assay using fluorescent DNA probes. J Clin Microbiol 1999; 37:165–170.

Sigler L: Miscellaneous opportunistic fungi: Microascaceae and other Sacomycetes, Hyphomycetes, Coelomycetes, and Basidiomycetes. *In* Howard DH (ed): Fungi Pathogenic for Humans and Animals, 2nd ed. New York, Marcel Dekker, 2003, pp 637–676.

Silveira F, Nucci M: Emergence of black moulds in fungal disease: epidemiology and therapy. Curr Opin Infect Dis 2001; 14:679–684.

Sivak-Callcott JA, Livesley N, Nugent RA, et al: Localised invasive sino-orbital aspergillosis: characteristic features. Br J Ophthalmol 2004; 88:681–687.

Sobel JD, Lundstrom T: Management of candiduria. Curr Urol Rep 2001; 2:321–325.

Steinbach WJ, Benjamin DK, Jr., Kontoyiannis DP, et al: Infections due to *Aspergillus terreus*: a multicenter retrospective analysis of 83 cases. Clin Infect Dis 2004; 39:192–198.

Steinbach WJ, Mitchell TG, Schell WA, et al: Status of medical mycology education. Med Mycol 2003a; 41:457–467.

Steinbach WJ, Perfect JR: *Scedosporium* species infections and treatments. J Chemother 2003b; 15 Suppl 2:16–27.

Stevens DA: Diagnosis of fungal infections: current status. J Antimicrob Chemother 2002; 49 (Suppl 1):11–19.

Stringer JR, Beard CB, Miller RF, Wakefield AE: A new name (*Pneumocystis jiroveci*) for *Pneumocystis* from humans. Emerg Infect Dis 2002; 8:891–896.

Sutton DA, Sanche SE, Revankar SG, et al: In vitro amphotericin B resistance in clinical isolates of *Aspergillus terreus*, with a head-to-head comparison to voriconazole. J Clin Microbiol 1999; 37:2343–2345.

Swisher BL, Chandler FW: Grocott-Gomori methenamine silver method for detecting fungi: practical considerations. Lab Med 1982; 13:568.

Thakar A, Sarkar C, Khiwakar M, et al: Allergic fungal sinusitis: expanding the clinicopathologic spectrum. Otolaryngol Head Neck Surg 2004; 130:209–216.

Thiele D, Bergmann A: Protothecosis in human medicine. Int J Hyg Environ Health 2002; 204:297–302.

Thomas I, Schwartz RA: Cutaneous manifestations of systemic cryptococcosis in immunosuppressed patients. J Med 2001; 32:259–266.

Thomas PA: Current perspectives on ophthalmic mycoses. Clin Microbiol Rev 2003; 16:730–797.
This paper is a comprehensive review of mycotic infections of the orbit and adjacent external ocular tissues.

Totet A, Pautard JC, Raccurt C, et al: Genotypes at the internal transcribed spacers of the nuclear rRNA

VII

operon of *Pneumocystis jiroveci* in nonimmunosuppressed infants without severe pneumonia. J Clin Microbiol 2003; 41:1173–1180.

Van Burik JA, Colven R, Spach DH: Cutaneous aspergillosis. J Clin Microbiol 1998; 36:3115–3121.

Vazquez JA, Sobel JD: Mucosal candidiasis. Infect Dis Clin North Am 2002; 16:793–820.

Veligandla SR, Hinrichs SH, Rupp ME, et al: Delayed diagnosis of osseous blastomycosis in two patients following environmental exposure in nonendemic areas. Am J Clin Pathol 2002; 118:536–541.

Vennewald I, Schonlebe J, Klemm E: Mycological and histological investigations in humans with middle ear infections. Mycoses 2003; 46:12–18.

Vilchez RA, Fung J, Kusne S: Cryptococcosis in organ transplant recipients: an overview. Am J Transplant 2002; 2:575–580.

Walsh TJ, Groll A, Hiemenz J, et al: Infections due to emerging and uncommon medically important fungal pathogens. Clin Microbiol Infect 2004b; 10(Suppl 1):48–66.

Walsh TJ, Shoham S, Petraitiene R, et al: Detection of galactomannan antigenemia in patients receiving piperacillin–tazobactam and correlations between in vitro, in vivo, and clinical properties of the drug–antigen interaction. J Clin Microbiol 2004a; 42:4744–4748.

Warnock DW, Hajjeh RA, Lasker BA: Epidemiology and prevention of invasive aspergillosis. Curr Infect Dis Rep 2001; 3:507–516.

Wazir JF, Ansari NA: *Pneumocystis carinii* infection. Update and review. Arch Pathol Lab Med 2004; 128:1023–1027.

Weems JJ, Jr.: *Candida parapsilosis:* epidemiology, pathogenicity, clinical manifestations, and antimicrobial susceptibility. Clin Infect Dis 1992; 14:756–766.

Weitzman I, Salkin IF, Rosenthal SA: Evaluation of *Trichophyton* agars for identification of *Trichophyton soudanense*. J Clin Microbiol 1983; 18:203–205.

Weitzman I, Whittier S, McKitrich JC, Della-Latta P: Zygospores: the last word in identification of rare or atypical zygomycetes isolated from clinical specimens. J Clin Microbiol 1995; 33:781–783.

Wheat LJ: Current diagnosis of histoplasmosis. Trends Microbiol 2003a; 11:488–494.

Wheat LJ: Rapid diagnosis of invasive aspergillosis by antigen detection. Transpl Infect Dis 2003c; 5:158–166.

Wheat LJ, Garringer T, Brizendine E, Connolly P: Diagnosis of histoplasmosis by antigen detection based upon experience at the histoplasmosis reference laboratory. Diagn Microbiol Infect Dis 2002; 43:29–37.

Wheat LJ, Kauffman CA: Histoplasmosis. Infect Dis Clin North Am 2003b; 17:1–19.

The paper provides an up-to-date clinical review of histoplasmosis, focusing on recognition, diagnosis, and management.

Wilkin A, Feinberg J: *Pneumocystis carinii* pneumonia: a clinical review. Am Fam Physician 1999; 60:1699–1708.

Wingard JR: Importance of *Candida* species other than *C. albicans* as pathogens in oncology patients. Clin Infect Dis 1995; 20:115–125.

Wolff AJ, O'Donnell AE: HIV-related pulmonary infections: a review of the recent literature. Curr Opin Pulmon Med 2003; 9:210–214.

Woods CW, McRill C, Plikaytis BD, et al: Coccidioidomycosis in human immunodeficiency virus-infected persons in Arizona, 1994–1997; incidence, risk factors, and prevention. J Infect Dis 2000; 181:1498–1434.

Woods GL, Schnadig VJ: Histopathology of fungal infections. *In* Anaissie E, McGinnis MR, Pfaller MA (eds): Clinical Mycology. Philadelphia, PA, Churchill Livingstone, 2003, pp 80–95.

Yeo SF, Wong B: Current status of nonculture methods for diagnosis of invasive fungal infections. Clin Microbiol Rev 2002; 15:465–484.

CHAPTER 61
Medical Parasitology

Thomas R. Fritsche, M.D., Ph.D., Rangaraj Selvarangan, B.V.Sc., Ph.D.

KEY POINTS

- Accurate diagnosis of parasitic infections usually depends on macroscopic or microscopic examination of specimens that have been appropriately collected and preserved. Thick and thin blood smears are useful to detect and characterize organisms found in the blood. Fecal specimens may either be fresh or placed into fixatives such as formalin and polyvinyl alcohol.

- Immunodiagnostic methods for parasitology include detection of both antibodies and antigens. Established enzyme immunoassays include antigen tests for *Plasmodium* spp. in blood or serum; *Giardia lamblia*, *Cryptosporidium* spp., and *Entamoeba histolytica* in feces; *Trichomonas vaginalis* in vaginal swabs. Direct fluorescent assays are also useful for identifying organisms in primary specimens.

- Molecular diagnostic methods are now emerging based on amplification techniques that offer high levels of sensitivity and specificity for both diagnosis and monitoring of parasitic diseases.

- The diagnosis of malaria should be considered in the differential diagnosis of unexplained fever with the history of travel in endemic geographic regions. Thick and thin blood smears are complementary for detecting and identifying the infecting *Plasmodium* spp. based on the varieties of developmental stages, presence of malarial pigment, and stippling seen in infected erythrocytes.

- Other protozoal infections include babesiosis and trypanosomiasis found in blood, leishmaniasis (causing cutaneous, mucocutaneous, and visceral forms of disease), and toxoplasmosis, often affecting the central nervous system following congenital infection and in patients with the acquired immunodeficiency syndrome (AIDS).

- Amebae are ingested as cysts, resulting in infection of the colon and passage of both cysts and trophozoites in the feces. The resulting diseases are amebic dysentery, amebic colitis, and liver abscesses. Diagnosis is made by microscopic examination of stool and by serological testing for antibodies in serum.

- Flagellates include *Giardia lamblia*, which causes diarrhea from ingestion of contaminated water and is diagnosed by finding trophozoites or cysts in feces. *Trichomonas vaginalis* can be detected in vaginal wet mounts by its characteristic motion.

- Coccidia (*Isospora*, *Cryptosporidium*, and *Cyclospora*) and microsporidia can cause protracted diarrhea in immunosuppressed individuals such as those with AIDS.

- Intestinal helminths include the nematodes (roundworms), cestodes (tapeworms), and trematodes (flukes). These organisms reside as adults in the gastrointestinal tract or in other locations (liver, lung, blood). Knowledge of their life cycles and zoogeography with intermediate hosts are critical for establishing the parasitic stage in presumed infection. Eggs, larvae, or adult forms (from 1 mm to >10 m in length, depending upon species) can be recovered from stool, urine, or sputum.

- Tissue helminths include filaria (larvae found in blood and also on skin biopsy), *Trichinella* (in muscle), *Strongyloides* (disseminated infection), and hydatidosis (large cystic lesions in the liver or lungs), among others.

- Arthropods cause disease through direct tissue invasion, envenomation, vesication, blood loss, transmission of infectious agents, hypersensitivity reactions, and psychological manifestations. Characteristics necessary for identification can be maintained by preserving the organisms in alcohol (ticks, mites, fleas, lice), by drying them (winged forms) after killing them with fumes of organic solvents, or killing with hot water (maggots) and subsequent storage in alcohol.

The study of parasitology has gained renewed importance in a world made smaller by the rapid movement of people, especially travelers to and migrants from areas endemic for parasitic disease, and by the appearance of emerging and re-emerging pathogens in individuals immunocompromised for a variety of reasons. Parasitic diseases of humans and domestic animals place a tremendous burden on limited health care resources, and adversely affect economic and societal development in many countries around the world. While the types of organism classified as parasites constitute a large group, those infecting humans are more limited in number and are composed mostly of protozoa, helminths, and arthropods (Table 61–1).

Clinicians in the United States and elsewhere are increasingly being confronted with unusual diagnostic problems associated with parasitic infections. Likewise, laboratorians have been challenged with the development of new technologies to accurately and rapidly diagnose such parasites as *Cryptosporidium parvum, Cryptosporidium hominis, Cyclospora cayetanensis, Toxoplasma gondii,* and microsporidia in both immuno-competent and immunocompromised hosts. The worldwide resurgence of malaria and other parasitic diseases has also required laboratorians to strengthen their expertise in the identification of the usual blood, intestinal, and tissue protozoa and helminths.

Once diagnosed, additional problems may be encountered in the management of these diseases owing to lack of effective therapies or the emergence of resistance to traditional therapy. Many parasites require arthropod vectors for their transmission, and the irregular application of vector control efforts has, in some instances, resulted in the emergence of insecticide resistance. Malaria has made a tremendous resurgence in many areas because of a relaxation in control efforts and the emergence of drug-resistant parasites and insecticide-resistant mosquitoes. Schistosomiasis has spread to many new areas secondary to an increase in irrigation as a result of population growth and the need to expand agricultural production.

Because of the chronic nature and generally long prepatent periods (time between infection and appearance of diagnostic stages) of many parasitic diseases, physicians may not consider them in a differential diagnosis unless the patient voluntarily offers information or specific inquiry is made about travel history or other possible exposure. Malaria is one parasitic disease that often presents as an acute, febrile illness and may have lethal consequences unless it is considered in the differential diagnosis and a history of travel to an endemic area is elicited.

Various estimates for the prevalence and related mortality figures of parasitic infections on a worldwide basis have been made (Table 61–2). The actual incidence of parasitic infections seen in the United States is unknown, however, because most infections are not reported to public health officials. *Giardia lamblia,* other intestinal protozoa, and intestinal roundworms are reported most frequently (7.2%, 10%, and 3.5%, respectively) by state laboratories, but other parasites, including *Cryptosporidium, Cyclospora,* and microsporidia, probably occur more frequently but are underdiagnosed (Kappus, 1994).

This chapter provides an overview of the general approach laboratorians use to recover and identify parasitic protozoa and helminths from human specimens. Discussion of the individual species of parasites focuses on essential clinical and biological information necessary to assist in diagnosis and management. For more extensive coverage of specific parasites, a number of excellent texts are available (Beaver, 1984; Warren, 1990; Lane, 1993; Guerrant, 1999; Garcia, 1999, 2001; Markell, 1999; Strickland, 2000; Cook, 2002; Mullen, 2002; among others). Parasitology atlases are also important resources for any laboratorian performing parasitology examinations and should be readily available (Spencer, 1982; Brooke, 1984; Ash, 1987, 1997; Sun, 1988; Peters, 1989; Isenberg, 2004; Murray, 2003). Several texts specifically address pathologic aspects of parasitic infections (Marcial-Rojas, 1971; Binford, 1976; Sun, 1982; Von Lichtenberg, 1991; Woods, 1993; Orihel, 1995; Connor, 1997; Gutierrez, 2000). Parasitic infections that are problematic in immunocompromised patients also have been reviewed (Walzer, 1989).

Laboratory Methods

Numerous methods have been described for the recovery and identification of parasites in clinical specimens, some of which are useful for detection of a variety of species whereas others detect only a particular species. It is preferable for the laboratory to offer a limited number of procedures competently performed than to offer a larger variety of infrequently performed tests that may prove problematic. Analyses of blood and fecal specimens comprise the largest share of clinician requests for parasitologic evaluation. A variety of additional specimens are submitted to the laboratory less frequently, including urogenital specimens, sputum, aspirates, and biopsy material. As newer information becomes available

Table 61–1 A Summary of the More Commonly Found Human Parasites and Their Primary Sites of Infection

Subkingdom Protozoa	Subkingdom Metazoa
Phylum Sarcomastigophora	**Phylum Platyhelminthes (flatworms)**
Subphylum Sarcodina (amebae)	**Class Cestoidea (tapeworms)**
Entamoeba histolytica (I)*	*Diphyllobothrium* spp. (I)*
E. dispar (I)	*Dipylidium caninum* (I)*
E. hartmanni (I)	*Echinococcus granulosus* (H)*
E. coli (I)	*E. multilocularis* (H)*
Iodamoeba butschlii (I)	*Hymenolepis nana* (I)*
Endolimax nana (I)	*H. diminuta* (I)*
Naegleria fowleri (T, C)*	*Taenia saginata* (I)*
Acanthamoeba spp. (T, C, E)*	*T. solium* (I, T)*
Balamuthia mandrillaris (T, C)*	**Class Trematoda (flukes)**
Blastocystis hominis (I)	*Clonorchis sinensis* (H)
Subphylum Mastigophora (flagellates)	*Fasciola hepatica* (H)*
Giardia lamblia (I)*	*Fasciolopsis buski* (I)
Dientamoeba fragilis (I)*	*Heterophyes heterophyes* (I)
Chilomastix mesnili (I)	*Metagonimus yokagawai* (I)
Retortamonas intestinalis (I)	*Nanophyetus salmincola* (I)*
Enteromonas hominis (I)	*Opisthorchis viverrini* (H)
Trichomonas hominis (I)	*Paragonimus* spp. (L)*
T. vaginalis (V)*	*Schistosoma haematobium* (B)
Leishmania tropica (T)	*S. japonicum* (B)
L. major (T)	*S. mekongi* (B)
L. aethiopica (T)	*S. mansoni* (B)
L. mexicana (T)*	**Phylum Nematoda (roundworms)**
L. braziliensis (T)	**Class Adenophorea (Aphasmidia)**
L. donovani (T)	*Trichinella spiralis* (T, I)*
Trypanosoma gambiense (B, C)	*Trichuris trichiura* (I)*
T. rhodesiense (B, C)	*Capillaria philippinensis* (I)
T. cruzi (B, T)*	**Class Secernentia (Phasmidia)**
Phylum Ciliophora (ciliates)	*Enterobius vermicularis* (I)*
Balantidium coli (I)*	*Ascaris lumbricoides* (I)*
Phylum Apicomplexa (apicomplexans)	*Ancylostoma duodenale* (I)
Class Sporozoea	*Necator americanus* (I)*
Subclass Piroplasma	*Strongyloides stercoralis* (I)
Babesia spp. (B)*	*Trichostrongylus* spp. (I)*
Subclass Coccidia	*Anisakis* spp. (I)*
Plasmodium falciparum (B)	*Wuchereria bancrofti* (T, B)
P. malariae (B)	*Brugia malayi* (T, B)
P. ovale (B)	*Loa loa* (T, B)
P. vivax (B)	*Onchocerca volvulus* (T)
Cryptosporidium parvum (I)*	*Mansonella perstans* (T, B)
Cyclospora cayetanensis (I)*	*M. ozzardi* (T, B)
Isospora belli (I)*	*M. streptocerca* (T)
Toxoplasma gondii (T)*	*Dracunculus medinensis* (T)
Phylum Microspora (microsporidia)	*Angiostrongylus cantonensis* (T)
Encephalitozoon spp. (E, H, T)*	*A. costaricensis* (T)
E. intestinalis (I, T)*	
Enterocytozoon bieneusi (I)*	

* Pathogenic parasite that occurs naturally in the United States.

B = blood; C = spinal fluid; E = eye; H = liver; I = intestine; L = lung; T = tissue; V = vagina.

Source: adapted from Murray PR, Barron EJ, Pfaller M, et al: Manual of Clinical Microbiology, 6th ed. Washington, DC, ASM Press, 1995.

Table 61–2 Estimated Prevalence of Parasitic Infections Worldwide

Disease	Estimated Population Involved	Annual Number of Deaths
Protozoan		
Amebiasis	Up to 10% of world population	40 000–110 000
African trypanosomiasis	100 000 new cases/year	5000
American trypanosomiasis	24 million	60 000
Giardiasis	200 million	
Leishmaniasis	1.2 million	
Malaria	400–490 million	2.2–2.5 million
Helminthic		
Ascariasis	1.3 billion	1550
Cestodiases	65 million	
Clonorchiasis/opisthorchiasis	13.5 million	
Dracunculiasis	<100 000	
Fasciolopsiasis	10 million	
Lymphatic filariasis	128 million	
Hookworm	1.3 billion	
Onchocerciasis	17.7 million	
Paragonimiasis	2.1 million	
Schistosomiasis	150 million	500 000–1 million
Strongyloidiasis	35 million	
Trichostrongyliasis	5.5 million	
Trichuriasis	900 million	

Adapted from Markell EK, John DT, Krotoski WA: Markell and Voge's Medical Parasitology, 8th ed. Philadelphia, PA, WB Saunders, 1999.

on certain of the so-called emerging parasites, the laboratory may need to develop and use additional, highly specific test methodologies or find competent referral laboratories where such tests are performed.

The types of specimen collected for laboratory evaluation depend on the species and stage of the parasite suspected. Knowledge of the life cycle of the parasite aids in determining the type, number, and frequency of specimens required for diagnosis. Immunologic and molecular methods for the diagnosis of parasitic diseases also are useful in many instances, and may be the only methods available in certain circumstances. Complete descriptions of the general and esoteric laboratory procedures for the recovery and identification of parasites referred to here may be found in a variety of sources to which the reader is referred (Beaver, 1984; Ash, 1987; Balows, 1988; Price, 1994; Garcia, 1999, 2001, 2003; Isenberg, 2004; Murray, 2003).

Familiarity with the calibration and use of the ocular micrometer is necessary for any laboratory performing parasitologic examination (Clinical and Laboratory Standards Institute, 2005). Measurement of the size of protozoal trophozoites and cysts and of helminth eggs and larvae is often required to make an accurate identification. Differentiation of pathogenic and nonpathogenic amebae (specifically *Entamoeba histolytica* and *Entamoeba hartmanni*) can only be made with assurance by taking careful size measurements. Similarly, eggs of *Diphyllobothrium* spp., *Paragonimus westermani*, and *Fasciola/Fasciolopsis* may be readily differentiated on the basis of accurate measurements (Smith, 1979; Clinical and Laboratory Standards Institute, 2005).

Examination of Blood

Parasites that may be detected in blood specimens include the agents of malaria (*Plasmodium* spp.), babesiosis (*Babesia* spp.), trypanosomiasis (*Trypanosoma* spp.), leishmaniasis (*Leishmania donovani*), and filariasis (*Wuchereria bancrofti*, *Brugia malayi*, *Loa loa*, and *Mansonella* spp.). The most important techniques to be performed in the clinical laboratory to assist in the diagnosis of blood parasites are the preparation, staining, and examination of thick and thin blood films. Other techniques used less frequently include the buffy coat smear and various concentration techniques reserved for recovery of microfilariae (National Committee for Clinical Laboratory Standards, 2000).

Thick and Thin Blood Films

Examination of permanent stained blood films is required to make an identification of most blood parasites. Thin films are prepared in the same

manner as for hematologic differential evaluation; blood is spread over the slide in a thin layer, yielding intact, nonoverlapping cellular elements. Integrity of the blood cell membranes is important to determine the intracellular or extracellular nature of the infection. In the thick film, blood is concentrated in a small area that is many cell layers deep. During staining, the erythrocytes are dehemoglobinized and only leukocyte nuclei, platelets, and parasites (if present) are visible. The thick film is preferred for diagnosis, because it contains 16–30 times more blood per microscopic field than does the thin film, thus increasing the chances of detecting light parasitemia and decreasing the time needed for a reliable examination. The amount of blood examined in a thick film in 5 minutes using the 100× oil immersion objective would require at least 30 minutes when examining an equivalent amount in a thin film. While thick films increase the likelihood of detecting an infection, species identifications are usually performed by examination of thin films because morphology is often more definitive, especially for the malarial parasites. For routine examination, both thick and thin films should be prepared.

Preparation of Slides

Blood for examination may be obtained by fingerstick, earlobe puncture, or venipuncture. Fingerstick blood should flow freely to prevent dilution with tissue fluid, and it should not be contaminated with the alcohol disinfectant, which should be allowed to dry first. If obtained by venipuncture, the first drop of blood (anticoagulant-free) from the needle is used to prepare the films at the bedside. Use of anticoagulants is discouraged when malaria is suspected because they may cause distortion of the parasites and interfere with staining. In practice, however, blood usually is submitted to the laboratory in an anticoagulant, which may be the only practical method to ensure that high-quality smears can be prepared. Ethylenediaminetetraacetic acid (EDTA)-anticoagulated blood is preferred in such cases and should be transported to the laboratory within the hour to prevent deterioration of organism morphology. Anticoagulants do not interfere with the staining of microfilariae.

Both thin and thick films should be prepared on clean, grease-free slides. Thick films are prepared by puddling several small drops of blood into an area the size of a dime (1.5 cm) and allowing the blood to dry flat at room temperature, usually overnight. A proper thick film should be thin enough that newspaper print may be read through it. If it is too thick, the film may peel from the slide. Excess heat may fix erythrocytes and prevent dehemoglobinization.

Staining

Blood begins to lose its affinity for stain in about 3 days, and older thick films do not dehemoglobinize well. Best staining results are achieved when using Giemsa stain, because host cell and parasite chromatin stains vividly while the hemoglobin in erythrocytes is only a pale red, and it is the only stain that allows visualization of the erythrocyte stippling that occurs with infection by certain malarial parasites. Wright's stain may be used for thin films, but it stains parasites less well than Giemsa and it stains erythrocytes, producing a busier background. Because Wright's stain incorporates alcohol as its fixative, thick films must be lysed in water before staining.

The Giemsa staining procedure requires somewhat more attention to preparation of reagents and staining protocol than does the Wright's staining procedure, which is often automated. Generally, fresh Giemsa stain must be made each day of use by diluting stock solution into phosphate-buffered water. To achieve appropriate staining reactions, including appearance of Schüffner's stippling, buffered water must be maintained at pH 6.8–7.2. Each new lot of stock Giemsa stain must be checked to determine optimal staining time and dilution, because there is some variation from lot to lot (National Committee for Clinical Laboratory Standards, 2000).

Examination of Smears

Both thick and thin smears are examined in their entirety under the low-power (10×) objective to detect microfilariae, which rarely occur in large numbers. In particular, the feathered edge of thin smears should be examined, as microfilariae are often carried there during preparation of the smear. Examination using a 50× oil immersion objective may subsequently be used to screen blood films for protozoa, although thorough examination using the 100× oil immersion objective still is necessary to detect the smallest parasites such as *Plasmodium* spp., *Babesia* spp., and leishmanias. Again, examination of the feathered edge is important because the erythrocytes are drawn out into a single layer of cells, allowing thorough evaluation of their morphology and the presence of intracellular protozoa. An experienced microscopist should examine at least 100 oil immersion fields (requiring about 5 minutes) on the thick blood film and 200 fields (requiring at least 15 minutes) on the thin film using the 100× objective before issuing a negative report (Ash, 1987).

VII

A variety of special techniques have been described for the concentration of blood parasites, specifically leishmaniae, trypanosomes, and microfilariae, details of which may be found elsewhere (Beaver, 1984; Ash, 1987; National Committee for Clinical Laboratory Standards, 2000; Garcia, 2001, 1999; Isenberg, 2004).

Preparation of buffy coat smears, which most clinical laboratories can perform with existing resources, is helpful in the detection of *L. donovani*, trypanosomes, and microfilariae. Following centrifugation of an anticoagulated blood sample, the layer of cells between the plasma and packed erythrocytes is drawn off and used to prepare blood films for staining or for preparation of a wet mount to detect motile organisms (Ash, 1987; Strickland, 2000).

For detection of microfilariae, Knott's concentration or membrane filtration is helpful, particularly when the density of microfilariae in peripheral blood is very low. In the Knott technique, anticoagulated blood is lysed with 2% formalin and centrifuged to concentrate the microfilariae in the sediment, which may then be examined as a wet preparation or stained with Giemsa or hematoxylin stains. In the membrane filtration procedure, blood is lysed and passed through a 5 μm membrane filter, which is subsequently stained with hematoxylin to reveal any microfilariae (Ash, 1987; National Committee for Clinical Laboratory Standards, 2000).

Use of the fluorochrome acridine orange in a microhematocrit centrifuge format (QBC blood parasite detection method, Becton Dickinson, Franklin Lakes, NJ) allows detection of blood parasites and appears to be more sensitive than traditional thick and thin smears. Laboratories that encounter malaria infrequently may experience difficulty in interpreting results by this method, however, and are encouraged to retain expertise in performance of traditional blood film techniques (National Committee for Clinical Laboratory Standards, 2000).

Examination of Fecal Specimens

The presence of intestinal parasites is primarily identified through the direct examination of stool using wet mounts, concentration techniques, permanent stained smears and, less frequently, culture. Newer immunoassay methods using species-specific antibody reagents to detect antigens of *G. lamblia*, *Cryptosporidium* spp., and *E. histolytica* have become popular. Stages of helminths commonly recovered include eggs and larvae, although intact worms or portions thereof may occasionally be seen. Intestinal protozoan infections are diagnosed by detection of trophozoites, cysts, or oocysts. Routine methods for the identification of ova and parasites (O & P examination) should include procedures that permit recovery of both protozoa and helminths, with use of special procedures limited to specific requests. At a minimum, laboratories performing parasitologic examination should be capable of performing direct wet mount examination of fresh stool, a concentration procedure, and a permanent stain method. Many protozoan infections will be missed unless permanent stains are examined (Garcia, 1979, 1997, 2003; Price, 1994; Clinical and Laboratory Standards Institute, 2005).

Specimen Collection, Handling, and Preservation

Recovery and subsequent identification of parasites in fecal specimens requires proper collection and handling. Old, poorly preserved, or contaminated specimens are of little value. Specimens should not be collected for 1 week after the patient has ingested any materials that leave a crystalline residue, such as nonabsorbable antidiarrheal compounds, antacids, bismuth, barium, or antimalarial agents. Oily laxatives such as mineral oil may also interfere with examination. Use of antibiotics or contrast media may decrease the numbers of organisms, especially protozoa, in the intestinal tract for several weeks (Ash, 1987; Garcia, 2003).

Specimens may be submitted to the laboratory either fresh or in appropriate preservatives. All fresh specimens should be examined within 1 hour of passage, and liquid specimens should be examined within 30 minutes or placed immediately in preservatives to maintain the best yield. This method ensures that fragile protozoal trophozoites are not inadvertently destroyed. Specimens that cannot be processed immediately should be left at room temperature or refrigerated and should not be placed in an incubator, because this only speeds disintegration of parasites.

Specimens may be passed directly into clean, dry paper cartons or by having the patient squat over wax paper and transferring a portion to a container. Diarrheic specimens may also be collected in clean bedpans. Containers should have tight-fitting lids and should be placed in plastic bags before transport to the laboratory. Inadvertent introduction of urine or toilet water with the specimen may readily destroy protozoal trophozoites and should be avoided. Also, contamination with water or

Table 61–3 Stool Fixatives and Examination Techniques

Fixative	Examination Technique		
	Direct Wet Mount	Concentration Procedure	Permanent Stained Smear
None (fresh stool)	Yes	Yes	Yes
10% formalin	Yes	Yes	No
Schaudinn's fluid	No	No	Yes
Polyvinyl alcohol (PVA)	No	No*	Yes
Modified PVA[†]	No	No*	Yes
Merthiolate–iodine–formalin (MIF)	Yes	Yes	No[‡]
Sodium acetate–formalin (SAF)	Yes	Yes	Yes

* Although concentration techniques using PVA have been described, they are not widely used because of problems with recovery of some organisms. [†] Copper sulfate or zinc sulfate replaces the mercuric chloride. [‡] Smears prepared from MIF-preserved specimens may be stained with polychrome IV stain.

soil may accidentally introduce free-living organisms that may prove difficult to differentiate from parasitic ones.

Kits consisting of vials of preservatives appropriate for performing direct examinations, concentration procedures, and preparation of stained smears are available from a number of commercial sources at low cost. Aliquots of freshly passed stool should be immediately placed into these vials and mixed thoroughly. These kits are especially helpful for those patients who are unable to bring in a fresh sample in timely fashion or for those who will be collecting several specimens over the course of several days. With the two-vial technique, one portion of specimen is fixed in three parts of 5–10% buffered formalin and another portion in three parts of polyvinyl alcohol (PVA) fixative. Other preservation systems available include merthiolate–iodine–formalin (MIF) and sodium acetate–formalin (SAF) (Table 61–3). SAF has an advantage in that it can be used for permanent stains as well as for direct mounts and concentration procedures, and that it does not contain mercury, which is present in Schaudinn's and PVA fixatives. In addition to being poisonous, mercury presents disposal problems in an increasing number of states. However, the quality of permanent stains when using SAF is not as good as with Schaudinn's or PVA fixatives. Use of zinc-sulfate-based PVA and other newer commercial products are gaining popularity, and their use may be indicated when mercury chloride-based compounds cannot be used (Garcia, 1993, 1997, 2001; Clinical and Laboratory Standards Institute, 2005).

Examination of three specimens collected every other day is considered the minimum necessary to perform an adequate O & P evaluation (Garcia, 2003; Clinical and Laboratory Standards Institute, 2005). This procedure ensures an optimum interval for recovery of those parasites that are known to shed diagnostic forms intermittently, especially *G. lamblia* and *Strongyloides stercoralis*. Additional sensitivity may be achieved in detecting these parasites, as well as *E. histolytica*, using purgation. The laboratory must be notified prior to initiation of purgation, however, to have staff available for processing. Specimens should be collected in separate containers and submitted to the laboratory within minutes of collection. Saline purgatives such as sodium sulfate or buffered phosphosoda are recommended.

Macroscopic Examination

Fecal specimens should be examined grossly for consistency (formed, soft, loose, or watery), and for the presence of mucus, blood, larval or adult worms, and proglottids. Protozoan trophozoites are more likely to be found in watery or loose specimens, whereas cysts predominate in formed or soft specimens. Helminths or their eggs may be found in any type of fecal specimen. Most parasites are uniformly distributed in the stool as a result of the mixing action of the cecum, although some eggs (especially schistosomes) may enter the fecal stream in the lower colon and rectum and be unevenly distributed, as may pinworm and *Taenia* spp. eggs. Protozoal trophozoites may be more numerous in the last portion of stool evacuated and should be specifically sought in mucus (Garcia, 2003).

Microscopic Examination

Specimens may be examined microscopically by direct wet mounts of fresh or preserved material, wet mounts of concentrates, or permanent stains. Each procedure has specific advantages and limitations. Direct saline wet mounts of fresh feces allow detection and observation of motile protozoan trophozoites and helminth larvae. Direct mounts of preserved feces may allow detection of parasites that do not concentrate well.

Concentration procedures increase the examiner's ability to detect protozoan cysts and helminth eggs and larvae but are unsatisfactory for detecting protozoan trophozoites. Permanent stains are useful for detection and morphologic examination of protozoan trophozoites and cysts.

The circumstances under which each procedure is performed varies depending on the type of specimen (formed, soft, loose, or watery) submitted. Generally, a fresh soft, loose, or watery specimen should have all three procedures performed (Garcia, 2003). Watery specimens may be concentrated by simple centrifugation rather than by flotation or formalin–ethyl acetate concentration. The direct wet mount may be omitted if the specimen is submitted in preservatives (Clinical and Laboratory Standards Institute, 2005). At a minimum, formed specimens should be examined by a concentration procedure, although improved yield has been demonstrated when a permanent stain is added to the work-up (Garcia, 1979, 2001).

Direct Wet Mount

The direct wet mount is one of the most easily performed parasitologic tests, although proper interpretation requires careful examination and experience in using the microscope to full advantage. The test is most useful when fresh specimens, especially liquid stools or duodenal aspirates, are examined for motile trophozoites or helminth larvae. A small amount of stool is mixed with a drop of 0.85% saline and covered with a coverslip. The preparation should be dense enough that newspaper print can just be read through it.

Examination of the entire coverslip is performed systematically under the low-power (10×) objective with the microscope diaphragm closed down to increase contrast. Suspicious objects and those that are refractile, such as protozoal cysts, should then be examined with the high-power (40×) objective. Detection of motility of slow-moving amebae requires that an object be examined for at least 15 seconds. In the absence of suspicious objects, up to a third of the preparation should be examined using the 40× objective. Use of the oil immersion objective usually is not performed unless the coverslip has been sealed with nail polish or vaspar (a 50:50 mixture of petroleum jelly and paraffin).

A second preparation may be made in identical fashion except that a drop of a 1:5 dilution of Lugol's iodine or an equivalent preparation is added in place of the saline. Use of straight Lugol's or Gram's iodine causes clumping of material and is not recommended. Iodine is helpful in enhancing the visibility of nuclear structures in protozoal cysts and for detecting glycogen inclusions. Limitations, however, include loss of trophozoite motility and cyst refractility, and difficulty in recognizing chromatoid bodies.

Concentration Techniques

Concentration procedures, which may be performed on fresh or preserved specimens (Table 61–3), are more sensitive than direct wet mount examination for detection of protozoan cysts and helminth eggs and larvae because they decrease the amount of background material in the preparations and, in most circumstances, actually concentrate the organisms. Although a variety of methods and modifications have been described, some are useful only for specific parasites (Melvin, 1982; Ash, 1987; Garcia, 2001, 1999; Clinical and Laboratory Standards Institute, 2005). For routine use, a method should be selected that allows reliable detection of both protozoan cysts and helminth eggs. Concentration methods are based on sedimentation or flotation principles. In sedimentation the heavier parasites settle to the bottom as a result of gravity or centrifugation. In flotation the lighter parasite cysts and eggs rise to the surface of a solution of high specific gravity. The two most widely used concentration procedures in the United States are the zinc sulfate centrifugal flotation technique of Faust and the formalin ether sedimentation of Ritchie (or their modifications). In practice, ethyl acetate has replaced ether in the latter method because of the dangers associated with handling ether, and comparable results are achieved (Truant, 1981).

Formalin–ethyl acetate concentration is a biphasic sedimentation technique that is efficient in recovering most protozoan cysts and helminth eggs and larvae, including operculate eggs, and is moderately effective for schistosome eggs. Less distortion of protozoal cysts occurs with this technique than with zinc sulfate flotation. Eggs of *Hymenolepis nana* may be missed, however, and concentration of *G. lamblia* and *Iodamoeba bütschlii* cysts may not be very good. For proper concentration of coccidian oocysts and spores of microsporidia, attention must be paid to the recommended speed and time of centrifugation (Isenberg, 2004; Clinical and Laboratory Standards Institute, 2005). Despite these problems, the technique is widely used for both its simplicity and its suitability in most laboratory situations.

With the zinc sulfate flotation method, fresh stool is processed using zinc sulfate with a specific gravity of 1.18 and formalinized stool is processed with a solution of specific gravity of 1.20. Parasitic elements are recovered from the surface film of the solution following centrifugation. This method yields a cleaner preparation than does formalin–ethyl acetate concentration, but it is unreliable for the recovery of nematode larvae, infertile eggs of *Ascaris*, and the eggs of most trematodes and large tapeworms. Problems with recovery also occur with stool specimens containing excessive amounts of fats. Use of formalinized stool specimens rather than fresh stool helps clear the specimen and prevents popping of opercula and distortion of the parasites (Bartlett, 1978).

Permanent Stains

Use of stained slide preparations provides a permanent record of a patient's specimen and allows review by consultants should difficulties arise in identification. Of the methods described for studying fecal specimens, only the permanent stain is designed for analysis using the oil immersion objective (100×). The permanent stain is most useful for detection of protozoal trophozoites and cysts, which may be recognized when the direct and concentrated preparations are negative. Although generally not useful for detecting helminth eggs or larvae, permanent stains are inherently more sensitive for detecting protozoal infections, and their use has been recommended for every stool sample submitted for O & P examination (Clinical and Laboratory Standards Institute, 2005).

A variety of staining techniques and modifications have been described that have both advantages and disadvantages. The Wheatley trichrome stain and iron hematoxylin stain are all-purpose methods that allow detection of amebae and flagellates. Unfortunately, detection of most human-infecting coccidia and microsporidia requires the use of special stains. Technical problems may arise in the performance of any staining procedure; most are related to the age of the specimen, proper smear preparation and fixation, and quality of the reagents. Positive control slides of known staining quality should be run with each batch of slides stained. This is especially true in the performance of the more specific stains for coccidia and microsporidia. Less commonly used stains, such as polychrome IV stain for use with MIF-preserved specimens and chlorazol black E stain for use with fresh specimens are not reviewed here further, but details may be found elsewhere (Clinical and Laboratory Standards Institute, 2005; Garcia, 2001).

Wheatley's Trichrome Stain

In the United States, the Wheatley modification of the trichrome method continues to find widespread acceptance because of its simplicity, reliability, and cost-effectiveness. Details of the procedure are available from a number of sources (Melvin, 1982; Price, 1994; Isenberg, 2004; Clinical and Laboratory Standards Institute, 2005). Appropriate specimens include those that have been fixed in Schaudinn's fixative or PVA fixatives; SAF- or MIF-preserved specimens may be stained with trichrome, but results are less satisfactory.

Iron Hematoxylin Stain

Iron hematoxylin stains are technically more difficult to perform than the trichrome stain, but results generally are superior owing to enhanced definition of key nuclear and cytoplasmic characteristics (Price, 1994). A modified iron hematoxylin stain that may prove to be useful incorporates carbol fuchsin, allowing concurrent staining of acid-fast organisms such as *Cryptosporidium*, *Cyclospora*, and *Isospora* (Palmer, 1991; Clinical and Laboratory Standards Institute, 2005). Specimens fixed in Schaudinn's, PVA, or SAF fixatives may be stained with iron hematoxylin stains (the preferred stain for SAF).

Modified Acid-Fast Stains

Oocysts of *Cryptosporidium*, *Cyclospora*, and *Isospora* are difficult to recognize on trichrome- or iron-hematoxylin-stained smears, but their presence may be detected by using an acid-fast staining technique such as the modified Kinyoun method, modified acid-fast dimethyl sulfoxide (DMSO), or auramine-O (Ma, 1983; Bronsdon, 1984; Current, 1991; Clinical and Laboratory Standards Institute, 2005). Acid-fast stains are sensitive and cost-effective for detection of these protozoa, but they lack specificity. Close attention must be paid to defined morphologic criteria when using these stains, and the use of positive control material is mandatory. For laboratories in which *Cryptosporidium* is rarely encountered, use of the highly specific and sensitive commercially available immunoassay reagents is recommended. Stool, sputa, biliary tract, and other appropriate specimens that are fresh, formalin-fixed, or SAF-fixed may be used with acid-fast stains.

Stains for Microsporidia

Microsporidia (specifically *Enterocytozoon hieneusi* and *Encephalitozoon intestinalis*, along with a number of other species) have been implicated as

VII

common agents of diarrheal disease, especially in immunocompromised patients, although their detection has been problematic. Although biopsy and electron microscopy have been a mainstay in their diagnosis, staining procedures that may be performed in the clinical laboratory have been described. A modified trichrome stain using an increased (10-fold) concentration of chromotrope 2R combined with an increase in the staining time has gained acceptance as a specific test for the identification of microsporidial spores (Weber, 1992, 1994; Murray, 2003). Fluorescent staining methods using optical whitening agents such as Uvitek-2B and Calcofluor white are also useful for rapid and sensitive screening of stool and other clinical specimens for such spores (van Gool, 1993; DeGirolami, 1995; Didier, 1995; Luna, 1995). The small size (1.5–3 μm) of these organisms makes their detection difficult, and such studies should not be undertaken without appropriate control materials for comparison.

Additional Techniques for Examination of Enteric Parasites

Cellulose Tape Technique for Pinworms

The female pinworm, *Enterobius vermicularis*, migrates from the cecum to the perianal skin, where she deposits typical eggs that are fully embryonated. The eggs or, occasionally, adult worms may be detected on examination of clear, adhesive cellophane tape or commercial collection kits that have been pressed on to the perianal skin. Eggs or adults are rarely found in stool, which is considered to be an inappropriate specimen for detection of this parasite. Specimens should be collected late at night, when the worms are most active, or first thing in the morning before bathing or defecation. Several specimens taken on different days should be examined before ruling out infection.

Egg Studies

Estimation of worm burden occasionally is requested to assist in the evaluation of therapeutic efficacy or following rates of reinfection with intestinal nematodes (*Ascaris*, *Trichuris*, and hookworms) or, occasionally, schistosomes. Procedures include the direct smear method of Beaver, the Stoll dilution egg count, Kato's thick smear, and various modifications (Beaver, 1984; Ash, 1987; Clinical and Laboratory Standards Institute, 2005). Large variations in results are inherent when performing these tests, and levels of egg counts indicating clinical significance vary depending on the infecting species, person's age, and nutritional status (Beaver, 1984).

Egg hatching methods have been used in the analysis of schistosomiasis to detect their presence in light infections and to determine their viability. Schistosome eggs, which are fully embryonated when passed, contain a miracidium that hatches within several hours when eggs are placed in dechlorinated water. In practice, urine or stool is mixed in about 10 volumes of water, which is then placed in a sidearm or Erlenmeyer flask. All but the sidearm or the top of the flask is covered with foil wrap, and the unit is placed under a desk lamp. Hatched miracidia are positively phototropic and congregate near the light. Eggs, if available, may be examined directly for viability by examining for movement of cilia within flame (excretory) cells (Clinical and Laboratory Standards Institute, 2005).

Nematode Culture and Recovery Techniques

Several culture techniques (coproculture) assist in the detection and identification of certain nematode infections, including the Harada–Mori filter paper strip culture, filter paper/slant culture, and charcoal culture (Beaver, 1984; Ash, 1987; Clinical and Laboratory Standards Institute, 2005). Differentiation of hookworms and trichostrongyles on the basis of egg morphology is difficult, whereas infective-stage larvae are more readily identified. Such culture techniques may also prove useful in recovery of *Strongyloides* larvae, which may be few in number, and for differentiating them from those of hookworms. With all culture methods, feces are incubated in a humid environment to encourage egg hatching. In the Harada–Mori and filter paper/slant techniques, larvae migrate from the feces into a water phase, where they may be readily detected. In the charcoal culture, larvae first migrate into a dampened gauze pad, which is then placed in water, allowing the larvae to settle out.

The Baermann funnel technique is a sensitive and reliable method for recovery of *Strongyloides* and other nematode larvae from a stool specimen. In this assay, feces are placed on several layers of gauze on top of a wire screen that is suspended in a funnel. The bottom of the funnel is clamped off, and water is added to the level of the gauze. Larvae actively migrate through the gauze and settle to the bottom of the funnel where they may be drawn off for examination. Larval recovery may be improved over that of the culture techniques because a larger amount of feces is examined. In latent *Strongyloides* infection, in which few larvae are being shed, several

Table 61–4 Objects Recoverable from Stool That Resemble Enteric Parasites

Type of Artifact	Resemblance
Neutrophils	*Entamoeba histolytica* cysts
Macrophages	*Entamoeba histolytica* trophozoites
Columnar epithelial cells	Amebic trophozoites
Squamous epithelial cells	Amebic trophozoites
Yeasts	Protozoan cysts (especially *Endolimax nana*)
Fungal conidia	Helminth eggs
Mushroom spores	Helminth eggs
Plant cells	Protozoan cysts, helminth eggs
Plant hairs	Nematode larvae
Pollen grains	Helminth eggs (*Ascaris* or *Taenia*)
Diatoms	Helminth eggs
Starch granules, fat globules, air bubbles, mucus	Protozoan cysts
Ingested mite eggs	Helminth eggs
Ingested plant nematode eggs	Helminth eggs
Ingested plant nematode larvae	Nematode larvae

Adapted from Isenberg HE (ed): Clinical Microbiology Procedures Handbook, Vols 1 and 2, 2nd edn. Washington, DC, American Society for Microbiology, 2004.

examinations over a week's time may be required to demonstrate the infection (Ash, 1987; Garcia, 2003).

Objects Resembling Enteric Parasites

A large variety of objects that closely resemble various parasite life cycle stages may be seen in feces and other specimens sent for O & P examination. Careful differentiation of these objects from real parasites is necessary to prevent inappropriate or unnecessary treatment. White blood cells, macrophages, and squamous and columnar epithelial cells may resemble amebae; yeasts and starch granules may resemble protozoal cysts; pollen and fungal conidia may resemble helminth eggs; plant fibers may resemble nematode larvae; and pieces of vegetables or vegetable skins may resemble adult worms or proglottids (Table 61–4). Examples of artifacts and pseudoparasites have been reviewed elsewhere (Ash, 1997; Garcia, 2001; Isenberg, 2004; Clinical and Laboratory Standards Institute, 2005).

Examination of Urogenital and Other Specimens (Sputa, Aspirates, Biopsies)

Vaginal and urethral discharges, prostatic secretions, or urine may be submitted to the laboratory for detection of *Trichomonas vaginalis*. The most rapid and cost-effective method is the preparation of several wet mounts using a drop of specimen (urine should be centrifuged) diluted with a drop of saline, which is then covered with a coverslip. The slide is examined under the low-power (10×) objective using reduced lighting conditions for the motile trophozoites, which display a jerky movement. High-power examination may reveal the beating flagella and undulating membrane characteristic of the species. Use of culture, fluorescent antibody reagents, or DNA probe techniques improves sensitivity, if needed (Briselden, 1994). Demonstration of imidazole drug resistance requires culture of the organism (Meri, 2000).

A number of protozoal and helminthic parasites may be detected in sputa, and the appropriate examination technique depends on the suspected organism. Generally, the technique required to detect a parasite from its usual site of infection is applied to sputum and most commonly involves a wet mount. When amebae are suspected, permanent stains should be performed. Acid-fast or specific antibody-based stains are appropriate for *Cryptosporidium*, whereas modified trichrome or fluorochrome stains should be used for detection of spores of microsporidia. Identification techniques for *Pneumocystis jiroveci* (formerly *Pneumocystis carinii*) are described elsewhere.

Examination of aspirates requires the use of stains as appropriate for the implicated organism. In addition to the methods used for sputum, Giemsa staining is often appropriate when examining for protozoa, especially the hemoflagellates. Biopsy material should be submitted for routine histology after imprint smears are prepared for staining with Giemsa or other appropriate permanent stain. Culture for leishmanias and trypanosomes also can be performed on tissues and may be important for demonstrating those infections. Skin biopsies sent for *Onchocerca* or *Mansonella* examination should be teased apart in saline and the saline examined after 30–60 minutes for microfilariae. Muscle biopsy for *Trichinella spiralis* larvae may be examined by compressing the fresh specimen between two glass slides or by submitting it for routine histology. Likewise, rectal or bladder biopsies may be examined for schistosome eggs.

Parasite Culture Techniques

Culture methods have been described for a wide variety of protozoan parasites but few clinical laboratories undertake the effort because of infrequent requests and unfamiliarity with the methods. When culture requests are made, they are usually for *T. vaginalis*, *Leishmania* spp., *Trypanosoma cruzi*, *E. histolytica*, *Acanthamoeba* spp., or *Naegleria fowleri*. In addition, virology laboratories are occasionally asked to culture for *T. gondii*. Methods are reviewed elsewhere (Ash, 1987; Fritsche, 1989a; Garcia, 2001; Isenberg, 2004; Murray, 2003; Clinical and Laboratory Standards Institute, 2005).

Immunodiagnostic Methods

Several immunodiagnostic methodologies are available to identify the parasitic-antigen or the antibody that is produced in response to the parasitic infection. Some of the signals are amplified while others are direct detection methods. In general laboratory methods employed are enzyme immunoassay (EIA), immunofluorescence assay (IF), direct fluorescence antibody assay (DFA), Western blot, radioimmunoassay, and immunodiffusion, among others.

Antigen Detection

Antigen detection methods are commercially available for several parasitic diseases, including amebiasis, cryptosporidiosis, giardiasis, malaria, and trichomoniasis (Table 61–5), and these methods may be useful for initial testing or in those instances in which traditional tests are negative, yet a high index of clinical suspicion remains. These tests have the advantage of detecting current infection and can often be performed by someone other than an experienced morphologist (Wilson, 1995).

Antigen detection in stool samples is usually performed using fecal immunoassays. A number of published studies have suggested that these assays have good sensitivity and specificity when compared with routine ova and parasite examination (Aldeen, 1995; Kehl, 1995; Zimmerman, 1995; Maraha, 2000; Hanson, 2001; Garcia, 2003). These immunoassays are easy to use, rapid, permit batch processing and do not require experienced microscopists. Given the current shortage of medical technologists and individuals with specialized training in parasitology, use of immunoassays appears to be an attractive alternative. However laboratories that use rapid immunoassays should be aware of the potential problems with false-positive results and closely monitor test performance. Currently, fecal immunoassays are marketed for *G. lamblia*, *C. parvum/C. hominis*, the *E. histolytica/E. dispar* group, and *E. histolytica*. Antigen detection tests using blood or serum are also available for *Plasmodium* spp. and *W. bancrofti*. A latex agglutination test for *T. vaginalis* antigen detection in vaginal swabs has also been introduced recently. Additional commercially-manufactured kits are under development for detection of *Dientamoeba fragilis* and the microsporidia. Immunoassays are usually available in three formats: EIA, DFA, and lateral flow (immunochromatography) cartridges. Fresh or preserved stool samples are appropriate for most antigen detection kits (Fedorko, 2000). While each kit has unique operating characteristics, most are generally comparable in performance (Garcia, 2000, 2003; Katanik, 2001).

Rapid antigen detection methods developed for malaria detect either histidine rich protein II (HRP-II) or parasite lactate dehydrogenase (pLDH), or both, in peripheral blood. The HRP-II tests are specific for *Plasmodium falciparum* while pLDH tests detect all four *Plasmodium* spp. Sensitivities of these assays are comparable to, or lower than, traditional microscopic examination but have sensitivities of more than 90%. These tests are not currently approved by the Food and Drug Administration (FDA) for clinical diagnosis of malaria in the United States.

Detection of *T. vaginalis* antigens from vaginal samples may also be performed using rapid antigen tests. These tests can be used for rapid detection of *T. vaginalis* infection in the clinic setting and may replace wet mount examinations which generally have lower sensitivities, depending on the proficiency of the personnel performing the microscopic examination. Miller and colleagues demonstrated that the *T. vaginalis* rapid antigen test had comparable sensitivities to culture (Miller, 2003).

Most enzyme immunoassays are available in microwell format. The antigen from frozen, fresh, or 10%-formalin-preserved stool samples are

Table 61–5 Antigen-Based Detection Assays for Parasites.

Analyte	Test System	Manufacturer/Distributor	Format
Cryptosporidium spp.	Xpect™ Cryptosporidium	Remel	Cartridge
	Cryptosporidium	Wampole	EIA
	Crypto Cel	CeLLabs	IFA
	ProSpecT® Cryptosporidium	Remel	EIA
	Cryptosporidium TEST	TechLab	EIA
	Crypto CELISA	CeLLabs	EIA
	PARA-TECT™ Cryptosporidium	Medical Chemical Co.	EIA
Giardia lamblia	ProSpecT® Giardia Rapid Assay	Remel	Cartridge
	Giardia Cel	CeLLabs	IFA
	Xpect™ GIARDIA	Remel	Cartridge
	ProSpecT® Giardia	Remel	EIA
	PARA-TECT™ Giardia	Medical Chemical Co.	EIA
	GIARDIA II	TechLab	EIA
	GiardEIA™	Antibodies	EIA
	Giardia CELISA	CeLLabs	EIA
	Giardia	Wampole	EIA
Entamoeba histolytica	E. histolytica	Wampole	EIA
	Entamoeba CELISA PATH	CeLLabs	EIA
	E. histolytica II	TechLab	EIA
Cryptosporidium/ Giardia	Xpect® Giardia/ Cryptosporidium	Remel	Cartridge
	Immunocard STAT Cryptosporidium/Giardia	Meridian Bioscience	Cartridge
	MERIFLUOR Cryptosporidium/Giardia	Meridian Bioscience	IFA
	Crypto Giardia DFA	IVD Research Inc	IFA
	Crypto/Giardia Cel	CeLLabs	IFA
	PARA-TECT™ Cryptosporidium/Giardia DFA	Medical Chemical Co.	IFA
	ColorPAC™ Giardia/Cryptosporidium	Becton Dickinson	Cartridge
	ProSpecT® Giardia/Cryptosporidium	Remel	EIA
G. lamblia, C. parvum, and *E. histolytica/ dispar* combination	Biosite Triage® Parasite Panel	Biosite Diagnostics	Cartridge
Plasmodium spp.	NOW Malaria test	Binax	Cartridge
	OptiMAL	Flow	Dipstick
	Paracheck Pf	Orchid	Cartridge
	Rapimal MT Pf	CeLLabs	Dipstick
Wuchereria bancrofti	NOW Filariasis	Binax	Cartridge
	Filariasis -CELISA	CeLLabs	EIA
Trichomonas vaginalis	Light Diagnostic T. Vaginalis	Chemicon	DFA
	OSOM® Trichomonas Rapid Test	Genzyme	Dipstick
	XenoStrip-Tv™	Xenotope Diagnostics	Cartridge

Cartridge, Lateral flow cartridge; DFA, direct fluorescence antibody assay; EIA, Enzyme immunoassay; Dipstick, dipstick enzyme immunoassay; IFA, Immunofluorescence assay.

suitable for testing by this methodology. Concentrated or PVA samples are not suitable for testing with EIA kits. Parasite antigen is captured by immobilized antibodies coated on microwells and detected by an enzyme-conjugated secondary antibody that is capable of producing a colored reaction following the addition of substrate. Although the colored wells can be read either visually or using a spectrometer, the latter seems to be the preferred option because of occasional ambiguous results obtained with some kits (Kehl, 1995). In general EIA tests have good sensitivities and specificities. Garcia and colleagues evaluated nine immunoassay kits for detection of *G. lamblia* and *Cryptosporidium* spp. in comparison with a reference DFA test that visualizes the parasite directly in the sample and found that all the kits had high sensitivities, ranging from 94–99%, and 100% specificities (Garcia, 1997, 2003). However, published reports have suggested that occasional problems are found with some EIA kits that may produce false positive results and which have led to their recall (Doing, 1999). Hence, a strong QC program and participation in proficiency test programs are required to insure high-quality test results. Local epidemiology of the parasitic infection can help to determine whether additional confirmatory testing is required; consultation with local public health authorities may prove useful in characterizing which infections are being seen locally. Additionally for some diseases such as giardiasis, examination of two specimens by either EIA or microscopy may be necessary to achieve a diagnostic sensitivity of more than 90% (Hanson, 2001).

Lateral Flow cartridges are a popular immunoassay format of immunoassay because of their ease of use and the minimal performance time required. These kits can be stored conveniently at room temperatures and may be used in single or batch processing. The parasite antigen in the sample migrates through the membrane and binds to specific capture antibodies; use of a secondary reagent results in development of a colored reaction. These kits also have an internal control to ensure that the colloidal dye conjugates used in the assay are intact and that proper capillary flow has occurred. To ensure complete migration of the specimen only the supernatant of a well-mixed stool sample is used, while some samples may be diluted to a liquid state before testing. Any color visible at the reagent test zone (usually a band) is interpreted as positive. Some studies have demonstrated that cartridge assays are somewhat less sensitive than a microwell EIA plate assay (Pillai, 1999; Johnston, 2003). In such a situation it may be necessary to perform alternative O&P studies if patients' symptoms persist.

DFA testing allows direct visualization of the parasites in stool specimen using antibodies conjugated to fluorescent dyes. These assays are easy to perform and to interpret, permitting rapid screening of the slides when compared with some of the traditional stains used in parasitology (Zimmerman, 1995; Garcia, 2001, 2003). A fluorescence microscope is necessary for this procedure, a limiting factor in some laboratories. Currently, kits are available for detection of cysts of *G. lamblia* and oocysts of *Cryptosporidium* spp. Fixed stool specimens may be used for this procedure (10% formalin, SAF, or ECOFIX; Fedorko, 2000). Although fresh stool samples can be tested directly, the sensitivity of the assay can be improved by performing the test on centrifuged stool (500 *g* for 10 min). Occasionally fluorescing bacteria and yeast may be seen but these are readily distinguished from *Giardia* and *Cryptosporidium* on the basis of their size and shape. The edges of the wells should be carefully examined to avoid missing light infections. Given the recent recognition of additional *Cryptosporidium* spp. that may infect humans, studies relating to specificity of the various immunoassays are needed to determine actual sensitivity in detecting any *Cryptosporidium* infection (Graczyk, 1996; Coupe, 2005).

Serologic Diagnosis

Tests that are available from public health, hospital, or commercial laboratories to detect immunologic reactivity to parasitic diseases are summarized in Table 61–6. Historically, serologic procedures for parasitic diseases have been plagued by low sensitivity and specificity, primarily owing to the complex antigenic nature of parasites and the possibilities for cross-reactions from related species. The introduction of newer test methodologies combined with the use of more highly defined antigenic components are providing more accurate results with greater predictive values. Many of the newer tests use the EIA or immunoblot (Western blot) formats, although indirect immunofluorescence (IFA), indirect hemagglutination (IHA), complement fixation (CF), and bentonite flocculation (BF) methodologies remain popular.

Serologic diagnosis of parasitic infection is used as an adjunct to the usual diagnostics modalities or in special situations where identification of the parasite itself or its antigen or nucleic acid from host tissue or excreta is not possible. Parasitic infections such as toxoplasmosis and toxocariasis reside in deep tissues and cannot be readily diagnosed by morphologic means, and others such as cysticercosis and echinococcosis develop in organs, where invasive studies that may be required are not recommended in the initial patient evaluation. Other conditions such as filariasis, schistosomiasis, and strongyloidiasis may remain subclinical because of light infections or because the clinical evaluation occurred during the prepatent period. Other circumstances where serologic evaluation may prove useful are diagnosis of extraintestinal amoebiasis and trichinellosis. The chronic stages of trypanosomiasis are also preferably diagnosed by

Table 61–6 Serological Assays for Parasites Available from Reference Laboratories

Disease	Organism	Specimen type	Assay
Amoebiasis	*Entamoeba histolytica*	Serum	EIA, ID, IHA
Babesiosis	*Babesia microti, Babesia* sp. WA1	Serum	IFA
Chagas	*Trypanosoma cruzi*	Serum	IFA, EIA, CF
Cysticercosis	*Taenia solium*	Serum, CSF	EIA, IB
Echinococcosis	*Echinococcus granulosus*	Serum	EIA, IB, IHA, IFA
Fascioliasis	*Fasciola hepatica*	Serum	EIA, IB
Filariasis	*Wuchereria bancrofti*	Serum	EIA
Leishmaniasis	*Leishmania braziliensis, Leishmania donovani, Leishmania tropica*	Serum	IFA, EIA, CF
Malaria	*Plasmodium* spp.	Serum	IFA
Paragonimiasis	*Paragonimus westermani*	Serum	EIA, IB
Schistosomiasis	*Schistosoma* spp.	Serum	EIA, IB
Strongyloidiasis	*Strongyloides stercoralis*	Serum	EIA
Toxoplasmosis	*Toxoplasma gondii*	CSF, serum	IFA, EIA
Trichinellosis	*Trichinella spiralis*	Serum	EIA, BF

BF, bentonite flocculation; CF, complement fixation; EIA, enzyme immunoassay; IB, immunoblot; ID, immunodiffusion; IHA, indirect hemagglutination.

serology. Serological studies also help in the diagnosis of occult infections such as visceral larva migrans, cysticercosis and filariasis. Lastly, serological studies serve as a powerful tool to understand the epidemiology of diseases such as schistosomiasis, toxoplasmosis, amoebiasis, Chagas disease, malaria, and babesiosis. High antibody levels are useful for diagnostic purposes if they occur in a patient with no previous exposure to the parasite or recent history of travel to an endemic area. Unfortunately, positive antibody levels in persons living in endemic areas do not often help in the clinical diagnosis. Detection of antibodies, especially IgG, indicates evidence of infection but may not be able to differentiate active from past exposure. In some parasitic diseases the levels of antibodies may decline slowly following successful therapy or self-cure. Serologic tests for parasitic diseases generally evaluate IgG levels, with the exception of toxoplasmosis and babesiosis where IgM- and IgA-specific antibodies may be helpful to determine the age of infection (National Committee for Clinical Laboratory Standards, 2004).

Because serologic tests for parasitic diseases are infrequently requested, specimens generally are submitted to public (Centers for Disease Control and Prevention [CDC]) or private reference laboratories. Some of the more commonly requested tests, especially those that are available as commercial kits, are often available locally, including those for toxoplasmosis, amebiasis, and trichinosis.

Many of these assays are developed in-house and hence lack correlation with universal standards. Interpretive criteria are established by reagent manufacturers or by the center performing the test, and these criteria often vary from institution to institution. Individuals requesting such tests should inquire about the performance characteristics, including sensitivity and specificity, and should be aware that cross-reactions may occur. For example, antibody tests for Chagas' disease are known to crossreact with antibodies produced in response to *Leishmania* infections. However the reactivity to homologous antigen is higher and this test is useful in diagnosis of chronic stages of the disease when parasitemia is generally low. Usually serology for chronic Chagas' disease correlates well with molecular diagnostic methods (Weinberg, 2001). Helminthic parasites are well-known to cross-react in serologic assays that use crude antigen preparations, because of phylogenetic – hence antigenic – similarities.

Several factors that may influence the test performance of serologic assays include disease manifestation, test format, reagents used, and parasite viability to name a few. In amoebiasis the sensitivity of the test increases in patients with invasive amoebiasis but may be weak in intestinal amoebiasis with minimal tissue invasion, and absent for asymptomatic carriers. The type of serological assay format may also determine the sensitivity, as in the diagnosis of toxoplasmosis (National Committee for Clinical Laboratory Standards, 2004). The double sandwich IgM enzyme-linked immunosorbent assay (ELISA) is known to be more sensitive and specific than IgM immunofluorescence for detecting recently acquired and congenital toxoplasmosis. IHA has been the primary test for serodiagnosis of amoebiasis. The sensitivity of the assay is also dependent on the type or stage of parasite antigen used; for example the sensitivity of cutaneous leishmaniasis can be improved by using amastigote antigens in place of promastigote antigen in the IF test. Serologic assays are also affected by parasite viability; hydatid cysts occurring in the lung and dead or calcified cysts are less frequently detected than active cysts in the liver.

Molecular Diagnostic Methods

Diagnostic methods using DNA amplification and nucleic acid probe techniques have been described for most of the common parasitic diseases and offer high levels of sensitivity and specificity (Weiss, 1995; Wilson, 1995). For more complete details on the topic the reader is referred to a recent publication (Persing, 2004). Molecular methods offer some unique advantages such as rapid (automated) results, high sensitivity and specificity, and ability to detect and differentiate species variants, all independent of the patient's underlying immune status – a potentially limiting feature of serologic assays. Molecular techniques are prone to cross-contamination, however, if proper processing precautions are not strictly enforced.

While most of these applications have remained as tools for research laboratories and are not routinely available, several polymerase chain reaction (PCR) assays have been developed for parasites such as *Plasmodium* spp., *Babesia* spp., *T. gondii*, *Leishmania* spp., *Trypanosoma* spp., *G. lamblia*, *Cryptosporidium* spp., and *T. vaginalis* (Table 61–7). Some of these assays are available in real-time format, wherein the kinetics of the nucleic acid amplification reaction are recorded and analyzed by computer algorithms to allow detection of amplicons. In the last decade several real-time PCR methods have been developed for clinical diagnosis of some of the parasitic diseases (Table 61–7). The introduction of this technology has allowed rapid detection and avoided the fear of cross contamination due to steps involved in postamplification analysis. PCR also presents the opportunity to monitor success of anti-parasitic therapy (Lee, 2002; Bossolasco, 2003) or detect reactivation following therapy (Costa, 2000). By the innate nature of molecular methods being genotypic, PCR assays have the ability to accurately detect to the species level, depending upon the gene being targeted (Vallejo, 1999; Mahboudi, 2002). To date, the equipment and other resources needed, including personnel trained in molecular biology, have remained out of reach for most diagnostic laboratories because of fiscal limitations. Although a variety of commercial diagnostic kits are available for detection of viral and bacterial pathogens, only one kit has received approval for a parasite, that being for *T. vaginalis* (Briselden, 1994). Molecular methods may prove to have great importance in the identification of parasite-harboring vectors and contribute to disease prevention through control programs targeted to such vectors (Weiss, 1995).

Quality Assurance, Quality Improvement, and Safety

A quality assurance program for the parasitology section of the laboratory is similar to that for the other laboratory sections and covers all essential aspects of the operation including, among others, a well written and complete procedure manual that is reviewed annually, guidelines for maintaining all specimen and test result records, complete quality control program with appropriate technical supervision and review, and participation in an approved proficiency testing program. Laboratories also need to focus on customer satisfaction, using a variety of measures available, and participate in the team approach to identifying problems and generating solutions as part of a continuous quality improvement process.

The performance of individuals responsible for the parasitology section should be monitored periodically with both internal and external unknown specimens, and competency assessments should be up to date, especially for those laboratories that encounter positive specimens infrequently. A variety of reference materials should be readily available for use at the laboratory bench, including positive slides and fecal specimens, printed atlases, and slide atlases.

Unpreserved specimens for parasitologic examination should be considered potentially infectious, and all blood and body fluids should be handled according to Universal Precautions as defined by the Final Rule on Blood-borne Pathogens by the Occupational Safety and Health Administration as published in the Federal Register. In addition to blood-borne viral pathogens, malarial parasites and hemoflagellates may also remain infective in fresh stool

Table 61–7 Real-Time PCR for parasites

Parasite	Target	Specimen Type	Reference
Leishmania spp.	rDNA	Whole blood	Bossolasco, 2003
Plasmodium spp.	rDNA	Whole blood	Lee, 2002; de Monbrison 2003; Farcas, 2004; Perandin, 2004
Toxoplasma gondii	rDNA, and B1 gene	Amniotic fluid, blood, cerebrospinal fluid, tissue	Costa, 2000, 2001; Lin, 2000; Kupferschmidt, 2001; Buchbinder, 2003; Reischl, 2003
Entamoeba histolytica	rDNA	Stool	Blessmann, 2002; Verweij, 2004
Giardia lamblia	rDNA	Stool	Verweij, 2004
Cryptosporidium spp.	rDNA	Stool	Fontaine, 2002; Coupe, 2005
Cyclospora spp.	rDNA	Stool	Varma, 2003
Trichomonas vaginalis	β-tubulin gene	Vaginal samples	Hardick, 2003

specimens, including cysts of enteric protozoa, eggs of *Taenia solium*, *E. vermicularis*, and *H. nana*, and larvae of *S. stercoralis*. *Trichuris trichiura*, *Ascaris lumbricoides*, and hookworms may remain infective in older specimens, and *Ascaris* eggs can survive and embryonate while in 5% formalin. Fecal specimens also may contain pathogens such as *Salmonella*, *Shigella*, or viruses. Strict observance of proper specimen handling techniques and disposal is essential. Personal attention to hand washing is also necessary. Use of ethyl acetate in place of ether in the performance of concentration techniques is strongly recommended to guard against the possibility of explosion (Truant, 1981; Clinical and Laboratory Standards Institute, 2005).

Blood and Tissue Protozoa

Malaria

Malaria (from the Italian *mal' aria*, meaning 'bad air') is an acute and sometimes chronic infection of the blood stream characterized clinically by fever, anemia, and splenomegaly, and is caused by apicomplexan parasites of the genus *Plasmodium*. The defining clinical features of a malarial attack or paroxysm consist of, in order, shaking chills, fever (up to 40°C or higher), and generalized diaphoresis, followed by resolution of fever. The paroxysm occurs over 6–10 hours and is initiated by the synchronous rupture of erythrocytes with the release of new infectious blood stage forms known as merozoites. The disease generally occurs between 45° N and 40° South (World Health Organization, 1987) and is spread exclusively by female anopheline mosquitoes. The four species of plasmodia causing human malaria are *Plasmodium vivax*, *P. falciparum*, *Plasmodium malariae*, and *Plasmodium ovale*. *P. falciparum* infection occurs principally in tropical areas worldwide, whereas *P. vivax* infections occur in both tropical and temperate zones. *P. malariae* also occurs worldwide but to a much lesser extent than either *P. falciparum* or *P. vivax*. *P. ovale* is the least frequent of the malarias, with most cases being acquired in western Africa, India, or South America.

Because infection with falciparum malaria is potentially life-threatening, its presence must be considered in the differential diagnosis of unexplained fever, and history of travel in endemic geographic areas should always be sought. In an era of increasing world travel, the risk of acquiring malaria is not insignificant, and the rapid spread of drug-resistant strains poses particular problems when considering appropriate prophylaxis or therapy.

Laboratory evaluation of patients suspected of having malaria continues to rely on timely examination of thick and thin blood films to demonstrate the intraerythrocytic parasites. Although they are straightforward in their approach, performance of these techniques may be problematic. Reliable identification of organisms requires continuous training to maintain expertise; therefore, those laboratories that rarely see positive specimens may choose to refer specimens to reference laboratories, provided processing and reporting is timely.

More advanced laboratory methods, including acridine orange staining (see above under Laboratory Methods) or detection of parasite-specific DNA (Lanar, 1989; Weiss, 1995; Clinical and Laboratory Standards Institute, 2005) provide enhanced sensitivity and specificity but are

VII

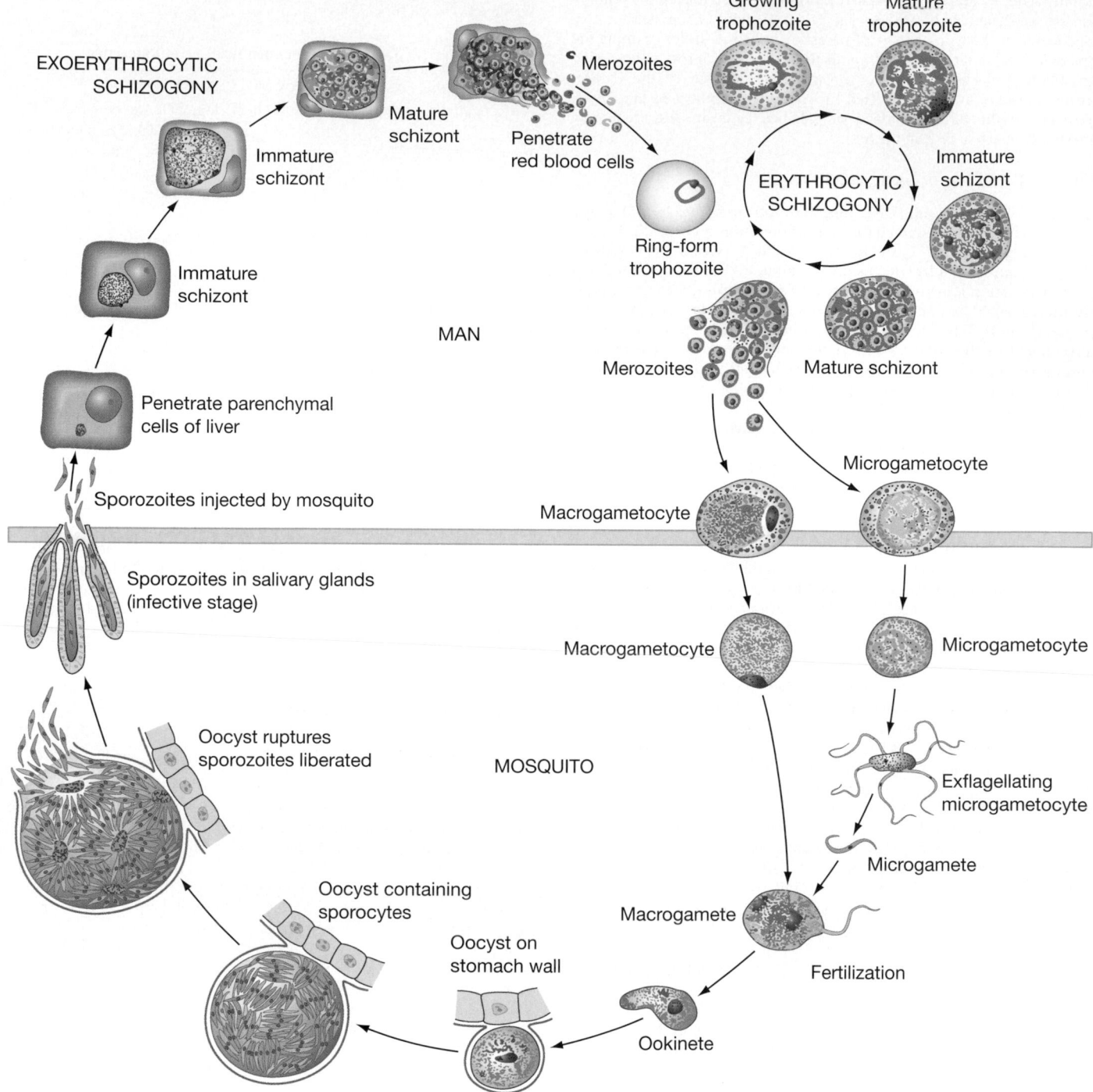

Figure 61–1 Life cycle of malarial parasites. (Courtesy of the Centers for Disease Control, Parasitology Training Branch, Atlanta, GA.)

generally not appropriate or available for smaller laboratories. The recent development of immunocapture assays for the detection of *Plasmodium*-specific lactate dehydrogenase or HRP-II appears to provide a high degree of sensitivity and specificity in the diagnosis of malaria. Several versions of these tests, configured as 'dipstick' methods, are especially promising in situations where ease of performance is critical and usual laboratory facilities are lacking (Palmer, 1998; Piper, 1999; Marx, 2005).

Life Cycle

Malarial parasites undergo a sexual phase (sporogony) in *Anopheles* mosquitoes that results in the production of infectious sporozoites and an asexual stage (schizogony) in humans that results in the production of schizonts and merozoites (Fig. 61–1). In the blood stream, some merozoites eventually differentiate into gametocytes (gametogony), which, when ingested by female anopheline mosquitoes, mature into the male microgametes and the female macrogametes. Fusion of a microgamete and a macrogamete results in the formation of the motile ookinete, which migrates to the outside of the stomach wall and forms an

oocyst. Within the oocyst, numerous spindle-shaped sporozoites are formed. The mature oocyst ruptures into the body cavity, releasing the sporozoites, which then migrate through the tissues to the salivary glands, from which they are injected into the vertebrate host as the mosquito feeds. The time required for development in the mosquito ranges from 8–21 days.

The sporozoites injected into the vertebrate host reach the hepatic parenchymal cells within minutes and initiate the proliferative phase known as exoerythrocytic schizogony. Release of merozoites from ruptured hepatic schizonts initiates the blood stream infection or erythrocytic schizogony and, eventually, the clinical symptoms of malaria. *P. vivax* and *P. ovale* differ from *P. falciparum* and *P. malariae* in that true disease relapses of the former species may occur weeks to months following subsidence of previous attacks. This occurs as a result of renewed exoerythrocytic and, eventually, erythrocytic schizogony from latent hepatic sporozoites, which are known as hypnozoites (Krotoski, 1982). Recurrences of disease due to *P. falciparum* or *P. malariae*, called recrudescences, arise from an increase in numbers of persisting blood stage forms to clinically

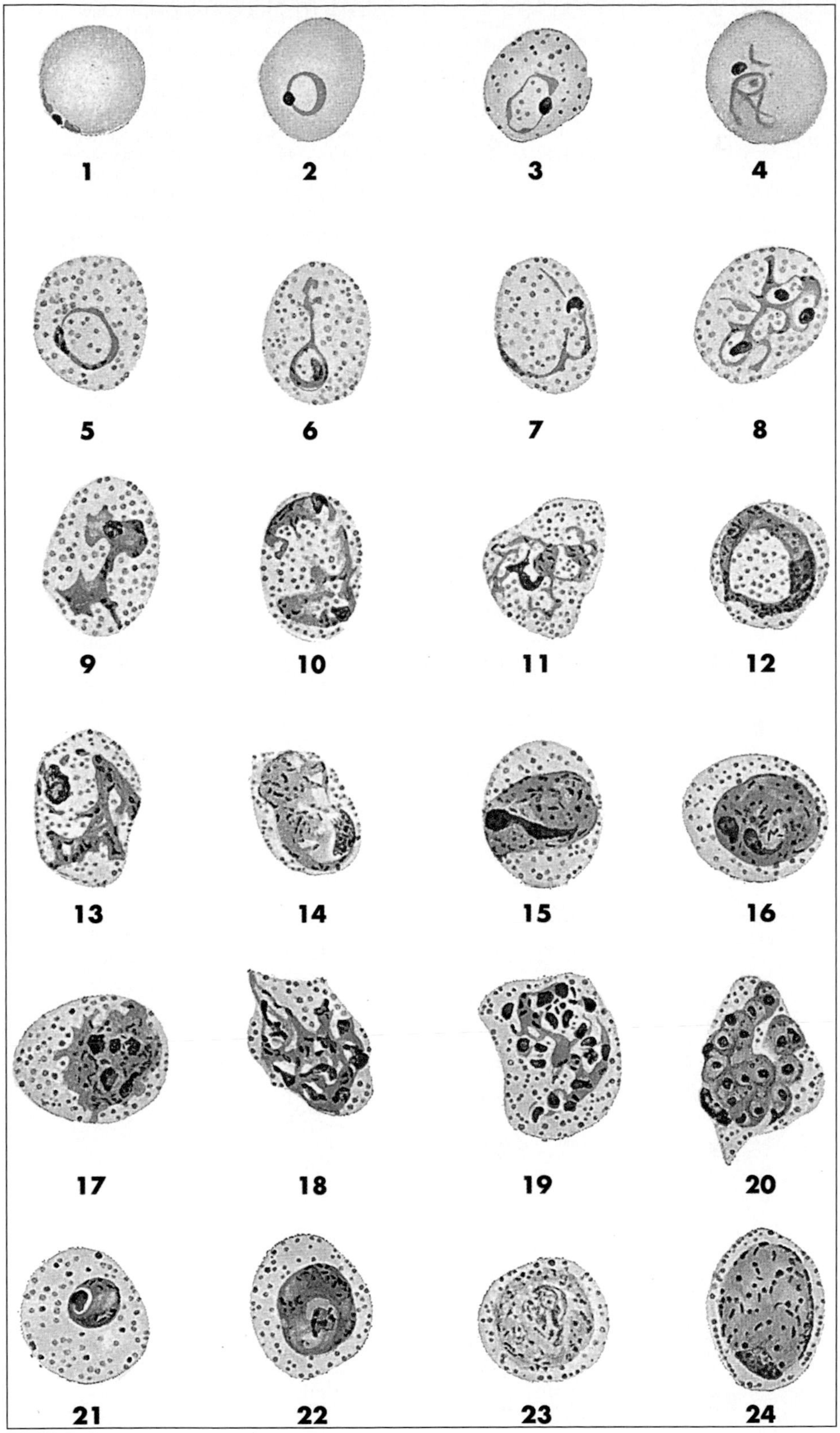

Figure 61–2 *Plasmodium vivax. 1*, Normal-size erythrocyte with marginal ring form trophozoite. *2*, Young signet ring form of trophozoite in macrocyte. *3*, Slightly older ring form trophozoite in erythrocyte showing basophilic stippling. *4*, Polychromatophilic erythrocyte containing young tertian parasite with pseudopodia. *5*, Ring form of trophozoite showing pigment in cytoplasm of an enlarged cell containing Schüffner's stippling. This stippling does not appear in all cells containing the growing and older forms of *Plasmodium vivax*, but it can be found with any stage from the fairly young ring form onward. *6* and *7*, Very tenuous medium trophozoite forms. *8*, Three ameboid trophozoites with fused cytoplasm. *9–13*, Older ameboid trophozoites in process of development. *10*, Two ameboid trophozoites in one cell. *14*, Mature trophozoite. *15*, Mature trophozoite with chromatin apparently in process of division. *16–19*, Schizonts showing progressive steps in division (presegmenting schizonts). *20*, Mature schizont. *21* and *22*, Developing gametocytes. *23*, Mature microgametocyte. *24*, Mature macrogametocyte. (From Wilcox A: Manual for the Microscopical Diagnosis of Malaria in Man. Bulletin No. 180, National Institute of Health, 1942.)

detectable levels, not from persisting liver stage forms. Liver cells are infected only by sporozoites from the mosquito; thus, transfusion-acquired *P. vivax* or *P. ovale* infection does not relapse.

Merozoites released from infected hepatocytes subsequently infect erythrocytes. Following amplification of parasites in the blood stream for a period of time, and the development of synchrony in their appearance, clinical attacks of malaria occur. *P. vivax* and *P. ovale* parasites primarily infect young erythrocytes, whereas *P. malariae* infects older erythrocytes and *P. falciparum* infects erythrocytes of all ages.

Morphologic stages seen in erythrocytes include trophozoites (growing forms), schizonts (dividing forms), and gametocytes (sexual forms) (Figs 61–2 to 61–5). The youngest trophozoites have a globose shape with a central vacuole, a red chromatin mass, and blue cytoplasm. In stained blood films, early trophozoites resemble signet rings and are generally referred to as rings or ring forms. Growing trophozoites beyond the ring stage retain a single chromatin mass but have more abundant cytoplasm, which may appear compact or be ameboid (irregular). Mature trophozoites still have only one chromatin mass but an increased amount of cytoplasm that partially fills the erythrocyte. Hemozoin (hematin) pigment, a breakdown product of hemoglobin, is characteristic of all erythrocytes containing mature stages of malarial parasites but is not evident in ring forms. Immature schizonts have two or more chromatin masses and

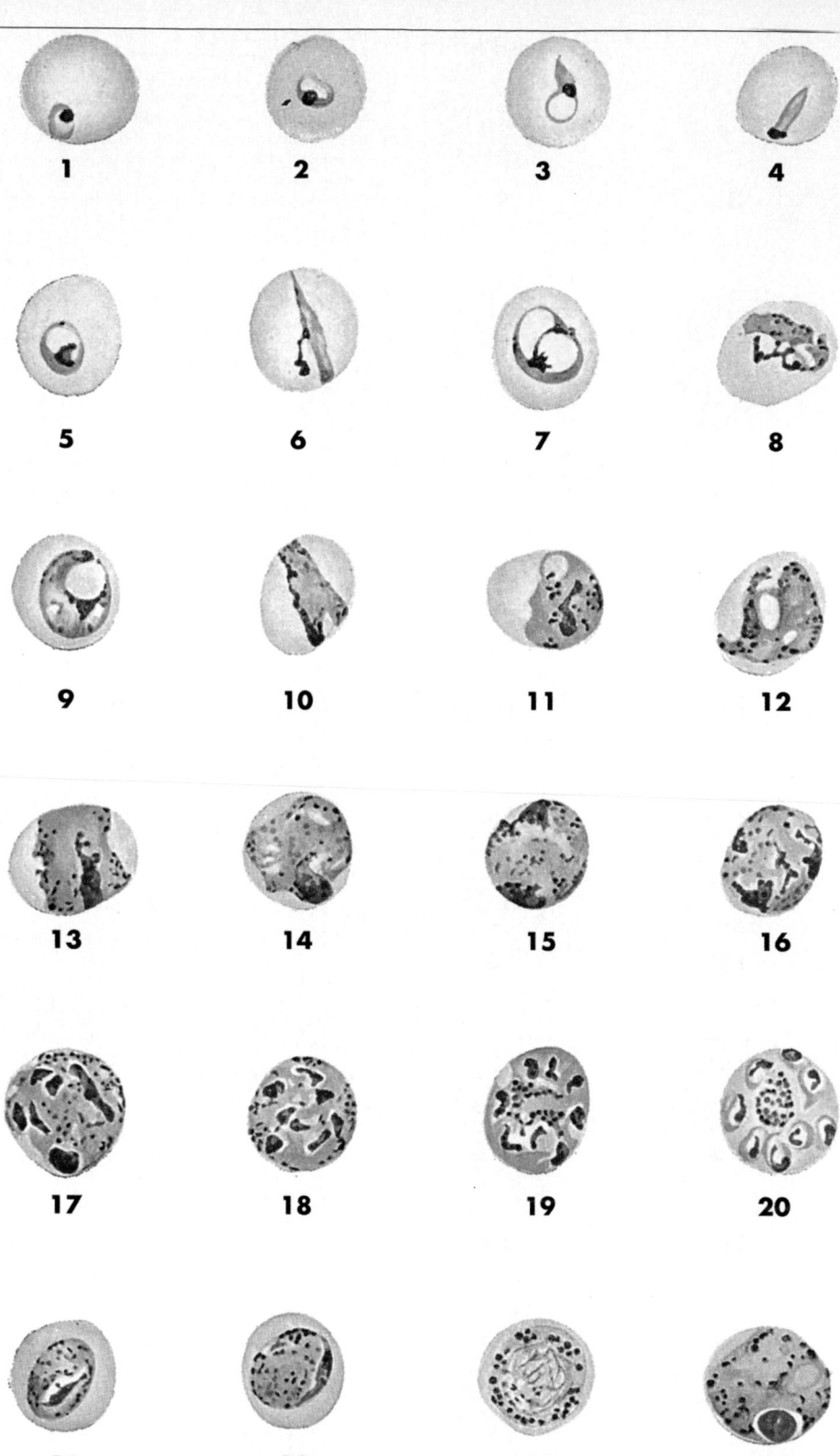

Figure 61–3 *Plasmodium malariae.* *1,* Young ring form trophozoite of quartan malaria. *2–4,* Young trophozoite forms of the parasite showing gradual increase of chromatin and cytoplasm. *5,* Developing ring form of trophozoite showing pigment granule. *6,* Early band form of trophozoite – elongated chromatin, some pigment apparent. *7–12,* Some forms that the developing trophozoite of quartan malaria may take. *13* and *14,* Mature trophozoites – one a band form. *15–19,* Phases in the development of the schizont (presegmenting schizonts). 20, Mature schizont. *21,* Immature microgametocyte. 22, Immature macrogametocyte. *23,* Mature microgametocyte. 24, Mature macrogametocyte. (From Wilcox A: Manual for the Microscopical Diagnosis of Malaria in Man. Bulletin No. 180, National Institute of Health, 1942.)

undivided cytoplasm, whereas mature schizonts have both cytoplasm and chromatin completely divided so that individual merozoites are evident. The mature schizont ruptures the erythrocyte, releasing merozoites and initiating a new cycle of infection. The erythrocytic cycle takes approximately 48 hours (tertian periodicity) for *P. falciparum,* *P. ovale,* and *P. vivax* infections and 72 hours (quartan periodicity) in *P. malariae* infections. At some point during the infection, a subpopulation of merozoites develops into gametocytes. Those of *P. vivax, P. malariae,* and *P. ovale* are rounded, whereas those of *P. falciparum* are elongated (sausage-shaped). Macrogametocytes (female) characteristically have a compact chromatin mass, whereas microgametocytes (male) have chromatin that is more dispersed. Developing gametocytes are more compact than growing trophozoites.

Epidemiology

Endemic transmission of malaria requires a reservoir of infection, an appropriate mosquito vector, and a susceptible host. Control of malaria is directed at elimination of mosquito hosts, treatment of active cases, and prophylaxis of susceptible persons. However, emergence of mosquitoes resistant to insecticides, development of resistance to prophylaxis and therapy by *P. falciparum* and, more recently, *P. vivax* (Murphy, 1993), and lack of adequate funding have made control difficult in many areas.

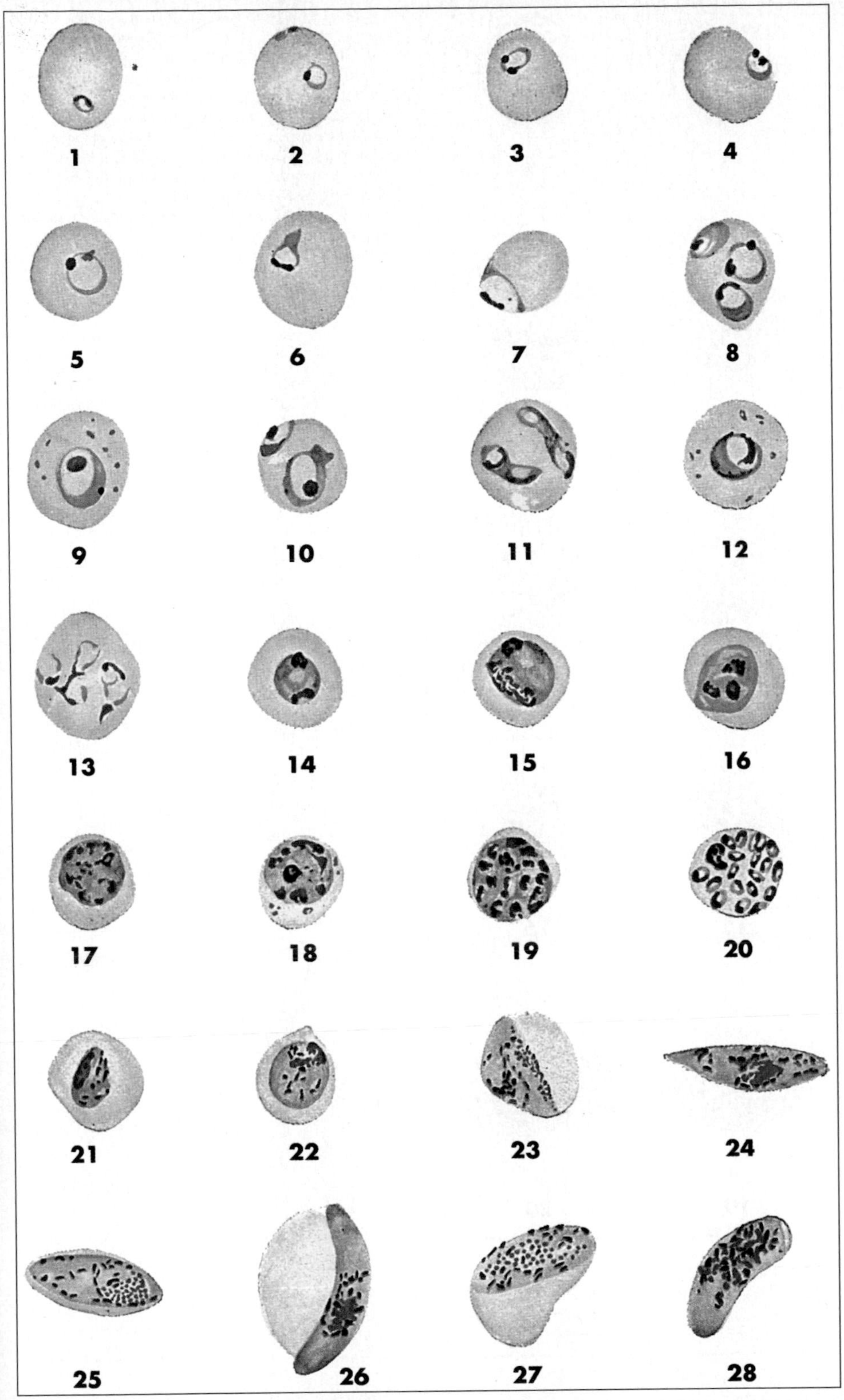

Figure 61–4 *Plasmodium falciparum. 1,* Very young ring-form trophozoite. *2,* Double infection of single cell with young trophozoites, one a 'marginal form,' the other 'signet ring' form. *3* and *4,* Young trophozoites showing double chromatin dots. *5–7,* Developing trophozoite forms. *8,* Three medium trophozoites in one cell. *9,* Trophozoite showing pigment, in a cell containing Maurer's dots. *10* and *11, Two* trophozoites in each of two cells, showing variation of forms that parasites may assume. *12,* Almost mature trophozoite showing haze of pigment throughout cytoplasm. Maurer's dots in the cell. *13,* Estivo-autumnal 'slender forms.' *14,* Mature trophozoite, showing clumped pigment. *15,* Parasite in the process of initial chromatin division. *16–19,* Various phases of the development of the schizont (presegmenting schizonts). *20,* Mature schizont. *21–24,* Successive forms in the development of the gametocyte – usually not found in the peripheral circulation. *25,* Immature macrogametocyte. *26,* Mature macrogametocyte. *27,* Immature microgametocyte. *28,* Mature microgametocyte. (Courtesy of National Institute of Health, USPHS.)

Black people with sickle cell trait are less susceptible to *P. falciparum* malaria, and persons who lack certain Duffy blood group determinants are protected against *P. vivax* infections (Miller, 1976). Glucose-6-phosphate dehydrogenase (G6PD) deficiency has been associated with protection from malaria, but the evidence is less striking than with these other genetic abnormalities.

Transfusion-induced malaria may occur when blood donors have subclinical malaria and may prove fatal for the recipient. Similarly, congenital malaria may occur in infants born to mothers from endemic areas. The infant acquires the infection at birth as a result of rupture of placental blood vessels with maternal–fetal transfusion. Neither transfusion nor congenital malaria is expected to relapse because exoerythrocytic schizogony does not occur. The number of civilian cases of malaria reported in the United States increased from 151 in 1970 to 1838 in 1980 but dropped to 1411 in 1993 (Centers for Disease Control and Prevention, 1988, 1993). Species causing infection in 1987 were *P. vivax* (44%), *P. falciparum* (43%), *P. malariae* (4%), *P. ovale* (3%), and undetermined (6%). Interval between arrival in the United States and onset of illness was less than 1 month for 25% of *P. vivax* and 80% of *P. falciparum* cases. Only 3% of patients became ill more than 1 year after arrival. United States citizens acquired the infection in Africa (63%), Asia (18%), Western Hemisphere (14%), or Oceania (4%).

Clinical Disease

Most patients who develop *P. falciparum* infection become symptomatic within 1 month of exposure, whereas there may be a delay of up to 6

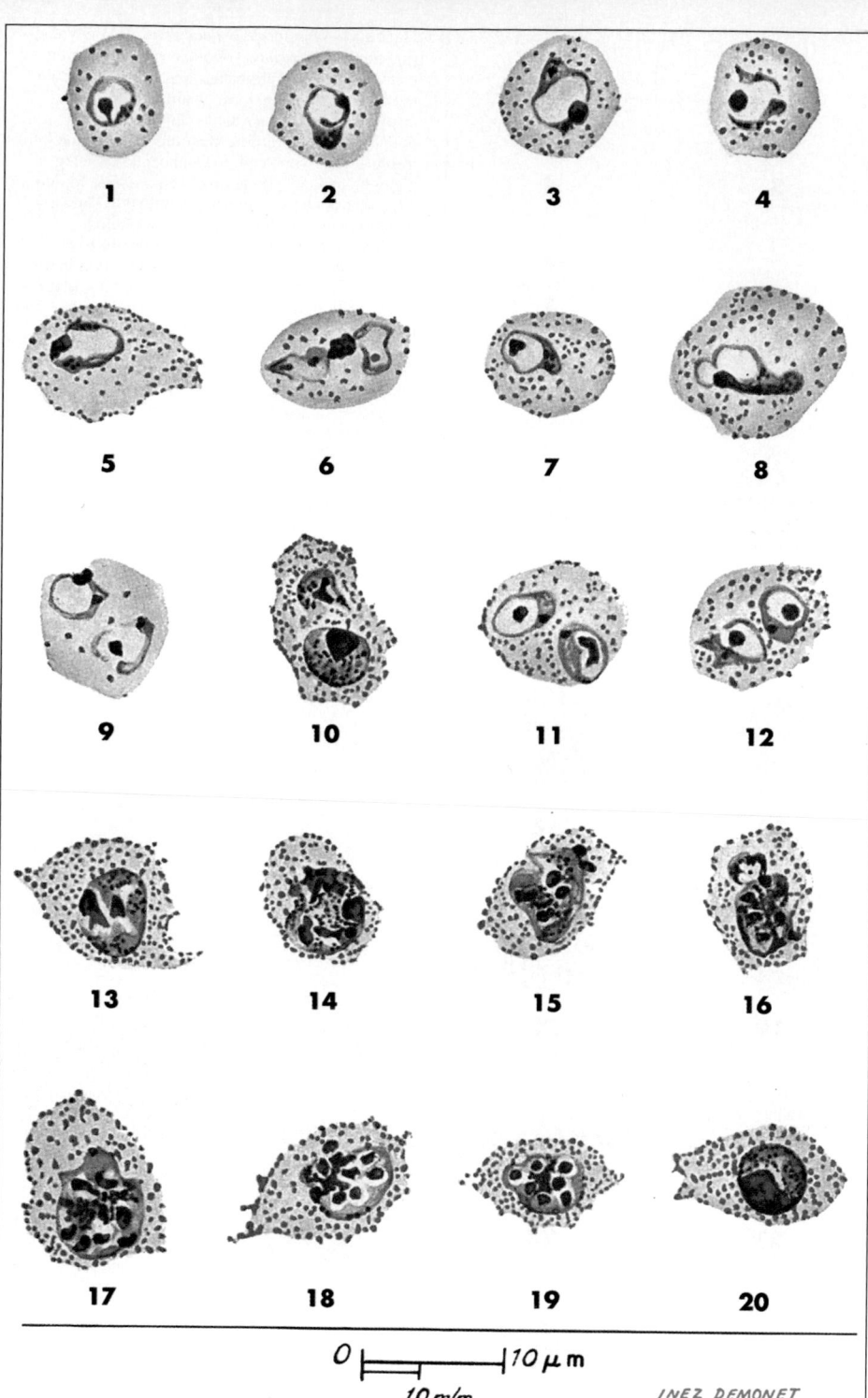

Figure 61–5 *Plasmodium ovale. 1,* Young ring-shaped trophozoite. *2–5,* Older ring-shaped trophozoites. *6–8,* Older ameboid trophozoites. *9, 11,* and *12,* Doubly infected cells, trophozoites. *10,* Doubly infected cell, young gametocytes. *13,* First stage of the schizont. *14–19,* Schizonts, progressive stages. *20,* Mature gametocyte. Free translation of legend accompanying original plate in *Guide pratique d'examen microscopique du sang appliqué au diagnostic du paludisme'* by Georges Villain. Reproduced with permission from *Biologie Medicale* supplement, 1935. (Courtesy of Aimee Wilcox, National Institutes of Health Bulletin No. 180, USPHS.)

months or more with the other *Plasmodium* species. The common presenting symptoms of malaria include chills and fever, which are often associated with splenomegaly. In the early stages of the disease, the febrile episodes occur irregularly but eventually become more synchronous, assuming the usual tertian (*P. vivax, P. falciparum,* and *P. ovale*) or quartan (*P. malariae*) periodicity. Patients with malaria may develop anemia and may have other manifestations, including diarrhea, abdominal pain, headache, and muscle aches and pains. *P. falciparum* malaria can result in high (50%) parasitemias, which can lead to severe hemolysis with hemoglobinuria and profound anemia. Erythrocytes infected with growing trophozoites and schizonts of *P. falciparum* become sequestered in small vessels of the body and may lead to occlusion of these vessels, causing symptoms related to capillary obstruction and tissue anoxia. Involvement of the brain is known as cerebral malaria, in which the patient becomes disoriented, progressing to delirium, coma, and often

death. Exchange transfusion may be lifesaving in severe *P. falciparum* infections (Nielson, 1979; Powell, 2002).

The course of untreated malaria depends on the species. Most fatal cases of malaria are due to *P. falciparum.* In nonfatal cases, the febrile paroxysms become less severe with time and the disease gradually subsides. Patients with *P. vivax* or *P. ovale* infection may have relapses after many months or, occasionally, years. Persons with *P. falciparum* and *P. malariae* infection may have symptom-free periods but suffer from sporadic recrudescences owing to persisting low-grade parasitemia. Relapses and recrudescences may be associated with changes in the host's defense mechanisms or possibly with antigenic changes in the infecting organisms.

Peripheral smears may show leukocytes that contain malaria pigment. Increased reticulocyte counts occur commonly and are associated with the rapid erythrocyte turnover. The presence of greatly enlarged platelets also may be noted on peripheral blood films and occur as a result of their rapid

Table 61–8 Comparison of Plasmodium Species Affecting Humans

Species	Appearance of Erythrocyte Size	Schüffner's Stippling	Parasite Cytoplasm	Appearance of Parasite Pigment	Number of Merozoites	Stages Found in Circulating Blood
Plasmodium vivax	Enlarged. Maximum size (attained with mature trophozoites and schizonts) may be 1–2 times normal erythrocyte diameter	+ With all stages except early ring forms	Irregular, ameboid in trophozoites. Has 'spread-out' appearance	Golden brown, inconspicuous	12–24; average is 16	All stages. Wide range of stages may be seen on any given film
Plasmodium malariae	Normal	– (Ziemann's dots rarely seen)	Rounded, compact trophozoites with dense cytoplasm. Band-form trophozoites occasionally seen.	Dark brown, coarse, conspicuous	6–12; average is 8; 'rosette' schizonts occasionally seen	All stages. Wide variety of stages usually not seen. Relatively few rings or gametocytes generally present
Plasmodium ovale	Enlarged. Maximum size maybe 1 1/4–1 1/2 times normal red blood cell diameter. Approximately 20% or more of infected red blood cells are oval and/or fimbriated (border has irregular projections)	+ With all stages except early ring forms	Rounded, compact trophozoites. Occasionally slightly ameboid. Growing trophozoites have large chromatin mass	Dark brown, conspicuous	6–14; average is 8	All stages
Plasmodium falciparum	Normal. Multiply-infected red blood cells are common	– (Maurer's dots occasionally seen)	Young rings are small, delicate, often with double chromatin dots. Gametocytes are crescent or elongate	Black; coarse and conspicuous in gametocytes	6–32: average is 20–24	Rings and/or gametocytes. Other stages develop in blood vessels of internal organs but are not seen in peripheral blood except in severe infections

Source: with permission from Smith JW, Melvin DM, Orihel TC, et al: Diagnostic Parasitology – Blood and Tissue Parasites. Chicago, IL, American Society of Clinical Pathologists, 1976.

turnover secondary to splenic sequestration. Malarial infections may interfere with certain serologic tests, producing false-positive results, especially those for syphilis.

Therapy and prophylaxis of malaria have become highly complex topics because of the widespread appearance of resistance by *P. falciparum* to chloroquine and other antimalarials and, to a lesser extent, resistance by *P. vivax* to chloroquine. Also, persons who have acquired *P. vivax* or *P. ovale* malaria, or who have spent extended time in areas highly endemic for these parasites, require treatment with primaquine to eradicate hepatic hypnozoites and prevent relapse. Use of primaquine may be dangerous in patients who have G6PD deficiency and screening of at-risk patients may be necessary prior to initiating therapy.

Diagnosis

Malaria should be included in the differential diagnosis of fever in patients who have a history of travel to or residence in endemic areas, drug addiction, or blood transfusion. Diagnosis usually is established by demonstrating parasites in thick and thin blood films. Blood specimens are ideally collected just prior to the next anticipated fever spike or at the onset of a fever. Specimens drawn several hours apart sometimes may be required to demonstrate infection or to diagnose the species, because the number and morphologic stages of parasites vary during the cycle. Careful examination of thick films should reveal the presence of the parasites in almost all patients with clinically apparent malaria.

Identification of malarial parasites in thin blood films requires a systematic approach. There are three major factors to consider: appearance of infected erythrocytes, appearance of parasites, and stages found. Table 61–8 summarizes diagnostic characteristics of the species, which are illustrated in Figures 61–2 to 61–5. Erythrocytes infected by *P. vivax* or *P. ovale* parasites often appear enlarged compared with adjacent, uninfected cells, whereas *P. malariae* and *P. falciparum* parasites are usually found in erythrocytes of normal size. 20% or more of erythrocytes infected with *P. ovale* are often oval or fimbriated (having irregular projections of the cell margins), whereas less than 6% of erythrocytes infected with *P. vivax* are oval. Schüffner's stippling, numerous small uniform pink granules in the erythrocyte, is usually seen in cells infected with *P. vivax* and *P. ovale*, although it may not be evident in cells infected with early ring forms or in slides that have not been stained at the appropriate pH (see earlier under Laboratory Methods). The presence of Schüffner's

stippling is helpful because it is not seen in *P. malariae* or *P. falciparum* infection.

As trophozoites grow in the infected cells, the amount of hemoglobin in the erythrocyte decreases and hemozoin pigment accumulates. The amount and appearance of the pigment vary among the species. Ring forms of all parasites may have a similar appearance and, if only occasional ring forms are found, the species may not be identifiable. Young rings of *P. falciparum* are smaller than those of the other species (one sixth the diameter of the red blood cell, compared with one third the diameter of the red blood cell for the other species). Rings of *P. falciparum* that have grown are similar in size to those of the other species. Trophozoites that appear to be lying on the surface of the erythrocyte or protruding from it are called appliqué or accolé forms, and are most often seen in *P. falciparum* infections. The presence of doubly infected cells and double chromatin dots in ring trophozoites occurs most commonly in *P. falciparum* infections but can occur with the other species.

Growing trophozoites of *P. vivax* have irregular shapes and are termed ameboid. Those of *P. malariae* and *P. ovale* remain compact. Mature trophozoites and schizonts of *P. falciparum* are usually sequestered in capillary beds secondary to cytoadherence to endothelial cells and are not seen in the peripheral blood except in very severe infections. When schizonts are identified in the peripheral blood, determining the number of merozoites is helpful in identifying the various species. The gametocytes of *P. falciparum* are readily identified by their characteristic sausage shape. Gametocytes of *P. vivax*, *P. malariae*, and *P. ovale* have a similar shape and so are difficult to differentiate, although characteristics of infected red cells can aid identification.

The varieties of developmental stages in the peripheral blood aid in diagnosis. In *P. falciparum* infections, ring forms predominate, and finding numerous ring forms without more mature stages is evidence for *P. falciparum* infection. In *P. vivax*, *P. malariae*, and *P. ovale* infections, various stages of parasites are found with some predominance of one stage depending on the phase of the cycle.

Thick films are preferred for detecting malaria infections because a greater quantity of blood is examined (see above under Laboratory Methods). Ring forms often have the appearance of punctuation marks rather than complete rings, and the presence of red chromatin and blue cytoplasm should be required to identify them as parasites. Schüffner's stippling may still be a helpful identifying characteristic, and it may be

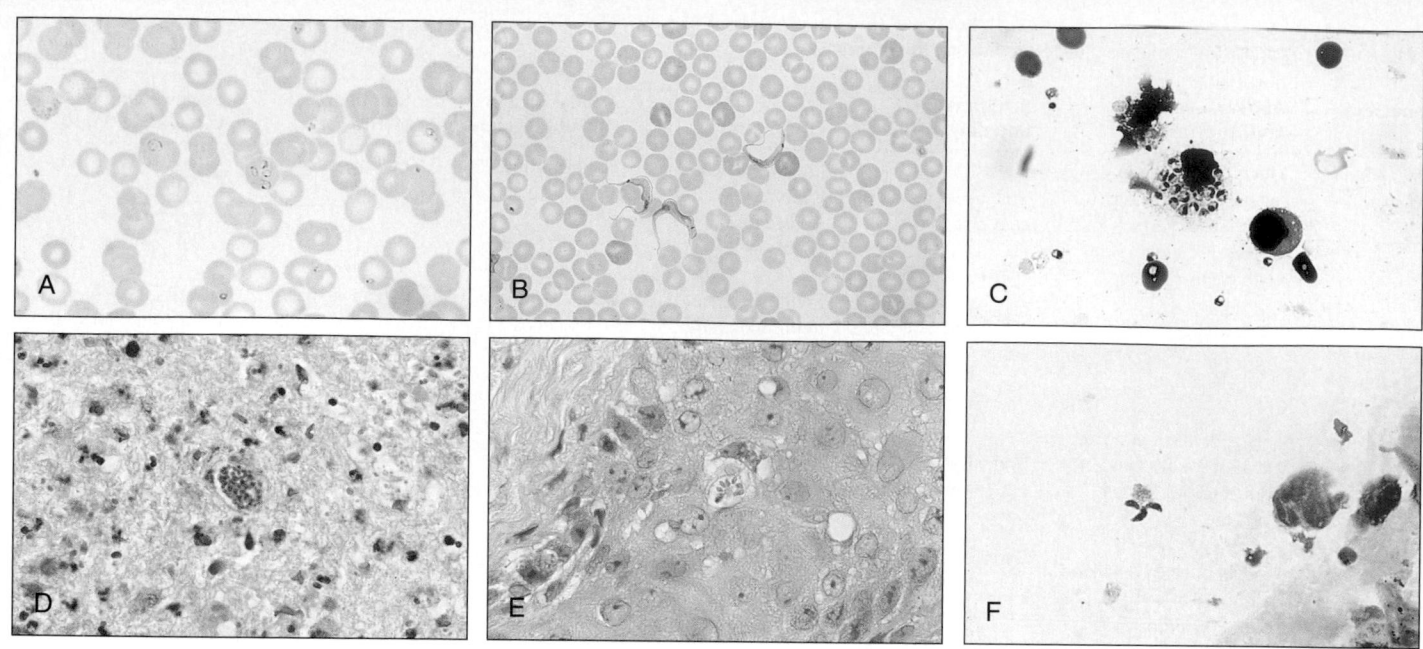

Figure 61–6 *A*, Human infection with *Babesia microti*; note high parasitemia and multiple-infected red cell (oil immersion). *B*, *Trypanosoma* sp. in stained blood film; note nucleus, kinetoplast, and undulating membrane (oil immersion). *C*, *Leishmania mexicana* amastigotes in impression smear of thigh lesion; Giemsa stain (oil immersion). *D*, Pseudocyst of *Toxoplasma gondii* in brain tissue (hematoxylin and eosin [H&E]; oil immersion). *E*, Cutaneous rosette of *T. gondii* tachyzoites in an immunocompromised patient (H&E; oil immersion). *F*, Tachyzoites of *T. gondii* recovered from a bronchoalveolar lavage specimen from an individual infected with the human immunodeficiency virus (Giemsa stain; oil immersion).

recognized around growing trophozoites as a pink halo rather than the distinct granules seen in thin films. The ameboid character of *P. vivax* trophozoites is not as evident in thick films, but the number of merozoites in mature schizonts is helpful. Macro- and microgametocytes cannot usually be differentiated. The distinctive sausage shape of *P. falciparum* gametocytes is still evident, although they may be more stubby than in thin films. Gametocytes of the other species can be detected and are easily differentiated from host cell nuclei by the presence of refractile hemozoin pigment.

Mixed infections occur occasionally (about 5% of the time) but caution should be used in making such diagnoses unless there is definite evidence of two separate populations of parasites. The most common mixed infections are *P. falciparum* and *P. vivax*. Finding gametocytes of *P. falciparum* in a person obviously infected with *P. vivax* is diagnostic.

There are multiple artifacts that may be confused with malarial parasites in thick and thin films. The most common artifact in thin films are blood platelets superimposed on red blood cells. These platelets should be readily identified because they do not have a true ring form, do not show differentiation of the chromatin and cytoplasm, and do not contain pigment. Clumps of bacteria or platelets may be confused with schizonts. At times, masses of fused platelets may resemble gametocytes of *P. falciparum* but do not show the differential staining or the pigment. Precipitated stain and contaminating bacteria, fungi, or spores may also be confused with these parasites.

Species-specific serologic tests for malaria are particularly useful for epidemiologic surveys and for detection of infected blood donors. Such tests do not reliably differentiate current from past infection, however. Sensitive and specific IFA tests using antigens from the four human species are available from the CDC (Wilson, 1995). Assays for the direct detection of malarial antigens in blood are especially promising (see Laboratory Methods).

Babesiosis

Like malarial parasites, the etiologic agents of babesiosis or piroplasmosis are apicomplexan protozoa found worldwide that infect erythrocytes, often producing a febrile illness of variable severity. Unlike malaria, babesiosis is transmitted by ticks and is found in a variety of animal species that serve as reservoirs (Krause, 2002).

Human infections in the United States occur predominantly in the northeastern and midwestern states, where the rodent parasite *Babesia microti* is responsible for infection (Homer, 2000). *Ixodes scapularis* is the usual tick vector. Recent studies have implicated another, as yet unnamed, *Babesia* species (tentatively known as WA1) as being responsible for disease in the western United States. This parasite, associated with disease in Washington state and California, is thought to be transmitted by the western black-legged tick, *Ixodes pacificus* (Quick, 1993; Persing, 1995). In Europe, the canine

parasite *Babesia divergens*, transmitted by *Ixodes ricinus*, infects humans and a recent report of a *B. divergens*-like infection in Washington State expands the range of known human cases (Herwaldt, 2004).

The spectrum of babesiosis varies from latent, subclinical infection to fulminant, hemolytic disease. Fatalities have been reported, especially in splenectomized or immunocompromised individuals. Immunocompetent persons may experience symptoms similar to those of malaria, including fever, chills, malaise, and anemia, although without recognizable periodicity. Investigation of an outbreak caused by *B. microti* on Nantucket Island in New England showed that some symptomatic patients harbored the parasite for months and others showed serologic evidence of infection without a history of clinical disease (Ruebush, 1980). Other evidence is accumulating indicating that chronic subclinical infections may not be uncommon (Persing, 1995).

Babesia parasites multiply in erythrocytes by schizogony but do not produce gametocytes. Although trophozoites of many species appear pear-shaped at some point in their development, those of *B. microti* usually appear as delicate ring forms that may be easily confused with those of malarial parasites, especially *P. falciparum* (Fig. 61–6*A*) (Healy, 1980; Homer, 2000). *Babesia* trophozoites can be differentiated from those of malarial parasites by the presence of multiple rings in one cell that may form a tetrad (Maltese cross) and the absence of large, growing trophozoites and gametocytes. Also, *Babesia*-infected cells lack hemozoin pigment, which is present in *Plasmodium*-infected cells. History of residence in or travel to endemic areas, or of a recent tick bite, might suggest *Babesia* infection. Serologic tests (IFA) for both *B. microti* and WA1 are available from the CDC on referral from state health departments. Serology tests for malaria are negative in babesiosis, although patients with malaria may cross-react in the *Babesia* serologies (Wilson, 1995).

Hemoflagellates

The hemoflagellates of humans and animals are members of the order Kinetoplastida and are characterized by the presence of a large mitochondrion known as a kinetoplast, which contains enough DNA to be seen by light microscopy when treated with Giemsa stain. Two genera important in human disease are *Trypanosoma* and *Leishmania*. Members of both genera are transmitted by arthropod vectors and have animal hosts that serve as reservoirs.

The kinetoplastida assume different morphologic forms depending on their presence in vertebrate hosts, including humans, or their insect vectors (Fig. 61–7). The amastigote stage is spherical, 2–5 μm in diameter, and displays a nucleus and kinetoplast. By definition an external flagellum is lacking, although an axoneme (the intracellular portion of the flagellum) is apparent at the ultrastructural level. Amastigotes may be found in human or animal hosts infected with either *T. cruzi* or *Leishmania* spp.,

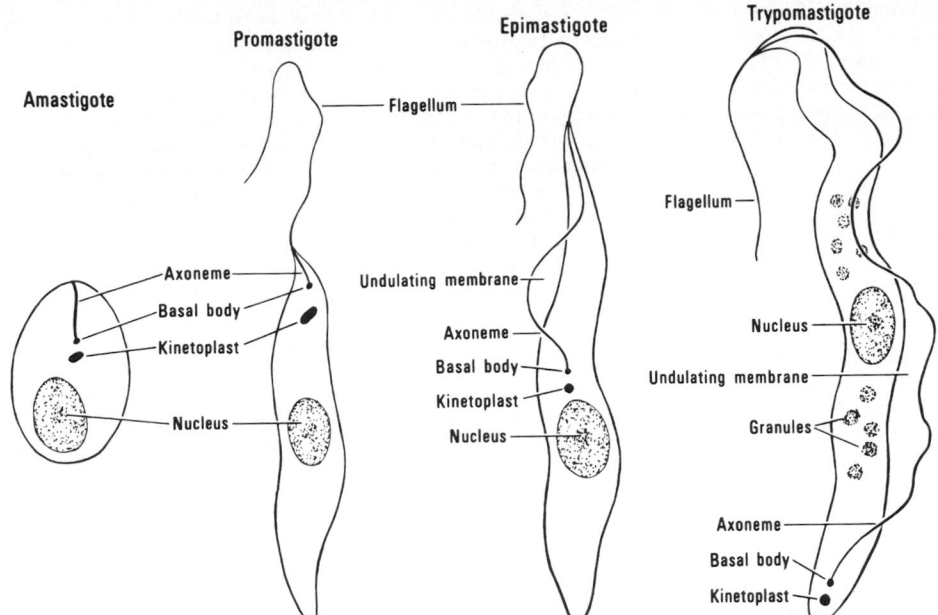

Figure 61–7 Morphology of hemoflagellates.

where they multiply exclusively within cells. The promastigote is an elongated and slender organism with a central nucleus, an anteriorly located kinetoplast and axoneme, and a free flagellum extending from the anterior end. This stage occurs in the insect vectors of *Leishmania* and is the stage detected in culture. The epimastigote is similar to the promastigote, but the kinetoplast is found closer to the nucleus and has a small undulating membrane that becomes a free flagellum. All species of *Trypanosoma* that infect humans assume an epimastigote stage in the insect vector or in culture. In the trypomastigote, the kinetoplast is found at the posterior end and the flagellum forms an undulating membrane that extends the length of the cell, emerging as a free flagellum at the anterior end. Trypomastigote forms occur predominantly in the blood stream of mammalian hosts infected with the various *Trypanosoma* spp. The infectious stages found in appropriate insect vectors following transformation from the epimastigote form are known as metacyclic trypomastigotes.

Trypanosoma

Infections with trypanosomes include those caused by *Trypanosoma brucei* (African or Old World trypanosomiasis) and *T. cruzi* (American or New World trypanosomiasis, or Chagas' disease). Both are of great importance in endemic areas but are rarely seen in the United States. A third species, *Trypanosoma rangeli*, has been described in humans in the Americas but does not cause clinical illness. Blood stream trypomastigotes of the *T. brucei* group (Fig. 61–6B) are up to 30 µm long with graceful curves and a small kinetoplast. Those of *T. cruzi* are shorter (20 µm), assume S and C shapes in stained blood films, and display a larger kinetoplast.

In equatorial Africa, parasites of the *T. brucei* group infect both animals and humans and are transmitted by the bite of tsetse flies in the genus *Glossina*. Multiplication of the organisms at the bite site often produces a transient chancre. East African trypanosomiasis is caused by *T. brucei rhodesiense*, which has a number of animal reservoir hosts. The disease is characterized by a rapidly progressive acute febrile illness with lymphadenopathy. Patients die before central nervous system (CNS) involvement is prominent.

The infection in western Africa is caused by *T. brucei gambiense*, which is responsible for classic African sleeping sickness. The disease has a more chronic course that begins with intermittent fevers, night sweats, and malaise. Lymphadenopathy, especially of the cervical lymph nodes (Winterbottom's sign), may be pronounced. Involvement of the CNS becomes prominent with time. Somnolence, confusion, and fatigue progress, leading to stupor, coma, and eventual death. Humans are the primary reservoir for this disease (World Health Organization, 1986).

The diagnosis is suspected on the basis of geographic history and clinical findings. Patients show high total immunoglobulin M (IgM) levels in blood and cerebrospinal fluid (CSF). There is pleocytosis with 50–500 mononuclear cells per microliter in CSF. The diagnosis is established by demonstrating the parasites in thick and thin films of peripheral blood, buffy coat preparations, aspirates of lymph nodes or bone marrow, or in spun CSF that is stained with Giemsa (Van Meirvenne, 1985; Cattand, 1988; National Committee for Clinical Laboratory Standards, 2000). Culture or animal inoculation may also be helpful, if it is available.

American trypanosomiasis, or Chagas' disease, is caused by *T. cruzi*. In its sylvatic form, the parasite occurs in the United States, Central America, and most of South America. Human infections are common in parts of Mexico and Central and South America, where they are transmitted by kissing bugs of the family Reduviidae. Genera and species involved in transmission vary from one country to another and among different ecologic niches. Some reduviids are responsible for maintaining the sylvatic cycle in animal reservoirs, whereas others are adapted to a domiciliary life in which they infest poorly constructed houses, usually in rural areas. At the time of feeding, the reduviid bug defecates. The bug feces contain infective trypomastigotes that, as a result of scratching or rubbing, enter the body at the bite site or through intact mucosa of the mouth or conjunctiva. The infective forms actively enter nearby tissue cells, where they transform into dividing amastigotes. When the infected cell is filled with amastigotes, transformation to trypomastigotes occurs, followed by cell rupture. Trypomastigotes are released into the peripheral blood and reach distant tissues, where they can start the reproductive cycle de novo.

Chagas' disease may cause acute or chronic infections. Acute disease is most common in children under the age of 5 years and is characterized by malaise, chills, fever, hepatosplenomegaly, and myocarditis. Swelling of the tissues around the eye (Romaña's sign) may be present if inoculation of the organisms occurs on the face. Swelling of tissues at other locations following the bite of an infected reduviid is called a chagoma. In older individuals, the acute course is milder or often asymptomatic. In either case, the patient remains infected for life. Chronic manifestations of the infection, including megaesophagus, megacolon, and alterations in the conduction system of the heart, are related to destruction of the effector cells of the parasympathetic system by autoantibodies. The infection can be transmitted by blood transfusion, and quiescent infections may be exacerbated by immunosuppression.

Diagnosis in the acute stage is established by demonstrating the parasite in thick and thin blood films, in buffy coat smears, or in aspirates of chagomas or enlarged lymph nodes. Aspirates, blood, and biopsy specimens can also be cultured using Novy–MacNeal–Nicolle medium (Ash, 1987; Visvesvara, 2004b; National Committee for Clinical Laboratory Standards, 2000; Garcia, 2001). In endemic areas, xenodiagnosis (examination of the gut contents of laboratory-raised reduviids that have been allowed to feed on a patient) may be used. In the chronic stage, serodiagnosis is the method of choice. EIA, IFA, and CF tests are available, although they cannot differentiate between acute and chronic disease, and cross-reactions may occur in patients with leishmaniasis.

Leishmania

Leishmaniasis is a disease of the reticuloendothelial system caused by kinetoplastid protozoa of the genus *Leishmania*. All species that infect humans have animal reservoirs and are transmitted by sandflies belonging to the genera *Phlebotomus* in the Old World and *Lutzomyia* in the New World. The parasites assume the amastigote form in mammalian hosts and the promastigote form in insect vectors. Species of *Leishmania* cannot be differentiated by examination of either amastigotes or promastigotes. Leishmaniasis may assume many different clinical forms: cutaneous, mucocutaneous, and visceral disease are the best known. The form and severity of disease vary with the infecting species, the particular host's immune status, and prior exposure (Peters, 1987; Cook, 2002).

Cutaneous Leishmaniasis

Old World cutaneous leishmaniasis (oriental sore) occurs in southern Europe, northern and eastern Africa, the Middle East, Iran, Afghanistan, India, and southern Russia. Infections are caused by *Leishmania tropica*, *Leishmania major*, and *Leishmania aethiopica*, although *L. donovani* and *Leishmania infantum* may also produce cutaneous lesions. *L. tropica* produces the urban or dry ulcer, which is more long lived than the rural or wet ulcer of *L. major*. Ulcers caused by these species usually develop on an exposed area of the body and heal spontaneously. Infection produces long-lasting immunity. *L. tropica* may become viscerotropic, as was demonstrated recently in military personnel who participated in Operation Desert Storm (Magill, 1993). *L. aethiopica* causes a more aggressive cutaneous infection, which in some individuals metastasizes to produce mucosal lesions or diffuse cutaneous leishmaniasis, the latter of which is characterized by multiple skin nodules resembling lepromatous leprosy.

Cutaneous leishmaniasis of the New World is caused by many species, including *Leishmania mexicana*, *Leishmania braziliensis*, *Leishmania amazonensis*, *Leishmania venezuelensis*, *Leishmania garnhami*, *Leishmania pifanoi*, *Leishmania peruviana*, *Leishmania panamensis*, and *Leishmania guyanensis*. Lesions produced by *L. mexicana* often involve the earlobe (chiclero ulcer), are self-limiting, and are not known to metastasize to the mucosa. However, *L. mexicana* and *L. amazonensis* may produce diffuse cutaneous lesions similar to those produced by *L. aethiopica*. A focus of cutaneous leishmaniasis exists in the southern part of Texas, where infections are caused by one or more species (Gustafson, 1985). *L. peruviana*, which has been found on the western slopes of the Peruvian Andes, causes an infection called uta, a benign cutaneous lesion occurring predominantly in children. *L. peruviana* is acquired in the home, where the main reservoirs are domestic dogs. This epidemiologic situation contrasts with other cutaneous leishmaniases, which are usually acquired in forests and have wild animals as reservoir hosts.

Mucocutaneous Leishmaniasis

Mucocutaneous leishmaniasis (espundia) is caused primarily by *L. braziliensis* and rarely by other species, which produce typical cutaneous lesions that are generally more aggressive, last longer, and often disseminate to mucous membranes, especially in the nasal, oral, or pharyngeal areas. In these locations, they may produce disfiguring lesions secondary to erosions of soft tissues and cartilage. *L. braziliensis* is distributed in Mexico and Central and South America.

Visceral Leishmaniasis

Visceral leishmaniasis of the Old World occurs sporadically over a wide geographic area and is caused by either *L. donovani* or by *L. infantum*. *L. donovani* predominates in Africa, India, and Asia, and *L. infantum* predominates in the Mediterranean region and the Middle East, although overlapping ranges occur. New World visceral leishmaniasis is caused by *L. chagasi* and occurs sporadically throughout Central and South America. Some species that cause cutaneous disease, on occasion, also have been responsible for visceral disease, as demonstrated recently in some troops who participated in Operation Desert Storm (Magill, 1993). In some areas, humans may serve as the disease reservoir, although a variety of animals, including dogs and cats, usually assume this role.

The infection usually is benign and often subclinical, although some individuals, especially young children and malnourished individuals, have marked involvement of the viscera, especially liver, spleen, bone marrow, and lymph nodes. In some cases, death occurs after months to years unless it is treated appropriately. The infection is called kala-azar in India, in reference to the darkening of the skin. Visceral leishmaniasis also is an opportunistic infection in individuals with concurrent human immunodeficiency virus (HIV) disease, and the condition responds poorly to therapy in such circumstances (Medrano, 1992; Strickland, 2000).

Diagnosis of Leishmaniasis

The diagnosis usually is established by visualization of amastigotes in smears, imprints, or biopsies, or by growth of promastigotes in culture. In integumentary leishmaniasis, the border of the most active lesion should be biopsied, and the fresh biopsy should be used to make imprints. A smear should also be prepared by making a 2–3 mm incision at the border of the ulcer and recovering small amounts of tissue from the cut surfaces with the scalpel blade. Both the imprint and the smear should be treated with Giemsa stain. Specimens that may be submitted when visceral leishmaniasis is suspected include buffy coat preparations, lymph node and bone marrow aspirates, and spleen and liver biopsies (Garcia, 2001).

A culture is desirable because it is more sensitive and allows determination of the species or subspecies, a practice that may help with the clinical management of the patient. Biopsy or aspirate specimens collected aseptically are cultured in Novy–MacNeal–Nicolle medium or in Schneider's *Drosophila* medium supplemented with fetal calf serum (Visvesvara, 2004b). Cultures usually begin to show promastigotes in 2–5 days but should be held for 4 weeks.

Amastigotes found in imprints, smears, and tissue sections are recognized by their size (2–4 µm), the presence of delicate cytoplasm, a nucleus, and a kinetoplast (Fig. 61–6C). In tissue sections, they may appear smaller because of shrinkage during fixation. Amastigotes must be differentiated from other intracellular organisms, including yeast cells of *Histoplasma capsulatum* and trophozoites of *T. gondii*. *Leishmania* spp. have a kinetoplast and do not have a cell wall. In contrast, *Histoplasma* lack the kinetoplast and the cell wall stains with periodic-acid–Schiff (PAS) and methenamine silver stains. According to one study (Weigle, 1987), the sensitivity of histologic sections stained with hematoxylin-eosin is 14%; imprints, 19%; cultures, 58%; and all methods combined, 67%.

Toxoplasma gondii

T. gondii is a protozoan parasite of the phylum Apicomplexa that has a worldwide distribution in humans and in domestic and wild animals, especially carnivores. Infection in immunocompetent persons is generally asymptomatic or mild, but immunocompromised patients may experience serious complications. Infection in utero may result in serious congenital infection with sequelae or stillbirth (Remington, 2005).

The sexual stage in the life cycle of this coccidian parasite is completed in the intestinal epithelium of cats and other felines, which serve exclusively as definitive hosts. During this enteroepithelial cycle, asexual schizogony and sexual gametogony occur, leading to the development of immature oocysts that are passed in the feces. Oocysts mature to the infective stage (which contain two sporocysts with four sporozoites each) in the environment in 2–21 days. Ingestion of infective oocysts may lead to infection of a wide variety of susceptible vertebrate hosts in which the actively growing trophozoites (tachyzoites) may infect any nucleated cells. Proliferation of tachyzoites results in cell death and injury to the host during acute infection. Once immunity has developed, the organisms form tissue cysts that may eventually contain hundreds or thousands of slowly growing bradyzoites. Presence of tissue cysts is characteristic of chronic infections. All stages of the life cycle occur in felines, but only the trophozoite and cyst stages occur in humans and other intermediate hosts.

Humans acquire infection with *T. gondii* by ingestion of inadequately cooked meat, especially lamb or pork, that contains tissue cysts or by ingestion of infective oocysts from material contaminated by cat feces. Outbreaks have occurred from inhaling contaminated dust in an indoor riding stable (Teutch, 1979) and from drinking contaminated water or unpasteurized goat's milk (Benenson, 1982; Sacks, 1982). Transmission via blood transfusion and through organ transplantation also can occur.

Most acute infections are asymptomatic or mimic other infectious diseases in which fever and lymphadenopathy are prominent. Congenital infection may occur when the mother develops acute infection during gestation. Risk of infection to the neonate is unrelated to the presence or absence of symptoms in the mother, but severity of infection depends on the stage of gestation when it is acquired. Intrauterine death, microcephaly, or hydrocephaly with intracranial calcifications may develop if infection is acquired in the first half of pregnancy. Infections in the second half of pregnancy are usually asymptomatic at birth, although fever, hepatosplenomegaly, and jaundice may appear. Chorioretinitis, psychomotor retardation, and convulsive disorders may appear months or years later (Remington, 2005).

In immunosuppressed individuals, especially those with the acquired immunodeficiency syndrome (AIDS), infections with *T. gondii* usually present with CNS involvement (Luft, 1988). Other possible clinical and pathologic manifestations include pneumonitis, myocarditis, retinitis, pancreatitis, or orchitis (Luft, 1989; Schnapp, 1992). Toxoplasmosis may be difficult to diagnose clinically and is often discovered at autopsy (Gutierrez, 2000). These infections usually result from reactivation of a latent infection, acquired months or years before, but occasionally result from a primary infection.

Diagnosis of toxoplasmosis may be established by examination of tissues, blood, or body fluids (Wilson, 2003). Demonstration of tachyzoites or tissue cysts is definitive but may prove difficult to demonstrate in hematoxylin and eosin (H&E)-stained sections; fluorescent or immuno-

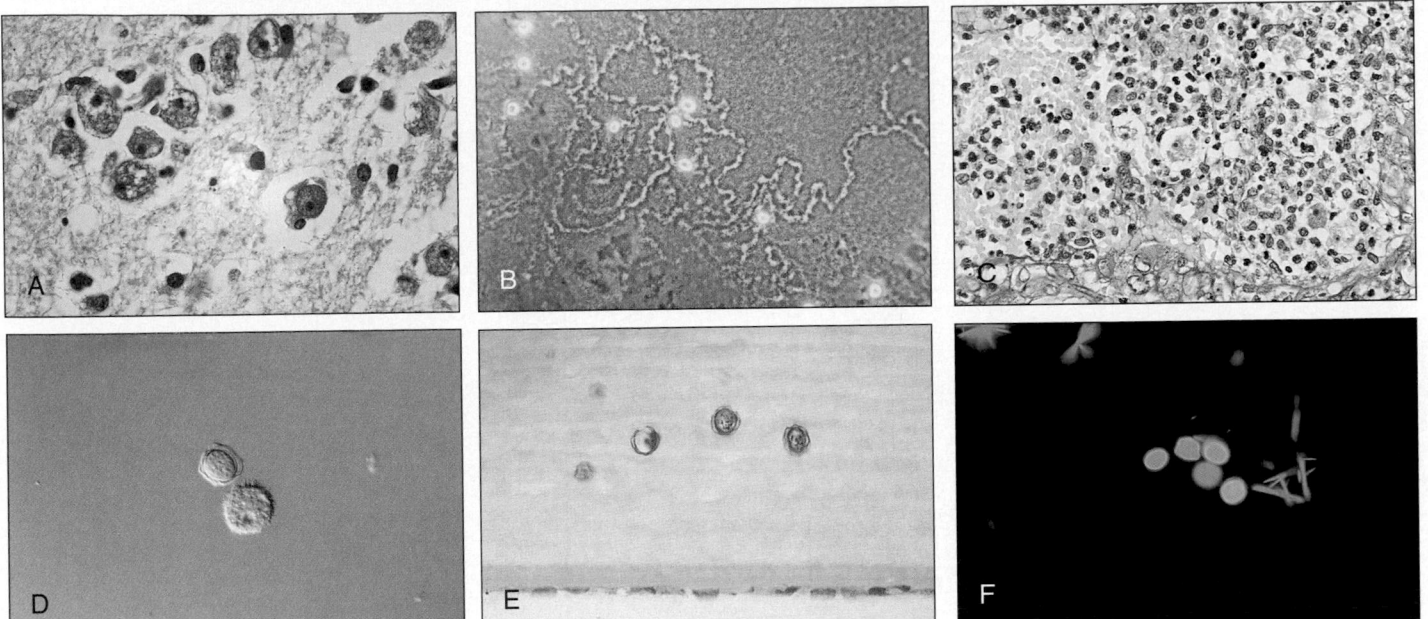

Figure 61–8 *A, Naegleria fowleri* trophozoites in primary amebic meningoencephalitis (H&E; oil immersion). *B, Acanthamoeba* sp. culture showing trails left by motile trophozoites on a lawn of *Escherichia coli* (phase contrast microscopy; ×100). *C, Acanthamoeba* sp. trophozoites within a cutaneous lesion in an individual infected with the human immunodeficiency virus (Giemsa stain; oil immersion). *D, Acanthamoeba* sp. trophozoite and cyst (differential interference contrast microscopy; ×400). *E,* Doubled walled cysts of *Acanthamoeba* sp. within corneal stroma (H&E; oil immersion). *F,* Cysts of *Acanthamoeba* sp. stained with Calcofluor white (epifluorescence microscopy; ×400).

peroxidase stains, if available, are useful. Giemsa is good for staining smears of body fluids and tissue imprints. Organisms may be demonstrated by inoculating appropriate material into tissue culture or uninfected mice. Recovery in routine viral cultures also has been described but requires extended incubation (Shepp, 1985). Isolation of organisms from blood or body fluid is evidence for acute infection, whereas recovery from tissues may reflect chronic infection. In smears, tachyzoites are crescent-shaped or oval, measuring approximately 3×7 μm; cysts measure up to 30 μm in diameter and are usually spherical, except in muscle fibers, where they appear elongated (Fig. 61–6*D, E,* and *F*).

Use of PCR technology is highly sensitive and specific in detecting toxoplasmic encephalitis, disseminated disease, and intrauterine infection (Cazenave, 1991; Grover, 1990; Parmley, 1992; Weiss, 1995). These procedures are not widely available, however, and require careful quality control to avoid false-positive results.

Serology remains the primary approach to establish a diagnosis of toxoplasmosis (Wilson, 2003; National Committee for Clinical Laboratory Standards, 2004). The Sabin–Feldman dye test and IFA test are standards to which other methods are compared, although the former is performed in only a few centers. Many EIA tests are commercially available and generally provide results similar to those of IFA. Antibodies appear in 1–2 weeks, and titers peak at 6–8 weeks. Tests for IgM-specific antibodies are especially useful for diagnosis of congenital and acute infection, but knowledge of test limitations, specifically the occurrence of false-positive reactions, is extremely important. The persistence of IgM-specific antibodies, sometimes for a year or more, also is problematic and must be interpreted in conjunction with IgG antibody results. Because many persons have had asymptomatic infections, low IgG titers have little significance. Titers in patients with chronic ocular infections may also be low. Immunocompromised patients such as those with AIDS who have active *Toxoplasma* infections almost always have pre-existing specific IgG antibodies, although titers may be low, and IgM activity is infrequently seen. Interpretation of IgG and IgM antibody titers varies by test methodology and by manufacturer. The laboratory performing the test should provide the necessary interpretive criteria (National Committee for Clinical Laboratory Standards, 2004).

Opportunistic Free-Living Amebae

Amebae of the genera *Naegleria, Acanthamoeba,* and *Balamuthia* are inhabitants of soil, water, and other environmental substrates, where they feed on other microscopic organisms, especially bacteria and yeasts. All three genera have been associated with opportunistic infection of the CNS and *Acanthamoeba* cause keratitis (Martinez, 1985; Marciano-Cabral, 1988; Ubelaker, 1991; Kilvington, 1994; Visvesvara, 2003).

Primary amebic meningoencephalitis, caused by the ameboflagellate *Naegleria fowleri,* typically affects children and young adults who have been swimming or diving in warm, freshwater lakes or pools. The ameboflagellate enters the brain via the cribriform plate and olfactory bulbs and reaches the frontal lobes, where it produces an acute hemorrhagic meningoencephalitis that is usually fatal within 1 week of onset of symptoms. The disease has an extremely poor prognosis, despite vigorous therapeutic intervention. Diagnosis is usually established at autopsy examination by finding trophozoites (cysts are rarely seen) in tissue sections (Fig. 61–8*A*). Antemortem diagnosis is made occasionally by identifying typical trophozoites in CSF either on direct wet mounts, stained preparations, or in culture. Trophozoites measure 10–35 μm; have large, round, central karyosomes; and if exposed to warm distilled water, convert to flagellated forms in 1–2 hours. Cysts are spherical, measuring 7–15 μm in diameter. Culture usually is performed on non-nutrient agar plates (1.5% agar, 0.5% sodium chloride, pH 6.6–7.0) seeded with a lawn of heat-killed or living *Escherichia coli* (Visvesvara, 2003). Amebae ingest the bacteria, leaving tracks in the bacterial lawn, which may be seen under low-power magnification using reduced light (Fig. 61–8*B*).

Granulomatous amebic meningoencephalitis (GAE) may be caused by several species of *Acanthamoeba,* including *Acanthamoeba castellani, Acanthamoeba culbertsoni, Acanthamoeba polyphaga,* and *Acanthamoeba astronyxis,* among others (Marciano-Cabral, 2003). It is usually a subacute or chronic opportunistic infection of chronically ill, debilitated, and immunosuppressed individuals, leading to death weeks to months following onset of symptoms. Infection is thought to spread hematogenously from primary foci in skin, pharynx, or the respiratory tract. Systemic infections occur in individuals with AIDS, and may present as ulcerative skin lesions, subcutaneous abscesses, or erythematous nodules (Fig. 61–8*C*) (Tan, 1993). Exposure to fresh water is not necessary because cysts of *Acanthamoeba* readily become airborne and may be recovered from the throat and nasal passages (Wang, 1967; Lawande, 1979). The pathologic reaction in tissues is granulomatous, with trophozoites predominating in viable tissue and cysts predominating in areas of necrosis. Diagnosis usually is established at autopsy, but organisms may be recognized in brain biopsies or recovered using the culture technique described for *Naegleria. Acanthamoeba* trophozoites are somewhat larger than *Naegleria,* measuring 15–45 μm, and display needle-like filamentous projections from the cell known as acanthopodia. Cysts measure 10–25 μm and are double-walled, displaying a wrinkled outer wall (ectocyst) and a polygonal, stellate, or round inner wall (endocyst) (Fig. 61–8*D*). Identification to the species level is problematic and reflects uncertainty as to the validity of the 18 or more described species. Use of immunofluorescence and immunoperoxidase techniques may prove useful in differentiating species and are available from the CDC (Visvesvara, 2003).

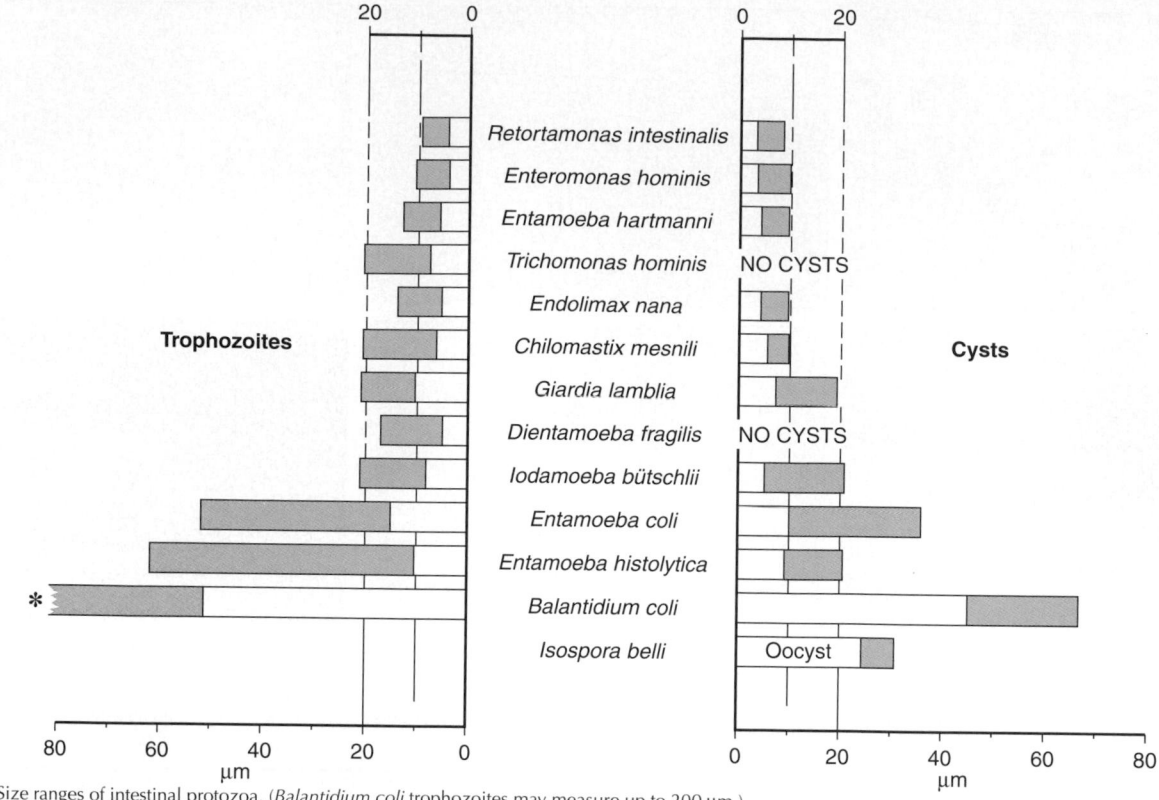

Figure 61–9 Size ranges of intestinal protozoa. (*Balantidium coli* trophozoites may measure up to 200 μm.)

GAE may also be caused by leptomyxid amebae, specifically *Balamuthia mandrillaris* (Visvesvara, 1993). Morphologically, *Balamuthia* cannot be differentiated from *Acanthamoeba* by routine histology, although differences may be detected at the ultrastructural level. These organisms are antigenically distinct and may be identified using specific monoclonal or polyclonal antisera in immunofluorescence or immunoperoxidase assays (Visvesvara, 2003). *Balamuthia* do not grow on agar plates used for *Naegleria* and *Acanthamoeba*, but have been recovered in tissue culture using mammalian cell lines.

Acanthamoeba keratitis is an increasingly recognized painful infection of the cornea that is most likely to occur in persons who use daily-wear or extended-wear soft contact lenses or who have experienced trauma to the cornea (Anuran, 1987; Kilvington, 1994; Marciano-Cabral, 2003). Incomplete or infrequent disinfection and use of homemade saline are known risk factors for acquiring the infection (Stehr-Green, 1990). The disease is characterized by development of a paracentral ring infiltrate of the corneal stroma, which progresses to ulceration and possible perforation, with loss of the eye. The infection may be confused with fungal, bacterial, or herpetic keratitis but is characteristically refractory to commonly used antimicrobials. Keratoplasty has been used routinely in the management of this disease, although recent advances in medical therapy have been reported (Varga, 1993). Diagnosis usually is established by demonstrating amebic trophozoites or cysts in corneal scrapings or biopsies (Fig. 61–8E). A variety of permanent stains can be used including Giemsa, PAS, and trichrome. Use of the fluorochrome Calcofluor white is especially helpful in recognizing amebic cysts (Fig. 61–8F) (Marines, 1987). Cultures (described earlier) increase sensitivity.

Intestinal and Urogenital Protozoa

Protozoal groups inhabiting the intestinal tract of humans include the amebae, flagellates, ciliates, coccidia, and microsporidia, not all of which are pathogens. In a review of fecal specimens submitted to state health department laboratories, *G. lamblia* was present in 7.2%, *E. histolytica* in 0.9%, *D. fragilis* in 0.5%, and *Cryptosporidium* spp. in 0.2% of specimens. Nonpathogenic protozoa were found in approximately 10.7% of specimens (Kappus, 1994). Most intestinal infections are acquired by fecal–oral contamination, either directly, from food handlers, or indirectly via contaminated water.

For most laboratorians, identification of intestinal protozoa is one of the more difficult aspects of parasitology. Protozoal parasites are small, and the pathogenic species must be differentiated from the nonpathogenic species and from inflammatory cells, epithelial cells, yeasts, pollen, and other confusing objects. There are a number of characteristics that assist in identifying intestinal protozoa. Size is helpful (Fig. 61–9), and a properly calibrated ocular micrometer must be available. Differentiation of amebae from flagellates in wet mounts of fresh material is relatively easy because of the typical pseudopod extension seen with amebae, whereas flagellates move more rapidly and in a so-called falling leaf, darting, or tumbling fashion.

Number and size of nuclei and pattern of chromatin distribution, best seen in permanent stained preparations, are also useful. Cytoplasmic characteristics include fibrils and other special structures typical of flagellates, ingested materials in amebic trophozoites, and glycogen masses and chromatoid bodies in amebic cysts. Flagellates generally are elongate and tapered, with a nucleus or nuclei at one end.

When examined by any method, both nuclear and cytoplasmic characteristics should be assessed from a number of individual organisms to complete the identification. When reporting the presence of two or more species in a sample, the observer should be able to define distinct populations of organisms, to prevent confusion from an occasional organism with an atypical appearance.

Trophozoites predominate in liquid stool but degenerate within an hour after passage unless they are placed into preservatives. Cysts predominate in formed stool and are more resistant to degeneration. Both forms may be seen in direct wet mounts prepared from fresh feces. Formalin does not preserve trophozoites well, and they may be missed unless permanent stained smears are prepared. Definitive identification should be made on examination of permanent stained slides.

Amebae and *Blastocystis hominis*

Three genera of amebae may inhabit the intestinal tract of humans: *Entamoeba*, *Endolimax*, and *Iodamoeba*. Cysts are ingested and excyst in the small intestine. The resulting trophozoites proliferate by binary fission in the lumen of the colon. Both cysts and trophozoites may be passed in feces, but only mature cysts are infective. *E. histolytica* is the only amebic species capable of invading tissues and causing disease.

The genus *Entamoeba*, characterized by the presence of chromatin on the nuclear membrane, includes *E. histolytica*, the etiologic agent of amebiasis, *E. dispar*, a nonpathogenic species morphologically identical to *E. histolytica*, *E. hartmanni* and *Entamoeba coli*, which are commonly found commensal species, and *Entamoeba polecki*, which is occasionally found in people who have contact with pigs (Fig. 61–10) (Levin, 1970; Gay, 1985). *Entamoeba gingivalis*, which does not have a known cyst stage, may inhabit the oral cavity of people with poor oral hygiene (Dao, 1983). *E. polecki* and *E. gingivalis* are seen infrequently and are not described further.

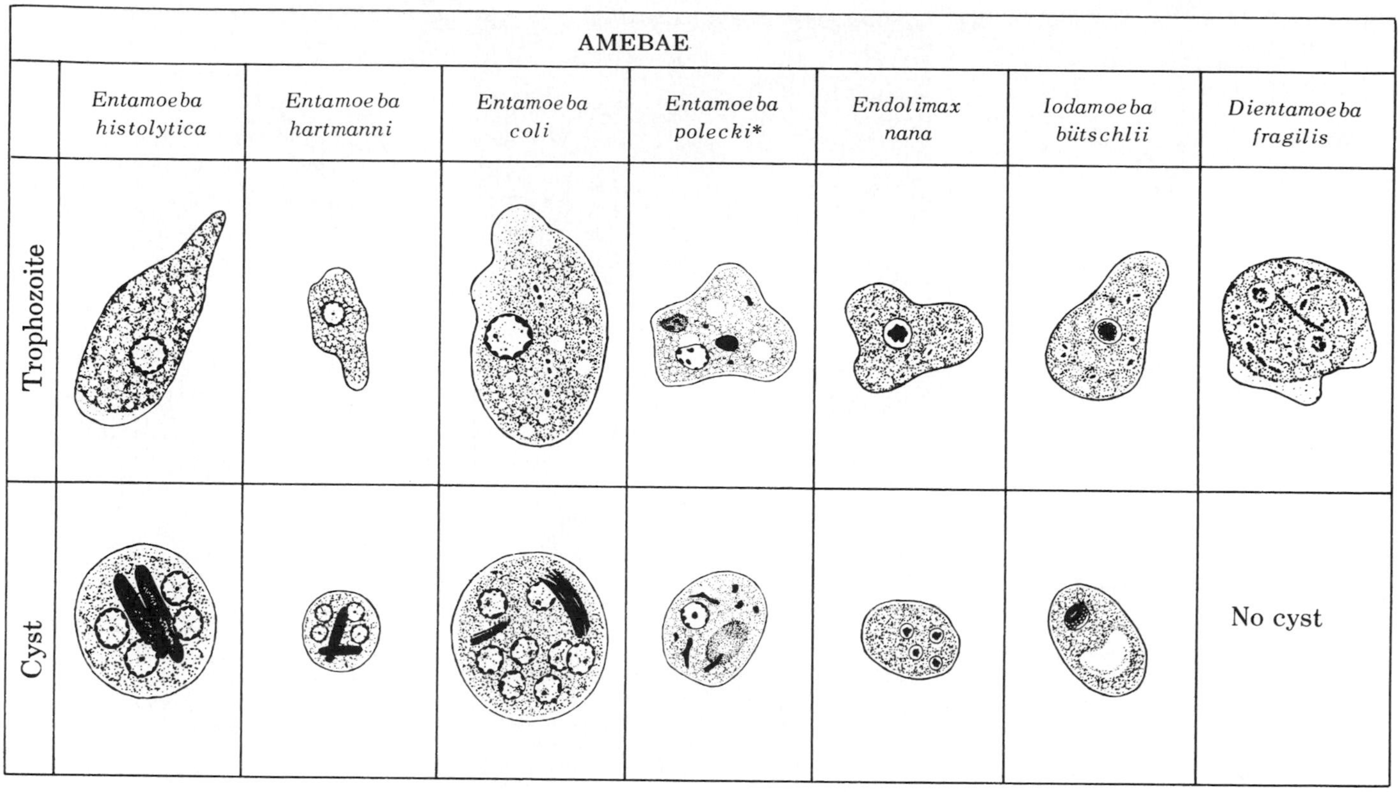

AMEBAE						
Entamoeba histolytica	*Entamoeba hartmanni*	*Entamoeba coli*	*Entamoeba polecki**	*Endolimax nana*	*Iodamoeba bütschlii*	*Dientamoeba fragilis*
Trophozoite						
Cyst						No cyst

*Rare, probably of animal origin

Figure 61–10 Amebae found in human stool specimens. (*Dientamoeba fragilis* is a flagellate.)

Endolimax nana and *I. bütschlii* are nonpathogenic species. *Dientamoeba fragilis* now is recognized as a flagellate, although it lacks external flagella, and is discussed with the flagellates in the text but may be found with the amebae in tables and figures because it is morphologically similar to the amebae (Murray, 2003).

Entamoeba histolytica

E. histolytica may cause various clinical diseases, most commonly amebic dysentery, amebic colitis, and liver abscesses (Beaver 1984; Ravdin, 1988; Strickland, 2000). General host defense mechanisms, previous contact with the parasite, diet, and the strain of *E. histolytica* influence the severity of infection. Analysis of isoenzyme patterns (zymodemes) has shown that only certain strains can cause invasive disease and that most infections remain undetected (Bruckner, 1992; Murray, 2003). Genetic and biochemical differences between invasive and noninvasive strains have been identified, and it has been proposed that nonpathogenic strains be named *Entamoeba dispar* (Diamond, 1993).

Amebic dysentery, which occurs infrequently in the United States, is an acute disease characterized by bloody diarrhea with abdominal cramping. Invasion of the intestinal mucosa occurs, producing ulceration that may lead to perforation and peritonitis. The more common form of disease seen in this country is amebic colitis, which may mimic ulcerative colitis and other forms of inflammatory bowel disease. Symptoms are generally less severe than in amebic dysentery but may include nonbloody diarrhea, constipation, abdominal cramping, and weight loss. Small, pinpoint mucosal ulcerations may develop and expand within the submucosa to form flask-shaped ulcers. All of the colon may be involved or only a portion, most commonly the cecum, rectosigmoid, or ascending colon.

Amebic liver abscess is the most common form of extraintestinal amebiasis, occurring in approximately 5% of patients with a history of intestinal amebiasis. Symptoms include fever and right upper quadrant pain. These liver abscesses are usually diagnosed by radiographic scans, ultrasound, and serologic tests. Amebae are present in the stool in less than half of patients at the time liver abscess is manifest. Amebic hepatitis, characterized by an enlarged, tender liver in someone with intestinal amebiasis, may occur in some cases. Its pathogenesis is poorly understood. Rarely, amebic abscesses appear in other organs, such as the lung, brain, or skin, either by hematogenous spread from the intestine or by contiguous spread from a liver abscess. Masses of granulomatous tissue, known as amebomas, may form in response to the presence of amebae, which in the intestine may cause a so-called napkin ring lesion that could be mistaken for a carcinoma.

Epidemiology

Most infections with *E. histolytica* are acquired by ingestion of contaminated food or water, although one outbreak was caused by a contaminated colonic irrigation machine (Istre, 1982). Pseudo-outbreaks of amebiasis result from laboratory misidentification of inflammatory cells, other amebae, and fecal debris as *E. histolytica* (Krogstad, 1978; Centers for Disease Control and Prevention, 1985). Although *E. histolytica* is an endemic parasite in the United States, many citizens acquire infections while traveling through or residing in foreign countries.

Diagnosis

Examination of a series of stool specimens should be sufficient for diagnosis of intestinal amebiasis in most cases. If the patient has been given antibiotics or contrast media, the amebic infection may be masked for a period of time. Aspirated material from liver abscesses can be examined microscopically to detect trophozoites. The last material aspirated is most likely to contain trophozoites and may be examined by direct microscopic examination or permanently stained slides. If tissue is available, sections may show organisms that stain prominently with PAS (Fig. 61–11C).

Culture procedures (Diamond, 1988; Visvesvara, 2004a; Clinical and Laboratory Standards Institute, 2005) are not widely used for diagnosis but are useful for research and are essential to determine pathogenicity based on zymodemes. EIA antigen detection tests that are both specific, sensitive, and able to differentiate *E. histolytica* from *E. dispar* are commercially available (Table 61–5; Garcia, 2003; Clinical and Laboratory Standards Institute, 2005). Use of PCR amplification techniques and DNA probes are also useful for differentiating *E. histolytica* from *E. dispar* (Samuelson, 1989; Bendall, 1993; Weiss, 1995), but none are commercially available at this time.

Serologic tests (Table 61–6) are most useful for diagnosis of extraintestinal infections because approximately 95% of patients with amebic liver abscess are seropositive. This decreases to 70% for patients with active intestinal infection and to 10% in asymptomatic carriers. Detectable titers may persist for months or years after successful treatment (Rosenblatt, 1995; Wilson, 1995).

Trophozoites of *E. histolytica* vary from 10–60 μm in diameter, with the commensal forms usually 15–20 μm and the invasive forms over 20 μm in greatest dimension (Table 61–9; Figs 61–9 to 61–12). In direct wet mounts, trophozoites show progressive motility via rapidly formed hyaline pseudopodia that demonstrate a sharp demarcation between

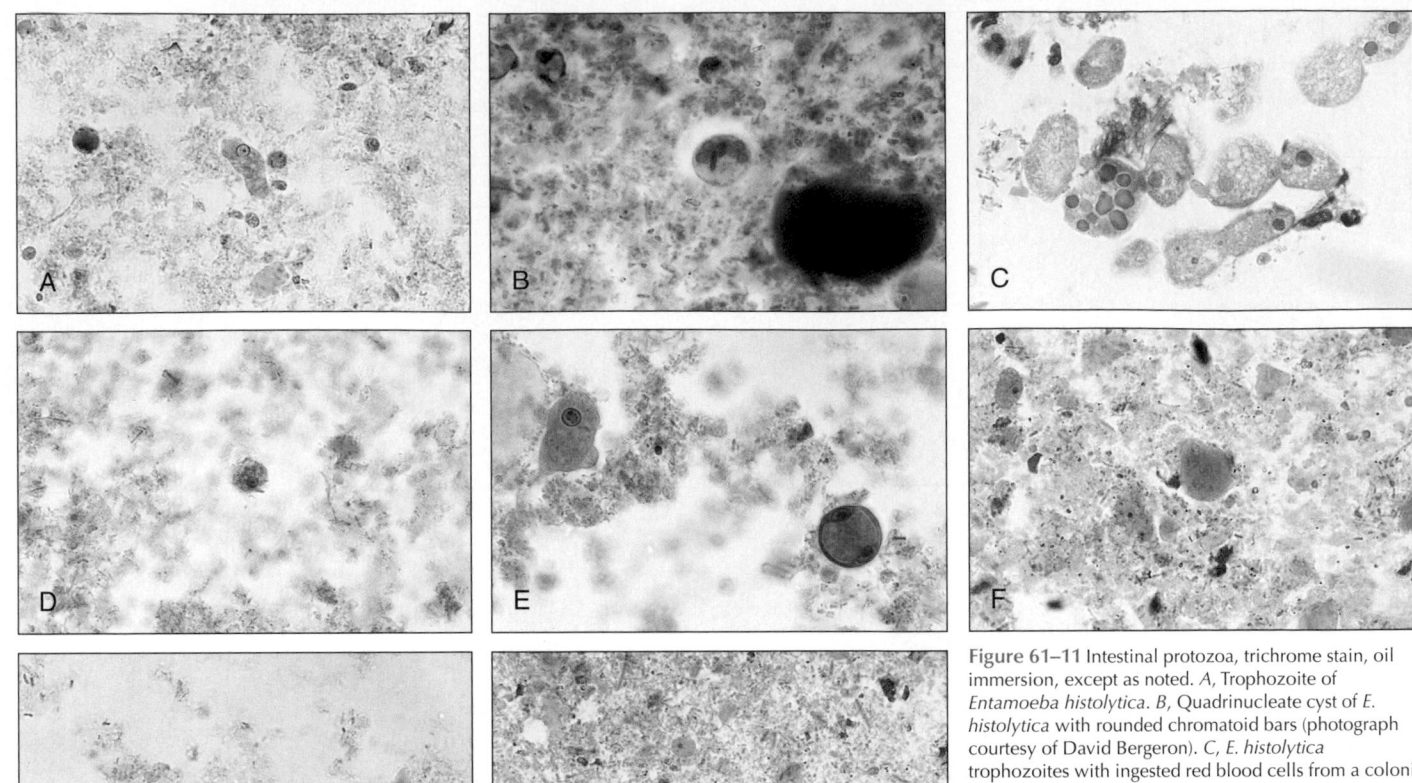

Figure 61–11 Intestinal protozoa, trichrome stain, oil immersion, except as noted. *A*, Trophozoite of *Entamoeba histolytica*. *B*, Quadrinucleate cyst of *E. histolytica* with rounded chromatoid bars (photograph courtesy of David Bergeron). *C*, *E. histolytica* trophozoites with ingested red blood cells from a colonic lesion (H&E). *D*, Trophozoite of *E. hartmanni*. *E*, Trophozoite and binucleate cyst of *E. coli*. *F*, Multinucleate cyst of *E. coli*. *G*, Cyst of *Iodamoeba bütschlii* with characteristic glycogen vacuole. *H*, Binucleate trophozoites typical for *Dientamoeba fragilis*.

endoplasm and ectoplasm; unstained nuclei are not visible. In invasive disease, some trophozoites contain ingested erythrocytes (Fig. 61–11C), a feature diagnostic of *E. histolytica* infection. In stained preparations, the peripheral nuclear chromatin is evenly distributed along the nuclear membrane as fine granules. The karyosome is small and often centrally located, with fine fibrils, which generally are not visible, attaching it to the nuclear membrane. Variations in nuclear structure occur, with some karyosomes being located eccentrically and peripheral chromatin irregularly distributed. The only characteristic that is pathognomonic for *E. histolytica* is phagocytosis of erythrocytes, which very rarely occurs with other species. The cytoplasm is finely granular, and in invasive organisms, there are either no inclusions or only erythrocyte inclusions. Noninvasive organisms may contain ingested bacteria. In degenerating organisms, the cytoplasm may become vacuolated and nuclei may show abnormal chromatin clumping.

Cysts of *E. histolytica* are spherical and measure 10–20 µm (usually 12–15 µm) in diameter (Table 61–10; Figs 61–9, 61–10, and 61–12). The rounded precyst stage has a single nucleus but does not have a refractile cyst wall. As it matures, the cyst develops four nuclei, each approximately one sixth the diameter of the cyst. Cyst nuclei appear similar to those of trophozoites, but their smaller size makes them less useful as differentiating features. The cyst cytoplasm may contain glycogen vacuoles and chromatoid bodies with blunted or rounded ends. The number and size of nuclei and the appearance of chromatoid bodies are important diagnostic criteria for identifying cysts.

Those laboratories who do not use one of the immunologic or molecular methods to differentiate *E. histolytica* from *E. dispar*, and who rely exclusively on morphologic analysis, must use a reporting format that takes the differing technologies into consideration. Thus, a report of '*E. histolytica*/*E. dispar*' would be most appropriate in the latter circumstance.

Nonpathogenic Amebae

Laboratory personnel must be able to differentiate the nonpathogenic or commensal intestinal amebae from *E. histolytica*/*E. dispar* and *D. fragilis* (a flagellate), which are potential pathogens. Identification characteristics, best visualized in permanent stained sections, are summarized in Tables 61–9 and 61–10 and Figures 61–9, 61–10, and 61–12. Identification of

trophozoites is based on size and nuclear and cytoplasmic characteristics; identification of cysts is based on size, number and characteristics of nuclei, and presence and character of chromatoid bodies and glycogen masses.

E. hartmanni has morphologic characteristics similar to those of *E. histolytica*, except trophozoites have a maximum diameter of 12 µm and cysts have a maximum diameter of 10 µm, and cysts often have a single nucleus. Historically, *E. hartmanni* has been called the small race of *E. histolytica*. Differentiation requires careful measurement of a representative sample of organisms with a properly calibrated ocular micrometer.

Entamoeba coli, a common lumen-dwelling ameba, may be difficult to differentiate from *E. histolytica*. The cytoplasm stains somewhat more darkly than the cytoplasm of *E. histolytica* and is more vacuolated, containing numerous ingested bacteria, yeasts, and other materials. Although nuclear characteristics differ from those of *E. histolytica* (Fig. 61–12), significant overlap may occur, especially in specimens that have not been promptly preserved. Mature cysts of *E. coli* contain eight nuclei, although occasional cysts contain 16 or more. Immature cysts, which are not common, have four nuclei that are larger (one fourth the diameter of the cyst) than nuclei of *E. histolytica* (one sixth the diameter of the cyst) and may contain glycogen. Distribution of peripheral chromatin and karyosomes should not be given great emphasis in identification of *Entamoeba* cysts. Chromatoid bodies, when present, are irregular in shape with splintered or pointed ends, rather than the rounded ends seen in *E. histolytica*.

Endolimax nana is the smallest ameba to infect humans. Trophozoites often have atypical nuclei that contain a triangular chromatin mass, a band of chromatin across the nucleus, or two discrete masses of chromatin on opposite sides of the nuclear membrane (Fig. 61–12). A clear halo or karyolymph space surrounds the karyosome and extends to the nuclear membrane. The atypical nuclear forms may be helpful in differentiating *E. nana* from *I. bütschlii*, which is similar in appearance, but larger. Cysts of *Endolimax* usually contain four nuclei, although smaller numbers may be seen. Glycogen, when present, occurs diffusely in the cytoplasm rather than as a discrete mass. Cysts are easily differentiated from those of other amebae but may be confused with *Blastocystis hominis* organisms. The nuclei of *B. hominis*, however, lack the halos that are typically seen with *E. nana* cysts.

Table 61–9 Morphology of Trophozoites of Intestinal Amebae

Species	Size (in Diameter or Length)	Motility	Nucleus Numbers[‡]	Peripheral Chromatin	Karyosomal Chromatin	Cytoplasm Appearance	Inclusions
Entamoeba histolytica/E. dispar	10–60 µm; usual range, 15–20 µm commensal form[*]; over 20 µm for invasive form[†]	Progressive, with hyaline, finger-like pseudopods	1 Not visible in unstained preparations	Fine granules; usually evenly distributed and uniform in size	Small, discrete; usually central but occasionally eccentric	Finely granular	Erythrocytes occasionally in invasive forms. Noninvasive contain bacteria
Entamoeba hartmanni	5–12 µm; usual range 8–10 µm	Usually nonprogressive but may be progressive occasionally	1 Not visible in unstained preparations	Similar to *E. histolytica*	Small, discrete, often eccentric	Finely granular	Bacteria
Entamoeba coli	15–50 µm; usual range 20–25 µm	Sluggish, nonprogressive with blunt pseudopods	1 Often visible in unstained preparation	Coarse granules, irregular in size and distribution	Large, discrete, usually eccentric	Coarse, often vacuolated	Bacteria, yeasts, other materials
Endolimax nana	6–12 µm; usual range 8–10 µm	Sluggish, usually nonprogressive with blunt pseudopods	1 Visible occasionally in unstained preparations	None	Large, irregularly shaped	Granular, vacuolated	Bacteria
Iodamoeba bütschlii	8–20 µm; usual range 12–15 µm	Sluggish, usually nonprogressive	1 Not usually visible in unstained preparations	None	Large, usually central. Surrounded by refractile, achromatic granules. These granules are often not distinct even in stained slides	Coarsely granular, vacuolated	Bacteria, yeasts, or other material
Dientamoeba fragilis[§]	5–15 µm; usual range 9–12 µm	Pseudopods are angular, serrated, or broad lobed and hyaline, almost transparent	2 (In approximately 20% of organisms only 1 nucleus is present.) Nuclei invisible in unstained preparations	None	Large cluster of 4–8 granules	Finely granular, vacuolated	Bacteria

[*] Usually found in asymptomatic or chronic cases; may contain bacteria. [†] Usually found in acute cases; often contain red blood cells. [‡] Visibility is for unfixed material. Nuclei may sometimes be visible in fixed material. [§] A flagellate (see text).

Source: adapted from Brooke MM, Melvin DM: Morphology of Diagnostic Stages of Intestinal Parasites of Man. USDHEW PHS Publication No. 1966, 1969.

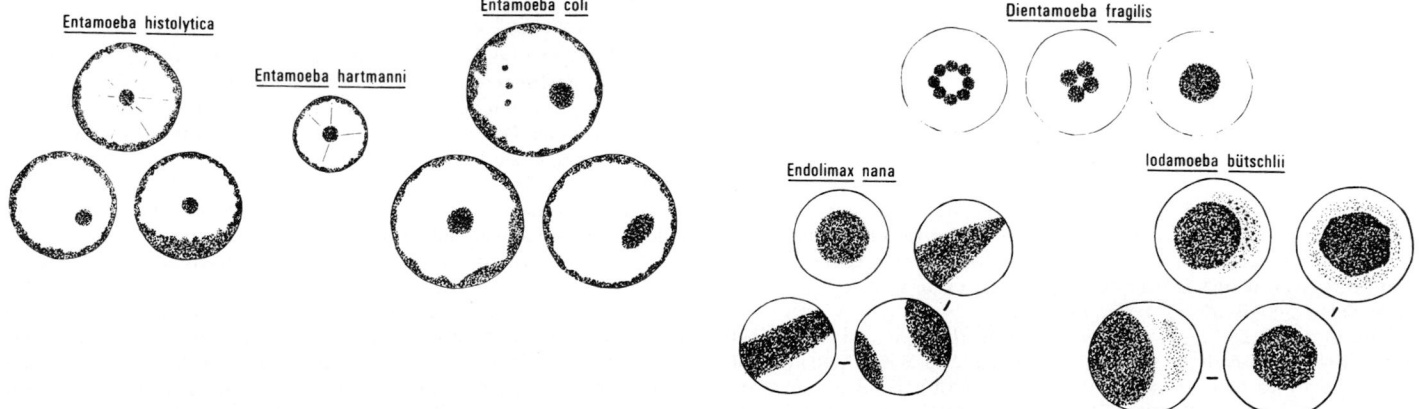

Figure 61–12 Nuclei of amebae. This drawing shows some of the various appearances of amebic nuclei in stained preparations. (*Dientamoeba fragilis* is a flagellate; see text.)

The nuclei of *I. bütschlii* trophozoites and cysts have a large, centrally located karyosome frequently surrounded by achromatic granules that may not be distinct but appear only as a muddy karyolymph space or halo. In some nuclei, the halo is clear without evident achromatic granules, making the organism indistinguishable from *E. nana*. Cysts of *I. bütschlii* contain a single nucleus, in which the karyosome is often eccentric with a nearby crescent of achromatic granules (see Figs. 61–9, 61–10, and 61–12). The cyst is characterized by a prominent vacuole of glycogen that stains reddish brown in iodine-stained wet mounts, thus the name of the

organism. Glycogen is dissolved by aqueous fixatives and may not be demonstrable in material that has been stored.

Blastocystis hominis

B. hominis is an ameba-like protozoan that inhabits the large bowel and is frequently found in stool specimens of asymptomatic individuals. Some studies have linked heavy infections to symptomatic intestinal disease, although this remains controversial (Markell, 1986; Sheehan, 1986; Miller, 1988; Zierdt, 1991; Stenzel, 1996). *Blastocystis* may assume one of

VII

Table 61–10 Morphology of Cysts of Intestinal Amebae

Species	Size	Shape	Nucleus Number	Peripheral Chromatin	Karyosomal Chromatin	Cytoplasm Chromatoid Bodies	Glycogen
Entamoeba histolytica/ E. dispar	10–20 μm; usual range 12–15 μm	Usually spherical	4 in mature cyst. Immature cysts with 1 or 2 occasionally seen	Peripheral chromatin present. Fine, uniform granules, evenly distributed	Small, discrete, usually central	Present. Elongated bars with bluntly rounded ends	Usually diffuse. Concentrated mass often present in young cysts. Stains reddish brown with iodine.
Entamoeba hartmanni	5–10 μm; usual range 6–8 μm	Usually spherical	4 in mature cyst. Immature cysts with 1 or 2 often seen	Similar to *E. histolytica*	Similar to *E. histolytica*	Present. Elongated bars with bluntly rounded ends	Similar to *E. histolytica*
Entamoeba coli	10–35 μm; usual range 15–25 μm	Usually spherical. Occasionally oval, triangular, or of another shape	8 in mature cyst. Occasionally supernucleate cysts with 16 or more are seen. Immature cysts with 2 or more occasionally seen	Peripheral chromatin present. Coarse granules irregular in size and distribution, but often appear more uniform than in trophozoites	Large, discrete, usually eccentric, but occasionally central	Present. Usually splinter-like with pointed ends	Usually diffuse, but occasionally well-defined mass in immature cysts. Stains reddish brown with iodine
Endolimax nana	5–10 μm; usual range 6–8 μm	Spherical, ovoid, or ellipsoidal	4 in mature cysts. Immature cysts with less than 4 rarely seen	None	Large, usually centrally located	Occasionally, granules or small oval masses seen, but bodies as seen in *Entamoeba* species are not present	Usually diffuse. Concentrated mass seen occasionally in young cysts. Stains reddish brown with iodine
Iodamoeba bütschlii	5–20 μm; usual range 10–12 μm	Ovoid, ellipsoidal, triangular, or of another shape	1 in mature cyst	None	Large, usually eccentric. Refractile, achromatic granules on one side of karyosome	Granules occasionally present, but bodies as seen in *Entamoeba* species are not present	Compact, well-defined mass. Stains dark brown with iodine

Source: adapted from Brooke MM, Melvin DM: Morphology of Diagnostic Stages of Intestinal Parasites of Man. USDHEW PHS Publication No. 1966, 1969.

three forms: vacuolated, which is seen most commonly; ameboid; or granular. The vacuolated form, also known as the central vacuolar form, usually is spherical and variable in size (5 to 20 μm), with a central clear area and two to four peripheral nuclei (Figs 61–13*A* and 61–14*G*). Ameboid forms with bizarre shapes may predominate in heavy infections. Presence of *Blastocystis* should be reported, especially when they are numerous (five or more per 400× field) (Sheehan, 1986; Stenzel, 1996).

Flagellates

Dientamoeba fragilis

D. fragilis is an ameboid pathogen that infects the colon and has been associated with diarrheal disease, especially in young children (Yang, 1977; Spencer 1979; Turner, 1985; Preiss, 1991; Johnson, 2004). Although similar in appearance to amebae, *Dientamoeba* has been reclassified as a flagellate on the basis of ultrastructural details and antigenic similarities. Also, no cyst stage has been described. Because of the similarity of *Dientamoeba* to amebae at the light microscope level, this species has traditionally been included in tables and figures for amebae (see Table 61–9, Figs. 61–9, 61–10; 61–11*H*, and 61–12).

Symptoms of *D. fragilis* infection include diarrhea and abdominal distention. Recent evidence suggests that dientamebiasis is a more frequent cause of diarrhea than previously thought: 4.3% of patients in one study harbored this organism (Spencer, 1979; Murray, 2003). Approximately 25% of persons infected with this parasite have symptomatic disease. In contrast to amebiasis, this infection is usually not associated with other fecal protozoa but does show a 10– 20 times greater than expected association with enterobiasis (pinworm infection, discussed later). This association and some experimental evidence suggest that *D. fragilis* infection may be spread by ingestion of pinworm eggs infected with *D. fragilis* (Burrows, 1956; Johnson, 2004). *D. fragilis* infection will be overlooked unless permanently stained slides are examined. Multiple specimens may need to be submitted because shedding varies from day to day. When preparing smears, the last portion of the stool evacuated should be examined because the number of parasites found there tends to be greater. Two thirds to four fifths of the organisms contain two nuclei that consist of a cluster of four to eight karyosomal granules, which may appear as one large irregular karyosome (Fig. 61–12). Uninucleate *D. fragilis* may be confused with trophozoites of *E. nana* or *I. bütschlii*. The cytoplasm is finely granular and often contains ingested bacteria. Trophozoites are delicate and may be easily overlooked, so stained slides must be carefully examined. An immunofluorescence method has been described that may help in the detection of this parasite, but it is not commercially available (Chan, 1993).

Giardia lamblia

G. lamblia is a pathogenic intestinal protozoan that causes both endemic and epidemic disease worldwide and, in the United States, it is especially problematic for travelers, campers, children attending day-care, and homosexual men (Wolfe, 1992). It frequently causes disease in individuals drinking contaminated water, and a number of large water-borne outbreaks have been described from places such as Aspen, Colorado; Leningrad, Russia; and Rome, New York (Craun, 1986). Pathogenic protozoa are not killed by the usual concentrations of chlorine in municipal water supplies and therefore, unless the water supply is filtered, it may serve as a source of infection, as it did in the Rome, New York, outbreak.

G. lamblia trophozoites multiply in the small bowel and attach to the mucosa by a ventral concave sucking disk. Infection may be asymptomatic or it may cause disease ranging from mild diarrhea with vague abdominal complaints to a malabsorption syndrome with diarrhea and steatorrhea, similar to that of sprue. Pathogenesis is not fully understood, although disruption of the integrity of the brush border with resulting disaccharidase deficiency may occur from direct or indirect effects of the organism's presence (Wolfe, 1992). Giardiasis should be considered in any patient presenting with diarrhea of more than 10 days' duration.

Diagnosis is established by demonstration of *Giardia* trophozoites or cysts, or both, in fecal specimens. Trophozoites predominate in diarrheic stool, whereas infectious cysts are more likely to be found in formed stool. The passage of organisms varies from day to day; therefore, examination of multiple specimens, collected on different days, may be necessary. Direct wet mounts are particularly helpful for demonstrating trophozoites, with their so-called falling-leaf motility, in a diarrheic or aspirate specimen. Cysts can be seen in both direct wet mounts and concentration techniques,

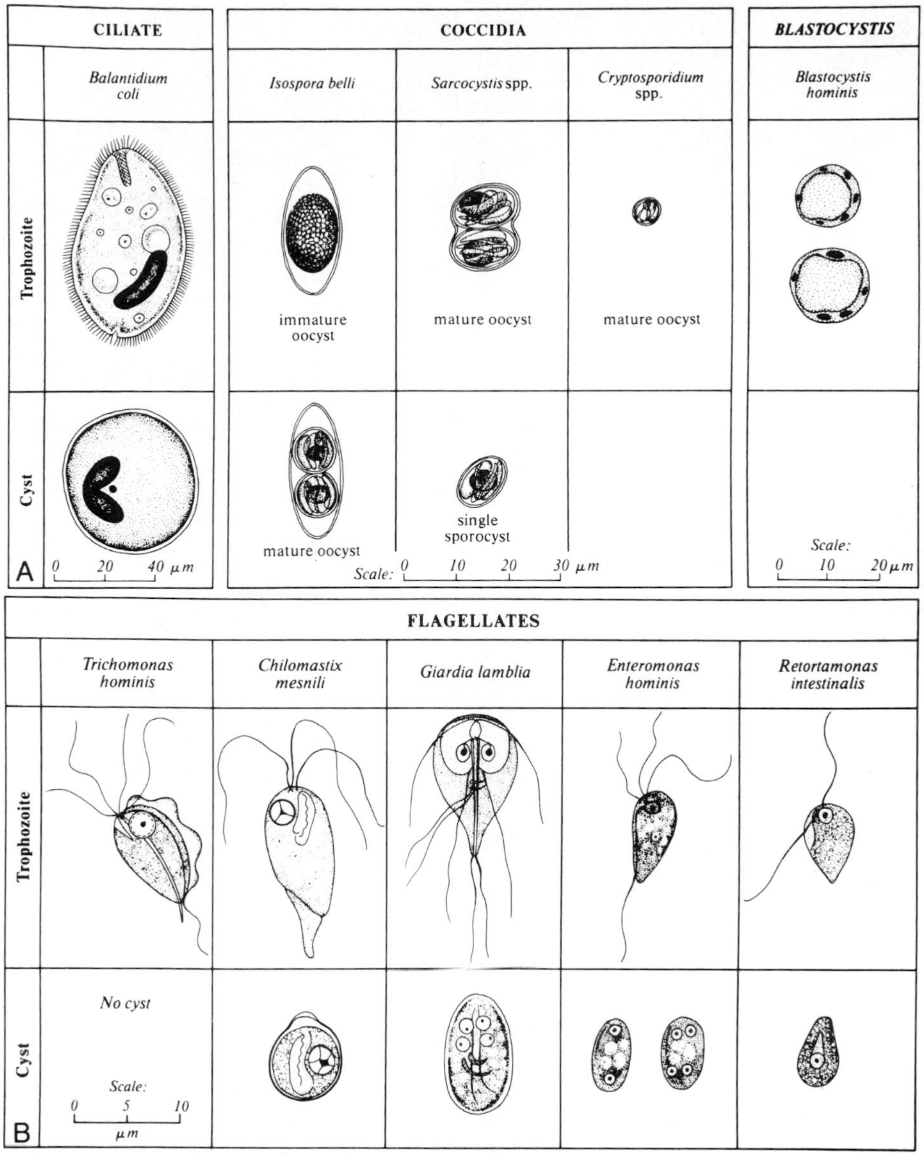

CILIATE	COCCIDIA			BLASTOCYSTIS
Balantidium coli	*Isospora belli*	*Sarcocystis* spp.	*Cryptosporidium* spp.	*Blastocystis hominis*

Trophozoite: immature oocyst (*Isospora belli*); mature oocyst (*Sarcocystis* spp.); mature oocyst (*Cryptosporidium* spp.)

Cyst: mature oocyst (*Isospora belli*); single sporocyst (*Sarcocystis* spp.)

Scale (Ciliate): 0 20 40 μm
Scale (Coccidia): 0 10 20 30 μm
Scale (Blastocystis): 0 10 20 μm

FLAGELLATES

Trichomonas hominis	*Chilomastix mesnili*	*Giardia lamblia*	*Enteromonas hominis*	*Retortamonas intestinalis*

Trophozoite row and **Cyst** row. For *Trichomonas hominis*: No cyst.

Scale: 0 5 10 μm

Figure 61–13 *A*, Ciliate, *Coccidia*, and *Blastocystis* spp. found in stool specimens of humans. *B*, Flagellates found in stool specimens of humans. (Adapted from Brooke MM, Melvin DM: Morphology of Diagnostic Stages of Intestinal Parasites of Man. Publication No. [CDC] 848116. Washington, DC, United States Department of Health and Human Services, 1984.)

and both trophozoites and cysts may be demonstrated in permanently stained slides. In some cases, the organisms cannot be demonstrated in fecal specimens, and small bowel aspirates or so-called string test specimens may be required. In such instances, the laboratory should be advised in advance so personnel will be available to perform a direct wet mount examination immediately on receipt of the specimen.

Many antigen detection methods based on immunofluorescence or EIA are commercially available (Garcia, 2001, 2003; Clinical and Laboratory Standards Institute, 2005). They appear to have good sensitivity and specificity, and may detect some infections not found by morphologic examination of stools. They also could be particularly helpful in epidemiologic investigations but they cannot replace the need for traditional morphologic examination of the specimen to detect other pathogenic parasites.

When viewed in their broadest dimension, *Giardia* trophozoites are pear-shaped with a tapered posterior end, and have two nuclei that give the appearance of a smiling face with prominent eyes (Table 61–11, Figs 61–13*B* and 61–14*C* to *E*). When viewed from the side, the anterior end of the organism is thicker and tapers posteriorly; the anterior half to three quarters consists of the sucking disk on the ventral surface. The four lateral, two ventral, and two caudal flagella usually are not evident in wet mounts or in stained preparations. Cysts are oval and usually quadrinucleate. Below the nuclei are dark-staining median bodies that cross longitudinal fibrils, providing distinctive internal characteristics. The cytoplasm often is retracted from the cyst wall.

Chilomatix mesnili

Chilomatix mesnili (Table 61–11, Figs 61–13*B* and 61–14*F*) is a nonpathogenic lumen-dwelling flagellate of humans that must be differentiated from trophozoites of amebae and *Giardia* in stained smears. The consistent location of the single nucleus at one end of the organism and the tapering of the end opposite the nucleus are helpful. If multiple organisms are examined, the cytostome and spiral groove are visible in some. The three external flagella are usually not visible in stained or formalin-fixed preparations. The lemon-shaped cysts contain various curved cytostomal fibers with a safety-pin-like appearance.

Pentatrichomonas hominis

Pentatrichomonas hominis, known previously as *Trichomonas hominis* (Table 61–11, Fig. 61–13*B*) is an infrequently seen nonpathogenic intestinal flagellate that may be confused with *E. hartmanni* or small *E. histolytica* trophozoites. Organisms do not stain particularly well and often are distorted in permanent smears. Several organisms may have to be examined in stained preparations in order to demonstrate the single *Entamoeba*-like nucleus, undulating membrane and associated costa, and flagella. A prominent rod-like object, the axostyle, runs through the organism and protrudes from the posterior end. No cyst stage has been described.

Trichomonas vaginalis

T. vaginalis is a common cause of vaginitis, characterized by inflammation, itching, vaginal discharge, and occasionally, dysuria. The infection usually is spread by sexual intercourse, often by males who have an asymptomatic infection. Occasionally, males may have symptomatic prostatitis or urethritis. *T. vaginalis* infections are usually diagnosed in the physician's office by direct wet mount examination of vaginal fluid, prostatic fluid, or sediments of freshly passed urine. Morphologically, *T. vaginalis* resembles *P. hominis* but is larger (up to 23 μm), and the undulating membrane extends only half the length of the body. Because of the difference in

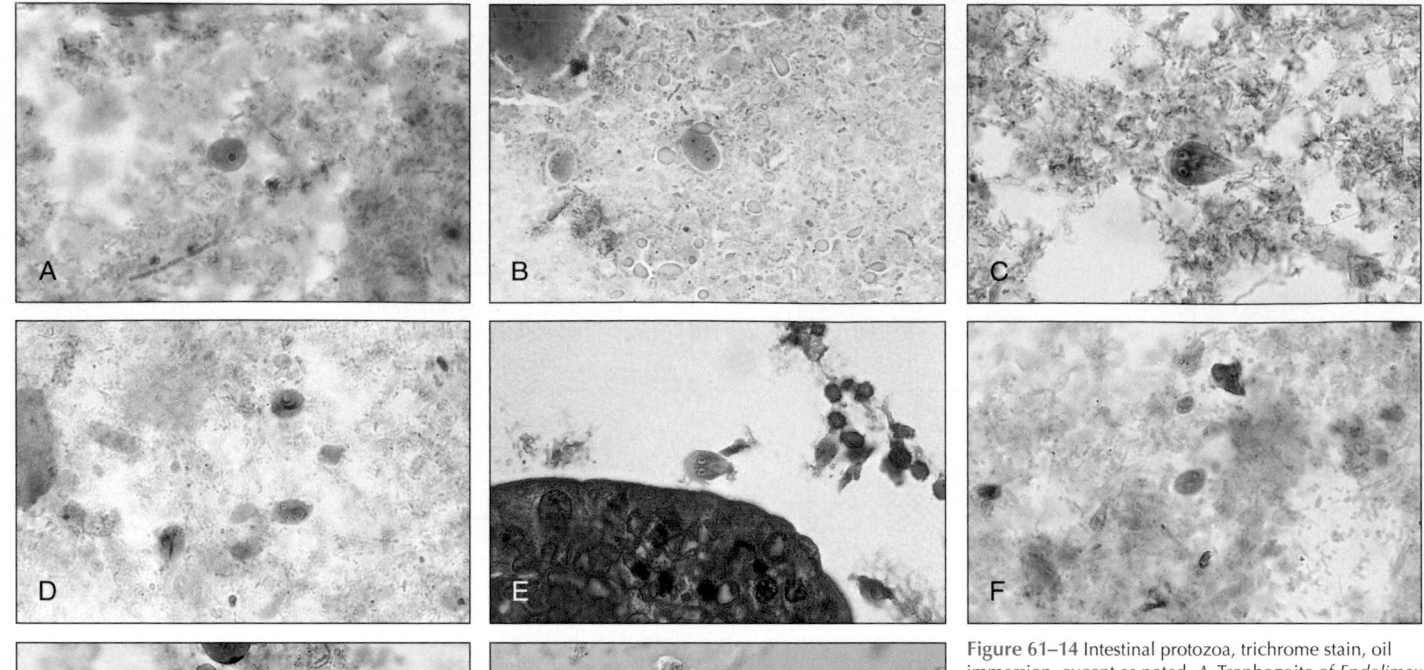

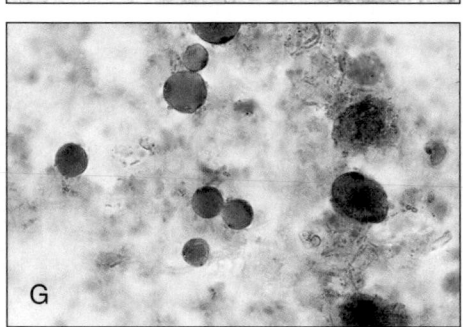

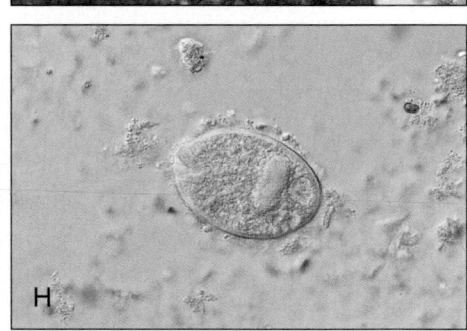

Figure 61–14 Intestinal protozoa, trichrome stain, oil immersion, except as noted. *A,* Trophozoite of *Endolimax nana. B,* Quadrinucleate cysts of *E. nana. C,* Trophozoite of *Giardia lamblia* displaying prominent nuclei, median bodies, flagellae and a tapered posterior end. *D,* Cysts of *G. lamblia* with nuclei and fibrils. *E,* Duodenal biopsy demonstrating a *G. lamblia* trophozoite (H&E). *F,* A lemon-shaped cyst of *Chilomastix mesnili* with visible nucleus and hyaline cap. *G,* Multiple central-vacuolar forms of *Blastocystis hominis. H,* Trophozoite of *Balantidium coli* in wet mount; note cilia covering the cell, cytostome, and macronucleus.

habitat, it generally is not necessary to differentiate these trichomonads morphologically.

Direct wet mount examination may be insensitive, and the use of culture or commercially available immunoassay techniques is recommended when the infection is not readily diagnosed (Garcia, 2001; Murray, 2003). Cultures, including use of a convenient 'pouch' system, have a sensitivity of about 90% (Krieger, 1988; Schmid, 1989; Beal, 1992; Levi, 1997), as do immunofluorescent and EIA techniques that use monoclonal antibodies (Krieger, 1988; Lisi, 1988; Wilson, 1995). Papanicolaou-stained gynecologic smears may reveal *T. vaginalis* on occasion but have poor sensitivity and specificity.

Other Flagellates

Enteromonas hominis and *Retortamonas intestinalis* are small, nonpathogenic, intestinal flagellates that are seen infrequently but, when present, may occur in large numbers. Morphologic characteristics are reviewed in Table 61–11 (see also Fig. 61–13*B*). *Trichomonas tenax* is a trichomonad that is occasionally recovered from the oral cavity but does not cause disease.

Ciliates

Balantidium coli

The ciliate *Balantidium coli* (Figs 61–13*A* and 61–14*H*) may cause a dysentery-like syndrome with colonic ulcerations similar to that of amebiasis, but does not produce liver abscesses or other systemic lesions. Human infection, rare in the United States, is usually acquired from hogs, which are commonly infected. *B. coli* is the largest protozoon to infect humans. Trophozoites are between 40 μm and over 200 μm in greatest dimension (most being 50–100 μm) and are uniformly covered with cilia that are slightly longer at the anterior end adjacent to the cytostome. There is a large macronucleus, which is readily seen in stained preparations, and a smaller micronucleus, which is infrequently visible. Numerous food vacuoles and contractile vacuoles are present in the cytoplasm. Cysts are rounded, measuring 50–70 μm in length. Cilia may be seen within younger cysts and nuclear characteristics are similar to those of trophozoites. Stool specimens that have been contaminated with stagnant

water may contain free-living ciliates, which usually can be distinguished from *B. coli* by differences in their ciliary pattern.

Coccidia

The coccidia comprise a large group of apicomplexan parasites that have a sexual stage in the intestinal tract of invertebrate and vertebrate animals. Some species also develop asexually in extraintestinal sites in host tissues. Genera infecting the intestine of humans, such as *Isospora, Sarcocystis, Cryptosporidium,* and *Cyclospora,* generally produce self-limited diarrheal disease in immunocompetent persons. Severe protracted diarrhea may develop in immunocompromised hosts following infection with *Isospora, Cryptosporidium,* and *Cyclospora.*

Isospora belli

Isospora belli undergoes both asexual and sexual development in the cytoplasm of small intestine epithelial cells (Fig. 61–15*A*). Sexual development results in the production of oocysts, which are passed in the stool and mature to the infective stage in the environment. Human infections cause diarrhea and malabsorption but are generally self-limited. In patients with AIDS or other immunosuppressive disorders, disease may persist for months or years, and may contribute to death (DeHovitz, 1986; Mannheimer, 1994; Murray, 2003). Diagnosis is established by finding the unsporulated oocysts measuring 12 × 30 μm in fecal specimens, usually in direct wet mounts or concentration preparations (Fig. 61–15*B*). If the unfixed specimen is left at room temperature for 24 to 48 hours, sporulation occurs. The infectious oocyst contains two sporocysts, each with four sporozoites (Fig. 61–13*A*). The oocysts, like those of *Cryptosporidium,* stain acid-fast.

Sarcocystis species

Sarcocystis spp. are typical two-host coccidia in which the sexual phase develops in the intestinal mucosa of carnivorous animals and the asexual, extraintestinal phase occurs in the muscles and tissues of various intermediate hosts. Humans may serve as either definitive or intermediate hosts, depending on the species of *Sarcocystis.* Intestinal infection with *Sarcocystis hominis* and *Sarcocystis suihominis* is acquired by ingestion of raw or incompletely cooked beef or pork, respectively, that contains tissue cysts

Table 61–11 Morphology of Intestinal Flagellates

Species	Size (Length)	Shape	Motility	Number of Nuclei	Number of Flagella*	Other Features
Trophozoites						
Pentatrichomonas hominis†	8–20 μm; usual range 11–12 μm	Pear shaped	Rapid, jerking	1 Not visible in unstained	3–5 anterior; 1 posterior	Undulating membrane extending length of body
Chilomastix mesnili	6–24 μm; usual range 10–15 μm	Pear shaped	Stiff, rotary	1 Not visible in unstained mounts	3 anterior; 1 in cytostome	Prominent cytostome extending 1/3–1/2. Spiral groove across ventral surface
Giardia lamblia	10–20 μm; usual range 12–15 μm	Pear shaped	Falling leaf	2 Not visible in unstained mounts	4 lateral; 2 ventral; 3 caudal	Sucking disk occupying 1/2–3/4 of ventral surface
Enteromonas hominis	4–10 μm; usual range 8–9 μm	Oval	Jerking	1 Not visible in unstained mounts	3 anterior; 1 posterior	One side of body flattened. Posterior flagellum extending free, posteriorly or laterally
Retortamonas intestinalis	4–9 μm; usual range 6–7 μm	Pear shaped or oval	Jerking	1 Not visible in unstained mounts	1 anterior 1 posterior	Prominent cytostome extending approximately 1/2 length of body

Species	Size	Shape	Number of Nuclei	Other Features
Cysts				
Chilomastix mesnili	6–10 μm; usual range 8–9 μm	Lemon shaped, with anterior hyaline knob or 'nipple'	1 Not visible in unstained preparations	Cytostome with supporting fibrils. Usually visible in stained preparations
Giardia lamblia	8–13 μm; usual range 11–12 μm	Oval or ellipsoidal	Usually 4. Not distinct in unstained preparations. Usually located at one end	Fibrils or flagella longitudinally in cyst. Cytoplasm often retracts from a portion of cell wall
Enteromonas hominis	4–10 μm; usual range 6–8 μm	Elongated or oval	1–4, usually 2 lying at opposite ends of cyst. Not visible in unstained mounts	Resembles *E. nana* cyst. Fibrils or flagella are usually not seen
Retortamonas intestinalis	4–9 μm; usual range 4–7 μm	Pear shaped or slightly lemon shaped	1 Not visible in unstained mounts	Resembles *Chilomastix* cyst. Shadow outline of cytostome with supporting fibrils extends above nucleus

* Not a practical feature for identification of species in routine fecal examinations. † *Pentatrichomonas hominis* does not have a cyst form.

Source: adapted from Brooke MM, Melvin DM: Morphology of Diagnostic Stages of Intestinal Parasites of Man. USDHEW PHS Publication No. 1966, 1969.

(sarcocysts). Infection usually is asymptomatic, but occasional patients have transient diarrhea, abdominal pain, or anorexia. Intestinal infection is self-limited because asexual multiplication occurs in the intermediate host and is not repeated in the definitive host. Oocyst production is limited by the number of organisms ingested in the form of sarcocysts. The diagnosis is established by detection of sporulated 25 × 33 μm sporocysts in the stools (Fig. 61–13A). Each mature sporocyst contains four sporozoites. The oocyst wall is thin and often not detectable, or has already ruptured, releasing the two sporocysts. These forms, best seen in wet mounts or acid-fast-stained smears, appear larger than oocysts of *Cryptosporidium*. Trichrome stains are of little value in detecting these parasites. Humans also may serve as intermediate hosts for several unnamed animal species of *Sarcocystis* (known collectively as *Sarcocystis lindemanni*), in which case cysts are found in skeletal and cardiac muscles (Beaver, 1979; Strickland, 2000).

Cryptosporidium species

Cryptosporidium spp. use a single host in their life cycle but may infect humans (predominantly *C. hominis* and *C. parvum*) and a wide variety of animals, including cattle and sheep (Coupe, 2005). Parasites develop in the brush border of epithelial cells of the small and large intestine and occasionally spread to other sites such as the gallbladder, the pancreas, and the respiratory tract (Figs 61–13A and 61–15C and D). *Cryptosporidium* is a common cause of acute, self-limited diarrhea in normal persons, especially in children who attend day-care. The epidemiology of cryptosporidiosis is similar to that of giardiasis. One of the largest known outbreaks of water-transmitted infection occurred in Milwaukee, Wisconsin, in 1993. In that outbreak, an estimated 400 000 individuals became ill from tap water contaminated with farm runoff following heavy rains (MacKenzie, 1994). Like cysts of *Giardia*, *Cryptosporidium* oocysts are refractory to usual chlorination levels of drinking water, and unless a community's water supply from a surface source is filtered, epidemics may occur. In patients with AIDS, *Cryptosporidium* may cause chronic secretory diarrhea that can last for months to years and may contribute to death. The incubation period is about 8 days and, in previously healthy persons,

the illness lasts 9–23 days. Patients may have malaise, fever, anorexia, abdominal cramps, and diarrhea (Current, 1991; Mannheimer, 1994).

Diagnosis usually is established by stool examination. Various concentration methods including formalin-ethyl acetate sedimentation and Sheather's sugar flotation work well (Garcia, 2001; Clinical and Laboratory Standards Institute, 2005). The availability of the formalin–ethyl acetate method makes this technique attractive, although centrifugation speed and times must be increased to maximize recovery (Isenberg, 2004; Clinical and Laboratory Standards Institute, 2005). A smear is prepared from the sediment and stained with an acid-fast stain or immunofluorescent reagents. Several acid-fast staining methods, including auramine-O, have been evaluated, but a modified cold Kinyoun method is most widely used. The spherical oocysts measure 4–6 μm in diameter and, when stained by the modified Kinyoun procedure, appear a deep fuchsia, although there is some unevenness of staining intensity and variability in the percentage of cysts that stain positive. Positive control slides must be used with every run.

Commercial immunofluorescent and EIA reagents, which provide good sensitivity and specificity (Garcia, 2003; Murray, 2003; Clinical and Laboratory Standards Institute, 2005), are especially good for laboratories where *Cryptosporidium* is infrequently encountered and where there is difficulty in maintaining expertise in the interpretation of the acid-fast stains.

The need to examine stool specimens for *Cryptosporidium* depends on the populations served and the goals, interests, and abilities of the individual laboratory. Some laboratories perform examination for *Cryptosporidium* only on specific request, and others evaluate all specimens from immunocompromised patients.

Cyclospora cayetanensis

Cyclospora cayetanensis is a recently described coccidian parasite responsible for diarrheal disease in immunocompetent and immunocompromised individuals (Ortega, 1994; Murray, 2003). The parasite has been recovered from patients in several countries, including the United States, and was initially described as a blue-green alga, cyanobacterium-like body, or coccidian-like body, among others (Ortega, 1993; Shields, 2003). Infection

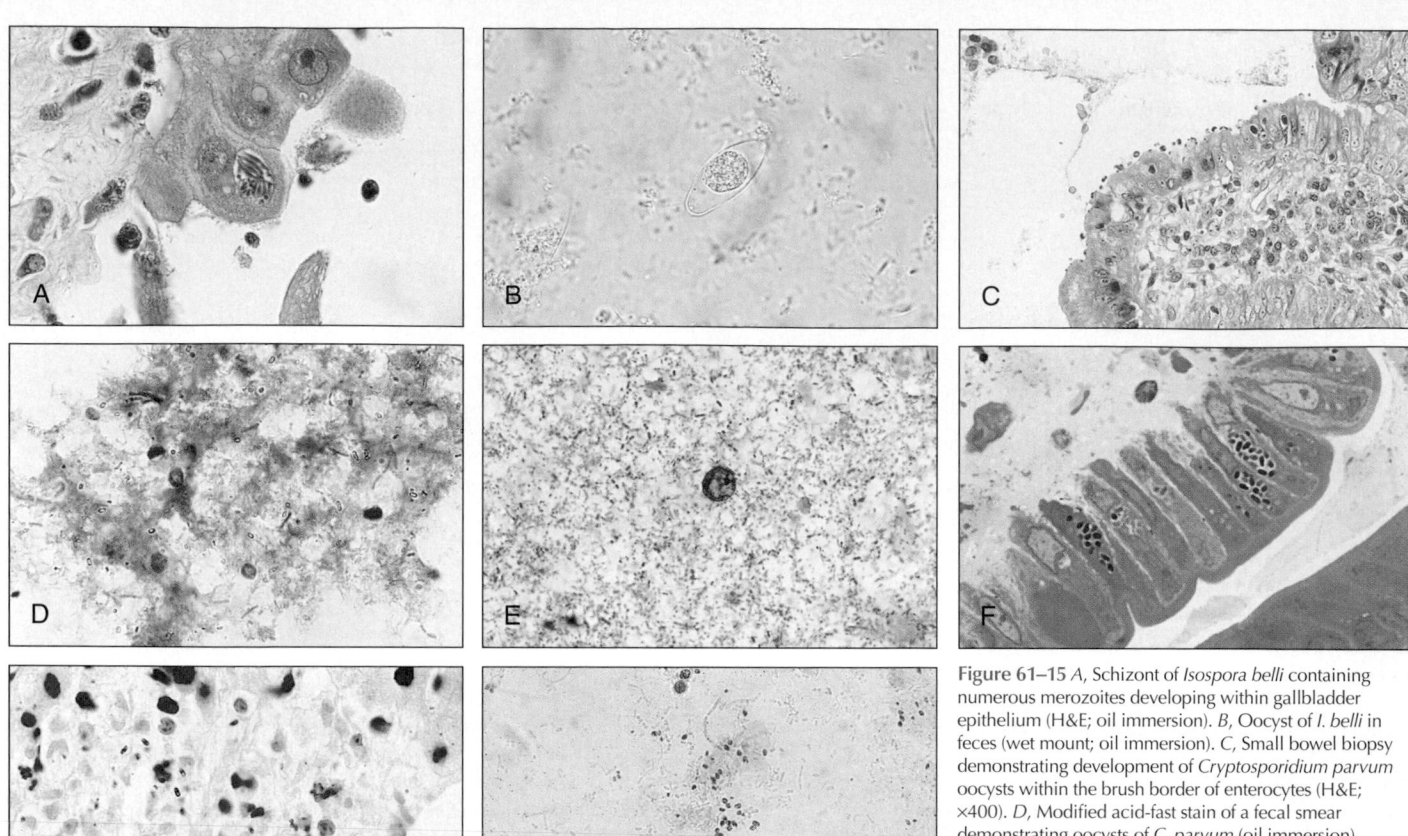

Figure 61–15 *A*, Schizont of *Isospora belli* containing numerous merozoites developing within gallbladder epithelium (H&E; oil immersion). *B*, Oocyst of *I. belli* in feces (wet mount; oil immersion). *C*, Small bowel biopsy demonstrating development of *Cryptosporidium parvum* oocysts within the brush border of enterocytes (H&E; ×400). *D*, Modified acid-fast stain of a fecal smear demonstrating oocysts of *C. parvum* (oil immersion). *E*, Modified acid-fast stain of a fecal smear demonstrating an oocyst of *Cyclospora cayetanensis* (oil immersion). *F*, Small bowel biopsy demonstrating development of microsporidial spores within enterocytes (epoxy-embedded section stained with toluidine blue; oil immersion). *G*, Microsporidial spores seen in liver parenchyma in an individual infected with the human immunodeficiency virus (Brown and Brenn stain; oil immersion). *H*, Numerous microsporidial spores in feces stained with the modified trichrome stain (oil immersion).

causes a flu-like illness with nausea, vomiting, weight loss, and explosive watery diarrhea lasting 1–3 weeks. Oocysts, passed unsporulated, appear as nonrefractile spheres 8–10 μm in diameter that contain a cluster of refractile globules enclosed within a membrane when viewed by light microscopy. 1–2 weeks are required for sporulation, after which the mature oocyst contains two sporocysts, each with two sporozoites. In trichrome-stained smears, the oocysts appear as clear, round, and somewhat wrinkled objects. Oocysts autofluoresce bright green to intense blue under ultraviolet epifluorescence and stain acid fast using modified acid-fast or auramine-O staining techniques. They must be differentiated from oocysts of *Cryptosporidium*, which stain in an identical fashion but are smaller (4–6 μm) (Fig. 61-15*E*).

Microsporidia

Microsporidia are obligate intracellular, spore-forming protozoan parasites in the phylum Microspora that infect a variety of animals, including humans (Shadduck, 1989; Franzen, 1999). They are serious pathogens in immunocompromised hosts, especially those with AIDS, in whom they are responsible for a large percentage (up to 30% in some studies) of otherwise unexplained diarrheal disease (Curry, 1993). *Enterocytozoon bieneusi* and *Encephalitozoon intestinalis*, the two species implicated most commonly in human intestinal infection, may cause protracted diarrhea and weight loss in AIDS patients similar to that caused by *Cryptosporidium*. *E. intestinalis* may also cause disseminated disease (Cali, 1993; Willson, 1995; Murray, 2003).

The organisms multiply intracellularly (merogony) and form resistant spores (sporogony) that eventually rupture the host cell and infect adjacent cells or are passed out of the body. The spore contains a coiled polar tubule, which is forcefully extruded under appropriate environmental stimuli and penetrates the membrane of the recipient cell. The parasite's sporoplasm is injected through the tubule into the host cell cytoplasm, where multiplication ensues. Reservoir hosts have not been identified. Occasionally, patients have been infected by other genera of microsporidia,

including *Encephalitozoon* (hepatitis, ocular infections, CNS disease), *Nosema* (disseminated infections), and *Pleistophora* (myositis) (Shadduck, 1989; Curry, 1993), among others (Franzen, 1999).

Until recently, diagnosis required examination of tissues submitted for routine light (Fig. 61-15*F* and *G*) and electron microscopy. Development of a modified trichrome staining method for examination of stool specimens for spores has been a significant advance in detecting infection (Weber, 1992). With this method, the small (1.5–3 μm), elliptical spores stain red against a faint green background, and some display a characteristic midbody cross-band (Fig. 61-15*H*). Modifications of this method have also been described. Fluorochrome stains such as Uvitex 2B and Calcofluor white appear to be more sensitive in detecting spores and may be useful in the initial screening of specimens (van Gool, 1993; DeGirolami, 1995; Luna, 1995). The small size of the spores makes detection by any method a challenge (Clinical and Laboratory Standards Institute, 2005).

Intestinal Helminths

Intestinal helminths covered here include those nematodes (roundworms), cestodes (tapeworms), and trematodes (flukes) that either reside as adults in the gastrointestinal tract or live in other locations (liver, lung, or blood) and produce eggs that exit the human body via the intestinal tract. Sizes for adult helminths vary from 1 mm to over 10 m in length; sizes for eggs range from 25–150 μm (Fig. 61–16).

An understanding of helminth life cycles and zoogeography is critical in knowing which parasite stages may be present in a presumed infection, what organs or tissues may be involved, and when diagnostic stages may be expected to appear following exposure. Although diagnosis usually depends on finding and identifying an appropriate developmental stage (egg, larva, or adult), some parasitic infections may be diagnosed chiefly on clinical grounds or on the basis of serologic evidence, or both.

Certain species have developmental cycles whereby infectious stages may be transmitted directly from person to person (*Enterobius* and *H.*

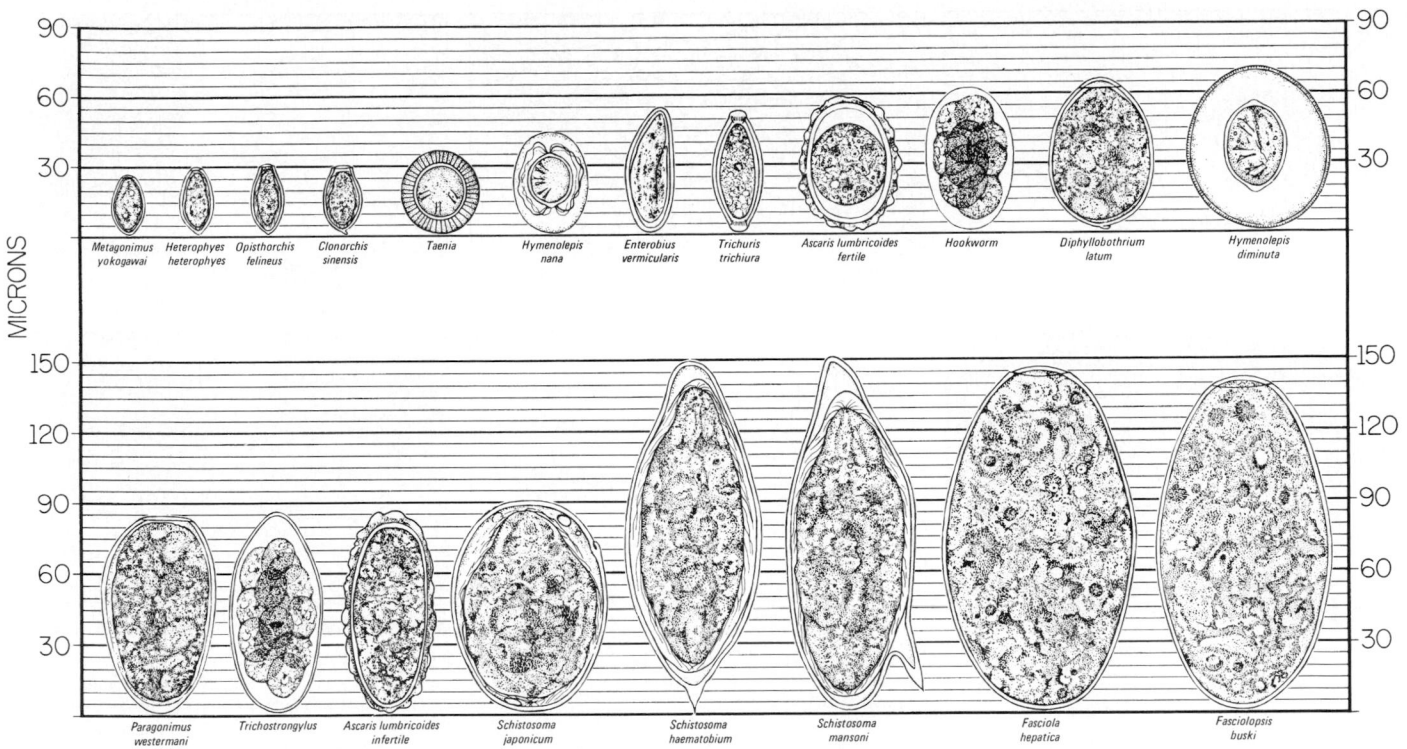

Figure 61–16 Relative sizes of helminth eggs. (Courtesy of Centers for Disease Control, Parasitology Training Branch, Atlanta, GA.)

nana). In others (*Trichuris*, *Ascaris*, and *Trichostrongylus*), an additional maturation period outside of the host is required before the parasite egg or larvae (in the latter case) is infectious. Ingestion of infective stages may also occur incidentally along with parasite vectors (*Dipylidium*, *Hymenolepis*), plants (*Fasciolopsis*, *Fasciola*), or animal tissues (*Trichinella*, *Taenia*, *Diphyllobothrium*, *Clonorchis*, *Opisthorchis*, *Paragonimus*, *Heterophyes*, *Metagonimus*, and *Nanophyetus*). In some cases, larval parasite stages may directly penetrate the skin (hookworms, *Strongyloides*, and schistosomes).

Recovery and identification of helminth eggs and larvae in stool, urine, or sputum requires a systematic approach and appropriate training of the individuals performing the evaluations. The size of the eggs and larvae is an especially important characteristic and often requires use of a properly calibrated ocular micrometer. External characteristics of eggs that should be noted include their shape, wall thickness, and the presence or absence of a mamillated covering, operculum, opercular shoulders, abopercular knob, polar plugs, or spines. Egg development (embryonated, unembryonated) and the presence or absence of hooklets, which are characteristic of cestodes, should also be noted. The examiner also needs to have an appreciation for the large variety of artifacts detected in human feces that may mimic parasite eggs and larvae (Table 61–4).

Nematodes

Enterobius vermicularis

Enterobiasis or oxyuriasis is the most common helminthic infection in children of all social strata in the United States. Although it is primarily a parasite of young children, rapid maturation of the egg allows it to be readily transmitted from child to child and from child to adult, in both family and institutional settings. Male and female worms reside primarily in the cecum and adjacent areas. Females measure up to 13 mm in length and have a pointed posterior end that gives rise to their common name, the pinworm. Both sexes have prominent lateral alae that are seen in cross-section and a prominent esophageal bulb (Fig. 61–17A to C).

Although males are rarely seen, females may be found on the surface of a stool specimen or on the perianal skin, especially at night, where eggs are deposited. Eggs are colorless, ovoid with one side flattened, and measure 20–40 μm wide by 50–60 μm long (Fig. 61–17B). They are infective within hours and, when ingested, complete development to the gravid adult stage within 1 month (the prepatent period).

Although infection may be asymptomatic, children often suffer from pruritus ani, irritability, and loss of sleep. Enterobiasis should be ruled out early in the evaluation of enuresis. Adult worms may also migrate to unusual sites such as the vagina, fallopian tubes, or peritoneal cavity. Their

ultimate death in these locations may provoke inflammatory, granulomatous reactions (Symmers, 1950; Garcia, 2003).

Recovery of eggs or, less commonly, adults from the perianal skin is usually done using the cellulose tape technique after the child has gone to sleep or first thing in the morning (Ash, 1987; Garcia, 2001). Only 5–10% of cases are detected using routine stool examination. Diagnosis may require examination of several samples taken on different days before eggs can be detected (Sadun, 1956).

Trichuris trichiura

Trichuriasis is common worldwide in tropical and subtropical regions. Adult worms are found in the large intestine, especially the cecum, but in heavy infections they can be found throughout the colon and rectum. Males and females measure up to 50 mm in length and remain attached to the intestinal mucosa by the long, slender anterior end, while the thicker posterior end hangs free in the lumen. Female worms are elongate, whereas the tails on males are coiled (Fig. 61–17D). *Trichuris* has a direct life cycle in which eggs are passed in stool unembryonated and require several weeks under appropriate soil conditions to mature to the infective stage. When embryonated eggs are ingested, larvae are released and mature into adults in the colon, where they attach and survive up to 10 years.

Light infections usually are asymptomatic, but when larger numbers (>300 worms) are present, diarrhea or symptoms of dysentery may develop in association with dehydration and anemia (Beaver, 1984; Strickland, 2000). Rectal prolapse, a life-threatening complication, may occur in heavily infected children (Cooper, 1988).

Diagnosis is made by finding the typical eggs in direct fecal smears or with concentration techniques. The eggs are barrel-shaped with refractile plugs at both ends and usually measure 50–55 μm long by 22–24 μm wide (Fig. 61–17E). Occasionally, humans may become infected with the dog whipworm, *Trichuris vulpis*, which has eggs that are larger, wider, and more barrel shaped than those of *Trichuris trichiura*. Egg quantitation techniques may occasionally be requested to assess infection intensity, therapeutic efficacy, and reacquisition rate of parasites.

Capillaria philippinensis

This parasite, normally found in fish-eating birds, infects humans who ingest raw or incompletely cooked fish that contain infective larvae in their flesh. Although first described in persons from the Philippines, and later Thailand, occasional cases have also been reported elsewhere in Asia, the Middle East, and South America (Cross, 1992; Murray, 2003). The parasites may cause chronic diarrhea, and infected individuals may pass eggs, larvae, and even adult worms in their feces. Eggs resemble those of *Trichuris*, although they measure 36–45 μm in length by 21 μm in width; have thick, radially striated shells; and mucoid plugs, which are inconspicuous.

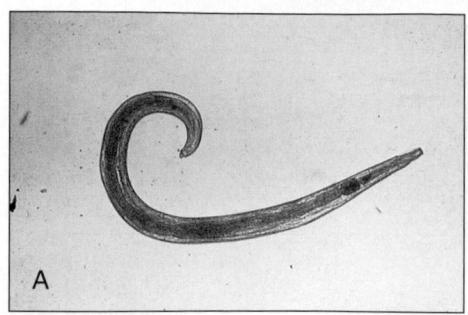
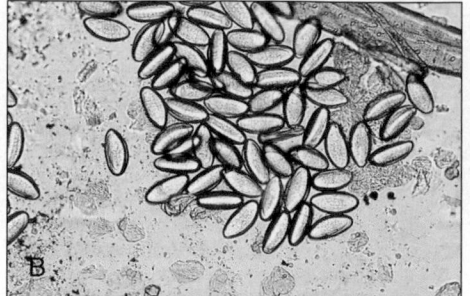
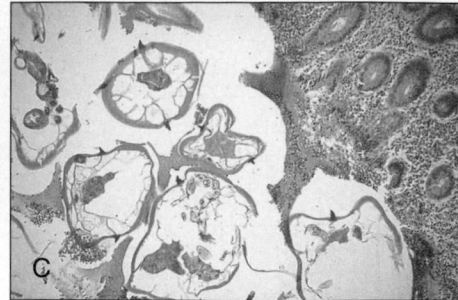
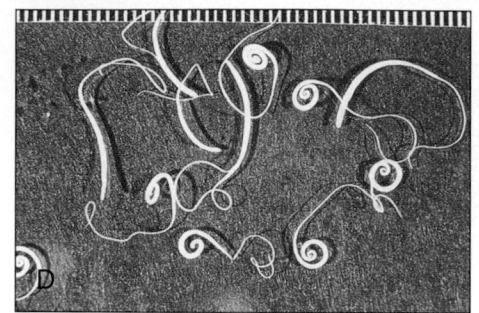
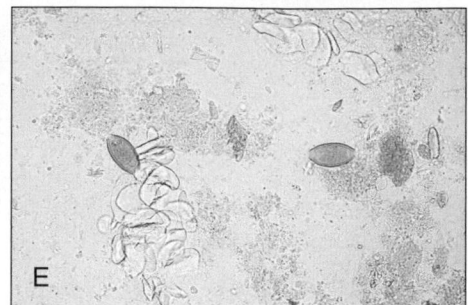
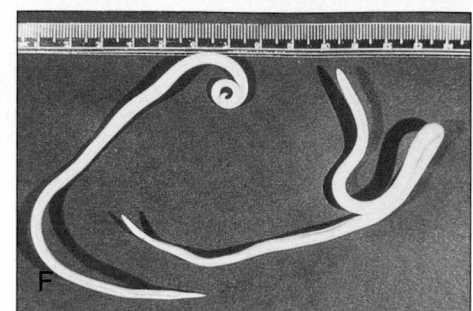
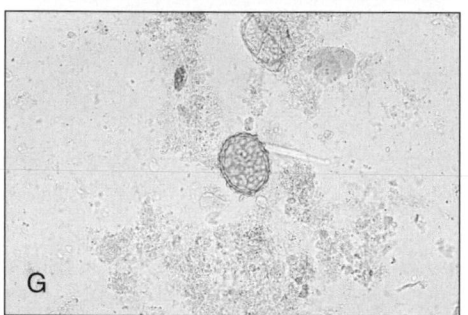
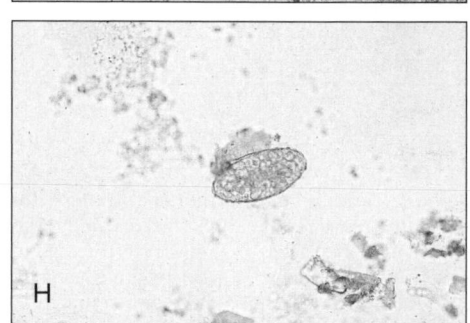

Figure 61–17 All direct examination with brightfield illumination except as noted. *A,* Adult male pinworm, *Enterobius vermicularis,* with curved posterior end; note prominent esophageal bulb (×4). *B,* Numerous eggs of *E. vermicularis* as seen on a Cellophane tape preparation (×400). *C,* Adult *E. vermicularis* in the appendix; note characteristic lateral alae (×100). *D,* Adult whipworms, *Trichuris trichiura;* note females with straight tails and males with coiled tails. *E,* Eggs of *T. trichiura* (×400). *F,* Adult female and male *Ascaris lumbricoides,* the large human roundworm. *G,* Fertile, unembryonated egg of *A. lumbricoides* (×400). *H,* Infertile and decorticate egg of *A. lumbricoides* (×400). (*D* and *F* from *A Pictorial Presentation of Parasites: A cooperative collection,* prepared and/or edited by H. Zaiman.)

Ascaris lumbricoides

This is the largest nematode that infects the intestinal tract of humans and is probably the most common of the intestinal roundworms, infecting an estimated 1.3 billion individuals worldwide (Markell, 1999). Infection occurs primarily in areas with little or no sanitation and, like *Trichuris,* is especially common in children, who are also more likely to harbor heavy infections.

Adult *Ascaris* live primarily in the duodenum and proximal jejunum. Females measure up to 35 cm in length by 6 mm in diameter. The male is somewhat smaller and has a ventrally curved tail, unlike the female (Fig. 61–17*F*). Both adult and immature worms can be identified by the presence of three prominent lips at the anterior end.

Females produce approximately 200 000 eggs per day, which are unembryonated when passed and require 4–6 weeks in a satisfactory environment to become infective. Following ingestion, eggs hatch in the intestine and larvae penetrate the mucosa to gain access to the blood stream. They are carried to the lungs and mature briefly in the alveolar capillary bed before entering the alveoli. Respiratory clearance mechanisms move the larvae to the epiglottis, where they are then swallowed and grow to adulthood in the small bowel. Development from embryonated egg to adult takes approximately 2 months.

Symptoms of ascariasis vary from asymptomatic infection to severe disease. Migration of large numbers of larvae through the lungs can cause *Ascaris* pneumonitis or Löffler syndrome, characterized by bilateral diffuse, mottled pulmonary infiltrates and mild bronchitis associated with peripheral eosinophilia. The syndrome is rare and usually occurs in individuals who have been previously exposed to *Ascaris* antigens.

The presence of a few worms in the intestine is rarely noticed, whereas heavy infections may produce varying degrees of abdominal pain and diarrhea. Intestinal obstruction may also occur with a mass of worms, especially in children. Even a small number of worms is cause for concern because of their ability to invade ectopic sites such as the common bile duct and liver, appendix, and stomach. Fever or drug therapy may stimulate migration. In endemic areas, anthelmintics often are prescribed prior to the use of anesthetics in elective surgery.

Infection is diagnosed by demonstrating eggs in feces or on recovery of an adult that has been passed or vomited. The large number of eggs produced every day makes detection of even a single worm probable. A count of fewer than 20 eggs per slide (2 mg of feces) indicates light infection, and a count of over 100 eggs per slide indicates heavy infection.

Fertile *Ascaris* eggs are round to slightly oval with a yellow-brown, irregular external mamillated layer and a thick shell. Eggs that have lost their mamillated layer are called decorticate and may superficially resemble hookworm eggs. They are passed unembryonated and measure approximately 55–75 μm long by 35–50 μm wide (Fig. 61–17*G* and *H*). Single females may produce unfertilized eggs, which are larger and more elongate (up to 90 μm in length) and have a thinner shell with irregular mamillations. These eggs are filled with irregularly sized fat globules.

Trichostrongylus spp.

Human disease caused by *Trichostrongylus* spp. represents a zoonotic infection because these parasites principally infect large herbivores such as sheep, cattle, and goats. Several species may infect humans, including *Trichostrongylus colubriformis, Trichostrongylus orientalis, Trichostrongylus axei,* and *Trichostrongylus brevis,* which are found in many parts of the world. Adult worms inhabit the small bowel and produce eggs that mature outside of the body. Larvae emerge and crawl about on soil and vegetation, where they are available to be ingested by definitive hosts. Unlike hookworms, they do not invade skin directly, nor does the life cycle involve a migratory phase through the lungs. Infections usually are light and asymptomatic, but heavy infections may produce abdominal pain and diarrhea, usually with eosinophilia. Eggs resemble those of hookworms but are longer and narrower, measuring 78–98 μm by 40–50 μm, and are slightly tapered at one end.

Hookworms

Hookworms, which are among the more common helminths known to infect humans, occur in tropical and subtropical regions and some temperate areas. *Necator americanus* is found in the United States and other areas of the world and frequently overlaps in distribution with *Ancylostoma duodenale,* which does not occur in the United States.

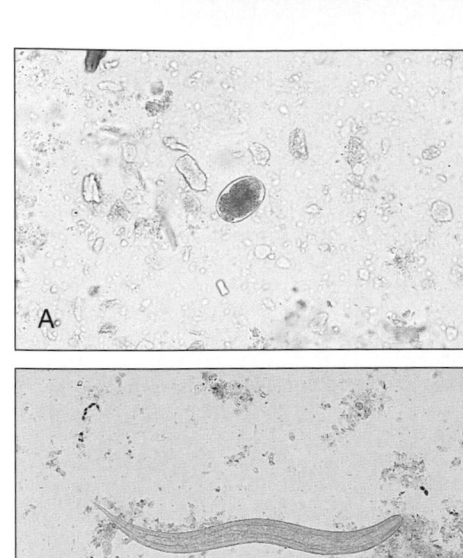
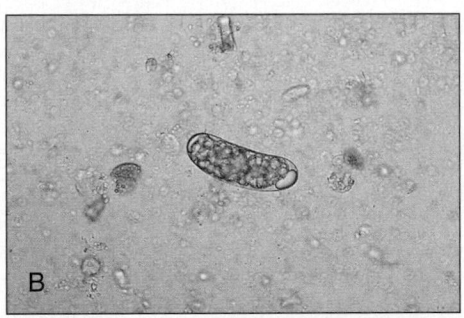
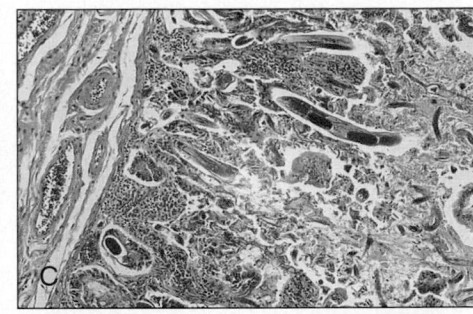
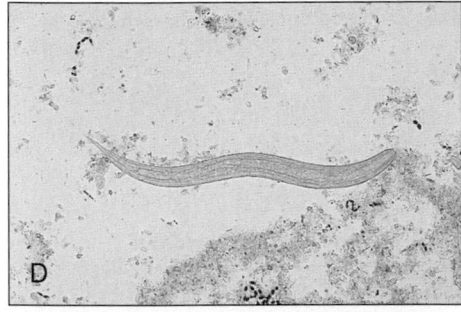
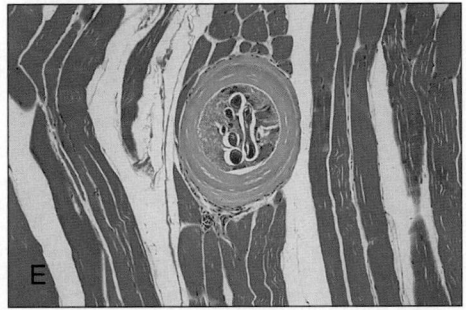
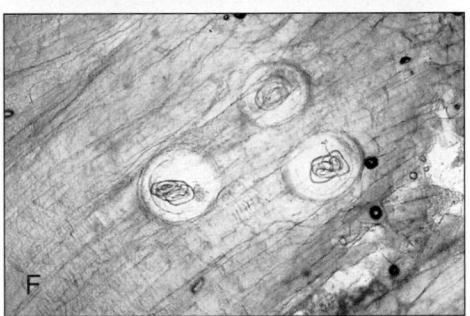
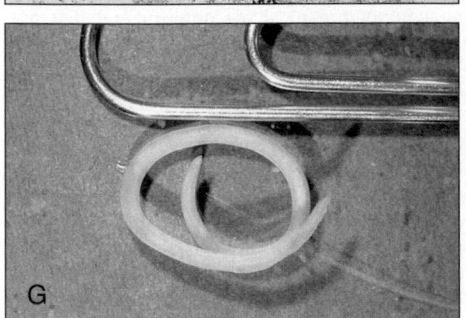
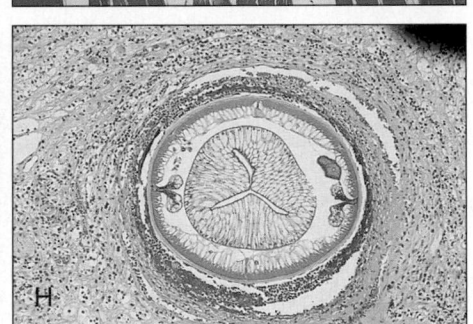

Figure 61–18 *A*, Hookworm (*Ancylostoma duodenale* or *Necator americanus*) egg (×400) *B*, Egg of *Heterodera* sp., a group of plant nematodes occasionally found as artifacts in human stool following ingestion of infected vegetables (×400). *C*, Massive *Strongyloides stercoralis* infection in the duodenal mucosa; note presence of adult female, eggs and larvae (H&E; ×100). *D*, *S. stercoralis* noninfectious rhabditiform larva (iodine stain, ×100). *E*, *Trichinella spiralis*, cross-section of a larva in gastrocnemius muscle (H&E; ×100). *F*, Multiple *T. spiralis* larvae in bear meat (compressed wet muscle preparation; ×100). *G*, Regurgitated *Pseudoterranova* sp. following fish dinner (×4). *H*, *Anisakis* sp., cross-section of larva found in small bowel following surgery for acute obstruction (H&E; ×400).

Adult females measure up to 12 mm in length and the males slightly less. Males are readily distinguished by the fan-shaped copulatory bursa at the posterior end. The anterior end of hookworms is modified into a buccal capsule that contains either teeth or cutting plates. Both sexes attach to the mucosa of the small intestine, where they may reside for up to 18 years (Beaver, 1988; Garcia, 2001).

Eggs are passed in feces and develop rapidly, depending on prevailing conditions. Rhabditiform larvae are released and develop into the infective filariform stage in about 7 days. On contact with an appropriate host, the larvae penetrate the skin, gain access to the host's circulation, travel to the lungs, and move up the tracheobronchial tree to be swallowed. On maturation in the small intestine, oviposition begins. Although the life cycles of both species are similar, *Ancylostoma* can mature directly to the adult stage in the intestine if the infective larvae are ingested.

Hookworms can produce disease in the skin, at the site of larval penetration. This condition, known as ground itch, is characterized by inflammation, redness, and blister formation, along with intense itching. Migration of large numbers of larvae through the lungs may produce Löffler syndrome, as described earlier for *Ascaris*. Depending on the worm burden, intestinal infection can result in gastroenteritis with abdominal pain, diarrhea, and nausea. Hookworms are best known, however, for their ability to produce chronic blood loss with secondary iron deficiency anemia. The presence of each adult *A. duodenale* can result in the loss of 0.15–0.25 mL of blood per day, compared with 0.03 mL for each *N. americanus*. Development of children can be severely affected with chronic infections. Blood loss and number of hookworms present correlate with the number of eggs per gram of stool, which may help determine when to initiate therapy in individuals living in endemic areas (Layrisse, 1964a, 1964b; Cook, 2002).

Diagnosis is made by finding the characteristic thin-shelled eggs in feces. The eggs are partially embryonated when passed and measure 58–76 μm in length by 36–40 μm wide (Fig. 61–18*A*). Embryonated eggs or free rhabditiform larvae may be found in unpreserved specimens that are not examined promptly. Hookworm rhabditiforms can be differentiated from those of *S. stercoralis* because the former have a longer buccal chamber and inconspicuous genital primordium (Fig. 61–19). Continued maturation of

larvae results in the appearance of infective filariforms, which have a pointed posterior end and an esophagus approximately one fourth the length of the larva. Hookworm eggs may need to be differentiated from those of *Trichostrongylus* spp. (which are longer and more pointed) and those of plant parasitic nematodes, especially *Heterodera* spp. (which are longer, have blunt ends, and are often asymmetric) (Fig. 61–18*B*).

Although adult hookworms can be differentiated on the basis of their mouth parts and the copulatory bursa in males, eggs of human hookworms are indistinguishable. In direct wet mounts, egg counts of fewer than five eggs per coverslip denote light infections that are unlikely to result in anemia, whereas more than 25 denote heavy infections that are likely to be associated with symptoms.

Strongyloides stercoralis

Strongyloidiasis occurs in many areas in the tropics and subtropics but the infection also occurs in temperate zones and has historically been endemic in areas of the southeastern United States. Adult females are 2–3 mm long and live buried in the mucosa of the duodenum, where they reproduce parthenogenetically (Fig. 61–18*C*). Parasitic males do not occur in the vertebrate phase of the cycle. The eggs hatch primarily in the small bowel, releasing first-stage or rhabditoid larvae, which are then passed in the feces (eggs are almost never found). In this direct cycle, the rhabditoid larvae metamorphose into infective third-stage filariform larvae in the soil. These infective larvae readily penetrate the skin of exposed individuals and migrate via the circulatory system to the lungs and then move up the bronchial tree and are swallowed. Development to the adult stage is then completed in the small intestine. Under appropriate soil conditions of high humidity, an indirect cycle may appear transiently in which the newly deposited larvae develop into a free-living generation consisting of reproductive males and females. Eggs produced by this generation develop into filariform larvae that are again infective for humans. A third variation in the life cycle of *Strongyloides* involves autoinfection, in which maturation to the filariform stage is completed within the intestinal tract, with subsequent reinvasion of bowel mucosa or perianal skin.

Disease presentation is variable and may depend on the strain acquired (Genta, 1989). Early migration of filariform larvae may produce irritation,

VII

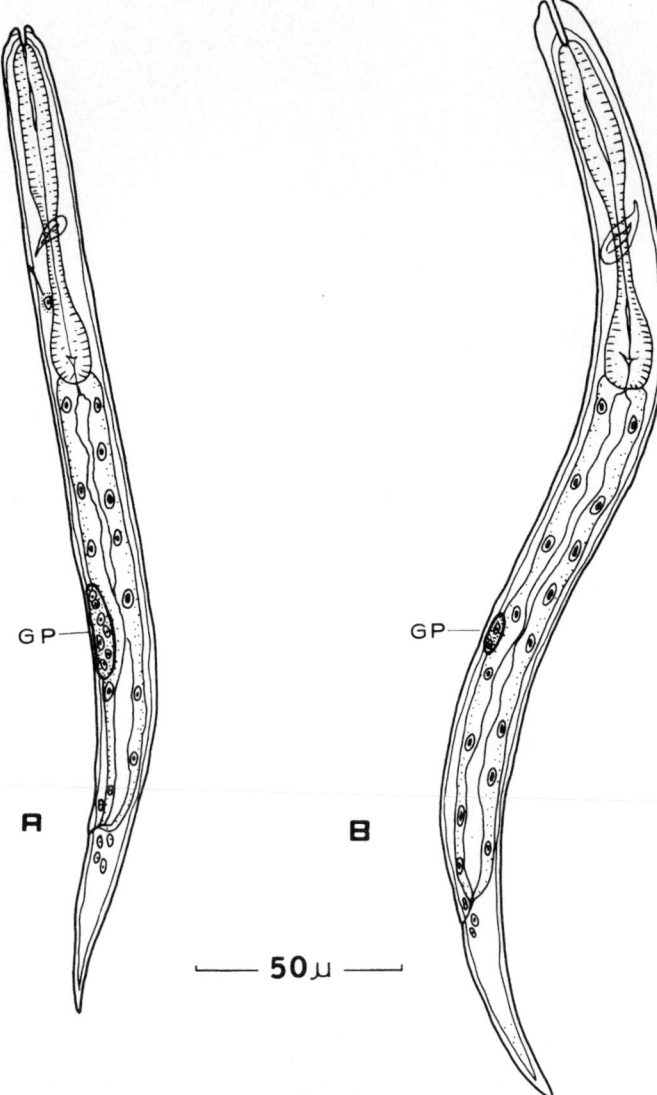

GP

GP

A

B

——— **50 μ** ———

Figure 61–19 Hookworm and *Strongyloides stercoralis* larvae. *A, S. stercoralis* rhabditoid larva in human stools. Note the short size of the buccal cavity and the large genital primordium (GP). *B,* Hookworm rhabditoid larva as seen in a few instances in stools left for at least 24 hours at room temperature. The buccal cavity is longer, and the genital primordium is smaller.

redness, and pruritus at the site of entry, whereas later migration through the lungs may produce Löffler syndrome (Purtilo, 1974). The presence of intestinal symptoms is related to the intensity of the infection. The affected individual may have symptoms of peptic ulcer, abdominal pain, and diarrhea. A malabsorption syndrome has been reported with chronic infection.

The ability of the parasite to autoinfect may result in persistence of the infection for decades, as was recognized in allied troops who were held as prisoners of war in south-east Asia during World War II (Gill, 1979). In otherwise healthy patients, autoinfection may produce larva currens (linear urticarial lesions). In immunocompromised, alcoholic, or malnourished patients, autoinfection may result in a life-threatening hyperinfection syndrome from the rapid multiplication of the parasite (Maayen, 1987; Genta, 1992). Severe pneumonia is often a presenting manifestation of hyperinfection, followed by marked diarrhea, enteritis, and septicemia. Patients who have lived in endemic areas should be screened for *Strongyloides* prior to receiving immunosuppressive therapy (Strickland, 2000).

Diagnosis is made on recovery and identification of typical rhabditiform larvae in stool specimens, although the routine O & P examination does not always reveal their presence (Fig. 61–18*D*) (Pelletier, 1988; Genta, 1989; Garcia, 2001). *Strongyloides* rhabditiform larvae must be differentiated from those of hookworms and are characterized by having a short buccal cavity and a prominent genital primordium (Fig. 61–19). *Strongyloides* filariform larvae have a notched tail and an esophagus approximately half the length of the body. Either stage of larvae are readily

seen in fresh saline wet mounts under low power. If the infective filariform larvae are detected in a recently passed specimen, then the diagnosis of superinfection is warranted (Eveland, 1975).

Examination of duodenal aspirates or string test specimens may be helpful in suspicious cases in which routine stool examinations are nonproductive. The Baermann funnel concentration method or one of the coproculture techniques (see earlier under Laboratory Methods) may also demonstrate the infection (Ash, 1987; Genta, 1989; Garcia, 1999; Clinical and Laboratory Standards Institute, 2005). Larvae may be found in sputum or other pulmonary specimens, especially in the hyperinfection syndrome. Serologic tests are useful when infection is suspected but cannot be demonstrated by other methods. EIA and other tests display good sensitivity and specificity, although crossreactions may appear with filariasis and some other nematode infections. These tests generally do not differentiate between past and current infection but may be useful in monitoring therapy (Wilson, 1995).

Anisakiasis

See below under Tissue Helminths.

Cestodes

The cestodes or tapeworms are ribbon-like platyhelminths that live in the intestinal tract of vertebrates as adults and in the tissues or body cavities of various intermediate hosts as larvae. They attach to intestinal mucosa by means of a scolex, or attachment organ, at the anterior end that may display suckers, grooves (bothria), or a rostellum with hooks, depending on the species. The body of the worm, or strobila, is comprised of an actively growing neck region and a series of proglottids that undergo sequential development through immature, mature, and finally, gravid stages at the posterior end. Each proglottid has a complete set of male and female gonads and is capable of producing fertile eggs. Eggs of most cestodes infecting humans (*Diphyllobothrium* being an exception) may be readily differentiated from those of other helminths by the presence in each of a six-hooked embryo. Depending on the species, eggs are released directly into the fecal stream or passed in intact proglottids. It is not uncommon in some species for long lengths of strobila to be passed intact or for proglottids to actively migrate out of the anus. The large species of *Taenia* and *Diphyllobothrium* may grow in length to 25 feet or more and live for 20 years.

Cestode larval stages develop to the infective stage in either invertebrate or vertebrate hosts, depending on the species, and complete their life cycle when ingested by a definitive host. Larval stages of several species may infect humans causing cysticercosis, hydatidosis, sparganosis, and coenurosis. These conditions are covered more fully below under Tissue Helminths.

Taenia saginata

Humans are the sole definitive host for *Taenia saginata*, the beef tapeworm. Although it is distributed worldwide, the worm is especially common in the Middle East, Africa, Europe, Asia, and Latin America. It occurs rarely and sporadically in the United States. Larval cysticerci (*Cysticercus bovis*) develop in the tissues of cattle that graze on land contaminated with human waste. When humans ingest infected raw or incompletely cooked beef, the cysticercus develops into a reproductive adult in the small intestine in 2–3 months. Symptoms are rare but may include abdominal discomfort and diarrhea. Unlike *T. solium*, the eggs of *T. saginata* are not infectious to humans and their ingestion does not result in cysticercosis.

Diagnosis is made by finding eggs in the stool, using direct or concentration techniques, or in the perianal folds, using the Cellophane tape technique. Eggs are spherical and measure 31–43 μm in diameter (Fig. 61–20*A*). The shell is thick, radially striated, and contains a six-hooked embryo. Eggs of all *Taenia* species are indistinguishable and should be reported only as *Taenia* eggs.

Species identification may be made on recovery of proglottids or, more rarely, the scolex. Proglottids of taeniids have a characteristic lateral protrusion known as the genital pore. Careful injection of India ink through the genital pore, using a tuberculin needle and syringe, may succeed in outlining the uterus. The gravid uterus of *T. saginata* has 15–20 lateral branches, whereas that of *T. solium* has 7–13 lateral branches (Figs 61–20*B* and 61–21). Proglottids may also be cleared overnight in glycerol or stained with carmine or hematoxylin using published procedures (Ash, 1987). If recovered, the scolex of *T. saginata* can be identified by the presence of four suckers and the absence of hooks on the crown or rostellum.

Taenia solium

T. solium, the pork tapeworm, is most common in Europe, especially eastern Europe, Latin America, China, Pakistan, and India. It is encountered in the

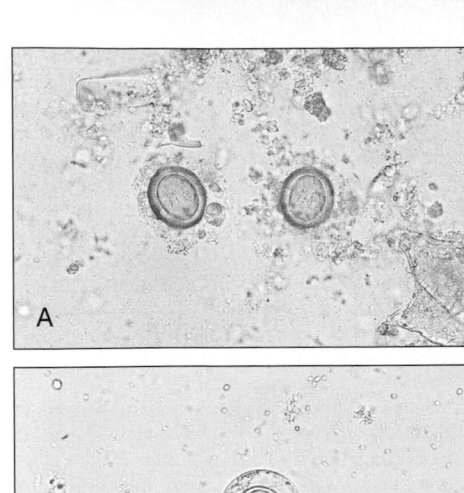
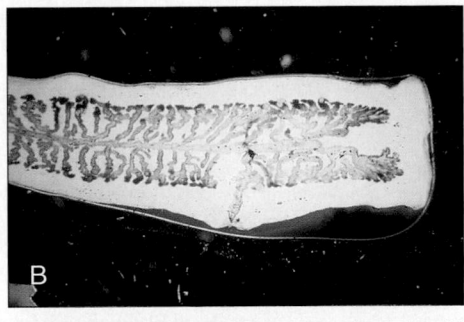
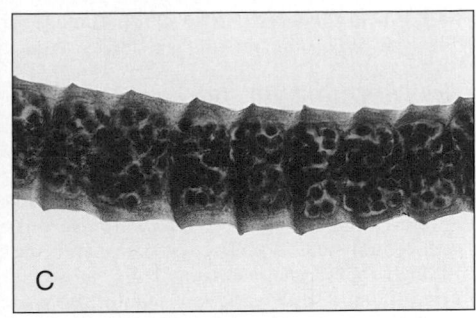
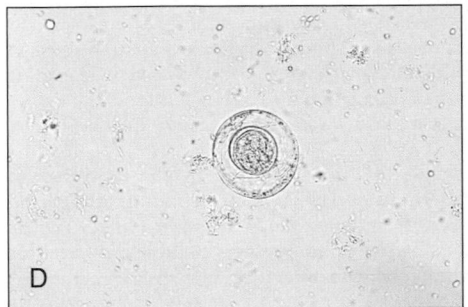
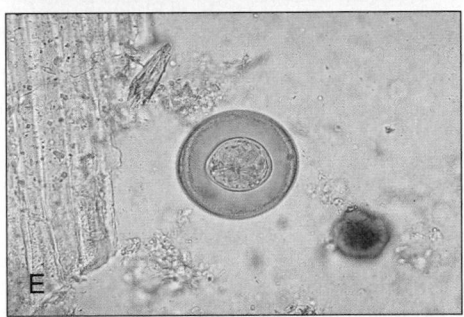
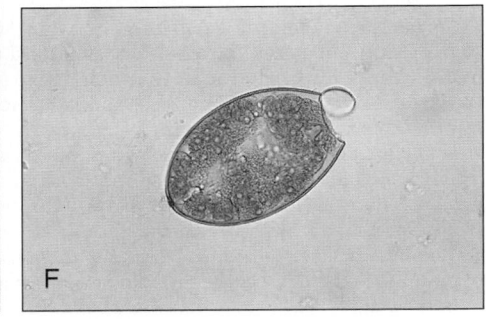
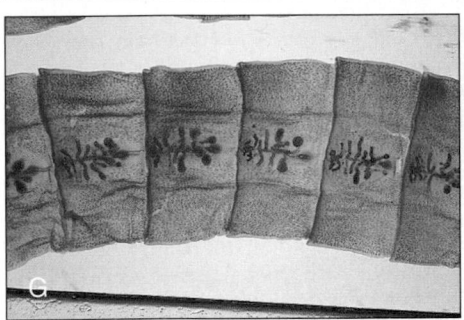
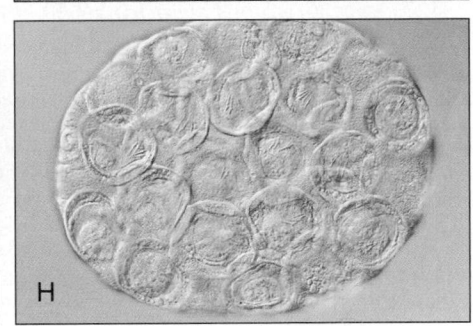

Figure 61–20 *A*, Eggs of *Taenia saginata* (indistinguishable from those of *Taenia solium*; ×400). *B*, Gravid proglottid of *T. saginata* injected through the genital pore with India ink. C, Gravid proglottids of *Hymenolepis nana* stained with acetocarmine (×100). *D*, Egg of *H. nana*; note presence of hooklets and polar filaments (×400). *E*, Egg of *Hymenolepis diminuta*; note lack of polar filaments (×400). *F*, Egg of *Diphyllobothrium* sp.; note open operculum and small terminal knob (×400). *G*, Gravid proglottids of *Diphyllobothrium* sp. stained with acetocarmine (×2). *H*, Egg packet of *Dipylidium caninum* (differential interference contrast microscopy, ×400).

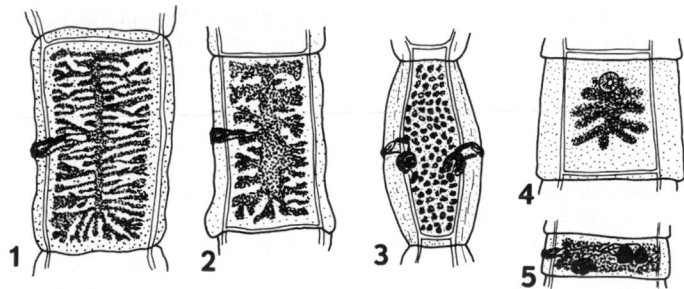

Figure 61–21 Gravid proglottids of different human tapeworms. *1, Taenia saginata. 2, Taenia solium. 3, Dipylidium caninum. 4, Diphyllobothrium latum. 5, Hymenolepis* spp.

United States on occasion, mostly in recent immigrants. Infection with the adult tapeworm is acquired by eating raw or incompletely cooked pork containing cysticerci (*Cysticercus cellulosae*). Symptoms, if present, are identical to those of *T. saginata* infection. More importantly, the accidental ingestion of *T. solium* eggs, either from one's own adult tapeworm or from contaminated food, may result in cysticercosis (Schantz, 1992). Further details on cysticercosis may be found below under Tissue Helminths.

Procedures used for diagnosis of intestinal *T. solium* infection are identical to those used for *T. saginata* infections, although certain morphologic differences are apparent. The scolex of *T. solium* has four suckers and, unlike *T. saginata*, a rostellum armed with two rows of hooks. Gravid proglottids have 7–13 lateral uterine branches (Fig. 61–21).

Hymenolepis nana

H. nana, known as the dwarf tapeworm, has worldwide distribution and is the most frequently recovered cestode species seen in the United States. It is a common parasite in mice and the smallest to infect humans, measuring up to 4.0 cm in length. The scolex has an armed rostellum and the proglottids have their genital pores all located on the same side of the strobila (Figs. 61–20C and 61–21). The life cycle may be either direct,

through the ingestion of infectious eggs, or indirect, through the ingestion of intermediate hosts (usually grain beetles) containing cysticercoid larvae. In the former instance, eggs may be passed directly from person to person, usually among children, or ingested in food, especially grain products that are contaminated with rodent droppings.

Eggs hatch in the intestine and the embryos penetrate the mucosa, where they mature as cysticercoid larvae. They subsequently emerge and reattach to the intestinal wall to complete their development into adult tapeworms in 2–3 weeks. Ingestion of grain beetles containing the cysticercoid larvae occurs much less frequently. Internal autoinfection may occur in some individuals in whom eggs hatch shortly after being discharged from the worm and rapidly invade the intestinal wall without leaving the body. Such a mechanism is thought to be responsible for the occasional case of massive infection.

Symptomatic infection, characterized by abdominal pain, diarrhea, anorexia, and irritability, may develop in patients with large numbers of worms. Diagnosis is made by recovery from stool of the oval, thin-shelled, colorless eggs, which measure 30–47 μm in diameter (Fig. 61–20D). They contain a centrally located, six-hooked embryo (oncosphere), which is separated from the outer shell by a clear space. The embryo displays two polar thickenings from which thin filaments arise and extend into the clear space between embryo and outer shell. Occasionally, intact strobila may be recovered if the stool is closely examined.

Hymenolepis diminuta

The rat tapeworm, *Hymenolepis diminuta*, is cosmopolitan in distribution and occasionally infects humans. Infections are rare, however, because of the obligate need for an arthropod intermediate host, in which the cysticercoid larvae develop. Human infection usually occurs following the accidental ingestion of infected beetles that contaminate grain or cereal products. Adult tapeworms develop in the small intestine, where they may grow to 60 cm in length. Like those of *H. nana*, the proglottids all have genital pores on one side but, unlike that species, the scolex lacks an armed rostellum. Infections usually are asymptomatic because of the small number of worms likely to infect one individual, although intestinal symptoms have been reported. Diagnosis is made by finding moderately thick-shelled, slightly ovoid, yellow-brown eggs measuring 70–85 μm by

60–80 μm in the feces (Fig. 61–20F). The eggs are most easily confused with those of *H. nana* but, unlike that species, lack polar filaments.

Diphyllobothrium spp.

Humans may be infected with one of several species of the fish tapeworm *Diphyllobothrium*, which normally infect piscivorous mammals and, possibly, birds (Curtis, 1991; Connor, 1997). These parasites are widely distributed in the temperate zones, especially northern Europe, Scandinavia, the former USSR, and Japan. Infections also occur in Canada, and in the north central states, Pacific coast states, and Alaska in the United States. Although *Diphyllobothrium latum* is the most common species known to infect humans, differentiation cannot be made on the basis of egg morphology.

The parasite inhabits the small intestine, where it can reach a length of 10 m or more and persist for years. Eggs are passed unembryonated in the feces and must reach a freshwater stream or lake to continue development. Following several weeks of embryonation, a ciliated larval form, the six-hooked coracidium, hatches and is ingested by a copepod, a type of zooplankton. The coracidium develops into a procercoid larva, which is infective for the second intermediate host, a fish. In fish, the procercoid migrates into the tissues and develops into the plerocercoid larva. Plerocercoids may be passed up the food chain unchanged and accumulate in larger fish. Humans acquire these larvae through ingestion of raw or incompletely cooked fish that have spent at least part of their life in fresh water.

Adult worms mature and initiate egg production in approximately 1 month. Infection may be asymptomatic, with passage of a length of strobila being the initial complaint. In others, a variable degree of abdominal discomfort and diarrhea may be present. Rarely, intestinal obstruction occurs. In endemic areas in northern Europe, a small percentage of patients develop vitamin B$_{12}$ deficiency and associated megaloblastic anemia.

Diagnosis is made by finding the typical brown, oval-shaped operculate eggs in feces using standard recovery techniques. Eggs measure 58–76 μm by 40–51 μm and, in addition to the operculum, have a small, round, knob-like projection on the abopercular end (Fig. 61–20F). Presence of the operculum is unique among those cestodes infecting humans, and care must be taken not to confuse these eggs with those of trematodes, especially *Paragonimus* or *Nanophyetus*. Identification to the genus level is possible when a length of strobila or an intact worm is passed. The scolex is elongated and displays a pair of longitudinal grooves known as bothria, which replace the usual suckers. Gravid proglottids are wider than they are long and have their genital pores located midventrally adjacent to a centrally located rosette-shaped uterus (Figs 61–20G and 61–21).

Dipylidium caninum

Dipylidium caninum is a common tapeworm of dogs and cats in most parts of the world and not infrequently infects humans, especially children. In the usual life cycle, tapeworm eggs are ingested by flea larvae, which infest areas frequented by dogs or cats. The cysticercoid larvae persist as the flea undergoes metamorphosis to the adult stage. Accidental ingestion of the adult flea containing the infectious cysticercoid results in infection. Children are at highest risk for infection because of their close contact with pets. Worms mature in the small intestine and grow up to 70 cm in length. Infections produce few symptoms, and generally cause concern only on detection of the actively moving proglottids.

Detection is based on finding characteristic eggs, egg packets, or proglottids in the feces. Spherical eggs, each containing a six-hooked embryo, measure from 24–40 μm in diameter and occur either singly or in packets (Fig. 61–20H). The scolex is somewhat elongate with four suckers and a small, retractable rostellum. Proglottids are barrel-shaped and possess two genital pores, one on each lateral margin, which give rise to the common name double-pored tapeworm (Fig. 61–21).

Trematodes

The trematodes, or flukes, are dorsoventrally flattened helminths (platyhelminths) that include both hermaphroditic forms (intestinal, liver, and lung flukes) and those with separate sexes (blood flukes or schistosomes). All species that infect humans are characterized by the presence of an oral sucker, through which the digestive tract opens, and a ventral sucker used for attachment. Adults vary in length from 1 mm (*Metagonimus*) to 70 mm (*Fasciola gigantica*).

Eggs reach the environment by being passed in the feces, sputum, or urine, depending on the species. The hermaphroditic flukes produce operculate eggs, which are not embryonated (*Clonorchis* and *Opisthorchis* being exceptions). Schistosome eggs are not operculated, and each contains a mature larva when passed. Trematode larvae, or miracidia, are ciliated and capable of penetrating the tissues of a molluscan host. Each species of trematode uses a particular species of snail as the first intermediate host. A complex asexual multiplication process within the snail results in the production of numerous free-swimming larvae called cercariae. Schistosome cercariae are capable of penetrating human skin directly, resulting in the disease schistosomiasis. Those of the hermaphroditic flukes encyst on aquatic vegetation or invade the tissues of second intermediate hosts such as fish or crabs, depending on the species. Ingestion of these encysted larval stages, known as metacercariae, results in human infection.

Human trematode infections occur in many tropical and subtropical regions. Their presence depends on a lack of sewage treatment, availability of appropriate intermediate hosts and, in the case of the hermaphroditic species, dietary customs associated with ingestion of infective metacercariae. Some of these diseases, especially schistosomiasis, are spreading because of the increased use of irrigation in endemic areas. Symptoms vary depending on the number of worms parasitizing the host at a given time, the tissues and organs involved, and host responses. Many infections are asymptomatic.

The diagnosis of trematode infections is made by the recovery and identification of the characteristic eggs in stool, sputum, urine, and occasionally, tissues. Direct mounts and formalin–ethyl acetate concentration methods are most useful for recovery of these eggs, whereas zinc sulfate flotation methods are less satisfactory.

Fasciolopsis buski

This intestinal trematode is the largest species to infect humans, varying from 20–75 mm in length and 8–20 mm in breadth. It occurs in many parts of China, Southeast Asia, and India and is frequently found in pigs, which serve as a natural reservoir. Infection is acquired by ingesting infectious metacercariae on aquatic food plants such as water chestnuts and water caltrop. Worms attach to the wall of the duodenum and jejunum, where they mature to egg-laying adults in about 3 months. Symptoms including diarrhea, epigastric pain, and nausea may develop if enough worms are present to produce ulceration of the superficial mucosa. Eosinophilia may be present, even in those who are asymptomatic.

Diagnosis is made by finding the large (130–140 μm by 80–85 μm), brown, oval, and thin-shelled eggs (Fig. 61–22A). The operculum may be inconspicuous, and the eggs are passed unembryonated. Differentiation from *Fasciola* eggs generally is not possible, although these infections may be differentiated on the basis of geographic history and symptoms. Eggs of echinostome trematodes, which occasionally infect humans, are similar but smaller (Beaver, 1984).

Heterophyes and Metagonimus

These two genera include a number of species of minute (1–3 mm in length) intestinal worms that infect humans. *Heterophyes heterophyes* and *Metagonimus yokogawai* are common parasites in Asia but, along with other species, are found in other parts of the world as well. Infections are acquired by ingestion of metacercariae in raw or incompletely cooked freshwater fish. Although they are of minor medical importance, infection with these worms may produce diarrhea and abdominal pain. Infections are self-limited because the worms have a life span of only a few months.

Diagnosis is established by finding the embryonated, operculate eggs, which measure 20–30 μm in length by 15–17 μm in width (Fig. 61–22B). Differentiation of these eggs from those of *Clonorchis* and *Opisthorchis* is difficult, although the operculum is more deeply seated with *Opisthorchis*. Such differentiation may be important, however, for medical reasons.

Nanophyetus salmincola

Nanophyetus salmincola is a small (0.8–1.1 mm) intestinal fluke that has been reported in humans in areas of far eastern Siberia and the Pacific north-west coast of the United States (Eastburn, 1987; Fritsche, 1989b). These worms are acquired by ingesting raw, incompletely cooked, or home-smoked salmon or trout that contain infectious metacercariae. The occurrence of symptoms is related to the number of worms present and may include abdominal pain and diarrhea, with or without eosinophilia. Eggs, 60–80 μm by 34–50 μm, are broadly ovoid, operculate, and yellowish brown (Eastburn, 1987). There is a thickening of the shell at the abopercular end, which should be differentiated from the knob seen on eggs of *Diphyllobothrium*. This fluke is the vector for a rickettsia that produces a highly lethal infection in canines known as 'salmon-poisoning' disease.

Fasciola hepatica

Cattle, sheep, and goats in many parts of the world are infected with the liver fluke *Fasciola hepatica* and, less commonly, with the related species

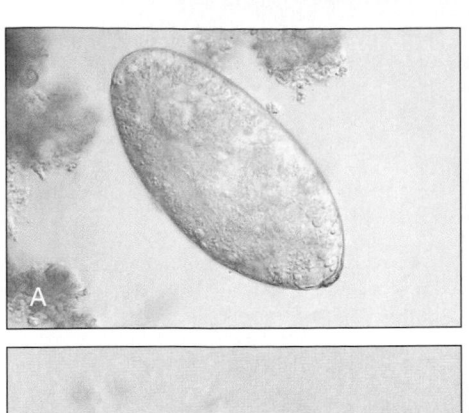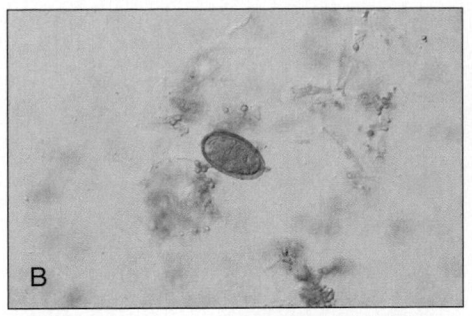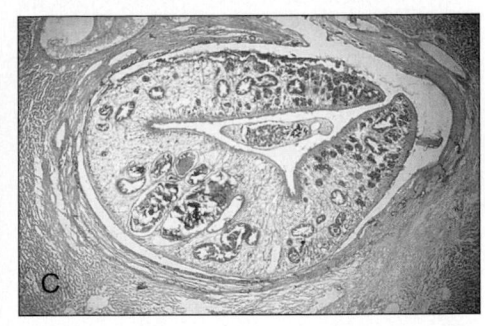
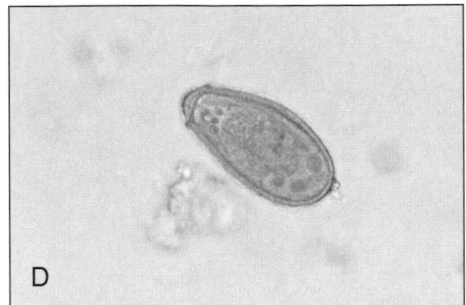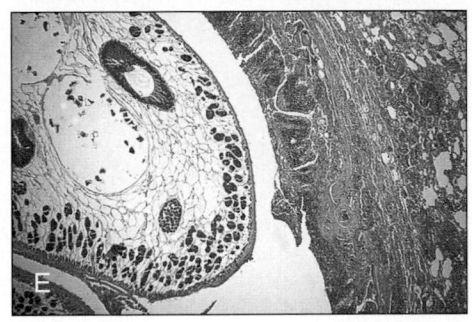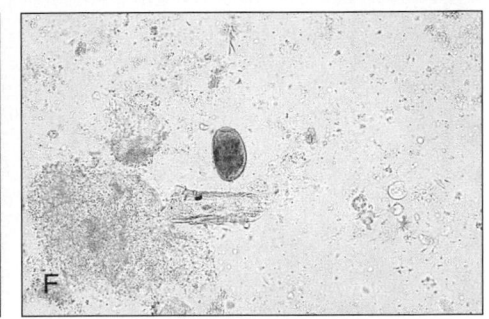

Figure 61–22 *A*, Egg of *Fasciolopsis buski*, indistinguishable from that of *Fasciola hepatica*, in stool (×400). *B*, Egg of *Heterophyes* sp. in stool (×400). *C*, Adult *Clonorchis sinensis* in bile duct (H&E; ×100). *D*, Egg of *C. sinensis* in stool (×1000). *E*, Pair of adult *Paragonimus* sp. in lung tissue with surrounding inflammatory reaction (H&E; ×10). *F*, Egg of *Paragonimus* sp. in stool; note prominent operculum (×100).

Fasciola gigantica. Adult parasites live in the biliary tree and lay eggs that are passed in the feces. Cercariae shed from the snail intermediate host encyst on aquatic vegetation, where infectious metacercariae are then available to herbivorous hosts. Humans usually acquire the infection by eating watercress. Once ingested, the larvae penetrate the intestinal wall and migrate through the peritoneal cavity to the liver. They burrow through the capsule and parenchyma, coming to reside within the bile ducts, where egg laying is initiated in about 2 months. Migration of the larvae through the liver elicits a painful inflammatory reaction both in the tissue and, later, in the bile ducts, which eventually become fibrosed. Clinical manifestations include colic, obstructive jaundice, abdominal pain and tenderness, cholelithiasis, and eosinophilia.

Diagnosis is made by finding eggs in the stool. The unembryonated, yellowish brown, operculate eggs, 130–150 μm by 63–90 μm, cannot easily be distinguished from those of *Fasciolopsis* (Fig. 61–22*A*). Spurious infections, which occur by ingesting infected cattle or sheep liver, are diagnosed by obtaining a good history and performing a follow-up stool examination to look for elimination of the eggs.

Clonorchis sinensis and Opisthorchis viverrini

Clonorchis sinensis, the Oriental liver fluke, and a closely related species, *Opisthorchis viverrini*, inhabit the biliary system of humans and other piscivorous animals, including cats and dogs. *C. sinensis* occurs mainly in China, Taiwan, Korea, Japan, and Vietnam, whereas *O. viverrini* is found primarily in south-east Asia, especially northern Thailand. Human infections are also known to occur with *Opisthorchis felineus* in Europe and *Amphimerus pseudofelineus* (same as *Opisthorchis guayaquilensis*) in Ecuador.

All these parasites are acquired by the ingestion of infectious metacercariae in raw or uncooked freshwater fish. Larvae migrate up the common duct into the liver bile ducts, where they live up to 20 years and grow up to 25 mm in length (Fig. 61–22*C*). They produce small eggs that are shed into the bile and subsequently passed in stools.

Infections are often asymptomatic, although large numbers of flukes and repeated infections may cause inflammation of the bile ducts and subsequent hyperplasia, fibrosis, and hepatic cirrhosis. Development of cholangiocarcinoma has been linked epidemiologically with longstanding infections.

Diagnosis is made by recovering the small brown, embryonated, operculate eggs from stools (Fig. 61–22*D*). Eggs of *Clonorchis* cannot be readily differentiated from those of *Opisthorchis*. Both measure 25–35 μm by 12–20 μm and have a prominent, seated opercula and a small knob at the abopercular end. These eggs are difficult to differentiate from those of the *Heterophyes*/*Metagonimus* group, although the latter species do not have the prominent, seated opercula or a small knob at the abopercular end. When specific identification is not possible, the laboratory report should reflect this (i.e., should state '*Clonorchis/Opisthorchis/Heterophyes/Metagonimus* eggs').

Paragonimus spp.

Several species of *Paragonimus* may parasitize the lungs of cats, dogs, and other carnivores, including humans. *Paragonimus westermani* is problematic in many areas of Asia, whereas in Central and South America several species have been implicated, including *Paragonimus mexicanus*, *Paragonimus caliensis*, and *Paragonimus ecuadoriensis*. *Paragonimus kellicotti* has occasionally been implicated in cases from North America, and other species have been described from Africa (Pachucki, 1984; Mariano, 1986; Strickland, 2000; Cook, 2002).

Adult worms measure up to 12 mm by 6 mm and often are found in pairs in lung parenchyma, where they reside in a fibrotic capsule produced by the host (Fig. 61–22*E*). The capsule communicates with the bronchi, through which eggs pass to be eventually expelled in sputa or feces. Although a specific snail serves as the first intermediate host, freshwater crabs or crayfish serve as second intermediates for the infectious metacercariae. Ingestion of uncooked, or marinated, crustacea may result in infection. Larvae are released in the stomach and migrate through the intestinal wall into the peritoneal cavity, eventually reaching the lungs after penetrating the diaphragm. Maturation takes approximately 5–6 weeks, and worms may live for many years.

Symptoms, when present, may be caused by larvae migrating through tissues or by adults established in the lungs. Not infrequently, worms develop in ectopic sites, including the peritoneum, subcutaneous tissues, and brain. The onset of lung infection is usually associated with fever, chills, and the appearance of eosinophilia. Once established, symptoms include chronic coughing with abundant mucus production, and episodes of hemoptysis. Radiographs may show nodular shadows, calcifications, or patchy infiltrates. Eggs remaining in the lung tissues or in ectopic sites may cause extensive granulomatous reaction.

Diagnosis is made by finding the typical eggs either in stools, sputum or, occasionally, tissues. Eggs of the different *Paragonimus* species cannot be readily differentiated, and specific identification may be inferred from the area of origin. The operculate, unembryonated eggs measure 80–120 μm by 45–70 μm and have a moderately thick, yellow-brown shell (Fig. 61–22*F*). The operculum is flattened and usually is set off from the rest of the shell by prominent shoulders. The abopercular end is somewhat thickened but does not have a knob. *Paragonimus* eggs may be differentiated from those of *Diphyllobothrium* and *Fasciola/Fasciolopsis*, which they superficially resemble, by size.

Schistosoma spp.

Schistosomiasis, or bilharzia, is among the most important parasitic diseases worldwide, afflicting 200–300 million individuals. Adult male and female blood flukes inhabit veins of the mesentery or bladder. The most important species infecting humans are *Schistosoma mansoni*, *Schistosoma japonicum*, *Schistosoma mekongi*, *Schistosoma haematobium*, and *Schistosoma intercalatum*; other species infect humans less frequently.

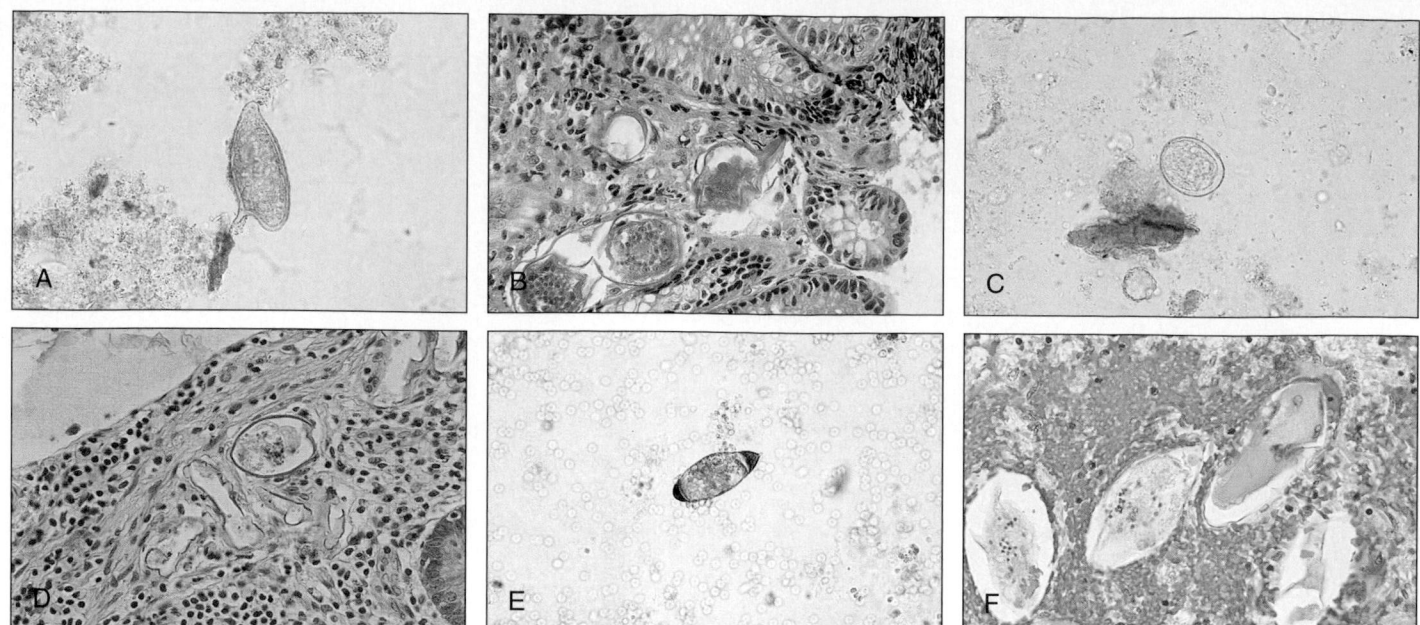

Figure 61–23 *A*, Egg of *Schistosoma mansoni*; note prominent lateral spine (×400). *B*, Eggs of *S. mansoni* in an intestinal biopsy; note presence of lateral spine (H&E; ×400). *C*, Egg of *Schistosoma japonicum*; note presence of small lateral spine ×400). *D*, Eggs of *S. japonicum* in a small bowel biopsy (H&E; ×400). *E*, Egg of *Schistosoma haematobium* found in urine sediment; note presence of a terminal spine (×400). *F*, Eggs of *S. haematobium* seen in a vulvar granuloma; note presence of a terminal spine (H&E; ×400).

Adult female schistosomes are slender, measuring up to 26 mm by 0.5 mm. Males, which are slightly shorter, enfold a female using the lateral margins of the body (the gynecophoral canal) to assist in sperm transfer. When examined in situ, schistosomes are often found in copula. In their preferred locations, blood flukes elicit little or no inflammatory response. Eggs are deposited in the smallest venule that can accommodate the female worm, where they elicit a strong granulomatous response that results in extrusion of the egg into the intestinal lumen or the bladder. Pathology is primarily related to the sites of egg deposition, numbers deposited, and host reaction to egg antigens.

Eggs are fully embryonated when passed and readily hatch when deposited in fresh water. The miracidia penetrate an appropriate species of snail host, where they undergo transformation and extensive asexual multiplication. After about 4 weeks, large numbers of fork-tailed cercariae emerge from the mollusk. Cercariae swim actively about for hours and readily penetrate the skin of susceptible hosts, including humans. After penetration, the cercariae, now called schistosomules, enter the circulation and pass through the lungs before reaching the mesenteric-portal vessels.

Symptoms of schistosomiasis result primarily from penetration of cercariae (cercarial dermatitis), initiation of egg laying (acute schistosomiasis or Katayama fever), and as a late-stage complication of tissue proliferation and repair (chronic schistosomiasis). In a matter of hours after cercarial penetration, a papular rash associated with pruritus may develop. This is a sensitization phenomenon resulting from prior exposure to cercarial antigens. The most severe form of dermatitis occurs in individuals who are repeatedly exposed to cercariae of nonhuman (primarily avian) schistosomes. Cercarial dermatitis or swimmer's itch occurs worldwide and is a well-recognized entity in the United States (Hoeffler, 1974).

Initiation of egg laying by mature worms 5–7 weeks after infection may result in acute schistosomiasis, or Katayama fever, a serum-sickness-like syndrome that occurs with heavy primary infections, especially those of *S. japonicum*. The antigenic challenge to the host is thought to result in immune complex formation (Boros, 1989).

Chronic infection results in continued egg deposition, many of which remain in the body. Granulomas produced around these eggs in the intestine and bladder are gradually replaced by collagen, resulting in fibrosis and scarring. Eggs trapped in the liver may induce pipe-stem fibrosis with obstruction to portal blood flow. Occasionally, eggs are deposited in ectopic sites, such as the spinal cord, lungs, or brain (Cook, 2002).

Diagnosis is established by demonstrating eggs in feces or urine by direct wet mount or formalin–ethyl acetate concentration methods. Zinc sulfate concentration is not satisfactory for recovery of the heavy schistosome eggs. Eggs also may be detected in biopsies of rectal, bladder and, occasionally, liver tissues either by crush preparation or in histologic section (Fig. 61–23). Use of egg hatching methods may occasionally be requested to determine viability or, less commonly, to detect light infections. Feces mixed with distilled water are placed in a flask that is covered with foil to keep out light, with only the neck or a sidearm exposed to a bright light. Miracidia, if present, actively swim to the light and can be detected using a hand lens.

Serologic tests may be helpful in screening persons who have traveled to endemic areas, those with negative urine or stool examinations who are at risk for infection, or for monitoring response to therapy. Although not widely available, a limited number of reference laboratories and the CDC provide testing. Generally, serologic testing varies with the antigens used and test methodologies employed. The CDC uses the Falcon assay screening test in a kinetic enzyme-linked immunosorbent assay (FAST-ELISA). Sera that are positive by the screening test are further evaluated by immunoblot to improve specificity (Wilson, 1995).

Schistosoma mansoni

S. mansoni occurs in Africa, especially in the tropical areas and the Nile delta, southern Africa, and Madagascar, Brazil, Venezuela, Surinam, and certain Caribbean islands, including Puerto Rico. Adult *S. mansoni* live primarily in the portal vein and in the distribution of the inferior mesenteric vein. Initial deposition of eggs in the large intestine may produce abdominal pain and dysentery, with abundant blood and mucus in the stool. Eggs may be detected in feces at this time. Chronic infection may result in liver fibrosis and portal hypertension, depending on the number of worms present; eggs may be more difficult to find in feces during this stage.

Eggs, 116–180 µm by 45–58 µm, are oval, with a large distinctive lateral spine that protrudes from the side of the egg near one end (Fig. 61–23*A* and *B*). If the spine is not visible, the egg may be rotated by gently tapping the coverslip. Movement of the miracidium within the egg may be evident in unfixed material if the larva is viable. Concentration techniques may be required to detect eggs, because individuals with limited exposure or with chronic infection may pass few of them.

Schistosoma japonicum

S. japonicum, which occurs in China, Southeast Asia, and the Philippines, causes disease that is clinically similar to that of *S. mansoni* but often more serious because many more (up to 10 times as many) eggs are produced by *S. japonicum*. The disease has been essentially eliminated from Japan, although animal reservoirs still exist. Adult worms live primarily in the distribution of the superior mesenteric vein, and eggs readily reach the liver, inducing fibrosis and portal hypertension as a common complication of chronic infection. The smaller size of the eggs predisposes them to dissemination, especially to the brain and spinal cord. The eggs are broadly oval, measuring 75–90 µm by 60–68 µm, and have an inconspicuous lateral spine, which may be difficult to demonstrate (Fig. 61–23*C* and *D*).

Schistosoma mekongi

This species occurs in humans and animal reservoirs in countries along the Mekong River, especially Cambodia and Laos (Bruce, 1980). It is similar to

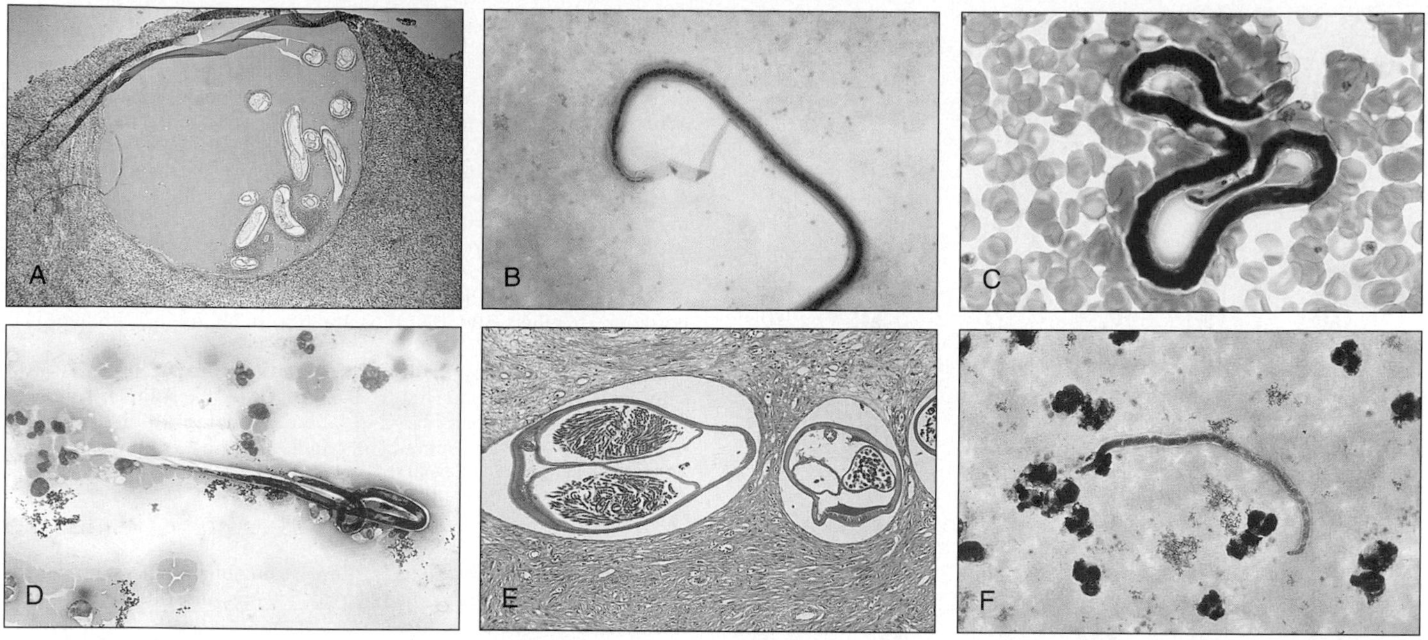

Figure 61–24 *A, Wuchereria bancrofti,* cross-section of adult in human lymph node; note extensive inflammatory reaction (H&E; ×100). *B,* Sheathed microfilaria of *W. bancrofti;* cell nuclei do not extend to the tip of the tail (Giemsa stain; ×1000). *C,* Sheathed microfilaria of *Brugia malayi;* two solitary cell nuclei are seen in the tail tip (Giemsa stain; ×1000). *D,* Sheathed microfilaria of *Loa loa;* cell nuclei extend to the tail tip (Giemsa stain; ×1000). *E, Onchocerca volvulus,* cross-section of adult in skin nodule (H&E; ×100). *F,* Unsheathed microfilaria of *Mansonella perstans;* cell nuclei extend to the tail tip (Giemsa stain; ×1000).

S. japonicum but is differentiated from that species by several biological characteristics and smaller eggs (60–70 μm by 52–61 μm), which otherwise are indistinguishable from those of *S. japonicum.*

Schistosoma haematobium

Urinary schistosomiasis occurs in many parts of Africa, the Middle East, and Madagascar. Parasites migrate via the hemorrhoidal veins to the venous plexuses of the urinary bladder, prostate, uterus, and vagina. One of the earliest and most common symptoms of infection is hematuria, especially at the end of micturition. Chronic infection may cause pelvic pain and bladder colic, with an increased desire to urinate. Accumulation of eggs in the tissues may result in hypertrophy of the urothelium, squamous metaplasia, and marked fibrosis, which may progress to obstruction and, ultimately, renal failure. Urinary schistosomiasis also has been associated with squamous cell carcinoma of the bladder (Badawi, 1992).

Eggs are recovered from the urine by examining a spun sediment. They are elongate, measuring 112–180 μm by 40–70 μm, and have a characteristic terminal spine (Fig. 61–23*E* and *F*). Occasionally, they may be detected in feces or in a rectal biopsy.

Schistosoma intercalatum

This species occurs in many parts of central and western Africa and produces intestinal schistosomiasis. Eggs have a terminal spine and so resemble those of *S. haematobium,* but they occur primarily in the feces and are larger (140–240 μm by 50–85 μm).

Tissue Helminths

Nematodes

Filaria

Filarial nematodes, also known as threadworms, are common arthropod-transmitted parasites of vertebrate animals. Adult male and female worms are long and slender, measuring up to 100 mm in length, and are known to inhabit a variety of tissues, including subcutaneous tissues, lymphatics, blood vessels, peritoneal and pleural cavities, heart, and brain. All species produce larvae known as microfilariae, which may be recovered from either blood or skin, depending on the species. The microfilariae of some species circulate in the blood with a well defined periodicity (either diurnal or nocturnal), whereas others do not. Microfilariae continue their development only in the appropriate arthropod vector, usually a mosquito or fly, where they mature to the infective stage. Such larvae are then deposited in the tissues of a definitive host when the vector takes another blood meal.

Diagnosis of filariasis usually is made by finding microfilariae in the blood or skin, because adult stages are often sequestered in the tissues. The use of Giemsa or hematoxylin-stained thick smears of peripheral blood is routine, although more sensitive procedures such as membrane filter, Knott's concentration, or saponin lysis may also be required (National Committee for Clinical Laboratory Standards, 2000). Microfilariae may be seen moving in direct mounts of blood or tissue fluid.

Species identification is important because pathogenicity varies. The principal characteristics that are used for identification of microfilariae include the presence or absence of a sheath and its staining characteristics, the shape of the tail and distribution of cell nuclei within, and the size of the cephalic space and appearance of its nuclear column. Because microfilariae of *Wuchereria* and *Brugia* usually display a nocturnal periodicity, blood from patients suspected to be infected with these filaria should be drawn between the hours of 10 pm and 2 am. *Loa loa* displays diurnal periodicity, so blood should preferably be drawn around noon. *Mansonella ozzardi* and *Mansonella perstans* are characteristically nonperiodic. Microfilariae of *Mansonella streptocerca* and *Onchocerca volvulus* are present in the skin and are detected by examination of skin snips or punch biopsies.

Serologic tests for the diagnosis of lymphatic filariasis may prove helpful in select patients, especially those who are not native to endemic areas. Such methods are limited in their ability to distinguish between past exposure and current infection, however, and infection with other nematode species may result in the appearance of crossreacting antibodies. Antigen detection tests also may be of value in the diagnosis of lymphatic filariasis but are not generally available (Wilson, 1995).

Wuchereria bancrofti

This species, responsible for bancroftian filariasis, is the most common filarial species to infect humans. Endemic areas include central and northern Africa, India, south-east Asia, certain south Pacific islands, and portions of Central and South America and the West Indies. Adult worms reside in the lymphatic system, where chronic infection and reinfection result in lymphadenopathy and lymphangitis, which may progress to lymphedema and obstructive fibrosis (Fig. 61–24*A*). Severe involvement of the lower extremities and genitalia may result in elephantiasis.

In most areas, microfilariae circulate in peripheral blood with a nocturnal periodicity that corresponds with the feeding activities of the usual vectors *Culex, Aedes,* and *Anopheles* mosquitoes. Infections originating in the South Pacific are essentially without periodicity. The microfilariae are sheathed, although this may not always be obvious with Giemsa staining. The tail is pointed, and there are no nuclei in the tip. The cephalic space is not as long as it is wide, and the nuclei in the nuclear column are distinct (Figs 61–24*B* and 61–25). Concentration procedures

VII

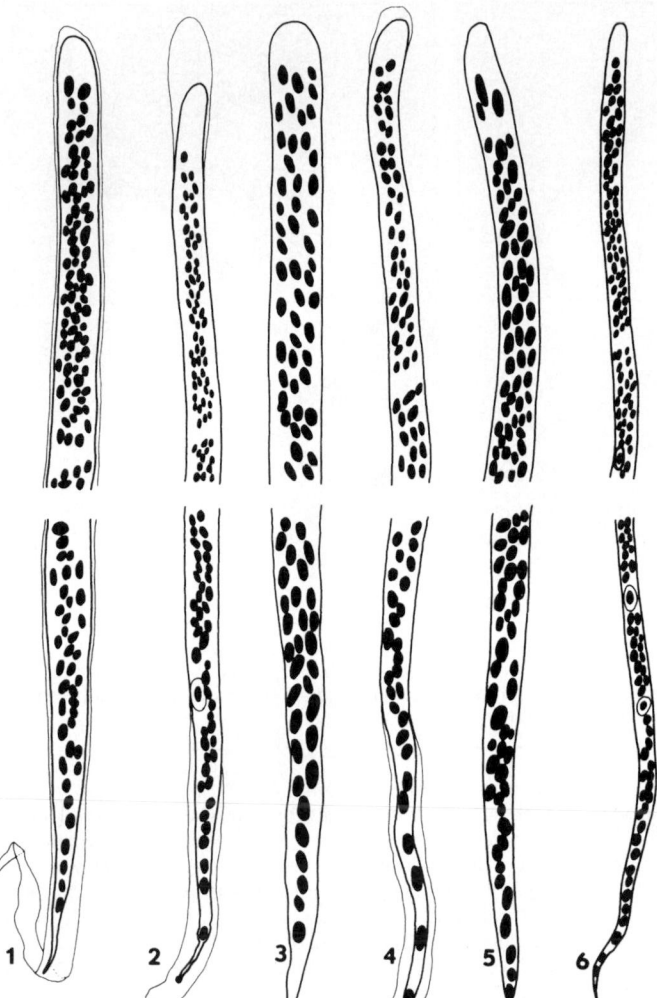

Figure 61–25 Anterior and posterior ends of microfilariae most commonly found in humans. *1, Wuchereria bancrofti. 2, Brugia malayi. 3, Onchocerca volvulus. 4, Loa loa. 5, Mansonella perstans. 6, Mansonella ozzardi.* All camera lucida drawings.

Onchocerca volvulus

Onchocerciasis is a leading cause of blindness in endemic areas, which include central Africa, Central America (Mexico and Guatemala), and northern South America. Vectors are black flies of the genus *Simulium*. Adult worms live in hard, fibrous nodules in subcutaneous and deeper tissues that can grow to be 40 mm in diameter (Fig. 61–24E). Nodules tend to occur on the upper half of the body in patients from central America and in the lower half in those from Africa. Adult worms produce microfilariae that migrate continuously through the skin. Complications arise from the migratory activities of the microfilariae, resulting in several forms of dermatitis. Movement of microfilariae through the surface of the eye may result in keratitis, corneal opacity, and damage to the anterior and posterior chambers and iris, thus leading to blindness with repeated infections over time.

Diagnosis is made by finding the typical microfilariae in teased skin snips or skin biopsies, preferably taken from over the scapular region or from the iliac crest, when placed in saline. Alternatively, fluids expressed from scarified skin or aspirates of nodules may be examined (Beaver, 1984; Garcia, 2001). Microfilariae in stained preparations lack both a sheath and nuclei in the tail tip (Fig. 61–25).

Mansonella spp.

Several species of *Mansonella* infect humans, but all are generally regarded as causing little pathology. Microfilariae, however, must be differentiated from the truly pathogenic filarial species. *M. ozzardi* is found in Central and South America, and some areas of the Caribbean. Adult parasites reside in subcutaneous tissues. *M. perstans* occurs in many areas of tropical Africa and sporadically in South America. Adults are thought to reside primarily in body cavities and the mesenteries. Microfilariae of both species are unsheathed and circulate in peripheral blood without evidence of periodicity. *M. ozzardi* microfilariae have a thin, pointed tail without nuclei, whereas the tail of *M. perstans* is broad and blunt with nuclei extending to the tip (Figs 61–24F and 61–25). *M. streptocerca*, which is found in tropical Africa, may be confused with *O. volvulus*, because both adult and microfilarial stages occur in skin and subcutaneous tissues. Also, dermatitis may be produced by this species. Microfilariae of this species, which may be recovered in skin snips, are unsheathed and have a crook in the tail with nuclei extending to the tip. All species of *Mansonella* are transmitted by gnats of the genus *Culicoides*.

Zoonotic Filariae

Certain filarial nematodes of the genera *Dirofilaria* and *Brugia* that naturally parasitize wild and domestic mammals sporadically infect humans. *Dirofilaria immitis*, commonly known as the canine heartworm, is widely distributed and human infections are well documented. The mosquito-transmitted larval stage migrates to the right side of the heart. When the worm dies it is swept into a small pulmonary artery, producing a granulomatous nodule that appears as a coin lesion on a chest radiograph. Diagnosis usually is made by histologic examination of the nodule.

Other species of *Dirofilaria*, including *Dirofilaria tenuis*, *Dirofilaria repens*, and *Dirofilaria ursi*, commonly cause subcutaneous nodules in humans but fail to produce microfilariae. Such nodules have been reported from many body sites, including the face, conjunctiva, and breast, and are usually removed surgically. Histologic examination often reveals a prominent mixed inflammatory reaction surrounding a dead worm. Criteria for identification of the zoonotic filariae in tissue sections may be found elsewhere (Orihel, 1995; Connor, 1997; Gutierrez, 2000).

Other
Dracunculus medinensis

Adult Guinea worms live in subcutaneous tissues and become clinically evident when the female worm migrates to the skin surface and produces a blister, usually on the lower extremities. When the extremity is immersed in water, the blister ruptures, releasing swarms of motile larvae from the female worm into the water. Specific zooplankton (i.e., copepods) ingest the larvae, which then mature to the infective stage and are transmitted back to humans when copepods are accidentally swallowed in drinking water.

The disease is endemic to areas of Africa, the Middle East, and Asia, and may be responsible for disfiguring cutaneous scars and more serious secondary bacterial infections. Extensive control efforts have been made in recent years to eradicate this parasite (Centers for Disease Control and Prevention, 1992; Cairncross, 2002).

Diagnosis is made by finding the female worm emerging at the skin surface and larvae in the discharge fluid. The worm may be gently extracted over a period of days, but care must be taken not to damage it

may be necessary for recovery because microfilariae may be present in small numbers.

Brugia malayi

This species produces disease similar to that of *W. bancrofti*, although it is often milder and more frequently involves the lymphatics of the upper extremities. The parasite occurs mainly in India, south-east Asia, Korea, the Philippines, and Japan. Human infections with related zoonotic species are encountered periodically in the United States.

The microfilariae circulate in the blood and are primarily periodic. Microfilarial sheaths of *Brugia malayi* stain well with Giemsa stain. The tail has a swelling at the tip and has two solitary nuclei located beyond the end of the nuclear column (termed subterminal and terminal nuclei). The cephalic space may be much longer than it is wide (Figs 61–24C and 61–25). *Brugia timori* is a distinct species occurring in the eastern end of the Indonesian archipelago, especially on the islands of Timor and Flores. Microfilariae are very similar to those of *B. malayi*, although somewhat larger.

Loa loa

Known as the eye worm, *Loa loa* lives in subcutaneous tissues. The nematodes migrate continuously, producing transient (2–3 days) local inflammatory reactions known as Calabar or fugitive swellings. Their occasional appearance in the conjunctiva allows them to be surgically excised. Loiasis occurs primarily in west and central Africa, where deer flies of the genus *Chrysops* serve as vector.

The parasite elicits strong eosinophilia and has occasionally been seen in the United States in people with a history of travel to Africa. The microfilariae, which circulate in the blood with diurnal periodicity, are sheathed, although the sheath does not stain with Giemsa's stain. Nuclei in the tail extend to the rounded tip. The nuclear column is distinct, and the cephalic space is short (Figs 61–24D and 61–25; National Committee for Clinical Laboratory Standards, 2000; Garcia, 2001).

during removal. Should the worm die in situ, pronounced inflammatory reactions and secondary bacterial infections may disable the affected individual.

Angiostrongylus cantonensis and *Angiostrongylus costaricensis*

Human eosinophilic meningoencephalitis, caused by *Angiostrongylus cantonensis*, occurs both in epidemics and sporadically in many areas of the south Pacific, south-east Asia, and Taiwan. The mature parasite is normally found in the pulmonary arteries of rats. Larvae migrate up the trachea and are passed in the feces. They develop to the infective stage in slugs or land snails and, when eaten by the usual rodent host, migrate through the brain before maturing in the pulmonary arteries. Humans acquire the infection by eating large edible snails; raw or incompletely cooked shrimp or crabs, which may serve as transport hosts; or vegetables contaminated with infected mollusks. In humans, the *A. cantonensis* larvae migrate to the central nervous system, producing a generally nonfatal meningitis with a high spinal fluid eosinophilia (Alicata, 1991). Diagnosis is established both clinically and historically, although larvae have occasionally been recovered from spinal fluid (Kubersky, 1979; Strickland, 2000; Cook, 2002).

Angiostrongylus costaricensis occurs widely in Central and South America (Loria-Cortez, 1980). The parasite, which is responsible for the intestinal form of angiostrongyliasis, normally resides in the mesenteric arteries of the ileum and cecum of rodents. Human infection occurs in the same anatomic location, but often results in granulomatous inflammation and symptoms of acute abdomen. Diagnosis is made by histologic examination of surgical specimens and finding adults or eggs in the tissues (Strickland, 2000).

Trichinella spiralis

Human trichinosis occurs worldwide, although its incidence in the United States has been in steady decline, with fewer than 100 cases reported each year. Humans acquire the infection through the ingestion of raw or incompletely cooked pork, pork products or, less commonly, bear meat that contains infective larvae. Ingested worms mature in the small intestine, where gravid females produce new larvae for 2–3 weeks. During this stage, gastrointestinal symptoms occur, lasting several days. Larvae subsequently enter lymphatics and venules, thus reaching the general circulation. They primarily invade the skeletal musculature, where they undergo further development and encapsulation. During the migratory and encapsulation phases, fever, muscle pain, respiratory difficulties, periorbital edema, and eosinophilia may develop, depending on the inoculating dose. After the parasites have encysted, there are few symptoms. Encysted larvae may remain viable for several years, although they eventually become calcified.

Diagnosis is usually made on the basis of history and clinical symptoms and is confirmed by the demonstration of trichinella cysts in skeletal muscle biopsy, particularly the gastrocnemius or deltoid muscles (Fig. 61–18E and F). Indirect tests include creatine phosphokinase, which is often elevated, and detection of antibodies by bentonite flocculation or EIA. Of these latter tests, creatine phosphokinase is more specific, and EIA is more sensitive (Wilson, 1995).

Larva Migrans

Larva migrans is caused by the prolonged wandering through body tissues of larvae of certain hookworms, ascarids, and *Strongyloides* species that normally infect wild or domestic animals. The syndrome varies with the species involved, the number of worms, and the tissues parasitized.

Cutaneous larva migrans (CLM), or ground itch, is produced by the cutaneous wanderings of cat or dog hookworms of the genus *Ancylostoma*, which penetrate the skin but cannot mature in the usual pattern. Serpiginous, erythematous, and pruritic tracks are apparent on the skin in areas where there has been contact with the ground. This is particularly problematic in warmer, humid climates, where eggs and larvae of these hookworms survive longer. Some species of *Strongyloides* that parasitize wild animals may cause a similar dermatitis (Beaver, 1984).

Visceral larva migrans (VLM) is produced primarily by the random wanderings of the dog ascarid *Toxocara canis* and, to a lesser degree, by *Toxocara cati* from the domestic cat. Children are usually infected following the accidental or intentional ingestion of soil contaminated with dog or cat feces. After hatching, the larvae are unable to complete their usual cycle and instead begin a prolonged migration through various tissues and organs. Children may present with failure to thrive and display fever, hepatomegaly, pneumonitis, hypereosinophilia, and hypergamma-globulinemia. An inflammatory reaction in the retina from ocular larva migrans may mimic retinoblastoma, a malignant tumor, from which it must be differentiated. Diagnosis of VLM is usually made on clinical grounds, because the parasite is rarely recovered. Serologic tests may be helpful in confirming a presumptive diagnosis, and the currently recommended procedure is an EIA that uses larval stage excretory–secretory antigens (Wilson, 1995; Garcia, 2001).

A VLM-like syndrome may also be caused by species of *Gnathostoma* that infect the stomach of various mammals. Human infections are most common in south-east Asia but have been reported in Mexico and Ecuador. These parasites use a copepod for the first intermediate host and fish and amphibians as secondary hosts. A variety of reptiles, birds, and mammals may serve as paratenic hosts. The larvae may migrate through subcutaneous tissues, causing transient swellings, and to deeper tissues, and eventually invade the CNS. The occurrence of migratory lesions and a history of eating raw fish may be helpful in establishing a clinical diagnosis.

Capillaria hepatica

Although normally a parasite common to rodents, this species occasionally causes human disease, especially in children, in whom it may mimic VLM, hepatitis, amebic liver abscess, and other diseases. In the usual rodent host, eggs are ingested and the resulting larvae migrate to the liver, where they mature and deposit eggs directly in the parenchyma. When the liver is eaten by a predator, the eggs are passed out in the feces and contaminate soil. Children are at particular risk of acquiring the eggs if they eat dirt. In endemic areas, diagnosis is made by examination of liver biopsies or tissue obtained at autopsy. Eggs are readily recognized in tissue biopsies by having thick striated walls and plugs at both ends.

Anisakis, Pseudoterranova, and *Eustrongylides* spp.

The ingestion of raw fish, although considered by many to be a delicacy, has resulted in an increase in the number of reported cases of fish nematode infections. *Anisakis* and *Pseudoterranova* are common gastrointestinal parasites of marine mammals, and the infective stages are found in various saltwater fish, salmon, and squid intermediate hosts. Small shrimp-like crustaceans (krill) serve as first intermediate host. When ingested, these larvae may penetrate the wall of the stomach or small bowel, causing acute abdominal pain. Anisakiasis may be presumptively diagnosed based on an appropriate history and clinical findings, and the condition may be confirmed by the recovery of an intact worm at endoscopy or by the presence of an eosinophilic granuloma containing an identifiable nematode in a surgical specimen. Species of *Anisakis* appear to be more prone to produce invasive disease, whereas *Pseudoterranova* spp. tend to be coughed up or vomited intact (Fig 61–18G and H) (Sakanari, 1989). The species level of larval anisakids is difficult to identify (Binford, 1976).

A small number of infections with *Eustrongylides* spp. have been reported in individuals who had eaten live minnows or home-prepared sushi. These parasites usually infect fish-eating birds but, in humans, the bright red larvae invade the abdominal cavity, requiring surgical removal (Wittner, 1989).

Cestodes

Several species of cestode infect humans in their larval stages and may produce serious disease. The more commonly encountered ones are readily distinguishable from each other and have unique patterns of transmission. When seen in tissue sections, larval and adult stages of cestodes contain basophilic-staining laminated bodies known as calcareous corpuscles, which are an important aid in their recognition.

Cysticercosis

Human infection with the larval stage of the pork tapeworm, *T. solium*, is found worldwide and occurs following the unintentional ingestion of the eggs of an adult tapeworm. The disease is especially prevalent in Mexico and the rest of Latin America, Europe, Africa, India, and Asia. Most cases in the United States originate from highly endemic areas, although, in recent years, the number of locally acquired cases has increased (Richards, 1985; Carabin, 2005).

Eggs may be ingested accidentally with contaminated food or water and subsequently hatch in the gastrointestinal tract. Embryos penetrate the intestinal mucosa and disseminate via the blood stream to distant sites, especially the skeletal muscle, and also to the heart, brain, or eye, where symptoms of infection and inflammation may become especially apparent. Seizures are a common complication in endemic areas and are often the presenting symptom (Fig. 61–26A).

The diagnosis is usually made on clinical grounds in endemic areas but may be much more difficult to establish in nonendemic settings. Use of computed tomographic (CT) scans is very helpful but generally not available in most endemic areas. Radiographs are helpful in recognizing the presence of calcified cysts but not in recognizing recent infections. Recovery of an intact cysticercus at surgery confirms the diagnosis. The cysticercus, or

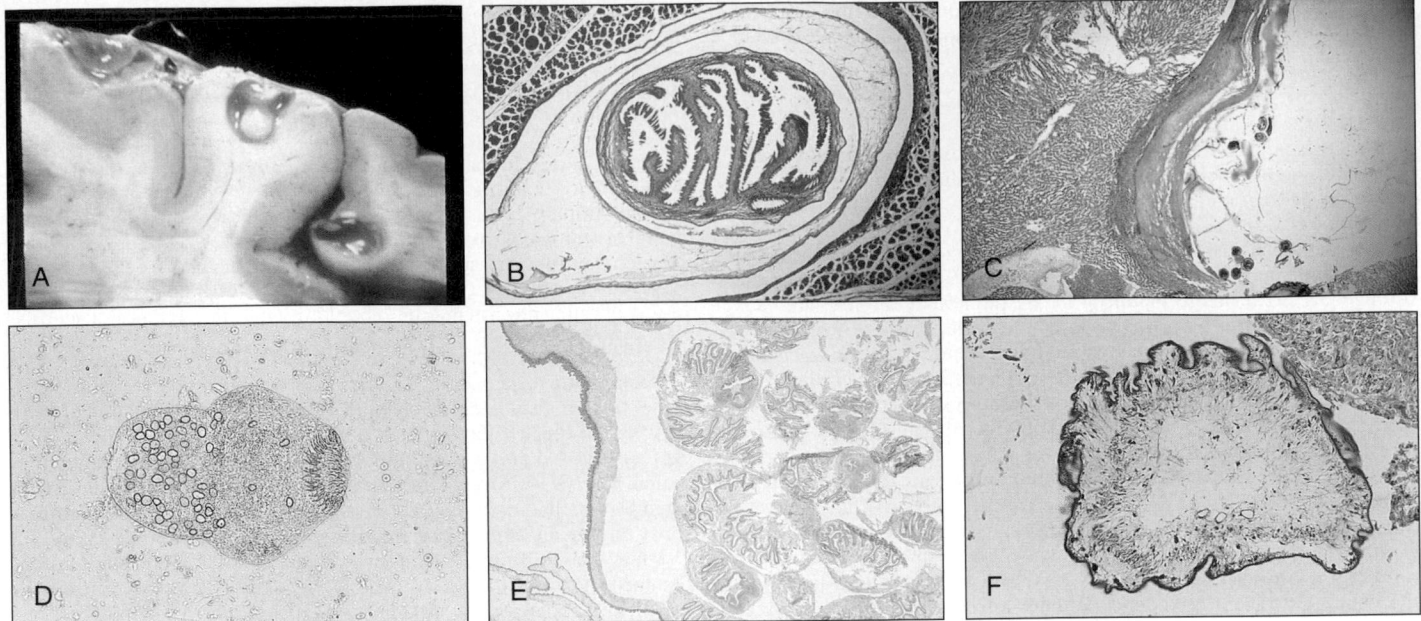

Figure 61–26 *A*, Neurocysticercosis. (Photograph from *A Pictorial Presentation of Parasites: A cooperative collection* prepared and/or edited by H. Zaiman.) *B*, Bladder worm (*Taenia solium* cysticercus) in muscle (H&E; ×10). *C*, Hydatid cyst in the liver; note presence of protoscolices, a thin germinal membrane, a thick laminated membrane, and fibrotic host reaction (×10). *D*, Protoscolex found in aspirate fluid from a hepatic hydatid cyst; note rostellar hooks and calcareous corpuscles (×400). *E*, Human infection with a coenurus larva; note thin bladder membrane and numerous developing protoscolices (×10). (Courtesy of Dr Heike Duebner.) *F*, Sparganum (larva of *Spirometra* spp.) found in a retro-orbital lesion (Giemsa stain; ×100).

bladder worm, is a translucent, fluid-filled, oval sac containing a single inverted scolex that measures 5 mm or more in diameter (Fig. 61–26*B*).

Among serologic assays, the glycoprotein immunoblot assay available from the CDC has high sensitivity and specificity, outperforming several EIAs with which it was compared (Diaz, 1992). Unfortunately, these assays do not distinguish between active and inactive infections, and thus are not useful in monitoring response to therapy.

The occurrence of cysticercosis in someone from a nonendemic area and without an appropriate travel history should be investigated for accidental exposure to individuals involved in food preparation, or for the possibility of infection with a different *Taenia* species (Schantz, 1992).

Hydatidosis

Human infection with larval stages of tapeworms of the genus *Echinococcus* may take one of three forms: unilocular hydatid disease caused by *Echinococcus granulosus*, multilocular or alveolar hydatid disease caused by *Echinococcus multilocularis*, and polycystic hydatid disease caused by *Echinococcus vogeli* (Thompson, 1995). Members of the dog family are definitive hosts for these minute tapeworms. What they lack in size they make up for in numbers, with many hundreds or thousands of worms producing large numbers of eggs in one host. Eggs are passed in the stools and ingested by the intermediate hosts, which include sheep, cattle, pigs, rodents, and other herbivorous animals. Humans, especially children, are infected following the accidental ingestion of eggs from the environment.

Eggs hatch in the intestine, and the embryos penetrate the intestinal wall and then enter the blood stream. Although most hydatids develop in the liver, some disseminate to other sites. Development of the cysts is slow and may take many years to form a cyst of 10–15 cm in diameter. In the usual secondary hosts, the cysts contain numerous protoscoleces, which proliferate from a germinal membrane.

E. granulosus, the most important species producing human disease, is common in many sheep- and cattle-raising areas of the world, including the United States, where dogs are the usual definitive host. Unilocular hydatids develop as single cysts in the liver and secondarily in the lungs or other locations. The cysts are filled with clear fluid and contain brood capsules and numerous protoscoleces, which can number in the thousands (Fig. 61–26*C* and *D*). Symptoms in humans are those of a slowly growing mass lesion, although infections in the CNS become apparent earlier than in other sites. The diagnosis is suggested based on clinical presentation and history plus the use of radiography, CT scans, and ultrasonography. Serologic tests are very useful in confirming a diagnosis and usually involve a screening test such as EIA or IHA followed, if positive, by a confirmatory assay such as immunoblot or gel diffusion (Wilson, 1995). Sensitivity varies from 60–90% depending on the characteristics of the case. False-positive reactions may occur with cysticercosis, although

disease presentation should prevent confusion. Aspiration of cyst contents is potentially dangerous because spillage of cyst contents may result in dissemination of disease or possibly anaphylactic shock; but if aspiration is performed, cyst contents usually reveal hydatid sand, a mixture of protoscoleces, disintegrating brood capsules, hooklets, and calcareous corpuscles.

E. multilocularis produces multilocular or alveolar hydatid disease in the northern regions of Europe and Russia, and in Alaska, Canada, and the northern tier of states in the United States. Intermediate hosts include several genera of small rodents; foxes, wolves, and dogs are definitive hosts. Human infection occurs in the liver, where the hydatid develops as an invasive cyst that insinuates itself within the tissue in an alveolar pattern. Although the germinal membrane proliferates in the human liver, protoscoleces fail to develop. The pathologic picture is reminiscent of hepatic carcinoma. Serologic assays that use *E. granulosus* antigens are useful in the diagnosis of this disease. The differential use of antigens from both parasites shows promise of discrimination between the two diseases (Wilson, 1995).

E. vogeli produces a polycystic hydatid cyst in humans that is invasive but, unlike *E. multilocularis*, produces both brood capsules and protoscoleces. The disease is limited to Latin America, where rodents, specifically the paca, and bush dogs complete the life cycle (D'Alessandro, 1979). Polycystic hydatid disease in South America may also be caused by *Echinococcus oligarthus*, a parasite of felids and rodents. This species is similar morphologically to *E. vogeli*, and cases have been misidentified in the past (D'Alessandro, 1995).

Sparganosis

Sparganosis is caused by larval cestodes of the genus *Spirometra*, which are closely related to *Diphyllobothrium* spp. Adult stages commonly parasitize cats and dogs and their relatives in Asia (*Spirometra mansoni*) and North America (*Spirometra mansonoides*). Life cycles are similar to those of *Diphyllobothrium*: copepods serve as first intermediate hosts for the procercoid larvae and fish serve as second intermediate hosts for plerocercoid larvae. Humans become infected with these larval stages (the sparganum) through ingestion of copepods in drinking water or ingestion of raw or incompletely cooked fish. Use of frogs and snakes as poultices may also result in the transfer of larvae to the human host. Sparganosis usually presents as localized or migratory subcutaneous swellings associated with erythema and pain, although brain infections occur. Surgical exploration may reveal a delicate, slender, ivory-colored worm varying from a few to many centimeters in length. Cross-sections demonstrate a thick tegument with deep folds and parenchyma with prominent muscle bundles. There is no body cavity seen, as in the nematodes, and calcareous corpuscles are numerous (Fig. 61–26*F*) (Orihel, 1995; Gutierrez, 2000).

Coenurosis

Intestinal *Taenia* spp. of cats and dogs (primarily *Taenia multiceps* and *Taenia serialis*) produce a larval stage in intermediate hosts known as a coenurus. This stage consists of a large (up to 10 cm) transparent sac containing numerous scoleces that bud off from a germinal membrane and invaginate into the fluid-filled cyst (Fig. 61–26E). Sheep are the usual intermediate hosts for *T. multiceps* and rodents, hares, and rabbits for *T. serialis*, although humans serve in this role through accidental ingestion of eggs originating from domestic cats and dogs. Like cysticerci, coenuri may develop in any organ, producing a similar disease. Diagnosis is usually made by examination of the excised cyst or its demonstration in tissue sections. The presence of multiple invaginated scoleces within a single bladder differentiates the coenurus from other larval cestodes.

Trematodes

All the liver, lung, and blood-inhabiting trematodes that mature in humans produce eggs that usually exit the body via stool, urine, or sputum. Because of their extraintestinal location, these flukes and their eggs may be found in tissues either incidentally or associated with symptoms.

Adult *F. hepatica*, *C. sinensis*, and *O. viverrini* may be found in hepatic and biliary tissues, and occasionally in ectopic locations. The presence of typical eggs either free in the tissues or within the uterus of the helminth often provides a definitive identification. Adult *Paragonimus* spp. primarily reside in the lung but may be found in ectopic sites such as brain and subcutaneous tissue, where they produce abscesses, often associated with large numbers of eggs. Adult schistosomes reside in blood vessels, primarily in the distribution of the inferior mesenteric vein (*S. mansoni*), superior mesenteric vein (*S. japonicum* and *S. mekongi*), and in the vesical plexus (*S. haematobium*). Although the adult stages are rarely encountered in tissue sections, eggs may be found in large numbers in the tissues of the intestine, liver, and bladder (Fig. 61–23B, D, F). Eggs also may disseminate via the blood stream to other sites, including the brain, spinal cord, lungs, heart, kidneys, and spleen. The eggs of *S. japonicum* are especially prone to disseminate because of their smaller size and the large numbers typically produced. Identification of eggs is dependent on recognition of their typical sizes and morphologic characteristics in appropriate tissues.

Medically Important Arthropods

Arthropods comprise a large and diverse group of organisms, few of which have clinical or economic significance. Those that do, however, are important causes of morbidity and mortality in humans and their domestic animals, and are responsible for serious economic losses to agriculture. Although perhaps best known among clinicians for their abilities to transmit various infectious agents, including viruses, bacteria (rickettsia, spirochetes, others), protozoa, and certain helminths, arthropods also cause serious disease by direct tissue invasion, envenomation, vesication, blood loss, and allergic reactions. Exaggerated fears of arthropods (entomophobia) and delusions of infestation (delusory parasitosis) are not uncommon neuroses, which may be disabling to some individuals. Species directly or indirectly responsible for human disease include representatives of all the major arthropod classes (Table 61–12).

In this section, an approach that the clinical laboratory may use when evaluating clinical specimens containing arthropods is presented, followed by a brief discussion of each of the arthropod groups of medical importance. A variety of general and specialized texts and guides are available for more complete coverage of the field of medical entomology (Beaver, 1984; Garcia, 2001; Goddard, 2002; Lane, 1993; Mullen, 2002; National Communicable Disease Center, 1969; Strickland, 2000).

Biological Characteristics

Arthropods are characterized by a bilaterally symmetric, segmented body; several pairs of jointed appendages; and a rigid chitinous exoskeleton that is molted repeatedly during growth. Development proceeds from egg to adult through either gradual (egg, nymph, and adult stages) or complete (egg, larva, pupa, and adult stages) metamorphosis. Bedbugs, kissing bugs, lice, and cockroaches are examples of insects that undergo gradual metamorphosis. Flies and mosquitoes; fleas; ants, bees, and wasps; and beetles undergo complete metamorphosis: worm-like larval forms pupate to emerge as adults. Arachnids undergo developmental changes most similar to the process of gradual metamorphosis. The larval stages of those arthropods that undergo complete metamorphosis often prove to be the most difficult for clinical laboratorians to identify and should be referred to a specialist.

Table 61–12 Classification of Arthropods of Medical Importance

Class Insecta (insects)
Order Anoplura (sucking lice)
Order Siphonaptera (fleas)
Order Dictyoptera (cockroaches)
Order Hemiptera (bedbugs, kissing bugs)
Order Hymenoptera (ants, wasps, bees)
Order Coleoptera (beetles)
Order Lepidoptera (moths, butterflies, caterpillars)
Order Diptera (flies, mosquitoes, midges)

Class Arachnida (arachnids)
Subclass Scorpiones (scorpions)
Subclass Araneae (spiders)
Subclass Acari (ticks, mites, chiggers)

Class Diplopoda (millipedes)

Class Chilopoda (centipedes)

Class Crustacea (crustaceans)
Order Copepoda (copepods)
Order Decapoda (crabs, crayfish)

Class Pentastomida (tongue worms)

Mechanisms of Injury

Direct Tissue Invasion

Invasion of superficial tissues (referred to as infestation) may occur with a variety of arthropods, of which scabies mites, chigoe fleas, and some dipteran larvae (maggots) are most common. Invasion of deeper body tissues and cavities (referred to as infection) occurs primarily with maggots and, rarely, pentastomid larvae. Tissue invasion by dipteran larvae is referred to as myiasis and may occur in either living or devitalized tissues, depending on the involved species.

Envenomation

Many arthropods are capable of injecting either saliva or venom with their bites or stings. For most individuals, these compounds cause only local tissue reactions, but serious, life-threatening reactions such as anaphylaxis may occur, often as a result of previous sensitization to the particular toxin. Hymenopteran (ants, bees, and wasps) and scorpion stings are among the greatest offenders (Reisman, 1994). The bites of certain arthropods, especially the centipedes; mosquitoes, flies, and biting midges; bedbugs, kissing bugs, and assassin bugs; sucking lice; fleas; and ticks and mites may also be toxic, causing either local or systemic reactions. Almost all spiders are venomous, but only a few groups (widow spiders, violin spiders, and certain tarantulas) pose significant health risks to humans. Less common but recognized causes of envenomation result from exposure to the urticating hairs of certain caterpillars and beetle larvae.

Vesication

Certain of the larger tropical millipedes are capable of spraying a vesicating (blister-causing) chemical substance from glands located on each body segment. These compounds are especially irritating should they reach the conjunctiva. Blister beetles are so named from their ability to discharge vesicating fluids (cantharidin, the active ingredient in the aphrodisiac Spanish fly) from their body when handled.

Blood Loss

Arthropods responsible for producing significant irritation or blood loss to humans and domestic animals include bedbugs, kissing bugs, lice, fleas, flies, mosquitoes, biting midges, ticks, and mites. Although these activities are rarely life-threatening, the concurrent transmission of infectious agents may be.

Transmission of Infectious Agents

Many arthropods play an integral role in either the mechanical or biological transmission of infectious disease agents. The common housefly, *Musca domestica*, may be responsible for the mechanical transmission of the agents of bacillary dysentery, cholera, typhoid, viral diarrhea, amebic dysentery, giardiasis, pinworms, and tapeworms. Mechanisms involved in the biological transmission of infectious agents vary from simple organism amplification in the arthropod vector to more complex life-cycle changes of the involved parasite. Ticks and mites are involved in the transmission of certain bacteria (*Rickettsia*, *Ehrlichia*, spirochetes, others), protozoa (*Babesia*), and viruses. Among the insects, lice are involved in the transmission of bacteria (*Rickettsia*, *Bartonella*, and *Borrelia*); kissing bugs transmit trypanosomes; fleas transmit the agents of plague, typhus, and canine tapeworm; and dipterans transmit arboviruses, malarial parasites, trypanosomes, leishmanias, filarial worms, and bacteria.

Hypersensitivity Reactions

Most of the serious reactions to arthropod bites and stings result from allergic hypersensitivities. Hymenopteran stings alone are responsible for most arthropod-related deaths and usually result from the development of hypersensitivity following repeated exposure to venom (Reisman, 1994). Allergies may also be exacerbated following exposure to the saliva, excrement, or body parts of mites, ticks, lice, bedbugs, caterpillars, moths, and butterflies. Asthma and hay fever may also develop in response to the presence of the large variety of house, dust, and animal mites in the environment (Frazier, 1980).

Psychological Manifestations

Entomophobia refers to an unreasonable or excessive fear of seeing or touching arthropods. Although this fear may occasionally result in the disruption of a person's normal activities, it rarely becomes incapacitating. Delusory parasitosis is a more serious emotional disorder in which an individual is convinced that he or she is infected with parasites or arthropods despite objective evidence to the contrary. As the delusion progresses, the individual may report loss of employment, divorce, repeated use of pesticide services, and movement from house to house. Visits to health-care providers are usually numerous, although unsatisfactory. The problem may originate either in the home or workplace and be transferable from one to the other. The delusion may be so convincing that other family members or friends may believe it or acquire it themselves. The patient may submit numerous specimens such as skin, fabric, lint, hair, and mucus to the laboratory. It is incumbent on the laboratory personnel to examine these materials to rule out true infestation. The mysterious onset of irritation and itching may be due to bites from unrecognized scabies mites, lice, fleas, or bedbugs, or from insects and mites questing from an abandoned rodent or bird nest in an area of human habitation. Before dismissing such causes, they must be looked for and their presence excluded (Lynch, 1993; Murray, 2004).

Laboratory Approaches to Arthropod Identification

Arthropod specimens are often directed to the clinical laboratory by both clinicians and patients with the expectation that they can be accurately identified, but few laboratory personnel receive more than a cursory exposure to entomology during training. Nonetheless, laboratorians should have access to texts and dichotomous keys, which should allow limited identification of the more commonly encountered medically important groups, especially ectoparasites (fleas, lice, mites, and ticks). Of more importance is the ability of the laboratory personnel to recognize those rare situations in which outside expertise should be sought. This specifically relates to those occasions when significant clinical decisions regarding therapy and prognosis are being made. State or local public health laboratories often have the expertise available or know of individuals trained in medical entomology at regional educational institutions, museums, or other public or private agencies, including the CDC.

Specimens submitted to the laboratory are most often intact organisms, skin scrapings, tissues, sputum, urine, or stool. Inanimate objects, including foodstuffs, water, clothing, bedding, and carpeting, among others, may also be submitted. It is not uncommon for patients to submit arthropods recovered from the toilet bowl following urination or a bowel movement. In most cases, the presence of such organisms is coincidental and not related to infection.

Proper killing and preservation of arthropods is important to preserve those characteristics necessary for identification. Small, nonwinged arthropods, especially ectoparasites (lice, fleas, ticks and mites), larval forms (maggots, grubs, and caterpillars), spiders, and scorpions should be placed directly into 70–80% ethyl alcohol. Large larval forms are best killed in hot (not boiling) water to extend their bodies and prevent contraction before immersion in alcohol. Attached tissue or other debris should be gently removed or washed away prior to preservation. The smaller forms (mites, small ticks, fleas, and sandflies) may be prepared as permanent slide mounts.

Winged insects, especially adult mosquitoes, midges, and flies, should be killed by exposure to the fumes of ethyl acetate or chloroform and preserved dry to retain the taxonomic information contained in the body and wing scales. Such arthropods usually are pinned and dried, followed by storage in tight-fitting boxes protected with naphthalene or dichlorobenzene. Further details regarding the collection, preservation, and preparation of arthropod specimens for examination are found elsewhere (Beaver, 1984; Steyskal, 1987; Lane, 1993; Garcia, 2001).

Insects

Insects comprise more than 90% of all described arthropod species, although few are responsible for human disease. Members of this class are distinguished from other arthropods by having a body divided into three parts (head, thorax, abdomen); one pair of antennae; three pairs of legs; and one, two, or no pairs of wings. This is the only arthropod class in which flight has developed.

Sucking Lice

Sucking lice are dorsoventrally flattened, wingless insects that have characteristic claws on the ends of each leg that allow attachment to body hairs or clothing (Fig. 61–27A and B). All species suck blood intermittently and may cause unexplained dermatitis. Eggs, known as nits, are deposited on either hair shafts or clothing, depending on the species. Although named for their primary site of attachment, they do not always remain confined to that location. The head louse, *Pediculus capitis*, and the body louse, *Pediculus humanus*, are indistinguishable to the nonspecialist. They are longer than they are wide, and grow to about 3 mm in length. Biological differences are apparent; only *P. humanus* transmits the agents of epidemic typhus, trench fever, and relapsing fever (Kim, 1986). Infestations with both species occur among people living in crowded conditions who have little opportunity for bathing and laundering. Children of school age are at particular risk for acquiring head lice through the sharing of caps, clothing, and combs (Orkin, 1985). Nits of head lice are deposited primarily on hair shafts, and those of body lice are deposited on clothing. Because objects such as hair casts, dander, hair spray, and fungal hair infections may mimic nits, differentiation is important. Nits are typically 1 mm long and, when unhatched, have intact opercula (Fig. 61–27C). Transmission occurs primarily through the sharing of infested clothing and bedding, because body lice tend to lay their eggs in clusters, especially along seams or waistbands. The pubic louse, *Phthirus pubis*, is distinctly different from the others; it is rounder (measuring up to 2 mm in diameter), the abdomen is more crab-like, and the first pair of legs is significantly smaller and more slender than the other pairs (Fig. 61–27B). Pubic lice and their nits are found primarily on pubic hairs but may extend to the chest, armpit, and facial hair. Transmission occurs primarily during sexual intercourse.

Fleas

Fleas are small (1–2 mm), laterally compressed, wingless ectoparasites capable of sucking blood (Fig. 61–27D). Long, muscular legs are adapted for jumping great distances. All fleas that attack humans are parasites of other mammals or poultry and include both blood-sucking pests (many species) and tissue-penetrating jiggers. Infestations commonly occur with exposure to domestic animals and pets; the most pestiferous species are the dog flea (*Ctenocephalides canis*), the cat flea (*Ctenocephalides felis*), and the human flea (*Pulex irritans*). Some individuals become highly sensitized to flea bites, whereas others are unaffected. Cat and dog fleas also are the usual intermediate hosts for the tapeworm *D. caninum* and less frequently for *H. diminuta* and *H. nana*. Because larvae of these species often develop in an animal's bedding, or in carpets and furniture, eradication may require fumigation and cleaning of those articles. The Oriental rat flea, *Xenopsylla cheopis*, is an extremely important species because it transmits the plague bacillus and the agent of murine typhus. Although normally parasitizing several species of rats, this flea readily attacks humans should the rodent host die. The jigger or chigoe flea *Tunga penetrans* is found in both Central and South America and regions of tropical Africa. The female flea attaches to and imbeds itself in the skin, especially between the toes and under the toenails, where it grows to the size of a small pea. After eggs are discharged, the flea dies, prompting an inflammatory response and possible secondary bacterial infection. Tungiasis is diagnosed by identifying the dark portion of the flea's abdomen (displaying the spiracles) protruding from the skin surface of an enlarging lesion (Beaver, 1984; Lane, 1993; Goddard, 2002).

Cockroaches

Cockroaches have closely adapted themselves to human habitation, sharing our food, shelter, and warmth. Although they are primarily nuisance pests, cockroaches are potential carriers of fecal pathogens owing to their ability to move quickly from sewers and drains to food preparation areas. In addition to transmitting pathogenic bacteria, they

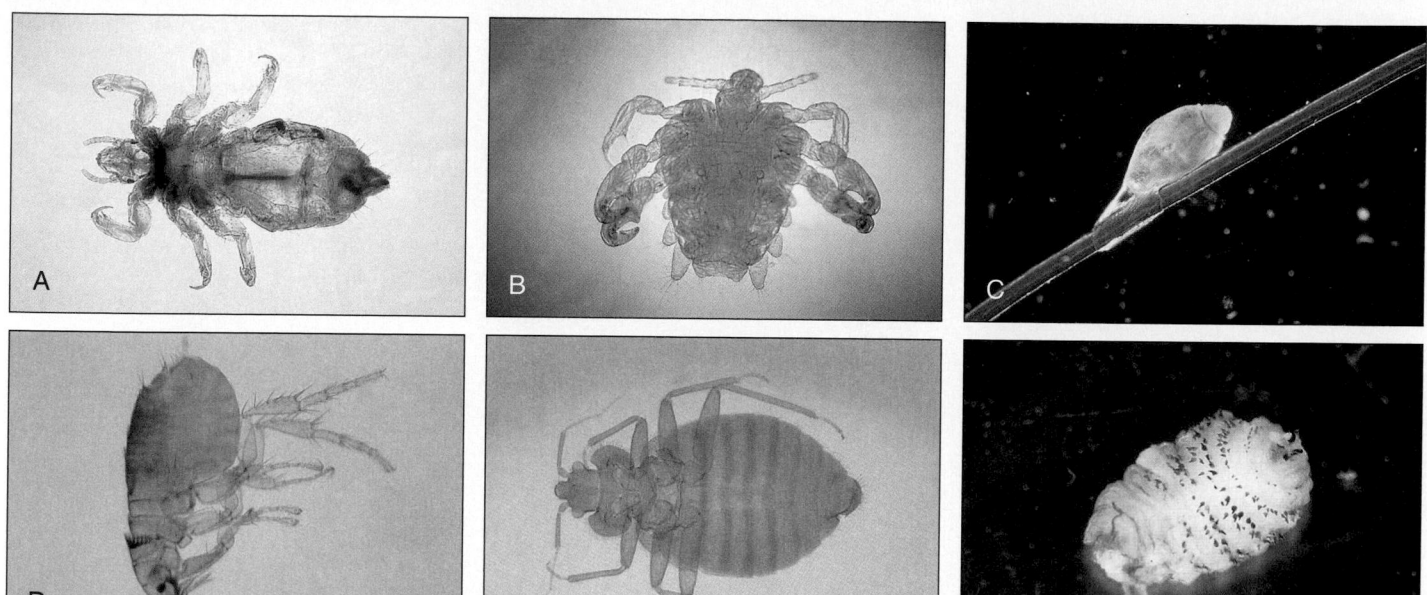

Figure 61–27 Medically important insects. *A, Pediculus capitis*, the head louse. *B, Phthirus pubis*, the crab louse. *C*, Empty egg case (nit) of *P. capitis*. *D, Ctenocephalides canis*, the common dog flea; note powerful hind legs. *E, Cimex lectularius*, the common bedbug. *F*, Larva of *Dermatobia hominis*, the human botfly; note the two sclerotized hooks at the anterior end and numerous body spines (×10). (*A, B*, and *E* with permission from ASM Press.)

may also spread hepatitis and polioviruses; intestinal protozoa, including *E. histolytica*; and several species of enteric nematode. Allergies and asthma may develop in some individuals following exposure to the excreta, cast skins, or body parts of cockroaches (Goddard, 2002).

Bedbugs and Kissing Bugs

Bedbugs (family Cimicidae) and kissing bugs (family Reduviidae) are blood-sucking insects that have a long, narrow proboscis that is folded underneath the body when not in use. Bedbugs (*Cimex lectularius* and *Cimex hemipterus*) are reddish brown, dorsoventrally flattened wingless insects approximately 5 mm in length (Fig. 61–27E). They are cosmopolitan in distribution and attack most any mammal, feeding primarily at night. During daylight hours, they hide under mattresses, loose wallpaper, and floorboards. Although they are not known to transmit disease, bedbug bites may cause painful weals or bullae, depending on an individual's sensitivity to their saliva.

Kissing bugs (*Triatoma, Rhodnius, Panstrongylus*) have a cone-shaped head on a narrow neck and an abdomen that is widened in the middle. These insects are black or brown and some have orange and black markings on the abdomen. They average 1–3 cm in length and, unlike bedbugs, have well developed wings for flight. Like bedbugs, kissing bugs are relatively painless feeders on vertebrates and produce similar skin reactions. In Mexico and Central and South America, they transmit the agent of Chagas disease, *T. cruzi*, in the feces, which are secondarily inoculated into the skin by the human host while scratching (Goddard, 2002; Lane, 1993).

Bees, Wasps, and Ants

Hymenopterans are social insects that readily defend their nests when disturbed. In nonreproductive females, the ovipositor is modified as a stinger capable of injecting venom for use in the capture of prey or for defense. The venom of bees, wasps, hornets, and yellow jackets causes only transient swelling and discomfort in most individuals but may be responsible for systemic reactions, including anaphylaxis, in others who were previously sensitized (Reisman, 1994). Up to 100 people in the United States die each year from hymenopteran stings. The Africanized honey bee is now present in North America following its introduction into Brazil in 1956. These bees, which are more easily provoked than other honey bees, exhibit massive stinging behavior. Many species of ant are problematic for humans because of their ability to bite, and some groups, such as harvester and fire ants, are capable of giving painful stings.

Beetles

Although beetles are perhaps best known as pests of agricultural crops, some species may give a painful bite, and others, especially the blister beetles, may exude vesicating fluids (cantharidin) that cause dermatitis or blister formation. The larvae of certain larder beetles have urticating hairs that may be responsible for dermatitis or, if ingested, irritation of the gastrointestinal tract. Larval and adult larder and grain beetles also may serve as intermediate hosts for the rodent and human tapeworms *H. diminuta* and *H. nana*.

Moths and Butterflies

Certain larvae (caterpillars) of lepidoptera possess urticating hairs or spines capable of injecting venom when handled. Although most effects of these toxins remain localized to the skin, systemic effects including shock and paralysis have been reported (Goddard, 2002). Adult tussock and gypsy moths are known to have urticating scales and hairs that may cause dermatitis, eye irritation, or respiratory tract irritation, especially among forestry workers (Shama, 1982).

Flies, Mosquitoes, and Midges

Diptera are characterized by the presence of a single pair of membranous wings. Among all arthropods, they are responsible for the greatest share of human disease through blood-sucking activities, biological or mechanical transmission of infectious agents, and direct tissue invasion by larval forms (myiasis). Bites from a variety of flies, mosquitoes and biting midges often cause local irritation from sensitivity to the saliva and, in some individuals, systemic reactions. In addition to blood-sucking activities, the repeated attacks themselves may be physically and psychologically damaging. Certain blood-sucking species are also responsible for the transmission of important human pathogens, including the agents of malaria, filariasis, and arboviral disease by mosquitoes; onchocerciasis by blackflies; loiasis by deer flies; leishmaniasis and bartonellosis by sand flies; and African trypanosomiasis by tsetse flies. Other viral, bacterial, and parasitic agents are readily transmitted mechanically by nonbiting flies such as house flies, flesh flies, and blow flies, which can easily contaminate human food.

Myiasis may occur in an accidental, facultative, or obligatory fashion. The housefly, *Musca domestica*, has no requirement for developing in mammalian tissue, yet may be found occasionally in dead tissue or under plaster casts. This type of accidental myiasis is not uncommon but is rarely clinically significant. Facultative myiasis is most often caused by blowflies and flesh flies, which ordinarily feed on dead tissues but may move into adjacent viable tissues. Obligatory myiasis is caused by certain species that develop only in living tissues. Those species that infect humans are all of zoonotic origin. The human botfly, *Dermatobia hominis*, develops in boil-like subcutaneous lesions, with the posterior end of the maggot appearing at the skin surface (Fig. 61–27F). This species is most commonly found in individuals who have spent time in Central or South America or, less frequently, Africa, and is unusual in that its eggs are mechanically transported to the host by other flying insects, usually mosquitoes. The tumbu fly (*Cordylobia anthropophaga*), found in sub-Saharan Africa, also causes a furuncular type of myiasis. Eggs of this species usually are laid on the ground or on hanging laundry, and larvae rapidly penetrate the skin

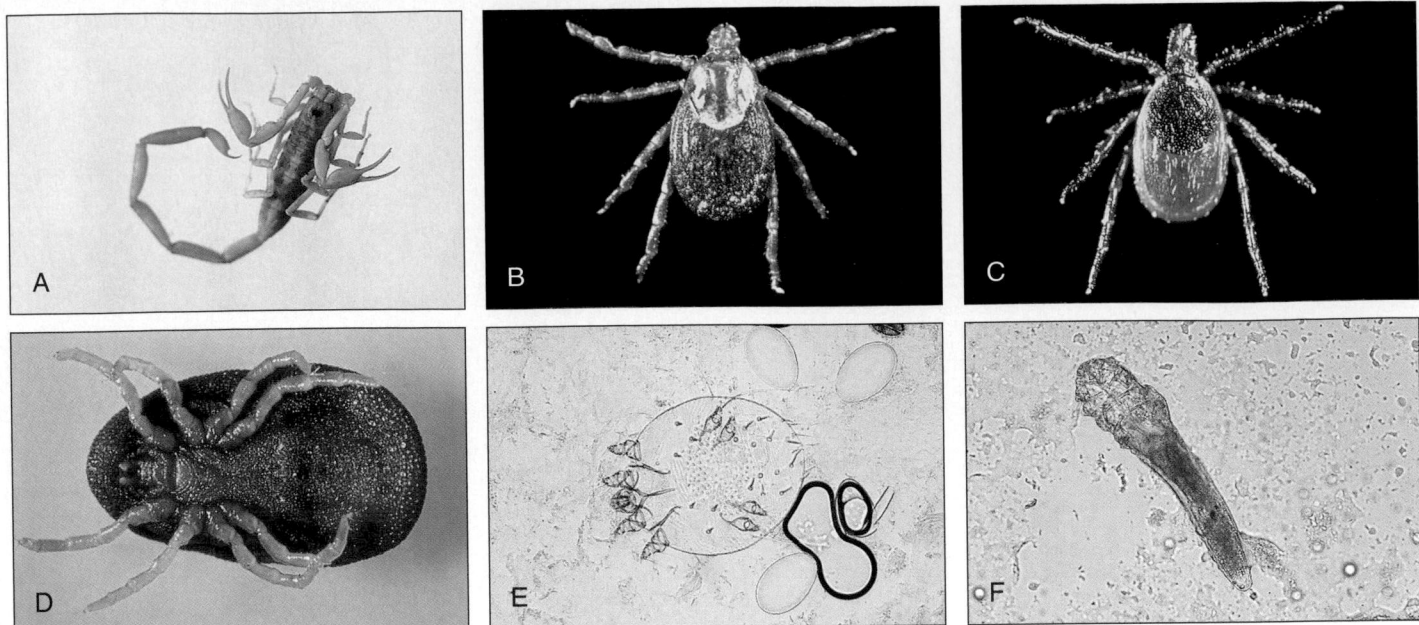

Figure 61–28 Medically important arachnids. *A,* Scorpion; note forward-directed pincher claws and stinger on the tail tip. *B, Dermacentor variabilis* (dog tick) nonengorged adult female. *C, Ixodes scapularis* (black-legged tick or deer tick) nonengorged adult female. *D, Ornithodoros* sp. (soft tick) nonengorged adult, ventral view. *E, Sarcoptes scabei* (itch mite) adult; note presence of adjacent eggs in skin scrapings. *F, Demodex folliculorum* (follicle mite) adult. (*A* with permission from ASM Press; *B* and *C* with permission from Northwest Infectious Disease Consultants; *E* with permission from *New England Journal of Medicine* 1994; 331:777.)

on contact. The most serious obligatory myiasis is caused by the Old World screwworm, *Chrysomya bezziana,* and the New World screwworm, *Cochliomyia hominivorax.* These species lay their eggs directly on their cattle hosts, usually on wounds or near the nostrils. The larvae actively feed on and move through living tissues. Human infections may be particularly destructive if the larvae invade the eye, nose, or mouth. Other species may also be responsible for traumatic, obligatory myiasis in humans (Lane, 1993).

Arachnids

Medically important arachnids include the scorpions, spiders, ticks, and mites. Scorpions and spiders have two body segments, the cephalothorax and the abdomen, whereas the ticks and mites have only one. Members of the group have four pair of legs as nymphs and adults; larval ticks and mites have three pair of legs. All lack antennae, mandibles, and wings. Scorpions and spiders are best known for their ability to inject poisonous venoms, whereas ticks and mites are best known as vectors for viral, bacterial, and protozoal pathogens.

Scorpions

Unlike other arachnids, scorpions have a pair of forward-directed pincer claws that impart a crab-like appearance and a segmented tail with a bulbous stinging apparatus in the tip (Fig. 61–28*A*). They are predatory in nature and paralyze their intended victim with venom from the sting, which may also be used for defensive purposes. Toxicity to humans varies depending on the species; many elicit no more reaction than that of a bee sting but some are deadly, causing over 1000 deaths annually. Poisonous species occur in the Western Hemisphere, Europe, Africa, and the Middle East (Beaver, 1984; Goddard, 2002).

Spiders

Spiders lack a tail with an attached stinger but instead have fang-like chelicerae among their mouthparts, through which venom can be expressed. Although the majority of spiders are venomous, few have chelicerae capable of penetrating human skin. Most spider bites cause only transitory irritation and pain. The widow spiders (genus *Lactrodectus*) are one group responsible for systemic arachnidism through the action of a potent neurotoxin capable of producing weakness, myalgia, paralysis, convulsions and, occasionally, death. Published mortality rates vary from less than 1% to 6%. Five closely related species occur in the United States; the black widow (*Lactrodectus mactans*) is the most widespread. Female black widow spiders are glossy black with a characteristic red or orange hourglass-shaped marking on the underside of the abdomen and have a leg span of 3–4 cm. They live in protected locations such as woodsheds, basements, and outdoor privies (Strickland, 2000).

Violin spiders (genus *Loxosceles*) are responsible for necrotic arachnidism or loxoscelism. In the United States the brown recluse or fiddleback spider (*Loxosceles reclusa*) is most often involved, although other species are present. This species is 1–2 cm long, tan to dark brown, and has a darkened violin-shaped marking oriented base forward on the dorsum of the cephalothorax. When present in homes they are reclusive in their habits, preferring undisturbed areas such as closets, basements, and under porches. Their bite is painless and often goes unrecognized until several hours later, when the area becomes red, swollen, and painful. The venom is dermonecrotic and hemolytic, producing cutaneous necrosis and sloughing of the involved skin over several days. The resulting lesion may be difficult to heal and subject to secondary infection. Systemic reactions such as hemolysis and acute renal failure are rare. Other spider genera have also been implicated in producing necrotic arachnidism (Fisher, 1994).

Ticks

Unlike spiders and scorpions, ticks have a fused cephalothorax and abdomen, and a characteristic toothed hypostome for feeding. Tick development progresses through four stages: egg, larva, nymph, and adult. Following hatching, a blood meal is required for progression to the subsequent stage. Humans usually acquire ticks in grassy or brushy areas in close proximity to the usual animal hosts. All species are obligate blood-sucking ectoparasites and are important vectors of viral, bacterial, and protozoal pathogens to humans and domestic animals. Their feeding activities also may produce local tissue damage and blood loss, especially to livestock and wildlife, or tick paralysis, a syndrome caused by a neurotoxin secreted by a tick's salivary glands that produces ascending flaccid paralysis and toxemia. Symptoms may closely mimic those of Guillain–Barré syndrome, poliomyelitis, or botulism. Removal of the attached tick usually results in resolution of symptoms within hours to days.

Species affecting humans include members of the family Ixodidae (hard ticks) and Argasidae (soft ticks). Hard ticks have anteriorly directed mouthparts and a sclerotized plate, or scutum, on the dorsum. The scutum covers the entire dorsum of the male but only the anterior portion in the female, allowing the body to swell when engorged (Fig. 61–28*B* and *C*). Argasid ticks have a soft leathery body lacking a scutum and ventrally directed mouthparts that are not visible when viewed from above (Fig. 61–28*D*). Unengorged ticks are generally 2–5 mm long but may enlarge to several times that size following engorgement. Engorged hard ticks may mimic soft ticks, so care must be exercised in their identification (Sonenshine, 1991, 1993).

Most ticks found crawling on or imbedded in human skin are hard ticks. Soft ticks tend to feed only briefly and then often at night. Important species of hard ticks in North America include *Dermacentor variabilis* (American dog tick), *Dermacentor andersoni* (Rocky Mountain wood tick),

Amblyomma americanum (Lone Star tick), *Rhipicephalus sanguineus* (brown dog tick), *Ixodes scapularis* (black-legged or deer tick), and *Ixodes pacificus* (western black-legged or deer tick). *Dermacentor* and *Amblyomma* ticks are called ornate ticks because of the presence of white markings on their scuta; the other species are inornate ticks.

Dermacentor ticks transmit Rocky Mountain spotted fever and possibly tularemia, Q fever, and Colorado tick fever. *Ixodes* ticks are vectors of Lyme disease, babesiosis, and ehrlichiosis, and in other parts of the world, these ticks are responsible for the transmission of certain arboviruses. *Amblyomma* ticks are capable of transmitting Rocky Mountain spotted fever, as well as tularemia and possibly Lyme disease. All these genera are capable of causing tick paralysis. *Rhipicephalus* ticks have been implicated in the transmission of Rocky Mountain spotted fever and ehrlichiosis in North America, and of boutonneuse fever in the Mediterranean area. Soft ticks of the genus *Ornithodoros* occur in many parts of the world, including the United States, and are important vectors of the relapsing fever spirochetes (*Borrelia recurrentis* and related forms) (Spach, 1993; Murray, 2003).

Mites

Mites are microscopic-sized (usually <1 mm) arachnids that are widely distributed in the environment. Medically important species may attack humans directly, serve as vectors for infectious diseases, or cause dust allergies. Humans are commonly infested with both *Demodex folliculorum* and *Demodex brevis*, the follicle mites, and *Sarcoptes scabei*, the itch or mange mite. Follicle mites are minute (0.1–0.4 mm), elongate parasites with stubby legs that can be recovered from hair follicles and sebaceous glands (Fig. 61–28F). They are common incidental findings on histologic skin preparations. Although their presence has been associated with various skin conditions, they are commonly found in healthy individuals as well, which makes their significance hard to assess (Burns, 1992).

Sarcoptes scabei mites are of greater medical importance because of their ability to create serpiginous tunnels through the upper layers of the epidermis. Transmitted through personal contact, these mites are found primarily in the interdigital spaces and the flexor surfaces of the wrists and forearms and less commonly in other areas, including the breasts, buttocks, and external genitalia. Inflammation and intense itching results from the tunneling activity and from the deposition of eggs and excreta. Clinical manifestations vary depending on the degree of sensitization to the parasites and their products. Lesions often become secondarily infected. A generalized dermatitis occurring in the presence of thousands of mites, typically in elderly or immunocompromised individuals, is known as crusted or Norwegian scabies.

The diagnosis is made by placing skin scrapings collected from tunneled areas in 20% potassium hydroxide or mineral oil for clearing and examining under the microscope. Detection of eggs, six-legged larvae, and eight-legged nymphs or adults is diagnostic but may be difficult to demonstrate (Figs 61–28E and 61–29). The diagnosis of scabies in an institutional or school setting may result in pseudoepidemics, in which numerous individuals develop itching without evidence of disease. Care must be exercised to properly diagnose the disease to identify real cases and differentiate them from cases of delusory parasitosis (Orkin, 1985; Lynch, 1993).

A number of animal mite species may attack humans for a blood meal, either as larval forms or as adults, when the normal mammalian or bird hosts are not available. Larval chigger mites (family Trombiculidae) are problematic in many parts of the world because their saliva can produce large weal-and-flare reactions with intense itching. Often red in color, these tiny six-legged larvae commonly attach to the skin in areas where clothing is restrictive, such as at the ankles, waistline, armpits, and wrists. In parts of Asia and Australia, trombiculid mites are vectors for the transmission of the agent of scrub typhus (Lane, 1993).

Certain nonbiting mites play a role in allergic rhinitis, asthma, and some skin conditions. The secretions, excreta, and body parts of *Dermatophagoides farinae* and *Dermatophagoides pteronyssinus* are potent allergens that may occur in great numbers in the household environment (Frazier, 1980). Routine testing by an allergist may identify the offending agent.

Classes of Lesser Medical Importance

Millipedes

Millipedes are worm-like arthropods with numerous apparent body segments, each with two pairs of legs, that are commonly found in and under decaying vegetation. Although they lack mouthparts capable of

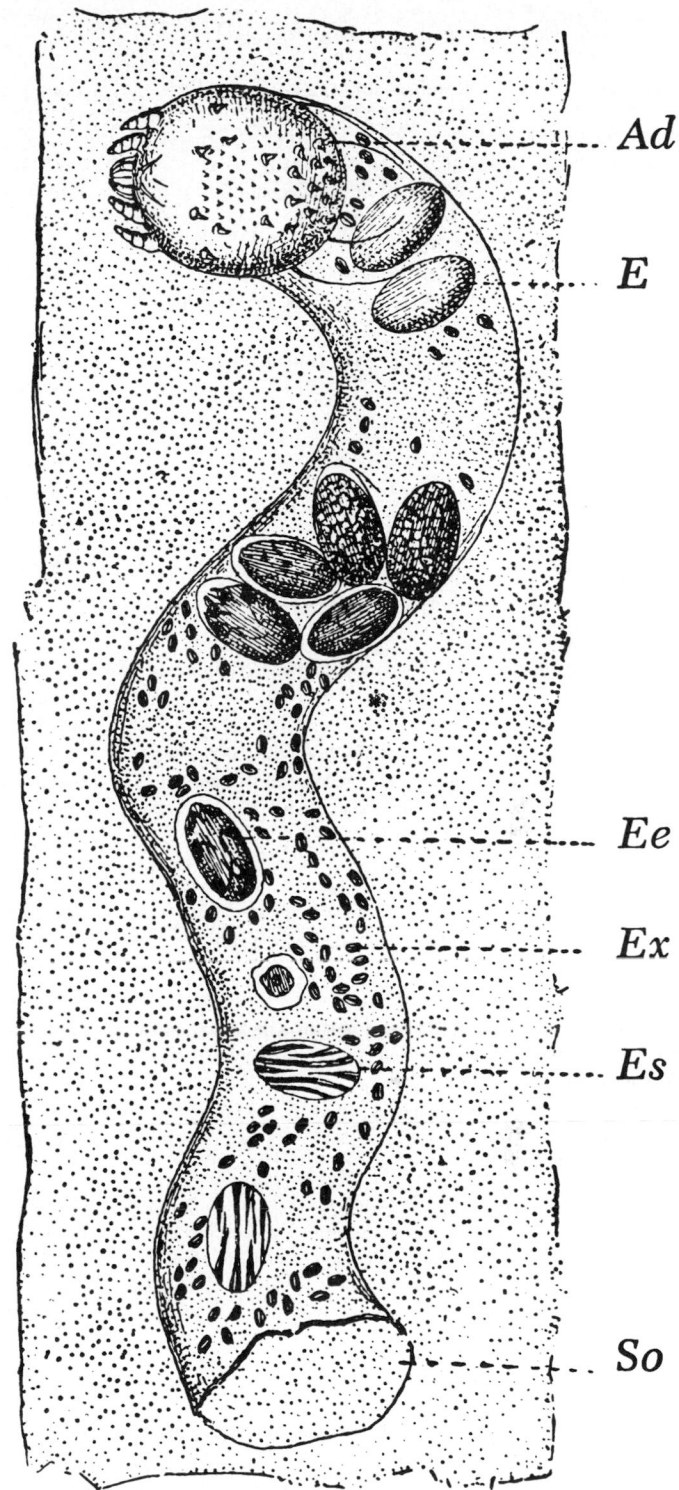

Figure 61–29 *Sarcoptes scabiei*. Diagram of a subcutaneous burrow. (Ad = adult female; E = eggs; Ee = embryo egg; Ex = excrement; Es = egg shell; So = skin orifice.)

producing serious bites, many species produce vesicating secretions from glands located on each body segment. When handled roughly, the larger tropical species are capable of squirting these fluids over a distance of several centimeters. Exposure of the skin or mucous membranes to these fluids may produce a burning sensation and blister formation.

Centipedes

Centipedes are flatter than millipedes, have only one pair of legs per body segment, and display long antennae. They are fast moving and can inflict a painful sting from a pair of forward-directed pincers that are modified from the first pair of legs. Although they are rarely responsible for serious injury to humans, the larger species (26–45 cm) found in the southern United States and in tropical regions are able to penetrate human skin when handled, giving a painful, burning sting with local tissue reaction.

Table 61–13 Parasitic Infections in Compromised Hosts

Infection	Predisposing Host Abnormalities	Comments	References
Intestinal Protozoa			
Cryptosporidiosis	AIDS (especially CD4+ <200/μL), transplantation, antineoplastic chemotherapy	Severe protracted diarrhea (up to 17 L/day.) May have extraintestinal involvement including pancreas, biliary tract, and lungs. Limited therapy available, is not curative	Wittner, 1993; Thielman, 1998
Isosporiasis	AIDS, transplantation, antineoplastic chemotherapy	Severe protracted diarrhea. Extraintestinal involvement of regional lymph nodes may be seen. Effective therapy is available	Wittner, 1993; Thielman, 1998
Cyclosporiasis	AIDS, probably other immunosuppression	Severe protracted diarrhea clinically similar to cryptosporidiosis and isosporiasis. Responds to trimethoprim–sulfamethoxazole	Wittner, 1993; Thielman, 1998
Microsporidiosis	AIDS, other severe immunosuppression	Various syndromes: 1. Multisystem disease 2. Enteritis with severe diarrhea (most frequent) 3. Ocular infection 4. Hepatobiliary with granulomas, hepatic necrosis or cholangitis 5. Skeletal muscle disease Examination of urinary sediment with appropriate stain may allow diagnosis on nonenteric syndromes and some cases of enteric disease	Wittner, 1993; Thielman, 1998
Giardiasis	Common variable immunodeficiency, X-linked agammaglobulinemia	Prolonged diarrhea with malabsorption. AIDS is *not* a predisposing condition	Thielman, 1998
Blood and Tissue Protozoa			
Granulomatous amebic encephalitis	AIDS and other immunocompromised states	Usually caused by amebae of the genera *Acanthamoeba* or *Balamuthia*. Produces subacute or chronic central nervous system infection but may be acute in severely immunosuppressed hosts with dissemination	Martinez, 1997
Toxoplasmosis	AIDS with CD4+ usually <100/μL and other immunocompromised states. Heart transplant, donor seropositive and recipient seronegative	Usually result of reactivation of cysts from previous infections. Often disseminated disease with multiorgan involvement or multifocal CNS lesions. Can cause pneumonitis resembling that caused by *Pneumocystis jiroveci*. May cause chorioretinitis. Can occur after transplantation of bone marrow but usually mild. Heart transplant with donor serologically positive and recipient serologically negative may lead to severe, often fatal toxoplasmosis	McCabe, 1993
Leishmaniasis	AIDS, other immunosuppression	Limited influence on cutaneous leishmaniasis. Susceptibility to visceral leishmaniasis increased but not disease severity. More likely to relapse after treatment	Herwaldt, 1999
American trypanosomiasis (Chagas disease)	AIDS, lymphoblastic lymphoma, cardiac transplantation, other immunosuppression	In AIDS – central nervous system often involved, myocarditis, skin lesions	Mileno, 1998; Markell, 1999
Babesiosis	Splenectomy	Usually subclinical infection in those with intact host defenses. Splenectomized patients usually develop clinically evident disease which can be fatal	Mileno, 1998; Markell, 1999
Helminth			
Strongyloidiasis	Immunosuppression for transplantation or by cancer chemotherapy or adrenal corticosteroids or lymphoma. AIDS is *not* a major predisposing factor	Because of endogenous autoinfection; hyperinfection or disseminated infection can develop and present as pneumonia or severe intestinal disease. Gram-negative sepsis or Gram-negative meningitis can result from translocation of intestinal bacteria via invading larvae. Should check for strongyloidiasis before immunosuppressing patient from highly endemic areas	Mileno, 1998; Markell, 1999
Arthropod			
Scabies	Malignancy, transplant immunosuppression, antineoplastic therapy,	AIDS Leads to 'Norwegian' or crusted scabies with widespread involvement by thick, crusted lesions. Sometimes has severe itching. Patient has numerous mites and is therefore highly contagious. Often less responsive to therapy	Mileno, 1998; Markell, 1999

AIDS = acquired immunodeficiency syndrome; CNS = central nervous system.

Although systemic reactions may occur in individuals who have been previously sensitized, fatalities are rare (Goddard, 2002).

Crustaceans

Crustaceans of medical importance are primarily those species that serve as hosts for larval stages of several different helminths. Several genera of crabs and crayfish are intermediate hosts for the metacercariae of various species of lung fluke (*Paragonimus* spp.) found around the world. Copepods are common microscopic zooplankton, certain species of which serve as first intermediate hosts for the nematodes *D. medinensis* and *Gnathostoma spinigerum* and for cestodes of the genera *Diphyllobothrium* and *Spirometra*.

Pentastomids

Pentastomes, or tongue worms, are arthropods of uncertain affinities owing to a lack of morphologic characteristics. Adult stages are worm-like organisms that live in the nasal passages of certain predatory reptiles, birds, and mammals. Larval stages resemble mites and reside in rodents, herbivores, and freshwater fish. Human liver and lung infections with larval stages have been reported from Asia and Africa. Adult stages have been recovered from the nasopharynx of individuals from the Middle East and Africa, where they are responsible for an obstructive condition known as halzoun (Beaver, 1984; Strickland, 2000).

Parasitic Infections and the Immunocompromised Host

Immunocompromised hosts are hosts who have abnormalities in their humoral or cellular immune systems resulting from disease, therapy, or congenital abnormality. Severe malnutrition may also compromise host defenses. In most instances the predisposing host abnormalities are primarily of the cellular (T cell) immune system and result from AIDS, malignancies, chemotherapy of malignancies, immunosuppression for transplantation, corticosteroid therapy, or a combination of these. For giardiasis the predisposing immune defect is with humoral immunity and for babesiosis it is with splenectomy.

With the worldwide epidemic of HIV infection and AIDS being particularly severe in underdeveloped countries with a high incidence of parasitic infections such as malaria, schistosomiasis, ascariasis, amebiasis, and filariasis, it is fortunate that these infections do not cause particularly severe disease in AIDS patients; however, as comorbidities their contribution to health-care costs is enormous.

Some parasitic infections such as cryptosporidiosis, toxoplasmosis, and strongyloidiasis are more severe in immunocompromised hosts, but there are differences. For example, while cryptosporidiosis and toxoplasmosis are particularly problematic in AIDS patients, strongyloidiasis is not a major problem in this population but is a problem in transplant recipients and patients receiving antineoplastic chemotherapy.

Table 61–13 lists parasitic infections that are more severe and/or frequent in immunocompromised patients. Clinical manifestations may be different than those seen in the general population, as is noted in the comment section.

References

Aldeen WE, Hale D, Robison AJ, et al: Evaluation of a commercially available ELISA assay for detection of *Giardia lamblia* in fecal specimens. Diagn Microbiol Infect Dis 1995; 21:77.

Alicata JE: The discovery of *Angiostrongylus cantonensis* as a cause of human eosinophilic meningitis. Parasitol Today 1991; 7:151.

Anuran JD, Starr MB, Jakobiec FA: *Acanthamoeba* keratitis: a review of the literature. Cornea 1987; 6:2.

Ash LR, Orihel TC: Parasites: A Guide to Laboratory Procedures and Identification. Chicago, IL, ASCP Press, 1987.

Ash LR, Orihel TC: Atlas of Human Parasitology, 4th ed. Chicago, IL, ASCP Press, 1997.

Badawi AF, Mostafa MH, O'Connor PJ: Involvement of alkylating agents in schistosome-associated bladder cancer: The possible basic mechanisms of induction. Cancer Lett 1992; 63:171.

Balows A, Hausler WJ Jr, Ohashi M, Turano A: Laboratory Diagnosis of Infectious Diseases. Principles and Practice, Vol 1. Bacterial, Mycotic and Parasitic Diseases. New York, Springer-Verlag, 1988.

Bartlett MS, Harper K, Smith N, et al: Comparative evaluation of a modified zinc sulfate flotation technique. J Clin Microbiol 1978; 7:524.

Beal C, Goldsmith M, Kotby M, et al: The plastic envelope method, a simplified technique for culture diagnosis of trichomoniasis. J Clin Microbiol 1992; 30:2265.

Beaver PC: Light long-lasting *Necator* infection in a volunteer. Am J Trop Med Hyg 1988; 39:369.

Beaver PC, Gadgil RK, Morera P: *Sarcocystis* in man: a review and report of five cases. Am J Trop Med Hyg 1979; 28:819.

Beaver PC, Jung RC, Cupp EW: Clinical Parasitology, 9th ed. Philadelphia, PA, Lea & Febiger, 1984.

Bendall RP, Chiodini PL: New diagnostic methods for parasitic infections. Curr Opin Infect Dis 1993; 6:318.

Benenson MW, Takafuji ET, Lemon SM, et al: Oocyst-transmitted toxoplasmosis associated with ingestion of contaminated water. N Engl J Med 1982; 307:666.

Binford CH, Connor DH: Pathology of Tropical and Extraordinary Diseases. Washington, DC, Armed Forces Institute of Pathology, 1976.

Blessmann, J, Buss H, Nu PA, et al: Real-time PCR for detection and differentiation of *Entamoeba histolytica* and *Entamoeba dispar* in fecal samples. J Clin Microbiol 2002; 40:4413.

Boros DL: Immunopathology of *Schistosoma mansoni* infection. Clin Microbiol Rev 1989; 2:250.

Bossolasco S, Gaiera G, Olchini D, et al: Real-time PCR assay for clinical management of human immunodeficiency virus-infected patients with visceral leishmaniasis. J Clin Microbiol 2003; 41:5080.

Briselden AM, Hillier SL: Evaluation of Affirm VP Microbial Identification Test for *Gardnerella vaginalis* and *Trichomonas vaginalis*. J Clin Microbiol 1994; 32:148.

Bronsdon MA: Rapid dimethyl sulfoxide-modified acid-fast stain of *Cryptosporidium* oocyst in stool specimens. J Clin Microbiol 1984; 19:952.

Brooke MM, Melvin DM: Morphology of diagnostic stages of intestinal parasites of man (Publication No. [CDC] 848116). Washington, DC, United States Department of Health and Human Services, 1984.

Bruce JI, Sornmani S: The Mekong schistosome. Malacological Review, Suppl. 2. Whitmore Lake, MI, 1980.

Bruckner DA: Amebiasis. Clin Microbiol Rev 1992; 5:356.

Buchbinder S, Blatz R, Rodloff AC: Comparison of real-time PCR detection methods for B1 and P30 genes of *Toxoplasma gondii*. Diagn Microbiol Infect Dis 2003;45:269.

Burns DA: Follicle mites and their role in disease. Clin Exp Dermatol 1992; 17:152.

Burrows RB, Swerdlow MA: *Enterobius vermicularis* as a probable vector of *Dientamoeba fragilis*. Am J Trop Med Hyg 1956; 5:258.

Cairncross S, Muller R, Zagaria N: Dracunculiasis (Guinea worm disease) and the eradication inititative. Clin Microbiol Rev 2002; 15:223.

Cali A, Kotler DP, Orenstein JM: *Septata intestinalis* N.G. N.Sp., an intestinal microsporidian associated with chronic diarrhea and dissemination in AIDS patients. J Eukaryot Microbiol 1993; 40:101.

Carabin H, Budke CM, Cowan LD, Willingham AL III, Torgerson PR: Methods for assessing the burden of parasitic zoonoses: echinococcosis and cysticercosis. Trends Parasitol 2005; 21:327.

Cattand P, Miezan BT, de Raadt P: Human African trypanosomiasis: Use of double centrifugation of cerebrospinal fluid to detect trypanosomes. Bull WHO 1988; 66:83.

Cazenave J, Cheyrou A, Blouin P, et al: Use of polymerase chain reaction to detect *Toxoplasma*. J Clin Pathol 1991; 44:1037.

Centers for Disease Control and Prevention: Pseudooutbreak of intestinal amebiasis, California. Morbid Mortal Wkly Rev 1985; 34:125.

Centers for Disease Control and Prevention: Malaria surveillance. Annual Summary. 1987, Issued November 1988.

Centers for Disease Control and Prevention: Surveillance for dracunculiasis. Morbid Mortal Wkly Rev 1992; 41:1.

Centers for Disease Control and Prevention: Summary of notifiable diseases, United States, 1993. Morbid Mortal Wkly Rev 1993; 42:1.

Chan FT, Guan MX, MacKenzie AMR: Application of indirect immunofluorescence to detection of *Dientamoeba fragilis* trophozoites in fecal specimens. J Clin Microbiol 1993; 31:1710.

Clinical and Laboratory Standards Institute: Procedures for the recovery and identification of parasites from the intestinal tract; approved guideline. CLSI Document M28-A2. Wayne, PA, CLSI, 2005.

This consensus document contains a detailed, up-to-date presentation on the processing of gastrointestinal specimens for parasitic infections, including use of immunoassays and test characteristics.

Connor DH, Chandler FW, Schwartz DA, et al: Pathology of Infectious Diseases. Stamford, CT, Appleton & Lange, 1997.

Cook GC (ed): Manson's Tropical Diseases, 21st ed. Philadelphia, PA, WB Saunders, 2002.

Cooper ES, Bundy DAP: *Trichuris* is not trivial. Parasitol Today 1988; 4:301.

Costa JM, Ernault P, Gautier E, et al: Prenatal diagnosis of congenital toxoplasmosis by duplex real-time PCR using fluorescence resonance energy transfer hybridization probes. Prenat Diagn 2001; 21:85.

Costa JM, Pautas C, Ernault P, et al: Real-time PCR for diagnosis and follow-up of Toxoplasma reactivation after allogeneic stem cell transplantation using fluorescence resonance energy transfer hybridization probes. J Clin Microbiol 2000; 38:2929.

Coupe S, Sarfati C, Hamane S, Derouin F: Detection of *Cryptosporidium* and identification to the species level by nested PCR and restriction fragment length polymorphism. J Clin Microbiol 2005; 43:1017.

Craun G: Waterborne giardiasis in the United States 1965–1984. Lancet 1986; 2:513–514.

Cross JH: Intestinal capillariasis. Clin Microbiol Rev 1992; 5:120.

Current WL, Garcia LS: Cryptosporidiosis. Clin Microbiol Rev 1991; 4:325.

Curry A, Caning E: Human microsporidiosis. J Infect 1993; 27:229.

Curtis MA, Bylund G: Diphyllobothriasis: fish tapeworm disease in the circumpolar north. Arctic Med Res 1991; 50:18.

D'Alessandro A, Ramirez LE, Chapadeiro E, et al: Second recorded case of human infection by *Echinococcus oligarthrus*. Am J Trop Med Hyg 1995; 52:29.

D'Alessandro A, Rausch RL, Cuello C, et al: *Echinococcus vogeli* in man, with a review of polycystic hydatid disease in Columbia and neighboring countries. Am J Trop Med Hyg 1979; 28:303.

Dao AH, Robinson DP, Wong SW: Frequency of *Entamoeba gingivalis* in human gingival scrapings. Am J Clin Pathol 1983; 80:380.

DeGirolami PC, Ezratty CR, Desai G, et al: Diagnosis of intestinal microsporidiosis by examination of stool and duodenal aspirate with Weber's modified trichrome and Uvitex 2B stains. J Clin Microbiol 1995; 33:805.

DeHovitz JA, Pape JW, Boncy J, et al: Isosporiasis in AIDS. N Engl J Med 1986; 315:87.

De Monbrison F, Angei C, Staal A, et al: Simultaneous identification of the four human *Plasmodium* species and quantification of *Plasmodium* DNA load in human blood by real-time polymerase chain reaction. Trans R Soc Trop Med Hyg 2003; 97:387.

Diamond LS: Cultivation of *Entamoeba histolytica* in vitro. In Ravdin JI (ed): Amebiasis: Human Infection by *Entamoeba histolytica*. New York, John Wiley & Sons, 1988, p 27.

Diamond LS, Clark CG: A redescription of *Entamoeba histolytica* Schaudinn, 1903 (emended Walker, 1911) separating it from *Entamoeba dispar* Brumpt, 1925. J Eukaryot Microbiol 1993; 40:340.

Diaz JF, Verastegui M, Gilman RH, et al: Immunodiagnosis of human cysticercosis (*Taenia solium*): a field comparison of an antibody-enzyme-linked immunosorbent assay (ELISA), an antigen-ELISA, and an enzyme-linked immunoelectrotransfer blot (EITB) assay in Peru. Am J Trop Med Hyg 1992; 46:610.

Didier ES, Orenstein JM, Aldras A, et al: Comparison of three staining methods for detecting microsporidia in fluids. J Clin Microbiol 1995; 33:3138.

Doing KM, Hamm JL, Jellison JA, et al: False-positive results obtained with the Alexon ProSpecT Cryptosporidium enzyme immunoassay. J Clin Microbiol 1999; 37:1582.

Eastburn RL, Fritsche TR, Terhune CA Jr: Human intestinal infection with Nanophyetus salmincola from salmonid fishes. Am J Trop Med Hyg 1987; 36:586.

Eveland LK, Kenney M, Yermakov V: Laboratory diagnosis of autoinfection in strongyloidiasis. Am J Clin Pathol 1975; 63:421.

Farcas GA, Zhong KJ, Mazzulli T, et al: Evaluation of the RealArt Malaria LC real time PCR assay for malaria diagnosis. J Clin Microbiol 2004; 42:636.

Fedorko DP, Williams EC, Nelson NA, et al: Performance of three enzyme immunoassays and two direct fluorescence assays for detection of Giardia lamblia in stool specimens preserved in ECOFIX. J Clin Microbiol 2000; 38:2781.

Fisher RG: Necrotic arachnidism. West J Med 1994; 160:570.

Fontaine M, Guillot E: Development of a TaqMan quantitative PCR assay specific for Cryptosporidium parvum. FEMS Microbiol Lett 2002; 214:13.

Franzen C, Müller A: Molecular techniques for detection, species differentiation, and phylogenetic analysis of microsporidia. Clin Microbiol Rev 1999; 12:243.

The species of microsporidia known to infect humans is increasing rapidly; this review focuses on the known species that have been studied using traditional and molecular phylogenetic techniques.

Frazier CA, Brown PA: Insects and Allergy and What to Do About Them. Norman, OK, University of Oklahoma Press, 1980.

Fritsche TR: Pathogenic protozoa: an overview of in vitro cultivation and susceptibility to chemotherapeutic agents. Clin Lab Med 1989a; 9:287.

Fritsche TR, Eastburn RL, Wiggins LH, et al: Praziquantel for treatment of human Nanophyetus salmincola (Troglotrema salmincola) infection. J Infect Dis 1989b; 160:896.

Garcia LS: Practical Guide to Diagnostic Parasitology. Washington, DC, American Society for Microbiology, 1999.

Garcia LS: Diagnostic Medical Parasitology, 4th ed. Washington, DC, American Society for Microbiology, 2001.

Garcia LS, Brewer TC, Bruckner DA: A comparison of the formalin-ether concentration and trichrome-stained smear methods for the recovery and identification of intestinal protozoa. Am J Med Technol 1979; 45:932.

Garcia LS, Shimizu RY: Evaluation of nine immunoassay kits (enzyme immunoassay and direct fluorescence) for detection of Giardia lamblia and Cryptosporidium parvum in human fecal specimens. J Clin Microbiol 1997; 35:1526.

Garcia LS, Shimizu RY: Detection of Giardia lamblia and Cryptosporidium parvum antigens in human fecal specimens using the ColorPAC combination rapid solid-phase qualitative immunochromatographic assay. J Clin Microbiol 2000; 38:1267.

Garcia LS, Shimizu RY, Shum A, et al: Evaluation of intestinal protozoan morphology in polyvinyl alcohol preservative: comparison of zinc sulfate- and mercuric chloride-based compounds for use in Schaudinn's fixative. J Clin Microbiol 1993; 31:307.

Garcia LS, Smith JW, Fritsche TR: Selection and use of laboratory procedures for diagnosis of parasitic infections of the gastrointestinal tract. CUMITECH 30A. Washington, DC, ASM Press, 2003.

This Cumitech reviews clinical aspects of the selection of laboratory tests for diagnosis of gastrointestinal parasites and limitations inherent to particular tests.

Gay JD, Abell TL, Thompson JH Jr, et al: Entamoeba polecki infection in southeast Asian refugees: multiple cases of a rarely reported parasite. Mayo Clin Proc 1985; 60:523.

Genta RM: Dysregulation of strongyloidiasis: a new hypothesis. Clin Microbiol Rev 1992; 5:345.

Genta RM, Walzer PD: Strongyloidiasis. In Walzer PD, Genta RM (eds): Parasitic Infections in the Compromised Host. New York, Marcel Dekker 1989; pp 463–525.

Gill GV, Bell DR: Strongyloides stercoralis infection in former Far East prisoners of war. Br Med J 1979; 2:572.

Goddard J: Physician's Guide to Arthropods of Medical Importance, 4th ed. Boca Raton, FL, CRC Press, 2002.

Graczyk TK, Cranfield MR, Fayer R: Evaluation of commercial enzyme immunoassay (EIA) and immunofluorescent antibody (FA) test kits for detection of Cryptosporidium oocysts of species other than Cryptosporidium parvum. Am J Trop Med Hyg 1996; 54:274.

Grover CM, Thulliez P, Remington JS, et al: Rapid prenatal diagnosis of congenital Toxoplasma infection by using polymerase chain reaction and amniotic fluid. J Clin Microbiol 1990; 28:2297.

Guerrant RL, Walker DH, Weller PF (eds): Tropical Infectious Diseases: Principles, Pathogens and Practice. Philadelphia, PA, Churchill Livingstone, 1999.

Gustafson RL, Reed CM, McGreevy PB, et al: Human cutaneous leishmaniasis acquired in Texas. Am J Trop Med Hyg 1985; 34:58.

Gutierrez Y: Diagnostic Pathology of Parasitic Infections with Clinical Correlations, 2nd ed. New York, Oxford University Press, 2000.

Hanson KL Cartwright CP: Use of an enzyme immunoassay does not eliminate the need to analyze multiple stool specimens for sensitive detection of Giardia lamblia. J Clin Microbiol 2001; 39:474.

Hardick J, Yang S, Lin S, et al: Use of the Roche LightCycler instrument in a real-time PCR for Trichomonas vaginalis in urine samples from females and males. J Clin Microbiol 2003; 41:5619.

Healy GR, Rubush TK: Morphology of Babesia microti in human blood smears. Am J Clin Pathol 1980; 73:107.

Herwaldt BL: Leishmaniasis. Lancet 1999; 335:1191.

Herwaldt BL, de Bruyn G, Pieniazek NJ, et al: Babesia divergens-like infection, Washington State. Emerg Infect Dis 2004; 10:622.

Hoeffler DF: Cercarial dermatitis, its etiology, epidemiology, and clinical aspects. JAMA 1974; 29:225.

Homer MJ, Aguilar-Delfin I, Telford SR III, et al: Babesiosis. Clin Microbiol Rev 2000; 13:451.

This paper reviews the common species producing babesiosis, clinical aspects of the disease, and diagnostic modalities, including molecular based studies that are an aid to diagnosis and epidemiology.

Isenberg HE 2nd ed: Clinical Microbiology Procedures Handbook, Vols 1 and 2. Washington, DC, American Society for Microbiology, 2004.

Istre GR, Kreiss K, Hopkins RS, et al: An outbreak of amebiasis spread by colonic irrigation at a chiropractic clinic. N Engl J Med 1982; 307:339.

Johnson EH, Windsor JJ, Clark CG: Emerging from obscurity: biological, clinical and diagnostic aspects of Dientamoeba fragilis. Clin Microbiol Rev 2004; 17:553.

Johnston SP, Ballard MM, Beach MJ, et al: Evaluation of three commercial assays for detection of Giardia and Cryptosporidium organisms in fecal specimens. J Clin Microbiol 2003 41:623.

Kappus KD, Lundgren RG, Juranek DD, et al: Intestinal parasitism in the United States: update on a continuing problem. Am J Trop Med Hyg 1994; 50:705.

Katanik MT, Schneider SK, Rosenblatt JE, et al: Evaluation of ColorPAC Giardia/Cryptosporidium rapid assay and ProSpecT Giardia/Cryptosporidium microplate assay for detection of Giardia and Cryptosporidium in fecal specimens. J Clin Microbiol 2001 39:4523.

Kehl KS, Cicirello H, Havens PL: Comparison of four different methods for detection of Cryptosporidium species. J Clin Microbiol 1995 33:416.

Kilvington S, White DG: Acanthamoeba: biology, ecology and human disease. Rev Med Microbiol 1994; 5:12.

Kim KC, Pratt HD, Stojanovich CJ: The Sucking Lice of North America. University Park, PA, Pennsylvania State University Press, 1986.

Krause PJ: Babesiosis. Med Clin North Am 2002; 86:361.

Krieger JN, Tam MR, Stevens CE, et al: Diagnosis of trichomoniasis: comparison of conventional wet-mount examination with cytologic studies, cultures, and monoclonal antibody staining of direct specimens. JAMA 1988; 259:1223.

Krogstad DJ, Spencer HC, Healy GR, et al: Amebiasis: epidemiologic studies in the United States. Ann Intern Med 1978; 88:89.

Krotoski WA, Garnham PCC, Krotoski DM, et al: Observations on early and late post-sporozoite tissue stages in primate malaria. I. Discovery of a new latent form of Plasmodium cynomolgi (the hypnozoite), and failure to detect hepatic forms within the first 24 hours after infection. Am J Trop Med Hyg 1982; 31:24.

Kubersky T, Bert RD, Briley JM, et al: Recovery of Angiostrongylus cantonensis from cerebrospinal fluid of a child with eosinophilic meningitis. J Clin Microbiol 1979; 9:629.

Kupferschmidt O, Kruger D, Held TK, et al: Quantitative detection of Toxoplasma gondii DNA in human body fluids by TaqMan polymerase chain reaction. Clin Microbiol Infect 2001 7:120.

Lanar DE, McLaughlin GL, Wirth DF, et al: Comparison of thick films, in vitro culture and DNA hybridization probes for detecting Plasmodium falciparum malaria. Am J Trop Med Hyg 1989; 40:3.

Lane RP, Crosskey RW: Medical Insects and Arthropods. London, Chapman & Hall, 1993.

Lawande RV, Abraham SN, John I, et al: Recovery of soil amebas from the nasal passages of children during the dusty harmattan period in Zaria. Am Soc Clin Pathol 1979; 71:201.

Layrisse M, Blumenfeld N, Carbonell L, et al: Intestinal absorption tests and biopsy of the jejunum in subjects with heavy hookworm infection. Am J Trop Med Hyg 1964a; 13:297.

Layrisse M, Roche M: The relationship between anemia and hookworm infection. Results of surveys of rural Venezuelan population. Am J Hyg 1964b; 79:279.

Lee MA, Tan CH, Aw LT, et al: Real-time fluorescence-based PCR for detection of malaria parasites. J Clin Microbiol 2002; 40:4343.

Levi MH, torres J, Pina C, Klein RS: Comparison of the InPouch TV culture system and Diamond's modified medium for detection of Trichomonas vaginalis. J Clin Microbiol 1997; 35:3308.

Levin RL, Armstrong DE: Human infection with Entamoeba polecki. Am J Clin Pathol 1970; 54:611.

Lin MH, Chen TC, Kuo TT, et al: Real-time PCR for quantitative detection of Toxoplasma gondii. J Clin Microbiol 2000; 38:4121.

Lisi PJ, Dondero RS, Kwiatkoski D, et al: Monoclonal-antibody based enzyme-linked immunosorbent assay for Trichomonas vaginalis. J Clin Microbiol 1988; 26:1684.

Loria-Cortez R, LoboSanahuja JF: Clinical abdominal angiostrongylosis. A study of 116 children with intestinal eosinophilic granuloma caused by Angiostrongylus costaricensis. Am J Trop Med Hyg 1980; 29:538.

Luft BJ: Toxoplasma gondii. In Walzer PD, Genta RM (eds): Parasitic Infections in the Compromised Host. New York, Marcel Dekker, 1989, p 179.

Luft BJ, Remingon JS: Toxoplasmic encephalitis. J Infect Dis 1988; 157:1.

Luna VA, Stewart BK, Bergeron DL, et al: Use of the fluorochrome calcofluor white in the screening of

CHAPTER 61: Medical Parasitology

stool specimens for spores of microsporidia. Am J Clin Pathol 1995; 103:656.

Lynch PJ: Delusions of parasitosis. Semin Dermatol 1993; 12:39.

Delusions of parasitosis are a common and complicated psychiatric process, and is taxing for all involved in the patient's care; this paper presents an overview of the syndrome along with management strategies.

Ma P, Soave R: Three-step stool examination for cryptosporidiosis in 10 homosexual men with protracted watery diarrhea. J Infect Dis 1983; 147:824.

Maayen S, Wormser GP, Widernorn J, et al: *Strongyloides stercoralis* hyperinfection in a patient with acquired immune deficiency syndrome. Am J Med 1987; 83:945.

McCabe R, Chirurgi V: Issues in toxoplasmosis. Infect Dis Clin North Am 1993; 7:587.

MacKenzie WR, Hoxie NJ, Proctor ME, et al: A massive outbreak in Milwaukee of *Cryptosporidium* infection transmitted through public water supply. N Engl J Med 1994; 331:161.

A detailed epidemiologic study is presented of the largest outbreak of cryptosporidiosis ever recorded.

Magill AJ, Grogl M, Gasser RA, et al: Visceral infection caused by *Leishmania tropica* in veterans of Operation Desert Storm. N Engl J Med 1993; 328:1384.

Mahboudi F, Abolhassani M, Tehrani SR, et al: Differentiation of old and new world leishmania species at complex and species levels by PCR. Scand J Infect Dis 2002; 34:756.

Mannheimer SB, Soave R: Protozoal infections in patients with AIDS. Cryptosporidiosis, isosporiasis, cyclosporiasis, and microsporidiosis. Infect Dis Clin North Am 1994; 8:483.

Maraha B, Buiting AG: Evaluation of four enzyme immunoassays for the detection of *Giardia lamblia* antigen in stool specimens. Eur J Clin Microbiol Infect Dis 2000; 19:485.

Marcial-Rojas RA: Pathology of Protozoal and Helminthic Diseases with Clinical Correlation. Baltimore, MD, Williams & Wilkins, 1971.

Marciano-Cabral F: Biology of *Naegleria* spp. Microbiol Rev 1988; 52:114.

Marciano-Cabral F, Cabral G: *Acanthamoeba* spp. as agents of disease in humans. Clin Microbiol Rev 2003; 16:273.

Mariano EG, Borja SR, Vruno MJ: A human infection with *Paragonimus kellicotti* (lung fluke) in the United States. Am J Clin Pathol 1986; 86:685.

Marines HM, Osato MS, Font RL: The value of calcofluor white in the diagnosis of mycotic and *Acanthamoeba* infections of the eye and ocular adnexa. Ophthalmology 1987; 94:23.

Markell EK, John DT, Krotowski WA: Markell and Voge's Medical Parasitology, 8th ed. Philadelphia, PA, WB Saunders, 1999.

Markell EK, Udkow MP: *Blastocystis hominis*: Pathogen or fellow traveler? Am J Trop Med Hyg 1986; 35:1023.

Martinez AJ, Visvesvara GS: Free living amphizoic and opportunistic amebas. Brain Pathol 1997; 7:583.

Martinez AJ: Free-living Amebas: Natural History, Prevention, Diagnosis, Pathology, and Treatment of Disease. Boca Raton, FL, CRC Press, 1985.

Marx A, Pewsner D, Egger M, et al: Meta-analysis: accuracy of rapid tests for malaria in travelers returning from endemic areas. Ann Intern Med 2005; 142:836.

Use of 'dipstick' immunochromatography methods for the rapid detection of malaria infections is becoming more popular; this paper reviews 21 published studies on the various methods, their clinical role in diagnosis, and limitations.

Medrano FJ, HernandezQuero J, Jimenez E, et al: Visceral leishmaniasis in HIV-infected individuals: a common opportunistic infection in Spain? AIDS 1992; 6:1499.

Melvin DM, Brooke MM: Laboratory Procedures for the Diagnosis of Intestinal Parasites, 3rd ed. (DHEW Publication [CDC] 828282). Atlanta, GA, Laboratory Training and Consultation Division, Centers for Disease Control, 1982.

Meri T, Sakari Jokiranta T, Suhonen, L, et al: Resistance of *Trichomonas vaginalis* to metronidazole: report of the first three cases from Finland and optimization of in vitro susceptibility testing under various oxygen concentrations. J Clin Microbiol 2000; 38:763.

Mileno MD, Bia FJ: The compromised traveler. Infect Dis Clin North Am 1998; 12:369.

Miller GA, Klausner JD, Coates TJ, et al: Assessment of a rapid antigen detection system for *Trichomonas vaginalis* infection. Clin Diagn Lab Immunol 2003; 10:1157.

Miller LH, Manson SJ, Clyde DF, et al: The resistance factor to *Plasmodium vivax* in blacks, the Duffy-blood-group genotype, FyFy. N Engl J Med 1976; 295:302.

Miller RA, Minshew BH: *Blastocystis hominis*: an organism in search of a disease. Rev Infect Dis 1988; 10:930.

Mullen G, Durden L: Medical and Veterinary Entomology, London, Academic Press, 2002.

Murphy GS, Basri H, Purnomo, et al: *Vivax malaria* resistant to treatment and prophylaxis with chloroquine. Lancet 1993; 341:96.

Murray WJ, Ash LR: Delusional parasitosis. Clin Microbiol Newslet 2004; 26:73.

Murray PR, Baron EJ, Jorgensen JH, et al: Manual of Clinical Microbiology, 8th ed. Washington, DC, ASM Press, 2003.

National Committee for Clinical Laboratory Standards: Laboratory diagnosis of blood borne parasitic diseases; approved guideline. NCCLS Document M15-A. Wayne, PA, NCCLS, 2000.

National Committee for Clinical Laboratory Standards: Clinical use and interpretation of serologic tests for *Toxoplasma gondii*: approved guideline M36-A. Wayne, PA, NCCLS, 2004.

This concensus guideline presents in an organized fashion the selection, interpretation and limitations of currently utilized serologic methods for the diagnosis of toxoplasmosis.

National Communicable Disease Center: Pictorial Keys: Arthropods, Reptiles, Birds, and Mammals of Public Health Significance. Atlanta, GA, Communicable Disease Center, 1969.

Nielson RL, Kohler RB, Chin W, et al: The use of exchange transfusions. A potentially useful adjunct in the treatment of fulminant falciparum malaria. Am J Med Sci 1979; 277:325.

Orihel TC, Ash LR: Parasites in Human Tissues. Chicago, IL, ASCP Press, 1995.

Orkin M, Maibach HI: Cutaneous Infestations and Insect Bites. New York, Marcel Dekker, 1985.

Ortega YR, Gilman RH, Sterling CR: A new coccidian parasite (Apicomplexa: Eimeriidae) from humans. J Parasitol 1994; 80:625.

Ortega YR, Sterling CR, Gilman RH, et al: *Cyclospora* species a new protozoan pathogen of humans. N Engl J Med 1993; 328:1308.

Pachucki CT, Levandowski RA, Brown VA, et al: American paragonimiasis treated with praziquantel. N Engl J Med 1984; 311:582.

Palmer CJ, Lindo JF, Klaskala WI, et al: Evaluation of the OptiMAL test for rapid diagnosis of *Plasmodium vivax* and *Plasmodium falciparum* malaria. J Clin Microbiol 1998; 36:203.

Palmer J: Modified iron hematoxylin/Kinyoun stain (letter). Clin Microbiol Newslett 1991; 13:39.

Parmley SF, Goebel FD, Remington JS: Detection of *Toxoplasma gondii* in cerebrospinal fluid from AIDS patients by polymerase chain reaction. J Clin Microbiol 1992; 30:3000.

Pelletier LL Jr, Baker CB, Gam AA, et al: Diagnosis and evaluation of treatment of chronic strongyloidiasis in ex-prisoners of war. J Infect Dis 1988; 157:573.

Perandin F, Manca N, Calderaro A, et al: Development of a real-time PCR assay for detection of *Plasmodium falciparum*, *Plasmodium vivax*, and *Plasmodium ovale* for routine clinical diagnosis. J Clin Microbiol 2004; 42:1214.

Persing DH, Herwaldt BL, Glaser C, et al: Infection with a *Babesia*-like organism in northern California. N Engl J Med 1995; 332:298.

Persing DH, Tenover FC, Versalovic, J, et al (eds): Molecular Microbiology: Diagnostic Principles and Practice. Washington, DC, American Society for Microbiology 2004.

Contains several chapters that provide a convenient overview of the current status on the use of molecular methods in the diagnosis of parasitic infections.

Peters W, Gilles HM: A Colour Atlas of Tropical Medicine and Parasitology, 3rd ed. London, Wolfe Medical, 1989.

Peters W, Killick-Kendrick R: The Leishmaniases in Biology and Medicine. London, Academic Press, 1987.

Pillai DR, Kain KC: Immunochromatographic strip-based detection of *Entamoeba histolytica–E. dispar* and *Giardia lamblia* coproantigen. J Clin Microbiol 1999; 37:3017.

Piper RC, LeBras J, Wentworth L, et al: Immuno-capture diagnostic assays for malaria utilizing *Plasmodium* lactate dehydrogenase (pLDH). Am J Trop Med Hyg 1999; 60:109.

Powell VI, Grima K: Exchange transfusion for malaria and *Babesia* infection. Transfus Med Rev 2002; 16:239.

Preiss U, Ockert G, Boremme S, et al: On the clinical importance of *Dientamoeba fragilis* infections in childhood. J Hyg Epidemiol Microbiol Immunol 1991; 35:27.

Price DL: Procedure Manual for the Diagnosis of Intestinal Parasites. Boca Raton, FL, CRC Press, 1994.

Purtilo DT, Meyers WM, Connor DH: Fatal strongyloidiasis in immunosuppressed patients. Am J Med 1974; 56:358.

Quick RE, Herwaldt BL, Thomford JW, et al: Babesiosis in Washington State: a new species of *Babesia*? Ann Intern Med 1993; 119:284.

Ravdin JI (ed): Amebiasis: Human Infection by *Entamoeba histolytica*. New York, John Wiley & Sons, 1988.

Reischl U, Bretagne S, Kruger D, et al: Comparison of two DNA targets for the diagnosis of toxoplasmosis by real-time PCR using fluorescence resonance energy transfer hybridization probes. BMC Infect Dis 2003 3:7.

Reisman RE: Insect stings. N Engl J Med 1994; 331:523.

Remington JS, Klein JO, Baker C et al (eds): Infectious Diseases of the Fetus and Newborn Infant, 6th ed. Philadelphia, PA, WB Saunders, 2005.

Richards FO, Schantz PM, RuizTiben E, et al: Cysticercosis in Los Angeles County. JAMA 1985; 254:444.

Rosenblatt JE, Sloan LM, Bestrom JE: Evaluation of an enzyme-linked immunoassay for the detection in serum of antibodies to *Entamoeba histolytica*. Diagn Microbiol Infect Dis 1995; 22:275.

Ruebush TK: Human babesiosis in North America. Trans R Soc Trop Med Hyg 1980; 74:149.

Sacks JJ, Roberto RR, Brooks NF: Toxoplasmosis infection associated with raw goat's milk. JAMA 1982; 248:1728.

Sadun EH, Melvin DM: The probability of detecting infections with *Enterobius vermicularis* by successive examination. J Pediatr 1956; 48:438.

Sakanari JA, McKerrow JH: Anisakiasis. Clin Microbiol Rev 1989; 2:278.

Samuelson J, Acuma-Soto R, Reed S, et al: DNA hybridization probe for clinical diagnosis of *Entamoeba histolytica*. J Clin Microbiol 1989; 27:672.

Schantz PM, Moore AC, Munoz JL, et al: Neurocysticercosis in an orthodox Jewish community in New York City. N Engl J Med 1992; 327:692.

Schmid GP, Matherny LC, Zaidi AA, et al: Evaluation of six media for the growth of *Trichomonas vaginalis* from vaginal secretions. J Clin Microbiol 1989; 27:1230.

Schnapp LM, Geaghan SM, Campagna A, et al: *Toxoplasma gondii* pneumonitis in patients infected with the human immunodeficiency virus. Arch Intern Med 1992; 152:1073.

Shadduck JA, Greeley E: Microsporidia and human infections. Clin Microbiol Rev 1989; 2:158.

VII

Shama SK, Etkind PH, Odell TM, et al: Gypsy-moth-caterpillar dermatitis. N Engl J Med 1982; 306:1300.

Sheehan DJ, Raucher BG, McKitriak JC: Association of *Blastocystis hominis* with signs and symptoms of human disease. J Clin Microbiol 1986; 24:548.

Shepp DH, Hackman RC, Conley FK, et al: *Toxoplasma gondii* reactivation identified by detection of parasitemia in tissue culture. Ann Intern Med 1985; 103:218.

Shields JM, Olson BH: *Cyclospora cayetanensis*: a review of an emerging parasitic coccidian. Int J Parasitol 2003; 33:371.

The recent emergence of Cyclospora from an obscure coccidian parasite of animals to a serious human pathogen is described.

Smith JW: Identification of fecal parasites in the special parasitology survey of the College of American Pathologists. Am J Clin Pathol 1979; 72(Suppl):371.

Sonenshine DE: Biology of Ticks, Vol 1. New York, Oxford University Press, 1991.

Sonenshine DE: Biology of Ticks, Vol 2. New York, Oxford University Press, 1993.

Spach DH, Liles WC, Campbell GL, et al: Tickborne diseases in the United States. N Engl J Med 1993; 329:936.

Spencer FM, Monroe LS: The Color Atlas of Intestinal Parasites, 2nd ed. Springfield, IL, Charles C Thomas, 1982.

Spencer MJ, Garcia LS, Chapin MR: *Dientamoeba fragilis*, an intestinal pathogen in children. Am J Dis Child 1979; 133:390.

Stehr-Green JK, Bailey TM, Visvesvara GS: The epidemiology of *Acanthamoeba* keratitis in the United States. Am J Ophthalmol 1990; 107:331.

Stenzel DJ, Boreham PFL: *Blastocystis hominis* revisited. Clin Microbiol Rev 1996; 9:563.

Steyskal GC, Murphy WL, Hoover EM: Insects and Mites: Techniques for Collection and Preservation. USDA Misc Publ No 1443, 1987.

Strickland GT (ed): Hunter's Tropical Medicine and Emerging Infectious Diseases, 7th ed. Philadelphia, PA, WB Saunders, 2000.

Sun TE: Pathology and Clinical Features of Parasitic Diseases. New York, Masson 1982.

Sun TE: Color Atlas and Textbook of Diagnostic Parasitology. New York, Igaku-Shoin, 1988.

Symmers WC Sr: Pathology of oxyuriasis, with special reference to granulomas due to the presence of *Oxyuris vermicularis* (*Enterobius vermicularis*) and its ova in tissues. Arch Pathol 1950; 50:475.

Tan B, WeldonLime CM, Rhone DP, et al: *Acanthamoeba* infection presenting as skin lesions in patients with the acquired immunodeficiency syndrome. Arch Pathol Lab Med 1993; 117:1043.

Teutch SM, Juranek DD, Sulzer A, et al: Epidemic toxoplasmosis associated with infected cats. N Engl J Med 1979; 300:695.

Thielman NM, Guerrant RL: Persistent diarrhea in the returned traveler. Infect Dis Clin North Am 1998; 12:489.

Thompson RCA, Lymbery AJ (eds): *Echinococcus* and Hydatid Disease. Wallingford, Oxfordshire, CAB International, 1995.

Truant AL, Elliott SH, Kelly MT, et al: Comparison of formalin-ethyl ether sedimentation, formalin-ethyl acetate sedimentation, and zinc sulfate flotation techniques for detection of intestinal parasites. J Clin Microbiol 1981; 13:882.

Turner JA: Giardiasis and infections with *Dientamoeba fragilis*. Pediatr Clin North Am 1985; 32:865.

Ubelaker HE: *Acanthamoeba* spp: 'opportunistic pathogens'. Trans Am Microsc Soc 1991; 110:289.

Vallejo GA, Guhl F, Chiari E, et al: Species specific detection of *Trypanosoma cruzi* and *Trypanosoma rangeli* in vector and mammalian hosts by polymerase chain reaction amplification of kinetoplast minicircle DNA. Acta Trop 1999; 72:203.

Van Gool T, Snijders F, Reis P, et al: Diagnosis of intestinal and disseminated microsporidial infections in patients with HIV by a new rapid fluorescent technique. J Clin Pathol 1993; 46:694.

Van Meirvenne N, le Ray D: Diagnoses of African and American trypanosomiases. Br Med Bull 1985; 41:156.

Varga JH, Wolf TC, Jensen HG, et al: Combined treatment of *Acanthamoeba* keratitis with propamidine, neomycin, and polyhexamethylene biguanide. Am J Ophthalmol 1993; 115:466.

Varma M, Hester JD, Schaefer III FW, et al: Detection of *Cyclospora cayetanensis* using a quantitative real-time PCR assay. J Microbiol Methods 2003; 53:27.

Verweij JJ, Blange RA, Templeton K, et al: Simultaneous detection of *Entamoeba histolytica*, *Giardia lamblia*, and *Cryptosporidium parvum* in fecal samples by using multiplex real-time PCR. J Clin Microbiol 2004; 42:1220.

Visvesvara GS: Pathogenic and opportunistic free-living amebae. *In* Murray PR, Barron EJ, Joregenson JH, et al (eds): Manual of Clinical Microbiology, 8th ed. Washington, DC, ASM Press 2003, p 1981.

Visvesvara GS: Parasite culture: *Entamoeba histolytica*. *In* Isenberg HD (ed): Clinical Microbiology Procedures Handbook, 2nd ed. Washington, DC, American Society for Microbiology, 2004a p 9.9.1.1.

Visvesvara GS: Parasite culture: *Leishmania* spp. and *Trypanosoma cruzi*. *In* Isenberg HD (ed): Clinical Microbiology Procedures Handbook, 2nd ed Washington, DC, American Society for Microbiology, 2004b p 9.9.5.1.

Visvesvara GS, Schuster FL, Marinez AJ: *Balamuthia mandrillaris* N.G., N. Sp., agent of amebic meningoencephalitis in humans and animals. J Eukaryot Microbiol 1993; 40:504.

Von Lichtenberg F: Pathology of Infectious Diseases. New York, Raven Press, 1991.

Walzer PD, Genta RM: Parasitic Infections in the Compromised Host. New York, Marcel Dekker, 1989.

Wang SS, Feldman HA: Isolation of *Hartmanella* species from human throats. N Engl J Med 1967; 277:1174.

Warren KS, Mahmoud AAF (eds): Tropical and Geographical Medicine, 2nd ed. New York, McGraw-Hill, 1990.

Weber R, Bryan RT, Owen RL, et al: Improved light-microscopical detection of microsporidia spores in stool and duodenal aspirates. N Engl J Med 1992; 326:161.

Weber R, Bryan RT, Schwartz DA, Owen RL: Human microsporidial infections. Clin Microbiol Rev 1994; 7:426.

Weigle KA, Davalos M, Heredia P, et al: Diagnosis of cutaneous and mucocutaneous leishmaniasis in Colombia: a comparison of seven methods. Am J Trop Med Hyg 1987; 36:489.

Weinberg GA: Laboratory diagnosis of ehrlichiosis and babesiosis. Pediatr Infect Dis J 2001; 20:435.

Weiss JB: DNA probes and PCR for diagnosis of parasitic infections. Clin Microbiol Rev 1995; 8:113.

World Health Organization: The Epidemiology and Control of African Trypanosomiasis. WHO Tech Rep Ser No 739. Geneva, WHO, 1986.

World Health Organization: The Biology of Malaria Parasites. WHO Tech Rep Ser No 743. Geneva, WHO, 1987.

Willson R, Harrington R, Stewart B, et al: Human immunodeficiency virus 1 associated necrotizing cholangitis caused by infection with *Septata intestinalis*. Gastroenterology 1995; 108:247.

Wilson M, Jones JL, McAuley JB: Toxoplasma. *In* Murray PR, Barron EJ, Joregenson JH, et al (eds): Manual of Clinical Microbiology, 8th ed. Washington, DC, ASM Press 2003, p 1970.

Wilson M, Schantz P, Pieniazek N: Diagnosis of parasitic infections: Immunologic and molecular methods. *In* Murray PR, Barron EJ, Pfaller MA, et al (eds): Manual of Clinical Microbiology, 6th ed. Washington, DC, ASM Press, 1995, p 1159.

Wittner M, Tanowitz HB, Weiss LM: Parasitic infections in AIDS patients. Infect Dis Clin North Am 1993; 7:569.

Wittner M, Turner JW, Jacquette G, et al: Eustrongylidiasis – a parasitic infection acquired by eating sushi. N Engl J Med 1989; 320:1124.

Wolfe MS: Giardiasis. Clin Microbiol Rev 1992; 5:93.

Woods GLY, Gutierrez DH, Walker DT, et al: Diagnostic Pathology of Infectious Diseases. Philadelphia, PA, Lea & Febiger, 1993.

Yang J, Scholten T: *Dientamoeba fragilis*: a review with notes on its epidemiology, pathogenicity, mode of transmission, and diagnosis. Am J Trop Med Hyg 1977; 26:16.

Zierdt CH: *Blastocystis hominis* past and future. Clin Microbiol Rev 1991; 4:61.

Zimmerman SK Needham CA: Comparison of conventional stool concentration and preserved-smear methods with Merifluor Cryptosporidium/Giardia Direct Immunofluorescence Assay and ProSpecT Giardia EZ Microplate Assay for detection of *Giardia lamblia*. J Clin Microbiol 1995 33:1942.

CHAPTER 62

Molecular Pathology of Infectious Diseases

Michael A. Pfaller MD

KEY POINTS

- Molecular diagnostic methods remain most valuable for the characterization of infectious agents that are difficult or impossible to detect and identify using conventional methods.

- When combined with modern serology, flow cytometry, and powerful tools such as electron microscopy and mass spectrometry, molecular techniques have markedly improved our capabilities to provide rapid (same day) and accurate detection of many emerging (new) and re-emerging pathogens as well as pathogens commonly encountered in medical practice.

- Molecular diagnostic methods are becoming more practical and cost-effective and the benefits to patient care are more widely recognized; however, this is still an expensive technology requiring skilled personnel and reimbursement issues are problematic.

- Fluorescent in situ hybridization technology uses fluorescent dyes linked to nucleic acid probes to produce a 'phylogenetic stain', allowing simultaneous detection and identification of an organism and at the same time preserving the organism's morphology and spatial localization in the tissue or clinical material.

- Commercial polymerase chain reaction (PCR) product development has focused primarily on systems for detection and quantitation of specific viral infections, detection of *Mycobacterium tuberculosis* and the leading agents of sexually transmitted diseases (*Chlamydia trachomatis* and *Neisseria gonorrhoeae*).

- The adaptability of real-time PCR has expanded the number of pathogens detectable by commercial systems to include the drug-resistant pathogens methicillin-resistant *Staphylococcus aureus* and vancomycin-resistant enterococci as well as selected emerging and re-emerging pathogens.

- A newly proposed nucleic acid amplification test (NAAT) should be validated by comparison with a sensitive culture and at least one validated PCR or other NAAT assay that targets a different gene or a different sequence of the same gene.

- In addition to assay performance, it is suggested that specimen throughput and volume requirements, limit of detection, ease of execution, instrument work space, and costs of reagent disposal all be considered when selecting a viral load assay.

- When applied in the settings of viral central nervous system infection and in acute respiratory tract infections in children, multiplex PCR has been shown to increase the diagnostic yield, reduce inappropriate antimicrobial therapy, promote more focused pathogen-specific therapy, facilitate the implementation of infection control precautions, and contribute to overall improved patient outcome.

- The availability of improved sequencing techniques, broader and more reliable databases, and more readily available kits and software, makes 16S rRNA sequence analysis a competitive alternative to routine microbial identification techniques for some groups of organisms.

The tremendous advances in biotechnology that have occurred in the latter half of the 1990s and early 2000s have resulted in the development and refinement of a remarkable array of modern techniques that are now applied for the diagnosis of infectious diseases (Table 62–1). Foremost among these techniques are the tools of molecular biology, which are used on a regular basis in clinical laboratories worldwide for diagnosis of disease, for guiding antimicrobial therapy, and for hospital epidemiology and infection control (Pfaller, 2001; Wolk, 2001; Raoult, 2004).

Molecular diagnostic methods remain most valuable for the characterization of infectious agents that are difficult or impossible to detect and identify using conventional methods. Likewise, when combined with modern serology, flow cytometry, and powerful tools such as electron microscopy and mass spectrometry, molecular techniques have markedly improved our capabilities to provide rapid (same-day) and accurate detection of many emerging (new) and re-emerging pathogens as well as pathogens commonly encountered in medical practice (Alvarez-Barrientos, 2000; Houpikian, 2002; Mezzasoma, 2002; Hazelton, 2003; Cockerill, 2004; Raoult, 2004). The principles of these techniques, as relevant to laboratory diagnosis, are covered in other chapters in this book. The present chapter will deal with the practical applications of these modern approaches to diagnosing and managing infectious diseases.

Molecular diagnosis of infectious diseases is largely nucleic acid based and requires the isolation of nucleic acids from microorganisms and clinical material and the use of restriction endonuclease enzymes, gel electrophoresis, and nucleic acid hybridization techniques. Increasingly, newer techniques for amplification of nucleic acids are applied to clinical material (Wolk, 2001). New platforms such as real-time polymerase chain reaction (PCR) combine nucleic acid amplification and fluorescent detection of the amplified product in the same closed system, resulting in a highly flexible, rapid, and accurate means by which to diagnose an ever-increasing spectrum of infectious diseases (Cockerill, 2004). DNA sequence analysis has become highly automated and is now practical for use in larger diagnostic and reference laboratories for the identification of a vast number of cultivatable, as well as noncultivatable, microorganisms (Aman, 1994; Wilson, 1994; Clarridge, 2004). Molecular array technology has been refined to the extent that it is now beginning to fulfill its considerable potential for the characterization of microorganisms in the clinical laboratory (Boriskin, 2004; Stöver, 2004; Zhou, 2004).

An important consideration in the more widespread application of molecular techniques is cost (Pfaller, 2001). In the area of diagnosis of

VII

Table 62–1 Modern Techniques Used To Diagnose Infectious Diseases

I. Direct Detection

A. Molecular detection
1. Nucleic acid probes
    a. liquid phase hybridization
    b. fluorescent in-situ hybridization (FISH)
2. Target amplification
3. Signal amplification

B. DNA microarrays

C. Flow cytometry

D. Electron microscopy (EM)

II. Modern Serology

A. Antigen microarrays

B. Synthetic antigens

III. Molecular Identification and Antimicrobial Resistance Testing

A. Nucleic-acid sequencing

B. DNA microarrays
1. Genus, species, and strain identification
2. Resistance genes
3. Gene mutation
4. Gene expression analysis

C. Molecular epidemiology typing

D. Mass spectrometry

Table 62–2 Selected Nucleic Acid Probe Method for Detection and Identification of Bacterial, Fungal, and Viral Pathogens

Organism(s)	Specimen type(s)	Method(s)
Bacteria		
Campylobacter spp.	Stool culture	Solution phase hybridization, chemiluminescent probe
Chlamydia trachomatis	Cervical and urethral swab; urine	Solution phase hybridization, chemiluminescent probe, hybrid capture
Enterobacteriaceae	Blood	FISH
Haemophilus influenzae	CSF or throat swab culture	Solution phase hybridization, chemiluminescent probe
Klebsiella pneumoniae	Blood culture	FISH
Listeria monocytogenes	Cultured isolate	Solution phase hybridization, chemiluminescent probe
Mycobacterium tuberculosis complex	Respiratory specimen culture	Solution phase hybridization, chemiluminescent probe
M. avium complex	Respiratory specimen culture	Solution phase hybridization, chemiluminescent probe
M. gordonae	Respiratory specimen culture	Solution phase hybridization, chemiluminescent probe
M. kansasii	Respiratory specimen culture	Solution phase hybridization, chemiluminescent probe
Neisseria gonorrhoeae	Urethral or cervical swab or culture	Solution phase hybridization, chemiluminescent probe, hybrid capture
Pseudomonas aeruginosa	Blood culture	FISH
Staphylococcus aureus	Blood culture	FISH using PNA probes
Methicillin-resistant *S. aureus*	Cultured organism	*mecA*-specific colorimetric cycling probe
Streptococcus spp.	Blood culture	FISH
S. pyogenes	Throat swab	Solution phase hybridization, chemiluminescent probe
Fungi		
Candida albicans	Blood culture	FISH using PNA probes
Coccidioides immitis	Cultured isolate	Solution phase hybridization, chemiluminescent probe
Blastomyces dermatitidis	Cultured isolate	Solution phase hybridization, chemiluminescent probe
Histoplasma capsulatum	Cultured isolate	Solution phase hybridization, chemiluminescent probe
Viruses		
Cytomegalovirus	Whole blood, WBC	Hybrid capture, In situ hybridization
Hepatitis B virus	Blood	Branched-chain DNA
Hepatitis C virus	Blood	Branched-chain DNA
Herpes simplex virus	Vesicle fluid	Hybrid capture
Human immunodeficiency virus	Blood	Branched-chain DNA
Human papilloma virus	Cervical swab or biopsy specimen	Hybrid capture, in situ hybridization
Epstein–Barr virus	CSF	In situ hybridization

List is not all inclusive.

CSF = cerebrospinal fluid; FISH = fluorescence in situ hybridization; PNA = peptide–nucleic acid; WBC = white blood cell.

infectious disease, improved patient outcome, and reduced cost of antimicrobials and duration of hospital stay may outweigh increased laboratory costs. Although difficult to quantify, there are now some excellent examples of the positive, and cost-effective, effects of the diagnostic applications of molecular methods (Shrestha, 2003a; Clarridge, 2004; Diekema, 2004; Scheuermann, 2004). In the case of communicable disease, the cost may be justified by improved infection control measures to protect patients and health-care workers (Cockerill, 2004). Molecular epidemiology may make a real contribution to detection and control of nosocomial spread of infection with potential to reduce nosocomial infection rates and the requirement for expensive antimicrobials used to treat resistant organisms (Hacek, 1999; Pfaller, 2001). Clearly, molecular diagnostic methods are becoming more practical and cost-effective and the benefits to patient care are more widely recognized; however, this is still an expensive technology requiring skilled personnel and reimbursement issues are problematic (Kant, 1995; Ross, 1999). Given these concerns, a facility's need for molecular diagnostic testing for infectious diseases should be examined critically by the affected clinical and laboratory services (Pfaller, 2001; Cockerill, 2004). In many instances, careful overseeing of test ordering and prudent use of a reference laboratory may be the most viable options.

Applications of Molecular Methods in Clinical Microbiology

The use of molecular methods for identification and direct detection of microorganisms in clinical microbiology is increasingly practical and several products are now available commercially (Tables 62–2 and 62–3). Nucleic acid probes are used for direct detection of organisms in clinical material or for identification of previously isolated organisms (Table 62–2). In addition, amplification-based techniques may be used for detection, quantification, and identification and to define selected characteristics (e.g. antibiotic resistance genes) of organisms (see Tables 62–3 to 62–7). Finally, molecular methods provide a powerful means of characterizing organisms as far as the subspecies level in epidemiologic investigations (see Table 62–8).

Detection of Pathogens Without Target Amplification

The detection of pathogenic microorganisms directly in specimens by nucleic acid probes has been investigated extensively using a variety of hybridization and signal-generating formats (Juretschko, 2004; Li, 2004). Commercial product development has focused on direct diagnosis of

sexually transmitted diseases and detection of respiratory pathogens using solution phase hybridization and acridinium-ester-labeled probes, although an increasing number of probes for detection of organisms in clinical material by fluorescent in-situ hybridization (FISH) are now available as well (Table 62–2).

Direct diagnosis by probe is rapid and free of the contamination problems associated with target amplification and is less susceptible to

Table 62–3 Commercial Nucleic Acid Amplification Systems for Diagnosis of Infectious Diseases

Organism	Specimen type(s)	Amplification technology	Amplicon detection
Bacillus anthracis	Human specimens and environmental samples	Real-time PCR*	FRET probes
Bordetella pertussis	Respiratory samples	Real-time PCR*	FRET probes
Chlamydia trachomatis	Cervical and urethral swabs; urine	PCR*	Microtiter capture probe
		NASBA[†]	Oligonucleotide probe attached to magnetic bead
		TMA[‡]	Acridinium ester probe
		SDA[¶]	Microwell capture probe
Neisseria gonorrhoeae	Cervical and urethral swabs	PCR*	Microtiter capture probe
		SDA[¶]	Microwell capture probe
Mycobacterium tuberculosis	Respiratory	PCR*	Microtiter capture probe
		TMA[‡]	Acridinium ester probe
		SDA[¶]	Microwell capture probe
Methicillin-resistant *S. aureus*	Nasal swab	Real-time PCR[∥]	Molecular beacon (fluorescence)
Vancomycin-resistant enterococci (*van*A & B)	Stool, rectal swab	Real-time PCR*	FRET probes
Cytomegalovirus	Blood, CSF	PCR*	Microtiter capture probe
		NASBA[†]	Oligonucleotide probe attached to magnetic bead
Epstein–Barr virus	CSF	PCR*	Microtiter capture probe
Hepatitis B virus	Blood	PCR*	Microtiter capture probe
Hepatitis C virus	Blood	RT-PCR*	Microtiter capture probe
		NASBA[†]	Oligonucleotide probe attached to magnetic bead
		TMA[§]	Acridinium ester probe
Human immunodeficiency virus	Blood	RT-PCR*	Microtiter capture probe
		NASBA[†]	Oligonucleotide probe attached to a magnetic bead
Human papilloma virus	Cervical swab and biopsies	PCR*	Line probe
		HCA**	Chemiluminescent hybrid capture
Herpes simplex virus	CSF, skin (vesicle), genital tract	PCR*	Microtiter capture probe
		Real-time PCR*	FRET probes
Enterovirus	CSF	PCR*	Microtiter capture probe
		Real-time PCR*	FRET probes
Varicella zoster virus	Skin lesion	Real-time PCR*	FRET probes
Variola virus	Skin lesion	Real-time PCR*	FRET probes
West Nile virus	CSF	Real-time PCR*	FRET probes
SARS coronavirus	Respiratory	Real-time PCR*	FRET probes

The table contains examples of available systems and is not intended to be all inclusive.

* Roche, Indianapolis, IN. [†] BioMérieux, St Louis, MO. [‡] Gen-Probe, San Diego, CA. [§] Bayer, Tarrytown, NY. [¶] Becton Dickinson, Cockeysville, MD. [∥] Infectio Diagnostic Sainte-Foy, Quebec. ** Digene, Silver Spring, MD.

CSF = cerebrospinal fluid; FRET = fluorescent resonance energy transfer; HCA = hybrid capture assay; LCR = ligase chain reaction; NASBA = nucleic acid strand-based amplification; PCR = polymerase chain reaction; SDA = strand displacement amplification; TMA = transcription-mediated amplification.

inhibition than many amplification procedures. A limitation of standard probe hybridization is the requirement for a 10^4 or greater number of copies of target nucleic acid for detection. For some applications, a convenient, rapid, non-culture-based method at this level of sensitivity might be of value, and signal amplification strategies can achieve detection of gene copy numbers as low as 500/μL (Shah, 1994; Murphy, 1999). However, even the most sophisticated signal amplification formats do not appear at present to match the analytical sensitivity of target amplification-based methods, which may detect fewer than 50 gene copies per microliter (Erali, 1999).

In infectious disease diagnostics, membrane-based probe hybridization (Southern blot, slot/dot blot) appears unlikely to be a significant tool in the clinical laboratory in the future. The membrane-based format is perhaps most applicable to batch processing of large numbers of specimens as in research applications. Classification of human papilloma virus (HPV) genotypes and reliable detection of HPV in diagnostic specimens was made possible initially by membrane-based DNA probe assays. A variety of whole genomic probes and oligonucleotide probes for the more common types of HPV (e.g. types 16 and 18, commonly associated with uterine cervical carcinoma, and types 6 and 11, associated with benign disease) have been described, and both isotopic and nonisotopic labeling have been used (Angel, 1992; Lorinez, 1992; Faulkner-Jones, 1993; Scheuermann, 2004). This approach has largely been replaced by the hybrid capture assay (HCA) and by PCR and sequencing (Scheuermann, 2004). Slot blot/dot blot formats have also been investigated for diagnosis of cerebral toxoplasmosis and falciparum malaria, among others, but have not been used to any degree in diagnostic laboratories.

An increasingly useful direct approach to visualization of microorganisms in clinical material is that of FISH (Jansen, 2000; Kempf, 2000; Hayden, 2001a, 2001b, 2002; Juretschko, 2004). FISH technology uses fluorescent dyes linked to nucleic acid probes to produce a 'phylogenetic stain,' allowing simultaneous detection and identification of an organism and at the same time preserving the organism's morphology and spatial localization in the tissue or clinical material (Juretschko, 2004). FISH is recognized as a rapid, cost-effective, and reliable method for both detection and identification of a wide array of bacterial, virus, fungal and protozoan species of clinical importance (Table 62–2) (Hogardt, 2000; Jansen, 2000; Kempf, 2000; Hayden, 2001a, 2001b, 2002; Oliveira, 2002, 2003; Chapin, 2003; Juretschko, 2004; Wilson, 2005). Individual probes specific for each pathogen may be derived from 16S and/or 18S rDNA sequence analysis and then used as the 'ultimate direct smear' to detect and identify pathogens prior to culture (Juretschko, 2004). Furthermore, FISH can be used to identify slow-growing and fastidious organisms that may be difficult to differentiate by biochemical assays. FISH may be coupled with confocal microscopy, flow cytometry, or immunological methods to provide detailed characterization of microorganisms (Juretschko, 2004). The recent development of peptide nucleic acid (PNA) probes has provided reagents for use in FISH that exhibit favorable hybridization characteristics (high specificities, strong affinities, and rapid kinetics) and an enhanced ability to penetrate the hydrophobic cell wall of organisms following preparation of a standard smear (Stender, 1999; Oliveira, 2002; Juretschko, 2004). This rapid, sensitive, and specific technology fits easily into the standard workflow of the clinical microbiology laboratory and should prove increasingly valuable as more reagents become available.

VII

Commercial probe systems have used solution-phase hybridization with nonisotopic labeling. Those that do not use signal amplification will be considered first. The acridinium-ester-labeled PACE2 products (Gen-Probe) with chemiluminescence detection are perhaps the most widely used. Gen-Probe assays use nonradioactive probe labeling, which permits a long shelf life. In addition, the formatting is relatively user-friendly and can be used for small or large numbers of specimens.

Nucleic acid probe hybridization assays target infectious processes in which the pathogens are present in sufficient concentration to permit current sampling methods to obtain enough organisms to be detected by the assays without further amplification. Gen-Probe (acridinium-ester-labeled) probes for detection of *Streptococcus pyogenes* (Group A β-hemolytic streptococcus) in throat swabs and for detection of *Chlamydia trachomatis* and *Neisseria gonorrhoeae* in cervical and urethral swabs are available commercially (Table 62–2). A single specimen can be used for detection of both *C. trachomatis* and *N. gonorrhoeae*. The reliability of the Gen-Probe kit for detection of *C. trachomatis* in clinical specimens has been evaluated relative to cell culture as well as to immunologic and target amplification methods. In contrast to culture, the immunologic and molecular methods were not dependent on the viability of the pathogen. In a direct comparison, the PACE2 Gen-Probe method was more sensitive than the Chlamydiazyme enzyme immunoassay (EIA) but less sensitive than a commercial target amplification assay (AMP-CT, Gen-Probe) (Wylie, 1998). The Gen-Probe assay for *N. gonorrhoeae* has been evaluated in a number of studies and the consensus opinion is that it may be most useful in situations where optimization of culture is difficult (Koumans, 1998). The fact that both gonococcal and chlamydial assays can be performed with a single swab collection is an important advantage and makes these assays more feasible, especially in a high-volume outpatient facility (Koumans, 1998; Li, 2004). It should be noted that culture for both *Chlamydia* and gonococci remains a requirement for mediocolegal purposes (Koumans, 1998).

Branched chain DNA (bDNA, Bayer) and hybrid capture assays (HCA, Digene) represent strategies of diagnostic probe tests that incorporate signal amplification (Wolk, 2001). HCAs for detection of HPV, herpes simplex virus (HSV), and cytomegalovirus (CMV) have been described (Scheuermann, 2004). The HCAs are reported to be more sensitive than culture for detection of both HSV and CMV. Modifications of the HPV assay have led to improved sensitivity (Poljak, 1999). The HCA system is, however, less sensitive than nucleic acid target amplification (Cope, 1997; Cullen, 1997; Barrett-Muir, 1998; Poljak, 1999).

Branched chain DNA (bDNA) probes (Bayer) have been developed for detection and quantitation of hepatitis C virus (HCV) and hepatitis B virus (HBV) (Urdea, 1991; Heerman, 1999), human immunodeficiency virus (HIV) (Murphy, 1999) and for detection of the *mec*A gene associated with oxacillin resistance in staphylococci (Kolbert, 1998). This probe hybridization assay is presented in an EIA-like format. The nucleic acids released from the organisms are captured to a solid surface by multiple capture probes. Target probes hybridize to both the microbial nucleic acid and the bDNA signal amplification multimer. Enzyme-labeled probes are bound to the bDNA, and detection occurs via a chemiluminescent process in which light is emitted in proportion to the original amount of target present (Wolk, 2001). The limit of detection of target nucleic acid is not as low as that achievable with target amplification (Zaaijer, 1994; Yen-Lieberman, 1996; Lunel, 1999). Quantitative results over a wide range of target concentrations may be useful for determination of viral load, prognosis, and monitoring response to therapy in a number of viral infections (Yen-Lieberman, 1996; Heerman, 1999; Lunel, 1999).

The ligase chain reaction (LCR, Abbott), Q-beta replicase amplification (Gene-Trak), Invader technology (ThirdWave Technologies) and Cycling Probe Technology (Velogene) represent probe amplification technologies, wherein the end product of the reaction is an amplified version of the original components used to detect the target (Wolk, 2001). Cycling probe technology is an isothermal and rapid reaction that has been used to detect *Mycobacterium tuberculosis* (Beggs, 1996), methicillin-resistant *Staphylococcus aureus* (MRSA) (Bekkaoui, 1999) and vancomycin-resistant enterococci (VRE) (Modrusan, 1999). It is more useful in identifying cultured organisms than detecting them directly in clinical specimens.

Nucleic Acid Probes for Culture Identification

DNA probes now have an established role in the identification of cultures of a number of microorganisms (Table 62–2). Culture identification by probe hybridization is not limited by a requirement to detect minute quantities of nucleic acid. The advantage of probe-based identification over nonmolecular methods is greatest for slow-growing organisms such as the mycobacteria or for organisms for which convenient commercial identification systems are not available. Another important role for molecular probes is the direct identification of microorganisms from blood cultures guided by the Gram stain morphology of the organism (Jansen, 2000; Kempf, 2000; Chapin, 2003; Oliveira, 2003; Lindholm, 2004; Wilson, 2005). Although identification by probe hybridization is more expensive than identification by conventional methods, a rapid (within 1 h of a positive culture) and accurate method for direct identification of pathogens from positive cultures may greatly improve antibiotic management and decrease the use of inappropriate antimicrobial agents.

Identification of cultured mycobacteria by conventional methods is slow and time consuming. Acridinium ester-labeled probes for identification of *M. tuberculosis* complex, the *Mycobacterium avium intracellulare* complex, *Mycobacterium gordonae*, and *Mycobacterium kansasii* are available commercially (Gen-Probe). The use of these probes permits identification from culture in one working day, and specificity and sensitivity (99% and 95.5%, respectively) are excellent (Goto, 1991; Walton, 1991; Richter, 1999; Scarparo, 2001; Li, 2004). Occasionally strains of *M. tuberculosis* may fail to react with the *M. tuberculosis* complex probe, and there appears to be a subspecies of *M. kansasii* that fails to react with the *M. kansasii* probe (Badak, 1999; Niemann, 1999).

Probes for identification from culture of *Histoplasma capsulatum*, *Blastomyces dermatitidis*, *Coccidioides immitis*, and *Cryptococcus neoformans* are also available (Stockman, 1993). Evaluations indicate that specificity is 100%, and a sensitivity of 97% or greater was reported for all species except *B. dermatitidis* (87.8%). With repeat testing the sensitivity improved to 97.3% for *B. dermatitidis* and 100% for all other species. Recently a commercially available peptide nucleic acid (PNA) FISH probe specific for *Candida albicans* was shown to be useful on aliquots taken directly from positive blood culture bottles to differentiate *C. albicans* from non-*C. albicans* yeast (Oliveira, 2001; Wilson, 2005).

The Gen-Probe *N. gonorrhoeae* probe system has been utilized for identification of cultured *N. gonorrhoeae* in addition to its use for direct application to clinical specimens (Young, 1993; Koumans, 1998). The *N. gonorrhoeae* probe (AccuProbe) compares favorably with a commercial rapid carbohydrate utilization system (Quadferm, BioMérieux) and a coagglutination system (Phadeback Monoclone GC test) for identification of cultured *N. gonorrhoeae*. Acridinium-ester-labeled nucleic acid probes for identification of a number of cultured bacteria, including *S. aureus*, *Streptococcus pneumoniae*, *Streptococcus pyogenes*, *Streptococcus agalactiae*, *Enterococcus* spp., *Listeria monocytogenes*, and *Haemophilus influenzae* are available (Table 62–2). These probes have been used to identify organisms harvested from positive blood cultures by centrifugation (Davis, 1991; Lindholm, 2004). Identification is simple to perform and results are available in approximately 30 minutes.

FISH technology has also been used to rapidly identify Gram-negative and Gram-positive bacteria, as well as *C. albicans*, directly from positive blood cultures (Jansen, 2000; Kempf, 2000; Oliveira, 2001, 2003; Chapin, 2003; Wilson, 2005). Both nucleic acid as well as PNA probes targeting 16S rRNA (18S rRNA for *C. albicans*) have been used and provide sensitive and specific results (97–100%) within 2.5 hours of blood culture positivity. The selection of probes was guided by the Gram morphology of the organisms in the blood culture broth. The FISH results were unaffected by the type of blood culture system or broth formulation (e.g. lytic medium, resin-, or charcoal-containing medium). This approach provided a time saving of 26–46 hours compared with conventional laboratory methods used for identification. It is likely that the costs of FISH (about $20 per positive blood culture specimen) can be justified by what might be saved in avoiding unnecessary antimicrobial therapy and possibly by a shortened hospital stay (Kempf, 2000). Furthermore, reducing unnecessary antimicrobial treatment may also have a favorable impact on the antimicrobial susceptibility profile of nosocomial pathogens thereby benefiting an even greater number of patients.

Nucleic Acid Amplification for Diagnosis

Nucleic acid amplification has the potential to overcome the principal limitation of diagnostic probe hybridization by selectively amplifying specific targets present in low concentrations to detectable levels. The PCR (Roche Molecular Systems) was the first amplification technique developed and remains the most widely investigated and applied method. Newer target amplification technologies, nucleic acid strand-based amplification (NASBA, BioMérieux), strand displacement amplification (SDA, Becton Dickinson), and transcription-mediated amplification (TMA, Gen-Probe) form the basis of additional systems now available (Wolk, 2001).

Several modifications of conventional PCR have been developed in efforts to expand and improve this technology (Wolk, 2001). Multiplex

Table 62–4 Applications of Multiplex PCR for Diagnosis of Infectious Diseases

Clinical Manifestation(s)	Specimen(s)	Targeted Pathogens
Meningitis, encephalitis, and/or meningoencephalitis	CSF	HSV, CMV, EBV, HHV-6 and EV EBV and *Toxoplasma gondii* *Neisseria meningitidis*, *Streptococcus pneumoniae*, and *Haemophilus influenzae*
Upper and lower respiratory infections	Throat, nose, and nasopharyngeal (NP) swabs; NP and endotracheal aspirates; bronchoalveolar lavage	Influenza, parainfluenza, RSV, adenovirus, and *Mycobacterium pneumoniae*, *Chlamydophila pneumoniae*, *M. pneumoniae* and adenovirus
Diarrheal disease	Stool, water	*Shigella* and diarrheagenic *Escherichia coli* *Campylobacter jejuni* and *C. coli*, *G. lamblia* and *Cryptosporidium parvum*
Genital infection	Genital swabs and scrapings	HSV, *Haemophilus ducreyi*, and *Treponema pallidum* HPV, HSV, and *Chlamydia trachomatis*, *N. gonorrhoeae* and *C. trachomatis*
Keratoconjunctivitis	Conjunctival and corneal swabs	Adenovirus, HSV, and *C. trachomatis*
Vesicular rashes	Vesicle fluids	HSV and VZV
Immunocompromised status	Blood	HIV-1 and –2, HTLV-1 and – 2
Malaria	Blood	*Plasmodium falciparum*, *P. vivax*, *P. malariae*, and *P. ovale*

CMV = cytomegalovirus; EBV = Epstein–Barr virus; EV = enterovirus; RSV = respiratory syncytial virus; HHV-6 = human herpes virus-6; HIV = human immunodeficiency virus; HPV = human papilloma virus; HSV = herpes simplex virus; HTLV = human T-cell lymphotrophic virus.

Source: adapted in part from Elnifro et al (2000). List not all inclusive.

PCR employs multiple primer sets and can be used to identify multiple organisms, or multiple targets, in a single reaction mix (Table 62–4). Nested PCR employs sequential amplification steps in order to enhance the sensitivity of the PCR. Reverse transcriptase PCR (RT-PCR) is used to detect RNA by using an enzyme with reverse transcriptase activity to create a complementary DNA (cDNA) from an RNA target. The cDNA may then be amplified by PCR. Quantitative PCR employs an internal standard and is used to assess the amount of a microbe present in a patient specimen.

Perhaps the most significant recent advance in PCR technology is the use of rapid-cycle nucleic acid amplification (PCR performed in 30 minutes versus hours to days with conventional PCR) coupled with simultaneous fluorescent amplicon detection carried out in a single closed system, otherwise known as real-time PCR (Wolk, 2001; Clinical and Laboratory Standards Institute, 2003; Cockerill, 2004). Real-time PCR minimizes the risk of amplicon cross-contamination and is a very flexible, rapid, and sensitive PCR platform (Table 62–5). Real-time PCR protocols couple melting curve determinations (sequence-dependent temperature at which half the strands become separated in solution) with specific internal fluorescent probes to ensure more specific hybridization and product identification (Wolk, 2001). A variety of internal probe formats exist, including hybridization probes such as fluorescence resonance energy transfer (FRET) probes, hydrolysis probes that use Taqman (Applied Biosystems) chemistry, and molecular beacon probes (Clinical and Laboratory Standards Institute, 2003; Wolk, 2001). Real-time PCR may be performed as a highly sensitive qualitative detection assay or used as a means of quantitating the amount of pathogen-specific nucleic acid in a specimen. Notably, real-time quantitative PCR assays often provide wider linear ranges than conventional quantitative PCR assays (Wolk, 2001). Several highly automated real-time PCR instruments are now available. These instruments include optical systems to excite and detect fluorescent emissions at a variety of wavelengths and have the potential to speed the results of PCR reactions and to improve the ability to multiplex PCR (Wolk, 2001). The available systems include the LightCycler instrument (Roche), the ABI Prism (Applied Biosystems), the SmartCycler instrument (Cepheid), and the iCycler instrument (Bio-Rad) (Wolk, 2001; Cockerill, 2004).

Commercial PCR product development has focused primarily on systems for detection and quantification of specific viral infections (HCV, HBV, HIV, CMV, EBV) and detection of *M. tuberculosis* complex and the leading agents of sexually transmitted diseases (*C. trachomatis* and *N. gonorrhoeae*) (Table 62–3). The adaptability of real-time PCR has expanded the number of pathogens detectable by commercial systems to include the drug-resistant pathogens MRSA and VRE (Cockerill, 2004; Diekema, 2004; Sakai, 2004; Warren, 2004) as well as selected emerging and re-emerging pathogens (Cockerill, 2004; Raoult, 2004). The commercial products are designed with a view to user acceptability, prevention of contamination, standardization of reagents and conditions, and potential for automation. A number of studies comparing two or more amplification methods have

Table 62–5 Advantages of Real-Time PCR

1. Rapid (30–40 min)
2. Closed system
   Simultaneous amplification and detection
   Limits contamination risk
3. Quantitative
4. Fluorescent detection (non gel-based)
5. Flexible
6. Improved standardization
   Availability of kits
   Analyte-specific reagents (ASRs)

been reported (Griffith, 1997; Schepetiuk, 1997; Stary, 1998; Brown, 1999; Van Dyck, 2001; Klein, 2004; Koenig, 2004), and in general, none of the newer methods (NASBA, TMA, SDA) has demonstrated a level of sensitivity greater than PCR. Factors in choosing between the systems may include the range of products available, suitability to the individual laboratory's work practices, and cost. It is probably most practical for a laboratory to choose a single amplification platform that can provide the full range of tests that it requires. The ability of some manufacturers of real-time PCR instruments to supply analyte specific reagents (ASR) for use with their instrument makes new assays easily adaptable for many clinical microbiology laboratories (Cockerill, 2004).

At present, molecular methods have an established role in the clinical diagnosis and management of a number of viral infections and in ensuring the safety of blood products (Roth, 1999; Smith, 2004). They are also considered essential for identifying potential agents of bioterrorism through the Laboratory Response Network and for diagnosing emerging (new) or re-emerging infectious diseases (Cockerill, 2004). In the case of many bacterial pathogens, evaluation of the role of molecular methods relative to culture or immunologic methods may be difficult to assess (Hall, 2004a; Hayden, 2004; Ieven, 2004). In most studies there are a number of specimens that test positive by amplification-based assays but negative by culture or immunologic methods. The classification of the results of these tests as false-positive by amplification or as false-negative by culture/antigen detection has important implications for purposes of calculating the sensitivity and specificity of the amplification-based assay and for judging the relative merits of these differing approaches to laboratory diagnosis. Many researchers have attempted to address this problem using the technique of discrepant analysis. The value and limitations of discrepant analysis remain controversial: proponents regard it as the most practical approach available (Schachter, 1998), whereas opponents believe that the process tends to bias results in favor of amplification-based assays (Hadgu, 1996; Miller, 1998). In addition to

VII

these concerns are those expressed by other authors regarding the highly variable quality of many published studies (Koumans, 1998). The use of an expanded gold standard or a battery of independent tests, in lieu of an absolute reference test (latent class analysis), has been suggested as a possible solution to this dilemma (Ieven, 2004). Ideally, a newly proposed nucleic acid amplification test (NAAT) should be validated by comparison with a sensitive culture and at least one validated PCR or other NAAT assay that targets a different gene or a different sequence of the same gene (Ieven, 2004).

Diagnosis of Viral Infection

The identification of HCV was made possible by the techniques of molecular biology; therefore, it is not surprising that PCR and other molecular methods have an important role in its diagnosis (Table 62–3). Serology allows detection of previous HCV infection but does not permit differentiation between current infection and patients who have spontaneously cleared the virus. As HCV is an RNA virus, reverse transcription into a cDNA is an essential preliminary step to amplification by PCR. A variety of 'home brew' PCR assays using reverse transcriptase and DNA polymerase have been described (Fiebelkorn, 2004). Roche Diagnostics markets a product (Amplicor RT-PCR) in which reverse transcription and amplification are performed by the same enzyme, Tth from *Thermus thermophilus*, and this process has been automated (COBAS Amplicor System) (Poljak, 1997; Pfaller, 2004a). Detection of the virus by molecular methods confirms current infection and has an established role in clinical diagnosis of HCV infection and in monitoring response to therapy (Fiebelkorn, 2004).

In diagnosis of HIV infection, virus-specific antibodies are detected by serologic testing and, because spontaneous clearance of HIV is not anticipated, unequivocal detection of these antibodies is generally accepted as evidence of current infection. In the case of the newborn, detection of antibodies may reflect transplacental transfer of maternal antibody, and a prolonged period of follow-up (up to 18 months) may be required to confirm infection by serologic methods alone. Detection of virus by molecular methods has a role in resolving the status of such infants and also in managing those patients whose serum is repeatedly indeterminate on serologic testing. HIV exists in blood both as RNA virus and as proviral DNA incorporated into the genome of peripheral blood mononuclear cells. Reverse transcriptase is not needed to detect the proviral DNA but is required for detection or quantitation of free HIV RNA. It has been reported that the Amplicor Monitor assay (Roche) is more sensitive than bDNA (Bayer)- or NASBA (BioMérieux)-based detection of HIV (Bootman, 1999) and levels of detection as low as 20 HIV RNA copies/ml of plasma can be achieved by specific RNA extraction protocols (Fischer, 1999, Murphy, 2000; Pfaller, 2004a).

PCR has also been studied extensively for diagnosis of CMV infection in transplant recipients, and commercial systems for detection by PCR (Long, 1998; Razonable, 2002; Pang, 2003; Smith, 2004), HCA (Mazzuli, 1999) and NASBA (Aono, 1998; Diaz-Mitoma, 2003) are now available. The problems of diagnosis of CMV disease differ from HCV and HIV infection in that the virus is ubiquitous and therefore its detection in blood by any method does not, per se, confirm clinical disease (Razonable, 2002). The challenge in CMV diagnosis has been to distinguish those immunocompromised patients who have or are likely to develop illness related to CMV from those in whom the CMV infection is not clinically significant (Patel, 1995; Pellegrin, 2000; Razonable, 2002). For these reasons, CMV was among the first viruses in which quantification of virus by PCR was investigated (Gerna, 1994; Boeckh, 1998; Caliendo, 2000; Diaz-Mitoma, 2003; Pang, 2003). Detection of CMV messenger RNA (using NASBA), which represents evidence of active transcription of the viral genome, has also been used to diagnose CMV disease and response to treatment but has not proved to be as useful as viral load determinations by PCR or HCA (Patel, 1995; Blok, 2000; Pellegrin, 2000; Diaz-Mitoma, 2003).

Quantification of virus by molecular methods is now recognized to be of significance in the diagnosis and management of HBV, HCV, HIV, CMV and EBV infections (Kimura, 1999; Murphy, 2000; Jabs, 2001; Diaz-Mitoma, 2003; Maurmann, 2003; Pang, 2003; Fiebelkorn, 2004). In addition to conventional quantitative PCR, bDNA, HCA, TMA, and real-time PCR approaches have been used.

Quantification of HCV viral load is important in disease prognosis and monitoring of therapy (Fiebelkorn, 2004). The most widely studied methods are the RT-PCR (Roche Monitor) and bDNA (Bayer) assays (Hawkins, 1997; Jacob, 1997; Lu, 1998; Fiebelkorn, 2004); however, NASBA (BioMérieux), TMA (Bayer), and the novel real-time PCR have been described as well (Lunel, 1999; Martel, 1999; Kleiber, 2000; Sawyer, 2000). The variety of the systems and the pace of development make definitive

statements about the relative values of the various systems difficult. Important issues to consider are the dynamic range (the range of concentrations of viral genomes within which the method is most accurate and reproducible) of the available systems, variation in their ability to detect and quantify the different HCV viral genotypes, and the difficulties in developing suitable standards for calibration. Currently, about 80% of laboratories participating in the College of American Pathologists (CAP) nucleic acid amplification proficiency testing program perform reverse-transcriptase PCR (RT-PCR) for HCV RNA using the Roche Amplicor HCV kits (Fiebelkorn, 2004).

Quantification of HIV viral load in plasma is a useful biological marker for assessing disease prognosis and outcome of antiretroviral therapy (Ledergerber, 1999). The technical approaches and problems associated with quantification of HIV RNA are generally similar to those noted previously for HCV (Garcia-Lerma, 1998; Erali, 1999; Triques, 1999; Murphy, 2000). A multicenter comparison of RT-PCR (Roche), NASBA (BioMérieux/Organon Teknika) and bDNA (Bayer) found the results from the three assays to be highly correlated; however, because differences in RNA measures between assays varied from patient to patient, the authors of this study recommended that RT-PCR, NASBA, and bDNA methods not be used interchangeably in patient monitoring (Murphy, 2000). In addition to assay performance, it is suggested that specimen throughput and volume requirements, limit of detection, ease of execution, instrument work space, and costs of reagent disposal all be considered when selecting a viral load assay (Murphy, 2000).

Nucleic acid amplification, especially real-time PCR, has been used for diagnosis of a variety of other viral infections including enterovirus (Rotbart, 1994; Pozo, 1998; Landry, 2003), HSV (Tremblay, 1997; Smith, 2004), JC virus (Garcia de Viedma, 1999), parvovirus (Jordan, 1998), VZV (Scheuermann, 2004), variola virus (Cockerill, 2004), West Nile virus (Cockerill, 2004), and SARS coronavirus (Cockerill, 2004; Drosten, 2004) among others (Tables 62–3 and 62–6). Amplification-based methods are becoming increasingly important in diagnosis and management of viral infection as the number of infections amenable to specific antiviral agents continues to increase and in particularly critical situations such as central nervous system infection (Read, 1997; Cockerill, 2004; Smith, 2004). Given the similar clinical presentations of a number of viral infections, there are several settings where multiplex PCR can be used rationally and effectively to improve diagnostic yield and to streamline day-to-day laboratory operations (Table 62–4) (Elnifro, 2000; Gruteke, 2004). The greatest application of multiplex PCR has been in diagnosing viral meningitis, encephalitis, and meningoencephalitis (Elnifro, 2000) and in acute respiratory tract infections in children (Gruteke, 2004). When applied in these settings, multiplex PCR has been shown to increase the diagnostic yield, reduce inappropriate antimicrobial therapy, promote more focused pathogen-specific therapy, facilitate the implementation of infection control precautions, and contribute to overall improved patient outcome (Elnifro, 2000; Cockerill, 2004; Gruteke, 2004; Smith, 2004).

Detection of Bacterial Pathogens

There are now several commercial amplification assays for the detection of *M. tuberculosis* complex (MTBC) in respiratory and non-respiratory specimens. These include PCR (Roche), TMA (Gen-Probe), and SDA (Becton Dickinson) (Table 62–3). In general, the sensitivity of these assays is excellent (95–100%) for specimens for which the smear for acid-fast bacilli (AFB) is positive, but is lower for specimens that are smear-negative (50–90%) (Ieven, 1997; Piersimoni, 1998, 2002; Pfyffer, 1999; Tortoli, 1999, Watterson, 2000; Woods, 2001; Dowdy, 2003; Hall, 2004a; Kivihya-Ndugga, 2004; Sloutsky, 2004; Thwaites, 2004).

In-house PCR methods, which use various procedures for specimen preparation and targets for amplification, are associated with lack of standardization, as illustrated by Noordhoek (1994), who documented great variations in the ability of laboratories to correctly detect MTBC in blinded specimens. For clinical laboratories, the problems of poor standardization are likely to be reduced by use of commercial assays with central control of reagent quality and standard operating procedures. In general, nucleic acid amplification assays for detection of MTBC are more sensitive than AFB smear but less sensitive than culture (Cloud, 2004; Kivihya-Ndugga, 2004; Thwaites, 2004). Currently, two commercial systems, Amplicor MTB ([PCR], Roche) and Amplified *Mycobacterium tuberculosis* Direct Test (AMTDT [TMA], Gen-Probe), are approved by the Food and Drug Administration (FDA) for use on AFB smear-positive respiratory tract specimens. In addition, AMTDT is approved for use on smear-negative respiratory samples. A number of studies have compared two or more amplification-based methods (Piersimoni, 1998, 2002; Brown, 1999; Tortoli, 1999; Cleary, 2003); however, none have been

Table 62–6 Clinically Important Microbial Pathogens Tested for by Non-Commercial Nucleic Acid Amplification-Based Tests

Organism(s)	Specimen Types(s)	Clinical Indication(s)
Ehrlichia spp.	Blood	Human granulocytic and monocytic ehrlichiosis
Chlamydophila pneumoniae	Respiratory	Atypical pneumonia
Legionella pneumophila	Respiratory	Atypical pneumonia
Mycoplasma influenzae	Respiratory	Atypical pneumonia
Haemophilus influenzae	CSF	Meningitis
Neisseria meningitidis	CSF	Meningitis
Streptococcus pneumoniae	CSF	Meningitis
Staphylococcus aureus	Nasal swab	Preoperative detection of carriage state
Helicobacter pylori	Gastric fluid, stool	Peptic ulcer disease
JC virus	CSF	Progressive multifocal leukoencephalopathy
Parvovirus B19	Amniotic fluid	Hydrops fetalis
	Serum	Anemia
Adenovirus	Urine, tissues, blood	Immunocompromised patients and transplant recipients
Human herpes virus 8	Lymphomatous effusions	Primary effusion lymphoma
Human metapneumovirus	Respiratory	Acute respiratory disease
Astroviruses and caliciviruses	Stool	Diarrhea
Aspergillus spp.	Respiratory and blood	Invasive aspergillosis
Candida spp.	Blood	Hematogenous candidiasis
Cryptosporidium spp.	Stool	Diarrhea
Plasmodium spp.	Blood	Malaria
Toxoplasma gondii	Blood, CSF, amniotic fluid	Congenital infection; toxoplasmosis in immunocompromised patients

All tests use polymerase chain reaction or reverse-transcriptase polymerase chain reaction. The list is not all-inclusive.

CSF = cerebrospinal fluid.

sufficiently comprehensive to permit a firm conclusion as to the relative merits of all systems. In general, the sensitivity and specificity of all of the commercial systems is comparable (Watterson, 2000). The sensitivity of all of these systems is lower, relative to culture, when testing specimens obtained after the inception of antituberculous therapy (Sloutsky, 2004; Thwaites, 2004) and when applied to non-respiratory specimens such as cerebrospinal fluid (CSF) (Woods, 2001; Piersimoni, 2002; Cloud, 2004; Thwaites, 2004). Nonspecific inhibition of amplification has been shown to affect all systems more or less equally (Carpentier, 1995; Lumb, 1999; Piersimoni, 2002). One advantage of the SDA-based BD ProbeTec ET *Mycobacterium tuberculosis* Complex Direct Detection Assay (Becton Dickinson) is the inclusion of an internal amplification control that is designed to detect the presence of inhibitory substances, thereby minimizing the reporting of false-negative test results (Piersimoni, 2002). Real-time PCR using ASR has been shown to be comparable in sensitivity and specificity to conventional PCR (Amplicor, Roche) and to TMA (AMTD) in testing clinical specimens (Lachnik, 2002; Cleary, 2003; Lemaitre, 2004). Potential advantages in favor of real-time PCR include more rapid time to results (1.5 h vs 3 h) and decreased susceptibility to inhibitors of amplification.

Culture retains its central role in the diagnosis of tuberculosis because the existing amplification assays do not detect all culture-positive specimens and it is necessary to isolate the organism for susceptibility testing (and epidemiologic typing, if indicated). Currently, the amplification tests cannot replace the AFB smear because the latter is used to determine the level of infectivity of patients (smear-positive patients are much more infectious than smear-negative patients) and in assessing initial response to therapy. There is not a similarly rich context in which to interpret the amplification-based methods. In addition, the amplification methods answer a much more specific question (is MTBC present?) than

does the smear (are AFB present?) and in doing so may miss important clues to the diagnosis of a specific infectious disease. At present, the role of amplification assays remains complementary to that of microscopy and culture in the diagnosis of tuberculosis and other mycobacterial infections (Watterson, 2000).

The amplification methods are highly specific in distinguishing MTBC from other mycobacteria (MOTT) in AFB-smear-positive specimens (Piersimoni, 2002; Cleary, 2003; Sloutsky, 2004), thus allowing initiation of appropriate therapy and infection control procedures (Watterson, 2000; Dowdy, 2003). However, cost-effectiveness remains a critical obstacle to the use of molecular amplification tests for the diagnosis of tuberculosis (Watterson, 2000; Dowdy, 2003). Arguably, no healthcare system could accommodate use of these methods on every specimen (Cantanzaro, 2000; Watterson, 2000). Furthermore, patient management is not always influenced by the test result, suggesting that the use of such tests be reserved for situations where clinical management will be aided by the inclusion of a molecular test (Cantanzaro, 2000; Watterson, 2000). A recent study found that the use of nucleic acid amplification testing (specifically the Gen-Probe TMA) of AFB smear-positive specimens is not cost-effective for most individual hospitals (Dowdy, 2003). The authors cautioned that several factors must be taken into account when considering cost-effectiveness estimates including the number of smear-positive specimens processed annually, the relative prevalence of *M. tuberculosis* in smear-positive specimens, and the marginal daily cost of respiratory isolation. Molecular testing is likely to be cost-effective mainly in those laboratories processing a large number of specimens and thus may be best accomplished by centralized reference laboratories.

Perhaps the greatest impact of rapid molecular tuberculosis (TB) diagnostics can be realized by applying this testing in TB suspects whose specimens are smear-negative (American Thoracic Society Workshop, 1997; Cantanzaro, 2000; Dowdy, 2003). Although smear-positive patients are well known to be infective, evidence is now emerging that smear-negative culture-positive TB patients can also be infectious (Sepkowitz, 1996). Thus, routine amplification-based testing of smear-negative specimens could play a very important role in disease-prevention efforts by identifying such individuals days or weeks before culture results are available (Dowdy, 2003). Given the fact that 50–90% of smear-negative but culture-positive specimens test positive by the various amplification-based tests for MTBC (Watterson, 2000), it has been demonstrated that molecular testing can be carried out on smear-negative specimens with high positive and negative predictive values, when combined with clinical judgment in identifying those patients at risk for TB (Cantanzaro, 2000). Further cost-justification of this strategy is necessary (Dowdy, 2003).

Nucleic acid amplification has also been applied to other bacterial pathogens of the respiratory tract (Cockerill, 2004; Ieven, 2004). *Legionella pneumophila* is a fastidious pathogen for which rapid diagnosis can be of critical importance. A commercially available conventional PCR assay (Legionella EnviroAmp system, Perkin Elmer) may have applications in rapid detection of *Legionella* in bronchoalveolar lavage samples (Weir, 1998); however, real-time PCR has been shown to be highly sensitive and specific for detection of *L. pneumophila* providing results in 1–2 hours, thus greatly accelerating the screening of clinical specimens (Hayden, 2001b; Rantakokko-Jalava, 2001). Similarly, *Bordetella pertussis*, *Chlamydia* (*Chlamydophila*) *pneumoniae*, and *Mycoplasma pneumoniae* present particular difficulties for the diagnostic laboratory that can be addressed effectively by PCR (Ieven, 1997, 2004; Farrell, 1999b; Grondahl, 1999; Cockerill, 2004). Multiplex PCR assays capable of detecting and discriminating among a wide range of potential respiratory pathogens (bacterial and viral) have been developed and offer promise for the future (Table 62–4) (Grondahl, 1999; Elnifro, 2000; Gruteke, 2004).

Diagnosis of sexually transmitted disease has also been an important area for the development and application of amplification assays. *N. gonorrhoeae* grows rapidly on appropriate conventional agar media, and culture has high sensitivity and specificity under optimal conditions (Koumans, 1998). *N. gonorrhoeae* is fastidious, however, and appropriate collection and transport and culture conditions are critical and may not be easily achieved in every setting. Culture of *C. trachomatis* is also demanding, requiring tissue culture facilities; therefore, nonculture methods for detection of *Chlamydia* antigen have been widely used.

Almost all the amplification methods have been applied to the detection of *C. trachomatis* in genital specimens (Schepetiuk, 1997; Stary, 1998; Morre, 1998; Pasternack, 1999; Vincelette, 1999; Van Dyck, 2001; Hall, 2004a; Koenig, 2004). In general, published evaluations indicate that the amplification-based methods are specific and more sensitive than cell culture or immunologic methods (Schepetiuk, 1997; Stary, 1998; Wylie, 1998; Vincelette, 1999; Van Dyck, 2001; Hall, 2004a). In a multicenter study of the automated COBAS Amplicor CT/NG PCR test (Roche), sensitivity and specificity varied with specimen type (Vincelette, 1999). The test showed a sensitivity of 100% and a specificity of 98.5% when male urethral swabs were tested; for endocervical swabs the sensitivity was 96.5% and specificity 99.4%, and for urine, sensitivity ranged from 94.4–95.1% and specificity from 99.8–100%. The performance of amplification assays on urine samples may facilitate screening for *C. trachomatis* infection, given the ease of obtaining a urine specimen compared to more invasive sampling methods. Several comparisons of the various amplification methods for *C. trachomatis* have been reported (Schepetiuk, 1997; Stary, 1998; Pasternack, 1999; Van Dyck, 2001; Koenig, 2004). Van Dyck and colleagues (2001) compared the performance of PCR (Roche), SDA (Becton Dickinson), and LCR (Abbott) for the detection of *C. trachomatis* in 396 endocervical swab specimens (50 culture-positive) and reported sensitivities and specificities of 98.0%, 94.0%, and 90.0% and 98.0%, 100%, and 98.6%, respectively. A recent study comparing SDA with real-time PCR found an overall agreement of 91.2% (Koenig, 2004). Notably, SDA results with a MOTA (method-other-than-acceleration) score between 2000 and 9999 (indeterminate) were not reproducible and tended to represent false-positives relative to PCR and culture. The available data suggest that comparable performance can be expected from the various systems for detection of *C. trachomatis*, with the caveat that repeat or confirmatory testing should be performed on specimens for which the results are 'indeterminate' (e.g. SDA MOTA scores between 2000 and 9999).

A single specimen may be used to detect both *C. trachomatis* and *N. gonorrhoeae* using PCR (Roche), SDA (Becton Dickinson), or TMB (Gen-Probe) (Vincelette, 1999; Koenig, 2004; Van Dyck, 2001). All three methods have been reported as being more sensitive than culture (88.9–95.2% versus 69.8%, respectively) in detecting *N. gonorrhoeae* in cervical specimens (Kehl, 1998; Van Dyck, 2001). As with *C. trachomatis*, false-positive results for *N. gonorrhoeae* have been reported in specimens with lower MOTA scores (2000–9999) as determined by SDA, suggesting the need for confirmatory testing (Koenig, 2004). These findings coupled with the potential for false-positive results with Amplicor PCR (Roche) in the presence of *Neisseria subflava* emphasize the continuing need for refinement of these technologies (Farrell, 1999a).

PCR has also been applied with excellent results in detecting agents of bacterial meningitis (Bryant, 2004; Parent du Châtelet, 2005; Robbins, 2005), enteropathogenic *Escherichia coli* and *Shigella* spp. (Aranda, 2004), and agents of bioterrorism such as *Bacillus anthracis* (Bode, 2004; Cockerill, 2004). The application of real-time PCR for the detection of *S. aureus* in nasal swab specimens was found to be a rapid, accurate, and cost-effective method for identifying *S. aureus* carriers for preoperative intervention (Shrestha, 2003a). Similarly, real-time PCR has proved useful in detecting the important nosocomial pathogens MRSA and VRE (Diekema, 2004; Warren, 2004). Early and accurate detection of MRSA and VRE carriers is necessary to focus isolation and prevention strategies. Application of real-time PCR for detection of VRE (*vanA* and *vanB* PCR) carriage (rectal swab or stool) in a university hospital reduced the mean time to detection of VRE in hospitalized patients from 3.4 to 1.3 days and allowed earlier isolation of VRE carriers and the earlier discharge of patients to long-term care and rehabilitation centers (Diekema, 2004).

PCR assays capable of amplifying ribosomal RNA genes (rRNA, rDNA) from essentially any bacterium and from a wide range of clinical specimens have been described and are now regularly applied in clinical microbiology and infectious diseases (Clarridge, 2004; Tang, 1998). Rapid sequencing of the amplified products and comparison of the sequence data with sequences in a DNA database has proven to be a powerful tool for the identification of a wide variety of microorganisms (Tang, 1998; Goldenberger, 1997; Hall, 2003a, 2003b, 2004a; Clarridge, 2004). This approach has also proven useful for the detection and identification of previously unrecognized or nonculturable pathogens (Fredericks, 1996; Clarridge, 2004; Cockerill, 2004). Broad range PCR coupled with molecular array technology further enhances the capabilities of molecular diagnostic microbiology (Belgrader, 1998; Marshall, 1998; Clarridge, 2004; Kolbert, 2004; Maiwald, 2004; Stöver, 2004).

Detection of Fungi

Invasive fungal infection is an important problem worldwide (Lin, 2001b; Marr, 2002; Pfaller, 2004b; Walsh, 2004). Serious life-threatening infections are being reported with an ever increasing array of pathogens, including the well-known opportunists *C. albicans*, *C. neoformans*, and *Aspergillus fumigatus* (Pfaller, 2004b; Walsh, 2004). Systemic fungal infection is difficult to diagnose in a timely fashion and this may contribute to the high mortality (Yeo, 2002).

PCR has been studied in greatest detail for the diagnosis of candidemia and invasive aspergillosis (Bougnoux, 1999; Latge, 1999; Yeo, 2002; Kawazu, 2004; Musher, 2004). Clinical specimens include serum or whole blood (*Candida* and *Aspergillus*), and respiratory samples (sputum or bronchoalveolar lavage [BAL] fluid) for aspergillosis (Yeo, 2002; Kawazu, 2004; Musher, 2004). Target sequences vary widely but most often include ribosomal genes (18S rRNA) or internal transcribed spacer (ITS) regions (Iwen, 2002; Yeo, 2002). Sensitivities range from 78–100% for candidiasis and from 33–100% in patients with proven invasive aspergillosis (Yeo, 2002). Specificities vary especially with PCR for aspergillosis where false-positives may be seen when BAL fluid is tested that are due to transient presence of conidia in the respiratory tract. Use of serum or plasma may be preferable over respiratory specimens, since contamination with conidia is much less likely. The combination of quantitative PCR and galactomannan antigen testing on BAL fluid has recently been shown to result in improved sensitivity and specificity when compared to either test alone in diagnosing invasive pulmonary aspergillosis (Musher, 2004). Likewise, antigen testing and real-time PCR using serum proved useful in weekly screening for invasive aspergillosis in patients with hematological disorders (Kawazu, 2004).

As with bacteria, the combination of broad range PCR to amplify a product (e.g. 18S rDNA) from all or most common fungi associated with human infection is a potentially important strategy (Van Burik, 1998; Yeo, 2002). Amplification followed by restriction endonuclease analysis, sequencing, or hybridization to a series of species- or genus-specific probes have all been shown to be viable options in an effort to broaden the diagnosis of fungal infections (Van Burik, 1998; Chemaly, 2004). At present, although promising reports continue to appear (Lin, 2001a), PCR for diagnosis of invasive fungal infection has not been widely used in clinical settings and it has not been shown convincingly that PCR can compensate for the limitations of culture in rapid diagnosis of invasive fungal infection in the immunocompromised host. Real-time PCR and microarray platforms coupled with fungal antigen detection will likely be required to significantly impact this difficult diagnostic problem.

Detection of Parasites

In clinical laboratories, diagnosis of infection with many protozoan parasites is dependent upon microscopy of feces, tissue, blood, or bone marrow smears. In the case of *Giardia lamblia*, *Entamoeba histolytica*, and *Cryptosporidium parvum*, detection of antigen in feces is an alternative. Microscopic examination of specimens is time-consuming, requires considerable skill, and has limited sensitivity for specimens containing few organisms (Petri, 2004). Likewise, culture is impractical for most parasitic infections because of the wide variety of potential pathogens and the highly specialized conditions required for each type of organism (Visvesvara, 2002). Given the limitations of conventional methods it would seem that there would be an even greater potential opportunity for the introduction of molecular diagnostic techniques into parasitology than into other areas of microbiology where conventional methods are much more productive (Petri, 2004). Despite these issues, and the fact that parasitologic expertise is declining in many clinical laboratories in North America, molecular testing for parasitic disease has been slow to develop. In order to be practical, molecular parasitology testing must be simple and cost-effective and at the same time capable of detecting multiple different parasites in a given specimen (Petri, 2004). These demands, coupled with the perception that the market for such testing, outside poor developing countries, is small, have conspired to limit development in this area.

Clearly, the application of PCR can improve the detection of protozoan parasites in clinical material. PCR amplification of the small subunit rRNA of *Plasmodium* has been shown to be more sensitive than microscopic examination of blood films by skilled microscopists for diagnosing falciparum malaria and for monitoring response to treatment (Ciceron, 1999; Moody, 2002). Real-time PCR amplification of an 18S rRNA gene subunit was both sensitive and specific in detecting four *Plasmodium* species (*Plasmodium falciparum*, *Plasmodium vivax*, *Plasmodium malariae*, and *Plasmodium ovale*) in blood (Rougemont, 2004). Quantitative measurement of the number of parasites using real-time PCR showed a rapid decline in parasitemia in response to therapy, paralleling that observed microscopically (Rougemont, 2004). Similarly encouraging results have been achieved in detection of *Babesia* spp. in blood and *Leishmania* parasites in bone marrow and blood (Krause, 1996, Katakura, 1998; Cascio, 2002). Detection of *Toxoplasma gondii* DNA in amniotic fluid can facilitate rapid diagnosis of congenital toxoplasmosis (Gratzl, 1998; Costa, 2001) and has been applied to CSF for diagnosis of cerebral toxoplasmosis in HIV-positive patients (Julander, 2001) and to blood for early detection of *T. gondii* reactivation in stem cell transplant recipients (Chandrasekar, 2005; Martino, 2005). Application of PCR to detection of intestinal parasites, including *Entamoeba histolytica*, *Cryptosporidium parvum*,

Giardia lamblia, and microsporidia has also been described (Haque, 1998; Morgan, 1998; Franzen, 1999; Ghosh, 2000; O'Connor, 2004). Although commercial amplification systems for diagnosis of parasitic diseases are not yet available, it is expected that molecular methods will gradually replace morphologic diagnosis, with resultant improvement in patient outcomes as parasitic diseases are accurately and sensitively diagnosed and then appropriately treated (Petri, 2004).

Identification of Cultures

The sensitivity of amplification-based methods facilitates their application to direct detection of pathogen-specific genomes in clinical material, but they are also valuable for identification of cultured microbes. A species-specific amplification reaction can identify a single species of particular importance, such as MTBC (Shrestha, 2003b). Alternatively, an amplification reaction may be designed to target a genus-specific or 'universal' target and restriction endonuclease digestion, hybridization with multiple probes, or sequence determination of the amplicon can be used to identify and discriminate among a variety of species (Watterson, 2000; Tortoli, 2001; Hall, 2003a, 2003b, 2004b; Clarridge, 2004). Identification of cultures by amplification was initially applied primarily to slow-growing mycobacteria (Hall, 2003a; Tortoli, 2001; Watterson, 2000) but also has applications for other unusual pathogens (Hall, 2003b, 2004b; Clarridge, 2004). It is logical and convenient for a laboratory using amplification for direct detection to use the same technology for culture identification where possible (Clarridge, 2004).

Species-specific amplification has been applied to rapid identification of cultured *M. tuberculosis*, *M. avium*, and *M. intracellulare* (Tortoli, 1998; Ninet, 1999; Watterson, 2000; Shrestha, 2003b). The application of these approaches to positive BACTEC vials with low growth index readings may reduce by 2–3 days the time to confirmation of tuberculosis. As with other bacteria, DNA sequencing of the 16S rRNA genes can be used for the reliable identification of mycobacterial species (Watterson, 2000). Amplification of the 16S–23S ribosomal spacer region with subsequent hybridization to probes bound to a nylon strip (INNO LiPA, Innogenetics) is the basis for a commercially available kit-based method for the identification of nine different mycobacterial species (Watterson, 2000; Tortoli, 2001). Another option is the PCR restriction enzyme assay (PRA), where a portion of the *hsp 65* gene is amplified and subsequently digested in two separate restriction enzyme digestions and the fragments analyzed by agarose gel electrophoresis (Watterson, 2000). This approach has been used to identify 34 mycobacterial species and subspecies (Devallois, 1997). Multiplex PCR has been reported as permitting differentiation among MTBC, *M. avium*, and other mycobacteria in a single PCR reaction (Cormican, 1995; Kulski, 1995).

Multiplex PCR has also been applied to rapid confirmation of toxigenicity in isolates of verocytotoxigenic *E. coli* (Paton, 1998; Aranda, 2004). Amplification and 16S rRNA gene sequence analysis has proved very useful in identifying poorly described, rarely isolated, or phenotypically aberrant strains (Tang, 1998; Clarridge, 2004). In its current state 16S rRNA sequence analysis allows bacterial identification that is more robust, reproducible, and accurate than that obtained by phenotypic testing. The availability of improved sequencing techniques, broader and more reliable databases, and more readily available kits and software, makes this technology a competitive alternative to routine microbial identification techniques for some groups of organisms (Clarridge, 2004). Technical and cost considerations (range $38–144 per isolate) limit the widespread use of 16S rRNA gene sequence analysis. The coupling of broad-range PCR with microarray analysis of the amplicon may make this technology more broadly applicable to microbiology laboratories in the future (Troesch, 1999; Stöver, 2004).

Detection of Antimicrobial Resistance

Resistance of microbes to antimicrobial agents is one of the major public health problems of this decade. Molecular methods have contributed substantially to our understanding of the genetics of antimicrobial resistance and the spread of resistance determinants. They also have the potential to contribute to prompt detection of resistance in clinical settings (Table 62–7) (Bergeron, 1998; Fluit, 2001; Diekema, 2004; Tenover, 2004). Standardized conventional antimicrobial susceptibility testing is growth-dependent and requires a pure culture of the pathogen and at least 18–24 hours before a result is available. Rapid automated systems such as Vitek may provide results within hours for certain organisms but may be less able to detect resistance mechanisms in which a period of induction in the presence of the antibiotic is required before the resistance is expressed.

Table 62–7 Application of Molecular Methods for Detection of Antimicrobial Resistance

Organism(s)	Antimicrobial Agent(s)	Gene(s)	Detection Method
Staphylococci	Methicillin or oxacillin	*mec*A	PCR, probe, bDNA
	Aminoglycosides	*aac*(6')-Ie+*aph*(2')	PCR, probe
	Macrolides	*erm*, *mef*, *msr*	PCR, probe
	Fluoroquinolones	Point mutations in *gyr*A, *grl*A	PCR and sequencing
	Mupirocin	*mup*A	PCR
	Vancomycin	*van*A	PCR
Enterococci	Vancomycin	*van*A, -B, -C, -D, -E, -G	PCR, probe
	Aminoglycosides	*aac*, *aph*, *ant*	PCR, probe
Streptococcus pneumoniae	β-lactams	*phbl*A, -2V, -2X	PCR
	Fluoroquinolones	Point mutations in *gyr*A and -B and *par*C and -E	PCR and sequencing
	Macrolides	*erm*, *mef*	PCR
Enterobacteriaceae	β-lactams	bla_TEM, bla_SHV	PCR, probe, sequencing
	Fluoroquinolones	Point mutations in *gyr*A and -B and *par*C and -E	PCR and sequencing
	Aminoglycosides	*ant*, *aac*	Probe, PCR
Mycobacterium tuberculosis	Rifamycins	Point mutations in *rpo*B	PCR and SSCP; PCR and sequencing
	Isoniazid	Point mutations in *kat*G, *inh*A, and *ahp*C	PCR and sequencing
	Ethambutol	Point mutations in *emb*B	PCR and SSCP
	Streptomycin	Point mutations in *rps* and *rrs*	PCR and sequencing
Helicobacter pylori	Macrolides	Point mutations in 23S rDNA	PCR and line probe (LiPA) or
Neisseria gonorrhoeae	Fluoroquinolones	Point mutations in *gyr*A and *par*C	PCR and sequencing
Candida albicans	Azoles	Mutation in *erg*11; over expression of ERG11, MDR1, CRD1 and –2	PCR and sequencing; quantitative RT-PCR; Northern blot
	Echinocandins	Point mutations in FKS genes	PCR and sequencing
	Flucytosine	Point mutation in uracil phosphoribosyl transferase gene	PCR and sequencing
Herpes viruses	Acyclovir and related drugs	Mutations or deletions in the *TK* (thymidine kinase) gene	PCR and sequencing
	Foscarnet	Point mutations in the DNA polymerase gene	PCR and sequencing
HIV	Nucleoside RT inhibitors	Point mutations in the *RT* gene	PCR and sequencing; PCR and LiPA
	Protease inhibitors	Point mutations in the *PROT* gene	PCR and sequencing

SSCP, single strand conformational polymorphism; TK, thymidine kinase; RT, reverse transcriptase; PROT, protease

VII

In the case of methicillin/oxacillin resistance in staphylococci, the resistance may be expressed in a very heterogeneous fashion, particularly in the coagulase-negative staphylococci, so that clinically relevant antimicrobial resistance may be difficult to detect by standardized susceptibility tests. Because of these difficulties, molecular detection of the *mec*A gene is considered the reference method against which phenotypic methods are compared. PCR, bDNA probes, and cycling probes have been extensively investigated for application in rapid detection of methicillin resistance in staphylococci (Vannuffel, 1995; Marshall, 1997; Kolbert, 1998; Ramotar, 1998; Bekkaoui, 1999; Diekema, 2004; Tenover, 2004; Warren, 2004). A real-time PCR assay for rapid detection of MRSA directly from nasal swab specimens is now commercially available (IDI-MRSA, Infectio Diagnostic) and has been shown to provide results within 1.5 hours with a sensitivity of 92% and a specificity of 94% when compared to culture-based methods (Warren, 2004). Application of this testing strategy should allow more efficient and effective use of infection control resources to control MRSA in healthcare facilities (Diekema, 2004; Warren, 2004).

Detection of drug resistance is especially problematic in slow-growing pathogens such as *M. tuberculosis* where weeks may elapse between submission of specimen and a final antimicrobial susceptibility report. For many years, this delay was not considered to be much of a problem, as tuberculosis was declining in incidence and antimicrobial resistance was uncommon. Susceptibility testing was performed primarily for confirmation of susceptibility and for monitoring for emergence of resistance. Since the late 1980s, timely laboratory guidance in relation to therapy of tuberculosis has become essential for a number of reasons (Watterson, 2000). These include the resurgence of tuberculosis globally (including in many developed countries), the emergence and spread of antimicrobial resistance in MTBC, and the emergence of a substantial population with the acquired immunodeficiency syndrome (AIDS) in whom tuberculosis can progress rapidly to death in the absence of appropriate therapy. In addition to improved detection of MTBC, rapid phenotypic and genotypic methods have been developed to aid in the screening for drug resistance mutations (Watterson, 2000). PCR amplification of DNA sequences from the *rpo*B (rifampin resistance), and the *kat*G, *inh*A, and *ahp*C genes (isoniazid resistance), followed by detection of mutations associated with resistance by sequencing or by single-strand conformational polymorphism, has a high sensitivity for detection of resistance to rifampin (>96%) and isoniazid (87%) (Table 62–7) (Telenti, 1997; Tenover, 2004). The INNO LiPA Rif. TB assay (Innogenetics) uses amplification and line-probe hybridization technology to simultaneously identify MTBC and screen for rifampin resistance mutations directly in smear-positive respiratory specimens and cultured isolates (Rossau, 1997). A similar application has been suggested for PCR coupled with high-density DNA microarrays (Troesch, 1999; Fluit, 2001). Rapid recognition of antimicrobial-resistant strains of MTBC is important in preventing spread of infection with such strains in susceptible patients and healthcare workers.

Molecular methods have applications in detection of drug resistance in a wider spectrum of organisms than just MTBC and MRSA (Table 62–7) (Tenover, 2004; Fluit, 2001). Detection of vancomycin resistance in enterococci, penicillin resistance in pneumococci, fluoroquinolone resistance in gonococci, and TEM β-lactamases in Gram-negative bacilli have been reported (Jones, 1997; Bergeron, 1998; Cockerill, 1999; Fluit, 2001; O'Neill,1999; Diekema, 2004; Grim, 2004; Tenover, 2004; Zhou, 2004). Rapid detection of specific resistant pathogens may prove to be very cost-effective. The use of real-time PCR to detect VRE has been shown to decrease the lengths of stay for patients discharged to long-term care by almost 2 days, saving one university hospital an estimated $205 000 annually (Diekema, 2004).

Detection of resistance to antiviral agents is increasingly important since drug resistance has been recognized as a significant barrier to effective chemotherapy of a number of viral infections. Phenotypic detection of drug resistance in HIV is complex and time-consuming and therefore impractical in most clinical situations (Petropoulos, 2004). Specific mutations in the HIV-1 reverse transcriptase (RT) gene and in the protease gene are associated with resistance to antiretroviral agents and are readily detected by a variety of molecular methods (Caliendo, 2004). Following reverse transcription and PCR amplification of the entire protease gene and most of the reverse transcriptase gene, the amplified products may be analyzed by one of several methods, including automated sequencing, DNA hybridization using high-density microarrays, and reverse hybridization using the line probe assay (LiPA) (Caliendo, 2004). The commercially available LiPA is designed to detect mutations associated with resistance at preselected codons in the *RT* and protease genes (Caliendo, 2004). Although this method does facilitate the more rapid detection of mutations associated with resistance, it does not provide information about the entire target gene sequence and thus may not be optimal for all significant mutations (Puchhammer-Stockl, 1999; Caliendo, 2004). Genotypic assays require not only detection of the resistance mutations but also an interpretation of how the mutations alter HIV-1 drug susceptibility. Given the complexities of this process it is important that both the technical and interpretive aspects of the testing are standardized.

Molecular methods for detection of resistance can be applied directly to clinical specimens and may therefore be appropriate for slow-growing bacteria, particularly urgent clinical situations, and detection of resistance in viruses (Tenover, 2004). In addition, they are applicable to nonviable organisms and may reduce biohazard risks associated with manipulation of viable pathogens such as *M. tuberculosis*. Molecular methods may also have particular advantages in relation to resistance mechanisms that are expressed only after prolonged induction, since phenotypic methods may not always be sufficiently reliable or timely in such cases. Despite these numerous advantages, molecular methods are not likely to substitute for phenotypic detection of resistance in most clinical situations in the near future.

Molecular methods for detection of antimicrobial resistance are limited in a number of respects (Bergeron, 1998; Fluit, 2001). First, absence of a known resistance gene does not exclude the possibility of resistance by another mechanism. In practical terms, molecular detection of antimicrobial resistance is based on detection of individual well characterized genes in a species or genus in which it is expected to occur. Molecular methods specific for one resistance mechanism will not detect new emerging resistance mechanisms and are unlikely to be applied to detection of expression of resistance genes in species in which that gene has not been observed previously. Furthermore, the already large number of known point mutations or genes leading to resistance and the labor-intensive nature of current amplification methods precludes any sort of 'molecular survey' for resistance. In contrast, phenotypic-based susceptibility testing allows for a practical 'survey' of resistance mechanisms by simultaneously testing several different classes of antimicrobial agent against a given pathogen. DNA microarray technology coupled with automated amplification techniques has the potential to address this issue (Grim, 2004; Zhou, 2004); however, the development of microarrays containing a broad range of resistance markers that are applicable to several different species is a considerable challenge that requires a much broader understanding of resistance mechanisms than is currently available (Fluit, 2001). A second limitation is that the presence of a gene for antimicrobial resistance need not result in the expression of the resistance phenotype. For example, *E. coli* possesses a chromosomal gene for an AmpC-like β-lactamase; however, it is almost never expressed and declaring a clinical isolate as 'resistant' to β-lactam agents on the basis of molecular detection of the AmpC gene would preclude the use of many agents with proven efficacy. In principle, this limitation is not insurmountable if assays to detect mRNA are used in preference to assays to detect the chromosomal gene. This is in fact an active area of investigation whereby gene expression profiles are used to detect drug resistance and to determine the mechanism of action of antimicrobial agents, as well as to discover new targets for drugs (Sturtevant, 2000; Frade, 2004; Hutter, 2004; Karababa, 2004). It seems likely that, for the present, molecular methods for detection of antimicrobial resistance will remain tools of investigation, drug discovery, and development, and of reference laboratories conducting studies monitoring resistance mechanisms and studies of the performance of phenotypic methods.

Molecular Epidemiology

The variety of molecular epidemiologic tools available at present is considerable (Table 62–8), and in particular there has been a proliferation of amplification-based methods (Hanage, 2004; Mathema, 2004; Rademaker, 2004; Soll, 2004). An exhaustive consideration of the relative merits of these approaches is beyond the scope of this chapter. It is important to emphasize that no one technique is universally applicable and that choice of a particular application is related to the species studied, the scope of the question posed, and the convenience of the technique (Soll, 2000, 2004). The techniques of molecular typing are useful in answering real clinical and infection control questions, and are not limited to research uses. Examples include clarifying the significance of multiple isolates of *Staphylococcus epidermidis* from a particular patient and predicting response to interferon in hepatitis C virus infection. Molecular evidence of identity between isolates of *S. epidermidis* obtained from culture at different times suggests that the isolate is clinically significant, and HCV genotypes 1b and 1a appear less likely to respond to interferon

Table 62–8 Molecular Methods for Epidemiologic Typing of Microorganisms

Method	Substrate	Principal characteristics	Examples
Plasmid analysis	Plasmid DNA	Potentially unstable owing to loss of plasmids. May be augmented by restriction endonuclease digestion	*Staphylococcus aureus*, coagulase-negative staphylococci, *Klebsiella*, *Serratia*, Enterobacteriaceae
Restriction endonuclease analysis of chromosomal DNA with conventional electrophoresis	Chromosomal DNA	Broadly applicable. Large numbers of bands. Not amenable to computer analysis	Enterococci, *S. aureus*, *Clostridium difficile*, *Candida* spp.
Pulsed-field gel electrophoresis	Chromosomal DNA	Broadly applicable. Uses infrequently cutting restriction enzymes to generate large DNA fragments (10–88 kb). Fewer bands. Excellent reproducibility and discriminatory power. Expensive equipment	Staphylococci, enterococci, Enterobacteriaceae, *Pseudomonas*, *Candida*
Genome restriction fragment length polymorphism analysis with DNA probes	Chromosomal DNA	Broadly applicable. Multistep process. Amenable to computer analysis. Includes IS6110 analysis of *Mycobacterium tuberculosis* and ribotyping	*M. tuberculosis*, *Candida* spp., Enterobacteriaceae, staphylococci, *Pseudomonas*
PCR-based methods: repetitive-element PCR spacer typing. Selective amplification of genome restriction fragments, multilocus allelic sequence-based typing	Chromosomal DNA	Broadly applicable. Rapid and moderately easy to perform. Crude extracts and small amounts of DNA may suffice	Enterobacteriaceae, *Acinetobacter*, staphylococci, *M. tuberculosis*, hepatitis C virus
Library probe genotypic hybridization schemes: multilocus probe dot blot patterns, high-density oligonucleotide patterns	Chromosomal DNA	Unambiguous yes–no result. Less discrimination than with other methods. Couple with DNA chip technology	*Burkholderia cepacia*, *S. aureus*, *M. tuberculosis*

This table contains examples of available methods and applications and is not intended to be all-inclusive.

PCR = polymerase chain reaction.

than other genotypes (Martinot-Peignoux, 1998; Vandelli, 1999). Molecular techniques are also helpful in detecting the emergence and spread of strains of an organism with unusual drug resistance patterns or pathogenicity, in determining the efficacy of infection control procedures, and in definition of source in outbreaks of infection related to food or therapeutic products (Diekema, 2003).

DNA-Dependent Molecular Typing Methods

The literature relating to DNA-dependent molecular typing, and in particular typing by amplification, has become a maze of acronyms and subtle variations. In order to impose some structure in this area it is helpful to consider two aspects of each method: the technical approach (amplification, restriction enzyme, probe, or a mixture of these) and the principle (arbitrary snapshot of the chromosome or focus on sequences that evolve rapidly). DNA-based typing methods are based on the progressive divergence that occurs in the sequence of identical bacterial cells over many generations of cell division. The more similar the sequence between two organisms isolated from different patients, the more likely it is that they originated from a common source in the recent past. The degree of divergence between organisms may be looked at over the entire sequence of the chromosome. The highest degree of resolution for such an approach would require sequencing of the entire chromosome; however, this is not practical. Therefore, most of the methods developed attempt to identify sequence variation at randomly distributed points throughout the chromosome. This snapshot is the basis for restriction fragment length polymorphism (RFLP), pulsed field gel electrophoresis (PFGE), and amplification typing using arbitrary primers. Sequence divergence does not occur at an equal rate at all points of the chromosome. Specific elements of the chromosome alter more rapidly with respect to the nucleotide sequence or with respect to the number of copies of the element and the distribution of the copies throughout the chromosome. Examples of rapidly evolving sequences include insertion sequences (IS), transposons (Tn), tandem repeat sequences, and integrons (In). A range of typing methods have exploited these highly variable sequences to study relationships between microbes. Some methods use a combination of whole chromosome digestion followed by probing for multicopy sequences. Critical variables to consider in relation to choice of a typing method for a particular application are its reproducibility both within and between laboratories, discriminatory power, speed, convenience, and cost (Soll, 2000). Increasingly, visual inspection and qualitative evaluation of the banding patterns produced by many of these typing methods is being complemented by use of more quantitative computerized analysis, and studies of the relative merits of the available analysis systems are appearing

(Gerner-Smidt, 1998; Olive, 1999; Soll, 2000, 2004; Barrett, 2004). The ability to transfer the digitized images of banding patterns rapidly to a central laboratory with the potential for rapid comparison of strains and the adoption of conventions in relation to designation of types can be expected to greatly increase the power of these techniques for tracking evolution and spread of specific strains at national and international levels. The difficulties to be overcome in terms of standardization of molecular typing methods are considerable (van Belkum, 1998).

Standard RFLP analysis with frequent cutting enzymes may generate a very large number of bands on gel electrophoresis. The method has been useful in typing of a great variety of organisms. For example, Bingen (1991) used RFLP to demonstrate that the vancomycin-resistant *Enterococcus faecium* isolates from a French hospital did not represent spread of a single resistant strain. Because of the complexity of the banding patterns that make analysis difficult, this method has been largely superseded.

One solution to the complexity of the patterns is to identify and analyze only a subset of bands that contain a specific sequence that occurs in multiple copies in the genome. This is achieved by transferring the DNA bands from the electrophoresis gel to a membrane (Southern blotting) and the subsequent application of DNA probes to the membrane. The most generally applicable multicopy sequence is the ribosomal RNA gene. This process, known as ribotyping, has been used to study relationships among strains of many species, and comparative studies of the value of ribotyping relative to traditional typing methods have been reported for some species. A fully automated, rapid system for performance of ribotyping with computer-assisted interpretation (Riboprinter, Qualicon, Wilmington, DE) is now available commercially (Pfaller, 2004c). The Riboprinter has been reported to be more discriminatory than arbitrarily primed PCR for *Salmonella enterica* (Hilton, 1998); however, in a comparison of the Riboprinter with PFGE for typing of *E. coli* and *Pseudomonas aeruginosa*, it was less discriminatory than PFGE (Pfaller, 1996). It has been suggested that the Riboprinter might be useful as a first-line typing tool but that strains that appear indistinguishable on ribotyping may be placed into distinct groups using PFGE (Pfaller, 2001, 2004c).

Probes that hybridize to multicopy sequences other than 16S rRNA are utilized in a similar fashion. Among the best studied of these applications is the use of a probe to the insertion sequence IS6110 to type MTBC. This method is relatively slow and has limited discriminatory power for MTBC strains with few copies of the IS6110 sequence (Yuen, 1993). It is well standardized and has proved very informative in defining the epidemiology of tuberculosis (van Embden, 1993; Bradford, 1998). More recently, a number of different typing methods for MTBC to supplement or substitute for the IS6110 typing have been described. Probing of RFLP digests with the multicopy polymorphic GC-rich sequences (PGRS) may be used to supplement IS6110 typing for strains with low IS6110 copy number (Bradford, 1998).

An adequate number of bands for analysis of most organisms (10–20 bands) can also be achieved by PFGE (Allardet-Servent, 1989; Goering, 2004). PFGE uses restriction enzymes to cut DNA at sequences that occur infrequently, producing a limited number of large DNA fragments. This approach requires that shearing forces resulting in random breaks in the bacterial chromosome are avoided in preparation of DNA for digestion. This is accomplished by imbedding the bacteria in agarose plugs before digestion of the cell wall. An electrophoresis system capable of separating the very large fragments of DNA must also be employed. Separation of large fragments is made possible by periodic alteration of the direction of the electric field operating in the electrophoresis chamber. PFGE permits separation of entire chromosomes so that for yeasts, which are eukaryotes, a karyotype may be generated without restriction enzyme digestion. PFGE is considered by some to be the most widely accepted and broadly applicable method for molecular typing. Principles for interpretation of PFGE gels have been proposed, and for many organisms it is the de facto standard for molecular typing against which other methods are compared (Tenover, 1995; Goering, 2004). The principal limitations of PFGE are that it is relatively slow and costly; however, some progress has been made in developing rapid protocols for PFGE (Matushek, 1996; Goering, 2004). PFGE is applicable to the study of the epidemiology of many of the pathogens, including MRSA (van Belkum, 1998), vancomycin-resistant *E. faecium* (Fridkin, 1998), penicillin-resistant *S. pneumoniae* (Rudolph, 1998), extended spectrum β-lactamase-producing *Klebsiella pneumoniae* (Liu, 1998), *E. coli* O157 (Grif, 1998), *Stenotrophomonas maltophilia* (Sader, 1994), and *Candida* spp., for which either karyotyping or RFLP analysis may be used (Cormican, 1996).

DNA amplification by PCR is applied to molecular typing in a variety of ways (Hanage, 2004; Mathema, 2004; Rademaker, 2004). One advantage of typing strategies utilizing PCR is the need for only small quantities of DNA. Additionally, the template DNA may be quite a crude preparation, which generally is not the case with restriction enzyme digest systems. At its simplest, PCR-based typing involves the use of one or a number of generic primers in nonstringent conditions that result in amplification of multiple fragments of varying sizes. The number and size of the amplified fragments are dependent on the sequence of the microbial genome, and a type-specific banding pattern is revealed by gel electrophoresis (NiRiain, 1994; Rademaker, 2004). This method, or variations of it, labeled random amplification of polymorphic DNA (RAPD) or DNA amplification fingerprinting (DAF), has broad applicability to a variety of contemporary pathogens, including *Enterobacter cloacae* and *Neisseria meningitidis* (NiRiain, 1994; Woods, 1994; Bart, 1998; Rademaker, 2004). Reproducibility of banding patterns using generic primers and nonstringent conditions can be problematic. Weak bands may appear and disappear from run to run; however, some groups appear to have overcome these difficulties (Bart, 1998). In general, these techniques may be most applicable to rapid and preliminary characterization of small numbers of strains within a single institution.

There is also emerging a variety of applications of PCR to typing of bacteria that exploit diversity of repetitive sequences such as the enterobacterial repetitive intergenic consensus (ERIC-PCR) and repetitive extragenic palindromic sequences (REPS). These approaches have proved valuable for typing *Acinetobacter* spp. and many other Gram-negative species (Vila, 1996). PCR has also been used in combination with restriction endonuclease digestion of whole chromosomal DNA as amplified fragment length polymorphism (AFLP) typing (Ahmed, 2004). In this approach, a subset of the fragments generated by digestion of chromosomal DNA with frequent cutting enzymes are amplified. In the case of *E. coli*, use of fluorescent labeled primers, precise sizing of fragments on an automated DNA sequencer, and the availability of the complete genome sequence for *E. coli* K-12 has resulted in a highly sophisticated typing method (Arnold, 1999). Knowledge of the entire genome sequence of *H. influenzae* strain Rd has similarly been exploited to develop a PCR typing method based on the variable number tandem repeat sequences (VNTRs) (van Belkum, 1997; Mathema, 2004). Spoligotyping of MTBC is another important PCR typing method, which is based on amplification of nonrepetitive spacer sequences located between small repetitive units (Sola, 1998).

PCR is also used to amplify regions of the microbial genome that evolve rapidly so that relatedness may be assessed by evaluation of products for sequence variation. Target sites include the spacer regions between genes for ribosomal RNA in *A. fumigatus* and the coagulase gene of *S. aureus* (Hookey, 1998; Radford, 1998). Sequence variation may be sought by evaluation of banding patterns produced on digestion of the amplified product with restriction enzymes or sequencing of the PCR product. Similar typing methods have proved valuable for typing of viruses. Typing

of HCV is of particular interest, as viral genotype is significant in predicting likely response to interferon-α therapy. HCV genotyping is most frequently based on detection of sequence variation in the conserved 5' untranslated region of the genome by RFLP, hybridization to genotype-specific probes (Line Probe Assay, Innogenetics), by sequencing or by cleavase fragment length polymorphism (Murphy, 1994; Davidson, 1995; Stuyver, 1996; Seme, 1997; Sreevatsan, 1998). The potential for misclassification of some strains where the distinction is based on a single nucleotide difference is recognized, and determination of the sequence in the core region also may be necessary for some subtypes (Seme, 1997). Direct sequencing of the PCR product obtained with the Roche Amplicor kit has been reported and may be a cost-effective approach to determination of HCV genotype (Holland, 1998). Similar approaches are applied to typing of HIV and other viruses (Peltola, 1998).

Plasmid profiles are much less widely used for molecular typing now than formerly, although study of plasmid DNA remains important in defining the epidemiology of dissemination of antimicrobial resistance mechanisms. Study of plasmid profiles in combination with typing based on chromosomal DNA has revealed that in some instances nosocomial spread of antimicrobial resistant strains may reflect simultaneous spread of strains harboring a plasmid and dissemination of a resistance plasmid among distinct strains (Liu, 1998).

Non-DNA-Dependent Molecular Typing

Several non-nucleic-acid-based typing methods have been applied to epidemiologic studies. Polyacrylamide gel electrophoresis (PAGE) of proteins has been applied to many bacteria but is no longer widely used (Mulligan, 1988). Multilocus enzyme electrophoresis (MLEE) is based on the electrophoretic mobility of a number of informative enzymes. Variations in the mobility of the enzymes are the basis of typing. MLEE is technically demanding and can be thought of as a way of examining relationships between organisms on a longer evolutionary time scale than is afforded by visual inspection of banding patterns in many of the DNA-based typing methods. Study of the electrophoretic mobility of the informative enzymes can be replaced by determination of the sequence of amplified fragments from the genes encoding the respective enzymes, a technique known as multilocus sequence typing (Vogel, 1998; Hanage, 2004). With use of computer-assisted analysis of the banding patterns obtained from DNA-based typing methods or of DNA sequence data, degrees of relationship over a longer evolutionary time scale can be defined in a manner similar to MLEE (Bart, 1998; Arnold, 1999; Hanage, 2004).

Standardization, Quality Control, and Proficiency Testing of Molecular Diagnostic Methods

As for all diagnostic pathology, the quality of results begins with the appropriateness of the test request and the quality of the specimen collection and transport. The laboratory must provide clinicians with guidelines as to what types of specimen may be submitted, how they should be collected and stored, and the time frame within which delivery to the laboratory is necessary (see Chs 1 and 63).

In the laboratory, the first step in quality testing is adequate validation of a particular test before it is introduced into diagnostic use, and, when in use, continuing attention must be paid to procedures to maintain quality standards. These issues have been comprehensively addressed in publications from the Association for Molecular Pathology (1999) and the Clinical and Laboratory Standards Institute (formerly National Committee for Clinical Laboratory Standards) (National Committee for Clinical Laboratory Standards, 1995; Clinical and Laboratory Standards Institute, 2003). Problems may occur at many levels. The design of the test may not allow for the full range of genetic diversity of the target taxon (misclassification of HCV subtype 2c as 2b [Seme, 1997]) or overlap of characteristics with related taxa (false-positive for MTBC in patients with pulmonary *M. kansasii* and *M. avium* infection [Jorgensen, 1999]). Problems in design may not be recognized, and performance may be overestimated in evaluations that do not use adequate reference tests (Koumans, 1998). Early reports of poor interlaboratory agreement on testing blinded specimens for MTBC and for HCV by PCR (Zaaijer, 1993; Noordhoek, 1994) suggested operational problems in diagnostic laboratories. In one study, four of 15 laboratories reported one or more false-positive results using in-house PCR for diagnosis of toxoplasmosis (Pelloux, 1998), and similar problems have been reported for detection of enteroviruses (Muir, 1999). The potential to improve interlaboratory agreement by standardization of reagents and protocols is emphasized by a report of much more satisfactory performance of a PCR assay for *C. trachomatis* with attention to these factors (Mahony, 1994), and increased use of commercial systems with standardized reagents and automated analysis has further reduced such problems.

Sample preparation is a critical issue in which a balance is sought between simplicity of preparation (for practicality, and to reduce risks of contamination) and thoroughness (to ensure release of nucleic acids and removal of inhibitory substances). Controls must be in place to detect contamination (e.g., duplicate testing, multiple negative controls) and to monitor for degradation of target or presence of inhibitors (positive control at the limits of detection, internal standard for amplification) (DuBois, 2004). It is essential that negative controls are adequate in number and processed through the specimen preparation procedure. A portion of a previously negative specimen is adequate for this purpose.

Selection of controls and standards is particularly problematic when the target infectious agent is highly diverse (HIV and HCV) and when quantitative results are required (DuBois, 2004). The complexity of these issues is evident in reports of commercial systems for quantification of HCV that may not detect genotypes 2 and 3 as efficiently as genotype 1 (Hawkins, 1997) and in differences in the hybridization efficiency of cloned and virion-derived DNA in assays for quantification of HBV DNA (Heerman, 1999). A detailed evaluation of parameters affecting outcome of assays for HIV RNA quantitation is available and many of the principles identified are generally applicable (Lew, 1998).

To ensure that reagents are of high quality and free of contamination it is convenient to purchase buffers prepared at a remote location. In this case, the manufacturer is responsible for providing data on the analytical quality of the reagents. An assessment of functional quality relative to previous lots may be adequate.

Contamination is a considerable problem for laboratories using diagnostic PCR. Interlaboratory studies have shown that negative samples may give positive results in some laboratories, and carryover of amplicons is the most likely explanation. Clearly, the consequences for patient care of a false-positive report for HCV, HIV, or MTBC are substantial. The foundation of carryover prevention in most laboratories at this point is physical separation of PCR reaction set-up and PCR product analysis areas with a strict unidirectional work flow (Mitchell, 2004). Automation of PCR may also aid in prevention of amplicon carryover (Wilke, 1995), and most of the manufacturers of commercial molecular diagnostic kits have developed, or are in the process of developing, automated or semiauto-mated systems to minimize potential for human error. False-positive results appear to be uncommon with the use of automated commercial test systems (Vincelette, 1999).

In addition to prevention of carryover, methods to prevent amplification of contaminating PCR products are available. The two principal methods are those using isopsoralen to modify amplicons to a nonamplifiable state and those using uracil DNA glycosylase to degrade amplicons before amplification (Rys, 1993). Whichever system is used, the impact of the technique on the limit of PCR detection should be determined. It is also important to demonstrate the effectiveness of the measure given the cost added to the procedure.

Functional checks on each new lot of enzyme is an appropriate check on the production and delivery procedure. For DNA polymerase, comparison with a previous lot of enzyme using specimens at the limit of detection may be appropriate. For restriction endonucleases, digestion of lambda phage DNA is recommended. The reproducibility of results in many molecular techniques is critically dependent on precise control of temperature and accurate reagent dispensing. The first essential of quality assurance is the acquisition of a high-quality instrument. Twice yearly, or more frequent, monitoring of temperature and performance of each well is recommended (Kopp, 1994). Pipettes should be calibrated twice yearly.

Quality laboratory service does not end with the generation of a result. Timely reporting is an essential element. Guidelines on the interpretation of the result are particularly important in relation to novel methods, since clinicians may not be familiar with the limitations of these methods. Guidance to appropriately limit test utilization is important for financial reasons, given the reimbursement issues involved. Only recently has the Health Care Financing Administration assigned payment codes for detection and identification of a limited number of specific pathogens (Association for Molecular Pathology, 1999). Furthermore, the extent to which these tests will be reimbursed is not fully known. Given past performance, it is unlikely that the level of reimbursement will completely cover the costs of testing in all instances.

Participation in proficiency testing programs is obviously an important and required aspect of maintaining quality molecular diagnostic services in the microbiology laboratory (Clinical and Laboratory Standards Institute, 2004; Versalovic, 2004). Proficiency testing for molecular methods used in the detection and identification of infectious agents is available for several different organisms. The College of American Pathologists (CAP) provides testing modules for nucleic acid probe-based detection and identification of *N. gonorrhoeae* and *C. trachomatis* (CAP Survey HC5); identification of cultures of mycobacteria (CAP Survey E); and amplification-based detection of a variety of organisms including HIV, HCV, CMV, MTBC, *C. trachomatis*, *N. gonorrhoeae*, and *Borrelia burgdorferi* (CAP Survey ID).

References

Ahmed N, Alam M, Rao KR, et al: Molecular genotyping of a large, multicentric collection of tubercle bacilli indicates geographical partitioning of strain variation and has implications for global epidemiology of *Mycobacterium tuberculosis*. J Clin Microbiol 2004; 42:3240–3247.

Allardet-Servent A, Bouziges N, Carles-Nurit MJ, et al: Use of low frequency cleavage restriction endonucleases for DNA analysis in epidemiological investigation of nosocomial bacterial infections. J Clin Microbiol 1989; 27:2057–2061.

Alvarez-Barrientos A, Arroyo J, Canton R, et al: Applications of flow cytometry to clinical microbiology. Clin Microbiol Rev 2000; 13:167–195.

Amann R, Ludwig W, Schleifer KH: Identification of uncultured bacteria: a challenging task for molecular taxonomists. ASM News 1994, 60:360–365.

American Thoracic Society Workshop: Rapid diagnostic tests for tuberculosis: what is the appropriate use? Am J Respir Crit Care Med 1997; 155:1804–1814.

Angel S, Maero E, Blanco JC. et al: Early diagnosis of *Toxoplasma* encephalitis in AIDS patients by dot blot hybridization analysis. J Clin Microbiol 1992; 30:3286–3287.

Aono T, Kondo K, Miyoshi H: Monitoring of human cytomegalovirus infections in pediatric bone marrow transplant recipients by nucleic acid sequence-based amplification. J Infect Dis 1998; 178:1244–1249.

Aranda KRS, Fagundes-Neto U, Scaletsky ICA: Evaluation of multiplex PCRs for diagnosis of infection with diarrheagenic *Escherichia coli* and *Shigella* spp. J Clin Microbiol 2004; 42:5849–5853.

Arnold C, Metherell L, Willshaw G, et al: Predictive fluorescent amplified-fragment length polymorphism analysis of *Escherichia coli*: high-resolution typing method with phylogenetic significance. J Clin Microbiol 1999; 37:1274–1279.

Association for Molecular Pathology: Association for Molecular Pathology Statement. Recommendations for in-house development and operation of molecular diagnostic tests. Am J Clin Pathol 1999; 111:449–462.
This is a key document for those laboratories that wish to establish a molecular diagnostic section using 'home brew' assays.

Badak FZ, Goksel S, Sertoz R: Use of nucleic acid probes for identification of *Mycobacterium tuberculosis* directly from MB/BacT bottles. J Clin Microbiol 1999; 37:1602–1605.

Barrett TJ, Ribot E, Swaminathan B: Molecular subtyping for epidemiology: issues in comparability of patterns and interpretation of data. *In* Persing DH, Tenover FC, Versalovic J, et al (eds): Molecular Microbiology: Diagnostic Principles and Practice, Washington, DC, ASM Press, 2004, pp 259–266.

Barrett-Muir WY, Aitken C, Templeton K, et al: Evaluation of the Murex hybrid capture cytomegalovirus DNA assay versus plasma PCR and shell vial assay for diagnosis of human cytomegalovirus viremia in immunocompromised patients. J Clin Microbiol 1998; 36:2554–2556.

Bart A, Schuurman IGA, Achtman M, et al: Randomly amplified polymorphic DNA genotyping of serogroup A meningococci yields results similar to those obtained by multilocus enzyme electrophoresis and reveals new genotypes. J Clin Microbiol 1998; 36:1746–1749.

Beggs ML, Cave MD, Marlowe C, et al: Characterization of *Mycobacterium tuberculosis* complex direct repeat sequence for use in cycling probe reaction. J Clin Microbiol 1996; 34:2985–2989.

Bekkaoui F, McNevin JP, Leung CH, et al: Rapid detection of the *mec*A gene in methicillin resistant staphylococci using a colorimetric cycling probe technology. Diagn Microbiol Infect Dis 1999; 34:83–90.

Belgrader P, Bennett W, Hadley D: Rapid pathogen detection using a microchip PCR array instrument. Clin Chem 1998; 44:2191–2194.

Bergeron MG, Ouellette M: Preventing antibiotic resistance through rapid genotypic identification of bacteria and of their antibiotic resistance genes in the clinical microbiology laboratory. J Clin Microbiol 1998; 36:2169–2172.

Bingen EH, Denamur E, Lambert-Zechovsky NY, Elion J: Evidence for the genetic unrelatedness or nosocomial vancomycin resistant *Enterococcus faecium* strains in a pediatric hospital. J Clin Microbiol 1991; 29:1888–1892.

Blok MJ, Lautenschlager I, Goossens VJ, et al: Diagnostic implications of human cytomegalovirus immediate early-1 and pp67 mRNA detection in whole-blood samples from liver transplant patients using nucleic acid sequence-based amplification. J Clin Microbiol 2000; 38:4485–4491.

Bode E, Hurtle W, Norwood D: Real-time PCR assay for a unique chromosomal sequence of *Bacillus anthracis*. J Clin Microbiol 2004, 42:5825–5831.

VII

Boeckh M, Boivin G: Quantitation of cytomegalovirus: methodologic aspects and clinical application. Clin Microbiol Rev 1998; 11:533–554.

Bootman J, Heath AB, Hughes P, Holmes H: An international collaborative study on the detection of an HIV-1 genotype B field isolate by nucleic acid amplification techniques. J Virol Methods 1999; 78:21–34.

Boriskin YS, Rice PS, Stabler RA, et al: DNA microarrays for virus detection in cases of central nervous system infection. J Clin Microbiol 2004; 42:5811–5818.

Bougnoux M, Dupont C, Mateo J: Serum is more suitable than whole blood for diagnosis of systemic candidiasis by nested PCR. J Clin Microbiol 1999; 37:925–930.

Bradford WZ, Koehler J, El-Hajj H: Dissemination of Mycobacterium tuberculosis across the San Francisco bay area. J Infect Dis 1998; 177:1104–1107.

Brown TJ, Power EGM, French GL: Evaluation of three commercial detection systems for Mycobacterium tuberculosis where clinical diagnosis is difficult. J Clin Pathol 1999; 52:193–197.

Bryant PA, Li HY, Zaia A, et al: Prospective study of a real-time PCR that is highly sensitive, specific, and clinically useful for diagnosis of meningococcal disease in children. J Clin Microbiol 2004; 42:2919–2925.

Caliendo AM, St George K, Kao SY, et al: Comparison of quantitative cytomegalovirus (CMV) PCR in plasma and CMV antigenemia assay: clinical utility of prototype Amplicor CMV Monitor test int ransplant recipients. J Clin Microbiol 2000; 38:2122–2127.

Caliendo AM, Yen-Lieberman B: Viral genotyping. In Persing DH, Tenover FC, Versalovic J, et al (eds). Molecular Microbiology: Diagnostic Principles and Practice, Washington, DC, ASM Press, 2004, pp 489–499.

Cantanzaro A, Perry S, Clarridge JE, et al: The role of clinical suspicion in evaluating a new diagnostic test for active tuberculosis: results of a multicenter prospective trial. JAMA 2000; 283:639–645.

An excellent discussion of key considerations when establishing molecular infectious disease testing services.

Carpentier E, Drouillard B, Dailloux M, et al: Diagnosis of tuberculosis by Amplicor Mycobacterium tuberculosis test: a multicenter study. J Clin Microbiol 1995; 33:3106–3110.

Cascio A, Calattini S, Colomba C, et al: Polymerase chain reaction in the diagnosis and prognosis of Mediterranean visceral leishmaniasis in immunocompetent children. Pediatrics 2002; 109:E27.

Chandrasekar PH: Real-time polymerase chain reaction for early diagnosis of toxoplasmosis in stem cell transplant recipients: ready for prime time? Clin Infect Dis 2005; 40:79–81.

Chapin K, Musgnug M: Evaluation of three rapid methods for the direct identification of Staphylococcus aureus from positive blood cultures. J Clin Microbiol 2003; 41:4324–4327.

Chemaly RF, Procop GW: Molecular detection and characterization of fungal pathogens. In Persing DH, Tenover FC, Versalovic J, et al (eds). Molecular Microbiology: Diagnostic Principles and Practice, Washington, DC, ASM Press, 2004, pp 551–559.

Ciceron L, Jaureguiberry G, Gay F, Danis M: Development of a Plasmodium PCR for monitoring efficacy of antimalarial treatment. J Clin Microbiol 1999; 37:35–38.

Clarridge JE III: Impact of 16S rRNA gene sequence analysis for identification of bacteria on clinical microbiology and infectious diseases. Clin Microbiol Rev 2004; 17:840–862.

State-of-the-art review of advantages and disadvantages of using gene sequencing to identify bacteria.

Cleary TJ, Roudel G, Casillas O, Miller N: Rapid and specific detection of Mycobacterium tuberculosis by using the Smart Cycler instrument and a specific fluorogenic probe. J Clin Microbiol 2003; 41:4783–4786.

Clinical and Laboratory Standards Institute: Quantitative molecular methods for infectious diseases. Approved Guideline. Wayne, PA, Clinical and Laboratory Standards Institute, 2003, MM6-A.

Clinical and Laboratory Standards Institute: Proficiency testing for molecular methods. Proposed Guideline. Wayne, PA, Clinical and Laboratory Standards Institute, 2004, MM14-P.

Cloud JL, Shutt C, Aldous W, Woods G: Evaluation of a modified Gen-Probe Amplified Direct Test for detection of Mycobacterium tuberculosis complex organism in cerebrospinal fluid. J Clin Microbiol 2004; 42:5341–5344.

Cockerill FR III: Genetic methods for assessing antimicrobial resistance. Antimicrob Agents Chemother 1999; 43:199–212.

Cockerill FR III, Smith TF: Response of the clinical microbiology laboratory to emerging (new) and reemerging infectious diseases. J Clin Microbiol 2004; 42:2359–2365.

Cope JU, Hildesheim A, Schiffman MH: Comparison of the hybrid capture tube test and PCR for detection of human papillomavirus DNA in cervical specimens. J Clin Microbiol 1997; 35:2262–2265.

Cormican M, Glennon M, NiRiain U, Flynn J: Multiplex PCR for identification of mycobacterial isolates. J Clin Pathol 1995; 48:203–205.

Cormican MG, Hollis RJ, Pfaller MA: DNA macrorestriction profiles and antifungal susceptibility of Candida (Torulopsis) glabrata. Diagn Microbiol Infect Dis 1996; 25:83–87.

Costa JM, Ernault P, Gautier E, Bretagne S: Prenatal diagnosis of congenital toxoplasmosis by duplex real-time PCR using fluorescence resonance energy transfer hybridization probes. Prenatal Diagn 2001; 21:85–88.

Cullen AP, Long CD, Lorincz AT: Rapid detection and typing of herpes simplex virus DNA in clinical specimens by the hybrid capture II signal amplification probe test. J Clin Microbiol 1997; 35:2275–2278.

Davidson FP, Simmonds JC, Ferguson LM: Survey of major genotypes and subtypes of hepatitis C virus using RFLP of sequences amplified from the 5′ non-coding region. J Gen Virol 1995; 76:1197–1204.

Davis TE, Fuller DD: Direct identification of bacterial isolates in blood cultures by using a DNA probe. J Clin Microbiol 1991; 29:2193–2196.

Devallois A, Goh KS, Rastogi N: Rapid identification of mycobacteria to species level by PCR-restriction fragment length polymorphism analysis of the hsp65 gene and proposition of an algorithm to differentiate 34 mycobacterial species. J Clin Microbiol 1997; 35:2969–2973.

Diaz-Mitoma F, Leger C, Miller H, et al: Comparison of DNA amplification, mRNA amplification, and DNA hybridization techniques for detection of cytomegalovirus in bone marrow transplant recipients. J Clin Microbiol 2003; 41:5159–5166.

Diekema DJ, Dodgson KJ, Sigurdardotter B, Pfaller MA: Rapid detection of antimicrobial-resistant organism carriage: an unmet clinical need. J Clin Microbiol 2004; 42:2879–2883.

A minireview discussing the potential (and real) benefits of 'real-time' detection of resistance genes in bacteria and in clinical specimens.

Diekema DJ, Pfaller MA: Infection control epidemiology and clinical microbiology. In Murray PR, Baron EJ, Jorgensen JH, et al (eds), Manual of Clinical Microbiology, 8th ed. Washington, DC, ASM Press, 2003, pp 129–138.

Dowdy DW, Maters A, Parrish N, et al: Cost-effectiveness analysis of the Gen-Probe Amplified Mycobacterium Tuberculosis Direct Test as used routinely on smear-positive respiratory specimens. J Clin Microbiol 2003; 41:948–953.

Drosten C, Doerr HW, Lim W, et al: SARS molecular detection external quality assurance. Emerg Infect Dis 2004; 10:2200–2203.

DuBois DB, Brown JT: Laboratory controls and standards. In Persing DH, Tenover FC, Versalovic J, et al (eds). Molecular Microbiology: Diagnostic Principles and Practice, Washington, DC, ASM Press, 2004, pp 697–703.

Elnifro EM, Ashshi AM, Cooper RJ, Klapper PE: Multiplex PCR: Optimization and application in diagnostic virology. Clin Microbiol Rev 2000; 13:559–570.

Erali M, Hillyard DR: Evaluation of the ultrasensitive Roche Amplicor HIV-1 monitor assay for quantitation of human immunodeficiency virus type 1 RNA. J Clin Microbiol 1999; 37:792–795.

Farrell DJ: Evaluation of Amplicor Neisseria gonorrhoeae PCR using cppB nested PCR and 16S rRNA PCR. J Clin Microbiol 1999a; 37:386–390.

Farrell DJ, Daggard G, Mukkur TK: Nested duplex PCR to detect Bordetella pertussis and Bordetella parapertussis and its applications in diagnosis of pertussis in nonmetropolitan Southeast Queensland, Australia. J Clin Microbiol 1999b; 37:606–610.

Faulkner-Jones BE, Tabrizi SN, Borg AJ: Detection of human papillomavirus DNA and mRNA using synthetic, type specific oligonucleotide probes. J Virol Methods 1993; 41:277–296.

Fiebelkorn KR, Nolte FS: RNA virus detection. In Persing DH, Tenover FC, Versalovic J, et al (eds). Molecular Microbiology: Diagnostic Principles and Practice, Washington, DC, ASM Press, 2004, pp 441–474.

Fischer M, Huber W, Kallivroussis A: Highly sensitive methods for quantitation of human immunodeficiency virus type 1 RNA from plasma, cells and tissues. J Clin Microbiol 1999; 37:1260–1264.

Fluit AD, Visser MR, Schmitz F-J: Molecular detection of antimicrobial resistance. Clin Microbiol Rev 2001; 14:836–871.

A more in depth review of methods for determining antimicrobial resistance genotypes.

Frade JP, Warnock DW, Arthington-Skaggs BA: Rapid quantification of drug resistance gene expression in Candida albicans by reverse transcriptase LightCycler PCR and fluorescent probe hybridization. J Clin Microbiol 2004; 42:2085–2093.

Franzen C, Muller A: Molecular techniques for detection, species differentiation, and phylogenetic analysis of microsporidia. Clin Microbiol Rev 1999; 12:243–285.

Fredericks DN, Relman DA: Sequence based identification of microbial pathogens: a reconsideration of Koch's postulates. Clin Microbiol Rev 1996; 9:18–33.

Fridkin SK, Yokoe DS, Whitney CG, et al: Epidemiology of a dominant clonal strain of vancomycin-resistant Enterococcus faecium at separate hospitals in Boston, Massachusetts. J Clin Microbiol 1998; 36:965–970.

Garcia de Viedma D, Alonso R, Miralles P, et al: Dual qualitative-quantitative nested PCR for detection of JC virus in cerebrospinal fluid: high potential for evaluation and monitoring of progressive multifocal leukoencephalopathy in AIDS patients receiving highly active antiretroviral therapy. J Clin Microbiol 1999; 37:724–728.

Garcia-Lerma JG, Yamamoto S, Gomez-Cano M: Measurement of human immunodeficiency virus type-1 plasma virus load based on reverse transcriptase (RT) activity: evidence of variabilities in levels of virion-associated RT. J Infect Dis 1998; 177:1221–1229.

Gerna G, Furione M, Baldanti F, Sarasini A: Comparative quantitation of human cytomegalovirus DNA in blood leukocytes and plasma of transplant and AIDS patients. J Clin Microbiol 1994; 32:2709–2717.

Gerner-Smidt P, Graves LM, Hunter S, Swaminathan B: Computerized analysis of restriction fragment length polymorphism patterns: comparative evaluation of two commercial software packages. J Clin Microbiol 1998; 36:1318–1323.

Ghosh S, Debnath A, Sil A, et al: PCR detection of Giardia lamblia in stool: targeting intergenic spacer region of multicopy rRNA gene. Mol Cell Probes 2000; 14:181–189.

Goering RV: Pulsed-field gel electrophoresis. *In* Persing DH, Tenover FC, Versalovic J, et al (eds). Molecular Microbiology: Diagnostic Principles and Practice, Washington, DC, ASM Press, 2004, pp 185–196.

Goldenberger D, Kunzli A, Vogt P, et al: Molecular diagnosis of bacterial endocarditis by broad-range PCR amplification and direct sequencing. J Clin Microbiol 1997; 35:2733–2739.

Goto M, Oka S, Okuzumi K, et al: Evaluation of acridinium ester labeled DNA probes for identification of *Mycobacterium tuberculosis* and *Mycobacterium avium-Mycobacterium intracellulare* complex in culture. J Clin Microbiol 1991; 29:2473–2476.

Gratzl R, Hayde M, Kohlhauser C: Follow-up of infants with congenital toxoplasmosis detected by polymerase chain reaction analysis of amniotic fluid. Eur J Clin Microbiol Infect Dis 1998; 17:853–858.

Grif K, Karch H, Schneider C: Comparative study of five different techniques for epidemiological typing of *Escherichia coli* O157. Diagn Microbiol Infect Dis 1998; 32:165–176.

Griffith BP, Rigsby MO, Garner RB, et al: Comparison of Amplicor HIV-1 monitor test and the nucleic acid sequence-based amplification assay for quantitation of human immunodeficiency virus RNA in plasma, serum and plasma subjected to freeze–thaw cycles. J Clin Microbiol 1997; 35:3288–3291.

Grimm V, Ezaki S, Susa M, et al: Use of DNA microarrays for rapid genotyping of TEM beta-lactamases that confer resistance. J Clin Microbiol 2004; 42:3766–3774.

Grondahl B, Puppe W, Hoppe A, et al: Rapid identification of nine microorganisms causing acute respiratory tract infections by a single tube multiplex reverse transcription-PCR: feasibility study. J Clin Microbiol 1999; 37:1–7.

Gruteke P, Glas AS, Dierdorp M, et al: Practical implementation of a multiplex PCR for acute respiratory tract infections in children. J Clin Microbiol 2004; 42:5592–5603.

Hacek DM, Suriano T, Noskin GA, et al: Medical and economic benefit of a comprehensive infection control program that includes routine determination of microbial clonality. Am J Clin Pathol 1999; 111:647–654.

Hadgu A: The discrepancy in discrepant analysis. Lancet 1996; 348:592–593.

Hall GS, Katanik M, Tuohy M, Sholtis M: Use of commercial amplification tests in the clinical microbiology laboratory: test selection and quality assurance. *In* Persing DH, Tenover FC, Versalovic J, et al (eds). Molecular Microbiology: Diagnostic Principles and Practice, Washington, DC, ASM Press, 2004a, pp 27–36.

Hall L, Doerr KA, Wohlfiel SL, Roberts GD: Evaluation of the MicroSeq system for identification of mycobacteria by 16S ribosomal DNA sequencing and its integration into a routine clinical mycobacteriology laboratory. J Clin Microbiol 2003a; 41:1447–1453.

Hall L, Wohlfiel S, Roberts GD: Experience with the MicroSeq D2 large-subuit riobosmal DNA sequencing kit for identification of commonly encountered, clinically important yeast species. J Clin Microbiol 2003b; 41:5099–5102.

Hall L, Wohlfiel S, Roberts GD: Experince with the MicroSeq D2 large-subunit ribosomal DNA sequencing kit identification of filamentous fungi encountered in the clinical laboratory. J Clin Microbiol 2004b; 42:622–626.

Hanage WP, Feil EJ, Brueggemann AB, Spratt BG: Mutilocus sequence typing: a strain characterization, population biology, and patterns of evolutionary descent. *In* Persing DH, Tenover FC, Versalovic J, et al (eds). Molecular Microbiology: Diagnostic Principles and Practice, Washington, DC, ASM Press, 2004, pp 235–243.

Haque R, Ali IK, Akther S, Petri WA Jr: Comparison of PCR, isoenzyme analysis, and antigen detection for diagnosis of *Entamoeba histolytica* infection. J Clin Microbiol 1998; 36:449–452.

Hawkins A, Davidson F, Simmonds P: Comparison of plasma virus loads among individuals infected with hepatitis C virus (HCV) genotypes 1, 2, and 3 by quantiplex HCV RNA assay and versions 1 and 2, Roche Monitor assay and an in house limiting dilution method. J Clin Microbiol 1997; 35:187–192.

Hayden RT: In vitro nucleic acid amplification techniques. *In* Persing DH, Tenover FC, Versalovic J, et al (eds). Molecular Microbiology: Diagnostic Principles and Practice, Washington, DC, ASM Press, 2004, pp 43–69.

Hayden RT, Qian X, Procop GD, et al: In situ hybridization for the identification of filamentous fungi in tissue section. Diagn Mol Pathol 2002; 11:119–126.

Hayden RT, Qian X, Roberts GD, Lloyd RV: In situ hybridization for the identification of yeast-like organisms in tissue section. Diagn Mol Pathol 2001a; 10:15–23.

Hayden RT, Uhl JR, Qian X, et al: Direct detection of *Legionella* species from bronchoalveolar lavage and open lung biopsy specimens: comparison of LightCycler PCR, in situ hybridization, direct fluorescence antigen detection, and culture. J Clin Microbiol 2001b; 39:2618–2626.

Hazelton PR, Gelderblom HR: Electron microscopy for rapid diagnosis of infectious agents in emergent situations. Emerg Infect Dis 2003; 9:294–303.

Heerman KH, Gerlich WH, Chudy M, et al, and the Eurohep Pathobiology Group: Quantitative detection of Hepatitis B virus DNA in two international reference plasma preparations. J Clin Microbiol 1999; 37:68–73.

Hilton AC, Penn CW: Comparison of ribotyping and arbitrarily primed PCR for molecular typing of *Salmonella enterica* and relationships between strains on the basis of these molecular markers. J Appl Microbiol 1998; 85:933–940.

Hogardt M, Trebesius K, Geiger AM, et al: Specific and rapid detection by fluorescent in situ hybridization of bacteria in clinical samples obtained from cystic fibrosis patients. J Clin Microbiol 2000; 38:818–825.

Holland J, Bastian I, Ratcliff RM: Hepatitis C genotyping by direct sequencing of the product from the Roche Amplicor test: methodology and application to a South Australian population. Pathology 1998; 30:192–195.

Hookey JV, Richardson JF, Cookson BD: Molecular typing of *Staphylococcus aureus* based on PCR restriction fragment length polymorphism and DNA sequence analysis of the coagulase gene. J Clin Microbiol 1998; 36:1083–1089.

Houpikian P, Raoult D: Traditional and molecular techniques for the study of emerging bacterial diseases: one laboratory's perspective. Emerg Infect Dis 2002; 8:122–131.
An excellent overview of the 'blending' of new and old technologies in a modern diagnostic microbiology laboratory.

Hutter B, Schaab C, Albrecht S, et al: Prediction of mechanisms of action of antibacterial compounds by gene expressing profiling. Antimicrob Agents Chemother 2004; 48:2838–2844.

Ieven M, Goossens H: Relevance of nucleic acid amplification techniques for diagnosis of respiratory tract infections in the clinical laboratory. Clin Microbiol Rev 1997; 10:242–256.

Ieven M, Loens K, Goossens H: Detection and characterization of bacterial pathogens by nucleic acid amplification: state-of-the-Art review. *In* Persing DH, Tenover FC, Versalovic J, et al (eds). Molecular Microbiology: Diagnostic Principles and Practice, Washington, DC, ASM Press, 2004, pp 323–348.

Iwen PC, Hinrichs SH, Rupp ME: Utilization of the internal transcribed spacer regions as molecular targets to detect and identify human fungal pathogens. Med Mycol 2002; 40:87–109.

Jabs WJ, Hennig H, Kittel M, et al: Normalized quantification by real-time PCR of Epstein–Barr virus load in patients at risk for past transplant lymphoproliferative disorders. J Clin Microbiol 2001; 39:564–569.

Jacob S, Baudy D, Jones E: Comparison of quantitative HCV RNA assays in chronic hepatitis C. Am J Clin Pathol 1997; 107:362–367.

Jansen GJ, Mooibroek M, Idema J, et al: Rapid identification of bacteria in blood cultures by using fluorescently labelled oligonucleotide probes. J Clin Microbiol 2000; 38:814–817.

Jones RN, Marshall SA, Pfaller MA: Nosocomial enterococcal blood stream infections in the SCOPE program: antimicrobial resistance, species occurrence, molecular testing results and laboratory testing accuracy. Diagn Microbiol Infect Dis 1997; 29:95–102.

Jordan J, Tiangco B, Kiss J, Koch W: Human parvovirus B19; prevalence of viral DNA in volunteer blood donors and clinical outcomes of transfusion recipients. Vox Sang 1998; 75:97–102.

Jorgensen JH, Salinas JR, Paxson R, et al: False-positive Gen-Probe direct *Mycobacterium tuberculosis* amplification test results for patients with pulmonary *M. kansasii* and *M. avium* infections. J Clin Microbiol 1999, 37:175–178.

Julander I, Martin C, Lappalainen M, et al: Polymerase chain reaction for diagnosis of cerebral toxoplasmosis in cerebrospinal fluid in HIV-positive patients. Scand J Infect Dis 2001; 33:538–541.

Juretschko S, Buccat AM, Fritsche TR: Applications of fluorescence in situ hybridization in diagnostic microbiology. *In* Persing DH, Tenover FC, Versalovic J, et al (eds). Molecular Microbiology: Diagnostic Principles and Practice, Washington, DC, ASM Press, 2004, pp 3–18.

Kant JA: Molecular diagnostics, reimbursement and other selected financial issues. Diagn Mol Pathol 1995; 4:79–81.

Karababa M, Coste AT, Rognon B, et al: Comparison of gene expression profiles of *Candida albicans* azole-resistant clinical isolates and laboratory strains exposed to drugs inducing multidrug transporters. Antimicrob Agents Chemother 2004; 48:3064–3079.

Katakura K, Kawazu S, Naya T: Diagnosis of kala-azar by nested PCR based on amplification of the *Leishmania* mini-exon gene. J Clin Microbiol 1998; 36:2173–2177.

Kawazu M, Kanda Y, Nannya Y, et al: Prospective comparison of the diagnostic potential of real-time PCR, double-sandwich enzyme-linked immunosorbent assay for galactomannan, and a (1–3)-β-D-glucan test in weekly screening for invasive aspergillosis in patients with hematological disorders. J Clin Microbiol 2004; 42:2733–2741.

Kehl SC, Georgakas K, Swain GR: Evaluation of Abbott LCx assay for detection of *Neisseria gonorrhoeae* in endocervical swab specimens from females. J Clin Microbiol 1998; 36:3549–3551.

Kempf VAJ, Trebesius K, Autenrieth IB: Fluorescent in situ hybridization allows rapid identification of microorganisms in blood cultures. J Clin Microbiol 2000; 38:830–838.

Kimura H, Morita M, Yabuta Y: Quantitative analysis of Epstein–Barr virus load by using a real-time PCR assay. J Clin Microbiol 1999; 37:132–136.

Kivihya-Ndugga L, van Cleeff M, Juma E, et al: Comparison of PCR with the routine procedure for diagnosis of tuberculosis in a population with high prevalences of tuberculosis and human immunodeficiency virus. J Clin Microbiol 2004; 42:1012–1015.

Kleiber J, Walter T, Habershausen G, et al: Performance characteristics of a quantitative, homogeneous TaqMan RT-PCR test for HCV RNA. J Mol Diagn 2000; 2:158–166.

Klein RS, El Khoury J: Emerging viral pathogens. *In* Persing DH, Tenover FC, Versalovic J, et al (eds). Molecular Microbiology: Diagnostic Principles and Practice, Washington, DC, ASM Press, 2004, pp 529–542.

VII

Koenig MG, Kosha SL, Doty BL, Heath DG: Direct comparison of the BD ProbeTec ET System with in-house LightCycler PCR assays for detection of *Chlamydia trachomatis* and *Neisserria gonorrhoeae* from clinical specimens. J Clin Microbiol 2004; 42:5751–5756.

Kolbert CP, Arruda J, Varga-Delmore P: Branched-DNA assay for detection of the *mecA* gene in oxacillin-resistant and oxacillin-sensitive staphylococci. J Clin Microbiol 1998; 36:2640–2644.

Kolbert CP, Rys PN, Hopkins M, et al: 16S ribosomal DNA sequence in analysis for identification of bacteria in a clinical microbiology laboratory. *In* Persing DH, Tenover FC, Versalovic J, et al (eds). Molecular Microbiology: Diagnostic Principles and Practice, Washington, DC, ASM Press, 2004, pp 361–378.

Kopp DW, Sansieri CA, Mifflin TE: Routine monitoring of temperatures inside thermal cycler blocks for quality control. Clin Chem 1994, 40:2117–2119.

Koumans EH, Johnson RE, Knapp JS, St. Louis ME: Laboratory testing for *Neisseria gonorrhoeae* by recently introduced nonculture tests; a performance review with clinical and public health considerations. Clin Infect Dis 1998; 27:1171–1180.

Krause PJ, Telford D III, Spielman A: Comparison of PCR with blood smear and inoculation of small animals for diagnosis of *Babesia microti* parasitemia. J Clin Microbiol 1996; 34:2791–2794.

Kulski J, Khinsoe C, Payle T, Christiansen K: Use of a multiplex PCR to detect and identify *Mycobacterium avium* and *M. intracellulare* in blood culture fluids in AIDS patients. J Clin Microbiol 1995, 33:668–674.

Lachnik J, Ackermann B, Bohrssen A, et al: Rapid-cycle PCR and fluorimetry for detection of mycobacteria. J Clin Microbiol 2002; 40:3364–3373.

Landry ML, Garner R, Ferguson D: Comparison of the NucliSens Basic Kit (nucleic acid sequence-based amplification) and the Argene Biosoft Enterovirus Consensus Reverse Transcription-PCR assays for rapid detection of enterovirus RNA in clinical specimens. J Clin Microbiol 2003; 41:5006–5010.

Latge JP: *Aspergillus fumigatus* and aspergillosis. Clin Microbiol Rev 1999; 12:310–350.

Ledergerber B, Egger M, Opravil M: Clinical progression and virological failure on highly active antiretroviral therapy in HIV-1 patients: A prospective cohort study. Lancet 1999; 353:863–868.

Lemaitre N, Armand S, Vachee A, et al: Comparison of the real-time PCR method and the Gen-Probe Amplified *Mycobacterium tuberculosis* Direct Test for detection of *Mycobacterium tuberculosis* in pulmonary and nonpulmonary specimens. J Clin Microbiol 2004; 42:4307–4309.

Lew J, Reichelderfer P, Fowler M: Determination of levels of human immunodeficiency virus type 1 RNA in plasma: Reassessment of parameters affecting assay outcome. J Clin Microbiol 1998; 36:1471–1479.

Li J, Hanna BA: DNA probes for culture confirmation and direct detection of bacterial infections: a review of technology. *In* Persing DH, Tenover FC, Versalovic J, et al (eds). Molecular Microbiology: Diagnostic Principles and Practice, Washington, DC, ASM Press, 2004, pp 19–26.

Lin MT, Lu HC, Chen WL: Improving efficacy of antifungal therapy by polymerase chain reaction-based strategy among febrile patients with neutropenia and cancer. Clin Infect Dis 2001a; 33:1621–1627.

Lin S, Schranz J, Teutsch S: Aspergillosis case-fatality rate: systematic review of the literature. Clin Infect Dis 2001b; 32:358–366.

Lindholm L, Sarkkinen H: Direct identification of gram-positive cocci from routine blood cultures by using AccuProbe tests. J Clin Microbiol 2004; 42:5609–5613.

Liu PYF, Tung JC, Ke SC, Chen SL: Molecular epidemiology of extended spectrum β-lactamase-producing *Klebsiella pneumoniae* isolates in a district hospital in Taiwan. J Clin Microbiol 1998; 36:2759–2762.

Long CM, Drew L, Miner R, et al: Detection of cytomegalovirus in plasma and cerebrospinal fluid specimens from human immunodeficiency virus infected patients by the Amplicor CMV test. J Clin Microbiol 1998; 36:2434–2438.

Lorinez AT: Diagnosis of human papillomavirus infection by the new generation of molecular DNA assays. Clin Immunol Newslett 1992, 12:8.

Lu RH, Hwang SJ, Chan CY, et al: Quantitative measurement of serum HCV RNA in patients with chronic hepatitis C: comparison between Amplicor HCV monitor system and branched DNA signal amplification assay. J Clin Lab Anal 1998; 12:121–125.

Lumb R, Davies K, Dawson D, et al: Multicenter evaluation of the Abbott LCx *Mycobacterium tuberculosis* ligase chain reaction assay. J Clin Microbiol 1999; 37:3102–3107.

Lunel F, Cresta P, Vitour D: Comparative evaluation of hepatitis C virus RNA quantitation by branched DNA, NASBA and monitor assays. Hepatology 1999; 29:528–535.

Mahony JB, Luinstra KE, Waner J, et al: Interlaboratory agreement study of a double set of PCR plasmid primers for detection of *Chlamydia trachomatis* in a variety of genitourinary specimens. J Clin Microbiol 1994; 32:87–91.

Maiwald M: Broad-range PCR for detection and identification of bacteria. *In* Persing DH, Tenover FC, Versalovic J, et al (eds). Molecular Microbiology: Diagnostic Principles and Practice, Washington, DC, ASM Press, 2004, pp pp 379–390.

Marr KA, Carter RA, Crippa F, et al: Epidemiology and outcome of mould infections in hematopoetic stem cell transplant recipients. Clin Infect Dis 2002; 34:909–917.

Marshall A, Hodgson J: DNA chips: An array of possibilities. Nature Biotechnol 1998; 16:27–31

Marshall SA, Wilke WW, Pfaller MA, Jones RN: *Staphylococcus aureus* and coagulase negative staphylococci from blood stream infections: frequency of occurrence, antimicrobial susceptibility and molecular (mecA) characterization of oxacillin resistance in the SCOPE program. Diagn Microbiol Infect Dis 1997; 30:205–214.

Martel M, Gomez J, Esteban JL: High-throughput real-time reverse transcription-PCR quantitation of hepatitis C virus RNA. J Clin Microbiol 1999; 37:327–332.

Martino R, Bretagne S, Einsele H, et al: Early detection of *Toxoplasma* infection by molecular monitoring of *Toxoplasma gondii* in peripheral blood samples after allogeneic stem cell transplantation. Clin Infect Dis 2005; 40:67–78.

Martinot-Peignoux M, Boyer N, Pouteau M: Predictors of sustained response to alpha interferon therapy in chronic hepatitis C. J Hepatol 1998; 29:214–223.

Mathema B, Kreisworth BN: Genotyping bacteria by using variable-number tandem repeats. *In* Persing DH, Tenover FC, Versalovic J, et al (eds). Molecular Microbiology: Diagnostic Principles and Practice, Washington, DC, ASM Press, 2004, pp 223–233.

Matushek MG, Bonten MJM, Hayden MK: Rapid preparation of bacterial DNA for pulsed-field gel electrophoresis. J Clin Microbiol 1996; 34:2598–2600.

Maurmann S, Fricke L, Wagner H-J, et al: Molecular parameters for precise diagnosis of asymptomatic Epstein–Barr virus reactivation in healthy carriers. J Clin Microbiol 2003; 41:5419–5428.

Mazzulli T, Drew LW, Yen-Lieberman B, et al: Multicenter comparison of the Digene Hybrid Capture CMV DNA Assay (Version 2.0), the pp65 antigenemia assay, and cell culture for detection of cytomegalovirus viremia. J Clin Microbiol 1999; 37:958–963.

Mezzasoma L, Bacarese-Hamilton T, DiCristina M, et al: Antigen microaarrays for serodiangosis of infectious diseases. Clin Chem 2002; 48:121–130.

Miller WC: Can we do better than discrepant analysis for new diagnostic test evaluation? Clin Infect Dis 1998; 27:1186–1193.

Mitchell PS, Germer JJ, Patel R: Nucleic acid amplification methods: laboratory design and operations. *In* Persing DH, Tenover FC, Versalovic J, et al (eds). Molecular Microbiology: Diagnostic Principles and Practice, Washington, DC, ASM Press, 2004, pp 85–93.

Modrusan Z, Marlowe C, Wheeler D, et al: Detection of vancomycin resistant genes *vanA* and *vanB* by cycling probe technology. Mol Cell Probes 1999; 13:223–231.

Moody A: Rapid diagnostic tests for malaria parasites. Clin Microbiol Rev 2002; 15:66–78.

Morgan UM, Pallant L, Dwyer BW, et al: Comparison of PCR and microscopy for detection of *Cryptosporidium parvum* in human fecal specimens: Clinical trial. J Clin Microbiol 1998; 36:995–998.

Morre SA, Sillekens PT, Jacobs M: Monitoring of *Chlamydia trachomatis* infections after antibiotic treatment using RNA detection by nucleic acid sequence based amplification. Mol Pathol 1998; 51:149–154.

Muir P, Ras A, Klaper PE: Multicenter quality assessment of PCR methods for detection of enteroviruses. J Clin Microbiol 1999; 37:1409–1414.

Mulligan ME, Peterson LE, Kwok RYY, et al: Immunoblots and plasmid fingerprints compared with serotyping and polyacrylamide gel electrophoresis for typing *Clostridium difficile*. J Clin Microbiol 1988; 26:41–46.

Murphy DG, Cote L, Fauvel M, et al: Multicenter comparison of Roche COBAS AMPLICOR MONITOR version 1.5, Organon Teknika NucliSens QT with Extractor, and Bayer Quantiplex version 3.0 for quantification of human immunodeficiency virus type 1 RNA in plasma. J Clin Microbiol 2000; 38:4034–4041.

Murphy D, Gonin P, Fauvel M: Reproducibility and performance of the second-generation branched-DNA assay in routine quantification of human immunodeficiency virus type 1 RNA in plasma. J Clin Microbiol 1999; 37:812–814.

Murphy D, Willems B, Delage G: Use of the 5' noncoding region for genotyping hepatitis C virus. J Infect Dis 1994; 169:473–475.

Musher B, Fredricks D, Leisenring W, et al: *Aspergillus* galactomannan enzyme immunoassay and quantitative PCR for diagnosis of invasive aspergillosis with bronchoalveolar lavage fluid. J Clin Microbiol 2004; 42:5517–5522.

National Committee for Clinical Laboratory Standards: Molecular diagnostic methods for infectious disease. Approved Guideline. Villanova, PA, National Committee for Clinical Laboratory Standards, 1995, MM3-A.

Niemann S, Richter E, Rusch-Gerdes S: Stability of *Mycobacterium tuberculosis* IS6110 restriction fragment length polymorphism patterns and spoligotypes determined by analyzing serial isolates from patients with drug-resistant tuberculosis. J Clin Microbial 1999; 37:409–412.

Ninet B, Rohner P, Metral C, Auckenthaler R: Assessment of use of the COBAS Amplicor system with BACTEC 12B cultures for rapid detection of frequently identified mycobacteria. J Clin Microbiol 1999; 37:782–784.

NiRiain U, Cormican M, Flynn J, et al: PCR based fingerprinting of *Enterobacter cloacae*. J Hosp Infect 1994; 27:237–240.

Noordhoek GT, Kolk AHJ, Bjune G: Sensitivity and specificity of PCR for detection of *Mycobacterium tuberculosis*: a blind comparison study among seven laboratories. J Clin Microbiol 1994; 32:277–284.

O'Connor RM, Mackay MR, Ward H: Molecular approaches for detection, species identification, and genotyping of *Cryptosporidium*. *In* Persing DH, Tenover FC, Versalovic J, et al (eds). Molecular Microbiology: Diagnostic Principles and Practice, Washington, DC, ASM Press, 2004, pp 583–601.

O'Neill AM, Gillespie SH, Whitting GC: Detection of penicillin susceptibility in *Streptococcus pneumoniae* by pbp2b PCR-restriction fragment length polymorphism analysis. J Clin Microbiol 1999; 37:157–160.

Olive DM, Bean P: Principles and applications of methods for DNA based typing of microbial organisms. J Clin Microbiol 1999; 37:1661–1669.

Oliveira K, Brecher SM, Durbin A, et al: Direct identification of *Staphylococcus aureus* from positive blood culture bottles. J Clin Microbiol 2003; 41:889–891.

Oliveira K, Haase G, Kurtzman C, et al: Differentiation between *Candida albicans* and *Candida dubliniensis* by fluorescence in situ hybridization using peptide nucleic acid probes. J Clin Microbiol 2001; 39:4138–4141.

Oliveira K, Procop GW, Wilson D, et al: Rapid identification of *Staphylococcus aureus* directly from blood cultures by fluorescence in situ hybridization with peptide nucleic acid probes. J Clin Microbiol 2002; 40:247–251.

Pang XL, Chui L, Fenton J, et al: Comparison of LightCycler-based PCR, COBAS Amplicor CMV Monitor, and pp65 antigenemia assays for quantitative measurement of cytomegalovirus viral load in peripheral blood specimens from patients after solid organ transplantation. J Clin Microbiol 2003; 41:3167–3174.

Parent du Châtelet I, Traore Y, Gessner BD, et al: Bacterial meningitis in Burkina Faso: surveillance using field-based polymerase chain reaction testing. Clin Infect Dis 2005; 40:17–25.
A recent study demonstrating the value of multiplex PCR in diagnosing bacterial meningitis.

Pasternack R, Vuorinen P, Miettinen A: Comparison of a transcription-mediated amplification assay and polymerase chain reaction for detection of *Chlamydia trachomatis* in first-void urine. Eur J Clin Microbiol Infect Dis 1999; 18:142–144.

Patel R, Smith TF, Espy M, et al: A prospective comparison of molecular diagnostic techniques for the early detection of cytomegalovirus in liver transplant recipients. J Infect Dis 1995; 171:1010–1014.

Paton AW, Paton JC: Detection and characterization of Shiga toxigenic *Escherichia coli* by using multiplex PCR assays for stx1, stx2, eaeA enterohaemorrhagic *E. coli* hlyA, rfbO111, and rfbO157. J Clin Microbiol 1998; 36:598–602.

Pellegrin I, Garrigue I, Ekouevi D, et al: New molecular assay to predict occurrence of cytomegalovirus disease in renal transplant recipients. J Infect Dis 2000; 182:36–42.

Pelloux H, Guy E, Angelici MC: A second European collaborative study on polymerase chain reaction for *Toxoplasma gondii*, involving 15 teams. FEMS Microbiol Lett 1998; 165:231–237.

Peltola H, Leinikki P: Rubella gene sequencing as a clinician's tool. Lancet 1998; 352:1799–1800.

Petri WA Jr: Overview of the development, utility, and future of molecular diagnostics for parsitic disease. *In* Persing DH, Tenover FC, Versalovic J, et al (eds). Molecular Microbiology: Diagnostic Principles and Practice, Washington, DC, ASM Press, 2004, pp 579–582.

Petropoulos CJ: Phenotypic testing of human immunodeficiency virus type 1 drug susceptibility. *In* Persing D, Tenover FC, Versalovic J, et al (eds). Molecular Microbiology: Diagnostic Principles and Practice, Washington, DC, ASM Press, 2004, pp 501–528.

Pfaller MA: Molecular approaches to diagnosing and managing infectious diseases: practicality and costs. Emerg Infect Dis 2001; 7:312–318.

Pfaller MA, Caliendo AM, Versalovic J: Molecular biology. *In* Isenberg HD (ed.): Clinical Microbiology Procedures Handbook, 2nd ed. Washington, DC, ASM Press, 2004a, pp 12.1.1–12.6.1.

Pfaller MA, Diekema DJ: Rare and emerging opportunistic fungal pathogens: concern for resistance beyond *Candida albicans* and *Aspergillus fumigatus*. J Clin Microbiol 2004b; 42:4419–4431.

Pfaller MA, Hollis RJ: Automated ribotyping. *In* Persing DH, Tenover FC, Versalovic J, et al (eds).

Molecular Microbiology: Diagnostic Principles and Practice, Washington, DC, ASM Press, 2004c, pp 245–258.

Pfaller MA, Wendt C, Hollis RJ: Comparative evaluation of an automated ribotyping system versus pulsed field gel electrophoresis for epidemiological typing of clinical isolates of *Escherichia coli* and *Pseudomonas aeruginosa* from patients with recurrent gram-negative bacteremia. Diagn Microbiol Infect Dis 1996; 25:1–8.

Pfyffer GE, Funke-Kissling P, Rundler E, Weber R: Performance characteristics of the BDProbeTec system for direct detection of *Mycobacterium tuberculosis* complex in respiratory specimens. J Clin Microbiol 1999; 37:137–140.

Piersimoni C, Callegaro A, Scarparo C: Comparative evaluation of the new Gen-Probe *Mycobacterium tuberculosis* amplified direct test and the semi-automated Abbott LCx *Mycobacterium tuberculosis* assay for direct detection of *Mycobacterium tuberculosis* complex in respiratory and extrapulmonary specimens. J Clin Microbiol 1998; 36:3601–3604.

Piersimoni C, Scarparo C, Piccoli P, et al: Performance assessment of two commercial amplification assays for direct detection of *Mycobacterium tuberculosis* complex from respiratory and extrapulmonary specimens. J Clin Microbiol 2002; 40:4138–4142.

Poljak M, Brencic A, Vince A, Marin IJ: Comparative evaluation of first and second generation Digene hybrid capture assays of human papillomaviruses associated with high or intermediate risk for cervical cancer. J Clin Microbiol 1999; 37:796–797.

Poljak M, Seme K, Koren S: Evaluation of the automated COBAS AMPLICOR hepatitis C virus PCR system. J Clin Microbiol 1997; 35:2983–2984.

Pozo F, Casas I, Tenorio A, et al: Evaluation of a commercially available reverse transcription-PCR assay for diagnosis of enteroviral infection in archival and prospectively collected cerebrospinal fluid specimens. J Clin Microbiol 1998; 36:1741–1745.

Puchhammer-Stockl E, Schmied B, Mandl CW, et al: Comparison of line probe assay (LIPA) and sequence analysis for detection of HIV-1 drug resistance. J Med Virol 1999; 57:283–289.

Rademaker JLW, Savelkoul P: PCR amplification-based microbial typing. *In* Persing DH, Tenover FC, Versalovic J, et al (eds). Molecular Microbiology: Diagnostic Principles and Practice, Washington, DC, ASM Press, 2004, pp 197–221.

Radford SA, Johnson EM, Leeming JP: Molecular epidemiological study of *Aspergillus fumigatus* in a bone marrow transplantation unit by PCR amplification of ribosomal intergenic spacer sequences. J Clin Microbiol 1998; 36:1294–1299.

Ramotar K, Bobrowska M, Jessamine P, Toye B: Detection of methicillin resistance in coagulase negative staphylococci initially reported as methicillin susceptible using automated methods. Diagn Microbiol Infect Dis 1998; 30:267–273.

Rantakokko-Jalava K, Jalava J: Development of conventional and real-time PCR assays for detection of *Legionella* DNA in respiratory specimens. J Clin Microbiol 2001; 39:2904–2910.

Raoult D, Fournier PE, Drancourt M: What does the future hold for clinical microbiology? Nat Rev Microbiol 2004; 2:151–159.

Razonable RR, Paya CV, Smith TF: Role of the laboratory in diagnosis and management of cytomegalovirus infection in hematopoetic stem cell and solid-organ transplant recipients. J Clin Microbiol 2002; 40:746–752.

Read SJ, Jeffery KJM, Bangham CRM: Aseptic meningitis and encephalitis: the role of PCR in the diagnostic laboratory. J Clin Microbiol 1997; 35:691–696.

Richter E, Niemann S, Gerdes R, Hoffner S: Identification of *Mycobacterium kansasii* by using a DNA probe (Accuprobe) and molecular techniques. J Clin Microbiol 1999; 37:964–970.

Robbins JB, Schneerson R, Gotschlich EC: Surveillance for bacterial meningitis by means of polymerase chain reaction. Clin Infect Dis 2005; 40:26–27

Ross JS: Financial determinants of outcomes in molecular testing. Arch Pathol Lab Med 1999; 123:1071–1075.

Rossau R, Traore H, De Beenhouwer H, et al: Evaluation of the INNO-LiPA Rif. TB assay, a reverse hybridization assay for the simultaneous detection of *Mycobacterium tuberculosis* complex and its resistance to rifampin. Antimicrob Agents Chemother 1997; 41:2093–2098.

Rotbart HA, Sawyer MH, Fast S: Diagnosis of enteroviral meningitis by using PCR with a colorimetric microwell detection assay. J Clin Microbiol 1994; 32:2590–2592.

Roth WK, Weber M, Seifried E: Feasibility and efficacy of routine PCR screening of blood donations for hepatitis C virus, hepatitis B virus and HIV-1 in the blood bank setting. Lancet 1999; 353:359–363.

Rougemont M, Van Saanen M, Sahli R, et al: Detection of four *Plasmodium* species in blood from humans by 18S rRNA gene subunit-based and species-specific real-time PCR assays. J Clin Microbiol 2004; 42:5636–5643.

Rudolph KM, Parkinson AJ, Roberts MC: Molecular analysis by pulsed-field gel electrophoresis and antibiogram of *Streptococcus pneumoniae* serotype 6B isolates from selected areas within the United States. J Clin Microbiol 1998; 36:2703–2707.

Rys PN, Persing DH: Preventing false positives: quantitative evaluation of three protocols for inactivation of polymerase chain reaction amplification products. J Clin Microbiol 1993; 31:2356–2360.

Sader H, Pignatari AC, Frei R, et al: Pulsed field gel electrophoresis of restriction-digested genomic DNA and antimicrobial susceptibility of *Xanthomonas maltophilia* strains from Brazil, Switzerland and the USA. J Antimicrob Chemother 1994; 33:615–618.

Sakai H, Procop GW, Kobayashi N, et al: Simultaneous detection of *Staphylococcus aureus* and coagulase-negative staphylococci in positive blood cultures by real-time PCR with two fluorescence resonance energy transfer probe sets. J Clin Microbiol 2004; 42:5739–5744.

Sawyer L, Leung I, Friesenhahn M, et al: Clinical laboratory evaluation of a new sensitive and specific assay for qualitative detection of hepatitis C virus RNA in clinical specimens. J Hepatol 2000; 32(Suppl 2):116A.

Scarparo C, Piccoli P, Rigon A, et al: Direct identification of mycobacteria from MB/BacT Alert 3D bottles: comparative evaluation of two commercial probe assays. J Clin Microbiol 2001; 39:3222–3227.

Schachter J: Two different worlds we live in. Clin Infect Dis 1998; 27:1181–1185.

Schepetiuk A, Kok T, Martin L, et al: Detection of *Chlamydia trachomatis* in urine samples by nucleic acid tests: comparison with culture and enzyme immunoassay of genital swab specimens. J Clin Microbiol 1997; 35:3355–3357.

Scheuermann RH, Domiati-Saad R, Rogers BB: DNA virus detection. *In* Persing DH, Tenover FC, Versalovic J, et al (eds). Molecular Microbiology: Diagnostic Principles and Practice, Washington, DC, ASM Press, 2004, pp 429–440.

Seme K, Poljak M, Koren S: Mistyping of two Slovenian hepatitis C virus subtype 2c isolates as subtype 2b by two 5′ noncoding region genotyping methods. J Clin Microbiol 1997; 35:3369.

Sepkowitz KA: How contagious is tuberculosis? Clin Infect Dis 1996;23:954–962.

Shah JS, Liu J, Smith J: Novel ultrasensitive, Q-beta replicase amplified hybridization assay for detection of *Chlamydia trachomatis*. J Clin Microbiol 1994; 32:2718–2724.

Shrestha NK, Shermock KM, Gordon SM, et al: Predictive value and cost-effectiveness analysis of a rapid polymerase chain reaction for preoperative detection of nasal carriage of *Staphylococcus aureus*. Infect Control Hosp Epidemiol 2003a; 24:327–333.
An example of how rapid detection of an important nosocomial pathogen can improve patient care and minimize nosocomial infection (and also save money).

VII

Shrestha NK, Tuohy MJ, Hall GS, et al: Detection and differentiation of *Mycobacterium tuberculosis* and nontuberculous mycobacterial isolates by real-time PCR. J Clin Microbiol 2003b; 41:5121–5126.

Sloutsky A, Han LL, Werner BG: Practical strategies for performance optimization of the enhanced Gen-Probe Amplified Mycobacterium Tuberculosis Direct Test. J Clin Microbiol 2004; 42:1547–1551.

Smith TF, Espy MJ, Jones MF: Molecular virology: current and future trends. *In* Persing DH, Tenover FC, Versalovic J, et al (eds). Molecular Microbiology: Diagnostic Principles and Practice, Washington, DC, ASM Press, 2004, pp 543–548.

Sola C, Horgen L, Maisetti J, et al: Spoligotyping followed by double-repetitive-element PCR as rapid alternative to IS6110 fingerprinting for epidemiological studies of tuberculosis. J Clin Microbiol 1998; 36:1122–1124.

Soll DR: The ins and outs of DNA fingerprinting the infectious fungi. Clin Microbiol Rev 2000; 13:332–370.

Soll DR, Lockhart SR, Pujol C: Laboratory procedures for epidemiological analysis of microorganisms. *In* Murray PR, Baron EJ, Jorgensen JH, et al (eds), Manual of Clinical Microbiology, 8th ed. Washington, DC, ASM Press, 2003, pp 139–161.

Sreevatsan S, Bookout JB, Ringpis FM: Algorithmic approach to high-throughput molecular screening for alpha interferon-resistant genotypes in hepatitis C patients. J Clin Microbiol 1998; 36:1895–1901.

Stary A, Schuh E, Kerschbaumer M, Gotz B, Lee H: Performance of transcription-mediated amplification and ligase chain reaction assays for detection in urogenital samples obtained by noninvasive methods. J Clin Microbiol 1998; 36:2666–2670.

Stender H, Mollerup TA, Lund K, et al: Direct detection and identification of *Mycobacterium tuberculosis* in smear-positive sputum samples by fluorescence in situ hybridization (FISH) using peptide nucleic acid (PNA) probes. Int J Tuberc Lung Dis 1999; 3:830–837.

Stockman L, Clark KA, Hunt JM, Roberts GD: Evaluation of commercially available acridinium ester-labeled chemiluminescent DNA probes for culture identification of *Blastomyces dermatitidis, Coccidioides immitis, Cryptococcus neoformans* and *Histoplasma capsulatum*. J Clin Microbiol 1993; 31:845–850.

Stöver AG, Jeffery E, Xu J, Persing DH: Hybridizaton array technology. *In* Persing DH, Tenover FC, Versalovic J, et al (eds). Molecular Microbiology: Diagnostic Principles and Practice, Washington, DC, ASM Press, 2004, pp 619–639.

Sturtevant J: Applications of differential-display reverse transcription-PCR to molecular pathogenesis and medical mycology. Clin Microbiol Rev 2000; 13:408–427.

Stuyver L, Wyseur A, van Arnhem W, et al: Second generation line probe assay for hepatitis C virus genotyping. J Clin Microbiol 1996; 34:2259–2266.

Tang YW, Ellis NM, Hopkins MK, et al: Comparison of phenotypic and genotypic techniques for identification of unusual aerobic pathogenic gram-negative bacilli. J Clin Microbiol 1998; 36:3674–3679.

Teltenti A, Honore N, Bernasconi C: Genotypic assessment of isoniazid and rifampicin resistance in *Mycobacterium tuberculosis*: a blind study at reference laboratory level. J Clin Microbiol 1997; 35:719–723.

Tenover F, Arbeit RD, Goering RV: Interpreting chromosomal DNA restriction patterns produced by pulsed field gel electrophoresis: Criteria for bacterial strain typing. J Clin Microbiol 1995; 33:2233–2239.

Tenover FC, Rasheed JK: Detection of antimicrobial resistance genes and mutations associated with antimicrobial resistance in microorganisms. *In* Persing DH, Tenover FC, Versalovic J, et al (eds). Molecular Microbiology: Diagnostic Principles and Practice, Washington, DC, ASM Press, 2004, pp 391–406.

Thwaites GE, Caws M, Hong TT, et al: Comparison of conventional bacteriology with nucleic acid amplification (Amplified Mycobacterium Direct Test) for diagnosis of tuberculous meningitis before and after inception of antituberculous chemotherapy. J Clin Microbiol 2004; 42:996–1002.

Tortoli E, Lavinia F, Simonetti MT: Early detection of *Mycobacterium tuberculosis* in BACTEC cultures by ligase chain reaction. J Clin Microbiol 1998; 36:2791–2792.

Tortoli E, Nanetti A, Piersimoni C, et al: Performance assessment of new multiplex probe assay for identification of mycobacteria. J Clin Microbiol 2001; 39:1079–1084.

Tortoli E, Tronci M, Tosi CP: Multicenter evaluation of two commercial amplification kits (Amplicor, Roche and LCx Abbott) for direct detection of *Mycobacterium tuberculosis* in pulmonary and extrapulmonary specimens. Diagn Microbiol Infect Dis 1999; 33:173–179.

Tremblay C, Coutlee F, Weiss J, et al: Evaluation of a non-isotopic polymerase chain reaction assay for detection in clinical specimens of herpes simples virus type 2 DNA. Clin Diagn Virol 1997; 8:53–62.

Triques K, Coste J, Perret JL: Efficiencies of four versions of the Amplicor HIV-1 monitor test for quantification of different subtypes of human immunodeficiency virus type 1. J Clin Microbiol 1999; 37:110–116

Troesch A, Nguyen H, Miyada CG: *Mycobacterium* species identification and rifampicin resistance testing with high-density DNA probe arrays. J Clin Microbiol 1999; 37:49–55.

Urdea MS, Horn T, Fultz T: Branched DNA amplification multimers for the sensitive, direct detection of human hepatitis viruses. Nucl Acids Res Symp Series 1991; 24:197–200.

Van Belkum A, Melchers WJG, Ijsseldijk C, et al: Outbreak of amoxicillin-resistant *Haemophilus influenzae* type B: variable number of tandem repeats as novel molecular markers. J Clin Microbiol 1997; 35:1517–1520.

Van Belkum A, van Leeluwen W, Kaufmann ME, et al: Assessment of resolution and intercenter reproducibility of results of genotyping *Staphylococcus aureus* by pulsed-field gel electrophoresis of *Sma*I macrorestriction fragments: a multicenter study. J Clin Infect Dis 1998; 36:1653–1659.

Van Burik JA, Myerson D, Schreckhise RW, Bowden RA: Panfungal PCR assay for detection of fungal infection in human blood specimens. J Clin Microbiol 1998; 36:1169–1175.

Vandelli C, Renzo F, Braun HB: Prediction of successful outcome in a randomized controlled trial of the long-term efficacy of interferon alpha treatment for chronic hepatitis C. J Med Virol 1999; 58:26–34.

Van Dyck E, Ieven M, Pattyn S, et al: Detection of *Chlamydia trachomatis* and *Neisseria gonorrhoeae* by enzyme immunoassay, culture, and three nucleic acid amplification tests. J Clin Microbiol 2001; 39:1751–1756.

Van Embden JDA, Cave MD, Crawford JT: Strain identification of *Mycobacterium tuberculosis* by DNA fingerprinting: recommendations for a standardized methodology. J Clin Microbiol 1993; 31:406–409.

Vannuffel P, Gigi J, Ezzedine H: Specific detection of methicillin resistant *Staphylococcus* species by multiplex PCR. J Clin Microbiol 1995; 33:2864–2867.

Versalovic J, Unger ER: External quality assessment and proficiency testing in diagnostic molecular microbiology. *In* Persing DH, Tenover FC, Versalovic J, et al (eds). Molecular Microbiology: Diagnostic Principles and Practice, Washington, DC, ASM Press, 2004, pp 691–696.

Vila J, Marcos MA, Jimenez de Anta MT: A comparative study of different PCR-based DNA fingerprinting techniques for typing *Acinetobacter calcoaceticus–A. baumannii* complex. J Med Microbiol 1996; 44:482–489.

Vincelette J, Schirm J, Bogard M: Multicenter evaluation of the fully automated COBAS amplicor PCR test for detection of *Chlamydia trachomatis* in urogenital specimens. J Clin Microbiol 1999; 37:74–80.

Visvesvara GS, Garcia LS: Culture of protozoan parasites. Clin Microbiol Rev 2002; 15:327–328.

Vogel U, Morrrelli G, Zurth K: Necessity of molecular techniques to distinguish between *Neisseria meningitidis* strains isolated from patients with meningococcal disease and from their healthy contacts. J Clin Microbiol 1998; 36:2465–2470.

Walsh TJ, Groll A, Hiemenz J, et al: Infections due to emerging and uncommon medically important fungal pathogens. Clin Microbiol Infect 2004; 10(Suppl 1):48–66.

Walton DT, Valesco M: Identification of *Mycobacterium gordonae* from culture by the Gen-Probe rapid diagnostic system: evaluation of 218 isolates and potential sources of false negative results. J Clin Microbiol 1991; 29:1850–1854.

Warren DK, Liao RS, Merz LR, et al: Detection of methicillin-resistant *Staphylococcus aureus* directly from nasal swab specimens by a real-time PCR assay. J Clin Microbiol 2004; 42:5578–5581.

Watterson SA, Drobniewski FA: Modern laboratory diagnosis of mycobacterial infections. J Clin Pathol 2000; 53:727–732.

A thorough discussion of molecular methods and other new technology applied to the diagnosis of mycobacterial infections.

Weir SC, Fischer SH, Stock F, Gill VJ: Detection of *Legionella* by PCR in respiratory specimens using a commercially available kit. Am J Clin Pathol 1998; 110:295–300.

Wilke WW, Sutton LD, Jones RN: Automation of polymerase chain reaction (PCR) tests as a mechanism to achieve acceptable contamination rates. Clin Chem 1995, 41:622–623.

Wilson DA, Joyce MJ, Hall LS, et al: Multicenter evaluation of *Candida albicans* peptide mucleic fluorescent in situ hybridization probe for characterization of yeast isolates from blood cultures. J Clin Microbiol 2005; 43:2909–2912.

Wilson KH: Detection of culture-resistant bacterial pathogens by amplification and sequencing of ribosomal DNA. Clin Infect Dis 1994; 18:958–962.

Wolk D, Mitchell S, Patel R: Principles of molecular microbiology testing methods. Infect Dis Clin N Amer 2001; 15:1157–1204.

Woods GL, Bergmann JS, Williams-Bouyer N: Clinical evaluation of the Gen-Probe Amplified Mycobacterium Tuberculosis Direct Test for rapid detection of *Mycobacterium tuberculosis* in select nonrespiratory specimens. J Clin Microbiol 2001; 39:747–749.

Woods JP, Kersulyte D, Tolan RW Jr, et al: Use of arbitrarily primed polymerase chain reaction analysis to type disease and carrier strains of *Neisseria meningitidis* isolated during a university outbreak. J Infect Dis 1994; 169:1384–1389.

Wylie JL, Moses S, Babcock R, et al: Comparative evaluation of Chlamydiazyme, PACE 2, and AMP-CT assays for detection of *Chlamydia trachomatis* in endocervical specimens. J Clin Microbiol 1998; 36:3488–3491.

Yen-Lieberman B, Brambilla D, Jackson B: Evaluation of a quality assurance program for quantitation of human immunodeficiency virus type I RNA in plasma by the AIDS clinical trials group virology laboratories. J Clin Microbiol 1996; 34:2695–2701.

Yeo SF, Wong B: Current status of nonculture methods for diagnosis of invasive fungal infections. Clin Microbiol Rev 2002; 15:465–484.

An excellent review of molecular immunologic, and biochemical approaches to the rapid diagnosis of invasive mycoses.

Young H, Moyes A: Comparative evaluation of Accuprobe culture identification test for *Neisseria gonorrhoeae* and other rapid methods. J Clin Microbiol 1993; 31:1996–1999.

Yuen LKW, Ross BC, Jackson KM, Dwyer B: Characterization of *Mycobacterium tuberculosis* strains from Vietnamese patients by Southern blot hybridization. J Clin Microbiol 1993; 31:1615–1618.

Zaaijer HL, Cuypers HTM, Reesink HW, et al: Reliability of polymerase chain reaction for detection of hepatitis C virus. Lancet 1993; 341:722–724.

Zaaijer HL, ter Borg F, Cuypers HTM, et al: Comparison of methods for detection of hepatitis B virus DNA. J Clin Microbiol 1994; 32:2088–2091.

Zhou W, Du W, Cao H, et al: Detection of *gyr*A and *par*C mutations associated with ciprofloxacin resistance in *Neisseria gonorrhoeae* by use of oligonucleotide biochip technology. J Clin Microbiol 2004: 42:5819–5824.

VII

CHAPTER 63

Specimen Collection and Handling for Diagnosis of Infectious Diseases

Ann C. Croft MT(ASCP), Gail L. Woods MD

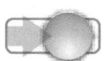

KEY POINTS

• Collect specimens from site of infection prior to initiation of therapy.

• Collect adequate volume of sample for testing required.

• For bacterial, fungal and viral cultures submit tissue, fluid or aspirate if possible, as these are always superior to a swab specimen.

• Use required collection and transport materials to preserve specimen integrity.

• Communicate clear orders and source information.

• Expedite the transport of specimens to the laboratory and do not allow them to sit in collection areas.

Appropriate specimen collection, transport and processing are crucial preanalytical steps in the accurate diagnosis of infectious diseases. Guidelines for specimen handling are discussed in this chapter. General principles are reviewed first, followed by discussion of the most common types of specimens submitted to the clinical microbiology laboratory for testing.

General principles

Timing of Specimen Collection

For optimal detection of the pathogen(s) responsible for an infectious disease, specimens should be collected at a time when the likelihood of recovering the suspected agent is greatest. For example, the likelihood of recovering most viruses is greatest in the acute phase of the illness. Specimens for recovery of bacteria should ideally be collected before antimicrobial therapy is started.

Specimen Volume

The volume of specimen collected must be adequate for performance of the microbiological studies requested. If insufficient volume is received, the physician or ward nurse should be notified; either additional sample can be obtained, or the physician must prioritize the requests. If a swab is used to collect the specimen, a polyester-tipped swab on a plastic shaft is acceptable for most organisms. Calcium alginate should be avoided for collection of samples for viral culture, because it could inactivate herpes simplex virus (HSV); cotton may be toxic to *Neisseria gonorrhoeae*; and wooden shafts should be avoided, because the wood may be toxic to *Chlamydia trachomatis*. Swabs are not optimal for detection of anaerobes, mycobacteria, or fungi, and should not be used when these organisms are suspected. An actual tissue sample or fluid aspirate is always superior to a swab specimen for the recovery of pathogenic organisms.

Specimen Collection

Specimens should be obtained from the site of infection with minimal contamination from adjacent tissues and organ secretions and, with the exception of stool, should be collected in a sterile container. All specimens should be labeled with the name and identification number of the person from whom the specimen was collected, the source of the specimen, and the date and time it was collected.

Specimen Transport

After collection, specimens should be placed in a biohazard bag and transported to the laboratory as soon as possible. If a delay is unavoidable, urine, sputum and other respiratory specimens, stool, and specimens for detection of *C. trachomatis* or viruses should be refrigerated to prevent overgrowth of normal flora. Cerebrospinal fluid (CSF) and other body fluids, blood, and specimens collected for recovery of *N. gonorrhoeae* should be held at room temperature, because refrigeration adversely affects recovery of potential pathogens from these sources.

Unacceptable Specimens

Each laboratory director must establish criteria for rejecting specimens unsuitable for culture. Most clinical microbiologists agree that the following specimens should be rejected:
- Any specimen received in formalin
- 24-hour sputum collections
- Specimens in containers from which the sample has leaked
- Specimens that have been inoculated on to agar plates that have dried out or are outdated
- Specimens contaminated with barium, chemical dyes, or oily chemicals
- Foley catheter tips
- Duplicate specimens (except blood cultures) received in a 24-hour period
- Blood catheter tips submitted for patients without concomitant positive blood culture

The following specimens should be rejected for anaerobic culture:
- Gastric washings
- Urine other than suprapubic aspirate
- Stool (except for recovery of *Clostridium difficile* for epidemiologic studies or for diagnosis of bacteria associated with food poisoning [discussed below])
- Oropharyngeal specimens, except deep tissue samples obtained during a surgical procedure
- Sputum
- Swabs of ileostomy or colostomy sites
- Superficial skin specimens.

Universal Precautions

Universal precautions must be followed when handling all specimens. Appropriate barriers are used to prevent exposure of skin and mucous membranes to the specimen. Gloves and a lab coat must be worn at all times, and masks, goggles (or working behind a plastic shield), and impermeable gowns or aprons must be worn in situations in which there is risk of splashes or droplet formation. Optimally, all specimen containers but, at a minimum, those containing respiratory secretions and those submitted specifically for detection of mycobacteria or fungi should be opened in a biological safety cabinet. Specimens collected for virus isolation should be handled in a biological safety cabinet to prevent contamination of the cell cultures.

Referral Testing

When specimens or cultures must be shipped to a reference laboratory, they must be packaged according to dangerous goods shipping guidelines (see IATA website). Specimens must be limited to no more than 40 mL. Cultures of bacteria and fungi should be grown on solid media in tubes. The cap of the primary container (tube or vial) should be sealed with waterproof tape and inserted into a second container, surrounded by sufficient packing material to absorb the entire volume of the culture or specimen if the primary container were to leak or break. If several primary tubes are placed in a second container, they must be either individually wrapped or separated so as to prevent contact between them and there must be secondary packaging, which must be leakproof. The second container should be capped and placed in a shipping container made of corrugated fiberboard or hard plastic. An itemized list of contents must be enclosed between the secondary and outer packaging. The secondary and outer containers should be of sufficient strength to maintain their integrity at temperature and air pressures to which they will be subjected. If a specimen must be shipped on dry ice (which is considered to be a hazardous material), it must be marked 'Dry ice, frozen medical specimen.' The dry ice should be placed outside the second container with the packing material in such a way that the container does not become loose inside the outer container as the dry ice evaporates. All infectious shipping packages must be labeled with an official label containing the address and contents as well as the name and telephone number of the person responsible for the shipment.

Blood

Detection of blood-borne pathogens is one of the most important functions of the microbiology laboratory. Culture of blood is essential in identifying bacteria responsible for bacteremia, sepsis, infections of native and prosthetic valves, suppurative thrombophlebitis, mycotic aneurysms, and infections of vascular grafts. Blood cultures also are useful in diagnosing some viral infections and invasive or disseminated infections caused by certain fungi, especially species of *Candida*, *Cryptococcus neoformans*, species of *Fusarium*, and *Histoplasma capsulatum*. Parasites are detected in blood by microscopic examination of peripheral smears. In general, blood should be collected for culture before beginning antimicrobial therapy when any one or a combination of the following are present: fever (38°C or greater), hypothermia (36°C or lower), leukocytosis (especially with a left shift), granulocytopenia, or hypotension.

Specimen Collection

Timely detection and accurate identification of organisms in the blood depend on appropriate collection, transport, and processing of the specimen. Germane to the detection of all microorganisms in the blood is the phlebotomy technique. To minimize contamination of blood specimens by skin flora, the venipuncture site should be prepared with a bactericidal agent. The skin first is cleaned with alcohol (70% isopropyl or ethyl alcohol) and then with a 1–2% iodine solution, an iodophor, or chlorhexidine. For maximum antisepsis, the area should dry for 1–2 minutes prior to venipuncture of the selected peripheral vein.

Appropriate Timing for Detection of Bacteremia and Fungemia

The optimal time to draw blood for cultures when bacteremia or fungemia is suspected is just before a chill but, because this is not predictable, most blood cultures are collected after the onset of fever and chills. Blood is drawn with a needle and syringe and, without changing needles, is injected directly into bottles of culture media or other blood culture system (Krumholz, 1990). The inoculated bottles are immediately inverted several times to ensure mixing, and then transported to the laboratory at room temperature as soon after collection as possible. Blood cultures should never be refrigerated.

Specimen Volume

In adults with bacteremia, the number of colony-forming units (CFU) per milliliter of blood is frequently low. Therefore, for adults, collecting 20–30 mL of blood per culture set is strongly recommended (Ilstrup, 1983; Washington, 1986; Towns, 2002; Cockerill, 2004). In infants and children, the concentration of microorganisms in blood is higher, and collection of 1–5 mL of blood per culture is adequate.

Specimen Draws

Recommendations concerning the number of blood specimens to collect are based on the nature of the bacteremia: transient, intermittent, or continuous. Transient bacteremia follows manipulation of a focus of infection (e.g., an abscess, a furuncle, or cellulitis), instrumentation of a contaminated mucosal surface (as occurs during dental procedures, cystoscopy, urethral catheterization, suction abortion, or sigmoidoscopy), or a surgical procedure in a contaminated site (such as transurethral resection of the prostate, vaginal hysterectomy, colon resection, and debridement of infected burns). Transient bacteremia also occurs early in the course of many systemic and localized infections such as meningitis, pneumonia, pyogenic arthritis, and osteomyelitis. Most intermittent bacteremias are associated with an undrained abscess, whereas continuous bacteremia is the hallmark of intravascular infection, such as bacterial endocarditis, mycotic aneurysm, or an infected intravascular catheter. Continuous bacteremia also occurs during the first few weeks of typhoid fever and brucellosis.

The optimal number of blood cultures for detection of bacteremia in patients without endocarditis is controversial. Most authorities agree that two or three 20 mL blood samples drawn over a 24-hour period and equally distributed into aerobic and anaerobic blood culture bottles is sufficient to detect the majority of blood stream infections. One investigator demonstrated that a total of four blood cultures drawn within 24 hours increased the yield of potential pathogens by as much as 20% (Cockerill, 2004). The optimal time interval between cultures is unknown, but 30 to 60 minutes for the first two sets has been suggested, with another one to two sets drawn over the remaining 24 hours if symptoms of septicemia persist (Cockerill, 2004). However, if initiation of antimicrobial therapy is deemed urgent, cultures should be collected before therapy is begun, from separate sites within a few minutes.

Organisms such as the coagulase-negative staphylococci, viridans streptococci, corynebacteria, *Bacillus* species, and *Propionibacterium* species are frequent blood culture contaminants but may also be true pathogens. Collecting two sets of blood cultures per febrile episode helps distinguish probable pathogens from contaminants. The latter are generally present in only one bottle of one set of cultures, whereas pathogens are typically recovered from more than one set.

VII

Recovery of Microorganisms

Host factors such as antibodies, complement, phagocytic white blood cells, and antimicrobial agents may impede recovery of microorganisms from blood; therefore, various approaches have been used to counteract these factors. Diluting the blood specimen in broth medium in a 1:10 ratio provides optimal neutralization of the serum bactericidal activity (Washington, 1986). Incorporating 0.02–0.05% sodium polyanethol sulfonate in the blood culture medium inhibits coagulation, phagocytosis, and complement activation, and inactivates aminoglycosides. Methods that counteract the presence of antimicrobial agents include adding penicillinases to broth media to inactivate penicillins, using antibiotic-adsorbent resins, or using the lysis–centrifugation system (described under Manual Blood Cultures, below).

Blood Culture Systems

Several blood culture systems, each with advantages and disadvantages, are available (Wilson, 1996; Reimer, 1997). Automated detection systems are rapidly replacing manual systems, but many smaller laboratories still rely on manual methods. Both automated and manual systems use nutritionally enriched liquid media, which are capable of supporting growth of most bacteria. Traditionally, two bottles are inoculated, and one is vented to ensure recovery of aerobes. Given the decline in anaerobic bacteremias, this practice of one aerobic and one anaerobic bottle per set has been questioned (Sharp, 1991; Murray, 1992). Routine inoculation of two aerobic media and only selective use of anaerobic blood cultures may allow detection of more bacteremias and fungemias.

Manual Blood Cultures

Culture bottles are examined daily for 7 days for evidence of growth, indicated by turbidity, hemolysis, gas production, discrete colonies, or a combination of these. When growth is apparent, a smear of the broth is stained with Gram's stain and examined microscopically, and the broth is subcultured to appropriate agar media. Routine subculture of macroscopically negative broths should be performed from the vented bottle 6–18 hours after inoculation. Routine subculture of the anaerobic bottle is unnecessary. Advantages of conventional broth cultures are the low cost of materials and a low contamination rate. The major drawback is the time-consuming process of routine bottle examination and subculture.

A less labor-intensive manual blood culture system consists of a broth medium in a bottle to which a chamber containing agar media on a paddle is attached. To subculture this biphasic system, the bottle is tipped, allowing the blood–broth mixture to enter the chamber and flow over the agar media. Colonies on the agar medium are used for identification and susceptibility testing. For recovery of aerobic and facultative bacteria and yeasts, this system is comparable to or better than other systems (Murray, 1991). The yield of anaerobes from conventional broth systems, however, may be higher.

The lysis–centrifugation blood culture system consists of a tube containing reagents that inhibit coagulation and the complement cascade, lyse blood cells, and provide a cushion for the microorganisms during centrifugation. Blood is added to the tube, which is inverted several times to prevent clotting and transported to the laboratory as soon as possible. Ideally, the specimen is processed immediately, but processing can be delayed for up to 8 hours without adversely affecting recovery of microorganisms. To process the culture, the tube is centrifuged for 30 minutes at $3000 \times g$, the supernatant is discarded, and the sediment is mixed on a vortex mixer and plated onto agar media. Smaller tubes for low-volume samples, from infants and young children, are also available. Advantages of lysis–centrifugation include excellent recovery of *Staphylococcus aureus*, some Enterobacteriaceae, and fungi (it is the best system for recovery of moulds such as *H. capsulatum*), the direct availability of colonies for identification and susceptibility testing, and the ability to carry out quantitative cultures. Moreover, this system is flexible because special media can be inoculated to recover organisms with specific growth requirements, such as species of *Legionella* and mycobacteria. However, the system is labor-intensive, is less likely to recover *Streptococcus pneumoniae*, *Haemophilus influenzae* or anaerobes, and the risk for contamination is increased.

Automated Blood Culture Systems

Several automated continuously monitoring blood culture systems are available commercially (Wilson, 1996). Advantages of all such systems are elimination of the need for blind subculture and the shortening of the usual incubation period from 7 to 5 days (Woods, 1994; Reisner, 1999). One such system is based on the colorimetric detection of CO_2 produced during microbial growth (Thorpe, 1990). A CO_2 sensor is bonded to the bottom of each blood culture bottle and is separated from the broth medium by a membrane that is impermeable to most ions and to components of media

and blood but freely permeable to CO_2. Inoculated bottles are placed in cells in the instrument, which provides continuous rocking of both aerobic and anaerobic bottles. If bacteria are present, they generate CO_2, which is released into the broth medium; the pH then decreases, causing the sensor to change color from green to yellow. Color changes are monitored once every 10 minutes by a colorimetric detector. Media available for use with this system include routine aerobic and anaerobic media, which accommodate 5–10 mL of blood; Pedi-BacT, which accommodates 4 mL of blood or less; and FAN (fastidious antibiotic neutralization), which enhances recovery of fungi and recovery of bacteria from patients receiving antimicrobial agents.

A second continuous-monitoring system is based on fluorescent technology (Nolte, 1993). Bonded to the base of each vial is a CO_2 sensor that is impermeable to ions, medium components, and blood but freely permeable to CO_2. If organisms are present, they release CO_2 into the medium; it then diffuses into the sensor matrix and generates hydrogen ions. The subsequent decrease in pH increases the fluorescence output of the sensor, changing the signal transmitted to the optical and electronic components of the instrument. The computer generates growth curves, and data are analyzed according to growth algorithms. Inoculated bottles are placed in individual cells of the instrument, in which both aerobic and anaerobic bottles are continuously rocked. Aerobic and anaerobic low-volume (5–7 mL of blood) and high-volume (8 to 10 mL of blood) media, Peds-Plus medium (0.5 to 5 mL of blood), and the Myco F Lytic medium for recovery of fungi and mycobacteria are available (Waite, 1998).

A third system detects growth of organisms in broth by measuring gas consumption and/or gas production (Zwadyk, 1994). Each inoculated vial is fitted with a disposable connector that contains a recessed needle. The needle penetrates the bottle stopper and connects the bottle headspace to the sensor probe. The sensor monitors changes within the headspace in the consumption and/or production of all gases (CO_2, N_2, and H_2) by growing organisms and creates data points internally in the computer. Two basic types of medium are available: aerobic and anaerobic media that contain 80 mL of broth and accommodate 0.1–10 mL of blood, and EZ Draw (direct draw) aerobic and anaerobic bottles that contain 40 mL of broth and accommodate 0.1–5 mL of blood.

Detection of Rarely Encountered Organisms

Detection of some bacteria requires prolonged incubation or special media. For example, when brucellosis is suspected, blood should be collected early in the disease and cultures should be incubated for 2–3 weeks, although with the automated systems brucellas often grow in less than 1 week (Bannatyne, 1997). Infections with species of *Borrelia*, except *Borrelia burgdorferi* (the etiologic agent of Lyme disease, most commonly diagnosed serologically), are diagnosed by detecting spirochetes in the peripheral blood during febrile periods. Organisms are visualized in wet preparations made by mixing a drop of blood with a drop of sodium citrate, and examining it with light- or dark-field microscopy, and in thin and thick blood films stained with Wright's or Giemsa stains, examined by light microscopy. To isolate *Leptospira interrogans* from blood, a few drops of fresh or anticoagulated blood collected during the first week of illness are added to each of three to four tubes of leptospiral semisolid culture medium (Fletcher's medium or Ellinghausen–McCollough–Johnson–Harris medium).

Two methods may be used to recover mycobacteria from blood specimens. With the lysis–centrifugation technique, a concentrate is prepared; the sediment is inoculated to solid and/or liquid media; and the cultures are incubated for up to 8 weeks. An alternative and perhaps more rapid approach is direct inoculation of the Myco F Lytic medium (monitored for growth by the BACTEC 9000 instruments) or the 13 A medium (monitored by the BACTEC 460TB).

Detection and Notification of Positive Cultures

Positive blood cultures containing commonly isolated aerobic organisms are usually detected within 12–36 hours of incubation. The initial report will consist of a Gram stain report only. Identification and susceptibility results can be expected within 24–48 hours after the Gram stain report. Cultures containing anaerobes are usually not detected for 48–72 hours, and identification and susceptibility reports will not be available for another 3–4 days. Fastidious organisms, such as those found in the HACEK group (*Haemophilus/Actinobacillus/Cardiobacterium/Eikenella/Kingella*) may not be detected until 3–5 days.

Detection of Viruses

Blood specimens are useful in diagnosing infections with a limited number of viruses (Table 63–1). Viremia usually occurs during the incubation period or the first 1–2 days after symptoms begin; so blood should be

Table 63–1 Specimen Requirements for Optimal Detection of Viruses Found in Blood

| Virus | Blood Specimen Requirements | | |
	Type Collected	Fraction Used for Detection	Volume (mL)
Cytomegalovirus	With anticoagulant*	Leukocytes	5–10
Enteroviruses	With or without anticoagulant*	Serum or leukocytes	5–10
Human immunodeficiency virus†	EDTA	Mononuclear cells or plasma	2–5
Human herpesvirus-6	Heparinized	Mononuclear cells	5–10
Parvovirus B19	Without anticoagulant	Serum	5–10
Arthropod-borne viruses‡	With or without anticoagulant	Leukocytes or homogenized clot	5–10

* Heparin or EDTA may be used for cytomegalovirus; heparin, citrate, or EDTA for enteroviruses. † For monitoring HIV viral load in patients receiving antiretroviral therapy. ‡ Includes viruses of eastern, western, and Venezuelan equine encephalitis, St Louis and California encephalitis, yellow fever, dengue, and Colorado tick fever.

EDTA = ethylenediaminetetraacetic acid.

collected early in the illness. An exception is infection with human immunodeficiency virus (HIV), which is detected nearly continuously in peripheral blood mononuclear cells and plasma of most seropositive persons. One blood sample per 24-hour period collected from a peripheral vein or through an intravascular catheter is adequate for virus detection.

Specimen requirements differ for the different viruses (shown in Table 63–1). All blood samples should be transported to the laboratory as rapidly as possible. If a delay in processing is unavoidable, specimens may be stored overnight at 4°C, except specimens for detection of HIV RNA in plasma, which must be processed (i.e., plasma separated) within 6 hours of specimen collection. Those viruses detected routinely in most clinical virology laboratories – cytomegalovirus (CMV) and the enteroviruses – are discussed. For detection of other viruses listed in Table 63–1, specimens often are sent to a reference laboratory.

Detection of CMV and the enteroviruses in blood involves separation of the component most likely to contain the virus and inoculation of that fraction to cell monolayers that support viral replication or preparation of a smear for staining with monoclonal antibodies. CMV is detected most often in neutrophils but may be present in peripheral blood mononuclear cells; thus, for optimal detection, both neutrophils and mononuclear cells should be cultured or stained (Howell, 1979). The enteroviruses are recovered equally well from leukocytes, primarily mononuclear cells, and from serum (Prather, 1984).

To separate leukocytes, blood with anticoagulants must be collected. The anticoagulant used (citrate or sodium heparin is acceptable) is based on the leukocyte separation system (several are commercially available) (Woods, 1987a; Storch, 1994). To separate serum, the blood is collected in a tube without anticoagulant and allowed to clot at 4°C. When a firm clot forms, the sample is centrifuged at 2000 × g for 10 minutes at 4°C, and the serum is aseptically removed.

Cell monolayers inoculated for virus isolation are selected based on the virus expected to be present. To recover CMV, inoculating MRC-5 or other human fibroblast cell cultures is recommended. Incubating monolayers in maintenance medium containing 10^{-5} M dexamethasone for a minimum of 24 hours before inoculation increases the rate of detection of CMV and decreases the time for appearance of cytopathic effect (Thiele, 1988). For recovery of enteroviruses, MRC-5 and primary monkey kidney cells should be inoculated, and the rate of isolation may be increased by also inoculating Buffalo green monkey kidney and human rhabdomyosarcoma cells (Dagan, 1986). Serum specimens are inoculated, adsorbed, incubated, and examined for virus-specific cytopathic effect. For leukocyte suspensions, cell monolayers are inoculated with 0.5 mL of specimen, 1.0 mL of maintenance medium is added, and cell cultures are incubated overnight. The cell suspension then is removed, cell monolayers are washed with sterile phosphate buffered saline, 1.5 mL of maintenance medium is added, and cultures are reincubated.

In addition to conventional cell culture, centrifugation culture should be performed when detection of CMV is requested (Woods, 1987b). More sensitive methods for detecting CMV in blood are the antigenemia assay, performed by staining cytospin preparations of leukocytes with monoclonal antibodies against the viral matrix protein (pp 65) (Van Der Bij, 1988; Brumback, 1997), and quantitative polymerase chain reaction (PCR) (Herrmann, 2004; Kalpoe, 2004; Meyer-Koenig, 2004).

Detection of Parasites

Blood specimens are useful for diagnosis of malaria, babesiosis, trypanosomiasis, and some filariasis. Specimens should be collected in tubes with anticoagulant and transported promptly to the laboratory. If smears must be sent to a reference laboratory, they should be fixed in absolute alcohol soon after they are made. The techniques used in the laboratory for detecting the above parasites are the same and are discussed here in order of the simplest to the most complicated.

The simplest technique for detecting parasites in a sample of blood is the direct mount, prepared by placing one drop of blood on a glass slide, covering it with a cover glass, and examining it immediately. Direct mounts are excellent for diagnosis of trypanosomiasis or filariasis because the trypomastigotes and the microfilariae easily can be seen moving, often with low or medium power. The definitive diagnosis is made by staining smears.

The thin smear, made as for hematologic work and stained in a similar manner, is the standard preparation for determining the species of *Plasmodium*, *Babesia*, *Trypanosoma*, and microfilaria found. Thin smears for parasitologic work are fixed and then preferably stained manually with Giemsa stain, but automated hematologic staining is adequate. Smears are first scanned at low power to detect microfilariae, which are large objects (between 100 and 200 μm) and easily seen, usually at the lateral edges of the smear. After they are located, microfilariae should be studied under oil immersion for identification (see Ch. 61). Following scanning with low power, the smear is examined with a high dry objective, searching for trypanosomes; and finally under oil immersion, to find and identify *Plasmodium*, *Babesia*, and *Trypanosoma*.

Thick smears are useful for detecting all the parasites mentioned earlier, and are part of the minimum laboratory work-up for their diagnosis. A drop of blood is placed on a clean glass slide and, with the corner of another slide, is gently spread to cover 1 cm square. The preparation is allowed to dry and without fixation is stained with Giemsa stain, allowing for its dehemoglobinization.

Body Fluids

Cerebrospinal Fluid

CSF is collected to diagnose meningitis and, less frequently, viral encephalitis. Infectious meningitis, a medical emergency requiring early therapy to prevent death or serious neurologic sequelae, is divided into acute, subacute, and chronic clinical syndromes, based on duration of symptoms (Table 63–2). An acute presentation occurs in about 10% of cases and is most likely to be caused by pyogenic bacteria. Almost all persons with viral meningitis and about 75% of those with bacterial meningitis have a subacute presentation; the rest present with chronic meningitis (responsible pathogens are listed in Table 63–2). The enteroviruses are the agents most commonly responsible for meningitis, and they should be considered first in the differential diagnosis of meningitis in a child or adolescent during the late summer and early fall. The pyogenic bacteria responsible for meningitis vary with the age of the affected individual (Table 63–3).

VII

Table 63–2 Infectious Meningitis Syndromes

Syndrome	Onset/Duration	Probable Pathogens
Acute	<24 hours	Pyogenic bacteria
Subacute	1–7 days	Enteroviruses, pyogenic bacteria
Chronic	Persisting at least 4 weeks	*Mycobacterium tuberculosis*
		Treponema pallidum
		Brucella sp.
		Leptospira interrogans
		Borrelia burgdorferi
		Cryptococcus neoformans
		Coccidioides immitis
		Histoplasma capsulatum
		Candida sp.

Table 63–3 Common Bacterial Causes of Acute Meningitis by Age

Age	Organisms
Neonates–3 months	Group B streptococcus
	Escherichia coli
	Listeria monocytogenes[*]
	Streptococcus pneumoniae
4 months–6 years[†]	*Streptococcus pneumoniae*
6–45 years	*Neisseria meningitidis*
>45 years	*Streptococcus pneumoniae*
	Listeria monocytogenes
	Group B streptococcus

[*] May cause meningitis in immunocompromised individuals in all age groups.
[†] Incidence of meningitis due to *Haemophilus influenzae* type b in the United States has declined dramatically as a result of vaccination.

Table 63–4 Normal Cerebrospinal Fluid Parameters and Changes in Infectious Meningitis

Condition	WBCs (cells/μL)[*]		Protein (mg/dL)	Glucose (mg/dL)
Normal	5 (lymphocytes)		14–45	45–100 (²/₃ serum)
Meningitis				
Acute/subacute bacterial	500–200 000 (PMNs)	↑	↑	↓
Chronic bacterial	200–2000		↑	↓
tuberculous, fungal	(lymphocytes)		↑	↓
Enteroviral	200–2000 (PMNs early; lymphocytes later)	↑		Normal

↑ = increased; ↓ = decreased; PMNs = polymorphonuclear leukocytes; WBC = white blood cells.

[*] Cell type listed usually predominates.

Sample Collection and Transport

CSF is usually obtained by lumbar spinal puncture but sometimes it is aspirated from the ventricles or collected from a shunt. As when collecting blood for culture, careful skin antisepsis is essential for collection of CSF, which typically is submitted to the laboratory in three tubes. Suggestions for tests performed on fluid in each tube are: tube 1, cell counts and differential stains; tube 2, preparation of smears to stain with the Gram's stain or other stains and for culture; tube 3, protein and glucose and, if indicated, special tests such as the cryptococcal antigen, serologic test for syphilis, other serologic studies, and cytology. The parameters of normal CSF and the usual changes that occur during meningitis caused by different organisms are shown in Table 63–4.

CSF should be transported promptly to the laboratory and processed as rapidly as possible. If a brief delay in processing is unavoidable, the specimen should be held at room temperature unless viral culture is requested, in which case a portion (preferably 1 mL but no less than 0.5 mL) may be refrigerated for a short time. Specimen processing differs for bacteria, fungi, viruses, and parasites and is discussed separately for each group of organisms.

Sample Processing for Bacterial and Fungal Culture

Processing CSF for routine bacterial culture includes concentration (if 1 mL or more of specimen is received), preparation of a smear by cytocentrifugation for staining with Gram's stain, and culture. Concentrate the fluid by centrifugation at a minimum of $1500 \times g$ for 15 minutes. The supernatant is decanted into a sterile tube, leaving about 0.5 mL of sediment and fluid, which is thoroughly mixed on a vortex mixer or by forcefully aspirating up and down into a sterile pipette.

Diagnosis of chronic bacterial meningitis requires specific requests because the CSF is handled differently for each entity. To diagnose brucellosis, the CSF is processed as described earlier for routine bacterial culture, but the media are incubated for 2–3 weeks. For leptospirosis, *Leptospira interrogans* may be cultured from the CSF during the first few weeks of illness. Special media (listed earlier under blood) are inoculated with a few drops of CSF and incubated as outlined in Chapter 56.

The diagnosis of neurosyphilis is based on the following findings in the CSF: pleocytosis, elevated protein concentration, and a positive Venereal Disease Research Laboratory (VDRL) test (CSF VDRL), which currently is the only useful method for detecting antibodies to *Treponema pallidum* in the CSF (see Ch. 58). The CSF VDRL test is indicated only if the person has a positive serum test for syphilis (Albright, 1991a). The specimen should be refrigerated until it is tested. Involvement of the central nervous system by *B. burgdorferi* (Lyme disease) also is diagnosed serologically, by detection of specific IgM and IgG in CSF and serum.

Processing CSF for detection of mycobacteria is indicated only for samples with pleocytosis, or decreased glucose, or elevated protein values (Albright, 1991b). For optimal recovery, culture of at least 5 mL is recommended. The fluid is centrifuged at $3000–3600 \times g$ for 30 minutes, the supernatant is decanted, and the sediment is thoroughly mixed on a vortex mixer and used to prepare smears for staining and to inoculate appropriate media (see Ch. 59). Nucleic acid amplification, using a modification of a commercial assay, may be useful for direct detection of *Mycobacterium tuberculosis* complex in CSF (Cloud, 2004)

Processing CSF for detection of fungi is similar to that described for detection of bacteria. Organisms are concentrated by filtration or by centrifugation. A cytocentrifuge preparation or a smear of the sediment

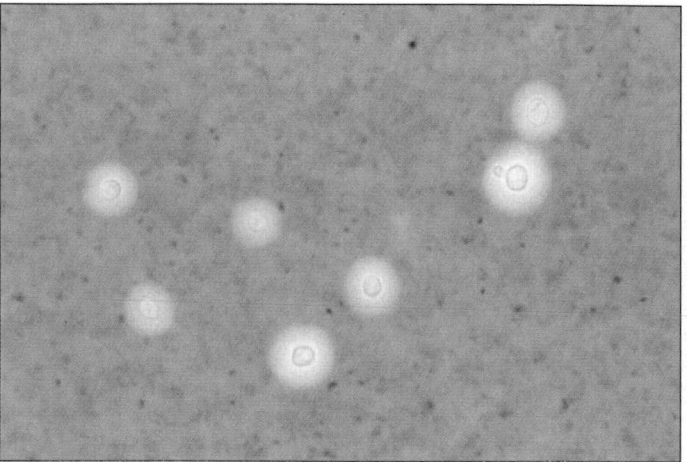

Figure 63–1 India ink preparation of cerebrospinal fluid shows encapsulated yeast forms of *Cryptococcus neoformans*. (×400.)

stained with the Gram's stain is examined, and appropriate media (such as brain–heart infusion or SABHI agar without antibiotics) are inoculated for culture.

Additional Diagnostic Tests

In addition to smears stained with the Gram's stain and bacterial culture, the supernatant of a centrifuged specimen or the original fluid may be used to perform latex agglutination tests for detection of antigens of group B streptococcus, *S. pneumoniae*, some serotypes of *Neisseria meningitidis*, *Escherichia coli* (the K1 capsular antigen cross-reacts with that of *N. meningitidis* type B), and *H. influenzae* type b. These latex tests are most useful in diagnosing partially treated meningitis (Bhisitkul, 1994; Maxson, 1994) and in confirming a positive Gram-stained smear. The routine use of latex tests should be discouraged because, compared with smears stained with Gram's stain, their sensitivity is not significantly greater and they are much more expensive (Kiska, 1995; Perkins, 1995).

Rapid tests are available for diagnosis of meningitis caused by *C. neoformans*. These include the India ink preparation, latex agglutination, and an enzyme-linked immunosorbent assay (ELISA). The latter two are specific for the capsular antigen. Encapsulated yeast cells of *C. neoformans* are visible in CSF mixed with India ink (one drop of CSF sediment with one drop of India ink, available at art supply stores) on a glass slide, coverslipped and examined under high-power magnification (Fig. 63–1). The sensitivity of the India ink stain is low, except in HIV-infected persons; therefore, the cryptococcal latex agglutination test or the ELISA, both of which are highly specific and have sensitivities of over 90%, is recommended for diagnosis. Supernatant of a centrifuged specimen, or unspun CSF can be used for these latter two tests. False-positive latex agglutination results occur, due to the presence of *Trichosporon asahii* or to the introduction of trace amounts of condensation from agar into the test fluid. To avoid the latter problem, the latex test should be performed before culture or, better, on a separate sample (Heelan, 1991).

Sample Processing for Viral Culture and Parasitology

Processing CSF for diagnosis of viral infections involves conventional cell culture (primarily for detection of enteroviruses) or, for viruses that cause encephalitis (western equine, eastern equine, Venezuelan equine, St Louis, Japanese, and La Crosse and West Nile), serologic tests. In addition, the PCR is a useful tool for detection of enteroviruses, HSV, and CMV nucleic acid in CSF (Lakeman, 1995; Mitchell, 1997; Jacques, 2003; Lai, 2003). Cell lines for isolation of enteroviruses are those discussed earlier for blood specimens.

CSF is occasionally sent to the laboratory for diagnosis of African trypanosomiasis (*Trypanosoma gambiense* and *Trypanosoma rhodesiense*) or infection with free-living amoebae (*Naegleria fowleri* and species of *Acanthamoeba*). Once the specimen is received in the laboratory, it should be processed immediately. Wet preparations are prepared directly from the specimen and from the sediment, prepared by first shaking the tube gently (a step necessary because the parasites often stick to the wall of the tube) and then centrifuging the specimen at $250 \times g$ for 10 minutes. Preparations are examined under the microscope with the condenser in a low position to allow visualization of trophozoites or, preferably, by phase contrast microscopy.

Cultures of free-living amoebae from CSF are done on non-nutrient agar plates covered with a suspension of *E. coli* or *Enterobacter aerogenes*. The fluid is centrifuged at $250 \times g$ for 10 minutes, the supernatant is removed with a sterile pipette, and the sediment is mixed with 0.5 mL of saline solution and poured at the center of the plate. The culture is incubated at 37°C and examined for amebas daily for 10 days using a microscope, under a 10× objective (Martinez, 1991).

Other Body Fluids

Fluid is collected from the pericardial, thoracic, or peritoneal cavity, or from joint spaces, by aspirating with a needle and syringe. A volume of 1–5 mL is adequate for isolating most bacteria, but 10–15 mL is optimal for recovery of mycobacteria and fungi, which are generally present in low numbers. Moreover, to diagnose peritonitis associated with chronic ambulatory peritoneal dialysis, collection of at least 50 mL of fluid may improve recovery of the responsible pathogen (Dawson, 1985). To transport the fluid, it is aspirated into a sterile container and delivered promptly to the laboratory. Alternatively, peritoneal fluid may be directly inoculated into blood culture bottles at the patient's bedside (Luce, 1988); however submission of fluid in blood culture bottles eliminates the possibility of direct Gram staining and delays the identification and susceptibility of any pathogens isolated.

Enteroviruses, primarily Coxsackie viruses A and B, are among the most common causes of infectious pericarditis. These viruses may be detected in pericardial fluid by conventional cell culture but, because they are not recovered in all cases, collection of throat washings and stool (which are more likely to yield the virus), in addition to pericardial fluid, is strongly recommended for virus isolation from persons with suspected enteroviral pericarditis. Other viruses (HSV, varicella zoster virus, CMV, Epstein–Barr virus, hepatitis B virus, mumps virus, and influenza virus) are infrequent agents of pericarditis and usually are not detected in pericardial fluid.

Sample Processing for Bacterial Culture

Processing fluid from body cavities for detection of bacteria involves preparing a smear for Gram's stain and inoculating appropriate media for culture. As mentioned previously, the sample may be inoculated into blood culture bottles at the bedside, although this is not optimal, or it may be processed in the laboratory. In the laboratory the fluid is centrifuged at $1500–2500 \times g$ for 20–30 minutes. The supernatant is removed, leaving about 0.5 mL fluid in addition to the sediment, which is mixed thoroughly and then used to prepare smears and inoculate media. Alternatively, a small volume of noncloudy, nonviscous fluid (about 0.1 mL) may be removed before centrifugation and used to prepare a cytocentrifuged smear.

Fluid specimens submitted for detection of mycobacteria are processed as described earlier for CSF. Fluids for fungal culture should be concentrated by centrifugation as described for bacteria. The supernatant is removed, leaving 1.5–2.0 mL, in which the sediment is thoroughly mixed. A smear of the sediment is prepared for staining with Gram's or Calcofluor white. Ideally, 0.5–1.0 mL of sediment is inoculated to primary fungal planting media (as for CSF), but lesser volumes are acceptable.

Parasitological Examination

Body fluids are rarely collected for detection of parasites; however, *Entamoeba histolytica* may be found in the pericardial, pleural, or peritoneal cavity as a result of rupture of an abscess of the liver (into the peritoneal, pleural, or pericardial cavity) or of the lungs (into the pleural or pericardial

cavity) or to perforation of amebic ulcers (into the peritoneal cavity). Hydatid cysts are infrequently diagnosed by examination of body cavity fluid, also due to rupture of a cyst into a viscus contiguous to the cavity in question. The fluid collected is usually clear and contains hydatid sand (see Ch. 61) but rarely is turbid because of superimposed bacterial infection. Uncommonly, in individuals with a filarial infection, examination of wet preparations of a body cavity fluid may demonstrate the microfilariae; and in patients with *Strongyloides* hyperinfection, larvae may be detected in body cavity fluids.

Tissues

Tissue specimens obtained surgically are procured at great expense and at considerable risk to the patient; therefore, it behooves the surgeon to obtain an amount of material that is adequate for both histopathologic and microbiological examination. Swabs are rarely adequate for this purpose. The histopathology of the lesion serves not only to differentiate between infection and malignancy but also to distinguish between a suppurative and a granulomatous process. In some cases, special stains are helpful in establishing the etiology of the process. In chronic lesions the differential diagnosis includes disease due to actinomycetes, brucellas, mycobacteria, and fungi, any one of which may be present only in small numbers, again emphasizing the need for obtaining adequate samples for examination and culture.

Specimen Collection and Processing

Tissue obtained surgically for culture should be placed into a sterile, wide-mouthed, screw-capped container. As a general rule, tissue should be bisected aseptically by the surgeon in the operating room and material representative of the pathologic process should be submitted for both histopathologic and microbiological examination. Good communication between histopathologist and microbiologist is important, especially in cases of fever of unknown origin for which an exploratory laparotomy is being performed and multiple biopsy specimens are taken.

Tissue received in the laboratory is finely minced with sterile scissors or scalpels, added to a small volume of broth, and then rendered homogeneous either in a tissue grinder, mortar and pestle, or stomacher to provide a 20% suspension. This suspension is used to inoculate all of the necessary culture media and is then stored under refrigeration for at least 2 weeks before being discarded.

Eye

Conjunctival Specimens

Conjunctival scrapings or swab specimens are collected to determine the etiologic agent of conjunctivitis. Bacteria are the most common etiologic agents of infectious conjunctivitis, and those most frequently implicated are *S. pneumoniae*, *Staphylococcus aureus*, and *Staphylococcus epidermidis* in adults; and *H. influenzae*, *S. pneumoniae*, and *S. aureus* in children. Trachoma, caused by *C. trachomatis*, is a leading cause of blindness worldwide. *C. trachomatis* also may cause inclusion conjunctivitis in newborns and, less commonly, in adults. Viruses are responsible for about 15–20% of cases of acute infectious conjunctivitis, and in the United States, most epidemics of viral conjunctivitis are caused by adenoviruses. Rarely, parasites are causes of conjunctivitis.

Specimen Collection and Processing

Conjunctival cells are obtained from the superior and inferior tarsal conjunctiva by using a swab moistened with broth or a sterile platinum spatula. Ideally, smears are prepared and, if a bacterial or fungal infection is suspected, culture media are inoculated directly by the individual collecting the sample. If direct preparation of smears and inoculation of media is not possible, swab specimens may be collected. Smears should be air-dried and promptly transported, with the inoculated media, to the laboratory. If viral culture is requested, a second sample (swab or scrapings) is collected, placed in viral transport medium, and delivered promptly to the laboratory, or refrigerated for a short time and then transported on wet ice. A rapid diagnosis may be provided by direct or indirect immunofluorescent staining of smears of conjunctival cells with virus-specific antibodies, but cell culture is the most sensitive method for detecting potential viral pathogens and always should be done.

To detect *C. trachomatis*, a smear prepared directly from conjunctival scrapings may be stained with the Giemsa stain and examined for epithelial cells with basophilic intracytoplasmic inclusions diagnostic of

For optimal detection of mycobacteria in sputum, collection of three samples on three separate days is recommended. Sputum and other respiratory secretions must be decontaminated to prevent the normal respiratory flora from overgrowing the slower-growing mycobacteria. This process and detection methods are discussed in Chapter 59. All specimens submitted for mycobacterial stain, culture, and molecular testing should be processed in a biological safety cabinet, preferably in an isolated room with negative air pressure (level 3 laboratory).

All specimens submitted for fungal culture should also be handled as described for mycobacteria. The quality of the specimens should be determined by screening with smears stained with Gram's stain (as described earlier for bacteria). Acceptable expectorated sputum, induced sputum, and tracheal aspirate specimens should be inoculated to culture media for recovery of fungi. In general, to culture fungi media with and without blood enrichment, and media containing antimicrobial agents should be used. However, when making media selection, the laboratory director also should consider cost and the types of fungus usually encountered in the patient population served by the laboratory.

Induced sputum specimens are useful for diagnosis of *Pneumocystis jiroveci* (previously *Pneumocystis carinii*) pneumonia in persons with the acquired immunodeficiency syndrome (AIDS) (Wolfson, 1990). First, a Gram-stained smear of the specimen is examined to determine whether it is representative of lower respiratory tract secretions. Acceptable specimens are treated with a mucolytic agent (such as *N*-acetyl-L-cysteine), and smears are prepared and stained for detection of *P. jiroveci* (see Ch. 60).

Bronchoscopy Specimens

Bronchoalveolar lavage fluid and protected brush specimens are useful for diagnosis of bacterial pneumonia in ventilated patients who have not received antimicrobial therapy, and for detection of opportunistic pathogens in immunocompromised patients with pneumonia (Baselski, 1994; Carroll, 2002). Data indicate that culture of bronchoalveolar lavage specimens is also useful for diagnosis of acute bacterial pneumonia (Baselski, 1994). All bronchoscopy specimens should be plated quantitatively to determine significance of potential pathogens recovered. Only protected brush specimens are suitable for anaerobic culture (Baselski, 1994). For culture of species of *Legionella*, sputum specimens are preferable because bronchoalveolar lavage samples are diluted with saline and may contain small amounts of the anesthetic used locally, which inhibits the organism.

Specimen Collection and Transport

The protected brush sample is collected with a small brush that holds 0.001–0.01 mL of secretions, placed in a catheter, within a double cannula. The outer cannula has a displaceable polyethylene glycol plug at the tip. To obtain a specimen, the cannula is inserted to the desired area via bronchoscopy, the inner cannula is pushed out, dislodging the protective plug (water-soluble), and the brush is extended even farther, beyond the inner cannula. Once the sample is taken, the brush is pulled back into the inner cannula, and both brush and inner cannula are pulled into the outer cannula to prevent contamination of the brush when the catheter is removed. The brush then is placed in 1 mL of sterile saline or broth. The specimen should be transported immediately to the laboratory and processed as soon as possible. If a delay is unavoidable, the specimen should be stored in the refrigerator.

To collect bronchoalveolar fluid, the tip of the bronchoscope is carefully wedged into an airway lumen. A volume of saline (usually >140 mL) in three to four aliquots is injected through the lumen, sampling an estimated 1 million alveoli. The total volume returned varies based on the volume instilled, but is typically 10–100 mL. The transport time to the laboratory should be minimal (<30 min) and, once it is in the laboratory, the specimen should be processed as soon as possible. If a delay cannot be avoided, the fluid should be stored in the refrigerator.

Specimen Processing

To process the protected brush specimen, the fluid in which the brush is suspended is agitated on a vortex mixer and the resulting suspension is used for a cytospin preparation and for culture inoculum. Using a calibrated 0.01 mL inoculating loop, the suspension is plated onto appropriate media and carefully streaked for isolation. Colony counts of more than 1000 CFU/ml of potential pathogens (corresponding to 10^6 organisms/mL of the original specimen) appear to correlate with infection (Baselski, 1994). The bronchoalveolar sample is inoculated onto agar media by using a 0.001 mL calibrated inoculating loop (as used for urine cultures, described in the following section). The presence of more than 10 000 CFU/ml of fluid correlates with disease. Staining cytocentrifuge

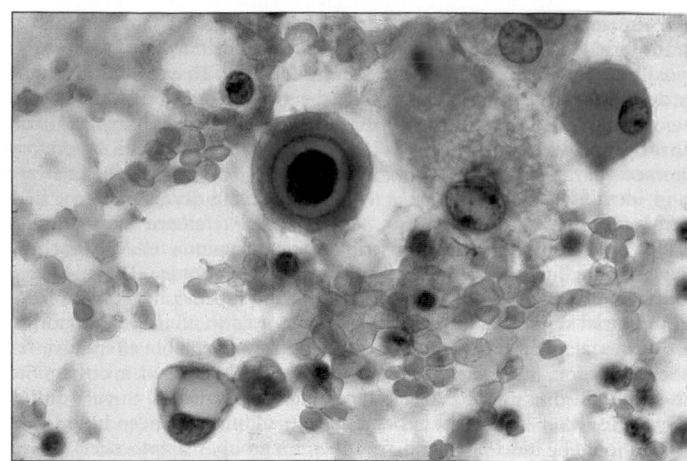

Figure 63–4 Cytologic preparation of bronchoalveolar lavage fluid shows an enlarged cell with intranuclear and intracytoplasmic inclusions, consistent with cytomegalovirus. (Papanicolaou's stain, × 250.) (Courtesy of Vicki J. Schnadig, M.D., Department of Pathology, University of Texas Medical Branch, Galveston, TX.)

preparations of the fluid with Gram's stain is recommended; visualizing one or more bacteria without squamous epithelial cells per oil immersion field strongly suggests acute bacterial pneumonia (Kahn, 1987; Baselski, 1994).

Processing bronchoalveolar lavage specimens for detection of viruses includes direct microscopic examination and conventional cell culture. Examination of cytocentrifuge preparations stained with the Papanicolaou stain allows detection of cytopathic changes, especially useful for diagnosis of CMV pneumonia (Fig. 63–4) (Woods, 1990). Cytospin preparations also may be stained with an acid-fast stain; with specific antibodies, such as those for detection of *Legionella* species or *P. jiroveci*; or with nonspecific stains for detection of *P. jiroveci* or other fungi (such as a silver stain, Calcofluor white, or Giemsa). For detection of mycobacteria, the specimen should be decontaminated and handled as described in Chapter 59. To recover fungi the sediment of a centrifuged specimen should be inoculated on to primary fungal media.

Urinary Tract

The urinary tract above the urethra is sterile in healthy humans but the urethra is normally colonized with many different bacteria, so urine specimens collected by a noninvasive method (such as the clean-catch, midstream specimen) become contaminated during their passage. Commensal bacteria are differentiated from potential pathogens by quantitative cultures of urine, a procedure initially promoted by Kass (1956). Originally, growth of $\geq 10^5$ CFU of bacteria per milliliter of urine was considered highly indicative of infection, but this criterion has been modified for different situations. For example, in young, sexually active women with the acute urethral syndrome (dysuria, frequency, and urgency), as few as 10^2 CFU/mL is considered significant in the presence of concomitant pyuria (Stamm, 1982). True urinary infections associated with fewer than 10^5 CFU/mL may occur in infants and children, in males, and in persons who are catheterized, were recently treated with antimicrobial agents, drink large amounts of fluids (which dilutes urine), have symptoms and concomitant pyuria, have urinary obstruction, or have pyelonephritis acquired from hematogenous spread (especially infections due to yeast and *S. aureus*) (Pezzlo, 1988; Baron, 1994). Consequently, proper interpretation of urine culture results requires communication between clinicians and laboratory personnel.

Specimen Collection and Transport

Acceptable methods of urine collection include midstream clean catch (preferably a first voided morning specimen), catheterization, and suprapubic aspiration. In general, 24 hour urine specimens should be rejected, except when detection of *Schistosoma haematobium* is requested specifically. Most commonly, the midstream flow of a clean-catch urine is collected. For women, the periurethral area and perineum is first cleansed with soapy sterile gauze pads in a front-to-back motion, rinsed with a moistened sterile gauze pad, and dried with a dry sterile gauze pad. For males, cleansing the genital area may not improve the detection of bacteriuria significantly and may not be necessary (Lipsky, 1984). During voiding, women should hold the labia apart and men who are not circumcised should hold back the foreskin. The first few milliliters of urine are passed into the toilet bowel or a bedpan, to flush out bacteria normally colonizing the urethra, and the midstream portion is collected in a sterile container with a wide mouth and tightly fitting lid.

Catheterization is associated with the risk of inducing a nosocomial infection and should therefore be restricted to persons who are unable to produce a midstream sample; for example, individuals with an altered sensorium or those unable to void for neurologic or urologic reasons. Using strict aseptic technique, the catheter is inserted into the urethra, the first few milliliters of urine passed are discarded to clear organisms that may have entered the tip of the catheter during placement, and the midportion of the sample is obtained for culture. Urine may be collected from an indwelling catheter by aspirating with a 28-gauge needle and syringe through the rubber connector between the catheter and the collecting tubing, taking care to first disinfect the puncture site. Urine should not be collected from catheter bags, and Foley catheter tips should not be accepted for culture because they almost always are contaminated with urethral organisms.

Suprapubic aspiration is used primarily for neonates. The procedure requires a full bladder; the overlying skin is disinfected, the bladder is punctured above the symphysis pubis with a 22-gauge needle on a syringe, and about 10 mL of urine is aspirated.

All urine specimens should be transported promptly to the laboratory and should be processed within 2 hours after collection. If a delay in transport or processing cannot be avoided, specimens may be refrigerated up to 24 hours. Collection kits containing preservatives to maintain the bacterial population stable for 24 hours at room temperature are commercially available but offer no advantage over refrigeration.

Specimen Processing

Quantitative bacterial culture of a urine specimen is done by inoculating appropriate media (see Ch. 56) with a measured amount of urine, most commonly with a plastic or wire calibrated loop designed to deliver a known volume. A 0.001 mL loop is used to inoculate all urine specimens except those collected from women with suspected acute urethral syndrome and suprapubic aspirates. Both the latter are inoculated with a 0.01 mL loop. The appropriate loop is inserted vertically into the well-mixed urine sample, and the loopful of urine removed is spread over the surface of the agar plate as illustrated in Figure 63–5. Without reflaming, the loop is again inserted vertically into the urine, and the sample removed is inoculated to a second plate.

Some bacteria are not detected by routine culture of urine and, when these pathogens are suspected, specific tests must be requested. For example, urine is an acceptable specimen for detection of *N. gonorrhoeae*

and *C. trachomatis* by nucleic acid amplification. The manufacturer's directions for urine collection and processing must be followed. *Leptospira interrogans* may be detected in urine after the first week of illness and for several months thereafter. Urine should be processed as soon as possible after collection, because acidity may harm the organisms. One or two drops of undiluted urine, and urine diluted 1:10 in broth, are inoculated to 5 mL of Fletcher's medium or Ellinghausen–McCullough–Johnson–Harris medium containing 5-fluorouracil. Culture of urine for mycobacteria is discussed in Chapter 59. Yeasts may be recovered from urine on the media plated for routine bacterial culture but, if fungal culture is specifically requested, the sediment of a centrifuged urine specimen should be plated on to media such as inhibitory mold or SABHI agar containing antibacterial agents.

When urine specimens are submitted for culture of viruses they should be submitted in liquid media containing antibiotics (e.g., penicillin, gentamicin, and amphotericin B), or antibiotics should be added to the sample when it is received in the laboratory, to minimize bacterial contamination of cell cultures. Cell lines are selected for inoculation based on the viruses most commonly isolated – CMV, adenovirus, and HSV.

Over half the urine specimens submitted to the clinical laboratory for culture yield no growth or have bacterial counts below levels considered clinically significant; therefore, screening tests that quickly identify urine samples yielding 'negative' culture results have been developed in an attempt to provide rapid results, eliminate negative specimens, and allow more time for positive specimens, thus improving efficiency and cost. Urine screen and culture results correlate well when 10^5 CFU/mL or greater is the reference, but they compare less favorably in the presence of lower colony counts (Pezzlo, 1988). Other issues to consider regarding the use of bacteriuria screens are the ability to detect pyuria and the cost. The latter is especially important when considering automation.

Screening urine specimens by staining with Gram's stain is rapid and economical. Finding one or more organisms per oil immersion field in a smear prepared from an uncentrifuged specimen correlates well with bacteriuria at 10^5 CFU/mL or greater (Rippin, 1995). The sensitivity of Gram's stain, however, decreases when compared with lower colony counts, and examination of smears is tedious and time-consuming. Commercially available dipstick tests that combine nitrate reductase (an enzyme present in most of the Gram-negative bacilli that cause urinary tract infections) and leukocyte esterase (an enzyme produced by neutrophils) are rapid, inexpensive, and simple to perform, but their sensitivity is too low for use as single screen for urinary tract infections (Pezzlo, 1988; Shaw, 1998; Semeniuk, 1999).

Several automated urine screening systems are commercially available. A colorimetric filtration system provides rapid results and detects over 90% of all positive samples (including those containing neutrophils and only 10^2 CFU/mL), but may yield false-negative results with enterococci and *P. aeruginosa* (Pezzlo, 1988; Shaw, 1997). Urine is forced through a filter paper that retains cells, and then a stain is passed through the filter. The intensity of the resulting color, read manually or with a photometer, correlates with the number of particles adhering to the filter.

A bioluminescent system is based on the reaction of adenosine triphosphate (present in all living cells) with luciferin and luciferase, which produces light that is measured by a luminometer. By selectively releasing adenosine triphosphate from bacteria alone, the number of CFU in a urine sample may be estimated. This technique compares favorably with culture at a level of 10^5 CFUs/mL or more but, because it requires an incubation step, results are not available for a few hours. Another system combines staining and video image analysis as a rapid screen. This method has greater than 92% sensitivity with colony counts of 10^4 CFU/ml or more.

Genital Tract

Specimens from genital sites are submitted for detection of microorganisms responsible for several clinical syndromes, each of which are associated with certain pathogens. The syndromes each have a distinctive clinical presentation and require specific collection, transport, and testing procedures. For many tests the manufacturer's collection and transport devices must be used for optimal detection of the responsible pathogen.

Vaginal Secretions

Vaginal secretions are useful in determining the etiologic agent of vulvovaginitis and bacterial vaginosis (so named because the condition is noninvasive). In postpubescent females, the most common pathogens are *Gardnerella vaginalis* (in association with anaerobes such as *Mobiluncus* spp.), species of *Candida*, and *Trichomonas vaginalis*. A wet-mount preparation is the most valuable diagnostic test and may be performed by

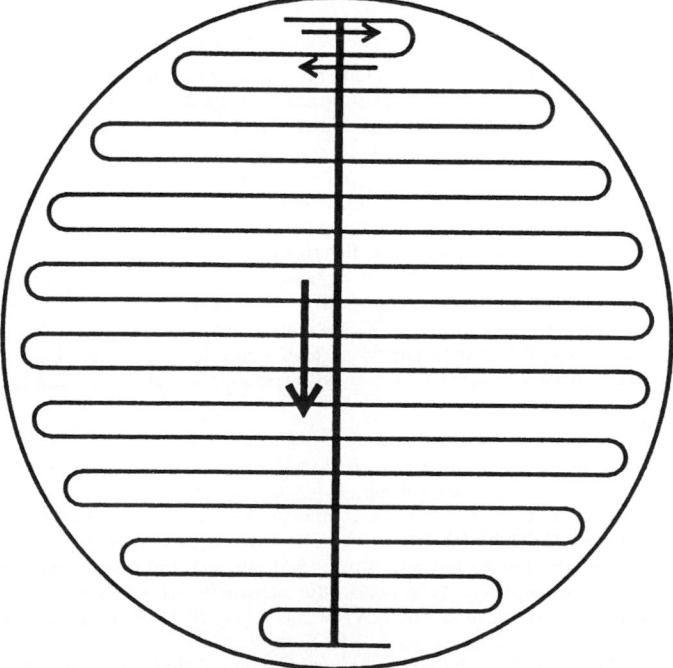

Figure 63–5 Technique for inoculating urine onto agar plates. (Redrawn from Woods GL, Gutierrez Y: Diagnostic Pathology of Infectious Diseases. Philadelphia, PA, Lea & Febiger, 1993.)

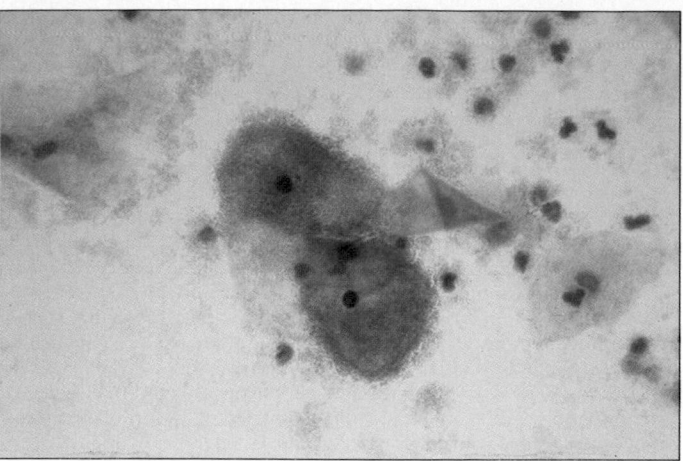

Figure 63–6 'Clue cells' in a smear of vaginal discharge. (Papanicolaou's stain, × 400.) (Courtesy of Vicki J. Schnadig, M.D., Department of Pathology, University of Texas Medical Branch, Galveston, TX.)

the attending physician; cultures are not necessary for diagnosis. A swab of the discharge is placed in a tube containing about 1 mL of normal saline and transported to the laboratory. Remove the swab from the saline and firmly press the swab tip several times against a glass slide to express liquid and cellular material. Coverslip the slide and examine it under low- and high-power magnifications, looking for 'clue cells' (epithelial cells covered with small coccobacillary bacteria) (Fig. 63–6), consistent with the diagnosis of nonspecific vaginosis; pseudohyphae, suggestive of vaginal candidiasis; and motile trichomonads. Detection of all three pathogens also can be accomplished with a commercial vaginal pathogens PCR test (Briselden, 1994). Swabs and transport tubes supplied by the test manufacturer must be used.

Other useful diagnostic tests are vaginal pH and the 'whiff test.' The vaginal pH is usually about 4.5 in women with vulvovaginal candidiasis but is above 4.5 in those with bacterial vaginosis or trichomoniasis. A positive whiff test is determined by the generation of a pungent, fishy odor after addition of 10% potassium hydroxide to a drop of vaginal discharge placed on a slide or on the speculum. This is associated predominantly with bacterial vaginosis but occasionally occurs with trichomoniasis.

Endocervical and Urethral Specimens

Endocervical specimens are collected to determine the etiologic agent(s) of cervicitis and to identify asymptomatic persons infected with an organism that causes sexually transmitted disease. Endocervical specimens are obtained after the cervix is visualized with the aid of a speculum moistened only with warm water, because lubricants may contain antibacterial agents. If a Papanicolaou smear is indicated, that sample should be collected first.

Specimens for microbiological studies are generally collected with a swab. As discussed earlier in this chapter, using a polyester-tipped swab with a plastic shaft is recommended. If a nonculture test kit is used for organism detection, the specimen must be collected with the swab supplied or specified by the manufacturer. Before collecting specimens for detection of *N. gonorrhoeae* and *C. trachomatis*, all secretions and discharge must be removed from the cervical os. The swab or brush then is inserted 1–2 cm into the endocervical canal (past the squamocolumnar junction), rotated firmly against the wall for 10–30 seconds, withdrawn without touching the surface of the vagina, and placed in the appropriate transport medium or tube system, used to prepare a slide for direct fluorescent antibody staining (for *C. trachomatis*), or used to immediately inoculate an agar medium for recovery of *N. gonorrhoeae*.

Specimen handling varies based on the organism sought. To isolate *N. gonorrhoeae*, direct inoculation of a selective agar medium, such as modified Thayer–Martin, within a container to which a CO_2-generating tablet is added, is optimal. Alternatively, the swab specimen can be placed in a tube transport system and delivered to the laboratory within 2 hours. If a delay in transport cannot be avoided, the swab should be left at room temperature, never refrigerated. If a DNA probe or nucleic acid amplification is used for detection of *N. gonorrhoeae*, the collection kit provided by the manufacturer must be used and the storage and transport instructions followed.

For detection of *C. trachomatis*, culture or non-culture methods may be used (see Ch. 55). For chlamydial culture, the specimen should be

transported in M4 media, which contains antibiotics to inhibit overgrowth of bacteria and fungi. To maintain the viability of *Chlamydia* organisms, the specimen should be transported to the laboratory immediately or stored in the refrigerator if immediate transport is not feasible. In the laboratory the specimen should be processed as soon as possible. If a delay in processing is unavoidable, specimens should be stored in the refrigerator if they can be processed within 48 hours. To detect chlamydial elementary bodies by DFA staining, the collection kit provided by the manufacturer must be used and the directions followed. The swab specimen is rolled over the microscope slide, allowed to dry, and the fixative provided is applied. For enzyme immunoassay, DNA probes, and nucleic acid amplification the collection kit/transport system provided by the manufacturer must be used, unless the manufacturer specifically states that an alternative transport system is acceptable. Manufacturers' guidelines concerning transport conditions, storage requirements, and time to processing must also be followed.

For optimal detection of HSV, cell culture is recommended. The swab specimen is placed in viral transport medium such as M4 and transported as soon as possible to the laboratory. If immediate delivery is not feasible, the specimen should be stored in the refrigerator. For patients who have visible lesions on the cervix, viral cytopathic changes may be seen in smears prepared from scrapings of the lesion base. Smears are fixed immediately and stained with Wright's or Giemsa stain (Tzanck preparation), which will not distinguish HSV and varicella zoster virus, or with a monoclonal antibody.

Genital tract infection with human papilloma virus (HPV) is thought to be the most common sexually transmitted disease in the United States, and infection with a high-risk type is the major risk factor for development of cervical carcinoma. Since it is not possible to culture the virus in vitro, other diagnostic methods must be used. Squamous cell changes can be visualized on exfoliated cell samples (Papanicolaou smear), but molecular techniques (e.g. nucleic acid hybridization with signal amplification and PCR) are more sensitive. Kit manufacturers' collection and transport instructions must be followed.

To detect *C. trachomatis* and *N. gonorrhoeae* in males, a urethral swab specimen or first-voided urine sample, depending on the detection method used, should be obtained. Optimally, urethral swab specimens are collected at least 2 hours after the patient has voided. Samples for *N. gonorrhoeae* are obtained first. The conditions concerning types of swab and specimen transport are the same as those described for endocervical swab specimens, although the smaller urogenital swabs are used. The swab is inserted into the urethra for 2–4 cm, rotated in one direction for 5 seconds, withdrawn, and placed in the appropriate transport medium or used to prepare smears for direct fluorescent antibody staining to detect *C. trachomatis* or for Gram's staining to diagnose gonorrhea (detection of intracellular Gram-negative diplococci in a smear of urethral discharge from symptomatic men provides a presumptive diagnosis).

Vesicles

Vesicular genital lesions are sampled to confirm HSV infection. The vesicle fluid is aspirated with a small-gauge needle on a tuberculin syringe. If only a small vesicle is present, it is unroofed and the base is firmly scraped with a Dacron swab or tongue depressor to ensure collection of cells. Vesicle fluid or swab specimens should be placed in a viral transport medium and processed for conventional cell culture. HSV may also be detected directly in clinical specimens by direct staining of smears, but this is less sensitive than culture and, if negative, should be followed by culture. To make a smear, cells collected with a tongue depressor or a Dacron swab are spread on a glass slide, and the material is fixed in acetone. The smear may be stained with the Papanicolaou, Wright's or Giemsa stain for detection of typical cytopathic changes typical of HSV (varicella zoster virus has an identical appearance) (Fig. 63–7), or with specific monoclonal antibodies.

Ulcers

Material from genital ulcers is collected to identify the responsible pathogen; HSV, *Haemophilus ducreyi*, *T. pallidum*, *C. trachomatis* (serogroups L_1, L_2, L_3), and *Calymmatobacterium granulomatis* should be considered in the differential diagnosis. Collection, transport, and processing of material from ulcerative lesions for detection of HSV are identical to the protocol discussed for vesicles. In general, the sensitivity of the direct tests previously described and recovery of the virus are lower in ulcerative lesions.

If infection with *H. ducreyi* is suspected, material from the base of the ulcer is collected on two cotton or Dacron swabs. One swab is used to inoculate a chocolate agar plate at the bedside. If bedside inoculation is not possible, the swab should be transported in modified Stuart's medium

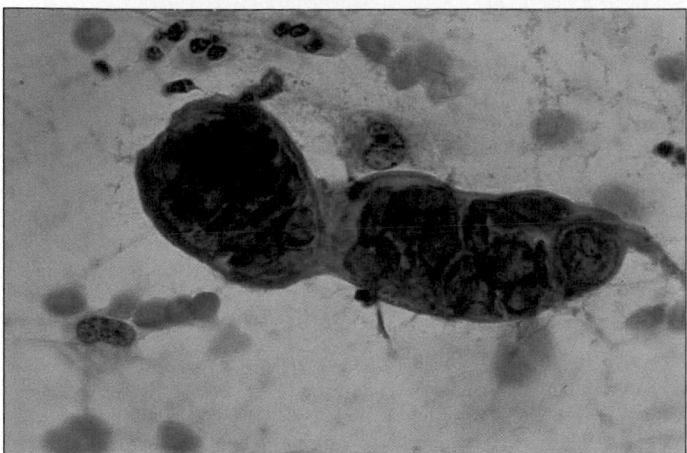

Figure 63–7 Multinucleate giant cell with intranuclear inclusions consistent with herpes simplex virus in a smear of endocervical cells. (Papanicolaou's stain, × 400.) (Courtesy of Vicki J. Schnadig, M.D., Department of Pathology, University of Texas Medical Branch, Galveston, TX.)

to the laboratory, and held at room temperature until processed. The second swab is used to prepare a smear for staining with Gram's stain. Observing many small pleomorphic Gram-negative coccobacilli arranged in groups of chains resembling a 'school of fish' suggests *H. ducreyi*. Culture, however, is more sensitive and is necessary for confirmation.

T. pallidum spirochetes may be detected in genital or other lesions but syphilis is usually diagnosed serologically. Gloves should be worn when examining lesions of suspected syphilis and when handling specimens obtained from those lesions. To collect the specimens, the surface of the lesion (if multiple lesions are present, the youngest should be selected) is cleaned with saline and blotted dry, and crusts are removed if present. The lesion is superficially abraded until slight bleeding occurs, and gentle pressure is applied to its base. The clear serum exudate from the subsurface is collected by touching the fluid with a glass slide or by using a capillary pipette and transferring the fluid to a glass slide. A coverslip is placed on the fluid and the specimen is examined immediately by dark-field microscopy. Alternatively, lesion material is aspirated with a 26-gauge needle inserted at the base, after which a drop of saline is drawn into the needle. The material then is expressed on to a glass slide, covered with a cover glass, and examined immediately by dark-field microscopy. The spirochetes of *T. pallidum* are 10–13 μm long by about 0.15 μm wide, have a regular tight coil, and are pointed at the ends.

Serogroups L_1, L_2, and L_3 of *C. trachomatis* may be detected by cell culture in a biopsy of the ulcerated lesion or in cellular material collected by first removing any exudate from the lesion and then firmly rotating a swab (on a plastic stick) against its base. Specimen transport and processing are the same as discussed for endocervical swab specimens. For optimal detection of *C. granulomatis*, subsurface tissue from an area of active granulation is biopsied and immediately transported to the laboratory in a sterile, dry container or in one containing a small amount of sterile saline without preservatives. Smears are prepared from a crushed piece of the tissue and stained with Giemsa or Dieterle's stain. The diagnosis is based on finding characteristic, encapsulated *C. granulomatis* organisms within macrophages.

Feces

Feces and, in some cases, rectal swab specimens are useful for determining the etiologic agent of infectious diarrhea or food poisoning, confirming the diagnosis of botulism, and diagnosing infections caused by adenoviruses, enteroviruses, some sexually transmitted pathogens, intestinal protozoa and helminths, and, in some instances, helminths of the respiratory and biliary tracts. Collection, transport, and processing of these specimens are different for viruses, bacteria, and parasites and are discussed separately for each group.

Viruses

Specimen Collection and Transport

Stool is preferred for detection of adenoviruses, enteroviruses, and the viruses responsible for gastroenteritis. Specimens should be collected in a clean container with a tight lid. If feces cannot be obtained, a swab is

inserted beyond the anal sphincter, rotated, withdrawn, and placed in M4 transport medium. Deliver specimens promptly to the laboratory; if not, refrigerate for a short time and transport on wet ice. If the specimen must be mailed to a reference laboratory, store at –70°C and ship on dry ice.

Specimen processing

Cell culture is recommended for detection of adenoviruses and enteroviruses, although an ELISA for detection of adenoviruses is available. Rotaviruses are responsible for most cases of viral gastroenteritis. Most commonly, rotavirus is detected by ELISA; latex agglutination kits also are available but appear to be less sensitive (Christensen, 1989). Specimens are processed according to the manufacturer's directions. Direct examination of stool specimens by electron microscopy is the reference method for detection of rotavirus and is useful for detection of caliciviruses, astroviruses, and noroviruses. Noroviruses also can be detected by PCR.

Bacterial Pathogens

Collection and Transport

Stool also is preferred for detection of bacteria responsible for infectious diarrhea but a rectal swab specimen is an acceptable alternative. Stool cultures for patients who have been hospitalized for more than 3 days are inappropriate. Stool specimens should be collected in a clean container with a tight lid, and the specimen should not be contaminated with urine, barium, or toilet paper. Rectal swab specimens, obtained as described earlier for viruses, are placed in a tube transport system containing modified Stuart's medium. Both specimen types should be transported promptly (within 2 hours) to the laboratory and processed as soon as possible, because the drop in pH that occurs as the stool cools may inhibit the growth of some pathogens, especially *Shigella*. If a delay in processing is unavoidable, or if the specimen must be mailed to a reference laboratory, transport of an aliquot of the specimen in transport media such as Cary Blair is required. For *C. difficile* culture or toxin testing, 20–50 mL of liquid stool should be submitted in a sterile container. The stool specimen is stable for 2 days, refrigerated, or frozen for 1 week.

Specimen Processing

Processing stool or rectal swab specimens for detection of bacteria is based on the organism or group of organisms expected to be present. Specimens received for 'routine' bacterial culture should be processed to allow recovery of *Shigella*, *Salmonella*, Shiga-like toxin producing *E. coli* (STEC), *Campylobacter jejuni/coli*, and *Aeromonas* species by plating to appropriate differential, inhibitory and non-inhibitory media (see Ch. 56). The prevalence of gastroenteritis caused by *Yersinia enterocolitica*, *Vibrio cholerae* or other *Vibrio* species, or *Plesiomonas shigelloides* is low in most parts of the United States; therefore, specific requests for their detection are most cost effective.

To detect STEC, the stool specimen is inoculated onto sorbitol–MacConkey agar (containing 1% D-sorbitol instead of lactose), a medium that differentiates isolates of STEC, which do not ferment sorbitol, from almost all other *E. coli*, which are sorbitol-positive. A more sensitive method than culture for detection of STEC is detection of toxin in the stool or stool filtrate by enzyme immunoassay or PCR (Gavin, 2004; Pulz, 2003).

When isolation of *Y. enterocolitica* is requested, CIN agar is inoculated and incubated at room temperature. The organism also can be recovered by inoculating media typically used for 'routine' bacterial culture (see Ch. 56). A MacConkey plate may be incubated at room temperature for 48 hours. Colonies of *Y. enterocolitica* are purple and pinhead in size.

Species of *Vibrio* frequently grow on the media used for 'routine' stool culture but, for their optimal recovery, thiosulfate citrate bile salts sucrose (TCBS) agar is inoculated. *Plesiomonas shigelloides* also grows on media used for 'routine' culture; but because up to 30% of *P. shigelloides* isolates ferment lactose, their colonies do not appear sufficiently distinct to be recognized on these media, and screening all colonies for *Plesiomonas* is not cost-effective. For this reason, culture of stool or rectal swab specimens for *P. shigelloides* should be requested specifically. Use of the selective–differential medium inositol brilliant green bile salts agar has been suggested but is not essential.

Rectal swab specimens submitted for detection of *C. trachomatis* are placed in transport medium and delivered promptly to the laboratory, or are refrigerated for a short time. Rectal swab specimens collected to diagnose gonorrhea are treated as discussed earlier for endocervical specimens.

Stool specimens or gastric contents collected from persons with short incubation food poisoning should be evaluated for *S. aureus* and *Bacillus*

VII

cereus. Processing includes preparation and examination of smears stained with Gram's stain, and culture. Because both organisms may be present normally in food, quantitative cultures must be performed. A series of dilutions (10^{-1}, 10^{-2}, 10^{-3}, 10^{-4}, and 10^{-5}) of the sample are prepared in buffered gelatin diluent, and 0.1 mL of the undiluted specimen and each one of the dilutions are plated on to colistin–nalidixic acid or phenylethyl alcohol blood agar (selective for Gram-positive organisms). In addition, to demonstrate endospore production by *B. cereus*, 1 mL of the original specimen is mixed with 1 mL of absolute ethanol and the mixture is allowed to stand for 1 hour at room temperature. Dilutions of the mixture are prepared as described above, and 0.1 mL of each dilution and of the undiluted mixture are plated onto sheep blood agar. All plates are incubated for 18–24 hours at 35–37°C in ambient air, and the colonies are counted. The presence of 10^5 CFU or more of *S. aureus* or *B. cereus* organisms per gram of specimen has potential significance, especially if found in samples from the majority of affected individuals. Testing for agents causing bacterial food poisoning as described above is normally conducted at public health laboratories and not in the clinical laboratory.

The clinical diagnoses of food-borne botulism and infant botulism may be confirmed by detecting botulinal toxin, *Clostridium botulinum*, or both in feces. Optimally, 25–50 mL of stool, 15–20 mL of serum, and a sample of the suspect food should be collected. Most clinical laboratories are not properly equipped to process specimens from persons with suspected botulism. In the United States, when a case of botulism is identified, investigators at the CDC should be notified to ensure appropriate diagnosis, treatment, and investigation of the potential outbreak.

Diseases associated with *C. difficile*, such as pseudomembranous colitis and antibiotic-associated diarrhea, are caused by the toxins produced by the organism and are diagnosed by detecting toxin A, B, or both in feces. The reference method for detection of the cytotoxin is cell culture assay. To extract toxin, the stool specimen is clarified by centrifugation at $2000 \times g$ for 20 minutes or $10\,000 \times g$ for 10 minutes and filtered through a 0.45 µm membrane filter. Serial dilutions are prepared and inoculated to cell monolayers, which are incubated for 24–48 hours. Alternatively, toxin A or both toxins A and B may be detected in stool samples by ELISA. This technique appears to be almost as sensitive as cell culture, and provides results within a few hours (Whittier, 1993; Merz, 1994). The sensitivity of different commercial ELISAs, however, varies (Lyerly, 1998; Fedorko, 1999; Turgeon, 2003; Wilkins, 2003). Tests for detection of the common antigen glutamate dehydrogenase (GDH) are also commercially available (Wilkins, 2003). These tests, like bacterial culture, do not distinguish isolates that produce toxin from those that do not. However, despite this, the common antigen, which has a turnaround time of 15–45 minutes, has been shown to be a useful screening test in certain institutions. Specimens yielding negative results require no further testing, whereas GDH-positive specimens should be tested for toxins.

For epidemiologic studies, *C. difficile* may be isolated from stool or from rectal swab specimens placed in an anaerobic transport system. Because many bacteria are present in stool, procedures that select for *C. difficile* must be used. The most effective medium for this purpose is cycloserine cefoxitin fructose egg yolk agar (CCFA), with or without horse blood. The organism grows more quickly and luxuriantly on formulations containing horse blood. The medium is incubated anaerobically for 48 hours and the plates are examined for colonies that have a peripheral fringe and a 'horse stable' odor. Alternatively, *C. difficile* may be isolated by using an alcohol spore selection procedure, where 1 mL of the original specimen is mixed with 1 mL of absolute ethanol. The mixture is allowed to stand for 1 hour at room temperature, followed by subculture to CCFA and incubation anaerobically.

Clostridium perfringens is one cause of long-incubation food poisoning (7–15 hours after eating contaminated food). It also may cause antibiotic-associated diarrhea, typically in hospitalized elderly patients, and enteritis necroticans. To diagnose food poisoning caused by *C. perfringens*, quantitative anaerobic culture of a stool specimen that was transported in an anaerobic transport collection system is performed. Ethanol-treated and untreated fecal material are diluted as described earlier for detection of bacteria associated with short-incubation food poisoning. Phenylethyl alcohol agar plates are inoculated and incubated anaerobically for 48 hours. A spore count of 10^5 or more per gram of stool may be significant, especially if demonstrated in samples from the majority of affected individuals. As previously noted, testing for agents of food poisoning is conducted primarily in public health laboratories and not in the clinical laboratory. The toxin may be detected in the original stool specimen but this test is usually performed in reference laboratories. Similar criteria are used to diagnose diarrhea produced by *C. perfringens* during antibiotic therapy.

In regard to mycobacterial culture, stool specimens usually are submitted for isolation of *Mycobacterium avium* complex (primarily from patients with AIDS), but *M. tuberculosis* and other species of *Mycobacterium* also may be recovered. Processing the specimen (1–2 g of formed stool or 5 mL of liquid stool) involves decontamination and concentration, preparation of smears, and inoculation of media as discussed in Chapter 59.

Parasites

The backbone of diagnostic parasitology in the clinical laboratory is examination of stool samples for parasitic protozoa and helminth eggs or larvae. Laboratories performing such tests should have adequate facilities for handling stool samples and a good microscope with a calibrated micrometer to measure the organisms found. Staining of fecal smears is also required for identification of intestinal protozoa.

Specimen Collection and Transport

The specimen (usually collected by the patient) can be collected in a clean, dry, wide-mouthed container. A portion of the sample is then aliquoted into two vials containing preservatives; one with modified polyvinyl alcohol (PVA) and the other with 10% formalin. Fecal specimens should not be collected from the toilet bowl and should not be contaminated with urine, water, mineral or caster oil, antidiarrheal compounds, or radiologic contrast medium. Once collected and preserved the sample should be delivered to the laboratory at the patient's convenience. The use of fresh stool is optimal for examination for *E. histolytica* trophozoites; however, it is usually very difficult to transport a fresh specimen to the laboratory and into the hands of the microbiologist within the 30–60 minutes after collection required to visualize motile trophozoites. Although it is rarely possible to perform wet mounts on fresh stools for motile trophozoites, they can still be identified on stained preparations, and the use of preserved specimens for examination minimizes the exposure of laboratory personnel to live organisms.

Several kits, most consisting of two vials, one with fixative (formalin) for helminth eggs and protozoan cysts, and the other with PVA for preparation of smears for staining, are commercially available for collection and transport of fecal samples. The question of how many fecal specimens are required for identification of all individuals with intestinal protozoa or helminths is still without a definitive answer. It has been advised that a minimum of three specimens should be collected on different days and examined (Proctor, 1991). However, some recommend collection of only one or two specimens. For cost containment, the clinician should request examination of only one specimen, because about 90% of all infections are diagnosed on the first sample (Montessori, 1987). If a parasite is not detected in the first sample, a second or third should be requested. If two or more specimens collected on different days are received in the laboratory at the same time, it has been suggested they be pooled and evaluated as one (Peters, 1988). This practice, however, is controversial. Stool examinations for parasites in patients who have been hospitalized for more than 3 days are inappropriate (Siegel, 1990).

Specimen processing

The examination of stool samples for parasites includes preparation of saline solution and of iodine (Lugol's)-stained wet mounts of freshly collected samples (i.e., those that can be examined within a few hours of collection). This is followed by concentration of cysts and helminth eggs, and finally by preparation of smears for staining with the trichrome stain. The wet preparations, if performed, should be made and examined before doing the concentration and trichrome staining. Even if a parasite is seen in the wet mount, examination of a concentrated specimen is recommended because specimens submitted for ova and parasite examination not uncommonly contain multiple parasites. In particular, helminth eggs are often only visible in the concentrate.

The standard fecal smear, which has about 2 mg of feces, is made from a fresh fecal sample as follows: one drop of saline solution is placed on a clear glass slide; with an applicator stick, a small amount of feces is picked up and with circular movements is mixed thoroughly with the saline (until enough sample is dissolved), and the mixture is covered with a 22 mm square cover glass. A good wet smear prepared as described, if placed on a paper with small print, should allow the print to be read through the smear. The smear stained with iodine is prepared in the same manner. Both the saline solution and the iodine solution wet preparations can be made on the same glass slide, at the same time mixing the feces with the saline solution first and then with the iodine solution. The saline solution smear will show trophozoites and cysts of protozoa, plus all the helminth eggs and larvae. The smear stained with iodine does not show trophozoites, because they are destroyed by the iodine unless the sample was previously fixed. The main advantage of the iodine stain is that it allows better visualization of some morphologic characteristics of cysts.

The saline solution shows movement of trophozoites, which is useful for their identification. To prepare wet mounts from formalin-fixed material, the contents are mixed well and one drop is placed directly on to the glass slide and on to a drop of iodine solution.

Examination of the saline solution smear is carried out with medium power (10 × objective) at first. Beginning at the left upper corner of the cover slide, the slide is moved horizontally from the right to the left. The operation is repeated until the entire 22 mm square cover glass is examined. All helminth eggs or larvae and all protozoan cysts should be noted. Examination with the high-power objective is done next for detection and identification of protozoa, looking randomly for about 5–10 minutes per preparation.

The concentration technique, which can be done both on fresh and fixed specimens, is particularly useful because it allows detection of organisms present in low numbers. The ideal method for routine evaluation is the formalin ether concentration, which has been made safer by the use of ethyl acetate or formalin Hemo-de rather than diethyl ether. The permanently stained fecal smear for diagnosis of infection with intestinal protozoa is considered the standard of good practice for North American clinical laboratories. Smears for staining are prepared by spreading a thin film of well-mixed fresh or PVA-preserved stool across half the surface of a slide with a flattened wooden applicator stick. Fresh stool smears are fixed in Schaudinn's solution before they are dried and stained Certain intestinal parasites – *Cryptosporidium*, microsporidia, and *Cyclospora* – require special stains for detection, as discussed in Chapter 61.

Skin and Subcutaneous Lesions

Vesicles, Bullae, and Pustules

Specimen Collection and Transport

Fluid is the optimal specimen and may be collected from a vesicle or bulla by aspirating with a needle and syringe, removing the needle, capping the syringe and transporting the syringe to the laboratory. If viral culture is desired inoculate a portion of the fluid into M4 transport medium. Vesicles and bullae may also be sampled by unroofing the lesion and vigorously rubbing the base with a swab, and then submitting the swab for testing. Pustules are similarly sampled with a swab after removing any crusted material. A minimum of two swab specimens should be collected, one for culture, the other for preparation of smears for staining. However, if detection of more than one group of organisms (e.g., viruses and bacteria, or bacteria and fungi) is requested, collecting at least three swab specimens is optimal. For suspected viral infection, the individual collecting the specimen should prepare a smear at the bedside by rolling the entire surface of the swab over a glass slide and allowing the material to air dry.

All swabs for bacterial or fungal testing may be placed in tube transport systems containing modified Stuart's medium; if anaerobic culture is ordered, place one swab in an anaerobic transport device. Transport smears, fluid, and swab specimens promptly to the laboratory.

Specimen processing

Processing specimens from vesicles or pustules for detection of viruses involves cell culture; and for varicella zoster virus, and possibly HSV, examination of stained smears is helpful. Specimens for culture are refrigerated for a short time until they are processed. Swab specimens received in viral transport medium are vigorously agitated on a vortex mixer, and then the swab is removed and discarded. Processing specimens for detection of bacteria and/or fungi involves preparation of a smear for staining with Gram's stain (for bacteria) or Calcofluor white (for fungi) and inoculation of appropriate media for culture, as discussed in Chapters 56 and 60.

Cutaneous Ulcers

Aspirates and swab specimens are collected from cutaneous ulcers for microbiological studies. Lesions may be primary (e.g., those caused by viruses, *Bacillus anthracis*, *C. diphtheriae*, *Francisella tularensis*, *P. aeruginosa*, mycobacteria, or fungi), or decubitus ulcers may become secondarily colonized or infected with aerobic and anaerobic bacteria.

Collection, transport, and processing of swab specimens obtained from cutaneous ulcers for detection of viruses are identical to what were described earlier for vesicles and pustules. Handling of specimens obtained from cutaneous ulcers differs for bacteria and fungi and is discussed separately for each of the organisms that cause primary lesions and for the bacteria associated with chronic ulcers.

B. anthracis causes anthrax, a rare disease in the United States, limited to persons working with raw imported wool and other animal products contaminated with spores of *B. anthracis* and persons exposed to spores through an act of bioterrorism. Cutaneous anthrax begins as a painless papule but becomes vesicular, then hemorrhagic, necrotic, and covered with an eschar. For optimal diagnosis, two swab specimens of the exudate are collected: one for culture, the other for preparation of smears for staining with Gram's stain and with fluorescent antibodies (the latter should be performed in a reference laboratory). Because of the hazardous nature of *B. anthracis*, sending specimens from persons with suspected anthrax to a reference laboratory should be considered. If specimens are processed in the clinical laboratory, they must be handled in a biological safety cabinet. The swab for culture is inoculated onto sheep blood agar, which is incubated in ambient air.

C. diphtheriae is the cause of cutaneous diphtheria, an ulcerative lesion covered with a layer of necrotic debris resembling a membrane. For optimal diagnosis, a smear for staining with methylene blue is prepared from material collected from the edge of the membrane, and two swab specimens from the membrane are collected. One swab is used for routine bacterial culture and the other for inoculation of media selective for *C. diphtheriae* (e.g. cysteine tellurite agar) if available.

Ecthyma gangrenosus is an ulcerative cutaneous lesion that almost always occurs during bacteremia with *P. aeruginosa* but rarely develops during bacteremia with other Gram-negative bacilli. Ideally, two swab specimens are collected from the ulcer base; one is used to prepare a smear for staining with Gram's stain and the other to inoculate media for culture.

The diagnosis of the ulceroglandular form of tularemia requires the collection of a swab specimen from material at the base of the ulcer. The swab is processed for routine bacterial culture and the plates are held for a full 7 days, as *F. tularensis* is a slowly growing bacterium, producing pinpoint colonies in 3–5 days on chocolate agar, but does not grow on sheep blood agar. Suspicious isolates should be referred immediately to the nearest public health laboratory for identification.

Mycobacteria that may be isolated from cutaneous ulcers include *Mycobacterium fortuitum*, *Mycobacterium abscessus*, *Mycobacterium chelonae*, *Mycobacterium marinum*, *Mycobacterium haemophilum*, *Mycobacterium ulcerans*, and uncommonly *M. tuberculosis*, *M. avium* complex, and *Mycobacterium kansasii*. Exudate aspirated with a needle and syringe or a tissue sample is optimal for recovery of mycobacteria. To transport the aspirate, the material is expelled into a sterile tube, which is tightly capped and delivered promptly to the laboratory. Tissue samples are placed on sterile, moist gauze in a sterile container, which is tightly capped. Swab samples are not acceptable for processing for mycobacteria, as mycobacteria become entrapped in the fibers of the swab and are difficult to dislodge. Specimens may be refrigerated for a short time until they are processed (see Ch. 59).

Many aerobic, facultative, and anaerobic bacteria colonize chronic skin ulcers. To identify the organisms responsible, cultures of deep tissues or a deep aspirate of purulent material collected with a needle and syringe provide the most useful bacteriologic information. To transport aspirated pus, remove and discard the needle, cap the syringe, and deliver it promptly to the laboratory. If transport will be delayed, inject a portion of the aspirate into an anaerobic gel transport tube. Tissue samples are transported in a sterile cup with moist sterile gauze to keep tissue from drying out. Processing the specimen involves preparing a smear for staining with Gram's stain and inoculating appropriate media for aerobic and anaerobic culture.

An aspirate of the exudate from the active margin of an ulcer (transported as described earlier for bacteria) or a tissue sample is optimal for detection of fungi. A swab specimen of the exudate is suboptimal and should be discouraged. Processing the specimen for detection of fungi involves preparing a smear for direct microscopic examination (potassium hydroxide or calcofluor white preparation) and inoculation of appropriate media for culture, such as brain-heart infusion, inhibitory mold, or SABHI agar containing antibiotics and cycloheximide.

Wound Infections and Abscesses

Ideally, purulent material is aspirated with a needle and syringe and transported as described earlier for ulcerative lesions. If an aspirate cannot be obtained, swab specimens of exudate collected from the deep portion of the lesion are acceptable. For routine bacterial culture, two swab specimens are optimal: one to prepare a smear for staining with Gram's stain and one for culture. To recover anaerobes, an additional swab specimen must be collected and placed in an anaerobic transport system. All specimens should be delivered promptly to the laboratory and processed as soon as possible. If a delay in processing is unavoidable, specimens may be stored in the refrigerator, except those for recovery of anaerobes, which should be maintained at room temperature.

VII

References

Albright RE Jr, Christenson RH, Emlet JL, et al: Issues in cerebrospinal fluid management. CSF Venereal Disease Research Laboratory Testing. Am J Clin Pathol 1991a; 95:397.

Albright RE Jr, Graham CB III, Christenson RH, et al: Issues in cerebrospinal fluid management. Acid-fast bacillus smear and culture. Am J Clin Pathol 1991b; 95:418.

Bannatyne RM, Jackson MC, Memish S: Rapid diagnosis of *Brucella* bacteremia by using the BACTEC 9240 system. J Clin Microbiol 1997; 35:2673.

Baron EJ, Peterson LR, Finegold SM (eds): Microorganisms encountered in the urinary tract. *In* Bailey and Scott's Diagnostic Microbiology, 9th ed. St Louis, MO, CV Mosby, 1994.

Baselski VS, Wunderink RG: Bronchoscopic diagnosis of pneumonia. Clin Microbiol Rev 1994; 7:533.

Bhisitkul DM, Hogan AE, Tanz RR: The role of bacterial antigen detection tests in the diagnosis of bacterial meningitis. Pediatr Emerg Care 1994; 10:67.

Bisno AL, Gerber MA, Gwaltney Jr. JM, et al: Practice guidelines for the diagnosis and management of group A streptococcal pharyngitis. Clin Infect Dis 2002; 35:113–125.

Reviews the advantages and limitations of the different tests for diagnosis of group A streptococcal pharyngitis. Also provides guidelines for management of group A streptococcal pharyngitis.

Briselden AM, Hillier SL: Evaluation of Affirm VP microbial identification test for *Gardnerella vaginalis* and *Trichomonas vaginalis*. J Clin Microbiol 1994; 32:148–152.

Brumback BG, Bolejack SN, Morris MV, et al: Comparison of culture and the antigenemia assay for detection of cytomegalovirus in blood specimens submitted to a reference laboratory. J Clin Microbiol 1997; 35:1819.

Carroll KC: Laboratory diagnosis of lower respiratory tract infections: controversy and conundrums. J Clin Microbiol 2002; 40:3115–3120.

Reviews microbiologic tests for diagnosis of lower respiratory tract infections, including acute bronchitis, community-acquired pneumonia, and nosocomial pneumonia.

Christensen ML: Human viral gastroenteritis. Clin Microbiol Rev 1989; 2:51.

Cloud JL, Shutt C, Aldous W, et al: Evaluation of a modified Gen-Probe Amplified Direct Test for detection of *Mycobacterium tuberculosis* complex organisms in cerebrospinal fluid. J Clin Microbiol 2004; 42:5341.

Cockerill III FR, Wilson JW, Vetter EA, et al: Optimal testing parameters for blood cultures. Clin Infect Dis 2004; 38:1724–1730.

Provides data regarding optimal testing parameters for blood cultures when using automated blood culture systems.

Dagan R, Menegus MA: A combination of four cell types for rapid detection of enterovirus in clinical specimens. J Med Virol 1986; 19:219.

Dawson MS, Harford AM, Garner BK, et al: Total volume culture technique for the isolation of microorganisms from continuous ambulatory peritoneal dialysis patients with peritonitis. J Clin Microbiol 22:391, 1985.

Fedorko DP, Engler HD, O'Shaughnessy EM, et al: Evaluation of two rapid assays for detection of *Clostridium difficile* toxin A in stool specimens. J Clin Microbiol 1999; 37:3044.

Flayhart D, Lema C, Borek A, Carroll KC: Comparison of the bbl chromagar staph aureus Agar Medium to Conventional Media for Detection of *Staphylococcus aureus* in respiratory samples. J Clin Microbiol 2004; 42:3566–3569.

Friedman RL: Pertussis: The disease and new diagnostic methods. Clin Microbiol Rev 1988; 1:365.

Gavin PJ, Peterson LR, Pasquariello AC, et al: Evaluation of performance and potential clinical impact of ProSpecT Shiga toxin *Escherichia coli* microplate assay for detection of Shiga toxin-producing *E. coli* in stool samples. J Clin Microbiol 2004; 42:1652–1656.

Gerber MA, Shulman ST: Rapid diagnosis of pharyngitis caused by group A streptococci. Clin Microbiol Rev 2004; 17:571–580.

Provides an in-depth review of the advantages and limitations of rapid tests for diagnosis of group A streptococcal pharyngitis. Also discusses possible reasons for false-positive and false-negative results and the cost effectiveness of using these tests.

Gilligan PH: Endotracheal aspirates: to screen or not to screen, is that even the question? Clin Microbiol Newslett 1999; 21:44.

Havlik D, Woods GL: Screening sputum specimens submitted for mycobacterial culture. Lab Med 1995; 26:411.

Heelan JS, Corpus L, Kessimian N: False-positive reactions in the latex agglutination test for *Cryptococcus neoformans* antigen. J Clin Microbiol 1991; 29:1260.

Herrmann B, Larsson VC, Rubin CJ, et al: Comparison of a duplex quantitative real-time PCR assay and the COBAS Amplicor CMV Monitor test for detection of cytomegalovirus. J Clin Microbiol 2004; 42:1909–1914.

Howell CL, Miller MJ, Martin WJ: Comparison of rates of virus isolation from leukocyte populations separated from blood by conventional and Ficoll-Paque/Macrodex methods. J Clin Microbiol 1979; 10:533.

Ilstrup DM, Washington JA II: The importance of volume of blood cultured in the detection of bacteremia and fungemia. Diagn Microbiol Infect Dis 1983; 1:107.

Ingram JG, Plouffe JF: Danger of sputum purulence screen in culture of *Legionella* species. J Clin Microbiol 1994; 32:209.

Jacques J, Carquin J, Brodard V, et al: New reverse transcription-PCR assay for rapid and sensitive detection of Enterovirus genomes in cerebrospinal fluid specimens of patients with aseptic meningitis. J Clin Microbiol 2003; 41:5726–5728.

Kahn FW, Jones JM: Diagnosing bacterial respiratory infection by bronchoalveolar lavage. J Infect Dis 1987; 155:862.

Kalpoe JS, Kroes AC, de Jong MD, et al: Validation of clinical application of cytomegalovirus plasma DNA load measurement and definition of treatment criteria by analysis of correlation to antigen detection. J Clin Microbiol 2004; 42:1498–1504.

Kass EH: Asymptomatic infections of the urinary tract. Trans Assoc Am Physicians 1956; 69:56.

Kiska DL, Jones MC, Mangum ME, et al: Quality assurance study of bacterial antigen testing of cerebrospinal fluid. J Clin Microbiol 1995; 33:1141.

Krumholz HM, Cummings S, York M: Blood culture phlebotomy: switching needles does not prevent contamination. Ann Intern Med 1990; 113:290.

Lai KK, Cook L, Wendt S, et al: Evaluation of real-time PCR versus PCR with liquid-phase hybridization for detection of Enterovirus RNA in cerebrospinal fluid. J Clin Microbiol 2003; 41:3133–3141.

Lakeman FD, Whitley RJ: Diagnosis of herpes simplex encephalitis: application of polymerase chain reaction to cerebrospinal fluid from brain-biopsied patients and correlation with disease. National Institute of Allergy and Infectious Disease Collaborative Antiviral Study Group. J Infect Dis 1995; 171:857–863.

Lipsky BA, Innuni TS, Plorde JJ, et al: Is the clean-catch midstream void procedure necessary for obtaining urine culture specimens from men? Am J Med 1984; 76:257.

Luce E, Nakagawa D, Lovell J, et al: Improvement in the bacteriologic diagnosis of peritonitis with the use of blood culture media. Trans Am Soc Artif Intern Organs 1982; 28:259.

Lyerly DM, Neville LH, Evans T, et al: Multicenter evaluation of the *Clostridium difficile* TOX A/B test. J Clin Microbiol 1998; 36:184.

McCarter YS, Robinson A: Quality evaluation of sputum specimens for mycobacterial culture. Am J Clin Pathol 1996; 105:769.

Mandell LA, Bartlett JG, Dowell SF, et al: Update of practice guidelines for the management of community-acquired pneumonia in immunocompetent adults. Clin Infect Dis 2003; 37:1405–1433.

Guidelines developed by the Infectious Diseases Society of America for managing community-acquired pneumonia in adults. Also provides recommendations regarding diagnostic tests.

Martinez AJ, Visvesvara GS: Diagnosis of pathogenic free-living amebas. Clin Lab Med 1991; 11:861.

Maxson S, Lewno MJ, Schutze GE: Clinical usefulness of cerebrospinal fluid bacterial antigen studies. J Pediatr 1994; 125:235.

Merz CS, Kramer C, Forman M, et al: Comparison of four commercially available rapid enzyme immunoassays with cytotoxin assay for detection of *Clostridium difficile* toxin(s) from stool specimens. J Clin Microbiol 1994; 32:1142.

Meyer-Koenig U, Weidmann M, Kirste G, Hufert FT: Cytomegalovirus infection in organ-transplant recipients: diagnostic value of pp65 antigen test, qualitative polymerase chain reaction (PCR) and quantitative Taqman PCR. Transplantation 2004; 77:1692–1698.

Mitchell PS, Espy MJ, Smith TF, et al: Laboratory diagnosis of central nervous system infections with herpes simplex virus by PCR performed with cerebrospinal fluid specimens. J Clin Microbiol 1997; 35:2873–2877.

Montessori GA, Bischoff L: Searching for parasites in stool: Once is usually enough. Can Med Assoc J 1987; 137:702.

Morris AJ, Tanner DC, Reller LB: Rejection criteria for endotracheal aspirates from adults. J Clin Microbiol 1027.; 1993; 31

Murray PR, Spizzo AW, Niles AC: Clinical comparison of the recoveries of bloodstream pathogens in Septi-Chek brain heart infusion broth with saponin, Septi-Chek tryptic soy broth, and the Isolator lysis-centrifugation system. J Clin Microbiol 1991; 29:901.

Murray PR, Traynor P, Hopson D: Clinical assessment of blood culture techniques: analysis of recovery of obligate and facultative anaerobes, strict aerobic bacteria, and fungi in aerobic and anaerobic blood culture bottles. J Clin Microbiol 1992; 30:1462.

Murray PR, Washington JA II: Microscopic and bacteriologic analysis of expectorated sputum. Mayo Clin Proc 1975; 50:339.

Nolte FS, Williams JM, Jerris RC, et al: Multicenter clinical evaluation of a continuous monitoring blood culture system using fluorescent-sensor technology (BACTEC 9240). J Clin Microbiol 1993; 31:552.

Perkins MD, Mirrett S, Reller LB: Rapid bacterial antigen detection is not clinically useful. J Clin Microbiol 1995; 33:1486.

Peters CS, Hernandez L, Sheffield N, et al: Cost containment of formalin-preserved stool specimens for ova and parasites from outpatients. J Clin Microbiol 1988; 26:1584.

Pezzlo M: Detection of urinary tract infections by rapid methods. Clin Microbiol Rev 1988; 1:268.

Prather SL, Dagan R, Jenista JA, et al: The isolation of enteroviruses from blood: a comparison of four processing methods. J Med Virol 1984; 14:221.

Proctor EM: Laboratory diagnosis of amebiasis. Clin Lab Med 1991; 11:829.

Pulz M, Matussek A, Monazahian M, et al: Comparison of a Shiga toxin enzyme-linked immunosorbent assay and two types of PCR for detection of Shiga toxin-producing *Escherichia coli* in human stool specimens. J Clin Microbiol 2003; 41:4671–4675.

Reimer LG, Wilson ML, Weinstein MP: Update on detection of bacteremia and fungemia. Clin Microbiol Rev 1997; 10:444.

Reisner BS, Woods GL: Times to detection of bacteria and yeasts in BACTEC 9240 blood culture bottles. J Clin Microbiol 1999; 37:2024–2026.

Rippin KP, Stinson WC, Eisenstadt J, Washington JA: Clinical evaluation of the slide centrifuge

(Cytospin) Gram's stained smear for the detection of bacteriuria and comparison with the FiltraCheck-UTI and UTIscreen. Am J Clin Pathol 1995; 103:316–319.

Semeniuk H, Church D: Evaluation of the leukocyte esterase and nitrite urine dipstick screening tests for detection of bacteriuria in women with suspected uncomplicated urinary tract infections. J Clin Microbiol 1999; 37:3051–3052.

Sharp SE. Routine anaerobic blood cultures: still appropriate today? Clin Microbiol Newslett 1991; 13:179.

Shaw KN, McGowan KL: Evaluation of a rapid screening filter test for urinary tract infection in children. Pediatr Infect Dis J 1997; 16:283.

Shaw KN, McGowan KL, Gorelick MH, Schwartz JS: Screening for urinary tract infection in infants in the Emergency Department: Which test is best? Pediatrics 1998; 101(6):E1.

Siegel DL, Edelstein PH, Nachamkin I: Inappropriate testing for diarrheal diseases in the hospital. JAMA 1990; 263:979.

Stamm WE, Counts GW, Running KR, et al: Diagnosis of coliform infection in acute dysuric women. N Engl J Med 1982; 307:463.

Storch GA, Gaudreault-Keener M, Welby PC: Comparison of heparin and EDTA transport tubes for detection of cytomegalovirus in leukocytes by shell vial assay, pp65 antigenemia assay, and PCR. Clin Microbiol 1994; 32:2581.

Thiele GM, Woods GL: The effect of dexamethasone on detection of cytomegalovirus in tissue culture and by immunofluorescence. J Virol Methods 1988; 22:319.

Thorpe TC, Wilson ML, Turner JE, et al: BacT/Alert: an automated colorimetric microbial detection system. J Clin Microbiol 1990; 28:1608.

Towns ML, Reller LB: Diagnostic methods; current best practices and guidelines for isolation of bacteria and fungi in infective endocarditis. Infect Dis Clin North Am 2002; 16:363–376.

Turgeon DK, Novicki TJ, Quick J, et al: Six rapid tests for direct detection of *Clostridium difficile* and its toxins in fecal samples compared with the Fibroblast Cytotoxicity Assay. J Clin Microbiol 2003; 41:667–670.

Van Der Bij W, Torensma R, van Son WJ, et al: Rapid immunodiagnosis of active cytomegalovirus infection by monoclonal antibody staining of blood leukocytes. J Med Virol 1988; 25:179.

Waite R, Woods GL: Evaluation of BACTEC Myco/F lytic medium for recovery of mycobacteria and fungi from blood. J Clin Microbiol 1998; 36:1176.

Washington JA II, Ilstrup DM: Blood cultures: Issues and controversies. Rev Infect Dis 1986; 8:792.

Whittier S, Shapiro DS, Kelly WS, et al: Evaluation of four commercially available enzyme immunoassays for laboratory diagnosis of *Clostridium difficile* associated diseases. J Clin Microbiol 1993; 31:2861.

Wilkins TD, Lyerly DM: *Clostridium difficile* testing: after 20 years, still challenging. J Clin Microbiol 2003; 41:531–534.

Reviews the tests currently available for diagnosis of C. difficile-associated diseases, with an emphasis on enzyme-linked immunosorbent assays for detection of toxin(s).

Wilson ML: Continuously monitoring blood culture systems: an update. American Society of Clinical Pathologists (ASCP) Check Sample 1996; 39:129.

Wolfson JS, Waldron MA, Sierra LS: Blinded comparison of a direct immunofluorescent monoclonal antibody staining method and a Giemsa staining method for identification of *Pneumocystis carinii* in induced sputum and bronchoalveolar lavage specimens of patients infected with human immunodeficiency virus. J Clin Microbiol 1990; 28:2136.

Woods GL: Optimal protocol for processing high-volume and Peds Plus™ blood cultures by the BACTEC NR860™. Am J Clin Pathol 1994; 101:162.

Woods GL, Proffitt MR: Comparison of plasmagel with LeucoPREP™-Macrodex methods for separation of leukocytes for virus isolation. Diagn Microbiol Infect Dis 1987a; 8:123.

Woods GL, Thompson AB, Rennard SL, et al: Detection of cytomegalovirus in bronchoalveolar lavage specimens: spin amplification and staining with a monoclonal antibody to the early nuclear antigen for diagnosis of cytomegalovirus pneumonia. Chest 1990; 98:568.

Woods GL, Young A, Johnson A, et al: Detection of cytomegalovirus by 24-well plate centrifugation assay using a monoclonal antibody to an early nuclear antigen and by conventional cell culture. J Virol Methods 1987b; 18:207.

Zwadyk P, Pierson CL, Young C: Comparison of Difco ESP and Organon Teknika BacT/Alert continuous-monitoring blood culture systems. J Clin Microbiol 1994; 32:1273.

CHAPTER 64

Bioterrorism: Microbiology

Judy A. Daly PhD

KEY POINTS

• Accepting nature as the constant reservoir and source of infectious agents puts bioterrorism preparedness in the most appropriate context of preparedness against infectious agents.

• The Laboratory Response Network (LRN) is a consortium and partnership of laboratories that provide immediate and sustained laboratory testing and communication in support of public health emergencies, particularly in response to acts of bioterrorism.

• Clinical laboratories (sentinel laboratories) play a critical role in the LRN: their heightened awareness to the possibility of recovering the agents of bioterrorism from patient specimens and referral of suspect isolates to the appropriate public health reference laboratory is crucial.

• United States, international, and commercial regulations mandate the proper packing, documentation, and safe shipment of dangerous goods in order to protect the public, airline workers, couriers, and other persons who work for commercial shippers and who handle the dangerous goods during the many segments of the shipping process.

• Based on the ease of transmission, severity of morbidity, mortality, and likelihood of use, biological agents can be classified into three categories (Table 64–3).

• Sentinel laboratories are clinical laboratories that follow biosafety level 2 (BSL-2) guidelines. Their primary responsibility is to recognize and rule out or refer suspicious agents by following standardized sentinel laboratory guidelines.

Infectious Agents as Tools of Mass Casualties

Accepting nature as the constant reservoir and source of infectious agents puts bioterrorism preparedness in the more appropriate context of preparedness against the infectious agents. By their very nature, infectious agents have the capability to spread fast. The past and the present efforts of the World Health Organization and many national agencies to strengthen global preparedness for defense against infectious disease threats is part and parcel of bioterrorism preparedness. Infectious agents have been, and in the foreseeable future will remain, potential tools of mass casualties. Historically, outbreaks (wars) of microbial species against the human species have killed far more people than war itself. Examples include: the death of 95% of pre-Columban Native American populations from

diseases such as smallpox, measles, plague, typhoid, and influenza; the death of 25 million Europeans (a quarter of the population) caused by bubonic plague in the 14th century; and 21 million deaths due to the influenza pandemic of 1918–1919 (Diamond, 1999). Advances in public health, diagnostic and pharmacological interventions are needed to protect the population from emerging and re-emerging infectious diseases, including those related to potential bioterrorism events.

Biowarfare Versus Bioterrorism

It is important to recognize that biological agents have been used in warfare from antiquity to the present. The intentional use of living organisms or infected materials derived from them has occurred over centuries during war and 'peace' time by armies, states, groups and individuals (Christopher, 1997; Eitzen, 1997; Tucker, 1999; Beeching, 2002). The use of catapults during medieval times introduced new technology to biological warfare. In 1346, the attacking Tartar force experienced an epidemic of plague during the siege of Kaffa. They catapulted the cadavers of their dead into the city to initiate a plague epidemic. An outbreak of plague did occur, followed by the retreat of the defending forces and the conquest of Kaffa.

In 1763, the introduction of a specific disease, smallpox, as a weapon in the North American Indian Wars became a significant milestone in the history of biological warfare, by handing blankets and a handkerchief from the smallpox hospital to the Native Americans. During World War I, Germany was accused of causing cholera in Italy, and plague in St Petersburg in 1915.

The modern era of biological weapons development began immediately before and during World War II (Table 64–1). The Allied Biological Weapons program had shifted from British research on anthrax (and the development of the World War II anthrax cattlecake retaliation weapon) to a large United-States-based research, development, and production capability. This offensive program was unilaterally abandoned in 1969, giving impetus to the creation of the Biological and Toxin Weapons Convention. Unfortunately, the number of countries engaged in biological weapons experimentation grew from four in the 1960s to 11 in the 1990s. It is estimated that at least 10 nations and possibly 17 possess biological warfare agents.

The Concept of 'Bioterrorism'

As the ease of cultivating microorganisms increased and technology became cheap, dissident groups and well financed organizations used these agents to terrorize civilians in order to accomplish political goals. Examples of these attempts are listed in Table 64–2.

Table 64–1 Chronology of Biodefense Actions

1910–1920s	The first use of chemical and biological weapons in combat led to efforts to ban their use.
1925	The use of biological and chemical weapons in war was prohibited by the Geneva Protocol. The United States signed but failed to ratify the treaty. The treaty contained no provision for verifications and inspection.
1950s–1970s	The Soviet Union and United States built arsenals of biological and chemical weapons. International pressures mounted to draw up new treaties to curb such weapons.
November 25, 1969	President Richard Nixon unilaterally renounced the use of biological weapons in war by the United States and restricted research to immunization and safety efforts. Three months later, he extended the ban to include toxins. The United States Army Medical Research Institute for Infectious Diseases (USARMIID) at Fort Detrick, MD, was established to conduct unclassified research on safety against potential agents of bioterrorism.
1972	A convention on the prohibition of the development, production, and stockpiling of bacteriological (biological) and toxin weapons and their destruction opened for signature at Washington, London, and Moscow on April 10, 1972.
1975	The United States Congress ratified the Biological and Toxin Weapons Convention (BWC) as well as the 1925 Geneva Protocol on January 22, 1975. The Biological and Toxin Weapons Convention entered into force March 26, 1975. (There are now 143 state parties to the convention and an additional 18 signatories. Article VI of the Convention has proved to be an inadequate mechanism for actions against noncompliance.)
1980s	Arms control initiatives failed to curb biological and chemical weapons proliferation.
1984	President Reagan's administration presented a draft treaty to ban the production and storage of chemical weapons to the Conference on Disarmament in Geneva.
1990s	Concerns over exposure to chemical and biological weapons during the Persian Gulf War increased support for international treaties.
May 13, 1991	Shortly after the Allied victory against Iraq, President George Bush announced that the United States would renounce the use of chemical weapons for any reason – and an international treaty banning them took effect.
April 1992	Russian President Boris Yeltsin declared that Russia's biological weapons program was being discontinued.
January 1993	President George Bush signed the Chemical Weapons treaty at the convention banning the production and use of chemical weapons.
January 7, 1997	The Presidential Advisory Committee on Gulf War veterans' illnesses found no conclusive evidence linking Gulf War syndrome to chemical or biological weapons.
April 15, 1997	New regulations aimed at limiting access to chemicals and pathogens that could be made into weapons came into effect under the 1996 Antiterrorism and Effective Death Penalty Act.
April 29, 1997	The Chemical Weapons Convention (CWC) went into effect. It has more than 160 signatories and 65 ratifications.
July 25, 2001	The United States rejected a protocol to strengthen the Biological Weapons Convention as well as the whole approach to it. As in the Chemical Weapons Conventions (CWC), a strong bioweapons protocol could add to the deterrence of bioweapons, which are a much greater threat than chemical weapons.
November 19, 2001	The fifth BWC Review Conference was held.

Table 64–2 Examples of Bioterrorism

- Bulgarian defector Georgi Markov was assassinated in London, UK (1978) using ricin-filled pellets and a spring-loaded device disguised in an umbrella. A similar device used against a second defector in the same area was unsuccessful.
- Sverdlovsk, Russia (1979): Accidental release of anthrax from Soviet bioweapons facility caused an epidemic of inhalational anthrax with at least 77 cases and 60 deaths.
- Rajneeshee Cult (1984): An Indian religious cult headed by Rajneeshee plotted to contaminate restaurant salad bars in Dalles, OR, with *Salmonella typhimurium*. The motivation was to incapacitate voters, win local elections, and seize political control of the county. The incident resulted in a large community outbreak of salmonellosis involving 751 patients and at least 45 hospitalizations. The plot was revealed when the cult collapsed and members turned informant.
- Aum Shinrikyo (1995): A New Age Doomsday cult seeking to establish a theocratic state in Japan attempted at least 10 times to use anthrax, botulinum toxin, Q fever agent and Ebola virus in aerosol form. All attempts with biological weapons failed. Multiple chemical weapon attacks with Sarin and hydrogen cyanide in Matsumato, Tokyo and assassination campaigns were conducted. The nerve gas Sarin killed 12 and injured 5500 in the Tokyo subway.
- Texas (1997): Intentional contamination of muffins and doughnuts with laboratory cultures of *Shigella dysenteriae*. Caused gastroenteritis in 45 laboratory workers; four were hospitalized.
- Unknown individual group (2001): Intentional dissemination of anthrax spores through the US postal system led to the death of five people, infection of 22 others and contamination of several government buildings. Investigation into the attacks has not so far led to any conclusions.

Although events like these do not reach the level of national or international security, they can have significant public health consequences and therefore require preparedness at the local level. Active surveillance and rapid response at the local level will fulfill the definition for bioterrorism preparedness – 'think locally, act globally.'

Potential Biological Weapons Threat: Repositories and Sources

Nations and dissident groups have the access to skills needed to selectively cultivate some of the most dangerous pathogens and to deploy them as agents of biological terrorism and war (Henderson, 1998). The Japanese cult, Aum Shinrikyo, that released the nerve gas Sarin in the Tokyo subway also had plans for biological terrorism (Daplan, 1996). They were in possession of large quantities of nutrient media, botulinum toxin, and anthrax cultures and flew aircraft equipped with spray tanks. Members of this group had traveled to Zaire in 1992 to obtain samples of Ebola virus. Aum Shinrikyo is an example of a large, well financed organization that was attempting to develop a biological weapons capability. Such organizations would be expected to cause the greatest harm, because of their access to scientific expertise, biological agents, and, most importantly, dissemination technology.

The status of one of Russia's largest and most sophisticated former bioweapons facilities, called Vector, in Koltsovo, Novosibirsk is of concern. The facility housed the smallpox virus, as well as work on Ebola, Marburg and the hemorrhagic fever viruses (e.g., Machupo and Crimean–Congo) (Henderson, 1998). A visit in 1997 found a half-empty facility protected by a handful of guards. No one is clear where the scientists have gone. The confidence that this is the only storage site for smallpox outside the Centers for Disease Control and Prevention (CDC) is lacking.

The Threat of Biological Weapons

Components

A biological weapons system comprises four components; a payload, munitions, delivery system, and dispersion system. The payload is the biological agent itself. The munition protects and carries the payload to maintain its potency during delivery. The delivery system can be a missile, vehicle (aircraft, boat, automobile, or truck), or an artillery shell. The dispersion system ensures dissemination of the payload at the target site.

For a biological weapon to be highly effective, certain conditions should be optimized. The biological agent should consistently produce the

Table 64–3 Potential Agents of Bioterrorism

Category A	Category B	Category C
Variola major (smallpox)	*Coxiella burnetii* (Q fever)	Nipah virus
Bacillus anthracis (anthrax)	*Brucella* species (brucellosis)	Hantaviruses
Yersinia pestis (plague)	*Burkholderia mallei* (glanders)	Tickborne hemorrhagic fever viruses
Clostridium botulinum toxin (botulism)	*Burkholderia pseudomallei* (melioidosis) alphaviruses:	Tickborne encephalitis viruses
Francisella tularensis (tularemia)	Venezuelan encephalomyelitis; eastern and western	Yellow fever
Filoviruses: Ebola hemorrhagic fever; Marburg hemorrhagic fever	equine encephalomyelitis	Multi-drug-resistant tuberculosis
Arenaviruses: Lassa (Lassa fever); Junin (Argentine hemorrhagic fever) and related viruses	Ricin toxin from *Ricinus communis* (castor beans)	
	Epsilon toxin of *Clostridium perfringens*	
	Staphylococcal enterotoxin B	
	Trichothecene mycotoxins	
	Food- or waterborne pathogens including, but not limited to:	
	Salmonella species; *Shigella dysenteriae*; *Escherichia coli* (0157:H7); *Vibrio cholerae*; and *Cryptosporidium parvum*	
	Rickettsia prowazekii (typhus fever)	
	Chlamydia psittaci (psittacosis)	

desired effect of death or disease. It should be highly contagious with a short and predictable incubation period, and infective in low doses. The disease should be difficult to identify and be suspected as an act of bioterrorism. The agents should be suitable for mass production, storage, and weaponization, and stable during dissemination. The target population should have little or no immunity and little or no access to treatment. The terrorists should have means to protect or treat their own forces and population against the infectious agents or the toxins (Beeching, 2002).

The agents with potential for biological terrorism include bacterial, fungal, and viral pathogens and toxins produced by living organisms. Infectious agents that could potentially be used include those causing anthrax (*Bacillus anthracis*), plague (*Yersinia pestis*), tularemia (*Francisella tularensis*), equine encephalitides (e.g. Venezuelan equine encephalitis viruses), hemorrhagic fevers (arenaviruses, filoviruses, flaviviruses, and bunyaviruses), and smallpox (variola virus). Toxins include botulinum toxin from *Clostridium botulinum*; ricin toxin from the castor bean *Ricinus communis*; trichothecene mycotoxins from *Fusarium*, *Myrotecium*, *Trichoderma*, *Stachybotrys*, and other filamentous fungi; staphylococcal enterotoxins from *Staphylococcus aureus*; and toxins from marine organisms such as dinoflagellates, shellfish, and blue-green algae. Depending on the agents, a lethal or incapacitating outcome may occur.

Types of Bioterrorism Attack

A bioterrorist attack may occur in two scenarios – overt and covert. Attacks with biological agents are more likely to be covert. The attack by a biological agent will not have an immediate impact because of the delay between exposure and the onset of illness (i.e., the incubation period). Therefore, the first victims of a bioterrorism action will need to be identified by physicians or other primary health-care providers. Based on the first wave of victims, public health officials will need to determine that an attack has occurred, identify the organism, and prevent more casualties through prevention strategies (e.g., mass vaccination, prophylactic treatment) and infection control procedures (Kaufman, 1997). The clues to a potential bioterrorist attack include an outbreak of diseases in a non-endemic area, a seasonal disease during an off-season time, a known pathogen with unusual resistance or unusual epidemiologic features, an unusual clinical presentation or age distribution, and a genetically identical pathogen emerging rapidly in different geographical areas (Centers for Disease Control and Prevention, 2000a).

Agents of Bioterrorism Attacks

Based on the ease of transmission, severity of morbidity, mortality, and likelihood of use, biological agents can be classified into three categories (Table 64–3). Table 64–4 summarizes the biological agents in category A. Table 64–5 summarizes the biological agents in category B.

Laboratory Response Network for Bioterrorism

The Laboratory Response Network (LRN) is a consortium and partnership of laboratories that provide immediate and sustained laboratory testing and communication in support of public health emergencies, particularly in response to acts of bioterrorism. The LRN is currently made up of local, state, and federal public health laboratories in addition to private and commercial clinical laboratories, and selected food, water, agricultural, military, and veterinary testing laboratories. Other key partners include the Federal Bureau of Investigation, the Department of Defense, the Environmental Protection Agency, the Department of Agriculture, the Department of Justice, the Department of Energy, the Food and Drug Administration, the Association of Public Health Laboratories, the National Institutes of Health, the American Association of Veterinary Laboratory Diagnosticians, and the American Society for Microbiology. All laboratories are regarded as partners and, in some cases, registered members of the LRN. Preliminary testing and screening are performed primarily in a distributed rather than a centralized fashion to ensure a prompt and rapid initial response; a system of triage and referral of specimens ensures transfer of appropriate materials to specialized laboratories where sophisticated equipment, technologies, and expertise are applied to specimen analysis.

The goals of the LRN are to:

1. ensure that the nation's public health, clinical and other select laboratories are prepared to detect and respond to a bioterrorism or chemical terrorism event in an appropriate and integrated manner
2. ensure that all member reference laboratories collectively maintain state-of-the-art biodetection and diagnostic capabilities and surge capacity as well as secure electronic communication of test results for the biological and chemical agents likely to be used in the commission of a biocrime or bioterrorism event
3. work with other departments and agencies to ensure a successful federal response to an act of bioterrorism and to facilitate and optimize the ability of states to competently respond independently to biocrimes or public health emergencies in the state
4. promote the CDC's and Human Health Services's bioterrorism research agenda and the CDC's internal response needs
5. enlist an optimal number of registered participating LRN laboratories throughout the United States as determined by the LRN working group.

The LRN maintains:

1. a registry and linkage of clinical and private laboratories in the United States that includes sentinel and reference laboratories
2. complete, accurate, and standardized protocols for all levels of testing for agents deemed critical and likely to be used in the commission of biocrimes or acts of bioterrorism
3. secure but accessible supply of standardized reagents and diagnostic technologies produced and maintained by the CDC
4. secure electronic laboratory reporting that integrates with key epidemiologic, surveillance, and emergency response components
5. training and proficiency testing essential to the diagnostic process.

Clinical laboratories play a critical role in the LRN. Their heightened awareness to the possibility of recovering the agents of bioterrorism from patient specimens and referral of suspect isolates to the appropriate public health reference laboratory is crucial.

Classification of LRN Laboratories

The classification of bioterrorism laboratories by the LRN (Fig. 64–1) was revised in 2003. The original designations of level A, B, C, and D laboratories

Table 64–4 Summary of Category A Biological Agents

Agents	Infective Dose	Incubation Period (d)	Mortality (%) Untreated	Treated	Diagnostic Sample	Diagnostic assays	Isolation	Treatment	Prophylaxis	Vaccines Availability
Anthrax	8000–50 000 spores	1–6	≈100	≈99	Blood	Gram stain Ag-ELISA Serology: ELISA	Standard	Ciprofloxacin 400 mg i.v. q. 12 h Doxycycline 100 mg i.v. q. 12 h and 1–2 additional antimicrobials	Ciprofloxacin, 500 mg p.o. twice daily ×60 d	Yes
Botulism	0.0001 g/kg (type A)	1–5	Outbreak: First patient: 25 Subsequent cases: 4 Overall: 5–10		Nasal swab (possibly)	Ag-ELISA Mouse neutral	Standard	Antitoxin available through CDC via state and local health departments. More Information at CDC 404-639-2888 (24 h/d)	Preventalent toxoid	Investigation
Tularemia	10–50 organisms	2–10	33	<4	Blood, sputum, serum, EM of tissue	Culture Serology: agglutination	Standard	Streptomycin 1 g i.m. q. 12 h ×10 d Gentamicin, 5 mg/kg/d i.m. or i.v. ×10–14 d	Doxycycline 100 mg p.o. q. 12 h ×14 days Tetracycline 500 mg p.o. q. 6 h ×7 d Ciprofloxacin 500 mg p.o. q. 12 h ×14 d	Investigation
Plague	100–500	2–3	40–70	5	Blood, sputum, lymph node aspirate	Gram or Wright–Giemsa stain Ag-ELISA Culture Serology: ELISA, IFA	Droplet until patients treated for 3 days	Streptomycin 15 mg/kg (max. 1 g) i.m. q. 12 h ×10 d Gentamicin, 5 mg/kg/d i.m. or i.v., or 2 mg/kg loading dose followed by 1.7 mg/kg i.m. or i.v. t.d.s. ×10 d Chloramphenicol 25 mg/kg initial dose followed by 60 mg/kg/d i.v. q. 6 h	Doxycycline 100 mg p.o. q. 12 h ×14 days Tetracycline 500 mg p.o. q. 6 h ×10 d Ciprofloxacin 500 mg p.o. q. 12 h ×7 d	Yes
Smallpox	10–100 particles	7–17	Variola minor: <1 Variola major: 20–50		Pharyngeal swab, scab material	ELISA PCR Virus isolation	Airborne	Cidofovir (effective in vitro)	Vaccinia immunoglobulin 0.6 mL/kg i.m. (within 3 d of exposure, best within 24 h)	Yes
Viral hemorrhagic fever (HF)	1–10 particles	4–21	53–88		Serum, blood	Viral isolation Ag-ELISA RT-PCR Serology: ELISA	Contact, consider additional precautions if massive hemorrhage	Ribavirin 30 mg/kg i.v. initial dose, 15 mg/kg i.v. q. 6 h ×4 d, 7.5 mg/kg q. 8 h ×6 d for Congo–Crimean HF arenavirus (CCHF) Antibody passive for Argentine HF, Bolivian HF, Lassa fever, and CCHF	N/A	Investigation

CDC = Centers for Disease Control and Prevention; ELISA = enzyme-linked immunosorbent assay; EM = electron micrograph; i.m. = intramuscularly; i.v. = intravenously; IFA = indirect fluorescent antibody assay; p.o. = by mouth; PCR = polymerase chain reaction.

Table 64–5 Category B Bioterrorism Agents

Bacteria	Viruses	Toxins
Coxiella burnetii (Q fever)	Alpha viruses	
Brucella species (brucellosis)	Venezuelan encephalomyelitis	Ricin toxin (*Ricinus communis*)
Burkholderia mallei (glanders)	Eastern equine encephalomyelitis	Epsilon toxin (*Clostridium perfringens*)
Burkholderia pseudomallei (melioidosis)	Western equine encephalomyelitis	Enterotoxin B (*Staphylococcus aureus*)
Rickettsia prowazekii (typhus fever)		Trichothecene mycotoxins*
Chlamydia psittaci (psittacosis)		

Food or Water Borne Pathogens

Salmonella species
Shigella dysenteriae
Escherichia coli 0157:H7
Vibrio cholerae
Cryptosporidium parvum

* Not listed under Centers for Disease Control category B agents.

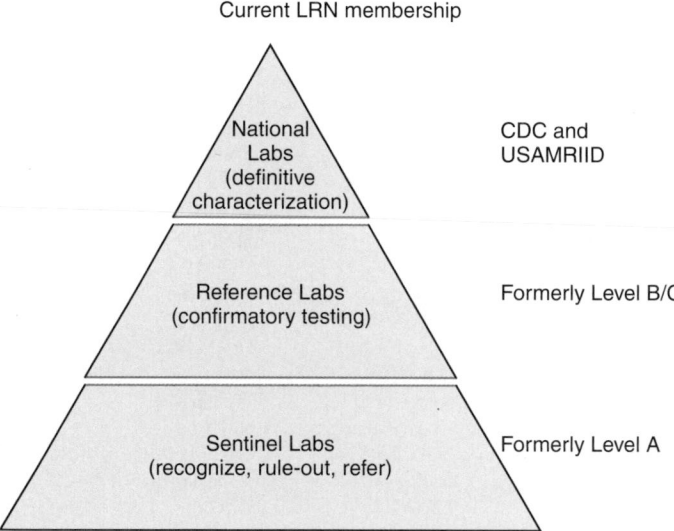

Figure 64–1 Classification of Laboratory Response Network (LRN) laboratories. CDC, Centers for Disease Control and Prevention; USAMRIID, United States Army Medical Research Institute for Infectious Diseases.

is no longer recognized and they are now designated as sentinel, reference, and national laboratories (Fig. 64–1).

Sentinel (formerly Level A)

Sentinel laboratories are clinical laboratories that follow biosafety level 2 (BSL-2) guidelines. Their primary responsibility is to recognize and rule out or refer suspicious agents by following standardized Sentinel Laboratory guidelines. Even though many Sentinel laboratories are capable of providing a 'presumptive identification' of some of the targeted organisms, they must refer isolates to an LRN reference laboratory.

Reference (formerly Levels B and C)

LRN reference laboratories are local and state public health laboratories, selected academic- or university-based laboratories, and designated specialty laboratories (veterinary, water, food, chemical, military, agricultural) that possess the reagents and technology for definitive confirmation of organisms, including toxin testing, referred by sentinel laboratories. LRN reference laboratories follow BSL-3 containment and practice guidelines.

National Laboratories (formerly Level D)

LRN national laboratories are Federal laboratories that have BSL-4 containment facilities and practice guidelines. The primary laboratory at this level is located at the CDC and specializes in the isolation and identification of BSL-4 agents such as Ebola, Marburg, and variola (smallpox) virus. This laboratory also possesses the capability of advanced genetic characterization and archiving of all bioterrorism agents.

The Clinical Laboratory's Responsibility

As members of the LRN, sentinel laboratories have access to the network and serve as 'sentinels' for the early detection of and raising of suspicion regarding a suspicious agent that cannot be ruled out as a possible bioterrorism-associated organism. Sentinel laboratories do not have access to the CDC secure website for Reference Laboratory Testing Protocols or reagents. Instead, sentinel laboratories must use conventional tests to facilitate the 'rule-out' or 'referral' of a suspicious isolate to an LRN reference laboratory.

The sentinel laboratory is not responsible for and should not make the decision that a bioterrorism event has occurred; that responsibility rests with local, state, and federal health and law enforcement officials. A designated individual within your facility (preferably the Infection Control Officer) should be notified of a suspicious agent, who in turn notifies the local public health officials. Under no circumstances should the laboratory contact law enforcement or public health officials. The exception is the need to contact the LRN reference laboratory for guidance in the disposition of the suspicious agent prior to referral for confirmatory testing.

Note: In no case should the sentinel laboratory accept environmental (powders, letters, packages), animal, food, or water specimens for examination, culture, or transport for bioterrorism-associated agents. Such specimens should be submitted directly to the nearest LRN reference laboratory.

Shipping and Handling of Infectious Materials Guidelines

United States, international, and commercial regulations mandate the proper packing, documentation, and safe shipment of dangerous goods in order to protect the public, airline workers, couriers, and other persons who work for commercial shippers and who handle the dangerous goods during the many segments of the shipping process. In addition, proper packing and shipping of dangerous goods will reduce the exposure of the shipper to the risks of criminal and civil liabilities associated with shipping dangerous goods, particularly infectious substances.

The process of properly packing and shipping an infectious substance, a diagnostic specimen, or a biological agent is composed of the following sequential steps:

1. Training of all persons involved in the shipping process
2. Determination of the applicability of the regulations
3. Determination of any applicable shipping limitations
4. Classification of the substance to be shipped
5. Identification of the substance to be shipped
6. Selection of the appropriate packing instructions to use
7. Selection of appropriate packaging
8. Marking and labeling the packaging
9. Documentation of the shipment.

Failure to follow governmental and commercial regulations for the packing and shipping of infectious substances and other dangerous goods can result in criminal prosecution and substantial financial penalties.

Potential Agents of Bioterrorism

Bacillus anthracis

Bacillus anthracis is an aerobic, spore-forming, nonmotile, large, Gram-positive rod.

Clinical Presentation

Humans can become infected with *B. anthracis* by handling products or consuming undercooked meat from infected animals. Infection may also result from inhalation of *B. anthracis* spores from contaminated animal products, such as wool, or the intentional release of spores. Human-to-human transmission has not been reported. Three forms of anthrax occur in humans: cutaneous, gastrointestinal, and inhalational (Lew, 2000).

Cutaneous Anthrax

Cutaneous infections occur when the bacterium or spore enters a cut or abrasion on the skin. Skin infection begins as a raised itchy bump or papule. Within 1–2 days, the bump develops into a fluid-filled vesicle, which ruptures to form a painless ulcer (called an eschar), usually 1–3 cm in diameter with a characteristic black, necrotic (dying) area in the center. Approximately 20% of untreated cases of cutaneous anthrax result in death, either because the infection becomes systemic or because of respiratory distress caused by edema in the cervical and upper thoracic regions.

Gastrointestinal Anthrax

The gastrointestinal form of anthrax may follow the consumption of contaminated meat from infected animals and is characterized by an acute inflammation of the intestinal tract. Initial signs of nausea, loss of appetite, vomiting, and fever are followed by abdominal pain, vomiting of blood, and severe bloody diarrhea. The mortality rate is difficult to determine for gastrointestinal anthrax, but is estimated to be 25–60% if not treated.

Inhalational Anthrax

Inhalational anthrax results from inhaling *B. anthracis* spores and is most likely following an intentional aerosol release of *B. anthracis*. After an incubation period of 1–6 days (depending on the number of inhaled spores), disease onset is gradual and nonspecific. Fever, malaise, and fatigue may be present initially, sometimes in association with a nonproductive cough and mild chest discomfort. These initial symptoms are often followed by a short period of improvement (ranging from several hours to days), followed by the abrupt development of severe respiratory distress with dyspnea (labored breathing), diaphoresis (perspiration), stridor (high-pitched whistling respiration), and cyanosis (bluish skin color). Shock and death usually occur within 24–36 h of the onset of respiratory distress and, in later stages, mortality approaches 100% despite aggressive treatment.

Specimen Selection and Testing

Refer to Table 64–6 for specimen selection for recovering *B. anthracis* (Logan, 1999).

Perform Gram's stain procedure/QC per standard laboratory protocol. *B. anthracis* is a large, Gram-positive rod ($1–1.5 \times 3–5\,\mu m$). Vegetative cells seen on Gram stain of blood and impression smears are in short chains of two to four cells that are encapsulated, which may be seen on the Gram stain as clear zones around the bacilli. Spores are not present in clinical samples unless exposed to low CO_2 levels, such as those found in ambient atmosphere; higher CO_2 levels within the body inhibit sporulation. The presence of large, encapsulated, Gram-positive rods in the blood is strongly presumptive of *B. anthracis* identification. *B. anthracis* forms oval, central-to-subterminal spores ($1 \times 1.5\,\mu m$) on sheep's blood agar (SBA) that do not cause significant swelling of the cell; it frequently occurs as long chains of bacilli. However, cells from growth on SBA, regardless of the incubation conditions (ambient atmosphere or CO_2-enriched), are not encapsulated (Gilchrist, 2000).

Inoculate and streak media for isolation of the respective specimen types (Table 64–6). After incubation of SBA plates for 15–24 h at 35–37°C, well isolated colonies of *B. anthracis* are 2–5 mm in diameter. The flat or slightly convex colonies are irregularly round, with edges that are slightly undulate (irregular, wavy border), and have a ground-glass appearance. There may be often comma-shaped projections from the colony edge, producing the 'Medusa-head' colony. *B. anthracis* grows well on SBA but does not grow on MAC. *B. anthracis* grows rapidly; heavily inoculated areas may show growth within 6–8 h and individual colonies may be detected within 12–15 h. *B. anthracis* is nonmotile. For presumptive identification criteria, refer to Table 64–7 and Figure 64–2. While hemolysis, Gram's stain morphology, or motility can be used for rule-out when the result provides clear evidence that the isolate is not *B. anthracis* (e.g., a clearly visible zone of β-hemolysis), a combination of two sentinel laboratory tests is recommended for rule-out. Immediately notify the State Public Health Laboratory Director (or designate) and State Public Health Department epidemiologist/health officer if *B. anthracis* cannot be ruled out and a bioterrorist event is suspected. Immediately notify physician/infection control according to internal policies if *B. anthracis* cannot be ruled out.

Brucella species

Brucella is a small, fastidious, aerobic, Gram-negative coccobacillus. In 1954 *Brucella suis* became the first biological agent to be weaponized by the United States in the days of its offensive biological warfare program. The infective dose for these organisms is very low if acquired via the inhalation route, which makes them a potentially effective bioterrorism agent and also makes them a hazard in the clinical microbiology laboratory.

Clinical presentation:

Brucella can cause both acute and chronic infections. The symptoms of brucellosis are nonspecific and systemic, with fever, sweats, headache, anorexia, back pain, and weight loss being frequent. The chronic form of the disease can mimic military tuberculosis, with suppurative lesions in the liver, spleen, and bone. The organism is often included in the differential diagnosis of fevers of unknown origin. It has a mortality of 5% in untreated individuals.

Specimen Selection and Testing

Refer to Table 64–8 for specimen selection for *Brucella* species. Aseptically inoculate liquid blood culture bottles with maximum amount of blood or body fluid, per manufacturers' instructions. Incubate at 35°C. Incubate nonautomated broth blood cultures for 21 days, with blind subculturing every 7 days, followed by terminal subculturing of negative blood cultures and holding sealed plates for 7 additional days. Incubate automated systems for 10 days and perform terminal subcultures at 7 days to increase yield. Isolation of *Brucella* is often delayed compared to other bloodstream pathogens, with peak isolation occurring at 3–4 days compared to 6–36 h for most other pathogens.

Although an incubation time of 21 days with weekly or terminal blind subculture is advocated, careful studies in *Brucella*-endemic areas using the BACTEC 9240 system (B D Division Instrument Systems, Sparks, MD) suggest that a maximum incubation time of 10 days is sufficient for reliable recovery of this organism, with 93% of 97 patient isolates being detected in 5 days (Bannatyne, 1997). For the BacT Alert system (BioMérieux, Inc., Hazelwood, MO), terminal subcultures at 7 days increased yield. Lysis-centrifugation has been shown to be less sensitive than broth-based systems for pediatric specimens. There is very limited published data with the ESP system (TREK Diagnostics, Westlake, OH), so its effectiveness in the recovery of *Brucella* is unknown. For tissues, inoculate blood agar plates (SBA), chocolate agar, and MacConkey agar or EMB agar (see Table 64–8) and incubate for up to 7 days at 35°C in a humidified incubator with 5–10% CO_2. Humidity may be maintained by placing a pan of water in the bottom of the incubator or by wrapping the plates with gas-permeable tape. *Brucella* has been responsible for many laboratory-acquired infections (Sewell, 1995; Fiori, 2000). If *Brucella* is suspected or the Gram stain shows a small, Gram-negative coccobacillus, avoid aerosols and perform subcultures in a biosafety cabinet (Schreckenberger, 1999). Plates should be taped shut and all further testing should be performed only in the biosafety cabinet, using biosafety level III practices. Brucellas are small ($0.4 \times 0.8\,\mu m$), Gram-negative coccobacilli that can be visualized directly from positive blood culture bottles or Gram stains of colonies from primary media. Subculture suspicious blood cultures to SBA, chocolate agar and MacConkey agar, or EMB agar. Incubate plates at 35°C in a humidified incubator with 5–10% CO_2. All oxidase, catalase and urea reactions are positive for *Brucella* spp. (Fig. 64–3).

Warning: The identification of *Brucella* species should not be attempted with commercial identification systems (Shapiro, 1999). *Haemophilus* can be confused with *Brucella*; however, *Haemophilus* does not grow on SBA. When in doubt, differentiate between these two genera by performing a satellite test. Inoculate a blood agar plate, followed by crossstreaking or spotting with *Staphylococcus aureus* ATCC 25923. After 24–48 h of incubation in 5% CO_2, *Haemophilus* demonstrates satellite growth around the *S. aureus*, while *Brucella* growth is not limited to the area around the staphylococcus.

Other organisms that can be confused with *Brucella* species because they are urease-positive are *Oligella ureolytica* (usually found only in the urine), *Psychrobacter phenylpyruvicus*, *Psychrobacter immobilis*, and *Bordetella bronchiseptica* (motile) (Table 64–9).

Brucella species will grow on subculture after 48 h of incubation in 5–10% CO_2 on chocolate agar and SBA. The organism does not grow on

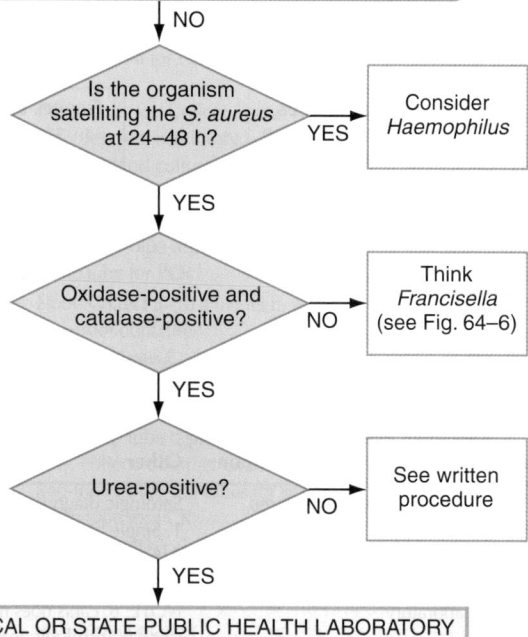

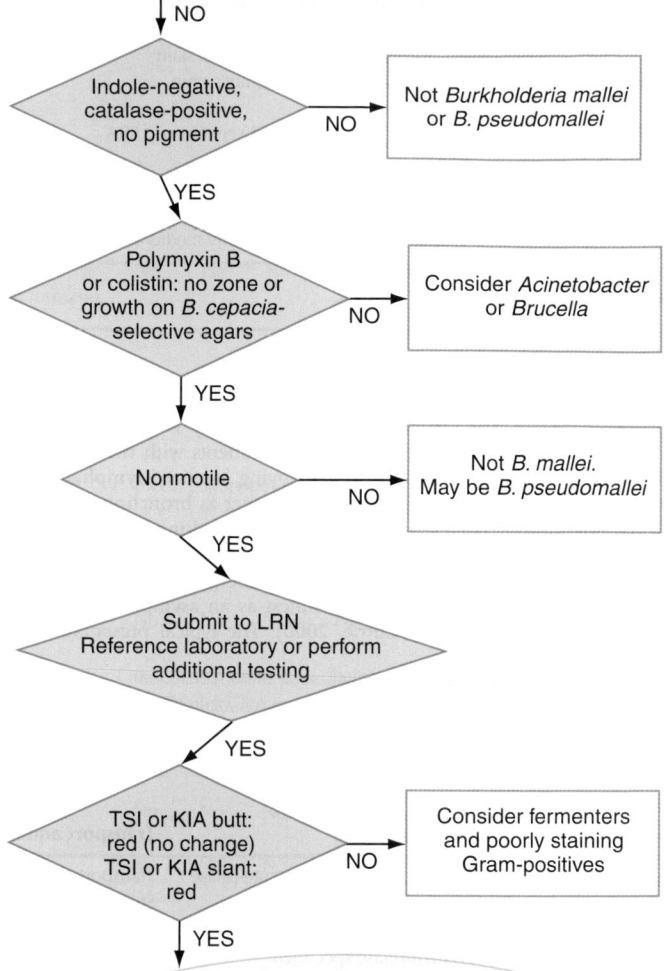

Figure 64–3 *Brucella*: Sentinel Laboratory flowchart.

Figure 64–4 *Burkholderia mallei*: Sentinel Laboratory flowchart. KIA = Kligler iron agar; TSI = triple sugar iron agar

acute infection is pneumonia. The incubation period of this infection is 2–5 days. The disease presents with high fever, dyspnea, and pleuritic chest pain. Subacute infections can mimic those of *Mycobacterium tuberculosis*. Patients can have low-grade fevers, malaise, anorexia, and weight loss, which occur over a period of months.

Chronic infection is similar to miliary tuberculosis in that the infection is disseminated, and granulomatous lesions can be seen in a variety of tissues. Patients may have minimal symptoms, but most have symptoms similar to miliary tuberculosis, including fever, cough, and weight loss.

Specimen Selection and Testing

Appropriate specimens include blood, bone marrow, sputum, abscess material, and wound swabs. *B. mallei* is a small, Gram-negative coccobacillus (Table 64–10). *B. pseudomallei* is a small, Gram-negative rod. The organisms may be observed in direct Gram stain from respiratory specimens or abscess material/wounds (Gilligan, 2003). They can also be seen in smears of positive blood culture bottles. Routine isolation media should be used (sheep blood agar [SBA], MacConkey agar, etc.). For improved isolation, a colistin disk or polymyxin B disk may be placed in the initial inoculation area of the SBA if isolation of *Burkholderia* spp. is specifically requested. On SBA, *B. mallei* shows smooth, gray, translucent colonies in 2 days, without pigment or distinctive odor. *B. mallei* will grow without any inhibition around the colistin or polymyxin B disk. On SBA, *B. pseudomallei* often reveals small, smooth creamy colonies in the first 1–2 days, which gradually change after a few days to dry, wrinkled colonies similar to *Pseudomonas stutzeri*. Colonies are neither yellow- nor violet-pigmented. *B. pseudomallei* will grow without any inhibition around the colistin or polymyxin B disk. 'Sniffing' of plates containing *B. pseudomallei* is dangerous and should not be done. However, the odor will be apparent without sniffing. Follow the isolation schemes shown in Figures 64–4 and 64–5 for screening and confirmation.

Further epidemiologic investigation is needed whenever a presumptive identification of *B. mallei* or *B. pseudomallei* is made. Within the hospital setting, the infectious disease service and/or infection control department should be notified so further investigation of the patient's history can be made so that naturally occurring infections can be ruled out. The State Laboratory Director (or designate) should be notified of the presumptive identification of *B. mallei* or *B. pseudomallei*. The State Public Health Laboratory Director will coordinate notification of the Centers for Disease Control and Prevention and State and Federal law enforcement agencies.

Table 64–9 Differentiation of *Brucella* from Other Urea-Positive, Oxidase-Positive Gram-Negative Coccobacilli

	Brucella	EO-2, EO-4 Psychrobacter immobilis	Psychrobacter phenylpyruvicus	Oligella ureolytica	Actinobacillus spp.	Bordetella bronchiseptica Ralstonia paucula (IV c2)	Bordetella hinaii	Haemophilus spp.[†]
Gram stain morphology	Tiny ccb, stains faintly	Small ccb, rods EO-2 in packets	Ccb	Tiny ccb	Ccb, rods	Ccb, rods	Ccb, rods	Ccb
Catalase	+	+	+	+	v	+	+	v
Oxidase	+	+	+	+	+	+	+	v
Urea[*]	+	v	+	+	+	+	14% pos.	v
Motility	–	–	–	+, delayed	–	+	+	–
PDA	–	–	+	+	–	v	–	–
Nitrate	+	v	68%	+	+	v	–	NA
Nitrite	–	v	–	+	–	–	–	NA
TSI	Alkaline	Alkaline	Alkaline	Alkaline	Acid/Acid	Alkaline	Alkaline	No growth
MAC – 48 h	–, poor	–, poor	–, poor	–, poor	–, poor	+	+	–

O. ureolytica is primarily a uropathogen. *Actinobacillus actinomycetemcomitans* is urea-negative and rarely oxidase-positive. Urea-positive actinobacilli are from animal sources.

[*] Use rapid urea test to increase sensitivity. [†] Only grows on chocolate; or on blood agar associated with a *Staphylococcus* colony.

NA = not applicable; v = variable; ccb = coccobacilli; PDA = phenylalanine deaminase; TSI = triple sugar iron agar; MAC = MacConkey's agar.

Table 64–10 Specimen Selection: Melioidosis and Glanders (*Burkholderia pseudomallei* and *B. mallei*)

Disease	Specimen Selection	Transport and Storage	SBA	CA	MAC	PC	Stain
Possible *B. pseudomallei* or *B. mallei* exposure in asymptomatic patient	No cultures or serology indicated						Follow public health instructions if advised to collect specimens
Clinical illness	Bone marrow	Transport within ≤2 h, at RT. Store ≤24 h at 4°C		X		Gram stain	*B. pseudomallei* is a small Gram-negative bacillus that may demonstrate bipolar morphology on stain. *B. mallei* is a small Gram-negative coccobacillus. Incubation should be at 35–37°C, ambient atmosphere; CO_2 incubation is acceptable
	Blood cultures: Collect 2 sets (1 set is 2 bottles) per institutional procedure for routine blood cultures OR collect lysis-centrifugation (e.g., isolator) blood cultures	Transport at RT. Incubate at 35–37°C per blood culture protocol	Blood culture bottles OR collect lysis-centrifugation (e.g., isolator) blood cultures and plate to: X				Cultures should be manipulated in a biological safety cabinet. Personal protective equipment includes gloves, gown, mask, and protective faceshield. All cultures should be taped shut during incubation. Incubation should be at 35–37°C, ambient atmosphere; CO_2 incubation is acceptable

CA = chocolate agar; MAC = MacConkey agar; PC = selective medium for *Burkholderia cepacia*; RT = room temperature; SBA = sheep's blood agar.

Coxiella burnetii

Coxiella burnetii is a pleomorphic coccobacillus that is Gram-negative, obligately intracellular, and 0.3–0.7 μm long. There is a sporelike form, the small-cell variant, which is remarkably stable in extracellular environments. A large-cell variant also exists that is the vegetative, metabolically active form. Mixtures of both forms are found in phagolysosomes. There is phase variation, similar to that in *Salmonella*, in which the lipopolysaccharide (LPS) varies chemically as either the virulent, phase I 'smooth' type LPS, or the phase II 'rough' LPS, associated with avirulent *C. burnetii*. *C. burnetii* is phylogenetically related to *Pseudomonas*, *Francisella*, and *Legionella*, within the *Legionella* group of the γ-Proteobacteria subdivision. It is more distantly related to *Rickettsia* (Heinzen, 1997).

Clinical presentation

The symptoms of Q fever are generally nonspecific. There are multiple presentations, most commonly pneumonia (47–63%), hepatitis (60%), or fever only (14%) (Raoult, 2001). It is estimated that self-limited febrile illness may, in fact, be the most common form of the disease. The incubation period is 2–3 weeks. The organisms proliferate in the lung following inhalation of contaminated aerosols and then invade the blood stream. Acute Q fever is characterized by sudden onset of high fever, headache, myalgias, arthralgias, cough, and, less frequently, rash or a meningeal syndrome. In addition to radiographic manifestations of pneumonia, patients often have elevated liver enzyme levels, elevated erythrocyte sedimentation rates, and thrombocytopenia. Development of chronic Q fever is a more serious disease, which can occur up to 20 years after the initial infection. The major complication of chronic Q fever is endocarditis. Overall, the mortality rate of Q fever is low, approximately 2.4% (Tissot-Dupont, 1992), but it may be as high as 65% among those with chronic Q fever (Raoult, 2001).

Specimen Selection and Testing

The laboratory diagnosis of Q fever is based mainly on serologic testing (Fournier, 1998). Patients with acute Q fever typically produce an antibody response primarily to *C. burnetii* phase II antigen, while chronic

Morphology: Gram-negative rod, small, straight or slightly curved, may demonstrate bipolar morphology at 24 h and peripheral staining, like endospores, when cultures are older.

Growth: Poor growth at 24 h; good growth of white colonies at 48 h on SBA, may develop wrinkled colonies in time, nonpigmented. Often demonstrates strong characteristic musty, earthy odor.

Reactions: Oxidase-positive, growth on MacConkey agar in 48 h, indole negative

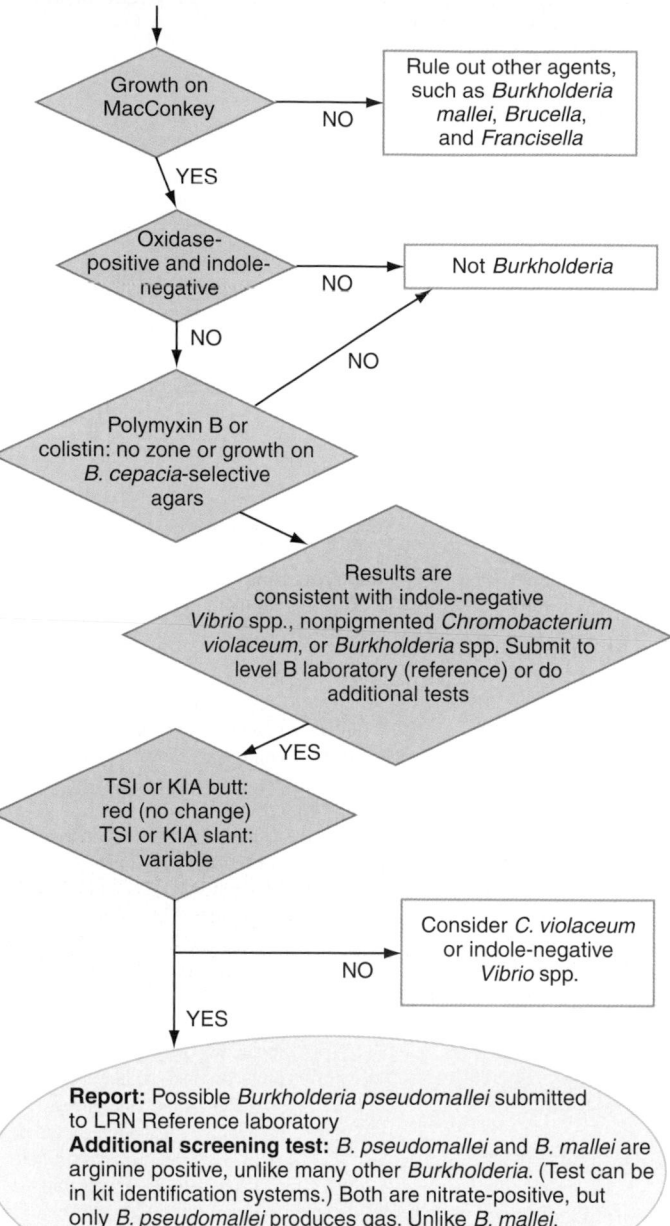

Figure 64–5 *Burkholderia pseudomallei*: Sentinel Laboratory flowchart. KIA = Kligler iron agar; SBA = sheep blood agar; TSI = triple sugar iron agar.

Table 64–11 Specimen Selection: Q fever (*Coxiella burnetii*)

Specimen Selection	Transport and Storage	Specimen Plating and Processing
Serum: collect 10 ml of serum (red-top, tiger-top, or gold-top tube) as soon as possible after onset of symptoms (acute) and with a follow-up specimen (convalescent) at ≥14 days for serological testing.	Transport within ≈6 h, at 4°C. Store at –20 to –70°C.	**Do not attempt tissue culture isolation**, as that could result in a very unsafe situation in which there is a significant amount of infectious organism. Sentinel laboratories should consult with State Public Health Laboratory Director (or designate) prior to or concurrent with testing if *C. burnetii* is suspected by the attending physician. Serology is available through commercial reference as well as public health laboratories.
Blood: Collect blood in EDTA (lavender) or sodium citrate (blue) and maintain at 4°C for storage and shipping for PCR or special cultures. If possible, collect specimens prior to antimicrobial therapy.	Transport within ≈6 h, at 4°C. Store at –4° C	
Tissue, body fluids, others, including cell cultures and cell supernatants: Specimens can be kept at 2–8°C if transported within 24 h. Store frozen at –70°C or on dry ice.	Transport within <24 h, at 2–8°C. Store at –70°C or on dry ice	

EDTA = ethylenediaminetetraacetic acid.

can be inadvertently isolated in conventional cell cultures in a wide variety of cell lines, including all fibroblast cell lines. After an incubation period of 5–15 days, *C. burnetii*-infected cells are detectable as cytoplasmic inclusions.

Collect serum (red-top or serum separator tube [SST], tiger-top tube) as soon as possible after onset of symptoms (acute phase) and with a follow-up specimen (convalescent phase) at 14 days for serological testing (Table 64–11). Collect blood in an ethylenediaminetetraacetic acid (EDTA) (lavender) or sodium citrate (blue) tube and maintain at 4°C for storage and shipping for PCR or special cultures. If possible, collect specimens prior to antimicrobial therapy. Tissue, body fluids, and others, including cell cultures and cell supernatants, can be kept at 2–8°C if transported within 24 h. Store frozen at –70°C or on dry ice.

Level A (sentinel) laboratories should consult with the State Public Health Laboratory Director (or designate) prior to or concurrent with testing if *C. burnetii* is suspected by the attending physician. Serology is available through commercial reference as well as public health laboratories. Report positive results to the patient's physician and hospital infection control and public health officials.

Francisella tularensis

Francisella tularensis is a tiny, pleomorphic, nonmotile, Gram-negative, facultative intracellular coccobacillus (0.2–0.5 × 0.7–1.0 μm). It is a fastidious organism and may require cysteine supplementation for good growth on general laboratory media (Wong, 1999).

Clinical presentation

The symptoms of tularemia are not unique. The incubation period is 2–10 days. There are multiple presentations, most commonly as ulceroglandular disease (45–80%). The bacteria replicate in the skin at the localized site of penetration, where an ulcer usually forms. From the penetration site(s), bacteria are transported by the lymphatic system to regional nodes and then may be disseminated to blood and other sites. Onset is sudden: typically, the patient has a temperature of 38–40°C accompanied by chills, headache, generalized body aches (often prominent in the low back), coryza, pharyngitis, cough, and chest pain or tightness. Without treatment, nonspecific symptoms usually persist for several weeks, and sweats, chills, progressive weakness, and weight loss characterize the illness. Other forms of tularemia may be complicated by

C. burnetii infections typically elicit a higher antibody response to phase I antigen. The diagnosis can by confirmed by (1) demonstration of fourfold or greater changes in antibody titer between paired acute- and convalescent-phase serum samples by immunofluorescence antibody testing, (2) detection of *C. burnetii* by polymerase chain reaction (PCR) or immunohistochemical staining of biopsy material from affected organs, or (3) culture of this material. Because of the highly infectious nature of this organism (BSL-3), specimens from suspected cases of Q fever should be immediately forwarded to a local or State Health Department for isolation and identification. Because of the extreme infectivity of *C. burnetii*, level A (sentinel) laboratories should not attempt to culture this organism but should be aware of the potential for inadvertent isolation of *C. burnetii* in cell culture systems designed for virus isolation. *C. burnetii*

Table 64–12 Specimen Selection: Tularemia (*Francisella tularensis*)

Disease	Specimen Selection	Transport and Storage	SBA	CA	MAC	Stain	Other
			Specimen Plating and Processing				
Possible *F. tularensis* exposure in asymptomatic patient	No cultures or serology indicated						Follow public health instructions if advised to collect specimens
Oculoglandular tularemia	Conjunctival scraping	≤24 h, 4°C	X	X	X	Gram stain; prepare smears for DFA referral	Add a BCYE plate and a plate selective for *Neisseria gonorrhoeae* such as modified Thayer–Martin. Manipulate cultures in a biological safety cabinet. Personal protective equipment includes gloves, gown, mask, and protective faceshield. All cultures should be taped shut during incubation
	Lymph node aspirate: Flushing with 1.0 ml of sterile saline may be needed to obtain material	Transport at RT, 4°C if transport is delayed. Store ≤24 h at 4°C	X	X	X	Gram stain; prepare smears for DFA referral	
	Blood cultures: Collect 2 sets (1 set is 2 bottles) per institutional procedure for routine blood cultures. Growth is more likely from aerobic bottle	Transport at RT, 4°C if transport is delayed. Store ≤24 h at 4°C.	Blood culture bottles; subculture the broth to BCYE plate and incubate aerobically				Cultures should be manipulated in a biological safety cabinet. Personal protective equipment includes gloves, gown, mask, and protective faceshield. All cultures should be taped shut during incubation
Ulceroglandular tularemia	Blood cultures: Collect 2 sets (1 set is 2 bottles) per institutional procedure for routine blood cultures. Growth is more likely from aerobic bottle	Transport at RT. Incubate at 35–37°C per blood culture protocol	Blood culture bottles; subculture the broth to BCYE plate and incubate aerobically				Cultures should be manipulated in a biological safety cabinet. Personal protective equipment includes gloves, gown, mask, and protective faceshield. All cultures should be taped shut during incubation
	Ulcer or tissue: Collect biopsy (best specimen), scraping or swab	≤24 h, 4°C	X	X	X	Gram stain	Add a BYCE plate and a plate selective for *Neisseria gonorrhoeae* such as modified Thayer–Martin. Prepare smears for DFA referral. Manipulate cultures in a biological safety cabinet. Personal protective equipment includes gloves, gown, mask and protective faceshield. All cultures should be taped shut during incubation
	Lymph node aspirate: Flushing with 1.0 ml of sterile saline may be needed to obtain material	Transport at RT; 4°C if transport is delayed. Store ≤24 h at 4°C	X	X	X	Gram stain	
Pneumonic tularemia	Sputum/throat: Collect routine throat culture using a swab or expectorated sputum collected into sterile, leakproof container	≤24 h, 4°C	X	X	X	Gram stain; prepare smears for DFA referral	Add a BYCE plate and a plate selective for *Neisseria gonorrhoeae* such as modified Thayer–Martin. Prepare smears for DFA referral. Manipulate cultures in a biological safety cabinet. Personal protective equipment includes gloves, gown, mask and protective faceshield. All cultures should be taped shut during incubation
	Bronchial/tracheal wash: Collect per institution's procedure in area dedicated to collecting respiratory specimens under isolation/containment circumstances, i.e., isolation chamber/ 'bubble'	≤24 h, 4°C	X	X	X	Gram stain	
	Blood cultures: Collect 2 sets (1 set is 2 bottles) per institutional procedure for routine blood cultures. Growth is more likely from aerobic bottle	Transport at RT. Incubate at 35–37°C per blood culture protocol	Blood culture bottles; Subculture the broth to BYCE plate and incubate aerobically				Cultures should be manipulated in a biological safety cabinet. Personal protective equipment includes gloves, gown, mask, and protective faceshield. All cultures should be taped shut during incubation
	2 red-top or gold-top tubes: For PCR and serology (acute and, if needed for diagnosis, convalescent serum in 14 days)	≤2 h RT; ≤24 h, 4°C	No				Positive serology test would meet presumptive criteria. Confirmation requires culture identification or a fourfold rise in titer

BCYE = buffered charcoal-yeast extract agar; CA = chocolate agar; DFA = direct fluorescent antibody; MAC = MacConkey agar; RT = room temperature; SBA = sheep's blood agar.

bacteremic spread, leading variously to tularemic pneumonia, sepsis, and meningitis (rare) (Overholt, 1961).

Specimen Selection and Testing

Acceptable specimens include blood, biopsied tissue or ulcer scraping or aspirate or involved tissue (Table 64–12). Perform Gram stain procedure/ quality control per standard laboratory protocol. Staining of *F. tularensis* often reveals the presence of tiny, 0.2–0.5 × 0.7–1.0 µm, pleomorphic, poorly staining, Gram-negative coccobacilli seen mostly as single cells. The Gram stain interpretation may be difficult because the cells are minute

and faintly staining. *F. tularensis* cells are smaller than *Haemophilus influenzae*. Bipolar staining is not a distinctive feature of *F. tularensis* cells. *F. tularensis* grows in commercial blood culture media. These organisms require cysteine supplementation; therefore, *F. tularensis* may at first grow on SBA, but upon subsequent passage will fail to grow on standard SBA. On cysteine supplemented agar plates, it is a gray-white, opaque colony, usually too small to be seen at 24 h on most general media such as chocolate agar, Thayer–Martin, and buffered charcoal-yeast extract agar. After incubation for 48 h or more, colonies are about 1–2 mm in diameter, white to gray to bluish-gray, opaque, flat, with an entire edge, smooth, and

VII

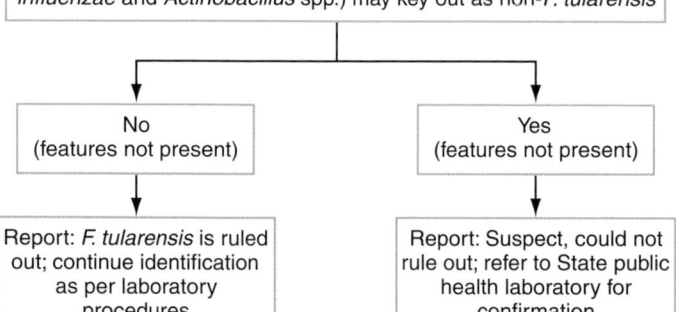

Morphology: Aerobic, pleomorphic, minute (0.2–0.5 × 0.7–1.0 μm), faintly staining, Gram-negative coccobacillus

Growth: Scant to no growth on SBA after > 48 h.
Produces 1–2 mm gray to grayish white colonies on chocolate agar after > 48 h.

↓

Perform all additional work in biosafety cabinet

↓

Oxidase: Negative
Catalase: Weak positive
β-lactamase: positive
Satellite: Negative
Urease: Negative

Warning: Automated identification systems (e.g., *Haemophilus influenzae* and *Actinobacillus* spp.) may key out as non-*F. tularensis*

No
(features not present)

Yes
(features not present)

Report: *F. tularensis* is ruled out; continue identification as per laboratory procedures

Report: Suspect, could not rule out; refer to State public health laboratory for confirmation

Figure 64–6 *Francisella tularensis*: Sentinel Laboratory flowchart. SBA = sheep blood agar

have a shiny surface. *F. tularensis* will not grow on MacConkey or EMB plates. As depicted in Figure 64–6, *F. tularensis* is also-oxidase negative, weakly catalase-positive, β-lactamase-positive, satellite- or XV-test-negative and urease-test-negative.

Immediately notify the State Public Health Laboratory Director (or designate) and State Public Health Department epidemiologist/health officer if *F. tularensis* cannot be ruled out and a bioterrorist event is suspected. Immediately notify physician/infection control according to internal policies if *F. tularensis* cannot be ruled out.

The most common misidentification of *F. tularensis* is *H. influenzae* (satellite- or XV-positive) and *Actinobacillus* species (β-lactamase-negative). Identification of isolates by using commercial identification systems is not recommended because of the high probability of misidentification. The Vitek NHI panel may give as high as 99% confidence to the identification of *Actinobacillus actinomycetemcomitans* with strains of *F. tularensis*.

Unknown Viruses

Viruses described as potential agents of bioterrorism include those listed in Tables 64–13 and 64–14. These viruses are possible candidates for receipt by the laboratory as an unknown virus if there is an outbreak (Henderson, 1999; Centers for Disease Control and Prevention, 2001). If a smallpox virus, filovirus, arenavirus, alphavirus, or Crimean–Congo hemorrhagic fever virus infection is suspected, contact public health

officials before specimen collection. Do not collect specimens and use viral transport medium unless specifically requested by public health officials. Do not accept environmental or animal specimens. Forward such specimens directly to the State health laboratory. Alert public health officials. Do not inoculate specimens received for ruling out a potential viral agent of bioterrorism into cell culture. Immediately inform the appropriate personnel designated by the hospital's bioterrorism readiness protocol. Medical personnel should initiate direct communication with the local or State department of health. Unidentifiable patterns of cytopathic effect (CPE) could be caused by a potential agent of bioterrorism. Consult the physician to see if the patient's clinical presentation is consistent with smallpox or a hemorrhagic viral infection. If the patient's history and/or disease is consistent, notify the Public Health Department and follow instructions to forward the culture and remaining specimens to the appropriate laboratory.

Smallpox

Transmission of variola virus occurs directly by inhalation of infective aerosols or by direct contact with contaminated materials (Ropp, 1999). Viral spread may occur with onset of fever (prodrome phase) but is greatest with the onset of rash. Infectivity diminishes with the onset of scab formation; however, the person is contagious to others until the eradication of all scabs. Symptoms develop approximately 12–14 days after a primary exposure. A period of approximately 2 weeks may ensue before detection of visible symptoms and confirmation of the diagnosis. The symptoms are typical of many viral infections and include fever and severe myalgias (Table 64–15). Initial presentation of vesicles occurs in the oropharynx within 72 h of the first symptoms. Lesions then spread, first to the face and then to the arms, hands, and feet, during the next 7–14 days. Vesicles are more abundant on the face, forearms, and lower legs and are sparser on the trunk. The smallpox rash initially presents as erythematous papules, which progress to form vesicles, then pustules, and finally scabs. Death may occur within 5–7 days in rapidly progressing infection or within 10–14 days in the more classical presentation of the infection.

The disease most commonly confused with smallpox is chickenpox. During the first 2–3 days of illness, the appearance of the rash of smallpox is indistinguishable from the rash of chickenpox. Several notable differences aid in the correct identification of the viral syndrome: (1) Smallpox lesions develop simultaneously, mature uniformly, and disperse in equal concentrations over infected body sites; in contrast, different developmental stages of lesions (crops) occur concurrently during chickenpox; (2) Smallpox vesicles are more abundant on the face, forearms, and lower legs and are sparser on the trunk. Chickenpox lesions often localize on the trunk and head.

Complications arise in some individuals after immunization with the smallpox vaccine. The currently described syndromes are as follows: (1) generalized vaccinia, a harmless infection typified by numerous lesions on the body; (2) progressive vaccinia (vaccinia necrosum) characterized by progressive necrosis of the vaccination site; (3) eczema vaccinatum, an often serious infection that occurs in individuals with eczema; (4) erythema multiforme, an erythematous rash possibly linked to an allergic reaction; and (5) postvaccinal encephalitis, a rare central nervous system infection in primary vaccines.

Alphaviruses

Most notably recognized as agents of equine encephalitis, the alphaviruses possess the capacity to cause epidemic human disease (Beaty, 1995; Centers for Disease Control and Prevention, 2001). In humans as well as horses, the viruses have a proclivity for the central nervous system. Generalized symptoms, such as fever, malaise, and headache, precede the onset of encephalitis. Depending on the etiologic agent, symptoms may progress to more serious neurological manifestations. Of the three viral syndromes, Venezuelan equine encephalitis (VEE) has a lower morbidity/mortality rate. Symptoms resembling a flu-like syndrome usually manifest after an

Table 64–13 Potential Viral Bioterrorism Agents

Poxviridae	Arenaviridae	Bunyaviridae	Flaviviridae	Filoviridae	Alphavirus
Variola virus (smallpox)	Lassa fever virus	Rift Valley fever virus	Kyasanur Forest disease virus	Ebola virus	Eastern equine encephalitis virus
	Junin virus (Argentinian HF)	Crimean–Congo HF virus	Omsk HF virus	Marburg virus	Western equine encephalitis virus
	Machupo virus (Bolivian HF)	Hantavirus (HF)	Dengue HF virus		Venezuelan equine encephalitis virus
	Guanarito virus (Venezuelan HF)		Yellow fever virus		

HF, hemorrhagic fever.

Table 64–14 Epidemiology of Viral Bioterrorism Agents

Virus family	Disease	Geographic Location	Transmission	Prevention
Poxviridae	Smallpox	Unknown*	Person–person	Vaccine
Arenaviridae	Lassa fever	West Africa	Rodent	Ribavirin
	South American hemorrhagic fevers	South America	Rodent	Vaccine/plasma[†]
Bunyaviridae	Crimean–Congo hemorrhagic fever	Asia, central Africa	Tick	
	Rift Valley fever	Africa	Mosquito; blood of infected animals (e.g., sheep)	
	Hantavirus hemorrhagic fever	South-east Asia	Rodent	
Flaviviridae	Yellow fever	South America, Africa	Mosquito	Vaccine
	Dengue hemorrhagic fever	Asia, Africa, Australia, Americas	Mosquito	Insect repellants (DEET)
	Kyasanur Forest disease	India	Tick	Vaccine
	Omsk hemorrhagic fever	Russia	Tick Muskrat–human	
Filoviridae	Ebola and Marburg hemorrhagic fever	Africa	Direct contact[‡]	
Alphavirus	Eastern equine encephalitis	Canada to South America, Caribbean	Mosquito	No human vaccine
	Western equine encephalitis	Canada to South America	Mosquito	No human vaccine
	Venezuelan equine encephalitis	South America	Mosquito	No human vaccine

* Smallpox was deemed eradicated worldwide in 1980. [†] Vaccine available for Junin virus only. Convalescent-phase plasma therapy useful with some South American hemorrhagic fevers. [‡] Direct contact with infected body fluids (including vomitus, urine, and stool) promotes transmission of arenaviruses or filoviruses. Airborne transmission is also a remote possibility.

Table 64–15 Diseases with Symptoms Compatible with Smallpox or Other Viral Bioterrorism Agents

Pre-exanthem	Early exanthem	Late exanthem
Influenza	Measles, rubella	Chickenpox
Sepsis	Varicella-zoster	Erythema multiforme
Central nervous system infection	Misc. viral exanthema*	Stevens-Johnson syndrome
	Drug eruptions	Scabies
Appendicitis	Syphilis	Impetigo
Pneumonia	Erythema multiforme	Drug eruptions
Leukemia	Insect bites	Pemphigus
Enteric fever	Meningococcemia[†]	Misc. viral exanthem*
		Meningococcemia[†]

* A miscellaneous viral exanthema (skin rash) would include infections caused by herpes simplex virus, varicella zoster virus, enteroviruses, or other poxviruses, such as the agents of vaccinia, molluscum contagiosum, or other poxviruses that can be passed from animals to humans, such as monkeypox. [†] Meningococcemia could be confused with hemorrhagic smallpox.

incubation period of less than 1 week. Only a small percentage of cases progress to neurological involvement, and the prospects for recovery surpass those for eastern equine encephalitis virus (EEE) or western equine encephalitis virus (WEE). Both EEE and WEE produce more serious effects that often develop into coma. Fatalities are higher with EEE, and infection often results in permanent sequelae. As with all arboviruses, either a mosquito or a rodent vector spreads alphaviruses in nature. Human transmission through infectious aerosols gives these viruses bioterrorism potential.

Viral Hemorrhagic Fever Viruses

Clinical symptoms will vary, depending on the virus and response of the patient (Borio, 2002). After incubation periods ranging from 2 days to 3 weeks, general symptoms include fever, headache, other central nervous system symptoms, malaise, muscle and joint pain, nausea, diarrhea, and cough. South American hemorrhagic fever (SAHF) virus produces petechiae over the palate and in the axillary regions. The filoviruses produce a maculopapular rash on the trunk. As the infection progresses, petechiae and hemorrhage of the mucous membranes develop, accompanied by blood in the urine and vomitus. Coagulopathy, microvascular damage, circulatory shock, and multiorgan failure characterize later stages of infection. Lassa fever and Rift Valley fever viruses produce less serious hemorrhagic manifestation than SAHF, Crimean–Congo hemorrhagic fever, and Ebola and Marburg hemorrhagic fever infections. Severe necrosis of the liver and retinitis are unique to Rift Valley fever. Depending on the pathogen, mortality rates range from low to very high (Ebola virus). The mode of transmission of Ebola and Marburg viruses involves intimate contact with infected fluid and tissue.

Clinical features

The recognition of the initial signs of a viral epidemic within a population varies, depending on a number of factors, including mode of transmission, incubation period, and clinical presentation. Viral shedding usually occurs before onset of symptoms and can continue through the course of the illness. Collection of specimens during early infection enhances the ability of the laboratory to recover or detect the virus. Transmission occurs either through direct contact with an infected individual (or animal), exposure to contaminated fomites, or through the bite of an insect vector. An epidemic propagated through person-to-person contact spreads more slowly through a population. Viral exposure through a common source, such as contaminated food, water, or aerosolized product, results in concurrent disease in a larger number of individuals. The laboratory must be alert to an unknown virus in a variety of specimens. Some viral infections disseminate from a primary infection site to a secondary location within the host. For example, smallpox is shed from the upper respiratory mucosa during the very early stages of infection, but is found in larger concentrations in the characteristic skin lesions that develop later. Differentiation of the unknown virus from other pathogens is important for infection control and rapid detection of an infection.

Specimen Selection and Testing

If smallpox, filovirus, arenavirus, alphavirus, or Crimean–Congo hemorrhagic fever virus infection is suspected, contact public health officials before collection of specimens for diagnostic testing. Do not inoculate specimens received for ruling out a potential viral agent of bioterrorism into cell culture. Immediately inform the appropriate personnel designated by the hospital's bioterrorism readiness protocol. Initiate direct communication with the local or State department of health. Sentinel laboratories should not accept environmental or animal specimens; such specimens should be forwarded directly to the State health laboratory. Smallpox specimens include skin lesions, vesicle fluid, scrapings and crusts (Table 64–16). Alphaviruses specimens include respiratory secretions, blood

VII

Table 64–16 Specimen Selection: Viral Diseases

Disease/Agent	Specimen Selection		Transport and Storage	Specimen Plating and Processing
Smallpox (variola virus)	See CDC document *Specimen Collection and Transport Guidelines* for detailed instructions: http://www.bt.cdc.gov/agent/smallpox/response-plan/index.asp#guidec (Click on 'Guide D'). NOTE: Only recently, successfully vaccinated personnel (within 3 years) wearing appropriate barrier protection (gloves, gown, and shoe covers) should be involved in specimen collection for suspected cases of smallpox. Respiratory protection is not needed for personnel with recent, successful vaccination. Masks and eyewear or faceshields should be used if splashing is anticipated. If unvaccinated personnel must be used to collect specimens, only those without contraindications to vaccination should be used, as they will require immediate vaccination if the diagnosis of smallpox is confirmed. Fit-tested N95 masks should be worn by unvaccinated individuals caring for suspected patients.			
	Rash	Biopsy specimens Scabs Vesicular fluid	See CDC document *Specimen Collection and Transport Guidelines* for detailed instructions (Guide D).	1. **A suspected case of smallpox should be reported immediately to the respective Local and State Health Departments for review.** 2. And if, after review, smallpox is still suspected, one of the following should be contacted immediately: A. CDC Emergency Response Hotline (24 hours): 770–488–7100 B. Poxvirus Section, Division of Viral and Rickettsial Diseases, NCID, CDC, Atlanta, Georgia 30333. Laboratory: 404–639–4931 C. Bioterrorism Preparedness and Response Program, NCID, CDC: 404–639–0385 or 404–639–2468. (8am to 5pm weekdays) **NOTE: Approval must be obtained prior to the shipment of potential smallpox patient clinical specimens to CDC** 3. At this time, review the packaging/shipping requirements with CDC and request assistance in coordinating a carrier for transport/shipment A. **Hand-carry all specimens and do not send specimens via pneumatic tube system** B. Do not attempt viral cultures: this is a Biosafety Level 4 agent, and this could result in a very unsafe situation in which there is a significant amount of infectious virus
	Posterior tonsillar tissue swab	Swab		
	Blood	Use plastic tubes		
	Autopsy	Portions of skin containing lesions, liver, spleen, lung, lymph nodes, and/or kidney		
Viral hemorrhagic fevers (various viruses including Ebola, Marburg, Lassa, Machupo, Junin, Guanarito, Sabia, Crimean–Congo hemorrhagic fever, Rift Valley fever, Omsk hemorrhagic fever, Kyasanur Forest disease virus, and others)	Serum for antibody testing: collect blood in red-top or gold-top tubes. Obtain convalescent serum at least 14 days after acute specimen is obtained. Use a Vacutainer or other sealed sterile dry tube for blood collection.		Transport within ≈2 h, at RT. Store at –20 to –70°C	Specific handling conditions are currently under development. Contact CDC to discuss proper collection and handling 1. Double-bag each specimen 2. Swab the exterior of the outside bag with disinfectant *before* removal from the patient's room 3. Do not use glass tubes 4. Hand carry all specimens and do not send specimens via pneumatic tube system **NOTE:** Disposable equipment and sharps go into rigid containers containing disinfectant that are then autoclaved or incinerated. Double-bag refuse. The exterior of the outside bag is to be treated with disinfectant and then autoclaved or incinerated. **Do not attempt tissue culture isolation**. This is only to be done in a Biosafety Level 4 facility In laboratory: 1. Strict barrier precautions are to be used. Personal protective equipment includes gloves, gown, mask, shoe covers, and protective faceshield 2. Handle specimens in biological safety cabinet if possible 3. Consider respiratory mask with HEPA filter 4. Specimens should be centrifuged at low speed
	Viral culture, blood: Collect serum, heparinized plasma (green-top tube), or whole blood during acute febrile illness.		Transport at RT. Store 4°C or frozen on dry ice or liquid nitrogen	
	Throat wash specimens: Mix with equal volume of viral transport medium.		Transport on wet ice. Store at –40°C or colder	
	Urine: Mix with equal volume of viral transport medium.		Transport on wet ice. Store at –40°C or colder	
	Cerebrospinal fluid, tissue, other specimens		As per discussion with CDC	
	Blood cultures: If clinical and travel history warrants, collect 2 sets (1 set is 2 bottles) of blood cultures per institutional procedure for routine blood cultures. Malaria smear of peripheral blood: If clinical and travel history warrants		Transport at RT. Incubate at 35–37°C per blood culture protocol. Lavender-top tube at RT	Bacteremia with disseminated intravascular coagulation and malaria due to *Plasmodium falciparum* are two life-threatening and treatable clinical entities that can present with prominent clinical findings of hemorrhage and fever in a patient with a travel history to areas with viral hemorrhagic fever. Handle with precautions noted above. Continue to use the same precautions as above.

Table 64–16 Specimen Selection: Viral Diseases (cont'd)

Disease/ Agent	Specimen Selection	Transport and Storage	Specimen Plating and Processing
Alphaviruses (includes eastern equine, western equine, Venezuelan equine encephalitis viruses and others)	Serum: Collect 10 ml of serum (red-top, tiger-top, or gold-top tube) as soon as possible after onset of symptoms (acute) and with a follow-up specimen (convalescent) at ≥14 d for serological testing.	Transport within ≈6 h, at 4°C. Store at −20 to −70°C.	**Do not attempt tissue culture isolation,** as that could result in a very unsafe situation in which there is a significant amount of infectious organism.
	Blood: Collect blood in EDTA (lavender) or sodium citrate (blue) and maintain at 4°C for storage and shipping for PCR or special studies.	Transport within ≈6 h, at 4°C. Store at −4° C	
	Cerebrospinal fluid: Specimens (greater than 1 ml) can be kept at 2–8°C if transported within 24 h. If frozen, store at −70°C and transport on dry ice.	Transport on wet ice. If already frozen, store at −70°C and transport on dry ice	
	Tissue, body fluids, others, including cell cultures and cell supernatants: Specimens can be kept at 2–8°C if transported within 24 h. If frozen, store at −70°C and transport on dry ice.	Transport on wet ice. If already frozen, store at −70°C and transport on dry ice	

CDC = Centers for Disease Control and Prevention; EDTA = ethylenediaminetetraacetic acid; RT = room temperature.

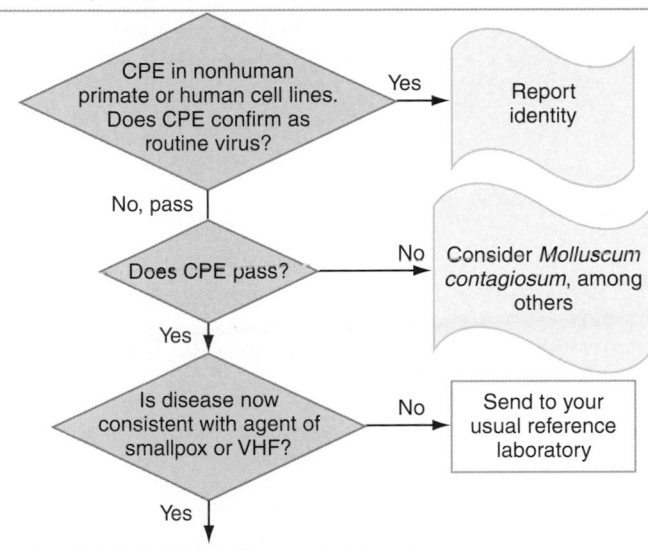

Figure 64–7 Unknown viruses: Sentinel Laboratory flowchart. CPE = cytopathic effect.

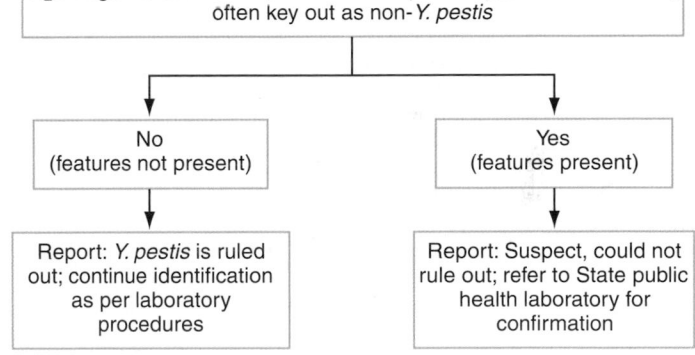

Figure 64–8 *Yersinia pestis*: Sentinel Laboratory flowchart.

and cerebrospinal fluid (Table 64–16). Viral hemorrhagic fever viruses specimens include serum, heparinized plasma (not EDTA, citrate, or oxalate), whole blood, throat washings, tissue, and urine (Table 64–16). Unknown virus specimens include any type of viral or bacterial sample from a clinically unrecognized case (Table 64–16).

Unidentifiable patterns of CPE could be caused by a potential agent of bioterrorism (Fig. 64–7). Consult the physician to see if the patient's clinical presentation is consistent with smallpox or a hemorrhagic viral infection. If the patient's history and/or disease is consistent, do not perform additional manipulations of the cell cultures. Notify the Public Health Department and follow instructions to forward the culture and remaining specimens to the appropriate laboratory.

Smallpox: The agent of smallpox (variola virus) will grow in cell lines used for herpesviruses. CPE is described as hypertrophic rounding of the cells in the monolayer. *Alphaviruses:* Cell lines that permit growth include MRC-5, A-549, Vero, LLCMK, and hamster kidney. CPE may only occur after passage. *Viral hemorrhagic fever virus:* Filoviruses, arenaviruses, and SAHF viruses are cultivable in nonhuman primate and human cell lines, such as Vero and MRC-5. Hemadsorption of specific types of human or

animal erythrocytes to the cell monolayer determines the presence of a hemagglutinin-producing virus. None of the currently identified viral bioterrorism agents would produce monolayer hemadsorption. If the virus is unidentifiable by standard methods, contact the patient's physician to confirm that the clinical history is consistent with a virus of bioterrorism. If the patient's history and/or disease is consistent with exposure to a viral bioterrorism agent, do not destroy specimens or cultures. Contact public health officials for instructions. If the patient's history and/or disease is not consistent with a viral agent of bioterrorism, follow routine laboratory protocols.

Yersinia pestis

Yersinia pestis is a nonmotile, slow-growing, facultative organism classified in the family Enterobacteriaceae. It appears as plump, Gram-negative coccobacilli that are seen mostly as single cells or pairs, and which may exhibit bipolar staining from a direct specimen.

Humans can acquire plague through the bite of infected fleas, direct contact with contaminated tissue, or inhalation (Perry, 1997). Clinically,

Table 64–17 Specimen Selection: Plague (*Yersinia pestis*)

Disease	Specimen Selection	Transport and Storage	SBA	CA	MAC	Stain	Other
Possible *Y. pestis* exposure in asymptomatic patient	No cultures or serology indicated						Follow public health instructions if advised to collect specimens
Bubonic plague	Blood cultures: Collect 2 sets (1 set is 2 bottles) per institutional procedure for routine blood cultures	Transport at RT. Incubate at 35–37°C per blood culture protocol	Blood culture bottles			Gram stain of positive cultures	If suspicion of plague is high, obtain an additional set for incubation at RT (22–28°C) without shaking
	Tiger-top, red-top, or gold-top tube: For serology (acute and, if needed for diagnosis, convalescent serum in 14 d) Green-top (heparin) tube: For PCR	≤24 h, 4°C	No			No	Patients with negative cultures having a single titer, ≥1:10, specific to F1 antigen by agglutination would meet presumptive criteria
	Lymph node (bubo) aspirate: Flushing with 1.0 ml of sterile saline may be needed to obtain material	Transport at RT, or 4°C if transport is delayed. Store ≤24 h at 4°C.	X	X	X	Gram stain, Giemsa, Wright's stain	Contact LRN reference lab or above laboratory to prepare smears for DFA
	Tissue: Collect in sterile container with 1–2 drops of sterile, nonbacteriostatic saline	Transport at RT, or 4°C if transport is delayed. Store ≤24 h at 4°C.	X	X	X	Gram stain, Giemsa, Wright's stain	Contact LRN reference lab or above laboratory to prepare smears for DFA
	Throat: Collect routine throat culture using a swab collected into sterile, leakproof container	≤24 h, 4°C	X	X	X	Gram stain	Contact LRN reference lab or above laboratory to prepare smears for DFA
Pneumonic plague	Sputum/throat: Collect routine throat culture using a swab or expectorated sputum collected into sterile, leakproof container	≤24 h, 4°C	X	X	X	Gram stain	Contact LRN reference lab or above laboratory to prepare smears for DFA
	Bronchial/tracheal wash: Collect per institution's procedure in area dedicated to collecting respiratory specimens under isolation/containment circumstances, i.e., isolation chamber/'bubble'	≤24 h, 4°C	X	X	X	Gram stain	Contact LRN reference lab or above laboratory to prepare smears for DFA
	Blood cultures: Collect 2 sets (1 set is 2 bottles) per institutional procedure for routine blood cultures	Transport at RT. Incubate at 35–37°C per blood culture protocol	Blood culture bottles			Gram stain of positive cultures	If suspicion of plague is high, obtain an additional set for incubation at RT (22–28°C) without shaking
	Tiger-top, red-top, or gold-top tube: For serology (acute and, if needed for diagnosis, convalescent serum in 14 d) Green-top (heparin) tube: For PCR	≤24 h, 4°C	No			No	Patients with negative cultures having a single titer, ≥1:10, specific to F1 antigen by agglutination would meet presumptive criteria

CA = chocolate agar; DFA = direct fluorescent antibody; LRN = Laboratory Response Network; MAC = MacConkey agar; RT = room temperature; SBA = sheep's blood agar.

plague may present in bubonic, septicemic, and pneumonic forms (Perry, 1997). Bubonic plague is characterized by sepsis that is accompanied by the sudden onset of fever, chills, weakness, headache, and the formation of painful buboes (swelling of regional lymph nodes of the groin, axilla, or neck). Septicemic plague is similar to bubonic plague but lacks the swelling of the lymph nodes. Pneumonic plague, the most deadly form of the disease and the form that can be transmitted rapidly, presents as fever and lymphadenopathy with cough, chest pain, and often hemoptysis. Secondary pneumonia from hematogenous spread of the organisms can occur (secondary pneumonic plague). The organism can also occasionally be passed from human to human by close contact as in primary pneumonic plague (Campbell, 1998). Primary pneumonic plague would probably be the form that would be seen if *Y. pestis* were used in a bioterrorism event.

Lower respiratory tract (pneumonic) specimens include bronchial wash or transtracheal aspirate (Table 64–17). For blood specimens (septicemic), collect appropriate blood volume and number of sets per established laboratory protocol. In suspected cases of plague, an additional blood or broth culture (general nutrient broth) should be incubated at room temperature (22–28°C), the temperature at which *Y. pestis* grows faster. Aspirate of involved tissue (bubonic) specimens include liver, spleen, bone marrow, and lung. Perform Gram stain procedure/quality control per standard laboratory protocol. Direct microscopic examination of specimens and cultures by Gram's stain can provide a rapid presumptive

identification. Stained specimens containing *Y. pestis* often reveal plump, Gram-negative rods, 1–2 × 0.5 µm, that are seen mostly as single cells or pairs and short chains in liquid media. Presence of bipolar cells in these smears should trigger the suspicion of plague. Wright's stain often reveals the bipolar staining characteristics of *Y. pestis*, whereas Gram's stain may not. Wayson's stain, another polychromatic stain, can be used instead of Wright–Giemsa. *Y. pestis* grows as gray-white, translucent colonies, usually too small to be seen as individual colonies at 24 h. After incubation for 48 h, colonies are about 1–2 mm in diameter, gray-white to slightly yellow, and opaque. There is little or no hemolysis of the sheep red blood cells. *Y. pestis* will grow as small, non lactose fermenting colonies on MacConkey or EMB agar.

Sentinel (level A) laboratories should consult with the State Public Health Laboratory Director prior to or concurrent with testing if *Y. pestis* is suspected by the physician. Immediately notify physician/infection control according to internal policies if *Y. pestis* cannot be ruled out.

Some of the automated identification systems do not identify *Y. pestis* adequately (Fig. 64–8). *Y. pestis* have been falsely identified as *Yersinia pseudotuberculosis*, *Shigella*, H_2S-negative *Salmonella*, or *Acinetobacter* (Chu, 2000). *Y. pestis* is alkaline slant/acid butt in triple sugar iron. In most conventional biochemical or commercial identification systems, the organism appears relatively inert, making further biochemical testing of little value.

References

Bannatyne RM, Jackson MC, Memish Z: Rapid detection of *Brucella bacteremia* by using the Bactec 9240 system. J Clin Microbiol 1997; 35: 2673–2674.

Beaty BJ, Calisher CH, Shope RE: Arbo viruses. *In* Lennette EH, Lennette DA, Lennette ET (eds): Viral Rickettsial and Chlamydial Infections, 7th ed. Washington, DC, American Public Health Association, 1995, pp 189–212.

Beeching NG, Dance D, Alastair, RO, et al: Biological warfare and bioterrorism. Br Med J 2002; 321:336–339.

Borio L., Inglesby T, Peters CJ, et al: Hemorrhagic fever viruses as biological weapons. Medical and public health management. JAMA 2002; 287:2391–2405.

Campbell GL, Dennis DT: Plague and other *Yersinia* infections. *In* Kasper DL, et al (eds): Harrison's Principles of Internal Medicine, 14th ed. New York, McGraw-Hill, 1998, pp 975–983.

Centers for Disease Control and Prevention: Biological and chemical terrorism: strategic plan for preparedness and response: recommendations of the CDC strategic planning workgroup. Morbid Mortal Wkly Rep 2000a; 49(RR-4): 1–26.

Centers for Disease Control and Prevention: Laboratory-acquired human glanders – Maryland. Morbid Mortal Wkly Rep 2000b; 49:532–535.

Centers for Disease Control and Prevention: Recognition of illness associated with the intentional release of a biological agent. Morbid Mortal Wkly Rep 2001; 50:893–897.

Christopher GW, Cieslak TJ, Pavlin JA, et al: Biological warfare. A historical perspective. JAMA 1997; 278:412–417.

Chu MC: Laboratory manual of plague diagnostic tests. Centers for Disease Control and Prevention, Atlanta, GA, 2000.

Currie BJ, Fisher DA, Anstey NM, Jacups SP: Melioidosis: acute and chronic disease, relapse and reactivation. Trans R Soc Trop Med Hyg 2000; 94:301–304.

Daplan E, Marchell A: The Cult at the End of the World. New York, Crown Publishing, 1996.

Diamond J: Guns, Germs and Steel. New York, Norton & Co., 1999.

Eitzen EM, Takafuji, ET: Historical overview of biological warfare. *In* Sidell FR, Takafujii EF, Franz DR (eds): Medical Aspects of Chemical and Biological Warfare. Washington, DC, Borden Institute, 1997, pp 415–423.

Fiori PL, Mastrandrea, Rapelli P: *Brucella abortus* infection acquired in microbiology laboratories. J Clin Microbiol 38:2005–2006, 2000.

Fournier PE, Marrie TG, Raoult D: Diagnosis of Q fever. J Clin Microbiol 1998; 36:1823–1834.

Gilchrist MJR, McKinney WP, Miller JM, Weissfeld AS: Cumitech 33, Laboratory Safety, management, and diagnosis of biological agents associated with bioterrorism. Snyder JW (coordinating ed.). Washington, DC, ASM Press, 2000.

Gilligan PH, Lum G, Vandamme P, Whittier S: *Burkholderia, Stenotrophomonas, Ralstonia, Brevundimonas, Comamonas,* and *Acidovorax. In* Murray PR, Baron EJ, Pfaller MA, et al (eds): Manual of Clinical Microbiology, 8th ed. Washington, DC, ASM Press, 2003, pp 729–748.

Heinzen RH: Intracellular development of *Coxiella burnetii. In* Anderson B, Friedman H, Bendinelli M (eds): Rickettsial Infection and Immunity. New York, Plenum Press, 1997, pp 99–130.

Henderson DA: Bioterrorism as a public health threat. Emerg Infect Dis 1998; 4:488–492.

Henderson, DA, Inglesby TV, Bartlett, JG, et al: Smallpox as a biological weapon: medical and public health management. JAMA 1999; 281:2127–2137.

Kaufman AF, Metzer MI, Schmid GP: The economic impact of a bioterrorism attack: are prevention and past attack intervention programs justifiable? Emerg Infect Dis 1997; 3:73–94.

Lew DP: *Bacillus anthracis* (anthrax). *In* Mandell GL, Bennett JE, Dolin R (eds): Principles and Practice of Infectious Disease, 5th ed. Philadelphia, PA, Churchill Livingstone, 2000, pp 2215–2220.

Logan NA, Turnbull, PC: Bacillus and recently derived genera. *In* Murray PR, Baron EJ, Pfaller MA, et al (eds): Manual of Clinical Microbiology, 7th ed. Washington, DC, ASM Press, 1999, pp 357–369.

Overholt EL, Tigertt WD, Kadull PJ, et al: An analysis of forty-two cases of laboratory-acquired tularemia. Am J Med 1961; 30:785–806.

Perry RD, Fetherston JD: *Yersinia pestis* – etiologic agent of plague. Clin Microbiol Rev 1997; 10:35–66.

Raoult, D, Mege JL, Marrie T: Q fever: queries remaining after decades of research. *In* Scheld WM, Craig WA, Hughes JM (eds): Emerging Infections. Washington, DC, ASM Press, 2001, pp 29–56.

Ropp SL, Esposito JJ, Loparev VN, Palumb GJ: Poxviruses infecting humans. *In* Murray PR, Baron EJ, Pfaller MA, et al (eds): Manual of Clinical Microbiology, 7th ed. Washington, DC, ASM Press, 1999, pp 1137–1144.

Schreckenberger PC, Von Coraevenitz A: *Acinetobacter, Achromobacter, Alcaligenes, Moraxella, Methylobacterium,* and other nonfermentative gram-negative rods. *In* Murray PR, Baron EJ, Pfaller MA, et al (eds): Manual of Clinical Microbiology, 7th ed. Washington, DC, ASM Press, 1999, pp 539–560.

Sewell, DL: Laboratory-associated infections and biosafety. Clin Microbio Rev 1995; 8:389–405.

Shapiro DS, Wong, JD: *Brucella. In* Murray PR, Baron EJ, Pfaller MA, et al (eds): Manual of Clinical Microbiology, 7th ed. Washington, DC, ASM Press, 1999, pp 625–631.

Tissot-Dupont H, Raoult D, Brouqui P, et al: Epidemiologic features and clinical presentation of acute Q fever in hospitalized patients 323 French cases. Am J Med 1992; 93:427–437.

Tucker JB: Historical trends related to bioterrorism: An empirical analysis. Emerg Infect Dis 1999; 5:498–504.

Wong JD, Shapiro DS: Francisella. *In* Murray PR, Baron EJ, Pfaller MA, et al (eds): Manual of Clinical Microbiology, 7th ed. Washington, DC, ASM Press, 1999, pp 647–651.

PART VIII

Molecular Pathology

Edited by

Elizabeth R. Unger MD PhD, Matthew R. Pincus MD PhD

CHAPTER 65

Introduction to Molecular Pathology

Elizabeth R. Unger MD PhD, Matthew R. Pincus MD PhD

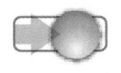

KEY POINTS

• The revolution in molecular biology has had a profound impact on the field of clinical pathology (diagnostic medicine).

• New techniques, including polymerase chain reaction and other amplification and hybridization methods, are capable of detecting DNA in very small quantities in tissue and body fluids.

• This enables detection of disease states, including cancer.

• The human genome project has created new high-throughput and highly sensitive genetic methods (such as microarrays) not only for detecting abnormal genes in patient specimens but also for establishing patterns of gene expression that are characteristic of specific diseases.

• New proteomic methods in detecting protein expression on serum samples from patients allow for diagnosis of different types of cancers.

• The new gene array and proteomic methodologies require sophisticated mathematical methods of pattern recognition that allow for detection of disease.

The Molecular Biology Revolution and Its Impact on the Practice of Pathology

Molecular pathology refers to the analysis of nucleic acids and proteins to diagnose disease, predict the occurrence of disease, predict the prognosis of diagnosed disease and guide therapy. Recent advances in molecular biology have revolutionized the practice of medicine, especially diagnostic medicine. These revolutionary changes result from our new abilities to clone disease-causing genes and the proteins that they encode; to detect the presence of these genes, which are present in minute quantities in body fluids and/or tissues, using amplification methods based on the polymerase chain reaction (PCR) and on new, highly sensitive DNA hybridization methods; and, using new, highly sensitive methods, based on such techniques as mass spectroscopy, to identify proteins that are implicated in causing disease (Pincus, 2003). Many of these techniques have been developed to the stage where they are employed in so-called 'high-throughput' processes that enable single patient samples to be analyzed for multiple genes or proteins. Some of these processes have already become completely automated.

A major consequence of the revolution in molecular biology has the mapping of the human genome in the Human Genome Project (Venter, 2001) and the genomes of a number of other species. These projects have identified numerous new genes of unknown function whose functions can now be determined and whose expressions can be monitored in different disease states. In addition, the techniques employed in these projects have

been proving exceptionally useful in studying patterns of gene expression in different disease states (see, for example, *Golub, 1999).

Discussion of Diagnostic Molecular Pathology

These new methods will now be described in Sections VIII and IX of this book. In Section VIII, we first discuss the principles that underlie the main diagnostic approaches used in clinical molecular biology. Chapter 66 describes the basic principles in gene hybridization, including use of Southern and Northern blots, and gene cloning, and Chapter 67 discusses amplification methodology, including PCR, that allows gene identification and quantification of gene expression. In the ensuing Chapter 68, we discuss how the expression of multiple genes – in fact, of whole genomes – can now be assayed on microarrays.

One of the motivations for detecting genetic abnormalities in specific diseases, especially in hematopoietic cancers such as chronic myelogenous leukemia, is the finding that, in many such disease states, there are well defined, reproducible chromosomal abnormalities. In fact, increasing numbers of these diseases can be identified on chromosomes using the newly developed technique of fluorescent in situ hybridization (FISH), which enables detection of gene rearrangements and gene deletions in a number of diseases, especially in cancers. Thus in Chapter 69 we discuss the cytogenetics of human diseases and show how FISH technology has enabled major advances in diagnosis of disease. All these diagnostic approaches constitute diagnostic or clinical molecular biology or molecular diagnostics. In Chapter 70, we therefore discuss how a molecular diagnostics laboratory is established. In the following two chapters, we then demonstrate how molecular biology techniques are used to diagnose specific diseases, first, in Chapter 71, for hematopoietic diseases, mainly the leukemias and lymphomas, and then, in Chapter 72, for many other disease states.

One of the consequences of the genetic revolution has been the ability to identify single gene mutations in patients' DNA that may either result in disease or may simply be polymorphisms. The latter can be taken advantage of in establishing the parentage of children and the investigation of crime. Consequently, there has been a dramatic increase in the use of the molecular diagnostics laboratory for forensic purposes. We thus describe, in Chapter 73, how single nucleotide polymorphisms are used to establish parentage and the identities of the victims and perpetrators of crime.

Another momentous consequence of the revolution in molecular biology has been the discovery that virtually all human cancers are caused by oncogenes, which are mutated forms of normally occurring genes (proto-oncogenes) produced by mutational events associated with, for instance, carcinogens and oncogenic viruses. These genes encode abnormally functioning mutated and/or overexpressed proteins. It is these mutated proteins that promote cell transformation. Many oncogenic proteins are critical components of so-called signal transduction pathways, in which ligands, such as growth factors, bind to cell membrane receptors, setting in motion a chain of protein activation cascades that are ultimately transmitted to the nucleus, resulting in increased transcription and ultimately high levels of expression of promitotic proteins such as the cyclins. When one or more of the proteins on mitogenic signal transduction pathways become mutated, the cells in which they are expressed become transformed into cancer cells. Once transformed, cancer cells express a number of proteins, in addition to the mutated or overexpressed oncoproteins, that are not expressed by normal cells even in growth phase.

These findings have been translated into new clinical diagnostic methods for the detection of these abnormal proteins in the early detection of cancer in patients. Therefore, Section IX of this book is devoted to the way in which these proteins are used in early tumor detection and to follow the efficacy of treatment of cancer. One of the major findings in this area has been that screening for cancer is most effective when multiple oncoproteins are assayed. A pathbreaking step in this area of multiple protein assays has been the development of new mass-spectroscopic techniques that enable detection of patterns of protein expression in serum that are unique to specific cancers, in a field known as proteomics that is showing great promise in screening for a number of different major human cancers.

A major impact of the human genome project has been the ability to study multiple gene expression, mainly using microarrays, in normal individuals and in specific disease states. Cancer is a major area in which the differential expression of specific genes characterizes particular tumors. Combination of gene expression with proteomics now allows for diagnosis of and screening for a number of different types of tumor, uniting molecular genetic and proteomic approaches. In Chapter 76 of Section IX, therefore, we discuss these approaches. We also discuss the methodologies used in mapping the genome since these approaches are involved in screening for different diseases. As the functions of more genes become known, it will become increasingly feasible to screen the genomes of patients for gene abnormalities, especially those causing or predisposing patients to develop cancer. To an increasing degree, clinical laboratories will be called upon to perform this type of analysis.

Implications of Molecular Diagnostics on the Practice of Pathology and Medicine

Re-defining Disease

The availability of the sequence of the human genome and the identification of all the human genes immediately change our understanding of health, disease susceptibility and precursors, and disease (Pandey, 2000). An ability to identify the gene expression pattern that makes a disease entity unique further allows the pathologist to delineate uniquely clinically different diseases that may be difficult or impossible to distinguish on the basis of morphology or other laboratory data alone (Heller, 1997; Golub, 1999). A poignant example of this phenomenon is the diagnosis of leukemias and lymphomas. Morphologically and even immunophenotypically it may prove difficult to distinguish among different types of each disease; however, specific gene rearrangements and patterns of gene expression now enable distinction of different types. In addition, the relationships among diseases are also more sharply defined, and sometimes radically changed, by comparisons among the diseases' gene expression profiles (Anbazhagan, 1999).

In the opposite direction, sequencing of disease genes and testing for mutations are demonstrating that diseases have broad spectrums of presentation that range from mild symptoms that are unrecognized as part of the disease, and may even include complexes not previously recognized in isolation as forms of the disease, to full manifestation of the disease. A compelling example of this marked expansion of the syndromes comprising a disease is cystic fibrosis (Friedman, 1999). In addition to the severe and milder pulmonary and pancreatic dysfunctions long accepted as cystic fibrosis, isolated examples of congenital bilateral absence of the vas deferens, chronic pancreatitis, and sinopulmonary complaints have been associated with mutations of the cystic fibrosis gene (CFTR). These mutations are frequently not associated with the severe classical form of the disease. Recognition of symptom complexes extending the definition of diseases on the basis of gene mutations will both focus appropriate patient management in the milder or atypical forms of the disease and define pathobiology, not only of whole genes but also of affected specific exons and introns.

Use of Molecular Biology in the Treatment of Disease

As noted in Chapter 73, genes and noncoding regions of genomes have polymorphisms which often have no clinical significance but are quite

useful in establishing parentage or identities of individuals. Mapping of the human genome reveals that these polymorphisms occur in the human genome approximately 1 per 1000 base pairs (bp). However, it has been found that some of these polymorphisms are in genes whose functions are important in response of individual patients to therapy (Evans, 1999). Genes for drug-metabolizing enzymes, both activating and inactivating, and genes for ligands and receptors may show polymorphisms that either decrease or increase the therapeutic effectiveness or toxicity of drugs already in wide use, accounting for some idiosyncratic responses previously not understood or predictable. As more polymorphisms are identified and correlated with individual patients' response to treatment, the pathologist will be called upon to profile common polymorphisms in patients who are beginning therapy for common diseases such as diabetes, hypertension, cancer, and infections. The laboratory's definition of the individual patient's genotype/phenotype will determine the specific drugs and doses suitable for that patient. This evolution puts the pathologist in a more definitive position to determine appropriate therapy than traditional prediction of disease behavior based on morphology of lesions or culture characteristics of infectious organisms.

In addition to phenotyping patients, the pathologist is now being called upon for genotyping of infectious agents such as human immunodeficiency virus (HIV). Different strains show markedly different drug susceptibilities. Thus determination of the genotypes of infectious agents has major therapeutic implications.

Proteomic approaches to cancer detection have likewise resulted in the development of new therapies. For example, many breast cancers express the neu/HER2 growth factor receptor, whose presence can be detected in serum by immunoassay. As described in Chapter 74, a cytotoxic antibody, Herceptin, to this receptor, which does not crossreact with the diagnostic antibodies, has been found to destroy breast cancer cells and is now used to treat neu/HER2-positive breast cancers effectively.

Data Analysis

To capitalize fully on the power of molecular pathology, wholly new approaches to data analysis and relating data to disease management are being developed. Pathologic investigation of disease and of basic biology has traditionally analyzed and related only one or a few markers such as antigens, enzymes, structural proteins, and the like. Molecular techniques are now producing data on many thousands of genes, including their expression and their sequences. Digesting all these data, organizing them into profiles of diseases or patients, and relating different profiles demand new approaches to bioinformatics. As discussed in Chapter 76, this involves the use of mathematical algorithms that allow pattern recognition, such as neural network theory (Khan, 2001). Thus the pathologist must work closely with mathematicians and must learn more sophisticated analytic approaches to diagnosis (Bitner, 1999).

Quality Assurance

As with all laboratory methods, excellent quality assurance programs are required to ensure that molecular pathologic results are accurate and useful. As discussed in Chapter 70, two essential components of quality assurance programs are standardization of methods and interlaboratory comparison of test results. Standardized methods for performance of the most common clinical molecular pathologic tests are published by the National Committee for Clinical Laboratory Standards (NCCLS), now known as the Clinical and Laboratory Standards Institute. Use of these guidelines ensures that the data generated in molecular pathology laboratories are produced by methods that are the standard of excellent practice. Interlaboratory comparison of test performance is provided by the College of American Pathologists (CAP) (www.cap.org). The CAP interlaboratory comparison surveys include molecular microbiology, genetics, hematology, parentage and identity, and general forensic applications.

Applying established standards of quality assurance and using molecular pathologic techniques with a thorough understanding of their respective strengths and weaknesses as presented in the following chapters, the pathologist will continue to capitalize on the opportunities these techniques offer for improved patient care and understanding of basic pathobiology.

Some Caveats

As will be seen throughout this section and the next, molecular diagnostic techniques provide new insights into disease, never before possible. However, these techniques must not be used alone but in coordination with traditional laboratory tests. For example, in the diagnostic work-up of leukemias, the traditional morphological and immunochemical testing must always be performed. Gene analysis becomes critical when there is a question as to the type of leukemia or the characterization of the types of gene rearrangement that have occurred. In cases of tissue pathology, the morphologic skills involved in histopathology and cytopathology must be employed to ensure that appropriate cells and tissues are analyzed molecularly. Otherwise, analysis of other than targeted cells/tissues, despite high-quality technical methods interpreted with skill and experience, can lead to erroneous, sometimes dangerously misleading, results.

On the other hand, rapid progress in the development of highly sensitive molecular biological and proteomic techniques are allowing some 'stand-alone' capabilities for molecular diagnostics. For example, use of FISH to detect bladder cancer in urine is now recognized as an excellent means of diagnosing this condition. Other, similar developments in molecular biological approaches are showing promise in screening for specific diseases.

In summary, molecular pathology is penetrating and permeating the entire clinical laboratory just as immunopathology did over two decades ago. Section boundaries or barriers will continue to break down and dissolve in this transformation of laboratory medicine through the impact of the new biology of medicine, 'cell and molecular biology.'

References

Anbazhagan R, Tihan T, Bornman DM, et al: Classification of small cell lung cancer and pulmonary carcinoid by gene expression profiles. Cancer Res 1999; 59:5119–5122.

Bitner M, Meltzer P, Trent J: Data analysis and integration: of steps and arrows. Nat Genet 1999; 22:213–214.

Evans WE, Relling MV: Pharmacogenomics: translating functional genomics into rational therapeutics. Science 1999; 286:487–491.

Friedman KJ, Silverman LM: Cystic fibrosis syndrome: a new paradigm for inherited disorders and implications for molecular diagnostics. Clin Chem 1999; 45:929–931.

Golub TR, Slonim DK, Tamayo P et al: Molecular classification of cancer: class discovery and class prediction by gene expression monitoring. Science 286:531–537, 1999.

This is a seminal paper that shows how analysis of multiple gene expression can be used to distinguish between different types of leukemia.

Heller RA, Schena M, Chai A, et al: Discovery and analysis of inflammatory disease-related genes using cDNA microarrays. Proc Natl Acad Sci USA 1997; 94:2150–2155.

Khan J, Wei JS, Ringner M et al: Classification and diagnostic prediction of cancers using gene expression profiling and artificial neural networks. Nat Med 2001; 7:673–679.

Pandey A, Mann M: Proteomics to study genes and genomes. Nature 2000; 405:837–846.

Pincus MR, Friedman FK: Oncoproteins in the detection of human malignancies. *In* Molecular Diagnostics. New York, Reed Business Information Publishers, 2003, vol 1, pp 23–38.

This paper reviews how multiple oncoproteins can be used serodiagnostically not only to screen for different types of cancer but in some cases to predict the future occurrence of cancers.

Venter JC, Adams MD, Myers EW et al: The sequence of the human genome. Science 2001; 291:1304–1351.

VIII

CHAPTER 66

Molecular Diagnostics: Basic Principles and Techniques

Martin Steinau, PhD Margaret A. Piper, PhD MPH Elizabeth R. Unger PhD MD

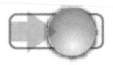

KEY POINTS
- Familiarity with the basics of nucleic acid biochemistry and biology is required to understand molecular diagnostic testing.
- The chemical stability of double-stranded DNA stands in contrast to the lability of RNA.
- Base-pairing of nucleic acids is dictated by achieving an energetically favorable state, and forms the basis for cellular DNA replication, RNA transcription and hybridization assays.
- The chemical similarity of nucleic acid molecules, regardless of their source, means that methods of extraction, storage, and handling are similar.
- Enzymes that synthesize and modify nucleic acids (polymerases, transcriptases, nucleases, ligases, etc.) may be harnessed as tools for molecular biology and molecular diagnostics.
- Nucleic acid analyses include electrophoresis, hybridization assays, amplification techniques, and polymorphism analyses. Complete assays or diagnostic tests often include several of these techniques, such as amplification, electrophoresis, and hybridization.
- Molecular diagnostics is now part of the mainstream of laboratory diagnostics

Nucleic acids are the critical molecules of life. Deoxyribonucleic acid (DNA) resides in the nucleus of eukaryotic cells and maintains all the information necessary for maintenance of the organism and for transfer of the information to successive generations. Ribonucleic acid (RNA) carries information from DNA to the cytoplasm of a cell and directs synthesis of the proteins necessary for the function of the organism. The normal state of health depends on the stability of DNA and on accurate DNA duplication and translation into protein. Modern cell biology seeks to determine the basic mechanisms of cell structure and function, and studies are increasingly focused at the level of the gene, the protein coding units of DNA. As a consequence, diagnostic methods are also being directed toward nucleic acid evaluation. The goal of this chapter is to provide the conceptual framework for diagnostic applications of nucleic acid analyses.

Nucleic Acid Biochemistry and Biology

Nucleic acid biochemistry is central to modern cell biology and dictates many aspects of diagnostic applications. Many of the enzymes associated with in vivo nucleic acid synthesis, degradation, and repair have become basic laboratory tools for manipulation and analysis of DNA and RNA. Cellular mechanisms that operate to direct and control DNA replication, transcription, and translation address the basic biology of the cell in health and disease. Diagnosis, therapy, and research are all increasingly directed at a molecular level of cellular function. This first section provides an overview of those aspects of nucleic acid biochemistry and biology that are required to understand the current diagnostic applications of molecular biology. Further details are available from textbooks of cell biology (Alberts, 2002).

Molecular Composition and Structure

DNA is a long, double-stranded polymeric molecule (dsDNA) that exists predominantly in the form of a right-handed double helix. Each single-stranded DNA molecule (ssDNA) is composed of a small number of building blocks. The backbone of the ssDNA polymer is the sugar deoxyribose connected by phosphate groups (Fig. 66–1A). Phosphodiester bonds between the 3' carbon of one sugar ring and the 5' carbon of the next give the backbone its invariant structure and its 5' to 3' directionality. Linked to the 1' carbon of each sugar is one of four possible bases: thymine (T) and cytosine (C) (pyrimidines); adenine (A) and guanine (G) (purines). The bases can occur in any sequence order, and thus form the variable portion of ssDNA. The building blocks of the single-stranded polymer are the four deoxyribonucleotide triphosphates (dTTP, dCTP, dATP, dGTP), each consisting of a sugar molecule, a triphosphate group, and one base. During DNA synthesis, nucleotides are first stripped of two phosphate groups and then enzymatically linked together by phosphodiester bonds to form a chain.

DNA is an extraordinarily stable molecule, losing its normal conformational structure only at extremes of heat, at extremes of pH, or in the presence of destabilizing agents. The double-stranded helix is the most energetically favorable state for DNA, and an examination of the components of DNA explains this fact. Both sugar and phosphate groups are hydrophilic, forming stable hydrogen bonds with surrounding water molecules in solution. Bases, however, are hydrophobic, and are not soluble in water at neutral pH. A stable molecule of DNA must ensure that the bases do not contact water. This is possible when two antiparallel ssDNA polymers (one running in the 3' to 5' direction, the other 5' to 3') twist around the same axis. This arrangement allows planar hydrogen bonds to form between adenine and thymine, and between guanine and cytosine (Fig. 66–1B). As long as the two chains have base sequences in complementary order, the strands of the helix have a ladder-like structure with rungs (base pairs [bp]) of consistent size. The flexibility of the carbon–oxygen linkages in the phosphodiester bond allows the ladder to

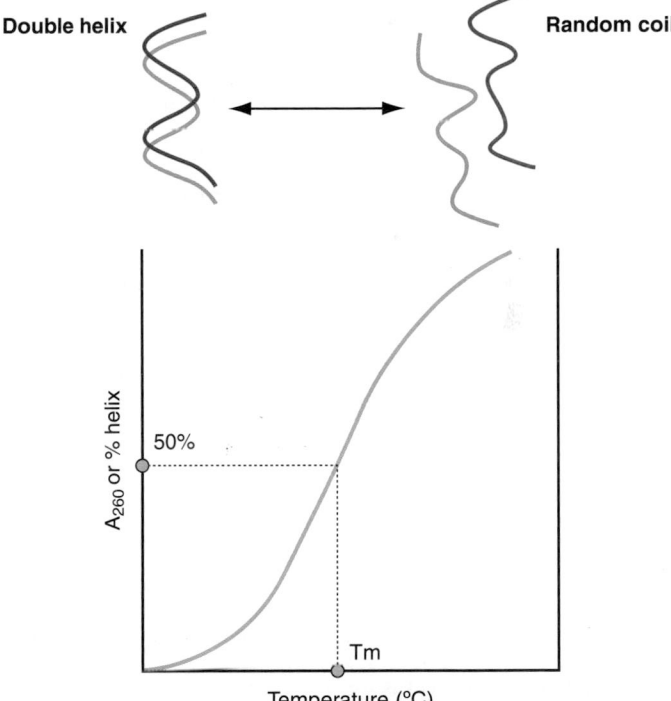

Figure 66–1 Repeating backbone of DNA and complementary base pairs. *A,* A single-stranded DNA chain. Repeating nucleotide units are linked by phosphodiester bonds that join the 5′-carbon of one sugar to the 3′-carbon of the next. (* In RNA, the sugar is ribose, which has a 2′-hydroxyl added to deoxyribose.) *B,* Purine and pyrimidine bases and the formation of complementary base pairs. Shaded bars indicate the formation of hydrogen bonds. († In RNA, thymine is replaced by uracil, which differs from thymine only in the lack of the methyl group.) (Adapted with permission from Piper MA, Unger ER: Nucleic Acid Probes: A Primer for Pathologists. Chicago, IL, ASCP Press, 1989.)

twist, forming a regular helix such that the planar base pairs are stacked on top of each other, leaving no room for water molecules in between. The polymeric series of base-pair hydrogen bonds holds the ssDNA chains tightly together, and the helical conformation protects the base pairs from water, exposing only the hydrophilic backbones.

Helical dsDNA is stable over a pH range of approximately 4–9. Solutions with pH outside these limits have the capacity to disrupt the base-pair bonds and cause the DNA helix to denature or unwind into two separate, random coils. Extreme heat, and hydrogen bond disrupters such as formamide, also have the same effect. This helix to coil transition can be followed spectrophotometrically at A_{260} (Fig. 66–2). The bases absorb ultraviolet light maximally at this wavelength but at a lower molar absorptivity in dsDNA; absorptivity increases 20–30% when dsDNA is converted to ssDNA. Because temperature is often used to effect this transition, the process has been referred to as *melting,* and the temperature at which 50% of dsDNA is converted to ssDNA is called the *melting point* or T_m of the DNA. The T_m of DNA molecules depends on the relative G–C versus A–T base-pair content, as the three hydrogen bonds of G–C base pairs require more energy to disrupt them than the two hydrogen bonds of A–T base pairs. The melting process can be reversed by lowering the temperature, and the two complementary strands can reform the original helix if the base pairs reform in the correct linear conformation.

The length of a fully extended eukaryotic DNA molecule would be about 3 m per genome, much longer than the cell itself. Undegraded purified DNA forms a stringy, viscous solution, reflecting the extreme length of genomic DNA (Fig. 66–3). In vivo, however, DNA is organized into highly compacted, regular units called chromosomes. A chromosome is composed of its DNA strand wound around DNA-associated proteins (chromatin) in a highly structured fashion. The chromosome structure involves several hierarchical levels of chromatin packing, from a 'beads-on-a-string' nucleosome (146 nucleotide pairs wound around a histone core) to highly condensed loops each containing about 100 000 bp of DNA. Each human cell nucleus contains two sets of 23 chromosomes of characteristic length and unique base-pair sequence. Together these chromosomes constitute the *human genome.* As a result of the Human Genome Project, the complete sequence of the 3 billion chemical base pairs that make up the human genome was finished in 2001.

RNA differs from DNA in chemical composition, structure, and function (Table 66–1). In RNA the sugar is ribose, containing a hydroxyl group at the 2′ position, and thymine is replaced by the methylated uracil (U). RNA exists predominantly as a single-stranded molecule and in much shorter lengths than DNA. The structure of RNA is more irregular, owing to the single-stranded nature of the molecule, but may contain some helical sections. RNA molecules of the same base sequence, however, will form

Figure 66–2 Melting/annealing curve of double-stranded helical nucleic acid. (Adapted with permission from Piper MA, Unger ER: Nucleic Acid Probes: A Primer for Pathologists. Chicago, IL, ACSP Press, 1989.)

the same three-dimensional structure as a result of adopting the most energetically favorable conformation. RNA is much less stable than DNA, not only because of the single-stranded, more random structure but also because of its susceptibility to alkaline hydrolysis via the 2′ hydroxyl group of the ribose moiety. RNA is also rapidly degraded by RNA-specific enzymes, which are ubiquitous.

Nucleic Acid-Associated Enzymes

DNA must be duplicated prior to cell division so that daughter cells retain an exact copy of the genetic information contained in parent chromosomes.

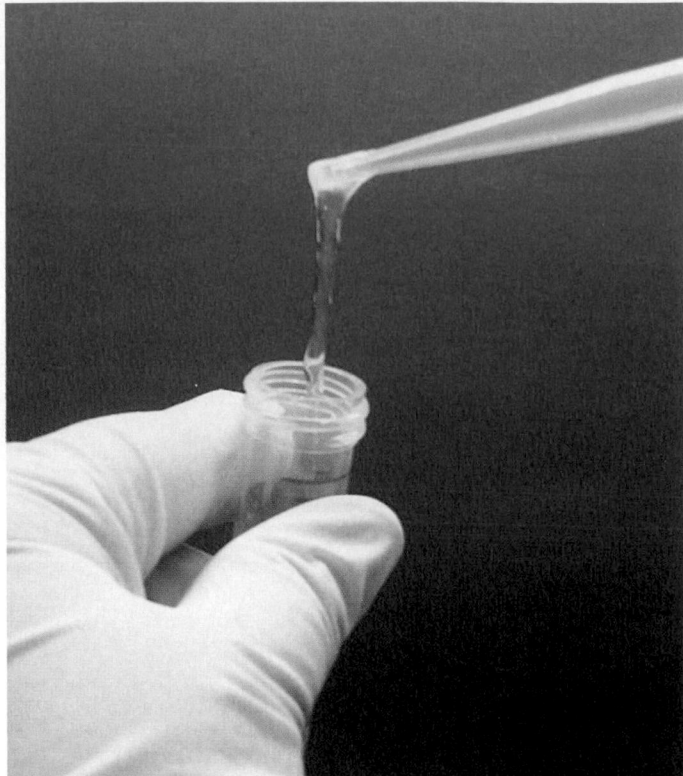

Figure 66–3 Photograph of purified DNA demonstrating stringy, viscous nature of minimally sheared genomic DNA.

Table 66–2 Nucleic Acid Enzymes and Associated Functions

Enzyme	In vivo Function
Polymerases DNA polymerases RNA polymerases	Polymerases join DNA or RNA nucleotides together to form a single-stranded daughter molecule using a stretch of single-stranded parent molecule as a template. These enzymes perform syntheses according to base-pair rules and proceed in the 5' to 3' direction
Reverse transcriptase	Mostly of viral origin, reverse transcriptase catalyzes the synthesis of DNA from either an RNA or a DNA template
DNA ligases	Joins DNA fragments formed by discontinuous synthesis in DNA replication or in DNA repair pathways
Nucleases DNases, RNases Endonucleases Exonucleases	Nucleases 'digest' nucleic acid molecules by breaking phosphodiester bonds Endonucleases digest nucleic acids from the middle of the molecule whereas exonucleases begin at a free end and may require a 3' or 5' end. Nucleases may have single-stranded, double-stranded, DNA, or RNA specificity. Some polymerases also have nuclease activity
Restriction endonucleases	Bacterial endonucleases that recognize specific short DNA base-pair sequences and cleave the DNA molecule only at the recognition site

Enzyme	Sequence cleaved

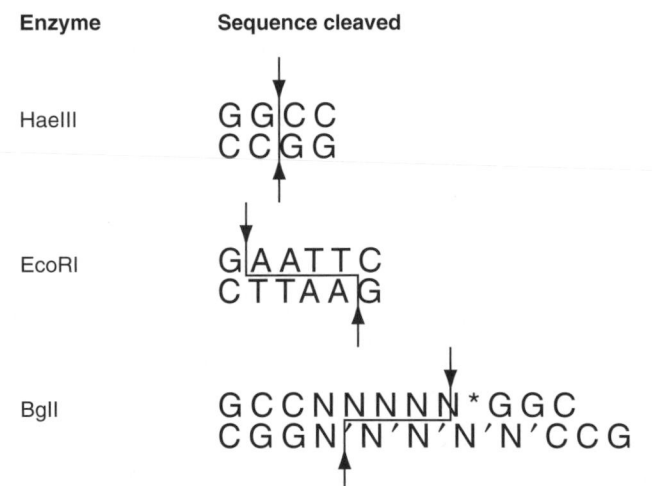

Figure 66–4 Examples of DNA restriction enzymes and their specificities. Enzymes are named for the bacteria from which they are isolated (*where N is any base and N' its pairing counterpart).

Table 66–1 Comparison of Key Features of DNA and RNA

Feature	DNA	RNA
Sugar	Deoxyribose	Ribose
Base pairs	Thymine–Adenine Cytosine–Guanine	Uracil–Adenine Cytosine–Guanine
Structure	Double-stranded Alpha helix	Single-stranded Random (see text)
Stability	Stable Degraded by DNase	Subject to base hydrolysis Degraded by RNase
Function	Maintains genetic information in nucleus	Carries genetic information to cytoplasm

RNA must be synthesized by all functioning cells to direct the synthesis of necessary proteins. DNA must be degraded during repair of damaged segments, and RNA is continually degraded and resynthesized. Enzymes that operate directly on nucleic acids affect these and other functions. Table 66–2 lists major categories of nucleic acid-specific enzyme and their in vivo functions. In vitro, purified enzymes have become laboratory tools for the molecular biologist, allowing genetic engineering and facilitating many nucleic acid assays.

Nucleic-acid-specific enzymes include polymerases, which catalyze the formation of phosphodiester bonds during synthesis; and nucleases, which hydrolyze these bonds. RNA-specific nucleases (RNases) are present virtually everywhere. Because of this, it requires much greater care in laboratory practice to work in vitro with RNA than with DNA. Restriction endonucleases are a special category of nucleases found only in bacteria, where they function to destroy foreign DNA. The recognition sites for restriction enzymes are located anywhere within the DNA molecules, are sequence-specific, and can vary from approximately 4 bp to 12 bp in length. At the recognition sequence or nearby, restriction endonucleases make specific asymmetric or blunt end cuts in DNA molecules (Fig. 66–4). Over 3000 restriction endonucleases have been discovered and categorized according to the structure of their corresponding sequence recognition sites (Pingoud, 2001). The in vivo function and in vitro utility of many of these nucleic-acid-specific enzymes will be discussed in the following sections.

Replication of DNA

The DNA duplication process, known as *semiconservative replication*, uses each strand of the parent molecule to direct the synthesis of a daughter strand (Virshup, 1990). Since the base sequence of the parent strand dictates the sequence of the daughter strand, replication is faithful and the replication products consist of two dsDNA molecules composed of one parent strand and one daughter strand each, with exactly the same base-pair sequence. Although this is conceptually simple, the process is complicated and involves a number of accessory proteins and enzymes. First, for synthesis to begin, a small single-stranded region must be produced. This is not energetically favorable, and must be effected with proteins that unwind and separate the strands of the helix. Next, a short RNA primer is synthesized complementary to the single-stranded sequence. DNA polymerase III proceeds with DNA synthesis and later the RNA primer is excised and replaced with DNA by DNA polymerase I. Chromosomal DNA contains many initiation sites for replication, and this process occurs simultaneously across the chromosome. Interestingly, DNA polymerase III is a directional enzyme, and can synthesize DNA only in the 5' to 3' direction because it requires a free 3'OH end. This means that only one daughter strand, called the leading strand, can be synthesized continuously. The opposite strand, called the lagging strand, is primed by RNA primase that does not require a free 3'OH end. It is synthesized discontinuously in short fragments (Okazaki fragments) as the replication fork is opened up. These fragments are then joined together by DNA ligase. DNA polymerase III is also unique in that it has proofreading and exonuclease activity. If an incorrect nucleotide is added to the growing chain, it is detected and excised by the nuclease portion of the enzyme, and the correct nucleotide is then added. This helps explain the extraordinary fidelity of the DNA replication process. Postsynthesis repair mechanisms also contribute to the accuracy of replication (see later under Mechanisms of DNA Repair).

Transcription of DNA to RNA

Sections of DNA that specify amino acid sequences of proteins are called genes; one gene contains the amino acid sequence code for one protein as well as DNA sequences necessary for the regulation of the production of that protein. Within the 6 billion nucleotides of the human genome, there are about 30 000–40 000 protein-coding genes. Although these coding sequences are of paramount importance to the cell and to the function of the organism as a whole, they actually make up less than 5% of the nucleotides. The vast majority of the human genome is composed of noncoding DNA regions and we are only beginning to understand the function of these regions. These sequences were sometimes called *junk DNA*, but it appears that much of it may well have some purpose, such as secondary regulatory roles in gene expression.

Protein synthesis begins with the activation of the appropriate gene. A copy of the gene is made from DNA in the form of RNA. Because the RNA copy carries the code from the DNA in the cell nucleus to the cytoplasm, where amino acid synthesis takes place, this type of RNA is called *messenger RNA* (mRNA). Messenger RNA is synthesized from only one strand of the DNA gene; the complementary DNA strand is not used. This is accomplished by a process called *transcription*. Synthesis of mRNA proceeds in much the same fashion as DNA replication, with the ssDNA sequence dictating the mRNA sequence using the same rules of base-pair complementarity (uracil base pairs with adenine). When the end of the gene is reached, mRNA synthesis is terminated. Some genes are always expressed, while others are only active in certain physiological situations. The rate of transcription also varies in different cells (see section on Transcriptional Control, below).

Post-Transcriptional Modification

Prior to export to the cytoplasm, the mRNA molecule is modified in several ways (Rosenthal, 1994). Messenger RNA contains both amino acid coding sequences (exons) and noncoding sequences (introns); introns are excised from the mRNA molecule prior to protein synthesis. A molecular complex called a spliceosome (Sharp, 1988), which is composed of both low-molecular-weight RNA and protein, recognizes mRNA sequences that identify the boundaries of an intron, joins the flanking exons, and releases the intron. Splicing must be exact, as the addition or subtraction of a single nucleotide at the splice junction would change the three-nucleotide reading frame in the nucleotide sequences that follow.

Further modifications to the mRNA molecule include the addition of 7-methyl guanosine residues to the 5′ end in a unique 5′–5′ phosphodiester bond. This is called a *cap* and aids in the binding of the ribosome to the mRNA molecule for initiation of protein synthesis. A poly-A *tail*, which may be necessary for stability and transport to the cytoplasm, is added to the 3′ end. The polyadenylation locus is specified in part by the sequence AAUAAA usually found in the 3′ untranslated region of the RNA transcript. At this point, the mRNA molecule is ready to direct the synthesis of its corresponding protein.

Translation of RNA to Protein

Protein synthesis requires translation from the language of nucleotides to that of amino acids. 21 different amino acids are used in protein synthesis; each amino acid is specified by one or more mRNA nucleotide triplets called *codons*. Because an amino acid can be encoded by more than one codon, the code is referred to as a *degenerate code*. For example, AAG is the codon for lysine and UCG is the triplet for serine. Thus, an amino-acid coding sequence is read in groups of three nucleotides running in the 5′ to 3′ direction; this is the *reading frame* of a protein coding sequence. Three specific codons (*stop* codons) do not code for amino acids but instead signal the end of a gene.

Translation from the mRNA nucleotide code to protein is mediated by ribosomes in the cytoplasm of the cell. A ribosome binds to the 5′ end of the mRNA and provides a stable chemical environment for all the molecules involved in protein synthesis. Amino acids are linked in the correct sequence by the action of small, adaptor RNA molecules called *transfer RNAs* (tRNAs). Each tRNA molecule contains a region that is complementary to a particular mRNA codon: the *anticodon*. Linked to one end of the tRNA is the amino acid that corresponds to the complementary

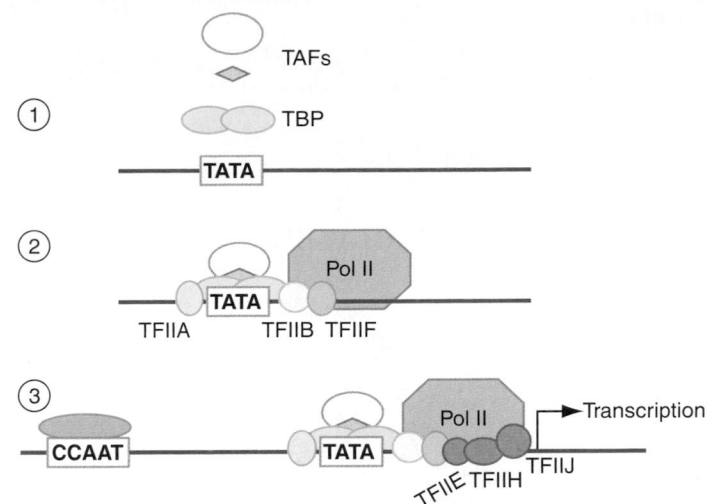

Figure 66–5 Assembly of the polymerase II transcription initiation complex. (1) The basal TFIID complex assembles as the TATA-box binding protein (TBP) and associated factors (TAFs) at the TATA box of the promoter region. (2) Additional transcription factors TFIIA and TFIIB are recruited to enable the polymerase II enzyme (Pol II) and TFIIF to bind. (3) The complex is stabilized with TFIIE, TFIIH and TFIIJ. Typically, binding of additional factors to upstream enhancer sites like CCAAT or GGGCGG are required for effective RNA transcription.

mRNA codon of the tRNA. A tRNA with the correct complementary anticodon binds to the first codon in the mRNA sequence, which is always AUG. When another specific tRNA binds to the next codon, ribosomal enzymes catalyze the formation of a peptide bond between the two amino acids linked to the tRNAs, removing the linkage between the first amino acid and its tRNA molecule. The first tRNA is ejected from the ribosome and a new tRNA binds to the next codon. As this process continues, the ribosome moves along the mRNA molecule, completing the synthesis of the amino acid chain. When the stop codon (UAG, UGA, or UAA) is reached, the ribosome detaches from the mRNA. In reality, several ribosomes can move along the same mRNA molecule, each translating the mRNA code into a new protein molecule.

Transcriptional Control

To allow for cellular differentiation and response to environmental stimuli, there must be mechanisms controlling the repertoire of gene transcription and protein translation. Some of these mechanisms operate at the level of DNA and control the transcription of mRNA (Rosenthal, 1994). For example, promoters are DNA sequences that are important for the initiation of mRNA transcription. Promoters are found upstream (toward the 5′ end) at a relatively invariant distance from the beginning of the protein coding sequence. There are several different kinds of promoter consensus sequences (nucleotide sequences that are found in many examples). The most common promoters are rich in adenine and thymine and have been called *TATA boxes*. Because A–T base pair bonds are weaker than G–C base-pair bonds, DNA unwinds more easily at repeat A–T sequences. Other recognized promoter sequences are the *GC box* and the *CAA motif*. After transcriptional activation, a local ssDNA region is produced and stabilized by the assembly of a complex of RNA polymerase and general transcription factors. Messenger RNA is synthesized from the local region of ssDNA and the mRNA is quickly ejected as the DNA returns to its more energetically favorable double-stranded helical state.

Enhancers are DNA sequences that can augment mRNA transcription and may be found in different locations relative to the gene that they affect. Gene-specific transcription factors are proteins that bind to enhancers and promoters and selectively stimulate or inhibit mRNA transcription (Papavassiliou, 1995). In eukaryotes, enhancers commonly contain multiple binding sites for several transcription factors, so it is the net effect of factors binding to these DNA elements that determines the activation and rate of expression (Fig. 66–5). The availability of transcription factors, in turn, are controlled by cellular events such as phosphorylation, or by other proteins such as hormones and growth factors. A network of intra- and extracellular chemical communications can thus select and control the synthesis of necessary proteins.

Because mRNA is far less stable than DNA, the half-life of mRNA is very short. New mRNA molecules are continually transcribed from DNA. As the cell responds to changes in transcriptional signals, the genes that are transcribed into mRNA can be quickly changed, resulting in the immediate

dsRNA

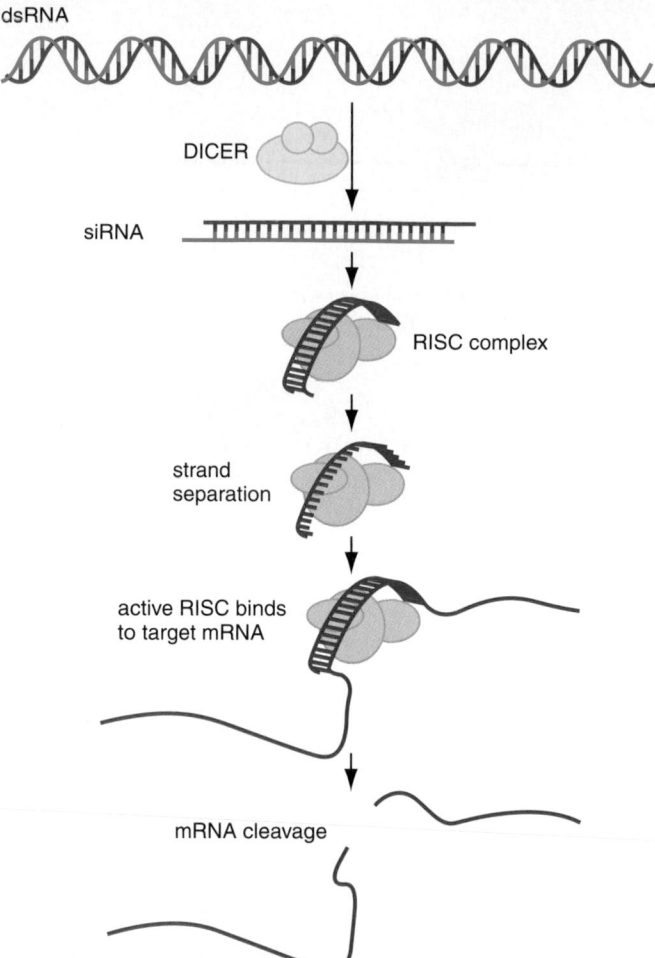

DICER

siRNA

RISC complex

strand separation

active RISC binds to target mRNA

mRNA cleavage

Figure 66–6 Diagram of the RNAi pathway: dsRNA is recognized by the DICER complex and processed into smaller siRNA molecules of 21–24 nucleotides. The RISC protein complex assembles with the siRNAs and unwinds the double strand. Active RISC binds to the target mRNA with complementary sequence and cleaves it, resulting in a nonfunctional message and a silent gene.

Table 66–3 DNA Repair Pathways

Direct repair	Repairs certain types of DNA damage in a single-step reaction
Mismatch repair	Checks for errors made when DNA is replicated. Any mispaired bases in the daughter strand are removed and replaced with the correct match
Base excision repair	Repairs small, non-helix-deforming adducts such as those produced by methylation, oxidation, reduction, or base fragmentation by ionizing radiation
Nucleotide excision repair	Removes bulky DNA adducts such as thymine dimers and certain photoproducts, as well as chemical adducts and crosslinks
Double-strand break repair	Repairs double-strand breaks that result from physiologic processes or from ionizing radiation and oxidative insults

for this, the proofreading activity of the polymerase can recognize the error, remove the incorrect base, and proceed again with synthesis. Together, the error avoidance mechanisms reduce base-pair mismatches to approximately 1 in 10 million (Radman, 1988). This represents a 100 000-fold increase in efficiency compared to the error rate of 1 in 100 bases for in vitro solid phase oligonucleotide synthesis.

In spite of remarkable error avoidance in DNA replication, occasional mistakes do occur. In addition, DNA can be damaged by normal biochemical reactions and by nonphysiologic agents such as ultraviolet light and environmental carcinogens. There are several repair mechanisms that mend damaged DNA (Yu, 1999) (Table 66–3).

Direct repair mechanisms repair lesions in a single-step reaction. For example, O^6-methylguanine DNA methyltransferase repairs alkylation lesions by transferring the alkyl group from the lesion to the active site of the enzyme. Other direct repair mechanisms characterized in *Escherichia coli* may also exist in human cells (Yu, 1999).

Mismatch repair (MMR) functions immediately after DNA replication to replace mismatched bases with the correct ones (Modrich, 1994). Several MMR proteins recognize the error in the newly synthesized daughter strand and excise a region that includes the mismatch. DNA polymerase III and ligase restore the correct sequence and integrity of the daughter strand. The importance of this mechanism in stabilizing the genome is evidenced by recent studies associating hereditary nonpolyposis colorectal cancer with defects in mismatch repair proteins.

Base excision repair targets small, non-helix-deforming adducts such as those produced by methylation, oxidation, reduction, or base fragmentation by ionizing radiation. Base excision leaves 3–4 nucleotide sequence gaps that are then filled with the correct nucleotides; nicks are sealed with ligase. Larger, bulky adducts or dimers that distort the DNA helix may be caused by UV radiation, carcinogens, and therapeutic drugs, among other agents. Such damage is removed by the nucleotide excision repair (NER) pathway, which utilizes an enzyme system composed of many proteins to excise a single-stranded oligonucleotide containing the lesion (Sancar, 1994). The gap is then filled in by DNA polymerase and ligated. There are two nucleotide excision repair pathways: one, in which lesions that block transcription are rapidly removed (transcription-coupled repair; Hanawalt, 1994) and a second, global pathway that repairs bulk DNA, including the nontranscribed strand of active genes. Some of the possible consequences of the loss of NER activity are exemplified by the disease xeroderma pigmentosum, which is caused by mutations in *NER*. Xeroderma pigmentosum results in extreme sensitivity to sunlight, with skin cancers occurring at an early age (Weeda, 1998).

Double-strand breaks occurring rarely or produced by ionizing radiation and oxidative damage present significant repair problems. If unresolved, replication and transcription of involved sequences will be blocked. To maintain local and overall genomic integrity, double-stranded breaks are repaired by nonhomologous or allelic recombinational repair mechanisms.

It is now clear that DNA repair plays a central role in the life of the cell. Recent evidence also indicates that several proteins that are primary repair proteins also function in transcription and in regulation of the cell cycle. Thus, the processes involving DNA appear to be highly integrated and are increasingly studied as a whole and in relation to human disease.

synthesis of new proteins. Thus, the cell has the ability to rapidly adjust its protein output in response to its environment.

Recently a novel method of post transcriptional gene suppression by short segments of RNA, called *RNA interference* or *RNAi* was discovered to be present in most eukaryotes. First discovered in the nematode *Caenorhabditis elegans* (Fire, 1998), RNAi results from the presence of dsRNA that triggers a cellular pathway consisting of two main phases (Fig. 66–6). First, dsRNA is recognized by a specific endonuclease termed the DICER. This enzyme cleaves the dsRNA molecule into shorter nucleotide duplexes of 21–24 bp. In the second phase, these small interference RNAs (siRNA) become incorporated into another enzyme complex – the RNA-induced silencing complex (RISC). Here, the two short siRNA strands are separated and target mRNAs with complementary sequences. Active RISC subsequently degrades the targeted mRNA molecules with a very high degree of specificity. It is thought that this mechanism is likely to be directed against viruses and other nucleotides with pathogenic potential. However RNAi is effective against both exogenous and endogenous nucleic acids and can be induced artificially to inhibit the expression of any genes of interest, including those involved in diseases such as cancer, diabetes or pathogenic infections (Dykxhoorn, 2005).

Mechanisms of DNA Repair

Errors in DNA replication and damage to DNA during the normal cellular lifetime must be minimized to preserve the health of the entire organism. Several mechanisms operate to maintain the normal DNA sequence. First, there are the error-avoidance mechanisms that operate during DNA replication. The DNA polymerase that synthesizes new DNA polymers selects each successive nucleotide monomer based on its complementarity to the next nucleotide in the template strand. Fidelity at this level is high and most errors in synthesis are avoided at this stage. Nevertheless, an occasional base may be incorrectly added to the growing strand. To adjust

DNA Mutations

In spite of extensive repair mechanisms, alterations in DNA base sequence (mutations) occur, and to some extent must occur for the process of evolution to continue. Yet, for an individual organism, some mutations are clearly harmful and can be associated with cancer and with inherited

Table 66–4 Types of DNA Mutation and Examples of Associated Diseases

Mutation	Description	Disease
Point	Single base-pair substitution	Sickle cell anemia
Deletion/insertion	Subtraction/addition of amino acid codons in multiples of three. Reading frame is retained	Becker muscular dystrophy
Deletion/insertion with frameshift	Subtraction/addition of amino acid codons not in multiples of three. Results in a shift of the reading frame and a completely different amino-acid coding sequence from the mutation on	Duchenne muscular dystrophy
Amplification/ trinucleotide repeat	Increase in the number of repeat sequences in microsatellite DNA. Results in disruption of gene expression	Fragile X syndrome
Translocation	Interchromosomal exchange of large chromosome segments. Results in a new protein with different function	Chronic myelogenous leukemia

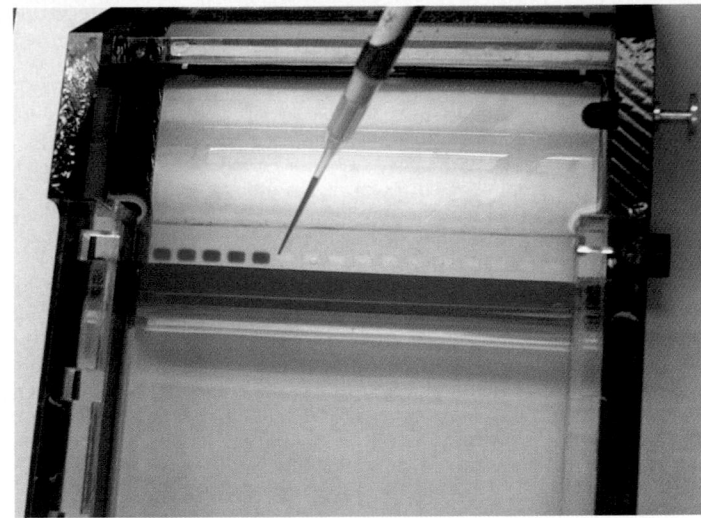

Figure 66–7 Photograph of loading sample and dye through buffer into wells of an agarose gel in a submarine gel electrophoresis apparatus.

genetic disease. Studies of these diseases have led to the characterization of the various types of mutation that occur in the human genome (Weatherall, 1987). These can be conceptually grouped into a few major categories (Table 66–4). A point mutation is found in the β-globin gene in sickle cell anemia (Kan, 1992). A thymine base replaces an adenine base, causing a critical change in the structure of hemoglobin. As described in Chapter 72, muscular dystrophy is caused by deletions in the gene for the muscle protein dystrophin. In the Becker form of the disease, the deletions do not disrupt the reading frame but, in most of the cases with the more severe Duchenne form, the reading frame is changed by the deletions, effectively abolishing the function of the protein (Liechti-Gallati, 1989).

Human DNA contains many short sequences of nucleotides (microsatellite DNA) that are sometimes grouped in tandem arrays and are repeated many times throughout the human genome. The number of tandem repeats at particular locations is a heritable trait. Some trinucleotide repeats have been found to increase in number in association with disease (Sutherland, 1994). In fragile X syndrome (Chapter 72), expression of the disease is associated with the amplification beyond a certain limit of the number of an intragenic trinucleotide repeat sequence. The expansion of the trinucleotides repeats beyond a critical number disrupts expression of the gene.

Translocations may not always be detectable by chromosomal karyotype analysis. At the gene level, a translocation may create a fusion gene, the combination of two different genes abnormally joined at the translocation site. This can not only create an altered gene transcript but may also bring the product of one gene under the transcriptional control of the other. For example, as discussed at length in Chapter 71, the Philadelphia chromosome, found in most cases of chronic myelogenous leukemia, results from a reciprocal translocation between the c-abl gene on chromosome 9 and a region termed the breakpoint cluster region (bcr) on chromosome 22. The fusion gene produced by this chromosomal rearrangement, consisting of most of the c-abl gene and a truncated bcr, codes for a c-Abl protein that is larger than the normal product, has increased enzymatic activity, and is thought to interfere with signal transduction pathways normally involved in the control of cell death and proliferation.

It is both the type of mutation as well as its location in relation to the gene that determines the ultimate effect on the protein product. Mutations may have no effect on protein expression or functional activity; many human proteins exist in detectable variants that have no disease association. Mutations occurring in intron regions presumably have no effect at all. Even small mutations, however, in regions that code for key functional domains (exons) may drastically alter or eliminate function. 'Nonsense mutations,' mutations that change an amino acid codon to a stop codon, or vice versa, result in abnormally short or long protein products, respectively. Missense mutations, those that change the code from one amino acid to another, may or may not alter protein function, depending on the change and the

function of the amino acid. Similarly, mutations within sequences that denote intron–exon splice sites could eliminate exons or introduce introns into the transcribed mRNA. Mutations may also occur in regulatory sequences, such as promoters or enhancers, producing dramatic effects on the levels of transcription.

Nucleic Acid Analyses

The unique biochemical properties of nucleic acids have been exploited to yield information about the biology or biochemistry of a system. While some of the assays, such as electrophoresis, are applicable to other biochemical building blocks such as proteins and lipids, the majority are particular to nucleic acids. The following sections briefly describe the principles of the basic categories of analyses used to characterize DNA and RNA: electrophoretic separations, hybridization assays, amplification techniques, and restriction fragment length polymorphisms. In practice, the categories are often combined to produce novel variations of the same theme; for example, a complete assay may involve amplification, electrophoresis, and hybridization.

Electrophoretic Separation

The repeating sugar–phosphate backbone of nucleic acids results in a net negative charge evenly distributed over these linear molecules. Therefore, movement of DNA or RNA in response to an electric field will be proportional to the molecular weight or length of the molecule. This property is used to characterize the size of nucleic acid fragments by electrophoretic separation. The format is analogous to that used for the separation of proteins according to size. Multiple samples are applied in separate wells at one end of a solid but porous separation medium. When a voltage is applied, the samples move toward the positive electrode in a linear fashion, each sample well forming one lane of migration. The solid electrophoretic medium and array of sample wells is known as a gel. Size standards, referred to as DNA or RNA ladders, are mixtures of nucleic acids of known fragment length that are analyzed in one or more lanes of the gel. Comparison of the distance of migration of an unknown sample with the ladder, either by 'eye' or by computer-assisted measurement, allows size determination.

The composition and concentration of the separation medium determines the size of the fragments, which may be separated into distinct bands. Other variables that contribute to resolution are the thickness of the gel, the length of the electrophoresis path, the time of electrophoresis, and the applied voltage. In practice, these factors are adjusted empirically and controlled as carefully as possible to ensure reproducibility from day to day. Agarose is the separation medium most often used, usually in conjunction with a horizontal electrophoresis bed in which the gel is submerged in buffer, the submarine gel. Samples are made heavy with sucrose or Ficoll and loaded into slots in the gel through the buffer (Fig. 66–7). Higher resolving power, allowing differentiation of a single base pair in length, is achieved with acrylamide, usually used in a vertical format, although increasingly capillary formats are being adopted, which decrease both the time of the separation and the amount of sample required. The simplest approach to visualizing the bands separated by electrophoresis is by staining with intercalating dyes (e.g., ethidium bromide), which insert between stacked bases, and viewing with ultraviolet transillumination. Direct visualization requires that the band achieves a significant concentration. In some applications the nucleic acid fragments may be detected by a radioactive or fluorescent tag, which can increase sensitivity.

The molecules in genomic DNA are reduced to fragments that may be resolved by electrophoresis through digestion with restriction enzymes. Restriction enzymes with a relatively simple recognition sequence produce fragments less than 50 kilobase pairs (kb) in length. Extremely large DNA fragments, measured in megabase pairs (Mbp), are produced from digestion with enzymes with a complex recognition sequence and must be separated in special electrophoretic systems utilizing a pulsed electrical field. Most applications of DNA electrophoresis utilize nondenaturing conditions (i.e., the fragments resolved into bands are double-stranded). By contrast, most RNA separations utilize denaturing conditions (either formamide or glyoxal) to eliminate secondary structure of the single-stranded molecules. RNA molecules, as transcripts of DNA, are 'presized' and relatively small, so that no digestion is required prior to electrophoresis.

Nucleic Acid Hybridization

Hybridization is a fundamental concept in nucleic acid biochemistry; it is defined as the interaction between two single-stranded nucleic acid molecules to form a duplex (double-stranded) molecule based on the complementary base pairing of their respective sequences. Hybridization is a direct consequence of the stable double-stranded structure of DNA under physiologic conditions. As discussed earlier, the helix is formed of two antiparallel strands of DNA held together by the combined strength of many specific hydrogen bonds between complementary base pairs, as well as by hydrophobic shielding of bases from an aqueous environment. Central to the hybridization reaction is the fact that the binding between separate, complementary molecules (strands) is both reversible and base-sequence-specific.

When neither DNA strand is labeled, the process of reforming the stable double-stranded structure is referred to as *annealing*. If one strand is labeled (i.e., has a marker that is capable of being detected in some fashion), the labeled strand is referred to as a *probe* and the process is called *hybridization* because a hybrid molecule is formed between a labeled and unlabeled strand. RNA molecules can also participate in the hybridization process. Base pairing may occur between complementary strands of DNA, between DNA and RNA, and between complementary strands of RNA, resulting in DNA–DNA, DNA–RNA, and RNA–RNA duplex structures. Duplex molecules with exact complementarity in base sequence form the most stable structures, but structures with varying degrees of base-pair mismatch may form, depending on the conditions. The relative instability of these mismatched duplexes will be reflected in the lowered temperature of their disassociation (lower T_m, see Fig. 66–2).

Environmental conditions can be manipulated to control the degree of base-pair mismatching that will be tolerated in a duplex structure (i.e., the *stringency* of the sequence match) (Fig. 66–8). Low stringency refers to conditions such as high salt, low temperature, and no formamide, which favor shielding of hydrophobic bases from the aqueous environment even without perfect alignment; the match need not be perfect. High-stringency conditions – high temperature (close to T_m), low salt, and high formamide – will only allow the most perfectly matched duplex structures to remain in a stable helix conformation.

Hybridization Assays: Basic Components

When the hybridization reaction is used to analyze the nucleic acid content of an unknown sample, the process is known as a *hybridization assay*. The property of complementary base pairing allows fragments of known composition (the probe) to interrogate an unknown for the presence of matching (complementary) sequences. All hybridization assays, therefore, require several basic elements: a probe, a sample, controlled conditions permissive of complementary base pairing, and a method for detecting specific probe–sample hybrids. Each of these elements will be briefly discussed below, as well as the variations in formats that have been developed to allow hybridization assays to be performed and interpreted.

Probe

The specificity of the hybridization reaction is determined by the probe; thus, the probe is central to a hybridization assay in the same way that the primary antibody is central to an immunoassay. A probe is a well-characterized fragment of nucleic acid, either DNA or RNA. In most assay formats it is the probe that carries the reporter group for detection of

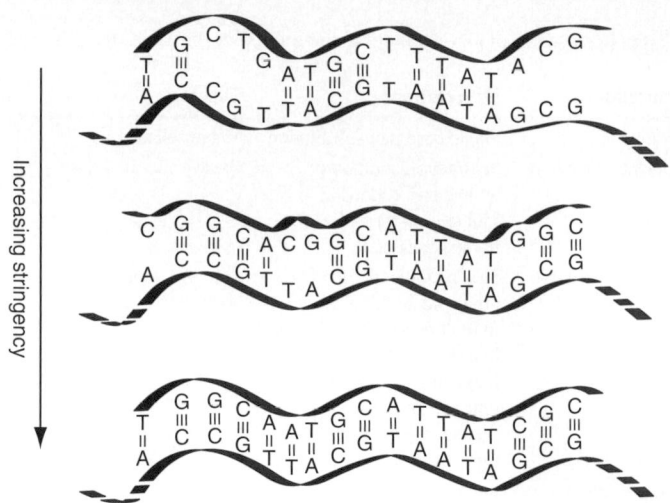

Figure 66–8 Illustration of stringency. As the stringency of the hybridization solution is increased, fewer mismatches are tolerated in a hybrid duplex. At very high stringency, even a single base-pair mismatch will disrupt the duplex.

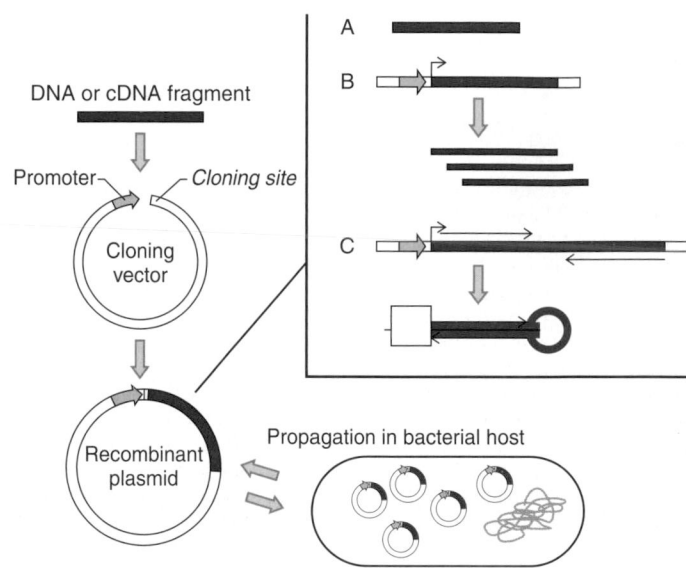

Figure 66–9 Production of cloned DNA or RNA. A DNA fragment or RNA that was converted into cDNA can be inserted into a cloning vector. The recombinant plasmid is transformed into a bacterial host, where it is rapidly propagated to millions of copies. The multiplied DNA fragment can either be isolated by excision through restriction enzymes, which recognize sequences at the borders of the insert (A), or used to initiate RNA in vitro transcription with a promoter sequence in the plasmid (B). Such systems are also used to produce double-stranded RNA by cloning two complementary sequences in sense and antisense direction, typically with a spacer that forms a stabilizing loop in the dsRNA fragment (C).

hybridized molecules into the reaction, although variations occur. Reporter groups may be radioactive or nonradioactive (i.e., affinity label).

Many probes are produced through recombinant nucleic acid technology, as illustrated in Figure 66–9. Plasmids – short, circular, double-stranded segments of DNA – are harnessed as vectors to propagate desired sequences in bacteria. The segment of interest is introduced into the plasmid using restriction enzyme digestion and ligation, resulting in a new 'recombined' molecule that retains the ability to be propagated in bacteria and includes the DNA sequence of interest. Bacteria containing the recombinant plasmid can be grown in culture, and the small circular plasmids can easily be separated from the bacterial genome on the basis of size. Many identical copies are obtained; thus, the DNA is often referred to as *cloned*. Purified plasmid may be used as probe in assays where vector sequences do not interfere with the specificity of the reaction. In many applications the inserted DNA sequence is separated from the vector sequence by digesting the isolated plasmid with the same restriction enzyme originally used in construction of the recombinant molecule. The probe resulting from either of these approaches is a double-stranded DNA molecule. Double-stranded probes must be denatured prior to use, and probe reannealing limits the extent of hybridization of probe with target.

A plasmid vector that does not contain cloned DNA is a commonly used negative control for this type of probe.

Plasmid vectors have been constructed to include RNA promoter regions adjacent to the inserted DNA sequence. These recombinant plasmids are used to produce RNA transcripts of the DNA insert. The result is a single-stranded RNA probe that will not undergo self-hybridization. Controlling the orientation of the DNA insert with respect to the RNA promoter allows production of transcripts in the *sense* (same as mRNA) or *antisense* (complementary to mRNA) direction. In many applications the sense transcripts form ideal negative control probes for hybridization reactions with antisense probes. Non-specifically-bound RNA probe (i.e., RNA not in a stable duplex structure) can be removed with the use of RNase specific for single-stranded RNA. The lability of RNA requires that the probes be handled with extreme care to prevent degradation (sterile technique, treated water and glassware.)

Recombinant probes, whether DNA or RNA, are genetically complex; that is, they may include many kilobases of genetic information. By contrast, probes produced by synthetic methods are relatively short segments of DNA. Oligonucleotide probes produced by automated chemical reactions are usually 15–45 bases in length synthesized to produce a specified base sequence. Probes with very high specificity of hybridization can be designed on the basis of sequence information available in data banks. They can be generated in a sense or antisense direction at a relatively low cost. These short probes are single-stranded, diffuse into target and hybridize rapidly because of their small size, and are extremely sensitive to even single base-pair mismatches. The final sensitivity achieved with oligonucleotide probes is lower than that achieved with recombinant probes because of their limited genetic complexity. Multiple oligonucleotide probes directed to different areas of the same target have in some instances been used to increase the sensitivity by increasing the representation of the target sequence in the probe mixture. This approach is analogous to the use of a blend of monoclonal antibodies that react to different epitopes of the same complex antigen.

Probes longer than those obtained by direct chemical synthesis may be generated with the polymerase chain reaction (PCR) or other amplification technology. These probes may be single-stranded or double-stranded depending on the conditions employed and may be as long as the product of the amplification reaction; in most cases 100 bp to 1 kb in length.

Sample

While probe selection and preparation are central to determining the sensitivity and specificity of the hybridization assay, the contribution of sample preparation to a successful assay cannot be overlooked. In clinical applications, samples of interest may be quite diverse. For example, a microbiology laboratory could anticipate testing specimens of blood, urine, stool, and sputum. Integrity of RNA targets may be difficult to maintain under such conditions and even DNA may be degraded with improper handling. The goal of sample preparation is to maintain nucleic acid integrity and make the target genetic information available for interaction with the probe. For some applications the requirement of target integrity will dictate immediate snap freezing or addition of lysis buffers containing potent RNase and DNase inhibitors. In other applications, more routine methods of sample collection will allow adequate target preservation.

The physical and chemical similarities of nucleic acids, regardless of source, allow for uniform methods of extraction and purification. For many assays it is preferable to extensively purify DNA or RNA to remove inhibitors of enzymes to be added to the assay (such as a restriction enzyme or polymerase) and to maximize accessibility of target to probe. Complete purification schemes, however, are time-consuming and require a relatively large amount of starting sample. In many applications, relatively abbreviated sample purifications can be used. Purifications commonly use cell lysis (mechanical, chemical, or both), protease treatment, and organic or inorganic extractions. Automated methods are now available to standardize and streamline sample extraction.

Controlled Conditions Permissive for Complementary Base Pairing

The sensitivity and specificity of the hybridization reaction are greatly influenced by the physical–chemical environment during the reaction and subsequent detection/collection of hybrid molecules. In practice, the hybridization cocktail is the medium used to control the environment of the hybridization reaction. Empirically designed, the *hybridization cocktail* is a mixture of reagents selected to favor interaction of nucleic acids through sequence-specific hydrogen bonds rather than via charge. The components vary widely but include buffers, salts, denaturants such as formamide, high-molecular-weight polymers, carrier DNA or RNA, and

various components added to reduce background (such as detergents, bovine serum albumin, Ficoll). Such a complex mixture is conveniently referred to as a *cocktail*. The ionic strength of both the hybridization cocktail and the subsequent washes is most often modulated by the concentration of a *saline sodium citrate* buffer (SSC), composed of 0.15 mol/L sodium chloride, 0.015 mol/L trisodium citrate, pH 7.0. The shorthand notation for these conditions refers to the strength of SSC; that is, $2 \times$ SSC, $0.1 \times$ SSC. The final stringency of the hybridization reaction is controlled by the formamide and salt concentration of the hybridization cocktail, the temperature of the hybridization reaction, and the temperature and salt concentration of the washing steps.

Detection of Hybrids

A wide variety of techniques have been applied to collection and analysis of specific hybrids, discussed briefly later under Hybridization Assay Formats. Once specific hybrids have been collected, methods of detection are obviously linked to methods of labeling. Many research applications and the first clinical applications of hybridization assays utilized radioactive labels such as phosphorus-32 (^{32}P), iodine-125 (^{125}I), sulfur-35 (^{35}S), carbon-14 (^{14}C), and tritium (^{3}H) with detection through autoradiography or scintillation counting. Specific activity of the label directly influenced the sensitivity of the detection. For clinical applications, alternatives to radioisotopic labeling were sought. Radioactive probes have a relatively short half-life, making one of the key reagents in the hybridization assay unstable. In addition, the hazard to laboratory personnel and cost of radioactive waste disposal contributed to the need for nonradioactive methods. Non-isotopically-labeled probes are stable reagents, greatly facilitating the commercial production and standardization that are crucial for assay reproducibility.

Nonisotopic labeling and detection methods for nucleic acids have many similarities to immunochemical assays developed for nonisotopic protein detection. In some applications, nucleic acids are directly linked to a signal-generating compound, usually a fluorochrome but occasionally an enzyme. This situation is analogous to immunoassays in which the primary antibody is labeled. More commonly, nucleic acids are indirectly detected in a multistep assay similar in concept to an indirect antibody reaction. Biotin, a commonly used affinity label for immunoassays, was the first affinity label introduced into nucleic acids (Langer, 1981). Biotin itself generates no signal, but is detected by high-affinity interaction with an avidin or streptavidin molecule that is in turn complexed or conjugated to a signal-generating enzyme, fluorochrome, or metallic particles detected by light scattering (Yguerabide, 2001). Many other functional groups have been developed as nonisotopic labels such as bromodeoxyuridine, digoxigenin, and sulfone. Detection in these cases is achieved with high-affinity antibodies directed against the functional group. These antibodies are usually directly linked to a signal-generating enzyme or fluorochrome, functioning like a labeled secondary antibody in an immunohistochemistry reaction. Biotin may also be detected with an antibiotin antibody rather than an avidin or streptavidin molecule.

Because affinity labels are detected with large, bulky proteins such as avidin or antibody, availability of the label to the detection reagent is a crucial factor in determination of sensitivity. Increasing the number of affinity tags will not necessarily increase the number of detecting molecules that will be bound to the nucleic acid. In addition, because affinity labels are themselves bulky, overincorporation into the nucleic acid molecule can lead to steric hindrance of the hybridization reaction. For these reasons, the specific activity of the affinity label does not directly control the sensitivity of the detection.

One advantage of the indirect detection of affinity labels is that a variety of detection methods can be used for the same label (Fig. 66–10). For example, biotin may be detected with avidin linked to an enzyme with subsequent color or chemiluminescent detection, or avidin with fluorescent tag. For all nonradioactive methods, the detection portion of the assay is crucial in obtaining optimal sensitivity. An effective hybridization reaction can be marred by detection reagents with poor background and suboptimal signal generation. The choice of the enzyme labels (peroxidase vs alkaline phosphatase), enzyme substrate (colorimetric vs chemiluminescent), and even source of reagents are critical for optimal results.

Hybridization Assay Formats

A wide variety of hybridization assay formats have been developed, each designed to solve the methodologic problems of the hybridization assay: conditions permitting specific complementary base pairing, a method to detect hybrids, and an interpretation of the result. Each method has particular strengths and weaknesses and selection of format is dictated by the clinical setting and the particular diagnostic question. There is no one

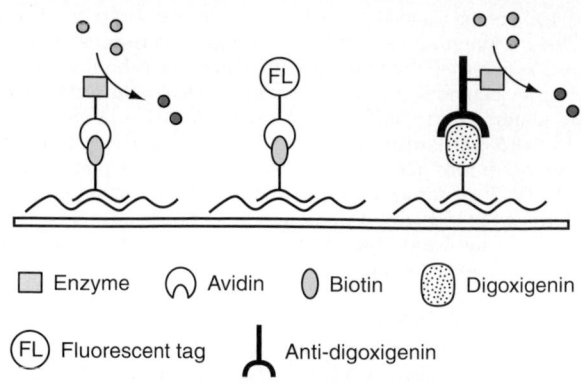

Enzyme   Avidin   Biotin   Digoxigenin

FL Fluorescent tag   Anti-digoxigenin

○ Substrate (colorimetric or chemiluminescent)

Figure 66–10 Examples of affinity-labeled probe detection systems. Dark blue circles represent the product of the enzyme-catalyzed reaction. (With permission from Unger ER, Piper MA: Nucleic acid biochemistry and diagnostic applications. *In* Burtis CA, Ashwood ER (eds): Tietz Textbook of Clinical Chemistry, 2nd ed. Philadelphia, PA, WB Saunders, 1994.)

perfect assay. Several of the basic formats will be briefly described, along with their particular strengths and weaknesses.

Each hybridization assay requires both positive and negative controls for validation. A positive sample control is one known to contain sequences complementary to the probe. This is used to establish that sample preparation is adequate to release target for the hybridization assay, and to ensure that probe will hybridize with the specific target under the assay conditions. The sample control may also be used to monitor the sensitivity of the assay if the positive control is chosen near the lower limits of detection. A negative sample control (i.e., one known not to contain sequences complementary to the probe) is used to monitor the specificity of the probe–target interactions. Controls for the probe include vector sequences or unrelated probes labeled, hybridized, and detected under identical assay conditions. These latter controls allow monitoring of the background signal generated by localization of probe through nonhybridized interactions such as charge or trapping. In clinical practice, additional controls may be employed to monitor each step of the hybridization assay.

Liquid or Solution Phase Hybridization

In liquid hybridization assays, both the sample and probe interact in solution, which maximizes the kinetics of the reaction. The sample nucleic acids are generally purified from contaminating proteins and lipids, which could interfere with the collection of hybrids at the end of the assay, and some sample degradation is tolerated by the assay. The sample is denatured and randomly sheared prior to addition of single-stranded probe lacking the ability to self-hybridize.

Hybridization may be detected by the specific binding of hybrids to a solid matrix such as hydroxyapatite, which binds only duplex structures. Once hybrids are bound, unhybridized probe may be efficiently removed by washing. Detection of the label on the bound probe permits quantitation of the hybridization reaction. In a variation of this approach, one commercial assay (Hybrid-Capture) uses an antibody specific for RNA–DNA hybrids to specifically bind duplex structures formed of the DNA target and RNA probe. An alternative analysis involves digestion of the hybridization reaction mixture with S1 nuclease, an enzyme that acts only on single-stranded nucleic acid. Duplex structures resistant to digestion may then be precipitated by treatment with trichloroacetic acid. In the hybridization protection assay, label on the probe is protected from chemical degradation only when the probe is involved in a duplex structure.

Many other variations of the solution-phase hybridization assay are in use. Optimal kinetics, toleration for abbreviated purification steps, and some sample degradation make the assay adaptable for clinical application. Quantification of the reaction product may be achieved, depending on the detection system. The solution phase format does not permit identification of the size of the hybridizing product. Low positive reactions are difficult to interpret, as low levels of specific target and high levels of weakly crossreacting target will yield similar results. Solution phase hybridization is adaptable to the 96-well format with an enzyme-linked immunosorbent assay (ELISA)-type read-out, and increasing automation of the assay can be anticipated.

Solid-Support Hybridization

Variations of the solid-support hybridization assays include dot or blot hybridization, Southern and Northern hybridization, microarray hybridiza-

tions ('DNA chips') and in situ hybridization. In these assays, the hybridization occurs in a biphasic environment, a solid phase (usually sample) and a liquid phase (usually probe). The kinetics of hybridization to a nucleic acid bound to a solid support is greatly slowed, and the extent of the hybridization reaction is limited. These disadvantages are often outweighed by the convenience of having a solid medium to carry through multiple steps of the assay.

Dot/Blot Hybridization

In this assay format, multiple samples are immobilized in a geometric array on a nitrocellulose or nylon membrane. The name of the assay comes from the shape of each sample on the membrane. When samples are applied by hand, the shape is more random (blot). With the use of commercially available manifolds, samples are usually applied with the use of suction, the sample shape is very regular – round (dot) or elongated (slot). The solid matrix allows multiple samples to be processed through all steps of the assay simultaneously. The fact that all samples and controls are exposed to exactly the same reagents and conditions increases the standardization of the assay.

The extent of sample preparation varies from complete purification of nucleic acids prior to application to the filter, to direct application of unpurified sample. Some degree of sample degradation is tolerated by the assay. Purified nucleic acids have the advantage of being most available for interaction with probe and having the least problems with background. Individual sample purification, however, is time-consuming and labor-intensive. Applications using direct application of unpurified sample take the entire array through an abbreviated purification procedure, which usually involves lysis and denaturation, protein digestion, and washing with detergent. The advantages of this approach are that it is applicable to small amounts of starting material and minimizes sample preparation time. However, the final sensitivity of the reaction is lower, and background from nonspecific probe interactions can make the assay unreliable.

Interpretation of the results of a dot/blot hybridization assay is relatively straightforward. If hybridization has occurred, a signal is generated in the specified spot. Depending on the label used for signal generation, results may be quantified; however, usually a simple yes/no interpretation is given (i.e., the sample has more or less signal than adjacent samples and known positive and negative controls). Weak signals, which may result from a very small amount of specific target or from a large amount of weakly cross-reacting target, may cause problems in interpretation. No information is available about the size of the hybridizing fragments.

One interesting variation of the dot/blot assay is known as the reverse dot/line blot assay. In this format, applied in situations where one sample must be tested with many different probes and sample may be limited, the label is carried into the assay by the sample. The unlabeled probes, or targets, are fixed to the solid support in a linear or matrix array. Areas of specific hybrid formation are identified and interpreted as in the standard dot blot assay. This assay format is a convenient means of identifying the product of an amplification assay (see below and Chapter 67), such as in HLA (Bugawan, 1994) or human papillomavirus typing (Gravitt, 1998).

Southern and Northern Hybridizations

Both Southern and Northern hybridizations combine electrophoretic separation of test nucleic acid with transfer to a solid support and subsequent hybridization. These assays, therefore, not only give information about the presence of hybridization but permit determination of the molecular weight of the hybridizing species.

The original procedure was termed Southern blot hybridization or Southern blotting, after its inventor, E. M. Southern (Southern, 1975). In this assay, the sample is DNA. Northern blotting was named by analogy for the technique using RNA samples. (Extending the analogy even further, the Western blot is a similar procedure in which proteins are subjected to electrophoresis and transfer; a south-western blot has been described for a technique separating and blotting DNA followed by incubation with protein solutions to permit evaluation of specific DNA-binding proteins.)

Sample preparation is time-consuming and labor-intensive for both of these techniques. Degradation of sample nucleic acids is not tolerated by the assays and a relatively large amount of starting material is required. For Southern hybridizations, the DNA must be purified with minimal shearing. This is because sizing of the DNA fragments is achieved through digestion with one or more restriction enzymes. Shearing and degradation introduce random breaks in the sample, reducing the quantity available to be specifically cut at appropriate recognition sequences. Impurities in the sample may interfere with the activity and sequence specificity of the restriction enzyme. Partially or improperly digested samples can produce spurious band sizes or result in such a reduced concentration of

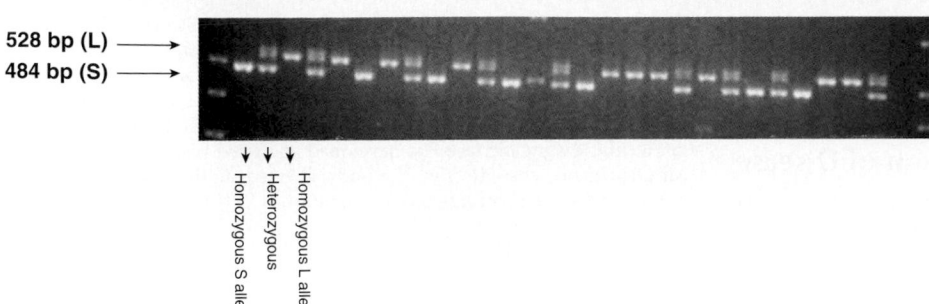

528 bp (L) →
484 bp (S) →

Homozygous S allele
Heterozygous
Homozygous L allele

Figure 66–11 Example of polymorphism analysis by gel electrophoresis (allelic typing of the serotonin transporter gene [5-HTTLPR]). A polymorphism consisting of a 44-base-pair insertion/deletion polymorphism in the 5′ regulatory region is suggested to be associated with major depressive disorder. The presence of the two different alleles can be screened using polymerase chain reaction primers upstream and downstream of the site producing fragments of distinct length. The amplicons are then separated by gel electrophoresis and stained with ethidium bromide. An individual is either homozygous for the long version (L allele = upper band), heterozygous with both alleles (two bands) or homozygous for the short version (S allele = lower band).

the specific band that it is no longer detected during hybridization. For Northern hybridizations, the starting material is RNA, and extreme care must be taken to avoid degradation during sample collection and preparation because of the ubiquitous nature of RNases. RNA is composed of fragment sizes determined by transcription and processing of message and ribosomal RNA. It is not digested prior to electrophoresis but is separated under denaturing conditions to remove secondary structure.

The size-separated fragments in the agarose gel are then transferred to a nylon or nitrocellulose filter. As originally designed, the transfer occurred passively through capillary action. Most current applications use vacuum or pressure to speed the transfer. After transfer, the nucleic acids are immobilized by baking or ultraviolet crosslinking and the entire membrane is hybridized with labeled probe.

Hybridization is followed by autoradiographic, colorimetric, or chemiluminescent detection of bands containing sequences complementary to the probe. Interpretation involves both detection of a hybridizing species and determination of the molecular weight of the molecule. These technically demanding assays require several days to perform but may be required in clinical applications in which the information cannot be obtained in any other format. The presence of bands at molecular weights different from normal or germ-line (developmentally unaltered) samples can indicate a change in the genetic material.

Microarray hybridization ('DNA chip technology')

Microarray hybridizations can be thought of as a variation of the dot/blot format in which the dotted material is arranged in a regular grid-like pattern with each feature reduced to a very small size so that hundreds to thousands of features can be placed on one solid surface, currently most often a glass microscope slide. By convention in these applications the sample is labeled and the arrayed features are referred to as probes. Microarrays allow genome wide transcription profiling or sequence determination in a single experiment. The technique and applications are described in greater detail in Chapter 69.

In Situ Hybridization

In situ hybridization is simply detection of specific genetic information within a morphologic context. This specialized type of solid-support assay involves taking morphologically intact tissue, cells, or chromosomes affixed to a glass microscope slide through the hybridization process. Autoradiographic, colorimetric, and fluorescent methods of detection have been applied. Evaluation of the final product is very analogous to evaluation of immunohistochemistry and requires experience in histopathology. The strength of the method lies in linking microscopic morphologic evaluation with detection of hybridization.

The method, discussed in Chapter 69, also has applications in cytogenetic analysis of metaphase chromosome spreads or of interphase nuclei. In this context, the detection is usually fluorescent, and the technique is referred to as fluorescent in situ hybridization (FISH). Detecting numerical aberrations or translocations of chromosomes can be achieved rapidly using probes for specific targets. FISH avoids some of the difficulties of conventional cytogenetics and may have greater sensitivity for some targets. Although FISH cannot completely replace karyotyping, it can complement and reduce the need for the frequency of cytogenetic analysis. Newer variations of FISH (Luke, 1998) are exploiting the possibilities of automation (fast-FISH) and expanding the information that can be obtained in a single assay. FICTION (fluorescence immunophenotyping and interphase cytogenetics as a tool for investigation of neoplasms) combines immunophenotyping with FISH; fiber FISH makes it possible to simultaneously detect and map chromosomal break points. FISH is considered in more detail in Chapter 69. In situ hybridization can be very

labor-intensive and tedious. Recent improvements resulting in automated processing of slides through the assay hold much promise for more widespread adoption of this technique.

Amplification Methods

It is virtually impossible to read any medical journal without encountering at least one application of PCR technology. The PCR has forever changed the scope of research questions that can be addressed by virtually eliminating the problem of limited sample size. The importance and elegance of the concept has been recognized through awarding of the Nobel Prize in Chemistry to its inventor, Kary Mullis, less than 10 years after publication of the first practical application of PCR (Saiki, 1985). There are now other methodologies that result in multiplication of target, probe, or signal. These may be grouped together as amplification technologies and are described in Chapter 67.

Polymorphism-Based Assays

Although more than 99% of the human genome is identical in all individuals, there are still millions of regions of DNA that vary between individuals. While most polymorphisms have no recognized functional consequence, changes in promoter or enhancer regions may result in altered transcription regulation, cause variation in the mRNA splice products if present in intron–exon junctions, or produce altered amino acid sequences if an exon is affected. The serotonin transporter gene (5-HTTLPR), for instance, exists in two alternative allelic variants characterized by a 44-base-pair insertion/deletion polymorphism in the promoter region. This polymorphism has been associated with major depressive disorders and the two allelic versions can be distinguished by PCR amplification of the relevant DNA region, resulting in two different-sized products (Fig. 66–11). Most of the variations occur in the form of an individual base change known as single nucleotide polymorphisms (SNPs). An example would be the alteration of a DNA fragment ACGT to ACTT by replacement of the third base from a guanine to a thymine. Two unrelated individuals will have approximately three million SNPs that differ between them.

The sequence-specific recognition features of restriction enzymes have been used since the 1970s for the detection of such sequence variations. In such assays, called restriction fragment length polymorphism (RFLP, 'riflip'), DNA is digested with a restriction enzyme and the fragments are analyzed by gel electrophoresis followed by band visualization or Southern blot analysis with a site-specific probe. Changes in the sequence of the DNA may result in alteration of the recognition sequence of the enzyme. A SNP alteration may introduce additional restriction enzyme sites, remove restriction sites, or insert or delete sequences between restriction sites. These changes will be reflected in a change in the band size visualized in a gel or hybridizing to the site-specific probe. Although the approach has been applied with considerable success in family studies, RFLP is a relatively crude method. Sequence polymorphism can only be detected if the distance between two restriction sites is directly affected and the majority of SNPs would not be detected.

Because of the tremendous potential of polymorphism assays to predict inheritance of altered alleles, considerable effort has been made in recent years to improve the speed, precision and cost effectiveness of these methods. The completion of the Human Genome Project in 2001 provided a reference against which all other sequencing data can be compared. Researchers are also systematically screening the genome to discover new SNPs. High-throughput SNP analysis methods have been developed which simultaneously scan thousands of SNPs in thousands of samples. Comprehensive mapping of an individual's SNP pattern is also termed genotyping. Genotyping is somewhat easier, since one form of the known gene sequence (allele) can be compared with an alternative form at a

VIII

specific predetermined site. A large variety of approaches for allelic discrimination are currently applied and typically use a combination of molecular techniques. More information can be found in Chen & Sullivan (Chen, 2002).

Relationship to Laboratory Evaluation of Disease

Subsequent chapters describe the current applications of molecular diagnostics. It is clear that this new technology has impacted all areas of laboratory diagnosis. Molecular methods also have the potential to redefine laboratory evaluation of disease to include issues beyond disease diagnosis.

Molecular Diagnosis

The advantages of a molecular approach to diagnosis will be described in detail for each aspect of current application. Increased automation and commercially designed methods have reduced costs and the level of technical expertise required to perform the tests. Increasingly, molecular technology is being integrated into the mainstream of laboratory testing.

Detecting mutations and associating them with disease is at the heart of the current explosion of information in medical science and of many applications in molecular diagnostics. One of the most important consequences of the revolution in molecular genetics has been the ability to locate a gene responsible for a disease without knowing the protein product. Termed *positional cloning*, this process uses RFLP linkage analysis of families that carry and express the disease to locate polymorphic markers closer and closer to the disease gene until it is ultimately located. Closely linked polymorphic markers that tend to segregate with disease may be useful in clinical diagnostic tests even before the gene is completely characterized and the protein product finally identified. In this scenario, molecular diagnostic tests are developed and used first, to be replaced by simpler, more cost-effective methods directed at the level of the gene product when the consequence of mutation is fully understood.

Beyond Diagnosis

Molecular analyses have the potential to greatly expand the role of the laboratory in areas beyond disease diagnosis. Molecular analysis of the somatic mutations in cancer has the potential to provide prognostic information, guide selection of optimal therapy, and monitor response to therapy. This is discussed in Chapters 71 and 76. The implications of using molecular markers to detect neoplastic cells in the absence of clinical or morphologic evidence of disease, known as *minimal residual disease*, are now being explored in a variety of malignancy types (see Ch. 71). This approach of using molecular markers for disease detection can also be anticipated to impact secondary methods of cancer prevention (screening) and assessment of adequacy of surgical resection (evaluation of margins). Gene therapy for inherited genetic disease as well as cancer is being introduced based on a detailed understanding of the underlying disease. Monitoring these patients for presence and activity of the introduced therapeutic gene will add another aspect to the laboratory evaluation of disease.

References

Alberts B, Johnson A, Lewis J, et al: Molecular Biology of the Cell, 4rd ed. New York, Garland Publishing, 2002.
An excellent, clearly written textbook of molecular biology. It is available in searchable format through the NCBI bookshelf web site:
http://www.ncbi.nlm.nih.gov/entrez/query.fcgi?db=Books

Bugawan TL, Apple R, Erlich H: A method for typing polymorphism as the HLA-A locus using PCR amplification and immobilized oligonucleotide probes. Tissue Antigens 1994; 44:137–147.

Chen X, Sullivan PF: Single nucleotide polymorphism genotyping: biochemistry, protocol, cost and thoughput. Pharmacogenomics J 2003; 3: 77–96.

Dykxhoorn DM, Lieberman J: The silent revolution: RNA interference as basic biology, research tool and therapeutic. Ann Rev Med 2005; 56: 401–423.
A review of the field of RNA interference; includes helpful diagrams and 114 references.

Fire A, Xu S, Montgomery MK, et al: Potent and specific genetic interference by double-stranded RNA in *Caenorhabditis elegans*. Nature 1998; 391:806–811.
First description of RNAi in animal cells.

Gravitt PE, Peyton CL, Apple RJ, Wheeler CM: Genotyping of 27 human papillomavirus types by using L1 consensus PCR products by a single-hybridization, reverse line blot detection method. J Clin Microbiol 1998; 36:3020–3027.

Hanawalt PC: Transcription-coupled repair and human disease. Science 1994; 266:1957–1958.

Kan YW: Development of DNA analyses for human diseases: sickle cell anemia and thalassemia as paradigm. JAMA 1992; 267:1532–1536.

Langer PR, Waldrop AA, Ward DC: Enzymatic synthesis of biotin-labeled polynucleotides: Novel nucleic acid affinity probes. Proc Natl Acad Sci USA 1981; 78:6633–6637.
First description of affinity-labeled nucleotides that achieved sensitivity of detection required for eventual replacement of radioactive methods.

Liechti-Gallati S, Koenig M, Kunkel LM, et al: Molecular deletion patterns in Duchenne and Becker type muscular dystrophy. Hum Genet 1989; 81:343–348.

Luke S, Shepelsky M: FISH: recent advances and diagnostic aspects. Cell Vis 1998; 5:49–53.

Modrich P: Mismatch repair, genetic stability, and cancer. Science 1994; 266:1959–1960.

Papavassiliou AG: Transcription factors. N Engl J Med 1995; 332:45–47.
From the 'Molecular Medicine' series in the New England Journal of Medicine, *a brief review of transcription factors and their importance in medicine.*

Pingoud A, Jeltsch A: Structure and function of type II restriction endonucleases. Nucl Acids Res 2001; 29:3705–3727.

Radman M, Wagner R: The high fidelity of DNA duplication. Sci Am 1988; 259:40–46.

Rosenthal N: Regulation of gene expression. N Engl J Med 1994; 331:931–933.
From the 'Molecular Medicine' series in the New England Journal of Medicine, *a brief review of the regulation of gene expression and relevance to disease.*

Saiki RK, Scharf S, Faloona F, et al: Enzymatic amplification of β-globin genomic sequences and restriction site analysis for the diagnosis of sickle-cell anemia. Science 1985; 230:1350–1354.
Original description of the polymerase chain reaction.

Sancar A: Mechanisms of DNA excision repair. Science 1994; 266:1954–1956.

Sharp PA: RNA splicing and genes. JAMA 1988; 260:3035–3041.

Southern EM: Detection of specific sequences among DNA fragments separated by gel electrophoresis. J Mol Biol 1975; 98:503–517.
Original description of electrophoretic separation of DNA fragments, transfer to filter and hybridization for identification.

Sutherland GR, Richards RI: Dynamic mutations. Sci Am 1994; 82:157–163.

Virshup DM: DNA replication. Curr Opin Cell Biol 1990; 2:453–460.

Weatherall DJ: Molecular pathology of single gene disorders. J Clin Pathol 1987; 40:959–970.

Weeda G, de Boer J, Donker I, et al: Molecular basis of DNA repair mechanisms and syndromes. Rec Results Cancer Res 1998; 154:147–155.

Yguerabide J, Yguerabide EE: Resonance light scattering particles as ultrasensitive labels for detection of analytes in a wide range of applications. J Cellular Biochem Suppl 2001;37:71–81.

Yu Z, Chen J, Ford BN, et al: Human DNA repair systems: an overview. Environ Mol Mutagen 1999; 33:3–20.

Polymerase Chain Reaction and Other Nucleic Acid Amplification Technology

Frederick S. Nolte PhD, Charles E. Hill MD PhD

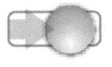

KEY POINTS

- Nucleic amplification technology has created new opportunities for the clinical laboratory to impact patient care.

- Although the polymerase chain reaction is the most mature and widely used nucleic acid amplification method, there are other methods that have diagnostic applications.

- Clinical applications of the technology cut across the traditional disciplines in laboratory medicine.

- An understanding of the basic principles and relative strengths and limitations of the nucleic amplification methods is important for all involved in the practice of clinical pathology.

The development of the polymerase chain reaction (PCR) by Mullis and colleagues (Saiki, 1988) was a milestone in biotechnology that heralded the beginning of molecular diagnostics. Although PCR is the most widely used nucleic acid amplification method, other approaches have been developed, and several have unique properties and advantages. These methods are based on target, probe, or signal amplification. Examples of each category will be discussed in the sections that follow. These techniques have analytical sensitivity unparalleled in laboratory medicine, creating new opportunities for the clinical laboratory to impact patient care.

Target Amplification Methods

Polymerase chain reaction, transcription-based amplification, and strand displacement amplification are all examples of target amplification methods. All these methods share certain fundamental characteristics. They are enzyme-mediated processes in which a single enzyme or multiple enzymes synthesize copies of target nucleic acid. The amplification products in all the techniques are defined by two oligonucleotide primers that bind to complementary sequences on opposite strands of double-stranded targets. All result in the production of millions to billions of copies of the targeted sequence in a matter of hours and, in each case, the amplification products can serve as templates for subsequent rounds of amplification. Because of this, all the techniques are sensitive to contamination with product molecules from previous amplifications, which can lead to false-positive reactions. However, special laboratory design, practices, and workflow have been developed to reduce the possibility of false-positive reactions to acceptable levels.

Polymerase Chain Reaction

PCR is a simple in vitro chemical reaction that permits the synthesis of essentially limitless quantities of a targeted nucleic acid sequence. This is accomplished through the action of a DNA polymerase that, under the right conditions, can copy a strand of DNA. At its simplest, a PCR consists of target DNA, a molar excess of two oligonucleotide primers, a heat-stable DNA polymerase, an equimolar mixture of deoxyribonucleotide triphosphates (dATP, dCTP, dGTP, and dTTP), $MgCl_2$, KCl, and a Tris-HCl buffer. The two primers flank the sequence to be amplified, are typically less than 100 bases long, and are complementary to opposite strands of the target.

To initiate a PCR, the reaction mixture is heated to separate the two strands of target DNA (denaturation) and then cooled to permit the primers to anneal to the target DNA in a sequence-specific manner (annealing) (Fig. 67–1). The DNA polymerase then initiates extension of each primer at its 3′ end (extension). The primer extension products are dissociated from the target DNA by heating. Each extension product, as well as the original target, can serve as a template for subsequent rounds of primer annealing and extension.

A PCR cycle consists of three steps: denaturation, annealing, and extension. At the end of each cycle, the PCR products are theoretically doubled. Thus, after n PCR cycles, the target sequence can be amplified 2^n-fold. The whole procedure is carried out in a programmable thermal cycler that precisely controls the temperature at which the steps occur, the length of time that the reaction is held at the different temperatures, and the number of cycles. Ideally, after 20 cycles of PCR, a millionfold amplification is achieved and, after 30 cycles, a billionfold. In practice, the amplification may not be completely efficient, because of failure to optimize the reaction conditions or the presence of inhibitors of the DNA polymerase. In such cases, the total amplification is best described by the expression $(1 + e)^n$ where e is the amplification efficiency ($0 = e = 1$) and n is the total number of cycles.

Reverse-Transcriptase Polymerase Chain Reaction

PCR as it was originally described was a technique for DNA amplification. Reverse-transcriptase PCR (RT-PCR) was developed to amplify RNA targets. In this process complementary DNA (cDNA) is first produced from RNA targets by reverse transcription, and then the cDNA is amplified by PCR. As originally described, RT-PCR employed two enzymes, a heat-labile RT such as avian myeloblastosis virus reverse transcriptase (AMV-RT) and a thermostable DNA polymerase. Because of the temperature requirements of the heat-labile enzyme, cDNA synthesis had to occur at lower temperatures. This presented problems both in terms of the nonspecific primer annealing and inefficient primer extension due to formation of RNA secondary structures. These problems have been largely overcome by the development of a thermostable DNA polymerase derived from *Thermus thermophilus* that under the proper conditions can function efficiently as both an RT and a DNA polymerase (Myers, 1991). RT-PCRs using this enzyme are more specific and efficient than previous protocols using conventional, heat-labile RT enzymes. Commercially available kits (AMPLICOR, Roche Diagnostics, Indianapolis, IN) employing this single-enzyme RT-PCR are available for detection of hepatitis C virus (HCV) RNA and for quantification of human immunodeficiency virus (HIV)-1 and HCV RNA in clinical specimens.

While the single enzyme RT-PCR has improved specificity and efficiency for problematic targets, there remain many applications that use a two-enzyme system. Modified heat-labile RT enzymes and optimized mixtures of reverse transcriptases with improved specificity and efficiency are now commercially available. Performing a separate RT reaction with random

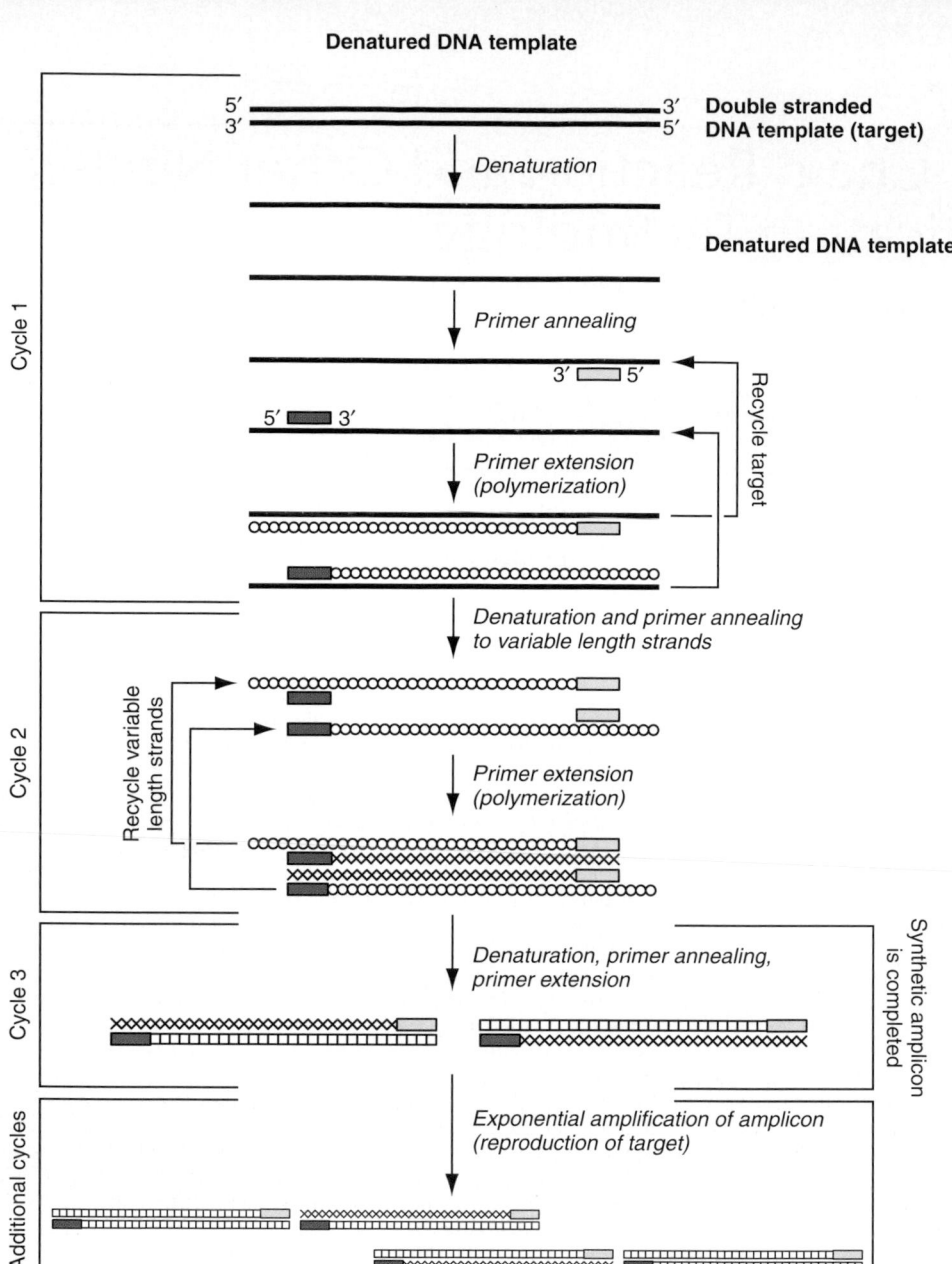

Figure 67–1 Polymerase chain reaction. (Redrawn from Wolk, 2001.)

sequence primers allows PCR analysis of multiple targets from a single RT reaction. The RT reaction may be performed with oligo-dT primers providing cDNA of the mRNAs only. This scheme also allows PCR to be performed for multiple targets from a single RT reaction.

Nested Polymerase Chain Reaction

Nested PCR was developed to increase both the sensitivity and specificity of PCR (Haqqi, 1988). It employs two pairs of amplification primers and two rounds of PCR. Typically, one primer pair is used in the first round of PCR of 15–30 cycles. The products of the first round of amplification are then subjected to a second round of amplification using the second set of primers, which anneal to a sequence internal to the sequence amplified by the first primer set. The increased sensitivity arises from the high total cycle number and the increased specificity arises from the annealing of the second primer set to sequences found only in the first-round products, thus verifying the identity of the first-round product. The major disadvantage of nested PCR is the high rate of contamination that can occur during the transfer of first-round products to the second tube for the second round of amplification. This can be avoided either by physically separating the first- and second-round amplification mixtures with a layer of wax or oil, or by designing single-tube amplification protocols. In practice, the enhanced sensitivity afforded by nested PCR protocols is rarely required in diagnostic applications, and the identity of an

amplification product is usually confirmed by hybridization with a nucleic acid probe.

Multiplex Polymerase Chain Reaction

In multiplex PCR, two or more primer sets, designed for amplification of different targets, are included in the same reaction mixture (Chamberlain, 1988). With this technique more than one target sequence in a clinical specimen can be coamplified in a single tube. The primers used in multiplexed reactions must be selected carefully to have similar annealing temperatures and must be noncomplementary to each other to avoid primer-dimers and inefficient reactions. Multiplex PCRs are more complicated to develop and are often less sensitive than single-primer-set PCR reactions, but allow multiple targets to be detected from a single specimen in one reaction.

End-Point Quantitative Polymerase Chain Reaction

A linear relationship should exist between the quantity of input template and the amount of amplification product. However, since the final amount of PCR product depends on exponential amplification of the initial quantity of template, minor differences in amplification efficiency may lead to very large and unpredictable differences in the final product yield (Clementi, 1993). The tube-to-tube differences may depend on sample preparation and nucleic acid purification procedures, presence of inhibitors, and thermal cycler performance. For these reasons, simple quantification of product accumulated at the end of the reaction and the use of external standard curves do not provide reliable quantification of the amount of template initially present in the sample.

A variety of PCR-based strategies have been developed to accurately quantify DNA and RNA targets in clinical specimens but the competitive PCR (cPCR) approach has proved reliable and robust for clinical applications (Gilliland, 1990; Piatak, 1993). The basic concept behind cPCR is the coamplification in the same reaction tube of two different templates of equal or similar lengths and with the same primer binding sequences. Since both templates are amplified with the same primer pair, identical thermodynamics and amplification efficiency are ensured. The amount of one of the templates must be known and, after amplification, products from both templates must be distinguishable. Different types of competitor have been used in cPCR but, in general, competitors similar in size and base composition to the target work most effectively. RNA competitors should be used in quantitative RT-PCRs to address the problem of variable RT efficiency.

The yield of PCR product is described by the equation, $Y = I(1 + e)^n$, where Y is the quantity of PCR product, I is the quantity of template at the beginning of the reaction, e is the efficiency of the reaction, and n is the number of cycles. In cPCR this equation is written for both templates, as follows: competitor, $Y_c = I_c(1 + e)^n$; and target, $Y_t = I_t(1 + e)^n$. Since e and n are the same for both the competitor and target, the relative product ratio Y_c/Y_t directly depends on their initial concentration ratio I_c/I_t and the function $Y_c/Y_t = I_c/I_t$ is linear.

A single concentration of competitor is sufficient, in theory, to quantify an unknown amount of target without the use of a standard curve. However, because analysis of two template species present in a sample at widely different amounts may be difficult and imprecise in practice, cPCR using several concentrations of competitor within the expected concentration range of the target were generally performed. However, this approach provided no more accurate results than the use of a single concentration of competitor in a study of different approaches to standardization of cPCR (Haberhausen, 1998). The commercially available, end-point quantitative PCR assays for HIV-1, and HCV (Amplicor Monitor Tests, Roche Diagnostics, Indianapolis, IN) use a single concentration of a competitor to determine the initial concentration of the target.

The next generation of quantitative PCR assays for the clinical laboratory will employ homogenous, kinetic (real-time) methods for product detection (Barbeau, 2004) (see next section). These methods provide for more precise measurements of initial template concentrations because the analysis is performed early in the log phase of product accumulation and, as a result, are less prone to error resulting from differences in sample-to-sample amplification efficiency.

Real-Time (Homogeneous, Kinetic) Polymerase Chain Reaction

Real-time PCR describes methods by which the target amplification and detection steps occur simultaneously in the same tube (homogeneous). These methods require special thermal cyclers with precision optics that can monitor the fluorescence emission from the sample wells. The computer software supporting the thermocycler monitors the data throughout the PCR at every cycle (kinetic) and generates an amplification plot for each reaction. A typical amplification plot is shown in Figure 67–2. The amplification plot shows the normalized fluorescence signal from the reporter (R_n) at each cycle number. In the initial cycles there is little change in the amount of fluorescence. This defines the baseline of the plot. An increase above the baseline indicates detection of accumulated PCR product. A fixed fluorescence threshold can be set above the baseline to call positive samples. The PCR cycle at which the sample fluorescence passes the threshold is defined as the cycle threshold (C_T). There is an inverse linear relationship between the log of the initial target concentration and the C_T. Alternatively, the cycle number corresponding to the maximal rate change in fluorescence, the second derivative maximum, has a similar relationship to initial target concentration.

In the simplest format, PCR product is detected as it is produced using fluorescent dyes that preferentially bind to double-stranded DNA. SYBR Green I is one such dye that has been used in this application (Morrison, 1998). In the unbound state, the fluorescence is relatively low but when bound to double-stranded DNA the fluorescence is greatly enhanced. The DNA-binding dye will bind to any double-stranded DNA and therefore will bind both specific and nonspecific PCR products equally well. The specificity of the detection can be improved through melting curve analysis. As the temperature is raised slowly, the two strands of the amplicon will melt apart and the amount of fluorescence will decrease. The data are

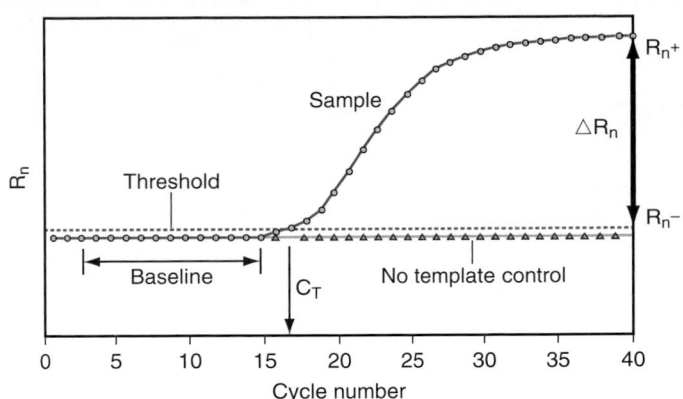

Figure 67–2 Real-time PCR amplification plot. (Redrawn from Applied Biosystems.)

transformed and analyzed by plotting the first derivative of fluorescence on the y-axis and temperature on the x-axis. The specific amplified product will have a characteristic melting peak at its predicted melting temperature (T_m), whereas the primer dimers and other nonspecific products should have a different T_m or give broader peaks (Ririe, 1997).

The specificity of real time PCR can also be increased by including hybridization probes in the reactions mixture. These probes are labeled with fluorescent dyes or with combinations of fluorescent and a quencher dye. In the 5′ nuclease (TaqMan) PCR assay, the 5′–3′ exonuclease activity of Taq DNA polymerase is used to cleave a nonextendable hybridization probe during the primer extension phase of PCR (Holland, 1991). This approach uses dual-labeled fluorogenic hybridization probes. One fluorescent dye serves as reporter and its emission spectrum is quenched by the second fluorescent dye. The nuclease degradation of the hybridization probe releases the reporter dye, resulting in an increase in its peak fluorescent emission (Fig. 67–3). The increase in fluorescent emission indicates that specific PCR product has been made and the intensity of fluorescence is related to the amount of product (Heid, 1996). Specificity is increased because signal is generated only when the primer and probe are bound to the same template strand.

Fluorescence resonance energy transfer (FRET) probes can also be used to detect PCR product as it is generated (Lay, 1997). This method requires two specially designed sequence-specific oligonucleotide probes. These hybridization probes are designed to hybridize next to each other on the product molecule. As shown in Figure 67–4, the 3′ end of one probe is labeled with a donor dye and the 5′ end of the other probe is labeled with an acceptor dye. The donor dye is excited by an external light source and, instead of emitting light, transfers its energy to the acceptor dye by a process called FRET. The excited acceptor dye emits light at a longer wavelength than the unbound donor dye and the intensity of the acceptor dye light emission is proportional to the amount of PCR product.

Real-time detection and quantification of PCR product can also be accomplished using molecular beacons (Tyagi, 1998). Molecular beacons are hairpin-shaped oligonucleotide probes with an internally quenched fluorophore whose fluorescence is restored when they bind to a target nucleic acid (Fig. 67–5). They are designed in such a way that the loop portion of the probe molecule is complementary to the target sequence. The stem is formed by the annealing of complementary arm sequences on the ends of the probe. A fluorescent dye is attached to one end of one arm and a quenching molecule is attached to the end of the other arm. The stem keeps the fluorophore and quencher in close proximity such that no light emission occurs. When the probe encounters a target molecule, it forms a hybrid that is longer and more stable than the stem, and undergoes a conformational change that forces the stem apart and causes the fluorophore and quencher to move away from each other, restoring fluorescence.

It is not absolutely necessary to have a stem loop structure to use nonhydrolyzable probes in real-time PCR applications. Dark quencher probes contain a fluorophore on the 5′ end, and a nonfluorescent quencher molecule on the 3′ end (Afonina, 2002). The fluorescence is quenched when the probe is in a random coil configuration and emitted when the probe anneals to the target sequence. Similar to molecular beacons or FRET probes, the DNA polymerase does not degrade these probes during target amplification. Since the dark quencher is not fluorescent, it does not contribute to background signal. This has the advantage of improved signal-to-noise ratio for the detection system, which may improve sensitivity. These probes also incorporate a hybridization-stabilizing compound, known as a minor groove binder. It is a small, crescent-shaped molecule that is

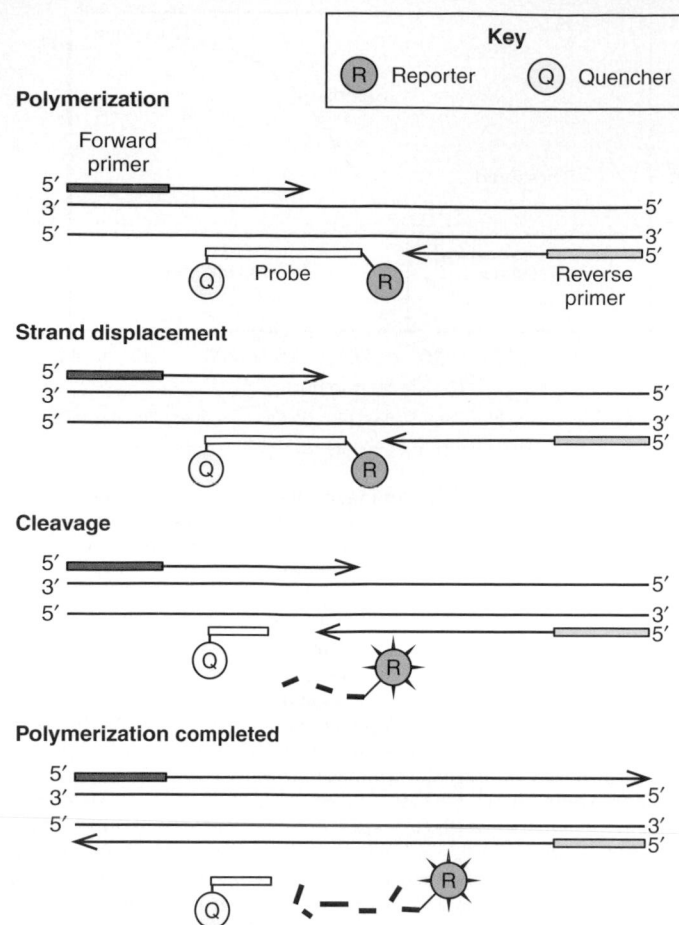

Figure 67–3 Mechanism of signal generation in 5' nuclease PCR assays. (Redrawn from Applied Biosystems.)

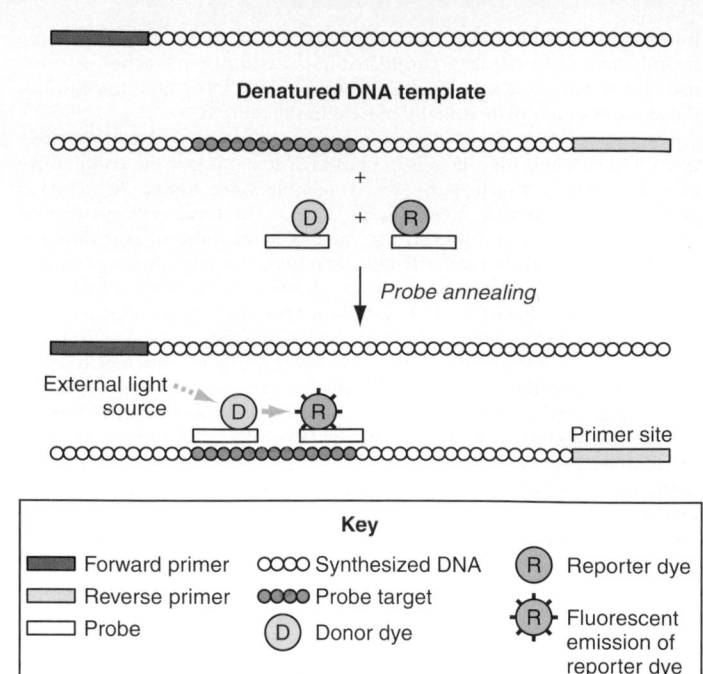

Figure 67–4 Fluorescence resonance energy transfer probes. (Redrawn from Wolk, 2001.)

covalently linked to 3' end of the probe that spans about 3–4 nt and snugly fits into the minor groove of DNA where it forms hydrogen bonds with the template. The minor groove binder allows the use of shorter probes and enables improved T_m leveling, which improves the specificity of the detection reaction (Kutyavin, 2000).

Real-time PCR methods decrease the time required to perform nucleic acid assays because there are no post-PCR processing steps. Also, since amplification and detection occur in the same closed tube, these methods eliminate the postamplification manipulations that can lead to laboratory contamination with amplicon. In addition, real-time PCR methods lend themselves well to quantitative applications because analysis is performed early in the log phase of product accumulation and as a result are less prone to error that may result from differences in amplification efficiency between samples.

Rapid-Cycle Polymerase Chain Reaction

While real-time PCR methods have had a significant impact on assay time, a great deal of emphasis continues to be placed on reducing the assay time for the various PCR formats. Rapid-cycle PCR is not chemically different from any of the standard PCR formats (Wittwer, 1991). The polymerases used in PCR are capable of incorporating 35–100 nucleotides per second. It is clear that most of the time consumed in performing PCR is temperature equilibration for the solution so that efficient annealing and extension occur, as well as a significant amount of time in changing the temperature. By reducing the thermal profile of the solution using thin-walled tubes or capillaries that force the reaction solution into thin columns or sheets of fluid, it is possible to improve thermal transfer rates as well as equilibration

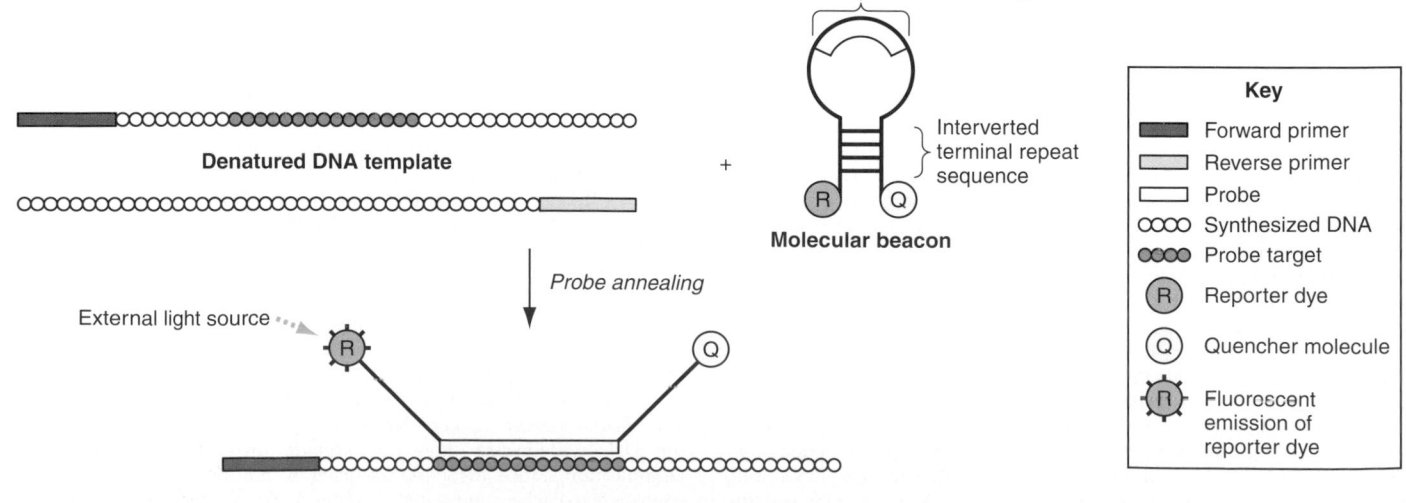

Figure 67–5 Molecular beacon probes. (Redrawn from Wolk, 2001.)

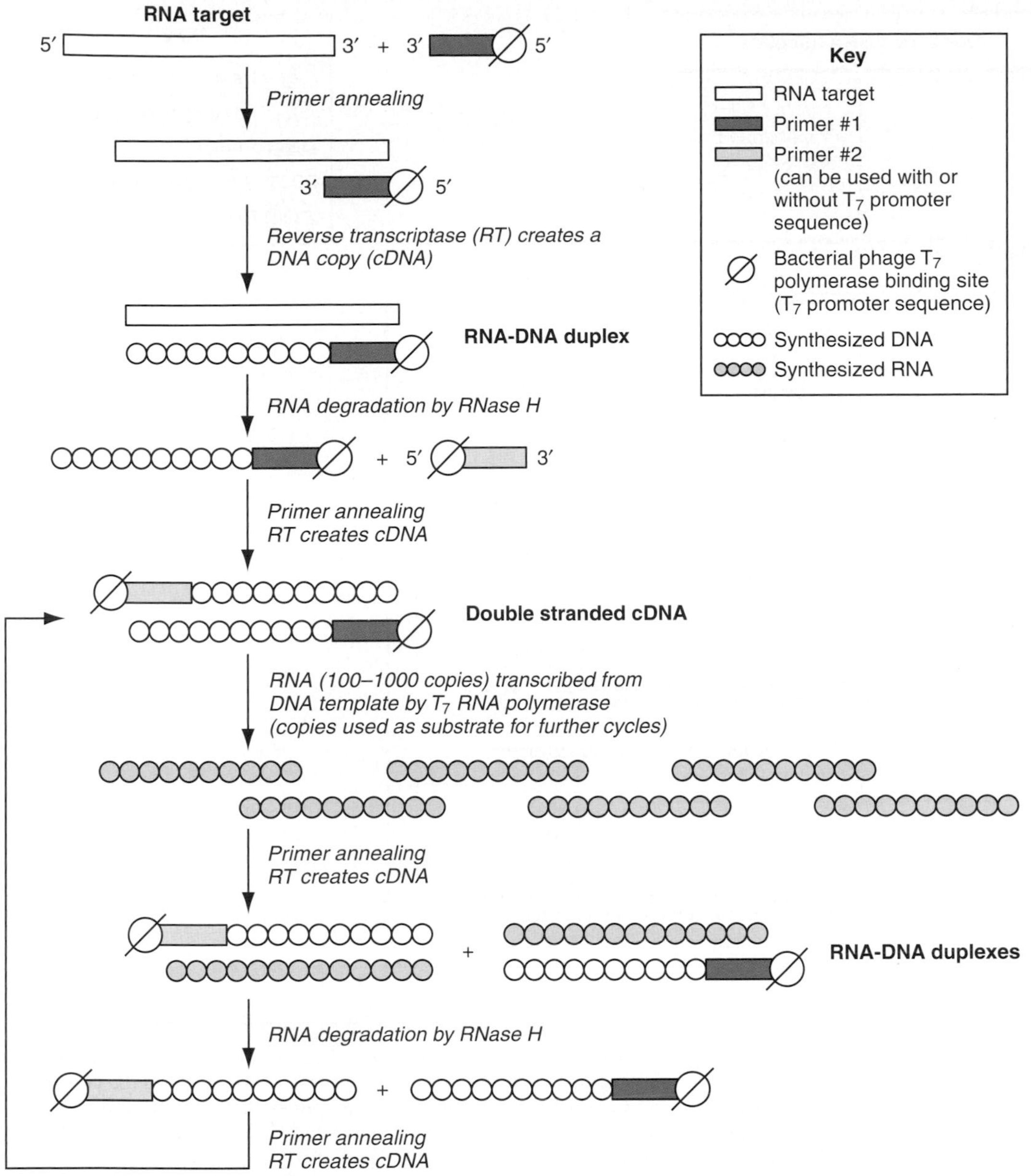

Figure 67–6 Transcription-based amplification. (Redrawn from Wolk, 2001.)

RNA target

5′ ▭ 3′ + 3′ ▮⌀ 5′

Primer annealing

3′ ▮⌀ 5′

Reverse transcriptase (RT) creates a DNA copy (cDNA)

RNA-DNA duplex

RNA degradation by RNase H

+ 5′ ⌀▭ 3′

Primer annealing RT creates cDNA

Double stranded cDNA

RNA (100–1000 copies) transcribed from DNA template by T7 RNA polymerase (copies used as substrate for further cycles)

Primer annealing RT creates cDNA

RNA-DNA duplexes

RNA degradation by RNase H

Primer annealing RT creates cDNA

Key

- ▭ RNA target
- ▮ Primer #1
- ▭ Primer #2 (can be used with or without T7 promoter sequence)
- ⌀ Bacterial phage T7 polymerase binding site (T7 promoter sequence)
- ○○○○ Synthesized DNA
- ●●●● Synthesized RNA

---

rates such that thermocycling time can be significantly reduced. In highly optimized systems, it is possible to approach the ideal processivity rate of the polymerase such that a 40 cycle PCR may be performed in 30 minutes or less using standard or real-time PCR chemistries.

Transcription-Based Amplification

Transcription-based amplification includes transcription-mediated amplification (TMA) and nucleic acid sequence-based amplification (NASBA). Both TMA and NASBA are isothermal nucleic acid amplification techniques that, although slightly different in practice, are identical in concept, and will be described together (Kwoh, 1989; Compton, 1991). TMA and NASBA are the intellectual properties of Gen-Probe, San Diego, CA, and BioMérieux, Durham, NC, respectively. These techniques essentially recapitulate retroviral replication in vitro, converting RNA into DNA and then using the DNA as a template for transcription of multiple copies of RNA.

The process begins with an RNA target, which in most cases will exist as a single-stranded entity, removing the need for thermal denaturation of the template prior to amplification (Fig. 67–6). A sequence-specific DNA primer binds to the RNA target. Reverse transcriptase then extends the primer, creating a DNA–RNA heteroduplex. The 5′ end of the sequence-specific primer contains the promoter for a T7 bacteriophage polymerase. The presence of this T7 promoter in the 5′ end of the primer results in the synthesis of a DNA strand complementary to the initial RNA target containing the T7 promoter at its 5′ end. In the case of TMA, the reverse-transcriptase enzyme itself degrades the initial RNA template as it synthesizes its complementary DNA. In NASBA, a separate enzyme, RNAse

H, degrades the initial RNA template. RNAse H selectively cleaves RNA, which is heteroduplexed to DNA, but not RNA alone. In either case, the resultant single-stranded, complementary DNA with the T7 promoter sequence binds to a second primer at its 3′ end. The DNA polymerase extends from this second primer, resulting in the synthesis of a double-stranded DNA molecule containing an intact T7 promoter. This DNA molecule can now serve as a template for T7 polymerase, a bacteriophage enzyme that specifically recognizes the T7 promoter and synthesizes multiple copies of RNA. Each of these newly synthesized RNA molecules is antisense to the initial target, allowing them to hybridize to the second primer. The reverse-transcriptase, second primer, RNAse H, and DNA polymerase then use this antisense RNA molecule as a template to synthesize new double-stranded DNA templates, which in turn make more RNA template. A 10^9-fold amplification of target RNA can be achieved with these methods in 2 hours or less.

TMA and NASBA have several distinct advantages over other RNA amplification techniques. Perhaps the most significant of these advantages is that no initial denaturation is required for the amplification to occur. Hence, ds DNA sequences are not denatured, and thus are incapable of binding to primers in the reaction. DNA contamination can be particularly problematic when techniques such as PCR are used to assay for the RNA transcripts of retroviral or intronless eukaryotic genes. NASBA and TMA eliminate the problem of DNA contamination giving a falsely elevated determination of RNA. A second advantage is that this technology uses isothermal processes that obviate the need for sophisticated thermocyclers. Combining this technology with molecular beacons or other sequence-specific probes that can be added directly to the

VIII

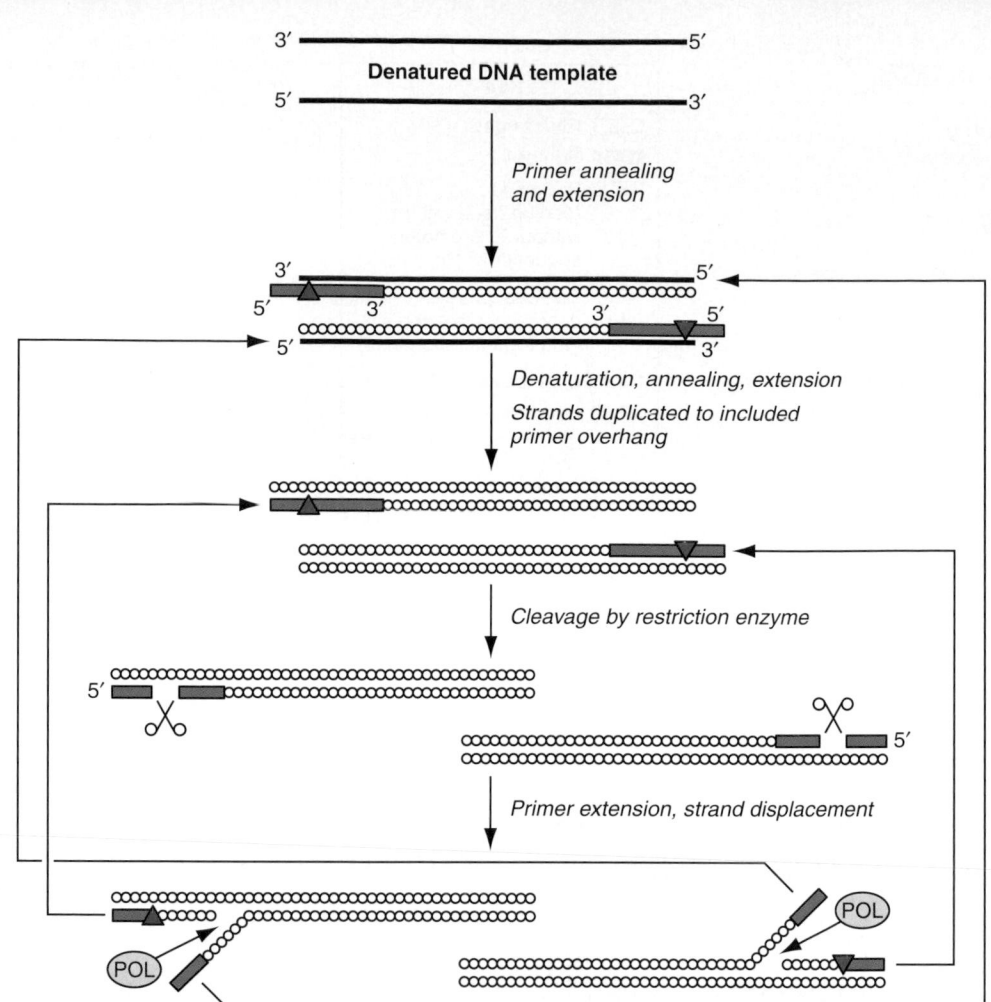

Figure 67–7 Strand displacement amplification. (Redrawn from Wolk, 2001.)

amplification mixture creates a closed-tube system, which aids in preventing amplicon cross-contamination in the laboratory.

NASBA and TMA have been used successfully in a wide variety of applications. They have been used to detect a number of pathogens, including viruses such as HIV, HCV, varicella zoster virus, cytomegalovirus (CMV), rhinovirus, enterovirus, measles, human papillomavirus, and bacteria such as *Mycobacterium tuberculosis*, *Neisseria gonorrhoeae*, *Chlamydia trachomatis*, *Mycoplasma pneumoniae*, and *Campylobacter jejuni*. In addition, quantitative tests for HIV and HCV have been developed using this technology. Furthermore, human genetic applications such as HLA typing and factor V Leiden mutation detection have been described.

In summary, TMA and NASBA are isothermal RNA amplification techniques with a widespread applicability and several unique advantages over other amplification methods, especially for the elimination of DNA contamination issues, particularly those related to retroviral and intronless genes. Combining these techniques with fluorescent probes allows one-step, closed-tube, real-time amplification without the need for thermal cycling.

Strand-Displacement Amplification

Strand-displacement amplification (SDA) is an isothermal template amplification technique that can be used to detect trace amounts of DNA or RNA of a particular sequence. SDA as it was first described was a conceptually straightforward amplification process with some technical limitations (Walker, 1992a, 1992b). Since its initial description, however, it has evolved into a highly versatile tool that is technically simple to perform but conceptually complex.

In its current iteration SDA occurs in two discrete phases, target generation and exponential target amplification (Little, 1999). Only the target amplification phase is shown in Figure 67–7. In the target generation phase, a double-stranded DNA target is denatured and hybridized to two different primer pairs, designated as bumper and amplification primers. The amplification primers include the single-stranded restriction endonuclease

enzyme sequence for *BsoB1* located at the 5′ end of the target binding sequence. The bumper primers are shorter and anneal to the target DNA just upstream of the region to be amplified. In the presence of *BsoB1*, an exonuclease-free DNA polymerase, and a dNTP mixture consisting of dUTP, dATP, dGTP, and thiolated dCTP (C_s), simultaneous extension products of both the bumper and amplification primers are generated. This process displaces the amplification primer products, which are available for hybridization with the opposite-strand products with the opposite-strand bumper and amplification primers.

The simultaneous extension of opposite-strand primers produces strands complementary to the products formed by extension of the first amplification primer with C_s incorporated into the *BsoB1* cleavage site. This product enters the exponential target amplification phase of the reaction. The *BsoB1* enzyme recognizes the double-stranded site, but because one strand contains C_s, it is nicked rather than cleaved by the enzyme. The DNA polymerase then binds to the nick and begins synthesis of a new strand while simultaneously displacing the downstream strand. This step recreates the double-stranded species with the hemimodified restriction endonuclease recognition sequence, and the iterative nicking and displacement process repeats. The displaced strands are capable of binding to opposite-strand primers, which produces exponential amplification of the target sequences.

These single-stranded products also bind to detector probes for real-time detection. The detector probes are single-stranded DNA molecules with fluorescein and rhodamine labels. The region between the labels includes a stem-loop structure. The loop contains the recognition site for the *BsoB1* enzyme. The target specific sequences are located 3′ to the rhodamine label. In the absence-specific target the stem-loop structure is maintained with the fluorescein and rhodamine labels in close proximity. The net effect is that very little emission for the fluorescein is detected after excitation. After SDA, the probe is converted to a double-stranded species, which is cleaved by *BsoB1*. The cleavage causes physical separation of the fluorescein and rhodamine labels, which results in an increase in emission from the fluorescein label.

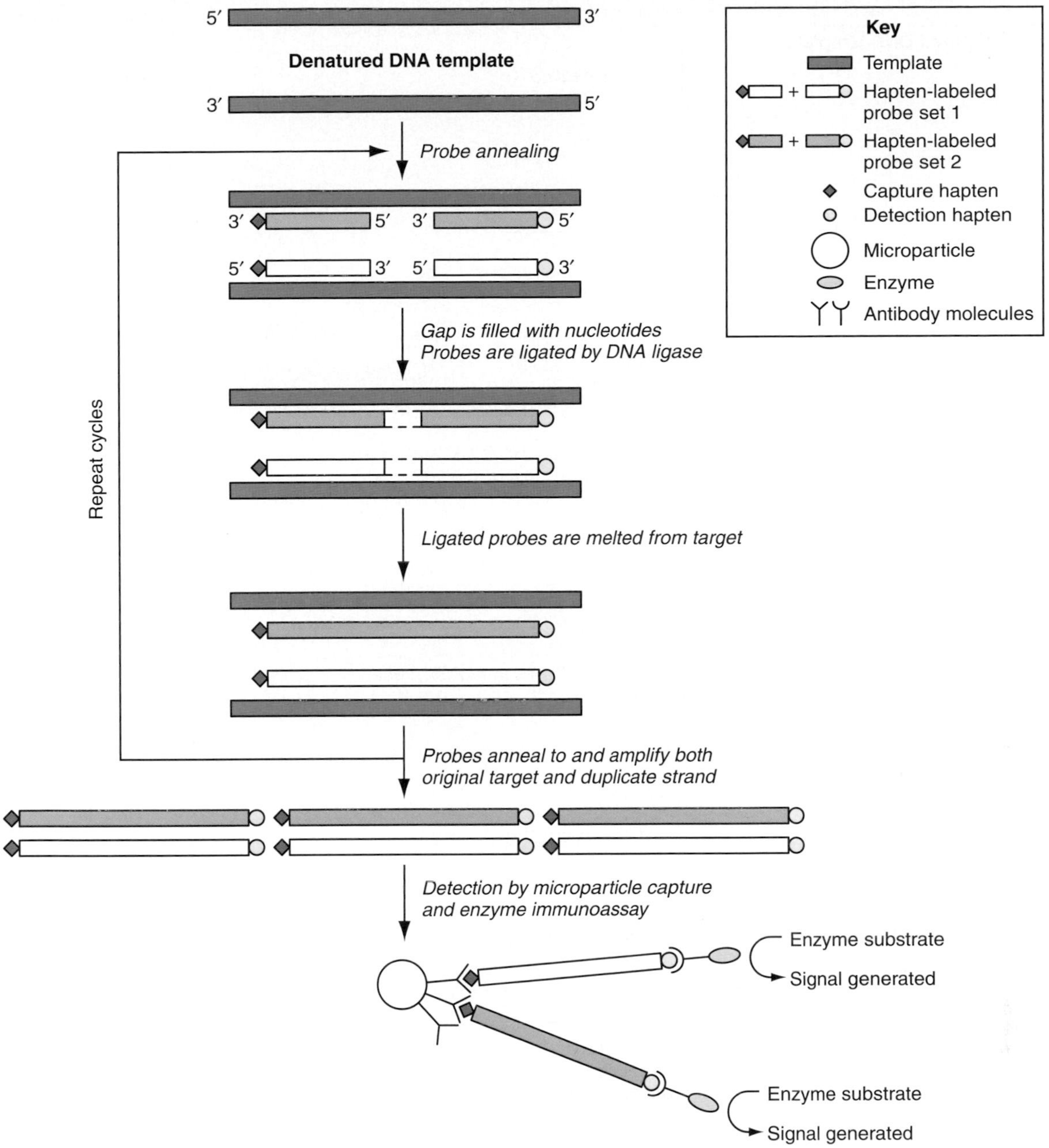

5′ ▮▮▮▮▮▮▮▮▮▮▮ 3′

Denatured DNA template

3′ ▮▮▮▮▮▮▮▮▮▮▮ 5′

Probe annealing

Key

Template

+ Hapten-labeled probe set 1

+ Hapten-labeled probe set 2

◆ Capture hapten

○ Detection hapten

◯ Microparticle

⬭ Enzyme

𝖄𝖄 Antibody molecules

3′ ◆▭▭▭ 5′ 3′ ▭▭▭○ 5′

5′ ◆▭▭▭ 3′ 5′ ▭▭▭○ 3′

Gap is filled with nucleotides
Probes are ligated by DNA ligase

◆▭▭▭┆┆▭▭▭○

◆▭▭▭┆┆▭▭▭○

Ligated probes are melted from target

◆▭▭▭▭▭○

◆▭▭▭▭▭○

Repeat cycles

Probes anneal to and amplify both
original target and duplicate strand

◆▭▭▭○ ◆▭▭▭▭▭○ ◆▭▭▭▭▭▭○
◆▭▭▭○ ◆▭▭▭○ ◆▭▭▭○

Detection by microparticle capture
and enzyme immunoassay

Enzyme substrate

Signal generated

Enzyme substrate

Signal generated

Figure 67–8 Gapped ligase chain reaction. (Redrawn from Wolk, 2001.)

The diagnostic applications of SDA include the direct detection of *M. tuberculosis*, *C. trachomatis*, and *N. gonorrhoeae* in clinical specimens. SDA has a reported sensitivity high enough to detect as few as 10–50 copies of a target molecule (Walker, 1992a). By using a primer set designed to amplify a repetitive sequence with 10 copies in the *M. tuberculosis* genome, the assay is sensitive enough to detect 1–5 genome copies of the bacterium. Recently, SDA has been adapted to quantify RNA by adding a reverse-transcriptase step (RT-SDA). In this case, a primer hybridizes to the target RNA and a reverse-transcriptase synthesizes a cDNA. This cDNA can then serve as a template for primer incorporation and strand displacement. The products of this strand displacement then feed into the amplification scheme described above. RT-SDA has been used for the determination of HIV viral load (Nycz, 1998).

The main advantage of SDA is that it is an isothermal process that, unlike PCR, can be performed at a single temperature after initial target denaturation. This eliminates the need for expensive thermocyclers. Furthermore, samples can be subjected to SDA in a single tube, with amplification times varying from 30 minutes to 2 hours. The main disadvantage of SDA lies in the fact that, unlike PCR, the relatively low temperature at which SDA is carried out (52.5°C) can result in nonspecific primer hybridization to sequences found in complex mixtures such as genomic DNA. Hence, when the target is in low abundance compared to background DNA, nonspecific amplification products can swamp the system, decreasing the sensitivity of the technique. However, the use of organic solvents to increase stringency at low

temperatures and the recent introduction of more thermostable polymerases capable of strand displacement have alleviated much of this problem.

Probe Amplification Methods

Probe amplification methods differ from target amplification in that the amplification products contain a sequence only present in the initial probes. Ligase amplification reaction and cleavase/invader technology are examples of probe amplification methods that have been used for diagnostic applications.

Ligase Amplification Reaction

In a standard ligase amplification reaction (LAR) two oligonucleotide probes hybridize adjacent to one another on each of the denatured target DNA strands such that a 'nick' is formed. A thermostable DNA ligase then seals the 'nick' by joining the 3′ end of one probe and the 5′ end of the other. Each ligated product, as well as the original target, can serve as a template in subsequent rounds of denaturation, annealing, and ligation, resulting in an exponential accumulation of products (Wu, 1989; Barany, 1991).

A modification of this technique called gapped ligase chain reaction (G-LCR) differs from standard LAR in that a short gap is formed after

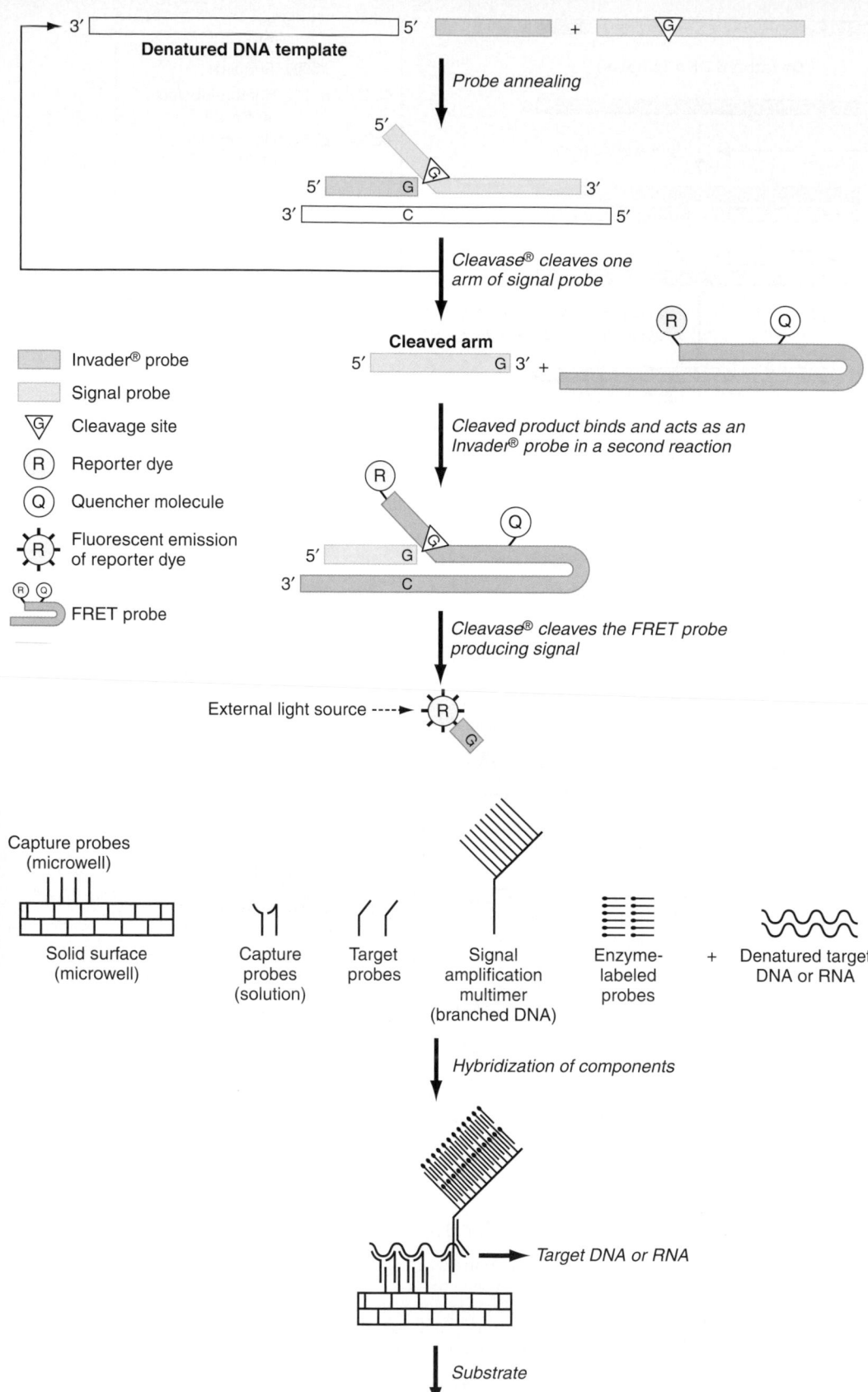

3′ [ ] 5′ **Denatured DNA template**

Probe annealing

5′

5′ ⬚ G ⬚ 3′

3′ [C] 5′

Cleavase® cleaves one arm of signal probe

Cleaved arm

5′ [G] 3′ +

R ⬚ Q

Cleaved product binds and acts as an Invader® probe in a second reaction

R

Q

5′ ⬚ G ⬚

3′ ⬚ C ⬚

Cleavase® cleaves the FRET probe producing signal

External light source ----▸ R ⬚ G

Invader® probe

Signal probe

Cleavage site

Reporter dye

Quencher molecule

Fluorescent emission of reporter dye

FRET probe

Figure 67–9 Invasive cleavage and detection of an oligonucleotide probe using a FEN-1 DNA polymerase. (Redrawn from Wolk, 2001.)

Figure 67–10 Branched DNA amplification. (Redrawn from Wolk, 2001.)

Capture probes (microwell)

Solid surface (microwell)

Capture probes (solution)

Target probes

Signal amplification multimer (branched DNA)

Enzyme-labeled probes

+ Denatured target DNA or RNA

Hybridization of components

▸ *Target DNA or RNA*

Substrate

Chemiluminescence

CHAPTER: **67** Polymerase Chain Reaction and Other Nucleic Acid Amplification Technology

annealing of the probes to the template (Fig. 67–8). The gap is filled by a thermostable DNA polymerase and the resulting nick is then ligated by the DNA ligase (Birkenmeyer, 1991). A combination G-LCR kit for detection of both *C. trachomatis* and *N. gonorrhoeae* in clinical specimens was commercially available (Abbott) but later was withdrawn from the US market. However, it is still available outside the United States. In this test the amplification products are captured by microparticles coated with antihapten antibody, which binds to the capture hapten present on one of the probes. The detection antibody is directed against a second hapten present on the other probe and is conjugated to alkaline phosphatase. The detection antibody binds only to amplification product captured by the microparticle. The bound product is detected by the addition of flurogenic substrate, which is dephosphorylated to yield a fluorescent molecule (Fig. 67–8).

Cleavase/Invader Technology

Cleavase/invader technology is a probe amplification method that relies on the specific recognition and cleavage of particular DNA structures by members of the FEN-1 family of DNA polymerases (Lyamichev, 1999). These polymerases will cleave the 5′ single-stranded flap of a branched base-paired duplex and are termed cleavases. This enzymatic activity probably plays an essential role in the elimination of complex nucleic acid structures that arise during DNA replication and repair in vivo. Since these structures may occur anywhere in the replicating genome, the enzyme recognizes the molecular structure of the substrate without regard to the sequence of the nucleic acids making up the DNA complex (Lieber, 1996). This enzymatic activity has proved to be a very useful tool for DNA analysis and is the basis of this technology.

In cleavase/invader assays two primers are designed that hybridize to the target sequence in an overlapping fashion (Fig. 67–9). Under the proper annealing conditions, signal and invader probes bind to the target sequence such that the invader hybridizes upstream of the signal probe with a region of overlap between the 3′ end of invader and the 5′ end of signal probe. Under the proper conditions, the overlap of binding sites for the primers results in a displacement equilibrium between the primers. Cleavase will only cleave 5′ flaps; thus the 5′ end of the signal probe is released. The target sequence acts as a scaffold upon which the proper DNA structure can form. Since the DNA structure that serves as the cleavase substrate will only occur in the presence of the target sequence, the generation of cleavage products indicates the presence of the target. The cleaved product is detected by binding to and serving as an invader probe for a FRET probe. The 5′ end of the FRET probe is cut by cleavase, releasing the reporter molecule in the same way that it releases the 5′ end of the signal probe.

Use of a thermostable cleavase enzyme allows the reactions to be run at high enough temperatures for a primer exchange equilibrium to exist. This allows multiple cleavase products to form from a single target molecule. Hence, the invader assay can be run under isothermal conditions, removing the need for thermal cycling. This technology has been used for detection, quantification, and characterization of a variety of microbial and human nucleic acid targets (Rosetti, 1997; Ryan, 1999).

The cleavase/invader technology has several inherent advantages over other amplification strategies. Because of the fact that the overlap in the invader probe need only be one base pair, this technology can easily be adapted to detect point mutations of interest by designing the overlap region to encompass the mutation to be detected. In addition, unlike target amplification techniques in which the target sequence itself is amplified, the invader assay does not increase the amount of the target sequence. Thus, the invader assay is less prone to problems of false positives due to amplicon crosscontamination.

In addition to the invader assay, cleavase can also be used to generate fragment-length polymorphisms (in a fashion analogous to restriction fragment-length polymorphism). By melting genomic DNA and cooling rapidly, highly reproducible hairpin loop secondary structures will form in the DNA that can serve as substrates for cleavase. Digestion of the DNA results in a distinct pattern that has been successfully employed to screen for interferon-α-resistant hepatitis C (Sreevatsan, 1998) and to detect specific mutations in human genes (Rosetti, 1997). Because of the fact that hairpin loops occur with a greater diversity than most restriction enzyme recognition sites, this offers a versatile fragmentation pattern analysis.

Thus, structure-specific endonucleases can be used to detect nucleic acid targets of a particular sequence, employed in assay for point mutations, and applied to generate diverse fragmentation patterns capable of distinguishing complex genotypes. These enzymes are powerful tools for nucleic acid analysis.

Signal Amplification Methods

In signal amplification methods, the concentration of probe or target does not increase. The increased analytical sensitivity comes from increasing the concentration of label molecules attached to the target nucleic acid. Multiple enzymes, multiple probes, multiple layers of probes, and reduction of background noise have been used to enhance target detection (Kricka, 1999). Target amplification systems generally have greater analytical sensitivity than signal amplification methods, but technological developments, particularly in branched DNA assays, have lowered the limits of detection to levels that may rival target amplification assays in some applications (Kern, 1996).

Signal amplification assays have several advantages over target amplification assays. In signal amplification systems, the number of target

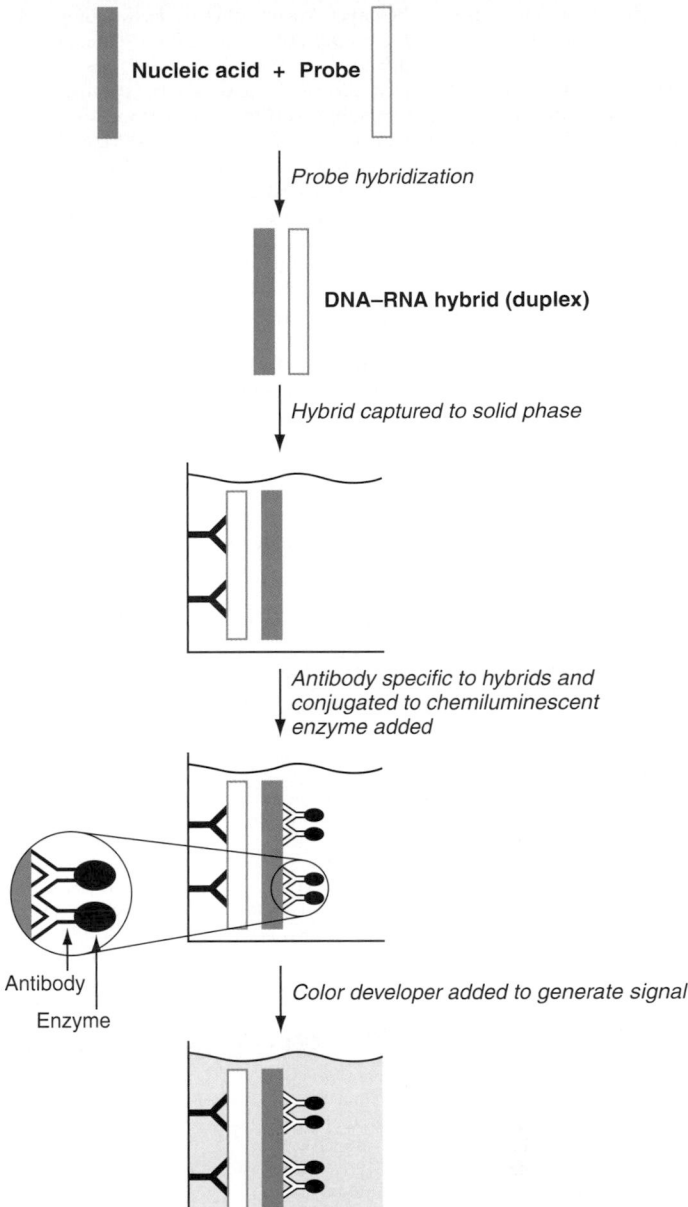

Figure 67–11 Hybrid capture amplification. (Redrawn from Wolk, 2001.)

molecules is not altered and, as a result, the signal is directly proportional to the amount of target sequence present in the clinical specimen. This reduces concerns about false positives due to crosscontamination and simplifies the development of quantitative assays. Since signal amplification systems are not dependent on enzymatic processes to amplify target sequences, they are not affected by the presence of enzyme inhibitors in clinical specimens. Consequently, less cumbersome nucleic acid extraction methods may be used. Typically, signal amplification systems employ either larger probes or more probes than target amplification systems and, consequently, are less susceptible to errors resulting from target sequence heterogeneity. Finally, RNA can be measured directly, without the synthesis of a cDNA intermediate. Branched DNA and hybrid capture are examples of signal amplification systems that have developed into diagnostic tests.

Branched DNA

The branched DNA (bDNA) is a solid-phase, sandwich hybridization assay incorporating multiple sets of synthetic oligonucleotide probes (Nolte, 1998). The key to this technology is the amplifier molecule; a DNA molecule with 15 identical branches, each of which can bind three labeled probes.

Multiple target-specific probes are used to capture the target nucleic acid on to the surface of a microtiter well (Fig. 67–10). A second set of target-specific probes also binds to the target. Preamplifier molecules bind to the second set of target probes and up to eight bDNA amplifiers. Three alkaline phosphatase-labeled probes hybridize to each branch of the amplifier. Detection of the bound labeled probes is achieved by incubating the complex with an enzyme-triggerable substrate, dioxetane, and then measuring the light emission in a luminometer. The resulting signal is directly proportional to the quantity of target in the sample. The quantity of target in the sample is determined from an external standard curve.

Nonspecific hybridization of any of the amplification probes and nontarget nucleic acids leads to amplification of the background signal. In order to reduce the hybridization potential to all nontarget, the nonnatural bases isocytidine (isoC) and isoguanosine (isoG) were incorporated into the amplification probes of the third-generation bDNA assays (Collins, 1995). IsoC and isoG bases pair with each other but not with any of the four naturally occurring bases (Piccirilli, 1990). The use of isoC and isoG probes in bDNA assays increases target-specific amplification without a concomitant increase in background, thereby greatly enhancing the detection limits. The detection limit of the third-generation bDNA assay for HIV-1 RNA is 50 copies/mL (Kern, 1996). bDNA assays for the quantification of HBV DNA, HCV RNA, and HIV-1 RNA are commercially available (Bayer Diagnostics). An instrument platform for bDNA assays automates the incubation, washing, reading, and data processing.

Hybrid Capture Assays

The hybrid capture system is a solution hybridization, antibody capture assay that uses chemiluminescent detection. The target DNA in the specimen is denatured and hybridized with a specific RNA probe (Fig. 67–11). The DNA–RNA hybrids are captured by antibodies specific for DNA–RNA hybrids that are coated on to the surface of a tube. Alkaline-phosphatase-conjugated antihybrid antibodies bind to the immobilized hybrids. The bound enzyme–antibody conjugate is detected with a chemiluminescent substrate and the light emitted is measured in a luminometer. Signal amplification results from the large number of antibody binding sites and the efficiency of the enzyme–substrate reaction. The intensity of the emitted light is proportional to the amount of target DNA in the specimen. Hybrid capture assays for detection of HPV (Cope, 1997) and CMV (Mazzulli, 1999) in clinical specimens are commercially available (Digene, Gaithersburg, MD).

Summary

In this chapter we have provided a basis for understanding the principles underlying the various nucleic acid amplification methods and their relative strengths and limitations. The technology has already had a tremendous impact on the diagnosis of infectious diseases and genetic disorders and promises to revolutionize the diagnosis and management of patients with cancer. The real power of the technology lies in its ability to cut across traditional disciplines in laboratory medicine. Consequently, a thorough understanding of the basic principles of nucleic acid amplification technology is important for all involved in the practice of laboratory medicine.

References

Afonina IA, Reed MW, Lusby E, et al: Minor groove binder-conjugated DNA probes for quantitative DNA detection by hybridization-triggered fluorescence. Biotechniques 2002; 32:940–944.
This paper describes the development of second-generation real-time PCR probes employing DNA minor groove binders and a dark quencher, and their use in single nucleotide polymorphism detection, viral load determination, and gene expression analysis.

Barany F: Genetic disease detection and DNA amplification using cloned thermostable ligase. Proc Natl Acad Sci USA 1991; 88:189–193.

Barbeau JM, Goforth J, Caliendo AM, Nolte FS: Performance characteristics of a quantitative TaqMan hepatitis C virus RNA analyte-specific reagent. J Clin Microbiol 2004; 42:3739–3746.

Birkenmeyer LG, Mushahwar IK: DNA probe amplification methods. J Virol Meth 1991; 35:117–126.

Chamberlain JS, Gibbs RA, Rainer JE, et al: Deletion screening of the Duchenne muscular dystrophy locus via multiplex DNA amplification. Nucleic Acids Res 1988; 16:1141–1156.

Clementi M, Menzo S, Bagnarelli P, et al: Quantitative PCR and RT-PCR in virology. PCR Methods Appl 1993; 2:191–196.

Collins ML, Zayati C, Detmer JJ, et al: Preparation and characterization of RNA standards for use in quantitative branched-DNA hybridization assays. Anal Biochem 1995; 226:120–129.

Compton J: Nucleic acid sequence-based amplification. Nature 1991; 350:91–92.

Cope JJ, Hildesheim A, Schiffman MH, et al: Comparison of the hybrid capture tube test and PCR for detection of human papillomavirus DNA in cervical specimens. J Clin Microbiol 1997; 35:2262–2265.

Gilliland G, Perrin S, Blanchard K, Bunn HF: Analysis of cytokine mRNA and DNA: detection and quantitation by competitive polymerase chain reaction. Proc Natl Acad Sci USA 1990; 887:2725–2729.

Haberhausen G, Pinsl J, Kuhn C-C, Markert-Hahn C: Comparative study of different standardization concepts in quantitative competitive reverse transcription-PCR assays. J Clin Microbiol 1998; 36:628–633.

Haqqi TM, Sarkar G, David CS, Sommer SS: Specific amplification with PCR of a refractory segment of genomic DNA. Nucleic Acids Res 1988; 16:11844.

Heid CA, Stevens J, Livak KJ, Williams PM: Real time quantitative PCR. Genome Res 1996; 6:986–994.

Holland PM, Abramson RD, Watson R, Gelfand DH: Detection of specific polymerase chain reaction product by utilizing the 5′ to 3′ exonuclease activity of *Thermus aquaticus* DNA polymerase. Proc Natl Acad Sci USA 1991; 88:7276–7280.
This paper describes how the 5′ exonuclease activity of a DNA polymerase can be used to detect PCR products, which was a key factor in the development of real-time PCR.

Kern D, Collins M, Fultz T, et al: An enhanced-sensitivity branched-DNA assay for quantification of human immunodeficiency virus type 1 RNA in plasma. J Clin Microbiol 1996; 34:3196–3202.

Kricka LJ: Nucleic acid detection technologies – labels, strategies, and formats. Clin Chem 1999; 45:453–458.

Kutyavin IV, Afonina IA, Mills A, et al: 3′-minor groove binder-DNA probes increase sequence specificity at PCR extension temperatures. Nucleic Acids Res 2000; 28:655–661.

Kwoh DY, David GR, Whitfield KM, et al: Transcription-based amplification system and detection of amplified human immunodeficiency virus type 1 with a bead-based sandwich hybridization format. Proc Natl Acad Sci USA 1989; 86:1173–1177.

Lay MJ, Wittwer CT: Real-time fluorescence genotyping of factor V Leiden during rapid cycle PCR. Clin Chem 1997; 43:2262–2267.

Lieber MR: The FEN-1 family of structure-specific nucleases in eukaryotic DNA replication, recombination and repair. BioEssays 1996; 19:233–240.

Little MC, Andrews J, Moore R, et al: Strand displacement amplification and homogeneous real-time detection incorporated in a second-generation DNA probe system, BDProbeTecET. Clin Chem 1999; 45:777–784.

Lyamichev V, Mast A, Hall JG, et al: Polymorphism identification and quantitative detection from genomic DNA by invasive cleavage of oligonucleotide probes. Nature Biotech 1999; 17:292–296.

Mazzulli T, Drew LW, Yen-Lieberman B, et al: Multicenter comparison of the Digene hybrid capture CMV DNA assay (version 2.0), the pp65 antigenemia assay, and cell culture for detection of cytomegalovirus viremia. J Clin Microbiol 1999; 37:958–963.

Morrison T, Weiss JJ, Wittwer CT: Quantification of low copy transcripts by continuous SYBR green I dye monitoring during amplification. BioTechniques 1998; 24:954–958.

Myers TW, Gelfand DH: Reverse transcription and DNA amplification by a *Thermus thermophilus* DNA polymerase. Biochemistry 1991; 30:7661–7666.
This paper is another milestone in the enzymology of PCR. It describes the use of a single thermostable enzyme to accomplish both the reverse-transcriptase and cDNA amplification, facilitating the development of one-step, closed-tube RT-PCR for RNA targets.

Nolte FS: Branched DNA signal amplification for direct quantitation of nucleic acid sequences in clinical specimens. Adv Clin Chem 1998; 33:201–235.

Nycz CM, Dean CH, Haaland PD, et al: Quantitative reverse transcription strand displacement amplification; quantitation of nucleic acids using an isothermal amplification technique. Anal Biochem 1998; 259:226–234.

Piatak M Jr, Luk K-C, Williams B, Lifson JD: Quantitative competitive polymerase chain reaction for accurate quantitation of HIV DNA and RNA species. BioTechniques 1993; 14:70–80.

Piccirilli JA, Krauch T, Moroney SE, Benner SA: Enzymatic incorporation of a new base pair into DNA and RNA extends the genetic alphabet. Nature 1990; 343:33–37.

Ririe K, Rasmussen RP, Wittwer CT: Product differentiation by analysis of DNA melting curves during the polymerase chain reaction. Anal Biochem 1997; 245:154–160.
This paper describes how melting curve analysis using a microvolume fluorometer integrated with a thermal cycler can be used to differentiate and identify PCR products by monitoring the double-stranded DNA binding dye SYBR green.

Rosetti S, Englisch S, Bresin E, et al: Detection of mutations in human genes by a new rapid method: cleavage fragment length polymorphism analysis (CFLPA). Mol Cell Probes 1997; 11:155–160.

Ryan D, Nuccie B, Arvan D: Non-PCR dependent detection of the factor V Leiden mutation for genomic DNA using a homogeneous invader microtiter plate assay. Mol Diagn 1999; 4:135–144.

Saiki RK, Gelfand DH, Stoffel S, et al: Primer-directed enzymatic amplification of DNA with a thermostable DNA polymerase. Science 1988; 239:487–491.

This seminal paper describes the use of a thermostable DNA polymerase to catalyze the polymerase chain reaction. This development made PCR much more 'user friendly' and paved the way for automation of the process.

Sreevatsan S, Bookout JB, Ringplis FM, et al: Algorithmic approach to high-throughput molecular screening for alpha interferon-resistant genotypes in hepatitis C patients. J Clin Microbiol 1998; 36:1895–1901.

Tyagi S, Bratu DP, Kramer FR: Multicolor molecular beacons for allele discrimination. Nature Biotech 1998; 16:49–53.

Walker GT, Little M, Nadeau J, Shank DD: Strand displacement amplification – an isothermal, in vitro DNA amplification technique. Nucleic Acid Res 1992a; 20:1691–1696.

Walker GT, Little MC, Nadeau JG, Shank DD: Isothermal in vitro amplification of DNA by a restriction enzyme/DNA polymerase system. Proc Natl Acad Sci USA 1992b; 89:392–396.

Wittwer CT, Garling DJ: Rapid cycle DNA amplification: time and temperature optimization. Biotechniques 1991; 10:76–83.

Wu DY, Wallace RB: The ligation amplification reaction (LAR) – amplification of specific DNA sequences using sequential rounds of template-dependent ligation. Genomics 1989; 4:560–569.

CHAPTER 68

Hybridization Array Technologies

Martin H. Bluth, M.D., Ph.D., Michael E. Zenilman, M.D.

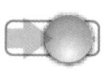

KEY POINTS

• Array technology provides a unique and powerful approach to screen a sample for dozens to thousands of genes.

• Many hybridization array platforms exist; however, currently glass-based microarrays are favored for high-density applications.

• Positive signals are generated when a tagged nucleic acid moiety hybridizes with its complementary probe localized on a solid support (i.e., 'chip').

• Care must be taken when performing and interpreting microarray experiments, as numerous factors must be considered in analysis.

• Numerous applications of array technology have been proposed in the past few years, ranging from molecular staging of tumors to the identification and characterization of microbial agents.

In only a few short years, hybridization array technology, which enables the performance of thousands of simultaneous hybridization reactions on a solid substrate within a single analytical procedure, has gone from theoretical construct to practical reality. Such massively parallel determinations offer previously unimaginable opportunities for diagnostic application, ranging from gene sequencing and detection of genetic polymorphisms to measurement of gene expression profiles in cancer cells. Microarray-based systems offer a platform for quantifying the expression of thousands of genes at the same time. Therefore, an unprecedented advantage of this technology affords analysis of whole cassettes of genes, or patterns of gene expression, rather than one, two, or three genes at a time. The general schema for microarray processing includes the generation of nucleic acid (i.e., DNA) complementary to genes of interest, which is laid out in microscopic quantities on solid surfaces at defined positions (the 'probe'), nucleic acid (DNA) from samples is added over the surface – complementary DNA binds and the presence of bound DNA is detected by fluorescence following laser excitation (for general review see Friend, 2002).

It is clear that hybridization array technology has revolutionized the way we approach the study of disease. The one-gene-one-protein-one-function approach is no longer the mainstay of scientific design. Array technology introduced a complicated mirror image of this approach, in other words, multiple functions, multiple proteins, multiple genes. The power of this technology lies in the 'screening' capability it provides. Under defined experimental conditions, one now has the ability to determine changes in the patterns of genes identifying multiple genes acting in concert. These patterns can then be 'mined' through various computer algorithms, grouped into functional categories (i.e. respiratory genes, inflammatory genes, etc.), and used to derive signatures diagnostic of disease or to generate novel hypotheses about pathogenesis and cell function. The relationship of these genes to one another (increased vs decreased expression) are determined and generally expressed as fold-change. Microarray findings of differential gene expression require confirmation by other techniques such as quantitative reverse-transcriptase polymerase chain reaction (RT-PCR) or additional independent microarray studies.

Once candidate genes or groups of genes are identified, classical approaches to gene function (i.e., gene knockout or gene knockdown) can then be employed to elucidate or validate gene function. More importantly, hybridization array technology, with subsequent data mining, allows for the consideration of unexpected genes that are not associated with the disease being studied, generating new paradigms for future study. Similar platforms can be used to sequence large genes and to scan the genome for single nucleotide polymorphisms and methylation sites. The purpose of this chapter is to review the theoretical basis for the various matrix hybridization platforms and to provide a perspective on their clinical application, both now and in the future.

Array technologies

A hybridization array is the molecular equivalent of a spreadsheet, where each cell or address reveals a specific piece of data, usually inferred from the binding of a ligand to its specific target. The first array-based methods were exploited in immunoassays (Ekins, 1987, 1999) and arrays also have been proposed for parallel studies of diverse targets such as proteins, lipids, carbohydrates, and small molecules (Fodor, 1991; Pirrung, 1992; Southern, 1996a; Guschin, 1997; Schena, 1998). Similar to antigen–antibody interactions on immunoarrays, the fundamental principle of nucleic acid arrays is detection of specific hybridization between complementary strands. The principles of nucleic acid hybridization and an overview of various platforms are covered in Chapter 66. The effectiveness of solid-support hybridization formats was pioneered with the use of nitrocellulose membranes (Gillespie, 1965) for dot blots (Kafatos, 1979), line probes, and Southern blots (Southern, 1975). Changing the labeled entity from the probe to the sample was first referred to as reverse line-blot (or dot blot) hybridization, and led to the beginning of interrogating one sample for multiple potential targets. Moving from dozens to thousands of targets has come about rapidly over the last few years, driven in part by the unique convergence of microfabrication, robotics, and bioinformatics technologies and the demand for high-throughput genetic analysis resulting from the human genome project.

The field is bursting with potential, and many investigators foresee diagnostic and prognostic applications in tumor classification, chemo-therapeutic responsiveness, pathogen detection, monitoring antibiotic resistance, and characterizing inflammatory responses. Array technology may make the dream of personalized molecular medicine, where the genes of an individual patient may be assessed for risk factors and disease susceptibility and to predict response to therapy, a reality. One such study is using gene expression profiling to predict which trauma and burns patients will develop sepsis and multisystem organ failure (www.gluegrant.org). However, challenges of reproducibility and laboratory quality control remain to be addressed before this enormous potential is realized.

Macroarrays

The term *macroarray* has been applied to formats in which areas of probe localization, often called features, are large enough to be visualized without magnification. These have been manufactured on nylon or nitrocellulose membranes or as plastic strips with linear arrays of bound target. Because of the size of the features, the density of macroarrays is much lower than microarrays, ranging from a few dozen to hundreds or even thousands of probes. They are usually deposited on to the membrane by printing or dot blotting, then dried and stored for future use.

Nylon, plastic and glass (silicon wafer) are standard supports to make macroarrays. Nylon suffers several drawbacks when compared to silicon, which is now becoming the preferred matrix for hybridization arrays. Besides its porous nature, nylon displays high autofluorescence, limiting the sensitivity of fluorescence-based detection because of high background values. The latter also precludes the possibility to develop ratiometric (or 'two-color') assays. This approach uses two targets, each labeled with a different fluor. Most commonly, one is a constant reference control used in direct comparison to the unknown sample, with results expressed as a ratio of the two emitted fluorescent signals (Duggan, 1999).

Macroarrays are currently used for targeted applications. For example, some commercial arrays target all the known cytokine genes or those within specific signal transduction pathways that are activated during infectious and inflammatory processes. Other arrays, targeting the genes altered during oncogenesis, have been used in cancer research (e.g., Atlas Human Arrays, Clontech, Palo Alto, CA, or GeneFilters, Research Genetics, Huntsville, AL). Other commercial applications, usually in kit format, are used to detect and type specific PCR products, such as in the cystic fibrosis mutation screen, human leukocyte antigen (HLA) typing or human papilloma virus (HPV) typing. The advantages of macroarrays include the ability to use standard hybridization equipment, simplified reading or scanning, and affordability.

Some groups have been successful in producing high-density nylon arrays on a custom basis for gene discovery purposes (Gress, 1992; Takahashi, 1995; Granjeaud, 1996; Pietu, 1996; Clark, 1999). Even in high-density configurations, the size of the nylon arrays requires a relatively large volume of hybridization fluid, a practical limitation with respect to generating probe from small amounts of diagnostic material. Because microarrays, rather than macroarrays, represent the high-density, high-throughput platform of choice, the bulk of this chapter focuses on applications of microarrays.

Microarrays

Assay miniaturization saves time while cutting costs in biomedical diagnostic applications and research. Working with smaller volumes reduces reagent consumption, increases sample concentration, and improves reaction kinetics. These improvements allow the investigator to determine hundreds or thousands of results in the time formerly required for a single experiment. Microarrays are now available from several commercial suppliers, along with reading and fabrication equipment for custom manufacture of dedicated arrays for specific research or diagnostic applications.

Microarray Substrates

A major distinction between microarrays and macroarrays consists of the choice of a nonporous solid support. By preventing diffusion of the target nucleic acids, nonporous surfaces (plastic, glass, or silicon substrates) allow faster hybridization kinetics and easier washing steps. In order to allow spatial discrimination of numerous reactions performed simultaneously, the molecular probes are bound to a solid surface in defined arrays. Deposition of probes on a solid substrate is also more amenable to automation and enables higher array densities with optimal image definition. These features apply to any type of microarray, from synthetic oligonucleotides to cloned cDNAs or PCR products (Southern, 1999). Most microarrays are now developed on glass. As opposed to plastic derivatives, glass transparency and lack of autofluorescence allows low-background, fluorescence-based detection. However, as materials science becomes more involved in array technologies, alternative substrates, including coated glass and plastic substrates, may become available.

Microarray Fabrication

3'-end functionalization (i.e., chemical modification) of nucleic acids – oligonucleotides, PCR products, cDNAs, or peptide nucleic acid oligomers

– is required to obtain covalent immobilization on either glass or polypropylene surfaces (Matson, 1995; Beier, 1999). For example, treatment of glass slides with silane allows amino-covered glass to bind amino-linked probes, using bifunctional molecules such as a dialdehyde or a diisothiocyanate (Case-Green, 1994; Guo, 1994). Alternatively, glass coating with a polycation (e.g., polylysine) allows direct charge-coupled binding of polyanionic DNA probes (Maskos, 1993a), an ultraviolet photo-crosslinking step adds covalent bonds to the ionic interaction. Covalent binding is essential to permit stringent washes and therefore accurate discrimination of hybridized species. Several protocols have been published to address surface activation (Maskos, 1992; Beattie, 1995; Matson, 1995; Beier, 1999). An interesting alternative consists of deposition of small patches of activated polyacrylamide to which presynthesized oligonucleotides are attached by microinjection (Khrapko, 1991; Yershov, 1996; Guschin, 1997).

Packing density of probes attached to solid surfaces will influence greatly the performance of hybridization matrices. Poor coupling efficiency, which is often encountered on glass matrices, can result in low probe density and low signal:noise ratios. On the other hand, overly dense packing of oligonucleotides on to a solid surface causes spatial hindrance. This problem may be even more formidable with longer biomolecules such as cDNAs. Hybridization yields can be increased by up to two orders of magnitude by introducing spacers between the surface and the oligonucleotides (Southern, 1999). The longer the spacer, the better the hybridization but, interestingly, there is an optimal spacer length beyond which hybridization yield declines (Shchepinov, 1997; Duggan, 1999). For example, a 40-carbon atom spacer provides a reported 150-fold hybridization enhancement (Shchepinov, 1997). The density of oligonucleotides is approximately 0.1 pmol/mm^2 on a glass surface, two orders of magnitude less than on aminated polypropylene. Thus, a potential advantage of glass over plastic matrices at present is an optimal oligonucleotide density associated with lower spatial hindrance (Southern, 1999). Improved surface chemistries may one day allow production of arrays on plastic sheets or films, which may dramatically reduce production costs.

The terminal composition (5' end) of the oligonucleotides influences their duplex yield as measured by relative intensity. As expected, G:C rich 5' extremities lead to a better yield than their homologues (same composition but different sequences) (Maskos, 1993b). Approaches to modify the 5' end of oligonucleotides (e.g., covalent addition of a degenerated linker) can therefore be considered to minimize this contribution. Alternatively, knowledge that mismatches at the ends are less destabilizing and therefore more difficult to discriminate by hybridization (Southern, 1999) has led to clever improvements for detection of hybridization events. As polymerases and ligases are most sensitive to terminal (as opposed to internal) mismatches, enzymatic methods have been developed with improved detection stringency (solid-phase minisequencing [Pastinen, 1997, 1998; Syvanen, 1999], genetic-bit analysis [Nikiforov, 1994], or ligation-assays [Landegren, 1988; Nickerson, 1990]).

Commercially available arrays have been previously reviewed by Marshall (1998). Fabrication of microarrays falls into two broad categories – those made by direct probe delivery on to the solid surface and those made by in situ synthesis. A third method, developed by Nanogen (San Diego, CA), consists of prefabricated oligonucleotides captured onto electroactive spots on silicon wafers (Edman, 1997; Sosnowski, 1997; Cheng, 1998; Heller, 1998). Modification of the electric field through independent, spatially addressable electrodes can speed up hybridization and, when the polarity is reversed, provide stringent washing (Edman, 1997).

Delivery Technologies

Deposition of presynthesized biomolecules was initiated by Pat Brown and colleagues (Schena, 1995; Shalon, 1996). Biochemical substances (e.g., proteins, peptides, oligonucleotides, cDNAs) are prepared, purified, and stored in microtiter plates. Small quantities of molecules are mechanically delivered on precisely defined locations on a solid surface, using different precision robotic systems. This method is very flexible in terms of biochemical composition, microarray topology (e.g., size and density of the spots, replicate spots for each molecule), and ease of prototyping, allowing for design alteration for different applications. Mechanical methods allow the synthesis of moderate- to high-density microarrays (up to about 16 000 probes/cm^2 [Graves, 1999]). It is the method of choice when large numbers of microarrays are needed with the same composition, as well as for long sequences using PCR products. Several companies are now manufacturing and selling premanufactured arrays (e.g., MicroMax, NEN Life Science, Boston, MA) or arrayers based on deposition (Cheung, 1999) as an alternative to building an arrayer (Brown, 2000).

Delivery procedures consist of different microprinting systems. Most arrayers use fountain pen-like microdispensing tips (e.g., Cartesian Technologies, Irvine, CA), but some original systems such as the pin-and-

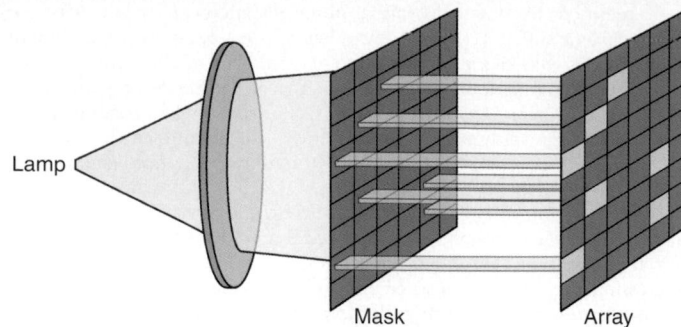

Figure 68–1 Photolithographic synthesis. Ultraviolet light is transmitted through a photolithographic mask, allowing localized photodeprotection of specific chemical building blocks. (Courtesy of Affymetrix.)

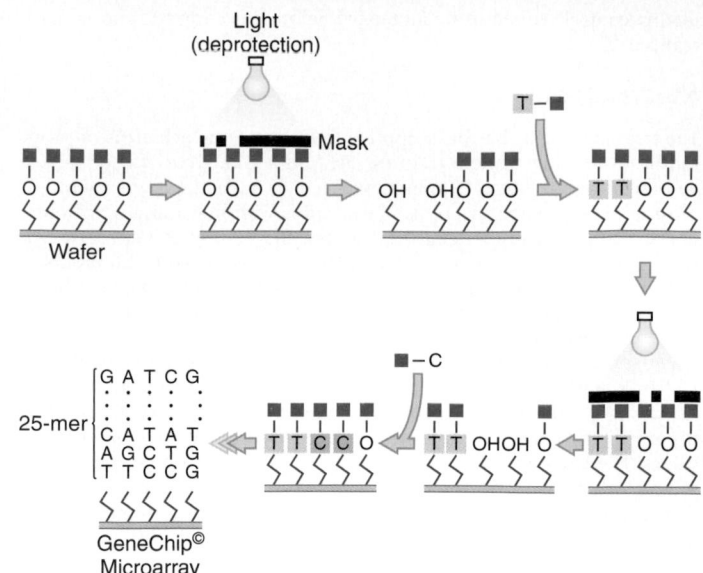

Figure 68–2 Diagram of GeneChip® array manufacture using a unique combination of photolithography and combinatorial chemistry. (Courtesy of Affymetrix.)

ring technique have been developed (Genetic MicroSystems, Woburn, MA). In general, because of surface tension, static, and other effects, the reproducibility of printed arrays is lower than in situ synthesis and must be corrected by separate experiments (repeats), replicate spots (on the same slide), multicolor fluorescence detection, and/or other specific detection algorithms (Chen, 1997). Because of its flexibility and availability, printed array technology will probably have the largest impact on research and clinical laboratories over the next few years.

In Situ Synthesis

In situ synthesis allows higher yields, lower chip-to-chip variation, and higher probe densities. These methods also permit the manufacture of true 'random access' arrays, meaning that each oligonucleotide in any position can have any chosen sequence (Southern, 1999). Combinatorial strategies refer to methods developed to make microarrays containing all sequences of a given length (also referred to as 'generic arrays'). Combinatorial arrays have been promoted mostly to study large-scale hybridization behavior (Southern, 1994) or for solid-state nucleic acid sequencing (Drmanac, 1993a, 1993b, 1999, 1998; Lipshutz, 1993; Macevicz, 1991; Strezoska, 1991).

Manufacturing techniques include photolithographic masks to control chemical activation by photodeprotection steps (Fodor, 1991), ink-jet deposition (Stimpson, 1998), as well as physical barriers to sequential flooding of precursors (Maskos, 1993c). Affymetrix has coupled photochemical deprotection to solid-phase DNA synthesis by adapting techniques from the semiconductor industry (Pease, 1994; Lockhart, 1996; Lipshutz, 1999). Synthetic linkers modified with photochemically removable protecting groups are attached to silicon wafers. By shining ultraviolet light through a photolithographic mask, localized photodeprotection occurs and permits specific chemical building blocks (hydroxyl-protected deoxynucleosides) to react with the deprotected groups (Fodor, 1991) (Fig. 68–1). Cycles alternating photodeprotection and incubation with different chemical building blocks allow light-directed synthesis of polydeoxynucleotides (Fig. 68–2). The synthesized oligonucleotides have a maximum practical length because of the limited efficiency of the photodeprotection (80–95% at each cycle) (Forman, 1999). Therefore, the proportion of 20-mers displaying the predefined sequence is between 1% and 36% ($0.8E20–0.95E20$) (Fodor, 1991).

Mechanical masks or barriers permit confinement of surface areas before flooding with defined precursors. Physical masks of different shapes (circular, diamond) allow in situ synthesis of a given precursor in known locations. Sequential displacement of masks followed by the flooding of another precursor allows synthesis of large combinatorial deoxynucleotide arrays (Southern, 1992, 1996b; Maskos, 1993c). To date, Affymetrix is able to synthesize up to 400 000 different polydeoxynucleotides in a 1.6 cm² area (Fodor, 1991). Critical to this step is the precise alignment of the mask with the wafer before each synthesis step. To ensure that this critical step is accurately completed, chrome marks on the wafer and on the mask are perfectly aligned. Although the process is highly efficient, some activated molecules fail to attach the new nucleotide. To prevent these 'outliers' from becoming probes with missing nucleotides, a capping step is used to truncate them. In addition, the side chains of the nucleotides are protected to prevent the formation of branched oligonucleotides (www.affymetrix.com). Despite high cost, this is the method of choice for large-scale differential gene expression studies because of sensitivity, reproducibility, and redundancy of information.

Ink-jet technologies owe their development to the printer industry and are currently being developed by several companies such as Incyte Pharmaceuticals (Palo Alto, CA), Protogene (Palo Alto, CA), and Rosetta

Inpharmatics (Kirkland, WA) (Blanchard, 1996). This technology is also commercially available (Ink-Jet, Packard Instruments, Meriden, CT; Piezoelectric pump, GeSiM, Grosserkmannsdorf, Germany). Such an approach offers versatility in the biomolecules being delivered and eliminates the need for physical contact with the surface of the array; this last property may be of relevance for the development of arrays coated with thin layers of metals and using different detection methods (Heyse, 1998; Schmid, 1998). Light scattering from microparticles tagging target sequences can be detected as an evanescent wave immediately above the surface of the glass. This method allows real-time affinity measurement with a very low background (Stimpson, 1996).

Oligonucleotide Microarrays

Thermodynamics, kinetics of hybridization, and quantitative aspects of oligonucleotide hybridization have been extensively studied (reviewed by Wetmur, 1991; Hoheisel, 1996). Oligonucleotide arrays have a lower sensitivity than cDNA arrays for detection of rare messages or hybridization targets, and poor predictability of hybridization characteristics because hybridization potential, and therefore the expected signal intensity, do not correlate well with the G:C content or the melting temperature (Graves, 1999; Lockhart, 1996). On the other hand, oligonucleotide arrays are easier to construct using deposition of synthesized product or in situ synthesis described above. In addition, hybridization conditions can be more homogenous than on a cDNA array, provided that the array is designed with oligonucleotides of equivalent sizes.

Oligonucleotide arrays have applications in gene expression profiling as well as in DNA sequencing. For sequencing applications, they can be divided into two fields: generic arrays (representing a random oligonucleotide matrix) or dedicated arrays (for molecular variants of a predetermined target). Generic arrays have been proposed as an inexpensive alternative to sequencing. Using all possible combinations of an *n*-mer allows 'walking' at every position along a nucleotide sequence. This type of array is the only one capable of detecting sequences that are lacking in large electronic libraries. Hyseq (Sunnyvale, CA) claims a leadership position in the field of sequencing by hybridization. This approach is described more fully below under Sequencing Arrays. In contrast, dedicated arrays are used for repetitive sequencing (resequencing) of the same target for detection of nucleotide polymorphisms or functional mutations. This implies knowledge of the targets and their most frequent variants, in order to incorporate predetermined sets of oligonucleotides on the diagnostic array. This approach has been used for detection of genetic polymorphisms associated with human immunodeficiency virus (HIV) drug resistance as well as other polymorphisms. Oligonucleotide arrays can also be used to define single nucleotide polymorphisms (Guo, 1994), even by comparing two samples with multicolor fluorescence (Chee, 1996). Further examples of these applications are described below.

The search for oligomers of higher affinity has opened the way for chemical modifications of the oligonucleotide probe and template in order to improve the kinetics and thermodynamics of binding. Peptide nucleic acid probes (PNAs) allow hybridization to be performed at a higher stringency, because of the high-stability of PNA–DNA duplexes (Corey, 1997). Methylated RNA probes (Corey, 1998) display relatively similar affinities. However, PNAs display more rapid hybridization conditions than their nucleic acid counterparts, primarily because of their neutral backbone structure (Freeman, 1999). Overall, it can be said that, although the reduction of the hybridization time from hours to minutes would be a clear asset, the problem of unpredictability of the melting points of these high-affinity oligomers must be overcome before implementation on microarrays (Weiler, 1997). In addition to probes, targets can be chemically modified to locally enhance signals. Pyrimidine-rich target regions can generate higher hybridization signal by incorporating 5-methyluridine during in vitro transcription (Woski, 1998).

cDNA Microarrays

Microarrays of cDNA sequences allow hybridization-based monitoring of the expression of the cognate genes. Therefore, this strategy implies access to clones or the possibility of generating PCR products. To date, the best strategies use two-color fluorescence detection to discriminate between a sample and its control and check for differential level of expression. This method has been pioneered and validated by Pat Brown and colleagues at Stanford University (Schena, 1995, 1996; Shalon, 1996). Advantages of this approach are calculating a ratio on every probe, to control for the quality of the probe, the specific hybridization properties of each target/probe pair, and the labeling efficacy. Synteni (a subsidiary of Incyte, Palo Alto, CA) has developed its Gene Expression Micro-arrays (GEMs) for this purpose (Schena, 1998). NEN Life Science is now selling glass slides prespotted with 2400 known human genes (MicroMax).

Although they appear to be inherently less reproducible, cDNA microarrays currently offer the greatest versatility in terms of probe deposition and accessibility of the technology. Several companies now offer equipment for array manufacture and reading of hybridized matrices. It is likely that cDNA arrays and high-density oligonucleotide arrays will play complementary roles in research laboratories over the next few years; high-density arrays will be used primarily for the discovery of diagnostically relevant loci and dedicated arrays will be used increasingly for the medium- to low-density analysis of diagnostically relevant loci discovered by high-density array analysis.

Sequencing arrays

Nucleic acid sequence data are fundamental to modern molecular biology. Conventional methods (Maxam, 1977; Sanger, 1977) are time consuming, labor intensive, and costly. Alternative sequencing methods using solid-phase hybridization were proposed on a theoretical basis (Bains, 1988; Khrapko, 1989) within 15 years of the discovery of these methods (Southern, 1975). The theoretical articles were followed shortly by data confirming the principles of array-based sequencing for short artificial templates (Southern, 1992; Pease, 1994; Parinov, 1996). A well-written review of microarray sequencing methods was published in 1999 (Hacia, 1999). The reader might note, however, that much of the work published and cited in this area is provided by researchers with some financial interest in one or more of the proprietary devices evaluated in these publications. Rather than endorsing a particular device or method, this chapter acquaints the reader with basic principles involved in the assay.

Any nucleic acid sequence can in theory be broken down into subsets of length n. All the possible oligonucleotides of length n (n-mers) can then be placed at fixed locations on a solid surface. Nucleic acid to be sequenced (the template) is amplified if necessary, labeled with a direct (fluorescent, luminescent, radioactive) or indirect (affinity) label, and allowed to hybridize to the bound collection of n-mers. Detection of label allows the sequencer to verify a match with an n-mer at a particular locus on the solid surface. The intensity of signal at that locus should be directly proportional to the number of domains in the template corresponding to the n-mer at that locus. Methods for all these steps are outlined in preceding sections of this chapter.

For sequencing applications, the n-mers that match the template are then assembled into a definite order by analysis of n-mers with overlapping sequence, similar in principle to the arrangement of contigs by large-scale sequencing programs. Consider a nonanucleotide template that, under stringent conditions, is bound only to the loci containing the following four tetramers on an array with all 256 possible tetramers:

Tetramer	Intensity
5'ACTG	2
5'CTGA	2
5'TGAC	1
5'GACT	1

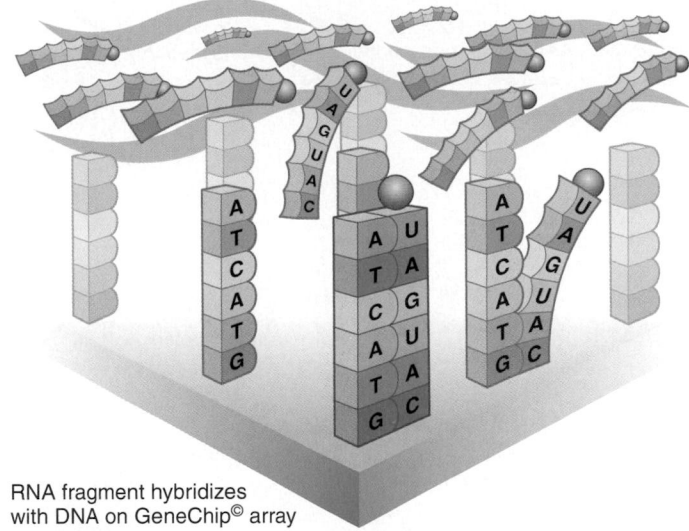

RNA fragments with fluorescent tags from sample to be tested

RNA fragment hybridizes with DNA on GeneChip© array

Figure 68–3 Cartoon depicting hybridization of tagged probes to Affymetrix GeneChip® microarray. (Courtesy of Affymetrix.)

It is trivial to reason from the areas of overlap that the nonanucleotide template was 5'ACTGACTGA. Computational analysis of this kind is straightforward. Since the computation, the scanning of the array to detect label, the labeling itself, and to some extent even the extraction and amplification of the DNA can be automated, it is lovely to envision a 'black box' that accomplishes all this in an afternoon. Consider, however, a nonanucleotide that binds to loci containing the following tetramers:

Tetramer	Intensity
5'TCTA	1
5'CTAC	1
5'TACT	1
5'ACTT	1
5'CTTC	1
5'TTCT	1

This could represent 5'TCTACTTCT or 5'TTCTACTTC; there is no computational way to resolve it. Where n is less than half the length of the template, repeats of the same length as $n/2$ can render the data ambiguous. Computation becomes increasingly difficult as template length becomes an increasingly higher multiple of n; hence, it is desirable to have as long an n as possible for sequencing unknown domains. The practical length of n remains limited by technology, however, since 4^n (the number of loci required for universal representation) exceeds 1 million for $n = 10$. This approaches the current limits of the number of distinct oligonucleotides that can be differentiated on a photolithographic chip (Lipshutz, 1999).

Hybridization, Detection, and Image Analysis

A critical component of microarray assays is the quality and labeling of the probe. Because sample carries the label, sample-to-sample variation in probe preparation and labeling can be anticipated. When microarrays are used for gene expression profiling, this step is even more critical because of the difficulties in obtaining high quality mRNA. Insufficient, degraded, or poor-quality RNA can deliver erroneous results that lead, after data mining, to improper conclusions (Russo, 2003). Although there are many protocols available for high yield of RNA, a final yield of at least a few micrograms of mRNA per experiment is desirable in most applications, although protocols have used smaller amounts of RNA with subsequent amplification using cDNA intermediates that incorporate an RNA promoter and allow amplification with an RNA polymerase. Initial approaches (Auffray, 1980) converted mRNA to a fluorescent cDNA probe with direct incorporation of fluorescent nucleotides. Currently most approaches use total RNA and there are numerous variations of incorporation of label into cDNA or RNA probes, including indirect affinity labels such as biotin with detection using antibody/avidin/streptavidin tagged with fluors or light-scattering gold particles (Figs 68–3 and 68–4). Each step of probe preparation from extraction through labeling must be carefully controlled to assure reproducible results.

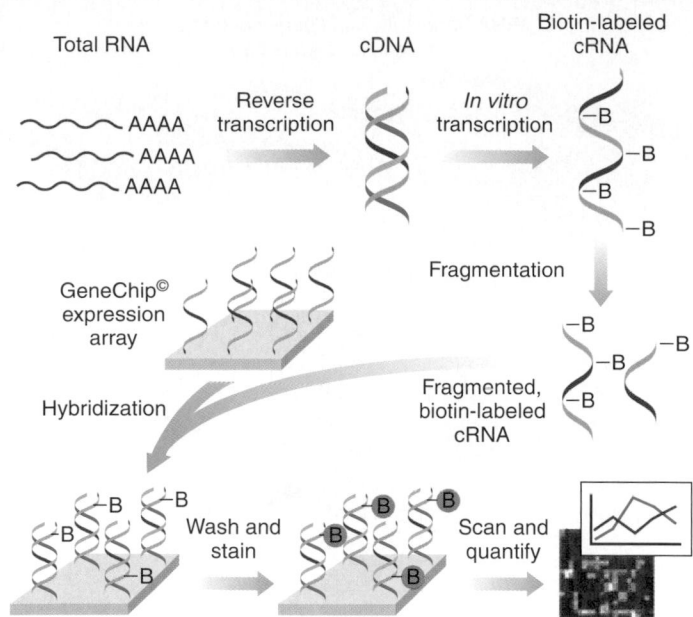

Figure 68–4 Standard eukaryotic gene expression assay. Labeled cDNA or cRNA targets derived from the mRNA of an experimental sample are hybridized to nucleic acid probes attached to the solid support. By monitoring the amount of label associated with each DNA location, it is possible to infer the abundance of each mRNA species represented. (Courtesy of Affymetrix.)

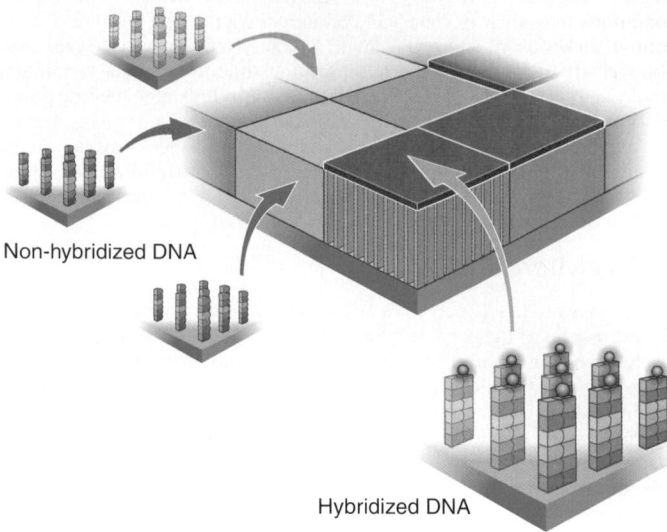

Figure 68–5 Cartoon depicting scanning of tagged and un-tagged probes on an Affymetrix GeneChip® microarray. (Courtesy of Affymetrix.)

The usual consideration of time, temperature, stringency, and probe concentration determine the conditions of the microarray hybridization. Arrays often include negative control probes to allow optimal stringency to be determined. Because of the extremely high complexity of the probe used in gene expression profiling, hybridization times are generally extended to allow low-abundance messages to hybridize. Washes are designed to remove nonspecifically bound probe and reduce background. All steps need to be optimized and standardized. After a successful hybridization, labeled nucleic acid is bound to complementary sequences that are tethered to the array (Fig. 68–5). Some form of image analysis is used to capture signal. In most approaches, the entire slide is scanned (fluorescence, autoradiographic or light scattering) and an algorithm is used to link features with intensities and gene lists. Software associated with the scanner can generate a 'mask' to align image with grid used to construct the array. Data acquisition generates large datasets (one image uses typically 10–50 megabytes) that have to be stored under standard formats (BMP, GIF, JPG). Image processing software will become increasingly automated to ensure proper grid adjustment, detect artifacts, and identify features to extract meaningful information. Various algorithms are available to determine signal intensity and correct for background. After intensities are assigned to each feature, the data are ready for analysis (see Bioinformatics, below).

Bioinformatics

The most challenging aspect of microarrays starts here, when large datasets have been assembled and purged of artifacts and await analysis (Draghici, 2003; Parmigiana, 2003). The approach depends on the nature of the question and design of the experiment. An initial exploration of the data set is used to evaluate the quality, usually including an assessment of background and mean intensity of the features on the array. To facilitate statistical comparisons between arrays, intensities are commonly log transformed and arrays are 'normalized' to each other.

A popular approach to normalizing gene expression is predicated on the assumption that the conditions being compared (i.e. normal versus tumor, or infected versus non-infected) would affect the gene expression of relatively few genes, leaving most unaffected. In the absence of systematic bias, the median intensity of all features on the array should be unchanged. Thus, a common normalization method is to divide each intensity measurement on the array by the median intensity of the array (Kano, 2003). These assumptions are reasonable when the array contains a large number of genes that represent a wide range of biological function.

One caveat of the total intensity normalization methods arises from its implicit assumption that systematic variation is constant across the entire range of expression intensities of the array. However, as data from technical replicate arrays show, systematic variation is often intensity-dependent, or nonlinear. In other words, systematic variation observed at low expression intensities differs from systematic variation observed at medium and high intensities (Simon, 2005). Thus, linear adjustments, such as dividing each measurement on an array with the median intensity of the array, would not be appropriate for some genes. For perhaps 80% of the arrays, systematic variation is close enough to linear so that total intensity normalization methods are sufficient. However, for the remaining 20% of the arrays, non-linear normalization methods are required (Genomics and Bioinformatics Group, 2005).

Quantile normalization is a nonlinear normalization method that is often performed on microarrays. In addition to assuming that most genes are unchanged in their expression across experimental conditions, quantile normalization also makes the strong assumption that the distribution of gene expression intensities must also be invariant across the arrays (Irizarry, 2003). Thus, not only should the median intensity be the same for each array, the intensity at every quantile of the array should be the same. Given this assumption, quantile normalization sorts all intensity values on the array by increasing intensity values and adjusts the intensities so that the smallest intensity value on each array is identical, the second smallest values are identical, and so forth. Note that the gene with the smallest intensity value on one array may be different from the gene with the smallest intensity value on another array.

Intensity-dependent systematic variation has also been shown for two-color technology arrays. Intensity-dependent dye bias was first identified by Terry Speed's laboratory, where it was observed that low-abundance genes appear to be upregulated in the Cy5 channel and moderately expressed genes appear to be upregulated in the Cy3 channel (Yang, 2002). This systematic artifact can be effectively corrected by performing a locally weighted linear regression (lowess) (Fig. 68–6). The validity of using housekeeping genes for normalization has been called into question in the past few years. In this method, it is assumed that the expression levels of housekeeping genes are constant across experimental conditions. Thus, intensity measurements of an array can be normalized to the mean intensities of these genes. However, the expression levels of some housekeeping genes have been shown to vary considerably across some experimental conditions (Thellin, 1999).

Once data have been normalized, quality control is performed at both the sample level and gene level. Sample-level quality control assesses sample data globally to identify outliers or, in cases where replicate reproducibility is generally observed, one or a few samples that may represent outliers. Potential outliers may be identified as those that do not cluster with replicate samples or those that do not correlate highly with replicate samples. Hierarchical clustering, principal component analysis, class prediction algorithms, and similarity metrics are often used to perform sample-level quality control (Grewal, 2003).

Gene-level quality control filters out genes for which the large proportion of measurements fall within the noise range, to create a restricted set of genes for further analysis. Genes that are removed correspond to those that are not expressed in the tissue(s) of concern or whose expression levels are so low

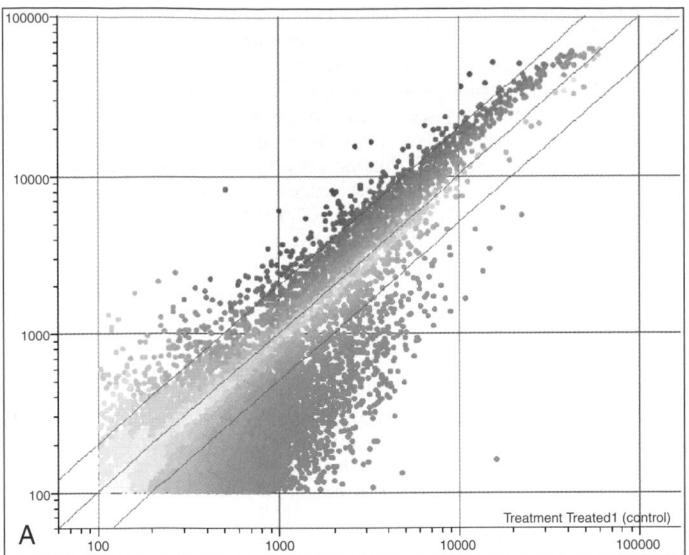

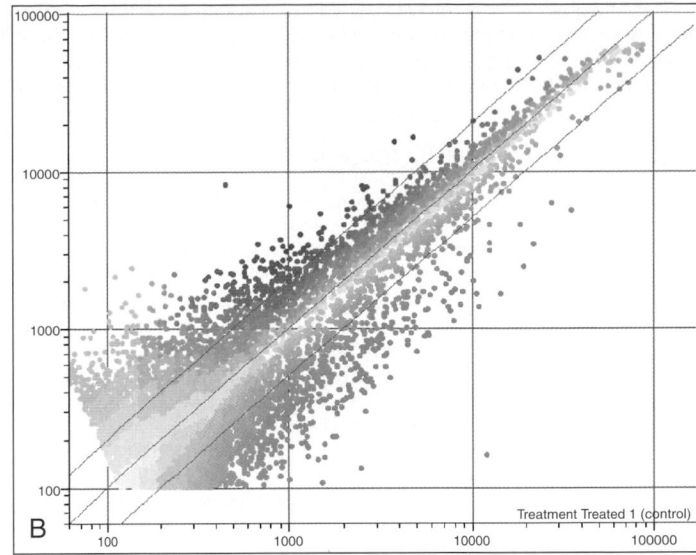

Figure 68–6 Lowess intensity-dependent normalization is used for two-color data. It is a type of within-slide normalization scheme that adjusts for intensity-dependent variation due to dye properties. Dye bias is caused by inconsistencies in the relative fluorescence intensity between Cy5 and Cy3. These inconsistencies often result in nonlinear relationship between the two dyes and a curve will occur in a scatter plot. *A*, Data before normalization. *B*, By applying lowess normalization a locally weighted regression is fitted to the data to adjust the control value for each measurement. As a result, the plot of signal versus control value will be linear. (Courtesy of Agilent Technologies.)

that the technology is not sufficiently sensitive to detect differences in expression. Removal of such genes generally reduces noise, the likelihood of false positives in subsequent differential expression filters, and the severity of multiple testing corrections required in downstream statistical analyses.

Once normalization and quality control of imported data have been completed, one can perform analyses to isolate the genes of interest. One basic objective in a microarray experiment is to identify genes that may be differentially expressed among the different experimental conditions. Researchers rely on many different variants of common statistical tests to identify differentially expressed genes. One caveat to using statistical tests to identify differentially expressed genes is that the number of false positives from the statistical analysis is proportional to the number of tests that are performed. Because hundreds or thousands of genes are often tested at once, the number of false positives from the analysis can potentially dominate the list of candidate genes that are thought to be differentially expressed. Thus, it is important to limit the number of false positives in a statistical analysis by performing multiple testing correction. Two categories of multiple testing correction are those that determine the 'family-wise error rate' (FWER) and those that determine the 'false discovery rate' (FDR). FWER tests control the overall chance that at most one gene is incorrectly identified as being differentially expressed after the statistical analysis and after performing the multiple testing correction (Grewal 2003). Examples of FWER tests are the Bonferroni, Holms–Bonferroni step-down, and Westfall and Young Permutation. FDR tests confine the probability of false positives to be proportional to the number of genes that pass the statistical test instead of the total number of genes tested by the statistical analysis. An example of a FDR test is the Benjamini and Hochberg false discovery rate (Benjamini, 1995). There are several excellent statistical packages available on line, such as BRB Tools, SAM, Focus, D Chip, R Bioconductor Library, PAM, etc.

Clustering analysis (Fig. 68–7) is suitable for grouping genes that behave similarly across multiple conditions of an experiment. Clustering has many applications in expression data analysis. It allows one to infer the previously unknown function of a gene from the functions of the genes that it clusters with. This is based on the assumption that genes that share similar functions share similar expression behavior across experimental conditions. Clustering may also be useful in finding genes that may be co-regulated. This is based on the assumption that genes that are co-regulated share similar expression profiles. Thus, it may be useful to analyze the promoter regions of genes that cluster together to find common regulatory elements (Grewal, 2003).

The generated genes of interest can then be integrated with known biology. The ability to crossreference gene lists from differential expression analysis and/or clustering analysis against gene ontology or other gene function lists to ascertain significance of overlap is available in some programs (e.g., GeneSpring). In addition, genes can be referenced to known biological pathways, and/or public (NCBI) databases (GenBank, LocusLink, UniGene, SAGE).

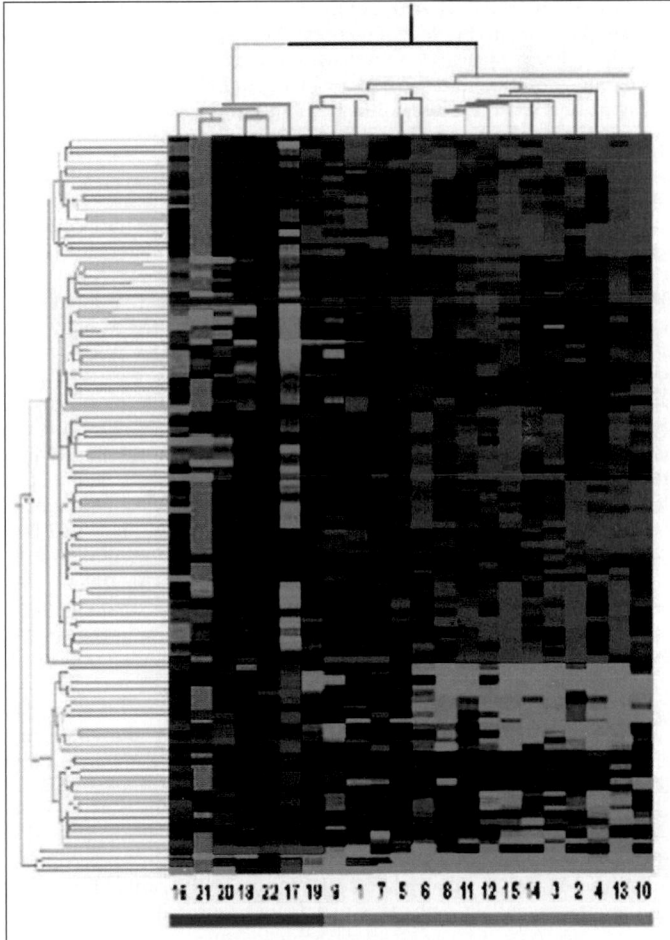

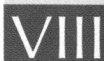

Figure 68–7 Hierarchical clustering dendrogram of duodenal genes from different celiac disease (orange bar) and control (blue) biopsies. Clustering of 109 genes across 22 samples clusters the seven control samples (blue bar) separately from the 15 celiac disease patients (orange bar). Each column represents a celiac disease or a control sample and each row represents an individual gene. For each gene, a green signal represents underexpression, black signals denote similarly expressed genes, a red signal represents overexpressed genes, and grey signals denote missing data. (Adapted with permission of the BMJ Publishing Group from Diosdado B, Wapenaar MC, Franke L, et al: A microarray screen for novel candidate genes in coeliac disease pathogenesis. Gut 2004; 53: 944.)

Thus, because of the intensive need for pattern recognition, multidimensional data interpretation, and crossplatform comparison, microarray technology will enjoy a close relationship with bioinformatics, and coevolution of both hardware and software appears to be inevitable (see Chapter 76).

Intellectual Property Issues

Microarray technology is a rapidly moving field with fierce competition. It is therefore important to emphasize that numerous patents have been filed and that some are directly relevant to clinical diagnosis. For instance, Affymetrix (Santa Clara, CA) possesses broad patent rights on high-density oligonucleotide arrays (Chee, 1998; Holmes, 1998), regardless of the means by which they are made. Assuming that a laboratory decides to develop in-house moderate-density arrays for tumor testing, and charge for such a service, this array might infringe Affymetrix's patents if it exceeds 400 features/cm^2, irrespective of the synthesis method (Fodor, 1998). Array technologies using micromatrices of polyacrylamide gel pads (three-dimensional gel elements) represent a new approach that might not infringe Affymetrix claims (Khrapko, 1991; Yershov, 1996; Guschin, 1997). It is hoped that, as occurred with nucleic acid amplification technologies, competition between manufacturers will bring down costs of high- and medium-density arrays and allow for the democratization of this powerful technology.

Clinical Applications of Array Technology

Numerous applications of microarray technology have been proposed in the past few years, ranging from molecular staging of tumors to the identification and characterization of microbial agents. This has led many to speculate that array technology represents the 'next wave' of technological advances to have a practical impact on the diagnosis of human disease, second only to PCR as a core technology in the clinical molecular diagnostics laboratory. This section focuses on current and future applications of array technology.

Array Technology in the Clinical Laboratory

Clinical laboratory utility of array technology, although not currently widespread, appears to be on the horizon. Roth and colleagues (Roth, 2004) have recently employed array analysis to detect common respiratory pathogens and compared this with conventional culture from middle ear fluid samples. The sensitivities of the array assay compared to culture for *Haemophilus influenzae*, *Moraxella catarrhalis*, *Streptococcus pyogenes*, and *Streptococcus pneumoniae* were 96% (93% for culture), 73% (93% for culture), 93% (80% for culture), and 100% (78% for culture), respectively. Furthermore, tissue based microarray has been used as a tool for internal quality control to improve the interpretation of immunohistochemical staining (Packeisen, 2002; Gulmann, 2004). Small-scale, automated, microfluidic array instruments that have the ability to detect RNA species at a frequency of 1:100 000 with a short turnaround time and low coefficient of variation (0.09–0.11) have also been described (Baum, 2003), which help to characterize this technology on a technical level with regard to dynamic range, discrimination power, and reproducibility. However, methodological consistency, quality control, and disease-specific application will probably have to be overcome prior to implementation as a routine test into the clinical laboratory. Furthermore, the FDA has recently granted 501(k) clearance to Roche Molecular Systems to market its AmpliChip CP450 Genotyping test for use on the Affymetrix instrumentation system (Malone, 2005). This will allow determination of a patient's cytochrome P450 2D6 and 2C19 genotypes, genes that code for liver enzymes that are important in drug metabolism and allow the clinician to optimize drug dosing and minimize potential side-effects on the basis of individual genotype. This is the first time a microarray chip has been given marketing clearance as a diagnostic device for use in the clinical laboratory, heralding the potentially new era of personalized medicine.

Array Technology in Clinical Disease

Microarray technology has provided the ability to screen genes that are differentially regulated in experimental and clinical disease and allow further correlation of select genes with their function. For example Ji and colleagues (Ji, 2003) used microarray technology to screen for genes that are upregulated in the early stage of acute pancreatitis using two different experimental models of the disease. Many genes were upregulated in both experimental systems, suggesting their importance in the human condition. However, one gene in particular, *EGR1*, was further analyzed through classical approaches (gene knockout) and was shown to be a key regulator in disease that may be important in the development of early acute pancreatitis. Others (Iacobuzio-Donahue, 2003) have performed a comprehensive evaluation and comparison of gene expression profiles of 39 samples of pancreatic cancer and identified between six and 40 genes that were highly expressed when examined by multiple methods (oligonucleotide arrays, cDNA arrays, or serial analysis of gene expression [SAGE]), which may eventually be translated into clinically useful targets.

Microarray analysis of cells and tissues as a means to identify key therapeutic candidates continues to evolve. Malignancies or their tissue components that have been analyzed in the quest for identifying key targets, diagnostic or prognostic indicators, or novel pathways include melanoma (Nambiar, 2004), leukemias (Moos, 2002; Jaakson, 2003), lymphomas (Hedvat, 2002; Kobayashi, 2003), myelodysplastic syndromes (Pellagatti, 2004), prostate (Pettus, 2004), bladder (Dyrskjot, 2003), renal (Moch, 1999), colorectal (Frederiksen, 2003), breast (Jeffrey, 2002; Wilson, 2004), ovarian (Rosen, 2004), and endometrial (Saidi, 2004) carcinoma.

Other clinical applications that utilize the gene screening capability of microarray technology include the study of the effect of ionizing radiation (Amundson, 1999), detection of hepatitis D virus (Sun, 2004), identification of central nervous system pathogens (Hanson, 2004), karyotyping of cell-free DNA in amniotic fluid (Larrabee, 2004), viral diagnosis (Striebel, 2003), providing molecular markers for allergic (Jahn-Schmid, 2003) and inflammatory disorders (Bennett, 2003), Alzheimer's disease (Pasinetti, 2001), multiple sclerosis (Whitney, 1999), diabetes (Sreekumar, 2002; Mootha, 2003), transplant rejection (Flechner, 2004) and pulmonary hypertension (Geraci, 2001). The ability to predict adverse drug reactions (Guzey, 2002), response to therapy (Sotiriou, 2002), drug sensitivity (Stein, 2004), and toxicity profiles (Waring, 2001), among others (Cox, 2001), have also been reported. Because of the potential for speed and automation, microarray sequencing is attractive as an alternative to classical phenotypic methods, notably drug resistance screening.

Limitations

Despite the excitement and increase in the potential clinical application of microarray technology care must be taken in its interpretation. Clinical application will require procedures for quality control and quality assurance. The approach to ensuring reproducibility for high-density data presented in microarrays is unprecedented in the clinical laboratory. Each of the large number of steps from sample extraction, labeling, hybridization, image analysis, and data analysis, contributes to difficulties in data reproducibility, and can differ in commercially available systems (Kothapalli, 2002). Even relatively minor changes, such as varying the method used for nucleic acid isolation (Feezor, 2004) can affect results of gene expression profiling.

Approaches to prevent such inconsistencies include: verification of each clone sequence prior to printing the microarray; performing experiments in duplicate or triplicate where possible; and verification of candidate genes by classical methods (PCR, Northern blotting, RNase protection assay, etc.). Some investigators (Rajeevan, 2001) have shown that the majority of array results were qualitatively accurate in cross-validation experiments using real-time RT-PCR. However, for genes showing less than a fourfold difference on the arrays, consistent crossvalidation with real-time RT-PCR was not achieved. It is also very important to determine whether the difference in mRNA expression translates to a difference in the expression levels of the corresponding protein products. Currently, how frequently a difference in mRNA level translates to a difference in protein expression level is not clear.

Caution must also be exercised in interpreting differentially regulated genes during tumor progression (staging microarray). Any nucleic acid source derived from biopsy tissue is made up of many different cell populations and may represent homogeneous tissue only after the tumor mass has reached a large enough size (i.e., late stage). While certain methods are available to isolate specific cells of interest in smaller tumors (e.g., laser capture microdissection), they are technically demanding, time-consuming and not universally available.

Like all sequencing strategies, microarrays have limited sensitivity for minority alleles. The example of sequence-based identification of drug resistance in HIV will be particularly instructive. Microarray sequencing of clinical isolates can correctly predict some instances of drug resistance on the basis of specific mutations (Race, 1998), and is already evolving toward standard practice (Perez-Olmeda, 1999). Even making the optimistic assumption that sequencing can detect a resistance allele when represented in 1% of the viral population or more, however, there is reason to doubt the predictive value of a test negative for resistance. Few virologists would argue that 0.5% prevalence of drug resistance is unimportant in a virus that generates over a billion copies a day. Therefore, it should be understood that the power of this technology currently lies in its ability to screen for the regulation of genes in defined parameters (Russo, 2003).

Further advances in diagnosis, classification, and prognosis await discovery by microarray-based methods in the near future. As emphasized earlier, it is not merely improvements in apparatus that make this possible, but more sophisticated analytic strategies, which evolve to keep up with the more complex data generated by these devices (Bassett, 1999).

References

Amundson SA, Bittner M, Chen Y, et al: Fluorescent cDNA microarray hybridization reveals complexity and heterogeneity of cellular genotoxic stress responses. Oncogene 1999; 18:3666.

Auffray C, Rougeon F: Purification of mouse immunoglobulin heavy-chain messenger RNAs from total myeloma tumor RNA. Eur J Biochem 1980; 107:303

Bains W, Smith GC: A novel method for nucleic acid sequence determination. J Theor Biol 1988; 135:303.

Bassett DE Jr, Eisen MB, Boguski MS: Gene expression informatics – it's all in your mine. Nat Genet 1999; 21:51–55.

Baum M, Bielau S, Rittner N, et al: Validation of a novel, fully integrated and flexible microarray benchtop facility for gene expression profiling. Nucleic Acids Res 2003; 31:e151.

Beattie WG, Meng L, Turner SL, et al: Hybridization of DNA targets to glass-tethered oligonucleotide probes. Mol Biotechnol 1995; 4:213.

Beier M, Hoheisel JD: Versatile derivatisation of solid support media for covalent bonding on DNA-microchips. Nucl Acids Res 1999; 27:1970.

Benjamini Y, Hochberg Y: Controlling the false discovery rate: a practical and powerful approach to multiple testing. J R Statist Soc B 1995; 57:2889.

Bennett L, Palucka AK, Arce E, et al: Interferon and granulopoiesis signatures in systemic lupus erythematosus blood. J Exp Med 2003; 197:711.

Blanchard AP, Kaiser RJ, Hood LE: High-density oligonucleotide arrays. Biosens Bioelectron 1996; 11:687.

Brown MP, Grundy WN, Lin D, et al: Knowledge-based analysis of microarray gene expression data by using support vector machines. Proc Natl Acad Sci USA 2000; 97:262–267.

Case-Green SC, Southern EM: Studies on the base pairing properties of deoxyinosine by solid phase hybridisation to oligonucleotides. Nucl Acids Res 1994; 22:131.

Chee M, et al: Arrays of nucleic acid probes on biological chips. Nov 17, 1998; Patent US1995000441887.

Chee M, Yang R, Hubbell E, et al: Accessing genetic information with high-density DNA arrays. Science 1996; 274:610.

Chen Y, Dougherty ER, Bittner ML: Ratio-based decisions and the quantitative analysis of cDNA microarray images. Biomed Optics 1997; 2:364.

Cheng J, Sheldon EL, Wu L, et al: Preparation and hybridization analysis of DNA/RNA from E. coli on microfabricated bioelectronic chips. Nat Biotechnol 1998; 16:541.

Cheung VG, Morley M, Aguilar F, et al: Making and reading microarrays. Nat Genet 1999; 21(Suppl 1):1.

Clark MD, Panopoulou GD, Cahill DJ, et al: Construction and analysis of arrayed cDNA libraries. Methods Enzymol 1999; 303:205.

Corey DR: Peptide nucleic acids: expanding the scope of nucleic acid recognition. Trends Biotechnol 1997; 15:224.

Corey DR: DNA/RNA Diagnostics. Washington, DC, Cambridge Healthtech Institute, 19–21 May 1998.

Cox JM: Applications of nylon membrane arrays to gene expression.analysis. J Immunol Meth 2001; 250:3.

Diosdado B., Wapenaar M., Franke L., et al: A microarray screen for novel candidate genes in coeliac disease pathogenesis. Gut 2004; 53: 944.

Draghici, S: Data analysis tools for DNA microarrays. Boca Raton, FL, Chapman & Hall/CRC Press, 2003.

Drmanac R, Crkvenjakov R: Method of sequencing of genomes by hybridization of oligonucleotide probes. Apr 13, 1993b; Patent US5667972. Available on line at: http://www.freepatentsonline.com/5667972.html.

Drmanac R, Drmanac S: cDNA screening by array hybridization. Methods Enzymol 1999; 303:165–178.

Drmanac R, Drmanac S, Strezoska Z, et al: DNA sequence determination by hybridization: A strategy for efficient large-scale sequencing. Science 1993a; 260:1649.

Drmanac S, Kita D, Labat I, et al: Accurate sequencing by hybridization for DNA diagnostics and individual genomics. Nat Biotechnol 1998; 16:54.

Duggan DJ, Bittner M, Chen Y, et al: Expression profiling using cDNA microarrays. Nat Genet 1999; 21:10.

Dyrskjot L. Clasification of bladder cancer by microarray expression profiling: towards a general clinical use of microarrays in clinical diagnostics. Expert Rev Mol Diagn 2003; 3:635.

Edman CF, Raymond DE, Wu DJ, et al: Electric field directed nucleic acid hybridization on microchips. Nucl Acids Res 1997; 25:4907.

Ekins RP, Jackson TM: Free Ligand Assay. UK Patent no CA1227425 8 803 000. 1987.

Ekins RP, Chu FW: Microarrays: Their origins and applications. Trends Biotechnol 1999; 17:217.

Feezor RJ, Baker HV, Mindrinos M, et al: Whole blood and leukocyte RNA isolation for gene expression analysis. Physiol Genomics 2004; 19:247.

Flechner SM, Kurian SM, Head SR, et al: Kidney transplant rejection and tissue injury by gene profiling of biopsies and peripheral blood lymphocytes. Am J Transplant 2004; 4:1475.

Fodor SP, Read JL, Pirrung MC, et al: Light-directed, spatially addressable parallel chemical synthesis. Science 1991; 251:767.

Fodor SP, Stryer L, Read J, et al: Arrays of materials attached to a substrate. Apr 28, 1998; Patent US1995000466632. Available on line at: http://www.freepatentsonline.com/5744305.html.

Forman JE, Walton ID, Stern D, et al: Molecular modeling of nucleic acids. Washington, DC, American Chemical Society, 1999.

Frederiksen CM, Knudsen S, Laurberg S, et al: Classification of Dukes' B and C colorectal cancers using expression arrays. J Cancer Res Clin Oncol 2003; 129:263.

Freeman WM, Gioia L: The maturation of nucleic acid technologies. Trends Biotechnol 1999; 17:44.

Friend SH, Stoughton RB: The magic of microarrays. Sci Am 2002; 286:44.

Geraci MW, Moore M, Gessell T, et al: Gene expression patterns in the lungs of patients with primary pulmonary hypertension: a gene microarray analysis. Circ Res 2001; 88:555–562.

Genomics and Bioinformatics Group: Microarray Data Analysis. Low-Level Analysis of Affymetrix Chips. Bethesda, MD, National Institute of Health, 2005. Available on line at: http://discover.nci.nih.gov/microarrayAnalysis/Affymetrix.Preprocessing.jsp.

Gillespie D, Spiegelman SA: A quantitative assay for DNA-RNA hybrids with DNA immobilized on a membrane. J Mol Biol 1965; 12:829.

Granjeaud S, Nguyen C, Rocha D, et al: From hybridization image to numerical values: a practical, high throughput quantification system for high density filter hybridizations. Genet Anal 1996; 12:151.

Graves DJ: Powerful tools for genetic analysis come of age. Trends Biotechnol 1999; 17:127.

Gress TM, Hoheisel JD, Lennon GG, et al: Hybridization fingerprinting of high-density cDNA-library arrays with cDNA pools derived from whole tissues. Mamm Genome 1992; 3:609.

Grewal A, Lambert P, Stockton J. Current Protocols in Bioinformatics. New York: John Wiley, 2003, p 7.1.1.

Gulmann C, Loring P, O'Grady A, Kay E: Miniature tissue microarrays for HercepTest® standardisation and analysis. J Clin Pathol. 2004; 57:1229.

Guo Z, Guilfoyle RA, Thiel AJ, et al: Direct fluorescence analysis of genetic polymorphisms by hybridization with oligonucleotide arrays on glass supports. Nucl Acids Res 1994; 22:5456.

Guschin D, Yershov G, Zaslavsky A, et al: Manual manufacturing of oligonucleotide, DNA, and protein microchips. Anal Biochem 1997; 250:203.

Guzey C, Spigset O. Genotyping of drug targets: a method to predict adverse drug reactions? Drug Saf 2002; 25:553.

Hacia JG: Resequencing and mutational analysis using oligonucleotide microarrays. Nat Genet 1999; 21:42.

Hanson EH, Neimeyer DM, Folio L, et al: Potential use of microarray technology for rapid identification of central nervous system pathogens. Mil Med 2004; 169: 594.

Hedvat CV, Hegde A, Chaganti RS, et al: Application of tissue microarray technology to the study of non-Hodgkin's and Hodgkin's lymphoma. Hum Pathol 2002; 33:968.

Heller MJ, O'Connell J P, Juncosa R D, et al: Methods for hybridization analysis utilizing electronically controlled hybridization. Dec 15, 1998; Patent US5849486. Available on line at: http://www.freepatentsonline.com/5849486.html.

Heyse S, Ernst OP, Dienes Z, et al: Incorporation of rhodopsin in laterally structured supported membranes: observation of transducin activation with spatially and time-resolved surface plasmon resonance. Biochemistry 1998; 37:507.

Hoheisel JD: Sequence-independent and linear variation of oligonucleotide DNA binding stabilities. Nucl Acids Res 1996; 24:430.

Holmes CP: Cyclic nucleic acid and polypeptide arrays. Jun 23, 1998; Patent US1996000647618.

Iacobuzio-Donahue CA, Ashfaq R, Maitra A, et al: Highly expressed genes in pancreatic ductal adenocarcinomas: a comprehensive characterization and comparison of the transcription profiles obtained from three major technologies. Cancer Res 2003; 63:8614.

Irizarry RA, Bolstad BM, Collin F, et al: Summaries of Affymetrix GeneChip probe level data. Nucleic Acids Res 2003; 31:e15.

Jaakson K Zernant J, Kulm M, et al: Genotyping microarray (gene chip) for the ABCR (ABCA4) gene. Hum Mutat 2003; 22:395.

Jahn-Schmid B, Harwanegg C, Hiller R, et al: Allergen microarray: comparison of microarray using recombinant allergens with conventional diagnostic methods to detect allergen-specific serum Immunoglobulin E. Clin Exp Allergy 2003; 33:1443.

Jeffrey SS, Fero MJ, Borresen-Dale AL, et al: Expression array technology in the diagnosis and treatment of breast cancer. Mol Interv 2002; 2:101.

Ji, B, Chen, XQ, Misek DE, et al: Pancreatic gene expression during the initiation of acute pancreatitis: identification of EGR-1 as a key regulator. Physiol Genomics 2003; 14:59.

An example of how microarray is employed to screen for regulation of gene expression in two models of experimental pancreatitis with subsequent validation of select genes (EGR-1) by conventional methods.

Kafatos FC, Jones CW, Efstratiadis A: Determination of nucleic acid sequence homologies and relative concentrations by a dot hybridization procedure. Nucl Acids Res 1979; 7:1541.

Kano M, Kashima H, Shibuya T, et al: A method for normalization of gene expression data. Genome Informatics 2003; 14:336.

Khrapko KR, Lysov YP, Khorlin AA, et al: A method for DNA sequencing by hybridization with oligonucleotide matrix. DNA Seq 1991; 1:375.

VIII

CHAPTER 69

Applications of Cytogenetics in Modern Pathology

Constance K. Stein PhD

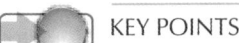

KEY POINTS

• Identification of chromosomal abnormalities often correlates to disease and phenotypic abnormalities that will aid in clinical diagnosis and treatment.

• Standard morphology and a specific banding pattern have been established for all human chromosomes. A variety of different staining technologies are used to uniquely identify chromosomes and determine if anomalies exist.

• Fluorescence in situ hybridization (FISH), a unique diagnostic tool combining technologies from both cytogenetics and molecular genetics, can provide important information on the status of genes.

• The two basic categories of cytogenetic abnormality are numerical and structural.

• Cytogenetic abnormalities may be either de novo or inherited. Detection may occur at any stage of a person's life from prenatal to adulthood.

• Identification of a cytogenetically abnormal clone in a cancer can provide information on diagnosis, prognosis, treatment, and disease progression.

• Many syndromes have been specifically linked to particular chromosomal anomalies; for example, trisomy 21 in Down syndrome, 45,X in Turner syndrome, and deletion of 22q11.2 in velocardiofacial syndrome.

• Microdeletion syndromes may require a combination of karyotype analysis, FISH, and clinical evaluation for diagnosis.

• Cytogenetic analysis can be used in nearly every medical specialty and is an important element in clinical laboratory medicine.

Introduction

Genetics is broadly defined as the scientific study of heredity but, in clinical laboratory medicine, interest is focused on two subspecialties of this field: (1) human genetics, the study of heredity in man; and (2) medical genetics, the study of human genetic variation of medical significance. Medical genetics can be further subdivided into five groups, two primarily clinical fields (clinical genetics and genetic counseling) and three laboratory sciences (cytogenetics, molecular genetics, and biochemical genetics).

Groundbreaking discoveries in the field of medicine can be attributed to genetics. Research, including the information obtained from the Human Genome Project (as described in Chapter 76) continues to identify new genes and mutations directly related to disease. Knowing the underlying cause of a disease provides new opportunities for diagnosis, and, opens up the possibility for gene therapy and the likelihood of curing some genetic diseases in the future. Currently, there is a growing demand for ways to use this information to benefit individual patients. This has led to new laboratory techniques in molecular genetics and cytogenetics that are providing improved methods of diagnosis and treatment. The major emphasis of this chapter is cytogenetics, and discussion of molecular diagnostics can be found in Chapter 72.

Definitions

As in all areas of medicine, genetics relies on the proper use of specific terms for communication. The following definitions provide a basic vocabulary for this field.

Gene: a sequence of nucleotides that represents a functional unit of inheritance; a region of DNA that codes for a product, either RNA or protein.

Chromosome: a highly ordered structure composed of DNA and proteins that carries the genetic information. In humans, there are 46 chromosomes ordered in pairs.

Autosome: all chromosomes other than the X and Y chromosomes, which are designated the *sex chromosomes*.

Homologous chromosomes or *homologs*: sister chromosomes, the members of a pair of chromosomes in which one is inherited from the mother and the other from the father.

Locus: the position of a gene on a chromosome.

Allele: an alternative form of a gene occupying the same locus. An allele may be the result of a mutation. There is a maximum of two alleles per diploid chromosome complement (one allele per chromosome), but multiple alleles may exist within a population.

Mutation: a permanent heritable change in the sequence of genomic DNA. This may manifest at both the molecular and cytogenetic levels. Not all mutations are negative events. Many are benign (e.g., blue eye color) and some have positive effects (e.g., sickle cell trait in countries with a significant risk of malaria). Individuals with a *constitutional mutation* (i.e., a mutation present in every cell of the body) may pass that mutation on to their progeny by germ-line transmission. In some cases, notably cancer, an *acquired mutation* may arise in a single somatic cell, which then divides mitotically, giving rise to a new clone of cells. The mutation will be limited to this clone and will not be transmitted to progeny of the individual. In rare instances of *gonadal mosaicism*, a de novo acquired mutation may arise in the gonads, resulting in a mixed population of normal and mutant gametes. Progeny receiving the new mutation may display a phenotype not present in either parent.

Karyotype: the chromosome constitution of an individual. *Karyogram*: a figure showing the paired chromosomes from a cell arrayed in a standard sequence.

Diploid: the presence of two copies of each unique chromosome per cell. In humans, the chromosomes occur in pairs and the diploid (2N) number is 46.

Haploid: one copy of each unique chromosome. In humans, the gametes are haploid (N = 23).

Homozygous: both alleles at a locus are the same. (In the ABO system, an AA complement represents homozygosity.)

Heterozygous: the two alleles at a locus are different. (In the ABO system, an AO complement represents heterozygosity.)

Hemizygous: the presence of only one chromosome or chromosome segment rather than the usual two; applies to males with a single X chromosome.

Genotype: the genetic constitution of an individual or organism (i.e., what alleles are present). (In the ABO system, AA, AO, BB, BO, AB, and OO are genotypes.)

Phenotype: the appearance of an individual that results from the interaction of environment and genotype. (In the ABO system, A, B, and O blood types represent the phenotypic expression of the alleles for a given individual.)

Dominant allele: an allele that is expressed when present in only a single dose (i.e., it 'dominates' over the other allele present). (In the ABO system, A is dominant over O such that an AO genotype results in an A blood type phenotype. Similarly, the presence of pigment (T) is dominant to the absence of pigment (t) (i.e., albinism), such that Tt results in pigmentation.)

Recessive allele: in a diploid organism, an allele that is only expressed when homozygous. (In the ABO system, the O blood group is only seen with a OO genotype; O is recessive to A and B. Similarly, albinism (t) is recessive to pigmentation (T), and an albino phenotype only occurs with a tt genotype.)

Codominant alleles: in a diploid organism, alleles that show no dominance or recessivity to each other but, when present together, are both fully expressed. (In the ABO system, A and B are codominant such that an AB genotype expresses both A and B antigens.)

Independent assortment: random assortment of chromosomes (paternal and maternal) in the gametes; 50:50 chance of inheriting a given chromosome from one parent.

Linkage: the presence of two or more genes on the same chromosome that tend to be inherited together.

Crossing over: the physical exchange of genetic material between homologous chromosomes.

Recombination: the generation of new allelic combinations on chromosomes, usually by crossing over.

Mitosis: somatic cell division in which the DNA replicates and is evenly distributed to two equal daughter cells.

Meiosis: cell division in the gonads that produces the gametes. A single DNA replication is followed by two cell divisions which reduces the total DNA content of a cell from $2N$ to N. Recombination occurs to increase genetic diversity within a population.

Nondisjunction: failure of chromosomes or chromatids to separate to opposite poles in cell division. Usually results in one too many or one too few chromosomes in a cell.

Cytogenetics

Cytogenetics is defined as the science that combines the methods and findings of cytology and genetics to allow the investigation of heredity at the cellular level. This involves careful evaluation of the chromosomes, structures composed of double-stranded DNA that is complexed with histone and nonhistone proteins. Chromosomes were first observed in tumor cells by Walther Fleming in 1882, only 16 years after Mendel established genetics as a new field of science, making cytogenetics one of the oldest fields of genetics. Just after the turn of the century, the importance of the sex chromosomes was established and in 1959, cytogenetic studies were first utilized in clinical laboratory studies. The ability to detect changes in chromosome structure and directly correlate them to disease and phenotypic anomalies in individuals proved a major advancement in clinical diagnosis. Over the years, the number and types of studies have grown and many of the tests performed have become the 'gold standard' for diagnosis. In today's world, with a growing number of disease genes being cloned, there is an increasing emphasis on developing molecular direct mutation analyses (see Chapter 72). These studies work well when a diagnosis is known or suspected but, in the absence of a known disorder, cytogenetics still retains its position as the only clinical laboratory test to be able to survey the cellular genetic constitution of an individual with a single assay. Consequently, clinical applications for cytogenetic analysis can be found in all age groups and range from prenatal diagnosis to cancer evaluation.

Chromosomes

In order to recognize abnormalities, it is first important to understand what comprises a 'normal' chromosome set. The human chromosome

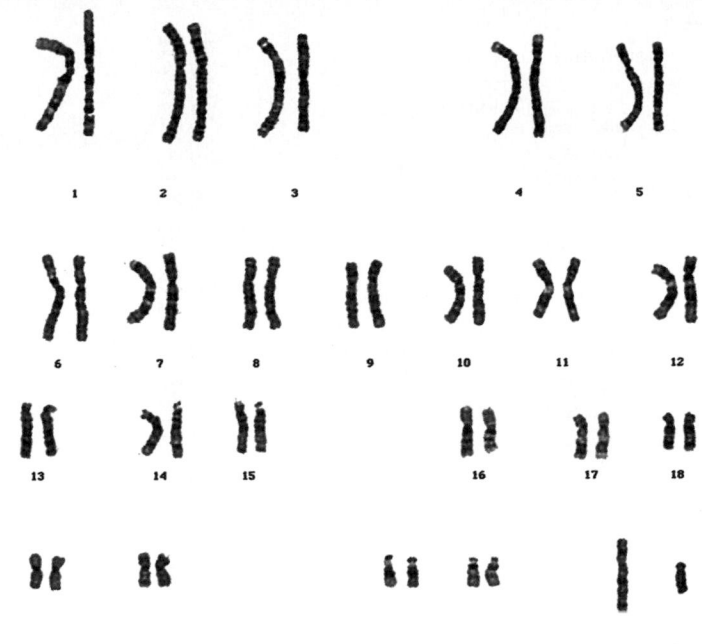

Figure 69–1 Karyotype of male human chromosome complement; 46 total chromosomes are ordered in pairs. Note the nonhomologous pair of sex chromosomes with one X and one Y chromosome (lower right).

complement includes 46 chromosomes ordered in 23 pairs (Fig. 69–1). One member of each pair is inherited from an individual's mother and the other comes from the father. 22 pairs are known as autosomes and appear as homologs of each other (i.e., they are indistinguishable from each other). The 23rd pair includes the sex chromosomes, which are homologous in a female, who has two X chromosomes, and are non-homologous (structurally different) in a male, with one X and one Y chromosome (Fig. 69–1). Genes are encoded in the DNA and are arrayed along the length of the chromosomes. During the cell cycle, the absolute length of the chromosomes will vary but the most condensed form is reached in metaphase, at which time chromosomes can most easily be observed. Because of this, metaphase chromosomes are the basis for most cytogenetic studies.

Chromosome Structure

A single metaphase chromosome is composed of two DNA double helices. Each double helix is termed a *chromatid* and the two chromatids are held together by an as yet unreplicated region of DNA known as the *centromere* or primary constriction. In addition to its function in cell division, the centromere acts as a landmark and divides the chromosome into two distinct regions known as arms (Fig. 69–2A). The shorter of the two arms is designated the p arm and the longer arm is known as the q arm. When the centromere is approximately equidistant from both ends, the chromosome is said to be metacentric but if it is closer to one end than the other, the chromosome is submetacentric (Fig. 69–2B). Five pairs of acrocentric chromosomes have modified short arms with stalks containing only multiple copies of rRNA genes that are capped by a modified telomere termed a *satellite* (Fig. 69–2A).

The end of a chromosome is the *telomere*. These regions are known to be composed of tandemly repeated DNA with the sequence $(TTAGGG)_n$ that functions to stabilize the chromosomes. The mechanics of DNA replication are such that not all of the telomere DNA can be replicated at each division so there is a shortening of the telomeres over time. It has been postulated that total loss of the telomeres leads to an increase in chromosomal aberrations that may, in part, be responsible for the human aging process (Harley, 1990; Wright, 1992; de Lange, 1998).

Cell Culture

To obtain metaphase cells for a chromosome analysis, cells from a patient must be cultured in vitro. The average human cell divides once every 24 hours, so only about 1% of the cell population is dividing at any given time. However, some cells, such as lymphocytes in a normal healthy individual, do not divide at all. Special culture techniques have therefore been developed to stimulate the cells to divide and increase the yield of metaphase cells.

A

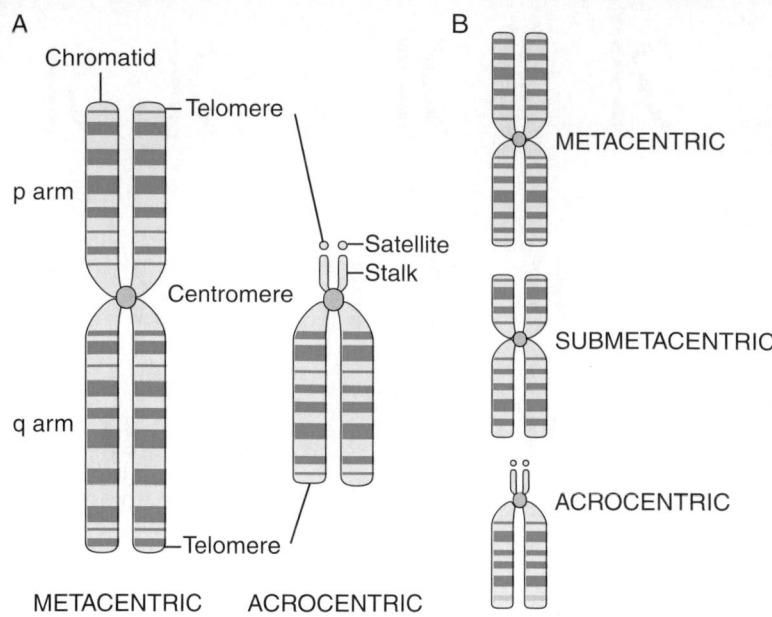

Chromatid

Telomere

p arm

Satellite
Stalk

Centromere

q arm

Telomere

METACENTRIC   ACROCENTRIC

B

METACENTRIC

SUBMETACENTRIC

ACROCENTRIC

Figure 69–2 Chromosome structure. *A,* Schematic of metaphase chromosome anatomy showing major landmarks. Each chromosome is composed of two chromatids held together by the centromere. The telomere is the end structure of the chromosome. A typical metacentric form is contrasted with an acrocentric having a modified short arm structure composed of stalks and satellites. In all cases, the shorter, or p, arm is oriented up and the longer, or q, arm is oriented down. *B,* The relative position of the centromere can vary, resulting in metacentric (centromere near the middle), submetacentric (centromere closer to one end), and acrocentric (modified short arm) chromosomes.

Specimens

Virtually any viable, nucleated cell sample can be used for cytogenetic analysis. However, certain types of cells are easier to obtain and culture, and are therefore favored for chromosomal preparations. For routine cytogenetic studies of adults and children, heparinized peripheral blood is the preferred specimen. Obtaining a sample via standard phlebotomy is usually easy to arrange and relatively painless for the patient. In hematologic disorders, the best results are obtained from bone marrow samples, since this is the origin of the disease. Fibroblast cultures from skin biopsies or skin punches provide an adequate source of metaphase cells. Tissues such as liver, kidney, lung, and muscle are not routinely used because of the invasive nature of acquiring such specimens; however, these tissues frequently provide an excellent resource if obtained soon after death during autopsy or from a fetal loss. Products-of-conception samples may contain a mix of maternal and fetal tissue and so require extra care in establishing a culture (De Martinville, 1984).

The most common specimen for prenatal analysis is amniotic fluid collected by amniocentesis. This procedure is performed under ultrasound guidance in order to avoid the fetus as the physician passes a needle through the mother's abdomen and uterus into the amniotic sac. This is typically done between 16 and 18 weeks of gestation, at which time 20–30 mL of amniotic fluid (fetal urine) can be withdrawn without endangering the fetus. Cells present in the sample are derived from the fetus and provide a source of material for cytogenetic, molecular genetic, and biochemical assays. The fluid itself contains α-fetoprotein (AFP) as well as other proteins and enzymes and forms the substrate for other prenatal assays. The risk of fetal loss due to amniocentesis is approximately 0.5%.

Another prenatal procedure is chorionic villus sampling, which provides tissue from the developing placenta (chorionic villi) (Blakemore, 1988; Rhoads, 1989). The transabdominal or transvaginal procedure is performed at 10–14 weeks' gestation and has a risk of fetal loss of approximately 1%. Since no amniotic fluid is collected, no AFP or related testing can be done, although standard cytogenetic, biochemical, and molecular analyses are possible.

Cordocentesis or percutaneous umbilical blood sampling results in a fetal blood specimen that can be used for rapid karyotyping or molecular studies. This procedure is done at later gestational ages (≥20 weeks) and carries a higher risk of fetal loss (2–5%).

All clinical samples for cytogenetic analysis must be collected in as sterile a manner as possible. The presence of bacteria or fungi will severely compromise the study, since the prokaryotic cells will usually outcompete and overgrow any human cells present. To maximize the number of viable cells, specimens should be transported to the laboratory as soon as possible after collection. Blood, bone marrow, amniotic fluid, and chorionic villi should be maintained at room temperature, whereas solid tissue is transported on wet ice. The difference in temperature of transport is due to the native conditions of the sample. Blood, bone marrow, and amniotic fluid cells occur as individual cells in a fluid substrate, and the integrity of the sample will not be compromised as long as this relationship is maintained at a temperature near that of the body. However, tissue collection requires cells to be excised from the body, leaving broken and dying cells at the periphery of the sample. The release of lysosomal enzymes facilitates degradation of the dead cells and will attack adjacent living cells under the proper conditions. If the temperature is dropped to near 4°C, enzyme activity will be inhibited and the viability of the sample is maintained.

Cell Culture Technique

Depending on the cell type, either a suspension (floating) or monolayer (fixed to a surface) culture technique may be employed. Blood and bone marrow cells are grown in suspension and are simply aliquoted directly into an appropriate culture medium. Bone marrow is typically cultured for 24–48 hours, whereas lymphocytes require 3–4 days in culture for maximum yield. Furthermore, since lymphocytes do not normally divide in culture, they must be induced using a mitogen, usually phytohemagglutinin, and the resultant metaphase cells can then be collected by use of a mitotic inhibitor such as colcemid. Amniotic fluid cells, chorionic villi, and solid tissue are all grown as a monolayer in situ. Tissue and chorionic villi are first disaggregated using a mild collagenase treatment, and the individual cells are then seeded on to glass coverslips and covered with culture medium. In an amniotic fluid sample, the cells must be separated from the fluid by centrifugation before being plated in dishes and allowed to form in situ colonies. Typical culture times are 5–10 days for chorionic villi and amniocytes and up to 2 weeks for solid tissue culture.

Once maximum growth has been achieved, all cell types are harvested using similar techniques. The cells are swelled hypotonically (to the point that the cell membrane is stretched but not broken) and are then fixed. Gentle blowing on the coverslip containing fixed cells from in situ cultures results in the rupture of the cell membrane and a spreading of the metaphase chromosomes. Although most laboratories still perform these steps manually, an automated robotic harvester has been developed that can process large numbers of cultures quite efficiently. For suspension cultures, the fixed cells must be dropped on to a clean microscope slide, which mechanically breaks the membranes and leaves the chromosomes separated slightly from each other but in a discrete region occupied by a single cell (Fig. 69–3). After air drying, the slides are suitable for staining. In some cases, artificial aging of the cells at 65°C for 30–60 minutes improves the quality of the staining.

Staining

Chromosomes are routinely stained using Giemsa or Wright's stain, positively charged dyes that bind to the negatively charged DNA molecule. Mild trypsinization of the chromosomes prior to staining apparently weakens the DNA–protein interactions, yielding a defined pattern of alternating light and dark regions after the stain is applied. This is called the banding pattern (G-banding for Giemsa banding) (Yunis, 1973; Burkholder, 1977; Holmquist, 1982). Each pair of chromosomes has a unique band pattern that is schematically represented as an ideogram (ISCN, 2005) (Fig. 69–4), and this is used to identify each chromosome and the chromosomal subregions.

G-banding, which allows a permanently stained preparation (Sumner, 1973). The current major application of Q-banding is for rapid identification of the Y chromosome. The distal end of the long arm of the Y chromosome is composed of heterochromatin and is the most brightly fluorescent region in a human metaphase (Fig. 69–5A). In cases of ambiguous genitalia, a quick Q-banded preparation can usually answer the question of the presence or absence of a Y chromosome in the patient. C-banding, constitutive or centromere banding, is used to evaluate constitutive heterochromatin or to determine if a chromosome has two centromeres (dicentric). Normally, a centromere appears as a single dark spot on an overall pale-staining chromosome (Holmquist, 1979). In the case of a dicentric chromosome, the presence of two dark regions will clearly identify the two centromeres (Fig. 69–5B). R-banding, or reverse banding, results in chromosomes with the same banding pattern as that seen in G-banding, but the light and dark bands are reversed, hence the name. Because the telomeres of the chromosomes tend to be small, light-staining bands, a deletion may not be easily detected using standard G-banding. In R-banding, however, the telomeres should appear as dark bands and their absence as the result of a deletion is more obvious.

Karyotype Analysis

To perform a cytogenetic (karyotype) analysis, it is essential to be able to rapidly and accurately identify each chromosome and determine when chromosome abnormalities are present. The first step is to count the number of chromosomes present in the cell being evaluated. The number of active centromeres defines the total number of chromosomes and will total 46 in a normal human diploid cell. Too many or too few chromosomes indicate a potential numerical abnormality. In vitro culture can result in culture artifacts, so no single cell is used to define a patient's chromosome complement. Therefore, a typical clinical study requires analysis of 15–20 cells. In cases of mosaicism or for other special situations 10–30 additional cells may be evaluated.

Individual chromosomes are identified based on the overall size of each chromosome, the position of its centromere, and the banding pattern. Any variation in chromosome structure should be detected at this time. In most circumstances, routine G-banding of metaphase chromosomes is sufficient for clinical diagnostic purposes. However, some disorders are associated with very small deletions of chromosomal material that may not be resolved at this level, so high-resolution analysis is used. Special culture conditions are employed, and the cells are harvested at a slightly

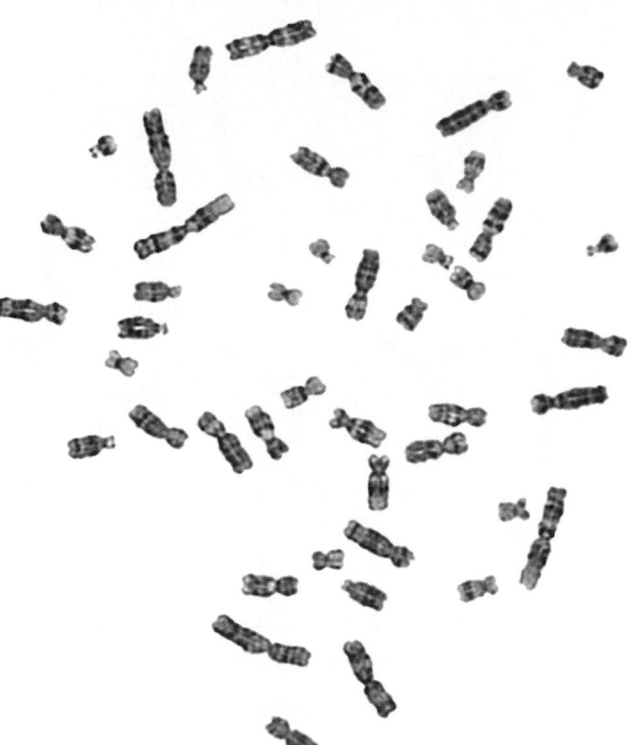

Figure 69–3 Metaphase chromosome spread. Chromosomes from a single cell as seen on a microscope slide.

Although standard G-banding is adequate for most situations, additional information about chromosome structure can be obtained with other special staining technologies. The most common special stains include Q-banding, C-banding, and R-banding. Q-banding or quinacrine fluorescence staining was originally used in routine karyotyping (Comings, 1975). However, because the fluorescence is transient, it has now been replaced by

Figure 69–4 Examples of ideograms for chromosomes 1, 7, 14, and Y showing the expected pattern of alternating light and dark bands.

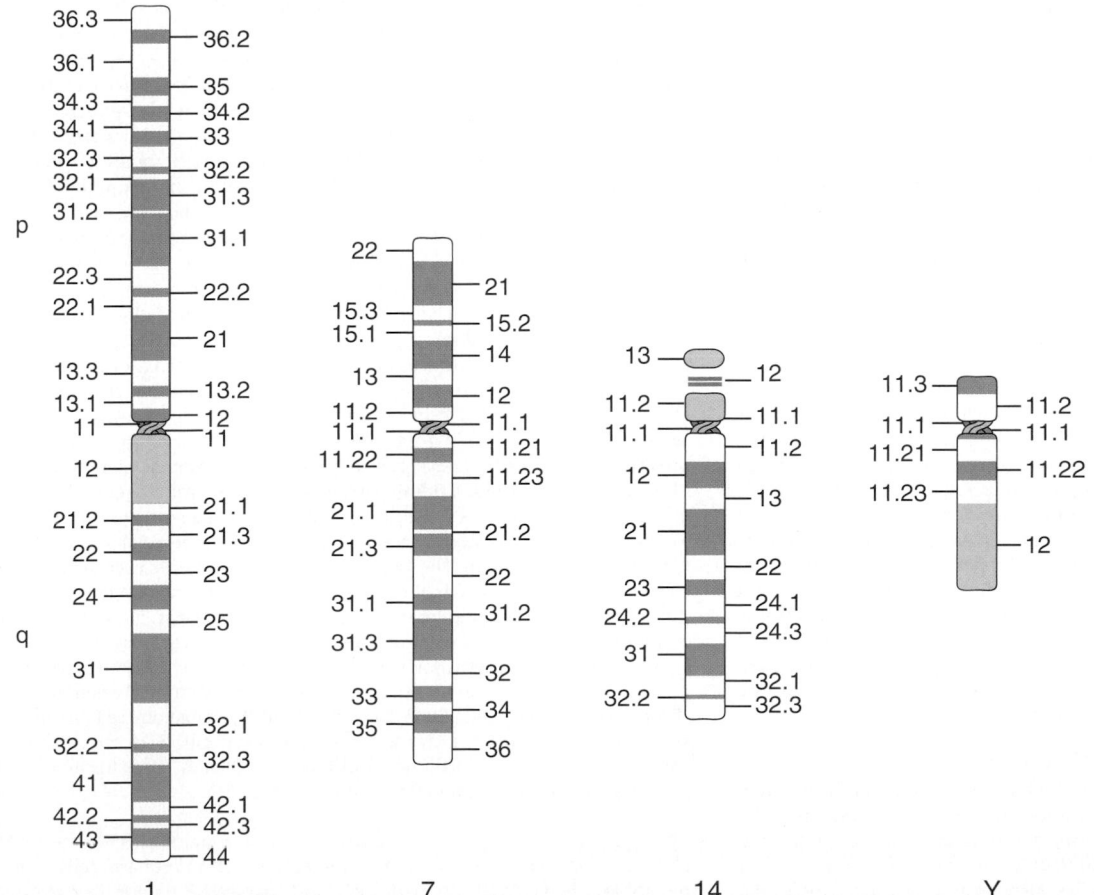

VIII

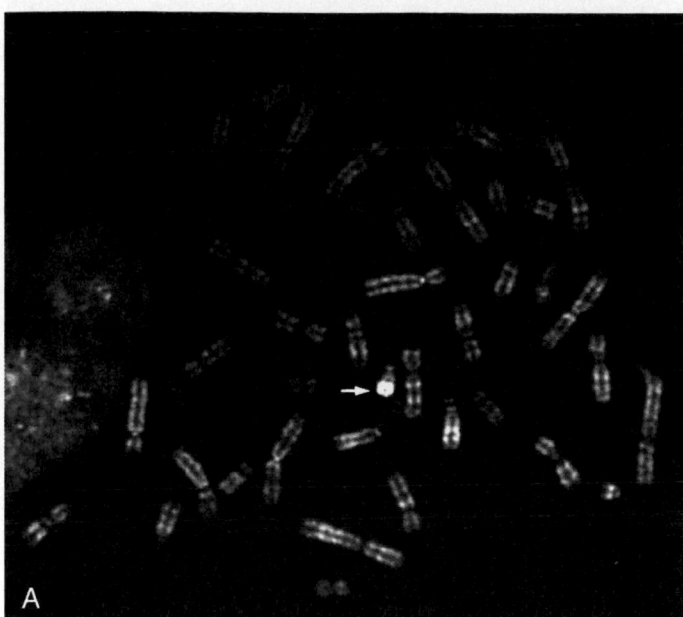

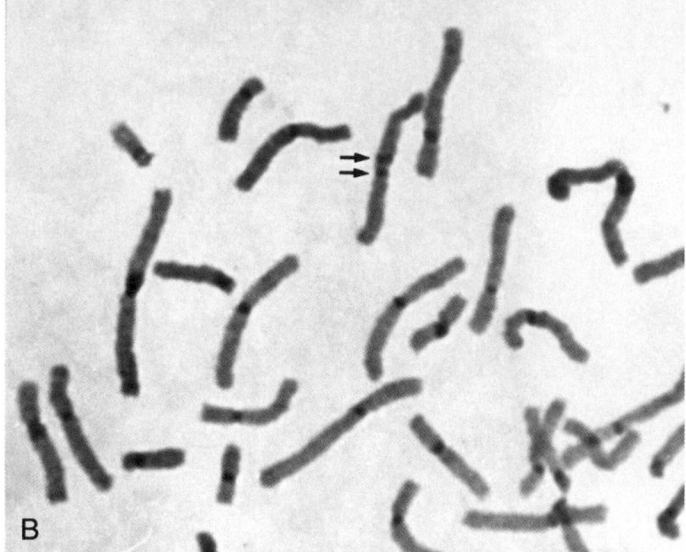

Figure 69–5 *A*, Q-banded metaphase showing bright fluorescence of the Y chromosome (arrow). *B*, C-banded chromosomes showing the dark staining centromeres. A dicentric chromosome was detected with two dark bands (two arrows).

earlier stage of cell division, prometaphase. At this point in the cell cycle, the chromosomes are less condensed and physically longer, making the presence of small abnormalities easier to detect.

The analysis is performed by a technologist viewing the cells at the microscope and, once the study is complete, a determination is made as to whether the chromosome complement is 'normal' or 'abnormal.' For documentation, representative metaphase cells are captured and karyograms (illustrations of the chromosomes of a given cell, Fig. 69–1) are prepared. Traditionally, the capture has been performed by photography using a 35 mm camera mounted on the microscope. The film is then developed and photographic prints are made. The chromosomes can be cut out and attached to a sheet of paper. The homologous pairs are arrayed from large to small with special placement for the pair of sex chromosomes. By convention, the shorter arm, the p arm, is oriented up, and the longer q arm is oriented down.

Computer-Assisted Imaging

Currently, most cytogenetics laboratories have moved to computer-assisted imaging. Although photographic prints give a high-resolution image, the technique requires significant time and effort. It is now possible to mount a charge-coupled device (CCD) video camera on the microscope in place of the 35 mm camera. Using specially designed software, an image of a metaphase cell is captured using a standard frame grabber, digitized, and displayed on the computer monitor. At this point, the software allows the image to be modified by lightening, darkening, or changing the contrast, and a variety of manipulations of the chromosomes are possible, including straightening and importing chromosomes from other fields. A karyogram can then be generated using a pattern-recognition subroutine that will automatically identify the chromosomes and place them in their proper places on a karyogram form. Depending on the software and the quality of the image, the accuracy of this process can vary from 10% to 85%. After the computer has taken its 'best guess,' a trained cytogenetic technologist must make the appropriate corrections. Once the chromosomes are properly positioned, additional cosmetic enhancements are possible to eliminate ragged edges or bits of background. The final version of the karyogram is then printed out directly by a high-resolution printer. Although the overall quality is not as high as a photographic rendering, there is a tremendous saving of time using the computerized system. A routine karyogram from capture to printing should take a trained technologist on average 15–20 minutes. Another major advantage of the computer-assisted system is in fluorescence microscopy.

Fluorescence In Situ Hybridization

The classical cytogenetic staining discussed above is the result of dyes that bind to the DNA or protein of a chromosome and allow visualization by light microscopy. In situ hybridization, a combination of molecular and cytogenetic technologies, opened another door that has allowed further investigation of chromosome anomalies. Here, instead of a dye, a molecular probe (i.e., a fragment of DNA) binds to the chromosome. In early studies, the probe was labeled with a radioactive compound (usually tritium) such that after 5–10 days of exposure to X-ray film, a pattern of silver grains could be detected identifying the chromosomal location of that probe. This technique facilitated gene mapping by identifying gene loci (Trask, 1991).

Autoradiography was useful, but only one probe at a time could be used, it required a significant length of time for exposure, and there was a degree of scatter of the silver grains that necessitated statistical analysis of the data obtained. In the mid-1980s, a variation of the technique was developed that has proven to be extremely useful in clinical applications. The new technology, fluorescence in situ hybridization (FISH), is quicker, more specific, and allows the use of multiple probes in a single hybridization procedure. Furthermore, instead of radioactively labeled probes, a fluorescent dye is used that is visualized using fluorescence microscopy (Ledbetter, 1989).

In clinical applications of FISH, the most common goal is to determine if a gene, a specific mutation, or a particular chromosomal rearrangement is present, so the molecular probe(s) used must be well characterized and specific to the locus in question. There are three basic types of probe. *Chromosome painting* probes are actually a cocktail of many unique DNA fragments from along the entire length of a chromosome such that, following hybridization, the entire chromosome fluoresces (Fig. 69–6A). *Repeat sequence* probes are isolated from telomere or centromere regions. Centromere probes are usually used in chromosome enumeration (i.e., to detect the gain or loss of specific chromosomes) (Figs. 69–6C and D) (Lichter, 1990). A true telomere probe recognizes the six base repeat present at the ends of all chromosomes and will confirm the presence or absence of the telomeric regions. A *unique sequence* probe is usually isolated from cloned DNA of a disease-causing gene or a fragment of DNA of known location associated with a particular gene. This type of probe is used to identify the presence or absence of the gene, gene region, or chromosomal rearrangement of interest (Cherif, 1989; Lindsay, 1993). *Subtelomere* probes are a subset of this category. Research revealed that there are unique sequences just proximal to the telomere of each chromosome arm that can be used for specific identification of each arm. The subtelomere probes that have been generated have become very valuable in characterizing cryptic rearrangements by determining if all subtelomeres are present and located on the correct chromosome arms and, if not, if a rearrangement has occurred (Fig. 69–6B). Furthermore, it has been shown that 3–5% of patients with unexplained mental retardation have a cytogenetically undetectable terminal deletion of a chromosome (Flint, 1995, 2003; Rosenberg, 2001). Subtelomere FISH now allows identification of such deletions and localization to the specific chromosome affected (National Institutes of Health and Institute of Molecular Medicine Collaboration, 1996; Irons, 2003).

Technique

FISH can be performed on either metaphase or interphase cells. For metaphase FISH, cells are cultured and harvested as for a routine

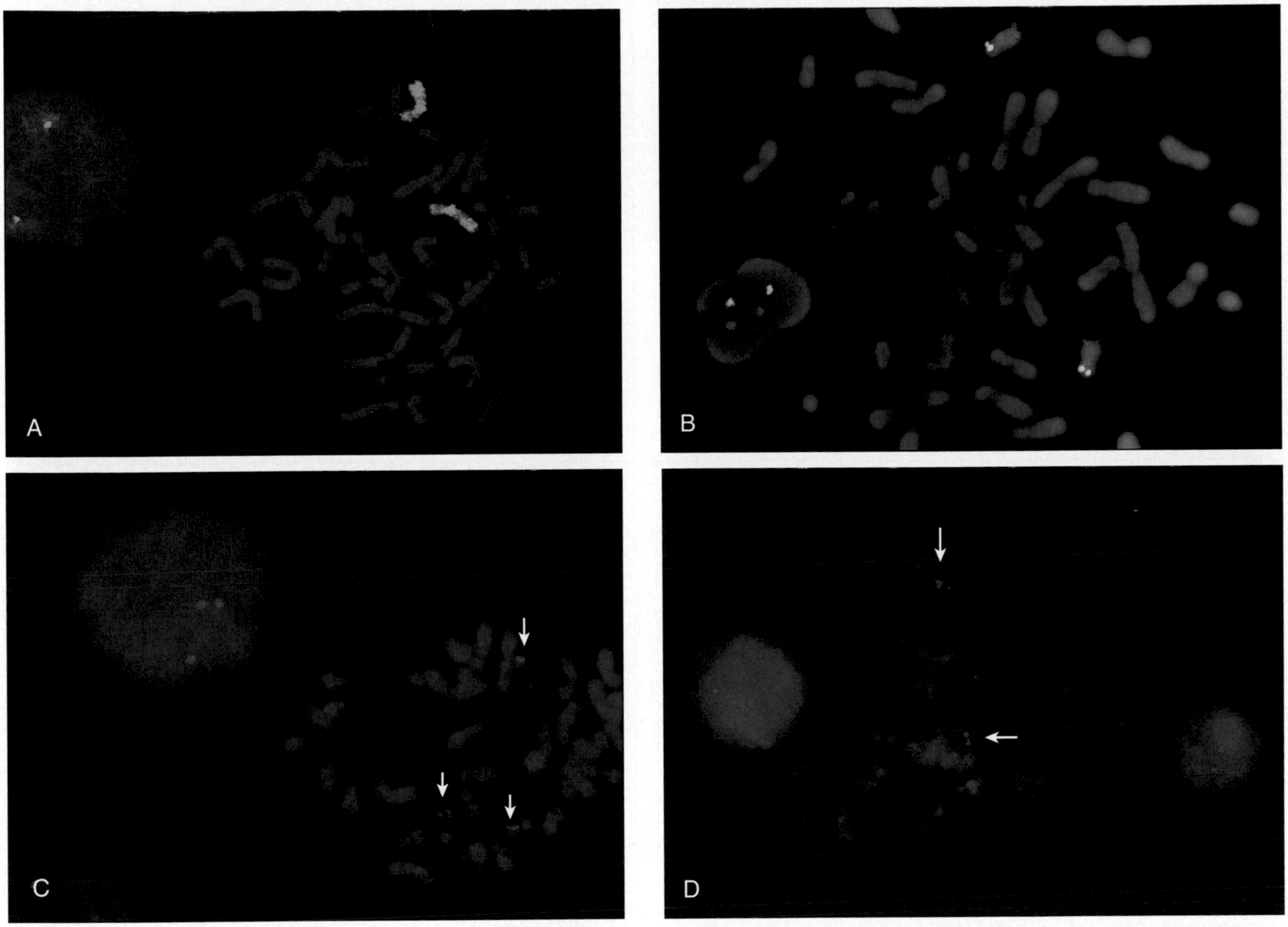

Figure 69–6 Fluorescence in situ hybridization (FISH). *A*, Whole chromosome paint probe highlighting the two X chromosomes in a female cell. *B*, Chromosomes showing hybridization with subtelomere probes. The p or short arm subtelomere is indicated by the green signals, and the q or long arm subtelomere is indicated by the red signals. Paired red and green signals are seen in the interphase nucleus to the left. *C* and *D*, Repeat sequence centromere probe for chromosome 21. *C*, Trisomy 21 seen at left in an interphase nucleus and at right in a metaphase (arrows). *D*, Normal complement of two copies of chromosome 21 (arrows) seen in interphase (left and right) and in a metaphase (center).

karyotype analysis, but no culture is required for interphase FISH. Fixed cells are collected and slides are made as described above for karyotyping. The DNA on the slides is then denatured and a fluorescently labeled single-stranded molecular probe is allowed to hybridize to the chromosomal DNA using an annealing temperature that favors hybridization of homologous regions of DNA (Fig. 69–7A). After an appropriate period of hybridization, excess probe is washed away and the nonhybridized DNA is counterstained with another fluorochrome to allow visualization of the entire chromosome complement. A fluorescent microscope with light from a 100 W mercury bulb in combination with appropriate sets of exciter filters allows evaluation of the cells. Due to the optical limitations of the glass filters, a maximum of three colors can be visualized on a typical fluorescent microscope. For documentation, a 35 mm camera attached to the microscope can be used, although superior results are obtained using a computer-assisted system to acquire the fluorescent images. Appropriate software packages will also allow enhancement of weak signals and sharpening of the image.

One of the most critical elements in FISH is the selection of a specific probe or probes that will help to answer a clinical question. For example, one of the most useful clinical applications of FISH is the detection of microdeletions too small to be seen using classical cytogenetics (Fig. 69–7B to D). The gene must be known and the probe used must be homologous to the critical region of the gene that is usually deleted. Hybridization with the probe should result in a fluorescent signal only at the target locus. If a signal is present, DNA complementary to the probe is present, so there is no deletion (Fig. 69–7B). However, the absence of signal indicates that a deletion exists (i.e., there is no DNA sequence present on the chromosome that is complementary to the probe, so no hybridization can occur) (Fig. 69–7D). A control probe to a different region of the chromosome being tested is usually used as a hybridization control (Fig. 69–7C). An

unaffected individual should have two signals per cell for each autosomal gene, one signal for each chromosome of the pair (Fig. 69–8A). An affected individual with a deletion should have a single signal per cell, showing one normal and one deleted chromosome (Fig. 69–8B). The control probe should show two signals per cell in all cells that are scored. In a metaphase cell, the chromosomes may be short and condensed, with each chromatid individually visible, resulting in a discrete FISH signal on each chromatid. In these cells, there may appear to be two signals per chromosome for a total of four signals but, in actual scoring, only complete chromosomes are considered so a signal on one or both chromatids would be counted as just one positive signal.

One of the problems with this detection system is that the lack of signal is the positive indication of a deletion. Technical failure of hybridization may also result in absence of signal. To eliminate this as a source of error, a minimum of 20 cells must be evaluated and all cells must agree in signal count. If mosaicism is suspected, additional cells may be surveyed. In addition, unique sequence probes are currently used in combination with a control probe (Fig. 69–7C). The secondary probe is localized to the same arm of the chromosome as the deletion locus. It may be labeled with the same fluorochrome as the deletion locus probe but it has been found that the interpretation of the hybridization results is easier if the control site probe is labeled with a different-color fluorochrome. In all cells evaluated, two clear control signals must be seen, and then the corresponding signals for the disease locus can be recorded. This provides a hybridization control as well as a marker for the chromosome of interest (Fig. 69–7D). If a dual color system is used, results may be obtained in interphase as well as metaphase cells.

Chromosome painting probes are most useful in identifying complex rearrangements or marker chromosomes. If a patient has an abnormal chromosome with extra material of unknown origin, it may be possible to

VIII

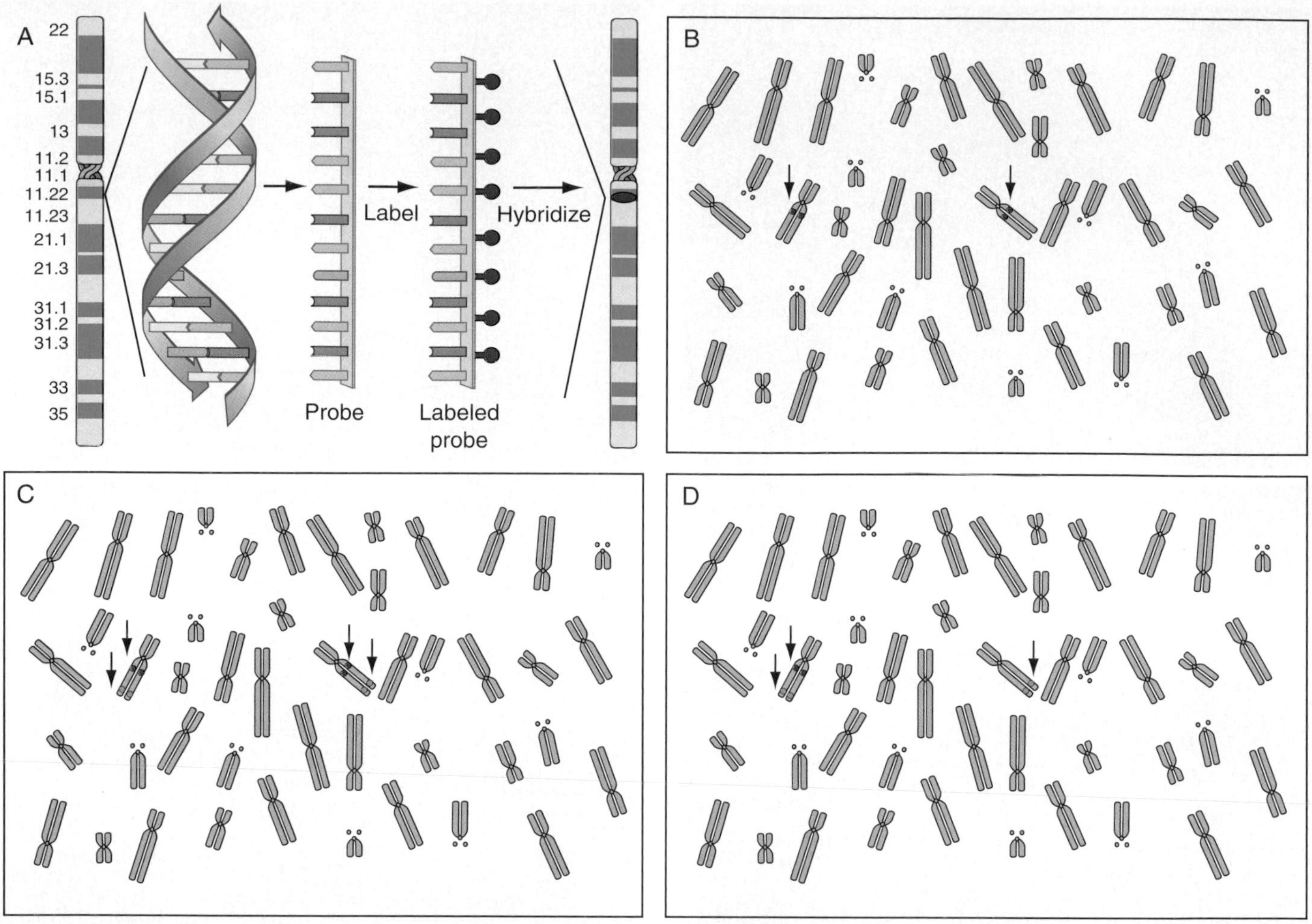

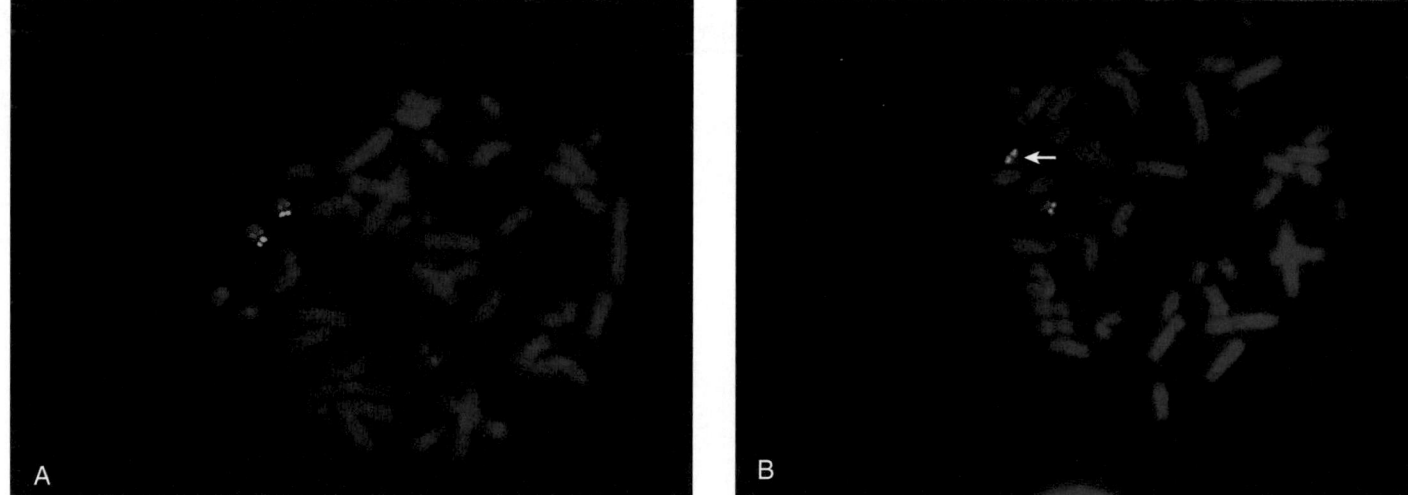

Figure 69–7 *A*, Schematic of FISH technology. DNA derived from a known gene is rendered single stranded, labeled with a fluorescent tag, then hybridized back to the chromosomes of a metaphase cell. *B* to *D*, Depiction of a metaphase cell with 46 chromosomes that has been processed using FISH technology. The labeled probes hybridized to targets are indicated with arrows. *B*, Dual signals indicating hybridization to both alleles of target gene. *C*, Target gene indicated by red signal and a control probe indicated in green. Complete hybridization to all alleles. *D*, Hybridization of both controls (green) but presence of only a single target gene indicating deletion of one allele.

Figure 69–8 FISH detection of a microdeletion of chromosome 22 associated with velocardiofacial syndrome. *A*, An individual with no deletion showing the presence of one red (gene locus) and one green (control locus) signal for each chromosome 22. *B*, Patient with a deletion seen as a chromosome with only a single green (control) signal. The homologous chromosome 22 is 'normal' with one red and one green signal.

use chromosome painting to identify the source of the extra DNA. This may help in either diagnosis or prognosis of the individual. For example, in the case of a patient with only one identifiable X chromosome and a small, unidentified marker chromosome, it will be important to determine if the origin of the marker is an X or a Y chromosome. This can be accomplished using chromosome paints for the X and Y chromosomes labeled with different fluorochromes.

FISH probes are most informative when evaluated in metaphase cells where it is possible to identify the specific chromosome to which the probe hybridizes. However, in some cell preparations, very few metaphase cells may be present and, in these cases, information may be obtained with unique sequence or repeat sequence probes in interphase nuclei. Here, the technical problems are increased as a result of random loss of signal, extra signals, and overlapping signals in cells, so additional cells (a

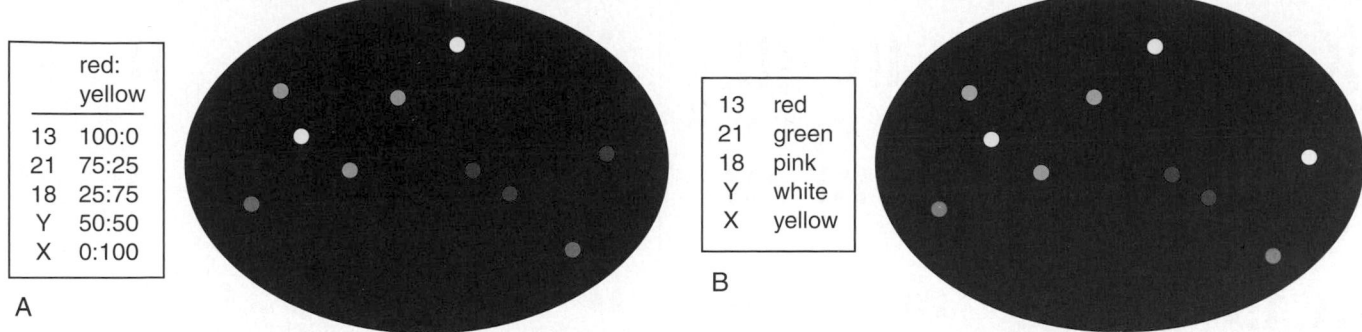

red: yellow	
13	100:0
21	75:25
18	25:75
Y	50:50
X	0:100

A

13	red
21	green
18	pink
Y	white
X	yellow

B

Figure 69–9 Multicolor FISH. *A,* Diagram of the staining pattern for five combination probes (chromosomes 13, 18, 21, X, and Y) in an interphase cell. Table at the left shows relative proportions of the red and yellow fluorochromes used for each probe. *B,* The same cell depicted in A, now showing the computer-derived artificial color assignments (key shown in box to left). This cell can now be interpreted as having two copies each for chromosomes 13, 21, and X, three copies of chromosome 18, and one Y chromosome.

total of 50–200) must be counted to obtain a statistically significant result.

Multicolor Fluorescence In Situ Hybridization

Another advantage of FISH is the ability to hybridize multiple probes to a single slide to obtain a better understanding of chromosome rearrangements (Schrock, 1996; Speicher, 1996). For most FISH probes, the maximum number of colors is three (one target sequence, one control sequence, and one counterstain), and this can be handled by a typical fluorescent microscope. However, if more than three colors are needed, a computer-assisted imaging system is required. This is because a fluorescent image is the result of the light from the mercury bulb passing through an exciter filter, hitting the fluorochrome on the slide, and transmitting an image of the appropriate color to the eyepiece for viewing. Each fluorochrome requires its own filter so, for each additional color desired, the light must pass through additional thicknesses of glass. The optical properties of glass and light limit the total number of viewable colors to three. However, with a computer-assisted system, detection of multiple colors becomes possible. The computer does not actually 'see' more colors but it can detect subtle differences in shades better than the human eye. In a relatively simple example, two fluorochromes are used and mixed in varying proportions to give a range of colors. In the example in Figure 69–9A, a red fluorochrome is mixed with a yellow fluorochrome generating intermediate colors from red to yellow. Eight signals are seen, but as viewed through the microscope, it is impossible to be absolutely sure which signal corresponds to a particular chromosome. Although difficult to distinguish by the human eye, the computer can register each color as a different shade of gray and then the software assigns a unique color to that shade for display on the computer monitor. Figure 69–9B shows the final multi-color version using many different colors now easily distinguishable but very different from the original presentation (Fig. 69–9A). Using the key to the left, the following chromosomes are detected: two each for chromosomes 13, 21, and X; three chromosomes 18, and one Y chromosome. This cell is therefore trisomic for chromosome 18 with an XXY sex chromosome complement. Combinations of fluorochromes have been developed that allow detection of each of the 24 different chromosomes followed by a unique color assignment by the computer (Reid, 1992a, 1992b; Divane, 1994).

Chromosome Abnormalities

Clinical cytogenetic testing is an integral part of clinical medicine. Finding a particular chromosome anomaly may explain a physical problem or phenotypic abnormality in the patient and be directly associated with a disease diagnosis. It is therefore critical to determine if an affected individual has a chromosome complement that differs from the standard pattern of 23 pairs of chromosomes with known morphology. There are two basic categories of cytogenetically detectable variation: (1) numerical and (2) structural change.

Numerical Abnormalities

In humans and other mammals, the chromosomes occur in pairs, so of the 46 human chromosomes there are only 23 uniquely different chromosomes. A set of 23 comprises the haploid (N) number of chromosomes, which is the number of chromosomes in a gamete. At fertilization, two haploid complements join to form a zygote with 46 chromosomes, the diploid ($2N$) complement. Errors in division can give rise to chromosome complements that have more or less than 46 chromosomes. Exact multiples of the

haploid set of chromosomes is called *euploidy.* Gain or loss of one or a few chromosomes is known as *aneuploidy.*

Euploidy

Diploidy, the normal state of human cells, is a form of euploidy. Abnormal euploidies include triploidy ($3N$ = 69 chromosomes) and tetraploidy ($4N$ = 92 chromosomes), which are not compatible with life and are detected primarily in spontaneous abortus tissues. Triploidy (Fig. 69–10A) may be due to the failure in gametogenesis of one of the meiotic divisions, giving rise to a $2N$ gamete that, when fertilized by a haploid gamete from the other parent, produces a triploid zygote. Alternatively, a $3N$ complement may be derived from dispermy, the fertilization of a haploid egg by two sperm, and this generally results in a partial hydatidiform mole. Tetraploidy, on the other hand, is usually a postmeiotic event and presents as a duplication of a diploid complement (XXXX or XXYY), most probably due to failure of an early mitotic cleavage division in the zygote.

Aneuploidy

More common are nondisjunctional errors resulting in aneuploidy. Here, a single pair of chromosomes fails to disjoin properly in division, giving rise to one extra chromosome or one missing chromosome per cell. Occasionally, more than one pair of chromosomes may be involved, but these cases are extremely rare. Nondisjunction errors may occur in either meiosis or mitosis. Early mitotic nondisjunction in a zygote may result in an individual with the aberrant chromosome complement in all cells of the body, but a latter division error usually produces a *mosaic,* an individual with two cell lines that differ only by a single chromosome.

In normal meiosis, one DNA replication is followed by two cell divisions resulting in four haploid (N) gametes (one copy of each chromosome) (Fig 69–11A). The first meiotic division is the reduction division, in which the total number of chromosomes per cell is reduced by half. The second meiotic division is a simple mitotic type of division with a separation of the centromeres and distribution of the chromosomes to daughter cells. Meiotic errors may result in gametes with either an extra or missing chromosome (Angell, 1994). A nondisjunction error in the first meiotic division (Fig. 69–11B) leads to two gametes that are disomic for one chromosome and two gametes that are missing that chromosome (nullosomic). When fertilized, the former will give a trisomic conception for the nondisjoined chromosome (example: trisomy 21 in Fig. 69–10B), and the latter will result in a monosomy. Similarly, Fig. 69–11C shows an error in the second meiotic division resulting in two normal haploid gametes, one disomic gamete and one nullosomic gamete.

Trisomy or monosomy may occur for any chromosome, but most of these are incompatible with life and will terminate spontaneously. Trisomy 16, for example, is the most commonly detected trisomy in spontaneous abortus tissue but is not reported in liveborn individuals. Liveborn autosomal trisomies include chromosomes 13, 18, and 21. Infrequently, patients with a mosaic chromosome complement for trisomies 8, 9, or 22 are identified. Sex chromosome trisomies are viable and well documented (see below). The only viable monosomy is of the X chromosome (45,X). Examples of clinically significant aneuploidies will be discussed later in this chapter.

Since trisomies and monosomies are largely incompatible with life, it had been assumed that these would result in fetal wastage. However, molecular analyses have shown that a small fraction of these aneuploid conceptions are 'rescued' and go on to produce liveborn children. In the case of a monosomy, the rescue is accomplished by duplication of the single

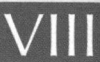

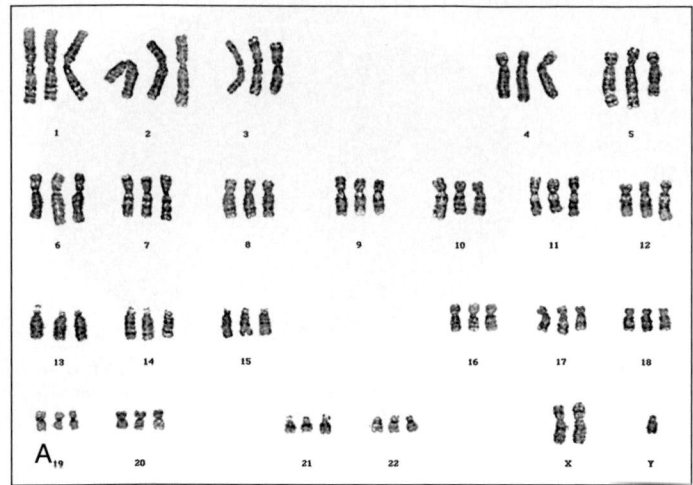
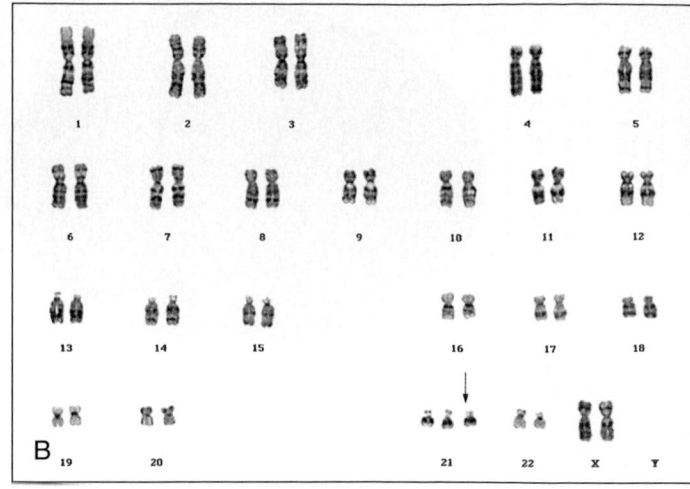

Figure 69–10 Numerical chromosome abnormalities. *A*, Triploid (3*n*) chromosome complement with three copies of each chromosome (69,XXY). *B*, Trisomy 21 (47,XX,+21) with one extra chromosome 21 (arrow).

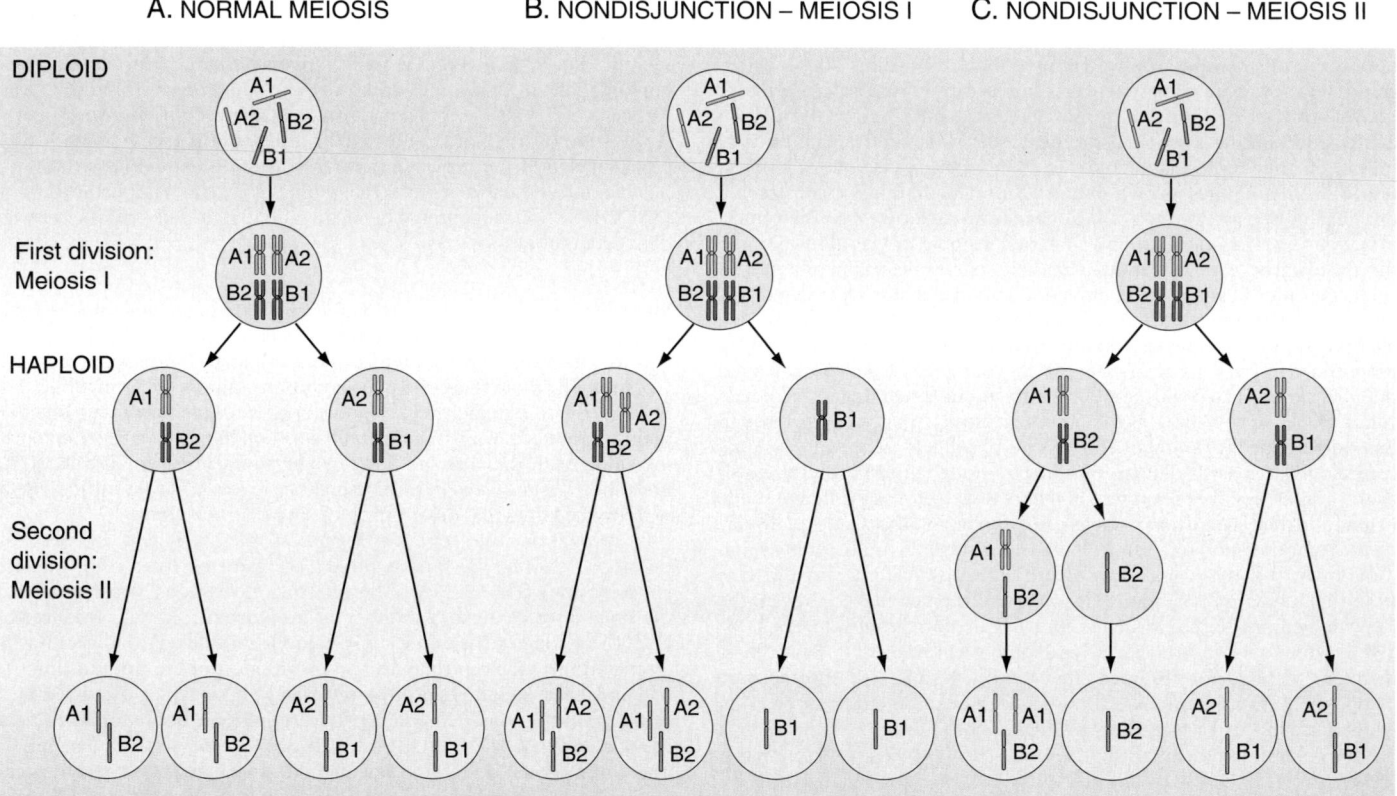

Figure 69–11 Meiosis and meiotic nondisjunction errors resulting in aneuploid gametes. *A*, Normal meiosis generating four gametes with a haploid chromosome set. *B*, Nondisjunction in meiosis I leading to an extra copy of chromosome 'A' (heterodisomy) in two gametes (far left) but the lack of any 'A' chromosome (nullosomy) in the remaining two gametes (right). *C*, Nondisjunction in meiosis II results in two gametes with a normal chromosome complement (right), one gamete missing an 'A' chromosome (left center), and one gamete with an extra duplicated chromosome (two copies of 'A1' resulting in isodisomy for chromosome 'A1'(left).

existing chromosome, resulting in a chromosome complement with *uniparental isodisomy* for that chromosome (two copies of the same chromosome inherited from one parent) (Fig. 69–12, right) (Ledbetter, 1995). This is exemplified by several reported cases in the literature in which a child affected with cystic fibrosis (CF) was shown to be homozygous for the ΔF508 mutation, although molecular tests on both parents revealed that only one was a carrier of ΔF508 (Spence, 1988; Voss, 1989). The interpretation is that the conception was a nonviable monosomy 7 rescued by duplication of the existing chromosome 7 that happened to be carrying the mutation for cystic fibrosis. A similar situation is possible in the case of a trisomy. Again, most trisomies are nonviable but, if one of the

three chromosomes is lost, a disomy for that chromosome pair is reinstated (Fig. 69–12, left). In a set of three chromosomes, loss of a single chromosome will result in a complement with one maternal and one paternal chromosome (*biparental heterodisomy*) two out of three times. One third of the time, the two remaining chromosomes are from a single parent (i.e., uniparental disomy). In this situation, it makes a difference in which meiotic division the error occurred. A first-division nondisjunction will result in heterodisomy, which is two homologous but heterozygous chromosomes (one grandmaternal and one grandpaternal); however, a second division error will result in duplicate copies of a single chromosome, isodisomy (Figs 69–11B and C and 69–13). Although it

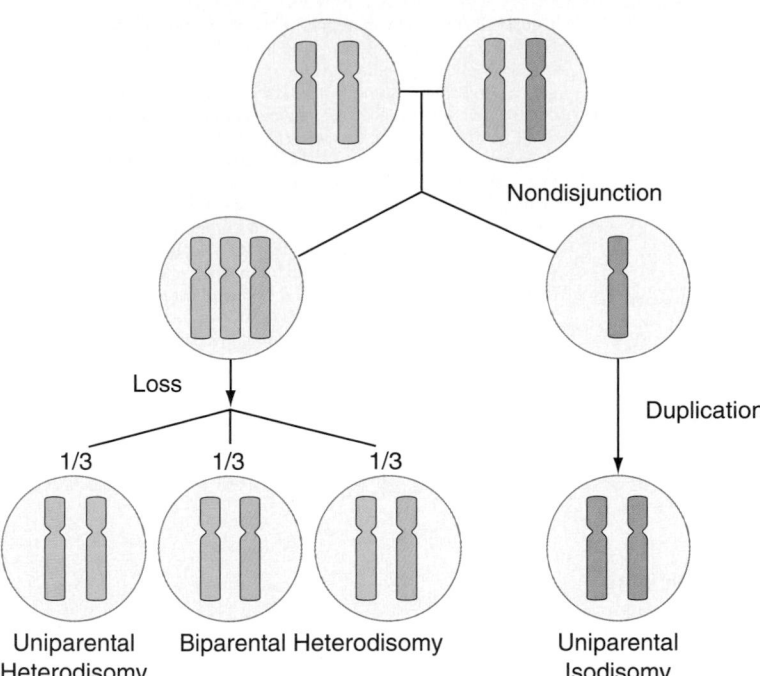

Figure 69–12 Generation of uniparental disomy from nondisjunction errors. To the left of the diagram, heterodisomy resulting from reduction of a trisomy to a disomy is illustrated. On the right, isodisomy as the result of monosomy rescue (duplication of a single existing chromosome) is seen.

used to be thought that having two chromosomes per pair was sufficient, the data strongly indicate that, in some cases, it is essential for the pairs to comprise one maternal and one paternal chromosome. This issue, including the problems of uniparental versus biparental disomy and isodisomy versus heterodisomy, is of major importance in understanding issues of *imprinting*, a topic discussed in detail in Chapter 72 (Nicholls, 1998; Hall, 1990, Cassidy, 1992; Petersen, 1992).

Structural Chromosome Abnormalities

Chromosomes are not static structures but undergo recombination in both meiosis and mitosis. This is a natural process that is critical in generating variation in the species, so a highly developed regulatory system is in place to prevent error from occurring. Nevertheless, errors do occur, sometimes resulting in chromosome rearrangements that change the structure of one or more chromosomes. Such abnormalities are quite varied and are often patient-specific. Rearrangements may be (1) *balanced*, if all the chromosomal material is present and functional but simply arranged in a different conformation; or (2) *unbalanced*, if there is loss and/or duplication of some chromosomal material. Balanced rearrangements are usually clinically benign and tend to be stably transmitted but may increase the risk of errors in meiosis resulting in chromosomal imbalances in fetuses or liveborn children. Unbalanced chromosome complements are generally associated with an abnormal clinical phenotype that often includes developmental delay and mental retardation.

A *deletion* is the loss of a part of a chromosome and leads to partial monosomy of the chromosome involved (Fig. 69–14B). Deletions vary in size from quite large to very small and may be *terminal* (left), loss of a portion of the chromosome including the telomere; or *interstitial* (right), loss of an internal piece of chromosome. Chromosome breakage, unequal crossing over, or nondisjunction errors involving chromosome rearrangements may result in a deletion. In general, larger deletions result in more severe clinical abnormalities because of the greater number of gene loci that are missing.

A *duplication* is the presence of an additional copy of a chromosome segment that leads to partial trisomy for that chromosome (Fig. 69–14C). This anomaly may also be *terminal* or *interstitial*. True duplications appear to be quite rare and are usually sporadic. Duplications are generated by the same mechanisms as deletions and may be the reciprocal outcome of those processes. As is true of deletions, the larger the duplicated piece of chromosome, the more severe the clinical abnormalities tend to be.

An *inversion* is a reversal of a chromosomal segment with respect to the normal gene arrangement and requires a minimum of two breaks in one chromosome (Fig. 69–14D). Inversions are classified as either (1) *paracentric*, where the two breaks occur on the same side of the centromere (i. e., in the same arm); or (2) *pericentric*, where the breaks occur on opposite sides of the centromere and the inversion involves both arms (Fig. 69–15A). The majority of inversions are balanced but, if the chromosome breaks within

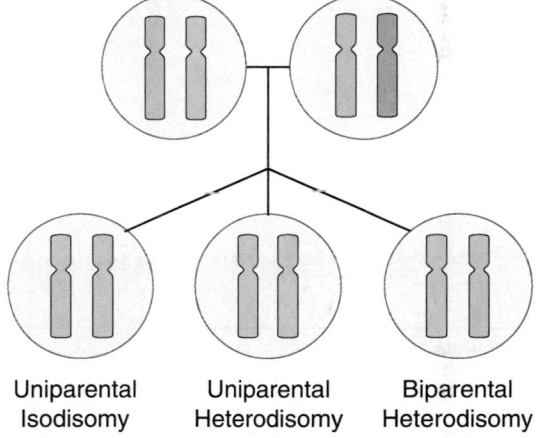

Figure 69–13 Isodisomy versus heterodisomy. The expected conformation of a cell is biparental heterodisomy (right), i.e., one chromosome from each parent. Division errors can result in an aberrant distribution of parental chromosomes such that two copies of one chromosome from one parent (uniparental isodisomy) (left) or two different chromosomes from the same parent (uniparental heterodisomy) (center) occur.

a gene and disrupts normal production of a required gene product, clinical abnormalities may be detected. There is an increased risk of meiotic error, and inversion carriers frequently exhibit infertility or early spontaneous fetal loss due to unbalanced chromosome products.

For an inversion carrier, meiosis begins as normal, with the pairing of the homologous chromosomes. The process is a little more complex for an inverted chromosome, which must form a structure known as an inversion loop (Fig. 69–15B) in order for the homologous loci to pair (i.e., A to a, B to b, C to c, etc.). If no recombination occurs while the loop is present and the chromosomes separate normally, the gametes will not be negatively impacted. However, crossing over within the inversion loop can lead to unbalanced meiotic products. For a paracentric inversion, the results of recombination are usually nonviable acentric and dicentric chromosomes, so there is an apparent suppression of recombination (i.e., the only viable gametes produced are from nonrecombined chromosomes) (Fig. 69–15B). For pericentric inversions, it is possible that gametes with chromosome duplication and/or deletion may be derived. In general, larger pericentric inversions result in smaller duplications/deficiencies and increase the likelihood that a child will be live born with a chromosome imbalance and probably phenotypic abnormalities. Once an inversion carrier has been identified, prenatal diagnosis can be utilized to assess the chromosomes for each conception.

NORMAL:

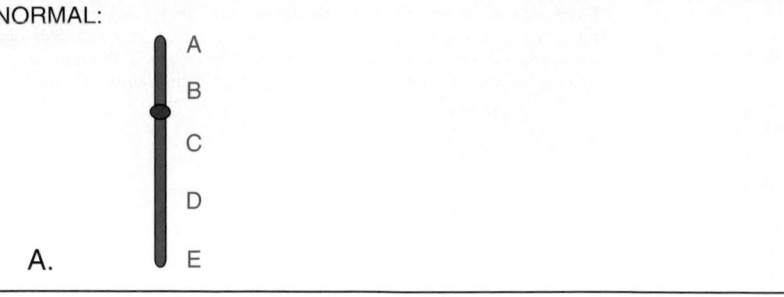

A.

DELETION:

Terminal   Interstitial

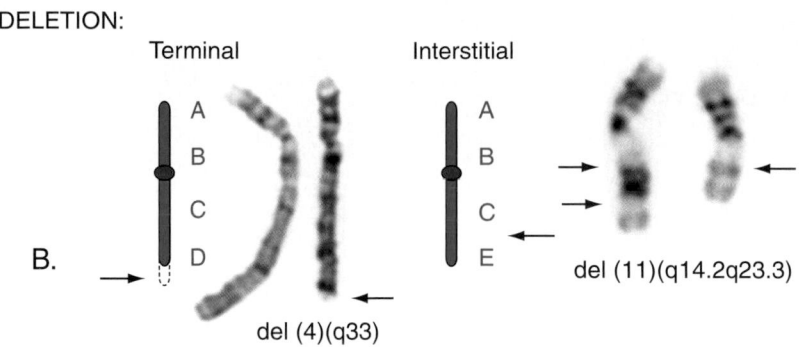

B.   del (4)(q33)   del (11)(q14.2q23.3)

DUPLICATION:

Terminal   Interstitial

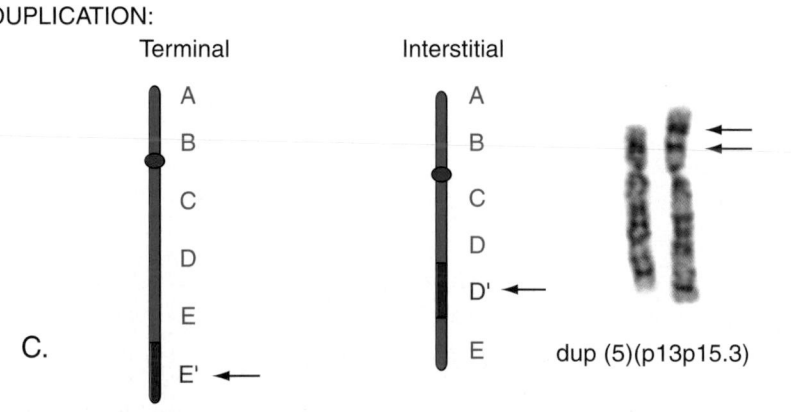

C.   dup (5)(p13p15.3)

INVERSION:

Pericentric   Paracentric

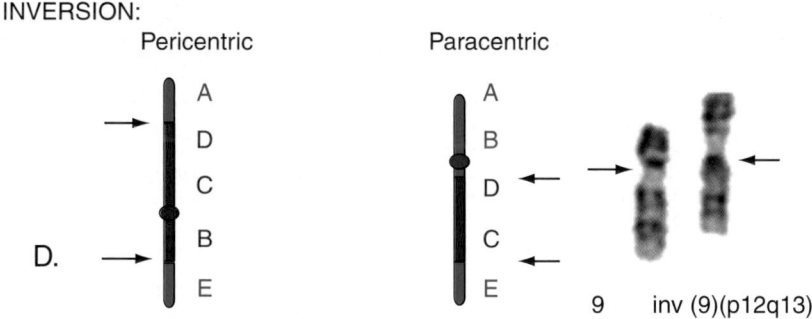

D.   9   inv (9)(p12q13)

Figure 69–14 Schematic representations of different structural chromosome anomalies described in the text associated with examples of each anomaly. *A,* The normal configuration of a generalized chromosome, where A to E represent different gene loci and the centromere is represented by a dot located between the B and C loci. *B, Deletion:* Chromosome deletion showing terminal (loss of E locus) and interstitial (loss of D locus) configurations. Examples: terminal deletion of the long arm of chromosome 4 (del[4][q33]), and an interstitial deletion of the long arm of chromosome 11 (del[11][q14.2q23.3]). *C, Duplication:* Chromosome duplication showing terminal (gain of E′) and interstitial (gain of D′) configurations. Example: terminal duplication of the short arm of chromosome 5 (double arrows indicate duplicated band). *D, Inversion:* Chromosome inversion showing pericentric and paracentric forms. Example: pericentric inversion of chromosome 9 (arrows indicate centromeres).

Translocations are rearrangements involving two or more nonhomologous chromosomes. Each chromosome breaks once and the pieces exchange places, establishing two (or more) derivative chromosomes (Fig. 69–14E). As with inversions, the majority of translocations are balanced, and only when an important structural gene is disrupted does the translocation have clinical ramifications.

The primary danger of a balanced translocation is that carriers are at increased risk for chromosomally abnormal liveborn children. In the first meiotic division, translocated chromosomes assume a cross-shaped structure in order for all alleles to pair properly (Fig. 69–16). At anaphase, the alternate chromosomes must segregate together to generate balanced gametes. Up to one third of the time, the chromosomes will not segregate in this manner and the resulting gametes will be unbalanced. The most common errors are termed adjacent-1 and adjacent-2 segregation. Although both of these patterns result in duplication/deficiency of chromosomal material in the gametes, adjacent-2 is more deleterious, since it is characterized by the unnatural occurrence of homologous centromeres in a single cell. Viability of a fetus receiving an unbalanced gamete is dependent on the chromosomes and genes involved in the translocation and the size of the duplication/deletion. Chromosomes may also follow a 3:1 segregation pattern, in which three chromosomes separate to one cell with the remaining chromosome in the second cell. This results in gross imbalances of chromosomal material and is usually lethal in utero. Once a translocation carrier has been identified, prenatal diagnosis is possible.

Robertsonian translocations are a variation of the classic translocation. They occur only between two acrocentric chromosomes and appear to be a fusion of the long arms at the centromere, with the resulting loss of both short arms (Fig. 69–14E). Loss of the acrocentric short arms is not deleterious, since multiple copies of the rRNA genes are located on all acrocentric chromosomes. An individual who is a Robertsonian translocation carrier has a chromosome count of 45 because two chromosomes have functionally become one and share one centromere. These individuals are at increased risk for meiotic nondisjunction errors resulting in children who are trisomic for one of the rearranged chromosomes. The most common example of this is an individual with a Robertsonian translocation involving chromosomes 13 and 14 who has liveborn children with trisomy 13 (Fig. 69–17). The affected

TRANSLOCATION:

Reciprocal –

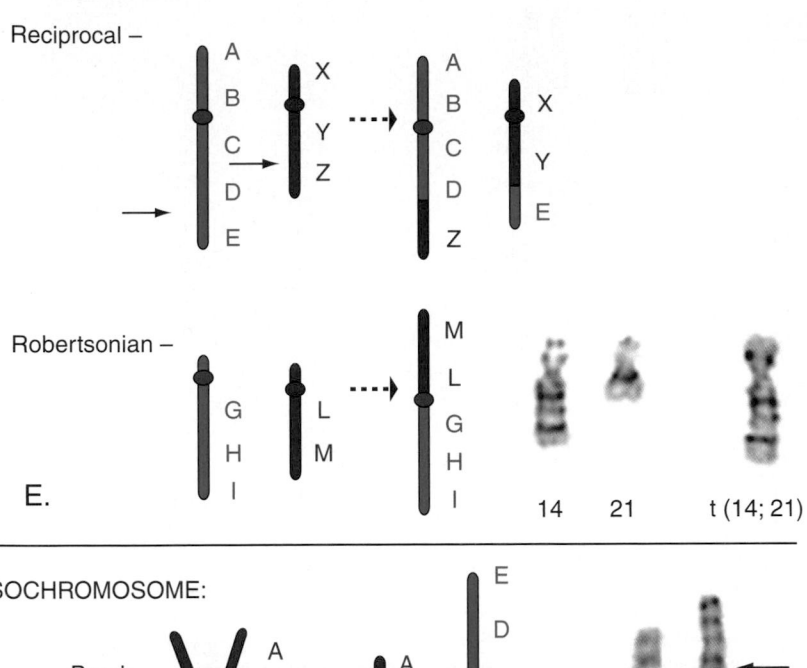

Robertsonian –

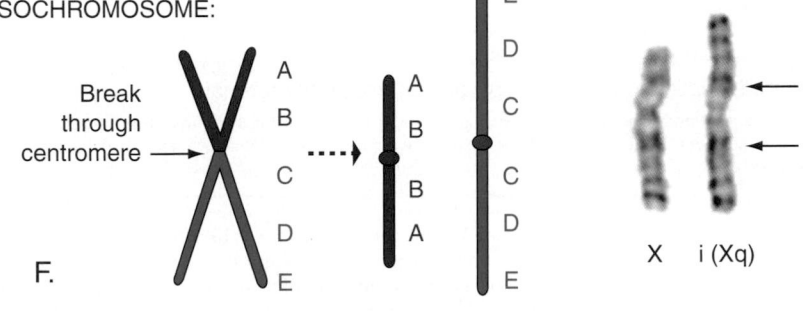

E.

14   21   t (14; 21)

ISOCHROMOSOME:

Break through centromere →

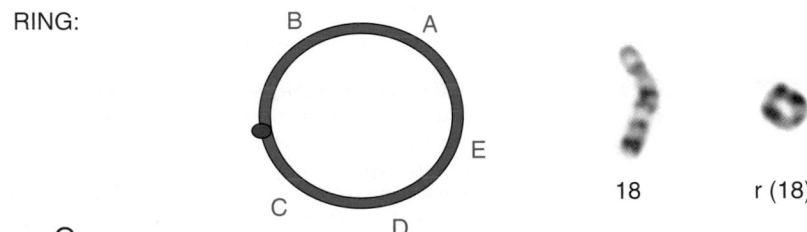

F.

X   i (Xq)

RING:

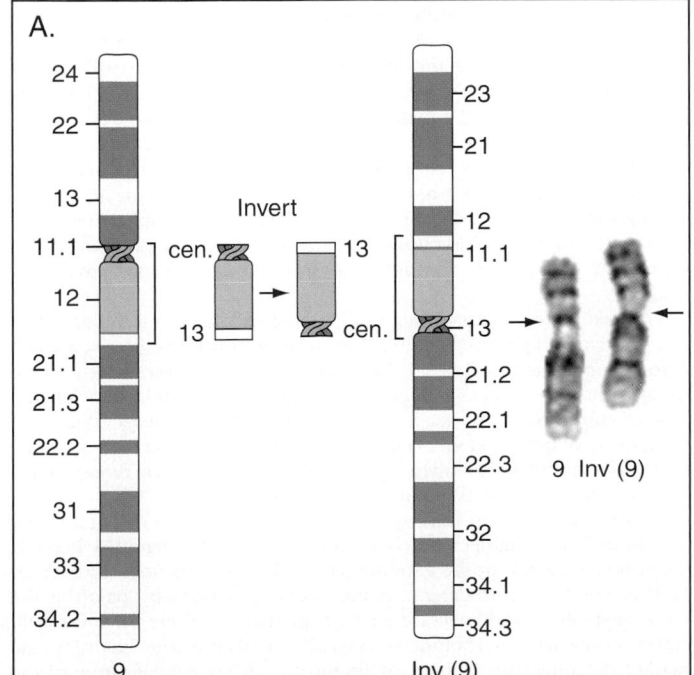

G.

18   r (18)

Figure 69–14 *(cont'd) E, Translocation*: Reciprocal translocation where the E and Z loci exchange places. A Robertsonian translocation shown by the fusion of two acrocentric chromosomes at the centromere. Example: chromosomes 14 and 21 followed by the 14;21 Robertsonian translocation. *F, Isochromosome*: results from a misdivision of the centromere generating inverted duplications of the long and short arms of the original chromosome. Example: isochromosome of the long arm of the X chromosome. *G, Ring chromosome*. Example: chromosome 18 and ring 18.

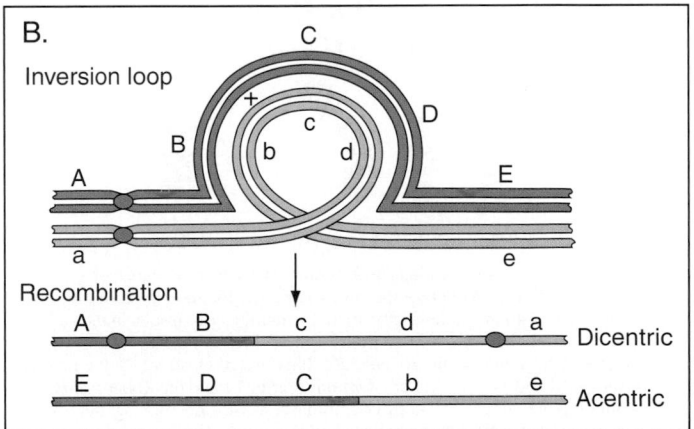

Figure 69–15 Chromosome inversion. *A,* Diagram of a pericentric inversion of chromosome 9 using ideograms to illustrate the mechanism of inversion. Banded chromosomes demonstrating this inversion are shown to the right. *B,* Inversion loop showing the pairing of homologs in meiosis for one normal chromosome (dark green) and one with a paracentric inversion (light green). If recombination occurs at the point indicated by the X in the loop, recombinant chromosomes would be generated as shown at the bottom. In the case of a paracentric inversion, the recombined chromosomes produced would be either dicentric or acentric.

VII

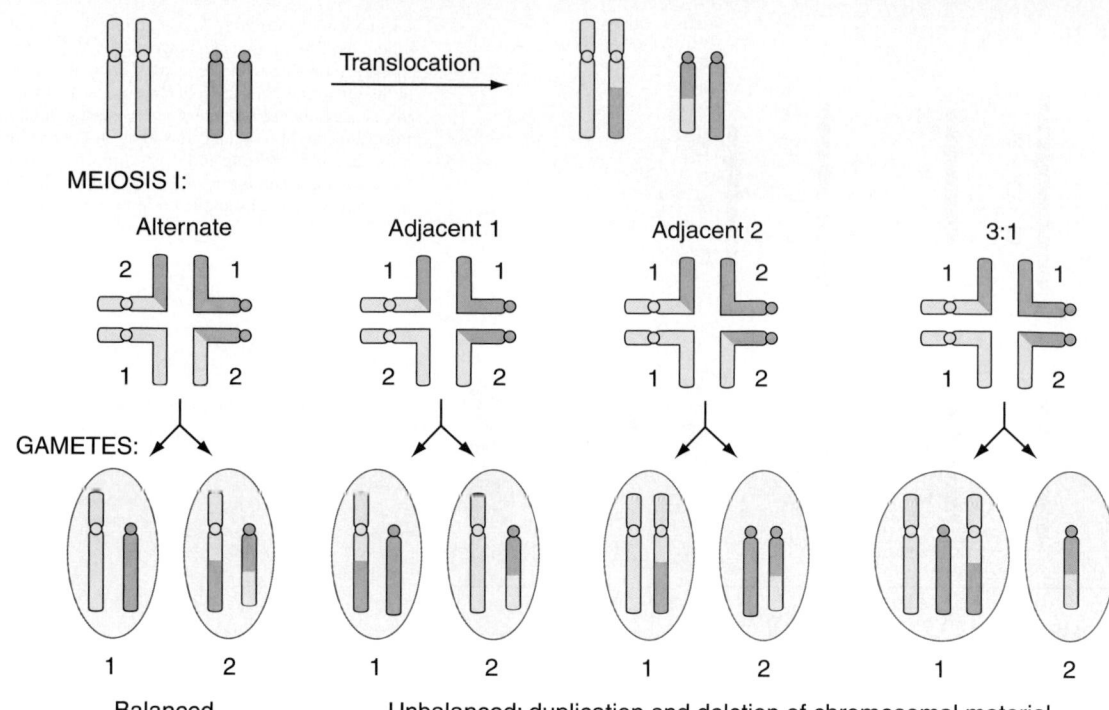

Translocation

MEIOSIS I:

Alternate	Adjacent 1	Adjacent 2	3:1

GAMETES:

1	2	1	2	1	2	1	2

Balanced   Unbalanced: duplication and deletion of chromosomal material

Figure 69–16 Chromosome translocation. Generation of gametes from a hypothetical translocation in meiosis is diagrammed. The chromosomes pair in a cross-shaped configuration in meiosis I. Alternate segregation will result in balanced gametes. Adjacent 1, adjacent 2, or 3:1 segregation will produce unbalanced gametes, which may give rise to an abnormal liveborn child. (Only one of several possible 3:1 segregations is shown).

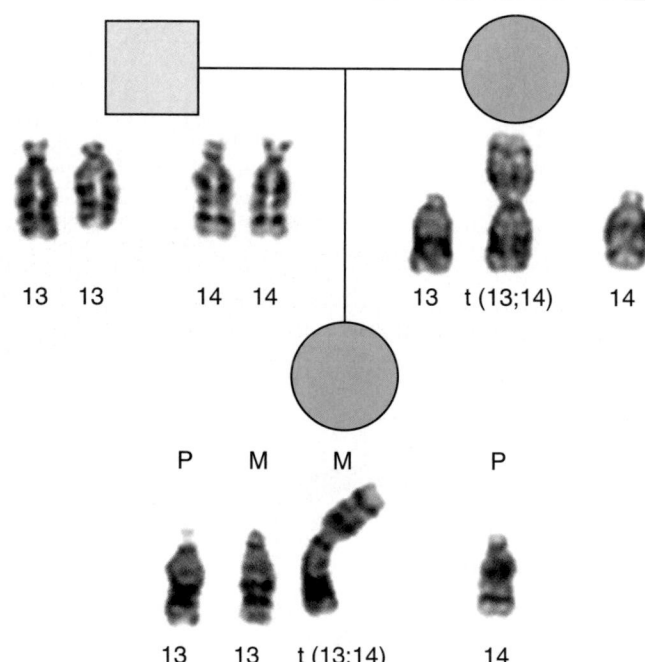

13   13   14   14   13   t (13;14)   14

P   M   M   P

13   13   t (13;14)   14

Figure 69–17 Pedigree and banded chromosomes showing inheritance of a Robertsonian translocation of chromosomes 13 and 14. The mother carries the translocation (t(13;14)) in a balanced form, but a meiotic error results in the transmission of both the Robertsonian translocation chromosome and the chromosome 13 from the mother to the child. The child has trisomy 13 (P = paternal chromosomes 13 and 14; M = maternal chromosomes 13 and the Robertsonian translocation). *Note*: the second copy of chromosome 14 is not missing, but is present as part of the Robertsonian rearrangement.

child will have 46 chromosomes, including two free copies of chromosomes 13 and the Robertsonian translocation. Another common rearrangement is a Robertsonian 14;21 translocation (Fig. 69–14E), which could give rise to trisomy 21 progeny.

Although the most common Robertsonian translocations occur between nonhomologous acrocentric chromosomes, it is possible to have such a rearrangement between homologous chromosomes. For example, an individual with a Robertsonian 21;21 translocation would have a total of

45 chromosomes including the translocation in which the two 21s are joined at the centromere. This type of rearrangement is virtually always de novo, since carriers of the abnormality are unlikely to have normal progeny. Possible gametes include: (1) a cell with the Robertsonian translocation (two copies of chromosome 21), which, if fertilized, will give rise to a Down syndrome child; or (2) a cell with no copies of chromosome 21, which, if fertilized, will result in a monosomy 21, which is not compatible with life.

A chromosome that is the result of misdivision of the centromere during cell division, resulting in two copies of one chromosome arm but missing the other arm, is an *isochromosome* (Fig. 69–14F). This mechanism can result in two derivative chromosomes – one with an inverted duplication of the short arm and one with an inverted duplication of the long arm. If both derivative chromosomes are retained in the cell, it would be trisomic for that chromosome, a condition that is usually lethal. In a living individual, therefore, it is most common that one of the two derivative chromosomes is lost, resulting in a carrier who is trisomic for only one duplicated arm and monosomic for the other arm. The best known example is the isochromosome of the long arm of the X. A patient with Turner syndrome (see below under Sex Chromosome Aneuploidies) may have one intact X chromosome and one isochromosome Xq (trisomy for the long arm but a monosomy for the short arm of the X). Since two functional copies of the X short arm are required for normal female development, this chromosome arrangement results in abnormal development. Acrocentric chromosomes may also form isochromosomes (inverted duplication of the long arm), but the resulting homozygosity of all loci present could lead to expression of recessive disorders that would otherwise not have been evident.

A *ring chromosome* occurs when both telomeres of a chromosome are lost and the remaining portion of the chromosome circularizes to re-establish chromosome stability (Fig. 69–14G). Unfortunately, these constructs are usually unstable because replication can result in interlinked circles that lead to chromosome breakage and loss when the homologs attempt to separate at anaphase. Under certain circumstances, however, rings can be stably transmitted in cell lines. This usually occurs when the ring contains genetic material that is essential for normal cell function.

A *marker* chromosome is a chromosome with a centromere that is stably transmitted to daughter cells but cannot be clearly identified because either it is too small or the banding pattern is too ambiguous. Multicolor FISH is a useful tool to determine the origin of markers. By 'painting' the entire metaphase and generating an image with a unique color for each chromosome pair, it should be possible to identify the origin of the marker chromosome, as its color should match the color for one of the other known chromosomes of the set.

Table 69–1 Common Abbreviations for Chromosome Abnormalities

Abbreviation	Meaning
cen	Centromere
del	Deletion
dup	Duplication
ins	Insertion
inv	Inversion
i	Isochromosome
mar	Marker
r	Ring
rob	Robertsonian translocation
t	Translocation

Conclusions

Chromosome abnormalities, either numerical or structural, that result in an unbalanced chromosome complement are usually associated with some type of abnormal clinical finding, and the size of the imbalance tends to be proportional to the severity of the problem. Most individuals who are diagnosed as having a constitutional chromosome abnormality have only a single chromosome defect. However, there are rare instances in which one person may have two or more chromosomal errors. Acquired chromosome abnormalities (seen in cancer cells) may be more complex and may have multiple numerical and structural changes in a single cell line.

Nomenclature

With such a broad range of chromosome variation, it was necessary to develop a system of classification that would allow each individual's chromosome complement to be succinctly described and understood worldwide. The first cytogenetic nomenclature provided a framework, and the 'language' has been evolving ever since. Currently, the International System of Cytogenetic Nomenclature (ISCN) is recognized as the standard.

The nomenclature describing a chromosome complement can be broken down into three basic parts: (1) the total number of chromosomes, (2) the sex chromosome complement, and (3) any chromosome abnormalities. These units are listed in order, separated by commas. So, an apparently normal female would be coded as 46,XX and a male would be 46,XY. If two or more cell lines are present, they are listed sequentially, separated by a slant line, with a normal diploid clone, if present, always listed last (45,X/46,XX). Other clones are ordered by size, with the largest clone placed first. The number of cells in each clone is indicated by a number enclosed in brackets (45,X[15]/47,XXX[3]/46,XX[12]). For numerical anomalies, the total number of chromosomes would be increased or decreased to indicate the overall change, and the specific chromosome gained or lost would be noted at the end. For example, trisomy 13 in a female would be written as 47,XX,+13 and monosomy 8 in a male would be written 45,XY,−8. However, for a sex chromosome variation that is known to be constitutional, it is not necessary to use a + or − sign, since the change in chromosome complement can be noted directly. Monosomy X becomes 45,X and gain of a sex chromosome would be 47,XXY, 47,XXX, or 47,XYY. On the other hand, if the sex chromosome change is acquired, as in some cancer cell lines, a + or − indicating this would be required (e.g., 45,X,−Y for a male whose Y chromosome has been lost as a result of his disease).

Structural changes in the chromosomes do not affect the total number of chromosomes present but should be noted at the end of the nomenclature to clarify the status of the rearranged chromosome(s). In order to streamline the nomenclature, a series of abbreviations for the common structural anomalies has been generated that shortens the overall nomenclature (Table 69–1). A structural abnormality is indicated by the abbreviation of the abnormality followed by the chromosome involved and breakpoint(s) on the chromosome(s). For rearrangements in which two chromosomes are involved, a first set of parentheses gives the chromosomes (lowest numbered or sex chromosome first) followed by the breakpoints of the rearrangement in the same relative order; that is, t(4;9)(q21.2;p22) is a translocation between chromosomes 4 and 9 with breakpoints 4q21.2 and 9p22.

Examples include the following:

Deletion:	46,XX,del(4)(p15)	Terminal deletion of the short arm of 4 at band 15
Duplication:	46,XX,dup(11)(q13q23)	Interstitial duplication of the long arm of 11

Table 69–2 Chromosome Abnormalities in Spontaneous Fetal Losses and in Liveborn Infants

Abnormality	Chromosome	Spontaneous Fetal Losses (%)	Incidence in Live Births
45,X		18.0	1/4000
Triploidy		17.0	1/60 000
Tetraploid		6.0	0
Trisomy	16	16.4	0
	22	5.7	0
	21	4.7	1/830
	15	4.2	0
	14	3.7	0
	18	3.0	1/7500
	13	2.0	1/5000
	Other	12.3	1/10 000
Unbalanced rearrangement		3.0	1/2000
Balanced rearrangement		4.0	3/1000

Source: data from Hook, 1977; Jacobs, 1992; Nussbaum, 2004; Turnpenny, 2005)

Translocation:	46,XY,t(4;9)(q21.2;p22)	Translocation between 4q and 9p
Inversion:	46,XY,inv(9)(p11q21.1)	Pericentric inversion in 9 between bands p11 and q21.1

Clinical

Clinical Applications

Cytogenetic abnormalities may be found in apparently 'normal' individuals as well as in patients with phenotypic anomalies or with a diagnosed genetic disorder. Diagnosis may occur at any stage of life. When the same set of features is seen in several unrelated individuals, it may be possible to establish a syndrome. The characteristics associated with a syndrome are assumed to have a common basis, which can often be shown to be a specific chromosome abnormality. However, although a syndrome is defined by a certain set of characters, there is variability in affected individuals and not all will show an identical phenotype.

Prenatal Cytogenetics

Studies have shown that 1 in 13 conceptuses has a chromosomal abnormality but, of these, only 6 in 1000 are live born, indicating that most errors are recognized and biologically eliminated. For example, of all 45,X conceptions, 95% will spontaneously terminate. Similar frequencies of termination are recorded for the liveborn trisomies (90% of trisomy 13 conceptions, 80% of trisomy 18 conceptions, and 65% of trisomy 21 conceptions terminate). On average, 15% of all recognized pregnancies end in a spontaneous fetal loss, with 80% of these occurring in the first trimester. Of all spontaneous abortions, 60% are chromosomally abnormal (Table 69–2), and of these, 52% are autosomal trisomies. The most common trisomy seen in abortus material is trisomy 16 but the most frequent class of chromosome error in spontaneous losses is 45,X.

One of the most important statistics is the direct correlation between advanced maternal age and births with chromosomal abnormalities. Although the exact reason for the phenomenon is unclear, population studies have shown that women over the age of 35 have an increased risk for a chromosomally abnormal conception (Hassold, 1985) with the most common abnormality being Down syndrome (trisomy 21) (Figs 69–10B and 69–18). This becomes important in a society in which women are delaying childbearing until later in life, so prenatal diagnosis has become a major area of clinical cytogenetic study. In addition to screening for an age-related risk, other common reasons for referral include a family history of or previous child with a chromosome abnormality, abnormal levels of AFP in a screening test, and an abnormality detected on ultrasound.

The most common chromosome abnormalities detected in prenatal testing are the liveborn trisomies and the sex chromosome aneuploidies. Because these are usually the result of a meiotic nondisjunction error, there is a very low risk of recurrence. Occasionally, a child with a balanced

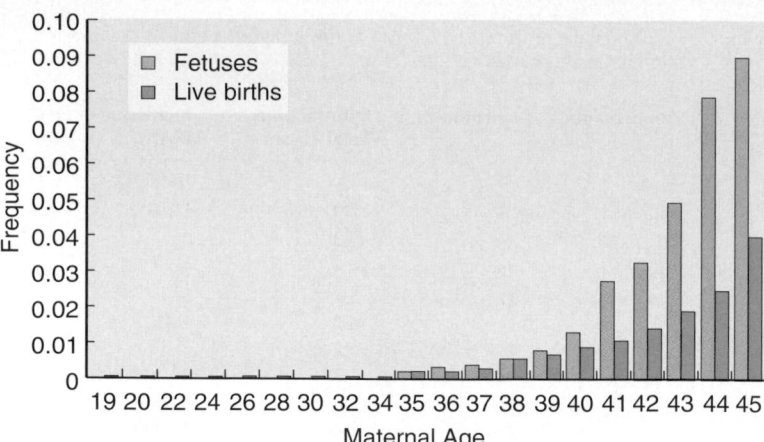

Figure 69–18 Increased risk of a Down syndrome conception with increased maternal age. The number of live births is lower at older ages due to the intervention of prenatal diagnosis followed by termination of abnormal pregnancies.

or unbalanced structural chromosome abnormality will be identified. In these circumstances, karyotype analysis on both biological parents is used to differentiate between an inherited rearrangement and a de novo anomaly in the child. For example, a child with an inherited balanced translocation has a less than 1% risk that the chromosome rearrangement will pose any problem. However, if the apparently balanced translocation seen in the fetus is not detected in either biological parent, it must have arisen de novo in the child, and there is a 5–10% risk of related impairment for the infant. Unfortunately, finding an *unbalanced* translocation in a fetus, regardless of the carrier status of the parents, is a serious situation and almost always results in some type of genetic defect for the child. Follow-up to determine if one of the parents is a balanced translocation carrier will provide information about recurrence risk for future pregnancies.

Postnatal

Approximately 0.6% of newborns have a chromosome abnormality. If an infant presents with signs or symptoms of a defined syndrome, karyotype analysis may confirm a diagnosis. If the newborn has clinical anomalies unrelated to a specific disorder, karyotype analysis may provide information on a chromosome abnormality related to the clinical findings. Ambiguous genitalia may be related to an abnormal sex chromosome complement but, if the chromosomes are shown to be normal, the physician knows that another cause for the patient's abnormality must be sought. If the child dies shortly after birth, cytogenetic analysis may provide information critical in understanding the demise, and these data should be correlated with autopsy results to substantiate a diagnosis.

Childhood and Adult

A common misconception about genetic disorders is that, because they are inherited, the diagnosis will be obvious at birth. In fact, the full clinical presentation of many disorders takes time to develop and may not be fully expressed until later in life. Consequently, some of the most difficult diagnostic problems occur in children and adults. In addition to considering the full range of cytogenetic possibilities, molecular and biochemical options must also be taken into account.

Cancer Genetics

Another area of medicine in which cytogenetics is increasingly important is oncology. Although the range of variability in the karyotypic findings of most solid tumors makes treatment decisions difficult, excellent clinical data exist for leukemias and lymphomas, including specific chromosome rearrangements that are directly associated with tumorigenesis (Table 69–3; see Ch. 71; Block, 1998). Karyotype findings were originally used primarily as confirmation of a clinical diagnosis, but the role of genetics in patient management changed dramatically in 2001 when the World Health Organization (WHO) published a revised classification for leukemias and lymphomas (Jaffe, 2001). The new methodology is based on data collected by clinical study groups that had shown a direct correlation between the presence of various chromosomal abnormalities and patients' response to therapy. Therefore, in the revised classification system, genetic findings, either cytogenetic or molecular, became a requirement for final diagnosis in most hematological disorders. Cytogenetics had suddenly been pushed to the forefront of testing for oncology patients.

In addition to diagnosis, karyotype analysis can provide other valuable information regarding a cancer patient's disease. Once a chromosome abnormality has been detected, the progress of the disease can be monitored.

If treatment is successful, most chromosome abnormalities are no longer evident in the bone marrow and, as long as the karyotype appears to be 'normal,' the patient is said to be in cytogenetic remission. However, if the treatment does not eliminate the aberrant cell line completely, remission may be merely an interlude in which the disease-causing cells are suppressed to such low levels that they are not detectable by routine karyotype analysis. Then at relapse, the same chromosome anomalies will reappear and may be accompanied by additional abnormalities and/or more complex cell lines, findings consistent with disease progression. An increase in complexity over time is known as karyotype evolution. In general, poor prognosis and severity of disease is directly correlated to the number and type of chromosome abnormalities seen.

FISH has become a valuable tool in clinical oncology studies with many probes commercially available (Cremer, 1988; Anastasi, 1991). Studies can be done on either interphase or metaphase cells, with the choice resting on the type of data desired. Using interphase cells is often preferred since it provides a much larger sample that can be quickly assayed giving results with a higher level of statistical significance (Werner, 1997).

For translocations, combination FISH probes have been developed that hybridize to the opposite sides of the translocation breakpoints. There are two common strategies employed to detect a translocation. Splitting of the signals may occur if the translocation separates two probes generating two different-colored signals in place of the original single-color signal. Alternatively, fusion may occur if the translocation results in relocation of the probes, bringing two different probes into proximity and generating a two-color fusion that creates a new color. For example, FISH fusion technology has been used to identify the 9;22 translocation in leukemia. This rearrangement is characterized by a translocation between the *ABL* proto-oncogene on chromosome 9 (9q34.1) and the *BCR* gene on chromosome 22 (22q11.2) (Fig. 69–19A), which produces a disease-associated chimeric gene on the derivative chromosome 22, also known as the Philadelphia chromosome (Ph') (see also Chapter 71). The translocation is seen in chronic myeloid leukemia (CML), acute myeloid leukemia (AML), and acute lymphoblastic leukemia (ALL) (Table 69–3), and, cytogenetically, it appears to be the same in all diseases. However, at the molecular level, the translocation can be separated into two classes: (1) the major breakpoint (*M-bcr*) rearrangement that results in a chimeric protein of 210 kD (most common in CML), and (2) the minor breakpoint (*m-bcr*) rearrangement that results in a chimeric protein of 190 kD (seen in some adults and about 50% of childhood ALL). A FISH assay has been engineered to detect both rearrangements (Vysis, Inc.). A pair of probes is used: (1) red – localized to the *ABL* locus on chromosome 9, and (2) green – located at the *BCR* locus (chromosome 22) encompassing the m-bcr breakpoint but proximal to the M-bcr breakpoint. When no translocation is present, two green signals (detecting each *ABL* allele) and two red signals (detecting each *BCR* allele) should be present in each cell (Fig. 69–19B and C). When the M-bcr rearrangement occurs, the translocation breaks chromosome 22 distal to the probe recognition site such that the entire green signal remains on chromosome 22. On chromosome 9, the translocation splits the red *ABL* signal such that a small red signal is left on the derivative chromosome 9 and the remainder of the red signal moves to chromosome 22. This brings one green and one red signal adjacent to one another on the derivative chromosome 22 (Ph'), and, with the resolution of the light microscope, the two signals merge, giving a single yellow fusion signal. Therefore, a cell with a M-bcr translocation will have four signals: one green (chromosome 22), one large red (chromosome 9), one small red (the rearranged chromosome 9),

Table 69–3 Common Cytogenetic Rearrangements in Leukemia and Lymphoma

Disorder	Chromosome Rearrangement(s)	Genes Involved	FAB Classification (If Different)
Chronic myeloproliferative disease			
Chronic myelogenous leukemia (chronic)	t(9;22)(q34.1;q11.2)	ABL; BCR	
Chronic myelogenous leukemia (accelerated or blast phase)	+8, i(17q), +19, + Ph'		
Polycythemia vera	+8, +9, del(20q), del(13q)		
Chronic idiopathic myelofibrosis	+8, −7, del(7q), del(11q), del(13q), del(20q)		
Essential thrombocythemia	+8, del(13q)		
Myelodysplastic syndromes			
Myelodysplastic syndrome with isolated del(5q)	del(5)(q13q33), del(5)(q22q33)		5q− syndrome
Chronic myelomonocytic leukemia	−7, del(7q),+8, abnormalities of 12p		
Refractory anemia, refractory anemia with ringed sideroblasts, refractory anemia with excess blasts	−5, del(5q), −7, del(7q), +8, del(20q)		
Acute myeloid leukemia (AML) with recurrent cytogenetic abnormalities			
AML with t(8;21)	t(8;21)(q22;q22)	AML1; ETO	AML-M2
AML with inversion or translocation 16	inv(16)(p12q22), t(16;16)(p13;q22)	CBFβ; MYH11	AML-M4Eo
Acute promyelocytic leukemia	t(15;17)(q22;q12)	PML; RARα	AML-M3
AML with 11q23 (MLL) abnormalities	t(9;11)(p21;q23), t(11;19)(q23;p13.1), t(11;19)(q23;p13.3),	AF9; MLL MLL; ENL	AML-M5
AML with multilineage dysplasia	−5, del(5q), −7, del(7q), +8, del(11q), del(20q), +21, translocations involving 3q21 and 3q26, t(9;22)(q34.1;q11.2)		AML-M1, AML-M6
Precursor B-lymphoblastic leukemia/lymphoma			ALL-L1/L2
	t(1;19)(q23;p13.3)	PBX; E2A	
	t(9;22)(q34;q11.2)	ABL; BCR	
	11q23 rearrangements, including:	MLL	
	t(1;11)(p32;q23)	AF1P; MLL	
	t(4;11)(q21;q23)	AF4; MLL	
	t(11;19)(q23;p13)	MLL; ENL	
	t(12;21)(p13q22)	TEL; AML	
	Hyperdiploidy (modal number 50–56)		
Precursor T-lymphoblastic leukemia/lymphoma			ALL-L1/L2
	Rearrangements at 14q11.2, 7q35, and 7p14–15	T-cell receptor loci	
	del(9p)	CDKN2A	
	translocations at 1p32	TAL1	
Mature B-cell neoplasms			
Chronic lymphocytic leukemia/small lymphocytic leukemia	+12, del13q, del11q23–24, 14q+, del17p13		
Lymphoplasmacytic lymphoma/ Waldenström's macroglobulinemia	t(9;14)(p13;q32)	PAX5; IGH	
Plasma cell myeloma	t(11;14)(q13;q32)	CCND1; BCL1	
Marginal zone B-cell lymphoma (MALT)	+3, t(11;18)(q21;q21)		
Follicular lymphoma	t(14;18)(q32;q21), t(18;22)(q21;q11.2), +7, +18, del(6q), del/t(3)(q27)	IGH; BCL2 BCL2; IGL	
Mantle cell lymphoma	t(11;14)(q13;q32)	CCND1; BCL1	
Burkitt's lymphoma	t(8;14)(q24;q32)	MYC; IGH	
	t(2;8) (p12;q24)	IGK; MYC	
	t(8;22)(q24;q11.2)	MYC; IGL	

and one yellow fusion signal detecting the Ph' chromosome (Fig. 69–19*B* and *D*). The m-bcr rearrangement is slightly different. Chromosome 22 is broken within the green probe recognition site, such that one portion of the green signal will stay on chromosome 22 but the second section will move to the derivative chromosome 9. The red probe site on chromosome 9 is split as described above, with one portion remaining on chromosome 9 and a second section moving to chromosome 22. This reciprocal translocation thus results in two yellow fusion signals (derivative 9 is red fused to green, and derivative 22 is green fused to red). The net result of the m-bcr FISH assay is four probe signals: one green (chromosome 22), one red (chromosome 9), and two yellow fusion signals detecting the 9;22 translocation (Figs. 69–19*B* and *E*). Being able to determine which of the two rearrangements is present in a patient sample simplifies the diagnosis and leads to the most appropriate treatment methodology for the individual. Other FISH detection assays using other disease gene specific probes can be designed to evaluate for a wide array of different cancer related chromosome rearrangements.

In addition, chromosomal aneuploidies in cancer cells can be easily detected. For example: (1) use of a chromosome 12-specific centromere probe to screen an interphase cell population for trisomy 12 cells indicative of CLL, (2) use of a chromosome 7 probe to detect monosomy 7 in myelodysplastic syndrome and AML, and (3) use of a chromosome 8 probe to identify trisomy 8 in both chronic and acute disorders. The use of different-colored X and Y probes in evaluating the success of a bone marrow transplant when the donor and recipient are of opposite sexes has also been highly successful. Following transplantation, a male who has received female donor cells should have an XX complement. Failure of the engraftment may be signaled by the presence of a high frequency of XY cells. The FISH can be repeated at regular intervals to monitor the progress and provide an early warning if the patient's leukemic cell population begins to proliferate.

Initially, clinicians were concerned about apparently discrepant results from karyotype analysis and FISH on the same patient sample. By karyotype, a patient with CML may show all cells with a t(9;22), but only

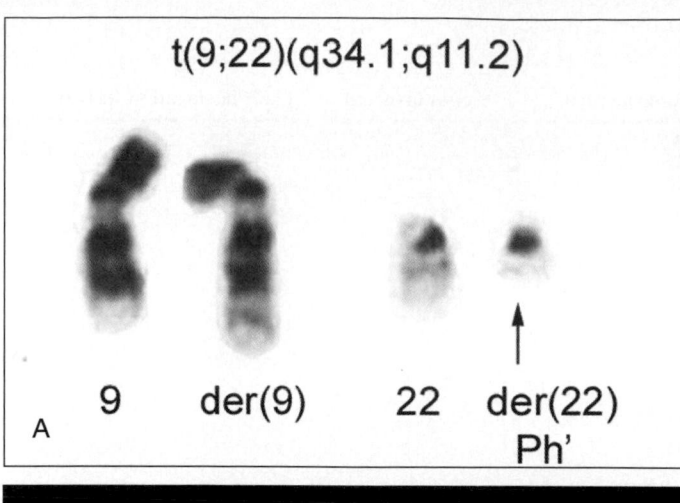

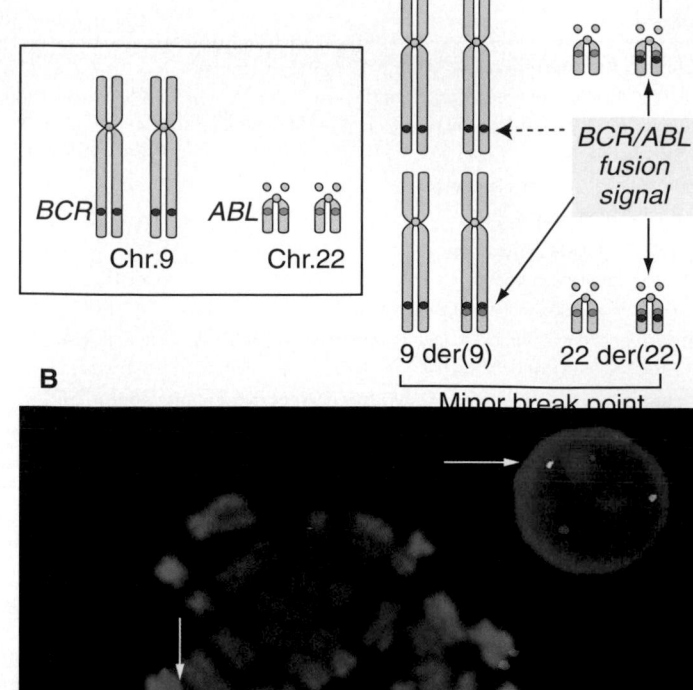

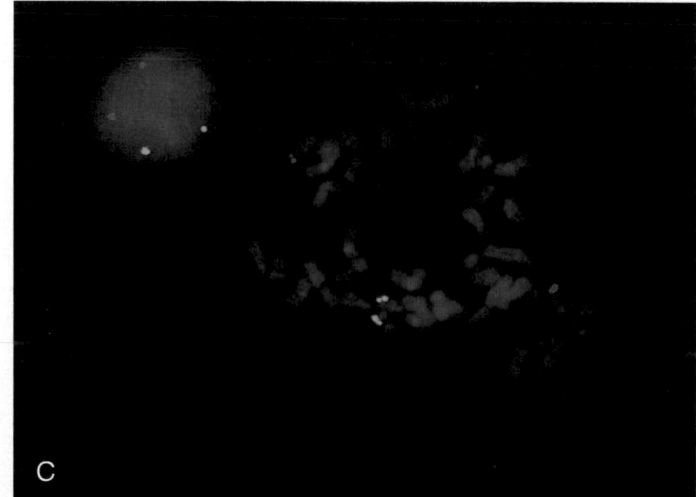

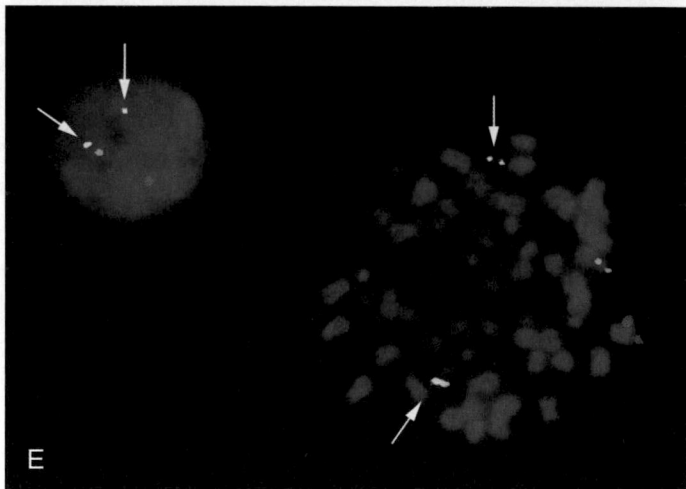

Figure 69–19 FISH detection of the 9;22 translocation in CML. *A*, Banded chromosomes showing the 9;22 translocation. The derivative chromosome 22 is known as the Ph' or Philadelphia chromosome. *B*, Diagram showing FISH detection for a normal cell with no translocation (left) and for both the major (M-bcr) and minor (m-bcr) breakpoint rearrangements. Upper right shows the signal pattern for the M-bcr translocation: chr. 9 – red signal, der(9) – partial red signal with chromosome 22 material below (yellow) (dashed arrow), chr. 22 – green signal, and the der(22), the Ph' chromosome with a green-red *BCR-ABL* fusion signal and chromosome 9 material below. The lower right shows the m-bcr signal pattern: chr. 9 – red signal, der(9) – red-green fusion signal and chromosome 22 material below, chr. 22 – green signal, and the der(22) – green-red fusion signal with chromosome 9 material below. *C to D.* Actual FISH images. *C*, No translocation is present as seen by two copies each of the chromosome 9 (red) and chromosome 22 (green) probes in both interphase (left) and metaphase (right) cells. *D*, Cells with a M-bcr translocation as detected by the single yellow fusion signal (arrow) plus one green, one large red, and one small red signal (metaphase on the left and interphase on the right). *E*, Cells with a m-bcr translocation as detected by two yellow fusion signals (arrows) plus one green and one red signal (metaphase on the right and interphase on the left).

30% of cells will be positive for the translocation by interphase FISH. These data are actually consistent. Karyotype can only be performed on dividing cells and, since cancer cells tend to divide frequently, a karyotype analysis would typically show 100% leukemic cells. FISH, on the other hand, detects all nucleated cells, but not all cells in a bone marrow sample are from the disease clone. An affected individual will also have a normal cell population. Interphase FISH can quantify the relative numbers of normal and disease cells, thus providing a more accurate estimate of disease involvement within the total population. This can be used advantageously to monitor a patient's response to treatment. Testing sequential samples over time can show a reduction in the disease cell population, and relapse will be reflected by a rise in the leukemic cell population. Thus, it is important to perform both karyotype analysis and FISH on a diagnosis specimen. The karyotype will define the chromosomal abnormalities present, and the FISH will establish the baseline frequency of the leukemic clone(s). These data can then be used as a reference point for all future testing for the patient.

Multicolor FISH has also been used to evaluate leukemic cell lines. The data being collected suggest that cancer cells actually undergo a significantly greater degree of chromosome rearrangement than was previously appreciated. It is hoped that some of the new rearrangements being detected will give clues to new cancer-related genes (Veldman, 1997).

Cytogenetic Disorders

Chromosomal Aneuploidy Syndromes

Autosomal Aneuploidies

The most common cause of mental retardation is trisomy 21 or Down syndrome. This disorder has a birth incidence of 1 in 700 and is characterized by hypotonia, flat facies, slanted palpebral fissures, small ears, protruding tongue, transverse palmar crease, heart defects, and hypogonadism. Approximately 92.5% of all Down syndrome individuals have 47 chromosomes including three copies of chromosome 21 resulting

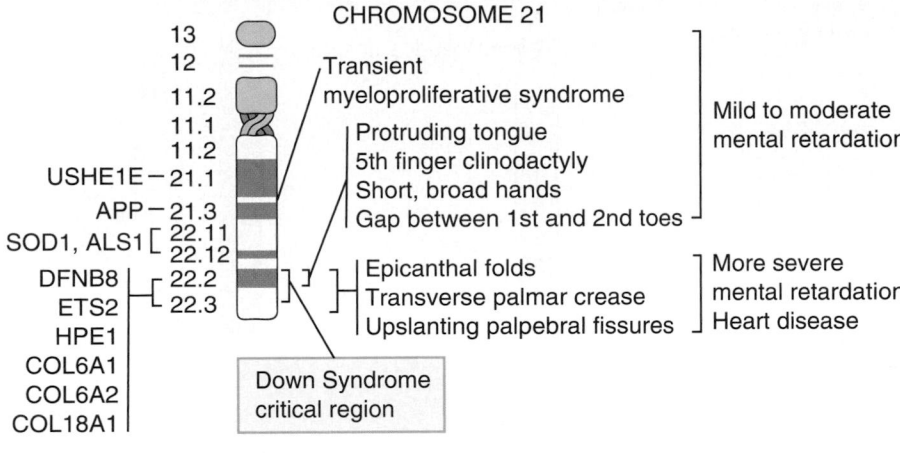

CHROMOSOME 21

13
12
11.2
11.1
11.2
USHE1E — 21.1
APP — 21.3
SOD1, ALS1 [22.11
          22.12
DFNB8 [22.2
ETS2 [22.3
HPE1
COL6A1
COL6A2
COL18A1

Transient
myeloproliferative syndrome

Protruding tongue
5th finger clinodactyly
Short, broad hands
Gap between 1st and 2nd toes

Mild to moderate
mental retardation

Epicanthal folds
Transverse palmar crease
Upslanting palpebral fissures

More severe
mental retardation
Heart disease

Down Syndrome
critical region

Figure 69–20 Map of chromosome 21 showing the Down syndrome critical region and relative positions of loci associated with various clinical features to the right. On the left, other mapped loci are shown. ALS1 = amyotrophic lateral sclerosis; APP = amyloid β-precursor protein (associated with Alzheimer's disease); COL6A1/COL6A2/COL18A1 = collagen genes; DFNB8 = deafness 8; ETS2 = oncogene *ETS-2*; HPE1 = alobar holoprosencephaly-1; SOD1 = superoxide dismutase-1; USH1E = Usher syndrome. (Source: data from Korenberg, 1990; Delabar, 1993; OMIM, 1999.)

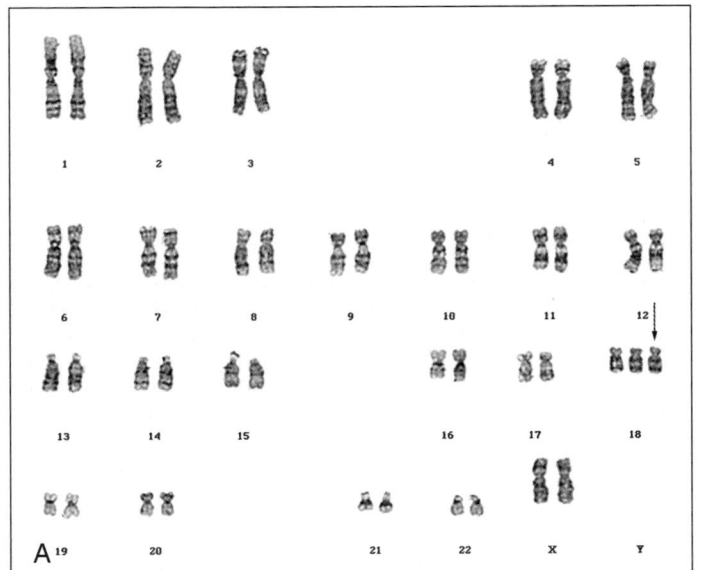

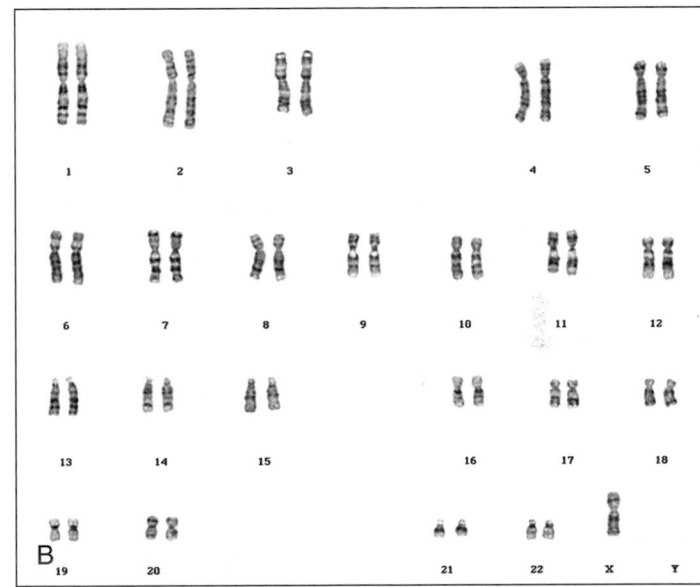

Figure 69–21 Karyotypes from numerical chromosome syndromes. *A*, Edwards syndrome (trisomy 18): 47,XX,+18. *B*, Turner syndrome (monosomy X): 45,X.

from a nondisjunction error in parental meiosis. Just under 3% of patients tend to express a milder phenotype and have been shown to be mosaics with two cell lines (47,XX,+21/46,XX or 47,XY,+21/46,XY), and about 5% of Down syndrome patients have only 46 chromosomes, since the extra 21 is part of a Robertsonian or other translocation. A child with a translocation is often indicative of the presence of a translocation carrier parent so, in these cases, karyotype analysis of both parents is appropriate to determine if the couple is at increased risk of having additional Down syndrome children in future pregnancies. Although it is most common for a Down syndrome patient to have three complete copies of chromosome 21, molecular studies of individuals with chromosome 21 rearrangements have clearly shown that it is only necessary to have three copies of the region of chromosome 21 encompassing bands 21q22.12–21q22.3, the Down syndrome critical region (Fig. 69–20) (Korenberg, 1990; Delabar, 1993).

The other two liveborn trisomies are trisomy 13 and trisomy 18. *Trisomy 13*, Patau syndrome, with a birth incidence of 1 in 4000 to 1 in 10 000, is characterized by a small head, cleft lip and/or cleft palate, cyclopia, transverse palmar crease, polydactyly of the hands and/or feet, prominent heel, ventricular septal defect, and punched-out scalp. *Trisomy 18*, or Edwards syndrome (Fig. 69–21*A*), is seen in approximately 1 in 8000 newborns with features including a low birth weight, small mouth and jaw, ventricular septal defect, hypoplasia of the muscles, a prominent occiput, low-set malformed ears, rocker bottom feet, and crossed fingers.

Despite its often severe clinical consequences, Down syndrome is usually quite manageable, and patients live into the second or third decade of life. Trisomy 13 and trisomy 18 are considerably less compatible with life, and patients usually die within the first month of life. If an individual survives the first year, the outlook is bleak, since patients do not learn to talk, walk, or care for themselves. Because of this, counseling for prenatally diagnosed cases of trisomy 13 and 18 includes the option of termination of pregnancy.

Sex Chromosome Aneuploidies

Sex chromosome aneuploidies are relatively common (overall frequency of 1 in 500 births), and are phenotypically milder than autosomal aneuploidies because of the effect of X inactivation and the limited number of genes present on the Y chromosome. Four disorders, including three trisomies and one monosomy, account for the majority of cases. All are the result of nondisjunction errors in meiosis and, except for XYY which is exclusively paternal, the other disorders may result from either maternal or paternal error.

The aberrant karyotypes of individuals with three X chromosomes (47,XXX females) or with one X and two Y chromosomes (47,XYY males) often go undetected throughout life. The birth incidence is relatively high, 1 in 1000, but other than being somewhat taller than average, there are no striking features that would indicate a chromosomal abnormality. Some individuals have generalized learning difficulties and so may be identified by school screening programs. XXX females and XYY males are also detected in infertility clinics, although the cytogenetic abnormality is not related to the reason for referral, since comprehensive evaluations have shown that these individuals are fully fertile and generally have chromosomally normal children. XYY males do have an increased risk of behavioral problems, and early studies suggested that they also had criminal tendencies because there was a higher than expected incidence of XYY in inmates of penal institutions (Jacobs, 1968; Price, 1970). However, subsequent work has shown that: (1) the conclusions of the original study were biased because of a sampling error, (2) criminality is most probably due to a combination of multiple causes, and (3) XYY males are no more prone to a criminal behavior than any other male (Witkin, 1976; Pitcher, 1982; Theilgaard, 1984).

Klinefelter syndrome (47,XXY) males tend to be tall and thin with relatively long legs, although early in life these findings seldom set them apart from their peers. Some individuals are identified in school because

Table 69–4 Distribution of Different Chromosome Complements that Give Rise to Turner Syndrome

Occurrence (%)	Chromosome Anomaly
50	45,X
20	46,X,i(Xq)
15	X chromosome deletions or rings, or the presence of a Y chromosome
10	Mosaics: 45,X/46,XX; 45,X/46,XY

of their learning difficulties but the most common reason for referral is postpubertal hypogonadism; female-like breast development; and infertility due to small testicles, hyalinized testicular tubules, and azoospermia. A milder form of Klinefelter syndrome with the potential for fertility due to normal testicular development is seen in individuals with a mosaic chromosome complement including a 46,XY cell line (47,XXY/46,XY). The relative proportion of XY and XXY cells during sex determination in the early zygote and in the testes is the key for fertility. An excess of XXY cells will push the individual toward a true Klinefelter, whereas higher numbers of XY cells should moderate the phenotype and increase the likelihood of fertility.

The most commonly recognized sex chromosome aneuploidy presenting with a female phenotype is 45,X: *Turner syndrome* (Fig. 69–21B). In sex determination, normal female development is dependent on the presence of two active X chromosomes. The critical region for female differentiation has been narrowed to a region of the short arm of the X just proximal to the centromere. If that region is missing or inactive, an individual with Turner syndrome will result. About half of all Turner syndrome patients have the classic 45,X chromosome complement, which represents the only viable liveborn monosomy. The single X chromosome is usually maternal in origin, indicating that a paternal meiotic nondisjunction is the most common source of error. In addition to 45,X, more complex karyotypes are also possible (Table 69–4) (Palmer, 1976). The greatest concern is for individuals who possess a complete or partial Y chromosome in at least one cell line, who are at increased risk for gonadoblastoma.

The phenotype for Turner syndrome is highly variable. Affected individuals are typically short (<150 cm) with gonadal dysgenesis and learning difficulties. Other common features include webbed neck resulting from cystic hygroma in utero, low posterior hairline, heart and renal anomalies, cubitus valgus (increased carrying angle of the elbow), and shield chest. At birth, patients may present with edema of the hands and feet. Turner syndrome patients are usually of normal intelligence, although this can vary and some individuals have significant mental handicaps. Furthermore, although infertility used to be accepted as the standard in Turner syndrome, it is now known that some patients, usually those with mosaic karyotypes, can reproduce successfully. Furthermore, using donor egg technologies, a Turner syndrome patient can complete a full pregnancy and deliver a normal child. Therefore, because of this great diversity of presentation, prenatal counseling for a couple with an identified Turner syndrome fetus is extremely difficult. In general, however, most liveborn Turner syndrome patients can live productive lives, and mildly affected individuals may not know that they are affected with the disorder until puberty.

Other Sex Chromosome Abnormalities

Sex determination in humans is the result of a complex biochemical pathway involving the interaction of proteins produced by genes present on the autosomes and the X and Y chromosomes. The default sex in humans is female so, in the absence of any male-determining stimuli, a female individual will develop. The primary trigger for male development is a gene located on the short arm of the Y chromosome designated *TDF*, the testes determining factor, which is located in the sex-determining region of the Y chromosome (*SRY*) (Fig. 69–22). The protein produced by *TDF* initiates the male developmental pathway. A number of disorders associated with mutations in different genes within this pathway have been identified and can result in ambiguous genitalia or genotype/phenotype mismatch (phenotypic male with an XX sex chromosome complement or a phenotypic female with an XY complement).

An XX male can usually be attributed to one of two causes. The more common of the two is virilization of a female fetus as a result of the autosomal recessive disorder congenital adrenal hyperplasia (CAH). The defect in CAH is the lack of the enzyme 21-hydroxylase. Without this enzyme, the normal biosynthetic pathway is blocked and androgens

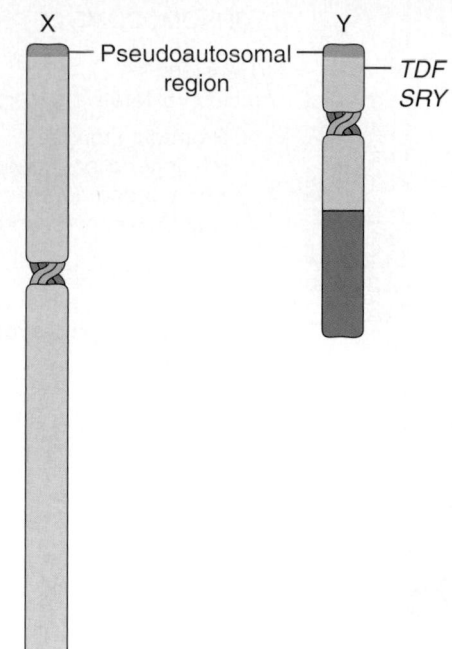

Figure 69–22 Diagram of relative locations of *TDF, SRY*, and the pseudoautosomal regions of the X and Y chromosomes.

accumulate in the body. Excessive levels of male hormones in the female circulation may result in a male-appearing infant despite a female chromosome complement. Furthermore, since androgens are capable of crossing the placenta, a normal female fetus may develop ambiguous genitalia due to exposure from excess hormones from a CAH-affected mother.

A phenotypic male with an XX sex chromosome complement may also result from a cryptic translocation between the X and Y chromosomes. The distal ends of the short arms of the X and Y chromosomes are homologous and comprise what is termed the pseudoautosomal regions (Fig. 69–22). This is the primary site of X and Y chromosome pairing during meiosis, and recombination may occur between X and Y alleles. Rarely, a recombination event outside the boundaries of the pseudoautosomal region takes place resulting in the transfer of unique Y loci, including *SRY*, to the tip of the X chromosome. The amount of chromosome material involved in such an exchange is extremely small and cannot be cytogenetically detected. In a male with such a balanced translocation, there would be no clinical abnormalities, since the genes are all present, although in alternate locations. However, if this male transmits his rearranged X chromosome to an offspring who has received an X from the mother, the resultant child will have an apparent XX chromosome complement but a male or Klinefelter male phenotype due to the presence of the *TDF* gene that triggers the male developmental pathway.

The reciprocal of the above-described translocation may result in a Turner female with an apparent XY complement. The male developmental pathway will not be initiated in an individual with a Y chromosome that has no *TDF/SRY*, and sex determination will default to female. However, the lack of two intact copies of the proximal X short arm will prevent 'normal' female development, and a Turner syndrome individual should result. This situation is quite rare. The more common finding for an XY female is androgen insensitivity, also known as 'testicular feminization.' In these individuals, the Y chromosome is intact, and *TDF* is present and functional. The problem is a mutation of the androgen receptor gene located on the long arm of the X chromosome (Xq21.3) that results in no androgen receptor protein being produced. *TDF* will initiate male development, but the pathway will be blocked at the point where the androgen receptor protein is required to form a complex between testosterone and dihydrotestosterone. Without this critical step, further male differentiation is not possible, and the phenotype will default back to female. However, these individuals are infertile because of the lack of any functional internal genitalia, and commonly present with a blind vagina and testes in the abdomen or inguinal canal.

Structural Chromosome Anomalies

A reasonable number of syndromes directly related to a structural chromosome abnormality have been described. Most of these are quite rare. The following is a discussion of some of the more common syndromes (see also Jones, 2006).

Table 69–5 Microdeletion and Contiguous Gene Syndromes

Disorder	Location	Genes	Clinical findings
Angelman syndrome	15q11.2	UBE3A	Severe MR, developmental delay, large mouth, prognathia, ataxia, seizures
DiGeorge syndrome	22q11.2, 10p, 4q, 6q	?GCSL + others?	Characteristic facies, cleft palate, heart defect, hypoplasia of the thymus and parathyroids, severe hypocalcemia, seizures
Ichthyosis	Xp22.32	STS	Scaly skin, short stature, hypogonadism, MR
Kallmann syndrome	Xp22.3	KAL1	Hypogonadism, inability to smell
Langer–Giedion syndrome	8q24.11–q24.13	TRPSI TRPSII EXT	Craniofacial dysmorphism, skeletal abnormalities, mild to severe mental deficiency
Lissencephaly	17p13.3	LIS1	Smooth brain, profound retardation, seizures
Miller–Dieker syndrome	17p13.3	LIS1 ?other(s)	Lissencephaly, microcephaly, high forehead, small nose, micrognathia, low-set ears
Prader–Willi syndrome	15q11.2	SNRPN	Hypotonia at birth, almond-shaped eyes, moderate to severe MR, absent sense of satiation leading to overeating, small hands and feet, hypogonadism
Retinoblastoma	13q14.1-q14.2	Rb1	Tumors of the retinoblast cells of the eye
Rubinstein–Taybi syndrome	16p13.3	CBP	Beaked nose, prominent columella, hypoplastic maxilla, downslanted palpebral fissures, broad thumbs and first toes, MR, speech delay
Smith–Magenis syndrome	17p11.2		Brachycephaly, midface hypoplasia, broad nasal bridge, prominent jaw, short broad hands, hyperactivity, delayed speech, self destructive behavior, MR
Velocardiofacial syndrome	22q11.2	?GCSL	Palatal defects, hypoplastic alae nasi with long nose, learning disability, congenital heart disease
WAGR	11p13.3	WT1 AN2 ? others	Wilm's tumor, aniridia, genitourinary defects, and mental retardation
Williams syndrome	7q11.2	ELN	Low IQ, hypersensitivity to sound, blue eyes with stellate pattern in the iris, prominent lips, hoarse voice, supravalvular aortic stenosis or other cardiac defect, hypercalcemia, premature aging of the skin

MR = mental retardation.

Wolf–Hirschhorn syndrome, also known as 4p– syndrome, is due to a terminal deletion of the short arm of chromosome 4, del(4)(p16). Clinical findings include microcephaly, micrognathia, hypotonia, epicanthal folds, and developmental delay. The characteristic facial appearance has been likened to a Greek warrior's helmet because of the arched eyebrows and long nose. Individuals with this disorder require special education and are at increased risk of seizures.

Cri-du-chat or 5p– syndrome, del(5)(p15), is characterized by a distinctive high-pitched, cat-like cry in infancy. Other features include low birth weight and subsequent slow growth, hypotonia, microcephaly, hypertelorism, epicanthal folds, cardiac anomalies, and mental retardation. Affected children have delayed development and may reach the cognitive and social level of a 5- or 6-year-old.

Microdeletion Syndromes and Contiguous Gene Syndromes

By definition, a microdeletion is a very small deletion, usually only a fraction of a single chromosome band. Microdeletions can be confused with molecular deletions, so it is important to recognize that, although microdeletions are small, they are significantly larger (>500 kb) than the typical molecular deletion (1 base pair [bp] to several hundred bp), which can only be resolved by molecular technology (see Chapter 72). The actual size of a microdeletion can vary from patient to patient, and some may be large enough to identify by karyotype analysis, although most will require FISH for detection. Although originally thought to be deletions within single genes, it has now been shown that certain syndromes are actually due to deletions that encompass portions of several adjacent, unrelated genes. The clinical presentation may therefore be a combination of features due to the absence of several different gene products. The size of the deletion and number of genes affected may vary, such that the phenotype expressed may differ significantly between individuals. Collectively, these are called *contiguous gene syndromes*. Included in this group are many of the microdeletion syndromes (Table 69–5) as well as the larger, classic deletion syndromes such as Wolf–Hirshhorn and cri-du-chat.

Miller–Dieker syndrome clearly illustrates the overlap between microdeletion and contiguous gene syndromes. The disorder has been associated with a microdeletion of the distal short arm of chromosome 17 (17p13.3), and the cardinal clinical features are lissencephaly (smooth brain) and craniofacial anomalies. Isolated lissencephaly has also been recognized as an independent entity, so Miller–Dieker syndrome is a more complex presentation that couples the brain defect with characteristic facial features. Molecular analysis has shown there are at least two genes involved in Miller–Dieker syndrome, so it is a true contiguous gene syndrome resulting from a microdeletion. A smaller deletion of the *LIS1* gene only would result in isolated lissencephaly (Ledbetter, 1992).

Prader–Willi syndrome and *Angelman syndrome* are the best-known microdeletion syndromes. Both share the same interstitial deletion of the proximal long arm of chromosome 15, del(15)(q11.2q11.2), but the clinical presentations are significantly different. Prader–Willi patients are small and hypotonic at birth but change within the first year of life and begin to gain weight rapidly. If not placed on a controlled diet, they can become quite obese through overeating. Other characteristics include small hands and feet, hypogonadism, and a bad temper. Although they are developmentally delayed, most do well in special education classes. Because of their temper and difficulty in controlling their diet, Prader–Willi patients may be placed in special group homes that provide the proper environment. Angelman syndrome patients, on the other hand, are severely mentally retarded. Although they are friendly, they usually cannot carry on a normal conversation, and discourse is often punctuated by bursts of inappropriate laughter. The disorder is also characterized by hyperactivity, short stature, microcephaly, seizures, and ataxia.

By routine or high-resolution cytogenetic analysis, the 15q deletion can be detected in about 60% of Prader–Willi individuals but only 10–20% of Angelman syndrome patients. Use of FISH has provided a much better diagnostic tool and, for both syndromes, deletions can now be established in 80–85% of cases. Although it was accepted that not all deletions would be visible at the cytogenetic level, it was considered odd that FISH was unable to detect a deletion in 100% of cases. This, in addition to the fact that Prader–Willi syndrome and Angelman syndrome appear to share the same deletion but have such entirely different phenotypes, suggested that there might be another cause for the disorders. It is now known that Prader–Willi syndrome and Angelman syndrome are examples of genetic imprinting, and that the mutational processes resulting in the diseases are much more complex than a simple deletion of DNA (Nicholls, 1989; Robinson, 1991) (see Chapter 72 for a discussion of imprinting and molecular detection of imprinted genes).

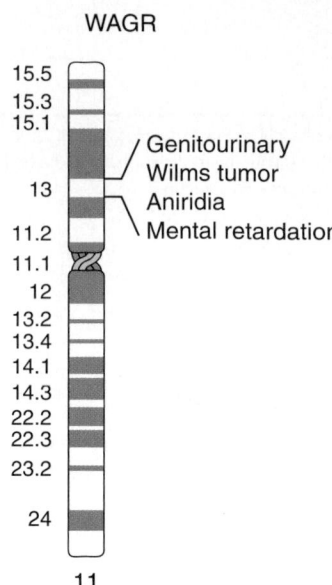

WAGR

Genitourinary
Wilms tumor
Aniridia
Mental retardation

11

Figure 69–23 Diagram of the contiguous gene syndrome WAGR showing relative positions of the different genes on the short arm of chromosome 11.

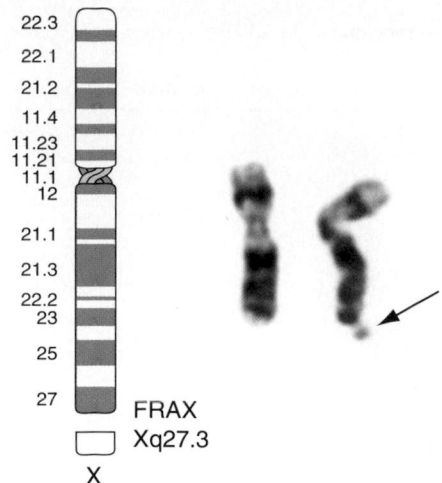

FRAX
Xq27.3

X

Figure 69–24 Fragile X. Ideogram of the fragile X (left) and a representative pair of G-banded chromosomes showing the fragile X on the right.

Williams syndrome has been associated with a deletion of the elastin gene *(ELN)* on the proximal long arm of chromosome 7 (7q11.23). The disorder is characterized by cardiac abnormalities, hypertension, hoarse voice, premature aging of the skin, and behavioral anomalies. Since elastin is known to be an important protein lending elasticity to tissues such as the heart, blood vessels, skin, and vocal cords, its absence explains many of the physical anomalies associated with this syndrome. The behavioral problems, however, could not be attributed to the lack of elastin, so it is currently believed that Williams syndrome is actually a contiguous gene syndrome and that the variability of the phenotype is related to the number of adjacent genes deleted in combination with *ELN*.

A very well characterized contiguous gene syndrome is located on the short arm of chromosome 11 (11p13) and is known as WAGR (*W*ilms tumor, *a*niridia, *g*enitourinary defects, and mental *r*etardation). Except for the genitourinary defects, which appear to be due to a variant mutation in the Wilms tumor locus, each of the other three anomalies has been associated with a particular gene and these are arranged in tandem on the short arm of chromosome 11 (Fig. 69–23). The phenotype of an affected individual will vary depending on the size of the deletion. Statistically, about 1 in 3 children diagnosed with aniridia will also develop Wilms tumor. Conversely, only 1 in 50 Wilms patients has aniridia. With larger deletions, mental retardation and genitourinary defects may also be seen.

Velocardiofacial syndrome is possibly the most common microdeletion syndrome in humans but it is often not recognized because it has a broad spectrum of clinical features and a presentation that can be quite mild. The disorder is usually diagnosed in the newborn period because of feeding difficulties, cardiac defects, and characteristic facial dysmorphologies. Learning disabilities, short stature, and conductive hearing loss are noted as the individual ages. Interestingly, 10–15% of patients will have a much more mildly affected parent with the same deletion. The 3 Mb deletion on the proximal long arm of chromosome 22 (22q11.2q11.2) is thought to be due to recombination between direct repeats that flank the common deletion region. Such intrachromosomal recombination would generate a loop structure that would be detected as a chromosomal defect by cell maintenance enzymes. Cellular repair enzymes would then excise the DNA in the loop and reseal the linear portion of the chromosome, resulting in the chromosomal deletion and loss of all associated genes, which could lead to disease (McDermid, 2002). A similar mechanism resulting in the classic Williams syndrome deletion has also been reported (Bayes, 2003), suggesting the possibility that this is a new mutation strategy that could explain deletion formation in a variety of other diseases.

Other Cytogenetic Phenomena

Fragile X Syndrome

Fragile X syndrome is the second leading cause of mental retardation and is the primary cause of inherited mental retardation. The disorder was first described by Herbert Lubs in 1969, when he noted the correlation between retardation and a 'marker' X in affected family members (Lubs, 1969). The marker X has subsequently become known as the fragile X, a break or gap in the structure of the X chromosome that can be detected cytogenetically (Fig. 69–24) by culturing cells in the appropriate induction medium. Unfortunately, not all affected individuals express the fragile X cytogenetically, so the clinical test is flawed. Nevertheless, it was the only assay available for many years and provided much-needed confirmation of diagnosis in many individuals. In 1991, the gene associated with fragile X syndrome was cloned and the mutation was identified as an amplification of a trinucleotide repeat sequence, something that had never before been seen or associated as a disease-causing mechanism. Fortunately, this mutation is detectable at the molecular level, and a highly proficient clinical test has been developed to allow direct mutation detection for fragile X syndrome (Rousseau, 1991; Verkerk, 1991) (see Chapter 72) so the cytogenetic test is no longer used.

Breakage Syndromes

Chromosomal breakage syndromes (Table 69–6) are a set of autosomal recessive disorders that were originally grouped together because of the common finding of chromosome instability or fragility (Arlett, 1978). Because of this, cytogenetic testing was possible as an aid in diagnosis. Molecular studies have shown an additional commonality among the disorders in that the primary mutation in each is a defect in a DNA repair gene. This helped to explain the other features of the syndromes, since inability to repair the DNA can lead to (1) breakage or increased recombination that can be characterized by chromosome instability, and (2) widespread mutation and defect in DNA sequences that can lead to cancer.

Summary

Cytogenetics is a relatively old, labor-intensive laboratory science, and it is still performed in much the same way it always has been, although the advent of the computer-assisted karyotyping system and the robotic harvester has added an element of advanced technology to the laboratory. Although it was once predicted that molecular diagnostics would eliminate the need for cytogenetics, that has not occurred, and cytogenetics is still the only clinical assay that can provide a quick overview of the entire human genome. Karyotype analysis continues to be important in assessing numerical and structural chromosome anomalies and is the gold standard for diagnosis of many disorders. Determination of the cytogenetic lesion is currently required for diagnosis of many cancers. To meet new challenges, cytogenetics has added new testing and new technologies. Use of FISH has bridged the gap between cytogenetics and molecular diagnostics such that the two areas provide complementary information in many cases. Thus, for the present, cytogenetics continues to hold an important place in clinical laboratory medicine.

Table 69–6 Chromosome Breakage Syndromes

Disorder	Clinical Features	Gene Locus	Cytogenetic Manifestation	Type of Cancer	DNA Repair Defect	Misc
Fanconi anemia	Pancytopenia, pre- or postnatal growth retardation, hypoplastic or missing thumbs, possible arm deformation, brownish pigmentation of skin	1. Group A: 16q24.3 2. Group C – 9q22.3 3. Group D -3p22–p26 4. Group E – 6p21–p22 5. Groups B, F, H unmapped	Increased chromosome breakage detected by treatment with mitomycin C and diepoxybutane	Increased risk of AML, and progressive bone marrow failure		Current therapy: Bone marrow transplantation
Bloom syndrome	Growth retardation, butterfly rash on face, possible malignancy	15q26.1	Increased sister chromatid exchange in response to UV light or BrdU incorporation		Abnormal DNA ligase I activity	High frequency in Ashkenazi Jewish population: 1/110 carrier frequency
Ataxia telangiectasia	Ataxia with degeneration of central nervous system, telangiectasia on face, deficiency in cellular immunity, degenerative, growth retardation	11q22.3	Increased spontaneous breakage, increased rings, triradials, and translocations, particularly with 7 and 14, induced with bleomycin or ionizing radiation	Various leukemias and solid tumors		
Xeroderma pigmentosum	Sensitivity to sun, neurological abnormalities, ataxia and spasticity	Incidence: 1 in 250,000 1. A: 9q22.3 2. C: 653p25 3. D: 19q13.2–q13.3 4. E: 11p11–p12 5. F: 16p13.1–13.2, 16p13.13–p13.3 6. G: 13q33	Increase in SCE and chromosome rearrangement in response to UV light	Increased incidence of skin cancer	1. Lack of excision of thymine dimers 2. Postreplication repair defect	
Cockayne syndrome	Dwarfism, premature aging, microdephaly, neurologic deficit, pigmentary degeneration, deafness, sensitivity to sunlight, MR	Chr. 5	UV sensitivity	Increased incidence of skin cancer	Possible DNA ligase deficiency or defect of transcription coupled repair	

AML = acute myeloid leukemia; MR = mental retardation; UV = ultraviolet.

References

Anastasi J: Interphase cytogenetic analysis in the diagnosis and study of neoplastic disorders. Am J Clin Pathol 1991; 95(Suppl 1): S22–S28.

Angell RR, Xian J, Deith J, et al: First meiotic division abnormalities in human oocytes: mechanism of trisomy formation. Cytogenet Cell Genet 1994; 65:194–202.

Arlett CF, Lehmann AR: Human disorders showing increased sensitivity to the induction of genetic damage. Ann Rev Genet 1978; 12:95–115.

Bayes M, Magano LF, Rivera N, et al: Mutation mechanisms of Williams–Beuren syndrome deletions. Am J Hum Genet 2003; 73:131–151.

Blakemore KJ: Prenatal diagnosis by chorionic villus sampling. Obstet Gynecol Clin North Am 1988; 15:179–213.

Block, AW: Cancer cytogenetics. In Gersen S, Keagle M (eds): The Principles of Clinical Cytogenetics. Totowa, NJ, Humana Press, 1998, p 345.
An excellent reference covering cytogenetic aspects of oncology. Figures and tables are invaluable aides in interpreting patient results.

Burkholder GC, Weaver MG: DNA–protein interactions and chromosome banding. Exp Cell Res 1977; 110:251–262.

Cassidy SB, Lai L-W, Erickson RP, et al: Trisomy 15 with loss of the paternal 15 as a cause of Prader–Willi syndrome due to maternal disomy. Am J Hum Genet 1992; 51:701–708.

Cherif D, Bernard O, Berger R: Detection of single-copy genes by nonisotopic in situ hybridization on human chromosomes. Hum Genet 1989; 81:358–362.

Comings DE, Kovacs BW, Avelino E, et al: Mechanism of chromosome banding. V. Quinacrine banding. Chromosoma 1975; 50:111–145.

Cremer T, Lichter P, Borden J, et al: Detection of chromosome aberrations in metaphase and interphase tumor cells by in situ hybridization using chromosome-specific library probes. Hum Genet 1988; 80:235–246.

Delabar J-M, Theophile D, Rahmani Z, et al: Molecular mapping of the twenty-four features of Down syndrome on chromosome 21. Eur J Hum Genet 1993; 1:114–124.

De Lange T: Telomeres and senescence: ending the debate. Science 1998; 279:334–335.

De Martinville B, Blakemore KJ, Mahoney MJ, et al: DNA analysis of first-trimester chorionic villous biopsies: test for maternal contamination. Am J Hum Genet 1984; 36:1357–1368.

Divane A, Carter NP, Spathas DH, et al: Rapid prenatal diagnosis of aneuploidy from uncluttered amniotic fluid cells using five-colour fluorescence in situ hybridization. Prenat Diagn 1994; 14:1056–1069.

Flint J, Knight S: The use of telomere probes to investigate submicroscopic rearrangements associated with mental retardation. Curr Opin Genet Devel 2003; 13: 310–316.

Flint J, Wilke AOM, Buckle VJ, et al: The detection of subtelomeric chromosomal rearrangements in idiopathic mental retardation. Nat Genet 1995; 9:132–139.

Hall JG: Genomic imprinting: review and relevance to human diseases. Am J Hum Genet 1990; 46:857–873.

Harley CB, Futcher AB, Greider CW: Telomeres shorten during ageing of human fibroblasts. Nature 1990; 345:458–460.

Hassold T, Chiu D: Maternal age-specific rates of numerical chromosome abnormalities with special reference to trisomy. Hum Genet 1985; 70:11–17.

Holmquist G: The mechanism of C-banding: depurination and beta-elimination. Chromosoma 1979; 72:203–224.

Holmquist G, Gray M, Porter T, et al: Characterization of Giemsa dark- and light-band DNA. Cell 1982; 31:121–129.

Hook EB, Hamerton JL: The frequency of chromosome abnormalities detected in consecutive newborn studies – differences between studies – results by sex and by severity of phenotypic involvement. In Hook EB, Porter IH (eds): Population Cytogenetics. New York State Department of Health, Birth Defects Institute Symposium 1975. New York, Academic Press, 1977, p 63.

Irons M: Use of subtelomeric fluorescence in situ hybridization in cytogenetic diagnosis. Curr Opin Pediatr 2003; 15:594–597.

ISCN 2005: An International System for Human Cytogenetic Nomenclature. Basel, S Karger, 2005.
This reference provides the standard ideograms, the accepted cytogenetic nomenclature and how it is to be applied, and examples of usage of terminology.

Jacobs PA, Browne C, Gregson N, et al: Estimates of the frequency of chromosome abnormalities detectable in unselected newborns using moderate levels of banding. J Med Genet 1992; 29:103–108.

Jacobs PA, Price WH, Court Brown WM: Chromosome studies on men in a maximum security hospital. Ann Hum Genet 1968; 31:339–358.

Jaffe ES, Harris NL, Stein H, and Vardiman JW: Pathology and Genetics: Tumours of Haematopoietic and Lymphoid Tissues. Lyon, IARC Press, 2001.
This text is an important guide, providing the pathology (i.e., descriptions and findings) associated with leukemias and lymphomas. It includes the current WHOclassification for hematological disorders.

Jones KL (ed): Smith's Recognizable Patterns of Human Malformation, 6th ed. Philadelphia, PA, Elsevier Saunders, 2006.

VII

Korenberg JR, Kawashima H, Pulst S-M, et al: Molecular definition of a region of chromosome 21 that causes features of the Down syndrome phenotype. Am J Hum Genet 1990; 47:236–246.

Ledbetter DH, Cavenee WK: Molecular cytogenetics: interface of cytogenetics and monogenic disorders. In The Metabolic Basis of Inherited Disease, 6th ed. New York, McGraw-Hill, 1989, pp 343–371.

Ledbetter DH, Engel E: Uniparental disomy in humans: development of an imprinting map and its implications for prenatal diagnosis. Hum Mol Genet 1995; 4:1757–1764.

Ledbetter SA, Kuwano A, Dobyns WB, et al: Microdeletions of chromosome 17p13 as a cause of isolated lissencephaly. Am J Hum Genet 1992; 50:182–189.

Lichter P, Jauch A, Cremer T, et al: Detection of Down syndrome by in situ hybridization with chromosome 21 specific DNA probes. In Patterson D (ed): Molecular Genetics of Chromosome 21 and Down Syndrome. New York, Wiley-Liss, 1990.

Lindsay EA, Halford S, Wadey R, et al: Molecular cytogenetic characterization of the DiGeorge syndrome region using fluorescence in situ hybridization. Genomics 1993; 17:403–407.

Lubs HA: A marker X chromosome. Am J Hum Genet 1969; 31:231–244.

McDermid HE, Morrow BE: Genomic disorders on 22q11. Am J Hum Genet 2002; 70:1077–1088.

National Institutes of Health and Institute of Molecular Medicine Collaboration: A complete set of human telomeric probes and their clinical application. Nat Genet 1996; 14:86–89.

Nicholls RD, Knoll JHM, Butler MG, et al: Genetic imprinting suggested by maternal heterodisomy in non-deletion Prader–Willi syndrome. Nature 1989; 342:281–285.

Nicholls RD, Saitoh S, Horsthemke B: Imprinting in Prader–Willi and Angelman syndromes. Trends Genet 1998; 14:194–198.

Nussbaum RL, McInnes RR, Willard HF: Thompson and Thompson – Genetics in Medicine, 6th ed. Philadelphia, PA, WB Saunders, 2004.

Excellent textbook covering all aspects of medical genetics. It provides a basic introduction to the field followed by detailed descriptions of subspecialties including cytogenetics, molecular genetics, cancer genetics, immunogenetics, prenatal genetics, and genetic counseling.

OMIM (Online Mendelian Inheritance in Man). http://www.ncbi.nlm.nih.gov/Omim/.

The best source of information on genes related to diseases. Each entry includes data on the discovery of the gene, cytogenetic and molecular aspects of the disorder, possible genetic testing, related diseases, and references to the scientific literature.

Palmer CG, Reichmann A: Chromosomal and clinical findings in 110 females with Turner syndrome. Hum Genet 1976; 35:35–49.

Petersen MB, Bartsch O, Adelsberger PA, et al: Uniparental isodisomy due to duplication of chromosome 21 occurring in somatic cells monosomic for chromosome 21. Genomics 1992; 13:269–274.

Pitcher DR: Chromosome and violence. Practitioner 1982; 226:497–501.

Price WH, Jacobs PA: The 47,XXY male with special reference to behavior. Semin Psychol 1970; 2:30–39.

Reid T, Baldini A, Rand TC, et al: Simultaneous visualization of seven different DNA probes by in situ hybridization using combinatorial fluorescence and digital imaging microscopy. Proc Natl Acad Sci USA 1992a; 89:1388–1392.

Reid T, Landes G, Dackowski W, et al: Multicolor fluorescence in situ hybridization for the simultaneous detection of probe sets for chromosomes 13, 18, 21, X and Y in uncultured amniotic fluid cells. Hum Mol Genet 1992b; 1: 307–313.

Rhoads GG, Jackson LG, Sachslesselman SE, et al: The safety and efficacy of chorionic villus sampling for early prenatal diagnosis of cytogenetic abnormalities. N Engl J Med 1989; 320:609–617.

Robinson WP, Bottani A, Yagang X, et al: Molecular, cytogenetic and clinical investigations of Prader–Willi syndrome patients. Am J Hum Genet 1991; 49:1219–1234.

Rosenberg MJ, Killoran C, Dziadzio L, et al: Scanning for telomeric deletions and duplications and uniparental disomy using genetic markers in 120 children with malformations. Hum Genet 2001; 109:311–318.

Rousseau F, Heitz D, Biancalana V, et al: Direct diagnosis by DNA analysis of the fragile X syndrome of mental retardation. N Engl J Med 1991; 325:1673–1681.

Schrock E, du Manoir S, Veldman T, et al: Multicolor spectral karyotyping of human chromosomes. Science 1996; 273:494–497.

Speicher MR, Ballard SG, Ward DC: Karyotyping human chromosomes by combinatorial multi-fluor FISH. Nat Genet 1996; 12:368–375.

Spence EJ, Perciaccante RG, Greig GM, et al: Uniparental disomy as a mechanism for human genetic disease. Am J Hum Genet 1988; 42:217–226.

Sumner AT, Evans HJ, Buckland RA: Mechanisms involved in the banding of chromosome with quinacrine and Giemsa I. The effects of fixation in methanol–acetic acid. Exp Cell Res 1973; 81:214–222.

Theilgaard A: A psychological study of the personalities of XYY- and XXY-men. Acta Psychiatr Scand Suppl 1984; 315:1–133.

Trask BJ: Fluorescence in situ hybridization: applications in cytogenetics and gene mapping. Trends Genet 1991; 7:149–154.

Turnpenny P, Ellard S: Emery's Elements of Medical Genetics, 12th ed., Edinburgh, Churchill Livingstone, 2005.

Veldman T, Vignon C, Schrock E, et al: Hidden chromosome abnormalities in haematological malignancies detected by multicolour spectral karyotyping. Nat Genet 1997; 15:406–410.

Verkerk AJMH, Pieretti M, Sutcliffe JS, et al: Identification of a gene (FMR-1) containing a CGG repeat coincident with a breakpoint cluster region exhibiting length variation in fragile X syndrome. Cell 1991; 65:905–914.

Voss R, Ben-Simon E, Avital A, et al: Isodisomy of chromosome 7 in a patient with cystic fibrosis: could uniparental diasomy be common in humans? Am J Hum Genet 1989; 45:373–380.

Vysis, Inc. http://www.vysis.com.

Developer and manufacturer of FISH probes. The website provides information on the probes available and the biology behind the detection assay.

Werner M, Ewig M, Nasarek A: Value of fluorescence in situ hybridization for detecting the bcr/abl gene fusion in interphase cells of routine bone marrow specimens. Diagn Mol Pathol 1997; 6:282–287.

Witkin HA, Mednick SA, Schulsinger F, et al: Criminality in XYY and XXY men. Science 1976; 193:547–555.

Wright WE, Shay JW: Telomere positional effects and the regulation of cellular senescence. Trends Genet 1992; 8:193–197.

Yunis JJ, Sanchez O: G-banding and chromosome structure. Chromosoma 1973; 44:15–23.

Further Reading

Borgaonkar D: Chromosomal Variation in Man: A Catalog of Chromosomal Variants and Anomalies, 5th ed. New York, Wiley-Liss, 1989.

De Grouchy J, Turleau C: Clinical Atlas of Human Chromosomes, 2nd ed. New York, John Wiley & Sons, 1984.

Gelehrter T, Collins FC, Ginsburg D: Principles of Medical Genetics, 2nd ed. Baltimore, MD, Williams & Wilkins, 1998.

Heim S, Mitelman F: Cancer Cytogenetics, 2nd ed. New York, Wiley-Liss, Inc, 1995.

This is an excellent source of information covering all aspects of cancer genetics. It includes molecular, cytogenetic, and clinical aspects of all known leukemias, lymphomas, and solid tumors.

McKusick V: Mendelian Inheritance in Man: Catalogs of Autosomal Dominant, Autosomal Recessive, and X-linked Phenotypes, 11th ed. Baltimore, MD, Johns Hopkins Press, 1983.

Mitelman F: Catalog of Chromosome Aberrations in Cancer, 5th ed. New York, Wiley-Liss, Inc, 1994.

Rooney DE, Czepulkowski BH: Human Cytogenetics, A Practical Approach. Oxford, IRL Press, 1992.

Verma R, Babu A: Human Chromosomes – Principles and Techniques, 2nd ed. New York, McGraw-Hill, 1995.

CHAPTER 70

Establishing a Molecular Diagnostics Laboratory

Andrea Ferreira-Gonzalez PhD, David S. Wilkinson MD PhD, Carleton T. Garrett MD PhD

KEY POINTS

• Molecular diagnostic testing requires separate facilities to eliminate or control contamination, especially for nucleic acid amplification techniques that have exquisite sensitivity and specificity, but are susceptible to false positive signals from miniscule amounts of amplified products, carryover from different specimens, or other environmental sources. Essential equipment is unique and not usually found in typical clinical laboratories. Personnel must be trained in the procedures and precautions of molecular diagnostic procedures with specific certification now provided by professional organizations.

• The format for molecular diagnostic testing has traditionally been 'home-brew' assays that require extensive validation by the laboratory performing them. A growing number of assays are available commercially in which the kit manufacturer provides reagents (including quality control specimens) for each step of an assay, or the laboratory can combine reagents from different kits for particular clinical uses. Automation has been applied to various stages of assays from extraction of nucleic acid through analytic performance with homogeneous assays emerging for use as closed systems.

• Factors influencing test selection in a molecular diagnostics laboratory include clinical need for rapid turn-around time of results, cost-effectiveness compared to alternative methods such as microbiologic culture, level of reimbursement achieved from health insurance plans, and the feasibility of licensing patented processes.

• Establishing and offering a molecular diagnostic test requires optimization of each step of the analytic process followed by a validation process that entails standardization (whenever possible) with reference materials (e.g., from a national or international organization), definition of analytical sensitivity, accuracy, imprecision, linearity, effects of pre-analytic variables/interferences, and clinical sensitivity, efficacy, and interpretation. Use of analyte-specific reagents (ASR) requires a statement in the result report that the laboratory has determined the assay's performance characteristics. Genetic test reports should also be accompanied by statements that qualify the sensitivity or predictive value of the result.

• Each step of the testing process for molecular diagnostics requires quality control to monitor reagent preparation, specimen collection, specimen processing and aliquotting, and performance of the assay. In-house-developed assays have a critical need for quality control to establish the strength, purity, and performance of each reagent. Equipment such as thermocyclers require temperature checks, and pipetters require quality control and maintenance. Quality assurance programs monitor compliance with standards of training, competence, equipment, safety, and other laboratory issues plus an evaluation of overall results of patient testing services. Laboratory accreditation is based on these practices plus successful proficiency testing and checklists designed for molecular pathology.

During the past decade a vast amount of knowledge has been gained regarding genes and their role in human disease. This knowledge has allowed us to better understand many disease processes. As a consequence, diseases are increasingly being defined in terms of their molecular pathogenesis. This has led to the development of new clinical molecular assays for use in diagnosis, prognosis, selection of therapeutic modalities, and monitoring of disease. Clinical molecular assays represent a collection of techniques and reagents in which the main analyte is nucleic acid. The nucleic acid can be DNA or RNA. There are many applications of this technology to different areas of the clinical laboratory. One of the major advantages of using nucleic acid as the analyte is that it represents nature's most specific marker of all living organisms, i.e., the order of the nucleotides comprising the organism's genome. The number of distinct arrangements of the four different nucleotides, which can be present in a DNA molecule that is only as large as the smallest virus, is many times greater than the total number of different types of living organisms on this planet, allowing the DNA sequence of each living organism to contain unique information that can be used to identify it. In addition to the identification of specific organisms, individual changes in DNA sequences are the cause of genetic and malignant diseases and thus provide important diagnostic and prognostic information. Until the development of simple and robust methods for detecting differences in nucleic acid sequences, analysis of these analytes at the sequence level in the clinical laboratory was not practical. Recent advances in new technology and instrumentation, and efforts in standardization, have overcome many of these limitations.

Laboratory Facilities

The power of molecular diagnostics is derived from the exquisite sensitivity and specificity given by the use of nucleic acid as the analyte. The high sensitivity is derived from in vitro amplification of specific nucleic acid target sequences present in a patient's specimen. In vitro amplification creates millions or billions of copies of the target sequence and thus enables detection of as little as a single target molecule in the patient specimen. At the same time, however, this high sensitivity poses major challenges for the

VIII

use of this technology. Thus, one of the major advantages of this technology is also one of its major limitations. Opening and closing the microcentrifuge tubes containing amplified product can aerosolized microdroplets that can carry 10–100 copies of the amplified target sequence. These microdroplets can subsequently be deposited on bench tops, instruments, furniture, floor, dust, hair, exposed skin, virtually any and every surface. Another important source of contamination can be the target nucleic acid itself. Sample handling procedures must always protect against crosscontamination of patient specimens. A source of contamination by nucleic acid that is sometimes overlooked results from processing patient samples in an environment in which the target nucleic acid has been amplified biologically either by cloning or culturing the cell or microorganism. Thus, it is necessary to design the molecular diagnostics laboratory facility carefully to assure sufficient and adequate space for personnel and equipment, but also to minimize the potential problem of specimen contamination with natural nucleic acid or template and/or nucleic acid from in vitro amplification (amplicon).

Laboratory Design

Laboratory space should be designed to minimize the risk of contamination and maximize work flow. Barrier containment through the use of physically separate work areas for reagent preparation, specimen accessioning, nucleic acid extraction and analysis of the amplified material is highly desirable. An ideal laboratory is composed of three completely independent rooms or areas. Two of these rooms are considered clean rooms, since all tasks and duties before in vitro amplification are performed in these laboratories. These rooms are called preamplification rooms. The third room is considered a dirty room, since it is dedicated to in vitro amplification and analysis of the amplified material. This room is called the postamplification room. The air handling systems for each of these rooms should be completely independent of one another. If this is not possible, it is highly recommended that the preamplification laboratories are located closest to the source of air in reference to both laboratories. The preamplification laboratories should be under positive air pressure. This will impede the entrance of any airborne contaminant into the preamplification laboratory when the door is opened. In addition, the postamplification laboratory should be under negative air pressure to impede anything from coming out of this laboratory and contaminating the surrounding environment. Construction of an anteroom into each laboratory is an inexpensive way of creating differential pressures for the laboratory. A positive pressurized anteroom for a preamplification laboratory can be created by use of a fan in the ceiling of the anteroom that draws air from inside the laboratory and blows it into the anteroom. This positively pressurized anteroom serves much the same purpose as having the entire laboratory under positive pressure. Similarly, an anteroom for the postamplification room can be easily made into a negatively pressurized room by having the fan draw air out of the anteroom and blow it into the laboratory. There should be a seal around the door separating the anteroom from the laboratory to avoid air within the laboratory from going back into the anteroom. It is important to emphasize that the door leading into the anteroom from the outside and the door into the laboratory should never be opened at the same time. An additional safety feature is to place sticky mats at the entrance of each anteroom or laboratory. The size of the anteroom is determined by the activities that will be carried out in it. In addition, if dedicated disposable laboratory coats, hats and booties are used, space will be needed for storing these items.

Different activities are carried out in each of the three rooms/areas. In vitro amplification is never carried out in the two preamplification laboratories. One of these rooms is dedicated to reagent preparation and the other to specimen accessioning, specimen preparation, and reaction set-up. In the event of limited space, the two preamplification rooms can be combined into one laboratory. The use of dead air boxes for reagent preparation and reaction set up is highly recommended and it is more critical in the event that both laboratories must be combined. The use of dead air boxes provides a tightly controlled environment where reagent and reaction preparation can be carried out. It is important to try to locate this area in a section of the laboratory with low traffic. No genomic or plasmid DNA, RNA or patient specimen should be introduced into the dead air box where reagent preparation takes place. This dead air box should be furnished with an ultraviolet light connected to a timer. The surface areas of the dead air boxes should be treated with ultraviolet light, wiped with 10% freshly made sodium hypochlorite solution and finally wiped with 75% ethanol solution before and after working in this area. For the reasons already stated, these areas should contain dedicated equipment and instrumentation that is not shared with any other area. Some of the dedicated instruments are pipetter, vortex, tips, tubes, etc. It is recommended that dedicated laboratory wear and gloves be put on before starting work in this environment.

The second clean room or area within the preamplification laboratory is where specimen accessioning, specimen processing, and addition of nucleic acid to the appropriate reaction tube is carried out. This area should be furnished with at least one environmental biosafety cabinet for specimen processing and nucleic acid extraction in addition to dedicated laboratory equipment that is used solely for this purpose. Another completely separate environmental biosafety cabinet should be available if any tissue culture is carried out in this laboratory and separate laboratory equipment should be dedicated to this function. Also, if organic nucleic acid extractions are used in the laboratory, a chemical safety cabinet should be available for handling the phenol and chloroform steps during the extraction procedure. If both DNA and RNA extraction are carried out in the same preamplification laboratory, one should perform these procedures in separate areas of the laboratory and have dedicated instruments, pipettes, and filtered tips for each procedure. In circumstances where space is a major issue and it is not possible to dedicate two completely separated areas, extraction of DNA and RNA should be performed at different times or on different days after thoroughly cleaning the areas before working. As already described, all areas should be wiped with a 10% solution of daily-prepared sodium hypochlorite and with a solution of 75% ethanol.

The postamplification laboratory is where in vitro amplification and analysis of nucleic acid is carried out. Instruments used in this laboratory should not be shared with the preamplification areas. If thermocyclers are used in in vitro amplification of nucleic acid, it is recommended that they be placed in this laboratory. If thermocyclers are placed in the preamplification laboratory, under no circumstances can reaction tubes be opened after amplification in this room. In addition, thermocyclers should be plugged into dedicated power lines with their own circuit breaker to avoid any fluctuation in electricity that could affect their performance. Normally this laboratory will require more space than the preamplification laboratories since instrumentation for analysis of amplified product tends to be more extensive than that required for reagent preparation and nucleic acid extraction. Gel electrophoresis, for example, frequently requires significant open bench space. A darkroom with a dedicated automatic film processor and a freezer is highly recommended. It is, however, preferable to place the dark room outside the postamplification laboratory so as to have access to it without having to go into the postamplification laboratory.

Real-time technology has recently been introduced in the clinical laboratory, with major success. One of the great benefits of these instruments is that, as they perform in vitro amplification, they can simultaneously detect the amplified product. This allows detection and quantification of specific nucleic acid sequences without further manipulation or opening of test tubes and dramatically reduces the risk of amplicon contamination. For assays developed and performed using these types of instrument, the risks of amplicon contamination are significantly reduced. However, at this juncture, molecular diagnostics laboratories must continue to rely on standard 'open' platforms for many tests, particularly those developed in-house using analyte-specific reagents. For these assays, the risk of amplicon contamination still remains a significant issue that must be addressed through laboratory design and practices to minimize the risk.

Practices to Aid in Contamination Control

The introduction of simple practices in the daily routine can aid in the control of amplicon and target contamination. Unidirectional work-flow must be strictly adhered to, whereby personnel perform tasks in the clean rooms first and only after completing their tasks there move on into the post-amplification room. No personnel who have worked in the postamplification laboratory should return to the preamplification area before showering and changing their clothes. Use of disposable laboratory coats, booties, and hats is recommended. If cloth lab coats are used it is necessary to keep dedicated lab coats for each laboratory and they should be kept inside the laboratories and not worn in the office space. Use of different-colored lab coats for each area is one way to remind personnel of the strict work-flow.

Another extremely important factor in laboratory workflow is house-keeping. Control of work-flow of housekeeping personnel is likewise important. The safest approach is to have laboratory staff perform some of the housekeeping duties by bagging the trash from each laboratory and placing it outside the laboratory for pickup by housekeeping staff. If this is not done, housekeeping personnel must be instructed to remove trash first from the preamplification room, then from the office space and last from the postamplification room.

Protection of counter tops with absorbent plastic backed paper is not recommended as paper, if not changed often, can collect dust and with it amplified material. If used, this type of paper should be discarded immediately after each use. The use of bleach (hypochlorite) appears to be the most generally accepted method for decontaminating surfaces.

Decontamination of counter tops, laboratory equipment and furniture should be performed by wiping with a freshly made 10% solution of bleach and then with a 75% ethanol solution, or even water, to dilute the bleach, which could corrode the surfaces. All pipette tips should contain a hydrophobic filter in order to avoid any contamination of the tip of the pipetter with template or amplified material. Evaluation of the effectiveness of the hydrophobic barrier can be assessed by setting the pipette beyond its upper limit and drawing fluid from a colored solution into the disposable pipette tip that contains the hydrophobic barrier. If the tip of the pipette becomes stained by the fluid then the barrier is inadequate. After use, disposable pipette tips should be placed into zip-lock bags, making sure that the bags are completely sealed before discarding them. Gloves should be changed periodically or as soon any contamination is suspected.

Another approach to preventing amplicon contamination is to treat amplicon chemically so that it will not be able to support amplification even if accidentally added to another sample. Amplicon can be destroyed by different means. The most widely used means is ultraviolet irradiation. Ultraviolet treatment of DNA induces crosslinking of the two strands of DNA by forming thymidine dimers. This crosslinked DNA can no longer serve as an effective template. One disadvantage of ultraviolet treatment is that it is most effective in sequences over 700 nucleotides in length. In most clinical assays, the length of the amplicon is less than 700 bp.

A chemical means of inactivating or sterilizing amplicon is through the incorporation of deoxyuridine triphosphate instead of deoxythymidine triphosphate into the amplicon during the amplification procedure. After amplification, if this uracil-containing amplicon contaminates another sample by accident, it can be destroyed prior to amplification by treating the sample with uracil-N-glycosylase (UNG). The uracil-containing amplicon is the substrate for UNG, while the thymidine-containing template is not. The mechanism behind this chemical reaction is that UNG removes uracil residues from the amplicon, still leaving an intact phosphodiester backbone on the amplicon. During the first denaturation step of the amplification procedure, the phosphodiester bonds break at the sites where the uracil residues were located. The fragmented amplicon is no longer able to act as a template. Use of deoxyuridine triphosphate and UNG have been shown to be effective in controlling contamination if amplification of the uracil-containing amplicon does not exceed 10^6–10^7 copies per reaction.

Another method of sterilization uses the photochemical treatment of isopsoralen compounds. These are added to the reaction mixture prior to amplification. Following polymerase chain reaction (PCR) but before the reaction tube is opened, the vessel is exposed to ultraviolet light (300–400 nm), which activates the isopsoralens to form adductors between the pyrimidines on the amplicons. These adductors stop Taq polymerase from processing along the amplicons and thus prevent subsequent reamplification of any of these contaminating amplicons.

Transfer of paper, such as written procedures or notes regarding specific samples, between laboratories and office is also a concern. This should be reduced as much as possible, especially paperwork used in the post-amplification laboratory. It is highly recommended that a computer network be put in place in the laboratory with a number of computer terminals throughout the different laboratories and office areas in order to reduce or eliminate the movement of paper throughout the laboratory and back into the office area. It is important that the network server be backed up daily.

Equipment

Laboratory equipment necessary for successfully conducting current typical molecular diagnostics tests can include instrumentation not generally found in the typical clinical laboratory. Even where there is overlap in the type of equipment that is used it is important that the molecular diagnostic laboratory contains its own equipment for purposes of contamination control. A comprehensive list of laboratory equipment is given in Table 70–1. Some additional specialized equipment not included in the list that might be useful, depending on the scope of the testing menu, includes an automatic DNA sequencer, real-time thermocyclers, capillary electrophoresis instruments and even high-performance liquid chromatography. A large number of these specialized instruments are very expensive, which can make implementation of testing that requires these instruments difficult. More recently, a new method of acquisition of instrumentation has become possible through reagent rental agreements with some of the manufacturers of in vitro diagnostic tests and analyte-specific reagents. This funding mechanism has been in use for many years in other areas of the clinical laboratory but is new in molecular diagnostics.

Personnel

Laboratories performing molecular diagnostic testing are classified as high-complexity testing laboratories under the Clinical Laboratory Improvement

Table 70–1 Capital Equipment Requirements

Description	Quantity
DNA thermal cycler(s)	2
Laminar flow environmental hoods	2
Freezer/refrigerator	2
–20°C manual defrost freezer	2
–70°C freezer	1
Angle-head microcentrifuge, 14 000 rpm	2
Horizontal microcentrifuge, 14 000 rpm	1
Electronic balance	2
pH meter	2
Heating/stir plate	2
Water bath	1
Electrophoresis power supplies	3
Mini PAGE electrophoresis apparatus	2
Photodocumentation system	1
Agarose gel electrophoresis apparatus	4
Automated X-ray film processor	1
Autoradiography cassettes (17 × 14 in)	4
Autoradiography cassettes (8 × 10 in)	4
Standard micropipetters (three sizes)	18
Dead air box	2
Real time instrument	1
Vortex mixers	3
Pneumatic pipette aid	4
Counter-top radioactive counter	1
Ultraviolet-spectrophotometer	1
Geiger counter	1
Dry water bath	4
Refrigerated microcentrifuge	2
Hybridization oven	1
Table-top refrigerated centrifuge	1
Incubator	2

Amendment of 1988 (CLIA'88) (Bachner, 1988). This imposes specific educational and training requirements for personnel working in these laboratories. In addition, it is important to keep in mind that not only are these tests more complex than standard laboratory tests but some have been developed in-house. Moreover, because of the introduction of new technology, these assays are constantly being modified to improve specificity, sensitivity, turn around time, work flow, etc.

Laboratory Director

As per CLIA'88, directors of high-complexity testing laboratories must either: (1) be an MD or DO with training in Clinical or Anatomical Pathology; (2) be an MD or DO with 2 years of experience in directing or supervising a high-complexity testing laboratory; or (3) hold a doctorate in one of the biological sciences and have 2 years of experience in supervising a high-complexity laboratory.

The responsibilities of the laboratory director are test selection, implementation, and resolution of technical difficulties. The laboratory director is also responsible for developing laboratory programs for analytical and clinical validation of new molecular tests and development of management guidelines and practices that ensure reliable performance of clinical testing. In addition, the laboratory director must also be responsible for the development, implementation, and review of the laboratory quality assurance and control programs.

Technical Supervisor

As per CLIA'88 a technical supervisor must meet one of the following criteria to qualify for this position. The individual must possess: (1) an MD or DO with 1 year of experience in a high-complexity testing laboratory; (2) a master's degree with 2 years of experience; or (3) a bachelor's degree with 4 years of experience.

Medical Technologists and Molecular Biology Technician

Medical technologists and molecular biology technicians are responsible for tasks and duties necessary for the daily operation of the laboratory testing agenda. These individuals are responsible for specimen accessioning and processing, performing daily testing, maintaining appropriate testing and quality control records, adhering to written procedures and quality control policies, identifying problems, and documenting equipment maintenance. Record keeping for laboratory procedures is complicated by the fact that assays developed in-house are constantly being modified to improve the testing process. In addition, some laboratory instruments are used solely for molecular diagnostic testing and there is little clinical laboratory experience with them. Because of these factors, it is important that technical staff and in particular senior technical staff have a high sense of professional commitment and display constant interest and effort in improving their education and training. It is also important that they acquire as many advanced laboratory skills as possible and that they are crosstrained in most or all of the different tests used in the laboratory. It is crucial that the technical personnel fully understand the scientific basics of the methodology and the clinical applications and implications of the different molecular tests.

Residents, Fellows and Graduate Students

Involvement of residents, fellows, and graduate students can contribute significantly to the success of a molecular diagnostics laboratory. The value of these individuals comes from their high level of professional commitment and their insight into the clinical utility of individual tests. If such individuals are given time to work in the molecular diagnostics laboratory, they are frequently able to rapidly develop and validate a new molecular assay. In return, these individuals gain expertise in an area of laboratory medicine that is rapidly growing and this may provide them with an advantage when seeking future employment. As part of their training in molecular diagnostics, it is important for residents, fellows, and graduate students to gain experience in each of the different areas of testing, including infectious disease, genetic disease, and cancer. Training should include the basic principles of molecular biology; hands-on experience in optimizing, validating, and performing molecular diagnostic testing; test result interpretation; and preparation of reports for review. In addition, it is recommended that laboratory directors familiarize trainees with the different issues involved in laboratory management.

Certification of Personnel in Molecular Diagnostics

Certification of doctoral level personnel working in molecular diagnostic laboratories can follow several different routes depending on the type of doctoral degree as well as other training experience. One avenue open to individuals with either an MD or PhD is provided by the American Board of Medical Genetics (ABMG) and is intended for individuals who provide services in medical genetics. The ABMG is a member of the American Board of Medical Specialties, which is the parent organization for boards that provide certification in pathology, pediatrics, internal medicine, surgery, and other medical specialties. Certification consists of a general examination followed by a subspecialty examination in clinical genetics, medical genetics, clinical cytogenetics, clinical biochemical genetics, or clinical molecular genetics. To be eligible for certification by the ABMG, an individual must meet the criteria in the desired area of certification. The requirements for certification in clinical molecular genetics will be discussed here. In addition to possessing the appropriate doctoral degree, the candidate for the clinical molecular genetics board must complete 2 years of training in a fully accredited program. The candidate must present a logbook of 150 clinical molecular cases and a completed clinical molecular genetics test and method competency list signed by the laboratory director, with half of the time of the training spent at the bench. The examination is offered every 3 years.

Recently, the American Board of Medical Specialties approved the application from the American Board of Pathology and the ABMG to create a joint subspecialty certification in molecular genetic pathology. Candidates for this certification must hold an MD or DO degree, have been certified by their respective boards, have a valid unrestricted license to practice medicine or osteopathy in the United States, and have completed a year of training in an accredited program. Today, there are 11 programs that have received full accreditation by the ABGM and 12 programs that have either received provisional accreditation or are in the process of seeking accreditation. Standards for training in molecular diagnostics are being defined by the different organizations involved in certification. The candidate must present a logbook of 150 clinical molecular cases. The examination is offered every other year.

In addition, the American Board of Clinical Chemistry (ABCC) has approved a certification program in molecular diagnostics that was offered for the first time in June 2000. The ABCC is an independent, not-for-profit-corporation that certifies doctoral level professionals in clinical chemistry and toxicological chemistry. The rules and regulations of the ABCC for certification in molecular diagnostics have recently been established. Prior to admission to examination the applicant must have a certification from any of the following boards: the ABCC, the American Board of Medical Microbiology, the American Board of Pathology, the American Board of Medical Laboratory Immunology, the American Board of Bioanalysis or the American Board of Histocompatibility and Immunogenetics. Applicants must meet education and experience requirements in addition to three letters of recommendation to attest to familiarity with the applicant's professional expertise, length of experience in the field, etc. The examination is offered once a year.

Subspecialty certification in molecular diagnostics is being offered to non-doctoral-level individuals, including medical technologists and molecular biology technicians, through the National Credentialing Agency for Laboratory Personnel, Inc. (NCA). NCA is a nongovernmental, nonprofit organization that conducts certification of laboratory personnel. Medical technologists and molecular biology technicians are certified as laboratory specialists in molecular biology (LSp[MB]). There are seven routes for eligibility:

1. Successfully complete a National Accrediting Agency for Clinical Laboratory Sciences-accredited baccalaureate or postbaccalaureate program in molecular diagnostics or molecular biotechnology.
2. Successfully complete a baccalaureate or a postbaccalaureate program in a molecular biology program sponsored by an accredited college or university that includes the equivalent of 6 months of full-time experience in a full-service molecular biology laboratory.
3. Successfully complete a NAACLS-accredited or NAACLS-approved baccalaureate-level education program in a clinical laboratory science (clinical laboratory sciences, medical technology, cytogenetics) and complete the equivalent of 6 months of full-time experience gained within the last year in a full-service molecular biology laboratory.
4. Be certified as a clinical laboratory scientist or equivalent, a clinical laboratory specialist in cytogenetics, or an advanced registered technologist (Canadian Society for Medical Laboratory Science), and complete the equivalent of 6 months of full-time work experience gained with the last year in a full-service in a full-service molecular biology laboratory.
5. Have a baccalaureate degree in the biological, chemical and/or medical sciences from an accredited college or university and complete the equivalent of 1 year of full-time work experience within the last 2 years in a full-service molecular biology laboratory.
6. Have a baccalaureate degree from an accredited college or university and complete 36 semester hours in the biological, chemical, and/or medical sciences (in addition to or part of the baccalaureate degree) and complete the equivalent of 1 year of full-time work experience gained within the last 2 years in a full-service molecular biology laboratory.
7. Be certified as a registered technologist by the Canadian Society for Medical Laboratory Science and complete the equivalent of 2 years of full-time work experience gained within the last 4 years in a full-service molecular biology laboratory.

A full-service molecular biology laboratory is defined as one capable of providing individuals with knowledge and practical experience in all aspects of molecular analysis including, but not limited to, recombinant DNA technologies, polymerase chain reaction, and hybridization techniques.

A number of different universities and colleges have started offering baccalaureate and masters programs with a molecular specialty. Not every program provides eligibility for the NCA examination upon completion. A list of the different degree programs and eligibility for NCA examination is listed at www.amp.org. This examination is offered twice a year in over 80 test centers throughout the country and even in a few foreign centers.

More recently, the American Society for Clinical Pathologists (ASCP; www.ascp.org) has introduced a new certification for technologists with emphasis on molecular diagnostics. This molecular diagnostics certification enables technical personnel working in this area to achieve recognition. To be eligible for this examination category, an applicant must satisfy the requirements of at least one of the following routes:

1. ASCP certified as a technologist or specialist and a baccalaureate degree from a regionally accredited college/university.
2. Baccalaureate degree from a regionally accredited college/university, including courses in biological science, chemistry and mathematics and successful completion of a NAACLS-approved baccalaureate molecular diagnostics or molecular biotechnology program.
3. Baccalaureate degree in biological or chemical science from a regionally accredited college/university and 12 months acceptable clinical laboratory experience in molecular diagnostics in a CLIA-regulated, accredited clinical laboratory in the past 5 years.
4. Graduate-level degree (masters or doctorate) in the natural sciences or medical laboratory sciences from a regionally accredited college/university and 6 months acceptable clinical laboratory experience in molecular diagnostics in a CLIA regulated, accredited clinical laboratory within the last 5 years.

Table 70–2 Automatic Nucleic Acid Extractors

Manufacturer	Technology	Instruments	Type of Sample	Sample/Run	Run Duration	Hands on Time
Qiagen	Magnetic particles/silica extraction	BioRobot 9604	Blood, buffy coat, tissue, buccal swab, paraffin-embedded sections, urine, cerebral spinal fluid, dried blood, plasma, serum	96	<2.5 h	20 min
		BioRobot 48	Blood, buffy coat, tissue, buccal swab, paraffin-embedded sections, urine, cerebral spinal fluid, dried blood, plasma, serum	48 (multiples of 6)	20 min/6 samples 2.5 h/48 samples	35 min/24 samples
		BioRobot EZ1	Blood, buffy coat, tissue, buccal swab, paraffin-embedded sections, urine, cerebral spinal fluid, dried blood, plasma, serum	1–6	20 min	
Roche Diagnostics	Magnetic particles/ specific oligonucleotide capture probes	MagNA Pure LC	Blood, buffy coats, cells, fungi, bacteria, cerebrospinal fluid, urine, paraffin-embedded sections, buccal swabs, plasma, serum	32 (multiples of 8)	2 h/24 samples	35 min/24 samples
		MagNA Pure Compact	Blood, buffy coats, cells, fungi, bacteria, cerebrospinal fluid, urine, paraffin-embedded sections, buccal swabs, plasma, serum	1–8		30 min/24 samples
	Filter-based/silica extraction	Ampliprep	Plasma, serum	72	2.5 h	
BioMérieux	Magnetic particles/silica extraction	Nuclisens extractor		10	45 min	20 min
		Nuclisens EasyMag (in development)		24	1 h	<20 min
Gentra Systems	Modified salting out method	AutoPure LS	Whole blood, buffy coat, packed cells, lysates for compromised samples, buccal swabs, cultured cells	96 (multiples of 8)	8 h/96 samples 4 h/48 samples	35 min

Clinical Test Formats

There are basically two test formats in use in the majority of laboratories performing molecular diagnostic testing. The two formats are tests developed in-house by each laboratory, also known as home-brew assays, and reagents provided in kit format by medical device manufacturers.

Tests Developed In-House

Tests developed in-house consist of those assays that have been fully developed and validated by the laboratory performing them. They are also referred to as 'home brew' tests. Usually these assays use a combination of reagents that are purchased separately from a variety of manufacturers. Each laboratory determines the performance characteristics of the assay for a clinical condition in a particular patient population. The analytical and clinical validation of the entire testing process is the responsibility of each laboratory.

Kit-based Manual Methods

There are two general categories of kit-based manual methods used in molecular diagnostics. In the first category the kit manufacturer provides quality-controlled reagents for every step required to carry out the entire molecular test. An example of this type of kit would be the set of reagents provided by Roche Molecular Systems for quantifying human immuno-deficiency virus (HIV)-1 in the plasma of patients diagnosed with acquired immunodeficiency syndrome (AIDS). These kits include the reagents necessary for nucleic acid isolation, amplification, and detection. They also include information about sensitivity, specificity, and tolerance limits for the particular clinical condition. These kits may be labeled by the manufacturers as US Food and Drug Administration (FDA)-approved, FDA-cleared, for research use only, or for investigation use only. Analytical and clinical validation of these kits differs drastically depending upon the labeling. Validation procedures will be discussed below.

The second category of kit-based manual methods includes kits developed by a manufacturer to provide quality-controlled reagents for performing a particular step in molecular testing. For example, kits are commercially available for nucleic acid extraction, kits containing amplification reagents, including controls, in vitro amplified nucleic acid detection systems, etc. With these, the laboratory develops a particular molecular test by combining two or more kits from the same or even from different manufacturers for a particular clinical condition in a given patient population. Analytical and clinical validation of each step and the entire procedure will be discussed below.

Automated Platforms for Molecular Testing

In recent years the development and introduction of automated platforms for molecular diagnostic testing has become more common (Espy, 2001; Germer, 2003; Cook, 2004; Dalesio, 2004). Automated devices that consume less time, handle small volumes, and, in theory, allow for better precision have replaced many molecular diagnostic tests that were historically performed as a series of manual pipetting steps. A large number of these platforms have been developed by different reagent manufacturers to provide automation for a single step or several steps of the testing process. The evolution of molecular diagnostics automation has occurred in stages. For the purposes of discussion, we will group these devices according to the criterion of function.

Single-function automated instruments have been in use for some time in the molecular diagnostics laboratory. The typical single function automated instrument is a thermocycler, since it provides automated amplification of nucleic acid by performing all steps necessary for the amplification of nucleic acids. Nucleic acid extractors represent another early example of a single-function device that converts a six-step procedure into a single step process. These early nucleic acid extractors were based upon phenol/chloroform extraction and mimicked the corresponding manually performed method by using nearly the same reagents and protocols. These and other single step automated instruments – including robots for reagent preparation and aliquoting, automatic DNA sequencers, etc. – have been incorporated into molecular diagnostics laboratories. Development of new procedures for nucleic acid extraction has completely revolutionized the design of automatic nucleic acid extractors. The use of magnetic beads has dramatically changed how laboratories process and isolate nucleic samples from patients' specimens. A representative list of newer automatic extractors is provided in Table 70–2. Molecular diagnostic laboratories are rapidly embracing these automatic nucleic acid extractors, as this specific step in the testing process is one of the most labor-intensive of the entire process. These devices provide higher throughput capabilities, greater precision, and personnel savings.

More recently automated instruments that perform more than a single function have been developed and introduced into molecular diagnostic laboratories. The Roche Molecular Systems COBAS Amplicor analyzer is an example of one such automated platform. This instrument contains a thermocycler for nucleic acid amplification, a three-dimensional cartesian arm with a gripper, heating blocks, wash stations, and even a colorimeter reader. With the development of fluorescently labeled probes that only become detectable when they have bound to their target sequence, PCR thermal cyclers have evolved into multifunction devices. These probes incorporate two fluorescent dyes, generally at either end of the probe, rather than just a single fluorescent dye. The dyes are matched in terms of excitation and emission requirements such that the dye being excited by the external fluorescent source emits at a wavelength that is absorbed by the second dye. This process is referred to as fluorescence energy transfer and works so long as the two dyes are relatively close to each other. This technique is described in Chapter 67. During the PCR process, either the bound probe becomes degraded, allowing the two dyes to separate, or the structure of the probe changes, resulting in an increased distance between the dyes. The net result is that the fluorescent signal increases proportionally to the amount of product created in the PCR reaction. This process is referred to as real-time PCR. In order to detect the increase in PCR product, optics have been incorporated into the thermocycler that allow signal acquisition as the PCR is actually being performed.

A number of different manufacturers have developed and marketed different types of real time instrument (Roche's Lightcycler, Taq96 and Taq48; BioRad's iCycler; ABI's TaqMan). The great benefit of these instruments is that they can perform the PCR reaction and simultaneously acquire the signal, permitting qualitative and quantitative analysis of the PCR reaction as it occurs and eliminating the need for postamplification processing for detection and quantification of the target sequence. This feature allows a dramatic reduction of the turnaround time for molecular diagnostics tests from days to hours. The throughput of these devices is greatly enhanced and molecular diagnostics laboratories now use them routinely for diagnostic testing.

It is anticipated that fully automated instruments that execute the entire analytical process from nucleic extraction to amplification, detection, and quantification in a self-contained, walk-away operation will be available in the near future. Two examples of such automated platforms are the Ampliprep-TaqMan from Roche Molecular Systems and the TIGRIS from Gen-Probe. These integrated automated instruments are designed for use with homogeneous systems that permit amplification and detection in the same tube without having to open reaction tubes for any kind of postamplification manipulation.

The increasing availability of these commercial devices poses many opportunities for clinical laboratories to adopt automation. One core issue in this decision will be economics. While the cost of manually performing molecular testing is substantial, the cost of acquiring automated instruments to perform these steps/tests may also be significant. Laboratories must evaluate the cost–benefit of these automated devices wisely in relation to the anticipated revenue from implementation and the cost of the instruments. More recently, a number of manufacturers have started offering reagent rental programs for many of these automated platforms. Careful comparison of the cost of performing the test manually versus the cost of performing it by automated means must be carried out.

Test Selection

As with any other clinical laboratory, the primary goal of the molecular diagnostics laboratory is to provide reliable and timely tests that produce results for analytes deemed by the medical community to be important for patient care. Test selection is critical for the success of the molecular diagnostic laboratory. Several key considerations are important in test selection (Association for Molecular Pathology, 1999). Any new test should provide a less expensive or more effective avenue for diagnosis and/or management of the patient. It is also important not just to make decisions about test selection solely on the basis of the cost of performing it but to also determine how the new test could impact the overall care and management of the patient. In some circumstances molecular testing might appear at first to increase the cost of managing the patient by adding a new test to the existing battery used for a particular clinical condition. However, by introducing the new test, patient management could be made more effective. One example would be the use of HIV-1 viral load testing to monitor disease progression and the effectiveness of drug therapy in infected individuals. Many patients infected with HIV-1 are currently treated with a combination or cocktail of different drugs including protease inhibitors and nonnucleoside and nucleoside reverse transcriptase inhibitors. These drugs have proved very effective in reducing morbidity and mortality in a large number of HIV-1 infected patients but they are expensive and the virus does become resistant to them. Thus, even though addition of this test added cost to managing HIV infected patients, the test provides a means of rapidly and accurately determining the effectiveness of the expensive drug treatment regimens.

Another consideration might be the introduction of a molecular test to replace an existing laboratory test where the molecular test is more cost-effective. Even if the actual cost of the molecular test is greater than that of the test being replaced, increased sensitivity, increased specificity, or reduced turnaround time might result in significant savings in managing patients. An example here would be the management of patients with a presumptive diagnosis of *Mycobacterium tuberculosis*. During the time when this diagnosis cannot be ruled out, the patients are treated with potentially hepatotoxic drugs or placed in isolation. The standard laboratory test of directly observing an acid-fast stain of the patient's sputum for the presence of *M. tuberculosis* lacks sensitivity but is extremely rapid. On the other hand, culture is extremely sensitive but could take up to 6 weeks to produce a result. Given this situation, a molecular test that allows for a more rapid diagnosis with a high degree of sensitivity and specificity would allow rapid discontinuation of drug therapy or isolation for patients who do not in fact have the disease.

Identifying molecular tests that would be potentially useful at the medical center is a responsibility of the medical and technical directors. Sometimes this can be aided by reviewing the medical center's list of send out tests. Clinicians and pathologists can be a valuable source for identifying the testing needs for the medical center. It is important that, during the process of test selection, the technical capabilities of the laboratory are realistically matched against the real-world clinical needs in terms of test volume, required turnaround time and the associated costs of performing the assay.

Once a particular analyte has been identified for testing by molecular means, it is important to consider the various testing approaches that are available. For example, for some analytes one could use Southern hybridization, in vitro nucleic acid amplification, cytogenetics, or FISH. Before selecting a particular methodology, it is important to keep in mind the clinical condition in question and the advantages and disadvantages of each of the different methodologies for diagnosing that condition.

Introduction of the new test in association with a clinical trial period allows for evaluation of the clinical utility of the test and may provide a useful marketing opportunity. If carefully designed, this approach allows the laboratory to work directly with the end user of the test and provides an avenue for end-users to understand the clinical utility of the test and its limitations and eventually to utilize the particular test more effectively. It is important to clearly define metrics that can be evaluated by the end of the clinical trial and that can be used to justify either implementing the test or discarding it.

Reimbursement for Molecular Diagnostic Tests

Reimbursement for laboratory tests is a complex process that can be broken down into three phases. The three phases are coverage, coding, and payment for services rendered by the laboratory. Coverage decisions are usually determined by each of the different healthcare plans. In the United States, health insurance coverage is provided by public programs such as Medicare and Medicaid or by private health plans purchased individually or through an employer. In general, the scope of coverage provided by a health plan is outlined in broad benefits categories; decisions about specific services are made on a case-by-case basis during claims processing. Health plans may develop formal coverage policies that describe whether a particular service is covered and the conditions under which it will be covered. Medical directors, the federal and state governments, medical policy advisory committees, employers, and unions are among some of the entities involved in making coverage decisions. Medical necessity is the primary criterion used by health plans when making coverage decisions, although the definition of medical necessity is subject to differing interpretations. One of the primary criteria is that the technology must have final approval from the appropriate government regulatory body. In addition, the scientific evidence must permit conclusions to be drawn concerning the effect of the technology on health outcomes.

Billing for molecular diagnostics tests follows the same procedure as any other laboratory tests. Generally, a Current Procedural Terminology (CPT) code and International Classification of Disease (ICD-9) diagnostic code facilitates the billing process by conveying what services or procedures were performed and why. Beyond this, the reimbursement process is usually institution-specific and relies on the computerized and manual billing procedures in place at each institution. It is important to determine in

Table 70–3 Molecular Current Procedural Terminology Codes

Molecular Diagnostics Infectious Disease Analyte-Specific Codes

Infectious agent by nucleic acid (DNA or RNA) (87470–87752)

   Direct probe technique

   Amplified probe technique

   Quantification

Infectious agent not otherwise specified (NOS) (87797–87799)

   Direct probe technique

   Amplified probe technique

   Quantification

HIV Genotyping RT + PR (87901)

HCV Genotyping (87902)

Molecular Diagnostics Procedure Specific Codes

83890 Molecular isolation or extraction

83891 Isolation or extraction of highly purified nucleic acid

83892 Enzymatic digestion

83893 Dot/slot blot production

83894 Separation by gel electrophoresis (e.g.. agarose, polyacrylamide)

83896 Nucleic acid probe, each

83897 Nucleic acid transfer (e.g., Southern, Northern)

83898 Amplification of patient nucleic acid (e.g., PCR, LCR) single primer pair, each primer pair

83901 Amplification of patient nucleic acid, multiplex, each reaction

83902 Reverse transcription

83903 Mutation scanning, by physical properties, heteroduplex, denaturing gradient gel electrophoresis (DGGE), RNAase A, single segment, each

83904 Mutation identification by sequencing, single segment, each segment

83905 Mutation identification by allele specific transcription., single segment, each segment

83912 Interpretation and report

Table 70–4 Current Procedural Terminology Code Billing for Molecular Tests

Test Name	Code	Number of Times Code Billed	Name of Procedure or Test
Factor V Leiden by Real Time Technology	83890	1	Nucleic Acid Isolation
	83898	1	Amplification
	83896	2	Probe each
	83912	1	Interpretation and Report
T(9;22) by Real Time RT-PCR	83891	1	Nucleic Acid Isolation
	83902	2	Reverse Transcription
	83898	2	Amplification
	83894	2	Probe each
	83912	1	Interpretation and Report
HIV-1 Viral Load	87536	1	HIV quantitative
CMV Viral Load	87497	1	CMV quantitative
HCV Viral Load	87522	1	HCV quantitative

CMV = cytomegalovirus; HCV = hepatitis C virus; HIV = human immunodeficiency virus; RT-PCR = reverse transcriptase polymerase chain reaction.

advance the requirements in terms of documentation and computer access for generating a bill. Until recently, there were only a few CPT codes specific for molecular diagnostics (Table 70–3). These were procedure-specific CPT codes used for billing for nucleic acid extraction, enzymatic digestion, in vitro amplification, and so on. More recently, many new CPT codes specific for microbiology molecular diagnostics have been added to the growing list. These new infectious agent codes are global codes that include test procedure, interpretation, and report. Over 60 of these new codes are analyte-specific and are used for molecular microbiology tests. There are usually three different codes for each analyte, one for the direct probe technique, another for the in vitro amplification technique, and another for quantification, regardless of the technology used. For those organisms without CPT codes, three generic codes have been added, called 'Not otherwise specified' (NOS.)

For all other molecular tests without an analyte-specific CPT code, a combination of procedural CPT codes can be used. In addition to the procedure specific codes, there is a specific code for interpretation and report that may be reported at the technical level or the professional level but not both. Table 70–4 lists examples of billing for analyte-specific CPT codes and procedure-specific CPT codes. because of the limited nature and description of the procedure CPT codes, there is a lack of consistency in interpretation of code intent. Furthermore, there is a lack of representation of newer technologies such as bead array, real-time PCR, microarray, etc., which are widely used by a large number of clinical laboratories. In lieu of these, laboratories might be forced to undercode.

More recently, a new set of alpha-numeric modifiers have been devised for the procedure-specific CPT codes. The purpose of these is to help third-party payers identify the services for which they are paying. The new system uses these modifiers to identify neoplasia (solid tumors), neoplasia (lymphoid/hematopoietic), non-neoplastic hematology/coagulation, histocompatibility/blood typing, neurologic non-neoplastic, muscular non-neoplastic, metabolic, other; metabolic transport, metabolic–pharmacogenetics, and dysmorphology. For now, these alpha-numeric modifiers are not mandatory and, if they become required, one can envision that this might actually reduce payment for tests that identify a significant number of mutations in the testing.

Reimbursement levels for any individual test are set by third-party payers and may bear little relationship to the actual cost of performing the test. Some third-party payers reimburse at very high levels but others follow set laboratory schedule fees set by Medicare and Medicaid for the specific CPT codes. FDA approval is not required for billing for these tests and a disclaimer for those tests that are not FDA-cleared should be added to the final report to reflect this issue. This will be further discussed below. Some third-party payers refuse to reimburse for tests bearing such disclaimers, since they believe that the cost of such testing should be born through research grants, even though the performance characteristics and clinical utility of the test has been validated by the clinical laboratory.

Patent Issues

The vast majority of in vitro amplification procedures are patented processes and a license agreement for their use must be obtained or the laboratory using the procedure is liable to prosecution for infringement of patent. Traditionally, a license for a particular procedure is obtained by purchasing an FDA-approved set of reagents sold by a manufacturer who holds the patent to the amplification process. This approach is very limited for molecular diagnostic tests since only a very few tests have been approved by the FDA. Thus, a laboratory using a particular patented process for clinical use must first negotiate a license agreement with the patent holder. It is extremely important to realize that, depending in the complexity of the institution seeking the agreement and the complexity of the agreement, it can take between 3 months and a full year to obtain a license to perform and bill the procedure for clinical purposes.

Almost identical considerations apply to the use of sequence information required to design an assay. Sequences of newly discovered genes, for example human genes or virus genomes, are frequently patented by their discoverers, and use of the sequence information without a licensing agreement runs the same risk of liability for patent infringement. Unfortunately, the current environment and the diversity of sources for sequence information means that it is not always clear whether the sequence has been patented or even, if it has been, who owns the patent. It is therefore advisable, before undertaking the development of any test on published sequences for which a major commitment of resources is planned, to check with the investigators who first described the sequence whether there are any patent issues involved.

Analytical and Clinical Validation of Molecular Assays

As with any other area of the clinical laboratory, the introduction of a new test requires proper validation (Clinical and Laboratory Standards Institute, 1995, 2003; Niesters, 2001, 2002; Prence, 1999). Validation of a clinical test is a complex process that can be divided in two phases: analytical and clinical validation. A number of different organizations have provided guidelines and standards for molecular diagnostics testing. A list of these guidelines is provided in Table 70–5. The parameters that must be assessed during the analytical validation phase are sensitivity, specificity, accuracy, precision and, for quantitative assays, assay linearity.

Table 70–7 Documentation Checklist for Assay Validation

Name of test	State the name of the test including technology used. Be sure that the name identifies the particular organism and/or disease/condition to be tested
Intended use	What the test measures and for what purpose. Identify the particular microorganism and parameter(s) tested, and indicate the use of the test (e.g., diagnosis, prognosis, monitoring response to treatment, guiding therapy, etc.)
Indications for use	Provide clinical condition(s). Use reference standard definitions as found in OMIM
Method category	Identify methodology used for the test
Testing procedure	Information with regard to specimen types, specimen handling and transport procedures, nucleic acid isolation and storage, description of the test procedure, data reports, expected results, technical interpretation of results. All these parameters should be included in policies and procedures for the particular test
Test results	Examples of results
Analytical verification	Analytical sensitivity, specificity, precision, dynamic range, crossreactivity, interfering substances, etc.
Quality control and quality assurance	Delineate quality control and quality assurance program. Identify informal proficiency program if no HHS-approved program exists
Assay limitations	Clearly explain and/or discuss potential limitations of the assay
Clinical data	Primary objective of the study, clinical condition evaluated, patient population, demographics, sample size estimate
Clinical verification	Clinical sensitivity, specificity, positive and negative predictive value
Reporting of test results	Clinical interpretation
Clinical utility	Potential clinical benefit to patient

HHS = Department of Health and Human Services; OMIM = Online Mendelian Inheritance in Man (http://www.ncbi.nlm.nih.gov/Omim/).

developed and its performance characteristics determined by (laboratory name). It has not been cleared by the US Food and Drug Administration.' But at the same time the FDA has allowed laboratories to add in the report that ASRs do not require FDA approval, that the test using the particular ASR can be used for clinical purposes and that the laboratory is certified under CLIA'88 to perform high-complexity testing.

In addition to the definition of ASRs, the FDA proposed a set of controls and restrictions to be applied to their use to ensure their quality and consistency and to clarify that laboratories that set up in-house-developed assays are responsible for the performance of the test. Interestingly, these controls applied to both the laboratory developing in-house assays that use ASRs and the manufacturers of these types of reagent. Laboratories are required to meet CLIA'88 high-complexity certification requirements and determine the performance characteristics of the in-house assay following CLIA'88 regulations. Manufacturers of ASRs are required to register with the FDA, follow Good Manufacturing Practice, and restrict the sale of this type of reagent to laboratories certified under CLIA for high-complexity testing. In addition, they are responsible for reporting to the FDA any adverse effects due to failure in the manufacturing process.

Special Constraints Relevant to Genetic Testing

Genetic tests are performed for diagnostic and/or prognostic purposes, prenatal diagnosis, newborn screening, determination of carrier status, diagnosis, prognosis, presymptomatic, and predictive testing. A number of limitations must be considered when offering genetic testing. The first is that a test might not detect all the possible mutations that could be present in a particular gene that causes a disease. A single gene can have a host of different mutations. A negative result cannot completely guarantee that the person tested does not carry a mutation in a particular gene. At the same time, a positive test result may pose different risks for different people. In addition, another limitation of genetic testing is related to the complexity of the development of certain genetic diseases. This poses challenges mainly for genetic testing for predictive purposes. Penetrance may be less than 100% and/or the disease may be caused by an as yet unknown genetic change in addition to the known mutations in the gene(s) being tested. Thus, predictive testing cannot provide answers with certainty for every individual who might be at risk for a disease.

Quality Control and Quality Assurance

Quality Control of the Testing Process

Establishment of molecular diagnostic tests, particularly amplification assays, requires development of controls for each step of the testing process, including reagent preparation, specimen collection, specimen aliquoting, and performance of the actual assay (Neumaier, 1998; McGovern, 1999; Mulcahy, 1999; Schwartz, 1999; Carter, 2001; Dequeker,

2001; Commission on Laboratory Accreditation, 2005). There are a number of quality control considerations that apply to all molecular assays and are important to guarantee reliable results. Table 70–8 provides a list of the different parameters that need to be part of the quality assurance/quality control program. As with any laboratory test, a well-thought-out and well-written laboratory procedure is key to ensuring the reproducible performance of the assay. It is one of the most important aids during hands-on training of new personnel or when the procedure is not performed very often. The procedure protocol should be written following specific guidelines set up by the National Committee for Clinical Laboratory Standards and described in the clinical laboratory technical procedure manuals.

A careful selection of control reagents is vital for the correct interpretation of test results. Several types of controls are used throughout the execution of an assay to assure appropriate performance. Negative and positive controls are required by CLIA'88 regulations and must be processed in every clinical test. Failure to obtain the correct result for any of the controls invalidates the entire test and requires retesting of all samples. Whenever possible, positive and negative control reagents should resemble a patient specimen as much as possible. Furthermore, a positive control should represent a clinically relevant level of the nucleic acid target sequence against a background of negative nucleic acid target sequence. The negative control should contain 'background' nucleic acid sequences expected to be present in the patient's sample. In addition to the negative and positive controls, a blank control should be included with every assay that contains all the components of the reaction mixture except nucleic acid.

In addition to these controls, it is imperative in some instances to include an internal control to check for the presence of inhibitors in the individual patient samples. If this latter control is not used then, when a negative result is obtained, it is not clear if the absence of amplicon is due to the absence of the target sequence in the patient specimen or to the presence of inhibitors that inhibited the amplification reaction. In order to avoid this situation, amplification of an internal positive control sequence is recommended. The internal positive control can be an endogenous nucleic acid sequence that is unrelated to the target sequence of the clinical assay but is constitutively present in the sample. Alternatively, it may represent a sequence that is 'spiked' into the clinical sample at some step in the testing process. The former endogenous internal positive control generally requires a separate set of primers and may require a separate reaction. The spiked control is generally a sequence that is designed to be amplified by the same primers used for the clinical target and is usually amplified in the same reaction tube as the clinical sample. As is the case with the external clinical positive control, the internal control should be used at a concentration relevant to the clinical testing process. The internal positive controls are also very valuable to assess the presence of amplifiable nucleic acid, the absence of inhibitors, and that the amplification and detection reactions are performed according to the specifications.

The use of a series of positive controls at different concentrations of target sequence can be very helpful in monitoring the assay for changes in

Table 70–8 Conducting the Clinical Testing Process

Activity		Considerations
Reagent preparation	1	Perform in cleanest environment
	2	Store working stock solutions in single use aliquots
	3	Quality control each new set of reagents prior to use in clinical testing. Use low copy number sample for sensitivity evaluation
	4	Preparation of master mixes to reduce variability and errors
Specimen collection	1	Establish acceptable tolerance limits for each specimen type to be tested (storage temperature, transport time, anticoagulant, etc.)
	2	Distribute protocols for proper specimen handling to all potential users
	3	Capture clinical and analytical information on requisition
Specimen processing	1	Specimen must be received and stored in preamplification (clean) laboratory
	2	Develop guidelines to ensure against specimen mix-up and to preserve integrity of target sequence
Analysis of specimen		
A. Extraction procedure	1	Evaluate extraction procedures for presence of inhibitors and factors that decrease yield of target
	2	Internal control added to the sample at the time of extraction to determine false negatives due to inhibitors or determine this rate by some other means. If an internal control is not to be evaluated with each patient sample, then the rate of false negatives should be stated on the report in a disclaimer in case of negative results
B. Assay set-up, amplification and detection	1	Optimize concentration of primers, $MgCl_2$, dNTPs; volume; cycling conditions and detection system
	2	Develop guidelines to minimize possibility of contamination by template nucleic acid or amplicon (see sections on Quality control)
	3	Controls must be processed in the same manner as patient specimens
	4	Develop guidelines to set up assay to avoid crosscontamination of specimens and controls
Interpretation and report	1	Develop guidelines for interpretation and report
	2	Interpretation should be performed by at least two individuals independently
	3	Develop guidelines for report distribution

sensitivity over time. In addition, inclusion of a positive control where the concentration of target sequence is below the detection threshold of the assay can be very useful for detecting low levels of amplicon.

It is extremely important for in-house-developed assays to implement a quality control program for validating the strength, purity, and performance of every critical reagent in the testing process. Every critical reagent should be tested before being approved for clinical testing. Tolerance limits should be established for every critical reagent. Whenever possible, these limits should be established using a quantitative measurement to avoid subjective evaluation of the quality of the critical reagent.

Quality Control of Equipment

All equipment used in the molecular diagnostic laboratory must have a written quality control procedure that describes equipment maintenance procedures and calibration checks. The quality control procedure must be written in accordance with guidelines published in 1992 as the *Clinical Laboratory Technical Procedure Manual* by the National Committee for Clinical Laboratory Standards (now the Clinical and Laboratory Standards Institute). As with any other clinical laboratory equipment, tolerance limits for acceptable performance and calibration checks for all laboratory equipment used during the testing process should be clearly defined and monitored in a regular fashion to assure continued production of accurate and reliable test results. When performance or calibration checks fall outside the tolerance limit defined for any particular instrument, the latter should be immediately taken out of service for repair. After repair the equipment should be calibrated before being placed back in use. As part of the quality control program developed by each laboratory, documentation of all maintenance, performance checks, and calibration or repair for each piece of equipment should be maintained and kept according to the laboratory policy for document retention.

Thermocyclers are a crucial item in any molecular diagnostic laboratory. Any change in the performance of thermocyclers has a direct impact in the sensitivity and precision of the assay performed in that piece of equipment. Maintenance, quality control, and calibration of this instrument, as for any other, should follow the manufacturer's recommendations. Briefly, as part of the performance monitoring for thermocyclers, determination and documentation of the cycling time, verification of the set point error, and any error messages should be recorded. Cycling times between different runs should not differ by more than 2 minutes. Fluctuations in the cycling time are a warning sign that the thermocycler needs to be adjusted and restored to its original condition. In addition, it is recommended that the chiller, heater, and block temperature uniformity tests be performed according to the manufacturer's recommendations. The block temperature uniformity check can be accomplished by using a thermocouple with a temperature probe.

Another important equipment item that is used daily in a molecular diagnostics laboratory is the pipetter. Pipettes are used for almost every step of the testing procedure. Special emphasis should be placed on the quality control and maintenance of the pipettes since they could be a major source of error. All other pieces of equipment should be quality controlled and maintained according to the manufacturer's recommendation. Whenever possible, calibration of the equipment should be performed by using certified standards or reference materials.

Quality Assurance

Every molecular diagnostics laboratory should develop a comprehensive written quality assurance program. The objective of the quality assurance program is to monitor and evaluate, objectively and systematically, the quality and appropriateness of the test results. The quality assurance program should address every aspect of the testing process from preanalytic, through analytic, to postanalytic process. The program must include written policies and documentation for education and training of personnel, continuing medical education, proficiency testing, internal and external inspections, including documentation of corrective actions for deficiencies cited, and quality control programs for clinical testing, equipment performance, and safety.

The quality assurance program monitors aspects of clinical testing that do not directly bear on the analytic validity of the test result and thus are generally not part of the quality control program for clinical testing. Some of these parameters are monthly turnaround times, monthly review of normal and abnormal results, development of specimen rejection criteria, review of the log of rejected specimens, and indicators of test quality. In addition, the laboratory must participate in proficiency survey programs. There are a number of tests for which proficiency programs have been developed by different professional associations. The College of American Pathologists (CAP) offers a variety of independent and combined programs for molecular diagnostics in infectious disease, oncology, and genetics. This last program is offered in combination with the American College of Medical Genetics. Recently, the CDC has made available a Performance Evaluation Program for *M. tuberculosis* and for HIV-1. For those tests where there is no official proficiency program offered, informal proficiency programs must be established through the exchange of samples between laboratories offering the same service or through other means as may be available to the laboratory.

Laboratory Accreditation

Laboratories performing testing on human specimens for the purposes of diagnosis, prevention or treatment of a disease are subject to federal regulation imposed by CLIA'88. As described in Chapters 1 and 9, CLIA'88 set standards designed to improve quality in laboratory practices and also expanded federal oversight to almost every clinical laboratory in the United States. It is important to point out that laboratories performing research are not subject to CLIA'88 unless the research laboratory reports specific results to the individuals tested, their families, and/or treating

VIII

physician. This applies even if there is a disclaimer in the final report that states that the test results should be used for research purposes only and/or there is no charge for the test. CLIA'88 describes very specific standards in all areas of the testing process, personnel training, proficiency testing, quality control, and quality assurance. The federal regulation establishes a registry, sanctions, and enforcement procedures to ensure that the standards defined in the federal regulation are maintained. The regulations for implementing CLIA'88 were developed by the Department of Health and Human Services (HHS) through the Public Health Service. At that time, the CDC was assigned to categorize analytes and supervise implementation of standards. The FDA was assigned to review and guarantee the safety and efficacy of tests, and the Health Care Finance Administration was to collect fees, issue permits, survey laboratories and initiate punitive actions when necessary.

Under CLIA'88, tests are categorized as waived provider-performed microscopy, moderate complexity, and high complexity. Tests are placed into moderate- and high-complexity testing categories on the basis of a numerical scoring system. The scoring system takes into account some of the following factors: knowledge required for performing the test, training and expertise, availability of calibrators, quality control, proficiency testing, operational characteristics, degree of interpretation and judgment, etc. A test is considered to be moderately complex if the score is 13 or less. A test with a score above 13 is considered to be complex.

Molecular diagnostic tests are considered to be high-complexity testing and as such laboratories performing this testing must seek accreditation from the HHS. HHS has granted the College of American Pathologists the status of an enforcement agency for those regulations by accepting their accreditation program as being equivalent to or more stringent in the areas of quality control assurance than the standards described in CLIA'88. Thus, most laboratories performing molecular diagnostic testing are CLIA'88-accredited through the CAP. CAP introduced a molecular pathology checklist in 1993 and it has been updating yearly since then. In addition, the molecular pathology checklist is a great resource when developing a molecular diagnostic laboratory for the development of quality control, quality assurance programs, specimen requisition, reporting, etc.

Laboratories performing DNA identity testing as a part of forensic DNA casework must also seek accreditation for this purpose. One approach is through a program offered by the American Society of Criminalist Laboratory Directors (ASCLD). ASCLD offers a Crime Laboratory Accreditation Program. This accreditation is a voluntary program in which any crime laboratory performing DNA analysis can participate to demonstrate that management operations, personnel, procedures, equipment, physical plant security, and safety comply with the guidelines proposed by the Technical Working Group on DNA Analysis Methods (TWGDAM). The National Forensic Science Technology Center offers assistance to crime laboratories that are preparing for ASCLD/Lab accreditation in addition to provide certification to DNA laboratories that comply with TWGDAM guidelines. For parentage testing, the American Association of Blood Banks has developed guidelines for paternity testing utilizing DNA and offers accreditation through their Parentage Testing Accreditation Program. There are over 40 AABB accredited parentage-testing laboratories. This accreditation helps laboratories achieve quality performance.

References

Association for Molecular Pathology: Recommendations for in-house development and operation of molecular diagnostic tests. Am J Clin Pathol 1999; 111:449–463.

Bachner P. Hamlin W: Federal regulation of clinical and the clinical laboratory improvement amendments of 1988 – Part II. Clin Lab Med 1993; 13: 987–994.

Carter MA: Ethical aspects of genetic testing. Biol Res Nurs 2001; 3:24–32.

Clinical and Laboratory Standards Institute: MM3-A Molecular diagnostics method for infectious diseases: approved guideline. Wayne, PA, CLSI/NCCLS, 1995.

Clinical and Laboratory Standards Institute: MM6-A Quantitative molecular methods for infectious diseases: approved guideline. Wayne, PA, CLSI, 2003.

This is a very comprehensive guideline that provides valuable information regarding the verification of new molecular quantitative assays in the clinical laboratory.

Commission on Laboratory Accreditation: Molecular pathology inspection checklist, 2005 edition. Commission on Laboratory Accreditation, College of American Pathologists, Northfield, IL, 2005.

Cook L, Ng KW, Bagabag A, et al: Use of the MagNA pure LC automated nucleic acid extraction system followed by real-time reverse transcription-PCR for ultrasensitive quantitation of hepatitis C virus RNA. J Clin Microbiol 2004; 42:4130–4136.

Dalesio N, Marsiglia V, Quinn A, et al: Performance of the MagNA pure LC robot for extraction of *Chlamydia trachomatis* and *Neisseria gonorrhoeae* DNA from urine and swab specimens. J Clin Microbiol 2004; 42:3300–3302.

Dequeker E, Ramsden S, Grody WW, et al: Quality control in molecular genetic testing. Nat Rev Genet 2001; 2:717–723.

Espy MJ, Rys PN, Wold AD, et al: Detection of herpes simplex virus DNA in genital and dermal specimens by LightCycler PCR after extraction using the IsoQuick, MagNA Pure, and BioRobot 9604 methods. J Clin Microbiol 2001; 39:2233–2236.

Food and Drug Administration Modernization Act 1997: Washington, DC, Public Law 105–115, 111 Statute 2296, 1997.

Germer JJ, Lins MM, Jensen ME, et al: Evaluation of the MagNA pure LC instrument for extraction of hepatitis C virus RNA for the COBAS AMPLICOR Hepatitis C Virus Test, version 2.0. J Clin Microbiol 2003; 41:3503–3508.

Kaul K, Leonard DGB, Gonzalez A, Garrett CT: Oversight of genetic testing: an update. J Mol Diagn 2001; 3:85–91.

McGovern MM, Benach MO, Wallenstein S, et al: Quality assurance in molecular genetic testing laboratories. JAMA 1999; 281:835–840.

Medical Device Amendments 1976: Washington, DC, Public Law 94–295, 90 Statute 539, 1976.

Medical Devices: classification/reclassification; restricted devices; analyte specific reagents. Federal Register 1997; 62:62243–66260.

Mulcahy GM: The integration of molecular diagnostic methods into the clinical laboratory. Ann Clin Lab Sci 1999; 29:43–54.

Neumaier M, Braun A, Wagener C: Fundamentals of quality assessment of molecular amplification methods in clinical diagnostics. International Federation of Clinical Chemistry Scientific Division Committee on Molecular Biology Techniques. Clin Chem 1998; 44:12–26.

Niesters HG: Clinical virology in real time. J Clin Virol 2002; 25(Suppl 3):3–12.

This article reviews current advances in technology that have been introduced in the clinical molecular virology laboratory in recent years. It provides a good perspective on the future technological advances that are likely to apply to the clinical laboratory.

Niesters HG: Quantitation of viral load using real-time amplification techniques. Methods 2001; 25:419–429.

Prence EM: A practical guide for the validation of genetic tests. Genet Test 1999; 3:201–205.

Safe Medical Device Act 1990: Washington, DC, Public Law 101–629, 104 Statute 4523, 1990.

Schwartz MK: Genetic testing and the clinical laboratory improvement amendments of 1988: present and future. Clin Chem 1999; 45:739–745.

Swanson PE: Labels, disclaimers, and rules (Oh my!). Analyte-specific reagents and practice of immunohistochemistry. Am J Clin Pathol 1999; 111:445–448.

Molecular Diagnosis of Hematopoietic Neoplasms

David S. Viswanatha MD FRCPC, Richard S. Larson MD PhD

KEY POINTS

- Molecular diagnosis is an established and increasingly integral component of the classification of hematolymphoid disorders and provides prognostic information as well as specific markers for sensitive minimal residual disease (MRD) monitoring.

- While several complementary laboratory techniques are utilized to identify specific tumor genetic anomalies, these have varying sensitivities and the choice of methodology depends on the phase of disease (i.e., diagnosis versus post-treatment), as well as the type of sample obtained. Polymerase chain reaction (PCR) methods are highly sensitive and specific but must be rigorously quality-controlled.

- Characteristic genetic abnormalities are highly associated with or definitive of specific pathologic entities among the leukemias and myeloproliferative diseases; the presence of these specific associations serves to more accurately classify these diseases but also has prognostic value and therapeutic implications.

- Despite the large and unpredictable genomic breakpoint-fusion regions in individual leukemias generated by recurrent chromosomal translocations, reverse transcription PCR (RT-PCR) can be successfully employed to detect the resultant unique chimeric gene fusion mRNA species.

- Numerical and structural genetic aberrations are employed in rational risk stratification schema for the optimal management of childhood acute lymphoblastic leukemias.

- Specific chromosomal translocations in childhood leukemia patients can be traced back to birth, implying that initial genetic lesions predisposing to many childhood leukemias may originate in utero; however, the finding of these translocations in random neonatal cord blood samples suggests that secondary genetic events are required to produce overt leukemia in a susceptible individual.

- Rearrangements of the immunoglobulin and T-cell receptor genes serve as powerful molecular markers for demonstrating the presence or absence of clonality in lymphoid populations. Southern blot hybridization (SBH) and PCR are the two molecular techniques used to demonstrate clonotypic rearrangements of these genetic loci.

- While SBH is a 'gold standard' for lymphoid clonality detection, it is laborious, technically demanding, and time-intensive, thus increasingly favoring PCR technique in the clinical setting; however, PCR is prone to both false-negative and false-positive results and the interpreting molecular pathologist requires a broad knowledge of the technical aspects and limitations of these assays.

- Non-Hodgkin lymphomas are also frequently associated with recurrent genetic aberrations, particularly chromosomal translocations. In addition to more accurately classifying lymphoma subtypes, these markers can also provide evidence of lymphoid clonality in situations where the differential diagnosis includes an atypical reactive process.

- Chromosomal translocations in the non-Hodgkin lymphomas generally result in overexpression of a particular gene (in contrast to the formation of a chimeric gene, mRNA and novel fusion protein as with many leukemias). DNA-based PCR methods may therefore have suboptimal clinical sensitivity in diagnostic specimens, as a result of the very large regions of genomic DNA spanning the break-fusion regions. Fluorescence in situ hybridization provides a rapid alternative for initial diagnosis in this setting, with high detection rates.

- Post-therapy MRD monitoring of hematolymphoid neoplasms is becoming increasingly refined and more reproducible with the widespread use of automated quantitative 'real time' PCR (Q-PCR) platforms.

- Evaluation of MRD status is important for determining therapeutic efficacy, risk of relapse, and the necessity and timing of additional treatment interventions.

VIII

• At present, the most informative clinical scenarios for Q-PCR assessment of MRD in hematopoietic cancers include chronic myeloid leukemia, acute promyelocytic leukemia, and childhood acute lymphoblastic leukemia.

• Although knowledge of characteristic single genetic markers has revolutionized our definition and understanding of hematolymphoid tumors, further progress in the elucidation of disease pathogenesis, prognostic prediction, and identification of potential therapeutic targets is being derived from global genomic and proteomic analyses. One such example is the substantial body of information emerging from gene expression microarray technology, as exemplified by the delineation of distinct phenotypic and clinical subgroups within the otherwise histopathologically homogeneous category of diffuse large B-cell lymphoma.

Introduction: Role of Clinical Molecular Diagnostics in Hematologic Cancers

The diagnosis of hematolymphoid neoplasms continues to undergo a dramatic transformation with the advent and application of new technologies. While traditional morphologic (light microscopic) evaluation of glass slides still occupies the centerpiece of pathologic diagnosis, the judicious application of ancillary methods, such as special cytochemistry, immunohistochemistry, flow cytometry, cytogenetics (including fluorescence in situ hybridization [FISH]) and molecular genetics, has allowed for much improved diagnostic reproducibility and refinement. The relative ease of sampling sites such as the lymph nodes and bone marrow, as well as the provision of easily disaggregated viable cell samples for analysis have driven this paradigm of diagnostic evaluation. The nature of the hematolymphoid system is also conducive to relatively easy monitoring of disease status following therapy, which represents another important facet in the management of patients with these illnesses.

Given this plethora of diagnostic tools, what role does molecular genetic evaluation or molecular diagnostics play? There are perhaps four major scenarios in which molecular diagnostic analysis of a hematolymphoid proliferation is important. First, molecular investigation can establish a diagnosis in situations wherein morphologic details and results of other laboratory tests are inconclusive for malignancy. The presence of specific genetic abnormalities, or the demonstration of tumor genetic 'homogeneity' of a cell population (e.g., by antigen receptor gene rearrangement studies) can establish the presence of a clonal pathologic process. Second, molecular methods are utilized to subclassify disease entities. To this end, the current World Health Organization (WHO) classification of hematologic neoplasms includes molecular characterization as a defining feature of many leukemias and lymphomas (Jaffe, 2001). Next, specific genetic anomalies in hematolymphoid malignancies have important prognostic value, which in turn can influence the initial treatment of certain tumors to produce an optimal clinical outcome. Finally, being potentially of high sensitivity, molecular techniques can be used to assess patients after the onset of therapy, by monitoring for the presence and extent of minimal residual disease (MRD). Table 71–1 summarizes some of the key instances in which molecular diagnostic evaluation is sought in hematopathology practice. As the synergy between expanding basic biologic information and rapidly progressing technology continues unabated, the future holds promise for many additional applications of molecular diagnostics in the pathology laboratory, including the prediction of disease susceptibility, severity, or treatment response based on polygenic factors; pharmacogenomic profiling of patients to determine drug sensitivity and toxicity profiles; and the assessment of individual responses to increasingly 'targeted' therapies.

This chapter focuses on the background, clinical rationale, and fundamental technical considerations underlying the molecular diagnostic evaluation and monitoring of hematologic and lymphoid tumors. As the large majority of these laboratory assays are polymerase chain reaction (PCR)-based, the emphasis is accordingly placed on methods concerning either DNA or RNA (i.e., reverse-transcription) PCR techniques. Of note, it is apparent that the detection of tumor-specific genetic abnormalities can be achieved by different analytic means, for example cytogenetics, FISH, or PCR. Although at first glance these various methods may seem redundant, these laboratory techniques should be considered to be complementary and the choice of methodology is determined by a number of factors, including knowledge of the detection rates and limitations of various techniques, level of interpretive experience and expertise with these procedures, the type of sample, and the phase of the disease under investigation. In the last case, sensitivity issues become paramount and PCR-

Table 71–1 Indications for Molecular Diagnostic Investigation in Hematologic and Lymphoid Neoplasia

Indication	Examples
Diagnosis	Determination of a clonal B-cell population in a morphologically equivocal tissue proliferation or when other ancillary investigations are noninformative
	Determination of T-cell clonality
	Small tissue biopsy or type of sample not amenable to other investigative technique
Subclassification	Identification of specific subtypes of acute myeloid and lymphoid leukemia, e.g., t(8;21)/AML1–ETO in acute myeloid leukemia with maturation
	Distinction between small B-lymphocyte non-Hodgkin lymphomas with overlapping morphologic features, e.g., mantle cell lymphoma vs small lymphocytic lymphoma
Prognosis	Identification of 'favorable'-outcome acute leukemia subtypes with possibility of specific therapy, e.g., t(15;17)/PML–RARα in acute promyelocytic leukemia and use of all *trans* retinoic acid (atRA) with chemotherapy
	Identification of 'unfavorable'-outcome acute leukemia subtypes, e.g., t(9;22)/BCR–ABL1 in Ph+ acute lymphoblastic leukemia
	Identification of prognostic subsets in B-cell tumors, e.g., somatic hypermutation status in chronic lymphocytic leukemia; t(11;18)/API2–MALT1 in antibiotic therapy unresponsive extranodal marginal zone B-cell lymphomas
Minimal residual disease	Utility in monitoring chronic myeloid leukemia, acute promyelocytic leukemia and childhood acute lymphoblastic leukemia following initiation of therapy
	Assessment of patient samples prior to autologous transplantation for non-Hodgkin lymphoma

based assays are likely to be required to identify residual disease. Table 71–2 indicates comparative analytic sensitivities of the principal modalities used to detect hematolymphoid-tumor-related genetic abnormalities.

The increasingly ubiquitous need for molecular genetic evaluation of hematopoietic cancers has initiated earnest attempts to address and achieve better interlaboratory standardization, and such efforts can be expected to continue to improve the benchmarks of sensitivity and specificity in this field. Nonetheless, in the application and interpretation of molecular diagnostic tests, one caveat that cannot be emphasized enough is that the results of these investigations must never be considered in isolation but rather in conjunction with the salient clinical, morphologic, and additional laboratory data concerning the individual patient. Regardless of the remarkable specificity and sensitivity of molecular markers, the evident complexity of hematolymphoid neoplasia mandates such a fully integrated approach in order to diminish the possibility of diagnostic error.

Molecular Diagnosis of the Leukemias

Gene Fusion Concept in Leukemia and the Basis for Reverse-Transcriptase Polymerase Chain Reaction Analysis

The leukemias are hematologic cancers with a diverse pathogenesis and pathobiology. However, a significant proportion of these tumors are characterized by nonrandom, (usually) balanced chromosomal translocations, resulting in the formation of fusion, or chimeric, genes. In general, although two such fusions are created in this abnormal event (i.e., one on each reciprocal translocated chromosome), typically only one of these derivative loci gives rise to a leukemogenic 'hybrid' gene. At the molecular level, the intronic breakpoint and fusion sites in the involved genes are highly variable among patients with the same type of leukemia, although there may be evidence of clustered breakpoint 'hotspots' in certain types of leukemia-related rearranging genes. Despite the variability in breakpoint sites in both of the involved genes, a consistent feature of the leukemic gene fusion is the production of a chimeric mRNA molecule. This abnormal transcript is further translated to a fusion protein, presumed to be operative in disrupting many cellular pathways involved in regulating normal proliferative capacity, differentiation, and

Table 71–2 Relative Sensitivities of Major Techniques used to Detect Leukemia or Lymphoma-Associated Translocation Fusion Genes

Method	Analytic Sensitivity (%)*	Notes
Cytogenetics	5	Global genomic assessment Requires fresh, sterile cells Detects numerical and structural chromosome aberrations Difficult or impossible to detect subtle alterations in DNA
Fluorescence in situ hybridization	1–5	Targeted assessment of large genomic abnormalities Technically straightforward and rapid; can frequently be performed on interphase nuclei Applicable to a variety of tissue sources Requires rigorous quality standards to avoid false-positive results at low levels of the abnormality in question
Southern blot hybridization	5–10	Targeted assessment for structural abnormalities in genomic DNA Technically laborious and time-intensive Requires samples with preserved high-molecular-weight DNA (e.g., fresh or frozen cells)
Polymerase chain reaction (PCR)	10^{-2}–10^{-4}	Targeted assessment of small genomic or mRNA abnormalities Detection of unique chimeric fusion gene mRNA species is highly sensitive Technically straightforward and rapid but may require post-PCR detection procedures Applicable to a broad range of sample types, including fixed paraffin-embedded tissues Useful for high sensitivity minimal residual disease monitoring

* Analytic sensitivity is defined as the minimum number of tumor cells that can be detected in a background of nontumor cells, expressed as a percentage. These dilutional levels are generally attainable with the indicated molecular methods, although several technical or biologic factors may influence the lower limits of detection.

survival in immature (i.e., precursor) marrow stem or progenitor cells. Although the formation of a translocation fusion gene is known to be necessary for disease production, results from animal models have suggested that, at least for some types of leukemia, this may not be a sufficient event, requiring additional secondary, incompletely characterized genetic insults as well.

One practical aspect of the chimeric gene concept is that, regardless of the variable location of the genomic (DNA-level) breakpoints in a given translocation gene fusion, the presence of this abnormality can be confirmed by detecting the corresponding invariant chimeric mRNA species. In the molecular diagnostic laboratory, we can thus use the reverse-transcription polymerase chain reaction (RT-PCR) method to first convert the fusion mRNA transcript to its complementary DNA (cDNA), and then amplify this specific molecule. The ability to perform RT-PCR analysis obviates the difficulties imposed by the often very large flanking regions of intronic DNA surrounding the genomic breakpoint-fusion loci, which would normally not be amenable to amplification by standard DNA-based PCR approaches. Furthermore, the presence of such an aberrant mRNA species is highly specific for the disease, as it should not theoretically be present in normal cells. Table 71–3 provides a list of the major leukemia-associated translocations along with their resultant fusion gene and mRNA products.

Two related concepts are important in the further understanding of chimeric genes and transcripts. 'Breakpoint heterogeneity' refers to the presence of two (or possibly more) common breakpoint loci in a particular gene, which can be targeted by the translocation event. In some examples, different breakpoint sites may be correlated with a presenting disease phenotype or particular clinical features (e.g., the BCR–ABL1 fusion in chronic myeloid leukemia [CML] versus acute lymphoblastic leukemia [ALL]), but this is not always the case. Secondly, alternative exon splicing

of a single chimeric transcript may occur, such that additional, related mRNA products may be observed during PCR amplification of the principal target (e.g., the TEL–AML1 fusion in pediatric ALL). RT-PCR-based assays require fresh bone marrow aspirate or blood cells, although cryopreserved tissue or cells can also be used effectively for RNA isolation. RNA extraction and RT-PCR from paraffin tissue block samples has also been successfully described; however, fixed cellular material is often degraded or compromised by the presence of PCR inhibitors resulting in a higher failure rate of PCR detection. Finally, given the highly sensitive nature of PCR amplification, these laboratory assays must be carefully controlled to avoid false-positive contamination artifacts. The following sections describe the molecular genetic and diagnostic features of the most common, prognostically important leukemic diseases.

Chronic Myeloid Leukemia and Ph⁺ Acute Lymphoblastic Leukemia: t(9;22)/*BCR–ABL1* Abnormality

Chronic myeloid leukemia, although an uncommon hematologic neoplasm, is prototypic of the leukemic diseases. CML is a clonal marrow stem cell disease resulting predominantly in hyperproliferation of granulocytic cells at all stages of maturation. The natural course of CML is typified by a protracted 'chronic phase', often for several years, followed by a rapid transformation to an aggressive acute myeloid or lymphoid 'blast crisis', with a fatal outcome. The decades-long investigation and treatment of this disorder has led from the association of a karyotypic abnormality with the disease phenotype to the unraveling of its molecular genetic and biologic pathogenesis and, currently, to the development and introduction of a novel targeted pharmacologic therapy in the form of imatinib mesylate (Gleevec, Novartis Corporation) (Goldman, 2003). CML is characterized by the presence of the t(9;22)(q34;q11) chromosomal translocation, initially observed as an abnormal 22q– abnormality termed the Philadelphia chromosome (Ph) (Nowell, 1960; Rowley, 1973). This translocation leads to juxtaposition of the ABL1 tyrosine kinase gene (9[q34]) with the BCR gene (22[q11]) on the derivative chromosome 22q, with formation of the BCR–ABL1 fusion gene and mRNA, and production of a chimeric BCR–ABL protein (Melo, 1996; Deininger, 2000). Notably, the t(9;22)/BCR–ABL1 is pathognomonic not only of CML as it also occurs in 20–25% of adult and approximately 3% of pediatric cases of ALL (i.e., Ph⁺ ALL) that have highly aggressive disease behavior. Although the functional role of the normal BCR gene product is not completely understood, this abnormal genetic fusion disrupts the localization and regulated activity of the ABL tyrosine kinase, producing complex effects on cellular signal transduction pathways, proliferation, apoptosis control, and cell adhesion (Deininger, 2000). Intriguingly, in vivo topographic studies of the BCR and ABL1 genes in cycling normal hematopoietic progenitor cells, as well as the surprising demonstration of very low levels of BCR–ABL transcripts in the blood of many healthy subjects, suggest that the t(9;22) may occur relatively frequently in normal human bone marrow cells (Biernaux, 1995; Bose, 1998; Neves, 1999). The complex interplay of host response to these abnormal genetic rearrangements and the acquisition of other initiating or potentiating genetic lesions leading to the overt development of CML (or Ph⁺ ALL) is yet to be determined. Definitive treatment for patients with CML is achieved by allogeneic bone marrow or stem cell transplantation, although the frontline management of CML has now been significantly altered with the advent of the tyrosine kinase inhibitor imatinib mesylate (Druker, 2001; O'Brien, 2003). Ph⁺ ALL is associated with very poor overall outcome in response to conventional high-dose chemotherapy, necessitating consideration of marrow or stem cell transplantation. The addition of novel agents like imatinib mesylate may also offer benefit for these patients.

At the DNA level the BCR–ABL1 gene fusion exhibits features of breakpoint heterogeneity, with three main recognized breakpoint loci in the BCR gene, as well as some alternatively spliced transcript variation (Fig. 71–1) (Deininger, 2000; Melo, 1996). In virtually all cases of CML, the BCR gene breakpoints are situated in the so-called 'major' breakpoint cluster region, or M-BCR. These break sites occur in a relatively small 5.8 kb genomic region spanning BCR exons b1–b5 (also known as exons e12-e16), specifically between the b2 and b3, or the b3 and b4 exons. In contrast, the breakpoints in the ABL1 gene are distributed over a very large region of intronic DNA 5′ to exon a2. In CML therefore, two types of BCR–ABL1 fusion mRNA transcripts can arise from M-BCR locus gene fusions, namely the b2–a2, or b3–a2 forms (Fig. 71–1). These two products encode a novel protein of 210 kD (p210). While most cases of CML harbor either a b2–a2 or b3–a2 transcript type, occasional tumors may demonstrate alternative splicing of the latter form to produce both transcripts simultaneously.

CHAPTER: 71 Molecular Diagnosis of Hematopoietic Neoplasms

Table 71–3 Common Leukemia-associated Translocations and Resultant Fusion Genes and mRNA Species

Genetic Abnormality	Disease Associations	Basic Molecular Pathogenesis	Detection
t(9;22)/*BCR–ABL1*	• Chronic myeloid leukemia (100%) • Ph$^+$ adult acute lymphoblastic leukemia (ALL) (20–25%) • Ph$^+$ pediatric acute lymphoblastic leukemia (3%)	Chimeric fusion protein with deregulation of ABL tyrosine kinase; effects on cell proliferation, apoptosis, adhesion	RT-PCR; FISH
del 4q12/*FIP1L1–PDGFRA*	Hypereosinophilic syndrome/chronic eosinophilic leukemia (subset of cases)	Deregulation of PDGFRα receptor tyrosine kinase	FISH > RT-PCR
t(15;17)/*PML-RARα*	Acute promyelocytic leukemia (100%)	Chimeric fusion protein; interference with myeloid maturation and differentiation	RT-PCR; FISH
t(8;21)/*AML1–ETO* inv(16) or t(16;16)/*CBFB-MYH11*	Acute myeloid leukemia (AML) (10%) Acute myelomonocytic leukemia with abnormal eosinophils (AMML-Eo)	Chimeric fusion protein affecting the core binding factor (CBF) transcriptional regulatory pathway; aberrant effects on myeloid cell proliferation and differentiation	RT-PCR; FISH
FLT3 mutations	Acute myeloid leukemia (20–30%)	Internal tandem duplication (ITD) or point mutation resulting in constitutive activity of FLt3 tyrosine kinase and cell proliferation	DNA PCR
JAK2 mutation	Chronic myeloproliferative disorders excluding CML: P.vera (~90%), chronic idiopathic myelofibrosis, essential thrombocytosis (~50%); rarely in myelodysplastic syndrome or atypical MDS/MPD	Single G>T point mutation producing V617F amino acid substitution; results in loss of autoinhibition and constitutive activation of Jak2 tyrosine kinase	DNA PCR
t(12;21)/*TEL–AML1*	Childhood B-precursor acute lymphoblastic leukemia (20%)	Chimeric fusion protein; disruption of CBF transcriptional regulatory pathway; abnormal effects on Tel transcriptional function	RT-PCR; FISH
t(1;19)/*E2A-PBX1*	Childhood pre-B cell ALL (3%)	Chimeric fusion protein; interference with normal early B-cell development	RT-PCR
11q23/*MLL* translocations	• Childhood (mainly infant) B-lineage ALL (5%) • Adult de novo AML, usually monocytic (subset of cases) • Subset of secondary AML (after DNA topoisomerase II agent exposure)	Chimeric fusion proteins; disruption of MLL-mediated regulation of hematopoiesis	FISH; RT-PCR

FISH = fluorescence in situ hybridization; RT-PCR = reverse-transcriptase polymerase chain reaction.

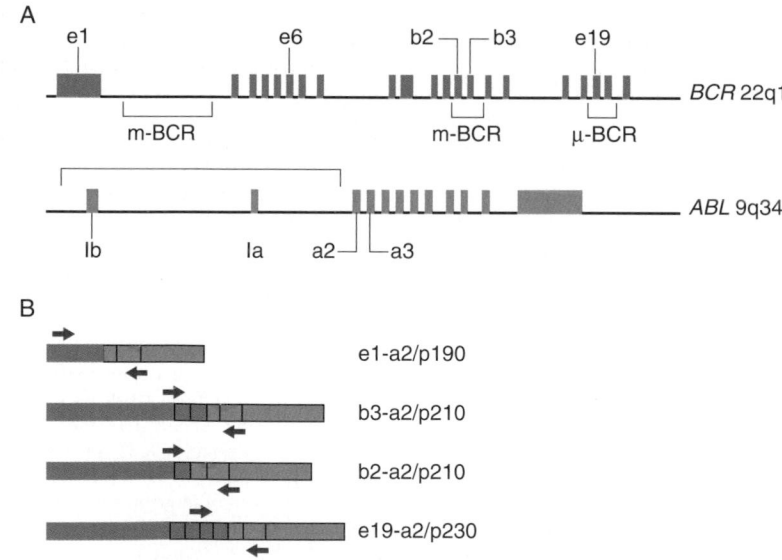

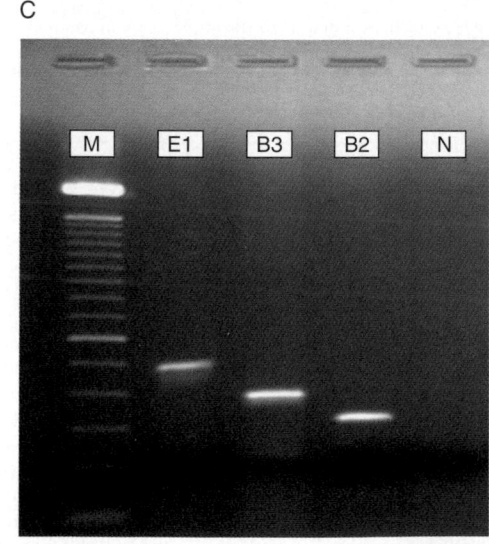

Figure 71–1 t(9;22)/*BCR–ABL1* abnormality in chronic myeloid leukemia (CML) and Philadelphia-chromosome-positive acute lymphoblastic leukemia (Ph$^+$ ALL). *A,* Exon map of the translocated *BCR* and *ABL1* genes (not to scale). Three major breakpoint regions are recognized in the *BCR* gene: the minor breakpoint cluster region (m-BCR), the major breakpoint cluster region (M-BCR) and the μ-BCR. The M-BCR is involved in essentially all cases of CML and approximately one third of de novo adult Ph$^+$ ALL. A small percentage of pediatric Ph$^+$ ALL may have *BCR* breakpoints at this site as well. The m-BCR is typically associated with the vast majority of pediatric Ph$^+$ ALL and most adult Ph$^+$ ALL. Breakpoints at the μ-BCR have been associated with the entity chronic neutrophilic leukemia. For the *ABL1* gene, breakpoints are distributed throughout a large region 5' of exon 2 (a2) encompassing the first exon region. *B,* The principal *BCR–ABL1* chimeric transcripts arising from these various translocation fusion gene breakpoints. The exon–exon fusions are indicated for these transcripts and the corresponding chimeric protein product sizes are shown in kilodaltons (e.g., e1–a2/p190). The orange arrows indicate relative positions of polymerase chain reaction (PCR) primers used to detect these forms in reverse-transcriptase (RT)-PCR assays. *C,* Typical RT-PCR gel electrophoresis results for detection of the m-BCR and M-BCR transcripts: M = molecular size marker (100 bp); E1 = e1–a2 product; B3 = b3–a2 product; B2 = b2–a2 product; N = no template control.

There appears to be no clinical or prognostic significance to the type of M-BCR locus *BCR–ABL1* fusion in CML. A second common breakpoint locus is present in the *BCR* gene, designated as the 'minor' breakpoint cluster region, or m-BCR (Fig. 71–1). Translocations involving this locus result in the formation of an e1–a2 *BCR–ABL1* fusion transcript, encoding a 190 kD

BCR–ABL protein (p190). The e1–a2 type *BCR–ABL1* is highly characteristic of Ph$^+$ ALL. However, the subdivision of M-BCR and m-BCR fusions as 'CML-associated' and 'ALL-associated' is not so straightforward, despite these general correlations between *BCR–ABL1* breakpoint–fusion location and disease phenotype. While the vast majority of pediatric Ph$^+$ ALL cases are of e1–a2 (m-BCR) type, approximately 30–40% of adult Ph⁺ ALL patients demonstrate b3–a2 or b2–a2 (M-BCR) BCR–ABL1 fusions. In the latter situation, distinction of true de novo Ph⁺ ALL from CML in lymphoid blast crisis is important. In addition, it is well known that a significant proportion of classic CML with the expected b3–a2 or b2–a2 transcript types will also demonstrate concurrent low abundance e1–a2 mRNA, because of a minimal degree of alternative splicing of the longer M-BCR-derived transcript (Saglio, 1996; van Rhee, 1996). Potentially more confusing is the finding of rare Ph⁺ chronic leukemias with the e1–a2 fusion that manifest a predominantly monocytic phenotype (rather than the typical myeloid cell predominance of CML). These foregoing observations underscore the pathobiologic variability associated with BCR–ABL1 expression in different myeloid and lymphoid progenitor cells. The third cluster region for BCR–ABL1 gene fusions has been called the μ-BCR (Fig. 71–1) and results in formation of an e19–a2 transcript. This fusion transcript is predicted to result in translation of a 230 kD protein (p230) and, although somewhat controversial, this type of BCR–ABL1 event has been associated with at least some cases of the very rare myeloproliferative disease described as chronic neutrophilic leukemia (CNL).

Figure 71–1 also indicates the placement of oligonucleotide PCR primers to specifically amplify the M-BCR (b3–a2, b2–a2), m-BCR (e1–a2) and μ-BCR (e19–a2) fusion transcripts following reverse transcription of total mRNA. Although gel electrophoresis sizing of PCR products is nominally sufficient to distinguish these BCR–ABL1 variants (Fig. 71–1), many diagnostic laboratories perform a post-PCR confirmatory assay, such as Southern blot hybridization using a junction-specific, labeled oligonucleotide probe, or related methods. Rarely occurring CML and Ph⁺ ALL cases involving the use of alternate, adjacent BCR or ABL exons have been encountered, generating b3–a3, b2–a3, e1–a3, or e6–a2 transcript forms (Melo, 1996; Deininger, 2000). In general, RT-PCR assays can be appropriately modified or constructed to detect these infrequent variants as well (Chasseriau, 2004). Genomic Southern blot methods to detect rearrangements of the BCR genomic locus have also been described but are of limited utility in relation to the rapidity, specificity, and relative simplicity of FISH and RT-PCR techniques. FISH analysis may have some additional utility for identifying concurrent large genomic deletions occurring on the derivative 9q or 22q chromosomes, which have been associated with inferior outcome in this subgroup of CML patients (Sinclair, 2000).

Molecular detection of these abnormal BCR–ABL1 mRNA chimeric transcripts is valuable in the diagnosis of CML and Ph⁺ ALL. For example, although approximately 98% of CML cases are BCR–ABL-positive, a small number of morphologic mimickers will lack this genetic abnormality. These leukemic disorders fall into an ill-defined subset including 'atypical' CML, chronic myelomonocytic leukemia (CMML), and other chronic myeloproliferative or myelodysplastic disorders. Clearly, the therapeutic options and outcome for such patients will be different from those for true CML. Conversely, atypical myeloproliferative presentations of CML are not infrequently encountered and the demonstration of BCR-ABL in these situations is critical for correct diagnosis and management. Similarly, detection of the BCR-ABL1 abnormality in adult and pediatric ALL identifies these subsets of patients who are at high risk of conventional chemotherapy failure and may benefit from more intensive treatment regimens. Molecular diagnostic evaluation for BCR-ABL is also important to resolve complex cytogenetic presentations masking the t(9;22), and to delineate the specific BCR-ABL1 fusion mRNA type for subsequent molecular residual disease detection following allogeneic transplantation or more conservative treatment modalities such as chemotherapy or imatinib mesylate therapy (discussed below in the section on Molecular Monitoring of Residual Disease.)

Acute Myeloid Leukemias

Acute myeloid leukemias (AMLs) can be broadly classified as being of relatively 'favorable,' 'intermediate,' or 'poor' prognosis types, based on the degree of cytogenetic complexity or the nature of specific genetic markers. For example, extensive numerical and structural karyotypic abnormalities, or the presence of 'myelodysplasia-background' genetic findings (e.g., abnormalities of chromosomes 5 or 7), are indicative of very aggressive subtypes of AML. Several nonrandom, recurring chromosomal translocations characterize another significant subset of AML and can be detected by PCR-based molecular diagnostic techniques. These translocations usually occur without additional cytogenetic findings, often show distinct genotype–phenotype correlations, and many are associated with relatively favorable outcome. In particular, the t(15;17), t(8;21) and inv(16) or related t(16;16) translocations together account for about 25–30% of de novo AML in both adults and children. By contrast, comparatively little is known regarding the molecular pathogenesis of a large subgroup of 'diploid' (normal) karyotype AML.

Nonetheless, recent data have shown that internal structural rearrangements or point mutations of the FLT3 gene represent one of the most frequent molecular findings in de novo AML with a diploid karyotype, and FLT3 abnormalities are associated with adverse outcome. The importance of these tumor genetic markers is reflected in the present WHO classification (Jaffe, 2001), in which acute myeloid leukemias are increasingly defined by their characteristic genetic abnormalities in relation to phenotypic features, prognosis and clinical outcome (Table 71–3). The identification of specific genetic markers can thus establish a definitive AML subclassification, provide important prognostic information, guide therapeutic intervention, and reveal insights into tumor biology. This section focuses on the common AML-related molecular genetic abnormalities that are currently considered to be the most clinically relevant because of their frequency of occurrence and impact on therapy or prognosis.

Acute Promyelocytic Leukemia: t(15;17)/PML–RARα Abnormality

Acute promyelocytic leukemia (APL), or AML-M3 (according to the previous French–American–British [FAB] classification of AML) accounts for 5–10% of de novo AML. Patients typically present with symptoms from peripheral blood cytopenias and have a high propensity for life-threatening coagulopathy. Morphologically, APL consists of a proliferation of hypergranular promyelocytes and myeloblasts; however, a 'microgranular' variant form is also frequently encountered (Brunning, 2001). APL is genetically defined by the presence of the t(15;17)(q22;q21) abnormality, resulting in the fusion of the retinoic acid receptor-alpha gene, RARα [17(q21)] with the PML gene [15(q22)] to form a PML–RARα chimeric gene on the derivative chromosome 15q (Grignani, 1994). The RARα gene product is a subunit of a heterodimeric nuclear receptor for the naturally occurring ligand retinoic acid, or vitamin A. The retinoid nuclear receptor pathway function in many aspects of normal cell proliferation and differentiation (Chambon, 1996). PML encodes a DNA-binding zinc finger protein and associates with several other proteins in a macromolecular complex, forming discrete nuclear bodies (Dyck, 1994; Weis, 1994). This interesting protein appears to have multiple possible cellular functions, including transcriptional regulation, apoptosis, and possibly immune surveillance (Quignon, 1998; Wang, 1998; Grimwade, 1999; Zhong, 2000).

The hybrid PML–RARα protein is clearly involved in disrupting numerous intracellular processes, primarily resulting in a failure of neoplastic myeloid precursors to differentiate beyond the promyelocytic stage. The significance of APL as a 'therapeutic paradigm' for leukemia resides in the ability of pharmacologic doses of all-trans retinoic acid (atRA) to induce leukemic cell differentiation in vivo. When used in combination with cytotoxic chemotherapy, the synergistic effects of atRA induce durable clinical remissions in the majority of patients (Tallman, 1997, 2002). This remarkable finding has intensified efforts to identify other avenues for 'cytodifferentiative' therapy in AML. While the effect of atRA would seem superficially related to the interaction with the RARα moiety in the abnormal PML–RARα protein, further investigations have unraveled the basic molecular mechanisms underlying the success of this agent. The normal retinoic acid receptor, when not bound to its retinoic acid ligand, associates with histone deacetylase (HDAC) in a nuclear protein co-repressor complex (Guidez, 1998; Melnick, 1999). This interaction serves to reduce the accessibility of chromatin to transcription factors (and thus locus-specific transcriptional activity), yet is reversible in normal marrow cells upon exposure to physiologic concentrations of retinoic acid. The PML–RARα oncoprotein stabilizes and enhances the state of transcriptional repression by this multiprotein complex, however, therapeutic doses of atRA appear to overcome this abnormal condition and relieve the cellular differentiation block (Melnick, 1999).

The molecular anatomy of the PML–RARα fusion gene and mRNA products in APL is summarized diagrammatically in Figure 71–2. The PML gene exhibits breakpoint heterogeneity in that one of three possible break sites can be encountered in any given patient, involving intron 3, intron 6, or occurring within exon 6 (Grignani, 1994; Gallagher, 1995). In contrast, the RARα breakpoints are uniformly distributed in intron 2 of the gene. Thus one of three possible PML–RARα chimeric mRNAs can result from this genetic fusion: PML exon 6/RARα exon 3 (long (L)-form, or BCR1), PML exon 3/RARα exon 3 (short [S] form, or BCR3) and PML exon 6Δ/RARα exon 3 (variable [V] form, or BCR2). The V-form transcript is unique in that the PML break occurs within exon 6 and a variable proportion of this exon is retained, although additional nucleotides may be added or deleted (Gallagher, 1995). Notably, an in-frame fusion mRNA is produced in each case of APL, underscoring the critical requirement for the PML–RARα protein in leukemogenesis. The L-form (BCR1) and S-form (BCR3) PML–RARα fusions are most commonly found in APL (≈45–50% of cases each), whereas the V

VIII

A

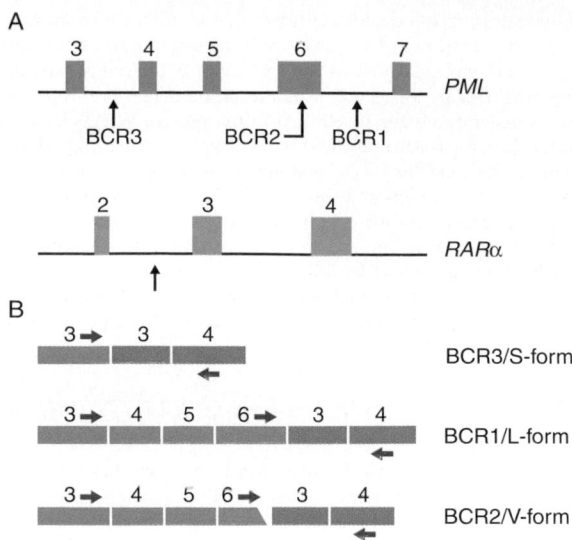

B

C

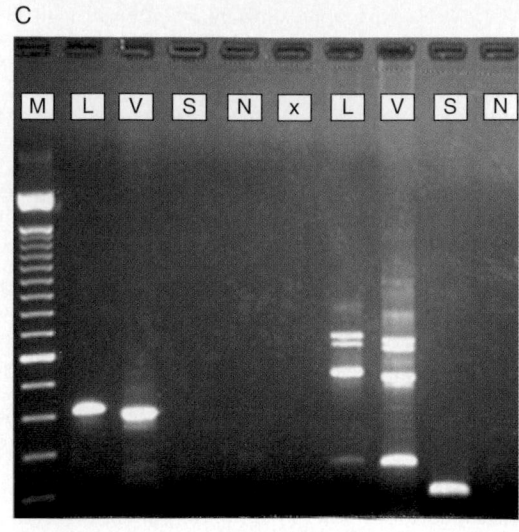

Figure 71–2 t(15;17)/*PML–RAR*α abnormality in acute promyelocytic leukemia. *A*, Partial schematic of *PML* and *RAR*α genomic exon configurations. Vertical black arrows indicate the three breakpoint sites in the *PML* gene (BCR1, BCR2, BCR3) and the intron2 breakpoint region in the *RAR*α gene. Note that the BCR2 breakpoint occurs within exon 6 of the *PML* gene. *B*, Representations of *PML–RAR*α mRNA transcript derived from the each of the three breakpoint–fusion events. The three transcripts are alternatively named according to the length of the chimeric species: long (L)-form for BCR1, short (S)-form for BCR3 and variable (V)-form for BCR2. Again, the BCR2/V-form fusion contains only a portion of *PML* exon 6, although extra nucleotides may be added or deleted at the junction to maintain an intact *PML–RAR*α reading frame. Orange arrows indicate the relative positions of polymerase chain reaction (PCR) primers to detect these chimeric transcripts by reverse-transcriptase (RT)-PCR technique. Panel C illustrates representative RT-PCR results detecting the t(15;17)/*PML–RAR*α abnormality: M = molecular size marker (100 bp); L = long form/BCR1; V = V-form/BCR2; S = S-form/BCR3; N = no template control; x = empty lane. The gel bands on the left side (up to the empty lane, x) indicate PCR products for L-form/BCR1 and V-form/BCR2 detected with primers situated in *PML* exon 6 and *RAR*α exon 4. Because exon 6 is not present in the S-form/BCR3 transcript, no PCR product is generated, as shown in the corresponding lane. Gel bands to the right of empty lane x show results obtained with a *PML* exon 3 primer and the same *RAR*α primer. In this case, a more complex banding pattern is seen for L-form/BCR1 and V-form/BCR2 products due to alternative splicing out of *PML* exon 5 and exons 5 and 6. The S-form/BCR3 fusion is readily detected with this primer set. Note that for the rare V-form/BCR2 type *PML–RAR*α, the PCR products are slightly smaller than the L-form/BCR1 species, because of the loss of some of *PML* exon 6.

form (*BCR2*) is only rarely encountered (≈5% of APL). The strategy for RT-PCR amplification of these *PML–RAR*α transcripts is depicted in Figure 71–2, as well as a representative diagnostic PCR assay. Of note, the L-form (*BCR1*) and V-form (*BCR2*)-type transcripts show alternative splicing out of exons 5 and 6, producing three major amplified products when a *PML* exon 3 primer is employed (Fig. 71–2).

The clinical relevance of detecting the *PML–RAR*α fusion abnormality in cases of suspected APL is evident from the efficacy of administering specific therapy (i.e., chemotherapy + atRA) with a high possibility of long-term remission and survival. To this end, despite the tight correlation between the t(15;17)/*PML–RAR*α and APL morphology, it is recognized that other rare APL-like myeloid leukemias do occur. These morphologic mimics harbor alternative translocations involving the *RAR*α gene with fusion partner genes other than *PML*. Examples of these variants include the t(11;17)/*PLZF–RAR*α, t(11;17)/*NuMA–RAR*α and the t(5;17)/*NPM–RAR*α acute myeloid leukemias (Melnick, 1999; Grimwade, 2000; Sainty, 2000). *PLZF-RAR*α-positive leukemias, in particular, are not responsive to the differentiating effects of atRA, and are associated with a less favorable outcome. Other morphologic AML subtypes characterized by increased promyelocytes are similarly atRA-unresponsive and also require distinction from true *PML–RAR*α-positive APL.

Several studies have assessed the possible clinical significance of the *PML–RAR*α transcript type in APL patients. Both the S-form (*BCR3*) and rare V-form (*BCR2*) *PML–RAR*α fusions have been associated with adverse features such as higher white blood cell count at presentation, poor atRA response, and possibly shorter remission duration (Vahdat, 1994; Gallagher, 1995, 1997; Jurcic, 2001); however, the independent prognostic value of molecular subclassification in APL remains to be definitively established. The *PML–RAR*α transcript also serves as a valuable molecular disease marker to follow therapeutic response. Given an array of additional treatment options for APL, including second-line intervention with arsenic trioxide (As$_2$O$_3$), or allogeneic marrow or stem cell transplantation, molecular residual disease assessment forms an integral aspect of the management of APL patients. Although this will be discussed further in the section on Molecular Monitoring of Residual Disease, the initial molecular investigation of the individual with APL is critical in order to define the type of *PML–RAR*α transcript for subsequent post-therapy evaluation.

Core-Binding-Factor-Related Acute Myeloid Leukemia: t(8;21)/AML1–ETO and Inv(16) or t(16;16)/CBFβ–MYH11 Abnormalities

Acute myeloid leukemias with the t(8;21)(q22;q22) and inv(16)(p13q22) or related t(16;16)(p13;q22) cytogenetic abnormalities together account

for approximately 20% of de novo cases (Brunning, 2001). While the t(8;21) is generally associated with AML showing maturation (FAB type AML-M2), the inv(16) and t(16;16) are highly correlated with acute myelomonocytic leukemia with abnormal eosinophils (FAB type AML-M4Eo) (Brunning, 2001). Clinically, these genetically defined AML subtypes are responsive to chemotherapy (especially high-dose cytarabine regimens) and are considered to be prognostically favorable in comparison to AML in general.

Although different respective leukemia phenotypes derive from these translocations, a remarkable and common pathobiologic feature of the t(8;21) and inv(16) or t(16;16) leukemias is disruption of the core binding factor (CBF) transcriptional regulatory pathway (Fig. 71–3) (Speck, 1999). CBF is a heterodimeric transcription factor that consists of a DNA binding α-subunit (CBFα) and a peptide-interacting β-subunit (CBFβ), which acts to stabilize CBFα at sites of DNA interaction. In normal cells, CBF acts at 'core' enhancer sequences in a number of genes required for proper myeloid and lymphoid cell differentiation or maturation (Fig. 71–3). The binding of CBF facilitates the access of other transcription factor complexes to these chromatin sites, in part through increased acetylation of DNA-bound histone proteins by histone acetyltransferases (Lorsbach, 2001). In human acute myeloid leukemias with the t(8;21), the *AML1* gene (also designated *RUNX1*, or *CBFA2*) encoding an isoform of CBFα, is joined to a putative transcription factor, *ETO* (or *MTG8*) to form the *AML1–ETO* fusion (Downing, 1999). In the case of the inv(16) or t(16;16), the gene producing CBFβ (i.e., *CBFB*) is juxtaposed to a smooth muscle myosin heavy chain gene *MYH11* to form the hybrid *CBFB–MYH11* (Liu, 1995). In either case, profound disruption of the normal cellular differentiation program is thought to be central to the causation of acute leukemia. The prominence of CBF pathway alterations in leukemogenesis is additionally emphasized by the finding of *AML1* gene translocations in several other types of leukemia and myelodysplasia, including the t(12;21)/*TEL–AML1* abnormality (Fig. 71–3), the most common single genetic abnormality in pediatric ALL. From a mechanistic viewpoint, the AML1-ETO leukemic fusion protein is thought to act in a dominant negative manner to normal AML1 (i.e., CBFα) by recruiting or stabilizing elements of transcriptional repression, including histone deacetylase complexes, at critical DNA sites (Lorsbach, 2001). In contrast, the CBFβ-MYH11 chimeric protein sequesters normal CBFα protein in the cytosol, thereby abrogating heterodimeric CBF assembly in the nucleus. In either case, the resultant inhibition of transcription at key genes alters the genetic program for normal proliferation and differentiation in hematolymphoid stem or progenitor cells. However, in keeping with the concept that an individual genetic aberrancy is of itself not likely to be sufficient for carcinogenesis, recent

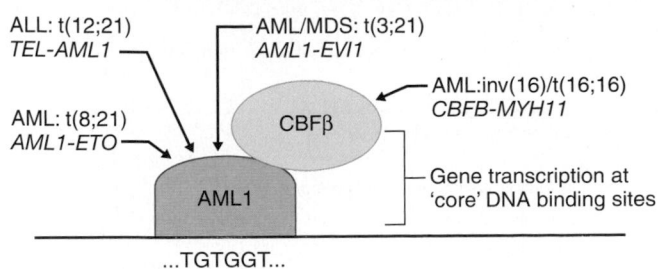

Figure 71–3 Disruption of the core binding factor transcriptional pathway in leukemogenesis. The schematic illustrates the central role of the core binding factor (CBF) transcriptional pathway in leukemogenesis. Both components of the heterodimeric CBF are targeted for disruption in a variety of acute lymphoblastic and myeloblastic leukemias. Of these, the t(8;21)/*AML1–ETO* and inv(16) or t(16;16)/*CBFB–MYH11* account for nearly 20% of de novo cases of acute myeloid leukemia, whereas the t(12;21)/*TEL–AML1* is found in 20% of pediatric acute lymphoblastic leukemias. Alternative gene nomenclature: *AML1 = CBFA2; ETO = MTG8; TEL = ETV6*. See text for further details.

data from transgenic mice genetically engineered to conditionally express an *AML1–ETO* oncogene have shown that an acute myeloid leukemia state develops only on subsequent exposure to a promoting mutagen (Lorsbach, 2001). The latter findings suggest that further investigation is required to more completely understand the definitive pathogenesis of these leukemias.

The molecular rearrangements underlying the *AML1–ETO* fusion are such that the breakpoint–fusion sites invariably involve the same intron regions in both genes, resulting in a consistent AML1-ETO mRNA molecule in each patient with this type of AML. In contrast, standard RT-PCR detection of the CBFB-MYH11 chimeric transcript is complicated by the potential for marked breakpoint heterogeneity, mainly in the *MYH11* gene, as well as by rare alternate breakage sites described in *CBFB*. In all, more than eight *CBFB–MYH11* fusion transcript forms have been identified to date (Liu, 1995; Viswanatha, 1998; Kadkol, 2004). Despite this complexity, the *CBFB–MYH11* gene fusion can be readily detected by RT-PCR, since nearly 95% of these tumors harbor the so-called 'type A' chimeric mRNA, characterized by fusion of *CBFB* nucleotide 495 to *MYH11* nucleotide 1921 to form a transcript of relatively short length. More comprehensive PCR strategies have also emerged to detect the majority of the other rare *CBFB–MYH11* fusion types, each of which account for fewer than 5% of cases of inv(16) or t(16;16) AML (Kadkol, 2004). RT-PCR analysis for the *CBFB–MYH11* abnormality is particularly advantageous, since standard cytogenetic interpretation may be uninformative in some cases (Merchant, 2004). Given the generally more favorable clinical outcome for both of these AML subtypes, molecular diagnosis can thus play a significant role both in initial identification and in disease monitoring following treatment.

Acute Myeloid Leukemia with FLT3 Gene Abnormalities

A relatively large number of AML cases with diploid karyotype are encountered for which little is known regarding fundamental pathogenesis. The clinical behavior of diploid AML is accordingly heterogeneous. Expression of the *FLT3* gene (FMS-like tyrosine kinase; also known as *FLK2* and *STK1*) produces a membrane-spanning signal transduction protein of the receptor tyrosine kinase (RTK) type III family, whose members also include the platelet-derived growth factor receptor genes and the *c-kit* gene (Agnes, 1994). FLT3 receptor–ligand interactions are important for the maintenance and propagation of early progenitor cells in normal myeloid and lymphoid hematopoiesis. Not surprisingly, the wild-type receptor protein is also expressed in the majority of AML and B-lineage ALLs, emphasizing its role in the survival and proliferation of immature hematopoietic cells (Gilliland, 2002; Stirewalt, 2003). Genetic alterations of the *FLT3* gene in AML were first described in the form of internal tandem duplications (ITDs) of part of the coding region for the juxtamembrane portion of this tyrosine kinase (Nakao, 1996b). The resultant molecular defect is predicted to produce a dominant, constitutive activation of the abnormal *FLT3* gene, an observation supported by the finding that all ITDs preserve an intact reading frame, despite the introduction of additional nucleotides at the DNA and mRNA level. Since then, *FLT3* gene ITD mutations have been shown to occur in 20–30% of de novo AML, with many patients being of younger age (<65 years) and having a diploid tumor karyotype (Gilliland, 2002). The presence of *FLT3* ITD is only rarely encountered in ALL.

A second type of activating lesion in the *FLT3* gene comprising 5–10% of AML cases has been elucidated recently, namely a point mutation affecting

the amino acid site Asp835 in the 'activation loop' (Yamamoto, 2001). The Asp835 mutation, in which aspartic acid at this site is replaced by another amino acid residue, is also thought to cause deregulation of FLT3 protein by direct effects on the activity of the kinase portion of the molecule. These *FLT3* gene mutations are together estimated to occur in at least 30% of adult AML (as well as a smaller number of pediatric AML, secondary AML and myelodysplasias), and appear to be distributed among all morphologic subtypes; *FLT3* is consequently the most common recurrent abnormal genetic finding encountered in AML. Most cases of AML with *FLT3* abnormalities involve only one allele of the gene with preservation of the remaining wild-type locus; however, occasional biallelic mutations have been noted. In contrast to the situation for translocation fusion genes with chimeric mRNA transcripts, *FLT3* ITDs can be detected by PCR amplification of genomic DNA. Amplification of exons 14 and 15 of *FLT3* (previously designated as exons 11 and 12) can identify the ITD, as these are variably larger in fragment size than expected for this region in the wild type gene. The presence of an ITD can be established by PCR product sizing, single-strand conformation analysis, or DNA sequencing. Different molecular approaches are used to detect the Asp835 mutation, including DNA PCR followed by amplicon digestion with informative restriction endonucleases, direct sequencing, or other sequence-specific methods.

Although the presence of *FLT3* gene mutations in AML has been associated with poor prognosis, the data are most compelling in the pediatric population (Zwaan, 2003; also reviewed in Stirewalt, 2003). Among adults with AML, the strength of an independent association between *FLT3* mutations and adverse outcome continues to be defined. Interestingly, *FLT3* ITD mutations are frequently observed in APL (FAB AML-M3), suggesting a cooperative role for this genetic aberration in the pathophysiology of a subset of this generally more favorable type of AML (Kiyoi, 1997). APL patients with *FLT3* mutations do not have a significantly different outcome than those without; however, *FLT3* gene abnormalities are associated with proliferative features, such as leukocytosis. Conversely, many other AML patients with mutated *FLT3* have aggressive biologic behavior and shortened survival; some of these leukemias harbor coexisting unfavorable genetic lesions, although most do not. A clue to the apparently more diverse effects of *FLT3* mutation in normal-karyotype AML has come from the observation that a high 'gene dosage' or ratio of *FLT3* ITDs relative to wild-type allele may be correlated with poor clinical outcome (Thiede, 2002). Elevated ITD:wild-type ratios in these cases of AML could possibly arise from gene amplification of the ITD, or from the presence of a more prevalent subclone of leukemic cells with the *FLT3* ITD (Stirewalt, 2003).

Regardless of the specific mechanism underlying *FLT3* activation, high expression of this altered gene seems to be associated with poor prognosis in many cases of AML. Assays to evaluate *FLT3* gene status, relative mRNA quantity, or protein expression levels will thus contribute an additional aspect to the diagnosis, classification, and prognosis of AML. With an increasing pharmacologic focus on the development of class-specific RTK inhibitors as anticancer agents, the mutated *FLT3* gene product represents another potentially important therapeutic target and further provides a tumor-specific molecular marker for minimal disease detection.

Acute Lymphoblastic Leukemias

Significant biologic and clinical differences exist between adult- and childhood-onset ALL. Comparatively little is known about the pathogenesis of adult ALL, which overall is associated with a relatively unfavorable outcome. As such, cytogenetic and molecular genetic anomalies in adult ALL are incompletely characterized, with the exception of the very poor-prognosis t(9;22)/*BCR–ABL1* (i.e., Ph⁺ ALL). Beyond detection of the *BCR–ABL1* gene fusion, molecular diagnosis is currently of limited utility in the management of adult ALL. In marked contrast, the molecular diagnostic evaluation of pediatric ALL is of substantial value in the stratification of patients to 'risk-adapted' treatment strategies. Over the past 20 years, the improvement in therapeutic regimens for these children, coupled with a more profound understanding of ALL tumor biology, has resulted in cure rates approaching 80% overall (Pui, 2004). In turn, this has led to the concept of tailoring therapy to defined subsets of patients based on a combination of presenting clinical and biologic features, including early treatment response and tumor genetics. The aim in childhood ALL has thus evolved to balance the highest probability of long-term remission with the lowest chance of therapy-related adverse events. While clinical features (e.g., age, degree of leukocytosis, central nervous system involvement, etc.) are initially used to separate 'standard' from 'high'-risk individuals, tumor genetics are also an integral component of the initial (i.e., pretreatment) evaluation of childhood ALL patients. Broadly, both numerical and structural chromosomal abnormalities are considered in

Table 71–4 Genetic Risk Stratification in Pediatric B-lineage Acute Lymphoblastic Leukemia

Abnormality	Prognostic Significance	Notes
High hyperdiploidy (> 52 chromosomes)	Favorable	Hyperdiploid tumors with particular trisomic chromosomes (e.g., +4,+10,+17) associated with very favorable outcome
t(12;21)/TEL–AML1	Favorable	Very favorable outcome but appreciable incidence of late relapses
t(1;19)/E2A-PBX1	Unfavorable	Intermediate-prognosis abnormality; intensive therapy results in good outcome
t(9;22)/BCR–ABL1	Unfavorable	Very high risk for relapse/refractory disease
11q23/MLL gene rearrangements	Unfavorable	Very high risk for infant acute lymphoblastic leukemia; also considered high risk factor for older children
Hypodiploidy (< 40 chromosomes)	Unfavorable	Very high risk for relapse/refractory disease

Tumor genetic features are considered in conjunction with clinical and laboratory findings, including age, presenting blast count, evidence of extramedullary disease, etc. These genetic risk factors therefore modify and refine traditional parameters. Other risk predictors, such as end of induction marrow blasts, have not been included (e.g., 'M3' marrow with >20% residual blasts as a very high risk feature of primary treatment failure).

this process (Table 71-4). In the former instance, 'high hyperdiploidy,' or tumor aneuploidy with a chromosome number in excess of 52, has been associated with more favorable treatment response and outcome, particularly if certain chromosomal trisomies (e.g., +4, +10, +17) are present (Harris, 1992; Heerema, 2000; Moorman, 2003). Conversely, tumor hypodiploidy, especially less than 40 chromosomes, is associated with a very high propensity for treatment failure (Heerema, 1999). Among the structural rearrangements, four chromosomal translocations account for approximately one-third of pediatric ALL cases, each with prognostic importance: the t(9;22)/BCR–ABL1, t(1;19)/E2A–PBX1, t(12;21)/TEL–AML1, and rearrangements involving the 11(q23)/MLL locus (Bartolo, 2000; Harrison, 2001; Pui, 2004). In general, the numerical and structural abnormalities occur exclusive to one another in any given case of childhood ALL; however, occasionally these abnormalities can coexist.

Major Translocation Fusion Gene Abnormalities In Childhood Acute Lymphoblastic Leukemia

The t(9;22)(q34;q11)/BCR–ABL1 is found in approximately 3% of childhood ALL. Typically, these patients present with markedly elevated lymphoblast counts and other adverse clinical features. The structure and molecular diagnostic aspects of the BCR–ABL1 gene fusion were discussed above; however, in pediatric ALL, it is noted that the minor breakpoint cluster region (m-BCR) or e1–a2 type chimeric mRNA is detected in approximately 80–90% of cases. The presence of the BCR–ABL1 in childhood ALL is an independently poor prognostic factor, placing these patients among those at the very highest risk of primary treatment failure and relapse (Fletcher, 1991; Gaynon, 1997). The majority of BCR–ABL1 positive ALL patients are candidates for more aggressive therapy, including early allogeneic transplantation; however, the introduction of imatinib mesylate may represent an additional therapeutic modality in this disease. Molecular analysis of the BCR–ABL1 transcript is critical for risk prediction in childhood ALL, as well as providing a marker for residual disease monitoring.

Pediatric ALL characterized by the t(1;19)(q23;p13) abnormality are uncommon, accounting for less than 5% of cases. This translocation is strongly associated with 'pre-B' immunophenotypic features, typified by the presence of cytoplasmic IgM production in the tumor cells. Following its initial recognition in childhood ALL, the t(1;19) was associated with poor outcome. However, it has become apparent that more intensive treatment protocols largely negate the adverse effects of this genotype, resulting in stable remissions for most of these individuals. Recognition of this translocation is thus required for appropriate therapy. The t(1;19) almost always occurs as an unbalanced form of translocation (with resultant loss of some genetic material) and produces the chimeric E2A–PBX1 gene fusion (Hunger, 1991). The E2A gene encodes a series of basic helix–loop–helix transcription factors, which are involved in myocyte and B-lymphocyte development. PBX1 is a DNA-binding transcription factor that is not normally expressed in lymphoid cells. The fusion E2A–PBX1 protein replaces the DNA binding and protein dimerization motifs of E2A with the DNA binding region of PBX1, predisposing the progenitor B-cell to neoplastic proliferation. The location of genomic breakpoints within E2A and PBX1 introns is consistent in essentially all cases, resulting in the formation of a single E2A–PBX1 transcript (Hunger, 1991), with only few reported variants. This fusion mRNA is readily amenable to RT–PCR detection and can also serve as a disease-specific marker for sensitive detection in the bone marrow. Of note, rare cytogenetically detectable ALL cases may occur with a balanced

t(1;19), but these lack the E2A–PBX1 and appear to be associated with an inferior outcome (Privitera, 1992).

Overall, 20–25% of pediatric ALLs are characterized by the presence of the t(12;21)(p13;q22) abnormality, establishing this lesion as the most common recurrent genetic findings in this disease. In fact, the t(12;21) is cytogenetically cryptic in almost all cases, instead often being suggested by an apparent deletion of the short arm of one chromosome 12. Although patients with t(12;21) ALL are found distributed among different clinical risk groups, in general, these individuals are between the ages of 2 and 10 and have diploid karyotype tumors (Rubnitz, 1997b). The t(12;21) results in the joining of the 12p locus TEL gene (also known as ETV6) with the AML1 (or RUNX1, CBFA2) gene on 21q to form the chimeric gene fusion, TEL–AML1 on the derivative chromosome 12 (Romana, 1995). Pediatric patients with TEL–AML1-positive ALL have a favorable outcome, with excellent disease-free remissions approaching 80–90% (similar to the aforementioned high-hyperdiploid group with specific chromosomal trisomies) (Shurtleff, 1995; Borkhardt, 1997; Rubnitz, 1997a, 1997b). However, reports of a substantial late relapse rate among some TEL–AML1 ALL patients have refocused attention on more clearly defining the risk characteristics of this group, even though many such relapsed patients remain responsive to 'salvage therapy' protocols (Harbott, 1997; Seeger, 1998; Ford, 2001). The molecular pathology of TEL–AML1 ALL is related to disruption of normal core binding factor (CBF) activity leading to enhanced transcriptional repression of many target genes, as similarly discussed for the AML1–ETO abnormality in AML (Fig. 71–3) (Zelent, 2004). In a large number of TEL–AML1 ALL cases, the remaining TEL allele is partially or completely deleted in a subclonal manner, suggesting that this event may be an important secondary event for leukemogenic transformation, through complete loss of normal TEL function (Raynaud, 1996). At the DNA level, TEL and AML1 break-sites in ALL occur most often in the same genomic regions of TEL intron 5 and AML1 intron 1 (Romana, 1995), with evidence of some propensity for breakpoint clustering. A second minor variant with breakpoints situated in AML1 intron 2 is also described. The in-frame transcribed TEL–AML1 mRNA thus encompasses a novel region joining TEL exon 5 to AML1 exon 2 (most cases), or TEL exon 5 to AML1 exon 3 (fewer cases) (Nakao, 1996a). Additional complexity is present in this gene fusion as a result of alternative splicing out of AML1 exons 2 and/or 3, with the possibility of detecting up to four TEL-AML1 amplified transcript forms by RT-PCR in any given case (Fig. 71–4). Molecular (RT-PCR) detection of the TEL–AML1 is frequently employed in pediatric ALL, given the inability to diagnose the t(12;21) by standard cytogenetics. The chimeric mRNA further represents a highly specific molecular marker for residual disease assessment.

Translocations involving the 'mixed lineage leukemia' (MLL) gene, located on chromosome 11(q23), are observed in approximately 5% of pediatric ALL cases overall and are disproportionately represented in infants less than one year of age (Bartolo, 2000). The presence of MLL gene translocations is associated with a poor outcome for these very young children and is considered an adverse finding in older children as well, particularly in the setting of a poor prednisone response (Pui, 2003). Infant MLL-positive leukemias are of B-lineage, lack CD10 positivity, and demonstrate aberrant expression of some myeloid-associated markers (Chen, 1993). Clinically, these patients have high initial leukocyte counts, organomegaly and a tendency for involvement of the central nervous system. Translocations involving 11(q23)/MLL also occur in de novo AML and secondary (therapy-related) AML (Table 71–3), in either case characterized by monocytic morphologic features (i.e., FAB AML-M4 or M5 types).

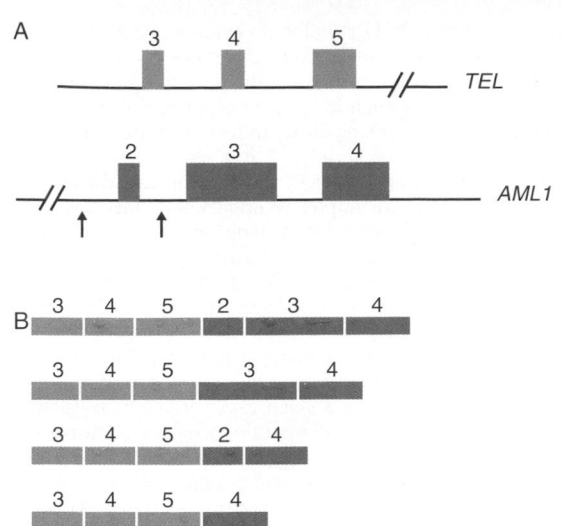

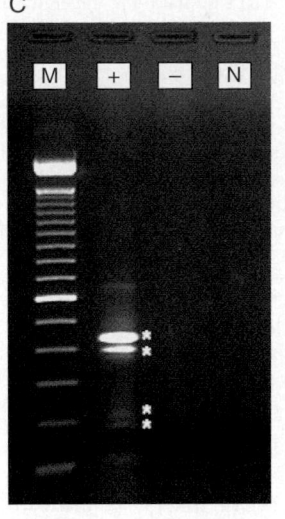

Figure 71–4 t(12;21)/*TEL–AML1* abnormality in childhood B-cell acute lymphoblastic leukemia. *A,* Partial schematic of *TEL* and *AML1* genomic exon configurations. For the *TEL* gene, breakpoints occur in intron 5, whereas for *AML1,* breakpoints can occur either in intron 1, or in a smaller number of cases, in intron 2 (shown by vertical black arrows). The most common primary mRNA transcript resulting from the *TEL–AML1* fusion is thus TEL exon 5- AML1 exon 2, as illustrated in *B.* However, additional complexity can occur as a result of alternative splicing out of the relatively short AML1 exon 2, exon 3 or both of these, in any given case of *TEL–AML1*-positive acute lymphoblastic leukemia. These alternative transcript forms are also indicated in panel B. Note that in the less frequent setting of a primary TEL exon 5- AML1 exon 3 fusion, only one additional alternative transcript would be expected. *C,* Typical reverse-transcriptase polymerase chain reaction results as revealed on an ethidium-bromide-stained agarose gel. M = molecular size marker (100 bp); + = leukemia sample positive for *TEL–AML1* fusion; – = leukemia sample negative for *TEL–AML1* fusion; N – no template control. The four possible TEL–AML1 transcript forms arising from the single gene fusion in this positive case are indicated by asterisks and the band intensities demonstrate that the full length transcript type is typically most abundant.

In de novo adult AML, *MLL* gene rearrangements, specifically the t(9;11) abnormality, may not represent a high-risk tumor genotype. In contrast, secondary AML arises in subsets of both pediatric and adult patients who have had prior dose-intensive chemotherapy with DNA topoisomerase II inhibitors (e.g., epipodophyllotoxins and anthracyclines); these tumors occur abruptly within a few months to years after exposure and have a very aggressive, treatment-resistant course (Super, 1993; Smith, 1994). The pathobiology underlying *MLL* gene translocations in these different types of de novo and secondary acute lymphoid and myeloid leukemia is becoming better understood. The MLL protein is a large (≈430 kD) DNA-binding protein that is characterized by several functional domains, indicating its role as a multifunctional transcriptional factor (Li, 2005). *MLL* is known to regulate several *HOX* (homeobox) genes involved in the coordination of proper skeletal development during mammalian embryogenesis (Yu, 1995). Several *HOX* genes also appear to be central to the development and maintenance of myeloid and lymphoid progenitor cells, thus establishing a tight link for *MLL* in the genetic control of normal hematopoiesis as well (Ernst, 2004a, 2004b; Hess, 2004). *MLL* gene translocations produce an altered functional form of the protein; in each instance, the N-terminal 'A–T hook' DNA binding motif of MLL is retained in the chimeric protein, typically with fusion to a portion of another transcription factor (Waring, 1997). Recent data indicate that abnormal expression of MLL fusion proteins can constitutively deregulate certain *HOX* genes, leading to hematopoietic progenitor cell immortalization and predisposition to leukemogenesis (Armstrong, 2003; Hess, 2004). Nonetheless, the basic molecular mechanisms leading to abnormal genetic program regulation in hemato-poietic cells by *MLL* translocations is an ongoing focus of study (Li, 2005).

Some additional key biologic insights have emerged from the structural analysis of *MLL* gene breakpoints in different subsets of leukemias. The majority of de novo AML with *MLL* translocations have break sites situated 5' in the *MLL* breakpoint cluster region, whereas the preponderance of secondary AMLs occur in a more distal (3') segment of this locus (Stissel-Broeker, 1996). Infant ALL cases strikingly also tend to associate with the 3' genomic region, suggesting a commonality in pathogenesis with secondary AML. This 3' 'hotspot' area contains a strong consensus binding site for DNA topoiso-merase II, as well as an adjacent 'scaffold attachment region' that is highly susceptible to cleavage by endonucleases. Although the presence of the topoisomerase II site presents an attractive explanation for the basis of developing secondary AML (e.g., via double strand break induction by topoisomerase II inhibitors and subsequent *MLL* translocation rearrange-ments), the hypersensitive 3' scaffold site of the gene has received further attention, since it too appears to be particularly prone to double-strand breaks in experimental models (Stissel-Broeker, 1996). The latter *MLL* locus is in fact targeted during diverse apoptogenic stimuli (e.g., following cellular stress or DNA damage) (Betti, 2001, 2003; Sim, 2001; Greaves, 2003a). These recent investigations imply that exposure to agents that can induce this site-specific *MLL* breakage potentially set the stage for *MLL* gene fusions, leading to the very aggressive forms of leukemia observed in infants and after distinct types of chemotherapy. In turn, as the causal etiology is already identified for secondary AML with *MLL* translocations, current studies in infant ALL seek to discover possible exogenous or naturally occurring transplacental factors that may predispose developing fetal hematopoietic stem cells to *MLL* gene breakage and illegitimate recombination. The implications of these and other studies are outlined generally in the next section.

The *MLL* gene is involved in translocation events with more than 30 known partner genes; however, the t(4;11)/*MLL-AF4* abnormality is the most frequently encountered in infant ALL (75% of cases). *MLL* gene locus breakpoints are distributed over an 8.3 kb region of DNA encompassing exons 5–11. This marked breakpoint heterogeneity may also occur in the translocated gene (e.g., *AF4*), resulting in the possibility of several *MLL* hybrid gene products, one of which is typically expressed in any given patient with this leukemia. RT-PCR can be used to identify the MLL-AF4 chimeric mRNA as well as other MLL fusion gene transcripts; however, the combination of multiple rearranging gene partners in these leukemias and the potential for substantial genomic breakpoint variability requires comprehensive and technically challenging labora-tory approaches, such as multiplex PCR assays (Pallisgaard, 1998; Andersson, 2001). *MLL* gene locus rearrangements have also been successfully detected by Southern blot analysis, although the FISH technique now provides a rapid, less cumbersome, and equally efficacious alternative for this purpose (Cuthbert, 2000). RT-PCR, even with the limitations described, nevertheless retains an important place in the diagnosis and monitoring of these leukemias, since the specific fusion gene type can be specifically and more sensitively identified, in contrast to other analytic methods.

Prenatal Origins of Childhood Leukemias

Major advances have been made in understanding the molecular basis of the pediatric acute leukemias. These efforts span the realms of basic science, translational research, and, increasingly, population-based methods. Studies of concordant ALL occurring in monozygotic twins first demonstrated that the leukemias arising in each paired affected individual were genetically identical, based on molecular analysis of the genomic breakpoint sequences of involved *MLL, TEL–AML1,* or clonotypic immunoglobulin or T-cell receptor gene rearrangements (summarized in Greaves, 2003b). Notably, the concordance rates are different for leukemic subtypes in twins, approaching 100% for *MLL* translocation ALL and only 10% for *TEL–AML1* ALL, suggesting a variable transforming potential for these different gene fusions in vivo and raising the issue of the nature and timing of secondary genetic insults. The impact of these investigations has been corroborated using similar experimental techniques to 'backtrack' leukemia-specific DNA markers to respective, archived neonatal blood samples of individual (non-twin) children of different ages with genetically-defined subtypes of ALL or AML (Cuthbert, 1997; Wiemels, 1999, 2002a; Fasching, 2000; Yagi, 2000; Greaves, 2003a, 2003b).

Together, these data strongly suggest that many pediatric ALL (and some AML) have origins in utero; in other words, prenatal acquisition of potentially leukemogenic translocation events or other genetic abnor-malities can occur during the time of active fetal hematopoiesis, but in most cases additional, later occurring genetic alterations in susceptible individuals are required in order to produce overt leukemia. The rapid evolution of *MLL*-associated ALL versus the longer latency (i.e., older age at onset) of *TEL–AML1* ALL indicates that both the biologic effects of the primary (predisposing) genetic lesion and the timing and type of promoting insult(s) are heterogeneous, although, within defined subtypes of leukemia, it may now be possible to better elucidate the molecular pathways resulting in tumorigenesis.

Not all types of pediatric ALL, however, can be traced back to a prenatal clonal cell origin. The retrospective neonatal blood data for the t(1;19)/E2A–PBX1 ALL subgroup instead support the concept that the majority of these patients develop this genetic aberration in the postnatal period (Wiemels, 2002b).

Prospective RT-PCR and FISH screening of blood samples from healthy newborn children has subsequently revealed a detection frequency of 1% for the TEL–AML1 abnormality and 0.2% for the AML1–ETO fusion transcript, markedly higher than the incidence of either of these leukemia subtypes in childhood (Mori, 2002). These data demonstrate that the occurrence of at least some chromosomal translocation fusion genes is a common event in utero; however the presence of such an abnormality is clearly insufficient to cause overt leukemia in the vast majority of individuals. Although the translocation-type acute leukemias are karyotypically characterized in most instances by an apparent 'single genetic anomaly,' it is becoming evident that these tumors also conform to the 'two-hit' hypothesis of Knudson proposed for solid tissue cancers (Knudson, 1992), as discussed in further detail in Chapter 75. In this concept, the initiating translocation event must be stable enough in a long-lived progenitor hematopoietic cell to confer some advantage in survival or proliferation; the acquisition of one or more subsequent genotoxic events in a susceptible individual would then lead to complete malignant transformation.

The fate of such silent 'translocation-positive' cells is thus an important parameter, not only for understanding disease pathogenesis but also in a practical setting for the appropriate interpretation of molecular diagnostic assays in the context of detecting minimal residual disease. While much research remains directed at the basic molecular and cell biology of childhood acute leukemias, molecular epidemiologic methods will play an increasing role in identifying the interplay between environmental factors and host genetic polymorphisms that underlie the predisposition to this disease in some individuals. The possibility of developing strategies to decrease the risk of childhood leukemia in utero is thus a goal of these efforts.

Continuing Impact of Molecular Characterization of Hematopoietic Tumors: FIP1L1–PDGFRA and Disorders of Primary Eosinophilia; Jak2 Gene Mutation and Chronic Myeloproliferative Disorders

As is evident from the description of FLT3 gene mutations in AML, the paradigm of disease classification continues to shift as knowledge concerning leukemia molecular biology expands. In this regard, the recent discovery of the FIP1L1-PDGFRA gene fusion abnormality in a significant subset of cases of idiopathic hypereosinophilic syndrome/chronic eosinophilic leukemia (HES/CEL) is particularly illuminating (**Cools, 2003**). This genetic anomaly may also be highly associated with presentations characterized as systemic mastocytosis with eosinophilia (SMCD-eos), although the distinction from classical HES/CEL may not be clear by clinical and pathologic criteria in many cases (**Pardanani, 2004; Bain, 2004**).

The FIP1L1–PDGFRA chimeric gene is formed on chromosome 4(q12). At the molecular level, these genes are juxtaposed following an interstitial deletion or translocation of the intervening CHIC2 gene. Whereas RT-PCR can identify a fusion gene transcript in many cases, FISH methods targeting CHIC2 deletion are more informative in revealing the FIP1L1–PDGFRA. Remarkably, its presence confers tumor responsiveness to imatinib mesylate (Gleevec[R]) therapy, introducing a novel treatment option for this rare and otherwise intractable neoplastic disorder (**Gotlib, 2004**). In contrast, systemic mastocytosis, which may show overlapping phenotypic features with FIP1L1–PDGFRA disease, is characterized by a point mutation in the cKIT gene (D816V), and is unresponsive to imatinib administration (**Pardanani, 2003**).

Early in 2005, four research groups independently described a novel single point mutation abnormality in the JAK2 (Janus kinase 2) gene, occurring in the classically defined chronic myeloproliferative disorders exclusive of CML (**Baxter, 2005; Levine, 2005; James, 2005; Kralovics, 2005**). This mutation, producing a V617F amino acid substitution (phenylalanine for valine), is thought to be central to the pathophysiologic cell proliferation in these disorders by constitutively activating the Jak2 tyrosine Kinase. Strikingly, each major investigative group arrived at this finding by very different experimental approaches. In subset analyses of these and other series, JAK2 mutations have been found in the majority of polycythemia vera cases, but rather variable proportions (e.g. one-third to one-half) of chronic idiopathic myelofibrosis (CIMF) and essential thrombocytosis (ET). The mutation has also been encountered in a small number of atypical myeloproliferative/myelodysplastic tumors and some myelodysplasias, but is absent in lymphoblastic leukemias and lymphoid tumors. Of note, most of the myeloproliferative disorders with this abnormality show a heterozygous mutation pattern, although a minority of cases (most notably in polycythemia vera) demonstrated homozygous mutations in the tumor cells arising from mitotic duplication of the mutated JAK2 allele.

Although the clinical significance of JAK2 mutation in this category of myeloid diseases is at present incompletely understood, this discovery refines the diagnostic classification of a large percentage of such neoplasms previously defined mainly by morphologic criteria. The presence of JAK2 gene mutations in chronic myeloproliferative disorders can be detected by a variety of methods including allele-specific PCR, PCR with melting curve analysis, allele-specific fluorescent probe hybridization, restriction enzymatic digestion and direct sequencing. The latter two methods may be of limited analytic sensitivity for detecting small percentages of JAK2 mutated cells in a given case, although in general, sequencing is performed for molecular diagnostic confirmation of patient samples identified as mutation positive by other methods.

These foregoing recently identified genetic lesions associations are significant in two profoundly critical aspects: first, that targeted pharmacologic and clinico-pathologic therapies (such as imatinib or other small molecule inhibitors) may have more broad spectrum effects against particular classes of oncogenic proteins, thus offering additional therapeutic avenues to certain patients; and second, that the ongoing elucidation of genetic anomalies like FIP1L1-PDGFRA or JAK2 mutation will further recast historically described hematologic tumors such as HES/CEL and the chronic myeloproliferative diseases in a new, molecularly-defined manner. As such, these advances are serving to continually reshape our current conceptualization of myeloproliferative disease classification schema.

Molecular Diagnosis of Non-Hodgkin Lymphoma

Rationale for Molecular Genetic Analysis in the Lymphoid Disorders

The non-Hodgkin lymphomas and chronic lymphoid leukemias encompass relatively common adult malignancies, and the incidence of these diseases is increasing (Ries, 1994; Chiu, 2003; Liu, 2003). A central paradigm for the diagnosis of lymphoma is the demonstration of clonality, which is highly correlated with the malignant state. In many instances, clonality can be suggested or established with the aid of immunophenotypic studies, by demonstrating light-chain restriction in the case of B-cell neoplasms, or aberrant antigen expression in the setting of T-cell proliferations. However, there are several instances in which the foregoing analyses may be insufficient and the determination of lymphoid clonality remains a key diagnostic issue. In these situations, which include samples with uninformative phenotypic features, small tissue biopsies, partially degraded specimens, and paraffin-embedded tissues, molecular assessment of clonal antigen receptor gene rearrangement is extremely valuable. Standard molecular clonality detection methods are also employed to resolve the definitive diagnosis of lymphoid neoplasms with features potentially mimicking benign hyperplasias (e.g., follicular lymphoma or extranodal marginal zone B-cell lymphoma), to assign cell lineage in undifferentiated hematopoietic tumors (i.e., B- vs T-cell) and to aid in the diagnosis of atypical T-cell lymphoproliferations.

Along with characteristic light microscopic tumor cell features and phenotypic cell marker profiling (e.g., by flow cytometry and immuno-peroxidase), the identification of recurrent, nonrandom tumor genetic abnormalities most commonly produced by chromosomal translocation events has also markedly improved the diagnostic precision and subclassification of the non-Hodgkin lymphomas. Indeed, cytogenetic and molecular genetic data of this type now form an integral part of the current WHO lymphoma classification (Jaffe, 2001). The following sections detail the molecular approaches to the determination of B- and T-cell clonality, and the detection and significance of common recurrent lymphoma translocations.

Antigen Receptor Gene Rearrangements for Clonality Determination

Mechanism of Antigen Receptor Gene Rearrangements

The antigen receptor genes are rearranged early in the development of B and T lymphocytes in the bone marrow and thymus, respectively. The process

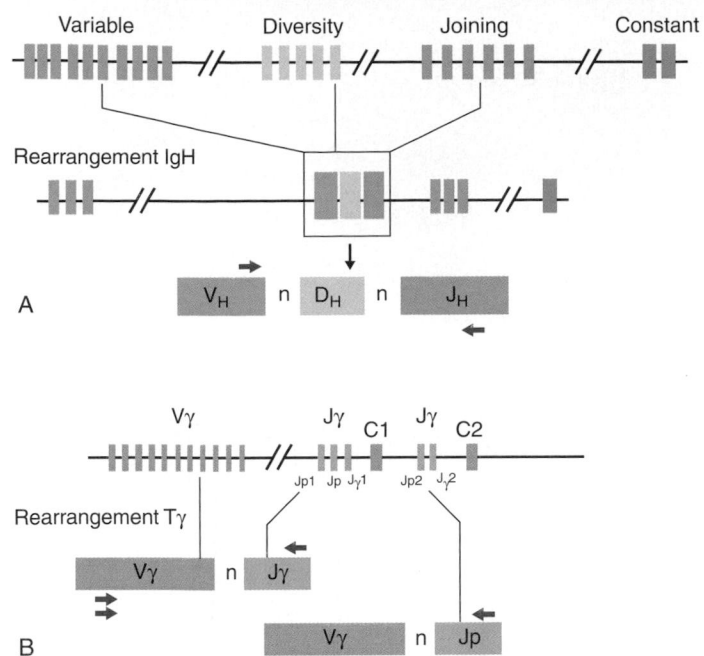

A

B

Figure 71–5 Somatic gene segment rearrangement of immunoglobulin and T-cell receptor genes. *A*, The basic process of somatic rearrangement of the immunoglobulin heavy chain (*IgH*) locus at chromosome 14q32 occurring in developing B-cells. Selection and rearrangement of IgH diversity (D$_H$) and joining (J$_H$) gene segments first occurs over a large region of intervening DNA, followed by the recruitment of a variable region (V$_H$) exon to complete a VDJ coding cassette. Substantial diversity is generated at the nucleotide level because of the recombination potential of the many V, D and J segments. In addition, the activity of the enzyme terminal deoxynucleotidyl transferase (TdT), which inserts a random number of 'nontemplated' (N) nucleotides at the rearranged junctions, adds to this diversity. The VDJ rearranged segment is then joined with the constant region (C$_H$) to complete the heavy chain gene-coding unit. Similar genetic recombination events occur at the immunoglobulin light chain genes (κ and λ) in sequence following the *IgH* gene process. If genetic rearrangements fail to produce a functional immunoglobulin protein at one allele, the mechanism proceeds at the second allele. The T-cell receptor gamma gene (*Tγ*) depicted in *B* shares similar structural and rearrangement features with the *IgH* gene. The *Tγ* gene located at chromosome 7p15 is less complex having only 11 Vγ segments capable of functional rearrangements and no D segments, although there are two J-segment loci (Jp and Jγ) and two constant regions. The presence of shared sequence homology among many V gene segments in the *IgH* and *Tγ* genes, along with the highly homologous nature of the respective J-segments at these loci, permits the detection of most rearrangements occurring in B- or T-cell lymphocytes by polymerase chain reaction methods employing flanking 'consensus' oligonucleotide primers. This concept is depicted by orange arrows and is detailed further in Figure 71–6.

of DNA rearrangement, or genetic recombination, essentially involves the splicing and fusion of one of numerous *variable* (V) gene segments with a joining (J) exon. At some loci, notably the immunoglobulin heavy-chain and T-cell-receptor-β genes, an additional diversity (D) segment is interposed between V and J segments. The assembled V–J or V–D–J segment is subsequently joined with the constant (C) region of the antigen receptor gene to produce an intact coding sequence capable of translation to a functional antigen receptor protein (Fig. 71–5) (Macintyre, 1999; Bassing, 2002). Immune cells incapable of producing functional receptor proteins undergo deletion by apoptosis. For immature B cells, the immunoglobulin heavy-chain gene on chromosome 14(q32) is the first to undergo this segmental rearrangement, followed in turn by the κ light chain gene on 2(p12). If the latter attempt is nonproductive at both alleles, the λ locus on 22(q11) is selected in order to generate the final tetrameric immunoglobulin molecule. For T cells, the T-cell receptor δ (Tδ) (14[q11]) and γ (Tγ) (7[p15]) loci initiate this process in the thymus; however, many of these gene rearrangements fail to produce a functional heterodimeric receptor protein. Thus, rearrangement continues essentially simultaneously at the T-cell receptor α (Tα) and β (Tβ) loci, located on chromosomes 14(q11) and 7(q34), respectively, generating a Tαβ receptor in the large majority (85–90%) of T cells. As an important point related to molecular analysis (discussed below), nearly all mature Tαβ cells still retain a Tγ locus gene rearrangement.

Enormous diversity exists among the immunoglobulin and T-cell receptors, arising from the potential for genetic recombination between numerous V, (D) and J gene segments at these loci. In addition, the activity of the enzyme terminal deoxynucleotidyl transferase (TdT) adds random nontemplated ('N') nucleic acid bases at the junctions of the rearranged gene segments in immature B and T cells, further increasing sequence diversity (Fig. 71–5). As a result of this entire process, individual B and T lymphocytes harbor specific gene rearrangement sequences and express correspondingly unique antigen receptor immune proteins on their cell surfaces. In a polyclonal lymphoid expansion, a highly variable distribution of antigen receptor gene rearrangements is generally present, whereas a monoclonal population is characterized by a single identical gene rearrangement in each cell. This concept is exploited in both Southern blot hybridization (SBH) analysis and PCR technique, to distinguish polyclonal ('benign') from monoclonal ('malignant') proliferations.

Techniques to Detect Antigen Receptor Gene Rearrangements

Southern Blot Hybridization

Genomic SBH technique can be considered a relatively 'large-scale' molecular approach, involving restriction endonuclease enzyme digestions of a high-molecular-weight DNA sample, followed by fragment separation, immobilization on a nylon or nitrocellulose membrane, and specific radioisotope (or nonisotopic) labeled probe detection of one or more

relatively large target DNA fragments (Cossman, 1988; Beishuizen, 1993; Langerak, 1999; Macintyre, 1999; Medeiros, 1999; Arber, 2000). A schematic summary and example of genomic SBH as applied to the diagnosis of lymphoma is shown in Figure 71–6. To briefly summarize, for a structurally unaltered (non-rearranged) region of the target DNA, SBH analysis will reveal a certain pattern of fragment sizes or bands, termed a 'germline' configuration, based on the distribution of particular restriction enzyme sites flanking or within the locus in question. If this region of DNA is rearranged, as in the case of the B- and T-cell antigen receptor loci, a different banding pattern will be produced (as a result of shifts in the locations of germline restriction enzyme sites) and these changes can be readily recognized by hybridization with a specific probe. The sensitivity of SBH is such that at least 5% of a population of cells must contain the same nongermline rearrangement in order to be detected (Table 71–2). In a polyclonal lymphocyte population, individual B or T cells carry unique rearrangements of their antigen receptor genes and would theoretically be expected to generate a 'ladder' or broad distribution of rearrangements when analyzed by SBH with the appropriate probes. In practice, however, no such rearrangement pattern is seen in polyclonal proliferations, since even highly selected and expanded groups of reactive lymphoid cells do not typically constitute up to 5% of the total cells in these situations. In contrast, each cell in a monoclonal population contains an identical antigen receptor gene rearrangement, and SBH will identify distinct, rearranged (non-germline) bands (Fig. 71–6).

The successful application of SBH technique to detect lymphoid clonality is dependent on several factors. First, the locus being interrogated must be structurally favorable for study by enzyme digestion and probe hybridization. Certain loci, such as the Tα gene, are very large and difficult to adequately assess with high sensitivity using a practical number of restriction enzyme digests and probes. Conversely, the Tγ locus, as discussed further below, is relatively small and of limited diversity, resulting in poor specificity and generally precluding its use for SBH. Second, hybridization probes must be easily available for use in the clinical diagnostic setting. Probes may be produced from either cloned genomic DNA or cDNA complementary to the region of interest, and several are available commercially. Finally, SBH method requires the use of high-molecular-weight, nondegraded DNA from fresh or frozen tissue sources. Of note, since a consistent amount of DNA is used per enzymatic digest (e.g., 5 μg), the relative proportion of clonal cells in a given sample can be estimated by SBH analysis.

For determination of B-cell clonality by SBH, both the immunoglobulin heavy-chain (IgH) and the light-chain genes have been used. The *IgH* gene is frequently assessed with a J-region probe (Cossman, 1988; Beishuizen, 1993; Medeiros, 1999). The *IgH* J region (J$_H$) is highly informative, since this locus is relatively compact, easily defined by restriction enzyme digestions, and always involved in recombination events in B cells (Fig. 71–6). With the use of a Jκ probe, the κ light chain gene can also be

VII

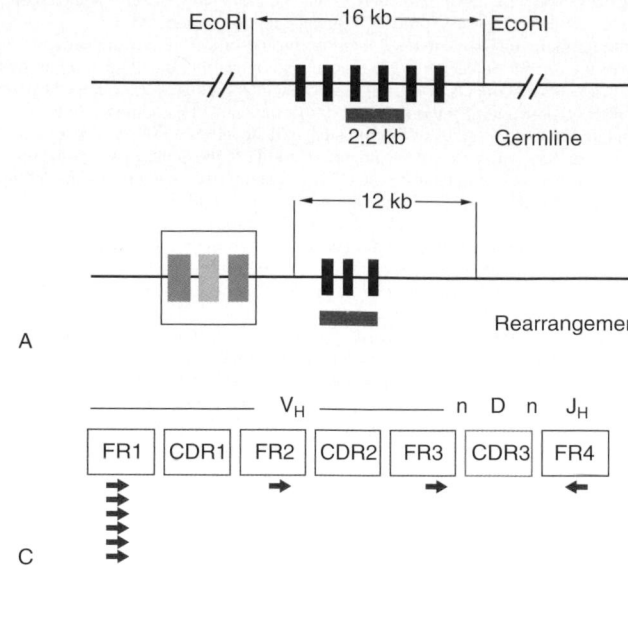

A

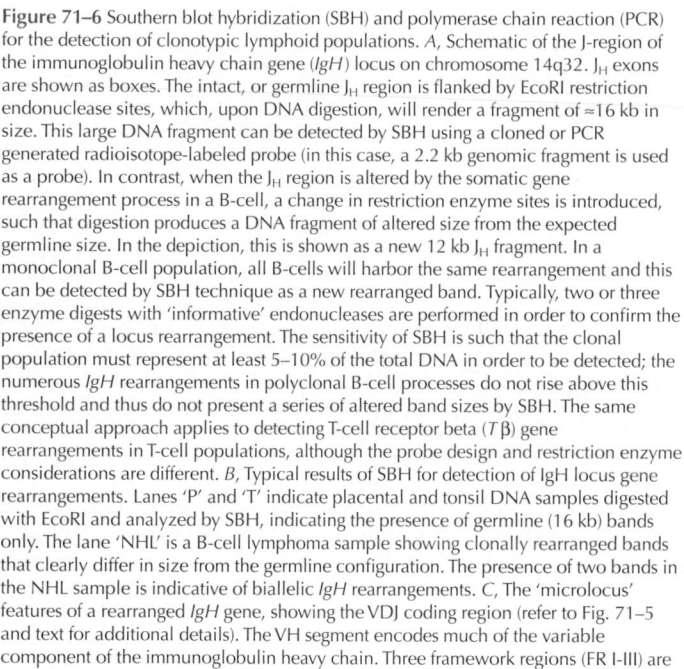

C

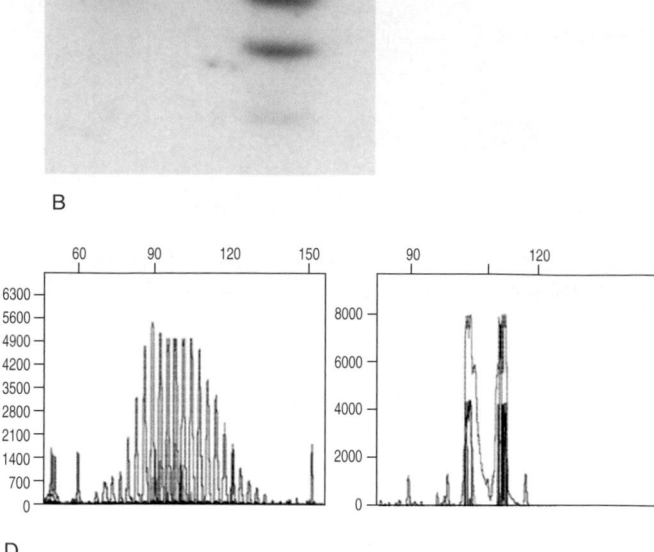

B

D

Figure 71–6 Southern blot hybridization (SBH) and polymerase chain reaction (PCR) for the detection of clonotypic lymphoid populations. *A*, Schematic of the J-region of the immunoglobulin heavy chain gene (*IgH*) locus on chromosome 14q32. J_H exons are shown as boxes. The intact, or germline J_H region is flanked by EcoRI restriction endonuclease sites, which, upon DNA digestion, will render a fragment of ≈16 kb in size. This large DNA fragment can be detected by SBH using a cloned or PCR generated radioisotope-labeled probe (in this case, a 2.2 kb genomic fragment is used as a probe). In contrast, when the J_H region is altered by the somatic gene rearrangement process in a B-cell, a change in restriction enzyme sites is introduced, such that digestion produces a DNA fragment of altered size from the expected germline size. In the depiction, this is shown as a new 12 kb J_H fragment. In a monoclonal B-cell population, all B-cells will harbor the same rearrangement and this can be detected by SBH technique as a new rearranged band. Typically, two or three enzyme digests with 'informative' endonucleases are performed in order to confirm the presence of a locus rearrangement. The sensitivity of SBH is such that the clonal population must represent at least 5–10% of the total DNA in order to be detected; the numerous *IgH* rearrangements in polyclonal B-cell processes do not rise above this threshold and thus do not present a series of altered band sizes by SBH. The same conceptual approach applies to detecting T-cell receptor beta (*Tβ*) gene rearrangements in T-cell populations, although the probe design and restriction enzyme considerations are different. *B*, Typical results of SBH for detection of IgH locus gene rearrangements. Lanes 'P' and 'T' indicate placental and tonsil DNA samples digested with EcoRI and analyzed by SBH, indicating the presence of germline (16 kb) bands only. The lane 'NHL' is a B-cell lymphoma sample showing clonally rearranged bands that clearly differ in size from the germline configuration. The presence of two bands in the NHL sample is indicative of biallelic *IgH* rearrangements. *C*, The 'microlocus' features of a rearranged *IgH* gene, showing the VDJ coding region (refer to Fig. 71–5 and text for additional details). The VH segment encodes much of the variable component of the immunoglobulin heavy chain. Three framework regions (FR I-III) are

identified as well as two complementary determining regions (CDR I and II). The third and most variable region of nucleotide sequence is comprised of the junction between V, D, and J segments, along with non-templated (N) nucleotide insertions mediated by the enzyme TdT; this region is termed CDR III and represents a highly unique nucleotide sequence in each B-cell. Given the shared sequence homology between V_H segments in the framework regions and also between J_H segments, 'consensus' PCR primers can be designed to amplify the short stretches of nucleotides comprising the CDR III. Most commonly, this is accomplished with paired FR III and J_H consensus primers, as depicted by the respective orange arrows. Other PCR approaches include the use of a FR II consensus primer, or a family of FR I-specific primers (these alternatives are also indicated by orange arrows). Note that as the FR primer is moved more 5', the size of the generated PCR products also increases. *D*, Typical results of IgH PCR using FR III and J_H consensus primers. In a polyclonal B-cell population, a range of VDJ rearrangement sizes exists, defined by the nature of V, D, and J segments used and the number of inserted N-nucleotides. This fragment size range is normally distributed, as shown in the left side panel. In contrast, a monoclonal B-cell population is characterized by a single (or dual, if bi-allelic) rearrangement(s), as demonstrated in the right hand panel. (The PCR data were generated with one primer fluorescently-labeled and analysis performed by capillary electrophoresis; the y-axis represents relative fluorescence intensity of the PCR products and the x-axis shows software-deduced base pair size of the amplicons relative to the red sizing markers.) Similar technical approaches and results are obtained with T-cell gamma (Tγ) receptor gene PCR (not shown). Consensus primer PCR, while rapid and extremely useful for lymphoid clonality detection, suffers from a false negative rate due to occasional occurrences of primer-template inhomology, or somatic hypermutation in the primer binding site. The latter situation is encountered mostly with germinal center-associated B-cell lymphomas (e.g., follicular and diffuse large B-cell types). The sensitivity of consensus primer PCR (1–5%) is better than SBH, but can be compromised when an abundant polyclonal lymphocyte background obscures a clonal population.

targeted for SBH analysis, although a minority of lymphoma cases (mainly those with λ light chain rearrangements) may be missed due to site-specific deletions of the rearranged κ loci encompassing the Cκ and sometimes the Jκ regions (Medeiros 1999; Cossman 1998). Rearrangements of the λ light chain gene can be assessed with a constant region (Cλ) probe; however, this locus is highly polymorphic with typically used restriction enzyme digests and banding results are more difficult to interpret (Saueracker, 1992).

The T-cell β locus (*Tβ*) has proved to be most useful for detection of T-cell clonality by SBH, and this region shares structural features with the *IgH* gene. The complexity of the *Tβ* locus is notably greater because of the presence of two Dβ, Jβ, and Cβ regions available at each allele for recombination with a large repertoire of Vβ region segments. However, since the two Cβ regions are nearly identical in sequence, *Tβ* gene rearrangements can be identified by SBH using a common Cβ genomic probe and appropriate restriction digests of the target DNA (Langerak, 1999; Medeiros, 1999). The use of specific Jβ region probes has also been described to detect clonality at the *Tβ* locus and may offer some advantages in conjunction with Cβ probes (Langerak, 1999). In contrast, the *Tγ* locus is generally less favorable for SBH analysis because of the relatively small number of rearranging Vγ and Jγ region segments. This limited capacity for segmental recombination creates a relatively small pool of functional *Tγ* gene

rearrangements. Thus, in a polyclonal T-cell population, SBH with a Jγ region probe may potentially resolve several prominent bands in addition to the expected germline fragments, in contrast to SBH analysis at the *Tβ* locus, in which rearrangements from expanded individual benign reactive lymphocyte subsets do not rise above the threshold of detection sensitivity (Cossman, 1988; Medeiros, 1999). This situation leads to the possibility of miscalling such 'pseudoclonal' bands in reactive T-cell processes as true monoclonal rearrangements or, conversely, may obscure the identification of a true monoclonal *Tγ* gene rearrangement in the presence of coexistent benign T cells.

Polymerase Chain Reaction

Rearrangements of the immunoglobulin and T-cell-receptor genes can be identified by PCR methods as well. In contrast to SBH, which detects relatively large structural genomic alterations on the basis of changes in restriction enzyme sites, PCR is designed to amplify short regions of DNA encompassing the immediate area of gene segment fusion in the rearranged antigen receptor genes. Under standard PCR conditions, a germline antigen receptor gene configuration is amplified at poor efficiency or not amplified at all, because of the very large intervening areas of DNA between primer sites. However, when coding V, (D), and J

Table 71–5 Southern Blot Hybridization versus Polymerase Chain Reaction Method for Lymphoid Clonality Analysis

	Advantages	Disadvantages
Southern blot	Essentially no false negative results Can detect nature of uncommon rearrangements (e.g., partial D–J) Can detect presence of oligoclonal gene rearrangement patterns	Cost, labor, technical difficulty Time-intensive (requires 1–2 weeks) Use of radionuclide-labeled probes Requirement for high-molecular-weight DNA Large amount of DNA required (5 µg per enzymatic digestion) Limited analytic sensitivity (can detect 5–10% of a monoclonal population in background cells)
Polymerase chain reaction	Rapid (24–48 h), inexpensive, technically straightforward Use of DNA from many sources, including paraffin tissues Requires minimal DNA (≈0.5–1 µg per reaction) Sensitive (nominally 1–5%, can be augmented) Can combine different PCR strategies to increase clonality detection rate	False-positive risk (contamination) False-negative risk (detection rate not 100%) Cannot detect uncommon (partial) rearrangements (unless special primer sets are used) May miss oligoclonal populations Analytic sensitivity can be adversely affected by prominent polyclonal lymphocyte background when using consensus primers

segments are juxtaposed in a rearranged gene, amplification of the region between the now closely apposed primers is readily accomplished by PCR. The two most widely used loci for PCR determination of lymphoid clonality are the *IgH* and *Tγ* genes.

A schematic depiction of PCR directed at the *IgH* locus is demonstrated in Figure 71–6. Several approaches have been described for *IgH* PCR. The most commonly applied technique involves amplification across the third complementary determining region (CDR III) of the rearranged *IgH* gene (Slack, 1993; Segal, 1994; Derksen, 1999; Medeiros, 1999; Macintyre, 1999). The CDR III encompasses the site at which the V, D, and J exons are joined in the rearranged *IgH* gene. The V_H gene region comprises approximately 100 discrete coding or functional segments that can be grouped into six 'families' based on sequence similarities. The D_H and J_H regions contain approximately 15–20 and six gene segments, respectively. Recombination of these many potential exon segments thus creates significant *IgH* diversity, augmented substantially by the addition of junctional nontemplated ('N') nucleotides by the enzyme TdT (Figs 71–5 and 71–6). While the more 5' complementary determining regions (CDR I and CDR II) also show relative sequence variability among B-cells, the CDR III is most informative in this regard, as it is produced from the junction of diverse V, (D) and J segments, along with the random introduction of N-nucleotides. As a result, the CDR III is unique in any given B cell and can be used as a powerful 'fingerprint' marker of clonality in B-cell neoplasia.

Although the CDR III is highly variable between B lymphocytes, PCR methods targeting this region are fortunately simplified by the use of 'consensus' primers. The 3' end of the flanking V_H-region, known as framework region (FR) III, exhibits nucleotide sequences that are highly conserved among the majority of V_H gene segments (Fig. 71–6). Similarly, the J_H exons each contain segments with an identical nucleotide sequence. Complementary FR III and J_H PCR primers can thus be designed that flank and can therefore amplify the CDR III in the DNA of most B-cells. Identification of amplified rearrangements is achieved by gel electrophoresis (e.g., agarose or polyacrylamide), or more commonly now by capillary electrophoresis following PCR amplification with fluorescent primers (Beaubier, 2000; Greiner, 2002). In a polyclonal B-cell proliferation, many hundreds or thousands of individual CDR III rearrangements can be expected. Since none of these reactive B-cell subpopulations is typically present above the sensitivity threshold of standard PCR analysis (nominally 1–2%), a smear or faint multiple-band ladder pattern is visualized by gel electrophoresis or is rendered as a series of normally distributed peaks by capillary electrophoresis (Fig. 71–6). In a monoclonal B-cell process, all cells harbor an identical CDR III rearrangement that is preferentially amplified during the PCR, producing one distinct clonal band or peak profile during post-PCR analysis. Occasionally, a second amplified band or peak may be present, indicative of biallelic *IgH* rearrangements.

The *Tγ* locus, though not well suited for SBH, has nonetheless been successfully utilized for the determination of T-cell clonality by PCR (Slack, 1993; Beaubier, 2000; Greiner, 2002; Lawnicki, 2003). *Tγ* gene rearrangement occurs early in developing thymic T lymphocytes and this genetic event is retained, even though the vast majority of developing T cells continues to rearrange the *Tα* and *Tβ* loci and ultimately develop a *Tαβ* receptor phenotype. The *Tγ* locus therefore provides a global marker for clonality assessment in suspected T-cell neoplasia. The *Tγ* locus encompasses 11 coding *Vγ* region segments, grouped into four families based on sequence similarities. Five *Jγ* region segments are present,

including the highly conserved *Jγ1* and *Jγ2* exons as well as *Jp*, *Jp1* and *Jp2* exons (Fig. 71–5) (Greiner, 2002). *Tγ* PCR also relies on the unique nature of junctional rearrangements in individual T lymphocytes; the technique is very informative despite the limited segmental diversity of this locus, with some caveats in mind (discussed in the following section). Consensus primers complementary to sequences of shared homology in the T-cell gamma V and J segments can be used to simplify the PCR procedure. Analogous to the case for *IgH* PCR, amplification products from polyclonal T cells tend to produce a smear or bell-shaped peak pattern by electrophoresis of PCR products, whereas monoclonality is evident as one or two discrete bands or peaks.

Advantages and Shortcomings of Southern Blot Hybridization and Polymerase Chain Reaction for Lymphoid Clonality Assessment

The decision to use PCR versus SBH requires knowledge of several factors such as tissue source, type of lymphoproliferative disorder being investigated, sensitivity of the respective assays, and false-positive and -negative rates. The advantages and disadvantages of the respective techniques are summarized in Table 71–5. In general, the PCR technique has gained wide popularity for clonality determination, principally because of its rapidity and relative ease of performance. The SBH method, in contrast, is very labor-intensive, more costly and requires approximately 1–2 weeks for completion. In addition, SBH is usually performed with radioactively labeled probes. Further disadvantages of SBH include the requirement for fresh or frozen tissue of good quality (for high-molecular-weight DNA) and a relatively low sensitivity, in the range of 5–10%. PCR is advantageous in that the turnaround time is within days, it is cheaper, and it requires a far smaller quantity of starting DNA (i.e., 0.5–1 µg) than SBH. PCR has a nominal sensitivity of 1–2%, although a prominent polyclonal B- or T-cell background can significantly worsen this level and reduce the ability of the technique to detect a coexistent monoclonal lymphocyte population. The sensitivity of antigen-receptor PCR can be further extended to between 0.1% and 0.01% in specially modified and optimized applications such as residual lymphoma or leukemia detection. Moreover, PCR can be performed from fresh samples or fixed paraffinized tissue sources, although certain fixatives (e.g., B5), or substances commonly used in lymph node or bone marrow processing, may inhibit the PCR.

Although PCR methods are more 'simplistic' by comparison, the technique is very liable to 'micromolecular' alterations in the regions targeted by oligonucleotide primers. Thus, the use of consensus primers will not amplify uncommon *IgH* or *Tγ* rearrangements involving gene segments lacking the conserved, complementary sites for these primer sequences. Perhaps more significantly, nucleotide base mutations or deletions in the template DNA may abrogate efficient binding of the complementary primer sequences, leading to PCR failure. Such situations occur more commonly in certain B-lymphoid tumors that have undergone somatic nucleotide hypermutations of the CDR and adjacent regions. Examples include follicular lymphomas, some diffuse large B-cell lymphomas, and lymphomas with plasmacytoid differentiation, where the detection of clonality can vary from only 35% to 60% using standard *IgH* CDR III PCR (Segal, 1995; Lombardo, 1996; Derksen, 1999). The detection rate of clonality in small B-lymphocyte tumors of presumed 'pregerminal center' association (e.g., small lymphocytic lymphoma, mantle cell lymphoma) is in contrast nearly 100%. B-cell ALLs and

Table 71–6 Common Lymphoma-associated Translocations and Resultant Fusion Genes

Genetic Abnormality	Disease Associations	Basic Molecular Pathogenesis	Detection*
t(14;18)/BCL2-IgH	Follicular lymphoma (90%) Diffuse large B-cell lymphoma (20–30%)	Overexpression of antiapoptotic Bcl-2 protein	FISH > PCR
t(11;14)/BCL1–IgH	Mantle cell lymphoma (≈100%)	Overexpression of G1-phase cell cycle protein cyclin D1	FISH >> PCR
t(8;14)/c-myc-IgH and variant c-myc translocations	Burkitt leukemia/lymphoma (100%)	Overexpression of potent early response mitogenic transcriptional factor c-Myc	FISH
t(11;18)/API2–MALT1 t(14;18)/MALT1–IgH	Extranodal marginal zone lymphomas (≈20–30%)	Upregulation of NF-κB signal transduction pathway activity	FISH; RT-PCR (for API2–MALT1 mRNA)
t(2;5)/NPM–ALK and variant ALK translocations	T-cell anaplastic large cell lymphoma (~80–90%)	Constitutive activation and abnormal localization of Alk tyrosine kinase	FISH (all variants); RT-PCR (for NPM–ALK mRNA)

* Detection by molecular techniques indicated; specific diagnosis can also be established in some tumors by detecting specific protein over-expression (e.g., cyclin D1 in mantle cell lymphoma, Alk in T-anaplastic large cell lymphoma)

lymphomas may occasionally harbor a clonal D–J rearrangement alone, or undergo V$_H$ gene region deletions and substitutions, also precluding the success of standard CDR III PCR approaches in a minority of cases (Beishuizen, 1994; Height, 1996; Szczepanski, 2002).

Different problems exist for Tγ clonality assessment. Despite the unique junctional nature of each Tγ V-J segment rearrangement in individual T-cells, the rather limited exon diversity at this locus may result in PCR amplicons with very similar size and even sequence characteristics. This may on occasion create difficulty in resolving a monoclonal T-cell population when background polyclonal T-cells are present, since amplified sequences of like but nonhomologous nature may create 'heteroduplexes' with the target amplicons during gel electrophoresis, thereby masking the ability to detect the monoclonal population. Conversely, a limited or skewed reactive T-cell population may demonstrate a highly selected pattern of Tγ gene segment usage, producing a 'pseudoclonal' amplification result resembling a clonotypic T-cell population. (The latter complications are in general less common with IgH PCR, given the greater degree of recombination potential provided by the more numerous rearranging V, D and J segments, and a correspondingly more extended amplicon fragment size range.)

Given these shortcomings of the PCR technique, SBH may still be required to resolve a difficult issue of clonality in a lymphoid proliferation. Because SBH assesses the structure of larger genomic regions, the technique is not prone to the difficulties addressed above for PCR. SBH is considered the 'gold standard' for clonality determination in this diagnostic setting and fortunately, since PCR is a very rapid method, one can subsequently revert to SBH analysis should the PCR results be inconclusive. However, the requirement for adequate amounts of DNA from fresh or frozen tissue often cannot be met, and this sample limitation has stimulated improvements to PCR techniques and post-PCR analysis. For example, alternative primer sets have been used to circumvent amplification failure due to alterations in the CDR III or FR III regions not infrequently encountered in IgH locus PCR. An upstream consensus framework region II (FR II) primer or a number of FR I 'family-specific' V$_H$ primers can be combined with the consensus J$_H$ primer (Fig. 71–6) (Deane, 1991; Ramasamy, 1992; Aubin, 1995; Derksen, 1999). Similarly, rearrangements at the immunoglobulin light-chain genes can be analyzed by PCR methods (Gong, 1999; Diss, 2002; Pai, 2005). These maneuvers serve to increase the overall success of clonality detection from approximately 65% (with standard IgH CDR III PCR alone) to nearly 90%, although at the expense of somewhat greater technical labor and complexity.

The use of comprehensive PCR primer sets has been emphasized to maximize clonality detection at the Tγ locus (Lawnicki, 2003). Changes to gel analysis can also significantly affect the resolution and hence detection of clonal PCR products. Use of polyacrylamide gel electrophoresis is generally more informative than agarose gel analysis and modifications to the gel composition can have important effects. In the case of Tγ PCR, resolution of true monoclonal populations can be substantially augmented by 'heteroduplex' pretreatment of the PCR products prior to (nondenaturing) gel electrophoresis; in this procedure, rapidly migrating monoclonal homoduplex bands can be clearly distinguished from slowly moving heteroduplexes in the gel, allowing separation of potentially similar amplicons on the basis of both size and sequence characteristics (Bottaro, 1994; Chhanabhai, 1997; Langerak, 1997). The advent of high-resolution capillary electrophoresis instrumentation and better standardization of associated interpretation criteria represent further improvements

in evaluating PCR products for clonal lymphoid populations (Lee, 2000; Lawnicki, 2003). Capillary electrophoresis, in contrast to standard gel approaches, resolves denatured single-stranded fluorescently labeled PCR products according to precise amplicon length (Fig. 71–6).

Lastly, as a footnote, the demonstration of recurrent chromosomal translocations in subsets of non-Hodgkin lymphomas by PCR technique provides yet another marker, if the initial antigen receptor gene rearrangement PCR is not informative. This aspect is discussed in the following section.

To summarize, PCR and SBH are key and complementary techniques for the determination of clonality in B- and T-cell lymphoid disorders. In general, PCR methods are considered 'front-line,' with SBH being reserved for those cases with adequate material and in which a negative PCR result is deemed inconsistent with other clinical or pathologic findings. In this regard, it is important to bear in mind the concepts of 'detection rate' and 'sensitivity,' as related to PCR technique. The detection rate of IgH or Tγ PCR will be dependent on a number of previously described factors, such as the subtype of lymphoproliferative disease, the PCR methodology (simple vs comprehensive primer sets), and the type of post-PCR analysis employed. PCR will not detect clonal rearrangements in all cases of malignant lymphoid tumors. Thus, knowledge of the overall detection rate of a certain PCR approach (i.e., the expected false-negative frequency) or improvements to enhance this approach are valuable for interpretation of results. An example is in the detection of follicular lymphoma, typically associated with a 40–60% clonal IgH detection rate using IgH CDR III PCR method alone (Segal, 1995; Derksen, 1999). By combining the IgH PCR with a PCR assay to identify BCL2 gene rearrangements, up to 80–85% of cases can be detected (Segal, 1995). Similar improvements can be gained by introducing additional IgH primers or targeting light-chain gene loci.

On the other hand, the capability of a given PCR assay to resolve minute amounts of a molecular target, or its analytic sensitivity, is often exploited in specialized circumstances such as the monitoring of minimal residual disease (i.e., lymphoma or leukemia) during or following a course of treatment. Sensitivity is usually measured in a dilutional manner and is optimized by sequencing the unique junctional region of a rearranged clonal antigen receptor gene and designing tumor 'allele-specific' primers or probes for use in monitoring subsequent post-therapy samples from a given patient. Nevertheless, for routine clinical molecular diagnosis, the nominal sensitivity of a diagnostic PCR assay using consensus (non-optimized) primers should be determined in each laboratory and the factors adversely influencing that basic sensitivity level (e.g., increased polyclonal background lymphoid cells) should be clearly understood. Importantly, because diagnostic PCR-based molecular assays are capable of achieving high levels of sensitivity, great care must be taken to minimize and eliminate the possibility of sample contamination in the laboratory: even a minute amount of extraneous, contaminating template may convert a truly polyclonal PCR result to a false-positive interpretation of monoclonality, with correspondingly serious clinical consequences.

Molecular Detection and Significance of Common Lymphoma-Associated Chromosomal Translocations

Our growing understanding of the biology of non-Hodgkin lymphoma has been substantially furthered by the identification of recurrent chromosomal translocations associated with particular neoplasms (Table 71–6) (Vega,

2003). Identification of these genetic abnormalities is not only very useful for diagnosis (establishment of clonality and lymphoma classification) but often provides prognostic information or reveals a specific tumor marker for residual disease detection. In general, chromosome translocations in the non-Hodgkin lymphomas result in the fusion of two genetic loci, most commonly involving the *IgH* locus on chromosome 14(q32) in B-cell neoplasms. Consequently, a normally highly regulated proto-oncogene becomes constitutively activated, leading to marked overexpression of an oncogenic protein. In other cases, for example, the t(2;5) in anaplastic large T-cell lymphoma, a chimeric fusion gene is produced and expressed as a hybrid mRNA and protein. In either case, interference with normal lymphoid cell growth, homeostasis, or death (apoptosis) is thought to play a central role in lymphomagenesis. Lymphoma-associated translocation events are thought in many tumors to be linked to aberrant consequences of the recombinase (RAG)/DNA breakage–repair enzyme systems active during the time of normal antigen receptor gene rearrangement.

The exact mechanisms underlying translocation events in leukemias and lymphomas are incompletely understood, but may involve nonrandom spatial proximity of genes during cell cycling, fragile sites such as single-stranded intermediates of DNA prone to breakage and recombination, and others (Neves, 1999; Roix, 2003; Raghavan, 2004). As alluded to earlier, it is noteworthy that many of the known chromosomal translocations associated with hematolymphoid malignancies are detectable at low levels in the hematopoietic or lymphoid cells from healthy individuals, indicating that these events are relatively common but most probably insufficient to cause overt disease without additional promoting genetic lesions. While most leukemia-associated translocations are detected by the presence of their fusion mRNA species, many of the gene fusion abnormalities in the lymphomas are amenable to PCR detection directly from genomic DNA because of a greater degree of break-site clustering within the rearranged genes and relatively short intervening genomic regions. The latter features allow the use of consensus sequence primers flanking the gene fusion site for detection of these lymphoma-associated translocations in standardized DNA PCR assays. Nonetheless, the overall detection rate of lymphoma-specific translocations by PCR technique is often limited by breakpoint heterogeneity, and additional analyses, such as FISH or immuno-histochemistry, play vital roles in the specific diagnosis and subclassification of the non-Hodgkin lymphomas.

Follicular and Diffuse Large B-cell Lymphomas and the t(14;18)/BCL2–IgH Abnormality

The t(14;18) abnormality is the most common translocation encountered in B-lineage lymphoma. At the molecular level, this translocation results in the juxtaposition of the *BCL2* gene with the J-region of the immunoglobulin heavy-chain locus (J_H) (Bakhshi, 1985; Cleary, 1985; Tsujimoto, 1985; Weiss, 1987). As a consequence, the *BCL2* gene is brought under the control of the highly active IgH enhancer element, leading to marked over-expression of BCL2 protein. The gene product of *BCL2* is a prototypic antiapoptotic molecule capable of abrogating the normal process of programmed cell death, thereby protecting cells from a variety of lethal genetic or cytotoxic events (Hockenberry, 1990; Yang, 1996; Adams, 1998). *BCL2* gene rearrangements are present in 85–90% of follicular lymphomas, approximately 25% of diffuse large B-cell lymphomas (DLBCLs), and rarely in other B-lymphoproliferative disorders (Weiss, 1987; Horsman, 1995). The partial genomic structure of the *BCL2* gene locus is illustrated in Figure 71–7. The largest proportion (60–65%) of break–fusion sites in the *BCL2* gene occur in a tightly clustered area of approximately 150 base pairs (bp) in the 3' non-coding segment of exon 3 known as the major breakpoint region (MBR) (Cleary, 1985). A smaller number of breakpoints (15–20%) occur far downstream in a second area termed the minor cluster region (mcr) (Cleary, 1986; Ngan, 1989). Rarely, a 5' region of *BCL2* described as the 'variant cluster region' (VCR) is rearranged in B-cell chronic lymphocytic leukemias; typically, the VCR locus is involved in translocations with the immunoglobulin light-chain genes (Adachi, 1990; Dyer, 1994).

BCL2 gene rearrangements can be detected by SBH technique using cloned MBR and mcr locus DNA probes, although this is typically a laborious approach (Horsman, 1995). FISH has also proved highly effective in the molecular cytogenetic identification of the t(14;18) (Poetsch, 1996; Vega, 2003). However, as a result of the relatively tight clustering of genomic breakpoints in the MBR and (to a lesser extent) mcr loci, rapid PCR methods can also be employed to detect the majority of *BCL2–IgH* fusions (Ladanyi, 1992; Liu, 1993; Horsman, 1995; Aster, 2002; Hsi, 2002; Iqbal, 2004). In the majority of situations, the intervening region of genomic DNA between the opposing primers is sufficiently short to allow successful amplification. This strategy is accomplished using MBR

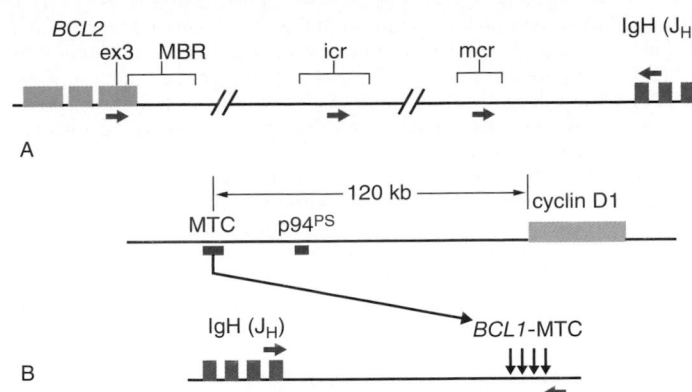

Figure 71–7 The t(14;18)/*BCL2-IgH* and t(11;14)/*BCL1–IgH* genetic abnormalities in non-Hodgkin lymphoma. *A,* The consequences of the t(14;18) abnormality in follicular and diffuse large B-cell lymphomas. Most genomic breakpoints are relatively tightly clustered in the 3' aspect of the non-coding exon 3 of the *BCL2* gene, in a region termed the major breakpoint region (MBR). Two additional *BCL2* breakpoint clusters have been described: the minor cluster region (mcr) and the intermediate cluster region (icr). For the *IgH* gene, breakpoints occur within the J_H segment region. Because of the clustered nature of breakpoints and the relatively short intervening distances between *BCL2* and J_H in the rearranged configuration, consensus *BCL2* and J_H polymerase chain reaction (PCR) primers (orange arrows) can be used to detect most *BCL2–IgH* gene fusions arising from the t(14;18). Note that a closely related t(14;18) variant occurs in extranodal marginal zone B-cell lymphomas resulting in a *MALT1–IgH* gene fusion. Although karyotypically identical, molecular techniques (e.g., PCR or fluorescence in situ hybridization [FISH]) are required to distinguish this entity from the *BCL2–IgH* anomaly. *B,* The result of the t(11;14) translocation in mantle cell lymphoma, causing a genetic rearrangement between the *BCL1* locus on 11q13 and the *IgH* J-region. As shown, the *BCL1* locus is situated far 5' from the cyclin D1 gene (nomenclature *CCND1*), which nonetheless is the target for deregulation by the *IgH* enhancer element. The majority (50%) of *BCL1* breakpoints occur at the major translocation cluster (MTC) located approximately 120 kb from *CCND1*. Two genomic probes (MTC and p94^{PS}) are illustrated that can identify 50–60% *BCL1* locus rearrangements by Southern blot technique; however, this molecular approach is now seldom used. Because of tight clustering at the MTC (small vertical black arrows), PCR using *BCL1*–MTC and J_H consensus primers (orange arrows) can be employed, although this approach detects only about 40–50% of *BCL1–IgH* rearrangements overall (and an even lower fraction when using paraffin tissue sources). Given the greater degree of breakpoint heterogeneity at the *BCL1* locus, FISH technique is a highly attractive method for detecting the presence of the t(11;14).

and mcr oligonucleotide primers placed upstream of the clustered break-site regions, in combination with a consensus J_H primer (Fig. 71–7). Overall, a standard PCR technique such as this can identify approximately two-thirds of all *BCL2–IgH* gene fusions arising from the t(14;18) in non-Hodgkin lymphoma (Horsman, 1995). In contrast to SBH, PCR can be performed from fixed, archival tissue material, although DNA extracted from paraffin-embedded sources may be compromised as a consequence of crosslinking and degradation. As a result, the *BCL2–IgH* detection rates for both MBR and mcr locus fusions are usually lower in paraffin tissue specimens than in fresh or frozen tissue samples. The application of 'long-distance' DNA PCR (LD-PCR) technique to identify and further characterize the molecular anatomy of *BCL2–IgH* fusions has also been recently described using high-molecular-weight DNA (Akasaka, 1998a; Albinger-Hegyi, 2002). Analysis of LD-PCR products has revealed extended break-sites occurring throughout the region 3' to MBR and 5' of mcr, largely accounting for the remainder of *BCL2–IgH* fusions not identified by standard PCR techniques. Evidence for a third cluster site, the intermediate cluster region (icr) has emerged from some of these investigations (Fig. 71–7) (Albinger-Hegyi, 2002).

The identification of *BCL2* gene rearrangements in neoplastic lymphoid proliferations is very useful in several clinical contexts, including diagnosis and disease subclassification. As previously mentioned, clonal immuno-globulin gene rearrangements are frequently not detected by standard *IgH* PCR techniques in many follicular lymphomas and a subset of diffuse large B-cell lymphomas (Segal, 1995; Derksen, 1999). However, the *BCL2–IgH* abnormality can often be detected by PCR in these cases, providing an alternative clonal marker to distinguish follicular lymphoma from an atypical or florid but benign follicular hyperplasia, for example. Furthermore, PCR analysis for the *BCL2–IgH* fusion can be used to differentiate subtypes of low-grade non-Hodgkin lymphoma with potentially overlapping morphologic patterns, such as follicular lymphoma versus lymphomas of mantle or extranodal marginal zone (ENMZL) type; this distinction may be quite critical in the setting of ENMZL, as described below in the section on abnormalities of the *MALT1* gene. One molecular diagnostic caveat to be bear in mind concerns the minor proportion of follicular lymphomas that lack the t(14;18). In general, many of these *BCL2–IgH*-negative follicular lymphomas are of higher grade (e.g., WHO 2/3 or 3/3) and are often characterized by alternative genetic anomalies, such as *BCL6* gene rearrangements.

As indicated, the presence of *BCL2* gene rearrangements in follicular lymphomas is almost always correlated with BCL2 protein overexpression. Conversely, it is important to note that many B-cell lymphomas and leukemias are associated with deregulated BCL2 protein expression in the absence of structural *BCL2* gene alterations, presumably via different genetic or possibly epigenetic mechanisms. In this regard, the demonstration of BCL2 protein expression in a nonfollicular type of B-cell lymphoma does not connote the presence of a *BCL2* gene rearrangement. Among DLBCLs, the presence of the t(14;18)/*BCL2-IgH* has been associated with a 'germinal center' phenotype. While increasing evidence supports the concept that germinal center type DLBCL has a relatively favorable clinical outcome, the prognostic value of the t(14;18) itself in DLBCL remains controversial (Gascoyne, 1997; Barrans, 2003).

Mantle Cell Lymphoma and the t(11;14)/BCL1–IgH Abnormality

The t(11;14) is essentially uniformly present in mantle cell lymphoma (MCL), although it has been occasionally described in cases of prolymphocytic leukemia, splenic marginal zone lymphoma (previously referred to as splenic lymphoma with 'villous lymphocytes,' or SLVL), and chronic lymphocytic leukemia (CLL). However, critical reappraisal of the clinical and pathologic spectrum of MCL has led to the conclusion that many, if not nearly all of these other t(11;14)-positive B-cell tumors are in fact atypical presentations of MCL. The t(11;14) places the *BCL1* locus in proximity to the J_H region of the *IgH* gene. The cyclin D1 gene or *CCND1* is located at a great distance telomeric to the majority of 11(q13)/*BCL1* break sites, but nonetheless is the target of transcriptional deregulation by the *IgH* gene in *BCL1–IgH* fusions. Cyclin D1 is an early G1-phase cell cycle protein normally required for the activity of cyclin-dependent kinases (cdk)4 and 6; these holoenzyme complexes promote progression through the G_1/S transition of the cell cycle in proliferating cells principally through phosphorylation of the retinoblastoma protein (Sherr, 1999). Oncogenic overexpression of D1 type cyclin is thus thought to play a major role in the pathogenesis of MCL. The tight correlation between cyclin D1 abnormalities and MCL has been aptly demonstrated by both mRNA and protein analyses (Rimokh, 1993; Bosch, 1994; Oka, 1994; Yang, 1994; Alkan, 1995; de Boer, 1995, 1997; Zukerberg, 1995; Soslow, 1997; Vasef, 1997). From the molecular diagnostic viewpoint, detection of *BCL1* genetic locus rearrangements implies *CCND1* (cyclin D1) overexpression and is diagnostic of MCL.

Identification of the t(11;14) or *BCL1* genetic rearrangements in MCL is variable depending on the methodology employed and ranges from less than 50% to 100%. The *BCL1* locus encompasses a large region on chromosome band 11(q13). Approximately one-half of *BCL1* breakpoints occur in a well defined area, referred to as the major translocation cluster region (MTC) (Williams, 1991, 1993a; Chibbar, 1998). The MTC is located nearly 120 kilobases (kb) centromeric of the *CCND1* gene (Fig. 71–7). Other breakpoints have been defined by SBH and are either more distal to the MTC or located in the immediate 5' region of the cyclin D1 gene (Williams, 1991, 1993b). SBH method using a single MTC region probe will detect nearly all *BCL1* MTC break-site rearrangements, accounting for 50% of cases overall (Williams, 1993a). With the use of multiple genomic probes, an additional number of non-MTC-related breakpoints can also be identified, increasing the SBH detection rate to 70% (Williams, 1991). However, this technical complexity, as well as the lack of commonly available genomic probes for the multiple *BCL1* regions, renders SBH impractical for routine diagnostic purposes. PCR technique has been successfully used to identify the subset of *BCL1–IgH* fusions occurring in the tightly clustered MTC region, accounting for an overall *BCL1* rearrangement detection rate of approximately 40% (Fig. 71–7) (Pinyol, 1996; Chibbar, 1998).

It is thus evident that the large and widely distributed breakpoint region encompassed by the *BCL1* locus presents substantial difficulties for these molecular diagnostic approaches. To this end, FISH assays have emerged as the method of choice for resolving t(11;14)/*BCL1–IgH* fusions in MCL (Coignet, 1996; Remstein, 2000b; Belaud-Rotureau, 2002). Commercially available FISH probes detect the t(11;14) span large genomic regions of both the *BCL1* and *IgH* loci; in an experienced laboratory this technique therefore detects essentially 100% of *BCL1* rearrangements in MCL. Some investigators have also described the use of quantitative 'real time' RT-PCR evaluation of cyclin D1 mRNA levels to assist in the diagnosis of MCL

(Elenitoba-Johnson, 2002; Thomazy, 2002; Jones, 2004). Finally, cyclin D1 protein overexpression can be readily detected by immunohistochemical technique, providing an additional rapid, widely applicable, and complementary method in the diagnosis of MCL (Yang, 1994; Alkan, 1995; de Boer, 1995; Zukerberg, 1995; Soslow, 1997; Vasef, 1997; Belaud-Rotureau, 2002). It should be noted that recent rare cases of morphologically and phenotypically classical MCL lack the t(11;14) and cyclin D1 overexpression but have been associated with deregulation of other D-type cyclins (Rosenwald, 2003).

Clinically, MCL is an aggressive B-cell lymphoma, despite having the morphology of an 'indolent' small B-lymphocyte lymphoma (Argatoff, 1997; Samaha, 1998; Weisenburger, 1999; Campo, 1999). Given overlapping anatomic distribution and morphologic features in common with several low-grade B-cell lymphomas, distinguishing MCL is therefore critical for prognostic and treatment purposes. Although the molecular mechanisms of transformation by deregulated cyclin D1 have not been completely elucidated at the present time, the application of gene expression microarray technology is providing new insights into the pathogenesis of this type of non-Hodgkin lymphoma (Rosenwald, 2003).

Extranodal Marginal Zone B-cell Lymphomas and Abnormalities of the MALT1 Gene

Extranodal marginal zone B-cell lymphomas, also referred to as mucosa-associated lymphoid tissue lymphomas ('MALTomas'), are uncommon and unusual tumors. In addition to neoplastic growth in many diverse extranodal tissue sites (stomach, lung, salivary gland, thyroid, etc.), these tumors are often characterized by the presence of predisposing inflammatory conditions and a preceding or coexistent reactive lymphoid component. Gastric ENMZL is prototypic of these lymphomas and a large number of gastric tumors are related to the presence of *Helicobacter pylori* infection, which appears to play a key role in the pathogenesis of early disease (Zucca, 2000; Isaacson, 2004).

While a proportion of these lymphomas in all sites may have a normal karyotype or recurrent numerical chromosome changes (e.g., trisomies of 3 or 18), specific translocation abnormalities have recently been identified among subsets of ENMZL and the pathobiology of the latter lesions is now becoming better understood. The t(11;18)/*API2–MALT1* abnormality was the first to be described and is characterized by fusion of an inhibitor-of-apoptosis gene (*API2*, or *IAP2*) to a gene encoding a paracaspase-like protein (*MALT1*, also known as *MLT1*) (Dierlamm, 1999; Rosenwald, 1999; Baens, 2000; Motegi, 2000; Remstein, 2000a; Yonezumi, 2001; Ye, 2003a, 2003b). *API2–MALT1*-positive tumors have a predilection for gastric and lung sites, with infrequent occurrences elsewhere. A second translocation event occurring in ENMZL is characterized by the *MALT1–IgH* gene fusion (Murga Penas, 2003; Sanchez-Izquierdo, 2003; Streubel, 2003, 2004; Remstein, 2004; Ye, 2005). *MALT1* is situated slightly centromeric to the *BCL2* locus on chromosome 18q and as such these two t(14;18)-associated gene fusions are indistinguishable by standard cytogenetics, requiring instead specific molecular analyses (e.g., FISH) for differentiation. Intriguingly, *MALT1–IgH*-positive lymphomas are distributed in orbital, parotid, lung, and cutaneous sites and are very uncommonly encountered in the stomach. A third rare translocation described mainly in gastric ENMZL is the t(1;14)/*BCL10–IgH* anomaly (Wotherspoon, 1990; Willis, 1999).

Despite the apparent complexity of translocation genotypes and tissue distribution, a fundamental pathogenesis links these events in the development of ENMZL. Through overexpression of either MALT1 or BCL10 proteins, or by expression of an abnormally active chimeric MALT1 (i.e., from the *API2–MALT1* rearrangement), constitutive activation of the NF-κB signal transduction pathway is induced, leading to profoundly altered effects on cell growth, immunity and apoptosis regulation (Isaacson, 2004).

Detection of these translocation events is generally best accomplished by FISH techniques. RT-PCR analysis for the *API2–MALT1* transcript has been described and represents an alternative method to evaluate for the t(11;18); however, owing to substantial breakpoint heterogeneity in both genes, comprehensive primers (and sufficient RNA) need to be employed for PCR detection. Nuclear BCL10 protein overexpression is observed most consistently and strongly with the t(1;14) abnormality, although it is also seen in the majority of t(11;18)-positive tumors (Ye, 2000; Liu, 2001a; Maes, 2002). Although prone to subjective interpretation, it has been suggested that aberrant patterns of BCL10 positivity, as determined by immunohistochemistry, can potentially be used to indicate the presence of such translocation events in ENMZL and may provide additional diagnostic information to differentiate a malignant lesion from a benign lymphoid proliferation (Liu, 2001a; Ye, 2005). The clinical significance of recognizing these ENMZL subsets is exemplified by the observation that *API2–MALT1*-positive gastric lymphomas do not respond to broad-spectrum antibiotic eradication of *H. pylori*, a therapeutic option that is often successful in inducing tumor regression in a significant subset of translocation-negative gastric ENMZL (Liu, 2001b, 2002). Furthermore, by elucidating the molecular pathogenesis of these related genetic subtypes of ENMZL, targeted pharmacologic therapies can potentially be developed.

To complete the discussion of gastric ENMZL in particular, the use of *IgH* PCR for assessing minimal residual disease following therapy deserves consideration. The significance of detecting clonal B-cells using by PCR technique in post-treatment biopsies from patients with gastric ENMZL has been controversial, with some reports suggesting prolonged persistence of monoclonality after histologic eradication of lymphoma, and others paradoxically showing the presence of clonotypic B-cell populations in benign gastric lymphoid proliferations (Bertoni, 2002; Wundisch, 2003). While many of these studies have employed PCR techniques with differing sensitivities, it appears that the decrease in PCR-detected clonotypic B-cells generally lags behind the histologic normalization of gastric tissue in successfully treated patients. These findings suggest caution in the interpretation of molecular clonality investigations and careful correlation with morphologic findings in this clinical setting.

Diffuse Large B-cell Lymphomas and Abnormalities of the BCL6 Gene

Cytogenetic aberrations of chromosome 3(q27) and the *BCL6* gene have been relatively recently characterized in a subset of non-Hodgkin B-cell lymphomas. In contrast to other lymphoma-associated translocations, fusions of the *BCL6* gene can involve a large number of partner genes, many of which are unrelated to the antigen receptor genes (Ohno, 1997, 2004; Ohshima, 1997; Chen, 1998). A number of cases will demonstrate the classic t(3;14)(q27;q32) abnormality, joining the *BCL6* gene to the *IgH* locus, while others may involve the immunoglobulin light-chain genes. The apparent 'promiscuity' of *BCL6* gene translocations has led to the concept of heterologous promoter substitution as a mechanism for *BCL6* deregulation and resultant overproduction of the BCL6 protein (Chen, 1998). Expression of BCL6 is, however, present in normal germinal center lymphocytes and murine *BCL6* gene 'knockout' models have shown that this gene product is vital for the formation of the normal germinal center reaction and for T-cell-dependent antibody responses (Dent, 1997; Ye, 1997). Furthermore, BCL6 appears necessary for control of Th2-type cytokine-induced inflammatory responses by normally downregulating the expression of a class of signal transduction molecules, the STAT proteins (Dent, 1997; Ye, 1997). The transcriptional repression role of BCL6 is mediated via recruitment of co-repressor factors (Polo, 2004). Recently, BCL6 has been shown to downregulate the p53 tumor suppressor protein, suggesting that BCL6 may function to protect germinal center B cells from apoptotic signaling arising from physiologic DNA double-strand breakage during the somatic mutation process (Phan, 2004). Importantly, BCL6 is not expressed in normal pregerminal center ('naïve') B cells and is rapidly downregulated in B cells exiting the germinal center environment. Accordingly, the presence of BCL6 protein expression is observed in the majority of large B-cell lymphomas, follicular lymphomas, and Burkitt's lymphomas, tumors presumed to derive from related germinal center counterparts, but not in other B-cell lymphoma subtypes (Cattoretti, 1995; Onizuka, 1995; Pittaluga, 1996; Falini, 1997).

Not unexpectedly, aberrant *BCL6* gene rearrangements are also found predominantly in germinal-center-associated lymphomas, principally diffuse large B-cell (30–40%) or follicular (10–15%) types (Otsuki, 1995; Ohno, 1997, 2004; Ohshima, 1997; Chen, 1998). In addition, a sizable proportion of these lymphomas demonstrate somatic hypermutations of the *BCL6* 5' regulatory (noncoding) region, which may or may not be associated with detectable structural gene abnormalities (Migliazza, 1995). The significance of *BCL6* mutational alterations in the absence of *BCL6* gene rearrangement is not completely understood at present, since a proportion of normal germinal center and memory B cells (with intact *BCL6* alleles) also display this finding. The latter findings in turn suggest that *BCL6* mutations occur in many reactive lymphocytes during the process of normal germinal center activation in conjunction with the physiologic immunoglobulin gene somatic mutation process (Shen, 1998). Some evidence has shown that at least a subset of 5' *BCL6* mutations in B-cell lymphomas are distributed differentially to mutations in normal B-cells, implying that, despite a common molecular mechanism

for induction of these mutations, the regions targeted result in divergent biologic effects (Pasqualucci, 2003).

Nonetheless, the overexpression of BCL6 protein appears to be integrally related to the pathogenesis of diffuse large B-cell lymphomas and this situation can be induced by *BCL6* translocation, or by other mechanisms without rearrangement of the *BCL6* gene itself (Allman, 1996). In addition, *BCL6* gene alterations may be related to the pathogenesis of distinct subtypes of follicular lymphoma, particularly those characterized by high cytologic grade (e.g., grade '3B' tumors) and absence of the t(14;18)/*BCL2–IgH* (Katzenberger, 2004). Abnormalities of the *BCL6* gene have also been described among post-transplant large B-cell lymphomas and in some of the aggressive lymphomas arising in the setting of human immunodeficiency virus (HIV)/acquired immunodeficiency syndrome (AIDS). While the exact molecular mechanisms predisposing to the development of large B-cell lymphoma continue to be defined, it is evident that deregulation of *BCL6* 'immortalizes' these lymphoid cells in a germinal center state, thus creating an environment conducive to additional lymphomagenic genetic derangements.

The detection of *BCL6* gene rearrangements arising from translocations can be accomplished by several methods. SBH analysis has been utilized, as the majority of these cases exhibit breakpoint clustering spanning the near 5' region, the first noncoding exon and intron 1 of the *BCL6* gene (Offit, 1994). More recent applications include long-distance DNA PCR specifically for the t(3;14) abnormality and FISH technique (Akasaka, 1996; Ueda, 1997; Sanchez-Izquierdo, 2001). However, the clinical significance of *BCL6* genetic abnormalities in lymphoma currently remains incompletely understood and controversial. Some studies have implied an adverse prognosis for large B-cell lymphomas with *BCL6* gene rearrangements, perhaps pertaining to tumors with non-immunoglobulin gene translocations (Akasaka, 2000; Barrans, 2002), whereas other investigations have shown either opposite findings, or no convincing prognostic effect (Jerkeman, 2002). As BCL6 protein is expressed in a large number of large B-cell lymphomas, the presence of this marker on its own has not been independently associated with disease outcome. Nonetheless, the clinical significance of BCL6 expression in diffuse large B-cell lymphomas is emerging in combination with other gene and protein markers defining a 'germinal center' phenotype. The latter studies, performed either by gene expression microarray analyses or by corroborative quantitative PCR and immunohistochemical methods, have established a relationship between this gene expression 'signature' and favorable patient survival (discussed further below in the section on Gene Expression Profiling). In this regard, the determination of BCL6 expression status in large B-cell lymphomas in concert with other key germinal center markers now appears to be of prognostic value, while the molecular pathogenesis of *BCL6* gene alterations in these malignancies continues to be studied.

Burkitt Lymphoma/Leukemia and Abnormalities of the c-myc Gene

Genetic alteration of the *c-myc* locus is classically associated with Burkitt's lymphoma/leukemia; however, this gene is also implicated in the pathogenesis of other lymphoid tumors, including high-grade (secondary) transformations of indolent lymphomas, HIV/AIDS-associated lymphomas, and occasional aggressive post-transplant lymphoproliferative disorders. Most commonly, the *c-myc* gene is translocated to the *IgH* locus as a result of the t(8;14) abnormality. In other instances, *c-myc* may be brought adjacent to the Igκ (2[p12]) or Igλ (22[q11]) light-chain genes. In each case, *c-myc* is placed under the strong transcriptional influence of the immunoglobulin enhancer element leading to overexpression of the gene. *c-myc* is normally a highly regulated gene involved in 'early' nuclear response to cytoplasmic growth-inducing signals. The c-Myc gene product forms a DNA-binding complex with a protein partner, Max, to initiate transcription of several downstream genes required for entry into the cell cycle and cell proliferation (Blackwood, 1991). Max is in turn regulated through dimerization with other proteins such as Mad and these alternate complexes act to repress transcriptional activity (Ayer, 1993; 1995; Zervos, 1993). As a result of *c-myc* translocation in lymphoma, overproduction of c-Myc leads to an increase in c-Myc/Max dimers and potent transactivation of multiple cognate target genes, ultimately driving uncontrolled cellular proliferation (Amati, 1993; Hecht, 2000). As a corollary, Burkitt's disease is among the most rapidly dividing and aggressive of human neoplasms.

The molecular anatomy of *c-myc* region breakpoints has been well studied in Burkitt's lymphoma with the t(8;14) (Neri, 1988; Hecht, 2000; Blum, 2004). In so-called endemic Burkitt's lymphoma, *c-myc* break-sites occur far upstream of the gene and primarily involve the *IgH* J_H locus on 14(q32). In contrast, sporadic type Burkitt's lymphomas demonstrate *c-myc*

VIII

breaks closer to the 5′ region of the gene and typically are associated with fusion to the immunoglobulin isotype switch region. These data indicate that translocation events involving c-myc in these Burkitt's lymphoma variants occur at slightly different stages of maturation in a developing B cell. Clinically, however, these differences appear to be insignificant. Rearrangements of the c-myc locus or the presence of the t(8;14) can be detected by SBH analysis, FISH, or long-distance DNA PCR approaches (Akasaka, 1998b; Siebert, 1998). Detection of c-myc translocations by standard PCR approaches is not possible because of the breakpoint heterogeneity in c-myc and the long intervening spans of DNA; FISH or karyotype analysis thus currently remain the best options for identifying these abnormalities. Practically, the diagnosis of Burkitt's lymphoma/leukemia can usually be suspected with a high degree of probability using a combination of clinical, morphologic, and targeted immunohistochemical studies (Braziel, 2001).

T-cell Anaplastic Large Cell Lymphoma and Alterations of the ALK Gene

Anaplastic large cell lymphoma (ALCL) is a unique subtype of peripheral T-cell non-Hodgkin lymphoma that may present as a primary cutaneous disease or, more commonly, as a systemic form involving lymph nodes, visceral organs, and skin. A phenotypic hallmark in nearly all cases of ALCL is strong expression of the CD30 (Ki-1) antigen, an activation marker and member of the tumor necrosis factor family (Smith, 1993). Although classical ALCL tumors are known to be of T-cell lineage, some examples fail to express lineage-associated T-cell markers ('null' cell type), but these cases can usually be confirmed as being of T-cell origin, based on T-cell-receptor gene clonality studies. T-cell ALCL is characterized by translocations involving the anaplastic lymphoma kinase (ALK) gene located on chromosome 2(p23). The ALK gene encodes a novel tyrosine kinase that is not normally expressed in lymphoid cells (Morris, 1997). The t(2;5) abnormality is the most commonly encountered translocation in ALCL and results in joining of the ALK gene to the NPM gene on chromosome 5(q35) (Kaneko, 1989; Rimokh, 1989; Mason, 1990; Stein, 2000). The normal NPM gene product, nucleophosmin, is a ubiquitously expressed nucleolar phosphoprotein thought to be important in ribosome assembly. As a result of the NPM–ALK gene fusion, the tyrosine kinase activity of ALK becomes deregulated, contributing to lymphomagenesis through increased target protein phosphorylation and signal transduction (Falini, 2001). The cellular sublocalization of this fusion kinase activity is abnormally mediated by the NPM moiety. Unlike the more typical gene overexpression consequences of most lymphoma-associated translocations, the NPM–ALK fusion differs in that a chimeric mRNA and protein are produced, although overproduction of the normally silent ALK gene in a T lymphocyte appears to be the principal mechanism involved in malignant transformation. In addition to NPM–ALK, less common variant genetic rearrangements of ALK are also described in this lymphoma, including the t(1;2), t(2;3), and inv(2) abnormalities, all giving rise to ALK gene deregulation (Stein, 2000; Delsol, 2001).

Genomic breakpoints in cases of t(2;5)-positive ALCL lie consistently within the same intron regions in both NPM and ALK genes, resulting in the generation of a single, unique NPM–ALK chimeric mRNA. As a result, RT-PCR technique can be used to detect the fusion transcript with high specificity and sensitivity (Ladanyi, 1994; Downing, 1995; Elmberger, 1995; Weiss, 1995; Wellmann, 1995; Lamant, 1996; Yee, 1996). In addition, long distance PCR has also been successfully employed to identify the genomic NPM–ALK abnormality (Ladanyi, 1996; Sarris, 1998). The latter approach requires high-molecular-weight DNA but obviates the need for RNA isolation and reverse transcription. FISH methodology is an attractive alternative to other molecular techniques in the setting of a possible ALCL, since rearrangements of the ALK locus can be targeted irrespective of the partner gene involved. Since classical cytogenetics is technically demanding and infrequently performed on tissue biopsies, these molecular methods have served to simplify and augment the detection rate of this genetic lesion. Finally, as with other specific gene overexpression phenomena in non-Hodgkin lymphomas, ALCL can be readily diagnosed with monoclonal antibodies directed to the ALK protein; immunohistochemical localization of ALK is an important diagnostic adjunct and also correlates to some extent with the type of translocation event resulting in ALK overexpression (Falini, 1999a; Stein, 2000).

Clinically, the identification of ALK positivity in a lymphoma suspected to be ALCL is very important, since this subset of T-cell neoplasms carries a significantly better prognosis than ALK-negative T-cell lymphomas with anaplastic morphology, or peripheral T-cell lymphomas in general (Falini, 1999b; Gascoyne, 1999). Earlier reports suggested that rare cases of Hodgkin lymphoma might be ALK-positive; however, current consensus is that such cases probably represent true ALCL with morphologically overlapping features. Such occurrences serve to highlight the difficulties in subclassifying so-called 'gray zone' lymphomas at the interface of Hodgkin's disease and non-Hodgkin lymphoma. The demonstration of molecular or immunohistochemical evidence for ALK gene dysregulation thus represents a significant advance in the accurate diagnosis of ALCL and its distinction from Hodgkin lymphoma. From a diagnostic perspective, it is critical to recall that ALCL can present with variable morphologic features or, in occasional cases, lack uniform CD30 positivity, necessitating an appropriate threshold of suspicion for pursuing the presence of ALK gene abnormalities. While some controversy has existed regarding the presence of ALK fusion proteins in primary cutaneous ALCL, the preponderance of data supports the view that ALK positivity in an apparent primary skin lesion most probably indicates the presence of systemic disease requiring thorough clinical and radiologic examination. Finally, several reports have recently documented the presence of the t(2;17)/CLTC–ALK, or NPM–ALK fusions in very rare and unusual occurrences of diffuse large B-cell lymphoma with plasmablastic features (de Paepe, 2003; Gascoyne, 2003). The latter tumors are not associated with the favorable outcome of T-ALCL but serve to highlight the role of disordered ALK gene function in other subsets of lymphoma.

Molecular Monitoring of Residual Disease

Background and Caveats in Minimal Residual Disease Analysis

Traditionally and to date, the evaluation of residual hematolymphoid disease following the initiation of therapy has been accomplished by morphologic assessment predicated on a microscopic level of disease less than 5% in the bone marrow. The advent of sensitive molecular biologic techniques capable of detecting tumor-specific markers has provided unprecedented opportunities to more precisely quantify and monitor tumor disease burden following initiation of therapy. Although minimal residual disease (MRD) can be demonstrated at various levels using a variety of genetic techniques, the applicability of cytogenetics or even standard FISH is relatively limited for highly sensitive detection. While the latter methods can be used to confirm remission status at disease levels of approximately 1–5%, the presence and temporal change in low level MRD appear to be important parameters associated with patient outcome in several hematolymphoid cancers. To this end, sensitive and reproducible PCR-based technologies have taken center stage in MRD detection and form an integral aspect of enhanced clinical management for patients with these disorders (Paietta, 2002). It should be noted that low-level MRD can also be identified by flow cytometric assays designed to detect aberrant cell marker expression profiles characteristic of various leukemias and lymphomas. Although immunophenotypic approaches (i.e., flow cytometry) also have substantial and often equivalent merit in MRD evaluation, this discussion is outside the scope of this section.

Until recently, the quantitation of small amounts of residual disease was achieved by laborious and technically challenging competitive PCR assays. These experiments have been valuable in confirming the relationship between precise measurement of MRD and its effect on clinical outcome. Serial measurements were shown to be capable of defining a 'disease-course picture,' with the ability to predict relapse risk in many patients. However, competitive PCR methods rely upon end-point detection; that is, the quantity of an amplified, specific target is determined following the completion of all PCR cycles. This feature is problematic because factors limiting amplification efficiency late in the 'plateau phase' of the PCR (e.g., exhaustion of reagents, preferential re-annealing of PCR product strands preventing primer binding, etc.) can create profound effects on accurate quantification as related to the initial amount of specific target. These problems have now been largely obviated by the development of 'real time' quantitative fluorescent PCR methods (referred to as Q-PCR here). Two similar proprietary technical platforms, TaqMan (Applied Biosystems Inc., Foster City, CA) and LightCycler (Roche Diagnostics, Indianapolis, IN), have dramatically changed the laboratory measurement of MRD by PCR technique (Heid, 1996; Wittwer, 1997; Gibson, 1999; van der Velden, 2003); these techniques are discussed at length in Chapter 67. Notably, quantitative data can be highly correlated using either format for a given MRD target (Eckert, 2003). The culmination of these efforts as applied to the hematolymphoid malignancies is most aptly demonstrated by the recent comprehensive publications of the Europe Against Cancer (EAC) consortium regarding MRD monitoring in the leukemias (Beillard, 2003; Gabert, 2003).

In addition to the foregoing technical concerns, the general discussion of molecular MRD assessment would not be complete without consideration of the broad range of clinical and tumor biologic factors that influence successful PCR analysis. Timing of sample collection for MRD analysis is a paramount issue. For some types of leukemia, positivity for a tumor-specific marker at the end of induction therapy may not have significant prognostic value, whereas the opposite may be true for a different type of neoplasm. Related to timing is the choice between single (or static) time-point MRD measurements versus serial assessments over a time course. The latter approach may be associated with additional patient morbidity (e.g., repeated bone marrow samplings) but will provide more refined data on tumor burden and biological behavior. Furthermore, since 'threshold' levels of MRD indicative of disease cure have not been reliably established for hematolymphoid malignancies, the great value of Q-PCR lies in its ability to sensitively monitor the changes in disease level with time. For most situations, bone marrow is preferred over blood for MRD evaluation, since detection in marrow samples is often significantly enhanced. However, some leukemias derived from early progenitor or 'stem cell' origin show multilineage differentiation capacity (e.g., CML) and detection of MRD from blood samples is equally sensitive. An important consideration in developing MRD assays is the interpretation of positive values in relation to potentially confounding 'rare event' occurrences. For some patients, the detection of very low-level disease-specific chimeric transcripts may nonetheless be compatible with long-term stable remission status. Such is the case in a number of patients with t(8;21)/AML1–ETO-positive acute myeloid leukemia treated with either chemotherapy or transplantation (Kusec, 1994; Jurlander, 1996), and this situation has been observed in successfully treated patients with other leukemias. These findings suggest that for at least some (or perhaps many) individuals apparently cured of hematologic disease, complete eradication of very low-level MRD may not be possible with currently available therapies. Minor populations of remaining tumor cells may reside in a 'dormant' or nonproliferative state. Again, the distinct advantage of Q-PCR rests in the ability of sequential assays to determine the 'activity' of residual cells as a surrogate for assessing the biologic potential for disease relapse.

Finally, recent studies have demonstrated the occurrence of leukemia or lymphoma-associated translocation fusion genes, such as the t(9;22)/BCR–ABL1 and the t(14;18)/BCL2–IgH, in the blood or tissues of healthy individuals, suggesting that aberrant genetic recombination may be a relatively common event. This implies that single genetic events in isolation are likely insufficient to result directly in a hematolymphoid malignancy (Limpens, 1995; Biernaux, 1995; Dolken, 1996; Bose, 1998). However, these genetic lesions in normal subjects have been detected at very low levels, requiring highly sensitive PCR assays. Although rare event detection in 'innocent bystander' cells would appear to have implications for MRD monitoring in post-therapy leukemia or lymphoma patients, the reproducible sensitivity limits of current Q-PCR technologies are generally constructed to optimize for MRD detection within a clinically relevant range, without significant risk of identifying such anomalous cells. In conclusion, it is evident that the utility of PCR for MRD monitoring is dependent on several factors, including the type of hematopoietic disease, the timing and frequency of monitoring, the sensitivity levels of the assays in use, and the effect of clinical interventions. A thorough understanding of these interrelationships is required to design meaningful MRD assays and the application of automated, fluorescent Q-PCR methods is a significant advance in establishing highly accurate and reproducible standards for clinical use.

Clinical Applications of Minimal Residual Disease Analysis

The concepts and utility of MRD evaluation are effectively demonstrated in the current management of several specific hematolymphoid diseases. With the continuing emergence of novel therapeutic agents or strategies, MRD detection plays a prominent role in gauging treatment response, timing alternative interventions, and predicting risk of relapse. The application of MRD technology has been most fully realized in the post-therapeutic setting for CML. Therapeutic responses are initially evaluated by clinical (hematologic) and cytogenetic standards. Molecular MRD assessment is pertinent in three situations in CML: postallogeneic marrow or stem cell transplant (ABM/SCT), interferon (IFN)-α therapy, and imatinib mesylate therapy. Qualitative, high-sensitivity end-point RT-PCR analysis for BCR–ABL1 fusion transcript has shown value for risk prediction in CML patients following ABM/SCT. Early PCR positivity (i.e., <6 months post-transplant) is not predictive of subsequent relapse risk, probably because of ongoing graft versus leukemia effect during this period. However, later conversion to PCR-positive status (6–12 months after transplant), or persistent PCR detection of BCR–ABL1 is associated with an appreciable statistical risk of relapse (Radich, 1995). This risk diminishes as the interval from transplant increases, but PCR positivity at later time-points remains a significant risk factor for relapse. Conversely, patients remaining PCR-negative more than a year from transplant have a good prognosis.

These data are generally supportive of the use of RT-PCR assessment for BCR–ABL1 in the post-transplant setting; however, some patients with PCR positivity in the most predictive monitoring interval maintain remission from disease, and a small number of long-term survivors continue to demonstrate low levels of BCR–ABL1 mRNA. Q-PCR studies have more clearly refined the ability to identify patients at highest risk of treatment failure. The quantitative level of BCR–ABL1 transcript (expressed as the ratio of BCR–ABL/ABL) in the early post-transplant period has been strongly correlated with risk of relapse (Olavarria, 2001; Faderl, 2004). Other data similarly suggest the Q-PCR technique improves outcome prediction in PCR-positive patients further out from transplantation (Radich, 2001). Q-PCR for BCR–ABL has also proven worthwhile in evaluating treatment response to IFN-α, despite the observation that molecular remissions with this agent are very uncommon. In this setting, reduction of the BCR–ABL/ABL ratio below a certain threshold has been shown to correlate with a low relapse rate, whereas those with higher BCR–ABL levels have a markedly elevated risk of treatment failure.

The largest impact of Q-PCR monitoring of BCR–ABL in CML, however, has come with the widespread use of targeted therapy with imatinib. Imatinib as a single agent is capable of inducing hematologic and cytogenetic remissions in the majority of patients within 6–12 months; a minority of patients will also attain molecular remission status. Data derived from the large International Randomized Study of Interferon and STI-571 (IRIS) clinical trial have demonstrated that the kinetics of BCR–ABL reduction with imatinib therapy (previously known as STI-571) is related to progression-free survival. 'Major molecular responders' (defined as those achieving a >3 log reduction in BCR–ABL from baseline level at diagnosis within 1 year) tended to have continuous clinical and cytogenetic remission, whereas failure to manifest more than 2 log reduction in BCR–ABL level by 6 months was correlated with an elevated risk of disease progression (Hughes, 2003; Faderl, 2004). Q-PCR has also proved valuable in predicting patients with resistance to imatinib therapy: individuals with serially increasing BCR–ABL levels were shown to have a strong association with the presence of mutations in the translocated ABL gene that conferred resistance to the drug, whereas those with stable low levels of transcript had an exceedingly low incidence of imatinib resistance due to such mutations (Branford, 2004). Although universal guidelines for post-therapeutic BCR–ABL monitoring in CML are still being defined, Q-PCR methodology has become a new standard for ongoing MRD evaluation in this disease (Faderl, 2004). Notably for serial BCR–ABL MRD assessments in CML patients, peripheral blood can be substituted for bone marrow samples with equivalent efficacy, thereby reducing patient morbidity.

Patients with acute promyelocytic leukemia (APL) treated with combination chemotherapy and atRA have a relatively favorable prognosis, yet disease relapses occur frequently. The use of qualitative RT-PCR methods to detect the PML–RARα fusion mRNA (with a typical sensitivity of 10^{-3}–10^{-4}) has been established as a very powerful tool for predicting relapse risk in individual patients (Jurcic, 2001; Grimwade, 2002; Lo Coco, 2002). The timing, or phase of disease therapy, is an important consideration in this leukemia. Patients evaluated for PML–RARα at the end of induction are often found to be positive so the predictive value at this time-point is not significant. By the end of consolidation therapy however, PCR positivity is strongly predictive of relapse in patients who have apparently achieved clinical complete remission, as nearly all such patients will progress to hematologic relapse within months. The positive predictive value for overt relapse is also high in patients repeatedly testing positive by PCR on consecutive occasions. Thus, a major therapeutic goal in APL is the achievement of 'molecular remission' (i.e., PCR-negative) status.

Despite the indispensable contribution of qualitative PCR for PML–RARα assessment following therapy initiation, it is recognized that a significant number of patients with a negative PCR assessment at the end of consolidation therapy will also suffer relapse. Thus, recent advances in this area have focused on increasing the precision of PML–RARα detection, while also improving assay sensitivity (Choppa, 2003). More frequent molecular monitoring (e.g., after each chemotherapy course) and, by

VIII

extension, measurement of the rate of $PML-RAR\alpha$ reduction are important goals in this disease that may be achieved with routine analysis by Q PCR. To this end, several APL study groups have reported results of serial $PML-RAR\alpha$ monitoring using Q-PCR techniques. This approach has shown benefit in detecting low-level molecular disease and in predicting relapse (Grimwade, 2002; Gallagher, 2003).

In concert with improvements in molecular monitoring in APL, attention has similarly been directed toward treating persistent MRD or 'molecular relapse,' before hematologic relapse develops. Preliminary trials have suggested a significantly improved overall survival in patients treated for molecular MRD only (Lo Coco, 2002). The availability of several 'second-line' therapeutic options for relapsed or primary treatment-refractory APL (e.g., arsenic trioxide [As_2O_3]), allogeneic transplantation, and possibly anti-CD33 antibody therapy (Mylotarg, Wyeth Ayerst, Inc.)] is clearly an impetus for these interventional efforts. Although no guidelines have been firmly established for $PML-RAR\alpha$ monitoring in APL, common sampling time-points include the end of induction, end of consolidation, then every 2–3 months for the first year after therapy, as this is the window during which most relapses occur. Of note, $PML-RAR\alpha$ detection by Q-PCR (or qualitative RT-PCR assays for that matter) must be performed on bone marrow aspirate samples, since the sensitivity of detection in peripheral blood after treatment onset is markedly lower.

As described for childhood ALL, sophisticated clinical and tumor genetic classifications have been developed for predicting patient outcome at diagnosis. Useful as these parameters have been for the early stratification of patients to optimized therapy arms, a significant minority of these children (20–30%) experience treatment failure and leukemic relapse. In the quest for better surrogate markers of biologic response and disease clearance, MRD assessment has emerged as a very powerful method of post-therapeutic prediction, providing a more 'individualized' approach to risk evaluation. Levels of molecular MRD as high as $10^{-2}-10^{-3}$ at the end of induction therapy have been shown to be strongly and independently correlated with risk of relapse; lower levels of MRD are apparently also associated with some degree of increased risk compared to MRD negative status (Cave, 1998; van Dongen, 1998; Pui, 2000; Goulden, 2001; Nyvold, 2002).

The common pediatric ALL-associated translocation fusion gene abnormalities are present in slightly less than one-third of de novo B-lineage ALL and recurrent translocation abnormalities in T-cell ALL are less prevalent still. Attention has thus been focused on developing highly sensitive and precise DNA-based Q-PCR assays directed at clonotypic rearrangements of the antigen receptor genes, including the immunoglobulin heavy- and light-chain genes (IgH, $Ig\kappa$) and the T-cell receptor loci ($T\gamma$, $T\beta$, and $T\delta$) (summarized in van der Velden, 2003). These clonotypic gene rearrangements serve as individual, tumor-specific signatures or 'fingerprints' for MRD detection. Notably in B-lineage ALL, crosslineage gene rearrangements occur frequently at the T-cell receptor genes, such that most B-cell ALL tumors have at least one and as many as two or three unique gene rearrangements available for MRD monitoring. These highly specific DNA sequences, formed by the recombination of V, (D), and J segments along with nontemplated (N) nucleotide insertions, can be sequenced for the design and synthesis of patient tumor-specific PCR primers and probes for use in Q-PCR. This can be accomplished by employing one consensus region primer and consensus fluorescent probe, along with an 'allele-specific' oligonucleotide (ASO) primer complementary to the region of unique clonotypic sequence in the gene rearrangement of interest.

Typical sensitivities for antigen receptor gene Q-PCR are in the range of $10^{-2}-10^{-5}$, depending on the characteristics of the particular target gene sequence and the degree of nonspecific competition for primers by potentially homologous rearrangements in background B or T cells. Accordingly, multiple antigen receptor gene targets may have to be assessed and possibly multiple primer/probe sequences made and evaluated for obtaining the best dilutional sensitivity in a given case of ALL. Quantification of MRD in pediatric ALL relies upon serial dilutions of the patient's diagnostic leukemia DNA in a background DNA source (e.g., pooled donor WBC) and the bone marrow MRD sample value is then determined from a standard curve generated from these dilutions. The timing of MRD assessment is critical in pediatric ALL. The end of induction therapy is a significant and highly informative time-point, although ongoing serial measurements can further increase the predictive value (van Dongen, 1998). MRD positivity later in therapy (e.g., following consolidation) also has prognostic value for relapse risk prediction, however, the sensitivity of antigen receptor gene Q-PCR for lower levels of MRD is poorer at these intervals, emphasizing the importance of earlier evaluation.

The multi-institutional BIOMED-2 European group has published detailed descriptions of optimized primer/probe sets for the initial detection of clonotypic antigen receptor gene markers for application in subsequent high sensitivity molecular MRD protocols (van Dongen, 2003). This comprehensive work represents a major step toward creating uniformity in Q-PCR data collection between testing centers involved in pediatric ALL trials. With these advances, some ALL cooperative study groups have begun to incorporate MRD data from early therapeutic time-points as a routine component of risk assessment, such that 'high risk' MRD-positive patients are rapidly stratified into more intensive therapy arms.

Clonotypic IgH and $BCL2$ gene rearrangements has also been described for monitoring MRD status in blood or marrow after intensive therapies such as high-dose chemotherapy and autologous stem cell rescue for non-Hodgkin B-cell lymphomas (Bowman, 2004). Typically, these are 'small B-lymphocyte' B-cell neoplasms (e.g., MCL, CLL, follicular lymphoma) with a propensity for widespread dissemination, including the bone marrow. In each of these clinical settings, the utility of MRD evaluation for lymphoma in the bone marrow must be interpreted in the context of other follow-up parameters (especially imaging studies), to exclude extramedullary sites of relapse. In another application, detection of clonal B cells in stem cell collections prior to autologous transplant has been correlated with increased risk of disease relapse after transplant, compared to patients receiving PCR negative samples.

Emerging Technologies: The Role of Gene Expression Profiling Using Microarray Technology in Hematolymphoid Neoplasia

Since its introduction, microarray analysis of global gene expression has been a promising tool for biomedical research. Although microarray analysis is not yet routinely used in the clinical laboratory, it is a powerful emerging technology that has led to a number of clinically-important observations (Levene, 2003; Hubank, 2004). Microarrays contain oligonucleotide or cDNA targets on a 'chip' surface. These targets represent a large component of the genome or the entire genome and are designed to determine the mRNA expression levels of many genes in parallel from a single sample. Detailed overviews of the various options for array-based expression analyses, as well as techniques related to their analysis and interpretation, are discussed elsewhere in this book (Chapters 68 and 76). Recent studies on hematopoietic neoplasms have provided insights into 'class prediction' (prediction of a tumor type on the basis of specific gene expression profiles of selected informative genes) as well as 'class discovery' (discovery of new subentities within tumor groups formerly regarded as a homogenous entity). Class discovery is not solely limited to identification of new subtypes of leukemia, for instance, but includes definition of prognostically differing groups, which are anticipated to influence therapeutic strategies. As a result of these early successes in class discovery and prediction, it seems a realistic goal that response to therapy, relapse risk, and even risk of developing a secondary malignancy may be predicted from microarray analysis. Here, we will briefly focus on the observations that have provided insight into classification, diagnosis, and prognosis of leukemias and lymphomas using microarrays.

Distinguishing Acute Myeloid Leukemia from Acute Lymphoblastic Leukemia on the Basis of Gene Expression

The distinction between ALL and AML is a critical part of daily routine practice and an absolute necessity for therapeutic decisions. This distinction is currently based on morphologic review, enzyme cytochemistries, immunophenotyping, and tumor karyotyping. The work of Golub and co-investigators was a key event in demonstrating the applicability of microarrays to hematopoietic neoplasms (Golub, 1999). These efforts showed that the separation of AML and ALL is possible solely on the basis of microarray analysis. These investigators studied 38 cases of acute leukemia (27 patients with ALL and 11 patients with AML) and identified 50 discriminatory genes that distinguished AML from ALL. In 36 of the 38 cases, the diagnosis of leukemia type was correctly made by the microarray data alone. In a subsequent set of 34 unknown samples that had not been used to build the prediction model, the gene set correctly classified 29 (85%) of the cases. Moos and co-workers confirmed that a discriminatory set of genes could distinguish AML from ALL in 51 pediatric cases as well

(Moos, 2002). Although not superior to current comprehensive pathologic analysis, these studies represent a major step toward the molecular diagnosis of leukemia.

Acute Lymphoblastic Leukemia

With regard to ALL, the pivotal discrimination of unselected ALL and AML samples based on their gene expression signature inspired a number of follow-up studies. In one milestone study, subtypes of pediatric ALL were correlated with unique gene expression profiles (Yeoh, 2002). This study further proposed subsets of marker genes suitable for initial diagnosis as well as candidate gene profiles as predictors of clinical outcome. More specifically, 327 patients were classified according to their immunologic and tumor genetic nature: T-lineage ALL and *E2A–PBX1*, *BCR–ABL1*, *TEL–AML1*, *MLL* and hyperdiploid types of B-lineage ALL. The expression signature of some cases did not allow for their classification into one of these categories, and a novel subgroup of ALL was proposed. Of particular interest, these investigators identified specific gene signatures in ALL blasts at diagnosis which appeared to indicate an increased propensity for developing therapy-induced AML after successful treatment of the ALL. These observations were extended in a microarray analysis study that compared cases of acute leukemia with *MLL* gene aberrations to other ALL and AML cases, showing a clear separation of all three groups (Armstrong, 2002).

Acute Myeloid Leukemia

A number of studies have been performed correlating microarray findings with classification of AML. Haferlach addressed whether French–American–British (FAB) subtypes could be correlated with gene expression profiles (Haferlach, 2002a, 2002b, 2002c). This group studied 130 cases of AML classified by FAB using morphology, cytochemistry, and cytogenetics. Immunophenotyping was also carried out on all AML-M0 cases. Based on a limited gene expression signature, cases of classical APL (AML-M3), microgranular APL (AML-M3v), acute myelomonocytic leukemia with abnormal eosinophils (AML-M4eo), and acute erythroleukemia (AML-M6) could be distinguished from all other subtypes with 100% accuracy. The comparison between acute myeloid leukemia with maturation (AML-M2) and acute myelomonocytic leukemia (AML-M4) produced the lowest accuracy (85%), a finding very similar to the concordance obtained by morphologic review (and compatible with the arbitrary threshold of greater than 20% positivity for nonspecific esterase cytochemistry used to traditionally distinguish these leukemias). Comparisons among other AML subcategories ranged between 86% and 95% accuracy. In addition, microarray analysis separated 28 cases of acute myeloid leukemia with maturation (AML-M2) into three cytogenetic subgroups: t(8;21)/ *AML1–ETO*, normal karyotype, and complex abnormal karyotype. Overall, these results indicate that AML-M3, AML-M3v, AML-M4eo, AML-M6, and subtypes of AML-M2 are indeed distinct entities with respect to their gene expression profiles while other AML subcategories defined or described by FAB classification features are more heterogeneous.

Microarray data have also been directly compared with flow cytometric and cytogenetic data in AML. This is critical since, in many clinical trials, the karyotype of the leukemic blasts has been shown to be the most important independent prognostic parameter with respect to treatment response and survival in AML. Schoch et al demonstrated that the cytogenetically defined subtypes of AML with t(8;21)/*AML1–ETO*, AML with t(15;17)/*PML–RAR*α and AML with inv(16)/*CBFB–MYH11* are characterized by different and specific gene expression profiles; a minimum set of only 13 genes was sufficient to accurately predict these karyotypes (Schoch, 2002). These findings are consistent with the comparative FAB studies cited above, since the t(8;21), t(15;17), and inv(16) anomalies are highly correlated with AML-M2, AML-M3/M3v, and AML-M4eo morphologic subtypes, respectively. Fewer studies have been performed that correlate microarray analysis with clinical outcome. Two recent efforts focused mainly on adult AML have confirmed previously identified genotype–expression relationships, but have revealed further novel biologic clusters and the ability to construct 'predictor' gene sets that correlate with clinical outcome (Bullinger, 2004; Valk, 2004).

Non-Hodgkin Lymphomas and Chronic Leukemias

Class discovery and prediction studies have also been performed using samples from patients with lymphomas. Gene expression profiling studies of DLBCL have shown that this diagnostic category encompasses at least two genetically distinct diseases that differ in oncogenic mechanism and clinical outcome (Alizadeh, 2000; Rosenwald, 2002; Dybkaer, 2004). One of these DLBCL subgroups has been termed the germinal center B-cell-like group (GCB) and expresses a high frequency of germinal center associated marker genes. The other subgroup is termed the activated B-cell-like group (ABC) and expresses genes associated with mitogenic activation. Although differences between microarray studies related to reproducibility of similar gene sets remain problematic, validation experiments, such as those described by Lossos et al have generally confirmed the existence of distinct biologic types of DLBCL (Lossos, 2004). Intriguingly, further investigation of the ABC type of DLBCL has revealed that the NF-κB signal transduction pathway is constitutively activated and NF-κB has been suggested as a therapeutic target in this subgroup of DLBCL (Davis, 2002).

Gene expression microarray studies of CLL have also led to identification of two subtypes that exhibit different clinical outcomes and also segregate with respect to the presence or absence of somatic mutations of the immunoglobulin heavy chain (*IgH*) gene. *IgH* mutational status is difficult to analyze in the routine diagnostic laboratory setting, however, the results of microarray analyses uncovered expression of the *ZAP-70* gene as a strong surrogate marker. High *ZAP-70* mRNA levels correlated with unmutated *IgH* genes and consequently poorer outcome (Rosenwald, 2001). This has led preliminarily to efforts to assess ZAP-70 protein in CLL as a possible indicator of disease aggressiveness. Microarray studies in MCL have also led to unique insights into the 'proliferation signature' of these typically treatment-refractory lymphomas, generating potential therapeutic targets for novel pharmaceuticals (Rosenwald, 2003).

Natural killer (NK)-cell lymphoproliferative diseases are rare entities characterized by a proliferation of CD3⁻/CD56⁺ lymphocytes, which can be divided into two distinct categories: aggressive NK cell leukemia and chronic NK lymphocytosis. In a study of 19 such cases, 15 genes were identified that could clearly distinguish these entities with nearly 80% accuracy (Choi, 2004). Finally, the capability of gene expression profiling in identifying the role of non-neoplastic cells within a tumor was recently emphasized in a study of 191 biopsy specimens obtained from patients with untreated follicular lymphoma (Dave, 2004). Two multigene expression signatures allowed patients to be separated into four quartiles with differing median survival independent of clinical prognostic variables. Most intriguingly, the length of survival among these follicular lymphoma patients correlated with the molecular profile of the nonmalignant tumor infiltrating immune cells.

It is thus evident that microarray technology is beginning to reshape many of our concepts of tumor classification and will certainly add novel contributions to the understanding of tumor biology. Global gene expression analysis in hematolymphoid neoplasms holds promise for guiding clinicians and investigators toward further refinements in diagnosis, classification and prognostication, as well as the identification of potential new therapeutic targets. While microarray methodology in its current format is not readily applicable to the clinical molecular diagnostic laboratory, key aspects or offshoots of this approach will undoubtedly show impact in the form of multigene Q-PCR or multiantigen immunophenotyping analyses.

Acknowledgments

The authors wish to kindly acknowledge the expert assistance of A. A. Magotra, M. Grady and A. M. B. Viswanatha in the preparation of this chapter.

References

Adachi M, Tefferi A, Greipp PR, et al: Preferential linkage of BCL-2 to immunoglobulin light chain gene in chronic lymphocytic leukemia. J Exp Med 1990; 171:559–564.

Adams JM, Cory S. The Bcl-2 protein family: arbiters of cell survival. Science 1998; 281:1322–1326.

Agnes F, Shamoon B, Dina C, et al: Genomic structure of the downstream part of the human FLT3 gene: exon/intron structure conservation among genes encoding receptor tyrosine kinases (RTK) of subclass III. Gene 1994; 145:283–288.

Akasaka T, Akasaka H, Yonetani N, et al: Refinement of the BCL2/immunoglobulin heavy chain fusion gene in t(14;18) (q32;q21) by polymerase chain reaction amplification for long targets. Genes Chromosomes Cancer 1998a; 21:17–29.

Akasaka T, Muramatsu M, Ohno H, et al: Application of long-distance polymerase chain reaction to detection of junctional sequences created by chromosomal translocation in mature B-cell neoplasms. Blood 1996; 88: 985–994.

Akasaka T, Ueda C, Kurata M, et al: Nonimmunoglobulin (non-Ig)/BCL6 gene fusion in diffuse large B-cell lymphoma results in worse prognosis than Ig/BCL6. Blood 2000; 96:2907–2909.

Akasaka T, Yonetani N, Akasaka H: Detection of t(8;14)(q24;q32) by polymerase chain reaction for long DNA targets: a report of two patients with B-cell non-Hodgkin's lymphoma. Int J Hematol 1998b; 67:75–79.

Albinger-Hegyi A, Hochreutener B, Abdou M-T, et al: High frequency of t(14;18)-translocation breakpoints outside of major breakpoint and minor cluster regions in follicular lymphomas. Improved polymerase chain reaction protocols for their detection. Am J Pathol 2002; 160:823–832.
This is a comprehensive molecular analysis of additional breakpoint regions in the BCL2 gene, with strategies to improve the molecular diagnostic detection of the t(14;18)/BCL2-IgH.

Alizadeh AA, Eisen MB, Davis RE, et al: Distinct types of diffuse large B-cell lymphoma identified by gene expression profiling. Nature 2000; 403:503–511.
A landmark paper that initially identified intrinsic biologic and clinical groups of 'germinal center' and 'activated' B-cell signatures among large B-cell lymphomas by gene expression microarray technique.

Alkan S, Schnitzer B, Thompson JL: Cyclin D1 protein expression in mantle cell lymphoma. Ann Oncol 1995; 6:567–570.

Allman D, Jain A, Dent A, et al: BCL-6 expression during B-cell activation. Blood 1996; 87:5257–5268.

Amati B, Brooks MW, Levy N: Oncogenic activity of the c-Myc protein requires dimerization with Max. Cell 1993; 72:233.

Andersson A, Hoglund M, Johansson B, et al: Paired multiplex reverse-transcriptase polymerase chain reaction (PMRT-PCR) analysis as a rapid and accurate diagnostic tool for the detection of MLL fusion genes in hematologic malignancies. Leukemia 2001; 15:1293–1300.

Arber DA. Molecular diagnosis approach to non-Hodgkin's lymphoma. J Mol Diag 2000; 2:178–190.

Argatoff LH, Connors JM, Klasa RJ: A clinicopathologic study of 80 cases. Blood 1997; 89:2067–2078.

Armstrong SA, Golub TR, Korsmeyer SJ. MLL-rearranged leukemias: insights from gene expression profiling. Sem Hematol 2003; 40:268–273.

Armstrong SA, Staunton JE, Silverman LB, et al: MLL translocations specify a distinct gene expression profile that distinguishes a unique leukemia. Nat Genet 2002; 30:41–47.

Aster JC, Longtine JA. Detection of BCL2 rearrangements in follicular lymphoma. Am J Pathol 2002; 160:759–763.

Aubin J, Davi F, Nguyen-Salomon F, et al: Description of a novel FR1 IgH PCR strategy and its comparison with three other strategies for the detection of clonality in B cell malignancies. Leukemia 1995; 9:471–479.

Ayer DE, Kretzner L, Eisenman RN: Mad: a heterodimeric partner for Max that antagonizes Myc transcriptional activity. Cell 1993; 72:211.

Ayer DE, Lawrence QA, Eisenman RN: Mad–Max transcriptional repression is mediated by ternary complex formation with mammalian homologs of yeast repressor Sin3. Cell 1995; 80:767–776.

Baens M, Maes B, Steyls A, et al: The product of the t(11;18), an API2–MLT fusion, marks nearly half of gastric MALT type lymphomas without large cell proliferation. Am J Pathol 2000; 156:1433–1439.

Bakhshi A, Jensen JP, Goldman P, et al: Cloning the chromosomal breakpoint of t(14;18) human lymphomas: clustering around JH on chromosome 14 and near a transcriptional unit on 18. Cell 1985; 41:899–906.

Bain BJ. Relationship between idiopathic hypereosinophilic syndrome, eosinophilic leukemia, and systemic mastocytosis. Am J Hematol 2004; 77:82–85.

Barrans SL, O'Connor SJ, Evans PA, et al: Rearrangement of the BCL6 locus at 3q27 is an independent poor prognostic factor in nodal diffuse large B-cell lymphoma. Br J Haematol 2002; 117:322–332.

Barrans SL, Evans PAS, O'Connor SJM, et al: The t(14;18) is associated with germinal center-derived diffuse large B-cell lymphoma and is a strong predictor of outcome. Clin Cancer Res 2003; 9:2133–2139.

Bartolo C, Viswanatha DS. Molecular diagnosis in pediatric acute leukemias. Clin Lab Med 2000; 20:139–182.

Bassing CH, Swat W, Alt FW. The mechanism and regulation of chromosomal V(D)J recombination. Cell 2002; 109:S45–S55.

Baxter EJ, Scott LM, Campbell PJ, et al: Acquired mutation of the tyrosine kinase JAK2 in human myeloproliferative disorders. Lancet 2005; 365:1054–1061

Beaubier NT, Hart AT, Bartolo C, et al: Comparison of capillary electrophoresis and polyacrylamide gel electrophoresis for the evaluation of T and B cell clonality by polymerase chain reaction. Diagn Mol Pathol 2000; 9:121–131.

Beillard E, Pallisgaard N, van der Velden VHJ, et al: Evaluation of candidate control genes for diagnosis and residual disease detection in leukemic patients using 'real-time' quantitative reverse-transcriptase polymerase chain reaction (RQ-PCR) – a Europe against cancer program. Leukemia 2003; 17:2474–2486.

Beishuizen A, Verhoeven M-AJ, Mol EJ, et al: Detection of immunoglobulin heavy-chain gene rearrangements by Southern blot analysis: recommendations for optimal results. Leukemia 1993; 7:2045–2053.

Beishuizen A, Verhoeven MA, van Wering ER, et al: Analysis of Ig and T-cell receptor genes in 40 childhood acute lymphoblastic leukemias at diagnosis and subsequent relapse: implications for the detection of minimal residual disease by polymerase chain reaction analysis. Blood 1994; 83:2238–2247.

Belaud-Rotureau MA, Parrens M, Dubus P, et al: A comparative analysis of FISH, RT-PCR, PCR, and immunohistochemistry for the diagnosis of mantle cell lymphomas. Mod Pathol 2002; 15:517–525.

Bertoni F, Conconi A, Capella C, et al: Molecular follow-up in gastric mucosa-associated lymphoid tissue lymphomas: early analysis of the LY03 cooperative trial. Blood 2002; 99:2541–2544.

Betti CJ, Villalobos MJ, Diaz MO, et al: Apoptopic stimuli initiate MLL-AF9 translocations that are transcribed in cells capable of division. Cancer Res 2003; 63:1377–1381.

Betti CJ, Villalobos MJ, Diaz MO, Vaughan AT. Apoptotic triggers initiate translocations within the MLL gene involving the nonhomologous end joining repair system. Cancer Res 2001; 61:4550–4555.

Biernaux C, Loos M, Sels A, et al: Detection of major bcr-abl gene expression at a very low level in blood cells of some healthy individuals. Blood 1995; 86:3118–3122.

Blackwood EM, Eisenman RN: Max: A helix-loop-helix zipper protein that forms a sequence-specific DNA-binding complex with Myc. Science 1991; 251:1211–1217.

Blum KA, Lozanski G, Byrd JC. Adult Burkitt leukemia and lymphoma. Blood 2004; 104:3009–3020.

Borkhardt A, Cazzaniga G, Viehmann S, et al: Incidence and clinical relevance of TEL/AML1 fusion genes in children with acute lymphoblastic leukemia enrolled in German and Italian multicenter therapy trials. Blood 1997; 90:571–577.

Bosch F, Jares P, Campo E: PRAD1/cyclin d1 gene overexpression in chronic lymphoproliferative disorders: a highly specific marker of mantle cell lymphoma. Blood 1994; 84:2726–2732.

Bose S, Deininger M, Gora-Tybor J, et al: The presence of typical and atypical BCR–ABL fusion genes in leukocytes of normal individuals: biologic significance and implications for the assessment of minimal residual disease. Blood 1998; 92:3362–3367.

Bottaro M, Berti E, Biondi A, et al: Heteroduplex analysis of T-cell receptor γ gene rearrangements for diagnosis and monitoring of cutaneous T-cell lymphomas. Blood 1994; 83:3271–3278.

Bowman A, Jones D, Medeiros LJ, et al: Quantitative PCR detection of t(14;18) bcl2/JH fusion sequences in follicular lymphoma patients. J Mol Diagn 2004; 6:396–400.

Branford S, Rudzki Z, Parkinson I, Grigg A, et al: Real-time quantitative PCR analysis can be used as a primary screen to identify patients with CML treated with imatinib who have BCR–ABL kinase domain mutations. Blood 2004; 104:2926–2932.

Braziel RM, Arber DA, Slovak ML, et al: The Burkitt-like lymphomas: a Southwest Oncology Group study delineating phenotypic, genotypic, and clinical features. Blood 2001; 97:3713–3720.

Brunning RD, Matutes E, Flandrin G, et al: Acute myeloid leukaemia with recurrent genetic abnormalities. *In* Jaffe E, Harris N, Stein H, et al (eds): Pathology and Genetics: Tumours of the Haematopoietic and Lymphoid Tissues. World Health Organization Classification of Tumours. Lyon, France: IARC Press; 2001.

Bullinger L, Dohner K, Bair E, et al: Use of gene-expression profiling to identify prognostic subclasses in adult actue myeloid leukemia. N Engl J Med 2004; 350:1605–1616.

Campo E, Raffeld M, Jaffe E: Mantle-cell lymphoma. Semin Hematol 1999; 36:115–127.

Cattoretti G, Chang CC, Cechova K, et al: BCL-6 protein is expressed in germinal-center B cells. Blood 1995; 86:45–53.

Cave H, van der Werf ten Bosch J, Suciu S, et al: Clinical significance of minimal residual disease in childhood acute lymphoblastic leukemia. N Engl J Med 1998; 339:591–598.

Chambon P. A decade of molecular biology of retinoic acid receptors. FASEB J 1996; 10:940–954.

Chasseriau J, Rivet J, Bilan F, et al: Characterization of the different BCR–ABL transcripts with a single multiplex RT-PCR. J Mol Diagn 2004; 6:343–347.

Chen W, Iida S, Louie DC, et al: Heterologous promoters fused to BCL6 by chromosomal translocations affecting band 3q27 cause its deregulated expression during B-cell differentiation. Blood 1998; 91:603–607.

Chen C-S, Sorensen PHB, Domer PH, et al: Molecular rearrangements on chromosome 11q23 predominant in infant acute lymphoblastic leukemia and are associated with specific biologic variables and poor outcome. Blood 1993; 81:2386–2393.

Chhanabhai M, Adomat SA, Gascoyne RD, Horsman DE: Clinical utility of heteroduplex analysis of TCR gamma gene rearrangements in the diagnosis of T-cell lymphoproliferative disorders. Am J Clin Pathol 1997; 108:295–301.

Chibbar R, Leung K, McCormick S, et al: bcl-1 gene rearrangements in mantle cell lymphoma: a comprehensive analysis of 118 cases, including B-5 fixed tissue, by polymerase chain reaction and Southern transfer analysis. Mod Pathol 1998; 11:1089–1097.

Chiu BC, Weisenburger DD. An update of the epidemiology of non-Hodgkin's lymphoma. Clin Lymphoma 2003; 4:161–168.

Choi YL, Makishima H, Ohashi J, et al: DNA microarray analysis of natural killer cell-type lymphoproliferative disease of granular lymphocytes with purified CD3⁻CD56⁺ fractions. Leukemia 2004; 18:556–565.

Choppa PC, Gomez J, Vall HG, et al: A novel method for the detection, quantitation, and breakpoint cluster region determination of t(15;17) fusion transcripts using a one-step real-time multiplex RT-PCR. Am J Clin Pathol 2003; 119:137–144.

Cleary ML, Galili N, Sklar J: Detection of a second t(14;18) breakpoint cluster region in follicular lymphomas. J Exp Med 1986; 164:315–320.

Cleary ML, Sklar J: Nucleotide sequence of t(14;18) chromosomal translocation breakpoint in follicular lymphoma and demonstration of a breakpoint cluster region near a transcriptionally active locus on chromosome 18. Proc Natl Acad Sci USA 1985; 82:7439–7443.

Coignet LJA, Schuuring E, Kibbelaar RE: Detection of 11q13 rearrangements in hematologic neoplasias by double-contour fluorescence in situ hybridization. Blood 1996; 87:1512–1519.

Cools J, DeAngelo DJ, Gotlib J, et al: A tyrosine kinase created by fusion of the PDGFRA and FIP1L1 genes as a therapeutic target of imatinib in idiopathic hypereosinophilic syndrome. N Engl J Med 2003; 348:1201–1214.

Cossman J, Uppenkamp M, Sundeen J, et al: Molecular genetics and the diagnosis of lymphoma. Arch Pathol Lab Med 1988; 112:117–127.

Cuthbert G, Thompson K, Breese G, et al: Sensitivity of FISH in detection of MLL gene rearrangements. Genes Chromosomes Cancer 2000; 29:180–185.

Cuthbert KB, Ford AM, Repp R, et al: Backtracking leukemia to birth: identification of clonotypic gene fusion sequences in neonatal blood spots. Proc Natl Acad Sci USA 1997; 94:13950–13954.

Dave SS, Wright G, Tan B, et al: Prediction of survival in follicular lymphoma based on molecular features of tumor-infiltrating immune cells N Engl J Med 2004; 351: 2159–2169.

Davis RE, Staudt LM: Molecular diagnosis of lymphoid malignancies by gene expression profiling. Curr Opin Hematol 2002; 9:333–338.

Deane M, McCarthy KP, Weidemann LM, Norton JD: An improved method for detection of B-lymphoid clonality by polymerase chain reaction. Leukemia 1991; 5:726–730.

De Boer CJ, Schuuring E, Dreef E, Peters G: Cyclin D1 protein analysis in the diagnosis of mantle cell lymphoma. Blood 1995; 86: 2715–2723.

De Boer CJ, van Krieken JM, Schuuring E, Kluin PM: Bcl-1/cyclin D1 in malignant lymphoma. Ann Oncol 1997; 8(Suppl 2): S109–S117.

Deininger MW, Goldman JM, Melo JV: The molecular biology of chronic myeloid leukemia. Blood 2000; 96:3343–3356.

A comprehensive and concise review of the molecular biology of chronic myeloid leukemia.

Delsol G, Ralfkiaer E, Stein H, et al: Anaplastic large cell lymphoma. In Jaffe E, Harris N, Stein H, et al (eds): Pathology and Genetics: Tumours of the Haematopoietic and Lymphoid Tissues. World Health Organization Classification of Tumours. Lyon, France: IARC Press; 2001, pp 230–235.

Dent AL, Shaffer AL, Yu X, et al: Control of inflammation, cytokine expression, and germinal center formation by BCL-6. Science 1997; 276:589–592.

De Paepe P, Baens M, van Krieken H, et al: ALK activation by the CLTC-ALK fusion is a recurrent event in large B-cell lymphoma. Blood 2003; 102:2638–2641.

Derksen PWB, Langerak AW, Kerkhof E, et al: Comparison of different polymerase chain reaction-based approaches for clonality assessment of immunoglobulin heavy-chain gene rearrangements in B-cell neoplasia. Mod Pathol 1999; 12:794–805.

By comparing a variety of oligonucleotide primer methods, this effort helps in the rational application of PCR to B-cell clonality determination in the clinical setting.

Dierlamm J, Baens M, Wlodarska I, et al: The apoptosis inhibitor gene API2 and a novel 18q gene, MLT, are recurrently rearranged in the t(11;18)(q21;q21) associated with mucosa-associated lymphoid tissue lymphomas. Blood 1999; 93:3601–3609.

Diss TC, Liu HX, Du MQ, Isaacson PG: Improvements to B cell clonality analysis using PCR amplification of immunoglobulin light chain genes. J Clin Pathol Mol Pathol 2002; 55:98–101.

Dolken G, Illerhaus G, Hirt C, Metelsmann R: BCL-2/JH rearrangements in circulating B cells of healthy blood donors and patients with non-malignant diseases. J Clin Oncol 1996; 14:1333–1344.

Downing JR: The AML1-ETO chimaeric transcription factor in acute myeloid leukaemia: biology and clinical significance. Br J Haematol 1999; 106:296–308.

Downing JR, Shurtleff SA, Zielenska M, et al: Molecular detection of the (2;5) translocation of non-Hodgkin's lymphoma by reverse transcriptase-polymerase chain reaction. Blood 1995; 85:3416–3422.

Druker BJ, Talpaz M, Resta DJ, et al: Efficacy and safety of a specific inhibitor of the BCR–ABL tyrosine kinase in chronic myeloid leukemia. N Engl J Med 2001; 344:1031–1037.

Dybkaer K, Iqbal J, Zhou G, Chan WC: Molecular diagnosis and outcome prediction in diffuse large B-cell lymphoma and other subtypes of lymphoma Clin Lymphoma 2004; 5:19–28.

Dyck J, Maul GG, Miller WH, et al: A novel macromolecular structure is a target of the promyelocytic-retinoic acid receptor oncoprotein. Cell 1994; 76:333–343.

Dyer MJS, Zani BJ, Lu WZ, et al: BCL2 translocations in leukemia of mature B cells. Blood 1994; 83:3682–3688.

Eckert C, Scrideli CA, Taube T, et al: Comparison between TaqMan and LightCycler technologies for quantification of minimal residual disease by using immunoglobulin and T-cell receptor genes consensus probes. Leukemia 2003; 17:2517–2524.

Elenitoba-Johnson KSJ, Bohling SD, Jenson SD, et al: Fluorescence PCR quantification of cyclin D1 expression. J Mol Diagn 2002; 4:90–96.

Elmberger PG, Lozano MD, Weisenburger DD, et al: Transcripts of the npm–alk fusion gene in anaplastic large cell lymphoma, Hodgkin's disease, and reactive lymphoid lesions. Blood 1995; 86:3517–3521.

Ernst P, Fisher JK, Avery W, et al: Definitive hematopoiesis requires the mixed-lineage leukemia gene. Dev Cell 2004a; 6:437–443.

Ernst P, Mabon M, Davidson AJ, et al: An Mll-dependent Hox program drives hematopoietic expansion. Curr Biol 2004b; 14:2063–2069.

Faderl S, Hochhaus A, Hughes T. Monitoring of minimal residual disease in chronic myeloid leukemia. Hematol Oncol Clin N Am 2004; 18:657–670.

A concise summary of the application of current state-of-the-art molecular methods to chronic myeloid leukemia management following therapy.

Falini B: Anaplastic large cell lymphoma: pathological, molecular and clinical features. Br J Haematol 2001; 114:741–760.

A comprehensive examination of the complex interplay between morphologic and genetic variants in this unique T-cell lymphoma.

Falini B, Fizzotti M, Pileri S, et al: Bcl-6 protein expression in normal and neoplastic lymphoid tissue. Ann Oncol 1997; 8(Suppl 2):S101–S104.

Falini B, Pileri S, Zinzani PL, et al: ALK⁺ lymphoma: clinico-pathological findings and outcome. Blood 1999b; 93:2697–2706.

Falini B, Pulford K, Pucciarini A, et al: Lymphomas expressing ALK fusion protein(s) other than NPM-ALK. Blood 1999a; 10:3509–3515.

Fasching K, Panzer S, Haas OA, et al: Presences of clone-specific antigen receptor gene rearrangements at birth indicates an in utero origin of diverse types of early childhood acute lymphoblastic leukemia. Blood 2000; 95:2722–2724.

Fletcher JA, Lynch EA, Kimball VM, et al: Translocation (9;22) is associated with extremely poor prognosis in intensively treated children with acute lymphoblastic leukemia. Blood 1991; 77:435–439.

Ford AM, Fasching K, Panzer-Grumayer, et al: Origins of 'late' relapse in childhood acute lymphoblastic leukemia with TEL–AML1 fusion genes. Blood 2001; 98:558–564.

Gabert J, Beillard E, van der Velden VHJ, et al: Standardization and quality control studies of 'real-time' quantitative reverse transcriptase polymerase chain reaction of fusion gene transcripts for residual disease detection in leukemia – a Europe Against Cancer Program. Leukemia 2003; 17:2318–2357.

This landmark collaborative effort describes experimental design and validation of quantitative PCR (Q-PCR) methods to detect the major recurrent leukemia-associated translocation fusion genes. The study is significant in its scope, as well as in the dedication to establishing more universal standards for performance of Q-PCR for minimal residual disease monitoring.

Gallagher RE, Li Y-P, Rao S, et al: Characterization of acute promyelocytic leukemia cases with PML–RARα break/fusion sites in PML exon 6: Identification of a subgroup with decreased in vitro responsiveness to all-trans retinoic acid. Blood 1995; 86:1540–1547.

Gallagher RE, Willman CL, Slack JL, et al: Association of PML–RARα type with pretreatment hematologic characteristics but not treatment outcome in acute promyelocytic leukemia: an intergroup molecular study. Blood 1997;90:1656–1663.

Gallagher RE, Yeap BY, Bi W et al: Quantitative real-time RT-PCR analysis of PML–RARα mRNA in acute promyelocytic leukemia: assessment of prognostic significance in adult patients from intergroup protocol 0129. Blood 2003; 101:2521–2528.

Gascoyne RD, Adomat SA, Krajewski S, et al: Prognostic significance of Bcl-2 protein expression and Bcl-2 gene rearrangement in diffuse aggressive non-Hodgkin's lymphoma. Blood 1997; 90:244–251.

Gascoyne RD, Aoun P, Wu D, et al: Prognostic significance of anaplastic lymphoma kinase (ALK) protein expression in adults with anaplastic large cell lymphoma. Blood 1999; 93:3913–3921.

Gascoyne RD, Lamant L, Martin-Subero JI, et al: ALK-positive diffuse large B-cell lymphoma is associated with Clathrin-ALK rearrangements: report of 6 cases. Blood 2003; 102:2568–2573.

Gaynon PS, Crotty ML, Sather HN, et al: Expression of BCR-ABL, E2A-PBX1 and MLL-AF4 fusion transcripts in newly diagnosed children with acute lymphoblastic leukemia: a Children's Cancer Group initiative. Leuk Lymphoma 1997; 26:57–65.

Gibson UEM, Heid CA, Williams PM: A novel method for real time quantitative RT-PCR. Genome Res 1999; 6:995–1001.

Gilliland DG, Griffin JD: The roles of FLT3 in hematopoiesis and leukemia. Blood 2002; 100:1532–1542.

Goldman JM, Melo, JV: Chronic myeloid leukemia – advances in biology and new approaches to treatment. N Engl J Med 2003; 349: 1451–1464.

An excellent review encompassing basic science to current and evolving clinical management in chronic myeloid leukemia.

Golub TR, Slonim DK, Tamayo P, et al: Molecular classification of cancer: class discovery and class prediction by gene expression monitoring. Science 1999; 286:531–537.

Gong JZ, Zheng S, Chiarle R, et al: Detection of immunoglobulin κ light chain rearrangements by polymerase chain reaction. An improved method for detecting clonal B-cell lymphoproliferative disorders. Am J Pathol 1999; 155:355–363.

Gotlib J, Cools J, Malone III JM, et al: The FIP1L1–PDGFRα fusion tyrosine kinase in hypereosinophilic syndrome and chronic eosinophilic leukemia: implications for diagnosis, classification, and management. Blood 2004; 103:2879–2891.

Goulden N, Oakhill A, Steward C. Practical application of minimal residual disease assessment in childhood acute lymphoblastic leukaemia. Br J Haematol 2001; 112:275–281.

Greaves MF, Maia AT, Wiemels JL, Ford AM: Leukemia in twins: lessons in natural history. Blood 2003b; 102:2321–2333.

Greaves MF, Wiemels J: Origins of chromosome translocations in childhood leukemia. Nat Rev Cancer 2003a; 3:1–11.

An outstanding summation of the intriguing issue that many, if not most pediatric leukemias can be traced to an initial genetic event occurring in utero. The implications for our understanding of childhood leukemogenesis are presented.

Greiner TC, Rubocki RJ: Effectiveness of capillary electrophoresis using fluorescent-labeled primers in detecting T-cell receptor γ gene rearrangements. J Mol Diagn 2002; 4:137–143.

Grignani F, Fagioli M, Alcalay M, et al: Acute promyelocytic leukemia: from genetics to treatment. Blood 1994; 83:10–25.

Grimwade D: The pathogenesis of acute promyelocytic leukaemia: evaluation of the role of molecular diagnosis and monitoring in the management of the disease. Br J Haematol 1999; 106:591–613.

Grimwade D, Biondi A, Mozziconacci M, et al: Characterization of acute promyelocytic leukemia cases lacking the classic t(15;17): results of the European Working Party. Blood 2000; 96:1297–1308.

Grimwade D, Lo Coco F: Acute promyelocytic leukemia: a model for the role of molecular diagnosis and residual disease monitoring in directing treatment approach in acute myeloid leukemia. Leukemia 2002; 16:1959–1973.

Summarizes the compelling data for PCR monitoring of minimal residual disease in acute promyelocytic leukemia, with an important discussion of interpretive caveats.

Guidez F, Ivins S, Zhu J, et al: Reduced retinoic acid-sensitivities of nuclear receptor corepressor binding to PML- and PLZF-RARα underlie molecular pathogenesis and treatment of acute promyelocytic leukemia. Blood 1998; 91:2634–2642.

Haferlach T, Kohlmann A, Dugas M, et al: Gene expression profiling is able to reproduce different phenotypes in AML as defined by the FAB classification. Blood 2002a; 100:195a.

Haferlach T, Kohlmann A, Dugas M, et al: The diagnosis of 14 specific subtypes of leukemia is possible based on gene expression profiles: a study on 263 patients with AML, ALL, CML, or CLL. Blood 2002b; 100:139a.

Haferlach T, Schnittger S, Kohlmann A, et al: Genetic profiling in acute monoblastic versus mature monocytic leukemia: A gene expression study on 22 patients. Blood 2002c; 100:195a.

Harbott J, Viehmann S, Borkhardt A, et al: Incidence of *TEL/AML1* fusion gene analyzed consecutively in children with acute lymphoblastic leukemia in relapse. Blood 1997; 90:4933–4937.

Harris MB, Shuster JJ, Carroll A, et al: Trisomy of leukemic cell chromosomes 4 and 10 identifies children with B-progenitor cell acute lymphoblastic leukemia with a very low risk of treatment failure: a Pediatric Oncology Group study. Blood 1992; 79:3316–3324.

Harrison CJ: The detection and significance of chromosomal abnormalities in childhood acute lymphoblastic leukaemia. Blood Rev 2001; 15:49–59.

Hecht JL, Aster JC: Molecular biology of Burkitt's lymphoma. J Clin Oncol 2000; 18:3707–3721.

Heerema NA, Nachman JB, Sather HN, et al: Hypodiploidy with less than 45 chromosomes confers adverse risk in childhood acute lymphoblastic leukaemia: a report from the Children's Cancer Group. Blood 1999; 94:4036–4046.

Heerema NA, Sather HN, Sensel MG, et al: Prognostic impact of trisomies 10, 17 and 5 among children with acute lymphoblastic leukaemia and high hyperdiploidy (>50 chromosomes). J Clin Oncol 2000; 18:1876–1887.

Heid CA, Stevens J, Livak KJ, Williams PM: Real time quantitative PCR. Genome Res 1996; 6:986–994.

Height SE, Swansbury GJ, Matutes E, et al: Analysis of clonal rearrangements of the Ig heavy chain locus in acute leukemia. Blood 1996; 87:5242–5250.

Hess JL: MLL: a histone methyltransferase disrupted in leukemia. Trends Mol Med 2004; 10:500–507.

Hockenberry D, Nunez G, Milliman C, et al: Bcl-2 is an inner mitochondrial membrane protein that blocks programmed cell death. Nature 1990; 348:334–336.

Horsman DE, Gascoyne RD, Coupland RW, et al: Comparison of cytogenetic analysis, Southern analysis, and polymerase chain reaction for the detection of t(14;18) in follicular lymphoma. Am J Clin Pathol 1995; 103:472–478.

Hsi ED, Tubbs RR, Lovell MA, et al: Detection of bcl-2/J$_H$ translocation by polymerase chain reaction. A summary of the experience of the Molecular Oncology Survey of the College of American Pathologists. Arch Pathol Lab Med 2002; 126:902–908.

Hubank M: Gene expression profiling and its application in studies of haematological malignancy. Br J Haematol 2004; 124:577–594.

Succinct overview of gene expression profiling technology and its applications to several types of hematologic and lymphoid cancer.

Hughes TP, Kaeda J, Branford S, et al: Frequency of major molecular responses to imatinib or interferon alfa plus cytarabine in newly diagnosed chronic myeloid leukemia. N Engl J Med 2003; 349:1423–1432.

This important paper not only establishes the benefit of monitoring chronic myeloid leukemia patients using quantitative (Q)-PCR but also derives some important parameters related to the success or failure of imatinib therapy.

Hunger SP, Galili N, Carroll AJ, et al: The t(1;19)(q23;p13) result in consistent fusion of E2A and PBX1 coding sequences in acute lymphoblastic leukemias. Blood 1991; 77:687–693.

Iqbal S, Jenner MJR, Summers, KE, et al: Reliable detection of clonal IgH/Bcl2 MBR rearrangement in follicular lymphoma: methodology and clinical significance. Br J Hematol 2004; 124:325–328.

Isaacson PG, Du M-Q. MALT lymphoma: from morphology to molecules. Nat Rev Cancer 2004; 4:644–653.

Excellent and comprehensive summary of the rapid progress made in our understanding of the genetics and pathogenesis of extranodal marginal zone B-cell lymphomas.

Jaffe ES, Harris N, Stein H, et al: Pathology and Genetics: Tumours of the Haematopoietic and Lymphoid Tissues. World Health Organization Classification of Tumours. Lyon, France, IARC Press, 2001.

James C, Ugo V, Le Couedic JP, et al : A unique clonal JAK2 mutation leading to constitutive signalling causes polycythaemia vera. Nature 2005; 434:1144–1148.

Jerkeman M, Aman P, Cavallin-Stahl E, et al: Prognostic implications of BCL6 rearrangement in uniformly treated patients with diffuse large B-cell lymphoma – a Nordic Lymphoma Group study. Int J Oncol 2002; 20:161–165.

Jones CD, Darnell KH, Warnke RA, et al: CyclinD1/CyclinD3 ratio by real-time PCR improves specificity for the diagnosis of mantle cell lymphoma. J Mol Diagn 2004; 6:84–89.

Jurcic JG, Nimer SD, Scheinberg DA, et al: Prognostic significance of minimal residual disease detection and PML/RAR-α isoform type: long-term follow-up in acute promyelocytic leukemia. Blood 2001; 98:2651–2656.

Jurlander J, Caligiuri MA, Ruutu T, et al: Persistence of the AML/ETO fusion transcript in patients treated with allogeneic bone marrow transplantation for t(8;21) leukemia. Blood 1996; 88:2183–2191.

Kadkol S, Bruno A, Dodge C, et al: Comprehensive analysis of *CBFβ-MYH11* fusion transcripts in acute myeloid leukemia by RT-PCR analysis. J Mol Diag 2004; 6:22–27.

Kaneko Y, Frizzera G, Edamura S, et al: A novel translocation, t(2;5)(p23;q35), in childhood phagocytic large T-cell lymphoma mimicking malignant histiocytosis. Blood 1989; 73: 806–813.

Katzenberger T, Ott G, Klein T, et al: Cytogenetic alterations affecting BCL6 are predominantly found in follicular lymphomas grade 3B with a diffuse large B-cell component. Am J Pathol 2004; 165:481–490.

Kiyoi H, Naoe T, Yokota S, et al: Internal tandem duplication of FLT3 associated with leukocytosis in acute promyelocytic leukemia. Leukemia Study Group of the Ministry of Health and Welfare (Kohseisho). Leukemia 1997; 11:1447–1452.

Knudson AG: Stem cell regulation, tissue ontogeny, and oncogenic events. Semin Cancer Biol 1992; 3:99–106.

Kralovics R, Passamonti F, Buser A, et al: A gain-of-function mutation of JAK2 in myeloproliferative disorders. N Engl J Med 2005; 352:1779–1790.

Kusec R, Laczika K, Knobl P, et al: AML1/ETO fusion mRNA can be detected in remission blood samples of all patients with t(8;21) acute myeloid leukemia after chemotherapy or autologous bone marrow transplantation. Leukemia 1994; 8:735–739.

Ladanyi M, Cavalchire G: Detection of the NPM-ALK genomic rearrangement of Ki-1 lymphoma and isolation of the involved NPM and ALK introns. Diagn Mol Pathol 1996; 5:154–158.

Ladanyi M, Cavalchire G, Morris SW, et al: Reverse transcriptase polymerase chain reaction for the Ki-1 anaplastic large cell lymphoma-associated t(2;5) translocation in Hodgkin's disease. Am J Pathol 1994; 145:1296–1300.

Ladanyi M, Wang S: Detection of rearrangements of the BCL2 major breakpoint region in follicular lymphomas. Correlation of polymerase chain reaction results with Southern blot analysis. Diagn Mol Pathol 1992; 1 :31–35.

Lamant L, Meggetto F, Saati TA, et al: High incidence of the t(2;5)9p23;q35) translocation in anaplastic large cell lymphoma and its lack of detection in Hodgkin's disease. Comparison of cytogenetic analysis, reverse transcriptase-polymerase chain reaction, and P-80 immunostaining. Blood 1996; 87:284–291.

Langerak AW, Szczepanski T, van der Burg M, et al: Heteroduplex PCR analysis of rearranged T cell receptor genes for clonality assessment in suspect T cell proliferations. Leukemia 1997; 11:2192–2199.

Langerak AW, Walvers-Tettero ILM, van Dongen JJM: Detection of T cell receptor beta (TCRB) gene rearrangement patterns in T cell malignancies by Southern blot analysis. Leukemia 1999; 13:965–974.

Lawnicki LC, Rubocki RJ, Chan WC, et al: The distribution of gene segments in T-cell receptor γ gene rearrangements demonstrates the need for multiple primer sets. J Mol Diagn 2003; 5:82–87.

A key publication that systematically examines the utility of multiple primers to detect clonotypic T-cell gamma gene rearrangements. Data are provided on the use of V and J gene segments in T-cell neoplasms, as well as proper primer design and post-PCR analysis by capillary electrophoresis.

Lee S-C, Berg KD, Racke FK, et al: Pseudo-spikes are common in histologically benign lymphoid tissues. J Mol Diagn 2000; 2:145–152.

Levene AP, Morgan GJ, Davies FE: The use of genetic microarray analysis to classify and predict prognosis in haematological malignancies. Clin Lab Haem 2003; 25:209–220.

Levine RL, Wadleigh M, Cools J, et al: Activating mutation in the tyrosine kinase JAK2 in polycythemia vera, essential thrombocytopenia, and agnogenic myeloid metaplasia. Cancer Cell 2005; 7:387–397.

Li Z-Y, Liu D-P, Liang C-C. New insight into the molecular mechanisms of *MLL*-associated leukemia. Leukemia 2005; 19:183–190.

Limpens J, Stad R, Vos C, et al: Lymphoma-associated translocation t(14;18) in blood B cells or normal individuals. Blood 1995; 85:2528–2536.

Liu H, Ye H, Dogan A, et al: T(11;18)(q21;q21) is associated with advanced mucosa-associated lymphoid tissue lymphoma that expresses nuclear BCL10. Blood 2001a; 98:1182–1187.

Liu H, Ruskon-Fourmestraux A, Lavergne-Slove A, et al: Resistance of t(11;18) positive gastric mucosa-associated lymphoid tissue lymphoma to *Helicobacter pylori* eradication therapy. Lancet 2001b; 357:39–40.

Liu H, Ye H, Ruskone-Fourmestraux A, et al: T(11;18) is a marker for all stage gastric MALT lymphomas that will not respond to *H. pylori* eradication. Gastroenterology 2002; 122:1286–1294.

Liu J, Johnson RM, Traweek ST: Rearrangement of the *BCL-2* gene in follicular lymphoma. Detection by PCR in both fresh and fixed tissue samples. Diagn Mol Pathol 1993; 2:241–247.

Liu PP, Hajra A, Wijmenga C et al: Molecular pathogenesis of the chromosome 16 inversion in the M4Eo subtype of acute myeloid leukemia. Blood 1995; 9:2289–2302.

Liu S, Semenciw R, Mao Y: Increasing incidence of non-Hodgkin's lymphoma in Canada, 1970–1996: age-period-cohort analysis. Hematol Oncol 2003; 21:57–66.

Lo Coco F, De Santis S, Esposito A, et al: Molecular monitoring of hematologic malignancies: current and future issues. Sem Hematol 2002; 39 Suppl 1:14–17.

Lombardo JF, Hwang TS, Maiese RL, Segal GH: Optimal primer selection for clonality assessment by polymerase chain reaction analysis: III. Intermediate and high grade B-cell neoplasms. Hum Pathol 1996; 27:373–380.

Lorsbach RB, Downing JR: The role of the AML1 transcription factor in leukemogenesis. Int J Hematol 2001; 74:258–265.

Lossos IS, Czerwinski DK, Alizadeh AA, et al:

Prediction of survival in diffuse large-B-cell lymphoma based on the expression of six genes. N Engl J Med 2004; 350:1828–1837.

Macintyre EA, Delbesse E: Molecular approaches to the diagnosis and evaluation of lymphoid malignancies. Sem Hematol 1999; 36:373–389.

Presents a concise overview of the theory and application of major molecular techniques used to evaluate lymphoid proliferations.

Maes B, Demunter A, Peeter B, De Wolf-Peeters C: BCL10 mutation does not represent an important pathogenic mechanism in gastric MALT-type lymphoma, and the presence of the API2-MLT fusion is associated with aberrant nuclear BCL10 expression. Blood 2002; 99:1398–1404.

Mason DY, Bastard C, Rimokh R, et al: CD30-positive large cell lymphomas (`Ki-1 lymphoma') are associated with a chromosomal translocation involving 5q35. Br J Haematol 1990; 74:161.

Medeiros LJ, Carr J: Overview of the role of molecular methods in the diagnosis of malignant lymphomas. Arch Pathol Lab Med 1999; 123:1189–1207.

A comprehensive article reviewing the pros and cons of commonly employed molecular methods in lymphoma diagnosis.

Melnick A, Licht JD: Deconstructing a disease: RARα, its fusion partners, and their roles in the pathogenesis of acute promyelocytic leukemia. Blood 1999; 93:3167–3215.

A very thorough examination of the key molecular mechanisms involved in the pathogenesis of acute promyelocytic leukemia and related 'APL-like' tumors. This extensive review also emphasizes the concept of all trans retinoic acid efficacy in t(15;17)/PML–RARα-positive APL, as compared to other myeloid leukemias with variant translocations of the RARα gene.

Melo JV: The diversity of BCR–ABL fusion proteins and their relationship to leukemia phenotype. Blood 1996; 88:2375–2384.

Merchant SH, Haines S, Hall B, et al: Fluorescence in-situ hybridization identifies cryptic t(16;16)(p13;q22) masked by del(q22) in a case of AML-M4Eo. J Mol Diagn 2004; 6:271–274.

Migliazza A, Martinotti S, Chen W, et al: Frequent somatic hypermutation of the 5' noncoding region of the *BCL6* gene in B-cell lymphoma. Proc Natl Acad Sci USA 1995; 92:12520–12524.

Moorman AV, Richards SM, Martineau M, et al: Outcome heterogeneity in childhood high-hyperdiploid acute lymphoblastic leukemia. Blood 2003; 102:2756–2762.

Moos PJ, Raetz EA, Carlson MA, et al: Identification of gene expression profiles that segregate patients with childhood leukemia. Clin Cancer Res 2002; 8:3118–313.

Mori H, Colman SM, Xiao Z, et al: Chromosome translocations and covert leukemic clones are generated during normal fetal development. Proc Natl Acad Sci USA 2002; 99:8242–8247.

Morris SW, Naeve C, Mathew P, et al: ALK, the chromosome 2 gene locus altered by the t(2;5) in non-Hodgkin's lymphoma, encodes a novel neural receptor tyrosine kinase that is highly related to leukocyte tyrosine kinase (LTK). Oncogene 1997; 14:2175–2188.

Motegi M, Yonezumi M, Suzuki H, et al: API2-MALT1 chimeric transcripts involved in mucosa-associated lymphoid tissue type lymphoma predict heterogeneous products. Am J Pathol 2000; 156:807–812.

Murga Penas EM, Hinz K, Röser K, et al: Translocations t(11;18)(q21;q21) and t(14;18)(q32;q21) are the main chromosomal abnormalities involving *MLT/MALT1* in MALT lymphomas. Leukemia 2003; 17:2225–2229.

Nakao M, Yokota S, Horiike S, et al: Detection and quantification of TEL/AML1 fusion transcripts by polymerase chain reaction in childhood acute lymphoblastic leukemia. Leukemia 1996a; 10:1463–1470.

Nakao M, Yokota S, Iwai T, et al: Internal tandem duplication of the flt3 gene found in acute myeloid leukemia. Leukemia 1996b; 10:1911–1918.

Neri A, Barriga F, Knowles DM, et al: Different regions of the immunoglobulin heavy-chain locus are involved in chromosomal translocations in distinct pathogenetic forms of Burkitt lymphoma. Proc Natl Acad Sci USA 1988; 85:2748–2752.

Neves H, Ramos C, da Silva MG, et al: The nuclear topography of *ABL*, *BCR*, *PML*, and *RARα* genes: evidence for gene proximity in specific phases of the cell cycle and stages of hematopoietic differentiation. Blood 1999; 93:1197–1207.

Ngan B, Nourse J, Cleary ML: Detection of chromosomal translocation t(14;18) within the minor cluster region of bcl-2 by polymerase chain reaction and direct genomic sequencing of the enzymatically amplified DNA in follicular lymphomas. Blood 1989; 73:1759–1762.

Nowell PC, Hungerford DA: A minute chromosome in human chronic granulocytic leukemia. Science 1960; 132:1497.

Nyvold C, Madsen HO, Ryder LP, et al: Precise quantification of minimal residual disease at day 29 allows identification of children with acute lymphoblastic leukemia and an excellent outcome. Blood 2002; 99:1253–1258.

O'Brien SG, Guilhot F, Larson RA, et al: Imatinib compared with interferon and low-dose cytarabine for newly diagnosed chronic-phase chronic myeloid leukemia. N Engl J Med 2003; 348:994–1004.

Key paper documenting the superiority of imatinib therapy over interferon-based therapy for patients with chronic myeloid leukemia.

Offit K, Lo Coco F, Louie DC, et al: Rearrangement of the Bcl-6 gene as a prognostic marker in diffuse large cell lymphoma. N Engl J Med 1994; 331: 74–80.

Ohno H: Pathogenetic role of *BCL6* translocation in B-cell non-Hodgkin's lymphoma. Histol Histopathol 2004; 19:637–650.

Ohno H, Fukuhara S: Significance of rearrangement of the BCL6 gene in B-cell lymphoid neoplasms. Leuk Lymphoma 1997; 27:53–63.

Ohshima A, Miura I, Hashimoto K, et al: Rearrangements of the BCL6 gene and chromosome aberrations affecting 3q27 in 54 patients with non-Hodgkin's lymphoma. Leuk Lymphoma 1997; 27:329–334.

Oka K, Ohno H, Kita K: PRAD1 gene overexpression in mantle cell lymphoma but not in other low grade B-cell lymphomas, including extranodal lymphoma. Br J Haematol 1994; 86:786–791.

Olavarria E, Kanfer E, Szydlo R, et al: Early detection of BCR–ABL transcripts by quantitative reverse transcriptase-polymerase chain reaction predicts outcome after allogeneic stem cell transplantation for chronic myeloid leukemia. Blood 2001; 97:1560–1565.

Onizuka T, Moriyama M, Yamochi T, et al: BCL-6 gene product, a 92- to 98-kD nuclear phosphoprotein, is highly expressed in germinal center B cells and their neoplastic counterparts. Blood 1995; 86:28–37.

Otsuki T, Yano T, Clark HM, et al: Analysis of LAZ3 (BCL-6) status in B-cell non-Hodgkin's lymphomas: results of rearrangement and gene expression studies and a mutational analysis of coding region sequences. Blood 1995; 85: 2877–2884.

Pai RK, Chakerian AE, Binder JM, et al: B-cell clonality determination using an immunoglobulin kappa light chain polymerase chain reaction method. J Mol Diagn 2005; 7:300–307.

Paietta, E: Assessing minimal residual disease (MRD) in leukemia: a changing definition and concept? Bone Marrow Transplant 2002; 29:459–465.

Pallisgaard N, Hokland P, Riishoj DC, et al: Multiplex reverse transcription-polymerase chain reaction for simultaneous screening of 29 translocations and chromosomal aberrations in acute leukemia. Blood 1998; 92:574–588.

Pardanani A, Brockman SR, Paternoster SF, et al: *FIP1L1–PDGFRA* fusion: prevalence and clinicopathologic correlates in 89 consecutive patients with moderate to severe eosinophilia. Blood 2004; 104:3038–3045.

Pardanani A, Ketterling RP, Brockman SR, et al: *CHIC2* deletion, a surrogate for *FIP1L1–PDGFRA* fusion, occurs in systemic mastocytosis associated with eosinophilia and predicts response to imatinib therapy. Blood 2003; 102:3093–3096.

Pasqualucci L, Migliazza A, Basso K, et al: Mutations of the BCL6 proto-oncogene disrupt its negative autoregulation in diffuse large B-cell lymphoma. Blood 2003; 101:2914–2923.

Phan RT, Dalla-Favera R: The BCL6 proto-oncogene suppresses p53 expression in germinal center B cells. Nature 2004; 432:635–639.

Pinyol M, Campo E, Nadal A: Detection of the bcl-1 rearrangement at the major translocation cluster in frozen and paraffin-embedded tissues of mantle cell lymphomas by polymerase chain reaction. Am J Clin Pathol 1996; 105: 532–537.

Pittaluga S, Ayoubi TAY, Wlodarska I, et al: BCL-6 expression in reactive lymphoid tissue and in B-cell non-Hodgkin's lymphomas. J Pathol 1996; 179: 145–150.

Poetsch M, Weber-Matthison K, Plendl JJ, et al: Detection of the t(14;18) chromosomal translocation by interphase cytogenetics with yeast-artificial-chromosome probes in follicular lymphoma and nonneoplastic lymphoproliferation. J Clin Oncol 1996; 14:963–969.

Polo JM, Dell'oso T, Ranuncolo SM, et al: Specific peptide interference reveals BCL6 transcriptional and oncogenic mechanisms in B-cell lymphoma cells. Nat Med 2004; 10:1329–1335,

Privitera E, Kamps MP, Hayashi Y, et al: Different molecular consequences of the 1;19 chomosomal translocation in childhood B-cell precursor acute lymphoblastic leukemia. Blood 1992; 79:1781–1788.

Pui C-H, Campana D: New definition of remission in childhood acute lymphoblastic leukemia. Leukemia 2000; 14:783–785.

Pui C-H, Chessels JM, Camitta B, et al: Clinical heterogeneity in childhood acute lymphoblastic leukemia with 11q23 rearrangements. Leukemia 2003; 17:700–706.

Pui C-H, Relling MV, Downing JD: Acute lymphoblastic leukemia. N Engl J Med 2004; 350:1535–1548.

This concise review details the advances made in understanding the biology of pediatric ALL, with an emphasis on some of the more recent molecular pathway prognostic factors and pharmacogenomics.

Quignon F, De Bels F, Koken M, et al: PML induces a novel caspase-independent death process. Nat Genet 1998; 20:259–265.

Radich JP, Gehly G, Gooley T, et al: Polymerase chain reaction detection of the BCR–ABL fusion transcript after allogeneic marrow transplantation for chronic myeloid leukemia: Results and implications in 346 patients. Blood 1995; 85: 2632–2638.

Radich JP, Gooley T, Bryant E et al: The significance of *BCR-ABL* molecular detection in chronic myeloid leukemia patients 'late,' 18 months or more after transplantation. Blood 2001; 98:1701–1707.

Raghavan SC, Swanson PC, Wu X, et al: A non-B-DNA structure at the Bcl-2 major breakpoint region is cleaved by the RAG complex. Nature 2004; 428:88–93.

Ramasamy I, Brisco M, Morley A: Improved PCR method for detecting monoclonal immunoglobulin heavy chain rearrangement in B cell neoplasms. J Clin Pathol 1992; 43:770–775.

Raynaud SD, Cave H, Baens M, et al: The 12;21 translocation involving TEL and deletion of the other TEL allele: two frequently associated alterations found in childhood actue lymphoblastic leukemia. Blood 1996; 87:2891–2899.

Remstein ED, James CD, Kurtin PJ: Incidence and subtype specificity of *API2–MALT1* fusion translocations in extranodal, nodal, and splenic marginal zone lymphomas. Am J Pathol 2000a; 156:1183–1188.

Remstein ED, Kurtin PJ, Buno I, et al: Diagnostic utility of fluorescence in situ hybridization in mantle-cell lymphoma. Br J Haematol 2000b; 110:856–862.

Remstein ED, Kurtin PJ, Einerson RR, et al: Primary pulmonary MALT lymphomas show frequent and heterogeneous cytogenetic abnormalities, including aneupolidy and translocations involving API2 and MALT1 and IGH and MALT1. Leukemia 2004; 18:156–160.

Ries LAG, Miller BA, Hankey BF: SEER Cancer Statistics Review, 1973–1991: tables and graphs. NIH Publ No 94–2789. Bethesda, MD, National Cancer Institute, 1994.

Rimokh R, Berger F, Bastard C: Rearrangement and overexpression of the BCL-1/PRAD-1 gene in intermediate lymphocytic lymphomas and in t(11q13)-bearing leukemias. Blood 1993; 81:3063–3067.

Rimokh R, Magaud JP, Berger F, et al: A translocation involving a specific breakpoint (q35) on chromosome 5 is characteristic of anaplastic large cell lymphoma (`Ki-1 lymphoma). Br J Haematol 1989; 71:31–36.

Roix JJ, McQueen PG, Munson PJ, et al: Spatial proximity of translocation-prone gene loci in human lymphomas. Nat Genet 2003; 34:287–291.

Romana SP, Mauchauffe M, Le Coniat M, et al: The t(12;21) of acute lymphoblastic leukemia results in a *TEL–AML1* gene fusion. Blood 1995; 85:3662–3670.

Rosenwald A, Alizadeh AA, Widhopf G, et al: Relation of gene expression phenotype to immunoglobulin mutation genotype in B-cell chronic lymphocytic leukemia. J Exp Med 2001; 194:1639–1647.

Rosenwald A, Ott G, Stilgenbauer S, et al: Exclusive detection of the t(11;18)(q21;q21) in extranodal marginal zone B cell lymphomas (MZBL) of MALT type in contrast to other MZBL and extranodal large B cell lymphomas. Am J Pathol 1999; 155:1817–1821.

Rosenwald A, Wright G, Chan WC, et al: The use of molecular profiling to predict survival after chemotherapy for diffuse large-B-cell lymphoma. N Engl J Med 2002; 346:1937–1947.

Rosenwald A, Wright G, Wiestner A, et al: The proliferation gene expression signature is a quantitative integrator of oncogenic events that predicts survival in mantle cell lymphoma. Cancer Cell 2003; 3:185–197.

Rowley JD: A new consistent chromosomal abnormality in chronic myelogenous leukaemia identified by quinacrine fluorescence and Giemsa staining. Nature 1973; 243:290–293.

Rubnitz JE, Behm FG, Pui CH, et al: Genetic studies of childhood acute lymphoblastic leukemia with emphasis on p16, MLL, and ETV6 gene abnormalities: results of St Jude Total Therapy Study XII. Leukemia 1997b; 11:1201–1206.

Rubnitz JE, Downing JR, Pui CH, et al: TEL gene rearrangement in acute lymphoblastic leukemia: a new genetic marker with prognostic significance. J Clin Oncol 1997a; 15:1150–1157.

Saglio G, Pane F, Gottardi E, et al: Consistent amounts of acute leukemia-associated P190BCR/ABL transcripts are expressed by chronic myelogenous leukemia patients at diagnosis. Blood 1996; 87:1075–1080.

Samaha H, Dumontel C, Ketterer N, Moullett I: Mantle cell lymphoma: a retrospective study of 121 cases. Leukemia 1998; 12:1281–1287.

Sanchez-Izquierdo D, Buchonnet G, Siebert R, et al: MALT1 is deregulated by both chromosomal translocation and amplification in B-cell non-Hodgkin lymphoma. Blood 2003; 101:4539–4546.

Sanchez-Izquierdo D, Siebert R, Harder L, et al: Detection of translocations affecting the BCL6 locus in B cell non-Hodgkin's lymphoma by interphase fluorescence in situ hybridization. Leukemia 2001; 15:1475–1484.

Sainty D, Liso V, Cantu-Rajnoldi A, et al: A new morphological classification system for acute promyelocytic leukemia distinguishes cases with underlying *PLZF-RARA* rearrangements. Blood 2000; 96:1287–1296.

Sarris AH, Luthra R, Cabanillas F, et al: Genomic DNA amplification and the detection of t(2;5)(p23;q35) in lymphoid neoplasms. Leuk Lymphoma 1998; 29:507–514.

Saueracker EA, Kay PH, Spagnolo DV: Distinguishing between monoclonal rearrangements and allelic forms of the immunoglobulin lambda light chain constant region genes: Significance in the diagnosis of non-Hodgkin's lymphoma. Diagn Mol Pathol 1992; 1:109–117.

Schoch C, Kohlmann A, Schnittger S, et al: Acute myeloid leukemias with reciprocal rearrangements can be distinguished by specific gene expression profiles Proc Natl Acad Sci USA 2002; 99:10008–10013.

Seeger K, Adams HP, Buchwald D, et al: *TEL–AML1* fusion transcript in relapsed childhood acute lymphoblastic leukemia. The Berlin-Frankfurt-Munster Study Group. Blood 1998; 91:1716–1722.

Segal GH, Jorgensen T, Masih AS, Braylan RC: Optimal primer selection for clonality assessment by polymerase chain reaction analysis: I. Low grade B-cell lymphoproliferative disorders of nonfollicular center cell type. Hum Pathol 1994; 25:1269–1275.

Segal GH, Jorgensen T, Scott M, Braylan RC: Optimal primer selection for clonality assessment by polymerase chain reaction analysis: II. Follicular lymphomas. Hum Pathol 1995; 25:1276–1282.

Shen HM, Peters A, Baron B, et al: Mutation of BCL-6 gene in normal B cells by the process of somatic hypermutation of Ig genes. Science 1998; 280:1750–1752.

Sherr CJ, Roberts JM: CDK inhibitors: positive and negative regulators of G_1-phase progression. Genes Devel 1999; 13:1501–1512.

Shurtleff SA, Buijs A, Behm FG, et al: *TEL/AML1* fusion resulting from a cryptic t(12;21) is the most common genetic lesion in pediatric ALL and defines a subgroup of patients with an excellent prognosis. Leukemia 1995; 9:1985–1989.

Siebert R, Matthiesen P, Harder S, et al: Application of interphase fluorescence in situ hybridization for the detection of the Burkitt translocation t(8;14)(q24;q32) in B-cell lymphoma. Blood 1998; 91: 984–990.

Sim SP, Liu LF: Nucleolytic cleavage region during apoptosis. J Biol Chem 2001; 276:31590–31595.

Sinclair PB, Nacheva EP, Leversha N, et al: Large deletions at the t(9;22) breakpoint are common and may identify a poor-prognosis subgroup of patients with chronic myeloid leukemia. Blood 2000; 95:738–744.

Slack DN, McCarthy KP, Wiedemann LM, Sloane JP: Evaluation of sensitivity, specificity and reproducibility of an optimized method for detecting clonal rearrangements of immunoglobulin and T-cell receptor genes in formalin-fixed, paraffin-embedded sections. Diagn Mol Pathol 1993; 2: 223–232.

Smith CA, Gruss HJ, Davis T, et al: CD30 antigen, a marker for Hodgkin's lymphoma, is a receptor whose ligand defines an emerging family of cytokines with homology to TNF. Cell 1993; 73:1349–1360.

Smith MA, Rubinstein L, Ungerleider RS: Therapy-related acute myeloid leukemia following treatment with epipodophyllotoxins: estimating the risk. Med Pediatr Oncol 1994; 23:86–98.

Soslow RA, Zukerberg LR, Harris NL, Warnke RA: BCL-1 (PRAD1/cyclin D1) overexpression distinguishes the blastoid variant of mantle cell lymphoma from B-lineage lymphoblastic lymphoma. Mod Pathol 1997; 10:810–817.

Speck NA, Stacy T, Wang Q, et al: Core-binding factor:

A central player in hematopoiesis and leukemia. Cancer Res (Suppl) 1999; 59:1789s–1793s.

Stein H, Foss H-D, Dürkopp H, et al: CD30+ anaplastic large cell lymphoma: a review of its histopathologic, genetic and clinical features. Blood 2000; 96:3681–3695.

Stirewalt DL, Radich JP: The role of FLT3 in haematopoietic malignancies. Nat Rev Cancer 2003; 3:650–665.

This comprehensive review covers the molecular and cell biology of FLT3 in normal hematopoiesis, as well as the association of FLT3 gene mutations (and their significance) in acute leukemia.

Stissel-Broeker PL, Super HG, Thirman MJ, et al: Distribution of 11q23 breakpoints within the MLL breakpoints cluster region in de novo acute leukemia and in treatment-related acute myeloid leukemia: correlation with a scaffold attachment regions and topoisomerase II consensus binding sites. Blood 1996; 87:1912–1922.

Streubel B, Lamprecht A, Dierlamm J, et al: T(14;18)(q32;q21) involving IGH and MALT1 is a frequent chromosomal aberration in MALT lymphoma. Blood 2003; 101:2335–2339.

Streubel B, Simonitsch-Klupp I, Mullauer L, et al: Variable frequencies of MALT lymphoma-associated genetic aberrations in MALT lymphomas of different sites. Leukemia 2004; 18:1722–1726.

A comprehensive 'mapping' type study using fluorescence in situ hybridization to outline the prevalence and distribution of major MALT lymphoma-associated translocations.

Super HJ, McCabe NR, Thirman MJ, et al: Rearrangements of the MLL gene in therapy-related acute myeloid leukemia in patients previously treated with agents targeting DNA-topoisomerase II. Blood 1993; 82:3705–3711.

Szczepanski T, Willemse MJ, Brinkhof B, et al: Comparative analysis of Ig and TCR gene rearrangements at diagnosis and at relapse of childhood precursor-B-ALL provides improved strategies for selection of stable PCR targets for monitoring of minimal residual disease. Blood 2002; 99:2315–2323.

Tallman MS, Andersen JW, Schiffer CA, et al: All *trans*-retinoic acid in acute promyelocytic leukemia. N Engl J Med 1997; 337:1021–1028.

Tallman MS, Nabhan C, Feusner JH, Rowe JM: Acute promyelocytic leukemia: evolving therapeutic strategies. Blood 2002; 99:759–767.

Thiede C, Steudel C, Mohr B, et al: Analysis of FLT3-activating mutations in 979 patients with acute myelogenous leukemia: association with FAB subtypes and identification of subgroups with poor prognosis. Blood 2002; 99:4326–4335.

Thomazy VA, Luthra R, Uthman MO, et al: Determination of cyclin D1 and CD20 mRNA levels by real-time quantitative RT-PCR from archival tissue sections of mantle cell lymphoma and other non-Hodgkin's lymphomas. J Mol Diagn 2002; 4:201–208.

Tsujimoto Y, Cossman J, Jaffe E, Croce CM: Involvement of the *bcl-2* gene in human follicular lymphomas. Science 1985; 228:1440–1443.

Ueda Y, Nishida K, Miki T, et al: Interphase detection of BCL6/IgH fusion gene in non-Hodgkin lymphoma by fluorescence in situ hybridization. Cancer Genet Cytogenet 1997; 99:102–107.

Vahdat L, Maslak P, Miller WH Jr, et al: Early mortality and the retinoic acid syndrome in acute promyelocytic leukemia: Impact of leukocytosis, low-dose chemotherapy, PMN/RARα isoform, and CD13 expression in patients treated with all-*trans* retinoic acid. Blood 1994; 84:3843–3849.

Valk PJM, Verhaak RGW, Beijen A, et al: Prognostically useful gene-expression profiles in acute myeloid leukemia. N Engl J Med 2004; 350:1617–1628.

Van der Velden VHJ, Hochhaus A, Cazzaniga G, et al: Detection of minimal residual disease in hematologic malignancies by real-time quantitative PCR: principles, approaches, and laboratory aspects. Leukemia 2003; 17:1013–1034.

A complete and elegant technical appraisal of the state-of-the-art in minimal residual disease detection by quantitative PCR-based techniques.

Van Dongen JJM, Langerak AW, Bruggemann M, et al: Design and standardization of PCR primers and protocols for detection of clonal immunoglobulin and T-cell receptor gene recombinations in suspect lymphoproliferations: report of the BIOMED-2 Concerted Action BMH4-CT98–3936. Leukemia 2003; 17:2257–2317.

As with the Gabert et al paper, this European contribution is remarkable in its complete evaluation of multiple antigen receptor gene loci and lymphoid tumor-associated genetic abnormalities for the development of diagnostic PCR assays. The implication is that better and more comprehensive genetic marker characterization will lead to improved minimal residual disease detection approaches by quantitative PCR molecular techniques.

Van Dongen JJM, Seriu T, Panzer-Grumayer ER, et al: Prognostic value of minimal residual disease in acute lymphoblastic leukaemia in childhood. Lancet 1998; 352:1731–1738.

Van Rhee F, Hochhaus A, Lin F, et al: p190 BCR–ABL mRNA is expressed at low levels in p210-positive chronic myeloid and acute lymphoblastic leukemias. Blood 1996; 87:5213–5217.

Vasef MA, Medeiros LJ, Koo C: Cyclin D1 immunohistochemical staining is useful in distinguishing mantle cell lymphoma from other low-grade B-cell neoplasms in bone marrow. Am J Clin Pathol 1997; 108:302–307.

Vega F, Medeiros J: Chromosomal translocations involved in non-Hodgkin lymphomas. Arch Pathol Lab Med 2003; 127:1148–1160.

Viswanatha DS, Chen IM, Liu PP, et al: Characterization and use of an antibody detecting the CBFB/SMMHC fusion protein in inv 16(16)(16) associated acute myeloid leukemias. Blood 1998; 91:1882–1890.

Wang ZG, Ruggero D, Ronchetti S, et al: Pml is essential for multiple apoptotic pathways. Nat Genet 1998; 20:266–272.

Waring PM, Cleary ML: Disruption of a homolog of trithorax by 11q23 translocations: Leukemogenic and transcriptional implications. Curr Top Microbiol Immunol 1997; 220:1–23.

Weis K, Rambaud S, Lavau C, et al: Retinoic acid regulates aberrant nuclear localization of PML–RARα in acute promyelocytic leukaemia cells. Cell 1994; 76:345–356.

Weisenburger DD, Armitage JO: Mantle cell lymphoma – an entity comes of age. Blood 1999; 87:4483–4494.

Weiss LM, Lopategui JR, Sun LH, et al: Absence of the t(2;5) in Hodgkin's disease. Blood 1995; 85:2845–2847.

Weiss LM, Warnke RA, Sklar J, Cleary ML: Molecular analysis of the t(14;18) chromosomal translocation in malignant lymphomas. N Engl J Med 1987; 317:1185–1189.

Wellmann A, Otsuki T, Vogelbruch M, et al: Analysis of the t(2;5)(p23;q35) translocation by reverse transcription-polymerase chain reaction in CD30+ anaplastic large-cell lymphomas, in other non-Hodgkin's lymphomas of T-cell phenotype, and in Hodgkin's disease. Blood 1995; 86:2321–2328.

Wiemels JL, Cazzaniga G, Daniotti M, et al: Prenatal origin of acute lymphoblastic leukaemia in children. Lancet 1999; 354:1499–1503.

Wiemels JL, Leonard B, Wang Y, et al: Site-specific translocation and evidence of post-natal origin of the t(1;19) E2A-PBX1 translocation in childhood acute lymphoblastic leukemia. Proc Natl Acad Sci USA 2002b; 99:15101–15106.

Wiemels JL, Xiao Z, Buffler PA, et al: In utero origin of t(8;21) AML1–ETO translocations in childhood actue myeloid leukemia. Blood 2002a; 99:3801–3805.

Williams ME, Meeker TC, Swerdlow SH: Rearrangement of the chromosome 11 bcl-1 locus in centrocytic lymphoma: Analysis with multiple breakpoint probes. Blood 78:493–498.

Williams ME, Swerdlow SH, Meeker TC: Chromosome t(11;14)(q13;q32) breakpoints in centrocytic lymphoma are highly localized at the bcl-1 major translocation cluster. Leukemia 1993a; 7:1437–1440.

Williams ME, Swerdlow SH, Rosenberg CL, Arnold A: Chromosome 11 translocation breakpoints at the PRAD1/cyclin D1 gene locus in centrocytic lymphoma. Leukemia 1993b; 7:241–245.

Willis TG, Jadayel DM, Ju MQ, et al: Bcl10 is involved in t(1;14)(p22;q32) of MALT B-cell lymphoma and mutated in multiple tumor types. Cell 1999; 96:35–45.

Wittwer CT, Ririe KM, Andrew RV, et al: The LightCycler: a microvolume multisample fluorimeter with rapid temperature control. Biotechniques 1997; 22:176–181.

Wotherspoon AC, Soosay GN, Diss TC, Isaacson PG: Low-grade primary B-cell lymphoma of the lung. An immunohistochemical, molecular, and cytogenetic study of a single case. Am J Clin Pathol 1990; 94:655–660.

Wundisch T, Neubauer A, Stolte M, et al: B-cell monoclonality is associated with lymphoid follicles in gastritis. Am J Surg Pathol 2003; 27:882–887.

Yagi T, Hibi S, Tabata Y, et al: Detection of clonotypic IGH and TCR rearrangements in the neonatal blood spots of infants and children with B-cell precursor acute lymphoblastic leukemia. Blood 2000; 96:264–268.

Yamamoto Y, Kiyoi H, Nakano Y, et al: Activating mutation of D835 within the activation loop of FLT3 in human hematologic malignancies. Blood 2001; 97:2434–2439.

Yang E, Korsmeyer SJ: Molecular thanatopsis: a discourse on the BCL2 family and cell death. Blood 1996; 88:386–401.

Yang WI, Zukerberg LR, Motokura T: Cyclin D1 (Bcl-1, PRAD1) protein expression in low-grade B-cell lymphomas and reactive hyperplasia. Am J Pathol 1994; 145:86–96

Ye BH, Cattoretti G, Shen Q, et al: The BCL-6 proto-oncogene controls germinal-centre formation and Th2-type inflammation. Nat Genet 1997; 16:161–170.

Ye H, Dogan A, Karran L, et al: BCL10 expression in normal and neoplastic lymphoid tissue. Nuclear localization in MALT lymphoma. Am J Pathol 2000; 157:1147–1154.

Ye H, Gong L, Liu H, et al: MALT lymphoma with t(14;18)(q32;q21)/IGH-MALT1 is characterized by strong cytoplasmic MALT1 and BCL10 expression. J Pathol 2005; 205:293–301.

Ye H, Liu H, Attygalle A, et al: Variable frequencies of t(11;18)(q21;q21) in MALT lymphomas of different sites: significant association with CagA strains of H. pylori in gastric MALT lymphomas. Blood 2003a; 102:1012–1018.

Ye H, Liu H, Raderer M, et al: High incidence of t(11;18)(q21;q21) in Helicobacter pylori-negative gastric MALT lymphomas. Blood 2003b; 101:2547–2550.

Yee HT, Ponzoni M, Merson A, et al: Molecular characterization of the (2;5)(p23;q35) translocation in anaplastic large cell lymphoma (Ki-1) and Hodgkin's disease. Blood 1996; 87:1081–1088.

Yeoh EJ, Ross ME, Shurtleff SA, et al: Classification, subtype discovery, and prediction of outcome in pediatric acute lymphoblastic leukemia by gene expression profiling. Cancer Cell 2002; 1:133–143.

A landmark publication in gene expression microarray analysis of pediatric acute lymphoblastic leukemias.

Yonezumi M, Suzuki R, Suzuki H, et al: Detection of AP12-MALT1 chimaeric gene in extranodal and nodal marginal zone B-cell lymphoma by reverse transcription polymerase chain reaction (PCR) and genomic long and accurate PCR analyses. Br J Haematol 2001; 115:588–594.

Yu BD, Hell JL, Horning SE, et al: Altered Hox empression and segmental identity in MLL-mutant mice. Nature 1995; 378:505–508.

VIII

Zelent A, Greaves M, Enver T: Role of the *TEL–AML1* fusion gene in the molecular pathogenesis of childhood acute lymphoblastic leukemia. Oncogene, 2004; 23:4275–4283.

Zervos AS, Gyuris J, Brent R: Mxi1, a protein that specifically interacts with Max to bind Myc-Max recognition sites. Cell 1993; 72:223–232.

Zhong S, Salomoni P, Pandofi PP: The transcriptional role of PML and the nuclear body. Nature Cell Biol 2000; 2:E85–E90.

Zucca E, Bertoni F, Roggero E, Cavalli F: The gastric marginal zone B-cell lymphoma of MALT type. Blood 2000; 96:410–419.

Zukerberg LR, Yang WI, Arnold A, Harris NL: Cyclin D1 expression in non-Hodgkin's lymphomas:

detection by immunohistochemistry. Am J Clin Pathol 1995; 103:756–760.

Zwaan CM, Meshinchi S, Radich JP, et al: FLT3 internal tandem duplication in 234 children with acute myeloid leukemia: prognostic significance and relation to cellular drug resistance. Blood 2003; 102:2387–2394.

Molecular Diagnosis of Genetic Diseases

Wayne W. Grody MD PhD, Walter W. Noll MD

KEY POINTS

- Molecular testing for inherited disorders may be the most rapidly growing area of molecular pathology, owing to the plethora of disease genes discovered through the Human Genome Project.

- The mutations for single-gene disorders, whether dominant or recessive, can be detected by a variety of molecular diagnostic techniques, either specific to the mutation in question, if it is known, or by comprehensive gene sequencing or mutation scanning approaches if the mutation is not known.

- Certain disorders, such as cystic fibrosis, have sufficiently high mutation carrier frequencies that they have become targets for large-scale population screening programs.

- Late-onset dominant disorders, such as Huntington's disease and familial cancers, are now targets of presymptomatic testing.

- Each of these applications carries with it a variety of ethical concerns involving genetic privacy, informed consent, pregnancy termination, potential stigmatization, and theoretic risk of insurance discrimination.

Probably the fastest growing, and perhaps most controversial, area of molecular pathology, diagnostic molecular genetics holds promise of becoming the most powerful diagnostic and screening tool of the 21st century. With the rapidly accelerating pace of identification of new disease genes after completion of the human genome sequence and the recognition that virtually all diseases, including neoplastic and even infectious ones, have some genetic component, the clinical utility of this subspecialty can only continue to expand. Moreover, its unique capability to diagnose disease both prenatally and presymptomatically should confer on it a primary role in preventive medicine, a focus of increasing urgency in the present era of medical care cost containment. Even beyond that, diagnostic molecular genetics leads naturally into therapeutic molecular genetics, since essentially the same normal gene sequences used to detect molecular genetic defects by DNA hybridization could theoretically be used to correct such defects by gene replacement therapy. As the latter activity increases in scope and range of uses, it will become even further intertwined with the activities of the molecular diagnostic laboratory, to which will fall the responsibility for monitoring proper insertion and expression of the replacement gene.

Yet such progress does not come unencumbered by appreciable obstacles. Aside from the considerable technical sophistication and complexity of these procedures, they are inextricably bound up with a number of thorny ethical dilemmas. Dissecting a patient's most fundamental constitutional makeup, and the inborn defects therein, raises problematic questions about genetic discrimination, stigmatization, ethnic differences, privacy, informed consent, and confidentiality. Since at the molecular genetic level everything becomes a 'pre-existing condition,' the very definition of insurability may need to be revised; and instances of insurance and employment discrimination as a result of genetic testing, although rare (Hall, 2000), have been reported (Billings, 1992). Furthermore, discovery of any such heritable mutations in an individual has profound implications far beyond the immediate patient who requested the DNA test (the 'proband'), extending to all the other members of that person's family, none of whom may have consented to exploring or revealing this type of information. Indeed, with the almost unlimited power of DNA testing afforded by amplification techniques such as the polymerase chain reaction (PCR), it becomes quite easy to perform genetic analysis without the patient's consent or even knowledge, since the testing can be done on minute portions of tissue or fluid samples obtained for other unrelated purposes. Prenatal diagnosis – and, by extension, preconception genetic carrier screening of couples – becomes caught up in the passionate ethical and religious debates over abortion. And gene therapy, despite general consensus that it should be directed only at somatic, rather than germline, cellular targets (and even this notion is beginning to change), raises the specter of eugenics among those who do not have to remember back all that far to times when such notions were not only accepted but actively espoused.

Much of diagnostic molecular genetics involves the assessment of risk for occurrence or recurrence of a disorder in an individual or family. For reasons to be described more fully in this chapter, the test results obtained are often expressed not in terms of a numerical concentration or a yes/no answer but as a probability, which sometimes is derived by multifactorial Bayesian analysis (Ojino, 2004). The accurate and meaningful conveyance of such complex uncertainties to patients and even referring physicians can be quite difficult and time-consuming. For this reason, and owing to the serious ethical implications of these tests as described above, this area of laboratory medicine, perhaps more than most others, requires very close communication between the laboratory and the referring clinician or genetic counselor. In fact, many of these tests should only be ordered through a medical geneticist or genetic counselor, since these are the specialists best qualified to assess the appropriateness of the test and explain the results to the patient. Some large reference laboratories specializing in this type of testing even employ their own genetic counselors on staff as a further safeguard for appropriate use and communication with primary care physicians who may not be well-versed in these matters.

Choice of Techniques

With so many genetic disease genes, loci, and mutational mechanisms known, diagnostic molecular genetics must take advantage of the entire spectrum of modern molecular biological techniques available. These include PCR, Southern blotting, allele-specific probe hybridization, DNA sequencing, real-time PCR, nucleic acid microarrays, Invader assay, amplification refractory mutation system (ARMS), oligonucleotide ligation assay (OLA), mutation scanning methods such as denaturing gradient gel electrophoresis (DGGE) and single-strand conformation polymorphism (SSCP), mass spectrometry, and others. The choice of which technique to use in a particular case will depend, to a large extent, on two factors: (1) the present knowledge of the gene(s) associated with the disease in question, and (2) its degree of molecular heterogeneity. The first criterion roughly divides all genetic diseases into two categories: those for which the causative gene has been isolated and those for which it has not. Those in the first category can often be approached by direct gene/mutation analysis; those in the latter can only be approached by linkage analysis using polymorphic DNA markers nearby on the same chromosome, provided the disease has been mapped to that rather crude level. The second concept, heterogeneity, refers to the number of different genes, or the variety of mutations within a single gene, that can cause the same disease. The greater the heterogeneity, the more difficult, labor-intensive, and expensive the DNA test becomes (and the more complex the results reporting). Indeed, the mutations responsible for some disorders are so numerous and spread across such large genes that direct detection of all of them is not feasible and one must revert back to linkage analysis even though the causative gene has been identified and cloned. In other disorders, one or more mutations may be of sufficiently high frequency in particular ethnic populations that screening for those few, while ignoring the many rarer mutations reported, can provide a test of sufficient yield to justify the direct approach.

To make such tests practical and of reasonable cost, a number of multiplexing strategies for simultaneous mutation detection have been devised, as described below. Yet the reader should keep in mind that all of these involve some compromise as to overall test sensitivity. Indeed, the field of diagnostic molecular genetics tolerates, by necessity, a number of screening tests with clinical sensitivities noticeably below those that would be considered acceptable in other areas of the clinical laboratory. The decision of just how low the acceptable sensitivity cut-off should be often comes down to public health considerations. Most geneticists have reasoned that, at least for screening tests, the potential public health benefits of offering a test of suboptimal sensitivity outweigh the arguments for withholding it, as long as sufficient education and counseling are provided to patients so that they understand the residual risk inherent in a negative test result. It is important to keep in mind that we are speaking here about clinical sensitivity, not analytical sensitivity. It is assumed that the test is capable of detecting a given mutation whenever it is present; it is just that many rarer mutations will not be targeted by the assay, so that some proportion of carriers will be 'missed' – a sort of 'clinical false negative' (Palomaki 2004).

Direct mutation tests have been simplified immeasurably by the advent of PCR. Through the judicious choice of primers, this technique allows the laboratory to hone in on the precise mutation of interest, or a 'hot spot' within a gene containing several possible mutation sites, using minute amounts of starting material. Once the region containing the suspected mutation is amplified, it can be analyzed by gel or capillary electrophoresis, sequencing, or DNA probe hybridization. For a deletion that would be expected to alter the length of the amplicon, accurate molecular sizing of the PCR products by electrophoresis will be sufficient. Alternatively, if the deletion or point mutation disrupts (or creates) a restriction endonuclease

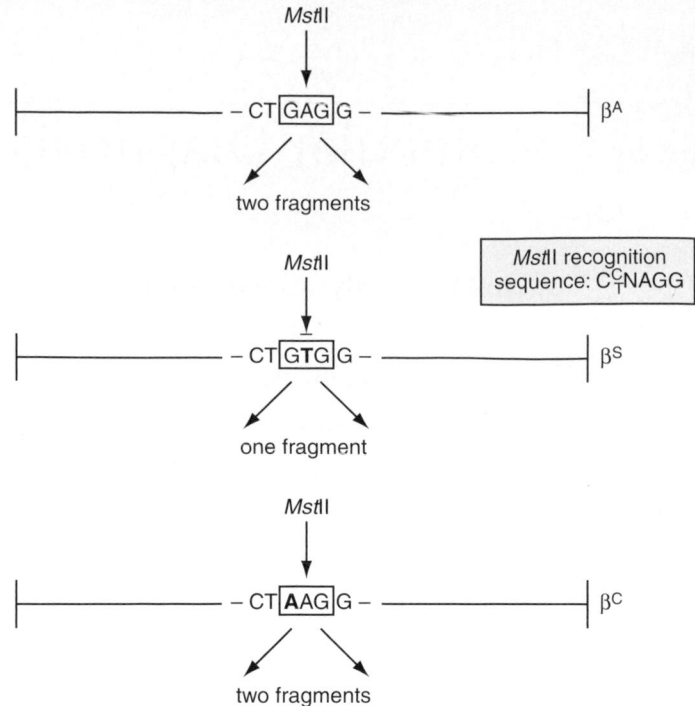

Figure 72–1 Schematic example of detection of a point mutation by differential cleavage with a restriction enzyme. In this case, the sickle cell mutation, substitution of T for A in codon 6 of the β-globin gene destroys an MstII cleavage site so that digestion of a polymerase chain reaction product from the region will produce two DNA fragments in normals but only one fragment in HbS homozygotes. Mutation of the first nucleotide in this codon, found in hemoglobin-C disease, does not destroy the MstII site (since the enzyme can accommodate any nucleotide in this position) and thus cannot be detected by this method.

cleavage site, it can be detected by electrophoretic analysis of PCR products digested with that enzyme (Fig. 72–1). Another option is to hybridize the PCR products with allele-specific oligonucleotide (ASO) probes, short DNA fragments that are precisely complementary to either the normal or mutant target sequence. As discussed in Chapter 66, if the hybridization, usually in a dot or line blot format, is performed under sufficiently stringent conditions, target DNA containing the mutation will hybridize only with the mutant probe, and vice versa for normal target DNA. Several mutation hot spots in a gene can be amplified together by multiplex PCR. As a variation on this approach, any number of allelic probes can be spread out on a solid support for subsequent hybridization with the specimen DNA (or amplicons) in the form of a microarray or in suspension on microbeads. Lastly, a number of commercial reagents and instruments are available that detect point mutations by differential probe/quencher hybridization or by capillary electrophoresis and other sophisticated techniques, as described in Chapters 68 and 76.

To scan a disease gene for unknown mutations that may lie anywhere within it, several screening techniques that cast a wider net are available. SSCP, DGGE, denaturing high-performance liquid chromatography (dHPLC), and other variations of the same principle can theoretically detect point mutations anywhere within a gene because of the altered topology the substituted nucleotides induce in single-stranded or mismatched double-stranded DNA. These approaches obviate the need for separate and specific ASO probes for every possible mutation, although they can only be performed on limited, PCR-amplified stretches of the gene (usually single exons or parts of exons) at one time and they are not 100% sensitive. The protein truncation test detects mutations causing premature termination of the gene's polypeptide product; it requires an involved in vitro transcription/translation approach, and will only pick up 'stop' mutations (and some frameshifts and splicing variants), while overlooking common single nucleotide substitutions (missense mutations). The only technique that should be 100% sensitive in detecting all possible point mutations, at least in theory, is complete DNA sequencing of the gene, although even it will miss mutations that lie outside the usual coding region targets (e.g., in introns, promoters, or enhancer regions).

Disorders due to gene expansion by a trinucleotide repeat mutation can be diagnosed by Southern blot or PCR, in either case by observing a larger-than-normal target DNA fragment. Disorders due to large deletions may be diagnosed by Southern blot by observing loss or decrease in size of a

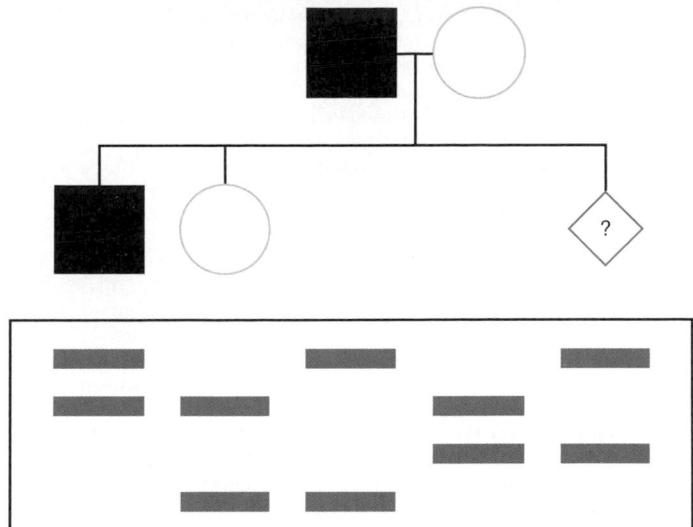

Figure 72–2 Example of restriction fragment length polymorphism analysis for prenatal diagnosis of an autosomal dominant disorder. In this Southern blot, the upper band from the father is the one that co-segregates with the disease phenotype, as seen in the affected son. Because the fetus (?) has also inherited this band, it is predicted to be affected. The precise risk depends on the map distance between the disease gene and the restriction fragment length polymorphism (RFLP) marker.

target fragment, or by PCR, through loss of a product normally amplified from that site or appearance of a new 'junction' fragment.

For those disorders with too many unknown mutations, or an unknown gene, predictive diagnosis by linkage analysis is possible in certain families. Because the analysis requires comparative testing of other affected and unaffected siblings and parents, not every family will be accessible or informative by this approach. Also required is knowledge of closely linked, preferably flanking or even intragenic, polymorphic DNA markers that can be observed to co-segregate consistently with either the normal or disease phenotype within the family. Traditionally, the markers used have been restriction fragment length polymorphisms (RFLPs) detected by Southern blot. More recently, microsatellite polymorphisms – tandem oligonucleotide sequences of variable repeat length – detectable by PCR and gel or capillary electrophoresis have become favored because of their abundance throughout the genome, the multiallelic nature of their polymorphisms, and the relative ease of the testing methodology. Very large genes, such as those for neurofibromatosis and Duchenne muscular dystrophy (DMD), will usually have intragenic microsatellites that can be accessed, minimizing the chances of recombination between the mutation and the marker.

Linkage techniques are less favored than the direct mutation detection approach because of the need to test multiple family members and because meiotic recombination between the gene and the marker can disrupt the apparent phase of linkage between parent and offspring, leading to false-positive or false-negative interpretation of results. For each centimorgan of map distance between the two loci, 1% recombination can be expected (1 cM = 1 million base pairs [bp]). For example, in Figure 72–2 the fetus is predicted to be affected, having inherited the same upper RFLP fragment as the previously affected son. But if the polymorphic restriction endonuclease site being tested is 5 cM away from the disease gene, one can only conclude that the fetus is at 95% risk of being affected.

Choice of Applications

To some extent, the choice of technique will also depend on the application or clinical indication. In medical genetics, these applications fall in five major areas: carrier screening, newborn screening, diagnostic testing, presymptomatic DNA testing, and prenatal testing.

Carrier screening is the term applied to detection of recessive mutations in healthy individuals for purposes of genetic counseling and family planning. This application is further subdivided into screening of those individuals with a family history of the disorder and population-based screening of large numbers of individuals who have negative family history but who may be at risk of the disorder because of its prevalence within their ethnic group or in the population at large. In either case, the ultimate purpose is to identify couples at risk (i.e., both the man and the woman are heterozygous for mutations within the gene) who would then have a 25%

chance of having an affected child with each pregnancy. But the testing strategies chosen for the two groups will differ. Obviously, a person whose sibling has the disorder is at much higher risk of being a carrier than someone in the general population. That person may therefore warrant more aggressive testing (e.g., screening for a greater number of mutations or possibly linkage analysis or even complete gene sequencing) than would be cost-effective for a member of the general population. On the other hand, access to the affected sibling's DNA may allow prior identification of the mutation, which would render subsequent testing of other family members much easier. Population-based screening, in contrast, typically strives to keep the testing procedure as rapid and inexpensive as possible, focusing on perhaps a few of the more prevalent mutations, sacrificing clinical test sensitivity for cost-effectiveness and expediency. And, of course, with negative family history there are no affected family members to make either single-site mutation testing or linkage analysis an option.

Like population-based carrier screening, *newborn screening* aims to identify relatively prevalent (as genetic diseases go) inherited defects in otherwise asymptomatic individuals. And, indeed, the most important disease targets, such as phenylketonuria, galactosemia, sickle cell disease, and cystic fibrosis, are likewise autosomal recessive disorders. In this case, however, the goal is to ascertain affected babies early in life so that treatment (dietary or pharmaceutical) can be initiated before irreversible damage occurs. At the time of this writing, molecular genetic methods in this setting are employed mainly as a backup for confirmation of positives ascertained by less expensive and more comprehensive biochemical or enzymatic methods, but this situation could reverse itself in the future as molecular methods become increasingly automated.

Diagnostic genetic testing is, by definition, performed on a symptomatic individual. Since the DNA tests for genetic disease are absolutely disease-specific and the diseases themselves quite rare, these procedures do not cast a wide enough net to be used for extensive differential diagnosis; the symptoms must be sufficiently suggestive of the disorder in question to justify ordering the test. Also, one must weigh the DNA test against more traditional methods with regard to cost, convenience, and utility. For example, hemoglobin electrophoresis may be more convenient and comprehensive for sorting out a suspected hemoglobinopathy than the specific DNA test for the sickle cell disease mutation. On the other hand, molecular testing may be more advantageous for early or atypical clinical presentations. For example, molecular testing for cystic fibrosis mutations can be performed in the newborn period when traditional sweat chloride analysis is either inconvenient or unreliable. DNA tests also have the advantage of working well post-mortem, when classical biochemical analytes can no longer be assessed.

Presymptomatic DNA testing is applied primarily to late-onset dominant disorders, in which the offspring of an affected parent are aware that they are at 50% risk of having inherited the disease gene and desire to know their status prior to its clinical onset in order to make informed reproductive, employment, and lifestyle decisions or initiate surveillance or preventive interventions. The prototypic disorders in this group are Huntington's disease and the heritable cancer syndromes, although such diseases as neurofibromatosis, Marfan syndrome, adult polycystic kidney disease, and tuberous sclerosis are also relevant. This sort of testing has been the most problematic, from a psychosocial and ethical standpoint, of any in diagnostic molecular genetics, with the risk of severe adverse consequences of results reporting, including suicide. Because of this, established testing protocols include stipulations for informed consent, concurrent clinical assessment, extensive pre- and post-test genetic counseling, and psychosocial support (Huntington's Disease Society of America, 1989; American College of Medical Genetics, 1999).

Finally, there is the clinical application most distinctive of medical genetics: *prenatal testing,* or the detection of disease in the fetus. With a few exceptions (such as hydrops fetalis in homozygous β-thalassemia, thanatophoric dwarfism, and type I osteogenesis imperfecta), most mendelian disorders, especially inborn errors of metabolism, are not expressed either symptomatically or biochemically in the fetus, so predictive diagnosis can only be made at the DNA level. Even for those disorders that might be detected biochemically, DNA often proves to be a far more accessible substrate, from an obstetric point of view, than the affected protein products or metabolic substrates. While molecular analysis can be performed on minute amounts of amniotic fluid or chorionic villus samples collected by routine methods, even if obtained for other purposes, unless the protein product is expressed in fibroblasts (and thus amniocytes), biochemical analysis will require invasive biopsy of deep fetal tissues. For example, assay of phenylalanine hydroxylase activity to diagnose phenylketonuria would require fetal liver biopsy, and quantification of dystrophin to diagnose DMD would require fetal muscle biopsy.

It goes without saying that the primary objective in prenatal diagnosis is the identification of an affected fetus in a timely manner so that a practical option of pregnancy termination can be offered to the couple. While some may argue an advantage for obtaining diagnosis prenatally so that therapy can be instituted promptly at birth, or for psychological reassurance of a couple if the fetus is found to be unaffected, it is difficult to justify the risk of miscarriage from amniocentesis and chorionic villus sampling (CVS) performed for these other purposes. For an affected fetus, unless one intends to initiate therapy in utero, provisional treatment at birth while awaiting neonatal testing is perfectly acceptable.

While prenatal genetic counseling is always nondirective, with moral and/or religious objections to abortion respected, both the clinical counselor and the DNA testing laboratory have a legitimate right and, indeed, responsibility to question the appropriateness of a prenatal test request, with its attendant risk and expense, from a couple for whom termination is not an option (the same would apply to requests coming too late in pregnancy for termination to be performed). It is because of these problems that invasive prenatal testing is not offered as a general population screening tool in women with no family history of the disorder in question. The power of PCR to enable single-cell genetic analysis has recently opened the way for preimplantation diagnosis, usually approached by performing in vitro fertilization and microdissection of a single blastomere from the early embryo. This strategy, initially applied to selected cases at risk for cystic fibrosis (Handyside, 1992) and other disorders, could potentially be offered to any at-risk couple for whom abortion is not an option, although it is not without its own ethical (and economic) objections.

Yet despite all these medical and moral dilemmas, when performed in appropriate circumstances prenatal molecular genetic testing can offer at-risk couples, many of whom have already suffered the trauma of at least one affected child, one of the most valuable services in all of clinical medicine.

Special Concepts Unique to Molecular Genetic Disorders

While the DNA analysis techniques discussed in this chapter for diagnosis of genetic disease are generally the same as those used for molecular diagnosis of cancer or infectious diseases, their application in the former has revealed a number of unusual phenomena that one must keep in mind when dealing with particular hereditary disorders. Some of these concepts were known since Mendel's time but can now be understood mechanistically at the DNA level; others have emerged much more recently as unexpected byproducts of the molecular dissection of specific disease genes.

Molecular Heterogeneity

Precious few genetic disorders are associated with a single mutation consistently identified in all affected cases (e.g., the missense mutation in codon 6 of the β-globin gene causing sickle cell disease). The vast majority of genetic disorders can be caused by more than one – sometimes hundreds – of different mutations within the disease gene (e.g., the *CFTR* gene of cystic fibrosis), and sometimes even by more than one gene (e.g., the *TSC1* and *TSC2* genes of tuberous sclerosis, or the *BRCA1* and *BRCA2* genes of familial breast/ovarian cancer). Obviously, identifying the causative mutations in such disorders is technically much more difficult or sometimes impossible. A corollary of such molecular heterogeneity is that not all of the mutations will produce equally severe disease: some may cause only mild forms or even related syndromes with little resemblance to the classical phenotype (e.g., isolated absence of the vas deferens caused by certain mutations in the *CFTR* gene, or either multiple endocrine neoplasia or Hirschsprung's disease caused by different mutations in the *RET* gene). All of this variability adds greatly to the complexity of genetic counseling and genetic testing.

Variable Penetrance and Expressivity

Penetrance refers to the proportion of individuals who, having inherited a mutant disease gene, will actually display the disease phenotype. Usually applied to dominant disorders, it can produce the striking appearance of 'generation-skipping' in disease pedigrees. This can complicate both molecular diagnostics and genetic counseling, since it may not be clear whether the propositus inherited the disease from a parent or instead represents a new mutation in the family. It is a feature of such relatively common genetic disorders as Marfan syndrome and neurofibromatosis, both of whose genes are identified but not yet easy enough to work with for routine direct mutation detection to replace linkage analysis or mutation scanning techniques in most cases.

Variable expressivity refers to the appearance of different signs and symptoms of a disorder in individuals inheriting the same mutation(s). Like penetrance, it is probably a reflection of differential gene effects within dissimilar genetic backgrounds (in other words, the modulation of phenotypic expression by other nonallelic genes). It, too, makes ascertainment and counseling difficult, and raises ethical issues in considering abortion for diseases of variable and unpredictable severity.

Crossing Over

This phenomenon of meiotic recombination between homologous chromosomes is, in addition to random mutation, the major driving force behind genetic diversity and evolution in sexually reproducing organisms. Its importance in diagnostic molecular genetics lies in its disruption of linkage between a disease gene and a nearby polymorphic marker, producing false-positive or false-negative diagnoses in those disorders tested by linkage analysis. As discussed earlier, the risk can be minimized by choosing markers that are more closely linked to or internal to the disease gene. This has become much more feasible as the human genomic map has become saturated with short tandem repeat polymorphisms that can be accessed easily with PCR primers.

Uniparental Disomy

This unusual cause of a recessive single-gene disorder was first discovered in a cystic fibrosis patient, only one of whose parents was a carrier (Spence, 1988). By DNA haplotyping using polymorphic markers, it was shown that the patient had inherited two copies of the carrier parent's chromosome 7 containing the mutant cystic fibrosis gene and no chromosome 7 from the other parent. The phenomenon has since been observed in other cases of cystic fibrosis and diseases involving other chromosomes as well. For some diseases, such as Prader–Willi and Angelman syndromes (see below), the incidence of uniparental disomy approaches that of classical mutation mechanisms in the molecular pathogenesis, justifying routine testing for this phenomenon.

Imprinting

Imprinting refers to the differential expression of a gene in an offspring, depending on whether it was inherited from the mother or the father, or sometimes on other epigenetic influences (Hall, 1999). Some genes are only expressed or, conversely, turned off, when they pass through the oocyte lineage, and others only when they pass through the spermatocyte line. If an individual inherits the normal allele through the nonexpressing parental line, it cannot counteract a recessive mutation inherited from the other parent. In at least some cases, the molecular mechanism appears to be differential methylation of chromosome regions and regulatory elements. This is the basis for both the deletional and uniparental disomy cases of Prader–Willi and Angelman syndromes (see below).

Anticipation

This term refers to a progressive increase in severity and/or age of onset of a genetic disorder in subsequent generations of a family. It is typically associated with the trinucleotide repeat disorders such as myotonic dystrophy and fragile X syndrome, in which the increasing severity can be correlated with further expansion of the repeat region. In the former disease, especially severe cases with childhood or infantile onset have been born to affected mothers, invoking an influence by imprinting as well (Lopez, 1994). The converse is seen in Huntington's disease, where expansion of the triplet repeat is more likely to occur when it is inherited from the father. It is for these reasons that accurate molecular sizing of trinucleotide repeat lengths is so important for diagnosis and genetic counseling in these disorders.

Epigenetic Influences and Nonmendelian Inheritance

Epigenetic changes are heritable but potentially reversible changes in gene expression that do not represent a change in the sequence of the cell's genomic DNA. The most striking examples of epigenetic inheritance are genomic imprinting (discussed above) and mammalian X-chromosome inactivation, both involving transcriptional silencing of genes by methylation of cytosines at CpG dinucleotides. The methylation status of DNA is maintained following DNA replication by methylases, which act on hemimethylated double-stranded DNA to methylate the newly synthesized DNA strand as well. The process is perpetuated indefinitely in succeeding cell divisions. Recent evidence suggests that de novo methylation of CpG doublets may take place in the promoters of some tumor suppressor genes, silencing these genes and in essence constituting one or both of the 'hits' in a tumor suppressor gene that leads to tumor development (Jones, 1999).

Another category of epigenetic inheritance that is less clearly understood involves the property of some proteins to influence the conformation of newly synthesized or assembled proteins in a self-perpetuating manner. The most notable examples in mammals are the prion diseases, responsible for scrapie and bovine spongiform encephalopathy in animals and kuru and Creutzfeldt–Jakob disease in humans. The disease-producing prion protein, which may result from a coding-sequence mutation in familial cases, is folded into an abnormal conformation and exerts an effect on newly synthesized prions in such a way that it perpetuates and proliferates the conformational abnormality that produces disease.

Allele Frequencies and Mass Population Screening

Reference has already been made to the application of carrier screening for recessive mutations on a population-wide basis. To justify, from a public health standpoint, the effort and expenditure required to perform a DNA test on thousands or millions of people, the incidence of the disease must be sufficiently high, either in the whole population or in the particular racial or ethnic group(s) being targeted for screening. For any autosomal recessive disease of appreciable incidence, the law of Hardy–Weinberg equilibrium predicts that the carrier frequency will be a good deal higher than the prevalence of affected individuals. In addition, the candidate disease target must be sufficiently severe and/or amenable to some medical intervention upon identification. Several disorders would now appear to fit these criteria. Mutations associated with hereditary hemochromatosis and activated protein C resistance (factor V-Leiden) are found in 5–10% of the Caucasian population, while the carrier frequency of the sickle cell mutation approaches 10% in the African American population. Unfortunately, controversies over disease penetrance in the first two and complex socioeconomic issues in the third have limited the application of these genes to screening (Grody, 2003a; Imperatore, 2003). Screening for thalassemia in Mediterranean and Asian populations, and for a panel of recessive disorders such as Tay–Sachs disease and Gaucher's disease in the Ashkenazi-Jewish population, is similarly justified by allele frequencies in the target group. Cystic fibrosis mutations, while of lower frequency, potentially place such a large majority of North American couples at risk that they have been chosen as the first target for general molecular genetic population screening in the United States (see below). This movement of molecular genetic testing out of the realm of rare or esoteric diseases and into the setting of common traits will have a profound effect on preventive medicine and public health, and will drive new developments in DNA test automation in the coming years.

Specific Disease Examples

Cystic Fibrosis

Because of its high carrier frequency in North America and northern Europe, its serious clinical nature, its straightforward mendelian (autosomal recessive) inheritance pattern, and its well studied although quite complex gene, cystic fibrosis has emerged as the paradigmatic disorder for large-scale molecular genetic screening. Within its scope can be found the full panoply of applicable molecular genetic techniques and the full spectrum of scientific and ethical dilemmas arising from the clinical variability of the disease, the extreme molecular heterogeneity of the causative mutations, and the anticipated advent of novel treatments, including gene replacement therapy. With a carrier frequency as high as 1 in 29 in Caucasians of northern European ancestry (and progressively less in southern European people, Hispanic people, African American people, and Asian people), there was ample motivation to screen relatives of patients and even the general population in order to identify couples at 1 in 4 risk of having an affected child with each pregnancy. But since carriers are asymptomatic and have normal sweat chloride levels, this had to await the isolation of the gene in 1989 (Kerem, 1989; Riordan, 1989). While it had been mapped to chromosome 7 some years earlier, allowing for prenatal diagnosis by linkage analysis in informative families, screening and testing in others, especially those with no family history of the disorder, could only be considered once the gene was cloned and the mutations identified.

Even with that laudable accomplishment, however, the history of DNA testing for cystic fibrosis has been fraught with problems and controversies. The gene is over 250 000 bp long and encodes a large ion channel protein called the cystic fibrosis transmembrane conductance regulator (CFTR)

Table 72–1 Recommended Core Mutation Panel for General Population Cystic Fibrosis Carrier Screening

ΔF508	ΔI507	G542X	G551D	W1282X	N1303K
R553X	621+1G>T	R117H	1717–1G>A	A455E	R560T
R1162X	G85E	R334W	R347P	711+1G>T	1898+1G>A
2184delA	1078delT*	3849+10kbC>T	2789+5G>A	3659delC	I148T*
3120+1G>A					

Panel recommended by the American College of Medical Genetics (Grody 2001a)

* Mutations subsequently removed from the panel (Watson 2004)

(Collins, 1992). Most notably, the spectrum of mutations observed is remarkably heterogeneous. While a three-nucleotide deletion of phenylalanine codon 508 (designated ΔF508) accounts for about 70% of the mutations in non-Hispanic Caucasians (and significantly less in other ethnic/racial groups), over 1300 additional mutations have so far been reported. Most of these are so rare that it is neither feasible nor cost-effective to include them in testing panels; only about seven (in addition to ΔF508) account for more than 1% each of cystic fibrosis mutations in most Caucasian populations (Tsui, 1992) (Table 72–1). The sensitivity of carrier screening with mutation panels of between six and 25 alleles ranges from a high of 97% in Ashkenazi Jews (Abeliovich, 1992) to 75–90% in non-Ashkenazi North American Caucasians, about 60% in Hispanic Americans, 50% in African Americans, and less than 10% in Asians (Ober, 1992; Grebe, 1994; Macek, 1997). Such variable and suboptimal sensitivity in an ethnically heterogeneous population like that of the United States, and the difficulties involved in counseling patients as to the residual carrier risk of testing negative, made population-based carrier screening for cystic fibrosis mutations a controversial subject (Wilfond, 1990; Grody, 1999). After much debate and several pilot screening studies, a consensus conference recommended that screening be offered to all pregnant couples and those planning pregnancy (NIH Consensus Statement Online, 1997). A steering committee representing the American College of Medical Genetics, the American College of Obstetricians and Gynecologists, and the National Human Genome Research Institute decided on a core screening panel of the 25 most prevalent mutations in the general mixed population (Grody 2001a). The same group produced accompanying educational materials providing guidance to obstetricians on how the screening test should be offered, patient education brochures, and tables for determining the residual risk in those who test negative.

With the launch of these guidelines in 2001, *CFTR* mutation analysis instantly became the highest-volume molecular genetic test and one of the highest in all of molecular diagnostics. Given such a market, reagent and instrumentation vendors soon came forward with a variety of assays and platforms, which have now largely replaced the in-house methods previously employed by individual laboratories. The commercial methods, which incorporate at least the core panel of 25 mutations, and sometimes more, include ASO probes on paper strips (Fig. 72–3), ARMS, OLA, Invader assay, microbeads, and microarrays (Richards, 2004). In addition, complete gene sequencing is offered by a few laboratories (Strom, 2003), although it is too expensive for general carrier screening and is used primarily to assist in diagnosis of atypical cystic fibrosis cases or to identify parental mutations in affected offspring in order to enable prenatal diagnosis in future pregnancies.

Even several years after launch, the cystic fibrosis carrier screening program continues to prove a challenge for both the referring obstetricians and the genetic testing laboratories. Questions remain about uptake, proper communication of results, the utility of offering extended mutation panels (especially for those couples that test positive–negative in the initial screen), and even which mutations should be included in the core panel. The panel has already been modified once, after early data from national screening indicated that one of the mutations (1078delT) was more rare than previously thought, and another one (I148T) was not a mutation at all but a benign polymorphism; both of these have since been dropped (Watson, 2004).

Another problem with genetic counseling for cystic fibrosis is the variable clinical severity of the disorder and the inconsistency of genotype–phenotype correlations. Beyond the finding that ΔF508 homozygotes tend to have pancreatic insufficiency, there is little about disease severity or complications that can be predicted reliably from knowing an affected individual's two mutations (Cystic Fibrosis Genotype–Phenotype Consortium, 1993). Even homozygotes for ΔF508, considered the prototypical 'severe' mutation, can show a wide range in their degree of pulmonary compromise (Burke, 1992). Conversely, there are mutations

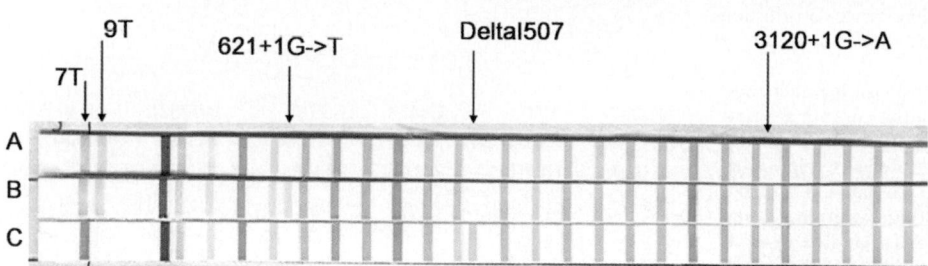

Figure 72–3 Reverse hybridization strips (Roche Molecular Diagnostics, Indianapolis, IN) containing allele specific oligonucleotide probes for the 25 *CFTR* mutations recommended by the American College of Medical Genetics and corresponding normal sequences, plus the intronic polyT tract alleles 5T, 7T and 9T. The genotypes are: A, wild-type 7T/9T; B, compound heterozygous 621+1G>T/3120+1G>A 7T/9T; C, heterozygous delta507 7T/7T.

that cause pulmonary disease yet maintain normal sweat chloride levels (Highsmith, 1994), and there are mutations and polymorphisms (such as R117H and an intronic polythymidine tract) that do not cause cystic fibrosis at all but rather male infertility due to congenital absence of the vas deferens (Anguiano, 1992; Gervais, 1993). Taken together with the ever-increasing median lifespan of cystic fibrosis patients and the eventual advent of effective gene replacement therapies, these factors render genetic counseling and parental decision-making for the disorder quite difficult. Given the molecular and clinical heterogeneity of most genetic disorders, these problems are likely to prove the rule rather than the exception in diagnostic molecular genetics.

Duchenne Muscular Dystrophy

This X-linked progressive myopathy was the first disorder whose causative gene was isolated by the process of positional cloning (Rowland, 1988). Prior to that discovery, the only tests that could be offered to at-risk families were detection of some (but not all) female carriers by the finding of elevated serum creatine phosphokinase levels, followed by prenatal sex determination with the option to terminate a male fetus (even though 50% of these pregnancies would be normal). Genetic counseling was rendered even more problematic because about one third of cases of DMD arise from new mutations.

Even after its discovery, translation to clinical application was not easy because the gene, dubbed 'dystrophin,' proved to be the largest yet discovered, spanning 2.4 million bp and composed of 79 exons (Ahn, 1993). Use of full-length or partial cDNA probes to detect the variety of deletions accounting for two thirds of cases was labor-intensive and time-consuming (Darras, 1988; Prior, 1991). It was only with the advent of multiplex PCR, described in Chapter 67, that a system was developed for rapid and inexpensive identification of more than 98% of dystrophin deletions and their localization to specific exons of the gene (Beggs, 1990; Multicenter Study Group, 1992). In this system a deletion is identified by absence of one or more of the multiple expected amplicons on ethidium-bromide-stained electrophoresis gels or capillary electrophoresis instruments (since a target gene deletion will abolish the hybridization site[s] of one or more primers, causing PCR failure) (Fig. 72–4). Such fine-structure mapping combined with sequencing has also revealed important insights into the molecular pathogenesis of DMD and the milder allelic variant, Becker muscular dystrophy (BMD). While both are most often caused by large dystrophin deletions, those in BMD typically preserve the correct reading frame in the resulting processed transcript, while deletions in Duchenne muscular dystrophy more often produce frameshift mutations and a more truncated protein product (Monaco, 1988).

The remaining one third of DMD patients and 15% of BMD patients in whom no deletion is detected usually have point mutations or microdeletions/insertions. Since the gene is so large, it is not an easy matter to identify these lesions directly, though gene scanning by conformational analysis (SSCP, DGGE) followed by sequencing has been used (Prior 1995; Mendell, 2001). If that fails, one must revert to linkage analysis. This approach is possible only in informative families in which DNA from previously affected individuals is available for study. Early protocols relied on RFLP markers flanking the dystrophin gene; more recently, intragenic microsatellite markers have led to more rapid and accurate PCR-based chromosome haplotyping (Darras, 1987), although there is still a risk of false results from crossover events, owing to the large size of the gene. Alternatively, studies at the protein level can be performed by observing decreased or absent dystrophin in DMD, and dystrophin of abnormal molecular weight in BMD, by Western blot or immunohistochemistry of muscle biopsy tissue (Hoffman, 1988). This procedure has limitations for prenatal diagnosis, for which a fetal muscle biopsy would be required, but it can be used in this setting as well as for proband diagnosis. Thus, the molecular diagnosis of DMD has come full circle: from identification of the gene without knowing the protein product ('reverse genetics') to

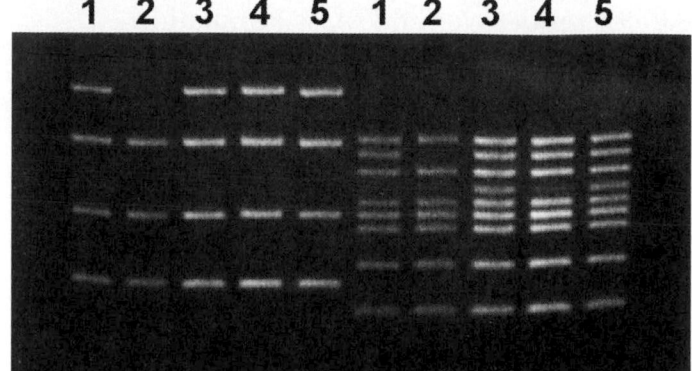

Figure 72–4 Multiplex polymerase chain reaction (PCR) analysis for dystrophin gene deletions in Duchenne muscular dystrophy. DNA samples from five patients were amplified simultaneously with five primer pairs (left half of gel) and nine primer pairs (right half of gel) and the products were analyzed by polyacrylamide gel electrophoresis. Absence of an expected PCR product band is indicative of a deletion. Patient 2 lacks the top band in the five-plex and the second-from-top band in the nine-plex; these correspond to deletions in exons 50 and 48, respectively, in the dystrophin gene. (Band 4 in the nine-plex is light but present in all of the samples.) (Courtesy of Dr Kathryn E. Kronquist.)

identification and diagnostic use of the protein product from knowing the gene. This sort of evolution can be expected in the laboratory diagnosis of many genetic diseases, since functional studies of a gene product are by definition more comprehensive than attempting to track down countless individual mutations at the DNA level.

Sickle Cell Anemia and Other Hemoglobinopathies

Given the long history of study of the protein product, diagnosis of molecular defects in the genes encoding the globin polypeptides did not come about through techniques of 'reverse genetics'; rather, these genes were cloned by classical methods, using antiglobin antibodies for polysome precipitation to isolate the relevant messenger ribonucleic acids (mRNAs). As such, hemoglobin mutations, and the one causing sickle cell anemia in particular, were among the very first to be diagnosed at the DNA level. As it happens, the sickle cell point mutation in codon 6 of the β-globin gene lies within (and thus destroys) a restriction endonuclease cleavage site (for *Ms*II or *Dde*I), providing a rapid method of detection using either Southern blot or restriction enzyme digestion of β-globin PCR products (Hatcher, 1992) (Fig. 72–1). Alternatively, the hemoglobin S and hemoglobin A sequences can be distinguished by dot blot using allele-specific oligonucleotide probes complementary to either the normal or mutant sequence (Conner, 1983). These DNA-based techniques can be used for diagnosis, carrier screening, or prenatal diagnosis on amniocytes, in the latter case obviating the need for invasive fetal blood sampling and classical hemoglobin electrophoresis. In addition, as more states initiate newborn screening programs for sickle cell disease, even if done by biochemical methods, the DNA test becomes important for backup confirmation of positives and ambiguous screening results, as in compound heterozygous states involving HbS and a thalassemia mutation. Several studies have shown that these DNA tests can be done on the same filter-paper blood spots collected for the initial newborn screening (McCabe, 2004). A different mutation in codon 6, causing hemoglobin C disease, does not abolish the restriction endonuclease recognition sequence (because it occurs at a flexible nucleotide position for the enzyme) and so must be distinguished by ASO probes (Maggio, 1993).

The thalassemias involve both qualitative and quantitative alterations in one or more globin chains, and their diagnosis at the molecular level is correspondingly more complex than that of sickle cell anemia. α-Thalassemia is the more straightforward, since it is usually caused by deletion of either or both of the two contiguous α genes on one or the other or both chromosomes 16. This can be detected by Southern blot or PCR, allowing differentiation of the silent carrier state (one α gene missing) from the very severe hydrops fetalis (all four genes missing) and the two intermediate states (Oron-Karni, 1998). Molecular diagnosis of β-thalassemia is more complicated because of the wide variety of promoter, termination, deletion, splice site, and frameshift mutations that have been documented. However, within each at-risk population (Mediterranean, Asian, African), a limited subset of mutations (usually 10 or less) accounts for the majority of cases and carriers. Therefore, testing with a panel of mutation-specific probes/primers, along the lines of cystic fibrosis screening, is reasonable (Naja, 2004). In addition, the β-globin gene is not that large, so sequencing or gene scanning can also be employed.

Hereditary Thrombophilias

Cystic fibrosis is not the only disorder with sufficiently high mutation frequency to consider population screening using molecular methods. Several other disease genes have revealed carrier frequencies at least an order of magnitude higher than that for cystic fibrosis. Included in this group are genes involved in the anticoagulant system, which, as discussed in Chapter 41, keeps the clotting cascade in check. The most notable such allele is the factor V-Leiden mutation, a single nucleotide change causing an amino acid substitution (R506Q) in the clotting factor V protein, rendering it resistant to cleavage by activated protein C (Bertina, 1994). The allele is carried in 5–7% of the Caucasian population and is responsible for over 90% of clinical activated protein C (APC) resistance, resulting in a tendency toward idiopathic venous thromboembolism (Ridker, 1997a). It produces a relative risk of thrombosis of about sevenfold in the heterozygous state and about 80-fold in the homozygous state. It is also associated with pregnancy complications such as recurrent miscarriage. Testing for the mutation is straightforward because, like the sickle cell mutation, it destroys a restriction endonuclease cleavage site (Fig. 72–5), and automated methods for higher throughput have been developed, such as real-time PCR (Louis, 2004) and the 'Invader' assay which relies on signal amplification by fluorescent resonance energy transfer (FRET) and a cleavage enzyme (Ryan, 1999), as described at length in Chapter 67.

As for cystic fibrosis, however, there are controversies over which patients should be offered screening. Despite the dramatically increased relative risk, the absolute risk conferred by this mutation is rather low, with a lifetime penetrance for thrombotic symptoms of about 10%. Most carriers, therefore, would not be candidates for anticoagulant therapy, with its risks of hemorrhage and stroke, and so it is uncertain whether such screening would alter patient management in a meaningful way. Some have proposed screening individuals with environmental risk factors known to act synergistically with the factor V-Leiden risk, such as women on oral contraceptives. Yet here too it could be argued that obligating such women who test positive to turn to less effective methods of birth control might cause more harm than good, increasing the pregnancy rate with its own attendant complications – some of which, ironically, are thrombotic in nature (Kupferminc, 1999). At present, most requests received by molecular genetics laboratories for factor V-Leiden testing are on patients who have already experienced an otherwise unexplained thromboembolic event, and two professional consensus statements, by the American College of Medical Genetics (ACMG) and the College of American Pathologists, have designated this as the primary unequivocal indication for testing (Grody 2001b; Press, 2002).

Along with factor V-Leiden, there are other inherited mutations of high allele frequency that confer thrombotic risk, as also discussed in Chapter 41. The prothrombin 20210A variant, a single nucleotide change in the 3′ untranslated region of the prothrombin gene, results in increased circulating prothrombin levels and a phenotype similar to that of factor V-Leiden; it is present in 1–2% of the general population (Poort, 1996). The 677C→T variant of methylenetetrahydrofolate reductase, an enzyme involved in the folate cycle of homocysteine metabolism, is carried by 30–40% of the general population and is associated with elevated plasma homocysteine levels and risk of vascular (including coronary artery) thrombosis. Indications for this test are even more nebulous, because not everyone with the variant has hyperhomocysteinemia, and not all hyper-homocysteinemia is caused by this variant. Thus, biochemical measurement of plasma homocysteine levels may be a more effective screening method. Also, folate fortification of foods may make the genetic factor less relevant by broadly reducing homocysteine levels in the population. Still, the mutations

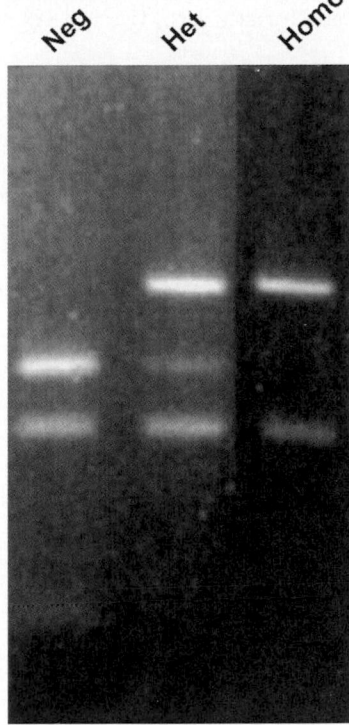

Figure 72–5 Example of polymerase chain reaction (PCR)-based electrophoretic analysis of the factor V-Leiden mutation. A PCR-amplified fragment of the factor V gene encompassing codon 506 will contain two *MnlI* restriction cleavage sites in normal DNA, but only one if the R506Q mutation, which destroys one of the sites, is present. The resulting restriction digest patterns will show two, three, or four bands, respectively, depending on whether the mutation is homozygous (right lane), absent (left lane), or heterozygous (middle lane). The shortest fragment, migrating near the bottom of the gel photo, is often difficult to see.

for each of these factors can act synergistically with one another, so that patients carrying two or even three of these defects, including also the more rare deficiencies of protein S and C, are at greatly increased risk (Koeleman, 1994; Ridker, 1997b). DNA tests for several of these thrombophilia mutations can be multiplexed in a single assay (Louis, 2004).

Trinucleotide Repeat Expansion Disorders

An important class of disease-causing mutations was revealed in 1991 with the discovery that X-linked spinal and bulbar muscular atrophy (Kennedy's disease, SBMA) and fragile X syndrome (FRAXA) are associated with amplification of unstable trinucleotide repeat sequences in the androgen receptor (*AR*) and *FMR1* ('fragile X mental retardation') genes, respectively. Since that time, similar disease-producing mutations have been associated with several additional neurologic and muscle disorders (summarized in Table 72–2), and in the process have provided a molecular classification of the spinocerebellar ataxias. The affected gene in each of these disorders normally contains a repeated sequence of 3 bp – for example, $(CGG)_n$ in the *FMR1* gene – where n is variable but normally limited in its range. In the disease state, however, the size of the triplet repeat is expanded outside the normal range, sometimes only slightly and in other instances markedly. The mechanisms by which these expanded repeat sequences produce disease are various, and include gene silencing and toxic gain of function by mutant proteins.

Fragile XA and Fragile XE Syndromes

FRAXA is the most common single-gene defect causing moderate to severe mental retardation in males. Affected males with this X-linked disorder typically also exhibit dysmorphic features including large ears, a long face, prominent jaw, and macroorchidism. Approximately 1 in 2500 females are heterozygous carriers of the FRAXA mutation, and one third of these may show evidence of mental impairment or learning disability in the absence of the classic dysmorphism seen in affected males.

As explained in Chapter 69, the cytogenetic hallmark of FRAXA is a 'fragile site' on the X chromosome at Xq27.3, resulting from a failure of normal chromatin condensation during mitosis. Although the inheritance pattern of the disease is clearly X-linked, it does not correspond clearly to either a recessive or dominant pattern of gene expression. The most puzzling feature has been the presence of phenotypically normal men ('transmitting males') who are obligate carriers of the genetic abnormality.

CHAPTER: 72 Molecular Diagnosis of Genetic Diseases

Table 72–2 Disorders Characterized by Unstable Expansions of DNA Trinucleotide Repeats

Disorder	Chromosome Location	Normal Alleles, Intermediate Alleles	Expanded Alleles	Anticipation	Transmission Sex Bias	Position of Repeat	Gene Product
Fragile site/mental retardation associated with CGG or GCC expansion (X-linked)							
Fragile X syndrome (CGG), FRAXA	Xq27	6–50 51–200	>200	Yes	Maternal, full mutation	5'-UTR	FMR-1
Fragile X syndrome (GCC), FRAXE	Xq28	6–25	>200			5'-UTR	FMR-2
Diseases associated with CAG repeat expansion (autosomal dominant except for X-linked Kennedy's disease)							
Spinobulbar muscular atrophy (Kennedy's disease)	Xq11–12	11–33	36–62			Coding	Androgen receptor
Huntington's disease	4p16	6–35 36–39	40–121	Marked in juvenile cases	Paternal, early onset	Coding	Huntingtin
Dentatorubral-pallidoluysian atrophy	12p13	3–35	49–85	Yes	Paternal	Coding	Atrophin
Spinocerebellar ataxia 1	6p23	6–44	40–81	Marked in juvenile cases	Paternal, early onset	Coding	Ataxin 1
Spinocerebellar ataxia 2	12q24	16–31	36–64	Yes	Paternal	Coding	Ataxin 2
Spinocerebellar ataxia 3 (Machado–Joseph disease)	l4q24–q31	12–41	55–84	Yes	Paternal	Coding	Ataxin 3
Spinocerebellar ataxia 6	19p13	6–17	21–30	Yes	Paternal	Coding	CACNA1A
Spinocerebellar ataxia 7	3p21–pl2	4–35 28–3	37–>200	Yes	Paternal	Coding	Ataxia-7
Spinocerebellar ataxia 12	5q31–q33	7–28	66–78	Yes	Paternal	5'-UTR	PPP2R2B
Spinocerebellar ataxia 17	6p27	25–42	45–63	Yes	Paternal	Coding	TBP
Diseases associated with CTG expansion (autosomal dominant)							
Myotonic dystrophy	19q13	5–35	50–>200	Yes	Maternal congenital form	3'-UTR	Myotonin protein kinase
Spinocerebellar ataxia 8	13q21	16–92	110–130	Yes	Maternal	Noncoding	
Disease associated with GAA expansion (autosomal recessive)							
Friedreich ataxia	9q13	6–36	200–>900	No		Intron	Frataxin

These men are sons of proven FRAXA carriers, they pass the carrier state to all of their daughters, and their daughters in turn transmit the fully expressed disease to a high proportion of their sons.

The discovery in 1991 of the genetic abnormality that causes FRAXA immediately clarified its unusual pattern of inheritance (Fu, 1991). The 5' untranslated region of the *FMR1* gene at chromosome Xq27.3 carries a $(CGG)_n$ triplet repeat of variable size. In normal individuals, *n* ranges up to about 50, but in individuals with clinically apparent FRAXA, *n* is greater than 200 (referred to as a 'full mutation'). Both men and women who carry an X chromosome where *n* is between 59 and about 200 (referred to as a 'premutation') do not show signs of classic fragile X syndrome, but are at risk of passing an allele of even larger size to their children. This is because of the 'instability' of the premutation alleles and their tendency to increase in size during the meiotic cell divisions that produce the male and female gametes. Alleles of normal size are not unstable and are passed unchanged. Thus it appears that there is a pool of small premutation alleles in the population, possibly of ancient origin, that is at risk of undergoing further expansion with each passage through another generation. As the premutation allele increases in size, the likelihood that it will expand further in the next generation increases, ranging from very low likelihood for repeats in the 60s to almost 100% for repeats above 100 (Nolin, 2003). Alleles with about 51–58 repeats have a tendency to expand into the higher permutation range but apparently not into the full mutation range. Interestingly, expansion to a full mutation only occurs in female meiosis, never in males, which corresponds to the observation that the daughters of normal transmitting males are always phenotypically normal. Figure 72–6B illustrates a family with FRAXA: a premutation allele is transmitted from the first to the second generation, and then expands to a full mutation in the third generation.

The mechanism by which the expanded triplet repeat in the 5' noncoding region of the *FMR1* gene produces the FRAXA phenotype is under active investigation. As the size of the repeat expands, there is progressive methylation of the regulatory region of the *FMR1* gene and decreased expression of FMR-1 protein. This RNA-binding protein is widely expressed in the developing brain and in other tissues. Its loss of expression in FRAXA presumably disturbs normal brain development and leads to mental retardation. Rare patients with typical fragile X syndrome do not have triplet repeat expansion or gene hypermethylation but do have inactivating point mutations leading to loss of FMR1 protein expression. Rare phenotypically

normal or high-functioning males with full *FMR1* gene repeat expansions and cytogenetically visible fragile sites, but with no gene hypermethylation and normal FMR1 protein expression, have also been described (Hagerman, 1994; Smeets, 1995). These findings all support the hypothesis that it is lack of FMR1 protein expression, usually caused by hypermethylation-related down-regulation of gene transcription, that is responsible for the disease phenotype.

Since the premutation is not methylated and the phenomenon of 'normal' transmitting males was widely observed, it was long assumed that these alleles had no direct phenotypic effect. It was therefore quite surprising when more recent studies documented cases of premature ovarian failure and an unusual tremor–ataxia–dementia syndrome in female and male premutation carriers, respectively. The penetrance appears to be about 20% for the former (Sherman, 2000) and as high as 75% for the latter (Jacquemont, 2004). The molecular mechanism may be related to higher *FMR1* mRNA levels in premutation carriers being translated less efficiently and/or interfering with translation of the normal allele or other interacting genes. Obviously, these revelations have made genetic counseling for fragile X syndrome even more complicated. They also raise additional ethical concerns regarding proposals to embark on population screening for fragile X premutations.

Rare families with X-linked mental retardation and a cytogenetically demonstrable fragile site at chromosome Xq27–28, but no hyper-methylation or expansion of the $(CGG)_n$ repeat in *FMR1*, led to the discovery of a second, more distal fragile site at Xq28 associated with hypermethylation and expansion of a $(GCC)_n$ repeat (FRAXE). Most affected males show only mild mental impairment without the dysmorphic features of FRAXA; this plus the extreme rarity of the condition have called into question the indications for testing and screening (Brown, 1996).

Neurodegenerative Disorders: Huntington's Disease, X-linked Spinal and Bulbar Muscular Atrophy, the Spinocerebellar Ataxias, and Dentatorubral-Pallidoluysian Atrophy

Huntington's disease; X-linked spinal and bulbar muscular atrophy (SBMA); the spinocerebellar ataxias (SCA) types 1, 2, 3, 6, 7, and 17; and dentatorubral-pallidoluysian atrophy (DRPLA) are autosomal dominant or X-linked (SBMA) diseases characterized by selective neuronal degeneration in the central nervous system (CNS). In each of these disorders

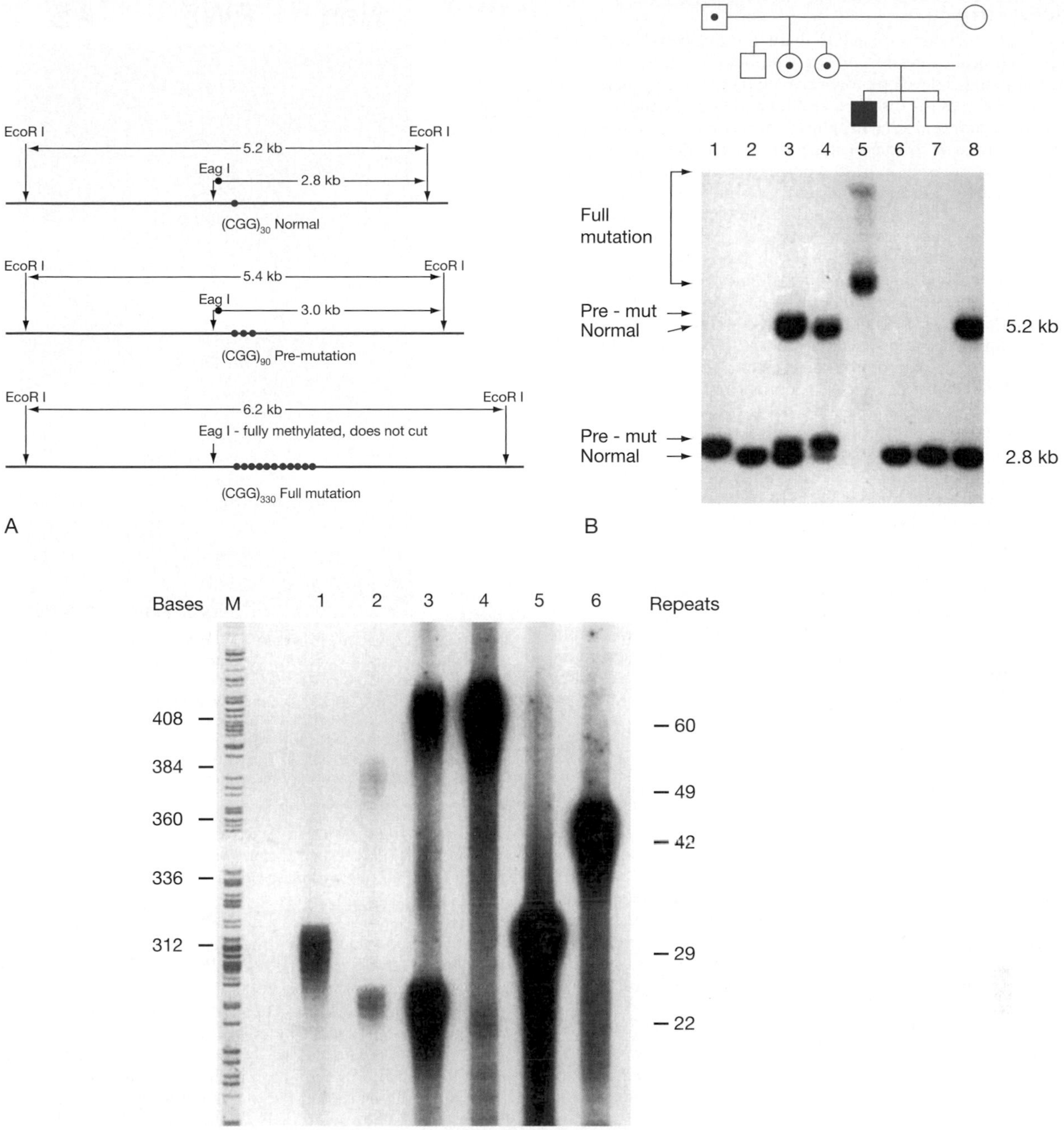

Figure 72–6 Detection of the (CGG)$_n$ repeat expansion in fragile X syndrome. *A*, Diagram of normal, premutation, and full-mutation alleles at the FRAXA locus. When expansion of the repeat to a full mutation occurs, the *Eag* I restriction enzyme site becomes methylated and does not cut with the enzyme. *B*, Family of a patient (darkened square) with fragile X syndrome. A Southern blot of *Eco*R I/*Eag* I-digested DNA from each individual in the pedigree was examined with a labeled DNA probe that hybridizes 3' to the repeat. The three individuals on the right of the figure are normal (open squares and circles). Note that the two males each have a single 2.8 kb band, while the female has both a 2.8 and a 5.2 kb band. This is the expected result. The 5.2 kb band in the female is from the normal inactive (and, therefore, methylated) X chromosome in each of her cells. Since the DNA on this chromosome is methylated, it is not cut by *Eag* I. The 2.8 kb band, however, is from the normal unmethylated active X chromosome (*Eag* I will cut the DNA in this case) in the female and in the males. The affected male has a greatly enlarged band. This is a consequence of marked expansion of the trinucleotide repeat as well as methylation of the *Eag* I restriction enzyme site. The three individuals marked by bold dots are carriers of premutation alleles. In the females, the distinction between normal and expanded alleles is seen most clearly in DNA from their active (unmethylated) X chromosomes. Here, there are distinct bands of 2.8 and 3.0 kb. Higher in the gel the resolution is not as good, and the 5.2 and 5.4 kb alleles are barely separated. Note that in this peripheral blood sample from the mother of the affected patient, X chromosome inactivation is skewed with respect to the repeat expansion: a greater proportion of normal X chromosomes in this cell population have randomly been inactivated compared to the X chromosomes carrying the premutation allele. *C*, Sizing of trinucleotide repeats by gel electrophoresis following amplification of the locus by the polymerase chain reaction (PCR) (Levinson, 1994). Lanes 1 through 6 represent six different individuals; lane M contains a size marker. The PCR products were labeled by incorporation of ^{32}P-dCTP during the amplification reaction and the dried gel was exposed to X-ray film. Heterozygous females show two alleles, males and homozygous females show single alleles. The multiple bands produced with each allele are due to 'slippage' of the DNA polymerase during the PCR reaction; the most intense band is taken as representative of the actual size of the allele. (*C*, courtesy of Dr Anne Maddalena, Genetics & IVF Institute, Fairfax, VA.)

there is expansion of a (CAG)$_n$ trinucleotide repeat in the coding region of a novel gene that produces abnormal elongation of a polyglutamine tract (two other SCA types, 8 and 12, exhibit triplet repeat expansions in untranslated regions of the genes and presumably act by other mechanisms). The resultant abnormal protein produces intranuclear neuronal inclusions. It is postulated that the expanded polyglutamine sequences in each of these proteins leads to alterations in their folding and binding characteristics and a gain in function that is toxic to neurons in a selective manner, causing apoptosis (Everett, 2004). Intranuclear neuronal inclusions, produced by these abnormal proteins, have been demonstrated in several of these disorders.

In common with the other triplet repeat disorders, the expanded repeats in the neurodegenerative disorders are unstable and tend to increase in size in subsequent generations. There is a positive, but not absolute, correlation between increasing repeat size, early disease onset, and clinical severity. In contrast to fragile X and myotonic dystrophy, where the most dramatic increases in repeat size occur in maternal meioses, paternal transmission produces the largest expansions in the exonic repeat neurodegenerative disorders. Consequently, juvenile-onset cases of Huntington's disease, DRPLA, and the SCAs are usually transmitted by the father.

Myotonic Dystrophy

Myotonic dystrophy is an autosomal dominant, multisystem disorder with a wide range of clinical expression. In late childhood or early adulthood, the most typical patients develop progressive myotonia and weakness and atrophy of the muscles of the distal extremities and face. Cataracts, cardiac conduction defects, and testicular atrophy are also common. However, the disease may be so mild as to consist solely of cataracts developing in old age, or so severe as to present at birth with marked muscle degeneration and mental retardation proceeding to early death. Sometimes the full spectrum of the disease can be observed in the same family, occurring in a pattern referred to by geneticists as 'anticipation': the disease becoming more severe, with an earlier age at onset, in succeeding generations. Anticipation is present in virtually all of the trinucleotide repeat disorders but is most striking in myotonic dystrophy, where the clinical phenotype can progress from cataracts to severe congenital disease in three generations.

Myotonic dystrophy is caused by expansion of a $(CTG)_n$ repeat in the 3' untranslated region of the myotonin protein kinase gene on chromosome 19q13.3 (Fu, 1992; Mahadevan, 1992). In normal individuals, this repeat ranges in size from 5 to 35 and is genetically stable. CTG repeats greater than 50 are genetically unstable and prone to expansion as they are passed to subsequent generations. In the range of 50–100 these repeats are often asymptomatic or produce minimal symptoms. When more than 100 repeats are present, the typical myotonic dystrophy phenotype is likely. Although there is a general correlation between repeat length and clinical severity, the size of the repeat is not a reliable prognostic indicator in the individual case. The extreme expansions to 1000–2000 repeats seen in congenital myotonic dystrophy occur only with female transmission of the unstable repeat; thus, congenital myotonic dystrophy is always inherited from the mother.

The mechanism by which the expanded trinucleotide repeat in the myotonin protein kinase gene produces the myotonic dystrophy phenotype is not known. Since the repeat is not located in the coding region of the gene, it is possible that protein expression is altered or that regulatory mRNA interactions are perturbed.

Friedreich Ataxia

Friedreich ataxia is the most common of the hereditary ataxias, with an incidence of 2 per 100 000. Unlike other trinucleotide repeat disorders, Friedreich ataxia is inherited as an autosomal recessive disease and shows no evidence of anticipation. The expanded $(GAA)_n$ repeat is located in the first intron of the *FRDA* gene and reduces the expression of frataxin, a mitochondrial-targeted protein, probably through some interference with transcription or RNA processing. Frataxin is involved in mitochondrial respiration, iron balance, and response to oxidative stress. Some 97% of *FRDA* alleles are due to $(GAA)_n$ expansions; the remaining alleles are due to other inactivating mutations, including point mutations (Lodi, 1999).

Laboratory Testing for Trinucleotide Repeat Disorders

Depending upon the length of the repeat segment, expansions of trinucleotide repeats are readily demonstrated by either Southern blot or PCR. PCR, followed by sizing of the products on an electrophoretic gel or capillary, is generally preferred for most of these disorders because of its speed, simplicity, and ability to resolve alleles differing in size by just one repeat unit. This is of particular importance when it is necessary to differentiate stable alleles at the upper size limit from small premutation or disease-causing alleles. For example, it is critically important to distinguish a 40-repeat from a 39-repeat in Huntington's disease because of the dramatically different clinical implications and the psychosocial impact of a positive result. PCR is also the method of choice for accurate sizing of FRAXA premutation alleles, which is necessary for graded risk counseling of female carriers. However, where triplet expansions are very large, as in fully expressed FRAXA or myotonic dystrophy, it may not be possible to amplify the greatly expanded DNA segment by PCR; in this case, Southern blotting is the preferred technique. Southern blotting is also helpful in determining the methylation status of FRAXA full mutations, through the use of methylation-sensitive restriction endonucleases, and in assuring that a large Huntington's disease or FRAXA allele has not been missed in a patient who appears homozygous 'normal' by PCR. Similarly, it will more reliably identify mosaic males whose cells show a mixture of premutation and full mutation alleles, a not infrequent finding because of the mitotic instability of the full mutation. Figure 72–6 illustrates the use of Southern blotting and PCR to detect full FRAXA mutations and FRAXA premutation alleles.

Prader–Willi and Angelman Syndromes

These two disorders, whose genes lie at approximately the same locus on chromosome 15, are almost always discussed together, even though they

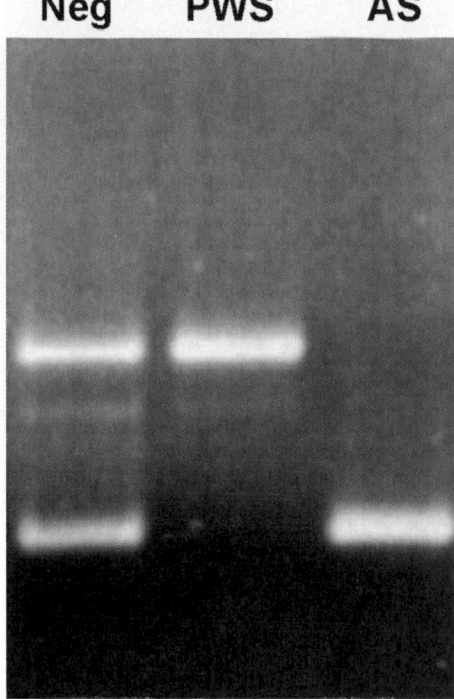

Figure 72–7 Polymerase-chain-reaction-based electrophoretic analysis of methylation patterns in Prader–Willi and Angelman syndromes using the sodium bisulfite method of Kosaki (1997). In Prader–Willi syndrome, only the methylated maternal allele (upper band) is present, due to either deletion of the paternal allele or uniparental disomy for the maternal allele. In Angelman syndrome, only the unmethylated paternal allele (lower band) is present, due to either deletion of the maternal allele or uniparental disomy for the paternal allele. Similar analysis can also be done by Southern blot using methylation-sensitive restriction enzymes.

are caused by two different genes and have almost nothing in common phenotypically. Prader–Willi syndrome (PWS) is characterized by obesity, mental retardation, hypoplastic genitalia, and dysmorphic features, while Angelman syndrome exhibits ataxia, puppet-like facies, mental retardation, paroxysmal laughter, and seizures. What they do share, remarkably, is a powerful imprinting mechanism determining disease expression. Both disorders are almost always sporadic. Prader–Willi syndrome, whose gene is not yet known, is most often caused by a deletion at 15q12 in the paternally inherited chromosome only; this is pathologic because only the paternal *PWS* gene is expressed. The opposite is true for Angelman syndrome, which is most often caused by deletion of a known gene (*UBE3A*) exclusively on the maternally inherited chromosome, which is the only allele normally expressed (Knoll, 1989; Matsuura, 1997). Alternatively, Prader–Willi syndrome can be caused by uniparental disomy for the maternal chromosome 15, which carries only the nonexpressing copy of the gene; likewise, Angelman syndrome can be caused by uniparental disomy for the paternal chromosome 15. These phenomena can be detected by fluorescence *in situ* hybridization (FISH), discussed in Chapter 69, chromosome haplotyping with microsatellite markers, or Southern blotting with methylation-sensitive restriction enzymes that can distinguish the methylated maternal critical region from the unmethylated paternal critical region. More recently, a differential PCR scheme was developed that amplifies either the methylated or unmethylated allele of the nearby *SNRPN* gene within the critical region, based on resistance of methylated cytosines to chemical modification by sodium bisulfite (Kosaki, 1997) (Fig. 72–7). It is important to keep in mind, however, that neither the Southern blot nor PCR method will distinguish between the deletional or uniparental disomy mechanisms, nor will they detect cases (more frequent in Angelman syndrome) due to point mutations within the causative gene. These methods also will not distinguish rare cases of Angelman syndrome or Prader–Willi syndrome due to primary imprinting defects (resulting from aberrant methylation caused by a mutation in the chromosome 15 imprinting center) (Burger, 1997), which would have a much higher recurrence risk.

Familial Cancers

All cancers are genetic disorders at the cellular level, caused by mutations in genes that control cell proliferation and differentiation. These genes may be divided broadly into two groups, those that promote proliferation

Table 72–3 Hereditary Cancer Syndromes

Disorder (OMIM Entry)	Associated Tumors	Population Incidence	Gene	Chromosome Location
Tumor suppressor genes (autosomal dominant mode of inheritance)				
Basal cell nevus (Gorlin) syndrome (109400)	Basal cell carcinoma, medulloblastoma	1/40 000	PTCH	9q22
Cowden syndrome (158350)	Breast, thyroid carcinoma	1/200 000	PTEN	10q23
Familial adenomatous polyposis (175100)	Colorectal, duodenal carcinoma	1/10 000	APC	5q21
Hereditary breast-ovarian cancer syndrome (113705, 600185)	Breast, ovarian, pancreatic, prostate carcinoma	1/300–1/500	BRCA1 BRCA2	17q21 13q12
Hereditary diffuse gastric carcinoma (137215)	Gastric carcinoma	Rare	CDH1	16q22
Hereditary leiomyomatosis and renal cell carcinoma (150800, 605839)	Cutaneous and uterine leiomyomas, papillary renal cell carcinoma	Rare	FH	1q42
Hereditary melanoma (600160, 606719)	Melanoma, pancreatic carcinoma	Unknown	CDKN2A (p16)	9p21
Hereditary paraganglioma (602690, 185470, 602413)	Paraganglioma, pheochromocytoma	Rare	SDHD SDHB SDHC	11q23 1p35–36 1q21
Juvenile polyposis syndrome (174900)	Gastrointestinal cancer	1/100 00	SMAD4 BMPR1A	18q21 10q22
Tumor suppressor genes (autosomal dominant mode of inheritance)				
Li–Fraumeni syndrome (151623)	Sarcomas, breast carcinoma, leukemia, brain tumors	Rare	p53	17p13
Multiple endocrine neoplasia, type 1 (MEN1) (131100)	Pancreatic islet cell, pituitary, parathyroid tumors	1/100 000	MEN1	11q13
Neurofibromatosis type 1 (162200)	Neurofibroma/sarcoma, pheochromocytoma	1/3 000	NF1	17q11
Neurofibromatosis, type 2 (101000)	Acoustic neuroma, meningioma	1/40 000	NF2	22q12
Peutz-Jeghers syndrome (175200)	Gastrointestinal tumors	1/200 000	STK11	19p13
Retinoblastoma, hereditary (180200)	Retinoblastoma, osteosarcoma	1/20 000	RB1	13q14
Von Hippel–Lindau disease (193300)	Hemangioblastoma, renal cell carcinoma, pheochromocytoma	1/40 000	VHL	3p25
Oncogenes (autosomal dominant mode of inheritance)				
Hereditary melanoma (123829)	Melanoma	Rare	CDK4	12q13
Multiple endocrine neoplasia type 2A and type 2B (171400, 162300)	Medullary thyroid carcinoma, pheochromocytoma, parathyroid hyperplasia/adenoma; multiple mucosal neuromas (type 2B)	1/30 000	RET	10q12
Hereditary papillary renal carcinoma (605074)	Papillary renal carcinoma	Rare	MET	7q31
DNA repair genes (autosomal dominant mode of inheritance)				
Hereditary nonpolyposis colorectal cancer (114500)	Colorectal, endometrial, ovarian carcinoma	1/400–1/700	MSH2 MLH1 MSH6 PMS2	2p16 3p21 2p16 7p22
DNA repair genes (autosomal recessive mode of inheritance)				
Ataxia telangiectasia (208900)	Lymphomas, others	1/40 000–1/100 000	ATM	11q22
Bloom syndrome (210900)	Various	Rare	BLM	15p26
Fanconi anemia (607139, 300515, 227645, 605724, 227646, 600901, 603467, 602956)	Acute myelogenous leukemia, others	1/100 000	FANCA-G	Various
MYH-associated polyposis (608456)	Colorectal carcinoma, duodenal polyposis	1/10 000	MYH	1p34
Xeroderma pigmentosum (278700, 133510, 278720, 278730, 278740, 133520, 133530, 603968)	Cutaneous basal carcinoma and squamous carcinoma	Rare	XPA-G, POLH	Various

Source: data from various sources, including Garber, 2005; GeneReviews, 2005.

(proto-oncogenes or, simply, oncogenes), and those that restrain cell growth (tumor suppressor genes). Both sets of these genes are discussed in Chapter 75. Most often, mutations in these genes occur in somatic cells, usually requiring alterations over many cell cycles in several oncogenes or tumor suppressor genes before a cancer develops. However, in some individuals the initial mutation in this progression may be a germline lesion, inherited from a parent and present in every cell of that individual's body.

Heritable cancer-causing mutations have been found most often in tumor suppressor genes, including several groups of genes that encode proteins with DNA repair functions, but have also been found in a few oncogenes (Table 72–3). The inherited mutation should be viewed as the initiating event in tumor development, not in itself sufficient to cause cancer but simply the first step in a series of mutations that ultimately lead to uncontrolled cell growth, analogous to the first somatic mutation that initiates tumor development in a sporadic cancer. It is likely that most of the heritable mutations that contribute to cancer development have not been identified, since they are by themselves not highly penetrant and require the interaction of other genetic and environmental factors to initiate tumor development – a complex situation that is difficult to unravel. However, a number of highly penetrant genes have been identified that are major initiators of tumor development in what are recognizable heritable cancer syndromes (Table 72–3).

In comparison with their sporadic counterparts, hereditary cancers often develop at an earlier age, are frequently multifocal, and appear bilaterally in paired organs. Noting these distinguishing features in sporadic retinoblastoma and familial retinoblastoma, Knudson postulated that at least two mutational events are necessary to produce a tumor (Knudson, 1971). In the case of a sporadic tumor, two independent mutational events in the same cell are necessary to initiate tumor development, whereas in the case of a hereditary tumor, the first mutation is already present at birth in every cell of the body, making it more likely that a second mutational event will occur at an earlier age and often in more than one cell. Knudson's 'two-hit' hypothesis is an important concept that has guided many studies of the genetic basis of cancer. Elucidation of the heritable mutations in the hereditary cancer syndromes has been enormously informative, not only in understanding these rare disorders but in understanding the fundamental changes responsible for common malignancies as well.

In the following discussion, some fundamental concepts of hereditary cancer syndromes are discussed in the context of a disorder caused by a tumor suppressor gene, retinoblastoma, and a disorder caused by an oncogene, multiple endocrine neoplasia type 2. This is followed by descriptions of hereditary breast–ovarian cancer and hereditary colorectal cancer, the most common hereditary cancer syndromes, for which more than a million individuals in the United States are at risk. Table 72–3 lists these disorders and a number of other hereditary cancer syndromes. The section ends with a discussion of current approaches to genetic testing for these disorders. For further information, the reader is directed to two recent reviews of hereditary cancer syndromes (Nagy, 2004; Garber, 2005).

Tumor Suppressor Genes: Retinoblastoma as a Paradigm

Although familial cancer syndromes due to mutations in tumor suppressor genes follow a dominant pattern of inheritance, at the cellular level the changes often appear recessive, since tumorigenesis is initiated (in most cases) only when both copies of the tumor suppressor gene are inactivated. Loss of the normal gene inherited from the unaffected parent may occur as the result of a second novel pathogenic mutation, by large-scale deletion, by replacement with a duplicated copy of the mutant gene inherited from the affected parent by genetic mechanisms such as chromosomal nondisjunction or mitotic recombination, or by gene silencing due to hypermethylation. These events occur in retinoblastoma, a tumor of the retina caused by functional loss of both copies of the *RB1* gene, which encodes the RB protein that is involved in cell cycle and transcriptional regulation. In most cases, both of these mutational events occur somatically and a solitary, sporadic tumor develops. But in approximately one third of the cases, the first *RB1* mutation is present in the germline of the affected child, having been inherited from a similarly affected parent or occurring as a new mutation during gametogenesis. When this is the case, the likelihood that the remaining normal *RB1* gene will undergo mutation in at least one retinal precursor cell is greater than 90%. As Knudson observed, in most patients with familial disease the tumors are bilateral and multifocal (Knudson, 1971), implying that several cells have sustained additional *RB1* mutations. It is not known if *RB1* mutations alone are sufficient for tumorigenesis, but they certainly appear to be the initiating event.

Familial retinoblastoma has served as a model in guiding important cancer research. This has led to the discovery of a large number of tumor suppressor genes that are key determinants of the pathogenesis of several hereditary cancer syndromes, including hereditary breast-ovarian cancer and hereditary colorectal cancer. These tumor suppressor genes are also critical to the development of many common sporadic cancers.

Oncogenes: Multiple Endocrine Neoplasia Type 2 as a Paradigm

There are just a few familial cancer syndromes that are known to be caused by a heritable mutation in an oncogene (Table 72–3). Of these, multiple endocrine neoplasia type 2A (MEN 2A) and its variants, familial medullary thyroid carcinoma (FMTC) and multiple endocrine neoplasia type 2B (MEN 2B), are best known. Single, activating mutations in just one allele of the proto-oncogene *RET* are sufficient to initiate tumorigenesis in these disorders (Eng, 1999).

All three of these syndromes are characterized by hyperplasia of thyroid C cells and medullary thyroid carcinoma. In families afflicted with MEN 2A, pheochromocytomas and/or parathyroid adenomas or parathyroid hyperplasia are also present. MEN 2B is further characterized by the presence of multiple mucosal neuromas of the lips, mouth, and gastrointestinal tract, a marfanoid habitus, a particularly aggressive clinical course, and a high proportion of affected individuals due to new *RET* mutations.

RET is a signaling molecule with extracellular receptor and intracellular tyrosine kinase domains. With few exceptions, the known FMTC and MEN 2A mutations are single base substitutions in one of five codons in the extracellular domain, in each case producing substitution of a cystine by another amino acid. More than 95% of the MEN 2B mutations are identical, consisting of a single base substitution producing a missense mutation in the tyrosine kinase domain. Mutations have not been found in fewer than 5% of the families affected with one of these disorders (Eng, 1999).

Hereditary Breast–Ovarian Cancer

Hereditary breast–ovarian cancer (HBOC) affects more individuals than any other hereditary cancer syndrome (Narod, 2004). It is caused by germline mutations in *BRCA1* and *BRCA2*, autosomal tumor suppressor genes with roles in DNA repair, transcription regulation, and cell cycle control. The combined carrier prevalence of abnormal variants of these two genes in the general US population is generally estimated to be 1/500–1/300. Three founder mutations in Ashkenazi Jews are responsible for increasing the prevalence 10-fold (1/40) in this population. HBOC accounts for 5–10% of female breast cancer cases and 12% of ovarian cancer cases. Whereas the lifetime risk to women of developing breast or ovarian cancer in the general population is 7% and 1%, respectively, the risk to mutation carriers is 56–87% for breast cancer (the risk of a second, contralateral cancer approaches 60%) and 23–54% for ovarian cancer. Other cancers, especially breast cancer in men, pancreatic cancer and prostate cancer are more prevalent as well. Characteristically, tumors occur at an earlier age than their sporadic counterparts, with average age of diagnosis of breast cancer in the 40s compared to the average age of diagnosis of sporadic breast cancer at age 64. Development of breast cancer at an early age is one of the strongest predictors of the presence of HBOC.

BRCA1 and *BRCA2* are both large genes, encoding proteins of 1863 amino acids and 3418 amino acids, respectively. Disease-causing mutations, mostly frameshift or nonsense mutations which cause protein truncation, are distributed widely across both genes. To date, more than 700 unique deleterious *BRCA1* mutations and almost 800 deleterious *BRCA2* mutations have been identified. Although the presence of founder mutations permits a targeted approach to mutation identification in Ashkenazi Jews, whole-gene sequencing or gene scanning techniques are required for mutation detection in the heterogeneous general US population.

Genetic testing for *BRCA1* and *BRCA2* mutations in high-risk patients and family members has moved into clinical practice. Effective cancer prevention strategies for mutation carriers (increased surveillance, chemoprevention, prophylactic surgery) have markedly reduced the incidence of ovarian cancer and of primary and secondary breast cancers (Narod, 2004). Individuals at high risk can be identified by their personal history of ovarian or early-onset breast cancer in women or breast cancer in men, and/or by a family history of these cancers in either the paternal or maternal lineages (National Comprehensive Cancer Network, 2005). Since HBOC is an autosomal dominant disorder, first-degree relatives of mutation carriers have a 50% risk of carrying the same mutation.

The Hereditary Colorectal Cancer Syndromes

Hereditary nonpolyposis colorectal cancer (HNPCC, or Lynch syndrome), as its name implies, is a hereditary colorectal cancer syndrome that is not associated with an abundance of adenomatous polyps. In contrast, familial adenomatous polyposis (FAP) and MYH-associated polyposis (MAP) are hereditary disorders in which variable and sometimes large numbers of adenomatous polyps may be present. This useful, if imperfect, clinical distinction is an important guide to the evaluation of individuals who are at risk for these disorders.

Hereditary Nonpolyposis Colorectal Cancer

HNPCC is the second most common hereditary cancer syndrome, affecting almost as many individuals as are affected by hereditary breast–ovarian cancer. However, since it is almost equally penetrant in both sexes, its public health impact is equivalent to that of HBOC. Notably, and often unrecognized, endometrial cancer is a prominent part of the syndrome, with more affected women developing endometrial cancer than colorectal cancer. HNPCC accounts for 3–5% of all colorectal cancers and 2–3% of all endometrial cancers. The disease is caused by germline mutations in one of five DNA mismatch repair genes, *MSH2*, *MLH1*, *MSH6*, *PMS2* and *PMS1*, each contributing roughly 50%, 40%, 10%, <1% and <1%, respectively, to the overall incidence of the disorder. The combined carrier prevalence of abnormal variants of *MSH2* and *MSH1*, which account for approximately 90% of HNPCC, is estimated to be between 1/700 and 1/400. Colorectal cancer in HNPCC is characterized by early age of onset (average 44 years, compared to 72 years for sporadic colorectal cancer), occurs predominantly on the right side of the colon, and may occur as multiple primary tumors simultaneously or over a period of time. The lifetime risk to men and women of developing colorectal cancer is approximately 80% (compared to a 2% lifetime general population risk), while the lifetime risk of endometrial cancer is 40–60% (compared to a 1.5% lifetime general population risk). The lifetime risks of gastric cancer, 13%, and of ovarian cancer, 12% (compared to 1% for the general population), are also increased.

A number of guidelines for identifying individuals at risk for HNPCC have been described that use a combination of personal and family history of cancer, for example, the Amsterdam Criteria and Bethesda Guidelines (Giardiello, 2001; GeneReviews, 2005). Early-onset colorectal cancer and/or endometrial cancer are the strongest predictors of the disorder, particularly when they are seen together in an individual or family, are accompanied by other tumors associated with the disease, and occur in more than one generation of the family.

Another predictor of HNPCC in a patient is the presence of 'microsatellite instability' in the DNA of that individual's colorectal cancer. The term describes an alteration in the length of repeat DNA sequences (microsatellites) in the tumor due to mismatch repair errors during DNA replication. Microsatellite instability is highly sensitive but has low specificity in detecting colorectal cancer due to HNPCC, but when combined with immunohistochemistry to detect absence of one or more of the mismatch repair proteins, is a useful indicator that germline genetic testing for HNPCC is indicated (GeneReviews, 2005).

The DNA mismatch repair genes are moderately large genes, with MSH2 encoding a protein of 935 amino acids and MLH1 encoding a protein of 757 amino acids. Although there are a few mutations that have a high relative prevalence in some populations due to founder effects, the vast majority are distributed widely across both genes. Most mutations are frameshift or nonsense mutations that cause loss of gene expression due to RNA instability, protein instability or protein truncation. In addition, large deletions of single or multiple exons account for approximately one third of the mutations present in MSH2 and for a smaller fraction of the mutations in MLH1.

Genetic testing for MSH2 and MLH1 mutations in high-risk patients and family members has moved into clinical practice in a manner similar to that which has occurred for BRCA1 and BRCA2 testing for HBOC. For those individuals who are identified as carrying deleterious mutations, complete colonoscopy, beginning at an early age and at regular intervals, is very effective at identifying premalignant adenomatous polyps, while endometrial biopsy and transvaginal ultrasound may identify early endometrial cancer. If colorectal cancer does develop, subtotal colectomy may be considered as an alternative to segmental resection because of the high rate of synchronous and metachronous tumors in patients with HNPCC. Prophylactic hysterectomy–bilateral salpingo-oophorectomy may be considered in women who have completed their families. As in all autosomal dominant disorders, first-degree family members of mutation carriers have a 50% risk of also carrying that mutation.

Two reviews of HNPCC that discuss genetic testing are recommended (Giardiello, 2001; GeneReviews, 2005).

Familial Adenomatous Polyposis and Attenuated Familial Adenomatous Polyposis

Familial adenomatous polyposis is a hereditary colorectal cancer syndrome that can present with a striking phenotype in the colon – multifocal colorectal cancer in a background of thousands of adenomatous polyps. It is now recognized that the FAP phenotype is diverse and the number of colonic polyps can vary markedly. Accordingly, 'classical' FAP is now diagnosed when an individual develops at least 100 adenomatous polyps over his/her lifetime, while 'attenuated' FAP (AFAP) is the term applied to a patient whose lifetime polyp burden is in the range of 20–100 polyps. The distinction is entirely clinical, since both disorders are caused by germline mutations in the APC (adenomatous polyposis coli) gene, a tumor suppressor gene with several important cellular functions and a likely initiator of sporadic colorectal cancer development as well. Germline APC mutations are carried by 1/10 000–1/5 000 individuals; most of these mutations have been inherited from a similarly affected parent but 20–30% are de novo mutations. Accordingly, FAP or AFAP cannot be ruled out because of an absence of a positive family history, which is particularly important to keep in mind when assessing a patient with a low polyp burden.

Early onset colorectal cancer (average age 39 years for FAP, ≈50 years for AFAP) requires early diagnosis and close clinical monitoring for individuals determined to be at risk by family history and/or genetic testing. Screening sigmoidoscopies should be started at age 10 and prophylactic colectomy performed when polyps have developed. For individuals at risk for the less florid AFAP, screening may begin later in the teens, but colonoscopy is advised because polyps preferentially develop in the right side of the colon. Colectomy is performed when the polyp burden is no longer manageable by polypectomy. Upper gastrointestinal surveillance is also indicated since gastric and small bowel polyps also develop. This is particularly important in the duodenum, especially in the periampullary region, where the lifetime risk of progression to cancer is 5–12% for FAP.

Patients with FAP and AFAP are also at higher risk for a number of other cancers (gastric, pancreatic, biliary tract, thyroid) and frequently have other clinical findings: desmoid tumors, osteomas, dental abnormalities, epidermoid cysts, and congenital hypertrophy of the retinal pigmented epithelium (CHRPE). Of these, desmoid tumors, affecting approximately 10% of patients with FAP, are the most important. These clonal proliferations of myofibroblasts form in the abdominal wall or the abdominal cavity where they are locally invasive, compress abdominal organs, and may cause serious morbidity and mortality.

APC is a large gene, encoding a protein of 2843 amino acids. Most disease-causing mutations are frameshift or nonsense mutations producing protein truncation. These mutations are distributed widely along the gene. Some genotype–phenotype correlations are possible: mutations that produce extraintestinal features tend to map to particular regions of the gene, while those that are associated with AFAP cluster in the 5' and 3'-most regions of the gene.

Genetic testing for APC mutations is appropriate for members of families in which this disorder is known to occur as well as for individuals without a significant family history who have a large number of adenomatous polyps, since 20–30% of FAP/AFAP patients have de novo mutations.

Two reviews of FAP that discuss genetic testing are recommended (Giardiello, 2001; GeneReviews, 2005).

MYH-associated Polyposis

MYH-associated polyposis is a recently recognized autosomal recessive hereditary cancer syndrome caused by mutations in the human homolog of the bacterial mutY gene, MYH (Al-Tassan, 2002; Wang, 2004). The clinical phenotype is very similar to that of AFAP or the less florid variants of FAP, that is, a polyp burden in the tens to hundreds, not thousands. As with FAP/AFAP, patients are at risk for duodenal polyposis and some have been reported to have some of the extraintestinal manifestations, CHRPE and osteomas, as well. Because of the autosomal recessive nature of this disorder, MAP families typically show no evidence of vertical transmission of the disease, as would be true for the autosomal dominant FAP/AFAP, but might include affected siblings. It is estimated that the carrier frequency for mutant MYH alleles is approximately 2%, which implies a 1/10 000 frequency of biallelic (affected) individuals. This is very similar to the number of patients who have FAP/AFAP.

The close similarity of the MAP and FAP/AFAP phenotypes, and the fact that as many as 30% of individuals with FAP have no evidence of vertical transmission in the family because they carry de novo APC mutations, can make diagnosis difficult, especially when the polyp burden is not large. In many cases it is necessary to perform mutation analysis for both APC and MYH to arrive at a diagnosis.

MYH is one of a group of base excision repair genes that recognize and repair the misincorporation of 8-oxoguanosine during DNA replication. In the absence of repair, G:C→T:A mutations occur. Biallelic inactivation of MYH allows these mutations to accumulate and, in the colonic epithelium, leads to biallelic inactivating mutations in APC. This initiates a series of mutational events that result in a clinical phenotype very similar to AFAP or FAP (Al-Tassan et al, 2002).

The mutation spectrum in MYH has just begun to be explored. There are two common mutations in European populations, Y165C and G382D, that account for most of the known deleterious mutations in that population. Importantly, in the few non-European individuals with polyposis syndromes in which biallelic mutations were detected, neither of these mutations was present. Accordingly, effective detection strategies are still being developed. Whole gene sequencing is one approach. Another approach, which has been used in individuals of European descent, is initial screening for the two common mutations, followed by whole gene sequencing if just one of the common mutations is detected.

Laboratory Testing for Familial Cancer Mutations

DNA analysis for heritable, cancer-predisposing mutations has enormous potential for disease prevention and early treatment. If a very high proportion of the cancer-causing mutations in a particular gene are known, and these mutations are relatively few in number, direct analysis for these mutations may be simple and inexpensive. Fortunately, this may sometimes be the case with an oncogene, since activation of the gene can only be achieved in a limited number of ways. As mentioned above, the spectrum of mutations in RET that are responsible for MEN 2 is quite small, with just a handful of well-defined mutations accounting for more than 95% of the total.

If, on the other hand, the gene is large, and cancer-causing mutations are numerous and widely dispersed (which is commonly the case with tumor suppressor genes, since they can be inactivated in many different ways), then mutation analysis must of necessity be less targeted and be capable of screening large stretches of DNA. In that case, direct DNA sequencing or gene scanning techniques such as DHPLC, SSCP, or heteroduplex analysis must be used. In addition, whole exon deletions or duplications, or even whole gene deletions that are not detectable by sequencing or gene scanning may constitute a significant percentage of the deleterious mutations in a particular gene. In this case, techniques that are capable of assessing gene dosage, such as Southern blotting, some variation of quantitative PCR, or a hybridization platform that is capable of measuring sequence dosage in a comparative way, must be used.

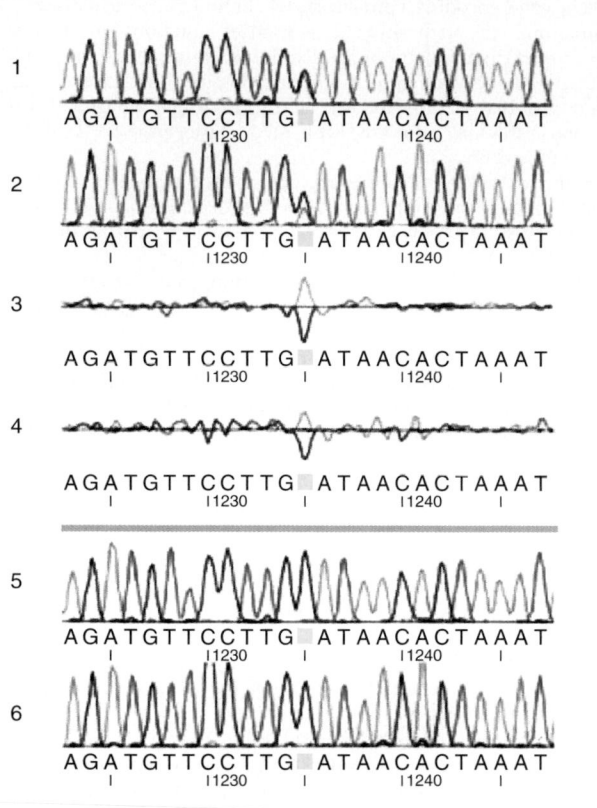

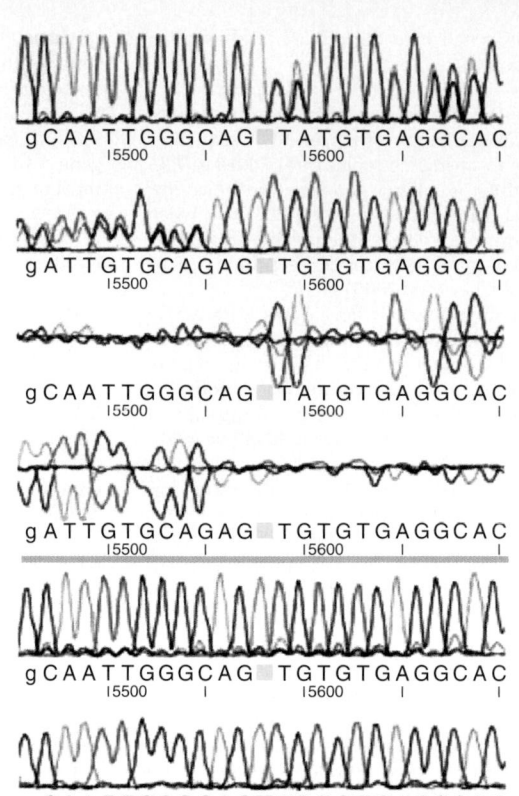

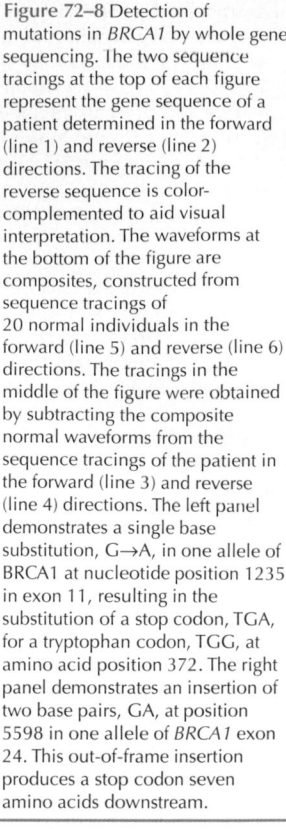

Figure 72–8 Detection of mutations in *BRCA1* by whole gene sequencing. The two sequence tracings at the top of each figure represent the gene sequence of a patient determined in the forward (line 1) and reverse (line 2) directions. The tracing of the reverse sequence is color-complemented to aid visual interpretation. The waveforms at the bottom of the figure are composites, constructed from sequence tracings of 20 normal individuals in the forward (line 5) and reverse (line 6) directions. The tracings in the middle of the figure were obtained by subtracting the composite normal waveforms from the sequence tracings of the patient in the forward (line 3) and reverse (line 4) directions. The left panel demonstrates a single base substitution, G→A, in one allele of BRCA1 at nucleotide position 1235 in exon 11, resulting in the substitution of a stop codon, TGA, for a tryptophan codon, TGG, at amino acid position 372. The right panel demonstrates an insertion of two base pairs, GA, at position 5598 in one allele of *BRCA1* exon 24. This out-of-frame insertion produces a stop codon seven amino acids downstream.

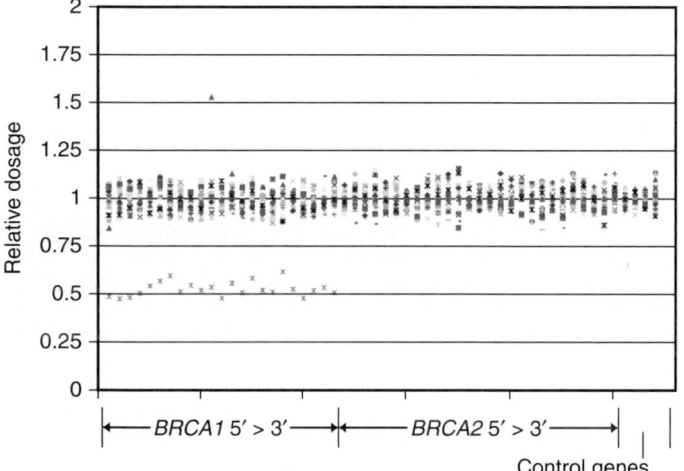

Figure 72–9 Detection of large deletions and duplications in *BRCA1* and *BRCA2*. 23 genomic regions in *BRCA1* and 26 regions in *BRCA2* were interrogated at at least two separate loci in a series of multiplex polymerase chain reactions designed to assess relative dosage. Data from these loci were combined into a single data point. Each multiplex reaction consisted of approximately equal numbers of targets in *BRCA1* and *BRCA2*. The scatterplot illustrates gene dosage across all exons of *BRCA1* and *BRCA2* (displayed 5'–3'), and four control loci in 32 patient samples. A value of 1.0 indicates a normal complement of two genomic copies. A value of 0.5 indicates the presence of just one genomic copy (a deletion). A value of 1.5 indicates the presence of three genomic copies (a duplication). Data points from each patient are represented by unique symbols. In this figure, one patient carries a deletion of the entire *BRCA1* gene, represented by symbols (blue x) from all 23 exons clustering near the 0.5 relative dosage line. A second patient carries a duplication of BRCA1 exon 13, represented by the single symbol (red triangle) at the 1.5 relative dosage line. The remaining 12 patients have normal dosage at each locus.

acids downstream, again resulting in a truncated, nonfunctional protein. Figure 72–9 illustrates a multiplex PCR-based assessment of relative sequence dosage across all exons of BRCA1 and BRCA2. Each exon is interrogated at at least two separate loci and the data are combined into a single data point. A whole gene deletion of BRCA1 is represented as one-half normal dosage along the entire length of BRCA1, while a duplication of BRCA1 exon 13 is represented by a single data point at one and a half times normal dosage. While these approaches can be time-consuming and costly, once a mutation is identified in an affected individual, subsequent testing of other members of the family is relatively simple and inexpensive, since it can be directed specifically at that abnormality.

A further complication of mutational analysis of cancer predisposition genes relates to the functional significance of some mutations that may be found. Whereas protein-truncating and splice site mutations in tumor suppressor genes are usually significant, missense mutations that produce a conservative amino acid substitution are likely to be benign. And yet this cannot be concluded with certainty, since even synonymous mutations (base changes that do not cause an amino acid substitution) may affect RNA splicing, particularly if they occur close to the exon–intron boundary. So other lines of evidence must be used as well, such as co-segregation of the mutation with cancer in families, case control studies, amino acid conservation across species, and functional analyses. Since each single line of evidence may not in itself allow accurate mutation classification, means must be found to integrate these data into a clinically useful prediction. In clinical laboratory practice, mutation classification often presents a greater challenge than the analytical methods used to obtain the data.

Finally, genetic testing for cancer risk is especially useful if the results can positively affect clinical management. Fortunately, as discussed above, effective measures can be taken to prevent or minimize the risk of cancer development in many hereditary cancer syndromes, including those that most frequently affect a large number of individuals.

Hemochromatosis

Hereditary hemochromatosis, first recognized in its full clinical expression as the triad of cirrhosis, diabetes mellitus, and bronzing of the skin, was originally thought to be a rare disorder of iron overload affecting about 1 in 5000 or fewer Caucasians. However, when genetic studies linked the disease-causing gene to the HLA locus on chromosome 6, and biochemical tests of iron overload (principally transferrin saturation) were utilized, it was recognized that the underlying genetic predisposition to iron overload was extremely common. Indeed, hereditary hemochromatosis is now recognized as an autosomal recessive disorder with a carrier frequency as high as one in eight in people of northern European descent, making it the most

Figure 72–8 illustrates the sequence tracings of two examples of deleterious mutations in *BRCA1*. The left side of the figure demonstrates a single base substitution, G→A in one allele of *BRCA1* at nucleotide position 1235, resulting in the substitution of a stop codon, TGA, for tryptophan, TGG, at amino acid position 372 in exon 11. This mutation produces a truncated, nonfunctional protein, or may result in an unstable RNA that is degraded. The right side of the figure demonstrates an insertion of two base pairs, GA, at position 5598 in one allele of *BRCA1* exon 24. This out-of-frame insertion produces a stop codon seven amino common genetic disorder in the US Caucasian population. The incidence of at-risk homozygotes is 1 in 250, but only a fraction of these accumulate sufficient excess iron to produce the tissue injury associated with the classical disorder.

Our understanding of hereditary hemochromatosis entered a new era with the identification of the *HFE* gene (initially called *HLA-H*) within the major histocompatibility locus on chromosome 6 (Feder, 1996). The HFE protein, although it is a major histocompatibility complex class I-like molecule, does not bind and present endogenous peptides and is not thought to have an immunologic function. Rather, as discussed in Chapter 21, evidence is accumulating that the HFE protein interacts with the transferrin receptor and modulates enteric absorption of dietary iron (Waheed, 1999). Mutations in *HFE* impair this regulatory function, leading to excess iron absorption and storage in tissues.

As noted in Chapter 21, a single missense mutation in *HFE*, C282Y, which results in a tyrosine substitution for cystine at amino acid 282 in the HFE protein, is present in the homozygous state in 80–90% of Caucasians with hemochromatosis. An additional small percentage of hemochromatosis patients are compound heterozygotes, carrying one chromosome with a C282Y mutation and another with an H63D mutation. H63D is a common polymorphism, with a carrier frequency of approximately 20%, and its association with iron overload is very low (1–2%) in the compound heterozygous state and probably even lower when homozygous (Gochee, 2002). Recently the penetrance of the C282Y homozygous state has also been questioned, and may be appreciably lower than the 80% earlier quoted, perhaps as low as 10% or even 1% (Beutler, 2002; Pietrangelo, 2004). For this reason, population screening of individuals with no clinical or biochemical signs of hemochromatosis for these mutations has not been recommended. As for factor V-Leiden, the DNA test is best reserved for differential diagnosis in patients already exhibiting the clinical disorder or elevated transferring saturation detected on biochemical screening.

The C282Y and H63D mutations are single-nucleotide substitutions and may be analyzed easily by a variety of PCR, real-time PCR, microarray, microplate, or sequencing methods.

Spinal Muscular Atrophy

Spinal muscular atrophy is an autosomal recessive motor neuron disorder characterized by proximal muscle weakness and wasting. The most severe form, type I (also called Werdnig–Hoffmann disease), presents with hypotonia in infancy and early childhood death due to respiratory failure. Intermediate and atypical forms are also described. The disease is caused by mutations in the *SMN1* gene on chromosome 5q13. With a carrier frequency of 1 in 50, spinal muscular atrophy is one of the more common lethal recessive disorders, approaching the incidence of cystic fibrosis.

The majority (95%) of affected patients exhibit loss of the *SMN1* gene, either through complete gene deletion or through a gene conversion event involving sequences in the adjacent *SMN2* gene which differs by a single nucleotide in exon 7. The *SMN2* gene is believed to be nonessential since both alleles are absent in 5–10% of normal individuals, yet is partially protective as demonstrated by the finding of higher *SMN2* copy number in patients with less severe forms of the disease (Mailman, 2002). The presence of this closely homologous gene has necessitated the development of meticulously designed allele-specific PCR/restriction endonuclease assays to determine homozygous deletion of *SMN1* in the presence of *SMN2*. Identification of carriers, based on *SMN1* gene dosage analysis, is even more challenging, and requires the use of quantitative or real-time PCR methods (Ojino, 2004b). The small percentage of patients not showing loss or conversion of both *SMN1* genes usually carry a small intragenic mutation in one allele, of which a large number have been reported. These can be detected by sequencing or by multiplex allele-specific PCR assays (Mailman, 2002).

Mitochondrial DNA Disorders

In addition to the 6 billion bp of DNA that comprise the human nuclear diploid genome, vital genetic information is also encoded in DNA molecules carried by the mitochondria. These 16 500 bp, double-stranded circular DNA molecules are present in 2–10 copies in each of the up to several hundred mitochondria of the cell. Mitochondrial DNA codes for 13 of the proteins of the respiratory chain and adenosine triphosphate (ATP) synthase, 22 transfer RNAs required for their translation, and two ribosomal RNAs. Mitochondrial DNA is self-replicating and is transmitted strictly by maternal inheritance, since the mitochondria of a spermatozoon are not incorporated into the zygote upon fertilization of an ovum.

Disease-causing abnormalities of mitochondrial DNA may result from several different mechanisms (Servidei, 2002). Single large deletions (and, rarely, duplications) that apparently occur sporadically in oogenesis are typical of Kearns–Sayre syndrome, a myopathy characterized principally by

progressive external ophthalmoplegia and pigmentary retinopathy. A wide range of disorders are characterized by multiple small deletions and show typical mendelian autosomal dominant or autosomal recessive patterns of inheritance, apparently because they are due to undefined defects in nuclear genes important for mitochondrial DNA replication. Most distinctive from a genetic point of view are the disorders that follow a pattern of strict maternal inheritance, never showing transmission from an affected male and passing from an affected female equally to her sons and daughters. These diseases are most often due to point mutations in one of the genes encoding a transfer RNA (e.g., myoclonic epilepsy and ragged red fibers [*MERRF*) and mitochondrial myopathy, encephalopathy, lactic acidosis, and stroke-like episodes [*MELAS*]) or a mitochondrial protein (e.g., Leber's hereditary optic neuropathy [*LHON*]). In addition to the inherited encephalomyopathies, there is growing evidence that tissue-specific accumulations of somatic mitochondrial mutations may contribute to the development of many common late-onset degenerative disorders, and perhaps to aging itself.

Laboratory confirmation of the large mitochondrial DNA deletions often present in Kearns–Sayre syndrome is easily accomplished by Southern blot analysis of mitochondrial DNA from affected tissues using labeled whole mitochondrial DNA as a probe. Point mutations in other disorders may be analyzed by a number of techniques. Often the clinical presentation will guide the choice of mutation panel testing in a stepwise fashion, as particular mutations are associated with each of the major syndromes (e.g., missense mutations G11778A, T14484C, and G3460A with LHON). If these tests are negative, one can proceed to a second-tier panel or to complete mtDNA sequencing. The situation is complicated by the finding that some mutations are found in more than one syndrome, and by the phenomenon of heteroplasmy – the occurrence of different proportions of mutant and normal mitochondria in different tissues. For this latter reason, mitochondrial DNA testing may require biopsy of the involved tissue (e.g., muscle) since the mutation may not be represented highly enough in blood to be detectable.

Other Targets of Molecular Genetic Testing and Screening

The specific disease examples covered in this chapter were chosen because they are among those tested most widely by molecular genetics laboratories, a market that is reflected by their inclusion in the College of American Pathologists/American College of Medical Genetics proficiency testing programs. This in turn has been dictated largely by their mutation carrier frequency or disease prevalence in the general population, and by their clinical severity. As already described, if the carrier frequency of a recessive mutation is sufficiently high in the target population, general screening may be justified. For these and other disorders, the application of the test to differential diagnosis, prenatal diagnosis, or presymptomatic diagnosis may also be of value. With over 10 000 genetic diseases catalogued, there are obviously many others that could be considered, and in fact at the time of this writing there are over 1000 different molecular genetic disease tests available as listed in the useful online database, GeneClinics.org. Many of these are esoteric and offered by only one or a few laboratories. Tests for extremely rare, or 'orphan,' genetic diseases may only be available in the research laboratory that cloned the gene. This has led to some difficulty since such laboratories, while performing a vital service to the small number of families at risk, are not CLIA-certified and therefore should not be releasing test results for medical management. A number of solutions have been proposed, such as modifying certain CLIA requirements for such settings, partnering of the research laboratory with a clinical laboratory in their own institution, or establishing a network of dedicated orphan disease laboratories.

Some disorders, which are rare in the general population, are sufficiently prevalent in a particular racial or ethnic group to justify limited population screening. For example, a number of laboratories offer an Ashkenazi-Jewish screening panel to include any or all of the following autosomal recessive diseases, which have carrier frequencies ranging from 1/100 to 1/15: Tay–Sachs disease, Gaucher's disease, Canavan's disease, cystic fibrosis, familial dysautonomia, Niemann–Pick disease A, Fanconi anemia C, Bloom syndrome, and connexin-26-related hearing loss. Screening of just the first four of these diseases has a positive yield of 1 in 6 in this population (Eng 1997).

Beyond the driver of service to a particular indigenous patient population, the choice of molecular genetic test menu from the large and ever-expanding universe of known disease genes will depend on both intellectual and economic factors (Amos, 2004). Development of a molecular test may be spurred by a clinical colleague's interest in a particular disease and accrual of a stable of patients and at-risk relatives. A molecular test may be needed as back-up to a biochemical test done at the same institution, as for hemoglobinopathies, alpha-1-antitrypsin deficiency, or congenital adrenal

CHAPTER 73

Identity Analysis: Use of DNA Polymorphisms in Parentage and Forensic Testing

Herbert F. Polesky MD, Rhonda K. Roby MPH

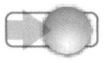

KEY POINTS
- DNA markers have nearly replaced other systems for identity testing.

- Standardized marker systems with known allelic polymorphisms are used in panels. Alleles with short tandem repeats (STR) form the basis of commercially available kits.

- Forensic testing requires documentation of all steps taken during collection, extraction, and testing so results can withstand legal challenges.

- DNA can be obtained from any sample that contains cellular material. The stability of DNA allows it to withstand harsh environmental conditions and long post-mortem intervals. Care must be taken to exclude contamination with DNA from other sources.

- Mitochondrial DNA can be extracted from bone and teeth after hundreds of years because it is small and present at hundreds to thousands of copies per cell. Mitochondrial DNA is maternally inherited and can be useful for identifying remains.

- DNA is used in identification of remains and can be used to link a suspect to a crime, to exculpate falsely accused suspects, to recognize serial crimes, and to distinguish copycat crimes, or to aid in accident reconstruction (for example, to determine who was driving a car by the identification of the bloodstains on the left-hand side of the windshield).

- Pathology laboratories can use DNA testing to resolve specimen mix-ups such as when samples are inadvertently switched or pathologic material floats on to a histologic or cytologic slide.

- Standards and quality assurance guidelines for parentage and forensics laboratories have been developed by the American Association of Blood Banks and the FBI's DNA Advisory Board, respectively.

In previous editions of this text, parentage (relatedness) and forensic (criminalistics) testing were treated as separate subjects. In the past decade DNA testing has become the dominant method in both areas. Except for analysis of test results and the source of samples, the similarities are greater than the differences. In parentage testing, samples obtained from multiple individuals are compared for inherited similarities while most often in forensic DNA testing, crime scene samples are evaluated for an exact match with a suspect.

A frequently quoted early reference to disputed parentage appears in the Bible (1 Kings 3:16–27), in which Solomon makes a decision about the maternity of a disputed child by threatening to use his sword to provide each claimant with a portion of the child. When paternity is in dispute, the arbiter of truth often is faced with the dilemma similar to that faced by Solomon: lack of witnesses to the event and the likelihood that the principals might not know or tell the truth. Similarly, short of eyewitnesses or confession, identifying a person at a crime scene is difficult to accomplish and most evidence merely suggests a suspect linkage. The availability of biologic evidence, such as DNA, provides information that can lead to clear resolution of disputed facts.

Historical Background

The discovery of the ABO blood group system by Landsteiner in 1900 (Landsteiner, 1901) and the recognition that these measurable characteristics followed the genetic rules described by Gregor Mendel (Mendel, 1866) provided objective laboratory evidence that could be used by courts to aid in deciding when a person had been falsely accused of paternity. In the United States, laws addressing the use of genetic markers for proving nonpaternity were enacted in 1935 (Schatkin, 1952). In the ensuing years, knowledge about useful genetic marker systems increased dramatically. By 1976, joint guidelines developed by an American Medical Association–American Bar Association (AMA-ABA) committee recommended seven systems for routine blood group investigations in cases of disputed parentage (ABO, Rh, MNSs, Kell, Duffy, Kidd, and HLA) (Miale, 1976). Other genetic systems such as polymorphic serum proteins and red cell enzymes were also recognized as useful. Many of these same genetic markers have also been used to match crime scene evidence with suspects or victims.

In 1980, DNA restriction fragment length polymorphism (RFLP) was described by Botstein (Botstein, 1980). Sir Alec Jeffreys is credited with the first report in the scientific literature to suggest that DNA typing might be useful for forensic identification, and coined the term 'DNA fingerprint' in his *Nature* article in 1985 (Jeffreys, 1985a, 1985b). Commercial laboratories began parentage and criminalistics casework using DNA testing in 1986

(Forensic Science Associates in 1986, Lifecodes in 1986, Cellmark in 1987) and then government crime laboratories began in 1989 (FBI, December 1989, Virginia, March 1989). In 1990 when the first edition of *Standards for Parentage Testing Laboratories* (American Association of Blood Banks, 1990) was published, specific requirements for RFLP testing were included along with those for what are now referred to as classical systems (red blood cell surface antigens, human leukocyte antigens, red cell enzymes, and serum protein genetic markers). DNA testing has virtually replaced traditional serology. The forensic DNA testing community has endured many iterations of DNA methods and technologies, and has standardized its testing with a set of 13 core short tandem repeat (STR) loci as the current mainstay of testing in order to build its international offender databases. This core set of loci is supplemented by other DNA testing, gender analysis (Amelogenin),Y chromosome markers, and mitochondrial DNA sequencing. Capillary electrophoresis is the main instrument platform and few laboratories still use slab gel electrophoresis.

Advantages of DNA

DNA permits the direct identification of the individual source because it is personal and manifests biological variation. DNA is useful as an identity marker because it is: (1) present throughout all cells of the body (except mature red cells); (2) the same in all cells of the body (except haploid sex gametes); (3) the same throughout life from the time of conception (except that a progenitor stem cell transplantation can result in the presence of donor characteristics rather than the recipient's inherited DNA); and (4) different in all individuals (except identical twins). DNA evidence is considered evidence of positive identification, rather than merely statistical evidence of identification. The FBI now considers a DNA profile result with a discriminatory power of 1:10 times the US population as evidence that a given individual is the source of a given DNA specimen.

DNA tests have a sensitivity that is far superior to traditional serologic markers. Polymerase chain reaction (PCR)-based testing can be accomplished on minute samples and even invisible trace DNA deposits. DNA is a robust molecule resistant to strong acids, alkalis, detergents, and environmental factors (Kobilinsky, 1992). The typing information from DNA is found within the sequence of nucleotides that are independent of the shape of the molecule. Consequently, DNA tests can be successfully performed on specimens that are older and have been exposed to greater environmental insults than is the case with traditional markers.

The bulk of the casework for crime laboratories in the United States is from sexual assaults. Vaginal swabs will contain bacteria and female epithelial cells as well as the male sperm. DNA from sperm can be separated from nonsperm DNA by a differential lysis procedure because of the protective capsule of spermatozoa (see later under DNA Extraction). This allows for individualization of the source of the semen without the confounding data of the non-semen evidence. DNA probes are also generally human- or primate-specific so the presence of bacterial DNA is of no consequence.

Choosing Genetic Markers

Polymorphisms

The model genetic system for testing would be one in which the individual has a unique marker. In determining relationships, this marker can be found in both the child and the putative parent. At present, short of gene sequencing, none of the marker systems provide such specific findings. Thus, multiple genetic systems that meet certain criteria are used for parentage and identity testing. Ideally, the system should have multiple alleles distributed in the population so that there is a high power of exclusion and the least common phenotype has a frequency that can be determined reliably. All markers in the system should be expressed (no null alleles) as co-dominant, mutation rates should be known and low, and phenotypes should be stable under usual storage conditions. Methods for detecting the markers should be reliable, reproducible, and feasible for a large number of laboratories. The genetics of the system must be known and follow established inheritance patterns (mendelian laws). The system should be independent of other markers routinely tested. If the system is intended for calculating estimates of paternity or identity, the gene frequencies in various populations must be established (Budowle, 2001).

The DNA from every human (except identical twins) is unique, because of the presence of 'polymorphisms', differences in the DNA between individuals. However, the vast preponderance of the DNA sequence is identical between individuals. On average, only 1 in 1000 nucleotide pairs differs between individuals. Nonetheless, this amounts to an average of 3 million pairs that differ between any two individuals and accounts for the tremendous genetic variation among individuals. Although the diversity in the coding regions of DNA (genes) is great, the noncoding regions of DNA also give rise to a great deal of diversity.

Length-based polymorphisms are found in repetitive DNA. Over 90% of the human genome is composed of noncoding or 'junk' DNA, of which approximately 20–30% is composed of repetitive regions. Many of the repetitive regions vary in the number of core repeats between different individuals; so-called variable number of tandem repeat (VNTR) loci. DNA fragments containing VNTRs will vary in length and are thus useful for analysis. Dinucleotide repeats are most common, but larger core repeats are more useful for forensic purposes. RFLP, amplified DNA fragment-length polymorphisms (AmpFLPs), and STRs are examples of fragment-length analytic techniques. Sequence polymorphisms exist within the DNA sequence of similarly sized DNA fragments. Sequence polymorphisms consist of difference changes in one or more bases in DNA sequence at a particular location in the genome. Sequence variations can be manifest as regions of alternative alleles or base substitutions, additions, or deletions. Most sequence polymorphisms are mere point mutations within repetitive and nonrepetitive regions and are known as single nucleotide polymorphisms (SNPs). SNPs, sequence-specific oligonucleotides (e.g. reverse dot blots), and mitochondrial DNA tests are examples of sequence-based tests.

Samples and Specimen Collection

The ideal sample is one collected from the individual to be tested. For parentage testing and entering information into DNA databases, fresh whole blood, blood stains on filter paper and/or buccal swabs are most frequently used. Results from testing are often used in legal proceedings. Thus, all aspects of the procedures used should be well documented, since they may be subject to challenge by one of the parties. It is very important to ensure documentation of the identification of the tested individuals, the collection, and the labeling of samples. Although many parentage disputes are civil actions, some jurisdictions require documents showing the chain of custody of samples similar to those used in criminal matters. American Association of Blood Banks (AABB)-accredited laboratories are required to obtain a history of any recent transfusion (in the preceding 3 months) or a hematopoietic stem cell transplant. A photographic identification and appropriate informed consent must also accompany each sample. The consent for a minor should be from an individual with legal rights to the custody of the child.

Proper specimen collection at a crime scene is very important. The evidence must be recognized before it can be properly collected. This is often accomplished with the help of chemicals and/or alternate light sources to make blood stains visible. Blood spatter pattern analysis is also employed to help the investigator interpret and intelligently collect specimens from a plethora of bloodstains. Adequate chain-of-custody documentation, packaging and sealing, and preservation of the specimen are as important as the initial collection.

Biological fluids shed on to items that can be collected (e.g., blood onto a piece of clothing) should simply be collected and packaged separately. When biological fluid has been deposited on to a surface or an item that cannot be collected, the fluid should be collected by swabbing with clean sterile swabs moistened with sterile distilled water, until the entire stain is collected. For bite marks on bodies, a technique has been described (Sweet, 1997) that involves swabbing with a wet swab followed by a dry swab. A control swab should be collected from an unstained area adjacent to the fluid stain. The stain and control swabs should be air-dried and packaged separately.

Ethylenediaminetetraacetic acid (EDTA) and citrate-phosphate-dextrose (CPD) remain the anticoagulants of choice for DNA testing. Heparin-anticoagulated blood is not recommended for DNA testing. Even though mature red blood cells are devoid of DNA (both nuclear and mitochondrial), ample DNA is present from circulating white cells for testing. Despite inhibition of the PCR reaction by heme, blood is a good source of DNA for PCR testing because the heme inhibitory activity can easily be diluted away.

However, sources of DNA other than blood are preferred in postmortem settings if there is significant putrefaction. Virtually any tissue may be successfully used for DNA typing purposes. Some tissues that may be intuitively thought to be better sources of DNA because they are more densely cellular and hence contain higher concentrations of DNA are, in fact, less optimal because of higher rates of postmortem degradation (Kobilinsky, 1992). Among soft tissues, liver DNA appears to degrade

Table 73–1 Systems Used by Participants in CAP Proficiency Surveys

System	1999 (% of Respondents)		2004 (% of Respondents)	
	Forensic Labs	Parentage Labs	Forensic Labs	Parentage Labs
*CSF1PO	52	47	88	90
D2S1338			11	43
*D3S1358	43	41	89	89
*D5S818	52	53	89	91
*D7S820	53	58	89	91
*D8S1179	33	39	89	90
*D13S317	53	58	89	92
*D16S539	44	33	89	88
*D18S51	37	39	89	87
D19S433			11	42
*D21S11	37	41	89	90
FES/FPS	14	27		16
*FGA	43	67	89	91
PENTA E			32	28
*TH01	53	55	89	92
*TPOX	51	51	89	85
*vWA31/A	56	67	89	97
Amelogenin	52	43	89	90
Y-STRs			6	31
RFLPs	43	44	0	6

* CODIS loci.

An exact mtDNA sequence match can be traced through the maternal lineage of a family for many generations. However, the discriminatory power of mtDNA sequencing is limited – on the order of one in a few hundred. Also, this testing is very expensive. Few laboratories are performing this kind of testing at this time.

Other Systems

A very small number of laboratories use classical test systems, RFLP testing and dot blot tests. Although not routinely used in parentage or forensic identity testing, test systems using combinations of gene amplification by PCR with sequence-specific primers, sequence-specific oligonucleotide probes (SSOP), and direct sequencing have been described for studies of the genes at the MHC locus (Allen, 1994; Bunce, 1995).

Methods to detect single-nucleotide polymorphisms, also know as SNPs, are used to determine a single base change in a sequence at a specific location. Because of the limited variability at these loci, as many as 70 SNPs need to be tested to get the same level of information about relatedness provided by a multiplex of several STR loci. These markers have been used in the identification of highly degraded samples such as those that were obtained at the World Trade Center site.

Analysis and Use of Test Data

DNA in the Crime Laboratory

DNA testing has become routine in the crime lab (National Research Council, 1996) and DNA evidence is now routinely admitted into court. In the United States, approximately three quarters of criminal DNA tests involve sexual assault; a significant proportion involve homicide. Approximately one third of DNA tests exonerate wrongfully accused suspects (Fig. 73–3), one quarter are inconclusive, and somewhat less than half result in a match of the suspect to a crime. Only a fraction of the cases in which DNA evidence is tested are actually litigated, as most cases result in a plea bargain. In the criminalistics context, DNA can be used to link a suspect to a crime, to exculpate falsely accused suspects, to recognize serial crimes and distinguish copycat crimes, or to aid in accident reconstruction (e.g., to determine who was driving a car by the identification of the bloodstains on the left-hand side of the windshield). In addition to the use of DNA for associative evidence at scenes of crimes, DNA is used in identification of remains.

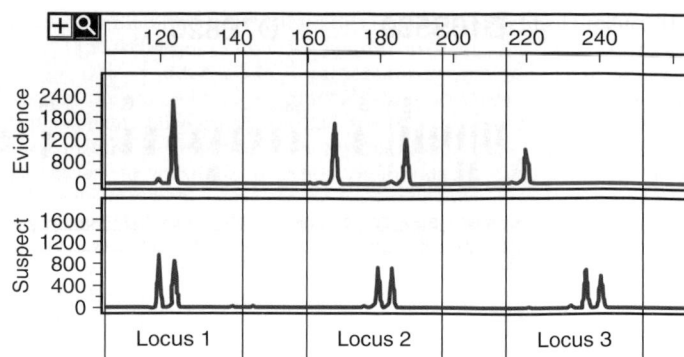

Figure 73–3 Exclusion of suspect when compared to crime scene evidence. The profile for the evidence at Locus 1, Locus 2, and Locus 3 is clearly different from the suspect's profile. The evidence could not be contributed by the suspect.

Table 73–2 Identification of Possible 'Floater'

STR Locus	Floater	Tissue Block	Patient Sample	Frequency of Patient's Phenotype
CSF1PO	10,12	10,12	10,12	0.191
D3S1358	15,16	16,17	16,17	0.099
D5S818	11	11,12	11,12	0.024
D7S820	9,11	11	11	0.0529
D8S1179	13	12,14	12,14	0.0976
D13S317	11	11	11	0.0798
D16S539	9,11	11,12	11,12	0.1764
D18S51	14,15	14,15	14,15	0.0477
D21S11	30	28, 31.2	28, 31.2	0.0341

Shaded results indicate the floater is not identical to patient or tissue block. The chance that the tissue block has the same genetic markers as the patient compared to a random Caucasian individual $>1.86 \times 10^{10}$.

DNA in the Pathology Laboratory

DNA identity tests can be used to resolve specimen mix-ups (Weedn, 1993) such as when samples are inadvertently switched or pathologic material floats on to a histologic or cytologic slide. Urine drug tests that have been challenged on the basis of alleged sample switching may be resolved by DNA testing. Testing may be used to confirm or refute mislabeling of biopsy specimens. A small fragment of cancerous tissue ('floater') on a glass microscope slide can be determined to be from someone other than the patient (Table 73–2).

STR markers are also used to evaluate engraftment of marrow after transplantation. In cases where the donor is related to the recipient, testing of multiple markers may be required to find an informative locus.

Exclusion of Parentage

The primary goal of genetic marker testing in cases of disputed parentage is to identify the biological parent of a given child. Although this cannot be done with absolute certainty, genetic marker tests can provide objective evidence of nonparentage. By using multiple genetic systems, it is possible to exclude most (>99%), but not all nonparents.

In systems that follow the rules of mendelian genetics, exclusions are identified by finding exceptions to the expected inheritance pattern. Interpretation of test results when paternity is in question usually depends on assuming that the sample defined as maternal is from the child's biological mother. The child's and mother's phenotypes should be compared to determine whether results are consistent with expected inheritance patterns. An allele present in the child but not in the mother is referred to as the obligatory paternal gene (OG). If both alleles in the child and mother are identical, then there are alternative (two) possibilities for the paternal gene.

If the tested male does not have the possibility of passing the OG and the marker for the gene is absent in the presumed mother, the exclusion observed is termed direct (Table 73–3). This type of exclusion in one of the classical systems was usually enough to conclude that the tested male is not the biological father of the child in question. In DNA systems, because the rate of mutation is orders of magnitude greater than observed in classical systems, an exclusion at a single locus is not considered enough

Table 73–3 Exclusion of Parentage: Phenotype (*Genotype*)

Type of Exclusion	Child	Mother	Tested Man	Obligatory Gene(s)
Direct	AB (*ab*)	A (*aa, a?*)	C (*cc, c?*)	*b*
	AC (*ac*)	AB (*ab*)	AD (*ad*)	*c*
	AB (*ab*)	C (*cc, c?*)	AC (*ac*)	*b* (maternal)
Two-haplotype	A (*aa, a?*)	A (*aa, a?*)	BC (*bc*)	*a* or ?
	A (*aa, a?*)	AB (*aa, ab*)	BC (*bc*)	*a* or ?
	AB (*ab*)	AB (*ab*)	CD (*cd*)	*a* or *b*
	AB (*ab*)	Not available	CD (*cd*)	*a* or *b*
Indirect*	A (*aa, a?*)	A (*aa, a?*)	B (*bb, b?*)	*a* or ?
	B (*bb, b?*)	AB (*ab*)	A (*aa, a?*)	*b* or ?
	B (*bb, b?*)	C (*cc, c?*)	AB (*ab*)	*b* or ? (maternal)
	B (*bb, b?*)	Not available	A (*aa, a?*)	*b* or ?

* Mutation must be considered.

Table 73–4 Power of Exclusion (*A*): Selected Test System

System	A
Classical	
ABO	0.166
RH	0.283
ACP	0.239
Restriction fragment length polymorphism	
D2S44	0.95
D10S28	0.96
Short tandem repeats	
D7S820	0.523
D13S317	0.417
vWA31/A	0.65

Values vary in different populations

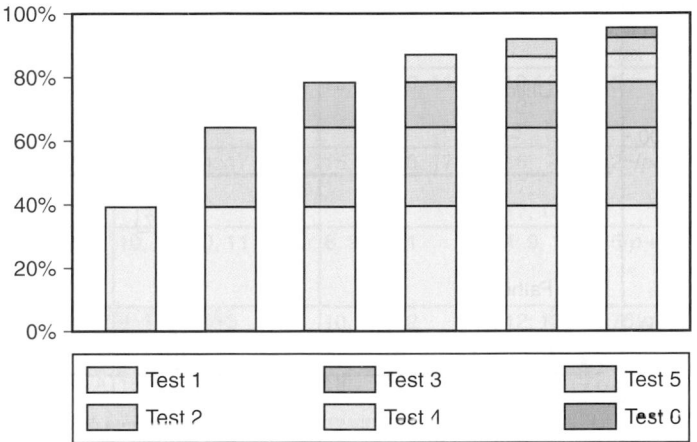

Figure 73–4 Cumulative power of exclusion (each added test: *A* = 0.4). The percentage of the population excluded by each additional test becomes smaller and smaller. The overall exclusion probability of the six tests is 95.3%. If a seventh test with *A* = 0.5 was performed; only an additional 2.4% of the population would be excluded ([1–0.953] × 0.5 = 0.0235).

evidence to establish nonpaternity (Standards for Relationship Testing Laboratories, 2005). A direct exclusion also occurs when the child or the tested male is heterozygous and the two markers are absent in the other person. This type of direct exclusion sometimes is referred to as a two-haplotype exclusion. In cases in which only the child and one alleged parent are available for testing, if the tested individual or child has two haplotypes, neither of which is in the other, it is possible to establish nonparentage.

Absence of an expected genetic marker in the child when the parent in question appears to be homozygous for the gene is called an indirect exclusion. This is sometimes called reverse homozygosity. One indirect exclusion is not sufficient evidence to conclude that the tested individual is not the parent. Interpretation of reverse homozygosity as an indirect exclusion presumes that the tested subjects both have two identical alleles at the locus. In PCR testing of STRs this absence of expected allele may occur if there is a binding site mutation (Harrison, 2004) in one of the tested individuals or it is possible that a rare null allele(or other undetected allele) or mutation is present in the child as well as the parent in question. The finding of indirect exclusions in at least two independent systems usually is sufficient evidence to reach a conclusion of non-paternity.

Power of Exclusion

Prior to testing, it is possible to provide an estimate of the average chance that testing will prove nonparentage if the accused is not the parent. This is referred to as the power of exclusion. For each genetic system, an average power of exclusion (*A*) can be calculated based on the gene frequencies (*p, q*) for the alleles in the system. The general equation, $A = pq(1 - pq)$, for a two-allele system was reported by Wiener in 1930. When a system has multiple alleles, more complex formulas are required (Walker, 1978). The general equation has also been adapted (Brenner, 1990) to determine *A* for systems that do not have discrete alleles, such as DNA RFLP systems as follows:

$$A = h^2(1 - hH^2),$$

where *H* is the percentage homozygosity and *h* the percentage heterozygosity observed at the locus. Table 73–4 shows *A* values for selected systems. A highly polymorphic system has a greater power of exclusion than a system with only a few alleles or one that has one or two common alleles and many rare alleles (Table 73–4).

Cumulative Probability of Exclusion

When testing includes several independent genetic systems, a cumulative probability of exclusion can be calculated by using the following formula:

CPE = 1 – (1ts}– P1) (1ts}– P2) (1ts}– P3) … (1ts}– Pn),

where *P* is the *A* for each system used. As shown in Figure 73–4, as more and more systems are used, fewer and fewer individuals are excluded by each additional test. With an appropriately selected battery of DNA marker systems, a CPE of 0.995 or greater is easily achieved.

Inclusion of Parentage

If, after testing multiple independent systems, the parent in dispute is not excluded (Fig. 73–5), then an estimate of the possibility that the tested person could be the biological parent should be calculated.

In providing estimates of inclusion of paternity, appropriate gene frequency tables should be used. In general, this means that a population of random persons of the same race has been phenotyped, that the size of the sample is large enough to provide gene frequencies with minimum errors of estimation for the alleles in the system, and that the tested male and biological father are from the same population. When multiple systems have been tested, the differences observed in gene frequencies in populations from various geographic locations become unimportant in calculations of the likelihood of paternity (Hummel, 1981). In cases in which the tested male is of mixed racial background or from a population for which there are inadequate frequency tables, it may be impossible to provide a precise estimate of paternity. However, when multiple systems with a high power of exclusion have been used and the paternity index value using a reference population is high, there is a minimal chance that frequencies from a more defined population will have a significant effect on the conclusion of parentage. In these situations, comparisons with frequencies for several defined racial groups may also be helpful.

If the tested male is not excluded, it always can be argued that the amount of testing was inadequate, that evidence for exclusion will be found by testing another genetic system, or that the true parent is a close relative of the tested man. This line of reasoning could be correct only if the tested male has been falsely accused. In addition to the average power of exclusion described above, it also is possible to calculate the frequency with which a random male will not be excluded (RMNE) based on a mother–child pair exhibiting the observed phenotypes (Salmon, 1983). This value is related to the actual power of exclusion for the tests performed.

Paternity Index Calculation

In cases where a trio has been tested, a general approach referred to as the 'comparison of sperm method' is usually used (Walker, 1978). This

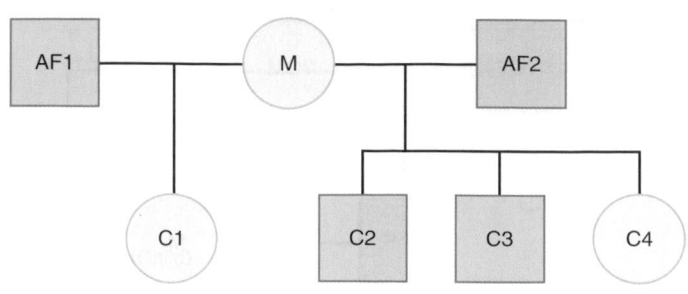

System	AF1	AF2	Child 1	Child 2	Child 3	Child 4
CSF1PO	10, 11	11, 12	10, **14**	12, **14**	**9**, 12	11, **14**
D3S1358	15, 17	15, 17	**14**, **17**	**17**	**14**, 16	**14**, 15
D5S818	13, 14	11, 12	**10**, 14	**10**, **12**	**12**	**12**
D7S820	8, 9	10, 13	8, **11**	10, **11**	10, **14**	13, **14**
D13S317	11, 12	8, 10	12, **14**	8, **10**	10, **14**	**10**
D16S539	12, 15	9, 11	**8**, 15	**8**, 11	11, **13**	9, **13**
vWA31/A	14, 20	16, 17	**15**, 20	**15**, 17	16, **18**	17, **18**
TH01	8, 9	6, 9	8, **9.3**	6, **9.3**	8, **9.3**	9, **9.3**
TPOX	8, 11	8, 10	**8**	**8**, 12	**8**, 12	**8**
Amelogenin	Male	Male	Female	Male	Male	Female
DYS390	23	23			23	23	
DYS391	10	11			11	11	

Figure 73–7 Family study – presumed mother (M) is deceased: All four children in this family study could have the same mother. The probable maternal marker in each system is shown in bold and underlined. Note: in some systems either marker could be maternal in one of the children (D3S1358 in child 1). Alleged father (AF) 1 shares a marker with child 1 in all systems and is excluded as the possible father of children 2, 3, and 4 in several systems. AF 2 is excluded as the father of child 1 in every system except D3S1358 and TPOX. AF 2 is also excluded as the father of child 3 in two systems (D3S1358 and TH01). The finding of a possible match in nine of 11 systems, including two Y-STRs, suggests that the true father of child 3 might be a relative of AF 2, or two mutations have occurred.

participate in proficiency testing programs. The possibility of significant judicial scrutiny of every step of the procedures and practices used from collection of samples to reporting of results is to be expected. Challenges to the validation of the methods used, the source of the data bases used in statistical reports, and the qualification of the personnel are not uncommon. There is general agreement as to proper laboratory procedures that should be used in DNA testing and, although the DNA typing methods are not specifically standardized, procedures are remarkably uniform.

The FBI's Technical Working Group on DNA Analysis Methods, now known as the Scientific Working Group on DNA Analysis Methods, promulgated early guidelines for DNA analytic procedures that became de facto standards (Technical Working Group, 1989, 1995). These standards were modified by the FBI's DNA Advisory Board and adopted by the FBI Director pursuant to the DNA Identification Act, a component of the Crime Bill passed in 1994 (Federal Bureau of Investigation, 1998). These standards apply to crime laboratories that submit DNA results to the FBI's National DNA Index System or that accept certain federal grants. The American Society of Crime Laboratory Directors has an accreditation program for crime labs. The American Board of Criminalists certifies criminalists and has a subspecialty category for DNA analysts. Analysts who work on casework samples must have college credit (or equivalent) in genetics, biochemistry, and molecular biology and 1 year of forensic biology experience. Each of these standards calls for proficiency testing by each analyst twice a year.

The American Association of Blood Banks, now known as AABB, began developing standards and accrediting parentage testing laboratories in 1984. The 7th edition, renamed *Standards for Relationship Testing Laboratories*, was published in 2005. All aspects of parentage testing from laboratory organization to process control and improvement are covered. The Standards include requirements for documents and records, report content, and interpretation of results. Laboratories are required to participate in graded proficiency testing.

Conclusion

Scientific evidence that will aid in resolving cases of disputed parentage, questions of relatedness, and identity can be obtained from testing multiple DNA systems. Current technology provides test results that exclude more than 99.9% of falsely accused individuals in parentage and criminal cases. It is not possible to prove paternity or guilt by laboratory tests. The mathematical estimates derived from genetic marker tests when no exclusion is found or there is a match between sample and suspect are a significant source of data that can be used to establish parentage or guilt.

Acknowledgment

The authors would like to thank Victor Weedn, M.D., J.D. for material from Chapter 68 in the last edition.

References

Alford RL, Hammond HA, Coto I, Caskey CT: Rapid and efficient resolution of parentage by amplification of short tandem repeats. Am J Hum Genet 1994; 55:190–195.

Allen M, Lui L, Gyllensten U: A comprehensive polymerase chain reaction oligonucleotide typing system for the HLA class I A locus. Hum Immunol 1994; 40:25–32.

American Association of Blood Banks. Standards for parentage testing laboratories. Arlington, VA, AABB, 1990.

Botstein D, White RL, Skolnick M, Davis RW: Construction of a genetic linkage map in man using restriction fragment polymorphisms. Am J Hum Genet 1980; 32:314–331.

Brenner CH: A note on paternity computation in cases lacking a mother. Transfusion 1993; 33:51–54.

Brenner CH, Morris JW: Paternity index calculations in single locus hypervariable DNA probes: Validation and other studies. *In* International Symposium on Human Identification, 1989. Madison, WI, Promega Corporation, 1990, pp 21–53.

Budowle B, Shea B, Niezgoda S, Chakraborty R: CODIS STR loci data from 41 sample populations. J Forensic Sci 2001; 46: 453–489.
Reference for the frequency data used to calculate parentage results as well as population frequencies for the chance that a matching sample is from a random individual. Several manufacturers also have websites with frequency tables based on results from their reagents.

Bunce M, Fanning GC, Welsh KI: Comprehensive, serologically equivalent DNA typing for HLA-B by PCR using sequence-specific primers (PCAR-SSP). Tissue Antigens 1995; 45:81–90.

Butler JM, Reeder DJ: Short Tandem Repeat DNA Internet DataBase. Available on line at: http://www.cstl.nist.gov/biotech/strbase.
This website, supported by the National Institute of Standards and Technology (NIST) has updated information on STR loci including new variants. It also contains links to other useful sites.

Butler JM, Levin BC: Forensic applications of mitochondrial DNA. Trends Biotechnol 1998; 16:158–162.

Crouse CA, Ban JD, D'Alessio JK: Extraction of DNA from forensic-type sexual assault specimens using simple, rapid sonication procedures. Biotechniques 1993, 15.641–646.

DNA Advisory Board. Quality assurance standards for forensic DNA testing laboratories (approved July 1998). Forensic Sci Comm 2000; 2. Available on line at: www.fbi.gov/programs/lab/fsc/current/codis2.htm.
Basic QA/QC requirements for forensic testing laboratories.

Essen-Möller E: Die Beweiskraft der Ähnlichkeit in Vaterschaftsnachweis: theoretische Grundlagen. Mitt Anthrop Ges (Wien) 1938; 68:9–53.

Foster EA, Jobling MA, Taylor PG, et al: Jefferson fathered slave's last child. Nature 1998; 396:27–28; also see Nature 1998; 396:13–14.

Harrison C, Allen R, Eisenberg A, et al: Phenotype versus genotype reporting for DNA polymorpisms. Prog Forensic Genet 10 2004; 526–528.

Holland MM, Parsons TJ: Mitochondrial DNA sequence analysis – validation and use for forensic casework. Forensic Sci Rev 1999; 11:21–50.

Hummel K, Claussen M: Exclusion efficiency and biostatistical value of conventional blood group systems in European and non-European populations; suitability of Central European tables from non-German speaking populations. *In* Hummel K, Gerchow J (eds): Biomathematical Evidence of Paternity. Berlin, Springer-Verlag, 1981, pp 97–108.

Ivanov P, Wadhams M, Roby R, et al: Mitochondrial DNA sequence heteroplasmy in the Grand Duke of Russia Georgij Romanov establishes the authenticity of the remains of Tsar Nicholas II. Nat Genet 1996:12:417–420.

Jeffreys AJ, Wilson V, Thein SL: Hypervariable 'minisatellite' regions in human DNA. Nature 1985a; 314:67–73.

Jeffreys AJ, Wilson V, Thein SL: Individual specific 'fingerprints' of human DNA. Nature 1985b; 316:76–79.

Kobilinsky L: Recovery and stability of DNA in samples of forensic science significance. Forensic Sci Rev 1992; 4:67–87.

Landsteiner K: Über Agglutinationserscheinungen normalen menschlichen Blutes. Wien Klin Wochenschr 1901; 14; 1132–1134.

Mayr WR: Paternity testing with unavailable putative father or mother. *In* Walker RH (ed): Inclusion Probabilities in Parentage Testing. Arlington, VA, American Association of Blood Banks, 1983, pp 373–379.

Mendel G: Versuche über Pflanzen-Hybriden. Verhandlung Nat Forsch Verein Brunn 1866; 4;3–47.

Miale JB, Jennings ER, Rettberg WAH, et al: Joint AMA-ABA guidelines: present status of serologic testing in problems of disputed parentage. Family Law Q 1976; 10:247–285.

National Research Council: The Evaluation of Forensic DNA Evidence. Washington, DC, National Academy of Sciences, 1996.

This monograph is a comprehensive evaluation of testing and statistical evaluation of data intended for use in legal proceedings.

Parentage Act: Minnesota Statutes 2004, 257.55 Presumption of paternity.

Parsons TJ, Weedn VW: Preservation and recovery of DNA in postmortem specimens and trace samples. *In* Haglund WD, Sorg MH (eds): Forensic Taphonomy: The Postmortem Fate of Human Remains. Boca Raton, FL, CRC Press, 1997.

Salmon D: The random man not excluded expression in paternity testing. *In* Walker RH (ed): Inclusion Probabilities in Parentage Testing. Arlington, VA, American Association of Blood Banks, 1983, pp 281–292.

Schatkin SB: Disputed Paternity Proceedings, 3rd ed. Albany, NY, Banks & Co, 1952, pp 233–234.

Standards for Relationship Testing Laboratories, 7th ed. Bethesda, MD, American Association of Blood Banks, 2005.

The AABB periodically provides standards for accredited parentage testing laboratories that include key elements of QA/QC, testing, reporting and validation requirements. With each edition of Standards a companion Guidance for Standards is published that has detailed explanations of the requirements, and appendices with useful tables and formulas.

Sweet D, Lorente M, Lorente JA, et al: An improved method to recover saliva from human skin: the double swab method. J Forensic Sci 1997; 42:320–322.

Technical Working Group on DNA Analysis Methods: Guidelines for a quality assurance program for DNA restriction fragment length polymorphism analysis. Crime Lab Dig 1989; 17:40–59.

Technical Working Group on DNA Analysis Methods: Guidelines for a quality assurance program for DNA Analysis. Crime Lab Dig 1995; 22:21–43.

Traver M: Paternity calculations: special situations. *In* Statistics Workshop. Madison, WI, Promega Corporation, 1996.

Walker RH: Probability in the analysis of paternity test results. *In* Silver H (ed): Paternity Testing. Washington, DC, American Association of Blood Banks, 1978, pp 69–135.

The proceedings of the Airlie Conference contains numerous papers dealing with methods of calculating data from paternity testing using the classical systems. Though pre DNA testing, the principles apply to STR systems.

Walsh PS, Metzger DA, Higuchi R: Chelex 100 as a medium for simple extraction of DNA for PCR-based typing from forensic material. Biotechniques 1991; 10:506–518.

Weber JL, May PE: Abundant class of human DNA polymorphisms which can be typed using the polymerase chain reaction. Am J Hum Genet 1989; 44:388–396.

Weedn VW: Where did this come from? Identification of sample mix-ups by DNA testing. Am J Clin Pathol 1993; 100:592–593.

Wenk RE, Traver M, Chiafari FA: Determination of sibship in any two persons. Transfusion 1986; 36:259–262.

Wiener AS, Lederer M, Polayes SH: Studies in isohemagglutination. IV: On the chance of proving non-paternity, with special reference to blood groups. J Immunol 1930; 19:259–282.

CHAPTER 74

Diagnosis and Management of Cancer Using Serologic Tumor Markers

Peng Lee MD PhD, Matthew R. Pincus MD PhD, Richard A. McPherson MD

KEY POINTS

- This chapter discusses the use of proteins, whose serum levels are often elevated in patients with malignancies, in the diagnosis and management of cancer.

- Many of these are so-called oncofetal antigens, i.e., proteins that are expressed in fetal tissue during development but are not normally found in the tissues of adults. These include α-fetoprotein (AFP) and carcinoembryonic antigen (CEA), whose serum levels are frequently elevated in hepatocellular and colon cancers, respectively.

- Other proteins, such as CA 19-9, CA 125, and CA 15-3, are expressed in epithelial cells and are also often present in the sera of patients with pancreatic, ovarian, and breast cancers, respectively.

- Since these 'tumor marker' proteins are not tissue-specific and can also be expressed in diseases other than cancer, their sensitivities and specificities are not sufficiently high that they can be used as cancer-screening proteins. Their use is predominantly in following patients who are being treated for known malignancies.

- The exception to this is prostate-specific antigen (PSA), a chymotrypsin-like enzyme that is expressed almost exclusively in prostate tissue and is elevated in the sera of most patients with prostate cancer. Elevated serum PSA levels therefore have a high sensitivity for diagnosing prostate cancer; since PSA is also elevated in other prostate diseases, such as benign prostatic hyperplasia, it has a lower specificity but nonetheless can still be used very effectively to screen patients for this disease.

- New developments in the field of early tumor detection using serum markers are also introduced in this chapter. These include use of mitogenic proteins, such as HER-2/Neu, known to function as signal transduction proteins whose levels are elevated in many types of cancers; detection of genes encoding these proteins in body fluids; and proteomic approaches involving patterns of expression of multiple proteins that typify specific cancers.

Despite the advancement of multidisciplinary treatment modalities, cancer mortality has not been significantly reduced for the last 50 years. This is in contrast to dramatic decreases in mortality due to cardiovascular and infectious disease. Studies have shown that early detection of cancer can lead to superior long-term survival. Thus, there is an urgent need to search for cancer biomarkers with high sensitivity and specificity to allow for early cancer detection, effective treatment, and decreased mortality. Therefore, much effort has been devoted to the discovery, characterization, and clinical application of tumor markers to detect the presence of cancer at an early stage. As a result, increasing numbers of biomarkers have been identified and employed as markers with prognostic value in the daily clinical management of cancer patients. These markers can be used not only to classify cancers but also to monitor response to neoadjuvant therapy. For example, estrogen receptor (ER), progesterone receptor (PR) and HER2/neu oncogene are used in the diagnosis and management of cancer patients using surgical specimens. ER has been shown to be a prognostic marker for breast cancer and a predictive marker for hormonal treatment (Jensen, 2003). HER2/neu amplification and overexpression were shown to be associated with poor prognosis and to be a predictor for therapeutic response in breast cancer (Wilmanns, 2004). PR has been shown to be associated with a good prognosis in ovarian cancer (Munstedt, 2000; Lee, 2005).

Among these markers are a number of tumor markers present in circulating body fluids, including blood. Broadly, body fluid tumor biomarkers (principally serum and urine) are divided into three categories: tumor associated proteins such as the oncofetal antigens, which seem to be polyclonal antibodies. For example, CA 19-9, CA 125, and CA 15-3 are much more sensitive and specific than CEA for pancreatic, ovarian, and breast carcinomas, respectively. These markers are recommended to replace the polyclonal CEA test for the diagnosis and management of patients with the above-mentioned carcinomas. Various tumor markers derived from different tumors also share many tumor-associated epitopes. For example, CA 19-9, CA 15-3, and CA 125 are expressed by almost all carcinomas in varying degrees. In addition to the sharing of any given epitope by more than one carcinoma, it is also possible for a single molecule to express more than one epitope (Yu, 1991). For example, it is likely that CA 15-3 and CA 125 are expressed by the same mucin molecule.

Clinical Applications

The serum tumor markers are currently used for screening, diagnosing, and predicting prognosis and treatment response. Use of tests for screening of disease, even those with high sensitivity and specificity, should be confined as much as possible to populations at risk for the disease. This is because the positive predictive value (PPV) depends on the prevalence of the disease. Since, as noted above, most of the tumor markers described in this chapter are expressed both in neoplastic and benign conditions, their use is confined to following possible tumor recurrence in patients being treated for specific types of tumor.

Screening

The recommendation of screening for prostate cancer by the measurement of serum PSA in combination with a digital rectal examination (DRE) in men over age 50 is due to the high tissue specificity of PSA (Wu, 1994) and the high prevalence of prostate cancer. Combination of the PSA test and DRE provides the least costly approach to the early detection of prostate cancer (Littrup, 1993). PSA screening is especially recommended for African American men because the incidence of prostate cancer for African Americans is nearly twice that of the general population and the death rate is up to three times higher. Screening permits the treatment of organ-confined, potentially curable prostate cancer discovered in men with a life expectancy of longer than 10 years.

Although not approved for screening for hepatocellular carcinoma in the United States, AFP has been used to screen for primary hepatocellular carcinoma in China because of the high incidence of liver cancer in that country. The diagnosis of ovarian cancer has traditionally relied on imaging and discovery at surgery, e.g., exploratory laparotomy. However, in most cases, at the time of detection, the tumor has advanced to a stage at which the possibility of cure is low. The feasibility of screening for ovarian cancer in women by measuring serum CA 125 is still being investigated.

Diagnosis

Several approaches have been suggested recently to improve the diagnostic yield of many tumor markers. The use of multiple markers is one approach that has received wide acceptance. As is also noted in the Chapter 75, specific patterns of multiple tumor markers seem to be associated with individual malignant diseases. Another approach to improving both the specificity and sensitivity of a tumor markers, as in the case of serum PSA test, involves the measurement of the velocity (the rate of increase in PSA concentration over time) and the density (e.g., by dividing the serum PSA concentration by the volume of the prostate gland, determined by transrectal ultrasound) (Benson, 1992). These efforts are aimed at a better discrimination between the following scenarios: a mildly elevated serum PSA level associated with a small prostate gland may indicate cancer, whereas the same PSA value in a patient with a large gland may indicate BPH.

Prognosis: Recurrence, Metastasis and Survival

The assessment of tumor aggressiveness and the prognosis for the outcome of a cancer patient has received much attention in recent years. The knowledge of tumor aggressiveness helps in the development of a proper therapy for the patient. For example, the detection of tumor markers, highly associated with malignancy and metastases, will suggest a more rigorous and systemic treatment. Monitoring tumor markers for the detection of recurrence following the surgical removal of the tumor is the second most useful application of tumor markers. It is well known that the appearance of most of the circulating tumor markers has a lead time of several months (3–6 months) prior to the stage at which many of the physical procedures could be used for the detection of cancer. The specificity of tumor markers does not present a problem for this application. The ease of drawing blood and the sensitivity of tumor marker tests make this noninvasive monitoring process now widely accepted.

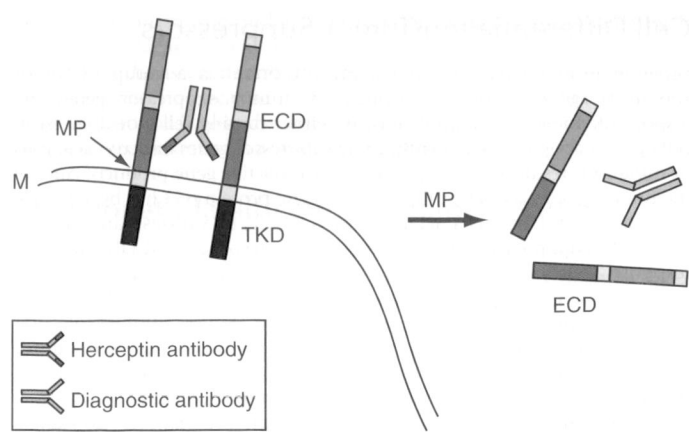

Figure 74–2 HER2/*neu* monoclonal antibodies are used both therapeutically and diagnostically in breast cancer. Humanized HER2 monoclonal antibody trastuzumab (Herceptin), shown with a dark blue complementarity determining region (CDR), reacts with a specific region of HER2 epitope (dark blue), causes the death of malignant breast cells, and is often effective in the treatment of breast cancer. On the other hand, different monoclonal antibodies, which do not crossreact with the trastuzumab determinant, recognize the extracellular domain (ECD) of HER2/*neu* in serum after it is cleaved off this growth factor receptor by metalloprotease. Because trastuzumab and diagnostic monoclonal antibodies recognize different epitopes of HER2, there is no interference in detecting serum levels of HER2 in trastuzumab-treated patients. ECD = extracellular domain; M = cell membrane; MP = metalloprotease; TKD = tyrosine kinase domain

Most tumor markers become increasingly elevated when the tumor metastasizes. Unfortunately, very few tumor markers have a clear-cut boundary between benign and malignant stages. Proteins that reflect the risk factors associated with the process of tumor metastases, such as proteases and adhesion molecules, are usually better markers for predicting prognosis. However, most of these markers are still measured in tumor tissues and tissue cytosols. The finding of the extracellular domain of c-*erb*B-2 protein in the serum (Fig. 74–2) and the correlation of the serum extracellular domain with the levels of other serum tumor markers is encouraging. In the near future, it is hoped that it will become possible to measure these serum prognostic factors in the blood. Another area of intensive study is to explore the use of serum marker surrogates in the prediction of cancer patient survival.

Monitoring Treatment Response

One of the most useful applications of tumor markers involves monitoring the course of the disease, especially during treatment. The serum level of tumor markers reflects the success of surgery or the efficacy of chemotherapy. Detecting elevated levels of a tumor marker after surgery would indicate either incomplete removal of the tumor, recurrence, or the presence of metastases. The measurement of serum tumor markers during chemotherapy also gives an indication of the effectiveness of the antitumor drug used and a guide for the selection of the most effective drug for each individual case.

Recommendations for Ordering Tumor Marker Tests

When ordering tumor markers as an adjunct diagnostic test for managing cancer patients, the following recommendations should be kept in mind in order to avoid misinterpretation of the test results.

Never Rely on the Result of a Single Test. Because of low specificity associated with most tumor markers, it is difficult to differentiate between malignant and benign diseases on the basis of the result of a single test result. Most tumor marker elevations found in nonmalignant diseases may be transient, whereas with cancer the level often either remains elevated or rises continuously. Ordering serial testing can help to detect falsely elevated levels due to transient elevation. For example, elevated serum AFP can be detected in patients with either primary hepatocellular carcinoma or benign liver disease. However, on a subsequent testing 2 weeks later, the serum AFP will remain elevated in patients with cancer, whereas in patients with benign conditions the serum AFP may return to normal levels.

When Ordering Serial Testing, be Certain to Order Every Test from the Same Laboratory Using the Same Assay Kit. Each different commercial kit may generate different results even though all are designed for the same tumor marker. Ordering from the same laboratory also ensures a more consistent performance. It is important to ensure that any change observed during the monitoring process is due to a change of tumor volume or other tumor activities and not to laboratory variability.

Be Certain that the Tumor Marker Selected for Monitoring Recurrence was Elevated in the Patient Prior to Surgery. Because none of the tumor markers are 100% sensitive to the detection of any particular cancer, it is important to be certain that the tumor marker ordered to detect recurrence was elevated before surgery. Otherwise, multiple markers should be measured prior to the surgery in order to select the tumor marker showing the highest elevation as the marker for monitoring the disease activity. Multiple markers may be used to monitor the therapeutic effects for increased sensitivity.

Consider the Half-Life of the Tumor Marker when Interpreting the Test Result. Prior to surgery, estimate the time required for the level to decline to the normal or, in the case of PSA, to an undetectable level, based on the known half-life of the tumor marker. It is important that the success of surgical removal of a tumor as determined by tumor marker concentrations is not assessed earlier than 2 weeks postoperatively. If possible it is preferable to wait one whole month to allow the pre-existing tumor marker in the serum adequate time to decline to lower levels. For example, the half-life of serum PSA is approximately 3–4 days. Therefore, it will take 30 days for a serum PSA at 50 ng/mL to drop to an undetectable level following successful surgery.

Consider How the Tumor Marker is Removed from or Metabolized in the Blood Circulation. Elevated serum tumor markers are frequently detected in patients with renal or liver disease, depending on whether the tumor marker is removed through the kidney or metabolized by the liver. For example, serum CEA is often elevated in patients with liver disease because the impaired liver fails to remove CEA efficiently from the blood circulation, whereas an elevated serum β_2-microglobulin (β_2M) has been frequently found in patients with renal failure in which even the small β_2M molecule has difficulty passing through the glomerular membrane in a normal fashion.

Consider Ordering Multiple Markers to Improve Both the Sensitivity and the Specificity for Diagnosis. Tumors are made of heterogeneous types of cell. Some may still be normal while others may be heterogeneous tumor cells as a result of different sequences of multiple mutations. Each type of cell may express a single marker or a number of characteristic tumor markers. The same marker may also be produced by different types of cell. Some cells may never produce any unique marker. Certain types of cancer are heterogeneous in their cellular composition. Consequently, more than one tumor marker may be required to provide a high sensitivity of detection. The heterogeneity in cell composition and the percentage cell distribution of each tumor explains why a number of tumor markers may be required to reach a high (>90%) detection sensitivity and the reason that the sensitivity of an individual marker differs among cancer patients. Multiple tumor markers associated with individual malignant diseases are listed in Table 74–2; the appearance of individual tumor markers in various malignancies is listed in Table 74–3. This explains why none of the tumor markers presently employed are 100% sensitive and specific, and why the use of multiple markers will improve the sensitivity of detection. However, a unique pattern of multiple markers may be identified with tumors derived from the same tissues. Therefore, ordering multiple tumor markers may also improve the test specificity. For example, a specific pattern seems to be associated with colon, breast, ovarian, and pancreatic carcinomas when all four MAb-defined tumor markers, CEA, CA 19-9, CA 15-3, and CA 125, are measured simultaneously. This information is clinically important, since more than 60% of diagnosed human cancers are epithelial-cell-derived carcinomas (Wu, 1989). Multiple markers were used to develop a more specific screening strategy for ovarian cancer. The use of CA 15-3 and CA72.4 in combination with CA 125 can increase the apparent specificity of the CA 125 assay for distinguishing malignant from benign ovarian disease (Bast, 1991). Another example is the combination of CEA, CA19-9 and CA72-4. Use of this combination improves the diagnostic accuracy of gastrointestinal cancers (Carpelan-Holmstrom, 2002). During the selection of multiple tumor markers, only markers that are complementary to each other should be selected. Many tumor markers, which run parallel to each other when correlated with tumor activities, should not be selected for this purpose.

Be Aware of the Presence of Ectopic Tumor Markers. The expression of tumor markers is under genetic regulation. For benign tumors, the markers produced by the tumor are usually cell-specific and are related to normal cell products at an elevated concentration (Fig. 74–1). If a benign tumor becomes malignant, synthesis of the marker proteins may no longer occur. In addition, proteins that are normally found at an early fetal stage and not at normal cell regulatory mechanisms may become constitutively expressed. This is the reason that carcinoembryonic proteins and ectopic tumor markers are usually expressed in advanced malignant diseases. In other words, the appearance of ectopic tumor markers is associated with poor prognosis or metastases. For example, elevated serum concentrations of AFP may be detected in patients with cancers of the gastrointestinal tract involving metastases even though the liver function tests are normal. Table 74–4 lists some of the known ectopic markers and their associated malignant diseases.

One should be aware of the recent guidelines on gastrointestinal and breast cancer marker use published by the American Society of Clinical Oncology (Smith, 1999). They recommend monthly breast self-examination, annual mammography of the preserved and contralateral breast, and a careful history and physical examination every 3–6 months for 3 years, then every 6–12 months for 2 years, and annually thereafter. They do not recommend the use of tumor markers (such as CEA, CA 15-3, and CA 27.29) for screening, nor do they recommended routine bone scans, chest radiographs, hematologic blood counts, liver ultrasonograms, or computed tomography for screening. The American College of Physicians has also published clinical guidelines concerning the early detection of prostate cancer. They emphasize the importance of both screening PSA and performing DRE for the early detection of prostate cancer. Even though DRE is not as sensitive as PSA screening, it can detect cancer that would otherwise be missed by PSA measurement (Coley, 1997a, 1997b).

Heterophilic Antibody. The use of MAbs in immunoassays and the increasing clinical application of mouse MAbs for targeted imaging and immunotherapy create a new problem. Treated individuals apparently produce heterophilic antibodies against murine antibodies that interfere with many of the immunoassays for tumor markers (Nahm, 1990) although this is not a common encounter. The interference by the heterophilic antibodies in human sera can either increase or decrease the results of an immunoassay. These antibodies react in a way similar to antigens in terms of binding to both solid-phase-associated and signal-labeled antibodies. These heterophilic antibodies may bind to a site other than the analyte-binding site, crosslinking the signal antibody with the capture antibody, and thus generate a false assay response. It is known that as many as 15–40% of individuals may have one or more heterophilic antibodies. The standard approach for reducing heterophilic antibody interference is to include in the assay excess mouse sera or nonspecific mouse immunoglobulins in the immunoassay.

Individual Tumor Markers

α-Fetoprotein

AFP is a major fetal serum protein and is also one of the major carcino-embryonic proteins. AFP resembles albumin in many physical and chemical properties. In the fetus, AFP is synthesized by the yolk sac and the fetal hepatocytes and to a lesser extent by the fetal gastrointestinal tract and kidneys. Elevated AFP can be found in patients with primary hepatocellular carcinoma and yolk-sac-derived germ cell tumors and is the most useful serum marker for the diagnosis and management of hepatocellular carcinoma (HCC) and germ cell tumors (Lamerz, 1997). However, AFP is also transiently elevated during pregnancy and in many benign liver diseases. Because of the high prevalence of liver cancer in China and other countries in south-east Asia, AFP testing has been used successfully in screening for hepatocellular carcinoma in that region of the world. Tests for both AFP and hCG are helpful in reducing clinical staging errors in patients with some testicular tumors and aid in the differential diagnosis of various germ cell tumors. Because an increase of fucosylation of AFP (hence the lentil lectin reactivity of serum AFP) has been found in primary hepatocellular carcinoma, the determination of lentil lectin reactivity of serum AFP was found helpful not only in order to differentiate between primary hepatocellular carcinoma and benign liver diseases but also to provide an early signal indicating that hepatocellular carcinoma may begin to develop in patients with liver disease. Although the necessity for routine AFP screening needs further study, one study indicates that combined screening with AFP and ultrasonography results in increased sensitivity from 75% to near 100% in detecting hCC of patients with hepatitis B and C (Izzo, 1998; Gebo, 2002). Lastly, AFP is currently offered for prenatal screening for neural tube defects and, in conjunction with free β-hCG and unconjugated estriol, for Down syndrome (Cuckle, 2000; Yamamoto, 2001).

Angiogenic Factors

Angiogenesis is the formation of blood vessels in situ, involving the orderly migration, proliferation, and differentiation of vascular cells.

IX

Table 74–2 Serological Tumor Markers Associated with Individual Malignant Diseases

Malignant Disease	Major Marker	Other Markers
Neuronal Tumors		
Brain tumor	Desmosterol	Polyamines
Neuroblastoma	VMA	HVA, NSE, cystathionine, ferritin, metanephrines
Head and neck tumors		
Squamous cell carcinoma	CYFRA 21-1	
Endocrine System		
Pituitary tumors	Growth hormone	IGF-I
Adrenal pituitary tumors	Cortisol	Free catecholamines, DHEA, 17-ketosteroids, prolactin
Cushing syndrome	ACTH	Endorphin, lipotropin
Hypercalcemia of malignancy	PTH-related peptide	
Endocrine pancreatic tumors:	Pancreatic polypeptide:	Chromogranin AC-peptide, IGF-I binding protein I
Gastrinoma	Gastrin	
Glucagonoma	Glucagon	
Insulinoma	Insulin	
Medullary carcinoma of thyroid	Calcitonin	NSE
Microadenomas (pituitary)	Prolactin	
Multiple endocrine neoplasias	Chromogranin A	
Papillary and follicular thyroid cancer	Thyroglobulin	
Parathyroid tumors	PTH-intact	
Zollinger–Ellison syndrome	Gastrin	
Pheochromocytoma	Metanephrine	Chromogranin A, plasma catecholamines
Pituitary tumors	Free βhCG	FSH, LH, prolactin, TSH
Bone and Skeletal Muscle System		
Osteosarcomas	Alkaline phosphatase	
Breast Cancer		
Breast cancer	HER2/*neu*, CA 15-3	CYFRA 21-1, CEA, calcitonin
Pulmonary System		
Bronchogenic carcinoma	Prolactin	
Lung cancer (NSC)	CYFRA 21-1, NSE	ACTH, CK-BB, calcitonin, CA 72-4, CEA, AFP, Ferritin, LASA-P, TPA
Carcinoid tumors	Histamine, ADH, bradykinin	
Oat-cell cancer	ACTH, ADH, CEA, CK-BB, NSE, bombesin, calcitonin	
Gastrointestinal System		
Colorectal cancer	CEA	CA 19-5, CA 19-9, CA 72-4, NSE
Gastric carcinoma	CA 72-4	CA 19-9, CA 50, CEA, ferritin, CK-BB, hCG, LASA-P, pepsinogen II
Hepatocellular carcinoma	AFP	CEA, ferritin, rGT, ALP, TPA, γ-glutamyltransferase
Pancreatic carcinoma	CA 19-9	CA 19-5, CA 50, CA 72-4, CEA, CK-BB, ADH, ALP
Vipoma (pancreas)	VIP	
Genitourinary System		
Bladder cancer	T-antigen, urokinase inhibitor, TPA, cytokeratins	Glycosaminoglycans, uroplakins
Nonseminomatous testicular tumor	AFP	hCG
Prostate carcinoma	PSA	PAP, racemase
Renal cell carcinoma	Renin, erythropoietin, IL-4, PGA	
Testicular cancer	hCG	PLAP, Oct3/4
Gynecological Tumors		
Cervical cancer	SCC	CA 125, CEA, TPA
Ovarian carcinoma	CA 125	UGF, inhibin, AFP, amylase isoenzyme, CEA, CK-BB, hCG
Choriocarcinoma	hCG	
Placental tumors	hCG	Free α-hCG, CA 15-3, PTH, NSE, prolactin
Uterine cancer	SCC	
Teratoblastoma	AFP	hCG, ferritin
Hematology Malignancies and Lymphomas		
B-cell chronic lymphocytic leukemia	TdT	Serum β₂M, LASA-P
B-cell malignancies	β₂M	
Multiple Myeloma	Bence–Jones protein	β₂M
Chronic myelogenous leukemia	TdT	
Hairy cell leukemia	IL-2 receptor	
Hodgkin's disease	LASA-P, ferritin	
Leukemia	TdT	ALP, β₂M, ferritin, LDH, myelin basic protein, adenosine deaminase, PNP
Lymphoma	β₂M	TdT, Ki-67, LASA-P

Table 74–2 Serological Tumor Markers Associated with Individual Malignant Diseases (*cont'd*)

Malignant Disease	Major Marker	Other Markers
Multiple myeloma	Immunoglobulin heavy and light chain	Bence–Jones protein, β_2M, IgA
Waldenström's disease	IgM immunoglobulins	β_2M
Melanoma		
Melanoma antigen	Melanoma-associated LASA-P, L-dopa	C-reactive protein
Endoreticular System		
Spleen tumors	Ferritin	
Other		
Sarcoma	β_2M	

β_2M = β_2-microglobulin; ACTH = adrenocorticotropic hormone; ADH = antidiuretic hormone; AFP = α-fetoprotein; ALP = alkaline phosphatase; CEA = carcinoembryonic antigen; CK-BB = creatine kinase isoenzyme BB; DHEA = dehydroepiandrosterone; FSH = follicle-stimulating hormone; hCG = human chorionic gonadotropin; IGF = insulin-like growth factor; IL = interleukin; LASA-P = lipid-associated sialic acid in plasma; LDH = lactate dehydrogenase; LH = luteinizing hormone; NSC = non-small-cell; NSE = neuron-specific enolase; PAP = prostatic acid phosphatase; PGA = prostaglandin A; PLAP = placental alkaline phosphatase; PNP = purine nucleoside phosphorylase; PTH = parathyroid hormone; rGT = ; SCC = squamous cell carcinoma; TPA = tissue plasminogen activator; TSH = thyroid-stimulating hormone; VIP = vasoactive intestinal polypeptide; UGF = uterine growth factor; VMA = vanillylmandelic acid.

Table 74–3 Malignant Disease Associated with Individual Serologic Tumor Markers

Tumor Marker	Associated Malignant Disease Major Disease	Minor Disease
α-Fetoprotein	Primary hepatocellular carcinoma	Teratoblastomas of the ovary and testes
β-hCG	Pituitary tumors	
β_2-Microglobulin	B-cell neoplasias	Multiple myeloma, B-cell lymphoma, B-cell chronic lymphocytic leukemia and reticulum cell, sarcoma; Waldenström's macroglobulinemia
β-Human chorionic gonadotropin	Choriocarcinoma	Testicular cancers (nonseminomatous), trophoblastic tumors
Bence–Jones protein	Multiple myeloma	
Bombesin	Oat-cell cancer	
C-reactive protein	Melanoma	
CA 15-3	Breast cancer	Various carcinomas
CA 19-9	Pancreatic and gastric carcinoma	Various carcinomas
CA 72-4	Gastric carcinoma	Various carcinomas
CA 125	Ovarian carcinoma	Various carcinomas
CA 549	Breast cancer	
CA M26	Breast cancer	
Calcitonin	Medullary carcinoma	Cancer of the thyroid, liver cancer, renal cancer
Carcinoembryonic antigen	Colorectal carcinoma	Various carcinomas
c-*erb*B-2 oncoprotein	Breast carcinoma	Various carcinomas
Chromogranin A	Pheochromocytoma, neuroblastoma	Multiple endocrine neoplasias, small cell lung cancer, carcinoid tumors
CYFRA 21-1	Squamous cell carcinoma of the lung	
DHEA	Adrenal/pituitary cancer	
Ferritin	Acute myelocytic leukemia	Hodgkin's lymphoma, neuroblastoma and various carcinomas, teratoblastoma
Galactosyltransferase	Ovarian cancer	
Galactosyltransferase isoenzyme II	Pancreatic cancer	
Gastrin	Gastrinoma	Zollinger-Ellison syndrome
Her2/*neu*	*See* c-*erb*B-2 oncoprotein	
Human chorionic gonadotropin	Choriocarcinoma	Gastric, ovarian, and breast carcinoma, trophoblastic or germ cell tumors, testicular cancer
Hyaluronic acid	Mesothelioma	
Immunoglobulin A	Multiple myeloma	
Insulin-like growth factor-I	Pituitary cancer	Insulinoma
Interleukin-2 receptor	Leukemia	
Immunoglobulins	Multiple myeloma	Mediterranean lymphoma, Waldenström's macroglobulinemia, malignant lymphoma
Inhibin	Granulosa-cell tumors	
17-ketosteroids	Adrenal/pituitary cancer	

Blood vessel formation is also important in the pathogenesis of rapid growth and metastasis of solid tumors. Several angiogenic factors have been identified including acidic and basic fibroblast growth factor (bFGF), described in Chapter 75, angiogenin and vascular endothelial growth factor (VEGF) (Folkman, 1992). Both angiogenic and antiangiogenic factors have been found in the serum of patients with malignant disease (Morelli, 1998). Serum levels of bFGF and VEGF reflect their expression in individual tumors (Poon, 2003; Granato, 2004). The significance of elevated serum VEGF in cancer patients has been evaluated in several studies including breast, ovarian, hepatocellular, colorectal, and renal cell carcinomas and soft tissue sarcoma. Elevated serum VEGF values in ovarian cancer patients were correlated with cancer differentiation, metastasis, and, more significantly, shorter average survival time (Alvarez Secord, 2004; Harlozinska, 2004; Li, 2004). Further more, elevated serum VEGF has been associated with shorter survival in renal cell carcinoma (Ljungberg, 2003) and colon carcinoma (De Vita, 2004).

IX

Table 74–4 Ectopic Tumor Markers

Marker	Tumor
α-Fetoprotein	Gastrointestinal, renal, bladder, and ovarian carcinoma
Calcitonin	Endocrine tumors (islet cell, carcinoid, medullary thyroid, pheochromocytoma); lung, breast, and ovary carcinoma
Chromogranin A	Endocrine tumors (islet cell, carcinoid, medullary thyroid, pheochromocytoma), prostate cancer
Free α-hCG	Colorectal carcinoma and pancreatic endocrine tumors
hCG	Gastric and pancreatic carcinoma, hepatoma, ovarian carcinoma, germ cell tumor of testis
Thyroglobulin	Differentiated thyroid carcinoma

hCG = human chorionic gonadotropin.

β$_2$-Microglobulin

β$_2$M is the constant light chain of the human histocompatibility locus antigen (HLA) expressed on the surface of most nucleated cells. The molecular weight of β$_2$M is only 11.8 kDa. β$_2$M is shed into the extracellular fluid and is elevated not only in solid tumors but also in lympho-proliferative diseases (including B-cell chronic lymphocytic leukemia, non-Hodgkin's lymphoma, and, importantly, multiple myeloma) (Wu, 1986). Serum concentration of β$_2$M correlates with lymphocyte activity, making β$_2$M a good marker for lymphoid malignancies of the B-cell line. It has been used as an indicator of the patient's response to treatment (Haferlach, 1997). CSF levels of β$_2$M are useful for detecting metastases in the central nervous system (CNS). It is reported that serum β$_2$M level is elevated in 75% of multiple myeloma patients (Kyle, 2003) and is useful in following the efficacy of the treatment of this disease.

Carcinoembryonic Antigen

CEA is a glycoprotein with a molecular weight of approximately 200 kDa. It is the first of the so-called carcinoembryonic proteins and was discovered by Gold and Freedman in 1965. CEA is still the most widely used tumor marker for gastrointestinal cancer today, but most CEA assays have replaced polyclonal with monoclonal anti-CEA antibodies.

CEA was originally thought to be a specific marker for colorectal cancer but turned out to be a nonspecific marker on further studies. CEA levels can be elevated in breast, lung, and liver cancers, among others. CEA studies demonstrated that tumor markers could be used to follow patients during therapy and to detect recurrence after successful surgery. The association between highly elevated serum tumor marker concentration and metastases and poor prognosis was also discovered through CEA studies. Elevated CEA levels prior to resection of colon cancer may suggest a worse prognosis. Declining levels during therapy suggests response to therapy, while increasing levels suggest disease progression. However, clinical decisions regarding management of disease cannot be based on CEA levels alone (Mitchell, 1998). As the liver metabolizes CEA, liver damage can impair CEA clearance and lead to increased levels in the blood circulation. Increased CEA concentrations have been observed in some patients following radiation treatment and chemotherapy. It was recommended that CEA should form part of the AJCC staging system (Compton, 2000). CEA can be used as a marker for monitoring colorectal cancer (Bast, 2001). However, a low positive predictive value for diagnosis in asymptomatic patients limits its widespread use in screening.

Other genetic tumor markers are becoming used with increased frequency. For example, transforming growth factor (TGF)-α, fibroblast growth factor, and Ras oncoprotein are all increased in colorectal cancer and decreased after surgical resection. More recently, mutations of DNA mismatch repair genes (e.g. hMSH2, hMLH1 and hMSH6) are shown to be associated with hereditary nonpolyposis colorectal cancer. Further clinical studies to correlate the serum levels of expression and mutation in these genes might yield a better diagnostic/prognostic tool.

CA 15-3 and CA27.29

These antigens correspond to sequences of mucins called polymorphic epithelial mucins (PEMs), which are often overexpressed on the cell surfaces of malignant glandular cells such as occur in breast cancer, and increasing amounts are shed into the circulation where they can be detected, making them useful as tumor markers. The polypeptide core of PEM contains a 69-amino acid cytoplasmic domain and a much larger extracellular domain, consisting of 20 amino acid tandem repeats that vary between individuals, and different alleles of the human MUC1 gene may code for between 25 and 100 or more tandem repeats. A large part of the molecule is carbohydrate and the degree of glycosylation is variable, making PEM very heterogeneous in structure (Klee, 2004).

The CA 15-3 determinant is identified by two distinct monoclonal antibodies. The assay uses a solid-phase conjugated MAb, MAb 115D8, to capture the MAM-6 antigen in human plasma, and a labeled MAb DF3 as detecting antibody. MAb 115D8 was prepared against human defatted milk fat globule and MAb DF3 was prepared against the breast carcinoma cell line MCF-7. The CA 15-3 antigen is present in a variety of adenocarcinomas including breast, colon, lung, ovary, and pancreas.

CA 15-3 is a more sensitive and specific marker for monitoring the clinical course of patients with metastatic breast cancer (Canizares, 2001). CA 15-3 levels increase with higher stages of breast cancer stage (Bast, 2001). In addition, CA 15-3 can be used to predict adverse outcomes in breast cancer patients (Gion, 2002; Kumpulainen, 2002; Duffy, 2004). However, the relative low sensitivity (23%) and specificity (69%) (Chan, 2001) in detecting breast cancer has limited its usage. CA 15-3 can also be elevated in chronic hepatitis, liver cirrhosis, sarcoidosis, tuberculosis, and systemic lupus erythematosus, and in patients who smoke (Tondini, 1988). CA 27.29, another mucin marker MUC1-associated antigen, is a slightly more sensitive breast cancer marker than CA 15.3. The US Food and Drug Administration (FDA) has approved both CA 15-3 and CA 27.29 for monitoring therapy of advanced or recurrent breast cancer.

CA 19-9, CA 50, and CA 19-5

CA 19-9 is the first tumor marker of a group of new epitopes, including CA 125, CA 15-3, and CEA, defined by monoclonal antibodies. These new monoclonal kits detect newly discovered epitopes and were designed to replace polyclonal CEA measurements for various carcinomas. The assay for CA 19-9 measures a carbohydrate antigenic determinant expressed on a high-molecular-weight mucin. CA 19-9 is an epitope, defined as sialylated lacto-N-fucopentaose II, recognized by the MAb 1116NS-199. The molecule, carrying the CA 19-9 epitope, appears as mucin in the sera of cancer patients but as a ganglioside in tumor cells. CA 19-9 is also related to Lewis blood group substances. Only serum antigen from cancer patients belonging to the Le (a$^-$b$^+$) or Le (a$^+$b$^-$) blood group will be CA 19-9-positive. In addition to CA 19-9, CA 19-5 and CA50 have also been defined by monoclonal antibodies that are only slightly different from CA 19-9. CA 19-9 can be elevated in patients with colorectal cancer, gastric cancer, and pancreatic cancer. The epitope related to CA 50 is very similar to that of CA 19-9 but lacks a fucose residue, the same epitope found in Lewis-negative Le (a$^-$b$^-$) individuals. Serum CA 19-9 concentrations not only are frequently highly elevated in both gastric and pancreatic carcinomas but also are useful for monitoring the success of therapy and for detecting recurrence in these cancer patients. However, it has been reported that CA 19-9 and CA 50 complement each other in pancreatic and other carcinomas: their simultaneous use will improve the sensitivity in detecting these malignant diseases. CA 19-5 is detected by mouse MAb CC3C-195 and reacts with both Le^a and sialyl-Le^a epitopes. CC3C-195 binds with high affinity to the sialylated Le^a blood group antigen but exhibits a lower affinity to the nonsialylated form. Elevated serum levels of CA 50 and CA 19-5 can also be found in patients with colon, pancreatic, and hepatocellular carcinomas. False positives may occur in patients with benign liver disease and may be due to cholestasis in these patients (Wu, 1992).

CA 125

CA 125 is another antigenic determinant defined by a MAb and is also associated with a high-molecular-weight (>200 kDa) mucin-like glycoprotein. CA 125 is expressed by more than 80% of nonmucinous epithelial ovarian carcinomas and is found in most serous, endometrioid, and clear cell carcinomas of the ovary (Jacobs, 1989). However, patients undergoing chemotherapy may show a false decline of CA 125 antigen and a negative result does not always rule out tumor recurrence. CA 125 is also used clinically for follow-up on uterine tumors (>60% are elevated) and benign tumors, including endometriosis. Recent studies showed greatly improved sensitivity of serum CA125 in combination with other markers using proteomics techniques, shown by several studies (discussed in detail in succeeding chapters) (Jacobs, 2004; Lu, 2004; Zhang, 2004). Studies for the application of serum CA125 in other cancerous (e.g. non-Hodgkin's lymphoma, lung cancer) and non-malignant (e.g. liver cirrhosis) diseases have been performed (Ando, 2003; Xiao, 2003; Zidan, 2004) and showed increased levels of CA125 in the sera of these patients.

CA 72-4

The CA 72-4 assay detects a mucin-like human adenocarcinoma-associated antigen, TAG-72, which is a high-molecular-weight (>10⁶ Da) mucin-like complex molecule. Because the TAG-72 can be detected in both fetal epithelia and sera from patients with various carcinomas, it is also considered to be a carcinoembryonic protein. However, only moderately elevated serum CA 72-4 are found in most carcinomas. Currently, CA 72-4 is considered to be useful marker for the management of patients with gastric and colorectal carcinoma. CA 72-4 has been proposed as a specific marker for tumor occurrence of resectable gastric cancer (Marrelli, 2001) and a prognostic marker for survival (Gaspar, 2001). CA 72-4 has been reported to be an independent prognostic marker for survival in colorectal cancer (Louhimo, 2002) in multivariate analysis together with β-hCG and CEA.

Calcitonin

Calcitonin is one of the circulating peptide hormones that may become elevated in patients with increased bone turnover rate associated with skeletal metastases. Calcitonin can be ectopically elevated in bronchogenic carcinomas and is also elevated in medullary carcinoma of the thyroid.

Chromogranin A

Chromogranin A is a major soluble protein of the chromaffin granule. Chromogranin A and catecholamines are released from the adrenal medulla upon stimulation of the splanchnic nerve. However, chromogranin A is not confined to chromaffin cells of the adrenal medulla and sympathetic neurons. It is also present in various neuroendocrine organs. Elevated serum chromogranin A levels can be detected in pheochromocytoma (Giovanella, 2002), medullary carcinoma of thyroid, and small-cell lung carcinoma (Ma, 2003). Interestingly, increased serum chromogranin A levels are detected in epithelial cancers with neuroendocrine differentiation, including prostate, breast, ovary, pancreas, and colon (Wu, 2000).

Prostate cancer with neuroendocrine differentiation has been an active area of study. Higher levels of serum chromogranin A is associated with poorly differentiated prostate cancer (Isshiki, 2002). It is also increased after androgen blockade therapy and systemic radionucleotide therapy (Ferrero-Pous, 2001) for prostate cancer. Furthermore, an association between increased chromogranin A and prostate cancer metastasis has been observed (Tarle, 2002). Intermittent androgen deprivation therapy can reduce the levels of chromogranin A, and thus the neuroendocrine differentiation of prostate cancer (Sciarra, 2003).

Cytokeratin 19 Fragment

Cytokeratin 19 fragment (CYFRA 21-1) is a fragment of the cytokeratin 19 intermediate filament found in the serum. It is a subunit of a cytokeratin intermediate filament expressed in simple epithelia and their malignant counterparts. Studies of elevated serum CYFRA 21-1 have concentrated on breast cancer and squamous cell carcinoma of the lung. CYFRA 21-1 was reported to have a sensitivity of 60%, 64.2%, and 89% for the detection of stage IV breast cancer, recurrence, and metastasis respectively. Probability of survival for primary cancer patients, recurrence after surgery and response after chemotherapy were correlated with elevated preoperative serum CYFRA 21-1 in breast cancer patients (Nakata, 2000, 2004). CYFRA 21-1 was also shown to reflect the tumor mass in multiple studies with correlation to tumor stage, survival, predictive role in surgical treatment for early stage disease and chemotherapy for advanced stage non-small cell lung cancer. In one study of head and neck squamous cell carcinoma (SCC), increased postradiotherapeutic or chemotherapeutic CYFRA 21-1 has been explored as an early indicator for distant metastasis (Kuropkat, 2002). CYFRA 21-1 is not increased in patients with non-neoplastic lung disease including pneumoconiosis and obstructive airway disease (Schneider, 2003).

Human Chorionic Gonadotropin

Human chorionic gonadotropin, a member of the glycoprotein hormone family, is synthesized and secreted by trophoblast cells of the placenta and is a heterodimeric hormone composed of noncovalently linked α and β subunits internally linked by disulfide bonds. The current assays using monoclonal antibodies are available to detect intact hCG, 'nicked' hCG or hCGn (which is partially degraded hCG missing peptide bonds between amino acids 44–45 or 47–48), hCG α subunit, hCG β subunit and hCG β core (residual hCG β, residues 6–40 joined by disulfide bond to hCG β, residues 55–92) (Berger, 2002, Birken, 2003). Both malignant and nonmalignant trophoblast cells synthesize and secrete not only the

biologically active α and β-dimer but also the uncombined (or free) α and β subunits. In addition to the intact dimer, a free β subunit of hCG has been detected in the serum of women during early pregnancy and in patients with malignant tumors (detailed in Chapter 25).

Measurement of the free β-subunit is useful for the detection of recurrence or metastasis for choriocarcinoma when the intact hCG may remain normal. Analysis of serum hCG subunits is especially useful for managing patients with germ cell tumors (von Eyben, 2003). However, elevated hCG can be found in trophoblastic tumors, choriocarcinoma, and testicular tumors. More than 60% of patients with nonseminomatous germ cell tumors and 10–30% with seminomas have elevated free β-hCG.

Seminomatous testicular cancer contains both intact hCG and β-hCG or free α subunits in equal amounts. Therefore, only one assay is needed for monitoring these patients. On the other hand, only hCG or β-hCG subunits may be found in patients with nonseminomatous cancers. The measurement of both free subunits and intact hCG will increase the test sensitivity for these patients with nonseminomatous cancers.

Ectopic free β-hCG production occurs in approximately 30% of patients with other cancers including urothelial cancer, but only the free β-hCG and its respective breakdown product, β-core, has been detected in these clinical samples. Ectopic α-hCG is a marker of malignancy in pancreatic endocrine tumors (Ma, 2003). Recent efforts in preparation of new World Health Organization reference reagent for hCG (HCG, hCG-α and hCG-β) and its related molecules may decrease the non-specific reaction and increased accuracy of clinical hCG testing (Bristow, 2005).

HER2/*neu* (c-*erb*B-2) Oncoprotein

The HER2/*neu* (c-*erb*B-2) oncogene is a 185 kDa transmembrane protein of the tyrosine kinase receptor family and is discussed extensively in Chapter 75. It shows structural and functional homology with the epidermal growth factor receptor (EGFR) containing intracellular, transmembrane, and extracellular domains (Fig. 74–2). HER2/*neu* has been found to be elevated in the sera of patients with a number of different epithelial cell cancers, including breast, lung, colorectal, and ovarian cancers. Enzyme-linked immunosorbent assay (ELISA) measures the levels of the circulating c-*erb*B-2, referred to as p105 or serum HER2 constituting the ectodomain (Fig. 74–2). Here we emphasize that, in patients with breast cancer, serum HER2/*neu* is more important as a prognostic and predictive marker. At the time of initial diagnosis, serum HER2/*neu* is elevated in only 5–10% of breast cancer patients. Increased serum HER2/*neu* before adjuvant therapy has been shown to be associated with increased tumor size, tumor grade, and positive lymph nodes. Pre- and postchemotherapy HER2/*neu* levels could serve as a prognostic marker for disease-free survival and overall survival (Hayes, 2001; Saghatchian, 2004). In addition, serum HER2/*neu* levels correlate with response to chemotherapy (that includes chemotherapeutic agents and hormone antagonists and Herceptin (Trastuzumab), an anti-HER2/*neu* antibody); higher levels predict shorter treatment response while low levels suggest longer or complete treatment responses (Colomer, 2000; Harris, 2001; Lipton, 2002; Bethune-Volters, 2004; Luftner, 2004). HER2/*neu* is also overexpressed and/or amplified in ovarian cancer, prostate, gastric cancer and bronchial carcinomas so it can be used as a therapeutic target in these cancers (Agus, 2000).

There are two currently FDA-approved ELISA assays for serum circulating HER2 using monoclonal antibodies, one for microtiter plate assay (Oncogene Science) and one for an automated instrument (Bayer Diagnostics). More importantly, the serum HER2/*neu* test is not interfered by heterophile antibodies and more significantly the therapeutic MAb trastuzumab because different antigen epitopes are targeted (Fig. 74–2).

p53

p53 (detailed in Chapter 75) is a 53 kDa nuclear phosphoprotein and a negative regulator of cell growth. It functions as a tumor suppressor by inducing the expression of gene products that are responsible for inhibiting or arresting cell growth and proliferation. The ability of p53 protein to regulate transcription of its target genes is based on its sequence-specific DNA binding activity and the presence of a domain that can activate transcription when attached to the DNA-binding domain of p53 target protein. It is the DNA-binding domain that appears to be sensitive to disruption by mutation, and most lesions associated with human cancers occur within this domain. The encoding gene for p53 has been found to be mutated in about half of almost all types of cancer arising from a wide spectrum of tissues. Because of its short half-life (20 minutes), the wild-type p53 protein in the blood circulation is not detectable (Malkin, 1990; Harris, 1993). However, current molecular techniques such as PCR/SSCP (detailed in Section VIII) can detect serum p53 gene mutations. The presence of p53 antibody in serum facilitated the

IX

detection of abnormal p53 serologically. Significantly, the presence of p53 antibody in serum is associated with expression of p53 mutations and positively correlates with the degree of cancer malignancy (discussed in Chapter 75).

Parathyroid Hormone-Related Peptide

Plasma concentrations of parathyroid hormone-related peptide (PTH-RP) are elevated in the majority of patients with cancer-associated hypercalcemia. PTH-RP is secreted by tumors associated with hypercalcemia. The circulatory forms of PTH-RP in these patients include both a large amino-terminal peptide and a carboxyl terminal peptide with close sequence homology to parathyrin (PTH). The mechanism by which PTH-RP induces hypercalcemia involves binding and activating receptors that also bind PTH. Measuring the concentrations of PTH-RPs may be useful in the differential diagnosis of hypercalcemia related to malignancy and associated either with primary hyperparathyroidism, sarcoidosis, vitamin D toxicity, or various malignancies (including squamous cell, renal, bladder, and ovarian carcinomas). It should be noted that patients with impaired renal function but without hypercalcemia or cancer may have increased plasma concentrations of PTH-RP (Burtis, 1990).

Prostate-Specific Antigen

PSA is a member of the kallikrein family of serine proteases that is synthesized uniquely in the epithelial cells of the prostate gland. Its expression in these cells is regulated by the androgen receptor. Because of its high degree of tissue specificity, it is perhaps the most widely used tumor marker discovered thus far. The normal reference range is 0–4 ng/ml. The cancer sensitivity and tissue specificity of PSA makes it the most useful tumor marker available for the screening and management of prostate cancer. Lack of cancer specificity, in distinguishing prostate cancer and nonmalignant prostate lesions, is the main drawback with PSA. Benign conditions such as BPH, acute prostatitis, and infarction can also be correlated with elevated serum PSA levels.

PSA serves as an excellent cancer marker in prostate cancer screening, diagnosis, prediction of cancer risk, and recurrence. Since its discovery in prostate cancer serum in 1980 (Papsidero, 1980), PSA has been subjected to intensive research and clinical usage in the screening, detection, and monitoring of prostate cancer. PSA and its various forms are used to guide clinical decisions for further tissue biopsy diagnosis, resulting in increased prostate cancer detection, especially in young men. Use of PSA in prostate cancer detection has also resulted in a reduction in the number of prostate cancers discovered only at late stages in which metastases occurred, from about 30% of all newly diagnosed cases to about 10% of all such cases (Cooperberg, 2004). Annual PSA screening is recommended both by the American Urological Association and the American Cancer Society for all men over the age of 50. In addition, because of its tissue specificity, the PSA assay is particularly useful for monitoring the success of surgical prostatectomy. Complete removal of the prostate should result in an undetectable PSA level, while incomplete resection of the gland (not persistent disease) might result in measurable levels of PSA. However, it should remain unchanged on extended follow-up. Any increase in measurable PSA after a successful radical prostatectomy would indicate prostate cancer recurrence or metastasis. It should be noted that a transient and modest increase of PSA may occur during radiation therapy, which should not be misinterpreted as disease progression.

Multiple studies suggest that over 80% (in some studies, >90%, e.g., DeSoto-LaPaix, 2003) of patients with prostate cancer are diagnosed with this condition from serum PSA levels that are above 4 ng/ml. Because BPH and acute prostatitis also induce elevated serum PSA levels, approximately half of patients with PSA values above 4 ng/ml are not found to have prostate cancer on biopsy even at significantly elevated levels, i.e., over 10 ng/ml. These studies therefore suggest that PSA has a sensitivity of a minimum of 80% and a specificity of around 50%. However, it has also been found that about 20% of initially negative biopsies, when repeated over a 3-year period, become positive (DeSoto-LaPaix, 2003). Thus the specificity of PSA may be higher, assuming that the biopsies missed a malignant lesion and that a new malignancy did not occur over the 3 year time period.

On the other hand, the cutoff value of 4.0 ng/ml does not sufficiently distinguish patients with and without prostate cancer, including aggressive ones (Schroder, 2000; Horninger, 2002; Punglia, 2003; Thompson, 2004). In a recent study (Thompson, 2004), it was found that, in a large group of over 1000 patients who were followed annually with serum PSA levels and prostate biopsies, over 25% were found to have prostate cancer, some of them with high Gleason scores, with serum PSA levels that were less than 4 ng/ml, many of then having PSA levels of less than 2 ng/ml. This result

suggests that using the 4 ng/ml cutoff value for PSA limits its sensitivity to around 75%, which is close to the 80% value obtained in other studies. This study could not reveal whether the PSA values in the 25% group with biopsy-proven but serum-PSA-negative prostate cancer would rise, and, if so, over what time interval. Ironically, as discussed above, first biopsies also miss detection of prostate cancer approximately 20% of the time. In fact, repeat biopsies are often performed as a result of elevated and rising PSA values.

One solution to the dilemma of detecting prostate cancer in patients whose serum PSA levels are less than 4 ng/ml is to change the cutoff to lower values (Punglia, 2003) and, in fact, many commercial PSA test kits now available are capable of detecting serum PSA below 0.1 ng/ml. Unfortunately, this has the effect of substantially diminishing the specificity of PSA, consequently diminishing its positive predictive value and its ability to be used to screen patients for this disease.

There are several approaches that have been developed both to increase the sensitivity and specificity of PSA in detecting prostate cancer. First, as noted previously, use of serum PSA in combination with either DRE or transrectal ultrasound of the prostate results in increases in both sensitivity and specificity (Catalona, 1991; Brawer, 1992). In addition, the PSA fractions, i.e., free and bound, have been used to increase the sensitivity and specificity of elevated serum PSA in the diagnosis of prostate cancer.

Free PSA, Complex PSA, and percentage of free PSA

PSA is capable of complexing with various endogenous protease inhibitors, including α_1-antichymotrypsin (ACT) and α_2-macroglobulin (to which it binds covalently). Consequently, serum PSA exists in the serum largely (up to 90% of total PSA) (Vessella, 1997) in the form of a PSA-ACT (PSA–α_1-antichymotrypsin) complex (Christensson, 1993).

It has been found that, in prostate cancer, there is generally an increase in the serum concentration of bound PSA and a corresponding decrease in unbound or free PSA (Parsons, 2004). Thus, immunoassays have been developed that quantify either bound or free PSA. Based on these assays, it has been found that measuring complex PSA (with ACT) directly not only eliminates many technical problems associated with PSA assays but also improves the differentiation of BPH from prostate cancer (Wu 1994, 1998), thereby increasing test specificity (Parsons, 2004). Conversely, measurement of free PSA (fPSA) and the calculation of percentage of fPSA (%fPSA = [fPSA/total PSA] × 100), which has an inverse relationship with prostate cancer risk (Polascik, 1999), have been used to help to differentiate BPH from prostate cancer, also increasing test specificity and reducing unnecessary biopsies for BPH patients. More importantly, the free PSA ratio improves the specificity for prostate cancer detection in men with PSA between 4–10 ng/ml, also reducing unnecessary biopsies. In addition, free PSA may be useful as a prostate cancer morbidity predictor (Polascik, 1999; Ito, 2003). Some studies also showed that %fPSA can be used to predict prostate cancer in patients with PSA less than 4.0 ng/ml (Djavan, 1999, Horninger, 2002). One caveat is that free PSA is subject to quick degradation at 4°C or above. The recommended time interval from sample collection and assay should be less than 3 hours and the sample should be stored and shipped at −70°C (Woodrum, 1996). Overall, prostatic cancer is associated with elevated complexed PSA and low %fPSA (<6%) (Catalona, 1995), and higher ratios of free PSA (>23%) are usually associated with BPH.

There are several different assays for free and complexed PSA, some of which are summarized in Figure 74–3. When PSA is bound, certain antigenic determinants are 'buried' by the protein to which it binds (mainly, ACT). These are, of course, exposed on free PSA, so that antibodies to the 'buried' determinants of complexed PSA will detect only free PSA. On the other hand, there are determinants that are exposed on both free and complexed PSA and can be detected by antibodies to these determinants, allowing for determination of total PSA. Finally, antibodies to the buried PSA determinant are available that also block the common exposed determinant. These antibodies react only with free PSA by binding to the buried determinant but also block the exposed common site. Now, in the presence of this blocking antibody, another antibody is added that reacts only with the common exposed determinant. The only available common exposed determinants are on complexed PSA. Thus this double antibody approach, using a blocking antibody and a detection antibody, quantifies the level of complexed PSA.

PSA Doubling Time, Velocity and Density

The time required for the PSA value to double is known as the PSA doubling time. It has been shown that the PSA doubling time can predict recurrence after radical prostatectomy in androgen-independent prostate cancer patients (Lee, 2003; Loberg, 2003).

The rate of PSA increase over time, PSA velocity (Carter, 1992), is the PSA difference divided by the number of year(s). It has been shown that a

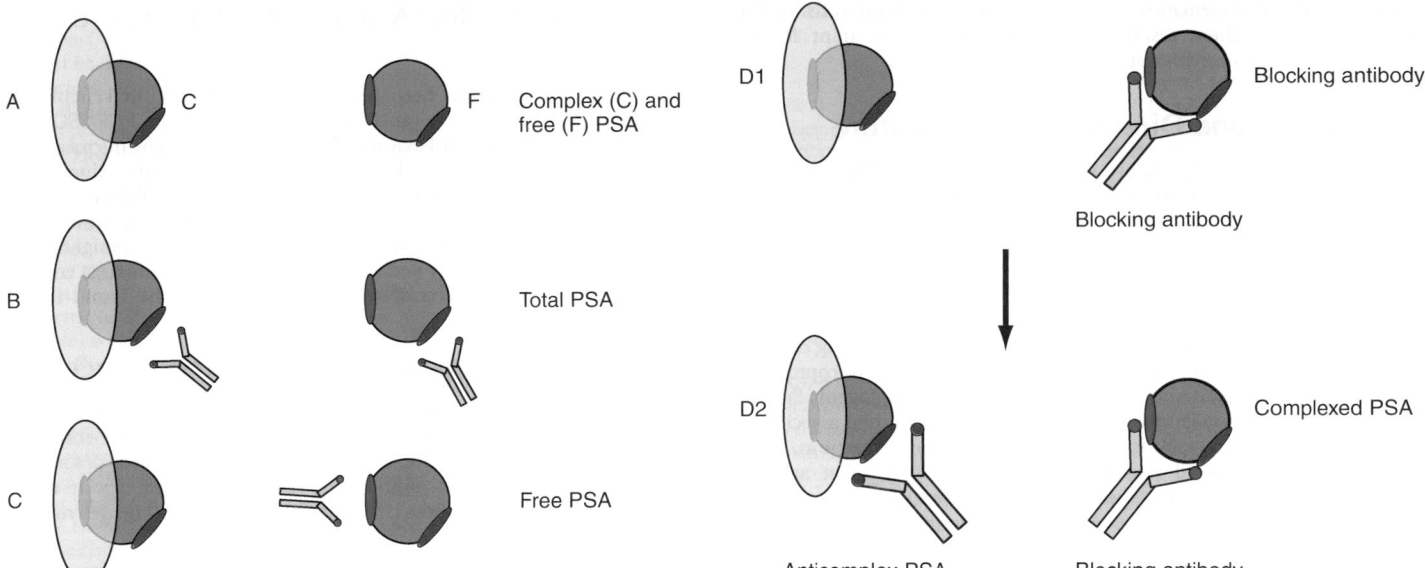

Figure 74–3 Three different assays for prostate-specific antigen (PSA). In *A*, PSA is shown to exist in the free (F) or complexed (C) states. Some of its antigenic determinants (blue in the figure) are buried in the complexed state. These are exposed in the free state. On the other hand, as shown in *B*, there are common determinants, red in the figure, that are exposed in both complexed and free PSA. Antibodies to these common determinants will detect total PSA (free + complexed). Since the blue determinants are exposed only in free PSA, as shown in *C*, antibodies to these determinants will detect only free PSA. Finally, as shown in *D1*, antibodies have been developed against the blue determinant of free PSA that also block the red determinant. Thus antibodies to the red determinant, which is common to both free and complexed PSA, will react only with complexed PSA as shown in *D2*. This is the basis for the Bayer assay for complexed PSA.

PSA velocity of 0.75 ng/year or above is a strong predictor of cancer with a specificity of 95% (Carter, 1992). More recently, it has been shown that PSA velocity may be useful in predicting prostate cancer risk when PSA levels are between 2.0 and 4.0 ng/ml (Fang, 2002). This is especially useful in predicting the risk of cancer and guiding the necessity of prostate biopsy in patients with low/normal PSA value (2.0–4.0 ng/ml). In a recent study, it has been shown that patients with a preoperative PSA velocity above 2.0 ng/ml may have a relatively high risk of death from prostate cancer (D'Amico, 2004). This is a notable finding because prostate cancer causes significant mortality, although a large number of prostate cancer patients die from other causes. While these studies demonstrate a method of identifying aggressive forms of prostate cancer, randomized larger cohort studies are needed to validate these observations. Preoperative PSA velocity is not a good parameter for prostate cancer grade, stage, or recurrence (Freedland, 2001). *PSA density* is a measure of the ratio of total PSA to prostate gland volume as measured by transurethral ultrasonography; PSA densities of greater than 0.15 indicate an increased probability of prostate cancer as opposed to BPH (Polascik, 1999).

PSA, therefore, is a useful biomarker for prostate cancer, and can be made even more useful diagnostically both by employing it in conjunction with other methods such as DRE and by quantifying its fractions (complexed and free).

Fecal Occult Blood Testing and Mutant Protein Markers in Stool

Perhaps the most familiar test to screen for cancer in patients is the fecal occult blood test, which is performed in the physician's office on stool samples obtained from a DRE. It is performed routinely on most patients as part of annual check-ups. In the hospital outpatient setting, it is more common to have the patient obtain a stool sample for testing after a bowel movement. The idea, of course, is that if blood is discovered in the stool, there is the chance that a colonic tumor is the cause, and further work-up, such as colonoscopy, is therefore strongly recommended. The actual test for occult blood is based on the ability of the heme moiety of hemoglobin to catalyze the oxidation of the colorless compound guaiaconic acid (hence the name, guaiac test) in the presence of H_2O_2 to a highly conjugated blue-colored quinone. Usually, the guaiaconic acid is impregnated on a strip or solid support, and the stool specimen is placed on a discrete section of the strip. It is obvious that this is a nonspecific test since blood in stool can be caused by a number of nonmalignant causes such as hemorrhoids, colitis, diverticulitis, and local trauma to the perianal area, diminishing the specificity of this test. False positives for this test are also caused by exogenous factors such as meat fibers from meat ingestion and bismuth, present in antacid preparations such as Pepto-Bismol. In addition, the ability of this method to detect the presence of colon cancer depends on

such factors as whether and to what extent a cancer hemorrhages, its location (the closer to the rectum, the greater the likelihood of detection) and its pattern of growth (e.g., exophytic tumors are more likely to be detected than nonexophytic ones). The sensitivity of the fecal occult blood test is between 15% and 30%. It is much less effective than colonoscopy, the definitive mode of colon cancer detection. However, it offers the advantage of being noninvasive although now, with 'virtual colonoscopy' based on CT scanning of the colon, this advantage is diminished.

As a result, there has been an effort to devise new noninvasive tests on stool specimens that have higher sensitivity and specificity than fecal occult blood tests. As discussed in the following chapter, several mutant genes that code for proteins that are involved with control of the cell cycle have been strongly implicated as vitally important causative factors of colon cancer. These include mutant *ras* (of the Kirsten or K-variety), mutant p53, the adenomatous polyposis coli (*APC*) gene and the gene product BAT-26, associated with microsatellite instability. All of these mutant genes are oncogenes in colon cancer. Standardized reverse-transcriptase polymerase chain reaction (RT-PCR) techniques, discussed in Section VIII, are available to detect mutations in any or all of these proteins. In addition, 'long' DNA, thought to result from disordered apoptosis of cancer cells in colon cancer, has also been found to occur in a number of colon cancers. If sufficient numbers of cancer cells from a colon cancer are sloughed off into the lumen, one or more of the above mutant genes (and/or long DNA) can be discovered, allowing for the noninvasive detection of colon cancer.

Using this approach, a cooperative study, involving the Colorectal Cancer Study Group, has recently been completed in which over 5000 patients were entered and over 2000 were completely evaluated for colon cancer using fecal occult blood testing, multioncogene testing on stool and colonoscopy (Imperiale, 2004). All patients were 50 years of age or older (mean, 69.5 years). The results showed that the genetic RT-PCR-based methodology results in significantly higher rates of detection than fecal occult blood testing. Overall, the rate of detection of adenocarcinoma was 51.6% for the genetic screening while it was 12.9% for fecal occult blood screening. Interestingly, advanced adenomas were detected in 15.1% of cases in the genetic screening and 10.7% in the fecal occult blood screening. Since this condition may be regarded as a precursor for frank malignancy, both methods seem to have similar rates of early detection. On the other hand, the rate of detection of TNM stage I colon cancer by genetic screen was 53.3% while that for fecal, occult blood screening was 6.7%, suggesting that genetic screening is substantially more effective in detecting true colon cancer in its early stages. Surprisingly, both tests were found to have similar apparent false positivity rates in conditions of minor polyps (7.6% vs 4.8% for genetic and occult blood tests, respectively) and the condition of no polyps found on colonoscopy (5.6% vs 4.8% for genetic and occult blood tests, respectively). Although this study has certain drawbacks, such as too few patients with cancers and advanced adenomas with high-grade dysplasia, skewing of the age of the population to 65 years of age and

biomarker discovery and detection. Urol Oncol 2004; 22:322–328.

Polascik TJ, Oesterling JE, Partin AW: Prostate specific antigen: a decade of discovery – what we have learned and where we are going. J Urol 1999; 162:293–306.

Poon RT, Lau CP, Cheung ST, et al: Quantitative correlation of serum levels and tumor expression of vascular endothelial growth factor in patients with hepatocellular carcinoma. Cancer Res 2003; 63:3121–3126.

Punglia RS, D'Amico AV, Catalona WJ, et al: Effect of verification bias on screening for prostate cancer by measurement of prostate-specific antigen. N Engl J Med 2003; 349:335–342.

Rai AJ, Chan DW: Cancer proteomics: serum diagnostics for tumor marker discovery. Ann N Y Acad Sci 2004; 1022: 286–294.
Serves as an example and summary of the identification of biomarkers using current serum proteomics technology and will be the trend for future biomarkers.

Saghatchian M, Guepratte S, Hacene K, et al: Serum HER-2 extracellular domain: relationship with clinicobiological presentation and prognostic value before and after primary treatment in 701 breast cancer patients. Int J Biol Markers 2004; 19:14–22.
Provides evidence that serum HER2/neu may be useful in prognosis and monitoring treatment of breast cancer patients.

Sangrajrang S, Arpornwirat W, Cheirsilpa A, et al: Serum p53 antibodies in correlation to other biological parameters of breast cancer. Cancer Detect Prev 2003; 27: 182–186.

Schlichtholz B, Legros Y, Gillet D, et al: The immune response to p53 in breast cancer patients is directed against immunodominant epitopes unrelated to the mutational hot spot. Cancer Res 1992; 52:6380–6384.

Schneider J, Philipp M, Velcovsky HG, et al: Pro-gastrin-releasing peptide (ProGRP), neuron specific enolase (NSE), carcinoembryonic antigen (CEA) and cytokeratin 19-fragments (CYFRA 21-1) in patients with lung cancer in comparison to other lung diseases. Anticancer Res 2003; 23:885–893.

Schroder FH, van der Cruijsen-Koeter I, de Koning HJ, et al: Prostate cancer detection at low prostate specific antigen. J Urol 2000; 163:806–812.

Sciarra A, Monti S, Gentile V, et al: Variation in chromogranin A serum levels during intermittent versus continuous androgen deprivation therapy for prostate adenocarcinoma. Prostate 2003; 55:168 179.

Sheen-Chen SM, Eng HL, Huang CC, Chen WJ: Serum levels of soluble E-selectin in women with breast cancer. Br J Surg 2004; 91:1578–1581

Smith TJ, Davidson NE, Schapira DV, et al: American Society of Clinical Oncology 1998 update of recommended breast cancer surveillance guidelines. J Clin Oncol 1999; 17:1080–1082.

Soussi T: p53 Antibodies in the sera of patients with various types of cancer: a review. Cancer Res 2000; 60:1777–1788.

Soussi T, Beroud C: Assessing TP53 status in human tumours to evaluate clinical outcome. Nat Rev Cancer 2001; 1:233–240.

Syrigos KN, Salgami E, Karayiannakis AJ, et al: Prognostic significance of soluble adhesion molecules in Hodgkin's disease. Anticancer Res 2004; 24:1243–1247.

Tarle M, Ahel MZ, Kovacic K: Acquired neuroendocrine-positivity during maximal androgen blockade in prostate cancer patients. Anticancer Res 2002; 22:2525–2529.

Thompson IM, Pauler DK, Goodman PJ, et al: Prevalence of prostate cancer among men with a prostate-specific antigen level < or =4.0 ng per milliliter. N Engl J Med 2004; 350:2239–2246.

Tondini C, Hayes DF, Gelman R, et al: Comparison of CA15-3 and carcinoembryonic antigen in monitoring the clinical course of patients with metastatic breast cancer. Cancer Res 1988; 48:4107–4112.

Vessella RL, Lange PH: Issues in the assessment of prostate-specific antigen immunoassays. An update. Urol Clin North Am 1997; 24:261–268.

Von Eyben FE: Laboratory markers and germ cell tumors. Crit Rev Clin Lab Sci 2003; 40:377–427.

Von Knobloch R, Brandt H, Hofmann R: Molecular serological diagnosis in transitional cell bladder cancer. Ann N Y Acad Sci 2004; 1022:70–75.

Wilmanns C, Grossmann J, Steinhauer S, et al: Soluble serum E-cadherin as a marker of tumour progression in colorectal cancer patients. Clin Exp Metastasis 2004; 21:75–78.

Woodrum D, French C, Shamel LB: Stability of free prostate-specific antigen in serum samples under a variety of sample collection and sample storage conditions. Urology 1996; 48(Suppl):33–39.

Wooster R, Neuhausen SL, Mangion J, et al: Localization of a breast cancer susceptibility gene, BRCA2, to chromosome 13q12–13. Science 1994; 265:2088–2090.

Wu JT: Expression of monoclonal antibody-defined tumor markers in four carcinomas. Ann Clin Lab Sci 1989; 19:17–26.

Wu JT: Serum alpha-fetoprotein and its lectin reactivity in liver diseases: a review. Ann Clin Lab Sci 1990; 20:98–105.

Wu JT: Assay for prostate specific antigen (PSA): problems and possible solutions. J Clin Lab Anal 1994; 8:51–62.

Wu JT, Carlisle P: Low frequency and low level of elevation of serum CA 72-4 in human carcinomas in comparison with established tumor markers. J Clin Lab Anal 1992; 6:59–64.

Wu JT, Clayton F, Myers S, Knight J: A simple radial immunodiffusion method for assay of β 2-microglobulin in serum. Clin Chem 1986; 32:2070–2073.

Wu JT, Erickson AJ, Tsao KC, et al: Elevated serum chromogranin A is detectable in patients with carcinomas at advanced disease stages. Ann Clin Lab Sci 2000; 30:175–178.

Wu JT, Liu GH: Advantages of replacing the total PSA assay with the assay for PSA-alpha 1-antichymotrypsin complex for the screening and management of prostate cancer. J Clin Lab Anal 1998; 12:32–40.

Xiao WB, Liu YL: Elevation of serum and ascites cancer antigen 125 levels in patients with liver cirrhosis. J Gastroenterol Hepatol 2003; 18:1315–1316.

Yamamoto H, Lambert-Messerlian GM, Silver HM, et al: Maternal serum levels of type I and type III procollagen peptides in pre-eclamptic pregnancy. J Matern Fetal Med 2001; 10:40–43.

Yu YH, Schlossman DM, Harrison CL, et al: Coexpression of different antigenic markers on moieties that bear CA 125 determinants. Cancer Res 1991; 51:468–475.

Zhang Z, Bast RC Jr, Yu Y, et al: Three biomarkers identified from serum proteomic analysis for the detection of early stage ovarian cancer. Cancer Res 2004; 64:5882–5890.
Serves as an example and summary of the identification of biomarkers using current serum proteomics technology and will be the trend for future biomarkers.

Zidan J, Hussein O, Basher W, Zohar S: Serum CA125: a tumor marker for monitoring response to treatment and follow-up in patients with non-Hodgkin's lymphoma. Oncologist 2004; 9:417–421.

CHAPTER 75

Oncoproteins and Early Tumor Detection

Matthew R. Pincus MD PhD, Paul W. Brandt-Rauf MD PhD DPH,
Martin H. Bluth MD PhD

KEY POINTS

- As a result of the vast progress that has been made very recently in sequencing the entire human genome and in illuminating pathways that are involved in tumorigenesis, it has become clear that the malfunctioning of mutant proteins is the central cause of human cancers.

- These proteins – growth factors, growth factor receptors, G-proteins such as p21^{ras}, the mitogen-activated protein kinases (MAPKs), and nuclear proteins such as Myc, Fos, Jun and p53 – are critical on signal transduction pathways in which proliferation signals from growth factors at the cell membrane are transduced to the nucleus and stimulate cell division.

- The mutations in these proteins result in amino acid substitutions or deletions that cause them to be permanently activated. Mutations in regulatory domains of the genes encoding these proteins can result in protein overexpression, which can also result in continuous mitogenic signaling.

- These proteins and antibodies to them can be used to detect the presence at early stages – and even to predict the future occurrence – of cancers in patients.

- Detection of these mutated proteins can be readily accomplished using enzyme-linked immunoassays (ELISA), Western blotting and mass spectroscopy.

- This has given rise to a whole new field of proteomics, i.e., detection of these proteins, and the DNA encoding them, in the blood and other body fluids of patients.

- Although mutated signal transduction proteins are involved in many different human cancers, it appears that there are patterns of expression of mutated proteins that typify specific cancers.

As a result of the vast progress that has been very recently made in sequencing the entire human genome and in illuminating pathways that are involved in tumorigenesis, it has become clear that the malfunctioning of mutant proteins is the central cause of human cancers. This has given rise to a whole new field of proteomics, i.e., detection of these aberrant proteins in the blood and other body fluids of patients. This chapter explains these new approaches and emphasizes that many of these aberrant proteins are actually involved in the transmission of proliferation signals on signal transduction pathways, the more prominent of which are discussed. The fundamental aims of this chapter are to explain our understanding of the signal transduction pathways in cell proliferation, how different mutant proteins on these pathways can cause abnormal, continuous proliferation signaling leading to cell transformation, how these proteins and antibodies to them can be used to detect the presence – and even to predict the future occurrence – of cancers in patients and how new proteins, that are strongly associated with different types of cancer have been discovered and can be used to detect these cancers at early stages.

Cell Biology and Mitogenesis

Control of the process of cell division in eukaryotic cells, especially in the higher forms of life, is vital to the processes of cell proliferation and

IX

differentiation. The fine balance between these two processes is regulated by numerous proteins that interact in the cell to ensure that this balance is maintained. Virtually all these proteins, many of which are critical in regulating the cell cycle, are encoded by oncogenes. Mutations in oncogenes can result in the production of proteins that either become permanently activated in stimulating cell growth and proliferation (such as the *ras*-gene-encoded p21 protein) or become inactive in inhibiting cell proliferation (such as the p53 protein). Both events give rise to malignant tumor cells. Knowledge not only of the existence of these oncogenes and their encoded oncoproteins but also of the mechanisms by which they exert their effects has resulted in a new series of highly sensitive assays for both mutated oncogenes and their encoded mutant proteins. Assays using amplification methods such as polymerase chain reaction (PCR) for mutated oncogenes are discussed in Section VIII. In this chapter, we discuss how detection of oncogenic proteins, or oncoproteins, that occur in the serum of patients with malignant tumors enables the diagnosis of malignancy to be made, often at an early stage of tumor development. Because the finding of elevated levels of any of these oncoproteins or mutated forms of these proteins in human serum indicates the likely presence of a malignant tumor, these proteins are also referred to in this chapter as tumor markers.

Oncogenesis, the process by which normal cells become malignant, involves multiple steps, which can be broadly classified into tumor initiation and tumor promotion. Mitogenesis itself is a multistep process that commences at the cell membrane as a result of the activation of a growth factor receptor, which then activates other membrane and cytosolic proteins and second-messenger molecules that transduce the mitogenic 'signal' to the nucleus.

Signal Transduction Pathways

A number of the steps on the signal transduction pathway that are invoked in the transduction of the growth factor-initiated signal to the nucleus has become elucidated, but many of the steps that are involved are not fully understood. One well-established pathway, for the *ras*-oncogene-induced mitogenic signaling pathway, is summarized in Figure 75–1. This figure shows that, when a growth factor receptor is activated by its growth factor, it in turn activates several intermediary proteins (Grb-2 and SOS) that activate the all-important G-protein (i.e., guanosine triphosphate [GTP]-binding protein), p21^{ras}. This membrane-bound 21 kDa protein, containing 189 amino acids, is activated when the SOS protein induces it to bind GTP in place of GDP. In its activated (GTP-bound) state p21^{ras} directly activates *raf* (Moodie, 1993; Stokoe, 1994), which, in turn, induces a sequential protein kinase cascade beginning with the kinase, MEK (formerly called MAP kinase kinase) and mitogen activated protein (MAP) kinase encoded by the *ERK* gene, as shown in Figure 75–1.

MAP kinase directly activates nuclear transcription factors, one of these being Fos. This important protein forms a heterodimeric complex with another nuclear transcription factor, Jun, which is directly activated by Jun kinase (JNK). The Fos–Jun complex, also called AP1, binds to specific regions of genomic DNA, inducing the transcription of mitogenic proteins such as the cyclins. Transcription of these proteins is blocked by the antioncogene p53 protein (Fig. 75–1), which further induces the transcription of antimitotic proteins such as Bax and Waf that induce apoptosis.

Also shown in Figure 75–1 are several other important nuclear oncogene-encoded proteins such as Myc, a 75 kDa protein that is overexpressed in Burkitt's lymphoma. This oncogene protein is not directly on the *ras* signal transduction pathway. Interestingly, there are cell lines that when transfected either with the *ras* oncogene or with the *myc* oncogene do not undergo cell transformation but when transfected with both oncogenes simultaneously do undergo cell transformation. These results indicate that *ras* and *myc* may be interdependent and are an excellent prototypical example of the multistage nature of oncogenesis.

A central feature of the signal transduction events summarized in Figure 75–1 is that the activation cascades are ordered and are under tight regulatory control. Thus, for example, while SOS activates Ras-p21, GTPase-activating protein (GAP) induces hydrolysis of GTP bound to Ras-p21, causing its inactivation (Fig. 75–1). Activated MEK downregulates SOS, diminishing GDP/GTP exchange by Ras-p21 (Holt, 1996).

If one or more proteins on pathways such as the one shown in Figure 75–1 become mutated so that they cannot be downregulated, continuous mitogenic signaling becomes possible, leading ultimately to neoplasia. The more such mutations occur, the more likely it is that the cell will undergo malignant transformation. Thus, progressive lesions in the mitogenic pathway may correspond to the multiple steps in carcinogenesis.

Table 75–1 summarizes the mechanisms by which each type of signal transduction element has been found to induce cell transformation,

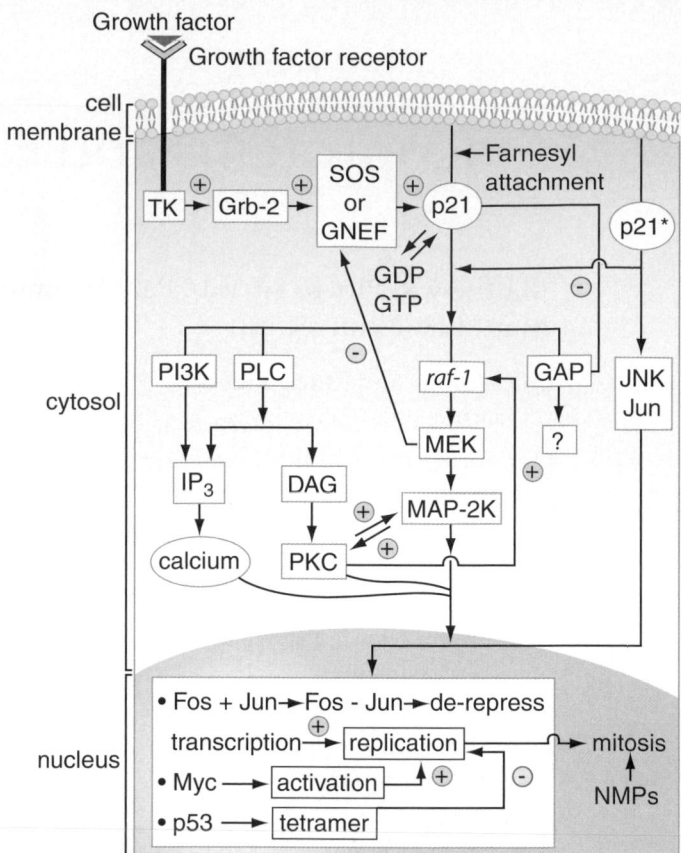

Figure 75–1 Scheme of some of the known components of the *ras* signal transduction pathway beginning (top, left) when a growth factor binds to its cell receptor. The remainder of events is explained in the text. DAG = diacylglycerol; GAP = GTPase-activating protein, which promotes hydrolysis of GTP to GDP bound to p21; grb-2 = the adaptor protein that concurrently binds p21 and the guanine nucleotide exchange protein or factor, SOS; PI3K = phosphoinositol-3-hydroxy kinase, an enzyme that induces synthesis of IP3 and is involved in many aspects of mitogenic signal transduction; IP3 = inositol triphosphate; MAP-2 kinase = mitogen-activated protein kinase or microtubule-associated protein kinase-2 (MAP-2K in the figure, also called ERK); *myc*, *fos*, and *jun* = nuclear oncogenes that code for nuclear proteins; NMP = nuclear matrix proteins; PKC = protein kinase C; PLC = phospholipase C; Raf-1 = the oncogene-encoded p74 protein, which functions as a kinase that phosphorylates another kinase of molecular mass 43 kDa, called MAP-2 kinase kinase, MEK (as in the figure, or MAP-KK in the figure; *ras*-p21 protein, p21^{ras}, defined in the text.

Table 75–1 Mechanisms for Induction of Carcinogenesis by Mitogenic Pathway Elements

Pathway Element	Mechanism of Action
1. Growth factors	a. Overproduction by cell into surroundings
	b. Interaction of growth factors with high affinity receptors
2. Growth factor receptors	a. Overexpression leading to high concentration of dimers
	b. Loss of extracellular domain resulting in permanent dimerization of growth factor receptor and continuous signaling
	c. Amino acid substitutions in transmembrane domain leading to permanent dimerization
3. Cytosolic proteins	a. Overexpression of normal G-proteins and protein kinases
	b. Amino acid substitutions that permanently change conformation to activated form
	c. Mutations that remove regulatory domains of kinases
4. Nuclear oncoproteins	a. Overexpression of transcription and replication proteins
	b. Mutations in antioncogene proteins that inactivate them
	c. Mutations that remove regulatory domains

Table 75–2 Summary of Some Important Oncogenes and Their Protein Products

Oncogene	Protein Product	Function
1. *erbB**	EGF receptor	Binds to EGF; dimerizes; activates tyrosine kinases in signal transduction. May work through *ras*
2. *erbB-2**	GF receptor	Very similar to EGF receptor but uses different GF. May work through *ras*
3. *sis**	β-chain of PDGF	Growth factor receptor. May work through *ras*
4. *src*	Tyrosine kinase	Transduces signal through *ras*
5. *ras**	p21 proteins; H-, K-, and N- forms	G-proteins; bind to cell membrane and transduce signals through second messengers and *raf*, GAP(?), JNK, PKC and PLC
6. *rap-1A*	Anti-*ras* oncogene; in *ras* family	Blocks *ras* action in cells
7. *raf**	74 kDa protein	Phosphorylates MAP kinase kinase, which then phosphorylates MAP kinase
8. *erk-1* and *erk-2**	MAP kinase family 43 kDa proteins	Involved in cytoskeletal rearrangements and nuclear signaling.
9. *myc**	62/64 kDa nuclear protein	Turns on transcription factors involved in replication.
10. *jun*	Nuclear protein	Forms complex with *fos*
11. *fos*	Nuclear protein	Forms complex with *jun*. *fos–jun* complex activates transcription factors
12. p53*	53 kDa nuclear anti-oncogene protein	Forms tetramers, then binds DNA segments to block transcription and replication.
13. *NMP22**	236 kDa nuclear matrix protein	Involved in mitotic spindle formation

Only a few of the many (more than 50) oncogenes are listed in this table. The ones that are listed here encode proteins for which assays have been developed or are closely related to these proteins. No growth factors except PDGF are included in this table. The following abbreviations are used: GF, growth factor; EGF, epidermal growth factor; PKC, protein kinase C; PLC, phospholipase C; GAP, GTPase activating protein; MAP kinase, mitogen-activated protein kinase; NMP22, nuclear matrix protein 22. The names of the oncogenes are commonly used and relate to the sources from which they were originally discovered. For example, *ras* is an abbreviation for **ra**t **s**arcoma viral oncogene.

* Oncogene-encoded proteins for which assays have been performed on human serum.

beginning with growth factors, progressing to growth factor receptors, then to G proteins and the kinase cascades, and finally to nuclear proteins. These mechanisms are discussed in more detail in each section of this chapter devoted to these different signal transduction proteins.

Oncoproteins in Tumor Detection

Detection of mutated signal transduction proteins or high levels of the wild-type proteins in serum or body fluids is strongly suggestive of neoplasia. Therefore, many assays for different oncoproteins are now available in kit form, including enzyme-linked immunosorbent assay (ELISA) assays for the growth factors transforming growth factor (TGF)-α and fibroblast growth factor (FGF), the growth factor receptor proteins EGFr and HER-2/Neu, Ras-p21, and the nuclear proteins p53, Myc, and NMP22 from such companies as Oncogene Science (Uniondale, NY), Triton Bioscience (Houston, TX) and Matritech (Newton, MA). A number of studies also employ the technique of Western blotting or immunoblotting, as described elsewhere in this book.

Numerous studies have documented alterations in oncogene, oncoprotein, or growth factor expression in terms of messenger RNA (mRNA) or protein in tumor tissue compared with normal tissue (Pimentel, 1989; Brandt-Rauf, 1998; Pincus, 2003). Several studies have examined oncoprotein or growth factor expression in biological fluids such as urine or effusions and demonstrated the feasibility of using these peptides and proteins as markers for the presence of neoplasia (Niman, 1985; Yeh, 1989). Succeeding studies have confirmed these initial findings, resulting in the clinical use of these markers to detect the presence of neoplasia.

Recent studies have now revealed that oncogenes themselves can be detected in the body fluids of patients with different types of cancer. With the advent of microarray techniques both for gene expression and for protein detection, it is now possible to assay for the presence of multiple oncogenes and oncoproteins in the body fluids, especially serum, of cancer patients. A new, parallel approach for screening for cancer has been developed in which serum samples are subjected to mass spectroscopy and pattern analysis that detects the presence of proteins expressed uniquely in the blood of cancer patients.

The focus of this chapter will therefore be on the identification of different oncoproteins and growth factors, the genes encoding these proteins, in serum, plasma, or urine in patients with cancer or at-risk for the development of cancer.

A summary of some of the many (>50) known oncogenes and their functions in the cell is given in Table 75–2. Those for which commercial assays are available are labeled with an asterisk.

Growth Factors

Since various growth factors are believed to play a role in influencing cellular proliferation during tumorigenesis and since growth factors are actively secreted into the extracellular environment, they are potentially attractive targets for detection in blood during cancer development. Several studies to date have been able to demonstrate differences in blood levels of growth factors in cancer patients and non-cancer controls.

Transforming Growth Factors-α and -β

TGF-α is a polypeptide with 50 amino acids that binds to the EGF receptor, which dimerizes upon binding to EGF. TGF-β is a family of proteins labeled β_1–β_5. TGF-β_1 is a homodimer of two 12 kDa subunits linked together by disulfide bonds. While TGF-β has been found to be elaborated by many different types of human malignant tumors, elevated serum levels of this growth factor have been found predominantly in cancers of the liver and bladder. Interestingly, TGF-β has been found to inhibit mitosis in specific cell lines in culture, such as mink bronchial epithelial cells. Thus, the serum of patients who have tumors elaborating this growth factor can be assayed for it by measuring the extent of inhibition of cell growth.

TGF-β activity, determined using this technique, has been found to be markedly elevated in patients with hepatocellular carcinoma but not in age-matched controls (Shirai, 1992). In the sera of patients who have undergone surgical resection of these tumors, the activity of TGF-β is barely detectable, suggesting that the tumor was the source of the elevated levels of growth factor in serum. Interestingly, in many patients with hepatocellular carcinoma, TGF-β has been found to be elevated in urine (Tsai, 1997).

Use of an ELISA with a monoclonal antibody directed against TGF-β_2 has revealed that TGF-β_2 is elevated in a high proportion of patients with invasive bladder cancer but not in patients with noninvasive bladder cancers or in cancer-free patients (Klocker, 1994; Brandt-Rauf, 1998; Pincus, 2003). Recently, a new tumor marker for bladder cancer that appears to be more accurate in diagnosing both noninvasive and invasive bladder cancer is the nuclear matrix protein NMP22, detected in urine, as discussed below.

Thus, serum assays for TGF-β are highly useful in diagnosing and following hepatocellular carcinoma. They are less useful in the diagnosis of carcinoma of the bladder, although for invasive bladder cancer this growth factor has a high sensitivity and specificity.

TGF-α has been found to be elevated in a large number of patients with epithelial cell tumors (Katoh, 1990; Chakrabarty, 1994), predominantly

gene and of its encoded p21 protein have been found in approximately one of three common human epithelial cell tumors, in over 90% of human pancreatic tumors and 75% of human colon cancers (Almoguera, 1988; Forester, 1987).

One of the consequences of amino acid substitutions in p21 and presumably in other signal-transducing proteins is the abnormal activation of alternate, unregulated signal transduction pathways. Oncogenic p21^{ras} protein (p21 in Fig. 75–1) has been found to bind directly to Jun, the nuclear transcription factor and its activating kinase, Jun kinase (JNK). This binding process results in the direct activation of these nuclear transcription-inducing proteins, thereby bypassing the normal cellular controls. This bypass or short-circuit pathway is shown on the right side of Figure 75–1 for p21 (Adler, 1995; Amar, 1997). In addition, oncogenic p21^{ras} protein requires activation of protein kinase C as a downstream event on its signal transduction pathway (Pincus, 1992), as illustrated in Figure 75–1.

As noted previously, the ras-oncogene-encoded p21 proteins are 21 kDa membrane-associated G proteins that have been implicated in the growth signal transduction process from the cell membrane to cytoplasmic kinases. Qualitative (i.e., point mutations) and quantitative (i.e., over-expression) changes in p21 have been identified as contributing to human carcinogenesis (Barbacid, 1987). By as yet undefined mechanisms, p21 proteins gain access to the extracellular environment. Thus, increased amounts of p21 or point-mutated forms of p21 can be detected by immunoblotting with monoclonal antibodies in the supernatant of cells in culture known to overexpress p21 or to express mutant p21, respectively (Brandt-Rauf, 1991, 1998; Pincus, 2003).

Similarly, mice bearing tumors that overexpress p21 or express mutant p21 are found by immunoblotting to have increased amounts of p21 or mutant forms of p21 in their serum, respectively (Hamer, 1991). These results suggest that the detection of increased p21 or mutant p21 in blood is possible in humans.

Because of its central role in mitogenic signal transduction, overexpressed and/or mutated p21 protein might be expected to be present in a wide variety of human tumors. Indeed, elevated serum p21 has been identified in the serum of up to 68% of patients with many different cancers, including breast, prostate, colon, lung, and liver cancer. On the other hand, only a small percentage of normal individuals have been found to have detectable serum levels (Weissfeld, 1994).

A very high incidence of the occurrence of the oncogenic form of the K-ras gene has been found in human pancreatic and colonic cancers. New assays based on reverse-transcriptase (RT)-PCR have detected the ras oncogene in the stool of a high percentage of patients with colonic cancer (Pincus, 2004). Further similarly encouraging results have been obtained using the sputum of patients with lung cancer. Parallel results have now been obtained using the ELISA for the p21 protein using the serum of patients with lung and colonic carcinoma. Elevated levels (five times more than controls) of serum p21^{ras} have been found in up to 83% of lung cancer patients, while only low levels were found in the sera of normal individuals (Brandt-Rauf, 1991, 1998). In addition, studies have been carried out in which PCR for K-ras mutant genes with base changes at codons 12 and 13 has been performed concurrently on tumor tissue and serum from patients with different stages of colorectal cancer (de Kok, 1997). In over 90% of the patients with specific mutant ras genes found in tumor tissue, the same mutated ras gene was discovered in their sera, irrespective of the stage of the tumor.

Previously, in the discussion of the HER-2/neu-oncogene-encoded p185 protein, it was noted that elevations of the serum levels of this protein were found in patients with pneumoconioses who then progressed to develop frank malignancies. A parallel study has been performed on patients with pneumoconioses in which assays were carried out for p21^{ras} in their sera. For patients with this predisposing condition, 39% have been found by immunoblotting (Western blotting) to have elevated serum levels of the p21 protein. Almost all of these patients developed a malignant lung tumor subsequent to the observed elevations of the p21 protein. Thus, like p185 ECD, elevated serum p21 is a biomarker of early malignant disease in patients with a known predisposition. An obvious study that is yet to be performed is to assay the sera of these patients for both HER-2/neu and p21^{ras} to increase the sensitivity of the assays.

The preceding studies are concerned with detecting elevated serum levels of p21 in serum as an indicator of malignancy. As noted previously, a major mechanism for oncogenesis induced by the p21^{ras} protein is amino acid substitutions in its sequence that result in its permanent activation. Identification of mutant ras genes by PCR and direct sequencing of DNA isolated from the serum or plasma of three patients with pancreatic cancer has been described (Sorenson, 1994) but until recently the direct detection of mutant p21 protein had not been reported in human blood (de Kok, 1997). Now, however, oncogenic amino acid substitutions in the

p21 protein can be identified through the use of monoclonal antibodies that recognize specific oncogenic substitutions.

Mutated p21 has been found in the serum of patients with a known history of exposure to the carcinogen vinyl chloride. This chemical has been shown to predispose individuals to developing angiosarcomas (Brandt-Rauf, 1998). Tissue studies of these angiosarcomas reveal that a mutant ras gene that codes for aspartic acid in place of the normally occurring glycine at position 13 in the polypeptide chain is present in the tumor cells. A monoclonal antibody that recognizes the Asp13 form of the p21 protein has been obtained (Oncogene Science). This mutant p21 protein has been identified in the sera of 80% of patients with vinyl-chloride-induced angiosarcoma of the liver but not in normal individuals (DeVivo, 1994). There is a direct correlation, moreover, between the degree of exposure of patients to vinyl chloride and the probability of discovering the oncogenic form of the protein in their serum.

A number of other highly specific antimutant p21 monoclonal antibodies have been obtained that recognize specific amino acid substitutions at positions 12, 13, 59, and 61. Use of these antibodies on the sera of patients with known risk factors for cancer appears to offer much promise for early tumor detection.

Cytosolic Mitogenic Kinases: raf

As shown in Figure 75–1 and Table 75–2, Raf is a 74 kDa protein that is a critical target of p21^{ras}. It directly activates MEK, which, in turn, activates MAPK (ERK) (Fig. 75–1, Table 75–2). It is involved in cell growth, proliferation, apoptosis, and differentiation. There are several different isoforms of Raf, such as Raf A and Raf B, which may differ in their exact cellular functions. Over 30 mutations of the B-raf gene associated with human cancers have been identified (Wan, 2004). Western blot analysis showed that activated Raf was overexpressed in tissues obtained from cirrhosis and hepatocellular carcinoma patients (91.2% and 100% respectively) (Hwang, 2004). B-raf mutations have also been found in colon cancer, although less frequently than K-ras (Monstein, 2004). However Raf is found minimally to not at all in tissues from patients with bladder or endometrial carcinoma (Mutch, 2004; Stoehr, 2004). Its role in melanoma is less clear, as Raf is also found in a majority of benign nevi (Wellbrock, 2004). These results suggest that Raf may be a useful and specific marker for both colon and hepatocellular carcinomas.

Nuclear Oncoproteins

As noted previously, two important nuclear proteins that appear to play critical roles in the regulation of cell growth and division are the tumor suppressor gene protein, p53, and the p62/75 protein encoded by the c-myc oncogene for which serum assays have been developed. Furthermore, nuclear skeletal or matrix proteins are the targets of signal transducing kinases such as MAP kinase, as indicated in Figure 75–1.

p53 and c-myc Proteins

The protein p53 is known to function as a homotetramer and, in this form, binds to specific sequences of DNA. The effect is to repress the mitotic process. In addition, activation of p53 in transformed cells results in apoptosis via activation of proapoptotic proteins such as Bax, waf^{p21}, and caspases. Thus, p53 is an antioncogene protein. Mutations can occur in p53 that inactivate it. This inactivation can itself be oncogenic because the vital control that this protein exerts over mitogenesis is removed. Among the inactivating mutations are deletions of the whole gene, as has been found in a number of colon cancers, and mutations in the gene resulting in amino acid substitutions in the encoded p53 protein. These substitutions cause conformational changes in the protein that result in its inability to perform its antioncogenic function in the cell (Brandt-Rauf, 1996).

Many different point mutations in p53 have been identified in human tumors (Soussi, 1994). The effect of these mutations is to cause a loss of the normal growth-inhibitory function of p53 and, at the same time, some of these mutations result in p53 proteins with considerably increased half-lives so that the mutant proteins accumulate in the transformed cells (Soussi, 1994).

The c-myc oncoprotein is activated to cause cell transformation by overexpression, so it, too, accumulates in transformed cells (Field, 1990). Thus, for both p53 and p62/75 myc, increased levels of the proteins can be detected in transformed cells and human tumors (Field, 1990; Soussi, 1994). This overexpression apparently results in leakage of the proteins into the extracellular environment. Not only can these proteins therefore be detected in serum and other body fluids but these normally sequestered proteins are recognized as foreign, so that some cancer patients develop antibodies to p53 or p62/75 *myc*. As a result, increased concentrations of p53 or p62/75 or of antibodies to these proteins in blood are excellent markers for the study of human carcinogenesis.

Detection of Malignancies by Assaying for p53 Protein

Hepatocellular Carcinoma

Increased levels of mutant p53 in serum by ELISA (>0.3 ng/mL, the upper limit of 100 normals) have been found in 20% of patients with hepatocellular carcinoma and 30% of patients with cirrhosis, a group known to be at increased risk for the development of hepatocellular carcinoma (Virji, 1992). Since patients with cirrhosis have high levels of p53 in their sera and a known risk factor for developing hepatocellular carcinoma, the elevated p53 levels may be an early indicator of tumorigenesis.

Breast and Lung Cancers

There have been few studies on p53 as a tumor marker in the sera of patients with breast and lung cancers. Elevated serum mutant p53 levels determined by ELISA have been reported in 8% of breast cancer patients, with levels decreasing following surgical resection of the tumors (Rosanelli, 1993), indicating that the tumors were the source of the elevated p53. Elevations of p53 protein have not been observed in the sera of any normal individuals.

For lung cancer, elevated serum mutant p53 levels determined by ELISA and immunoblotting have been found in up to 34% of lung cancer patients but not in normal individuals (Fontanini, 1994). For these patients, immunohistochemical staining of subsequently obtained biopsy tissue showed elevated p53 levels, correlating with the serum findings.

Colon Cancer

An important mechanism believed to be operative in the development of colonic carcinoma is the deletion of the normal *p53* gene or mutation of the gene leading to a nonfunctional antioncogenic protein. Elevated serum mutant p53 determined by ELISA has been found in about one in five patients with colon carcinomas and in approximately one in ten patients with colon adenomas. Normal individuals were found to be negative for serum p53 protein. These results show relatively low sensitivity of this marker for colon cancer, possibly because deletion of the *p53* gene occurred in a high percentage of the tumors studied.

Bladder Cancer

Studies on the urine of patients with bladder cancer using PCR for *p53* on shed cells in urine samples found that the *p53* gene was mutated in a high proportion of these patients (Sidransky, 1991), supporting the use of p53 in screening for this disease in a completely noninvasive manner. As discussed further below, p53, together with several other promising markers, may result in a set of tests that have a high positive predictive value.

Circulating Anti-p53 Antibodies in Tumor Detection

Serum antibodies against p53 have been reported to be a frequent occurrence in patients with several types of cancer. Production of antibodies to p53 and other oncoproteins has been attributed to their accumulation in necrotic cells and their subsequent release into the circulation, where they are recognized as foreign (Pincus, 2003). For p53, there is another cause for the development of antibodies to oncogenic p53. Like oncogenic p21^{ras}, mutant p53 proteins containing single amino acid substitutions at critical positions in the polypeptide chain themselves become oncogenic. These amino acid substitutions induce major changes in the conformation of the p53 protein (Brandt-Rauf, 1996; Adler, 1998). Among these changes is the exposure of specific antigenic determinants that are not normally exposed (Pincus, 2003). If the protein diffuses into the circulation, antibodies against these determinants often develop.

In several major studies (including a large study of 1392 cancer patients), elevated serum levels of anti-p53 antibodies were found in patients with ovarian and colon cancers (15%); lung cancers, including small cell tumors (up to 25%); and breast cancers, including intraductal carcinoma (up to 15%). Normal individuals did not have elevated serum levels of these antibodies (Angelopoulou, 1994). In a significant number of patients who have been followed for the presence of anti-p53 antibodies in their sera, the appearance of these antibodies has been found to precede the occurrence of malignant tumors. Anti-p53 antibodies are also found to occur in over 20% of patients with bladder cancer (mostly at more advanced stages), in a high proportion of patients with pancreatic and hepatocellular carcinomas, and in childhood lymphomas.

Continuing follow-up studies on anti-p53 antibodies in patients with different cancers reveal that up to half of the patients with hepatocellular carcinoma, regardless of the size, have markedly elevated serum levels of anti-p53 (Ryder, 1996). These elevated levels correlate with the known elevation of p53 in the sera of patients with this type of cancer, as discussed above. Furthermore, anti-p53 antibodies have been found in the serum of patients with oral lesions, and many of these patients were found to have premalignant lesions (Kaur, 1997), indicating that anti-p53 antibodies are markers for early detection of oral cancer. Anti-p53 has also been found to be elevated in over 50% of patients with esophageal squamous cell carcinoma (Shimada, 1998).

In a prospective study of patients with carcinoma of the lung, serum anti-p53 levels were found in 100% of patients with large cell carcinoma, 28% with adenocarcinomas, 55% with squamous cell carcinomas, and 71% with small-cell carcinomas (Segawa, 1998). These results demonstrate that elevated serum anti-p53 levels are tumor-type-specific for carcinoma of the lung, showing high positivity rates for large- and small-cell lung carcinomas.

A recent retrospective study (Li, 2004) of 103 patients with a known prolonged exposure to asbestos whose serum was banked between the years 1980 and 1988 has been performed. These patients were all followed until the end of 2001. Assays for anti-p53 antibodies were performed on the banked sera. It was found that, of 49 patients who developed cancer, 13 (26.5%) had significantly elevated levels of anti-p53 antibodies in their sera while four of 54 (7.4%) individuals who did not develop cancer were found to have these antibodies. In all four cases, the antibody levels were found to be marginally above the cut-off for positivity and in all four, subsequent banked serum samples were found to be antibody-negative. In contrast, in all 13 cancer patients for whom multiple samples were available, all samples were positive for these antibodies. Statistical analysis of these results show that the presence of anti-p53 antibodies is an independent predictor of cancer occurrence and that survival in anti-p53-antibody-free patients is significantly greater than in anti-p53-antibody-positive patients.

myc-Oncogene-Encoded Protein in Tumor Detection

The *myc* gene codes for a protein of molecular mass 75 kDa that functions as a transcription factor. When activated, it derepresses expression of other genes that encode proteins involved in replication. This oncogene is overexpressed in a number of tumors, including Burkitt's lymphoma wherein the *myc* gene on chromosome 8 is translocated to a long-terminal-repeat-like region of an immunoglobulin-coding region of chromosome 14. Long terminal repeat regions allow constitutive expression of genes that are adjacent to them.

c-*myc*-related proteins and antibodies to the c-*myc* protein have, like p53 and antibodies to it, been identified in the serum of cancer patients. Detection of this 62/75 kDa protein is hampered by its short half-life in serum. However, it is possible to detect a specific c-*myc*-related p40 protein in the serum of these patients, using immunoblotting. The highest frequencies of occurrence of *myc* protein in human serum has been found to occur in breast (about 20%) and colon cancer. Treatment of both types of cancer results in marked diminution in the serum levels of this protein. Recurrences result in elevated levels; c-*myc* protein is therefore useful in following the course of malignant tumors. It has not been detected in the sera of normal individuals.

Serum Anti-c-*myc* Protein Antibodies in Tumor Detection

High serum levels of anti-c-*myc* antibodies have been found in the sera of patients with colorectal cancer (55% to 65%) and in the sera of patients with both myeloid leukemias and Burkitt's lymphoma. Lower occurrences of elevated antibodies have been reported in patients with breast cancer (around 10%) and ovarian cancers (10%). Anti-c-*myc* antibodies have not been found in the sera of normal individuals.

Nuclear Matrix Proteins – Detection of Bladder Cancer

As noted in Figure 75–1, important targets of oncogene-encoded proteins are nuclear matrix proteins (NMPs), also referred to as nuclear skeletal proteins, and nuclear mitotic apparatus proteins. These 236 kDa proteins are vital for correct mitotic spindle formation. They contain a globular head and tail separated by a central rod-like α-helical core domain consisting of heptad repeat sequences. These proteins vary by cell type, stage of differentiation, and cell cycle. Crucially, a number of tumor-associated NMPs has been identified, each specific for one of five tumor types (bladder, prostate, breast, colon, and bone). The best studied is one strongly associated with transitional cell carcinoma of the bladder, NMP22, which functions as a nuclear mitotic apparatus protein, involved with chromosomal separation during mitosis (Hughes, 1999). The amount of this protein in malignant transitional epithelial cells is 10–20 times that in normal cells.

Antibodies that are specific for this NMP have been developed and are now used in a commercial ELISA on urine (Matritech, Newton, MA). The basis for the assay is that, since malignant urothelial cells are sloughed off into the urine, and this NMP is specific for bladder cancer cells, elevation of this protein in urine can be detected in patients with bladder cancer. Multiple studies of patients who have bladder cancers of a variety of different stages reveal that the sensitivity is close to 90% in malignant, invasive cancer and 75% in carcinoma in situ. The latter result is highly encouraging, since this stage is the earliest detectable one. For malignant papillary, noninvasive carcinoma, the sensitivity is 62%. The overall specificity for this marker is over 90%.

Comparison of the sensitivity of NMP22 ELISA with that of cytology reveals that the two methods are about 83% sensitive for invasive carcinoma, but for grade I transitional cell carcinoma, NMP22 is 61% sensitive while cytology is only 17% sensitive (Landman, 1998). For grades II and III cancers, the NMP22 ELISA is more sensitive at 78% and 93% as compared with cytologic sensitivities of 50% and 87%, respectively (Landman, 1998).

This method has been approved by the US Food and Drug Administration, both for screening for the presence of bladder cancer and for the follow-up of bladder cancer in patients who have been treated for this disease. With respect to the latter use of this method, clinical studies have been performed in which the NMP22 ELISA was performed on the urine of patients who have been treated for transitional cell carcinoma, 20–60 days following treatment, who were then subjected to cystoscopy 2–6 months following treatment. Using a cutoff of 10 U/mL, 86% of patients with negative (<10 U/mL) NMP22 values were found to have negative cystoscopic results and 71% of patients with values greater than 10 U/mL were found to have positive cystoscopic findings. These results, combined with those of other studies, suggest that this methodology may well obviate the necessity for performing cystoscopy on many patients who are being followed for tumor recurrence (Miyanaga, 1997).

NMP22 can be used to monitor the recurrence or bladder cancer after resection. However, since recurrent tumors are smaller than initial tumors, cutoff values should be altered in these cases as the sensitivity of this test increases from 19% to 49% when the cutoff value is reduced to 5.0 U/ml (Miyanaga, 2003).

Bladder Tumor Antigen

Several other biomarkers for bladder cancer are also being used to aid in the diagnosis and follow-up of this disease. Prominent among these is the so-called bladder tumor antigen, which measures a human complement H protein that is produced by malignant but not by normal transitional epithelial cells. This marker has a somewhat lower sensitivity than that for NMP-22 and also has a lower specificity due to false-positive results from trauma to the urothelial tract. However, use of NMP-22 together with bladder tumor antigen and a number of other markers, including urokinase-type plasminogen activator, can improve the overall sensitivity of bladder cancer detection (Shariat, 2003). It should be further noted that other tests on urine, such as those for mutant or absent p53 as discussed above and for homozygous deletion of the 9p21 chromosome, discussed below, also have high diagnostic yields. Since these tests are relatively simple to perform, it is conceivable that they can be placed on a chip, to be discussed below, that will allow for simultaneous evaluations. A positive result on one or more test would be diagnostic of bladder cancer.

Use of Multiple Oncoprotein Markers in the Diagnosis of Cancer

In view of the success in detecting the presence of cancer using single oncoprotein markers, it is surprising that there have been few studies using multiple oncoprotein markers to detect cancers. When such studies have been performed, it has been found that the diagnostic yield is definitely increased.

Multiple Oncoprotein Assay in Patients at Risk for Tumor Development

In a prospective study, 46 patients with a history of exposure to carcinogens and with attendant pneumoconiosis participated in a study in which their sera were assayed for elevated levels of five oncoproteins: p21^{ras}, Fes, Myb, PDGF and Int-1. Eighteen of these patients were found to have cancer, including 13 with lung cancer or mesothelioma, at the time the assays were performed. Of these 18 patients, 13 were found to have markedly elevated levels of at least one of the five oncoproteins assayed for. Eight of these patients were found to have elevations of at least two of these proteins. Another seven patients were found to have elevations of at least two of these oncoproteins but were not found to have cancer. Although some of these latter patients were lost to follow-up, long term follow-up revealed the subsequent development of cancer in all the remaining patients. Importantly, several of the patients with only one elevated marker were found to have elevations of different tumor markers in their serum, emphasizing the importance of assaying for as many different oncoproteins as possible (Qin, 2002).

Oncoprotein Arrays Likewise Hold Promise in Detecting Antioncoprotein Antibodies in Patients' Sera

Based on the findings discussed above that many patients with cancers are found to have antibodies to a variety of oncoproteins, such as p53 and Myc, studies have been performed to detect one or more such antibodies in patients' sera. In one such study, a miniarray of up to seven full length recombinant oncoproteins was prepared and included such oncoproteins as Myc and p53.

This array was employed to detect antibodies in 527 sera from patients with six different types of cancer (Zhang, 2003). The antibody frequency to any one oncoprotein was on the order of 15–20%, but inclusion of all seven oncoproteins resulted in detection of up to 68%. Furthermore, distinct patterns of antibody expression were found for patients with breast, lung, and prostate cancer although no discrete patterns were found for patients with gastric, colorectal, and hepatocellular carcinomas.

These encouraging results can easily be enhanced by the inclusion of more oncoproteins. Given the results discussed above on results in detection of single oncoproteins, it would seem even more effective to construct arrays with the antibodies to the large number of known oncoproteins in cancer patients to assay for the presence of increased levels of these and/or mutated forms.

Proteomic Approaches to Early Detection of Cancer in Serum

The above approaches to tumor detection are based on using known onco-proteins that are expressed in uncontrolled cell proliferation. Alternatively, other approaches, mainly the so-called proteomic approach, described extensively in the next chapter, have been developed over the past several years to search for the expression of multiple proteins (hence the term 'proteomic') that occur uniquely in human cancers and not in normal and nonmalignant cells. These proteins are then used to detect tumors at an early stage. These techniques involve two-dimensional polyacrylamide gel electrophoresis on protein extracts, from tissue and serum, which are first labeled with different fluorochromes (Wulfkuhle, 2003). The resulting gels from cancer patients are compared with those from normals to detect differences in fluorescent labeling. Bands that differ are eluted and subjected to mass spectrometry to determine molecular weight and fragmentation patterns.

Ultimately, mass spectroscopy, the principles of which are described in Chapters 4 and 23, can be used to obtain sequence information on these proteins. Using this technique, the RS/DI-1 protein that regulates protein–RNA interactions has been identified as a circulating protein in the sera of breast cancer patients but not in normal individuals. Likewise the protein PGP9.5 has been found to occur in the sera of patients with lung cancer (Wulfkuhle et al, 2003).

This approach has therefore shown promise in identifying unique markers for different types of cancer. However, it requires high concentrations of proteins to enable detection on the two-dimensional gels and is quite time-consuming. Nonetheless, it is a powerful method for the discovery of proteins that are unique to specific types of tumor.

Within the past 2 years, another, more direct and more sensitive approach has been designed that enables detection of cancer in the serum of affected patients. In this method the sera of patients is directly applied to a chip, which allows for the partial separation of the proteins in the sample. The chip is then subjected to surface-enhanced laser desorption ionization time of flight (SELDI-TOF) mass spectrometry, as described in Chapter 4. This produces a complex pattern of protein and protein ion fragments with different mass-to-charge ratios (Wulfkuhle et al, 2003).

The patterns for the sera of patients with cancer are compared with those from normal individuals using computer pattern-recognition algorithms (some of them based on neural network theory) that can distinguish cancer patterns from normal ones. Importantly, the normal sera provide a 'training set' of patterns that defines the normal pattern while a second set of sera from known cancer patients defines the cancer training set (Wulfkuhle et al, 2003). The idea of profiling patients with different tumor types is consistent with the discussion above, in which it was noted that certain patterns of antioncoprotein antibody occurrence in serum appear to characterize specific cancers.

The proteomic pattern-recognition approach was applied to 25 patients with ovarian cancers at all stages and a group of unaffected individuals. The sera were analyzed in a blind study. The method resulted in detecting 100% of the patients with ovarian cancer, including 18 who had stage I (early) disease. All the sera from the unaffected patients were identified as being negative for ovarian cancer (Wulfkuhle et al, 2003). On the other hand, the sera from patients with other types of cancer could not be classified by the algorithm, suggesting that ovarian cancer has a unique protein 'profile.'

Similar results have been obtained now for patients with breast and prostate cancers. In one study, using an algorithm that incorporated a decision tree classification system, the method had a sensitivity of 83% and a specificity of 97% in distinguishing sera from patients with prostate cancer from sera from patients with non-cancerous conditions like benign prostatic hypertrophy (BPH) or with no disease. The sensitivity could be raised to 100% by incorporation of a more robust algorithm (Wulfkuhle et al, 2003).

As noted in Chapter 74, prostate specific antigen (PSA) is the marker used in the diagnosis of prostate cancer; the upper limit of normal for PSA is taken to be 4 ng/ml but the 4–10 ng/ml range encompasses many false-positive results. Thus this method was applied to patients found to have serum PSA levels of 4–10 ng/ml. It was found that it could accurately predict the occurrence of cancer in 95% of patients with PSA values in this range and could detect 70% (107 of 153 patients) with benign disease but PSA levels above 4 ng/ml (upper reference range) (Wulfkuhle et al, 2003).

The proteomic approach thus appears to be highly promising. Drawbacks include the absence of identity of many of the proteins in the training sets. In the case of prostate cancer detection, different groups who have analyzed the sera of prostate cancer patients and unaffected individuals have obtained different diagnostic protein patterns in none of which PSA has been identified (Diamandis, 2003). Yet PSA is known to be elevated in over 90% of patients with prostate cancer. Further questions have been raised as to whether important protein molecules such as PSA are present in sufficiently high concentration in a serum sample to be detected by the method and whether the actual patterns really characterize prostate tissue. With identification of the proteins in the training sets, these questions should be resolved.

Detection of Oncogenes in Serum and Other Body Fluids

Cell-Free Nucleic Acid Testing in Cancer

Protein tumor markers and histopathologic staging have been the cornerstones of diagnosis and prognosis of malignancy. Over the past decade, the discovery of cell-free nucleic acids in serum, plasma, urine, or other body fluids has promoted investigation of oncogenes encoding oncoproteins as a means to detect malignancy in a variety of cancers with potentially greater sensitivity (Schmidt, 2004), including melanoma (Kopreski, 1999), lung (Fleishhacker, 2001; Schmidt, 2004), colon (Silva, 2002), breast (Chen, 2000; Gal, 2001), prostate (Goessl, 2001, 2002), ovary (Hickey, 1999), EBV-positive lymphomas (Lechowicz, 2002; Lei, 2002), intracranial neoplasms (Rhodes, 1994) and bladder (Goessl, 2001, 2002; Utting, 2002).

The basic concept is that tumor-derived nucleic acid can be detected in cell-free sources, such as serum, plasma, urine, lavage fluid, etc., using amplification methods such as RT-PCR. Normally, DNA is isolated from tissue through standard procedures using phenol chloroform extraction followed by ethanol precipitation. However, DNA can also be obtained directly from serum, plasma, or other body fluids by centrifugation, separating it from cells and platelets. The methodology of cell-free nucleic-

acid-based detection includes detection of gene mutations, microsatellite alterations, and promoter hypermethylation.

Gene Mutations

These normally involve nucleic acid sequencing and can detect single base changes in genomic or mitochondrial DNA (gDNA and mtDNA, respectively). mtDNA can have 20–200 copies of DNA compared with two copies of gDNA. Mutated mtDNA was detected in 3/3 patients (100%) with prostate cancer (Jeronimo, 2001) whereas others have reported a lower mtDNA detection rate in patients with colorectal cancer (Anker, 1997; Hibi, 2001). Tumor and plasma DNA of 25 patients with breast or small cell lung cancer were analyzed for the presence of p53 gene mutations. Six patients had detectable mutations in their tissue and three of these six (50%) had mutations detected in their plasma (Silva, 1999). Furthermore, although gene mutations have been detected in tissue obtained from malignant and healthy patients, the same is not true for plasma. Mutations detected in plasma are very specific for malignancy (Johnson, 2002).

Microsatellite Alterations

These are polymorphic repetitive nucleic acid sequences, varying from 2–6 base pairs, that form variable stretches of DNA that appear as loss of heterozygosity (LOH) and are detectable by microsatellite analysis using PCR. A panel of four to six appropriate markers to detect these microsatellites can be used to profile tumors. Loss of heterozygosity requires at least 20% of tumor DNA within normal DNA. Microsatellite instability refers to detection of additional PCR products and requires a ratio of tumor to normal DNA of greater than 0.5% (Goessl, 2001, 2002). Microsatellite alterations performed on cell-free bronchial lavage specimens from lung cancer patients revealed tumor-associated genes in 47% if DNA was used as the source material ($n = 30$) and in 100% if RNA was used ($n = 25$) (Schmidt, 2004). In addition, four microsatellite loci were detected in the sera of 17/34 breast cancer patients; loss of heterozygosity at various loci was observed in 16 patients and microsatellite instability was detected in one patient (Schwarzenbach, 2004). However, no correlation was found between circulating tumor DNA and the level of tumor-associated protein marker CA 15-3 (Schwarzenbach, 2004) (see chapter on tumor markers). Plasma loss of heterozygosity was has also been found in patients with recurrent bladder cancer, for which it appears to be a reliable marker (Dominguez, 2002).

Promoter Hypermethylation

Methylation of CpG islands, located in the promoter region of many genes, is associated with their transcriptional inactivation. Thus, aberrant hypermethylation of key tumor suppressor genes can permit expression of otherwise quiescent oncogenes. Promoter hypermethylation can be detected by methylation-specific PCR (MSP), and the reduced protein expression can be determined by immunohistochemistry. MSP requires a ratio of tumor to normal DNA of 0.1–0.001% (Goessl, 2001, 2002; Bearzatto, 2002). Aberrant methylation of at least one of four tumor suppressor genes was detected in tissue biopsies from 15 of 22 (68%) patients with non-small-cell lung cancer. Of the 15 patients with positive non-small-cell lung cancer, 11 (73%) also had abnormal methylated DNA in their serum samples (Esteller, 1999). In addition, 17/27 patients (63%) of bladder cancer patients displayed alterations in tumor suppressor genes in cell- and serum-derived DNA (Dominguez, 2002).

Interpretation of results obtained from cell-free testing warrants caution as results may vary depending on the detection method (promoter hypermethylation, gene rearrangements, microsatellite alterations, PCR, RT-PCR, the sample tested (Lee, 2001), and the nucleic acid source used (RNA, DNA) (Fleishhacker, 2001; Garcia, 2001; Johnson, 2002; Schmidt, 2004). Nonetheless this remains a promising new modality for early cancer detection (Chan, 2002; Lechowicz, 2002).

Gene Arrays Detecting Oncoprotein Abnormalities

We have noted that circulating DNA from mutated oncogenes can be readily detected in the serum of cancer patients (Sorenson et al, 1994; de Kok, 1997) and that use of PCR methodology has successfully identified $p21^{ras}$ in the stool of patients with colorectal cancer, altered p53 in the urine of patients with bladder cancer (Sidransky, 1991), and ras, neu/HER2, and PDGF in the bile of patients with biliary tract cancer (Su et al, 2001). Given the existence now of microchips that contain entire genomes that can be hybridized with the total RNA of cells to detect different levels of gene expression, studies using such chips on which different oncogenes are present may be effective in detecting expression of specific oncogenes present in body fluids from patients with different cancers.

That these types of studies are feasible has been demonstrated in a recent study on the tissue of 20 squamous cell esophageal carcinomas (Arai, 2003). A total of 57 oncogenes were present on the array and included many of the oncogenes discussed here, including *FGF*, *erb*-B2 (*neu*/HER2) and *myc*. In nine of the 20 specimens, expression of eight oncogenes, including *erb*-B2 and *myc*, was two to four times higher than in normal, control tissue. Comparison of these results with those obtained using conventional hybridization methods revealed that, frequently, this gene amplification was found not to be due to an increase in copy number. As noted above, the p53 gene is frequently overexpressed and/or mutated in squamous cell carcinomas of the esophagus and in head and neck squamous cell carcinomas. Unfortunately, p53 was not included on this array. In addition, this study did not include hybridization assays for mutant genes.

Nonetheless, these studies illustrate that oncogenes are frequently overexpressed in human cancers and can be detected on gene arrays. The earlier PCR studies on body fluids illustrate that gene amplification and mutation can also be readily detected in these body fluids. Therefore gene arrays containing large numbers of different oncogenes, allowing for rapid assays, appear to hold great promise in tumor detection on body fluids.

Cell DNA Testing for Cancer Using Fluorescence In Situ Hybridization

This technique is described in Chapter 69 on Cytogenetics. In brief, DNA oligonucleotide probes containing sequences known to occur uniquely on specific chromosomes are incubated with cells concentrated from body fluids, including blood and urine. These probes are so constructed that they hybridize either to specific normally occurring DNA sequences on specific chromosomes or to known abnormally occurring spliced chromosomal sequences (usually the result of translocations). The latter often produce either overexpressed mitogenic proteins or mutated constitutively activated mitogenic proteins.

An example of the application of this technique is in the diagnosis of bladder cancer for which a new test, the Vysis-Abbott Urovision detection system, has been developed and has recently been FDA-approved. A critical and common chromosomal lesion in this disease is the 9p21 homozygous deletion, perhaps the most constant genetic finding in bladder cancer. This results in deletion of a tumor suppressor gene that codes for the p16 antioncogene protein, again resulting in loss of control of mitotic rate (Halling, 2002, 2003).

An oligonucleotide probe, labeled with a gold fluorescent dye, has been developed to a sequence of 9p21. In addition, several other oligonucleotide probes have been prepared, linked to other colored fluorescent dyes, that hybridize to specific sequences in the centromeres of other 'control' chromosomes. A mixture of these probes is incubated with cells obtained from the urinary sediments of patients and subjected to fluorescence microscopy. If the cells are normal, duplicate colored spots, from diploid normal chromosomes, appear in these cells.

On the other hand, absence of one or both yellow spots for chromosome 9p21 but the presence of duplicate fluorescent spots for the control probes is a strong indication of 9p21 deletion and the presence of urothelial (most probably, bladder) cancer. It should be noted that this hybridization procedure is also capable of detecting malignant aneuploid bladder epithelial cells (with multiple copies of chromosomes) directly.

This method has a sensitivity of 36% for grade 1 cancers, 76% for grade 2, and almost 100% for grade 3 cancers and an overall specificity of 97 (Halling, 2002, 2003). It therefore has great potential in detecting bladder cancer, especially if it is combined with probes for other genetic lesions known to occur in this disease as discussed in the bladder cancer markers section above. In addition, multiple probes for known chromosomal lesions in a variety of lymphomas and leukemias have been prepared and are promising for the detection of these diseases in body fluids and tissue.

Evaluation and Conclusions

Well-defined pathways for mitogenic signal transduction exist between the membrane and the nucleus of cells. These pathways consist mainly of proteins, mutations in or overexpression of which can give rise to uncontrolled mitogenic signaling and cancer.

Diagnostic Efficacy of Serum Oncoproteins

The results of assays for the different oncoproteins discussed above in serum and urine (NMP-22) are summarized in Figure 75–3 for different tumor types. The figure shows three-dimensional graphs of tumor type (y-axis), tumor marker (x-axis) and percentage of cases of each tumor type successfully detected by each marker. The results for each marker is given as a specifically colored three-dimensional bar graph. From Figure 75–3, it is clear that, of the proteins studied thus far, high positivity rates occur in certain cancers, while the control groups, given adjacent to each tumor type with an 'N' in parenthesis, show very low positivity rates. Interestingly, although the oncoproteins studied are from signal transduction pathways that are involved in many different types of cell, there seems to be some specificity of expression of particular oncoproteins for certain types of cancer.

For example, the growth factor TGF-α is elevated in a large proportion of colorectal, brain, and ovarian cancers while TGF-β is elevated in hepatocellular, lung, and bladder cancers; the p185 ECD (*neu*) protein is elevated in the sera of many patients with breast (at more advanced stages) carcinomas (Fig.; p21^{ras} protein is elevated in colorectal and hepatocellular carcinomas, angiosarcomas of the liver and lung cancers; p53 is elevated in colorectal and lung cancers and is elevated uniquely in oropharyngeal cancers. In addition, it is elevated in a high proportion of lymphomas. Anti-Myc antibody is elevated in many colon cancers and, interestingly, in a high proportion of prostate cancers. This latter finding suggests the need for further investigation. For example, elevated serum anti-Myc may aid in the definitive diagnosis of prostate cancer in patients with elevated serum PSA.

It should be noted that, for these proteins, the sensitivity for disease detection is high and exceeds that for any of the oncofetal antigens. Also, in every study performed to date, on several thousand patients, the frequency of occurrence of these growth factors and oncoproteins is very low in the sera of individuals who do not have cancer. Therefore, the specificity of using growth factors and oncoproteins as tumor markers is also relatively high. This conclusion does not imply that absence of a given oncoprotein in the serum of a patient implies absence of a malignancy. Because of the multistep nature of carcinogenesis, there are many potential oncoproteins that may become abnormal. Any one or group of other oncoproteins may therefore be present in the patient's serum.

Indeed, Figure 75–3 also indicates that the frequency of detection of certain oncoproteins in the sera of patients who have a given type of tumor can be relatively low. For example, from Figure 75–3A, c-Myc has been found to be elevated in the sera of about 8% of patients with breast cancer. The low rates of detection of this oncoprotein in this tumor type results from the large number of possible steps on the pathway where aberrant proteins or growth factors can be produced. Thus, the tumors that occur in a given tissue may have a multiplicity of different causes, leading to the production of different aberrant proteins in the chain.

The next step, therefore, in using these oncoprotein markers in the early diagnosis of cancer is to assay for multiple markers on a given patient's serum, since discovery of at least one aberrant component of the signal transduction pathway is much more likely. If at least one positive result is found, the patient can be followed for signs of the development of a tumor.

As discussed above, progress has been made in this area. Protein and gene arrays for multiple oncoproteins and oncogenes have been constructed and have succeeded in increasing the rate of positive diagnoses for cancer in patients. Furthermore, the advent of the proteomic/pattern recognition approach to cancer detection is proving to be successful in studies in which it has been thus far tested, i.e., in the diagnosis of ovarian, prostate, and breast cancers. Combination of these two methods would result in high diagnostic yields; use of both would be feasible in that each can be performed rapidly.

Origins of Malignancies

Figure 75–3 indicates that discovery of an elevated level of an oncoprotein in the serum of a patient does not generally give conclusive information as to the source of the malignancy. For example, although p21^{ras} has been found to be elevated, with some specificity, in colon, lung, and angiosarcomas of the liver; and *neu*/HER-2 (c-*erbB*-2) p185 ECD has been found to be elevated in colon, lung, and breast cancers, elevation of one of these oncoproteins in a patient's serum would not allow identification of exactly the tissue of origin of a malignancy. Because the signal transduction pathways in most cells are remarkably similar to one another, a rise in any oncoprotein can signify malignancy in a number of different cell types. On the other hand, using the proteomic approach, serum protein patterns on SELDI-TOF mass spectrometry are uniquely characteristic of specific tumors so that this approach can identify the tissue of origin of the tumor.

Additionally, many studies on the correlations between the presence of tumors and serum levels of oncoproteins remain to be performed. For

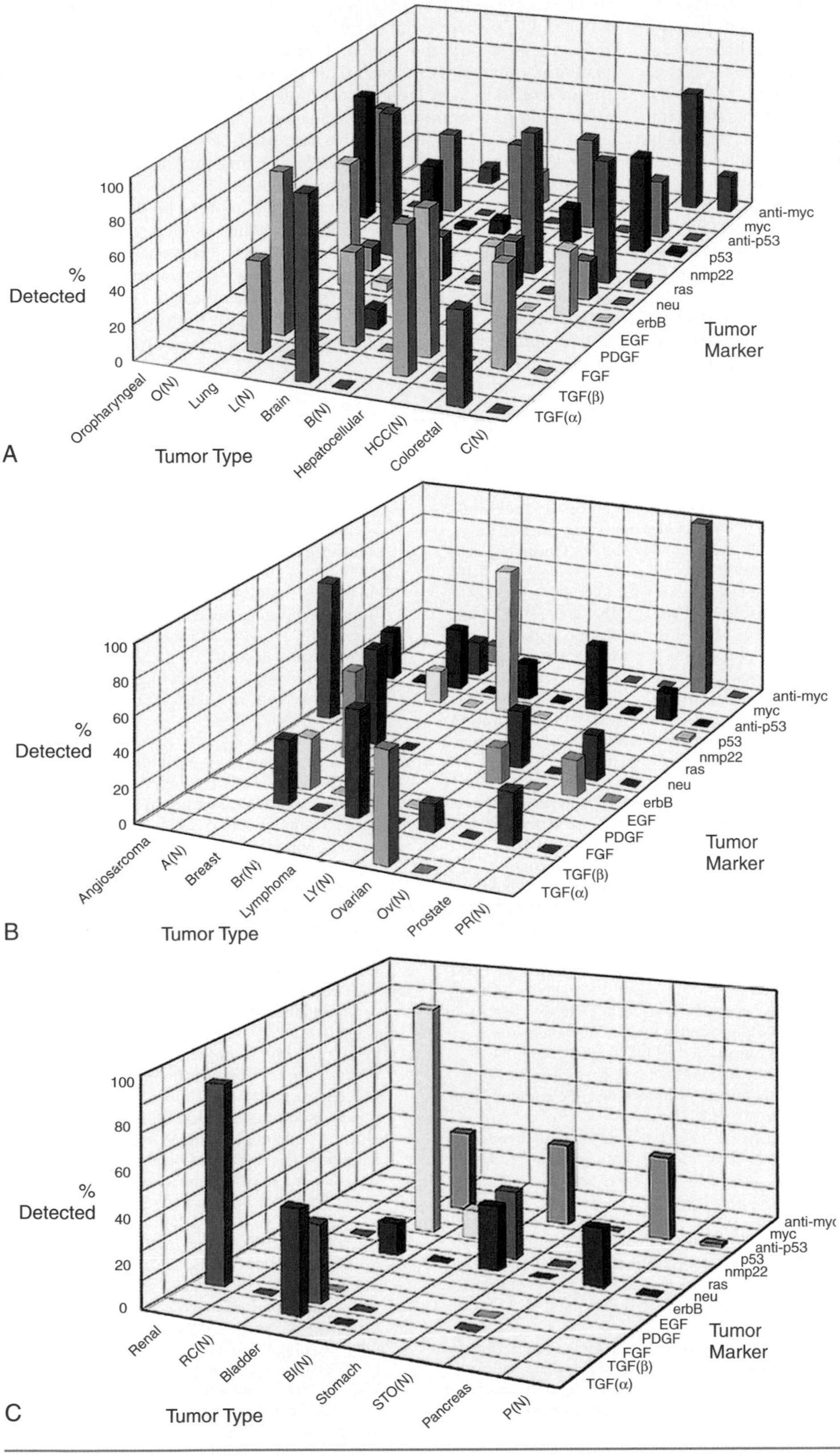

TUMOR MARKERS

A — Tumor Type: Oropharyngeal, O(N), Lung, L(N), Brain, B(N), Hepatocellular, HCC(N), Colorectal, C(N); Tumor Marker: anti-myc, myc, anti-p53, p53, nmp22, ras, neu, erbB, EGF, PDGF, FGF, TGF(β), TGF(α); % Detected

B — Tumor Type: Angiosarcoma, A(N), Breast, Br(N), Lymphoma, LY(N), Ovarian, Ov(N), Prostate, PR(N); Tumor Marker: anti-myc, myc, anti-p53, p53, nmp22, ras, neu, erbB, EGF, PDGF, FGF, TGF(β), TGF(α); % Detected

C — Tumor Type: Renal, RC(N), Bladder, Bl(N), Stomach, STO(N), Pancreas, P(N); Tumor Marker: anti-myc, myc, anti-p53, p53, nmp22, ras, neu, erbB, EGF, PDGF, FGF, TGF(β), TGF(α); % Detected

Figure 75–3 Summary of results of serum assays for different components of mitogenic signaling pathways. These are three-dimensional plots of tumor type on the X axis, pathway component on the Y axis and the percentage detected or the frequency of finding each of the pathway components elevated in the serum of patients with each tumor type on the perpendicular Z axis. Next to the results for each tumor type, the results for control groups are labeled as 'N' for 'normals,' i.e., age- and sex-matched controls who were tumor-free. The controls for patients with each tumor type are abbreviated with a single letter (with 'N' in parentheses) for each tumor type, such as 'B' for brain in A. TGF$_\alpha$ = transforming growth factor α; TGF$_\beta$ = transforming growth factor β; FGF = fibroblast growth factor; PDGF = platelet-derived growth factor; EGF = epidermal growth factor; erbB = epidermal growth factor (EGF) receptor; Neu = the p185 protein that is similar to the erbB protein and is also called erbB-2 and HER-2; Ras = the p21 protein; NMP-22 = nuclear matrix protein number 22; p53 = an antioncogene protein; anti-p53 = anti-p53 antibody; myc = a nuclear oncogene that encodes the Myc protein; anti-Myc = antibody to the Myc protein.

example, there are no published data on the occurrence of detectable forms of mutant p21^{ras} protein in the serum of patients with pancreatic carcinoma with control groups consisting of age- and sex-matched control individuals and with groups containing patients with pancreatitis but no tumors. This is a vitally needed study, because over 90% of pancreatic cancers express oncogenic p21^{ras} (Almoguerra, 1988).

One manner of using serum oncoproteins to detect specific tumors at an early stage in tumor progression is on populations known to be at risk for developing specific cancers from a history of exposure to carcinogens or mutagens as in occupational exposure or from pre-existing medical conditions as seen from the examples of vinyl chloride exposure associated with angiosarcoma of the liver and pneumoconioses associated with lung cancer. Both conditions are associated with elevated serum levels of p21^{ras} protein; the latter is also associated with elevated serum levels of p185^{neu}.

Tumor Size and Oncoprotein Levels

Currently, there is little information on the minimum size of a tumor that gives rise to serum elevations of oncoproteins. However, there are indications that small lesions may give rise to significant levels of certain oncoproteins. First, in a significant number of patients with known cancer risks, oncoproteins were discovered in their sera prior to the development of detectable cancer. Thus, in patients with asbestosis, the ECD of the p185[erbB] protein became elevated before lung tumors were diagnosed. Overexpression of the p185 ECD occurred in a number of patients prior to the diagnosis of breast cancer. East Asian patients who had high serum levels of p185 ECD went on to develop hepatocellular carcinoma. Patients with pneumoconioses were found to have elevated levels of p185 ECD and/or p21 protein and subsequently developed lung carcinomas. Mutant (Asp 13-) p21 protein was discovered in the serum of a very high percentage of patients with vinyl chloride exposure who subsequently developed angiosarcoma. Anti-p53 antibodies were found in the sera of individuals who subsequently developed angiosarcomas or lung cancers. All these studies suggest that malignant lesions that are undetectable by conventional techniques may be detected by measuring the serum levels of oncoproteins or antibodies to oncoproteins, especially in patients with known exposures or risk factors for cancer.

Second, there appears to be a good correlation in some patients between serum levels of marker oncoproteins and tumor size and/or level of expression of the marker in the tumor tissue itself. In this regard, some small adenomas (<1 cm) have been found to give rise to elevated levels of p185 ECD or p21[ras] in these patients' sera. For both p21[ras] protein and p185[erbB] ECD, there is an excellent correlation between serum level of these markers and the pre- and post-treatment clinical status of the patient. Nonetheless, substantially more correlation studies between tumor size and serum level of oncoproteins remain to be performed. One confounding factor may be that a small tumor may produce large amounts of the marker, while larger tumors may produce smaller amounts. In this respect, oncoproteins become elevated in a large proportion of carcinomas *in situ* as evidenced by elevated serum levels of p185[neu] protein in incipient breast cancer and NMP22 in carcinoma in situ of the bladder.

Despite the foregoing caveats in interpretations of elevations of serum levels of oncoproteins or the detection of abnormal forms of these proteins in serum and the need for further correlation studies to be performed, assays for the presence of oncoproteins in serum show exceptional promise for detection of malignant tumors at an early stage and for monitoring their progression, response to therapy, remission, and recurrence.

References

Adler V, Pincus MR, Brandt-Rauf PW, Ronai Z: Complexes of *ras*-p21 with *jun*-N-kinase and c-*jun* proteins. Proc Natl Acad Sci USA 1995; 92:10585–10589.

Adler V, Pincus MR, Minamoto T, et al: Conformation-dependent phosphorylation of p53. Proc Natl Acad Sci USA 1998; 94:1686–1691.

Almoguera C, Shibata D, Forrester K, et al: Most human carcinomas of the endocrine pancreas contain mutant c-K-*ras* genes. Cell 1988; 53:549–554.

Amar S, Glozman A, Chung DL, et al: Selective inhibition of oncogenic ras-p21 *in vivo* by agents that block its interaction with *jun*-N-kinase (JNK) and *jun* proteins. Implications for the design of selective chemotherapeutic agents. Cancer Chemother Pharmacol 1997; 41:79–85.

Angelopoulou K, Diamandis EP, Sutherland DJ, et al: Prevalence of serum antibodies against the p53 tumor suppressor gene protein in various cancers. Int J Cancer 1994; 58:480–487.

Anker P, Lefort F, Vasioukhin V, et al: K-ras mutations are found in DNA extracted from the plasma of patients with colorectal cancer. Gastroenterology 1997; 112:1114–1120.

Arai H, Ueno T, Tangoku A, et al: Detection of amplified oncogenes by genome DNA microarrays in human primary esophageal squamous cell carcinoma: comparison with conventional comparative genomic hybridization analysis. Cancer Genet Cytogenet 2003; 146:16–21.

Ariad S, Seymour L, Bezwoda WR: Platelet-derived growth factor (PDGF) in plasma of breast cancer patients: correlation with stage and rate of progression. Breast Cancer Res Treat 1991; 20:11–17.

Barbacid M: Ras genes. Ann Rev Biochem 1987; 56:779–827.

Bearzatto A, Conte D, Frattini M, et al: p16[INK4A] hypermethylation detected by fluorescent methylation-specific PCR in plasmas from non-small cell lung cancer. Clin Cancer Res 2002; 8:3782–3787.

Bhatavdekar JM, Patel DD, Vora HH, et al: Circulating markers and growth factors as prognosticators in men with advanced tongue cancer. Tumour Biol 1993; 14: 55–58.

Brandt-Rauf PW: Oncogene proteins as biomarkers in the molecular epidemiology of occupational carcinogenesis: the example of the *ras* oncogene-encoded p21 protein. Int Arch Occup Environ Health 1991; 63:1–8.

Brandt-Rauf PW, Chen JM, Marion M-J, et al: Conformational effects in the p53 protein of mutations induced during chemical carcinogenesis: molecular dynamic and immunologic analyses. J Protein Chem 1996; 15:367–375.

Brandt-Rauf PW, Luo JC, Carney WP, et al: The detection of increased amounts of the extracellular domain of the c-*erbB-2* oncoprotein in serum during pulmonary carcinogenesis in humans. Int J Cancer 1994a; 56:383–386.

Brandt-Rauf PW, Pincus MR, Carney WP: The c-*erbB-2* protein in oncogenesis: molecular structure to molecular epidemiology. Crit Rev Oncog 1994b; 5:313–329.

Brandt-Rauf PW, Pincus MR: Molecular markers of carcinogenesis. Pharmacol Ther 1998; 77:135–148.
This is a review of the relevant oncoproteins that either have proved to be markers for early tumor detection or that show great promise as biomarkers for early cancer detection.

Brandt-Rauf PW, Rackovsky S, Pincus MR: Correlation of the transmembrane domain of the *neu* oncogene-encoded p185 protein with its function. Proc Natl Acad Sci USA 1990; 87:8660–8675.

Brandt-Rauf PW, Smith S, Hemminki K, et al: Serum oncoproteins and growth factors in asbestosis and silicosis patients. Int J Cancer 1992; 50:881–885.

Brattstrom D, Bergvist M, Larsson A, et al: Basic fibroblast growth factor and vascular endothelial growth factor in sera from non-small cell lung cancer patients. Anticancer Res 1998; 18:1123–1127.

Breuer B, DeVivo I, Luo JC, et al: *erbB-2* and myc oncoproteins in sera and tumors of breast cancer patients. Cancer Epidemiol Biomarkers Prev 1994; 3:63–66.

Breuer B, Luo JC, DeVivo I, et al: Detection of elevated c-*erbB-2* oncoprotein in the serum and tissue in breast cancer. Med Sci Res 1993; 21:383–384.

Carney WP, Hamer PJ, Petit D, et al: Detection and quantitation of the human neu oncoprotein. Tumor Marker Oncol 1991; 6:53.

Chakrabarty S, Huang S, Moskal TL, et al: Elevated serum levels of transforming growth factor-alpha in breast cancer patients. Cancer Lett 1994;79:157–160.

Chan KC, Lo YM: Circulating nucleic acids as a tumor marker. Histol Histopathol 2002; 17:937–943.

Chen XQ, Bonnefoi H, Pelte MF, et al: Telomerase RNA as a detection marker in the serum of breast cancer patients. Clin Cancer Res 2000; 6:3823–3826.

Coltrera MD, Wang J, Porter PL, Gown AM: Expression of platelet-derived growth factor B-chain and the platelet-derived growth factor receptor beta subunit in human breast tissue and breast carcinoma. Cancer Res 1995; 55:2703–2708.

De Kok JB, van Solinge WW, Ruers TJ, et al: Detection of tumor DNA in serum of colorectal cancer patients. Scand J Clin Lab Invest 1997; 57:601–604.

DeVivo I, Marion MJ, Smith SJ, et al: Mutant c-Ki-*ras* p21 protein in chemical carcinogenesis in humans exposed to vinyl chloride. Cancer Causes Control 1994; 5:273–278.

Diamandis, E.P. Point: Proteomic patterns in biological fluids: do they represent the future of cancer diagnostics? Clin Chem 2003; 49: 1272–1275.

Dominguez G, Carballido J, Silva J, et al: p14ARF promoter hypermethylation in plasma DNA as an indicator of disease recurrence in bladder cancer patients. Clin Cancer Res 2002; 8:980–985.

Esteller M, Sanchez-Cespedes M, Rosell R, et al: Detection of aberrant promoter hypermethylation of tumor suppressor genes in serum DNA from non-small cell lung cancer patients. Cancer Res 1999; 59:67–70.

Field JK, Spandidos DA: The role of *ras* and *myc* oncogenes in human solid tumours and their relevance in diagnosis. Anticancer Res 1990; 10:1–22.

Fleischhacker M, Beinert T, Ermitsch M, et al: Detection of amplifiable messenger RNA in the serum of patients with lung cancer. Ann NY Acad Sci 2001; 945:178–188.

Fontanini G, Fiore L, Bigini D, et al: Levels of p53 antigen in serum of non-small lung cancer patients correlate with positive p53 immunohistochemistry on tumor sections, tumor necrosis and nodal involvement. Int J Oncol 1994; 5:553.

Forester K, Almoguera C, Han K, et al: Detection of high incidence of K-*ras* oncogenes during human colon tumorigenesis. Nature 1987; 327:298–303.

Fujimoto K, Ichimori Y, Kakizoe T, et al: Increased serum levels of basic fibroblast growth factor in patients with renal cell carcinoma. Biochem Biophys Res Commun 1991; 180:386–392.

Gal S, Fidler C, Lo YM, et al: Detection of gammaglobin mRNA in the plasma of breast cancer patients. Ann N Y Acad Sci 2001; 945:192–194.

Garcia JM, Silva JM, Domiguez G, et al: Heterogeneous tumour clones as an explanation of discordance between plasma DNA and tumor DNA alterations. Genes Chromosomes Cancer 2001; 31:300–301.

Geddert H, Zerioub M, Wolter M, et al: Gene amplification and protein overexpression of c-erb-b2 in Barrett carcinoma and its precursor lesions. Am J Clin Pathol 2002; 118:60–66.

Goessl C, Muller M, Heicappell R, et al: DNA-based detection of prostate cancer in blood, urine, and ejaculates. Ann NY Acad Sci 2001; 945:51–58.

Goessl C, Muller M, Straub B, et al: DNA alterations in body fluids as molecular tumor markers for urological malignancies. Eur Urol 2002; 41:668–676.

Halling KC, King W, Sokolova IA, et al: A comparison of BTA stat, hemoglobin dipstick, telomerase and Vysis UroVysion assays for the detection of urothelial carcinoma in urine. J Urol 2002; 167:2001–2006.
This is a comprehensive review and assessment of different markers for bladder cancer. It emphasizes the value of using FISH as a method for detection of bladder cancer.

Halling KC: Vysis UroVysion for the detection of urothelial cancer. Expert Rev Mol Diagn 2003; 3:507–519.

Hamer PJ, LaVecchio J, Ng S, et al: Activated Val-12 ras p21 in cell culture fluids and mouse plasma. Oncogene 1991; 6:1609–1615.

Hibi K, Nakayama H, Yamazaki T, et al: Detection of mitochondrial DNA alterations in primary tumors and corresponding serum of colorectal cancer patients. Int J Cancer 2001; 94:429–431.

Hickey KP, Boyle KP, Jepps HM, et al: Molecular detection of tumour DNA in serum and peritoneal fluid from ovarian cancer patients. Br J Cancer 1999; 80:1803–1808.

Hioki O, Watanabe A, Minemura M, et al: Clinical significance of serum hepatocyte growth factor levels in liver diseases. J Med 1993; 24:35–46.

Holt KH, Kasson BG, Pessin JE: Insulin stimulation of MEK-dependent but ERK-independent SOS protein kinase. Mol Cell Biol 1996; 16:577–583.

Hughes JH, Cohen MB: Nuclear matrix proteins and their potential applications to diagnostic pathology. Am J Clin Pathol 1999; 111:267–274.

Hwang YH, Choi JY, Kim S, et al: Over-expression of c-raf-1 proto-oncogene in liver cirrhosis and hepatocellular carcinoma. Hepatol Res 2004; 29:113–121.

Ii M, Yoshida H, Aramaki Y, et al: Improved enzyme immunoassay for human basic fibroblast growth factor using a new enhanced chemiluminescence system. Biochem Biophys Res Commun 1993; 193:540–545.

Jeronimo C, Nomoto S, Caballero OL, et al: Mitochondrial mutations in early stage prostate cancer and bodily fluids. Oncogene 2001; 20:5195–5198.

Johnson PJ, Lo YM: Plasma nucleic acids in the diagnosis and management of malignant disease. Clin Chem 2002; 48:1186–1193.

Kath R, Hoffken K, Otte C, et al: The neu-oncogene product in serum and tissue of patients with breast carcinoma. Ann Onco 1993;l 4:585–590.

Katoh M, Inagaki H, Kurosawa-Ohsawa K, et al: Detection of transforming growth factor alpha in human urine and plasma. Biochem Biophys Res Commun 1990; 167:1065–1072.

Kaur J, Srivastava A, Ralhan R: Serum p53 antibodies in patients with oral lesions: correlation with p53/HSP70 complexes. Int J Cancer 1997; 74:609–613.

Klocker EI, Stenzl A, Cronauer MV, et al: Quantitative determination of transforming growth factor-alpha in serum and urine in patients with bladder cancer and its expression in malignant and non-malignant primary epithelial cells. Proc Am Assoc Cancer Res 1994; 35:A261.

Kopreski MS, Benko FA, Kwak LW, et al: Detection of tumor messenger RNA in the serum of patients with malignant melanoma. Clin Cancer Res 1999; 5:1961–1965.

Kurobe M, Takei Y, Ezawa H, et al: Increased level of basic fibroblast growth factor (bFGF) in sera of patients with malignant tumors. Horm Metab Res 1993; 25:395–396.

Landman J, Chang Y, Kavaler E, et al: Sensitivity and specificity of NMP-22, telomerase and BTA in the detection of human bladder cancer. Urology 1998; 52:398–402.

Lechowicz MJ, Lin L, Ambinder RF: Epstein–Barr virus DNA in body fluids. Curr Opin Oncol 2002; 14:533–537.

Lee TH, Montalvo L, Chrebtow V, et al: Quantitation of genomic DNA in plasma and serum samples: higher concentrations of genomic DNA found in serum than in plasma. Transfusion 2001; 41:276–282.

Lei KI, Chan LY, Chan WY, et al: Diagnostic and prognostic implications of circulating cell-free Epstein-Barr virus DNA in natural killer/T-cell lymphoma. Clin Cancer Res 2002; 8:29–34.

Li Y, Karjalainen A, Koskinen H, et al: p53 Autoantibodies predict subsequent development of cancer. Int J Cancer 2004; 114:157–160.

Lindmark G, Sundberg C, Glimelius B, et al: Stromal expression of platelet-derived growth factor beta-receptor and platelet-derived growth factor B-chain in colorectal cancer. Lab Invest 1993; 69:682–689.

Luo JC, Yu MW, Chen CJ, et al: Serum c-erbB-2 oncopeptide in hepatocellular carcinogenesis. Med Sci Res 1993; 21:305.

Miyanaga N, Akaza H, Ishikawa S, et al: Clinical evaluation of nuclear matrix protein 22 (NMP22)

in urine as a novel marker for urothelial cancer. Eur Urol 1997; 31:163–168.

Miyanaga N, Akaza H, Tsukamoto S, et al: Usefulness of urinary NMP22 to detect tumor recurrence of superficial bladder cancer after transurethral resection. Int J Clin Oncol 2003; 8:369–373.

Molina R, Jo J, Filella X, et al: C-erb-B oncoprotein in the sera and tissue of patients with breast cancer. Utility in prognosis. Anticancer Res 1996; 16:2295–2300.

Monstein HJ, Fransen K, Dimberg J, et al: K-ras and B-raf gene mutations are not associated with gastrin- and CCK2-receptor mRNA expression in human colorectal tumour tissues. Eur J Clin Invest 2004; 34:100–106.

Moodie SA, Willumsen BM, Weber MJ, Wolfman A: Complexes of Ras-GTP with Raf-1 and mitogen-activated protein kinase kinase. Science 1993; 260:1658–1661.

Mori S, Mori Y, Mukaiyama T, et al: In vitro and in vivo release of soluble erbB-2 protein from human carcinoma cells. Jpn J Cancer Res 1990; 81:489–494.

Mutch DG, Powell MA, Mallon MA, et al: RAS/RAF mutation and defective DNA mismatch repair in endometrial cancers. Am J Obstet Gynecol 2004; 190:935–942.

Nedvidkova J, Nemec J, Stolba P, et al: Epidermal growth factor (EGF) in serum of patients with differentiated carcinoma of thyroids. Neoplasma 1992; 39:11–14.

Niman HL, Thompson AM, Yu A, et al: Anti-peptide antibodies detect oncogene-related proteins in urine. Proc Natl Acad Sci USA 1985; 82:7924–7928.

Pawlikowski M, Cicslak D, Stepien H, et al: Elevated blood serum levels of epidermal growth factor in some patients with gastric cancer. Endokrynol Pol 1989; 40:149–153.

Pimentel E: Oncogenes, 2nd ed. Boca Raton, FL, CRC Press, 1989.

Pincus MR, Brandt-Rauf PW, Michl J, et al: ras-p21-induced cell transformation: Unique signal transduction pathways and implications for the design of new chemotherapeutic agents. Cancer Invest 18:39–50, 2000.

Pincus MR: Development of new anti-cancer peptides from conformational energy analysis of the oncogenic Ras-p21 protein and its complexes with target proteins. Front Biosci 2004; 9:3486–3509.

Pincus MR, Chung D, Dykes DC, et al: Pathways for activation of the ras-oncogene-encoded p21 protein. Ann Clin Lab Sci 1992; 22:323–342.

Pincus MR, Friedman FK: Oncoproteins in the detection of human malignancies. Mol Diagn 2003; 1:23–38.
This is a review of oncoproteins as markers for early tumor detection with an emphasis on oncoproteins as elements of signal transduction pathways.

Qin LX, Tang ZY: The prognostic molecular markers in hepatocellular carcinoma. World J Gastroenterol 2002; 8: 385–392.

Rhodes CH, Honsinger C, Sorenson GD: Detection of tumor-derived DNA in cerebrospinal fluid. J Neuropathol Exp Neurol 1994; 53:375–368.

Rosanelli GP, Wirnsberger GH, Purstner P, et al: DNA flow cytometry and immunohistochemical demonstration of mutant p53 protein versus TPS and mutant p53 protein serum levels in human breast cancer. Proc Am Assoc Cancer Res 1993; 34:A1353.

Ryder SD, Rizzi PM, Volkmann M, et al: Use of a specific ELISA for the detection of antibodies directed against p53 protein in patients with hepatocellular carcinoma. J Clin Pathol 1996; 4:295–299.

Schmidt B, Carstensen T, Engel E, et al: Detection of cell-free nucleic acids in bronchial lavage fluid supernatants from patients with lung cancer. Eur J Cancer 2004; 40:452–460.

Schwarzenbach H, Muller V, Stahmann N, et al: Detection and characterization of circulating microsatellite-DNA in blood of patients with breast cancer. Ann N Y Acad Sci 2004; 1022:25–32.

Segawa Y, Kageyama M, Suzuki S, et al: Measurement and evaluation of serum anti-p53 antibody levels in patients with lung cancer at its initial presentation: a prospective study. Br J Cancer 1998; 78:667–672.
This is a valuable study on the use of anti-p53 antibodies as a means for detecting lung cancers.

Shariat SF, Casella R, Monoski MA, et al: The addition of urinary urokinase-type plasminogen activator to urinary nuclear matrix protein 22 and cytology improves the detection of bladder cancer. J Urol 2003; 170:2244–2247.

Shimada H, Nakajima K, Ochiai T, et al: Detection of serum p53 antibodies in patients with esophageal squamous cell carcinoma: Correlation with clinicopathological features and tumor markers. Oncol Rep 1998; 5:871–874.

Shirai Y, Kawata S, Ito N, et al: Elevated levels of plasma transforming growth factor-beta in patients with hepatocellular carcinoma. Jpn J Cancer Res 1992; 83:676–679.

Sidransky D, Von Eschenbach A, Tsai YC, et al: Identification of p53 gene mutation in bladder cancers and urine samples. Science 1991; 252:706–709.

Silva JM, Gonzalez R, Dominguez G, et al: TP53 gene mutations in plasma DNA of cancer patients. Genes Chromosomes Cance 1999;r 24:160–161.

Silva JM, Rodriguez R, Garcia JM, et al: Detection of epithelial tumour RNA in the plasma of colon cancer patients is associated with advanced stages and circulating tumour cells. Gut 2002; 50:530–534.

Slamon DJ, Godolphin W, Jones LA, et al: Studies on the HER-2/neu proto-oncogene in human breast and ovarian cancer. Science 1989; 244:707–712.
This is a landmark paper that established HER-2/neu as an important factor in breast cancer causation and its use as a pronostic factor for disease progression.

Sorenson GD, Pribish DM, Valone FH, et al: Soluble normal and mutated DNA sequences from single-copy genes in human blood. Cancer Epidemiol Biomarkers Prev 1994; 3:67–71.

Soussi T, Legros Y, Lubin R, et al: Multifactorial analysis of p53 alteration in human cancer: a review. Int J Cancer 1994; 57:1–9.

Stoehr R, Brinkmann A, Filbeck T, et al: No evidence for mutation of B-RAF in urothelial carcinomas of the bladder and upper urinary tract. Oncol Rep 2004; 11:137–141.

Stokoe D, MacDonald SG, Cadwallader K, et al: Activation of Raf as a result of recruitment to the plasma membrane. Science 1994; 275:1463–1467.

Su WC, Shiesh SC, Liu HS, et al: Expression of oncogene products, HER2/Neu and Ras and fibrosis-related factors bFGF, TGF-beta and PDGF in bile from biliary malignancies and inflammatory disorders. Dig Dis Sci 2001; 46: 1387–1392.

Tomiya T, Fujiwara, K: Serum transforming growth factor-alpha level as a marker of hepatocellular carcinoma complicating cirrhosis. Cancer 1996; 77:1056–1060.

Tsai JF, Jeng JE, Chuang LY, et al: Urinary transforming growth factor-beta 1 in relation to serum alpha-fetoprotein in hepatocellular carcinoma. Scand J Gastroenterol 1997; 32:254–260.

Utting M, Werner W, Dahse R, et al: Microsatellite analysis of free tumor DNA in urine, serum, and plasma of patients: a minimally invasive method for the detection of bladder cancer. Clin Cancer Res 2002; 8:35–40.

Virji MA, Rosendale B, Piper M, et al: Circulating levels of a mutant p53 protein in patients with hepatocellular carcinoma. Proc Am Assoc Cancer Res 1992; 33:A1508.

Vlasoff DM, Baschinsky DY, De Young BR, et al: C-erb B2 (Her2/neu) is neither overexpressed nor amplified in hepatic neoplasms. Appl Immunohistochem Mol Morphol 2002; 10:237–241.

Wan PT, Garnett MJ, Roe SM, et al: Mechanism of activation of the RAF-ERK signaling pathway by oncogenic mutations of B-RAF. Cell 2004; 116:855–867.

IX

Weissfeld JL, Larsen RD, Niman HL, et al: Evaluation of oncogene-related proteins in serum. Cancer Epidemiol Biomarkers Prev 1994; 3:57–62.

Wellbrock C, Ogilvie L, Hedley D, et al: V599EB-RAF is an oncogene in melanocytes. Cancer Res 2004; 75:2338–2342.

Wu JT, Astill ME, Zhang P: Detection of the extracellular domain of c-erbB-2 oncoprotein in sera from patients with various carcinomas: correlation with tumor markers. J Clin Lab Anal 1993; 7:31–40.

Wulfkuhle JD, Liotta LA, Petricoin EF: Proteomic applications for the early detection of cancer. Nat Rev Cancer 2003; 3: 267–275.

This is a clearly written review of different proteomic approaches in detecting cancer in blood samples and explains the bases for these approaches that enable a good understanding of each method.

Yazici H, Altun M, Hafiz G, et al: Serum and tissue c-erb B2, bcl-2, and mutant p53 oncoprotein levels in nasopharyngeal cancer. Cancer Invest 2001; 19:773–778.

Yeh J, Yeh JC: Transforming growth factor-alpha and human cancer. Biomed Pharmacother 1989; 43:651–659.

Yu MW, Chen CJ, Luo JC, et al: Correlations of chronic hepatitis B virus infection and cigarette smoking with elevated expression of neu oncoprotein in the development of hepatocellular carcinoma. Cancer Res 1994a; 54:5106–5110.

Yu MW, Luo JC, Brandt-Rauf PW, et al: Correlations of chronic hepatitis B virus infection and cigarette smoking with elevated expression of the neu oncoprotein in the development of hepatocellular carcinoma. Proc Am Assoc Cancer Res 1994b; 35:A1754.

Zhang JY, Casiano CA, Peng XX, et al: Enhancement of antibody detection in cancer using panel of recombinant tumor-associated antigens. Cancer Epidemiol Biomarkers Prev 2003; 12:136–143.

This is an important paper showing that using panels of oncoproteins on blood and body fluids is more effective than using single oncoproteins alone in detecting cancer.

CHAPTER 76

Diagnostic and Prognostic Impact of High-Throughput Genomic and Proteomic Technologies in the Post-Genomic Era

Jennifer Beane BA BE, Aran Kadar MD, Charles DeLisi PhD, Martin H. Bluth MD PhD, Avrum Spira MD PhD

KEY POINTS

- Recent completion of the human genome project has provided scientists with a detailed map of the human genome and predicted coding regions that have facilitated the emergence of high-throughput genomic and proteomic technologies.

- A number of mature platforms exist for high-throughput profiling of gene expression in human tissue, including serial analysis of gene expression (SAGE), DNA microarrays and real competitive polymerase chain reaction.

- Emerging proteomic technologies, including mass spectrometry and protein arrays, have begun to explore the dynamic and complex protein composition of healthy and diseased human tissue.

- DNA microarray and SAGE technologies have identified diagnostic gene expression signatures for a number of hematologic and solid malignancies that are often difficult to distinguish using traditional histological analysis.

- Prognostic gene and protein expression profiles have been identified in a large number of cancer settings, including lymphoma, lung cancer, breast cancer, and acute myeloid leukemia.

- Validation in large clinical trials and standardization of the techniques, controls, and inclusion of analytical standards is needed prior to widespread clinical implementation of these technologies.

Introduction

With the complete sequence of the human and other genomes recently elucidated, we have witnessed an explosion of information and high-throughput tools that are profoundly altering biomedical research and the culture of science. This revolution, which began in the mid-1980s, emerged from developments in three areas: molecular biology, most notably the breakthroughs in rapid DNA sequencing; information technology, in particular the ability to store and analyze unprecedented quantities of data; and – most importantly – progress in human genetics, especially the identification of thousands of single-gene human disorders. The convergence of these technological and scientific advances raises promise for the rapid identification of disease-related genes, leading to improved diagnostic tests and more effective therapies.

Detailed maps of human and other genomes provide the information to chart a course toward understanding and treating many diseases, but that course remains a long and difficult one. While progress will come most readily for disorders following mendelian patterns of inheritance, even these disorders will pose significant difficulties. For example, although the biology and genetics of sickle-cell anemia have been reasonably well understood for more than half a century – a single valine replaces glutamic acid at position 6 in the beta-hemoglobin chain – effective treatment has been slow to develop. The penetrance of genetic diseases thought to be due to single mutations often relies on more complex interactions between the mutation and a variety of concurrent gene polymorphisms, such as those seen in the genes encoding surface proteins on postcapillary venule endothelial cells that in part account for sickle cell disease severity.

Many common diseases, in particular cardiovascular disease, mental illness, and almost all cancers, stem from multigenic causes. In addition, these diseases invariably have strong environmental components, presenting a substantial challenge to the development of effective and economical diagnostic and prognostic tests. Even in the absence of a confounding environmental influence, linking the quantifiable phenotype of a disease to a set of distinct alleles is a complex undertaking. Further complicating matters, many disorders do not have sharply defined, quantifiable phenotypes.

In a chapter filled with promising technologies, we make these sobering remarks to emphasize that greater understanding never guarantees cures or therapies. However, greater understanding does aid the development of rational strategies to detect and control disease. The reference genome allows us to rapidly characterize polymorphisms across the human population, and it also enables molecular fingerprinting technologies that permit identification of the precursors and consequences of normal and pathological changes in gene and protein expression. We can feel confident that the power of genomic technologies is well beyond anything previously available and that it will make possible during the next several decades a host of new diagnostics and therapeutics for cancer and other common diseases, profoundly altering the practice of medicine.

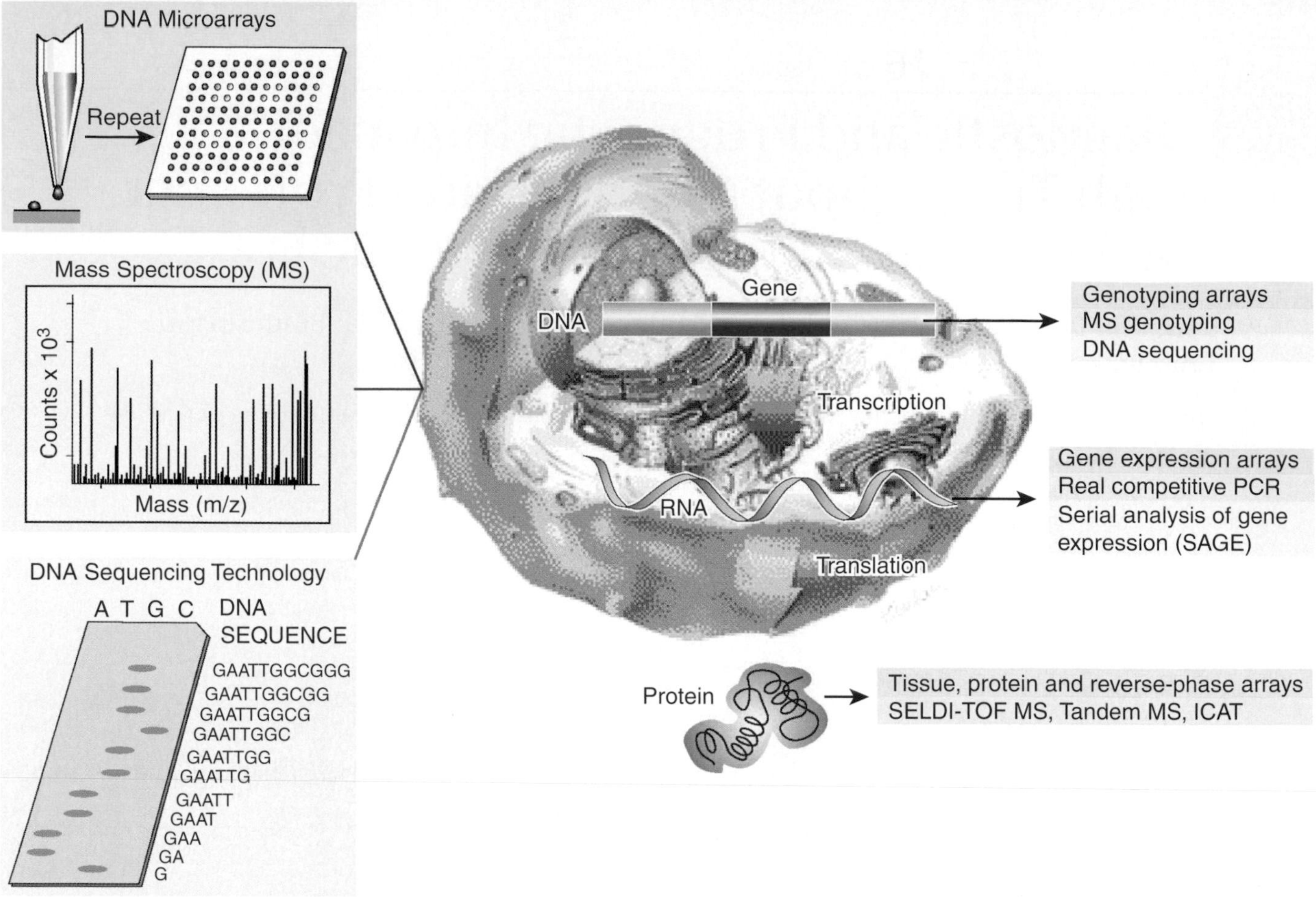

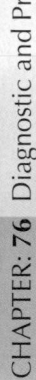

Figure 76–1 High throughput platforms and the central dogma of biology. The three major technologies responsible for rapid analysis of biological systems include mass spectrometry, sequencing, and microarrays. Examples of each technology have been listed as applied to each broad stage of biological information – DNA, RNA, and protein. MS = mass spectroscopy; SELDI–TOF = surface-enhanced laser desorption ionization, time-of-flight mass spectroscopy; ICAT = isotope-coded affinity tags. (Adapted with permission from Kufe DW, Holland JF: Cancer Medicine, 6th ed. Hamilton, Ontario, BC Decker, 2003; Wilson J, Hunt T: Molecular biology of the cell, 4th ed. New York, Garland Science, 2003; Brown TA Genomes, 2nd ed. New York, John Wiley & Sons, 2002.)

This chapter will focus on a number of high-throughput genomic and proteomic technologies that have the potential to impact disease classification and prognostication (Fig. 76–1). These molecular tools have affected virtually all forms of human pathology; however, given the public health implications and preponderance of recent publications in the field, we will concentrate on diagnostic and prognostic applications related to cancer. Following a brief overview of the human genome project and the resulting high-throughput technologies, we will discuss examples of applications in the setting of a number of hematological and solid malignancies. The scope of the chapter has been constrained to focus on high-throughput technologies and therefore does not represent a comprehensive overview of all technologies being used in clinical genomic and proteomic studies. In addition, within the technologies presented, some are highlighted in greater detail because of their widespread use. As more data are produced using the technologies, strategies combining datasets may become powerful approaches to developing accurate clinical tools. In addition to measuring gene and protein expression levels, understanding human genetic variation in DNA will be important in elucidating disease markers and mechanisms. A discussion of high-throughput genotyping technologies to assay single nucleotide polymorphisms is, however, beyond the scope of this chapter (for a review, see Syvanen, 2001.)

The Human Genome Project

Public Sequencing Effort (Hierarchical Shotgun Sequencing)

The sequencing of the human genome was a 15-year, $3 billion project, initiated in 1990 as a joint effort between the US Department of Energy and the National Institutes of Health (Collins, 2003). From the project's inception through 1995, genetic and physical maps of the human and mouse genomes were constructed and the yeast and worm genomes were

sequenced. These initial projects, coupled with advances in sequencing technology and sequence data analysis, outlined cost effective strategies and techniques while demonstrating the feasibility of sequencing the human genome. In March 1999, the effort to sequence the human genome commenced in earnest and was set to be completed in two phases – the first phase would include the completion of a draft sequence and the second would be a finishing phase to resolve misassembled regions and fill in sequence gaps. By June 2000, the centers involved in the project were producing raw sequence data at a rate of about 1000 nucleotides per second, 24 hours a day, 7 days a week (Lander, 2001).

The first phase of the Human Genome Project, a collaborative endeavor of 20 groups in six countries, was completed and published in February 2001 in the journal *Nature* (Genome International Sequencing Consortium, 2001; Lander, 2001). The draft sequence covered about 96% of the euchromatic part (gene-rich) of the human genome and 94% of the entire genome with an average of fourfold coverage (i.e. each base sequenced an average of four times). The International Human Genome Sequencing Consortium employed a sequencing strategy referred to as hierarchical shotgun sequencing (also known as map-based, BAC-based, or clone by clone sequencing) (Olson, 2001). Genomic DNA obtained from volunteers from a variety of racial and ethnic backgrounds was partially digested with restriction endonucleases. Fragments of 1–2 Mb in length were cloned into bacterial artificial chromosomes (BACs). Eight DNA libraries containing overlapping insert clones were created, representing 65-fold coverage of the genome (each base is represented on average 65 times if all eight libraries are examined).

The BACs containing fragments of the human genome are inserted into bacteria and replicated as the bacteria grow and divide. Each BAC clone is completely digested with a restriction enzyme to produce a unique pattern of DNA fragments, known as a fingerprint. The fingerprints from different BAC clones can be compared to select a set of overlapping BAC clones that cover a portion of the genome (a large region of the genome covered by overlapping clones is called a contig). The contigs can be positioned along the chromosome by using known markers from previously constructed genetic and physical maps of the human genome. The selected BAC clones are sheared into smaller overlapping fragments, subcloned, and sequenced. Subcloning is necessary because each sequencing reaction can only reliably read about 500 bp. The sequence of the BAC clone can be reconstructed from the set of sequences obtained from the subclones, and the BAC fingerprints guide the assembly of several BAC clones into contigs.

Draft sequences were required to have an average of fourfold coverage and have 99% accuracy as determined by software (i.e., PHRED and PHRAP) that assigns base quality scores and assembles sequences according to the scores. Throughout the duration of the project, sequences greater than 2 kb in length were required to be deposited in public databases within 24 hours (the data are available from the University of California at Santa Cruz's Genome Browser, www.genome.ucsc.edu, the National Center for Biotechnology Information's GenBank, www.ncbi.nih.gov, and the European Bioinformatics Institute's and the Sanger Centre's Ensembl, www.ensembl.org). The assembly of the draft sequence was a three part process that involved filtering the sequence data to eliminate bacterial and mitochondrial sequences, constructing a layout of the clones along the genome, and merging the overlapping clones to produce a draft sequence.

The hierarchical shotgun sequencing approach was chosen by the public consortium for several reasons. Dividing up the work among sequencing centers was straightforward using clones. Also, the assembly of clones to produce a draft sequence would probably be more accurate because approximately 46% of the human genome is comprised of repeat sequences and contains widespread individual sequence variation. In addition, the approach could also deal with cloning bias, and underrepresented sequences could be targeted for sequencing.

Private Sequencing Effort (Whole Genome Shotgun Sequencing)

In 1998, a private company, Celera Genomics, lead by Craig Venter, announced its intention of sequencing the human genome in 3 years using a different approach known as whole-genome shotgun sequencing. Celera's draft of the human genome sequence was reported in the February 2001 issue of *Science* (Venter, 2001). Celera generated 14.8 billion base pairs of DNA sequence in 9 months to produce a 2.91 billion bp consensus sequence of the euchromatic part of the human genome with an average of fivefold coverage. The company used genomic DNA obtained from three females and two males of the following ethno-geographic groups: African American, Asian-Chinese, Hispanic-Mexican, and Caucasian. 16 different DNA libraries were constructed with three different insert sizes: 2 kb, 10 kb, and 50 kb. Both ends of the insert from clones chosen at random were sequenced to produce 'mate pair' sequencing reads. The average distance between mate pairs was known because the range of insert sizes for a clone taken from a particular library could be characterized by calculating the distance between mate pairs in previously sequenced stretches of the genome. Celera generated a set of 27.26 million reads with an average length of 543 bp.

Celera combined its sequence data with all the data from the publicly funded effort available up to September 2000 in GenBank and pursued two different assembly strategies. The whole genome assembly strategy involved 'shredding' the publicly funded sequences into small fragments, combining these fragments with Celera's reads, identifying overlapping sequences, and joining them to produce long, continuous consensus sequences. These contigs were ordered and gaps between contigs were quantified using the information obtained from the mate pair reads. A variant of the above process, known as compartmentalized shotgun assembly, yielded slightly better results because sequences were first clustered, based on mapping information, to a region of the chromosome before performing the process described above.

Analyses of the draft sequences performed by the two groups yielded similar results. Some genes were derived from bacteria or transposable elements, and large segmental duplications were also apparent throughout the genome. The distribution of genes, CpG islands, recombination sites, and repeats were found to be highly variable across the genome. Widespread genetic variation was apparent and about 2.1 million single nucleotide polymorphisms, one per 1250 bp, were discovered. One of the most surprising results revealed by the completion of the draft sequence was the estimate that the genome contained about 30 000 protein-coding genes, considerably less than the 100 000 or more that had been postulated. The number is only one-third greater than that of the worm; however, there are probably a much larger number of different proteins because of alternative splicing (Claverie, 2001). Scientists used many gene prediction methods to arrive at the gene estimate of 30 000. Gene prediction algorithms predict the location of unknown genes in the genome using sequence characteristics learned from known genes, including codon and nucleotide composition within coding regions and conserved sequences at exon/intron boundaries and within promoter regions. The human genome sequence has a low signal to noise ratio because the coding regions only represent about 3% of the genome and, therefore, algorithms produce a large number of false positives. Most algorithms, however, use two other important sources of information – similarity to known human proteins and expressed transcripts, and homology to proteins and sequences characterized in other organisms (for a review on gene prediction algorithms, see Mathe, 2002).

Finishing the Sequence of the Human Genome

Most recently, in October 2004 in the journal *Nature*, the International Human Genome Sequencing Consortium published an article entitled, 'Finishing the euchromatic sequence of the human genome' (International Human Genome Sequencing Consortium, 2004) The article reported that the draft sequence was missing about 10% of the euchromatic portion of the genome, contained about 150 000 gaps, and had many sequence segments that had not been assigned an order or orientation. The current sequence contains 2.35 billion nucleotides, covers about 99% of the genome, and has only 341 gaps (with an error of one mistake every 100 000 bases). The sequence revision predicts between 20 000 and 25 000 protein-coding genes and the discrepancy in numbers is due to differences in gene prediction algorithms. The newly published sequence reveals that segmental duplications cover about 5.3% of the euchromatic portion, providing insights into the evolution of the human genome and aiding the study of diseases caused by deletions and rearrangements of these regions (e.g., DiGeorge syndrome) (Stankiewicz, 2002). The recently published sequence also makes it possible to trace the birth and death of genes – genes recently born as a result of gene duplication, and genes lost as a result of mutation.

The sequencing of the human genome is a monumental achievement and 'holds an extraordinary trove of information about human development, physiology, medicine, and evolution' (Lander, 2001). It has provided the infrastructure for sequencing other genomes and for understanding the structure and complexity of human genetic variation. This detailed map of the human genome and the predicted coding regions has facilitated the emergence of a number of high-throughput technologies through which scientists have begun to explore the complete set of gene and protein expression in healthy and diseased human tissue. These technologies promise to revolutionize the classification of human disease and usher in an era of individualized molecular medicine.

High-Throughput Technologies

Genomic

An intimate understanding of cellular machinery represents the first step to unraveling the complexity of human disease. Important insights into the function of a gene can be deduced by determining the cell type and conditions under which a gene is expressed and by quantifying the level of message transcribed. A common technique used to assay the level of expression of a single gene (represented by mRNA) across a few different conditions is a Northern blot. This 'gene by gene' approach began to change in the early 1990s as a result of the success of the Human Genome Project and various technological advances that enabled the development of high-throughput gene expression analyses where several genes could be assayed simultaneously. Three different genomic high-throughput technologies will be discussed. Serial analysis of gene expression (SAGE) (Velculescu, 1995) and DNA microarrays (Schena, 1995, Lockhart, 1996) were both developed in the 1990s and are currently in widespread use, while real competitive polymerase chain reaction (PCR) using matrix assisted laser desorption ionization time of flight mass spectroscopy (MALDI-TOF-MS) was first published in 2003 (Ding, 2003). The basic principles underlying DNA microarrays are discussed in Chapter 68 while those underlying real competitive PCR are discussed in Chapter 67.

Depending on the experimental design, samples are obtained from cell cultures or surgical tissues and total RNA is isolated. Techniques such as laser capture microdissection (Emmert-Buck, 1996) are often used before RNA isolation to obtain a homogeneous population of cells from tissue specimens. After total RNA or mRNA is obtained and reverse transcribed to make cDNA, each technology uses a different protocol to rapidly measure the transcript levels of the genes in each sample. The principles of each method as well as their corresponding advantages and disadvantages will be outlined below.

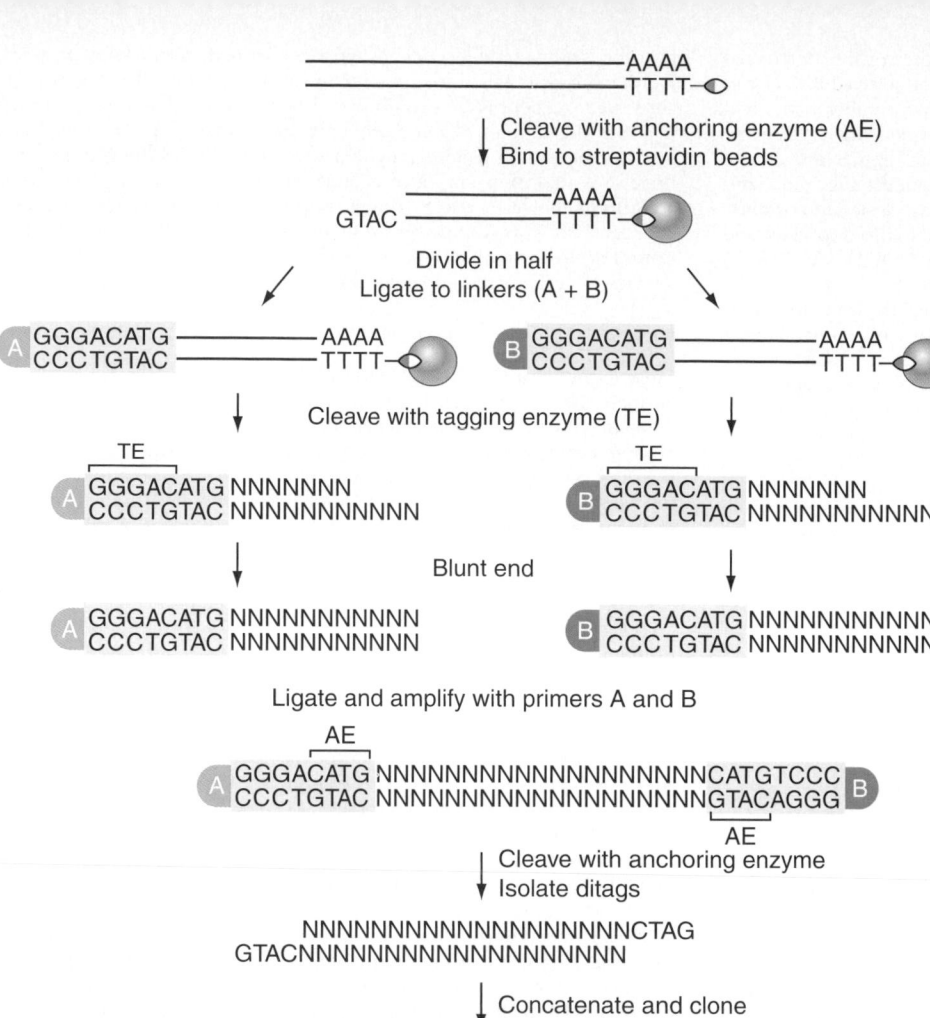

Figure 76–2 Serial analysis of gene expression (SAGE) is a technique that measures the expression levels of genes in a sample of interest. RNA is isolated from the sample, cDNA is synthesized, and several thousand short base pair tags are isolated. SAGE uses two types of restriction enzyme: one, called an anchoring enzyme (i.e., *NlaIII*), recognizes a specific 4 bp sequence and cleaves DNA every 256 bps, immediately 5′ of the sequence tag. The second enzyme, called the tagging enzyme (i.e., *BsmFI*), behaves differently and cleaves DNA 14–15 bps immediately 3′ of its recognition sequence. First, the cDNA fragments are cut with the anchoring enzyme, captured using streptavidin–biotin affinity chromatography, purified, and split into two pools, A and B. Second, two different linkers (A and B) are ligated to the 5′ ends of the cDNA fragments in their respective pools. The cDNA fragments in each pool are then cut with the tagging enzyme, resulting in a new fragment that contains the linker plus a short 10 bp region of the cDNA, known as a tag. The two pools of cDNA fragments are ligated together, creating 'ditags.' The ditags are amplified by PCR using primers designed based on sequences in linkers A and B. After amplification, the anchoring enzyme is used to cleave the linkers off the ends of the ditags. Ditags from different reactions are ligated together to form strings of 10–50 tags. The concatenated strings of ditags are cloned into plasmids and sequenced. The sequences of the tags are used to identify the corresponding genes and are a measure of the transcript abundance. (Adapted with permission from Yamamoto M, Wakatsuki T, Hada A, Ryo A: Use of serial analysis of gene expression (SAGE) technology. J Immunol Methods 2001;250:45–66.)

Serial Analysis of Gene Expression

Serial Analysis of Gene Expression (SAGE) measures the expression level of genes in a sample by isolating and sequencing several thousand short 10–14 bp tags isolated from cDNA. Two important pieces of information can be deduced from the output: the sequences of the tags usually allow identification of their corresponding genes and the number of times a particular tag is sequenced is a measure of transcript abundance. The ability to uniquely identify a transcript using as short a sequence as 9 bp resides in the probability of defining this sequence from others. Such a sequence can distinguish 262 144 transcripts (4^9), which is greater than current estimates of the number of transcripts in the human genome (Velculescu, 1995; Pennisi, 2000).

The SAGE protocol involves isolating RNA from a sample of interest. The RNA is converted to double-stranded cDNA using a biotinylated oligo (dT) primer for first strand synthesis. SAGE then uses two types of restriction enzymes. The first one, called an *anchoring* enzyme, recognizes a specific 4 bp sequence (e.g., *NlaIII*). Any 4 bp-recognizing enzyme may be used because, on average, they cleave every 256 bp (4^4). The anchoring enzyme leaves a short, overhanging, single-stranded piece of DNA at the 5′ end of the site of cleavage. The biotinylated fragment, which represents the 3′ end of the gene, is then bound to streptavidin beads, capturing only the digested cDNA fragments containing a portion of the poly(A⁺) tail. The captured fragments are purified and randomly split equally into two pools.

The second enzyme, called the *tagging* enzyme, behaves differently and cleaves DNA 14–15 bp immediately 3′ of its recognition sequence (e.g., *BsmFI*). The recognition sequence for the tagging enzyme is engineered into the sequence of the linkers described below.

After the purified fragments are split into two pools, two different oligonucleotide linkers, each containing a different PCR primer sequence (for purposes of discussion the linkers will be labeled A and B), the tagging enzyme recognition sequence, and a single-stranded DNA overhang that is part of the anchoring enzyme recognition sequence are designed and synthesized. Linker A is ligated to the 5′ ends of the cDNA fragments in one

pool and linker B is ligated to the 5′ ends of the cDNA fragments in the other pool. The ligation proceeds by means of base pairing between the complementary single-stranded overhanging DNA ends on both the cDNA fragments and linkers, creating an intact anchoring enzyme recognition sequence. The cDNA fragments in each pool are then cut with the tagging enzyme, resulting in a new fragment that contains the linker plus a short 10 bp region of the cDNA, known as a *tag* (the remaining cDNA fragment and the poly(A⁺) portion of the tail are removed). The two pools of cDNA fragments are ligated together, creating 'ditags' (the new sequences are as follows: linker A–tag–tag–linker B). The ditags are amplified by PCR using primers designed based on sequences in linkers A and B.

The creation of the ditags is important for several reasons. First, the ditags can be amplified by PCR for subsequent cloning steps. Second, each tag within a ditag is linked tail to tail and flanked by anchoring enzyme recognition sequences, providing important orientation information used to identify the genes corresponding to each tag. Finally, even if tags are in high abundance the probability of creating identical ditags is extremely low. As a result, the occurrence of identical ditags indicates PCR bias, and these ditags are excluded from the final analysis to ensure accurate quantification of transcript abundance (Velculescu, 1995; Yamamoto, 2001).

After amplification, the anchoring enzyme is used to cleave the linkers from the ditags. Ditags from different reactions are ligated together to form strings of 10–50 tags. The concatenated strings of ditags are cloned into plasmids and sequenced. Typically about 50 000 tags are sequenced for each sample of interest, using a high-throughput sequencer (for more details on the methodology, see the review by Madden, 2000). The absolute expression levels of genes in the sample are quantified by counting the number of tags sequenced that correspond to each gene. Figure 76–2 provides a visual scheme of the procedure.

The National Cancer Institute's Cancer Genome Anatomy Project has chosen SAGE technology to sequence over 5 million tags across more than 100 different human cell types. The data are stored in a public database known as SAGEmap (Lal, 1999; Lash, 2000), and there are several tools such as SAGE Genie (Boon, 2002) available for reliably assigning tags to

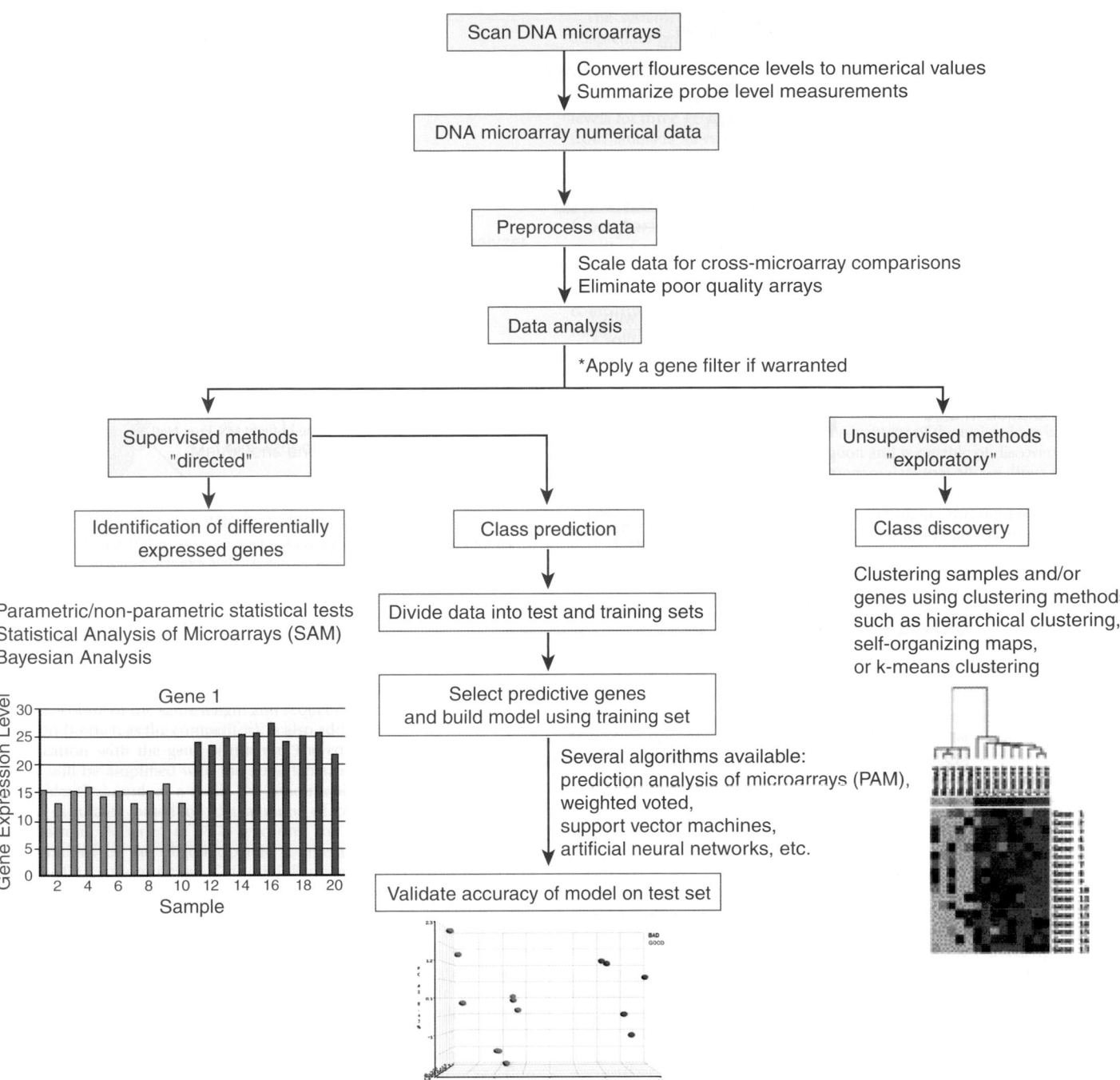

Figure 76–3 Analysis of DNA microarray data. The schematic diagram outlines the various steps required in the analysis of DNA microarray data. Image files are converted to numerical values and normalized, poor quality arrays are removed from the analysis, and genes that are not accurately detected by the array or genes that show little variation across samples are filtered out. Downstream computational and statistical analysis of the data can be divided into two categories – supervised and unsupervised methods. Supervised methods, such as class prediction algorithms, use predefined groups of samples to identify genes that can distinguish between groups and accurately classify unknown samples. Unsupervised methods, also known as class discovery methods, try to find previously unknown classes, such as novel cancer subtypes, within a dataset.

genes and for data analysis and visualization. Additional information and details can be obtained on line at http://cgap.nci.nih.gov/SAGE or http://www.sagenet.org.

DNA Microarrays

DNA microarrays are orderly arrays of spots, each composed of DNA representing a single gene, immobilized on to a solid support such as a glass slide as described in Chapter 68. DNA microarrays take advantage of Watson–Crick base pairing and, therefore, only strands of DNA that are complementary will hybridize and produce a signal that can be used as a measure of gene expression. The production and use of microarrays requires several steps including the creation of probes, array fabrication, target hybridization, fluorescence scanning, and image processing to produce a numerical readout of gene expression. Throughout the chapter, a probe will refer to a nucleic acid sequence that is attached to a solid support and the target will be a complementary free sequence of nucleic acids being measured for its abundance using microarrays (Phimister,

1999). A detailed description regarding the fabrication of cDNA and oligonucleotide arrays, along with how the RNA is prepared and hybridized to these platforms, can be found in Chapter 68.

DNA microarray experiments can produce millions of data points, which require a suite of data processing steps to select relevant genes. Although there is no standard protocol, the following steps are usually present in the analyses of a DNA microarray experiment (Fig. 76–3). The image files are converted to numerical values that are normalized and summarized using a software program (there are freely available and commercial programs [Affymetrix, 2001; Li, 2001; Irizarry, 2003]), poor quality arrays are removed from the analysis, genes that are not accurately detected by the array or genes that show little variation across samples are filtered out, and a variety of computational and statistical analyses are performed. Exploratory data analyses, including classification and the identification of differentially expressed genes can be divided into two categories – supervised and unsupervised methods. Supervised methods, such as class prediction algorithms, use predefined groups of samples

Mass Spectrometry

Mass spectrometry (MS) represents the major tool used to investigate the protein composition of complex biological samples. The principles of mass spectroscopy are discussed in Chapters 4 and 23, and the use of MS for detection of cancer-related proteins is discussed in Chapter 75. Prior to the discoveries that made MS protein analysis feasible, protein identification depended on more labor-intensive techniques such as Edman sequencing or antibody-based assays. The major obstacle to high-throughput protein analysis using MS has been the technical difficulty of ionizing proteins. The innovations of John Fenn, working with electrospray ionization, and Koichi Tanaka, who developed laser desorption ionization, opened the door to the field of proteomics. For their contributions to the field, both scientists shared half of the 2002 Nobel Prize in Chemistry. Electrospray ionization creates small, charged droplets of protein in solution. As the droplets move towards a vacuum chamber, the liquid evaporates, leaving behind a charged protein moiety. In laser desorption, a protein is placed in a chemical solution (called a matrix) which, when energized by a burst of energy, imparts ions to that protein. Once ionized, the weight-to-charge (m/z) ratio can be determined by the response of the protein to variations in an electromagnetic field.

Further analytic problems arise from the elaborate structure of proteins as well as the sheer abundance seen in most biological samples. With its secondary, tertiary, and quaternary structure, as well as post-translational modifications, protein structure is much more complex and less predictable than DNA or RNA. Advances in protein analysis have allowed for more rapid identification; however, many of these methods are subject to variations due to the context in which the protein is found, in particular its shape and the protein environment in which it is analyzed. Separation remains an important step in reducing complex biological specimens into more manageable samples. The bulk of proteomic experiments rely on separation of constituent proteins over a two-dimensional gel, a time- and labor-intensive method that slows the discovery process and requires relatively large amounts of starting sample. Other techniques to improve the resolution of data include proteomic analysis of whole cell lysate, usually separated by high-pressure liquid chromatography, or multidimensional liquid chromatography.

While the quantity of a peptide in a sample can increase the amplitude of the m/z spike seen on MS, other factors such as propensity of a peptide to ionize or the surrounding ions at the time of measurement also affect amplitude, making it difficult to comparatively quantify similar samples from different experimental conditions. The use of isotope-coded affinity tags (ICAT) allows quantitative comparison of samples. The tag consists of a biotin marker and a link, which contains either eight hydrogens or eight deuteriums. In order to compare the amount of a single protein from two different samples, one would label one sample with the light marker, the other with a heavy marker. This is done prior to MS analysis, which would then show a series of paired peaks for individual peptide fragments, with the heavy tag samples having an m/z 8 units greater than the sample with the light tag. One can then compare the relative amplitude of the two samples.

Multidimensional protein identification technology (MudPIT) allows identification of proteins from a digested sample. Protein fragments are introduced from high-pressure liquid chromatography into a tandem mass spectrometer. The m/z ratio for each peptide is measured in the first MS chamber, after which the peptide is fragmented. By comparing the relative weights of these fragments, one can determine the amino acid responsible for the change, in effect sequencing the peptide. These measured peptide sequences are matched to predicted fragments of known proteins, generating the identity of a large number of proteins from a complex biological sample.

Protein Arrays

Tissue microarrays produce a compact arrangement of sections from frozen or paraffin-embedded tissue, combining the samples on to a single platform. Prior to the sampling advances described by Kononen, the number of sections that could be arranged in parallel limited the simultaneous investigation of multiple tissue sections. Currently, a tissue microarray can hold up to a thousand samples, which can be tagged and labeled via in situ hybridization or immunohistochemical assays (Kononen, 1998; Russo, 2003). The potential for such large-scale parallel inquiry provides a more rapid means of answering questions about the biological mechanisms involved in progression from normal tissue to neoplasia (Kononen, 1998) or the pathways related to variable prognosis among tumors of similar histology (Bubendorf, 1999), as well as providing a ready means of validating results from other genomic or proteomic experiments (Chen, 2003).

Paweletz and associates have pioneered the development of reverse-phase protein microarrays. Rather than spotting small sections of tissue, these slides hold arrays of whole cell lysate from a specific cellular portion of tissue (Paweletz, 2001) Under the microscope, scientists can 'hand pick'

those cells of interest, capturing them with a small focused laser that binds cells to an overlying transfer film.

In contrast to arrays containing a tissue or cells of interest, arrays can also hold material designed to bind proteins from a sample applied to the surface of the array. Antibodies, DNA, RNA, and ribosomes – any substance with an affinity for a protein – can be used as a probe on the surface of the array. Manufacturing of these slides uses similar spotting technology to that described for oligonucleotide arrays (see above).

Molecular Markers for the Diagnosis of Human Neoplasia

Genomic

One clinically relevant application of genomic high-throughput technologies is the identification of diagnostic molecular markers for human diseases such as cancer. Histologic analysis complemented by immunohistochemistry, electron microscopy, and molecular analysis of chromosomal abnormalities is frequently used to classify cancers. Definitive diagnoses can often be difficult to determine but are important because they often influence patient treatment, response, and prognosis. The first paper to use DNA microarrays in clinical samples in order to develop gene expression profiles for cancer classification was published in 1999 by Todd Golub (Golub, 1999). Since that time, DNA microarrays have been extensively used across a wide range of malignant and normal tissue specimens in an attempt to develop diagnostic and prognostic tests.

AML/ALL: A Novel Paradigm

As mentioned in Chapter 71, a pioneering study has been performed using DNA microarrays to distinguish acute myeloid leukemia (AML) from acute lymphoblastic leukemia (ALL). In this study, Affymetrix GeneChips containing approximately 6800 human genes were employed to measure gene expression of bone marrow mononuclear cells obtained from patients with either of these diseases (Golub, 1999). The choice of acute leukemias, a hematological malignancy, in this study was important for several reasons. Previous DNA microarray experiments had produced reproducible results on cell lines; however, clinical specimens introduce additional noise that may obscure differences. Mononuclear cells reduce noise because they are a relatively homogeneous cancer cell population, in contrast to biopsies of solid tumors with varying amounts of surrounding stromal cells. In addition, distinction between acute leukemia subtypes is difficult using existing techniques, and the discovery of additional molecular markers would increase the accuracy of diagnosis and ultimately impact the choice of a therapeutic regime.

In order to explore whether differences in gene expression could be detected between the 27 ALL and 11 AML samples in this study, a method called 'neighborhood analysis' was used. The method ranks genes whose expression patterns across patients are highly correlated to the class of the sample (ALL or AML). A gene that is expressed at high levels across all ALL patients but at low levels in AML patients, for example, will be highly ranked. The significance, or how likely the correlation is by chance, is assessed by randomly assigning class labels to each of the samples and repeating the analysis. Approximately 1100 genes were significantly correlated with the class labels, and the top 50 genes were subsequently used in a weight-voted class prediction algorithm that predicts the class of unknown samples. Each of the 50 genes casts a vote indicating the class of the new sample. Each gene's 'vote,' either AML or ALL, is determined by calculating whether the expression value for the gene in the unknown sample is closer to the mean expression value for the gene across all ALL or all AML patients. The votes are then weighted according to the strength of the correlation between the gene expression levels and the class vector. The votes for each class are summed, and the unknown sample is assigned to the class with the larger total vote. An additional metric, known as the prediction strength, can be calculated to determine the margin of victory (for additional details, see http://www.broad.mit.edu/cancer/software/genecluster2/gc2.html and Reich, 2004). The accuracy of the prediction method was evaluated by 'leave one out' crossvalidation, where one of the 38 samples is withheld, the analysis is repeated, and the class of the left out sample is predicted. Using this approach, this study found that 36 of the 38 samples were classified correctly and two were classified as uncertain on crossvalidation. The predictor was also tested on an independent set of 34 additional samples and correctly classified in 29 of the 34 samples. The committee of 50 genes contained known markers of lymphoid versus myeloid cell lineage as well as genes related to carcinogenesis.

In addition to identifying markers capable of distinguishing AML and ALL, Golub and colleagues used an unsupervised clustering method known as self-organizing maps (SOM) to evaluate whether the two subtypes of leukemia could be found within the gene expression data without prior knowledge of the two leukemia classes. SOMs group samples into a user-defined number of clusters based on gene expression pattern similarities. Two-cluster SOM produced one cluster containing 24 of the 25 ALL samples and another cluster with 10 of the 13 AML samples. A four-cluster SOM was also capable of distinguishing among T-lineage ALL, B-lineage ALL, and AML. The success of this initial experiment and its exciting implications, as well as improvements in DNA microarray technology, analysis, and availability, has resulted in an exponential increase of clinical studies using microarrays. The results of several of these recent studies will be presented below.

Small Round Blue Cell Tumors of Childhood: Shifting the Paradigm to Solid Tumors

Another cancer that is difficult to accurately diagnose using a variety of histological and specialized molecular analyses is small, round blue cell tumors (SRBT) of childhood, which include neuroblastoma, rhabdomyosarcoma, non-Hodgkin lymphoma, and the Ewing family of tumors (EWS). Khan and colleagues were among the first to identify molecular markers predictive of the SRBT subtypes (Khan, 2001). Predictive genes were chosen using artificial neural networks (ANN), which are pattern recognition computer programs modeled after the neural structure and behavior of the human brain. Similar to the human brain, ANNs are capable of learning from experience. A neuron can accept many inputs but has only one output and, in an analogous manner, artificial neurons output a signal based on several inputs. ANNs are several connected artificial neurons that can recognize patterns in training data through optimization of several parameters (the weights assigned to the links between neurons) to accurately predict the tumor type of unknown samples.

Khan and colleagues used cDNA microarray containing 6567 genes to measure the gene expression of 63 samples, which included both tumor biopsies (13 EWS and 10 rhabdomyosarcoma) and cell lines (10 EWS, 10 rhabdomyosarcoma, 12 neuroblastoma, and 8 Burkitt lymphomas, a subset of non-Hodgkin lymphoma). Using a filtered set of 2308 genes, the 63 samples representing four SRBT diagnostic categories were used to train linear ANN models. 96 probes corresponding to 93 genes were selected based on the ANN models because they minimized the misclassification error rate to 0%. The algorithm was validated on a test set of 25 samples that were a mixture of cell lines, tumor biopsies, and five non-SRBTs. 17 SRBT test samples were classified correctly and the remaining three SRBTs, along with the five non-SRBTs, could not be assigned a subtype. Interestingly, even though data from only neuroblastoma cell lines were used in the training set, the model accurately predicted neuroblastoma tumor biopsy specimens in the test set. The results suggest that the use of cell lines may be beneficial in reducing noise created by stromal contamination of the tumor specimens.

Many of the 96 predictive genes reported in the above study were expressed at high levels in one, two, or three of the four diagnostic categories. One marker, MIC2, is currently used to diagnose EWS. However, MIC2 was highly expressed in EWSs and in some rhabdomyosarcomas, suggesting that the marker may lack specificity if used alone. Another molecular marker, FGFR4, a tyrosine kinase receptor related to myogenesis and upregulated only in rhabdomyosarcoma samples was investigated by immunostaining across a variety of tissues. FGFR4 was found to be upregulated in some other cancers and normal tissues, providing clues to its potential biological importance while reducing its potential as a specific molecular marker. The finding illustrates that a compendium of genes, instead of a single molecular marker, may increase the diagnostic sensitivity and specificity. This complements the conclusions of Chapter 76 on oncoproteins in tumor diagnosis: arrays of oncoproteins are more effective in early tumor detection than single individual oncoproteins.

Additional Diagnostic Cancer Applications

In addition to these studies, several other DNA microarray and SAGE experiments have been conducted to develop diagnostic tests for human cancers that are difficult to classify with conventional histological methods (see also Chapter 68). Barrett's esophagus, where the lining of the esophagus is replaced with a metaplastic columnar lining, is a condition associated with gastroesophageal reflux disease that can lead to the development of either squamous cell carcinoma or adenocarcinoma. Esophageal cancer is usually difficult to detect at an early stage and has a high mortality rate. Hierarchal clustering and ANNs were used to discover gene expression profiles measured by cDNA microarrays that could distinguish between esophageal cancer and Barrett's metaplasia specimens (Selaru, 2002; Xu, 2002). The expression levels of a small subset of predictor genes were quantified with Taqman quantitative reverse-transcriptase (RT) PCR (AppliedBiosystems, Inc.) on 39 patients with either Barrett's metaplasia or esophageal cancer to assess their clinical usefulness (Brabender, 2004).

New diagnostic molecular markers are also needed to distinguish between follicular-patterned thyroid lesions. Papillary thyroid carcinoma is usually diagnosed with a fine-needle aspiration after detection of a thyroid nodule; however, the test cannot differentiate between follicular thyroid adenoma (FTA) and follicular thyroid carcinoma (FTC), and a more invasive surgical biopsy is usually warranted. Cerutti and colleagues have attempted to develop a preoperative diagnostic test by constructing and analyzing three SAGE libraries using a FTA, a FTC, and a normal thyroid specimen (Cerutti, 2004). Over 360 000 tags were sequenced among the three libraries, and 305 genes were significantly differentially expressed between the three groups. A subset of these genes was chosen for validation with RT-PCR on independent samples that included 10 FTAs, 13 FTCs, and eight patient-matched normal thyroid tissues. RT-PCR was performed on a subset of the 305 genes: 12 of the most highly expressed genes in FTC and five of the most highly expressed genes in FTA/normal thyroid were chosen for validation with RT-PCR. Four genes (DDIT3, ARG2, ITM1, and C1orf24) validated the SAGE results and were able to predict 19 out of the 23 samples correctly on leave-one-out crossvalidation. In addition, immunohistochemistry was performed on 32 FTA and 27 FTC paraffin-embedded tissues using antibodies against two of the four genes, DDIT3 and ARG2. DDIT3 and ARG2 showed staining for FTCs, and negative staining for ARG2 in most samples, suggesting that these markers might improve the preoperative diagnosis of thyroid nodules.

Histological identification of the primary tumor site in patients presenting with metastatic adenocarcinoma can also be difficult. SAGE datasets suggested that primary and metastatic adenocarcinomas clustered together according to their site of origin, and a variety of RNA quantification methods, including DNA microarrays and SAGE, as well as the literature were used to select tumor- and site-specific molecular markers (Dennis, 2002). Buckhaults and colleagues analyzed a set of 11 SAGE libraries of ovarian, breast, pancreatic, and colon adenocarcinomas to select five genes that were able to discriminate these carcinomas of different tissue origins (Buckhaults, 2003). A class prediction algorithm, known as a two-dimensional gene-expression-based classification map, was able to correctly classify the tissue origin in 81% of the 62 independent samples of ovarian, breast, pancreatic, and colorectal carcinomas based on RT-PCR data of the five genes. A related study, aimed at identifying molecular markers of metastasis in primary tumors, compared gene expression profiles of unpaired primary adenocarcinomas and metastatic nodules from different individuals across a broad spectrum of tumor types. 128 genes were identified whose expression patterns could distinguish primary from metastatic adenocarcinoma (Ramaswamy, 2003). Ramaswamy and colleagues demonstrated that a subset of the 128 genes were associated with metastasis in independent datasets from primary lung, breast, and prostate adenocarcinomas as well as medulloblastomas and large B-cell lymphomas. The findings challenge the hypothesis that metastatic potential arises in a few cells in the primary tumor, and suggests that the ability to metastasize pre-exists in the primary tumor. If this is correct, gene expression patterns in primary tumors could predict future risk of distant metastasis.

High-throughput genomic technologies have also been used in a variety of other diseases including bladder carcinoma (Dyrskjot, 2003), central nervous system embryonal tumors (Pomeroy, 2002), ovarian cancer (Sawiris, 2002), breast cancer (Perou, 2000, Porter, 2001, 2003a), pancreatic cancer (Iacobuzio-Donahue, 2002), lung cancer (Bhattacharjee, 2001), and colorectal cancer (Buckhaults, 2001) to aid in disease diagnosis and the identification of novel disease subtypes. The use of high-throughput genomic technologies to develop disease diagnostics is an inherently difficult problem because predictive genes identified by a training set are based on histopathological diagnoses. The histological methods for classification of certain cancers, however, may be imperfect, making it difficult to assess the true accuracy of the molecular markers. In addition, it is difficult to verify the existence of novel disease subtypes found in DNA microarray experiments if no complementary histological evidence is available. In the future, pathologists will probably use high-throughput genomic technology to facilitate accurate diagnosis in difficult cases. A majority of studies using genomic high-throughput studies have chosen, therefore, to focus on identifying gene expression profiles predictive of disease prognosis given the limited number histological or clinical indicators for disease outcome (see below).

Proteomic

In Chapter 75, a new approach for the early detection of several different types of cancer based on patterns of protein expression, called proteomics, was discussed as showing great potential. This approach does not search

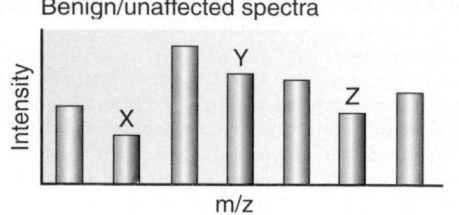

Benign/unaffected spectra

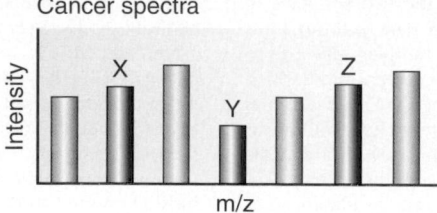

Cancer spectra

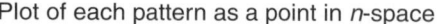

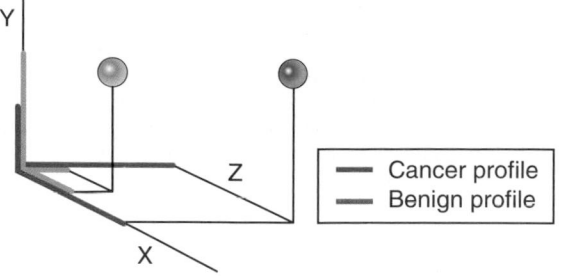

Plot of each pattern as a point in *n*-space

Figure 76–6 Proteomic pattern diagnostics. Pattern analysis identifies m/z ratios with the 'most fit' combination of proteins for distinguishing between clinical states of interest. (Redrawn from Petricoin EF et al. Nature Reviews Drug Discovery 1, 683–695 (2002).)

for specific known proteins but rather for differences in patterns of protein expression (the identity of many of these proteins is unknown) based on the use of MS. We discuss this approach further here to illustrate the power of high throughput postgenomic methods in cancer detection. As noted, this approach does not identify the proteins involved but relies instead on the varying amplitudes of several different m/z ratios present across samples (Fig. 76–6). Given the more favorable prognosis seen with malignancies diagnosed at earlier stages, there has been a great deal of interest in using proteomic tools to search for diagnostic markers in readily available biological samples such as blood, urine, or saliva (Chapter 75).

Ovarian Cancer: A New Paradigm for Early Detection

Patients with ovarian cancer frequently suffer a worse prognosis than those with other malignancies, in part due to the advanced stage of disease at diagnosis. In an attempt to develop a screening test for high risk women, Liotta and colleagues used a MS-based platform to analyze serum samples of patients with ovarian cancer compared to controls and found that their model was able to distinguish between serum of women with and without ovarian cancer with a remarkably high degree of accuracy (Petricoin, 2002).

Their method utilizes SELDI-TOF MS: surface-enhanced laser desorption ionization (SELDI) coupled with a mass spectrometer that measures the time of flight (TOF) of the ionized proteins from laser to the detector. Serum samples are placed on a chip with embedded weak cations, which provide the 'surface enhancement' of SELDI. Excess serum is washed off, and proteins bound to the weak cations remain on the chip, where they are combined with a matrix solution and ionized when exposed to a laser.

Each serum sample results in approximately 15 000 m/z values of varying amplitude. The bioinformatic tools used to parse through such a complicated data set rely on class prediction using a genetic algorithm. The class prediction involves a 'training' set of known cancer and noncancer samples. The genetic algorithm selects a panel of m/z values and tests its ability to differentiate between cancer and control. The 'genetics' of a genetic algorithm represent a biological analogy describing the repeated mixing and matching of the most successful m/z values, allowing 'survival of the fittest' values in successive generations of testing, ultimately producing the most discriminatory panels, which are tested on a masked group of patients and controls.

Although the panel used in this study resulted in a test with 100% sensitivity and 95% specificity, validation in a more realistic clinical setting remains to be done. The idea of studying a group of markers in parallel would seem appropriate, given the complexity of tumor biology and its interaction with the host. The absence of protein identification with this technique constrains the test. It is not clear if the values included represent participants in tumor biology shed into the bloodstream or nonspecific markers of inflammation. With 15 000 data points to choose from in each serum sample, there is a significant risk of overfitting any model so that it would have little clinical utility in a practical setting.

Additional Cancers

Liotta's paper represents one of the most significant early attempts at harnessing MS in the search for a clinically useful biomarker, and has been followed by numerous similar studies in patients with breast (Kuerer, 2002),

prostate (Ornstein, 2004b), and lung cancer (Chen, 2003). By applying these techniques of detection and analysis to prostate cancer, preliminary data from men with an indeterminate elevation of prostate specific antigen (PSA) suggest that there is an 'ion signature' that distinguishes between men with prostate cancer and those with benign prostatic hypertrophy with 100% sensitivity and 67% specificity (Ornstein, 2004a).

Because the serum represents a particularly complicated specimen for two-dimensional polyacrylamide gel electrophoresis (2D-PAGE)-based proteomic analysis, other specimens in proximity to the tissue in question may be more readily available and simpler to work with. Nipple aspirate fluid is easily obtained and, in the case of unilateral disease, allows for a simple paired sample from the unaffected breast. Kuerer and colleagues used 2D-PAGE in an initial descriptive study comparing protein expression in the nipple aspirate from both breasts in patients with unilateral breast cancer and a healthy volunteer (Kuerer, 2002). Their results showed highly concordant protein electrophoresis patterns when nipple aspirate fluid was compared from each breast in the control subject, as opposed to the samples obtained from patients with breast cancer, which exhibited a larger number of proteins unique to the affected breast compared to the unaffected breast in the same patient. The finding suggests that localized breast malignancy significantly alters the protein expression in the nipple aspirate fluid, raising the possibility of a diagnostic marker.

Prognostic Molecular Markers of Disease

Genomic

Patients diagnosed with the same type of cancer and treated using similar protocols often respond quite differently and have varying survival rates. Several clinical and histological variables such as age, serum protein levels, and stage or grade of tumor can be used to assess a patient's prognosis with variable accuracy. Many studies have utilized genomic high-throughput technologies, especially DNA microarrays, as described at length in Chapter 68, to identify gene expression signatures that predict patient survival or relapse rates. Instead of comparing two different disease states, as detailed above in the diagnostics section, the experimental design for the development of molecular prognostic indicators usually attempts to stratify a particular cancer into subtypes according to outcome, using either unsupervised or supervised computational approaches (Fig. 76–3). The marker associated with poor prognosis may provide clues about the biological mechanisms underlying resistance to chemotherapeutics and aid the identification of new drug targets.

Diffuse Large B-cell Lymphoma

Identifying molecular markers that predict patient survival involves distinguishing subtle differences between specimens and, as above in the diagnostics section, many studies have been conducted on hematological malignancies where a homogenous population of cells can easily be isolated. Diffuse large B-cell lymphoma (DLBCL) is the most common adult lymphoid neoplasm and comprises 30–40% of all non-Hodgkin lymphoma. Response to chemotherapy is highly variable and less than half of the patients treated achieve long-term remission. Currently, the

International Prognostic Index (IPI) is used to approximate the outcome of patients diagnosed with DLBCL based on several clinical factors such as serum lactate dehydrogenase and stage. Alizadeh and colleagues constructed a specialized cDNA microarray, known as the Lymphochip, with 17 856 probes chosen from germinal center B-cells, DLBCL, and other lymphoma cDNA libraries (Alizadeh, 2000). 128 Lymphochips were used to assay 96 normal and malignant samples from leukemia and lymphoma cell lines and from patients with DLBCL, follicular lymphoma, and chronic lymphocytic leukemia. Hierarchical clustering of the microarrays revealed three subgroups of DLBCL samples based on genes related to proliferation, T cells, lymph-node biology, and germinal center B-cells. DLBCLs are thought to arise at different stages of B-cell differentiation, and hierarchical clustering of just the DLBCL samples across the genes related to germinal center B cells separated the sample into two distinct clusters – germinal center B-cell-like DLBCL and activated B-cell-like DLBCL. The two subtypes were shown to have statistically different overall survival (72% of germinal cell B-cell-like DLBCL subjects were alive after 5 years in comparison to 16% of activated B-cell-like DLBCL subjects) and these two classes could be used to further stratify patients identified as low-risk by the IPI. This study was one of the first to relate tumor subtypes identified by global gene expression profiling to patient outcome. Use of DNA microarray in diagnosing this condition and further subtyping it into the germinal center B-cell-like group and the activated B-cell-like group is discussed in Chapter 71.

A follow-up study by Shipp and colleagues tested whether a gene expression profile could be identified, without prior discovery of subtypes, that predicted survival in DLBCL patients (Shipp, 2002). Affymetrix HuGeneFL microarrays containing approximately 6800 probes were used to measure global gene expression profiles across 58 patients with DLBCL (32 patients with cured disease, 26 patients with refractory/fatal disease). The weighted voted class prediction algorithm with crossvalidation was used to identify a gene expression signature of 13 genes capable of distinguishing between patients with cured and fatal disease. The prediction model was also able to stratify patients into good and poor prognosis groups within categories defined by the IPI. As additional validation, the current study was compared to previous findings reported by Alizadeh's group. The studies used microarray platforms that interrogated two different but overlapping sets of genes. Genes used to distinguish the two subtypes of DLBCL in the Alizadeh study that were also present on the HuGeneFL microarray separated the 58 DLBCLs into two groups, but the groups did not correlate with overall survival rates. However, three out of the 13 predictive genes identified by Shipp and colleagues were present on the Lymphochip and correlated with survival across the patients in the Alizadeh study.

In a related study, Rosenwald and colleagues used the Lymphochip to study 240 patients with untreated DLBCL that subsequently received anthracycline-based chemotherapy (Rosenwald, 2002). Using a training set of 160 samples, gene expression levels were correlated with survival times using the Cox proportional hazards model. 670 genes had expression patterns that were significantly correlated with prognosis, and these genes were clustered to identify sets of genes with similar expression patterns. The highly correlated genes were involved in similar biological processes, and four sets of correlated genes related to proliferation, major histocompatibility complex (MHC) class II, lymph-node biology, and germinal center B cells were used to develop a class prediction model. The gene expression levels of genes within each set were averaged, and these composite values were used to build a multivariate prediction model. The model was capable of assigning each sample in the test set a score related to the risk of succumbing to the disease. Scores assigned by the model to the entire set of samples were stratified into quartiles, with a 5-year survival of 73% in the first group compared to 15% in the fourth group.

Follicular Lymphoma

A similar survival prediction model was used to predict the prognosis of patients with follicular lymphoma, a cancer similarly arising from germinal center B cells (Dave, 2004). Treatments may involve chemotherapy, immunological therapy, or hematopoietic stem-cell transplantation; however, there is no consensus as to which regime is superior, and outcome is highly variable. Tumor biopsies from 191 patients with follicular lymphoma were divided into a training and test set. Using the Cox proportional hazards model to correlate genes with survival, two highly correlated sets of genes were chosen to build a multivariate predictive model. The set associated with a favorable prognosis contained genes highly expressed in T cells and macrophages, whereas the set associated with poor prognosis contained genes expressed in macrophages and dendritic cells. In further experiments on biopsy specimens separated into malignant and nonmalignant fractions, the two sets of genes were highly expressed only in the nonmalignant fractions. The results suggest that the tumor microenvironment significantly influences prognosis.

The above lymphoma studies demonstrate that microarrays may be successful in accurately predicting patient prognosis and may complement currently used methods such as the IPI. The results imply that biopsies obtained at the time of diagnosis can be used to predict prognosis and could influence treatment decisions. As noted above, however, there is disagreement between studies as a result of several factors, including the DNA microarray platform used, patient population, differences in treatment regimes, sample size, the variable quality of long term follow-up data, and choice of prediction methodology (see Pitfalls section, below). The follicular lymphoma study also demonstrates the importance of the tumor microenvironment, something that is not typically explored in DNA microarray studies.

Acute Myeloid Leukemia

Despite the potential problems, many other studies have been conducted on a wide-range of tumor types. In 2004, two studies published in the *New England Journal of Medicine* identified gene expression profiles that can be used as prognostic indicators in AML (Bullinger, 2004; Valk, 2004). Bullinger's group used cDNA microarrays (≈39 000 probes) to obtain global gene expression profiles for 116 patients with AML and Valk's group used Affymetrix human U133A microarrays (≈22 000 probes) to assay 285 patients with AML. Unsupervised hierarchical clustering in both studies revealed clusters that correlated with cytogenetic and molecular abnormalities present in the tumors. Using the Cox proportional hazards model implemented in Significance Analysis of Microarray (SAM) software (Tusher, 2001), Bullinger and colleagues identified gene expression patterns that correlated with survival. K-means clustering was used to divide the training samples into two groups, representing good and bad outcome, based on the genes selected by SAM. The Prediction Analysis of Microarrays (PAM) algorithm was used to develop an outcome predictor using 133 genes based on the two identified groups in the training set. The prediction algorithm was applied to the test samples and was able to separate them into two groups that differed significantly in survival times. Valk's group used similar methods to identify genes that could classify samples into disease subgroups previously identified by clustering analysis. The subgroups were associated with cytogenetic and molecular abnormalities as well as patient prognosis. Both studies demonstrate the usefulness of global gene expression analysis in dissecting the heterogeneity that exists within tumors of the same type. The high degree of overlapping results between these two studies demonstrates the potential microarray technology has to distinguish between subtle tumor subtypes and add prognostic information to current clinical practice.

Breast Cancer

While similar prognostic biomarker studies have been carried out in prostate cancer (Dhanasekaran, 2001), lung adenocarcinoma (Beer, 2002), and multiple myeloma (Tian, 2003b), the identification of prognostic biomarkers in breast cancer, however, best demonstrates how successful high-throughput genomic studies can translate into important clinical tools. Prognostic molecular markers were identified from gene expression studies using primary breast cancer biopsies from patients under 55 years old with sporadic node-negative disease that did and did not develop metastases within 5 years. The predictive power of these molecular markers was deemed to be greater than other clinical and histological factors such as tumor grade, size, angio-invasion, or estrogen receptor status (van't Veer, 2002). Similar studies on breast cancer have subsequently been conducted (van de Vijver, 2002; Huang, 2003, Sotiriou, 2003) and a recent paper describes the development of a predictive model that uses gene expression, clinical, and histological data to more accurately estimate prognosis (Pittman, 2004).

One bottleneck to performing DNA microarray studies is the dearth of snap-frozen tissues from patients with long-term follow-up. Snap-freezing tissue preserves the integrity of the RNA and is ideal for DNA microarray experiments; however, most tissue banks or clinical trials have collected paraffin-embedded tissue. Paraffin embedded tissue contains partially degraded RNA that is usually insufficient to obtain high-quality DNA microarray results (although advances in this area are ongoing). Technologies such as real competitive PCR and real-time PCR are being used to measure gene expression levels in these tissues, but the amount of RNA obtained from tissue blocks often limits assays to a few hundred genes. Using RT-PCR, Paik and colleagues studied 21 genes (16 cancer-related and five reference genes for normalization) chosen from the breast cancer DNA microarray studies outlined above. Samples included 675 paraffin-embedded tissue blocks obtained from patients enrolled in the National Surgical Adjuvant Breast and Bowel Project B-14 trials (Paik, 2004). All tissue blocks were obtained from tamoxifen-treated patients that had node-negative, estrogen-receptor positive primary breast cancer. The expression levels of the 16 cancer-related genes were used to calculate a score representing the risk of cancer reoccurrence at a distant site. The patients

IX

were stratified into low-, intermediate-, and high-risk groups based on the reoccurrence score. The reoccurrence score provided significant predictive information beyond tumor grade, age, and tumor size. The simplified 21 gene assay can be more easily translated into a clinical prognostic test designed to help physicians decide which tamoxifen-treated, node-negative, ER-positive breast cancer patients should receive chemotherapy.

Prognostic molecular markers for breast cancer have also been identified using SAGE technology. SAGE, unlike DNA microarrays, cannot be used to assay hundreds of clinical samples; however, it is not restricted to known genes or limited by the selection of probes on a microarray. SAGE is capable of identifying novel transcripts that have not previously been described, possibly because of their tissue-specific expression (an advantage in developing therapeutics). Two studies using SAGE libraries obtained from normal, ductal carcinoma in situ (DCIS), invasive, and metastatic breast tumors were used to identify transcripts that changed between each of the disease states (Porter, 2001, 2003a). Several DCIS or invasive/metastatic 'specific' genes were assayed by mRNA in situ hybridization using 18 frozen DCIS and invasive breast cancer samples and by immunohistochemistry using 769 DCIS, invasive, and metastatic breast tumor samples. S100A7, a member of the S100 family of calcium binding proteins, was preferentially expressed in DCIS (with highest levels restricted to high-grade comedo DCIS) versus normal or invasive/metastatic tumors. Although S100A7 is expressed less strongly in invasive tumors, the levels are higher in ER-negative, poorly differentiated, lymph-node-positive tumors, suggesting that its expression in DCIS may be a useful prognostic indicator. In a follow-up study, Porter et al. further characterized dermcidin, identified in the previous studies as preferentially expressed in invasive and metastatic tumors. Dermcidin is a newly characterized gene expressed in sweat glands and the pons of the brain (Porter, 2003b). The marker was expressed in a subset of invasive tumors by immunohistochemistry and its expression correlated with larger tumor size and presence of metastatic lymph nodes. In a subset of cases, higher expression levels were attributable to gene amplification at the gene locus on chromosome 12. Dermcidin was shown to enhance cell growth and survival and may be a promising prognostic indicator of overall and distant metastatic-free survival.

Integrating Genomics and Proteomics: Lung Cancer as the New Paradigm

The development of high-throughput technology allows one not only to look at how multiple genes or proteins might predict a clinical feature of interest but also to study overlap in transcriptional activity and protein translation. Beer and colleagues have looked at the ability of genetic profiling and protein translation in lung adenocarcinoma to predict survival (Chen, 2003). After filtering low abundance genes, they found approximately 5000 genes consistently expressed across a cohort of 86 adenocarcinoma samples and 10 normal tissue samples. Hierarchical clustering and leave-one-out crossvalidation generated a list of the 50 genes most effective at dividing patients into high- and low-risk groups for mortality over several years of follow-up. Of particular interest was the observation that stage I patients, those most likely to experience a surgical cure of their disease, could also be divided into high- and low-risk groups, potentially identifying a novel group that would benefit from adjuvant chemotherapy.

A total of 76 of the tumor samples underwent both microarray and proteomic analysis. In the examples of genes found along with their corresponding protein product, correlation peaked at 0.39. While statistically significant, the low degree of correlation underlines the point that the oversimplified model of transcription and translation is in reality a much more elaborate system of translational regulation, glycosylation, phosphorylation, and further downstream modifications. As the authors conclude, many of the transcripts probably do not correlate well with their protein counterparts as a result of this continued post-translational development.

The extension of their investigation to include genomics and proteomics uncovered a significant cohort of genes and proteins involved in the glycolytic pathway and upregulated among patients with a high risk of mortality, suggesting that this integration of genomics and proteomics has particular value in shedding light on the molecular pathogenesis of disease states.

Pitfalls of Molecular Markers for both Prognostics and Diagnostics

Disagreement Between Related DNA Microarray Datasets

The diffuse large B-cell lymphoma studies by Alizadeh and Shipp identified subsets of genes that specified two subtypes of DLBCL patients

that differed in survival. Shipp and colleagues also identified two subtypes of DLBCL patients; however, they did not correlate with survival. The above example illustrates one of many DNA microarray studies where there is little or no overlap of the results. There are several potential causes in experimental design and analyses of DNA microarray results that may account for the widespread discrepancies (Simon, 2003). Two different studies performed using similar tissue samples may have slightly different patient populations and sample sizes. Tissue heterogeneity is also a problem – biopsies obtained from different locations have varying numbers of normal cells contaminating the tumor samples. Additionally, there is no 'standard' for preprocessing and analyzing microarray data. New computational approaches are continually emerging and two groups analyzing the same dataset will often produce disparate gene lists. Finally, methodologies to compare datasets generated using different DNA microarray platforms are currently being developed, and similar studies with nonoverlapping results may have employed inadequate methods of comparison (see also Chapter 68).

'Overfitting' the Predictor

Traditionally, clinical studies aim to associate a handful of variables across several hundred patients whereas DNA microarray studies contain thousands of variables (gene expression levels) across relatively small numbers of patients (typically 20–200 patients). Many class prediction algorithms yield accurate results for the samples in the study that they were derived from but, when applied to an independent patient sample, performance drops significantly – a phenomenon known as overfitting (Ransohoff, 2004). The results of DNA microarray studies are therefore the most robust when the data is divided into a training and test or validation set (Ntzani, 2003). In addition to the need for independent sample validation, it is also important to validate the gene expression levels using a different technology. In order to realize the true promise of these technologies, it is critical to develop methods to combine several gene expression studies to identify markers that are consistently correlated with disease class or outcome, and then validate these markers using a different technology and cohort of patients.

The 'Bystander' Effect

Miklos and colleagues compared DNA microarray studies measuring prefrontal cortex gene expression in patients with and without schizophrenia to non-microarray studies that included genetic, RNA, and protein measurements using a variety of approaches (Miklos, 2004). Little overlap was found between the DNA microarray and the nonmicroarray experiments. One reason may be that genes identified using DNA microarray studies are 'bystander', not involved in the pathogenesis of the disease state. Genes identified by genetic linkage studies are usually causally related to a disease; however, expression levels of these genes may remain constant because the genetic alteration only affects mRNA splicing or posttranscriptional regulation. Also, DNA microarray technologies may not be sensitive enough to accurately measure gene expression changes in genes expressed at low levels.

Despite the above cautions, DNA microarray studies in the recent literature have begun to explore the biological significance and therapeutic potential of promising genes in greater depth using in vitro and in vivo models. For example, using DNA microarrays Tian and colleagues identified a gene, DKK1, that was differentially expressed in multiple myeloma patients with and without focal bone lesions (Tian, 2003a). Patients with bone lesions expressed higher levels of DKK1 RNA and protein. DKK1 is involved in bone formation through the Wnt signaling pathway, and marrow plasma from patients with bone lesions was shown to block osteoblast differentiation in vitro, indicating a causal role in disease progression and a potential therapeutic target. Another study, using cDNA microarrays to study liver samples from patients with hepatitis-B-positive hepatocellular carcinomas with and without intrahepatic metastases found that paired primary and metastatic tumors had similar gene expression patterns (Ye, 2003). Many differentially expressed genes, however, were identified between primary carcinomas that did and did not metastasize. Osteopontin, a glycoslyated phosphoprotein that acts as a cytokine, was overexpressed in primary tumors with metastasis. Further experimental studies showed that cellular invasiveness was reduced in hepatoma-derived cell lines treated with neutralizing osteopontin antibody. In addition, nude mice injected with hepatocellular carcinoma cells had a reduced incidence of metastasis if treated with osteopontin-specific antibody.

Limitations of Proteomic Techniques

Proteomic studies suffer from similar problems to those outlined above for DNA microarrays, including tissue heterogeneity, overfitting of predictive models, and the identification of causative disease proteins. Specific criticism of proteomic techniques for the diagnosis of cancer focuses largely on the SELDI-TOF MS technique. Diamandis has been the most widely published critic of this approach, and has outlined several shortcomings of the technology (Diamandis, 2004a, 2004b). While several papers have published impressive diagnostic yields using a panel of mass spectra, or 'ion signatures,' there have been few positive identifications of proteins responsible for those peaks Some of those proteins identified have been studied previously as tumor markers but dismissed as acute phase reactants. The absence of more positive protein identification limits the interpretation of published results, which potentially record differences attributable to something other than the underlying cancer, such as generalized inflammation.

The narrow dynamic detection range of the mass spectroscopy technology also limits proteomic studies. In the case of serum samples, there is generally minimal preprocessing prior to MS analysis, involving surface enhancement through incubation on a weakly cationic protein chip – a nonspecific process that would likely only bind to the most abundant proteins in the sample, failing to detect potentially informative low-abundance proteins. One would likely not expect the proteins shed from a malignancy such as prostate cancer to be the most abundant protein in a serum sample. By some estimates, SELDI-TOF MS could not detect proteins at less than 1 μg/dL, a concentration many times higher than that of most known tumor markers (Diamandis, 2003).

Conclusions and Future Challenges

The recent completion of the human genome project and advances within the biotechnology sector offer unprecedented opportunities for identification of biomarkers associated with cancer and other pathologies. Genome sequence data combined with high-throughput biomarker discovery will facilitate the correlation of genetic variation with disease diagnosis and biological outcomes. The emerging fields of functional genomics and functional proteomics offer the opportunity to translate these advances into a full comprehension of the pathophysiology of cancer and other complex multigenic diseases.

High-throughput genomic and proteomic technologies have the potential to transform clinical practice and are likely to lead to the supplementation or replacement of traditional diagnostic and prognostic biomarkers. Many of the studies detailed in this chapter have demonstrated the utility of gene expression profiles for the classification of tumors into distinct, clinically relevant subtypes and the prediction of clinical outcomes. In addition, emerging proteomics platforms have just begun to add another layer of molecular information to the study of human disease. These technologies should lead to a new era of individualized molecular medicine, whereby each patient will be treated on the basis of the genetic changes in their tumor and their own genetic make-up, resulting in more effective and less toxic therapy.

While these high-throughput platforms offer the promise of impacting the practice of medicine, a number of obstacles remain to widespread clinical implementation of these technologies. Genomic and proteomic biomarkers are an emerging class of laboratory tests that present special implementation challenges for the clinical laboratory, including analytical, bioinformatics, and bioethical issues. Considerable efforts are required to provide the necessary clinical laboratory infrastructure for standard high-throughput analyzers capable of detecting genomic and proteomic alterations within a variety of biological samples, high-performance computing, and advanced data management capabilities. Significant improvements in analytical tools are needed, as are efforts to standardize the techniques, controls, and reference standards. The application of such information to medical diagnosis and treatment will require considerable changes in the training of physicians. The most pressing need, however, is for extensive independent validation of the profiles described in the sections above using large, statistically powered datasets. Inclusion of genomic and proteomic-based molecular profiling techniques into clinical trial protocols will be needed to realize the potential of this technology to improve diagnosis and tailored treatment of human disease.

References

Affymetrix I: Affymetrix Microarray Suite User Guide, version 5. Santa Clara, CA, Affymetrix Technical Report, 2001.

Alizadeh AA, Eisen MB, Davis RE, et al: Distinct types of diffuse large B-cell lymphoma identified by gene expression profiling. Nature 2000; 403:503–511.
This study analyzed diffuse large B cell lymphoma patient samples using DNA microarrays and was one of the first to relate tumor subtypes identified by global gene expression profiling to patient outcome.

Anderson NL, Anderson NG: The human plasma proteome: history, character, and diagnostic prospects. Mol Cell Proteomics 2002; 1:845–867.

Beer DG, Kardia SL, Huang CC, et al: Gene-expression profiles predict survival of patients with lung adenocarcinoma. Nat Med 2002; 8:816–824.

Bhattacharjee A, Richards WG, Staunton J, et al: Classification of human lung carcinomas by mRNA expression profiling reveals distinct adenocarcinoma subclasses. Proc Natl Acad Sci USA 2001; 98:13790–13795.

Boon K, Osorio EC, Greenhut SF, et al: An anatomy of normal and malignant gene expression. Proc Natl Acad Sci USA 2002; 99:11287–11292.

Brabender J, Marjoram P, Salonga D, et al: A multigene expression panel for the molecular diagnosis of Barrett's esophagus and Barrett's adenocarcinoma of the esophagus. Oncogene 2004; 23:4780–4788.

Brown MP, Grundy WN, Lin D, et al: Knowledge-based analysis of microarray gene expression data by using support vector machines. Proc Natl Acad Sci USA 2000; 97:262–267.

Bubendorf L, Kolmer M, Kononen J, et al: Hormone therapy failure in human prostate cancer: analysis by complementary DNA and tissue microarrays. J Natl Cancer Inst 1999; 91:1758–1764.

Buckhaults P, Rago C, St Croix B, et al: Secreted and cell surface genes expressed in benign and malignant colorectal tumors. Cancer Res 2001; 61:6996–7001.

Buckhaults P, Zhang Z, Chen YC, et al: Identifying tumor origin using a gene expression-based classification map. Cancer Res 2003; 63:4144–4149.

Bullinger L, Dohner K, Bair E, et al: Use of gene-expression profiling to identify prognostic subclasses in adult acute myeloid leukemia. N Engl J Med 2004; 350:1605–1616.

Cerutti JM, Delcelo R, Amadei MJ, et al: A preoperative diagnostic test that distinguishes benign from malignant thyroid carcinoma based on gene expression. J Clin Invest 2004; 113:1234–1242.

Chen G, Gharib TG, Wang H, et al: Protein profiles associated with survival in lung adenocarcinoma. Proc Natl Acad Sci USA 2003; 100:13537–13542.
Analyzes resected lung tumors which underwent both DNA microarray and proteomic analysis, and gene and protein expression levels and were mostly poorly correlated. However, the integration of the two techniques revealed components of the glycolysis pathway associated with poor patient survival.

Claverie JM: Gene number. What if there are only 30 000 human genes? Science 2001; 291:1255–1257.

Collins FS, Morgan M, and Patrinos A: The Human Genome Project: lessons from large-scale biology. Science 2003; 300:286–290.

Datson NA, van der Perk-de Jong, van den Berg MP, et al: MicroSAGE: a modified procedure for serial analysis of gene expression in limited amounts of tissue. Nucleic Acids Res 1999; 27:1300–1307.

Dave SS, Wright G, Tan B, et al: Prediction of survival in follicular lymphoma based on molecular features of tumor-infiltrating immune cells. N Engl J Med 2004; 351:2159–2169.

Dennis JL, Vass JK, Wit EC, et al: Identification from public data of molecular markers of adenocarcinoma characteristic of the site of origin. Cancer Res 2002; 62:5999–6005.

Dhanasekaran SM, Barrette TR, Ghosh D, et al: Delineation of prognostic biomarkers in prostate cancer. Nature 2001; 412:822–826.

Diamandis EP: Point: Proteomic patterns in biological fluids: do they represent the future of cancer diagnostics? Clin Chem 2003; 49:1272–1275.

Diamandis EP: Analysis of serum proteomic patterns for early cancer diagnosis: drawing attention to potential problems. J Natl Cancer Inst 2004a; 96:353–356.

Diamandis EP: Mass spectrometry as a diagnostic and a cancer biomarker discovery tool: opportunities and potential limitations. Mol Cell Proteomics 2004b; 3:367–378.

Ding C, Cantor CR: A high-throughput gene expression analysis technique using competitive PCR and matrix-assisted laser desorption ionization time-of-flight MS. Proc Natl Acad Sci USA 2003; 100:3059–3064.

Ding C, Maier E, Roscher AA, et al: Simultaneous quantitative and allele-specific expression analysis with real competitive PCR. BMC Genet 2004; 5:8.

Dudoit S: FJST: comparison of discrimination methods for the classification of tumors using gene expression data. J Am Statistical Assoc 2002; 97:77–87.

Dyrskjot L, Thykjaer T, Kruhoffer M, et al: Identifying distinct classes of bladder carcinoma using microarrays. Nat Genet 2003; 33:90–96.

Eisen MB, Spellman PT, Brown PO, et al: Cluster analysis and display of genome-wide expression patterns. Proc Natl Acad Sci USA 1998; 95:14863–14868.

Emmert-Buck MR, Bonner RF, Smith PD, et al: Laser capture microdissection. Science 1996; 274:998–1001.

Genome International Sequencing Consortium: Initial sequencing and analysis of the human genome. Nature 2001; 409:860–921. Available on line at: http://www.nature.com/genomics/human/index.html.

Golub TR, Slonim DK, Tamayo P, et al: Molecular classification of cancer: class discovery and class prediction by gene expression monitoring. Science 1999; 286:531–537.
Describes the first use of DNA microarrays to assay the gene expression of thousands of genes in clinical samples (human acute leukemias) to both identify new cancer classes and to predict the class of unknown samples.

Huang E, Cheng SH, Dressman H, et al: Gene expression predictors of breast cancer outcomes. Lancet 2003; 361:1590–1596.

Iacobuzio-Donahue CA, Maitra A, Shen-Ong GL, et al: Discovery of novel tumor markers of pancreatic cancer using global gene expression technology. Am J Pathol 2002; 160:1239–1249.

International Human Genome Sequencing Consortium: Finishing the euchromatic sequence of the human genome. Nature 2004; 431:931–945.

Irizarry RA, Bolstad BM, Collin F, et al: Summaries of Affymetrix GeneChip probe level data. Nucleic Acids Res 2003; 31:e15.

Kaminski N, Friedman N: Practical approaches to analyzing results of microarray experiments. Am J Respir Cell Mol Biol 2002; 27:125–132.

Khan J, Wei JS, Ringner M, et al: Classification and diagnostic prediction of cancers using gene expression profiling and artificial neural networks. Nat Med 2001; 7:673–679.

Kononen J, Bubendorf L, Kallioniemi A, et al: Tissue microarrays for high-throughput molecular profiling of tumor specimens. Nat Med 1998; 4:844–847.

Kuerer HM, Goldknopf IL, Fritsche H, et al: Identification of distinct protein expression patterns in bilateral matched pair breast ductal fluid specimens from women with unilateral invasive breast carcinoma. High-throughput biomarker discovery. Cancer 2002; 95:2276–2282.

Lal A, Lash AE, Altschul SF, et al: A public database for gene expression in human cancers. Cancer Res 1999; 59:5403–5407.

Lander ES, Linton LM, Birren B, et al: Initial sequencing and analysis of the human genome. Nature 409:860–921, 2001.

A thorough presentation of the history of the human genome project, the methodology used by the public consortium, the quality of the draft sequence, and the biological insights revealed by the initial analyses.

Lash AE, Tolstoshev CM, Wagner L, et al: SAGEmap: a public gene expression resource. Genome Res 2000; 10:1051–1060.

Leung YF, Cavalieri D: Fundamentals of cDNA microarray data analysis. Trends Genet 2003; 19:649–659.

Li C, Wong WH: Model-based analysis of oligonucleotide arrays: expression index computation and outlier detection. Proc Natl Acad Sci USA 2001; 98:31–36.

Lockhart DJ, Dong H, Byrne MC, et al: Expression monitoring by hybridization to high-density oligonucleotide arrays. Nat Biotechnol 1996; 14:1675–1680.

Madden SL, Wang CJ, Landes G: Serial analysis of gene expression: from gene discovery to target identification. Drug Discov Today 2000; 5:415–425.

Mathe C, Sagot MF, Schiex T, et al: Current methods of gene prediction, their strengths and weaknesses. Nucleic Acids Res 2002; 30:4103–4117.

Miklos GL, Maleszka R: Microarray reality checks in the context of a complex disease. Nat Biotechnol 2004; 22:615–621.

Ntzani EE, Ioannidis JP: Predictive ability of DNA microarrays for cancer outcomes and correlates: an empirical assessment. Lancet 2003; 362:1439–1444.

Oh P, Li Y, Yu J, et al: Subtractive proteomic mapping of the endothelial surface in lung and solid tumours for tissue-specific therapy. Nature 2004; 429:629–635.

Olson MV: The maps. Clone by clone by clone. Nature 2001; 409:816–818.

Ornstein DK, Rayford W, Fusaro VA, et al: Serum proteomic profiling can discriminate prostate cancer from benign prostates in men with total

prostate specific antigen levels between 2.5 and 15.0 ng/ml. J Urol 2004a; 172:1302–1305.

Ornstein DK, Rayford W, Fusaro VA, et al: Serum proteomic profiling can discriminate prostate cancer from benign prostates in men with total prostate specific antigen levels between 2.5 and 15.0 ng/ml. J Urol 2004b; 172:1302–1305.

Paik S, Shak S, Tang G, et al: A multigene assay to predict recurrence of tamoxifen-treated, node-negative breast cancer. N Engl J Med 2004; 351:2817–2826.

Paweletz CP, Charboneau L, Bichsel VE, et al: Reverse phase protein microarrays which capture disease progression show activation of pro-survival pathways at the cancer invasion front. Oncogene 2001; 20:1981–1989.

Pennisi E: And the gene number is…? Science 2000; 288:1146–1147

Perou CM, Sorlie T, Eisen MB, et al: Molecular portraits of human breast tumours. Nature 2000; 406:747–752.

Petricoin EF, Ardekani AM, Hitt BA, et al: Use of proteomic patterns in serum to identify ovarian cancer. Lancet 2002; 359:572–577.

Describes how a mass spectrometry based platform is used to analyze proteins present in serum samples of patients with and without ovarian cancer to develop a model capable of accurately distinguishing between the two disease states.

Phimister B: Going global. Nat Genet Suppl 1999; 21:1.

Pittman J, Huang E, Dressman H, et al: Integrated modeling of clinical and gene expression information for personalized prediction of disease outcomes. Proc Natl Acad Sci USA 2004; 101:8431–8436.

Pomeroy SL, Tamayo P, Gaasenbeek M, et al: Prediction of central nervous system embryonal tumour outcome based on gene expression. Nature 2002; 415:436–442.

Porter D, Lahti-Domenici J, Keshaviah A, et al: Molecular markers in ductal carcinoma in situ of the breast. Mol Cancer Res 2003a; 1:362–375.

Porter D, Weremowicz S, Chin K, et al: A neural survival factor is a candidate oncogene in breast cancer. Proc Natl Acad Sci USA 2003b; 100:10931–10936.

Porter DA, Krop IE, Nasser S, et al: A SAGE (serial analysis of gene expression) view of breast tumor progression. Cancer Res 2001; 61:5697–5702.

Quackenbush J: Computational analysis of microarray data. Nat Rev Genet 2001; 2:418–427.

Ramaswamy S, Ross KN, Lander ES, et al: A molecular signature of metastasis in primary solid tumors. Nat Genet 2003; 33:49–54.

Ransohoff DF: Rules of evidence for cancer molecular-marker discovery and validation. Nat Rev Cancer 2004; 4:309–314.

Reich M, Ohm K, Angelo M, et al: GeneCluster 2.0: an advanced toolset for bioarray analysis. Bioinformatics 2004; 20:1797–1798.

Rosenwald A, Wright G, Chan WC, et al: The use of molecular profiling to predict survival after chemotherapy for diffuse large-B-cell lymphoma. N Engl J Med 2002; 346:1937–1947.

Russo G, Zegar C, Giordano A: Advantages and limitations of microarray technology in human cancer. Oncogene 2003; 22:6497–6507.

Sawiris GP, Sherman-Baust CA, Becker KG, et al: Development of a highly specialized cDNA array for the study and diagnosis of epithelial ovarian cancer. Cancer Res 2002; 62:2923–2928.

Schena M, Shalon D, Davis RW, et al: Quantitative monitoring of gene expression patterns with a complementary DNA microarray. Science 1995; 270:467–470.

Selaru FM, Zou T, Xu Y, et al: Global gene expression profiling in Barrett's esophagus and esophageal cancer: a comparative analysis using cDNA microarrays. Oncogene 2002; 21:475–478.

Shipp MA, Ross KN, Tamayo P, et al: Diffuse large B-cell lymphoma outcome prediction by gene-expression profiling and supervised machine learning. Nat Med 2002; 8:68–74.

Simon R, Lam AP: BRB ArrayTools, 2004.

Simon R, Radmacher MD, Dobbin K, et al: Pitfalls in the use of DNA microarray data for diagnostic and prognostic classification. J Natl Cancer Inst 2003; 95:14–18.

Sotiriou C, Neo SY, McShane LM, et al: Breast cancer classification and prognosis based on gene expression profiles from a population-based study. Proc Natl Acad Sci USA 2003; 100:10393–10398.

Spira A, Beane J, Schembri F, et al: Noninvasive method for obtaining RNA from buccal mucosa epithelial cells for gene expression profiling. Biotechniques 2004; 36:484–487.

Stankiewicz P, Lupski JR: Genome architecture, rearrangements and genomic disorders. Trends Genet 2002; 18:74–82.

Syvanen AC: Accessing genetic variation: genotyping single nucleotide polymorphisms. Nat Rev Genet 2001; 2:930–942.

Tian E, Zhan F, Walker R, et al: The role of the Wnt-signaling antagonist DKK1 in the development of osteolytic lesions in multiple myeloma. N Engl J Med 2003a; 349:2483–2494.

Tian E, Zhan F, Walker R, et al: The role of the Wnt-signaling antagonist DKK1 in the development of osteolytic lesions in multiple myeloma. N Engl J Med 2003b; 349:2483–2494.

Tibshirani R, Hastie T, Narasimhan B, et al: Diagnosis of multiple cancer types by shrunken centroids of gene expression. Proc Natl Acad Sci USA 2002; 99:6567–6572.

Tumor Analysis Best Practices Working Group: Expression profiling – best practices for data generation and interpretation in clinical trials. Nat Rev Genet 2004; 5:229–237.

Tusher VG, Tibshirani R, Chu G: Significance analysis of microarrays applied to the ionizing radiation response. Proc Natl Acad Sci USA 2001; 98:5116–5121.

Valk PJ, Verhaak RG, Beijen MA, et al: Prognostically useful gene-expression profiles in acute myeloid leukemia. N Engl J Med 2004; 350:1617–1628.

Van de Vijver MJ, He YD, van't Veer LJ, et al: A gene-expression signature as a predictor of survival in breast cancer. N Engl J Med 2002; 347:1999–2009.

Van't Veer LJ, Dai H, van de Vijver MJ, et al: Gene expression profiling predicts clinical outcome of breast cancer. Nature 2002; 415:530–536.

Velculescu VE, Zhang L, Vogelstein B, et al: Serial analysis of gene expression. Science 1995; 270:484–487.

Venter JC, Adams MD, Myers EW, et al: The sequence of the human genome. Science 2001; 291:1304–1351. The paper and other information can be accessed on line at http://www.sciencemag.org/content/vol291/issue5507/.

Xu Y, Selaru FM, Yin J, et al: Artificial neural networks and gene filtering distinguish between global gene expression profiles of Barrett's esophagus and esophageal cancer. Cancer Res 2002; 62:3493–3497.

Yamamoto M, Wakatsuki T, Hada A, Ryo A: Use of serial analysis of gene expression (SAGE) technology. J Immunol Methods 2001; 250:45–66

Ye QH, Qin LX, Forgues M, et al: Predicting hepatitis B virus-positive metastatic hepatocellular carcinomas using gene expression profiling and supervised machine learning. Nat Med 2003; 9:416–423.

APPENDIX 1

Physiologic Solutions, Buffers, Acid–Base Indicators, Standard Reference Materials, and Temperature Conversions

Physiologic Solutions

A physiologic solution is one that contains various salts in concentrations that closely approximate the composition of fluids in the human body. The simplest of these is physiologic saline, which has the same osmotic pressure as the blood. There are more elaborate solutions – for example, to maintain tissues in a metabolically active state for longer periods of time. Table A1–1 gives formulas of some solutions that are isotonic with respect to blood.

Buffers*

Buffers have the ability to resist changes in pH. Buffers usually consist of a weak acid and its salt or a weak base and its salt. The Henderson–Hasselbalch equation:

$$pH = pK + \log [salt]/[acid] \qquad (1)$$

is useful in calculating the acid (or base) to salt ratio required to establish a desired pH from a buffer system.

Example 1.

If the pH of a 0.1 M acetate buffer is known to be 4.90, calculate the concentration of acetic acid and sodium acetate in the buffer (pK for acetic acid = 4.76).

Substituting values of pH and pK in equation 1:

log[acetate]/[acetic acid] = 4.90 − 4.76 = 0.14
[acetate]/[acetic acid] = 1.38
[acetate] = 1.38[acetic acid]

Because the total buffer/L concentrations is 0.1 M,

$$[acetate] + [acetic acid] = 0.1 \ M \qquad (2)$$

Substituting the value of acetate in Equation 2:

1.38[acetic acid] + [acetic acid] = 0.1 M

Hence
[acetic acid] = 0.042 M
[acetic acid] = 2.52 g/L
[acetate] = 0.058 M
= 4.76 g/L

Example 2.

If 648 mL of 0.025 molar diethylbarbituric acid and 10 mL of 0.5 molar sodium diethylbarbiturate are mixed and diluted to 1 L, calculate the pH

of the solution (pK for diethylbarbituric acid = 7.98 and molar concentration = moles/liter).

The following relationship exists between molarity and volume of a solution:

$$M1V1 = M2V2 \qquad (3)$$

where:
M1 = molarity of the initial solution
V1 = volume of the initial solution
M2 = molarity of the final solution
V2 = volume of the final solution.

Use Equation 3 to calculate changes in salt and acid concentrations after dilution to 1 L:

[Sodium diethylbarbiturate] = 0.025 × 0.648
= 0.0162 mol/L
[Diethylbarbituric acid] = 0.5 × 0.01
= 0.005 mol/L

Calculate pH of the solution using Equation 1:

pH = 7.98 − log(0.0162/0.005)
= 7.98 − log 3.24
= 7.98 − 0.51
= 7.47

The maximum buffering capacity is at the pK value of the weak acid or base. For instance, for acetic acid with a pH value of 4.76, more acid is required to change the pH of an acetate buffer from 4.76 to 4.66 than from 4.20 to 4.10. Efficient buffering capacity covers a pH range of about 1 unit on either side of the pK value of the weak acid or base. For acetic acid, this would be from about pH 3.8–5.8.

Sorensen's Phosphate Buffers

These buffer solutions are generally useful, because the range of the mixtures is from pH 5–8.

Prepare 0.1 molar solutions of monobasic potassium phosphate (13.6 g/L) and dibasic sodium phosphate (14.2 g/L). Mix solutions in the ratio indicated in Table A1–2 to obtain the buffer of desired pH.

Table A1–1 Physiologic Solutions

	Saline	Locke's solution	Ringer's solution	Tyrode's solution
Sodium chloride	0.85 g	0.9 g	0.7 g	0.8 g
Calcium chloride		0.024 g	0.0026 g	0.02 g
Potassium chloride		0.042 g	0.035 g	0.02 g
Sodium bicarbonate		0.01–0.03 g		0.1 g
D-Glucose		0.01–0.25 g		0.1 g
Magnesium chloride				0.01 g
Monosodium phosphate				0.005 g
Distilled water	100 mL	100 mL	100 mL	100 mL

For a comprehensive discussion, including preparation of buffer solutions of a definite ionic strength, consult Bates RG: Determination of pH – Theory and Practice, 2nd ed. New York, John Wiley & Sons, 1973.

Table A1–2 Sorensen's Table of Buffer Mixtures

Na₂HPO₄ solution (mL)	KH₂PO₄ solution (mL)	pH
0.25	9.75	5.288
0.5	9.5	5.589
1.0	9.0	5.906
2.0	8.0	6.239
3.0	7.0	6.468
4.0	6.0	6.643
5.0	5.0	6.813
6.0	4.0	6.979
7.0	3.0	7.168
8.0	2.0	7.381
9.0	1.0	7.731
9.5	0.5	8.043

Table A1–3 Tris(hydroxymethyl)aminomethane Buffer

mL 0.1 N HCl added	Resulting pH at 23°C	Resulting pH at 37°C
5.0	9.10	8.95
7.5	8.92	8.78
10.0	8.74	8.60
12.5	8.62	8.48
15.0	8.50	8.37
17.5	8.40	8.27
20.0	8.32	8.18
22.5	8.23	8.10
25.0	8.14	8.00
27.5	8.05	7.90
30.0	7.96	7.82
32.5	7.87	7.73
35.0	7.77	7.63
37.5	7.66	7.52
40.0	7.54	7.40
42.5	7.36	7.22
45.0	7.20	7.05

Table A1–4 Acid–Base Indicators

Indicator	pH range	Quantity of indicator per 10 mL	Color Acid	Color Alkaline
Thymol blue (A)*†	1.2–2.8	1–2 drops 0.1% soln. in aq.	Red	Yellow
Methyl orange (B)	3.1–4.4	1 drop 0.1% soln. in aq.	Red	Orange
Bromphenol blue (A)†	3.0–4.6	1 drop 0.1% soln. in aq.	Yellow	Blue-violet
Bromcresol green (A)†	4.0–5.6	1 drop 0.1% soln. in aq.	Yellow	Blue
Methyl red (A)†	4.4–6.2	1 drop 0.1% soln. in aq.	Red	Yellow
Bromcresol purple (A)†	5.2–6.8	1 drop 0.1% soln. in aq.	Yellow	Purple
Bromthymol blue (A)†	6.2–7.6	1 drop 0.1% soln. in aq.	Yellow	Blue
Phenol red (A)†	6.4–8.0	1 drop 0.1% soln. in aq.	Yellow	Red
Neutral red (B)	6.8–8.0	1 drop 0.1% soln. in 70% alc.	Red	Yellow
Thymol blue (A)†‡	8.0–9.6	1–5 drops 0.1% soln. in aq.	Yellow	Blue
Phenolphthalein (A)	8.0–10.0	1–5 drops 0.1% soln. in 70% alc.	Colorless	Red
Thymolphthalein (A)	9.4–10.6	1 drop 0.1% soln. in 90% alc.	Colorless	Blue

The letters A or B after the name of the indicator signify, respectively, that the compound is an indicator *acid* or *base*.

* For the acid range.

† Sodium salt.

‡ For the alkaline range.

Tris(hydroxymethyl)aminomethane Buffer*

Tris(hydroxymethyl)aminomethane buffer can be used for a pH range between 7.0–9.0, but its best buffer capacity is between 7.5–8.5. It is practically ineffective below pH 7.0 and above pH 9.0. One advantage of the buffer is its excellent stability. The buffer can be prepared by weighing the desired amount of tris(hydroxymethyl)aminomethane,

* If buffers of a higher molarity are desired, the 0.1 N HCl may have to be replaced by 1.0 N HCl.

Table A1–5 Commonly Used Acids and Alkalies*

Solution	Mol. weight	Spec. gravity†	g/L†	Molarity†	Normality†	Approx. number of mL required to make 1000 mL of 1N solution
Conc. HCl	36.46	1.19	440	12	12	83
Conc. H_2SO_4	98.08	1.84	1730	18	36	28
Conc. HNO_3	63.02	1.42	990	16	16	64
Conc. lactic acid	90.08	1.21	1030	11	11	87
Glacial acetic acid	60.08	1.06	1060	17.5	17.5	57
Conc. NH_4OH	35.05	0.90	250	15	15	67

* Commercially available.

† Figures may vary slightly according to the lot or manufacturer.

Table A1–6 Standard Reference Materials (SRM) for Clinical Measurements

SRM #	SRM type	Stoichiometric purity mass fraction in %	Certified use	Unit size (in g)
40h	Sodium oxalate	99.972	Reductometric standard	60
83d	Arsenic trioxide	99.9926	Reductometric standard	60
84k	Potassium hydrogen phthalate	99.9911	Acidimetric standard	60
136e	Potassium dichromate	99.984	Oximetric standard	60
350a	Benzoic acid	99.9958	Acidimetric standard	30
723c	Tris(hydroxymethyl) aminomethane	99.901	Acidimetric standard	50
911b	Cholesterol	99.8	Identity and purity	2.0
912a	Urea	99.9	Identity and purity	25
913	Uric acid	99.7	Identity and purity	10
914a	Creatinine	99.7	Identity and purity	10
915a	Calcium carbonate	99.9	Identity and purity	20
916a	Bilirubin	98.3	Identity and purity	0.1
917a	D-Glucose (dextrose)	99.7	Identity and purity	25
918a	Potassium chloride	99.9817	Identity and purity	30
919a	Sodium chloride	99.89	Identity and purity	30
930e	Glass filters, transmittance		Wavelength range (440–635 nm)	3 filters
931f	Liquid filters, absorbance		Wavelength range (302–678 nm)	Ampules
934	Clinical laboratory thermometers (0, 25, 30, 37)		Temperature	One each
937	Iron metal	99.90		50
955b	Lead in blood			Set of 4 ampules

Table A1–7 Temperature Conversions

Centigrade	Fahrenheit	Centigrade	Fahrenheit
110°	230°	38°	100.4°
100	212	37.5	99.5
95	203	37	98.6
90	194	36.5	97.7
85	185	36	96.8
80	176	35.5	95.9
75	167	35	95
70	158	34	93.2
65	149	33	91.4
60	140	32	89.6
55	131	31	87.8
50	122	30	86
45	113	25	77
44	111.2	20	68
43	109.4	15	59
42	107.6	10	50
41	105.8	+5	41
40.5	104.9	0	32
40	104	−5	23
39.5	103.1	−10	14
39	102.2	−15	+5
38.5	101.3	−20	−4

$$1°F = −17.2°C$$
$$1°C = 33.8°F$$

To convert Fahrenheit into centigrade, subtract 32 and multiply by 0.555.

To convert centigrade to Fahrenheit, multiply by 1.8 and add 32.

dissolving it in water, and adjusting the pH to the desired value with HCl. For example, if 100 mL of 0.05 M buffer is desired, place 0.6057 g of tris(hydroxymethyl)aminomethane into a 100-mL volumetric flask. This is dissolved in approximately 50 mL of distilled water. Add 0.1 N HCl, as indicated in Table A1–3, and fill up to the mark with distilled water. The table shows the pH values obtained when 0.6057 g of tris(hydroxymethyl)aminomethane dissolved in water is mixed with the indicated amounts of 0.1 N HCl and diluted to 100 mL.

Acid–Base Indicators*

An acid–base indicator is a weak acid or a weak base, the undissociated form of which has a color and constitution other than the iogenic form. Color change takes place over a certain narrow range of hydrogen ion concentrations. This range is called the color change interval and is expressed in terms of pH (the negative logarithm of the hydrogen ion concentration). A great number of substances show indicator properties, although relatively few of them are practically applied for neutralization reactions and pH determinations. Some commonly used acid–base indicators are shown in Table A1–4. In general, weak acids should be titrated in the presence of indicators that change in slightly alkaline solutions. Weak bases should be titrated in the presence of indicators that change in slightly acid solutions. Some commonly used acids and alkalis are listed in Table A1–5.

The availability of precision pH meters allows titration to a selected end point (pH) and may replace use of indicators for several applications.

Dean JA (ed): Handbook of Chemistry, 13th ed. New York, McGraw-Hill, 1985.

Fasman GD (ed): Handbook of Biochemistry and Molecular Biology, 3rd ed. Cleveland, CRC Press, 1976.

Meinke WW: Standard Reference Materials for Clinical Measurements. Anal Chem 1971; 43:28A.

The Merck Index: An Encyclopedia of Chemicals and Drugs. 12th ed. Whitehouse Station, NJ, Merck and Co., 1996.

* Based on Dean JA (ed): Handbook of Chemistry, revised 13th ed. New York, McGraw-Hill, 1985.

APPENDIX 2

Desirable Weights, Body Surface Area, and Body Mass Index (BMI)

Table A2–1 Comparison of the Weight-For-Height Tables from Actuarial Data: Non-Age-Corrected Metropolitan Life Insurance Company and Age-Specific Gerontology Research Center Recommendations

Height (ft and in)		Metropolitan 1983 weights* (25–59 years)		Gerontology Research Center* (age-specific weight range for men and women)				
		Men	Women	20–29 years	30–39 years	40–49 years	50–59 years	60–79 years
4	10		100–131	84–111	92–119	99–127	107–135	115–142
4	11		101–134	87–115	95–123	103–131	111–139	119–147
5	0		103–137	90–119	98–127	106–135	114–143	123–152
5	1	123–145	105–140	93–123	101–131	110–140	118–148	127–157
5	2	125–148	108–144	96–127	105–136	113–144	122–153	131–163
5	3	127–151	111–148	99–131	108–140	117–149	126–158	135–168
5	4	129–155	114–152	102–135	112–145	121–154	130–163	140–173
5	5	131–159	117–156	106–140	115–149	125–159	134–168	144–179
5	6	133–163	120–160	109–144	119–154	129–164	138–174	148–184
5	7	135–167	123–164	112–148	122–159	133–169	143–179	153–190
5	8	137–171	126–167	116–153	126–163	137–174	147–184	158–196
5	9	139–175	129–170	119–157	130–168	141–179	151–190	162–201
5	10	141–179	132–173	122–162	134–173	145–184	156–195	167–207
5	11	144–183	135–176	126–167	137–178	149–190	160–201	172–213
6	0	147–187		129–171	141–183	153–195	165–207	177–219
6	1	150–192		133–176	145–188	157–200	169–213	182–225
6	2	153–197		137–181	149–194	162–206	174–219	187–232
6	3	157–202		141–186	153–199	166–212	179–225	192–238
6	4			144–191	157–205	171–218	184–231	197–244

* Values in this table are for height without shoes and weight without clothes. The Metropolitan Life Insurance Company (1983 Metropolitan Height and Weight Tables. Stat Bull Metropol Life Ins Co, 1983; 64[Jan–Jun]:2) presented a table for nude heights and weights (Table 4) as well as a table for heights and weights clothed (Table 1).

From Andres R: Mortality and obesity: The rationale for age-specific height–weight tables. *In* Hazzard WR, Bierman EL, Blass JP, Ettinger WH Jr, Halter JB (eds): Principles of Geriatric Medicine and Gerontology, 3rd ed. New York, McGraw-Hill, 1994, p 847, with permission.

Table A2–2 Body Mass Index (BMI) Table

To use this table, find the appropriate height in the left hand column. Move across to a given weight.
The number at the top of the column is the BMI at the height and weight. Pounds have been rounded off.

BMI	19	20	21	22	23	24	25	26	27	28	29	30	31	32	33	34	35
							Body weight (lb)										
Height (in) 58	91	96	100	105	110	115	119	124	129	134	138	143	148	153	158	162	167
59	94	99	104	109	114	119	124	128	133	138	143	148	153	158	163	168	173
60	97	102	107	112	118	123	128	133	138	143	148	153	158	163	168	174	179
61	100	106	111	116	122	127	132	137	143	148	153	158	164	169	174	180	185
62	104	109	115	120	126	131	136	142	147	153	158	164	169	175	180	186	191
63	107	113	118	124	130	135	141	146	152	158	163	169	175	180	186	191	197
64	110	116	122	128	134	140	145	151	157	163	169	174	180	186	192	197	204
65	114	120	126	132	138	144	150	156	162	168	174	180	186	192	198	204	210
66	118	124	130	136	142	148	155	161	167	173	179	186	192	198	204	210	216
67	121	127	134	140	146	153	159	166	172	178	185	191	198	204	211	217	223
68	125	131	138	144	151	158	164	171	177	184	190	197	203	210	216	223	230
69	128	135	142	149	155	162	169	176	182	189	196	203	209	216	223	230	236
70	132	139	146	153	160	167	174	181	188	195	202	209	216	222	229	236	243
71	136	143	150	157	165	172	179	186	193	200	208	215	222	229	236	243	250
72	140	147	154	162	169	177	184	191	199	206	213	221	228	235	242	250	258
73	144	151	159	166	174	182	189	197	204	212	219	227	235	242	250	257	265
74	148	155	163	171	179	186	194	202	210	218	225	233	241	249	256	264	272
75	152	160	168	176	184	192	200	208	216	224	232	240	248	256	264	272	279
76	156	164	172	180	189	197	205	213	221	230	238	246	254	263	271	279	287

BMI	36	37	38	39	40	41	42	43	44	45	46	47	48	49	50	51	52
							Body weight (lb)										
Height (in) 58	172	177	181	186	191	196	201	205	210	215	220	224	229	234	239	244	248
59	178	183	188	193	198	203	208	212	217	222	227	232	237	242	247	252	257
60	184	189	194	199	204	209	215	220	225	230	235	240	245	250	255	261	266
61	190	195	201	206	211	217	222	227	232	238	243	248	254	259	264	269	275
62	196	202	207	213	218	224	229	235	240	246	251	256	262	267	273	278	284
63	203	208	214	220	225	231	237	242	248	254	259	265	270	278	282	287	293
64	209	215	221	227	232	238	244	250	256	262	267	273	279	285	291	296	302
65	216	222	228	234	240	246	252	258	264	270	276	282	288	294	300	306	312
66	223	229	235	241	247	253	260	266	272	278	284	291	297	303	309	315	322
67	230	236	242	249	255	261	268	274	280	287	293	299	306	312	319	325	331
68	236	243	249	256	262	269	276	282	289	295	302	308	315	322	328	335	341
69	243	250	257	263	270	277	284	291	297	304	311	318	324	331	338	345	351
70	250	257	264	271	278	285	292	299	306	313	320	327	334	341	348	355	362
71	257	265	272	279	286	293	301	308	315	322	329	338	343	351	358	365	372
72	265	272	279	287	294	302	309	316	324	331	338	346	353	361	368	375	383
73	272	280	288	295	302	310	318	325	333	340	348	355	363	371	378	386	393
74	280	287	295	303	311	319	326	334	342	350	358	365	373	381	389	396	404
75	287	295	303	311	319	327	335	343	351	359	367	375	383	391	399	407	415
76	295	304	312	320	328	336	344	353	361	369	377	385	394	402	410	418	426

Source; http://www.nhlbi.nih.gov/guidelines/obesity/bmi_tbl.htm

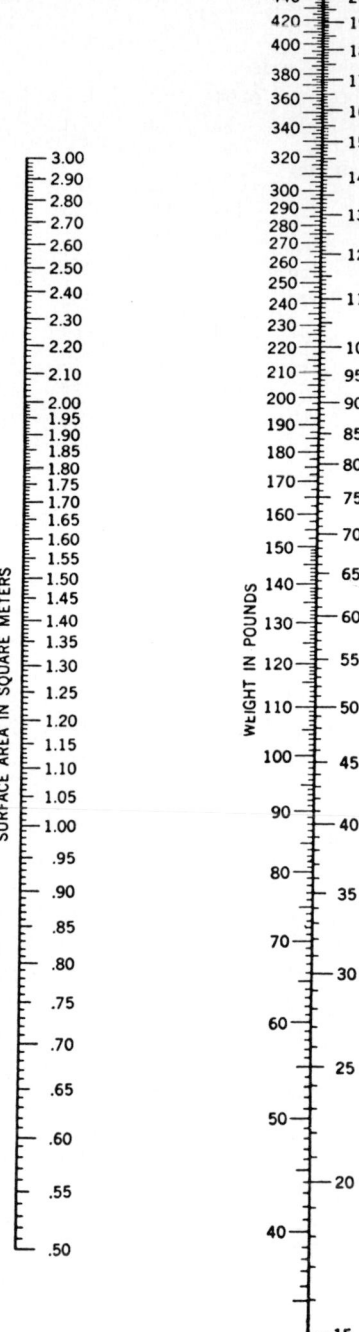

Figure A2–1 Nomogram for the determination of body surface area of children and adults. (From Boothby WM, Sandiford RB: Boston Med Surg J 1921; 185:337, with permission.)

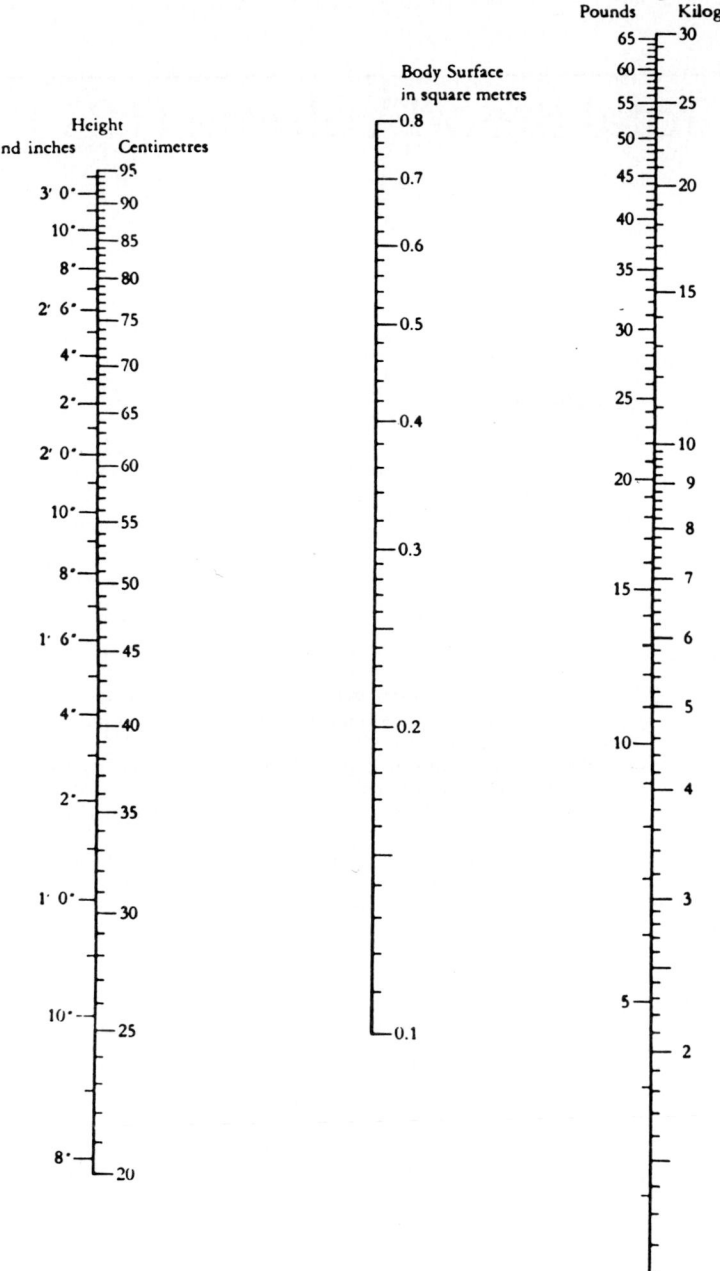

Figure A2-2 Nomogram for the determination of body surface area of children. (From DuBois EF: Basal Metabolism in Health and Disease. Philadelphia, Lea & Febiger, 1936.)

APPENDIX 3

Approximations of Total Blood Volume (TBV)

When estimating a patient's total blood volume (TBV), a commonly used approximation is 70 mL of TBV per kilogram body weight. While useful in many patients, in others, particularly children and overweight or thin adults, this figure offers only a poor approximation of actual TBV. In these patients, other methods of estimation of TBV are more appropriate.

Adults

The COBE Spectra uses the Nadler and Allen formula to calculate approximate TBV for patients (COBE Spectra Apheresis System Operator's Manual, 1997). This formula uses patient height, weight, and sex to calculate TBV. Specifically, the formula is:

Males: $TBV(mL) = 604 + [367 \times height^3 (m)] + [32.2 \times weight (kg)]$

Females: $TBV(mL) = 183 + [356 \times height^3 (m)] + [33.1 \times weight (kg)]$

TBV can also be approximated using the patient's calculated body surface area (Shoemaker, 1989):

Males: $TBV = 2740 \ mL/m^2$

Females: $TBV = 2370 \ mL/m^2$

Another relatively simple approximation uses Gilcher's so-called 'rule of fives,' reproduced below, as an estimate of blood volume which is more tailored to the individual patient than the 70 mL/kg rule (Gilcher, 1996).

	Fat	Thin	Normal	Muscular
Males	60	65	70	75
Females	55	60	65	70

Children

The Nadler and Allen calculation can be particularly inaccurate in children, especially prepubertal boys, in whom it has been recommended that the female gender be entered to improve the estimation (Kim, 2000). The following values for TBV per kilogram body weight can be used (Oski, 1993):

Premature infants	89–105mL/kg
Term newborns	82–86mL/kg
Infants and preschoolers	73–82mL/kg

COBE® Spectra™ Apheresis System Operator's Manual: Lakewood, CO, Gambro® BCT™, 1997, p 1.

Gilcher RO: Apheresis: Principles and practices. *In* Rossi EC, Simon TL, Moss GS, Gould SA (eds): Principles of Transfusion Medicine, 2nd ed. Baltimore, Williams & Wilkins, 1996, p 542.

Kim HC: Therapeutic pediatric apheresis. J Clin Apheresis 2000; 15:129–157.

Oski FA: The erythrocyte and its disorders. *In* Nathan DG, Oski FA (eds): Hematology of Infancy and Childhood, 4th ed. Philadelphia, WB Saunders Company, 1993, p 28.

Shoemaker WC: Fluids and electrolytes in the acutely ill adult. *In* Shoemaker WC, Ayres S, Grenvik A, et al. (eds): Textbook of Critical Care, 2nd ed. Philadelphia, WB Saunders Company, 1989, p 1130.

APPENDIX 4

Periodic Table of the Elements

Table A4–1 Periodic Table of the Elements

KEY TO CHART

Atomic Number → **50** +2 ← Oxidation State
Symbol → **Sn** +4
1989 Atomic Weight → 118.71
18 18 4 ← Electron Configuration

1 Group IA	2 IIA	New notation → Previous IUPAC form → CAS version →										13 IIIB IIIA	14 IVB IVA	15 VB VA	16 VIB VIA	17 VIIB VIIA	18 VIIIA	Shell
1 +1 **H** −1 1.00794 1																	**2** 0 **He** 4.0020602 2	K
3 +1 **Li** 6.941 2-1	**4** +1 **Be** 9.012182 2-2											**5** +3 **B** 10.811 2-3	**6** +2 +4 −4 **C** 12.011 2-4	**7** +1 +2 +3 +4 +5 −1 −2 −3 **N** 14.00674 2-5	**8** −2 **O** 15.9994 2-6	**9** −1 **F** 18.998403 2	**10** 0 **Ne** 20.1797 2-8	K-L
11 +1 **Na** 22.989768 2-8-1	**12** +2 **Mg** 24.3050 2-8-2	3 IIIA IIIB	4 IVA IVB	5 VA VB	6 VIA VIB	7 VIIA VIIB	8	9 VIIIA VIII	10	11 IB	12 IIB	**13** +3 **Al** 26.981539 2-8-3	**14** +2 +4 −4 **Si** 28.0855 2-8-4	**15** +3 +5 −3 **P** 30.97362 2-8-5	**16** +3 +5 −2 **S** 32.066 2-8-6	**17** +1 +5 +7 −1 **Cl** 35.4527 2-8-7	**18** 0 **Ar** 39.948 2-8-8	K-L-M
19 +1 **K** 39.0983 -8-8-1	**20** +2 **Ca** 40.078 -8-8-2	**21** +3 **Sc** 44.955910 -8-9-2	**22** +2 +3 +4 **Ti** 47.88 -8-10-2	**23** +2 +3 +4 +5 **V** 50.9415 -8-11-2	**24** +2 +3 +6 **Cr** 51.9961 -8-13-1	**25** +2 +3 +4 +7 **Mn** 54.93085 -8-13-2	**26** +2 +3 **Fe** 55.847 -8-14-2	**27** +2 +3 **Co** 58.93320 -8-15-2	**28** +2 +3 **Ni** 58.6934 -8-16-2	**29** +1 +2 **Ni** 63.546 -8-18-1	**30** +2 **Zn** 65.39 -8-18-2	**31** +3 **Ga** 69.723 -8-18-3	**32** +2 +4 **Ge** 72.61 -8-18-4	**33** +2 +3 −3 **As** 74.92159 -8-18-5	**34** +4 +6 −2 **Se** 78.96 -8-18-6	**35** +1 +5 −1 **Br** 79.904 -8-18-7	**36** 0 **Kr** 83.80 -8-18-8	-L-M-N
37 +1 **Rb** 85.4678 -18-8-1	**38** +2 **Sr** 87.62 -18-8-2	**39** +3 **Y** 88.90585 -18-9-2	**40** +4 **Zr** 91.224 -18-12-1	**41** +3 +5 **Nb** 92.90638 -18-10-2	**42** +6 **Mo** 95.94 -18-13-1	**43** +4 +6 +7 **Tc** (98) -18-13-2	**44** +3 **Ru** 101.07 -18-15-1	**45** +3 **Rh** 102.90550 -18-16-1	**46** +2 +4 **Pd** 106.42 -18-18-0	**47** +1 **Ag** 107.8682 -18-18-1	**48** +2 **Cd** 112.411 -18-18-2	**49** +3 **In** 114.818 -18-18-3	**50** +2 +4 **Sn** 118.710 -18-18-4	**51** +3 +5 −3 **Sb** 121.757 -18-18-5	**52** +4 +6 −2 **Te** 127.60 -18-18-6	**53** +1 +5 +7 −1 **I** 126.90447 -18-18-7	**54** 0 **Xe** 131.29 -18-18-8	-M-N-O
55 +1 **Cs** 132.90543 -18-8-1	**56** +2 **Ba** 137.327 -18-8-2	**59*** +3 **La** 139.9055 -18-9-2	**72** +4 **Hf** 178.49 -32-10-2	**73** +5 **Ta** 180.9479 -32-11-2	**74** +6 **W** 183.84 -32-12-2	**75** +4 +6 +7 **Re** 186.207 -32-13-2	**76** +3 +4 **Os** 190.23 -32-14-2	**77** +3 +4 **Ir** 192.22 -32-15-2	**78** +2 +4 **Pt** 195.08 -32-16-2	**79** +1 +3 **Au** 196.96654 -32-18-1	**80** +1 +2 **Hg** 200.59 -32-18-2	**81** +1 +3 **Tl** 204.3833 -32-18-3	**82** +2 +4 **Pb** 207.2 -32-18-4	**83** +3 +5 **Bi** 208.98037 -32-18-5	**84** +2 +4 **Po** (209) -32-18-6	**85** **At** (210) -32-18-7	**86** 0 **Rn** (222) -32-18-8	-N-O-P
87 +1 **Fr** (223) -18-8-1	**88** +2 **Ra** 226.025 -18-8-2	**89**** **Ac** +3 227.08 -18-9-2	**104** **Unq** +4 (261) -32-10-2	**105** **Unp** (262) -32-11-2	**106** **Unh** (263) -32-12-2	**107** **Uns** (262) -32-13-2												O P Q

*Lanthanides	**58** +3 +4 **Ce** 140.115 -19-9-2	**59** +3 **Pr** 140.90765 -21-8-2	**60** +3 **Nd** 144.24 -22-8-2	**61** +3 **Pm** (145) -23-8-2	**62** +2 +3 **Sm** 150.36 -24-8-2	**63** +2 +3 **Eu** 151.965 -25-8-2	**64** +3 **Gd** 157.25 -25-9-2	**65** +3 **Tb** 158.92534 -27-8-2	**66** +3 **Dy** 162.50 -28-8-2	**67** +3 **Ho** 164.93032 -29-8-2	**68** +3 **Er** 167.26 -30-8-2	**69** +3 **Tm** 168.93421 -31-8-2	**70** +2 +3 **Yb** 173.04 -32-8-2	**71** +3 **Lu** 174.967 -32-9-2	N O P
**Actinides	**90** +4 **Th** 232.0381 -18-10-2	**91** +4 +5 **Pa** 231.03588 -20-9-2	**92** +3 +4 +5 +6 **U** 238.0289 -21-9-2	**93** +3 +4 +5 +6 **Np** 237.048 -22-9-2	**94** +3 +4 +5 +6 **Pu** (244) -24-8-2	**95** +3 +4 +5 +6 **Am** (243) -25-8-2	**96** +3 **Cm** (247) -25-9-2	**97** +3 +4 **Bk** (247) -27-8-2	**98** +3 **Cf** (251) -28-8-2	**99** +3 **Es** (252) -29-8-2	**100** +3 **Fm** (257) -30-8-2	**101** +2 +3 **Md** (258) -31-8-2	**102** +2 +3 **No** (259) -32-8-2	**103** +3 **Lr** (260) -32-9-2	O P Q

The new IUPAC format numbers the groups from 1 to 18. The previous IUPAC numbering system and the system used by Chemical Abstracts Service (CAS) are also shown.

For radioactive elements that do not occur in nature, the mass number of the most stable isotope is given in parentheses.

From Lide DR, Frederikse HPR: CRC Handbook of Chemistry and Physics, 74th ed. 1993–1994. Boca Raton, FL, CRC Press, 1993.

Leigh GJ (ed): Nomenclature of Inorganic Chemistry, Oxford, Blackwell Scientific Publications, 1990.

Chemical and Engineering News, 1985, 63:27.

APPENDIX 5

SI Units

H. Peter Lehmann PhD, John Bernard Henry MD

The SI consists of seven dimensionally independent base units, which are listed in Table A5–1, along with the symbols to be used to denote these units. Table A5–2 lists a number of derived units of the SI that are used in the clinical laboratory. There are two kinds of derived unit: coherent units, which are derived directly from the base units without the use of conversion factors; and noncoherent units, which are constructed from the base units and contain a numerical factor in order to make the numbers more convenient to use. The prefixes to denote fractions or multiples of base and derived SI units are given in Table A5–3. A complete description of the SI and its application in medicine may be found in the World Health Organization publication *The SI for the Health Professions* (World Health Organization, 1977). A comprehensive list of quantities and their internationally recommended SI units are given in Tietz, 1995.

In making the conversion to recommend SI units (Tables A5–4 to A5–13), the following guidelines were followed:

1. All reference intervals have been converted to SI units except in cases in which the measurements are not quantitative.
2. Chemical names have not been changed; e.g., urea is retained instead of changing to carbamide.
3. Factors are those published by the American National Metric Council (Lundberg, 1986; Beeler, 1987; Young, 1987), based on the Metric Commission of Canada (1981) factors.
4. Factors are calculated to the base unit for volume of 1 L.
5. The order of magnitude of the factors is calculated to make the values in SI units convenient numbers–i.e., with prefixes, a number not greater than 1000 or smaller than 0.001.
6. The number in recommended SI units is equal to the number in conventional units times the factor.
7. For compounds for which relative molecular masses are not definitely known (e.g., proteins), reference intervals are converted to mass amounts per liter.
8. For mixtures of indeterminate composition (e.g., phospholipids), reference intervals are converted to mass amounts per liter or are based on a given standard – e.g., DHEA for 17-ketosteroids.
9. Quantities of a relative nature that are usually expressed as percentages – e.g., fractions of LD isoenzymes–are given as fractions.
10. Enzyme units are given as the International Unit per liter (U/L). Although the coherent SI unit for catalytic activity (including enzymes), the katal, has been defined as the number of moles of substrate converted per second under defined conditions, its adoption is limited.
11. The pH scale is retained for measurement of hydrogen ion concentrations.
12. It is recommended that the unit millimeters of mercury (mmHg) be retained for pressure (P_{CO_2}, P_{O_2}) at the present time.
13. Percentages are expressed as fractions in the SI, where a fraction is a dimensionless quantity given by the number of defined particles constituting a specified component divided by the total number of defined particles in the system.

Table A5–2 SI Derived Units

Quantity	Unit Name	Unit Symbol
Area	square meter*	m^2
Volume	cubic meter*	m^3
	liter†	$L = dm^{3‡}$
Concentration		
Mass	kilogram/liter†	kg/L
Substance	mole/liter†	mol/L
Molality	mole/kilogram	mol/kg
Density	kilogram/liter†	kg/L
Mass fraction	kilogram/kilogram	kg/kg
Mole fraction	mole/mole	mol/mol
Number concentration	number/liter	L^{-1}
Temperature	degree celsius*	$°C = °K - 273.15$
Pressure	pascal*	$Pa = kg/m^2$
Frequency	hertz*	Hz = 1 cycle/s
Clearance	liter/second†	L/s
Electrical potential	volt*	$V = kg\ m^2/s^3A$
Energy	joule*	$J = kg\ m^2/s^2$

* Derived coherent unit. † Derived noncoherent unit. ‡ Both 'L' and 'l' are symbols for the liter.

Table A5–3 Prefixes

Prefix	Prefix Symbol	Factor
exa	E	10^{18}
peta	P	10^{15}
tera	T	10^{12}
giga	G	10^9
mega	M	10^6
kilo	k	10^3
hecto	h	10^2
deca	da	10^1
deci	d	10^{-1}
centi	c	10^{-2}
milli	m	10^{-3}
micro	µ	10^{-6}
nano	n	10^{-9}
pico	p	10^{-12}
femto	f	10^{-15}
atto	a	10^{-18}

Table A5–1 SI Base Units

Quantity	Name	Symbol
Length	meter	m
Mass	kilogram	kg
Time	second	s
Electric current	ampere	A
Thermodynamic temperature	kelvin	K
Luminous intensity	candela	cd
Amount of substance	mole	mol

References

Beeler MF: SI units and the AJCP. Am J Clin Pathol 1987; 87:140.

Lundberg GD, Iverson C, Radulescu G: Now read this: the SI units are here. JAMA 1986; 255:2329.

Metric Commission of Canada: The SI Manual in Health Care. Ottawa, Sector 9.10 Health and Welfare, Metric Commission of Canada, 1981.

Tietz NW (ed): Clinical Guide to Laboratory Tests, 3rd ed. Philadelphia, PA, WB Saunders, 1995.

World Health Organization: The SI for the Health Professions. Geneva, WHO, 1977.

Young DS: Implementation of SI units for clinical laboratory data: style specifications and conversion tables. Ann Intern Med 1987, 106:114.

Table A5–4 Whole Blood, Serum, and Plasma Chemistry

Component	System	Typical Reference Intervals		
		Conventional Units	Factor*	Recommended SI Units†
Acetoacetic acid				
qualitative	Serum	Negative	–	Negative
quantitative	Serum	0.2–1.0 mg/dL	97.95	20–100 µmol/L
Acetone				
qualitative	Serum	Negative	–	Negative
quantitative	Serum	0.3–2.0 mg/dL	172.95	20–340 µmol/L
Albumin				
qualitative	Serum	3.2–4.5 g/dL (salt fractionation)	10	32–45 g/L
		3.2–5.6 g/dL (electrophoresis)		32–56 g/L
		3.8–5.0 g/dL (dye binding)		38–50 g/L
Alcohol, ethyl	Serum or whole blood	Negative–but presented as mg/dL	0.2171	Negative–but presented as mmol/L
Aldolase	Serum			
adults		3–8 Sibley-Lehninger U/dL at 37°C	7.4	22–59 mU/L at 37°C
children		Approximately 2× adult levels	–	Approximately 2× adult levels
newborn		Approximately 4× adult levels	–	Approximately 4× adult levels
α-Amino acid nitrogen	Serum	3.6–7.0 mg/dL	0.7139	2.6–5.0 mmol/L
δ-Aminolevulinic acid	Serum	0.01–0.03 mg/dL	76.26	0.8–2.3 µmol/L
Ammonia	Plasma	20–120 µg/dL (diffusion)	0.5872	12–70 µmol/L
		40–80 µg/dL (enzymatic method)		23–47 µmol/L
		12–48 µg/dL (resin method)		7–28 µmol/L
Amylase	Serum	16–120 Somogyi units/dL	1.85	30–220 U/L
Argininosuccinate lyase	Serum	0–4 U/dL	10	0–40 U/L
Arsenic†	Whole blood	<7 µg/dL	0.05055	<0.4 µmol/L
Ascorbic acid (vitamin C)	Plasma	0.6–1.6 mg/dL	56.78	34–91 µmol/L
	Whole blood	0.7–2.0 mg/dL		40–114 µmol/L
Barbiturates	Serum, plasma, or whole blood	Negative	–	Negative
Base excess	Whole blood			
male		−3.3 to +1.2 mEq/L	1	−3.3 to +1.2 mmol/L
female		−2.4 to +2.3 mEq/L		−2.4 to +2.3 mmol/L
Base, total	Serum	145–160 mEq/L	1	145–160 mmol/L
Bicarbonate	Plasma	21–28 mmol/L	1	21–28 mmol/L
Bile acids	Serum	0.3–3.0 mg/dL	10	3.0–30.0 mg/L
Bilirubin				
direct (conjugated)	Serum	<0.3 mg/dL	17.10	<5 µmol/L
indirect (unconjugated)	Serum	0.1–1.0 mg/dL		2–17 µmol/L
total	Serum	0.1–1.2 mg/dL		2–21 µmol/L
newborns total	Serum	1.0–12.0 mg/dL		17–205 µol/L
Blood gases (see Ch. 15)				
pH	Whole blood	7.38–7.44 (arterial)	1	7.38–7.44
		7.36–7.41 (venous)		7.36–7.41
P_{CO_2}	Whole blood	35–40 mm Hg (arterial)	0.1333	4.7–5.3 kPa
		40–45 mm Hg (venous)		5.3–6.0 kPa
P_{O_2}	Whole blood	95–100 mm Hg (arterial)	0.1333	12.7–13.3 kPa
Bromide	Serum	<5 mg/dL	0.125	<0.63 mmol/L
Calcium		4.0–4.8 mg/dL	0.2500	1.00–1.20 mmol/L
ionized	Serum	2.0–2.4 mEq/L	0.5000	
		30–58% of total	0.01	0.30–1.58 of total
total	Serum	9.2–11.0 mg/dL	0.2500	2.30–2.74 mmol/L
		4.6–5.5 mEq/L	0.5000	
Carbon dioxide (CO_2 content)	Whole blood (arterial)	19–24 mmol/L	1	19–24 mmol/L
	Plasma or serum (arterial)	21–28 mmol/L		21–28 mmol/L
Carbon dioxide	Whole blood (venous)	22–26 mmol/L	1	22–26 mmol/L
	Plasma or serum (venous)	24–30 mmol/L		24–30 mmol/L
CO_2 combining power	Plasma or serum (venous)	24–30 mmol/L	1	24–30 mmol/L
CO_2 partial pressure (P_{CO_2})	Whole blood (arterial)	35–40 mm Hg	0.1333	4.7–5.3 kPa
	Whole blood (venous)	40–45 mm Hg		5.3–6.0 kPa

Table A5–4 Whole Blood, Serum, and Plasma Chemistry (cont'd)

Component	System	Conventional Units	Factor*	Recommended SI Units†
			Typical Reference Intervals	
Carbonic acid (H$_2$CO$_3$)	Whole blood (arterial)	1.05–1.45 mmol/L	1	1.05–1.45 mmol/L
	Whole blood (venous)	1.15–1.50 mmol/L		1.15–1.50 mmol/L
	Plasma (venous)	1.02–1.38 mmol/L		1.02–1.38 mmol/L
Carboxyhemoglobin (carbon monoxide hemoglobin)	Whole blood suburban nonsmokers	<1.5% saturation of hemoglobin	0.01	Fraction hemoglobin saturated: <0.015
	smokers	1.5–5.0% saturation		0.015–0.050
	heavy smokers	5.0–9.0% saturation		0.050–0.090
Carotene, beta	Serum	40–200 µg/dL	0.01863	0.7–3.7 µmol/L
Ceruloplasmin	Serum	23–50 mg/dL	10	230–500 mg/L
Chloride	Serum	95–103 mEq/L	1	95–103 mmol/L
Cholesterol				
total (see Ch. 17)	Serum	150–250 mg/dL (varies with diet, sex, and age)	0.02586	3.88–6.47 mmol/L
esters	Serum	65–75% of total cholesterol	0.01	Fraction of total cholesterol: 0.65–0.75
Cholinesterase (pseudocholinesterase)	Erythrocytes	0.65–1.3 pH units	1	0.65–1.3 units§
	Plasma	0.5–1.3 pH units	1	0.5–1.3 units
		8–18 U/L at 37°C		
Citrate	Serum or plasma	1.7–3.0 mg/dL	52.05	88–156 µmol/L
Copper	Serum, plasma			
	male	70–140 µg/dL	0.1574	11–22 µmol/L
	female	80–155 µg/dL		13–24 µmol/L
Cortisol	Plasma			
	8 am–10 am	5–23 µg/dL	27.59	138–635 nmol/L
	4 pm–6 pm	3–13 µg/dL	83–359 nmol/L	
Creatine	Serum or plasma			
	male	0.1–0.4 mg/dL	76.25	8–31 µmol/L
	female	0.2–0.7 mg/dL		15–53 µmol/L
Creatine kinase (CK)	Serum			
	male	55–170 U/L at 37°C	1	55–170 U/L at 37°C
	female	30–135 U/L at 37°C	1	30–135 U/L at 37°C
Creatinine (see Ch. 15)	Serum or plasma	0.6–1.2 mg/dL (adult)	88.40	53–106 µmol/L
		0.3–0.6 mg/dL (children <2 y)		27–53 µmol/L
Creatinine clearance (endogenous) (see Ch. 14)	Serum or plasma and urine			
	male	107–139 mL/min	0.01667	1.78–2.32 mL/s
	female	87–107 mL/min		1.45–1.78 mL/s
Cryoglobulins	Serum	Negative	–	Negative
Electrophoresis, protein	Serum			
albumin		52–65% of total protein	0.01	Fraction of total protein: 0.52–0.65
α-1		2.5–5.0% of total protein	0.01	0.025–0.05
α-2		7.0–13.0% of total protein	0.01	0.07–0.13
β		8.0–14.0% of total protein	0.1	0.08–0.14
γ		12.0–22.0% of total protein	0.01	0.12–0.22
	Serum	Concentration		
albumin		3.2–5.6 g/dL	10	32–56 g/L
α-1		0.1–0.4 g/dL		1–4 g/L
α-2		0.4–1.2 g/dL		4–12 g/L
β		0.5–1.1 g/dL		5–11 g/L
γ		0.5–1.6 g/dL		5–16 g/L
Fats, neutral (see Triglycerides)				
Fatty acids				
total (free and esterified)	Serum	9–15 mmol/L	1	9–15 mmol/L
free (nonesterified)	Plasma	300–480 µEq/L	1	300–480 µmol/L
Ferritin	Serum			
male		15–200 ng/mL	1	15–200 µg/L
female		12–150 ng/mL	1	15–150 µg/L
Fibrinogen	Plasma	200–400 mg/dL	0.01	2.00–4.00 g/L
Fluoride	Whole blood	<0.05 mg/dL	0.5263	<0.027 mmol/L
Folate	Serum			11–57 nmol/L
		≥3.5 ng/mL (radioassay)	2.266	>5 nmol/L
	Erythrocytes	166–640 ng/mL (bioassay)		376–1450 nmol/L
		>140 ng/mL (radioassay)		>317 nmol/L
Galactose	Whole blood			
adults		None	–	None
children		<20 mg/dL	0.05551	<1.11 mmol/L
Gamma globulin	Serum	0.5–1.6 g/dL	10	5–16 g/L
Globulins, total	Serum	2.3–3.5 g/dL	10	23–35 g/L

Table A5–4 Whole Blood, Serum, and Plasma Chemistry (*cont'd*)

Component	System	Typical Reference Intervals		
		Conventional Units	Factor*	Recommended SI Units†
Glucose, fasting	Serum or plasma	70–110 mg/dL	0.05551	3.9–6.1 mmol/L
	Whole blood	60–100 mg/dL		3.3–5.6 mmol/L
Glucose tolerance	Serum or plasma			
oral	fasting	70–110 mg/dL	0.05551	3.9–6.1 mmol/L
	30 min	30–60 mg/dL above fasting		1.7–3.3 mmol/L above fasting
	60 min	20–50 mg/dL above fasting		1.1–2.8 mmol/L above fasting
	120 min	5–15 mg/dL above fasting		0.3–0.8 mmol/L above fasting
	180 min	Fasting level or below	–	Fasting level or below
intravenous	Serum or plasma			
	fasting	70–110 mg/dL	0.05551	3.9–6.1 mmol/L
	5 min	Maximum of 250 mg/dL		Maximum of 13.9 mmol/L
	60 min	Significant decrease	–	Significant decrease
	120 min	Below 120 mg/dL	0.05551	Below 6.7 mmol/L
	180 min	Fasting level	–	Fasting level
Glucose-6-phosphate dehydrogenase (G6PD)	Erythrocytes	250–5000 units/10^6 cells	1	250–5000 μunits/cell
		1200–2000 mU/mL packed erythrocytes	1	1200–2000 U/L packed erythrocytes
γ-Glutamyltransferase	Serum	5–40 U/L	1	5–40 U/L at 37°C
Glutathione	Whole blood	24–37 mg/dL	0.03254	0.78–1.20 mmol/L
Growth hormone	Serum	<10 ng/mL	1	<10 μg/L
Guanase	Serum	<3 nmol/mL/min	1	<3 U/L at 37°C
Haptoglobin	Serum	60–270 mg/dL	0.01	0.6–2.7 g/L
Hemoglobin	Serum or plasma			
qualitative		Negative	–	Negative
quantitative		0.5–5.0 mg/dL	10	5–50 mg/L
	Whole blood			
female		12.0–16.0 g/dL	10	120–160 g/L
male		13.5–18.0 g/dL		135–180 g/L
α-Hydroxybutyrate dehydrogenase	Serum	140–350 U/mL	1	140–350 kU/L
17-Hydroxycorticosteroids	Plasma			
male		7–19 μg/dL	25.59§	193–524 mmol/L
female		9–21 μg/dL		248–579 mmol/L
after 24 USP units of ACTH intramuscularly		35–55 μg/dL		966–1517 nmol/L
Immunoglobulins:	Serum			
IgG		800–1801 mg/dL	0.01	8.0–18.0 g/L
IgA		113–563 mg/dL		1.1–5.6 g/L
IgM		54–222 mg/dL		0.5–2.2 g/L
IgD		0.5–3.0 mg/dL	10	5.0–30.0 mg/L
IgE		0.01–0.04 mg/dL		0.1–0.4 mg/L
Insulin	Plasma bioassay	11–240 μU/mL	7.175‡	79–1722 pmol/L
	radioimmunoassay	4–24 μU/mL		29–172 pmol/L
Insulin tolerance	Serum			
(0.1 unit/kg)	Fasting	Glucose of 70–110 mg/dL	0.05551	Glucose of 3.9–6.1 mmol/L
	30 min	Fall to 50% of fasting level	0.01	Fall to 0.5 of fasting level
	90 min	Fasting level	–	Fasting level
Iron, total	Serum	60–150 μg/dL	0.1791	10.7–26.9 μmol/L
Iron-binding capacity	Serum	250–400 μg/dL	0.1791	44.8–71.6 μmol/L
Iron saturation	Serum	20–55%	0.01	Fraction of total iron-binding capacity: 0.20–0.55
Isocitric dehydrogenase	Serum	50–240 U/mL at 25°C (Wolfson–Williams Ashman units)	0.0166	0.83–4.18 U/L at 25°C
Ketone bodies	Serum	Negative	–	Negative
17-Ketosteroids	Plasma	25–125 μg/dL	34.67**	866–4334 nmol/L
Lactic acid (as lactate)	Whole blood			
venous		5–20 mg/dL	0.1110	0.6–2.2 mmol/L
arterial		3–7 mg/dL		0.3–0.8 mmol/L
Lactate dehydrogenase (LD)	Serum	(lactate → pyruvate) 80–120 units at 30°C	0.48	38–62 U/L at 30°C
		(pyruvate → lactate) 185–640 units at 30°C	0.48	90–310 U/L at 30°C
		(lactate → pyruvate) 100–190 U/L at 37°C	1	100–190 U/L at 37°C
Lactate dehydrogenase isoenzymes	Serum			Fraction of total LD
LD_1 (anode)		17–27%	0.01	0.17–0.27
LD_2		27–37%		0.27–0.37
LD_3		18–25%		0.18–0.25
LD_4		3–8%		0.03–0.08
LD_5 (cathode)		0–5%		0.00–0.05

Table A5–4 Whole Blood, Serum, and Plasma Chemistry (cont'd)

Component	System	Typical Reference Intervals		
		Conventional Units	**Factor***	**Recommended SI Units†**
Lactate dehydrogenase (heat stable)	Serum	30–60% of total	0.01	Fraction of total LD: 0.30–0.60
Lactose tolerance	Serum	Serum glucose changes similar to glucose tolerance test	–	Serum glucose changes similar to glucose tolerance test
Lead	Whole blood	<50 μg/dL	0.04826	<2.41 μmol/L
Leucine aminopeptidase (LAP)	Serum			
male		80–200 U/mL (Goldbarg–Rutenberg)	0.24	19.2–48.0 U/L
female		75–185 U/mL (Goldbarg–Rutenberg)		18.0–44.4 U/L
Lipase	Serum	0–1.5 U/mL (Cherry–Crandall)	278	0–417 U/L
		14–280 mU/mL	1	14–280 U/L
Lipids, total	Serum	400–800 mg/dL	0.01	4.00–8.00 g/L
cholesterol (see Ch. 17)		150–250 mg/dL	0.02586	3.88–6.47 mmol/L
triglycerides (see Ch. 17)		10–90 mg/dL	0.01129††	0.11–2.15 mmol/L
phospholipids		150–380 mg/dL	0.01	1.50–3.80 g/L
fatty acids (free)		9.0–15.0 mmol/L	1	9.0–15.0 mmol/L
phospholipid phosphorus		8.0–11.0 mg/dL	0.3229	2.58–3.55 mmol/L
Lithium	Serum	Negative	–	Negative
therapeutic interval		0.5–1.4 mEq/L	1	0.5–1.4 mmol/L
Long-acting thyroid-stimulating hormone (LATS)	Serum	None detected	–	None detected
Luteinizing hormone (LH)	Serum			
male		6–30 mU/mL	1	6–30 U/L
female		Midcycle peak: 3× baseline value	–	Midcycle peak: 3× baseline value
		Premenopausal <30 mU/mL	1	Premenopausal <30 U/L
		Postmenopausal >35 mU/mL		Postmenopausal >35 U/L
Macroglobulins, total	Serum	70–430 mg/dL	0.01	0.7–4.3 g/L
Magnesium	Serum	1.3–2.1 mEq/L	0.5000	0.65–1.05 mmol/L
		1.8–3.0 mg/dL	0.4114	0.74–1.23 mmol/L
Methemoglobin	Whole blood	<0.24 g/dL	10	<2.4 g/L
		<1% of total hemoglobin	0.01	Fraction of total hemoglobin <0.01
Mucoprotein	Serum	80–200 mg/dL	0.01	0.8–2.0 g/L
Muramidase	Serum	4–13 mg/L	1	4–13 mg/L
Myoglobin	Serum	<90 μg/L	1	<90 μg/L
Nonprotein nitrogen (NPN)	Serum or plasma	20–35 mg/dL	0.7139	14.3–25.0 mmol/L
	Whole blood	25–50 mg/dL		17.8–35.7 mmol/L
5'-Nucleotidase	Serum	0–1.6 units at 37°C	1	0–1.6 units at 37°C
Ornithine carbamyl transferase	Serum	8–20 mU/mL at 37°C	1	8–20 U/L at 37°C
Osmolality	Serum	280–295 mOsm/kg	1	280–295 mmol/kg
Oxygen (see Ch. 14)				
pressure (Po₂)	Whole blood (arterial)	95–100 mmHg	0.1333	12.7–13.3 kPa
content	Whole blood (arterial)	15–23 volume	0.01	Volume fraction: 0.15–0.23
saturation	Whole blood (arterial)	94–100%	0.01	Fraction saturated: 0.94–1.00
pH	Whole blood (arterial)	7.38–7.44	1	7.38–7.44
	Whole blood (venous)	7.36–7.41		7.36–7.41
	Serum or plasma (venous)	7.35–7.45		7.35–7.45
Phenylalanine	Serum			
adults		<3.0 mg/dL	60.54	<182 μmol/L
newborns (term)		1.2–3.5 mg/dL		73–212 μmol/L
Phosphatase				
acid phosphatase	Serum	0.13–0.63 U/L at 37°C (p-nitrophenylphosphate)	16.67	2.2–10.5 U/L at 37°C
alkaline phosphatase	Serum	20–130 U/L at 37°C (p-nitrophenylphosphate in AMP buffer)	1	20–130 U/L at 37°C
Phospholipid phosphorus (see Lipids, total)				
Phospholipids (see Lipids, total)				
Phosphorus, inorganic	Serum			
adults		2.3–4.7 mg/dL	0.3229	0.74–1.52 mmol/L
children		4.0–7.0 mg/dL		1.29–2.26 mmol/L
Potassium	Plasma	3.8–5.0 mEq/L	1	3.8–5.0 mmol/L
Prolactin	Serum			
female		1–25 ng/mL	1	1–25 μg/L
male		1–20 ng/mL		1–20 μg/L

Table A5–4 Whole Blood, Serum, and Plasma Chemistry (cont'd)

Component	System	Typical Reference Intervals		
		Conventional Units	Factor*	Recommended SI Units†
Proteins (see Ch. 19)	Serum			
total		6.0–7.8 g/dL	10	60–78 g/L
albumin		3.2–4.5 g/dL		32–45 g/L
globulin		2.3–3.5 g/dL		23–35 g/L
Protein fractionation, see Electrophoresis				
Protoporphyrin	Erythrocytes	15–50 mg/dL	0.01777	0.27–0.89 µmol/L
Pyruvate	Whole blood	0.3–0.9 mg/dL	113.6	34–102 µmol/L
Salicylates	Serum	Negative	–	Negative
therapeutic interval		15–30 mg/dL	0.07240	1.08–2.17 mmol/L
Sodium	Plasma	136–142 mEq/L	1	136–142 mmol/L
Sulfate, inorganic	Serum	0.2–1.3 mEq/L	0.5	0.10–0.65 mmol/L
		0.9–6.0 in mg/dL as SO_4^-	0.1042	0.09–0.63 mmol/L as SO_4^-
Sulfhemoglobin	Whole blood	Negative	–	Negative
Sulfonamides	Serum or whole blood	Negative	–	Negative
Testosterone	Serum or plasma			
male		300–1200 ng/dL	0.03467	10.4–41.6 nmol/L
female		30–95 ng/dL		1.0–3.3 mmol/L
Thiocyanate	Serum	Negative	–	Negative
Thyroid hormone tests (see Ch. 24)	Serum			
thyroxine, total (T_4)		5.5–12.5 µg/dL	12.87	71–161 nmol/L
thyroxine, free (FT_4)		0.9–2.3 ng/dL	12.87	12–30 pmol/L
T_3 resin uptake		25–38 relative % uptake	0.01	Relative uptake fraction: 0.25–0.38
thyroxine-binding globulin (TBG)	Serum	10–26 µg/dL	10	100–260 µg/L
thyrotropin (TSH)	Serum	0.5–5 µU/mL	1	0.5–5 µU/L
triiodothyronine (T_3)		80–200 mg/dL	0.0154	1.23–3 of nmol/L
Transferases				
aspartate amino transferase (AST or SGOT)	Serum	8–33 U/L at 37°C	1	8–33 U/L at 37°C
alanine amino transferase (ALT or SGPT)	Serum	4–36 U/L at 37°C	1	4–36 U/L at 37°C
γ glutamyl transferase (GGT)		5–40 U/L at 37°C	1	5–40 U/L at 37°C
Triglycerides (see Ch. 17)	Serum	10–190 mg/dL	0.01129††	0.11–2.15 mmol/L
Troponin I	Serum	<2.0 mg/mL		0–0.6 µg/L
				0–0.1 µg/L
Urea nitrogen	Serum	8–23 mg/dL	0.357	2.9–8.2 mmol/L
Urea clearance	Serum and urine			
maximum clearance		64–99 mL/min	0.01667	1.07–1.65 L/s
standard clearance		41–65 mL/min, or more than 75% of normal clearance		0.68–1.08 L/s or more than 0.75 of normal clearance
Uric acid	Serum			
male		4.0–8.5 mg/dL	0.05948	0.24–0.51 mmol/L
female		2.7–7.3 mg/dL		0.16–0.43 mmol/L
Vitamin A	Serum	15–60 µg/dL	0.03491	0.52–2.09 µmol/L
Vitamin A tolerance	Serum	15–60 µg/dL	0.03491	0.52–2.09 µmol/L
	fasting 3 h or 6 h after 5000 units vitamin A/kg	200–600 µg/dL	0.03491	6.98–20.95 µmol/L
	24 h	Fasting values or slightly above	–	Fasting values or slightly above
Vitamin B_{12}	Serum	160–950 pg/mL	0.7378	118–701 pmol/L
Unsaturated vitamin B_{12}-binding capacity	Serum	1000–2000 pg/mL	0.7378	738–1475 pmol/L
Vitamin C	Plasma	0.6–1.6 mg/dL	56.78	34–91 µmol/L
Xylose absorption	Serum normal in malabsorption	25–40 mg/dL 1–2 h	0.06661	1.67–2.66 mmol/L 1–2 h
		Maximum ≈10 mg/dL		Maximum ≈0.67 mmol/L
		Dose: adult 25 g D-xylose children 0.5 g D-xylose/kg		
Zinc	Serum	50–150 µg/dL	0.1530	7.7–23.0 µmol/L

* Factor = number factor (note that units are not presented). † Value in SI units = value in conventional units × factor. ‡ Usually not measured in blood (preferred specimen is urine, hair, or nails except in acute cases, when gastric contents are used). § Unit based on hydrogen ion concentration. ¶As cortisol. ‖ 1 International Unit of insulin corresponds to 0.04167 mg of the 4th International Standard (a mixture of 52% beef insulin and 48% pig insulin). ** As DHEA. †† As triolein.

Table A5–5 Urine

Component	Type of Urine System	Conventional Units	Factor*	Recommended SI Units†
Acetoacetic acid	Random	Negative	–	Negative
Acetone	Random	Negative	–	Negative
Addis count	12 h collection	WBC and epithelial cells:		
		1 800 000/12 h	1	1.8×10^6 12 h
		RBC 500 000/12 h	1	0.5×10^6 12 h
		Hyaline casts: <5000/12 h	1	$<5.0 \times 10^3$ 12 h
Albumin				
qualitative	Random	Negative	–	Negative
quantitative	24 h	15–150 mg/d	0.001	0.015–0.150 g/d
Aldosterone	24 h	2–26 µg/d	2.774	6–72 nmol/d
Alkapton bodies	Random	Negative	–	Negative
α-Amino acid nitrogen	24 h	100–290 mg/d	0.07139	7.1–20.7 mmol/d
δ-Aminolevulinic acid	Random			
adults		0.1–0.6 mg/dL	76.26	8–46 µmol/L
children		<0.5 mg/dL		<38 µmol/L
	24 h	1.5–7.5 mg/d	7.626	11–57 µmol/d
Ammonia nitrogen	24 h	20–70 mEq/d	1	20–70 mmol/d
		500–1200 mg/d	0.07139	35.6–85.7 mmol/d
Amylase	2 h	35–260 Somogyi units/h	0.1850	6.5–48.1 U/h
Arsenic	24 h	<50 µg/L	0.01335	<0.67 µmol/L
Ascorbic acid	Random	1–7 mg/dL	56.78	57–397 µmol/L
	24 h	>50 mg/d	5.678	>284 µmol/d
Bence Jones protein	Random	Negative	–	Negative
Beryllium	24 h	<0.05 µg/d	111.0	<5.55 nmol/d
Bilirubin, qualitative	Random	Negative	–	Negative
Blood, occult	Random	Negative	–	Negative
Borate	24 h	<2 mg/L	16.44	<32 µmol/L
Calcium				
qualitative (Sulkowitch)	Random	1 + turbidity	1	1 + turbidity
quantitative	24 h			
average diet		100–240 mg/d	0.02495	2.5–6.0 mmol/d
low-calcium diet		<150 mg/d		<3.7 mmol/d
high-calcium diet		240–300 mg/d		6.0–7.5 mmol/d
Catecholamines	Random	<14 µg/dL	59.11*	<828 nmol/L
	24 h	<100 µg/d (varies with activity)	5.911*	<591 nmol/d
epinephrine		<10 ng/d	5.458	<55 nmol/d
norepinephrine		<100 ng/d	5.911	<591 nmol/d
total free catecholamines		4–126 µg/d	5.911*	24–745 nmol/d
total metanephrines		0.1–1.6 mg/d	5.458†	0.5–8.7 µmol/d
Chloride	24 h	140–250 mEq/d	1	140–250 nmol/d
Concentration test (Fishberg)	Random – after fluid restriction			
specific gravity		>1.025	1	>1.025
osmolality		>850 mOsm/kg	1	>850 mmol/kg
Copper	24 h	<50 µg/d	0.01574	<0.8 µmol/d
Coproporphyrin	Random			
adult		3–20 µg/dL	15.27	46–305 nmol/L
	24 h			
adult		50–160 µg/d	1.527	76–244 nmol/d
children		<80 µg/d		<122 nmol/d
Creatine	24 h			
male		<40 mg/d	7.625	<305 µmol/d
female		<100 mg/d		<763 µmol/d
		Higher in children and during pregnancy	–	Higher in children and during pregnancy
Creatinine	24 h			
male		20–26 mg/kg/d	8.840	177–230 µmol/kg/d
		1.0–2.0 g/d	8.840	8.8–17.7 mmol/d
female		14–22 mg/kg/d	8.840	124–195 µmol/kg/d
		0.8–1.8 g/d	8.840	7.1–15.9 mmol/d
Cystine, qualitative	Random	Negative	–	Negative
Cystine and cysteine	24 h	10–100 mg/d	4.161†	42–416 µmol/d
Dehydroepiandrosterone	24 h			
male		0.2–2.0 mg/d	3.467	0.7–6.9 µmol/d
female		0.2–1.8 mg/d		0.7–6.2 µmol/d

Table A5–5 Urine (*cont'd*)

Component	Type of Urine System	Typical Reference Intervals		
		Conventional Units	Factor*	Recommended SI Units†
Diacetic acid	Random	Negative	–	Negative
Epinephrine	24 h	<20 µg/d	5.458	<109 nmol/d
Estrogens, total	24 h			
	male	5–18 µg/d	3.468‡	17–62 nmol/d
	female			
	ovulation	28–100 µg/d	3.468	97–347 nmol/d
	luteal peak	22–80 µg/d		76–364 nmol/d
	at menses	4–25 µg/d		14–87 nmol/d
	pregnancy	Up to 45 000 µg/d	0.003468	Up to 156 µmol/d
	postmenopausal	Up to 10 µg/d	3.468	Up to 35 nmol/d
Estrogens, fractionated	24 h, nonpregnant, midcycle			
estrone (E₁)	–	2–25 µg/d	3.699	7–93 nmol/d
estradiol (E₂)	–	<10 µg/d	3.671	<37 nmol/d
estriol (E₃)	–	2–30 µg/d	3.468	7–104 nmol/d
Etiocholanolone	24 h			
	male	1.4–5.0 mg/d	3.443	4.8–17.2 µmol/d
	female	0.8–4.0 mg/d		2.8–13.8 µmol/d
Fat, qualitative	Random	Negative	–	Negative
FIGLU	24 h	<3 mg/d	5.740	<7.2 µmol/d
(*N*-formiminoglutamic acid)	after 15 g of L-histidine	4 mg/8 h		23.0 µmol/8 h
Fluoride	24 h	<1 mg/d	52.63	<53 µmol/d
Follicle-stimulating	24 h			
hormone (FSH)	adult	4–25 U/L	1	4–25 U/L
	prepubertal	4–30 U/L	1	4–30 U/L
	postmenopausal	40–50 U/L	1	40–50 U/L
	midcycle	2 × baseline	1	2 × baseline
Fructose	24 h	30–65 mg/d	0.005551	0.17–0.36 mmol/d
Glucose, qualitative	Random	Negative	–	Negative
Glucose, quantitative	24 h			
copper-reducing substances		0.5–1.5 g/d	1	0.5–1.5 g/d
total sugars		Average 250 mg/d	1	Average 250 mg/d
glucose		Average 130 mg/d	0.005551	Average 0.72 mmol/d
Gonadotropins, pituitary (FSH and LH)	24 h	10–50 U/L	1	10–50 U/d
11-Hydroxyandrosterone	24 h			
	male	0.1–0.8 mg/d	3.263	0.3–2.6 µmol/d
	female	<0.5 mg/d		<1.6 µmol/d
11-Hydroxyetiocholanolone	24 h			
	male	0.2–0.6 mg/d	3.26	0.7–2.0 µmol/d
	female	0.1–1.1 mg/d		0.3–3.63 µmol/d
11-Ketoandrosterone	24 h			
	male	0.2–1.0 mg/d	3.274	0.7–3.3 µmol/d
	female	0.2–0.8 mg/d		0.7–2.6 µmol/d
11-Ketoetiocholanolone	24 h			
	male	0.2–1.0 mg/d	3.274	0.7–3.3 µmol/d
	female	0.2–0.8 mg/d		0.7–2.6 µmol/d
Lactose	24 h	14–40 mg/d	2.291	41–117 µmol/d
Lead	24 h	<100 µg/d	0.004826	<0.48 µmol/d
Magnesium	24 h	6.0–8.5 mEq/d	0.5000	3.0–4.3 mmol/d
Melanin, qualitative	Random	Negative	–	Negative
Mucin	24 h	100–150 mg/d	1	100–150 mg/d
Muramidase (lysozyme)	24 h	1.3–36 mg/d	1	1.3–36 mg/d
Myoglobin				
qualitative	Random	Negative	–	Negative
quantitative	24 h	<4 mg/L	1	<4 mg/L
Osmolality	Random	500–800 mOsm/kg water	1	500–800 mmol/kg
Pentoses	24 h	2–5 mg/kg/d	1	2–5 mg/kg/d
pH	Random	4.6–8.0	1	4.6–8.0
Phenolsulfonphthalein (PSP)	Urine timed after 6 mg PSP IV			Fraction dye excreted:
	15 min	20–50% dye excreted	0.01	0.20–0.50
	30 min	16–24% dye excreted		0.16–0.24
	60 min	9–17% dye excreted		0.09–0.17
	120 min	3–10% dye excreted		0.03–0.10

Table A5–5 Urine (*cont'd*)

Component	Type of Urine System	Typical Reference Intervals		
		Conventional Units	Factor*	Recommended SI Units†
Phenylpyruvic acid, qualitative	Random	Negative	–	Negative
Phosphorus	Random	0.9–1.3 g/d	32.29	29–42 mmol/d
Porphobilinogen				
qualitative	Random	Negative	–	Negative
quantitative	24 h	<1.0 mg/d	4.420	<4.4 μmol/d
Potassium	24 h	40–80 mEq/d	1	40–80 mmol/d
Pregnancy tests	Concentrated morning specimen	Positive in normal pregnancies or with tumors producing chorionic gonadotropin	–	Positive in normal pregnancies or with tumors producing chorionic gonadotropin
Pregnanediol	24 h			
male		<1.5 mg/d	3.120	<4.7 μmol/d
female		1–8 mg/d	3.120	3–25 μmol/d
peak		1 week after ovulation	–	1 week after ovulation
pregnancy		<50 mg/d	3.120	<156 μmol/d
children		Negative	–	Negative
Pregnanetriol	24 h			
male		0.4–2.4 mg/d	2.972	1.2–7.0 μmol/d
female		0.5–2.0 mg/d		1.5–5.9 μmol/d
children		Up to 1 mg/d		Up to 3 μmol/d
Protein, qualitative	Random	Negative	–	Negative
	24 h	40–150 mg/d	1	40–150 mg/d
Reducing substances, total	24 h	0.5–1.5 mg/d	1	0.5–1.5 mg/d
Sodium	24 h	75–200 mEq/d	1	75–200 mmol/d
Solids, total	24 h	55–70 g/d	1	55–70 g/d
		Decreases with age to 30 g/d	–	Decreases with age to 30 g/d
Specific gravity	Random			Relative density (U 20°C/water 20°C):
		1.016–1.022 (normal fluid intake)	1	1.016–1.022 (normal fluid intake)
		1.001–1.035 (range)		1.001–1.035 (range)
Sugars (excluding glucose)	Random	Negative	–	Negative
Titratable acidity	24 h	20–50 mEq/d	1	20–50 mmol/d
Urea nitrogen	24 h	6–17 g/d	35.70	214–607 mmol/d
Uric acid	24 h	250–750 mg/d	0.005948	1.5–4.5 mmol/d
Urobilinogen	2 h	0.3–1.0 Ehrlich units	1	0.3–1.0 U
	24 h	0.05–2.5 mg/d or	1.693	0.1–4.2 μmol/d
		0.5–4.0 Ehrlich units/d	1	0.5–4.0 U/d
Uropepsin	Random	15–45 units/h (Anson)	7.37	111–332 U/h
	24 h	1500–5000 units/d (Anson)		11–37 kU/h
Uroporphyrins				
qualitative	Random	Negative	–	Negative
quantitative	24 h	10–30 μg/d	1.204	12–36 nmol/d
Vanillylmandelic acid (VMA)	24 h	1.5–7.5 mg/d	5.046	7.6–37.9 μmol/d
Volume, total	24 h	600–1600 mL/d	0.001	0.6–1.6 L/d
Zinc	24 h	0.15–1.2 mg/d	15.30	2.3–18.4 μmol/d

* As norepinephrine. † As normetanephrine. ‡ Based on cystine. § Based on estriol.

Table A5–6 Synovial Fluid

Component	Typical Reference Intervals		
	Conventional Units	Factor	Recommended SI Units
Blood-serum-synovial fluid glucose difference	<10 mg/dL	0.05551	<0.56 mmol/l
Differential cell count	Granulocytes <25% of nucleated cells	0.01	Granulocyte number fraction: <0.25 of nucleated cells
Fibrin clot	Absent	–	Absent
Mucin clot	Abundant	–	Abundant
Nucleated cell count	<200 cells/μL	10^6	<200 × 10^6 cells/L
Viscosity	High	–	High
Volume	<3.5 mL	0.001	<0.0035 L

Component	Typical Reference Intervals		
	Conventional Units	**Factor**	**Recommended SI Units**
Liquefaction	Within 20 min		Within 20 min
Sperm morphology	>70% normal, mature spermatozoa	0.01	Number fraction: >0.70 normal, mature spermatozoa
Sperm motility	>60%	0.01	Number fraction: >0.60
pH	>7.0 (average 7.7)	1	>7.0 (average 7.7)
Sperm count	$60–150 \times 10^6$/mL	10^3	$60–150 \times 10^9$/L
Volume	1.5–5.0 mL	0.001	0.0015–0.005 L

Component	Typical Reference Intervals		
	Conventional Units	**Factor**	**Recommended SI Units**
Fasting residual volume	20–100 mL	0.001	0.02–0.10 L
pH	<2.0	1	<2.0
Basal acid output (BAO)*	0–6 mEq/h	1	0–6 mmol/h
Maximum acid output (MAO) (after histamine stimulation)	5–40 mEq/h	1	5–40 mmol/h
BAO/MAO ratio	<0.4	1	<0.4

* Varies between male and female and ages

Component	Typical Reference Intervals		
	Conventional Units	**Factor**	**Recommended SI Units**
Red cell volume			
male	20–36 mL/kg body weight	0.001	0.020–0.036 L/kg body weight
female	19–32 mL/kg body weight		0.019–0.032 L/kg body weight
Plasma volume			
male	25–43 mL/kg body weight	0.001	0.025–0.043 L/kg body weight
female	28–45 mL/kg body weight		0.028–0.045 L/kg body weight
Coagulation and hemostatic tests			
bleeding time	Depends on location and orientation of cut and on particular device, typically 2–8 min		
Activated partial thromboplastin time (APTT)	Depends on activator and phospholipid reagents used, typically 25–35 s		
Antithrombin III			
immunologic	20–30 mg/dL	10	200–300 mg/L
functional	80–120 U/dL	10	800–1200 U/L
Clot lysis time			
euglobulin factor	1½–4 h at 37°C		
whole blood	None by 24 h at 37°C		
Clot retraction	Complete by 4 h at 37°C		
Coagulation factors	0.50–1.50 µ/mL	1000	500–1500 U/L
Factor XIII (screening test)	Clot insoluble in 5 mol/L urea at 24 h		
Fibrinogen	200–400 mg/dL	0.01	2.0–4.0 g/L
Fibrin(ogen) degradation products			
serum FDP	<10 µg/mL	1	<10 mg/L
plasma D-dimers	<200 ng/mL	1	<200 µg/L
Plasminogen			
immunologic	10–20 mg/dL	10	100–200 mg/L
functional	80–120 U/dL	10	800–1200 U/L
Protein C	0.7–1.4 µ/mL	10	700–1400 U/L
Protein S (total)	0.7–1.4 µ/mL	10	700–1400 U/L
Prothrombin time	Depends on thromboplastin reagent used, typically 10–13 s		
Thrombin time	Depends on concentration of thrombin reagent used, typically 17–25 s		
Von Willebrand factor			
immunologic	50–150 U/dL	10	500–1500 U/L
ristocetin cofactor activity	50–150 U/dL		500–1500 U/L

Table A5–9 Hematology (cont'd)

Component	Typical Reference Intervals		
	Conventional Units	Factor	Recommended SI Units
Complete blood count (CBC)			
Hematocrit			Volume fraction:
male	41.5–50.4%	0.01	0.415–0.504
female	35.9–44.6%		0.359–0.446
Hemoglobin			
male	14.0–17.5 g/dL	10	140–175 g/L
female	12.3–15.3 g/dL		123–153 g/L
Red cell count			
male	$4.5–5.9 \times 10^6/\mu L$	10^6	$4.5–5.9 \times 10^{12}/L$
female	$4.5.–5.1 \times 10^6/\mu L$		$4.1–5.1 \times 10^{12}/L$
White cell count	$4.4–11.0 \times 10^3/\mu L$	10^6	$4.4–11.3 \times 10^9/L$
Erythrocyte indices			
Mean corpuscular volume (MCV)	80–96 μm^3	1	80–96 fL
Mean corpuscular hemoglobin (MCH)	27.5–33.2 pg	1	27.5–33.2 pg
Mean corpuscular hemoglobin concentration (MCHC)	33.4–35.5%	0.01	Concentration fraction: 0.334–0.355

White blood cell differential (adult)	Mean %	Range of absolute counts		Mean number fraction*	Range of absolute counts
segmented neutrophils	56	1800–7800/µL	10^6	0.56	$1.8–7.8 \times 10^9/L$
bands	3	0–700/µL		0.03	$0–0.70 \times 10^9/L$
eosinophils	2.7	0–450/µL		0.027	$0–0.45 \times 10^9/L$
basophils	0.3	0–200/µL		0.003	$0–0.20 \times 10^9/L$
lymphocytes	34	1000–4800/µL		0.34	$1.0–4.8 \times 10^9/L$
monocytes	4	0–800/µL		0.04	$0–0.80 \times 10^9/L$

Component	Conventional Units	Factor	Recommended SI Units
Hemoglobin A_2	1.5–3.5% of total hemoglobin	0.01	Mass fraction: 0.015–0.035 of total hemoglobin
Hemoglobin F	<2%	0.01	Mass fraction: <0.02

Osmotic fragility

% (w/v) NaCl	% Lysis Fresh	% Lysis 24 h at 37°C	Factor	NaCl mmol/L	Lysed Fraction Fresh	Lysed Fraction 24 h at 37°C
0.2	–		% NaCl – 171 % Lysis – 0.01	34.2	–	0.95–1.00
0.3	97–100	95–100		51.3	0.97–1.00	0.85–1.00
0.35	90–99	85–100		59.8	0.90–0.99	0.75–1.00
0.4	50–95	75–100		68.4	0.50–0.95	0.65–1.00
0.45	5–45	65–100		77.0	0.05–0.45	0.55–0.95
0.5	0.6	55–95		85.5	0–0.06	0.40–0.85
0.55	–	40–85		94.1	0	0.15–0.70
0.6	–	15–70		102.6	–	0–0.40
0.65	–	0–40		111.2	–	0–0.10
0.7	–	0–10		119.7	–	0–0.05
0.75	–	0–5		128.3	–	0

Component	Conventional Units	Factor	Recommended SI Units
Platelet count	150 000–450 000/µL	10^6	$150–450 \times 10^9/L$
Reticulocyte count	0.5–1.5%	0.01	Number fraction: 0.005–0.015
	25 000–75 000 cells/µL	10^6	$25–75 \times 10^9/L$
Sedimentation rate (ESR) (Westergren)			
men under 50 years	<15 mm/h		
men 50–85 years	<20 mm/h		
men over 85 years	<30 mm/h		
women under 50 years	<20 mm/h		
women 50–85 years	<30 mm/h		
women over 85 years	<42 mm/h		
Viscosity	1.4–1.8 times water	1	1.4–1.8 times water
Zeta sedimentation ratio	41–54%	0.01	fraction: 0.41–0.54

* All percentages are multiplied by 0.01 to give fraction.

Table A5–10 Amniotic Fluid

Component	Typical Reference Intervals		
	Conventional Units	Factor	Recommended SI Units
Appearance			
early gestation	Clear	–	Clear
term	Clear or slightly opalescent	–	Clear or slightly opalescent
Albumin			
early gestation	0.39 g/dL	10	3.9 g/L
term	0.19 g/dL		1.9 g/L

Table A5–10 Amniotic Fluid (cont'd)

Component	Typical Reference Intervals		
	Conventional Units	Factor	Recommended SI Units
Bilirubin			
early gestation	<0.075 mg/dL	17.10	<1.3 µmol/L
term	<0.025 mg/dL		<0.41 µmol/L
Chloride			
early gestation	Approximately equal to serum chloride	–	Approximately equal to serum chloride
term	Generally 1–3 } mEq/L lower than serum chloride	1	Generally 1–3 mmol/L lower than serum chloride
Creatinine			
early gestation	0.8–1.1 mg/dL	88.40	71–97 µmol/L
term	1.8–4.0 mg/dL (generally >2 mg/dL)		159–354 µmol/L (generally >177 µmol/L)
Estriol			
early gestation	<10 µg/dL	3.468	<347 nmol/L
term	<60 µg/dL		>2081 nmol/L
Lecithin:sphingomyelin			
early (immature)	<1:1	1	<1:1
term (mature)	>2:1		>2:1
Osmolality			
early gestation	Approximately equal to serum osmolality	–	Approximately equal to serum osmolality
term	230–270 mOsm/kg	1	230–270 mmol/kg
P_{CO_2}			
early gestation	33–55 mm Hg	0.1333	4.4–7.3 kPa
term	42–55 mm Hg (increases toward term)		5.6–7.3 kPa (increases toward term)
pH			
early gestation	7.12–7.38	1	7.12–7.38
term	6.91–7.43 (decreases toward term)		6.91–7.43
Protein, total			
early gestation	0.60 ± 0.24 g/dL	10	60 ± 2.4 g/L
term	0.26 ± 0.19 g/dL		2.6 ± 1.9 g/L
Sodium			
early gestation	Approximately equal to serum sodium	–	Approximately equal to serum sodium
term	7–10 mEq/L lower than serum sodium	1	7–10 mmol/L lower than serum sodium
Staining, cytologic			
Oil Red O			
early gestation	Stained fraction: <10%	0.01	Stained fraction: <0.1
term	Stained fraction: >50%		>0.5
Nile blue sulfate			
early gestation	Stained fraction: 0	0.01	Stained fraction: <0.0
term	Stained fraction: >20%		>0.2
Urea			
early gestation	18.0 ± 5.9 mg/dL	0.1665	3.00 ± 0.98 mmol/L
term	30.3 ± 11.4 mg/dL		5.04 ± 1.90 mmol/L
Uric acid			
early gestation	3.72 ± 0.96 mg/dL	59.48	221 ± 57 µmol/L
term	9.90 ± 2.23 mg/dL		589 ± 133 µmol/L
Volume			
early gestation	450–1200 mL	0.001	0.45–1.2 L
term	500–1400 mL (increases toward term)		0.5–1.4 L (increases toward term)

Table A5–11 Cerebrospinal Fluid

Component	Typical Reference Intervals		
	Conventional Units	Factor	Recommended SI Units
Albumin	<10–30 mg/dL	10	100–300 mg/L
Cell count	<5 cells/µL	10^6	$<5 \times 10^6$/L
Glucose	40–80 mg/dL	0.05551	2.8–4.4 mmol/L
Lactate dehydrogenase (LD)	Approximately 10% of serum level	–	Activity fraction: approximately 0.1 of serum level
Proteins	12–60 mg/dL	10	120–600 mg/L
Protein electrophoresis			Fraction:
prealbumin	2–7%	0.01	0.2–0.07
albumin	56–76%		0.56–0.76
α-1 globulin	2–7%		0.02–0.07
α-2 globulin	4–12%		0.04–0.12
β globulin	8–18%		0.08–0.18
γ globulin	3–12%		0.03–0.12
Xanthochromia	Negative	–	Negative

Table A5–12 Miscellaneous

Component	Typical Reference Intervals			
	Specimen	**Conventional Units**	**Factor**	**Recommended SI Units**
Bile, qualitative	Random stool	Negative in adults	–	Negative in adults
		Positive in children	–	Positive in children
Chloride	Sweat	4–60 mEq/L	1	4–60 mmol/L
Clearances	Serum and urine (timed)			
creatinine, endogenous		115 ± 20 mL/min	0.01667	1.92 ± 0.33 mL/s
Diodrast		600–720 mL/min		10.00–12.00 mL/s
inulin		100–150 mL/min		1.67–2.50 mL/s
PAH		600–750 mL/min		10.00–12.50 mL/s
Diagnex blue (tubeless gastric analysis)	Urine	Free acid present	–	Free acid present
Fat	Stool, 72 h			
total fat		<5 g/24 h	1	<5 g/d
		10–25% of dry matter	0.01	Mass fraction: 0.1–0.25 of dry matter
neutral fat		1–5% of dry matter		0.01–0.05 of dry matter
free fatty acids		5–13% of dry matter		0.05–0.13 of dry matter
combined fatty acids		5–15% of dry matter		0.05–0.15 of dry matter
Nitrogen, total	Stool, 24 h	10% of intake		Mass fraction: 0.1 of intake
		1–2 g/24 h	71.39	71–143 mmol/d
Sodium	Sweat	10–80 mEq/L	1	10–80 mmol/L
Trypsin activity	Random, fresh stool	Positive (2+ to 4+)	–	Positive (2+ to 4+)
Thyroid iodine-131 uptake		7.5–25% in 6 h	0.01	Fraction uptake: 0.075–0.25 in 6 h
Urobilinogen				
qualitative	Random stool	Positive	–	Positive
quantitative	Stool, 24 h	40–200 mg/24 h	1.693	68–339 µmol/d
		80–280 Ehrlich units/24 h		

Table A5–13 Selected Pediatric Reference Values

Parameter	Value		
S-Acid phosphatase			
newborn	7.4–19.4 U/L		
2–13 y	6.4–15.2 U/L		
S-Aldolase			
newborn	to 4× adult value		
child	to 2× adult value		
S-Alkaline phosphatase			
newborn	40–300 U/L		
child	60–270 U/L		
S-α-fetoprotein			
newborn	Up to 100 mg/L		
2 wk	Undetectable		
S-Amylase			
newborn	Little, if any, amylase activity		
1 y	Adult values		
S-Aspartate aminotransferase			
newborn	16–74 U/L		
1–3 y	6–30 U/L		
S-Bilirubin, newborn	Preterm	Full-term	
24 h	17–103 µmol/L (10–60 mg/L)	34–103 µmol/L (20–60 mg/L)	
48 h	17–103 µmol/L (10–60 mg/L)	103–120 µmol/L (60–70 mg/L)	
3–5 d	171–257 µmol/L (100–150 mg/L)	68–205 µmol/L (40–120 mg/L)	
S-Calcium			
preterm, first week	1.50–2.50 mmol/L (60–100 mg/L)		
full-term, first week	1.75–3.00 mmol/L (70–120 mg/L)		
1–2 years	2.50–3.00 mmol/L (100–120 mg/L)		
2–16 years	2.25–2.87 mmol/L (90–115 mg/L)		
U-Catecholamines	Norepinephrine	Epinephrine	
1 year	30–90 nmol/d (5.4–15.9 µg/d)	1–23 nmol/d (0.1–4.3 µg/d)	
1–5 years	50–180 nmol/d (8.1–30.8 µg/d)	4–50 nmol/d (0.8–9.1 µg/d)	
6–15 years	110–420 nmol/d (19.0–71.1 µg/d)	7–339 nmol/d (1.3–10.5 µg/d)	
>15 years	200–510 nmol/d (34.4–87.0 µg/d)	19–72 nmol/d (3.5–13.2 µg/d)	

Table A5–13 Selected Pediatric Reference Values (cont'd)

Parameter	Value
U-Chloride (varies with chloride intake)	
infant	1.7–8.5 mmol/d
child	17–34 mmol/d
S-Cholesterol	
cord blood	1.2–2.5 mmol/L (460–980 mg/L)
1–2 years	1.8–4.9 mmol/L (700–1900 mg/L)
2–16 years	3.5–6.5 mmol/L (1350–2500 mg/L)
U-Cortisol (free)	
4 months–10 years	6–74 nmol/d (2–27 µg/d)
11–20 years	2–152 nmol/d (0.7–55 µg/d)
S-Creatine kinase	
newborn	3× adult values
3 weeks–3 months	1.5× adult values
>1 year	Adult values
S-Creatinine	Upper reference value:
up to 5 years	44 µmol/L (5.0 mg/L)
up to 6 years	53 µmol/L (6.0 mg/L)
up to 7 years	62 µmol/L (7.0 mg/L)
up to 8 years	71 µmol/L (8.0 mg/L)
up to 9 years	80 µmol/L (9.0 mg/L)
up to 10 years	88 µmol/L (10.0 mg/L)
>10 years	106 µmol/L (12.0 mg/L)
S-Estradiol	
0–2 years	0–26 pmol/L (0–7 pg/mL)
2–4 years	0–26 pmol/L (0–7 pg/mL)
4–6 years	0–51 pmol/L (0–14 pg/mL)
6–8 years	0–37 pmol/L (0–10 pg/mL)
8–10 years	0–367 pmol/L (0–100 pg/mL)
10–12 years	0–367 pmol/L (0–100 pg/mL)
12–14 years	0–367 pmol/L (0–100 pg/mL)
14–16 years	26–385 pmol/L (7–105 pg/mL)
16–26 years	26–1175 pmol/L (7–320 pg/mL)
Fecal fat	
pre-term newborn	Up to 0.40 excreted
full-term newborn	Up to 0.20 excreted
3 months–1 year	Up to 0.15 excreted
1 year	Up to 0.085 excreted
P-Nonesterified fatty acids	
newborn	0–1845 mmol/L
4 months–10 years	300–1100 mmol/L
S-Glucose	
preterm newborn	1.1–3.6 mmol/L (200–656 mg/L)
full-term newborn	1.1–6.1 mmol/L (200–1100 mg/L)
child	3.3–5.8 mmol/L (600–1050 mg/L)
S-γ-Glutamyltransferase	
premature newborn	56–233 U/L
newborn–3 weeks	10–103 U/L
3 weeks–3 months	4–111 U/L
1–5 years	2–23 U/L
6–15 years	2–23 U/L
16 years–adult	2–35 U/L
S-Haptoglobin	
newborn	Detectable haptoglobin in only 0.1–0.2
≥1 year	Adult values
S-Immunoglobulin IgG	
0–5 weeks	7500–15,000 mg/L
6 months	1500–7000 mg/L
1 year	1400–10,300 mg/L
5 years	3700–15,000 mg/L
10 years	4400–15,500 mg/L
S-Immunoglobulin IgA	
0–5 weeks	None
6 months	200–1300 mg/L
1 year	200–1300 mg/L
5 years	300–2000 mg/L
10 years	500–2300 mg/L

Table A5–13 Selected Pediatric Reference Values (*cont'd*)

Parameter	Value		
S-Immunoglobulin IgM			
0–5 weeks	<200 mg/L		
6 months	300–600 mg/L		
1 year	300–1600 mg/L		
5 years	200–2200 mg/L		
10 years	300–1700 mg/L		
Inulin clearance			
<1 month	29–88 mL/min per 1.73 m² of body surface		
1–6 months	40–112 mL/min per 1.73 m² of body surface		
6–12 months	62–121 mL/min per 1.73 m² of body surface		
>1 year	78–164 mL/min per 1.73 m² of body surface		
U-17-Ketosteroids*			
0–3 days	0–0.2 µmol/d (0–0.5 mg/d)		
1–3 years	<7.0 µmol/d (<2.0 mg/d)		
3–6 years	2–10 µmol/d (0.5–3.0 mg/d)		
6–9 years	3–14 µmol/d (0.8–4.0 mg/d)		
	Male		**Female**
10–12 years	2–21 µmol/d (0.7–6.0 mg/d)		2–17 µmol/d (0.7–5.0 mg/d)
Adolescent	10–52 µmol/d (3–15 mg/d)		10–42 µmol/d (3–12 mg/d)
S-Lactate dehydrogenase			
1–3 days	Up to 2× → ult values		
S-Phosphorus (inorganic)			
	Preterm		**Full-term**
newborn	1.81–2.58 mmol/L (56.0–80.0 mg/L)		1.61–2.52 mmol/L (50.0–78.0 mg/L)
6–10 days	1.97–3.78 mmol/L (61–117 mg/L)		1.58–2.87 mmol/L (49–89 mg/L)
4 months	1.55–2.62 mmol/L (48–81 mg/L)		
1 year	1.26–1.94 mmol/L (39–60 mg/L)		
2–16 years	0.84–1.61 mmol/L (26–50 mg/L)		
S-Potassium			
preterm newborn	4.5–7.2 mmol/L		
full-term newborn	5.0–7.7 mmol/L		
2 days–2 weeks	4.0–6.4 mmol/L		
2 weeks–3 months	4.0–6.2 mmol/L		
3 months–1 year	3.7–5.6 mmol/L		
1–16 years	3.6–5.2 mmol/L		
S-Testosterone	**Male**		**Female**
0–2 years	0.14–1.28 nmol/L (0–0.4 ng/mL)		0.24–0.62 nmol/L (0.1–0.2 ng/mL)
2–4 years	0.17–5.55 nmol/L (0–1.6 ng/mL)		0.24–0.69 nmol/L (0.1–0.2 ng/mL)
4–6 years	0.28–1.39 nmol/L (0.1–0.4 ng/mL)		0.35–0.69 nmol/L (0.1–0.2 ng/mL)
6–8 years	0.21–9.72 nmol/L (0.1–2.8 ng/mL)		0.52–1.04 nmol/L (0.1–0.3 ng/mL)
8–10 years	0.31–1.74 nmol/L (0.1–0.5 ng/mL)		0.69–1.39 nmol/L (0.2–0.4 ng/mL)
10–12 years	0.29–10.06 nmol/L (0.1–2.9 ng/mL)		0.69–1.74 nmol/L (0.2–0.5 ng/mL)
12–14 years	0.17–26.37 nmol/L (0–7.6 ng/mL)		1.04–2.43 nmol/L (0.3–0.7 ng/mL)
14–16 years	3.12–19.43 nmol/L (0.9–5.6 ng/mL)		1.21–3.30 nmol/L (0.3–1.0 ng/mL)
16–18 years	9.02–25.33 nmol/L (2.6–7.3 ng/mL)		1.39–3.30 nmol/L (0.4–1.0 ng/mL)
18–20 years	13.88–24.98 nmol/L (4.0–7.2 ng/mL)		1.39–3.30 nmol/L (0.4–1.0 ng/mL)
20–25 years	11.80–38.86 nmol/L (3.4–11.2 ng/mL)		1.39–3.30 nmol/L (0.4–1.0 ng/mL)
S-Thyroxine			
1–3 days	142–296 nmol/L (11.0–23.0 µg/dL)		
1 week–1 month	116–232 nmol/L (9.0–18.0 µg/dL)		
1–4 months	97–212 nmol/L (7.5–16.5 µg/dL)		
4–12 months	71–187 nmol/L (5.5–14.5 µg/dL)		
1–6 years	71–174 nmol/L (5.5–13.5 µg/dL)		
6–10 y	64–161 nmol/L (5.0–12.5 µg/dL)		

Information based on Meites S (ed): Pediatric Clinical Chemistry. Washington, DC, American Association for Clinical Chemistry, 1977.

* As DHEA

P = plasma; S = serum; U = urine.

APPENDIX 6

Common Chimeric Genes Identified in Human Malignancies

Naif Z. Abraham Jr MD PhD

Tables A6-1 and A6-2 give well known examples of common recurrent translocations identified in a number of malignancies. Table A6-1 correlates the specific translocation and genes involved with the respective malignancy. For example, in chronic myelogenous leukemia (CML), the typical chromosomal translocation present is t(9;22)(q34q11), where typically the long arms of chromosome 22 and 9 are involved in a reciprocal translocation or genetic fusion. The bcr gene is located on chromosome 22q11, while the able oncogene resides on chromosome 9q34. This translocation produces an abnormal bcr/abl fusion gene. This gene, in turn, is transcribed into an abnormal bcr/abl fusion mRNA, which in turn is translated into the leukemia producing bcr/abl protein molecule. This fusion protein possesses an abnormally increased tyrosine kinase activity which is involved in malignant transformation of hematopoietic cells to produce CML.

Table A6-2 indicates the genes and their chromosomal locations, their apparent protein product, and the abbreviation or nomenclature used in the research and medical literature to identify them. For example, in transformation to CML, key genes involved are bcr and abl where the nomenclature 'bcr' stands for *B*reakpoint *C*luster *R*egion and 'abl' refers to the human homolog of the oncogene of the *Abe*lson murine *l*eukemia virus or v-*abl*. It is hoped that these tables with their 'explanations' of the gene nomenclature will be helpful in clarifying to the student of molecular and clinical pathology the function and/or particular research history of these genes and protein products. All information contained within these tables was located and identified in references listed at the end of Appendix 6.

Table A6–1 Common Recurrent Chromosome Changes with Common Chimeric Genes and Protein Fusions Identified in Malignancies

Malignancy	Translocation, genes/proteins involved
Hematopoietic malignancies	
Chronic myelogenous leukemia	t(9;22)(q34q11), BCR/ABL
Acute myeloid leukemia	t(8;21)(q22;q22), AML1/ETO
Acute promyelocytic leukemia	t(15;17)(q22;q12), PML/RAR alpha
AML with abnormal eosinophils	t(16;16)(p13;q22) or inv(16)(p13q22), CBFb/MYH11
Burkitt lymphoma	t(8;14)(q24;q32), c-MYC/Ig heavy chain locus
Precursor B ALL/lymphoma	t(9;22)(q34;q11.2), BCR/ABL
	t(4;11)(q21;q23), AF4/MLL
	t(1;19)(q23;p13.3), PBX/E2A
	t(12;21)(p13;q22), TEL/AML1
Mantle cell lymphoma	t(11;14)(q13;q32), Ig heavy chain locus/BCL1
Follicular lymphoma	t(14;18)(q32;q21), BCL2 rearranged
MALT lymphoma	t(11;18)(q21;q21), API2/MLT
Anaplastic large cell lymphoma	t(2;5)(p23;q35), ALK/NPM
T cell prolymphocytic leukemia	t(14;14)(q11;q32), TCR alpha/TCL1
	inv14q(q11;q32), TCR alpha/TCL1
Mesenchymal malignancies	
Alveolar soft part sarcoma	t(X;17)(p11;q25), ASPL/TFE3
Alveolar rhabdomyosarcoma	t(2;13)(q35;q14), PAX3/FKHR
Congenital fibrosarcoma	t(12;15)(p13;q25), ETV6/NTRK3
Dermatofibrosarcoma protuberans	t(17;22)(q22;q13), COLIA1/PDGFB
Desmoplastic small round cell tumor	t(11;22)(p13q;12), EWS/WT1
Ewing's sarcoma/peripheral primitive neuroectodermal tumor	t(11;22)(q24;q12), EWS/FLI1
Extraskeletal myxoid chondrosarcoma	t(9;22)(q22;q12), EWS/TEC
Malignant melanoma of soft parts/clear cell sarcoma	t(12;22)(q13;q12), EWS/ATF1
Myxoid/round cell liposarcoma	t(12;16)(q13;p11), TLS/CHOP
Synovial sarcoma	t(X;18)(p11.23;q11), SYT/SSX1
Carcinomas	
Renal cell carcinoma, papillary type	t(X;1)(p11;q21), TFE3/PRCC
	t(X;1)(p11;p34), TFE3/PSF
Papillary carcinoma of thyroid	2 protooncogenes identified in some cancers: RET and NTRK1 fused to the amino-terminus of different gene products

Sources: Alberti, 2003; Barone, 1994; Beckmann, 1990; Bernard, 1996; Bongarzone, 2003; Bursen, 2004; Cooper, 2002; Deng, 1993; DiMartino, 1999; Ernst, 2002; Hart, 2002; Hisaoka, 2004; Jaffe, 2001; Kundu, 2002; Labelle, 1995; Lasota, 2003; Lerman, 1983; Mathur, 2003; Oikawa, 2003; Patton, 1993; Pekarsky, 2001a,b; Pierotti, 1995, 2001; Ponder, 2002; Pulford, 1997; Ro, 1991; Rosenwald, 2004; Santoro, 1995, 2004; Schaefer, 2004; Sidhar, 1996; Soulez, 1999; Takahashi, 1985, 1987; Thayer, 1983; Thompson, 2004; Tong, 1986; Whitman, 2001; Yonezumi, 2001.

Table A6–2 Genes and Proteins Involved in Malignancies

Hematopoietic malignancies

BCR	**B**reakpoint **c**luster **r**egion gene, codes for a putative serine/threonine kinase, maps to chromosome 22q11
ABL	Human homologue of the oncogene of the **Ab**elson murine **l**eukemia *v*irus, or *v-abl*, codes for a non-receptor tyrosine kinase, maps to chromosome 9q34
AML1	**A**cute **m**yelogenous **l**eukemia-**1** gene, codes for a transcription factor, maps to chromosome 21q22; also known as core binding factor alpha 2 or CBF alpha 2, RUNX1, PEBP2 alpha B
ETO	**E**ight-**t**wenty-**o**ne gene, codes for a transcription factor, maps to chromosome 21q22
PML	**Pro**myelocytic **l**eukemia gene, codes for a nuclear factor which may influence transcription, maps to chromosome 15q22_
RAR alpha	**R**etinoic **a**cid **r**eceptor **alpha** gene, codes for a ligand-dependent nuclear retinoic acid receptor with transcription factor activity, maps to chromosome 17q21
CBF beta	**C**ore **b**inding **f**actor **beta**, codes for a transcription factor, maps to chromosome 16q22; also known as *PEBP*2B or *p*olyoma enhancer *b*inding *protein*
MYH11	**M**yosin **h**eavy chain **11** gene, codes for smooth muscle myosin heavy chain, maps to chromosome 16p13
c-MYC	**C**ellular homologue of the v-***myc*** oncogene from the avian *my*elocytomatosis retrovirus, codes for a transcription factor, maps to chromosome 8q24
Ig heavy chain locus	Codes for the principal constituent (i.e., the heavy or H chain) of the immunoglobulin molecule and determines the class (IgA, IgD, IgE, IgG, IgM) of the molecule, maps to chromosome 14q32
AF4	**A**LL-1 **f**used gene on chromosome **4**, codes for a putative transcription factor, maps to chromosome 4q21; also known as FEL
MLL	**M**ixed **l**ineage **l**eukemia or **m**yeloid/**l**ymphoid **l**eukemia gene, codes for a transcriptional regulator, maps to chromosome 11q23; also known as HRX and ALL-1
PBX1	**P**re-**B** cell leukemic homeobo**x** **1** gene, codes for a transcriptional activator, maps to chromosome 1q23
E2A	**E**nhancer binding **A** gene (encoding two proteins that bind to the kappa **E2** site in the enhancer region of the kappa light chain gene), codes for a transcription factor required in B cell development, maps to chromosome 19p13.3
TEL	**T**ranslocated **E***TS* (**E**26-*t*ransformation *s*pecific) **l**eukemia gene, codes for a transcription factor, maps to chromosome 12p13; also known as ETV6
BCL1	**B** cell **l**eukemia/lymphoma **1** gene, codes for a growth factor sensor protein involved in regulation of cell cycle division, maps to chromosome 11q13; also known as PRAD1/CCND1 or cyclin D1
BCL2	**B** cell **l**eukemia/lymphoma **2** gene, codes for BCL-2 protein which inhibits apoptosis (programmed cell death), maps to chromosome 18q21.3
API2	**Ap**optosis **i**nhibitor **2** gene, codes for an inhibitor of apoptosis, maps to chromosome 11q21; also known as c-IAP2, HIAP1, MIHC
MLT	**M**ALT (*m*ucosa-associated *l*ymphoid *t*issue) lymphoma-associated **t**ranslocation, codes for protein of unknown function, maps to chromosome 18q21
ALK	**A**naplastic **l**ymphoma **k**inase gene, codes for a receptor tyrosine kinase (expressed in neural tissue), maps to chromosome 2p23
NPM	**N**ucleo**p**hos**m**in (a nonribosomal nucleolar phosphoprotein involved in transporting ribosomal components between the nucleus and the cytoplasm for ribosomal assembly), coded by the NPM gene, maps to chromosome 5q35
TCR	**T** **c**ell antigen **r**eceptor, a T cell membrane/surface receptor for antigen, composed of polypeptide chains from the alpha/delta (chromosome 14q11), beta (chromosome 7q34), and/or gamma (chromosome 7p) gene sets
TCL1	**T** **c**ell **l**eukemia/lymphoma **1** gene, codes for a protein of unknown function, but may be involved in lymphoid cell proliferation and/or survival, maps to chromosome 14q32.1

Mesenchymal malignancies

ASPL	**A**lveolar **s**oft **p**art sarcoma **l**ocus, function unknown, maps to chromosome 17q25
TFE3	Gene codes for a **t**ranscription **f**actor which binds to the IgH intronic enhancer mu*E*3 DNA region, maps to chromosome Xp11.2
PAX3	**Pa**ired bo**x** transcription factor **3** gene, codes for a transcription factor, maps to chromosome 2q35
FKHR	**F**or**kh**ead-**r**elated gene, codes for a transcription factor, maps to chromosome 13q14; also known as FOXO1A
ETV6	**Et**s **v**ariant **6** gene, codes for a transcription factor, maps to chromosome 12p13; also known as TEL
NTRK3	**N**eurotrophin **t**ransmembrane **r**eceptor tyrosine **k**inase **3** gene, codes for a receptor that induces the release of neurotrophins, maps to chromosome 15q25; also known as TRKC or *t*ransmembrane *r*eceptor tyrosine *k*inase *C*
COL1A1	**Col**lagen type **1** **alpha** **1** chain gene, codes for an extracellular matrix protein, maps to chromosome 17q22
PDGFB	**P**latelet-**d**erived **g**rowth **f**actor **beta** chain gene, codes for a growth factor or mitogen, maps to chromosome 22q13; a human homologue of v-*sis* (*si*mian *s*arcoma virus) oncogene
EWS	**Ew**ing **s**arcoma gene, a putative nuclear RNA binding protein, maps to chromosome 22q12
WT1	**W**ilms' **t**umor protein **1** gene, codes for a transcription factor, maps to chromosome 11p13
FLI1	**F**reund's **l**eukemia **i**ntegration site **1** gene and an ETS family gene, codes for a transcriptional regulator protein, maps to chromosome 11q
TEC	**T**ranslocated in **e**xtraskeletal **c**hondrosarcoma, codes for a steroid nuclear receptor/transcription factor thought to be involved in control of cellular proliferation and apoptosis, maps to chromosome 9q22; also known as CHN (*chon*drosarcoma), NOR1 (*n*euron derived *o*rphan *r*eceptor *1*)—a receptor is termed an *orphan* when its ligand has not been isolated
ATF1	**A**ctivating **t**ranscription **f**actor **1** gene, codes for a transcription factor, maps to chromosome 12q13
TLS	**T**ranslocated in **l**ipo**s**arcoma gene, a putative nuclear RNA binding protein, maps to chromosome 16p11; also known as FUS or *fusion*
CHOP	**C**/EBP **ho**mologous **p**rotein—where C/EBP refers to *C*CAAT/enhancer-*b*inding *p*rotein—codes for a transcription factor, maps to chromosome 12q13; also known as GADD153, DDIT3
SYT	**SY**novial sarcoma **t**ranslocation gene, a putative transcriptional activator, maps to chromosome 18q11
SSX1	**S**ynovial **s**arcoma **X** chromosome breakpoint gene **1**, a putative transcriptional repressor/DNA binding factor, maps to chromosome Xp11

Carcinomas

TFE3	Gene codes for a **t**ranscription **f**actor which binds to the IgH intronic enhancer mu*E*3 DNA region, maps to chromosome Xp11.2
PRCC	**P**apillary **r**enal **c**ell **c**arcinoma gene, a ubiquitously expressed nuclear protein, maps to chromosome 1q21.2

Table A6–2 Genes and Proteins Involved in Malignancies (cont'd)

PSF	**P**TB-associated **s**plicing **f**actor gene where PTB = *p*olypyrimidine *tract-b*inding protein, codes for a ubiquitously expressed, putative multifunctional, nuclear protein possibly involved in transcription, maps to chromosome 1p34
RET	**R**earranged du**r**ing **t**ransfection, codes for a tyrosine kinase receptor, maps to chromosome 10q11
NTRK1	**N**eurotrophin **t**ransmembrane **r**eceptor tyrosine **k**inase **1** gene, codes for a tyrosine kinase receptor for nerve growth factor, maps to chromosome 1q21-22; also known as TRKA or *transmembrane receptor tyrosine kinase A*

Sources: Alberti, 2003; Barone, 1994; Beckmann, 1990; Bernard, 1996; Bongarzone, 2003; Bursen, 2004; Cooper, 2002; Deng, 1993; DiMartino, 1999; Ernst, 2002; Hart, 2002; Hisaoka, 2004; Jaffe, 2001; Kundu, 2002; Labelle, 1995; Lasota, 2003; Lerman, 1983; Mathur, 2003; Oikawa, 2003; Patton, 1993; Pekarsky, 2001a,b; Pierotti, 1995, 2001; Ponder, 2002; Pulford, 1997; Ro, 1991; Rosenwald, 2004; Santoro, 1995, 2004; Schaefer, 2004; Sidhar, 1996; Soulez, 1999; Takahashi, 1985, 1987; Thayer, 1983; Thompson, 2004; Tong, 1986; Whitman, 2001; Yonezumi, 2001.

Alberti L, Carniti C, Miranda C, et al: RET and NTRK1 proto-oncogenes in human diseases. J Cell Physiol 2003; 195:168–186.

Barone MV, Crozat A, Tabaee A, et al: CHOP (GADD153) and its oncogenic variant, TLS-CHOP, have opposing effects on the induction of G1/S arrest. Genes Dev 1994; 8:453–464.

Beckmann H, Su LK, Kadesch T: TFE3: A helix-loop-helix protein that activates transcription through the immunoglobulin enhancer muE3 motif. Genes Dev 1990; 4:167–179.

Bernard OA, Romana SP, Poirel H, Berger R: Molecular cytogenetics of t(12;21)(p13;q22). Leuk Lymphoma 1996; 23:459–465.

Bongarzone I, Pierotti MA: The molecular basis of thyroid epithelial tumorigenesis. Tumori 2003; 89:514–516.

Bursen A, Moritz S, Gaussmann A, et al: Interaction of AF4 wild-type and AF4-MLL fusion protein with SIAH proteins: Indication for t(4;11) pathobiology? Oncogene 2004; 23:6237–6249.

Cooper CS (ed): Translocations in Solid Tumors. Georgetown, Texas, Landes Bioscience, 2002.

Deng Z, Liu P, Marlton P, et al: Smooth muscle myosin heavy chain locus (*MYH11*) maps to 16p13.13-p13.12 and establishes a new region of conserved synteny between human 16p and mouse 16. Genomics 1993; 18:156–159.

DiMartino JF, Cleary ML: MLL rearrangements in haematological malignancies: lessons from clinical and biological studies. Br J Haematol 1999; 106: 614–626.

Ernst P, Wang J, Korsmeyer SJ: The role of MLL in hematopoiesis and leukemia. Curr Opin Hematol 2002; 9:282–287.

Hart SM, Foroni L: Core binding factor genes and human leukemia. Haematologica 2002; 87:1307–1323.

Hisaoka M, Ishida T, Imamura T, Hashimoto H: TFG is a novel fusion partner of NOR1 in extraskeletal myxoid chondrosarcoma. Genes Chromosomes Cancer 2004; 40:325–328.

Jaffe ES, Harris NL, Stein H, Vardiman JW (eds): WHO Classification of Tumours. Pathology and Genetics of Tumours of Haematopoietic and Lymphoid Tissues. Lyon, IARC Press, 2001.

Kundu M, Chen A, Anderson S, et al: Role of *Cbfb* in hematopoiesis and perturbations resulting from expression of the leukemogenic fusion gene *Cbfb-MYH11*. Blood 2002; 100:2449–2456.

Labelle Y, Zucman J, Stenman G, et al: Oncogenic conversion of a novel orphan nuclear receptor by chromosome translocation. Hum Mol Genet 1995; 4:2219–2226.

Lasota J: Genetics of soft tissue tumors. *In* Miettinen M: Diagnostic Soft Tissue Pathology. New York, Churchill Livingstone, 2003, pp 99–142.

Lerman MI, Thayer RE, Singer MF: Kpn I family of long interspersed repeated DNA sequences in primates: Polymorphism of family members and evidence for transcription. Proc Natl Acad Sci U S A 1983; 80:3966–3970.

Mathur M, Das S, Samuels HH: PSF-TFE3 oncoprotein in papillary renal cell carcinoma inactivates TFE3 and p53 through cytoplasmic sequestration. Oncogene 2003; 22:5031–5044.

Oikawa T, Yamada T: Molecular biology of the Ets family of transcription factors. Gene 2003; 303:11–34.

Patton JG, Porro EB, Galceran J, et al: Cloning and characterization of PSF, a novel pre-mRNA splicing factor. Genes Dev 1993; 7:393–406.

Pekarsky Y, Hallas C, Croce CM: Molecular basis of mature T-cell leukemia. JAMA 2001a; 286:2308–2314.

Pekarsky Y, Hallas C, Croce CM: The role of *TCL1* in human T-cell leukemia. Oncogene 2001b; 20: 5638–5643.

Pierotti MA: Chromosomal rearrangements in thyroid carcinomas: A recombination or death dilemma. Cancer Lett 2001; 166:1–7.

Pierotti MA, Bongarzone I, Borrello MG, et al: Rearrangements of TRK proto-oncogene in papillary thyroid carcinomas. J Endocrinol Invest 1995; 18:130–133.

Ponder BAJ: Multiple endocrine neoplasia type 2. *In* Vogelstein B, Kinzler KW (eds): The Genetic Basis of Human Cancer, 2nd ed. New York, McGraw-Hill, 2002, pp 501–513.

Pulford K, Lamant L, Morris SW, et al: Detection of anaplastic lymphoma kinase (ALK) and nucleolar protein nucleophosmin (NPM)-ALK proteins in normal and neoplastic cells with the monoclonal antibody ALK1. Blood 1997; 89:1394–1404.

Ro HS, Roncari DAK: The C/EBP-binding region and adjacent sites regulate expression of the adipose P2 gene in human preadipocytes. Mol Cell Biol 1991; 11:2303–2306.

Rosenwald A, Staudt LM, Duyster JG, Morris SW: Molecular aspects of non-Hodgkin lymphomagenesis. *In* Greer JP, Foerster J, Lukens JN, et al: (eds): Wintrobe's Clinical Hematology, 11th edition. Philadelphia, Lippincott Williams & Wilkins, 2004, pp 2325–2361.

Santoro M, Grieco M, Melillo RM, et al: Molecular defects in thyroid carcinomas: Role of the RET oncogene in thyroid neoplastic transformation. Eur J Endocrinol 1995; 133:513–522.

Santoro M, Melillo RM, Carlomagno F, et al: RET: Normal and abnormal functions. Endocrinology 2004 145:5448–5451; Epub 2004, Aug 26.

Schaefer KL, Brachwitz K, Wai DH, et al: Expression profiling of t(12;22) positive clear cell sarcoma of soft tissue cell lines reveals characteristic up-regulation of potential new marker genes including *ERBB3*. Cancer Res 2004; 64:3395–3405.

Sidhar SK, Clark J, Gill S, et al: The t(X;1)(p11.2;q21.2) translocation in papillary renal cell carcinoma fuses a novel gene *PRCC* to the *TFE3* transcription factor gene. Hum Mol Genet 1996; 5:1333–1338.

Soulez M, Saurin AJ, Freemont PS, Knight JC: SSX and the synovial-sarcoma-specfic chimaeric protein SYT-SSX co-localize with the human polycomb group complex. Oncogene 1999; 18:2739–2746.

Takahashi M, Cooper GM: Ret transforming gene encodes a fusion protein homologous to tyrosine kinases. Mol Cell Biol 1987; 7:1378–1385.

Takahashi M, Ritz J, Cooper GM: Activation of a novel human transforming gene, ret, by DNA rearrangement. Cell 1985; 42:581–588.

Thayer RE, Singer MF: Interruption of an alpha-satellite array by a short member of the KpnI family of interspersed, highly repeated monkey DNA sequences. Mol Cell Biol 1983; 3:967–973.

Thompson MA: Molecular genetics of acute leukemia. *In* Greer JP, Foerster J, Lukens JN, et al: (eds): Wintrobe's Clinical Hematology, 11th ed. Philadelphia, Lippincott Williams & Wilkins, 2004, pp 2045–2062.

Tong BD, Levine SE, Jaye M, et al: Isolation and sequencing of a cDNA clone homologous to the v-sis oncogene from human endothelial cells. Mol Cell Biol 1986; 6:3018–3022.

Whitman SP, Strout MP, Marcucci G, et al: The partial nontandem duplication of the MLL (ALL1) gene is a novel rearrangement that generates three distinct fusion transcripts in B-cell acute lymphoblastic leukemia. Cancer Res 2001; 61:59–63.

Yonezumi M, Suzuki R, Suzuki H, et al: Detection of API2-MALT1 chimaeric gene in extranodal and nodal marginal zone B-cell lymphoma by reverse transcription polymerase chain reaction (PCR) and genomic long and accurate PCR analyses. Br J Haematol 2001; 115:588–594.

Index

GUIDELINES FOR ORDERING BLOOD FOR ELECTIVE SURGERY

Also referred to as Maximum Surgical Blood Order Schedule (MSBOS)

These guidelines present a range in numbers of units of blood to be ordered as practiced at three different institutions: University Hospital SUNY Upstate Medical Center at Syracuse, NY; Virginia Commonwealth University Medical Center, Richmond, VA; University of Michigan Hospitals, Ann Arbor, MI. Each institution should set its own guidelines for ordering blood products to take into account varying medical needs and practices in collaboration with the hospital medical and surgical staff.

KEY: 0 = no testing required
T&S = type & screen
1-6 = number of units crossmatched
AO = as ordered
* = varies with purpose

Cardiopulmonary/Cardiothoracic

A-V canal repair	3
Angioplasty	T&S
Aortic or ventricular aneurysm repair	4
Aortic dissection	6
Aortic valve replacement	2 to 3
Atrial septal defect repair	3
Atrial septectomy	3
Blalock-Taussig shunt	1
Bidirectional Glenn's shunt	2
CABG (coronary vein graft)	2 to 4
Coarctation repair	3
Esophagogastrectomy	2
Esophageal hernia/hiatal	0 or T&S
Esophagoscopy	0
Fontan's procedure	3 to 4
Great vessel switch	3
Lobectomy	T&S or 1
Mediastinoscopy	0 or T&S
Mitral commissurotomy	3
Mitral valvuloplasty	2
Mitral valve annuloplasty	3
Mitral valve replacement	2 to 3
Mustard procedure	3
Open lung biopsy	T&S
Pacemaker insertion	0
Patent ductus arteriosus ligation	T&S
Pericardectomy	2
Pericardial window	0 or T&S
Pneumonectomy	T&S to 2
Pulmonary valve replacement	2 to 3
Pulmonary valvulotomy	3
Redo and repair	6
Septectomy	2
Sternal wire removal	0
Tetralogy of Fallot	3 to 4
Thoracotomy/lobectomy	1
Thoracoscopy	0
Transposition repair	3
Ventricular septal defect repair	3
Wedge resection	T&S

General Surgery

Abdominoperineal resection	T&S to 3
Amputations	T&S
Appendectomy	0
Bronchoscopy	0 or T&S
Catheter insertion/removal	0
Cholecystojejunostomy	T&S
Cholecystectomy	T&S
Colon resection	T&S to 2
Colostomy closure/takedown	T&S
Debridement (wound, burn)	AO
Denver peritoneal shunt insertion	0
Denver shunt revision	0
Dressing change	0
Exploratory laparotomy	T&S to 2
Gastric bypass	T&S
Gastrostomy tube insertion	0 or T&S
Hemicolectomy	2
Hemorrhoidectomy	0
Hepatic lobectomy	3 to 6
Hernia repair, inguinal	0 or T&S
Ileostomy	T&S
Iliac profunda bypass	1
Jejunostomy tube placement	0
Lumpectomy, breast mass	0
Mastectomy, simple	0
Mastectomy, modified radical	T&S
Mediastinoscopy	0 or T&S
Myotomy (pyloric)	0
Parotidectomy	0 or T&S
Pilonidal cyst	0
Portocaval shunt	4 to 6
Pseudoaneurysm repair	6
Rib resection	0
Sigmoidectomy	T&S
Sigmoidoscopy	0
Small bowel resection	T&S
Splenectomy	T&S to 2
Sympathectomy	T&S
Thyroidectomy	0 or T&S
Total colon resection	T&S
Vagotomy	0 or T&S
Vein stripping	T&S
Whipple's procedure	2

Gynecology

Anterior-posterior repair	T&S to 1
Cone biopsy (CO$_2$ laser)	0
Dilation and curettage (D&C)	0 to 2
Ectopic pregnancy	T&S to 2
Endometrium ablation	0
Examine under anesthesia (EUA)	0
Exploratory laparotomy	T&S to 2
Exenteration procedure	4
Groshong's catheter insertion	0
Hysterectomy, total abdominal	T&S to 2
Hysteroscopy	0
Laparoscopy	0
Laser vaporization	0
Neosalpingostomy	T&S
Oophorectomy	T&S
Ovarian wedge resection	T&S
Salpingo-oophorectomy	T&S
Uterine suspension	0
Tubal ligation	0
Tuboplasty	0 or T&S
Vaginectomy	T&S to 2
Vulvectomy	T&S to 2

Neurosurgery

Aneurysm clipping	2 to 6
Biopsy (cervical/brain)	T&S to 1
Burr hole	T&S
Carpal tunnel release	0
Cervical decompression	T&S to 2
Cervical discectomy	0 or T&S
Cordotomy	T&S
Cordectomy	1
Craniectomy	2
Cranioplasty	T&S to 2
Craniotomy	2
Endarterectomy, carotid	2
Hypophysectomy	T&S to 1
Laminectomy	T&S to 2
Lobectomy	2
Neuroma removal	T&S
Nerve repair	T&S
Pituitary tumor resection	1
Spinal fusion	T&S to 1
Stereotactic brain biopsy	0 or T&S
Stereotactic hematoma	T&S
Ulnar nerve transplant	0
Ventricular-peritoneal shunt insertion	0 or T&S

Orthopedics

Acromioplasty	0
Amputation	T&S
Arthroscopy	0 or T&S
Arthroplasty	T&S
Arthrotomy	0
Biopsy, excisional	0
Bipolar transfer	T&S
Carpal tunnel release	0
Closed reduction	0
Debridement	AO
Decompression laminectomy	T&S
Diskectomy	T&S
Fractures	0
*Fusions, other	T&S to 2
Hardware removal	0
Hip revision	2 to 4
Hip screw and nailing	T&S
Lumbar laminectomy	T&S
Meniscectomy	0
Nerve transposition	0
Neuroma excision	0
Open reduction	T&S to 2
Osteotomy	0
Posterior rod fusion	2
Prosthesis removal	T&S
Releases	0
Revascularization and exploration	T&S
Rodding (Grosse and Kempf)	T&S
Rotator cuff repair	T&S
Shoulder replacement	T&S
Shoulder repair	0
Spinal fusions	1 to 3
Tendon repair	0
Total elbow	T&S
Total hip	2 to 3
Total knee	T&S

Otorhinolaryngology/Head and Neck Surgery

Antrotomy	0
Atticoantrotomy	0
Bronchoscopy	0
Caldwell-Luc	0 or T&S
Cochlear implant	0
Composite resection	4